SCHWARTZ'S
PRINCIPLES OF SURGERY

SCHWARTZ'S
PRINCIPLES OF SURGERY

Ninth Edition

Editor-in-Chief

F. Charles Brunicardi, MD, FACS

DeBakey/Bard Professor and Chairman, Michael E. DeBakey
Department of Surgery, Baylor College of Medicine,
Houston, Texas

Associate Editors

Dana K. Andersen, MD, FACS

Professor and Vice-Chair, Department of Surgery,
Johns Hopkins University School of Medicine,
Surgeon-in-Chief, Johns Hopkins Bayview Medical Center,
Baltimore, Maryland

Timothy R. Billiar, MD, FACS

George Vance Foster Professor and Chairman of Surgery,
Department of Surgery, University of Pittsburgh School of
Medicine, Pittsburgh, Pennsylvania

David L. Dunn, MD, PhD, FACS

Vice President for Health Sciences, State University
of New York, Buffalo, Buffalo, New York

John G. Hunter, MD, FACS

Mackenzie Professor and Chair,
Department of Surgery, Oregon Health and Science
University, Portland, Oregon

Jeffrey B. Matthews, MD, FACS

Dallas B. Phemister Professor and Chairman,
Department of Surgery, University of Chicago,
Chicago, Illinois

Raphael E. Pollock, MD, PhD, FACS

Head, Division of Surgery, Professor and Chairman,
Department of Surgical Oncology, Senator A.M. Aiken, Jr.,
Distinguished Chair, University of Texas M.D.
Anderson Cancer Center, Houston, Texas

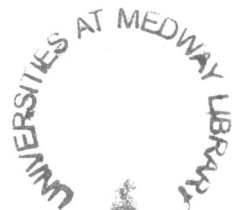

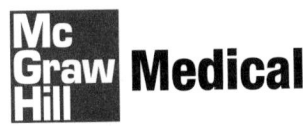

New York   Chicago   San Francisco   Lisbon   London   Madrid   Mexico City
Milan   New Delhi   San Juan   Seoul   Singapore   Sydney   Toronto

Schwartz's Principles of Surgery, Ninth Edition

3 4 5 6 7 8 9 10 DOW/DOW 14 13 12 11 10

Set ISBN 978-0-07-154769-7
Set MHID 0-07-154769-X
Book ISBN 978-0-07-1547703
Book MHID 0-07-154770-3
DVD ISBN 978-0-07-154771-0
DVD MHID 0-07-154771-1

This book was set in Minion Pro by Silverchair Science + Communications.
The editors were Marsha S. Loeb and Christie Naglieri.
The production supervisor was Catherine H. Saggese.
Project management was provided by Basia Jones at Silverchair Science + Communications.
The illustration manager was Armen Ovsepyan.
The interior designer was Alan Barnett; the cover designer was David Dell'Accio.
The index was prepared by Linda Hallinger.
RR Donnelley was the printer and binder.

This book is printed on acid-free paper.

McGraw-Hill books are available at special quantity discounts to use as premiums and sales promotions, or for use in corporate training programs. To contact a representative please e-mail us at bulksales@mcgraw-hill.com.

Library of Congress Cataloging-in-Publication Data

Schwartz's principles of surgery / editor-in-chief, F. Charles Brunicardi ; associate editors, Dana K. Andersen ... [et al.]. -- 9th ed.
    p. ; cm.
Includes bibliographical references and index.
ISBN-13: 978-0-07-154769-7 (set : alk. paper)
ISBN-10: 0-07-154769-X (set : alk. paper)
ISBN-13: 978-0-07-154770-3 (hardcover : alk. paper)
ISBN-10: 0-07-154770-3 (hardcover : alk. paper)
[etc.]
1. Surgery. I. Schwartz, Seymour I., 1928- II. Brunicardi, F. Charles. III. Title: Principles of surgery.
    [DNLM: 1. Surgery. 2. Surgical Procedures, Operative. WO 100 S399 2009]
RD31.P88 2009
617--dc22
                              2008044963

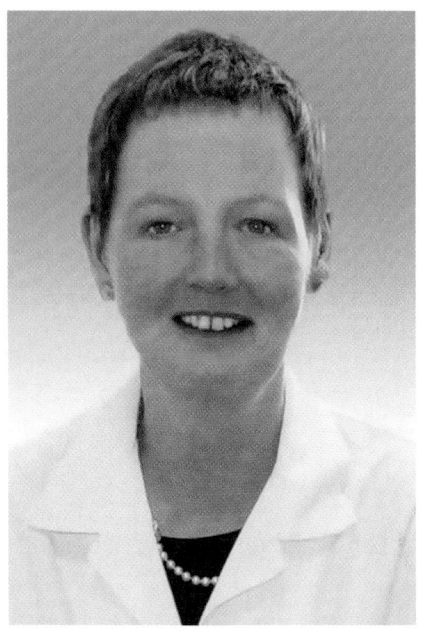

Margrét Oddsdóttir, MD (1955–2009)

The Editors of *Schwartz's Principles of Surgery* wish to dedicate this ninth edition to the memory of Margrét Oddsdóttir, the primary author of the "Gallbladder and Bile Ducts" chapter in these last two editions. Dr. Oddsdóttir was born in Isafjördur, Iceland, a small fishing village above the Arctic Circle in northern Iceland. She received her undergraduate and medical education, and performed a surgical internship at the University of Iceland. She completed her general surgery training at Yale University in 1994, and then became the first fellow in laparoscopic surgery under the direction of John Hunter at Emory. Following completion of her training, she returned to the University of Iceland, where she established herself as an expert gastrointestinal surgeon specializing in advanced minimally invasive surgery. In 2002, she became Professor and Chief of General Surgery in the same institution.

Margrét and her husband Jon had two sons who were born during her training years in the U.S. They frequently traveled with her to surgical meetings in this country, and Margrét became the close friend of many surgeons. She was relentless in identifying the brightest young Icelandic surgical trainees whom she then sent for training in this country, and was vigorous in her pursuit of the highest standards for her own department. Sadly, Margrét's death from advanced breast cancer was preceded 18 months before by the death of Jon from pancreatic cancer.

Immensely proud of her Viking heritage, Dr. Oddsdóttir was fond of quoting from the Hávamál, an ancient Viking poem. One quote that she was particularly fond of was "a man who has personal integrity is better placed than one whose life is spent impressing others. Nothing can take such a man's life away, for although death is inescapable, his posthumous reputation will never die."

Oddur and Siggi, we dedicate this book in honor of your mother, a surgeon of international renown, universally loved and respected by those of us lucky enough to have known her. Her memory will stay with us, her reputation as a leader in surgery will live on, and her words will be preserved in this most respected textbook of surgery.

The Editors of *Schwartz's Principles of Surgery*, Ninth Edition

To my wife, Melissa, my children, Isaac and Jackson, my mother, Rose, and my late father, Edward Brunicardi, for their love and support.

F.C.B.

To my wife, Cindy, and my children, Ashley, Lauren, Kathryn, Thomas, and Olivia.

D.K.A.

To my wife, Edith and our children Isabel and Alex.

T.R.B.

To my wife Kelli, and my children Edward, Julia, Evelyn, and Michael, my sister Diane, and my late parents for instilling in me a strong work ethic and the importance of academic excellence.

D.L.D.

To my wife Laura, my children, Sarah, Sam, and Jillian, and the residents, fellows and surgical faculty at OSHU who have created a community of health, collegiality, and open minded intellectual rigor.

J.G.H.

To Joan and our boys Jono, David, and Adam, for their love and support, and to the memory of my grandfather Dr. Benjamin Banks who continues to inspire me.

J.B.M.

To Dina and our children: Jessica, Sam, Eden, Noam, and Omer

R.E.P.

CONTENTS

Louis H. Alarcon, MD
Assistant Professor of Surgery, Department of Surgery, University of Pittsburgh School of Medicine, Pittsburgh, Pennsylvania
Chapter 13, Physiologic Monitoring of the Surgical Patient

Dana K. Andersen, MD, FACS
Professor and Vice-Chair, Department of Surgery, Johns Hopkins University School of Medicine, Surgeon-in-Chief, Johns Hopkins Bayview Medical Center, Baltimore, Maryland
Chapter 33, Pancreas

Peter Angelos, MD
Professor of Surgery and Chief of Endocrine Surgery, University of Chicago Medical Center, Chicago, Illinois
Chapter 48, Ethics, Palliative Care, and Care at the End of Life

Peter B. Angood, MD
Senior Advisor for Patient Safety, National Quality Forum, Washington, DC
Chapter 12, Patient Safety

Stanley W. Ashley, MD
Frank Sawyer Professor of Surgery, Department of Surgery, Harvard Medical School, Boston, Massachusetts
Chapter 28, Small Intestine

Samir S. Awad, MD
Associate Professor, Michael E. DeBakey Department of Surgery, Baylor College of Medicine, Houston, Texas
Chapter 1, Accreditation Council for Graduate Medical Education Core Competencies

Adrian Barbul, MD
Professor of Surgery, Department of Surgery, Johns Hopkins Medical Institutions, Baltimore, Maryland
Chapter 9, Wound Healing

Joel A. Bauman, MD
Resident Physician, Department of Neurosurgery, University of Pennsylvania, Philadelphia, Pennsylvania
Chapter 42, Neurosurgery

Carlos Bechara, MD
Assistant Professor of Surgery, Division of Vascular Surgery and Endovascular Therapy, Michael E. DeBakey Department of Surgery, Baylor College of Medicine, Houston, Texas
Chapter 23, Arterial Disease

Greg J. Beilman, MD
Professor of Surgery and Anesthesia, Chief of Surgical Critical Care/Trauma, University of Minnesota, Minneapolis, Minnesota
Chapter 6, Surgical Infections

Richard H. Bell Jr., MD
Assistant Executive Director, American Board of Surgery, Philadelphia, Pennsylvania
Chapter 33, Pancreas

Robert L. Bell, MD, MA, FACS
Director, Minimally Invasive Surgery, Director, Bariatric Surgery, Associate Professor of Surgery, Department of Surgery, Yale University School of Medicine, New Haven, Connecticut
Chapter 35, Abdominal Wall, Omentum, Mesentery, and Retroperitoneum

Arie Belldegrun, MD
Director, Institute of Urologic Oncology at UCLA, Professor and Chief, Division of Urologic Oncology, Roy and Carol Doumani Chair in Urologic Oncology, David Geffen School of Medicine at UCLA, Los Angeles, California
Chapter 40, Urology

Peleg Ben-Galim, MD
Assistant Professor, Department of Orthopedic Surgery, Baylor College of Medicine, Houston, Texas
Chapter 43, Orthopedic Surgery

David H. Berger, MD
Professor and Vice Chair, Michael E. DeBakey Department of Surgery, Baylor College of Medicine, Houston, Texas
Chapter 1, Accreditation Council for Graduate Medical Education Core Competencies
Chapter 30, The Appendix

Walter L. Biffl, MD
Associate Professor, Department of Surgery, Denver Health Medical Center/University of Colorado-Denver, Denver, Colorado
Chapter 7, Trauma

Timothy R. Billiar, MD, FACS
George Vance Foster Professor and Chairman of Surgery, Department of Surgery, University of Pittsburgh School of Medicine, Pittsburgh, Pennsylvania
Chapter 5, Shock

Kirby I. Bland, MD
Fay Fletcher Kerner Professor and Chairman, Department of Surgery, University of Alabama at Birmingham, Birmingham, Alabama
Chapter 17, The Breast

Mary L. Brandt, MD
Professor and Vice Chair, Michael E. DeBakey Department of Surgery, Baylor College of Medicine, Houston, Texas
Chapter 1, Accreditation Council for Graduate Medical Education Core Competencies

F. Charles Brunicardi, MD, FACS
DeBakey/Bard Professor and Chairman, Michael E. DeBakey Department of Surgery, Baylor College of Medicine, Houston, Texas
Chapter 1, Accreditation Council for Graduate Medical Education Core Competencies
Chapter 15, Molecular and Genomic Surgery
Chapter 33, Pancreas
Chapter 37, Inguinal Hernias

Jamal Bullocks, MD
Assistant Professor, Division of Plastic Surgery, Michael E. DeBakey Department of Surgery, Baylor College of Medicine, Houston, Texas
Chapter 16, The Skin and Subcutaneous Tissue

Catherine Cagiannos, MD
Assistant Professor of Surgery, Division of Vascular Surgery and Endovascular Therapy, Baylor College of Medicine, Houston, Texas
Chapter 23, Arterial Disease

Joanna M. Cain, MD
Chace/Joukowsky Chair of Obstetrics and Gynecology, Department of Obstetrics and Gynecology, Brown University, Portland, Oregon
Chapter 41, Gynecology

Rakesh K. Chandra, MD
Assistant Professor, Department of Otolaryngology, Head and Neck Surgery, Northwestern University, Chicago, Illinois
Chapter 18, Disorders of the Head and Neck

Catherine L. Chen, MPH
Fellow, Department of Surgery, Johns Hopkins University School of Medicine, Baltimore, Maryland
Chapter 12, Patient Safety

Changyi J. Chen, PhD
Molecular Surgery Endowed Chair, Professor of Surgery and Molecular and Cellular Biology, Michael E. DeBakey Department of Surgery, Baylor College of Medicine, Houston, Texas
Chapter 23, Arterial Disease

Orlo H. Clark, MD
Professor of Surgery, Department of Surgery, UCSF/Mt. Zion Medical Center, San Francisco, California
Chapter 38, Thyroid, Parathyroid, and Adrenal

Patrick Cole, MD
Resident, Division of Plastic Surgery, Michael E. DeBakey Department of Surgery, Baylor College of Medicine, Houston, Texas
Chapter 16, The Skin and Subcutaneous Tissue

Edward M. Copeland III, MD
Emeritus Distinguished Professor of Surgery, Department of Surgery, University of Florida, College of Medicine, Gainesville, Florida
Chapter 17, The Breast

Janice N. Cormier, MD
Associate Professor of Surgery, Department of Surgical Oncology, University of Texas M.D. Anderson Cancer Center, Houston, Texas
Chapter 36, Soft Tissue Sarcomas

Joseph S. Coselli, MD
Professor and Cullen Foundation Endowed Chair, Division of Cardiothoracic Surgery, Michael E. DeBakey Department of Surgery, Baylor College of Medicine, Houston, Texas
Chapter 22, Thoracic Aneurysms and Aortic Dissection

C. Clay Cothren, MD
Associate Professor of Surgery, Department of Surgery, University of Colorado, Denver, Denver, Colorado
Chapter 7, Trauma

Gregory A. Crooke, MD
Assistant Professor of Cardiothoracic Surgery, New York University School of Medicine, New York, New York
Chapter 21, Acquired Heart Disease

Daniel T. Dempsey, MD
Professor and Chair, Department of Surgery, Temple University School of Medicine, Philadelphia, Pennsylvania
Chapter 26, Stomach

Robert S. Dorian, MD
Chairman and Program Director, Department of Anesthesia, Saint Barnabas Medical Center, Livingston, New Jersey
Chapter 47, Anesthesia of the Surgical Patient

David L. Dunn, MD, PhD, FACS
Vice President for Health Sciences, State University of New York, Buffalo, Buffalo, New York
Chapter 6, Surgical Infections
Chapter 11, Transplantation

Geoffrey P. Dunn, MD
Medical Director, Department of Surgery, Hamot Medical Center, Erie, Pennsylvania
Chapter 48, Ethics, Palliative Care, and Care at the End of Life

Kelli M. Bullard Dunn, MD
Associate Professor of Surgery, Department of Surgical Oncology, State University of New York, Buffalo, Buffalo, New York
Chapter 29, Colon, Rectum, and Anus

David T. Efron, MD
Associate Professor of Surgery, Chief, Division of Trauma, Critical Care, and Emergency Surgery, Johns Hopkins Hospital, Baltimore, Maryland
Chapter 9, Wound Healing

Wafic M. ElMasri, MD
Cancer Research Training Award Postdoctoral Fellow, Medical Oncology Branch, Molecular Signaling Section, National Institutes of Health, National Cancer Institute, Bethesda, Maryland
Chapter 41, Gynecology

Fred W. Endorf, MD
Clinical Associate Professor, Department of Surgery, University of Minnesota, St. Paul, Minnesota
Chapter 8, Burns

Xin-Hua Feng, PhD
Professor, Michael E. DeBakey Department of Surgery, Baylor College of Medicine, Houston, Texas
Chapter 15, Molecular and Genomic Surgery

William E. Fisher, MD
Professor, Michael E. DeBakey Department of Surgery, Baylor College of Medicine, Houston, Texas
Chapter 33, Pancreas

Henri R. Ford, MD
Vice President and Surgeon-in-Chief, Children's Hospital Los Angeles, Professor of Surgery and Vice Dean for Medical Education, Keck School of Medicine, University of Southern California, Los Angeles, California
Chapter 39, Pediatric Surgery

Aubrey C. Galloway, MD
Seymour Cohn Professor, Chairman Department of Cardiothoracic Surgery, Department of Cardiothoracic Surgery, New York University School of Medicine, New York, New York
Chapter 21, Acquired Heart Disease

Francis H. Gannon, MD
Associate Professor of Pathology and Orthopedic Surgery, Staff Pathologist, DeBakey VA Medical Center, Baylor College of Medicine, Houston, Texas
Chapter 43, Orthopedic Surgery

David A. Geller, MD
Richard L. Simmons Professor of Surgery, Thomas E. Starzl Transplantation Institute, University of Pittsburgh, Pittsburgh, Pennsylvania
Chapter 31, Liver

Nicole S. Gibran, MD
Professor, Department of Surgery, Harborview Medical Center, Seattle, Washington
Chapter 8, Burns

Michael Gimbel, MD
Assistant Professor of Surgery, Division of Plastic and Reconstructive Surgery, University of Pittsburgh Medical Center, Pittsburgh, Pennsylvania
Chapter 45, Plastic and Reconstructive Surgery

Carlos D. Godinez Jr., MD
Fellow and Clinical Instructor, Minimally Invasive Surgery, Department of Surgery, University of Maryland School of Medicine, Baltimore, Maryland
Chapter 34, Spleen

Ernest A. Gonzalez, MD
Assistant Professor of Surgery, Department of Surgery, University of Texas Health Science Center, Houston, Texas
Chapter 4, Hemostasis, Surgical Bleeding, and Transfusion

John A. Goss, MD
Professor of Surgery, Michael E. DeBakey Department of Surgery, Baylor College of Medicine, Houston, Texas
Chapter 31, Liver

M. Sean Grady, MD
Charles Harrison Frazier Professor, Department of Neurosurgery, University of Pennsylvania School of Medicine, Philadelphia, Pennsylvania
Chapter 42, Neurosurgery

Tom Gregory, MD
Associate Professor, Department of Obstetrics and Gynecology, Division of Urogynecology, Oregon Health and Science University, Portland, Oregon
Chapter 41, Gynecology

Tracy C. Grikscheit, MD
Assistant Professor of Surgery, Department of Pediatric Surgery, Keck School of Medicine, University of Southern California, Los Angeles, California
Chapter 39, Pediatric Surgery

Eugene A. Grossi, MD
Professor of Cardiothoracic Surgery, New York University School of Medicine, New York, New York
Chapter 21, Acquired Heart Disease

David J. Hackam, MD, PhD
Roberta Simmons Associate Professor of Pediatric Surgery, University of Pittsburgh School of Medicine, Pittsburgh, Pennsylvania
Chapter 39, Pediatric Surgery

Daniel E. Hall, MD
Division of Trauma and General Surgery, University of Pittsburgh Medical Center, Pittsburgh, Pennsylvania
Chapter 48, Ethics, Palliative Care, and Care at the End of Life

Rosemarie E. Hardin, MD
Resident Cardiothoracic Surgery, University of Pittsburgh Medical Center, Pittsburgh, Pennsylvania
Chapter 46, Surgical Considerations in the Elderly

Michael H. Heggeness, MD, PhD
Chairman, Division of Orthopedic Surgery, Baylor College of Medicine, Houston, Texas
Chapter 43, Orthopedic Surgery

Lior Heller, MD
Associate Professor, Division of Plastic Surgery, Michael E. DeBakey Department of Surgery, Baylor College of Medicine, Houston, Texas
Chapter 16, The Skin and Subcutaneous Tissue

Daniel B. Hinshaw, MD
Veterans Administration Medical Center
Chapter 48, Ethics, Palliative Care, and Care at the End of Life

John B. Holcomb, MD
Professor, Department of Surgery and Director, Center for Translational Injury Research, University of Texas Health Science Center, Houston, Texas
Chapter 4, Hemostasis, Surgical Bleeding, and Transfusion

Larry H. Hollier, MD
Professor, Division of Plastic Surgery, Michael E. DeBakey Department of Surgery, Baylor College of Medicine, Houston, Texas
Chapter 16, The Skin and Subcutaneous Tissue

Abhinav Humar, MD
Professor of Surgery, Department of Surgery, University of Minnesota, Minneapolis, Minnesota
Chapter 11, Transplantation

Kelly K. Hunt, MD
Professor of Surgery, Department of Surgical Oncology, University of Texas M.D. Anderson Cancer Center, Houston, Texas
Chapter 17, The Breast

John G. Hunter, MD, FACS
Mackenzie Professor and Chair, Department of Surgery, Oregon Health and Science University, Portland, Oregon
Chapter 14, Minimally Invasive Surgery, Robotics, and Natural Orifice Transluminal Endoscopic Surgery
Chapter 25, Esophagus and Diaphragmatic Hernia
Chapter 32, Gallbladder and the Extrahepatic Biliary System

Tam T. Huynh, MD
Associate Professor of Surgery, Division of Vascular Surgery and Endovascular Therapy, Michael E. DeBakey Department of Surgery, Baylor College of Medicine, Houston, Texas
Chapter 23, Arterial Disease

Bernard M. Jaffe, MD
Professor Emeritus, Department of Surgery, Tulane University School of Medicine, New Orleans, Louisiana
Chapter 30, The Appendix

Badar V. Jan, MD
PGY-4 Surgical Resident, Department of Surgery, UMDNJ-Robert Wood Johnson Medical School, New Brunswick, New Jersey
Chapter 2, Systemic Response to Injury and Metabolic Support

Kenneth M. Jastrow, MD
Surgery Resident, Department of Surgery, University of Texas Health Science Center, Houston, Texas
Chapter 4, Hemostasis, Surgical Bleeding, and Transfusion

Blair A. Jobe, MD
Associate Professor of Surgery, The Heart, Lung and Esophageal Surgery Institute, University of Pittsburgh, Pittsburgh, Pennsylvania
Chapter 14, Minimally Invasive Surgery, Robotics, and Natural Orifice Transluminal Endoscopic Surgery
Chapter 25, Esophagus and Diaphragmatic Hernia

Tara B. Karamlou, MD, MSc
Cardiothoracic Surgery Fellow, University of Michigan, Ann Arbor, Michigan
Chapter 20, Congenital Heart Disease

Elise C. Kohn, MD
Senior Investigator and Section Head, Department of Molecular Signaling Section, Medical Oncology Branch, National Cancer Institute, Bethesda, Maryland
Chapter 41, Gynecology

Panagiotis Kougias, MD
Assistant Professor, Department of Surgery, Baylor College of Medicine, Houston, Texas
Chapter 23, Arterial Disease

Rosemary A. Kozar, MD
Associate Professor of Surgery, Department of Surgery, Memorial Hermann Hospital, Houston, Texas
Chapter 4, Hemostasis, Surgical Bleeding, and Transfusion

Jeffrey La Rochelle, MD
Fellow and Clinical Instructor, David Geffen School of Medicine at UCLA, Los Angeles, California
Chapter 40, Urology

Geeta Lal, MD
Assistant Professor of Surgery, University of Iowa Health Care, Carver College of Medicine, Department of Surgery, Division of Surgical Oncology and Endocrine Surgery, Iowa City, Iowa
Chapter 38, Thyroid, Parathyroid, and Adrenal

Thu Ha Liz Lee, MD
Assistant Professor of Surgery, Department of Surgery, University of Cincinnati, Cincinnati, Ohio
Chapter 1, Accreditation Council for Graduate Medical Education Core Competencies

Scott A. LeMaire, MD
Associate Professor and Director of Research, Division of Cardiothoracic Surgery, Michael E. DeBakey Department of Surgery, Baylor College of Medicine, Houston, Texas
Chapter 22, Thoracic Aneurysms and Aortic Dissection

Timothy K. Liem, MD
Associate Professor of Surgery, Adjunct Associate Professor of Radiology, Division of Vascular Surgery, Oregon Health and Science University, Portland, Oregon
Chapter 24, Venous and Lymphatic Disease

Scott D. Lifchez, MD
Assistant Professor, Department of Surgery, Division of Plastic Surgery, Johns Hopkins Medical Institutions, Baltimore, Maryland
Chapter 44, Surgery of the Hand and Wrist

Peter H. Lin, MD
Associate Professor of Surgery, Division of Vascular Surgery and Endovascular Therapy, Michael E. DeBakey Department of Surgery, Baylor College of Medicine, Houston, Texas
Chapter 23, Arterial Disease

Xia Lin, MD
Associate Professor, Michael E. DeBakey Department of Surgery, Baylor College of Medicine, Houston, Texas
Chapter 15, Molecular and Genomic Surgery

Joseph E. Losee, MD
Associate Professor of Surgery and Pediatrics, University of Pittsburgh Medical Center, Pittsburgh, Pennsylvania
Chapter 45, Plastic and Reconstructive Surgery

Stephen F. Lowry, MD
Professor and Chair, Department of Surgery, UMDNJ-Robert Wood Johnson Medical School, New Brunswick, New Jersey
Chapter 2, Systemic Response to Injury and Metabolic Support

James D. Luketich, MD
Henry T. Bahnson Professor of Cardiothoracic Surgery, Chief, The Heart, Lung and Esophageal Surgery Institute, Department of Surgery, Division of Thoracic and Foregut Surgery, University of Pittsburgh, Pittsburgh, Pennsylvania
Chapter 19, Chest Wall, Lung, Mediastinum, and Pleura

James R. Macho, MD
Emeritus Professor of Surgery, Department of Surgery, University of California, San Francisco, San Francisco, California
Chapter 37, Inguinal Hernias

Michael A. Maddaus, MD
Professor of Surgery, Department of Surgery, Division of General Thoracic and Foregut Surgery, University of Minnesota, Minneapolis, Minnesota
Chapter 19, Chest Wall, Lung, Mediastinum, and Pleura

Martin A. Makary, MD
Mark Ravitch Chair in General Surgery, Associate Professor of Health Policy, Department of Surgery, Johns Hopkins University School of Medicine, Baltimore, Maryland
Chapter 12, Patient Safety

Jeffrey B. Matthews, MD, FACS
Dallas B. Phemister Professor and Chairman, Department of Surgery, University of Chicago, Chicago, Illinois

Funda Meric-Bernstam, MD
Associate Professor, Department of Surgical Oncology, University of Texas M.D. Anderson Cancer Center, Houston, Texas
Chapter 10, Oncology

Gregory L. Moneta, MD
Professor of Surgery, Division of Vascular Surgery, Department of Surgery, Oregon Health and Science University, Portland, Oregon
Chapter 24, Venous and Lymphatic Disease

Ernest E. Moore, MD
Vice Chairman and Professor, Department of Surgery, University of Colorado, Denver, Denver, Colorado
Chapter 7, Trauma

Katie S. Nason, MD
Assistant Professor, Division of Thoracic Surgery, Department of General Surgery, University of Pittsburgh Medical Center, Pittsburgh, Pennsylvania
Chapter 19, Chest Wall, Lung, Mediastinum, and Pleura

Kurt D. Newman, MD
Professor of Surgery and Pediatrics, Division of Surgery, George Washington University School of Medicine, Washington, DC
Chapter 39, Pediatric Surgery

Lisa A. Newman, MD
Professor, Department of Surgery, University of Michigan Comprehensive Cancer Center, Ann Arbor, Michigan
Chapter 17, The Breast

Margrét Oddsdóttir, MD*
Professor of Surgery, Chief of General Surgery, Landspitali-University Hospital, Reykjavik, Iceland
Chapter 32, Gallbladder and the Extrahepatic Biliary System

Adrian E. Park, MD
Campbell and Jeanette Plugge Professor and Vice Chair, Division of General Surgery, University of Maryland Medical Center, Baltimore, Maryland
Chapter 34, Spleen

Timothy M. Pawlik, MD
Johns Hopkins University, Baltimore, Maryland
Chapter 48, Ethics, Palliative Care, and Care at the End of Life

Andrew B. Peitzman, MD
Mark M. Ravitch Professor and Vice Chairman, Department of Surgery, University of Pittsburgh School of Medicine, Pittsburgh, Pennsylvania
Chapter 5, Shock

Jeffrey H. Peters, MD
Chairman, Department of Surgery, University of Rochester Medical Center, Rochester, New York
Chapter 25, Esophagus and Diaphragmatic Hernia

Thai H. Pham, MD
Fellow, Department of General Surgery, Oregon Health and Science University, Portland, Oregon
Chapter 32, Gallbladder and the Extrahepatic Biliary System

Raphael E. Pollock, MD, PhD, FACS
Head, Division of Surgery, Professor and Chairman, Department of Surgical Oncology, Senator A.M. Aiken, Jr., Distinguished Chair, University of Texas M.D. Anderson Cancer Center, Houston, Texas
Chapter 10, Oncology
Chapter 36, Soft Tissue Sarcomas

Charles A. Reitman, MD
Associate Professor, Department of Orthopedic Surgery, Baylor College of Medicine, Houston, Texas
Chapter 43, Orthopedic Surgery

David A. Rothenberger, MD
Professor and Deputy, Department of Surgery, University of Minnesota, Minneapolis, Minnesota
Chapter 29, Colon, Rectum, and Anus

J. Peter Rubin, MD
Associate Professor of Surgery (Plastic), University of Pittsburgh Medical Center, Pittsburgh, Pennsylvania
Chapter 45, Plastic and Reconstructive Surgery

Ashok K. Saluja, PhD
Professor and Vice Chair, Department of Surgery, University of Minnesota, Minneapolis, Minnesota
Chapter 33, Pancreas

Philip R. Schauer, MD
Chief of Minimally Invasive General Surgery, Cleveland Clinic, Cleveland, Ohio
Chapter 27, The Surgical Management of Obesity

Bruce Schirmer, MD
Stephen H. Watts Professor of Surgery, University of Virginia Health System, Charlottesville, Virginia
Chapter 27, The Surgical Management of Obesity

Charles F. Schwartz, MD
Assistant Professor of Cardiothoracic Surgery, New York University School of Medicine, New York, New York
Chapter 21, Acquired Heart Disease

Subhro K. Sen, MD
Clinical Assistant Professor, Division of Plastic & Reconstructive Surgery, Department of Surgery, Stanford University Medical Center, Palo Alto, California
Chapter 44, Surgery of the Hand and Wrist

Neal E. Seymour, MD
Professor, Department of Surgery, Tufts University School of Medicine, Chief of General Surgery, Baystate Medical Center, Springfield, Massachusetts
Chapter 35, Abdominal Wall, Omentum, Mesentery, and Retroperitoneum

Mark L. Shapiro, MD
Associate Professor of Surgery, Associate Director Trauma Services, Department of Surgery, Duke University Medical Center, Durham, North Carolina
Chapter 12, Patient Safety

Kapil Sharma, MD
Assistant Professor, Division of Cardiothoracic Surgery, Michael E. DeBakey Department of Surgery, Baylor College of Medicine, Houston, Texas
Chapter 22, Thoracic Aneurysms and Aortic Dissection

Vadim Sherman, MD, FRCSC
Assistant Professor of Surgery, Director, Comprehensive Bariatric Surgery Center, Program Director, Minimally Invasive Fellowship, Michael E. DeBakey Department of Surgery, Baylor College of Medicine, Houston, Texas
Chapter 37, Inguinal Hernias

G. Tom Shires III, MD
Chair, Surgical Services, Presbyterian Hospital of Dallas, Dallas, Texas
Chapter 3, Fluid and Electrolyte Management of the Surgical Patient

Brian Shuch, MD
Chief Resident, Department of Urology, David Geffen School of Medicine, Los Angeles, California
Chapter 40, Urology

Michael L. Smith, MD
Assistant Professor, Department of Neurosurgery, Albert Einstein College of Medicine, Bronx, New York
Chapter 42, Neurosurgery

Samuel Stal, MD
Professor, Division of Plastic Surgery, Michael E. DeBakey Department of Surgery, Baylor College of Medicine, Houston, Texas
Chapter 16, The Skin and Subcutaneous Tissue

Ali Tavakkolizadeh, MB BS
Assistant Professor of Surgery, Department of Surgery, Harvard Medical School, Boston, Massachusetts
Chapter 28, Small Intestine

*Deceased.

Allan Tsung, MD
Assistant Professor, Department of Surgery, University of Pittsburgh, Pittsburgh, Pennsylvania
Chapter 31, Liver

Ross M. Ungerleider, MD
Professor of Surgery, Department of Surgery, Oregon Health and Science University, Portland, Oregon
Chapter 20, Congenital Heart Disease

Christopher G. Wallace, MD
Clinical and Research Microsurgery Fellow, Department of Plastic and Reconstructive Surgery, Chang Gung Memorial Hospital, Chang Gung University and Medical College, Taipei, Taiwan
Chapter 45, Plastic and Reconstructive Surgery

Kasper S. Wang, MD
Assistant Professor of Surgery, Department of Pediatric Surgery, Keck School of Medicine, University of Southern California, Los Angeles, California
Chapter 39, Pediatric Surgery

Randal S. Weber, MD
Professor and Hubert L. and Olive Stringer Distinguished Professor for Cancer Research and Chairman, Department of Head and Neck Surgery, University of Texas M.D. Anderson Cancer Center, Houston, Texas
Chapter 18, Disorders of the Head and Neck

Fu-Chan Wei, MD, FACS
Professor and Chancellor, Department of Plastic Surgery, College of Medicine, Chang Gung University, Chang Gung Memorial Hospital, Taipei, Taiwan
Chapter 45, Plastic and Reconstructive Surgery

Richard O. Wein, MD
Assistant Professor, Department of Otolaryngology-Head and Neck Surgery, Tufts New England Medical Center, Boston, Massachusetts
Chapter 18, Disorders of the Head and Neck

Jacob Weinberg, MD
Assistant Professor, Department of Orthopedic Surgery, Baylor College of Medicine, Houston, Texas
Chapter 43, Orthopedic Surgery

Karl F. Welke, MD
Assistant Professor, Division of Cardiothoracic Surgery, Oregon Health and Science University, Portland, Oregon
Chapter 20, Congenital Heart Disease

Edward E. Whang, MD
Associate Professor of Surgery, Department of Surgery, Harvard Medical School, Boston, Massachusetts
Chapter 28, Small Intestine

Michael E. Zenilman, MD
Clarence and Mary Dennis Professor and Chairman, Department of Surgery, SUNY Downstate Medical Center, Brooklyn, New York
Chapter 46, Surgical Considerations in the Elderly

Michael J. Zinner, MD
Moseley Professor of Surgery, Department of Surgery, Harvard Medical School, Boston, Massachusetts
Chapter 28, Small Intestine

Brian S. Zuckerbraun, MD
Assistant Professor of Surgery, Department of Surgery, University of Pittsburgh School of Medicine, Pittsburgh, Pennsylvania
Chapter 5, Shock

VIDEO CONTRIBUTORS

Daniel Albo, MD, PhD
Chief, General Surgery and Surgical Oncology, Director, Colorectal Cancer Center, Michael E. DeBakey VAMC, Houston, Texas
Hand Assisted Laparoscopic LAR
Hand Assisted Laparoscopic Right Hemi-Colectomy

John Bozinovski, MD, MSc, FRCSC
Attending Cardiac Surgeon, Department of Surgery, Royal Jubilee Hospital, Victoria, British Columbia, Canada
Open Surgical Treatment of Extent IV Thoracoabdominal Aortic Aneurysms

F. Charles Brunicardi, MD, FACS
DeBakey/Bard Professor and Chairman, Michael E. DeBakey Department of Surgery, Baylor College of Medicine, Houston, Texas
Knot Tying
Suturing
Laparoscopic Cholecystectomy on a Patient with Biliary Colic and Gall Stones
Laparoscopic Nissen Fundoplication
Laparoscopic Distal Pancreatectomy
Totally Extra-Peritoneal (TEP) Hernia Repair
Laparoscopic Adjustable Gastric Band and Hiatal Hernia Repair
Laparoscopic Sleeve Gastrectomy

Joseph F. Buell, MD
Professor of Surgery, University of Louisville, Louisville, Kentucky
Laparoscopic Left Hepatic Lobectomy for Benign Liver Mass

Orlo H. Clark, MD
Professor of Surgery, Department of Surgery, UCSF/Mt. Zion Medical Center, San Francisco, California
Bilateral Exploration Parathyroidectomy

Steven D. Colquhoun, MD
Surgical Director, Liver Transplantation, Comprehensive Transplant Center, Cedars-Sinai Medical Center, Associate Professor of Medicine, David Geffen School of Medicine, University of California, Los Angeles, Los Angeles, California
Right-Lobe Living-Donor Liver Transplantation

Joseph S. Coselli, MD
Professor and Cullen Foundation Endowed Chair, Division of Cardiothoracic Surgery, Michael E. DeBakey Department of Surgery, Baylor College of Medicine, Houston, Texas
Open Surgical Treatment of Extent IV Thoracoabdominal Aortic Aneurysms

David A. Geller, MD
Richard L. Simmons Professor of Surgery, Thomas E. Starzl Transplantation Institute, University of Pittsburgh, Pittsburgh, Pennsylvania
Laparoscopic Left Hepatic Lobectomy for Hepatocellular Carcinoma

Carlos D. Godinez, MD
Fellow and Clinical Instructor, Minimally Invasive Surgery, Department of Surgery, University of Maryland School of Medicine, Baltimore, Maryland
Laparoscopic Splenectomy

Marlon Guerrero, MD
Assistant Professor and Director of Endocrine Surgery, Department of Surgery, University of Arizona, Tucson, Arizona
Bilateral Exploration Parathyroidectomy

Shahzeer Karmali, BSc, MD, FRCSC
Assistant Professor of Surgery, Minimally Invasive and Bariatric Surgery, University of Alberta, Edmonton, Alberta, Canada
Laparoscopic Sleeve Gastrectomy
Laparoscopic Adjustable Gastric and Hiatal Hernia Repair

Geeta Lal, MD
Assistant Professor of Surgery, University of Iowa Health Care, Carver College of Medicine, Department of Surgery, Division of Surgical Oncology and Endocrine Surgery, Iowa City, Iowa
Bilateral Exploration Parathyroidectomy

Scott A. LeMaire, MD
Associate Professor and Director of Research, Division of Cardiothoracic Surgery, Michael E. DeBakey Department of Surgery, Baylor College of Medicine, Houston, Texas
Open Surgical Treatment of Extent IV Thoracoabdominal Aortic Aneurysms

Richard E. Link, MD
Associate Professor of Urology, Director, Division of Endourology and Minimally Invasive Surgery, The Scott Department of Urology, Baylor College of Medicine, Houston, Texas
Robotic-Assisted Laparoscopic Partial Nephractomy
Robotic-Assisted Laparoscopic Radial Prostatectomy

Paul Martin, MD
Professor of Medicine, Chief, Division of Hepatology, Schiff Liver Institute/Center for Liver Dieseases, University of Miami Miller School of Medicine, Miami, Florida
Right-Lobe Living Donor Liver Transplantation

Jeffrey B. Matthews, MD, FACS
Dallas B. Phemister Professor and Chair, Department of Surgery, University of Chicago, Chicago, Illinois
Laparoscopic Cystogastrostomy for Pancreatic Pseudocyst

Nicholas N. Nissen, MD
Assistant Surgical Director of the Multi-Organ Transplant Program, Center for Liver Diseases and Transplantation, Ceders-Sinai Medical Center, University of California, Los Angeles, Los Angeles, California
Right-Lobe Living-Donor Liver Transplantation

Adrian E. Park, MD
Campbell and Jeanette Plugge Professor and Vice Chair, Division of General Surgery, University of Maryland Medical Center, Baltimore, Maryland
Laparoscopic Splenectomy

Fred Poordad, MD
Chief, Hepatology and Liver Transplantation, Comprehensive Transplant Center, Cedars-Sinai Medical Center, Associate Professor of Medicine, David Geffen School of Medicine, University of California, Los Angeles, Los Angeles, California
Right-Lobe Living-Donor Liver Transplantation

Vivek N. Prachand, MD
Assistant Professor of Surgery, Department of Surgery, University of Chicago, Chicago, Illinois
Laparoscopic Cystogastrostomy for Pancreatic Pseudocyst

Steven Rudich, MD, PhD
Associate Professor of Surgery, Department of Surgery, University of Cincinnati, Cincinnati, Ohio
Laparoscopic Left Hepatic Lobectomy for Benign Liver Mass

Christopher R. Shackleton, MD
Principal, QV Research Consultancy, Formerly Professor, Department of Surgery, David Geffen School of Medicine, University of California, Los Angeles, Los Angeles, California
Right-Lobe Living-Donor Liver Transplantation

Vadim Sherman, MD, FRCSC
Assistant Professor of Surgery, Director, Comprehensive Bariatric Surgery Center, Program Director, Minimally Invasive Fellowship, Michael E. DeBakey Department of Surgery, Baylor College of Medicine, Houston, Texas
Laparoscopic Sleeve Gastrectomy
Totally Extra-Peritoneal (TEP) Hernia Repair
Laparoscopic Adjustable Gastric and Hiatal Hernia Repair

Amit D. Tevar, MD
Assistant Professor of Surgery, Department of Surgery, University of Cincinnati, Cincinnati, Ohio
Laparoscopic Left Hepatic Lobectomy for Benign Liver Mass

Mark C. Thomas, MD
Assistant Professor, Department of Surgery, University of Cincinnati, Cincinnati, Ohio
Laparoscopic Left Hepatic Lobectomy for Benign Liver Mass

Tram Tran, MD
Assisant Professor of Medicine, Geffen (UCLA) School of Medicine, Comprehensive Transplant Center, Cedars-Sinai Medical Center, Los Angeles, California
Right-Lobe Living-Donor Liver Transplantation

John Moore Vierling, MD
Professor, Michael E. DeBakey Department of Surgery, Baylor College of Medicine, Houston, Texas
Right-Lobe Living-Donor Liver Transplantation

Scott Weldon, MA, CMI
Supervisor, Medical Illustrator, Division of Cardiothoracic Surgery, Michael E. DeBakey Department of Surgery, Baylor College of Medicine, Houston, Texas
Open Surgical Treatment of Extent IV Thoracoabdominal Aortic Aneurysms

Steve Woodle, MD
Professor, Chief, Division of Transplant Surgery, University of Cincinnati, Cincinnati, Ohio
Laparoscopic Left Hepatic Lobectomy for Benign Liver Mass

INTERNATIONAL ADVISORY BOARD

Gaurav Agarwal, MS (Surgery), FACS
Additional Professor, Department of Endocrine and Breast Surgery, Sanjay Gandhi Postgraduate Institute of Medical Sciences, Lucknow, India

Äke Gösta Andrén-Sandberg, MD
Chief, Department of Surgery, Karolinska University Hospital at Huddinge, Stockholm, Sweden

Claudio Bassi, MD, FRCS
Professor, Surgical and Gastroenterological Department, University of Verona, Verona, Italy

Jacques Belghiti, MD
Professor, Department of Surgery, University of Paris VII, Hospital Beaujon, Clichy, France

Kent-Man Chu, MD

Professor of Surgery, Chief, Division of Upper Gastrointestinal Surgery, Department of Surgery, The University of Hong Kong, Queen Mary Hospital, Pokfulam, Hong Kong, China

Eugen H. K. J. Faist, MD

Department of Surgery, Ludwig-Maximilians University, Campus Grosshadern, Munich, Germany

Mordechai Gutman, MD

Head, Department of General Surgery, Meir Hospital, Kfar Saba, Israel

Serafin C. Hilvano, MD, FPCS, FACS

Professor and Chair, Department of Surgery, College of Medicine-Philippine General Hospital, University of the Philippines, Manila, Manila, Philippines

Jamal J. Hoballah, MD, MBA

Professor and Chairman, Department of Surgery, American University of Beirut Medical Center, Hamra District, Beirut, Lebanon

Seon-Hahn Kim, MD

Director of Robotic and MIS Center, Head of Colorectal Division, Professor, Department of Surgery, Korea University Anam Hospital, SungBook-gu, Seoul, South Korea

Yuko Kitagawa, MD

Professor, Department of Surgery, Keio University School of Medicine, Shinjuku-ku, Tokyo, Japan

J. E. J. Krige, MD, FRCS, FACS, FCS (SA)

Professor of Surgery, Surgical Gastroenterology, Department of Surgery, University of Cape Town, Cape Town, South Africa

Miguel Angel Mercado Diaz, MD

Professor and Chairman, Department of General Surgery, National Institute of Medical Science and Nutrition, Mexico DF, Mexico

Gerald C. O'Sullivan, MD, FRCSI, FACS (Hon)

Professor of Surgery, University College Cork, Mercy University Hospital, Cork, Ireland

Ori D. Rotstein, MD

Surgeon-in-Chief, St. Michael's Hospital, Professor, Department of Surgery, University of Toronto, Toronto, Ontario, Canada

John F. Thompson, MD

Melanoma Institute Australia, Royal Prince Alfred and Mater Hospitals, Sydney, Australia, Discipline of Surgery, The University of Sydney, Sydney, Australia

Garth Warnock, MD, MSc, FRCSC

Professor and Head, Department of Surgery, Universtiy of British Columbia, Surgeon-in-Chief, Vancouver Teaching Hospitals, Vancouver, British Columbia, Canada

Liwei Zhu, MD

Department of Surgery, Tianjin Medical University Hospital, Tianjin, China

Four decades have elapsed between the initial publication of *Principles of Surgery* and the ninth edition. Those four decades have witnessed an extraordinary improvement in the appreciation of disease processes, diagnosis, innovations in surgical techniques, and complementary therapeutic approaches.

The mapping of the human genome was associated with an amplification of the number of diseases with a genetic influence. The discovery of the *Helicobacter* bacillus and its causative role on ulcer diathesis has completely transformed the treatment of that disease. What had been one of the most common surgical procedures performed in one's senior surgical residency during my training—namely the anti-acid operations of partial gastric, vagotomy, and drainage—are now rarities.

Improvements in ultrasonography, computed tomography, and magnetic resonance imaging have markedly refined diagnosis, as have the advancements in endoscopy. Minimally invasive surgery has become the standard for many intra-abdominal and intrathoracic operations, and this has been refined by the employment of robotic techniques with visual enhancement. Natural orifice translaparoscopic enteric surgery (NOTES) has arrived on the scene.

Endovascular approaches have completely transformed the surgical management of peripheral vascular diseases, both arterial and venous. Cardiac surgery expanded geometrically—left ventricular assist devices and the ultimate of an artificial heart became realities. Perhaps the most dramatic technical successes were achieved in organ transplantation, which witnessed expected success in kidney, liver, small intestine, heart, and lung orthotopic replacement.

Improved appreciation of fluid and electrolyte and nutritional needs and the more liberal application of intravascular nutritional therapy have allowed for several of these technical expansions. Spectacular refinements in radiation therapy and chemotherapy have resulted in previously unanticipated resectability and improved survival rates for cancer patients. To complete the panoramic landscape, humanism has been featured, with considerations of ethical issues and concern with issues of an aging population, palliation, and end-of-life management.

The six editors who shepherded the production of the first publication could never have imagined all these changes. The two editors, Frank C. Spencer and I, who have been blessed with the longevity to witness the production of the current editors, enjoy a unique element of parental pride.

Seymour I. Schwartz, MD, FACS

When I was asked to serve as editor-in-chief of this historic textbook of surgery, my goal was to preserve its excellent reputation, honoring the commitment of Dr. Seymour Schwartz and previous co-editors and contributors who upheld the highest standard for seven prior editions. I would like to thank all who helped achieve this goal, namely the outstanding contributions by the individual chapter authors and the meticulous dedication of the editorial board, all of whom share a passion for patient care, teaching, and surgery.

It is this shared passion that has been channeled now into the creation of this new ninth edition; updating, improving, and fine-tuning it to secure its place as a leading international textbook of surgery. Each chapter has either been fastidiously updated or created anew by leaders in their respective surgical fields to ensure the highest quality of surgical teaching. Additionally, each chapter has been outfitted with quick-reference key points; highlighted evidenced-based references; and full-color illustrations, images, and information tables. Two new chapters have been added to this edition: *Accreditation Council for Graduate Medical Core Competencies* and *Ethics, Palliative Care, and Care at the End of Life.*

One new component of this edition is the inclusion of a digital video disc of surgical videos. Many students already augment their more traditional classroom and practical education through the breadth of information available in the electronic realm, such as that available on AccessSurgery.com. This collection of operative and instructional videos, generously provided by chapter authors and editors, provides accurate visual instruction and technique to round out students' surgical training. It is the sincere hope of all who have contributed to this textbook that the knowledge of craft contained within will provide a solid foundation for the acquisition of skill, a haven for the continuation of education, and motivation for the pursuit of excellence.

I wish to thank all of those responsible for the publication of this new edition, including the newest member of the editorial board, Dr. Jeffrey Matthews, as well as those who fearlessly signed on as contributors to our newly established international editorial board to provide regional perspective and commentary. I extend many thanks and gratitude to Marsha Loeb, Christie Naglieri, and all at McGraw-Hill for their guidance and knowledge throughout this process. I wish to thank Katie Elsbury for her dedication to the organization and editing of this textbook. I would also like to thank our families, whose love and support *continue* to make this book possible.

F. Charles Brunicardi, MD, FACS

The raison d'être for a new textbook in a discipline which has been served by standard works for many years was the Editorial Board's initial conviction that a distinct need for a modern approach in the dissemination of surgical knowledge existed. As incoming chapters were reviewed, both the need and satisfaction became increasingly apparent and, at the completion, we felt a sense of excitement at having the opportunity to contribute to the education of modern and future students concerned with the care of surgical patients.

The recent explosion of factual knowledge has emphasized the need for a presentation which would provide the student an opportunity to assimilate pertinent facts in a logical fashion. This would then permit correlation, synthesis of concepts, and eventual extrapolation to specific situations. The physiologic bases for diseases are therefore emphasized and the manifestations and diagnostic studies are considered as a reflection of pathophysiology. Therapy then becomes logical in this schema and the necessity to regurgitate facts is minimized. In appreciation of the impact which *Harrison's Principles of Internal Medicine* has had, the clinical manifestations of the disease processes are considered in detail for each area. Since the operative procedure represents the one element in the therapeutic armamentarium unique to the surgeon, the indications, important technical considerations, and complications receive appropriate emphasis. While we appreciate that a textbook cannot hope to incorporate an atlas of surgical procedures, we have provided the student a single book which will satisfy the sequential demands in the care and considerations of surgical patients.

The ultimate goal of the Editorial Board has been to collate a book which is deserving of the adjective "modern." We have therefore selected as authors dynamic and active contributors to their particular fields. The au courant concept is hopefully apparent throughout the entire work and is exemplified by appropriate emphasis on diseases of modern surgical interest, such as trauma, transplantation, and the recently appreciated importance of rehabilitation. Cardiovascular surgery is presented in keeping with the exponential strides recently achieved.

There are two major subdivisions to the text. In the first twelve chapters, subjects that transcend several organ systems are presented. The second portion of the book represents a consideration of specific organ systems and surgical specialties.

Throughout the text, the authors have addressed themselves to a sophisticated audience, regarding the medical student as a graduate student, incorporating material generally sought after by the surgeon in training and presenting information appropriate for the continuing education of the practicing surgeon. The need for a text such as we have envisioned is great and the goal admittedly high. It is our hope that this effort fulfills the expressed demands.

Seymour I. Schwartz, MD, FACS

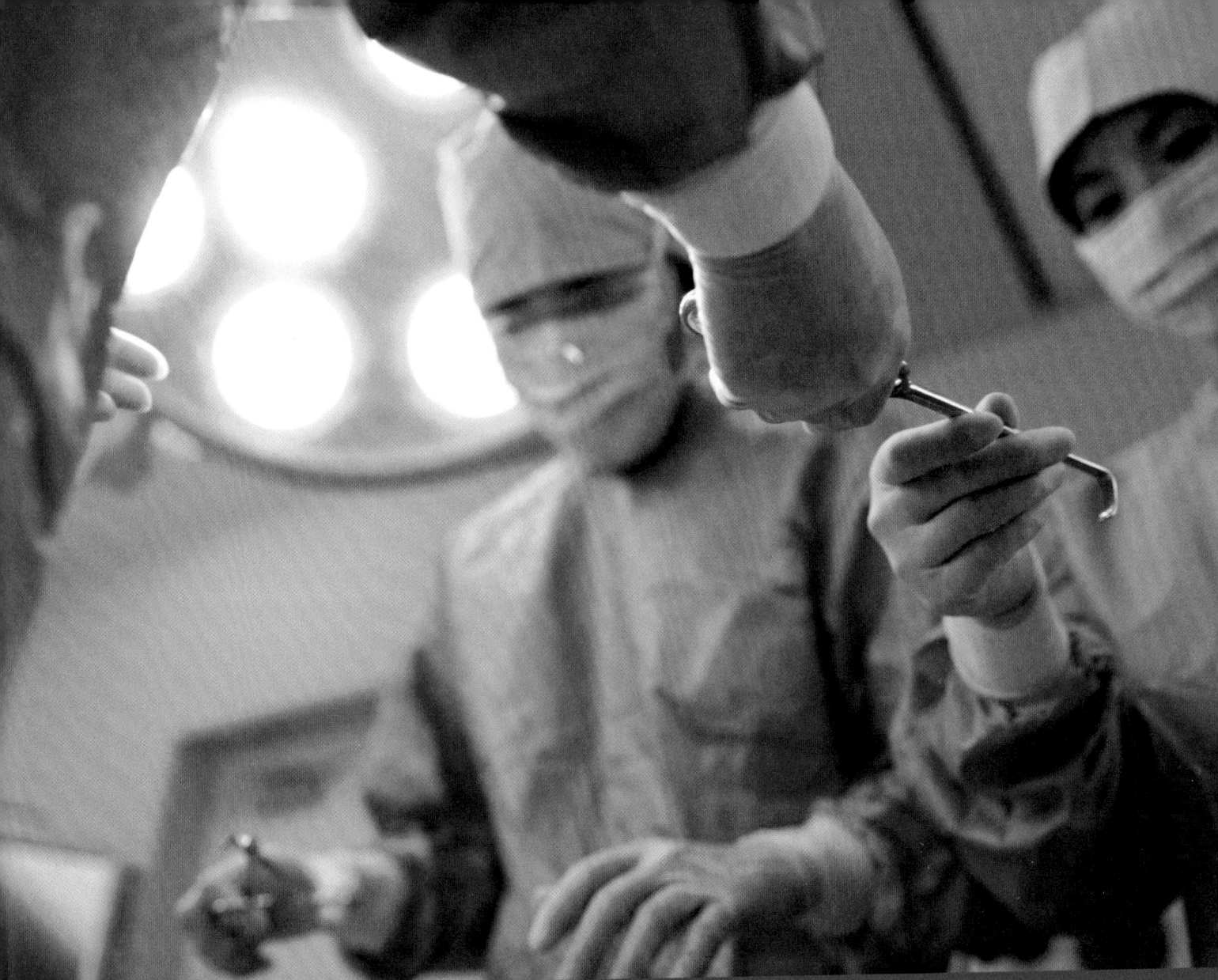

PART I

Basic Considerations

Accreditation Council for Graduate Medical Education Core Competencies

Thu Ha Liz Lee, David H. Berger, Samir S. Awad,
Mary L. Brandt, and F. Charles Brunicardi

ACCREDITATION COUNCIL FOR GRADUATE MEDICAL EDUCATION OUTCOMES PROJECT

Technologic and molecular advances have fundamentally changed the way medicine is practiced. The Internet has revolutionized the way both physicians and patients learn about diseases. In addition, political and economic pressures have altered the way society views and reimburses medical care. The end result of these changes is that access to medical care, access to information about medical care, and the very nature of the doctor-patient relationship has changed.[1] In response to this situation, the Accreditation Council for Graduate Medical Education (ACGME) Outcomes Project was developed. Dr. Leach stated that this initiative was based on three principles: (1) whatever we measure we tend to improve; (2) focusing on outcomes instead of processes allows programs flexibility to adapt based on their needs and resources; and (3) the public deserves to have access to data demonstrating that graduating physicians are competent.[2] This initiative changed the focus of graduate medical education from how programs were *potentially* educating residents by complying with the accreditation requirements to how programs are *actually* educating residents through assessment of the program's outcomes. In 1999, the Outcomes Project identified six core competencies that would provide a conceptual framework to train residents to competently and compassionately treat patients in today's changing health care system. The six core competencies as designated by the ACGME are patient care, medical knowledge, practice-based learning and improvement, interpersonal and communication skills, professionalism, and systems-based practice (Table 1-1).[3] Starting in July 2001, the ACGME implemented a 10-year timeline to implement these concepts into medical education. The timeline was divided into four phases, allowing flexibility for individual programs to meet these goals (Table 1-2).[4]

CORE COMPETENCIES

The core competencies include six specific areas that have been designated as critical for general surgery resident training. Each surgical training program must provide an environment that is conducive to learning the core competencies, establish a curriculum that addresses each of the competencies, and assess that learning has taken place (see Table 1-1). The six core competencies are as follows[5]:

1. Patient Care. Residents must be able to provide patient care that is compassionate, appropriate, and effective for the treatment of health problems and the promotion of health. Residents:
   a. Will demonstrate manual dexterity appropriate for their level;
   b. Will develop and execute patient care plans appropriate for the resident's level, including management of pain;
   c. Will participate in a program that must document a clinical curriculum that is sequential, comprehensive, and organized from basic to complex. The clinical assignments should be carefully structured to ensure that graded levels of responsibility, continuity in patient care, a balance between education and service, and progressive clinical experience are achieved for each resident.
2. Medical Knowledge. Residents must demonstrate knowledge of established and evolving biomedical, clinical, epidemiological, and social-behavioral sciences, as well as the application of this knowledge to patient care. Residents:
   a. Will critically evaluate and demonstrate knowledge of pertinent scientific information, and
   b. Will participate in an educational program that should include the fundamentals of basic science as applied to clinical

TABLE 1-1	Accreditation Council for Graduate Medical Education core competencies
Core Competency	**Description**
Patient care	To be able to provide compassionate and effective health care in the modern-day health care environment
Medical knowledge	To effectively apply current medical knowledge in patient care and to be able to use medical tools (i.e., PubMed) to stay current in medical education
Practice-based learning and improvement	To critically assimilate and evaluate information in a systematic manner to improve patient care practices
Interpersonal and communication skills	To demonstrate sufficient communication skills that allow for efficient information exchange in physician-patient interactions and as a member of a health care team
Professionalism	To demonstrate the principles of ethical behavior (i.e., informed consent, patient confidentiality) and integrity that promote the highest level of medical care
Systems-based practice	To acknowledge and understand that each individual practice is part of a larger health care delivery system and to be able to use the system to support patient care

surgery, including applied surgical anatomy and surgical pathology; the elements of wound healing; homeostasis, shock and circulatory physiology; hematologic disorders; immunobiology and transplantation; oncology; surgical endocrinology; surgical nutrition, fluid and electrolyte balance; and the metabolic response to injury, including burns.

3. Practice-Based Learning and Improvement. Residents must demonstrate the ability to investigate and evaluate their care of patients, to appraise and assimilate scientific evidence, and to continuously improve patient care based on constant self-evaluation and life-long learning. Residents are expected to develop skills and habits to be able to meet the following goals:
   a. Identify strengths, deficiencies, and limits in one's knowledge and expertise;
   b. Set learning and improvement goals;
   c. Identify and perform appropriate learning activities;
   d. Systematically analyze practice using quality improvement methods, and implement changes with the goal of practice improvement;
   e. Incorporate formative evaluation feedback into daily practice;
   f. Locate, appraise, and assimilate evidence from scientific studies related to their patients' health problems;
   g. Use information technology to optimize learning;
   h. Participate in the education of patients, families, students, residents and other health professions;
   i. Participate in mortality and morbidity conferences that evaluate and analyze patient care outcomes; and
   j. Utilize an evidence-based approach to patient care.

4. Interpersonal and Communication Skills. Residents must demonstrate interpersonal and communication skills that result in effective exchange of information and collaboration with patients, their families, and health professionals. Residents are expected to:
   a. Communicate effectively with patients, families, and the public, as appropriate, across a broad range of socioeconomic and cultural backgrounds;
   b. Communicate effectively with physicians, other health professionals, and health related agencies;
   c. Work effectively as a member or leader of a health care team or other professional group;
   d. Act in a consultative role to other physicians and health professionals;
   e. Maintain comprehensive, timely, and legible medical records, if applicable.
   f. Counsel and educate patients and families; and
   g. Effectively document practice activities.

5. Professionalism. Residents must demonstrate a commitment to carrying out professional responsibilities and an adherence to ethical principles. Residents are expected to demonstrate:
   a. Compassion, integrity, and respect for others;
   b. Responsiveness to patient needs that supersedes self-interest;
   c. Respect for patient privacy and autonomy;
   d. Accountability to patients, society and the profession;
   e. Sensitivity and responsiveness to a diverse patient population, including but not limited to diversity in gender, age, culture, race, religion, disabilities, and sexual orientation;
   f. High standards of ethical behavior; and
   g. A commitment to continuity of patient care.

6. Systems-Based Practice. Residents must demonstrate an awareness of and responsiveness to the larger context and system of health care, as well as the ability to call effectively on other resources in the system to provide optimal health care. Residents are expected to:
   a. Work effectively in various health care delivery settings and systems relevant to their clinical specialty;
   b. Coordinate patient care within the health care system relevant to their clinical specialty;
   c. Incorporate considerations of cost awareness and risk-benefit analysis in patient and/or population-based care as appropriate;

KEY POINTS

1. The Accreditation Council for Graduate Medical Education (ACGME) Outcomes Project changes the focus of graduate medical education from how programs are *potentially* educating residents to how programs are *actually* educating residents through assessment of competencies.

2. The six core competencies are patient care, medical knowledge, practice-based learning and improvement, interpersonal and communication skills, professionalism, and systems-based practice.

3. The Residency Review Committee recognizes the importance of simulators for technical training and mandated that all training programs have a skills laboratory by July 2008. A Surgical Skills Curriculum Task Force has developed a National Skills Curriculum to assist programs with training and assessing competency through simulators.

4. The ACGME has developed a professional development tool called the *ACGME Learning Portfolio*. This interactive web-based portfolio can be used as a tool for residents, faculty, and programs directors to allow for reflection, competency assessment, and identification of weaknesses.

5. There is much to be learned still, and programs should continue to share their experiences to identify benchmark programs.

TABLE 1-2	Accreditation Council for Graduate Medical Education timeline			

Phase	Dates	Program Focus	Accreditation Focus
1. Forming an initial response to changes in requirements	July 2001–June 2002	• Define objectives for residents to demonstrate learning the competencies • Review current approaches to evaluation of resident learning • Begin integrating the teaching and learning of competencies into residents' didactic and clinic experience	• Develop operational definitions of compliance • Provide constructive citations and recommendations with no consequences
2. Sharpening the focus	July 2002–June 2006	• Provide learning opportunities in all six competencies • Improve evaluation process to obtain accurate resident performance on the six core competencies • Provide aggregated resident performance data for the program's GMEC internal review	• Review evidence that programs are teaching and assessing the competencies • Provide constructive citations early in the phase and transition to citations with consequences later • Review evidence that GMECs' internal reviews of programs include consideration of aggregated performance data
3. Full integration	July 2006–June 2011	• Use resident performance data as basis for improvement and provide evidence for accreditation review • Use external measures to verify resident and program performance levels	• Review evidence that programs are making data-driven improvements • Review external program performance measures and input from GMECs as evidence for achieving educational goals
4. Expansion	July 2011–beyond	—	• Identify benchmark programs • Adapt and adopt generalizable information about models of excellence • Invoke community about building knowledge about good graduate medical education

GMEC = graduate medical education committee.

d. Advocate for quality patient care and optimal patient care systems;

e. Work in inter-professional teams to enhance patient safety and improve patient care quality;

f. Participate in identifying system errors and implementing potential systems solutions;

g. Practice high quality, cost effective patient care;

h. Demonstrate knowledge of risk-benefit analysis; and

i. Demonstrate an understanding of the role of different specialists and other health care professionals in overall patient management.

The goal of any surgical training program is to train physicians to provide the highest quality of patient care. The core competency mandates have set into motion changes in education that result in measurable outcome-based training. The challenge of the surgical educator is to develop innovative and focused learning techniques to accomplish this mandate within an 80-hour work week.

Patient Care

Patient care is the foundation for the practice of clinical medicine and must be addressed early and continuously during residency. Historically, patient care has been taught by an apprenticeship model; in other words, by the residents' spending time with attending physicians on the wards or in the operating rooms.[6] However, this training method has to be re-evaluated as a result of the ever-increasing constraints and changes in our health care system. Increasing public awareness of medical legal errors has resulted in heightened scrutiny with regard to patient safety issues.[1] In addition, there are increasing concerns related to the perceived financial setback and medical-legal impact of resident training in the operating room.[7] Even with the inherent flexibility provided by the ACGME, all of these factors, coupled with the work hour restrictions,[8] make surgical training in the modern health care system an especially challenging endeavor. Not only must educators impart the medical knowledge of caring for patients and new advances in patient care, but they must also impart the technical skills necessary to perform complex surgical procedures.

One of the subcompetencies under patient care is that residents "will demonstrate manual dexterity appropriate for their level."[5]

Traditionally, the operating room has been used to train residents in the technical aspects of patient care by "see one, do one, and teach one." A study by Velmahos and colleagues evaluated the knowledge and technical skills of residents who were randomly assigned either to training using the traditional approach or to training in a surgical skills laboratory using the principles of cognitive task analysis. This study revealed that the residents who trained using the laboratory approach had improved medical knowledge and technical skills.[9] Multiple studies like the one previously mentioned have revealed improved performance with simulators and advocated their use in technical skills training.[10–12] Having recognized the importance of incorporating simulation training into today's residency, the Residency Review Committee (RRC) mandated that all surgery programs be required to have a surgical skills laboratory by July 2008 to maintain their accreditation.[13] To assist programs, the Surgical Skills Curriculum Task Force, a joint project of the American College of Surgeons (ACS) and the Association of Program Directors in Surgery, developed a standardized skills curriculum.[14,15] This curriculum was developed in three phases (Table 1-3): phase I with modules for junior residents, phase II for senior residents, and phase III for team training. Another resource that programs may use in developing a surgical skills curriculum is the Fundamentals of Laparoscopic Surgery (FLS) program. This program is endorsed by the ACS and the Society of Gastrointestinal and Endoscopic Surgeons. The FLS consists of a comprehensive curriculum with hands-on skills training and an assessment tool designed to teach and assess the fundamentals of laparoscopic surgery.[16] Future goals for surgical education include a method to ensure that residents are "certified" and deemed competent to perform a procedure in a simulator environment before

TABLE 1-3	National skills curriculum phases and launch dates	
Phase		**Dates**
I	Basic/core skills and tasks	July 2007
II	Advanced procedures	January 2008
III	Team-based skills	July 2008

allowing residents to perform that particular procedure in the operating room.[17]

The RRC has mandated that all residency programs develop a surgical skills laboratory, and the majority of program directors feel that this is an important part of residency training. However, a study by Korndorffer and associates just before the mandate was issued revealed that only 55% of the 162 programs that replied to the survey had a surgical skills laboratory facility.[18] The average cost to develop a laboratory has been reported as $133,000 to $450,000, but the cost can range from $300 to $3 million.[18,19] Kapadia and colleagues surveyed 40 programs with surgical skills laboratories in place and found that funding came from industry (68%), surgery departments (64%), hospitals (46%), and other sources (29%). They also found a wide variation in the size of the facility, location, availability of simulators, protected time for skills training, and curriculum. This study also revealed that 65% of the programs believed that it was somewhat difficult to recruit faculty members to staff the laboratory; however, this could be related to the fact that 69% of the laboratories did not offer any faculty incentive to teach.[19] These studies suggest that although most surgical educators believe that surgical skills laboratories are important for resident education, there is still much room for improvement and standardization.

In addition to technical competency, residents are expected to "develop and execute patient care plans appropriate for the resident's level, including management of pain."[5] This can be reinforced during attendance at rounds and integrated into many of the conferences that are currently available in many surgery programs, such as grand rounds and the morbidity and mortality conference.[20,21] Prince and others demonstrated in an institutional study that use of an interactive format for the morbidity and mortality conference improved the educational value of the conference for residents at all levels.[22] Rosenfeld restructured the morbidity and mortality conference to make it more competence based. For example, each patient case was further divided into separate categories such as patient communication, ethical dilemmas, system problems, and practice-based improvement to enhance patient care.[20] Stiles and associates developed a morning report conference after the implementation of the night float system to improve patient sign-out procedures. They found that this forum not only helped to improve communication but also allowed for teaching, discussion of patient care plans, and direct evaluation of resident competence.[23]

Medical Knowledge

The ACGME has mandated that "residents must demonstrate knowledge of established and evolving biomedical, clinical, epidemiological, and social-behavioral sciences, as well as the application of this knowledge to patient care."[5] Surgery has undergone an exponential growth in new procedures and technology. With this explosion in medical innovation, training programs are posed with the daunting task of not only teaching the technical aspects of surgery, but also imparting the basic science and fundamentals of surgical diseases. Furthermore, development of the field of molecular biology and its application to surgical diseases has mandated that surgeons understand the basic molecular mechanisms of each disease process.[24,25] The new era of molecular biology requires understanding the complex science that can lead to advances such as molecular fingerprinting techniques to tailor treatments that are specific for each individual patient. Other, more cognitive tools such as how to critically review literature and how to logically evaluate the relevance of a study must also be imparted to residents so that they can correctly apply findings of the latest medical studies to each individual patient.

The ACGME mandates that residents "will participate in an educational program that should include the fundamentals of basic science as applied to clinical surgery, including applied surgical anatomy and surgical pathology; the elements of wound healing; homeostasis, shock and circulatory physiology; hematologic disorders; immunobiology and transplantation; oncology; surgical endocrinology; surgical nutrition, fluid and electrolyte balance; and the metabolic response to injury, including burns."[5] The ability of a surgical program to adequately meet this educational challenge can be improved by using innovative learning techniques. Educational systems such as the SQR3 (Survey, Question, Read, Recite, and Review) system of studying,[26] the Pimsleur model,[27] and Rosetta Stone learning techniques[28] are all tools that can aid in the understanding and application of advances in a rapidly changing surgical field. The authors' surgery residency program combined adult learning principles with some of these learning techniques into a problem-based learning program that met weekly after grand rounds. This mandatory, focused curriculum for the residents incorporated both basic science and its clinical application in an interactive and collaborative format. This educational format led to high resident satisfaction and also a sustainable increase in resident American Board of Surgery In-Training Examination scores.[29,30]

Residents are also expected to "critically evaluate and demonstrate knowledge of pertinent scientific information."[5] Residents can be taught early how to critically review the literature using the format of a journal club. The journal club is a widely used technique through which to disseminate the latest in medical knowledge. Even as early as the late 1980s, a study in the *Journal of the American Medical Association* found that residents who participated in a journal club had improved reading habits and improved medical knowledge compared with their peers who did not participate in a journal club.[31] The wide use of journal clubs in surgery education can be seen as a necessary foundation for medical education. In one survey, over 65% of general surgery residency programs have a journal club that meets at least once a month to discuss relevant surgical and medical topics.[32] MacRae and others took this approach a step further by evaluating the effect of a multifaceted Internet-based journal club and found that this learning format improved the skills of the surgical residents to critically appraise the medical literature.[33] Many online resources are available for residents that provide an abundant amount of material for study, reference, and interactive learning.[34-36] In particular, AccessSurgery provides an extensive online resource with medical data and operative techniques, with a core curriculum organized around the ACGME mandates (Fig. 1-1).[34] Finally, and perhaps most importantly, it must be conveyed to surgical trainees that surgery is a lifelong learning process, and the ability to continue building on one's medical knowledge is critical for a successful surgical career.

Practice-Based Learning and Improvement

The third ACGME mandate states that "residents must demonstrate the ability to investigate and evaluate their care of patients, to appraise and assimilate scientific evidence, and to continuously improve patient care based on constant self-evaluation and life-long learning."[5] This mandate comes from the increasing public demand for accountability and increased demand for data regarding outcomes for specific surgeon.[2] Practice-based learning and improvement involves a cycle of four steps: identify areas for improvement, engage in learning, apply the new knowledge and skills to a practice, and check for improvement.[37] This ability to critically and impartially analyze one's practice patterns to continually improve patient care should start early during training, so that this behavior becomes second nature for residents when they become practicing surgeons.

In residency training, the simplest example of practice-based learning is the surgical morbidity and mortality conference. This conference traditionally allows for in-depth discussions of surgical cases and adverse patient outcomes. Complications are categorized (preventable, probably preventable, possibly preventable, and unpreventable) and areas of improvement are identified. Rosenfeld as well as Williams and Dunnington have reformatted this conference to make it more competence based by having residents assess themselves. Residents are required to fill out a practice-based improvement form and identify areas of improvement.[20,38] Another

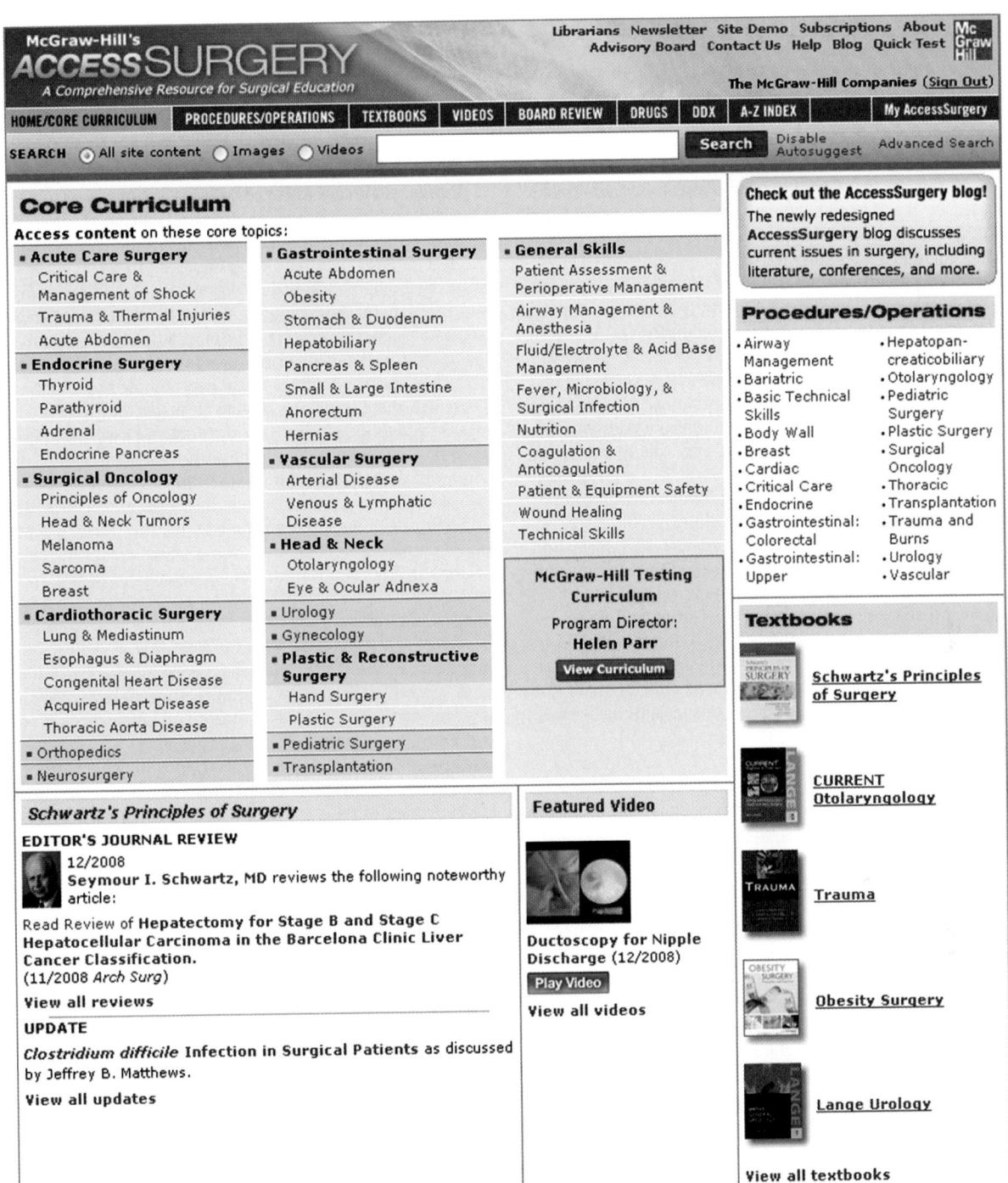

FIG. 1-1. AccessSurgery, a comprehensive resource for surgical education, is an online resource that provides extensive medical data and operative techniques, with a core curriculum organized around the ACGME mandates.

innovative modality to teach practice-based learning was described by Canal and colleagues, who developed a 6-week curriculum in continuous quality improvement for surgery residents that included a specific project. In this project, the residents identified a need for quality improvement, implemented a plan for improvement, and developed a method to measure the improvement. These residents scored significantly higher in knowledge of and experience in quality improvement after completing this curriculum and felt that it was an effective and formal way to teach them the science of practice-based improvement.[39]

Clearly, for surgeons to identify areas of improvement, there has to be some method to allow for comparison and reflection. An interesting Internet-based learning portfolio called *Computerized Obstetrics and Gynecology Automated Learning Analysis (KOALA)*

was developed for the obstetrics and gynecology residents in Canada. This portfolio encouraged self-analysis and self-directed learning by allowing residents to log patient encounters, list critical events and questions derived from these events, look up data used to answer these questions, and state how their practice patterns would be altered based on their reflections. Residents who used this method to reflect and critically analyze their performance scored significantly higher on the Self-Directed Learning Readiness Scale, looked forward to learning for life, and had a strong desire to learn new things.[40] An avenue currently available for practicing surgeons and residents to analyze their outcomes is the ACS Case Log System. This system was developed to support practice-based learning and improvement by allowing surgeons to voluntarily report their own results and compare them to those of other surgeons enrolled in the system. This allows surgeons to critically evaluate their practice outcomes and identify areas that need improvement.[41]

To further improve practice patterns, the ACGME has mandated that trainees must understand the use of information technology systems to manage patient information and support clinical care. Technology is rapidly improving, and hospitals are increasing their efficiency by using electronic medical records. One of the best examples of this is the Computerized Patient Record System (CPRS) used by the Veterans Affairs (VA) hospital system. This fully computerized patient database allows easy access to all patient clinical data, including laboratory tests, radiographic studies, physician notes, and appointment times. Use of this central core information system also has allowed the VA health system to develop the National Surgical Quality Improvement Program (NSQIP).[42] Using information from the CPRS, nurse reviewers are able to gather and input information into the NSQIP system. NSQIP has been the first prospective risk-adjusted outcomes-based program for comparing and improving surgical outcomes across multiple institutions. This program has revolutionized the reporting and quality control of surgical services within the VA system.

Practice-based learning is complex and involves many components, including self-awareness, critical thinking, problem solving, self-directed learning, analysis of outcomes, use of information technology, and focus on evidence-based medicine to improve practice outcomes and patient care.[5] This competency is multifaceted, and an extensive literature review by Ogrinc and associates found little instruction on how to impart these important skills to our residents. Much work appears to be needed before an ideal curriculum can be developed. Future plans should be made for faculty to develop these skills and for programs to continually share their experiences.[43]

Interpersonal and Communication Skills

The fourth competency mandated by the ACGME is that "residents must demonstrate interpersonal and communication skills that result in effective exchange of information and collaboration with patients, their families, and health professionals."[5] Effective communication between physicians, patients, and other health care professionals is essential to the successful and competent practice of medicine and patient care. Studies reveal that physicians with good communication and interpersonal skills have improved patient outcomes and are subject to less medical litigation.[44–46] In support of this, a root cause analysis by the Joint Commission identified breakdown in communication as the leading cause of wrong-site operations and other sentinel events.[47] The ACS has developed a Task Force on Communication and Interpersonal Skills to specifically address this issue and encourage practicing surgeons to develop these important skills.[48] The goal of this task force is to appropriately address the core competency of interpersonal skills and communication and to use novel educational techniques to improve these skills. Certain areas, such as palliative care and patient mortality, have not been a focus for surgeons or surgical trainees but are critical in the surgeon-patient relationship. Four areas in which surgeons can improve their communication skills have been identified in palliative care: the preoperative visit, and discussion of a poor prognosis, surgical complications, and death.[49] These are situations that all surgeons will face at some point in their careers, and the ability to communicate effectively and compassionately with patients during these stressful times is an important skill to develop. Fortunately, multiple techniques for imparting this particular skill have been described in the literature. The group at Southern Illinois University had teams of senior surgical faculty and a faculty member from the Department of Medical Humanities develop a case-based ethics curriculum that covered topics such as resource allocation, research ethics, substituted consent, competition of interests, truth telling, and communication.[17] Other methods to teach communication skills have relied on the use of standardized patients.[38,50,51] Yudkowsky and associates assessed the use of a patient-based communication skills examination. Their conclusion was that the use of a patient-based examination was able to demonstrate consistent results and that verbal feedback was beneficial for resident education on improvement of communication skills.[50] Other recommended teaching strategies include observation with real-time feedback, role modeling, self-assessment, and videotaping.[52]

Residents also are expected to "work effectively as a member or leader of a health care team or other professional group"[5] (Fig. 1-2). This is particularly important for surgeons, because caring for surgical patients requires a team approach to safely get the patient from the preoperative evaluation process, to the operating room, and through the postoperative course. Surgeons are typically the leaders of such teams; hence, it is important for residents to develop the necessary leadership skills during training. With less time spent in the hospital, the ability to learn from real-life situations is limited. Therefore, these principles need to be taught through other creative means such as didactic lectures or problem-based learning. Studies have revealed that formal leadership training not only improves communication skills[53,54] but also helps to develop conflict resolution skills.[55] Awad and colleagues instituted a formal collaborative leadership training program and found that this format significantly increased the residents' views of leadership in the areas of alignment, communication, and integrity.[56] Having recognized leadership training as a necessity for surgeons to thrive in today's medical environment, the ACS offers a course called "Surgeons as Leaders: From Operating Room to Boardroom," whose purpose is to provide surgeons with the skills needed for effective leadership.[57]

A subcompetency under communication and interpersonal skills is to "maintain comprehensive, timely, and legible medical records."[5] Not only does communication occur in person, but physicians commonly communicate their plans and thoughts in the medical record. One of the predominant issues in health care is medical errors related to poor communication. The consequences of poor communication have been shown to cause delays in patient care, improper use of resources, and serious adverse events that lead to significant morbidity and mortality.[58] This is especially important now, as many programs have instituted the night float system to maintain compliance with the work hour restrictions. For this system to work effectively, communication is integral for safe patient care during shift changes.[59,60] One example of a creative approach to this new challenge of information transfer is a web-based system that allows for secure storage of patient information, maintenance of patient lists, access to laboratory values and vital sign data, and

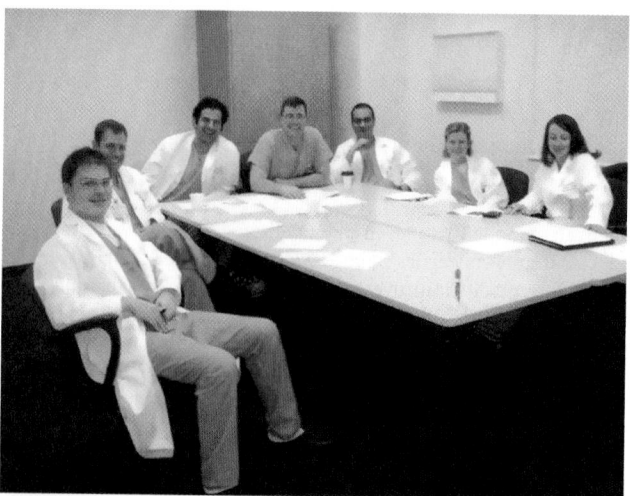

FIG. 1-2. Establishing interpersonal and communication skills equips residents with the necessary tools to communicate effectively with both patients and health professionals.

ability to compile this information to a sign-out list that can be passed on to a coverage team.[61] The residents that participated in the study of this system reported better sign-out quality, decreased time collecting data on prerounds, increased patient contact time, and improved continuity of care. Other medical centers also have begun to institute the use of computerized web-based systems for resident sign-out, and this format may become more widespread as the efficiency and safety of these systems become more apparent.

Not only should surgeons be technically competent and medically knowledgeable, but interpersonal and communication skills are also vital to patient care. The inherent nature of surgery often requires the bearing of bad news, disclosure of complications, and discussion of end-of-life issues. Learning and harnessing the skill of doing these things well during residency will provide a lifelong tool to effectively and compassionately care for patients.

Professionalism

The core competency of professionalism is expressed as follows: "residents must demonstrate a commitment to carrying out professional responsibilities, adherence to ethical principles, and sensitivity to a diverse patient population."[5] The trainee should demonstrate respect, compassion, and integrity while involved in patient care. In addition, residents should understand that their patients' needs supersede their own self-interest and that they are to be held accountable to their patients, society, and the profession.[5]

The ACS endorsed the Charter of Medical Professionalism as its Code of Professional Conduct in 2002.[62,63] This model of professionalism is based on three principles. First, the physician should be dedicated to the patient's welfare. This should supersede all financial, societal, and administrative forces. Second, the physician should have respect for the patient's autonomy. This entails being honest and providing the patient with all the necessary information to make an informed decision. Third, the medical profession should promote justice in the health care system by removing discrimination due to any societal barriers.[64] The ACS also has developed a Task Force on Professionalism to address the competency of professionalism for practicing surgeons and surgical residents. In 2004, this task force stated that professionalism is not just a desirable trait for surgeons to acquire peripherally but is the "central core" of the profession of surgery. The task force has stated the principles of professionalism and defined the responsibility of surgeons to commit to excellence.[65] In addition, it also has created a multimedia program geared toward teaching residents and surgeons about the principles of professionalism through clinical vignettes and discussions.[66] Kumar and associates evaluated this learning tool and found that residents who watched the ACS DVD had improved conceptual understanding of professionalism and scored higher on tests that evaluated these concepts than their peers who had not watched the video.[67]

Professionalism also has been taught by various other methods reported in the literature. A training program at the University of Washington set out to see if professionalism was teachable, learnable, and measurable. This group defined professionalism, developed a curriculum to teach professionalism, and evaluated these traits by a previously validated tool known as the *Global Resident Competency Rating Form*. They found that, after implementation of the curriculum, residents evaluated by the faculty were given significantly higher scores for traits that demonstrate professionalism such as (a) demonstrating respect, compassion, integrity, and reliability; (b) showing commitment to ethical principles; and (c) displaying sensitivity to patient culture, age, sex, and disabilities.[68] Rosenfeld also described a curriculum for professionalism taught by leaders in the community. This 2-year course on professionalism dealt with various topics such as ethics, communication, professional development, respect, sensitivity, and health care delivery. The topics were presented in various formats via lectures, discussion panels, small groups, and videos. The residents were then assessed for competency through quizzes on clinical vignettes and 360-degree evaluations. The preliminary results revealed that residents were treating their

patients and other health care workers in a more professional manner.[69] Heru described the use of role playing and instructional videotapes in teaching professionalism to residents. The residents who were taught using this format showed an increased awareness of unprofessional behavior and increased sensitivity to others, and were able to better deal with conflict.[70] Teaching residents how to navigate through difficult situations and manage conflict is also another important aspect of professionalism, which can further promote an environment of integrity and mutual respect. Fisher and Ury have described four principles for successful conflict resolution: (a) maintain objectivity by not focusing on the participants but focusing on the problem, (b) relinquish the position of power and inflexibility to concentrate more on individual interests, (c) create outcomes in which both parties will have gains, and (d) make sure there are objective criteria for the negotiating process. All of these principles are related to maintaining an open mind and dialogue and yielding to principles, not pressure.[71] These four principles can be integrated into a curriculum through various teaching techniques to help residents deal with conflict in a nonhostile and productive manner.

The ACS has set standards on professional behavior in the Code of Professional Conduct. With these standards used as a conceptual framework, the development of professionalism should be a continuous process for any physician. Surgeons should constantly analyze and reflect on their behavior and continue to work toward actions based on integrity, honesty, respect, altruism, compassion, accountability, excellence, and leadership. This is an area in which surgical educators, acting as mentors and role models through daily interactions with their patients, residents, and peers, may be the most powerful teaching tool (Fig. 1-3).[72,73]

Systems-Based Practice

The ACGME has mandated that "residents must demonstrate an awareness of and responsiveness to the larger context and system of health care, as well as the ability to call effectively on other resources in the system to provide optimal health care."[5] In today's medical world, resources and finances are limited, and each health care provider must understand that the business aspect of medicine is closely interrelated with the effective delivery of care. As health care costs have grown, so have health care management organizations. Learning how to interact with these organizations is crucial for the improvement of health care delivery and allocation of resources. Some reports have demonstrated that surgeons feel deficient in the understanding of public health and the business aspects of surgery.[74]

The ACS has developed a Task Force on Systems-Based Practice to specifically address this particular competency.[75] Systems-based practice is not inherently integrated into the surgical curriculum; therefore, it may be more challenging to incorporate and teach. Several methods for educating residents about systems-based practice have been described in the literature. Dunnington and Williams have arranged for residents to participate in hospital committees that focus on quality improvement and patient safety. The residents keep a journal of the issues that are discussed during the meetings and reflect on how these issues will affect the way that they practice medicine in the future. Both committee members and residents have found this to be a constructive learning process.[17] Davison and colleagues described a longitudinal systems-based practice into their 3-year-long core curriculum which included group discussions (risk management, discharge planning, patient relations), didactic lectures (structure of health care, pathway to surgery, current procedural terminology, governance, contract negotiations), and hospital training sessions. Personnel with expertise in health care delivery systems and health care management were enlisted to teach some of these courses.[76] Englander and associates applied systems-based practice by involving residents in the process of cost-reduction efforts. The residents identified a project that was cost inefficient then identified key issues, devised improvement plans, and subsequently implemented them. This educational exercise saved the hospital over $500,000 per year. The authors concluded that involving residents in

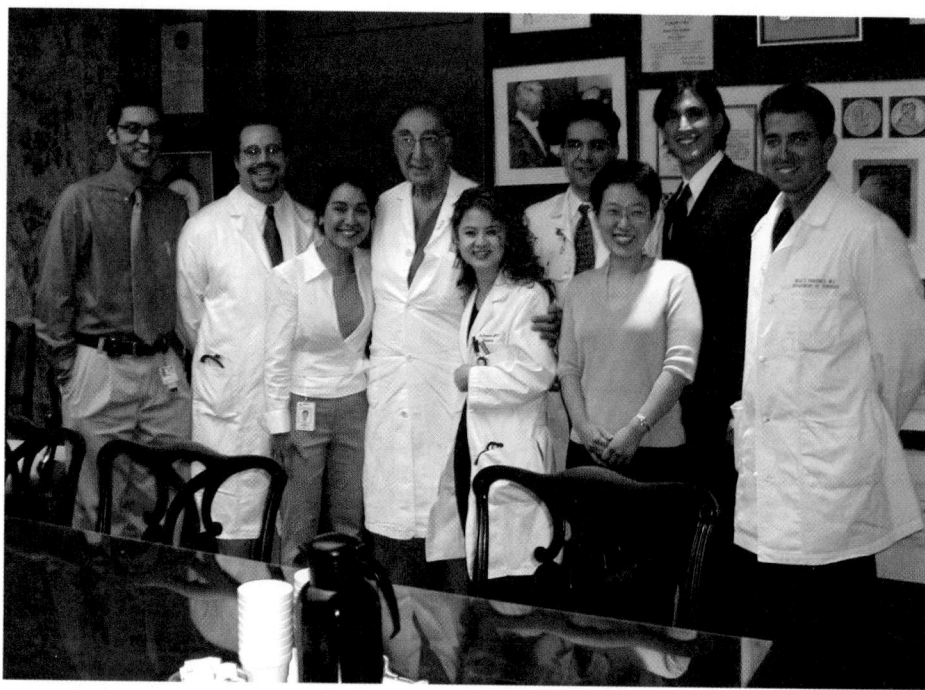

FIG. 1-3. Dr. Michael E. DeBakey, a surgical pioneer and transformational health care leader, served as a mentor and role model to generations of residents and inspired professionalism and the pursuit of excellence. He is pictured here with a group of chief residents at the Baylor College of Medicine.

cost-reduction efforts helps to teach and assess the skill of systems-based practice.[77] Conferences such as grand rounds, morbidity and mortality conferences, and morning reports have also been modified to teach the principles of systems-based practice.[20,21,23]

Given today's changing health care economics, surgeons are faced with the need to understand the business aspects of medicine to care optimally for patients. This involves being able to work effectively in different health care settings, incorporating cost awareness and risk-benefit analysis in patient care, improving patient safety and quality of care, and identifying system errors and implementing solutions (Fig. 1-4).[5] Unfortunately, this has not been an inherent part of surgical training, and many physicians do not feel that they have an adequate understanding of these concepts.[74] However, there are

strides in the right direction with various novel methods to incorporate systems-based practice into surgical curriculums.

ASSESSMENT AND THE ACCREDITATION COUNCIL FOR GRADUATE MEDICAL EDUCATION LEARNING PORTFOLIO

The ACGME not only has mandated the teaching of the six core competencies but also has stated that residents must be evaluated to ensure that they have acquired these necessary skills. There is little doubt that, in the future, these or similar core competencies will be used to assess practicing surgeons as well. Hence, the need to

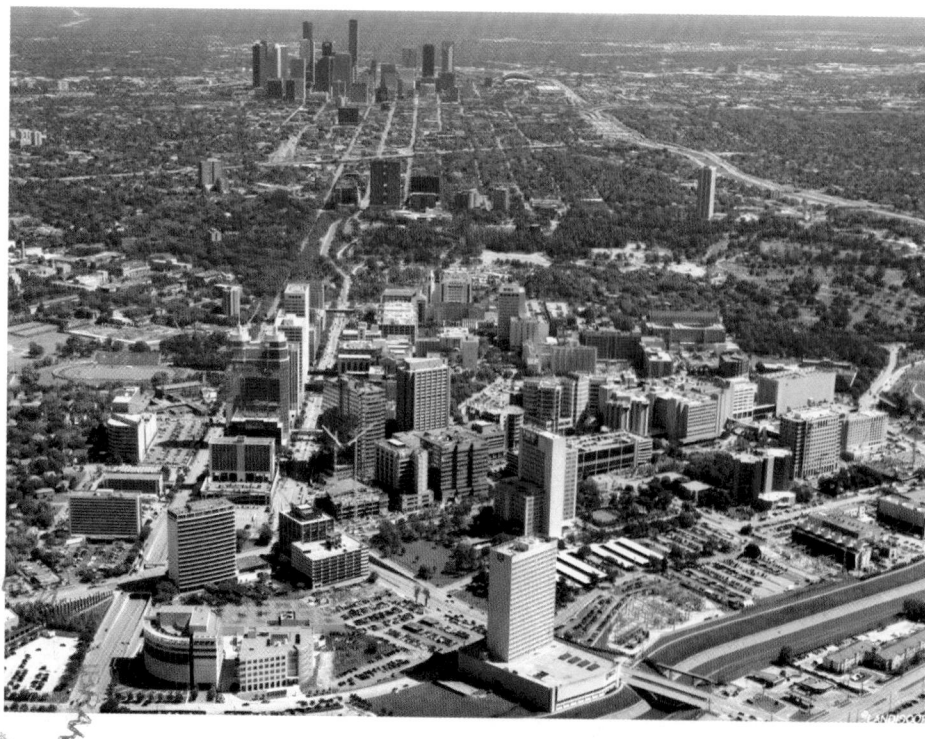

FIG. 1-4. One of the ACGME core competencies requires that residents demonstrate an awareness of and responsiveness to the larger context and system of health care, as well as the ability to call effectively on other resources in the system to provide optimal health care. The Texas Medical Center in Houston, Texas, encompasses 740 acres and 42 member institutions where residents must learn to navigate, comprehend, and utilize the larger health care system as a whole.

document the acquisition and maintenance of these competencies is important to all surgeons, not just those in training.

Competence has been defined as "the ability to do something well measured against a standard, especially ability acquired through training."[78] Miller has described a model of competency that consists of four levels: "knows," "knows how," "shows how," and "performs." Residents, early in their training, would most likely attain the level of "knows" and "knows how." This would be comparable to a resident's understanding the pathology and clinical diagnosis of appendicitis and the appropriate treatment algorithms. The "shows how" level would be demonstrated by a resident who could demonstrate how to perform an appendectomy while being supervised by faculty on a simulator or animal model. The "performs" level is the competence level at which the surgeon could perform this operation without any supervision or assistance in a real-life clinical situation. The levels of competency are not based on postgraduate year but are based on the ability to specifically meet a defined objective set forth by a surgical curriculum.[79]

The most pressing question is how to implement a competency-based curriculum and, perhaps even more of a challenge, how to assess the six core competencies. An assessment tool should ideally be reliable, valid, reproducible, and also practical.[80] The two most common evaluation tools in surgical programs have been the American Board of Surgery In-Training Examination (ABSITE) and the ward evaluation. The ABSITE is administered once a year and attempts to test the general medical knowledge and patient care knowledge of surgical trainees. A direct linear correlation has been described between the ABSITE score and the American Board of Surgery Qualifying Examination score,[81] which emphasizes the need to perform at an adequate level on the ABSITE. ABSITE scores also have been found to be higher in programs that have instituted mandatory reading programs and focused problem-based learning education programs.[29,82] Overall, the ABSITE remains a tried and true method of assessing the basic medical knowledge of surgical trainees.

The second method of evaluation has been the ward evaluation. These evaluations are typically performed at the end of the rotation and are subject to biases related to factors such as memory and the general impression of the surgery faculty of the given resident. These evaluations often consist of subjective terms that globally define the residents, for example, *excellent, good,* and *very good.* However, these ratings do not provide any objective data on competence.[83] Even though the ward evaluation provides general information on achievement of educational goals, the new ACGME mandates will require either revising these evaluations to make them more competence based or developing new methods for measuring outcomes.

A number of programs have instituted novel evaluation tools to assess for competency in patient care and medical knowledge. The Operative Performance Rating System (OPRS) is an innovative tool used to assess the competence of patient care that was developed by Larson and colleagues. It is an Internet-based system for evaluating sentinel procedures performed by residents that assesses not only technical skills but also the intraoperative decision-making process. They found this to be a feasible and reliable method. The authors concluded that this may be a way to evaluate competence in patient care, track the development of surgical skills, identify problems early on, and certify competence in a particular procedure.[84] Schell and Flynn described a web-based program for teaching and assessing medical knowledge and patient care. Residents were allowed to follow a self-paced curriculum by viewing a CD-ROM didactic lesson and participating in a minimally invasive skills laboratory to assess competency in the basics of minimally invasive surgery. They found that residents showed significant improvement in their surgical skills, and the trainees described a high satisfaction with this program and felt that it should be an integral component of their education.[10] The Objective Structured Assessment of Technical Skills (OSATS) test was developed at the University of Toronto to assess technical competency. The test is administered in stations that simulate tasks performed in the operating room, such as a small-bowel anastomosis, placement of a T tube, control of inferior vena cava hemorrhage, and so on. The participants are graded by a surgical evaluator who completes two standardized grading forms for each station. One grading form covers the specific steps and technical points of the station (i.e., correct suture, use of forceps, etc), whereas the second form is a global rating scale that evaluates the flow of operation and more subjective but important aspects of an operation. The authors concluded that this method has high reliability and construct validity for assessing competency in technical skills.[85] Furthermore, the OSATS examination has been validated in a number of studies as accurately representing the technical skills of a surgical trainee when compared with performance in carrying out a procedure on a live patient.[86,87] Virtual simulators have also been used effectively to teach and assess surgical skills, medical knowledge, and practice-based learning and improvement in a controlled environment.[12,88]

Other competencies, such as communication and professionalism, may require a more interactive and direct means for true assessment. The methods most described in the literature involve standardized patients and the 360-degree evaluations. Yudkowsky and colleagues described a method to assess communication and interpersonal skills, patient care, and professionalism known as the *Communication and Interpersonal Skills Objective Structured Clinical Assessment (CIS-OSCE) examination.* This examination was administered to residents in multiple specialties at the University of Illinois at Chicago and consisted of resident interaction with standardized patients on various matters such as obtaining informed consent, relaying bad news, and discussing domestic violence. They found this method of evaluation to be valid and feasible.[50] The Patient Assessment and Management Examination (PAME) to access competencies such as patient care, communication and interpersonal skills, and professionalism has also been described. This examination consists of six stations with standardized patients. It entails an initial assessment, ordering and interpretation of test, discussion of the findings with the patient, and evaluation of a higher level of thinking with implementation of a treatment plan. These interactions are observed by a staff physician, which allows for direct assessment of competencies.[38,51] The 360-degree evaluation to assess communication and professionalism has been described for various specialties. This process involves evaluation of the resident by various people who have had interactions with the resident, including patients as well as nurses and other ancillary staff. The resident's ability to communicate effectively and behave in a professional manner is evaluated based on a scale. This method has been found to be a valid and reliable method to assess for the competencies; however, it can be difficult to carry out.[89–91]

Practice-based learning and systems-based practice have been assessed through existing conferences. Rosenfeld as well as Williams and Dunnington revised their morbidity and mortality conference to allow for assessment of practice-based learning by having residents fill out a practice-based learning log. This allowed staff to determine whether the residents were able to identify key issues and implement improved practice patterns.[20,38] Stiles and associates developed a competency-based morning report format and felt that this was an ideal environment in which to directly assess many of the core competencies, including systems-based practice and practice-based learning, through direct interactions with the residents.[23]

In 2004, the Association of Program Directors and the ACS worked together to develop a web-based system to evaluate all of the core competencies at the end of residents' rotations. This evaluation system was studied throughout multiple institutions and found to be both a reliable and valid method to assess the core competencies.[92] In addition, the ACGME has developed a professional developmental tool called the *ACGME Learning Portfolio.* This portfolio is an interactive web-based portfolio that allows residents to record, organize, and reflect back on their learning experiences. Residents, faculty, and program directors can use this portfolio as a tool to allow for constructive feedback, to monitor a resident's progress, and to identify areas of weakness. It will also enable program directors to evaluate the quality of their curriculums and isolate deficiencies that require improvement.[93] Both of these tools use the web for data collection and evaluation, which allows for centralization and ease in interpretation of the data, permits use of real-time data to identify strengths and weaknesses, and may allow programs to provide competency-based performance data for the RRC. The number of assessment tools for the core competencies continues to increase as programs learn from trial and error. Programs should continue to share their work through publications to identify programs with models of excellence that can be adopted at other institutions (see Table 1-2).

CONCLUSION

The goal of the ACGME core competency mandate has been to ensure that patient care continues to improve into the twenty-first century with the development of benchmark programs and best educational practices. The goal of the modern surgical educator is to develop a better means to ensure that the material is properly taught and, even more importantly, truly learned. The defined core competencies provide an excellent framework for surgical education. This supplies an exciting foundation for the introduction of new educational initiatives and the development of novel educational programs through collaboration. These innovations should serve to move surgical education forward and allow for improved training of the surgeons of the future.

REFERENCES

Entries highlighted in bright blue are key references.

1. Nahrwold D: Why the 6 general competencies? *Surgery* 135:4, 2004.
2. Leach DC: A model for GME: Shifting from process to outcomes. A progress report from the Accreditation Council for Graduate Medical Education. *Med Educ* 38:12, 2004.
3. http://www.acgme.org/outcome/project/OPintrorev1_7-05.ppt#256: The ACGME Outcome Project: An Introduction, 2005, Accreditation Council for Graduate Medical Education [accessed January 15, 2008].
4. http://www.acgme.org/outcome/project/timeline/TIMELINE_index_frame.htm: Timeline—Working Guidelines, 2003, Accreditation Council for Graduate Medical Education [accessed January 15, 2008].
5. http://www.acgme.org/acWebsite/downloads/RRC_progReq/440general surgery01012008.pdf: ACGME Program Requirements for Graduate Medical Education in Surgery, 2007, Accreditation Council for Graduate Medical Education [accessed January 15, 2008].
6. Hamdorf JM, Hall JC: Acquiring surgical skills. *Br J Surg* 87:28, 2000.
7. Bridges M, Diamond DL: The financial impact of teaching surgical residents in the operating room. *Am J Surg* 177:28, 1999.
8. http://www.acgme.org/acWebsite/dutyHours/dh_Lang703.pdf: Duty Hours Language, 2007, Accreditation Council for Graduate Medical Education [accessed January 22, 2008].
9. Velmahos GC, Toutouzas KG, Sillin LF, et al: Cognitive task analysis for teaching technical skills in an inanimate surgical skills laboratory. *Am J Surg* 187:114, 2004.
10. Schell SR, Flynn TC: Web-based minimally invasive surgery training: Competency assessment in PGY 1-2 surgical residents. *Curr Surg* 61:120, 2004.
11. Park J, MacRae H, Musselman LJ, et al: Randomized controlled trial of virtual reality simulator training: Transfer to live patients. *Am J Surg* 194:205, 2007.
12. Andreatta PB, Woodrum DT, Birkmeyer JD, et al: Laparoscopic skills are improved with LapMentor training: Results of a randomized, double-blinded study. *Ann Surg* 243:854, 2006.
13. Bell RH: Surgical council on resident education: A new organization devoted to graduate surgical education. *J Am Coll Surg* 204:341, 2007.
14. Scott DJ, Dunnington GL: New ACS/APDS skills curriculum: Moving the learning curve out of the operating room. *J Gastrointest Surg* 12:213, 2008. Epub October 10, 2007.
15. http://www.facs.org/education/surgicalskills.html: Surgical Skills Curriculum Information, 2008, American College of Surgeons, Division of Education [accessed January 18, 2008].
16. http://www.flsprogram.org: Fundamentals of Laparoscopic Surgery, 2003–2008, Society of American Gastrointestinal and Endoscopic Surgeons [accessed January 18, 2008].
17. Dunnington GL, Williams RG: Addressing the new competencies for residents' surgical training. *Acad Med* 78:14, 2003.
18. Korndorffer JR Jr., Stefanidis D, Scott DJ: Laparoscopic skills laboratories: Current assessment and a call for resident training standards. *Am J Surg* 191:17, 2006.
19. Kapadia MR, DaRosa DA, MacRae HM, et al: Current assessment and future directions of surgical skills laboratories. *J Surg Educ* 64:260, 2007.
20. Rosenfeld JC: Using the morbidity and mortality conference to teach and assess the ACGME general competencies. *Curr Surg* 62:664, 2005.
21. Kravet SJ, Howell E, Wright SM: Morbidity and mortality conference, grand rounds, and the ACGME's core competencies. *J Gen Intern Med* 21:1192, 2006.
22. Prince JM, Vallabhaneni R, Zenati MS, et al: Increased interactive format for morbidity and mortality conference improves educational value and enhances confidence. *J Surg Educ* 64:266, 2007.
23. Stiles BM, Reece TB, Hedrick TL, et al: General surgery morning report: A competency-based conference that enhances patient care and resident education. *Curr Surg* 63:385, 2006.
24. Jiang Y, Casey G, Lavery IC, et al: Development of a clinically feasible molecular assay to predict recurrence of stage ii colon cancer. *J Mol Diagn* 10:346, 2008. Epub June 13, 2008.
25. Tamada K, Wang XP, Brunicardi FC: Molecular targeting of pancreatic disorders. *World J Surg* 29:325, 2005.
26. http://www.studygs.net/texred2.htm: The SQ3R Reading Method, Study Guides and Strategies [accessed January 28, 2008].
27. http://www.sybervision.com/pimsleurphp/ppimsleur.htm: The Pimsleur Foreign Language Learning System, SyberVision [accessed January 28, 2008).
28. http://www.rosettastone.com: Rosetta Stone, 1999–2008, Rosetta Stone Limited [accessed January 28, 2008].
29. Nguyen L, Brunicardi FC, Dibardino DJ, et al: Education of the modern surgical resident: Novel approaches to learning in the era of the 80-hour workweek. *World J Surg* 30:1120, 2006.
30. Lee L, Brunicardi C, Berger D, et al: Impact of a novel education curriculum on surgical training. *J Surg Res* 145:308, 2008. Epub February 11, 2008.
31. Linzer M, Brown JT, Frazier LM: Impact of a medical journal club on house-staff reading habits, knowledge, and critical appraisal skills. A randomized control trial. *JAMA* 260:2537, 1988.
32. Crank-Patton A, Fisher JB, Toedter LJ: The role of the journal club in surgical residency programs: A survey of APDS program directors. *Curr Surg* 58:101, 2001.
33. MacRae HM, Regehr G, McKenzie M, et al: Teaching practicing surgeons critical appraisal skills with an Internet-based journal club: A randomized, controlled trial. *Surgery* 136:641, 2004.
34. http://www.accesssurgery.com/index.aspx: McGraw-Hill's AccessSurgery, McGraw-Hill [accessed January 28, 2008].
35. http://www.mdconsult.com: MD Consult, 2008, Elsevier [accessed January 28, 2008].
36. http://www.uptodate.com: Tap into the World's Largest Clinical Community, 2008, UpToDate [accessed January 28, 2008].
37. Sachdeva AK: Surgical education to improve the quality of patient care: The role of practice-based learning and improvement. *J Gastrointest Surg* 11:1379, 2007. Epub August 15, 2007.
38. Williams RG, Dunnington GL: Accreditation Council for Graduate Medical Education core competencies initiative: The road to implementation in the surgical specialties. *Surg Clin North Am* 84:1621, 2004.
39. Canal DF, Torbeck L, Djuricich AM: Practice-based learning and improvement: A curriculum in continuous quality improvement for surgery residents. *Arch Surg* 142:479, 2007.
40. Fung MF, Walker M, Fung KF, et al: An Internet-based learning portfolio in resident education: The KOALA multicentre programme. *Med Educ* 34:474, 2000.
41. http://www.facs.org/members/pbls.html: Practice-Based Learning System, 2007, American College of Surgeons [accessed January 30, 2008].

42. Khuri SF, Daley J, Henderson W, et al: The Department of Veterans Affairs' NSQIP: The first national, validated, outcome-based, risk-adjusted, and peer-controlled program for the measurement and enhancement of the quality of surgical care. National VA Surgical Quality Improvement Program. *Ann Surg* 228:491, 1998.

43. Ogrinc G, Headrick LA, Mutha S, et al: A framework for teaching medical students and residents about practice-based learning and improvement, synthesized from a literature review. *Acad Med* 78:748, 2003.

44. Stewart MA: Effective physician-patient communication and health outcomes: A review. *Can Med Assoc J* 152:1423, 1995.

45. Ambady N, Laplante D, Nguyen T, et al: Surgeons' tone of voice: A clue to malpractice history. *Surgery* 132:5, 2002.

46. Nolin CE: Malpractice claims, patient communication, and critical paths: A lawyer's perspective. *Qual Manag Health Care* 3:65, 1995.

47. *http://www.jointcommission.org/SentinelEvents/SentinelEventAlert/sea_24.htm:* [accessed November 21, 2008].

48. *http://www.facs.org/education/tfinterpersonal.html:* Task Force on Interpersonal and Communication Skills, 2007, American College of Surgeons, Division of Education [accessed June 18, 2008].

49. Bradley CT, Brasel KJ: Core competencies in palliative care for surgeons: Interpersonal and communication skills. *Am J Hosp Palliat Care* 24:499, 2007–2008.

50. Yudkowsky R, Alseidi A, Cintron J: Beyond fulfilling the core competencies: An objective structured clinical examination to assess communication and interpersonal skills in a surgical residency. *Curr Surg* 61:499, 2004.

51. MacRae HM, Cohen R, Regehr G, et al: A new assessment tool: The patient assessment and management examination. *Surgery* 122:335; discussion 343, 1997.

52. Rider EA, Keefer CH: Communication skills competencies: Definitions and a teaching toolbox. *Med Educ* 40:624, 2006.

53. Itani KM, Liscum K, Brunicardi FC: Physician leadership is a new mandate in surgical training. *Am J Surg* 187:328, 2004.

54. Schwartz RW: Physician leadership: A new imperative for surgical educators. *Am J Surg* 176:38, 1998.

55. Schwartz RW, Pogge C: Physician leadership: Essential skills in a changing environment. *Am J Surg* 180:187, 2000.

56. Awad SS, Hayley B, Fagan SP, et al: The impact of a novel resident leadership training curriculum. *Am J Surg* 188:481, 2004.

57. *http://www.facs.org/education/surgeons_as_leaders.pdf:* Surgeons as Leaders, American College of Surgeons, Division of Education [accessed January 31, 2008].

58. Williams RG, Silverman R, Schwind C, et al: Surgeon information transfer and communication: Factors affecting quality and efficiency of inpatient care. *Ann Surg* 245:159, 2007.

59. Goldstein MJ, Kim E, Widmann WD, et al: A 360 degrees evaluation of a night-float system for general surgery: A response to mandated work-hours reduction. *Curr Surg* 61:445, 2004.

60. Lefrak S, Miller S, Schirmer B, et al: The night float system: Ensuring educational benefit. *Am J Surg* 189:639, 2005.

61. Van Eaton EG, Horvath KD, Lober WB, et al: A randomized, controlled trial evaluating the impact of a computerized rounding and sign-out system on continuity of care and resident work hours. *J Am Coll Surg* 200:538, 2005.

62. Gruen R, Arya J, Cosgrove E, et al: Professionalism in surgery. *J Am Coll Surg* 197:605, 2003.

63. ACS Task Force on Professionalism: Code of professional conduct. *J Am Coll Surg* 197:603, 2003.

64. Medical professionalism in the new millennium: A physician charter. *Ann Intern Med* 136:243, 2002.

65. Barry L, Blair P, Cosgrove E, et al: One year, and counting, after publication of our ACS "Code of Professional Conduct." *J Am Coll Surg* 199:736, 2004.

66. *https://web2.facs.org/timssnet464/acspub/frontpage.cfm?product_class=keepcur:* Keeping Current, American College of Surgeons [accessed February 5, 2008].

67. Kumar AS, Shibru D, Bullard MK, et al: Case-based multimedia program enhances the maturation of surgical residents regarding the concepts of professionalism. *J Surg Educ* 64:194, 2007.

68. Joyner BD, Vemulakonda VM: Improving professionalism: Making the implicit more explicit. *J Urol* 177:2287; discussion 2291, 2007.

69. Rosenfeld JC: Utilizing community leaders to teach professionalism. *Curr Surg* 60:222, 2003.

70. Heru AM: Using role playing to increase residents' awareness of medical student mistreatment. *Acad Med* 8:35, 2003.

71. Fisher R, Ury W: *Getting to Yes, 2nd ed.* Boston: Houghton Mifflin, 1991, p 1.

72. Wilkes M, Raven B: Understanding social influence in medical education. *Acad Med* 77:481, 2002.

73. Kalet A, Krackov S, Rey M: Mentoring for a new era. *Acad Med* 77:1171, 2002.

74. Satiani B: Business knowledge in surgeons. *Am J Surg* 188:13, 2004.

75. *http://www.facs.org/education/tfsbpractice.html:* Task Force on Systems-Based Practice, 2007, American College of Surgeons, Division of Education [accessed February 6, 2008].

76. Davison S, Cadavid J, Spear S: Systems based practice: Education in plastic surgery. *Plast Reconstr Surg* 119:415, 2007.

77. Englander R, Agostinucci W, Zalneraiti E, et al: Teaching residents systems-based practice through a hospital cost-reduction program: A "win-win" situation. *Teach Learn Med* 18:150, 2006.

78. *http://encarta.msn.com/dictionary_/competence.html:* Competence, in MSN Encarta Dictionary, 2008, Microsoft [accessed November 21, 2008].

79. Miller GE: The assessment of clinical skills/competence/performance. *Acad Med* 65(9 Suppl):S63, 1990.

80. Sidhu RS, Grober ED, Musselman LJ, et al: Assessing competency in surgery: Where to begin? *Surgery* 135:6, 2004.

81. Garvin PJ, Kaminski DL: Significance of the in-training examination in a surgical residency program. *Surgery* 96:109, 1984.

82. de Virgilio C, Stabile BE, Lewis RJ, et al: Significantly improved American Board of Surgery In-Training Examination scores associated with weekly assigned reading and preparatory examinations. *Arch Surg* 138:1195, 2003.

83. Williams RG, Klamen DA, McGaghie WC: Cognitive, social and environmental resources of bias in clinical competence ratings. *Teach Learn Med* 15:270, 2003.

84. Larson JL, Williams RG, Ketchum J, et al: Feasibility, reliability and validity of an operative performance rating system for evaluating surgery residents. *Surgery* 138:640; discussion 647, 2005.

85. Reznick R, Regehr G, MacRae H, et al: Testing technical skill via an innovative "bench station" examination. *Am J Surg* 173:226, 1997.

86. Martin JA, Regehr G, Reznick R, et al: Objective structured assessment of technical skill (OSATS) for surgical residents. *Br J Surg* 84:273, 1997.

87. Datta V, Bann S, Beard J, et al: Comparison of bench test evaluations of surgical skill with live operating performance assessments. *J Am Coll Surg* 199:603, 2004.

88. Aggarwal R, Ward J, Balasundaram I, et al: Proving the effectiveness of virtual reality simulation for training in laparoscopic surgery. *Ann Surg* 246:771, 2007.

89. Wood J, Collins J, Burnside ES, et al: Patient, faculty, and self-assessment of radiology resident performance: A 360-degree method of measuring professionalism and interpersonal/communication skills. *Acad Radiol* 11:931, 2004.

90. Joshi R, Ling F, Jaeger J: Assessment of a 360-degree instrument to evaluate residents' competency in interpersonal and communication skills. *Acad Med* 79:458, 2004.

91. Larkin G, McKay M, Angelos P: Six core competencies and seven deadly sins: A virtues-based approach to the new guidelines for graduate medical education. *Surgery* 138:490, 2005.

92. Tabuenca A, Welling R, Sachdeva AK, et al: Multi-institutional validation of a web-based core competency assessment system. *J Surg Educ* 64:390, 2007.

93. *http://www.acgme.org/acwebsite/portfolio/cbpac_faq.pdf:* ACGME Learning Portfolio: A Professional Development Tool, 2008, Accreditation Council for Graduate Medical Education [accessed June 18, 2008].

Systemic Response to Injury and Metabolic Support

Badar V. Jan and Stephen F. Lowry

INTRODUCTION

The immune system has developed to respond to and neutralize pathogenic micro-organisms as well as coordinate tissue repair. The inflammatory response to injury or infection involves cell signaling, cell migration, and mediator release. Minor host insults instigate a local inflammatory response that is transient and in most cases beneficial. Major host insults may propagate reactions that can become amplified, resulting in systemic inflammation and potentially detrimental responses. This topic is highly relevant because systemic inflammation is a central feature[1] of both sepsis and severe trauma. Understanding the complex pathways that regulate local and systemic inflammation is necessary to develop therapies to intervene during overwhelming sepsis or after severe injury. Sepsis, defined by a systemic inflammatory response to infection, is a disease process with an increasing incidence of over 900,000 cases per year. Trauma is the leading cause of mortality and morbidity for individuals under 50 years of age.

This chapter reviews the autonomic, cellular, and hormonal responses to injury. These facets of the inflammatory response to injury and infection are discussed in reference to the specific response being considered.

SYSTEMIC INFLAMMATORY RESPONSE SYNDROME

The systemic inflammatory response syndrome (SIRS) is characterized by a sequence of host phenotypic and metabolic responses to systemic inflammation that includes changes in heart rate, respiratory rate, blood pressure, temperature regulation, and immune cell activation (Table 2-1). The systemic inflammatory response includes two general phases: (1) an acute proinflammatory state resulting from innate immune system recognition of ligands, and (2) an anti-inflammatory phase that may serve to modulate the proinflammatory phase. Under normal circumstances, these coordinated responses direct a return to homeostasis[2] (Fig. 2-1).

CENTRAL NERVOUS SYSTEM REGULATION OF INFLAMMATION

Afferent Signals to the Brain

The central nervous system (CNS) plays a key role in orchestrating the inflammatory response. The CNS influences multiple organs through both neurohormonal and endocrine signals. Injury or infection signals are recognized by the CNS through afferent signal

TABLE 2-1	Clinical spectrum of infection and systemic inflammatory response syndrome (SIRS)
Term	**Definition**
Infection	Identifiable source of microbial insult
SIRS	Two or more of following criteria are met:
	Temperature ≥38°C (100.4°F) or ≤36°C (96.8°F)
	Heart rate ≥90 beats per minute
	Respiratory rate ≥20 breaths per minute or $PaCO_2$ ≤32 mmHg or mechanical ventilation
	White blood cell count ≥12,000/μL or ≤4000/μL or ≥10% band forms
Sepsis	Identifiable source of infection + SIRS
Severe sepsis	Sepsis + organ dysfunction
Septic shock	Sepsis + cardiovascular collapse (requiring vasopressor support)

$PaCO_2$ = partial pressure of arterial carbon dioxide.

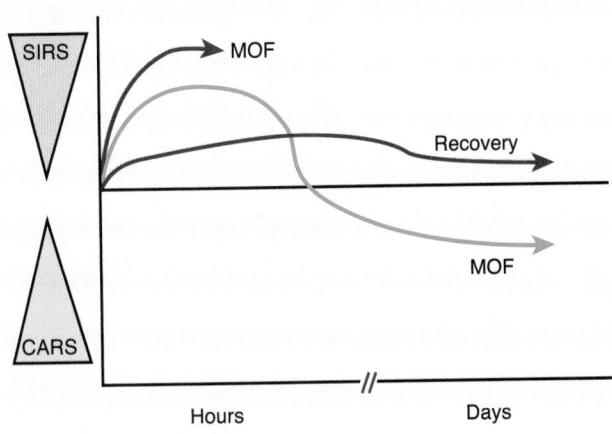

FIG. 2-1. Schematic representation of the systemic inflammatory response syndrome (SIRS) after injury, followed by a period of convalescence mediated by the counterregulatory anti-inflammatory response syndrome (CARS). Severe inflammation may lead to acute multiple organ failure (MOF) and early death after injury (*dark blue arrow*). A lesser inflammatory response followed by excessive CARS may induce a prolonged immunosuppressed state that can also be deleterious to the host (*light blue arrow*). Normal recovery after injury requires a period of systemic inflammation followed by a return to homeostasis (*red arrow*). (*Adapted with permission from Guirao X, Lowry SF: Biologic control of injury and inflammation: Much more than too little or too late.* World J Surg *20:437, 1996. With kind permission from Springer Science + Business Media.*)

pathways (Fig. 2-2). The CNS may respond to peripheral inflammatory stimuli through both circulatory and neuronal pathways. Inflammatory mediators activate CNS receptors and establish phenotypic responses such as fever and anorexia. The vagus nerve has been described as highly influential in mediating afferent sensory input to the CNS.[3]

Cholinergic Anti-Inflammatory Pathways

The vagus nerve exerts several homeostatic influences, including enhancing gut motility, reducing heart rate, and regulating inflammation. Central to this pathway is the understanding of neurally controlled anti-inflammatory pathways of the vagus nerve. Parasympathetic nervous system activity transmits vagus nerve efferent signals primarily through the neurotransmitter acetylcholine. This neurally mediated anti-inflammatory pathway allows for a rapid response to inflammatory stimuli and also for the potential regulation of early proinflammatory mediator release, specifically tumor necrosis factor (TNF).[4] Vagus nerve activity in the presence of systemic inflammation may inhibit cytokine activity and reduce injury from disease processes such as pancreatitis, ischemia and

reperfusion, and hemorrhagic shock. This activity is primarily mediated through nicotinic acetylcholine receptors on immune mediator cells such as tissue macrophages. Furthermore, enhanced inflammatory profiles are observed after vagotomy, during stress conditions.[4] Experimental trials have studied this pathway to develop therapeutic interventions. Specifically, nicotine, which also activates nicotinic acetylcholine receptors on immune cells, has been shown to reduce cytokine release after endotoxemia in animal models.[5]

HORMONAL RESPONSE TO INJURY

Hormone Signaling Pathways

Hormones are chemical signals that are released to modulate the function of target cells. Humans release hormones in several chemical categories, including polypeptides (e.g., cytokines, glucagon, and insulin), amino acids (e.g., epinephrine, serotonin, and histamine), and fatty acids (e.g., glucocorticoids, prostaglandins, and leukotrienes). Hormone receptors are present on or within the target cells and allow signal transduction to progress intracellularly mostly through three major pathways: (1) receptor kinases such as insulin and insulin-like growth factor (IGF) receptors, (2) guanine nucleotide-binding or G-protein receptors such as neurotransmitter and prostaglandin receptors, and (3) ligand-gated ion channels that permit ion transport when activated. On activation, the signal is then amplified through the action of secondary signaling molecules. Intracellular signaling leads to downstream effects such as protein synthesis and further mediator release. Protein synthesis is mediated through intracellular receptor binding either by hormone ligands or through subsequently released secondary signaling molecules. These, together with the targeted DNA sequences, activate transcription. The prototype of the intracellular hormone receptor is the glucocorticoid receptor (Fig. 2-3). This receptor is regulated by the stress-induced protein known as *heat shock protein (HSP)*, which maintains the glucocorticoid receptor in the cytosol; however, on ligand binding, HSP is released, and the receptor-ligand complex is transported to the nucleus for DNA transcription.[6]

Virtually every hormone of the hypothalamic-pituitary-adrenal axis influences the physiologic response to injury and stress (Table 2-2), but some with direct influence on the inflammatory response or immediate clinical impact are highlighted here.

Adrenocorticotropic Hormone

Adrenocorticotropic hormone (ACTH) is a polypeptide hormone released by the anterior pituitary gland. ACTH binds with receptors in the zona fasciculata of the adrenal gland, which mediate intracellular signaling and subsequent cortisol release. ACTH release follows circadian rhythms in healthy humans; however, during times of stress this diurnal pattern becomes blunted because ACTH release is elevated in proportion to the severity of injury. Several important stimuli for ACTH release are present in the injured

KEY POINTS

1. Systemic inflammation is characterized by exaggerated immune responses to either a sterile or infectious process. The cause of inflammatory activation needs to be addressed to resolve the dysregulated immune state.

2. An understanding of the signaling mechanisms and pathways underlying systemic inflammation can help guide therapeutic interventions in injured and/or septic patients.

3. Management of such patients is optimized with the use of evidence-based and algorithm-driven therapy.

4. Nutritional assessments, whether clinical or laboratory guided, and intervention should be considered at an early juncture in all surgical and critically ill patients.

5. Excessive feeding should be avoided in an effort to limit complications, including ventilator dependency, aspiration events, and infections.

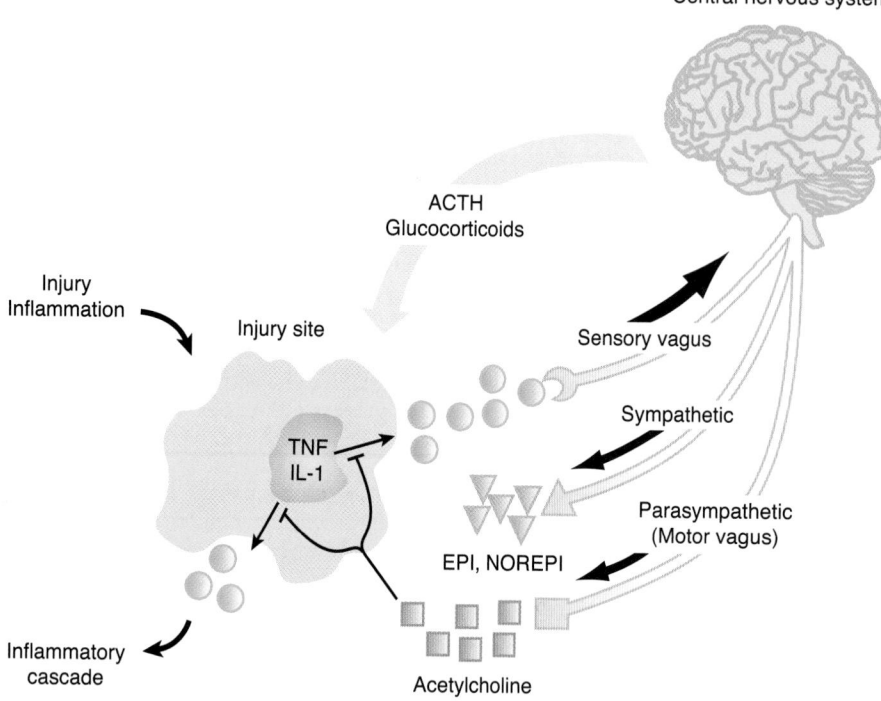

FIG. 2-2. Neural circuit relaying messages of localized injury to the brain (nucleus tractus solitarius). The brain follows with a hormone release (adrenocorticotropic hormone [ACTH], glucocorticoids) into the systemic circulation and by sympathetic response. The vagal response rapidly induces acetylcholine release directed at the site of injury to curtail the inflammatory response elicited by the activated immunocytes. This vagal response occurs in real time and is site specific. EPI = epinephrine; IL-1 = interleukin-1; NOREPI = norepinephrine; TNF = tumor necrosis factor. (*Adapted and re-created with permission from Macmillan Publishers Ltd. Tracey KJ: The inflammatory reflex.* Nature 420:853, 2002. *Copyright © 2002.*)

patient, including corticotropin-releasing hormone, pain, anxiety, vasopressin, angiotensin II, cholecystokinin, vasoactive intestinal polypeptide, catecholamines, and proinflammatory cytokines. Within the zona fasciculata of the adrenal gland, ACTH signaling activates intracellular pathways that lead to glucocorticoid production (Fig. 2-4). Conditions of excess ACTH stimulation result in adrenocortical hypertrophy.[7]

Cortisol and Glucocorticoids

Cortisol is a glucocorticoid steroid hormone released by the adrenal cortex in response to ACTH. Cortisol release is increased during times of stress and may be chronically elevated in certain disease processes. For example, burn-injured patients may exhibit elevated levels for 4 weeks.

Metabolically, cortisol potentiates the actions of glucagon and epinephrine that manifest as hyperglycemia. Cortisol acts on liver

enzymes by decreasing glycogenesis, while increasing gluconeogenesis. In skeletal muscle, cortisol facilitates the breakdown of protein and amino acids, and mediates the release of lactate. Subsequently, these substrates are used by the liver for gluconeogenesis. In adipose tissue cortisol stimulates the release of free fatty acids, triglycerides, and glycerol to increase circulating energy stores. Wound healing also is impaired, because cortisol reduces transforming growth factor beta (TGF-β) and insulin-like growth factor I (IGF-I) in the wound. This effect can be partially ameliorated by the administration of vitamin A.

Adrenal insufficiency represents a clinical syndrome highlighted largely by inadequate amounts of circulating cortisol and aldosterone. Classically, adrenal insufficiency is described in patients with atrophic adrenal glands caused by exogenous steroid administration who undergo a stressor such as surgery. These patients subsequently manifest signs and symptoms such as tachycardia, hypotension, weakness, nausea, vomiting, and fever. Critical illness may be associ-

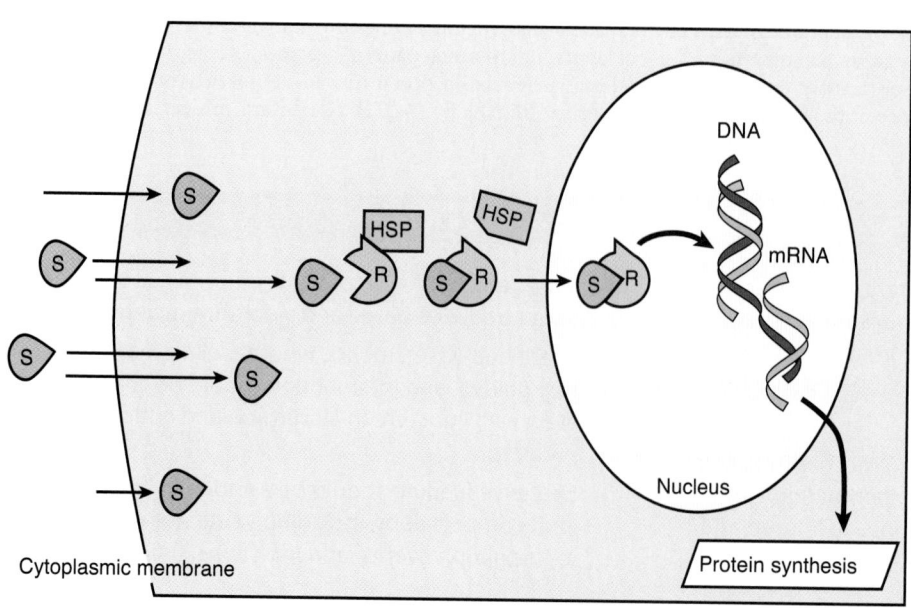

FIG. 2-3. Simplified schematic of steroid transport into the nucleus. Steroid molecules (S) diffuse readily across cytoplasmic membranes. Intracellularly the receptors (R) are rendered inactive by being coupled to heat shock protein (HSP). When S and R bind, HSP dissociates, and the S-R complex enters the nucleus, where the S-R complex induces DNA transcription, resulting in protein synthesis. mRNA = messenger RNA.

TABLE 2-2	Hormones regulated by the hypothalamus, pituitary, and autonomic system

Hypothalamic Regulation
Corticotropin-releasing hormone
Thyrotropin-releasing hormone
Growth hormone–releasing hormone
Luteinizing hormone–releasing hormone
Anterior Pituitary Regulation
Adrenocorticotropic hormone
Cortisol
Thyroid-stimulating hormone
Thyroxine
Triiodothyronine
Growth hormone
Gonadotrophins
Sex hormones
Insulin-like growth factor
Somatostatin
Prolactin
Endorphins
Posterior Pituitary Regulation
Vasopressin
Oxytocin
Autonomic System
Norepinephrine
Epinephrine
Aldosterone
Renin-Angiotensin System
Insulin
Glucagon
Enkephalins

ated with a relative adrenal insufficiency such that the adrenal gland cannot mount an effective cortisol response to match the degree of injury. Laboratory findings in adrenal insufficiency include hypoglycemia from decreased gluconeogenesis, hyponatremia from impaired renal tubular sodium resorption, and hyperkalemia from diminished kaliuresis. Diagnostic tests include baseline cortisol levels and ACTH-stimulated cortisol levels, both of which are lower than normal during adrenal insufficiency. Treatment strategies are controversial; however, they include low-dose steroid supplementation.[8]

Glucocorticoids have immunosuppressive properties that have been used when needed, as in organ transplantation. Immunologic changes associated with glucocorticoid administration include thymic involution, depressed cell-mediated immune responses reflected by decreases in T-killer and natural killer cell function, T-lymphocyte blastogenesis, mixed lymphocyte responsiveness, graft-versus-host reactions, and delayed hypersensitivity responses. In addition glucocorticoids inhibit leukocyte migration to sites of inflammation by inhibiting the expression of adhesion molecules. In monocytes, glucocorticoids inhibit intracellular killing while maintaining chemotactic and phagocytic properties. Glucocorticoids inhibit neutrophil superoxide reactivity, suppress chemotaxis, and normalize apoptosis signaling mechanisms but maintain neutrophil phagocytic function. In clinical settings manifested by hypoperfusion, such as septic shock, trauma, and coronary artery bypass grafting, glucocorticoid administration is associated with attenuation of the inflammatory response.

Macrophage Migration–Inhibiting Factor

Macrophage migration–inhibiting factor (MIF) is a neurohormone that is stored and secreted by the anterior pituitary and by intracellular pools within macrophages. MIF is a counterregulatory mediator that potentially reverses the anti-inflammatory effects of cortisol. During times of stress, hypercortisolemia, and host immunosuppression, MIF may modulate the inflammatory response by inhibiting the immunosuppressive effect of cortisol on immunocytes and thereby increasing their activity against foreign pathogens.[9]

Growth Hormones and Insulin-Like Growth Factors

Growth hormone (GH) is a neurohormone expressed primarily by the pituitary gland that has both metabolic and immunomodulatory effects. GH promotes protein synthesis and insulin resistance, and enhances the mobilization of fat stores. GH secretion is upregulated by hypothalamic GH–releasing hormone and downregulated by somatostatin. GH primarily exerts its downstream effects through direct interaction with GH receptors and secondarily through the enhanced hepatic synthesis of IGF-I. IGF circulates primarily bound to various IGF-binding proteins and also has anabolic effects, including increased protein synthesis and lipogenesis. In the liver, IGF stimulates protein synthesis and glycogenesis; in adipose tissue, it increases glucose uptake and lipid utilization; and in skeletal muscles, it mediates glucose uptake and protein synthesis.

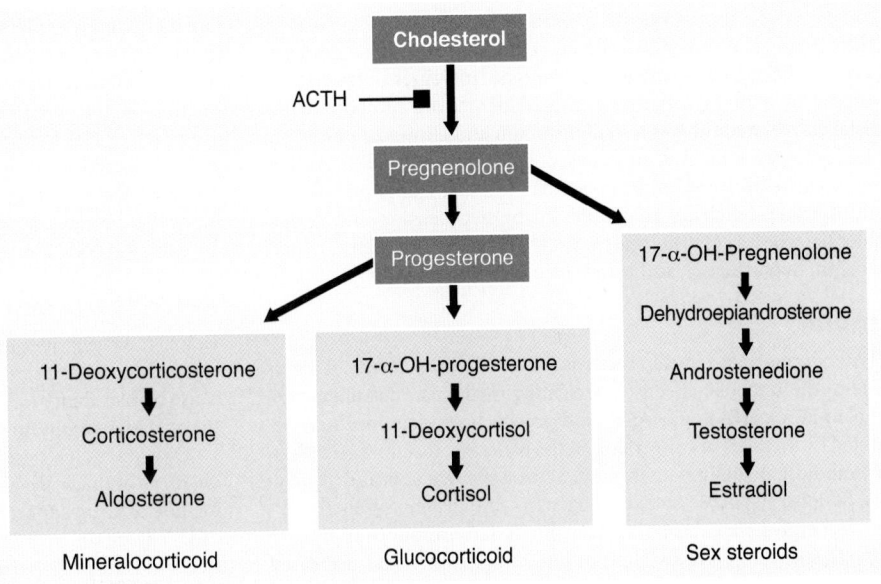

FIG. 2-4. Steroid synthesis from cholesterol. Adrenocorticotropic hormone (ACTH) is a principal regulator of steroid synthesis. The end products are mineralocorticoids, glucocorticoids, and sex steroids.

Critical illness is associated with an acquired GH resistance and contributes to decreased levels of IGF. This effect in part mediates the overall catabolic phenotype manifested during critical illness. In addition, GH enhances phagocytic activity of immunocytes through increased lysosomal superoxide production. GH also increases the proliferation of T-cell populations.[10] Exogenous GH administration has been studied in critically ill patients and may be associated with worse outcomes, including increased mortality, prolonged ventilator dependence, and increased susceptibility to infection.[11] The mechanisms through which GH is associated with these outcomes are unclear, although GH-induced insulin resistance and hyperglycemia may contribute.

Catecholamines

Catecholamines are hormones secreted by the chromaffin cells of the adrenal medulla and function as neurotransmitters in the CNS. The most common catecholamines are epinephrine, norepinephrine, and dopamine, which have metabolic, immunomodulatory, and vasoactive effects. After severe injury, plasma catecholamine levels are increased threefold to fourfold, with elevations lasting 24 to 48 hours before returning toward baseline levels.

Catecholamines act on both alpha and beta receptors, which are widely distributed on several cell types, including vascular endothelial cells, immunocytes, myocytes, adipose tissue, and hepatocytes. Epinephrine has been shown to induce a catabolic state and hyperglycemia through hepatic gluconeogenesis and glycogenolysis as well as by peripheral lipolysis and proteolysis. In addition epinephrine promotes insulin resistance in skeletal muscle. Catecholamines also increase the secretion of thyroid hormone, parathyroid hormones, and renin, but inhibit the release of aldosterone.

Epinephrine also has immunomodulatory properties mediated primarily through the activation of beta$_2$ receptors on immunocytes. Epinephrine has been shown to inhibit the release of inflammatory cytokines, including TNF, interleukin-1, and interleukin-6, while also enhancing the release of the anti-inflammatory mediator interleukin-10.[12] Similar to cortisol, epinephrine increases leukocyte demargination with resultant neutrophilia and lymphocytosis. The immunomodulatory sequelae of catecholamines in patients during septic shock have yet to be clearly elucidated.

Catecholamines exert several hemodynamic effects, including increased cardiac oxygen demand, vasoconstriction, and increased cardiac output. Catecholamines are used to treat systemic hypotension during septic shock. Because of the increased cardiac stress induced by catecholamines, however, cardioprotective strategies, including beta blockade for patients undergoing surgery, have shown significant benefit in reducing cardiac-related deaths.

Aldosterone

Aldosterone is a mineralocorticoid released by the zona glomerulosa of the adrenal cortex. Aldosterone increases intravascular volume by acting on the renal mineralocorticoid receptor of the distal convoluted tubules to retain sodium and eliminate potassium and hydrogen ions. Aldosterone secretion is stimulated by ACTH, angiotensin II, decreased intravascular volume, and hyperkalemia. Aldosterone deficiency is manifested by hypotension and hyperkalemia, whereas aldosterone excess is manifested by edema, hypertension, hypokalemia, and metabolic alkalosis.

Insulin

Hyperglycemia and insulin resistance are hallmarks of critical illness due to the catabolic effects of circulating mediators, including catecholamines, cortisol, glucagon, and growth hormone. Insulin is secreted by the islets of Langerhans in the pancreas. Insulin mediates an overall host anabolic state through hepatic glycogenesis and glycolysis, peripheral glucose uptake, lipogenesis, and protein synthesis.[13]

Hyperglycemia during critical illness has immunosuppressive effects, including glycosylation of immunoglobulins and decreased phagocytosis and respiratory burst of monocytes, and thus is associated with an increased risk for infection. Insulin therapy to manage hyperglycemia has grown in favor and has been shown to be associated with both decreased mortality and a reduction in infectious complications in select patient populations; however, caution should be exercised to avoid the deleterious sequelae of hypoglycemia from overaggressive glycemic control.[14] The ideal blood glucose range within which to maintain critically ill patients and avoid hypoglycemia has yet to be determined.

ACUTE PHASE PROTEINS

Acute phase proteins are a class of proteins produced by the liver that manifest either increased or decreased plasma concentration in response to inflammatory stimuli such as traumatic injury and infection. Specifically, C-reactive protein has been studied as a marker of proinflammatory response in many clinical settings, including appendicitis, vasculitis, and ulcerative colitis. Importantly, C-reactive protein levels do not show diurnal variations and are not modulated by feeding. Acute phase protein levels may be unreliable as an index of inflammation in the setting of hepatic insufficiency.

MEDIATORS OF INFLAMMATION

Cytokines

Cytokines are a class of protein signaling compounds that are essential for both innate and adaptive immune responses. Cytokines mediate a broad sequence of cellular responses, including cell migration, DNA replication, cell turnover, and immunocyte proliferation (Table 2-3). When functioning locally at the site of injury and infection, cytokines mediate the eradication of invading microorganisms and also promote wound healing. However, an exaggerated proinflammatory cytokine response to inflammatory stimuli may result in hemodynamic instability (i.e., septic shock) and metabolic derangements (i.e., muscle wasting).

Anti-inflammatory cytokines also are released, at least in part as an opposing influence to the proinflammatory cascade. These anti-inflammatory mediators also may result in immunocyte dysfunction and host immunosuppression. Cytokine signaling after an inflammatory stimulus is manifested by a fluctuating and counterregulated balance of opposing influences and should not be oversimplified into dichotomic proinflammatory and anti-inflammatory responses.[2]

Heat Shock Proteins

Heat shock proteins (HSPs) are a group of intracellular proteins that are increasingly expressed during times of stress, such as burn injury, inflammation, and infection. HSPs participate in many physiologic processes, including protein folding and protein targeting. The formation of HSPs requires gene induction by the heat shock transcription factor. HSPs bind both autologous and foreign proteins and thereby function as intracellular chaperones for ligands such as bacterial DNA and endotoxin. HSPs are presumed to protect cells from the deleterious effects of traumatic stress[15] and, when released by damaged cells, alert the immune system of the tissue damage.

Reactive Oxygen Species

Reactive oxygen species (ROS) are small molecules that are highly reactive due to the presence of unpaired outer orbit electrons. They can cause cellular injury to both host cells and invading pathogens through the oxidation of unsaturated fatty acids within cell membranes.

Oxygen radicals are produced as a by-product of oxygen metabolism as well as by anaerobic processes. Potent oxygen radicals include oxygen, superoxide, hydrogen peroxide, and hydroxyl radicals. The main areas of ROS production include mitochondrial electron transport, peroxisomal fatty acid metabolism, cytochrome

TABLE 2-3	Cytokines and their sources	
Cytokine	**Source**	**Comment**
TNF	*Macrophages/monocytes* Kupffer cells Neutrophils NK cells Astrocytes Endothelial cells T lymphocytes Adrenal cortical cells Adipocytes Keratinocytes Osteoblasts Mast cells Dendritic cells	Among earliest responders after injury; half-life <20 min; activates TNF receptors 1 and 2; induces significant shock and catabolism
IL-1	*Macrophages/monocytes* B and T lymphocytes NK cells Endothelial cells Epithelial cells Keratinocytes Fibroblasts Osteoblasts Dendritic cells Astrocytes Adrenal cortical cells Megakaryocytes Platelets Neutrophils Neuronal cells	Two forms (IL-1α and IL-1β); similar physiologic effects as TNF; induces fevers through prostaglandin activity in anterior hypothalamus; promotes β-endorphin release from pituitary; half-life <6 min
IL-2	*T lymphocytes*	Promotes lymphocyte proliferation, immunoglobulin production, gut barrier integrity; half-life <10 min; attenuated production after major blood loss leads to immunocompromise; regulates lymphocyte apoptosis
IL-3	*T lymphocytes* Macrophages Eosinophils Mast cells	
IL-4	*T lymphocytes* Mast cells Basophils Macrophages B lymphocytes Eosinophils Stromal cells	Induces B-lymphocyte production of IgG4 and IgE, mediators of allergic and anthelmintic response; downregulates TNF, IL-1, IL-6, IL-8
IL-5	*T lymphocytes* Eosinophils Mast cells Basophils	Promotes eosinophil proliferation and airway inflammation
IL-6	*Macrophages* B lymphocytes Neutrophils Basophils Mast cells Fibroblasts Endothelial cells Astrocytes Synovial cells Adipocytes Osteoblasts Megakaryocytes Chromaffin cells Keratinocytes	Elicited by virtually all immunogenic cells; long half-life; circulating levels proportional to injury severity; prolongs activated neutrophil survival
IL-8	*Macrophages/monocytes* T lymphocytes Basophils Mast cells Epithelial cells Platelets	Chemoattractant for neutrophils, basophils, eosinophils, lymphocytes

(Continued)

TABLE 2-3	Cytokines and their sources (continued)	
Cytokine	**Source**	**Comment**
IL-10	*T lymphocytes* B lymphocytes Macrophages Basophils Mast cells Keratinocytes	Prominent anti-inflammatory cytokine; reduces mortality in animal sepsis and ARDS models
IL-12	*Macrophages/monocytes* Neutrophils Keratinocytes Dendritic cells B lymphocytes	Promotes T_H1 differentiation; synergistic activity with IL-2
IL-13	*T lymphocytes*	Promotes B-lymphocyte function; structurally similar to IL-4; inhibits nitric oxide and endothelial activation
IL-15	*Macrophages/monocytes* Epithelial cells	Anti-inflammatory effect; promotes lymphocyte activation; promotes neutrophil phagocytosis in fungal infections
IL-18	*Macrophages* Kupffer cells Keratinocytes Adrenal cortical cells Osteoblasts	Similar to IL-12 in function; levels elevated in sepsis, particularly gram-positive infections; high levels found in cardiac deaths
IFN-γ	*T lymphocytes* NK cells Macrophages	Mediates IL-12 and IL-18 function; half-life of days; found in wounds 5–7 d after injury; promotes ARDS
GM-CSF	*T lymphocytes* Fibroblasts Endothelial cells Stromal cells	Promotes wound healing and inflammation through activation of leukocytes
IL-21	*T lymphocytes*	Preferentially secreted by T_H2 cells; structurally similar to IL-2 and IL-15; activates NK cells, B and T lymphocytes; influences adaptive immunity
HMGB1	*Monocytes/lymphocytes*	High mobility group box chromosomal protein; DNA transcription factor; late (downstream) mediator of inflammation (ARDS, gut barrier disruption); induces "sickness behavior"

ARDS = acute respiratory distress syndrome; GM-CSF = granulocyte-macrophage colony-stimulating factor; IFN = interferon; Ig = immunoglobulin; IL = interleukin; NK = natural killer; T_H1 = helper T cell subtype 1; T_H2 = helper T cell subtype 2; TNF = tumor necrosis factor.

P-450 reactions, and the respiratory burst of phagocytic cells. Host cells are protected from the damaging effects of ROS through the activity of endogenous antioxidants such as superoxide dismutase, catalase, and glutathione peroxidase. Under normal physiologic conditions ROS are balanced by antioxidative enzymes. During times of stress or ischemia, however, enzymatic clearance mechanisms are consumed, and on restoration of perfusion, the unbalanced production of ROS leads to reperfusion injury.[16]

Eicosanoids

Eicosanoids are derived primarily by oxidation of the membrane phospholipid arachidonic acid (eicosatetraenoic acid) and are composed of subgroups, including prostaglandins, prostacyclins, hydroxy-eicosatetraenoic acids (HETEs), thromboxanes, and leukotrienes. The synthesis of arachidonic acid from phospholipids requires the enzymatic activation of phospholipase A2 (Fig. 2-5). Products of the COX pathway include all of the prostaglandins and thromboxanes. The lipoxygenase pathway generates leukotrienes and HETE. Eicosanoids are not stored within cells but are instead generated rapidly in response to many stimuli, including hypoxic injury, direct tissue injury, endotoxin (lipopolysaccharide, or LPS), norepinephrine, vasopressin, angiotensin II, bradykinin, serotonin, acetylcholine, cytokines, and histamine. Eicosanoid pathway activation also leads to the formation of the anti-inflammatory compound lipoxin, which inhibits chemotaxis and nuclear factor κB (NF-κB) activation. Glucocorticoids, NSAIDs, and leukotriene inhibitors block the end products of eicosanoid pathways.

Eicosanoids have a broad range of physiologic roles, including neurotransmission, vasomotor regulation, and immune cell regulation (Table 2-4). Eicosanoids mostly generate a proinflammatory

response with deleterious host effects and are associated with acute lung injury, pancreatitis, and renal failure. Leukotrienes are potent mediators of capillary leakage as well as leukocyte adherence, neutrophil activation, bronchoconstriction, and vasoconstriction. Experimental models of sepsis have shown a benefit to inhibiting eicosanoid production. However, human sepsis trials have failed to show a mortality benefit using NSAIDs.[17]

Eicosanoids also have several recognized metabolic effects. Cyclooxygenase pathway products inhibit pancreatic β-cell release of insulin, whereas lipoxygenase pathway products stimulate β-cell activity. Prostaglandins such as prostaglandin E_2 can inhibit gluconeogenesis through the binding of hepatic receptors and also can inhibit hormone-stimulated lipolysis.[18]

Fatty Acid Metabolites

Fatty acid metabolites function as inflammatory mediators and as such have significant roles in the inflammatory response. As previously discussed, eicosanoids participate in inflammatory signaling; however, dietary omega-3 and omega-6 fatty acids also influence inflammation. Eicosanoids are produced primarily through two major pathways: (1) with arachidonic acid (omega-6 fatty acid) as substrate and (2) eicosapentaenoic acid (omega-3 fatty acid) as substrate. Many lipid preparations are soy based and are primarily composed of omega-6 fatty acids. Nutritional supplementation with either omega-6 or omega-3 fatty acid can significantly modulate the inflammatory response, because omega-6 substrate is associated with increased downstream mediator production. Omega-3 fatty acids have specific anti-inflammatory effects, including inhibition of NF-κB activity, TNF release from hepatic Kupffer cells, as well as leukocyte adhesion and migration. The anti-inflammatory effects of

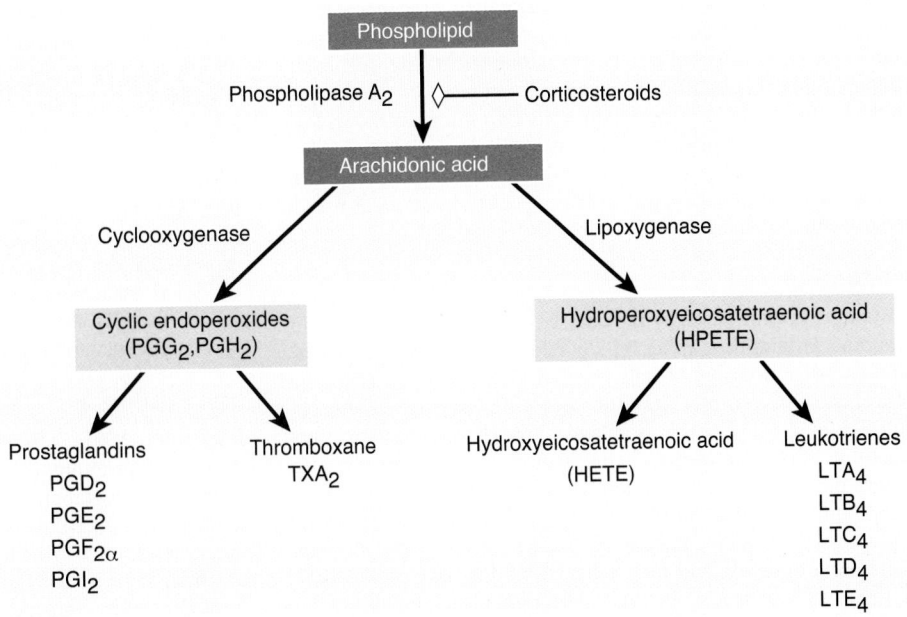

FIG. 2-5. Schematic diagram of arachidonic acid metabolism. LT = leukotriene; PG = prostaglandin; TXA$_2$ = thromboxane A$_2$.

TABLE 2-4	Systemic stimulatory and inhibitory actions of eicosanoids	
Organ/Function	**Stimulator**	**Inhibitor**
Pancreas		
Glucose-stimulated insulin secretion	12-HPETE	PGE$_2$
Glucagon secretion	PGD$_2$, PGE$_2$	
Liver		
Glucagon-stimulated glucose production	PGE$_2$	
Fat		
Hormone-stimulated lipolysis	PGE$_2$	
Bone		
Resorption	PGE$_2$, PGE-m, 6-K-PGE$_1$, PGF$_{1\alpha}$, PGI$_2$	
Pituitary		
Prolactin	PGE$_1$	
Luteinizing hormone	PGE$_1$, PGE$_2$, 5-HETE	
Thyroid-stimulating hormone	PGA$_1$, PGB$_1$, PGE$_1$, PGE$_1$	
Growth hormone	PGE$_1$	
Parathyroid		
Parathyroid hormone	PGE$_2$	PGF$_2$
Lung		
Bronchoconstriction	PGF$_{2\alpha}$, TXA$_2$, LTC$_4$, LTD$_4$, LTE$_4$	PGE$_2$
Kidney		
Stimulation of renin secretion	PGE$_2$, PGI$_2$	
Gastrointestinal system		
Cytoprotective effect	PGE$_2$	
Immune response		
Suppression of lymphocyte activity	PGE$_2$	
Hematologic system		
Platelet aggregation	TXA$_2$	PGI$_2$

5-HETE = 5-hydroxyeicosatetraenoic acid; 12-HPETE = 12-hydroxyperoxyeicosatetraenoic acid; 6-K-PGE$_1$ = 6-keto-prostaglandin E$_1$; LT = leukotriene; PG = prostaglandin; PGE-m = 13,14-dihydro-15-keto-PGE$_2$ (major urine metabolite of PGE$_2$); TXA$_2$ = thromboxane A$_2$.

omega-3 fatty acids on chronic autoimmune diseases such as rheumatoid arthritis, psoriasis, and lupus have been documented in both animals and humans. In experimental models of sepsis, omega-3 fatty acids inhibit inflammation, ameliorate weight loss, increase small-bowel perfusion, and may increase gut barrier protection. In human studies, omega-3 supplementation is associated with decreased production of TNF, interleukin-1β, and interleukin-6 by endotoxin-stimulated monocytes. In a study of surgical patients, preoperative supplementation with omega-3 fatty acid was associated with reduced need for mechanical ventilation, decreased hospital length of stay, and decreased mortality with a good safety profile.[19]

Kallikrein-Kinin System

The kallikrein-kinin system is a group of proteins that contribute to inflammation, blood pressure control, coagulation, and pain responses. Prekallikrein is activated by stimuli such as Hageman factor, trypsin, plasmin, factor XI, glass surfaces, kaolin, and collagen to produce the serine protease kallikrein, which subsequently plays a role in the coagulation cascade. High molecular weight kininogen is produced by the liver and is metabolized by kallikrein to form bradykinin.

Kinins mediate several physiologic processes, including vasodilation, increased capillary permeability, tissue edema, pain pathway activation, inhibition of gluconeogenesis, and increased bronchoconstriction. They also increase renal vasodilation and consequently reduce renal perfusion pressure. Decreased renal perfusion leads to activation of the renin-angiotensin-aldosterone system, which acts on the nephron to actively resorb sodium and subsequently increase intravascular volume.

Bradykinin and kallikrein levels are increased during gram-negative bacteremia, hypotension, hemorrhage, endotoxemia, and tissue injury. The degree of elevation in the levels of these mediators has been associated with the magnitude of injury and mortality. Clinical trials using bradykinin antagonists have shown some benefit in patients with gram-negative sepsis.[20]

Serotonin

Serotonin is a monoamine neurotransmitter (5-hydroxytryptamine) derived from tryptophan. Serotonin is synthesized by neurons in the CNS as well as by enterochromaffin cells of the GI tract and platelets.

This neurotransmitter stimulates vasoconstriction, bronchoconstriction, and platelet aggregation. Serotonin also increases cardiac inotropy and chronotropy through nonadrenergic cyclic adenosine monophosphate (cAMP) pathways. Serotonin receptors are located in the CNS, GI tract, and monocytes.[21] Ex vivo study has shown that serotonin receptor blockade is associated with decreased production of TNF and interleukin-1 in endotoxin-treated monocytes. Serotonin is released at sites of injury, primarily by platelets; however, its role in inflammatory modulation has yet to be clearly defined.

Histamine

Histamine is synthesized by the decarboxylation of the amino acid histidine. Histamine is either rapidly released or stored in neurons, skin, gastric mucosa, mast cells, basophils, and platelets. There are four histamine receptor (H) subtypes with varying physiologic roles. H_1 binding mediates vasodilation, bronchoconstriction, intestinal motility, and myocardial contractility. H_2 binding stimulates gastric parietal cell acid secretion. H_3 is an autoreceptor found on presynaptic histamine-containing nerve endings and leads to downregulation of histamine release. H_4 is expressed primarily in bone marrow, eosinophils, and mast cells. H_4 binding interactions have not been fully delineated but have been associated with eosinophil and mast cell chemotaxis. Increased histamine release has been documented in hemorrhagic shock, trauma, thermal injury, endotoxemia, and sepsis.[22]

CYTOKINE RESPONSE TO INJURY

Tumor Necrosis Factor

Tumor necrosis factor alpha (TNF) is a cytokine that is rapidly mobilized in response to stressors such as injury and infection, and is a potent mediator of the subsequent inflammatory response. TNF is primarily synthesized by macrophages, monocytes, and T cells, which are abundant in peritoneum and splanchnic tissues. Although the circulating half-life of TNF is brief, the activity of TNF elicits many metabolic and immunomodulatory activities. TNF stimulates muscle breakdown and cachexia through increased catabolism, insulin resistance, and redistribution of amino acids to hepatic circulation as fuel substrates. In addition, TNF also mediates coagulation activation, cell migration, and macrophage phagocytosis, and enhances the expression of adhesion molecules, prostaglandin E_2, platelet-activating factor, glucocorticoids, and eicosanoids.[23]

Tumor necrosis factor receptors (TNFRs) are composed of two subtypes: TNFR-1 and TNFR-2. TNFR-1 is ubiquitously expressed in most tissues and, on ligand binding, mediates apoptosis through proteolytic caspases. TNFR-2 is expressed primarily on immunocytes and, on ligand binding, leads to NF-κB activation and subsequent amplification of the inflammatory signal. TNFRs exist in both transmembrane and soluble form. In response to inflammatory stimuli such as injury and infection, TNFRs are proteolytically cleaved from cell membranes and are readily detectable in soluble form. This may represent a mechanism of inflammatory regulation, because soluble TNFRs maintain their affinity for TNF and thereby compete with and limit the activation of transmembrane TNFR.[24]

Interleukin-1

Interleukin-1 (IL-1) is represented by two active subtypes, IL-1α and IL-1β. IL-1α is primarily membrane associated and functions through cellular contact. IL-1β is readily detectable in soluble form and mediates an inflammatory sequence similar to that of TNF. IL-1 is primarily synthesized by monocytes, macrophages, endothelial cells, fibroblasts, and epidermal cells. IL-1 is released in response to inflammatory stimuli, including cytokines (TNF, IL-2, interferon-γ [IFN-γ]) and foreign pathogens, and requires the formation of the inflammasome in the cell for processing and release. High doses of either IL-1 or TNF are associated with profound hemodynamic compromise. Interestingly, low doses of both IL-1 and TNF com-

bined elicit hemodynamic events similar to those elicited by high doses of either mediator, which suggests a synergistic effect. IL-1 is an endogenous pyrogen because it acts on the hypothalamus by stimulating prostaglandin activity and thereby mediates a febrile response.

IL-1 is autoregulated by endogenous IL-1 receptor antagonists, which are released in response to inflammatory stimuli and compete with IL-1 at receptor binding sites. There are two primary receptor types for IL-1: IL-1R1 and IL-1R2. IL-1R1 is widely expressed and mediates inflammatory signaling on ligand binding. IL-1R2 is proteolytically cleaved from the membrane surface to soluble form on activation and thus serves as another mechanism for competition and regulation of IL-1 activity.[25]

Interleukin-2

Interleukin-2 (IL-2) is upregulated in response to IL-1 and is primarily a promoter of T-lymphocyte proliferation and differentiation, immunoglobulin production, and gut barrier integrity. IL-2 binds to IL-2 receptors, which are expressed on leukocytes. Partly due to its short half-life of <10 minutes, IL-2 is not readily detectable after acute injury. IL-2 receptor blockade induces immunosuppressive effects and can be pharmacologically used for organ transplantation. Attenuated IL-2 expression observed during major injury or blood transfusion may contribute to the relatively immunosuppressed state of the surgical patient.[26]

Interleukin-4

Interleukin-4 (IL-4) is released by activated helper T cells and stimulates the differentiation of T cells, and also stimulates T-cell proliferation and B-cell activation. It is also important in antibody-mediated immunity and in antigen presentation. IL-4 induces class switching of differentiating B lymphocytes to produce predominantly immunoglobulin G4 and immunoglobulin E, which are important immunoglobulins in allergic and antihelmintic responses. IL-4 has anti-inflammatory effects on macrophages, exhibited by an attenuated response to proinflammatory mediators such as IL-1, TNF, interleukin-6, and interleukin-8. In addition, IL-4 appears to increase macrophage susceptibility to the anti-inflammatory effects of glucocorticoids.

Interleukin-6

Interleukin-6 (IL-6) release by macrophages is stimulated by inflammatory mediators such as endotoxin, TNF, and IL-1. IL-6 is increasingly expressed during times of stress, as in septic shock. After injury, IL-6 levels in the circulation are detectable by 60 minutes, peak between 4 and 6 hours, and can persist for as long as 10 days. Plasma levels of IL-6 are proportional to the degree of injury during surgery. Interestingly, IL-6 has counterregulatory effects on the inflammatory cascade through the inhibition of TNF and IL-1. IL-6 also promotes the release of soluble tumor necrosis factor receptors and IL-1 receptor antagonists, and stimulates the release of cortisol. High plasma IL-6 levels have been associated with mortality during intra-abdominal sepsis.[27]

Interleukin-8

Interleukin-8 (IL-8) is synthesized by macrophages as well as other cell lines such as endothelial cells. Critical illness as manifested during sepsis is a potent stimulus for IL-8 expression. IL-8 stimulates the release of IFN-γ and functions as a potent chemoattractant for neutrophils. Elevated plasma IL-8 also has been associated with disease severity and end organ dysfunction during sepsis.[28]

Interleukin-10

Interleukin-10 (IL-10) is an anti-inflammatory cytokine synthesized primarily by monocytes; however, it is also released by other lymphocytes. IL-10 is increasingly expressed during times of systemic inflammation, and its release is specifically enhanced by TNF and IL-1. IL-10 inhibits the secretion of proinflammatory cytokines, including TNF and IL-1, partly through the downregulation of NF-κB and thereby functions as a negative feedback regulator of the inflammatory cascade. Experimental models of inflammation have shown that neutralization of IL-10 increases TNF production and mortality, whereas restitution of circulating IL-10 reduces TNF levels and subsequent deleterious effects. Increased plasma levels of IL-10 also have been associated with mortality and disease severity after traumatic injury. IL-10 may significantly contribute to the underlying immunosuppressed state during sepsis through the inhibition and subsequent anergy of immunocytes.[29]

Interleukin-12

Interleukin-12 (IL-12) has been described as a regulator of cell mediated immunity. IL-12 is released by activated phagocytes, including monocytes, macrophages, neutrophils, and dendritic cells, and is increasingly expressed during endotoxemia and sepsis. IL-12 stimulates lymphocytes to increase secretion of IFN-γ with the costimulus of interleukin-18 and also stimulates natural killer cell cytotoxicity and helper T cell differentiation. IL-12 release is inhibited by IL-10. IL-12 deficiency inhibits phagocytosis in neutrophils. In experimental models of inflammatory stress, IL-12 neutralization conferred a mortality benefit in mice during endotoxemia. However, in a cecal ligation and puncture model of intraperitoneal sepsis, IL-12 blockade was associated with increased mortality. Furthermore, later studies of intraperitoneal sepsis observed no difference in mortality with IL-12 administration; however, IL-12 knockout mice exhibited increased bacterial counts and inflammatory cytokine release, which suggests that IL-12 may contribute to an antibacterial response. IL-12 administration in chimpanzees is capable of stimulating the release of proinflammatory mediators such as IFN-γ and also anti-inflammatory mediators, including IL-10, soluble TNFR, and IL-1 receptor antagonists. In addition, IL-12 enhances coagulation as well as fibrinolysis. Despite evidence of both proinflammatory and anti-inflammatory pathway activation, most evidence suggests that IL-12 contributes to an overall proinflammatory response.[30]

Interleukin-13

Interleukin-13 (IL-13) exerts many of the same immunomodulatory effects as does IL-4. IL-13 inhibits monocyte release of TNF, IL-1, IL-6, and IL-8, while increasing the secretion of IL-1R antagonist. However, unlike IL4, IL-13 has no identifiable effect on T lymphocytes and only has influence on selected B-lymphocyte populations. Increased IL-13 expression is observed during septic shock and mediates neutropenia, monocytopenia, and leukopenia. In addition, IL-13 inhibits leukocyte interaction with activated endothelial surfaces. Similar to IL-4 and IL-10, IL-13 has a net anti-inflammatory effect.[31]

Interleukin-15

Interleukin-15 (IL-15) is synthesized in many cell types, including macrophages and skeletal muscle after endotoxin administration. IL-15 stimulates natural killer cell activation as well as B-cell and T-cell proliferation and thus functions as a regulator of cellular immunity. IL-15 has immunomodulatory effects similar to those of IL-2, in part due to shared receptor subunits. Furthermore, IL-15 acts as a potent inhibitor of lymphocyte apoptosis by enhancing the expression of antiapoptotic molecules such as Bcl-2.[32]

Interleukin-18

Interleukin-18 (IL-18), formerly IFN-γ–inducing factor, is synthesized primarily by macrophages. IL-18 and its receptor complex are members of the IL-1 superfamily. As with IL-1, macrophages release IL-18 in response to inflammatory stimuli, including endotoxin, TNF, IL-1, and IL-6. IL-18 level also is elevated during sepsis. IL-18 activates NF-κB through an Myeloid differentiation primary response gene (88) (MyD88)-dependent pathway with subsequent proinflammatory mediator release. IL-18 regulation is in part mediated through IL-18–binding protein (IL-18BP). This molecule is not a soluble receptor isoform but rather a specific endogenous antagonist. IL-18 also mediates hepatotoxicity associated with Fas ligand and TNF. The viral skin pathogen molluscum contagiosum secretes an IL-18BP–like protein, which neutralizes IL-18 and thereby inhibits the inflammatory response. IL-18 and IL-12 act synergistically to release IFN-γ from T cells. In a murine model of systemic inflammation, IL-18 neutralization reduced lethal endotoxemia. IL-18 signaling also is associated with increased expression of intercellular adhesion molecule-1. Interestingly, in a murine model of systemic inflammation, a reversal of left ventricular dysfunction was observed with IL-18 blockade, which suggests that IL-18 may contribute to the hemodynamic compromise during septic shock.[33]

Interferons

Interferons were first recognized as soluble mediators that inhibited viral replication through the activation of specific antiviral genes in infected cells. Interferons are categorized into two major subtypes based on receptor specificity and sequence homology. Type I interferons include IFN-α, IFN-β, and IFN-ω, which are structurally related and bind to a common receptor, IFN-α receptor. Type I interferons are expressed in response to many stimuli, including viral antigens, double-stranded DNA, bacteria, tumor cells, and LPS. Type I interferons influence adaptive immune responses by inducing the maturation of dendritic cells and by stimulating class I MHC expression. IFN-α and IFN-β also enhance immune responses by increasing the cytotoxicity of natural killer cells both in culture and in vivo. In murine models, the absence of IFN-α receptor results in greater susceptibility to viral infection as well as diminished LPS-induced lethality. Furthermore, type I interferons have also been studied as therapeutic agents in hepatitis C and relapsing multiple sclerosis.

Many of the physiologic effects observed with increased levels of IL-12 and IL-18 are mediated through IFN-γ. IFN-γ is a type II interferon secreted by T lymphocytes, natural killer cells, and antigen-presenting cells in response to bacterial antigens, IL-2, IL-12, and IL-18. IFN-γ stimulates the release of IL-12 and IL-18. Negative regulators of IFN-γ include IL4, IL-10, and glucocorticoids. IFN-γ binding with a cognate receptor activates the Janus kinase/signal transducer and activator of transcription (JAK/STAT) pathway, leading to subsequent induction of biologic responses. Macrophages stimulated by IFN-γ demonstrate enhanced phagocytosis and microbial killing, and increased release of oxygen radicals, partly through a nicotinamide adenosine dinucleotide phosphate-dependent phagocyte oxidase. IFN-γ mediates macrophage stimulation and thus may contribute to acute lung injury after major surgery or trauma. Diminished IFN-γ level, as seen in knockout mice, is associated with increased susceptibility to both viral and bacterial pathogens. IFN-γ regulates trafficking of immunocytes to sites of inflammation via upregulation of chemoattractants [e.g., monokine induced by IFN-γ (MIG), macrophage inflammatory protein 1-alpha and 1-beta] and adhesion molecules (e.g., intercellular adhesion molecule-1, vascular cell adhesion molecule-1). In addition, IFN-γ promotes differentiation of T cells to the helper T cell subtype 1 and also enhances B-cell isotype switching to immunoglobulin G.[34]

Granulocyte-Macrophage Colony-Stimulating Factor

Granulocyte-macrophage colony-stimulating factor (GM-CSF), as the name suggests, upregulates both granulocyte and monocyte cell lines from hematopoietic bone marrow stem cells. GM-CSF plasma levels are low to undetectable but rapidly increase in response to inflammatory stimuli such as TNF. GM-CSF inhibits both monocyte and neutrophil apoptosis and enhances macrophage cytokine release in response to inflammatory stimuli. GM-CSF also potentiates the release of neutrophil superoxide as well as the cytotoxicity of monocytes. Administration of GM-CSF has proven beneficial during the treatment of fungal infections in immunocompromised patients. GM-CSF may potentiate acute lung injury during critical illness, because GM-CSF blockade has been found to be associated with decreased alveolar macrophage activity and NF-κB intensity. This growth factor is effective in promoting the maturation and recruitment of functional leukocytes necessary for normal inflammatory cytokine responses and also may be effective in wound healing.[35]

High Mobility Group Box 1

High mobility group box 1 (HMGB1) is a DNA transcription factor that facilitates the binding of regulatory protein complexes to DNA. HMGB1 is actively secreted by macrophages, natural killer cells, and enterocytes. Endotoxin, TNF, and IFN-γ promote the release of HMGB1, and in a murine model of intraperitoneal sepsis, increased circulating HMGB1 was associated with increased mortality. HMGB1 also appears to have cytokine-like activities, because it promotes the release of TNF from monocytes. Interestingly, elevation of plasma HMGB1 levels after experimental induction of endotoxemia is delayed relative to that of other inflammatory mediators, with levels peaking at 16 hours and remaining elevated beyond 30 hours. This response contrasts with that of acute inflammatory mediators such as TNF, which peaks at 1 to 2 hours and becomes undetectable by 12 hours. Furthermore, HMGB1 blockade is associated with decreased mortality even when initiated 4 to 24 hours after the inflammatory stimulus.[36]

HMGB1 is passively released by necrotic cells. Thus, HMGB1 alone or in combination with other molecules may contribute to the regulation of inflammation after tissue injury. Receptors for HMGB1 are receptors for advanced glycation end products and toll-like receptor 4. Binding leads to the proinflammatory response through the activation of NF-κB. Clinical trials have demonstrated increased plasma HMGB1 during systemic inflammation, as in sepsis, hemorrhagic shock, pancreatitis, myocardial infarction, and major surgery.

CELLULAR RESPONSE TO INJURY

Gene Expression and Regulation

Many genes are regulated at the point of DNA transcription and thus influence whether messenger RNA (mRNA) and its subsequent product are expressed (Fig. 2-6). These mRNA transcripts are also regulated by modulation mechanisms, including (a) splicing, which can cleave mRNA and remove noncoding regions; (b) capping, which modifies the 5' ends of the mRNA sequence to inhibit breakdown by exonucleases; (c) and the addition of a polyadenylated tail, which adds a noncoding sequence to the mRNA, effectively increasing the half-life of the transcript. Once out of the nucleus, the mRNA can be inactivated or translated to form proteins. Many protein products are also further modified for specific function or trafficking.

Gene expression relies on the coordinated action of transcription factors and coactivators (i.e., regulatory proteins), which are complexes that bind to highly specific DNA sequences upstream of the target gene known as the *promoter region*. Enhancer sequences of DNA mediate gene expression, whereas repressor sequences are noncoding regions that bind proteins to inhibit gene expression. During systemic inflammation, transcription factors are highly important, because regulation of cytokine gene expression may have profound effects on the clinical phenotype.

CELL SIGNALING PATHWAYS

G-Protein Receptors

G-protein receptors (GPRs) are a large family of transmembrane receptors. They bind a multitude of ligands (e.g., epinephrine, brady-

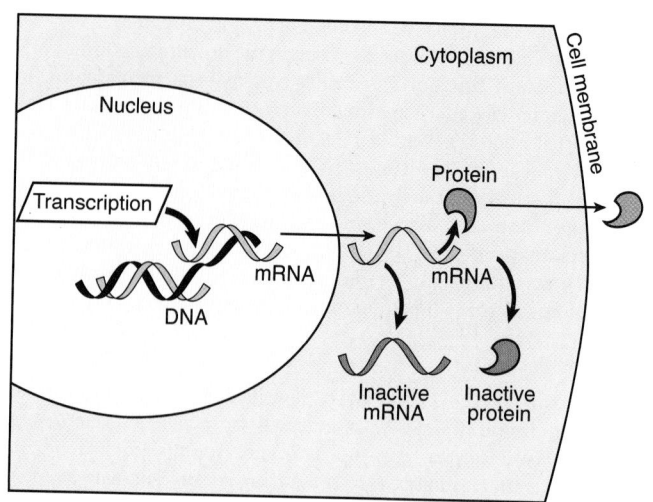

FIG. 2-6. Gene expression and protein synthesis can occur within a 24-hour period. The process can be regulated at various stages: transcription, messenger RNA (mRNA) processing, or protein packaging. At each stage, it is possible to inactivate the mRNA or protein, rendering these molecules nonfunctional.

kinin, leukotriene) and are involved in signal transduction during the inflammatory response. Extracellular ligands bind to GPR, which result in a conformational change and activation of associated proteins. The two major second messengers of the G-protein pathway are (1) cAMP, and (2) calcium, released from the endoplasmic reticulum (Fig. 2-7). Increased intracellular cAMP can activate gene transcription through the activity of intracellular signal transducers such as protein kinase A. Increased intracellular calcium can activate the intracellular signal transducer phospholipase C with further subsequent downstream effects. GPR binding also can promote the activity of protein kinase C, which can subsequently stimulate NF-κB as well as other transcription factors.

Ligand-Gated Ion Channels

Ligand-gated ion channels (LGICs) are transmembrane receptors that allow the rapid influx of ions (e.g., sodium, calcium, potassium, chloride) and are central to the signal transduction of neurotransmitters. On ligand binding LGICs effectively convert a chemical signal into an electrical signal. The prototypical LGIC is the nicotinic acetylcholine receptor (Fig. 2-8).

Receptor Tyrosine Kinases

Receptor tyrosine kinases (RTKs) are transmembrane receptors that are involved in cell signaling for several growth factors, including platelet-derived growth factor, insulin-like growth factor, epidermal growth factor, and vascular endothelial growth factor. On ligand binding, RTKs dimerize with adjacent receptors, undergo autophosphorylation, and recruit secondary signaling molecules (e.g., phospholipase C) (Fig. 2-9). Activation of RTK is important for gene transcription as well as cell proliferation and may have influence in the development of many types of cancer.

Janus Kinase/Signal Transducer and Activator of Transcription Signaling

The Janus kinases (JAKs) represent a family of tyrosine kinases that mediate signal transduction of several cytokines, including IFN-γ, IL-6, IL-10, IL-12, and IL-13. JAKs bind to cytokines, and on ligand binding and dimerization, activated JAKs recruit and phosphorylate signal transducer and activator of transcription (STAT) molecules (Fig. 2-10). Activated STAT proteins further dimerize and translocate into the nucleus and modulate the transcription of target genes. Interestingly, STAT-DNA binding can be observed

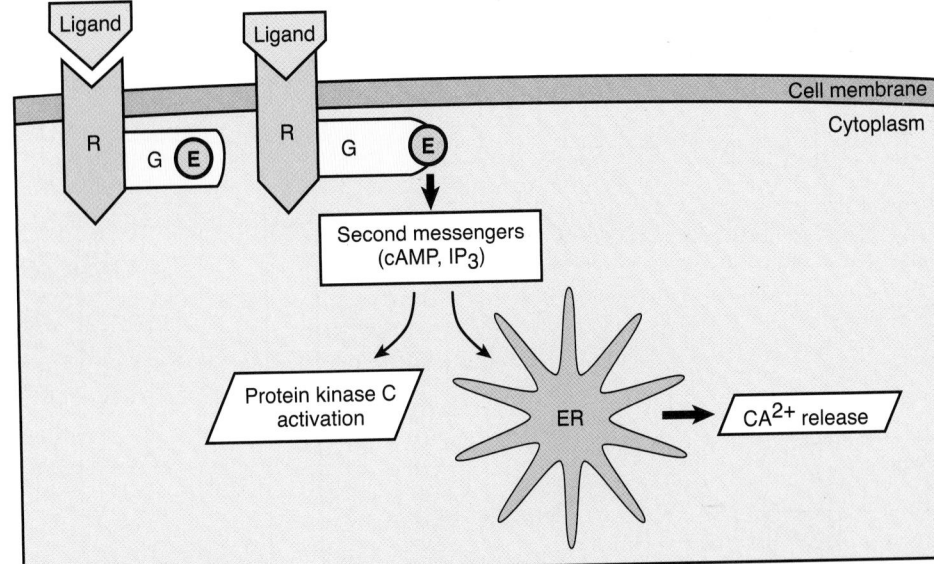

FIG. 2-7. G-protein–coupled receptors are transmembrane proteins. The G-protein receptors respond to ligands such as adrenaline and serotonin. On ligand binding to the receptor (R), the G protein (G) undergoes a conformational change through guanosine triphosphate–guanosine diphosphate conversion and in turn activates the effector (E) component. The E component subsequently activates second messengers. The role of inositol triphosphate (IP$_3$) is to induce release of calcium from the endoplasmic reticulum (ER). cAMP = cyclic adenosine triphosphate.

within minutes of cytokine binding. The JAK/STAT system is a rapid pathway for membrane to nucleus signal transduction. The JAK/STAT pathway is inhibited by the action of phosphatase, the export of STATs from the nucleus, as well the interaction of antagonistic proteins.[37]

Suppressors of Cytokine Signaling

Suppressor of cytokine signaling (SOCS) molecules are a group of cytokine-induced proteins that function as a negative feedback loop by downregulating the JAK/STAT pathway. SOCSs exert an inhibitory effect partly by binding with JAK and thus competing with STAT. A deficiency of SOCS activity may render a cell hypersensi-

tive to certain stimuli, such as inflammatory cytokines and growth hormones. Interestingly, in a murine model, SOCS knockout resulted in a lethal phenotype in part because of unregulated interferon-γ signaling. An example of this pathway is highlighted by an attenuated IL-6 response in macrophages via suppressor of cytokine signaling 3 (SOCS-3) inhibition of signal transducer and activator of transcription 3 (STAT3).[38]

Mitogen-Activated Protein Kinases

Pathways mediated through mitogen-activated protein kinase (MAPK) contribute to inflammatory signaling and regulation of cell proliferation and cell death (Fig. 2-11). MAPK pathways involve sequential stages of mediator phosphorylation resulting in the activation of downstream effectors, including c-Jun N-terminal kinase

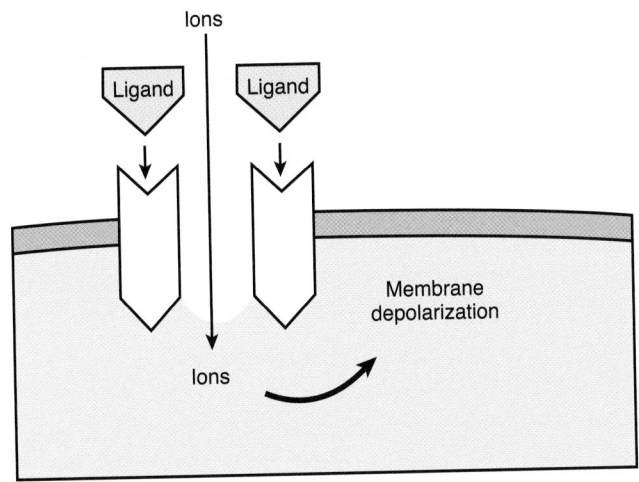

FIG. 2-8. Ligand-gated ion channels convert chemical signals into electrical signals, inducing a change in cell membrane potential. On activation of the channel, millions of ions per second influx into the cell. These channels are composed of many subunits, and the nicotinic acetylcholine receptor is one such example.

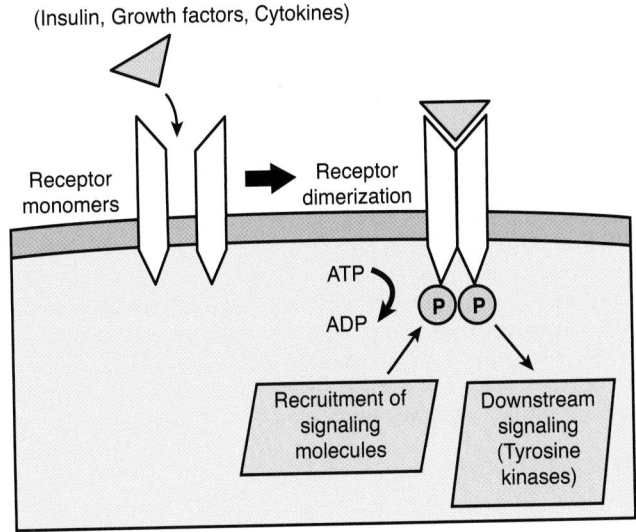

FIG. 2-9. The receptor tyrosine kinase requires dimerization of monomeric units. These receptors possess intrinsic enzymatic activity that requires multiple autophosphorylation steps to recruit and activate intracellular signaling molecules. ADP = adenosine diphosphate; ATP = adenosine triphosphate; P = phosphate.

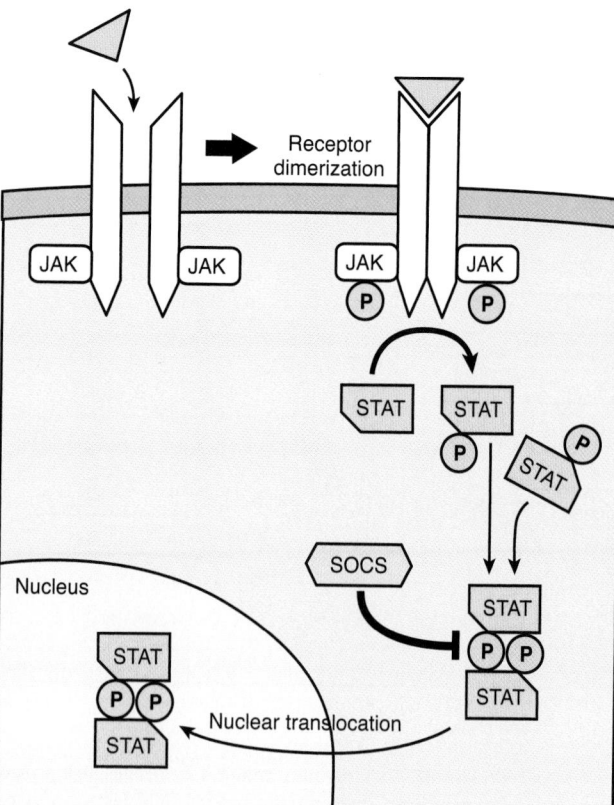

FIG. 2-10. The Janus kinase/signal transducer and activator of transcription (JAK/STAT) signaling pathway also requires dimerization of monomeric units. STAT molecules possess "docking" sites that allow for STAT dimerization. The STAT complexes translocate into the nucleus and serve as gene transcription factors. JAK/STAT activation occurs in response to cytokines (e.g., interleukin-6) and cell stressors, and has been found to induce cell proliferation and inflammatory function. Intracellular molecules that inhibit STAT function, known as *suppressors of cytokine signaling (SOCSs)*, have been identified. P = phosphate.

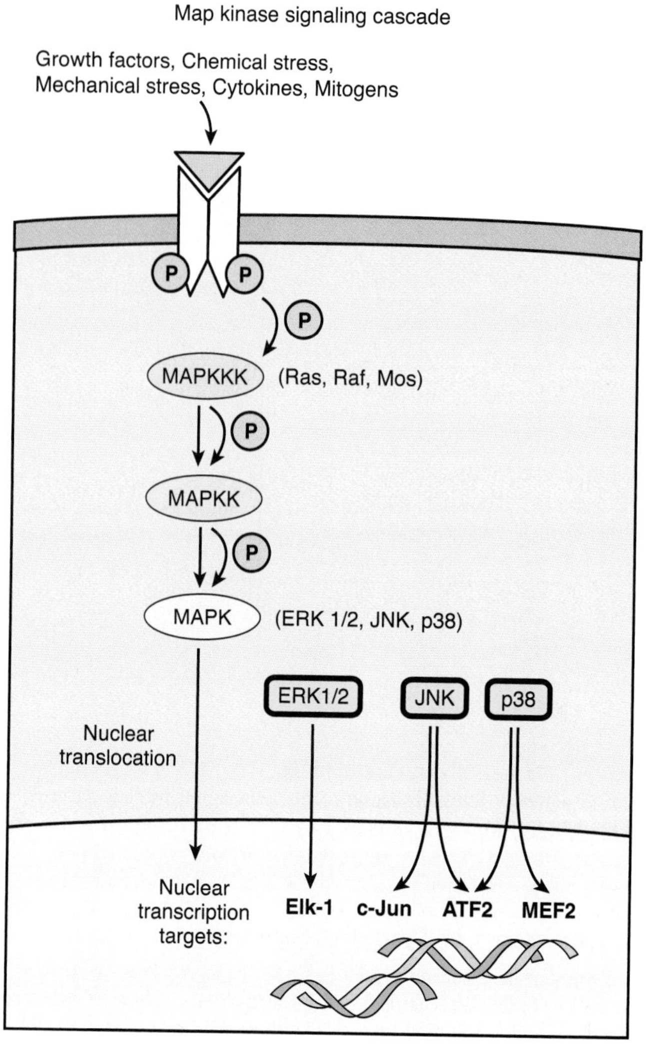

FIG. 2-11. The mitogen-activated protein kinase (MAPK) signaling pathway requires multiple phosphorylation steps. Ras, Raf, and Mos are examples of the MAPK kinase kinase (MAPKKK) and are upstream molecules. Well-characterized downstream kinases are extracellular signal regulated kinases 1 and 2 (ERK 1/2), c-Jun N-terminal kinases (JNKs) or stress-activated protein kinases (SAPKs), and p38 MAPKs that target specific gene transcription sites in the nucleus. ATF2 = activating transcription factor 2; MAPKK = mitogen-activated protein kinase kinase; MEF2 = myocyte-enhancing factor 2; P = phosphate.

(JNK), extracellular signal regulated protein kinase (ERK), and p38 kinase, with subsequent gene modulation. Dephosphorylation of MAPK pathway mediators inhibit their function. Activated JNK phosphorylates c-Jun, which dimerizes to form the transcription factor activated protein 1. The protein MAP/ERK kinase kinase (MEKK) has several functions, including protein kinase and ubiquitin ligase, and also has been shown to downregulate MAPK pathways. JNK is activated by TNF and IL-1 and is a regulator of apoptosis. Pharmacologic blockade of JNK was associated with decreased pulmonary injury and TNF and IL-1 secretion in an ischemia/reperfusion model. The p38 kinase is activated in response to endotoxin, viruses, IL-1, IL-2, IL-7, IL-17, IL-18, and TNF. The p38 also plays a role in immunocyte development, because p38 inactivation is a critical step in the differentiation of thymic T cells. These MAPK isoforms do not function independently but rather exhibit significant counteraction and cosignaling, which can influence the inflammatory response.[39]

Nuclear Factor κB

Nuclear factor κB (NF-κB) is a transcription factor that has a central role in regulating the gene products expressed after inflammatory stimuli (Fig. 2-12). NF-κB is composed of two smaller polypeptides, p50 and p65. NF-κB resides in the cytosol in the resting state primarily through the inhibitory binding of inhibitor of κB (I-κB). In response to an inflammatory stimulus such as TNF, IL-1, or endotoxin, a sequence of intracellular mediator phosphory-

lation reactions leads to the degradation of I-κB and subsequent release of NF-κB. On release, NF-κB travels to the nucleus and promotes gene expression. NF-κB also stimulates the gene expression for I-κB, which results in negative feedback regulation. In clinical appendicitis, for example, increased NF-κB activity was associated with initial disease severity, and levels returned to baseline within 18 hours after appendectomy in concert with resolution of the inflammatory response.[40]

Toll-Like Receptors and CD14

The innate immune system responds to pathogen-associated molecular patterns (PAMPs) such as microbial antigens and LPS. Toll-like receptors (TLRs) are a group of pattern recognition receptors activated by PAMPs that function as effectors of the innate immune system and belong to the IL-1 superfamily. Immunocyte recognition of LPS is mediated primarily by TLR4. LPS-binding proteins chaperone LPS to the CD14/TLR4 complex, which sets into effect cellular mechanisms that activate MAPK, NF-κB, and cytokine gene expres-

NF-κB activation

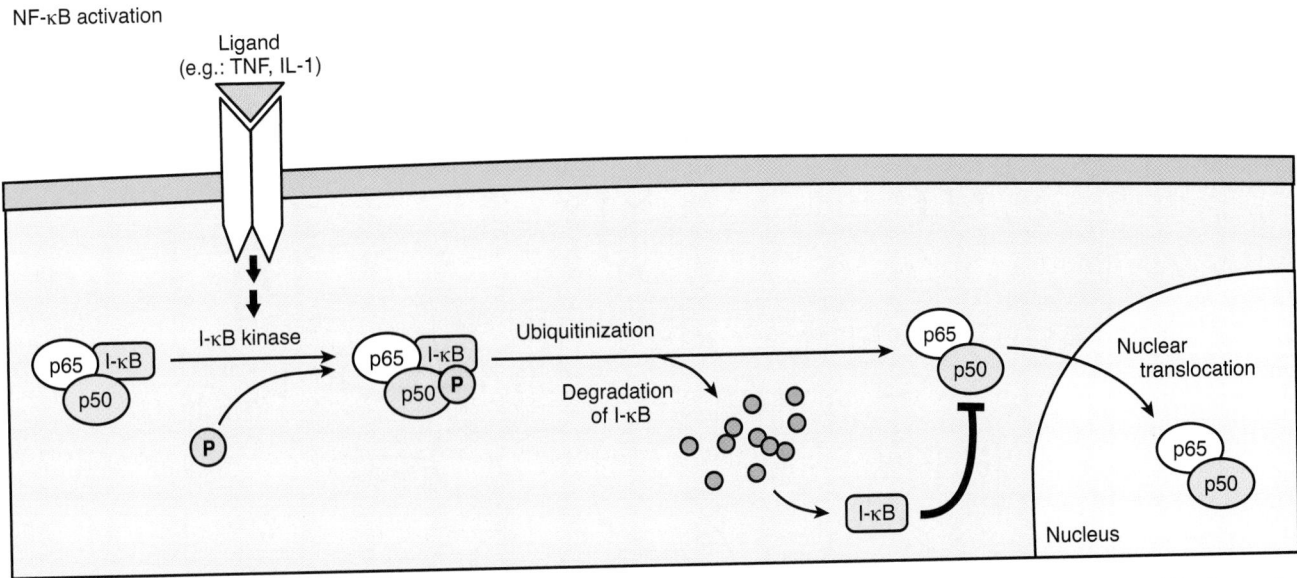

FIG. 2-12. Inhibitor of κB (I-κB) binding to the p50-p65 subunits of nuclear factor κB (NF-κB) inactivates the molecule. Ligand binding to the receptor activates a series of downstream signaling molecules, of which I-κB kinase is one. The phosphorylated NF-κB complex further undergoes ubiquitinization and proteosome degradation of I-κB, activating NF-κB, which translocates into the nucleus. Rapid resynthesis of I-κB is one method of inactivating the p50-p65 complex. IL-1 = interleukin-1; P = phosphate; TNF = tumor necrosis factor.

sion (Fig. 2-13). In contrast to TLR4, TLR2 recognizes PAMPs from gram-positive bacteria, including lipoproteins, lipopeptides, peptidoglycans, and phenol-soluble modulin from *Staphylococcus* species. Interestingly, loss-of-function single nucleotide polymorphisms of TLR are associated with an increased risk of infection in susceptible critically ill patients.[41] As multiligand receptors, TLRs also bind damage-associated molecular pattern molecules (DAMPs), which are endogenous cellular products released during times of stress or injury. DAMPs include products such as HMGB1, heat shock proteins, and hyaluronic acid. Innate immune activation by DAMPs stimulates the recruitment of inflammatory cells to the site of injury and also mediates proinflammatory signaling.[42]

APOPTOSIS

Apoptosis (regulated cell death) is an energy-dependent, organized mechanism for clearing senescent or dysfunctional cells, including macrophages, neutrophils, and lymphocytes, without promoting an inflammatory response. Conversely, cell necrosis results in a disorganized sequence of intracellular molecular releases with subsequent immune activation and inflammatory response. Systemic inflammation modulates apoptotic signaling in active immunocytes, which subsequently influences the inflammatory response through the loss of effector cells.

Apoptosis proceeds primarily through two pathways: the extrinsic pathway and the intrinsic pathway. The extrinsic pathway is activated through the binding of death receptors (e.g., Fas, TNFR), which leads to the recruitment of Fas-associated death domain protein and subsequent activation of caspase 3 (Fig. 2-14). On activation, caspases are the effectors of apoptotic signaling because they mediate the organized breakdown of nuclear DNA. The intrinsic pathway proceeds through protein mediators (e.g., Bcl-2, Bcl-2-associated death promoter, Bcl-2–associated X protein, Bim) that influence mitochondrial membrane permeability. Increased membrane permeability leads to the release of mitochondrial cytochrome C, which ultimately activates caspase 3 and thus induces apoptosis. These pathways do not function in a

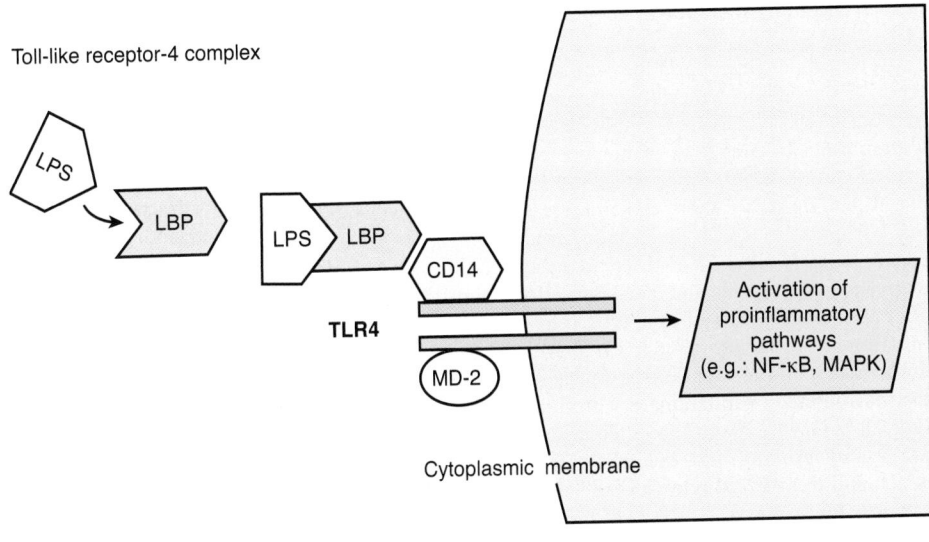

FIG. 2-13. Lipopolysaccharide (LPS) recognition by immune cells is primarily by the toll-like receptor-4 (TLR4)/CD14/MD-2 complex. LPS is transported by LPS-binding protein (LBP) to the cell surface complex. Other cell surface LPS sensors include ion-gated channels, CD11b/ CD18, and macrophage scavenger receptors. MAPK = mitogen-activated protein kinase; NF-κB = nuclear factor B.

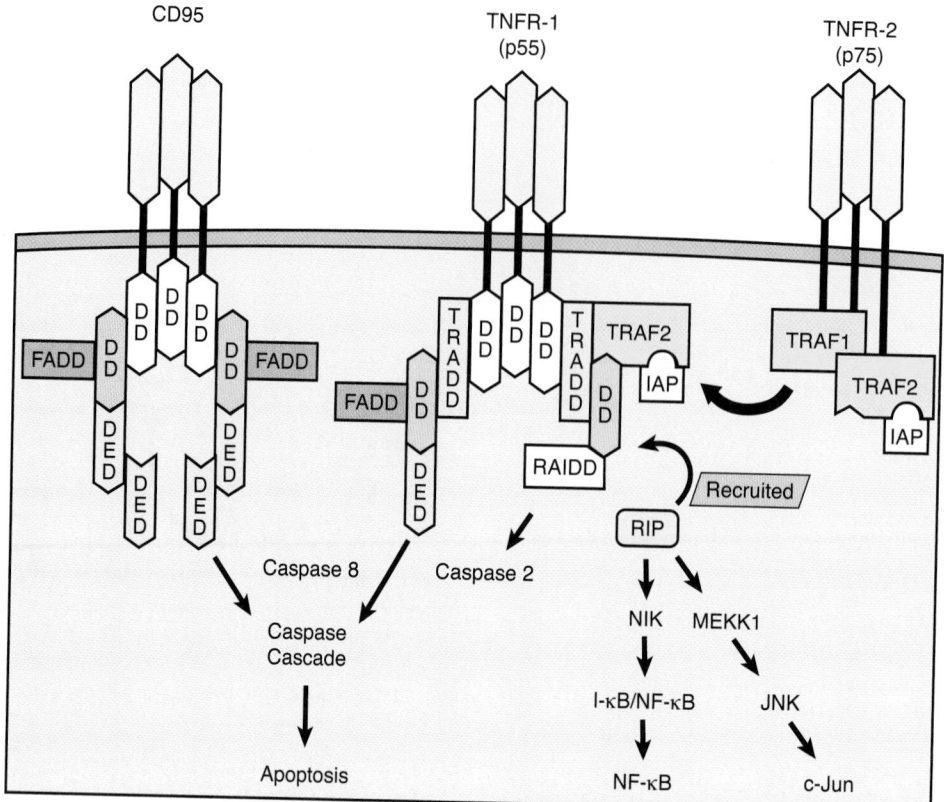

FIG. 2-14. Signaling pathway for tumor necrosis factor receptor 1 (TNFR-1) (55 kDa) and TNFR-2 (75 kDa) occurs by the recruitment of several adapter proteins to the intracellular receptor complex. Optimal signaling activity requires receptor trimerization. TNFR-1 initially recruits TNFR-associated death domain (TRADD) and induces apoptosis through the actions of proteolytic enzymes known as *caspases,* a pathway shared by another receptor known as *CD95 (Fas).* CD95 and TNFR-1 possess similar intracellular sequences known as *death domains (DDs),* and both recruit the same adapter proteins known as *Fas-associated death domains (FADDs)* before activating caspase 8. TNFR-1 also induces apoptosis by activating caspase 2 through the recruitment of receptor-interacting protein (RIP). RIP also has a functional component that can initiate nuclear factor κB (NF-κB) and c-Jun activation, both favoring cell survival and proinflammatory functions. TNFR-2 lacks a DD component but recruits adapter proteins known as TNFR-associated factors 1 and 2 (TRAF1, TRAF2) that interact with RIP to mediate NF-κB and c-Jun activation. TRAF2 also recruits additional proteins that are antiapoptotic, known as inhibitor of apoptosis proteins (IAPs). DED = death effector domain; I-κB = inhibitor of κB; I-κB/NF-κB = inactive complex of NF-κB that becomes activated when the I-κB portion is cleaved; JNK = c-Jun N-terminal kinase; MEKK1 = mitogen-activated protein/extracellular regulatory protein kinase kinase kinase-1; NIK = NF-κB–inducing kinase; RAIDD = RIP-associated interleukin-1b-converting enzyme and ced-homologue-1–like protein with death domain, which activates proapoptotic caspases. *(Adapted with permission from Lin E, Calvano SE, Lowry SF: Tumor necrosis factor receptors in systemic inflammation, in Vincent J-L (series ed), Marshall JC, Cohen J (eds): Update in Intensive Care and Emergency Medicine: Vol. 31: Immune Response in Critical Illness. Berlin: Springer-Verlag, 1999, p 365. With kind permission from Springer Science + Business Media.)*

completely autonomous manner, because there is significant interaction and crosstalk between mediators of both extrinsic and intrinsic pathways. Apoptosis is modulated by several regulatory factors, including inhibitor of apoptosis proteins and regulatory caspases (e.g., caspases 1, 8, 10).

Apoptosis during sepsis may influence the ultimate competency of the acquired immune response. In a murine model of peritoneal sepsis, increased lymphocyte apoptosis was associated with mortality, which may be due to a resultant decrease in IFN-γ release. In postmortem analysis of patients who expired from overwhelming sepsis, there was an increase in lymphocyte apoptosis, whereas macrophage apoptosis did not appear to be affected. Clinical trials have observed an association between the degree of lymphopenia and disease severity in sepsis. In addition, after the phagocytosis of apoptotic cells by macrophages, anti-inflammatory mediators such as IL-10 are released that may exacerbate immune suppression during sepsis. Neutrophil apoptosis is inhibited by inflammatory products, including TNF, IL-1, IL-3, IL-6, GM-CSF, and IFN-γ. This retardation in regulated cell death may prolong and exacerbate secondary injury through neutrophil free radical release as the clearance of senescent cells is delayed.[28]

CELL-MEDIATED INFLAMMATORY RESPONSE

Platelets

Platelets are nonnucleated structures containing both mitochondria and mediators of coagulation and inflammatory signaling. Platelets are derived from bone marrow megakaryocytes. Platelets are critically important in the hemostatic response and are activated by several factors, including exposed collagen. Activated platelets at the site of injury release inflammatory mediators that serve as the principal chemoattractant for neutrophils and monocytes. The migration of platelets and neutrophils through the vascular endothelium occurs within 3 hours of injury and is enhanced by serotonin release, platelet-activating factor, and prostaglandin E$_2$. Platelets are an important source of eicosanoids and vasoactive mediators. A hallmark of the septic response includes thrombocytopenia; however, the mechanism is unclear and likely multifactorial. Pharmaceutical agents such as NSAIDs inhibit platelet function through the blockade of COX.[43]

Lymphocytes and T-Cell Immunity

Lymphocytes are circulating immune cells composed primarily of B cells, T cells, and natural killer cells. As mediators of adaptive

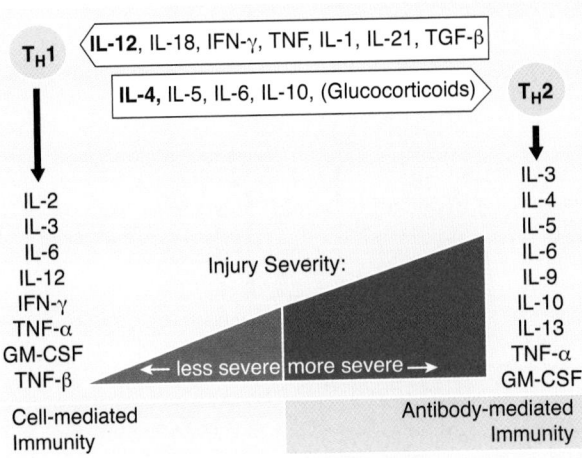

FIG. 2-15. Specific immunity mediated by helper T lymphocytes subtype 1 (T$_H$1) and subtype 2 (T$_H$2) after injury. A T$_H$1 response is favored in lesser injuries, with intact cell-mediated and opsonizing antibody immunity against microbial infections. This cell-mediated immunity includes activation of monocytes, B lymphocytes, and cytotoxic T lymphocytes. A shift toward the T$_H$2 response from naïve helper T cells is associated with injuries of greater magnitude and is not as effective against microbial infections. A T$_H$2 response includes the activation of eosinophils, mast cells, and B-lymphocyte immuno-globulin 4 and immunoglobulin E production. (Primary stimulants and principal cytokine products of such responses are in **bold** characters.) Interleukin-4 (IL-4) and IL-10 are known inhibitors of the T$_H$1 response. Interferon-γ (IFN-γ) is a known inhibitor of the T$_H$2 response. Although not cytokines, glucocorticoids are potent stimulants of a T$_H$2 response, which may partly contribute to the immunosuppressive effects of cortisol. GM-CSF = granulocyte-macrophage colony-stimulating factor; IL = interleukin; TGF = transforming growth factor; TNF = tumor necrosis factor. (*Adapted with permission from Lin E, Calvano SE, Lowry SF: Inflammatory cytokines and cell response in surgery. Surgery 127:117, 2000. Copyright Elsevier.*)

immunity, T lymphocytes are recruited to sites of injury. Helper T lymphocytes are broadly categorized into two groups: T$_H$1 and T$_H$2. T$_H$1 cells favor cellular immune responses and secrete IFN-γ, IL-2, and IL-12, whereas T$_H$2 cells favor humoral responses and produce IL-4, IL-5, IL-6, IL-9, IL-10, and IL-13. T$_H$1 activation is paramount in the defense against bacterial pathogens; however, during critical illness induced by severe trauma or sepsis, there appears to be a predominance of T$_H$2 over T$_H$1 cytokine responses, which may exacerbate immune dysregulation through amplified cytokine signaling (Fig. 2-15). In burn injury, T regulatory cells are associated with T-cell suppression via the release of transforming growth factor beta (TGF-β), which can downregulate T-cell function. Nutritional supplementation may confer a benefit in T-cell responses, because arginine is essential for T-cell proliferation and receptor function.[44]

Eosinophils

Eosinophils are immunocytes whose primary functions are antihelmintic. Eosinophils are found mostly in tissues such as the lung and GI tract, which may suggest a role in immune surveillance. Eosinophils can be activated by IL-3, IL-5, GM-CSF, chemoattractants, and platelet-activating factor. Eosinophil activation can lead to subsequent release of toxic mediators, including reactive oxygen species, histamine, and peroxidase.[45]

Mast Cells

Mast cells are important in the primary response to injury because they are located in tissues. TNF release from mast cells has been found to be crucial for neutrophil recruitment and pathogen clear-

ance. Mast cells are also known to play an important role in the anaphylactic response to allergens. On activation from stimuli including allergen binding, infection, and trauma, mast cells produce histamine, cytokines, eicosanoids, proteases, and chemokines, which leads to vasodilatation, capillary leakage, and immunocyte recruitment. Mast cells are thought to be important cosignaling effector cells of the immune system via the release of IL-3, IL-4, IL-5, IL-6, IL-10, IL-13, and IL-14, as well as macrophage migration–inhibiting factor.[46]

Monocytes

Monocytes are mononuclear phagocytes that circulate in the blood-stream and can differentiate into macrophages, osteoclasts, and dendritic cells on migrating into tissues. Macrophages are the main effector cells of the immune response to infection and injury, primarily through mechanisms that include phagocytosis of microbial pathogens, release of inflammatory mediators, and clearance of apoptotic cells. In humans, downregulation of monocyte and neutrophil TNFR expression has been demonstrated experimentally and clinically during systemic inflammation. In clinical sepsis, nonsurviving patients with severe sepsis have an immediate reduction in monocyte surface TNFR expression with failure to recover, whereas surviving patients have normal or near-normal receptor levels from the onset of clinically defined sepsis. In patients with congestive heart failure, there is also a significant decrease in the amount of monocyte surface TNFR expression compared with control patients. In experimental models, endotoxin has been shown to differentially regulate over 1000 genes in murine macrophages with approximately 25% of these corresponding to cytokines and chemokines. During sepsis, macrophages undergo phenotypic reprogramming highlighted by decreased surface human leukocyte antigen DR (a critical receptor in antigen presentation), which also may contribute to host immunocompromise during sepsis.[47]

Neutrophils

Neutrophils are among the first responders to sites of infection and injury and as such are potent mediators of acute inflammation. Chemotactic mediators from a site of injury induce neutrophil adherence to the vascular endothelium and promote eventual cell migration into the injured tissue. Neutrophils are circulating immunocytes with short half-lives (4 to 10 hours). On activation by inflammatory stimuli, including TNF, IL-1, and microbial pathogens, neutrophils are able to phagocytose, release lytic enzymes, and generate large amounts of toxic reactive oxygen species.[48]

ENDOTHELIUM-MEDIATED INJURY

Vascular Endothelium

Under physiologic conditions, vascular endothelium has overall anticoagulant properties mediated via the production and cell surface expression of heparin sulfate, dermatan sulfate, tissue factor pathway inhibitor, protein S, thrombomodulin, plasminogen, and tissue plasminogen activator. Endothelial cells also perform a critical function as barriers that regulate tissue migration of circulating cells. During sepsis, endothelial cells are differentially modulated, which results in an overall procoagulant shift via decreased production of anticoagulant factors, which may lead to microthrombosis and organ injury.

Neutrophil-Endothelium Interaction

The regulated inflammatory response to infection facilitates neutrophil and other immunocyte migration to compromised regions through the actions of increased vascular permeability, chemoattractants, and increased endothelial adhesion factors referred to as *selectins* that are elaborated on cell surfaces (Table 2-5). Prolonged and unremitting neutrophil activation and mediator release can

TABLE 2-5 Molecules that mediate leukocyte-endothelial adhesion, categorized by family

Adhesion Molecule	Action	Origin	Inducers of Expression	Target Cells
Selectins				
L-selectin	Fast rolling	Leukocytes	Native	Endothelium, platelets, eosinophils
P-selectin	Slow rolling	Platelets and endothelium	Thrombin, histamine	Neutrophils, monocytes
E-selectin	Very slow rolling	Endothelium	Cytokines	Neutrophils, monocytes, lymphocytes
Immunoglobulins				
ICAM-1	Firm adhesion/transmigration	Endothelium, leukocytes, fibroblasts, epithelium	Cytokines	Leukocytes
ICAM-2	Firm adhesion	Endothelium, platelets	Native	Leukocytes
VCAM-1	Firm adhesion/transmigration	Endothelium	Cytokines	Monocytes, lymphocytes
PECAM-1	Adhesion/transmigration	Endothelium, platelets, leukocytes	Native	Endothelium, platelets, leukocytes
β_2-(CD18) Integrins				
CD18/11a	Firm adhesion/transmigration	Leukocytes	Leukocyte activation	Endothelium
CD18/11b (Mac-1)	Firm adhesion/transmigration	Neutrophils, monocytes, natural killer cells	Leukocyte activation	Endothelium
CD18/11c	Adhesion	Neutrophils, monocytes, natural killer cells	Leukocyte activation	Endothelium
β_1-(CD29) Integrins				
VLA-4	Firm adhesion/transmigration	Lymphocytes, monocytes	Leukocyte activation	Monocytes, endothelium, epithelium

ICAM-1 = intercellular adhesion molecule-1; ICAM-2 = intercellular adhesion molecule-2; Mac-1 = macrophage antigen 1; PECAM-1 = platelet-endothelial cell adhesion molecule-1; VCAM-1 = vascular cell adhesion molecule-1; VLA-4 = very late antigen-4.

lead to tissue injury through the production of toxic oxygen metabolites and lysosomal enzymes that degrade tissue basal membranes, cause microvascular thrombosis, and activate myeloperoxidases. In response to inflammatory stimuli, including chemokines, thrombin, IL-1, histamine, and TNF, vascular endothelium increases surface expression of the adhesion molecule P-selectin, which is observable in 10 to 20 minutes and mediates neutrophil rolling (Fig. 2-16). After 2 hours, however, cell surface expression favors E-selectin expression. L-selectin and P-selectin glycoprotein ligand-1

(PSGL-1) are responsible for over 85% of monocyte-to-monocyte and monocyte-to-endothelium adhesion activity. Endothelial selectins interact with leukocyte selectins (PSGL-1, L-selectin) to mediate leukocyte rolling, which allows targeted immunocyte migration. Also important are secondary leukocyte-leukocyte interactions in which PGSL-1 and L-selectin binding facilitates further leukocyte tethering. Although there are distinguishable properties among individual selectins in leukocyte rolling, effective rolling most likely involves a significant degree of functional overlap.[49]

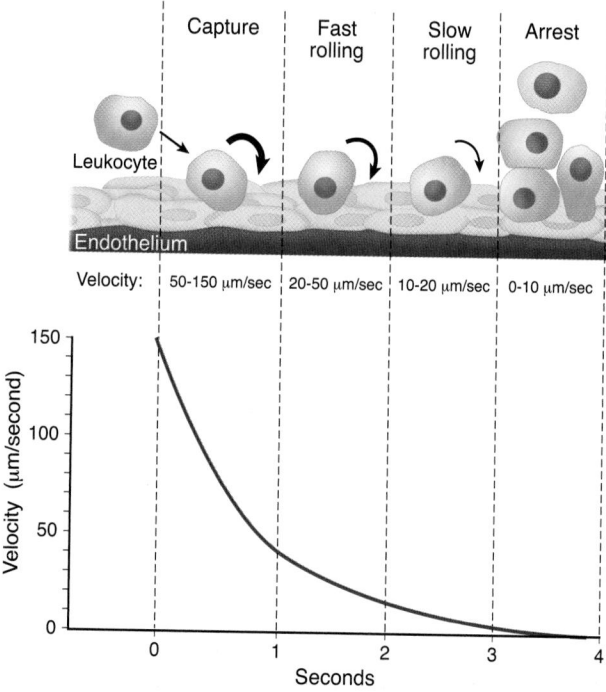

FIG. 2-16. Simplified sequence of selectin-mediated neutrophil-endothelium interaction after an inflammatory stimulus. *CAPTURE* (tethering), predominantly mediated by cell L-selectin with contribution from endothelial P-selectin, describes the initial recognition between leukocyte and endothelium, in which circulating leukocytes marginate toward the endothelial surface. *FAST ROLLING* (20 to 50 μm/s) is a consequence of rapid L-selectin shedding from cell surfaces and formation of new downstream L-selectin to endothelium bonds, which occur in tandem. *SLOW ROLLING* (10 to 20 μm/s) is predominantly mediated by P-selectins. The slowest rolling (3 to 10 μm/s) before arrest is predominantly mediated by E-selectins, with contribution from P-selectins. *ARREST* (firm adhesion) leading to transmigration is mediated by β-integrins and the immunoglobulin family of adhesion molecules. In addition to interacting with the endothelium, activated leukocytes also recruit other leukocytes to the inflammatory site by direct interactions, which are mediated in part by selectins. *(Adapted with permission from Lin E, Calvano SE, Lowry SF: Selectin neutralization: Does it make biological sense?* Crit Care Med 27:2050, 1999.)

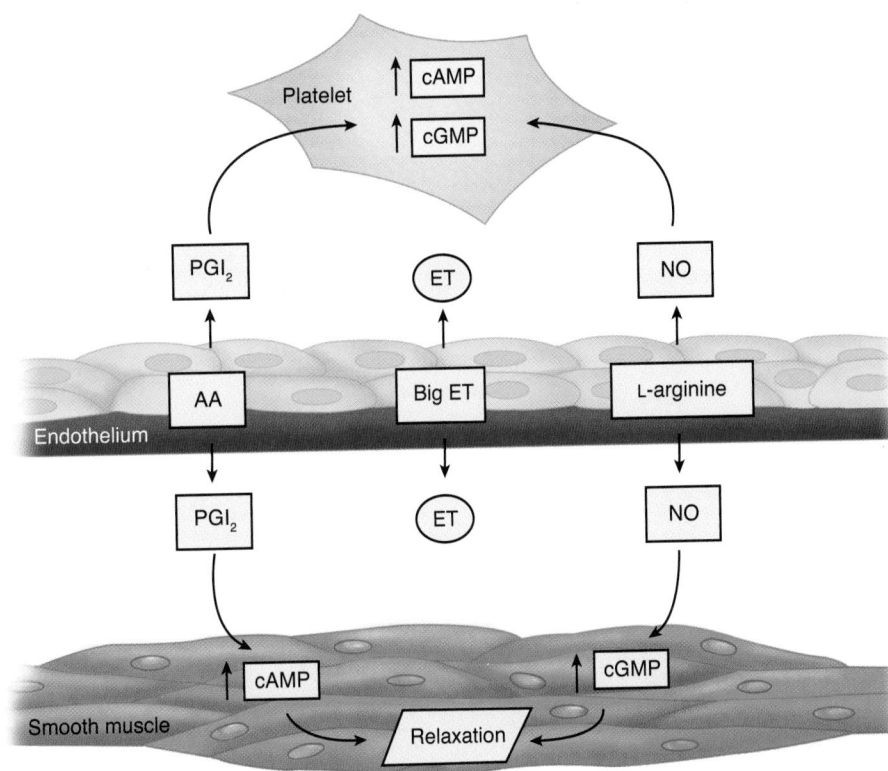

FIG. 2-17. Endothelial interaction with smooth muscle cells and with intraluminal platelets. Prostacyclin (prostaglandin I₂, or PGI₂) is derived from arachidonic acid (AA), and nitric oxide (NO) is derived from L-arginine. The increase in cyclic adenosine monophosphate (cAMP) and cyclic guanosine monophosphate (cGMP) results in smooth muscle relaxation and inhibition of platelet thrombus formation. Endothelins (ETs) are derived from "big ET," and they counter the effects of prostacyclin and NO.

Nitric Oxide

Nitric oxide (NO) was initially known as *endothelium-derived relaxing factor* due to its effect on vascular smooth muscle and has important functions in both physiologic and pathologic control of vascular tone. Normal vascular smooth muscle relaxation is maintained by a constant output of NO and subsequent activation of soluble guanylyl cyclase. NO also can reduce microthrombosis by reducing platelet adhesion and aggregation (Fig. 2-17). NO easily traverses cell membranes and has a short half-life of a few seconds and is oxidized into nitrate and nitrite. NO is constitutively expressed by endothelial cells; however, inducible NO synthase, which is normally not expressed, is upregulated in response to inflammatory stimuli, which increases NO production. Increased NO is detectable in septic shock and in response to TNF, IL-1, IL-2, and hemorrhage. NO mediates hypotension observed during septic shock; however, a clinical trial of a nonselective NOS inhibitor showed increased organ dysfunction and mortality.[50]

Prostacyclin

Prostacyclin is a member of the eicosanoid family and is primarily produced by endothelial cells. Prostacyclin is an effective vasodilator and also inhibits platelet aggregation. During systemic inflammation, endothelial prostacyclin expression is impaired, and thus the endothelium favors a more procoagulant profile. Prostacyclin therapy during sepsis has been shown to reduce the levels of cytokines, growth factors, and adhesion molecules through a cAMP-dependent pathway. In clinical trials, prostacyclin infusion is associated with increased cardiac output, splanchnic blood flow, and oxygen delivery and consumption with no significant decrease in mean arterial pressure. However, further study is required before the widespread use of prostacyclin is recommended.[51]

Endothelins

Endothelins (ETs) are potent mediators of vasoconstriction and are composed of three members: ET-1, ET-2, and ET-3. ETs are 21-amino-acid peptides derived from a 38-amino-acid precursor molecule. ET-1, synthesized primarily by endothelial cells, is the most potent endogenous vasoconstrictor and is estimated to be 10 times more potent than angiotensin II. ET release is upregulated in response to hypotension, LPS, injury, thrombin, TGF-β, IL-1, angiotensin II, vasopressin, catecholamines, and anoxia. ETs are primarily released to the abluminal side of endothelial cells, and very little is stored in cells; thus a plasma increase is associated with a marked increase in production. The half-life of plasma ET is between 4 and 7 minutes, which suggests that ET release is primarily regulated at the transcriptional level. Three endothelin receptors, referred to as ET_A, ET_B, and ET_C, have been identified and function via the G-protein–coupled receptor mechanism. ET_B receptors are associated with increased NO and prostacyclin production, which may serve as a feedback mechanism. Atrial ET_A receptor activation has been associated with increased inotropy and chronotropy. ET-1 infusion is associated with increased pulmonary vascular resistance and pulmonary edema and may contribute to pulmonary abnormalities during sepsis. At low levels, in conjunction with NO, ETs regulate vascular tone. However, at increased concentrations, ETs can disrupt the normal blood flow and distribution and may compromise oxygen delivery to the tissue. In addition, increased plasma ET concentration correlates with the severity of injury after major trauma or major surgical procedures, and in patients with cardiogenic or septic shock.[52]

Platelet-Activating Factor

Another endothelium-derived product is platelet-activating factor (PAF), a natural phospholipid constituent of cell membranes that is minimally expressed under normal physiologic conditions. During acute inflammation, PAF is released by neutrophils, platelets, mast cells, and monocytes, and is expressed at the outer leaflet of endothelial cells. PAF can further activate neutrophils and platelets, and increase vascular permeability. Antagonists to PAF receptors have been experimentally shown to mitigate the effects of ischemia and reperfusion injury. Human sepsis is associated with a reduction in levels of PAF-acetylhydrolase, which is the endogenous inhibitor of PAF. Indeed, PAF-acetylhydrolase administration in patients

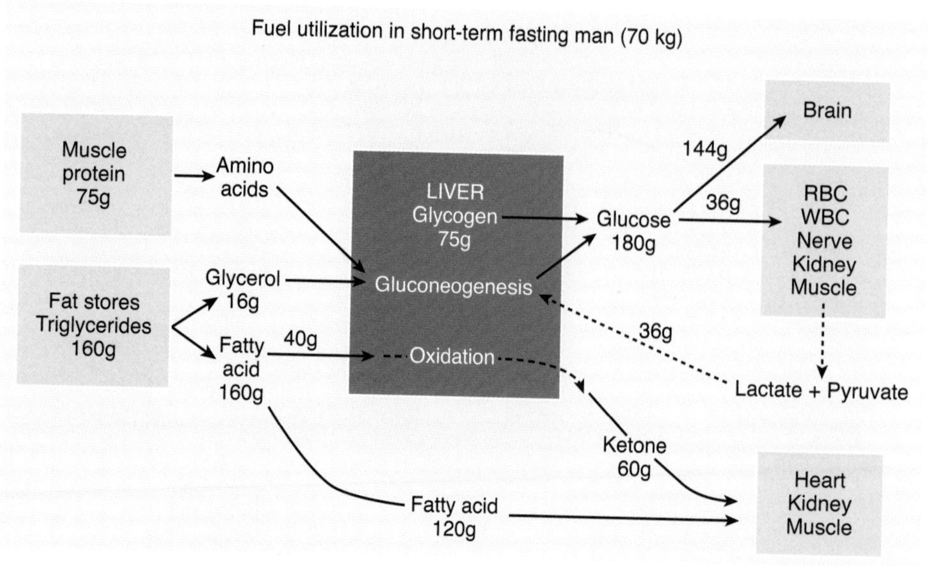

Fuel utilization in short-term fasting man (70 kg)

FIG. 2-18. Fuel utilization in a 70-kg man during short-term fasting with an approximate basal energy expenditure of 1800 kcal. During starvation, muscle proteins and fat stores provide fuel for the host, with the latter being most abundant. RBC = red blood cell; WBC = white blood cell. *(Adapted with permission from Cahill GF: Starvation in man. N Engl J Med 282:668, 1970. Copyright © Massachusetts Medical Society. All rights reserved.)*

with severe sepsis has yielded some reduction in multiple organ dysfunction and mortality.[53]

Atrial Natriuretic Peptides

Atrial natriuretic peptides (ANPs) are a family of peptides that are released primarily by atrial tissue but are also synthesized by the gut, kidney, brain, adrenal glands, and endothelium. They induce vasodilation as well as fluid and electrolyte excretion. ANPs are potent inhibitors of aldosterone secretion and prevent reabsorption of sodium. There is some experimental evidence to suggest that ANP can reverse acute renal failure or early acute tubular necrosis.

SURGICAL METABOLISM

The initial hours after surgical or traumatic injury are metabolically associated with a reduced total body energy expenditure and urinary nitrogen wasting. On adequate resuscitation and stabilization of the injured patient, a reprioritization of substrate use ensues to preserve vital organ function and to support repair of injured tissue. This phase of recovery also is characterized by functions that participate in the restoration of homeostasis, such as augmented metabolic rates and oxygen consumption, enzymatic preference for readily oxidizable substrates such as glucose, and stimulation of the immune system.

Understanding of the collective alterations in amino acid (protein), carbohydrate, and lipid metabolism characteristic of the surgical patient lays the foundation upon which metabolic and nutritional support can be implemented.

Metabolism during Fasting

Fuel metabolism during unstressed fasting states has historically served as the standard to which metabolic alterations after acute injury and critical illness are compared (Fig. 2-18). To maintain basal metabolic needs (i.e., at rest and fasting), a normal healthy adult requires approximately 22 to 25 kcal/kg per day drawn from carbohydrate, lipid, and protein sources. This requirement can be as high as 40 kcal/kg per day in severe stress states, such as those seen in patients with burn injuries.

In the healthy adult, principal sources of fuel during short-term fasting (<5 days) are derived from muscle protein and body fat, with fat being the most abundant source of energy (Table 2-6). The normal adult body contains 300 to 400 g of carbohydrates in the form of glycogen, of which 75 to 100 g are stored in the liver. Approximately 200 to 250 g of glycogen are stored within skeletal, cardiac, and smooth muscle cells. The greater glycogen stores within the muscle are not readily available for systemic use due to a deficiency in glucose-6-phosphatase but are available for the energy needs of muscle cells. Therefore, in the fasting state, hepatic glyco-

TABLE 2-6	A. Body fuel reserves in a 70-kg man and B. Energy equivalent of substrate oxidation

A. Component	Mass (kg)	Energy (kcal)	Days Available
Water and minerals	49	0	0
Protein	6.0	24,000	13.0
Glycogen	0.2	800	0.4
Fat	15.0	140,000	78.0
Total	70.2	164,800	91.4

B. Substrate	O_2 Consumed (L/g)	CO_2 Produced (L/g)	Respiratory Quotient	kcal/g	Recommended Daily Requirement
Glucose	0.75	0.75	1.0	4.0	7.2 g/kg per day
Dextrose	—	—	—	3.4	—
Lipid	2.0	1.4	0.7	9.0	1.0 g/kg per day
Protein	1.0	0.8	0.8	4.0	0.8 g/kg per day

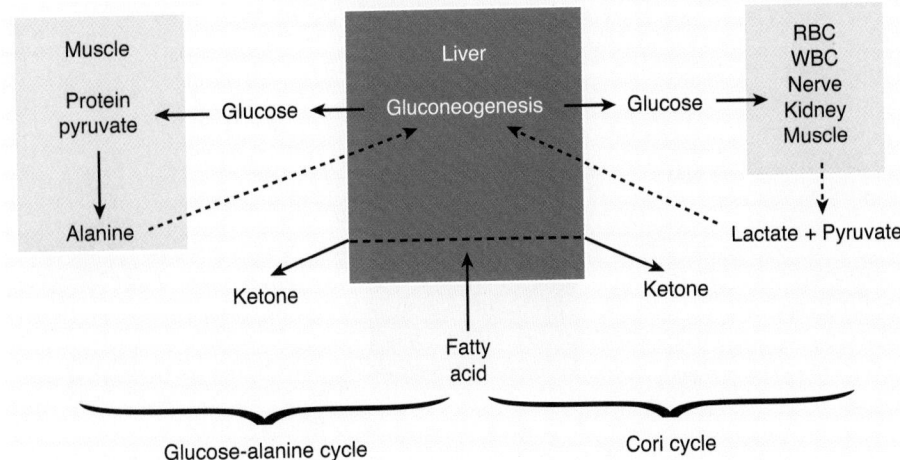

FIG. 2-19. The recycling of peripheral lactate and pyruvate for hepatic gluconeogenesis is accomplished by the Cori cycle. Alanine within skeletal muscles can also be used as a precursor for hepatic gluconeogenesis. During starvation, such fatty acid provides fuel sources for basal hepatic enzymatic function. RBC = red blood cell; WBC = white blood cell.

gen stores are rapidly and preferentially depleted, which results in a fall of serum glucose concentration within hours (<16 hours).

During fasting, a healthy 70-kg adult will utilize 180 g of glucose per day to support the metabolism of obligate glycolytic cells such as neurons, leukocytes, erythrocytes, and the renal medullae. Other tissues that use glucose for fuel are skeletal muscle, intestinal mucosa, fetal tissues, and solid tumors.

Glucagon, norepinephrine, vasopressin, and angiotensin II can promote the utilization of glycogen stores (glycogenolysis) during fasting. Although glucagon, epinephrine, and cortisol directly promote gluconeogenesis, epinephrine and cortisol also promote pyruvate shuttling to the liver for gluconeogenesis. Precursors for hepatic gluconeogenesis include lactate, glycerol, and amino acids such as alanine and glutamine. Lactate is released by glycolysis within skeletal muscles, as well as by erythrocytes and leukocytes. The recycling of lactate and pyruvate for gluconeogenesis is commonly referred to as the *Cori cycle*, which can provide up to 40% of plasma glucose during starvation (Fig. 2-19).

Lactate production from skeletal muscle is insufficient to maintain systemic glucose needs during short-term fasting (simple star-

vation). Therefore, significant amounts of protein must be degraded daily (75 g/d for a 70-kg adult) to provide the amino acid substrate for hepatic gluconeogenesis. Proteolysis during starvation, which results primarily from decreased insulin and increased cortisol release, is associated with elevated urinary nitrogen excretion from the normal 7 to 10 g per day up to 30 g or more per day.[54] Although proteolysis during starvation occurs mainly within skeletal muscles, protein degradation in solid organs also occurs.

In prolonged starvation, systemic proteolysis is reduced to approximately 20 g/d and urinary nitrogen excretion stabilizes at 2 to 5 g/d (Fig. 2-20). This reduction in proteolysis reflects the adaptation by vital organs (e.g., myocardium, brain, renal cortex, and skeletal muscle) to using ketone bodies as their principal fuel source. In extended fasting, ketone bodies become an important fuel source for the brain after 2 days and gradually become the principal fuel source by 24 days.

Enhanced deamination of amino acids for gluconeogenesis during starvation consequently increases renal excretion of ammonium ions. The kidneys also participate in gluconeogenesis by the use of glutamine and glutamate, and can become the primary source of

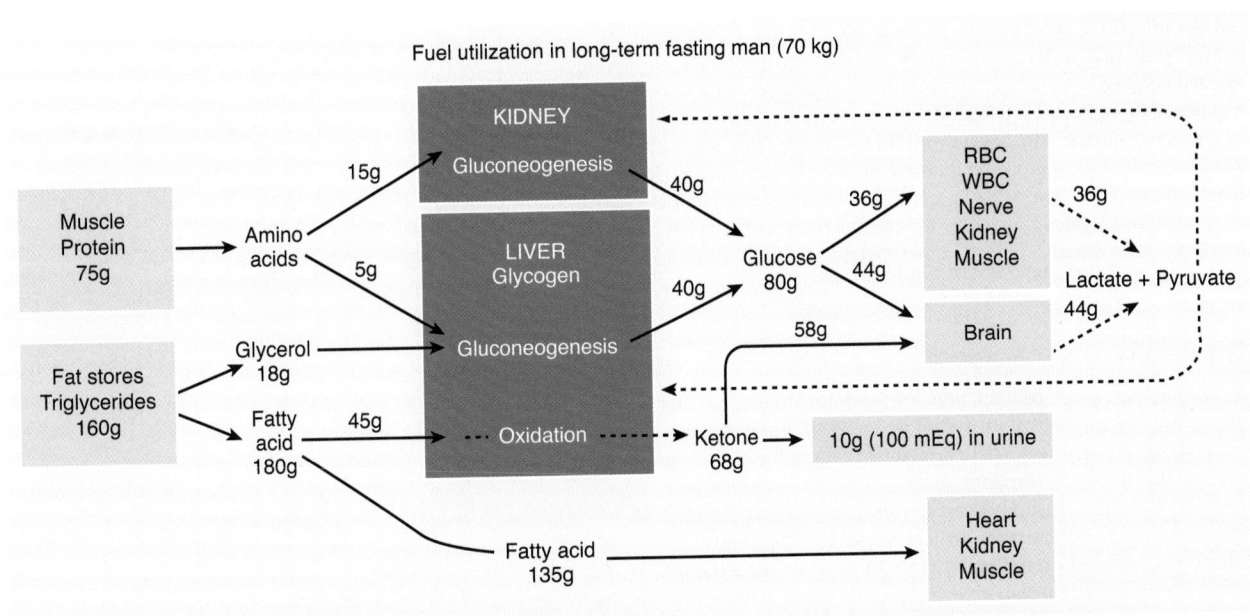

Fuel utilization in long-term fasting man (70 kg)

FIG. 2-20. Fuel utilization in extended starvation. Liver glycogen stores are depleted, and there is adaptive reduction in proteolysis as a source of fuel. The brain uses ketones for fuel. The kidneys become important participants in gluconeogenesis. RBC = red blood cell; WBC = white blood cell. *(Adapted with permission from Cahill GF: Starvation in man. N Engl J Med 282:668, 1970. Copyright © Massachusetts Medical Society. All rights reserved.)*

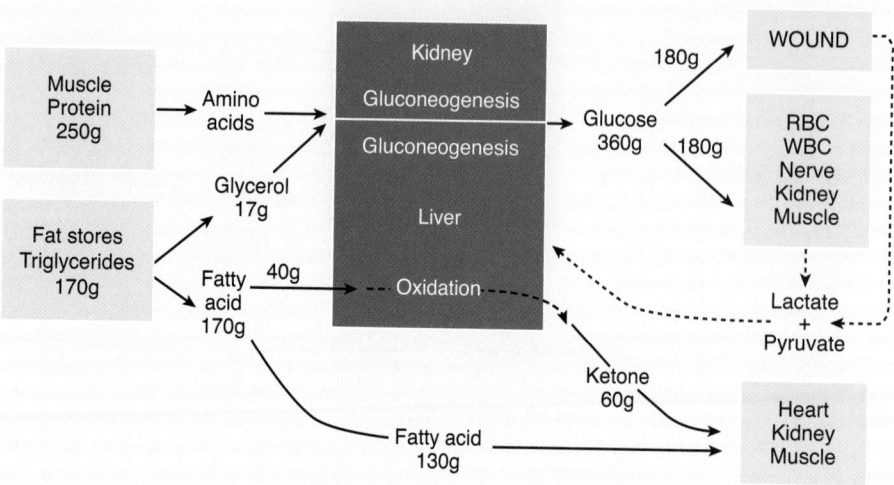

Fuel utilization following trauma

FIG. 2-21. Acute injury is associated with significant alterations in substrate utilization. There is enhanced nitrogen loss, indicative of catabolism. Fat remains the primary fuel source under these circumstances. RBC = red blood cell; WBC = white blood cell.

gluconeogenesis during prolonged starvation, accounting for up to one half of systemic glucose production.

Lipid stores within adipose tissue provide 40% or more of caloric expenditure during starvation. Energy requirements for basal enzymatic and muscular functions (e.g., gluconeogenesis, neural transmission, and cardiac contraction) are met by the mobilization of triglycerides from adipose tissue. In a resting, fasting, 70-kg person, approximately 160 g of free fatty acids and glycerol can be mobilized from adipose tissue per day. Free fatty acid release is stimulated in part by a reduction in serum insulin levels and in part by the increase in circulating glucagon and catecholamine. Such free fatty acids, like ketone bodies, are used as fuel by tissues such as the heart, kidney (renal cortex), muscle, and liver. The mobilization of lipid stores for energy importantly decreases the rate of glycolysis, gluconeogenesis, and proteolysis, as well as the overall glucose requirement to sustain the host. Furthermore, ketone bodies spare glucose utilization by inhibiting the enzyme pyruvate dehydrogenase.

Metabolism after Injury

Injuries or infections induce unique neuroendocrine and immunologic responses that differentiate injury metabolism from that of unstressed fasting (Fig. 2-21). The magnitude of metabolic expenditure appears to be directly proportional to the severity of insult, with thermal injuries and severe infections having the highest energy demands (Fig. 2-22). The increase in energy expenditure is mediated in part by sympathetic activation and catecholamine release, which has been replicated by the administration of catecholamines to healthy human subjects. Lipid metabolism after injury is intentionally discussed first, because this macronutrient becomes the primary source of energy during stressed states.[55]

Lipid Metabolism after Injury

Lipids are not merely nonprotein, noncarbohydrate fuel sources that minimize protein catabolism in the injured patient. Lipid metabolism potentially influences the structural integrity of cell membranes as well as the immune response during systemic inflammation. Adipose stores within the body (triglycerides) are the predominant energy source (50 to 80%) during critical illness and after injury. Fat mobilization (lipolysis) occurs mainly in response to catecholamine stimulus of the hormone-sensitive triglyceride lipase. Other hormonal influences which potentiate lipolysis include adrenocorticotropic hormone (ACTH), catecholamines, thyroid hormone, cortisol, glucagon, growth hormone release, reduction in insulin levels, and increased sympathetic stimulus.[56]

Lipid Absorption Although the process is poorly understood, adipose tissue provides fuel for the host in the form of free fatty acids and glycerol during critical illness and injury. Oxidation of 1 g of fat yields approximately 9 kcal of energy. Although the liver is capable of synthesizing triglycerides from carbohydrates and amino acids, dietary and exogenous sources provide the major source of triglycerides. Dietary lipids are not readily absorbable in the gut but require pancreatic lipase and phospholipase within the duodenum to hydrolyze the triglycerides into free fatty acids and monoglycerides. The free fatty acids and monoglycerides are then readily absorbed by gut enterocytes, which resynthesize triglycerides by esterification of the monoglycerides with fatty acyl coenzyme A (acyl-CoA) (Fig. 2-23). Long-chain triglycerides (LCTs), defined as those with 12 carbons or more, generally undergo this process of

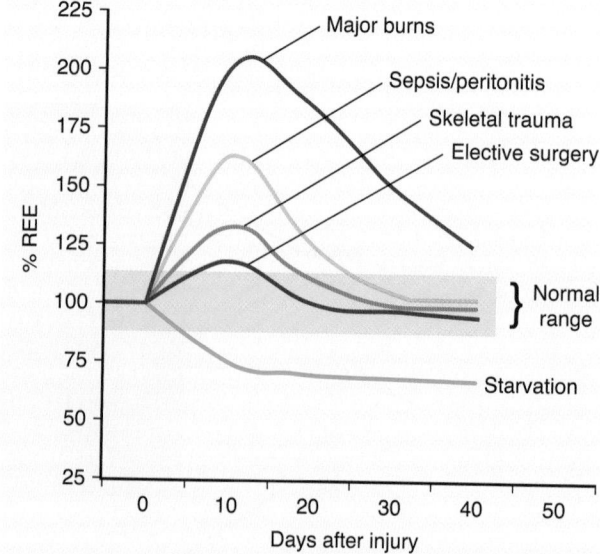

FIG. 2-22. Influence of injury severity on resting metabolism (resting energy expenditure, or REE). The shaded area indicates normal REE. (*Adapted with permission from Long CL et al: Metabolic response to injury and illness: Estimation of energy and protein needs from indirect calorimetry and nitrogen balance.* JPEN J Parenter Enteral Nutr *3:452, 1979.*)

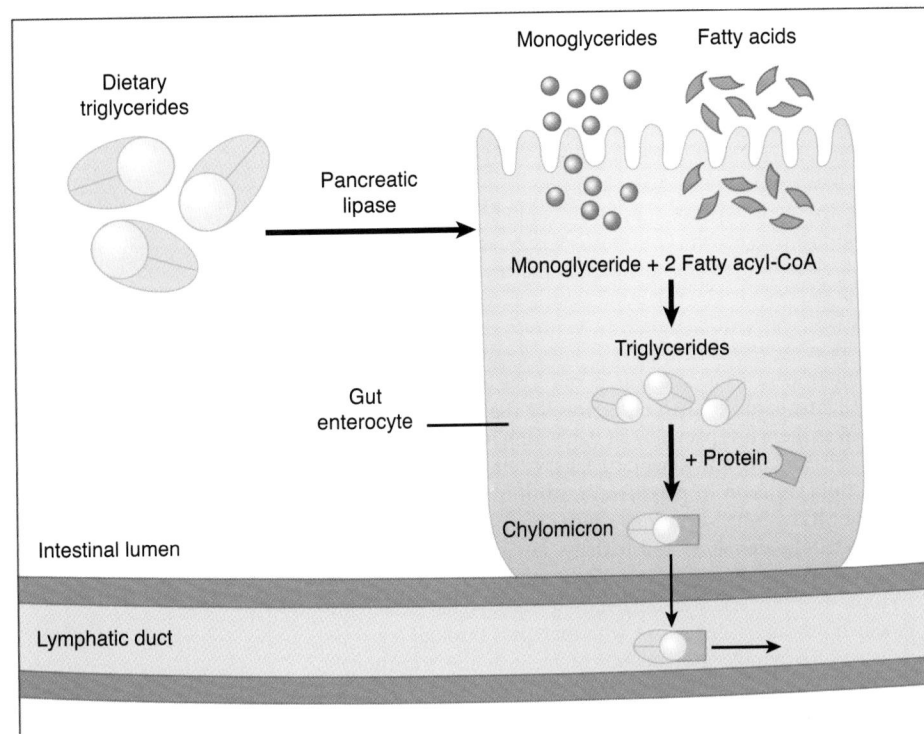

FIG. 2-23. Pancreatic lipase within the small intestinal brush borders hydrolyzes triglycerides into monoglycerides and fatty acids. These components readily diffuse into the gut enterocytes, where they are re-esterified into triglycerides. The resynthesized triglycerides bind carrier proteins to form chylomicrons, which are transported by the lymphatic system. Shorter triglycerides (those with <10 carbon atoms) can bypass this process and directly enter the portal circulation for transport to the liver. CoA = coenzyme A.

esterification and enter the circulation through the lymphatic system as chylomicrons. Shorter fatty acid chains directly enter the portal circulation and are transported to the liver by albumin carriers. Hepatocytes use free fatty acids as a fuel source during stress states but also can synthesize phospholipids or triglycerides (i.e., very-low-density lipoproteins) during fed states. Systemic tissue (e.g., muscle and the heart) can use chylomicrons and triglycerides as fuel by hydrolysis with lipoprotein lipase at the luminal surface of capillary endothelium.[57] Trauma or sepsis sup-

presses lipoprotein lipase activity in both adipose tissue and muscle, presumably mediated by TNF.

Lipolysis and Fatty Acid Oxidation Periods of energy demand are accompanied by free fatty acid mobilization from adipose stores. This is mediated by hormonal influences (e.g., catecholamines, ACTH, thyroid hormones, growth hormone, and glucagon) on triglyceride lipase through a cAMP pathway (Fig. 2-24). In adipose tissues, triglyceride lipase hydrolyzes triglycerides into free fatty

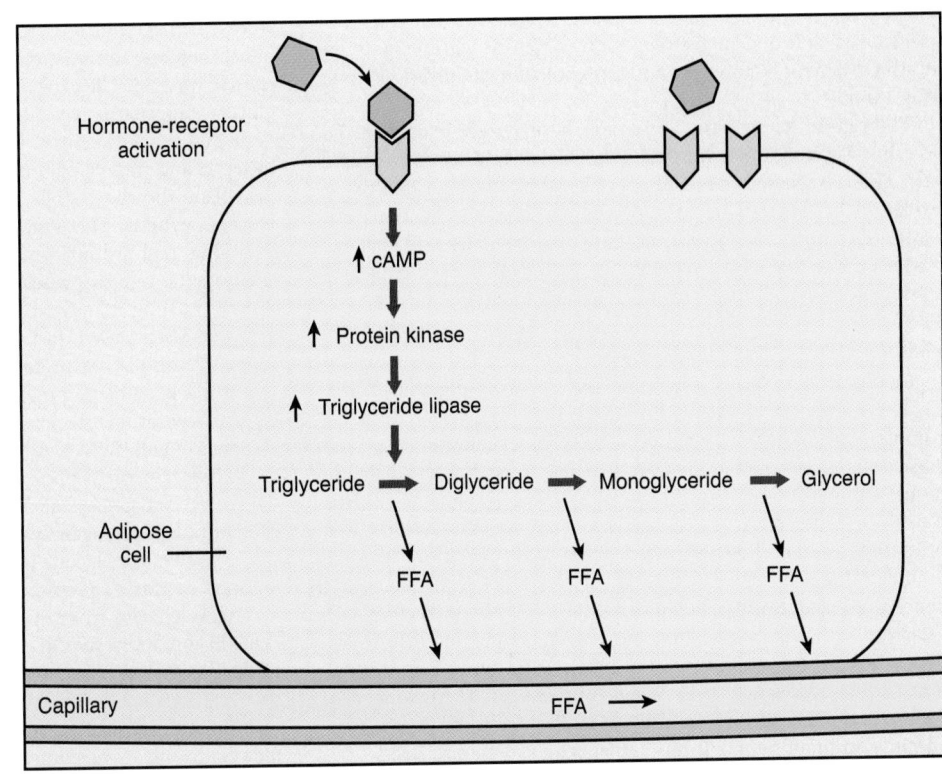

FIG. 2-24. Fat mobilization in adipose tissue. Triglyceride lipase activation by hormonal stimulation of adipose cells occurs through the cyclic adenosine monophosphate (cAMP) pathway. Triglycerides are serially hydrolyzed with resultant free fatty acid (FFA) release at every step. The FFAs diffuse readily into the capillary bed for transport. Tissues with glycerokinase can use glycerol for fuel by forming glycerol-3-phosphate. Glycerol-3-phosphate can esterify with FFAs to form triglycerides or can be used as a precursor for renal and hepatic gluconeogenesis. Skeletal muscle and adipose cells have little glycerokinase and thus do not use glycerol for fuel.

acids and glycerol. Free fatty acids enter the capillary circulation and are transported by albumin to tissues requiring this fuel source (e.g., heart and skeletal muscle). Insulin inhibits lipolysis and favors triglyceride synthesis by augmenting lipoprotein lipase activity as well as intracellular levels of glycerol-3-phosphate. The use of glycerol for fuel depends on the availability of tissue glycerokinase, which is abundant in the liver and kidneys.

Free fatty acids absorbed by cells conjugate with acyl-CoA within the cytoplasm. The transport of fatty acyl-CoA from the outer mitochondrial membrane across the inner mitochondrial membrane occurs via the carnitine shuttle (Fig. 2-25). Medium-chain triglycerides (MCTs), defined as those 6 to 12 carbons in length, bypass the carnitine shuttle and readily cross the mitochondrial membranes. This accounts in part for the fact that MCTs are more efficiently oxidized than LCTs. Ideally, the rapid oxidation of MCTs makes them less prone to fat deposition, particularly within immune cells and the reticuloendothelial system—a common finding with lipid infusion in parenteral nutrition.[58] However, exclusive use of MCTs as fuel in animal studies has been associated with higher metabolic demands and toxicity, as well as essential fatty acid deficiency.

Within the mitochondria, fatty acyl-CoA undergoes beta oxidation, which produces acetyl-CoA with each pass through the cycle. Each acetyl-CoA molecule subsequently enters the tricarboxylic acid (TCA) cycle for further oxidation to yield 12 adenosine triphosphate (ATP) molecules, carbon dioxide, and water. Excess acetyl-CoA molecules serve as precursors for ketogenesis. Unlike glucose metabolism, oxidation of fatty acids requires proportionally less oxygen and produces less carbon dioxide. This is frequently quantified as the ratio of carbon dioxide produced to oxygen consumed for the reaction and is known as the *respiratory quotient (RQ)*. An RQ of 0.7 would imply greater fatty acid oxidation for fuel, whereas an RQ of 1 indicates greater carbohydrate oxidation (overfeeding). An RQ of 0.85 suggests the oxidation of equal amounts of fatty acids and glucose.

Ketogenesis

Carbohydrate depletion slows the entry of acetyl-CoA into the TCA cycle secondary to depleted TCA intermediates and enzyme activity. Increased lipolysis and reduced systemic carbohydrate availability during starvation diverts excess acetyl-CoA toward hepatic ketogenesis. A number of extrahepatic tissues, but not the liver itself, are capable of using ketones for fuel. Ketosis represents a state in which hepatic ketone production exceeds extrahepatic ketone utilization.

The rate of ketogenesis appears to be inversely related to the severity of injury. Major trauma, severe shock, and sepsis attenuate ketogenesis by increasing insulin levels and by causing rapid tissue oxidation of free fatty acids. Minor injuries and infections are associated with modest elevations in plasma free fatty acid concentrations and ketogenesis. However, in minor stress states ketogenesis does not exceed that in nonstressed starvation.

Carbohydrate Metabolism

Ingested and enteral carbohydrates are primarily digested in the small intestine, where pancreatic and intestinal enzymes reduce the complex carbohydrates to dimeric units. Disaccharidases (e.g., sucrase, lactase, and maltase) within intestinal brush borders dismantle the complex carbohydrates into simple hexose units, which are transported into the intestinal mucosa. Glucose and galactose are primarily absorbed by energy-dependent active transport coupled to the sodium pump. Fructose absorption, however, occurs by concentration-dependent facilitated diffusion. Neither fructose and galactose within the circulation nor exogenous mannitol (for neurologic injury) evokes an insulin response. Intravenous administration of low-dose fructose in fasting humans has been associated with nitrogen conservation, but the clinical utility of fructose administration in human injury remains to be demonstrated.

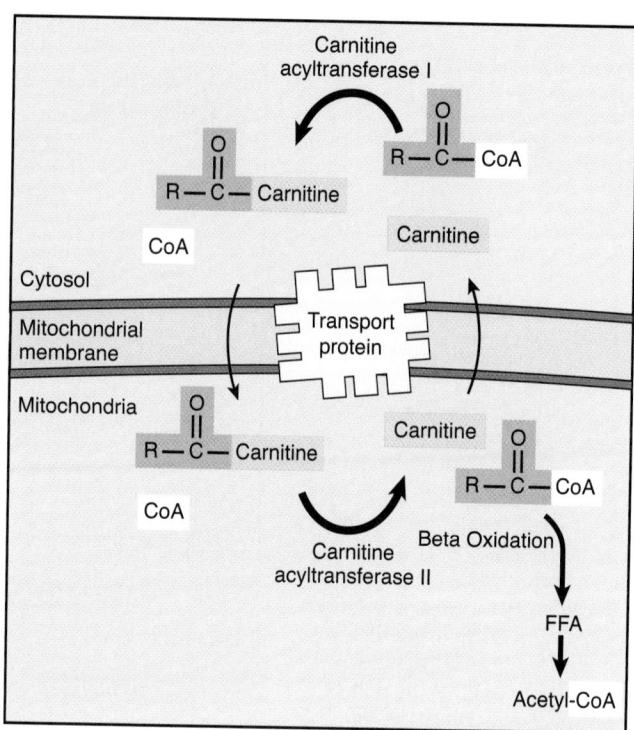

FIG. 2-25. Free fatty acids (FFAs) in the cells form fatty acyl coenzyme A (CoA) with CoA. Fatty acyl-CoA cannot enter the inner mitochondrial membrane and requires carnitine as a carrier protein (carnitine shuttle). Once inside the mitochondria, carnitine dissociates and fatty acyl-CoA is re-formed. The carnitine molecule is transported back into the cytosol for reuse. The fatty acyl-CoA undergoes beta oxidation to form acetyl-CoA for entry into the tricarboxylic acid cycle. "R" represents a part of the acyl group of acyl-CoA.

Discussion of carbohydrate metabolism primarily refers to the utilization of glucose. The oxidation of 1 g of carbohydrate yields 4 kcal, but sugar solutions such as those found in intravenous fluids or parenteral nutrition provide only 3.4 kcal/g of dextrose. In starvation, glucose production occurs at the expense of protein stores (i.e., skeletal muscle). Hence, the primary goal for maintenance glucose administration in surgical patients is to minimize muscle wasting. The exogenous administration of small amounts of glucose (approximately 50 g/d) facilitates fat entry into the TCA cycle and reduces ketosis. Unlike in starvation in healthy subjects, in septic and trauma patients provision of exogenous glucose never has been shown to fully suppress amino acid degradation for gluconeogenesis. This suggests that during periods of stress, other hormonal and proinflammatory mediators have a profound influence on the rate of protein degradation and that some degree of muscle wasting is inevitable. The administration of insulin, however, has been shown to reverse protein catabolism during severe stress by stimulating protein synthesis in skeletal muscles and by inhibiting hepatocyte protein degradation. Insulin also stimulates the incorporation of elemental precursors into nucleic acids in association with RNA synthesis in muscle cells.

In cells, glucose is phosphorylated to form glucose-6-phosphate. Glucose-6-phosphate can be polymerized during glycogenesis or catabolized in glycogenolysis. Glucose catabolism occurs by cleavage to pyruvate or lactate (pyruvic acid pathway) or by decarboxylation to pentoses (pentose shunt) (Fig. 2-26).

Excess glucose from overfeeding, as reflected by RQs >1.0, can result in conditions such as glucosuria, thermogenesis, and conversion to fat (lipogenesis). Excessive glucose administration results in elevated carbon dioxide production, which may be deleterious in patients with suboptimal pulmonary function, as well as hyperglycemia, which may contribute to infectious risk and immune suppression.

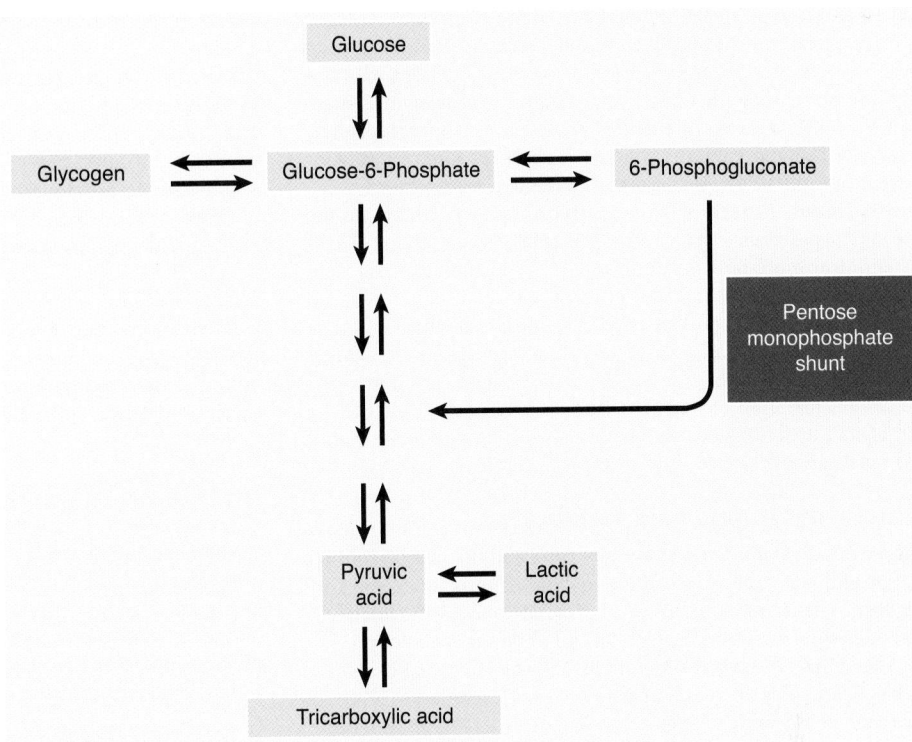

FIG. 2-26. Simplified schema of glucose catabolism through the pentose monophosphate pathway or by breakdown into pyruvate. Glucose-6-phosphate becomes an important "crossroad" for glucose metabolism.

Injury and severe infections acutely induce a state of peripheral glucose intolerance, despite ample insulin production at levels severalfold above baseline. This may occur in part due to reduced skeletal muscle pyruvate dehydrogenase activity after injury, which diminishes the conversion of pyruvate to acetyl-CoA and subsequent entry into the TCA cycle. The three-carbon structures (e.g., pyruvate and lactate) that consequently accumulate are shunted to the liver as substrate for gluconeogenesis. Furthermore, regional tissue catheterization and isotope dilution studies have shown an increase in net splanchnic glucose production by 50 to 60% in septic patients and a 50 to 100% increase in burn patients.[59] The increase in plasma glucose levels is proportional to the severity of injury, and this net hepatic gluconeogenic response is believed to be under the influence of glucagon. Unlike in the nonstressed subject, in the hypermetabolic, critically ill patient the hepatic gluconeogenic response to injury or sepsis cannot be suppressed by exogenous or excess glucose administration but rather persists. Hepatic gluconeogenesis, arising primarily from alanine and glutamine catabolism, provides a ready fuel source for tissues such as those of the nervous system, wounds, and erythrocytes, which do not require insulin for glucose transport. The elevated glucose concentrations also provide a necessary energy source for leukocytes in inflamed tissues and in sites of microbial invasions.

The shunting of glucose away from nonessential organs such as skeletal muscle and adipose tissues is mediated by catecholamines. Experiments with infusing catecholamines and glucagon in animals have demonstrated elevated plasma glucose levels as a result of increased hepatic gluconeogenesis and peripheral insulin resistance. Interestingly, although glucocorticoid infusion alone does not increase glucose levels, it does prolong and augment the hyperglycemic effects of catecholamines and glucagon when glucocorticoid is administered concurrently with the latter.

Glycogen stores within skeletal muscles can be mobilized by epinephrine activation of beta–adrenergic receptors, GTP-binding proteins (G-proteins), which subsequently activates the second messenger, cAMP. The cAMP activates phosphorylase kinase, which in turn leads to conversion of glycogen to glucose-1-phosphate. Phosphorylase kinase also can be activated by the second messenger, calcium, through the breakdown of phosphatidylinosi-

tol phosphate, which is the case in vasopressin-mediated hepatic glycogenolysis.[60]

Glucose Transport and Signaling

Hydrophobic cell membranes are relatively impermeable to hydrophilic glucose molecules. There are two distinct classes of membrane glucose transporters in human systems. These are the facilitated diffusion glucose transporters (GLUTs) that permit the transport of glucose down a concentration gradient (Table 2-7) and the Na^+/glucose secondary active transport system (SGLT), which transports glucose molecules against concentration gradients by active transport.

Five functional human GLUTs have been cloned since 1985. GLUT1 is the transporter in human erythrocytes. It is expressed on several other tissues, but little is found in the liver and skeletal muscle. Importantly, it is a constitutive part of the endothelium in the blood-brain barrier. GLUT2 is predominantly expressed in the sinusoidal membranes of liver, renal tubules, enterocytes, and insulin-secreting β-cells of the pancreas. GLUT2 is important for rapid export of glucose resulting from gluconeogenesis. GLUT3 is highly expressed in neuronal tissue of the brain, the kidney, and placenta, but GLUT3 mRNA has been detected in almost every human tissue. GLUT4 is significant to human metabolism because it is the primary glucose transporter of insulin-sensitive tissues, adipose tissue, and

TABLE 2-7	Human facilitated diffusion glucose transporter (GLUT) family	
Type	**Amino Acids**	**Major Expression Sites**
GLUT1	492	Placenta, brain, kidney, colon
GLUT2	524	Liver, pancreatic β-cells, kidney, small intestine
GLUT3	496	Brain, testis
GLUT4	509	Skeletal muscle, heart muscle, brown and white fat
GLUT5	501	Small intestine, sperm

skeletal and cardiac muscle. These transporters are usually packaged as intracellular vesicles, but insulin induces rapid translocation of these vesicles to the cell surface. GLUT4 function has important implications in the physiology of patients with insulin-resistant diabetes. GLUT5 has been identified in several tissues but is primarily expressed in the jejunum. Although it possesses some capacity for glucose transport, it is predominantly a fructose transporter.[61]

SGLTs are distinct glucose transport systems found in the intestinal epithelium and in the proximal renal tubules. These systems transport both sodium and glucose intracellularly, and glucose affinity for this transporter increases when sodium ions are attached. SGLT1 is prevalent on brush borders of small intestine enterocytes and primarily mediates the active uptake of luminal glucose. In addition, SGLT1 within the intestinal lumen also enhances gut retention of water through osmotic absorption. SGLT1 and SGLT2 are both associated with glucose reabsorption at proximal renal tubules.

Protein and Amino Acid Metabolism

The average protein intake in healthy young adults ranges from 80 to 120 g/d, and every 6 g of protein yields approximately 1 g of nitrogen. The degradation of 1 g of protein yields approximately 4 kcal of energy, similar to the yield in carbohydrate metabolism.

After injury the initial systemic proteolysis, mediated primarily by glucocorticoids, increases urinary nitrogen excretion to levels in excess of 30 g/d, which roughly corresponds to a loss in lean body mass of 1.5% per day. An injured individual who does not receive nutrition for 10 days can theoretically lose 15% lean body mass. Therefore, amino acids cannot be considered a long-term fuel reserve, and indeed excessive protein depletion (i.e., 25 to 30% of lean body weight) is not compatible with sustaining life.[62]

Protein catabolism after injury provides substrates for gluconeogenesis and for the synthesis of acute phase proteins. Radiolabeled amino acid incorporation studies and protein analyses confirm that skeletal muscles are preferentially depleted acutely after injury, whereas visceral tissues (e.g., the liver and kidney) remain relatively preserved. The accelerated urea excretion after injury also is associated with the excretion of intracellular elements such as sulfur, phosphorus, potassium, magnesium, and creatinine. Conversely, the rapid utilization of elements such as potassium and magnesium

during recovery from major injury may indicate a period of tissue healing.

The net changes in protein catabolism and synthesis correspond to the severity and duration of injury (Fig. 2-27). Elective operations and minor injuries result in lower protein synthesis and moderate protein breakdown. Severe trauma, burns, and sepsis are associated with increased protein catabolism. The rise in urinary nitrogen and negative nitrogen balance can be detected early after injury and peak by 7 days. This state of protein catabolism may persist for as long as 3 to 7 weeks. The patient's prior physical status and age appear to influence the degree of proteolysis after injury or sepsis.

Activation of the ubiquitin-proteosome system in muscle cells is one of the major pathways for protein degradation during acute injury. This response is accentuated by tissue hypoxia, acidosis, insulin resistance, and elevated glucocorticoid levels.

NUTRITION IN THE SURGICAL PATIENT

The goal of nutritional support in the surgical patient is to prevent or reverse the catabolic effects of disease or injury. Although several important biologic parameters have been used to measure the efficacy of nutritional regimens, the ultimate validation for nutritional support in surgical patients should be improvement in clinical outcome and restoration of function.

Estimation of Energy Requirements

Overall nutritional assessment is undertaken to determine the severity of nutrient deficiencies or excess and to aid in predicting nutritional requirements. Pertinent information is obtained by determining the presence of weight loss, chronic illnesses, or dietary habits that influence the quantity and quality of food intake. Social habits predisposing to malnutrition and the use of medications that may influence food intake or urination should also be investigated. Physical examination seeks to assess loss of muscle and adipose tissues, organ dysfunction, and subtle changes in skin, hair, or neuromuscular function reflecting frank or impending nutritional deficiency. Anthropometric data (i.e., weight change, skinfold thickness, and arm circumference muscle area) and biochemical determinations (i.e., creatinine excretion, albumin level, prealbumin level, total lym-

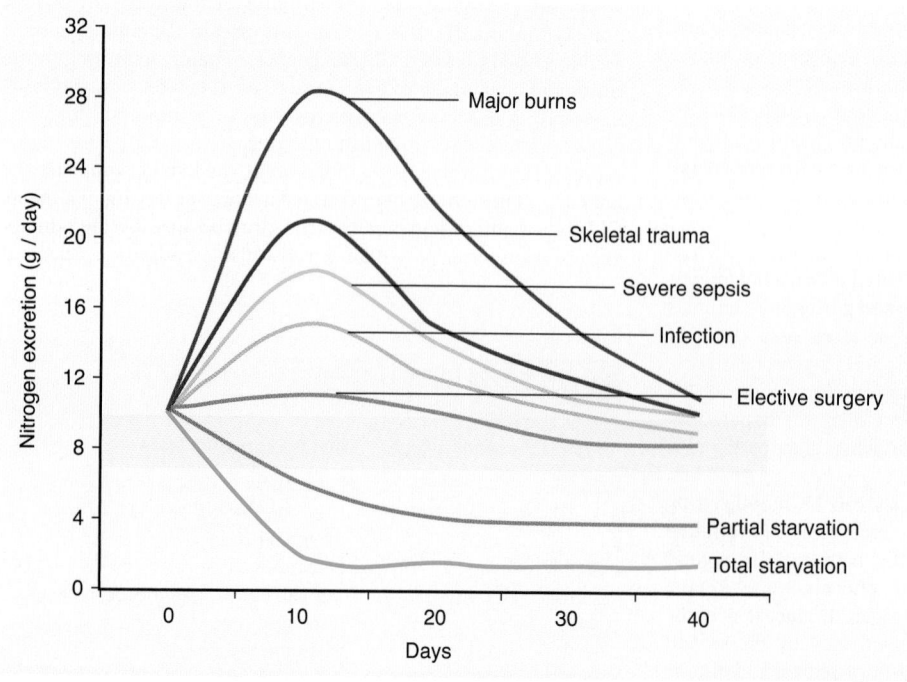

FIG. 2-27. The effect of injury severity on nitrogen wasting. (*Adapted with permission from Long CL et al: Metabolic response to injury and illness: Estimation of energy and protein needs from indirect calorimetry and nitrogen balance. JPEN J Parenter Enteral Nutr 3:452, 1979.*)

phocyte count, and transferrin level) may be used to substantiate the patient's history and physical findings. It is imprecise to rely on any single or fixed combination of the aforementioned findings to accurately assess nutritional status or morbidity. Appreciation for the stresses and natural history of the disease process, in combination with nutritional assessment, remains the basis for identifying patients in acute or anticipated need of nutritional support.

A fundamental goal of nutritional support is to meet the energy requirements for metabolic processes, core temperature maintenance, and tissue repair. Failure to provide adequate nonprotein energy sources will lead to consumption of lean tissue stores. The requirement for energy may be measured by indirect calorimetry and trends in serum markers (e.g., prealbumin level) and estimated from urinary nitrogen excretion, which is proportional to resting energy expenditure.[60] However, the use of indirect calorimetry, particularly in the critically ill patient, is labor intensive and often leads to overestimation of caloric requirements.

Basal energy expenditure (BEE) may also be estimated using the Harris-Benedict equations:

$$\text{BEE (men)} = 66.47 + 13.75\ (W) + 5.0\ (H) - 6.76\ (A)\ \text{kcal/d}$$

$$\text{BEE (women)} = 655.1 + 9.56\ (W) + 1.85\ (H) - 4.68\ (A)\ \text{kcal/d}$$

where W = weight in kilograms; H = height in centimeters; and A = age in years.

These equations, adjusted for the type of surgical stress, are suitable for estimating energy requirements in the majority of hospitalized patients. It has been demonstrated that the provision of 30 kcal/kg per day will adequately meet energy requirements in most postsurgical patients, with a low risk of overfeeding. After trauma or sepsis, energy substrate demands are increased, necessitating greater nonprotein calories beyond calculated energy expenditure (Table 2-8). These additional nonprotein calories provided after injury are usually 1.2 to 2.0 times greater than calculated resting energy expenditure, depending on the type of injury. It is seldom appropriate to exceed this level of nonprotein energy intake during the height of the catabolic phase.

The second objective of nutritional support is to meet the substrate requirements for protein synthesis. An appropriate nonprotein-calorie:nitrogen ratio of 150:1 (e.g., 1 g N = 6.25 g protein) should be maintained, which is the basal calorie requirement provided to limit the use of protein as an energy source. There is now greater evidence suggesting that increased protein intake, and a lower calorie:nitrogen ratio of 80:1 to 100:1, may benefit healing in selected hypermetabolic or critically ill patients. In the absence of severe renal or hepatic dysfunction precluding the use of standard nutritional regimens, approximately 0.25 to 0.35 g of nitrogen per kilogram of body weight should be provided daily.[64]

Vitamins and Minerals

The requirements for vitamins and essential trace minerals usually can be met easily in the average patient with an uncomplicated postoperative course. Therefore, vitamins usually are not given in the absence of preoperative deficiencies. Patients maintained on elemen-

tal diets or parenteral hyperalimentation require complete vitamin and mineral supplementation. Commercial enteral diets contain varying amounts of essential minerals and vitamins. It is necessary to ensure that adequate replacement is available in the diet or by supplementation. Numerous commercial vitamin preparations are available for intravenous or intramuscular use, although most do not contain vitamin K and some do not contain vitamin B_{12} or folic acid. Supplemental trace minerals may be given intravenously via commercial preparations. Essential fatty acid supplementation also may be necessary, especially in patients with depletion of adipose stores.

Overfeeding

Overfeeding usually results from overestimation of caloric needs, as occurs when actual body weight is used to calculate the BEE in patient populations such as the critically ill with significant fluid overload and the obese. Indirect calorimetry can be used to quantify energy requirements but frequently overestimates BEE by 10 to 15% in stressed patients, particularly if they are receiving ventilatory support. In these instances, estimated dry weight should be obtained from preinjury records or family members. Adjusted lean body weight also can be calculated. Overfeeding may contribute to clinical deterioration via increased oxygen consumption, increased carbon dioxide production and prolonged need for ventilatory support, fatty liver, suppression of leukocyte function, hyperglycemia, and increased risk of infection.

ENTERAL NUTRITION

Rationale for Enteral Nutrition

Enteral nutrition generally is preferred over parenteral nutrition based on the lower cost of enteral feeding and the associated risks of the intravenous route, including vascular access complications.[65] Laboratory models have long demonstrated that luminal nutrient contact reduces intestinal mucosal atrophy compared with parenteral or no nutritional support. Studies comparing postoperative enteral and parenteral nutrition in patients undergoing gastrointestinal surgery have demonstrated reduced infectious complications and acute phase protein production in those fed by the enteral route. Yet prospectively randomized studies of patients with adequate nutritional status (albumin ≥4 g/dL) undergoing gastrointestinal surgery demonstrate no differences in outcome and complications between those administered enteral nutrition and those given maintenance intravenous fluids alone in the initial days after surgery.[66] Furthermore, intestinal permeability studies in well-nourished patients undergoing upper gastrointestinal cancer surgery demonstrated normalization of intestinal permeability and barrier function by the fifth postoperative day.[67] At the other extreme, meta-analysis of studies involving critically ill patients demonstrates a 44% reduction in infectious complications in those receiving enteral nutritional support compared with those receiving parenteral nutrition. Most prospectively randomized studies in patients with severe abdominal and thoracic trauma demonstrate significant reductions in infectious

TABLE 2-8	Caloric adjustments above basal energy expenditure (BEE) in hypermetabolic conditions			
Condition	**kcal/kg per Day**	**Adjustment above BEE**	**Grams of Protein/kg per Day**	**Nonprotein Calories: Nitrogen**
Normal/moderate malnutrition	25–30	1.1	1.0	150:1
Mild stress	25–30	1.2	1.2	150:1
Moderate stress	30	1.4	1.5	120:1
Severe stress	30–35	1.6	2.0	90–120:1
Burns	35–40	2.0	2.5	90–100:1

complications in patients given early enteral nutrition compared with those who were unfed or received parenteral nutrition. The exception has been in studies of patients with closed-head injury, in which no significant differences in outcome were demonstrated between early jejunal feeding and other nutritional support modalities. Moreover, early gastric feeding after closed-head injury was frequently associated with underfeeding and calorie deficiency due to the difficulties in overcoming gastroparesis and the high risk of aspiration.

The early initiation of enteral feeding in burn patients, while sensible and supported by retrospective analysis, is an empiric practice supported by limited prospective trials.

Recommendations for instituting early enteral nutrition in surgical patients with moderate malnutrition (albumin level of 2.9 to 3.5 g/dL) can only be made by inference due to a lack of data directly pertaining to this population. For these patients, it is prudent to offer enteral nutrition based on measured energy expenditure of the recovering patient, or if complications arise that may alter the anticipated course of recovery (e.g., anastomotic leaks, return to surgery, sepsis, or failure to wean from the ventilator). Other clinical scenarios for which the benefits of enteral nutritional support have been substantiated include permanent neurologic impairment, oropharyngeal dysfunction, short-bowel syndrome, and bone marrow transplantation.

Collectively, the data support the use of early enteral nutritional support after major trauma and in patients who are anticipated to have prolonged recovery after surgery. Healthy patients without malnutrition undergoing uncomplicated surgery can tolerate 10 days of partial starvation (i.e., maintenance intravenous fluids only) before any clinically significant protein catabolism occurs. Earlier intervention is likely indicated in patients with poorer preoperative nutritional reserves.

Initiation of enteral nutrition should occur immediately after adequate resuscitation, most readily determined by adequate urine output. The presence of bowel sounds and the passage of flatus or stool are not absolute prerequisites for initiation of enteral nutrition, but in the setting of gastroparesis feedings should be administered distal to the pylorus. Gastric residuals of 200 mL or more in a 4- to 6-hour period or abdominal distention requires cessation of feeding and adjustment of the infusion rate. Concomitant gastric decompression with distal small-bowel feedings may be appropriate in certain patients such as closed-head injury patients with gastroparesis. There is no evidence to support withholding enteric feedings for patients after bowel resection or for those with low-output enterocutaneous fistulas of <500 mL/d, but low-residue formulations may be preferred. Enteral feeding should also be offered to patients with short-bowel syndrome or clinical malabsorption, but necessary calories, essential minerals, and vitamins should be supplemented using parenteral modalities.

Enteral Formulas

The functional status of the gastrointestinal tract determines the type of enteral solutions to be used. Patients with an intact gastrointestinal tract will tolerate complex solutions, but patients who have not been fed via the gastrointestinal tract for prolonged periods are less likely to tolerate complex carbohydrates such as lactose. In patients with malabsorption, such as in inflammatory bowel diseases, absorption may be improved by provision of dipeptides, tripeptides, and MCTs. However, MCTs are deficient in essential fatty acids, which necessitates supplementation with some LCTs.

Factors that influence the choice of enteral formula include the extent of organ dysfunction (e.g., renal, pulmonary, hepatic, or gastrointestinal), the nutrients needed to restore optimal function and healing, and the cost of specific products. There are still no conclusive data to recommend one category of product over another, and nutritional support committees typically develop the most cost-efficient enteral formulary for the most commonly encountered disease categories within the institution.

Low-Residue Isotonic Formulas

Most low-residue isotonic formulas provide a caloric density of 1.0 kcal/mL, and approximately 1500 to 1800 mL are required to meet daily requirements. These low-osmolarity compositions provide baseline carbohydrates, protein, electrolytes, water, fat, and fat-soluble vitamins (some do not have vitamin K) and typically have a nonprotein-calorie:nitrogen ratio of 150:1. These contain no fiber bulk and therefore leave minimum residue. These solutions usually are considered to be the standard or first-line formulas for stable patients with an intact gastrointestinal tract.

Isotonic Formulas with Fiber

Isotonic formulas with fiber contain soluble and insoluble fiber, which is most often soy based. Physiologically, fiber-based solutions delay intestinal transit time and may reduce the incidence of diarrhea compared with nonfiber solutions. Fiber stimulates pancreatic lipase activity and is degraded by gut bacteria into short-chain fatty acids, an important fuel for colonocytes. There are no contraindications for using fiber-containing formulas in critically ill patients.

Immune-Enhancing Formulas

Immune-enhancing formulas are fortified with special nutrients that are purported to enhance various aspects of immune or solid organ function. Such additives include glutamine, arginine, branched-chain amino acids, omega-3 fatty acids, nucleotides, and beta carotene.[68] Although several trials have proposed that one or more of these additives reduce surgical complications and improve outcome, these results have not been uniformly corroborated by other trials.[69] The addition of amino acids to these formulas generally doubles the amount of protein (nitrogen) found in standard formula; however, their cost can be prohibitive.[70]

Calorie-Dense Formulas

The primary distinction of calorie-dense formulas is a greater caloric value for the same volume. Most commercial products of this variety provide 1.5 to 2 kcal/mL and therefore are suitable for patients requiring fluid restriction or those unable to tolerate large-volume infusions. As expected, these solutions have higher osmolality than standard formulas and are suitable for intragastric feedings.

High-Protein Formulas

High-protein formulas are available in isotonic and nonisotonic mixtures and are proposed for critically ill or trauma patients with high protein requirements. These formulas have nonprotein-calorie:nitrogen ratios between 80:1 and 120:1.

Elemental Formulas

Elemental formulas contain predigested nutrients and provide proteins in the form of small peptides. Complex carbohydrates are limited, and fat content, in the form of MCTs and LCTs, is minimal. The primary advantage of such a formula is ease of absorption, but the inherent scarcity of fat, associated vitamins, and trace elements limits its long-term use as a primary source of nutrients. Due to its high osmolarity, dilution or slow infusion rates usually are necessary, particularly in critically ill patients. These formulas have been used frequently in patients with malabsorption, gut impairment, and pancreatitis, but their cost is significantly higher than that of standard formulas.

Renal-Failure Formulas

The primary benefits of renal formulas are the lower fluid volume and concentrations of potassium, phosphorus, and magnesium needed to meet daily calorie requirements. This type of formulation almost exclusively contains essential amino acids and has a high nonprotein-calorie:nitrogen ratio; however, it does not contain trace elements or vitamins.

Pulmonary-Failure Formulas

In pulmonary-failure formulas, fat content is usually increased to 50% of the total calories, with a corresponding reduction in carbohydrate content. The goal is to reduce carbon dioxide production and alleviate ventilation burden for failing lungs.

Hepatic-Failure Formulas

Close to 50% of the proteins in hepatic-failure formulas are branched-chain amino acids (e.g., leucine, isoleucine, and valine). The goal of such a formula is to reduce aromatic amino acid levels and increase the levels of branched-chain amino acids, which can potentially reverse encephalopathy in patients with hepatic failure.[71] The use of these formulas is controversial, however, because no clear benefits have been proven by clinical trials. Protein restriction should be avoided in patients with end-stage liver disease, because such patients have significant protein energy malnutrition that predisposed them to additional morbidity and mortality.[72]

ACCESS FOR ENTERAL NUTRITIONAL SUPPORT

The available techniques and repertoire for enteral access have provided multiple options for feeding the gut. Presently used methods and preferred indications are summarized in Table 2-9.[73]

Nasoenteric Tubes

Nasogastric feeding should be reserved for those with intact mentation and protective laryngeal reflexes to minimize risks of aspiration. Even in intubated patients, nasogastric feedings often can be recovered from tracheal suction. Nasojejunal feedings are associated with fewer pulmonary complications, but access past the pylorus requires greater effort to accomplish. Blind insertion of nasogastric feeding tubes is fraught with misplacement, and air instillation with auscultation is inaccurate for ascertaining proper positioning. Radiographic confirmation is usually required to verify the position of the nasogastric feeding tube.

Several methods have been recommended for the passage of nasoenteric feeding tubes into the small bowel, including use of prokinetic agents, right lateral decubitus positioning, gastric insufflation, tube angulation, and application of clockwise torque. However, the successful placement of feeding tubes by these methods is highly variable and operator dependent. Furthermore, it is time consuming, and success rates for intubation past the duodenum into the jejunum by these methods are <20%. Fluoroscopy-guided intubation past the pylorus has a >90% success rate, and more than half of these intubations result in jejunal placement. Similarly, endoscopy-guided placement past the pylorus has high success rates, but attempts to advance the tube beyond the second portion of the duodenum using a standard gastroduodenoscope is unlikely to be successful.

Small-bowel feeding is more reliable for delivering nutrition than nasogastric feeding. Furthermore, the risks of aspiration pneumonia can be reduced by 25% with small-bowel feeding compared with nasogastric feeding. The disadvantages of the use of nasoenteric feeding tubes are clogging, kinking, and inadvertent displacement or removal of the tube, and nasopharyngeal complications. If nasoenteric feeding will be required for longer than 30 days, access should be converted to a percutaneous one.[74]

Percutaneous Endoscopic Gastrostomy

The most common indications for percutaneous endoscopic gastrostomy (PEG) include impaired swallowing mechanisms, oropharyngeal or esophageal obstruction, and major facial trauma. It is frequently used for debilitated patients requiring caloric supplementation, hydration, or frequent medication dosing. It is also appropriate for patients requiring passive gastric decompression. Relative contraindications for PEG placement include ascites, coagulopathy, gastric varices, gastric neoplasm, and lack of a suitable abdominal site. Most tubes are 18F to 28F in size and may be used for 12 to 24 months.

Identification of the PEG site requires endoscopic transillumination of the anterior stomach against the abdominal wall. A 14-gauge angiocatheter is passed through the abdominal wall into the fully insufflated stomach. A guidewire is threaded through the angiocatheter, grasped by snares or forceps, and pulled out through the mouth. The tapered end of the PEG tube is secured to the guidewire and is pulled into position out of the abdominal wall. The PEG tube is secured without tension against the abdominal wall, and many have reported using the tube within hours of placement. It has been the practice of some to connect the PEG tube to a drainage bag for passive decompression for 24 hours before use, allowing more time for the stomach to seal against the peritoneum.

If endoscopy is not available or technical obstacles preclude PEG placement, the interventional radiologist can attempt the procedure percutaneously under fluoroscopic guidance by first insufflating the stomach against the abdominal wall with a nasogastric tube. If this also is unsuccessful, surgical gastrostomy tube placement can be considered, particularly with minimally invasive methods. When surgery is contemplated, it may be wise to consider directly accessing the small bowel for nutrition delivery.

Although PEG tubes enhance nutritional delivery, facilitate nursing care, and are superior to nasogastric tubes, serious complications occur in approximately 3% of patients. These complications include wound infection, necrotizing fasciitis, peritonitis, aspiration, leaks, dislodgment, bowel perforation, enteric fistulas, bleeding, and aspiration pneumonia.[75] For patients with significant gastroparesis or gastric outlet obstruction, feedings through PEG tubes are hazardous. In such cases, the PEG tube can be used for

TABLE 2-9	Options for enteral feeding access
Access Option	**Comments**
Nasogastric tube	Short-term use only; aspiration risks; nasopharyngeal trauma; frequent dislodgment
Nasoduodenal/ nasojejunal tube	Short-term use; lower aspiration risks in jejunum; placement challenges (radiographic assistance often necessary)
Percutaneous endoscopic gastrostomy (PEG)	Endoscopy skills required; may be used for gastric decompression or bolus feeds; aspiration risks; can last 12–24 mo; slightly higher complication rates with placement and site leaks
Surgical gastrostomy	Requires general anesthesia and small laparotomy; procedure may allow placement of extended duodenal/jejunal feeding ports; laparoscopic placement possible
Fluoroscopic gastrostomy	Blind placement using needle and T-prongs to anchor to stomach; can thread smaller catheter through gastrostomy into duodenum/ jejunum under fluoroscopy
PEG-jejunal tube	Jejunal placement with regular endoscope is operator dependent; jejunal tube often dislodges retrograde; two-stage procedure with PEG placement, followed by fluoroscopic conversion with jejunal feeding tube through PEG
Direct percutaneous endoscopic jejunostomy (DPEJ)	Direct endoscopic tube placement with enteroscope; placement challenges; greater injury risks
Surgical jejunostomy	Commonly carried out during laparotomy; general anesthesia; laparoscopic placement usually requires assistant to thread catheter; laparoscopy offers direct visualization of catheter placement
Fluoroscopic jejunostomy	Difficult approach with injury risks; not commonly done

decompression and allow access for converting the PEG tube to a transpyloric feeding tube.

Percutaneous Endoscopic Gastrostomy-Jejunostomy and Direct Percutaneous Endoscopic Jejunostomy

Although gastric bolus feedings are more physiologic, patients who cannot tolerate gastric feedings or who have significant aspiration risks should be fed directly past the pylorus. In the percutaneous endoscopic gastrostomy-jejunostomy (PEG-J) method, a 9F to 12F tube is passed through an existing PEG tube, past the pylorus, and into the duodenum. This can be achieved by endoscopic or fluoroscopic guidance. With weighted catheter tips and guidewires, the tube can be further advanced past the ligament of Treitz. However, the incidence of long-term PEG-J tube malfunction has been reported to be >50% as a result of retrograde tube migration into the stomach, kinking, or clogging.

Direct percutaneous endoscopic jejunostomy (DPEJ) tube placement uses the same techniques as PEG tube placement but requires an enteroscope or colonoscope to reach the jejunum. DPEJ tube malfunctions are probably less frequent than PEG-J tube malfunctions, and kinking or clogging is usually averted by placement of larger-caliber catheters. The success rate of DPEJ tube placement is variable because of the complexity of endoscopic skills required to locate a suitable jejunal site. In such cases where endoscopic means are not feasible, surgical jejunostomy tube placement is more appropriate, especially when minimally invasive techniques are available.

Surgical Gastrostomy and Jejunostomy

For a patient undergoing complex abdominal or trauma surgery, thought should be given during surgery to the possible routes for subsequent nutritional support, because laparotomy affords direct access to the stomach or small bowel. The only absolute contraindication to feeding jejunostomy is distal intestinal obstruction. Relative contraindications include severe edema of the intestinal wall, radiation enteritis, inflammatory bowel disease, ascites, severe immunodeficiency, and bowel ischemia. Needle-catheter jejunostomies also can be done with a minimal learning curve. The biggest drawback usually is possible clogging and knotting of the 6F catheter.[76]

Abdominal distention and cramps are common adverse effects of early enteral nutrition. Some have also reported impaired respiratory mechanics as a result of intolerance to enteral feedings. These are mostly correctable by temporarily discontinuing feedings and resuming at a lower infusion rate.

Pneumatosis intestinalis and small-bowel necrosis are infrequent but significant problems in patients receiving jejunal tube feedings. Several contributing factors have been proposed, including the hyper-osmolarity of enteral solutions, bacterial overgrowth, fermentation, and accumulation of metabolic breakdown products. The common pathophysiology is believed to be bowel distention and consequent reduction in bowel wall perfusion. Risk factors for these complications include cardiogenic and circulatory shock, vasopressor use, diabetes mellitus, and chronic obstructive pulmonary disease. Therefore, enteral feedings in the critically ill patient should be delayed until adequate resuscitation has been achieved. As alternatives, diluting standard enteral formula, delaying the progression to goal infusion rates, or using monomeric solutions with low osmolality requiring less digestion by the gastrointestinal tract all have been successfully used.

PARENTERAL NUTRITION

Parenteral nutrition is the continuous infusion of a hyperosmolar solution containing carbohydrates, proteins, fat, and other necessary nutrients through an indwelling catheter inserted into the superior vena cava. To obtain the maximum benefit, the calorie:protein ratio must be adequate (at least 100 to 150 kcal/g nitrogen), and both carbohydrates and proteins must be infused simultaneously. When the sources of calories and nitrogen are given at different times, there is a significant decrease in nitrogen utilization. These nutrients can be given in quantities considerably greater than the basic caloric and nitrogen requirements, and this method has proved to be highly successful in achieving growth and development, positive nitrogen balance, and weight gain in a variety of clinical situations. Clinical trials and meta-analysis of studies of parenteral feeding in the perioperative period have suggested that preoperative nutritional support may benefit some surgical patients, particularly those with extensive malnutrition. Short-term use of parenteral nutrition in critically ill patients (i.e., duration of <7 days) when enteral nutrition may have been instituted is associated with higher rates of infectious complications. After severe injury, parenteral nutrition is associated with higher rates of infectious risks than is enteral feeding (Table 2-10). Clinical studies have demonstrated that parenteral feeding with complete bowel rest results in augmented stress hormone and inflammatory mediator response to an antigenic challenge. However, parenteral feeding still is associated with fewer infectious complications than no feeding at all. In cancer patients, delivery of parenteral nutrition has not been shown to benefit clinical response, prolong survival, or ameliorate the toxic effects of chemotherapy, and infectious complications are increased.

Rationale for Parenteral Nutrition

The principal indications for parenteral nutrition are malnutrition, sepsis, or surgical or traumatic injury in seriously ill patients for whom use of the gastrointestinal tract for feedings is not possible. In

	Blunt Trauma		Penetrating Trauma		Total	
	TEN	**TPN**	**TEN**	**TPN**	**TEN**	**TPN**
Complication	**n = 48**	**n = 44**	**n = 38**	**n = 48**	**n = 44**	**n = 84**
Abdominal abscess	2	1	2	6	4	7
Pneumonia	4	10	1	2	5	12
Wound infection	0	2	3	1	3	3
Bacteremia	1	4	0	1	1	5
Urinary tract	1	1	0	1	1	2
Other	5	4	1	1	6	5
Total complications	**13**	**22**	**7**	**12**	**20**	**34**
% Complications per patient group	**27%**	**50%**	**18%**	**30%**	**23%**	**39%**

TABLE 2-10 Incidence of septic morbidity in parenterally and enterally fed trauma patients

TEN = total enteral nutrition; TPN = total parenteral nutrition.
Source: Reproduced with permission from Moore FA, Feliciano DV, Andrassy RJ et al: Early enteral feeding, compared with parenteral, reduces postoperative septic complications. *Ann Surg* 216(2):172–183, 1992.

some instances, intravenous nutrition may be used to supplement inadequate oral intake. The safe and successful use of parenteral nutrition requires proper selection of patients with specific nutritional needs, experience with the technique, and an awareness of the associated complications. As with enteral nutrition, the fundamental goals are to provide sufficient calories and nitrogen substrate to promote tissue repair and to maintain the integrity or growth of lean tissue mass. The following are patient groups for whom parenteral nutrition has been used in an effort to achieve these goals:

1. Newborn infants with catastrophic gastrointestinal anomalies, such as tracheoesophageal fistula, gastroschisis, omphalocele, or massive intestinal atresia
2. Infants who fail to thrive due to gastrointestinal insufficiency associated with short-bowel syndrome, malabsorption, enzyme deficiency, meconium ileus, or idiopathic diarrhea
3. Adult patients with short-bowel syndrome secondary to massive small-bowel resection (<100 cm without colon or ileocecal valve, or <50 cm with intact ileocecal valve and colon)
4. Patients with enteroenteric, enterocolic, enterovesical, or high-output enterocutaneous fistulas (>500 mL/d)
5. Surgical patients with prolonged paralytic ileus after major operations (>7 to 10 days), multiple injuries, or blunt or open abdominal trauma, or patients with reflex ileus complicating various medical diseases
6. Patients with normal bowel length but with malabsorption secondary to sprue, hypoproteinemia, enzyme or pancreatic insufficiency, regional enteritis, or ulcerative colitis
7. Adult patients with functional gastrointestinal disorders such as esophageal dyskinesia after cerebrovascular accident, idiopathic diarrhea, psychogenic vomiting, or anorexia nervosa
8. Patients with granulomatous colitis, ulcerative colitis, or tuberculous enteritis in which major portions of the absorptive mucosa are diseased
9. Patients with malignancy, with or without cachexia, in whom malnutrition might jeopardize successful use of a therapeutic option
10. Patients in whom attempts to provide adequate calories by enteral tube feedings or high residuals have failed
11. Critically ill patients who are hypermetabolic for >5 days or for whom enteral nutrition is not feasible

Patients in whom hyperalimentation is *contraindicated* include the following:

1. Patients for whom a specific goal for patient management is lacking or for whom, instead of extending a meaningful life, inevitable dying would be delayed
2. Patients experiencing hemodynamic instability or severe metabolic derangement (e.g., severe hyperglycemia, azotemia, encephalopathy, hyperosmolality, and fluid-electrolyte disturbances) requiring control or correction before hypertonic intravenous feeding is attempted
3. Patients for whom gastrointestinal tract feeding is feasible; in the vast majority of instances, this is the best route by which to provide nutrition
4. Patients with good nutritional status
5. Infants with <8 cm of small bowel, because virtually all have been unable to adapt sufficiently despite prolonged periods of parenteral nutrition
6. Patients who are irreversibly decerebrate or otherwise dehumanized

Total Parenteral Nutrition

TPN, also referred to as *central parenteral nutrition,* requires access to a large-diameter vein to deliver the entire nutritional requirements of the individual. Dextrose content of the solution is high (15 to 25%), and all other macronutrients and micronutrients are deliverable by this route.

Peripheral Parenteral Nutrition

The lower osmolarity of the solution used for peripheral parenteral nutrition (PPN), secondary to reduced levels of dextrose (5 to 10%) and protein (3%), allows its administration via peripheral veins. Some nutrients cannot be supplemented because they cannot be concentrated into small volumes. Therefore, PPN is not appropriate for repleting patients with severe malnutrition. It can be considered if central routes are not available or if supplemental nutritional support is required. Typically, PPN is used for short periods (<2 weeks). Beyond this time, TPN should be instituted.

Initiation of Parenteral Nutrition

The basic solution for parenteral nutrition contains a final concentration of 15 to 25% dextrose and 3 to 5% crystalline amino acids. The solutions usually are prepared in sterile conditions in the pharmacy from commercially available kits containing the component solutions and transfer apparatus. Preparation in the pharmacy under laminar flow hoods reduces the incidence of bacterial contamination of the solution. Proper preparation with suitable quality control is absolutely essential to avoid septic complications.

The proper provision of electrolytes and amino acids must take into account routes of fluid and electrolyte loss, renal function, metabolic rate, cardiac function, and the underlying disease state.

Intravenous vitamin preparations also should be added to parenteral formulas. Vitamin deficiencies are rare occurrences if such preparations are used. In addition, because vitamin K is not part of any commercially prepared vitamin solution, it should be supplemented on a weekly basis. During prolonged parenteral nutrition with fat-free solutions, essential fatty acid deficiency may become clinically apparent and manifests as dry, scaly dermatitis and loss of hair. The syndrome may be prevented by periodic infusion of a fat emulsion at a rate equivalent to 10 to 15% of total calories. Essential trace minerals may be required after prolonged TPN and may be supplied by direct addition of commercial preparations. The most frequent presentation of trace mineral deficiencies is the eczematoid rash developing both diffusely and at intertriginous areas in zinc-deficient patients. Other rare trace mineral deficiencies include a microcytic anemia associated with copper deficiency, and glucose intolerance presumably related to chromium deficiency. The latter complications are seldom seen except in patients receiving parenteral nutrition for extended periods. The daily administration of commercially available trace mineral supplements will obviate most such problems.

Depending on fluid and nitrogen tolerance, parenteral nutrition solutions generally can be increased over 2 to 3 days to achieve the desired infusion rate. Insulin may be supplemented as necessary to ensure glucose tolerance. Administration of additional intravenous fluids and electrolytes may occasionally be necessary in patients with persistently high fluid losses. The patient should be carefully monitored for development of electrolyte, volume, acid-base, and septic complications. Vital signs and urinary output should be measured regularly, and the patient should be weighed regularly. Frequent adjustments of the volume and composition of the solutions are necessary during the course of therapy. Samples for measurement of electrolytes are drawn daily until levels are stable and every 2 or 3 days thereafter. Blood counts, blood urea nitrogen level, levels of liver function indicators, and phosphate and magnesium levels are determined at least weekly.

The urine or capillary blood glucose level is checked every 6 hours and serum glucose concentration is checked at least once daily during the first few days of the infusion and at frequent intervals thereafter. Relative glucose intolerance, which often manifests as glycosuria, may occur after initiation of parenteral nutrition. If blood glucose levels remain elevated or glycosuria persists, the dextrose concentration may be decreased, the infusion rate slowed, or regular insulin added to each bottle. The rise in blood glucose concentration observed after initiating parenteral nutrition may be temporary, as the normal pancreas increases its output of insulin in response to the continuous carbohydrate infusion. In patients with diabetes mellitus, additional insulin may be required.

Potassium is essential to achieve positive nitrogen balance and replace depleted intracellular stores. In addition, a significant shift of potassium ion from the extracellular to the intracellular space may take place because of the large glucose infusion, with resultant hypokalemia, metabolic alkalosis, and poor glucose utilization. In some cases as much as 240 mEq of potassium ion daily may be required. Hypokalemia may cause glycosuria, which would be treated with potassium, not insulin. Thus, before giving insulin, the serum potassium level must be checked to avoid exacerbating the hypokalemia.

Patients with insulin-dependent diabetes mellitus may exhibit wide fluctuations in blood glucose levels while receiving parenteral nutrition. This may require protocol-driven intravenous insulin therapy. In addition, partial replacement of dextrose calories with lipid emulsions may alleviate these problems in selected patients.

Lipid emulsions derived from soybean or safflower oils are widely used as an adjunctive nutrient to prevent the development of essential fatty acid deficiency. There is no evidence of enhanced metabolic benefit when >10 to 15% of calories are provided as lipid emulsions. Although the administration of 500 mL of 20% fat emulsion one to three times a week is sufficient to prevent essential fatty acid deficiency, it is common to provide fat emulsions on a daily basis to provide additional calories. The triple mix of carbohydrate, fat, and amino acids is infused at a constant rate during a 24-hour period. The theoretical advantages of a constant fat infusion rate include increased efficiency of lipid utilization and reduction in the impairment of reticuloendothelial function normally identified with bolus lipid infusions. The addition of lipids to an infusion bag may alter the stability of some micronutrients in a dextrose–amino acid preparation.

INTRAVENOUS ACCESS METHODS

Temporary or short-term access can be achieved with a 16-gauge percutaneous catheter inserted into a subclavian or internal jugular vein and threaded into the superior vena cava. More permanent access with the intention of providing long-term or home parenteral nutrition can be achieved by placement of a catheter with a subcutaneous port for access by tunneling a catheter with a substantial subcutaneous length or threading a long catheter through the basilic or cephalic vein into the superior vena cava.

COMPLICATIONS OF PARENTERAL NUTRITION

Technical Complications

One of the more common and serious complications associated with long-term parenteral feeding is sepsis secondary to contamination of the central venous catheter. Contamination of solutions should be considered, but is rare when proper pharmacy protocols have been followed. This problem occurs more frequently in patients with systemic sepsis and in many cases is due to hematogenous seeding of the catheter with bacteria.[77] One of the earliest signs of systemic sepsis may be the sudden development of glucose intolerance (with or without temperature increase) in a patient who previously has been maintained on parenteral alimentation without difficulty. When this occurs, or if high fever (>38.5°C [101.3°F]) develops without obvious cause, a diligent search for a potential septic focus is indicated. Other causes of fever should also be investigated. If fever persists, the infusion catheter should be removed and submitted for culture. If the catheter is the cause of the fever, removal of the infectious source is usually followed by rapid defervescence. Some centers are now replacing catheters considered at low risk for infection over a guidewire. Should evidence of infection persist over 24 to 48 hours without a definable source, the

catheter should be replaced into the opposite subclavian vein or into one of the internal jugular veins and the infusion restarted. It is prudent to delay reinserting the catheter by 12 to 24 hours, especially if bacteremia is present.[78]

Other complications related to catheter placement include the development of pneumothorax, hemothorax, hydrothorax, subclavian artery injury, thoracic duct injury, cardiac arrhythmia, air embolism, catheter embolism, and cardiac perforation with tamponade. All of these complications may be avoided by strict adherence to proper techniques.

The use of multilumen catheters may be associated with a slightly increased risk of infection. This is most likely associated with greater catheter manipulation and intensive use. The rate of catheter infection is highest for those placed in the femoral vein, lower for those in the jugular vein, and lowest for those in the subclavian vein. When catheters are indwelling for <3 days, infection risks are negligible. If indwelling time is 3 to 7 days, the infection risk is 3 to 5%. Indwelling times of >7 days are associated with a catheter infection risk of 5 to 10%. Strict adherence to barrier precautions also reduces the rate of infection.

Metabolic Complications

Hyperglycemia may develop with normal rates of infusion in patients with impaired glucose tolerance or in any patient if the hypertonic solutions are administered too rapidly. This is a particularly common complication in patients with latent diabetes and in patients subjected to severe surgical stress or trauma. Treatment of the condition consists of volume replacement with correction of electrolyte abnormalities and the administration of insulin. This complication can be avoided with careful attention to daily fluid balance and frequent monitoring of blood glucose levels and serum electrolytes.

Increasing experience has emphasized the importance of not overfeeding the parenterally nourished patient. This is particularly true for the depleted patient in whom excess calorie infusion may result in carbon dioxide retention and respiratory insufficiency. In addition, excess feeding also has been related to the development of hepatic steatosis or marked glycogen deposition in selected patients. Cholestasis and formation of gallstones are common in patients receiving long-term parenteral nutrition. Mild but transient abnormalities of serum transaminase, alkaline phosphatase, and bilirubin levels occur in many parenterally nourished patients. Failure of the liver enzymes to plateau or return to normal over 7 to 14 days should suggest another etiology.

Intestinal Atrophy

Lack of intestinal stimulation is associated with intestinal mucosal atrophy, diminished villous height, bacterial overgrowth, reduced lymphoid tissue size, reduced immunoglobulin A production, and impaired gut immunity. The full clinical implications of these changes are not well realized, although bacterial translocation has been demonstrated in animal models. The most efficacious method to prevent these changes is to provide at least some nutrients enterally. In patients requiring TPN, it may be feasible to infuse small amounts of feedings via the gastrointestinal tract.

SPECIAL FORMULATIONS

Glutamine and Arginine

Glutamine is the most abundant amino acid in the human body, comprising nearly two thirds of the free intracellular amino acid pool. Of this, 75% is found within the skeletal muscles. In healthy individuals, glutamine is considered a nonessential amino acid, because it is synthesized within the skeletal muscles and the lungs. Glutamine is a necessary substrate for nucleotide synthesis in most dividing cells and hence provides a major fuel source for entero-

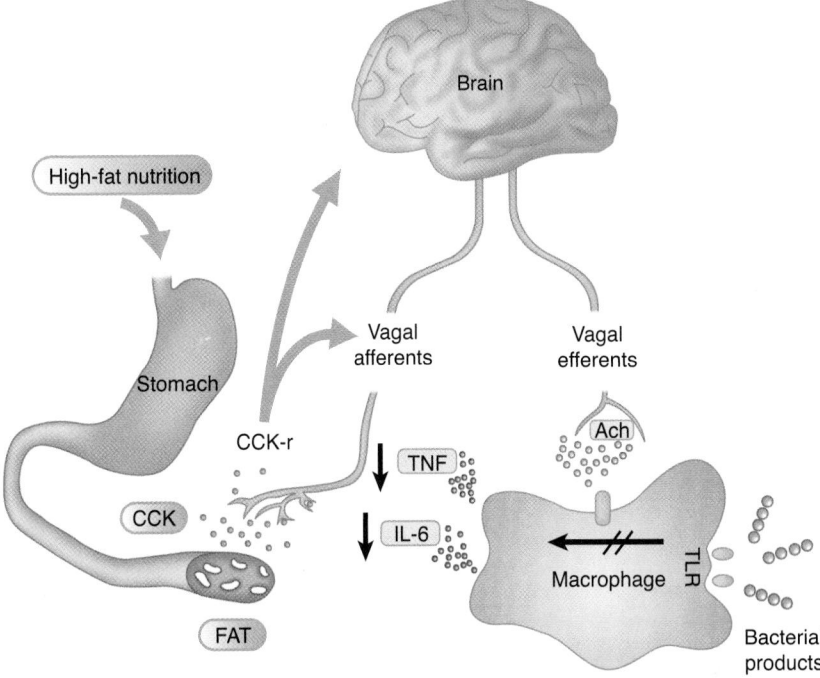

FIG. 2-28. Vagal afferent system senses peripheral inflammatory focus and also responses to intestinal luminal substrates, in this case enteral lipid signaling via cholecystokinin receptors (CCK-r). Efferent vagal signals limit proinflammatory cytokine production via activation of cholinergic nicotinic receptors on visceral immune cells. Clinical conditions that disrupt the integrity of this circuit may enhance inflammatory responses. Ach = acetylcholine; CCK = cholecystokinin; IL-6 = interleukin-6; TLR = toll-like receptor; TNF = tumor necrosis factor. *(Adapted with permission from Luyer MD, et al. Nutritional stimulation of cholecystokinin receptors inhibits inflammation via the vagus nerve.* J Exp Med *202:1023, 2005. By copyright permission of The Rockefeller University Press.)*

cytes. It also serves as an important fuel source for immunocytes such as lymphocytes and macrophages, and is a precursor for glutathione, a major intracellular antioxidant. During stress states such as sepsis, or in tumor-bearing hosts, peripheral glutamine stores are rapidly depleted, and the amino acid is preferentially shunted as a fuel source toward the visceral organs and tumors, respectively. These situations create, at least experimentally, a glutamine-depleted environment, with consequences including enterocyte and immunocyte starvation.

Glutamine metabolism during stress in humans, however, may be more complex than is indicated in previously reported animal data. Advanced methods of detecting glutamine traffic in patients with gastrointestinal cancer have not demonstrated more sequestration of glutamine in tumors than in normal intestine. There are data demonstrating decreased dependency on TPN in severe cases of short-bowel syndrome when glutamine therapy with modified diets and growth hormones are used. However, in patients with milder forms of short-bowel syndrome and better nutritional status, glutamine supplementation did not lead to appreciable enhancement in intestinal absorption. Although it is hypothesized that provision of glutamine may preserve immune cell and enterocyte function and enhance nitrogen balance during injury or sepsis, the clinical evidence in support of these phenomena in human subjects remains inconclusive.[79]

Arginine, also a nonessential amino acid in healthy subjects, first attracted attention for its immunoenhancing properties, wound-healing benefits, and association with improved survival in animal models of sepsis and injury. As with glutamine, the benefits of experimental arginine supplementation during stress states are diverse. In clinical studies involving critically ill and injured patients and patients who have undergone surgery for certain malignancies, enteral administration of arginine has led to net nitrogen retention and protein synthesis, whereas isonitrogenous diets have not. Some of these studies also provide in vitro evidence of enhanced immunocyte function. The clinical utility of arginine supplementation in improving overall patient outcome remains an area of investigation.

Omega-3 Fatty Acids

The provision of omega-3 polyunsaturated fatty acids (canola oil or fish oil) displaces omega-6 fatty acids in cell membranes, which theoretically reduces the proinflammatory response from prostaglandin production.[80]

Nucleotides

RNA supplementation in solutions is purported, at least experimentally, to increase cell proliferation, provide building blocks for DNA synthesis, and improve helper T cell function.

NUTRITION-INDUCED INFLAMMATORY MODULATION

Studies have demonstrated that the mode of nutritional supplementation, either enteral or parenteral, may influence stress-induced inflammatory responses. Intravenously fed subjects demonstrate a heightened response to proinflammatory stimuli such as endotoxin. Enteral feedings have been regarded as the feeding mode of choice when possible, and although advantages have been suggested, including improved GI barrier function, the mechanisms through which enteral feedings mediate efficacious effects have yet to be fully determined.

Providing further insight into the benefit of enteral feedings, Luyer and colleagues have demonstrated that enteral fat maintains both afferent and efferent vagal pathway signaling via intestinal cholecystokinin receptor activation. They observed that consumption of a high-density fat meal before stress induced by hemorrhage resulted in reduced systemic inflammation and improved outcome.[81] Thus, enteral nutrients may act as agonists for endogenous neuroendocrine anti-inflammatory pathways (Fig. 2-28).[82]

REFERENCES

Entries highlighted in bright blue are key references.

1. Bone RC: The pathogenesis of sepsis. *Ann Intern Med* 115:457, 1991.
2. Lowry SF: Human endotoxemia: A model for mechanistic insight and therapeutic targeting. *Shock* 24 Suppl 1:94, 2005.
3. Borovikova LV, Ivanova S, Zhang M, et al: Vagus nerve stimulation attenuates the systemic inflammatory response to endotoxin. *Nature* 405:458, 2000.

4. Czura CJ, Tracey KJ: Autonomic neural regulation of immunity. *J Intern Med* 257:156, 2005.

5. Wang H, Yu M, Ochani M, et al: Nicotinic acetylcholine receptor alpha7 subunit is an essential regulator of inflammation. *Nature* 421:384, 2003.

6. Heitzer MD, Wolf IM, Sanchez ER, et al: Glucocorticoid receptor physiology. *Rev Endocr Metab Disord* 8:321, 2007.

7. Venkataraman S, Munoz R, Candido C, et al: The hypothalamic-pituitary-adrenal axis in critical illness. *Rev Endocr Metab Disord* 8:365, 2007.

8. Dellinger RP, Levy MM, Carlet JM, et al: Surviving Sepsis Campaign: International guidelines for management of severe sepsis and septic shock: 2008. *Crit Care Med* 36:296, 2008.

9. Flaster H, Bernhagen J, Calandra T, et al: The macrophage migration inhibitory factor-glucocorticoid dyad: Regulation of inflammation and immunity. *Mol Endocrinol* 21:1267, 2007.

10. Agnese DM, Calvano JE, Hahm SJ, et al: Insulin-like growth factor binding protein-3 is upregulated in LPS-treated THP-1 cells. *Surg Infect (Larchmt)* 3:119; discussion 25, 2002.

11. Takal J, Ruokonen E, Webster NR et al: Increased mortality associated with growth hormone treatment in critically ill adults. *N Engl J Med* 341(11):785, 1999.

12. van der Poll T, Coyle SM, Barbosa K, et al: Epinephrine inhibits tumor necrosis factor-alpha and potentiates interleukin 10 production during human endotoxemia. *J Clin Invest* 97:713, 1996.

13. Van den Berghe G: How does blood glucose control with insulin save lives in intensive care? *J Clin Invest* 114:1187, 2004.

14. Van den Berghe G, Wouters P, Weekers F, et al: Intensive insulin therapy in the critically ill patients. *N Engl J Med* 345:1359, 2001.

15. Quintana FJ, Cohen IR: Heat shock proteins as endogenous adjuvants in sterile and septic inflammation. *J Immunol* 175:2777, 2005.

16. Crimi E, Sica V, Slutsky AS, et al: Role of oxidative stress in experimental sepsis and multisystem organ dysfunction. *Free Radic Res* 40:665, 2006.

17. Bernard GR, Wheeler AP, Russell JA et al: The effects of ibuprofen on the physiology and survival of patients with sepsis. The Ibuprofen in Sepsis Study Group. *N Engl J Med* 336(13):912, 1997.

18. Cook JA: Eicosanoids. *Crit Care Med* 33(12 Suppl):S488, 2005.

19. Calder PC: n-3 fatty acids, inflammation, and immunity—relevance to postsurgical and critically ill patients. *Lipids* 39:1147, 2004.

20. Schmaier AH: The kallikrein-kinin and the renin-angiotensin systems have a multilayered interaction. *Am J Physiol Regul Integr Comp Physiol* 285:R1, 2003.

21. Faerber L, Drechsler S, Ladenburger S, et al: The neuronal 5-HT3 receptor network after 20 years of research—evolving concepts in management of pain and inflammation. *Eur J Pharmacol* 560:1, 2007.

22. de Esch IJ, Thurmond RL, Jongejan A, et al: The histamine H4 receptor as a new therapeutic target for inflammation. *Trends Pharmacol Sci* 26:462, 2005.

23. Clark IA: How TNF was recognized as a key mechanism of disease. *Cytokine Growth Factor Rev* 18:335, 2007.

24. Khalil AA, Hall JC, Aziz FA, et al: Tumour necrosis factor: Implications for surgical patients. *ANZ J Surg* 76:1010, 2006.

25. Stylianou E, Saklatvala J: Interleukin-1. *Int J Biochem Cell Biol* 30:1075, 1998.

26. Bachmann MF, Oxenius A: Interleukin 2: From immunostimulation to immunoregulation and back again. *EMBO Rep* 8:1142, 2007.

27. Song M, Kellum JA: Interleukin-6. *Crit Care Med* 33(12 Suppl):S463, 2005.

28. Jean-Baptiste E: Cellular mechanisms in sepsis. *J Intensive Care Med* 22:63, 2007.

29. Scumpia PO, Moldawer LL: Biology of interleukin-10 and its regulatory roles in sepsis syndromes. *Crit Care Med* 33(12 Suppl):S468, 2005.

30. Weijer S, Florquin S, van der Poll T: Endogenous interleukin-12 improves the early antimicrobial host response to murine *Escherichia coli* peritonitis. *Shock* 23:54, 2005.

31. Socha LA, Gowardman J, Silva D, et al: Elevation in interleukin 13 levels in patients diagnosed with systemic inflammatory response syndrome. *Intensive Care Med* 32:244, 2006.

32. Hiromatsu T, Yajima T, Matsuguchi T, et al: Overexpression of interleukin-15 protects against *Escherichia coli*–induced shock accompanied by inhibition of tumor necrosis factor-alpha–induced apoptosis. *J Infect Dis* 187:1442, 2003.

33. Dinarello CA, Fantuzzi G: Interleukin-18 and host defense against infection. *J Infect Dis* 187(Suppl 2):S370, 2003.

34. Schroder K, Hertzog PJ, Ravasi T, et al: Interferon-gamma: An overview of signals, mechanisms and functions. *J Leukoc Biol* 75:163, 2004.

35. Hamilton JA, Anderson GP: GM-CSF Biology. *Growth Factors* 22:225, 2004.

36. Fink MP: Bench-to-bedside review: High-mobility group box 1 and critical illness. *Crit Care* 11:229, 2007.

37. Leonard WJ, O'Shea JJ: Jaks and STATs: Biological implications. *Annu Rev Immunol* 16:293, 1998.

38. Yoshimura A, Naka T, Kubo M: SOCS proteins, cytokine signalling and immune regulation. *Nat Rev Immunol* 7:454, 2007.

39. Cuevas BD, Abell AN, Johnson GL: Role of mitogen-activated protein kinase kinase kinases in signal integration. *Oncogene* 26:3159, 2007.

40. Zingarelli B: Nuclear factor-kappaB. *Crit Care Med* 33(12 Suppl):S414, 2005.

41. Agnese DM, Calvano JE, Hahm SJ, et al: Human toll-like receptor 4 mutations but not CD14 polymorphisms are associated with an increased risk of gram-negative infections. *J Infect Dis* 186:1522, 2002.

42. Lotze MT, Zeh HJ, Rubartelli A, et al: The grateful dead: Damage-associated molecular pattern molecules and reduction/oxidation regulate immunity. *Immunol Rev* 220:60, 2007.

43. Levi M: Platelets. *Crit Care Med* 33(12 Suppl):S523, 2005.

44. Ochoa JB, Makarenkova V: T lymphocytes. *Crit Care Med* 33(12 Suppl):S510, 2005.

45. Afshar K, Vucinic V, Sharma OP: Eosinophil cell: Pray tell us what you do! *Curr Opin Pulm Med* 13:414, 2007.

46. Bachelet I, Levi-Schaffer F: Mast cells as effector cells: A co-stimulating question. *Trends Immunol* 28:360, 2007.

47. Cavaillon JM, Adib-Conquy M: Monocytes/macrophages and sepsis. *Crit Care Med* 33(12 Suppl):S506, 2005.

48. Alves-Filho JC, Tavares-Murta BM, Barja-Fidalgo C, et al: Neutrophil function in severe sepsis. *Endocr Metab Immune Disord Drug Targets* 6:151, 2006.

49. Ley K, Laudanna C, Cybulsky MI, et al: Getting to the site of inflammation: The leukocyte adhesion cascade updated. *Nat Rev Immunol* 7:678, 2007.

50. Cauwels A: Nitric oxide in shock. *Kidney Int* 72:557, 2007.

51. Zardi EM, Zardi DM, Dobrina A, et al: Prostacyclin in sepsis: A systematic review. *Prostaglandins Other Lipid Mediat* 83:1, 2007.

52. Magder S, Cernacek P: Role of endothelins in septic, cardiogenic, and hemorrhagic shock. *Can J Physiol Pharmacol* 81:635, 2003.

53. Zimmerman GA, McIntyre TM, Prescott SM, et al: The platelet-activating factor signaling system and its regulators in syndromes of inflammation and thrombosis. *Crit Care Med* 30(5 Suppl):S294, 2002.

54. Mitch WE, Price SR: Mechanisms activating proteolysis to cause muscle atrophy in catabolic conditions. *J Ren Nutr* 13:149, 2003.

55. Guirao X: Impact of the inflammatory reaction on intermediary metabolism and nutrition status. *Nutrition* 18:949, 2002.

56. Souba WW: Nutritional support. *N Engl J Med* 336:41, 1997.

57. Bistrian BR: Clinical aspects of essential fatty acid metabolism: Jonathan Rhoads Lecture. *JPEN J Parenter Enteral Nutr* 27:168, 2003.

58. Kono H, Fujii H, Asakawa M, et al: Protective effects of medium-chain triglycerides on the liver and gut in rats administered endotoxin. *Ann Surg* 237:246, 2003.

59. Dahn MS, Mitchell RA, Lange MP et al: Hepatic metabolic response to injury and sepsis. *Surgery* 117(50):520, 1995.

60. Vidal-Puig A, O'Rahilly S: Metabolism. Controlling the glucose factory. *Nature* 413:125, 2001.

61. Brown GK: Glucose transporters: Structure, function and consequences of deficiency. *J Inherit Metab Dis* 23:237, 2000.

62. Volpi E, Sheffield-Moore M, Rasmussen BB, et al: Basal muscle amino acid kinetics and protein synthesis in healthy young and older men. *JAMA* 286:1206, 2001.

63. McClave SA, Lowen CC, Kleber MJ, et al: Clinical use of the respiratory quotient obtained from indirect calorimetry. *JPEN J Parenter Enteral Nutr* 27:21, 2003.

64. Chernoff R: Normal aging, nutrition assessment, and clinical practice. *Nutr Clin Pract* 18:12, 2003.

65. Heslin MJ, Brennan MF: Advances in perioperative nutrition: Cancer. *World J Surg* 24:1477, 2000.

66. Heslin MJ, Latkany L, Leung D, et al: A prospective, randomized trial of early enteral feeding after resection of upper gastrointestinal malignancy. *Ann Surg* 226:567; discussion 77, 1997.

67. Brooks AD, Hochwald SN, Heslin MJ, et al: Intestinal permeability after early postoperative enteral nutrition in patients with upper gastrointestinal malignancy. *JPEN J Parenter Enteral Nutr* 23:75, 1999.

68. Exner R, Tamandl D, Goetzinger P, et al: Perioperative GLY-GLN infusion diminishes the surgery-induced period of immunosuppression: Accelerated restoration of the lipopolysaccharide-stimulated tumor necrosis factor-alpha response. *Ann Surg* 237:110, 2003.

69. Lin E, Goncalves JA, Lowry SF: Efficacy of nutritional pharmacology in surgical patients. *Curr Opin Clin Nutr Metab Care* 1:41, 1998.

70. Heyland DK: Immunonutrition in the critically ill patient: Putting the cart before the horse? *Nutr Clin Pract* 17:267, 2002.

71. Btaiche IF: Branched-chain amino acids in patients with hepatic encephalopathy. 1982. *Nutr Clin Pract* 18:97, 2003.

72. Patton KM, Aranda-Michel J: Nutritional aspects in liver disease and liver transplantation. *Nutr Clin Pract* 17:332, 2002.

73. DiSario JA, Baskin WN, Brown RD, et al: Endoscopic approaches to enteral nutritional support. *Gastrointest Endosc* 55:901, 2002.

74. Heyland DK, Drover JW, Dhaliwal R, et al: Optimizing the benefits and minimizing the risks of enteral nutrition in the critically ill: Role of small bowel feeding. *JPEN J Parenter Enteral Nutr* 26(6 Suppl):S51; discussion S6, 2002.

75. Scolapio JS: Methods for decreasing risk of aspiration pneumonia in critically ill patients. *JPEN J Parenter Enteral Nutr* 26(6 Suppl):S58; discussion S61, 2002.

76. Vanek VW: Ins and outs of enteral access. Part 2: Long term access—esophagostomy and gastrostomy. *Nutr Clin Pract* 18:50, 2003.

77. Polderman KH, Girbes AR: Central venous catheter use. Part 2: Infectious complications. *Intensive Care Med* 28:18, 2002.

78. Kovacevich DS, Papke LF: Guidelines for the prevention of intravascular catheter–related infections: Centers for Disease Control and Prevention. *Nutr Clin Pract* 18:95, 2003.

79. Gore DC, Wolfe RR: Glutamine supplementation fails to affect muscle protein kinetics in critically ill patients. *JPEN J Parenter Enteral Nutr* 26:342; discussion 9, 2002.

80. Foitzik T, Eibl G, Schneider P, et al: Omega-3 fatty acid supplementation increases anti-inflammatory cytokines and attenuates systemic disease sequelae in experimental pancreatitis. *JPEN J Parenter Enteral Nutr* 26:351, 2002.

81. Luyer MD, Greve JW, Hadfoune M et al: Nutritional stimulations of cholecystokinin receptors inhibits inflammation via the vagus nerve. *J Exp Med* 202:1023, 2005.

82. Lowry SF: A new model of nutrition influenced inflammatory risk. *J Am Coll Surg* 205(4 Suppl):S65, 2007.

CHAPTER 2

Systemic Response to Injury and Metabolic Support

Fluid and Electrolyte Management of the Surgical Patient

G. Tom Shires III

INTRODUCTION

Fluid and electrolyte management is paramount to the care of the surgical patient. Changes in both fluid volume and electrolyte composition occur preoperatively, intraoperatively, and postoperatively, as well as in response to trauma and sepsis. The sections that follow review the normal anatomy of body fluids, electrolyte composition and concentration abnormalities and treatments, common metabolic derangements, and alternative resuscitative fluids. These concepts are then discussed in relationship to management of specific surgical patients and their commonly encountered fluid and electrolyte abnormalities.

BODY FLUIDS

Total Body Water

Water constitutes approximately 50 to 60% of total body weight. The relationship between total body weight and total body water (TBW) is relatively constant for an individual and is primarily a reflection of body fat. Lean tissues such as muscle and solid organs have higher water content than fat and bone. As a result, young, lean males have a higher proportion of body weight as water than elderly or obese individuals. Deuterium oxide and tritiated water have been used in clinical research to measure TBW by indicator dilution methods. In an average young adult male 60% of total body weight is TBW, whereas in an average young adult female it is 50%.[1] The lower percentage of TBW in females correlates with a higher percentage of adipose tissue and lower percentage of muscle mass in most. Estimates of percentage of TBW should be adjusted downward approximately 10 to 20% for obese individuals and upward by 10% for malnourished individuals. The highest percentage of TBW is found in newborns, with approximately 80% of their total body weight comprised of water. This decreases to approximately 65% by 1 year of age and thereafter remains fairly constant.

Fluid Compartments

TBW is divided into three functional fluid compartments: plasma, extravascular interstitial fluid, and intracellular fluid (Fig. 3-1). The extracellular fluids (ECF), plasma and interstitial fluid, together comprise about one third of the TBW and the intracellular compartment the remaining two thirds. The extracellular water comprises 20% of the total body weight and is divided between plasma (5% of body weight) and interstitial fluid (15% of body weight). Intracellular water makes up approximately 40% of an individual's total body weight, with the largest proportion in the skeletal muscle mass. ECF is measured using indicator dilution methods. The distribution volumes of NaBr and radioactive sulfate have been used to measure

ECF in clinical research. Measurement of the intracellular compartment is then determined indirectly by subtracting the measured ECF from the simultaneous TBW measurement.

Composition of Fluid Compartments

The normal chemical composition of the body fluid compartments is shown in Fig. 3-2. The ECF compartment is balanced between sodium, the principal cation, and chloride and bicarbonate, the principal anions. The intracellular fluid compartment is comprised primarily of the cations potassium and magnesium, and the anions phosphate and proteins. The concentration gradient between compartments is maintained by adenosine triphosphate–driven sodium-potassium pumps located with the cell membranes. The composition of the plasma and interstitial fluid differs only slightly in ionic composition. The slightly higher protein content (organic anions) in plasma results in a higher plasma cation composition relative to the interstitial fluid, as explained by the Gibbs-Donnan equilibrium equation. Proteins add to the osmolality of the plasma and contribute to the balance of forces that determine fluid balance across the capillary endothelium. Although the movement of ions and proteins between the various fluid compartments is restricted, water is freely diffusible. Water is distributed evenly throughout all fluid compartments of the body, so that a given volume of water increases the

% of Total body weight	Volume of TBW	Male (70 kg)	Female (60 kg)
Plasma 5%	Extracellular volume	14,000 mL	10,000 mL
Interstitial fluid 15%	Plasma	3500 mL	2500 mL
	Interstitial	10,500 mL	7500 mL
Intracellular volume 40%	Intracellular volume	28,000 mL	20,000 mL
		42,000 mL	30,000 mL

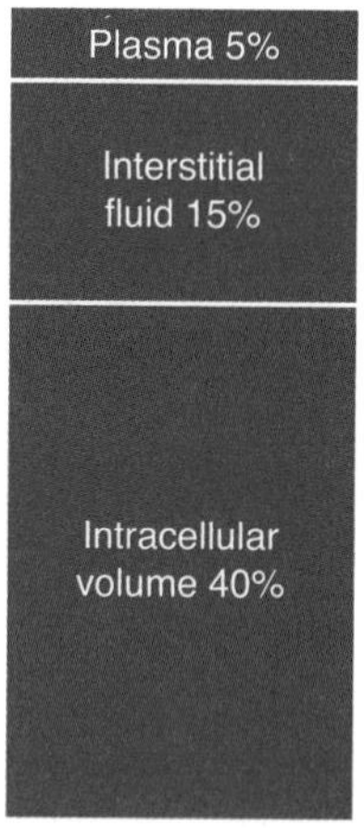

FIG. 3-1. Functional body fluid compartments. TBW = total body water.

KEY POINTS

1. Proper management of fluid and electrolytes facilitates crucial homeostasis that allows cardiovascular perfusion, organ system function, and cellular mechanisms to respond to surgical illness.

2. Knowledge of the compartmentalization of body fluids forms the basis for understanding pathologic shifts in these fluid spaces in disease states. Although difficult to quantify, a deficiency in the functional extracellular fluid compartment often requires resuscitation with isotonic fluids in surgical and trauma patients.

3. Alterations in the concentration of serum sodium have profound effects on cellular function due to water shifts between the intracellular and extracellular spaces.

4. Different rates of compensation between respiratory and metabolic components of acid-base homeostasis require frequent laboratory reassessment during therapy.

5. Most acute surgical illnesses are accompanied by some degree of volume loss or redistribution. Consequently, isotonic fluid administration is the most common initial IV fluid strategy, while attention is being given to alterations in concentration and composition.

6. Although active investigation continues, alternative resuscitation fluids have limited clinical utility, other than the correction of specific electrolyte abnormalities.

7. Some surgical patients with neurologic illness, malnutrition, acute renal failure, or cancer require special attention to well-defined, disease-specific abnormalities in fluid and electrolyte status.

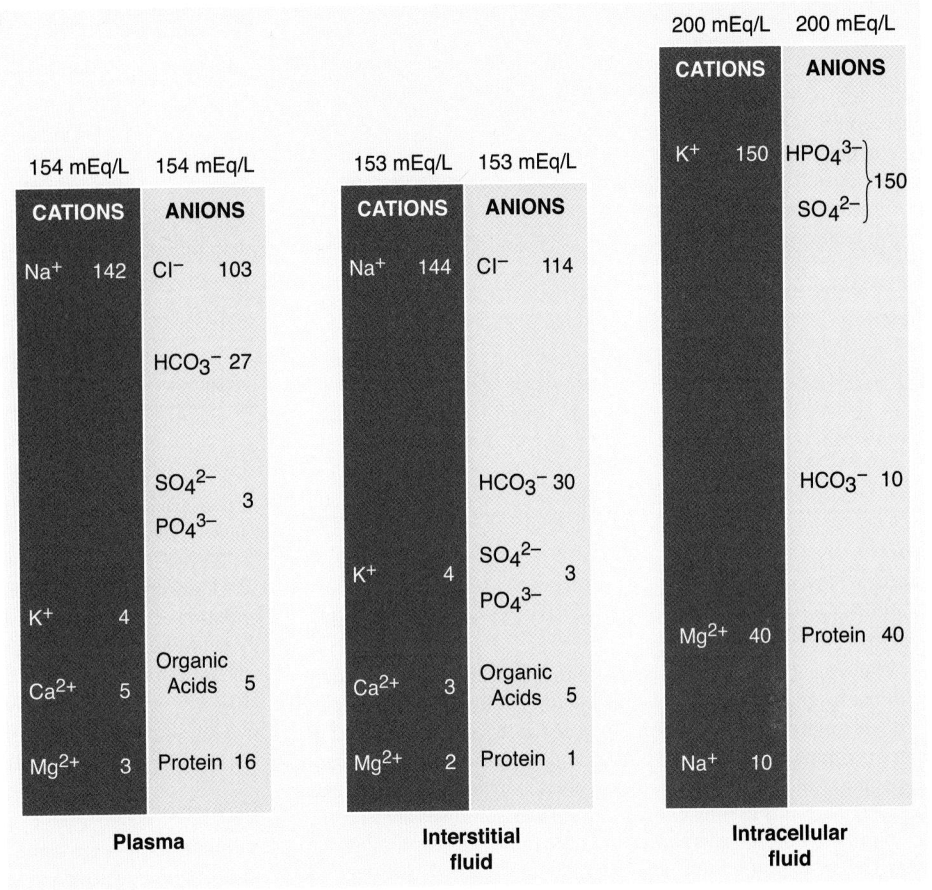

FIG. 3-2. Chemical composition of body fluid compartments.

volume of any one compartment relatively little. Sodium, however, is confined to the ECF compartment, and because of its osmotic and electrical properties, it remains associated with water. Therefore, sodium-containing fluids are distributed throughout the ECF and add to the volume of both the intravascular and interstitial spaces. Although the administration of sodium-containing fluids expands the intravascular volume, it also expands the interstitial space by approximately three times as much as the plasma.

Osmotic Pressure

The physiologic activity of electrolytes in solution depends on the number of particles per unit volume (millimoles per liter, or mmol/L), the number of electric charges per unit volume (milliequivalents per liter, or mEq/L), and the number of osmotically active ions per unit volume (milliosmoles per liter, or mOsm/L). The concentration of electrolytes usually is expressed in terms of the chemical combining activity, or equivalents. An equivalent of an ion is its atomic weight expressed in grams divided by the valence:

$$Equivalent = atomic weight (g)/valence$$

For univalent ions such as sodium, 1 mEq is the same as 1 mmol. For divalent ions such as magnesium, 1 mmol equals 2 mEq. The number of milliequivalents of cations must be balanced by the same number of milliequivalents of anions. However, the expression of molar equivalents alone does not allow a physiologic comparison of solutes in a solution.

The movement of water across a cell membrane depends primarily on osmosis. To achieve osmotic equilibrium, water moves across a semipermeable membrane to equalize the concentration on both sides. This movement is determined by the concentration of the solutes on each side of the membrane. Osmotic pressure is measured in units of osmoles (osm) or milliosmoles (mOsm) that refer to the actual number of osmotically active particles. For example, 1 mmol of sodium chloride contributes to 2 mOsm (one

from sodium and one from chloride). The principal determinants of osmolality are the concentrations of sodium, glucose, and urea (blood urea nitrogen, or BUN):

Calculated serum osmolality = 2 sodium + (glucose/18) + (BUN/2.8)

The osmolality of the intracellular and extracellular fluids is maintained between 290 and 310 mOsm in each compartment. Because cell membranes are permeable to water, any change in osmotic pressure in one compartment is accompanied by a redistribution of water until the effective osmotic pressure between compartments is equal. For example, if the ECF concentration of sodium increases, there will be a net movement of water from the intracellular to the extracellular compartment. Conversely, if the ECF concentration of sodium decreases, water will move into the cells. Although the intracellular fluid shares in losses that involve a change in concentration or composition of the ECF, an isotonic change in volume in either one of the compartments is not accompanied by the net movement of water as long as the ionic concentration remains the same. For practical clinical purposes, most significant gains and losses of body fluid are directly from the extracellular compartment.

BODY FLUID CHANGES

Normal Exchange of Fluid and Electrolytes

The healthy person consumes an average of 2000 mL of water per day, approximately 75% from oral intake and the rest extracted from solid foods. Daily water losses include 800 to 1200 mL in urine, 250 mL in stool, and 600 mL in insensible losses. Insensible losses of water occur through both the skin (75%) and lungs (25%), and can be increased by such factors as fever, hypermetabolism, and hyperventilation. Sensible water losses such as sweating or pathologic loss of GI fluids vary widely, but these include the loss of electrolytes as well as water (Table 3-1). To clear the products of metabolism, the kidneys

Routes	Average Daily Volume (mL)	Minimal (mL)	Maximal (mL)
H₂O gain:			
Sensible:			
Oral fluids	800–1500	0	1500/h
Solid foods	500–700	0	1500
Insensible:			
Water of oxidation	250	125	800
Water of solution	0	0	500
H₂O loss:			
Sensible:			
Urine	800–1500	300	1400/h
Intestinal	0–250	0	2500/h
Sweat	0	0	4000/h
Insensible:			
Lungs and skin	600	600	1500

TABLE 3-1 Water exchange (60- to 80-kg man)

TABLE 3-2 Signs and symptoms of volume disturbances

System	Volume Deficit	Volume Excess
Generalized	Weight loss	Weight gain
	Decreased skin turgor	Peripheral edema
Cardiac	Tachycardia	Increased cardiac output
	Orthostasis/hypotension	Increased central venous pressure
	Collapsed neck veins	Distended neck veins
		Murmur
Renal	Oliguria	—
	Azotemia	
GI	Ileus	Bowel edema
Pulmonary	—	Pulmonary edema

must excrete a minimum of 500 to 800 mL of urine per day, regardless of the amount of oral intake.

The typical individual consumes 3 to 5 g of dietary salt per day, with the balance maintained by the kidneys. With hyponatremia or hypovolemia, sodium excretion can be reduced to as little as 1 mEq/d or maximized to as much as 5000 mEq/d to achieve balance except in people with salt-wasting kidneys. Sweat is hypotonic, and sweating usually results in only a small sodium loss. GI losses are isotonic to slightly hypotonic and contribute little to net gain or loss of free water when measured and appropriately replaced by isotonic salt solutions.

Classification of Body Fluid Changes

Disorders in fluid balance may be classified into three general categories: disturbances in (a) volume, (b) concentration, and (c) composition. Although each of these may occur simultaneously, each is a separate entity with unique mechanisms demanding individual correction. Isotonic gain or loss of salt solution results in extracellular volume changes, with little impact on intracellular fluid volume. If free water is added or lost from the ECF, water will pass between the ECF and intracellular fluid until solute concentration or osmolarity is equalized between the compartments. Unlike with sodium, the concentration of most other ions in the ECF can be altered without significant change in the total number of osmotically active particles, producing only a compositional change. For instance, doubling the serum potassium concentration will profoundly alter myocardial function without significantly altering volume or concentration of the fluid spaces.

Disturbances in Fluid Balance

Extracellular volume deficit is the most common fluid disorder in surgical patients and can be either acute or chronic. Acute volume deficit is associated with cardiovascular and central nervous system signs, whereas chronic deficits display tissue signs, such as a decrease in skin turgor and sunken eyes, in addition to cardiovascular and central nervous system signs (Table 3-2). Laboratory examination may reveal an elevated blood urea nitrogen level if the deficit is severe enough to reduce glomerular filtration and hemoconcentration. Urine osmolality usually will be higher than serum osmolality, and urine sodium will be low, typically <20 mEq/L. Serum sodium concentration does not necessarily reflect volume status and therefore may be high, normal, or low when a volume deficit is present. The most common cause of volume deficit in surgical patients is a loss of GI fluids (Table 3-3) from nasogastric suction, vomiting, diarrhea, or enterocutaneous fistula. In addition, sequestration secondary to soft tissue injuries, burns, and intra-abdominal processes

such as peritonitis, obstruction, or prolonged surgery can also lead to massive volume deficits.

Extracellular volume excess may be iatrogenic or secondary to renal dysfunction, congestive heart failure, or cirrhosis. Both plasma and interstitial volumes usually are increased. Symptoms are primarily pulmonary and cardiovascular (see Table 3-2). In fit patients, edema and hyperdynamic circulation are common and well tolerated. However, the elderly and patients with cardiac disease may quickly develop congestive heart failure and pulmonary edema in response to only a moderate volume excess.

Volume Control

Volume changes are sensed by both osmoreceptors and baroreceptors. Osmoreceptors are specialized sensors that detect even small changes in fluid osmolality and drive changes in thirst and diuresis through the kidneys.[2] For example, when plasma osmolality is increased, thirst is stimulated and water consumption increases.[3] Additionally, the hypothalamus is stimulated to secrete vasopressin, which increases water reabsorption in the kidneys. Together, these two mechanisms return the plasma osmolality to normal. Baroreceptors also modulate volume in response to changes in pressure and circulating volume through specialized pressure sensors located in the aortic arch and carotid sinuses.[4] Baroreceptor responses are both neural, through sympathetic and parasympathetic pathways, and hormonal, through substances including renin-angiotensin, aldosterone, atrial natriuretic peptide, and renal prostaglandins. The net result of alterations in renal sodium excretion and free water reabsorption is restoration of volume to the normal state.

Concentration Changes

Changes in serum sodium concentration are inversely proportional to TBW. Therefore, abnormalities in TBW are reflected by abnormalities in serum sodium levels.

Hyponatremia

A low serum sodium level occurs when there is an excess of extracellular water relative to sodium. Extracellular volume can be high,

TABLE 3-3 Composition of GI secretions

Type of Secretion	Volume (mL/24 h)	Na (mEq/L)	K (mEq/L)	Cl (mEq/L)	HCO₃⁻ (mEq/L)
Stomach	1000–2000	60–90	10–30	100–130	0
Small intestine	2000–3000	120–140	5–10	90–120	30–40
Colon	—	60	30	40	0
Pancreas	600–800	135–145	5–10	70–90	95–115
Bile	300–800	135–145	5–10	90–110	30–40

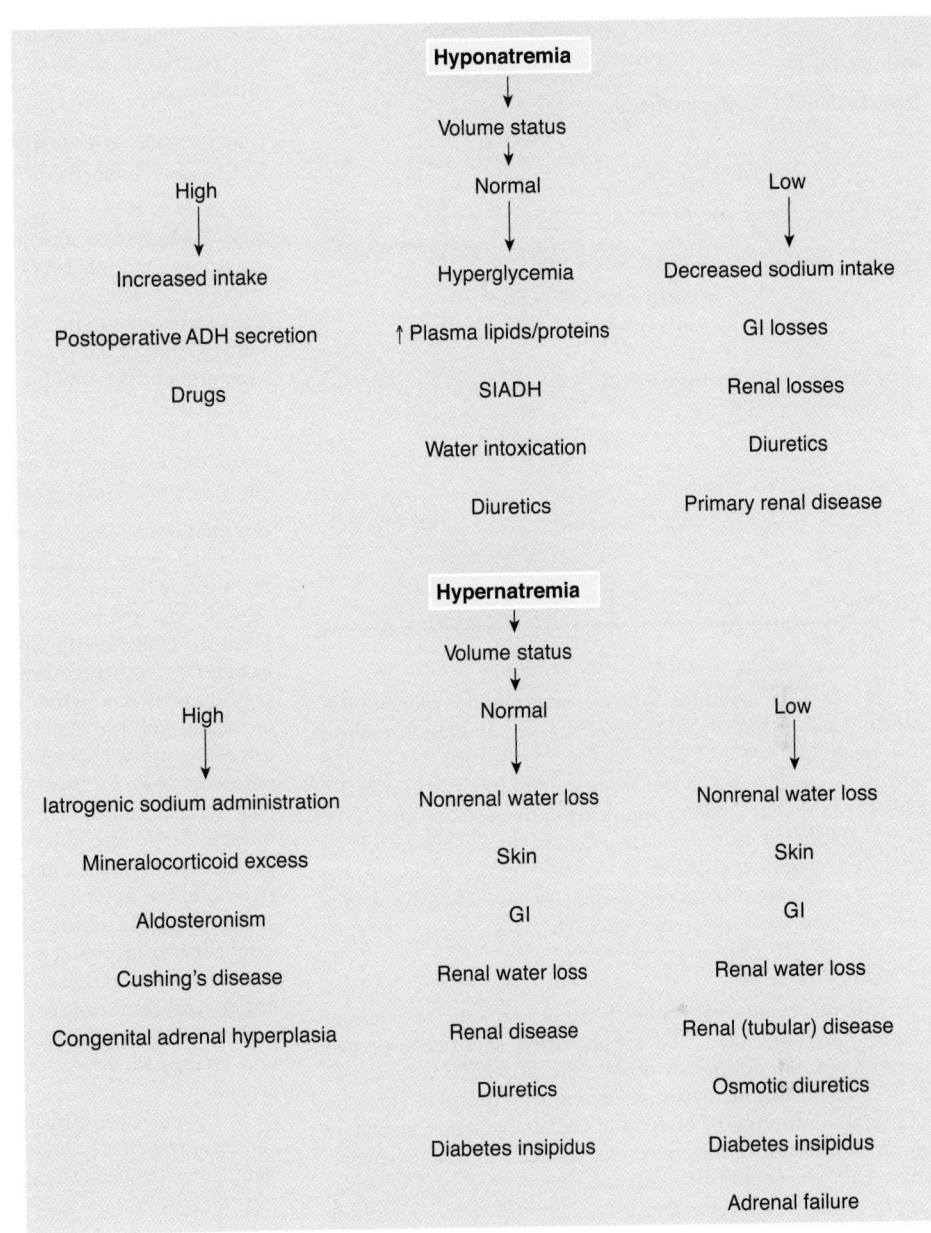

FIG. 3-3. Evaluation of sodium abnormalities. ADH = antidiuretic hormone; SIADH = syndrome of inappropriate secretion of antidiuretic hormone.

normal, or low (Fig. 3-3). In most cases of hyponatremia, sodium concentration is decreased as a consequence of either sodium depletion or dilution.[5] Dilutional hyponatremia frequently results from excess extracellular water and therefore is associated with a high extracellular volume status. Excessive oral water intake or iatrogenic IV excess free water administration can cause hyponatremia. Postoperative patients are particularly prone to increased secretion of antidiuretic hormone (ADH), which increases reabsorption of free water from the kidneys with subsequent volume expansion and hyponatremia. This is usually self-limiting in that both hyponatremia and volume expansion decrease ADH secretion. Additionally, a number of drugs can cause water retention and subsequent hyponatremia, such as the antipsychotics and tricyclic antidepressants as well as angiotensin-converting enzyme inhibitors. The elderly are particularly susceptible to drug-induced hyponatremia. Physical signs of volume overload usually are absent, and laboratory evaluation reveals hemodilution. Depletional causes of hyponatremia are associated with either a decreased intake or increased loss of sodium-containing fluids. A concomitant ECF volume deficit is common. Causes include decreased sodium intake, such as consumption of a low-sodium diet or use of enteral feeds, which are typically low in sodium; GI losses from vomiting, prolonged nasogastric suctioning, or diarrhea; and renal losses due to diuretic use or primary renal disease.

Hyponatremia also can be seen with an excess of solute relative to free water, such as with untreated hyperglycemia or mannitol administration. Glucose exerts an osmotic force in the extracellular compartment, causing a shift of water from the intracellular to the extracellular space. Hyponatremia therefore can be seen when the effective osmotic pressure of the extracellular compartment is normal or even high. When hyponatremia in the presence of hyperglycemia is being evaluated, the corrected sodium concentration should be calculated as follows:

For every 100-mg/dL increment in plasma glucose above normal, the plasma sodium should decrease by 1.6 mEq/L

Lastly, extreme elevations in plasma lipids and proteins can cause pseudohyponatremia, because there is no true decrease in extracellular sodium relative to water.

Signs and symptoms of hyponatremia (Table 3-4) are dependent on the degree of hyponatremia and the rapidity with which it occurred. Clinical manifestations primarily have a central nervous system origin and are related to cellular water intoxication and associated increases in intracranial pressure. Oliguric renal failure also can be a rapid complication in the setting of severe hyponatremia.

A systematic review of the etiology of hyponatremia should reveal its cause in a given instance. Hyperosmolar causes, including

TABLE 3-4	Clinical manifestations of abnormalities in serum sodium level

Body System	Hyponatremia
Central nervous system	Headache, confusion, hyperactive or hypoactive deep tendon reflexes, seizures, coma, increased intracranial pressure
Musculoskeletal	Weakness, fatigue, muscle cramps/twitching
GI	Anorexia, nausea, vomiting, watery diarrhea
Cardiovascular	Hypertension and bradycardia if significant increases in intracranial pressure
Tissue	Lacrimation, salivation
Renal	Oliguria
Body System	**Hypernatremia**
Central nervous system	Restlessness, lethargy, ataxia, irritability, tonic spasms, delirium, seizures, coma
Musculoskeletal	Weakness
Cardiovascular	Tachycardia, hypotension, syncope
Tissue	Dry sticky mucous membranes, red swollen tongue, decreased saliva and tears
Renal	Oliguria
Metabolic	Fever

hyperglycemia or mannitol infusion and pseudohyponatremia, should be easily excluded. Next, depletional versus dilutional causes of hyponatremia are evaluated. In the absence of renal disease, depletion is associated with low urine sodium levels (<20 mEq/L), whereas renal sodium wasting shows high urine sodium levels (>20 mEq/L). Dilutional causes of hyponatremia usually are associated with hypervolemic circulation. A normal volume status in the setting of hyponatremia should prompt an evaluation for a syndrome of inappropriate secretion of ADH.

Hypernatremia

Hypernatremia results from either a loss of free water or a gain of sodium in excess of water. Like hyponatremia, it can be associated with an increased, normal, or decreased extracellular volume (see Fig. 3-3). Hypervolemic hypernatremia usually is caused either by iatrogenic administration of sodium-containing fluids, including sodium bicarbonate, or mineralocorticoid excess as seen in hyperaldosteronism, Cushing's syndrome, and congenital adrenal hyperplasia. Urine sodium concentration is typically >20 mEq/L and urine osmolarity is >300 mOsm/L. Normovolemic hypernatremia can result from renal causes, including diabetes insipidus, diuretic use, and renal disease, or from nonrenal water loss from the GI tract or skin, although the same conditions can result in hypovolemic hypernatremia. When hypovolemia is present, the urine sodium concentration is <20 mEq/L and urine osmolarity is <300 to 400 mOsm/L. Nonrenal water loss can occur secondary to relatively isotonic GI fluid losses such as that caused by diarrhea, to hypotonic skin fluid losses such as loss due to fever, or to losses via tracheotomies during hyperventilation. Additionally, thyrotoxicosis can cause water loss, as can the use of hypertonic glucose solutions for peritoneal dialysis. With nonrenal water loss, the urine sodium concentration is <15 mEq/L and the urine osmolarity is >400 mOsm/L.

Symptomatic hypernatremia usually occurs only in patients with impaired thirst or restricted access to fluid, because thirst will result in increased water intake. Symptoms are rare until the serum sodium concentration exceeds 160 mEq/L but, once present, are associated with significant morbidity and mortality. Because symptoms are related to hyperosmolarity, central nervous system effects predominate (see Table 3-4). Water shifts from the intracellular to the extracellular space in response to a hyperosmolar extracellular space, which results in cellular dehydration. This can put traction on the cerebral vessels and lead to subarachnoid hemorrhage. Central nervous system symptoms can range from restlessness and irritability to seizures, coma, and death. The classic signs of hypo-

volemic hypernatremia, (tachycardia, orthostasis, and hypotension) may be present, as well as the unique findings of dry, sticky mucous membranes.

Composition Changes: Etiology and Diagnosis
Potassium Abnormalities

The average dietary intake of potassium is approximately 50 to 100 mEq/d, which in the absence of hypokalemia is excreted primarily in the urine. Extracellular potassium is maintained within a narrow range, principally by renal excretion of potassium, which can range from 10 to 700 mEq/d. Although only 2% of the total body potassium ($4.5 \text{ mEq/L} \times 14 \text{ L} = 63 \text{ mEq}$) is located within the extracellular compartment, this small amount is critical to cardiac and neuromuscular function; thus, even minor changes can have major effects on cardiac activity. The intracellular and extracellular distribution of potassium is influenced by a number of factors, including surgical stress, injury, acidosis, and tissue catabolism.

Hyperkalemia *Hyperkalemia* is defined as a serum potassium concentration above the normal range of 3.5 to 5.0 mEq/L. It is caused by excessive potassium intake, increased release of potassium from cells, or impaired potassium excretion by the kidneys (Table 3-5).[6] Increased intake can be either from oral or IV supplementation, or from red cell lysis after transfusion. Hemolysis, rhabdomyolysis, and crush injuries can disrupt cell membranes and release intracellular potassium into the ECF. Acidosis and a rapid rise in extracellular osmolality from hyperglycemia or IV mannitol can raise serum potassium levels by causing a shift of potassium ions to the extracellular compartment.[7] Because 98% of total body potassium is in the intracellular fluid compartment, even small shifts of intracellular potassium out of the intracellular fluid compartment can lead to a significant rise in extracellular potassium. A number of medications can contribute to hyperkalemia, particularly in the presence of renal insufficiency, including potassium-sparing diuretics, angiotensin-converting enzyme inhibitors, and NSAIDs. Spironolactone and angiotensin-converting enzyme inhibitors interfere with aldosterone activity, inhibiting the normal renal mechanism of potassium excretion. Acute and chronic renal insufficiency also impairs potassium excretion.

Symptoms of hyperkalemia are primarily GI, neuromuscular, and cardiovascular (Table 3-6). GI symptoms include nausea, vomiting, intestinal colic, and diarrhea. Neuromuscular symptoms

TABLE 3-5	Etiology of potassium abnormalities

Hyperkalemia
Increased intake
    Potassium supplementation
    Blood transfusions
    Endogenous load/destruction: hemolysis, rhabdomyolysis, crush injury, gastrointestinal hemorrhage
Increased release
    Acidosis
    Rapid rise of extracellular osmolality (hyperglycemia or mannitol)
Impaired excretion
    Potassium-sparing diuretics
    Renal insufficiency/failure
Hypokalemia
Inadequate intake
    Dietary, potassium-free intravenous fluids, potassium-deficient TPN
Excessive potassium excretion
    Hyperaldosteronism
    Medications
GI losses
    Direct loss of potassium from GI fluid (diarrhea)
    Renal loss of potassium (gastric fluid, either as vomiting or high nasogastric output)

TABLE 3-6 Clinical manifestations of abnormalities in potassium, magnesium, and calcium levels

	Increased Serum Levels		
System	**Potassium**	**Magnesium**	**Calcium**
GI	Nausea/vomiting, colic, diarrhea	Nausea/vomiting	Anorexia, nausea/vomiting, abdominal pain
Neuromuscular	Weakness, paralysis, respiratory failure	Weakness, lethargy, decreased reflexes	Weakness, confusion, coma, bone pain
Cardiovascular	Arrhythmia, arrest	Hypotension, arrest	Hypertension, arrhythmia, polyuria
Renal	—	—	Polydipsia

	Decreased Serum Levels		
System	**Potassium**	**Magnesium**	**Calcium**
GI	Ileus, constipation	—	—
Neuromuscular	Decreased reflexes, fatigue, weakness, paralysis	Hyperactive reflexes, muscle tremors, tetany, seizures	Hyperactive reflexes, paresthesias, carpopedal spasm, seizures
Cardiovascular	Arrest	Arrhythmia	Heart failure

range from weakness to ascending paralysis to respiratory failure. Early cardiovascular signs may be apparent from electrocardiogram (ECG) changes and eventually lead to hemodynamic symptoms of arrhythmia and cardiac arrest. ECG changes that may be seen with hyperkalemia include high peaked T waves (early), widened QRS complex, flattened P wave, prolonged PR interval (first-degree block), sine wave formation, and ventricular fibrillation.

Hypokalemia Hypokalemia is much more common than hyperkalemia in the surgical patient. It may be caused by inadequate potassium intake; excessive renal potassium excretion; potassium loss in pathologic GI secretions, such as with diarrhea, fistulas, vomiting, or high nasogastric output; or intracellular shifts from metabolic alkalosis or insulin therapy (see Table 3-5). The change in potassium associated with alkalosis can be calculated by the following formula:

Potassium decreases by 0.3 mEq/L for every
0.1 increase in pH above normal.

Additionally, drugs such as amphotericin, aminoglycosides, foscarnet, cisplatin, and ifosfamide that induce magnesium depletion cause renal potassium wastage.[8,9] In cases in which potassium deficiency is due to magnesium depletion,[10] potassium repletion is difficult unless hypomagnesemia is first corrected.

The symptoms of hypokalemia (see Table 3-6), like those of hyperkalemia, are primarily related to failure of normal contractility of GI smooth muscle, skeletal muscle, and cardiac muscle. Findings may include ileus, constipation, weakness, fatigue, diminished tendon reflexes, paralysis, and cardiac arrest. In the setting of ECF depletion, symptoms may be masked initially and then worsened by further dilution during volume repletion. ECG changes suggestive of hypokalemia include U waves, T-wave flattening, ST-segment changes, and arrhythmias (with digitalis therapy).

Calcium Abnormalities

The vast majority of the body's calcium is contained within the bone matrix, with <1% found in the ECF. Serum calcium is distributed among three forms: protein found (40%), complexed to phosphate and other anions (10%), and ionized (50%). It is the ionized fraction that is responsible for neuromuscular stability and can be measured directly. When total serum calcium levels are measured, the albumin concentration must be taken into consideration:

Adjust total serum calcium down by 0.8 mg/dL
for every 1-g/dL decrease in albumin.

Unlike changes in albumin, changes in pH will affect the ionized calcium concentration. Acidosis decreases protein binding, thereby increasing the ionized fraction of calcium.

Daily calcium intake is 1 to 3 g/d. Most of this is excreted via the bowel, with urinary excretion relatively low. Total body calcium balance is under complex hormonal control, but disturbances in

metabolism are relatively long term and less important in the acute surgical setting. However, attention to the critical role of ionized calcium in neuromuscular function often is required.

Hypercalcemia Hypercalcemia is defined as a serum calcium level above the normal range of 8.5 to 10.5 mEq/L or an increase in the ionized calcium level above 4.2 to 4.8 mg/dL. Primary hyperparathyroidism in the outpatient setting and malignancy in hospitalized patients, from either bony metastasis or secretion of parathyroid hormone–related protein, account for most cases of symptomatic hypercalcemia.[11] Symptoms of hypercalcemia (see Table 3-6), which vary with the degree of severity, include neurologic impairment, musculoskeletal weakness and pain, renal dysfunction, and GI symptoms of nausea, vomiting, and abdominal pain. Cardiac symptoms can be manifest as hypertension, cardiac arrhythmias, and a worsening of digitalis toxicity. ECG changes in hypercalcemia include shortened QT interval, prolonged PR and QRS intervals, increased QRS voltage, T-wave flattening and widening, and atrioventricular block (which can progress to complete heart block and cardiac arrest).

Hypocalcemia Hypocalcemia is defined as a serum calcium level below 8.5 mEq/L or a decrease in the ionized calcium level below 4.2 mg/dL. The causes of hypocalcemia include pancreatitis, massive soft tissue infections such as necrotizing fasciitis, renal failure, pancreatic and small bowel fistulas, hypoparathyroidism, toxic shock syndrome, abnormalities in magnesium levels, and tumor lysis syndrome. In addition, transient hypocalcemia commonly occurs after removal of a parathyroid adenoma due to atrophy of the remaining glands and avid bone remineralization, and sometimes requires high-dose calcium supplementation.[12] Additionally, malignancies associated with increased osteoclastic activity, such as breast and prostate cancer, can lead to hypocalcemia from increased bone formation.[13] Calcium precipitation with organic anions is also a cause of hypocalcemia and may occur during hyperphosphatemia from tumor lysis syndrome or rhabdomyolysis. Pancreatitis may sequester calcium via chelation with free fatty acids. Massive blood transfusion with citrate binding is another mechanism.[14,15] Hypocalcemia rarely results solely from decreased intake, because bone reabsorption can maintain normal levels for prolonged periods.

Asymptomatic hypocalcemia may occur when hypoproteinemia results in a normal ionized calcium level. Conversely, symptoms can develop with a normal serum calcium level during alkalosis, which decreases ionized calcium. In general, neuromuscular and cardiac symptoms do not occur until the ionized fraction falls below 2.5 mg/dL (see Table 3-6). Clinical findings may include paresthesias of the face and extremities, muscle cramps, carpopedal spasm, stridor, tetany, and seizures. Patients will demonstrate hyperreflexia and may exhibit positive Chvostek's sign (spasm resulting from tapping over the facial nerve) and Trousseau's sign (spasm resulting from pressure applied to the nerves and vessels of the upper extremity with a blood pressure cuff). Hypocalcemia may lead to

CHAPTER 3

Fluid and Electrolyte Management of the Surgical Patient

decreased cardiac contractility and heart failure. ECG changes of hypocalcemia include prolonged QT interval, T-wave inversion, heart block, and ventricular fibrillation.

Phosphorus Abnormalities

Phosphorus is the primary intracellular divalent anion and is abundant in metabolically active cells. Phosphorus is involved in energy production during glycolysis and is found in high-energy phosphate products such as adenosine triphosphate. Serum phosphate levels are tightly controlled by renal excretion.

Hyperphosphatemia Hyperphosphatemia can be due to decreased urinary excretion, increased intake, or endogenous mobilization of phosphorus. Most cases of hyperphosphatemia are seen in patients with impaired renal function. Hypoparathyroidism or hyperthyroidism also can decrease urinary excretion of phosphorus and thus lead to hyperphosphatemia. Increased release of endogenous phosphorus can be seen in association with any clinical condition that results in cell destruction, including rhabdomyolysis, tumor lysis syndrome, hemolysis, sepsis, severe hypothermia, and malignant hyperthermia. Excessive phosphate administration from IV hyperalimentation solutions or phosphorus-containing laxatives may also lead to elevated phosphate levels. Most cases of hyperphosphatemia are asymptomatic, but significant prolonged hyperphosphatemia can lead to metastatic deposition of soft tissue calcium-phosphorus complexes.

Hypophosphatemia Hypophosphatemia can be due to a decrease in phosphorus intake, an intracellular shift of phosphorus, or an increase in phosphorus excretion. Decreased GI uptake due to malabsorption or administration of phosphate binders and decreased dietary intake from malnutrition are causes of chronic hypophosphatemia. Most acute cases are due to an intracellular shift of phosphorus in association with respiratory alkalosis, insulin therapy, refeeding syndrome, and hungry bone syndrome. Clinical manifestations of hypophosphatemia usually are absent until levels fall significantly. In general, symptoms are related to adverse effects on the oxygen availability of tissue and to a decrease in high-energy phosphates, and can be manifested as cardiac dysfunction or muscle weakness.

Magnesium Abnormalities

Magnesium is the fourth most common mineral in the body and, like potassium, is found primarily in the intracellular compartments. Approximately one half of the total body content of 2000 mEq is incorporated in bone and is slowly exchangeable. Of the fraction found in the extracellular space, one third is bound to serum albumin. Therefore, the plasma level of magnesium may be a poor indicator of total body stores in the presence of hypoalbuminemia. Magnesium should be replaced until levels are in the upper limit of normal. The normal dietary intake is approximately 20 mEq/d and is excreted in both the feces and urine. The kidneys have a remarkable ability to conserve magnesium, with renal excretion <1 mEq/d during magnesium deficiency.

Hypermagnesemia Hypermagnesemia is rare but can be seen with severe renal insufficiency and parallel changes in potassium excretion. Magnesium-containing antacids and laxatives can produce toxic levels in patients with renal failure. Excess intake in conjunction with TPN, or rarely massive trauma, thermal injury, and severe acidosis, may be associated with symptomatic hypermagnesemia. Clinical examination (see Table 3-6) may find nausea and vomiting; neuromuscular dysfunction with weakness, lethargy, and hyporeflexia; and impaired cardiac conduction leading to hypotension and arrest. ECG changes are similar to those seen with hyperkalemia and include increased PR interval, widened QRS complex, and elevated T waves.

Hypomagnesemia Magnesium depletion is a common problem in hospitalized patients, particularly in the critically ill.[16] The kidney is primarily responsible for magnesium homeostasis through regula-

tion by calcium/magnesium receptors on the renal tubular cells that respond to serum magnesium concentrations.[17] Hypomagnesemia may result from alterations of intake, renal excretion, and pathologic losses. Poor intake may occur in cases of starvation, alcoholism, prolonged IV fluid therapy, and TPN with inadequate supplementation of magnesium. Losses are seen in cases of increased renal excretion from alcohol abuse, diuretic use, administration of amphotericin B, and primary aldosteronism, as well as GI losses from diarrhea, malabsorption, and acute pancreatitis. The magnesium ion is essential for proper function of many enzyme systems. Depletion is characterized by neuromuscular and central nervous system hyperactivity. Symptoms are similar to those of calcium deficiency, including hyperactive reflexes, muscle tremors, tetany, and positive Chvostek's and Trousseau's signs (see Table 3-6). Severe deficiencies can lead to delirium and seizures. A number of ECG changes also can occur and include prolonged QT and PR intervals, ST-segment depression, flattening or inversion of P waves, torsades de pointes, and arrhythmias. Hypomagnesemia is important not only because of its direct effects on the nervous system but also because it can produce hypocalcemia and lead to persistent hypokalemia. When hypokalemia or hypocalcemia coexists with hypomagnesemia, magnesium should be aggressively replaced to assist in restoring potassium or calcium homeostasis.

Acid-Base Balance
Acid-Base Homeostasis

The pH of body fluids is maintained within a narrow range despite the ability of the kidneys to generate large amounts of HCO_3^- and the normal large acid load produced as a by-product of metabolism. This endogenous acid load is efficiently neutralized by buffer systems and ultimately excreted by the lungs and kidneys.

Important buffers include intracellular proteins and phosphates and the extracellular bicarbonate–carbonic acid system. Compensation for acid-base derangements can be by respiratory mechanisms (for metabolic derangements) or metabolic mechanisms (for respiratory derangements). Changes in ventilation in response to metabolic abnormalities are mediated by hydrogen-sensitive chemoreceptors found in the carotid body and brain stem. Acidosis stimulates the chemoreceptors to increase ventilation, whereas alkalosis decreases the activity of the chemoreceptors and thus decreases ventilation. The kidneys provide compensation for respiratory abnormalities by either increasing or decreasing bicarbonate reabsorption in response to respiratory acidosis or alkalosis, respectively. Unlike the prompt change in ventilation that occurs with metabolic abnormalities, the compensatory response in the kidneys to respiratory abnormalities is delayed. Significant compensation may not begin for 6 hours and then may continue for several days. Because of this delayed compensatory response, respiratory acid-base derangements before renal compensation are classified as acute, whereas those persisting after renal compensation are categorized as chronic. The predicted compensatory changes in response to metabolic or respiratory derangements are listed in Table 3-7.[18] If the predicted change in pH is exceeded, then a mixed acid-base abnormality may be present (Table 3-8).

TABLE 3-7	Predicted changes in acid-base disorders
Disorder	**Predicted Change**
Metabolic	
Metabolic acidosis	$Pco_2 = 1.5 \times HCO_3^- + 8$
Metabolic alkalosis	$Pco_2 = 0.7 \times HCO_3^- + 21$
Respiratory	
Acute respiratory acidosis	$\Delta pH = (Pco_2 - 40) \times 0.008$
Chronic respiratory acidosis	$\Delta pH = (Pco_2 - 40) \times 0.003$
Acute respiratory alkalosis	$\Delta pH = (40 - Pco_2) \times 0.008$
Chronic respiratory alkalosis	$\Delta pH = (40 - Pco_2) \times 0.017$

Pco_2 = partial pressure of carbon dioxide.

TABLE 3-8 Respiratory and metabolic components of acid-base disorders

Type of Acid-Base Disorder	Acute Uncompensated			Chronic (Partially Compensated)		
	pH	PCO₂ (Respiratory Component)	Plasma HCO₃⁻ᵃ (Metabolic Component)	pH	PCO₂ (Respiratory Component)	Plasma HCO₃⁻ᵃ (Metabolic Component)
Respiratory acidosis	↓↓	↑↑	N	↓	↑↑	↑
Respiratory alkalosis	↑↑	↓↓	N	↑	↓↓	↓
Metabolic acidosis	↓↓	N	↓↓	↓	↓	↓
Metabolic alkalosis	↑↑	N	↑↑	↑	↑?	↑

ᵃMeasured as standard bicarbonate, whole blood buffer base, CO₂ content, or CO₂ combining power. The *base excess value* is positive when the standard bicarbonate is above normal and negative when the standard bicarbonate is below normal.

N = normal; PCO₂ = partial pressure of carbon dioxide.

Metabolic Derangements

Metabolic Acidosis Metabolic acidosis results from an increased intake of acids, an increased generation of acids, or an increased loss of bicarbonate (Table 3-9). The body responds by several mechanisms, including producing buffers (extracellular bicarbonate and intracellular buffers from bone and muscle), increasing ventilation (Kussmaul's respirations), and increasing renal reabsorption and generation of bicarbonate. The kidney also will increase secretion of hydrogen and thus increase urinary excretion of NH_4^+ ($H^+ + NH_3^+$ = NH_4^+). Evaluation of a patient with a low serum bicarbonate level and metabolic acidosis includes determination of the anion gap (AG), an index of unmeasured anions.

$$AG = (Na) - (Cl + HCO_3)$$

The normal AG is <12 mmol/L and is due primarily to the albumin effect, so that the estimated AG must be adjusted for albumin (hypoalbuminemia reduces the AG).[19]

$$Corrected\ AG = actual\ AG - [2.5(4.5 - albumin)]$$

Metabolic acidosis with an increased AG occurs either from ingestion of exogenous acid such as from ethylene glycol, salicylates, or methanol, or from increased endogenous acid production of the following:

β-Hydroxybutyrate and acetoacetate in ketoacidosis
Lactate in lactic acidosis
Organic acids in renal insufficiency

A common cause of severe metabolic acidosis in surgical patients is lactic acidosis. In circulatory shock, lactate is produced in the presence of hypoxia from inadequate tissue perfusion. The treatment is to restore perfusion with volume resuscitation rather than to attempt to correct the abnormality with exogenous bicarbonate.

TABLE 3-9 Etiology of metabolic acidosis

Increased Anion Gap Metabolic Acidosis
Exogenous acid ingestion
   Ethylene glycol
   Salicylate
   Methanol
Endogenous acid production
   Ketoacidosis
   Lactic acidosis
   Renal insufficiency
Normal Anion Gap
Acid administration (HCl)
Loss of bicarbonate
GI losses (diarrhea, fistulas)
Ureterosigmoidoscopy
Renal tubular acidosis
Carbonic anhydrase inhibitor

With adequate perfusion, the lactic acid is rapidly metabolized by the liver and the pH level returns to normal. The administration of bicarbonate for the treatment of metabolic acidosis is controversial, because it is not clear that acidosis is deleterious.[20] The overzealous administration of bicarbonate can lead to metabolic alkalosis, which shifts the oxyhemoglobin dissociation curve to the left; this interferes with oxygen unloading at the tissue level and can be associated with arrhythmias that are difficult to treat. An additional disadvantage is that sodium bicarbonate actually can exacerbate intracellular acidosis. Administered bicarbonate can combine with the excess hydrogen ions to form carbonic acid; this is then converted to CO_2 and water, which thus raises the partial pressure of CO_2 (PCO₂). This hypercarbia could compound ventilation abnormalities in patients with underlying acute respiratory distress syndrome. This CO_2 can diffuse into cells, but bicarbonate remains extracellular, which thus worsens intracellular acidosis. Clinically, lactate levels may not be useful in directing resuscitation, although lactate levels may be higher in nonsurvivors of serious injury.[21]

Metabolic acidosis with a normal AG results either from exogenous acid administration (HCl or NH_4^+), from loss of bicarbonate due to GI disorders such as diarrhea and fistulas or ureterosigmoidostomy, or from renal losses. In these settings, the bicarbonate loss is accompanied by a gain of chloride; thus, the AG remains unchanged. To determine if the loss of bicarbonate has a renal cause, the urinary [NH_4^+] can be measured. A low urinary [NH_4^+] in the face of hyperchloremic acidosis would indicate that the kidney is the site of loss, and evaluation for renal tubular acidosis should be undertaken. Proximal renal tubular acidosis results from decreased tubular reabsorption of HCO_3^-, whereas distal renal tubular acidosis results from decreased acid excretion. The carbonic anhydrase inhibitor acetazolamide also causes bicarbonate loss from the kidneys.

Metabolic Alkalosis Normal acid-base homeostasis prevents metabolic alkalosis from developing unless both an increase in bicarbonate generation and impaired renal excretion of bicarbonate occur (Table 3-10). Metabolic alkalosis results from the loss of fixed acids or the gain of bicarbonate and is worsened by potassium depletion. The majority of patients also will have hypokalemia, because extracellular potassium ions exchange with intracellular hydrogen ions and allow the hydrogen ions to buffer excess HCO_3^-. Hypochloremic, hypokalemic, and metabolic alkalosis can occur from isolated loss of gastric contents in infants with pyloric stenosis or adults with duodenal ulcer disease. Unlike vomiting associated with an open pylorus, which involves a loss of gastric as well as pancreatic, biliary, and intestinal secretions, vomiting with an obstructed pylorus results only in the loss of gastric fluid, which is high in chloride and hydrogen, and therefore results in a hypochloremic alkalosis. Initially the urinary bicarbonate level is high in compensation for the alkalosis. Hydrogen ion reabsorption also ensues, with an accompanied potassium ion excretion. In response to the associated volume deficit, aldosterone-mediated sodium reabsorption increases potassium excretion. The resulting hypokalemia leads to the excretion of hydrogen ions in the face of alkalosis, a paradoxic

TABLE 3-10 Etiology of metabolic alkalosis

Increased bicarbonate generation
1. Chloride losing (urinary chloride >20 mEq/L)
   Mineralocorticoid excess
   Profound potassium depletion
2. Chloride sparing (urinary chloride <20 mEq/L)
   Loss from gastric secretions (emesis or nasogastric suction)
   Diuretics
3. Excess administration of alkali
   Acetate in parenteral nutrition
   Citrate in blood transfusions
   Antacids
   Bicarbonate
   Milk-alkali syndrome

Impaired bicarbonate excretion
1. Decreased glomerular filtration
2. Increased bicarbonate reabsorption (hypercarbia or potassium depletion)

TABLE 3-11 Etiology of respiratory acidosis: hypoventilation

Narcotics
Central nervous system injury
Pulmonary: significant
  Secretions
  Atelectasis
  Mucus plug
  Pneumonia
  Pleural effusion
Pain from abdominal or thoracic injuries or incisions
Limited diaphragmatic excursion from intra-abdominal pathology
  Abdominal distention
  Abdominal compartment syndrome
  Ascites

aciduria. Treatment includes replacement of the volume deficit with isotonic saline and then potassium replacement once adequate urine output is achieved.

Respiratory Derangements

Under normal circumstances blood PCO_2 is tightly maintained by alveolar ventilation, controlled by the respiratory centers in the pons and medulla oblongata.

Respiratory Acidosis Respiratory acidosis is associated with the retention of CO_2 secondary to decreased alveolar ventilation. The principal causes are listed in Table 3-11. Because compensation is primarily a renal mechanism, it is a delayed response. Treatment of acute respiratory acidosis is directed at the underlying cause. Measures to ensure adequate ventilation are also initiated. This may entail patient-initiated volume expansion using noninvasive bilevel positive airway pressure or may require endotracheal intubation to increase minute ventilation. In the chronic form of respiratory acidosis, the partial pressure of arterial CO_2 remains elevated and the bicarbonate concentration rises slowly as renal compensation occurs.

Respiratory Alkalosis In the surgical patient, most cases of respiratory alkalosis are acute and secondary to alveolar hyperventilation. Causes include pain, anxiety, and neurologic disorders, including central nervous system injury and assisted ventilation. Drugs such as salicylates, fever, gram-negative bacteremia, thyrotoxicosis, and hypoxemia are other possibilities. Acute hypocapnia can cause an uptake of potassium and phosphate into cells and increased binding of calcium to albumin, leading to symptomatic hypokalemia, hypophosphatemia, and hypocalcemia with subsequent arrhythmias, paresthesias, muscle cramps, and seizures. Treatment should be directed at the underlying cause, but direct treatment of the hyperventilation using controlled ventilation may also be required.

FLUID AND ELECTROLYTE THERAPY

Parenteral Solutions

A number of commercially available electrolyte solutions are available for parenteral administration. The most commonly used solutions are listed in Table 3-12. The type of fluid administered depends on the patient's volume status and the type of concentration or compositional abnormality present. Both lactated Ringer's solution and normal saline are considered isotonic and are useful in replacing GI losses and correcting extracellular volume deficits. Lactated Ringer's is slightly hypotonic in that it contains 130 mEq of lactate. Lactate is used rather than bicarbonate because it is more stable in IV fluids during storage. It is converted into bicarbonate by the liver after infusion, even in the face of hemorrhagic shock. Evidence has suggested that resuscitation using lactated Ringer's may be deleterious because it activates the inflammatory response and induces apoptosis. The component that has been implicated is the D isomer of lactate, which unlike the L isomer is not a normal intermediary in mammalian metabolism.[22] However, subsequent in vivo studies showed significantly lower levels of apoptosis in lung and liver tissue after resuscitation with any of the various Ringer's formulations.[23]

Sodium chloride is mildly hypertonic, containing 154 mEq of sodium that is balanced by 154 mEq of chloride. The high chloride concentration imposes a significant chloride load on the kidneys and may lead to a hyperchloremic metabolic acidosis. Sodium chloride is an ideal solution, however, for correcting volume deficits associated with hyponatremia, hypochloremia, and metabolic alkalosis.

The less concentrated sodium solutions, such as 0.45% sodium chloride, are useful for replacement of ongoing GI losses as well as for maintenance fluid therapy in the postoperative period. This solution provides sufficient free water for insensible losses and enough sodium to aid the kidneys in adjustment of serum sodium levels. The addition of 5% dextrose (50 g of dextrose per liter) supplies 200 kcal/L, and

TABLE 3-12 Electrolyte solutions for parenteral administration

Solution	Electrolyte Composition (mEq/L)						
	Na	CL	K	HCO$_3^-$	Ca	Mg	mOsm
Extracellular fluid	142	103	4	27	5	3	280–310
Lactated Ringer's	130	109	4	28	3		273
0.9% Sodium chloride	154	154					308
D$_5$ 0.45% Sodium chloride	77	77					407
D$_5$W							253
3% Sodium chloride	513	513					1026

D$_5$ = 5% dextrose; D$_5$W = 5% dextrose in water.

TABLE 3-13 Alternative resuscitative fluids

Solution	Molecular Weight	Osmolality (mOsm/L)	Sodium (mEq/L)
Hypertonic saline (7.5%)	—	2565	1283
Albumin 5%	70,000	300	130–160
Albumin 25%	70,000	1500	130–160
Dextran 40	40,000	308	154
Dextran 70	70,000	308	154
Hetastarch	450,000	310	154
Hextend	670,000	307	143
Gelofusine	30,000	NA	154

NA = not available.

CHAPTER 3

Fluid and Electrolyte Management of the Surgical Patient

dextrose is always added to solutions containing <0.45% sodium chloride to maintain osmolality and thus prevent the lysis of red blood cells that may occur with rapid infusion of hypotonic fluids. The addition of potassium is useful once adequate renal function and urine output are established.

Alternative Resuscitative Fluids

A number of alternative solutions for volume expansion and resuscitation are available (Table 3-13).[24] Hypertonic saline solutions (3.5% and 5%) are used for correction of severe sodium deficits and are discussed elsewhere in this chapter. Hypertonic saline (7.5%) has been used as a treatment modality in patients with closed head injuries. It has been shown to increase cerebral perfusion and decrease intracranial pressure, thus decreasing brain edema.[25] However, there also have been concerns of increased bleeding, because hypertonic saline is an arteriolar vasodilator. A meta-analysis of the results of prospective randomized controlled trials in trauma patients suggests that hypertonic saline may be no better than standard-of-care isotonic saline.[26] In subgroup analysis, however, patients with shock and concomitant closed head injury did demonstrate benefit.

Colloids also are used in surgical patients, and their effectiveness as volume expanders compared with isotonic crystalloids has long been debated. Due to their molecular weight, they are confined to the intravascular space, and their infusion results in more efficient transient plasma volume expansion. However, under conditions of severe hemorrhagic shock, capillary membrane permeability increases; this permits colloids to enter the interstitial space, which can worsen edema and impair tissue oxygenation. The theory that these high molecular weight agents "plug" capillary leaks which occur during neutrophil-mediated organ injury has not been confirmed.[27,28] Four major types of colloids are available—albumin, dextrans, hetastarch, and gelatins—that are described by their molecular weight and size in Table 3-13. Colloid solutions with smaller particles and lower molecular weights exert a greater oncotic effect but are retained within the circulation for a shorter period of time than larger and higher molecular weight colloids.

Albumin (molecular weight 70,000) is prepared from heat-sterilized pooled human plasma. It is typically available as either a 5% solution (osmolality of 300 mOsm/L) or 25% solution (osmolality of 1500 mOsm/L). Because it is a derivative of blood, it can be associated with allergic reactions. Albumin has been shown to induce renal failure and impair pulmonary function when used for resuscitation in hemorrhagic shock.[29]

Dextrans are glucose polymers produced by bacteria grown on sucrose media and are available as either 40,000 or 70,000 molecular weight solutions. They lead to initial volume expansion due to their osmotic effect but are associated with alterations in blood viscosity. Thus dextrans are used primarily to lower blood viscosity rather than as volume expanders. Dextrans have been used, in association with hypertonic saline, to help maintain intravascular volume.

Hydroxyethyl starch solutions are another group of alternative plasma expanders and volume replacement solutions. Hetastarches are produced by the hydrolysis of insoluble amylopectin, followed by a varying number of substitutions of hydroxyl groups for carbon groups on the glucose molecules. The molecular weights can range from 1000 to 3,000,000. The high molecular weight hydroxyethyl starch hetastarch, which comes as a 6% solution, is the only hydroxyethyl starch approved for use in the United States. Administration of hetastarch can cause hemostatic derangements related to decreases in von Willebrand's factor and factor VIII:c, and its use has been associated with postoperative bleeding in cardiac and neurosurgery patients.[30,31] Hetastarch also can induce renal dysfunction in patients with septic shock and in recipients of kidneys procured from brain-dead donors.[32,33] Currently, hetastarch has a limited role in massive resuscitation because of the associated coagulopathy and hyperchloremic acidosis (due to its high chloride content). Hextend is a modified, balanced, high molecular weight hydroxyethyl starch that is suspended in a lactate-buffered solution, rather than in saline. A phase III clinical study comparing Hextend to a similar 6% hydroxyethyl starch in patients undergoing major abdominal surgery demonstrated no adverse effects on coagulation with Hextend other than the known effects of hemodilution.[34] Hextend has not been tested for use in massive resuscitation, and not all clinical studies show consistent results.[35]

Gelatins are the fourth group of colloids and are produced from bovine collagen. The two major types are urea-linked gelatin and succinylated gelatin (modified fluid gelatin, Gelofusine). Gelofusine has been used abroad with mixed results.[36] Like many other artificial plasma volume expanders, it has been shown to impair whole blood coagulation time in human volunteers.[37]

Correction of Life-Threatening Electrolyte Abnormalities[38]

Sodium

Hypernatremia Treatment of hypernatremia usually consists of treatment of the associated water deficit. In hypovolemic patients, volume should be restored with normal saline before the concentration abnormality is addressed. Once adequate volume has been achieved, the water deficit is replaced using a hypotonic fluid such as 5% dextrose, 5% dextrose in $\frac{1}{4}$ normal saline, or enterally administered water. The formula used to estimate the amount of water required to correct hypernatremia is as follows:

$$\text{Water deficit (L)} = \frac{\text{serum sodium} - 140}{140} \times \text{TBW}$$

Estimate TBW as 50% of lean body mass in men and 40% in women

The rate of fluid administration should be titrated to achieve a decrease in serum sodium concentration of no more than 1 mEq/h and 12 mEq/d for the treatment of acute symptomatic hypernatremia. Even slower correction should be undertaken for chronic hypernatremia (0.7 mEq/h), because overly rapid correction can lead to cerebral edema and herniation. The type of fluid used depends on the severity and ease of correction. Oral or enteral replacement is acceptable in most cases, or IV replacement with half- or quarter-normal saline can be used. Caution also should be exercised when using 5% dextrose in water to avoid overly rapid correction. Frequent neurologic evaluation as well as frequent evaluation of serum sodium levels also should be performed.

Hyponatremia Most cases of hyponatremia can be treated by free water restriction and, if severe, the administration of sodium. In patients with normal renal function, symptomatic hyponatremia does not occur until the serum sodium level is ≤20 mEq/L. If neurologic symptoms are present, 3% normal saline should be used to increase the sodium by no more than 1 mEq/L per hour until the serum sodium level reaches 130 mEq/L or neurologic symptoms are improved. Correction of asymptomatic hyponatremia should in-

TABLE 3-14	Treatment of symptomatic hyperkalemia

Potassium removal
  Kayexalate
    Oral administration is 15–30 g in 50–100 mL of 20% sorbitol
    Rectal administration is 50 g in 200 mL of 20% sorbitol
  Dialysis
Shift potassium
  Glucose 1 ampule of D_{50} and regular insulin 5–10 units IV
  Bicarbonate 1 ampule IV
Counteract cardiac effects
  Calcium gluconate 5–10 mL of 10% solution

D_{50} = 50% dextrose.

crease the sodium level by no more than 0.5 mEq/L per hour to a maximum increase of 12 mEq/L per day, and even more slowly in chronic hyponatremia. The rapid correction of hyponatremia can lead to pontine myelinolysis,[39] with seizures, weakness, paresis, akinetic movements, and unresponsiveness, and may result in permanent brain damage and death. Magnetic resonance imaging may assist in the diagnosis.[40]

Potassium

Hyperkalemia Treatment options for symptomatic hyperkalemia are listed in Table 3-14. The goals of therapy include reducing the total body potassium, shifting potassium from the extracellular to the intracellular space, and protecting the cells from the effects of increased potassium. For all patients exogenous sources of potassium should be removed, including potassium supplementation in IV fluids and enteral and parenteral solutions. Potassium can be removed from the body using a cation-exchange resin such as Kayexalate that binds potassium in exchange for sodium. It can be administered either orally, in alert patients, or rectally. Immediate measures also should include attempts to shift potassium intracellularly with glucose and bicarbonate infusion. Nebulized albuterol (10 to 20 mg) may also be used. Use of glucose alone will cause a rise in insulin secretion, but in the acutely ill this response may be blunted, and therefore both glucose and insulin may be necessary. Circulatory overload and hypernatremia may result from the administration of Kayexalate and bicarbonate, so care should be exercised when administering these agents to patients with fragile cardiac function. When ECG changes are present, calcium chloride or calcium gluconate (5 to 10 mL of 10% solution) should be administered immediately to counteract the myocardial effects of hyperkalemia. Calcium infusion should be used cautiously in patients receiving digitalis, because digitalis toxicity may be precipitated. All of the aforementioned measures are temporary, lasting from 1 to approximately 4 hours. Dialysis should be considered in severe hyperkalemia when conservative measures fail.

Hypokalemia Treatment for hypokalemia consists of potassium repletion, the rate of which is determined by the symptoms (Table 3-15). Oral repletion is adequate for mild, asymptomatic hypokalemia. If IV repletion is required, usually no more than 10 mEq/h is advisable in an unmonitored setting. This amount can be increased to 40 mEq/h when accompanied by continuous ECG monitoring, and even more in the case of imminent cardiac arrest from a malignant arrhythmia associated hypokalemia. Caution should be exercised when oliguria or impaired renal function is coexistent.

Calcium

Hypercalcemia Treatment is required when hypercalcemia is symptomatic, which usually occurs when the serum level exceeds 12 mg/dL. The critical level for serum calcium is 15 mg/dL, when symptoms noted earlier may rapidly progress to death. The initial treatment is aimed at repleting the associated volume deficit and then inducing a brisk diuresis with normal saline. Treatment of hypercalcemia associated with malignancies is discussed later in this chapter.

TABLE 3-15	Electrolyte replacement therapy protocol

Potassium
Serum potassium level <4.0 mEq/L:
  Asymptomatic, tolerating enteral nutrition: KCl 40 mEq per enteral access × 1 dose
  Asymptomatic, not tolerating enteral nutrition: KCl 20 mEq IV q2h × 2 doses
  Symptomatic: KCl 20 mEq IV q1h × 4 doses
  Recheck potassium level 2 h after end of infusion; if <3.5 mEq/L and asymptomatic, replace as per above protocol
Magnesium
Magnesium level 1.0–1.8 mEq/L:
  Magnesium sulfate 0.5 mEq/kg in normal saline 250 mL infused IV over 24 h × 3 d
  Recheck magnesium level in 3 d
Magnesium level <1.0 mEq/L:
  Magnesium sulfate 1 mEq/kg in normal saline 250 mL infused IV over 24 h × 1 d, then 0.5 mEq/kg in normal saline 250 mL infused IV over 24 h × 2 d
  Recheck magnesium level in 3 d
If patient has gastric access and needs a bowel regimen:
  Milk of magnesia 15 mL (approximately 49 mEq magnesium) q24h per gastric tube; hold for diarrhea
Calcium
Normalized calcium level <4.0 mg/dL:
  With gastric access and tolerating enteral nutrition: Calcium carbonate suspension 1250 mg/5 mL q6h per gastric access; recheck ionized calcium level in 3 d
  Without gastric access or not tolerating enteral nutrition: Calcium gluconate 2 g IV over 1 h × 1 dose; recheck ionized calcium level in 3 d
Phosphate
Phosphate level 1.0–2.5 mg/dL:
  Tolerating enteral nutrition: Neutra-Phos 2 packets q6h per gastric tube or feeding tube
  No enteral nutrition: $KPHO_4$ or $NaPO_4$ 0.15 mmol/kg IV over 6 h × 1 dose
  Recheck phosphate level in 3 d
Phosphate level <1.0 mg/dL:
  Tolerating enteral nutrition: $KPHO_4$ or $NaPO_4$ 0.25 mmol/kg over 6 h × 1 dose
  Recheck phosphate level 4 h after end of infusion; if <2.5 mg/dL, begin Neutra-Phos 2 packets q6h
  Not tolerating enteral nutrition: $KPHO_4$ or $NaPO_4$ 0.25 mmol/kg (LBW) over 6 h × 1 dose; recheck phosphate level 4 h after end of infusion; if <2.5 mg/dL, then $KPHO_4$ or $NaPO_4$ 0.15 mmol/kg (LBW) IV over 6 h × 1 dose

3 mmol $KPHO_4$ = 3 mmol Phos and 4.4 mEq K^+ = 1 mL
3 mmol $NaPO_4$ = 3 mmol Phos and 4 mEq Na^+ = 1 mL
Neutra-Phos 1 packet = 8 mmol Phos, 7 mEq K^+, 7 mEq Na^+
Use patient's lean body weight (LBW) in kilograms for all calculations.
Disregard protocol if patient has renal failure, is on dialysis, or has a creatinine clearance <30 mL/min.

Hypocalcemia Asymptomatic hypocalcemia can be treated with oral or IV calcium (see Table 3-15). Acute symptomatic hypocalcemia should be treated with IV 10% calcium gluconate to achieve a serum concentration of 7 to 9 mg/dL. Associated deficits in magnesium, potassium, and pH must also be corrected. Hypocalcemia will be refractory to treatment if coexisting hypomagnesemia is not corrected first. Routine calcium supplementation is no longer recommended in association with massive blood transfusions.[41]

Phosphorus

Hyperphosphatemia Phosphate binders such as sucralfate or aluminum-containing antacids can be used to lower serum phosphorus levels. Calcium acetate tablets also are useful when hypocalcemia is simultaneously present. Dialysis usually is reserved for patients with renal failure.

Hypophosphatemia Depending on the level of depletion and tolerance to oral supplementation, a number of enteral and parenteral repletion strategies are effective for the treatment of hypophosphatemia (see Table 3-15).

Magnesium

Hypermagnesemia Treatment for hypermagnesemia consists of measures to eliminate exogenous sources of magnesium, correct concurrent volume deficits, and correct acidosis if present. To manage acute symptoms, calcium chloride (5 to 10 mL) should be administered to immediately antagonize the cardiovascular effects. If elevated levels or symptoms persist, hemodialysis may be necessary.

Hypomagnesemia Correction of magnesium depletion can be oral if asymptomatic and mild. Otherwise, IV repletion is indicated and depends on severity (see Table 3-15) and clinical symptoms. For those with severe deficits (<1.0 mEq/L) or those who are symptomatic, 1 to 2 g of magnesium sulfate may be administered IV over 15 minutes. Under ECG monitoring, it may be given over 2 minutes if necessary to correct torsades de pointes (irregular ventricular rhythm). Caution should be taken when giving large amounts of magnesium, because magnesium toxicity may develop. The simultaneous administration of calcium gluconate will counteract the adverse side effects of a rapidly rising magnesium level and correct hypocalcemia, which is frequently associated with hypomagnesemia.

Preoperative Fluid Therapy

The administration of maintenance fluids should be all that is required in an otherwise healthy individual who may be under orders to receive nothing by mouth for some period before the time of surgery. This does not, however, include replenishment of a pre-existing deficit or ongoing fluid losses. The following is a frequently used formula for calculating the volume of maintenance fluids in the absence of pre-existing abnormalities:

For the first 0 to 10 kg	Give 100 mL/kg per day
For the next 10 to 20 kg	Give an additional 50 mL/kg per day
For weight >20 kg	Give an additional 20 mL/kg per day

For example, a 60-kg female would receive a total of 2100 mL of fluid daily: 1000 mL for the first 10 kg of body weight (10 kg × 100 mL/kg per day), 500 mL for the next 20 kg (10 kg × 50 mL/kg per day), and 80 mL for the last 40 kg (40 kg × 20 mL/kg per day).

An alternative approach is to replace the calculated daily water losses in urine, stool, and insensible loss with a hypotonic saline solution rather than water alone, which allows the kidney some sodium excess to adjust for concentration. Although there should be no "routine" maintenance fluid orders, both of these methods would yield an appropriate choice of 5% dextrose in 0.45% sodium chloride at 100 mL/h as initial therapy, with potassium added for patients with normal renal function. However, many surgical patients have volume and/or electrolyte abnormalities associated with their surgical disease. Preoperative evaluation of a patient's volume status and pre-existing electrolyte abnormalities is an important part of overall preoperative assessment and care. Volume deficits should be considered in patients who have obvious GI losses, such as through emesis or diarrhea, as well as in patients with poor oral intake secondary to their disease. Less obvious are those fluid losses known as *third-space* or *nonfunctional* ECF losses that occur with GI obstruction, peritoneal or bowel inflammation, ascites, crush injuries, burns, and severe soft tissue infections such as necrotizing fasciitis. The diagnosis of an acute volume deficit is primarily clinical (see Table 3-2), although the physical signs may vary with the duration of the deficit. Cardiovascular signs of tachycardia and orthostasis predominate with acute volume loss, usually accompanied by oliguria and hemoconcentration. Acute volume deficits should be corrected as much as possible before the time of operation.

Once a volume deficit is diagnosed, prompt fluid replacement should be instituted, usually with an isotonic crystalloid, depending on the measured serum electrolyte values. Patients with cardiovascular signs of volume deficit should receive a bolus of 1 to 2 L of isotonic fluid followed by a continuous infusion. Close monitoring during this period is imperative. Resuscitation should be guided by the reversal of the signs of volume deficit, such as restoration of acceptable values for vital signs, maintenance of adequate urine output ($^1/_2$ to 1 mL/kg per hour in an adult), and correction of base deficit. Patients whose volume deficit is not corrected after this initial volume challenge and those with impaired renal function and the elderly should be considered for more intensive monitoring in an intensive care unit setting. In these patients, early invasive monitoring of central venous pressure or cardiac output may be necessary.

If symptomatic electrolyte abnormalities accompany volume deficit, the abnormality should be corrected to the point that the acute symptom is relieved before surgical intervention. For correction of severe hypernatremia associated with a volume deficit, an unsafe rapid fall in extracellular osmolarity from 5% dextrose infusion is avoided by slowly correcting the hypernatremia with 0.45% saline or even lactated Ringer's solution rather than 5% dextrose alone. This will safely and slowly correct the hypernatremia while also correcting the associated volume deficit.

Intraoperative Fluid Therapy

With the induction of anesthesia, compensatory mechanisms are lost, and hypotension will develop if volume deficits are not appropriately corrected before the time of surgery. Hemodynamic instability during anesthesia is best avoided by correcting known fluid losses, replacing ongoing losses, and providing adequate maintenance fluid therapy preoperatively. In addition to measured blood loss, major open abdominal surgeries are associated with continued extracellular losses in the form of bowel wall edema, peritoneal fluid, and the wound edema during surgery. Large soft tissue wounds, complex fractures with associated soft tissue injury, and burns are all associated with additional third-space losses that must be considered in the operating room. These represent distributional shifts, in that the functional volume of ECF is reduced but fluid is not externally lost from the body. These functional losses have been referred to as *parasitic losses, sequestration,* or *third-space edema,* because the lost volume no longer participates in the normal functions of the ECF.

Until the 1960s saline solutions were withheld during surgery. Administered saline was retained and was felt to be an inappropriate challenge to a physiologic response of intraoperative salt intolerance. Basic and clinical research began to change this concept,[42,43] eventually leading to the current concept that saline administration is necessary to restore the obligate ECF losses noted earlier. Although no accurate formula can predict intraoperative fluid needs, replacement of ECF during surgery often requires 500 to 1000 mL/hr of a balanced salt solution to support homeostasis. The addition of albumin or other colloid-containing solutions to intraoperative fluid therapy is not necessary. Manipulation of colloid oncotic forces by albumin infusion during major vascular surgery showed no advantage in supporting cardiac function or avoiding the accumulation of extravascular lung water.[44]

Postoperative Fluid Therapy

Postoperative fluid therapy should be based on the patient's current estimated volume status and projected ongoing fluid losses. Any deficits from either preoperative or intraoperative losses should be corrected and ongoing requirements should be included along with maintenance fluids. Third-space losses, although difficult to measure, should be included in fluid replacement strategies. In the initial postoperative period, an isotonic solution should be administered. The adequacy of resuscitation should be guided by the restoration of acceptable values for vital signs and urine output and, in more complicated cases, by the correction of base deficit or lactate. If uncertainty exists, particularly in patients with renal or cardiac dysfunction, a central venous catheter or Swan-Ganz catheter may be inserted to help guide fluid therapy. After the initial 24 to 48 hours, fluids can be changed to 5% dextrose in 0.45% saline in patients unable to tolerate enteral nutrition. If normal renal function and adequate urine output are present, potassium may be added to the IV fluids. Daily fluid orders should begin with assessment of the patient's volume status and assessment of electrolyte abnormalities. There is rarely a need to check electrolyte levels in the first few days of an uncomplicated postoperative course. However, postoperative diuresis may require attention to replacement of urinary potassium loss. All measured losses, including losses through vomiting, nasogastric suctioning, drains, and urine output, as well as insensible losses, are replaced with the appropriate parenteral solutions as previously reviewed.

Special Considerations for the Postoperative Patient

Volume excess is a common disorder in the postoperative period. The administration of isotonic fluids in excess of actual needs may result in excess volume expansion. This may be due to the overestimation of third-space losses or to ongoing GI losses that are difficult to measure accurately. The earliest sign of volume overload is weight gain. The average postoperative patient who is not receiving nutritional support should lose approximately 0.25 to 0.5 lb/d (0.11 to 0.23 kg/d) from catabolism. Additional signs of volume excess may also be present as listed in Table 3-2. Peripheral edema may not necessarily be associated with volume overload, because overexpansion of total ECF may exist in association with a deficit in the circulating plasma volume.

Volume deficits also can be encountered in surgical patients if preoperative losses were not completely corrected, intraoperative losses were underestimated, or postoperative losses were greater than appreciated. The clinical manifestations are described in Table 3-2 and include tachycardia, orthostasis, and oliguria. Hemoconcentration also may be present. Treatment will depend on the amount and composition of fluid lost. In most cases of volume depletion, replacement with an isotonic fluid will be sufficient while alterations in concentration and composition are being evaluated.

ELECTROLYTE ABNORMALITIES IN SPECIFIC SURGICAL PATIENTS

Neurologic Patients

Syndrome of Inappropriate Secretion of Antidiuretic Hormone

The syndrome of inappropriate secretion of antidiuretic hormone (SIADH) can occur after head injury or surgery to the central nervous system, but it also is seen in association with administration of drugs such as morphine, nonsteroidals, and oxytocin, and in a number of pulmonary and endocrine diseases, including hypothyroidism and glucocorticoid deficiency. Additionally, it can be seen in association with a number of malignancies, most often small cell cancer of the lung but also pancreatic carcinoma, thymoma, and Hodgkin's disease.[45] SIADH should be considered in patients who are euvolemic and hyponatremic with elevated urine sodium levels and urine osmolality. ADH secretion is considered inappropriate when it is not in response to osmotic or volume-related conditions. Correction of the underlying problem should be attempted when possible. In most cases, restriction of free water will improve the hyponatremia. The goal is to achieve net water balance while avoiding volume depletion that may compromise renal function. Furosemide also can be used to induce free water loss. If hyponatremia persists after fluid restriction, the addition of isotonic or hypertonic fluids may be effective. The administration of isotonic saline may sometimes worsen the problem if the urinary sodium concentration is higher than the infused sodium concentration. The use of loop diuretics may be helpful in this situation by preventing further urine concentration. In chronic SIADH, when long-term

fluid restriction is difficult to maintain or is ineffective, demeclocycline and lithium can be used to induce free water loss.

Diabetes Insipidus

Diabetes insipidus (DI) is a disorder of ADH stimulation and is manifested by dilute urine in the case of hypernatremia. Central DI results from a defect in ADH secretion, and nephrogenic DI from a defect in end-organ responsiveness to ADH. Central DI is frequently seen in association with pituitary surgery, closed head injury, and anoxic encephalopathy.[46] Nephrogenic DI occurs in association with hypokalemia, administration of radiocontrast dye, and use of certain drugs such as aminoglycosides and amphotericin B. In patients tolerating oral intake, volume status usually is normal because thirst stimulates increased intake. However, volume depletion can occur rapidly in patients incapable of oral intake. The diagnosis can be confirmed by documenting a paradoxical increase in urine osmolality in response to a period of water deprivation. In mild cases, free water replacement may be adequate therapy. In more severe cases, vasopressin can be added. The usual dosage of vasopressin is 5 U SC every 6 to 8 hours. However, serum electrolytes and osmolality should be monitored to avoid excess vasopressin administration with resulting iatrogenic SIADH.

Cerebral Salt Washing

Cerebral salt wasting is a diagnosis of exclusion that occurs in patients with a cerebral lesion and renal wasting of sodium and chloride with no other identifiable cause.[47] Natriuresis in a patient with a contracted extracellular volume should prompt the possible diagnosis of cerebral salt wasting. Hyponatremia is frequently observed but is nonspecific and occurs as a secondary event, which differentiates it from SIADH.

Malnourished Patients: Refeeding Syndrome

Refeeding syndrome is a potentially lethal condition that can occur with rapid and excessive feeding of patients with severe underlying malnutrition due to starvation, alcoholism, delayed nutritional support, anorexia nervosa, or massive weight loss in obese patients.[48] With refeeding, a shift in metabolism from fat to carbohydrate substrate stimulates insulin release, which results in the cellular uptake of electrolytes, particularly phosphate, magnesium, potassium, and calcium. However, severe hyperglycemia may result from blunted basal insulin secretion. The refeeding syndrome can be associated with enteral or parenteral refeeding, and symptoms from electrolyte abnormalities include cardiac arrhythmias, confusion, respiratory failure, and even death. To prevent the development of refeeding syndrome, underlying electrolyte and volume deficits should be corrected. Additionally, thiamine should be administered before the initiation of feeding. Caloric repletion should be instituted slowly, at 20 kcal/kg per day, and should gradually increase over the first week.[49] Vital signs, fluid balance, and electrolytes should be closely monitored and any deficits corrected as they evolve.

Acute Renal Failure Patients

A number of fluid and electrolyte abnormalities are specific to patients with acute renal failure. With the onset of renal failure, an accurate assessment of volume status must be made. If prerenal azotemia is present, prompt correction of the underlying volume deficit is mandatory. Once acute tubular necrosis is established, measures should be taken to restrict daily fluid intake to match urine output and insensible and GI losses. Oliguric renal failure requires close monitoring of serum potassium levels. Measures to correct hyperkalemia as reviewed in Table 3-14 should be instituted early, including consideration of early hemodialysis. Hyponatremia is common in established renal failure as a result of the breakdown of proteins, carbohydrates, and fats, as well the administration of free water. Dialysis may be required for severe hyponatremia. Hypocalcemia, hypermagnesemia, and hyperphosphatemia also are associated with acute renal failure. Hypocalcemia should be verified by measuring ionized calcium, because many patients also are hypoalbuminemic. Phosphate binders can be used to control hyperphosphatemia, but dialysis may be required in more severe cases. Metabolic acidosis is commonly seen with renal failure, as the kidneys lose their ability to clear acid by-products. Bicarbonate can be useful, but dialysis often is needed. Although dialysis may be either intermittent or continuous, normalization of sodium, potassium, and bicarbonate levels may be best achieved using continuous therapy.[50]

Cancer Patients

Fluid and electrolyte abnormalities are common in patients with cancer. The causes may be common to all patient populations or may be specific to cancer patients and their treatment.[51] Hyponatremia is frequently hypovolemic due to renal loss of sodium caused by diuretics or salt-wasting nephropathy as seen with some chemotherapeutic agents such as cisplatin. Cerebral salt wasting also can occur in patients with intracerebral lesions. Normovolemic hyponatremia may occur in association with SIADH from cervical cancer, lymphoma, and leukemia, or from certain chemotherapeutic agents. Hypernatremia in cancer patients most often is due to poor oral intake or GI volume losses, which are common side effects of chemotherapy. Central DI also can lead to hypernatremia in patients with central nervous system lesions.

Hypokalemia can develop from GI losses associated with diarrhea caused by radiation enteritis or chemotherapy, or from tumors such as villous adenomas of the colon. Tumor lysis syndrome can precipitate severe hyperkalemia from massive tumor cell destruction.

Hypocalcemia can be seen after removal of a thyroid or parathyroid tumor or after a central neck dissection, which can damage the parathyroid glands. Hungry bone syndrome produces acute and profound hypocalcemia after parathyroid surgery for secondary or tertiary hyperparathyroidism because calcium is rapidly taken up by bones. Prostate and breast cancer can result in increased osteoblastic activity, which decreases serum calcium by increasing bone formation. Acute hypocalcemia also can occur with hyperphosphatemia, because phosphorus complexes with calcium. Hypomagnesemia is a side effect of ifosfamide and cisplatin therapy. Hypophosphatemia can be seen in hyperparathyroidism, due to decreased phosphorus reabsorption, and in oncogenic osteomalacia, which increases the urinary excretion of phosphorus. Other causes of hypophosphatemia in cancer patients include renal tubular dysfunction from multiple myeloma, Bence Jones proteins, and certain chemotherapeutic agents. Acute hypophosphatemia can occur as rapidly proliferating malignant cells take up phosphorus in acute leukemia. Tumor lysis syndrome or the use of bisphosphonates to treat hypercalcemia also can result in hyperphosphatemia.

Malignancy is the most common cause of hypercalcemia in hospitalized patients and is due to increased bone resorption or decreased renal excretion. Bone destruction occurs from bony metastasis as seen in breast or renal cell cancer but also can occur in multiple myeloma. With Hodgkin's and non-Hodgkin's lymphoma, hypercalcemia results from increased calcitriol formation, which increases both absorption of calcium from the GI tract and mobilization from bone. Humoral hypercalcemia of malignancy is a common cause of hypercalcemia in cancer patients. As in primary hyperparathyroidism, a parathyroid-related protein is secreted that binds to parathyroid receptors, stimulating calcium resorption from bone and decreasing renal excretion of calcium. The treatment of hypercalcemia of malignancy should begin with saline volume expansion, which will decrease renal reabsorption of calcium as the associated volume deficit is corrected. Once an adequate volume status has been achieved, a loop diuretic may be added. Unfortunately, these measures are only temporary, and additional treatment is often necessary. A variety of drugs are available with varying times of onset, duration of action, and side effects.[52] The bisphosphonates etidronate and pamidronate inhibit bone resorption and osteoclastic activity. They have a slow onset of action, but effects can last for 2 weeks. Calcitonin

also is effective, inhibiting bone resorption and increasing renal excretion of calcium. It acts quickly, within 2 to 4 hours, but its use is limited by the development of tachyphylaxis. Corticosteroids may decrease tachyphylaxis in response to calcitonin and can be used alone to treat hypercalcemia. Gallium nitrates are potent inhibitors of bone resorption. They display a long duration of action but can cause nephrotoxicity. Mithramycin is an antibiotic that blocks osteoclastic activity, but it can be associated with liver, renal, and hematologic abnormalities, which limits its use to the treatment of Paget's disease of bone. For patients with severe, refractory hypercalcemia who are unable to tolerate volume expansion due to pulmonary edema or congestive heart failure, dialysis is an option.

Tumor lysis syndrome results when the release of intracellular metabolites overwhelms the kidneys' excretory capacity. This rapid release of uric acid, potassium, and phosphorus can result in marked hyperuricemia, hyperkalemia, hyperphosphatemia, and hypocalcemia, and acute renal failure. It is typically seen with poorly differentiated lymphomas and leukemias but also can occur with a number of solid tumor malignancies. Tumor lysis syndrome most commonly develops during treatment with chemotherapy or radiotherapy. Once it develops, volume expansion should be undertaken and any associated electrolyte abnormalities corrected. In this setting, hypocalcemia should not be treated unless it is symptomatic to avoid metastatic calcifications. Dialysis may be required for management of impaired renal function or correction of electrolyte abnormalities.

REFERENCES

Entries highlighted in bright blue are key references.

1. Aloia JF, Vaswani A, Flaster E, et al: Relationship of body water compartment to age, race and fat-free mass. *J Lab Clin Med* 132:483, 1998.
2. Bourque CW, Oliet SHR: Osmoreceptors in the central nervous system. *Annu Rev Physiol* 59:601, 1997.
3. Sticker EM, Huang W, Sved AF: Early osmoregulatory signals in the control of water intake and neurohypophyseal hormone secretion. *Physiol Behav* 76:415, 2002.
4. Stauss HM: Baroreceptor reflex function. *Am J Physiol Regul Integr Comp Physiol* 283:R284, 2002.
5. Miller M: Syndromes of excess antidiuretic hormone release. *Crit Care Clin* 17:11, 2001.
6. Kapoor M, Chan G: Fluid and electrolyte abnormalities. *Crit Care Clin* 17:571, 2001.
7. Adrogue HJ, Lederer ED, Suki WN, et al: Determinants of plasma potassium in diabetic ketoacidosis. *Medicine* 65:163, 1986.
8. Swan S: Aminoglycoside nephrotoxicity. *Semin Nephrol* 17:27, 1997.
9. Cobos E, Hall RR: Effects of chemotherapy on the kidney. *Semin Nephrol* 13:297, 1993.
10. Kobrin SM, Goldfarb S: Magnesium deficiency. *Semin Nephrol* 10:525, 1990.
11. Fisken FA, Heath DA, Somers S, et al: Hypercalcemia in hospital patients: Clinical and diagnostic aspects. *Lancet* 1:202, 1981.
12. Cruz DN, Perazella MA: Biochemical aberrations in a dialysis patient following parathyroidectomy. *Am J Kidney Dis* 29:759, 1997.
13. Bushinsky DA, Monk RD: Calcium. *Lancet* 352:306, 1998.
14. Dunlay RW, Camp MA, Allon M, et al: Calcitriol in prolonged hypocalcemia due to tumor lysis syndrome. *Ann Intern Med* 110:162, 1989.
15. Reber PM, Heath H: Hypocalcemic emergencies. *Med Clin North Am* 19:93, 1995.
16. Wong ET, Rude RK, Singer FR, et al: A high prevalence of hypomagnesemia and hypermagnesemia in hospitalized patients. *Am J Clin Pathol* 79:348, 1983.
17. Quamme GA: Renal magnesium handling: New insights in understanding old problems. *Kidney Int* 52:1180, 1997.
18. Marino PL: Acid-base interpretations, in Marino PL (ed): *The ICU Book,* 2nd ed. Baltimore: Williams & Wilkins, 1998, p 581.
19. Gluck SL: Acid-base. *Lancet* 352:474, 1998.
20. Gauthier PM, Szerlip HM: Metabolic acidosis in the intensive care unit. *Crit Care Clin* 18:289, 2002.

21. Pal JD, Victorino GP, Twomey P, et al: Admission serum lactate levels do not predict mortality in the acutely injured patient. *J Trauma* 60:583, 2006.

22. Koustova E, Standon K, Gushchin V, et al: Effects of lactated Ringer's solution on human leukocytes. *J Trauma* 53:782, 2002.

23. Shires GT, Browder LK, Steljes TP, et al: The effect of shock resuscitation fluids on apoptosis. *Am J Surg* 189:85, 2005.

24. Roberts JS, Bratton SL: Colloid volume expanders: Problems, pitfalls, and possibilities. *Drugs* 55:621, 1998.

25. Shackford SR: Effects of small-volume resuscitation on intracranial pressure and related cerebral variables. *J Trauma* 42(5 Suppl):S48, 1997.

26. Wade CE, Kramer GC, Grady JJ, et al: Efficacy of 7.5% saline and 6% dextran-70 in treating trauma: A meta-analysis of controlled clinical studies. *Surgery* 122:609, 1997.

27. Ley K: Plugging the leaks. *Nat Med* 7:1105, 2001.

28. Conhaim RL, Watson KE, Potenza BM, et al: Pulmonary capillary sieving of hetastarch is not altered by LPS-induced sepsis. *J Trauma* 46:800, 1999.

29. Lucas CE: The water of life: A century of confusion. *J Am Coll Surg* 192:86, 2001.

30. de Jonge E, Levi M: Effects of different plasma substitutes on blood coagulation: A comparative review. *Crit Care Med* 291:1261, 2001.

31. Cope JT, Banks D, Mauney MC, et al: Intraoperative hetastarch infusion impairs hemostasis after cardiac operations. *Ann Thorac Surg* 63:78, 1997.

32. Schortgen F, Lacherade JC, Bruneel F, et al: Effects of hydroxyethylstarch and gelatin on renal function in severe sepsis: A multicenter randomized study. *Lancet* 357:911, 2001.

33. Cittanova ML, Leblance I, Legendre C, et al: Effect of hydroxyethylstarch in brain-dead kidney donors on renal function in kidney-transplant recipients. *Lancet* 348:1620, 1996.

34. Gan TJ, Bennett-Guerrero E, Phillips-Bute B, et al: Hextend, a physiologically balanced plasma expander for large volume use in major surgery: A randomized phase III clinical trial. *Anesth Analg* 88:992, 1999.

35. Boldt J, Haisch G, Suttner S, et al: Effects of a new modified, balanced hydroxyethyl starch preparation (Hextend) on measures of coagulation. *Br J Anaesth* 89:772, 2002.

36. Rittoo D, Gosling P, Bonnici C, et al: Splanchnic oxygenation in patients undergoing abdominal aortic aneurysm repair and volume expansion with eloHAES. *Cardiovasc Surg* 10:128, 2002.

37. Coats TJ, Brazil E, Heron M, et al: Impairment of coagulation by commonly used resuscitation fluids in human volunteers. *Emerg Med J* 23:846, 2006.

38. European Resuscitation Council: Part 8. Advanced challenges in resuscitation. Section 1: Life-threatening electrolyte abnormalities. *Resuscitation* 46:253, 2000.

39. Laureno R, Karp BI: Myelinolysis after correction of hyponatremia. *Ann Med* 126:67, 1997.

40. Chua GC, Sitoh YY, Lim CC, et al: MRI findings in osmotic myelinolysis. *Clin Radiol* 57:800, 2002.

41. American College of Surgeons: Shock, in *American College of Surgeons Advanced Trauma Life Support Manual,* 6th ed. Chicago: American College of Surgeons, 1997.

42. Shires GT, Williams J, Brown F: Acute changes in extracellular fluids associated with major surgical procedures. *Ann Surg* 154:803, 1961.

43. Shires GT, Jackson DE: Postoperative salt tolerance. *Arch Surg* 84:703, 1962.

44. Shires GT III, Peitzman AB, Albert SA, et al: Response of extravascular lung water to intraoperative fluids. *Ann Surg* 197:515, 1983.

45. Miller M: Syndromes of excess antidiuretic hormone release. *Crit Care Clin* 17:11, 2001.

46. Ober KP: Endocrine crises: Diabetes insipidus. *Crit Care Clin* 7:109, 1991.

47. Singh S, Bohn D, Carlotti APCP: Cerebral salt wasting: Truths, fallacies, theories, and challenges. *Crit Care Med* 30:2575, 2002.

48. Kozar RA, McQuiggan MM, Moore FA: Nutritional support in trauma patients, in Shikora SA, Martindale RG, Schwaitzberg SD (eds): *Nutritional Considerations in the Intensive Care Unit,* 1st ed. Dubuque, Iowa: Kendall/Hunt Publishing, 2002, p 229.

49. Crook MA, Hally V, Panteli JV: The importance of the refeeding syndrome. *Nutrition* 17:632, 2001.

50. Uchino S, Bellomo R, Ronco C: Intermittent versus continuous renal replacement therapy in the ICU: Impact on electrolyte and acid-base balance. *Intensive Care Med* 27:1037, 2001.

51. Kapoor M, Chan GZ: Fluid and electrolyte abnormalities. *Crit Care Clin* 17:503, 2002.

52. Barri YM, Knochel JP: Hypercalcemia and electrolyte disturbances in malignancy. *Hematol Oncol Clin North Am* 10:775, 1996.

CHAPTER 4

Hemostasis, Surgical Bleeding, and Transfusion

Ernest A. Gonzalez, Kenneth M. Jastrow,
John B. Holcomb, and Rosemary A. Kozar

BIOLOGY OF HEMOSTASIS

Hemostasis is a complex process whose function is to limit blood loss from an injured vessel. Four major physiologic events participate in the hemostatic process: vascular constriction, platelet plug formation, fibrin formation, and fibrinolysis. Although each tends to be activated in order, the four processes are interrelated so that there is a continuum and multiple reinforcements. The process is shown schematically in Fig. 4-1.

Vascular Constriction

Vascular constriction is the initial response to vessel injury. It is more pronounced in vessels with medial smooth muscles and is dependent on local contraction of smooth muscle. Vasoconstriction is subsequently linked to platelet plug formation. Thromboxane A_2 (TXA_2) is produced locally at the site of injury via the release of arachidonic acid from platelet membranes and is a potent constrictor of smooth muscle. Similarly, endothelin synthesized by injured

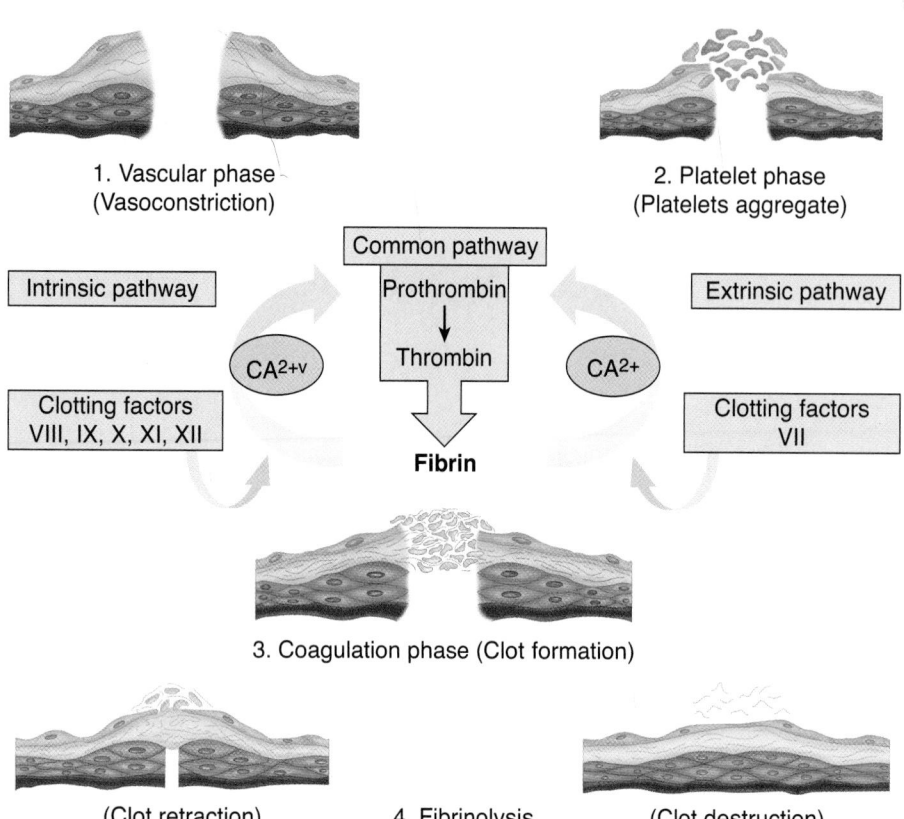

1. Vascular phase
(Vasoconstriction)

2. Platelet phase
(Platelets aggregate)

Intrinsic pathway

Common pathway
Prothrombin
↓
Thrombin

Extrinsic pathway

CA²⁺ᵛ

CA²⁺

Clotting factors
VIII, IX, X, XI, XII

Clotting factors
VII

Fibrin

3. Coagulation phase (Clot formation)

(Clot retraction)   4. Fibrinolysis   (Clot destruction)

FIG. 4-1. Biology of hemostasis. The four physiologic processes that interrelate to limit blood loss from an injured vessel are illustrated and include vascular constriction, platelet plug formation, fibrin clot formation, and fibrinolysis.

endothelium and serotonin (5-hydroxytryptamine) released during platelet aggregation are potent vasoconstrictors. Lastly, bradykinin and fibrinopeptides, which are involved in the coagulation scheme, also are capable of contracting vascular smooth muscle. The extent of vasoconstriction varies with the degree of vessel injury. A small artery with a lateral incision may remain open due to physical forces, whereas a similarly sized vessel that is completely transected may contract to the extent that bleeding ceases spontaneously.

Platelet Function

Platelets are anucleate fragments of megakaryocytes. The normal circulating number of platelets ranges between 150,000 and 400,000/μL. Up to 30% of circulating platelets may be sequestered in the spleen. If not consumed in a clotting reaction, platelets are normally removed by the spleen and have an average life span of 7 to 10 days.

Platelets play an integral role in hemostasis by forming a hemostatic plug and by contributing to thrombin formation (Fig. 4-2). Platelets do not normally adhere to each other or to the vessel wall but can form a plug that aids in cessation of bleeding when vascular disruption occurs. Injury to the intimal layer in the vascular wall exposes subendothelial collagen to which platelets adhere. This process requires von Willebrand's factor (vWF), a protein in the subendothelium that is lacking in patients with von Willebrand's disease. The vWF binds to glycoprotein I/IX/V on the platelet membrane. After adhesion, platelets initiate a release reaction that recruits other platelets from the circulating blood to seal the disrupted vessel. Up to this point, this process is known as *primary hemostasis.* Platelet aggregation is reversible and is not associated with secretion. Additionally, heparin does not interfere with this reaction, and thus hemostasis can occur in the heparinized patient. Adenosine diphosphate (ADP) and serotonin are the principal mediators in platelet aggregation.

Arachidonic acid released from the platelet membranes is converted by COX to prostaglandin G_2 (PGG₂) and then to prostaglandin H_2 (PGH₂), which, in turn, is converted to TXA₂. TXA₂ has potent vasoconstriction and platelet aggregation effects. Arachidonic acid may also be shuttled to adjacent endothelial cells and converted to prostacyclin (PGI₂), which is a vasodilator and acts to inhibit platelet aggregation. Platelet COX is irreversibly inhibited by aspirin and reversibly blocked by NSAIDs but is not affected by COX-2 inhibitors.

KEY POINTS

1. Therapeutic anticoagulation preoperatively and postoperatively is becoming increasingly more common. The patient's risk of intraoperative and postoperative bleeding should guide the need for reversal of anticoagulation therapy preoperatively and the timing of its reinstatement postoperatively.

2. The need for massive transfusion should be anticipated and guidelines should be in place to provide the simultaneous administration of blood, plasma, and platelets.

3. The acute coagulopathy of trauma results from a combination of activation of protein C and fibrinolysis. It is distinct from disseminated intravascular coagulation, is present on arrival to the emergency department, and is associated with an increase in mortality.

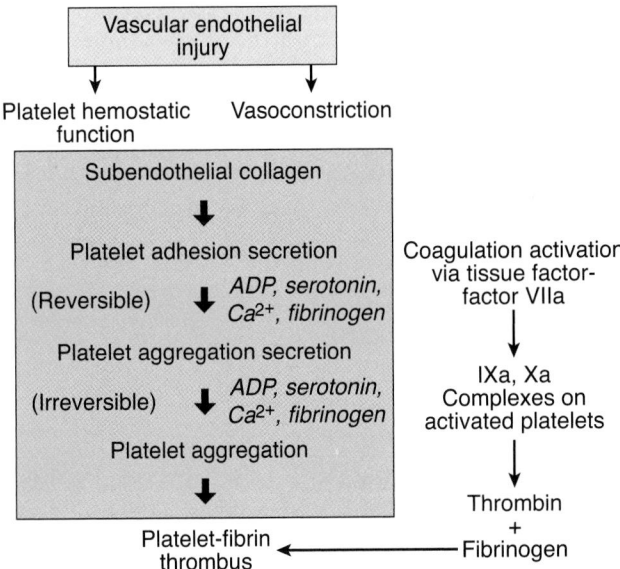

FIG. 4-2. Schematic of platelet activation and thrombus function. ADP = adenosine diphosphate.

adenosine monophosphate (cAMP), and by nitric oxide. As a consequence of the release reaction, alterations occur in the phospholipids of the platelet membrane that allow calcium and clotting factors to bind to the platelet surface, forming enzymatically active complexes. The altered lipoprotein surface (sometimes referred to as *platelet factor 3*) catalyzes reactions that are involved in the conversion of prothrombin (factor II) to thrombin (factor IIa) (Fig. 4-3) by activated factor X (Xa) in the presence of factor V and calcium, and it is involved in the reaction by which activated factor IX (IXa), factor VIII, and calcium activate factor X. Platelets may also play a role in the initial activation of factors XI and XII.

Coagulation

Under physiologic conditions, hemostasis is accomplished by a complex sequence of interactions between platelets, the endothelium, and multiple circulating or membrane-bound coagulation factors. As shown in Fig. 4-3, the coagulation cascade typically has been depicted as two intersecting pathways. The intrinsic pathway begins with factor XII and through a cascade of enzymatic reactions activates factors XI, IX, and VII in sequence. In the intrinsic pathway all of the components leading ultimately to fibrin clot formation are intrinsic to the circulating plasma and no surface is required to initiate the process. In contrast, the extrinsic pathway requires exposure of tissue factor on the surface of the injured vessel wall to initiate the arm of the cascade beginning with factor VII. The two arms of the coagulation cascade merge to a common pathway at factor X, and activation proceeds in sequence of factors II (prothrombin) and I (fibrinogen). Clot formation occurs after proteolytic conversion of fibrinogen to fibrin.

One convenient feature of depicting the coagulation cascade with two merging arms is that commonly used laboratory tests segregate abnormalities of clotting to one of the two arms (Table 4-1). An elevated activated partial thromboplastin time (aPTT) is associated with abnormal function of the intrinsic arm of the cascade, whereas an elevated prothrombin time (PT) is associated with the extrinsic arm. Vitamin K deficiency and warfarin use affect factors II, VII, IX, and X. Fibrinogen levels usually need to be <50 mg/dL to cause prolongation of the PT and aPTT. Recently, efforts have been made

In the second wave of platelet aggregation, a release reaction occurs in which several substances, including ADP, Ca²⁺, serotonin, TXA₂, and α-granule proteins are discharged. Fibrinogen is a required cofactor for this process, acting as a bridge for the glycoprotein IIb/IIIa receptor on the activated platelets. The release reaction results in compaction of the platelets into a plug, a process that is no longer reversible. Thrombospondin, another protein secreted by the α-granule, stabilizes fibrinogen binding to the activated platelet surface and strengthens the platelet-platelet interactions. Platelet factor 4 (PF4) and α-thromboglobulin also are secreted during the release reaction. PF4 is a potent heparin antagonist. The second wave of platelet aggregation is inhibited by aspirin and NSAIDs, by cyclic

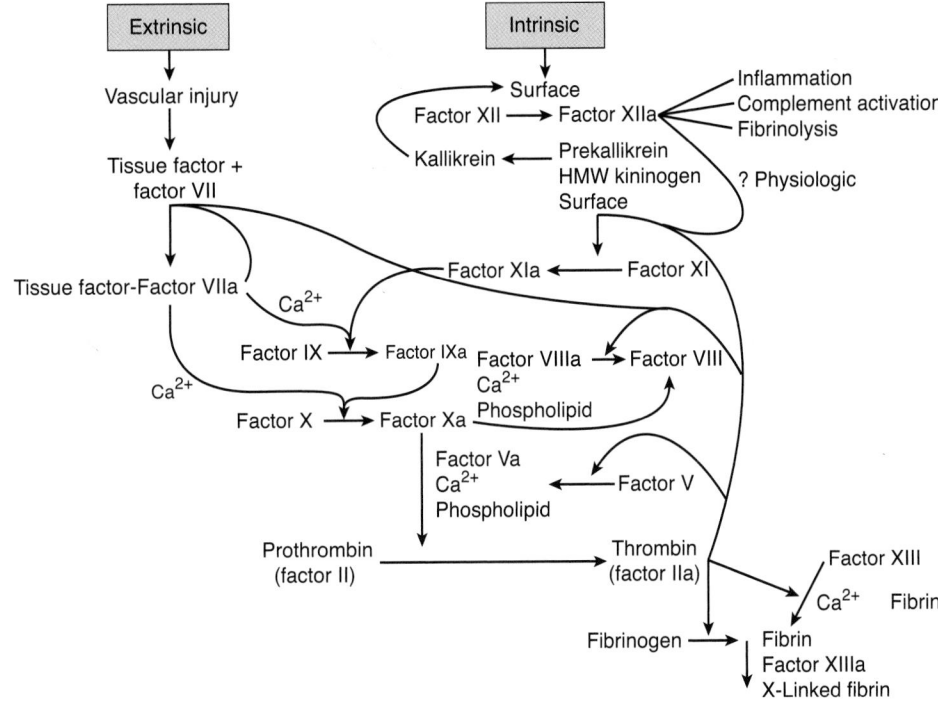

FIG. 4-3. Schematic of the coagulation system. HMW = high molecular weight.

TABLE 4-1	Coagulation factors tested by the PT and the aPTT

PT	aPTT
VII	XII
X	High molecular weight kininogen
V	Prekallikrein
II (prothrombin)	XI
Fibrinogen	IX
	VIII
	X
	V
	II
	Fibrinogen

aPTT = activated partial thromboplastin time; PT = prothrombin time.

to present the coagulation cascade in a more physiologically relevant format. The primary physiologic pathway for coagulation is initiated by the exposure of subendothelial tissue factor when the luminal surface of a vessel is injured. Propagation of the clotting reaction then ensues with a sequence of four enzymatic reactions, each of which involves a proteolytic enzyme that generates the next enzyme in the cascade by cleavage of a proenzyme and a phospholipid surface, such as a platelet membrane. Each reaction requires a helper protein. Factor VIIa binds to tissue factor on exposure of the latter molecule through injury to the vascular wall. The tissue factor VIIa complex catalyzes the activation of factor X to factor Xa. The reaction takes place on the phospholipid surface of activated platelets. This complex is four orders of magnitude more active at converting factor X than is factor VIIa alone and also activates factor IX to factor IXa. Factor Xa, together with factor Va and Ca^{2+} and phospholipid, comprises the prothrombinase complex that converts prothrombin to thrombin. Thrombin has multiple functions in the clotting process, including conversion of fibrinogen to fibrin and activation of factors V, VII, VIII, XI, and XIII, as well as activation of platelets.

Factor VIIIa combines with factor IXa to form the intrinsic factor complex, which is responsible for the bulk of the conversion of factor X to Xa. This intrinsic complex (VIIIa-IXa) is approximately 50 times more effective at catalyzing factor X activation than is the extrinsic (tissue factor VIIa) complex and five to six orders of magnitude more effective than is factor IXa alone.

Factor Xa combines with factor Va, also on the activated platelet membrane surface, to form the prothrombinase complex, which is responsible for converting prothrombin to thrombin. As with the VIIIa-IXa complex, the prothrombinase is significantly more effective at catalyzing its substrate than is factor Xa alone. Once formed, thrombin leaves the membrane surface and converts fibrinogen by two cleavage steps into fibrin and two small peptides termed *fibrinopeptides A* and *B*. Removal of fibrinopeptide A permits end-to-end polymerization of the fibrin molecules, whereas cleavage of fibrinopeptide B allows side-to-side polymerization of the fibrin clot. This latter step is facilitated by thrombin-activatable fibrinolysis inhibitor (TAFI), which acts to stabilize the resultant clot.

The coagulation system is exquisitely regulated. In addition to clot formation that must occur to prevent bleeding at the time of vascular injury, two related processes must exist to prevent propagation of the clot beyond the site of injury. First, there is a feedback inhibition on the coagulation cascade, which deactivates the enzyme complexes leading to thrombin formation. Second, mechanisms of fibrinolysis allow for breakdown of the fibrin clot and subsequent repair of the injured vessel with deposition of connective tissue.

Tissue factor pathway inhibitor (TFPI) blocks the extrinsic tissue factor–VIIa complex, eliminating this catalyst's production of factors Xa and IXa. Antithrombin III effectively neutralizes all of the

procoagulant serine proteases and only weakly inhibits the tissue factor–VIIa complex. The primary effect is to halt the production of thrombin. A third major mechanism of inhibition of thrombin formation is the protein C system. On its formation, thrombin binds to thrombomodulin and activates protein C to activated protein C (APC), which then forms a complex with its cofactor, protein S, on a phospholipid surface. The APC–protein S complex cleaves factors Va and VIIIa so they are no longer able to participate in the formation of tissue factor–VIIa or prothrombinase complexes. Of interest is an inherited form of factor V that carries a genetic mutation, called *factor V Leiden,* that is resistant to cleavage by APC and thus remains active (procoagulant). Patients with factor V Leiden are predisposed to venous thromboembolic events. As a result of the three systems described earlier, feedback inhibition of thrombin formation exists at upstream, intermediate, and downstream portions of the coagulation cascade to "turn off" thrombin formation once the procoagulant sequence is initially activated.

The same thrombin-thrombomodulin complex that leads to formation of APC also activates TAFI. In addition to stabilizing the clot, removal of the terminal lysine on the fibrin molecule by TAFI renders the clot more susceptible to lysis by plasmin. Degradation of fibrin clot is accomplished by plasmin, a serine protease derived from the proenzyme plasminogen. Plasmin formation occurs as a result of one of several plasminogen activators. Tissue plasminogen activator (tPA) is made by the endothelium and other cells of the vascular wall and is the main circulating form of this family of enzymes. The tPA is selective for fibrin-bound plasminogen so that endogenous fibrinolytic activity occurs predominantly at the site of clot formation. The other major plasminogen activator, urokinase plasminogen activator (uPA), also produced by endothelial cells as well as by urothelium, is not selective for fibrin-bound plasminogen.

Because of the complex nature of hemostasis, potential interference in the process can occur at many levels. Platelet number or function can be insufficient to adequately support coagulation. Alternatively, abnormalities in the clotting factors may underlie an abnormality of hemostasis, either from an intrinsic defect in one of the factors or as the result of pharmacotherapy.

Fibrinolysis

During the wound-healing process, the fibrin clot undergoes clot lysis, which permits restoration of blood flow. The main enzyme, plasmin, degrades the fibrin mesh at various places, which leads to the production of circulating fragments that are cleared by other proteases or by the kidney and liver. Fibrinolysis is initiated at the same time as the clotting mechanism under the influence of circulating kinases, tissue activators, and kallikrein, which are present in many organs, including the vascular endothelium. Fibrin is degraded by plasmin, a serine protease derived from the proenzyme plasminogen. Plasminogen may be converted by one of several plasminogen activators, including tPA and uPA. The tPA is synthesized by endothelial cells and released by the cells on thrombin stimulation as single-chain tPA. This is then cleaved by plasmin to form two-chain tPA. Bradykinin, a potent endothelium-dependent vasodilator cleaved from high molecular weight kininogen by kallikrein, causes contraction of nonvascular smooth muscle, increases vascular permeability, and enhances release of tPA. Both tPA and plasminogen bind to fibrin as it forms, and this trimolecular complex cleaves fibrin very efficiently. After plasmin is generated it cleaves fibrin, somewhat less efficiently, and it also will degrade fibrinogen. Fully cross-linked fibrin is also a relatively poor substrate for plasmin. Plasminogen activation may be initiated by activation of factor XII, which leads to the generation of kallikrein from prekallikrein and cleavage of high molecular weight kininogen by kallikrein.

Several characteristics of the enzymatic reactions ensure that fibrinolysis occurs at a controlled rate and preferentially at the site of clot formation. The tPA activates plasminogen more efficiently when it is bound to fibrin, so that plasmin is formed selectively on

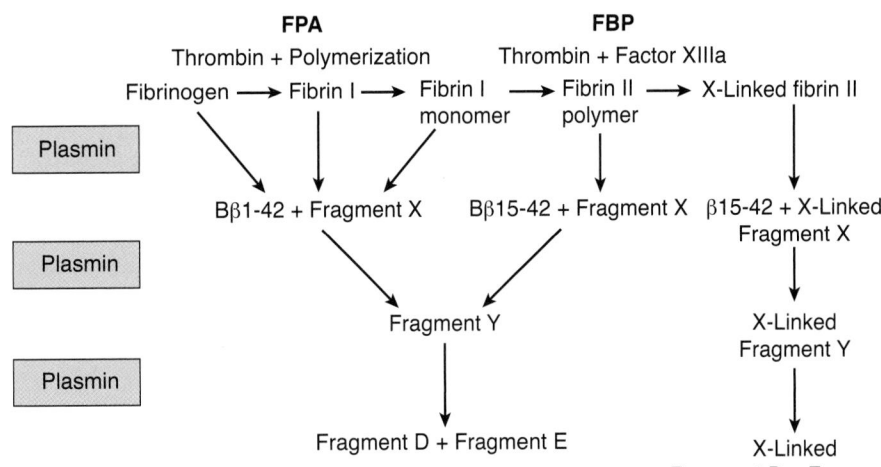

FIG. 4-4. Schematic of fibrin formation and dissolution. FBP = fibrin breakdown product; FPA = fibrinopeptide A.

the clot. Plasmin is inhibited by α_2-antiplasmin, a protein that is cross-linked to fibrin by factor XIII, which helps to ensure that clot lysis does not occur too quickly. Any circulating plasmin also is inhibited by α_2-antiplasmin and circulating tPA or urokinase. Clot lysis yields fibrin degradation products, including E-nodules and D-dimers. The smaller fragments interfere with normal platelet aggregation and the larger fragments may be incorporated into the clot in lieu of normal fibrin monomers. This may result in an unstable clot. Presence of D-dimers in the circulation may be a marker of thrombosis or other conditions in which a significant activation of the fibrinolytic system is present. The final inhibitor for the fibrinolytic system is TAFI, a procarboxypeptidase that is activated by the thrombin-thrombomodulin complex. The active enzyme removes lysine residues from fibrin that are essential for binding plasminogen. The sequence of fibrin formation and its dissolution by plasmin is presented in schematic form in Fig. 4-4.

CONGENITAL FACTOR DEFICIENCIES

Coagulation Factor Deficiencies

Inherited deficiencies of all of the coagulation factors are seen. However, the three most frequent are factor VIII deficiency (hemophilia A and von Willebrand's disease), factor IX deficiency (hemophilia B or Christmas disease), and factor XI deficiency. Hemophilia A and hemophilia B are inherited as sex-linked recessive disorders with males being affected almost exclusively. The clinical severity of hemophilia A and hemophilia B depends on the measurable level of factor VIII or factor IX in the patient's plasma. Plasma factor levels <1% of normal are considered severe disease, factor levels between 1 and 5% moderately severe, and levels of 5 to 30% mild disease. Patients with severe hemophilia have severe spontaneous bleeds, frequently into joints, which leads to crippling arthropathies. Intramuscular hematomas, retroperitoneal hematomas, and GI, genitourinary, and retropharyngeal bleeding are added clinical sequelae seen with severe disease. Intracranial bleeding and bleeding from the tongue or lingual frenulum may be life-threatening with severe disease. Patients with moderately severe hemophilia have less spontaneous bleeding but are likely to bleed severely after trauma or surgery. Those with mild disease do not bleed spontaneously and frequently have only minor bleeding after major trauma or surgery. Because platelet function is normal in individuals with hemophilia, patients may not bleed immediately after an injury or minor surgery because they have a normal response with platelet activation and formation of a platelet plug. At times, the diagnosis of hemophilia is not made in these patients until after their first minor procedure (e.g., tooth extraction or tonsillectomy).

Patients with hemophilia A or B are treated with factor VIII or factor IX concentrate, respectively. Recombinant factor VIII is strongly recommended for patients not treated previously and gener-

ally is recommended for patients who are both HIV and hepatitis C virus seronegative. For factor IX replacement, the preferred products are recombinant or high-purity factor IX, because of the risk of thrombosis with the intermediate factor IX (prothrombin complex) concentrates. Intermediate factor IX concentrates contain varying amounts of factors II, VII, and X and are reported to induce thrombosis when used in high doses. Furthermore, the cost of concentrates increases with the specific activity of factor VIII or factor IX.

Up to 20% of hemophiliac patients with factor VIII deficiency develop inhibitors. Some patients have low titers of the inhibitors and can be treated with higher dosages of factor VIII to achieve the desired plasma level. For patients with high titers of inhibitors alternate treatments must be used. These include porcine factor VIII, prothrombin complex concentrates, activated prothrombin complex concentrates, and recombinant factor VIIa. Factor VII is the most effective but must be given every 2 hours in situations with active bleeding and can be very expensive. Recombinant factor VIIa may be useful in factor IX–deficient patients with inhibitors. Additionally ε-aminocaproic acid, or Amicar, an inhibitor of fibrinolysis, is frequently a useful adjunct to factor VIII or IX or desmopressin acetate (DDAVP) in treatment of bleeding in patients with hemophilia. Excess ε-aminocaproic acid can lead to thrombosis, so the drug should be used with caution.

von Willebrand's Disease

von Willebrand's disease (vWD), the most common congenital bleeding disorder, is characterized by low levels of factor VIII. It is an autosomal dominant disorder, and the primary defect is a low level of vWF, a large glycoprotein responsible for carrying factor VIII and platelet adhesion. The latter is important for normal platelet adhesion to exposed subendothelium and for aggregation under high-shear conditions. Patients with vWD have bleeding that is characteristic of platelet disorders (i.e., easy bruising and mucosal bleeding). Menorrhagia is common in women. vWD is classified into three types. Type I is a partial quantitative deficiency, type II is a qualitative defect, and type III is total deficiency. One treatment for vWD is an intermediate-purity factor VIII concentrate such as Humate-P that contains vWF as well as factor VIII. The second treatment strategy is desmopressin acetate, which raises endogenous vWF levels by triggering release of the factor from endothelial cells. Desmopressin acetate is used once a day because time is needed for synthesis of new stores of vWF within the endothelial cells. Historically, patients with type I disease have been found to respond well to desmopressin acetate. Type II patients may respond, depending on the particular defect. Type III patients are usually unresponsive.

Factor XI Deficiency

Factor XI deficiency, an autosomal recessive inherited condition sometimes referred to as *hemophilia C*, is more prevalent in the

Ashkenazi Jewish population. Spontaneous bleeding is rare, but bleeding may occur after surgery, trauma, or invasive procedures. Patients with factor XI deficiency who present with bleeding or for whom surgery is planned and who are known to have bled previously are treated with fresh-frozen plasma (FFP). Each milliliter of plasma contains 1 unit of factor XI activity, so the volume needed depends on the patient's baseline level, the desired level, and the plasma volume. Recombinant factor VIIa treatment has been used successfully in children with severe factor XI deficiency who require major operations such as open heart surgery.[1] Desmopressin acetate also may be useful in the prevention of surgical bleeding in these patients.

Deficiency of Factors II (Prothrombin), V, and X

Inherited deficiencies of factors II, V, and X are rare. These deficiencies are inherited in an autosomal recessive pattern. Significant bleeding is encountered in homozygotes with <1% of normal activity. In any of these deficiencies, bleeding is treated with FFP. As with factor XI, FFP contains 1 unit of activity of each per milliliter. However, factor V activity is decreased because of its inherit instability. The half-life of prothrombin (factor II) is long (approximately 72 hours) and only approximately 25% of the normal level is needed for hemostasis. Prothrombin complex concentrates can be used to treat deficiencies of prothrombin or factor X. Daily infusions of FFP are used to treat bleeding in factor V deficiency, with a goal of 20 to 25% activity. Factor V deficiency may be coinherited with factor VIII deficiency. Treatment of bleeding in individuals with the combined deficiency requires factor VIII concentrate and FFP. Some patients with factor V deficiency also are lacking the factor V normally present in platelets and may need platelet transfusions as well as FFP.

Factor VII Deficiency

Inherited factor VII deficiency is a rare autosomal recessive disorder. Clinical bleeding can widely vary and does not always correlate with the level of factor VII coagulant activity in plasma. Bleeding is uncommon unless the level is <3%. The most common bleeding manifestations are easy bruising and mucosal bleeding, particularly epistaxis or oral mucosal bleeding. Postoperative bleeding is also common, reported in 30% of surgical procedures in such patients.[2] Treatment is with FFP or recombinant factor VIIa. The half-life of recombinant factor VIIa is only approximately 2 hours, but excellent hemostasis can be achieved with frequent infusions. The half-life of factor VII in FFP is up to 4 hours.

Factor XIII Deficiency

Congenital factor XIII deficiency, originally recognized by François Duckert in 1960, is a rare autosomal recessive disease usually associated with a severe bleeding diathesis.[3] The male:female ratio is 1:1. Although acquired factor XIII deficiency has been described in association with hepatic failure, inflammatory bowel disease, and myeloid leukemia, the only significant association with bleeding in children is the inherited deficiency.[4] Bleeding typically is delayed, because clots form normally but are susceptible to fibrinolysis. Umbilical stump bleeding is characteristic, and there is a high risk of intracranial bleeding. Spontaneous abortion is usual in women with factor XIII deficiency unless they receive replacement therapy. Replacement can be accomplished with FFP, cryoprecipitate, or a factor XIII concentrate. Levels of 1 to 2% are usually adequate for hemostasis.

Platelet Functional Defects

Inherited platelet functional defects include abnormalities of platelet surface proteins, abnormalities of platelet granules, and enzyme defects. The major surface protein abnormalities are thrombasthenia and Bernard-Soulier syndrome. Thrombasthenia or Glanzmann thrombasthenia is a rare genetic platelet disorder, inherited in an autosomal recessive pattern, in which the platelet glycoprotein IIb/IIIa complex is either lacking or present but dysfunctional. This

defect leads to faulty platelet aggregation and subsequent bleeding. The disorder was first described by Dr. Eduard Glanzmann in 1918.[5] Bleeding in thrombasthenic patients must be treated with platelet transfusions. The Bernard-Soulier syndrome, caused by a defect in the glycoprotein Ib/IX/V receptor for vWF, is necessary for platelet adhesion to the subendothelium. Transfusion of normal platelets is required to treat bleeding in these patients.

The most common intrinsic platelet defect is storage pool disease. It involves loss of dense granules [storage sites for ADP, adenosine triphosphate (ATP), Ca^{2+}, and inorganic phosphate] and α-granules. Dense granule deficiency is the most prevalent of these. It may be an isolated defect or occur with partial albinism in the Hermansky-Pudlak syndrome. Bleeding is variable, depending on the severity of the granule defect. Bleeding is caused by the decreased release of ADP from these platelets. An isolated defect of the α-granules is known as *gray platelet syndrome* because of the appearance of the platelets on Wright's stain preparations. A few patients have been reported who have decreased numbers of both dense and α-granules. They have a more severe bleeding disorder. Patients with mild bleeding as a consequence of a form of storage pool disease can be treated with desmopressin acetate. It is likely that the high levels of vWF in the plasma after desmopressin acetate administration somehow compensate for the intrinsic platelet defect. With more severe bleeding, platelet transfusion is required.

ACQUIRED HEMOSTATIC DEFECTS

Platelet Abnormalities

Acquired abnormalities of platelets may be quantitative or qualitative, although some patients have both types of defects. Quantitative defects may be a result of failure of production, shortened survival, or sequestration. Failure of production is generally a result of bone marrow disorders such as those caused by leukemia, myelodysplastic syndrome, severe vitamin B_{12} or folate deficiency, chemotherapeutic drug use, radiation therapy, acute ethanol intoxication, or viral infection. If a quantitative abnormality exists and treatment is indicated, either due to symptoms or the need for an invasive procedure, platelet transfusion is used. The etiology of both qualitative and quantitative defects is reviewed in Table 4-2.

Quantitative Defects

Failure of platelet production can occur when bone marrow production of platelets is affected by marrow-related disease such as leukemia or myelodysplasia, vitamin B_{12} or folate deficiencies, chemotherapy or radiation therapy, acute alcohol intoxication, or viral illnesses.

Shortened platelet survival is seen in immune thrombocytopenia, disseminated intravascular coagulation, and disorders characterized by platelet thrombi such as thrombotic thrombocytopenic purpura and hemolytic uremic syndrome. Immune thrombocytopenia may be idiopathic or associated with other autoimmune disorders or low-grade B-cell malignancies, and it may also be secondary to viral infections (including HIV infection) or use of certain drugs. Secondary immune thrombocytopenia often presents with a very low platelet count, petechiae and purpura, and epistaxis. Large platelets are seen on peripheral smear. Initial treatment consists of corticosteroids, IV gamma globulin, or anti-D immunoglobulin in patients who are Rh-positive. Effects of both gamma globulin and anti-D immunoglobulin are rapid in onset. Platelet transfusions usually are not needed unless central nervous system bleeding or active bleeding from other sites occurs. Survival of the transfused platelets is usually short.

Primary immune thrombocytopenia also is known as *idiopathic thrombocytopenic purpura* (ITP). In children it is usually acute and short lived, and typically follows a viral illness. In contrast, ITP in adults is gradual in onset, chronic, and has no identifiable cause. Because the circulating platelets in ITP are young and functional,

TABLE 4-2	Etiology of platelet disorders

A. Quantitative disorders
  1. Failure of production: related to impairment of bone marrow function
      a. Leukemia
      b. Myeloproliferative disorders
      c. Vitamin B_{12} or folate deficiency
      d. Chemotherapy or radiation therapy
      e. Acute alcohol intoxication
      f. Viral infections
  2. Decreased survival
      a. Immune-mediated disorders
          1) Idiopathic thrombocytopenia
          2) Heparin-induced thrombocytopenia
          3) Autoimmune disorders or B-cell malignancies
          4) Secondary thrombocytopenia
      b. Disseminated intravascular coagulation
      c. Disorders related to platelet thrombi
          1) Thrombocytopenic purpura
          2) Hemolytic uremic syndrome
  3. Sequestration
      a. Portal hypertension
      b. Sarcoid
      c. Lymphoma
      d. Gaucher's disease
B. Qualitative disorders
  1. Massive transfusion
  2. Therapeutic administration of platelet inhibitors
  3. Disease states
      a. Myeloproliferative disorders
      b. Monoclonal gammopathies
      c. Liver disease

TABLE 4-3	Management of idiopathic thrombocytopenic purpura (ITP) in adults

First Line
  a. Corticosteroids: The majority of patients respond, but only a few long term.
  b. IV immunoglobulin: Indicated with clinical bleeding, along with platelet transfusion, and when condition is steroid unresponsive. Response is rapid but transient.
  c. Anti-D immunoglobulin: Active only in Rh-positive patients before splenectomy. Response is transient.

Second Line
  a. Splenectomy: Open or laparoscopic. Criteria include severe thrombocytopenia, high risk of bleeding, and continued need for steroids. Treatment failure may be due to retained accessory splenic tissue.

Third Line
  a. Patients for whom first- and second-line therapies fail are considered to have chronic ITP. The objective in this subset of patients is to maintain the platelet count $>20-30 \times 10^9$/L and to minimize side effects of medications.
  b. Rituximab, an anti-CD20 monoclonal antibody: Acts by eliminating B cells.
  c. Alternative medications producing mixed results and a limited response: Danazol, cyclosporine A, dapsone, azathioprine, and vinca alkaloids.
  d. Thrombopoietic agents: A new class of drugs for patients with impaired production of platelets rather than accelerated destruction of platelets. Second-generation drugs still in clinical trials include AMG531 and eltrombopag.

bleeding is less for a given platelet count than when there is failure of platelet production. The pathophysiology of ITP is believed to involve both impaired platelet production and T cell–mediated platelet destruction.[6] Management options are summarized in Table 4-3. Treatment of drug-induced immune thrombocytopenia may simply entail withdrawal of the offending drug, but administration of corticosteroids, gamma globulin, and anti-D immunoglobulin may hasten recovery of the count.

Heparin-induced thrombocytopenia (HIT) is a form of drug-induced immune thrombocytopenia. It is an immunologic disorder in which antibodies against PF4 formed during exposure to heparin affect platelet activation and endothelial function with resultant thrombocytopenia and intravascular thrombosis.[7] The platelet count typically begins to fall 5 to 7 days after heparin has been started, but if it is a re-exposure, the decrease in count may occur within 1 to 2 days. HIT should be suspected if the platelet count falls to <100,000/μL or if it drops by 50% from baseline in a patient receiving heparin. Although HIT is more common with full-dose unfractionated heparin (1 to 3%), it also can occur with prophylactic doses or with low molecular weight heparins. Interestingly, approximately 17% of patients receiving unfractionated heparin and 8% of those receiving low molecular weight heparin develop antibodies against PF4, yet a much smaller percentage develop thrombocytopenia and even fewer clinical HIT.[8] In addition to the mild to moderate thrombocytopenia, this disorder is characterized by a high incidence of thrombosis, which may be arterial or venous. Importantly, the absence of thrombocytopenia in these patients does not preclude the diagnosis of HIT.

The diagnosis of HIT may be made by using either a serotonin release assay or an enzyme-linked immunosorbent assay (ELISA). The serotonin release assay is highly specific but not sensitive, so that a positive test result supports the diagnosis but a negative result does not exclude HIT.[7] On the other hand, the ELISA has a low specificity, so although a positive ELISA result confirms the presence of anti–heparin-PF4, it does not help in the diagnosis of clinical HIT. A negative ELISA result, however, essentially rules out HIT.

The initial treatment of suspected HIT is to stop heparin and begin an alternative anticoagulant. Stopping heparin without adding another anticoagulant is not adequate to prevent thrombosis in this setting. Alternative anticoagulants are primarily thrombin inhibitors. Those available in the United States are lepirudin, argatroban, and bivalirudin. In Canada and Europe, danaparoid also is available. Danaparoid is a heparinoid that has approximately 20% cross reactivity with HIT antibodies in vitro but a much lower cross reactivity in vivo. Because of warfarin's early induction of a hypercoagulable state, only once full anticoagulation with an alternative agent has been accomplished and the platelet count has begun to recover should warfarin be instituted.

There are also disorders in which thrombocytopenia is a result of platelet activation and formation of platelet thrombi. In thrombotic thrombocytopenic purpura (TTP), large vWF molecules interact with platelets, which leads to activation. These large molecules result from inhibition of a metalloproteinase enzyme, ADAMTS13, which cleaves the large vWF molecules.[9] TTP is classically characterized by thrombocytopenia, microangiopathic hemolytic anemia, fever, and renal and neurologic signs or symptoms. The finding of schistocytes on a peripheral blood smear aids in the diagnosis. The most effective treatment for TTP is plasmapheresis, although plasma infusion also has been attempted. A recent study comparing these two modalities reported a higher relapse rate and a higher mortality with plasma infusions. Platelet transfusions are contraindicated.[10] Additionally, rituximab, a monoclonal antibody against the CD20 protein on B lymphocytes, has shown promise as an immunomodulatory therapy directed against acquired TTP, which in the majority of cases is autoimmune mediated.[11]

Hemolytic uremic syndrome (HUS) often occurs secondary to infection by *Escherichia coli* 0157:H7 or other Shiga toxin–producing bacteria. The metalloproteinase is normal in these cases. HUS usually is associated with some degree of renal failure, with many patients requiring renal replacement therapy. Neurologic symptoms are less frequent. A number of patients develop features of both TTP and HUS. This may occur with autoimmune diseases, especially systemic lupus erythematosus, and HIV infection, or in association with certain drugs (such as ticlopidine, mitomycin C, gemcitabine), and immunosuppressive agents (such as cyclosporine and tacrolimus). Discontinuation of the involved drug is the mainstay of therapy. Plasmapheresis frequently is used, but it is not clear what etiologic factor is being removed by the pheresis.

Sequestration is another important cause of thrombocytopenia and usually involves sequestration of platelets in an enlarged spleen, typically related to portal hypertension, sarcoid, lymphoma, or Gaucher's disease. The total body platelet mass is essentially normal in patients with hypersplenism, but a much larger fraction of the platelets are in the enlarged spleen. Platelet survival is mildly decreased. Bleeding is less than anticipated from the count, because sequestered platelets can be mobilized to some extent and enter the circulation. Platelet transfusion does not increase the platelet count as much as it would in a normal person, because the transfused platelets are similarly sequestered in the spleen. Splenectomy is not indicated to correct the thrombocytopenia of hypersplenism caused by portal hypertension.

Thrombocytopenia is the most common abnormality of hemostasis that results in bleeding in the surgical patient. The patient may have a reduced platelet count as a result of a variety of disease processes as discussed earlier. In these circumstances, the marrow usually demonstrates a normal or increased number of megakaryocytes. By contrast, when thrombocytopenia occurs in patients with leukemia or uremia and in patients receiving cytotoxic therapy, there are generally a reduced number of megakaryocytes in the marrow. Thrombocytopenia also occurs in surgical patients as a result of massive blood loss and replacement with product deficient in platelets. Thrombocytopenia may also be induced by heparin administration in patients with cardiac and vascular disorders, as in the case of HIT, or may be associated with thrombotic and hemorrhagic complications. When thrombocytopenia is present in a patient for whom an elective operation is being considered, management is contingent on the extent and cause of platelet reduction. A count of >50,000/μL generally requires no specific therapy.

Prophylactic platelet administration has now become part of massive transfusion protocols. Platelets also are administered preoperatively to rapidly increase the platelet count in surgical patients with underlying thrombocytopenia. One unit of platelet concentrate contains approximately 5.5×10^{10} platelets and would be expected to increase the circulating platelet count by approximately 10,000/μL in the average 70-kg person. Fever, infection, hepatosplenomegaly, and the presence of antiplatelet alloantibodies decrease the effectiveness of platelet transfusions. In patients whose thrombocytopenia is refractory to standard platelet transfusion, the use of human leukocyte antigen (HLA)–compatible platelets coupled with special processors has proved effective.

Qualitative Platelet Defects

Impaired platelet function often accompanies thrombocytopenia. Impaired ADP-stimulated aggregation occurs with massive transfusion (>10 units of packed red blood cells). Uremia may be associated with increased bleeding time and impaired aggregation and can be corrected by hemodialysis or peritoneal dialysis. Defective aggregation and platelet secretion can occur in patients with thrombocythemia, polycythemia vera, or myelofibrosis.

Drugs that interfere with platelet function by design include aspirin, clopidogrel, dipyridamole, and the glycoprotein IIb/IIIa inhibitors. Both aspirin and clopidogrel irreversibly inhibit platelet function, clopidogrel through selective irreversible inhibition of ADP-induced platelet aggregation and aspirin through irreversible acetylation of platelet prostaglandin synthase. There are no prospective randomized trials in general surgical patients to guide the timing of surgery in patients taking aspirin and/or clopidogrel. The general recommendation is that, for each, a period of approximately 7 days is required from the time the drug is stopped until an elective procedure

can be performed.[12] Timing of urgent and emergent surgeries is even more unclear. Preoperative platelet transfusions may be beneficial, but again there are no good data to guide their administration. The problem is that accurate tests of platelet function are lacking. Other disorders associated with abnormal platelet function include uremia, myeloproliferative disorders, monoclonal gammopathies, and liver disease. In the surgical patient, platelet dysfunction of uremia often can be corrected by dialysis or the administration of desmopressin acetate. Platelet transfusion may not be helpful if the patient is uremic when the platelets are given. Platelet dysfunction in myeloproliferative disorders is intrinsic to the platelets and usually improves if the platelet count can be reduced to normal with chemotherapy. If possible, surgery should be delayed until the count has been decreased. These patients are at risk for both bleeding and thrombosis. Platelet dysfunction in patients with monoclonal gammopathies is a result of interaction of the monoclonal protein with platelets. Treatment with chemotherapy, or occasionally plasmapheresis, to lower the amount of monoclonal protein improves hemostasis.

Acquired Hypofibrinogenemia

Disseminated Intravascular Coagulation

The official definition of disseminated intravascular coagulation (DIC), as put forth by the Scientific Subcommittee on DIC of the Scientific and Standardization Committee of the International Society of Thrombosis and Haemostasis (SSC/ISTH), is that "DIC is an acquired syndrome characterized by the intravascular activation of coagulation with the loss of localization arising from different causes. It can originate from and cause damage to the microvasculature, which if sufficiently severe, can produce organ dysfunction."[13] Excessive thrombin generation leads to microthrombus formation, followed by consumption and depletion of coagulation factors and platelets, which leads to the classic picture of diffuse bleeding. The presence of an underlying condition that predisposes a patient to DIC is required for the diagnosis. Specific injuries include central nervous system injuries with embolization of brain matter, fractures with embolization of bone marrow, and amniotic fluid embolization. Embolized materials are potent thromboplastins that activate the DIC cascade.[14] Additional causes include malignancy, organ injury (such as severe pancreatitis), liver failure, certain vascular abnormalities (such as large aneurysms), snakebites, illicit drugs, transfusion reactions, transplant rejection, and sepsis.[13] DIC frequently accompanies sepsis and may be associated with multiple organ failure. As of yet, scoring systems for organ failure do not routinely incorporate DIC.[14] The important interplay between sepsis and coagulation abnormalities was demonstrated by Dhainaut and colleagues, who showed that administration of activated protein C was particularly effective in septic patients with DIC.[15] The diagnosis of DIC is made on the basis of an inciting cause with associated thrombocytopenia, prolongation of the PT, low fibrinogen level, and elevated levels of fibrin markers (fibrin degradation products, D-dimer, soluble fibrin monomers). A scoring system developed by the SSC/ISTH assigns a score between 0 and 1 to the measured value on each of these laboratory tests; a score of 5 or greater is considered to be overt DIC.[16]

The most important facets of treatment are relieving the patient's causative primary medical or surgical problem and maintaining adequate perfusion. If there is active bleeding, hemostatic factors should be replaced using FFP, which generally is sufficient to correct the hypofibrinogenemia, although cryoprecipitate and platelet concentrates also may be needed. Because microthrombi are generated during DIC, heparin therapy has been proposed. Most studies, however, have shown that heparin is not helpful in acute forms of DIC but may be indicated for purpura fulminans or venous thromboembolism.

Primary Fibrinolysis

An acquired hypofibrinogenic state in the surgical patient also can be a result of pathologic fibrinolysis. This may occur in patients after prostate resection when urokinase is released during surgical manipulation of the prostate or in patients undergoing extracorporeal bypass. The severity of fibrinolytic bleeding is dependent on the concentration of breakdown products in the circulation. The synthetic amino acid ε-aminocaproic acid interferes with fibrinolysis by inhibiting plasminogen activation.

Myeloproliferative Diseases

Polycythemia, particularly with marked thrombocytosis, presents a major surgical risk. In such patients, operations should be considered only for the most grave surgical emergencies. If possible, the operation should be deferred until medical management has restored normal blood volume, hematocrit level, and platelet count. Spontaneous thrombosis is a complication of polycythemia vera and can be explained in part by increased blood viscosity, increased platelet count, and an increased tendency toward stasis. Paradoxically, a significant tendency toward spontaneous hemorrhage also is noted in these patients. Myeloid metaplasia frequently represents part of the natural history of polycythemia vera. Approximately 50% of patients with myeloid metaplasia are postpolycythemic. Abnormalities in platelet aggregation and release have been demonstrated in these patients.

Thrombocytosis can be reduced by the administration of hydroxyurea or anagrelide. Elective surgical procedures should be delayed until the institution of appropriate treatment. Ideally, the hematocrit level should be kept below 48% and the platelet count under 400,000/μL. When an emergency procedure is required, phlebotomy and blood replacement with lactated Ringer's solution may be beneficial.

Coagulopathy of Liver Disease

The liver plays a key role in hemostasis because it is responsible for the synthesis of many of the coagulation factors (Table 4-4). The most common coagulation abnormalities associated with liver dysfunction are thrombocytopenia and impaired humoral coagulation function manifested as prolongation of the PT and increase in the International Normalized Ratio (INR).[17] Thrombocytopenia in patients with liver disease typically is related to hypersplenism, reduced production of thrombopoietin, and immune-mediated destruction of platelets. As noted earlier, in patients with hypersplenism the total body platelet mass is basically normal, but an abnormally high proportion of the platelets are found in the enlarged spleen. Less bleeding is seen than would be anticipated from the platelet count, because some of the sequestered platelets can be released into the circulation. Thrombopoietin, the primary stimulus for thrombopoiesis, may be responsible for some cases of thrombocytopenia in cirrhotic patients, although its role is not well delineated. Finally, immune-mediated thrombocytopenia may also occur in cirrhotic patients, especially those with hepatitis C and primary biliary cirrhosis.[18] Before any therapy to ameliorate thrombocytopenia is initiated, the actual need for correction should be strongly considered. In general, correction based solely on a low platelet count should be discouraged. Most often, treatment should be withheld for invasive procedures and surgery. Platelet transfusions are the mainstay of therapy; however, the effect typically lasts only several hours. Risks associated with transfusions in general,

| TABLE 4-4 | Coagulation factors synthesized by the liver |

Vitamin K–dependent factors: II (prothrombin factor), VII, IX, X
Fibrinogen
Factor V
Factor VIII
Factors XI, XII, XIII
Antithrombin III
Plasminogen
Protein C and protein S

and the development of antiplatelet antibodies in a patient population likely to need recurrent correction, should be considered. A potential alternative strategy is administration of interleukin-11, a cytokine that stimulates proliferation of hematopoietic stem cells and megakaryocyte progenitors.[16] Most studies using interleukin-11 have been in patients with cancer, although some evidence exists that it may be beneficial in cirrhotic patients as well. Significant side effects limit its usefulness.[19] A less well accepted option is splenectomy or splenic embolization to reduce hypersplenism. Not only are there risks associated with these techniques, but reduced splenic blood flow can reduce portal vein flow with subsequent portal vein thrombosis. Results are mixed after transjugular intrahepatic portosystemic shunt (TIPS). Therefore, treatment of thrombocytopenia should not be the primary indication for a TIPS procedure.

Decreased production or increased destruction of coagulation factors as well as a vitamin K deficiency can contribute to a prolonged PT and increased INR in patients with liver disease. As liver dysfunction worsens, so does the liver's synthetic function, which results in decreased production of coagulation factors. Additionally, abnormalities in laboratory results may mimic those of DIC. Elevated D-dimer levels have been reported to increase the risk of variceal bleeding.[20] The absorption of vitamin K is dependent on bile production. Therefore, patients with liver disease who have impaired bile production, such as those with cholestatic disease, may be at risk for vitamin K deficiency.

As with thrombocytopenia, correction of coagulopathy should be reserved for treatment of active bleeding and prophylaxis for invasive procedures and surgery. Coagulopathy caused by liver disease is most often treated with FFP, but because the coagulopathy generally is not a result of decreased levels of factor V, complete correction usually is not possible. If the fibrinogen level is <100 mg/dL, administration of cryoprecipitate may be helpful. Cryoprecipitate is also a source of factor VIII for the rare patient with a low factor VIII level.

Coagulopathy of Trauma

Traditionally recognized causes of traumatic coagulopathy include acidosis, hypothermia, and dilution of coagulation factors. However, a significant proportion of trauma patients arrive at the emergency department coagulopathic, and this early coagulopathy is associated with a significant increase in mortality.[21,22] Brohi and colleagues have demonstrated that only patients in shock arrive coagulopathic and that it is the shock that induces coagulopathy through systemic activation of anticoagulant and fibrinolytic pathways.[23] As shown in Fig. 4-5, hypoperfusion causes activation of thrombomodulin on the surface of endothelial cells. Circulating thrombin complexes with thrombomodulin. This complex not only induces an anticoagulant state through activation of protein C but also enhances fibrinolysis by deinhibition of tPA through the consumption of plasminogen activator inhibitor 1.

Lastly, the thrombin-thrombomodulin complex limits the availability of thrombin to cleave fibrinogen to fibrin, which may explain why injured patients rarely have low levels of fibrinogen.

Acquired Coagulation Inhibition

Among the most common acquired disorder of coagulation inhibition is the antiphospholipid syndrome (APLS), in which the lupus anticoagulant and anticardiolipin antibodies are present. These antibodies may be associated with either venous or arterial thrombosis, or both. In fact, patients who show recurrent thrombosis should be evaluated for APLS. The presence of antiphospholipid antibodies is very common in patients with systemic lupus erythematosus but also may be seen in association with rheumatoid arthritis and Sjögren's syndrome. There are also individuals who have no autoimmune disorders but develop transient antibodies in response to infections or who develop drug-induced APLS. The hallmark of APLS is a prolonged aPTT in vitro but an increased risk of thrombosis in vivo.[24]

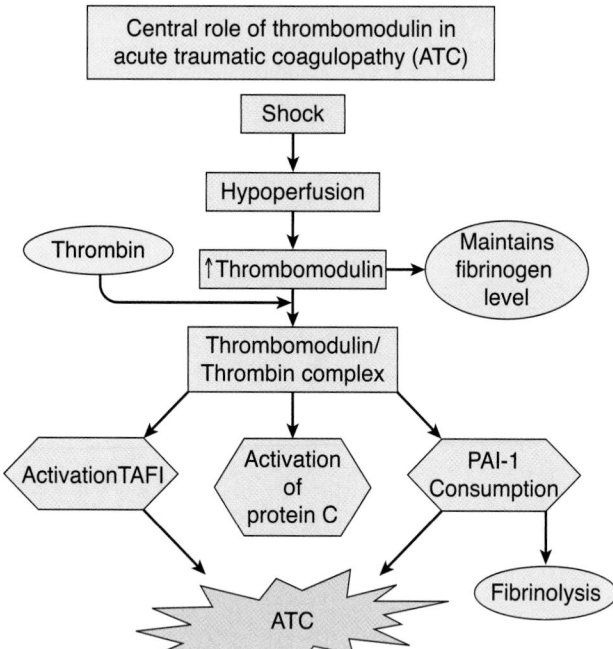

FIG. 4-5. Illustration of the pathophysiologic mechanism responsible for the acute coagulopathy of trauma. PAI-1 = plasminogen activator inhibitor 1; TAFI = thrombin-activatable fibrinolysis inhibitor.

Paraprotein Disorders

Paraprotein disorders are characterized by production of an abnormal globulin or fibrinogen that interferes with clotting or platelet function. This may be an immunoglobulin M in Waldenström's macroglobulinemia, an immunoglobulin G or immunoglobulin A in multiple myeloma, a cryoglobulin in liver disease (especially hepatitis C) or autoimmune diseases, or a cryofibrinogen. Chemotherapy usually is effective in lowering the level of paraproteins in macroglobulinemia and myeloma, although for rapid removal before surgery, plasmapheresis may be needed. Cryoglobulins and cryofibrinogens are usually removed by plasmapheresis.

Anticoagulation and Bleeding

Spontaneous bleeding can be a complication of anticoagulant therapy with either heparin, warfarin, low molecular weight heparins, or factor Xa inhibitors. The risk of spontaneous bleeding related to heparin administration is reduced when a continuous infusion technique is used. Therapeutic anticoagulation is more reliably achieved with a low molecular weight heparin. Laboratory testing is not routinely used to monitor dosing of these agents, which makes them attractive options for outpatient anticoagulation. If monitoring is needed for low molecular weight heparins (e.g., in the presence of renal insufficiency or severe obesity), the drug effect should be determined with an assay for anti-Xa activity.

Warfarin is used for long-term anticoagulation in various clinical conditions, including deep vein thrombosis, pulmonary embolism, valvular heart disease, atrial fibrillation, recurrent systemic embolism, and recurrent myocardial infarction, as well as in patients with prosthetic heart valves and prosthetic implants.[25–27] Due to the interaction of the P-450 system, the anticoagulant effect of the warfarin is reduced (e.g., higher dosage is required) in patients receiving barbiturates as well as in patients with diets low in vitamin K. Warfarin requirements also may be increased in patients taking contraceptives or estrogen-containing compounds, corticosteroids, or adrenocorticotropic hormone. A number of medications can alter warfarin requirements (Table 4-5).

Bleeding complications are frequent in patients taking anticoagulants. Examples include hematuria, soft tissue bleeding, intracere-

---

TABLE 4-5 Medications that can alter warfarin dosing

↓ Warfarin effect ↑ Warfarin requirements	Barbiturates, oral contraceptives, estrogen-containing compounds, corticosteroids, adrenocorticotropic hormone
↑ Warfarin effect ↓ Warfarin requirements	Phenylbutazone, clofibrate, anabolic steroids, L-thyroxine, glucagons, amiodarone, quinidine, cephalosporins

bral bleeding, skin necrosis, and abdominal bleeding. Bleeding into the abdominal cavity is by far the most common complication of warfarin therapy and may be either intraperitoneal, extraperitoneal, or retroperitoneal.[28–30] An intramural bowel hematoma is the most common cause of abdominal pain in patients receiving anticoagulation therapy.[31–33] Fortunately, most intramural bowel hematomas respond to nonoperative treatment. Bleeding secondary to anticoagulation therapy is also not an uncommon cause of rectus sheath hematomas. In most of these cases, reversal of anticoagulation is the only treatment that is necessary. Lastly, it is important to remember that one of the first symptoms of an underlying tumor may be bleeding in a patient who is receiving anticoagulation therapy.

Surgical intervention may prove necessary in patients receiving anticoagulation therapy. Increasing experience suggests that surgical treatment can be undertaken without discontinuing the anticoagulant program, depending on the procedure being performed.[34] Furthermore, the risk of thrombotic complications may be increased when anticoagulation therapy is discontinued abruptly. When the aPTT is <1.3 times the control value in a patient receiving heparin or when the INR is <1.5 in a patient taking warfarin, reversal of anticoagulation therapy may not be necessary. However, meticulous surgical technique is mandatory, and the patient must be observed closely throughout the postoperative period.

Certain surgical procedures should not be performed in concert with anticoagulation; this applies, in particular, to circumstances in which even minor bleeding can cause great morbidity, such as procedures involving the central nervous system or the eye. Emergency operations are occasionally necessary in patients who have been receiving heparin. The first step for these patients is to discontinue heparin. For more rapid reversal of anticoagulation, use of protamine sulfate is effective. However, significant adverse reactions may be encountered when administering protamine, especially in patients with severe fish allergies.[35,36] Symptoms include hypotension, flushing, bradycardia, nausea, and vomiting. Prolongation of the aPTT after heparin neutralization with protamine may also be a result of the anticoagulant effect of protamine. In a patient undergoing elective surgery who is receiving coumarin-derivative therapy sufficient to effect anticoagulation, the drug can be discontinued several days before the operation and the prothrombin concentration then checked (a level >50% is considered safe).[37] Rapid reversal of anticoagulation can be accomplished with FFP in an emergent situation. Parenteral administration of vitamin K also is indicated in elective surgical treatment of patients with biliary obstruction or malabsorption who may be vitamin K deficient. However, if low levels of factors II, VII, IX, and X (vitamin K–dependent factors) are a result of hepatocellular dysfunction, vitamin K administration is ineffective. For patients who were taking warfarin preoperatively and are at high risk for thrombosis, low molecular weight heparin should be administered while the INR is decreasing and should be restarted at prophylactic dosages as soon as possible after surgery. The perioperative management of patients receiving long-term oral anticoagulation therapy is an increasingly common problem. Firm evidence-based guidelines regarding which patients require perioperative "bridging" anticoagulation and the most effective way to bridge are lacking. IV unfractionated heparin and SC low molecular weight heparin in therapeutic dosages reduce the risk of venous thromboembolism but have not been proven to reduce the risk of arterial thromboembolism.[38] Bridging anticoagulation involves discontinuation of oral anticoagulation before surgery and the use of IV or SC agents for several days before and (sometimes) after surgery. Most studies have shown that preoperative bridging is associated with an acceptably low postoperative bleeding rate (1.8 to 5.8%). Not unexpectedly, the risk of bleeding can be substantially higher for procedures associated with intraoperative and postoperative bleeding.

Cardiopulmonary Bypass

The predisposing factors that are associated with excessive bleeding are prolonged perfusion times, prior use of oral anticoagulants or antiplatelet drugs, cyanotic heart disease, and hypothermia. Two factors triggering excessive bleeding associated with cardiopulmonary bypass are excessive fibrinolysis and platelet function defects, with the latter being more important.

The laboratory evaluation of patients with cardiopulmonary bypass hemorrhage should include INR, aPTT, complete blood count, platelet count, peripheral blood smear examination, and measurement of fibrin degradation products. The management entails empiric administration of platelets, and if hyperheparinemia is believed to be the major factor, 25% of the calculated dose of protamine should be administered and repeated every 30 to 60 minutes until the bleeding ceases. If there is laboratory evidence of excess fibrinolysis, ε-aminocaproic acid can be given at an initial dose of 5 to 10 g followed by 1 to 2 g/h until bleeding ceases. Aprotinin, a protease inhibitor that acts as an antifibrinolytic agent, has been shown to reduce transfusion requirements associated with cardiac surgery and orthotopic liver transplantation.[39]

Desmopressin acetate, which stimulates release of factor VIII from endothelial cells, also may be effective in reducing blood loss during cardiac surgery. Laboratory evidence of heparin-induced thrombocytopenia (HIT) often is found after cardiopulmonary bypass; however, clinically significant HIT is rare unless the patient has had previous heparin exposure or heparin continues to be administered in the postoperative period.

Local Hemostasis

Significant surgical bleeding usually is caused by ineffective local hemostasis. The goal is therefore to prevent further blood loss from a disrupted vessel that has been incised or transected. Hemostasis may be accomplished by interrupting the flow of blood to the involved area or by direct closure of the blood vessel wall defect.

Mechanical Procedures The oldest mechanical method of halting bleeding is digital pressure. When pressure is applied to an artery proximal to an area of bleeding, profuse bleeding may be reduced so that more definitive action is permitted. Application of an extremity tourniquet that occludes a major vessel proximal to the bleeding site and the Pringle maneuver for liver bleeding are good examples. Direct digital pressure over a bleeding site often is effective and has the advantage of being less traumatic than a hemostatic clamp. Even an "atraumatic" vascular clamp results in damage to the intimal wall of a blood vessel.

When a small vessel is transected, a simple ligature is sufficient. For large arteries with pulsation, a transfixion suture to prevent slipping is indicated. All sutures represent foreign material, and selection is based on their intrinsic characteristics and the state of the wound. Direct pressure applied by packs affords the best method of controlling diffuse bleeding from large areas, such as in the trauma situation. Bleeding from cut bone can be controlled by packing bone wax on the raw surface to achieve pressure.

The Harmonic scalpel is an instrument that cuts and coagulates tissue via vibration at 55 kHz. The device converts electrical energy into mechanical motion. The motion of the blade causes collagen molecules within the tissue to become denatured, forming a coagulum. No significant electrical current flows through the patient. The instrument has proved advantageous in performing thyroidectomy, hemorrhoidectomy, and transsection of the short gastric veins during splenectomy, and in transecting hepatic parenchyma.[40–42]

Thermal Agents Heat achieves hemostasis by denaturation of protein that results in coagulation of large areas of tissue. With cautery, heat is transmitted from the instrument by conduction directly to the tissue. When electrocautery is used, heating occurs by induction from an alternating current source. The amplitude setting should be high enough to produce prompt coagulation but not so high as to set up an arc between the tissue and the cautery tip. This avoids burns outside the operative field and prevents the exit of current through electrocardiographic leads, other monitoring devices, or permanent pacemakers or defibrillators. A negative grounding plate should be placed beneath the patient to avoid severe skin burns. Certain anesthetic agents (diethyl ether, divinyl ether, ethyl chloride, ethylene, and cyclopropane) cannot be used with electrocautery because of the hazard of explosion.

Use of direct current also can result in hemostasis. Because the protein moieties and cellular elements of blood have a negative surface charge, they are attracted to a positive pole, where a thrombus is formed. Direct currents in the 20- to 100-mA range have successfully controlled diffuse bleeding from raw surfaces, as has argon gas.

Topical Hemostatic Agents Topical hemostatic agents play an important role in common or complex general surgical procedures. These agents can be classified based on their mechanism of action and include physical or mechanical, caustic, biologic, and physiologic agents. Some agents induce protein coagulation and precipitation that results in occlusion of small cutaneous vessels, whereas others take advantage of later stages in the coagulation cascade, activating biologic responses to bleeding.[43] The ideal topical hemostatic agent has significant hemostatic action, shows minimal tissue reactivity, is nonantigenic, biodegrades in vivo, provides ease of sterilization, is low in cost, and can be tailored to specific needs.[44] Table 4-6 reviews only some of the commonly used products on the market.

Thrombin-derivative products direct the conversion of fibrinogen to fibrin, aiding in clot formation. Thrombin takes advantage of natural physiologic processes, thereby avoiding foreign body or inflammatory reactions, and the wound bed is not disturbed.[44] Caution must be taken in judging vessel caliber in the wound, because thrombin entry into larger-caliber vessels can result in systemic exposure to thrombin with a risk of disseminated intravascular clotting or death.

Fibrin sealants are prepared from cryoprecipitate (homologous or synthetic) and have the advantage of not promoting inflammation or tissue necrosis.[45] The sealant is administered using a dual syringe compartment system. In one compartment is fibrinogen, factor XIII, fibronectin, and fibrinolysis inhibitors. The second compartment contains thrombin and calcium chloride.[46] The use of fibrin glue is particularly helpful in patients who have received heparin or who have deficiencies in coagulation (e.g., hemophilia or von Willebrand's disease).[47–49]

Purified gelatin solution can be prepared into several vehicles, including powders, sponges or foams, and sheets or films.[43] Gelatin is hygroscopic, absorbing many times its weight in water or liquid. It is effectively metabolized and degraded by proteinases in the wound bed over a period of 4 to 6 weeks.[43] Gelfoam provides effective hemostasis for operative fields with diffuse small-vessel oozing.[50] Thrombin may be applied to this vehicle to boost hemostasis. Gelatin is relatively inexpensive, readily available, pliable, and easy to handle. Although relatively inert, the implanted gelatin can serve as a nidus for infection.[44]

These agents are not a substitute for meticulous surgical technique. The advantages and disadvantages of each agent must be weighed in selecting the correct agent to control bleeding. In general, the minimum amount of each topical hemostatic agent should be used to minimize toxic effects and adverse reactions, interference with wound healing, and procedural cost.

TABLE 4-6	Common hemostatic agents		
Hemostatic Agent	**Manufacturer**	**Cost**	**Comments**
Thrombin Products			
Floseal	Baxter	$1500 per 6 pack/5 mL	Disseminated intravascular coagulation may result from intra-
Thrombostat	Parke-Davis	$56–60/5000–10,000 vial	vascular exposure. Solution soaked in gauze or injected over
Thrombin-JMI	King Pharmaceuticals	$285/10,000 units	wound bed, forming attachment.
Fibrin Sealant			
Tisseel	Baxter	$135/2 mL	Useful in skin grafts or anticoagulated patients. Crosseal contains
Crosseal	Johnson & Johnson	$100–150/1 mL	no aprotinin, reduces anaphylaxis risk.
Gelatin Agents			
Gelfoam	Pfizer	$90/1 g	Forms hydrated meshwork to promote clotting. Can swell. May
Surgifoam	Johnson & Johnson	$8–14/gelatin square	cause granulomatous reaction.

TRANSFUSION

Background

Human blood replacement therapy was accepted in the late nineteenth century. This was followed by the introduction of blood grouping by Dr. Karl Landsteiner, who identified the major A, B, and O groups in 1900. In 1939 Dr. Philip Levine and Dr. Rufus Stetson followed with the concept of Rh grouping. These breakthroughs established the foundation from which the field of transfusion medicine has grown. Whole blood was considered the standard in transfusion until the late 1970s, when goal-directed component therapy began to take prominence. This change in practice was made possible by the development of improved collection strategies, testing for infection, and advances in preservative solutions and storage.

Replacement Therapy

Typing and Cross-Matching

Serologic compatibility for A, B, O, and Rh groups is established routinely. Cross-matching between donors' red blood cells and recipients' sera (the major cross-match) is performed. Rh-negative recipients should receive transfusions only of Rh-negative blood. However, this group represents only 15% of the population. Therefore, the administration of Rh-positive blood is acceptable if Rh-negative blood is not available. However, Rh-positive blood should not be transfused to Rh-negative females who are of childbearing age.

In emergency situations, type O-negative blood may be transfused to all recipients. O-negative and type-specific red blood cells are equally safe for emergency transfusion. Problems are associated with the administration of 4 or more units of O-negative blood, because there is a significant increase in the risk of hemolysis. In patients with clinically significant levels of cold agglutinins, blood should be administered through a blood warmer. If these antibodies are present in high titer, hypothermia is contraindicated.

In patients who have been transfused multiple times and who have developed alloantibodies or who have autoimmune hemolytic anemia with pan–red blood cell antibodies, typing and cross-matching is often difficult, and sufficient time should be allotted preoperatively to accumulate blood that might be required during the operation. Cross-matching should always be performed before the administration of dextran, because it interferes with the typing procedure.

The use of autologous transfusion is growing. Up to 5 units can be collected for subsequent use during elective procedures. Patients can donate blood if their hemoglobin concentration exceeds 11 g/dL or if the hematocrit is >34%. The first procurement is performed 40 days before the planned operation and the last one is performed 3 days before the operation. Donations can be scheduled at intervals of 3 to 4 days. Administration of recombinant human erythropoietin accelerates generation of red blood cells and allows for more frequent harvesting of blood.

Banked Whole Blood

Banked whole blood, once the gold standard, is rarely available. The shelf life is now around 6 weeks. At least 70% of the transfused erythrocytes remain in the circulation for 24 hours after transfusion and are viable. The age of red cells may play a significant role in the inflammatory response and incidence of multiple organ failure. The changes in the red blood cells that occur during storage include reduction of intracellular ADP and 2,3-diphosphoglycerate, which alters the oxygen dissociation curve of hemoglobin and results in a decrease in oxygen transport. Although all clotting factors are relatively stable in banked blood except for factors V and VIII, banked blood progressively becomes acidotic with elevated levels of lactate, potassium, and ammonia. The hemolysis that occurs during storage is insignificant.

Fresh Whole Blood

Fresh whole blood refers to blood that is administered within 24 hours of its donation. Advances in testing for infectious disease now make fresh whole blood another option. Recent evidence has shown that the use of fresh whole blood may improve outcomes in patients with trauma-associated coagulopathy in the combat situation,[51] and a civilian study will soon be under way. An advantage to the use of fresh whole blood is that it provides greater coagulation activity than equal units of component therapy.

Packed Red Blood Cells and Frozen Red Blood Cells

Packed red blood cells are the product of choice for most clinical situations. Concentrated suspensions of red blood cells can be prepared by removing most of the supernatant plasma after centrifugation. This preparation reduces, but does not eliminate, reaction caused by plasma components. It also reduces the amount of sodium, potassium, lactic acid, and citrate administered. Frozen red blood cells are not available for use in emergencies. They are used for patients who are known to have been previously sensitized. By freezing red blood cells viability is theoretically improved, and the ATP and 2,3-diphosphoglycerate concentrations are maintained. Little clinical outcome data are available to substantiate these findings.

Leukocyte-Reduced and Leukocyte-Reduced/Washed Red Blood Cells

Leukocyte-reduced and leukocyte-reduced/washed red blood cell products are prepared by filtration that removes approximately 99.9% of the white blood cells and most of the platelets (leukocyte-reduced red blood cells), and if necessary, by additional saline washing (leukocyte-reduced/washed red blood cells). Leukocyte reduction prevents almost all febrile, nonhemolytic transfusion reactions (fever and/or rigors), alloimmunization to HLA class I antigens, and platelet transfusion refractoriness as well as cytomegalovirus transmission. In most western nations, it is the standard red blood cell transfusion product. Opponents of universal leukoreduction believe that the additional costs associated with this process are not justified because they are of the opinion that transfused allogenic white blood cells have no significant immunomodulatory effects. Supporters of universal leukocyte reduction argue that allogenic transfusion of white cells predisposes to postoperative bacterial infection and multiorgan failure. Reviews of randomized trials and meta-analysis have not provided convincing evidence either way,[52,53] although a large Canadian retrospective study suggests a decrease in mortality and infections when leukocyte-reduced red blood cells are used.[54]

Platelet Concentrates

The indications for platelet transfusion include thrombocytopenia caused by massive blood loss and replacement with platelet-poor products, thrombocytopenia caused by inadequate platelet production, and qualitative platelet disorders. The shelf life of platelets is 120 hours from time of donation. One unit of platelet concentrate has a volume of approximately 50 mL. Platelet preparations are capable of transmitting infectious diseases and can provoke allergic reactions similar to those caused by blood transfusion. Therapeutic levels of platelets reached after therapy are in the range of 50,000 to 100,000/μL. However, there is a growing body of information suggesting that platelet transfusion thresholds can safely be lowered in patients who have no signs of hemostatic deficiency and who have no history of poor tolerance to low platelet counts. Prevention of HLA alloimmunization can be achieved by leukocyte reduction through filtration. In rare cases, such as in patients who have become alloimmunized through previous transfusion or patients who are refractory from sensitization through prior pregnancies, HLA-matched platelets can be used.

Fresh-Frozen Plasma

Fresh-frozen plasma (FFP) prepared from freshly donated blood is the usual source of the vitamin K–dependent factors and is the only source of factor V. However, FFP carries infectious risks similar to those of other component therapies. FFP has come to the forefront with the inception of damage control resuscitation in patients with trauma-associated coagulopathy. In an effort to increase the shelf life and avoid the need for refrigeration, lyophilized plasma is being tested. Preliminary animal studies suggest that this process preserves the beneficial effects of FFP.[55]

Concentrates and Recombinant DNA Technology

Technologic advancements have made the majority of clotting factors and albumin readily available as concentrates. These products are readily obtainable and carry no inherent infectious risks as do other component therapies.

Human Polymerized Hemoglobin (PolyHeme)

Human polymerized hemoglobin (PolyHeme) is a universally compatible, immediately available, disease-free, oxygen-carrying resuscitative fluid that has been successfully used in massively bleeding patients when red blood cells were not transfused. Advantages of an artificial oxygen carrier include the absence of blood-type antigens (no cross-match needed) and viral infections and long-term stability, which allows prolonged periods of storage. Disadvantages include shorter half-life in the bloodstream and the potential to increase cardiovascular complications. This product has not yet been approved for use in patients.

Indications for Replacement of Blood and Its Elements

General Indications

Improvement in Oxygen-Carrying Capacity Oxygen-carrying capacity is primarily a function of the red blood cells. Thus, transfusion of red blood cells should augment oxygen-carrying capacity. Additionally, hemoglobin is fundamental to arterial oxygen content and

thus oxygen delivery. Despite this obvious association, there is little evidence that actually supports the premise that transfusion of red blood cells equates with enhanced cellular delivery and utilization. The reasons for this apparent discrepancy are related to changes that occur with the storage of blood. The decrease in 2,3-diphosphoglycerate and p50 impair oxygen offloading, and deformation of the red cells impairs microcirculatory perfusion.[56]

Treatment of Anemia: Transfusion Trigger A 1988 National Institutes of Health Consensus Report challenged the dictum that a hemoglobin value of <10 g/dL or a hematocrit level of <30% indicates a need for preoperative red blood cell transfusion. This was verified in a prospective randomized controlled trial in critically ill patients that compared use of a restrictive transfusion threshold with use of a more liberal strategy and demonstrated that maintaining hemoglobin levels between 7 and 9 g/dL had no adverse effect on mortality. In fact, patients with Acute Physiology and Chronic Health Evaluation II (APACHE II) scores of 20 or less and patients 55 years or younger actually had a lower mortality.[57]

Despite these results, little has changed in transfusion practice. Critically ill patients frequently receive transfusions, with the hemoglobin level at which transfusion is initiated approaching 9 g/dL in a large observational study.[58]

One unresolved issue related to transfusion triggers is the safety of maintaining a hemoglobin level of 7 g/dL in a patient with ischemic heart disease. Data on this subject are mixed, and many studies have significant design flaws, including their retrospective nature. However, the majority of the published literature favors a restrictive transfusion trigger for patients with acute coronary syndrome without ST elevation, and many report worse outcomes in those patients receiving transfusions. Patients with acute myocardial infarctions with ST elevation may, however, benefit from receiving red blood cell transfusions for anemia.[56,58] Clearly, further investigation is warranted.

Volume Replacement The most common indication for blood transfusion in surgical patients is the replenishment of the blood volume, a deficit of which is difficult to evaluate.

Measurements of hemoglobin levels or hematocrit are frequently used to assess blood loss. These measurements can be misleading in the face of acute loss, because the levels can be normal in spite of severely contracted blood volume. Both the amount and the rate of bleeding are factors in the development of signs and symptoms of blood loss.[56] A healthy adult can lose up to 15% of total blood volume (class I hemorrhage or up to 750 mL) with only minor effects on the circulation. Loss of 15 to 30% of blood volume (class II hemorrhage or 750 to 1500 mL) is associated with tachycardia and decreased pulse pressure but, importantly, a normal blood pressure. Loss of 30 to 40% (class III hemorrhage or 1500 to 2000 mL) results in tachycardia, tachypnea, hypotension, oliguria, and changes in mental status. Class IV hemorrhage is loss of >40% of blood volume and is considered life-threatening.

Loss of blood in the operating room can be evaluated by estimating the amount of blood in the wound and on the drapes, weighing the sponges, and quantifying blood suctioned from the operative field. In patients with normal preoperative values, blood loss of up to 20% of total blood volume can be replaced with crystalloid solution. Blood loss above this amount may require the addition of packed red blood cells and, in the case of massive transfusion, the addition of FFP (detailed later in this chapter). Transfusion of platelets and/or FFP may be indicated in specific patients before or during an operative procedure (Table 4-7).

Damage Control Resuscitation

Current resuscitation algorithms are based on the sequence of crystalloid followed by red blood cells and then plasma and platelet transfusions and have been in widespread use since the 1970s. Recently, the damage control resuscitation (DCR) strategy, aimed at halting and/or preventing rather than treating the lethal triad of

TABLE 4-7 Replacement of clotting factors

Factor	Normal Level	Life Span In Vivo (Half-Life)	Fate during Coagulation	Level Required for Safe Hemostasis	Ideal Agent ACD Bank Blood [4°C (39.2°F)]	Ideal Agent for Replacing Deficit
I (fibrinogen)	200–400 mg/100 mL	72 h	Consumed	60–100 mg/100 mL	Very stable	Bank blood; concentrated fibrinogen
II (prothrombin)	20 mg/100 mL (100% of normal level)	72 h	Consumed	15–20%	Stable	Bank blood; concentrated preparation
V (proaccelerin, accelerator globulin, labile factor)	100% of normal level	36 h	Consumed	5–20%	Labile (40% of normal level at 1 wk)	Fresh-frozen plasma; blood under 7 d
VII (proconvertin, serum prothrombin conversion accelerator, stable factor)	100% of normal level	5 h	Survives	5–30%	Stable	Bank blood; concentrated preparation
VIII (antihemophilic factor, antihemophilic globulin)	100% of normal level (50–150% of normal level)	6–12 h	Consumed	30%	Labile (20–40% of normal level at 1 wk)	Fresh-frozen plasma; concentrated antihemophilic factor; cryoprecipitate
IX (Christmas factor, plasma thromboplastin component)	100% of normal level	24 h	Survives	20–30%	Stable	Fresh-frozen plasma; bank blood; concentrated preparation
X (Stuart-Prower factor)	100% of normal level	40 h	Survives	15–20%	Stable	Bank blood; concentrated preparation
XI (plasma thromboplastin antecedent)	100% of normal level	Probably 40–80 h	Survives	10%	Probably stable	Bank blood
XII (Hageman factor)	100% of normal level	Unknown	Survives	Deficit produces no bleeding tendency	Stable	Replacement not required
XIII (fibrinase, fibrin-stabilizing factor)	100% of normal level	4–7 d	Survives	Probably <1%	Stable	Bank blood
Platelets	150,000–400,000/μL	8–11 d	Consumed	60,000–100,000/μL	Very labile (40% of normal level at 20 h; 0 at 48 h)	Fresh blood or plasma; fresh platelet concentrate (not frozen plasma)

ACD = acid-citrate-dextrose.

Source: Reproduced with permission from Salzman EW: Hemorrhagic disorders, in Kinney JM, Egdahl RH, Zuidema GD (eds): *Manual of Preoperative and Postoperative Care*, 2nd ed. Philadelphia: WB Saunders, 1971, p 157. Copyright Elsevier.

coagulopathy, acidosis, and hypothermia, has challenged traditional thinking on early resuscitation strategies.

Rationale In civilian trauma systems nearly half of all deaths occur before a patient reaches the hospital, and few of these deaths are preventable.[59–61] Those patients who survive until arrival at an emergency center have a high incidence of truncal hemorrhage, and deaths in this group of patients may be potentially preventable. Truncal hemorrhage patients in shock often present with the early coagulopathy of trauma in the emergency department and are at significant risk of dying.[21,22,62]

Many of these patients receive a massive transfusion, generally defined as the administration of 10 or more units of packed red blood cells within 24 hours of admission. Although 25% of all trauma patients admitted receive a unit of blood early after admission, only a small percentage of patients receive a massive transfusion. In the military setting, however, the percentage of patients receiving a massive transfusion almost doubles.[63]

New Concepts in Resuscitation Strategies Standard advanced trauma life support guidelines start resuscitation with crystalloid, followed by packed red blood cells.[64] Only after liters of crystalloid have been transfused does transfusion of units of plasma or platelets begin. This conventional massive transfusion practice was based on a small uncontrolled retrospective study that used blood products containing increased amounts of plasma, which are no longer available.[65]

More recently, multiple retrospective studies have suggested that this standard resuscitation practice exacerbates the initial coagulopathy of trauma, thus increasing mortality, whereas transfusing a higher ratio of plasma and platelets to red blood cells is associated with improved survival.[66,67] An example of an adult massive transfusion clinical guideline specifying the early use of component therapy is shown in Fig. 4-6. Specific recommendations for the administration of component therapy during a massive transfusion are shown in Table 4-8. Recent data suggest that plasma should be given earlier to patients who are significantly injured and massively transfused, because they arrive in the intensive care unit coagulopathic.[68]

When one center modified its transfusion practice so that plasma was started when the first units of red cells were administered rather than waiting until after 6 units of red cells were transfused, a significant decrease in 30-day mortality was demonstrated.[69] This work documents the importance of starting increased amounts of plasma early and supports a 1:1 ratio of plasma to red cells in patients receiving massive transfusion. This is a shift from traditional resuscitation strategies that called for the early use of crystalloids followed by packed red cells and the administration of plasma only after large amounts of blood products were transfused or to treat the resultant coagulopathy. As noted earlier, this new strategy has been termed *damage control resuscitation* and represents an alternative to traditional resuscitation standards. The central tenet of DCR is transfusion of plasma and red blood cells in a 1:1 ratio, started within minutes of the patient's arrival to the emergency department. In Iraq and Afghanistan, DCR practices are demonstrating unprecedented success with improved overall survival.[70] Greater use of platelets recently has been added to the DCR approach, because survival is improved with their early and increased use. As an adjunct to DCR, recombinant activated factor VII is used by the military and many major civilian trauma centers. Retrospective studies in combat wounded reveals an association

A. Initial Transfusion of Red Blood Cells (RBCs):

1. Notify Blood Bank immediately of urgent need for RBCs.
   O Negative Uncrossmatched (available immediately).
   As soon as possible switch to O-negative for females and O-positive for males
   Type-Specific Uncrossmatched (available in approximately 5–10 minutes)
   Completely Crossmatched (available in approximately 40 minutes)
2. A blood sample must be sent to Blood Bank for a Type & Cross.
3. The Emergency Release of Blood form must be completed. If the blood type is not known and blood is needed immediately, O Negative RBCs should be issued.
4. RBCs will be transfused in the standard fashion. All patients must be identified (name and number) prior to transfusion.
5. Patients who are unstable or receive 1–2 RBCs and do not rapidly respond should be considered candidates for the massive transfusion (MT) guideline.

B. Adult Massive Transfusion Guideline:

1. The **Massive Transfusion Guideline (MTG)** should be initiated as soon as it is anticipated that a patient will require massive transfusion (≥10 U RBCs in 24 hours). The Blood Bank should strive to deliver plasma, platelets, and RBCs in a 1:1:1 ratio. To be effective and minimize further dilutional coagulopathy, the 1:1:1 ratio must be initiated early, ideally with the first 2 units of transfused RBCs. Crystalloid infusion should be minimized.
2. Once the MTG is activated, the Blood Bank will have 6 RBCs, 6 FFP, and a 6-pack of platelets packed in a cooler available for rapid transport. If 6 units of thawed FFP are not immediately available, the Blood Bank will issue units that are ready and notify appropriate personnel when the remainder is thawed. Every attempt should be made to obtain a 1:1:1 ratio of plasma:platelets:RBCs.
3. Once initiated, the MT will continue until stopped by the attending physician. MT should be terminated once the patient is no longer actively bleeding.
4. No blood components will be issued without a pickup slip with the recipient's medical record number and name.
5. Basic laboratory tests should be drawn immediately on ED arrival and optimally performed on point-of-care devices, facilitating timely delivery of relevant information to the attending clinicians. These tests should be repeated as clinically indicated (e.g., after each cooler of products has been transfused). Suggested laboratory values are:
   - CBC
   - INR, fibrinogen
   - pH and/or Base deficit
   - TEG, where available

FIG. 4-6. Adult transfusion clinical practice guidelines. ED = emergency department; CBC = complete blood count; INR = International Normalized Ratio; TEG = thromboelastography.

with decreased transfusions and improved 30-day survival.[71] However, some studies have reported increased thrombotic complications after administration of factor VII.[72]

To verify military and single-institution civilian data on DCR, a multicenter retrospective study of modern transfusion practices at 17 leading civilian trauma centers was recently completed.[73] There was significant variation among centers, with plasma:platelet:red blood cell ratios varying from 1:1:1 to 0.3:0.1:1 and corresponding survival rates ranging from 71 to 41%. Centers using ratios approximating 1:1:1 demonstrated significantly fewer truncal hemorrhagic deaths and significantly lower 30-day mortality without a concomitant increase in multiple organ failure as a cause of death. A prospective observational study will soon commence to study the practice of the early use of plasma.

Because only a small percentage of trauma patients require a massive transfusion and blood products in general are in short supply, attempts have been made to develop early prediction models. A comparison of results from both civilian and military studies

is shown in Table 4-9.[74-78] Although they are compelling, none of these algorithms has yet been prospectively validated.

Complications of Transfusion (Table 4-10)

Complications of transfusion are primarily related to blood-induced proinflammatory responses. Transfusion-related events are estimated to occur in approximately 10% of all transfusions, but <0.5% are serious. Transfusion-related deaths, although rare, do occur and are caused primarily by transfusion-related acute lung injury (16 to 22%), ABO hemolytic transfusion reactions (12 to 15%), and bacterial contamination of platelets (11 to 18%).[79]

Nonhemolytic Reactions

Febrile nonhemolytic reactions are defined as an increase in temperature [>1°C (1.8°F)] associated with a transfusion and are fairly common (approximately 1% of all transfusions). Preformed cytokines in donated blood and recipient antibodies reacting with donated anti-

TABLE 4-8	Component therapy administration during massive transfusion
Fresh-frozen plasma (FFP)	As soon as the need for massive transfusion is recognized. For every 6 units of red blood cells (RBCs), give 6 units of FFP (1:1 ratio).
Platelets	For every 6 units of RBCs and plasma, give one 6-pack of platelets. Six random-donor platelet packs = 1 apheresis platelet unit. Keep platelet counts >100,000 μ/L during active hemorrhage control.
Cryoprecipitate	After first 6 units of RBCs, check fibrinogen level. If ≤100 mg/dL, give 20 units of cryoprecipitate (2 g fibrinogen). Repeat as needed, depending on fibrinogen level.

TABLE 4-9	Comparison of massive transfusion prediction studies	
Authors	Variables	ROC AUC Value
McLaughlin et al[73]	SBP, HR, pH, Hct	0.839
Yücel et al[74]	SBP, HR, BD, Hgb, male gender, + FAST, long bone/pelvic fracture	0.892
Moore et al[75]	SBP, pH, ISS >25	0.804
Schreiber et al[76]	Hgb ≤11, INR >1.5, penetrating injury	0.80
Wade et al[77]	SBP, HR, pH, Hct	0.78

AUC = area under the curve; BD = base deficit; FAST = focused assessment by sonography in trauma; Hct = hematocrit; Hgb = hemoglobin level; HR = heart rate; INR = International Normalized Ratio; ISS = injury severity score; ROC = receiver operating characteristic; SBP = systolic blood pressure.

bodies are postulated causes. The incidence of febrile reactions can be greatly reduced by the use of leukocyte-reduced blood products. Pretreatment with acetaminophen reduces the severity of the reaction.

Bacterial contamination of infused blood is rare. Gram-negative organisms, especially *Yersinia enterocolitica* and *Pseudomonas* species, which are capable of growth at 4°C (39.2°F), are the most common cause. Most cases, however, are associated with the administration of platelets that are stored at 20°C (68°F) or even more commonly with apheresis platelets stored at room temperature. Bacterial contamination results in sepsis and death in up to 25% of patients.[80] Clinical manifestations include systemic signs such as fever and chills, tachycardia, and hypotension, and GI symptoms

(abdominal cramps, vomiting, and diarrhea). There also can be hemorrhagic manifestations such as hemoglobinemia, hemoglobinuria, and disseminated intravascular coagulation. If the diagnosis is suspected, the transfusion should be discontinued and the blood cultured. Emergency treatment includes administration of oxygen, adrenergic blocking agents, and antibiotics. Prevention includes avoidance of out-of-date platelets.

Allergic Reactions

Allergic reactions are relatively frequent, occurring in approximately 1% of all transfusions. Reactions usually are mild and consist of rash, urticaria, and fever occurring within 60 to 90 minutes of the

TABLE 4-10	Transfusion-related complications				
Abbreviation	Complication	Signs & Symptoms	Frequency	Mechanism	Prevention
NHTR	Febrile, nonhemolytic transfusion reaction	Fever	0.5–1.5% of transfusions	Preformed cytokines Host Ab to donor lymphocytes	Use leukocyte-reduced blood
	Bacterial contamination	High fever, chills Hemodynamic changes DIC Emesis, diarrhea Hemoglobinuria	<<0.05% of blood 0.05% of platelets	Infusion of contaminated blood	Store platelets <5 d
	Allergic reactions	Rash, hives Itching	0.1–0.3% of units	Soluble transfusion constituents	Provide antihistamine prophylaxis
TACO	Transfusion-associated circulatory overload	Pulmonary edema	? 1:200–1:10,00 of transfused patients	Large volume of blood transfused into an older patient with CHF	Increase transfusion time Administer diuretics Minimize associated fluids
TRALI	Transfusion-related acute lung injury	Acute (<6 h) hypoxemia Bilateral infiltrates ± Tachycardia, hypotension		Anti-HLA or anti-HNA Ab in transfused blood attacks circulatory and pulmonary leukocytes	Limit female donors
	Hemolytic reactions Acute	Fever Hypotension DIC Hemoglobinuria Hemoglobinemia Renal insufficiency	1:33,000–1:1,500,000 units	Transfusion of ABO incompatible blood Preformed IgM Ab to ABO Ag	Transfuse appropriately matched blood
	Delayed (2–10 d)	Anemia Indirect hyperbilirubinemia Elevated haptoglobin level Positive result on direct Coombs' test		IgG mediated	Identify patient's Ag to prevent recurrence

Ab = antibody; Ag = antigen; CHF = congestive heart failure; DIC = disseminated intravascular coagulation; HLA = human leukocyte antigen; HNA = anti–human neutrophil antigen; IgG = immunoglobulin G; IgM = immunoglobulin M.

start of the transfusion. In rare instances, anaphylactic shock develops. Allergic reactions are caused by the transfusion of antibodies from hypersensitive donors or the transfusion of antigens to which the recipient is hypersensitive. Allergic reactions can occur after the administration of any blood product. Treatment and prophylaxis consist of the administration of antihistamines. In more serious cases, use of epinephrine or steroids may be indicated.

Respiratory Complications

Respiratory compromise may be associated with transfusion-associated circulatory overload, which is an avoidable complication. It can occur with rapid infusion of blood, plasma expanders, and crystalloids, particularly in older patients with underlying heart disease. Central venous pressure monitoring should be considered whenever large amounts of fluid are administered. Overload is manifest by a rise in venous pressure, dyspnea, and cough. Rales generally can be heard at the lung bases. Treatment consists of initiating diuresis, slowing the rate of blood administration, and minimizing delivery of fluids while blood products are being transfused.

The *syndrome of transfusion-related acute lung injury (TRALI)* is defined as noncardiogenic pulmonary edema related to transfusion.[81] It can occur with the administration of any plasma-containing blood product. Symptoms are similar to those of circulatory overload with dyspnea and associated hypoxemia. However, TRALI is characterized as noncardiogenic and often is accompanied by fever, rigors, and bilateral pulmonary infiltrates on chest radiograph. It most commonly occurs within 1 to 2 hours after the onset of transfusion, but virtually always before 6 hours. The actual incidence is unknown, because most cases are not reported (or not diagnosed). The etiology is not well established, but TRALI is thought to be related to anti-HLA or anti–human neutrophil antigen antibodies in transfused blood that primes neutrophils in the pulmonary circulation. Multiparity of the donor is considered a major risk factor for the development of TRALI. In a recent study by Gajic and colleagues, critically ill patients who received high volumes of plasma had worsened gas exchange after transfusion of components from female but not male donors.[82] This association of TRALI with components from female donors has prompted the American Association of Blood Banks to propose the use of male-only donor plasma. Treatment of TRALI entails discontinuation of any transfusion, notification of the transfusion service, and provision of pulmonary support, which may vary from supplemental oxygen to mechanical ventilation.

Hemolytic Reactions

Hemolytic reactions can be classified as either acute of delayed. Acute hemolytic reactions occur with the administration of ABO-incompatible blood and are fatal in up to 6% of cases. Contributing factors include technical or clerical errors in the laboratory and administration of blood of the wrong blood type. Immediate hemolytic reactions are characterized by intravascular destruction of red blood cells and consequent hemoglobinemia and hemoglobinuria. DIC can be initiated activation of factor XII and complement by antibody-antigen complexes, which leads to initiation of the coagulation cascade. Finally, acute renal insufficiency results from the toxicity associated with free hemoglobin in the plasma, leading to tubular necrosis and precipitation of hemoglobin within the tubules.

Delayed hemolytic transfusion reactions occur 2 to 10 days after transfusion and are characterized by extravascular hemolysis, mild anemia, and indirect (unconjugated) hyperbilirubinemia. They occur when an individual has a low antibody titer at the time of transfusion but the titer increases after transfusion as a result of an anamnestic response. Reactions to non-ABO antigens involve immunoglobulin G–mediated clearance by the reticuloendothelial system.

If the patient is awake, the most common symptoms of acute transfusion reactions are pain at the site of transfusion, facial flushing, and back and chest pain. Associated symptoms include fever, respiratory distress, hypotension, and tachycardia. In anesthetized patients, diffuse bleeding and hypotension are the hallmarks. A high index of suspicion is needed to make the diagnosis. The laboratory criteria for a transfusion reaction are hemoglobinuria and serologic findings that show incompatibility of the donor and recipient blood. A positive Coombs' test result indicates the presence of transfused cells coated with patient antibody and is diagnostic. Delayed hemolytic transfusion reactions may also be manifested by fever and recurrent anemia. Jaundice and decreased haptoglobin levels usually occur, and low-grade hemoglobinemia and hemoglobinuria may be seen. The Coombs' test usually yields a positive result, and the blood bank must identify the antigen to prevent subsequent reactions.

If an immediate hemolytic transfusion reaction is suspected, the transfusion should be stopped immediately and a sample of the recipient's blood drawn and sent along with the suspect unit to the blood bank for comparison with the pretransfusion samples. Urine output should be monitored and adequate hydration maintained to prevent precipitation of hemoglobin within the tubules. Delayed hemolytic transfusion reactions do not usually require specific intervention.

Transmission of Disease

Among the diseases that have been transmitted by transfusion are malaria, Chagas' disease, brucellosis, and, very rarely, syphilis. Malaria can be transmitted by all blood components. The species most commonly implicated is *Plasmodium malariae*. The incubation period ranges from 8 to 100 days. The initial manifestations are shaking chills and spiking fever. Cytomegalovirus infection resembling infectious mononucleosis also has occurred.

Transmission of hepatitis C virus and HIV-1 has been dramatically minimized by the introduction of better antibody and nucleic acid screening for these pathogens. The infection rate for these pathogens is now estimated to be <1 per 1,000,000 units transfused. Hepatitis B virus transmission may still occur in about 1 in 100,000 transfusions in nonimmune recipients. Hepatitis A virus is very rarely transmitted because there is no asymptomatic carrier state. Recent concerns about the rare transmission of these and other pathogens, such as West Nile virus, are being addressed by current trials of "pathogen inactivation systems" that reduce infectious levels of all viruses and bacteria known to be transmittable by transfusion. Prion disorders (e.g., Creutzfeldt-Jakob disease) also are transmissible by transfusion, but there is currently no information on inactivation of prions in blood products for transfusion.

TESTS OF HEMOSTASIS AND BLOOD COAGULATION

The initial approach to assessing hemostatic function is a careful review of the patient's clinical history (including previous abnormal bleeding or bruising) and drug use, and basic laboratory testing. Common screening laboratory testing includes platelet count, PT or INR, and aPTT. Platelet dysfunction can occur at either extreme of platelet count. The normal platelet count ranges from 150,000 to 400,000/μL. Platelet counts >1,000,000/μL may be associated with bleeding or thrombotic complications. Increased bleeding complications may be seen with major surgical procedures when the platelet count is <100,000/μL and with minor surgical procedures when counts are <50,000/μL. Spontaneous hemorrhage can occur when the count falls below 20,000/μL.

The PT and aPTT are variations of plasma recalcification times initiated by the addition of a thromboplastic agent. The PT reagent contains thromboplastin and calcium that, when added to plasma, leads to the formation of a fibrin clot. The PT test measures the function of factors I, II, V, VII, and X. Factor VII is part of the extrinsic pathway and the remaining factors are part of the common pathway. Factor VII has the shortest half-life of the coagulation factors, and its synthesis is vitamin K dependent. The PT test is best suited to detection of abnormal coagulation caused by vitamin K deficiencies and warfarin therapy.

Due to variations in thromboplastin activity, it can be difficult to accurately assess the degree of anticoagulation on the basis of PT alone. To account for these variations, determination of the INR is now the method of choice for reporting PT values. The International Sensitivity Index (ISI) is unique to each batch of thromboplastin and is furnished by the manufacturer to the hematology laboratory. Human brain thromboplastin has an ISI of 1, and the optimal reagent has an ISI between 1.3 and 1.5.

The INR is a calculated number derived from the following equation:

$$INR = (\text{measured PT/normal PT})^{ISI}$$

The aPTT reagent contains a phospholipid substitute, activator, and calcium, which in the presence of plasma leads to fibrin clot formation. The aPTT measures function of factors I, II, and V of the common pathway and factors VIII, IX, X, and XII of the intrinsic pathway. Heparin therapy is often monitored by following aPTT values, with a therapeutic target range of 1.5 to 2.5 times the control value (approximately 50 to 80 seconds). Low molecular weight heparins are selective factor Xa inhibitors and may mildly elevate the aPTT, but therapeutic monitoring is not routinely recommended.

The bleeding time is used to evaluate platelet and vascular dysfunction, although not so frequently as in the past. Several standard methods have been described; however, the Ivy bleeding time is most commonly used. It is determined by placing a sphygmomanometer on the upper arm and inflating it to 40 mmHg and then making a 5-mm stab incision on the flexor surface of the forearm. The time is measured to cessation of bleeding, and the upper limit of normal bleeding time with Ivy's test is 7 minutes. A template aids in administering the test uniformly and adds to the reproducibility of the results. An abnormal bleeding time suggests either platelet dysfunction (intrinsic or drug induced), vWD, or certain vascular defects. Many laboratories are replacing the template bleeding time with an in vitro test in which blood is sucked through a capillary and the platelets adhere to the walls of the capillary and aggregate. The closure time in this system appears to be more reproducible than the bleeding time and also correlates with bleeding in patients with vWD, primary platelet function disorders, or other platelet dysfunction disorders and patients who are taking aspirin.

Additional medications may significantly impair hemostatic function, such as antiplatelet agents (clopidogrel and glycoprotein IIb/IIIa inhibitors), anticoagulant agents (hirudin, chondroitin sulfate, dermatan sulfate), and thrombolytic agents (streptokinase, tPA). If abnormal results on any of the coagulation studies cannot be explained by known medications, congenital abnormalities of coagulation or comorbid disease should be considered.

Thromboelastography (TEG) was originally described by Hartert in 1948.[83] Continuous improvements in this technique have made this test a valuable tool. TEG monitors hemostasis as a dynamic process rather than revealing isolated information as in conventional coagulation screens.[84] TEG measures the viscoelastic properties of blood as it is induced to clot in a low-shear environment (resembling sluggish venous flow). The patterns of change in shear elasticity allow the kinetics of clot formation and growth as well as the strength and stability of the formed clot to be determined. The strength and stability data provide information about the ability of the clot to perform the work of hemostasis, whereas the kinetic data determine the adequacy of quantitative factors available for clot formation. A sample of celite-activated whole blood is placed into a prewarmed cuvette. A suspended piston is then lowered into the cuvette, which is rotated through a 4.5-degree arc backwards and forwards. The normal clot goes through an acceleration and strengthening phase. The fiber strands that interact with activated platelets attach to the surface of the cuvette and the suspended piston. The clot forming in the cuvette transmits its

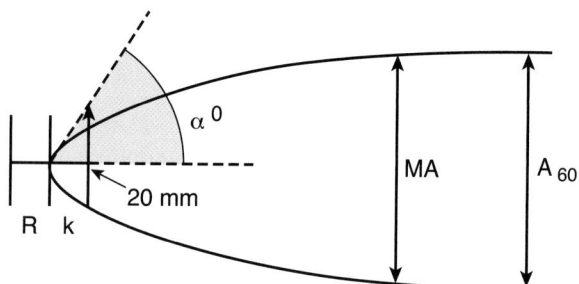

FIG. 4-7. Illustration of a thromboelastographic tracing. See text for explanation of parameters.

movement onto the suspended piston. A weak clot stretches and therefore delays the arc movement of the piston, which is graphically expressed as a narrow thromboelastogram. A strong clot, in contrast, will move the piston simultaneously and proportionally to the cuvette's movements, creating a thick thromboelastogram.[85]

The strength of a clot is graphically represented over time as a characteristic cigar-shaped figure (Fig. 4-7). There are five parameters of the TEG(r) tracing: R, k, alpha angle, MA, and MA60, all of which measure different stages of clot development.

R is the time from the commencement of the test to the initial fibrin formation.

k is a measure of the time from the beginning of clot formation until the amplitude of the TEG tracing reaches 20 mm and represents the dynamics of clot formation.

alpha angle is the angle between the line in the middle of the TEG(r) tracing and the line tangential to the developing body of the TEG(r) tracing. The alpha angle represents the acceleration (kinetics) of fibrin buildup and cross-linking.

MA is the maximum amplitude and reflects the strength of the clot, which is dependent on the number and function of platelets and the clot's interaction with fibrin.

MA60 is the rate of amplitude reduction 60 minutes after MA and represents the stability of the clot.

Examples of normal and abnormal TEG tracings are shown in Fig. 4-8. The usefulness of TEG has been sufficiently documented in general surgery,[86,87] cardiac surgery,[88] urologic surgery,[89] obstetrics,[90] pediatrics,[91] and liver transplantation.[92,93] It is the only test measuring all dynamic steps of clot formation until eventual clot lysis or retraction. Its role in evaluating coagulopathic patients is still being investigated.

EVALUATION OF HEMOSTATIC RISK IN THE SURGICAL PATIENT

Preoperative Evaluation of Hemostasis

Several hematologic disorders may have an impact on the outcome of surgery. The more common clinical situations faced by the surgeon are pre-existing anemia and oral anticoagulation therapy. Assessment of bleeding risk should also be considered in patients with liver or renal dysfunction.

When feasible, diagnostic evaluation of the patient with previously unrecognized anemia should be carried out before surgery, because certain types of anemia (particularly sickle cell disease and immune hemolytic anemias) may have implications for perioperative management. Hemoglobin levels below 7 or 8 g/dL appear to be associated with significantly more perioperative complications than higher levels.[94] Determination of the need for preoperative transfusion in an individual patient must consider factors other than the absolute hemoglobin level, including the presence of cardiopulmonary disease, the type of surgery, and the likelihood of surgical blood

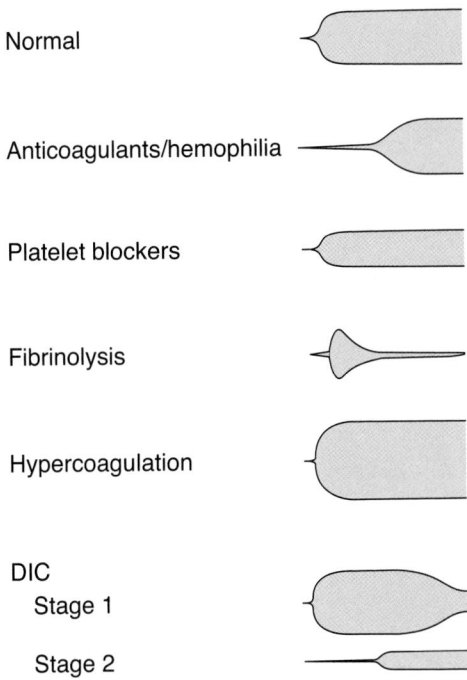

Normal

Anticoagulants/hemophilia

Platelet blockers

Fibrinolysis

Hypercoagulation

DIC
Stage 1

Stage 2

FIG. 4-8. Examples of normal and abnormal thromboelastographic tracings. DIC = disseminated intravascular coagulation.

antibody then destroys the recipient's own platelets. The resultant thrombocytopenia and bleeding may continue for several weeks. This uncommon cause of thrombocytopenia should be considered if bleeding follows transfusion by 5 or 6 days. Platelet transfusions are of little help in the management of this syndrome, because the new donor platelets usually are subject to the binding of antigen and damage from the antibody. Corticosteroids may be of some help in reducing the bleeding tendency. Posttransfusion purpura is self-limited, and the passage of several weeks inevitably leads to subsidence of the problem.

DIC is characterized by systemic activation of the blood coagulation system, which results in the generation and deposition of fibrin, leading to microvascular thrombi in various organs and contributing to the development of multiorgan failure. Consumption and subsequent exhaustion of coagulation proteins and platelets due to the ongoing activation of the coagulation system may induce severe bleeding complications.

Lastly, severe hemorrhagic disorders due to thrombocytopenia have occurred as a result of gram-negative sepsis. The pathogenesis of endotoxin-induced thrombocytopenia has been suggested to be related to lability of factor V, which appears necessary for this interaction. Defibrination and hemostatic failure also may occur with meningococcemia, *Clostridium perfringens* sepsis, and staphylococcal sepsis. Hemolysis appears to be one mechanism in sepsis leading to defibrination.

REFERENCES

Entries highlighted in bright blue are key references.

1. Avci Z, Malbora B, Gokdemir M, et al: Successful use of recombinant factor VIIa (NovoSeven) during cardiac surgery in a pediatric patient with congenital factor XI deficiency. *Pediatr Cardiol* 29:220, 2008.
2. Peyvandi F, Mannucci PM: Rare coagulation disorders. *Thromb Haemost* 82:1207, 1999.
3. Anwar R, Miloszewski KJ: Factor XIII deficiency. *Br J Haematol* 107:468, 1999.
4. Anwar R, Minford A, Gallivan L, et al: Delayed umbilical bleeding—a presenting feature for factor XIII deficiency: Clinical features, genetics, and management. *Pediatrics* 109:E32, 2002.
5. George JN, Caen JP, Nurden AT: Glanzmann's thrombasthenia: The spectrum of clinical disease. *Blood* 75:1383, 1990.
6. Stasi R, Evangelista ML, Stipa E, et al: Idiopathic thrombocytopenic purpura: Current concepts in pathophysiology and management. *Thromb Haemost* 99:4, 2008.
7. Baldwin ZK, Spitzer AL, Ng VL, et al: Contemporary standards for the diagnosis and treatment of heparin-induced thrombocytopenia (HIT). *Surgery* 143:305, 2008.
8. Amiral J, Peynaud-Debayle E, Wolf M, et al: Generation of antibodies to heparin-PF4 complexes without thrombocytopenia in patients treated with unfractionated or low-molecular-weight heparin. *Am J Hematol* 52:90, 1996.
9. Zimrin AB, Hess JR: Thrombocytopenic purpura: Going against the evidence. *Crit Care Med* 34:2247, 2006.
10. Darmon M, Azoulay E, Thiery G, et al: Time course of organ dysfunction in thrombotic microangiopathy in patients receiving either plasma or perfusion or plasma exchange. *Crit Care Med* 34:2127, 2006.
11. Fakhouri F, Vernant JP, Veyradier A, et al: Efficiency of curative and prophylactic treatment with rituximab in ADAMT13-deficient thrombotic thrombocytopenic purpura: A study of 11 cases. *Blood* 106:1932, 2005.
12. Lavelle WF, Lavelle EA, Uhl R: Operative delay for orthopedic patients on clopidogrel (Plavix): A complete lack of consensus. *J Trauma* 64:996, 2008.
13. Taylor FB, Toh CH, Hoots WK, et al: Towards definition, clinical and laboratory criteria, and a scoring system for disseminated intravascular coagulation. *Thromb Haemost* 86:1327, 2001.
14. Hess JR, Lawson JH: The coagulopathy of trauma versus disseminated intravascular coagulation. *J Trauma* 60:S12, 2006.
15. Dhainaut JF, Yan SB, Joyce DE, et al: Treatment effects of drotrecogin alfa (activated) in patients with or without overt disseminated intravascular coagulation. *J Thromb Haemost* 2:1924, 2004.

loss. Many patients have anemia postoperatively secondary to blood loss and hemodilution and do not necessarily require transfusion.

The most important component of the bleeding risk assessment is a directed bleeding history. A detailed patient history can provide meaningful clues to the presence of a bleeding tendency, such as easy bruising or a family history of bleeding problems. Patients who are reliable historians and who reveal no suggestion of abnormal bleeding on directed bleeding history and physical examination are at very low risk for having an occult bleeding disorder. Laboratory tests of hemostatic parameters in patients with low risk of bleeding are not required. When the directed bleeding history is unreliable or incomplete or when abnormal bleeding is suggested, a formal evaluation of hemostasis should be performed before surgery including measurement of the PT, the aPTT, and the platelet count.[95]

Evaluation of Excessive Intraoperative or Postoperative Bleeding

Excessive bleeding during or after a surgical procedure may be the result of ineffective hemostasis, blood transfusion, undetected hemostatic defect, consumptive coagulopathy, and/or fibrinolysis. Excessive bleeding from the operative field unassociated with bleeding from other sites usually suggests inadequate mechanical hemostasis.

Massive blood transfusion is a well-known cause of thrombocytopenia. Bleeding after massive transfusion can occur due to hypothermia, dilutional coagulopathy, platelet dysfunction, fibrinolysis, or hypofibrinogenemia. Another cause of hemostatic failure related to the administration of blood is hemolytic transfusion reaction. The first sign of a transfusion reaction may be diffuse bleeding. The pathogenesis of this bleeding is thought to be related to the release of ADP from hemolyzed red blood cells, resulting in diffuse platelet aggregation, after which the platelet clumps are removed out of the circulation.

Transfusion purpura occurs when the donor platelets are of the uncommon Pl(A1) group. This is an uncommon cause of thrombocytopenia and associated bleeding after transfusion. The platelets sensitize the recipient, who makes antibody to the foreign platelet antigen. The foreign platelet antigen does not completely disappear from the recipient circulation but attaches to the recipient's own platelets. The

16. Angstwurm MW, Dempfle CE, Spannagl M: New disseminated intravascular coagulation score: A useful tool to predict mortality in comparison with Acute Physiology and Chronic Health Evaluation II and Logistic Organ Dysfunction scores. *Crit Care Med* 34:314, 2006.

17. Trotter JF: Coagulation abnormalities in patients who have liver disease. *Clin Liver Dis* 10:665, 2006.

18. Feistauer SM, Penner E, Mayr WR, et al: Target platelet antigen of autoantibodies in patients with primary biliary cirrhosis. *Hepatology* 25:1343, 1997.

19. Ghalib R, Levine C, Hassan M, et al: Recombinant human interleukin-11 improves thrombocytopenia in patients with cirrhosis. *Hepatology* 37:1165, 2003.

20. Violl F, Basili S, Ferro D, et al: Association between high values of D-dimer and tissue plasminogen activator activity and first gastrointestinal bleeding in cirrhotic patients. CALC Group. *Thromb Haemost* 76:177, 1996.

21. Macleod J, Lynn M, McKenney MG, et al: Predictors of mortality in trauma patients. *Am Surg* 70:805, 2004.

22. Brohi K, Singh J, Heron M, et al: Acute traumatic coagulopathy. *J Trauma* 54:1127, 2003.

23. Brohi K, Cohen MJ, Ganter MT, et al: Acute coagulopathy of trauma: Hypoperfusion induces systemic anticoagulation and hyperfibrinolysis. *J Trauma* 64:1211, 2008.

24. Hoppensteadt DA, Fabbrini N, Bick RL, et al: Laboratory evaluation of the antiphospholipid syndrome. *Hematol Oncol Clin N Am* 22:19, 2008.

25. Singer DE, Albers GW, Dalen JE, et al: Antithrombotic therapy in atrial fibrillation: The Seventh ACCP Conference on Antithrombotic and Thrombolytic Therapy. *Chest* 126:429S, 2004.

26. Makris M, Watson HG: The management of coumarin-induced over-anticoagulation: Annotation. *Br J Haematol* 114:271, 2001.

27. Gibbar-Clements T, Shirrell D, Dooley R, et al: The challenge of warfarin therapy. *Am J Nurs* 100:38, 2000.

28. Morgan RJ, Bristol JB: Unusual finding in a patient taking warfarin. *Postgrad Med J* 75:299, 1999.

29. Wagner HE, Barbier PA, Schupfer G: Acute abdomen in patients under anticoagulant treatment. *Schweiz Med Wochenschr* 116:1802, 1986.

30. Acea Nebril B, Taboada Filgueira L, Sánchez González F, et al: Acute abdomen in anticoagulated patients: Its assessment the surgical indications. *Rev Clin Esp* 195:463, 1995.

31. Euhus DM, Hiatt JR: Management of the acute abdomen complicating oral anticoagulant therapy. *Am Surg* 56:581, 1990.

32. Polat C, Dervisoglu A, Guven H, et al: Anticoagulant-induced intramural intestinal hematoma. *Am J Emerg Med* 21:208, 2003.

33. Abbas MA, Collins JM, Olden KW, et al: Spontaneous intramural small-bowel hematoma: Clinical presentation and long-term outcome. *Arch Surg* 137:306, 2002.

34. Kearon C, Hirsh J: Management of anticoagulation before and after elective surgery. *N Engl J Med* 336:1506, 1997.

35. Horrow JC: Protamine: A review of its toxicity. *Anesth Analg* 64:348, 1985.

36. Lindblad B: Protamine sulfate: A review of its effects—hypersensitivity and toxicity. *Eur J Vasc Surg* 3:195, 1989.

37. Dentali F, Ageno W, Crowther M: Treatment of coumarin-associated coagulopathy: A systematic review and proposed treatment algorithms. *J Thromb Haemost* 4:1853, 2006.

38. Dunn A: Perioperative management of oral anticoagulation: When and how to bridge. *J Thromb Thrombolysis* 21:85, 2006.

39. Murkin JM, Lux J, Shannon NA, et al: Aprotinin significantly decreases bleeding and transfusion requirements in patients receiving aspirin and undergoing cardiac operations. *J Thorac Cardiovasc Surg* 107:554, 1994.

40. Gertsch P, Pellone A, Guerra A, et al: Initial experience with the Harmonic scalpel in liver surgery. *Hepatogastroenterology* 47:763, 2000.

41. Siperstein AE, Berber E, Morkoyun E: The use of the Harmonic scalpel vs. conventional knot tying vessel ligation in thyroid surgery. *Arch Surg* 137:137, 2000.

42. Chung CC, Ha JP, Tsang WW: Double-blind randomized trial comparing Harmonic scalpel hemorrhoidectomy, bipolar scissors hemorrhoidectomy, and scissors excision: Ligation technique. *Dis Colon Rectum* 45:789, 2002.

43. Palm M, Altman J: Topical hemostatic agents: A review. *Dermatol Surg* 34:431, 2008.

44. Larson PO: Topical hemostatic agents for dermatologic surgery. *J Dermatol Surg Oncol* 14:623, 1988.

45. Martinowitz U, Schulman S: Fibrin sealant in surgery of patients with a hemorrhagic diathesis. *Thromb Haemost* 74:486, 1995.

46. Bhanot S, Alex JC: Current applications of platelet gels in facial plastic surgery. *Facial Plast Surg* 18:27, 2002.

47. Thompson DF, Letassy NA, Thompson GD: Fibrin glue: A review of its preparation, efficacy, and adverse effects as a topical hemostat. *Drug Intell Clin Pharm* 22:946, 1988.

48. Currie LJ, Sharpe JR, Martin R: The use of fibrin glue in skin grafts and tissue-engineered skin replacements: A review. *Plast Reconstr Surg* 108:1713, 2001.

49. Morikawa T: Tissue sealing. *Am J Surg* 182:29S, 2001.

50. Parker RK, Dinehart SM: Hints for hemostasis. *Dermatol Clin* 12:601, 1994.

51. Spinella PC: Warm fresh whole blood transfusion for severe hemorrhage: U.S. military and potential civilian applications. *Crit Care Med* 36(7 Suppl):S340, 2008. [Review]

52. McAlister FA, Clark HD, Wells PS, et al: Perioperative allogeneic blood transfusion does not cause adverse sequelae in patients with cancer: A meta-analysis of unconfounded studies. *Br J Surg* 85:171, 1998.

53. Vamvakas EC, Blajchman MA: Universal WBC reduction: The case for and against. *Transfusion* 41:691, 2001.

54. Hebert PC, Fergusson D, Blajchman MA, et al: Clinical outcomes following institution of the Canadian universal leukoreduction program for red blood cell transfusions. *JAMA* 289:1941, 2003.

55. Sondeen JL, Prince MD, Medina L, et al: Comparison of lyophilized swine plasma to fresh frozen plasma plus two ratios of packed red blood cells in a cold, coagulopathic, poly trauma severe hemorrhage shock swine model. *Shock* 29(Suppl 1):13, 2008.

56. Gerber DR: Transfusion of packed red blood cells in patients with ischemic heart disease. *Crit Care Med* 36:1068, 2008.

57. Herbert PC, Wells GW, Blajchman MA, et al: A multicenter, randomized, controlled clinical trial of transfusion requirement in critical care. *N Engl J Med* 340:409, 1999.

58. Corwin HL, Gettinger A, Pearl RG, et al: The CRIT Study: Anemia and blood transfusion in the critically ill—current clinical practice in the United States. *Crit Care Med* 32:39, 2004.

59. Hoyt DB: A clinical review of bleeding dilemmas in trauma. *Semin Hematol* 41(1 Suppl 1):40, 2004.

60. Kauvar DS, Lefering R, Wade CE: Impact of hemorrhage on trauma outcome: An overview of epidemiology, clinical presentations, and therapeutic considerations. *J Trauma* 60(6 Suppl):S3, 2006.

61. Kauvar DS, Wade CE: The epidemiology and modern management of traumatic hemorrhage: US and international perspectives. *Crit Care* 9(Suppl 5):S1, 2005.

62. Niles SE, McLaughlin DF, Perkins J, et al: Traumatic coagulopathy in combat casualty care. *J Trauma* 64:1459, 2008.

63. Ferrara A, MacArthur JD, Wright HK, et al: Hypothermia and acidosis worsen coagulopathy in the patient requiring massive transfusion. *Am J Surg* 160:515, 1990.

64. Carrico CJ, Canizaro PC, Shires GT: Fluid resuscitation following injury: Rationale for the use of balanced salt solutions. *Crit Care Med* 4:46, 1976.

65. Harrigan C, Lucas CE, Ledgerwood AM, et al: Serial changes in primary hemostasis after massive transfusion. *Surgery* 98:836, 1985.

66. Gunter OL, Au BK, Mowery NT, et al: Optimizing outcomes in damage control resuscitation: Identifying blood product ratios associated with improved survival. *J Trauma* 63:1432, 2007.

67. Sperry J, Ochoa J, Gunn S, et al: FFP:PRBC transfusion ratio of 1:1.5 is associated with a lower risk of mortality following massive transfusion. *J Trauma* 64:247, 2008.

68. Gonzalez EA, Moore FA, Holcomb JB, et al: Fresh frozen plasma should be given earlier to patients requiring massive transfusion. *J Trauma* 62:112, 2007.

69. Gonzalez EA, Jastrow K, Holcomb JB, et al: Early achievement of a 1:1 ratio of FFP:RBC reduces mortality in patients receiving massive transfusion. *J Trauma* 64:247, 2008.

70. Borgman MA, Spinella PC, Perkins JG, et al: The ratio of blood products transfused affects mortality in patients receiving massive transfusions at a combat support hospital. *J Trauma* 63:805, 2007.

71. Spinella PC, Perkins JG, McLaughlin DF, et al: The effect of recombinant activated factor VII on mortality in combat-related casualties with severe trauma and massive transfusion. *J Trauma* 64:286, 2008.

72. Thomas GO, Dutton RP, Hemlock B, et al: Thromboembolic complications associated with factor VIIa administration. *J Trauma* 62:564, 2007.

73. Holcomb JB, Wade CE, Michalek JE, et al: Increased plasma and platelet to RBC ratios improve outcome in 466 massively transfused civilian trauma patients. *Ann Surg* 248:447, 2008.

74. McLaughlin DF, Niles SE, Salinas J, et al: A predictive model for massive transfusion in combat casualty patients. *J Trauma* 64(2 Suppl):S57, 2008.

75. Yücel N, Lefering R, Maegele M, et al: Trauma Associated Severe Hemorrhage (TASH) score: Probability of mass transfusion as surrogate for life threatening hemorrhage after multiple trauma. *J Trauma* 60:1228, 2006.

76. Moore FA, Nelson T, McKinley BA, et al: Massive transfusion in trauma patients: Tissue hemoglobin oxygen saturation predicts poor outcome. *J Trauma* 64:1010, 2008.

77. Schreiber MA, Perkins J, Kiraly L, et al: Early predictors of massive transfusion in combat casualties. *J Am Coll Surg* 205:541, 2007.

78. Wade CE, Holcomb JB, Chisholm GB, et al: Accurate and early prediction of massive transfusion in trauma patients [abstract]. *J Trauma.* In press.

79. Despotis GJ, Zhang L, Lublin DM: Transfusion risks and transfusion-related pro-inflammatory responses. *Hematol Oncol Clin N Am* 21:147, 2007.

80. Goodnough LT, Brecher ME, Kanter MH: Transfusion medicine: Blood transfusion. *N Engl J Med* 340:438, 1999.

81. Looney MR, Gropper MA, Matthay MA: Transfusion-related acute lung injury. *Chest* 126:249, 2004.

82. Gajic O, Murat Y, Iscimen R, et al: Transfusion from male-only versus female donors in critically ill recipients of high plasma volume components. *Crit Care Med* 35:1645, 2007.

83. Hartert H: Blutgerinnungsstudien mit der Thrombelastographie, einem neuen Untersuchungsverfahren. *Klin Wochenschr* 26:577, 1948.

84. Mallet SV, Cox DJA: Thrombelastography: A review article. *Br J Anaesth* 69:307, 1992.

85. *http://www.ispub.com/xml/journals/ija/vol1n3/qual.gif.* [accessed June 1, 2008].

86. Caprini JA, Arcelus JI, Laubach M, et al: Postoperative hypercoagulopathy and deep-vein thrombosis after laparoscopic cholecystectomy. *Surg Endosc* 9:304, 1995.

87. Arcelus JI, Traverso CI, Caprini JA: Thromboelastography for the assessment of hypercoagulability during general surgery. *Semin Thromb Hemost* 21(Suppl 4):21, 1995.

88. Shore-Lesserson L, Manspeizer HE, DePerio M, et al: Thromboelastography-guided transfusion algorithm reduces transfusions in complex cardiac surgery. *Anesth Analg* 88:312, 1999.

89. Bell CRW, Cox DJA, Murdock PJ, et al: Thrombelastographic evaluation of coagulation in transurethral prostatectomy. *Br J Urol* 78:737, 1996.

90. Beilin Y, Arnold I, Hossain S: Evaluation of the platelet function analyzer vs the thromboelastogram in the parturient. *Int J Obstet Anesth* 15:7, 2006.

91. Miller BE, Bailey JM, Mancuso TJ, et al: Functional maturity of the coagulation system in children: An evaluation using thromboelastography. *Anesth Analg* 84:745, 1997.

92. Kang Y: Thrombelastography in liver transplantation. *Semin Thromb Hemost* 21(Suppl 4):34, 1995.

93. Gillies BSA: Thromboelastography and liver transplantation. *Semin Thromb Hemost* 21(Suppl 4):45, 1995.

94. Shander A, Knight K, Thurer R, et al: Prevalence and outcomes of anemia in surgery: A systematic review of the literature. *Am J Med* 116(Suppl 7A):58S, 2004.

95. O'Donnell M, Kearon C: Perioperative management of oral anticoagulation. *Clin Geriatr Med* 22:199, 2006.

Shock

Brian S. Zuckerbraun, Andrew B. Peitzman, and Timothy R. Billiar

"Shock is the manifestation of the rude unhinging of the machinery of life."[1]

—Samuel V. Gross, 1872

EVOLUTION IN UNDERSTANDING SHOCK

Overview

Shock, at its most rudimentary definition and regardless of the etiology, is the failure to meet the metabolic needs of the cell and the consequences that ensue. The initial cellular injury that occurs is reversible; however, the injury will become irreversible if tissue perfusion is prolonged or severe enough such that, at the cellular level, compensation is no longer possible. Our evolution in the understanding of shock and the disease processes that result in shock made its most significant advances throughout the twentieth century as our appreciation for the physiology and pathophysiology of shock matured. Most notably, this includes the sympathetic and neuroendocrine stress responses on the cardiovascular system. The clinical manifestations of these physiologic responses are most often what lead practitioners to the diagnosis of shock as well as guide the management of patients in shock. However, hemodynamic parameters such as blood pressure and heart rate are relatively insensitive measures of shock, and additional considerations must be used to help aid in early diagnosis and treatment of patients in shock. The general approach to the management of patients in shock has been empiric: assuring a secure airway with adequate ventilation and restoration of vascular volume and tissue perfusion.

Historical Background

Integral to our understanding of shock is the appreciation that our bodies attempt to maintain a state of homeostasis. Claude Bernard suggested in the mid-nineteenth century that the organism attempts to maintain constancy in the internal environment against external forces that attempt to disrupt the *milieu interieur*.[2] Walter B. Cannon carried Bernard's observations further and introduced the term *homeostasis,* emphasizing that an organism's ability to survive was related to maintenance of homeostasis.[3] The failure of physiologic systems to buffer the organism against external forces results in organ and cellular dysfunction, what is clinically recognized as shock. He first described the *"fight or flight response,"* generated by elevated levels of catecholamines in the bloodstream. Cannon's observations on the battlefields of World War I led him to propose that the initiation of shock was due to a disturbance of the nervous system that resulted in vasodilation and hypotension. He proposed that secondary shock, with its attendant capillary permeability leak, was caused by a "toxic factor" released from the tissues.

In a series of critical experiments, Alfred Blalock documented that the shock state in hemorrhage was associated with reduced cardiac output due to volume loss, not a "toxic factor."[4] In 1934, Blalock proposed four categories of shock: hypovolemic, vasogenic, cardiogenic, and neurogenic. *Hypovolemic shock,* the most common type, results from loss of circulating blood volume. This may result from loss of whole blood (hemorrhagic shock), plasma, interstitial fluid (bowel obstruction), or a combination. *Vasogenic shock* results from decreased resistance within capacitance vessels, usually seen in sepsis. *Neurogenic shock* is a form of vasogenic shock in which spinal cord injury or spinal anesthesia causes vasodilation due to acute loss of sympathetic vascular tone. *Cardiogenic shock* results from failure of the heart as a pump, as in arrhythmias or acute myocardial infarction (MI).

TABLE 5-1	Classification of shock
Hypovolemic	
Cardiogenic	
Septic (vasogenic)	
Neurogenic	
Traumatic	
Obstructive	

This categorization of shock based on etiology persists today (Table 5-1). In recent clinical practice, further classification has described six types of shock: hypovolemic, septic (vasodilatory), neurogenic, cardiogenic, obstructive, and traumatic shock. *Obstructive shock* is a form of cardiogenic shock that results from mechanical impediment to circulation leading to depressed cardiac output rather than primary cardiac failure. This includes etiologies such as pulmonary embolism or tension pneumothorax. In *traumatic shock,* soft tissue and bony injury lead to the activation of inflammatory cells and the release of circulating factors, such as cytokines and intracellular molecules that modulate the immune response. Recent investigations have revealed that the inflammatory mediators released in response to tissue injury [damage-associated molecular patterns (DAMPs)] are recognized by many of the same cellular receptors [pattern recognition receptors (PRRs)] and activate similar signaling pathways as do bacterial products elaborated in sepsis (pathogen-associated molecular patterns), such as lipopolysaccharide.[5] These effects of tissue injury are combined with the effects of hemorrhage, creating a more complex and amplified deviation from homeostasis.

In the mid- to later twentieth century, the further development of experimental models contributed significantly to the understanding of the pathophysiology of shock. In 1947, Wiggers developed a sustainable, irreversible model of hemorrhagic shock based on uptake of shed blood into a reservoir to maintain a set level of hypotension.[6] G. Tom Shires added further understanding of hemorrhagic shock with a series of clinical studies demonstrating that a large extracellular fluid deficit, greater than could be attributed to

KEY POINTS

1. Shock is defined as a failure to meet the metabolic demands of cells and tissues and the consequences that ensue.

2. A central component of shock is decreased tissue perfusion. This may be a direct consequence of the etiology of shock, such as in hypovolemic/hemorrhagic, cardiogenic, or neurogenic etiologies, or may be secondary to elaborated or released molecules or cellular products that result in endothelial/cellular activation, such as in septic shock or traumatic shock.

3. Physiologic responses to shock are based upon a series of afferent (sensing) signals and efferent responses that include neuroendocrine, metabolic, and immune/inflammatory signaling.

4. The mainstay of treatment of hemorrhagic/hypovolemic shock includes volume resuscitation with blood products and fluids. In the case of hemorrhagic shock, timely control of bleeding is essential and influences outcome.

5. Prevention of hypothermia, acidemia, and coagulopathy are essential in the management of patients in hemorrhagic shock.

6. The mainstay of treatment of septic shock is fluid resuscitation, initiation of appropriate antibiotic therapy, and control of the source of infection. This includes drainage of infected fluid collections, removal of infected foreign bodies, and débridement of devitalized tissues.

7. A combination of physiologic parameters and markers of organ perfusion/tissue oxygenation are used to determine if patients are in shock and to follow the efficacy of resuscitation.

vascular refilling alone, occurred in severe hemorrhagic shock.[7,8] The phenomenon of fluid redistribution after major trauma involving blood loss was termed *third spacing* and described the translocation of intravascular volume into the peritoneum, bowel, burned tissues, or crush injury sites. These seminal studies form the scientific basis for the current treatment of hemorrhagic shock with red blood cells and lactated Ringer's solution or isotonic saline.

As resuscitation strategies evolved and patients survived the initial consequences of hemorrhage, new challenges of sustained shock became apparent. During the Vietnam War, aggressive fluid resuscitation with red blood cells and crystalloid solution or plasma resulted in survival of patients who previously would have succumbed to hemorrhagic shock. Renal failure became a less frequent clinical problem; however, a new disease process, acute fulminant pulmonary failure, appeared as an early cause of death after seemingly successful surgery to control hemorrhage. Initially called *DaNang lung* or *shock lung*, the clinical problem became recognized as acute respiratory distress syndrome (ARDS). This led to new methods of prolonged mechanical ventilation. Our current concept of ARDS is a component in the spectrum of multiple organ system failure.

Studies and clinical observations over the past two decades have extended the early observations of Canon, that "restoration of blood pressure prior to control of active bleeding may result in loss of blood that is sorely needed," and challenged the appropriate endpoints in resuscitation of uncontrolled hemorrhage.[9] Core principles in the management of the critically ill or injured patient include: (a) definitive control of the airway must be secured, (b) control of active hemorrhage must occur promptly (delay in control of bleeding increases mortality and recent battlefield data would suggest that in the young and otherwise healthy population commonly injured in combat, that control of bleeding is the paramount priority), (c) volume resuscitation with red blood cells, plasma, and crystalloid must occur while operative control of bleeding is achieved, (d) unrecognized or inadequately corrected hypoperfusion increases morbidity and mortality (i.e., inadequate resuscitation results in avoidable early deaths from shock), and (e) excessive fluid resuscitation may exacerbate bleeding (i.e., uncontrolled resuscitation is harmful). Thus both inadequate and uncontrolled volume resuscitation is harmful.

Current Definitions and Challenges

A modern definition and approach to shock acknowledges that shock consists of inadequate tissue perfusion marked by decreased delivery of required metabolic substrates and inadequate removal of cellular waste products. This involves failure of oxidative metabolism that can involve defects of oxygen (O_2) delivery, transport, and/or utilization. Current challenges include moving beyond fluid resuscitation based upon endpoints of tissue oxygenation, and using therapeutic strategies at the cellular and molecular level. This approach will help to identify compensated patients or patients early in the course of their disease, initiate appropriate treatment, and allow for continued evaluation for the efficacy of resuscitation and adjuncts.

Current investigations focus on determining the cellular events that often occur in parallel to result in organ dysfunction, shock irreversibility, and death. This chapter will review our current understanding of the pathophysiology and cellular responses of shock states. Current and experimental diagnostic and therapeutic modalities for the different categories of shock are reviewed, with a focus on hemorrhagic/hypovolemic shock and septic shock.

PATHOPHYSIOLOGY OF SHOCK

Regardless of etiology, the initial physiologic responses in shock are driven by tissue hypoperfusion and the developing cellular energy deficit. This imbalance between cellular supply and demand leads to neuroendocrine and inflammatory responses, the magnitude of which is usually proportional to the degree and duration of shock. The specific responses will differ based on the etiology of shock, as certain physiologic responses may be limited by the inciting pathology. For example, the cardiovascular response driven by the sympathetic nervous system is markedly blunted in neurogenic or septic shock. Additionally, decreased perfusion may occur as a consequence of cellular activation and dysfunction, such as in septic shock and to a lesser extent traumatic shock (Fig. 5-1). Many of the organ-specific responses are aimed at maintaining perfusion in the cerebral and coronary circulation. These are regulated at multiple levels including (a) stretch receptors and baroreceptors in the heart and vasculature (carotid sinus and aortic arch), (b) chemoreceptors, (c) cerebral

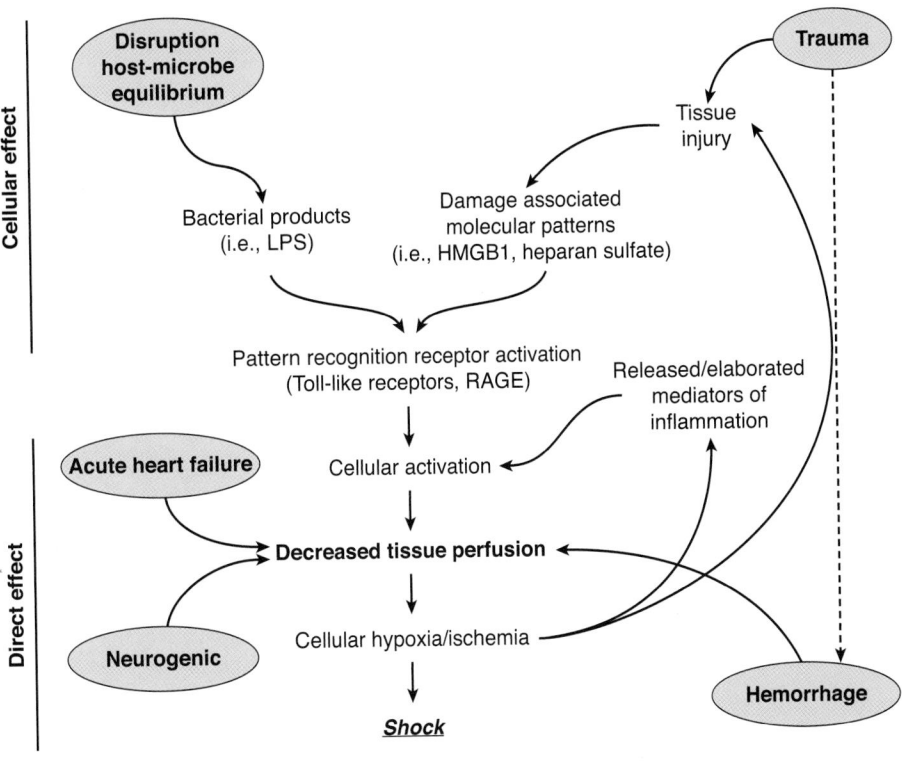

FIG. 5-1. Pathways leading to decreased tissue perfusion and shock. Decreased tissue perfusion can result directly from hemorrhage/hypovolemia, cardiac failure, or neurologic injury. Decreased tissue perfusion and cellular injury can then result in immune and inflammatory responses. Alternatively, elaboration of microbial products during infection or release of endogenous cellular products from tissue injury can result in cellular activation to subsequently influence tissue perfusion and the development of shock. HMGB1 = high mobility group box 1; LPS = lipopolysaccharide; RAGE = receptor for advanced glycation end products.

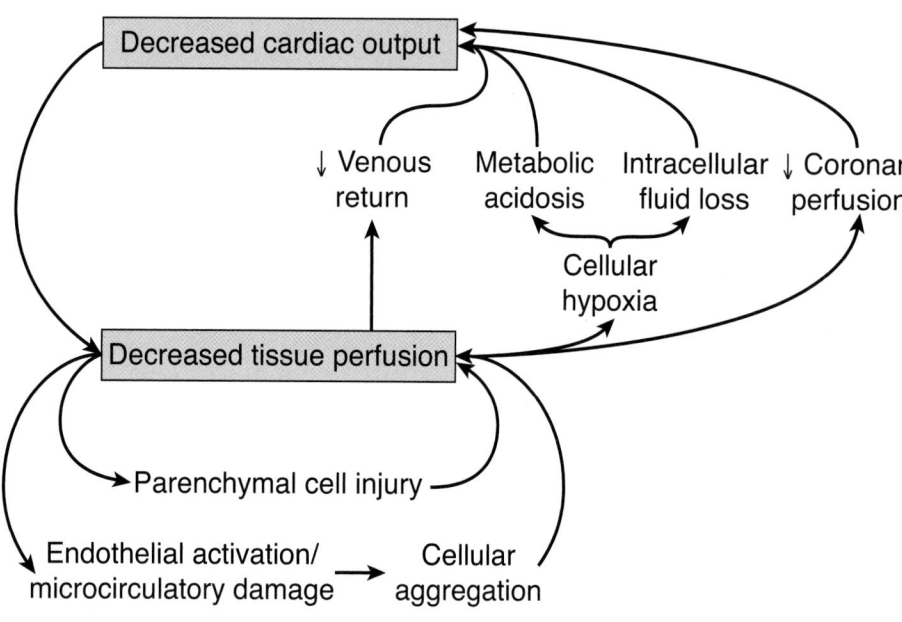

FIG. 5-2. The "vicious cycle of shock." Regardless of the etiology, decreased tissue perfusion and shock results in a feed-forward loop that can exacerbate cellular injury and tissue dysfunction.

ischemia responses, (d) release of endogenous vasoconstrictors, (e) shifting of fluid into the intravascular space, and (f) renal reabsorption and conservation of salt and water.

Furthermore, the pathophysiologic responses vary with time and in response to resuscitation. In hemorrhagic shock, the body can compensate for the initial loss of blood volume primarily through the neuroendocrine response to maintain hemodynamics. This represents the *compensated phase* of shock. With continued hypoperfusion, which may be unrecognized, cellular death and injury are ongoing and the *decompensation phase* of shock ensues. Microcirculatory dysfunction, parenchymal tissue damage, and inflammatory cell activation can perpetuate hypoperfusion. Ischemia/reperfusion injury will often exacerbate the initial insult. These effects at the cellular level, if untreated, will lead to compromise of function at the organ system level, thus leading to the "*vicious cycle*" of shock (Fig. 5-2). Persistent hypoperfusion results in further hemodynamic derangements and cardiovascular collapse. This has been termed the *irreversible phase* of shock and can

develop quite insidiously and may only be obvious in retrospect. At this point there has occurred extensive enough parenchymal and microvascular injury such that volume resuscitation fails to reverse the process, leading to death of the patient. In experimental animal models of hemorrhagic shock (modified Wiggers model), this is represented by the "uptake phase" or "compensation endpoint" when shed blood must be returned to the animal to sustain the hypotension at the set level to prevent further hypotension and death.[10] If shed blood volume is slowly returned to maintain the set level of hypotension, eventually the injury progresses to irreversible shock, where further volume will not reverse the process and the animal dies (Fig. 5-3).

Neuroendocrine and Organ-Specific Responses to Hemorrhage

The goal of the neuroendocrine response to hemorrhage is to maintain perfusion to the heart and the brain, even at the expense of

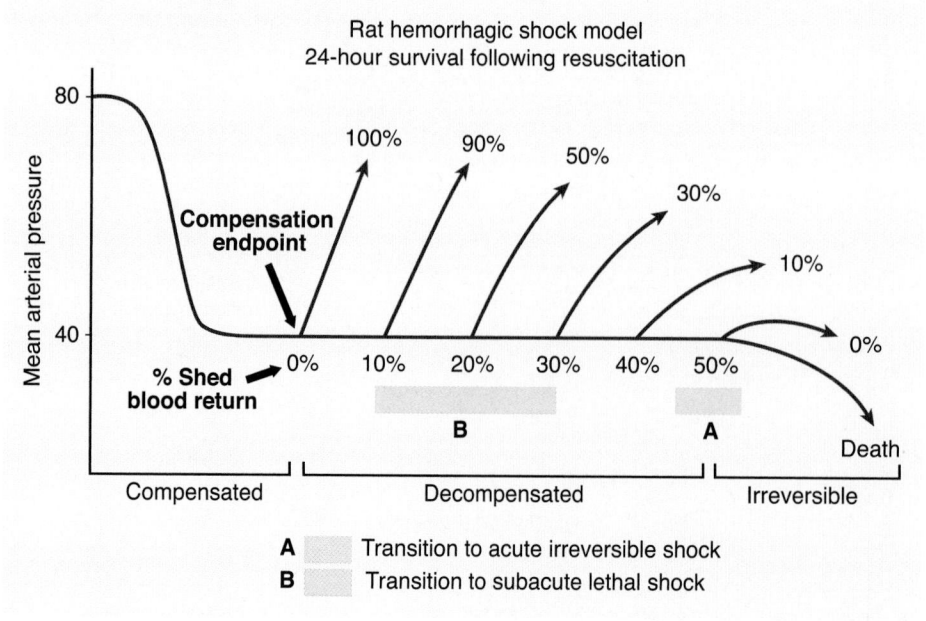

FIG. 5-3. Rat model of hemorrhagic shock through the phases of compensation, decompensation, and irreversibility. The percentages shown above the curve represent survival rates. *(From Shah et al,[10] with permission.)*

other organ systems. Peripheral vasoconstriction occurs, and fluid excretion is inhibited. The mechanisms include autonomic control of peripheral vascular tone and cardiac contractility, hormonal response to stress and volume depletion, and local microcirculatory mechanisms that are organ specific and regulate regional blood flow. The initial stimulus is loss of circulating blood volume in hemorrhagic shock. The magnitude of the neuroendocrine response is based on both the volume of blood lost and the rate at which it is lost.

Afferent Signals

Afferent impulses transmitted from the periphery are processed within the central nervous system (CNS) and activate the reflexive effector responses or efferent impulses. These effector responses are designed to expand plasma volume, maintain peripheral perfusion and tissue O_2 delivery, and restore homeostasis. The afferent impulses that initiate the body's intrinsic adaptive responses and converge in the CNS originate from a variety of sources. The initial inciting event usually is loss of circulating blood volume. Other stimuli that can produce the neuroendocrine response include pain, hypoxemia, hypercarbia, acidosis, infection, change in temperature, emotional arousal, or hypoglycemia. The sensation of pain from injured tissue is transmitted via the spinothalamic tracts, resulting in activation of the hypothalamic-pituitary-adrenal axis, as well as activation of the autonomic nervous system (ANS) to induce direct sympathetic stimulation of the adrenal medulla to release catecholamines.

Baroreceptors also are an important afferent pathway in initiation of adaptive responses to shock. Volume receptors, sensitive to changes in both chamber pressure and wall stretch, are present within the atria of the heart. They become activated with low volume hemorrhage or mild reductions in right atrial pressure. Receptors in the aortic arch and carotid bodies respond to alterations in pressure or stretch of the arterial wall, responding to larger reductions in intravascular volume or pressure. These receptors normally inhibit induction of the ANS. When activated, these baroreceptors diminish their output, thus disinhibiting the effect of the ANS. The ANS then increases its output, principally via sympathetic activation at the vasomotor centers of the brain stem, producing centrally mediated constriction of peripheral vessels.

Chemoreceptors in the aorta and carotid bodies are sensitive to changes in O_2 tension, H^+ ion concentration, and carbon dioxide (CO_2) levels. Stimulation of the chemoreceptors results in vasodilation of the coronary arteries, slowing of the heart rate, and vasoconstriction of the splanchnic and skeletal circulation. In addition, a variety of protein and nonprotein mediators are produced at the site of injury as part of the inflammatory response, and they act as afferent impulses to induce a host response. These mediators include histamine, cytokines, eicosanoids, and endothelins, among others that are discussed in greater detail later in this chapter in the Immune and Inflammatory Responses section.

Efferent Signals
Cardiovascular Response

Changes in cardiovascular function are a result of the neuroendocrine response and ANS response to shock, and constitute a prominent feature of both the body's adaptive response mechanism, and the clinical signs and symptoms of the patient in shock. Hemorrhage results in diminished venous return to the heart and decreased cardiac output. This is compensated by increased cardiac heart rate and contractility, as well as venous and arterial vasoconstriction. Stimulation of sympathetic fibers innervating the heart leads to activation of beta$_1$-adrenergic receptors that increase heart rate and contractility in this attempt to increase cardiac output. Increased myocardial O_2 consumption occurs as a result of the increased workload; thus, myocardial O_2 supply must be maintained or myocardial dysfunction will develop. The cardiovascular response in hemorrhage/hypovolemia differs from the responses elicited with the other etiologies of shock. These are compared in Table 5-2.

Direct sympathetic stimulation of the peripheral circulation via the activation of alpha$_1$-adrenergic receptors on arterioles induces vasoconstriction and causes a compensatory increase in systemic vascular resistance and blood pressure. The arterial vasoconstriction is not uniform; marked redistribution of blood flow results. Selective perfusion to tissues occurs due to regional variations in arteriolar resistance, with blood shunted away from less essential organ beds such as the intestine, kidney, and skin. In contrast, the brain and heart have autoregulatory mechanisms that attempt to preserve their blood flow despite a global decrease in cardiac output. Direct sympathetic stimulation also induces constriction of venous vessels, decreasing the capacitance of the circulatory system and accelerating blood return to the central circulation.

Increased sympathetic output induces catecholamine release from the adrenal medulla. Catecholamine levels peak within 24 to 48 hours of injury, and then return to baseline. Persistent elevation of catecholamine levels beyond this time suggests ongoing noxious afferent stimuli. The majority of the circulating epinephrine is produced by the adrenal medulla, while norepinephrine is derived from synapses of the sympathetic nervous system. Catecholamine effects on peripheral tissues include stimulation of hepatic glycogenolysis and gluconeogenesis to increase circulating glucose availability to peripheral tissues, an increase in skeletal muscle glycogenolysis, suppression of insulin release, and increased glucagon release.

Hormonal Response

The stress response includes activation of the ANS as discussed above in the Afferent Signals section, as well as activation of the hypothalamic-pituitary-adrenal axis. Shock stimulates the hypothalamus to release corticotropin-releasing hormone, which results in the release of adrenocorticotropic hormone (ACTH) by the pituitary. ACTH subsequently stimulates the adrenal cortex to release cortisol. Cortisol acts synergistically with epinephrine and glucagon to induce a catabolic state. Cortisol stimulates gluconeogenesis and insulin resistance, resulting in hyperglycemia as well as muscle cell protein breakdown and lipolysis to provide substrates for hepatic gluconeogenesis. Cortisol causes retention of sodium and water by the nephrons of the kidney. In the setting of severe hypovolemia, ACTH secretion occurs independently of cortisol negative feedback inhibition.

The renin-angiotensin system is activated in shock. Decreased renal artery perfusion, beta-adrenergic stimulation, and increased renal tubular sodium concentration cause the release of renin from the juxtaglomerular cells. Renin catalyzes the conversion of angiotensinogen (produced by the liver) to angiotensin I, which is then

TABLE 5-2	Hemodynamic responses to different types of shock					
Type of Shock	**Cardiac Index**	**SVR**	**Venous Capacitance**	**CVP/PCWP**	**Svo$_2$**	**Cellular/Metabolic Effects**
Hypovolemic	↓	↑	↓	↓	↓	Effect
Septic	↑↑	↓	↑	↑↓	↑↓	Cause
Cardiogenic	↓↓	↑↑	→	↑	↓	Effect
Neurogenic	↑	↓	→	↓	↓	Effect

The hemodynamic responses are indicated by arrows to show an increase (↑), severe increase (↑↑), decrease (↓), severe decrease (↓↓), varied response (↑↓), or little effect (→). CVP = central venous pressure; PCWP = pulmonary capillary wedge pressure; Svo$_2$ = mixed venous oxygen saturation; SVR = systemic vascular resistance.

converted to angiotensin II by angiotensin-converting enzyme (ACE) produced in the lung. While angiotensin I has no significant functional activity, angiotensin II is a potent vasoconstrictor of both splanchnic and peripheral vascular beds, and also stimulates the secretion of aldosterone, ACTH, and antidiuretic hormone (ADH). Aldosterone, a mineralocorticoid, acts on the nephron to promote reabsorption of sodium, and as a consequence, water. Potassium and hydrogen ions are lost in the urine in exchange for sodium.

The pituitary also releases vasopressin or ADH in response to hypovolemia, changes in circulating blood volume sensed by baroreceptors and left atrial stretch receptors, and increased plasma osmolality detected by hypothalamic osmoreceptors. Epinephrine, angiotensin II, pain, and hyperglycemia increase production of ADH. ADH levels remain elevated for about 1 week after the initial insult, depending on the severity and persistence of the hemodynamic abnormalities. ADH acts on the distal tubule and collecting duct of the nephron to increase water permeability, decrease water and sodium losses, and preserve intravascular volume. Also known as *arginine vasopressin,* ADH acts as a potent mesenteric vasoconstrictor, shunting circulating blood away from the splanchnic organs during hypovolemia.[11] This may contribute to intestinal ischemia and predispose to intestinal mucosal barrier dysfunction in shock states. Vasopressin also increases hepatic gluconeogenesis and increases hepatic glycolysis.

In septic states, endotoxin directly stimulates arginine vasopressin secretion independently of blood pressure, osmotic, or intravascular volume changes. Proinflammatory cytokines also contribute to arginine vasopressin release. Interestingly, patients on chronic therapy with ACE inhibitors are more at risk of developing hypotension and vasodilatory shock with open heart surgery. Low plasma levels of arginine vasopressin were confirmed in these patients.[12]

Circulatory Homeostasis
Preload

At rest, the majority of the blood volume is within the venous system. Venous return to the heart generates ventricular end-diastolic wall tension, a major determinant of cardiac output. Gravitational shifts in blood volume distribution are quickly corrected by alterations in venous capacity. With decreased arteriolar inflow, there is active contraction of the venous smooth muscle and passive elastic recoil in the thin-walled systemic veins. This increases venous return to the heart, thus maintaining ventricular filling.

Most alterations in cardiac output in the normal heart are related to changes in preload. Increases in sympathetic tone have a minor effect on skeletal muscle beds but produce a dramatic reduction in splanchnic blood volume, which normally holds 20% of the blood volume.

The normal circulating blood volume is maintained within narrow limits by the kidney's ability to manage salt and water balance with external losses via systemic and local hemodynamic changes and hormonal effects of renin, angiotensin, and ADH. These relatively slow responses maintain preload by altering circulating blood volume. Acute responses to intravascular volume include changes in venous tone, systemic vascular resistance, and intrathoracic pressure, with the slower hormonal changes less important in the early response to volume loss. Furthermore, the net effect of preload on cardiac output is influenced by cardiac determinants of ventricular function, which include coordinated atrial activity and tachycardia.

Ventricular Contraction

The Frank-Starling curve describes the force of ventricular contraction as a function of its preload. This relationship is based on force of contraction being determined by initial muscle length. Intrinsic cardiac disease will shift the Frank-Starling curve and alter mechanical performance of the heart. In addition, cardiac dysfunction has been demonstrated experimentally in burns and in hemorrhagic, traumatic, and septic shock.

Afterload

Afterload is the force that resists myocardial work during contraction. Arterial pressure is the major component of afterload influencing the ejection fraction. This vascular resistance is determined by precapillary smooth muscle sphincters. Blood viscosity also will increase vascular resistance. As afterload increases in the normal heart, stroke volume can be maintained by increases in preload. In shock, with decreased circulating volume and therefore diminished preload, this compensatory mechanism to sustain cardiac output is impeded. The stress response with acute release of catecholamines and sympathetic nerve activity in the heart increases contractility and heart rate.

Microcirculation

The microvascular circulation plays an integral role in regulating cellular perfusion and is significantly influenced in response to shock. The microvascular bed is innervated by the sympathetic nervous system and has a profound effect on the larger arterioles. Following hemorrhage, larger arterioles vasoconstrict; however, in the setting of sepsis or neurogenic shock, these vessels vasodilate. Additionally, a host of other vasoactive proteins, including vasopressin, angiotensin II, and endothelin-1, also lead to vasoconstriction to limit organ perfusion to organs such as skin, skeletal muscle, kidneys, and the GI tract to preserve perfusion of the myocardium and CNS.

Flow in the capillary bed often is heterogeneous in shock states, which likely is secondary to multiple local mechanisms, including endothelial cell swelling, dysfunction, and activation marked by the recruitment of leukocytes.[13] Together, these mechanisms lead to diminished capillary perfusion that may persist after resuscitation. In hemorrhagic shock, correction of hemodynamic parameters and restoration of O_2 delivery generally leads to restoration of tissue O_2 consumption and tissue O_2 levels. In contrast, regional tissue dysoxia often persists in sepsis, despite similar restoration of hemodynamics and O_2 delivery. Whether this defect in O_2 extraction in sepsis is the result of heterogeneous impairment of the microcirculation (intraparenchymal shunting) or impaired tissue parenchymal cell oxidative phosphorylation and O_2 consumption by the mitochondria is not resolved.[14] Interesting data suggest that in sepsis the response to limit O_2 consumption by the tissue parenchymal cells is an adaptive response to the inflammatory signaling and decreased perfusion.[15]

An additional pathophysiologic response of the microcirculation to shock is failure of the integrity of the endothelium of the microcirculation and development of capillary leak, intracellular swelling, and the development of an extracellular fluid deficit. Seminal work by Shires helped to define this phenomenon.[7,16] There is decreased capillary hydrostatic pressure secondary to changes in blood flow and increased cellular uptake of fluid. The result is a loss of extracellular fluid volume. The cause of intracellular swelling is multifactorial, but dysfunction of energy-dependent mechanisms, such as active transport by the sodium-potassium pump contributes to loss of membrane integrity.

Capillary dysfunction also occurs secondary to activation of endothelial cells by circulating inflammatory mediators generated in septic or traumatic shock. This exacerbates endothelial cell swelling and capillary leak, as well as increases leukocyte adherence. This results in capillary occlusion, which may persist after resuscitation, and is termed *no-reflow.* Further ischemic injury ensues as well as release of inflammatory cytokines to compound tissue injury. Experimental models have shown that neutrophil depletion in animals subjected to hemorrhagic shock produces fewer capillaries with no-reflow and lower mortality.[13]

METABOLIC EFFECTS

Cellular metabolism is based primarily on the hydrolysis of adenosine triphosphate (ATP). The splitting of the phosphoanhydride bond of the terminal or γ-phosphate from ATP is the source of energy for most processes within the cell under normal conditions. The majority of ATP is generated in our bodies through aerobic metabolism in the process of oxidative phosphorylation in the mitochondria. This process is dependent on the availability of O_2 as a final electron acceptor in the electron transport chain. As O_2 tension within a cell decreases, there is a decrease in oxidative phosphorylation, and the generation of ATP slows. When O_2 delivery is so severely impaired such that oxidative phosphorylation cannot be sustained, the state is termed *dysoxia*.[17] When oxidative phosphorylation is insufficient, the cells shift to anaerobic metabolism and glycolysis to generate ATP. This occurs via the breakdown of cellular glycogen stores to pyruvate. Although glycolysis is a rapid process, it is not efficient, allowing for the production of only 2 mol of ATP from 1 mol of glucose. This is compared to complete oxidation of 1 mol of glucose that produces 38 mol of ATP. Additionally, under hypoxic conditions in anaerobic metabolism, pyruvate is converted into lactate, leading to an intracellular metabolic acidosis.

There are numerous consequences secondary to these metabolic changes. The depletion of ATP potentially influences all ATP-dependent cellular processes. This includes maintenance of cellular membrane potential, synthesis of enzymes and proteins, cell signaling, and DNA repair mechanisms. Decreased intracellular pH also influences vital cellular functions such as normal enzyme activity, cell membrane ion exchange, and cellular metabolic signaling.[18] These changes also will lead to changes in gene expression within the cell. Furthermore, acidosis leads to changes in calcium metabolism and calcium signaling. Compounded, these changes may lead to irreversible cell injury and death.

Epinephrine and norepinephrine have a profound impact on cellular metabolism. Hepatic glycogenolysis, gluconeogenesis, ketogenesis, skeletal muscle protein breakdown, and adipose tissue lipolysis are increased by catecholamines. Cortisol, glucagon, and ADH also contribute to the catabolism during shock. Epinephrine induces further release of glucagon, while inhibiting the pancreatic β-cell release of insulin. The result is a catabolic state with glucose mobilization, hyperglycemia, protein breakdown, negative nitrogen balance, lipolysis, and insulin resistance during shock and injury. The relative underuse of glucose by peripheral tissues preserves it for the glucose-dependent organs such as the heart and brain.

Cellular Hypoperfusion

Hypoperfused cells and tissues experience what has been termed *oxygen debt*, a concept first proposed by Crowell in 1961.[19] The O_2 debt is the deficit in tissue oxygenation over time that occurs during shock. When O_2 delivery is limited, O_2 consumption can be inadequate to match the metabolic needs of cellular respiration, creating a deficit in O_2 requirements at the cellular level. The measurement of O_2 deficit uses calculation of the difference between the estimated O_2 demand and the actual value obtained for O_2 consumption. Under normal circumstances, cells can "repay" the O_2 debt during reperfusion. The magnitude of the O_2 debt correlates with the severity and duration of hypoperfusion. Surrogate values for measuring O_2 debt include base deficit and lactate levels, and are discussed later in the Hypovolemic/Hemorrhagic section.

In addition to induction of changes in cellular metabolic pathways, shock also induces changes in cellular gene expression. The DNA binding activity of a number of nuclear transcription factors is altered by hypoxia and the production of O_2 radicals or nitrogen radicals that are produced at the cellular level by shock. Expression of other gene products such as heat shock proteins, vascular endothelial growth factor, inducible nitric oxide synthase (iNOS), heme oxygenase-1, and cytokines also are clearly increased by shock.[20] Many of these shock-induced gene products, such as cytokines, have the ability to subsequently alter gene expression in specific target cells and tissues. The involvement of multiple pathways emphasizes the complex, integrated, and overlapping nature of the response to shock.

IMMUNE AND INFLAMMATORY RESPONSES

The inflammatory and immune responses are a complex set of interactions between circulating soluble factors and cells that can arise in response to trauma, infection, ischemia, toxic, or autoimmune stimuli.[20] The processes are well regulated and can be conceptualized as an ongoing surveillance and response system that undergoes a coordinated escalation following injury to heal disrupted tissue and restore host-microbe equilibrium, as well as active suppression back to baseline levels. Failure to adequately control the activation, escalation, or suppression of the inflammatory response can lead to systemic inflammatory response syndrome and potentiate multiple organ failure.

Both the innate and adaptive branches of the immune system work in concert to rapidly respond in a specific and effective manner to challenges that threaten an organism's well-being. Each arm of the immune system has its own set of functions, defined primarily by distinct classes of effector cells and their unique cell membrane receptor families. Alterations in the activity of the innate host immune system can be responsible for both the development of shock (i.e., septic shock following severe infection and traumatic shock following tissue injury with hemorrhage) and the pathophysiologic sequelae of shock such as the proinflammatory changes seen following hypoperfusion (see Fig. 5-1). When the predominantly paracrine mediators gain access to the systemic circulation, they can induce a variety of metabolic changes that are collectively referred to as the *host inflammatory response*. Understanding of the intricate, redundant, and interrelated pathways that comprise the inflammatory response to shock continues to expand. Despite limited understanding of how our current therapeutic interventions impact the host response to illness, inappropriate or excessive inflammation appears to be an essential event in the development of ARDS, multiple organ dysfunction syndrome (MODS), and posttraumatic immunosuppression that can prolong recovery.[21]

Following direct tissue injury or infection, there are several mechanisms that lead to the activation of the active inflammatory and immune responses. These include release of bioactive peptides by neurons in response to pain and the release of intracellular molecules by broken cells, such as heat shock proteins, mitochondrial peptides, heparan sulfate, high mobility group box 1, and RNA. Only recently has it been realized that the release of intracellular products from damaged and injured cells can have paracrine and endocrine-like effects on distant tissues to activate the inflammatory and immune responses.[22] This hypothesis, which was first proposed by Matzinger, is known as *danger signaling*. Under this novel paradigm of immune function, endogenous molecules are capable of signaling the presence of danger to surrounding cells and tissues. These molecules that are released from cells are known as *damage associated molecular patterns* (DAMPs, Table 5-3). DAMPs are recognized by cell surface

TABLE 5-3 Endogenous damage associated molecular pattern molecules

Hyaluronan oligomers
Heparan sulfate
Extra domain A of fibronectin
Heat shock proteins 60, 70, Gp96
Surfactant Protein A
β-Defensin 2
Fibrinogen
Biglycan
High mobility group box 1
Uric acid
Interleukin-1α
S-100s
Nucleolin

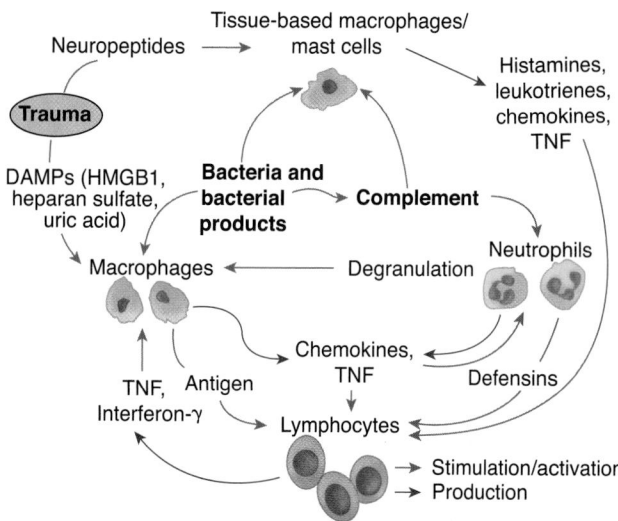

FIG. 5-4. A schema of information flow between immune cells in early inflammation following tissue injury and infection. Cells require multiple inputs and stimuli before activation of a full response. DAMPs = damage associated molecular patterns; HMGB1 = high mobility group box 1; TNF = tumor necrosis factor.

receptors to effect intracellular signaling that primes and amplifies the immune response. These receptors are known as *pattern recognition receptors (PRRs)* and include the Toll-like receptors (TLRs) and the receptor for advanced glycation end products. Interestingly, TLRs and PRRs were first recognized for their role in signaling as part of the immune response to the entry of microbes and their secreted products into a normally sterile environment. These bacterial products, including lipopolysaccharide, are known as *pathogen-associated molecular patterns.* The salutary consequences of PRR activation most likely relate to the initiation of the repair process and the mobilization of antimicrobial defenses at the site of tissue disruption. However, in the setting of excessive tissue damage, the inflammation itself may lead to further tissue damage amplifying the response both at the local and systemic level.[20] PRR activation leads to intracellular signaling and release of cellular products including cytokines (Fig. 5-4).

Before the recruitment of leukocytes into sites of injury, tissue-based macrophages or mast cells act as sentinel responders, releasing histamines, eicosanoids, tryptases, and cytokines (Fig. 5-5). Together these signals amplify the immune response by further activation of neurons and mast cells, as well as increasing the expression of adhesion molecules on the endothelium. Furthermore, these mediators cause leukocytes to release platelet-activating factor, further increasing the stickiness of the endothelium. Additionally, the coagulation and kinin cascades impact the interaction of endothelium and leukocytes.

Cytokines

The immune response to shock encompasses the elaboration of mediators with both proinflammatory and anti-inflammatory properties (Table 5-4). Furthermore, new mediators, new relationships between mediators, and new functions of known mediators are continually being identified. As new pathways are uncovered, understanding of the immune response to injury and the potential for therapeutic intervention by manipulating the immune response following shock will expand. What seems clear at present, however, is that the innate immune response can help restore homeostasis, or if it is excessive, promote cellular and organ dysfunction.

Multiple mediators have been implicated in the host immune response to shock. It is likely that some of the most important mediators have yet to be discovered, and the roles of many known mediators have not been defined. A comprehensive description of all of the mediators and their complex interactions is beyond the scope of this chapter. For a general overview, a brief description of the more extensively studied mediators, as well as some of the known effects of these substances, see the discussion below. A more comprehensive review can be found in Chap. 2.

Tumor necrosis factor alpha (TNF-α) was one of the first cytokines to be described, and is one of the earliest cytokines released in response to injurious stimuli. Monocytes, macrophages, and T cells release this potent proinflammatory cytokine. TNF-α levels peak within 90 minutes of stimulation and return frequently to baseline levels within 4 hours. Release of TNF-α may be induced by bacteria or endotoxin, and leads to the development of shock and hypoperfusion, most commonly observed in septic shock. Production of TNF-α also may be induced following other insults, such as hemorrhage and ischemia. TNF-α levels correlate with mortality in animal models of hemorrhage.[23] In contrast, the increase in serum TNF-α levels reported in trauma patients is far less than that seen in septic patients.[24] Once released, TNF-α can produce peripheral vasodilation, activate the release of other cytokines, induce procoagulant activity, and stimulate a wide array of cellular metabolic changes. During the stress response, TNF-α contributes to the muscle protein breakdown and cachexia.

Interleukin-1 (IL-1) has actions that are similar to those of TNF-α. IL-1 has a very short half-life (6 minutes) and primarily acts in a paracrine fashion to modulate local cellular responses. Systemically, IL-1 produces a febrile response to injury by activating prostaglandins in the posterior hypothalamus, and causes anorexia by activating the satiety center. This cytokine also augments the secretion of ACTH, glucocorticoids, and β-endorphins. In conjunction with TNF-α, IL-1 can stimulate the release of other cytokines such as IL-2, IL-4, IL-6, IL-8, granulocyte-macrophage colony-stimulating factor, and interferon-γ.

IL-2 is produced by activated T cells in response to a variety of stimuli and activates other lymphocyte subpopulations and natural killer cells. The lack of clarity regarding the role of IL-2 in the response to shock is intimately associated with that of understanding immune function after injury. Some investigators have postulated that increased IL-2 secretion promotes shock-induced tissue injury and the development of shock. Others have demonstrated that depressed IL-2 production is associated with, and perhaps contributes to, the depression in immune function after hemorrhage that may increase the susceptibility of patients who develop shock to suffer infections.[25,26] It has been postulated that overly exuberant proinflammatory activation promotes tissue injury, organ dysfunction, and the subsequent immune dysfunction/suppression that may be evident later.[21] Emphasizing the importance of temporal changes in the production of mediators, both the initial excessive production of IL-2 and later depressed IL-2 production are probably important in the progression of shock.

IL-6 is elevated in response to hemorrhagic shock, major operative procedures, or trauma. Elevated IL-6 levels correlate with mortality in shock states. IL-6 contributes to lung, liver, and gut injury after hemorrhagic shock.[27] Thus, IL-6 may play a role in the development of diffuse alveolar damage and ARDS. IL-6 and IL-1 are mediators of the hepatic acute phase response to injury, and enhance the expression and activity of complement, C-reactive protein, fibrinogen, haptoglobin, amyloid A, and alpha$_1$-antitrypsin, and promote neutrophil activation.[28]

IL-10 is considered an anti-inflammatory cytokine that may have immunosuppressive properties. Its production is increased after shock and trauma, and it has been associated with depressed immune function clinically, as well as an increased susceptibility to infection.[29] IL-10 is secreted by T cells, monocytes, and macrophages, and inhibits proinflammatory cytokine secretion, O_2 radical production by phagocytes, adhesion molecule expression, and lymphocyte activation.[29,30] Administration of IL-10 depresses cytokine production and improves some aspects of immune function in experimental models of shock and sepsis.[31,32]

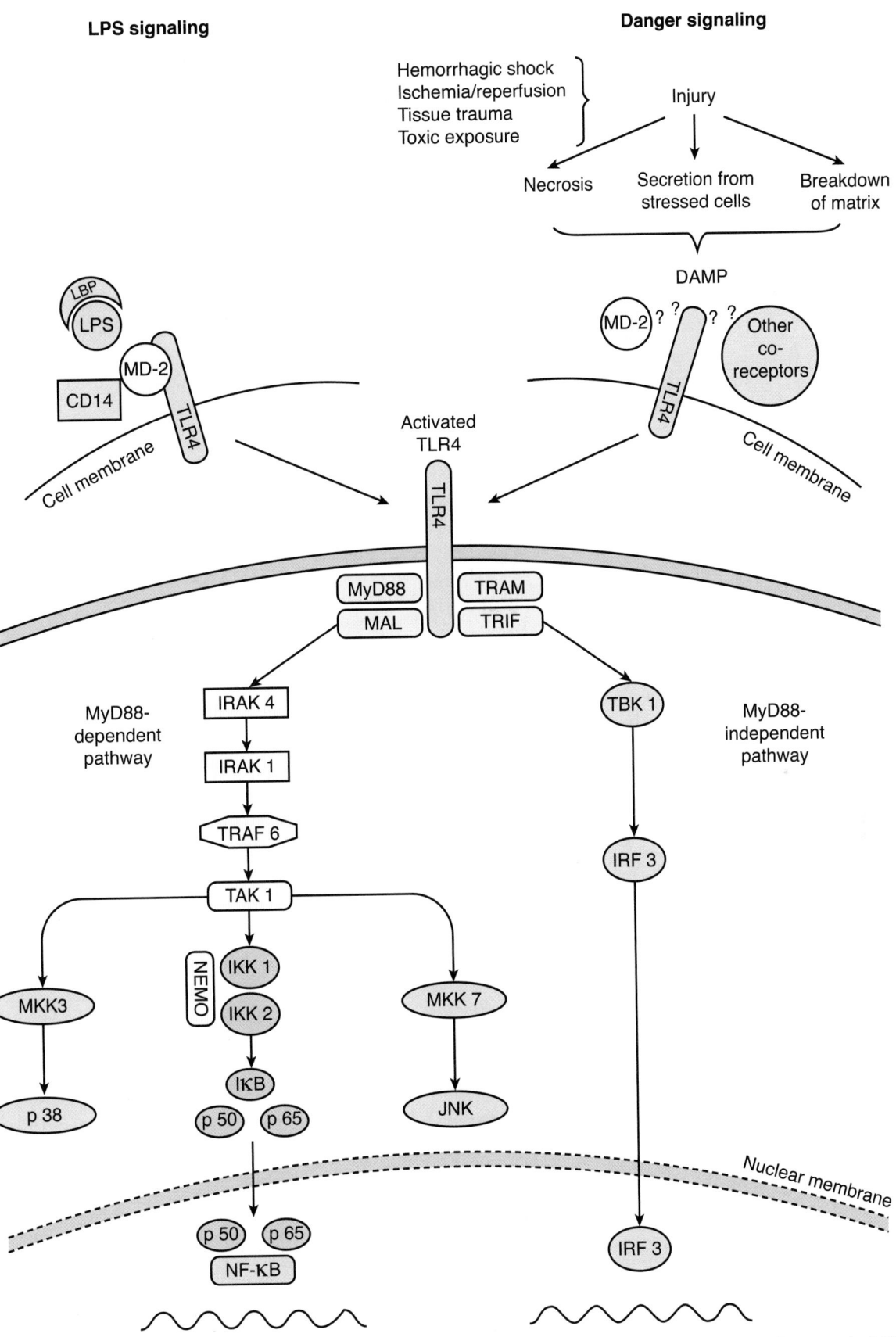

FIG. 5-5. Signaling via the pattern recognition receptor TLR4. LPS signaling via TLR4 requires the cofactors LPS binding protein (LBP), MD-2, and CD14. Endogenous danger signals released from a variety of sources also signal in a TLR4-dependent fashion, although it is as yet unknown what cofactors may be required for this activity. Once TLR4 is activated, an intracellular signaling cascade is initiated that involves both a MyD88-dependent and independent pathway. DAMP = damage associated molecular pattern; LPS = lipopolysaccharide; MD-2 = myeloid differentiation factor-2; MyD88 = myeloid differentiation primary response gene 88; NF-κB = nuclear factor κB; TLR4 = Toll-like receptor-4. (*From Mollen et al,*[74] *with permission.*)

CHAPTER 5

Shock

TABLE 5-4	Inflammatory mediators of shock

Proinflammatory	Anti-Inflammatory
Interleukin-1α/β	Interleukin-4
Interleukin-2	Interleukin-10
Interleukin-6	Interleukin-13
Interleukin-8	Prostaglandin E$_2$
Interferon	TGFβ
TNF	
PAF	

PAF = platelet activating factor; TGFβ = transforming growth factor beta; TNF = tumor necrosis factor.

Complement

The complement cascade can be activated by injury, shock, and severe infection, and contributes to host defense and proinflammatory activation. Significant complement consumption occurs after hemorrhagic shock.[33] In trauma patients, the degree of complement activation is proportional to the magnitude of injury and may serve as a marker for severity of injury. Patients in septic shock also demonstrate activation of the complement pathway, with elevations of the activated complement proteins C3a and C5a. Activation of the complement cascade can contribute to the development of organ dysfunction. Activated complement factors C3a, C4a, and C5a are potent mediators of increased vascular permeability, smooth muscle cell contraction, histamine and arachidonic acid by-product release, and adherence of neutrophils to vascular endothelium. Activated complement acts synergistically with endotoxin to induce the release of TNF-α and IL-1. The development of ARDS and MODS in trauma patients correlates with the intensity of complement activation.[34] Complement and neutrophil activation may correlate with mortality in multiply injured patients.

Neutrophils

Neutrophil activation is an early event in the upregulation of the inflammatory response; neutrophils are the first cells to be recruited to the site of injury. Polymorphonuclear leukocyte (PMNs) remove infectious agents, foreign substances that have penetrated host barrier defenses, and nonviable tissue through phagocytosis. However, activated PMNs and their products may also produce cell injury and organ dysfunction. Activated PMNs generate and release a number of substances that may induce cell or tissue injury, such as reactive O$_2$ species, lipid-peroxidation products, proteolytic enzymes (elastase, cathepsin G), and vasoactive mediators (leukotrienes, eicosanoids, and platelet-activating factor). Oxygen free radicals, such as superoxide anion, hydrogen peroxide, and hydroxyl radical, are released and induce lipid peroxidation, inactivate enzymes, and consume antioxidants (such as glutathione and tocopherol). Ischemia-reperfusion activates PMNs and causes PMN-induced organ injury. In animal models of hemorrhagic shock, activation of PMNs correlates with irreversibility of shock and mortality, and neutrophil depletion prevents the pathophysiologic sequelae of hemorrhagic and septic shock. Human data corroborate the activation of neutrophils in trauma and shock and suggest a role in the development of MODS.[35] Plasma markers of PMN activation, such as elastase, correlate with severity of injury in humans.

Interactions between endothelial cells and leukocytes are important in the inflammatory process. The vascular endothelium contributes to regulation of blood flow, leukocyte adherence, and the coagulation cascade. Extracellular ligands such as intercellular adhesion molecules, vascular cell adhesion molecules, and the selectins (E-selectin, P-selectin) are expressed on the surface of endothelial cells, and are responsible for leukocyte adhesion to the endothelium. This interaction allows activated neutrophils to migrate into the tissues to combat infection, but also can lead to PMN-mediated cytotoxicity and microvascular and tissue injury.

Cell Signaling

A host of cellular changes occur following shock. Although many of the intracellular and intercellular pathways that are important in shock are being elucidated, undoubtedly there are many more that have yet to be identified. Many of the mediators produced during shock interact with cell surface receptors on target cells to alter target cell metabolism. These signaling pathways may be altered by changes in cellular oxygenation, redox state, high-energy phosphate concentration, gene expression, or intracellular electrolyte concentration induced by shock. Cells communicate with their external environment through the use of cell surface membrane receptors which, once bound by a ligand, transmit their information to the interior of the cell through a variety of signaling cascades. These signaling pathways may subsequently alter the activity of specific enzymes, the expression or breakdown of important proteins, or affect intracellular energy metabolism. Intracellular calcium (Ca^{2+}) homeostasis and regulation represents one such pathway. Intracellular Ca^{2+} concentrations regulate many aspects of cellular metabolism; many important enzyme systems require Ca^{2+} for full activity. Profound changes in intracellular Ca^{2+} levels and Ca^{2+} transport are seen in models of shock.[36,37] Alterations in Ca^{2+} regulation may lead to direct cell injury, changes in transcription factor activation, alterations in the expression of genes important in homeostasis, and the modulation of the activation of cells by other shock-induced hormones or mediators.[38–40]

A proximal portion of the intracellular signaling cascade consists of a series of kinases that transmit and amplify the signal through the phosphorylation of target proteins. The O$_2$ radicals produced during shock and the intracellular redox state are known to influence the activity of components of this cascade, such as protein tyrosine kinases, mitogen activated kinases, and protein kinase C.[41–44] Either through changes in these signaling pathways, changes in the activation of enzyme systems through Ca^{2+}-mediated events, or direct conformational changes to oxygen-sensitive proteins, O$_2$ radicals also regulate the activity of a number of transcription factors that are important in gene expression, such as nuclear factor κB, APETALA1, and hypoxia-inducible factor 1.[45,46] It is therefore becoming increasingly clear that oxidant-mediated direct cell injury is merely one consequence of the production of O$_2$ radicals during shock.

The study of the effects of shock on the regulation of gene expression as an important biologic effect was stimulated by the work of Buchman and colleagues.[47] The effects of shock on the expression and regulation of numerous genes and gene products has been studied in both experimental animal models and human patients. These studies include investigations into single genes of interest as well as large-scale genomic and proteomic analysis.[48–50] Changes in gene expression are critical for adaptive and survival cell signaling. Polymorphisms in gene promoters that lead to a differential level of expression of gene products are also likely to contribute significantly to varied responses to similar insults.[51,52]

FORMS OF SHOCK

Hypovolemic/Hemorrhagic

The most common cause of shock in the surgical or trauma patient is loss of circulating volume from hemorrhage. Acute blood loss results in reflexive decreased baroreceptor stimulation from stretch receptors in the large arteries, resulting in decreased inhibition of vasoconstrictor centers in the brain stem, increased chemoreceptor stimulation of vasomotor centers, and diminished output from atrial stretch receptors. These changes increase vasoconstriction and peripheral arterial resistance. Hypovolemia also induces sympathetic stimulation, leading to epinephrine and norepinephrine release, activation of the renin-angiotensin cascade, and increased vasopressin release. Peripheral vasoconstriction is prominent, while lack of sympathetic effects on cerebral and coronary vessels and local autoregulation promote maintenance of cardiac and CNS blood flow.

TABLE 5-5 | Classification of hemorrhage

Parameter	Class I	II	III	IV
Blood loss (mL)	<750	750–1500	1500–2000	>2000
Blood loss (%)	<15	15–30	30–40	>40
Heart rate (bpm)	<100	>100	>120	>140
Blood pressure	Normal	Orthostatic	Hypotension	Severe hypotension
CNS symptoms	Normal	Anxious	Confused	Obtunded

bpm = beats per minute; CNS = central nervous system.

Diagnosis

Treatment of shock is initially empiric. A secure airway must be confirmed or established and volume infusion initiated while the search for the cause of the hypotension is pursued. Shock in a trauma patient and postoperative patient should be presumed to be due to hemorrhage until proven otherwise. The clinical signs of shock may be evidenced by agitation, cool clammy extremities, tachycardia, weak or absent peripheral pulses, and hypotension. Such apparent clinical shock results from at least 25 to 30% loss of the blood volume. However, substantial volumes of blood may be lost before the classic clinical manifestations of shock are evident. Thus, when a patient is significantly tachycardic or hypotensive, this represents both significant blood loss and physiologic decompensation. The clinical and physiologic response to hemorrhage has been classified according to the magnitude of volume loss. Loss of up to 15% of the circulating volume (700 to 750 mL for a 70-kg patient) may produce little in terms of obvious symptoms, while loss of up to 30% of the circulating volume (1.5 L) may result in mild tachycardia, tachypnea, and anxiety. Hypotension, marked tachycardia [i.e., pulse greater than 110 to 120 beats per minute (bpm)], and confusion may not be evident until more than 30% of the blood volume has been lost; loss of 40% of circulating volume (2 L) is immediately life threatening, and generally requires operative control of bleeding (Table 5-5). Young healthy patients with vigorous compensatory mechanisms may tolerate larger volumes of blood loss while manifesting fewer clinical signs despite the presence of significant peripheral hypoperfusion. These patients may maintain a near-normal blood pressure until a precipitous cardiovascular collapse occurs. Elderly patients may be taking medications that either promote bleeding (e.g., warfarin or aspirin), or mask the compensatory responses to bleeding (e.g., beta blockers). In addition, atherosclerotic vascular disease, diminishing cardiac compliance with age, inability to elevate heart rate or cardiac contractility in response to hemorrhage, and overall decline in physiologic reserve decrease the elderly patient's ability to tolerate hemorrhage. Recent data in trauma patients suggest that a systolic blood pressure (SBP) of less than 110 mmHg is a clinically relevant definition of hypotension and hypoperfusion based upon an increasing rate of mortality below this pressure (Fig. 5-6).[53]

In addressing the sensitivity of vital signs and identifying major thoracoabdominal hemorrhage, a study retrospectively identified patients with injury to the trunk and an abbreviated injury score of 3 or greater who required immediate surgical intervention and transfusion of at least 5 units of blood within the first 24 hours. Ninety-five percent of patients had a heart rate greater than 80 bpm at some point during their postinjury course. However, only 59% of patients achieved a heart rate greater than 120 bpm. Ninety-nine percent of all patients had a recorded blood pressure of less than 120 mmHg at some point. Ninety-three percent of all patients had a recorded SBP of less than 100 mmHg.[54] A more recent study corroborated that tachycardia was not a reliable sign of hemorrhage following trauma, and was present in only 65% of hypotensive patients.[55]

Serum lactate and base deficit are measurements that are helpful to both estimate and monitor the extent of bleeding and shock. The amount of lactate that is produced by anaerobic respiration is an indirect marker of tissue hypoperfusion, cellular O_2 debt, and the severity of hemorrhagic shock. Several studies have demonstrated that the initial serum lactate and serial lactate levels are reliable predictors of morbidity and mortality with hemorrhage following trauma (Fig. 5-7).[56] Similarly, base deficit values derived from arterial blood gas analysis provide clinicians with an indirect estimation of tissue acidosis from hypoperfusion. Davis and colleagues stratified the extent of base deficit into mild (–3 to –5 mmol/L), moderate (–6 to –9 mmol/L), and severe (less than –10 mmol/L), and from this established a correlation between base deficit upon admission with transfusion requirements, the development of multiple organ failure, and death (Fig. 5-8).[57] Both base deficit and lactate correlate with the extent of shock and patient outcome, but interestingly do not firmly correlate with each other.[58-60] Evaluation of both values may be useful in trauma patients with hemorrhage.

In management of trauma patients, understanding the patterns of injury of the patient in shock will help direct the evaluation and management. Identifying the sources of blood loss in patients with penetrating wounds is relatively simple because potential bleeding sources will be located along the known or suspected path of the wounding object. Patients with penetrating injuries who are in shock usually require operative intervention. Patients who suffer multisystem injuries from blunt trauma have multiple sources of potential hemorrhage. Blood loss sufficient to cause shock is gener-

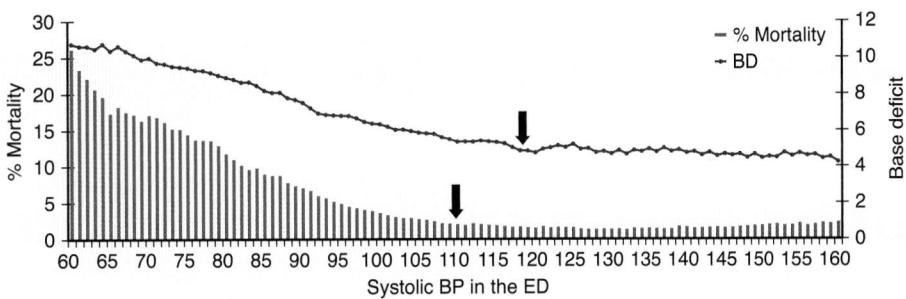

FIG. 5-6. The relationship between systolic blood pressure and mortality in trauma patients with hemorrhage. These data suggest that a systolic blood pressure of less than 110 mmHg is a clinically relevant definition of hypotension and hypoperfusion based upon an increasing rate of mortality below this pressure. Base deficit (BD) is also shown on this graph. ED = emergency department. (*From Eastridge et al,[53] with permission.*)

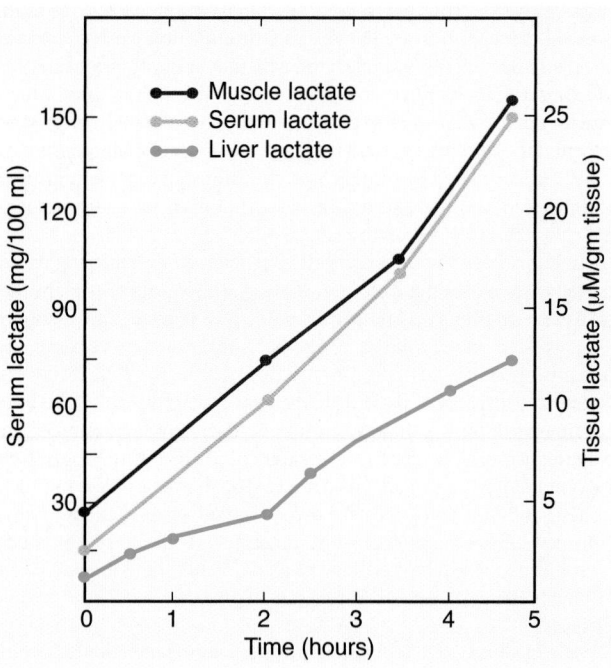

FIG. 5-7. Progressive increases in serum lactate, muscle lactate, and liver lactate in a baboon model of hemorrhagic shock. *(From Peitzman et al,[8] with permission.)*

wounds may cause massive blood loss rapidly. Direct pressure must be applied and sustained to minimize ongoing blood loss. Persistent bleeding from uncontrolled smaller vessels can, over time, precipitate shock if inadequately treated.

When major blood loss is not immediately visible in the setting of trauma, internal (intracavitary) blood loss should be suspected. Each pleural cavity can hold 2 to 3 L of blood and can therefore be a site of significant blood loss. Diagnostic and therapeutic tube thoracostomy may be indicated in unstable patients based on clinical findings and clinical suspicion. In a more stable patient, a chest radiograph may be obtained to look for evidence of hemothorax. Major retroperitoneal hemorrhage typically occurs in association with pelvic fractures, which is confirmed by pelvic radiography in the resuscitation bay. Intraperitoneal hemorrhage is probably the most common source of blood loss inducing shock. The physical exam for detection of substantial blood loss or injury is insensitive and unreliable; large volumes of intraperitoneal blood may be present before physical examination findings are apparent. Findings with intra-abdominal hemorrhage include abdominal distension, abdominal tenderness, or visible abdominal wounds. Hemodynamic abnormalities generally stimulate a search for blood loss before the appearance of obvious abdominal findings. Adjunctive tests are essential in the diagnosis of intraperitoneal bleeding; intraperitoneal blood may be rapidly identified by diagnostic ultrasound or diagnostic peritoneal lavage. Furthermore, patients that have sustained high-energy blunt trauma that are hemodynamically stable or that have normalized their vital signs in response to initial volume resuscitation should undergo computed tomography scans to assess for head, chest, and/or abdominal bleeding.

Treatment

Control of ongoing hemorrhage is an essential component of the resuscitation of the patient in shock. As mentioned in Diagnosis above, treatment of hemorrhagic shock is instituted concurrently with diagnostic evaluation to identify a source. Patients who fail to respond to initial resuscitative efforts should be assumed to have ongoing active hemorrhage from large vessels and require prompt operative intervention. Based on trauma literature, patients with ongoing hemorrhage demonstrate increased survival if the elapsed time between the injury and control of bleeding is decreased.

ally of a large volume, and there are a limited number of sites that can harbor sufficient extravascular blood volume to induce hypotension (e.g., external, intrathoracic, intra-abdominal, retroperitoneal, and long bone fractures). In the nontrauma patient, the GI tract must always be considered as a site for blood loss. Substantial blood loss externally may be suspected from prehospital medical reports documenting a substantial blood loss at the scene of an accident, history of massive blood loss from wounds, visible brisk bleeding, or presence of a large hematoma adjacent to an open wound. Injuries to major arteries or veins with associated open

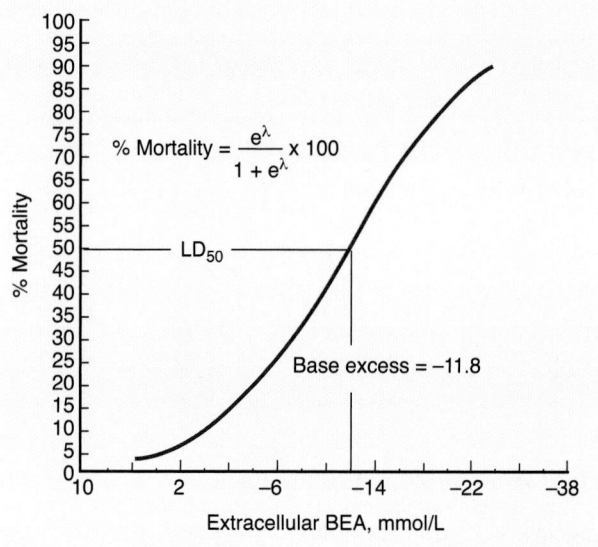

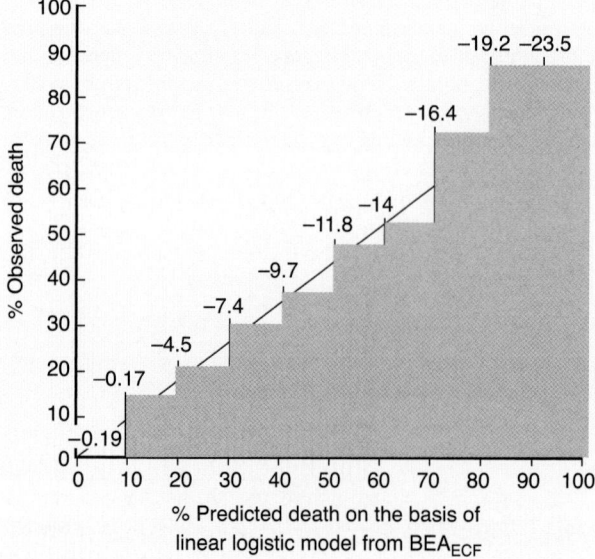

FIG. 5-8. The relationship between base deficit (negative base excess) and mortality in trauma patients. BEA = base excess arterial; ECF = extracellular fluid. *(Reproduced with permission from Siegel JH, Rivkind AI, Dalal S, et al: Early physiologic predictors of injury severity and death in blunt multiple trauma. Arch Surg 125:498, 1990. Copyright © 1990 American Medical Association. All rights reserved.)*

Although there are no randomized controlled trials, retrospective studies provide compelling evidence in this regard. To this end, Clarke and colleagues[61] demonstrated that trauma patients with major injuries isolated to the abdomen requiring emergency laparotomy had an increased probability of death with increasing length of time in the emergency department for patients who were in the emergency department for 90 minutes or less. This probability increased approximately 1% for each 3 minutes in the emergency department.

The appropriate priorities in these patients are (a) secure the airway, (b) control the source of blood loss, and (c) IV volume resuscitation. In trauma, identifying the body cavity harboring active hemorrhage will help focus operative efforts; however, because time is of the essence, rapid treatment is essential and diagnostic laparotomy or thoracotomy may be indicated. The actively bleeding patient cannot be resuscitated until control of ongoing hemorrhage is achieved. Our current understanding has led to the management strategy known as *damage control resuscitation*.[62] This strategy begins in the emergency department, continues into the operating room, and into the intensive care unit (ICU). Initial resuscitation is limited to keep SBP around 90 mmHg. This prevents renewed bleeding from recently clotted vessels. Resuscitation and intravascular volume resuscitation is accomplished with blood products and limited crystalloids, which is addressed further later in this section. Too little volume allowing persistent severe hypotension and hypoperfusion is dangerous, yet too vigorous of a volume resuscitation may be just as deleterious. Control of hemorrhage is achieved in the operating room, and efforts to warm patients and to prevent coagulopathy using multiple blood products and pharmacologic agents are used in both the operating room and ICU.

Cannon and colleagues first made the observation that attempts to increase blood pressure in soldiers with uncontrolled sources of hemorrhage is counterproductive, with increased bleeding and higher mortality.[3] This work was the foundation for the "hypotensive resuscitation" strategies. Several laboratory studies confirmed the observation that attempts to restore normal blood pressure with fluid infusion or vasopressors was rarely achievable and resulted in more bleeding and higher mortality.[63] A prospective, randomized clinical study compared delayed fluid resuscitation (upon arrival in the operating room) with standard fluid resuscitation (with arrival by the paramedics) in hypotensive patients with penetrating torso injury.[64] The authors reported that delayed fluid resuscitation resulted in lower patient mortality. Further laboratory studies demonstrated that fluid restriction in the setting of profound hypotension resulted in early deaths from severe hypoperfusion. These studies also showed that aggressive crystalloid resuscitation attempting to normalize blood pressure resulted in marked hemodilution, with hematocrits of 5%.[63] Reasonable conclusions in the setting of uncontrolled hemorrhage include: Any delay in surgery for control of hemorrhage increases mortality; with uncontrolled hemorrhage attempting to achieve normal blood pressure may increase mortality, particularly with penetrating injuries and short transport times; a goal of SBP of 80 to 90 mmHg may be adequate in the patient with penetrating injury; and profound hemodilution should be avoided by early transfusion of red blood cells. For the patient with blunt injury, where the major cause of death is a closed head injury, the increase in mortality with hypotension in the setting of brain injury must be avoided. In this setting, a SBP of 110 mmHg would seem to be more appropriate.

Patients who respond to initial resuscitative effort but then deteriorate hemodynamically frequently have injuries that require operative intervention. The magnitude and duration of their response will dictate whether diagnostic maneuvers can be performed to identify the site of bleeding. However, hemodynamic deterioration generally denotes ongoing bleeding for which some form of intervention (i.e., operation or interventional radiology) is required. Patients who have lost significant intravascular volume, but whose hemorrhage is controlled or has abated, often will respond to resuscitative efforts if the depth and duration of shock have been limited.

A subset of patients exists who fail to respond to resuscitative efforts despite adequate control of ongoing hemorrhage. These patients have ongoing fluid requirements despite adequate control of hemorrhage, have persistent hypotension despite restoration of intravascular volume necessitating vasopressor support, and may exhibit a futile cycle of uncorrectable hypothermia, hypoperfusion, acidosis, and coagulopathy that cannot be interrupted despite maximum therapy. These patients have deteriorated to decompensated or irreversible shock with peripheral vasodilation and resistance to vasopressor infusion. Mortality is inevitable once the patient manifests shock in its terminal stages. Unfortunately, this is all too often diagnosed in retrospect.

Fluid resuscitation is a major adjunct to physically controlling hemorrhage in patients with shock. The ideal type of fluid to be used continues to be debated; however, crystalloids continue to be the mainstay of fluid choice. Several studies have demonstrated increased risk of death in bleeding trauma patients treated with colloid compared to patients treated with crystalloid.[65] In patients with severe hemorrhage, restoration of intravascular volume should be achieved with blood products.[66]

Ongoing studies continue to evaluate the use of hypertonic saline as a resuscitative adjunct in bleeding patients.[67] The benefit of hypertonic saline solutions may be immunomodulatory. Specifically, these effects have been attributed to pharmacologic effects resulting in decreased reperfusion-mediated injury with decreased O_2 radical formation, less impairment of immune function compared to standard crystalloid solution, and less brain swelling in the multi-injured patient. The reduction of total volume used for resuscitation makes this approach appealing as a resuscitation agent for combat injuries and may contribute to a decrease in the incidence of ARDS and multiple organ failure.

Transfusion of packed red blood cells and other blood products is essential in the treatment of patients in hemorrhagic shock. Current recommendations in stable ICU patients aim for a target hemoglobin of 7 to 9 g/dL;[68,69] however, no prospective randomized trials have compared restrictive and liberal transfusion regimens in trauma patients with hemorrhagic shock. Fresh frozen plasma (FFP) should also be transfused in patients with massive bleeding or bleeding with increases in prothrombin or activated partial thromboplastin times 1.5 times greater than control. Civilian trauma data show that severity of coagulopathy early after ICU admission is predictive of mortality (Fig. 5-9).[70] Evolving data suggest more liberal transfusion of FFP in bleeding patients, but the clinical

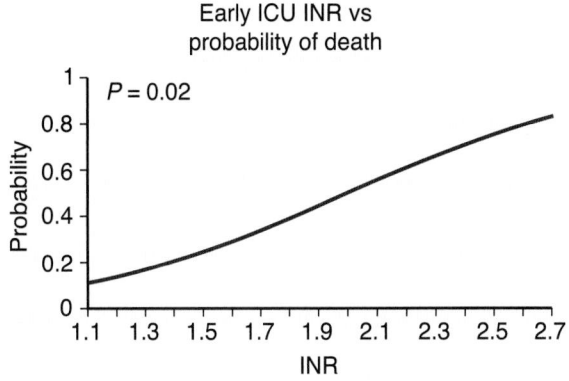

FIG. 5-9. The relationship between coagulopathy and mortality in trauma patients. Civilian trauma data show that severity of coagulopathy as determined by an increasing International Normalized Ratio (INR) early after intensive care unit (ICU) admission is predictive of mortality. (*From Gonzalez et al,*[70] *with permission.*)

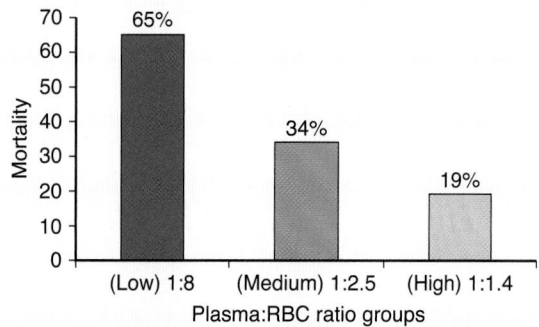

FIG. 5-10. Increasing ratio of transfusion of fresh frozen plasma to red blood cells improves outcome of trauma patients receiving massive transfusions. RBC = red blood cell. *(From Borgman et al,[71] with permission.)*

efficacy of FFP requires further investigation. Recent data collected from a U.S. Army combat support hospital in patients that received massive transfusion of packed red blood cells (>10 units in 24 hours) suggests that a high plasma to RBC ratio (1:1.4 units) was independently associated with improved survival (Fig. 5-10).[71] Platelets should be transfused in the bleeding patient to maintain counts above 50×10^9/L. There is a potential role for other blood products, such as fibrinogen concentrate of cryoprecipitate, if bleeding is accompanied by a drop in fibrinogen levels to less than 1 g/L. Pharmacologic agents such as recombinant activated coagulation factor 7, and antifibrinolytic agents such as ε-aminocaproic acid, tranexamic acid (both are synthetic lysine analogues that are competitive inhibitors of plasmin and plasminogen), and aprotinin (protease inhibitor) may all have potential benefits in severe hemorrhage but require further investigation.

Additional resuscitative adjuncts in patients with hemorrhagic shock include minimization of heat loss and maintaining normothermia. The development of hypothermia in the bleeding patient is associated with acidosis, hypotension, and coagulopathy. Hypothermia in bleeding trauma patients is an independent risk factor for bleeding and death. This likely is secondary to impaired platelet function and impairments in the coagulation cascade. Several studies have investigated the induction of controlled hypothermia in patients with severe shock based on the hypothesis of limiting metabolic activity and energy requirements, creating a state of "suspended animation." These studies are promising and continue to be evaluated in large trials.

Traumatic Shock

The systemic response after trauma, combining the effects of soft tissue injury, long bone fractures, and blood loss, is clearly a different physiologic insult than simple hemorrhagic shock. Multiple organ failure, including acute respiratory distress syndrome (ARDS), develops relatively often in the blunt trauma patient, but rarely after pure hemorrhagic shock (such as a GI bleed). The hypoperfusion deficit in traumatic shock is magnified by the proinflammatory activation that occurs following the induction of shock. In addition to ischemia or ischemia-reperfusion, accumulating evidence demonstrates that even simple hemorrhage induces proinflammatory activation that results in many of the cellular changes typically ascribed only to septic shock.[72,73] At the cellular level, this may be attributable to the release of cellular products termed *damage associated molecular patterns* (*DAMPs*, i.e., riboxynucleic acid, uric acid, and high mobility group box 1) that activate the same set of cell surface receptors as bacterial products, initiating similar cell signaling.[5,74] These receptors are termed *pattern recognition receptors* (*PRRs*) and include the TLR family of proteins. Examples of traumatic shock include small volume hemorrhage accompanied by soft tissue injury (femur fracture, crush injury), or any combination of hypovolemic, neurogenic, cardio-

genic, and obstructive shock that precipitate rapidly progressive proinflammatory activation. In laboratory models of traumatic shock, the addition of a soft tissue or long bone injury to hemorrhage produces lethality with significantly less blood loss when the animals are stressed by hemorrhage. Treatment of traumatic shock is focused on correction of the individual elements to diminish the cascade of proinflammatory activation, and includes prompt control of hemorrhage, adequate volume resuscitation to correct O_2 debt, débridement of nonviable tissue, stabilization of bony injuries, and appropriate treatment of soft tissue injuries.

Septic Shock (Vasodilatory Shock)

In the peripheral circulation, profound vasoconstriction is the typical physiologic response to the decreased arterial pressure and tissue perfusion with hemorrhage, hypovolemia, or acute heart failure. This is not the characteristic response in vasodilatory shock. Vasodilatory shock is the result of dysfunction of the endothelium and vasculature secondary to circulating inflammatory mediators and cells or as a response to prolonged and severe hypoperfusion. Thus, in vasodilatory shock, hypotension results from failure of the vascular smooth muscle to constrict appropriately. Vasodilatory shock is characterized by peripheral vasodilation with resultant hypotension and resistance to treatment with vasopressors. Despite the hypotension, plasma catecholamine levels are elevated, and the renin-angiotensin system is activated in vasodilatory shock. The most frequently encountered form of vasodilatory shock is septic shock. Other causes of vasodilatory shock include hypoxic lactic acidosis, carbon monoxide poisoning, decompensated and irreversible hemorrhagic shock, terminal cardiogenic shock, and postcardiotomy shock (Table 5-6). Thus, vasodilatory shock seems to represent the final common pathway for profound and prolonged shock of any etiology.[75]

Despite advances in intensive care, the mortality rate for severe sepsis remains at 30 to 50%. In the United States, 750,000 cases of sepsis occur annually, one third of which are fatal.[76] Sepsis accounts for 9.3% of deaths in the United States, as many yearly as MI.[77] Septic shock is a by-product of the body's response to disruption of the host-microbe equilibrium, resulting in invasive or severe localized infection.

In the attempt to eradicate the pathogens, the immune and other cell types (e.g., endothelial cells) elaborate soluble mediators that enhance macrophage and neutrophil killing effector mechanisms, increase procoagulant activity and fibroblast activity to localize the invaders, and increase microvascular blood flow to enhance delivery of killing forces to the area of invasion. When this response is overly exuberant or becomes systemic rather than localized, manifestations of sepsis may be evident. These findings include enhanced cardiac output, peripheral vasodilation, fever, leukocytosis, hyperglycemia, and tachycardia. In septic shock, the vasodilatory effects are due, in part, to the upregulation of the inducible isoform of nitric oxide synthase (iNOS or NOS 2) in the vessel wall. iNOS

TABLE 5-6	Causes of septic and vasodilatory shock

Systemic response to infection
Noninfectious systemic inflammation
    Pancreatitis
    Burns
Anaphylaxis
Acute adrenal insufficiency
Prolonged, severe hypotension
    Hemorrhagic shock
    Cardiogenic shock
    Cardiopulmonary bypass
Metabolic
    Hypoxic lactic acidosis
    Carbon monoxide poisoning

produces large quantities of nitric oxide for sustained periods of time. This potent vasodilator suppresses vascular tone and renders the vasculature resistant to the effects of vasoconstricting agents.

Diagnosis

Attempts to standardize terminology have led to the establishment of criteria for the diagnosis of sepsis in the hospitalized adult. These criteria include manifestations of the host response to infection in addition to identification of an offending organism. The terms *sepsis, severe sepsis,* and *septic shock* are used to quantify the magnitude of the systemic inflammatory reaction. Patients with *sepsis* have evidence of an infection, as well as systemic signs of inflammation (e.g., fever, leukocytosis, and tachycardia). Hypoperfusion with signs of organ dysfunction is termed *severe sepsis. Septic shock* requires the presence of the above, associated with more significant evidence of tissue hypoperfusion and systemic hypotension. Beyond the hypotension, maldistribution of blood flow and shunting in the microcirculation further compromise delivery of nutrients to the tissue beds.[78]

Recognizing septic shock begins with defining the patient at risk. The clinical manifestations of septic shock will usually become evident and prompt the initiation of treatment before bacteriologic confirmation of an organism or the source of an organism is identified. In addition to fever, tachycardia, and tachypnea, signs of hypoperfusion such as confusion, malaise, oliguria, or hypotension may be present. These should prompt an aggressive search for infection, including a thorough physical examination, inspection of all wounds, evaluation of intravascular catheters or other foreign bodies, obtaining appropriate cultures, and adjunctive imaging studies, as needed.

Treatment

Evaluation of the patient in septic shock begins with an assessment of the adequacy of their airway and ventilation. Severely obtunded patients and patients whose work of breathing is excessive require intubation and ventilation to prevent respiratory collapse. Because vasodilation and decrease in total peripheral resistance may produce hypotension, fluid resuscitation and restoration of circulatory volume with balanced salt solutions is essential. Empiric antibiotics must be chosen carefully based on the most likely pathogens (gram-negative rods, gram-positive cocci, and anaerobes) because the portal of entry of the offending organism and its identity may not be evident until culture data return or imaging studies are completed. Knowledge of the bacteriologic profile of infections in an individual unit can be obtained from most hospital infection control departments and will suggest potential responsible organisms. Antibiotics should be tailored to cover the responsible organisms once culture data are available, and if appropriate, the spectrum of coverage narrowed. Long-term, empiric, broad-spectrum antibiotic use should be minimized to reduce the development of resistant organisms and to avoid the potential complications of fungal overgrowth and antibiotic-associated colitis from overgrowth of *Clostridium difficile.* IV antibiotics will be insufficient to adequately treat the infectious episode in the settings of infected fluid collections, infected foreign bodies, and devitalized tissue. This situation is termed *source control* and involves percutaneous drainage and operative management to target a focus of infection. These situations may require multiple operations to ensure proper wound hygiene and healing.

After first-line therapy of the septic patient with antibiotics, IV fluids, and intubation if necessary, vasopressors may be necessary to treat patients with septic shock. Catecholamines are the vasopressors used most often. Occasionally, patients with septic shock will develop arterial resistance to catecholamines. Arginine vasopressin, a potent vasoconstrictor, is often efficacious in this setting.

The majority of septic patients have hyperdynamic physiology with supranormal cardiac output and low systemic vascular resistance. On occasion, septic patients may have low cardiac output despite volume resuscitation and even vasopressor support. Mortality in this group is high. Despite the increasing incidence of septic shock over the past several decades, the overall mortality rates have changed little. Studies of interventions, including immunotherapy, resuscitation to pulmonary artery endpoints with hemodynamic optimization (cardiac output and O_2 delivery, even to supranormal values), and optimization of mixed venous O_2 measurements up to 72 hours after admission to the ICU, have not changed mortality.

Over the past decade, multiple advances have been made in the treatment of patients with sepsis and septic shock (Fig. 5-11).[78,79] Negative results from previous studies have led to the suggestion that earlier interventions directed at improving global tissue oxygenation may be of benefit. To this end, Rivers and colleagues reported that goal-directed therapy of septic shock and severe sepsis initiated in the emergency department and continued for 6 hours significantly improved outcome.[80] This approach involved adjustment of cardiac preload, afterload, and contractility to balance O_2 delivery with O_2 demand. They found that goal-directed therapy during the first 6 hours of hospital stay (initiated in the emergency department) had significant effects, such as higher mean venous O_2 saturation, lower lactate levels, lower base deficit, higher pH, and decreased 28-day mortality (49.2 vs. 33.3%) compared to the standard therapy group. The frequency of sudden cardiovascular collapse was also significantly less in the group managed with goal-directed therapy (21.0 vs. 10.3%). Interestingly, the goal-directed therapy group received more IV fluids during the initial 6 hours, but the standard therapy group required more IV fluids by 72 hours. The authors emphasize that continued cellular and tissue decompensation is subclinical and often irreversible when obvious clinically. Goal-directed therapy allowed identification and treatment of these patients with insidious illness (global tissue hypoxia in the setting of normal vital signs).

Hyperglycemia and insulin resistance are typical in critically ill and septic patients, including patients without underlying diabetes mellitus. A recent study reported significant positive impact of tight glucose management on outcome in critically ill patients.[81] The two treatment groups in this randomized, prospective study were assigned to receive intensive insulin therapy (maintenance of blood glucose between 80 and 110 mg/dL) or conventional treatment (infusion of insulin only if the blood glucose level exceeded 215 mg/dL, with a goal between 180 and 200 mg/dL). The mean morning glucose level was significantly higher in the conventional treatment as compared to the intensive insulin therapy group (153 vs. 103 mg/dL). Mortality in the intensive insulin treatment group (4.6%) was significantly lower than in the conventional treatment group (8.0%), representing a 42% reduction in mortality. This reduction in mortality was most notable in the patients requiring longer than 5 days in the ICU. Furthermore, intensive insulin therapy reduced episodes of septicemia by 46%, reduced duration of antibiotic therapy, and decreased the need for prolonged ventilatory support and renal replacement therapy.

Another treatment protocol that has been demonstrated to increase survival in patients with ARDS investigated the use of lower ventilatory tidal volumes compared to traditional tidal volumes.[82] The majority of the patients enrolled in this multicenter, randomized trial developed ARDS secondary to pneumonia or sepsis. The trial compared traditional ventilation treatment, which involved an initial tidal volume of 12 mL/kg of predicted body weight and an airway pressure measured after a 0.5-second pause at the end of inspiration (plateau pressure) of 50 cm of water or less, with ventilation with a lower tidal volume, which involved an initial tidal volume of 6 mL/kg of predicted body weight and a plateau pressure of 30 cm of water or less. The trial was stopped after the enrollment of 861 patients because mortality was lower in the group treated with lower tidal volumes than in the group treated with traditional tidal volumes (31.0 vs. 39.8%, $P = .007$), and the number of days without ventilator use during the first 28 days after randomization was greater in this group (mean $\pm$ SD, 12

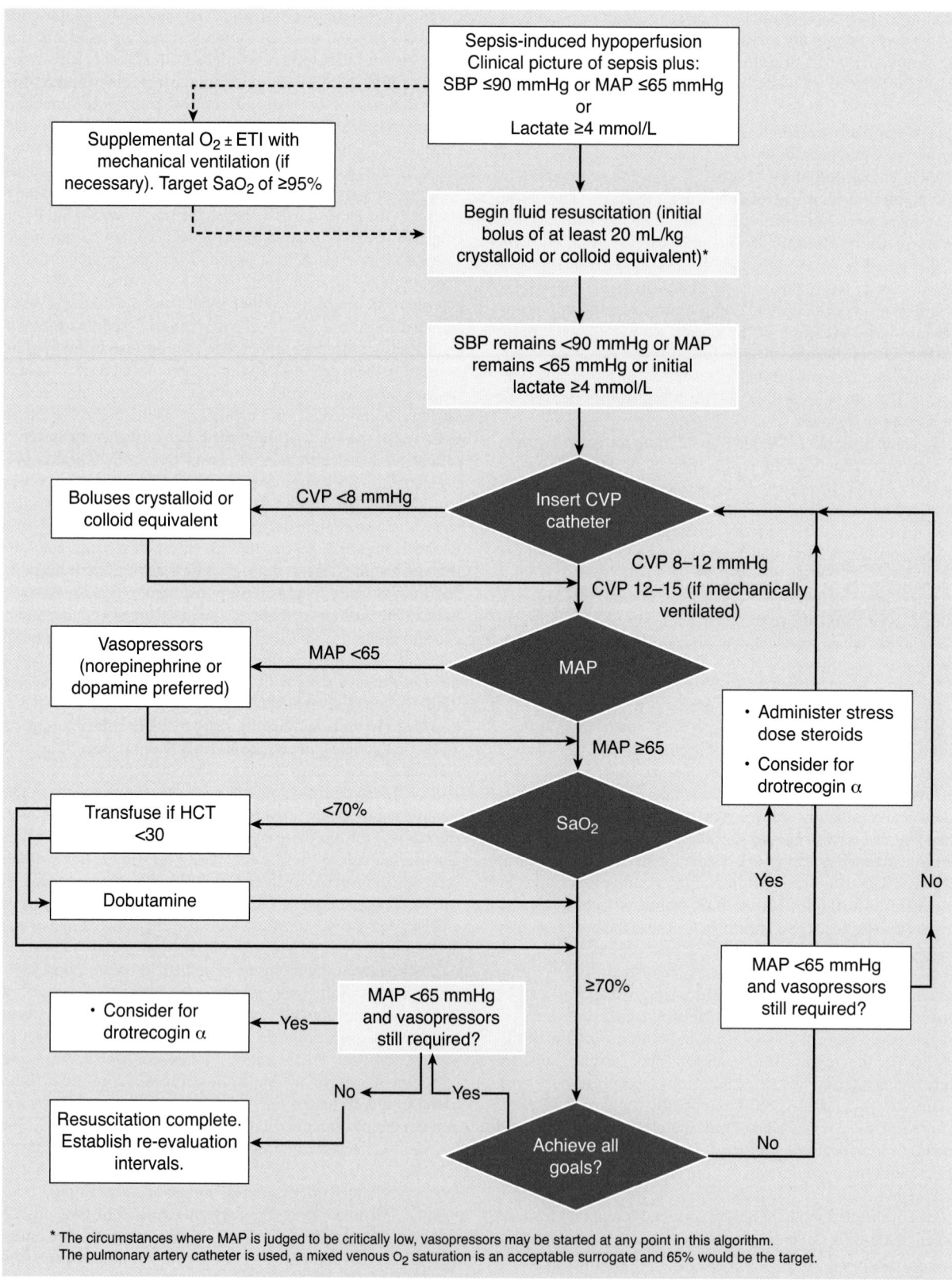

FIG. 5-11. An algorithm for the treatment of patients presenting with sepsis syndrome. CVP = central venous pressure; ETI = ejective time index; HCT = hematocrit; MAP = mean arterial pressure; O$_2$ = oxygen; SaO$_2$ = oxygen saturation; SBP = systolic blood pressure. *(From Cinel et al,[79] with permission.)*

± 11 vs. 10 ± 11; *P* = .007). The investigators concluded that in patients with acute lung injury and ARDS, mechanical ventilation with a lower tidal volume than is traditionally used results in decreased mortality and increases the number of days without ventilator use.

A recent study reported benefit from IV infusion of recombinant human activated protein C for severe sepsis.[83] Activated protein C is an endogenous protein that promotes fibrinolysis and inhibits thrombosis and inflammation. The authors conducted a randomized, prospective, multicenter trial assessing the efficacy of activated protein C in patients with systemic inflammation and organ failure due to acute infection. Treatment with activated protein C reduced the 28-day mortality rate from 31 to 25%; the reduction in relative risk of death was 19.4%. However, several follow-up studies have suggested that activated protein C may not improve mortality when patients are followed up to 6 months.

The use of corticosteroids in the treatment of sepsis and septic shock has been controversial for decades. The observation that severe sepsis often is associated with adrenal insufficiency or glucocorticoid receptor resistance has generated renewed interest in therapy for septic shock with corticosteroids. A single IV dose of 50 mg of hydrocortisone improved mean arterial blood pressure response relationships to norepinephrine and phenylephrine in patients with septic shock, and was most notable in patients with relative adrenal insufficiency. A more recent study evaluated therapy with hydrocortisone (50 mg IV every 6 hours) and fludrocortisone (50 μg orally once daily) vs. placebo for 1 week in patients with septic shock.[84] As in earlier studies, the authors performed corticotropin tests on these patients to document and stratify patients by relative adrenal insufficiency. In this study, 7-day treatment with low doses of hydrocortisone and fludrocortisone significantly and safely lowered the risk of death in patients with septic shock and relative adrenal insufficiency. In an international, multicenter, randomized trial of corticosteroids in sepsis (CORTICUS study; 499 analyzable patients), steroids showed no benefit in intent to treat mortality or shock reversal.[85] This study suggested that hydrocortisone therapy cannot be recommended as routine adjuvant therapy for septic shock. However, if SBP remains less than 90 mmHg despite appropriate fluid and vasopressor therapy, hydrocortisone at 200 mg/day for 7 days in four divided doses or by continuous infusion should be considered.

Additional adjunctive immune modulation strategies have been developed for the treatment of septic shock. These include the use of antiendotoxin antibodies, anticytokine antibodies, cytokine receptor antagonists, immune enhancers, a non–isoform-specific nitric oxide synthase inhibitor, and O_2 radical scavengers. These compounds are each designed to alter some aspect of the host immune response to shock that is hypothesized to play a key role in its pathophysiology. However, most of these strategies have failed to demonstrate efficacy in human patients despite utility in well-controlled animal experiments. It is unclear whether the failure of these compounds is due to poorly designed clinical trials, inadequate understanding of the interactions of the complex host immune response to injury and infection, or animal models of shock that poorly represent the human disease.

Cardiogenic Shock

Cardiogenic shock is defined clinically as circulatory pump failure leading to diminished forward flow and subsequent tissue hypoxia, in the setting of adequate intravascular volume. Hemodynamic criteria include sustained hypotension (i.e., SBP <90 mmHg for at least 30 minutes), reduced cardiac index (<2.2 L/min per square meter), and elevated pulmonary artery wedge pressure (>15 mmHg).[86] Mortality rates for cardiogenic shock are 50 to 80%. Acute, extensive MI is the most common cause of cardiogenic shock; a smaller infarction in a patient with existing left ventricular dysfunction also may precipitate shock. Cardiogenic shock complicates 5 to 10% of acute MIs. Conversely, cardiogenic shock is the most common cause of death in patients hospitalized with acute MI. Although shock may develop early after MI, it typically is not found on admission. Seventy-five percent of patients who have cardiogenic shock complicating acute MIs develop signs of cardiogenic shock within 24 hours after onset of infarction (average 7 hours).

Recognition of the patient with occult hypoperfusion is critical to prevent progression to obvious cardiogenic shock with its high mortality rate; early initiation of therapy to maintain blood pressure and cardiac output is vital. Rapid assessment, adequate resuscitation, and reversal of the myocardial ischemia are essential in optimizing outcome in patients with acute MI. Prevention of infarct extension is a

critical component. Large segments of nonfunctional but viable myocardium contribute to the development of cardiogenic shock after MI. In the setting of acute MI, expeditious restoration of cardiac output is mandatory to minimize mortality; the extent of myocardial salvage possible decreases exponentially with increased time to restoration of coronary blood flow. The degree of coronary flow after percutaneous transluminal coronary angioplasty correlates with inhospital mortality (i.e., 33% mortality with complete reperfusion, 50% mortality with incomplete reperfusion, and 85% mortality with absent reperfusion).[87] Inadequate cardiac function can be a direct result of cardiac injury, including profound myocardial contusion, blunt cardiac valvular injury, or direct myocardial damage (Table 5-7).[86–88] The pathophysiology of cardiogenic shock involves a vicious cycle of myocardial ischemia that causes myocardial dysfunction, which results in more myocardial ischemia. When sufficient mass of the left ventricular wall is necrotic or ischemic and fails to pump, the stroke volume decreases. An autopsy series of patients dying from cardiogenic shock have found damage to 40% of the left ventricle.[89] Ischemia distant from the infarct zone may contribute to the systolic dysfunction in patients with cardiogenic shock. The majority of these patients have multivessel disease, with limited vasodilator reserve and pressure-dependent coronary flow in multiple areas of the heart. Myocardial diastolic function is impaired in cardiogenic shock as well. Decreased compliance results from myocardial ischemia, and compensatory increases in left ventricular filling pressures progressively occur.

Diminished cardiac output or contractility in the face of adequate intravascular volume (preload) may lead to underperfused vascular beds and reflexive sympathetic discharge. Increased sympathetic stimulation of the heart, either through direct neural input or from circulating catecholamines, increases heart rate, myocardial contraction, and myocardial O_2 consumption, which may not be relieved by increases in coronary artery blood flow in patients with fixed stenoses of the coronary arteries. Diminished cardiac output may also decrease coronary artery blood flow, resulting in a scenario of increased myocardial O_2 demand at a time when myocardial O_2 supply may be limited. Acute heart failure may also result in fluid accumulation in the pulmonary microcirculatory bed, decreasing myocardial O_2 delivery even further.

Diagnosis

Rapid identification of the patient with pump failure and institution of corrective action are essential in preventing the ongoing spiral of

TABLE 5-7	Causes of cardiogenic shock

Acute myocardial infarction
    Pump failure
    Mechanical complications
        Acute mitral regurgitation
        Acute ventricular septal defect
        Free wall rupture
        Pericardial tamponade
Arrhythmia
End-stage cardiomyopathy
Myocarditis
Severe myocardial contusion
Left ventricular outflow obstruction
    Aortic stenosis
    Hypertrophic obstructive cardiomyopathy
Obstruction to left ventricular filling
    Mitral stenosis
    Left atrial myxoma
Acute mitral regurgitation
Acute aortic insufficiency
Metabolic
Drug reactions

decreased cardiac output from injury causing increased myocardial O_2 needs that cannot be met, leading to progressive and unremitting cardiac dysfunction. In evaluation of possible cardiogenic shock, other causes of hypotension must be excluded, including hemorrhage, sepsis, pulmonary embolism, and aortic dissection. Signs of circulatory shock include hypotension, cool and mottled skin, depressed mental status, tachycardia, and diminished pulses. Cardiac exam may include dysrhythmia, precordial heave, or distal heart tones. Confirmation of a cardiac source for the shock requires electrocardiogram and urgent echocardiography. Other useful diagnostic tests include chest radiograph, arterial blood gases, electrolytes, complete blood count, and cardiac enzymes. Invasive cardiac monitoring, which generally is not necessary, can be useful to exclude right ventricular infarction, hypovolemia, and possible mechanical complications.

Making the diagnosis of cardiogenic shock involves the identification of cardiac dysfunction or acute heart failure in a susceptible patient. In the setting of blunt traumatic injury, hemorrhagic shock from intra-abdominal bleeding, intrathoracic bleeding, and bleeding from fractures must be excluded, before implicating cardiogenic shock from blunt cardiac injury. Relatively few patients with blunt cardiac injury will develop cardiac pump dysfunction. Those who do generally exhibit cardiogenic shock early in their evaluation. Therefore, establishing the diagnosis of blunt cardiac injury is secondary to excluding other etiologies for shock and establishing that cardiac dysfunction is present. Invasive hemodynamic monitoring with a pulmonary artery catheter may uncover evidence of diminished cardiac output and elevated pulmonary artery pressure.

Treatment

After ensuring that an adequate airway is present and ventilation is sufficient, attention should be focused on support of the circulation. Intubation and mechanical ventilation often are required, if only to decrease work of breathing and facilitate sedation of the patient. Rapidly excluding hypovolemia and establishing the presence of cardiac dysfunction are essential. Treatment of cardiac dysfunction includes maintenance of adequate oxygenation to ensure adequate myocardial O_2 delivery and judicious fluid administration to avoid fluid overload and development of cardiogenic pulmonary edema. Electrolyte abnormalities, commonly hypokalemia and hypomagnesemia, should be corrected. Pain is treated with IV morphine sulfate or fentanyl. Significant dysrhythmias and heart block must be treated with antiarrhythmic drugs, pacing, or cardioversion, if necessary. Early consultation with cardiology is essential in current management of cardiogenic shock, particularly in the setting of acute MI.[86]

When profound cardiac dysfunction exists, inotropic support may be indicated to improve cardiac contractility and cardiac output. Dobutamine primarily stimulates cardiac beta$_1$ receptors to increase cardiac output but may also vasodilate peripheral vascular beds, lower total peripheral resistance, and lower systemic blood pressure through effects on beta$_2$ receptors. Ensuring adequate preload and intravascular volume is therefore essential prior to instituting therapy with dobutamine. Dopamine stimulates receptors (vasoconstriction), beta$_1$ receptors (cardiac stimulation), and beta$_2$ receptors (vasodilation), with its effects on beta receptors predominating at lower doses. Dopamine may be preferable to dobutamine in treatment of cardiac dysfunction in hypotensive patients. Tachycardia and increased peripheral resistance from dopamine infusion may worsen myocardial ischemia. Titration of both dopamine and dobutamine infusions may be required in some patients.

Epinephrine stimulates alpha and beta receptors and may increase cardiac contractility and heart rate; however, it also may have intense peripheral vasoconstrictor effects that impair further cardiac performance. Catecholamine infusions must be carefully controlled to maximize coronary perfusion, while minimizing myocardial O_2 demand. Balancing the beneficial effects of impaired cardiac performance with the potential side effects of excessive reflex tachycardia and peripheral vasoconstriction requires serial assessment of tissue perfusion using indices such as capillary refill, character of peripheral pulses, adequacy of urine output, or improvement in laboratory parameters of resuscitation such as pH, base deficit, and lactate. Invasive monitoring generally is necessary in these unstable patients. The phosphodiesterase inhibitors amrinone and milrinone may be required on occasion in patients with resistant cardiogenic shock. These agents have long half-lives and induce thrombocytopenia and hypotension, and use is reserved for patients unresponsive to other treatment.

Patients whose cardiac dysfunction is refractory to cardiotonics may require mechanical circulatory support with an intra-aortic balloon pump.[90] Intra-aortic balloon pumping increases cardiac output and improves coronary blood flow by reduction of systolic afterload and augmentation of diastolic perfusion pressure. Unlike vasopressor agents, these beneficial effects occur without an increase in myocardial O_2 demand. An intra-aortic balloon pump can be inserted at the bedside in the ICU via the femoral artery through either a cutdown or using the percutaneous approach. Aggressive circulatory support of patients with cardiac dysfunction from intrinsic cardiac disease has led to more widespread application of these devices and more familiarity with their operation by both physicians and critical care nurses.

Preservation of existing myocardium and preservation of cardiac function are priorities of therapy for patients who have suffered an acute MI. Ensuring adequate oxygenation and O_2 delivery, maintaining adequate preload with judicious volume restoration, minimizing sympathetic discharge through adequate relief of pain, and correcting electrolyte imbalances are all straightforward nonspecific maneuvers that may improve existing cardiac function or prevent future cardiac complications. Anticoagulation and aspirin are given for acute MI. Although thrombolytic therapy reduces mortality in patients with acute MI, its role in cardiogenic shock is less clear. Patients in cardiac failure from an acute MI may benefit from pharmacologic or mechanical circulatory support in a manner similar to that of patients with cardiac failure related to blunt cardiac injury. Additional pharmacologic tools may include the use of beta blockers to control heart rate and myocardial O_2 consumption, nitrates to promote coronary blood flow through vasodilation, and ACE inhibitors to reduce ACE-mediated vasoconstrictive effects that increase myocardial workload and myocardial O_2 consumption.

Current guidelines of the American Heart Association recommend percutaneous transluminal coronary angiography for patients with cardiogenic shock, ST elevation, left bundle-branch block, and age less than 75 years.[91] Early definition of coronary anatomy and revascularization is the pivotal step in treatment of patients with cardiogenic shock from acute MI.[92] When feasible, percutaneous transluminal coronary angioplasty (generally with stent placement) is the treatment of choice. Coronary artery bypass grafting seems to be more appropriate for patients with multiple vessel disease or left main coronary artery disease.

Obstructive Shock

Although obstructive shock can be caused by a number of different etiologies that result in mechanical obstruction of venous return (Table 5-8), in trauma patients this is most commonly due to the presence of tension pneumothorax. Cardiac tamponade occurs when sufficient fluid has accumulated in the pericardial sac to obstruct blood flow to the ventricles. The hemodynamic abnormalities in pericardial tamponade are due to elevation of intracardiac pressures with limitation of ventricular filling in diastole with resultant decrease in cardiac output. Acutely, the pericardium does not distend; thus small volumes of blood may produce cardiac tamponade. If the effusion accumulates slowly (e.g., in the setting of uremia, heart failure, or malignant effusion), the quantity of fluid producing cardiac tamponade may reach 2000 mL. The major determinant of the degree of hypotension is the pericardial pressure. With either cardiac tamponade or tension pneumothorax, reduced filling of the right side of the heart from either increased intrapleural pressure

TABLE 5-8 Causes of obstructive shock

Pericardial tamponade
Pulmonary embolus
Tension pneumothorax
IVC obstruction
    Deep venous thrombosis
    Gravid uterus on IVC
    Neoplasm
Increased intrathoracic pressure
    Excess positive end-expiratory pressure
    Neoplasm

IVC = inferior vena cava.

secondary to air accumulation (tension pneumothorax) or increased intrapericardial pressure precluding atrial filling secondary to blood accumulation (cardiac tamponade) results in decreased cardiac output associated with increased central venous pressure.

Diagnosis and Treatment

The diagnosis of tension pneumothorax should be made on clinical examination. The classic findings include respiratory distress (in an awake patient), hypotension, diminished breath sounds over one hemithorax, hyperresonance to percussion, jugular venous distention, and shift of mediastinal structures to the unaffected side with tracheal deviation. In most instances, empiric treatment with pleural decompression is indicated rather than delaying to wait for radiographic confirmation. When a chest tube cannot be immediately inserted, such as in the prehospital setting, the pleural space can be decompressed with a large caliber needle. Immediate return of air should be encountered with rapid resolution of hypotension. Unfortunately, not all of the clinical manifestations of tension pneumothorax may be evident on physical examination. Hyperresonance may be difficult to appreciate in a noisy resuscitation area. Jugular venous distention may be absent in a hypovolemic patient. Tracheal deviation is a late finding and often is not apparent on clinical examination. Practically, three findings are sufficient to make the diagnosis of tension pneumothorax: respiratory distress or hypotension, decreased lung sounds, and hypertympany to percussion. Chest x-ray findings that may be visualized include deviation of mediastinal structures, depression of the hemidiaphragm, and hypo-opacification with absent lung markings. As discussed above, definitive treatment of a tension pneumothorax is immediate tube thoracostomy. The chest tube should be inserted rapidly, but carefully, and should be large enough to evacuate any blood that may be present in the pleural space. Most recommend placement in the fourth intercostal space (nipple level) at the anterior axillary line.

Cardiac tamponade results from the accumulation of blood within the pericardial sac, usually from penetrating trauma or chronic medical conditions such as heart failure or uremia. Although precordial wounds are most likely to injure the heart and produce tamponade, any projectile or wounding agent that passes in proximity to the mediastinum can potentially produce tamponade. Blunt cardiac rupture, a rare event in trauma victims who survive long enough to reach the hospital, can produce refractory shock and tamponade in the multiply-injured patient. The manifestations of cardiac tamponade, such as total circulatory collapse and cardiac arrest, may be catastrophic, or they may be more subtle. A high index of suspicion is warranted to make a rapid diagnosis. Patients who present with circulatory arrest from cardiac tamponade require emergency pericardial decompression, usually through a left thoracotomy. The indications for this maneuver are discussed in Chap. 7. Cardiac tamponade also may be associated with dyspnea, orthopnea, cough, peripheral edema, chest pain, tachycardia, muffled heart tones, jugular venous distention, and elevated central venous pressure. Beck's triad consists of hypoten-

sion, muffled heart tones, and neck vein distention. Unfortunately, absence of these clinical findings may not be sufficient to exclude cardiac injury and cardiac tamponade. Muffled heart tones may be difficult to appreciate in a busy trauma center and jugular venous distention and central venous pressure may be diminished by coexistent bleeding. Therefore, patients at risk for cardiac tamponade whose hemodynamic status permits additional diagnostic tests frequently require additional diagnostic maneuvers to confirm cardiac injury or tamponade.

Invasive hemodynamic monitoring may support the diagnosis of cardiac tamponade if elevated central venous pressure, pulsus paradoxus (i.e., decreased systemic arterial pressure with inspiration), or elevated right atrial and right ventricular pressure by pulmonary artery catheter are present. These hemodynamic profiles suffer from lack of specificity, the duration of time required to obtain them in critically injured patients, and their inability to exclude cardiac injury in the absence of tamponade. Chest radiographs may provide information on the possible trajectory of a projectile, but rarely are diagnostic because the acutely filled pericardium distends poorly. Echocardiography has become the preferred test for the diagnosis of cardiac tamponade. Good results in detecting pericardial fluid have been reported, but the yield in detecting pericardial fluid depends on the skill and experience of the ultrasonographer, body habitus of the patient, and absence of wounds that preclude visualization of the pericardium. Standard two-dimensional or transesophageal echocardiography are sensitive techniques to evaluate the pericardium for fluid, and are typically performed by examiners skilled at evaluating ventricular function, valvular abnormalities, and integrity of the proximal thoracic aorta. Unfortunately, these skilled examiners are rarely immediately available at all hours of the night, when many trauma patients present; therefore, waiting for this test may result in inordinate delays. In addition, although both ultrasound techniques may demonstrate the presence of fluid or characteristic findings of tamponade (large volume of fluid, right atrial collapse, poor distensibility of the right ventricle), they do not exclude cardiac injury per se. Pericardiocentesis to diagnose pericardial blood and potentially relieve tamponade may be used. Performing pericardiocentesis under ultrasound guidance has made the procedure safer and more reliable. An indwelling catheter may be placed for several days in patients with chronic pericardial effusions. Needle pericardiocentesis may not evacuate clotted blood and has the potential to produce cardiac injury, making it a poor alternative in busy trauma centers.

Diagnostic pericardial window represents the most direct method to determine the presence of blood within the pericardium. The procedure is best performed in the operating room under general anesthesia. It can be performed through either the subxiphoid or transdiaphragmatic approach. Adequate equipment and personnel to rapidly decompress the pericardium, explore the injury, and repair the heart should be present. Once the pericardium is opened and tamponade relieved, hemodynamics usually improve dramatically and formal pericardial exploration can ensue. Exposure of the heart can be achieved by extending the incision to a median sternotomy, performing a left anterior thoracotomy, or performing bilateral anterior thoracotomies ("clamshell").

Neurogenic Shock

Neurogenic shock refers to diminished tissue perfusion as a result of loss of vasomotor tone to peripheral arterial beds. Loss of vasoconstrictor impulses results in increased vascular capacitance, decreased venous return, and decreased cardiac output. Neurogenic shock is usually secondary to spinal cord injuries from vertebral body fractures of the cervical or high thoracic region that disrupt sympathetic regulation of peripheral vascular tone (Table 5-9). Rarely, a spinal cord injury without bony fracture, such as an epidural hematoma impinging on the spinal cord, can produce neurogenic shock. Sympathetic input to the heart, which normally increases heart rate and cardiac contractility, and input to the adrenal medulla, which in-

TABLE 5-9	Causes of neurogenic shock

Spinal cord trauma
Spinal cord neoplasm
Spinal/epidural anesthetic

creases catecholamine release, may also be disrupted, preventing the typical reflex tachycardia that occurs with hypovolemia. Acute spinal cord injury results in activation of multiple secondary injury mechanisms: (a) vascular compromise to the spinal cord with loss of autoregulation, vasospasm, and thrombosis, (b) loss of cellular membrane integrity and impaired energy metabolism, and (c) neurotransmitter accumulation and release of free radicals. Importantly, hypotension contributes to the worsening of acute spinal cord injury as the result of further reduction in blood flow to the spinal cord. Management of acute spinal cord injury with attention to blood pressure control, oxygenation, and hemodynamics, essentially optimizing perfusion of an already ischemic spinal cord, seems to result in improved neurologic outcome. Patients with hypotension from spinal cord injury are best monitored in an ICU and carefully followed for evidence of cardiac or respiratory dysfunction.

Diagnosis

Acute spinal cord injury may result in bradycardia, hypotension, cardiac dysrhythmias, reduced cardiac output, and decreased peripheral vascular resistance. The severity of the spinal cord injury seems to correlate with the magnitude of cardiovascular dysfunction. Patients with complete motor injuries are over five times more likely to require vasopressors for neurogenic shock compared to those with incomplete lesions.[93] The classic description of neurogenic shock consists of decreased blood pressure associated with bradycardia (absence of reflexive tachycardia due to disrupted sympathetic discharge), warm extremities (loss of peripheral vasoconstriction), motor and sensory deficits indicative of a spinal cord injury, and radiographic evidence of a vertebral column fracture. Patients with multisystem trauma that includes spinal cord injuries often have head injuries that may make identification of motor and sensory deficits difficult in the initial evaluation. Furthermore, associated injuries may occur that result in hypovolemia, further complicating the clinical presentation. In a subset of patients with spinal cord injuries from penetrating wounds, most of the patients with hypotension had blood loss as the etiology (74%) rather than neurogenic causes, and few (7%) had the classic findings of neurogenic shock.[94] In the multiply injured patient, other causes of hypotension including hemorrhage, tension pneumothorax, and cardiogenic shock, must be sought and excluded.

Treatment

After the airway is secured and ventilation is adequate, fluid resuscitation and restoration of intravascular volume often will improve perfusion in neurogenic shock. Most patients with neurogenic shock will respond to restoration of intravascular volume alone, with satisfactory improvement in perfusion and resolution of hypotension. Administration of vasoconstrictors will improve peripheral vascular tone, decrease vascular capacitance, and increase venous return, but should only be considered once hypovolemia is excluded as the cause of the hypotension, and the diagnosis of neurogenic shock established. If the patient's blood pressure has not responded to what is felt to be adequate volume resuscitation, dopamine may be used first. A pure alpha agonist, such as phenylephrine, may be used primarily or in patients unresponsive to dopamine. Specific treatment for the hypotension is often of brief duration, as the need to administer vasoconstrictors typically lasts 24 to 48 hours. On the other hand, life-threatening cardiac dysrhythmias and hypotension may occur up to 14 days after spinal cord injury.

The duration of the need for vasopressor support for neurogenic shock may correlate with the overall prognosis or chances of improvement in neurologic function. Appropriate rapid restoration of blood pressure and circulatory perfusion may improve perfusion to the spinal cord, prevent progressive spinal cord ischemia, and minimize secondary cord injury. Restoration of normal blood pressure and adequate tissue perfusion should precede any operative attempts to stabilize the vertebral fracture.

ENDPOINTS IN RESUSCITATION

Shock is defined as inadequate perfusion to maintain normal organ function. With prolonged anaerobic metabolism, tissue acidosis and O_2 debt accumulate. Thus, the goal in the treatment of shock is restoration of adequate organ perfusion and tissue oxygenation. Resuscitation is complete when O_2 debt is repaid, tissue acidosis is corrected, and aerobic metabolism restored. Clinical confirmation of this endpoint remains a challenge.

Resuscitation of the patient in shock requires simultaneous evaluation and treatment; the etiology of the shock often is not initially apparent. Hemorrhagic shock, septic shock, and traumatic shock are the most common types of shock encountered on surgical services. To optimize outcome in bleeding patients, early control of the hemorrhage and adequate volume resuscitation, including both red blood cells and crystalloid solutions, are necessary. Expedient operative resuscitation is mandatory to limit the magnitude of activation of multiple mediator systems and to abort the microcirculatory changes, which may evolve insidiously into the cascade that ends in irreversible hemorrhagic shock. Attempts to stabilize an actively bleeding patient anywhere but in the operating room are inappropriate. Any intervention that delays the patient's arrival in the operating room for control of hemorrhage increases mortality, thus the important concept of *operating room resuscitation* of the critically injured patient.

Recognition by care providers of the patient who is in the compensated phase of shock is equally important, but more difficult based on clinical criteria. Compensated shock exists when inadequate tissue perfusion persists despite normalization of blood pressure and heart rate. Even with normalization of blood pressure, heart rate, and urine output, 80 to 85% of trauma patients have inadequate tissue perfusion, as evidenced by increased lactate or decreased mixed venous O_2 saturation.[56,95] Persistent, occult hypoperfusion is frequent in the ICU, with a resultant significant increase in infection rate and mortality in major trauma patients. Patients failing to reverse their lactic acidosis within 12 hours of admission (acidosis that was persistent despite normal heart rate, blood pressure, and urine output) developed an infection three times as often as those who normalized their lactate levels within 12 hours of admission. In addition, mortality was fourfold higher in patients who developed infections. Both injury severity score and occult hypotension (lactic acidosis) longer than 12 hours were independent predictors of infection.[96] Thus, recognition of subclinical hypoperfusion requires information beyond vital signs and urinary output.

Endpoints in resuscitation can be divided into *systemic* or *global parameters, tissue-specific parameters,* and *cellular parameters.* Global endpoints include vital signs, cardiac output, pulmonary artery wedge pressure, O_2 delivery and consumption, lactate, and base deficit (Table 5-10).

Assessment of Endpoints in Resuscitation

Oxygen Transport

Attaining supranormal O_2 transport variables has been proposed as a means to correct O_2 debt. Shoemaker and associates published the first randomized study examining supranormal O_2 consumption and delivery as endpoints in resuscitation.[97] The supranormal O_2 transport variables include O_2 delivery greater than 600 mL/min per square meter, cardiac index greater than 4.5 L/min per square meter, and O_2 consumption index greater than 170 mL/min per square meter. These authors reported a significant reduction in

TABLE 5-10	Endpoints in resuscitation

Systemic/global
  Lactate
  Base deficit
  Cardiac output
  Oxygen delivery and consumption
Tissue specific
  Gastric tonometry
  Tissue pH, oxygen, carbon dioxide levels
  Near infrared spectroscopy
Cellular
  Membrane potential
  Adenosine triphosphate

mortality in the patients achieving supranormal endpoints. More recent publications suggest that patients unable to increase O_2 delivery have a higher mortality, as opposed to it being a true benefit of the therapy.[98–100] This observation strongly correlates with age of the patient, with older patients less able to generate supranormal O_2 delivery. Gattinoni and colleagues reported effects of hemodynamic therapy in critically ill patients on 10,726 patients in 56 ICUs.[101] Seven hundred sixty-two patients met the predefined diagnostic categories and were assigned to one of three groups: control group, supranormal cardiac index group, and O_2 saturation group (with a goal of achieving normal venous O_2 saturation). The authors found that hemodynamic therapy aimed at reaching supranormal values for cardiac index or normal values for mixed venous O_2 saturation did not reduce morbidity or mortality among critically ill patients. In this paper's accompanying editorial, it was noted that failure to achieve both values is a relatively common problem, particularly among older or more severely ill patients. These results emphasize the importance of adequate volume replacement, maintenance of normal blood pressure, and the use of minor doses of inotropic drugs to maintain a normal cardiac output. In a recent paper from Shoemaker's group, supranormal values were achieved intentionally in 70% of the treatment group and spontaneously by 40% of the control group.[98] Mortality, incidence of organ failure and sepsis, and length of stay were no different between the treatment and control groups. Patients in each group who attained supranormal values had better outcomes than those who could not, and mortality was 30% in patients unable to reach supranormal values and 0% in patients with supranormal indices. Age younger than 40 years was the sole independent variable that predicted ability to reach these supraphysiologic endpoints. Thus, the evidence is insufficient to support the routine use of a strategy to maximize O_2 delivery in a group of unselected patients.

Inability to repay O_2 debt is a predictor of mortality and organ failure; the probability of death has been directly correlated to the calculated O_2 debt in hemorrhagic shock. Direct measurement of the O_2 debt in the resuscitation of patients is difficult. The easily obtainable parameters of arterial blood pressure, heart rate, urine output, central venous pressure, and pulmonary artery occlusion pressure are poor indicators of the adequacy of tissue perfusion. Therefore, surrogate parameters have been sought to estimate the O_2 debt; serum lactate and base deficit have been shown to correlate with O_2 debt.

Lactate

Lactate is generated by conversion of pyruvate to lactate by lactate dehydrogenase in the setting of insufficient O_2. Lactate is released into the circulation and is predominantly taken up and metabolized by the liver and kidneys. The liver accounts for approximately 50% and the kidney for about 30% of whole body lactate uptake. Elevated serum lactate is an indirect measure of the O_2 debt, and therefore an approximation of the magnitude and duration of the severity of shock. The admission lactate level, highest lactate level, and time interval to normalize the serum lactate are important prognostic indicators for survival. For example, in a study of 76 consecutive patients, 100% survival was observed among the patients with normalization of lactate within 24 hours, 78% survival when lactate normalized between 24 and 48 hours, and only 14% survivorship if it took longer than 48 hours to normalize the serum lactate.[56] In contrast, individual variability of lactate may be too great to permit accurate prediction of outcome in any individual case. Base deficit and volume of blood transfusion required in the first 24 hours of resuscitation may be better predictors of mortality than the plasma lactate alone.

Base Deficit

Base deficit is the amount of base in millimoles that is required to titrate 1 L of whole blood to a pH of 7.40 with the sample fully saturated with O_2 at 37°C (98.6°F) and a partial pressure of CO_2 of 40 mmHg. It usually is measured by arterial blood gas analysis in clinical practice as it is readily and quickly available. The mortality of trauma patients can be stratified according to the magnitude of base deficit measured in the first 24 hours after admission.[60] In a retrospective study of over 3000 trauma admissions, patients with a base deficit worse than 15 mmol/L had a mortality of 70%. Base deficit can be stratified into mild (3 to 5 mmol/L), moderate (6 to 14 mmol/L), and severe (15 mmol/L) categories, with a trend toward higher mortality with worsening base deficit in patients with trauma. Both the magnitude of the perfusion deficit as indicated by the base deficit and the time required to correct it are major factors determining outcome in shock.

Indeed, when elevated base deficit persists (or lactic acidosis) in the trauma patient, ongoing bleeding is often the etiology. Trauma patients admitted with a base deficit greater than 15 mmol/L required twice the volume of fluid infusion and six times more blood transfusion in the first 24 hours compared to patients with mild acidosis. Transfusion requirements increased as base deficit worsened and ICU and hospital lengths of stay increased. Mortality increased as base deficit worsened; the frequency of organ failure increased with greater base deficit.[57] The probability of trauma patients developing ARDS has been reported to correlate with severity of admission base deficit and lowest base deficit within the first 24 hours postinjury.[59] Persistently high base deficit is associated with abnormal O_2 utilization and higher mortality. Monitoring base deficit in the resuscitation of trauma patients assists in assessment of O_2 transport and efficacy of resuscitation.[58]

Factors that may compromise the utility of the base deficit in estimating O_2 debt are the administration of bicarbonate, hypothermia, hypocapnia (overventilation), heparin, ethanol, and ketoacidosis. However, the base deficit remains one of the most widely used estimates of O_2 debt for its clinical relevance, accuracy, and availability.

Gastric Tonometry

Lactate and base deficit indicate global tissue acidosis. Several authors have suggested that tissue-specific endpoints, rather than systemic endpoints, are more predictive of outcome and adequate resuscitation in trauma patients. With heterogeneity of blood flow, regional tissue beds may be hypoperfused. Gastric tonometry has been used to assess perfusion of the GI tract. The concentration of CO_2 accumulating in the gastric mucosa can be sampled with a specially designed nasogastric tube. With the assumption that gastric bicarbonate is equal to serum levels, gastric intramucosal pH (pHi) is calculated by applying the Henderson-Hasselbalch equation. pHi should be greater than 7.3; pHi will be lower in the setting of decreased O_2 delivery to the tissues. pHi is a good prognostic indicator; patients with normal pHi have better outcomes than those patients with pHi less than 7.3.[102–104] Goal-directed human studies, with pHi as an endpoint in resuscitation, have shown normalization of pHi to correlate with improved outcome in several studies, and with contradictory findings in other studies. Use of pHi as a singular endpoint in the resuscitation of critically ill patients remains controversial.[105]

Near Infrared Spectroscopy

Near infrared (NIR) spectroscopy can measure tissue oxygenation and redox state of cytochrome a,a_3 on a continuous, noninvasive basis. The NIR probe emits multiple wavelengths of light in the NIR spectrum (650 to 1100 nm). Photons are then either absorbed by the tissue or reflected back to the probe. Maximal exercise in laboratory studies resulted in reduction of cytochrome a,a_3; this correlated with tissue lactate elevation. NIR spectroscopy can be used to compare tissue oxyhemoglobin levels (indicating tissue O_2 supply to cytochrome a,a_3 with mitochondrial O_2 consumption), thus demonstrating flow-independent mitochondrial oxidative dysfunction and the need for further resuscitation. Trauma patients with decoupled oxyhemoglobin and cytochrome a,a_3 have redox dysfunction and have been shown to have a higher incidence of organ failure (89 vs. 13%).[106,107]

Tissue PH, Oxygen, and Carbon Dioxide Concentration

Tissue probes with optical sensors have been used to measure tissue pH and partial pressure of O_2 and CO_2 in subcutaneous sites, muscle, and the bladder. These probes may use transcutaneous methodology with Clark electrodes or direct percutaneous probes.[108,109] The percutaneous probes can be inserted through an 18-gauge catheter and hold promise as continuous monitors of tissue perfusion.

Right Ventricular End-Diastolic Volume Index

Right ventricular end-diastolic volume index (RVEDVI) seems to more accurately predict preload for cardiac index than does pulmonary artery wedge pressure.[110] Chang and colleagues reported that 50% of trauma patients had persistent splanchnic ischemia that was reversed by increasing RVEDVI. RVEDVI is a parameter that seems to correlate with preload-related increases in cardiac output. More recently, these authors have described left ventricular power output as an endpoint (LVP >320 mmHg·L/min per square meter), which is associated with improved clearance of base deficit and a lower rate of organ dysfunction following injury.[111]

REFERENCES

Entries highlighted in bright blue are key references.

1. Gross S: *A System of Surgery: Pathologic, Diagnostic, Therapeutic and Operative.* Philadelphia: Lea and Febiger, 1872.
2. Bernard C: *Lecons sur les Phenomenes de la Vie Communs aux Animaux et aux Vegetaux.* Paris: JB Ballieve, 1879.
3. Cannon W: *Traumatic Shock.* New York: D. Appleton and Co, 1923.
4. Blalock A: *Principles of Surgical Care, Shock and Other Problems.* St. Louis: CV Mosby, 1940.
5. Mollen KP, Levy RM, Prince JM, et al: Systemic inflammation and end organ damage following trauma involves functional TLR4 signaling in both bone marrow-derived cells and parenchymal cells. *J Leukoc Biol* 83:80, 2008.
6. Wiggers C: *Experimental Hemorrhagic Shock. Physiology of Shock.* New York: Commonwealth, 1950.
7. Carrico CJ, Canizaro PC, Shires GT: Fluid resuscitation following injury: Rationale for the use of balanced salt solutions. *Crit Care Med* 4:46, 1976.
8. Peitzman AB, Corbett WA, Shires GT 3rd, et al: Cellular function in liver and muscle during hemorrhagic shock in primates. *Surg Gynecol Obstet* 16:419, 1985.
9. Shaftan GW, Chiu CJ, Dennis C, et al: Fundamentals of physiologic control of arterial hemorrhage. *Surgery* 58:851, 1965.
10. Shah NS, Kelly E, Billiar TR, et al: Utility of clinical parameters of tissue oxygenation in a quantitative model of irreversible hemorrhagic shock. *Shock* 10:343, 1998.
11. Dunser MW, Wenzel V, Mayr AJ, et al: Management of vasodilatory shock: Defining the role of arginine vasopressin. *Drugs* 63:237, 2003.
12. Argenziano M, Chen JM, Choudhri AF, et al: Management of vasodilatory shock after cardiac surgery: Identification of predisposing factors and use of a novel pressor agent. *J Thorac Cardiovasc Surg* 116:973, 1998.
13. Barroso-Aranda J, Schmid-Schonbein GW, Zweifach BW, et al: Granulocytes and no-reflow phenomenon in irreversible hemorrhagic shock. *Circ Res* 63:437, 1988.
14. Ince C, Sinaasappel M: Microcirculatory oxygenation and shunting in sepsis and shock. *Crit Care Med* 27:1369, 1999.
15. Singer M, De Santis V, Vitale D, et al: Multiorgan failure is an adaptive, endocrine-mediated, metabolic response to overwhelming systemic inflammation. *Lancet* 364:545, 2004.
16. Shires T, Coln D, Carrico J, et al: Fluid therapy in hemorrhagic shock. *Arch Surg* 88:688, 1964.
17. Robin ED: Of men and mitochondria: Coping with hypoxic dysoxia. The 1980 J. Burns Amberson Lecture. *Am Rev Respir Dis* 122:517, 1980.
18. Stacpoole PW: Lactic acidosis and other mitochondrial disorders. *Metabolism* 46:306, 1997.
19. Crowell JW, Smith EE: Oxygen deficit and irreversible hemorrhagic shock. *Am J Physiol* 206:313, 1964.
20. Nathan C: Points of control in inflammation. *Nature* 420:846, 2002.
21. Sauaia A, Moore FA, Moore EE, et al: Early predictors of postinjury multiple organ failure. *Arch Surg* 129:39, 1994.
22. Matzinger P: The danger model: A renewed sense of self. *Science* 296:301, 2002.
23. Jiang J, Bahrami S, Leichtfried G, et al: Kinetics of endotoxin and tumor necrosis factor appearance in portal and systemic circulation after hemorrhagic shock in rats. *Ann Surg* 221:100, 1995.
24. Endo S, Inada K, Yamada Y, et al: Plasma endotoxin and cytokine concentrations in patients with hemorrhagic shock. *Crit Care Med* 22:949, 1994.
25. Puyana JC, Pellegrini JD, De AK, et al: Both T-helper-1- and T-helper-2-type lymphokines are depressed in posttrauma anergy. *J Trauma* 44:1037; discussion 1045, 1998.
26. Faist E, Schinkel C, Zimmer S, et al: Inadequate interleukin-2 synthesis and interleukin-2 messenger expression following thermal and mechanical trauma in humans is caused by defective transmembrane signalling. *J Trauma* 34:846; discussion 853, 1993.
27. Meng ZH, Dyer K, Billiar TR, et al: Essential role for IL-6 in postresuscitation inflammation in hemorrhagic shock. *Am J Physiol Cell Physiol* 280:C343, 2001.
28. Meng ZH, Dyer K, Billiar TR, et al: Distinct effects of systemic infusion of G-CSF vs. IL-6 on lung and liver inflammation and injury in hemorrhagic shock. *Shock* 14:41, 2000.
29. Neidhardt R, Keel M, Steckholzer U, et al: Relationship of interleukin-10 plasma levels to severity of injury and clinical outcome in injured patients. *J Trauma* 42:863; discussion 870, 1997.
30. Kasai T, Inada K, Takakuwa T, et al: Anti-inflammatory cytokine levels in patients with septic shock. *Res Commun Mol Pathol Pharmacol* 98:34, 1997.
31. Kahlke V, Dohm C, Mees T, et al: Early interleukin-10 treatment improves survival and enhances immune function only in males after hemorrhage and subsequent sepsis. *Shock* 18:24, 2002.
32. Karakozis S, Hinds M, Cook JW, et al: The effects of interleukin-10 in hemorrhagic shock. *J Surg Res* 90:109, 2000.
33. Younger JG, Sasaki N, Waite MD, et al: Detrimental effects of complement activation in hemorrhagic shock. *J Appl Physiol* 90:441, 2001.
34. Moore EE, Moore FA, Franciose RJ, et al: The postischemic gut serves as a priming bed for circulating neutrophils that provoke multiple organ failure. *J Trauma* 37:881, 1994.
35. Adams JM, Hauser CJ, Livingston DH, et al: Early trauma polymorphonuclear neutrophil responses to chemokines are associated with development of sepsis, pneumonia, and organ failure. *J Trauma* 51:452; discussion 456, 2001.
36. Lau YT, Hwang TL, Chen MF, et al: Calcium transport by rat liver plasma membranes during sepsis. *Circ Shock* 38:238, 1992.
37. Herman B, Gores GJ, Nieminen AL, et al: Calcium and pH in anoxic and toxic injury. *Crit Rev Toxicol* 21:127, 1990.
38. Somogyi R, Zhao M, Stucki JW: Modulation of cytosolic-[Ca2+] oscillations in hepatocytes results from cross-talk among second messengers. The synergism between the alpha 1-adrenergic response, glucagon and cyclic AMP, and their antagonism by insulin and diacylglycerol manifest themselves in the control of the cytosolic-[Ca2+] oscillations. *Biochem J* 286(Pt. 3):869, 1992.
39. Maki A, Berezesky IK, Fargnoli J, et al: Role of [Ca2+]i in induction of c-fos, c-jun, and c-myc mRNA in rat PTE after oxidative stress. *FASEB J* 6:919, 1992.
40. Trump BF, Berezesky IK: Calcium-mediated cell injury and cell death. *FASEB J* 9:219, 1995.

41. Khadaroo RG, Kapus A, Powers KA, et al: Oxidative stress reprograms lipopolysaccharide signaling via Src kinase-dependent pathway in RAW 264.7 macrophage cell line. *J Biol Chem* 278:47834, 2003.

42. Powers KA, Szaszi K, Khadaroo RG, et al: Oxidative stress generated by hemorrhagic shock recruits Toll-like receptor 4 to the plasma membrane in macrophages. *J Exp Med* 203:1951, 2006.

43. Suzuki YJ, Forman HJ, Sevanian A: Oxidants as stimulators of signal transduction. *Free Radic Biol Med* 22:269, 1997.

44. Mollen KP, McCloskey CA, Tanaka H, et al: Hypoxia activates c-Jun N-terminal kinase via Rac1-dependent reactive oxygen species production in hepatocytes. *Shock* 28:270, 2007.

45. Bertges DJ, Fink MP, Delude RL: Hypoxic signal transduction in critical illness. *Crit Care Med* 28(4 Suppl):N78, 2000.

46. Guillemin K, Krasnow MA: The hypoxic response: Huffing and HIF-ing. *Cell* 89:9, 1997.

47. Buchman TG, Cabin DE, Vickers S, et al: Molecular biology of circulatory shock. Part II. Expression of four groups of hepatic genes is enhanced after resuscitation from cardiogenic shock. *Surgery* 108:559, 1990.

48. Cobb JP, Laramie JM, Stormo GD, et al: Sepsis gene expression profiling: Murine splenic compared with hepatic responses determined by using complementary DNA microarrays. *Crit Care Med* 30:2711, 2002.

49. Cobb JP, O'Keefe GE: Injury research in the genomic era. *Lancet* 363:2076, 2004.

50. Wiegand G, Selleng K, Grundling M, et al: Gene expression pattern in human monocytes as a surrogate marker for systemic inflammatory response syndrome (SIRS). *Mol Med* 5:192, 1999.

51. Gray IC, Campbell DA, Spurr NK: Single nucleotide polymorphisms as tools in human genetics. *Hum Mol Genet* 9:2403, 2000.

52. Mira JP, Cariou A, Grall F, et al: Association of TNF2, a TNF-alpha promoter polymorphism, with septic shock susceptibility and mortality: A multicenter study. *JAMA* 282:561, 1999.

53. Eastridge BJ, Salinas J, McManus JG, et al: Hypotension begins at 110 mm Hg: Redefining "hypotension" with data. *J Trauma* 63:291; discussion 297, 2007.

54. Luna GK, Eddy AC, Copass M: The sensitivity of vital signs in identifying major thoracoabdominal hemorrhage. *Am J Surg* 157:512, 1989.

55. Victorino GP, Battistella FD, Wisner DH: Does tachycardia correlate with hypotension after trauma? *J Am Coll Surg* 196:679, 2003.

56. Abramson D, Scalea TM, Hitchcock R, et al: Lactate clearance and survival following injury. *J Trauma* 35:584; discussion 588, 1993.

57. Davis JW, Parks SN, Kaups KL, et al: Admission base deficit predicts transfusion requirements and risk of complications. *J Trauma* 41:769, 1996.

58. Kincaid EH, Miller PR, Meredith JW, et al: Elevated arterial base deficit in trauma patients: A marker of impaired oxygen utilization. *J Am Coll Surg* 187:384, 1998.

59. Rixen D, Raum M, Bouillon B, et al: Base deficit development and its prognostic significance in posttrauma critical illness: An analysis by the trauma registry of the Deutsche Gesellschaft fur unfallchirurgie. *Shock* 15:83, 2001.

60. Rutherford EJ, Morris JA Jr., Reed GW, et al: Base deficit stratifies mortality and determines therapy. *J Trauma* 33:417, 1992.

61. Clarke JR, Trooskin SZ, Doshi PJ, et al: Time to laparotomy for intra-abdominal bleeding from trauma does affect survival for delays up to 90 minutes. *J Trauma* 52:420, 2002.

62. Holcomb JB: Damage control resuscitation. *J Trauma* 62(6 Suppl):S36, 2007.

63. Marshall HP Jr., Capone A, Courcoulas AP, et al: Effects of hemodilution on long-term survival in an uncontrolled hemorrhagic shock model in rats. *J Trauma* 43:673, 1997.

64. Bickell WH, Wall MJ Jr., Pepe PE, et al: Immediate versus delayed fluid resuscitation for hypotensive patients with penetrating torso injuries. *N Engl J Med* 331:1105, 1994.

65. Human albumin administration in critically ill patients: Systematic review of randomised controlled trials. Cochrane Injuries Group Albumin Reviewers. *BMJ* 317:235, 1998.

66. Mann DV, Robinson MK, Rounds JD, et al: Superiority of blood over saline resuscitation from hemorrhagic shock: A 31P magnetic resonance spectroscopy study. *Ann Surg* 226:653, 1997.

67. Vassar MJ, Fischer RP, O'Brien PE, et al: A multicenter trial for resuscitation of injured patients with 7.5% sodium chloride. The effect of added dextran 70. The Multicenter Group for the Study of Hypertonic Saline in Trauma Patients. *Arch Surg* 128:1003; discussion 1011, 1993.

68. Hebert PC, Wells G, Blajchman MA, et al: A multicenter, randomized, controlled clinical trial of transfusion requirements in critical care. Transfusion Requirements in Critical Care Investigators, Canadian Critical Care Trials Group. *N Engl J Med* 34:409, 1999.

69. Hebert PC, Yetisir E, Martin C, et al: Is a low transfusion threshold safe in critically ill patients with cardiovascular diseases? *Crit Care Med* 29:227, 2001.

70. Gonzalez EA, Moore FA, Holcomb JB, et al: Fresh frozen plasma should be given earlier to patients requiring massive transfusion. *J Trauma* 62:112, 2007.

71. Borgman MA, Spinella PC, Perkins JG, et al: The ratio of blood products transfused affects mortality in patients receiving massive transfusions at a combat support hospital. *J Trauma* 63:805, 2007.

72. Roumen RM, Redl H, Schlag G, et al: Inflammatory mediators in relation to the development of multiple organ failure in patients after severe blunt trauma. *Crit Care Med* 23:474, 1995.

73. Leone M, Boutiere B, Camoin-Jau L, et al: Systemic endothelial activation is greater in septic than in traumatic-hemorrhagic shock but does not correlate with endothelial activation in skin biopsies. *Crit Care Med* 30:808, 2002.

74. Mollen KP, Anand RJ, Tsung A, et al: Emerging paradigm: Toll-like receptor 4-sentinel for the detection of tissue damage. *Shock* 26:430, 2006.

75. Landry DW, Oliver JA: The pathogenesis of vasodilatory shock. *N Engl J Med* 345:588, 2001.

76. Angus DC, Linde-Zwirble WT, Lidicker J, et al: Epidemiology of severe sepsis in the United States: Analysis of incidence, outcome, and associated costs of care. *Crit Care Med* 29:1303, 2001.

77. Linde-Zwirble WT, Angus DC: Severe sepsis epidemiology: Sampling, selection, and society. *Crit Care* 8:222, 2004.

78. Dellinger RP, Levy MM, Carlet JM, et al: Surviving Sepsis Campaign: International guidelines for management of severe sepsis and septic shock. *Crit Care Med* 36:296, 2008.

79. Cinel I, Dellinger RP: Advances in pathogenesis and management of sepsis. *Curr Opin Infect Dis* 20:345, 2007.

80. Rivers E, Nguyen B, Havstad S, et al: Early goal-directed therapy in the treatment of severe sepsis and septic shock. *N Engl J Med* 345:1368, 2001.

81. van den Berghe G, Wouters P, Weekers F, et al: Intensive insulin therapy in the critically ill patients. *N Engl J Med* 345:1359, 2001.

82. Ventilation with lower tidal volumes as compared with traditional tidal volumes for acute lung injury and the acute respiratory distress syndrome. The Acute Respiratory Distress Syndrome Network. *N Engl J Med* 342:1301, 2000.

83. Bernard GR, Vincent JL, Laterre PF, et al: Efficacy and safety of recombinant human activated protein C for severe sepsis. *N Engl J Med* 344:699, 2001.

84. Annane D, Sebille V, Charpentier C, et al: Effect of treatment with low doses of hydrocortisone and fludrocortisone on mortality in patients with septic shock. *JAMA* 288:862, 2002.

85. Sprung CL, Annane D, Keh D, et al: Hydrocortisone therapy for patients with septic shock. *N Engl J Med* 358:111, 2008.

86. Hollenberg SM, Kavinsky CJ, Parrillo JE: Cardiogenic shock. *Ann Intern Med* 131:47, 1999.

87. Webb JG, Lowe AM, Sanborn TA, et al: Percutaneous coronary intervention for cardiogenic shock in the SHOCK trial. *J Am Coll Cardiol* 42:1380, 2003.

88. Aji J, Hollenberg S: Cardiogenic shock: Giving the heart a break. *Crit Care Med* 34:1248, 2006.

89. Alonso DR, Scheidt S, Post M, et al: Pathophysiology of cardiogenic shock. Quantification of myocardial necrosis, clinical, pathologic and electrocardiographic correlations. *Circulation* 48:588, 1973.

90. Goldstein DJ, Oz MC: Mechanical support for postcardiotomy cardiogenic shock. *Semin Thorac Cardiovasc Surg* 12:220, 2000.

91. Gibbons RJ, Smith SC Jr., Antman E: American College of Cardiology/American Heart Association clinical practice guidelines: Part II: Evolutionary changes in a continuous quality improvement project. *Circulation* 107:3101, 2003.

92. Menon V, Hochman JS: Management of cardiogenic shock complicating acute myocardial infarction. *Heart* 88:531, 2002.

93. Levi L, Wolf A, Belzberg H: Hemodynamic parameters in patients with acute cervical cord trauma: Description, intervention, and prediction of outcome. *Neurosurgery* 33:1007; discussion 1016, 1993.

94. Zipnick RI, Scalea TM, Trooskin SZ, et al: Hemodynamic responses to penetrating spinal cord injuries. *J Trauma* 35:578; discussion 582, 1993.

95. Abou-Khalil B, Scalea TM, Trooskin SZ, et al: Hemodynamic responses to shock in young trauma patients: Need for invasive monitoring. *Crit Care Med* 22:633, 1994.

96. Claridge JA, Crabtree TD, Pelletier SJ, et al: Persistent occult hypoperfusion is associated with a significant increase in infection rate and mortality in major trauma patients. *J Trauma* 48:8; discussion 14, 2000.

97. Shoemaker WC, Appel PL, Kram HB, et al: Prospective trial of supranormal values of survivors as therapeutic goals in high-risk surgical patients. *Chest* 94:1176, 1988.

98. Velmahos GC, Demetriades D, Shoemaker WC, et al: Endpoints of resuscitation of critically injured patients: Normal or supranormal? A prospective randomized trial. *Ann Surg* 232:409, 2000.

99. Heyland DK, Cook DJ, King D, et al: Maximizing oxygen delivery in critically ill patients: A methodologic appraisal of the evidence. *Crit Care Med* 24:517, 1996.

100. McKinley BA, Kozar RA, Cocanour CS, et al: Normal versus supranormal oxygen delivery goals in shock resuscitation: The response is the same. *J Trauma* 53:825, 2002.

101. Gattinoni L, Brazzi L, Pelosi P, et al: A trial of goal-oriented hemodynamic therapy in critically ill patients. SvO2 Collaborative Group. *N Engl J Med* 333:1025, 1995.

102. Chang MC, Cheatham ML, Nelson LD, et al: Gastric tonometry supplements information provided by systemic indicators of oxygen transport. *J Trauma* 37:488, 1994.

103. Ivatury RR, Simon RJ, Havriliak D, et al: Gastric mucosal pH and oxygen delivery and oxygen consumption indices in the assessment of adequacy of resuscitation after trauma: A prospective, randomized study. *J Trauma* 39:128; discussion 134, 1995.

104. Maynard N, Beale R, Smithies M, et al: Gastric intramucosal pH in critically ill patients. *Lancet* 339:550, 1992.

105. Gomersall CD, Joynt GM, Freebairn RC, et al: Resuscitation of critically ill patients based on the results of gastric tonometry: A prospective, randomized, controlled trial. *Crit Care Med* 28:607, 2000.

106. Cairns CB, Moore FA, Haenel JB, et al: Evidence for early supply independent mitochondrial dysfunction in patients developing multiple organ failure after trauma. *J Trauma* 42:532, 1997.

107. Cohn SM, Crookes BA, Proctor KG: Near-infrared spectroscopy in resuscitation. *J Trauma* 54(5 Suppl):S199, 2003.

108. Knudson MM, Bermudez KM, Doyle CA, et al: Use of tissue oxygen tension measurements during resuscitation from hemorrhagic shock. *J Trauma* 42:608; discussion 614, 1997.

109. McKinley BA, Marvin RG, Cocanour CS, et al: Tissue hemoglobin O2 saturation during resuscitation of traumatic shock monitored using near infrared spectrometry. *J Trauma* 48:637, 2000.

110. Cheatham ML, Nelson LD, Chang MC, et al: Right ventricular end-diastolic volume index as a predictor of preload status in patients on positive end-expiratory pressure. *Crit Care Med* 26:1801, 1998.

111. Chang MC, Meredith JW, Kincaid EH, et al: Maintaining survivors' values of left ventricular power output during shock resuscitation: A prospective pilot study. *J Trauma* 49:26; discussion 34, 2000.

CHAPTER 6

Surgical Infections

Greg J. Beilman and David L. Dunn

HISTORICAL BACKGROUND

Although treatment of infection has been an integral part of the surgeon's practice since the dawn of time, the body of knowledge that led to the present field of surgical infectious disease was derived from the evolution of germ theory and antisepsis. Application of the latter to clinical practice, concurrent with the development of anesthesia, was pivotal in allowing surgeons to expand their repertoire to encompass complex procedures that previously were associated with extremely high rates of morbidity and mortality due to postoperative infections. However, until recently, the occurrence of infection related to the surgical wound was the rule rather than the exception. In fact, the development of modalities to effectively prevent and treat infection has occurred only within the last several decades.

A number of observations by nineteenth-century physicians and investigators were critical to our current understanding of the pathogenesis, prevention, and treatment of surgical infections. In 1846, Ignaz Semmelweis, a Magyar physician, took a post at the Allgemein Krankenhaus in Vienna. He noticed that the mortality from puerperal ("childbed") fever was much higher in the teaching ward (1:11) than in the ward where patients were delivered by midwives (1:29). He also made the interesting observation that women who delivered before arrival on the teaching ward had a negligible mortality rate. The tragic death of a colleague due to overwhelming infection after a knife scratch received during an autopsy of a woman who had died of puerperal fever led Semmelweis to observe that pathologic changes in his friend were identical to those of women dying from this postpartum disease. He then hypothesized that puerperal fever was caused by putrid material transmitted from patients dying of this disease by carriage on the examining fingers of the medical students and physicians who frequently went from the autopsy room to the wards. The low mortality noted in the midwives' ward, Semmelweis realized, was due to the fact that midwives did not participate in autopsies. Fired with the zeal of his revelation, he posted a notice on the door to the ward requiring all caregivers to rinse their hands thoroughly in chlorine water before entering the area. This simple intervention reduced mortality from puerperal fever to 1.5%, surpassing the record of the midwives. In 1861, he published his classic work on childbed fever based on records from his practice. Unfortunately, Semmelweis' ideas were not well accepted by the authorities of the time.[1] Despondent, he committed suicide in 1865 by intentionally cutting his finger during the autopsy of a woman who died of puerperal fever, presumably as the ultimate proof of his tenets.

Louis Pasteur performed a body of work during the latter part of the nineteenth century that provided the underpinnings of modern microbiology, at the time known as *germ theory*. His work in humans followed experiments identifying infectious agents in silkworms. He was able to elucidate the principle that contagious diseases are caused by specific microbes and that these microbes are foreign to the infected organism. Using this principle, he developed techniques of sterilization critical to oenology and identified several bacteria responsible for human illnesses, including *Staphylococcus*, *Streptococcus*, and pneumococcus.

Joseph Lister, the son of a wine merchant, was appointed professor of surgery at the Glasgow Royal Infirmary in 1859. In his early practice, he noted that more than 50% of his patients undergoing amputation died due to postoperative infection. After hearing of Pasteur's theory, Lister experimented with the use of a solution of carbolic acid, which he knew was being used to treat sewage. He first reported his findings to the British Medical Association in 1867 using dressings saturated with carbolic acid on 12 patients with compound fractures; 10 recovered without amputation, one survived with amputation, and one died of causes unrelated to the wound. In spite of initial resistance, his methods were quickly adopted throughout Europe.

From 1878 until 1880, Robert Koch was the District Medical Officer for Wollstein (then Prussia, now a part of Poland), which was an area in which anthrax was endemic. Performing experiments in his home, without the benefit of scientific equipment and academic contact, Koch developed techniques for culture of *Bacillus anthracis* and proved the ability of this organism to cause anthrax in healthy animals. He developed the following four postulates to identify the association of organisms with specific diseases: (a) the suspected pathogenic organism should be present in all cases of the disease and absent from healthy animals, (b) the suspected pathogen should be isolated from a diseased host and grown in a pure culture in vitro,

(c) cells from a pure culture of the suspected organism should cause disease in a healthy animal, and (d) the organism should be reisolated from the newly diseased animal and shown to be the same as the original. He used these same techniques to identify the organisms responsible for cholera and tuberculosis. During the next century, *Koch's postulates*, as they came to be called, became critical to our understanding of surgical infections and remain so today.[2]

The first intra-abdominal operation to treat infection via "source control" (i.e., surgical intervention to eliminate the source of infection) was appendectomy. This operation was pioneered by Charles McBurney at the New York College of Physicians and Surgeons, among others.[3] McBurney's classic report on early operative intervention for appendicitis was presented before the New York Surgical Society in 1889. Appendectomy for the treatment of appendicitis, previously an often fatal disease, was popularized after the 1902 coronation of King Edward VII of England was delayed due to his need for an appendectomy, which was performed by Sir Frederick Treves. The king desperately needed an appendectomy but strongly opposed going into the hospital, protesting, "I have a coronation on hand." However, Treves was adamant, stating, "It will be a funeral, if you don't have the operation." Treves carried the debate, and the king lived.

During the twentieth century, the discovery of effective antimicrobials added another tool to the armamentarium of modern surgeons. Sir Alexander Fleming, after serving in the British Army Medical Corps during World War I, continued work on the natural antibacterial action of the blood and antiseptics. In 1928, while studying influenza virus, he noted a zone of inhibition around a mold colony (*Penicillium notatum*) that serendipitously grew on a plate of *Staphylococcus*, and he named the active substance *penicillin*. This first effective antibacterial agent subsequently led to the

KEY POINTS

1. The incidence of surgical site infections can be reduced by appropriate patient preparation, timely perioperative antibiotic administration, maintenance of perioperative normothermia and normoglycemia, and appropriate wound management.

2. Principles relevant to appropriate antibiotic prophylaxis for surgery: (a) select an agent with activity against common organisms at the site of surgery, (b) the initial dose of the antibiotic should be given within 30 minutes of incision, (c) antibiotics should be redosed every 1 to 2 half-lives during surgery to ensure adequate tissue levels, and (d) antibiotics should not be continued for more than 24 hours after surgery for routine prophylaxis.

3. Source control is a key concept in the treatment of most surgically relevant infections. Infected or necrotic material must be drained or removed as part of the treatment plan in this setting. Delays in adequate source control are associated with worsened outcomes.

4. Sepsis is both the presence of infection and the host response to infection (systemic inflammatory response syndrome, SIRS). Sepsis is a clinical spectrum, ranging from sepsis (SIRS plus infection) to severe sepsis (organ dysfunction), to septic shock (hypotension requiring vasopressors). Outcomes in patients with sepsis are improved with an organized

approach to therapy that includes rapid resuscitation, antibiotics, and source control.

5. When using antimicrobial agents for therapy of serious infection, several principles should be followed: (a) identify likely sources of infection, (b) choose an agent (or agents) that covers likely organisms for these sources, (c) remember that inadequate or delayed antibiotic therapy results in increased mortality, so it is important to begin therapy with broader coverage, (d) when possible, obtain cultures early and use results to tailor therapy, (e) if there is no infection identified after 3 days, strongly consider discontinuation of antibiotics, and (f) stop antibiotics after an appropriate course of therapy.

6. The keys to good outcomes in patients with necrotizing soft tissue infection are early recognition and appropriate débridement of infected tissue with repeated débridement until no further signs of infection are present.

7. Transmission of HIV and other infections spread by blood and body fluid from patient to health care worker can be minimized by observation of universal precautions, which include routine use of barriers when anticipating contact with blood or body fluids, washing of hands and other skin surfaces immediately after contact with blood or body fluids, and careful handling and disposal of sharp instruments during and after use.

development of hundreds of potent antimicrobials, set the stage for their use as prophylaxis against postoperative infection, and became a critical component of the armamentarium to treat aggressive, lethal surgical infections.

Concurrent with the development of numerous antimicrobial agents were advances in the field of clinical microbiology. Many new microbes were identified, including numerous anaerobes; the autochthonous microflora of the skin, GI tract, and other parts of the body that the surgeon encountered in the process of an operation were characterized in great detail. However, it remained unclear whether these organisms, anaerobes in particular, were commensals or pathogens. Subsequently, the initial clinical observations of surgeons such as Frank Meleney, William Altemeier, and others provided the key, when they observed that aerobes and anaerobes could synergize to cause serious soft tissue and severe intra-abdominal infection.[4,5] Thus, the concepts that resident microbes were non-pathogenic until they entered a sterile body cavity at the time of surgery, and that many, if not most, surgical infections were polymicrobial in nature, became critical ideas and were promulgated by a number of clinician-scientists over the last several decades.[6,7] These tenets became firmly established after microbiology laboratories demonstrated the invariable presence of aerobes and anaerobes in peritoneal cultures obtained at the time of surgery for intra-abdominal infection due to a perforated viscus or gangrenous appendicitis. Clinical trials provided evidence that optimal therapy for these infections required effective source control, plus the administration of antimicrobial agents directed against both types of pathogens.

William Osler, a prolific writer and one of the fathers of American medicine, made an observation in 1904 in his treatise *The Evolution of Modern Medicine* that was to have profound implications for the future of treatment of infection: "Except on few occasions, the patient appears to die from the body's response to infection rather than from it."[8] The discovery of the first cytokines began to allow insight into the organism's response to infection, and led to an explosion in our understanding of the host inflammatory response. Expanding knowledge of the multiple pathways activated during the response to invasion by infectious organisms has permitted the design of new therapies targeted at modifying the inflammatory response to infection, which seems to cause much of the end-organ dysfunction and failure. Preventing and treating this process of multiple organ failure during infection is one of the major challenges of modern critical care and surgical infectious disease.

PATHOGENESIS OF INFECTION

Host Defenses

The mammalian host possesses several layers of endogenous defense mechanisms that serve to prevent microbial invasion, limit proliferation of microbes within the host, and contain or eradicate invading microbes. These defenses are integrated and redundant so that the various components function as a complex, highly regulated system that is extremely effective in coping with microbial invaders. They include site-specific defenses that function at the tissue level, as well as components that freely circulate throughout the body in both blood and lymph. Systemic host defenses invariably are recruited to a site of infection, a process that begins immediately upon introduction of microbes into a sterile area of the body. Perturbation of one or more components of these defenses (e.g., via immunosuppressants, chronic illness, and burns) may have substantial negative impact on resistance to infection.

Entry of microbes into the mammalian host is precluded by the presence of a number of barriers that possess either an epithelial (integument) or mucosal (respiratory, gut, and urogenital) surface. However, barrier function is not solely limited to physical characteristics: Host barrier cells may secrete substances that limit microbial proliferation or prevent invasion. Also, resident or commensal microbes (endogenous or autochthonous host microflora) adherent

to the physical surface and to each other may preclude invasion, particularly of virulent organisms (colonization resistance).[9]

The most extensive physical barrier is the integument or skin. In addition to the physical barrier posed by the epithelial surface, the skin harbors its own resident microflora that may block the attachment and invasion of noncommensal microbes. Microbes also are held in check by chemicals that sebaceous glands secrete and by the constant shedding of epithelial cells. The endogenous microflora of the integument primarily comprises gram-positive aerobic microbes belonging to the genera *Staphylococcus* and *Streptococcus*, as well as *Corynebacterium* and *Propionibacterium* species. These organisms, plus *Enterococcus faecalis* and *faecium*, *Escherichia coli*, and other Enterobacteriaceae, and yeast such as *Candida albicans*, can be isolated from the infraumbilical regions of the body. Diseases of the skin (e.g., eczema and dermatitis) are associated with overgrowth of skin commensal organisms, and barrier breaches invariably lead to the introduction of these microbes.

The respiratory tract possesses several host defense mechanisms that facilitate the maintenance of sterility in the distal bronchi and alveoli under normal circumstances. In the upper respiratory tract, respiratory mucus traps larger particles, including microbes. This mucus is then passed into the upper airways and oropharynx by ciliated epithelial cells, where the mucus is cleared via coughing. Smaller particles arriving in the lower respiratory tract are cleared via phagocytosis by pulmonary alveolar macrophages. Any process that diminishes these host defenses can lead to development of bronchitis or pneumonia.

The urogenital, biliary, pancreatic ductal, and distal respiratory tracts do not possess resident microflora in healthy individuals, although microbes may be present if these barriers are affected by disease (e.g., malignancy, inflammation, calculi, or foreign body), or if microorganisms are introduced from an external source (e.g., urinary catheter or pulmonary aspiration). In contrast, significant numbers of microbes are encountered in many portions of the GI tract, with vast numbers being found within the oropharynx and distal colorectum, although the specific organisms differ.

One would suppose that the entire GI tract would be populated via those microbes found in the oropharynx, but this is not the case. This is because after ingestion, these organisms routinely are killed in the highly acidic, low-motility environment of the stomach during the initial phases of digestion. Thus, small numbers of microbes populate the gastric mucosa [approximately 10^2 to 10^3 colony-forming units (CFU)/mL]; this population expands in the presence of drugs or disease states that diminish gastric acidity. Microbes that are not destroyed within the stomach enter the small intestine, in which a certain amount of microbial proliferation takes place, such that approximately 10^5 to 10^8 CFU/mL are present in the terminal ileum.

The relatively low-oxygen, static environment of the colon is accompanied by the exponential growth of microbes that comprise the most extensive host endogenous microflora. Anaerobic microbes outnumber aerobic species approximately 100:1 in the distal colorectum, and approximately 10^{11} to 10^{12} CFU/g are present in feces. Large numbers of facultative and strict anaerobes (*Bacteroides fragilis*, *distasonis*, and *thetaiotaomicron*, *Bifidobacterium*, *Clostridium*, *Eubacterium*, *Fusobacterium*, *Lactobacillus*, and *Peptostreptococcus* species) as well as several orders of magnitude fewer aerobic microbes (*E. coli* and other Enterobacteriaceae, *E. faecalis* and *faecium*, *C. albicans* and other *Candida* spp.) are present. Intriguingly, although colonization resistance on the part of this extensive, well-characterized host microflora effectively prevents invasion of enteric pathogens such as *Salmonella*, *Shigella*, *Vibrio*, and other enteropathogenic bacterial species, these same organisms provide the initial inoculum for infection should perforation of the GI tract occur. It is of great interest that only some of these microbial species predominate in established intra-abdominal infection.

Once microbes enter a sterile body compartment (e.g., pleural or peritoneal cavity) or tissue, additional host defenses act to limit and/or eliminate these pathogens. Initially, several primitive and relatively nonspecific host defenses act to contain the nidus of infection, which may include microbes as well as debris, devitalized tissue, and foreign bodies, depending on the nature of the injury. These defenses include the physical barrier of the tissue itself, as well as the capacity of proteins such as lactoferrin and transferrin to sequester the critical microbial growth factor iron, thereby limiting microbial growth. In addition, fibrinogen within the inflammatory fluid has the ability to trap large numbers of microbes during the process in which it polymerizes into fibrin. Within the peritoneal cavity, unique host defenses exist, including a diaphragmatic pumping mechanism whereby particles such as microbes within peritoneal fluid are expunged from the abdominal cavity via specialized structures on the undersurface of the diaphragm. Concurrently, containment by the omentum, the so-called *gatekeeper* of the abdomen and intestinal ileus, serves to wall off infection. However, the latter processes and fibrin trapping have a high likelihood of contributing to the formation of an intra-abdominal abscess.

Microbes also immediately encounter a series of host defense mechanisms that reside within the vast majority of tissues of the body. These include resident macrophages and low levels of complement (C) proteins and immunoglobulins (Ig, antibodies).[10] Resident macrophages secrete a wide array of substances in response to the above-mentioned processes, some of which appear to regulate the cellular components of the host defense response. Macrophage cytokine synthesis is upregulated. Secretion of tumor necrosis factor alpha (TNF-α), of interleukins (IL)-1β, 6, and 8; and of interferon-gamma (INF-γ) occurs within the tissue milieu, and, depending on the magnitude of the host defense response, the systemic circulation.[11] Concurrently, a counterregulatory response is initiated consisting of binding proteins (TNF-BP), cytokine receptor antagonists (IL-1ra) and anti-inflammatory cytokines (IL-4 and IL-10).

The interaction of microbes with these first-line host defenses leads to microbial opsonization (C1q, C3bi, and IgFc), phagocytosis, and both extracellular (C5b6-9 membrane attack complex) and intracellular microbial destruction (phagocytic vacuoles). Concurrently, the classic and alternate complement pathways are activated both via direct contact with and via IgM > IgG binding to microbes, leading to the release of a number of different complement protein fragments (C3a, C4a, C5a) that are biologically active, acting to markedly enhance vascular permeability. Bacterial cell wall components and a variety of enzymes that are expelled from leukocyte phagocytic vacuoles during microbial phagocytosis and killing act in this capacity as well.

Simultaneously, the release of substances to which polymorphonuclear leukocytes (PMNs) in the bloodstream are attracted takes place. These consist of C5a, microbial cell wall peptides containing *N*-formyl-methionine, and macrophage secretion of cytokines such as IL-8. This process of host defense recruitment leads to further influx of inflammatory fluid into the area of incipient infection, and is accompanied by diapedesis of large numbers of PMNs, a process that begins within several minutes and may peak within hours or days. The magnitude of the response and eventual outcome generally are related to several factors: (a) the initial number of microbes, (b) the rate of microbial proliferation in relation to containment and killing by host defenses, (c) microbial virulence, and (d) the potency of host defenses. In regard to the latter, drugs or disease states that diminish any or multiple components of host defenses are associated with higher rates and potentially more grave infections.

Definitions

Several possible outcomes can occur subsequent to microbial invasion and the interaction of microbes with resident and recruited host defenses: (a) eradication, (b) containment, often leading to the presence of purulence—the hallmark of chronic infection (e.g., a furuncle in the skin and soft tissue or abscess within the parenchyma of an organ or potential space), (c) locoregional infection (cellulitis, lymphangitis, and aggressive soft tissue infection) with or without distant spread of infection (metastatic abscess), or (d) systemic infection (bacteremia or fungemia). Obviously, the latter represents the failure of resident and recruited host defenses at the local level, and is associated with significant morbidity and mortality in the clinical setting. In addition, it is not uncommon that disease progression occurs such that serious locoregional infection is associated with concurrent systemic infection. A chronic abscess also may intermittently drain and/or be associated with bacteremia.

Infection is defined by identification of microorganisms in host tissue or the bloodstream, plus an inflammatory response to their presence. At the site of infection, the classic findings of rubor, calor, and dolor in areas such as the skin or subcutaneous tissue are common. Most infections in normal individuals with intact host defenses are associated with these local manifestations, plus systemic manifestations such as elevated temperature, elevated white blood cell (WBC) count, tachycardia, or tachypnea. The systemic manifestations noted above comprise the *systemic inflammatory response syndrome* (SIRS).

SIRS can be caused by a variety of disease processes, including pancreatitis, polytrauma, malignancy, and transfusion reaction, as well as infection (Fig. 6-1). Strict criteria for SIRS (tachycardia, tachypnea, fever, and elevated WBC count) have been broadened to include additional clinical indicators noted in Table 6-1.[12] SIRS caused by infection is termed *sepsis* and is mediated by the production of a cascade of proinflammatory mediators produced in re-

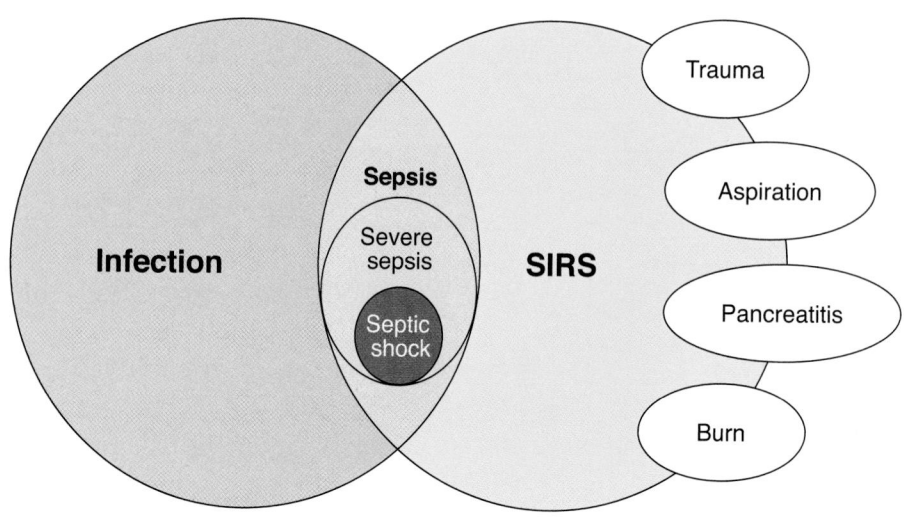

FIG. 6-1. Relationship between infection and systemic inflammatory response syndrome (SIRS). Sepsis is the presence both of infection and the systemic inflammatory response, shown here as the intersection of these two areas. Other conditions may cause SIRS as well (trauma, aspiration, etc.). Severe sepsis (and septic shock) are both subsets of sepsis.

TABLE 6-1	Criteria for systemic inflammatory response syndrome

General variables
　Fever [core temp >38.3°C (100.9°F)]
　Hypothermia [core temp <36°C (96.8°F)]
　Heart rate >90 bpm
　Tachypnea
　Altered mental status
　Significant edema or positive fluid balance (>20 mL/kg over 24 h)
　Hyperglycemia in the absence of diabetes
Inflammatory variables
　Leukocytosis (WBC >12,000)
　Leukopenia (WBC <4000)
　Bandemia (>10% band forms)
　Plasma C-reactive protein > 2 s.d. above normal value
　Plasma procalcitonin >2 s.d. above normal value
Hemodynamic variables
　Arterial hypotension (SBP <90 mmHg, MAP <70, or SBP decrease >40 mmHg)
　SvO_2 >70%
　Cardiac index >3.5 L/min per square meter
Organ dysfunction variables
　Arterial hypoxemia
　Acute oliguria
　Creatinine increase
　Coagulation abnormalities
　Ileus
　Thrombocytopenia
　Hyperbilirubinemia
Tissue perfusion variables
　Hyperlactatemia
　Decreased capillary filling

bpm = beats per minute; MAP = mean arterial pressure; SBP = systolic blood pressure; s.d. = standard deviations; SvO_2 = venous oxygen saturation; WBC = white blood cell count.

sponse to exposure to microbial products. These products include lipopolysaccharide (endotoxin) derived from gram-negative organisms; peptidoglycans and teichoic acids from gram-positive organisms; multiple cell wall components such as mannan from yeast and fungi; and many others. Patients have developed sepsis if they have met clinical criteria for SIRS and have evidence of a local or systemic source of infection.

Severe sepsis is characterized as sepsis (defined above) combined with the presence of new-onset organ failure. Severe sepsis is the most common cause of death in noncoronary critical care units, with a mortality rate of 51 cases/100,000 population per year in 2003.[13] A number of organ dysfunction scoring systems have been described.[14–16] With respect to clinical criteria, a patient with sepsis and the need for ventilatory support, with oliguria unresponsive to aggressive fluid resuscitation or with hypotension requiring vasopressors, should be considered to have developed severe sepsis. *Septic shock* is a state of acute circulatory failure identified by the presence of persistent arterial hypotension (systolic blood pressure <90 mmHg) despite adequate fluid resuscitation, without other identifiable causes. Septic shock is the most severe manifestation of infection, occurring in approximately 40% of patients with severe sepsis; it has an attendant mortality rate of 45 to 60%.[17,18]

Clinicians dedicated to improving the treatment of sepsis have recently developed a new classification scheme for this entity.[12] This scheme has borrowed from the tumor-node-metastasis staging scheme developed for oncology. The impetus for development of this scheme was related to the heterogeneity of the patient population developing sepsis, an example of which would include two patients, both in the intensive care unit (ICU), who develop criteria consistent with septic shock. Although both have infection and

sepsis-associated hypotension, one might expect a different outcome in a young, healthy patient who develops urosepsis than in an elderly, immunosuppressed lung transplant recipient who develops invasive fungal infection. The PIRO Staging System stratifies patients based on their predisposing conditions (P), the nature and extent of the infection (I), the nature and magnitude of the host response (R), and the degree of concomitant organ dysfunction (O). Current definitions using this system are listed in Table 6-2. Published trials using this classification system have confirmed the validity of this concept.[19] Further investigation is ongoing to evaluate the clinical utility of this scheme.

MICROBIOLOGY OF INFECTIOUS AGENTS

A partial list of common pathogens that cause infections in surgical patients is provided in Table 6-3.

Bacteria

Bacteria are responsible for the majority of surgical infections. Specific species are identified using Gram's stain and growth characteristics on specific media. The Gram's stain is an important evaluation that allows rapid classification of bacteria by color. This color is related to the staining characteristics of the bacterial cell wall: gram-positive bacteria stain blue and gram-negative bacteria stain red. Bacteria are classified based upon a number of additional characteristics including morphology (cocci and bacilli), the pattern of division [e.g., single organisms, groups of organisms in pairs (diplococci), clusters (staphylococci), and chains (streptococci)], and the presence and location of spores.

Gram-positive bacteria that frequently cause infections in surgical patients include aerobic skin commensals (*Staphylococcus aureus* and *epidermidis* and *Streptococcus pyogenes*) and enteric organisms such as *E. faecalis* and *faecium*. Aerobic skin commensals cause a large percentage of surgical site infections (SSIs), either alone or in conjunction with other pathogens; enterococci can cause nosocomial infections [urinary tract infections (UTIs) and bacteremia] in immunocompromised or chronically ill patients, but are of relatively low virulence in healthy individuals.

There are many pathogenic gram-negative bacterial species that are capable of causing infection in surgical patients. Most gram-negative organisms of interest to the surgeon are bacilli belonging to the family Enterobacteriaceae, including *E. coli*, *Klebsiella pneumoniae*, *Serratia marcescens*, and *Enterobacter*, *Citrobacter*, and *Acinetobacter* spp. Other gram-negative bacilli of note include *Pseudomonas* spp., including *P. aeruginosa* and *fluorescens* and *Xanthomonas* spp.

Anaerobic organisms are unable to grow or divide poorly in air, as most do not possess the enzyme catalase, which allows for metabolism of reactive oxygen species. Anaerobes are the predominant indigenous flora in many areas of the human body, with the particular species dependent on the site. For example, *Propionibacterium acnes* and other species are a major component of the skin microflora and cause the infectious manifestation of acne. As noted above, large

TABLE 6-2	PIRO classification scheme

Domain	Means of Classification
Predisposition	Premorbid illness that affects probability of survival (e.g., immunosuppression, age, genetics)
Insult (infection)	Type of infecting organisms, location of disease, intervention (source control)
Response	SIRS, other signs of sepsis, presence of shock, tissue markers (e.g., C-reactive protein, IL-6)
Organ dysfunction	Organ dysfunction as a number of failing organs or composite score

IL-6 = interleukin-6; SIRS = systemic inflammatory response syndrome.

TABLE 6-3	Common pathogens in surgical patients

Gram-positive aerobic cocci
   Staphylococcus aureus
   Staphylococcus epidermidis
   Streptococcus pyogenes
   Streptococcus pneumoniae
   Enterococcus faecium, E. faecalis
Gram-negative aerobic bacilli
   Escherichia coli
   Haemophilus influenzae
   Klebsiella pneumoniae
   Proteus mirabilis
   Enterobacter cloacae, E. aerogenes
   Serratia marcescens
   Acinetobacter calcoaceticus
   Citrobacter freundii
   Pseudomonas aeruginosa
   Xanthomonas maltophilia
Anaerobes
   Gram-positive
      Clostridium difficile
      Clostridium perfringens, C. tetani, C. septicum
      Peptostreptococcus spp.
   Gram-negative
      Bacteroides fragilis
      Fusobacterium spp.
Other bacteria
   Mycobacterium avium-intracellulare
   Mycobacterium tuberculosis
   Nocardia asteroides
   Legionella pneumophila
   Listeria monocytogenes
Fungi
   Aspergillus fumigatus, A. niger, A. terreus, A. flavus
   Blastomyces dermatitidis
   Candida albicans
   Candida glabrata, C. parapsilosis, C. krusei
   Coccidioides immitis
   Cryptococcus neoformans
   Histoplasma capsulatum
   Mucor/Rhizopus
Viruses
   Cytomegalovirus
   Epstein-Barr virus
   Hepatitis A, B, C viruses
   Herpes simplex virus
   HIV
   Varicella-zoster virus

numbers of anaerobes contribute to the microflora of the oropharynx and colorectum.

Infection due to *Mycobacterium tuberculosis* was once one of the most common causes of death in Europe, causing one in four deaths in the seventeenth and eighteenth centuries. In the nineteenth and twentieth centuries, thoracic surgical intervention often was required for severe pulmonary disease, now an increasingly uncommon occurrence in developed countries. This organism and other related organisms (*M. avium-intracellulare* and *M. leprae*) are known as *acid-fast bacilli*. Other acid-fast bacilli include *Nocardia* spp. These organisms typically are slow-growing, sometimes necessitating observation in culture for weeks to months before final identification, although DNA-based analysis is increasingly available to provide a means for preliminary, rapid detection.

Fungi

Fungi typically are identified by use of special stains (e.g., potassium hydroxide, India ink, methenamine silver, or Giemsa). Initial identification is assisted by observation of the form of branching and septation in stained specimens or in culture. Final identification is based on growth characteristics in special media, similar to bacteria, as well as on the capacity for growth at a different temperature [25 vs. 37°C (77 vs. 98.6°F)]. Fungi of relevance to surgeons include those that cause nosocomial infections in surgical patients as part of polymicrobial infections or fungemia (e.g., *C. albicans* and related species), rare causes of aggressive soft tissue infections (e.g., *Mucor*, *Rhizopus*, and *Absidia* spp.), and so-called *opportunistic pathogens* that cause infection in the immunocompromised host (e.g., *Aspergillus fumigatus, niger, terreus*, and other spp., *Blastomyces dermatitidis, Coccidioides immitis*, and *Cryptococcus neoformans*). Agents currently available for antifungal therapy are described in Table 6-4.

Viruses

Due to their small size and necessity for growth within cells, viruses are difficult to culture, requiring a longer time than is typically optimal for clinical decision making. Previously, viral infection was identified by indirect means (i.e., the host antibody response). Recent advances in technology have allowed for the identification of the presence of viral DNA or RNA using methods such as polymerase chain reaction. Similarly to many fungal infections, most viral infections in surgical patients occur in the immunocompromised host, particularly those receiving immunosuppression to prevent rejection of a solid organ allograft. Relevant viruses include adenoviruses, cytomegalovirus, Epstein-Barr virus, herpes simplex virus, and varicella-zoster virus. Surgeons must be aware of the manifestations of hepatitis B and C virus, as well as HIV infections, including their capacity to be transmitted to health care workers (see Blood-Borne Pathogens below). Prophylactic and therapeutic use of antiviral agents is discussed in Chap. 11.

TABLE 6-4	Antifungal agents and their characteristics

Antifungal	Advantages	Disadvantages	Approximate Daily Cost
Amphotericin B	Broad-spectrum, inexpensive	Renal toxicity, premeds, IV only	$11
Liposomal amphotericin B	Broad-spectrum	Expensive, IV only, renal toxicity	$600
Azoles			
Fluconazole	IV and PO availability	Narrow-spectrum, drug interactions	$21 (IV), <$1 (PO)
Itraconazole	IV and PO availability	Narrow-spectrum, no CSF penetration, drug interactions, decreased cardiac contractility	$200 (IV), $3 (PO)
Posaconazole	Broad-spectrum, zygomycete activity	PO only	$100
Voriconazole	IV and PO availability, broad-spectrum	IV diluent accumulates in renal failure, visual disturbances	$200 (IV), $70 (PO)
Echinocandins			
Anidulafungin, caspofungin, micafungin	Broad-spectrum	IV only, poor CNS penetration	$100–250

CSF = cerebrospinal fluid.

PREVENTION AND TREATMENT
OF SURGICAL INFECTIONS

General Principles

Maneuvers to diminish the presence of exogenous (surgeon and operating room environment) and endogenous (patient) microbes are termed *prophylaxis*, and consist of the use of mechanical, chemical, and antimicrobial modalities, or a combination of these methods.

As described above in Bacteria, the host resident microflora of the skin (patient and surgeon) and other barrier surfaces represent a potential source of microbes that can invade the body during trauma, thermal injury, or elective or emergent surgical intervention. For this reason, operating room personnel are versed in mild mechanical exfoliation of the skin of the hands and forearms using antibacterial preparations, and intraoperatively sterile technique is used. Similarly, application of an antibacterial agent to the skin of the patient at the proposed operative site takes place before creating an incision. Also, if necessary, hair removal should take place using a clipper rather than a razor; the latter promotes overgrowth of skin microbes in small nicks and cuts. Dedicated use of these modalities clearly has been shown to diminish the quantity of skin microflora, and although a direct correlation between praxis and reduced infection rates has not been demonstrated, comparison to infection rates before the use of antisepsis and sterile technique makes clear their utility and importance.

The aforementioned modalities are not capable of sterilizing the hands of the surgeon or the skin or epithelial surfaces of the patient, although the inoculum can be reduced considerably. Thus, entry through the skin, into the soft tissue, and into a body cavity or hollow viscus invariably is associated with the introduction of some degree of microbial contamination. For that reason, patients who undergo procedures that may be associated with the ingress of significant numbers of microbes (e.g., colonic resection) or in whom the consequences of any type of infection due to said process would be dire (e.g., prosthetic vascular graft infection) should receive an antimicrobial agent.

Source Control

The primary precept of surgical infectious disease therapy consists of drainage of all purulent material, débridement of all infected, devitalized tissue, and debris, and/or removal of foreign bodies at the site of infection, plus remediation of the underlying cause of infection.[20] A discrete, walled-off purulent fluid collection (i.e., an abscess) requires drainage via percutaneous drain insertion or an operative approach in which incision and drainage take place. An ongoing source of contamination (e.g., bowel perforation) or the presence of an aggressive, rapidly-spreading infection (e.g., necrotizing soft tissue infection) invariably requires expedient, aggressive operative intervention, both to remove contaminated material and infected tissue (e.g., radical débridement or amputation) and to remove the initial cause of infection (e.g., bowel resection). Other treatment modalities such as antimicrobial agents, albeit critical, are of secondary importance to effective surgery with regard to treatment of surgical infections and overall outcome. Rarely, if ever, can an aggressive surgical infection be cured only by the administration of antibiotics, and never in the face of an ongoing source of contamination. Also, it has been repeatedly demonstrated that delay in operative intervention, whether due to misdiagnosis or the need for additional diagnostic studies, is associated with increased morbidity and occasional mortality.[21-23]

Appropriate Use of Antimicrobial Agents

A classification of antimicrobial agents, mechanisms of action, and spectrum of activity is shown in Table 6-5. *Prophylaxis* consists of the administration of an antimicrobial agent or agents before initiation of certain specific types of surgical procedures to reduce the number of microbes that enter the tissue or body cavity. Agents are selected according to their activity against microbes likely to be present at the surgical site, based on knowledge of host microflora. For example, patients undergoing elective colorectal surgery should receive antimicrobial prophylaxis directed against skin flora, gram-negative aerobes, and amoebic bacteria. There are a wide variety of agents that meet these criteria.

By definition, prophylaxis is limited to the time before and during the operative procedure; in the vast majority of cases only a single dose of antibiotic is required, and only for certain types of procedures (see Surgical Site Infections below). However, patients who undergo complex, prolonged procedures in which the duration of the operation exceeds the serum drug half-life should receive an additional dose or doses of the antimicrobial agent. *Nota bene:* There is no evidence that administration of postoperative doses of an antimicrobial agent provides additional benefit, and this practice should be discouraged, as it is costly and is associated with increased rates of microbial drug resistance. Guidelines for prophylaxis are provided in Table 6-6.

Empiric therapy comprises the use of an antimicrobial agent or agents when the risk of a surgical infection is high, based on the underlying disease process (e.g., ruptured appendicitis), or when significant contamination during surgery has occurred (e.g., inadequate bowel preparation or considerable spillage of colon contents). Obviously, prophylaxis merges into empiric therapy in situations in which the risk of infection increases markedly because of intraoperative findings. Empiric therapy also often is used in critically ill patients in whom a potential site of infection has been identified and severe sepsis or septic shock occurs. Invariably, empiric therapy should be limited to a short course of drug (3 to 5 days), and should be curtailed as soon as possible based on microbiologic data (i.e., absence of positive cultures) coupled with improvements in the clinical course of the patient.

Similarly, empiric therapy merges into therapy of established infection in some patients as well. However, among surgical patients, the manner in which therapy is used, particularly in relation to the use of microbiologic data (culture and antibiotic sensitivity patterns), differs depending on whether the infection is monomicrobial or polymicrobial. Monomicrobial infections frequently are nosocomial infections occurring in postoperative patients, such as UTIs, pneumonia, or bacteremia. Evidence of SIRS (fever, tachycardia, tachypnea, or elevated leukocyte count) in such individuals, coupled with evidence of local infection (e.g., an infiltrate on chest roentgenogram plus a positive Gram's stain in bronchoalveolar lavage samples) should lead the surgeon to initiate empiric antibiotic therapy. Drug selection must be based on initial evidence (gram-positive vs. gram-negative microbes, yeast), coupled with institutional and unit-specific drug sensitivity patterns. It is important, however, to ensure that the antimicrobial coverage chosen is adequate, because delay in appropriate antibiotic treatment has been shown to be associated with increased mortality. Within 24 to 72 hours, culture and sensitivity reports will allow refinement of the antibiotic regimen to select the most efficacious agent. The clinical course of the patient is monitored closely, and in some cases (e.g., UTI) follow-up studies (urine culture) should be obtained after completion of therapy.

Although the primary therapeutic modality to treat polymicrobial surgical infections is source control as delineated above in Source Control, antimicrobial agents play an important role as well. Culture results are of lesser importance in managing these types of infections, as it has been repeatedly demonstrated that only a limited cadre of microbes predominate in the established infection, selected from a large number present at the time of initial contamination. Invariably, it is difficult to identify all microbes that comprise the initial polymicrobial inoculum. For this reason, the antibiotic regimen should not be modified solely on the basis of culture information, as it is less important than the clinical course of the patient. For example, patients who undergo appendectomy for gangrenous, perforated appendicitis, or bowel resection for intestinal perforation, should receive an antimicrobial agent or agents directed against aerobes and anaerobes for 3 to 5 days, occasionally longer. A survey

TABLE 6-5 Antimicrobial agents

Antibiotic Class, Generic Name	Trade Name	Mechanism of Action	Organism								
			S. pyogenes	MSSA	MRSA	S. epidermidis	Enterococcus	VRE	E. coli	P. aeruginosa	Anaerobes
Penicillins		Cell wall synthesis inhibitors (bind penicillin-binding protein)									
Penicillin G	—		1	0	0	0	±	0	0	0	1
Nafcillin	Nallpen, Unipen		1	1	0	±	0	0	0	0	0
Piperacillin	Pipracil		1	0	0	0	±	0	1	1	±
Penicillin/beta lactamase inhibitor combinations		Cell wall synthesis inhibitors/beta lactamase inhibitors									
Ampicillin-sulbactam	Unasyn		1	1	0	±	1	±	1	0	1
Ticarcillin-clavulanate	Timentin		1	1	0	±	±	0	1	1	1
Piperacillin-tazobactam	Zosyn		1	1	0	1	±	0	1	1	1
First-generation cephalosporins		Cell wall synthesis inhibitors (bind penicillin-binding protein)									
Cefazolin, cefalexin	Ancef, Keflex		1	1	0	±	0	0	1	0	0
Second-generation cephalosporins		Cell wall synthesis inhibitors (bind penicillin-binding protein)									
Cefoxitin	Mefoxin		1	1	0	±	0	0	1	0	1
Cefotetan	Cefotan		1	1	0	±	0	0	1	0	1
Cefuroxime	Ceftin		1	1	0	±	0	0	1	0	0
Third- and fourth-generation cephalosporins		Cell wall synthesis inhibitors (bind penicillin-binding protein)									
Ceftriaxone	Rocephin		1	1	0	±	0	0	1	0	0
Ceftazidime	Fortaz		1	±	0	±	0	0	1	1	0
Cefepime	Maxipime		1	1	0	±	0	0	1	1	0
Cefotaxime	Cefotaxime		1	1	0	±	0	0	1	±	0
Carbapenems		Cell wall synthesis inhibitors (bind penicillin-binding protein)									
Imipenem-cilastatin	Primaxin		1	1	0	1	±	0	1	1	1
Meropenem	Merrem		1	1	0	1	0	0	1	1	1
Ertapenem	Invanz		1	1	0	1	0	0	1	±	1
Aztreonam	Azactam	Cell wall synthesis inhibitor (bind penicillin-binding protein)	0	0	0	0	0	0	1	1	0
Aminoglycosides		Alteration of cell membrane, binding and inhibition of 30S ribosomal unit									
Gentamicin	—		0	1	0	±	1	0	1	1	0
Tobramycin, amikacin	—		0	1	0	±	0	0	1	1	0
Fluoroquinolones		Inhibit topoisomerase II and IV (DNA synthesis inhibition)									
Ciprofloxacin	Cipro		±	1	0	1	0	0	1	1	0
Levofloxacin	Levaquin		1	1	0	1	0	0	1	±	0
Glycopeptides		Cell wall synthesis inhibition (peptidoglycan synthesis inhibition)									
Vancomycin	Vancocin		1	1	1	1	1	0	0	0	0

Drug	Trade name	Mechanism							
Quinupristin-dalfopristin	Synercid	Inhibits two sites on 50S ribosome (protein synthesis inhibition)	1	1	1	1	1	0	±
Linezolid	Zyvox	Inhibits 50S ribosomal activity (protein synthesis inhibition)	1	1	1	1	1	0	±
Daptomycin	Cubicin	Binds bacterial membrane, results in depolarization, lysis	1	1	1	1	1	0	0
Rifampin	—	Inhibits DNA-dependent RNA polymerase	1	1	±	1	0	0	0
Clindamycin	Cleocin	Inhibits 50S ribosomal activity (protein synthesis inhibition)	1	0	0	0	0	0	1
Metronidazole	Flagyl	Production of toxic intermediates (free radical production)	0	0	0	0	0	0	1
Macrolides									
Erythromycin	—	Inhibit 50S ribosomal activity (protein synthesis inhibition)	1	±	±	0	0	0	0
Azithromycin	Zithromax		1	1	0	0	0	0	0
Clarithromycin	Biaxin		1	1	0	0	1	0	0
Trimethoprim-sulfamethoxazole	Bactrim, Septra	Inhibits sequential steps of folate metabolism	±	1	±	0	0	0	0
Tetracyclines									
Minocycline	Minocin	Bind 30S ribosomal unit (protein synthesis inhibition)	1	1	0	0	0	0	±
Doxycycline	Vibramycin		1	±	0	0	1	1	±
Tigecycline	Tygacil		1	1	1	1	0	0	1

E. coli = Escherichia coli; MRSA = methicillin-resistant Staphylococcus aureus; MSSA = methicillin-sensitive Staphylococcus aureus; P. aeruginosa = Pseudomonas aeruginosa; S. epidermidis = Staphylococcus epidermidis; S. pyogenes = Streptococcus pyogenes; VRE = vancomycin-resistant enterococcus.

1 = reliable activity; 0 = no activity.

± = variable activity.

The sensitivities presented are generalizations. The clinician should confirm sensitivity patterns at the locale where the patient is being treated because these patterns may vary widely depending on location.

TABLE 6-6 Prophylactic use of antibiotics

Site	Antibiotic	Alternative (e.g., penicillin allergic)
Cardiovascular surgery	Cefazolin, cefuroxime	Vancomycin
Gastroduodenal area	Cefazolin, cefotetan, cefoxitin, ampicillin-sulbactam	Fluoroquinolone
Biliary tract with active infection (e.g., cholecystitis)	Ampicillin-sulbactam, ticarcillin-clavulanate, piperacillin-tazobactam	Fluoroquinolone plus clindamycin or metronidazole
Colorectal surgery, obstructed small bowel	Cefazolin plus metronidazole, ertapenem, ticarcillin-clavulanate, piperacillin-tazobactam	Gentamicin or fluoroquinolone plus clindamycin or metronidazole
Head and neck	Cefazolin	Aminoglycoside plus clindamycin
Neurosurgical procedures	Cefazolin	Vancomycin
Orthopedic surgery	Cefazolin, ceftriaxone	Vancomycin
Breast, hernia	Cefazolin	Vancomycin

of several decades of clinical trials examining the effect of antimicrobial agent selection on the treatment of intra-abdominal infection revealed striking similarities in outcome among regimens that possessed aerobic and anaerobic activity (~10 to 30% failure rates): Most failures could not be attributed to antibiotic selection, but rather were due to the inability to achieve effective source control.[24]

Duration of antibiotic administration should be decided at the time the drug regimen is prescribed. As noted below in Surgical Site Infections, prophylaxis is limited to a single dose administered immediately before creating the incision. Empiric therapy should be limited to 3 to 5 days or less, and should be curtailed if the presence of a local site or systemic infection is not revealed.[25] This precept is highlighted by a study in which patients in whom SIRS was identified were closely monitored for the presence of infection: Less than half of them were found to harbor infection.[26]

Therapy for monomicrobial infections follows standard guidelines: 3 to 5 days for UTIs, 7 to 10 days for pneumonia, and 7 to 14 days for bacteremia. Longer courses of therapy in this setting do not result in improved care but are associated with increased risk of resistant organisms.[27,28] Antibiotic therapy for osteomyelitis, endocarditis, or prosthetic infections in which it is hazardous to remove the device consists of prolonged courses of an antibiotic or several agents in combination for 6 to 12 weeks. The specific agents are selected based on analysis of the degree to which the organism is killed in vitro using the minimum inhibitory concentration of a standard pure inoculum of 10^5 CFU/mL of the organism isolated from the site of infection or bloodstream. Sensitivities are reported in relation to the achievable blood level of each antibiotic in a panel of agents. The least toxic, least expensive agent to which the organism is most sensitive should be selected, although the latter parameter is of paramount importance. Serious or recrudescent infection may require therapy with two or more agents, particularly if a multidrug-resistant pathogen is causative, limiting therapeutic options to drugs to which the organism is only moderately sensitive. Commonly, an agent may be administered IV for 1 to 2 weeks, following which the treatment course is completed with oral drug. However, this should only be undertaken in patients who demonstrate progressive clinical improvement, and the oral agent should be capable of achieving high serum levels as well (e.g., fluoroquinolones).

The majority of studies examining the optimal duration of antibiotic therapy for the treatment of polymicrobial infection have focused on patients who develop peritonitis. Cogent data exist to support the contention that satisfactory outcomes are achieved with 12 to 24 hours of therapy for penetrating GI trauma in the absence of extensive contamination, 3 to 5 days of therapy for perforated or gangrenous appendicitis, 5 to 7 days of therapy for treatment of peritoneal soilage due to a perforated viscus with moderate degrees of contamination, and 7 to 14 days of therapy to adjunctively treat extensive peritoneal soilage (e.g., feculent peritonitis) or that occurring in the immunosuppressed host.[29] It bears repeating that the eventual outcome is more closely linked to the ability of the surgeon to achieve effective source control than to the duration of antibiotic administration.

In the later phases of postoperative antibiotic treatment of serious intra-abdominal infection, the absence of an elevated WBC count, lack of band forms of PMNs on peripheral smear, and lack of fever [<38.6°C (100.5°F)] provide close to complete assurance that infection has been eradicated.[30] Under these circumstances, antibiotics can be discontinued with impunity. However, the presence of one or more of these indicators does not mandate continuing antibiotics or altering the antibiotic(s) administered. Rather, a search for an extra-abdominal source of infection or a residual or ongoing source of intra-abdominal infection (e.g., abscess or leaking anastomosis) should be sought, the latter mandating maneuvers to effect source control.

Allergy to antimicrobial agents must be considered before prescribing them. First, it is important to ascertain whether a patient has had any type of allergic reaction in association with administration of a particular antibiotic. However, one should take care to ensure that the purported reaction consists of true allergic symptoms and signs, such as urticaria, bronchospasm, or other similar manifestations, rather than indigestion or nausea. Penicillin allergy is quite common, the reported incidence ranging from 0.7 to 10%. Although avoiding the use of any beta-lactam drug is appropriate in patients who manifest significant allergic reactions to penicillins, the incidence of cross reactivity appears highest for carbapenems, much lower for cephalosporins (~5 to 7%), and extremely small or nonexistent for monobactams.

Severe allergic manifestations to a specific class of agents, such as anaphylaxis, generally preclude the use of any agents in that class, except under circumstances in which use of a certain drug represents a lifesaving measure. In some centers, patients undergo intradermal testing using a dilute solution of a particular antibiotic to determine whether a severe allergic reaction would be elicited by parenteral administration. A pathway including such intradermal testing has been effective in reduction of vancomycin use to 16% in surgical patients with reported allergy to penicillin.[31] This type of testing is rarely used because it is simpler to select an alternative class of agent. Should administration of a specific agent to which the patient is allergic become necessary, desensitization using progressively higher doses of antibiotic can be undertaken, providing the initial testing does not cause severe allergic manifestations.

Misuse of antimicrobial agents is rampant in the inpatient and outpatient setting, and is associated with an enormous financial impact on health care costs, adverse reactions due to drug toxicity and allergy, the occurrence of new infections such as *Clostridium difficile* colitis, and the development of multiagent drug resistance among nosocomial pathogens. Each of these factors has been directly correlated with overall drug administration. It has been estimated that in the United States, in excess of $20 billion is spent on antibiotics each year, and the appearance of so-called *super bugs*—microbes sensitive to few if any agents—has been sobering.[32] The responsible practitioner limits prophylaxis to the period during the operative procedure, does not convert prophylaxis into empiric therapy except under well-defined conditions, sets the duration of antibiotic therapy from the outset, curtails antibiotic administration

TABLE 6-7	Risk factors for development of surgical site infections

Patient factors
    Older age
    Immunosuppression
    Obesity
    Diabetes mellitus
    Chronic inflammatory process
    Malnutrition
    Peripheral vascular disease
    Anemia
    Radiation
    Chronic skin disease
    Carrier state (e.g., chronic *Staphylococcus* carriage)
    Recent operation
Local factors
    Poor skin preparation
    Contamination of instruments
    Inadequate antibiotic prophylaxis
    Prolonged procedure
    Local tissue necrosis
    Hypoxia, hypothermia
Microbial factors
    Prolonged hospitalization (leading to nosocomial organisms)
    Toxin secretion
    Resistance to clearance (e.g., capsule formation)

wounds (class I) include those in which no infection is present; only skin microflora potentially contaminate the wound, and no hollow viscus that contains microbes is entered. Class ID wounds are similar except that a prosthetic device (e.g., mesh or valve) is inserted. *Clean/contaminated wounds* (class II) include those in which a hollow viscus such as the respiratory, alimentary, or genitourinary tracts with indigenous bacterial flora is opened under controlled circumstances without significant spillage of contents. Interestingly, while elective colorectal cases have classically been included as class II cases, a number of studies in the last decade have documented higher SSI rates (9 to 25%).[37–39] One study identified two thirds of infections presenting after discharge from hospital, highlighting the need for careful follow-up of these patients.[37] Infection is also more common in cases involving entry into the rectal space.[39] *Contaminated wounds* (class III) include open accidental wounds encountered early after injury, those with extensive introduction of bacteria into a normally sterile area of the body due to major breaks in sterile technique (e.g., open cardiac massage), gross spillage of viscus contents such as from the intestine, or incision through inflamed, albeit nonpurulent, tissue. *Dirty wounds* (class IV) include traumatic wounds in which a significant delay in treatment has occurred and in which necrotic tissue is present, those created in the presence of overt infection as evidenced by the presence of purulent material, and those created to access a perforated viscus accompanied by a high degree of contamination. The microbiology of SSIs is reflective of the initial host microflora such that SSIs following creation of a class I wound are invariable, due solely to skin microbes found on that portion of the body, while SSIs subsequent to a class II wound created for the purpose of elective colon resection may be caused by either skin microbes or colonic microflora, or both.

In the United States, hospitals are required to conduct surveillance for the development of SSIs for a period of 30 days after the operative procedure.[40] Such surveillance has been associated with greater awareness and a reduction in SSI rates, probably in large part based upon the impact of observation and promotion of adherence to appropriate care standards. Several different SSI risk stratification schemes have been developed via retrospective, multivariate analysis of large surveillance data sets. The National Nosocomial Infection Surveillance (NNIS) risk index is commonly used and assesses three factors: (a) American Society of Anesthesiologists Physical Status score greater than 2, (b) class III/IV wound, and (c) duration of operation greater than the 75th percentile for that particular procedure, to refine the risk of infection beyond that achieved by use of wound classification alone. Intriguingly, the risk of SSIs for class I wounds varies from approximately 1 to 2% for patients with low NNIS scores, to approximately 15% for patients with high NNIS scores (e.g., long operations and/or high American Society of Anesthesiologists scores), and it seems clear that additional refinements are required.[41]

SSIs are associated with considerable morbidity and occasional lethality, as well as substantial health care costs and patient inconvenience and dissatisfaction.[42] For that reason, surgeons strive to avoid SSIs by using the maneuvers described in the previous section Prevention and Treatment of Surgical Infections. Also, the use of prophylactic antibiotics may serve to reduce the incidence of SSI rates during certain types of procedures. For example, it is well accepted that a single dose of an antimicrobial agent should be

when clinical and microbiologic evidence does not support the presence of an infection, and limits therapy to a short course in every possible instance. The utility of prophylactic antibiotics to prevent infections related to thoracostomy tube insertion has been demonstrated,[33,34] but prolonged treatment while a thoracostomy tube remains in situ, or prolonged therapy of biliary, intra-abdominal, or abscess drain cultures is not to be condoned.

INFECTIONS OF SIGNIFICANCE IN SURGICAL PATIENTS

Surgical Site Infections

SSIs are infections of the tissues, organs, or spaces exposed by surgeons during performance of an invasive procedure. SSIs are classified into incisional and organ/space infections, and the former are further subclassified into superficial (limited to skin and subcutaneous tissue) and deep incisional categories.[35] The development of SSIs is related to three factors: (a) the degree of microbial contamination of the wound during surgery, (b) the duration of the procedure, and (c) host factors such as diabetes, malnutrition, obesity, immune suppression, and a number of other underlying disease states. Table 6-7 lists risk factors for development of SSIs. By definition, an incisional SSI has occurred if a surgical wound drains purulent material or if the surgeon judges it to be infected and opens it.

Surgical wounds are classified based on the presumed magnitude of the bacterial load at the time of surgery (Table 6-8).[36] *Clean*

TABLE 6-8	Wound class, representative procedures, and expected infection rates

Wound Class	Examples of Cases	Expected Infection Rates
Clean (class I)	Hernia repair, breast biopsy	1.0–5.4%
Clean/contaminated (class II)	Cholecystectomy, elective GI surgery (not colon)	2.1–9.5%
Clean/contaminated (class II)	Colorectal surgery	9.4–25%
Contaminated (class III)	Penetrating abdominal trauma, large tissue injury, enterotomy during bowel obstruction	3.4–13.2%
Dirty (class IV)	Perforated diverticulitis, necrotizing soft tissue infections	3.1–12.8%

TABLE 6-9	Quality improvement organizations of interest to surgeons in the United States	
Abbreviation	**Organization**	**Website**
SCIP	Surgical Care Improvement Project	*http://www.medqic.org* (Enter SCIP in search)
NSQIP	National Surgical Quality Improvement Program	*http://acsnsqip.org*
IHI	Institute for Healthcare Improvement	*http://www.ihi.org*
CMS	Center for Medicare and Medicaid Services	*http://www.hospitalcompare.hhs.gov*
NCQA	National Committee for Quality Assurance	*http://www.ncqa.org*

administered immediately before commencing surgery for class ID, II, III, and IV types of wounds.[43] It seems reasonable that this practice should be extended to patients in any category with high NNIS scores, although this remains to be proven. Thus the utility of prophylactic antibiotics in reducing the rate of wound infection subsequent to clean surgery remains controversial, and these agents should not be used under routine circumstances (e.g., in healthy young patients). However, because of the potential dire consequences of a wound infection after clean surgery in which prosthetic material is implanted into tissue, patients who undergo such procedures should receive a single preoperative dose of an antibiotic.

A number of health care organizations within the United States have become interested in evaluating performance of hospitals and physicians with respect to implementing standard of care therapies, one of which being reduction in SSIs, because the morbidity (and subsequent cost) of this complication is high. Several of these organizations are noted in Table 6-9. Appropriate guidelines in this area incorporating the principles discussed above in Prevention and Treatment of Surgical Infections have been developed and published.[44] However, adherence to these guidelines has been poor.[45] Driving incorporation of these guidelines into routine clinical practice is the belief that better adherence to evidence-based practice recommendations and more attention to designing systems of care with redundant safeguards will result in reduction of surgical complications and better patient outcomes. Importantly, the Center for Medicare and Medicaid Services, the largest third party payer in the United States, has required reporting by hospitals of many processes related to reduction of surgical infections, including appropriate use of perioperative antibiotics. This information, which is currently reported publicly by hospital, has led to significant improvement in reported rates of these process measures. The effects of this approach on SSIs are not known at this time.

Surgical management of the wound is also a critical determinant of the propensity to develop an SSI. In healthy individuals, class I and II wounds may be closed primarily, while skin closure of class III and IV wounds is associated with high rates of incisional SSIs (approximately 25 to 50%). The superficial aspects of these latter types of wounds should be packed open and allowed to heal by secondary intention, although selective use of delayed primary closure has been associated with a reduction in incisional SSI rates.[46] It remains to be determined whether NNIS-type stratification schemes can be used prospectively to target specific subgroups of patients who will benefit from the use of prophylactic antibiotic and/or specific wound management techniques. One clear example based on cogent data from clinical trials is that class III wounds in healthy patients undergoing appendectomy for perforated or gangrenous appendicitis can be primarily closed as long as antibiotic therapy directed against aerobes and anaerobes is administered. This practice leads to SSI rates of approximately 3 to 4%.[47]

Recent investigations have studied the effect of additional maneuvers in an attempt to further reduce the rate of SSIs. The adverse effects of hyperglycemia on WBC function have been well described.[48] A number of recent studies have reported the effects of hyperglycemia in vivo in diabetic patients, with increased SSI rates being associated with hyperglycemia in cardiac surgery patients

undergoing bypass.[49,50] On this basis, it is recommended that clinicians maintain appropriate blood sugar control in diabetic patients in the perioperative period to minimize the occurrence of SSIs.

The effects of the level of inhaled oxygen and prewarming of the wound on SSI rates also have been studied. Although an initial study provided evidence that patients who received high levels of inhaled oxygen during colorectal surgery developed fewer SSIs,[51] data to the contrary recently have been reported.[52,53] In another study, preoperative warming of the wound site for 30 minutes before surgery among patients undergoing clean surgery was associated with a decrease in SSIs (5% with warmed wounds vs. 14% without).[54] Unfortunately, several of the aforementioned studies report SSI rates among study patients that are higher than those reported and expected among similar groups of patients, making comparison difficult. Of note, stratification using the NNIS classification methodology was not used. Further evaluation via multicenter studies is needed before implementation of these modalities as standard therapies.

Effective therapy for incisional SSIs consists solely of incision and drainage without the addition of antibiotics. Antibiotic therapy is reserved for patients in whom evidence of significant cellulitis is present, or who manifest concurrent SIRS. The open wound often is allowed to heal by secondary intention, with dressings being changed twice a day. The use of topical antibiotics and antiseptics to further wound healing remains unproven, although anecdotal studies indicate their potential utility in complex wounds that do not heal with routine measures.[55] Despite a paucity of prospective studies,[56] vacuum-assisted closure is increasingly used in management of problem wounds and can be applied to complex wounds in difficult locations (Fig. 6-2). Although culture results are of epidemiologic interest, they rarely serve to direct therapy because antibiotics are not routinely withheld until results are known. The treatment of organ/space infections is discussed in Intra-Abdominal Infections, below.

Intra-Abdominal Infections

Microbial contamination of the peritoneal cavity is termed *peritonitis* or *intra-abdominal infection*, and is classified according to etiology. *Primary microbial peritonitis* occurs when microbes invade the normally sterile confines of the peritoneal cavity via hematogenous dissemination from a distant source of infection or direct inoculation. This process is more common among patients who retain large amounts of peritoneal fluid due to ascites, and in those individuals who are being treated for renal failure via peritoneal dialysis. These infections invariably are monomicrobial and rarely require surgical intervention. The diagnosis is established based on a patient who has ascites for medical reasons, physical examination that reveals diffuse tenderness and guarding without localized findings, absence of pneumoperitoneum on abdominal flat plate and upright roentgenograms, the presence of more than 100 WBCs/mL, and microbes with a single morphology on Gram's stain performed on fluid obtained via paracentesis. Subsequent cultures will typically demonstrate the presence of gram-positive organisms in patients receiving peritoneal dialysis. In patients without this risk factor organisms can include *E. coli*, *K. pneumo-*

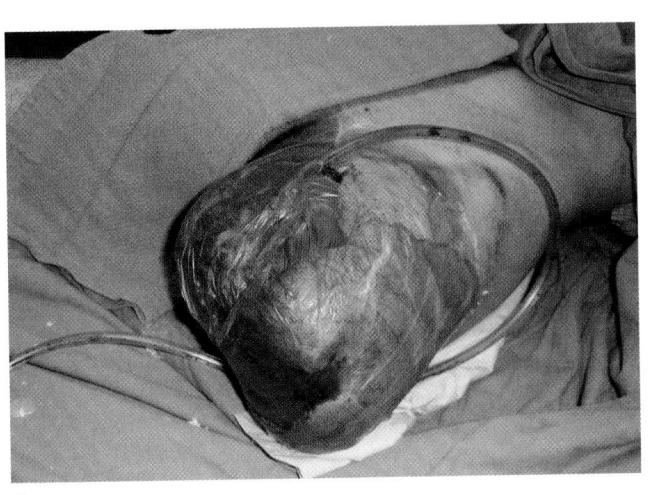
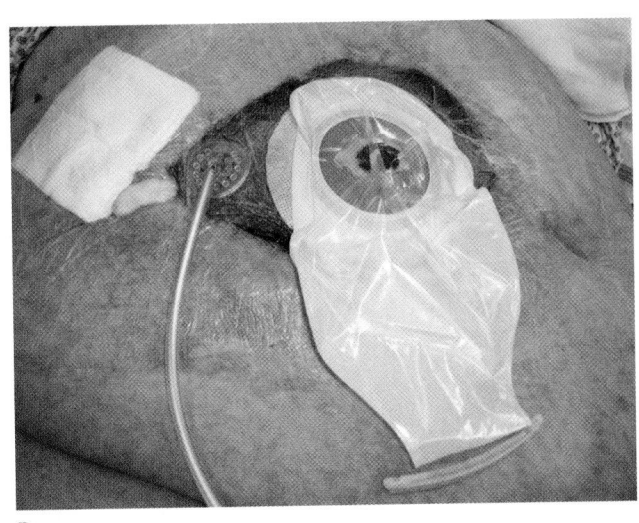

FIG. 6-2. Negative pressure wound therapy in a patient after amputation for wet gangrene (**A**), and in a patient with enterocutaneous fistula (**B**). It is possible to adapt these dressings to fit difficult anatomy and provide appropriate wound care while reducing frequency of dressing change. It is important to evaluate the wound under these dressings if patient demonstrates signs of sepsis with an unidentified source, because typical clues of wound sepsis, such as odor and drainage, are hidden by the suction apparatus.

niae, pneumococci, and others, although many different pathogens can be causative. Treatment consists of administration of an antibiotic to which the organism is sensitive; often 14 to 21 days of therapy are required. Removal of indwelling devices (e.g., peritoneal dialysis catheter or peritoneovenous shunt) may be required for effective therapy of recurrent infections.

Secondary microbial peritonitis occurs subsequent to contamination of the peritoneal cavity due to perforation or severe inflammation and infection of an intra-abdominal organ. Examples include appendicitis, perforation of any portion of the GI tract, or diverticulitis. As noted previously in Source Control, effective therapy requires source control to resect or repair the diseased organ; débridement of necrotic, infected tissue and debris; and administration of antimicrobial agents directed against aerobes and anaerobes.[57] This type of antibiotic regimen should be chosen because in most patients the precise diagnosis cannot be established until exploratory laparotomy is performed, and the most morbid form of this disease process is colonic perforation, due to the large number of microbes present. A combination of agents or single agents with a broad spectrum of activity can be used for this purpose; conversion of a parenteral to an oral regimen when the patient's ileus resolves will provide results similar to those achieved with IV antibiotics.[58] Effective source control and antibiotic therapy is associated with low failure rates and a mortality rate of approximately 5 to 6%; inability to control the source of infection leads to mortality greater than 40%.[59]

The response rate to effective source control and use of appropriate antibiotics has remained approximately 70 to 90% over the past several decades.[24,60] Patients in whom standard therapy fails develop an intra-abdominal abscess, leakage from a GI anastomosis leading to postoperative peritonitis, or *tertiary (persistent) peritonitis*. The latter is a poorly understood entity that is more common in immunosuppressed patients in whom peritoneal host defenses do not effectively clear or sequester the initial secondary microbial peritoneal infection. Microbes such as *E. faecalis* and *faecium*, *S. epidermidis*, *C. albicans*, and *P. aeruginosa* can be identified, typically in combination, and may be selected based on their lack of responsiveness to the initial antibiotic regimen, coupled with diminished activity of host defenses. Unfortunately, even with effective antimicrobial agent therapy, this disease process is associated with mortality rates in excess of 50%.[61,62]

Formerly, the presence of an intra-abdominal abscess mandated surgical re-exploration and drainage. Today, the vast majority of

such abscesses can be effectively diagnosed via abdominal computed tomographic (CT) imaging techniques and drained percutaneously. Surgical intervention is reserved for those individuals who harbor multiple abscesses, those with abscesses in proximity to vital structures such that percutaneous drainage would be hazardous, and those in whom an ongoing source of contamination (e.g., enteric leak) is identified. The necessity of antimicrobial agent therapy and precise guidelines that dictate duration of catheter drainage have not been established. A short course (3 to 7 days) of antibiotics that possess aerobic and anaerobic activity seems reasonable, and most practitioners leave the drainage catheter in situ until it is clear that cavity collapse has occurred, output is less than 10 to 20 mL/d, no evidence of an ongoing source of contamination is present, and the patient's clinical condition has improved.

Organ-Specific Infections

Hepatic abscesses are rare, currently accounting for approximately 15 per 100,000 hospital admissions in the United States. Pyogenic abscesses account for approximately 80% of cases, the remaining 20% being equally divided among parasitic and fungal forms.[63] Formerly, pyogenic liver abscesses were caused by pylephlebitis due to neglected appendicitis or diverticulitis. Today, manipulation of the biliary tract to treat a variety of diseases has become a more common cause, although in nearly 50% of patients no cause is identified. The most common aerobic bacteria identified in recent series include *E. coli*, *K. pneumoniae*, and other enteric bacilli, enterococci, and *Pseudomonas* spp., while the most common anaerobic bacteria are *Bacteroides* spp., anaerobic streptococci, and *Fusobacterium* spp. *C. albicans* and other similar yeasts cause the majority of fungal hepatic abscesses. Small (<1 cm), multiple abscesses should be sampled and treated with a 4- to 6-week course of antibiotics. Larger abscesses invariably are amenable to percutaneous drainage, with parameters for antibiotic therapy and drain removal similar to those mentioned above in Intra-Abdominal Infections. Splenic abscesses are extremely rare and are treated in a similar fashion. Recurrent hepatic or splenic abscesses may require operative intervention—unroofing and marsupialization or splenectomy, respectively.

Secondary pancreatic infections (e.g., infected pancreatic necrosis or pancreatic abscess) occur in approximately 10 to 15% of patients who develop severe pancreatitis with necrosis. The surgical treatment of this disorder was pioneered by Bradley and Allen, who

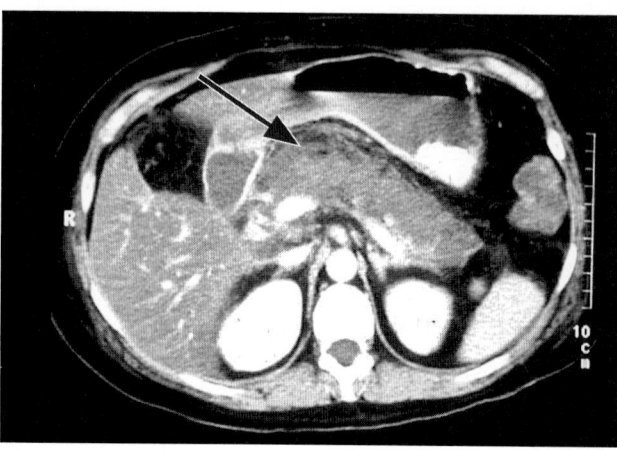

FIG. 6-3. Contrast-enhanced computed tomographic scan of pancreas with severe pancreatic necrosis. Note lack of IV contrast within the boggy pancreatic bed (*large black arrow*).

noted significant improvements in outcome for patients undergoing repeated pancreatic débridement of infected pancreatic necrosis.[64] Current care of patients with severe acute pancreatitis includes staging with dynamic, contrast-enhanced helical CT scan with 3-mm tomographs to determine the extent of pancreatic necrosis, coupled with the use of one of several prognostic scoring systems. Patients who exhibit significant pancreatic necrosis (grade greater than C, Fig. 6-3) should be carefully monitored in the ICU and undergo follow-up CT examination. A recent change in practice has been the elimination of the routine use of prophylactic antibiotics for prevention of infected pancreatic necrosis. Early results were promising;[65] however, several randomized multicenter trials have failed to show benefit and three meta-analyses have confirmed this finding.[66–68]

In two small studies, enteral feedings initiated early, using nasojejunal feeding tubes placed past the ligament of Treitz, have been associated with decreased development of infected pancreatic necrosis, possibly due to a decrease in gut translocation of bacteria. Recent guidelines support the practice of enteral alimentation in these patients, with the addition of parenteral nutrition if nutritional goals cannot be met by tube feeding alone.[69,70]

The presence of secondary pancreatic infection should be suspected in patients whose systemic inflammatory response (fever, elevated WBC count, or organ dysfunction) fails to resolve, or in those individuals who initially recuperate, only to develop sepsis syndrome 2 to 3 weeks later. CT-guided aspiration of fluid from the pancreatic bed for performance of Gram's stain and culture analysis is of critical importance. A positive Gram's stain or culture from CT-guided aspiration, or identification of gas within the pancreas on CT scan, mandate operative intervention.

Surgery for secondary pancreatic infection is designed to remove the infected inflammatory focus. It is the practice of the authors to expose the pancreatic bed through a transverse incision in the abdominal wall and lesser sac (Fig. 6-4). A jejunal feeding tube, gastrostomy tube, and cholecystectomy (if indicated) are all performed at the index operation if patient condition permits. The gastrocolic omentum is tacked to the abdominal wall on the peritoneal edges of the wound to sequester the intestines from the inflammatory process. After initial gentle débridement of necrotic tissue, the pancreatic bed is packed with gauze dressings and the abdomen closed temporarily with a permanent mesh or packed open. This mesh allows repeated reoperations without damage to the remaining fascia. In a similar fashion to surgery for necrotizing soft tissue infection, the surgeon should plan on scheduled relaparotomy and undertake débridement until necrotic tissue and purulence are absent and granulation tissue forms. Approximately 20 to 25% of patients will develop a GI fistula, which either heals or is amenable to surgical repair after resolution of the pancreatic infection. The laparoscopic approach to débridement first described in 1996 has been described using various techniqes.[71,72]

Infections of the Skin and Soft Tissue

Infections of the skin and soft tissue can be classified according to whether surgical intervention is required. For example, superficial skin and skin structure infections, such as cellulitis, erysipelas, and lymphangitis, invariably are effectively treated with antibiotics alone, although a search for a local source of infection should be undertaken. Generally, drugs that possess activity against the gram-positive skin microflora that are causative are selected. Furuncles or boils may drain spontaneously or require surgical incision and drainage.

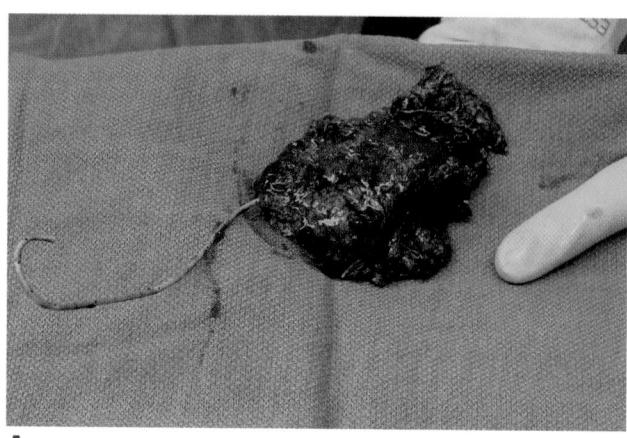

A

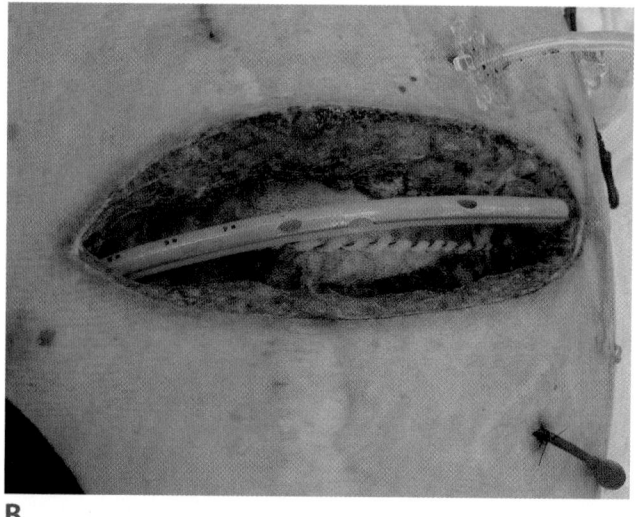

B

FIG. 6-4. Infected pancreatic necrosis. **A.** Necrosectomy specimen with pancreatic stent in situ. It is important to gently débride only necrotic pancreatic tissue, relying on repeated operation to ensure complete removal. **B.** Typical incision for infected pancreatic necrosis. Polypropylene mesh has been secured to fascia and is used for re-entry into the pancreatic bed. Note gastrostomy and feeding jejunostomy tubes. The chest tube in the wound is placed to allow closed continuous suction.

Antibiotics are prescribed if significant cellulitis is present or if cellulitis does not rapidly resolve after surgical drainage. Commonly acquired methicillin-resistant *S. aureus* infection should be suspected if infection persists after treatment with adequate drainage and antibiotics. These infections may require more aggressive drainage and altered antimicrobial therapy.[73]

Aggressive soft tissue infections are rare, difficult to diagnose, and require immediate surgical intervention plus administration of antimicrobial agents. Failure to do so results in an extremely high mortality rate (approximately 80 to 100%), and even with rapid recognition and intervention, current mortality rates remain high, approximately 16 to 25%.[74,75] Eponyms and classification in the past have been a hodgepodge of terminology, such as Meleney's synergistic gangrene, rapidly spreading cellulitis, gas gangrene, and necrotizing fasciitis, among others. Today, it seems best to delineate these serious infections based on the soft tissue layer(s) of involvement (e.g., skin and superficial soft tissue, deep soft tissue, and muscle) and the pathogen(s) that causes them.[76]

Patients at risk for these types of infections include those who are elderly, immunosuppressed, or diabetic; those who suffer from peripheral vascular disease; or those with a combination of these factors. The common thread among these host factors appears to be compromise of the fascial blood supply to some degree, and if this is coupled with the introduction of exogenous microbes, the result can be devastating. However, it is of note that over the last decade, extremely aggressive necrotizing soft tissue infections among healthy individuals due to streptococci have been described as well.

Initially, the diagnosis is established solely upon a constellation of clinical findings, not all of which are present in every patient. Not surprisingly, patients often develop sepsis syndrome or septic shock without an obvious cause. The extremities, perineum, and torso are most commonly affected, in that order. Careful examination should be undertaken for an entry site such as a small break or sinus in the skin from which grayish, turbid semipurulent material ("dishwater pus") can be expressed, as well as for the presence of skin changes (bronze hue or brawny induration), blebs, or crepitus. The patient often develops pain at the site of infection that appears to be out of proportion to any of the physical manifestations. Any of these findings mandates immediate surgical intervention, which should consist of exposure and direct visualization of potentially infected tissue (including deep soft tissue, fascia, and underlying muscle) and radical resection of affected areas. Radiologic studies should be undertaken only in patients in whom the diagnosis is not seriously considered, as they delay surgical intervention and frequently provide confusing information. Unfortunately, surgical extirpation of infected tissue frequently entails amputation and/or disfiguring procedures; however, incomplete procedures are associated with higher rates of morbidity and mortality (Fig. 6-5).

During the procedure, a Gram's stain should be performed on tissue fluid. Antimicrobial agents directed against gram-positive and gram-negative aerobes and anaerobes (e.g., vancomycin plus a carbapenem), as well as high-dose aqueous penicillin G (16,000 to 20,000 U/d), the latter to treat clostridial pathogens, should be administered. Approximately 50% of such infections are polymicrobial, the remainder being caused by a single organism such as *S. pyogenes*, *P. aeruginosa*, or *C. perfringens*. The microbiology of these polymicrobial infections is similar to that of secondary microbial peritonitis, with the exception that gram-positive cocci are more commonly encountered. Most should be returned to the operating room on a scheduled basis to determine if disease progression has occurred. If so, additional resection of infected tissue and débridement should take place. Antibiotic therapy can be refined based on culture and sensitivity results, particularly in the case of monomicrobial soft tissue infections. Adjunctive treatments, including treatment with hyperbaric oxygen or IV Ig, have been described with contradictory results. Hyperbaric oxygen therapy should be strongly considered in patients with infection caused by gas-forming organisms (e.g., *C. perfringens*). It may be reasonable to consider IV Ig in patients with group A streptococcal infection with toxic shock syndrome and in those patients with a high risk of death, such as the elderly or those with hypotension or bacteremia.[77]

Postoperative Nosocomial Infections

Surgical patients are prone to develop a wide variety of nosocomial infections during the postoperative period, which include SSIs, UTIs, pneumonia, and bacteremic episodes.[78] SSIs are discussed above in Surgical Site Infections, and the latter types of nosocomial infections are related to prolonged use of indwelling tubes and catheters for the purpose of urinary drainage, ventilation, and venous and arterial access, respectively.

The presence of a postoperative UTI should be considered based on urinalysis demonstrating WBCs or bacteria, a positive test for leukocyte esterase, or a combination of these elements. The diagnosis is established after more than 10^4 CFU/mL of microbes are identified by culture techniques in symptomatic patients, or more than 10^5 CFU/mL in asymptomatic individuals. Treatment for 3 to 5 days with a single antibiotic that achieves high levels in the urine is appropriate. Postoperative surgical patients should have indwelling urinary catheters removed as quickly as possible, typically within 1 to 2 days, as long as they are mobile.

Prolonged mechanical ventilation is associated with an increased incidence of pneumonia, and is frequently due to pathogens common in the nosocomial environment.[79] Frequently these organisms are highly resistant to many different agents.[80] The diagnosis of hospital-acquired pneumonia should be made using the presence of a purulent sputum, elevated leukocyte count, fever, and new chest x-ray abnormality. The presence of two of the clinical findings, plus chest x-ray findings, significantly increases the likelihood of ventilator-associated pneumonia.[81] Consideration should be given to performing bronchoalveolar lavage to obtain samples to assess by Gram's stain and obtaining a culture to assess for the presence of microbes. Surgical patients should be weaned from mechanical ventilation as soon as feasible, based on oxygenation and inspiratory effort.

Infection associated with indwelling intravascular catheters has become a common problem among hospitalized patients. Because of the complexity of many surgical procedures, these devices are increasingly used for physiologic monitoring, vascular access, drug delivery, and hyperalimentation. Among the several million catheters inserted each year in the United States, approximately 25% will become colonized, and approximately 5% will be associated with bacteremia. Duration of catheterization, insertion or manipulation under emergency or nonsterile conditions, use for hyperalimentation, and perhaps the use of multilumen catheters increase the risk of infection. Although no randomized trials have been performed, peripherally inserted central venous catheters have a similar catheter-related infection rate.[82]

Many patients who develop intravascular catheter infections are asymptomatic, often exhibiting an elevation in the blood WBC count. Blood cultures obtained from a peripheral site and drawn through the catheter that reveal the presence of the same organism increase the index of suspicion for the presence of a catheter infection. Obvious purulence at the exit site of the skin tunnel, severe sepsis syndrome due to any type of organism when other potential causes have been excluded, or bacteremia due to gram-negative aerobes or fungi should lead to catheter removal. Selected catheter infections due to low-virulence microbes such as *S. epidermidis* can be effectively treated in approximately 50 to 60% of patients with a 14- to 21-day course of an antibiotic, which should be considered when no other vascular access site exists.[83] The use of antibiotic-bonded catheters is associated with lower rates of colonization.[84] Routine, scheduled catheter changes over a guidewire are associated with slightly lower rates of infection, but an increase in the insertion-related complication rate.[85] The surgeon should carefully consider the need for any type of vascular access device, rigorously attend to

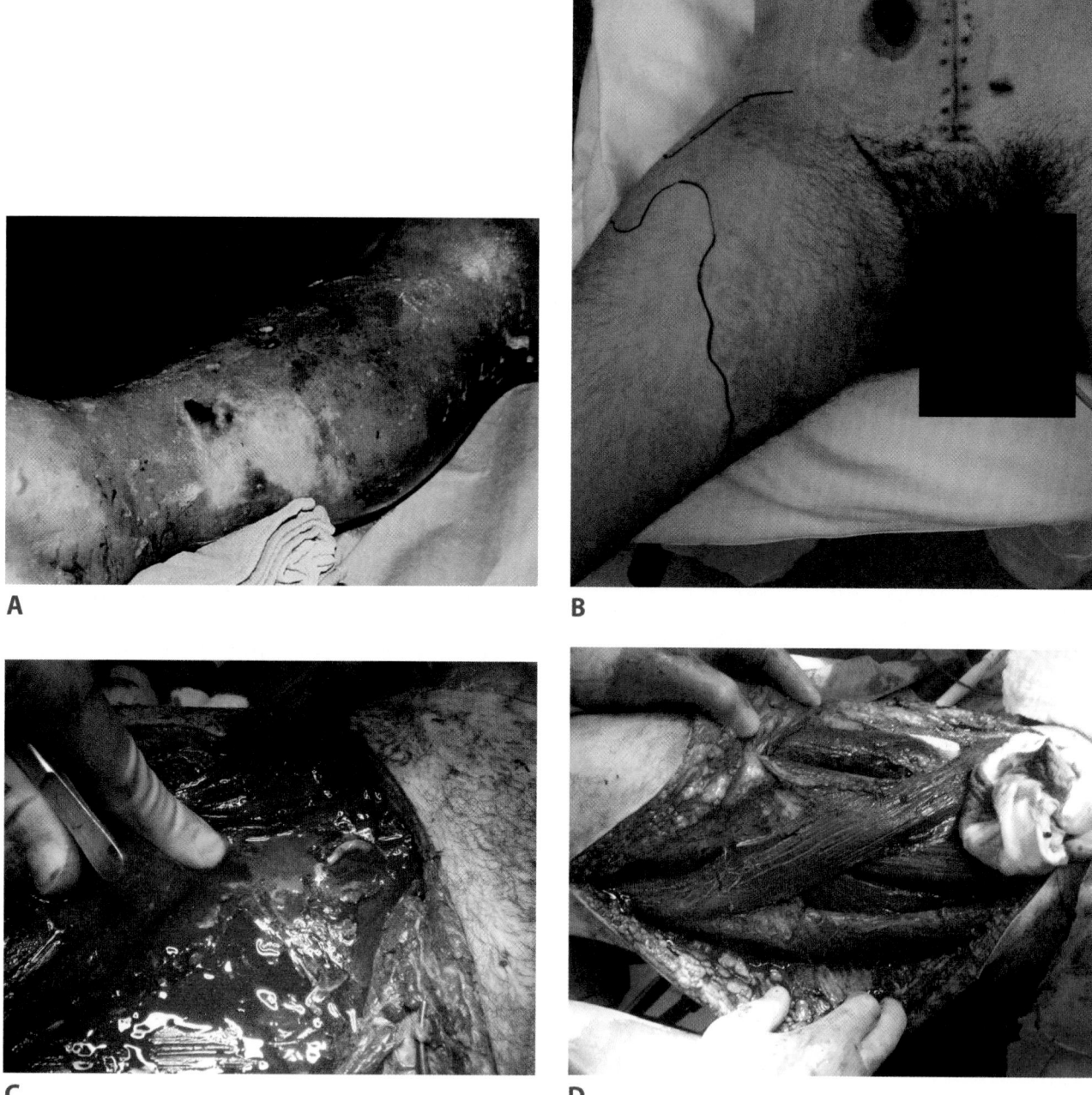

FIG. 6-5. Necrotizing soft tissue infection. **A.** This patient presented with hypotension due to severe late necrotizing fasciitis and myositis due to beta-hemolytic streptococcal infection. The patient succumbed to his disease after 16 hours despite aggressive débridement. **B.** This patient presented with spreading cellulites and pain on motion of his right hip 2 weeks after total colectomy. Cellulitis on right anterior thigh is outlined. **C.** Classic dishwater edema of tissues with necrotic fascia. **D.** Right lower extremity after débridement of fascia to viable muscle.

their maintenance to prevent infection, and remove them as quickly as possible. Use of antibacterial or antifungal agents to prevent catheter infection is of no utility and is contraindicated.

Sepsis

Severe sepsis is increasing in incidence, with over 750,000 cases estimated per year in the United States. This rate is expected to increase as the population of aged in the United States increases. The treatment of sepsis has improved dramatically over the last decade, with mortality rates dropping to under 30%.[86] Factors contributing

to this improvement in mortality relate both to recent randomized prospective trials demonstrating improved outcomes with new therapies, and to improvements in the process of care delivery to the sepsis patient. The "Surviving Sepsis Campaign," a multidisciplinary group that worked to develop treatment recommendations, has published guidelines incorporating evidence-based treatment strategies most recently in 2008.[87] These guidelines are summarized in Table 6-10.

Patients presenting with severe sepsis should receive resuscitation fluids to a central venous pressure target of 8 to 12 mmHg, with a goal of mean arterial pressure of 65 mmHg or greater and urine

TABLE 6-10	Summary of Surviving Sepsis Campaign guidelines

Initial evaluation and infection issues

Initial resuscitation: Begin resuscitation immediately in patients with hypotension or elevated serum lactate with resuscitation goal of CVP 8–12 mmHg, mean arterial pressure of ≥65 mmHg, and urine output of ≥0.5 mL/kg per hour.

Diagnosis: Obtain appropriate cultures before antibiotics but do not delay antibiotic therapy.

Antibiotic therapy: Begin IV antibiotic therapy as early as possible: Should be within the first hour after recognition of severe sepsis/septic shock; use broad-spectrum antibiotic regimen with penetration into presumed source; reassess regimen daily; discontinue antibiotics in 7–10 d for most infections; stop antibiotics for noninfectious issues.

Source control: Establish anatomic site of infection as rapidly as possible, implement source control measures as soon as possible after initial resuscitation. Remove intravascular access devices if potentially infected.

Hemodynamic support and adjunctive therapy

Fluid therapy: Fluid resuscitate using crystalloid or colloid, using fluid volumes of 1000 mL (crystalloid), target CVP of 8–12 mmHg.

Vasopressors/inotropic therapy: Maintain MAP of ≥65 mmHg; centrally administered norepinephrine or dopamine are first-line choices; dopamine should not be used for "renal protection"; insert arterial catheters for patients requiring vasopressors. Do not increase cardiac index to predetermined supranormal levels.

Steroids: Consider IV hydrocortisone (dose ≤300 mg/d) for adult septic shock when hypotension responds poorly to fluids and vasopressors.

Recombinant human activated protein C: Consider rhAPC in adult patients with sepsis-induced organ dysfunction and high risk of death if there are no contraindications.

Other supportive therapy

Blood product administration: Transfuse red blood cells when hemoglobin decreases to <7.0 g/dL.

Mechanical ventilation: Target an initial tidal volume of 6 mL/kg body weight and plateau pressure of ≤30 cm H_2O in patients with acute lung injury. Use PEEP to avoid lung collapse. Use a weaning protocol to evaluate the potential for discontinuing mechanical ventilation. Pulmonary artery catheter is not indicated for routine monitoring.

Glucose control: Use IV insulin to control hyperglycemia in patients with severe sepsis.

Prophylaxis: Use stress ulcer (proton pump inhibitor or H_2 blocker) and deep venous thrombosis (low-dose unfractionated or fractionated heparin) prophylaxis.

Limitation of support: Discuss advance care planning with patients and families and set realistic expectations.

CVP = central venous pressure; MAP = mean arterial pressure; PEEP = positive end-expiratory pressure; rhAPC = recombinant human activated protein C.
Source: Reproduced with permission from Dellinger et al.[87]

output of 0.5 mL/kg per hour or greater. Delaying this resuscitative step for as little as 3 hours until arrival in the ICU has been shown to result in poor outcome.[88] Typically, this goal necessitates early placement of central venous catheter.

A number of studies have demonstrated the importance of early empiric antibiotic therapy in patients who develop sepsis or nosocomial infection. This therapy should be initiated as soon as possible with broad-spectrum antibiotics directed against most likely organisms, because early appropriate antibiotic therapy has been associated with significant reductions in mortality,[89,90] and delays in appropriate antibiotic administration are associated with increased mortality.[91] Use of institutional and unit specific sensitivity patterns are critical in selecting an appropriate agent for patients with nosocomial infection. It is key, however, to obtain cultures of appropriate areas without delaying initiating antibiotics so that appropriate adjustment of antibiotic therapy can take place when culture results return.

Additionally, early identification and treatment of septic sources is key for improved outcomes in patients with sepsis. Although there are no randomized trials demonstrating this concept, repeated evidence in series including intra-abdominal infection, necrotizing soft tissue infection, and others demonstrate increased mortality with delayed treatment. A possible exception is that of infected pancreatic necrosis.

Multiple trials have evaluated the use of vasopressors and inotropes for treatment of septic shock. Current suggestions for first-line agents based on effects on splanchnic perfusion include norepinephrine, dopamine, and vasopressin.[92,93] It is important to titrate therapy based on other parameters such as mixed venous oxygen saturation and plasma lactate levels as well as mean arterial pressure to reduce the risk of vasopressor-induced perfusion deficits. Several recent randomized trials have failed to demonstrate benefit with use of pulmonary arterial catheterization, leading to a significant decrease in its use.

A number of other adjunctive therapies are useful in treatment of the patient with severe sepsis and septic shock. Corticosteroids, first evaluated unsuccessfully in the 1980s for treatment of sepsis (high dose), have recently been reintroduced to the armamentarium of the practitioner after the observation that many patients with septic shock have a relative adrenal insufficiency. Low-dose corticosteroids (hydrocortisone at 300 mg/d or less) can be used in patients with septic shock who are not responsive to fluids and vasopressors. However, a recent randomized trial failed to show survival benefit. Recombinant human activated protein C (drotrecogin alfa, Xigris) has been associated with significant survival benefit in patients with severe sepsis and at least one organ failure.[94] In surgical patients, this therapy should be reserved for patients with at least two organ failures or for patients with septic shock. Patients with acute lung injury associated with sepsis should receive mechanical ventilation with tidal volumes of 6 mL/kg and pulmonary airway plateau pressures of 30 cm H_2O or less. Finally, red blood cell transfusion should be reserved for patients with hemoglobin of less than 7 g/dL, with a more liberal transfusion strategy reserved for those patients with severe coronary artery disease, ongoing blood loss, or severe hypoxemia.

Blood-Borne Pathogens

Although alarming to contemplate, the risk of HIV transmission from patient to surgeon is low. By December 31, 2001, there had been six cases of surgeons with HIV seroconversion from a possible occupational exposure, from a total of 469,850 HIV cases to that date reported to the Centers for Disease Control and Prevention. Of the groups of health care workers with likely occupationally acquired HIV infection (n = 195), surgeons were one of the lower risk groups (compared to nurses at 59 cases and nonsurgeon physicians at 18 cases).[95] Transmission of HIV (and other infections spread by blood and body fluid) from patient to health care worker can be minimized by observation of universal precautions, which include the following: (a) routine use of barriers (such as gloves and/or goggles) when anticipating contact with blood or body fluids, (b) washing of hands and other skin surfaces immediately after contact with blood or body fluids, and (c) careful handling and disposal of sharp instruments during and after use. The current estimate of the risk of transmission is 0.3% after needlestick.

Postexposure prophylaxis for HIV has significantly decreased the risk of seroconversion for health care workers with occupational exposure to HIV. Steps to initiate postexposure prophylaxis should be initiated within hours rather than days for the most effective preventive therapy. Postexposure prophylaxis with a two- or three-drug regimen should be initiated for health care workers with significant exposure to patients with an HIV-positive status. If a patient's HIV status is unknown, it may be advisable to begin postexposure prophylaxis while testing is carried out, particularly if the patient is at high risk for infection due to HIV (e.g., IV narcotic use). Generally, postexposure prophylaxis is not warranted for exposure to sources with unknown status, such as deceased persons or needles from a sharps container.

The risks for surgeons of acquiring HIV infection have recently been evaluated by Goldberg and coauthors.[96] They noted that the risks are related to the prevalence of HIV infection in the population being cared for, the probability of transmission from a percutaneous injury suffered while caring for an infected patient, the number of such injuries sustained, and the use of postexposure prophylaxis. Annual calculated risks in Glasgow, Scotland, ranged from one in 200,000 for general surgeons not utilizing postexposure prophylaxis to as low as one in 10,000,000 with use of routine postexposure prophylaxis after significant exposures.

Hepatitis B virus (HBV) is a DNA virus that affects only humans. Primary infection with HBV generally is self-limited (~6% of those infected are over 5 years of age), but can progress to a chronic carrier state. Death from chronic liver disease or hepatocellular cancer occurs in roughly 30% of chronically infected persons. Surgeons and other health care workers are at high risk for this blood-borne infection and should receive the HBV vaccine; children are routinely vaccinated in the United States.[97] This vaccine has contributed to a significant decline in the number of new cases of HBV per year in the United States, from approximately 27,000 new cases in 1984 to 4700 new cases in 2006.[98] In the postexposure setting, hepatitis B immune globulin confers approximately 75% protection from HBV infection.[99]

Hepatitis C virus (HCV), previously known as non-A, non-B hepatitis, is a RNA flavivirus first identified specifically in the late 1980s. This virus is confined to humans and chimpanzees. A chronic carrier state develops in 75 to 80% of patients with the infection, with chronic liver disease occurring in three fourths of patients developing chronic infection. The number of new infections per year has declined since the 1980s due to the incorporation of testing of the blood supply for this virus. Fortunately, HCV virus is not transmitted efficiently through occupational exposures to blood, with the seroconversion rate after accidental needlestick reported to be approximately 2%.[100] To date, a vaccine to prevent HCV infection has not been developed. Experimental studies in chimpanzees with HCV Ig using a model of needlestick injury have failed to demonstrate a protective effect of this treatment in seroconversion after exposure, and no effective antiviral agents for postexposure prophylaxis are available. Early treatment of infection with INF-γ has been considered; however, this exposes patients who may not develop HCV infection–related sequelae to the side effects of this drug.[101]

BIOLOGIC WARFARE AGENTS

Several infectious organisms have been studied by the United States and the former Soviet Union and presumably other entities for potential use as biologic weapons. Programs involving biologic agents in the United States were halted by presidential decree in 1971. However, concern remains that these agents could be used by rogue states or terrorist organizations as alternatives to nuclear weapons as weapons of mass destruction, as they are relatively inexpensive to make in terms of infrastructure development. If so, all physicians including surgeons would need to familiarize themselves with the manifestations of infection due to these pathogens. The typical agent is selected for the ability to be spread via the inhalational route, as this is the most efficient mode of mass exposure. Some potential agents are discussed in the *Bacillus anthracis* (Anthrax), *Yersinia pestis* (Plague), Smallpox, and *Francisella tularensis* (Tularemia) sections that follow.

Bacillus anthracis (Anthrax)

Anthrax is a zoonotic disease occurring in domesticated and wild herbivores. The first identification of inhalational anthrax as a disease occurred among woolsorters in England in the late 1800s. The largest recent epidemic of inhalational anthrax occurred in Sverdlovsk, Russia, in 1979 after accidental release of anthrax spores from a military facility. Inhalational anthrax develops after a 1- to 6-day incubation period, with nonspecific symptoms including malaise, myalgia, and fever. Over a short period of time, these symptoms worsen, with development of respiratory distress, chest pain, and diaphoresis. Characteristic chest roentgenographic findings include a widened mediastinum and pleural effusions. A key aspect in establishing the diagnosis is eliciting an exposure history. Rapid antigen tests are currently under development for identification of this gram-positive rod. Drugs such as cephalosporins and trimethoprim-sulfamethoxazole are not active against this agent. Postexposure prophylaxis consists of administration of either ciprofloxacin or doxycycline.[102] If an isolate is demonstrated to be penicillin-sensitive, the patient should be switched to amoxicillin. Inhalational exposure followed by the development of symptoms is associated with a high mortality rate. Treatment options include combination therapy with ciprofloxacin, clindamycin, and rifampin, with clindamycin added to block production of toxin, and rifampin for its ability to penetrate the central nervous system and intracellular locations.

Yersinia pestis (Plague)

Plague is caused by the gram-negative organism *Yersinia pestis*. The naturally occurring disease in humans is transmitted via flea bites from rodents. It was the first biologic warfare agent, and was used in the Crimean city of Caffa by the Tartar army, whose soldiers catapulted bodies of plague victims at the Genoese. When plague is used as a biologic warfare agent, clinical manifestations include epidemic pneumonia with blood-tinged sputum if aerosolized bacteria were used, or bubonic plague if fleas were used as carriers. Individuals who develop a painful lesion termed a *bubo* associated with fever, severe malaise, and exposure to fleas should be suspected to have plague. Diagnosis is confirmed via aspirate of the bubo and a direct antibody stain to detect plague bacillus. Typical morphology for this organism is that of a bipolar safety-pin–shaped gram-negative organism. Postexposure prophylaxis for patients exposed to plague consists of doxycycline. Treatment of the pneumonic or bubonic/septicemic form includes administration of aminoglycosides, doxycycline, ciprofloxacin, and chloramphenicol.[103]

Smallpox

Variola, the causative agent of smallpox, was a major cause of infectious morbidity and mortality until its eradication in the late 1970s. During the European colonization of North America, British commanders may have used it against native inhabitants and the colonists by distribution of blankets from smallpox victims. Even in the absence of laboratory-preserved virus, the prolonged viability of variola virus has been demonstrated in scabs up to 13 years after collection; the potential for reverse genetic engineering using the known sequence of smallpox also makes it a potential biologic weapon.[104] This has resulted in the United States undertaking a vaccination program for key health care workers. Variola virus is highly infectious in the aerosolized form: After an incubation period of 10 to 12 days, clinical manifestations of malaise, fever, vomiting, and headache appear, followed by development of a characteristic centripetal rash (which is found to predominate on the face and extremities). The fatality rate may reach 30%. Postexposure prophylaxis with smallpox vaccine has been noted to be effective for up to 4 days postexposure. Cidofovir, an acyclic nucleoside phosphonate analogue, has demonstrated activity in animal models of poxvirus infections and may offer promise for the treatment of smallpox.[105]

Francisella tularensis (Tularemia)

The principal reservoir of this gram-negative aerobic organism is the tick. After inoculation, this organism proliferates within macrophages. This organism has been considered a potential bioterrorist threat due to a very high infectivity rate after aerosolization. Patients with tularemia pneumonia develop a cough and demonstrate pneumonia on chest roentgenogram. Enlarged lymph nodes are seen in approximately 85% of patients. The organism can be cultured from tissue samples, but this is difficult. Alternative diagnosis is based on acute-phase agglutination tests. Treatment of inhalational tularemia consists of administration of aminoglycosides or second-line agents such as doxycycline and ciprofloxacin.

REFERENCES

Entries highlighted in bright blue are key references.

1. Nuland SB: *The Doctors' Plague: Germs, Childbed Fever, and the Strange Story of Ignaz Semmelweis.* New York: WW Norton & Co., 2003, p 1.
2. Wangensteen OH, Wangensteen SD: Germ theory of infection and disease, in Wangensteen OH, Wangensteen SD: *The Rise of Surgery: From Empiric Craft to Scientific Discipline.* Minneapolis: University of Minnesota Press, 1978, p 387.
3. Rutkow E: Appendicitis: The quintessential American surgical disease. *Arch Surg* 133:1024, 1998.
4. Meleney F: Bacterial synergism in disease processes with confirmation of synergistic bacterial etiology of certain types of progressive gangrene of the abdominal wall. *Ann Surg* 94:961, 1931.
5. Altemeier WA: *Manual of Control of Infection in Surgical Patients.* Chicago: American College of Surgeons Press, 1976, p 1.
6. Bartlett JG: Intra-abdominal sepsis. *Med Clin North Am* 79:599, 1995.
7. Dunn DL, Simmons RL: The role of anaerobic bacteria in intra-abdominal infections. *Rev Infect Dis* 6:S139, 1984.
8. Osler W: *The Evolution of Modern Medicine.* New Haven, CT: Yale University Press, 1913, p 1.
9. Dunn DL: Autochthonous microflora of the gastrointestinal tract. *Perspect Colon Rectal Surg* 2:105, 1990.
10. Dunn DL, Meakins JL: Humoral immunity to infection and the complement system, in Howard RJ, Simmons RL, (eds): *Surgical Infectious Diseases*, 3rd ed. Norwalk, CT: Appleton & Lange, 1995, p 295.
11. Hack C, Aarden LA, Thijs LG: Role of cytokines in sepsis. *Adv Immuno* 66:101, 1997.
12. Levy MM, Fink MP, Marshall JC, et al: 2001 SCCM/ESICM/ACCP/ATS/SIS International Sepsis Definitions Conference. *Crit Care Med* 31:1250, 2003.
13. Dombrovskiy VY, Martin AA, Sunderram J, et al: Rapid increase in hospitalization and mortality rates for severe sepsis in the United States: A trend analysis from 1993 to 2003. *Crit Care Med* 35:1244, 2007.
14. Marshall JC, Cook DJ, Christou NV, et al: Multiple organ dysfunction score: A reliable descriptor of a complex clinical outcome. *Crit Care Med* 23:1638, 1995.
15. Ferreira FL, Bota DP, Bross A, et al: Serial evaluation of the SOFA score to predict outcome in critically ill patients. *JAMA* 286:1754, 2002.
16. Sauaia A, Moore FA, Moore EE, et al: Early risk factors for post injury multiple organ failure. *World J Surg* 20:392, 1996.
17. Valles J, Rello J, Ochagavia A, et al: Community-acquired bloodstream infection in critically ill patients. *Chest* 123:1615, 2003.
18. Esteban A, Frutos-Vivar F, Ferguson ND, et al: Sepsis incidence and outcome: Contrasting the intensive care unit with the hospital ward. *Crit Care Med* 35:1284, 2007.
19. Moreno RP, Metnitz V, Adler L, et al: Sepsis mortality prediction-based on predisposition, infection and response. *Intensive Care Med* 34:496, 2008.
20. Dunn DL: The biological rationale, in Schein M, Marshall JC (eds): *Source Control: A Guide to the Management of Surgical Infections.* New York: Springer-Verlag: 2003, p 9.
21. Rozycki GS, Tremblay L, Feliciano DV, et al: Three hundred consecutive emergent celiotomies in general surgery patients: Influence of advanced diagnostic imaging techniques and procedures on diagnosis. *Ann Surg* 235:681, 2002.
22. Cappendijk VC, Hazebroek FW: The impact of diagnostic delay on the course of acute appendicitis. *Arch Dis Child* 83:64, 2000.
23. Lee SL, Walsh AJ, Ho HS: Computed tomography and ultrasonography do not improve and may delay the diagnosis and treatment of acute appendicitis. *Arch Surg* 136:556, 2001.
24. Solomkin JS, Meakins JL Jr., Allo MD, et al: Antibiotic trials in intra-abdominal infections: A critical evaluation of study design and outcome reporting. *Ann Surg* 200:29, 1984.
25. Barie PS: Modern surgical antibiotic prophylaxis and therapy—less is more. *Surg Infect* 1:23, 2000.
26. Bossink AW, Groeneveld J, Hack CE, et al: Prediction of mortality in febrile medical patients: How useful are systemic inflammatory response syndrome and sepsis criteria? *Chest* 113:1533, 1998.
27. Hillier S, Roberts Z, Dunstan F, et al: Prior antibiotics and risk of antibiotic-resistant community-acquired urinary tract infection: A case-control study. *J Antimicrob Chemother* 60:92, 2007.
28. Chastre J, Wolff M, Fagon JY, et al: Comparison of 8 vs 15 days of antibiotic therapy for ventilator-associated pneumonia in adults: A randomized trial. *JAMA* 290:2588, 2003.
29. Bohnen JM. Duration of antibiotic treatment in surgical infections of the abdomen: Postoperative peritonitis. *Eur J Surg* 576:50, 1996.
30. Stone HH, Bourneuf AA, Stinson LD: Reliability of criteria for predicting persistent or recurrent sepsis. *Arch Surg* 120:17, 1985.
31. Park M, Markus P, Matesic D, et al: Safety and effectiveness of a preoperative allergy clinic in decreasing vancomycin use in patients with a history of penicillin allergy. *Ann Allergy Asthma Immunol* 97:681, 2006.
32. Turnidge J: Impact of antibiotic resistance on the treatment of sepsis. *Scand J Infect Dis* 35:677, 2003.
33. Nichols RL, Smith JW, Muzik AC, et al: Preventive antibiotic usage in traumatic thoracic injuries requiring closed tube thoracostomy. *Chest* 106:1493, 1994.
34. Gonzalez RP, Holevar MR: Role of prophylactic antibiotics for tube thoracostomy in chest trauma. *Am Surg* 64:617, 1998.
35. Mangram AJ, Horan TC, Pearson ML, et al: Guideline for prevention of surgical site infection, 1999. Hospital Infection Control Practices Advisory Committee. *Infect Control Hosp Epidemiol* 20:250, 1999.
36. Martone WJ, Nichols RL: Recognition, prevention, surveillance, and management of surgical site infections. *Clin Infect Dis* 33:S67, 2001.
37. Kobayashi M, Mohri Y, Inoue Y, et al: Continuous follow-up of surgical site infections for 30 days after colorectal surgery. *World J Surg* 32:1142, 2008.
38. Blumetti J, Luu M, Sarosi G, et al: Surgical site infections after colorectal surgery: Do risk factors vary depending on the type of infection considered? *Surgery* 142:704, 2007.
39. Konishi T, Watanabe T, Kishimoto J, et al: Elective colon and rectal surgery differ in risk factors for wound infection: Results of prospective surveillance. *Ann Surg* 244:758, 2006.
40. Weiss CA 3rd, Statz CL, Dahms RA, et al: Six years of surgical wound infection surveillance at a tertiary care center: Review of the microbiologic and epidemiological aspects of 20,007 wounds. *Arch Surg* 134:1041, 1999.
41. Roy MC, Herwaldt LA, Embrey R, et al: Does the Centers for Disease Control's NNIS system risk index stratify patients undergoing cardiothoracic operations by their risk of surgical-site infection? *Infect Control Hosp Epidemiol* 21:186, 2000.
42. Perencevich EN, Sands KE, Cosgrove SE, et al: Health and economic impact of surgical site infections diagnosed after hospital discharge. *Emerg Infect Dis* 9:196, 2003.
43. Page CP, Bohnen JM, Fletcher JR, et al: Antimicrobial prophylaxis for surgical wounds: Guidelines for clinical care. *Arch Surg* 128:79, 1993.
44. Bratzler DW, Houck PM: Surgical Infection Prevention Guidelines Writers Workgroup, et al: Antimicrobial prophylaxis for surgery: An advisory statement from the National Surgical Infection Prevention Project. *Clin Infect Dis* 38:1706, 2004.
45. Bratzler DW, Houck PM, Richards C, et al: Use of antimicrobial prophylaxis for major surgery: Baseline results from the National Surgical Infection Prevention Project. *Arch Surg* 140:174, 2005.
46. Cohn SM, Giannotti G, Ong AW, et al: Prospective randomized trial of two wound management strategies for dirty abdominal wounds. *Ann Surg* 233:409, 2001.
47. Margenthaler JA, Longo WE, Virgo KS, et al: Risk factors for adverse outcomes after the surgical treatment of appendicitis in adults. *Ann Surg* 238:59, 2003.

48. McManus LM, Bloodworth RC, Prihoda TJ, et al: Agonist-dependent failure of neutrophil function in diabetes correlates with extent of hyperglycemia. *J Leukoc Biol* 70:395, 2001.

49. Trick WE, Scheckler WE, Tokars JI, et al: Modifiable risk factors associated with deep sternal site infection after coronary artery bypass grafting. *J Thorac Cardiovasc Surg* 119:108, 2000.

50. Russo PL, Spellman DW: A new surgical-site infection risk index using risk factors identified by multivariate analysis for patients undergoing coronary artery bypass graft surgery. *Infect Control Hosp Epidemiol* 23:372, 2002.

51. Greif R, Akca O, Horn EP, et al: Supplemental perioperative oxygen to reduce the incidence of wound infection. *N Engl J Med* 342:161, 2000.

52. Pryor KO, Fahey TJ 3rd, Lien CA, et al: Surgical site infection and the routine use of perioperative hyperoxia in a general surgical population: A randomized controlled trial. *JAMA* 291:79, 2004.

53. Belda FJ, Aguilera L, Garcia de la Asuncion J, et al: Supplemental perioperative oxygen and the risk of surgical wound infection: A randomized controlled trial. *JAMA* 294:2035, 2005.

54. Melling AC, Ali B, Scott EM, et al: Effects of preoperative warming on the incidence of wound infection after clean surgery: A randomized controlled trial. *Lancet* 358:876, 2001.

55. Grubbs BC, Statz CL, Johnson EM, et al: Salvage therapy of open, infected surgical wounds: A retrospective review using Techni-Care. *Surg Infect* 1:109, 2000.

56. Gregor S, Maegele M, Sauerland S, et al: Negative pressure wound therapy: A vacuum of evidence? *Arch Surg* 143:189, 2008.

57. Solomkin JS, Mazuski JE, Baron EJ, et al: Infectious Diseases Society of America: Guidelines for the selection of anti-infective agents for complicated intra-abdominal infections. *Clin Infect Dis* 37:997, 2003.

58. Solomkin JS, Reinhart HH, Dellinger EP, et al: Results of a randomized trial comparing sequential intravenous/oral treatment with ciprofloxacin plus metronidazole to imipenem/cilastatin for intra-abdominal infections. The Intra-Abdominal Infection Study Group. *Ann Surg* 223:303, 1996.

59. Solomkin JS, Dellinger EP, Christou NV, et al: Results of a multicenter trial comparing imipenem/cilastatin to tobramycin/clindamycin for intra-abdominal infections. *Ann Surg* 212:58, 1990.

60. Solomkin JS, Yellin AE, Rotstein OD, et al: Protocol 017 Study Group. Ertapenem versus piperacillin/tazobactam in the treatment of complicated intra-abdominal infections: Results of a double-blind, randomized comparative phase III trial. *Ann Surg* 237:235, 2003.

61. Evans HL, Raymond DP, Pelletier SJ, et al: Tertiary peritonitis is not an independent predictor of mortality in surgical patients with intra-abdominal infection. *Surg Infect* 2:255, 2001.

62. Lamme V, Mahler CW, van Ruler O, et al: Clinical predictors of ongoing infection in secondary peritonitis: Systematic review. *World J Surg* 30:2170, 2006.

63. Leslie DB, Dunn DL: Hepatic abscess, in Cameron JL (ed): *Current Surgical Therapy*, 8th ed. Philadelphia, PA: Elsevier Health Sciences, 2004.

64. Bradley EL III, Allen K: A prospective longitudinal study of observation versus surgical intervention in the management of necrotizing pancreatitis. *Am J Surg* 161:19, 1991.

65. Pederzoli P, Bassi C, Vesentini S, et al: A randomized multicenter clinical trial of antibiotic prophylaxis of septic complications in acute necrotizing pancreatitis with imipenem. *Surg Gynecol Obstet* 176:480, 1993.

66. Nathens AB, Curtis JR, Beale RJ, et al: Management of the critically ill patient with severe acute pancreatitis. *Crit Care Med* 32:2524, 2004.

67. Mazaki T, Ishii Y, Takayama T: Meta-analysis of prophylactic antibiotic use in acute necrotizing pancreatitis. *Br J Surg* 93:674, 2006.

68. Villatoro E, Bassi C, Larvin M: Antibiotic therapy for prophylaxis against infection of pancreatic necrosis in acute pancreatitis. Cochrane Database. *Syst Rev* 18:CD002941, 2006.

69. Meier R, Beglinger C, Layer P, et al: ESPEN guidelines on nutrition in acute pancreatitis. European Society of Parenteral and Enteral Nutrition. *Clin Nutr* 21:173, 2002.

70. McClave SA, Chang WK, Dhaliwal R, et al: Nutrition support in acute pancreatitis: A systematic review of the literature. *JPEN J Parenter Enteral Nutr* 30:143, 2006.

71. el Yassini AE, Hoebeke Y, Keuleneer RD: Laparoscopic treatment of secondary infected pancreatic collections after an acute pancreatitis: Two cases. *Acta Chir Belg* 96:226, 1996.

72. Adamson GD, Cuschieri A: Multimedia article. Laparoscopic infracolic necrosectomy for infected pancreatic necrosis. *Surg Endosc* 17:1675, 2003.

73. Beilman GJ, Sandifer G, Skarda D, et al: Emerging infections with community-associated methicillin-resistant *Staphylococcus aureus* in outpatients at an Army Community Hospital. *Surg Infect (Larchmt)* 6:87, 2005.

74. Tillou A, St Hill CR, Brown C, et al: Necrotizing soft tissue infections: Improved outcomes with modern care. *Am Surg* 70:841, 2004.

75. Malangoni MA: Necrotizing soft tissue infections: Are we making any progress? *Surg Infect* 2:145, 2001.

76. Sawyer MD, Dunn DL: Serious bacterial infections of the skin and soft tissues. *Curr Opin Infect Dis* 8:293, 1995.

77. Kaul R, McGeer A, Norrby-Teglund A, et al: Intravenous immunoglobulin therapy for streptococcal toxic shock syndrome—a comparative observational study. The Canadian Streptococcal Study Group. *Clin Infect Dis* 28:800, 1999.

78. National Nosocomial Infections Surveillance System. National Nosocomial Infections Surveillance (NNIS) System Report, data summary from January 1992 to June 2002. *Am J Infect Control* 30:458, 2002.

79. Kollef MH. Treatment of ventilator-associated pneumonia: Get it right from the start. *Crit Care Med* 31:969, 2003.

80. Parker CM, Kutsogiannis J, Muscedere J, et al: Ventilator-associated pneumonia caused by multidrug-resistant organisms or pseudomonas aeruginosa: Prevalence, incidence, risk factors, and outcomes. *J Crit Care* 23:18, 2008.

81. Klompas M: Does this patient have ventilator-associated pneumonia? *JAMA* 297:1583, 2007.

82. Safdar N, Maki DG: Risk of catheter-related bloodstream infection with peripherally inserted central venous catheters used in hospitalized patients. *Chest* 128:489, 2005.

83. Marr KA, Sexton DJ, Conlon PJ, et al: Catheter-related bacteremia and outcome of attempted catheter salvage in patients undergoing hemodialysis. *Ann Intern Med* 127:275, 1997.

84. Rupp ME, Lisco SJ, Lipsett PA, et al: Effect of a second-generation venous catheter impregnated with chlorhexidine and silver sulfadiazine on central catheter-related infections: A randomized, controlled trial. *Ann Intern Med* 143:570, 2005.

85. Cobb D, High KP, Sawyer RG, et al: A controlled trial of scheduled replacement of central venous and pulmonary-artery catheters. *N Engl J Med* 327:1062, 1992.

86. Angus DC, Linde-Zwirble WT, Lidicker J, et al: Epidemiology of severe sepsis in the United States: Analysis of incidence, outcome, and associated costs of care. *Crit Care Med* 29:1303, 2001.

87. Dellinger RP, Levy MM, Carlet JM, et al: Surviving Sepsis Campaign: International guidelines for management of severe sepsis and septic shock: 2008. *Crit Care Med* 36:296, 2008.

88. Otero RM, Nguyen HB, Huang DT, et al: Early goal-directed therapy in severe sepsis and septic shock revisited: Concepts, controversies, and contemporary findings. *Chest* 130:1579, 2006.

89. Kumar A, Roberts D, Wood KE, et al: Duration of hypotension before initiation of effective antimicrobial therapy is the critical determinant of survival in human septic shock. *Crit Care Med* 34:1589, 2006.

90. Ibrahim EH, Sherman G, Ward S, et al: The influence of inadequate antimicrobial treatment of bloodstream infections on patient outcomes in the ICU setting. *Chest* 118:146, 2000.

91. Morrell M, Fraser VJ, Kollef MH: Delaying the empiric treatment of candida bloodstream infection until positive blood culture results are obtained: A potential risk factor for hospital mortality. *Antimicrob Agents Chemother* 49:3640, 2005.

92. De Backer D, Creteur J, Silva E, et al: Effects of dopamine, norepinephrine, and epinephrine on the splanchnic circulation in septic shock: Which is best? *Crit Care Med* 31:1659, 2003.

93. Russell JA, Walley KR, Singer J, et al: Vasopressin versus norepinephrine infusion in patients with septic shock. *N Engl J Med* 358:877, 2008.

94. Bernard GR, Vincent JL, Laterre PF, et al: Efficacy and safety of recombinant human activated protein C for severe sepsis. *N Engl J Med* 344:699, 2001.

95. Centers for Disease Control and Prevention. Updated U.S. Public Health Service guidelines for the management of occupational exposures to HBV, HCV, and HIV and recommendations for post-exposure prophylaxis. *MMWR Morb Mortal Wkly Rep* 50:23, 2001.

96. Goldberg D, Johnston J, Cameron S, et al: Risk of HIV transmission from patients to surgeons in the era of post-exposure prophylaxis. *J Hosp Infect* 44:99, 2000.

97. *http://www.cdc.gov/vaccines/recs/schedules/adult-schedule.htm*: Recommended Adult Immunization Schedule—United States [accessed April 30, 2008].

98. Wasley A, Grytdal S, Gallagher K: Surveillance for acute viral hepatitis—United States, 2006. *MMWR Morb Mortal Wkly Rep* 57(SS02):1, 2008.

99. ACIP. Immune globulins for protection against viral hepatitis. *MMWR Morb Mortal Wkly Rep* 30:423, 1981.

100. Puro V, Petrosillo N, Ippolito G, et al: Risk of hepatitis C seroconversion after occupational exposure in health care workers. *Am J Infect Control* 23:273, 1995.

101. Centers for Disease Control. Recommendations for the prevention and control of hepatitis C virus (HCV) infection and HCV-related chronic disease. *MMWR Morb Mortal Wkly Rep* 47:19, 1998.

102. Inglesby TV, O'Toole T, Henderson DA, et al: Anthrax as a biological weapon. *JAMA* 287:2236, 2002.

103. Inglesby TV, Dennis DT, Henderson DA, et al: Plague as a biological weapon. *JAMA* 283:2281, 2000.

104. Tucker JB: *Scourge. The Once and Future Threat of Smallpox.* New York: Grove Press, 2001, p 1.

105. DeClercq E: Cidofovir in the treatment of poxvirus infections. *Antiviral Res* 55:1, 2002.

CHAPTER 7

Trauma

C. Clay Cothren, Walter L. Biffl,
and Ernest E. Moore

INTRODUCTION

Trauma, or injury, is defined as cellular disruption caused by an exchange with environmental energy that is beyond the body's resilience. Trauma remains the most common cause of death for all individuals between the ages of 1 and 44 years and is the third most common cause of death regardless of age.[1] It is also the number one cause of years of productive life lost. The U.S. government classifies injury-related death into the following categories: accidents (unintentional injuries), intentional self-harm (suicide), assault (homicide), legal intervention or war, and undetermined causes. Unintentional injuries account for over 110,000 deaths per year, with motor vehicle collisions accounting for over 40%. Homicides, suicides, and other causes are responsible for another 50,000 deaths each year. However, death is a poor indicator of the magnitude of the problem, because most injured patients survive. For example, in 2004 there were approximately 167,000 injury-related deaths, but 29.6 million injured patients treated in emergency departments (EDs).[2] Injury-related medical expenditures are estimated to be $117 billion each year in the United States.[2] The aggregate lifetime cost for all injured patients is estimated to be in excess of $260 trillion. For these reasons, trauma must be considered a major public health issue. The American College of Surgeons Committee on Trauma addresses this issue by assisting in the development of trauma centers and systems. The organization of trauma systems has had a significant favorable impact on patient outcomes.[3-5]

INITIAL EVALUATION AND RESUSCITATION OF THE INJURED PATIENT

Primary Survey

The Advanced Trauma Life Support (ATLS) course of the American College of Surgeons Committee on Trauma was developed in the late 1970s, based on the assumption that appropriate and timely care can significantly improve the outcome for the injured patient.[6] ATLS provides a structured approach to the trauma patient with standard algorithms of care; it emphasizes the "golden hour" concept that timely prioritized interventions are necessary to prevent death. The ATLS format and basic tenets are followed throughout this chapter, with minor modifications. The initial management of seriously injured patients consists of the primary survey, concurrent resuscitation, the secondary survey, diagnostic evaluation, and definitive care. The first step in patient management is performing the primary survey, the goal of which is to identify and treat conditions that constitute an immediate threat to life. The ATLS course refers to the primary survey as assessment of the "ABCs" (*A*irway with cervical spine protection, *B*reathing, and *C*irculation). Although the concepts within the primary survey are presented in a sequential fashion, in reality they often proceed simultaneously. Life-threatening injuries must be identified (Table 7-1) and treated before advancing to the secondary survey.

Airway Management with Cervical Spine Protection

Ensuring a patent airway is the first priority in the primary survey. This is essential, because efforts to restore cardiovascular integrity will be futile unless the oxygen content of the blood is adequate. Simultaneously, all patients with blunt trauma require cervical spine immobilization until injury is excluded. This is typically accomplished by applying a hard collar or placing sandbags on both sides of the head with the patient's forehead taped across the bags to the backboard. Soft collars do not effectively immobilize the cervical spine.

In general, patients who are conscious, do not show tachypnea, and have a normal voice do not require early attention to the airway. Exceptions are patients with penetrating injuries to the neck and an expanding hematoma; evidence of chemical or thermal injury to the

KEY POINTS

1. Trauma remains the most common cause of death for all individuals between the ages of 1 and 44 years and is the third most common cause of death regardless of age.

2. The initial management of seriously injured patients consists of performing the primary survey (the "ABCs"—*A*irway with cervical spine protection, *B*reathing, and *C*irculation); the goals of the primary survey are to identify and treat conditions that constitute an immediate threat to life.

3. Patients with ongoing hemodynamic instability, whether "nonresponders" or "transient responders," require prompt intervention; one must consider the four categories of shock that may represent the underlying pathophysiology: hemorrhagic, cardiogenic, neurogenic, and septic.

4. All patients with blunt injury should be assumed to have unstable cervical spine injuries until proven otherwise; one must maintain cervical spine precautions and in-line stabilization.

5. Indications for immediate operative intervention for penetrating cervical injury include hemodynamic instability and significant external arterial hemorrhage; the management algorithm for hemodynamically stable patients is based on the presenting

6. symptoms and anatomic location of injury, with the neck being divided into three distinct zones.

6. Blunt injuries to the carotid and vertebral arteries are usually managed with systemic antithrombotic therapy.

7. The abdomen is a diagnostic black box. However, physical examination and ultrasound can rapidly identify patients requiring emergent laparotomy. Computed tomographic (CT) scanning is the mainstay of evaluation in the remaining patients to more precisely identify the site and magnitude of injury.

8. Manifestation of the "bloody vicious cycle" (the lethal combination of coagulopathy, hypothermia, and metabolic acidosis) is the most common indication for damage control surgery. The primary objectives of damage control laparotomy are to control bleeding and limit GI spillage.

9. The abdominal compartment syndrome may be primary (i.e., due to the injury of abdominal organs, bleeding, and packing) or secondary (i.e., due to reperfusion gut edema and ascites).

10. The gold standard for determining if there is a blunt descending torn aorta injury is CT scanning; indications are primarily based on injury mechanisms.

TABLE 7-1	Immediately life-threatening injuries to be identified during the primary survey

Airway
  Airway obstruction
  Airway injury
Breathing
  Tension pneumothorax
  Open pneumothorax
  Flail chest with underlying pulmonary contusion
Circulation
  Hemorrhagic shock
    Massive hemothorax
    Massive hemoperitoneum
    Mechanically unstable pelvis fracture
    Extremity losses
  Cardiogenic shock
    Cardiac tamponade
  Neurogenic shock
    Cervical spine injury
Disability
  Intracranial hemorrhage/mass lesion

mouth, nares, or hypopharynx; extensive subcutaneous air in the neck; complex maxillofacial trauma; or airway bleeding. Although these patients may initially have a satisfactory airway, it may become obstructed if soft tissue swelling, hematoma formation, or edema progresses. In these cases, elective intubation should be performed before evidence of airway compromise.

Patients who have an abnormal voice, abnormal breathing sounds, tachypnea, or altered mental status require further airway evaluation. Blood, vomit, the tongue, foreign objects, and soft tissue swelling can cause airway obstruction; suctioning affords immediate relief in many patients. In the comatose patient, the tongue may fall backward and obstruct the hypopharynx; this may be relieved by either a chin lift or jaw thrust. An oral airway or a nasal trumpet also can be helpful in maintaining airway patency, although the former is not usually tolerated by an awake patient. Establishment of a definitive airway (i.e., endotracheal intubation) is indicated in patients with apnea; inability to protect the airway due to altered mental status; impending airway compromise due to inhalation injury, hematoma, facial bleeding, soft tissue swelling, or aspiration; and inability to maintain oxygenation. Altered mental status is the most common indication for intubation. Agitation or obtundation, often attributed to intoxication or drug use, may actually be due to hypoxia.

Options for endotracheal intubation include nasotracheal, orotracheal, or surgical routes. Nasotracheal intubation can be accomplished only in patients who are breathing spontaneously. Although nasotracheal intubation is frequently used by prehospital providers, the primary application for this technique in the ED is in those patients requiring emergent airway support in whom chemical paralysis cannot be used. Orotracheal intubation is the most common technique used to establish a definitive airway. Because all patients are presumed to have cervical spine injuries, manual in-line cervical immobilization is essential.[6] Correct endotracheal placement is verified with direct laryngoscopy, capnography, audibility of bilateral breath sounds, and finally a chest film. The GlideScope, a video laryngoscope that uses fiberoptics to visualize the vocal cords, is being employed more frequently.[7] Advantages of orotracheal intubation include the direct visualization of the vocal cords, ability to use larger-diameter endotracheal tubes, and applicability to apneic patients. The disadvantage of orotracheal intubation is that conscious patients usually require neuromuscular blockade, which may result in inability to intubate,

aspiration, or medication complications. Those who attempt rapid-sequence induction must be thoroughly familiar with the procedure (see Chap. 13).

Patients in whom attempts at intubation have failed or who are precluded from intubation due to extensive facial injuries require surgical establishment of an airway. Cricothyroidotomy (Fig. 7-1) is performed through a generous vertical incision, with sharp division of the subcutaneous tissues and strap muscles. Visualization may be improved by having an assistant retract laterally on the neck incision using army-navy retractors. The cricothyroid membrane is verified by digital palpation through the space into the airway. The airway may be stabilized before incision of the membrane using a tracheostomy hook; the hook should be placed under the thyroid cartilage to elevate the airway. A 6.0 tracheostomy tube (maximum diameter in adults) is then advanced through the cricothyroid opening and sutured into place. In patients under the age of 8, cricothyroidotomy is contraindicated due to the risk of subglottic stenosis, and tracheostomy should be performed.

Emergent tracheostomy is indicated in patients with laryngotracheal separation or laryngeal fractures, in whom cricothyroidotomy may cause further damage or result in complete loss of the airway. This procedure is best performed in the OR where there is optimal lighting and availability of more equipment (e.g., sternal saw). In these cases, often after a "clothesline" injury, direct visualization and instrumentation of the trachea usually is done through the traumatic anterior neck defect or after a collar skin incision (Fig. 7-2). If the trachea is completely transected, a nonpenetrating clamp should be placed on the distal aspect to prevent tracheal retraction into the mediastinum; this is particularly important before placement of the endotracheal tube.

Breathing and Ventilation

Once a secure airway is obtained, adequate oxygenation and ventilation must be assured. All injured patients should receive supplemental oxygen and be monitored by pulse oximetry. The following conditions constitute an immediate threat to life due to inadequate ventilation and should be recognized during the primary survey: tension pneumothorax, open pneumothorax, and flail chest with underlying pulmonary contusion. All of these diagnoses should be made during the initial physical examination.

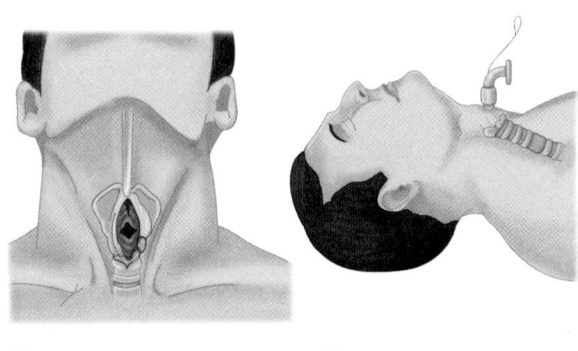

A   **B**

FIG. 7-1. Cricothyroidotomy is recommended for emergent surgical establishment of a patent airway. A vertical skin incision avoids injury to the anterior jugular veins, which are located just lateral to the midline. Hemorrhage from these vessels obscures vision and prolongs the procedure. When a transverse incision is made in the cricothyroid membrane, the blade of the knife should be angled inferiorly to avoid injury to the vocal cords. **A.** Use of a tracheostomy hook stabilizes the thyroid cartilage and facilitates tube insertion. **B.** A 6.0 tracheostomy tube or endotracheal tube is inserted after digital confirmation of airway access.

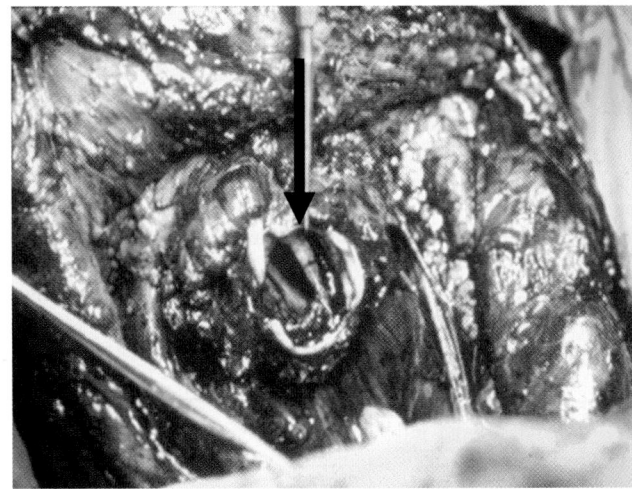

FIG. 7-2. A "clothesline" injury can partially or completely transect the anterior neck structures, including the trachea. With complete tracheal transection, the endotracheal tube is placed directly into the distal aperture, with care taken not to push the trachea into the mediastinum.

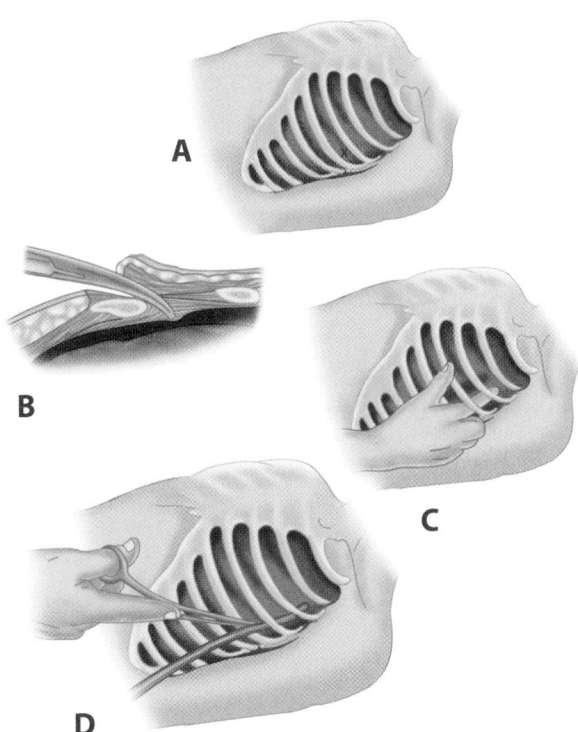

FIG. 7-3. A. Tube thoracostomy is performed in the midaxillary line at the fourth or fifth intercostal space (inframammary crease) to avoid iatrogenic injury to the liver or spleen. **B.** Heavy scissors are used to cut through the intercostal muscle into the pleural space. This is done on top of the rib to avoid injury to the intercostal bundle located just beneath the rib. **C.** The incision is digitally explored to confirm intrathoracic location and identify pleural adhesions. **D.** A 36F chest tube is directed superiorly and posteriorly with the aid of a large clamp.

The diagnosis of tension pneumothorax is implied by respiratory distress and hypotension in combination with any of the following physical signs in patients with chest trauma: tracheal deviation away from the affected side, lack of or decreased breath sounds on the affected side, and subcutaneous emphysema on the affected side. Patients may have distended neck veins due to impedance of the superior vena cava, but the neck veins may be flat due to systemic hypovolemia. Vital signs differentiate a tension pneumothorax from a simple pneumothorax; each can have similar signs, symptoms, and examination findings, but hypotension qualifies the pneumothorax as a tension pneumothorax. Although immediate needle thoracostomy decompression with a 14-gauge angiocatheter in the second intercostal space in the midclavicular line may be indicated in the field, tube thoracostomy should be performed immediately in the ED before a chest radiograph is obtained (Fig. 7-3). In cases of tension pneumothorax, the parenchymal tear in the lung acts as a one-way valve, with each inhalation allowing additional air to accumulate in the pleural space. The normally negative intrapleural pressure becomes positive, which depresses the ipsilateral hemidiaphragm and shifts the mediastinal structures into the contralateral chest. Subsequently, the contralateral lung is compressed and the heart rotates about the superior and inferior vena cava; this decreases venous return and ultimately cardiac output, which results in cardiovascular collapse.

An open pneumothorax or "sucking chest wound" occurs with full-thickness loss of the chest wall, permitting free communication between the pleural space and the atmosphere (Fig. 7-4). This compromises ventilation due to equilibration of atmospheric and pleural pressures, which prevents lung inflation and alveolar ventilation, and results in hypoxia and hypercarbia. Complete occlusion of the chest wall defect without a tube thoracostomy may convert an open pneumothorax to a tension pneumothorax. Temporary management of this injury includes covering the wound with an occlusive dressing that is taped on three sides. This acts as a flutter valve, permitting effective ventilation on inspiration while allowing accumulated air to escape from the pleural space on the untaped side, so that a tension pneumothorax is prevented. Definitive treatment requires closure of the chest wall defect and tube thoracostomy remote from the wound.

Flail chest occurs when three or more contiguous ribs are fractured in at least two locations. Paradoxical movement of this free-floating segment of chest wall may be evident in patients with

spontaneous ventilation, due to the negative intrapleural pressure of inspiration. Rarely the additional work of breathing and chest wall pain caused by the flail segment is sufficient to compromise ventilation. However, it is the decreased compliance and increased shunt fraction caused by the associated pulmonary contusion that is typically the source of postinjury pulmonary dysfunction. Pulmonary contusion often progresses during the first 12 hours. Resultant hypoventilation and hypoxemia may require presumptive intubation and mechanical ventilation. The patient's initial chest radiograph often underestimates the extent of the pulmonary parenchymal damage (Fig. 7-5); close monitoring and frequent clinical re-evaluation are warranted.

Circulation with Hemorrhage Control

With a secure airway and adequate ventilation established, circulatory status is the next priority. An initial approximation of the patient's cardiovascular status can be obtained by palpating peripheral pulses. In general, systolic blood pressure (SBP) must be 60 mmHg for the carotid pulse to be palpable, 70 mmHg for the femoral pulse, and 80 mmHg for the radial pulse. At this point in the patient's evaluation, any episode of hypotension (defined as a SBP <90 mmHg) is assumed to be caused by hemorrhage until proven otherwise. Blood pressure and pulse should be measured manually at least every 5 minutes in patients with significant blood loss until normal vital sign values are restored.

IV access for fluid resuscitation is obtained with two peripheral catheters, 16-gauge or larger in adults. Blood should be drawn simultaneously and sent for measurement of hematocrit level, as

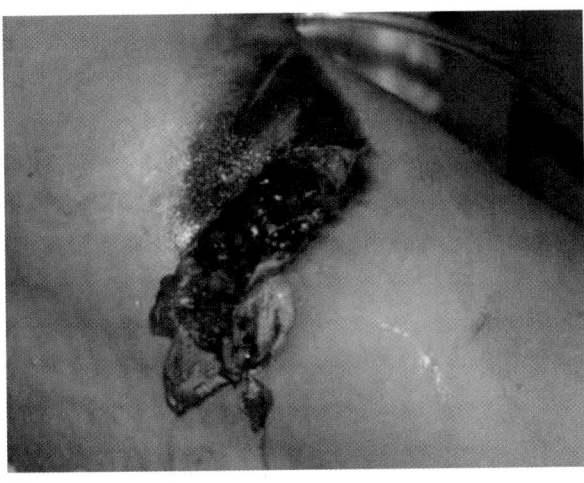
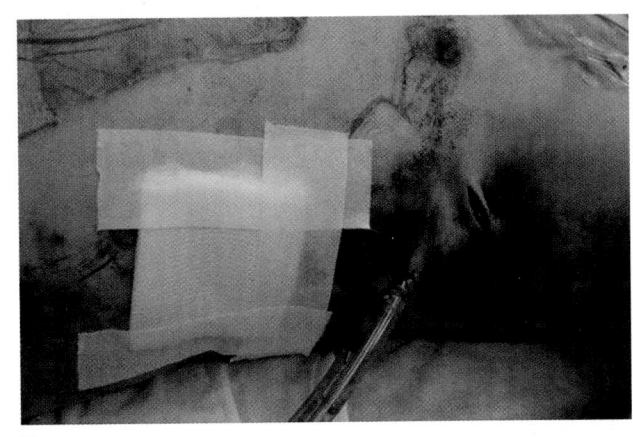

A   **B**

FIG. 7-4. **A.** Full-thickness loss of the chest wall results in an open pneumothorax. **B.** The defect is temporarily managed with an occlusive dressing that is taped on three sides, which allows accumulated air to escape from the pleural space and thus prevents a tension pneumothorax. Repair of the chest wall defect and tube thoracostomy remote from the wound is definitive treatment.

well as for typing and cross-matching for possible blood transfusion in patients with evidence of hypovolemia. According to Poiseuille's law, the flow of liquid through a tube is proportional to the diameter and inversely proportional to the length; therefore, venous lines for volume resuscitation should be short with a large diameter. If peripheral access with large-bore angiocatheters is inadequate, Cordis introducer catheters are preferred over triple-lumen catheters. In general, initial access in trauma patients is best secured in the groin or ankle, so that the catheter will not interfere with the performance of other diagnostic and therapeutic thoracoabdominal procedures. For patients requiring vigorous fluid resuscitation in whom peripheral angiocatheter access is difficult, saphenous vein cutdowns at the ankle provide excellent access (Fig. 7-6). The saphenous vein is reliably found 1 cm anterior and 1 cm superior to the medial malleolus. Standard 14-gauge catheters can be quickly placed, even in an exsanguinating patient with collapsed veins. Additional venous access often is obtained through the femoral or

subclavian veins with Cordis introducer catheters. A rule of thumb to consider is placement of femoral access for thoracic trauma and jugular or subclavian access for abdominal trauma. However, placement of jugular or subclavian central venous catheters provides a more reliable measurement of central venous pressure (CVP), which is helpful in determining the volume status of the patient and excluding cardiac tamponade. In hypovolemic patients under 6 years of age, an intraosseous needle can be placed in the proximal tibia (preferred) or distal femur of an unfractured extremity (Fig. 7-7). Flow through the needle should be continuous and does not require pressure. All medications administered IV may be administered in a similar dosage intraosseously. Although safe for emergent use, the needle should be removed once alternative access is established to prevent osteomyelitis.

External control of hemorrhage should be achieved promptly while circulating volume is restored. Manual compression of open wounds with ongoing bleeding should be done with a single 4 × 4

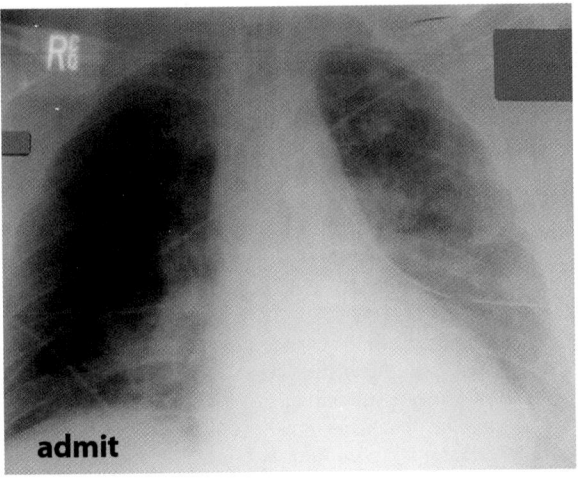
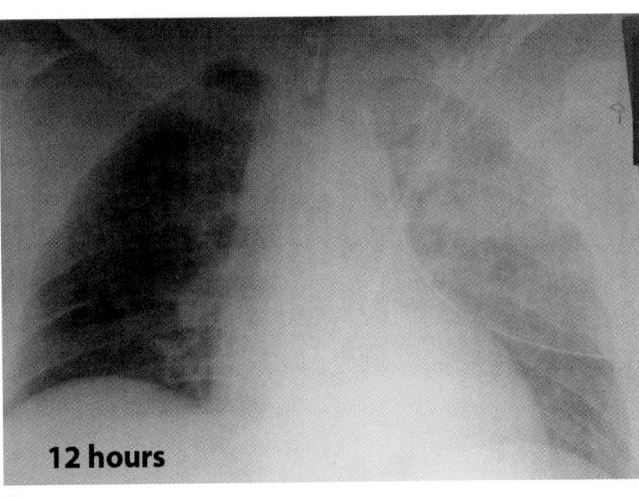

A   **B**

FIG. 7-5. **A.** Admission chest film may not show the full extent of the patient's thoracic injury. **B.** This patient's left pulmonary contusion blossomed 12 hours later, and its associated opacity is noted on repeat chest film.

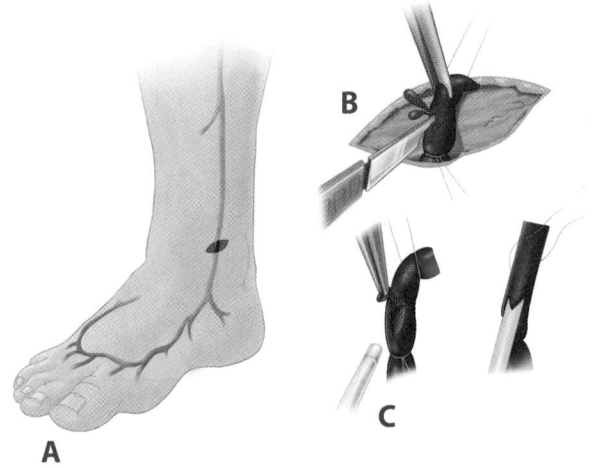

FIG. 7-6. Saphenous vein cutdowns are excellent sites for fluid resuscitation access. **A.** The vein is consistently found 1 cm anterior and 1 cm superior to the medial malleolus. **B.** Proximal and distal traction sutures are placed with the distal suture ligated. **C.** A 14-gauge IV catheter is introduced and secured with sutures and tape to prevent dislodgment.

gauze and a gloved hand. Covering the wound with excessive dressings may permit ongoing unrecognized blood loss that is hidden underneath the dressing. Blind clamping of bleeding vessels should be avoided because of the risk to adjacent structures, including nerves. This is particularly true for penetrating injuries of the neck, thoracic outlet, and groin, where bleeding may be torrential and arising from deep within the wound. In these situations, a gloved finger is placed through the wound directly onto the bleeding vessel and enough pressure is applied to control active bleeding. The surgeon performing this maneuver must then walk with the patient to the OR for open definitive treatment. For bleeding of the extremities

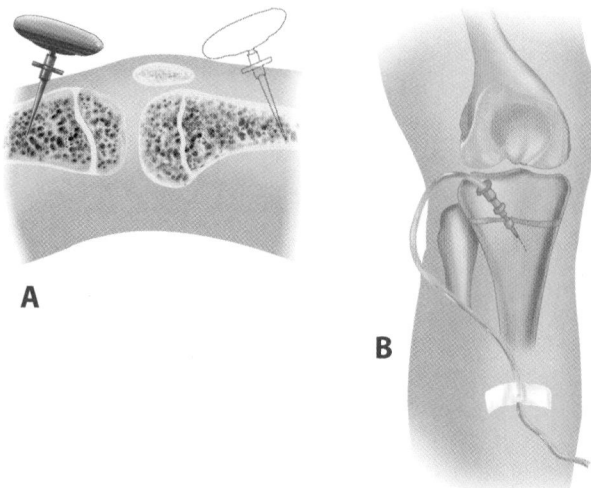

FIG. 7-7. Intraosseous infusions are indicated for children <6 years of age in whom one or two attempts at IV access have failed. **A.** The proximal tibia is the preferred location. Alternatively, the distal femur can be used if the tibia is fractured. **B.** The needle should be directed away from the epiphyseal plate to avoid injury. The position is satisfactory if bone marrow can be aspirated and saline can be easily infused without evidence of extravasation.

it is tempting to apply tourniquets for hemorrhage control, but digital occlusion will usually control the bleeding, and complete vascular occlusion risks permanent neuromuscular impairment. For patients with open fractures, fracture reduction with stabilization via splints will limit bleeding externally and into the subcutaneous tissues. Scalp lacerations through the galea aponeurotica tend to bleed profusely; these can be temporarily controlled with skin staples, Rainey clips, or a large full-thickness continuous running nylon stitch.

During the circulation section of the primary survey, four life-threatening injuries that must be identified are (a) massive hemothorax, (b) cardiac tamponade, (c) massive hemoperitoneum, and (d) mechanically unstable pelvic fractures. Massive hemoperitoneum and mechanically unstable pelvic fractures are discussed in "Emergent Abdominal Exploration" and "Pelvic Fractures and Emergent Hemorrhage Control," respectively. Three critical tools used to differentiate these in the multisystem trauma patient are chest radiograph, pelvis radiograph, and focused abdominal sonography for trauma (FAST) (see "Regional Assessment and Special Diagnostic Tests"). A massive hemothorax (life-threatening injury number one) is defined as >1500 mL of blood or, in the pediatric population, one third of the patient's blood volume in the pleural space (Fig. 7-8). Although it may be suspected on chest radiograph, tube thoracostomy is the only reliable means to quantify the amount of hemothorax. After blunt trauma, a hemothorax usually is due to multiple rib fractures with severed intercostal arteries, but occasionally bleeding is from lacerated lung parenchyma. After penetrating trauma, a systemic or pulmonary hilar vessel injury should be presumed. In either scenario, a massive hemothorax is an indication for operative intervention, but tube thoracostomy is critical to facilitate lung re-expansion, which may provide some degree of tamponade.

Cardiac tamponade (life-threatening injury number two) occurs most commonly after penetrating thoracic injuries, although occasionally blunt rupture of the heart, particularly the atrial appendage, is seen. Acutely, <100 mL of pericardial blood may cause pericardial tamponade. The classic diagnostic Beck's triad—dilated neck veins, muffled heart tones, and a decline in arterial pressure—often is not observed in the trauma bay because of the noisy environment and hypovolemia. Because the pericardium is not acutely distensible, the pressure in the pericardial sac will rise to match that of the injured chamber. When this pressure exceeds that of the right atrium, right atrial filling is impaired and right ventricular preload is reduced. This leads to decreased right ventricular output and increased CVP. Increased intrapericardial pressure also impedes myocardial blood flow, which leads to subendocardial ischemia and a further reduction in cardiac output.

Diagnosis is best achieved by bedside ultrasound of the pericardium (Fig. 7-9). Early in the course of tamponade, blood pressure and cardiac output will transiently improve with fluid administration. In patients with any hemodynamic disturbance, a pericardial drain is placed using ultrasound guidance (Fig. 7-10). Removing as little as 15 to 20 mL of blood will often temporarily stabilize the patient's hemodynamic status, prevent subendocardial ischemia and associated lethal arrhythmias, and allow transport to the OR for sternotomy. Pericardiocentesis is successful in decompressing tamponade in approximately 80% of cases; the majority of failures are due to the presence of clotted blood within the pericardium. Patients with a SBP <70 mmHg warrant emergency department thoracotomy (EDT) with opening of the pericardium to address the injury.

The utility of EDT has been debated for many years. Current indications are based on 30 years of prospective data (Table 7-2).[7] EDT is associated with the highest survival rate after isolated cardiac injury; 35% of patients presenting in shock and 20% without vital signs (i.e., pulse or obtainable blood pressure) are resuscitated after isolated penetrating injury to the heart. For all penetrating wounds, survival rate is 15%. Conversely, patient outcome is poor when EDT is done for blunt trauma, with 2% survival among patients in shock and <1% survival among those with no vital signs. Thus, patients undergoing cardiopulmonary resuscitation upon arrival to the ED

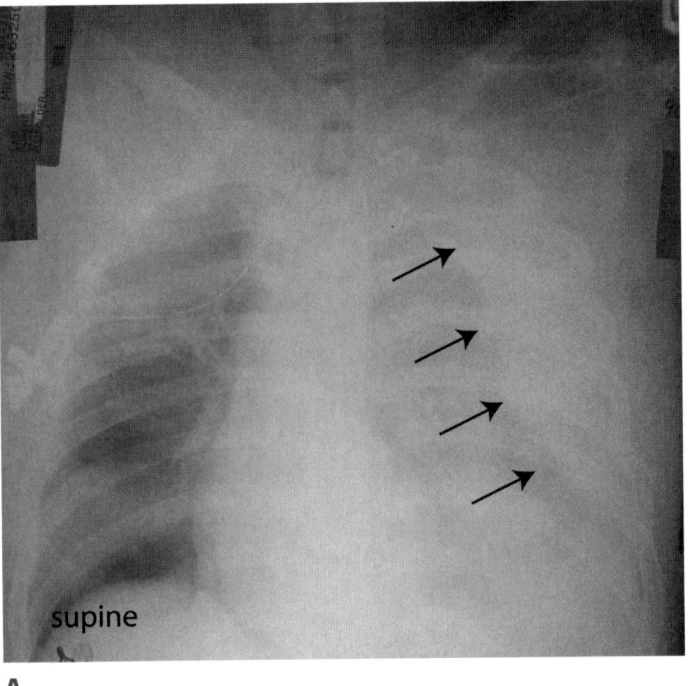

A

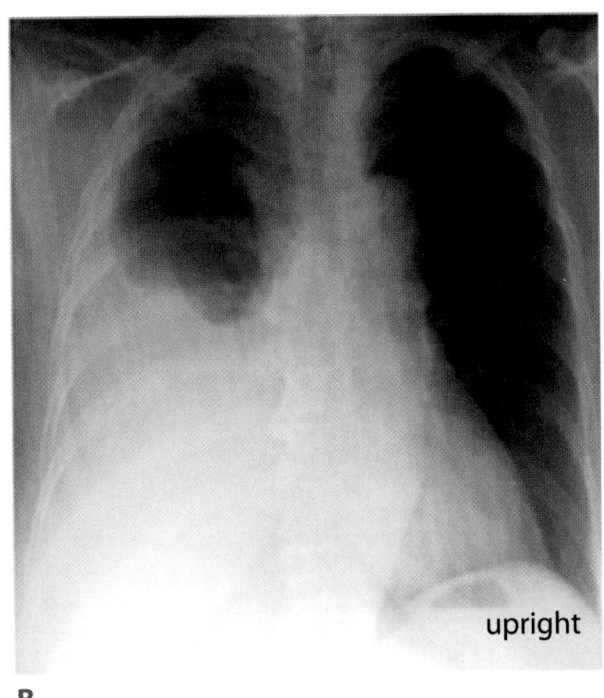

B

FIG. 7-8. More than 1500 mL of blood in the pleural space is a massive hemothorax. Chest film findings reflect the positioning of the patient. **A.** In the supine position, blood tracks along the entire posterior section of the chest and is most notable pushing the lung away from the chest wall. **B.** In the upright position, blood is visible dependently in the pleural space.

should undergo EDT selectively based on injury and transport time (Fig. 7-11). EDT is best accomplished using a left anterolateral thoracotomy, with the incision started to the right of the sternum (Fig. 7-12). A longitudinal pericardiotomy anterior to the phrenic nerve releases cardiac tamponade and allows access to the heart for cardiac repair and open cardiac massage. Cross-clamping of the aorta sustains central circulation, augments cerebral and coronary blood flow, and limits any abdominal blood loss (Fig. 7-13). The patient must sustain an SBP of 70 mmHg after EDT and associated interventions to be considered resuscitatable and hence transported to the OR.[8]

Disability and Exposure

The Glasgow Coma Scale (GCS) score should be determined for all injured patients (Table 7-3). It is calculated by adding the scores of the best motor response, best verbal response, and eye opening. Scores range from 3 (the lowest) to 15 (normal). Scores of 13 to 15

indicate mild head injury, 9 to 12 moderate injury, and <9 severe injury. The GCS is a quantifiable determination of neurologic function that is useful for both triage and prognosis.

Neurologic evaluation before administration of neuromuscular blockade for intubation is critical. Subtle changes in mental status can be caused by hypoxia, hypercarbia, or hypovolemia, or may be an early sign of increasing intracranial pressure. An abnormal mental status should prompt an immediate re-evaluation of the ABCs and consideration of central nervous system injury. Deterioration in mental status may be subtle and may not progress in a predictable fashion. For example, previously calm, cooperative patients may become anxious and combative as they become hypoxic. However, a patient who is agitated and combative from drugs or alcohol may become somnolent if hypovolemic shock develops. Seriously injured patients must have all of their clothing removed to avoid overlooking limb- or life-threatening injuries.

Shock Classification and Initial Fluid Resuscitation

Classic signs and symptoms of shock are tachycardia, hypotension, tachypnea, mental status changes, diaphoresis, and pallor (Table 7-4). The quantity of acute blood loss correlates with physiologic abnormalities. For example, although patients in class II shock may be tachycardic, they do not exhibit a reduction in blood pressure until over 1500 mL of blood loss, or class III shock. Physical findings should be viewed as a constellation and aid in the evaluation of the patient's response to treatment. The goal of fluid resuscitation is to re-establish tissue perfusion. Fluid resuscitation begins with a 2 L (adult) or 20 mL/kg (child) IV bolus of isotonic crystalloid, typically Ringer's lactate. For persistent hypotension, this is repeated once in an adult and twice in a child before red blood cells (RBCs) are administered. Patients who have a good response to fluid infusion (i.e., normalization of vital signs, clearing of the sensorium) and evidence of good peripheral perfusion (warm fingers and toes with normal capillary refill) are presumed to have adequate overall perfusion. Urine output is a quantitative, reliable indicator of organ perfusion. Adequate urine output is 0.5 mL/kg per hour in an adult,

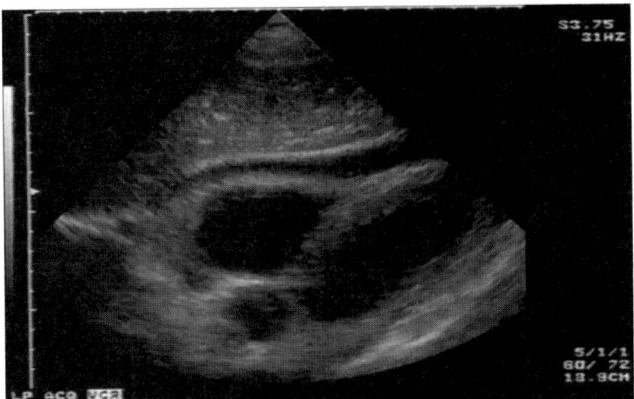

FIG. 7-9. Subxiphoid pericardial ultrasound reveals a large pericardial fluid collection.

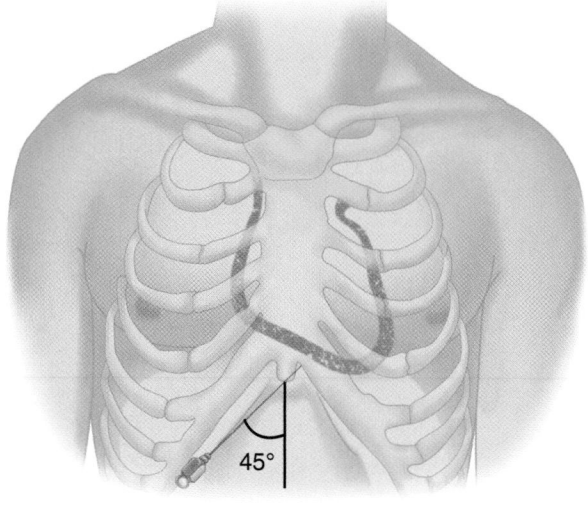

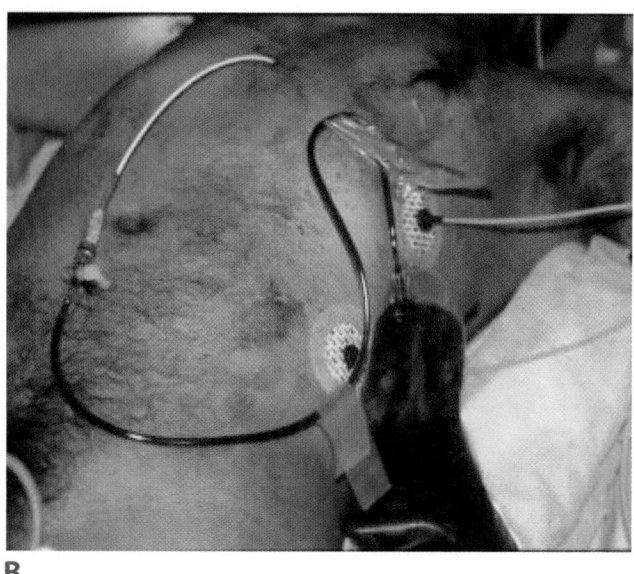

A

B

FIG. 7-10. Pericardiocentesis is indicated for patients with evidence of pericardial tamponade. **A.** Access to the pericardium is obtained through a subxiphoid approach, with the needle angled 45 degrees up from the chest wall and toward the left shoulder. **B.** Seldinger technique is used to place a pigtail catheter. Blood can be repeatedly aspirated with a syringe or the tubing may be attached to a gravity drain. Evacuation of unclotted pericardial blood prevents subendocardial ischemia and stabilizes the patient for transport to the operating room for sternotomy.

1 mL/kg per hour in a child, and 2 mL/kg per hour in an infant <1 year of age. Because measurement of this resuscitation-related variable is time dependent, it is more useful in the OR and intensive care unit (ICU) setting than in initial evaluation in the trauma bay.

There are several caveats to be considered and pitfalls to be avoided when evaluating the injured patient for shock. Tachycardia is often the earliest sign of ongoing blood loss. However, individuals in good physical condition with a resting pulse rate in the fifties may manifest a relative tachycardia in the nineties; although clinically significant, this does not meet the standard definition of tachycardia. Conversely, patients receiving cardiac medications such as beta blockers may not be capable of increasing their heart rate despite significant stress. Bradycardia occurs with severe blood loss; this is an ominous sign, often heralding impending cardiovascular collapse. Other physiologic stresses, aside from hypovolemia, may produce tachycardia, such as hypoxia, pain, anxiety, and stimulant drugs (cocaine, amphetamines). As noted previously, hypotension is not a reliable early sign of hypovolemia, because blood volume

must decrease by >30% before hypotension occurs. Additionally, younger patients with good sympathetic tone may surprise even the experienced clinician by maintaining SBP despite severe intravascular deficits until they are on the verge of cardiac arrest. Pregnant patients have a progressive increase in circulating blood volume over gestation; therefore, they must lose a relatively larger volume of blood before manifesting signs and symptoms of hypovolemia (see "Special Trauma Populations" below).

Based on the initial response to fluid resuscitation, hypovolemic injured patients can be separated into three broad categories: responders, transient responders, and nonresponders. Individuals who are stable or have a good response to the initial fluid therapy as evidenced by normalization of vital signs, mental status, and urine output are unlikely to have significant ongoing hemorrhage, and further diagnostic evaluation for occult injuries can proceed in an orderly fashion (see "Secondary Survey" below). At the other end of the spectrum are patients classified as "nonresponders" who have persistent hypotension despite aggressive resuscitation. These patients require immediate identification of the source of hypotension with appropriate intervention to prevent a fatal outcome. Patients considered as "transient responders" are those who respond initially to volume loading by an increase in blood pressure only to then hemodynamically deteriorate once more. This group of patients can be challenging to triage for definitive management.

TABLE 7-2	Current indications and contraindications for emergency department thoracotomy

Indications
  Salvageable postinjury cardiac arrest:
    Patients sustaining witnessed penetrating trauma with <15 min of prehospital CPR
    Patients sustaining witnessed blunt trauma with <5 min of prehospital CPR
  Persistent severe postinjury hypotension (SBP ≤60 mmHg) due to:
    Cardiac tamponade
    Hemorrhage—intrathoracic, intra-abdominal, extremity, cervical
    Air embolism
Contraindications
  Penetrating trauma: CPR >15 min and no signs of life (pupillary response, respiratory effort, motor activity)
  Blunt trauma: CPR >5 min and no signs of life or asystole

CPR = cardiopulmonary resuscitation; SBP = systolic blood pressure.

Persistent Hypotension

Patients with ongoing hemodynamic instability, whether "nonresponders" or "transient responders," require systematic evaluation and prompt intervention. The spectrum of disease in patients with persistent hypotension ranges from nonsurvivable multisystem injury to easily reversible problems such as a tension pneumothorax. One must first consider the four categories of shock that may be the underlying cause: hemorrhagic, cardiogenic, neurogenic, and septic. Except for patients transferred from outside facilities >12 hours after injury, few patients present in septic shock in the trauma bay. Patients with neurogenic shock as a component of hemodynamic instability often are recognized during the disability section of the primary survey to have paralysis, but those patients chemically paralyzed before physical examination may be misdiagnosed. In most cases, however,

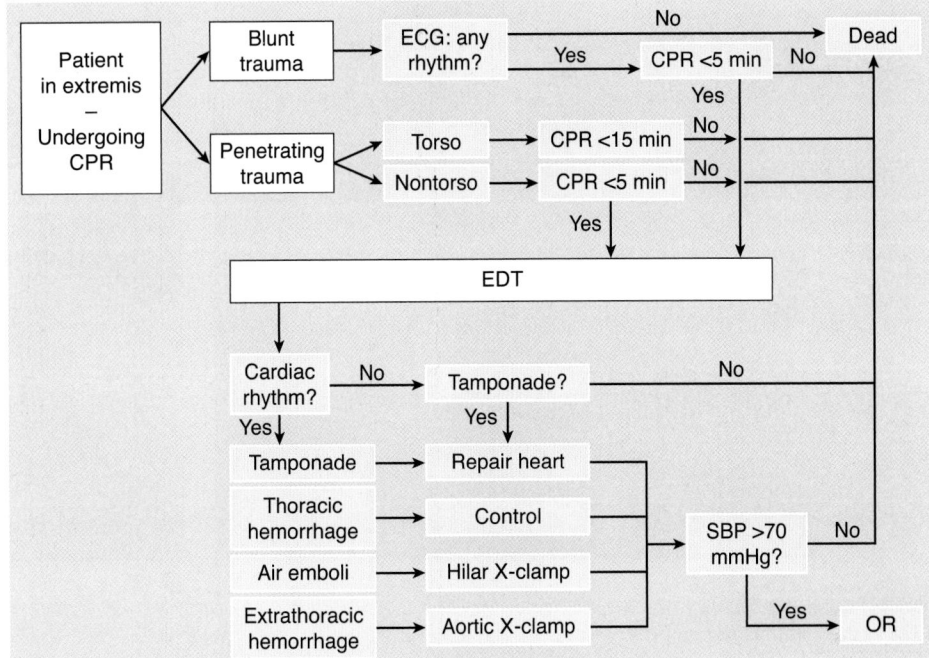

FIG. 7-11. Algorithm directing the use of emergency department thoracotomy (EDT) in the injured patient undergoing cardiopulmonary resuscitation (CPR). ECG = electrocardiogram; OR = operating room; SBP = systolic blood pressure.

the two broad categories of shock causing persistent hypotension are hemorrhagic and cardiogenic. An evaluation of the CVP will usually distinguish between these two categories. A patient with flat neck veins and a CVP of <5 cm H_2O is hypovolemic and is likely to have ongoing hemorrhage. A patient with distended neck veins or a CVP of >15 cm H_2O is likely to be in cardiogenic shock. The CVP may be falsely elevated, however, if the patient is agitated and straining, or fluid administration is overzealous; isolated readings must be interpreted with caution. Serial base deficit measurements also are helpful; a persistent base deficit of >8 mmol/L implies ongoing cellular shock.

Evolving technology, such as near infrared spectroscopy, will provide noninvasive monitoring of oxygen delivery to tissue.[9]

The differential diagnosis of cardiogenic shock in trauma patients is: (a) tension pneumothorax, (b) pericardial tamponade, (c) blunt cardiac injury, (d) myocardial infarction, and (e) bronchovenous air embolism. Tension pneumothorax, the most frequent cause of cardiac failure, and pericardial tamponade have been discussed earlier. Although as many as one third of patients sustaining significant blunt chest trauma experience blunt cardiac injury, few such injuries result in hemodynamic embarrassment. Patients with electrocardiographic

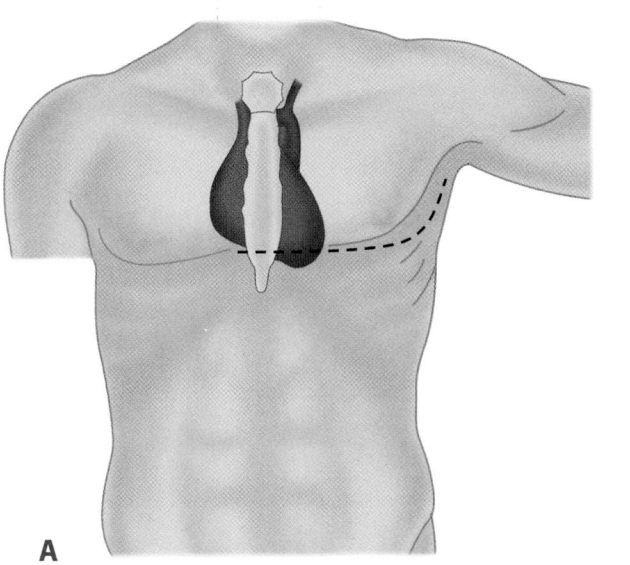

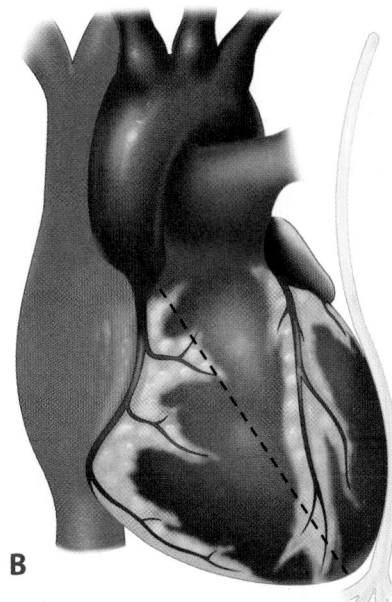

FIG. 7-12. A. Emergency department thoracotomy is performed through the fifth intercostal space using the anterolateral approach. **B** and **C.** The pericardium is opened anterior to the phrenic nerve, and the heart is rotated out for repair. **D.** Open cardiac massage should be performed with a hinged, clapping motion of the hands, with sequential closing from palms to fingers. The two-handed technique is strongly recommended because the one-handed massage technique poses the risk of myocardial perforation with the thumb. (*Continued*)

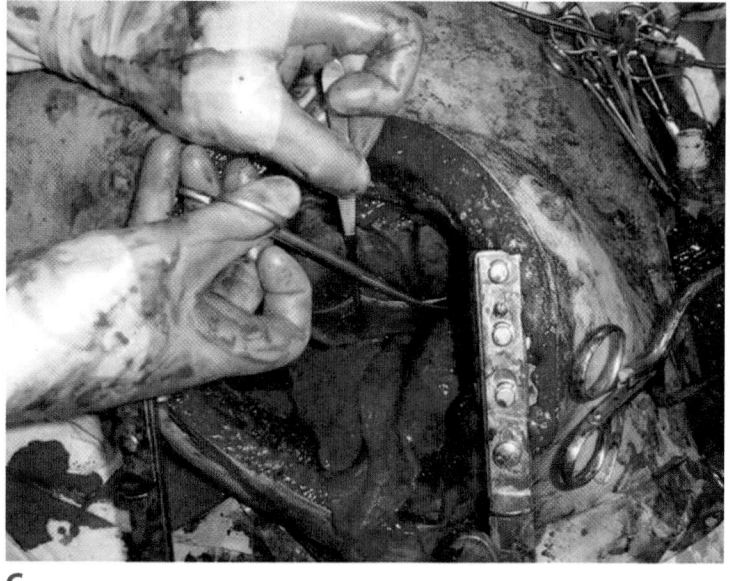

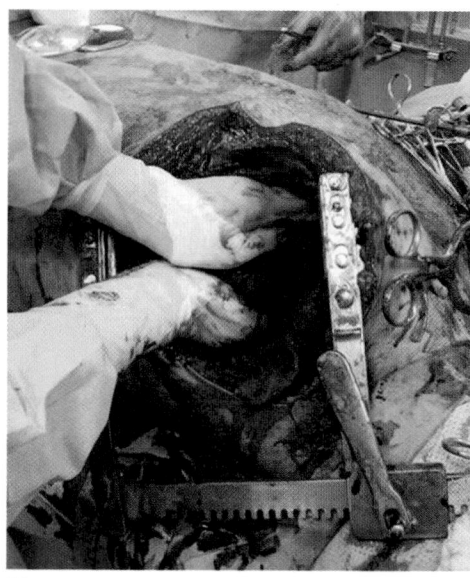

FIG. 7-12. *(Continued)*

(ECG) abnormalities or dysrhythmias require continuous ECG monitoring and antidysrhythmic treatment as needed. Unless myocardial infarction is suspected, there is no role for measurement of cardiac enzyme levels—they lack specificity and do not predict significant dysrhythmias.[10] The patient with hemodynamic instability requires aggressive resuscitation and may benefit from the placement of a pulmonary artery catheter to optimize preload and guide inotropic support. Echocardiography may be indicated to exclude pericardial tamponade or valvular or septal injuries. It typically demonstrates right ventricular dyskinesia but is less helpful in titrating treatment and monitoring the response to therapy unless done repeatedly. Patients with refractory cardiogenic shock may require placement of an intra-aortic balloon pump to decrease myocardial work and

enhance coronary perfusion. Acute myocardial infarction may be the cause of a motor vehicle collision or other trauma in older patients. Although optimal initial management includes treatment for the evolving infarction, such as lytic therapy and emergent angioplasty, these decisions must be individualized in accordance with the patient's other injuries.

Air embolism is a frequently overlooked or undiagnosed lethal complication of pulmonary injury. Air emboli can occur after blunt or penetrating trauma, when air from an injured bronchus enters an adjacent injured pulmonary vein (bronchovenous fistula) and returns air to the left heart. Air accumulation in the left ventricle impedes diastolic filling, and during systole air is pumped into the coronary arteries, disrupting coronary perfusion. The typical case is

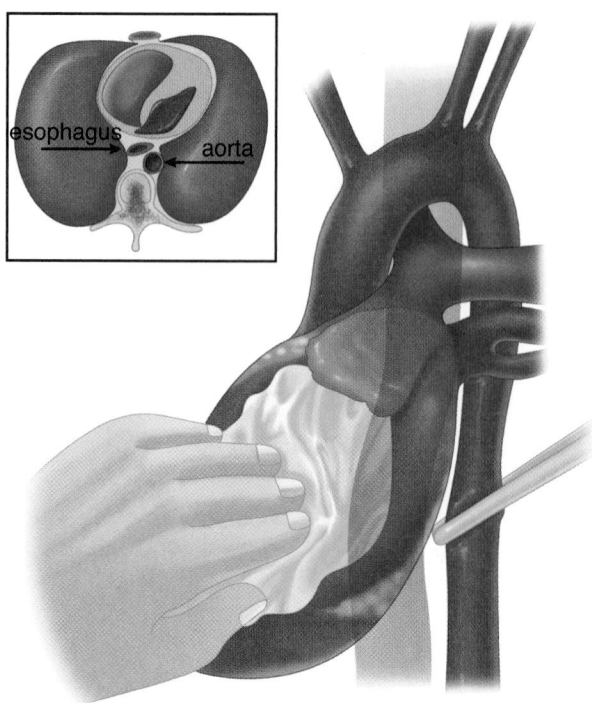

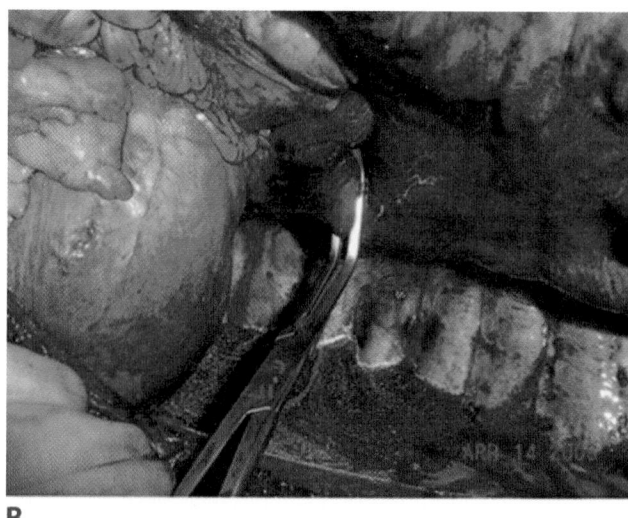

FIG. 7-13. Aortic cross-clamp is applied with the left lung retracted superiorly, below the inferior pulmonary ligament, just above the diaphragm. The flaccid aorta is identified as the first structure encountered on top of the spine when approached from the left chest.

TABLE 7-3 Glasgow Coma Scale[a]

		Adults	Infants/Children
Eye opening	4	Spontaneous	Spontaneous
	3	To voice	To voice
	2	To pain	To pain
	1	None	None
Verbal	5	Oriented	Alert, normal vocalization
	4	Confused	Cries but consolable
	3	Inappropriate words	Persistently irritable
	2	Incomprehensible words	Restless, agitated, moaning
	1	None	None
Motor response	6	Obeys commands	Spontaneous, purposeful
	5	Localizes pain	Localizes pain
	4	Withdraws	Withdraws
	3	Abnormal flexion	Abnormal flexion
	2	Abnormal extension	Abnormal extension
	1	None	None

[a]Score is calculated by adding the scores of the best motor response, best verbal response, and eye opening. Scores range from 3 (the lowest) to 15 (normal).

a patient with a penetrating thoracic injury who is hemodynamically stable but experiences arrest after being intubated and placed on positive pressure ventilation. The patient should immediately be placed in Trendelenburg's position to trap the air in the apex of the left ventricle. Emergency thoracotomy is followed by cross-clamping of the pulmonary hilum on the side of the injury to prevent further introduction of air (Fig. 7-14). Air is aspirated from the apex of the left ventricle and the aortic root with an 18-gauge needle and 50-mL syringe. Vigorous massage is used to force the air bubbles through the coronary arteries; if this is unsuccessful, a tuberculin syringe may be used to aspirate air bubbles from the right coronary artery. Once circulation is restored, the patient should be kept in Trendelenburg's position with the pulmonary hilum clamped until the pulmonary venous injury is controlled operatively.

Persistent hypotension due to uncontrolled hemorrhage is associated with high mortality. A rapid search for the source or sources of hemorrhage includes visual inspection with knowledge of the injury mechanism, FAST, and chest and pelvic radiographs. During diagnostic evaluation, type O RBCs (O-negative for women of childbearing age) and type-specific RBCs, when available, should be administered. In patients with penetrating trauma and clear indications for operation, essential films should be taken and the patient should be transported to the OR immediately. Such patients include those with massive hemothorax, those with initial chest tube output of >1 L with ongoing output of >200 mL/h, and those with abdominal trauma and ultrasound evidence of hemoperitoneum. In patients with gunshot wounds to the chest or abdomen, a chest and abdominal film, with radiopaque markers at the wound sites, should be obtained to determine the trajectory of the bullet or location of a retained fragment. For example, a patient with a gunshot wound to the upper abdomen should have a chest radiograph to ensure that the bullet did not traverse the diaphragm causing intrathoracic injury. Similarly, physical examination and chest radiograph of a patient with a gunshot wound to the right chest must evaluate the left hemithorax. If a patient has a penetrating weapon remaining in place, the weapon should *not* be removed in the ED, because it could be tamponading a lacerated blood vessel (Fig. 7-15). The surgeon should extract the offending instrument in the controlled environment of the OR, ideally once an incision has been made with adequate exposure. In situations in which knives are embedded in the head or neck, preoperative imaging may be useful to exclude arterial injuries. Blunt trauma patients with clear operative indications include hypotensive patients with massive hemothorax and those with a FAST examination documenting extensive free intraperitoneal fluid.

In patients without clear operative indications and persistent hypotension, one should systematically evaluate the five potential sources of blood loss: scalp, chest, abdomen, pelvis, and extremities. Significant bleeding at the scene may be noted by paramedics, but its quantification is unreliable. Examination should detect active bleeding from a scalp laceration that may be readily controlled with clips or staples. Thoracoabdominal trauma should be evaluated with a combination of chest radiograph, FAST, and pelvic radiograph. If the FAST results are negative and no other source of hypotension is obvious, diagnostic peritoneal aspiration should be entertained.[11] Extremity examination and radiographs should be used to search for associated fractures. Fracture-related blood loss, when additive, may be a potential source of the patient's hemodynamic instability. For each rib fracture there is approximately 100 to 200 mL of blood loss; for tibial fractures, 300 to 500 mL; for femur fractures, 800 to 1000 mL; and for pelvic fractures >1000 mL. Although no single injury may appear to cause a patient's hemodynamic instability, the sum of the injuries may result in life-threatening blood loss. The diagnostic measures advocated earlier are those that can be easily performed in the trauma bay. Transport of a hypotensive patient out of the ED for computed tomographic (CT) scanning may be hazardous; monitoring is compromised, and the environment is suboptimal for dealing with acute problems. The surgeon must accompany the patient and be prepared to abort the CT scan with direct transport to the OR. This dilemma is becoming less common in large trauma centers where CT scanning can be accomplished in the ED.

The role of treatment of hypotension in the ED remains controversial, and it is primarily relevant for patients with penetrating vascular injuries. Experimental work suggests that an endogenous sealing clot of an injured artery may be disrupted at an SBP of >90 mmHg[12]; thus, many believe that this should be the preoperative blood pressure target for patients with torso arterial injuries. On the other hand, optimal management of traumatic brain injury (TBI) includes maintaining the SBP at >90 mmHg.[13]

Secondary Survey

Once the immediate threats to life have been addressed, a thorough history is obtained and the patient is examined in a systematic fashion.

TABLE 7-4 Signs and symptoms of advancing stages of hemorrhagic shock

	Class I	Class II	Class III	Class IV
Blood loss (mL)	Up to 750	750–1500	1500–2000	>2000
Blood loss (%BV)	Up to 15%	15–30%	30–40%	>40%
Pulse rate	<100	>100	>120	>140
Blood pressure	Normal	Normal	Decreased	Decreased
Pulse pressure (mmHg)	Normal or increased	Decreased	Decreased	Decreased
Respiratory rate	14–20	20–30	30–40	>35
Urine output (mL/h)	>30	20–30	5–15	Negligible
CNS/mental status	Slightly anxious	Mildly anxious	Anxious and confused	Confused and lethargic

BV = blood volume; CNS = central nervous system.

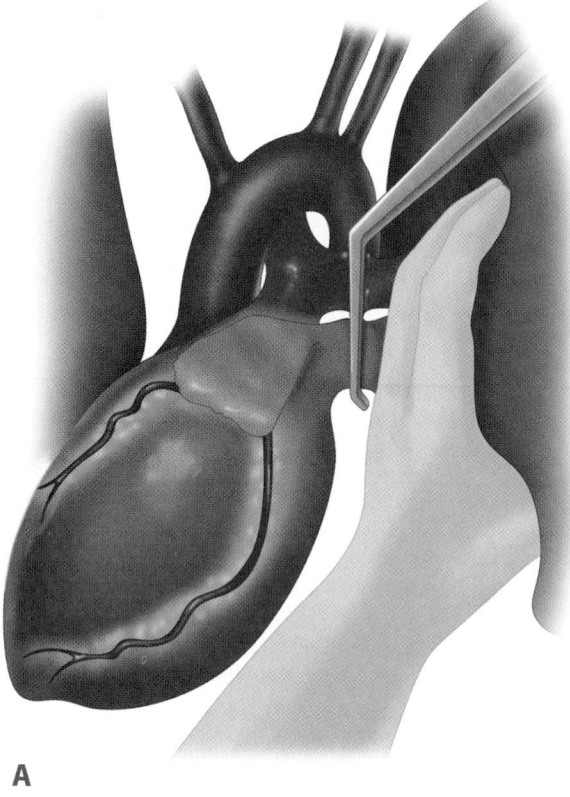 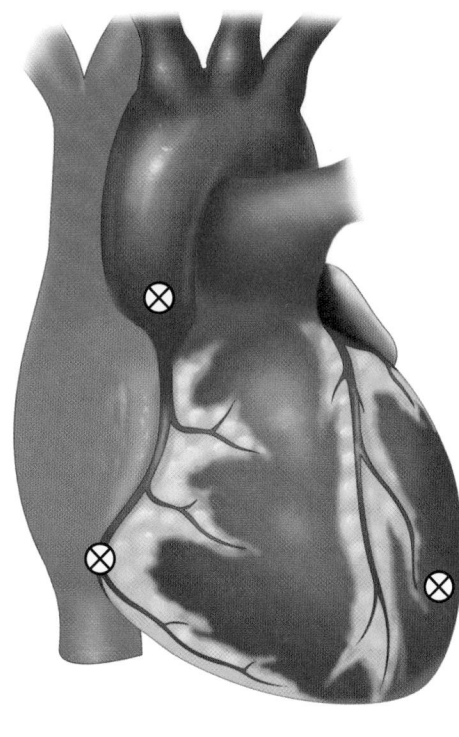

A **B**

FIG. 7-14. A. A Satinsky clamp is used to clamp the pulmonary hilum to prevent further bronchovenous air embolism. **B.** Sequential sites of aspiration include the left ventricle, the aortic root, and the right coronary artery.

The patient and surrogates should be queried to obtain an AMPLE history (*A*llergies, *M*edications, *P*ast illnesses or *P*regnancy, *L*ast meal, and *E*vents related to the injury). The physical examination should be head to toe, with special attention to the patient's back, axillae, and perineum, because injuries here are easily overlooked. All potentially seriously injured patients should undergo digital rectal examination to evaluate for sphincter tone, presence of blood, rectal perforation, or a high-riding prostate; this is particularly critical in patients with suspected spinal cord injury, pelvic fracture, or transpelvic gunshot wounds. Vaginal examination with a specu-

lum also should be performed in women with pelvic fractures to exclude an open fracture. Specific injuries, their associated signs and symptoms, diagnostic options, and treatments are discussed in detail later in this chapter.

Adjuncts to the physical examination include vital sign and CVP monitoring, ECG monitoring, nasogastric tube placement, Foley catheter placement, repeat FAST, laboratory measurements, and radiographs. A nasogastric tube should be inserted in all intubated patients to decrease the risk of gastric aspiration but may not be indicated in the awake patient. Nasogastric tube placement in

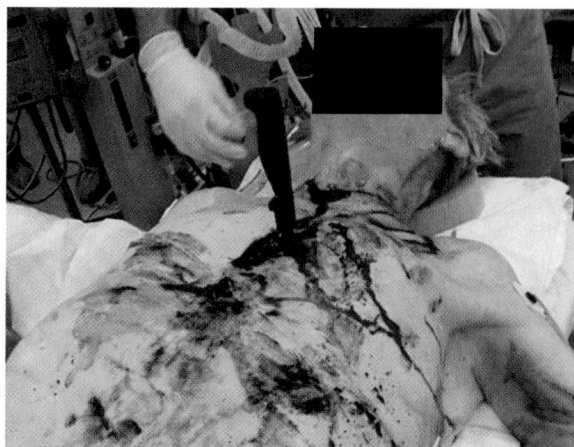 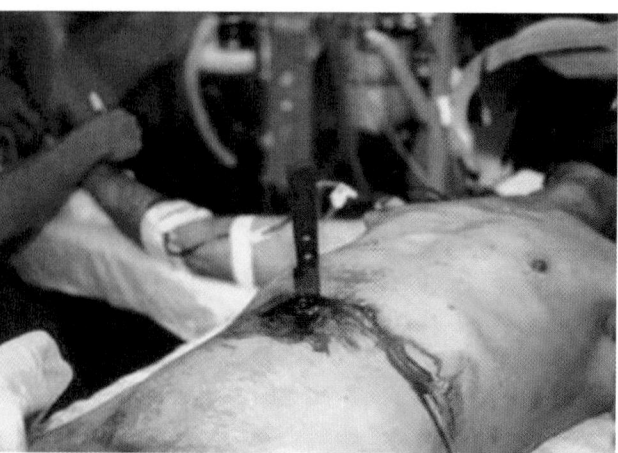

FIG. 7-15. If a weapon is still in place, it should be removed in the operating room, because it could be tamponading a lacerated blood vessel.

patients with complex facial fractures is contraindicated; rather, a tube should be placed orally if required. Nasogastric tube evaluation of stomach contents for blood may suggest occult gastroduodenal injury or the path of the nasogastric tube on a chest film may suggest a diaphragm injury. A Foley catheter should be inserted in patients unable to void to decompress the bladder, obtain a urine specimen, and monitor urine output. Gross hematuria demands evaluation of the genitourinary system for injury. Foley catheter placement should be deferred until urologic evaluation in patients with signs of urethral injury: blood at the meatus, perineal or scrotal hematomas, or a high-riding prostate. Although policies vary at individual institutions, patients in extremis with need for Foley catheter placement should undergo one attempt at catheterization; if the catheter does not pass easily, a percutaneous suprapubic cystostomy should be considered. Repeat FAST is performed if there are any signs of abdominal injury or occult blood loss.

Selective radiography and laboratory tests are done early in the evaluation after the primary survey. For patients with severe blunt trauma, lateral cervical spine, chest, and pelvic radiographs should be obtained, often termed *the big three*. For patients with truncal gunshot wounds, anteroposterior and lateral radiographs of the chest and abdomen are warranted. It is important to mark the entrance and exit sites of penetrating wounds with ECG pads, metallic clips, or staples so that the trajectory of the missile can be estimated. Limited one-shot extremity radiographs also may be taken. In critically injured patients, blood samples for a routine trauma panel (type and cross-match, complete blood count, blood chemistries, coagulation studies, lactate level, and arterial blood gas analysis) should be sent to the laboratory. For less severely injured patients only a complete blood count and urinalysis may be required. Because older patients may present in subclinical shock, even with minor injuries, routine analysis of arterial blood gases in patients over the age of 55 should be considered.

Many trauma patients cannot provide specific information about the mechanism of their injury. Emergency medical service personnel and police are trained to evaluate an injury scene and should be questioned. For automobile collisions, the speed of the vehicles involved, angle of impact (if any), use of restraints, airbag deployment, condition of the steering wheel and windshield, amount of intrusion, ejection or nonejection of the patient from the vehicle, and fate of other passengers should all be ascertained. For other injury mechanisms, critical information includes such things as height of a fall, surface impact, helmet use, and weight of an object by which the patient was crushed. In patients sustaining gunshot wounds, velocity, caliber, and presumed path of the bullet are important, if known. For patients with stab wounds, the length and type of object is helpful. Finally, some patients experience a combination of blunt and penetrating trauma. Do not assume that someone who was stabbed was not also assaulted; the patient may have a multitude of injuries and cannot be presumed to have only injuries associated with the more obvious penetrating mechanism. In sum, these details of information are critical to the clinician to determine overall mechanism of injury and anticipate its associated injury patterns.

Mechanisms and Patterns of Injury

In general, more energy is transferred over a wider area during blunt trauma than from a gunshot or stab wound. As a result, blunt trauma is associated with multiple widely distributed injuries, whereas in penetrating wounds the damage is localized to the path of the bullet or knife. In blunt trauma, organs that cannot yield to impact by elastic deformation are most likely to be injured, namely, the solid organs (liver, spleen, and kidneys). For penetrating trauma, organs with the largest surface area when viewed from the front are most prone to injury (small bowel, liver, and colon). Additionally, because bullets and knives usually follow straight lines, adjacent structures are commonly injured (e.g., the pancreas and duodenum).

Trauma surgeons often separate patients who have sustained blunt trauma into categories according to their risk for multiple injuries: those sustaining high energy transfer injuries and those sustaining low energy transfer injuries. Injuries involving high energy transfer include auto-pedestrian accidents, motor vehicle collisions in which the car's change of velocity (ΔV) exceeds 40 km/h or in which the patient has been ejected, motorcycle collisions, and falls from heights >20 ft.[14] In fact, for motor vehicle accidents the variables strongly associated with life-threatening injuries, and hence reflective of the magnitude of the mechanism, are death of another occupant in the vehicle, extrication time of >20 minutes, ΔV >40 km/h, lack of restraint use, and lateral impact.[14] Low-energy trauma, such as being struck with a club or falling from a bicycle, usually does not result in widely distributed injuries. However, potentially lethal lacerations of internal organs still can occur, because the net energy transfer to any given location may be substantial.

In blunt trauma, particular constellations of injury or injury patterns are associated with specific injury mechanisms. Frontal impact collisions typically produce multisystem trauma. When an unrestrained driver sustains a frontal impact, the head strikes the windshield, the chest and upper abdomen hit the steering column, and the legs or knees contact the dashboard. The resultant injuries can include facial fractures, cervical spine fractures, laceration of the thoracic aorta, myocardial contusion, injury to the spleen and liver, and fractures of the pelvis and lower extremities. When such patients are evaluated, the discovery of one of these injuries should prompt a search for others. Collisions with side impact also carry the risk of cervical spine and thoracic trauma, diaphragm rupture, and crush injuries of the pelvic ring, but solid organ injury usually is limited to either the liver or spleen based on the direction of impact. Not surprisingly, any time a patient is ejected from the vehicle or thrown a significant distance from a motorcycle, the risk of any injury increases.

Penetrating injuries are classified according to the wounding agent (i.e., stab wound, gunshot wound, or shotgun wound). Gunshot wounds are subdivided further into high- and low-velocity injuries, because the speed of the bullet is much more important than its weight in determining kinetic energy. High-velocity gunshot wounds (bullet speed >2000 ft/s) are infrequent in the civilian setting. Shotgun injuries are divided into close-range (<7 m) and long-range wounds. Close-range shotgun wounds are tantamount to high-velocity wounds because the entire energy of the load is delivered to a small area, often with devastating results. Long-range shotgun blasts result in a diffuse pellet pattern in which many pellets miss the victim, and those that do strike are dispersed and of comparatively low energy.

Regional Assessment and Special Diagnostic Tests

Based on mechanism, location of injuries identified on physical examination, screening radiographs, and the patient's overall condition, additional diagnostic studies often are indicated. However, the seriously injured patient is in constant jeopardy when undergoing special diagnostic testing; therefore, the surgeon must be in attendance and must be prepared to alter plans as circumstances demand. Hemodynamic, respiratory, and mental status will determine the most appropriate course of action. With these issues in mind, additional diagnostic tests are discussed on an anatomic basis.

Head

Evaluation of the head includes examination for injuries to the scalp, eyes, ears, nose, mouth, facial bones, and intracranial structures. Palpation of the head will identify scalp lacerations, which should be evaluated for depth, and depressed or open skull fractures. The eye examination includes not only pupillary size and reactivity, but also examination for visual acuity and for hemorrhage within the globe. Ocular entrapment, caused by orbital fractures with impingement on the ocular muscles, is evident when the patient cannot move his or her eyes through the entire range of motion. It is important to perform the eye examination early, because significant orbital swelling may prevent later evaluation. The tympanic membrane is visualized to identify hemotympanum, otorrhea, or rupture, which may signal an underlying head injury. Otorrhea, rhinorrhea, raccoon eyes, and Battle's sign (ecchymosis behind the ear) suggest a basilar skull fracture. Although such fractures may not require treatment, there is an association with blunt cerebrovascular injuries and a small risk of development of meningitis.

Anterior facial structures should be examined to rule out fractures. This entails palpating for bony step-off of the facial bones and instability of the midface (by grasping the upper palate and seeing if this moves separately from the patient's head). A good question to ask awake patients is whether their bite feels normal to them; abnormal dental closure suggests malalignment of facial bones and a possibility for a mandible or maxillary fracture. Nasal fractures, which may be evident on direct inspection or palpation, typically bleed vigorously. This may result in the patient's having airway compromise due to blood running down the posterior pharynx, or there may be vomiting provoked by swallowed blood. Nasal packing or balloon tamponade may be necessary to control bleeding. Examination of the oral cavity includes inspection for open fractures, loose or fractured teeth, and sublingual hematomas.

All patients with a significant closed head injury (GCS score <14) should undergo CT scanning of the head. For penetrating injuries, plain skull films may be helpful in the trauma bay to determine the extent of injury in hemodynamically unstable patients who cannot be transported for CT scan. The presence of lateralizing findings (e.g., a unilateral dilated pupil unreactive to light, asymmetric movement of the extremities either spontaneously or in response to noxious stimuli, or unilateral Babinski's reflex) suggests an intracranial mass lesion or major structural damage.

Such lesions include hematomas, contusions, hemorrhage into ventricular and subarachnoid spaces, and diffuse axonal injury (DAI). Epidural hematomas occur when blood accumulates between the skull and dura, and are caused by disruption of the middle meningeal artery or other small arteries in that potential space, typically after a skull fracture (Fig. 7-16). Subdural hematomas occur between the dura and cortex and are caused by venous disruption or laceration of the parenchyma of the brain. Due to associated parenchymal injury, subdural hematomas typically have a worse prognosis than epidural collections. Hemorrhage into the subarachnoid space may cause vasospasm and reduce cerebral blood flow. Intraparenchymal hematomas and contusions can occur anywhere within the brain. DAI results from high-speed deceleration injury and represents direct axonal damage. CT scan may demonstrate blurring of the gray and white matter interface and multiple small punctate hemorrhages, but magnetic resonance imaging is a more sensitive test. Although prognosis for these injuries is extremely variable, early evidence of DAI is associated with a poor outcome. Stroke syndromes should prompt a search for carotid or vertebral artery injury using standard four-vessel angiography or 16-slice CT angiography (Fig. 7-17).

Significant intracranial penetrating injuries usually are produced by bullets from handguns, but an array of other weapons or instruments can injure the cerebrum via the orbit or through the thinner temporal region of the skull. Although the diagnosis usually is obvious, in some instances wounds in the auditory canal, mouth, and nose can be elusive. Prognosis is variable, but most supratentorial wounds that injure both hemispheres are fatal.

Neck

All blunt trauma patients should be assumed to have cervical spine injuries until proven otherwise. During cervical examination one must maintain cervical spine precautions and in-line stabilization. During the primary survey, identification of penetrating injuries to the neck with exsanguination, expanding hematomas, and airway obstruction is a priority. A more subtle injury that may not be identified is a fracture of the larynx due to blunt trauma. Signs and

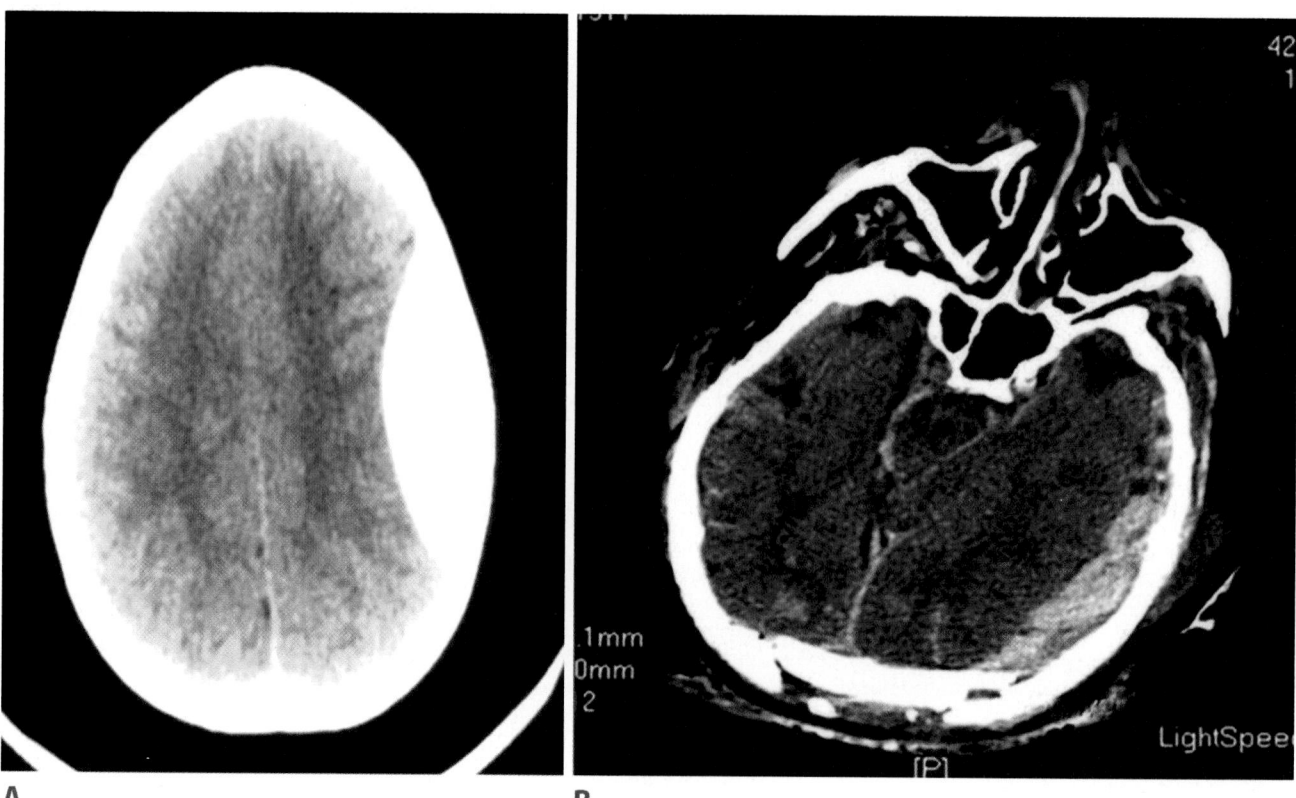

A　　　　　　　　　　　　　**B**

FIG. 7-16. Epidural hematomas (**A**) have a distinctive convex shape on computed tomographic scan, whereas subdural hematomas (**B**) are concave along the surface of the brain.

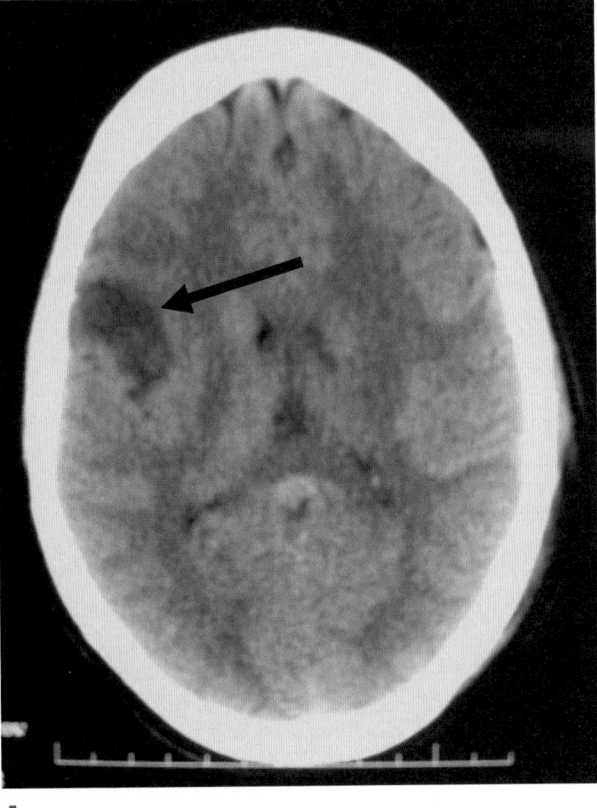

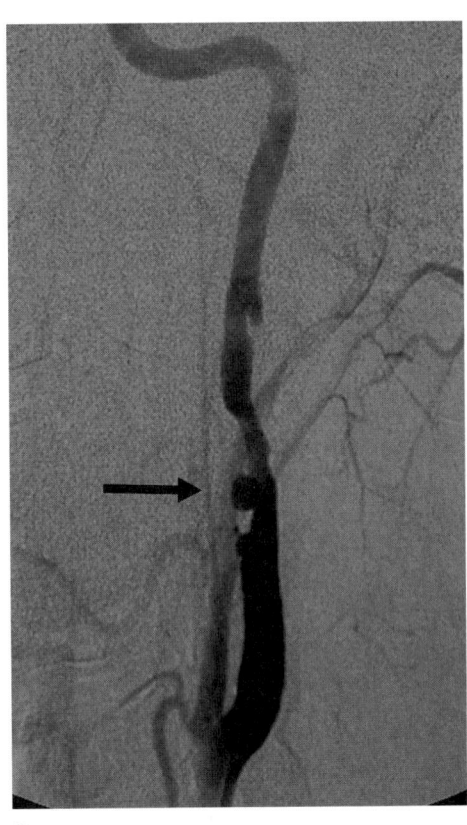

FIG. 7-17. A. A right middle cerebral infarct noted on a computed tomographic scan of the head. Such a finding should prompt imaging to rule out an associated extracranial cerebrovascular injury. **B.** An internal carotid artery pseudoaneurysm documented by angiography.

symptoms include hoarseness, subcutaneous emphysema (Fig. 7-18), and a palpable fracture.

Due to the devastating consequences of quadriplegia, a diligent evaluation for occult cervical spine injuries is mandatory. In the awake patient, the presence of posterior midline pain or tenderness should provoke a thorough radiologic evaluation. Additionally, intu-

bated patients, patients experiencing trauma associated with significant injury mechanisms, and patients with distracting injuries or another identified spine fracture should undergo imaging. Imaging options include CT scan or five plain radiograph views of the cervical spine: lateral view with visualization of C7 through T1, anteroposterior view, transoral odontoid views, and bilateral oblique views. If

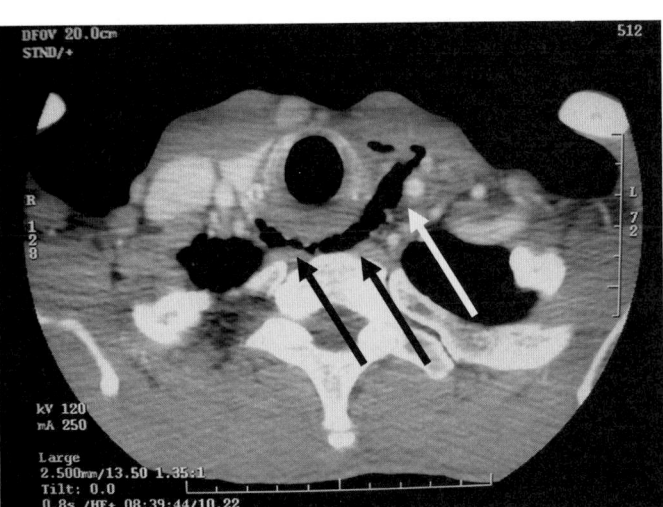

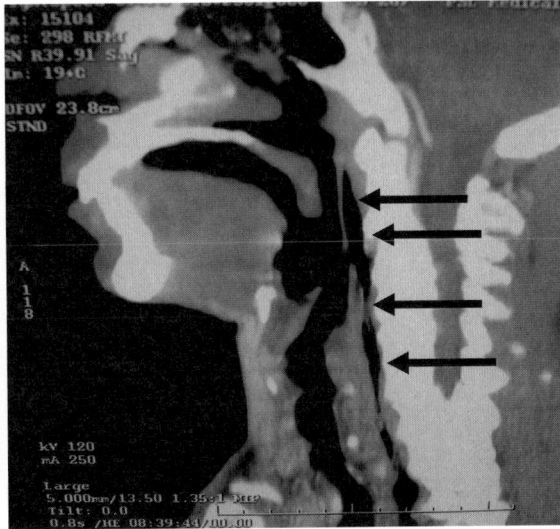

FIG. 7-18. A laryngeal fracture results in air tracking around the trachea along the prevertebral space (*arrows*).

pain or tenderness persists but no injuries are identified on plain radiographs, or if the patient cannot be examined in a timely manner, a CT scan should be performed. However, a ligamentous injury may not be visible with standard imaging techniques.[15] Flexion and extension views are typically obtained after a delay in patients with persistent pain but negative imaging findings. However, this should be done only in the presence of an experienced spinal surgeon, because patients can be rendered permanently quadriplegic when flexed and extended by inexperienced individuals.

Spinal cord injuries can be complete or partial. Complete injuries cause either permanent quadriplegia or paraplegia, depending on the level of injury. These patients have a complete loss of motor function and sensation two or more levels below the bony injury. Patients with high spinal cord disruption are at risk for shock due to physiologic disruption of sympathetic fibers. Significant neurologic recovery is rare. There are several partial or incomplete spinal cord injury syndromes. Central cord syndrome usually occurs in older persons who experience hyperextension injuries. Motor function and pain and temperature sensation are preserved in the lower extremities but diminished in the upper extremities. Some functional recovery usually occurs, but is often not a return to normal. Anterior cord syndrome is characterized by diminished motor function and pain and temperature sensation below the level of the injury, but position sensing, vibratory sensation, and crude touch are maintained. Prognosis for recovery is poor. Brown-Séquard syndrome is usually the result of a penetrating injury in which the right or left half of the spinal cord is transected. This rare lesion is characterized by the ipsilateral loss of motor function, proprioception, and vibratory sensation, whereas pain and temperature sensation are lost on the contralateral side.

Penetrating injuries of the anterior neck that violate the platysma are potentially life-threatening because of the density of critical structures in this region. Although presumptive exploration may be appropriate in some circumstances, selective nonoperative management is practiced in most centers (Fig. 7-19).[16,17] Indications for immediate operative intervention for penetrating cervical injury include hemodynamic instability or significant external hemorrhage. The management algorithm for hemodynamically stable patients is based on the presenting symptoms and anatomic location of injury, with the neck being divided into three distinct zones (Fig. 7-20). Zone I is between the clavicles and cricoid cartilage, zone II is between the cricoid cartilage and the angle of the mandible, and zone III is above the angle of the mandible. Due to technical difficulties of injury exposure and varying operative approaches, a precise preoperative diagnosis is desirable for symptomatic zone I and III injuries. Therefore, these patients should ideally undergo diagnostic imaging before operation if they remain hemodynamically stable. CT scanning of the neck and chest determines the injury track, and further studies are performed based on proximity to major structures.[18] Such additional imaging includes CT angiography, angiography of the great vessels, soluble contrast esophagram followed by barium esophagram, esophagoscopy, or bronchoscopy. Angiographic diagnosis, particularly of zone III injuries, may be followed by endovascular intervention for definitive treatment.

Patients with zone II wounds that do not penetrate the platysma can be discharged from the ED. Patients with zone II penetrating wounds are divided into those who are symptomatic and those who are not. Specific symptoms that should be elucidated include airway compromise, an expanding or pulsatile hematoma, dysphagia, hoarseness, and subcutaneous emphysema. Symptomatic patients should undergo emergent neck exploration. Asymptomatic patients with zone II injuries should be further divided into those with and those without a transcervical gunshot wound. Those without a transcervical component may be observed for 12 to 24 hours, whereas those with

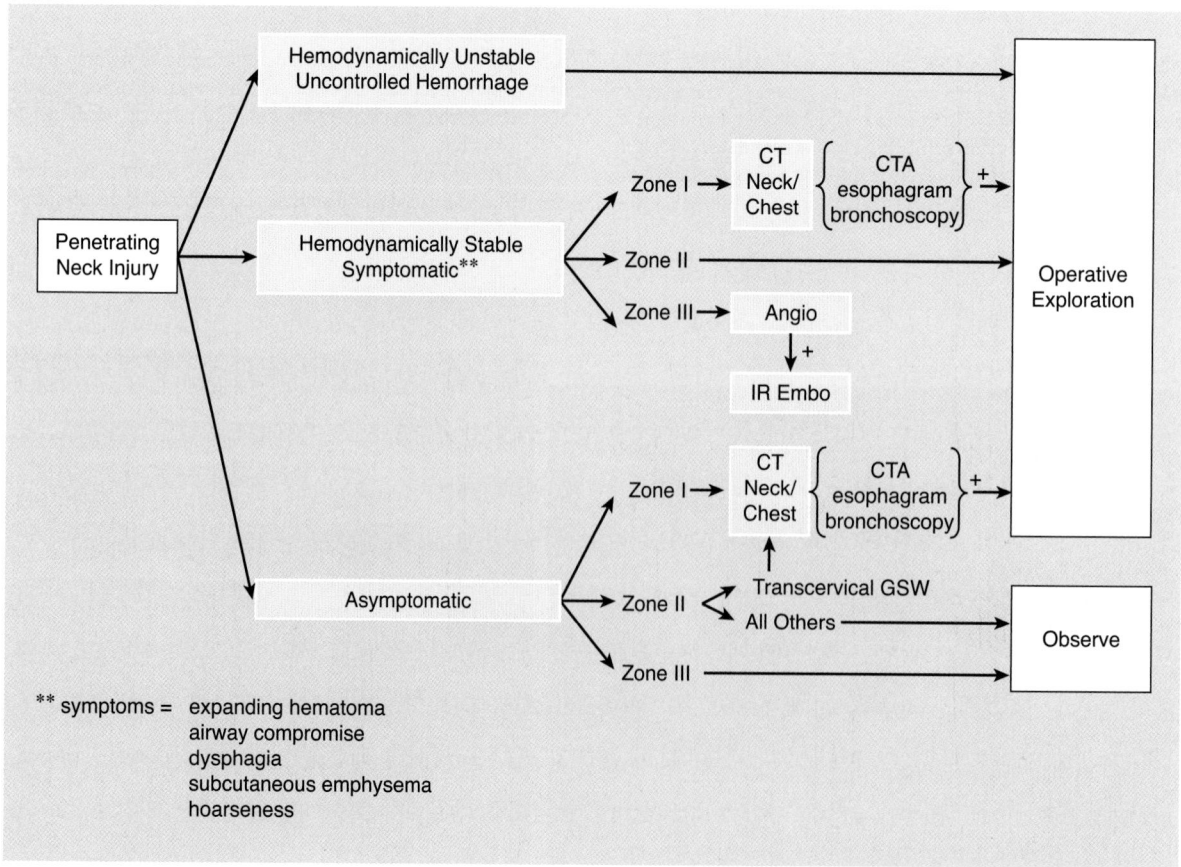

FIG. 7-19. Algorithm for the selective management of penetrating neck injuries. CT = computed tomography; CTA = computed tomographic angiography; GSW = gunshot wound; IR Embo = interventional radiology embolization.

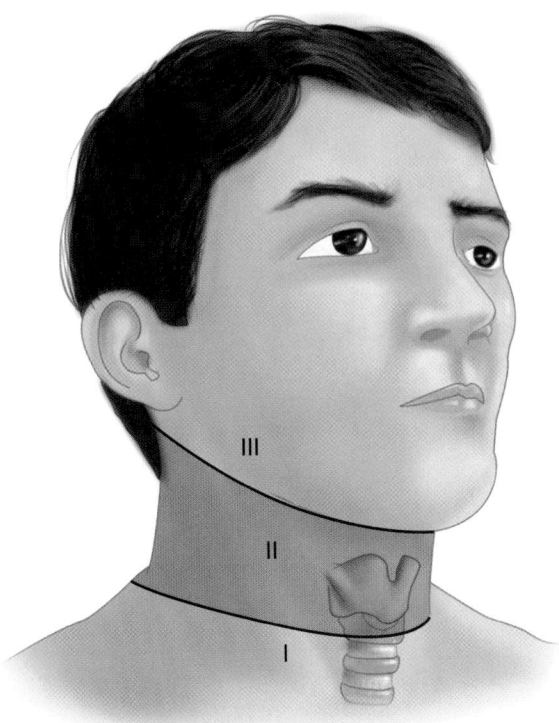

FIG. 7-20. For the purpose of evaluating penetrating injuries, the neck is divided into three zones. Zone I is up to the level of the cricoid and is also known as the *thoracic outlet.* Zone II is located between the cricoid cartilage and the angle of the mandible. Zone III is above the angle of the mandible.

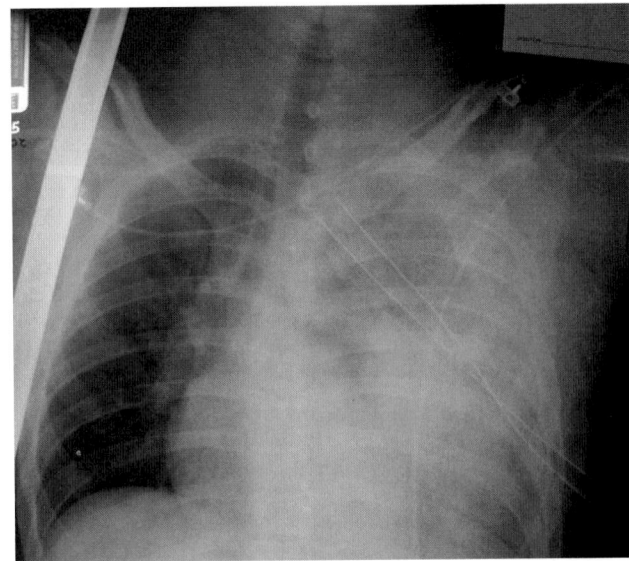

FIG. 7-21. Persistence of a hemothorax despite two tube thoracostomies is termed a *caked hemothorax* and is an indication for prompt thoracotomy.

transcervical gunshot wounds should undergo CT scanning to determine the track of the bullet. Based on location of the track and transfer of kinetic injury, further diagnostic imaging with angiography, esophagram, or bronchoscopy should be performed.

Chest

Blunt trauma to the chest may involve the chest wall, thoracic spine, heart, lungs, thoracic aorta and great vessels, and rarely the esophagus. Most of these injuries can be evaluated by physical examination and chest radiography, with supplemental CT scanning based on initial findings. Any patient who undergoes intervention—intubation, central line placement, tube thoracostomy—needs a repeat chest radiograph to document the adequacy of the procedure. This is particularly true in patients undergoing tube thoracostomy for a pneumothorax or hemothorax. Patients with persistent pneumothorax, large air leaks after tube thoracostomy, or difficulty ventilating should undergo fiber-optic bronchoscopy to exclude a bronchial injury or presence of a foreign body. Patients with hemothorax must have a chest radiograph documenting complete evacuation of the chest; a persistent hemothorax that is not drained by two chest tubes is termed a *caked hemothorax* and mandates prompt thoracotomy (Fig. 7-21).

Occult thoracic vascular injury must be diligently sought due to the high mortality of a missed lesion. Widening of the mediastinum on initial anteroposterior chest radiograph, caused by a hematoma around an injured vessel that is contained by the mediastinal pleura, suggests an injury of the great vessels. The mediastinal abnormality may suggest the location of the arterial injury (i.e., left-sided hematomas are associated with descending torn aortas, whereas right-sided hematomas are commonly seen with innominate injuries) (Fig. 7-22). Posterior rib fractures, sternal fractures, and laceration of small vessels also can produce similar hematomas. Other chest radiographic findings suggestive of an aortic tear are summarized in Table

7-5 (Fig. 7-23). However, at least 7% of patients with a descending torn aorta have a normal chest radiograph.[19] Therefore, screening spiral CT scanning is performed based on the mechanism of injury: high-energy deceleration motor vehicle collision with frontal or lateral impact, motor vehicle collision with ejection, falls of >25 ft, or direct impact (horse kick to chest, snowmobile or ski collision with tree).[20] In >95% of patients who survive to reach the ED, the aortic injury occurs just distal to the left subclavian artery, where it is tethered by the ligamentum arteriosum (Fig. 7-24). In 2 to 5% of patients the injury occurs in the ascending aorta, in the transverse arch, or at the diaphragm. Reconstructions with multislice CT scanning obviate the need for invasive angiography.[20]

For penetrating thoracic trauma physical examination, plain posteroanterior and lateral chest radiographs with metallic markings of entrance and exit wounds, pericardial ultrasound, and CVP measurement will identify the majority of injuries. Injuries of the esophagus and trachea are exceptions. Bronchoscopy should be performed to evaluate the trachea in patients with a persistent air leak from the chest tube or mediastinal air. Because esophagoscopy can miss injuries, patients at risk should undergo soluble contrast esophagraphy followed by barium examination to look for extravasation of contrast to identify an injury.[21] As with neck injuries, hemodynamically stable patients with transmediastinal gunshot wounds should undergo CT scanning to determine the path of the bullet; this identifies the vascular or visceral structures at risk for injury and directs angiography or endoscopy as appropriate. If there is a suspicion of a subclavian artery injury, brachial-brachial indices should be measured, but >60% of patients with an injury may not have a pulse deficit.[22] Therefore, CT angiography should be performed based on injury proximity to intrathoracic vasculature. Finally, despite entry wounds on the chest, penetrating trauma should not be presumed to be isolated to the thorax. Injury to contiguous body cavities (i.e., the abdomen and neck) must be excluded.

Abdomen

The abdomen is a diagnostic black box. Fortunately, with few exceptions, it is not necessary to determine in the ED which intra-abdominal organs are injured, only whether an exploratory laparotomy is necessary. Physical examination of the abdomen is unreliable in making this determination, and drugs, alcohol, and head and spinal cord injuries complicate clinical evaluation. However, the presence of abdominal rigidity or hemodynamic compromise is an indication for

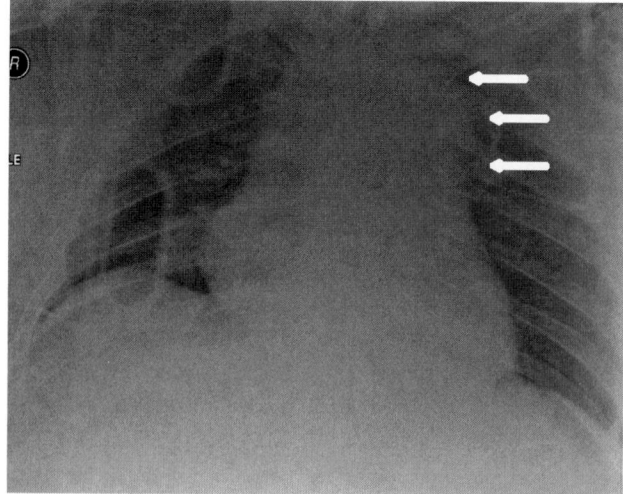

A

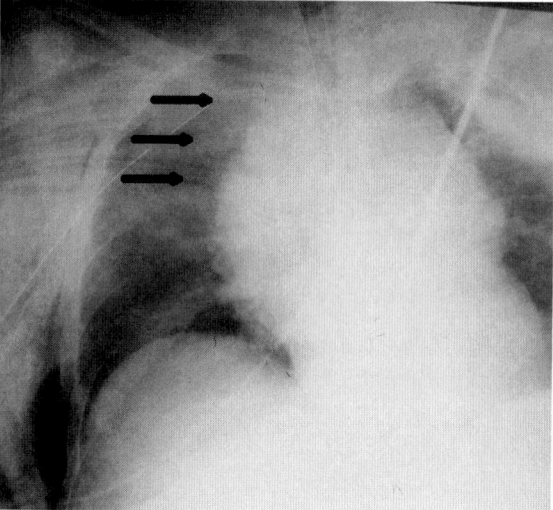

B

FIG. 7-22. Location of the hematoma within the mediastinal silhouette suggests the type of great vessel injury. A predominant hematoma on the left suggests the far more common descending torn aorta (**A**; *arrows*), whereas a hematoma on the right indicates a relatively unusual but life-threatening innominate artery injury (**B**; *arrows*).

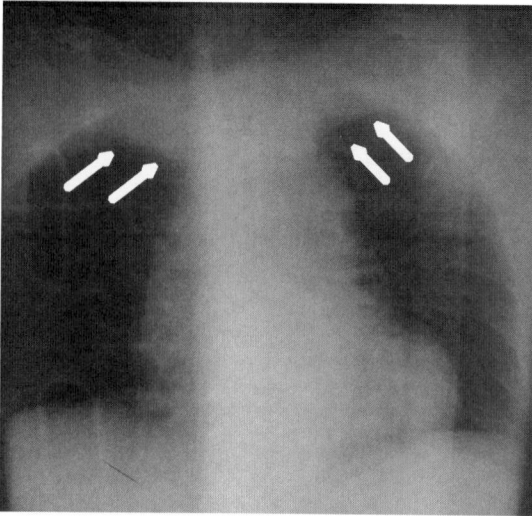

A

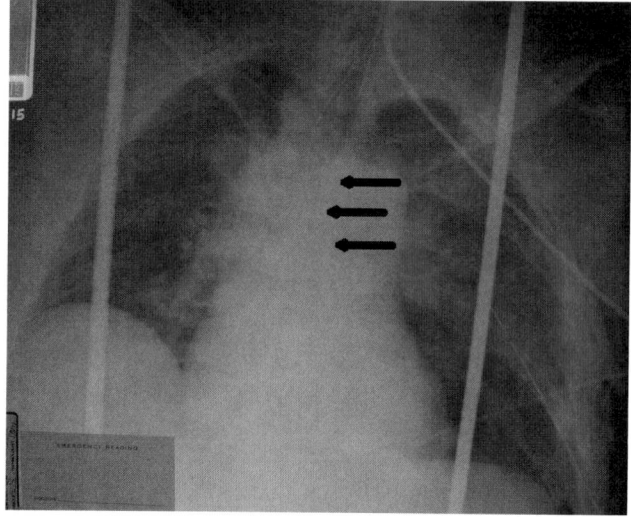

B

FIG. 7-23. Chest film findings associated with descending torn aorta include apical capping (**A**; *arrows*) and tracheal shift (**B**; *arrows*).

prompt surgical exploration. For the remainder of patients, a variety of diagnostic adjuncts are used to identify abdominal injury.

The diagnostic approach differs for penetrating trauma and blunt abdominal trauma. As a rule, minimal evaluation is required before

TABLE 7-5	Findings on chest radiograph suggestive of a descending thoracic aortic tear

1. Widened mediastinum
2. Abnormal aortic contour
3. Tracheal shift
4. Nasogastric tube shift
5. Left apical cap
6. Left or right paraspinal stripe thickening
7. Depression of the left main bronchus
8. Obliteration of the aorticopulmonary window
9. Left pulmonary hilar hematoma

laparotomy for gunshot or shotgun wounds that penetrate the peritoneal cavity, because over 90% of patients have significant internal injuries. Anterior truncal gunshot wounds between the fourth intercostal space and the pubic symphysis whose trajectory as determined by radiograph or entrance and exit wounds indicates peritoneal penetration should be operatively explored (Fig. 7-25). The exception is penetrating trauma isolated to the right upper quadrant; in hemodynamically stable patients with bullet trajectory confined to the liver by CT scan, nonoperative observation may be considered.[23,24] Gunshot wounds to the back or flank are more difficult to evaluate because of the retroperitoneal location of the injured abdominal organs. Triple-contrast CT scan can delineate the trajectory of the bullet and identify peritoneal violation or retroperitoneal entry, but may miss specific injuries.[25] Similarly, in obese patients, if the gunshot wound is thought to be tangential through the subcutaneous tissues, CT scan can delineate the track and exclude peritoneal violation. Laparoscopy is another option to assess peritoneal penetration and is followed by laparotomy to repair injuries if found. If there is doubt, it is always safer to explore the abdomen than to equivocate.

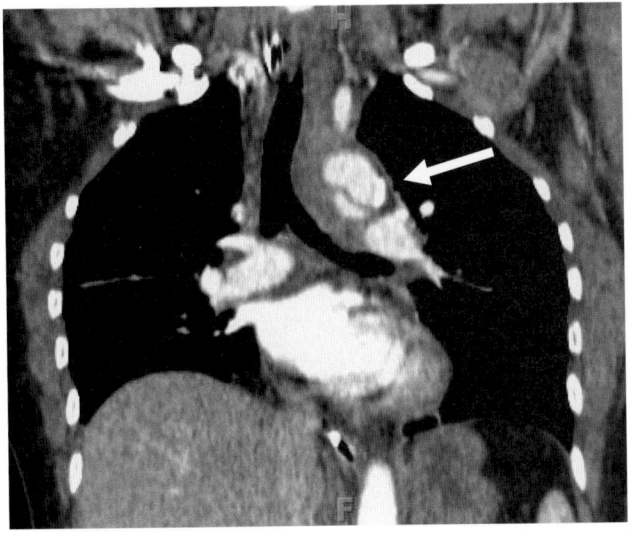

A

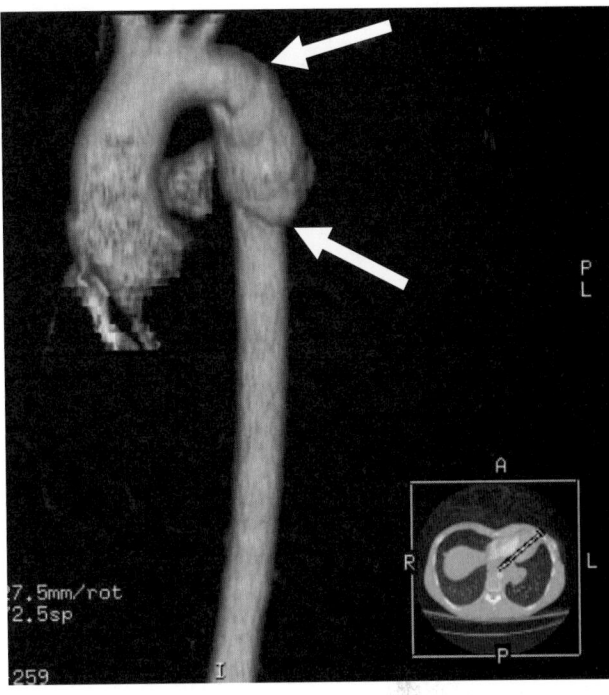

B

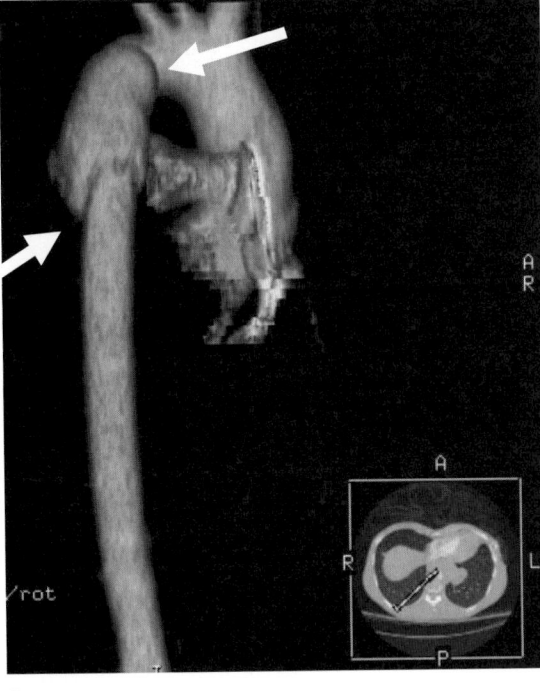

C

FIG. 7-24. Imaging to diagnose descending torn aorta includes computed tomographic angiography (**A**), with three-dimensional reconstructions (**B**, anterior; **C**, posterior) demonstrating the proximal and distal extent of the injury (*arrows*).

In contrast to gunshot wounds, stab wounds that penetrate the peritoneal cavity are less likely to injure intra-abdominal organs. Anterior abdominal stab wounds (from costal margin to inguinal ligament and bilateral midaxillary lines) should be explored under local anesthesia in the ED to determine if the fascia has been violated. Injuries that do not penetrate the peritoneal cavity do not require further evaluation, and the patient is discharged from the ED. Patients with fascial penetration must be further evaluated for intra-abdominal injury, because there is up to a 50% chance of requiring laparotomy. Debate remains over whether the optimal diagnostic approach is serial examination, diagnostic peritoneal lavage (DPL), or CT scanning.[26] If DPL is pursued, an infraumbilical approach is used (Fig. 7-26). After placement of the catheter, a 10-mL syringe is connected and the abdominal contents aspirated (termed a *diagnostic peritoneal aspiration*). The aspirate is considered to show positive findings if >10 mL of blood is aspirated. If <10 mL is withdrawn, a liter of normal saline is instilled. The effluent is withdrawn via siphoning and sent to the laboratory for RBC count, white blood cell (WBC) count, and deter-

mination of amylase, bilirubin, and alkaline phosphatase levels. Values representing positive findings are summarized in Table 7-6.

Abdominal stab wounds in three body regions require a unique diagnostic approach: thoracoabdominal stab wounds, right upper quadrant stab wounds, and back and flank stab wounds. Occult injury to the diaphragm must be ruled out in patients with stab wounds to the lower chest. For patients undergoing DPL evaluation, laboratory value cutoffs are different for those with thoracoabdominal stab wounds and for those with standard anterior abdominal stab wounds (see Table 7-6). An RBC count of >10,000/μL is considered a positive finding and an indication for laparotomy; patients with a DPL RBC count between 1000/μL and 10,000/μL should undergo laparoscopy or thoracoscopy. Patients with stab wounds to the right upper quadrant can undergo CT scanning to determine trajectory and confinement to the liver for potential nonoperative care.[23,24] Those with stab wounds to the flank and back should undergo triple-contrast CT to detect occult retroperitoneal injuries of the colon, duodenum, and urinary tract.[25]

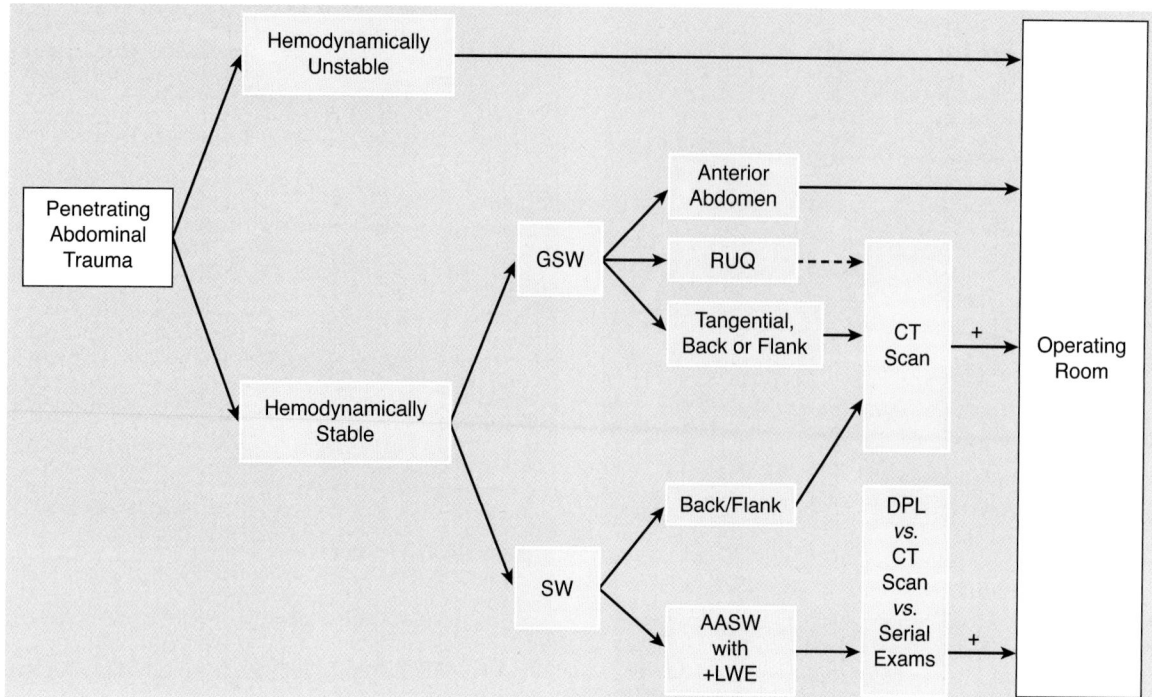

FIG. 7-25. Algorithm for the evaluation of penetrating abdominal injuries. AASW = anterior abdominal stab wound; CT = computed tomography; DPL = diagnostic peritoneal lavage; GSW = gunshot wound; LWE = local wound exploration; RUQ = right upper quadrant; SW = stab wound.

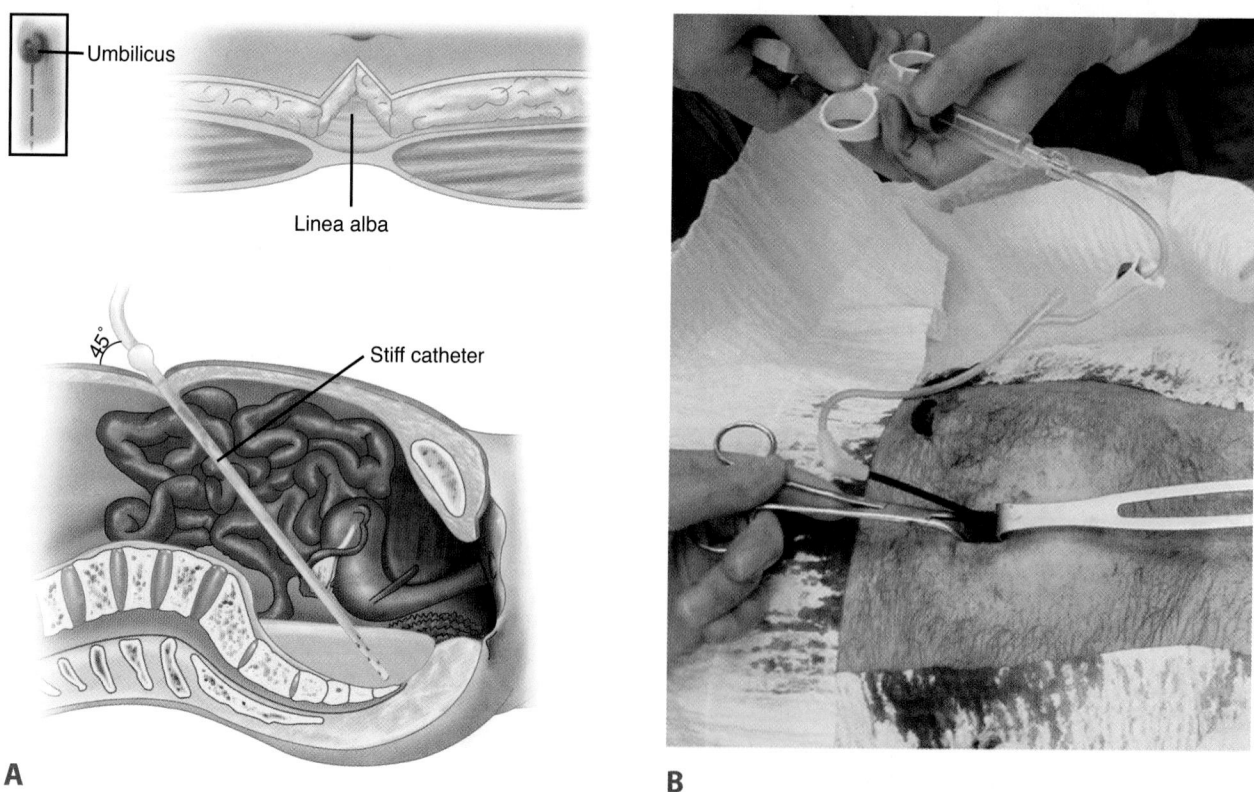

A   **B**

FIG. 7-26. Diagnostic peritoneal lavage is performed through an infraumbilical incision unless the patient has a pelvic fracture or is pregnant. **A.** The linea alba is sharply incised, and the catheter is directed into the pelvis. **B.** The abdominal contents should initially be aspirated using a 10-mL syringe.

TABLE 7-6	Criteria for "positive" finding on diagnostic peritoneal lavage	
	Anterior Abdominal Stab Wounds	**Thoracoabdominal Stab Wounds**
Red blood cell count	>100,000/mL	>10,000/mL
White blood cell count	>500/mL	>500/mL
Amylase level	>19 IU/L	>19 IU/L
Alkaline phosphatase level	>2 IU/L	>2 IU/L
Bilirubin level	>0.01 mg/dL	>0.01 mg/dL

Blunt abdominal trauma initially is evaluated by FAST examination in most major trauma centers, and this has largely supplanted DPL (Fig. 7-27).[27] FAST is not 100% sensitive, however, so diagnostic peritoneal aspiration is still advocated in hemodynamically unstable patients without a defined source of blood loss to rule out abdominal hemorrhage.[11] FAST is used to identify free intraperitoneal fluid (Fig. 7-28) in Morison's pouch, the left upper quadrant, and the pelvis. Although this method is exquisitely sensitive for detecting intraperitoneal fluid of >250 mL, it does not reliably determine the source of hemorrhage nor grade solid organ injuries.[28,29] Patients with fluid on FAST examination, considered a "positive FAST," who do not have immediate indications for laparotomy and are hemodynamically stable undergo CT scanning to quantify their injuries. Injury grading using the American Association for the Surgery of Trauma grading scale (Table 7-7) is a key component of nonoperative management of solid organ injuries. Additional findings that should be noted on CT scan in patients with solid organ injury include contrast extravasation (i.e., a "blush"), the amount of intra-abdominal hemorrhage, and presence of pseudoaneurysms (Fig. 7-29). CT also is indicated for hemodynamically stable patients for whom the physical examination is unreliable. Despite the increasing diagnostic accuracy of multislice CT scanners, CT still has limited sensitivity for identification of intestinal injuries. Bowel injury is suggested by findings of thickened bowel wall, "streaking" in the mesentery, free fluid without associated solid organ injury, or free intraperitoneal air.[30] Patients with free intra-abdominal fluid without solid organ injury are closely monitored for evolving signs of peritonitis; if patients have a significant closed head injury or cannot be serially examined, DPL should be performed to exclude bowel injury.

Pelvis

Blunt injury to the pelvis may produce complex fractures with major hemorrhage (Fig. 7-30). Plain radiographs will reveal gross abnormalities, but CT scanning may be necessary to determine the precise geometry. Sharp spicules of bone can lacerate the bladder, rectum, or vagina. Alternatively, bladder rupture may result from the direct blow to the torso if the bladder is full. CT cystography is performed if the urinalysis findings are positive for RBCs. Urethral injuries are suspected if examination reveals blood at the meatus, scrotal or perineal hematomas, or a high-riding prostate on rectal examination. Urethrograms should be obtained for stable patients before placing a Foley catheter to avoid false passage and subsequent stricture. Major vascular injuries causing exsanguination are uncommon in blunt pelvic trauma; however, thrombosis of either the arteries or veins in the iliofemoral system may occur, and CT angiography or formal angiography is diagnostic. Life-threatening hemorrhage can be associated with pelvic fractures and may initially preclude definitive imaging. Treatment algorithms for patients with complex pelvic fractures and hemodynamic instability are presented later in the chapter.

Extremities

Blunt or penetrating trauma to the extremities requires an evaluation for fractures, ligamentous injury, and neurovascular injury. Plain radiographs are used to evaluate fractures, whereas ligamentous injuries, particularly those of the knee and shoulder, can be imaged with magnetic resonance imaging. Physical examination often identifies arterial injuries, and findings are classified as either hard signs or soft signs of vascular injury (Table 7-8). In general, hard signs constitute indications for operative exploration, whereas soft signs are indications for further testing or observation. Bony fractures or knee dislocations should be realigned before definitive vascular examination. On-table angiography may be useful to localize the arterial injury and thus limit tissue dissection in patients with hard signs of vascular injury. For example, a patient with an absent popliteal pulse and femoral shaft fracture due to a bullet that entered the lateral hip and exited below the medial knee could have injured either the femoral or popliteal artery anywhere along its course (Fig. 7-31).

In management of vascular trauma, controversy exists regarding the treatment of patients with soft signs of injury, particularly those with injuries in proximity to major vessels. It is known that some of these patients will have arterial injuries that require repair. One approach has been to measure SBP using Doppler ultrasonography and compare the value for the injured side with that for the uninjured side, termed the *A-A index*.[31] If the pressures are within

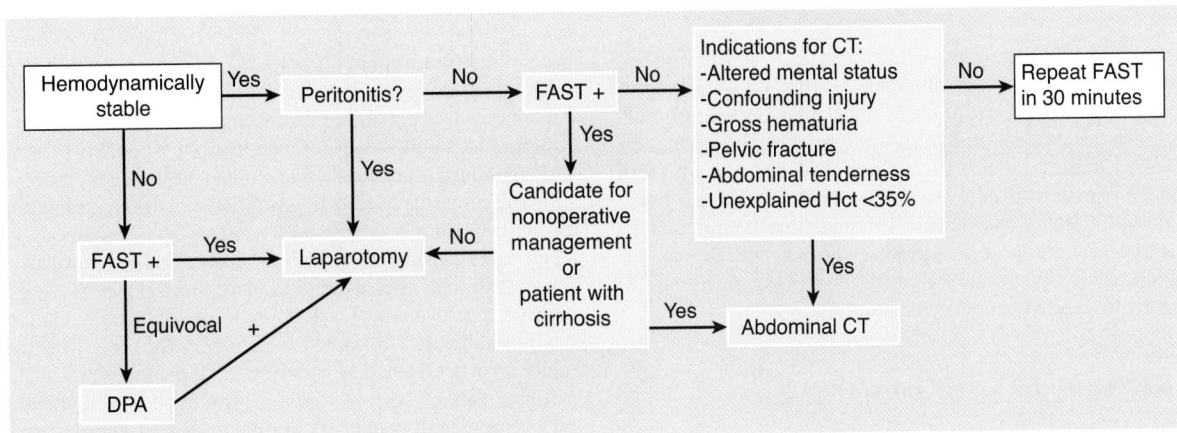

FIG. 7-27. Algorithm for the initial evaluation of a patient with suspected blunt abdominal trauma. CT = computed tomography; DPA = diagnostic peritoneal aspiration; FAST = focused abdominal sonography for trauma; Hct = hematocrit.

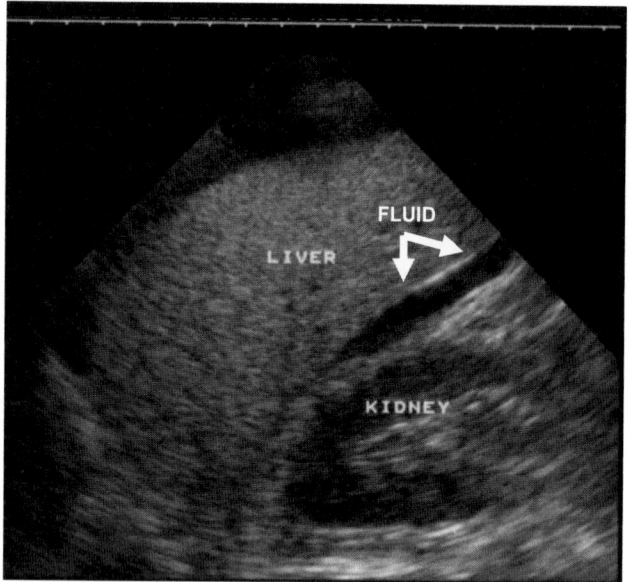

A

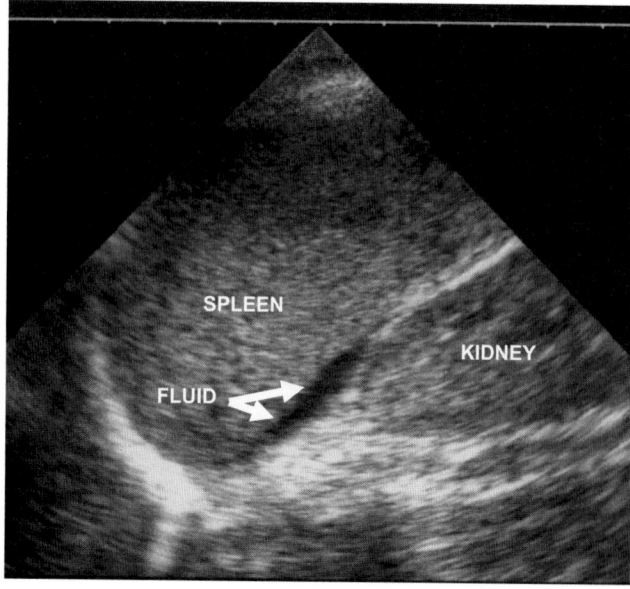

B

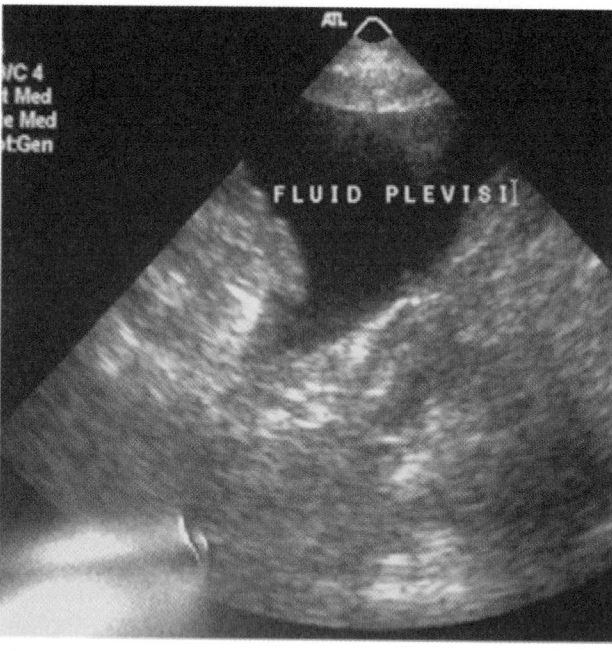

C

FIG. 7-28. Focused abdominal sonography for trauma imaging detects intra-abdominal hemorrhage. Hemorrhage is presumed when a fluid stripe is visible between the right kidney and liver (**A**), between the left kidney and spleen (**B**), or in the pelvis (**C**).

10% of each other, a significant injury is unlikely and no further evaluation is performed. If the difference is >10%, CT angiography or arteriography is indicated. Others argue that there are occult injuries, such as pseudoaneurysms or injuries of the profunda femoris or peroneal arteries, which may not be detected with this technique. If hemorrhage occurs from these injuries, compartment syndrome and limb loss may occur. Although busy trauma centers continue to debate this issue, the surgeon who is obliged to treat the occasional injured patient may be better served by performing CT angiography in selected patients with soft signs.

GENERAL PRINCIPLES OF MANAGEMENT

Over the past 20 years there has been a remarkable change in management practices and operative approach for the injured pa-

tient. With the advent of CT scanning, nonoperative management of solid organ injuries has replaced routine operative exploration. Those patients who do require operation may be treated with less radical resection techniques such as splenorrhaphy or partial nephrectomy. Colonic injuries, previously mandating colostomy, are now repaired primarily in virtually all cases. Additionally, the type of anastomosis has shifted from a double-layer closure to a continuous running single-layer closure; this method is technically equivalent to and faster than the interrupted multilayer techniques.[32] Adoption of damage control surgical techniques in physiologically deranged patients has resulted in limited initial operative time, with definitive injury repair delayed until after resuscitation in the surgical intensive care unit (SICU) with physiologic restoration.[33] Abdominal drains, once considered mandatory for parenchymal injuries and some anastomoses, have disappeared; fluid collections are managed by percutaneous techniques. Newer endovascular techniques such as

TABLE 7-7 American Association for the Surgery of Trauma grading scales for solid organ injuries

	Subcapsular Hematoma	Laceration
Liver Injury Grade		
Grade I	<10% of surface area	<1 cm in depth
Grade II	10–50% of surface area	1–3 cm
Grade III	>50% of surface area or >10 cm in depth	>3 cm
Grade IV	25–75% of a hepatic lobe	
Grade V	>75% of a hepatic lobe	
Grade VI	Hepatic avulsion	
Splenic Injury Grade		
Grade I	<10% of surface area	<1 cm in depth
Grade II	10–50% of surface area	1–3 cm
Grade III	>50% of surface area or >10 cm in depth	>3 cm
Grade IV	>25% devascularization	Hilum
Grade V	Shattered spleen Complete devascularization	

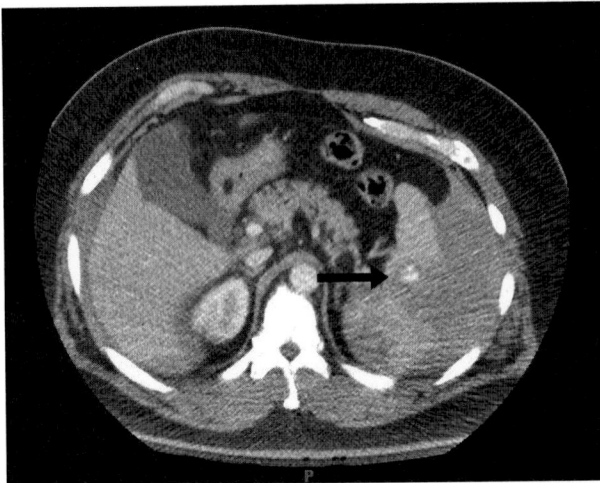

A

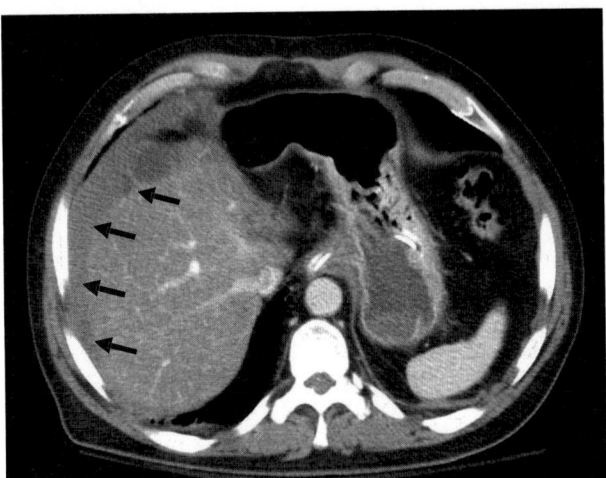

B

FIG. 7-29. Computed tomographic images reveal critical information about solid organ injuries, such as associated contrast extravasation from a grade IV laceration of the spleen (**A**; *arrows*) and the amount of subcapsular hematoma in a grade III liver laceration (**B**; *arrows*).

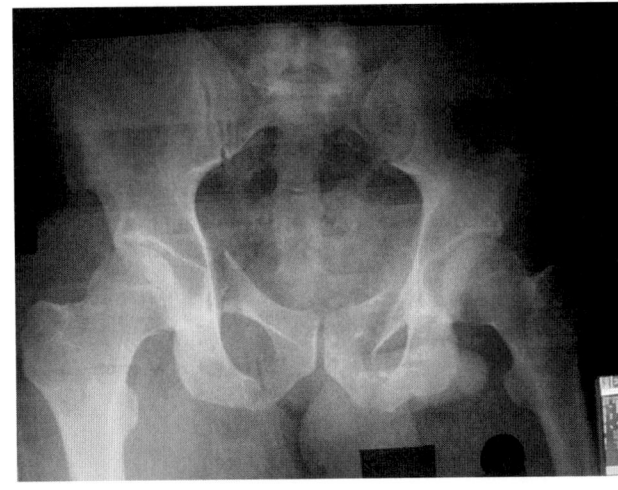

A

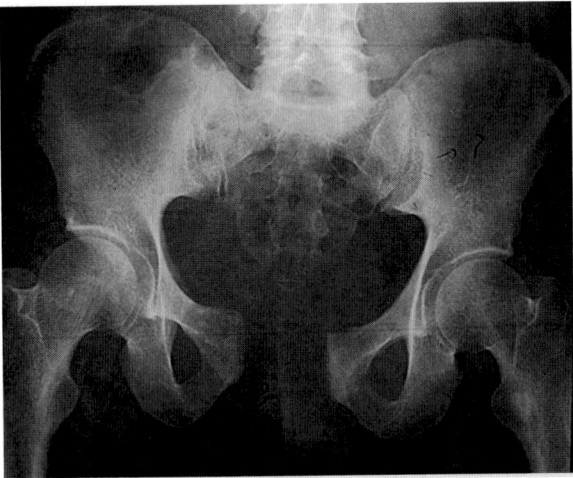

B

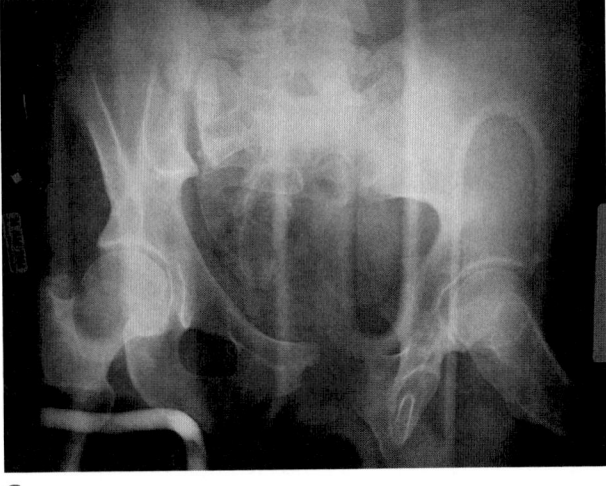

C

FIG. 7-30. The three types of mechanically unstable pelvis fractures are lateral compression (**A**), anteroposterior compression (**B**), and vertical shear (**C**).

TABLE 7-8	Signs and symptoms of peripheral arterial injury	
Hard Signs (Operation Mandatory)	**Soft Signs (Further Evaluation Indicated)**	
Pulsatile hemorrhage	Proximity to vasculature	
Absent pulses	Significant hematoma	
Acute ischemia	Associated nerve injury	
	A-A index of <0.9	
	Thrill or bruit	

A-A index = systolic blood pressure on the injured side compared with that on the uninjured side.

stenting of arterial injuries and angioembolization are routine adjuncts. Blunt cerebrovascular injuries have been recognized as a significant, preventable source of neurologic morbidity and mortality. The use of preperitoneal pelvic packing for unstable pelvic fractures as well as early fracture immobilization with external fixators are paradigm shifts in management. Finally, the institution of massive transfusion protocols balances the benefit of blood component therapy against immunologic risk. These conceptual changes have significantly improved survival of critically injured patients; they have been promoted and critically reviewed by academic trauma centers via forums such as the American College of Surgeons Committee on Trauma, the American Association for the Surgery of Trauma, the International Association of Trauma Surgery and Intensive Care, the Pan-American Trauma Congress, and other surgical organizations.

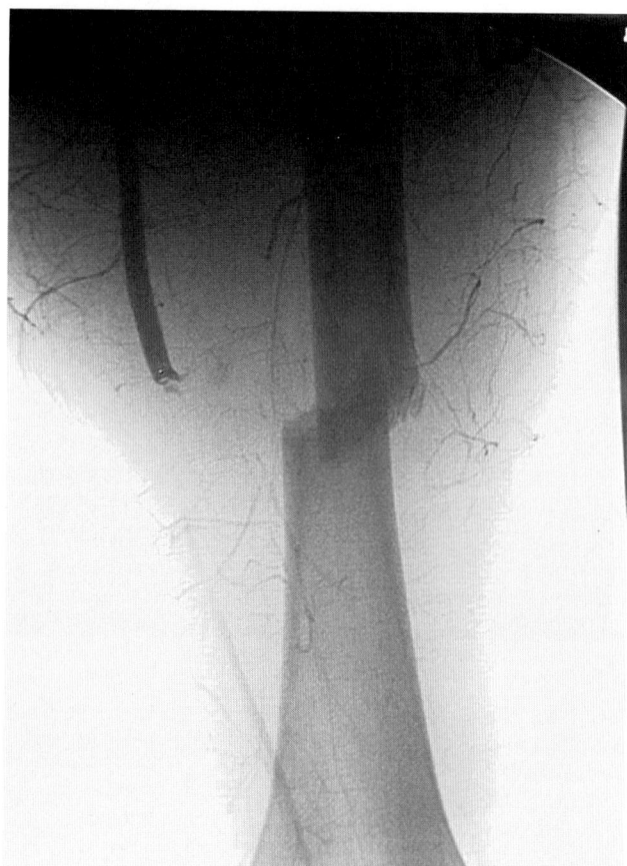

FIG. 7-31. On-table angiography in the operating room isolates the area of vascular injury to the superficial femoral artery in a patient with a femoral fracture.

Transfusion Practices

Injured patients with life-threatening hemorrhage may develop marked coagulopathy requiring clotting factor replacement. Fresh whole blood, arguably the optimal replacement, is no longer available in the United States. Rather, its component parts, packed red blood cells (PRBCs), fresh-frozen plasma, platelets, and cryoprecipitate, are administered. Specific transfusion triggers for individual blood components exist. Although current critical care guidelines indicate that PRBC transfusion should occur once the patient's hemoglobin level is <7 g/dL,[34] in the acute phase of resuscitation the endpoint is 10 g/dL.[35] Fresh-frozen plasma is transfused to keep the patient's International Normalized Ratio (INR) less than 1.5 and partial thromboplastin time (PTT) <45 seconds. Primary hemostasis relies on platelet adherence and aggregation to injured endothelium, and a platelet count of 50,000/μL is considered adequate if platelet function is normal. With massive transfusion, however, platelet dysfunction is common, and therefore a target of 100,000/μL is advocated. If fibrinogen levels drop below 100 mg/dL, cryoprecipitate should be administered. Such guidelines are designed to limit the transfusion of immunologically active blood components and decrease the risk of transfusion-associated lung injury and multiple organ failure.[36,37]

In the critically injured patient requiring large amounts of blood component therapy, a massive transfusion protocol should be followed (Fig. 7-32). This approach calls for administration of various components in a specific ratio during transfusion to achieve restoration of blood volume and correction of coagulopathy. Although the optimal ratio is yet to be determined,[38] the majority of trauma centers use a presumptive 1:1 or 1:2 red cell:plasma ratio in patients at risk for massive transfusion (10 units of PRBCs in 6 hours). Because complete typing and cross-matching takes up to 45 minutes, patients requiring emergent transfusions are given type O, type-specific, or biologically compatible RBCs. Blood typing, and to a lesser extent cross-matching, is essential to avoid life-threatening intravascular hemolytic transfusion reactions. Trauma centers and their associated blood banks must have the capability of transfusing tremendous quantities of blood components, because it is not unusual to have 100 component units transfused during one procedure and have the patient survive. Massive transfusion protocols, established preemptively, permit coordination of the activities of surgeons, anesthesiologists, and blood bank directors to facilitate transfusion at these rates should a crisis occur.

Postinjury coagulopathy is associated with core hypothermia and metabolic acidosis, termed the *bloody vicious cycle*.[33] The pathophysiology is multifactorial and includes inhibition of temperature-dependent enzyme-activated coagulation cascades, platelet dysfunction, endothelial abnormalities, and a poorly understood fibrinolytic activity. Such coagulopathy may be insidious, so the surgeon must be cognizant of subtle signs such as excessive bleeding from the cut edges of skin. Although the coagulopathic "ooze" may seem minimal compared with the torrential hemorrhage from a hole in the aorta, blood loss from the entire area of dissection can lead to exsanguination. Obtaining results for the usual laboratory tests of coagulation capability (i.e., INR, PTT, and platelet count) requires approximately 30 minutes. Such a delay is particularly troublesome for patients who have lost two blood volumes while waiting for the test results to return. Under such conditions, transfusion of fresh-frozen plasma and platelets must be empiric. Using damage control techniques to limit operative time and provide physiologic restoration in the SICU can be life saving (see "Damage Control Surgery" later).

Prophylactic Measures

All injured patients undergoing an operation should receive preoperative antibiotics. The type of antibiotic is determined by the anticipated source of contamination in the abdomen or other operative region; additional doses should be administered during the procedure based on blood loss and the half-life of the antibiotic. Extended postoperative antibiotic therapy is administered only for open fractures or significant intra-abdominal contamination. Tetanus prophylaxis is administered to all patients according to published guidelines.

Massive Transfusion Protocol

Trigger: Uncontrolled Hemorrhage/Anticipated Coagulopathy with SBP <90 mmHg Despite 3½ L Crystalloid (50 mL/kg)

Surgery & Anesthesia Response

Continued Treatment of Shock
Hemorrhage Control
Correct Hypothermia
Correct Acidosis
Normalize Ca^{2+}
Check labs q30m as needed
Consider Recombinant Factor VIIa therapy

Ongoing Component Therapy**
INR >1.5 or PTT >45 seconds → 4 units fresh frozen plasma
Platelet count <100,000/μL → 1 unit apheresis platelets
Fibrinogen <100 mg/dL → 10 units pooled cryoprecipitate

** If Rapid Thromboelastography (r-TEG) available:
ACT >125 seconds → 2 units FFP
MA <53 mm → 1 unit apheresis platelets
Angle <63 degrees → 10 units pooled cryoprecipitate
EPL >15% → consider fibrinolysis treatment

Blood Bank Response

Shipment	PRBCs	FFP	Platelets	Cryo
1	4	2		
2	4	2	1	10
3	4	2		
4	4	2	1	10

Shipments are delivered every 30 minutes until Massive Transfusion Protocol is terminated. Each shipment's quantity can be doubled at the request of Surgery or Anesthesia. Shipments >4 are determined by patient's clinical course and lab values.

FIG. 7-32. Denver Health Medical Center's Massive Transfusion Protocol. ACT = activated clotting time; Cryo = cryoprecipitate; EPL = estimated percent lysis; FFP = fresh-frozen plasma; INR = International Normalized Ratio; MA = maximum amplitude; PRBCs = packed red blood cells; PTT = partial thromboplastin time; SBP = systolic blood pressure.

Trauma patients are at risk for venous thromboembolism and its associated complications. In fact, pulmonary embolus can occur much earlier in the patient's hospital course than previously believed.[39] Patients at higher risk for venous thromboembolism are (a) those with multiple fractures of the pelvis and lower extremities, (b) those with coma or spinal cord injury, and (c) those requiring ligation of large veins in the abdomen and lower extremities. Morbidly obese patients and those over 55 years of age are at additional risk. Administration of low molecular weight heparin is initiated as soon as bleeding has been controlled and there is no intracranial pathology. In high-risk patients, removable inferior vena caval filters should be considered if there are contraindications to administration of low molecular weight heparin. Additionally, pulsatile compression stockings (also termed *sequential compression devices*) are used routinely unless there is a fracture.

A final prophylactic measure that is usually not considered is thermal protection. Hemorrhagic shock impairs perfusion and metabolic activity throughout the body, with resultant decrease in heat production and body temperature. Removing the patient's clothes causes a second thermal insult, and infusion of cold RBCs or room temperature crystalloid exacerbates the problem. As a result, injured patients can become hypothermic, with temperatures below 34°C (93.2°F) upon arrival in the OR. Hypothermia causes coagulopathy and myocardial irritability. Therefore, prevention must begin in the ED by maintaining a comfortable ambient temperature, covering stabilized patients with warm blankets, and administering warmed IV fluids and blood products. Additionally, in the OR a Bair Hugger warmer (the upper body or lower body blanket) and heated inhalation via the ventilatory circuit is instituted. For cases of severe hypothermia [temperature <30°C (86°F)], arteriovenous rewarming should be considered.

Operative Approaches and Exposure
Cervical Exposure

Operative exposure for midline structures of the neck (trachea, thyroid, bilateral carotid sheaths) is obtained through a collar incision; this is typically performed two finger breadths above the sternal notch, but can be varied based on the level of injury. After subplatysmal flap elevation, the strap muscles are divided in the midline to gain access to the central neck compartment. More superior and lateral structures are accessed by extending the collar incision upward along the sternocleidomastoid muscle; this may be done bilaterally if necessary. Unilateral neck exploration is done through an incision extending from the mastoid down to the clavicle, along the anterior border of the sternocleidomastoid muscle (Fig. 7-33). The carotid sheath, containing the carotid artery, jugular vein, and vagus nerve, is opened widely to examine these structures. The facial vein, which marks the carotid bifurcation, is usually ligated for exposure of the internal carotid artery.

Exposure of the distal carotid artery in zone III is difficult (see Fig. 7-33). The first step is division of the ansa cervicalis to facilitate mobilization of the hypoglossal nerve. Next, the posterior portion of the digastric muscle, which overlies the internal carotid, is transected. The glossopharyngeal and vagus nerves are mobilized and retracted as necessary. If accessible, the styloid process and attached muscles are removed. At this point anterior displacement of the mandible (subluxation) may be helpful. In desperate situations, the vertical ramus of the mandible may be divided. However, this maneuver often entails resection of the parotid gland and facial nerve for exposure of the distal internal carotid.

Thoracic Incisions

An anterolateral thoracotomy, with the patient placed supine, is the most versatile incision for emergent thoracic exploration. The location of the incision is in the fifth interspace, in the inframammary line (Fig. 7-34). If access is needed to bilateral pleural cavities, the original incision can be extended across the sternum with a Lebsche knife, into a "clamshell" thoracotomy (Fig. 7-35). If the sternum is divided, the internal mammary arteries should be ligated to prevent blood loss. The heart, lungs, descending aorta, pulmonary hilum, and esophagus are accessible with this approach. For control of the great vessels, the superior portion of the sternum may be opened and extension of the incision into the neck considered. A method advocated for access to the proximal left subclavian artery is through a fourth interspace anterolateral thoracotomy, superior sternal ex-

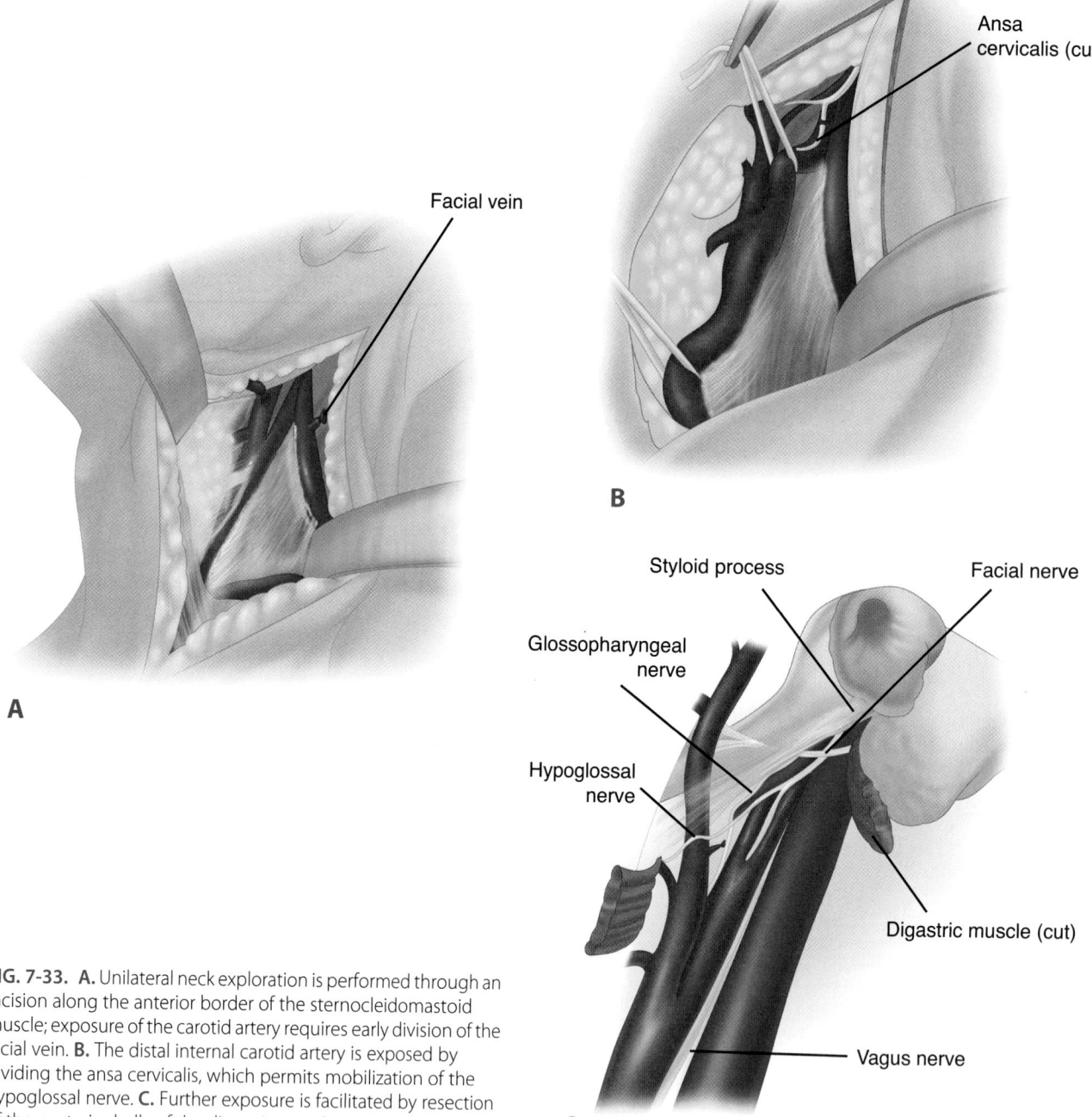

Facial vein

Ansa
cervicalis (cut)

A

B

Styloid process

Facial nerve

Glossopharyngeal
nerve

Hypoglossal
nerve

Digastric muscle (cut)

Vagus nerve

C

FIG. 7-33. A. Unilateral neck exploration is performed through an incision along the anterior border of the sternocleidomastoid muscle; exposure of the carotid artery requires early division of the facial vein. **B.** The distal internal carotid artery is exposed by dividing the ansa cervicalis, which permits mobilization of the hypoglossal nerve. **C.** Further exposure is facilitated by resection of the posterior belly of the digastric muscle.

tension, and left supraclavicular incision ("trap door" thoracotomy). Although the trap door procedure is appropriate after resuscitative thoracotomy, the proximal left subclavian artery can be accessed more easily via a sternotomy with a supraclavicular extension. If the left subclavian artery is injured outside the thoracic outlet, vascular control can be obtained via the sternotomy and definitive repair done through the supraclavicular incision. Median sternotomy is of limited utility in cases of cardiac trauma but can be used for anterior stab wounds to the heart. Typically, these patients have pericardial tamponade and undergo placement of a pericardial drain before a semiurgent median sternotomy is performed. Patients in extremis, however, should undergo anterolateral thoracotomy.

Median sternotomy with cervical extension may also be used for rapid exposure in patients with presumed proximal subclavian, innominate, or proximal carotid artery injuries. Care must be taken to avoid injury to the phrenic and vagus nerves that pass over the subclavian artery and to the recurrent laryngeal nerve passing posteriorly. Posterolateral thoracotomies are used for exposure of injuries to the posterior aspect of the trachea or main stem bronchi near the carina (right posterolateral thoracotomy), tears of the descending thoracic aorta (left posterolateral thoracotomy with left heart bypass), and intrathoracic esophageal injuries.

Emergent Abdominal Exploration

Abdominal exploration in adults is performed using a generous midline incision because of its versatility. For children under the age of 6, a transverse incision may be advantageous. Making the incision is faster with a scalpel than with an electrosurgical unit; incisional abdominal wall bleeding should be ignored until intra-abdominal sources of hemorrhage are controlled. Liquid and clotted blood is evacuated with multiple laparotomy pads and suction to identify the major source(s) of active bleeding. After blunt trauma the spleen and

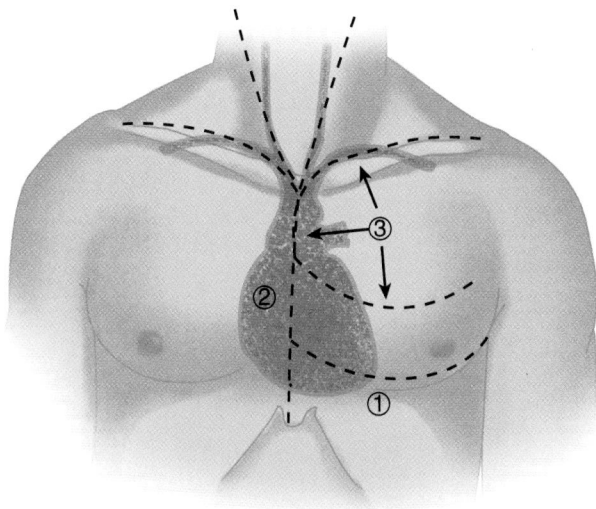

FIG. 7-34. Options for thoracic exposure include the most versatile incision, the anterolateral thoracotomy (*1*), as well as a median sternotomy (*2*) and a "trap door" thoracotomy (*3*). Any thoracic incision may be extended into a supraclavicular or anterior neck incision for wider exposure.

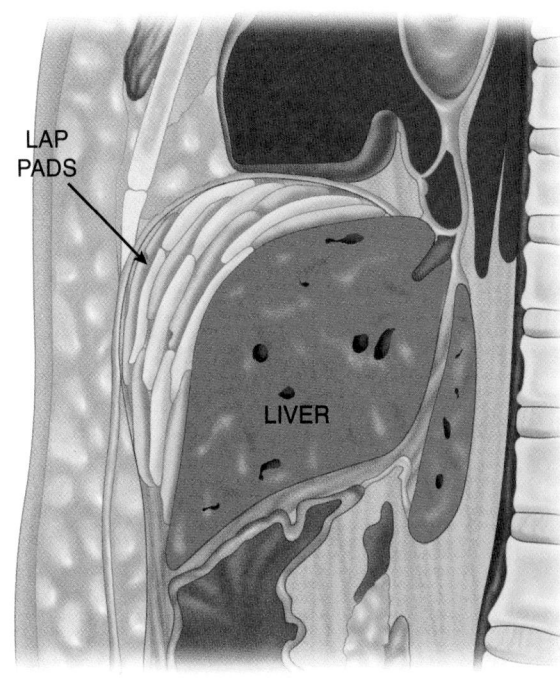

FIG. 7-36. A sagittal view of packs placed to control hepatic hemorrhage. Lap = laparotomy.

liver should be palpated and packed if fractured, and the infracolic mesentery inspected to exclude injury. In contrast, after a penetrating wound the search for bleeding should pursue the trajectory of the penetrating device. If the patient has an SBP of <70 mmHg when the abdomen is opened, digital pressure or a clamp should be placed on the aorta at the diaphragmatic hiatus. After the source of hemorrhage is localized, direct digital occlusion (vascular injury) or laparotomy pad packing (solid organ injury) is used to control bleeding (Fig. 7-36). If the liver is the source in a hemodynamically unstable patient, additional control of bleeding is obtained by clamping the hepatic pedicle (Pringle maneuver) (Fig. 7-37). Similarly, clamping

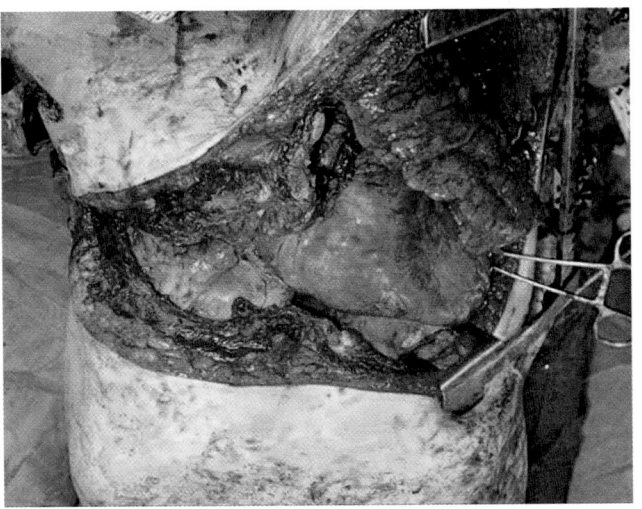

A

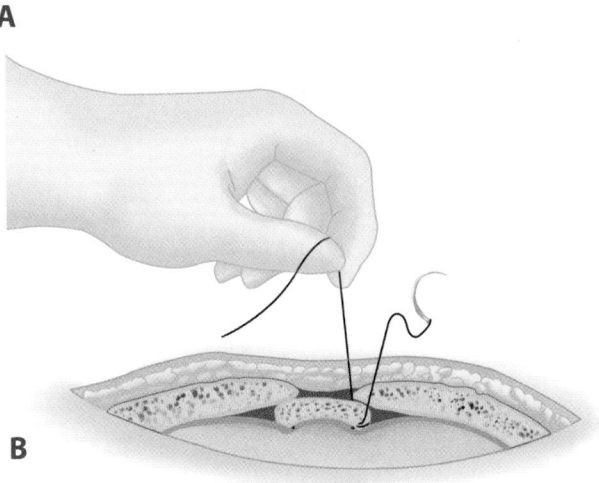

B

FIG. 7-35. A. A "clamshell" thoracotomy provides exposure to bilateral thoracic cavities. **B.** Sternal transection requires individual ligation of both the proximal and distal internal mammary arteries on the undersurface of the sternum.

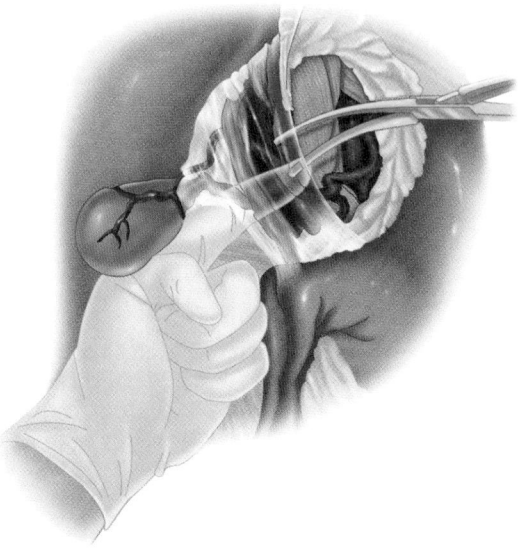

FIG. 7-37. The Pringle maneuver, performed with a vascular clamp, occludes the hepatic pedicle containing the portal vein, hepatic artery, and common bile duct.

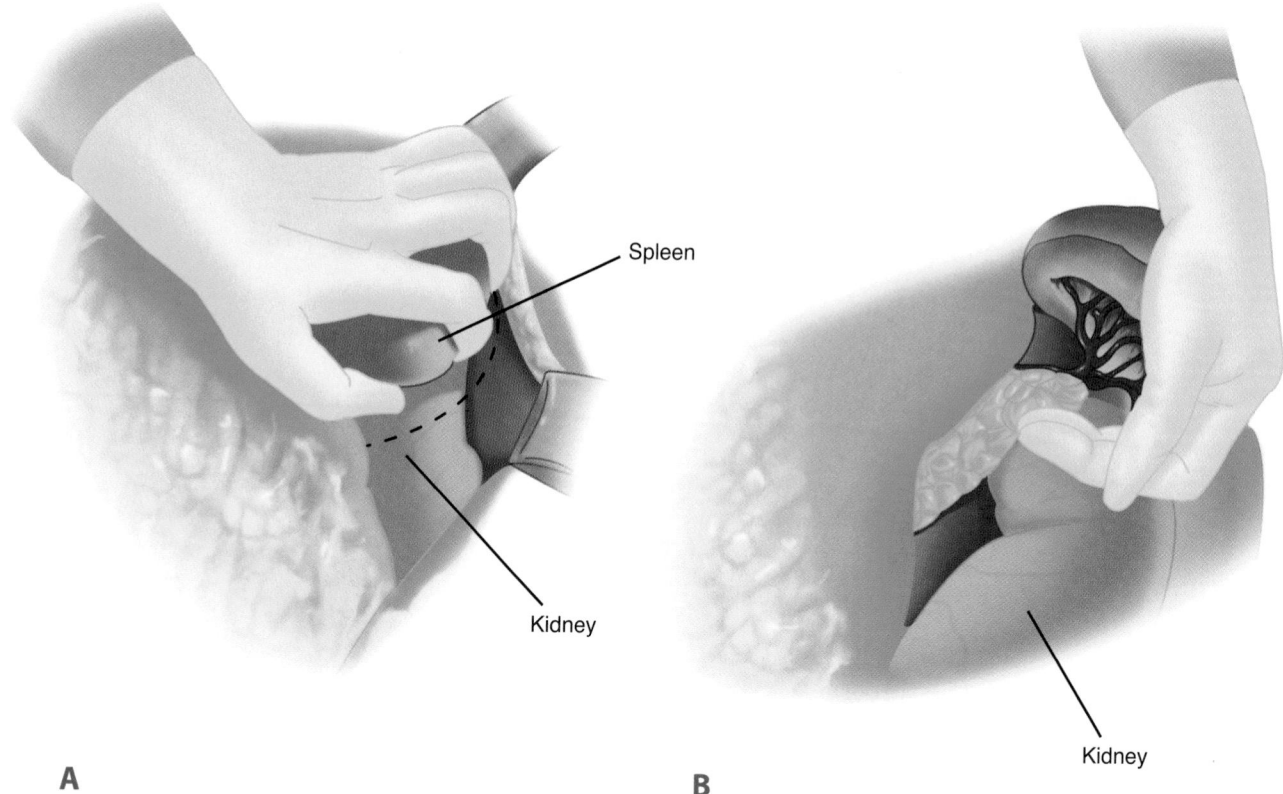

Spleen

Kidney

A

Kidney

B

FIG. 7-38. To mobilize the spleen, an incision is made into the endoabdominal fascia 1 cm lateral to the reflection of the peritoneum onto the spleen (**A**). While the spleen is gently rotated medially, a plane is developed between the pancreas and left kidney (**B**). With complete mobilization, the spleen can reach the level of the abdominal incision.

the splenic hilum may more effectively control bleeding than packing alone. When the spleen is mobilized, it should be gently rotated medially to expose the lateral peritoneum; this peritoneum and endoabdominal fascia are incised, which allows blunt dissection of the spleen and pancreas as a composite from the retroperitoneum (Fig. 7-38).

Rapid exposure of the intra-abdominal vasculature can prove challenging in the face of exsanguinating hemorrhage. The aorta, celiac axis, proximal superior mesenteric artery (SMA), and left renal arteries can be exposed with a left medial visceral rotation (Fig. 7-39). This is done by incising the lateral peritoneal reflection (white line of Toldt) beginning at the distal descending colon and extending the incision along the colonic splenic flexure, around the posterior aspect of the spleen, and behind the gastric fundus, ending at the esophagus. The left colon, spleen, pancreas, and stomach are then rotated toward the midline. The authors prefer to leave the kidney in situ when mobilizing the viscera because this exaggerates the separation of the renal vessels from the SMA. Proximal control of the aorta is obtained at the diaphragmatic hiatus; if an aortic injury is supraceliac, transecting the left crus of diaphragm or performing left thoracotomy may be necessary. Inferior vena cava injuries are approached by a right medial visceral rotation (Fig. 7-40). Proximal control is obtained just above the aortic bifurcation with direct pressure via a sponge stick; the injury is identified by cephalad dissection along the anterior surface of the inferior vena cava. The operative approach for SMA injuries is based on the level of injury. Fullen zone I SMA injuries, located posterior to the pancreas, can be exposed by a left medial visceral rotation. Fullen zone II SMA injuries, extending from the pancreatic edge to the middle colic branch, are approached via the lesser sac along the inferior edge of the pancreas at the base of the transverse mesocolon; the pancreatic body may be divided to gain proximal vascular access. More distal SMA injuries, Fullen zones III and IV, are approached directly within the mesentery. A venous

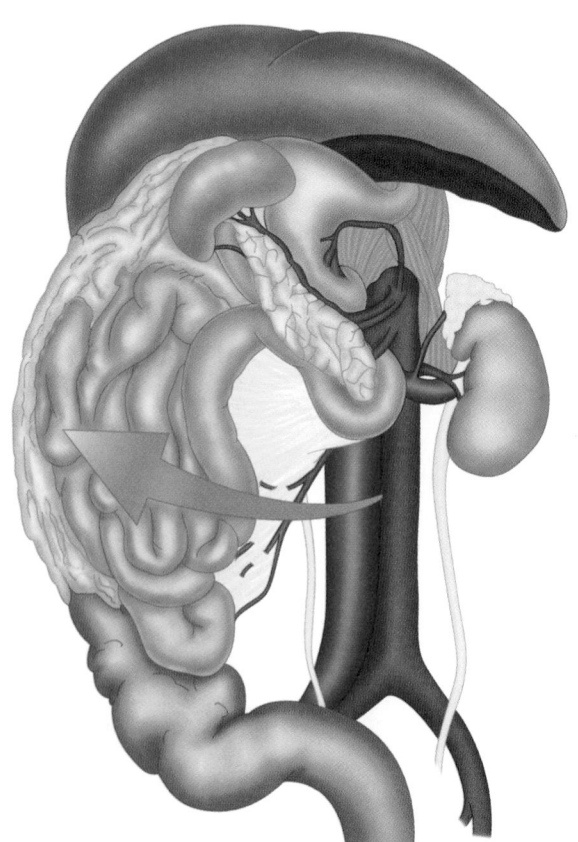

FIG. 7-39. A left medial visceral rotation is used to expose the abdominal aorta.

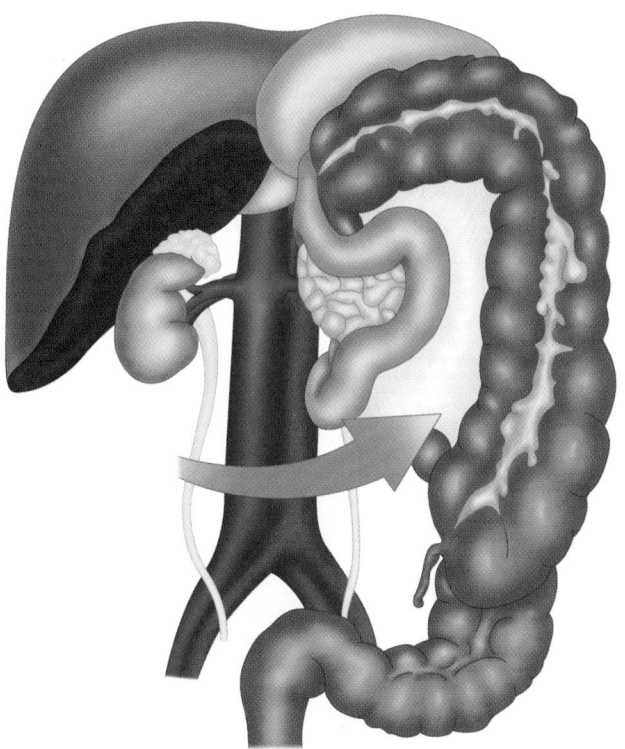

FIG. 7-40. A right medial visceral rotation is used to expose the infrahepatic vena cava.

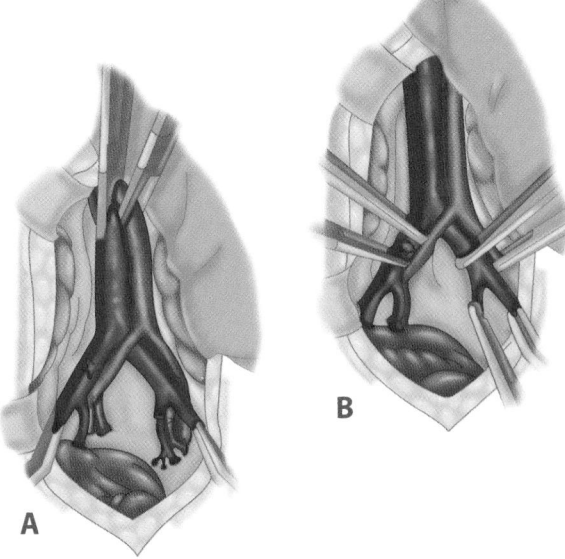

FIG. 7-41. Pelvic vascular isolation. **A.** Initially, clamps are placed on the aorta, inferior vena cava, and bilateral external iliac vessels. **B.** With continued dissection, the clamps can be moved progressively closer to the vascular injury to limit unwarranted ischemia.

injury behind the pancreas, from the junction of the superior mesenteric, splenic, and portal veins, is accessed by dividing the neck of the pancreas.

Injuries of the iliac vessels pose a unique problem for emergent vascular control due to the number of vessels, their close proximity, and cross circulation. Proximal control at the infrarenal aorta arrests the arterial bleeding and avoids splanchnic and renal ischemia; however, venous injuries are not controlled with aortic clamping. Tamponade with a folded laparotomy pad held directly over the bleeding site usually will establish hemostasis sufficient to prevent exsanguination. If hemostasis is not adequate to expose the vessel proximal and distal to the injury, sponge sticks can be strategically placed on either side of the injury and carefully adjusted to improve hemostasis. Alternatively, complete pelvic vascular isolation (Fig. 7-41) may be required to control hemorrhage for adequate visualization of the injuries. The right common iliac artery obscures the bifurcation of the vena cava and the right iliac vein; the iliac artery can be divided to expose venous injuries of this area (Fig. 7-42). The artery must be repaired after the venous injury is treated, however, because of limb-threatening ischemia.

Once overt hemorrhage is controlled, sources of enteric contamination are identified by serially running along the small and large bowel, looking at all surfaces. Associated hematomas should be

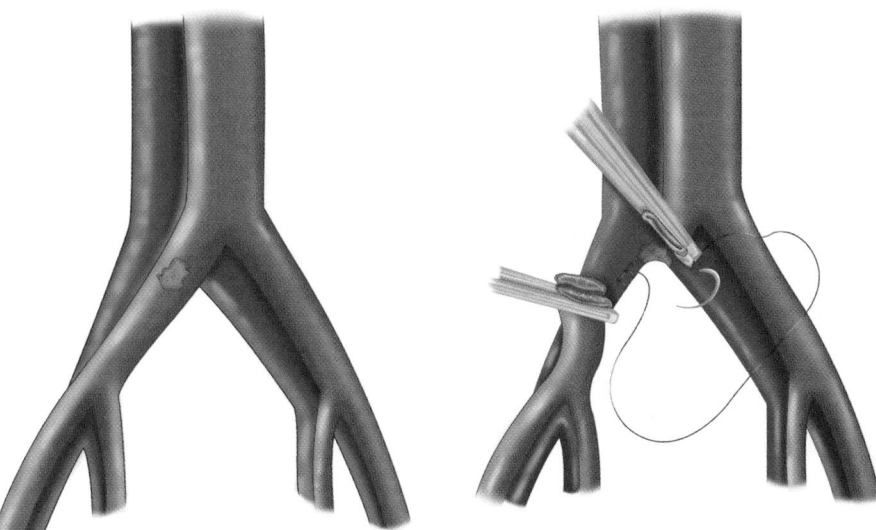

FIG. 7-42. The right common iliac artery can be divided to expose the bifurcation of the inferior vena cava and the right common iliac vein.

unroofed to rule out adjacent bowel injury. The anterior and posterior aspects of the stomach should be inspected, which requires opening the lesser sac for complete visualization. Duodenal injuries should be evaluated with a wide Kocher maneuver. During exploration of the lesser sac, visualization and palpation of the pancreas is done to exclude injury. Palpating the anterior surface is not sufficient, because the investing fascia may mask a pancreatic injury; mobilization, including evaluation of the posterior aspect, is critical. After injuries are identified, whether to use damage control techniques or perform primary repair of injuries is based on the patient's intraoperative physiologic status (see "Damage Control Surgery" and "Treatment of Specific Injuries" later). In a patient with multisystem trauma, enteral access via gastrostomy tube and needle-catheter jejunostomy should be considered. If abdominal closure is indicated after the patient's injuries are addressed, the abdomen is irrigated with warm saline and the midline fascia is closed with a running heavy suture. The skin is closed selectively based on the amount of intra-abdominal contamination.

Vascular Repair Techniques

Initial control of vascular injuries is accomplished digitally by applying enough direct pressure to stop the hemorrhage. Sharp dissection with fine scissors defines the injury and mobilizes sufficient length for proximal and distal control. Heparinized saline (50 units/mL) is injected into the proximal and distal ends of the injured vessel to prevent small clot formation on the exposed intima and media. Ragged edges of the injury site should be judiciously débrided using sharp dissection.

Options for the treatment of vascular injuries are listed in Table 7-9. Arterial repair should always be done for the aorta and the carotid, innominate, brachial, superior mesenteric, proper hepatic, renal, iliac, femoral, and popliteal arteries. In the extremities, at least one artery with distal runoff should be salvaged. Venous repair should be attempted for injuries of the superior vena cava, the inferior vena cava proximal to the renal veins, and the portal vein, although the portal vein may be ligated in extreme cases. Arterial injuries that may be treated conservatively include small pseudoaneurysms, intimal dissections, small intimal flaps, and small arteriovenous fistulas in the extremities. Follow-up imaging is performed 1 to 2 weeks after injury to confirm healing.

The type of operative repair for a vascular injury is based on the extent and location of injury. Lateral suture repair is preferred for arterial injuries with minimal loss of tissue. End-to-end primary anastomosis is performed if the vessel can be repaired without tension. Arterial defects of 1 to 2 cm often can be bridged by mobilizing the severed ends of the vessel after ligating small branches. The surgeon should not be reluctant to divide small branches to obtain additional length, because most injured patients have normal vasculature, and the preservation of potential collateral flow is not as important as in surgery for atherosclerosis. The aorta, subclavian artery, and

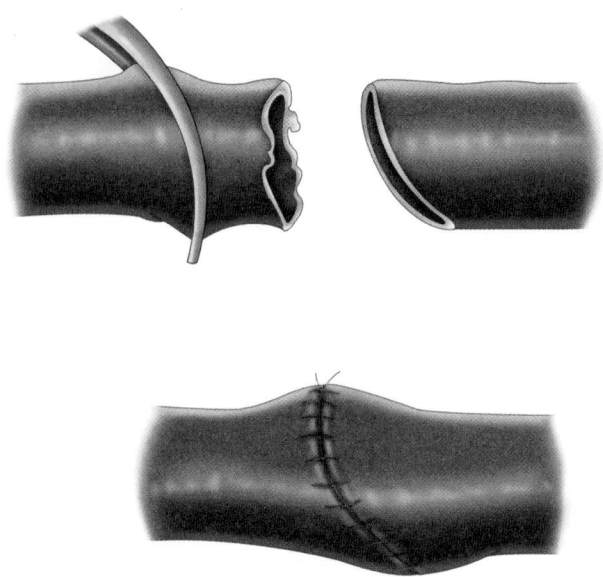

FIG. 7-43. Small arteries repaired with an end-to-end anastomosis are prone to stricture. Enlarging the anastomosis by beveling the cut ends of the injured vessel can minimize this problem. A curved hemostat is a useful adjunct to create the curve.

brachial artery, however, are difficult to mobilize for additional length. To avoid postoperative stenosis, particularly in smaller arteries, beveling or spatulation should be used so that the completed anastomosis is slightly larger in diameter than the native artery (Fig. 7-43). The authors emphasize the parachute technique to ensure precision placement of the posterior suture line (Fig. 7-44). If this technique is used, traction must be maintained on both ends of the suture, or leakage from the posterior aspect of the suture line may occur. A single temporary suture 180 degrees from the posterior row may be used to maintain alignment for challenging anastomoses.

TABLE 7-9	Options for the treatment of vascular injuries

Observation
Ligation
Lateral suture repair
End-to-end primary anastomosis
Interposition grafts
    Autogenous vein
    Polytetrafluoroethylene graft
    Dacron graft
Transpositions
Extra-anatomic bypass
Interventional radiology
    Stents
    Embolization

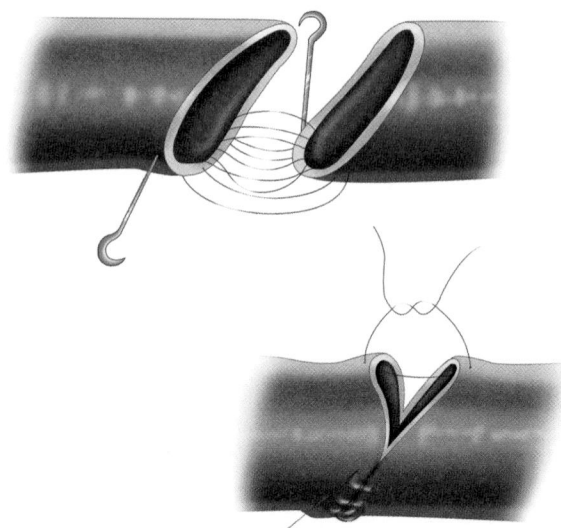

FIG. 7-44. The parachute technique is helpful for accurate placement of the posterior sutures of an anastomosis when the arterial end is fixed and an interposition graft is necessary. Traction must be maintained on both ends of the suture to prevent loosening and leakage of blood. Six stitches should be placed before the graft is pulled down to the artery.

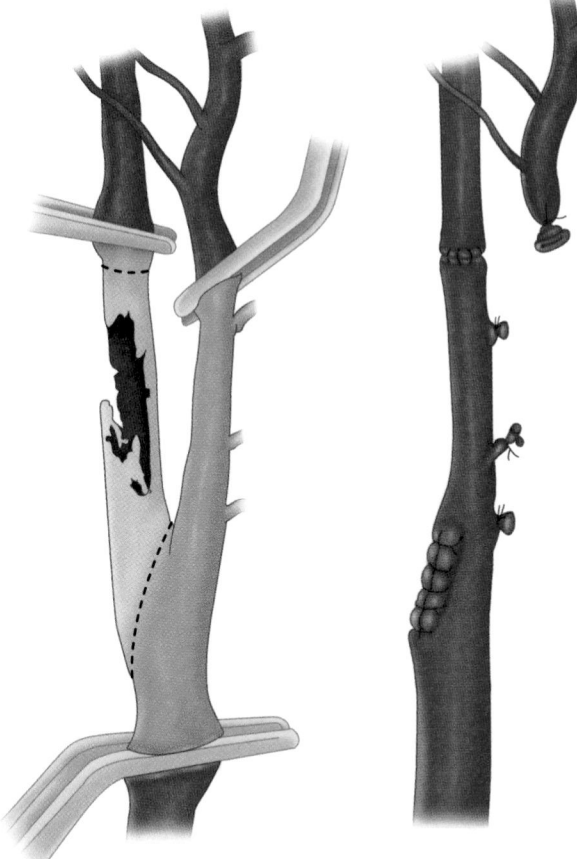

FIG. 7-45. Carotid transposition is an effective approach for treating injuries of the proximal internal carotid artery.

Interposition grafts are used when end-to-end anastomosis cannot be accomplished without tension despite mobilization. For vessels <6 mm in diameter (e.g., internal carotid, brachial, superficial femoral, and popliteal arteries), autogenous saphenous vein from the contralateral groin should be used, because polytetrafluoroethylene (PTFE) grafts of <6 mm have a prohibitive rate of thrombosis. Larger arteries (e.g., subclavian, innominate, aorta, common iliac) are bridged by PTFE grafts. Aortic or iliac arterial injuries may be complicated by enteric contamination from colon or small bowel injuries. There is a natural reluctance to place artificial grafts in such circumstances, but graft infections are rare and the time required to perform an axillofemoral bypass is excessive. Therefore, after the control of hemorrhage, bowel contamination is contained and the abdomen irrigated before placing PTFE grafts. After placement of the graft, it is covered with peritoneum or omentum before definitive treatment of the enteric injuries.

Transposition procedures can be used when an artery has a bifurcation and one vessel can safely be ligated. Injuries of the proximal internal carotid can be treated by mobilizing the adjacent external carotid, dividing it distal to the internal injury, and performing an end-to-end anastomosis between it and the distal internal carotid (Fig. 7-45). The proximal stump of the internal carotid is oversewn, with care taken to avoid a blind pocket where a clot may form. Injuries of the common and external iliac arteries can be handled in a similar fashion (Fig. 7-46), while maintaining flow in at least one internal iliac artery.

Venous injuries are inherently more difficult to reconstruct due to their propensity to thrombose. Small injuries without loss of tissue can be treated with lateral suture repair. More complex repairs with interposition grafts often fail; this typically does not occur acutely but rather gradually over 1 to 2 weeks. During this time adequate collateral circulation typically develops, which is sufficient to avoid acute venous hypertension. Therefore, it is reasonable to use PTFE for venous interposition grafting and accept a gradual, but eventual, thrombosis while allowing time for collateral circulation to develop. Such an approach is reasonable for venous injuries of the superior vena cava, suprarenal vena cava, and popliteal vein because ligation of these is associated with significant morbidity. In the remainder of venous injuries the vein may be ligated. In such patients, chronic venous hypertensive complications in the lower extremities often can be avoided by (a) temporary use of elastic bandages (Ace wraps) applied from the toes to the hips at the end of the procedure, and (b) temporary continuous elevation of the lower extremities to 30 to 45 degrees. These measures should be maintained for 1 week; if the

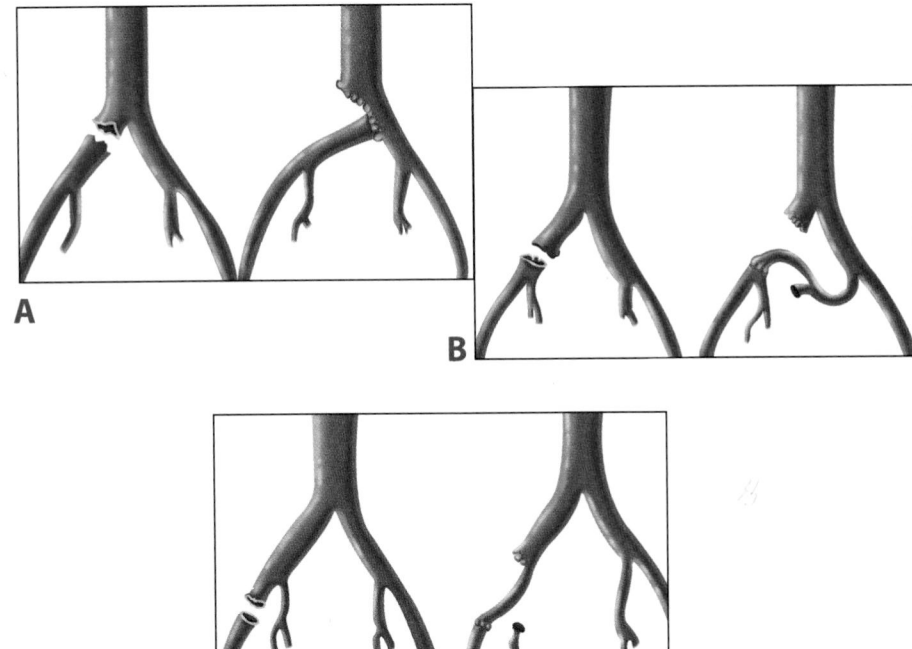

FIG. 7-46. Transposition procedures can be used for iliac artery injuries to eliminate the dilemma of placing an interposition polytetrafluoroethylene graft in the presence of enteric contamination. **A.** Right common iliac artery transposed to left common iliac artery. **B.** Left internal iliac artery transposed to the distal right common iliac artery. **C.** Right internal iliac artery transposed to the right external iliac artery.

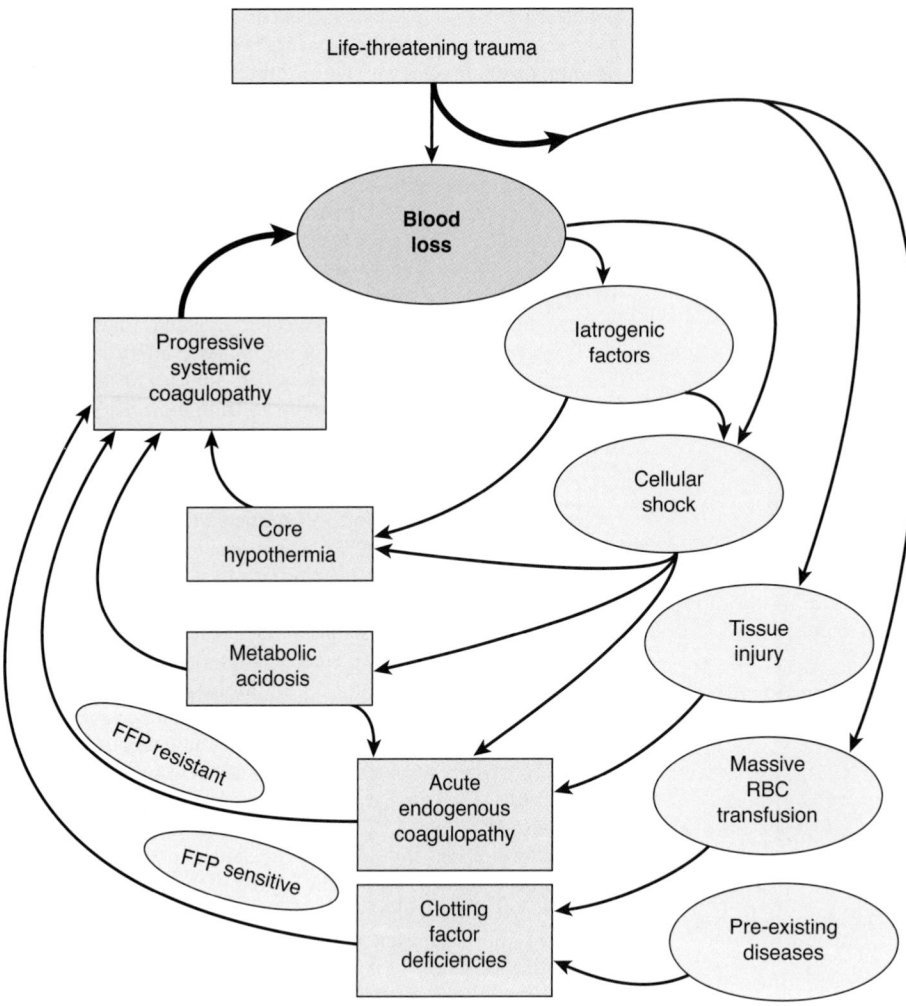

FIG. 7-47. The bloody vicious cycle. FFP = fresh-frozen plasma; RBC= red blood cell.

patient has no peripheral edema with ambulation, these maneuvers are no longer required.

Damage Control Surgery

The recognition of the bloody vicious cycle and the introduction of damage control surgery (DCS) have improved the survival of critically injured patients. The bloody vicious cycle, first described in 1981, is the lethal combination of coagulopathy, hypothermia, and metabolic acidosis (Fig. 7-47).[33] Hypothermia from evaporative and conductive heat loss and diminished heat production occurs despite the use of warming blankets and blood warmers. The metabolic acidosis of shock is exacerbated by aortic clamping, administration of vasopressors, massive transfusions, and impaired myocardial performance. Coagulopathy is caused by dilution, hypothermia, and acidosis. Once the cycle starts, each component magnifies the others, which leads to a downward spiral and ultimately a fatal arrhythmia. The purpose of DCS is to limit operative time so that the patient can be returned to the SICU for physiologic restoration and the cycle thus broken. Indications to limit the initial operation and institute DCS techniques include temperature <35°C (95°F), arterial pH <7.2, base deficit <15 mmol/L (or <6 mmol/L in patients over 55 years of age), and INR or PTT >50% of normal. The decision to abbreviate a trauma laparotomy is made intraoperatively as laboratory values become available and the patient's clinical course becomes clearer.

The goal of DCS is to control surgical bleeding and limit GI spillage. The operative techniques used are temporary measures, with definitive repair of injuries delayed until the patient is physiologically replete. Controlling surgical bleeding while preventing ischemia is of utmost importance during DCS. Aortic injuries must be repaired using an interposition PTFE graft. Although celiac artery injuries may be ligated, the SMA must maintain flow, and the insertion of an intravascular shunt is advocated. Similarly, perfusion of the iliac system and infrainguinal vessels can be restored with a vascular shunt, with interposition graft placement delayed until hours later. Venous injuries are preferentially treated with ligation in damage control situations, except for the suprarenal inferior vena cava and popliteal vein. For solid organ injuries to the spleen or one kidney, excision is indicated rather than an attempt at repair such as splenorrhaphy. For hepatic injuries, packing of the liver causes compression tamponade of bleeding (see Fig. 7-36). Translobar gunshot wounds of the liver are best controlled with balloon catheter tamponade, whereas deep lacerations can be controlled with Foley catheter inflation deep within the injury track (Fig. 7-48). For thoracic injuries requiring DCS several options exist. For bleeding peripheral pulmonary injuries, wedge resection using a gastrointestinal anastomosis (GIA) stapler is performed. In penetrating injuries, pulmonary tractotomy is used to divide the parenchyma (Fig. 7-49); individual vessels and bronchi are then ligated using a 3-0 polydioxanone (PDS) suture and the track left open. Patients who sustain more proximal injuries may require pulmonary lobectomy or pneumonectomy to control bleeding. Cardiac injuries may be temporarily controlled using a running 3-0 nonabsorbable polypropylene suture or skin staples. If this technique does not definitely control hemorrhage, pledgeted repair of the injury should be performed.

The second key component of DCS is limiting enteric content spillage. Small GI injuries (stomach, duodenum, small intestine, and colon) may be controlled using a rapid whipstitch of 2-0 nonabsorb-

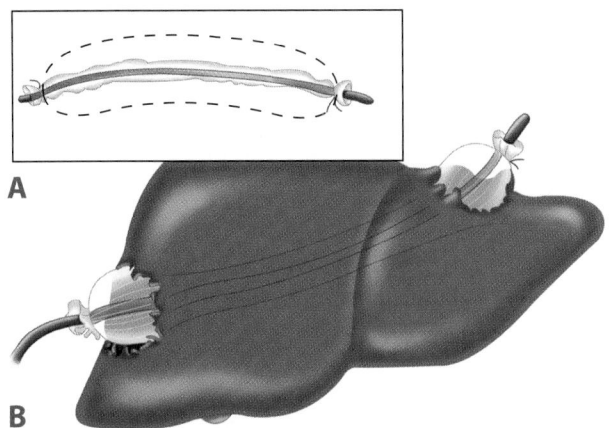

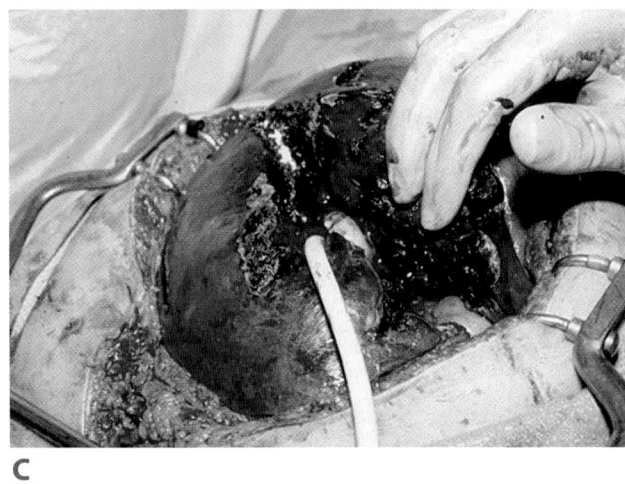

FIG. 7-48. A. An intrahepatic balloon used to tamponade hemorrhage from transhepatic penetrating injuries is made by placing a red rubber catheter inside a 1-inch Penrose drain, with both ends of the Penrose drain ligated. **B.** Once placed inside the injury track, the balloon is inflated with saline until hemorrhage stops. **C.** A Foley catheter with a 30-mL balloon can be used to halt hemorrhage from deep lacerations to the liver.

able polypropylene. Complete transection of the bowel or segmental damage is controlled using a GIA stapler, often with resection of the injured segment. Alternatively, open ends of the bowel may be ligated using umbilical tapes to limit spillage. Pancreatic injuries, regardless of location, are packed and the evaluation of ductal integrity postponed. Before the patient is returned to the SICU, the abdomen must be temporarily closed. Originally, penetrating towel clips were used to approximate the skin; however, the ensuing bowel edema often produced a delayed abdominal compartment syndrome. Currently, temporary closure of the abdomen is accomplished using an antimicrobial surgical incise drape (Ioban) (Fig. 7-50). In this technique, the bowel is covered with a fenestrated subfascial sterile drape (45 × 60 cm Steri-Drape), and two Jackson-Pratt drains are placed along the fascial edges; this is then covered using an Ioban drape, which allows

closed suction to control reperfusion-related ascitic fluid egress while providing adequate space for bowel expansion to prevent abdominal compartment syndrome. During the initial DCS stage, the subfascial sterile drape is not covered by a blue towel so that the status of the bowel and hemorrhage control can be assessed. Return to the OR in 12 to 24 hours is planned once the patient clinically improves, as evidenced by normothermia, normalization of coagulation test results, and correction of acidosis.

TREATMENT OF SPECIFIC INJURIES

Head Injuries

Intracranial Injuries

CT scanning, performed on all patients with a significant closed head injury (GCS score <14), identifies and quantitates intracranial lesions. Patients with intracranial hemorrhage, including epidural hematoma, subdural hematoma, subarachnoid hemorrhage, intracerebral hematoma or contusion, and diffuse axonal injury, are admitted to the SICU. In patients with abnormal findings on CT scans and GCS scores of ≤8, intracranial pressure (ICP) should be monitored using fiber-optic intraparenchymal devices or intraventricular catheters.[13] Although an ICP of 10 mmHg is believed to be the upper limit of normal, therapy is not initiated until ICP is >20 mmHg.[13] Indications for operative intervention to remove space-occupying hematomas are based on the clot volume, amount of midline shift, location of the clot, GCS score, and ICP.[13] A shift of >5 mm typically is considered an indication for evacuation, but this is not an absolute rule. Smaller hematomas that are in treacherous locations, such as the posterior fossa, may require drainage due to brain stem compression or impending herniation. Removal of small hematomas may also improve ICP and cerebral perfusion in patients with elevated ICP that is refractory to medical therapy. Patients with diffuse cerebral edema resulting in excessive ICP may require a decompressive craniectomy. Patients with open or depressed skull fractures, with or without sinus involvement, may require operative intervention. Penetrating injuries to the head require operative intervention for hemorrhage control, evacuation of blood, skull fracture fixation, or débridement.

General surgeons in communities without emergency neurosurgical coverage should have a working knowledge of burr hole placement in the event that emergent evacuation is required for a life-threatening epidural hematoma (Fig. 7-51).[40] The typical clinical course of an epidural hematoma is an initial loss of consciousness, a

FIG. 7-49. Pulmonary tractotomy divides the pulmonary parenchyma using either a transection/anastomosis (TA) or gastrointestinal anastomosis (GIA) stapler. The opened track permits direct access to injured vessels or bronchi for individual ligation.

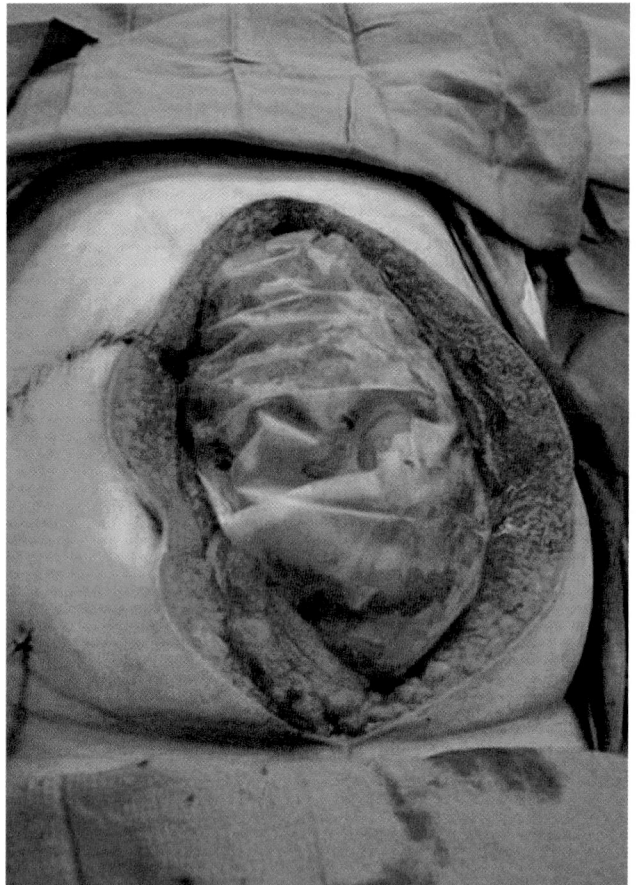

A

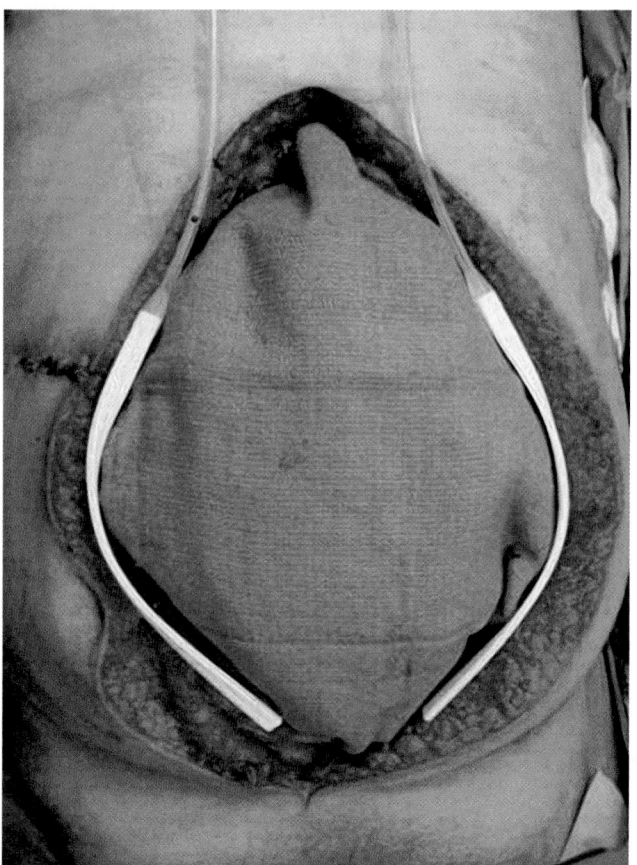

B

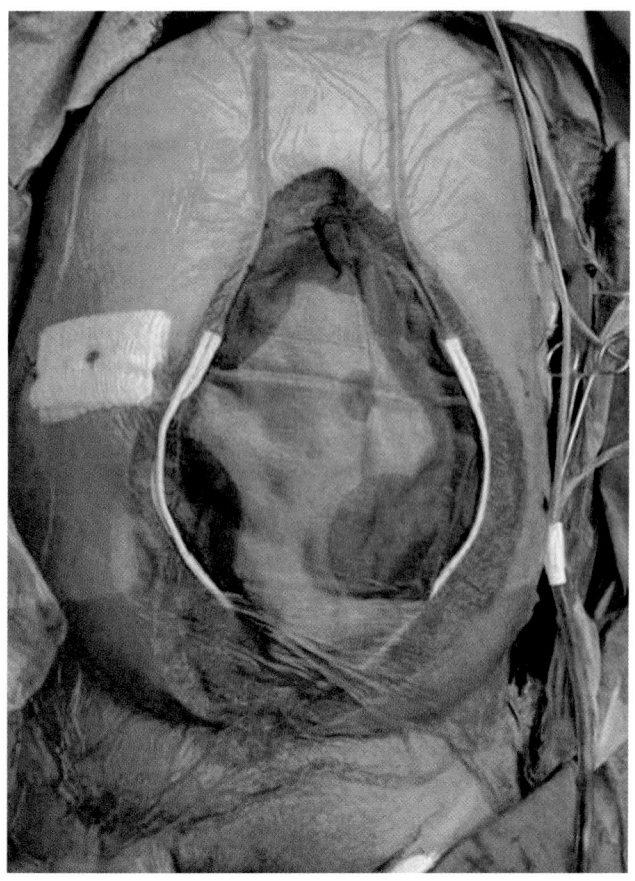

C

FIG. 7-50. Temporary closure of the abdomen entails covering the bowel with a fenestrated subfascial 45 × 60 cm sterile drape (**A**), placing Jackson-Pratt drains and a blue towel (**B**), and then occluding with an Ioban drape (**C**).

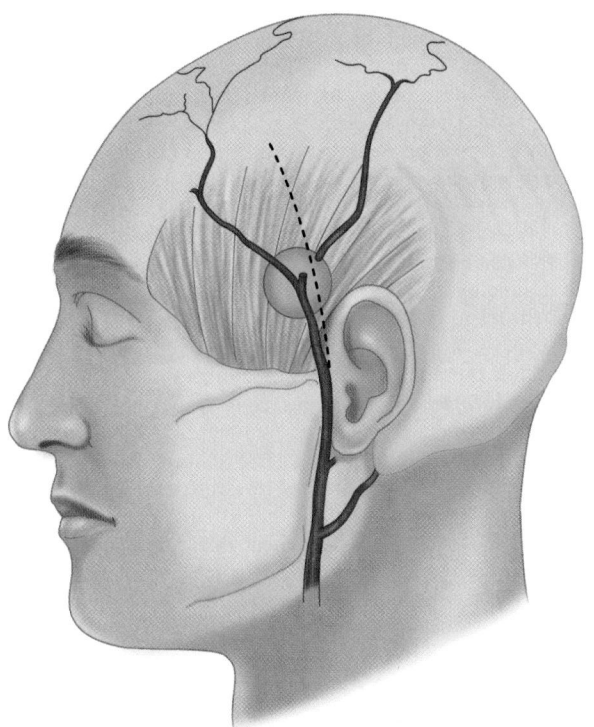

FIG. 7-51. A burr hole is made for decompression of an epidural hematoma as a life-saving maneuver. One or more branches of the external carotid artery usually must be ligated to gain access to the skull. No attempt should be made to control intracranial hemorrhage through the burr hole. Rather, the patient's head should be wrapped with a bulky absorbent dressing and the patient transferred to a neurosurgeon for definitive care.

lucid interval, recurrent loss of consciousness with an ipsilateral fixed and dilated pupil, and finally cardiac arrest. The final stages of this sequence are caused by blood accumulation that forces the temporal lobe medially, with resultant compression of the third cranial nerve and eventually the brain stem. The burr hole is made on the side of the dilated pupil to decompress the intracranial space. After stabilization, the patient is transferred to a facility with emergency neurosurgical capability for formal craniotomy.

In addition to operative intervention, postinjury care directed at limiting secondary injury to the brain is critical. The goal of resuscitation and management in patients with head injuries is to avoid hypotension (SBP of <90 mmHg) and hypoxia (partial pressure of arterial oxygen of <60 or arterial oxygen saturation of <90).[13] Attention, therefore, is focused on maintaining cerebral perfusion rather than merely lowering ICP. Resuscitation efforts aim for a euvolemic state and an SBP of >90 mmHg. Cerebral perfusion pressure (CPP) is equal to the mean arterial pressure minus the ICP, with a target range of 50 to 70 mmHg.[13] CPP can be increased by either lowering ICP or raising mean arterial pressure. Sedation, osmotic diuresis, paralysis, ventricular drainage, and barbiturate coma are used in sequence, with coma induction being the last resort. The partial pressure of carbon dioxide (PCO_2) should be maintained in a normal range (35 to 40 mmHg), but for temporary management of acute intracranial hypertension, inducing cerebral vasoconstriction by hyperventilation to a PCO_2 of <30 mmHg is occasionally warranted. Moderate hypothermia [32° to 33°C (89.6° to 91.4°F)] may decrease mortality risk and improve neurologic outcomes when maintained for at least 48 hours, but its ultimate role remains to be defined.[13] Patients with intracranial hemorrhage should be monitored for postinjury seizures, and prophylactic anticonvulsant therapy (e.g., phenytoin [Dilantin]) is indicated for 7 days after injury.[13]

Maxillofacial Injuries

Maxillofacial injuries are common with multisystem trauma and require coordinated management by the trauma surgeon and the specialists in otolaryngology, plastic surgery, ophthalmology, and oral and maxillofacial surgery. Delay in addressing these systems that control vision, hearing, smelling, breathing, eating, and phonation may produce dysfunction and disfigurement with serious psychologic impact. The maxillofacial complex is divided into three regions; the *upper face* containing the frontal sinus and brain, the *midface* containing the orbits, nose, and zygomaticomaxillary complex, and the *lower face* containing the mandible. High-impact kinetic energy is required to fracture the frontal sinus, orbital rims, and mandible, whereas low-impact forces will injure the nasal bones and zygoma.

The most common scenario, which at times may be life-threatening, is bleeding from facial fractures.[41] Temporizing measures include nasal packing, Foley catheter tamponade of posterior nasal bleeding, and oropharyngeal packing. Prompt angioembolization will halt exsanguinating hemorrhage. Fractures of tooth-bearing bone are considered open fractures and require antibiotic therapy and semiurgent repair to preserve the airway as well as the functional integrity of the occlusion (bite) and the aesthetics of the face. Orbital fractures may compromise vision, produce muscle injury causing diplopia, or change orbital volume to produce a sunken appearance to the orbit. Nose and nasoethmoidal fractures should be assessed carefully to identify damage to the lacrimal drainage system or to the cribriform plate producing cerebrospinal fluid rhinorrhea. After initial stabilization, a systematic physical examination of the head and neck should be performed that also includes cranial nerve examination and coronal and three-dimensional CT scanning of the maxillofacial complex (Fig. 7-52). Early consultation with the surgical specialists in this area is essential to prevent complications to these vital structures.

Neck and Cervical Spine Injuries

Blunt trauma can involve virtually every structure in the neck. Treatment of injuries to the cervical spine is based on the level of injury, the stability of the spine, the presence of subluxation, the extent of angulation, the level of neurologic deficit, and the overall

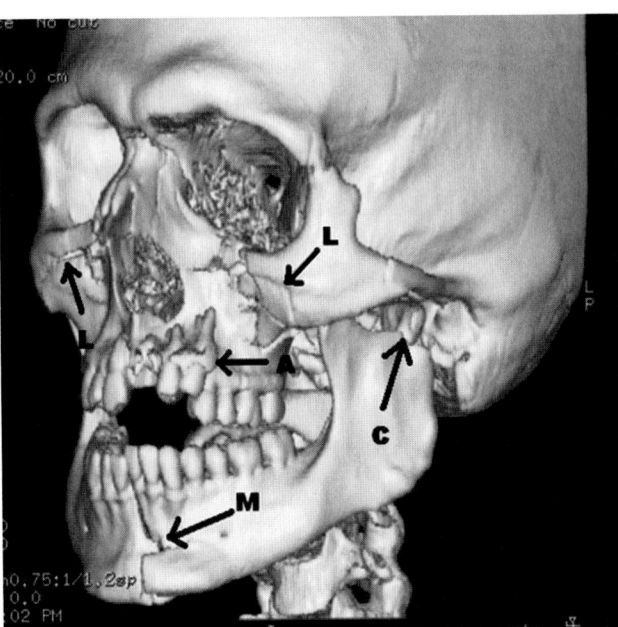

FIG. 7-52. Three-dimensional computed tomographic scan illustrating Le Fort II maxillary (*L*) and alveolar (*A*) fractures, and fracture of the mandible (*M*) at the midline and at the weaker condyle (*C*). (*Image courtesy of Vincent D. Eusterman, MD, DDS.*)

condition of the patient. In general, physician-supervised axial traction, via cervical tongs or the more commonly used halo vest, is used to reduce subluxations and stabilize the injury. Immobilization of injuries also is achieved with spinal orthoses (braces), particularly in those with associated thoracolumbar injuries. Surgical fusion typically is performed in patients with neurologic deficit, those with angulation of >11 degrees or translation of >3.5 mm, and those who remain unstable after external fixation. Indications for immediate operative intervention are deterioration in neurologic function and fractures or dislocations with incomplete deficit. Methylprednisolone generally is administered to patients with acute spinal cord injury. Although controversy exists, clinical data suggest initiating a 24-hour infusion if started within 3 hours and a 48-hour infusion if started 3 to 8 hours.[42] Current guidelines suggest an initial bolus of 30 mg/kg methylprednisolone followed by a 5.4-mg/kg infusion for 23 hours in patients with nonpenetrating injuries. The role and timing of operative surgical decompression after acute spinal cord injury is a matter of debate. However, evidence supports urgent decompression of bilateral locked facets in patients with incomplete tetraplegia or with neurologic deterioration. Urgent decompression in acute cervical spinal cord injury is safe. Performing surgery within 24 hours may decrease length of stay and complications.[43] Complete injuries of the spinal cord remain essentially untreatable. However, approximately 3% of patients who present with flaccid quadriplegia have concussive injuries, and these patients represent the very few who seem to have miraculous recoveries.

Subclinical fractures of the larynx and trachea may manifest as cervical emphysema, but fractures documented by CT scan often are repaired. Common injuries include thyroid cartilage fractures, rupture of the thyroepiglottic ligament, disruption of the arytenoids or vocal cord tears, and cricoid fractures. After necessary débridement of devitalized tissue, tracheal injuries are repaired end to end using a single layer of interrupted absorbable sutures. Associated injuries of the esophagus are common in penetrating injuries due to its close proximity. After débridement and repair, vascularized tissue is interposed between the repair and the injured trachea, and a closed suction drain is placed. The sternocleidomastoid muscle or strap muscles are useful for interposition and help prevent postoperative fistulas.

Cervical vascular injuries due to either blunt or penetrating trauma can result in devastating neurologic sequelae or exsanguination. Penetrating injuries to the carotid artery and internal jugular vein usually are obvious on operative neck exploration. The principles of vascular repair techniques (discussed previously) apply to carotid injuries, and options for repair include end-to-end primary repair (often possible with mobilization of the common carotid), graft interposition, and transposition procedures. All carotid injuries that can be repaired without undue physiologic ramifications should be. However, in patients who present in coma, particularly with a delay, ligation should be considered. In patients with uncontrolled hemorrhage, an alternative is temporary vascular control and revascularization using a Pruitt-Inahara shunt. Tangential wounds of the internal jugular vein should be repaired by lateral venorrhaphy, but extensive wounds are efficiently addressed by ligation. However, it is not advisable to ligate both jugular veins. Vertebral artery injuries due to penetrating trauma are difficult to control operatively because of the artery's protected location within the foramen transversarium. Although exposure from an anterior approach can be accomplished by removing the anterior elements of the bony canal and the tough fascia covering the artery between the elements, typically the most efficacious control of such injuries is angioembolization. Fogarty catheter balloon occlusion may be useful for controlling acute bleeding.

Blunt injury to the carotid or vertebral arteries may cause dissection, thrombosis, or pseudoaneurysm, typically in the surgically inaccessible distal internal carotid (Fig. 7-53).[44] Early recognition and

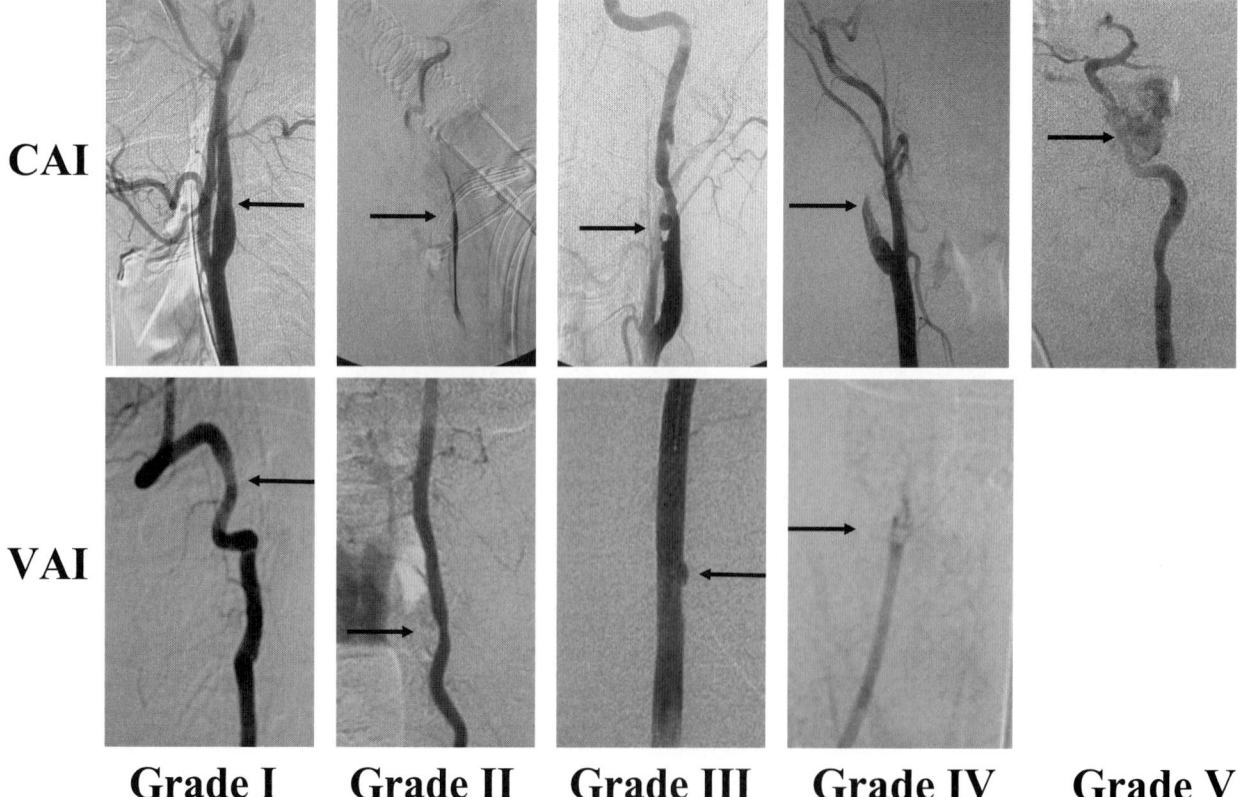

FIG. 7-53. The Denver grading scale for blunt cerebrovascular injuries. Grade I: irregularity of the vessel wall, dissection/intramural hematoma with <25% luminal stenosis. Grade II: visualized intraluminal thrombus or raised intimal flap, or dissection/intramural hematoma with 25% or more luminal narrowing. Grade III: pseudoaneurysm. Grade IV: vessel occlusion. Grade V: vessel transection. CAI = carotid artery injury; VAI = vertebral artery injury.

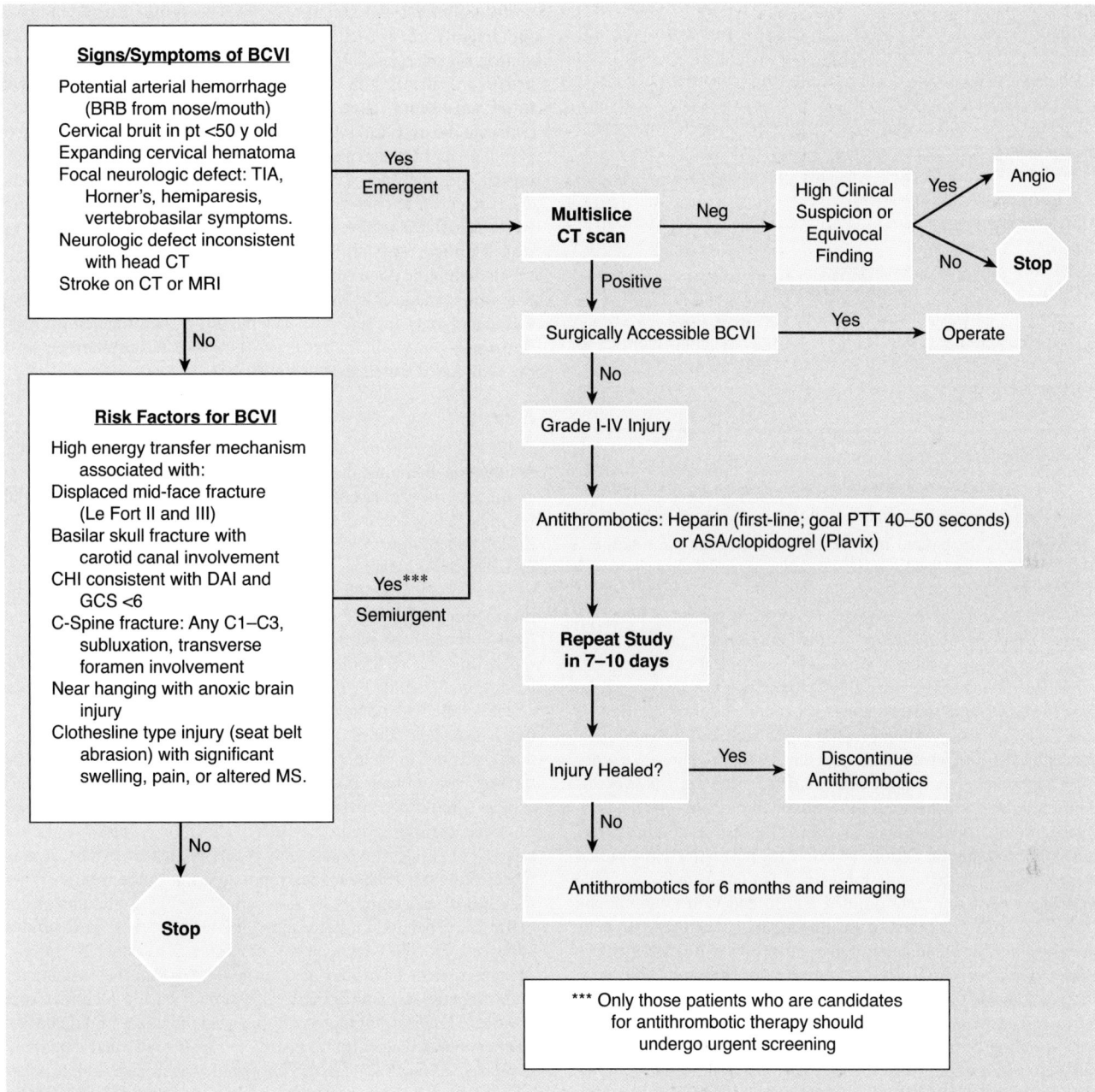

FIG. 7-54. Screening and treatment algorithm for blunt cerebrovascular injuries (BCVIs). Angio = angiography; ASA = acetylsalicylic acid; BRB = bright red blood; CHI = closed head injury; C-spine = cervical spine; CT = computed tomography; DAI = diffuse axonal injury; GCS = Glasgow Coma Scale score; MRI = magnetic resonance imaging; MS = mental status; Neg = negative; pt = patient; PTT = partial thromboplastin time; TIA = transient ischemic attack.

management of these injuries is paramount, because patients treated with antithrombotics have a stroke rate of <1% compared with stroke rates between 5 and 50% in untreated patients based on grade of injury. Because treatment must be instituted during the latent period between injury and onset of neurologic sequelae, diagnostic imaging is performed based on identified screening criteria (Fig. 7-54).[45] After identification of an injury, antithrombotics are administered if the patient does not have contraindications (intracranial hemorrhage, falling hemoglobin level with solid organ injury or pelvic fracture). Heparin, started without a loading dose at 15 units/kg per hour, is titrated to achieve a PTT between 40 and 50 seconds or antiplatelet agents are initiated (aspirin 325 mg/d and clopidogrel 75 mg/d). The types of antithrombotic treatment appear equivalent in published studies to date, and the duration of treatment is empirically recommended to be 6 months.[46,47] Thrombosis of the internal jugular veins

caused by blunt trauma can occur unilaterally or bilaterally and is often discovered incidentally, because most patients are asymptomatic. Bilateral thrombosis can aggravate cerebral edema in patients with serious head injuries; stent placement should be considered in such patients if ICP remains elevated.

Chest Injuries

The most common injuries from both blunt and penetrating thoracic trauma are hemothorax and pneumothorax. Few require operative intervention because >85% of patients can be definitively treated with a chest tube. The indications for thoracotomy include significant initial or ongoing hemorrhage from the tube thoracostomy and specific imaging-identified diagnoses (Table 7-10). One caveat concerns the patient who presents after a delay. Even when

TABLE 7-10	Indications for operative treatment of thoracic injuries

- Initial tube thoracostomy drainage of >1000 mL (penetrating injury) or >1500 mL (blunt injury)
- Ongoing tube thoracostomy drainage of >200 mL/h for 3 consecutive hours in noncoagulopathic patients
- Caked hemothorax despite placement of two chest tubes
- Selected descending torn aortas
- Great vessel injury (endovascular techniques may be used in selected patients)
- Pericardial tamponade
- Cardiac herniation
- Massive air leak from the chest tube with inadequate ventilation
- Tracheal or main stem bronchial injury diagnosed by endoscopy or imaging
- Open pneumothorax
- Esophageal perforation

the initial chest tube output is 1.5 L, if the output ceases and the lung is re-expanded, the patient may be managed through observation.

Great Vessels

Over 90% of thoracic great vessel injuries are due to penetrating trauma, although blunt injury to the innominate, subclavian, or descending aorta may cause a pseudoaneurysm or frank rupture.[22,48,49] Simple lacerations of the ascending or transverse aortic arch can be repaired with lateral aortorrhaphy. Repair of posterior injuries, or those requiring interposition grafting of the arch, call for cardiopulmonary bypass, and repair of complex injuries may require circulatory arrest. Innominate artery injuries are repaired using the bypass exclusion technique,[49] which avoids the need for cardiopulmonary bypass. Bypass grafting from the proximal aorta to the distal innominate with a prosthetic tube graft is performed before the postinjury hematoma is entered. The PTFE graft is anastomosed end to side from the proximal undamaged aorta and anastomosed end to end to the innominate artery (Fig. 7-55). The origin of the innominate is then oversewn at its base to exclude the pseudoaneurysm or other injury. Subclavian artery injuries can be repaired using lateral arteriorrhaphy or PTFE graft interposition; due to its multiple branches and tethering of the artery, end-to-end anastomosis is not advocated.

Descending thoracic aortic injuries may require urgent if not emergent intervention. However, operative intervention for intracranial or intra-abdominal hemorrhage or unstable pelvic fractures takes precedence. To prevent aortic rupture, pharmacologic therapy with an esmolol infusion should be instituted in the trauma bay, with a target SBP of <100 mmHg and heart rate of <100/min.[50] Open operative reconstruction of the thoracic aorta remains the mainstay of treatment,[19,51] although endovascular stenting is being used more frequently as the technology improves.[52] Endovascular techniques are particularly appealing in patients who cannot tolerate single lung ventilation, patients >65 years old who are at risk for cardiac decompensation with aortic clamping, or patients with uncontrolled intracranial hypertension. The major limitations are current endograft sizes, which are too large compared to the diameter of the thoracic aorta, and a lack of long-term follow-up data in young patients.

Open repair of the descending aorta entails placement of an interposition graft using partial left heart bypass.[53] With the patient in a right lateral decubitus position, the patient's hips and legs are rotated 45 degrees toward the supine position to gain access to the left groin for common femoral artery cannulation. Using a left posterolateral thoracotomy, the fourth rib is transected to expose the aortic arch and left pulmonary hilum. Partial left heart bypass is performed by cannulating the superior pulmonary vein with return through the left common femoral artery (Fig. 7-56). A centrifugal pump provides flow rates of 2.5 to 4 L/min to maintain a distal

perfusion pressure of >65 mmHg. This prevents ischemic injury of the spinal cord as well as the splanchnic bed, and reduces left ventricular afterload.[19] Heparinization is not required, a significant benefit in patients with multiple injuries, particularly in those with intracranial hemorrhage. Unless contraindicated, however, low-dose heparin (100 units/kg) typically is administered to prevent thromboembolic events. Once bypass is initiated, vascular clamps are applied on the aorta between the left common carotid and left subclavian arteries, on the left subclavian, and on the aorta distal to the injury. In most patients a short PTFE graft (usually 18 mm in diameter) is placed using a running 3-0 polypropylene suture. Primary arterial repair should be done when possible. Air and thrombus are flushed from the aortic graft before the final suture is tied, and the occluding vascular clamps are removed. The patient is then weaned from the centrifugal pump, the cannulas are removed, and primary repair of the cannulated vessels is performed.

Heart

Blunt and penetrating cardiac injuries have widely differing presentations and therefore disparate treatments. Survivable penetrating cardiac injuries consist of wounds that can be closed; most are stab wounds. Before repair of the injury is attempted, hemorrhage should be controlled; injuries to the atria can be clamped with a Satinsky vascular clamp, whereas digital pressure occludes the majority of ventricular wounds. Foley catheter occlusion of larger stellate lesions may be effective, but even minimal traction may enlarge the original injury. Temporary control of hemorrhage, and at times definitive repair, may be accomplished with skin staples for left ventricular lacerations. Definitive repair of cardiac injuries is performed with either running 3-0 polypropylene suture or interrupted, pledgeted 2-0 polypropylene suture (Fig. 7-57).[54] Use of pledgets may be particularly effective in the right ventricle to prevent sutures from pulling through the thinner myocardium. Injuries adjacent to coronary arteries should be repaired using horizontal mattress sutures, because use of running sutures results in coronary occlusion and distal infarction. Gunshot wounds may result in stellate lesions or contused, extremely friable myocardium adjacent to the wound. When the edges of such complex wounds cannot be fully approximated and hence the repair is not hemostatic, the authors have used surgical adhesive (BioGlue) to achieve hemostasis. Occasionally, interior structures of the heart may be damaged. Intraoperative auscultation or postoperative hemodynamic assessment usually identifies such injuries.[55] Echocardiography can diagnose the injury and quantitate its effect on cardiac output. Immediate repair of valvular damage or septal defects rarely is necessary and would require cardiopulmonary bypass, which is associated with a high mortality in this situation.

Patients with blunt cardiac injury typically present with persistent tachycardia or rhythm disturbances, but occasionally present with tamponade due to atrial or right ventricular rupture. There are no pathognomonic ECG findings, and cardiac enzyme levels do not correlate with the risk of cardiac complications.[10] Therefore, patients for whom there is high clinical suspicion of cardiac contusion and who are hemodynamically stable should be monitored for dysrhythmias for 24 hours by telemetry. Patients with hemodynamic instability should undergo echocardiography to evaluate for wall motion abnormalities, valvular dysfunction, chordae rupture, or diminished ejection fraction. If such findings are noted or if vasoactive agents are required, cardiac function can be continuously monitored using a pulmonary artery catheter. A precisely timed blow to the precordium can provoke sudden cardiac death, termed *commotio cordis*.[56] This phenomenon, affecting primarily adolescent males, usually is fatal unless cardiopulmonary resuscitation and defibrillation are instituted immediately.

Trachea, Bronchi, Pulmonary Parenchyma, and Esophagus

Fewer than 1% of all injured patients sustain intrathoracic tracheobronchial injuries, and only a small number require operative intervention. Although penetrating injuries may occur throughout the

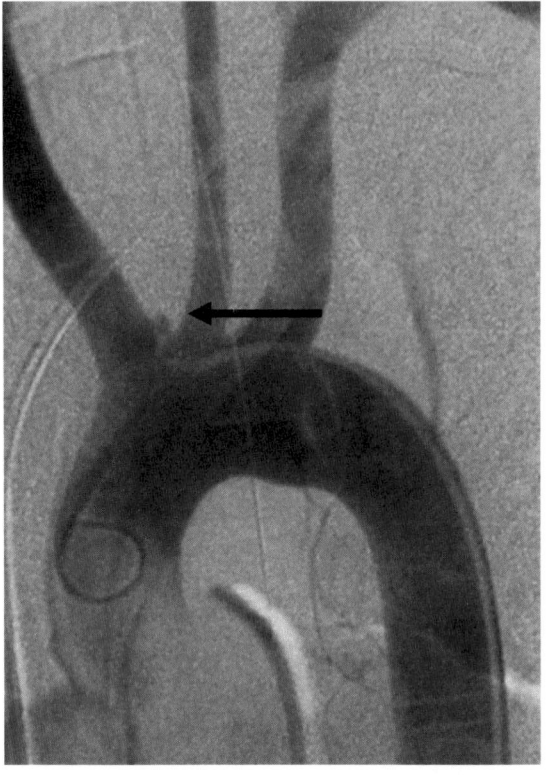

A

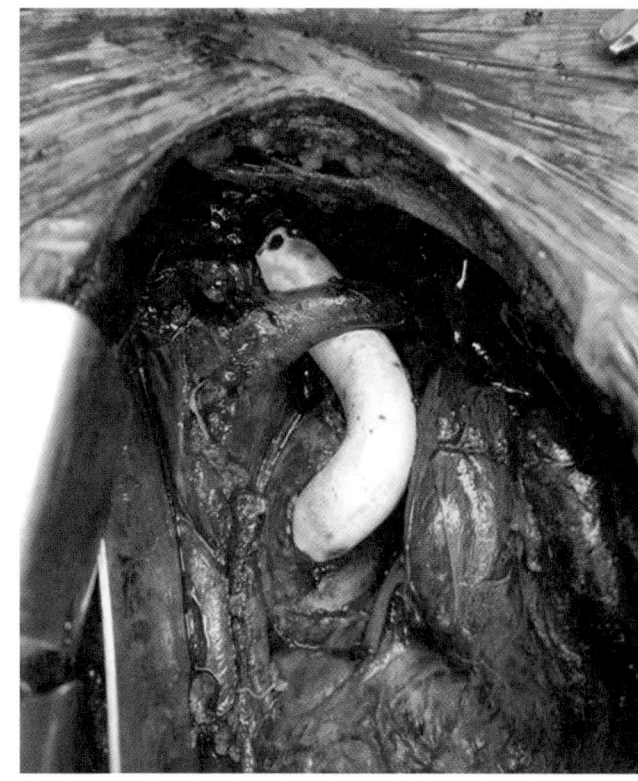

B

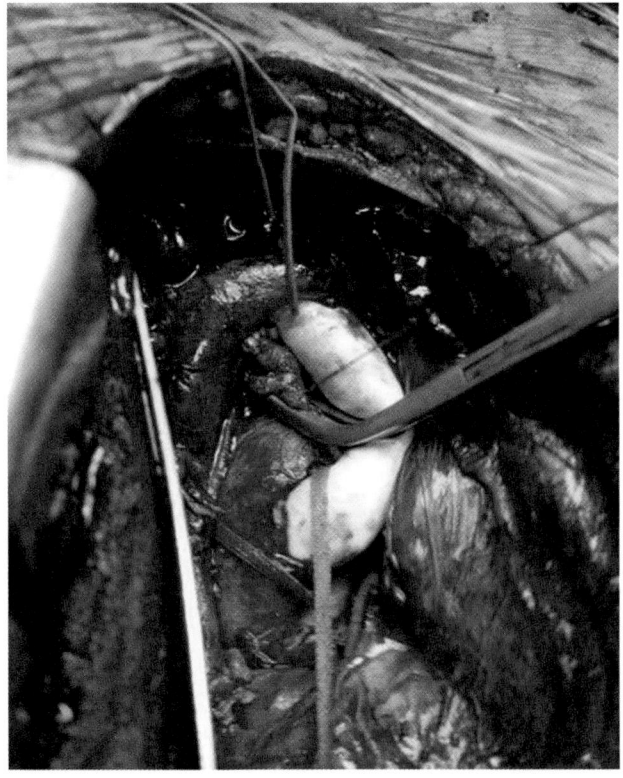

C

FIG. 7-55. A. Angiography reveals a 1-cm pseudoaneurysm of the innominate artery origin. **B.** In the first stage of the bypass exclusion technique, a 12-mm polytetrafluoroethylene graft is anastomosed end to side from the proximal undamaged aorta, tunneled under the vein, and anastomosed end to end to the innominate artery. **C.** The origin of the innominate is then oversewn at its base to exclude the pseudoaneurysm.

tracheobronchial system, blunt injuries occur within 2.5 cm of the carina. For patients with a massive air leak requiring emergent exploration, initial control of the injury to provide effective ventilation is obtained by passing an endotracheal tube either beyond the injury or into the contralateral mainstem bronchus. Principles of repair are similar to those for repair of cervical tracheal injuries. Devitalized tissue is débrided, and primary end-to-end anastomosis with 3-0 PDS suture is performed. Dissection should be careful and limited to the area of injury to prevent disruption of surrounding bronchial vasculature and ensuing ischemia and stricture. Suture

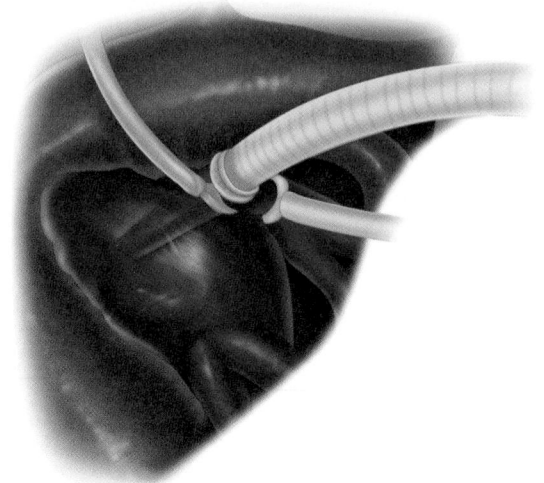
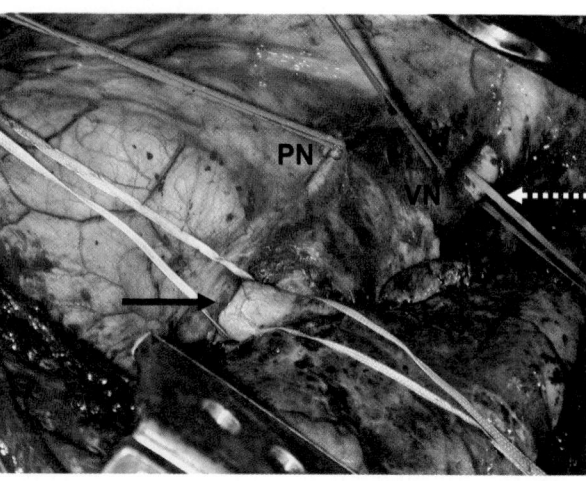

FIG. 7-56. When a tear of the descending thoracic aorta is repaired, perfusion of the spinal cord while the aorta is clamped is achieved by using partial left heart bypass. The venous cannula is inserted into the left superior pulmonary vein (*solid arrow*) because it is less prone to tearing than the left atrium. The subclavian artery (*dashed arrow*) is identified for vascular control. The phrenic nerve (PN) and vagus nerve (VN) should be identified during mediastinal exploration to prevent inadvertent injury.

lines should be encircled with vascularized tissue, either pericardium, intercostal muscle, or pleura. Expectant management is employed for bronchial injuries that are less than one-third the circumference of the airway and have no evidence of a persistent major air leak. In patients with peripheral bronchial injuries, indicated by persistent air leaks from the chest tube and documented by endoscopy, bronchoscopically directed fibrin glue sealing is occasionally required.

Injuries to the pulmonary parenchyma typically are discovered during exploration for a massive hemothorax after penetrating trauma. Peripheral lacerations with persistent bleeding can be managed with stapled wedge resection. More central injuries traditionally have been managed with pulmonary lobectomy or pneumonectomy. But current treatment relies on pulmonary tractotomy, which permits selective ligation of individual bronchioles and bleeders, prevents the development of an intraparenchymal hematoma or air embolism, and reduces the need for formal lobar resection (see Fig. 7-49).[57,58] A stapling device, preferably the longest GIA stapler available, is inserted directly into the injury track and positioned along the thinnest section of overlying parenchyma. The injury track is thus filleted open, which allows direct access to the bleeding vessels and leaking bronchi. The majority of injuries are definitively managed with selective ligation, and the defect is left open. Occasionally, tractotomy reveals a more proximal vascular injury that must be treated with formal lobectomy. Parenchymal injuries severe enough to mandate pneumonectomy usually are fatal because of right heart decompensation, and major pulmonary hilar injuries necessitating pneumonectomy are usually lethal in the field.[59]

One parenchymal injury that may be incidentally discovered during thoracic imaging is a posttraumatic pulmonary pseudocyst, colloquially termed a *pneumatocele*. Traumatic pneumatoceles typically follow a benign clinical course and are treated with aggressive pain management, pulmonary toilet, and serial chest radiography to monitor for resolution of the lesion. If the patient has persistent fever or leukocytosis, however, chest CT is done to evaluate for an evolving abscess, because up to 30% of pneumatoceles become infected. CT-guided catheter drainage may be required in such

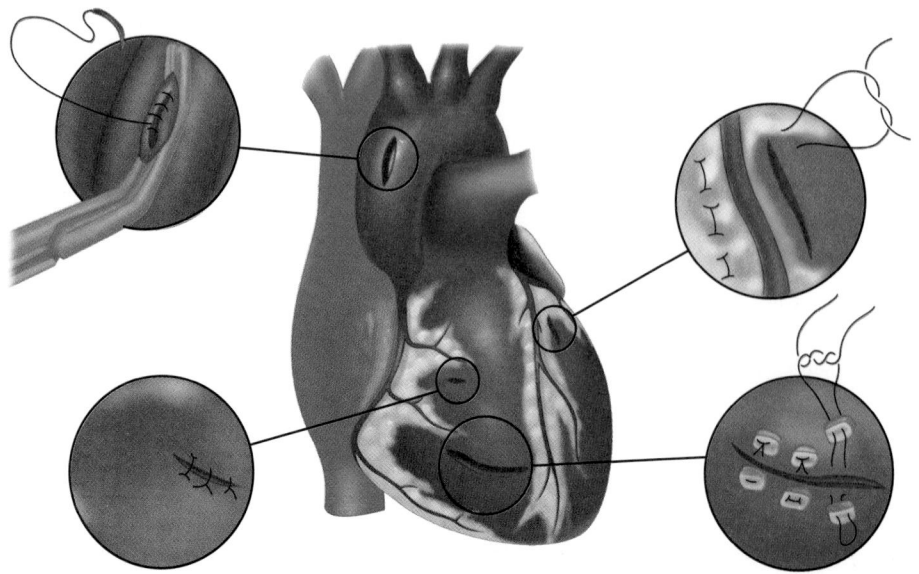

FIG. 7-57. A variety of techniques may be necessary to repair cardiac wounds. Generally, pledget support is used for the relatively thin-walled right ventricle.

cases, because 25% of patients do not respond to antibiotic therapy alone. Surgery, ranging from partial resection to anatomic lobectomy, is indicated for unresolving complex pneumatoceles or infected lesions refractory to antibiotic therapy and drainage.

The most common complication after thoracic injury is development of an empyema. Management is based on CT diagnostic criteria. Percutaneous drainage is indicated for single loculations without appreciable rind. Early decortication via video-assisted thoracic surgery is pursued in patients with multiple loculations or a pleural rind of >1 cm.[60] Antibiotic treatment is based on definitive culture results.

Due to the proximity of the structures, esophageal injuries often occur with tracheobronchial injuries, particularly in cases of penetrating trauma. Operative options are based on the extent and location of esophageal injury. With sufficient mobilization, a primary single-layer end-to-end anastomosis may be performed after appropriate débridement. As with cervical repairs, if there are two suture lines in close approximation (trachea or bronchi and esophagus) interposition of a vascularized pedicle will prevent fistula formation. Perforations close to the gastroesophageal junction may be best treated with segmental resection and gastric pull-up. With large destructive injuries or delayed presentation of injuries, esophageal exclusion with wide drainage, diverting loop esophagostomy, and placement of a gastrostomy tube should be considered.

Chest Wall and Diaphragm

Virtually all chest wall injuries, consisting of rib fractures and laceration of intercostal vessels, are treated nonoperatively with pain control, pulmonary toilet or ventilatory management, and drainage of the pleural space as indicated. Early institution of effective pain control is essential. The authors advocate rib blocks with 0.25% bupivacaine hydrochloride (Marcaine) in the trauma bay, followed by epidural placement supplemented with patient-controlled anesthesia. Persistent hemorrhage from a chest tube after blunt trauma most often is due to injured intercostal arteries; for unusual persistent bleeding (see Table 7-10), thoracotomy with direct ligation or angioembolization may be required to arrest hemorrhage. In rare cases of extensive flail chest segments or markedly displaced rib fractures, open reduction and internal fixation of the fracture with plates may be warranted. Chest wall defects, particularly those seen with open pneumothorax, are repaired using local approximation of tissues or tissue transfer for coverage. Scapular and sternal fractures rarely require operative intervention but are markers for significant thoracoabdominal force during injury. Careful examination and imaging should exclude associated injuries, including blunt cardiac injury and aortic tears. On the other hand, clavicle fractures often are isolated injuries and should be managed with pain control and immobilization. The exception is posterior dislocation of the clavicular head, which may injure the subclavian vessels.

Blunt diaphragmatic injuries result in a linear tear in the central tendon, whereas penetrating injuries are variable in size and location depending on the agent of injury. Regardless of the etiology, acute injuries are repaired through an abdominal incision or with thoracoscopy/laparoscopy. After delineation of the injury, the chest should be evacuated of all blood and particulate matter, and thoracostomy tube placed if not previously done. Allis clamps are used to approximate the diaphragmatic edges, and the defect is closed with a running No. 1 polypropylene suture. Occasionally, large avulsions or shotgun wounds with extensive tissue loss will require polypropylene mesh or acellular dermal matrix (AlloDerm) to bridge the defect. Alternatively, transposition of the diaphragm cephalad one to two intercostal spaces may allow repair without undue tension.[61]

Abdominal Injuries

Liver and Gallbladder

The liver's large size makes it the organ most susceptible to blunt trauma, and it is frequently involved in upper torso penetrating wounds. Nonoperative management of solid organ injuries is pursued in hemodynamically stable patients who do not have overt peritonitis or other indications for laparotomy. These patients should be admitted to the SICU with frequent hemodynamic monitoring, determination of hematocrit, and abdominal examination. The only absolute contraindication to nonoperative management is hemodynamic instability. Factors such as high injury grade, large hemoperitoneum, contrast extravasation, or pseudoaneurysms may predict complications or failure of nonoperative management. However, angioembolization and endoscopic retrograde cholangiopancreatography (ERCP) are useful adjuncts that can improve the success rate of nonoperative management.[62,63] The indication for angiography to control hepatic hemorrhage is transfusion of 4 units of RBCs in 6 hours or 6 units of RBCs in 24 hours without hemodynamic instability.

In the >10% of patients for whom emergent laparotomy is mandated, the primary goal is to arrest hemorrhage. Initial control of hemorrhage is best accomplished using perihepatic packing and manual compression. In either case, the edges of the liver laceration should be opposed for local pressure control of bleeding. Hemorrhage from most major hepatic injuries can be controlled with effective perihepatic packing. The right costal margin is elevated, and the pads are strategically placed over and around the bleeding site (see Fig. 7-36). Additional pads should be placed between the liver, diaphragm, and anterior chest wall until the bleeding has been controlled. Ten to 15 pads may be required to control the hemorrhage from an extensive right lobar injury. Packing of injuries of the left lobe is not as effective, because there is insufficient abdominal and thoracic wall anterior to the left lobe to provide adequate compression with the abdomen open. Fortunately, hemorrhage from the left lobe usually can be controlled by mobilizing the lobe and compressing it between the surgeon's hands. If the patient has persistent bleeding despite packing, injuries to the hepatic artery, portal vein, and retrohepatic vena cava should be considered. The Pringle maneuver can help delineate the source of hemorrhage. Hemorrhage from hepatic artery and portal vein injuries will halt with the application of a vascular clamp across the portal triad, whereas bleeding from the hepatic veins and retrohepatic vena cava will not.

Injuries of the portal triad vasculature should be addressed immediately. In general, ligation from the celiac axis to the level of the common hepatic artery at the gastroduodenal arterial branch is tolerated due to the extensive collaterals, but the proper hepatic artery should be repaired. The right or left hepatic artery, or in urgent situations the portal vein, may be selectively ligated; occasionally, lobar necrosis will necessitate delayed anatomic resection. If the right hepatic artery is ligated, cholecystectomy also should be performed. If the vascular injury is a stab wound with clean transection of the vessels, primary end-to-end repair is done. If the injury is destructive, temporary shunting should be performed followed by interposition reversed saphenous vein graft (RSVG). Blunt avulsions of the portal structures are particularly problematic if located at the hepatic plate, flush with the liver; hemorrhage control at the liver can be attempted with directed packing or Fogarty catheters. If the avulsion is more proximal, flush with the border of the pancreatic body or even retropancreatic, the pancreas must be transected to gain access for hemorrhage control and repair.

If massive venous hemorrhage is seen from behind the liver despite use of the Pringle maneuver, the patient likely has a hepatic vein or retrohepatic vena cava injury. If bleeding is controlled, the packing should be left undisturbed and the patient observed in the SICU. If bleeding continues despite repeat perihepatic packing, then direct repair, with or without hepatic vascular isolation, should be attempted. Three techniques have been used to accomplish hepatic vascular isolation: (a) isolation with clamps on the diaphragmatic aorta, the suprarenal vena cava, and the suprahepatic vena cava; (b) atriocaval shunt; and (c) Moore-Pilcher balloon shunt. All techniques are performed with an associated Pringle maneuver.

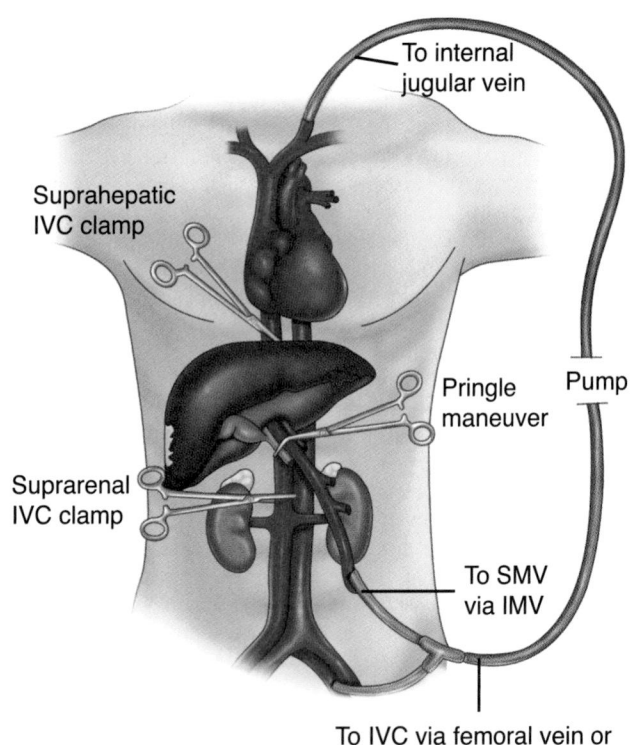

FIG. 7-58. Venovenous bypass permits hepatic vascular isolation with continued venous return to the heart. IMV = inferior mesenteric vein; IVC = inferior vena cava; SMV = superior mesenteric vein.

Even in experienced centers with readily available equipment, however, such techniques carry a mortality rate of >80%. Instead, recent efforts to control this highly lethal injury have used venovenous bypass (Fig. 7-58).[64]

Numerous methods for the definitive control of hepatic parenchymal hemorrhage have been developed. Minor lacerations may be controlled with manual compression applied directly to the injury site. Topical hemostatic techniques include the use of an electrocautery (with the device set at 100 watts), argon beam coagulator, microcrystalline collagen, thrombin-soaked gelatin foam sponge, fibrin glue, and BioGlue. Suturing of the hepatic parenchyma is an effective hemostatic technique. However, the "liver suture," blunt 0 chromic suture, may tear the liver capsule, and its use generally is discouraged due to the associated hepatic necrosis. A running suture is used to approximate the edges of shallow lacerations, whereas deeper lacerations are approximated using interrupted horizontal mattress sutures placed parallel to the edge of the laceration. When the suture is tied, tension is adequate when visible hemorrhage ceases or the liver blanches around the suture. This technique of placing large liver sutures controls bleeding through reapproximation of the liver laceration rather than direct ligation of bleeding vessels. Aggressive finger fracture to identify bleeding vessels followed by individual clip or suture ligation was advocated previously but currently has a limited role in hemostasis. Hepatic lobar arterial ligation may be appropriate for patients with recalcitrant arterial hemorrhage from deep within the liver and is a reasonable alternative to a deep hepatotomy, particularly in unstable patients. Omentum can be used to fill large defects in the liver. The tongue of omentum not only obliterates potential dead space with viable tissue but also provides an excellent source of macrophages. Additionally, the omentum can provide buttressing support for parenchymal sutures.

Translobar penetrating injuries are particularly challenging, because the extent of the injury cannot be fully visualized. As discussed later in "Damage Control Surgery," options include intraparenchymal tamponade with a Foley catheter or balloon occlusion (see Fig. 7-48).[65] If tamponade is successful with either modality, the balloon is left inflated for 24 to 48 hours followed by judicious deflation in the SICU and removal at a second laparotomy. Hepatotomy, using the finger fracture technique, with ligation of individual bleeders occasionally may be required. However, division of the overlying viable hepatic tissue may cause considerable blood loss in the coagulopathic patient. Finally, angioembolization is an effective adjunct in any of these scenarios and should be considered early in the course of treatment.

Several centers have reported patients with devastating hepatic injuries or necrosis of the entire liver who have undergone successful hepatic transplantation. Clearly this is dramatic therapy, and the patient must have all other injuries delineated, particularly those of the central nervous system, and have an excellent chance of survival excluding the hepatic injury. Because donor availability will limit such procedures, hepatic transplantation for trauma will continue to be performed only in extraordinary circumstances.

Cholecystectomy is performed for injuries of the gallbladder and after operative ligation of the right hepatic artery. Injuries of the extrahepatic bile ducts are a challenge due to their small size and thin walls. Because of the proximity of other portal structures and the vena cava, associated vascular injuries are common. These factors may preclude primary repair. Small lacerations with no accompanying loss or devitalization of adjacent tissue can be treated by the insertion of a T tube through the wound or by lateral suturing using 6-0 monofilament absorbable suture. Virtually all transections and any injury associated with significant tissue loss will require a Roux-en-Y choledochojejunostomy.[66] The anastomosis is performed using a single-layer interrupted technique with 4-0 or 5-0 monofilament absorbable suture. To reduce anastomotic tension, the jejunum can be sutured to the areolar tissue of the hepatic pedicle or porta hepatis. Injuries of the hepatic ducts are almost impossible to satisfactorily repair under emergent circumstances. One approach is to intubate the duct for external drainage and attempt a repair when the patient recovers. Alternatively, the duct can be ligated if the opposite lobe is normal and uninjured.

Patients undergoing perihepatic packing for extensive liver injuries typically are returned to the OR for pack removal 24 to 48 hours after initial injury. Earlier exploration may be indicated in patients with evidence of ongoing hemorrhage. Signs of rebleeding include a falling hematocrit, accumulation of blood clots under the temporary abdominal closure device, and bloody output from drains; the magnitude of hemorrhage is reflected in hemodynamic instability and the findings of metabolic monitoring. Patients with hepatic ischemia due to prolonged intraoperative use of the Pringle maneuver have an expected elevation but subsequent resolution of transaminases levels, whereas patients requiring hepatic artery ligation may have frank hepatic necrosis. Although patients should be evaluated for infectious complications, patients with complex hepatic injuries typically have intermittent "liver fever" for the first 5 days after injury.

The complications after significant hepatic trauma include delayed hemorrhage, bilomas, hepatic necrosis, arterial pseudoaneurysms, and various fistulas (Fig. 7-59). In patients requiring perihepatic packing, postoperative hemorrhage should be re-evaluated in the OR once the patient's coagulopathy is corrected. Alternatively, angioembolization is appropriate for complex injuries. Bilomas are loculated collections of bile, which may or may not be infected. If infected, they should be treated like an abscess via percutaneous drainage. Although small, sterile bilomas eventually will be reabsorbed, larger fluid collections should also be drained. Biliary ascites, due to the disruption of a major bile duct, often requires reoperation and wide drainage. Primary repair of the injured duct is unlikely to be successful. Resectional débridement is indicated for the removal of peripheral portions of nonviable hepatic parenchyma.

Pseudoaneurysms and biliary fistulas are rare complications in patients with hepatic injuries. Because hemorrhage from hepatic

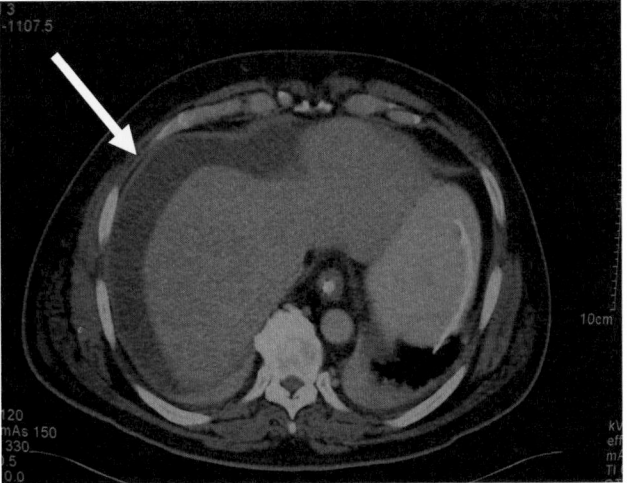

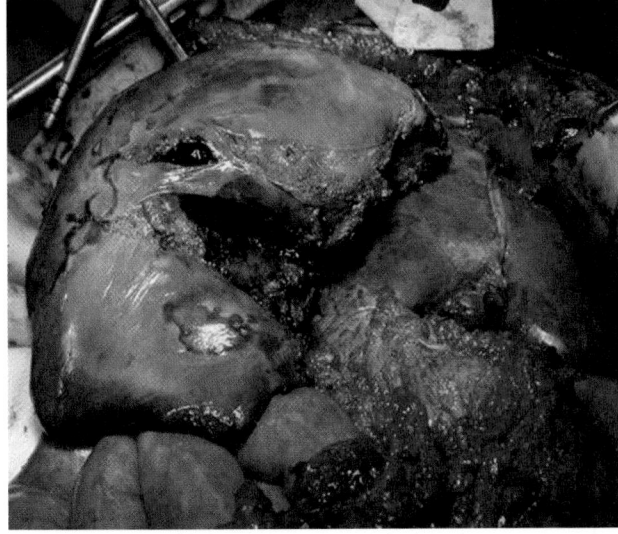

FIG. 7-59. Complications after hepatic trauma include bilomas (**A**; *arrow*), hepatic duct injuries (**B**), and hepatic necrosis after hepatic artery ligation or embolization (**C**).

injuries often is treated without isolating individual bleeding vessels, arterial pseudoaneurysms may develop, with the potential for rupture. Rupture into a bile duct results in hemobilia, which is characterized by intermittent episodes of right upper quadrant pain, upper GI hemorrhage, and jaundice. If the aneurysm ruptures into a portal vein, portal venous hypertension with bleeding esophageal varices may occur. Either scenario is best managed with hepatic arteriography and embolization. Biliovenous fistulas, causing jaundice due to rapid increases in serum bilirubin levels, should be treated with ERCP and sphincterotomy. Rarely, a biliary fistulous communication will form with intrathoracic structures in patients with associated diaphragm injuries, resulting in a bronchobiliary or pleurobiliary fistula. Due to the pressure differential between the biliary tract (positive) and the pleural cavity (negative), the majority require operative closure. Occasionally, endoscopic sphincterotomy with stent placement will effectively address the pressure differential, and the pleurobiliary fistula will close spontaneously.

Spleen

Until the 1970s, splenectomy was considered mandatory for all splenic injuries. Recognition of the immune function of the spleen refocused efforts on operative splenic salvage in the 1980s.[67,68] After success in pediatric patients, nonoperative management has become the preferred means of splenic salvage. The identification of contrast

extravasation as a risk factor for failure of nonoperative management led to liberal use of angioembolization. The true value of angioembolization in splenic salvage has not been rigorously evaluated. It is clear, however, that 20 to 30% of patients with splenic trauma deserve early splenectomy and that failure of nonoperative management often represents poor patient selection.[69,70] Unlike hepatic injuries, which rebleed in 24 to 48 hours, delayed hemorrhage or rupture of the spleen can occur up to weeks after injury. Indications for prompt laparotomy include initiation of blood transfusion within the first 12 hours and hemodynamic instability.

Splenic injuries are managed operatively by splenectomy, partial splenectomy, or splenic repair (splenorrhaphy), based on the extent of the injury and the physiologic condition of the patient. Splenectomy is indicated for hilar injuries, pulverized splenic parenchyma, or any injury of grade II or higher in a patient with coagulopathy or multiple injuries. The authors use autotransplantation of splenic implants (Fig. 7-60) to achieve partial immunocompetence in younger patients.[71] Drains are not used. Partial splenectomy can be employed in patients in whom only the superior or inferior pole has been injured. Hemorrhage from the raw splenic edge is controlled with horizontal mattress sutures, with gentle compression of the parenchyma (Fig. 7-61). As in repair of hepatic injuries, in splenorrhaphy hemostasis is achieved by topical methods (electrocautery; argon beam coagulation; application of thrombin-soaked gelatin foam sponges, fibrin glue, or BioGlue),

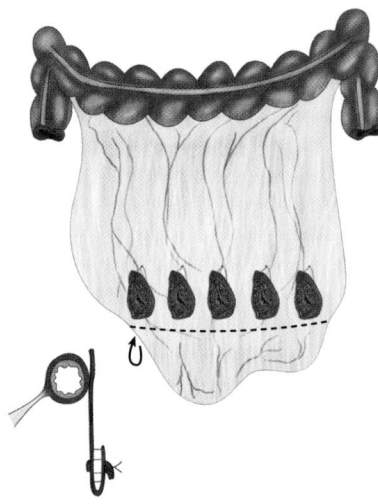 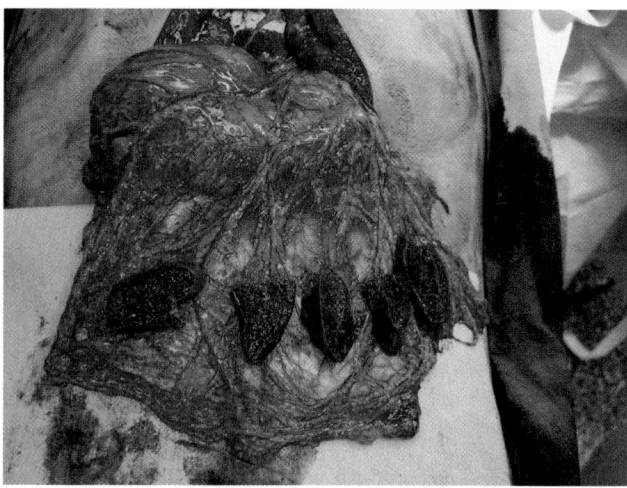

FIG. 7-60. Autologous splenic transplantation is performed by placing sections of splenic parenchyma, 40 × 40 × 3 mm in size, into pouches in the greater omentum.

envelopment of the injured spleen in absorbable mesh, and pledgeted suture repair.

After splenectomy or splenorrhaphy, postoperative hemorrhage may be due to loosening of a tie around the splenic vessels, an improperly ligated or unrecognized short gastric artery, or recurrent bleeding from the spleen if splenic repair was used. An immediate postsplenectomy increase in platelets and WBCs is normal; however, beyond postoperative day 5, a WBC count above 15,000/mm³ and a platelet/WBC ratio of <20 are strongly associated with sepsis and should prompt a thorough search for underlying infection.[72] A common infectious complication after splenectomy is a subphrenic abscess, which should be managed with percutaneous drainage. Additional sources of morbidity include a concurrent but unrecognized iatrogenic injury to the pancreatic tail during rapid splenectomy resulting in pancreatic ascites or fistula. Enthusiasm for splenic salvage was driven by the rare, but often fatal, complication of overwhelming postsplenectomy sepsis. Overwhelming postsplenectomy sepsis is caused by encapsulated bacteria, *Streptococcus pneumoniae*, *Haemophilus influenzae*, and *Neisseria meningitidis*, which are resistant to antimicrobial treatment. In patients undergoing splenectomy, prophylaxis against these bacteria is provided via vaccines administered optimally at 14 days.

Stomach and Small Intestine

Little controversy exists regarding the repair of injuries to the stomach or small bowel. Gastric wounds can be oversewn with a running single-layer suture line or closed with a transection/anastomosis (TA) stapler. If a single-layer closure is chosen, full-thickness bites should be taken to ensure hemostasis from the well-vascularized gastric wall. The most commonly missed gastric injury is the posterior wound of a through-and-through penetrating injury. Injuries also can be overlooked if the wound is located within the mesentery of the lesser curvature or high in the posterior fundus. To delineate a questionable injury, the stomach can be digitally occluded at the pylorus while methylene blue–colored saline is instilled via a nasogastric tube. Partial gastrectomy may be required for destructive injuries, with resections of the distal antrum or pylorus reconstructed using a Billroth I or II procedure. Patients with injuries that damage both Latarjet nerves or vagi should undergo a drainage procedure (see Chap. 26). Small intestine injuries can be repaired using a transverse running 3-0 PDS suture if the injury is less than one third the circumference of the bowel. Destructive injuries or multiple penetrating injuries occurring close together are treated with segmental resection followed by end-to-end anastomosis using a continuous, single-layer 3-0 polypropylene suture.[73] Mesenteric injuries may result in an ischemic segment of intestine, which mandates resection.

Following repair of GI tract injuries, there is an obligatory postoperative ileus. Return of bowel function is indicated by a decrease in gastrostomy or nasogastric tube output. The topic of nutrition is well covered in other chapters, but a few issues warrant mention. Multiple studies have confirmed the importance of early total enteral nutrition (TEN) in the trauma population, particularly its impact in reducing septic complications.[74] The route of enteral feedings (stomach vs. small bowel) tends to be less important, because gut tolerance appears equivalent unless there is upper GI tract pathology. Although early enteral nutrition is the goal, one should be wary with any bowel anastomoses; evidence of bowel function should be apparent before advancing to goal tube feedings. Overzealous jejunal feeding can lead to small bowel necrosis in the patient recovering from profound shock. Patients undergoing monitoring for nonoperative management of grade II or higher solid organ injuries should receive nothing by mouth for at least 48 hours in case they require an operation. Although there is general reluctance to initiate TEN in patients with an open abdomen, tube feeding by any route may be started within 24 hours of abdominal closure, because over 90% of patients will tolerate TEN. Moreover, in patients relegated to an open abdomen, TEN is frequently tolerated at low volumes—that is, trophic tube feeds (25 mL/h)—while active attempts are made to close fascia.

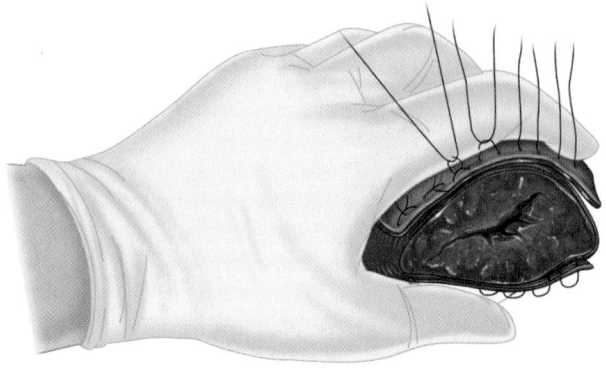

FIG. 7-61. Interrupted pledgeted sutures may effectively control hemorrhage from the cut edge of the spleen.

In general, wounds sustained from trauma should be examined daily for progression of healing and signs of infection. Complex soft tissue wounds of the abdomen, such as degloving injuries after blunt trauma (termed *Morel-Lavallee lesions*), shotgun wounds, and other destructive blast injuries, are particularly difficult to manage. Following initial débridement of devitalized tissue, wound care includes wet-to-dry dressing changes twice daily or application of a vacuum-assisted wound closure (VAC) device. Repeated operative débridement may be necessary, and early involvement of the reconstructive surgery service for possible flap coverage is advised. Midline laparotomy wounds are inspected 48 hours postoperatively by removing the sterile surgical dressing. If an ileostomy or colostomy was required, one should inspect it daily to ensure that it is viable. If the patient develops high-grade fever, the wound should be inspected sooner to exclude an early necrotizing infection. If a wound infection is identified—as evidenced by erythema, pain along the wound, or purulent drainage—the wound should be widely opened by removing skin staples. After ensuring that the midline fascia is intact with digital palpation, the wound is initially managed with wet-to-dry dressing changes. The most common intra-abdominal complications are anastomotic failure and abscess. The choice between percutaneous and operative therapy is based on the location, timing, and extent of the collection.

Duodenum and Pancreas

The spectrum of injuries to the duodenum includes hematomas, perforation (blunt blow-outs, lacerations from stab wounds, or blast injury from gunshot wounds), and combined pancreaticoduodenal injuries. The majority of duodenal hematomas are managed nonoperatively with nasogastric suction and parenteral nutrition. Patients with suspected associated perforation, suggested by clinical deterioration or imaging with retroperitoneal free air or contrast extravasation, should undergo operative exploration. A marked drop in nasogastric tube output heralds resolution of the hematoma, which typically occurs within 2 weeks; repeat imaging to confirm these clinical findings is optional. If the patient shows no clinical or radiographic improvement within 3 weeks, operative evaluation is warranted.

Small duodenal perforations or lacerations can be treated by primary repair using a running single-layer suture of 3-0 monofilament. The wound should be closed in a direction that results in the largest residual lumen. Challenges arise when there is a substantial loss of duodenal tissue. Extensive injuries of the first portion of the duodenum (proximal to the duct of Santorini) can be repaired by débridement and end-to-end anastomosis because of the mobility and rich blood supply of the distal gastric atrium and pylorus. In contrast, the second portion is tethered to the head of the pancreas by its blood supply and the ducts of Wirsung and Santorini; therefore, no more than 1 cm of duodenum can be mobilized away from the pancreas, and this does not effectively alleviate tension on the suture line. Moreover, suture repair using an end-to-end anastomosis in the second portion often results in an unacceptably narrow lumen. Therefore, defects in the second portion of the duodenum should be patched with a vascularized jejunal graft. Duodenal injuries with tissue loss distal to the papilla of Vater and proximal to the superior mesenteric vessels are best treated by Roux-en-Y duodenojejunostomy with the distal portion of the duodenum oversewn (Fig. 7-62). In particular, injuries in the distal third and fourth portions of the duodenum (behind the mesenteric vessels) should be resected, and a duodenojejunostomy performed on the left side of the superior mesenteric vessels.

Optimal management of pancreatic trauma is determined by where the parenchymal damage is located and whether the intrapancreatic common bile duct and main pancreatic duct remain intact. Patients with pancreatic contusions (defined as injuries that leave the ductal system intact) can be treated nonoperatively or with closed suction drainage if undergoing laparotomy for other indications. In contrast, pancreatic injuries associated with ductal disruption re-

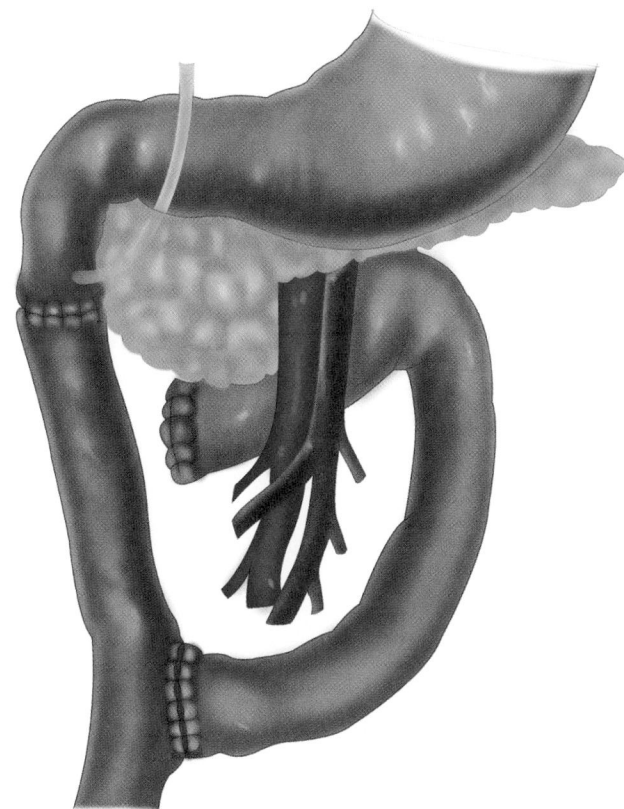

FIG. 7-62. Roux-en-Y duodenojejunostomy is used to treat duodenal injuries between the papilla of Vater and superior mesenteric vessels when tissue loss precludes primary repair.

quire intervention to prevent a pancreatic fistula or ascites. To determine the integrity of the pancreatic duct, several options exist. Direct exploration of the parenchymal laceration will often confirm the diagnosis of a ductal injury. Operative pancreatography can be performed through a duodenotomy by cannulating the duct using a 5F pediatric feeding tube. Under fluoroscopy, full-strength contrast material is slowly injected while observing for obstruction or extravasation. An alternative to pancreatography is to pass a 1.5- to 2.0-mm coronary artery dilator into the main duct via the papilla and observe the depth of the pancreatic wound. If the dilator is seen in the wound, a ductal injury is confirmed. Either technique requires the creation of a duodenal wound and hence the potential for anastomotic leak and a lateral duodenal fistula; this possibility may dampen a surgeon's enthusiasm for this approach. A third method for identifying pancreatic ductal injuries is endoscopic retrograde pancreatography. Although challenging to perform emergently in the OR, it can be performed postoperatively once resuscitation is accomplished and is particularly advantageous in stable patients or those with a delayed presentation.

Several options exist for treating injuries of the pancreatic body and tail when the pancreatic duct is transected. In stable patients, spleen-preserving distal pancreatectomy should be performed. An alternative, which preserves both the spleen and distal transected end of the pancreas, is either a Roux-en-Y pancreaticojejunostomy or pancreaticogastrostomy. If the patient is physiologically compromised, distal pancreatectomy with splenectomy is the preferred approach. Regardless of the choice of definitive procedure, the pancreatic duct in the proximal edge of transected pancreas should be individually ligated or occluded with a TA stapler. Application of fibrin glue over the stump may be advantageous.

Injuries to the pancreatic head add an additional element of complication because the intrapancreatic portion of the common bile

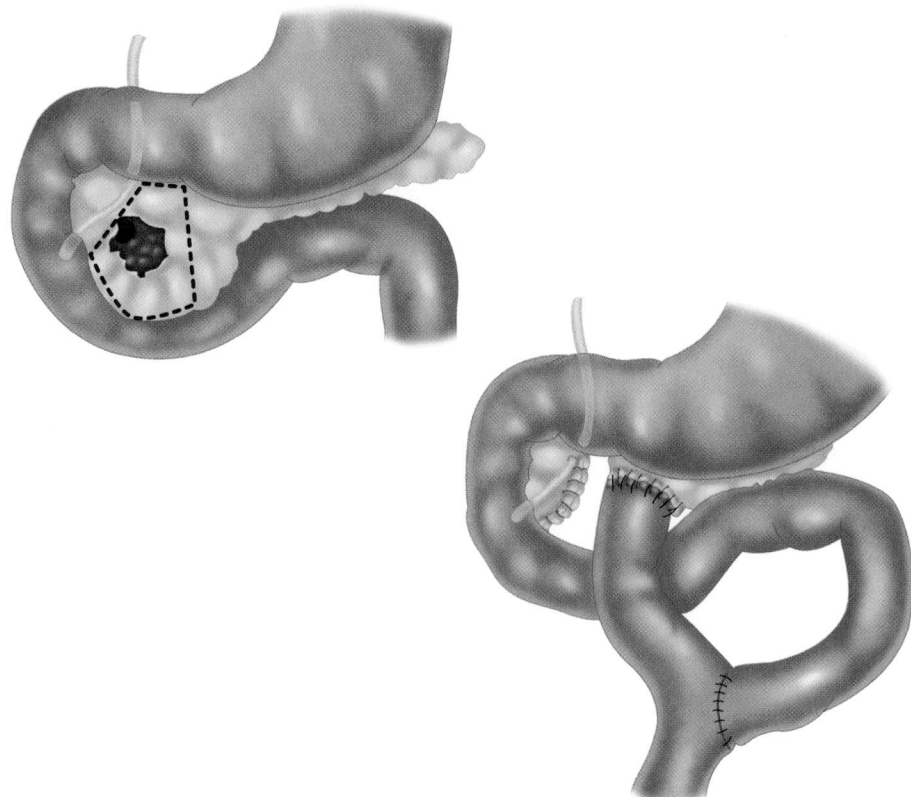

FIG. 7-63. For injuries of the pancreatic head that involve the pancreatic duct but spare the common bile duct, central pancreatic resection with Roux-en-Y pancreaticojejunostomy prevents pancreatic insufficiency.

duct traverses this area and often converges with the pancreatic duct. In contrast to diagnosis of pancreatic duct injuries, identification of intrapancreatic common bile duct disruption is relatively simple. The first method is to squeeze the gallbladder and look for bile leaking from the pancreatic wound. Otherwise, cholangiography, optimally via the cystic duct, is diagnostic. Definitive treatment of this injury entails division of the common bile duct superior to the first portion of the duodenum, with ligation of the distal duct and reconstruction with a Roux-en-Y choledochojejunostomy. For injuries to the head of the pancreas that involve the main pancreatic duct but not the intrapancreatic bile duct, there are few options. Distal pancreatectomy alone is rarely indicated due to the extended resection of normal gland and the resultant risk of pancreatic insufficiency. Central pancreatectomy preserves the common bile duct, and mobilization of the pancreatic body permits drainage into a Roux-en-Y pancreaticojejunostomy (Fig. 7-63). Although this approach avoids a pancreaticoduodenectomy (Whipple procedure), the complexity may make the pancreaticoduodenectomy more appropriate in patients with multiple injuries. Some injuries of the pancreatic head do not involve either the pancreatic or common bile duct; if no clear ductal injury is present, drains are placed. Rarely, patients sustain destructive injuries to the head of the pancreas or combined pancreaticoduodenal injuries that require pancreaticoduodenectomy. Examples of such injuries include transection of both the intrapancreatic bile duct and the main pancreatic duct in the head of the pancreas, avulsion of the papilla of Vater from the duodenum, and destruction of the entire second portion of the duodenum.

Pyloric exclusion often is used to divert the GI stream after high-risk, complex duodenal repairs (Fig. 7-64).[75] If the duodenal repair breaks down, the resultant fistula is an end fistula, which is easier to manage and more likely to close than a lateral fistula. To perform a pyloric exclusion, first a gastrostomy is made on the greater curvature near the pylorus. The pylorus is then grasped with a Babcock clamp, via the gastrostomy, and oversewn with an O polypropylene suture. A gastrojejunostomy restores GI tract continuity. Vagotomy is not

necessary because a risk of marginal ulceration has not been documented. Perhaps surprisingly, the sutures maintain diversion for only 3 to 4 weeks. Alternatively, the most durable pyloric closure is a double external staple line across the pylorus using a TA stapler.

Complications should be expected after such injuries. Delayed hemorrhage is rare but may occur with pancreatic necrosis or abdominal infection; this usually can be managed by angioembolization. If closed suction drains have been inserted for major pancreatic trauma, these should remain in place until the patient is tolerating an oral diet or enteral nutrition. Pancreatic fistula is diagnosed after postoperative day 5 in patients with drain output of >30 mL/d and a drain amylase level three times the serum value. Pancreatic fistula develops in over 20% of patients with combined injuries and should be managed similar to fistulas after elective surgery (see Chap. 33). Similarly, a duodenal fistula, presumptively an end fistula if a pyloric exclusion has been done, will typically heal in 6 to 8 weeks with adequate drainage and control of intra-abdominal sepsis. Pancreatic pseudocysts in patients managed nonoperatively suggest a missed injury, and ERCP should be done to evaluate the integrity of the pancreatic duct. Late pseudocysts may be a complication of operative management and are treated much like those in patients with pancreatitis (see Chap. 33). Intra-abdominal abscesses are common and routinely managed with percutaneous drainage.

Colon and Rectum

Currently, three methods for treating colonic injuries are used: primary repair, end colostomy, and primary repair with diverting ileostomy. Primary repairs include lateral suture repair or resection of the damaged segment with reconstruction by ileocolostomy or colocolostomy. All suturing and anastomoses are performed using a running single-layer technique (Fig. 7-65).[73] The advantage of definitive treatment must be balanced against the possibility of anastomotic leakage if suture lines are created under suboptimal conditions. Alternatively, although use of an end colostomy requires a second operation, an unprotected suture line with the potential for

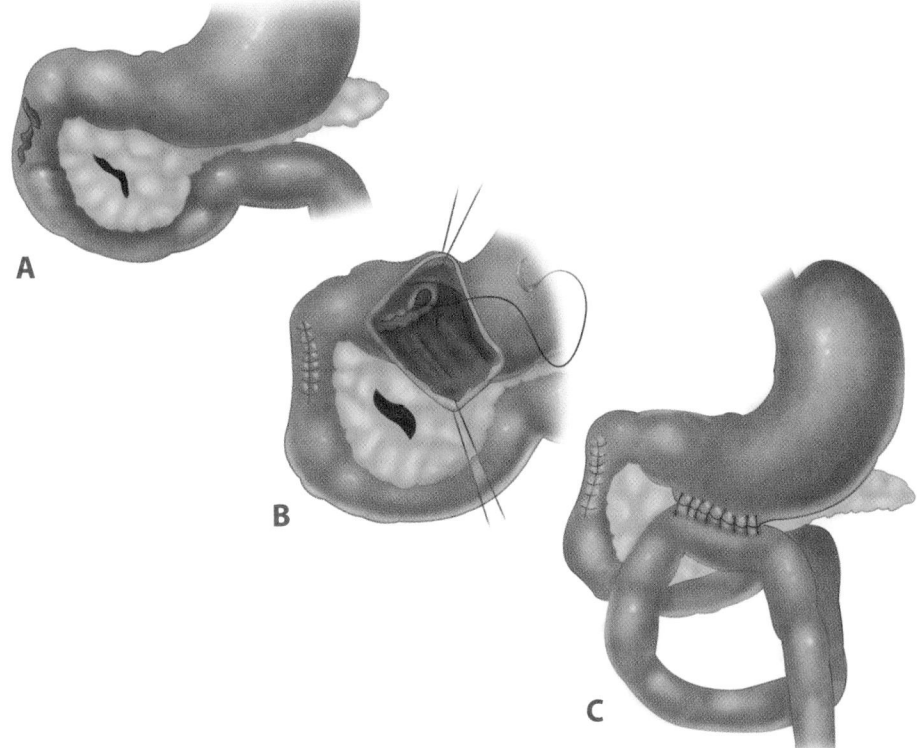

FIG. 7-64. A. Pyloric exclusion is used to treat combined injuries of the duodenum and the head of the pancreas as well as isolated duodenal injuries when the duodenal repair is less than optimal. **B** and **C.** The pylorus is oversewn through a gastrotomy, which is subsequently used to create a gastrojejunostomy. The authors frequently use needle-catheter jejunostomy tube feedings for these patients.

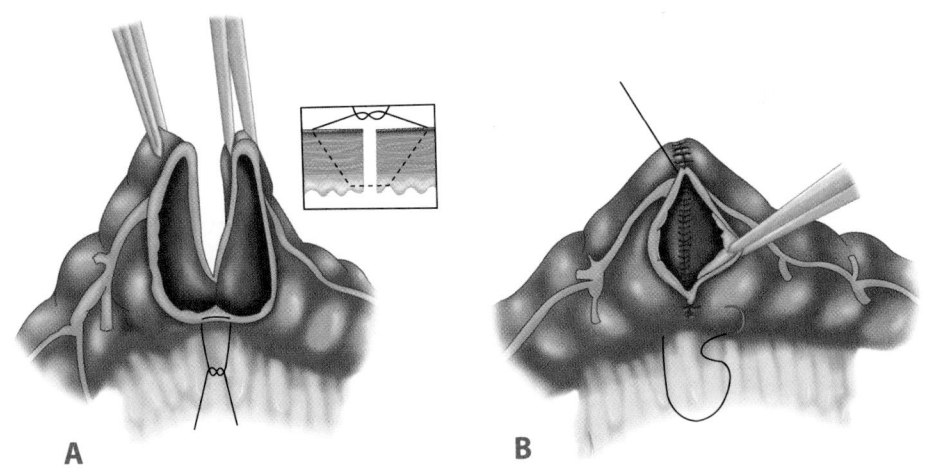

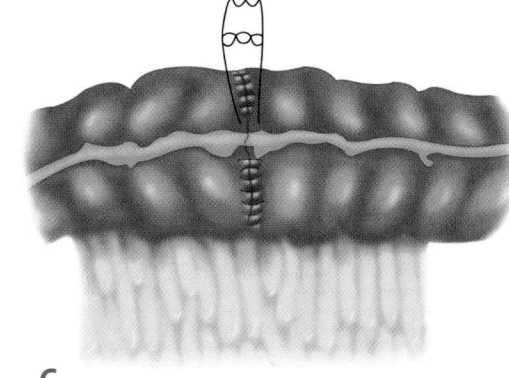

FIG. 7-65. Technique for bowel repair and anastomosis. **A.** The running, single-layer suture is started at the mesenteric border. **B.** Stitches are spaced 3 to 4 mm from the edge of the bowel and advanced 3 to 4 mm, including all layers except the mucosa. **C.** The continuous suture is tied near the antimesenteric border.

breakdown is avoided. Numerous large retrospective and several prospective studies have now clearly demonstrated that primary repair is safe and effective in virtually all patients with penetrating wounds.[76] Colostomy is still appropriate in a few patients, but the current dilemma is how to select which patients should undergo the procedure. Currently, the overall physiologic status of the patient, rather than local factors, directs decision making. Patients with devastating left colon injuries requiring damage control are clearly candidates for temporary colostomy. Ileostomy with colocolostomy, however, is used for most other high-risk patients.

Rectal injuries are similar to colonic injuries with respect to the ecology of the luminal contents, overall structure, and blood supply of the wall, but access to extraperitoneal injuries is limited due to the surrounding bony pelvis. Therefore, indirect treatment with intestinal diversion usually is required. The current options are loop ileostomy and sigmoid loop colostomy. These are preferred because they are quick and easy to perform, and provide essentially total fecal diversion. For sigmoid colostomy, technical elements include (a) adequate mobilization of the sigmoid colon so that the loop will rest on the abdominal wall without tension, (b) maintenance of the spur of the colostomy (the common wall of the proximal and distal limbs after maturation) above the level of the skin with a one-half-inch nylon rod or similar device, (c) longitudinal incision in the tenia coli, and (d) immediate maturation in the OR (Fig. 7-66). If the injury is accessible (e.g., in the posterior intraperitoneal portion of the rectum), repair of the injury should also be attempted. However, it is not necessary to explore the extraperitoneal rectum to repair a distal perforation. If the rectal injury is extensive, another option is to divide the rectum at the level of the injury, oversew or staple the distal rectal pouch if possible, and create an end colostomy (Hartmann's procedure). Extensive injuries may warrant presacral drainage with Penrose drains placed along Waldeyer's fascia via a perianal incision (see Fig. 7-66). In rare instances in which destructive injuries are present, an abdominoperineal resection may be necessary to avert lethal pelvic sepsis.

Complications related to colorectal injuries include intra-abdominal abscess, fecal fistula, wound infection, and stomal complications. Intra-abdominal abscesses occur in approximately 10% of patients, and most are managed with percutaneous drainage. Fistulas occur in 1 to 3% of patients and usually present as an abscess or wound infection with subsequent continuous drainage of fecal output; the majority will heal spontaneously with routine care (see Chap. 29). Stomal complications (necrosis, stenosis, obstruction, and prolapse) occur in 5% of patients and may require either immediate or delayed reoperation. Stomal necrosis should be carefully monitored, because spread beyond the mucosa may result in septic complications, including necrotizing fasciitis of the abdominal wall. Penetrating injuries that involve both the rectum and adjacent bony structures are prone to development of osteomyelitis. Bone biopsy is performed for diagnosis and bacteriologic analysis, and treatment entails long-term IV antibiotic therapy and occasionally débridement.

Abdominal Vasculature

Injury to the major arteries and veins in the abdomen are a technical challenge.[77-83] Although penetrating trauma indiscriminately affects all blood vessels, blunt trauma most commonly involves renal vasculature and rarely the abdominal aorta. Patients with a penetrating aortic wound who survive to reach the OR frequently have a contained hematoma within the retroperitoneum. Due to lack of mobility of the abdominal aorta, few injuries are amenable to primary repair. Small lateral perforations may be controlled with 4-0 polypropylene suture or a PTFE patch, but end-to-end interposition grafting with a PTFE tube graft is the most common repair. In contrast, blunt injuries are typically intimal tears of the infrarenal aorta and are readily exposed via a direct approach. To avoid future vascular-enteric fistulas, the vascular suture lines should be covered with omentum.

Penetrating wounds to the superior mesenteric artery (SMA) are typically encountered upon exploration for a gunshot wound, with "black bowel" and associated supramesocolic hematoma being pathog-

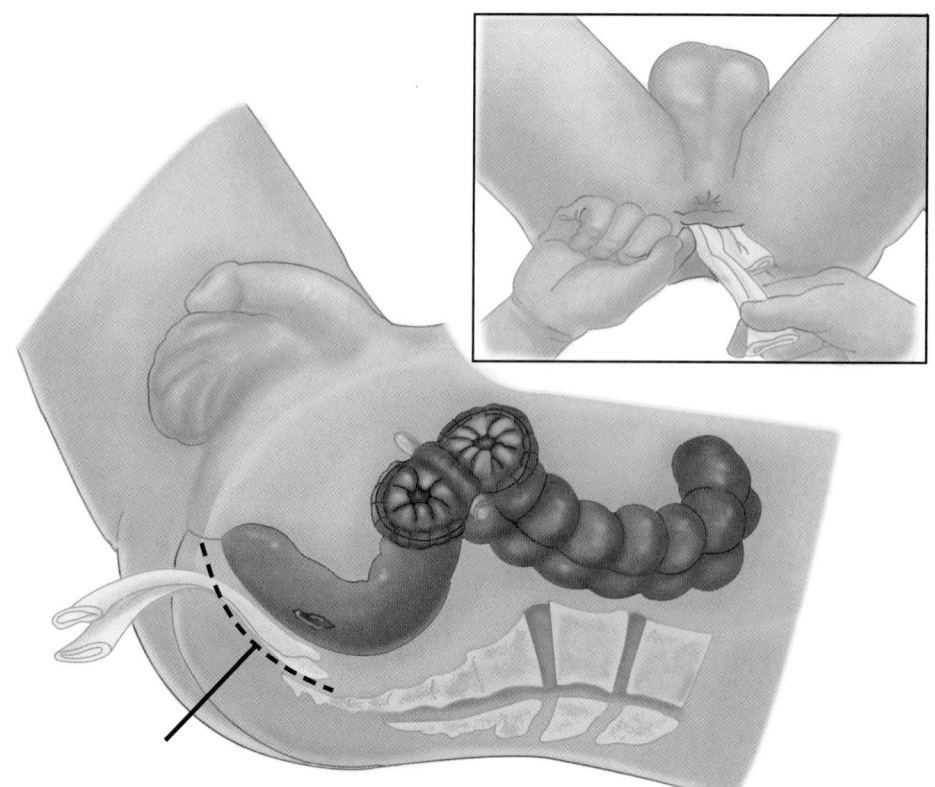

FIG. 7-66. Loop colostomy will completely divert the fecal flow, allowing the low rectal injury to heal. For extensive wounds, presacral drains are inserted through a perianal incision (*box*) and advanced along Waldeyer's fascia (*dashed line*).

nomonic. Blunt avulsions of the SMA are rare but should be considered in patients with a seat belt sign who have midepigastric pain or tenderness and associated hypotension. For injuries of the SMA, temporary damage control with a Pruitt-Inahara shunt can prevent extensive bowel necrosis; additionally, temporary shunting allows control of visceral contamination before placement of a PTFE graft. For definitive repair, end-to-end interposition RSVG from the proximal SMA to the SMA past the point of injury can be performed if there is no associated pancreatic injury. Alternatively, if the patient has an associated pancreatic injury, the graft should be tunneled from the distal aorta beneath the duodenum to the distal SMA. For proximal SMV injuries, digital compression for hemorrhage control is followed by attempted venorrhaphy; ligation is an option in a life-threatening situation, but the resultant bowel edema requires aggressive fluid resuscitation. Temporary abdominal closure and a second-look operation to evaluate bowel viability should be done.

Transpelvic gunshot wounds or blunt injuries with associated pelvic fractures are the most common scenarios in patients with iliac artery injuries. A Pruitt-Inahara shunt can be used for temporary shunting of the vessel for damage control. Definitive interposition grafting with excision of the injured segment is appropriate (see "Vascular Repair Techniques"). Careful monitoring for distal embolic events and reperfusion injury necessitating fasciotomy is imperative.

In general, outcome after vascular injuries is related to (a) the technical success of the vascular reconstruction and (b) associated soft tissue and nerve injuries. Vascular repairs rarely fail after the first 12 hours, whereas, soft tissue infection is a limb threat for several weeks. Following aortic interposition grafting, the patient's SBP should not exceed 120 mmHg for at least the first 72 hours postoperatively. Patients requiring ligation of an inferior vena cava injury often develop marked bilateral lower extremity edema. To limit the associated morbidity the patient's legs should be wrapped with elastic bandages from the toes to the hips and elevated at a 45- to 60-degree angle. For superior mesenteric vein injuries, either ligation or thrombosis after venorrhaphy results in marked bowel edema; fluid resuscitation should be aggressive and abdominal pressure monitoring routine in these patients. Prosthetic graft infections are rare compli-

cations, but prevention of bacteremia is imperative; administration of antibiotics perioperatively and treatment of secondary infections is indicated. Long-term arterial graft complications such as stenosis or pseudoaneurysms are uncommon, and routine graft surveillance rarely is performed. Consequently, long-term administration of anti-platelet agents or antithrombotics is not routine.

Genitourinary Tract

When undergoing laparotomy for trauma, the best policy is to explore all penetrating wounds to the kidneys. Parenchymal renal injuries are treated with hemostatic and reconstructive techniques similar to those used for injuries of the liver and spleen: topical methods (electrocautery; argon beam coagulation; application of thrombin-soaked gelatin foam sponge, fibrin glue, or BioGlue) and pledgeted suture repair. Two caveats are recognized, however: The collecting system should be closed separately, and the renal capsule should be preserved to close over the repair of the collecting system (Fig. 7-67). Renal vascular injuries are common after penetrating trauma and may be deceptively tamponaded, which results in delayed hemorrhage. Arterial reconstruction using graft interposition should be attempted for renal preservation. For destructive parenchymal or irreparable renovascular injuries, nephrectomy may be the only option; a normal contralateral kidney must be palpated, because unilateral renal agenesis occurs in 0.1% of patients.

Over 90% of all blunt renal injuries are treated nonoperatively. Hematuria typically resolves within a few days with bed rest, although rarely bleeding is so persistent that bladder irrigation to dispel blood clots is warranted. Persistent gross hematuria may require embolization, whereas urinomas can be drained percutaneously. Operative intervention after blunt trauma is limited to renovascular injuries and destructive parenchymal injuries that result in hypotension. The renal arteries and veins are uniquely susceptible to traction injury caused by blunt trauma. As the artery is stretched, the inelastic intima and media may rupture, which causes thrombus formation and resultant stenosis or occlusion. The success rate for renal artery repair approaches 0%, but an attempt is reasonable if the injury is <3 hours old or if the patient has a solitary kidney or bilateral injuries.[84] Reconstruction after blunt renal inju-

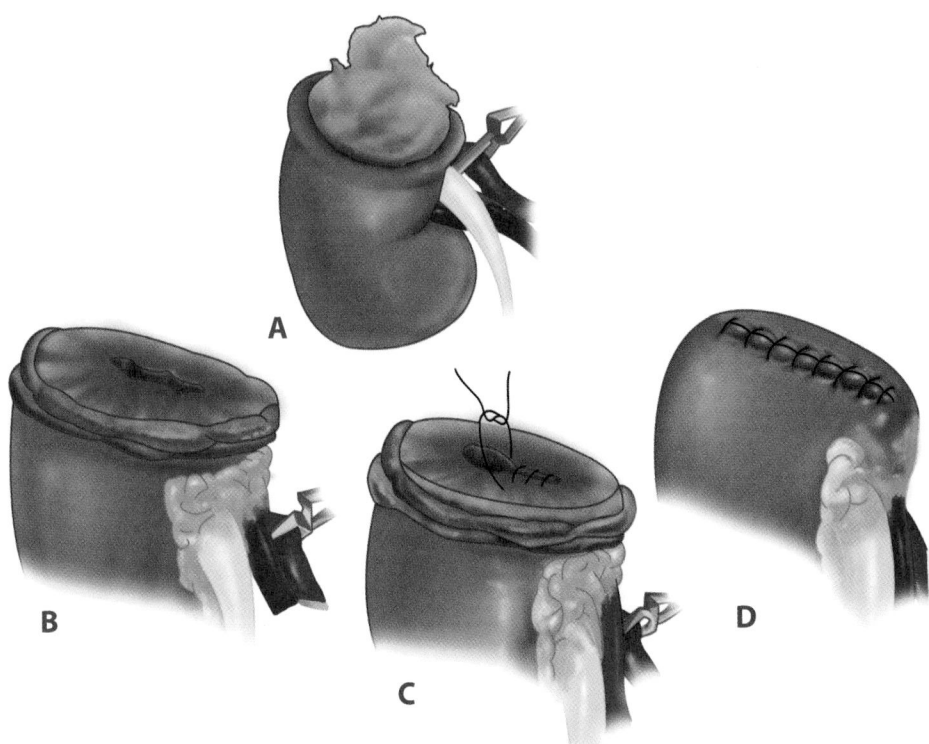

FIG. 7-67. When renorrhaphy is undertaken, effective repair is assisted by attention to several key points: **A.** Vascular occlusion controls bleeding and permits adequate visualization. **B.** The renal capsule is carefully preserved. **C.** The collecting system is closed separately with absorbable suture. **D.** The preserved capsule is closed over the collecting system repair.

ries may be difficult, however, because the injury is typically at the level of the aorta. If repair is not possible within this time frame, leaving the kidney in situ does not necessarily lead to hypertension or abscess formation. The renal vein may be torn or completely avulsed from the vena cava due to blunt trauma. Typically, the large hematoma causes hypotension, which leads to operative intervention. During laparotomy for blunt trauma, expanding or pulsatile perinephric hematomas should be explored. If necessary, emergent vascular control can be obtained by placing a curved vascular clamp across the hilum from an inferior approach. Techniques of repair and hemostasis are similar to those described earlier.

Injuries to the ureters are uncommon but may occur in patients with pelvic fractures and penetrating trauma. An injury may not be identified until a complication (i.e., a urinoma) becomes apparent. If an injury is suspected during operative exploration but is not clearly identified, methylene blue or indigo carmine is administered IV with observation for extravasation. Injuries are repaired using 5-0 absorbable monofilament, and mobilization of the kidney may reduce tension on the anastomosis. Distal ureteral injuries can be treated by reimplantation facilitated with a psoas hitch and/or Boari flap. In damage control circumstances, the ureter can be ligated on both sides of the injury and a nephrostomy tube placed.

Bladder injuries are subdivided into those with intraperitoneal extravasation and those with extraperitoneal extravasation. Ruptures or lacerations of the intraperitoneal bladder are operatively closed with a running, single-layer, 3-0 absorbable monofilament suture. Laparoscopic repair is becoming common in patients not requiring laparotomy for other injuries. Extraperitoneal ruptures are treated nonoperatively with bladder decompression for 2 weeks. Urethral injuries are managed by bridging the defect with a Foley catheter, with or without direct suture repair. Strictures are not uncommon but can be managed electively.

Female Reproductive Tract

Gynecologic injuries are rare. Occasionally the vaginal wall will be lacerated by a bone fragment from a pelvic fracture. Although repair is not mandated, it should be performed if physiologically feasible. More important, however, is recognition of the open fracture, need for possible drainage, and potential for pelvic sepsis. Penetrating injuries to the vagina, uterus, fallopian tubes, and ovaries are also uncommon, and routine hemostatic techniques are used. Repair of a transected fallopian tube can be attempted but probably is unjustified, because a suboptimal repair will increase the risk of tubal pregnancy. Transection at the injury site with proximal ligation and distal salpingectomy is a more prudent approach.

Pelvic Fractures and Emergent Hemorrhage Control

Patients with pelvic fractures who are hemodynamically unstable are a diagnostic and therapeutic challenge for the trauma team. These injuries often occur in conjunction with other life-threatening injuries, and there is no universal agreement among clinicians on management. Current management algorithms in the United States incorporate variable time frames for bony stabilization and fixation, as well as hemorrhage control by preperitoneal pelvic packing and/or angioembolization. Early institution of a multidisciplinary approach with the involvement of trauma surgeons, orthopedic surgeons, interventional radiologists, the director of the blood bank, and anesthesiologists is imperative due to high associated mortality rates (Fig. 7-68).

Evaluation in the ED focuses on identification of injuries mandating operative intervention (e.g., massive hemothorax, ruptured spleen) and injuries related to pelvic fracture that alter management (e.g., injuries to the iliac artery). Immediate temporary stabilization with sheeting of the pelvis or application of commercially available compression devices should be performed. If the patient's primary source of bleeding is the fracture-related hematoma, several options exist for hemorrhage control. Because 85% of bleeding due to pelvic

fractures is venous or bony in origin the authors advocate immediate external fixation and preperitoneal pelvic packing.[85] Anterior external fixation decreases pelvic volume, which promotes tamponade of venous bleeding and prevents secondary hemorrhage from the shifting of bony elements. Pelvic packing, in which six laparotomy pads (four in children) are placed directly into the paravesical space through a small suprapubic incision, provides tamponade for the bleeding (Fig. 7-69). Pelvic packing also eliminates the often difficult decision by the trauma surgeon: OR vs. Interventional Radiology? All patients can be rapidly transported to the OR and packing can be accomplished in under 30 minutes. In the authors' experience, this results in hemodynamic stability and abrupt cessation of the need for ongoing blood transfusion in the majority of cases. Patients also can undergo additional procedures such as laparotomy, thoracotomy, external fixation of extremity fractures, open fracture débridement, or craniotomy. Currently, angiography is reserved for patients with evidence of ongoing pelvic bleeding after admission to the SICU. Patients undergo standard posttrauma resuscitative SICU care, and the pelvic packs are removed within 48 hours, a time frame chosen empirically based on the authors' experience with liver packing. The authors elect to repack the patient's pelvis if there is persistent oozing and perform serial washouts of the preperitoneal space if it appears infected.

Another clinical challenge is the open pelvic fracture. In many instances the wounds are located in the perineum, and the risk of pelvic sepsis and osteomyelitis is high. To reduce the risk of infection, performance of a diverting sigmoid colostomy is recommended. The pelvic wound is manually débrided and then irrigated daily with a high-pressure pulsatile irrigation system until granulation tissue covers the wound. The wound is then left to heal by secondary intention with a wound VAC device.

Extremity Fractures, Vascular Injuries, and Compartment Syndromes

Patients with injured extremities often require a multidisciplinary approach with involvement of trauma, orthopedic, and plastic surgeons to address vascular injuries, fractures, soft tissues injuries, and compartment syndromes. Immediate stabilization of fractures or unstable joints is done in the ED using Hare traction, knee immobilizers, or plaster splints. In patients with open fractures the wound should be covered with povidone iodine (Betadine)–soaked gauze and antibiotics administered. Options for fracture fixation include external fixation or open reduction and internal fixation with plates or intramedullary nails. Vascular injuries, either isolated or in combination with fractures, require emergent repair. Common combined injuries include clavicle/first rib fractures and subclavian artery injuries, dislocated shoulder/proximal humeral fractures and axillary artery injuries, supracondylar fractures/elbow dislocations and brachial artery injuries, femur fracture and superficial femoral artery injuries, and knee dislocation and popliteal vessel injuries. On-table angiography in the OR facilitates rapid intervention and is warranted in patients with evidence of limb threat at ED arrival. Arterial access for on-table lower extremity angiography can be obtained percutaneously at the femoral vessels with a standard arterial catheter, via femoral vessel exposure and direct cannulation, or with superficial femoral artery (SFA) exposure just above the medial knee. Controversy exists regarding which should be done first, fracture fixation or arterial repair. The authors prefer placement of temporary intravascular shunts with arterial occlusions to minimize ischemia during fracture treatment, with definitive vascular repair following. Rarely, immediate amputation may be considered due to the severity of orthopedic and neurovascular injuries. This is particularly true if primary nerve transection is present in addition to fracture and arterial injury.[86] Collaborative decision making by the trauma, orthopedic, and plastic/reconstructive team is encouraged.

Operative intervention for vascular injuries should follow standard principles of repair (see "Vascular Repair Techniques"). For subclavian or axillary artery repairs, 6-mm PTFE graft and RSVG are

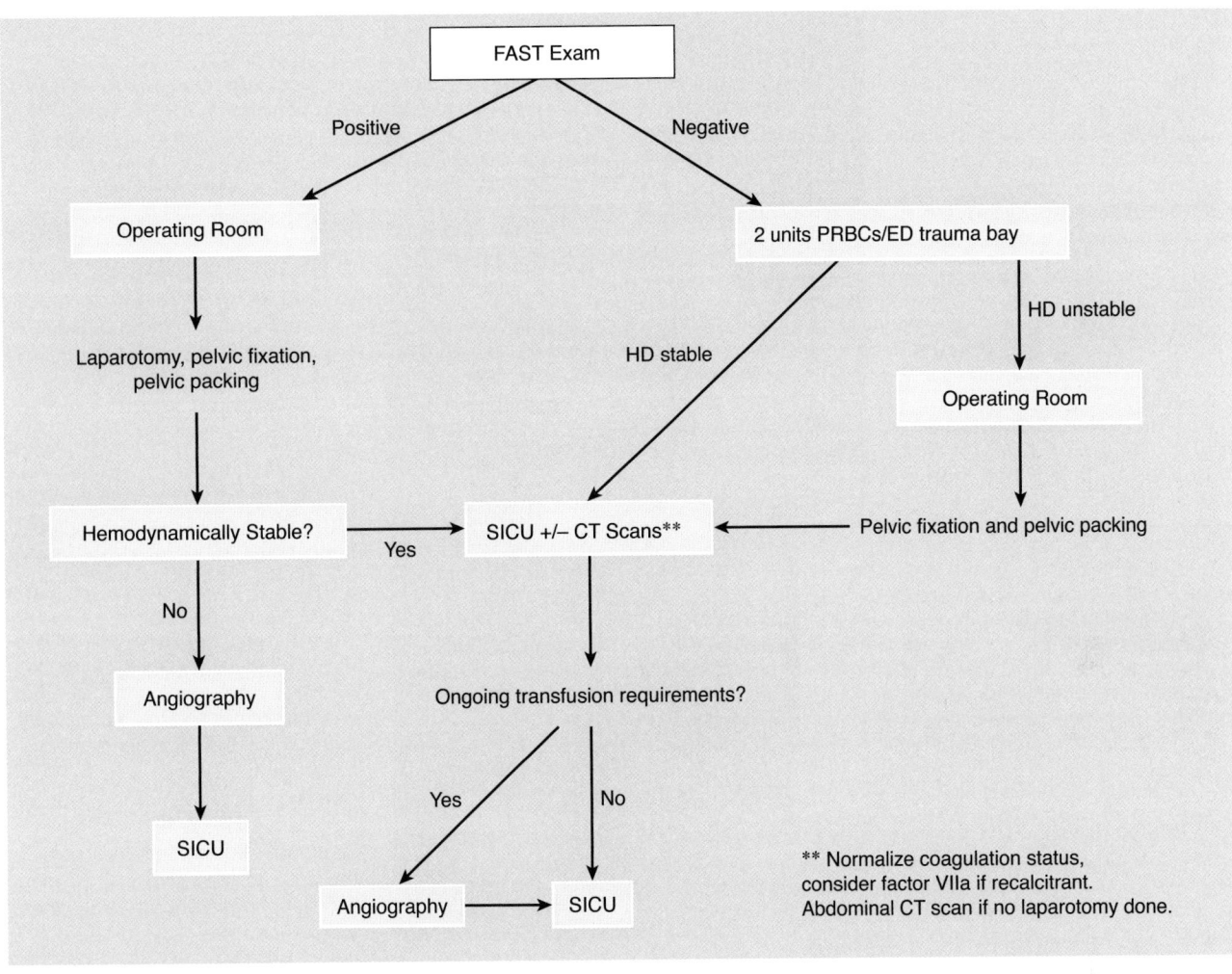

FIG. 7-68. Management algorithm for patients with pelvic fractures with hemodynamic instability. CT = computed tomography; ED = emergency department; FAST = focused abdominal sonography for trauma; HD = hemodynamic; PLT = platelets; PRBCs = packed red blood cells; SICU = surgical intensive care unit.

used. Because associated injuries of the brachial plexus are common, a thorough neurologic examination of the extremity is mandated before operative intervention. Operative approach for a brachial artery injury is via a medial upper extremity longitudinal incision; proximal control may be obtained at the axillary artery, and an S-shaped extension through the antecubital fossa provides access to the distal brachial artery. The injured vessel segment is excised, and an end-to-end interposition RSVG graft is performed. Upper extremity fasciotomy is rarely required unless the patient manifests preoperative neurologic changes or diminished pulse upon revascularization, or the time to operative intervention is extended. For SFA injuries, external fixation of the femur typically is performed, followed by end-to-end RSVG of the injured SFA segment. Close monitoring for calf compartment syndrome is mandatory. Preferred access to the popliteal space for an acute injury is the medial one-incision approach with detachment of the semitendinosus, semimembranosus, and gracilis muscles (Fig. 7-70). Another option is a medial approach with two incisions using a longer RSVG, but this requires interval ligation of the popliteal artery and geniculate branches. Rarely, with open wounds a straight posterior approach with an S-shaped incision can be used. If the patient has an associated popliteal vein injury, this should be repaired first with a PTFE interposition graft while the artery is shunted. For an isolated popliteal artery injury, RSVG is performed with an end-to-end anastomosis. Compartment syndrome is common, and presumptive four-compartment fasciotomies are warranted in patients with combined arterial and venous injury. Once the vessel is repaired and restoration of arterial flow

documented, completion angiography should be done in the OR if there is no palpable distal pulse. Vasoparalysis with verapamil, nitroglycerin, and papaverine may be used to treat vasoconstriction (Table 7-11).

Compartment syndromes, which can occur anywhere in the extremities, involve an acute increase in pressure inside a closed space, which impairs blood flow to the structures within. Causes of compartment syndrome include arterial hemorrhage into a compartment, venous ligation or thrombosis, crush injuries, and ischemia and reperfusion. In conscious patients, pain is the prominent symptom, and active or passive motion of muscles in the involved compartment increases the pain. Paresthesias may also be described. In the lower extremity, numbness between the first and second toes is the hallmark of early compartment syndrome in the exquisitely sensitive anterior compartment and its enveloped deep peroneal nerve. Progression to paralysis can occur, and loss of pulses is a late sign. In comatose or obtunded patients, the diagnosis is more difficult to secure. In patients with a compatible history and a tense extremity, compartment pressures should be measured with a hand-held Stryker device. Fasciotomy is indicated in patients with a gradient of <35 mmHg (gradient = diastolic pressure – compartment pressure), ischemic periods of >6 hours, or combined arterial and venous injuries. The lower extremity is most frequently involved, and compartment release is performed using a two-incision, four-compartment fasciotomy (Fig. 7-71). Of note, the soleus muscle must be detached from the tibia to decompress the deep flexor compartment.

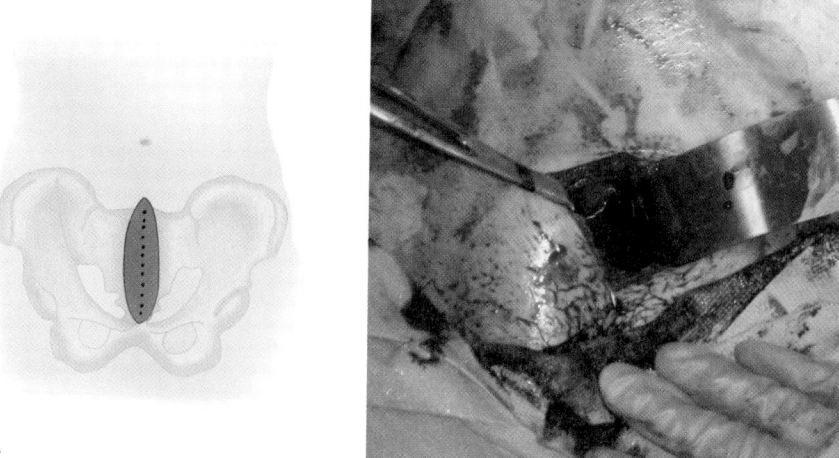

A

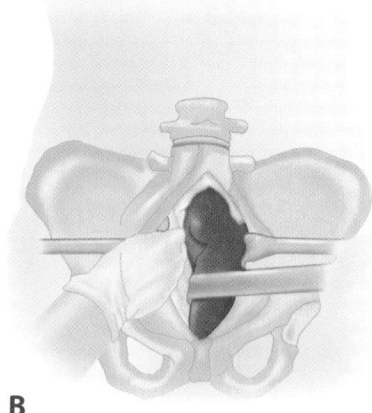

B

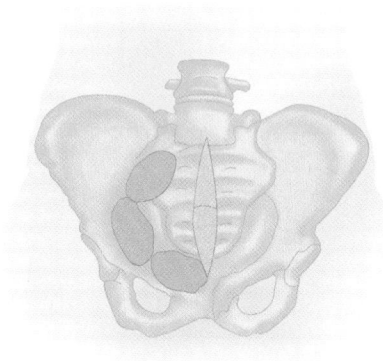

C

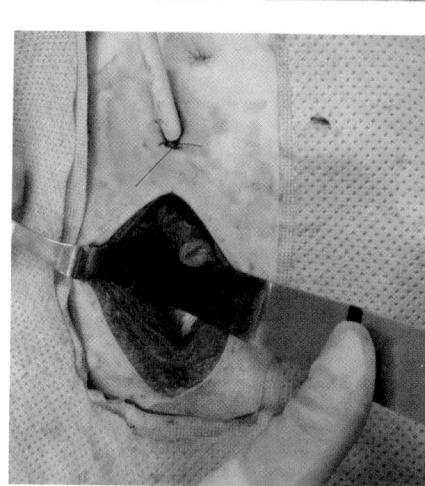

FIG. 7-69. A. Pelvic packing is performed through a 6- to 8-cm midline incision made from the pubic symphysis cephalad, with division of the midline fascia. **B.** The pelvic hematoma often dissects the preperitoneal and paravesical space down to the presacral region, which facilitates packing; alternatively, blunt digital dissection opens the preperitoneal space for packing. **C.** Three standard surgical laparotomy pads are placed on each side of the bladder, deep within the preperitoneal space; the fascia is closed with an O polydioxanone monofilament suture and the skin with staples.

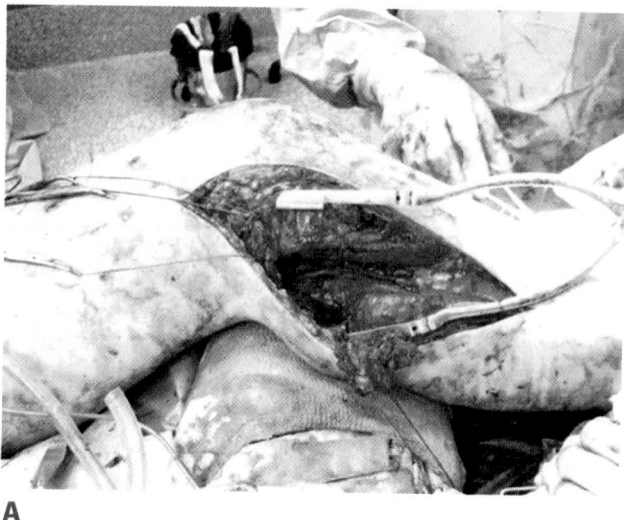

A

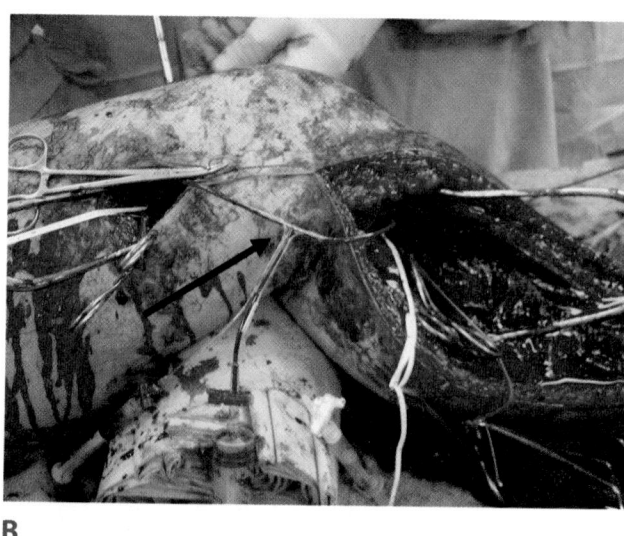

B

FIG. 7-70. A. The popliteal space is commonly accessed using a single medial incision (the detached semitendinosus, semimembranosus, and gracilis muscles are identified by different suture types). **B.** Alternatively, a medial approach with two incisions may be used. Insertion of a Pruitt-Inahara shunt (*arrow*) provides temporary restoration of blood flow, which prevents ischemia during fracture treatment.

TABLE 7-11 Arterial vasospasm treatment guideline

Step 1: Intra-arterial alteplase (tissue plasminogen activator) 5 mg/20 mL bolus
    If spasm continues, proceed to step 2.
Step 2: Intra-arterial nitroglycerin 200 *μ*g/20 mL bolus
    Repeat same dose once as needed.
        If spasm continues, proceed to step 3.
Step 3: Inter-arterial verapamil 10 mg/10 mL bolus
        If spasm continues, proceed to step 4.
Step 4: Inter-arterial papaverine drip 60 mg/50 mL given over 15 min

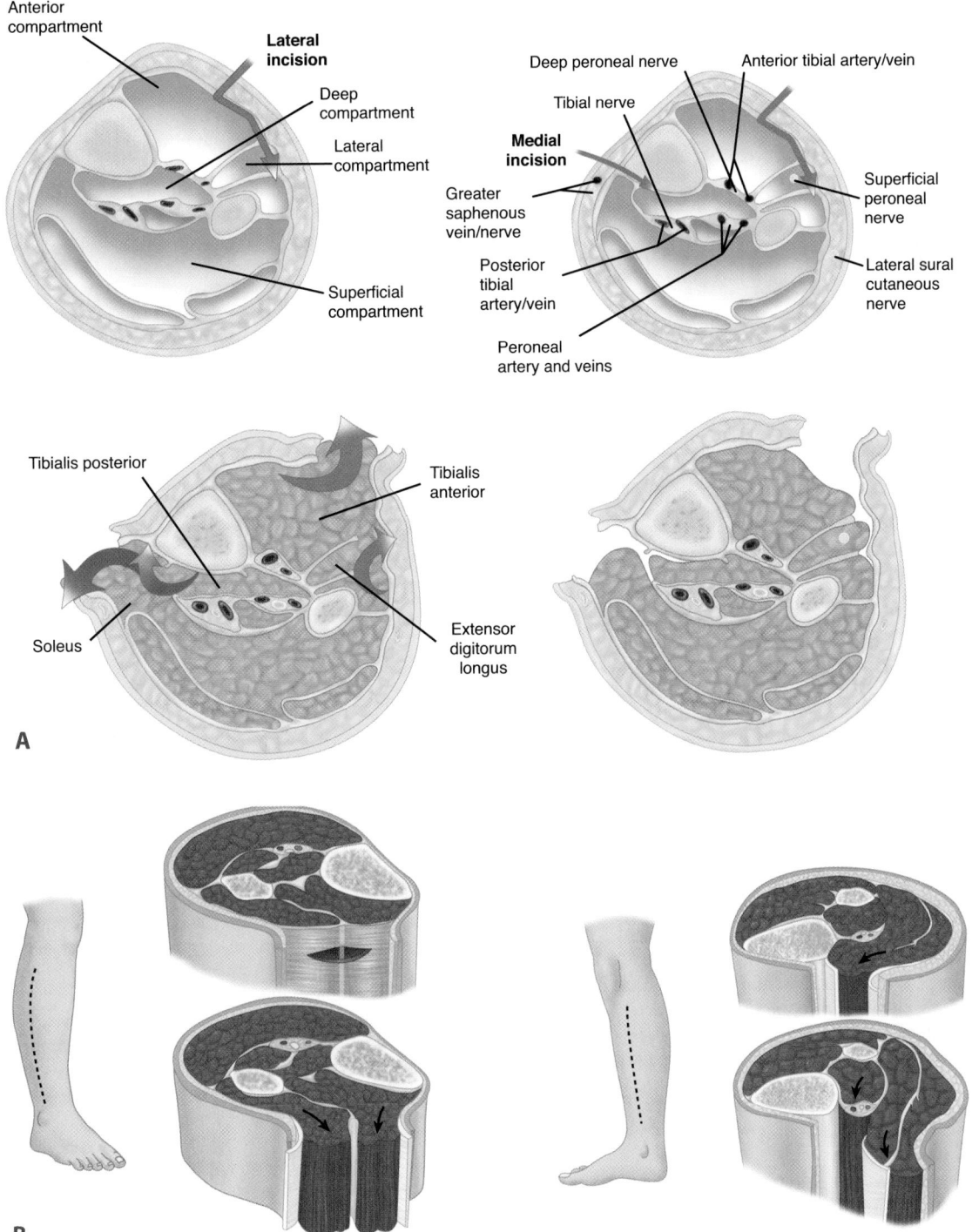

FIG. 7-71. A. The anterior and lateral compartments are approached from a lateral incision, with identification of the fascial raphe between the two compartments. Care must be taken to avoid the superficial peroneal nerve running along the raphe. **B.** To decompress the deep flexor compartment, which contains the tibial nerve and two of the three arteries to the foot, the soleus muscle must be detached from the tibia.

INTENSIVE CARE UNIT MANAGEMENT AND POSTOPERATIVE CONSIDERATIONS

Postinjury Resuscitation

ICU management of the trauma patient, either with direct admission from the ED or after emergent operative intervention, is considered in distinct phases, because there are differing goals and priorities. The period of acute resuscitation, typically lasting for the first 12 to 24 hours after injury, combines several key principles: optimizing tissue perfusion, ensuring normothermia, and restoring coagulation. There are a multitude of management algorithms aimed at accomplishing these goals, the majority of which involve goal-directed resuscitation with initial volume loading to attain adequate preload, followed by judicious use of inotropic agents or vasopressors.[87] Although the optimal hemoglobin level remains debated, during shock resuscitation a hemoglobin level of >10 g/dL is generally accepted to optimize oxygen delivery. After the first 24 hours of resuscitation, a more judicious transfusion trigger of a hemoglobin level of <7 g/dL in the euvolemic patient limits the adverse inflammatory effects of stored RBCs. The resuscitation of the severely injured trauma patient may require what appears to be an inordinate amount of crystalloid resuscitation. Infusion volumes of 10 L during the initial 6 to 12 hours may be required to attain an adequate preload. Although early colloid administration is appealing, evidence to date does not support this concept. In fact, optimizing crystalloid administration is a challenging aspect of early care (i.e., balancing cardiac performance against generation of an abdominal compartment syndrome and generalized tissue edema).

Invasive monitoring with pulmonary artery catheters is controversial but may be a critical adjunct in patients with multiple injuries who require advanced inotropic support. Not only do such devices allow minute-to-minute monitoring of the patient, but the added information on the patient's volume status, cardiac function, peripheral vascular tone, and metabolic response to injury permits appropriate therapeutic intervention. With added information on the patient's cardiac function, cardiac indices and oxygen delivery become important variables in the ongoing ICU management. Resuscitation to values of >500 mL/min per square meter for the oxygen delivery index and >3.8 L/min per square meter for the cardiac index are the goals. Pulmonary artery catheters also enable the physician to monitor response to vasoactive agents. Although norepinephrine is the agent of choice for patients with low systemic vascular resistance who are unable to maintain a mean arterial pressure of >60 mmHg, patients may have an element of myocardial dysfunction requiring inotropic support. The role of relative adrenal insufficiency is another controversial area.

Optimal early resuscitation is mandatory and determines when the patient can undergo definitive diagnosis as well as when the patient can be returned to the OR after initial damage control surgery. Specific goals of resuscitation before repeated "semielective" transport include a core temperature of >35°C (95°F), base deficit of <6 mmol/L, and normal coagulation indices. Although correction of metabolic acidosis is desirable, how quickly this should be accomplished requires careful consideration. Adverse sequelae of excessive crystalloid resuscitation include increased intracranial pressure, worsening pulmonary edema, and intra-abdominal visceral and retroperitoneal edema resulting in secondary abdominal compartment syndrome. Therefore, it should be the overall trend of the resuscitation rather than a rapid reduction of the base deficit that is the goal. Exogenous bicarbonate, occasionally given to improve cardiovascular function and response to vasoactive agents if the serum pH is below 7.2, obfuscates the base deficit trending, and lactate level is a more reliable indicator of adequate perfusion after the first 12 hours.

Abdominal Compartment Syndrome

Abdominal compartment syndrome is classified as intra-abdominal hypertension due to intra-abdominal injury (primary) or splanchnic reperfusion after massive resuscitation (secondary). Secondary ab-

TABLE 7-12	Abdominal compartment syndrome grading system	
	Bladder Pressure	
Grade	mmHg	cm H$_2$O
I	10–15	13–20
II	16–25	21–35
III	26–35	36–47
IV	>35	>48

dominal compartment syndrome may result from any condition requiring extensive crystalloid resuscitation, including extremity trauma, chest trauma, or even postinjury sepsis. The sources of increased intra-abdominal pressure include gut edema, ascites, bleeding, and packs, among others. A diagnosis of intra-abdominal hypertension cannot reliably be made by physical examination; therefore, it is obtained by measuring the intraperitoneal pressure. The most common technique is to measure a patient's bladder pressure. Fifty milliliters of saline is instilled into the bladder via the aspiration port of the Foley catheter with the drainage tube clamped, and a three-way stopcock and water manometer is placed at the level of the pubic symphysis. Bladder pressure is then measured on the manometer in centimeters of water (Table 7-12) and correlated with the physiologic impact of abdominal compartment syndrome. Conditions in which the bladder pressure is unreliable include bladder rupture, external compression from pelvic packing, neurogenic bladder, and adhesive disease.

Increased abdominal pressure affects multiple organ systems (Fig. 7-72). Abdominal compartment syndrome, as noted earlier, is defined as intra-abdominal hypertension and frequently manifests via such end-organ sequelae as decreased urine output, increased pulmonary inspiratory pressures, decreased cardiac preload, and increased cardiac afterload. Because any of these clinical symptoms of abdominal compartment syndrome may be attributed to the primary injury, a heightened awareness of this syndrome must be maintained. Organ failure can occur over a wide range of recorded bladder pressures. Generally, no specific bladder pressure prompts therapeutic intervention, except when the pressure is >35 mmHg. Rather, emergent decompression is carried out when intra-abdominal hypertension reaches a level at which end-organ dysfunction occurs. Mortality is directly affected by decompression, with 60% mortality in patients undergoing presumptive decompression, 70% mortality in patients with a delay in decompression, and nearly uniform mortality in those not undergoing decompression. Decompression is performed operatively either in the ICU if the patient is hemodynamically unstable or in the OR. ICU bedside laparotomy is easily accomplished, avoids transport of hemodynamically compromised patients, and requires minimal equipment (e.g., scalpel, suction device, cautery, and dressings for temporary abdominal closure). In patients with significant intra-abdominal fluid as the primary component of abdominal compartment syndrome, rather than bowel or retroperitoneal edema, decompression may be accomplished effectively via a percutaneous drain. This method is particularly applicable for nonoperative management of major liver injuries. These patients are identified by bedside ultrasound, and the morbidity of a laparotomy is avoided. When operative decompression is required with egress of the abdominal contents, temporary coverage is obtained using a subfascial 45 × 60 cm sterile drape and Ioban application (see Fig. 7-50).

The performance of damage control surgery and recognition of abdominal compartment syndrome have dramatically improved patient survival, but at the cost of an open abdomen. Several management points deserve attention. Despite having a widely open abdomen, patients can develop recurrent abdominal compartment syndrome, which increases their morbidity and mortality; therefore, bladder pressure should be monitored every 4 hours, with significant

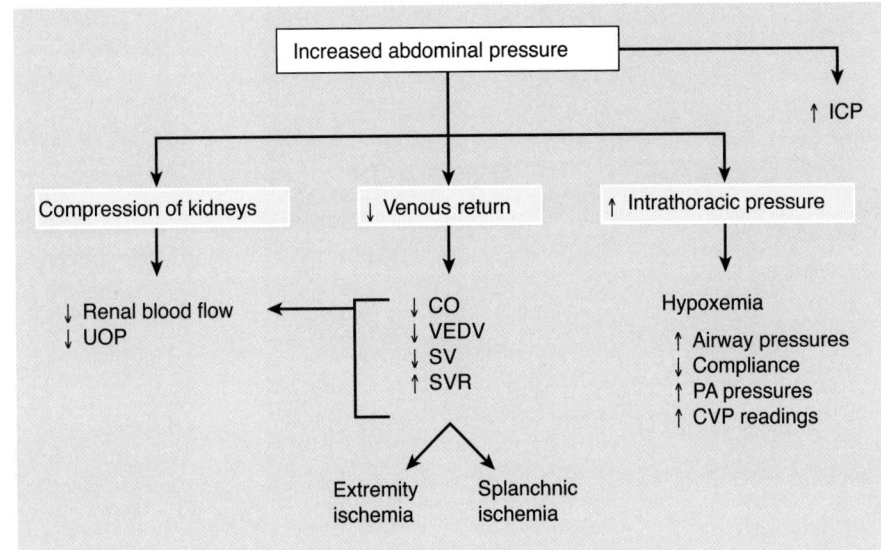

FIG. 7-72. Abdominal compartment syndrome is defined by the end organ sequelae of intra-abdominal hypertension. CO = cardiac output; CVP = central venous pressure; ICP = intracranial pressure; PA = pulmonary artery; SV = stroke volume; SVR = systemic vascular resistance; UOP = urine output; VEDV = ventricular end diastolic volume.

increases in pressures alerting the clinician to the possible need for repeat operative decompression. Patients with an open abdomen lose between 500 and 2500 mL per day of abdominal effluent. Appropriate volume compensation for this albumin-rich fluid remains controversial, with regard to both the amount administered (replacement based on clinical indices vs. routine $1/2$ mL replacement for every milliliter lost) as well as the type of replacement (crystalloid vs. colloid/blood products).

Following resuscitation and management of specific injuries, the goal of the operative team is to close the abdomen as quickly as possible. Multiple techniques have been introduced to obtain fascial closure of the open abdomen to minimize morbidity and cost of care. Historically, for patients who could not be closed at repeat operation, approximation of the fascia with mesh (prosthetic or biologic) was used, with planned reoperation. Another option was split-thickness

skin grafts applied directly to the exposed bowel for coverage; removal of the skin grafts was planned 9 to 12 months after the initial surgery, with definitive repair of the hernia by component separation. However, delayed abdominal wall reconstruction was resource invasive, with considerable patient morbidity. The advent of VAC technology has revolutionized fascial closure. The authors currently use a sequential closure technique with the wound VAC device that provides constant fascial tension and return to the OR every 48 hours until closure is complete (Fig. 7-73). The authors' success rate with this approach exceeds 95%. Among patients not attaining fascial closure, 20% suffer GI tract complications that prolong their hospital course. These include intra-abdominal abscess, enteric fistula, and bowel perforations (Fig. 7-74). Management includes operative or percutaneous drainage of abscesses, control of fistulas, and nutritional support for bowel complications.

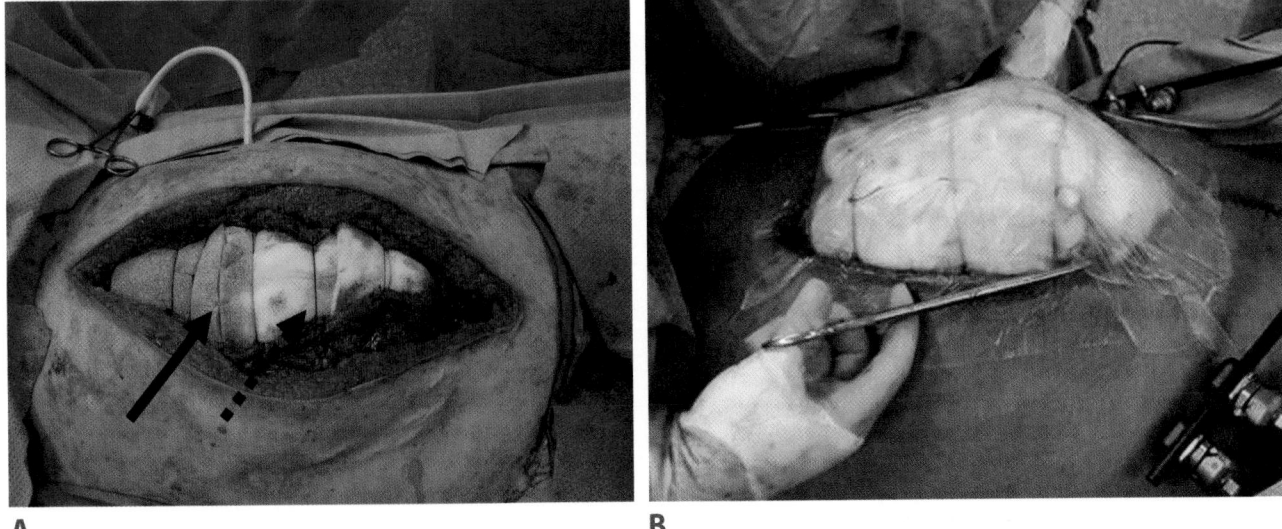

A   **B**

FIG. 7-73. The authors' sequential closure technique for the open abdomen. **A.** Multiple white sponges (*solid arrow*), stapled together, are placed on top of the bowel underneath the fascia. Interrupted No. 1 polydioxanone sutures are placed approximately 5 cm apart (*dashed arrow*), which puts the fascia under moderate tension over the white sponge. **B.** After the sticky clear plastic vacuum-assisted closure (VAC) dressing is placed over the white sponges and adjacent 5 cm of skin, the central portion is removed by cutting along the wound edges. (*Continued*)

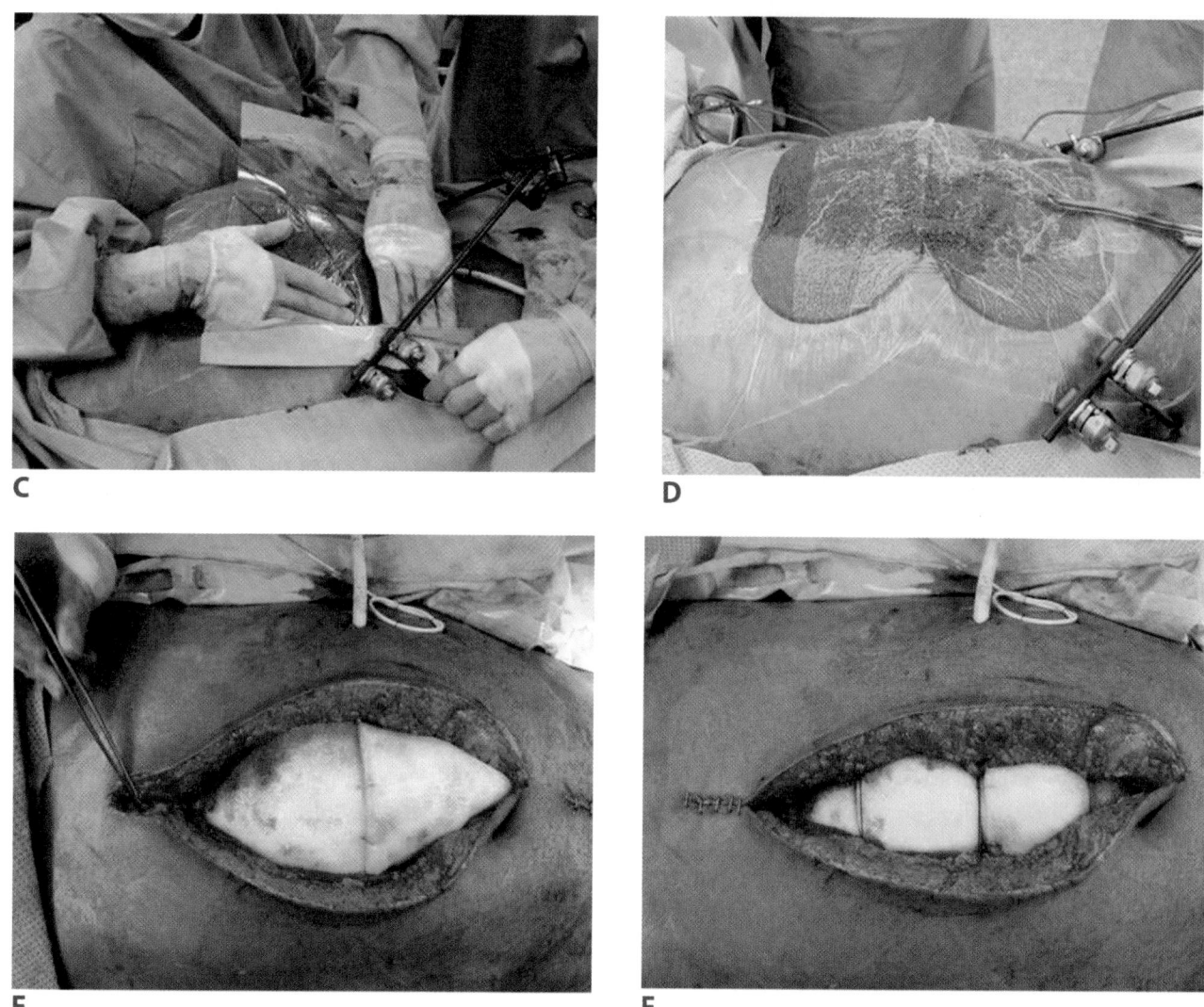

FIG. 7-73. (*Continued*) **C** and **D.** Black VAC sponges are placed on top of the white sponges and plastic-protected skin with standard occlusive dressing and suction. **E.** On return to the operating room (OR) 48 hours later, fascial sutures are placed from both the superior and inferior directions until tension precludes further closure; skin is closed over the fascial closure with skin staples. **F.** White sponges (fewer in number) are again applied and fascial retention sutures are placed with planned return to the OR in 48 hours.

SPECIAL TRAUMA POPULATIONS

Pregnant Patients

Seven percent of women are injured during their pregnancy. Motor vehicle collisions and falls are the leading causes of injury, accounting for 70% of cases. Fetal death after trauma most frequently occurs after motor vehicle collisions, but only 11% of fetal deaths are due to the death of the mother; therefore, early trauma resuscitation and management is directed not only at the mother but also at the fetus. Domestic violence is also common, affecting between 10 and 30% of pregnant women and resulting in fetal mortality of 5%.

Pregnancy results in physiologic changes that may impact postinjury evaluation (Table 7-13). Heart rate increases by 10 to 15 beats per minute during the first trimester and remains elevated until delivery. Blood pressure diminishes during the first two trimesters due to a decrease in systemic vascular resistance and rises again slightly during the third trimester (mean values: first = 105/60, second = 102/55, third = 108/67). Intravascular volume is increased by up to 8 L, which results in a relative anemia but also a relative hypervolemia. Consequently a pregnant woman may lose 35% of her blood volume before exhibiting signs of shock. Pregnant patients have an increase in tidal volume and minute ventilation but a decreased functional residual capacity; this results in a diminished PCO_2 reading and respiratory alkalosis. Also, pregnant patients may desaturate more rapidly, particularly in the supine position and during intubation. Supplemental oxygen is always warranted in the trauma patient but is particularly critical in the injured pregnant patient, because the oxygen dissociation curve is shifted to the left for the fetus compared to the mother (i.e., small changes in maternal oxygenation result in larger changes for the fetus because the fetus is operating in the steep portions of the dissociation curve). Anatomic changes contribute to these pulmonary functional alterations and are relevant in terms of procedures. With the gravid uterus enlarged, diagnostic peritoneal lavage (DPL) should be performed in a supraumbilical site with the catheter directed cephalad. In addition, the upward pressure on the diaphragm calls for caution when placing a thoracostomy tube; standard positioning may result in an intra-abdominal location or perforation of the diaphragm.

Other physiologic changes during pregnancy affect the GI, renal, and hematologic systems. The lower esophageal sphincter has decreased competency, which increases the risk for aspiration. Liver function test values increase, with the alkaline phosphatase level nearly doubling. The high levels of progesterone impair gallbladder contractions, which results in bile stasis and an increased incidence of gallstone formation; this may not affect the trauma bay evaluation

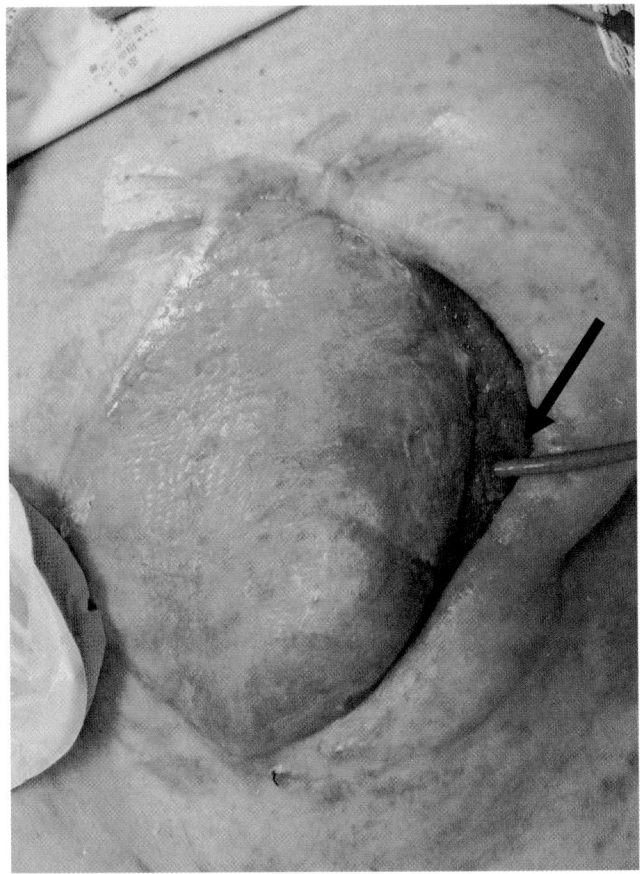

A

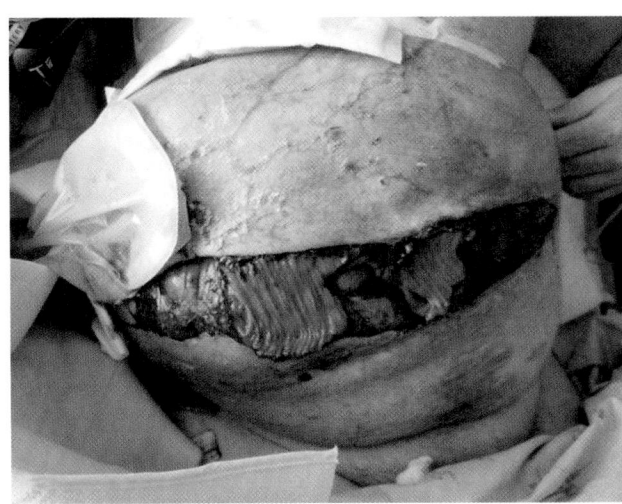

B

FIG. 7-74. Complications after split-thickness skin graft closure of the abdomen include enterocutaneous fistulas (intubated here with a red rubber catheter) (**A**; *arrow*) and rupture of the graft with exposure of the bowel mucosa (**B**).

but becomes important in a prolonged ICU stay. Plasma albumin level decreases from a normal of around 4.3 g/dL to an average of 3.0 g/dL. Renal blood flow increases by 30% during pregnancy, which causes a decrease in serum level of blood urea nitrogen and creatinine. The uterus may also compress the ureters and bladder, causing

TABLE 7-13	Physiologic effects of pregnancy

Cardiovascular
    Increase in heart rate by 10–15 bpm
    Decreased systemic vascular resistance resulting in:
        (a) Increased intravascular volume
        (b) Decreased blood pressure during the first two trimesters
Pulmonary
    Elevated diaphragm
    Increased tidal volume
    Increased minute ventilation
    Decreased functional residual capacity
Hematopoietic
    Relative anemia
    Leukocytosis
    Hypercoagulability
        (a) Increased levels of factors VII, VIII, IX, X, XII
        (b) Decreased fibrinolytic activity
Other
    Decreased competency of lower esophageal sphincter
    Increased enzyme levels on liver function tests
    Impaired gallbladder contractions
    Decreased plasma albumin level
    Decreased blood urea nitrogen and creatinine levels
    Hydronephrosis and hydroureter

hydronephrosis and hydroureter. Finally, as noted earlier there is a relative anemia during pregnancy, but a hemoglobin level of <11 g/dL is considered abnormal. Additional hematologic changes include a moderate leukocytosis (up to 20,000 mm³) and a relative hypercoagulable state due to increased levels of factors VII, VIII, IX, X, and XII and decreased fibrinolytic activity.

During evaluation in the ED, the primary and secondary surveys commence, with mindfulness that the mother always receives priority while conditions are still optimized for the fetus. This management includes provision of supplemental oxygen (to prevent maternal and fetal hypoxia), aggressive fluid resuscitation (the hypervolemia of pregnancy may mask signs of shock), and placement of the patient in the left lateral decubitus position (or tilting of the backboard to the left) to avoid caval compression. Assessment of the fetal heart rate is the most valuable information regarding fetal viability. Fetal monitoring should be performed with a cardiotocographic device that measures both contractions and fetal heart tones (FHTs). Because change in heart rate is the primary response of the fetus to hypoxia or hypotension, anything above an FHT of 160 is a cause for concern, whereas bradycardia (FHT of <120) is considered fetal distress. Ideally, if possible, a member of the obstetrics team will be present during initial evaluation to perform a pelvic examination using a sterile speculum. Vaginal bleeding can signal early cervical dilation and labor, abruptio placentae, or placenta previa. Amniotic sac rupture can result in prolapse of the umbilical cord with fetal compromise. Strong contractions are associated with true labor and should prompt consideration of delivery and resuscitation of the neonate. Focused prenatal history taking should elicit a history of pregnancy-induced hypertension, gestational diabetes, congenital heart disease, preterm labor, or placental abnormalities. Asking the patient when the baby first moved and if she is currently experiencing movement of the fetus is important. Determining fetal age is important for considerations of viability. Gestational age may be estimated by noting fundal height, with the fundus approximating the umbilicus at 20 weeks and the costal margin at 40 weeks. Discrepancy in dates and size may be due to uterine rupture or hemorrhage.

Initial evaluation for abdominopelvic trauma in pregnant patients should proceed in the standard manner. Ultrasound (FAST) of the abdomen should evaluate the four windows (pericardial, right and left upper quadrant, and bladder) and additionally assess FHTs, fetal movement, and sufficiency of amniotic fluid. DPL can be performed in pregnant women via a supraumbilical, open technique. Trauma radiography of pregnant patients presents a conundrum. Radiation damage has three distinct phases of damage and effect: preimplantation, during the period of organogenesis from 3 to 16 weeks, and after 16 weeks. Generally, it is accepted that "safe" doses of radiation from radiography are <5 rad.[88] A chest radiograph results in a dose of 0.07 mrad; CT scan of the chest, <1 rad; and CT scan of the abdomen, 3.5 rad. It is important, therefore, to limit radiographs to those that are essential and to shield the pelvis with a lead apron when possible. If clinically warranted, however, a radiograph should be obtained.

The vast majority of injuries are treated similarly whether the patient is pregnant or not. Following standard protocols for nonoperative management of blunt trauma avoids the risks associated with general anesthesia. A particular challenge in the pregnant trauma patient is a major pelvic fracture. Because uterine and retroperitoneal veins may dilate to 60 times their original size, hemorrhage from these vessels may be torrential. Fetal loss may be related to both maternal shock and direct injury to the uterus or fetal head. Penetrating injuries in this patient population also carry a high risk. The gravid uterus is a large target, and any penetrating injury to the abdomen may result in fetal injury depending on trajectory and uterine size. Gunshot wounds to the abdomen are associated with a 70% injury rate to the uterus and 35% mortality rate of the fetus. If the bullet traverses the uterus and the fetus is viable, cesarean section should be performed. On the other hand, stab wounds do not often penetrate the thick wall of the uterus. Indications for emergent cesarean section include (a) severe maternal shock or impending death (if the fetus is delivered within 5 minutes, survival is estimated at 70%), (b) uterine injury or significant fetal distress (anticipated survival rates of >70% if FHTs are present and fetal gestational age is >28 weeks).[89]

Any patient with a viable pregnancy should be monitored after trauma, with the length of monitoring determined by the injury mechanism and patient physiology. Patients who are symptomatic, defined by the presence of uterine irritability or contractions, abdominal tenderness, vaginal bleeding, or blood pressure instability, should be monitored in the hospital for at least 24 hours. In addition, patients at high risk for fetal loss (those experiencing vehicle ejection or involved in motorcycle or pedestrian collisions and those with maternal tachycardia, Injury Severity Score of >9, gestational period of >35 weeks, or history of prior assault) also warrant careful monitoring.[90] Patients without these risk factors who are asymptomatic can be monitored for 6 hours in the ED and sent home if no problems develop. They should be counseled regarding warning signs that mandate prompt return to the ED.

Geriatric Patients

Elderly trauma patients (>65 years of age) are hospitalized twice as often as those in any other age group, and this population accounts for one quarter of all trauma admissions. Although the physiology of aging separates older trauma patients from the younger generation (Table 7-14), treatment must remain individualized (some octogenarians look and physiologically act 50 years old, whereas others appear closer to 100 years). No chronologic age is associated with a higher morbidity or mortality, but a patient's comorbidities do impact the individual's postinjury course and outcome. For example, recognition that a patient is taking beta blockers affects the physician's evaluation of vital signs in the ED and impacts treatment course in the ICU, particularly if managing the patient's reflex tachycardia. These patients have limited cardio/physiologic reserve;

TABLE 7-14	Physiologic effects of aging

Cardiovascular
  Increased prevalence of heart disease
  Fatty deposition in the myocardium, resulting in:
    (a) Progressive stiffening and loss of elasticity
    (b) Diminished stroke volume, systolic contraction, and diastolic relaxation
  Decrease in cardiac output of 0.5% per year
  Atherosclerotic disease that limits cardiac response to stress
  Increased risk of coronary ischemia
  Thickening and calcification of the cardiac valves, which results in valvular incompetence
Pulmonary
  Loss of compliance
  Progressive loss of alveolar size and surface area
  Air trapping and atelectasis
Intracranial
  Loss of cerebral volume, resulting in:
    (a) Increased risk of tearing of bridging veins with smaller injuries
    (b) Accumulation of a significant amount of blood before symptoms occur
  Senescence of the senses
Other
  Decline in creatinine clearance by 80–90%
  Osteoporosis, which causes a greater susceptibility to fractures

---

early monitoring of arterial blood gas values will identify occult shock. A base deficit of >6 mmol/L is associated with a twofold higher risk of mortality in patients over the age of 55 than in younger patients (67% vs. 30%).[91]

Although the published literature on geriatric traumatic brain injury is relatively sparse and uncontrolled with regard to management, some interesting points are noted. First, outcomes are worse in this age group than in their younger counterparts. Based on data from the Traumatic Coma Databank, mortality in patients with severe head injury more than doubles after the age of 55. Moreover, 25% of patients with a normal GCS score of 15 had intracranial bleeding, with an associated mortality of 50%.[92] Just as there is no absolute age that predicts outcome, admission GCS score is a poor predictor of individual outcome. Therefore, the majority of trauma centers advocate an initial aggressive approach with re-evaluation at the 72-hour mark to determine subsequent care.

One of the most common sequelae of blunt thoracic trauma is rib fractures. In the aging population, perhaps due to osteoporosis, less force is required to cause a fracture. In fact, in one study, 50% of patients >65 years old sustained rib fractures from a fall of <6 ft, compared with only 1% of patients <65 years of age. Concurrent pulmonary contusion is noted in up to 35% of patients, and pneumonia complicates the injuries in 10 to 30% of patients with rib fractures, not surprisingly leading to longer ICU stays.[93,94] Additionally, mortality increases linearly with the number of rib fractures. Patients who sustain more than six rib fractures have pulmonary morbidity rates of >50% and overall mortality rates of >20%.

Chronologic age is not the best predictor of outcome, but the presence of pre-existing conditions, which affect a patient's physiologic age, is associated with increased mortality rates.[95,96] Injury Severity Score is probably the best overall predictor of patient outcome in the elderly[97]; however, for any given individual its sensitivity may not be precise, and there is a time delay in obtaining sufficient information to calculate the final score. In addition to pre-existing conditions and severity of injury, the occurrence of complications compounds the risk for mortality.

Pediatric Patients

Twenty million children, or almost one in four children, are injured each year, with an associated cost of treating the injured child of $16 billion per year. Injury is the leading cause of death among children over the age of 1 year, with 15,000 to 25,000 pediatric deaths per year. Disability after traumatic injury is more devastating, with rates 3 to 10 times that of the death rate. Pediatric trauma involves different mechanisms, different constellations of injury, and the potential for long-term problems related to growth and development. As with adult trauma, over 85% of pediatric trauma has a blunt mechanism, with boys injured twice as often as girls.[98] Falls are the most common cause of injury in infants and toddlers. In children, bicycle mishaps are the most common cause of severe injury, whereas motor vehicle–related injury predominates in adolescence. Although unintentional injuries are by far the most common type of injuries in childhood, the number of intentional injuries, such as firearm-related injury and child abuse, is increasing.

ED preparation for the pediatric trauma patient includes assembling age-appropriate equipment (e.g., intubation equipment; IV catheters, including intraosseous needles and 4F single-lumen lines), laying out the Broselow Pediatric Emergency Tape (which allows effective approximation of the patient's weight, medication doses, size of endotracheal tube, and chest tube size), and turning on heat lamps. Upon the pediatric patient's arrival, the basic tenets of the ABCs apply, with some caveats. In children, the airway is smaller and more cephalad in position compared with that of adults, and in children younger than 10 years, the larynx is funnel shaped rather than cylindrical as in adults. Additionally, the child's tongue is much larger in relation to the oropharynx. Therefore, a small amount of edema or obstruction can significantly reduce the diameter of the airway (thus increasing the work of breathing), and the tongue may posteriorly obstruct the airway, causing intubation to be difficult. During intubation, a Miller (straight) blade rather than a Macintosh (curved) blade may be more effective due to the acute angle of the cephalad, funnel-shaped larynx. Administration of atropine before rapid-sequence intubation will prevent bradycardia. Adequate ventilation is critical, because oxygen consumption in infants and young children is twice that in adults; onset of hypoxemia, followed by cardiac arrest, may be precipitous. Because gastric distension can inhibit adequate ventilation, placement of a nasogastric tube may facilitate effective gas exchange. Approximately one third of preventable deaths in children are related to airway management; therefore, if airway control cannot be obtained using a standard endotracheal method, surgical establishment of an airway should be considered. In children older than 11 years, standard cricothyroidotomy is performed. Due to the increased incidence of subglottic stenosis in younger patients, needle cricothyroidotomy with either a 14- or 16-gauge catheter is advocated, although it is rarely used. Alternatively, tracheostomy may be performed. In children, the standard physiologic response to hypovolemia is peripheral vasoconstriction and reflex tachycardia; this may mask significant hemorrhagic injury, because children can compensate for up to a 25% loss of circulating blood volume with minimal external signs. "Normal" values for vital signs should not necessarily make one feel more secure about the child's volume status. Volume restoration is based on the child's weight; two to three boluses of 20 mL/kg of crystalloid is appropriate.

After initial evaluation based on the trauma ABCs, identification and management of specific injuries proceeds. Acute traumatic brain injury is the most common cause of death and disability in any pediatric age group. Although falls are the most common mechanism overall, severe brain injury most often is due to child abuse (in children <2 years) or motor vehicle collisions (in those >2 years). Head CT should be performed to determine intracranial pathology, followed by skull radiography to diagnose skull fractures. As in adults, CPP is monitored, and appropriate resuscitation is critical to prevent the secondary insults of hypoxemia and hypovolemia. Although some data indicate that the pediatric brain recovers from traumatic injury better than the adult brain, this advantage may be eliminated if hypotension is allowed to occur.

As is true in adults, the vast majority of thoracic trauma is also blunt. However, because a child's skeleton is not completely calcified, it is more pliable. Significant internal organ damage may occur without overlying bony fractures. For example, adult patients with significant chest trauma have a 70% incidence of rib fractures, whereas only 40% of children with significant chest trauma do. Pneumothorax is treated similarly in the pediatric population; patients who are asymptomatic with a pneumothorax of <15% are admitted for observation, whereas those who have a pneumothorax of >15% or who require positive pressure ventilation undergo tube decompression. Presence of a hemothorax in this age group may be particularly problematic, because the child's chest may contain his or her entire blood volume. If the chest tube output is initially 20% of the patient's blood volume (80 mL/kg) or is persistently >1 to 2 mL/kg per hour, thoracotomy should be considered. Aortic injuries are rare in children, and tracheobronchial injuries are more amenable to nonoperative management. Thoracic injuries are second only to brain injuries as the main cause of death according to the National Pediatric Trauma Registry; however, the overall mortality rate of 15% correlates with the levels in many adult studies.

The evaluation for abdominal trauma in the pediatric patient is similar to that in the adult. FAST is valid in the pediatric age group to detect intra-abdominal fluid.[99] The mechanism of injury often correlates with specific injury patterns. A child sustaining a blow to the epigastrium (e.g., hitting the handlebars during a bike accident) should be evaluated for a duodenal hematoma and/or a pancreatic transection. After a motor vehicle collision in which the patient was wearing a passenger restraint, injuries comprising the "lap belt complex" or "seat belt syndrome" (i.e., abdominal wall contusion, small bowel perforation, flexion-distraction injury of the lumbar spine, diaphragm rupture, and occasionally abdominal aortic dissection) may exist. Nonoperative management of solid organ injuries, first used in children, is the current standard of care in the hemodynamically stable patient. If the patient shows clinical deterioration or hemodynamic lability, has a hollow viscus injury, or requires >40 mL/kg of packed RBCs, continued nonoperative management is not an option. Success rates of nonoperative management approach 95%, with an associated 10 to 23% transfusion rate. Blood transfusion rates are significantly lower in patients managed nonoperatively than in patients undergoing operation (13 vs. 44%).[100]

REFERENCES

Entries highlighted in bright blue are key references.

1. Minino AM, Heron MP, Murphy SL, et al: Deaths: Final data for 2004. *Natl Vital Stat Rep* 55, August 21, 2007. Available at *http://www.cdc.gov/nchs/data/nvsr/nvsr55/nvsr55_19.pdf* [accessed January 27, 2009].
2. National Center for Injury Prevention and Control: *CDC Injury Fact Book.* Atlanta: Centers for Disease Control and Prevention, November 2006. Available at *http://www.cdc.gov/ncipc/fact_book/InjuryBook2006.pdf* [accessed January 27, 2009].
3. Feliciano DV, Mattox KL, Moore EE (eds): *Trauma,* 6th ed. New York: McGraw-Hill, 2008.
4. Nathens AB, Jurkovich J, Maier RV, et al: Relationship between trauma center volume and outcomes. *JAMA* 285:1164, 2001.
5. Piontek FA, Coscia R, Marselle CS, et al: Impact of American College of Surgeons verification on trauma outcomes. *J Trauma* 54:1041, 2003.
6. American College of Surgeons: *Advanced Trauma Life Support,* 7th ed. Chicago: American College of Surgeons, 2004.
7. Xue FS, Zhang GH, Liu J, et al: The clinical assessment of GlideScope in orotracheal intubation under general anesthesia. *Minerva Anestesiol* 73:451, 2007.
8. Cothren CC, Moore EE: Emergency department thoracotomy for the critically injured patient: Objectives, indications, and outcomes. *World J Emerg Surg* 1:1, 2006.
9. Cohn SM, Nathens AB, Moore FA, et al: Tissue oxygen saturation predicts the development of organ dysfunction during traumatic shock resuscitation. *J Trauma* 62:44, 2007.

10. Biffl WL, Moore FA, Moore EE, et al: Cardiac enzymes are irrelevant in the patient with suspected myocardial contusion. *Am J Surg* 169:523, 1994.

11. Dolich MO, McKenney MG, Varela JE, et al: 2,576 ultrasounds for blunt abdominal trauma. *J Trauma* 50:108, 2001.

12. Sondeen JL, Coppes VG, Holcomb JB: Blood pressure at which rebleeding occurs after resuscitation in swine with aortic injury. *J Trauma* 54(Suppl):S110, 2003.

13. Brain Trauma Foundation, American Association of Neurological Surgeons, Congress of Neurological Surgeons: Guidelines for the management of severe traumatic brain injury. *J Neurotrauma* 24(Suppl):S1, 2007.

14. Ryb GE, Dischinger PC, Kufera JA, et al: Delta V, principal direction of force, and restraint use contributions to motor vehicle crash mortality. *J Trauma* 63:1000, 2007.

15. Diaz JJ Jr., Aulino JM, Collier B, et al: The early work-up for isolated ligamentous injury of the cervical spine: Does computed tomography scan have a role? *J Trauma* 59:897, 2005.

16. Biffl WL, Moore EE, Rehse DH, et al: Selective management of penetrating neck trauma based on cervical level of injury. *Am J Surg* 174:678, 1997.

17. Sekharan J, Dennis JW, Veldenz HC, et al: Continued experience with physical examination alone for evaluation and management of penetrating zone 2 neck injuries: Results of 145 cases. *J Vasc Surg* 32:483, 2000.

18. Inaba K, Munera F, McKenney M, et al: Prospective evaluation of screening multislice helical computed tomographic angiography in the initial evaluation of penetrating neck injuries. *J Trauma* 61:144, 2006.

19. Fabian TC, Richardson JD, Croce MA, et al: Prospective study of blunt aortic injury: Multicenter trial of the American Association for the Surgery of Trauma. *J Trauma* 42:374, 1997.

20. Dyer DS, Moore EE, Ilke DN, et al: Thoracic aortic injury: How predictive is mechanism and is chest computed tomography a reliable screening tool? A prospective study of 1,561 patients. *J Trauma* 48:673, 2000.

21. Flowers JL, Graham SM, Ugarte MA, et al: Flexible endoscopy for the diagnosis of esophageal trauma. *J Trauma* 40:261, 1996.

22. Cox CS Jr., Allen GS, Fischer RP, et al: Blunt versus penetrating subclavian artery injury: Presentation, injury pattern, and outcome. *J Trauma* 46:445, 1999.

23. Renz BM, Feliciano DV: Gunshot wounds to the right thoracoabdomen: A prospective study of nonoperative management. *J Trauma* 37:737, 1994.

24. Demetriades D, Hadjizacharia P, Constantinou C, et al: Selective nonoperative management of penetrating abdominal solid organ injuries. *Ann Surg* 244:620, 2006.

25. Boyle EM Jr., Maier RV, Salazar JD, et al: Diagnosis of injuries after stab wounds to the back and flank. *J Trauma* 42:260, 1997.

26. Biffl WL, Cothren CC, Brasel KJ, et al: A prospective observational multicenter study of the optimal management of patients with anterior abdominal stab wounds. *J Trauma* 64:250, 2008.

27. Rozycki GS, Ochsner MG, Schmidt JA, et al: A prospective study of surgeon-performed ultrasound as the primary adjuvant modality for injured patient assessment. *J Trauma* 39:492, 1995.

28. Branney SW, Wolfe RE, Moore EE, et al: Quantitative sensitivity of ultrasound in detecting free intraperitoneal fluid. *J Trauma* 39:375, 1995.

29. Ochsner MG, Knudson MM, Pachter HL, et al: Significance of minimal or no intraperitoneal fluid visible on CT scan associated with blunt liver and splenic injuries: A multicenter analysis. *J Trauma* 49:505, 2000.

30. Malhotra AK, Fabian TC, Katsis SB, et al: Blunt bowel and mesenteric injuries: The role of screening computed tomography. *J Trauma* 48:991, 2000.

31. Johansen K, Lynch K, Paun M, et al: Noninvasive vascular tests reliably exclude occult arterial trauma in injured extremities. *J Trauma* 31:515, 1991.

32. Burch JM, Franciose RJ, Moore EE, et al: Single-layer continuous versus two-layer interrupted intestinal anastomosis—a prospective randomized study. *Ann Surg* 231:832, 2000.

33. Moore EE: Staged laparotomy for the hypothermia, acidosis, and coagulopathy syndrome. *Am J Surg* 172:405, 1996.

34. Hebert PC, Wells G, Blajchman MA, et al: A multicenter, randomized, controlled clinical trial of transfusion requirements in critical care. *New Engl J Med* 340:409, 1999.

35. West MA, Shapiro MB, Nathens AB, et al: Inflammation and the host response to injury, a large-scale collaborative project: Patient-oriented research core-standard operating procedures for clinical care. IV. Guidelines for transfusion in the trauma patient. *J Trauma* 61:436, 2006.

36. Toy P, Popovsky MA, Abraham E, et al: Transfusion-related acute lung injury: Definition and review. *Crit Care Med* 33:721, 2005.

37. Moore FA, Moore EE, Sauaia A: Blood transfusion: An independent risk factor for postinjury multiple organ failure. *Arch Surg* 132:620, 1997.

38. Kashuk JL, Moore EE, Sauaia A, et al: Postinjury life-threatening coagulopathy: Is 1:1 the answer? *J Trauma* 65:261, 2008.

39. Menaker J, Stein DM, Scalea TM: Incidence of early pulmonary embolism after injury. *J Trauma* 63:620, 2007.

40. Rinker C, McMurry F, Groeneweg V, et al: Emergency craniotomy in a rural level III trauma center. *J Trauma* 44:984, 1998.

41. Cogbill T, Cothren CC, et al: Management of severe hemorrhage associated with maxillofacial injuries: A multicenter perspective. *J Trauma* 64:250, 2008.

42. Bracken MB, Shepard MJ, Holford TR, et al: Administration of methylprednisolone for 24 or 48 hours or tirilazad mesylate for 48 hours in the treatment of acute spinal cord injury. Results of the Third National Acute Spinal Cord Injury Randomized Controlled Trial. National Acute Spinal Cord Injury Study. *JAMA* 277:1597, 1997.

43. Fehlings MG, Perrin RG: The timing of surgical intervention in the treatment of spinal cord injury: A systematic review of recent clinical evidence. *Spine* 31:S28, 2006.

44. Biffl WL, Moore EE, Offner PJ, et al: Blunt carotid arterial injuries: Implications of a new grading scale. *J Trauma* 47:845, 1999.

45. Biffl WL, Moore EE, Ryu RK, et al: The unrecognized epidemic of blunt carotid arterial injuries: Early diagnosis improves neurologic outcome. *Ann Surg* 228:462, 1998.

46. Cothren CC, Moore EE, Biffl WL, et al: Anticoagulation is the gold standard therapy for blunt carotid injuries to reduce stroke rate. *Arch Surg* 139:540, 2004.

47. Edwards NM, Fabian TC, Claridge JA, et al: Antithrombotic therapy and endovascular stents are effective treatment for blunt carotid injuries: Results from long-term followup. *J Am Coll Surg* 204:1007, 2007.

48. Bladergroen M, Brockman R, Luna G, et al: A twelve-year study of cervicothoracic vascular injuries. *Am J Surg* 157:483, 1989.

49. Johnston RH, Wall MJ, Mattox KL: Innominate artery trauma: A thirty-year experience. *J Vasc Surg* 17:134, 1993.

50. Fabian TC, Davis KA, Gavant ML, et al: Prospective study of blunt aortic injury: Helical CT is diagnostic and antihypertensive therapy reduces rupture. *Ann Surg* 227:666, 1998.

51. Kim FJ, Moore EE, Moore FA, et al: Trauma surgeons can render definitive surgical care for major thoracic injuries. *J Trauma* 36:871, 1994.

52. Karmy-Jones R, Nicholls S, Gleason TG: The endovascular approach to acute aortic trauma. *Thorac Surg Clin* 17:109, 2007.

53. Moore EE, Burch JM, Moore JB: Repair of the torn descending thoracic aorta using the centrifugal pump with partial left heart bypass. *Ann Surg* 240:38, 2004.

54. Wall MJ, Mattox KL, Chen C, et al: Acute management of complex cardiac injuries. *J Trauma* 42:905, 1997.

55. Cothren CC, Moore EE: Traumatic ventricular septal defect. *Surgery* 142:776, 2007.

56. Maron BJ, Gohman TE, Kyle SB, et al: Clinical profile and spectrum of commotio cordis. *JAMA* 287:9, 2002.

57. Wall MJ Jr., Hirshberg A, Mattox KL: Pulmonary tractotomy with selective vascular ligation for penetrating injuries to the lung. *Am J Surg* 168:665, 1994.

58. Cothren C, Moore EE, Biffl WL, et al: Lung-sparing techniques are associated with improved outcome compared with anatomic resection for severe lung injuries. *J Trauma* 53:483, 2002.

59. Cryer HG, Mavroudis C, Yu J, et al: Shock, transfusion, and pneumonectomy: Death is due to right heart failure and increased pulmonary vascular resistance. *Ann Surg* 212:197, 1990.

60. de Souza A, Offner PJ, Moore EE, et al: Optimal management of complicated empyema. *Am J Surg* 180:507, 2000.

61. Bender JS, Lucas CE: Management of close-range shotgun injuries to the chest by diaphragmatic transposition: Case reports. *J Trauma* 30:1581, 1990.

62. Kozar RA, Moore FA, Cothren CC, et al: Risk factors for hepatic morbidity following nonoperative management: Multicenter study. *Arch Surg* 141:451, 2006.

63. Malhotra AK, Fabian TC, Croce MA, et al: Blunt hepatic injury: A paradigm shift from operative to nonoperative management in the 1990s. *Ann Surg* 231:804, 2000.

64. Biffl WL, Moore EE, Franciose RJ: Venovenous bypass and hepatic vascular isolation as adjuncts in the repair of destructive wounds to the retrohepatic inferior vena cava. *J Trauma* 45:400, 1998.

65. Poggetti RS, Moore EE, Moore FA, et al: Balloon tamponade for bilobar transfixing hepatic gunshot wounds. *J Trauma* 33:694, 1992.

66. Lillemoe KD, Melton GB, Cameron JL, et al: Postoperative bile duct strictures: Management and outcome in the 1990s. *Ann Surg* 232:430, 2000.

67. Pickhardt B, Moore EE, Moore FA, et al: Operative splenic salvage in adults: A decade perspective. *J Trauma* 29:1386, 1989.

68. Feliciano DV, Spjut-Patrinely V, Burch JM, et al: Splenorrhaphy: The alternative. *Ann Surg* 211:569, 1990.

69. McIntyre LK, Schiff M, Jurkovich GJ: Failure of nonoperative management of splenic injuries: Causes and consequences. *Arch Surg* 140:563, 2005.

70. Smith HE, Biffl WL, Majercik SD, et al: Splenic artery embolization: Have we gone too far? *J Trauma* 61:541, 2006.

71. Leemans R, Manson W, Snijder JA, et al: Immune response capacity after human splenic autotransplantation: Restoration of response to individual pneumococcal vaccine subtypes. *Ann Surg* 229:279, 1999.

72. Toutouzas KG, Velmahos GC, Kaminski A, et al: Leukocytosis after posttraumatic splenectomy: A physiologic event or sign of sepsis? *Arch Surg* 137:924, 2002.

73. Burch JM, Franciose RJ, Moore EE, et al: Single-layer continuous versus two-layer interrupted intestinal anastomosis: A prospective randomized trial. *Ann Surg* 231:832, 2000.

74. Todd SR, Kozar RA, Moore FA: Nutrition support in adult trauma patients. *Nutr Clin Pract* 21:421, 2006.

75. Vaughn GD, Frazier OH, Graham D, et al: The use of pyloric exclusion in the management of severe duodenal injuries. *Am J Surg* 134:785, 1977.

76. Nelson R, Singer M: Primary repair for penetrating colon injuries. *Cochrane Database Syst Rev* 3:CD002247, 2003.

77. Accola KD, Feliciano DV, Mattox KL, et al: Management of injuries to the superior mesenteric artery. *J Trauma* 26:313, 1986.

78. Asensio JA, Britt LD, Borzotta A, et al: Multi-institutional experience with the management of superior mesenteric artery injuries. *J Am Coll Surg* 193:354, 2001.

79. Burch JM, Richardson RJ, Martin RR, et al: Penetrating iliac vascular injuries: Experience with 233 consecutive patients. *J Trauma* 30:1450, 1990.

80. Mullins RJ, Lucas CE, Ledgerwood AM: The natural history following venous ligation for civilian injuries. *J Trauma* 20:737, 1980.

81. Pachter HL, Drager S, Godfrey N, et al: Traumatic injuries of the portal vein. *Ann Surg* 189:383, 1979.

82. Roth SM, Wheeler JR, Gregory RT, et al: Blunt injury of the abdominal aorta: A review. *J Trauma* 42:748, 1997.

83. Jurkovich GJ, Hoyt DB, Moore FA, et al: Portal triad injuries. *J Trauma* 39:426, 1995.

84. Knudson MM, Harrison PB, Hoyt DB, et al: Outcome after major renovascular injuries: A Western trauma association multicenter report. *J Trauma* 49:1116, 2000.

85. Cothren CC, Osborn PM, Moore EE, et al: Preperitoneal pelvic packing for hemodynamically unstable pelvic fractures: A paradigm shift. *J Trauma* 62:834, 2007.

86. Bosse MJ, MacKenzie EJ, Kellam JF, et al: An analysis of outcomes of reconstruction or amputation of leg-threatening injuries. *N Engl J Med* 347:1924, 2002.

87. Moore FA, McKinley BA, Moore EE, et al: Inflammation and the Host Response to Injury, a large-scale collaborative project: Patient-oriented research core—standard operating procedures for clinical care. III. Guidelines for shock resuscitation. *J Trauma* 61:82, 2006.

88. ACOG Committee on Obstetric Practice: ACOG Committee Opinion. Number 299, September 2004. Guidelines for diagnostic imaging during pregnancy. *Obstet Gynecol* 104:647, 2004.

89. Morris JA, Rosenbower TJ, Jurkovich GJ, et al: Infant survival after cesarean section for trauma. *Ann Surg* 223:481, 1996.

90. Curet MJ, Schermer CR, Demarest GB, et al: Predictors of outcome in trauma during pregnancy: Identification of patients who can be monitored for less than 6 hours. *J Trauma* 49:18, 2000.

91. Davis JW, Kaups KL: Base deficit in the elderly: A marker of severe injury and death. *J Trauma* 45:873, 1998.

92. Reynolds FD, Dietz PA, Higgins D, et al: Time to deterioration of the elderly, anticoagulated, minor head injury patient who presents without evidence of neurologic abnormality. *J Trauma* 54:492, 2003.

93. Bulger EM, Arneson MA, Mock CN, et al: Rib fractures in the elderly. *J Trauma* 48:1040, 2000.

94. Bergeron E, Lavoie A, Clas D, et al: Elderly trauma patients with rib fractures are at greater risk of death and pneumonia. *J Trauma* 54:478, 2003.

95. Morris JA, MacKenzie EJ, Damiano AM, et al: Mortality in trauma patients: The interaction between host factors and severity. *J Trauma* 30:1476, 1990.

96. Milzman DP, Boulanger BR, Rodriguez A, et al: Pre-existing disease in trauma patients: A predictor of fate independent of age and injury severity score. *J Trauma* 32:236, 1992.

97. Knudson MM, Lieberman J, Morris JA Jr., et al: Mortality factors in geriatric blunt trauma patients. *Arch Surg* 129:448, 1994.

98. Tepas JJ: The national pediatric trauma registry: A legacy of commitment to control childhood injury. *Semin Pediatr Surg* 13:126, 2004.

99. Partrick DA, Bensard DD, Moore EE, et al: Ultrasound is an effective triage tool to evaluate blunt abdominal trauma in the pediatric population. *J Trauma* 45:57, 1998.

100. Partrick DA, Bensard DD, Moore EE, et al: Nonoperative management of solid organ injuries in children results in decreased blood utilization. *J Pediatr Surg* 34:1695, 1999.

CHAPTER 8

Burns

Fred W. Endorf and Nicole S. Gibran

GROWING NEED FOR BURN EXPERTISE

Surgical care of the burn patient has evolved into a specialized field incorporating the interdisciplinary skills of burn surgeons, nurses, therapists, and other health care specialists. However, recent mass casualty events have been a reminder that health systems may be rapidly pressed to care for large numbers of burn patients. Naturally, general surgeons will be at the forefront in these events, so it is crucial that they are comfortable with the care of burned patients and well equipped to provide standard of care.

BACKGROUND

Burn injury historically carried a poor prognosis. With advances in fluid resuscitation[1] and the advent of early excision of the burn wound,[2] survival has become an expectation even for patients with severe burns. Continued improvements in critical care and progress in skin bioengineering herald a future in which functional and psychological outcomes are equally important as survival alone. With this shift in priority, the American Burn Association has emphasized referral to specialized burn centers after early stabilization. Specific criteria should guide transfer of patients with more complex injuries or other medical needs to a burn center (Table 8-1). The American Burn Association has published standards of care[3]

and created a verification process to ensure that burn centers meet those standards.[4] Because of increased prehospital safety measures, burn patients are being transferred longer distances to receive definitive care at regional burn centers; recent data from one burn center with a particularly wide catchment area confirmed that even transport times averaging 7 hours did not affect the long-term outcomes of burn patients.[5]

INITIAL EVALUATION

Initial evaluation of the burn patient involves four crucial assessments: airway management, evaluation of other injuries, estimation of burn size, and diagnosis of carbon monoxide and cyanide poisoning. With direct thermal injury to the upper airway or smoke inhalation, rapid and severe airway edema is a potentially lethal threat. Anticipating the need for intubation and establishing an early airway is critical. Perioral burns and singed nasal hairs are signs that the oral cavity and pharynx should be further evaluated for mucosal injury, but in themselves these physical findings do not indicate an upper airway injury. Signs of impending respiratory compromise may include a hoarse voice, wheezing, or stridor; subjective dyspnea is a particularly concerning symptom, and should trigger prompt elective endotracheal intubation. In patients with combined multiple trauma, especially oral trauma, nasotracheal

TABLE 8-1	Guidelines for referral to a burn center

Partial-thickness burns greater than 10% TBSA

Burns involving the face, hands, feet, genitalia, perineum, or major joints

Third-degree burns in any age group

Electrical burns, including lightning injury

Chemical burns

Inhalation injury

Burn injury in patients with complicated pre-existing medical disorders

Patients with burns and concomitant trauma in which the burn is the greatest risk. If the trauma is the greater immediate risk, the patient may be stabilized in a trauma center before transfer to a burn center.

Burned children in hospitals without qualified personnel for the care of children

Burn injury in patients who will require special social, emotional, or rehabilitative intervention

TBSA = total body surface area.

intubation may be useful but should be avoided if oral intubation is safe and easy.

Burn patients should be first considered trauma patients, especially when details of the injury are unclear. A primary survey should be conducted in accordance with advanced trauma life support guidelines. Concurrently with the primary survey, large-bore peripheral IV catheters should be placed and fluid resuscitation should be initiated; for a burn larger than 40% total body surface area (TBSA), two large-bore IVs are ideal. IV placement through burned skin is safe and effective but requires attention to securing the catheters. Central venous access may be necessary in the severely burned patient, and provides useful information as to volume status in the intensive care unit. Pediatric patients may require intraosseous access in emergent situations. An early and comprehensive secondary survey must be performed on all burn patients, but especially those with a history of associated trauma such as with a motor vehicle collision and a fire. Also, patients from structural fires in which the manner of egress is not known should be carefully evaluated for injuries from a possible jump or fall. Urgent radiology studies, such as a chest x-ray should be performed in the emergency department, but nonurgent skeletal evaluation (i.e., extremity x-rays) can be done in the intensive care unit to avoid hypothermia and delays in burn resuscitation. Hypothermia is one of the common prehospital complications that contributes to resuscitation failure. Patients should be wrapped with clean blankets in transport. Cooling blankets should be avoided in patients with moderate or large burns.

Patients with acute burn injuries should never receive prophylactic antibiotics. This intervention has been clearly demonstrated to promote development of fungal infections and resistant organisms and was abandoned in the mid-1980s. A tetanus booster should be administered in the emergency room.

Pain management for these patients has been widely recognized over the past 25 years. However, one must also consider treatment of the contribution of long-term anxiety. Therefore, it is important to administer an anxiolytic such as a benzodiazepine with the initial narcotics.

Most burn resuscitation formulas (Table 8-2) estimate fluid requirements using the burn size as a percent of TBSA burned. The "rule of nines" is a crude but quick and effective method of estimating burn size (Fig. 8-1). In adults, the anterior and posterior trunk each account for 18%, each lower extremity is 18%, each upper extremity is 9%, and the head is 9%. In children younger than 3 years old, the head accounts for a larger relative surface area and should be taken into account when estimating burn size. Diagrams such as the Lund and Browder chart give a more accurate accounting of the true burn size in children. The importance of an accurate burn size assessment cannot be overemphasized. Superficial or first-degree burns should not be included when calculating the percent of TBSA, and thorough cleaning of soot and debris is mandatory to avoid confusing areas of soiling with burns. Examination of referral data suggests that physicians inexperienced with burns tend to overestimate the size of small burns and underestimate the size of large burns, with potentially detrimental effects on pretransfer resuscitation.[6]

Another important contributor to early mortality in burns is carbon monoxide (CO) poisoning resulting from smoke inhalation. The affinity of CO for hemoglobin is approximately 200–250 times more than that of oxygen, which decreases the levels of normal oxygenated hemoglobin and can quickly lead to anoxia and death.[7] Unexpected neurologic symptoms should raise the level of suspicion, and an arterial carboxyhemoglobin level must be obtained because pulse oximetry is falsely elevated. Administration of 100% oxygen is the gold standard for treatment of CO poisoning, and reduces the half-life of CO from 250 minutes in room air to 40 to 60 minutes.[8] Some authors have proposed hyperbaric oxygen as an adjunctive therapy for CO poisoning.[9] However, the data are mixed regarding the success of hyperbaric oxygen, and its associated logistic difficulties and complications have limited its usefulness for patients with moderate or large burns.[10,11] Patients who sustain a cardiac arrest as a result of their CO poisoning have an extremely poor prognosis regardless of the success of initial resuscitation attempts.[12] Hydrogen cyanide toxicity may also be a component of smoke inhalation injury. Afflicted patients may have a persistent lactic acidosis or S-T elevation on electrocardiogram (ECG).[13] Cyanide inhibits cytochrome oxidase, which in turn inhibits cellular oxygenation.[14] Treatment consists of sodium thiosulfate, hydroxocobalamin, and 100% oxygen. Sodium thiosulfate works by transforming cyanide into a nontoxic thiocyanate derivative; however, it works slowly and is not effective for acute therapy. Hydroxocobalamin quickly complexes with cyanide and is excreted by the kidney, and is recommended for immediate therapy.[9] In the majority of patients, the lactic acidosis will resolve with ventilation and sodium thiosulfate treatment becomes unnecessary.[15]

KEY POINTS

1. Follow American Burn Association criteria for transfer of a patient to a regional burn center.

2. IV fluid resuscitation for patients with burns greater than 20% total body surface area (children with >15% total body surface area) should be titrated to mean arterial pressure (MAP) greater than 60 mmHg and urine output greater than 30 mL/h.

3. Never administer prophylactic antibiotics other than tetanus vaccination.

4. Patients with upper airway injury, partial pressure of arterial oxygen:fraction of inspired oxygen ratio less than 200 or carbon monoxide toxicity should be intubated for inhalation injury.

5. Early excision and grafting of full thickness and deep partial thickness burns improves outcomes.

TABLE 8-2	Burn resuscitation formulas		
	Electrolyte Solution	**Colloid Solution**	**D₅W**
Isotonic crystalloid formulas			
Parkland formula	Lactated Ringer's 4 mL/kg per % TBSA burn $^1/_2$ volume during first 8 h postinjury; $^1/_2$ during next 16 h postinjury		
Modified Brooke formula	Lactated Ringer's 2.0 mL/kg per % TBSA burn		
Haifa formula	Lactated Ringer's 1 mL/kg per % TBSA burn $^1/_2$ volume during first 8 h postinjury; $^1/_2$ during next 16 h postinjury	Fresh-frozen plasma 1.5 mL/kg per % TBSA burn $^1/_2$ volume during first 8 h postinjury; $^1/_2$ during next 16 h postinjury	
Hypertonic formulas			
Monafo formula	25 mEq/L NaCl Volume titrated to UOP 30 mL/h		

Warden formula	Lactated Ringer's plus 50 mEq NaHCO₃ (180 mEq Na/L)
	  titrated to UOP 30–50 mL/h for 8 h postinjury
	Lactated Ringer's titrated to UOP 30–50 mL/h beginning
	  8 h postburn		

Colloid formulas			
Evans formula	0.9% saline 1 mL/kg per % TBSA burn	Fresh-frozen plasma 1 mL/kg per % TBSA burn	2000 mL
Brooke formula	Lactated Ringer's 1.5 mL/kg per % TBSA burn	Fresh-frozen plasma 0.5 mL/kg per % TBSA burn	2000 mL
Slater formula	Lactated Ringer's 2000 mL/24 h	Fresh-frozen plasma 75 mL/kg per 24 h	

Demling formula	Dextran 40 in 0.9% NaCl
	2 mL/kg per hour for 8 h postinjury;
	Lactated Ringer's titrated to UOP >30 mL/h for next 18 h
	  postburn
		Fresh-frozen plasma
		0.5 mL/kg per hour starting 8 h postburn
		  continued for 18 h	

Note: Individual burn centers may modify these basic formulas for their own needs.

D₅W = 5% dextrose in water; NaCl = sodium chloride; NaHCO₃ = sodium bicarbonate; TBSA = total body surface area; UOP = urine output.

CLASSIFICATION OF BURNS

Burns are commonly classified as thermal, electrical, or chemical burns, with thermal burns consisting of flame, contact, or scald burns. Flame burns are not only the most common cause for hospital admission of burns, but also have the highest mortality. This is primarily related to their association with structural fires and the accompanying inhalation injury and/or CO poisoning.[16]

Electrical burns make up only 4% of U.S. hospital admissions but have special concerns, including the potential for cardiac arrhythmias and compartment syndromes with concurrent rhabdomyolysis. A baseline ECG is recommended in all patients with electrical injury, and a normal ECG in a low-voltage injury may preclude hospital admission. Because compartment syndrome and rhabdomyolysis are common in high-voltage electrical injuries, vigilance must be maintained for neurologic or vascular compromise, and fasciotomies should be performed even in cases of moderate clinical suspicion. Long-term neurologic and visual symptoms are not uncommon with high voltage electrical injuries, and ophthalmologic and neurologic consultation should be obtained to better define a patient's baseline function.[17]

Chemical burns are less common, but potentially are severe burns. The most important components of initial therapy are careful removal of the toxic substance from the patient and irrigation of the affected area with water for a minimum of 30 minutes. An exception to this is in cases of concrete powder or powdered forms of lye, which should be swept from the patient to avoid activating the aluminum hydroxide with water. The offending agents in chemical burns can be systemically absorbed and may cause specific metabolic derangements. Formic acid has been known to cause hemolysis and hemoglobinuria, and hydrofluoric acid causes hypocalcemia. Hydrofluoric acid is a particularly common offender due to its widespread industrial uses. Calcium-based therapies are the mainstay of treating hydrofluoric acid burns, with topical calcium gluconate applied to wounds,[18] and subcutaneous or IV infiltration of calcium gluconate for systemic symptoms. Intra-arterial infusion of calcium gluconate may be effective in the most severe cases.[19,20] Patients undergoing intra-arterial therapy need continuous cardiac monitoring. Persistent electrocardiac abnormalities or refractory hypocalcemia may signal the need for emergent excision of the burned areas.

BURN DEPTH

Burn wounds are commonly classified as superficial (first degree), partial thickness (second degree), full thickness (third degree), and fourth-degree burns, which affect underlying soft tissue. Partial-thickness burns are then classified as either superficial or deep partial thickness burns by depth of involved dermis. Clinically, first-degree burns are painful but do not blister, second-degree burns have dermal involvement and are extremely painful with weeping and blisters, and third-degree burns are hard, painless, and nonblanching. Jackson described three zones of tissue injury following burn injury.[21] The zone of coagulation is the most severely burned portion and is typically in the center of the wound. As the name implies, the affected tissue is coagulated and sometimes frankly necrotic, and will need excision and grafting. Peripheral to that is a zone of stasis, which has a local response of vasoconstriction and resultant ischemia. Appropriate resuscitation and wound care may help prevent conversion to a deeper wound, but infection or suboptimal perfusion may result in an increase in burn depth. This is clinically relevant because many superficial partial-thickness burns will heal with expectant manage-

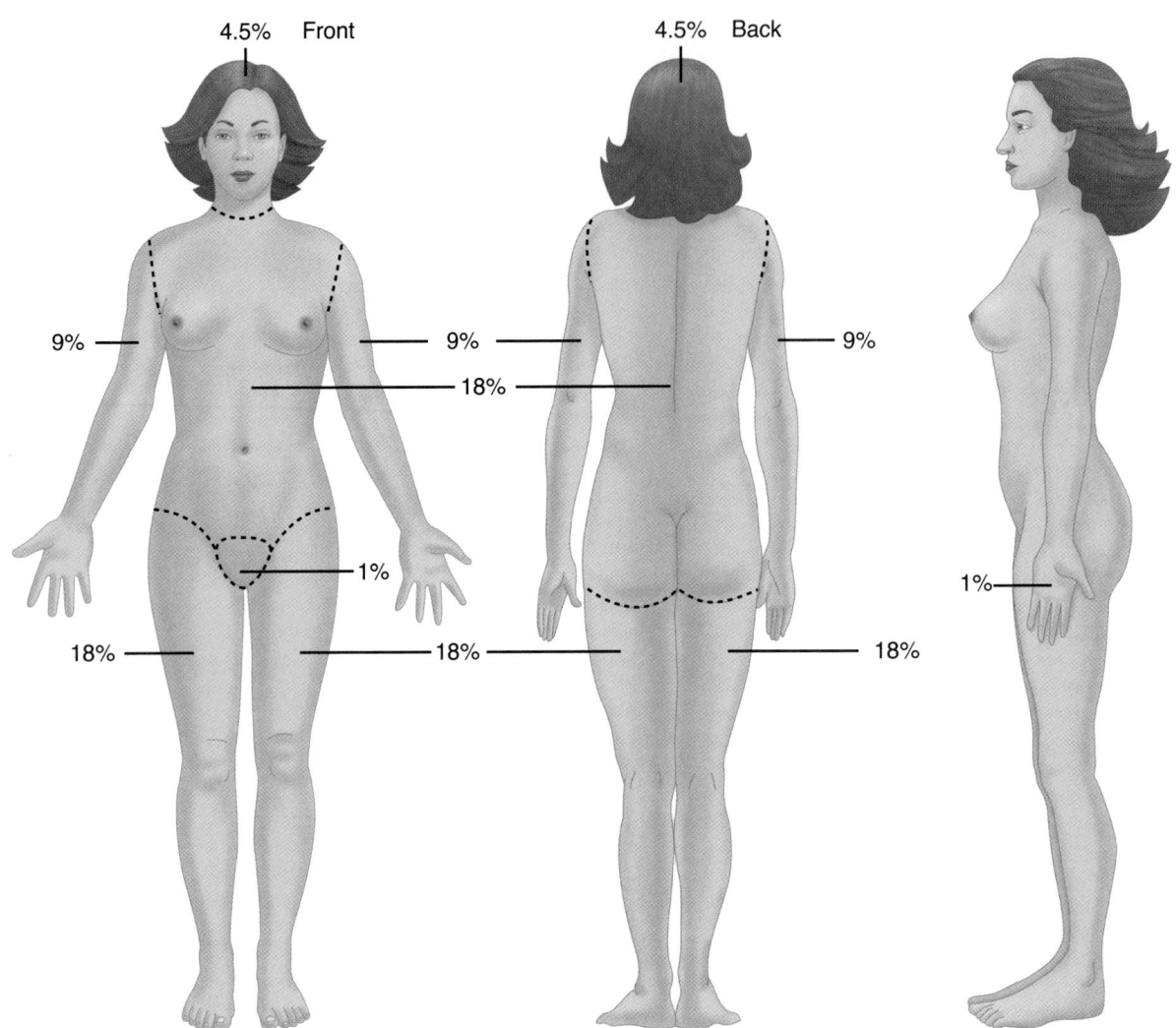

FIG. 8-1. The Rule of Nines can be used as a quick reference for estimating a patient's burn size by dividing the body into regions to which total body surface area is allocated in multiples of nine.

ment, while the majority of deep partial-thickness burns require excision and skin grafting. The last area of a burn is called the *zone of hyperemia*, which will heal with minimal or no scarring.

Unfortunately, even experienced burn surgeons have limited ability to accurately predict the healing potential of partial-thickness burns; one reason is that burn wounds evolve over 48–72 hours after a burn injury. Numerous techniques have been developed with the idea that better early prediction of burn depth will expedite appropriate surgical decision making. One of the most effective ways to determine burn depth is full-thickness biopsy, but this has several limitations. Not only is the procedure painful and potentially scarring, but accurate interpretation of the histopathology requires a specialized pathologist and may have slow turnaround times.[22] Laser Doppler can measure skin perfusion and use those measurements to predict burn depth, with a positive predictive value of up to 80% in some studies.[23,24] Noncontact ultrasound has been postulated as a painless modality to predict nonhealing wounds, and has the advantage of easily performed serial measurements.[25] Unfortunately, none of these newer therapies have proven adequately superior to justify their cost, and so have not yet substituted serial examination by experienced burn surgeons.

PROGNOSIS

The Baux score (mortality = age + percent TBSA) was used for many years to predict mortality in burns, and analysis of multiple risk factors for burn mortality validated age and percent TBSA as the strongest predictors of mortality.[26] Advancements in burn care have lowered overall mortality to the point that the Baux score may no longer be accurate. However, age and burn size, as well as inhalation injury, continue to be the most robust markers for burn mortality.[27] Age, even as a single variable, strongly predicts mortality in burns,[28] and inhospital mortality in elderly burn patients is a function of age regardless of other comorbidities.[29] In nonelderly patients, comorbidities such as preinjury HIV, metastatic cancer, and kidney or liver disease may influence mortality and length of stay.[30] A recent large database study of 68,661 burn patients found that the variables with the highest predictive value for mortality were age, percent TBSA, inhalation injury, coexistent trauma, and pneumonia.[31]

RESUSCITATION

A myriad of formulas exist for calculating fluid needs during burn resuscitation, suggesting that no one formula benefits all patients. The most commonly used formula, the Parkland or Baxter formula, consists of 3 to 4 mL/kg per percent burned of lactated Ringer's, of which half is given during the first 8 hours postburn, and the remaining half over the subsequent 16 hours. The concept behind the continuous fluid needs are simple. The burn (and/or inhalation injury) drives an inflammatory response that leads to capillary leak; as the plasma leaks into the extravascular space, crystalloid administration maintains the intravascular volume. Therefore, if a patient receives a large fluid bolus in a prehospital setting or emergency department, that fluid has likely leaked into the interstitium and the patient will still require ongoing burn resuscitation, according to the estimates. Continuation of fluid volumes should depend on the time since injury, urine output, and MAP; as the leak closes, the patient will require less volume to maintain these two resuscitation endpoints. Children under 20 kg have the additional requirement that they do not have sufficient glycogen stores to maintain an adequate glucose level in response to the inflammatory response. Specific pediatric formulas have been described, but the simplest approach is to add maintenance IV fluid with glucose supplementation in addition to the calculated resuscitation fluid with lactated Ringer's.

It is important to remember that any formula for burn resuscitation is merely a guideline, and fluid must be titrated based on appropriate measures of adequate resuscitation. A number of parameters are widely used to gauge burn resuscitation, but the most common remain the simple outcomes of blood pressure and urine output. As in any critically ill patient, the target MAP is 60 mmHg to ensure optimal end-organ perfusion. Goals for urine output should be 30 mL/h in adults and 1 to 1.5 mL/kg per hour in pediatric patients. Because blood pressure and urine output may not correlate perfectly with true tissue perfusion, the search continues for other adjunctive parameters that may more accurately reflect adequate resuscitation. Some centers have found serum lactate to be a better predictor of mortality in severe burns;[32,33] others have found that base deficit may be a better predictor of eventual organ dysfunction and mortality.[34,35] Burned patients with normal blood pressures and serum lactate levels may still have compromised gastric mucosal blood flow. However, continuous measurement of gastric mucosal pH is logistically difficult and has not been widely implemented.[36,37]

Invasive monitoring with pulmonary artery catheters typically results in significant excessive fluid administration without resulting in improved cardiac output or preload measurements, and the use of invasive monitoring seems to have variable effects on long-term outcomes.[38]

Actual administered fluid volumes typically exceed volumes predicted by standard formulas.[39] One survey of burn centers showed that 58% of patients receive more fluids than would be predicted by Baxter's formula.[40] A comparison of modern-day patients with historical controls shows that this over-resuscitation may be a relatively recent trend.[41] One theory is that increased opioid analgesic use results in peripheral vasodilation and hypotension and thus the need for greater volumes of bloused resuscitative fluids.[42] A classic study by Navar and associates showed that burned patients with inhalation injury required an average of 5.76 mL/kg per percent burned, versus 3.98 mL/kg per percent burned for patients without inhalation injury. This finding has been corroborated by subsequent studies.[43,44] Prolonged mechanical ventilation may also play a role in increased fluid needs.[45] A recent multicenter study found that age, weight, percent TBSA, and intubation on admission were significant predictors that the patient would receive more fluid during the resuscitation period. Those patients receiving higher fluid volumes were at increased risk of complications and death.[46] Common complications include abdominal compartment syndrome, extremity compartment syndrome, intraocular compartment syndrome, and pleural effusions. Monitoring bladder pressures can provide valuable information about the development of intra-abdominal hypertension.

The use of colloid as part of the burn resuscitation has generated much interest. In late resuscitation when the capillary leak has closed, colloid administration may decrease overall fluid volumes, and potentially may decrease associated complications such as intra-abdominal hypertension.[47] However, the use of albumin has never been shown to improve outcomes in burn patients and has controversial effects on mortality in critically ill patients.[48,49] Attempts to minimize fluid volumes in burn resuscitation have also led to the study of hypertonic solutions. Hypertonic solutions decrease initial resuscitation volumes as expected, but it appears to be a transient benefit and has the downside of causing hyperchloremic acidosis.[50]

Other adjuncts are being increasingly used during initial burn resuscitation. High-dose ascorbic acid (vitamin C) may decrease fluid volume requirements and ameliorate respiratory embarrassment during resuscitation.[51] Plasmapheresis may also decrease fluid requirements in patients who require higher volumes than predicted to maintain adequate urine output and MAP. It is postulated that plasmapheresis may filter out inflammatory mediators, thus decreasing ongoing vasodilation and capillary leak.[52]

TRANSFUSION

The role of blood transfusion in burns has undergone a re-evaluation in recent years. A large multicenter study found that increased numbers of transfusions were associated with increased infections and a higher mortality rate in burn patients, even when correcting for burn severity.[53] A follow-up study implanting a restrictive transfusion policy in burned children showed that a hemoglobin threshold of 7 g/dL had no more adverse outcomes versus a traditional transfusion trigger of 10 g/dL. In addition, costs incurred to the institution were significantly less.[54] These data, in concert with other reported complications such as transfusion-related lung injury,[55] have led to recommendations that blood transfusions be used only when there is an apparent physiologic need. Attempts to minimize blood transfusion in nonburned, critically ill patients have led to the use of erythropoietin by some centers. Unfortunately, a randomized study in burn patients showed that recombinant human erythropoietin did not effectively prevent anemia or decrease the number of transfusions given.[56]

INHALATION INJURY AND VENTILATOR MANAGEMENT

Inhalation injuries are commonly seen in tandem with burn injuries and are known to drastically increase mortality in burn patients.[57] Smoke inhalation is present in as many as 35% of hospitalized burn patients, and may triple the hospital stay compared to isolated burn injuries.[58] The combination of burns, inhalation injury, and pneumonia increases mortality by up to 60% over burns alone.[59] Subsequent development of the adult respiratory distress syndrome (ARDS) is common in these patients and may be caused in part by recruitment of alveolar leukocytes with an enhanced endotoxin-activated cytokine response.[60] When ARDS complicates burn and inhalation injury, it may result in mortality of up to 66%, and in one study, patients with 60% TBSA or greater in combination with inhalation injury and ARDS had 100% mortality.[61]

Smoke inhalation causes injury in two ways: by direct heat injury to the upper airways, and by inhalation of combustion products into the lower airways. Direct injury to the upper airway causes airway swelling that typically leads to maximal edema in the first 24 to 48 hours after injury, and will require a short course of endotracheal intubation for airway protection. Lower airway injury is caused by combustion products found in smoke, most commonly from synthetic substances burned in structural fires. These irritants cause direct mucosal injury, which in turn leads to mucosal sloughing, edema, reactive bronchoconstriction, and finally obstruction of the lower airways. Injury to both the epithelium and to pulmonary alveolar macrophages causes release of prostaglandins and chemokines, migration of neutrophils and other inflammatory mediators, a rise in tracheobronchial blood flow, and finally increased capillary permeability, leading to ARDS.

The physiologic effects of smoke inhalation are numerous. Inhalation injury decreases lung compliance[62] and increases airway resistance work of breathing.[63] Inhalation injury in the presence of burns will also increase overall metabolic demands.[64] The most common physiologic derangement seen with inhalation injury is an increase in fluid requirements during resuscitation of patients with burn injuries. Bronchoscopic findings, including carbon deposits, erythema, edema, bronchorrhea, and a hemorrhagic appearance, can be useful for confirmation of inhalation injury. Severe inhalation injury may result in mucosal sloughing with obstruction of smaller airways. Because bronchoscopy is an invasive test, attempts have been made to use other diagnostic modalities, such as thoracic computed tomographic scans[65] and xenon ventilation-perfusion scanning.[66] Many of these techniques do not change therapeutic protocols or outcomes,[67] and for this reason many centers still rely on a clinical diagnosis of inhalation injury.[68] A decreased partial pressure of arterial oxygen:fraction of inspired oxygen ratio <200 on admission may not only predict inhalation injury but also indicate increased fluid needs more accurately than bronchoscopic grading of the severity of inhalation.[69]

Treatment of inhalation injury consists primarily of supportive care. Aggressive pulmonary toilet and routine use of nebulized bronchodilators such as albuterol are recommended. Other nebulized agents have shown mixed results. Nebulized N-acetylcysteine is an antioxidant free-radical scavenger designed to decrease the toxicity of high oxygen concentrations. Aerosolized heparin aims to prevent formation of fibrin plugs and decrease the formation of airway casts. These agents seem to improve pulmonary toilet, but have no demonstrated effect on mortality.[70] Aerosolized tissue plasminogen activator[71] and recombinant human antithrombin[72] have shown promise in sheep models, but have not yet seen widespread clinical use. Administration of intrabronchial surfactant has been used as a salvage therapy in patients with severe burns and inhalation injury.[73] Inhaled nitric oxide may also be useful as a last effort in burn patients with severe lung injury for whom other means of ventilatory support have failed.[74] The use of steroids traditionally has been avoided due to worse outcomes in burn patients,[75] but new promising data in late ARDS have prompted scientific review of steroid use in this situation.[76]

New ventilator strategies have played an enormous role in improving the mortality of ARDS. Although ARDS still contributes to mortality in burn patients, treatments have improved so that mortality is primarily from multisystem organ failure rather than isolated respiratory causes.[77] The ARDS Network Study examined low tidal volume or "lung-protective ventilation" by comparing traditional tidal volumes of 12 mL/kg to low tidal volumes of 6 mL/kg. They found that patients on low tidal volume settings had a 22% lower mortality than patients with traditional tidal volumes.[78] A similar approach had previously been shown to improve outcomes in pediatric burn patients.[79] In patients with refractory hypoxemia despite lung-protective ventilation, prone positioning may help improve oxygenation, but has not shown a definitive effect on mortality.[80] No specific studies have examined prone positioning in burn patients, and caution must be used in patients with facial burns who are already at risk for loss of the endotracheal tube. High-frequency percussive ventilation (HFPV) is an alternative mode which has shown some early promise in patients with inhalation injury.[81] A recent study showed notable decreases in both morbidity and mortality with HFPV, especially in patients with less than 40% TBSA and inhalation injury.[82] A related technique is high-frequency oscillatory ventilation, which has been used primarily as a salvage modality in patients refractory to more conventional measure.[83] Extracorporeal membrane oxygenation also typically is reserved for salvage situations, and experience with this modality is limited to small numbers of patients.[84] A promising area of future study is arteriovenous carbon dioxide removal. This technique has proven superior to both low tidal volume ventilation and HFPV in a sheep model, but has not yet made the transition to clinical use.[85]

TREATMENT OF THE BURN WOUND

There are multitudes of topical therapies for the treatment of burn wounds. Of these, silver sulfadiazine is the most widely used in clinical practice. Silver sulfadiazine has a wide range of antimicrobial activity, primarily as prophylaxis against burn wound infec-

tions rather than treatment of existing infections. It has the added benefits of being inexpensive and easily applied, and has some soothing qualities. It is not significantly absorbed systemically and thus has minimal metabolic derangements. Silver sulfadiazine has a reputation for causing neutropenia, but this association is more likely to be a result of neutrophil margination due to the inflammatory response to the burn injury. True allergic reactions to the sulfa component of silver sulfadiazine are rare, and at-risk patients can have a small amount applied to identify a burning sensation or rash. Silver sulfadiazine will destroy skin grafts and is contraindicated on burns in proximity to newly grafted areas.

Mafenide acetate, either in cream or solution form, is an effective topical antimicrobial. It is effective even in the presence of eschar and can be used in both treating and preventing wound infections, and the solution form is an excellent antimicrobial for fresh skin grafts. The use of mafenide acetate may be limited by pain with application to partial-thickness burns. Mafenide is absorbed systemically, and a major side effect is metabolic acidosis resulting from carbonic anhydrase inhibition.

Silver nitrate is another topical agent with broad-spectrum antimicrobial activity. The solution used must be dilute (0.5%), and topical application can lead to electrolyte extravasation with resulting hyponatremia. A rare complication is methemoglobinemia. Although inexpensive, silver nitrate solution causes black stains and laundry costs may offset any fiscal benefit to the hospital.

For burns that are nearly healed, small or large, topical ointments such as bacitracin, neomycin, and polymyxin B can be used. These are also useful for superficial partial-thickness facial burns as they can be applied and left open to air without dressing coverage. Meshed skin grafts, in which the interstices are nearly closed, are another indication for use of these agents, preferably with greasy gauze to help retain the ointment in the affected area. All three have been rarely reported to cause nephrotoxicity and should not be used in large burns. The recent media fascination with methicillin-resistant *Staphylococcus aureus* has led to widespread use by community practitioners of mupirocin for new burns. Unless the patient has known risk factors for methicillin-resistant *S. aureus*, mupirocin should only be used in culture-positive burn wound infections to prevent encouragement of further resistance.

Silver-impregnated dressings such as Acticoat (Smith & Nephew, London, England) and Aquacel Ag (Convatec, Princeton, NJ) are increasingly being used for both donor sites and skin grafts, as well as for burns that are clearly partial-thickness on admission. These help reduce the number of dressing changes and may be more comfortable for the patient, but should not be used in wounds of heterogeneous depth, as they prevent serial examinations of the wound. Biologic membranes such as Biobrane (Dow-Hickham, Sugarland, TX) provide a prolonged barrier under which wounds may heal. Because of the occlusive nature of these dressings, these are typically used only on fresh superficial partial-thickness burns that are clearly not contaminated. Fig. 8-2 provides an algorithm that may assist in selecting the appropriate burn treatment.

NUTRITION

Nutritional support may be more important in patients with large burns than in any other patient population. Not only does adequate nutrition play a role in acute issues such as immune responsiveness, but the hypermetabolic response in burn injury may raise baseline metabolic rates by as much as 200%.[86] This can lead to catabolism of muscle proteins and decreased lean body mass that may delay functional recovery.[87] Early enteral feeding for patients with burns larger than 20% TBSA is not only safe, but it may help prevent loss of lean body mass,[88] slow the hypermetabolic response,[89] and result in more efficient protein metabolism.[90] If the enteral feeds are started within the first few hours after admission, gastric ileus can often be avoided. Adjuncts such as metoclopramide can promote GI motility; alternatively, advancing the tube into the small bowel with nasojeju-

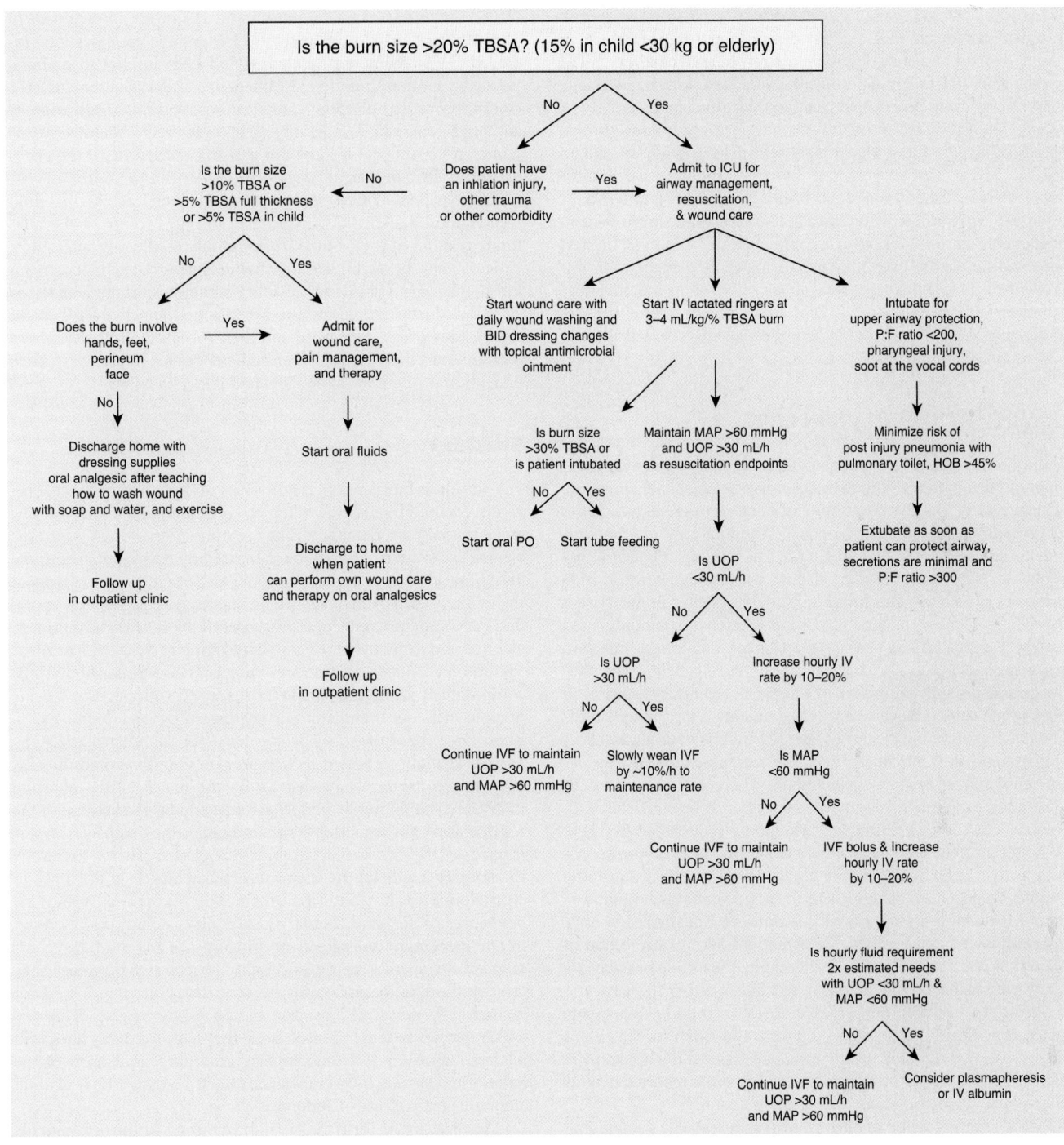

FIG. 8-2. Algorithm for burn treatment. HOB = head of bed; MAP = mean arterial pressure; P:F = partial pressure of arterial oxygen:fraction of inspired oxygen; TBSA = total body surface area; UOP = urine output.

nal feeding can be attempted if other measures for gastric feeding are unsuccessful.[91] In endotracheally intubated patients, trips to the operating room do not necessitate holding enteral feedings.[92] Immune modulating supplements such as glutamine may decrease infectious complications and mortality in burn patients,[93] likely via prevention of T-cell suppression in mesenteric lymph nodes.[94]

Calculating the appropriate caloric needs of the burn patient can be challenging. A commonly used formula in nonburned patients is the Harris-Benedict equation, which calculates caloric needs using factors such as gender, age, height, and weight. This formula uses an activity factor for specific injuries, and for burns the basal energy expenditure is multiplied by two. The Harris-Benedict equation may be inaccurate in burns of less than 40% TBSA, and in these patients,

the Curreri formula may be more appropriate. This formula estimates caloric needs = 25 kcal/kg per day + 40 kcal/% TBSA per day.[95] Indirect calorimetry also can be used to calculate resting energy expenditure, but in burn patients a "metabolic cart" has not been documented to be more beneficial than the predictive equations.[96] Titrating caloric needs closely is important because overfeeding patients will lead to storage of fat instead of muscle anabolism.[97]

Modifying the hypermetabolic response is an area of intense study with several recent findings. Beta blocker use in pediatric patients decreases heart rate and resting energy expenditure and abrogates protein catabolism, even in long-term use.[98] There may be benefits to beta blocker use in adult patients as well,[99] and many centers have begun using them routinely in the adult population.

The anabolic steroid oxandrolone has been extensively studied in pediatric patients as well, and has demonstrated improvements in lean body mass and bone density in severely burned children.[100] The weight gain and functional improvements seen with oxandrolone may persist even after stopping administration of the drug.[101] A recent double-blinded, randomized study of oxandrolone showed decreased length of stay, improved hepatic protein synthesis, and no adverse effects on the endocrine function, although the authors noted a rise in transaminases with unclear clinical significance.[102] Intensive insulin therapy in critically ill patients has shown benefit, presumably from avoidance of hyperglycemia.[103] However, in burn patients, the insulin itself may have a metabolic benefit, with improvements in lean body mass and amelioration of the inflammatory response to burn injury.[104,105] Oral hypoglycemic agents such as metformin also help to avoid hyperglycemia and may contribute to prevention of muscle catabolism.[106]

COMPLICATIONS IN BURN CARE

There are several complications commonly associated with treatment of burn patients. Although not always avoidable, maintaining vigilance for typical complications and using appropriate techniques for prevention may limit the frequency and severity of complications. Ventilator-associated pneumonia, as with all critically ill patients, is a significant problem in burn patients. However, it is so common in patients with inhalation injury, a better nomenclature may be postinjury pneumonia. Unfortunately, commonly used scores in critical illness such as the Clinical Pulmonary Infection Score have not been shown to be reliable in burn patients. Quantitative bronchoscopic cultures in the setting of clinical suspicion of pneumonia should guide treatment of pneumonia.[107] Simple measures such as elevating the head of the bed and maintaining excellent oral hygiene and pulmonary toilet are recommended to help decrease the risk of postinjury pneumonia. There is some question as to whether early tracheostomy will decrease infectious morbidity in burn patients, and whether it will affect long-term outcomes. There do not seem to be any major differences in the rates of pneumonia with early tracheostomy, although there may be less subglottic stenosis than in burn patients with prolonged endotracheal intubation.[108] It also appears that overall outcomes are not affected by early tracheostomy,[109] but practical considerations such as protection of facial skin grafts may play a role in deciding the timing of tracheostomy. One major consideration in deciding whether to perform a tracheostomy has been the presence of eschar at the insertion site, which complicates tracheostomy site care and increases the risk of airway infection. Bedside percutaneous dilatational tracheostomy is a facile method for performing tracheostomy and is reported to be as safe as open tracheostomy in the burn population.[110]

Massive resuscitation of burn patients may lead to an abdominal compartment syndrome characterized by increased airway pressures with hypoventilation, and decreased urine output and hemodynamic compromise. Decompressive laparotomy is the standard of care for refractory abdominal compartment syndrome but carries an especially lethal prognosis in burn patients.[111] Adjunctive measures such as minimizing fluid, performing truncal escharotomies, decreasing tidal volumes, and chemical paralysis should be initiated before resorting to decompressive laparotomy.

Deep vein thrombosis (DVT) has been commonly believed to be a rare phenomenon in burn patients, and there is a paucity of controlled studies regarding heparin prophylaxis in this population.[112] However, recent data show that 6 to 25% of burn patients may have DVT, and fatal pulmonary embolus has been reported in burn patients.[113,114] A large retrospective study in patients with routine prophylaxis found DVT in only 0.25% of patients, and reported no bleeding complications.[115] Thus, it appears that heparin prophylaxis is safe in burn patients and may help prevent thrombotic complications.

Unfortunately, the use of both prophylaxis and therapeutic heparin may be associated with heparin-induced thrombocytopenia

(HIT). One study of HIT in burn patients showed an incidence of 1.6% in heparinized burn patients. Thrombotic complications included DVT, pulmonary embolus, and even arterial thrombosis requiring limb amputation. Nonheparin anticoagulation for HIT commonly caused bleeding complications requiring transfusion.[116] Although rare, a high index of suspicion for HIT should be maintained in thrombocytopenic burn patients, particularly if the platelet counts drop in hospital days 7 to 10.

Burn patients often require central venous access for fluid resuscitation and hemodynamic monitoring. Because of the anatomic relation of their burns to commonly used access sites, burn patients may be at higher risk for catheter-related bloodstream infections. Because burn patients may commonly exhibit leukocytosis with a documented bloodstream infection, practice has been to rewire lines over a guidewire and then culture the catheter. However, this may increase the risk of catheter-related infections in burn patients and a new site should be used if at all possible.[117]

SURGERY

Full-thickness burns with a rigid eschar can form a tourniquet effect as the edema progresses, leading to compromised venous outflow and eventually arterial inflow. The resulting compartment syndrome is most common in circumferential extremity burns, but abdominal and thoracic compartment syndromes also occur. Warning signs of impending compartment syndrome may include paresthesias, pain, decreased capillary refill, and progression to loss of distal pulses; in an intubated patient, the surgeon should anticipate the compartment syndrome and perform frequent vascular evaluations. Abdominal compartment syndrome should be suspected with decreased urine output, increased ventilator airway pressures, and hypotension. Thoracic compartment syndrome may also be characterized by hypoventilation, increased airway pressures, and hypotension. Escharotomies are rarely needed within the first 8 hours following injury and should not be performed unless indicated because of the terrible aesthetic sequelae. When indicated, they usually are performed at the bedside preferably with electrocautery. Extremity incisions are made on the lateral and medial aspects of the limbs in an anatomic position and may extend onto thenar and hypothenar eminences of the hand. Digital escharotomies do not usually result in any meaningful salvage of functional tissue and are not recommended. Inadequate perfusion despite proper escharotomies may indicate the need for fasciotomy; however, this procedure should not be routinely performed as part of the eschar release. Thoracic escharotomies should be placed along the anterior axillary lines with bilateral subcostal and subclavicular extensions. Extension of the anterior axillary incisions down the lateral abdomen typically will allow adequate release of abdominal eschar.

The strategy of early excision and grafting in burned patients revolutionized survival outcomes in burn care. Not only did it improve mortality, but early excision decreased reconstruction surgery, improved hospital length of stay, and reduced costs of care.[118,119] After the initial resuscitation is complete and the patient is hemodynamically stable, attention should be turned to excising the burn wound. Burn excision and wound coverage should ideally start within the first several days, and in larger burns, serial excisions can be performed as the patient's condition allows. Excision is performed with repeated tangential slices using a Watson or Goulian blade until only nonburned tissue remains. It is appropriate to leave healthy dermis, which will appear white with punctate areas of bleeding. Excision to fat or fascia may be necessary in deeper burns. The downside of tangential excision is a high blood loss, though this may be ameliorated using techniques such as instillation of an epinephrine clysis solution underneath the burn. Pneumatic tourniquets are helpful in extremity burns, and compresses soaked in a dilute epinephrine solution are necessary adjuncts after excision. A fibrinogen and thrombin spray sealant (Tisseel Fibrin Sealant; Baxter, Deerfield, Illinois) also has beneficial effects on both hemostasis and graft adherence to the wound bed. The use of these techniques has markedly decreased the number of blood transfusions given during burn surgery.[120] For patients with clearly deep burns and concern for excessive blood loss, fascial excision may be used. In this technique, electrocautery is used to excise the burned tissue and the underlying subcutaneous tissue down to muscle fascia. This technique markedly decreases blood loss but results in a cosmetically inferior appearance due to the loss of subcutaneous tissue. For excision of burns in difficult anatomic areas such as the face, eyelids, or hands, a pressurized water dissector may offer more precision but is time consuming, has a steep learning curve, and is expensive.[121]

WOUND COVERAGE

Because full-thickness grafts are impractical for most burn wounds, split-thickness sheet autografts harvested with a power dermatome make the most durable wound coverings and have a decent cosmetic appearance. In larger burns, meshing of autografted skin provides a larger area of wound coverage. This also allows drainage of blood and serous fluid to prevent accumulation under the skin graft with subsequent graft loss. Areas of cosmetic importance such as the face, neck, and hands should be grafted with nonmeshed sheet grafts to ensure optimal appearance. Unfortunately, even extensive meshing of skin grafts in patients with limited donor sites may not provide adequate amounts of skin. Options for temporary wound coverage include human cadaveric allograft, which is incorporated into the wound but is rejected by the immune system and must be eventually replaced. This will allow time for donor sites to heal enough so that they may be reharvested. The search for a perfect permanent synthetic skin substitute remains elusive, but there are some products in use that help expedite removal of burn eschar and provide temporary wound coverage. Integra (Integra LifeSciences Corporation, Plainsboro, NJ) is a bilayer product with a porous collagen-chondroitin 6-sulphate inner layer that is attached to an outer sheet of silastic. The silastic barrier helps prevent fluid loss and infection, and the inner layer becomes vascularized, creating an artificial neodermis. At approximately 2 weeks, the silastic layer is removed and a thin autograft placed over the neodermis. This results in faster healing of the more superficial donor sites, and seems to have less hypertrophic scarring and improved joint function.[122] AlloDerm (LifeCell Corporation, The Woodlands, TX) is another dermal substitute consisting of cryopreserved acellular human dermis. This must also be used in combination with thin split-thickness skin grafts.[123]

Epidermal skin substitutes such as cultured epithelial autografts are an option in patients with massive burns and very limited donor sites.[124] Their clinical use has been limited by a long turnaround time for culturing, as well as the fragility of the cultured skin, which creates great difficulty with intraoperative handling and graft take. There are promising developments in skin culturing techniques, but none of the final products have yet become commercially available.[125]

Thighs make convenient anatomic donor sites, which are easily harvested and relatively hidden from an aesthetic standpoint. The thicker skin of the back is useful in older patients, who have thinner skin elsewhere and may have difficulty healing donor sites. The buttocks are an excellent donor site in infants and toddlers; Silvadene can be applied to the donor site with a diaper as coverage. The scalp is also an excellent donor site; the skin is thick and there are many hair follicles so it heals quickly. It has the added advantage of being completely hidden once hair regrows. Epinephrine clysis is necessary for harvesting the scalp, for both hemostasis of this hypervascular area and also to create a smooth surface for harvesting.

The list of commonly used donor site dressings is lengthy and includes simple transparent films to hydrocolloids, petrolatum gauzes, and silver-impregnated dressings. Donor sites close to fresh grafts may be dressed with a porous nonadherent gauze, and both the donor sites and grafts can be soaked with mafenide acetate for

ease of care. Principles behind choosing a dressing should balance ease of care, comfort, infection control, and cost. The choice of donor site dressing is largely institution dependent and few data support the clear superiority of any single treatment plan.

REHABILITATION

The rehabilitation of the burn patient is an integral part of their clinical care and should be initiated on admission. Immediate and ongoing physical and occupational therapy is mandatory to prevent loss of physical function. Patients that are unable to participate due to mechanical ventilation or other reasons should have passive range of motion done at least twice a day. This includes patients with burns over joints, such as with hand burns. Patients should be taught exercises they can do themselves to maintain full range of motion. Patients with foot and extremity burns should be instructed to walk independently without the help of crutches to prevent extremity swelling, desensitize the burned areas, and prevent disuse atrophy; when patients are not ambulating, they must elevate the affected extremity to minimize swelling. If postoperative immobilization is used for graft protection, the graft should be evaluated early and at frequent intervals so that active exercise can be resumed at the earliest possible occasion. The transition to outpatient care should also include physical and occupational therapy, with introduction of exercises designed to accelerate return to activities of daily living as well as specific job-related tasks. Tight-fitting pressure garments provide vascular support in burns that are further along in the healing process. However, they do provide vascular support that many patients find more comfortable.

Psychological rehabilitation is equally important in the burn patient. Depression, posttraumatic stress disorder, concerns about cosmetic appearance, and anxiety about returning to society constitute predictable barriers to progress in both the inpatient and outpatient setting. Psychological distress occurs in as many as 34% of burn patients, and persists in severity long after discharge.[126] Despite this, many patients will be able to quickly return to work or school, and goals should be set accordingly. The return to school for pediatric patients is typically prompt, averaging about 10 days after discharge. However, further study is needed to determine whether attendance and performance suffer despite early re-entry to school.[127] The involvement of clinical psychologists and psychiatrists is invaluable in providing guidance and coping techniques to lessen the significant psychological burden of burn injury.

PREVENTION

Despite many areas of progress in prevention, burns continue to be a common source of injury. Some successful initiatives have included community-based interventions targeting simple home safety measures. Smoke alarms are known to decrease mortality from structural fires, but not all homes are equipped with proper smoke alarms, particularly in low-income households. Mandatory smoke alarm installation via community initiatives can be successful, but appears to be contingent on close, long-term follow up to ensure proper maintenance and function.[128,129] Regulation of hot water heater temperatures has had some success, and may be even more effective in conjunction with community-based programs emphasizing education and in-home inspections.[130,131]

FUTURE AREAS OF STUDY

It has long been anecdotally noted that two patients of similar ages and burn size may have very divergent responses to their burn injuries. Attention is being increasingly turned to identifying genetic differences among burn patients and how they affect response to injury. Specific allele variants have been linked with increased mortality in burn patients.[132] It may be that genetic differences may predispose burn patients to severe sepsis,[133] perhaps by downregulating the immune response.[134] Inflammation and the Host Response to Injury is a prospective, multicenter, federally-funded study that aims to define specific genetic pathways that differ in the response to both burns and traumatic injury. Blood and tissue samples taken from a strictly defined patient population are analyzed using gene arrays to determine whether differential expression in certain genetic pathways affects clinical outcomes.[135]

With the progress achieved, the functional outcomes of burn survivors have become more important to clinical outcomes than survival. Since 1993, the National Institute of Disability and Rehabilitation Research has included burns as a model system for improving outcomes for survivors. These studies have been crucial for understanding the barriers that these patients face in returning to their communities, to the workplace, or to school.

REFERENCES

Entries highlighted in bright blue are key references.

1. Baxter CR, Shires T: Physiological response to crystalloid resuscitation of severe burns. *Ann N Y Acad Sci* 150:874, 1968.
2. Janzekovic Z: A new concept in the early excision and immediate grafting of burns. *J Trauma* 10(12):1103, 1970.
3. Practice Guidelines for Burn Care. *J Burn Care Rehabil* 22:1S, 2001.
4. Supple KG, Fiala SM, Gamelli RL: Preparation for burn center verification. *J Burn Care Rehabil* 18:58, 1997.
5. Klein MB, Nathens AB, Emerson D, et al: An analysis of the long-distance transport of burn patients to a regional burn center. *J Burn Care Res* 28:49, 2007.
6. Freiburg C, Igneri P, Sartorelli K, et al: Effects of differences in percent total body surface area estimation on fluid resuscitation of transferred burn patients. *J Burn Care Res* 28:42, 2007.
7. Prien T, Traber DL: Toxic smoke compounds and inhalation injury—a review. *Burns Incl Therm Inj* 14:451, 1988.
8. Crapo RO: Smoke-inhalation injuries. *JAMA* 246:1694, 1981.
9. Hampson NB, Mathieu D, Piantadosi CA, et al: Carbon monoxide poisoning: Interpretation of randomized clinical trials and unresolved treatment issues. *Undersea Hyperb Med* 28:157, 2001.
10. Juurlink DN, Stanbrook MB, McGuigan MA: Hyperbaric oxygen for carbon monoxide poisoning. *Cochrane Database Syst Rev* 2:CD002041, 2000.
11. Grube BJ, Marvin JA, Heimbach DM: Therapeutic hyperbaric oxygen: Help or hindrance in burn patients with carbon monoxide poisoning? *J Burn Care Rehabil* 9:249, 1988.
12. Hampson NB, Zmaeff JL: Outcome of patients experiencing cardiac arrest with carbon monoxide poisoning treated with hyperbaric oxygen. *Ann Emerg Med* 38:36, 2001.
13. Becker CE: The role of cyanide in fires. *Vet Hum Toxicol* 27:487, 1985.
14. Charnock EL, Meehan JJ: Postburn respiratory injuries in children. *Pediatr Clin N Am* 27:661, 1980.
15. Barillo DJ, Goode R, Esch V: Cyanide poisoning in victims of fire: Analysis of 364 cases and review of the literature. *J Burn Care Rehabil* 15:46, 1994.
16. http://www.ameriburn.org/resources_factsheet.php: American Burn Association, Burn Incidence and Treatment in the US: 2007 Fact Sheet [accessed January 6, 2008].
17. Arnoldo B, Klein M, Gibran NS: Practice guidelines for the management of electrical injuries. *J Burn Care Res* 27:439, 2006.
18. Chick LR, Borah G: Calcium carbonate gel therapy for hydrofluoric acid burns of the hand. *Plast Reconstr Surg* 86:935, 1990.
19. Hatzifotis M, Williams A, Muller M, et al: Hydrofluoric acid burns. *Burns* 30:156, 2004.
20. Dunser MW, Ohlbauer M, Rieder J, et al: Critical care management of major hydrofluoric acid burns: A case report, review of the literature, and recommendations for therapy. *Burns* 30:391, 2004.
21. Jackson D: The diagnosis of the depth of burning. *J British Surg* 40:588, 1953.
22. Watts AM, Tyler MP, Perry ME, et al: Burn depth and its histological measurement. *Burns* 27:154, 2001.
23. Bray R, Forrester K, Leonard C, et al: Laser Doppler imaging of burn scars: A comparison of wavelength and scanning methods. *Burns* 29:199, 2003.
24. Mileski WJ, Atiles L, Purdue G, et al: Serial measurements increase the accuracy of laser Doppler assessment of burn wounds. *J Burn Care Rehabil* 24:187, 2003.
25. Iraniha S, Cinat ME, VanderKam VM, et al: Determination of burn depth with noncontact ultrasonography. *J Burn Care Rehabil* 21:333, 2000.
26. Zawacki BE, Azen SP, Imbus SH, et al: Multifactorial probit analysis of mortality in burn patients. *Ann Surg* 189:1, 1979.
27. Ryan CM, Schoenfeld DA, Thorpe WP, et al: Objective estimates of the probability of death from burn injuries. *N Engl J Med* 362, 1998.
28. Moreau AR, Westfall PH, Cancio LC, et al: Development and validation of an age-risk score for mortality prediction after thermal injury. *J Trauma* 58: 967, 2005.
29. Pham TN, Kramer CB, Wang J, et al: Epidemiology and outcomes of older adults with burn injury: An analysis of the National Burn Repository. *J Burn Care and Research* [In Press]
30. Thombs BD, Singh VA, Halonen J, et al: The effects of preexisting medical comorbidities on mortality and length of hospital stay in acute burn injury: Evidence from a national sample of 31,338 adult patients. *Ann Surg* 245:629, 2007.
31. McGwin G, George RL, Cross JM, et al: Improving the ability to predict mortality among burn patients. *Burns* 34:320, 2008; Epub 2007, Sep 13.
32. Jeng JC, Jablonski K, Bridgeman A, et al: Serum lactate, not base deficit, rapidly predicts survival after major burns. *Burns* 28:161, 2002.
33. Cochrane A, Edelman LS, Saffle JR, et al: The relationship of serum lactate and base deficit in burn patients to mortality. *J Burn Care Res* 28:231, 2007.
34. Cartotto R, Choi J, Gomez M, et al: A prospective study on the implications of a base deficit during fluid resuscitation. *J Burn Care Rehabil* 24:75, 2003.
35. Andel D, Kamolz LP, Roka J, et al: Base deficit and lactate: Early predictors of morbidity and mortality in patients with burns. *Burns* 33:973, 2007; Epub 2007, Oct 24.
36. Venkatesh B, Meacher R, Muller MJ, et al: Monitoring tissue oxygenation during resuscitation of major burns. *J Trauma* 50:485, 2001.
37. Lorente JA, Ezpleta A, Esteban A, et al: Systemic hemodynamics, gastric intramucosal PCO2 changes, and outcome in critically ill burn patients. *Crit Care Med* 28:1728, 2000.
38. Holm C, Mayr M, Tegeler J, et al: A clinical randomized study on the effects of invasive monitoring on burn shock resuscitation. *Burns* 30:798, 2004.
39. Cartotto RC, Innes M, Musgrave MA, et al: How well does the Parkland formula estimate actual fluid resuscitation volumes? *J Burn Care Rehabil* 23:258, 2002.
40. Engrav LH, Colescott PL, Kemalyan N, et al: A biopsy of the use of the Baxter formula to resuscitate burns or do we do it like Charlie did it? *J Burn Care Rehabil* 21:91, 2000.
41. Friedrich JB, Sullivan SR, Engrav LH, et al: Is supra-Baxter resuscitation in burn patients a new phenomenon? *Burns* 30:464, 2004.
42. Sullivan SR, Friedrich JB, Engrav LH, et al: "Opioid creep" is real and may be the cause of "fluid creep." *Burns* 30:583, 2004.
43. Navar PD, Saffle JR, Warden GD: Effect of inhalation injury on fluid resuscitation requirements after thermal injury. *Am J Surg* 150:716, 1985.
44. Dai NT, Chen TM, Cheng TY, et al: The comparison of early fluid therapy in extensive flame burns between inhalation and noninhalation injuries. *Burns* 24:671, 1998.
45. Cancio LC, Chavez S, Alvarado-Ortega M, et al: Predicting increased fluid requirements during the resuscitation of thermally injured patients. *J Trauma* 56:404, 2004.
46. Klein MB, Hayden D, Elson C, et al: The association between fluid administration and outcome following major burn: A multicenter study. *Ann Surg* 245:622, 2007.
47. O'Mara MS, Slater H, Goldfarb IW, et al: A prospective, randomized evaluation of intra-abdominal pressures with crystalloid and colloid resuscitation in burn patients. *J Trauma* 58:1011, 2005.
48. Cochrane A, Morris SE, Edelman LS, et al: Burn patient characteristics and outcomes following resuscitation with albumin. *Burns* 33:25, 2007.
49. Perel P, Roberts I: Colloids versus crystalloids for fluid resuscitation in critically ill patients. *Cochrane Database Syst Rev* 4:CD000567, 2007.

50. Kinsky MP, Milner SM, Button B, et al: Resuscitation of severe thermal injury with hypertonic saline dextran: Effects on peripheral and visceral edema in sheep. *J Trauma* 49: 844, 2000.

51. Tanaka H, Matsuda T, Miyagantani Y, et al: Reduction of resuscitation fluid volumes in severely burned patients using ascorbic acid administration: A randomized, prospective study. *Arch Surg* 135:326, 2000.

52. Warden GD, Stratta RJ, Saffle JR, et al: Plasma exchange therapy in patients failing to resuscitate from burn shock. *J Trauma* 23:945, 1983.

53. Palmieri TL, Caruso DM, Foster KN, et al: Effect of blood transfusion on outcome after major burn injury: A multicenter study. *Crit Care Med* 34:1602, 2006.

54. Palmieri TL, Lee T, O'Mara MS, et al: Effects of a restrictive blood transfusion policy on outcomes in children with burn injury. *J Burn Care Res* 28:65, 2007.

55. Higgins S, Fowler R, Callum J, et al: Transfusion-related acute lung injury in patients with burns. *J Burn Care Res* 28:56, 2007.

56. Still JM Jr., Belcher K, Law EJ, et al: A double-blinded prospective evaluation of recombinant human erythropoietin in acutely burned patients. *J Trauma* 38:233, 1995.

57. Muller MJ, Pegg SP, Rule MR: Determinants of death following burn injury. *Br J Surg* 88:583, 2001.

58. Tredget EE, Shankowsky HA, Taerum TV, et al: The role of inhalation injury in burn trauma. A Canadian experience. *Ann Surg* 212:720, 1990.

59. Shirani KZ, Pruitt BA, Mason AD: The influence of inhalation injury and pneumonia on burn mortality. *Ann Surg* 205:82, 1987.

60. Wright MJ, Murphy JT: Smoke inhalation enhances early alveolar leukocyte responsiveness to endotoxin. *J Trauma* 59:64, 2005.

61. Darling GE, Keresteci MA, Ibanez D, et al: Pulmonary complications in inhalation injuries with associated cutaneous burn. *J Trauma* 40:83, 1996.

62. Jones WG, Barie PS, Madden M, et al: The use of compliance in predicting early mortality after inhalation injury. *Curr Surg* 45:309, 1988.

63. Mlcak R, Cortiella J, Desai M, et al: Lung compliance, airway resistance, and work of breathing in children after inhalation injury. *J Burn Care Rehabil* 18:531, 1997.

64. Demling R, Lalonde C, Youn YK, et al: Effect of graded increases in smoke inhalation injury on the early systemic response to a body burn. *Crit Care Med* 23:171, 1995.

65. Gore MA, Joshi AR, Nagarajan G, et al: Virtual bronchoscopy for diagnosis of inhalation injury in burnt patients. *Burns* 30:165, 2004.

66. Schall GL, McDonald HD, Carr LB, et al: Xenon ventilation-perfusion lung scans: The early diagnosis of inhalation injury. *JAMA* 240:2441, 1978.

67. Evidence-based surgery. *J Am Coll Surg* 196:308, 2003.

68. Heimbach DM, Waeckerle JF: Inhalation injuries. *Ann Emerg Med* 17:1316, 1988.

69. Endorf F, Gamelli RL: Inhalation injury, pulmonary perturbations, and fluid resuscitation. *J Burn Care Res* 28:80, 2007.

70. Ramzy PI, Barret JP, Herndon DN: Thermal Injury. *Crit Care Clin* 15:333, 1999.

71. Enkhbaatar P, Murakami K, Cox R, et al: Aerosolized tissue plasminogen inhibitor improves pulmonary function in sheep with burn and smoke inhalation. *Shock* 22:70, 2004.

72. Murakami K, McGuire R, Cox RA, et al: Recombinant antithrombin attenuates pulmonary inflammation following smoke inhalation and pneumonia in sheep. *Crit Care Med* 31:577, 2003.

73. Pallua N, Warbanow K, Noah EM, et al: Intrabronchial surfactant application in cases of inhalation injury: First results from patients with severe burns and ARDS. *Burns* 24:197, 1998.

74. Sheridan RL, Zapol WM, Ritz RH, et al: Low-dose inhaled nitric oxide in acutely burned children with profound respiratory failure. *Surgery* 126:856, 1999.

75. Moylan JA, Alexander LG Jr.: Diagnosis and treatment of inhalation injury. *World J Surg* 2:185, 1978.

76. Thompson BT: Glucocorticoids and acute lung injury. *Crit Care Med* 31:S253, 2003.

77. Hollingsed TC, Saffle JR, Barton RG, et al: Etiology and consequences of respiratory failure in thermally injured patients. *Am J Surg* 166:592, 1993.

78. The Acute Respiratory Distress Syndrome Network: Ventilation with lower tidal volumes as compared with traditional tidal volumes for acute lung injury and the acute respiratory distress syndrome. *N Engl J Med* 342:1301, 2000.

79. Sheridan RL, Kacmarek RM, McEttrick MM, et al: Permissive hypercapnia as a ventilatory strategy in burned children: Effect on barotrauma, pneumonia, and mortality. *J Trauma* 39:854, 1995.

80. Venet C, Guyomarc'h S, Migeot C, et al: The oxygenation variations related to prone positioning during mechanical ventilation: A clinical comparison between ARDS and non-ARDS hypoxemic patients. *Intensive Care Med* 27:1352, 2001.

81. Reper P, Van Bos R, Van Loey K, et al: High frequency percussive ventilation in burn patients: Hemodynamics and gas exchange. *Burns* 29:603, 2003.

82. Hall JJ, Hunt JL, Arnoldo BD, et al: Use of high-frequency percussive ventilation in inhalation injuries. *J Burn Care Res* 28:396, 2007.

83. Cartotto R, Ellis S, Gomez M, et al: High frequency oscillatory ventilation in burn patients with the acute respiratory distress syndrome. *Burns* 30:453, 2004.

84. Patton ML, Simone MR, Kraut JD, et al: Successful utilization of ECMO to treat an adult burn patient with ARDS. *Burns* 24:566, 1998.

85. Schmalstieg FC, Keeney SE, Rudloff HE, et al: Arteriovenous CO2 removal improves survival compared to high frequency percussive and low tidal volume ventilation in a smoke/burn sheep acute respiratory distress syndrome model. *Ann Surg* 246:512, 2007; discussion 521.

86. Hart DW, Wolf SE, Mlcak R, et al: Persistence of muscle catabolism after severe burn. *Surgery* 128:312, 2000.

87. Hart DW, Wolf SE, Chinkes DL, et al: Determinants of skeletal muscle catabolism after severe burn. *Ann Surg* 232:455, 2000.

88. Gottschlich MM, Jenkins ME, Mayes T, et al: The 2002 clinical research award: An evaluation of the safety of early vs. delayed enteral support and effects on clinical, nutritional, and endocrine outcomes after severe burns. *J Burn Care Rehabil* 23:401, 2002.

89. Hart DW, Wolf SE, Chinkes DL, et al: Effects of early excision and aggressive enteral feeding on hypermetabolism, catabolism, and sepsis after severe burn. *J Trauma* 54:755, 2003.

90. Jeschke MG, Herndon DN, Ebener C, et al: Nutritional intervention high in vitamins, protein, amino acids, and (omega)3 fatty acids improves protein metabolism during the hypermetabolic state after thermal injury. *Arch Surg* 136:1301, 2001.

91. Sefton EJ, Boulton-Jones JR, Anderton D, et al: Enteral feeding in patients with major burn injury: The use of nasojejunal feeding after the failure of nasogastric feeding. *Burns* 28:386, 2002.

92. Jenkins ME, Gottschlich MM, Warden GD: Enteral feeding during operative procedures in thermal injuries. *J Burn Care Rehabil* 15:199, 1994.

93. Garrel D, Patenaude J, Nedelec B, et al: Decreased mortality and infectious morbidity in adult burn patients given enteral glutamine supplements: A prospective, controlled, randomized clinical trial. *Crit Care Med* 31:2444, 2003.

94. Choudry MA, Haque F, Khan M, et al: Enteral nutritional supplementation prevents mesenteric lymph node T-cell suppression in burn injury. *Crit Care Med* 31:1764, 2003.

95. Curreri PW, Richmond D, et al: Dietary requirements of patients with major burns. *J Am Diet Assoc* 65:415, 1974.

96. Liusuwan RA, Palmieri TL, Kinoshita L, et al: Comparison of measured resting energy expenditure versus predictive equations in pediatric burn patients. *J Burn Care Rehabil* 26:464, 2005.

97. Hart DW, Wolf SE, Herndon DN: Energy expenditure and caloric balance after burn: Increased feeding leads to fat rather than lean mass accretion. *Ann Surg* 235:152, 2002.

98. Herndon DN, Hart DW, Wolf SE, et al: Reversal of catabolism by beta-blockade after severe burns. *N Engl J Med* 345:1223, 2001.

99. Arbabi S, Ahrns KS, Wahl WL, et al: Beta-blocker use is associated with improved outcomes in adult burn patients. *J Trauma* 56:265, 2004; discussion 269.

100. Murphy KD, Thomas S, Mlcak RP, et al: Effects of long-term oxandrolone administration in severely burned children. *Surgery* 136:219, 2004.

101. Demling RH, DeSanti L: Oxandrolone induced lean mass gain during recovery from severe burns is maintained after discontinuation of the anabolic steroid. *Burns* 29:793, 2003.

102. Jeschke MG, Finnerty CC, Suman OE, et al: The effect of oxandrolone on the endocrinologic, inflammatory, and hypermetabolic responses during the acute phase postburn. *Ann Surg* 246:351, 2007; discussion 360.

103. Van den Berghe G, Wouters P, Weekers F, et al: Intensive insulin therapy in critically ill patients. *N Engl J Med* 345:1359, 2001.

104. Thomas SJ, Morimoto K, Herndon DN, et al: The effect of prolonged euglycemic hyperinsulinemia on lean body mass after severe burn. *Surgery* 132:341, 2002.

105. Jeschke MG, Klein D, Herndon DN. Insulin treatment improves the systemic inflammatory reaction to severe trauma. *Ann Surg* 239:553, 2004.

106. Gore DC, Wolf SE, Sanford A, et al: Influence of metformin on glucose intolerance and muscle catabolism following severe burn injury. *Ann Surg* 241:334, 2005.

107. Pham TN, Neff MJ, Simmons JM, et al: The clinical pulmonary infection score poorly predicts pneumonia in patients with burns. *J Burn Care Res* 28:76, 2007.

108. Barret JP, Desai MH, Herndon DN: Effects of tracheostomies on infection and airway complications in pediatric burn patients. *Burns* 26:190, 2000.

109. Saffle JR, Morris SE, Edelman L: Early tracheostomy does not improve outcome in burn patients. *J Burn Care Rehabil* 23:431, 2002.

110. Gravvanis AI, Tsoutsos DA, Iconomou TG, et al: Percutaneous versus conventional tracheostomy in burned patients with inhalation injury. *World J Surg* 29:1571, 2005.

111. Hershberger RC, Hunt JL, Arnoldo BD, et al: Abdominal compartment syndrome in the severely burned patient. *J Burn Care Res* 28:708, 2007.

112. Faucher LD, Conlon KM: Practice guidelines for deep venous thrombosis prophylaxis in burns. *J Burn Care Res* 28:661, 2007.

113. Wibbenmeyer LA, Hoballah JJ, Amelon MJ, et al: The prevalence of venous thromboembolism of the lower extremity among thermally injured patients determined by duplex sonography. *J Trauma* 55:1162, 2003.

114. Wahl WL, Brandt MM, Ahrns KS, et al: Venous thrombosis incidence in burn patients: Preliminary results of a prospective study. *J Burn Care Rehabil* 23:97, 2002.

115. Fecher AM, O'Mara MS, Goldfarb IW, et al: Analysis of deep vein thrombosis in burn patients. *Burns* 30:591, 2004.

116. Scott JR, Klein MB, Gernsheimer T, et al: Arterial and venous complications of heparin-induced thrombocytopenia in burn patients. *J Burn Care Res* 28:71, 2007.

117. O'Mara MS, Reed NL, Palmieri TL, et al: Central venous catheter infections in burn patients with scheduled catheter exchange and replacement. *J Surg Res* 142:341, 2007; Epub 2007, Jul 12.

118. Engrav LH, Heimbach DM, Reus JL, et al: Early excision and grafting vs. nonoperative treatment of burns of indeterminant depth: A randomized prospective study. *J Trauma* 23:1001, 1983.

119. Thompson P, Herndon DN, Abston S, et al: Effect of early excision on patients with major thermal injury. *J Trauma* 27:205, 1987.

120. Sheridan RL, Tompkins RG: What's new in burns and metabolism. *J Am Coll Surg* 198:243, 2004.

121. Klein MB, Hunter S, Heimbach DM, et al: The Versajet water dissector: A new tool for tangential excision. *J Burn Care Rehabil* 26:483, 2005.

122. Jones I, Currie L, Martin R: A guide to biological skin substitutes. *Br J Plast Surg* 55:185, 2002.

123. Kearney JN: Clinical evaluation of skin substitutes. *Burns* 27:545, 2001.

124. Compton CC, Gill JM, Bradford DA, et al: Skin regenerated from cultured epithelial autografts on full-thickness burn wounds from 6 days to 5 years after grafting. A light, electron microscopic and immunohistochemical study. *Lab Invest* 60:600, 1989.

125. Boyce ST, Kagan RJ, Yakuboff KP, et al: Cultured skin substitutes reduce donor skin harvesting for closure of excised, full-thickness burns. *Ann Surg* 235:269, 2002.

126. Fauerbach JA, McKibben J, Bienvenu OJ, et al: Psychological distress after major burn injury. *Psychosom Med* 69:473, 2007.

127. Christiansen M, Carrougher GJ, Engrav LH, et al: Time to school re-entry after burn injury is quite short. *J Burn Care Res* 28:478, 2007; discussion 482.

128. Ballesteros MF, Jackson ML, Martin MW: Working toward the elimination of residential fire deaths: The Centers for Disease Control and Prevention's Smoke Alarm Installation and Fire Safety Education (SAIFE) Program. *J Burn Care Rehabil* 26:434, 2005.

129. DiGuiseppi C, Roberts I, Wade A, et al: Incidence of fires and related injuries after giving out free smoke alarms: Cluster randomised controlled trial. *Br Med J* 325:995, 2002.

130. Fallat ME, Rengers SJ: The effect of education and safety devices on scald burn prevention. *J Trauma* 34:560, 1993.

131. Cagle KM, Davis JW, Dominic W, et al: Results of a focused scald-prevention program. *J Burn Care Res* 27:859, 2006.

132. Barber RC, Aragaki CC, Chang LY, et al: CD14-159 C allele is associated with increased risk of mortality after burn injury. *Shock* 27:232, 2007.

133. Barber RC, Chang LY, Arnoldo BD, et al: Innate immunity SNPs are associated with risk for severe sepsis after burn injury. *Clin Med Res* 4:250, 2006.

134. Moore CB, Medina MA, van Deventer HW, et al: Downregulation of immune signaling genes in patients with large surface burn injury. *J Burn Care Res* 28:879, 2007.

135. Klein MB, Silver G, Gamelli RL, et al: Inflammation and the Host Response to Injury Investigators. Inflammation and the host response to injury: An overview of the multicenter study of the genomic and proteomic response to burn injury. *J Burn Care Res* 27:448, 2006.

Wound Healing

Adrian Barbul and David T. Efron

HISTORY OF WOUND HEALING

The earliest accounts of wound healing date back to about 2000 B.C., when the Sumerians employed two modes of treatment: a spiritual method consisting of incantations and a physical method of applying poultice-like materials to the wound. The Egyptians were the first to differentiate between infected and diseased wounds compared to noninfected wounds. The 1650 B.C. Edwin Smith Surgical Papyrus, a copy of a much older document, describes at least 48 different types of wounds. A later document (Ebers Papyrus, 1550 B.C.) relates the use of concoctions containing honey (antibacterial properties), lint (absorbent properties), and grease (barrier) for treating wounds. These same properties are still considered essential in contemporary daily wound management.

The Greeks, equipped with the knowledge bequeathed by the Egyptians, went even further and classified wounds as acute or chronic in nature. Galen of Pergamum (120–201 A.D.), appointed as the doctor to the Roman gladiators, had an enormous number of wounds to deal with after gladiatorial combats. He emphasized the importance of maintaining a moist environment to ensure adequate healing. It took almost 19 centuries for this important concept to be proven scientifically, when it was shown that the epithelialization rate increases by 50% in a moist wound environment when compared to a dry wound environment.[1]

The next major stride in the history of wound healing was the discovery of antiseptics and their importance in reducing wound infections. Ignaz Philipp Semmelweis, a Hungarian obstetrician (1818–1865), noted that the incidence of puerperal fever was much lower if medical students, after cadaver-dissection class and before attending childbirth, washed their hands with soap and hypochlorite. Louis Pasteur (1822–1895) was instrumental in dispelling the theory of spontaneous generation of germs and proving that germs were always introduced into the wound from the environment. Joseph Lister probably made one of the most significant contributions to wound healing. On a visit to Glasgow, Scotland, Lister noted that some areas of the city's sewer system were less murky than the rest. He discovered that the water from pipes that were dumping waste containing carbolic acid (phenol) was clear. In 1865, Lister began soaking his instruments in phenol and spraying the operating rooms, reducing the mortality rates from 50 to 15%. This practice led to the suspension of Lister, although subsequent confirmation of his results paved the way for his triumphant return to Edinburgh.

After attending an impressive lecture by Lister in 1876, Robert Wood Johnson left the meeting and began 10 years of research that would ultimately result in the production of an antiseptic dressing in the form of cotton gauze impregnated with iodoform. Since then, several other materials have been used to impregnate cotton gauze to achieve antisepsis.

Polymeric dressings were developed in the 1960s and 1970s. These polymeric dressings can be custom made to specific parameters, such as permeability to gases (occlusive vs. semiocclusive), varying degrees of absorbency, and different physical forms. Due to the ability to customize, the available range of materials that aid in wound care has grown exponentially to include an ever-expanding variety. Currently, the practice of wound healing encompasses manipulation and/or use of, among others, inflammatory cytokines, growth factors, and bioengineered tissue. It is the combination of all these modalities that enables optimal wound healing.

PHASES OF WOUND HEALING

As noted by John Hunter (1728–1793), a keen observer of biologic phenomena, "... the injury alone has in all cases a tendency to produce the disposition and the means of a cure."[2] Normal wound healing follows a predictable pattern that can be divided into overlapping phases defined by characteristic cellular populations and biochemical activities: (a) hemostasis and inflammation, (b) proliferation, and (c) maturation and remodeling. An approximate timeline of these events is depicted in Fig. 9-1. This sequence of events is fluid and overlapping, and in most circumstances spans the time from injury to resolution of acute wounds. All wounds need to progress through this series of cellular and biochemical events that characterizes the phases of healing to successfully re-establish tissue integrity.

Hemostasis and Inflammation

Hemostasis precedes and initiates inflammation, with the ensuing release of chemotactic factors from the wound site (Fig. 9-2A). Wounding by definition disrupts tissue integrity, leading to division of blood vessels and direct exposure of extracellular matrix to platelets. Exposure of subendothelial collagen to platelets results in platelet aggregation, degranulation, and activation of the coagulation cascade. Platelet α-granules release a number of wound-active substances, such as platelet-derived growth factor (PDGF), transforming growth factor beta (TGFβ), platelet-activating factor, fibronectin, and serotonin. In addition to achieving hemostasis, the fibrin clot serves as scaffolding for the migration into the wound of inflammatory cells such as polymorphonuclear leukocytes (PMNs, neutrophils) and monocytes.

Cellular infiltration after injury follows a characteristic, predetermined sequence (see Fig. 9-1). PMNs are the first infiltrating cells to enter the wound site, peaking at 24 to 48 hours. Increased vascular permeability, local prostaglandin release, and the presence of chemotactic substances, such as complement factors, interleukin-1 (IL-1), tumor necrosis factor alpha (TNF-α), TGFβ, platelet factor 4, or bacterial products, all stimulate neutrophil migration.

KEY POINTS

1. Wound healing is a complex cellular and biochemical cascade that leads to restitution of integrity and function.

2. Although individual tissues may have unique healing characteristics, all tissues heal by similar mechanisms, and the process undergoes phases of inflammation, cellular migration, proliferation, matrix deposition, and remodeling.

3. Factors that impede normal healing include local, systemic, and technical conditions that the surgeon must take into account.

4. Optimal outcome of acute wounds relies on complete evaluation of the patient and of the wound, and application of best practices and techniques.

5. Clinically, excess healing can be as significant a problem as impaired healing; genetic, technical, and local factors play a major role.

6. Future advances in growth factor understanding, tissue engineering, and dressing design are expected to increase the armamentarium in improving wound outcomes.

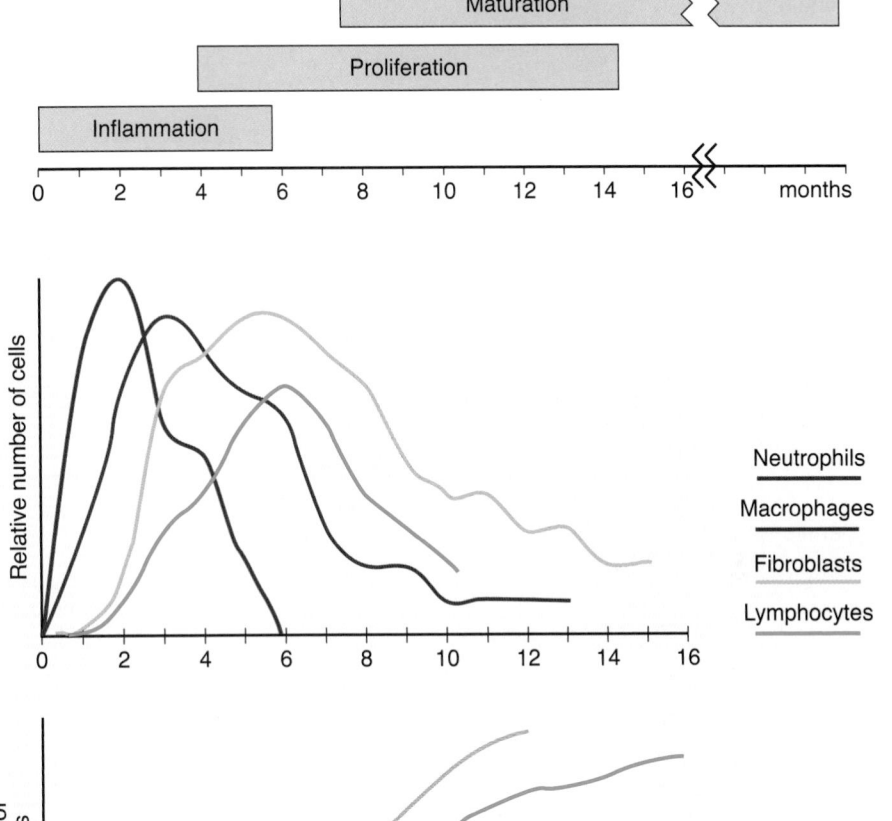

FIG. 9-1. The cellular, biochemical, and mechanical phases of wound healing.

The postulated primary role of neutrophils is phagocytosis of bacteria and tissue debris. PMNs are also a major source of cytokines early during inflammation, especially TNF-α,[3] which may have a significant influence on subsequent angiogenesis and collagen synthesis (see Fig. 9-2B). PMNs also release proteases such as collagenases, which participate in matrix and ground substance degradation in the early phase of wound healing. Other than their role in limiting infections, these cells do not appear to play a role in collagen deposition or acquisition of mechanical wound strength. On the contrary, neutrophil factors have been implicated in delaying the epithelial closure of wounds.[4]

The second population of inflammatory cells that invades the wound consists of macrophages, which are recognized as being essential to successful healing.[5] Derived from circulating monocytes, macrophages achieve significant numbers in the wound by 48 to 96 hours postinjury and remain present until wound healing is complete.

Macrophages, like neutrophils, participate in wound débridement via phagocytosis and contribute to microbial stasis via oxygen radical and nitric oxide synthesis (see Fig. 9-2C). The macrophage's most pivotal function is activation and recruitment of other cells via

mediators such as cytokines and growth factors, as well as directly by cell–cell interaction and intercellular adhesion molecules. By releasing such mediators as TGFβ, vascular endothelial growth factor (VEGF), insulin-like growth factor, epithelial growth factor, and lactate, macrophages regulate cell proliferation, matrix synthesis, and angiogenesis.[6,7] Macrophages also play a significant role in regulating angiogenesis and matrix deposition and remodeling (Table 9-1).

T lymphocytes comprise another population of inflammatory/immune cells that routinely invades the wound. Less numerous than macrophages, T-lymphocyte numbers peak at about 1 week postinjury and truly bridge the transition from the inflammatory to the proliferative phase of healing. Although known to be essential to wound healing, the lymphocytes' role in wound healing is not fully defined.[8] A significant body of data supports the hypothesis that T lymphocytes play an active role in the modulation of the wound environment. Depletion of most wound T lymphocytes decreases wound strength and collagen content,[9] whereas selective depletion of the CD8+ suppressor subset of T lymphocytes enhances wound healing. However, depletion of the CD4+ helper subset has no effect.[10] Lymphocytes also exert a downregulating effect on fibroblast collagen synthesis by cell-associated interferon-γ, TNF-α, and

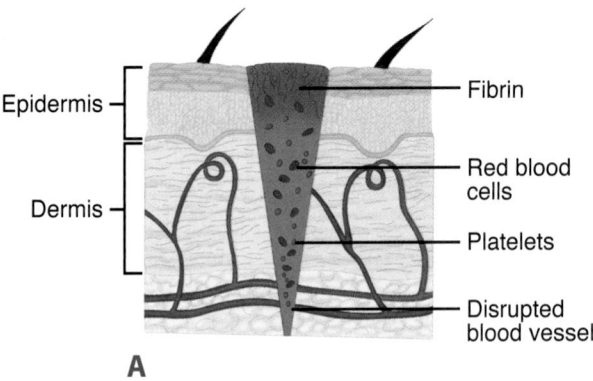

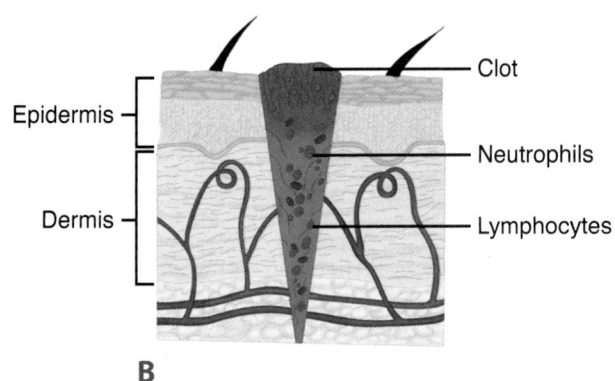

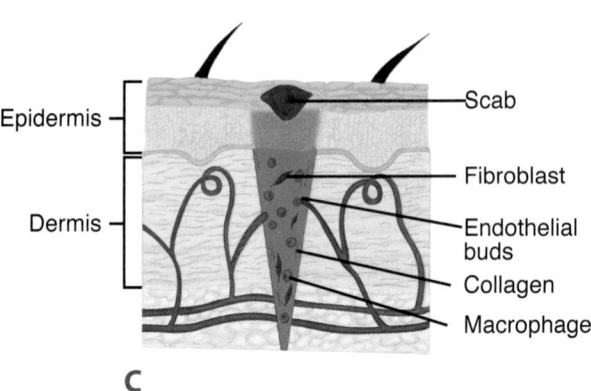

FIG. 9-2. The phases of wound healing viewed histologically. **A.** The hemostatic/inflammatory phase. **B.** Latter inflammatory phases reflecting infiltration by mononuclear cells and lymphocytes. **C.** The proliferative phase, with associated angiogenesis and collagen synthesis.

IL-1. This effect is lost if the cells are physically separated, suggesting that extracellular matrix synthesis is regulated not only via soluble factors but also by direct cell–cell contact between lymphocytes and fibroblasts.[11]

Proliferation

The proliferative phase is the second phase of wound healing and roughly spans days 4 through 12 (see Fig. 9-2C). It is during this phase that tissue continuity is re-established. Fibroblasts and endothelial cells are the last cell populations to infiltrate the healing wound, and the strongest chemotactic factor for fibroblasts is PDGF.[12,13] Upon entering the wound environment, recruited fibroblasts first need to proliferate, and then become activated, to carry out their primary function of matrix synthesis remodeling. This

TABLE 9-1	Macrophage activities during wound healing
Activity	**Mediators**
Phagocytosis	Reactive oxygen species
	Nitric oxide
Débridement	Collagenase, elastase
Cell recruitment and activation	Growth factors: PDGF, TGFβ, EGF, IGF
	Cytokines: TNF-α, IL-1, IL-6
	Fibronectin
Matrix synthesis	Growth factors: TGFβ, EGF, PDGF
	Cytokines: TNF-α, IL-1, IFN-γ
	Enzymes: arginase, collagenase
	Prostaglandins
	Nitric oxide
Angiogenesis	Growth factors: FGF, VEGF
	Cytokines: TNF-α
	Nitric oxide

EGF = epithelial growth factor; FGF = fibroblast growth factor; IGF = insulin-like growth factor; IFN-γ = interferon-γ; IL = interleukin; PDGF = platelet-derived growth factor; TGFβ = transforming growth factor beta; TNF-α = tumor necrosis factor alpha; VEGF = vascular endothelial growth factor.

activation is mediated mainly by the cytokines and growth factors released from wound macrophages.

Fibroblasts isolated from wounds synthesize more collagen than nonwound fibroblasts, they proliferate less, and they actively carry out matrix contraction. Although it is clear that the cytokine-rich wound environment plays a significant role in this phenotypic alteration and activation, the exact mediators are only partially characterized.[14,15] Additionally, lactate, which accumulates in significant amounts in the wound environment over time (~10 mmol), is a potent regulator of collagen synthesis through a mechanism involving adenosine 5′-diphosphate–ribosylation.[16,17]

Endothelial cells also proliferate extensively during this phase of healing. These cells participate in the formation of new capillaries (angiogenesis), a process essential to successful wound healing. Endothelial cells migrate from intact venules close to the wound. Their migration, replication, and new capillary tubule formation are under the influence of such cytokines and growth factors as TNF-α, TGFβ, and VEGF. Although many cells produce VEGF, macrophages represent a major source in the healing wound, and VEGF receptors are located specifically on endothelial cells.[18,19]

Matrix Synthesis
Biochemistry of Collagen

Collagen, the most abundant protein in the body, plays a critical role in the successful completion of adult wound healing. Its deposition, maturation, and subsequent remodeling are essential to the functional integrity of the wound.

Although there are at least 18 types of collagen described, the main ones of interest to wound repair are types I and III. Type I collagen is the major component of extracellular matrix in skin. Type III, which is also normally present in skin, becomes more prominent and important during the repair process.

Biochemically, each chain of collagen is composed of a glycine residue in every third position. The second position in the triplet is made up of proline or lysine during the translation process. The polypeptide chain that is translated from messenger RNA (mRNA) contains approximately 1000 amino acid residues and is called *protocollagen*. Release of protocollagen into the endoplasmic reticulum results in the hydroxylation of proline to hydroxyproline and of lysine to hydroxylysine by specific hydroxylases (Fig. 9-3). Prolyl hydroxylase requires oxygen and iron as cofactors, α-ketoglutarate as cosubstrate, and ascorbic acid (vitamin C) as an electron donor. In the endoplasmic reticulum, the protocollagen chain is also glycosylated by the linking of galactose and glucose at specific hydroxylysine

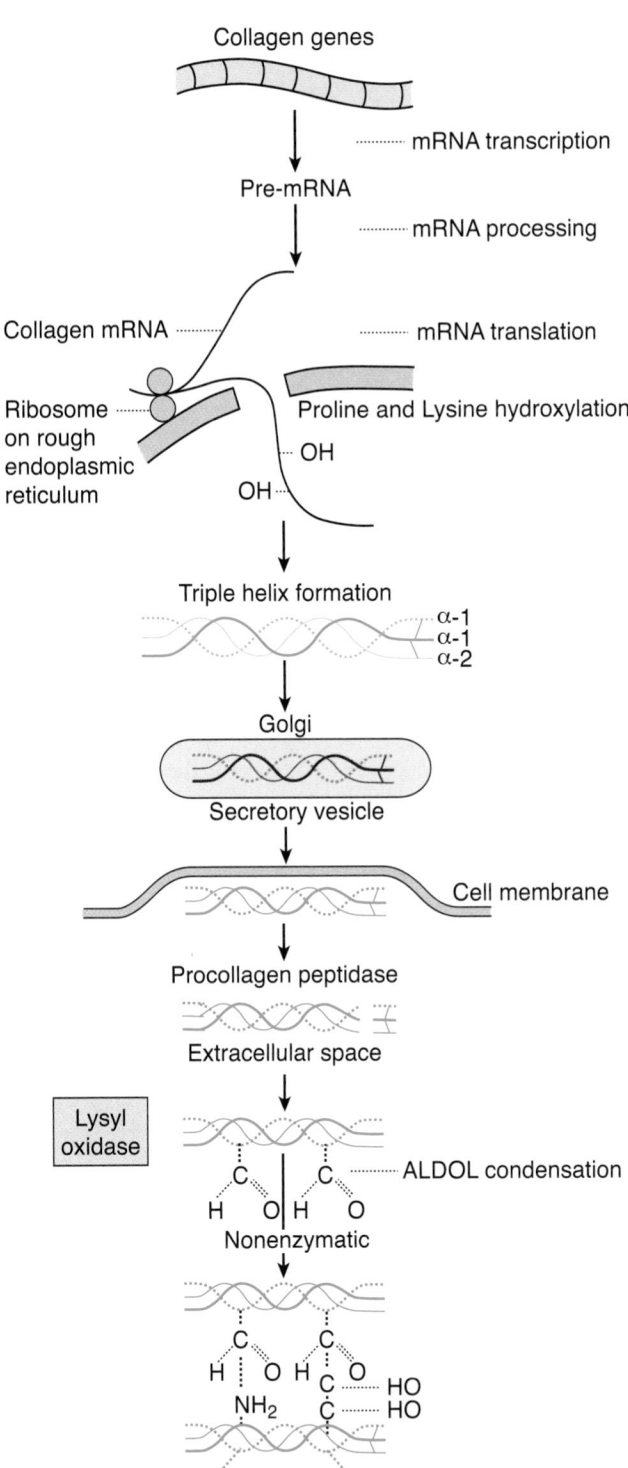

FIG. 9-3. The steps of collagen synthesis. mRNA = messenger RNA.

further polymerization and cross-linking. The resulting collagen monomer is further polymerized and cross-linked by the formation of intra- and intermolecular covalent bonds.

Collagen synthesis, as well as posttranslational modifications, is highly dependent on systemic factors such as an adequate oxygen supply, the presence of sufficient nutrients (amino acids and carbohydrates) and cofactors (vitamins and trace metals), and the local wound environment (vascular supply and lack of infection). Addressing these factors and reversing nutritional deficiencies can optimize collagen synthesis and deposition.

Proteoglycan Synthesis

Glycosaminoglycans comprise a large portion of the "ground substance" that makes up granulation tissue. Rarely found free, they couple with proteins to form *proteoglycans*. The polysaccharide chain is made up of repeating disaccharide units composed of glucuronic or iduronic acid and a hexosamine, which is usually sulfated. The disaccharide composition of proteoglycans varies from about 10 units in the case of heparan sulfate to as much as 2000 units in the case of hyaluronic acid.

The major glycosaminoglycans present in wounds are dermatan and chondroitin sulfate. Fibroblasts synthesize these compounds, increasing their concentration greatly during the first 3 weeks of healing. The interaction between collagen and proteoglycans is being actively studied. It is thought that the assembly of collagen subunits into fibrils and fibers is dependent on the lattice provided by the sulfated proteoglycans. Furthermore, it appears that the extent of sulfation is critical in determining the configuration of the collagen fibrils. As scar collagen is deposited, the proteoglycans are incorporated into the collagen scaffolding. However, with scar maturation and collagen remodeling, the content of proteoglycans gradually diminishes.

Maturation and Remodeling

The maturation and remodeling of the scar begins during the fibroplastic phase, and is characterized by a reorganization of previously synthesized collagen. Collagen is broken down by matrix metalloproteinases, and the net wound collagen content is the result of a balance between collagenolysis and collagen synthesis. There is a net shift toward collagen synthesis and eventually the re-establishment of extracellular matrix composed of a relatively acellular collagen-rich scar.

Wound strength and mechanical integrity in the fresh wound are determined by both the quantity and quality of the newly deposited collagen. The deposition of matrix at the wound site follows a characteristic pattern: Fibronectin and collagen type III constitute the early matrix scaffolding, glycosaminoglycans and proteoglycans represent the next significant matrix components, and collagen type I is the final matrix. By several weeks postinjury the amount of collagen in the wound reaches a plateau, but the tensile strength continues to increase for several more months.[20] Fibril formation and fibril cross-linking result in decreased collagen solubility, increased strength, and increased resistance to enzymatic degradation of the collagen matrix. Scar remodeling continues for many (6 to 12) months postinjury, gradually resulting in a mature, avascular, and acellular scar. The mechanical strength of the scar never achieves that of the uninjured tissue.

There is a constant turnover of collagen in the extracellular matrix, both in the healing wound, as well as during normal tissue homeostasis. Collagenolysis is the result of collagenase activity, a class of matrix metalloproteinases that require activation. Both collagen synthesis and lysis are strictly controlled by cytokines and growth factors. Some factors affect both aspects of collagen remodeling. For example, TGFβ increases new collagen transcription and also decreases collagen breakdown by stimulating synthesis of tissue inhibitors of metalloproteinase.[21] This balance of collagen deposition and degradation is the ultimate determinant of wound strength and integrity.

residues. These steps of hydroxylation and glycosylation alter the hydrogen bonding forces within the chain, imposing steric changes that force the protocollagen chain to assume an α-helical configuration. Three α-helical chains entwine to form a right-handed superhelical structure called *procollagen*. At both ends, this structure contains nonhelical peptide domains called *registration peptides*. Although initially joined by weak, ionic bonds, the procollagen molecule becomes much stronger by the covalent cross-linking of lysine residues.

Extracellularly, the nonhelical registration peptides are cleaved by a procollagen peptidase, and the procollagen strands undergo

Epithelialization

While tissue integrity and strength are being re-established, the external barrier must also be restored. This process is characterized primarily by proliferation and migration of epithelial cells adjacent to the wound (Fig. 9-4). The process begins within 1 day of injury and is seen as thickening of the epidermis at the wound edge. Marginal basal cells at the edge of the wound lose their firm attachment to the underlying dermis, enlarge, and begin to migrate across the surface of the provisional matrix. Fixed basal cells in a zone near the cut edge undergo a series of rapid mitotic divisions, and these cells appear to migrate by moving over one another in a leapfrog fashion until the defect is covered.[22] Once the defect is bridged, the migrating epithelial cells lose their flattened appearance, become more columnar in shape, and increase their mitotic activity. Layering of the epithelium is re-established, and the surface layer eventually keratinizes.[23]

Re-epithelialization is complete in less than 48 hours in the case of approximated incised wounds, but may take substantially longer in the case of larger wounds, in which there is a significant epidermal/dermal defect. If only the epithelium and superficial dermis are damaged, such as occurs in split-thickness skin graft donor sites or in superficial second-degree burns, then repair consists primarily of re-epithelialization with minimal or no fibroplasia and granulation tissue formation. The stimuli for re-epithelialization remain incompletely defined; however, it appears that the process is mediated by a combination of a loss of contact inhibition; exposure to constituents of the extracellular matrix, particularly fibronectin; and cytokines produced by immune mononuclear cells.[24,25] In particular, epithelial growth factor, TGFβ, basic fibroblast growth factor, PDGF, and insulin-like growth factor I have been shown to promote epithelialization.

Role of Growth Factors in Normal Healing

Growth factors and cytokines are polypeptides produced in normal and wounded tissue that stimulate cellular migration, proliferation, and function. They often are named for the cells from which they were first derived (e.g., platelet-derived growth factor, PDGF) or for their initially identified function (e.g., fibroblast growth factor). These names are often misleading, because growth factors have been demonstrated to have multiple functions. Most growth factors are extremely potent and produce significant effects in nanomolar concentrations.

They may act in an autocrine manner (in which the growth factor acts on the cell producing it), a paracrine manner (by release into the extracellular environment, where it acts on the immediately neighboring cells), or in an endocrine manner (in which the effect of the substance is distant to the site of release, and the substance is carried to the effector site through the bloodstream). The timing of release may be as important as concentration in determining the effectiveness of growth factors. As these polypeptides exert their effects by cell-surface receptor binding, the appropriate receptor on the responding cells must be present at the time of release for the biologic effect to occur. Table 9-2 summarizes the principal growth factors found in healing wounds and their known effects on cells participating in the healing process. Growth factors have divergent actions on different cells; they can be chemoattractive to one cell type while stimulating replication of a different cell type. Little is known about the ratio of growth factor concentrations, which may be as important as the absolute concentration of individual growth factors.

Growth factors act on cells via surface receptor binding. Various receptor types have been described, such as ion channels, G-protein linked, or enzyme linked. The response elicited in the cell is usually one of phosphorylation or dephosphorylation of second-messenger molecules through the action of phosphatases or kinases, resulting in activation or deactivation of proteins in the cytosol or nucleus of the target cell. Phosphorylation of nuclear proteins is followed by the initiation of transcription of target genes.[26] The signal is stopped by internalization of the receptor-ligand complex.

Wound Contraction

All wounds undergo some degree of contraction. For wounds that do not have surgically approximated edges, the area of the wound will be decreased by this action (healing by secondary intention); the shortening of the scar itself results in contracture. The myofibroblast has been postulated as being the major cell responsible for contraction, and it differs from the normal fibroblast in that it possesses a cytoskeletal structure. Typically this cell contains α-smooth muscle actin in thick bundles called *stress fibers*, giving myofibroblasts contractile capability.[27] The α-smooth muscle actin is undetectable until day 6, and then is increasingly expressed for the next 15 days of wound healing.[28] After 4 weeks this expression fades, and the cells are believed to undergo apoptosis.[29] A puzzling point is that the identification of myofibroblasts in the wound does not correspond directly to the initiation of wound contraction, which starts almost immediately after injury.

Fibroblasts placed in a collagen lattice in vitro actively move in the lattice and contract it without expressing stress fibers. It is postulated that the movement of cells with concomitant reorganization of the cytoskeleton is responsible for contraction.[30]

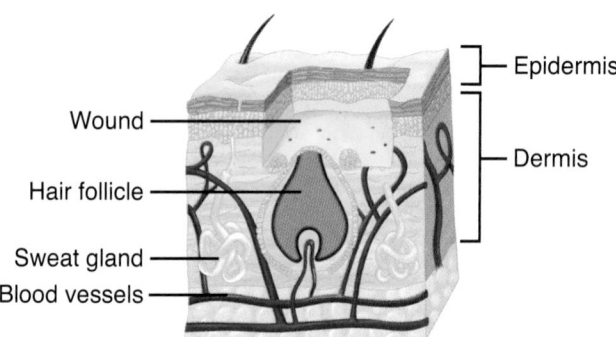

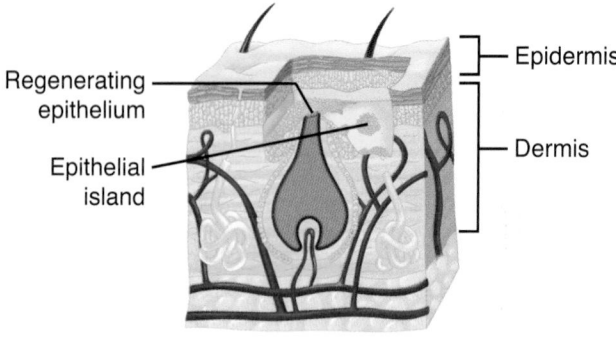

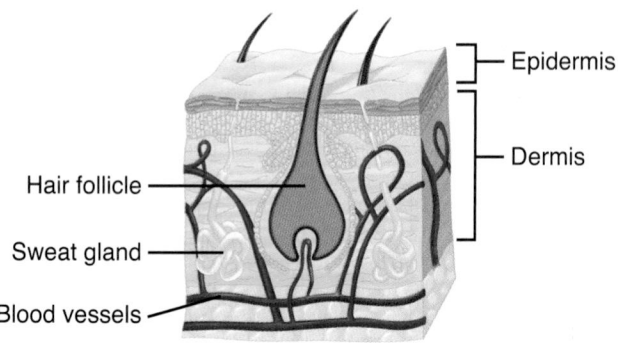

FIG. 9-4. The healing by epithelialization of superficial cutaneous wounds.

TABLE 9-2 Growth factors participating in wound healing

Growth Factor	Wound Cell Origin	Cellular and Biologic Effects
PDGF	Platelets, macrophages, monocytes, smooth muscle cells, endothelial cells	Chemotaxis: fibroblasts, smooth muscle, monocytes, neutrophils Mitogenesis: fibroblasts, smooth muscle cells Stimulation of angiogenesis Stimulation of collagen synthesis
FGF	Fibroblasts, endothelial cells, smooth muscle cells, chondrocytes	Stimulation of angiogenesis (by stimulation of endothelial cell proliferation and migration) Mitogenesis: mesoderm and neuroectoderm Stimulates fibroblasts, keratinocytes, chondrocytes, myoblasts
Keratinocyte growth factor	Keratinocytes, fibroblasts	Significant homology with FGF; stimulates keratinocytes
EGF	Platelets, macrophages, monocytes (also identified in salivary glands, duodenal glands, kidney, and lacrimal glands)	Stimulates proliferation and migration of all epithelial cell types
TGFα	Keratinocytes, platelets, macrophages	Homology with EGF; binds to EGF receptor Mitogenic and chemotactic for epidermal and endothelial cells Stimulates angiogenesis
TGFβ (three isoforms: β_1, β_2, β_3)	Platelets, T lymphocytes, macrophages, monocytes, neutrophils	TGFβ_1 stimulates wound matrix production (fibronectin, collagen glycosaminoglycans); regulation of inflammation TGFβ_3 inhibits scar formation
Insulin-like growth factors (IGF-I, IGF-II)	Platelets (IGF-I in high concentrations in liver; IGF-II in high concentrations in fetal growth); likely the effector of growth hormone action	Promote protein/extracellular matrix synthesis Increase membrane glucose transport
Vascular endothelial growth factor	Macrophages, fibroblasts, keratinocytes	Similar to PDGF Mitogen for endothelial cells (not fibroblasts) Stimulates angiogenesis
Granulocyte-macrophage colony-stimulating factor	Macrophage/monocytes, endothelial cells, fibroblasts	Stimulates macrophage differentiation/proliferation

EGF = epidermal growth factor; FGF = fibroblast growth factor; PDGF = platelet-derived growth factor; TGF = transforming growth factor.

HERITABLE DISEASES OF CONNECTIVE TISSUE

Heritable diseases of connective tissue consist of a group of generalized, genetically determined, primary disorders of one of the elements of connective tissue: collagen, elastin, or mucopolysaccharide. Five major types, Ehlers-Danlos syndrome (EDS), Marfan syndrome, osteogenesis imperfecta (OI), epidermolysis bullosa (EB), and acrodermatitis enteropathica (AE), are discussed, as each presents unique challenges to the surgeon.

Ehlers-Danlos Syndrome

EDS is a group of 10 disorders that present as a defect in collagen formation. Characteristics include thin, friable skin with prominent veins, easy bruising, poor wound healing, abnormal scar formation, recurrent hernias, and hyperextensible joints. GI problems include bleeding, hiatal hernia, intestinal diverticulae, and rectal prolapse. Small blood vessels are fragile, making suturing difficult during surgery. Large vessels may develop aneurysms, varicosities, arteriovenous fistulas, or may spontaneously rupture.[31–33] EDS must be considered in every child with recurrent hernias and coagulopathy, especially when accompanied by platelet abnormalities and low coagulation factor levels. Inguinal hernias in these children resemble those seen in adults. Great care should be taken to avoid tearing the skin and fascia. The transversalis fascia is thin, and the internal ring is greatly dilated. An adult-type repair with the use of mesh or felt may result in a lower incidence of recurrence.[34] Table 9-3 presents a description of EDS subtypes.

TABLE 9-3 Clinical, genetic, and biochemical aspects of Ehlers-Danlos subtypes

Type	Clinical Features	Inheritance	Biochemical Defect
I	Skin: soft, hyperextensible, easy bruising, fragile, atrophic scars; hypermobile joints; varicose veins; premature births	AD	Not known
II	Similar to type I, except less severe	AD	Not known
III	Skin: soft, not hyperextensible, normal scars; small and large joint hypermobility	AD	Not known
IV	Skin: thin, translucent, visible veins, normal scarring, no hyperextensibility; no joint hypermobility; arterial, bowel, and uterine rupture	AD	Type III collagen defect
V	Similar to type II	XLR	Not known
VI	Skin: hyperextensible, fragile, easy bruising; hypermobile joints; hypotonia; kyphoscoliosis	AR	Lysyl hydroxylase deficiency
VII	Skin: soft, mild hyperextensibility, no increased fragility; extremely lax joints with dislocations	AD	Type I collagen gene defect
VIII	Skin: soft, hyperextensible, easy bruising, abnormal scars with purple discoloration; hypermobile joints; generalized periodontitis	AD	Not known
IX	Skin: soft, lax; bladder diverticula and rupture; limited pronation and supination; broad clavicle; occipital horns	XLR	Lysyl oxidase defect with abnormal copper use
X	Similar to type II with abnormal clotting studies	AR	Fibronectin defect

AD = autosomal dominant; AR = autosomal recessive; XLR = X-linked recessive.
Source: Reproduced with permission from Phillips et al.[31] Copyright © Elsevier.

Marfan Syndrome

Patients with Marfan syndrome generally have tall stature, arachnodactyly, lax ligaments, myopia, scoliosis, pectus excavatum, and aneurysm of the ascending aorta. The genetic defect is in an extracellular protein, fibrillin, which is associated with elastic fibers. Patients who suffer from this syndrome also are prone to hernias. Surgical repair of a dissecting aneurysm is difficult, as the soft connective tissue fails to hold sutures. Skin may be hyperextensible, but shows no delay in wound healing.[35,36]

Osteogenesis Imperfecta

Characteristics of OI are brittle bones, osteopenia, low muscle mass, hernias, and ligament and joint laxity. OI is a result of a mutation in type I collagen. There are four major OI subtypes with mild to lethal manifestations. Patients experience dermal thinning and increased bruisability. Scarring is normal, and the skin is not hyperextensible. Surgery can be successful but difficult in these patients, as their bones fracture easily under minimal stress.[31,34] Table 9-4 lists the various features associated with the clinical subtypes of OI.

Epidermolysis Bullosa

EB is classified into three major subtypes: EB simplex, junctional EB, and dystrophic EB. The genetic defect involves impairment in tissue adhesion within the epidermis, basement membrane, or dermis, resulting in tissue separation and blistering with minimal trauma. Characteristic features of EB are blistering and ulceration. Management of nonhealing wounds in patients with EB is a challenge, as their nutritional status is compromised because of oral erosions and esophageal obstruction. Surgical interventions include esophageal dilation and gastrostomy tube placement. Dermal incisions must be meticulously placed to avoid further trauma to skin.[34,37] The skin requires nonadhesive pads covered by "bulky" dressing to avoid blistering.

Acrodermatitis Enteropathica

AE is an autosomal recessive disease of children that causes an inability to absorb sufficient zinc from breast milk or food. The AE mutation affects zinc uptake in the intestine by preventing zinc from binding to the cell surface and its translocation into the cell. Zinc deficiency is associated with impaired granulation tissue formation, as zinc is a necessary cofactor for DNA polymerase and reverse transcriptase, and its deficiency may impair healing due to inhibition of cell proliferation.

AE is characterized by impaired wound healing as well as erythematous pustular dermatitis involving the extremities and the areas around the bodily orifices. Diagnosis is confirmed by the presence of an abnormally low blood zinc level (>100 μg/dL). Oral supplementation with 100 to 400 mg zinc sulfate orally per day is curative for impaired healing.[38,39]

TABLE 9-4	Osteogenesis imperfecta: clinical and genetic features	
Type	**Clinical Features**	**Inheritance**
I	Mild bone fragility, blue sclera	Dominant
II	"Prenatal lethal"; crumpled long bones, thin ribs, dark blue sclera	Dominant
III	Progressively deforming; multiple fractures; early loss of ambulation	Dominant/recessive
IV	Mild to moderate bone fragility; normal or gray sclera; mild short stature	Dominant

HEALING IN SPECIFIC TISSUES

Gastrointestinal Tract

Healing of full-thickness injury to the GI tract remains an unresolved clinical issue. Healing of full-thickness GI wounds begins with a surgical or mechanical reapposition of the bowel ends, which is most often the initial step in the repair process. Sutures or staples are principally used, although various other means, such as buttons, plastic tubes, and various wrappings, have been attempted with variable success. Failure of healing results in dehiscence, leaks, and fistulas, which carry significant morbidity and mortality. Conversely, excessive healing can be just as troublesome, resulting in stricture formation and stenosis of the lumen. Repair of the GI tract is vital to restoring the integrity of the luminal structure, and to the resumption of motor, absorptive, and barrier functions.

The gross anatomic features of the GI tract are remarkably constant throughout most of its length. Within the lumen, the epithelium is supported by the lamina propria and underlying muscularis mucosa. The submucosa lies radially and circumferentially outside of these layers, is comprised of abundant collagenous and elastic fibers, and supports neural and vascular structures. Further toward the peritoneal surface of the bowel are the inner and outer muscle layers and, ultimately, a peritoneal extension, the serosa. The submucosa is the layer that imparts the greatest tensile strength and greatest suture-holding capacity, a characteristic that should be kept in mind during surgical repair of the GI tract. Additionally, serosal healing is essential for quickly achieving a watertight seal from the luminal side of the bowel. The importance of the serosa is underscored by the significantly higher rates of anastomotic failure observed clinically in segments of bowel that are extraperitoneal and lack serosa (i.e., the esophagus and rectum).

Injuries to all parts of the GI tract undergo the same sequence of healing as cutaneous wounds. However, there are some significant differences (Table 9-5). Mesothelial (serosal) and mucosal healing can occur without scarring. The early integrity of the anastomosis is dependent on formation of a fibrin seal on the serosal side, which achieves watertightness, and on the suture-holding capacity of the intestinal wall, particularly the submucosal layer. There is a significant decrease in marginal strength during the first week due to an early and marked collagenolysis. The lysis of collagen is carried out by collagenase derived from neutrophils, macrophages, and intraluminal bacteria. Collagenase activity occurs early in the healing process, and during the first 3 to 5 days collagen breakdown far exceeds collagen synthesis. The integrity of the anastomosis represents equilibrium between collagen lysis, which occurs early, and collagen synthesis, which takes a few days to initiate (Fig. 9-5). Collagenase is expressed postinjury in all segments of the GI tract, but it is much more marked in the colon compared to the small bowel. Collagen synthesis in the GI tract is carried out by both fibroblasts and smooth muscle cells. Colon fibroblasts produce greater amounts of collagen than skin fibroblasts, reflecting different phenotypic features, as well as different responses to cytokines and growth factors among these different fibroblast populations. Ultimate anastomotic strength is not always related to the absolute amount of collagen, and the structure and arrangement of the collagen matrix may be more important.[40]

Technical Considerations

Traditional teaching holds that in order for an anastomosis to heal without complications it must be tension-free, have an adequate blood supply, receive adequate nutrition, and be free of sepsis. Although sound principles for all wound healing, there are several considerations unique to anastomotic healing. From a technical viewpoint, the ideal method of suturing two ends of bowel together has not yet been identified. Although debate exists concerning methods of creating an anastomosis, clinically there has been no convincing evidence that a given technique has any advantage over another (i.e., hand-sutured vs. stapled, continuous vs. interrupted sutures,

		GI Tract	Skin
TABLE 9-5		Comparison of wound healing in the gastrointestinal tract and skin	
Wound environment	pH	Varies throughout GI tract in accordance with local exocrine secretions.	Usually constant except during sepsis or local infection.
	Microorganisms	Aerobic and anaerobic, especially in the colon and rectum; problematic if they contaminate the peritoneal cavity.	Skin commensals rarely cause problems; infection usually results from exogenous contamination or hematogenous spread.
	Shear stress	Intraluminal bulk transit and peristalsis exert distracting forces on the anastomosis.	Skeletal movements may stress the suture line but pain usually acts as a protective mechanism preventing excess movement.
	Tissue oxygenation	Dependent on intact vascular supply and neocapillary formation.	Circulatory transport of oxygen as well as diffusion.
Collagen synthesis	Cell type	Fibroblasts and smooth muscle cells.	Fibroblasts.
	Lathyrogens	D-Penicillamine has no effect on collagen cross-linking.	Significant inhibition of cross-linking with decreased wound strength.
	Steroids	Contradictory evidence exists concerning their negative effect on GI healing; increased abscess in the anastomotic line may play a significant role.	Significant decrease in collagen accumulation.
Collagenase activity	—	Increased presence throughout GI tract after transection and reanastomosis; during sepsis excess enzyme may promote dehiscence by decreasing suture-holding capacity of tissue.	Not as significant a role in cutaneous wounds.
Wound strength	—	Rapid recovery to preoperative level.	Less rapid than GI tissue.
Scar formation	Age	Definite scarring seen in fetal wound sites.	Usually heals without scar formation in the fetus.

absorbable vs. nonabsorbable sutures, or single- vs. two-layer closure). A recent meta-analysis revealed that stapled ileo-colic anastomoses have fewer leak rates than hand-constructed ones, but no data on colo-colic or small bowel anastomoses have been offered yet.[41] It is known, however, that hand-sutured everting anastomoses are at greater risk of leakage and cause greater adhesion formation, but have a lower incidence of stenosis. As no overall definite superiority of any one method exists, it is recommended that surgeons be familiar with several techniques and apply them as circumstances dictate.

Bone

After any type of injury to bone, several changes take place at the site of injury to restore structural and functional integrity. Most of the phases of healing resemble those observed in dermal healing, but some notable individual characteristics apply to bone injuries. The initial stage of hematoma formation consists of an accumulation of blood at the fracture site, which also contains devitalized soft tissue, dead bone, and necrotic marrow. The next stage accomplishes the liquefaction and degradation of nonviable products at the fracture site. The normal bone adjacent to the injury site can then undergo revascularization, with new blood vessels growing into the fracture site. This is similar to the formation of granulation tissue in soft tissue. The symptoms associated with this stage are characteristic of inflammation, with clinical evidence of swelling and erythema.

Three to 4 days after injury, soft tissue forms a bridge between the fractured bone segments in the next stage (soft callus stage). This soft tissue is deposited where neovascularization has taken place and serves as an internal splint, preventing damage to the newly laid blood vessels and achieving a fibrocartilaginous union. The soft callus is formed externally along the bone shaft and internally within the marrow cavity. Clinically, this phase is characterized by the end of pain and inflammatory signs.

The next phase (hard callus stage) consists of mineralization of the soft callus and conversion to bone. This may take up to 2 to 3 months and leads to complete bony union. The bone is now considered strong enough to allow weightbearing and will appear healed on radiographs. This stage is followed by the remodeling phase, in which the excessive callus is reabsorbed and the marrow cavity is recanalized. This remodeling allows for the correct transmission of forces and restores the contours of the bone.

As in dermal healing, the process of osseous union is mediated by soluble growth factors and cytokines. The most extensively studied group is the bone morphogenic proteins, which belong to the TGFβ superfamily. By stimulating the differentiation of mesenchymal cells into chondroblasts and osteoblasts, bone morphogenic proteins directly affect bone and cartilage repair. Other growth factors, such as PDGF, TGFβ, TNF-α, and basic fibroblast growth

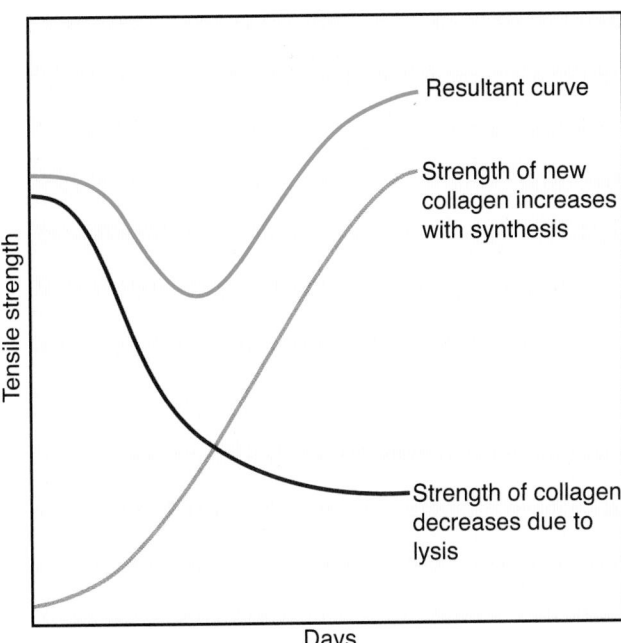

FIG. 9-5. Diagrammatic representation of the concept of GI wound healing as a fine balance between collagen synthesis and collagenolysis. The "weak" period when collagenolysis exceeds collagen synthesis can be prolonged or exacerbated by any factors that upset the equilibrium. *(Reproduced with permission from Hunt TK, Van Winkle W Jr: Wound healing: normal repair, in Dunphy JE (ed): Fundamentals of Wound Management in Surgery. New York: Chirurgecom, Inc., 1976, p. 29.)*

CHAPTER 9

Wound Healing

factor, also participate in bony repair by mediating the inflammatory and proliferative phases of healing.

Cartilage

Cartilage consists of cells (chondrocytes) surrounded by an extracellular matrix made up of several proteoglycans, collagen fibers, and water. Unlike bone, cartilage is very avascular and depends on diffusion for transmittal of nutrients across the matrix. Additionally, the hypervascular perichondrium contributes substantially to the nutrition of the cartilage. Therefore, injuries to cartilage may be associated with permanent defects due to the meager and tenuous blood supply.

The healing response of cartilage depends on the depth of injury. In a superficial injury, there is disruption of the proteoglycan matrix and injury to the chondrocytes. There is no inflammatory response, but an increase in synthesis of proteoglycan and collagen dependent entirely on the chondrocyte. Unfortunately, the healing power of cartilage is often inadequate and overall regeneration is incomplete. Therefore, superficial cartilage injuries are slow to heal and often result in persistent structural defects.

In contrast to superficial injuries, deep injuries involve the underlying bone and soft tissue. This leads to the exposure of vascular channels of the surrounding damaged tissue that may help in the formation of granulation tissue. Hemorrhage allows for the initiation of the inflammatory response and the subsequent mediator activation of cellular function for repair. As the granulation tissue is laid down, fibroblasts migrate toward the wound and synthesize fibrous tissue that undergoes chondrification. Gradually, hyaline cartilage is formed, which restores the structural and functional integrity of the injured site.

Tendon

Tendons and ligaments are specialized structures that link muscle and bone, and bone and bone, respectively. They consist of parallel bundles of collagen interspersed with spindle cells. Tendons and ligaments can be subjected to a variety of injuries, such as laceration, rupture, and contusion. Due to the mobility of the underlying bone or muscles, the damaged ends usually separate. Tendon and ligament healing progresses in a similar fashion as in other areas of the body (i.e., through hematoma formation, organization, laying down of reparative tissue, and scar formation). Matrix is characterized by accumulation of type I and III collagen along with increased water, DNA, and glycosaminoglycan content. As the collagen fibers are organized, transmission of forces across the damaged portion can occur. Restoration of the mechanical integrity may never be equal to that of the undamaged tendon.

Tendon vasculature has a clear effect on healing. Hypovascular tendons tend to heal with less motion and more scar formation than tendons with better blood supply. The specialized cells, tenocytes, are metabolically very active and retain a large regenerative potential, even in the absence of vascularity. Cells on the tendon surface are identical to those within the sheath and play a role in tendon healing as well.

Nerve

Nerve injuries are very common, with an estimated 200,000 repairs performed every year in the United States. Peripheral nerves are a complex arrangement of axons, nonneuronal cells, and extracellular elements. There are three types of nerve injuries: neurapraxia (focal demyelination), axonotmesis (interruption of axonal continuity but preservation of Schwann cell basal lamina), and neurotmesis (complete transection). After all types of injury, the nerve ends progress through a predictable pattern of changes involving three crucial steps: (a) survival of axonal cell bodies, (b) regeneration of axons that grow across the transected nerve to reach the distal stump, and (c) migration and connection of the regenerating nerve ends to the appropriate nerve ends or organ targets.

Phagocytes remove the degenerating axons and myelin sheath from the distal stump (wallerian degeneration). Regenerating axonal sprouts extend from the proximal stump and probe the distal stump and the surrounding tissues. Schwann cells ensheathe and help in remyelinating the regenerating axons. Functional units are formed when the regenerating axons connect with the appropriate end targets. Several factors play a role in nerve healing, such as growth factors, cell adhesion molecules, and nonneuronal cells and receptors. Growth factors include nerve growth factor, brain-derived neurotropic factor, basic and acidic fibroblastic growth factors, and neuroleukin. Cell-adhesion molecules involved in nerve healing include nerve-adhesion molecule, neuron-glia adhesion molecule, myelin adhesion glycoprotein, and N-cadherin. This complex interplay of growth factors and adhesion molecules helps in nerve regeneration.

Fetal Wound Healing

The main characteristic that distinguishes the healing of fetal wounds from that of adult wounds is the apparent lack of scar formation. Understanding how fetal wounds achieve integrity without evidence of scarring holds promise for the possible manipulation of unwanted fibrosis or excessive scar formation in adults. Although early fetal healing is characterized by the absence of scarring and resembles tissue regeneration, there is a phase of transition during gestational life when a more adult-like healing pattern emerges. This so-called "transition wound" occurs at the beginning of the third trimester, and during this period there is scarless healing; however, there is a loss of the ability to regenerate skin appendages.[42] Eventually a classic, adult-patterned healing with scar formation occurs exclusively, although overall healing continues to be faster than in adults.

There are a number of characteristics that may influence the differences between fetal and adult wounds. These include wound environment, inflammatory responses, differential growth factor profiles, and wound matrix.

Wound Environment

The fetus is bathed in a sterile, temperature-stable fluid environment, though this alone does not explain the observed differences. Experiments have demonstrated that scarless healing may occur outside of the amniotic fluid environment, and, conversely, scars can form in utero.[43,44]

Inflammation

The extent and robustness of the inflammatory response correlates directly with the amount of scar formation in all healing wounds. Reduced fetal inflammation due to the immaturity of the fetal immune system may partially explain the lack of scarring observed. Not only is the fetus neutropenic, but fetal wounds also contain lower numbers of PMNs and macrophages.[45]

Growth Factors

Fetal wounds are notable for the absence of TGFβ, which may have a significant role in scarring. Conversely, blocking TGFβ1 or TGFβ2 using neutralizing antibodies considerably reduces scar formation in adult wounds. Exogenous application of TGFβ3 downregulates TGFβ1 and TGFβ2 levels at the wound site with a resultant reduction in scarring.[46] Thus, the balance between the concentration and/or activity of TGFβ isoforms may be important for regulating scar production.

Wound Matrix

The fetal wound is characterized by excessive and extended hyaluronic acid production, a high molecular weight glycosaminoglycan that is produced primarily by fibroblasts. Although adult wounds also produce hyaluronic acid, its synthesis is sustained only in the fetal wound. Components of amniotic fluid, most specifically fetal urine, have a unique ability to stimulate hyaluronic acid production.[47] Fetal fibroblasts produce more collagen than adult fibroblasts, and the increased level of hyaluronic acid may aid in the orderly organization of collagen. As a result of these findings, hyaluronic acid is used topically to enhance healing and to inhibit postoperative adhesion formation.[48]

CLASSIFICATION OF WOUNDS

Wounds are classified as either acute or chronic. Acute wounds heal in a predictable manner and time frame. The process occurs with few, if any, complications, and the end result is a well-healed wound. Surgical wounds can heal in several ways. An incised wound that is clean and closed by sutures is said to heal by primary intention. Often, because of bacterial contamination or tissue loss, a wound will be left open to heal by granulation tissue formation and contraction; this constitutes healing by secondary intention. Delayed primary closure, or healing by tertiary intention, represents a combination of the first two, consisting of the placement of sutures, allowing the wound to stay open for a few days, and the subsequent closure of the sutures (Fig. 9-6).

The healing spectrum of acute wounds is broad (Fig. 9-7). In examining the acquisition of mechanical integrity and strength during healing, the normal process is characterized by a constant and continual increase that reaches a plateau at some point postinjury. Wounds with delayed healing are characterized by decreased wound-breaking strength in comparison to wounds that heal at a normal rate; however, they eventually achieve the same integrity and strength as wounds that heal normally. Conditions such as nutritional deficiencies, infections, or severe trauma cause delayed healing, which reverts to normal with correction of the underlying pathophysiology. Impaired healing is characterized by a failure to achieve mechanical strength equivalent to normally healed wounds. Patients with compromised immune systems, such as those with diabetes, chronic steroid usage, or tissues damaged by radiotherapy, are prone to this

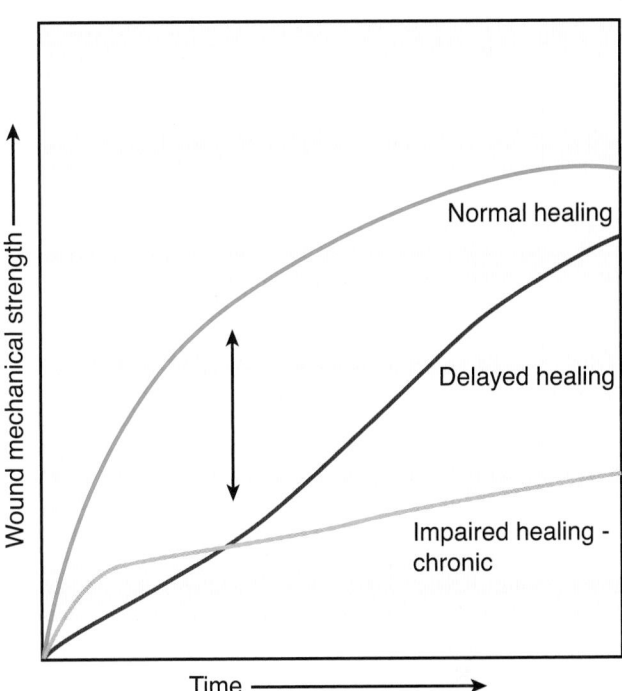

FIG. 9-7. The acquisition of wound mechanical strength over time in normal, delayed, and impaired healing.

type of impaired healing. The surgeon must be aware of these situations and exercise great care in the placement of incision and suture selection, postoperative care, and adjunctive therapy to maximize the chances of healing without supervening complications.

Normal healing is affected by both systemic and local factors (Table 9-6). The clinician must be familiar with these factors and should attempt to counteract their deleterious effects. Complications occurring in wounds with higher risk can lead to failure of healing or the development of chronic, nonhealing wounds.

Factors Affecting Wound Healing
Advanced Age

Most surgeons believe that aging produces intrinsic physiologic changes that result in delayed or impaired wound healing. Clinical experience with elderly patients tends to support this belief. Studies of hospitalized surgical patients show a direct correlation between

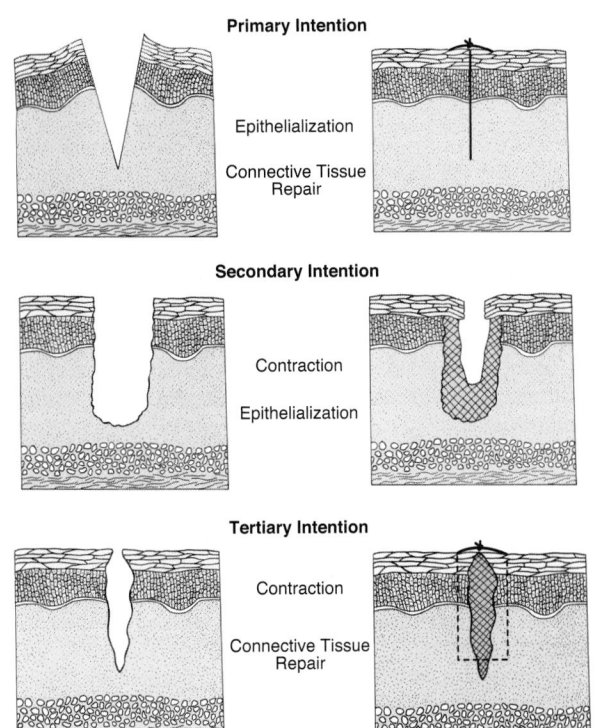

FIG. 9-6. Different clinical approaches to the closure and healing of acute wounds.

TABLE 9-6	Factors affecting wound healing
Systemic	
Age	
Nutrition	
Trauma	
Metabolic diseases	
Immunosuppression	
Connective tissue disorders	
Smoking	
Local	
Mechanical injury	
Infection	
Edema	
Ischemia/necrotic tissue	
Topical agents	
Ionizing radiation	
Low oxygen tension	
Foreign bodies	

older age and poor wound healing outcomes such as dehiscence and incisional hernia.[49,50] However, these statistics fail to take into account underlying illnesses or diseases as a possible source of impaired wound healing in the elderly. The increased incidence of cardiovascular disease, metabolic diseases (diabetes mellitus, malnutrition, and vitamin deficiencies), cancer, and the widespread use of drugs that impair wound healing may all contribute to the higher incidence of wound problems in the elderly. However, more recent clinical experience suggests that major operative interventions can be accomplished safely in the elderly.

The results of animal studies regarding the effects of aging on wound healing have yielded contradictory results. In healthy human volunteers there was a significant delay of 1.9 days in the epithelialization of superficial skin defects in those older than 70 years of age when compared to younger volunteers.[51] In the same volunteers, using a micro-model of fibroplasia, no difference in DNA or hydroxyproline wound accumulation could be demonstrated between the young and elderly groups; however, the young volunteers had a significantly higher amount of total α-amino nitrogen in their wounds, a reflection of total protein content of the wound. Thus, although wound collagen synthesis does not seem to be impaired with advanced age, noncollagenous protein accumulation at wounded sites is decreased with aging, which may impair the mechanical properties of scarring in elderly patients.

Hypoxia, Anemia, and Hypoperfusion

Low oxygen tension has a profoundly deleterious effect on all aspects of wound healing. Fibroplasia, although stimulated initially by the hypoxic wound environment, is significantly impaired by local hypoxia. Optimal collagen synthesis requires oxygen as a cofactor, particularly for the hydroxylation steps. Increasing subcutaneous oxygen tension levels by increasing the fraction of inspired oxygen (FiO_2) of inspired air for brief periods during and immediately after surgery results in enhanced collagen deposition and in decreased rates of wound infection after elective surgery.[52–54]

Major factors affecting local oxygen delivery include hypoperfusion either for systemic reasons (low volume or cardiac failure) or due to local causes (arterial insufficiency, local vasoconstriction, or excessive tension on tissues). The level of vasoconstriction of the subcutaneous capillary bed is exquisitely responsive to fluid status, temperature, and hyperactive sympathetic tone as is often induced by postoperative pain. Correction of these factors can have a remarkable influence on wound outcome, particularly on decreasing wound infection rates.[53–55] Mild to moderate normovolemic anemia does not appear to adversely affect wound oxygen tension and collagen synthesis, unless the hematocrit falls below 15%.[55]

Steroids and Chemotherapeutic Drugs

Large doses or chronic usage of glucocorticoids reduce collagen synthesis and wound strength.[56] The major effect of steroids is to inhibit the inflammatory phase of wound healing (angiogenesis, neutrophil and macrophage migration, and fibroblast proliferation) and the release of lysosomal enzymes. The stronger the anti-inflammatory effect of the steroid compound used, the greater the inhibitory effect on wound healing. Steroids used after the first 3 to 4 days postinjury do not affect wound healing as severely as when they are used in the immediate postoperative period. Therefore, if possible, their use should be delayed or, alternatively, forms with lesser anti-inflammatory effects should be administered.

In addition to their effect on collagen synthesis, steroids also inhibit epithelialization and contraction and contribute to increased rates of wound infection, regardless of the time of administration.[56] Steroid-delayed healing of cutaneous wounds can be stimulated to epithelialize by topical application of vitamin A.[56,57] Collagen synthesis of steroid-treated wounds also can be stimulated by vitamin A.

All chemotherapeutic antimetabolite drugs adversely affect wound healing by inhibiting early cell proliferation and wound DNA and protein synthesis, all of which are critical to successful repair. Delay in the use of such drugs for about 2 weeks postinjury appears to lessen the wound healing impairment.[58] Extravasation of most chemotherapeutic agents is associated with tissue necrosis, marked ulceration, and protracted healing at the affected site.[59]

Metabolic Disorders

Diabetes mellitus is the best known of the metabolic disorders contributing to increased rates of wound infection and failure.[60] Uncontrolled diabetes results in reduced inflammation, angiogenesis, and collagen synthesis. Additionally, the large- and small-vessel disease that is the hallmark of advanced diabetes contributes to local hypoxemia. Defects in granulocyte function, capillary ingrowth, and fibroblast proliferation all have been described in diabetes. Obesity, insulin resistance, hyperglycemia, and diabetic renal failure contribute significantly and independently to the impaired wound healing observed in diabetics.[61] In wound studies on experimental diabetic animals, insulin restores collagen synthesis and granulation tissue formation to normal levels if given during the early phases of healing.[62] In clean, noninfected, and well-perfused experimental wounds in human diabetic volunteers, type I diabetes mellitus was noted to decrease wound collagen accumulation in the wound, independent of the degree of glycemic control. Type II diabetic patients showed no effect on collagen accretion when compared to healthy, age-matched controls.[63] Furthermore, the diabetic wound appears to be lacking in sufficient growth factor levels, which signal normal healing. It remains unclear whether decreased collagen synthesis or an increased breakdown due to an abnormally high proteolytic wound environment is responsible.

Careful preoperative correction of blood sugar levels improves the outcome of wounds in diabetic patients. Increasing the inspired oxygen tension, judicious use of antibiotics, and correction of other coexisting metabolic abnormalities all can result in improved wound healing.

Uremia also has been associated with disordered wound healing. Experimentally, uremic animals demonstrate decreased wound collagen synthesis and breaking strength. The contribution of uremia alone to this impairment, rather than that of associated malnutrition, is difficult to assess.[61] The clinical use of dialysis to correct the metabolic abnormalities and nutritional restoration should impact greatly on the wound outcome of such patients.

Nutrition

The importance of nutrition in the recovery from traumatic or surgical injury has been recognized by clinicians since the time of Hippocrates. Poor nutritional intake or lack of individual nutrients significantly alters many aspects of wound healing. The clinician must pay close attention to the nutritional status of patients with wounds, as wound failure or wound infections may be no more than a reflection of poor nutrition. Although the full interaction of nutrition and wound healing is still not fully understood, efforts are being made to develop wound-specific nutritional interventions and the pharmacologic use of individual nutrients as modulators of wound outcomes.

Experimental rodents fed either a 0 or 4% protein diet have impaired collagen deposition with a secondary decrease in skin and fascial wound-breaking strength and increased wound infection rates. Induction of energy-deficient states by providing only 50% of the normal caloric requirement leads to decreased granulation tissue formation and matrix protein deposition in rats. Acute fasting in rats markedly impairs collagen synthesis while decreasing procollagen mRNA.[64]

Clinically, it is extremely rare to encounter pure energy or protein malnutrition, and the vast majority of patients exhibit combined protein-energy malnutrition. Such patients have diminished hydroxyproline accumulation (an index of collagen deposition) into subcutaneously implanted polytetrafluoroethylene tubes when compared to normally nourished patients (Fig. 9-8). Furthermore, malnutrition correlates clinically with enhanced rates of wound complications and

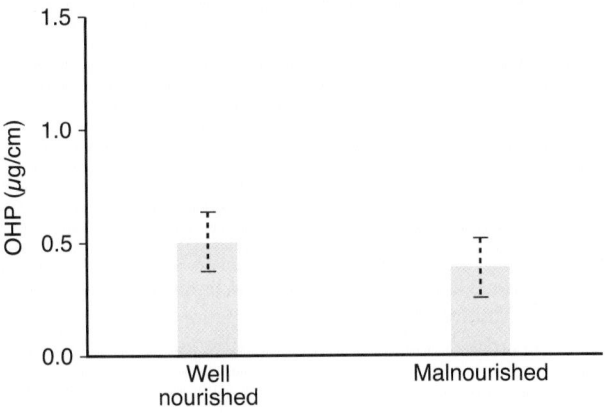

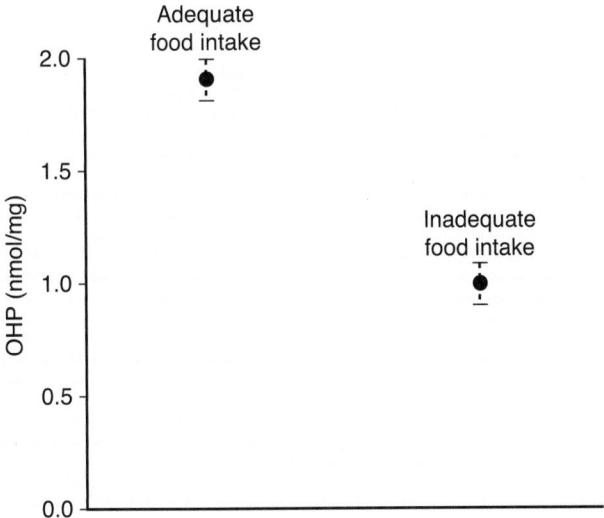

FIG. 9-8. Effect of malnutrition on collagen deposition in experimental human wounds. OHP = hydroxyproline.

tion with either 30 g of arginine aspartate (17 g of free arginine) or 30 g of arginine HCl (24.8 g of free arginine) daily for 14 days.[69] In a study of healthy older humans (aged 67 to 82 years), daily supplements of 30 g of arginine aspartate for 14 days resulted in significantly enhanced collagen and total protein deposition at the wound site when compared to controls given placebos. There was no enhanced DNA synthesis present in the wounds of the arginine-supplemented subjects, suggesting that the effect of arginine is not mediated by an inflammatory mode of action.[70] In this study, arginine supplementation had no effect on the rate of epithelialization of a superficial skin defect. This further suggests that the main effect of arginine on wound healing is to enhance wound collagen deposition. Recently, a dietary supplemental regimen of arginine, β-hydroxy-β-methylbutyrate, and glutamine was found to significantly and specifically enhance collagen deposition in elderly, healthy human volunteers when compared to an isocaloric, isonitrogenous supplement (Fig. 9-9).[71] As increases in breaking strength during the first weeks of healing are directly related to new collagen synthesis, arginine supplementation may result in an improvement in wound strength as a consequence of enhanced collagen deposition.

The vitamins most closely involved with wound healing are vitamin C and vitamin A. Scurvy, or vitamin C deficiency, leads to a defect in wound healing, particularly via a failure in collagen synthesis and cross-linking. Biochemically, vitamin C is required for the conversion of proline and lysine to hydroxyproline and hydroxylysine, respectively. Vitamin C deficiency has also been associated with an increased incidence of wound infection, and if wound infection does occur, it tends to be more severe. These effects are believed to be due to an associated impairment in neutrophil function, decreased complement activity, and decreased walling-off of bacteria secondary to insufficient collagen deposition. The recommended dietary allowance is 60 mg daily. This provides a considerable safety margin for most healthy nonsmokers. In severely injured or extensively burned patients this requirement may increase to as high as 2 g daily. There is no evidence that excess vitamin C is toxic;

increased wound failure after diverse surgical procedures. This reflects impaired healing response as well as reduced cell-mediated immunity, phagocytosis, and intracellular killing of bacteria by macrophages and neutrophils during protein-calorie malnutrition.[64]

Two additional nutrition-related factors warrant discussion. First, the degree of nutritional impairment need not be long-standing in humans, as opposed to the experimental situation. Thus, patients with brief preoperative illnesses or reduced nutrient intake in the period immediately preceding the injury or operative intervention will demonstrate impaired fibroplasias.[65,66] Second, brief and not necessarily intensive nutritional intervention, either via the parenteral or enteral route, can reverse or prevent the decreased collagen deposition noted with malnutrition or with postoperative starvation.[67]

The possible role of single amino acids in enhanced wound healing has been studied for the last several decades. Arginine appears most active in terms of enhancing wound fibroplasia. Arginine deficiency results in decreased wound-breaking strength and wound collagen accumulation in chow-fed rats. Rats that are given 1% arginine HCl supplementation, and are therefore not arginine-deficient, have enhanced wound-breaking strength and collagen synthesis when compared to chow-fed controls.[68] Studies have been carried out in healthy human volunteers to examine the effect of arginine supplementation on collagen accumulation. Young, healthy, human volunteers (aged 25 to 35 years) were found to have significantly increased wound collagen deposition after oral supplementa-

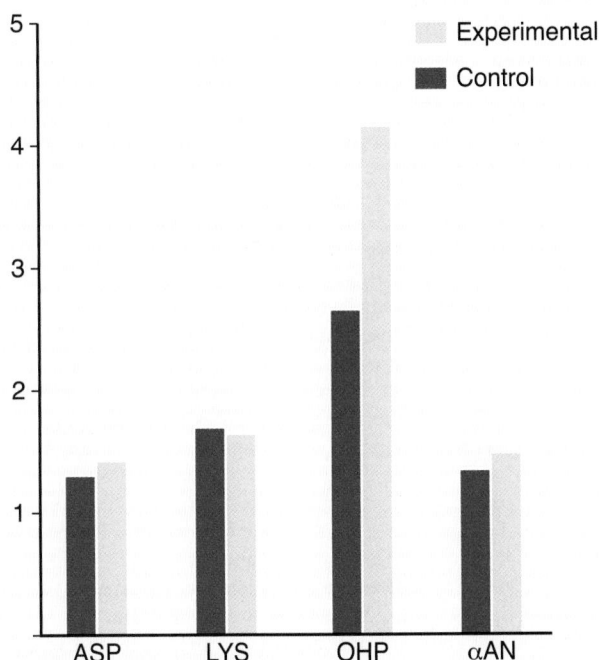

FIG. 9-9. Ratios of 14-day to 7-day values for aspartate (ASP), hydroxyproline (OHP), lysine (LYS), and α-amino nitrogen (αAN) in volunteers given dietary supplements of arginine, β-hydroxy-β-methylbutyrate, and glutamine. *$P < .05$. *(From Williams JZ, et al,[71] with permission.)*

however, there is no evidence that supertherapeutic doses of vitamin C are of any benefit.[72]

Vitamin A deficiency impairs wound healing, whereas supplemental vitamin A benefits wound healing in nondeficient humans and animals. Vitamin A increases the inflammatory response in wound healing, probably by increasing the lability of lysosomal membranes. There is an increased influx of macrophages, with an increase in their activation and increased collagen synthesis. Vitamin A directly increases collagen production and epidermal growth factor receptors when it is added in vitro to cultured fibroblasts. As mentioned in the section Steroids and Chemotherapeutic Drugs, supplemental vitamin A can reverse the inhibitory effects of corticosteroids on wound healing. Vitamin A also can restore wound healing that has been impaired by diabetes, tumor formation, cyclophosphamide, and radiation. Serious injury or stress leads to increased vitamin A requirements. In the severely injured patient, supplemental doses of vitamin A have been recommended. Doses ranging from 25,000 to 100,000 IU per day have been advocated.

The connections between specific minerals and trace elements and deficits in wound healing are complex. Frequently, deficiencies are multiple and include macronutrient deficiencies. As with some of the vitamins described above, the specific trace element may function as a cofactor or part of an enzyme that is essential for homeostasis and wound healing. Clinically, preventing deficiencies is often easier to accomplish than diagnosing them.

Zinc is the most well-known element in wound healing and has been used empirically in dermatologic conditions for centuries. It is essential for wound healing in animals and humans. There are more than 150 known enzymes for which zinc is either an integral part or an essential cofactor, and many of these enzymes are critical to wound healing.[73] With zinc deficiency there is decreased fibroblast proliferation, decreased collagen synthesis, impaired overall wound strength, and delayed epithelialization. These defects are reversed by zinc supplementation. To date, no study has shown improved wound healing with zinc supplementation in patients who are not zinc deficient.[74]

Infections

Wound infections continue to represent a major medical problem, both in terms of how they affect the outcome of surgical procedures (surgical site infections), and for their impact on the length of hospital stay and medical costs.[75] Many otherwise successful surgical operations fail because of the development of wound infections. The occurrence of infections is of major concern when implants are used, and their occurrence may lead to the removal of the prosthetic material, thus subjecting the patient to further operations and severe risk of morbidity and mortality. Infections can weaken an abdominal closure or hernia repair and result in wound dehiscence or recurrence of the hernia. Cosmetically, infections can lead to disfiguring, unsightly, or delayed closures.

Exhaustive studies have been undertaken that examine the appropriate prophylactic treatment of operative wounds. Bacterial contaminants normally present on skin are prevented from entry into deep tissues by intact epithelium. Surgery breaches the intact epithelium, allowing bacteria access to these tissues and the bloodstream. Antibiotic prophylaxis is most effective when adequate concentrations of antibiotic are present in the tissues at the time of incision, and assurance of adequate preoperative antibiotic dosing and timing has become a significant hospital performance measure.[76] Addition of antibiotics after operative contamination has occurred is clearly ineffective in preventing postoperative wound infections.

Studies that compare operations performed with and without antibiotic prophylaxis demonstrate that class II, III, and IV procedures (see below) treated with appropriate prophylactic antibiotics have only one third the wound infection rate of previously reported untreated series.[77] More recently, repeat dosing of antibiotics has been shown to be essential in decreasing postoperative wound infections in operations with durations exceeding the biochemical

half-life ($t_{1/2}$) of the antibiotic or in which there is large-volume blood loss and fluid replacement.[78,79] In lengthy cases, those in which prosthetic implants are used, or when unexpected contamination is encountered, additional doses of antibiotic may be administered for 24 hours postoperatively.

Selection of antibiotics for use in prophylaxis should be tailored to the type of surgery to be performed, operative contaminants that might be encountered during the procedure, and the profile of resistant organisms present at the institution where the surgery is performed. The continuing widespread appearance of methicillin-resistant *Staphylococcus aureus* and vancomycin-resistant enterococci has significantly restricted the selection of these agents for routine use. An example of surgery-specific treatment guidelines is provided in Table 9-7.[78]

Patients with prosthetic heart valves or any implanted vascular or orthopedic prostheses should receive antibiotic prophylaxis before any procedure in which significant bacteremia is anticipated. Dental procedures require prophylaxis with broad-spectrum penicillins or amoxicillin, whereas urologic instrumentation should be pretreated with a second-generation cephalosporin. Patients with prostheses who undergo GI surgery should receive anaerobic coverage combined with a cephalosporin.

The incidence of wound infection is about 5 to 10% nationwide and has not changed during the last few decades. Quantitatively, it has been shown that if the wound is contaminated with >10^5 microorganisms, the risk of wound infection is markedly increased, but this threshold may be much lower in the presence of foreign materials. The source of pathogens for the infection is usually the endogenous flora of the patient's skin, mucous membranes, or from hollow organs. The most common organisms responsible for wound infections, in order of frequency, are *Staphylococcus* species, coagulase-negative *Streptococcus,* enterococci, and *Escherichia coli.* The incidence of wound infection bears a direct relationship to the degree of contamination that occurs during the operation from the disease process itself (clean—class I, clean contaminated—class II, contaminated—class III, and dirty—class IV). Many factors contribute to the development of postoperative wound infections. Most surgical wound infections become apparent within 7 to 10 days postoperatively, although a small number manifest only years after the original operative intervention. With the hospital stay becoming shorter and shorter, many infections are detected in the outpatient setting, leading to underreporting of the true incidence of wound infections. There has been much debate about the actual definition of wound infection. The narrowest definition would include wounds that drain purulent material, with bacteria identified on culture. The more broad definition would include all wounds draining pus, whether or not the bacteriologic studies are positive; wounds that are opened by the surgeon; and wounds that the surgeon considers infected.[80]

Anatomically, wound infections can be classified as superficial or suprafascial and deep, involving fascia, muscle, or the abdominal cavity. About three fourths of all wound infections are superficial, involving skin and subcutaneous tissue only. Clinical diagnosis is easy when a postoperative wound looks edematous and erythematous and is tender. Often the presentation is more subtle, and development of postoperative fever (usually low-grade), development of a mild and unexplained leukocytosis, or the presence of undue incisional pain should direct attention to the wound. Inspection of the wound is most useful in detecting subtle edema around the suture or staple line, manifested as a waxy appearance of the skin, which characterizes the early phase of infection. If a wound infection is suspected, several stitches or staples around the most suspicious area should be removed with insertion of a cotton-tipped applicator into the subcutaneous area to open a small segment of the incision. This causes minimal if any discomfort to the patient. Presence of pus mandates further opening of the subcutaneous and skin layers to the full extent of the infected pocket. Samples should be taken for aerobic and anaerobic cultures, with very few patients requiring antibiotic therapy. Patients who are immunosuppressed (diabetics

TABLE 9-7 Antimicrobial prophylaxis for surgery

Nature of Operation	Common Pathogens	Recommended Antimicrobials	Adult Dosage before Surgery[a]
Cardiac	*Staphylococcus aureus, S. epidermidis*	Cefazolin *or*	1–2 g IV[c]
		Cefuroxime *or*	1.5 g IV[c]
		Vancomycin[b]	1 g IV
GI, esophageal, gastroduodenal	Enteric gram-negative bacilli, gram-positive cocci	High risk[d] only: cefazolin	1–2 g IV
Biliary tract	Enteric gram-negative bacilli, enterococci, clostridia	High risk[e] only: cefazolin	1–2 g IV
Colorectal	Enteric gram-negative bacilli, anaerobes, enterococci	Oral: neomycin + erythromycin base[f] *or* metronidazole[f]	—
Appendectomy, nonperforated[h]	—	Parenteral: cefoxitin[g] *or*	1–2 g IV
		Cefazolin +	1–2 g IV
		Metronidazole[g] *or*	0.5 g IV
		Ampicillin/sulbactam	3 g IV
Genitourinary[i]	—	High risk only: ciprofloxacin	500 mg PO or 400 mg IV
Gynecologic and obstetric	Enteric gram-negative bacilli, anaerobes, group B streptococci, enterococci	Cefoxitin[g] or cefazolin[g] *or*	1–2 g IV
Vaginal, abdominal, or laparoscopic hysterectomy		Ampicillin/sulbactam[g]	3 g IV
Cesarean section	Same as for hysterectomy	Cefazolin[g]	1–2 g IV after cord clamping
Abortion	Same as for hysterectomy	First trimester, high risk[i]: aqueous penicillin G *or*	2 million units IV
		Doxycycline	300 mg PO[k]
		Second trimester: cefazolin[g]	1–2 g IV
Head and neck surgery	Anaerobes, enteric gram-negative bacilli, *S. aureus*	Clindamycin +	600–900 mg IV
Incisions through oral or pharyngeal mucosa		Gentamicin *or*	1.5 mg/kg IV
		Cefazolin	1–2 g IV
Neurosurgery	*S. aureus, S. epidermidis*	Cefazolin *or*	1–2 g IV
		Vancomycin[b]	1 g IV
Ophthalmic	*S. epidermidis, S. aureus,* streptococci, enteric gram-negative bacilli, *Pseudomonas* spp.	Gentamicin, tobramycin, ciprofloxacin, gatifloxacin, levofloxacin, moxifloxacin, ofloxacin *or*	Multiple drops topically over 2 to 24 h
		Neomycin, gramicidin, polymyxin B or cefazolin	100 mg subconjunctivally
Orthopedic	*S aureus, S. epidermidis*	Cefazolin[l] *or*	1–2 g IV
		Cefuroxime[l] *or*	1.5 g IV
		Vancomycin[b,l]	1 g IV
Thoracic (noncardiac)	*S. aureus, S. epidermidis,* streptococci, enteric gram-negative bacilli	Cefazolin *or*	1–2 g IV
		Cefuroxime *or*	1.5 g IV
		Vancomycin[b]	1 g IV
Vascular	*S. aureus, S. epidermidis,* enteric gram-negative bacilli	Cefazolin *or*	1–2 g IV
Arterial surgery involving a prosthesis, the abdominal aorta, or a groin incision		Vancomycin[b]	1 g IV
Lower extremity amputation for ischemia	*S. aureus, S. epidermidis,* enteric gram-negative bacilli, clostridia	Cefazolin *or*	1–2 g IV
		Vancomycin[b]	1 g IV

[a]Parenteral prophylactic antimicrobials can be given as a single IV dose begun 60 min or less before the operation. For prolonged operations, (>4 h) or those with major blood loss, additional intraoperative doses should be given at intervals 1–2 times the half-life of the drug for the duration of the procedure in a patient with normal renal function. If vancomycin or a fluoroquinolone is used, the infusion should be started 60–120 min before the initial incision to minimize the possibility of an infusion reaction close to the time of induction of anesthesia and to have adequate tissue levels at the time of incision.

[b]Vancomycin is used in hospitals in which methicillin-resistant *Staphylococcus aureus* (MRSA) and *S. epidermidis* are a frequent cause of postoperative wound infection, for patients previously colonized with MRSA, or for those who are allergic to penicillin or cephalosporins. Rapid IC administration may cause hypotension, which could be especially dangerous during induction of anesthesia.

Even when the drug is given over 60 min, hypertension may occur; treatment with diphenhydramine (Benadryl and others) and further slowing of the infusion rate may be helpful. Some experts would give 15 mg/kg of vancomycin to patients weighing more than 75 kg up to a maximum of 1.5 g with a slower infusion rate (90 min for 1.5 g). To provide coverage against gram-negative bacteria, most Medical Letter consultants would also include cefazolin or cefuroxime in the prophylaxis regimen for patients not allergic to cephalosporins. Ciprofloxacin, levofloxacin, gentamicin, or aztreonam, each one in combination with vancomycin, can be used in patients who cannot tolerate a cephalosporin.

[c]Some consultants recommend an additional dose when patients are removed from bypass during open-heart surgery.

[d]Morbid obesity, esophageal obstruction, decreased gastric acidity, or gastrointestinal motility.

[e]Age >70 y, acute cholecystitis, nonfunctioning gallbladder, obstructive jaundice, or common duct stones.

[f]After appropriate diet and catharsis, 1 g of neomycin plus 1 g of erythromycin at 1 P.M., 2 P.M., and 11 P.M. or 2 g of neomycin plus 2 g of metronidazole at 7 P.M. and 11 P.M. the day before an 8 A.M. operation.

[g]For patients allergic to penicillin and cephalosporins, clindamycin with either gentamicin, ciprofloxacin, levofloxacin, or aztreonam is a reasonable alternative.

[h]For a ruptured viscous, therapy is often continued for about 5 days. Ruptured viscous in postoperative setting (dehiscence) requires antibacterial to include coverage of nosocomial pathogens.

[i]Urine culture positive or unavailable, preoperative catheter, transrectal prostatic biopsy, placement of prosthetic material.

[j]Patients with previous pelvic inflammatory disease, previous gonorrhea, or multiple sex partners.

[k]Divide into 100 mg 1 h before the abortion and 200 mg one half hour after.

[l]If a tourniquet is to be used in the procedure, the entire dose of antibiotic must be infused before its inflation.

Source: Reproduced with permission from Antimicrobial Prophylaxis for Surgery. *Treatment Guidelines from The Medical Letter* 4:84, 2006. The Medical Letter®, Inc. New Rochelle, New York.

and those on steroids or chemotherapeutic agents), who have evidence of tissue penetration or systemic toxicity, or who have had prosthetic devices inserted (vascular grafts, heart valves, artificial joints, or mesh) should be treated with systemic antibiotics.[80]

Deep wound infections arise immediately adjacent to the fascia, either above or below it, and often have an intra-abdominal component. Most intra-abdominal infections do not, however, communicate with the wound. Deep infections present with fever and leukocytosis. The incision may drain pus spontaneously or the intra-abdominal extension may be recognized after the drainage of what was thought to be a superficial wound infection, but pus draining between the fascial sutures will be noted. Sometimes wound dehiscence will occur. The most dangerous of the deep infections is necrotizing fasciitis. It results in high mortality, particularly in the elderly. This is an invasive process that involves the fascia and leads to secondary skin necrosis. Pathophysiologically, it is a septic thrombosis of the vessels between the skin and the deep layers. The skin demonstrates hemorrhagic bullae and subsequent frank necrosis, with surrounding areas of inflammation and edema. The fascial necrosis is usually wider than the skin involvement or than the surgeon estimates on clinical grounds. The patient is toxic, has high fever, tachycardia, and marked hypovolemia, which if uncorrected, progresses to cardiovascular collapse. Bacteriologically, this is a mixed infection, and samples should be obtained for Gram's stain smears and cultures to aid in diagnosis and treatment. As soon as bacteriologic studies have been sent, high-dose penicillin treatment needs to be started (20 to 40 million U/d IV). Cardiovascular resuscitation with electrolyte solutions, blood, and/or plasma is carried out as expeditiously as possible before induction of anesthesia. The aim of surgical treatment is thorough removal of all necrosed skin and fascia. If viable skin overlies necrotic fascia, multiple longitudinal skin incisions can be made to allow for excision of the devitalized fascia. Although removal of all necrotic tissue is the goal of the first surgical intervention, the distinction between necrotic and simply edematous tissue often is difficult. Careful inspection every 12 to 24 hours will reveal any new necrotic areas, and these need further débridement and excision. When all necrotic tissue has been removed and the infection has been controlled, the wounds may be covered with homo- or xenografts until definitive reconstruction and autografting can take place.

The mere presence of bacteria in an open wound, either acute or chronic, does not constitute an infection, because large numbers of bacteria can be present in the normal situation. Second, the bacteria grown may not be representative of the bacteria causing the actual wound infection. There seems to be confusion as to what exactly constitutes wound infection. For purposes of clarity, contamination, colonization, and infection should be differentiated. *Contamination* is the presence of bacteria without multiplication, *colonization* is multiplication without host response, and *infection* is the presence of host response in reaction to deposition and multiplication of bacteria. The presence of a host response helps to differentiate between infection and colonization as seen in chronic wounds. The host response that helps in diagnosing wound infection comprises cellulitis, abnormal discharge, delayed healing, change in pain, abnormal granulation tissue, bridging, and abnormal color and odor.

As discussed previously in the section Hemostasis and Inflammation, neutrophils play a major role in preventing wound infections. Chronic granulomatous disease (CGD) comprises a genetically heterogeneous group of diseases in which the reduced nicotinamide adenine dinucleotide phosphate–dependent oxide enzyme is deficient. This defect impairs the intracellular killing of microorganisms, leaving the patient liable to infection by bacteria and fungi. Afflicted patients have recurrent infections and form granulomas, which can lead to obstruction of the gastric antrum and genitourinary tracts and poor wound healing. Surgeons become involved when the patient develops infectious or obstructive complications.

The nitroblue tetrazolium reduction test is used to diagnose CGD. Normal neutrophils can reduce this compound, whereas neutrophils

from affected patients do not, facilitating the diagnosis via a colorimetric test. Clinically, patients develop recurrent infections such as pneumonia, lymphadenitis, hepatic abscess, and osteomyelitis. Organisms most commonly responsible are *Staphylococcus aureus, Aspergillus, Klebsiella, Serratia,* or *Candida.* When CGD patients require surgery, a preoperative pulmonary function test should be considered because such patients are predisposed to obstructive and restrictive lung disease. Wound complications, mainly infection, are common. Sutures should be removed as late as possible because the wounds heal slowly. Abscess drains should be left in place for a prolonged period until the infection is completely resolved.[81]

Chronic Wounds

Chronic wounds are defined as wounds that have failed to proceed through the orderly process that produces satisfactory anatomic and functional integrity or that have proceeded through the repair process without producing an adequate anatomic and functional result. The majority of wounds that have not healed in 3 months are considered chronic. *Skin ulcers,* which usually occur in traumatized or vascularly compromised soft tissue, are also considered chronic in nature, and proportionately are the major component of chronic wounds. In addition to the factors discussed in the preceding section that can delay wound healing, other causative mechanisms may also play a role in the etiology of chronic wounds. Repeated trauma, poor perfusion or oxygenation, and/or excessive inflammation contribute to the causation and the perpetuation of the chronicity of wounds.

Unresponsiveness to normal regulatory signals also has been implicated as a predictive factor of chronic wounds. This may come about as a failure of normal growth factor synthesis,[82] and thus an increased breakdown of growth factors within a wound environment that is markedly proteolytic because of overexpression of protease activity or a failure of the normal antiprotease inhibitor mechanisms.[83] Fibroblasts from chronic wounds also have been found to have decreased proliferative potential, perhaps because of senescence[84] or decreased expression of growth factor receptors.[85] Chronic wounds occur due to various etiologic factors, and several of the most common are discussed in the following sections.

Malignant transformation of chronic ulcers can occur in any long-standing wound (Marjolin ulcer). Any wound that does not heal for a prolonged period of time is prone to malignant transformation. Malignant wounds are differentiated clinically from non-malignant wounds by the presence of overturned wound edges. In patients with suspected malignant transformations, biopsy of the wound edges must be performed to rule out malignancy. Cancers arising de novo in chronic wounds include both squamous and basal cell carcinomas.

Ischemic Arterial Ulcers

Ischemic arterial ulcers occur due to a lack of blood supply and are painful at presentation. They usually are associated with other symptoms of peripheral vascular disease, such as intermittent claudication, rest pain, night pain, and color changes. These wounds commonly are present at the most distal portions of the extremities, such as the interdigital clefts, although more proximal locations are also encountered. On examination, there may be diminished or absent pulses with decreased ankle-brachial index and poor formation of granulation tissue. Other signs of peripheral ischemia, such as dryness of skin, hair loss, scaling, and pallor can be present. The wound itself usually is shallow with smooth margins, and a pale base and surrounding skin may be present. The management of these wounds is two-pronged and includes revascularization and wound care.[86] Nonhealing of these wounds is the norm unless successful revascularization is performed. After establishing adequate blood supply, most such wounds progress to heal satisfactorily.

A strategy of prevention is extremely important in the approach to patients with limb ischemia. In bedridden patients, especially those who are sedated (in the intensive care unit), demented, or with peripheral neural compromise (neuropathy or paraplegia), pressure ulcers develop rapidly and often unnecessarily. Removal of restrictive stockings (in patients with critical ischemia), frequent repositioning, and surveillance is vital to preventing these ulcers.[87]

Venous Stasis Ulcers

Although there is unanimous agreement that venous ulcers are due to venous stasis and hydrostatic back pressure, there is less consensus as to what are the exact pathophysiologic pathways that lead to ulceration and impaired healing. On the microvascular level, there is alteration and distention of the dermal capillaries with leakage of fibrinogen into the tissues; polymerization of fibrinogen into fibrin cuffs leads to perivascular cuffing that can impede oxygen exchange, thus contributing to ulceration. These same fibrin cuffs and the leakage of macromolecules such as fibrinogen and alpha$_2$-macroglobulin trap growth factors and impede wound healing. Another hypothesis suggests that neutrophils adhere to the capillary endothelium and cause plugging with diminished dermal blood flow. Venous hypertension and capillary damage lead to extravasation of hemoglobin. The products of this breakdown are irritating and cause pruritus and skin damage. The resulting brownish pigmentation of skin combined with the loss of subcutaneous fat produces characteristic changes called *lipodermatosclerosis*. Regardless of the pathophysiologic mechanisms, the clinically characteristic picture is that of an ulcer that fails to re-epithelialize despite the presence of adequate granulation tissue.

Venous stasis occurs due to the incompetence of either the superficial or deep venous systems. Chronic venous ulcers usually are due to the incompetence of the deep venous system and are commonly painless. Stasis ulcers tend to occur at the sites of incompetent perforators, the most common being above the medial malleolus, over Cockett's perforator. Upon examination, the typical location combined with a history of venous incompetence and other skin changes is diagnostic. The wound usually is shallow, with irregular margins and pigmented surrounding skin.

The cornerstone of treatment of venous ulcers is compression therapy, although the best method to achieve it remains controversial. Compression can be accomplished via rigid or flexible means. The most commonly used method is the rigid, zinc oxide–impregnated, nonelastic bandage. Others have proposed a four-layered bandage approach as a more optimal method of obtaining graduated compression.[88] Wound care in these patients focuses on maintaining a moist wound environment, which can be achieved with hydrocolloids. Other, more modern approaches include use of vasoactive substances and growth factor application, as well as the use of skin substitutes. Most venous ulcers can be healed with perseverance and by addressing the venous hypertension.[88] Unfortunately, recurrences are frequent in spite of preventative measures, largely because of patients' lack of compliance.[89,90]

Diabetic Wounds

Ten to 15% of diabetic patients run the risk of developing ulcers. There are approximately 50,000 to 60,000 amputations performed in diabetic patients each year in the United States. The major contributors to the formation of diabetic ulcers include neuropathy, foot deformity, and ischemia. It is estimated that 60 to 70% of diabetic ulcers are due to neuropathy, 15 to 20% are due to ischemia, and another 15 to 20% are due to a combination of both. The neuropathy is both sensory and motor, and is secondary to persistently elevated glucose levels. The loss of sensory function allows unrecognized injury to occur from ill-fitting shoes, foreign bodies, or other trauma. The motor neuropathy or Charcot foot leads to collapse or dislocation of the interphalangeal or metatarsophalangeal joints, causing pressure on areas with little protection. There is also severe micro- and macrovascular circulatory impairment.

Once ulceration occurs, the chances of healing are poor. The treatment of diabetic wounds involves local and systemic mea-

sures.[91] Achievement of adequate blood sugar levels is very important. Most diabetic wounds are infected, and eradication of the infectious source is paramount to the success of healing. Treatment should address the possible presence of osteomyelitis, and should employ antibiotics that achieve adequate levels both in soft tissue and bone. Wide débridement of all necrotic or infected tissue is another cornerstone of treatment. Off-loading of the ulcerated area by using specialized orthotic shoes or casts allows for ambulation while protecting the fragile wound environment. Topical application of PDGF and granulocyte-macrophage colony-stimulating factor has met with limited but significant success in achieving closure.[92] The application of engineered skin allograft substitutes, although expensive, has also shown some significant success.[93] Prevention and, specifically, foot care play an important role in the management of diabetics.[94]

Decubitus or Pressure Ulcers

The incidence of pressure ulcers ranges from 2.7 to 9% in the acute care setting, in comparison to 2.4 to 23% in long-term care facilities. A pressure ulcer is a localized area of tissue necrosis that develops when a soft tissue is compressed between a bony prominence and an external surface. Excessive pressure causes capillary collapse and impedes the delivery of nutrients to body tissues. Pressure ulcer formation is accelerated in the presence of friction, shear forces, and moisture. Other contributory factors in the pathogenesis of pressure ulcers include immobility, altered activity levels, altered mental status, chronic conditions, and altered nutritional status. The four stages of pressure ulcer formation are as follows: stage I, nonblanchable erythema of intact skin; stage II, partial-thickness skin loss involving epidermis or dermis, or both; stage III, full-thickness skin loss, but not through the fascia; and stage IV, full-thickness skin loss with extensive involvement of muscle and bone.

The treatment of established pressure ulcers is most successful when carried out in a multidisciplinary manner by involving wound care teams consisting of physicians, nurses, dietitians, physical therapists, and nutritionists. Care of the ulcer itself comprises débridement of all necrotic tissue, maintenance of a favorable moist wound environment that will facilitate healing, relief of pressure, and addressing host issues such as nutritional, metabolic, and circulatory status. Débridement is most efficiently carried out surgically, but enzymatic proteolytic preparations and hydrotherapy also are used. The wound bed should be kept moist by employing dressings that absorb secretions but do not desiccate the wound.[95] Operative repair, usually involving flap rotation, has been found to be useful in obtaining closure. Unfortunately, recurrence rates are extremely high, owing to the population at risk and the inability to fully address the causative mechanisms.[96,97]

EXCESS HEALING

Clinically, excess healing can be as significant as wound failure. It is likely that more operative interventions are required for correction of the morbidity associated with excessive healing than are required for wound failure. The clinical manifestations of exuberant healing are protean and differ in the skin (mutilating or debilitating scars, burn contractions), tendons (frozen repairs), the GI tract (strictures or stenoses), solid organs (cirrhosis, pulmonary fibrosis), or the peritoneal cavity (adhesive disease).

Hypertrophic scars (HTSs) and keloids represent an overabundance of fibroplasia in the dermal healing process. HTSs rise above the skin level but stay within the confines of the original wound and often regress over time. Keloids rise above the skin level as well, but extend beyond the border of the original wound and rarely regress spontaneously (Fig. 9-10). Both HTSs and keloids occur after trauma to the skin, and may be tender, pruritic, and cause a burning sensation. Keloids are 15 times more common in darker-pigmented ethnicities, with individuals of African, Spanish, and Asian ethnici-

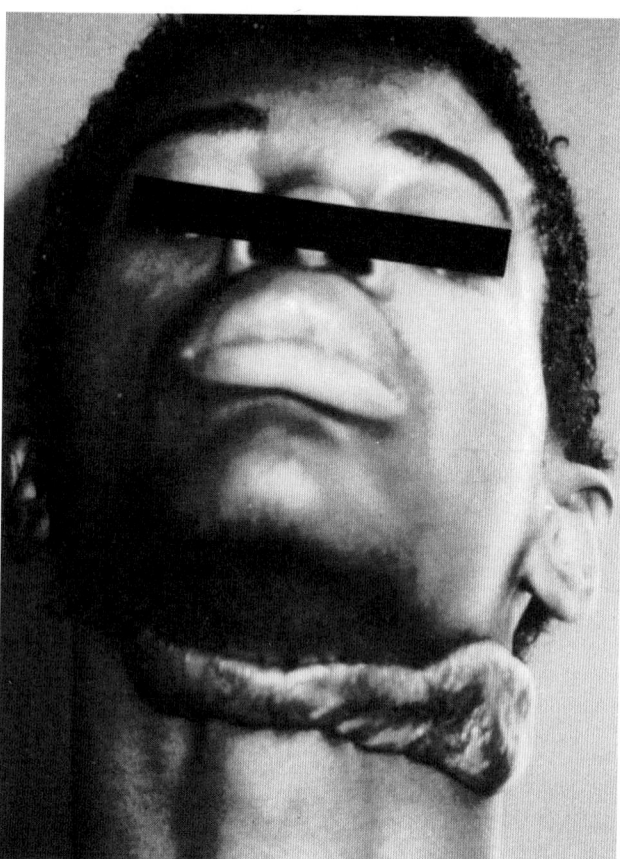

FIG. 9-10. Recurrent keloid on the neck of a 17-year-old patient that had been revised several times. *[Reproduced with permission from Murray JC, Pinnell SR: Keloids and excessive dermal scarring, in Cohen IK, Diegelmann RF, Lindblad WJ (eds):* Wound Healing: Bio-chemical and Clinical Aspects. *Philadelphia: WB Saunders, 1993.]*

ties being especially susceptible. Men and women are equally affected. Genetically, the predilection to keloid formation appears to be autosomal dominant, with incomplete penetration and variable expression.[98,99]

HTSs usually develop within 4 weeks after trauma. The risk of HTSs increases if epithelialization takes longer than 21 days, independent of site, age, and race. Rarely elevated more than 4 mm above the skin level, HTSs stay within the boundaries of the wound. They usually occur across areas of tension and flexor surfaces, which tend to be at right angles to joints or skin creases. The lesions are initially erythematous and raised, and over time may evolve into pale, flatter scars.

Keloids can result from surgery, burns, skin inflammation, acne, chickenpox, zoster, folliculitis, lacerations, abrasions, tattoos, vaccinations, injections, insect bites, ear piercing, or may arise spontaneously. Keloids tend to occur 3 months to years after the initial insult, and even minor injuries can result in large lesions. They vary in size from a few millimeters to large, pedunculated lesions with a soft to rubbery or hard consistency. Although they project above surrounding skin, they rarely extend into underlying subcutaneous tissues. Certain body sites have a higher incidence of keloid formation, including the skin of the earlobe as well as the deltoid, presternal, and upper back regions. They rarely occur on eyelids, genitalia, palms, soles, or across joints. Keloids rarely involute spontaneously, whereas surgical intervention can lead to recurrence, often with a worse result.

Histologically, both HTSs and keloids demonstrate increased thickness of the epidermis with an absence of rete ridges. There is an abundance of collagen and glycoprotein deposition. Normal skin has distinct collagen bundles, mostly parallel to the epithelial

surface, with random connections between bundles by fine fibrillar strands of collagen. In HTSs, the collagen bundles are flatter, more random, and the fibers are in a wavy pattern. In keloids, the collagen bundles are virtually nonexistent, and the fibers are connected haphazardly in loose sheets with a random orientation to the epithelium. The collagen fibers are larger and thicker and myofibroblasts are generally absent.[100]

Keloidal fibroblasts have normal proliferation parameters, but synthesize collagen at a rate 20 times greater than that observed in normal dermal fibroblasts, and 3 times higher than fibroblasts derived from HTSs. Abnormal amounts of extracellular matrix, such as fibronectin, elastin, and proteoglycans, also are produced. The synthesis of fibronectin, which promotes clot generation, granulation tissue formation, and re-epithelialization, decreases during the normal healing process; however, production continues at high levels for months to years in HTSs and keloids. This perturbed synthetic activity is mediated by altered growth factor expression. TGFβ expression is higher in HTSs, and both HTS- and keloid-derived fibroblasts respond to lower concentrations of TGFβ than do normal dermal fibroblasts. HTSs also express increased levels of insulin-like growth factor I, which reduces collagenase mRNA activity and increases mRNA for types I and II procollagen.

The underlying mechanisms that cause HTSs and keloids are not known. The immune system appears to be involved in the formation of both HTSs and keloids, although the exact relationship is unknown. Much is inferred from the presence of various immune cells in HTSs and keloids. For example, in both HTSs and keloids, keratinocytes express human leukocyte antigen-2 and intercellular adhesion molecule-1 receptors, which are absent in normal scar keratinocytes. Keloids also have increased deposition of immunoglobulin G (IgG), IgA, and IgM, and their formation correlates with serum levels of IgE. Antinuclear antibodies against fibroblasts, epithelial cells, and endothelial cells are found in keloids, but not HTSs. HTSs have higher T-lymphocyte and Langerhans cell contents. There also is a larger number of mast cells present in both HTSs and keloids compared to normal scars. Other mechanisms that may cause abnormal scarring include mechanical tension (although keloids often occur in areas of minimal tension) and prolonged irritation and/or inflammation that may lead to the generation of abnormal concentrations of profibrotic cytokines.

Treatment goals include restoration of function to the area, relief of symptoms, and prevention of recurrence. Many patients seek intervention due to cosmetic concerns. Because the underlying mechanisms causing keloids and HTSs remain unknown, many different modalities of treatment have been used without consistent success.

Excision alone of keloids is subject to a high recurrence rate, ranging from 45 to 100%. There are fewer recurrences when surgical excision is combined with other modalities such as intralesional corticosteroid injection, topical application of silicone sheets, or the use of radiation or pressure. Surgery is recommended for debulking large lesions or as second-line therapy when other modalities have failed. Silicone application is relatively painless and should be maintained for 24 hours a day for about 3 months to prevent rebound hypertrophy. It may be secured with tape or worn beneath a pressure garment. The mechanism of action is not understood, but increased hydration of the skin, which decreases capillary activity, inflammation, hyperemia, and collagen deposition, may be involved. Silicone is more effective than other occlusive dressings and is an especially good treatment for children and others who cannot tolerate the pain involved in other modalities.[101]

Intralesional corticosteroid injections decrease fibroblast proliferation, collagen and glycosaminoglycan synthesis, the inflammatory process, and TGFβ levels. When used alone, however, there is a variable rate of response and recurrence, therefore steroids are recommended as first-line treatment for keloids and second-line treatment for HTSs if topical therapies have failed. Intralesional injections are more effective on younger scars. They may soften, flatten, and give symptomatic relief to keloids, but they cannot make the lesions disappear nor can they narrow wide HTSs. Success is enhanced when used in combination with surgical excision. Serial injections every 2 to 3 weeks are required. Complications include skin atrophy, hypopigmentation, telangiectasias, necrosis, and ulceration.

Although radiation destroys fibroblasts, it has variable, unreliable results and produces poor results with 10 to 100% recurrence when used alone. It is more effective when combined with surgical excision. The timing, duration, and dosage for radiation therapy are still controversial, but doses ranging from 1500 to 2000 rads appear effective. Given the risks of hyperpigmentation, pruritus, erythema, paresthesias, pain, and possible secondary malignancies, radiation should be reserved for adults with scars resistant to other modalities.

Pressure aids collagen maturation, flattens scars, and improves thinning and pliability. It reduces the number of cells in a given area, possibly by creating ischemia, which decreases tissue metabolism and increases collagenase activity. External compression is used to treat HTSs, especially after burns. Therapy must begin early, and a pressure between 24 and 30 mmHg must be achieved in order to exceed capillary pressure, yet preserve peripheral blood circulation. Garments should be worn for 23 to 24 hours a day for up to 1 or more years to avoid rebound hypertrophy. Scars older than 6 to 12 months respond poorly.

Topical retinoids also have been used as treatment for both HTSs and keloids, with reported responses of 50 to 100%. Intralesional injections of interferon-γ, a cytokine released by T lymphocytes, reduce collagen types I, II, and III by decreasing mRNA and possibly by reducing levels of TGFβ. This treatment is experimental, and complications are frequent and dose-dependent. Intralesional injections of chemotherapeutic agents such as 5-fluorouracil have been used both alone and in combination with steroids. The use of bleomycin has been reported to achieve some success in older scars resistant to steroids.

Peritoneal Scarring

Peritoneal adhesions are fibrous bands of tissues formed between organs that are normally separated and/or between organs and the internal body wall. Most intra-abdominal adhesions are a result of peritoneal injury, either by a prior surgical procedure or due to intra-abdominal infection. Postmortem examinations demonstrate adhesions in 67% of patients with prior surgical procedures and in 28% with a history of intra-abdominal infection. Intra-abdominal adhesions are the most common cause (65 to 75%) of small bowel obstruction, especially in the ileum. Operations in the lower abdomen have a higher chance of producing small bowel obstruction. After rectal surgery, left colectomy, or total colectomy, there is an 11% chance of developing small bowel obstruction within 1 year, and this rate increases to 30% by 10 years. Adhesions also are a leading cause of secondary infertility in women and can cause substantial abdominal and pelvic pain. Adhesions account for 2% of all surgical admissions and 3% of all laparotomies in general surgery.[102]

Adhesions form when the peritoneal surface is damaged due to surgery, thermal or ischemic injury, inflammation, or foreign body reaction. The injury disrupts the protective mesothelial cell layer lining the peritoneal cavity and the underlying connective tissue. The injury elicits an inflammatory response consisting of hyperemia, fluid exudation, release and activation of white blood cells and platelets in the peritoneal cavity, activation of inflammatory cytokines, and the onset of the coagulation and complement cascades. Fibrin deposition occurs between the damaged but opposed serosal surfaces. These filmy adhesions often are transient and degraded by proteases of the fibrinolytic system, with restoration of the normal peritoneal surface. If insufficient fibrinolytic activity is present, permanent fibrous adhesions will form by collagen deposition within 1 week of the injury (Fig. 9-11).

Extensive research has been done on the effect of surgery and peritonitis on the fibrinolytic and inflammatory cascades within the peritoneal cavity. During normal repair, fibrin is principally degraded by the fibrinolytic protease plasmin, which is derived from

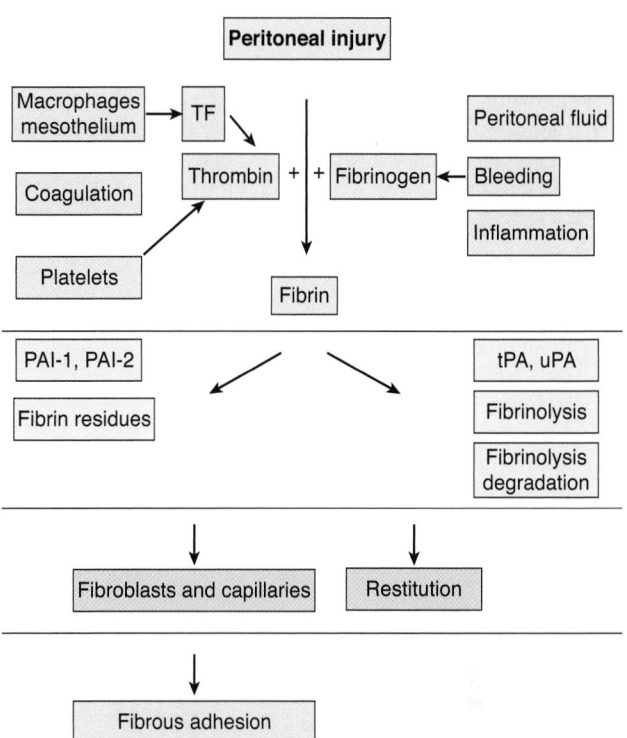

FIG. 9-11. Fibrin formation and degradation in peritoneal tissue repair and adhesion formation. PAI-1, -2 = types 1 and 2 plasminogen activator inhibitor; TF = tissue factor; tPA = tissue plasminogen activator; uPA = urokinase plasminogen activator.

inactive plasminogen through the action of two plasminogen activators: tissue-type plasminogen activator and urokinase-type plasminogen activator. Fibrinolytic activity in peritoneal fluid is reduced after abdominal surgery due to initial decreases in tissue-type plasminogen activator levels and later to increases in plasminogen activator inhibitor 1, which are induced by various cytokines, including TNF-α, IL-1, and IL-6.[103]

There are two major strategies for adhesion prevention or reduction. Surgical trauma is minimized within the peritoneum by careful tissue handling, avoiding desiccation and ischemia, and spare use of cautery, laser, and retractors. Fewer adhesions form with laparoscopic surgical techniques due to reduced tissue trauma. The second major advance in adhesion prevention has been the introduction of barrier membranes and gels, which separate and create barriers between damaged surfaces, allowing for adhesion-free healing. Modified oxidized regenerated cellulose and hyaluronic acid membranes or solutions have been shown to reduce adhesions in gynecologic patients, and have been investigated for their ability to prevent adhesion formation in patients undergoing bowel surgery.[104,105] Wrapping of the bowel suture area or placement in the proximity of the anastomoses with these substances is, however, contraindicated due to an elevated risk of leak.[106]

TREATMENT OF WOUNDS

Local Care

See Fig. 9-12. Management of acute wounds begins with obtaining a careful history of the events surrounding the injury. The history is followed by a meticulous examination of the wound. Examination should assess the depth and configuration of the wound, the extent of nonviable tissue, and the presence of foreign bodies and other contaminants. Examination of the wound may require irrigation and débridement of the edges of the wound, and is facilitated by use

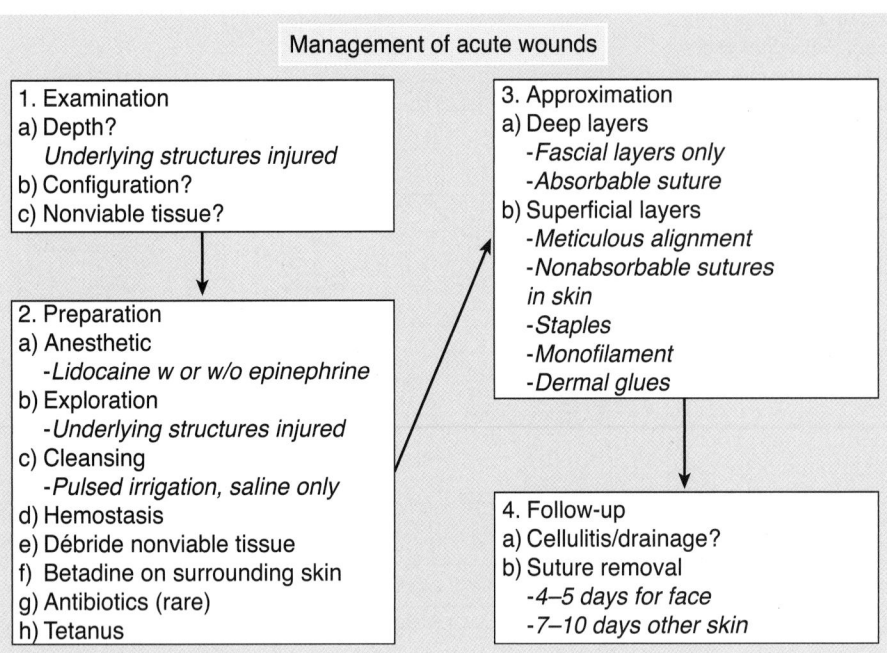

Management of acute wounds

1. Examination
a) Depth?
   Underlying structures injured
b) Configuration?
c) Nonviable tissue?

2. Preparation
a) Anesthetic
   -Lidocaine w or w/o epinephrine
b) Exploration
   -Underlying structures injured
c) Cleansing
   -Pulsed irrigation, saline only
d) Hemostasis
e) Débride nonviable tissue
f) Betadine on surrounding skin
g) Antibiotics (rare)
h) Tetanus

3. Approximation
a) Deep layers
   -Fascial layers only
   -Absorbable suture
b) Superficial layers
   -Meticulous alignment
   *-Nonabsorbable sutures
   in skin*
   -Staples
   -Monofilament
   -Dermal glues

4. Follow-up
a) Cellulitis/drainage?
b) Suture removal
   -4–5 days for face
   -7–10 days other skin

FIG. 9-12. Algorithm for management of acute wounds.

of local anesthesia. Antibiotic administration and tetanus prophylaxis may be needed, and planning the type and timing of wound repair should take place.

After completion of the history, examination, and administration of tetanus prophylaxis, the wound should be meticulously anesthetized. Lidocaine (0.5 to 1%) or bupivacaine (0.25 to 0.5%) combined with a 1:100,000 to 1:200,000 dilution of epinephrine provides satisfactory anesthesia and hemostasis. Epinephrine should not be used in wounds of the fingers, toes, ears, nose, or penis due to the risk of tissue necrosis secondary to terminal arteriole vasospasm in these structures. Injection of these anesthetics can result in significant initial patient discomfort, and this can be minimized by slow injection, infiltration of the subcutaneous tissues, and buffering the solution with sodium bicarbonate. Care must be observed in calculating the maximum dosages of lidocaine or bupivacaine to avoid toxicity-related side effects.

Irrigation to visualize all areas of the wound and remove foreign material is best accomplished with normal saline (without additives). High-pressure wound irrigation is more effective in achieving complete débridement of foreign material and nonviable tissues. Iodine, povidone-iodine, hydrogen peroxide, and organically based antibacterial preparations have all been shown to impair wound healing due to injury to wound neutrophils and macrophages, and thus should not be used. All hematomas present within wounds should be carefully evacuated and any remaining bleeding sources controlled with ligature or cautery. If the injury has resulted in the formation of a marginally viable flap of skin or tissue, these should be resected or revascularized before further wound repair and closure.

After the wound has been anesthetized, explored, irrigated, and débrided, the area surrounding the wound should be cleaned, inspected, and the surrounding hair clipped. The area surrounding the wound should be prepared with povidone-iodine or similar solution and draped with sterile towels. Having ensured hemostasis and adequate débridement of nonviable tissues and removal of any remaining foreign bodies, irregular, macerated, or beveled wound edges should be débrided in order to provide a fresh edge for reapproximation. Although plastic surgical techniques such as W- or Z-plasty are seldom recommended for acute wounds, great care must be taken to realign wound edges properly. This is particularly important for wounds that cross the vermilion border, eyebrow, or hairline. Initial sutures that realign the edges of these different tissue types will speed and greatly enhance the aesthetic outcome of the wound repair.

In general, the smallest suture required to hold the various layers of the wound in approximation should be selected in order to minimize suture-related inflammation. Nonabsorbable or slowly absorbing monofilament sutures are most suitable for approximating deep fascial layers, particularly in the abdominal wall. Subcutaneous tissues should be closed with braided absorbable sutures, with care to avoid placement of sutures in fat. Although traditional teaching in wound closure has emphasized multiple-layer closures, additional layers of suture closure are associated with increased risk of wound infection, especially when placed in fat. Drains may be placed in areas at risk of forming fluid collections.

In areas of significant tissue loss, rotation of adjacent musculocutaneous flaps may be required to provide sufficient tissue mass for closure. These musculocutaneous flaps may be based on intrinsic blood supply, or may be moved from distant sites as free flaps and anastomosed into the local vascular bed. In areas with significant superficial tissue loss, split-thickness skin grafting (placed in a delayed manner to assure an adequate tissue bed) may be required and will speed formation of an intact epithelial barrier to fluid loss and infection. Split-thickness skin grafts are readily obtained using manual or mechanical dermatomes, and the grafts may be "meshed" in order to increase the surface area of their coverage. It is essential to ensure hemostasis of the underlying tissue bed before placement of split-thickness skin grafts, as the presence of a hematoma below the graft will prevent the graft from taking, resulting in sloughing of the graft. In acute, contaminated wounds with skin loss, use of porcine xenografts or cadaveric allografts is prudent until the danger of infection passes.

After closing deep tissues and replacing significant tissue deficits, skin edges should be reapproximated for cosmesis and to aid in rapid wound healing. Skin edges may be quickly reapproximated with stainless steel staples or nonabsorbable monofilament sutures. Care must be taken to remove these from the wound before epithelialization of the skin tracts where sutures or staples penetrate the dermal layer. Failure to remove the sutures or staples by 7 to 10 days after repair will result in a cosmetically inferior wound. When wound cosmesis is important, the above problems may be avoided by placement of buried dermal sutures using absorbable braided sutures. This method of wound closure allows for a precise reapproximation of wound edges, and may be enhanced by application of wound closure tapes to the surface of the wound. Intradermal absorbable sutures do not require removal. Use of skin tapes alone is only recommended for closure of the smallest superficial wounds. Larger wounds generate sufficient lateral tension that the epithelial edges either separate or curl upward under the tapes, resulting in inadequate epithelial apposition and poor cosmesis.

The development of octyl-cyanoacrylate tissue glues has shown new promise for the management of simple, linear wounds with viable skin edges. These new glues are less prone to brittleness and have superior burst-strength characteristics. Studies have shown them to be suitable for use in contaminated situations without significant risk of infection. When used in the above types of wounds, these glues appear to provide superb cosmetic results and result in significantly less trauma than sutured repair, particularly when used in pediatric patients.

Antibiotics

Antibiotics should be used only when there is an obvious wound infection. Most wounds are contaminated or colonized with bacteria. The presence of a host response constitutes an infection and justifies the use of antibiotics. Signs of infection to look for include erythema, cellulitis, swelling, and purulent discharge. Indiscriminate use of antibiotics should be avoided to prevent emergence of multidrug-resistant bacteria.

Antibiotic treatment of acute wounds must be based on organisms suspected to be found within the infected wound and the patient's overall immune status. When a single specific organism is suspected, treatment may be commenced using a single antibiotic. Conversely, when multiple organisms are suspected, as with enteric contamination or when a patient's immune function is impaired by diabetes, chronic disease, or medication, treatment should commence with a broad-spectrum antibiotic or several agents in combination. Last, the location of the wound and the quality of tissue perfusion to that region will significantly impact wound performance after injury. Antibiotics can also be delivered topically as part of irrigations or dressings, although their efficacy is questionable.

Dressings

The main purpose of wound dressings is to provide the ideal environment for wound healing. The dressing should facilitate the major changes taking place during healing to produce an optimally healed wound. Although the ideal dressing is still not a clinical reality, technological advances are promising (Table 9-8).

Covering a wound with a dressing mimics the barrier role of epithelium and prevents further damage. In addition, application of compression provides hemostasis and limits edema. Occlusion of a wound with dressing material helps healing by controlling the level of hydration and oxygen tension within the wound. It also allows transfer of gases and water vapor from the wound surface to the atmosphere. Occlusion affects both the dermis and epidermis, and it has been shown that exposed wounds are more inflamed and develop more necrosis than covered wounds. Occlusion also helps in dermal collagen synthesis and epithelial cell migration and limits tissue desiccation. As it may enhance bacterial growth, occlusion is contraindicated in infected and highly exudative wounds.

TABLE 9-8	Desired characteristics of wound dressings

Promote wound healing (maintain moist environment)
Conformability
Pain control
Odor control
Nonallergenic and nonirritating
Permeability to gas
Safety
Nontraumatic removal
Cost-effectiveness
Convenience

Dressings can be classified as primary or secondary. A primary dressing is placed directly on the wound and may provide absorption of fluids and prevent desiccation, infection, and adhesion of a secondary dressing. A secondary dressing is one that is placed on the primary dressing for further protection, absorption, compression, and occlusion. Many types of dressings exist and are designed to achieve certain clinically desired endpoints.

Absorbent Dressings

Accumulation of wound fluid can lead to maceration and bacterial overgrowth. Ideally, the dressing should absorb without getting soaked through, as this would permit bacteria from the outside to enter the wound. The dressing must be designed to match the exudative properties of the wound and may include cotton, wool, and sponge.

Nonadherent Dressings

Nonadherent dressings are impregnated with paraffin, petroleum jelly, or water-soluble jelly for use as nonadherent coverage. A secondary dressing must be placed on top to seal the edges and prevent desiccation and infection.

Occlusive and Semiocclusive Dressings

Occlusive and semiocclusive dressings provide a good environment for clean, minimally exudative wounds. These film dressings are waterproof and impervious to microbes, but permeable to water vapor and oxygen.

Hydrophilic and Hydrophobic Dressings

Hydrophilic and hydrophobic dressings are components of a composite dressing. Hydrophilic dressing aids in absorption, whereas a hydrophobic dressing is waterproof and prevents absorption.

Hydrocolloid and Hydrogel Dressings

Hydrocolloid and hydrogel dressings attempt to combine the benefits of occlusion and absorbency. Hydrocolloids and hydrogels form complex structures with water, and fluid absorption occurs with particle swelling, which aids in atraumatic removal of the dressing. Absorption of exudates by the hydrocolloid dressing leaves a yellowish-brown gelatinous mass after dressing removal that can be washed off. Hydrogel is a cross-linked polymer that has high water content. Hydrogels allow a high rate of evaporation without compromising wound hydration, which makes them useful in burn treatment.

Alginates

Alginates are derived from brown algae and contain long chains of polysaccharides containing mannuronic and glucuronic acid. The ratios of these sugars vary with the species of algae used, as well as the season of harvest. Processed as the calcium form, alginates turn into soluble sodium alginate through ion exchange in the presence of wound exudates. The polymers gel, swell, and absorb a great deal of fluid. Alginates are being used when there is skin loss, in open surgical wounds with medium exudation, and on full-thickness chronic wounds.

Absorbable Materials

Absorbable materials are mainly used within wounds as hemostats and include collagen, gelatin, oxidized cellulose, and oxidized regenerated cellulose.

Medicated Dressings

Medicated dressings have long been used as a drug-delivery system. Agents delivered in the dressings include benzoyl peroxide, zinc oxide, neomycin, and bacitracin-zinc. These agents have been shown to increase epithelialization by 28%.

The type of dressing to be used depends on the amount of wound drainage. A nondraining wound can be covered with a semiocclusive dressing. Drainage of less than 1 to 2 mL/d may require a semiocclusive or absorbent nonadherent dressing. Moderately draining wounds (3 to 5 mL/d) can be dressed with a nonadherent primary layer plus an absorbent secondary layer plus an occlusive dressing to protect normal tissue. Heavily draining wounds (>5 mL/d) require a similar dressing to moderately draining wounds, but with the addition of a highly absorbent secondary layer.

Mechanical Devices

Mechanical therapy augments and improves on certain functions of dressings, in particular the absorption of exudates and control of odor. The vacuum-assisted closure system assists in wound closure by applying localized negative pressure to the surface and margins of the wound. The negative pressure therapy is applied to a special foam dressing cut to the dimensions of the wound and positioned in the wound cavity or over a flap or graft. The continuous negative pressure is very effective in removing exudates from the wound. This form of therapy has been found to be effective for chronic open wounds (diabetic ulcers and stages 3 and 4 pressure ulcers), acute and traumatic wounds,[107] flaps and grafts, and subacute wounds (i.e., dehisced incisions), although more randomized trials need to be carried out to confirm efficacy.

Skin Replacements

All wounds require coverage in order to prevent evaporative losses and infection and to provide an environment that promotes healing. Both acute and chronic wounds may demand use of skin replacement, and several options are available.

Conventional Skin Grafts

Skin grafts have long been used to treat both acute and chronic wounds. Split- or partial-thickness grafts consist of the epidermis plus part of the dermis, whereas full-thickness grafts retain the entire epidermis and dermis. Autologous grafts (autografts) are transplants from one site on the body to another; allogeneic grafts (allografts, homografts) are transplants from a living nonidentical donor or cadaver to the host; and xenogeneic grafts (heterografts) are taken from another species (e.g., porcine). Split-thickness grafts require less blood supply to restore skin function. The dermal component of full-thickness grafts lends mechanical strength and resists wound contraction better, resulting in improved cosmesis. Allogeneic and xenogeneic grafts require the availability of tissue, are subject to rejection, and may contain pathogens.

The use of skin grafts or bioengineered skin substitutes and other innovative treatments (e.g., topically applied growth factors, systemic agents, and gene therapy) cannot be effective unless the wound bed is adequately prepared. This may include débridement to remove necrotic or fibrinous tissue, control of edema, revascularization of the wound bed, decreasing the bacterial burden, and minimizing or eliminating exudate. Temporary placement of allografts or xenografts may be used to prepare the wound bed.

TABLE 9-9	Desired features of tissue-engineered skin

Rapid re-establishment of functional skin (epidermis/dermis)
Receptive to body's own cells (e.g., rapid "take" and integration)
Graftable by a single, simple procedure
Graftable on chronic or acute wounds
Engraftment without use of extraordinary clinical intervention (i.e., immunosuppression)

Skin Substitutes

Originally devised to provide coverage of extensive wounds with limited availability of autografts, skin substitutes also have gained acceptance as natural dressings. Manufactured by tissue engineering, they combine novel materials with living cells to provide functional skin substitutes, providing a bridge between dressings and skin grafts.

Skin substitutes have theoretical advantages of being readily available, not requiring painful harvest, and they may be applied freely or with surgical suturing. In addition, they promote healing, either by stimulating host cytokine generation or by providing cells that may also produce growth factors locally. Their disadvantages include limited survival, high cost, and the need for multiple applications (Table 9-9). Allografting, albeit with a very thin graft, may at times be required to accomplish complete coverage.

A variety of skin substitutes are available, each with its own set of advantages and disadvantages; however, the ideal skin substitute has yet to be developed (Table 9-10). The development of newer composite substitutes, which provide both the dermal and epidermal components essential for permanent skin replacement, may represent an advance toward that goal. The acellular (e.g., native collagen or synthetic material) component acts as a scaffold, promotes cell migration and growth, and activates tissue regeneration and remodeling. The cellular elements re-establish lost tissue and associated function, synthesize extracellular matrix components, produce essential mediators such as cytokines and growth factors, and promote proliferation and migration.

Cultured epithelial autografts (CEAs) represent expanded autologous or homologous keratinocytes. CEAs are expanded from a biopsy of the patient's own skin, will not be rejected, and can stimulate re-epithelialization as well as the growth of underlying connective tissue. Keratinocytes harvested from a biopsy roughly the size of a postage stamp are cultured with fibroblasts and growth factors and grown into sheets that can cover large areas and give the appearance of normal skin. Until the epithelial sheets are sufficiently expanded, the wound must be covered with an occlusive dressing or a temporary allograft or xenograft. The dermis regenerates very slowly, if at all, for full-thickness wounds, because the sheets are very fragile, difficult to work with, are susceptible to infection, and do not resist contracture well, leading to poor cosmetic results.

TABLE 9-10	Advantages and disadvantages of various bioengineered skin substitutes

Skin Substitute	Advantages	Disadvantages
Cultured allogeneic keratinocyte graft	No biopsy needed	Unstable
	"Off the shelf" availability	Does not prevent wound contracture
	Provides wound coverage	Inadequate cosmesis
	Promotes healing	Possibility of disease transmission
		Fragile
Bioengineered dermal replacement	Prevents contracture	Limited ability to drive re-epithelialization
	Good prep for graft application	Largely serves as temporary dressing
Cultured bilayer skin equivalent	More closely mimics normal anatomy	Cost
	Does not need secondary procedure	Short shelf life
	Easily handled	True engraftment questionable
	Can be sutured, meshed, etc.	

CEAs are available from cadavers, unrelated adult donors, or from neonatal foreskins. Fresh or cryopreserved cultured allogeneic keratinocytes can be left in place long enough to be superseded by multiplying endogenous skin cells because, unlike allografts containing epidermal Langerhans cells, they do not express major histocompatibility antigens. Cryopreserved CEAs are readily available "off the shelf," and provide growth factors that may aid healing. However, like autologous keratinocyte sheets, the grafts lack the strength provided by a dermal component and pose a risk of disease transmission.

Viable fibroblasts can be grown on bioabsorbable or nonbioabsorbable meshes to yield living dermal tissue that can act as a scaffold for epidermal growth. Fibroblasts stimulated by growth factors can produce type I collagen and glycosaminoglycans (e.g., chondroitin sulfates), which adhere to the wound surface to permit epithelial cell migration, as well as adhesive ligands (e.g., the matrix protein fibronectin), which promote cell adhesion. This approach has the virtue of being less time-consuming and expensive than culturing keratinocyte sheets. There are a number of commercially available, bioengineered dermal replacements approved for use in burn treatment as well as other indications.

Bioengineered skin substitutes have evolved from keratinocyte monolayers to dermal equivalents to split-thickness products with a pseudoepidermis and, most recently, to products containing both epidermal and dermal components that resemble the three-dimensional structure and function of normal skin (see Table 9-10). Indicated for use with standard compression therapy in the treatment of venous insufficiency ulcers and for the treatment of neuropathic diabetic foot ulcers, these bilayered skin equivalents also are being used in a variety of wound care settings.

Growth Factor Therapy

As discussed previously in the section Chronic Wounds, it is believed that nonhealing wounds result from insufficient or inadequate growth factors in the wound environment. A simplistic solution would be to flood the wound with single or multiple growth factors in order to "jump-start" healing and re-epithelialization. Although there is a large body of work demonstrating the effects of growth factors in animals, translation of these data into clinical practice has met with limited success. Growth factors for clinical use may be either recombinant or homologous/autologous. Autologous growth factors are harvested from the patient's own platelets, yielding an unpredictable combination and concentration of factors, which are then applied to the wound. This approach allows treatment with patient-specific factors at an apparently physiologic ratio of growth factor concentrations. Recombinant molecular biologic means permit the purification of high concentrations of individual growth factors. Current Food and Drug Administration–approved formulations, as well as those used experimentally, deliver concentrations approximately 10^3 times higher than those observed physiologically.

At present, only platelet-derived growth factor BB (PDGF-BB) is currently approved by the Food and Drug Administration for treatment of diabetic foot ulcers.[92] Application of recombinant human PDGF-BB in a gel suspension to these wounds increases the incidence of total healing and decreases healing time. Several other growth factors have been tested clinically and show some promise, but currently none are approved for use. A great deal more needs to be discovered about the concentration, temporal release, and receptor cell population before growth factor therapy is to make a consistent impact on wound healing.

REFERENCES

Entries highlighted in bright blue are key references.

1. Winter GD: Formation of the scab and the rate of epithelialisation of superficial wounds in the skin of the young domestic pig. *Nature* 193:293, 1962.
2. Gulliver G (ed): *The Works of John Hunter.* London: Longman, 1837.
3. Feiken E, Romer J, Eriksen J, et al: Neutrophils express tumor necrosis factor-alpha during mouse skin wound healing. *J Invest Dermatol* 105:120, 1995.
4. Dovi JV, He L-K, DiPietro LA: Accelerated wound closure in neutrophil-depleted mice. *J Leukoc Biol* 73:448, 2003.
5. Leibovich SJ, Ross R: The role of the macrophage in wound repair. A study with hydrocortisone and antimacrophage serum. *Am J Pathol* 78:71, 1975.
6. DiPietro LA: Wound healing: The role of the macrophage and other immune cells. *Shock* 4:233, 1995.
7. Zabel DD, Feng JJ, Scheuenstuhl H, et al: Lactate stimulation of macrophage-derived angiogenic activity is associated with inhibition of Poly(ADP-ribose) synthesis. *Lab Invest* 74:644, 1996.
8. Schäffer MR, Barbul A: Lymphocyte function in wound healing and following injury. *Br J Surg* 85:444, 1998.
9. Efron JE, Frankel HL, Lazarou SA, et al: Wound healing and T-lymphocytes. *J Surg Res* 48:460, 1990.
10. Barbul A, Breslin RJ, Woodyard JP, et al: The effect of in vivo T helper and T suppressor lymphocyte depletion on wound healing. *Ann Surg* 209:479, 1989.
11. Rezzonico R, Burger D, Dayer JM: Direct contact between T lymphocytes and human dermal fibroblasts or synoviocytes down-regulates types I and III collagen production via cell-associated cytokines. *J Biol Chem* 273:18720, 1998.
12. Grotendorst GR: Chemoattractants and growth factors, in Cohen K, Diegelmann RF, Lindblad WJ (eds): *Wound Healing, Biochemical and Clinical Aspects.* Philadelphia: WB Saunders, 1992, p 237.
13. Bonner JC, Osornio-Vargas AR, et al: Differential proliferation of rat lung fibroblasts induced by the platelet-derived growth factor-AA, -AB, and -BB isoforms secreted by rat alveolar macrophages. *Am J Respir Cell Mol Biol* 5:539, 1991.
14. Pricolo VE, Caldwell MD, Mastrofrancesco B, et al: Modulatory activities of wound fluid on fibroblast proliferation and collagen synthesis. *J Surg Res* 48:534, 1990.
15. Regan MC, Kirk SJ, Wasserkrug HL, et al: The wound environment as a regulator of fibroblast phenotype. *J Surg Res* 50:442, 1991.
16. Gimbel ML, Hunt TK, Hussain MZ: Lactate controls collagen gene promoter activity through poly-ADP-ribosylation. *Surg Forum* 51:26, 2000.
17. Ghani QP, Hussain MZ, Hunt TK: Control of procollagen gene transcription and prolyl hydroxylase activity by poly(ADP-ribose), in Poirier G, Moreaer A (eds): *ADP-Ribosylation Reactions.* New York: Springer-Verlag, 1992, p 111.
18. Xiong M, Elson G, Legarda D, et al: Production of vascular endothelial growth factor by murine macrophages: Regulation by hypoxia, lactate, and the inducible nitric oxide synthase pathway. *Am J Pathol* 153:587, 1998.
19. Ferrara N, Davis-Smith T: The biology of vascular endothelial growth factor. *Endocrine Rev* 18:4, 1997.
20. Levenson SM, Geever EF, Crowley LV, et al: The healing of rat skin wounds. *Ann Surg* 161:293, 1965.
21. Zhou LJ, Ono I, Kaneko F: Role of transforming growth factor-beta 1 in fibroblasts derived from normal and hypertrophic scarred skin. *Arch Dermatol Res* 289:645, 1997.
22. Stenn KS, Depalma L: Re-epithelialization, in Clark RAF, Hensen PM (eds): *The Molecular and Cellular Biology of Wound Repair.* New York: Plenum, 1988, p 321.
23. Johnson FR, McMinn RMH: The cytology of wound healing of the body surface in mammals. *Biol Rev* 35:364, 1960.
24. Woodley DT, Bachman PM, O'Keefe EJ: The role of matrix components in human keratinocyte re-epithelialization, in Barbul A, Caldwell MD, Eaglstein WH, et al (eds): *Clinical and Experimental Approaches to Dermal and Epidermal Repair. Normal and Chronic Wounds.* New York: Wiley-Liss, 1991, p 129.
25. Lynch SE: Interaction of growth factors in tissue repair, in Barbul A, Caldwell MD, Eaglstein WH, et al (eds): *Clinical and Experimental Approaches to Dermal and Epidermal Repair. Normal and Chronic Wounds.* New York: Wiley-Liss, 1991, p 341.
26. Jans DA, Hassan G: Nuclear targeting by growth factors, cytokines, and their receptors: A role in signaling? *Bioassays* 20:400, 1998.
27. Schmitt-Graff A, Desmouliere A, Gabbiani G: Heterogeneity of myofibroblast phenotypic features: An example of fibroblastic cell plasticity. *Virchows Arch* 425:3, 1994.

28. Darby I, Skalli O, Gabbiani G: Alpha-smooth muscle actin is transiently expressed by myofibroblasts during experimental wound healing. *Lab Invest* 63:21, 1990.

29. Desmouliere A, Redard M, Darby I, et al: Apoptosis mediates the decrease in cellularity during the transition between granulation tissue and scar. *Am J Pathol* 146:56, 1995.

30. Ehrlich HP: Wound closure: Evidence of cooperation between fibroblasts and collagen matrix. *Eye* 2:149, 1988.

31. Phillips C, Wenstrup RJ: Biosynthetic and genetic disorders of collagen, in Cohen IK, Diegelmann RF, Linblad WJ (eds): *Wound Healing: Biochemical and Clinical Aspects.* Philadelphia: WB Saunders, 1992, p 152.

32. Sidhu-Malik NK, Wenstrup RJ: The Ehlers-Danlos syndromes and Marfan syndrome: Inherited diseases of connective tissue with overlapping clinical features. *Semin Dermatol* 14:40, 1995.

33. Woolley MM, Morgan S, Hays DM: Heritable disorders of connective tissue. Surgical and anesthetic problems. *J Pediatr Surg* 2:325, 1967.

34. McEntyre RL, Raffensperger JG: Surgical complications of Ehlers-Danlos syndrome in children. *J Pediatr Surg* 13:531, 1977.

35. Hunt TK: Disorders of wound healing. *World J Surg* 4:271, 1980.

36. Anonymous: Heritable disorders of connective tissue. *JAMA* 224(5 Suppl):774, 1973.

37. Carter DM, Lin AN: Wound healing and epidermolysis bullosa. *Arch Dermatol* 124:732, 1988.

38. Kruse-Jarres JD: Pathogenesis and symptoms of zinc deficiency. *Am Clin Lab* 20:17, 2001.

39. Okada A, Takagi Y, Nezu R, et al: Zinc in clinical surgery—a research review. *Jpn J Surg* 20:635, 1990.

40. Thornton FJ, Barbul A: Healing in the gastrointestinal tract. *Surg Clin North Am* 77:549, 1997.

41. Choy PYG, Bissett IP, Docherty JG, et al: Stapled versus handsewn methods for ileocolic anastomoses. Cochrane Database of Systematic Reviews 2007, Issue 3. Art. No.: CD004320. DOI: 10.1002/14651858.CD004320.pub2.

42. Lorenz PH, Whitby DJ, Longaker MT, et al: Fetal wound healing. The ontogeny of scar formation in the non-human primate. *Ann Surg* 217:391, 1993.

43. Longaker MT, Whitby DJ, Ferguson MWJ, et al: Adult skin wounds in the fetal environment heal with scar formation. *Ann Surg* 219:65, 1994.

44. Lorenz HP, Longaker MT, Perkocha LA, et al: Scarless wound repair: A human fetal skin model. *Development* 114:253, 1992.

45. Adzick NS, Harrison MR, Glick PL, et al: Comparison of fetal, newborn and adult rabbit wound healing by histologic, enzyme-histochemical and hydroxyproline determinations. *J Pediatr Surg* 20:315, 1991.

46. Shah M, Foreman DM, Ferguson MWJ: Neutralizing antibody to TGF-β1,2 reduces cutaneous scarring in adult rodents. *J Cell Sci* 107:1137, 1994.

47. Longaker MT, Adzick NS: The biology of fetal wound healing: A review. *Plast Reconstr Surg* 87:788, 1990.

48. Seeger JM, Kaelin LD, Staples EM, et al: Prevention of postoperative pericardial adhesions using tissue-protective solutions. *J Surg Res* 68:63, 1997.

49. Halasz NA: Dehiscence of laparotomy wounds. *Am J Surg* 116:210, 1968.

50. Mendoza CB, Postlethwait RW, Johnson WD: Incidence of wound disruption following operation. *Arch Surg* 101:396, 1970.

51. Holt D, Kirk SJ, Regan MC, et al: Effect of age on wound healing in healthy humans. *Surgery* 112:293, 1992.

52. Jonson K, Jensen JA, Goodson WH III, et al: Tissue oxygenation, anemia and perfusion in relation to wound healing in surgical patients. *Ann Surg* 214:605, 1991.

53. Hopf HW, Hunt TK, West JM, et al: Wound tissue oxygen tension predicts the risk of wound infection in surgical patients. *Arch Surg* 132:997, 1997.

54. Greif R, Akca O, Horn EP, et al: Supplemental perioperative oxygen to reduce the incidence of surgical-wound infection. Outcomes Research Group. *N Engl J Med* 342:161, 2000.

55. Kurz A, Sessler D, Leonhardt R: Perioperative normothermia to reduce the incidence of surgical-wound infection and shorten hospitalization. *N Engl J Med* 334:1209, 1996.

56. Ehrlich HP, Hunt TK: Effects of cortisone and vitamin A on wound healing. *Ann Surg* 167:324, 1968.

57. Anstead GM: Steroids, retinoids, and wound healing. *Adv Wound Care* 11:277, 1998.

58. Ferguson MK: The effect of antineoplastic agents on wound healing. *Surg Gynecol Obstet* 154:421, 1982.

59. Larson DL: Alterations in wound healing secondary to infusion injury. *Clin Plast Surg* 17:509, 1990.

60. Cruse PJE, Foord RA: A prospective study of 23,649 surgical wounds. *Arch Surg* 107:206, 1973.

61. Yue DK, McLennan S, Marsh M, et al: Effects of experimental diabetes, uremia, and malnutrition on wound healing. *Diabetes* 36:295, 1987.

62. Goodson WH III, Hunt TK: Studies of wound healing in experimental diabetes mellitus. *J Surg Res* 22:221, 1977.

63. Black E, Vibe-Petersen J, Jorgensen LN, et al: Decrease in collagen deposition in wound repair in type I diabetes independent of glycemic control. *Arch Surg* 138:34, 2003.

64. Williams JZ, Barbul A: Nutrition and wound healing. *Surg Clin North Am* 83:571, 2003.

65. Goodson WH, Jensen JA, Gramja-Mena L, et al: The influence of a brief preoperative illness on postoperative healing. *Ann Surg* 205:250, 1987.

66. Windsor JA, Knight GS, Hill GL: Wound healing in surgical patients: Recent food intake is more important than nutritional status. *Br J Surg* 75:135, 1988.

67. Haydock DA, Hill GL: Improved wound healing response in surgical patients receiving intravenous nutrition. *Br J Surg* 74:320, 1987.

68. Seifter E, Rettura G, Barbul A, et al: Arginine: An essential amino acid for injured rats. *Surgery* 84:224, 1978.

69. Barbul A, Lazarou S, Efron DT, et al: Arginine enhances wound healing in humans. *Surgery* 108:331, 1990.

70. Kirk SJ, Regan MC, Holt D, et al: Arginine stimulates wound healing and immune function in aged humans. *Surgery* 114:155, 1993.

71. Williams JZ, Abumrad NN, Barbul A: Effect of a specialized amino acid mixture on human collagen deposition. *Ann Surg* 236:369, 2002.

72. Levenson SM, Seifter E, VanWinkle W: Nutrition, in Hunt TK, Dunphy JE (eds): *Fundamentals of Wound Management in Surgery.* New York: Appleton-Century-Crofts, 1979, p 286.

73. Jeejeebhoy KN, Cheong WK: Essential trace metals: Deficiencies and requirements, in Fischer JE (ed): *Nutrition and Metabolism in the Surgical Patient.* Boston: Little, Brown and Company, 1996, p 295.

74. Wilkinson EAJ, Hawke CI: Oral zinc for arterial and venous ulcers (Cochrane Review), in *The Cochrane Library,* 1:2002. Oxford: Update Software.

75. Robson MC: Wound infection: A failure of wound healing caused by an imbalance of bacteria. *Surg Clin North Am* 77:637, 1997.

76. Birkmeyer NJO, Birkmeyer JD: Strategies for improving surgical quality—should payers reward excellence or effort? *N Engl J Med* 354:864, 2006.

77. Classen DC, Evans RS, Pestotnik SL, et al: The timing of prophylactic administration of antibiotics and the risk of surgical-wound infection. *N Engl J Med* 326:281, 1992.

78. Anonymous: Antimicrobial prophylaxis in surgery. *The Medical Letter* 4:83, 2006.

79. Gupta N, Kaul-Gupta R, Carstens MM, et al: Analyzing prophylactic antibiotic administration in procedures lasting more than four hours: Are published guidelines being followed? *Am Surg* 69:669, 2003.

80. Arnold MA, Barbul A: Surgical site infections, in Cameron JL (ed): *Current Surgical Therapy,* 9th ed. St. Louis: Mosby-Elsevier, 2008, p 1152.

81. Liese JG, Jenrossek V, Jannson A, et al: Chronic granulomatous disease in adults. *Lancet* 347:220, 1996.

82. Falanga V, Eaglstein WH: The "trap" hypothesis of venous ulceration. *Lancet* 341:1006, 1993.

83. Lobmann R, Ambrosch A, Schultz G, et al: Expression of matrix-metalloproteinases and their inhibitors in the wounds of diabetic and non-diabetic patients. *Diabetologia* 45:1011, 2002.

84. Stanley A, Osler T: Senescence and the healing rates of venous ulcers. *J Vasc Surg* 33:1206, 2001.

85. Kim BC, Kim HT, Park SH, et al: Fibroblasts from chronic wounds show altered TGF-β-signaling and decreased TGF-β type II receptor expression. *J Cell Physiol* 195:331, 2003.

86. Hopf HW, Ueno C, Aslam R, et al: Guidelines for the treatment of arterial insufficiency ulcers. *Wound Repair Regen* 14:693, 2006.

87. Hopf HW, Ueno C, Aslam R, et al: Guidelines for the prevention of lower extremity arterial ulcers. *Wound Repair Regen* 16:175, 2008.

88. Robson MC, Cooper DM, Aslam R, et al: Guidelines for the treatment of venous ulcers. *Wound Repair Regen* 14:649, 2006.

89. Flour M: Venous ulcer management: Has research led to improved healing for the patient? in Cherry G (ed): *The Oxford European Wound Healing Course Handbook.* Oxford: Positif Press, 2002, p 33.

90. Robson MC, Cooper DM, Aslam R, et al: Guidelines for the prevention of venous ulcers. *Wound Repair Regen* 16:147, 2008.

91. Steed DL, Attinger C, Colaizzi T, et al: Guidelines for treatment of diabetic ulcers. *Wound Repair Regen* 14:680, 2006.

92. Smiell JM, Wieman TJ, Steed DL, et al. Efficacy and safety of becaplermin (recombinant human platelet-derived growth factor BB) in patients with non-healing, lower extremity diabetic ulcers: A combined analysis of four randomized trials. *Wound Repair Regen* 7:335, 1999.

93. Jeffcoate WJ, Harding KG: Diabetic foot ulcers. *Lancet* 361:1545, 2003.

94. Steed DL, Attinger C, Brem H, et al: Guidelines for the prevention of diabetic ulcers. *Wound Repair Regen* 16:169, 2008.

95. Whitney J, Phillips L, Aslam R, et al: Guidelines for the treatment of pressure ulcers. *Wound Repair Regen* 14:663, 2006.

96. Eaglstein WH, Falanga V: Chronic wounds. *Surg Clin North Am* 77:689, 1997.

97. Stechmiller JK, Cowan L, Whitney J, et al: Guidelines for the prevention of pressure ulcers. *Wound Repair Regen* 16:151, 2008.

98. Niessen FB, Spauwen PH, Schalkwijk J, et al: On the nature of hypertrophic scars and keloids: A review. *Plast Reconstr Surg* 104:1435, 1999.

99. Marneros AG, Norris JE, Olsen BR, et al: Clinical genetics of familial keloids. *Arch Dermatol* 137:1429, 2001.

100. Tredget EE, Nedelec B, Scott PG, et al: Hypertrophic scars, keloids, and contractures. *Surg Clin North Am* 77:701, 1997.

101. Mustoe TA: Evolution of silicone therapy and mechanism of action in scar management. *Aesthetic Plast Surg* 32:82, 2008.

102. Dijkstra FR, Nieuwenhuijzen M, Reijnen MM, et al: Recent clinical developments in pathophysiology, epidemiology, diagnosis and treatment of intra-abdominal adhesions. *Scand J Gastroenterol Suppl* 232:52, 2000.

103. Cheong YC, Laird SM, Shellton JB, et al: The correlation of adhesions and peritoneal fluid cytokine concentrations: A pilot study. *Hum Reprod* 17:1039, 2002.

104. Beck DE, Cohen Z, Fleshman JW, et al: A prospective, randomized multicenter, controlled study of the safety of Seprafilm adhesion barrier in abdominopelvic surgery of the intestine. *Dis Colon Rectum* 46:1310, 2003.

105. Fazio VW, Cohen Z, Fleshman JW, et al: Reduction in adhesive small-bowel obstruction by Seprafilm adhesion barrier after intestinal resection. *Dis Colon Rectum* 49:1, 2006.

106. Zeng Q, Yu Z, You J, et al: Efficacy and safety of Seprafilm for preventing postoperative abdominal adhesion: Systematic review and meta-analysis. *World J Surg* 31:2125, 2007.

107. Armstrong DG, Lavery L: Negative pressure wound therapy after partial diabetic foot amputation: A multicentre, ramdomised controlled trial. *Lancet* 366:1704, 2005.

CHAPTER 9

Wound Healing

CHAPTER 10

Oncology

Funda Meric-Bernstam and Raphael E. Pollock

ONCOLOGY AND SURGICAL PRACTICE

As the population ages, oncology is becoming a larger portion of surgical practice. The surgeon often is responsible for the initial diagnosis and management of solid tumors. Knowledge of cancer epidemiology, etiology, staging, and natural history is required for initial patient assessment, as well as to determination of the optimal surgical therapy.

Modern cancer therapy is multidisciplinary, involving the coordinated care of patients by surgeons, medical oncologists, radiation oncologists, reconstructive surgeons, pathologists, radiologists, and primary care physicians. *Primary* (or *definitive*) *surgical therapy* refers to en bloc resection of tumor with adequate margins of normal tissues and regional lymph nodes as necessary. *Adjuvant therapy* refers to radiation therapy and systemic therapies, including chemotherapy, immunotherapy, hormonal therapy, and, increasingly, biologic therapy. The primary goal of surgical and radiation therapy is local and regional control. On the other hand, the primary goal of systemic therapy is systemic control by treatment of distant foci of subclinical disease to prevent distant recurrence. Surgeons must be familiar with adjuvant therapies to coordinate multidisciplinary care and to determine the best sequence of therapy.

Recent advances in molecular biology are revolutionizing medicine. Nowhere has basic biology had a greater and more immediate impact than in oncology. New information is being translated rapidly into clinical use, with the development of new prognostic and predictive markers and new biologic therapies. It is therefore essential that surgeons understand the principles of molecular oncology to appropriately interpret these new contributions and incorporate them into practice.

EPIDEMIOLOGY

Basic Principles of Cancer Epidemiology

The term *incidence* refers to the number of new cases occurring; incidence usually is expressed as the number of new cases per 100,000 persons per year. *Mortality* refers to the number of deaths occurring and is expressed as the number of deaths per 100,000 persons per year. Incidence and mortality data are usually available through cancer registries. Mortality data are also available as public records in many countries where deaths are registered as vital statistics, often with the cause of death. In areas where cancer registries do not exist, mortality data are used to extrapolate incidence rates. However, these numbers are likely to be less accurate than registry data, because the relationship between incidence and cause-specific death is likely to vary significantly among countries owing to the variation in health care delivery.

The incidence of cancer varies by geography. This is due in part to genetic differences and in part to differences in environmental and dietary exposures. Epidemiologic studies that monitor trends in cancer incidence and mortality have tremendously enhanced our understanding of the etiology of cancer. Furthermore, analysis of trends in cancer incidence and mortality allows us to monitor the effects of different preventive and screening measures, as well as the evolution of therapies for specific cancers.

The two types of epidemiologic studies that are conducted most often to investigate the etiology of cancer and the effect of prevention modalities are cohort studies and case-control studies. Cohort studies follow a group of people who initially do not have a disease over time and measure the rate of development of a disease. In cohort studies, a group that is exposed to a certain environmental factor or intervention usually is compared to a group that has not been exposed (e.g., smokers vs. nonsmokers). Case-control studies compare a group of patients affected with a disease to a group of individuals without the disease for a given exposure. The results are expressed in terms of an odds ratio, or relative risk. A relative risk <1 indicates a protective effect of the exposure, whereas a relative risk >1 indicates an increased risk of developing the disease with exposure.

Cancer Incidence and Mortality in the United States

In the year 2008, an estimated 1.44 million new cancer cases were diagnosed in the United States.[1] In addition, over a million cases of basal and squamous cell carcinomas of the skin, 54,020 cases of melanoma in situ, and 67,770 cases of carcinoma in situ of the breast were predicted.[1] Furthermore, an estimated 565,650 people were expected to die of cancer in the United States in the same year.[1] The estimated new cancer cases and deaths by cancer type are shown in Table 10-1.[1] The most common causes of cancer death in men are cancers of the lung and bronchus, prostate, and colon and rectum; in women, the most common cancers are of the lung and bronchus, breast, and colon and rectum (Fig. 10-1).[1]

Trends in Cancer Incidence and Mortality

Cancer deaths accounted for 23% of all deaths in the United States in 2005, second only to deaths from heart disease.[1] As the life expectancy of the human population increases because of reductions in other causes of death such as infections and cardiovascular disease, cancer is becoming the leading cause of death. Cancer is the leading cause of death among women aged 40 to 79 years and among men aged 60 to 79 years.[1]

Cancer incidence stabilized in males between 1995 and 2003 but has increased by 0.3% per year in females during the period from 1987 to 2003.[1] The annual age-adjusted cancer incidence rates among

TABLE 10-1	Estimated new cancer cases and deaths, United States, 2007[a]					
	Estimated New Cases Both Sexes	**Estimated Deaths Both Sexes**			**Estimated New Cases Both Sexes**	**Estimated Deaths Both Sexes**
All cancers	**1,444,920**	**559,650**		**Genital system**	**306,380**	**55,740**
Oral cavity and pharynx	**34,360**	**7550**		Uterine cervix	11,150	3670
Digestive system	**271,250**	**134,710**		Uterine corpus	39,080	7400
Esophagus	15,560	13,940		Ovary	22,430	15,280
Stomach	21,260	11,210		Vulva	3490	880
Small intestine	5640	1090		Vagina and other genital, female	2140	790
Colon and rectum	112,340	52,180		Prostate	218,890	27,050
Anus, anal canal, and anorectum	4650	690		Testis	7920	380
Liver and intrahepatic bile duct	19,160	16,780		Penis and other genital, male	1280	290
Gallbladder and other biliary	9250	3250		**Urinary system**	**120,400**	**27,340**
Pancreas	37,170	33,370		Urinary bladder	67,160	13,750
Other digestive organs	4800	2200		Kidney and renal pelvis	51,190	12,890
Respiratory system	**229,400**	**164,840**		Ureter and other urinary organs	2050	700
Larynx	11,300	3660		**Eye and orbit**	**2340**	**220**
Lung and bronchus	213,380	160,390		**Brain and other nervous system**	**20,500**	**12,740**
Other respiratory organs	4720	790		**Endocrine system**	**35,520**	**2320**
Bones and joints	**2370**	**1330**		Thyroid	33,550	1530
Soft tissue (including heart)	**9220**	**3560**		Other endocrine	1970	790
Skin (excluding basal and squamous)	**65,050**	**10,850**		**Lymphoma**	**71,380**	**19,730**
				Multiple myeloma	**19,900**	**10,790**
Melanoma	59,940	8110		**Leukemia**	**44,240**	**21,790**
Other nonepithelial	5110	2740		**Other and unspecified primary sites[b]**	**32,100**	**45,230**
Breast	**180,510**	**40,910**				

[a]Excludes basal and squamous cell skin cancers and in situ carcinomas except those of urinary bladder.
[b]More deaths than cases suggest lack of specificity in recording underlying causes of death on death certificate.
Source: Modified with permission from Jemal et al.[1]

males and females for selected cancer types are shown in Fig. 10-2.[1] Prostate cancer rates rapidly increased and decreased between 1995 and 1998, but stabilized from 1998 to 2004. These trends are thought to be attributable to increased use of prostate-specific antigen (PSA) screening.[1] Age-adjusted incidence rate of breast cancer started to decrease from 2001 to 2004.[2] This decrease in breast cancer incidence has at least temporally been associated with the first report of the Women's Health Initiative, which documented an increased risk of coronary artery disease and breast cancer with the use of hormone replacement therapy; this was followed by a drop in the use of hormone replacement therapy by postmenopausal women in the United States.[2]

From 1993 to 2003, for all cancer types combined, cancer death rates decreased by 1.6% per year in males and by 0.8% per year in females. The 5-year survival rates for selected cancers are listed in Table 10-2.[1] Mortality for cancer at all four major sites has continued to decrease except for female lung cancer, for which rates increased by 0.3% per year from 1995 to 2003. The decrease in lung cancer death rates in men is thought to be due to a decrease in tobacco use, whereas the decreases in death rates from breast, colorectal cancer, and prostate cancer reflect advances in early detection and treatment.

Global Statistics on Cancer Incidence

It has been estimated that there were a total of 10.9 million new cancer cases around the world in 2002.[3] Lung cancer is the leading cancer in the world, accounting for 1.35 million new cases and 1.15 million deaths per year.[3] Breast cancer is now the second most common cancer (1.15 million cases per year) and the fifth most common cause of cancer death, after gastric cancer (934,000 cases, 700,000 deaths), colorectal cancer (1.03 million cases, 529,000 deaths), and liver cancer (626,000 cases, 598,000 deaths).[3]

Stomach Cancer

The incidence of stomach cancer varies significantly among different regions of the world. The age-adjusted incidence is highest in Japan (62.1 per 100,000 men, 26.1 per 100,000 women). In comparison, the rates are much lower in North America (7.4 per 100,000

KEY POINTS

1. The following alterations are critical for malignant cancer growth: self-sufficiency of growth signals, insensitivity to growth-inhibitory signals, evasion of apoptosis, potential for limitless replication, angiogenesis, and invasion and metastasis.

2. Understanding cancer biology is essential to successfully implement personalized cancer therapy.

3. Modern cancer therapy is multidisciplinary, involving coordinated care by surgeons, medical oncologists, radiation oncologists, reconstructive surgeons, pathologists, radiologists, and primary care physicians.

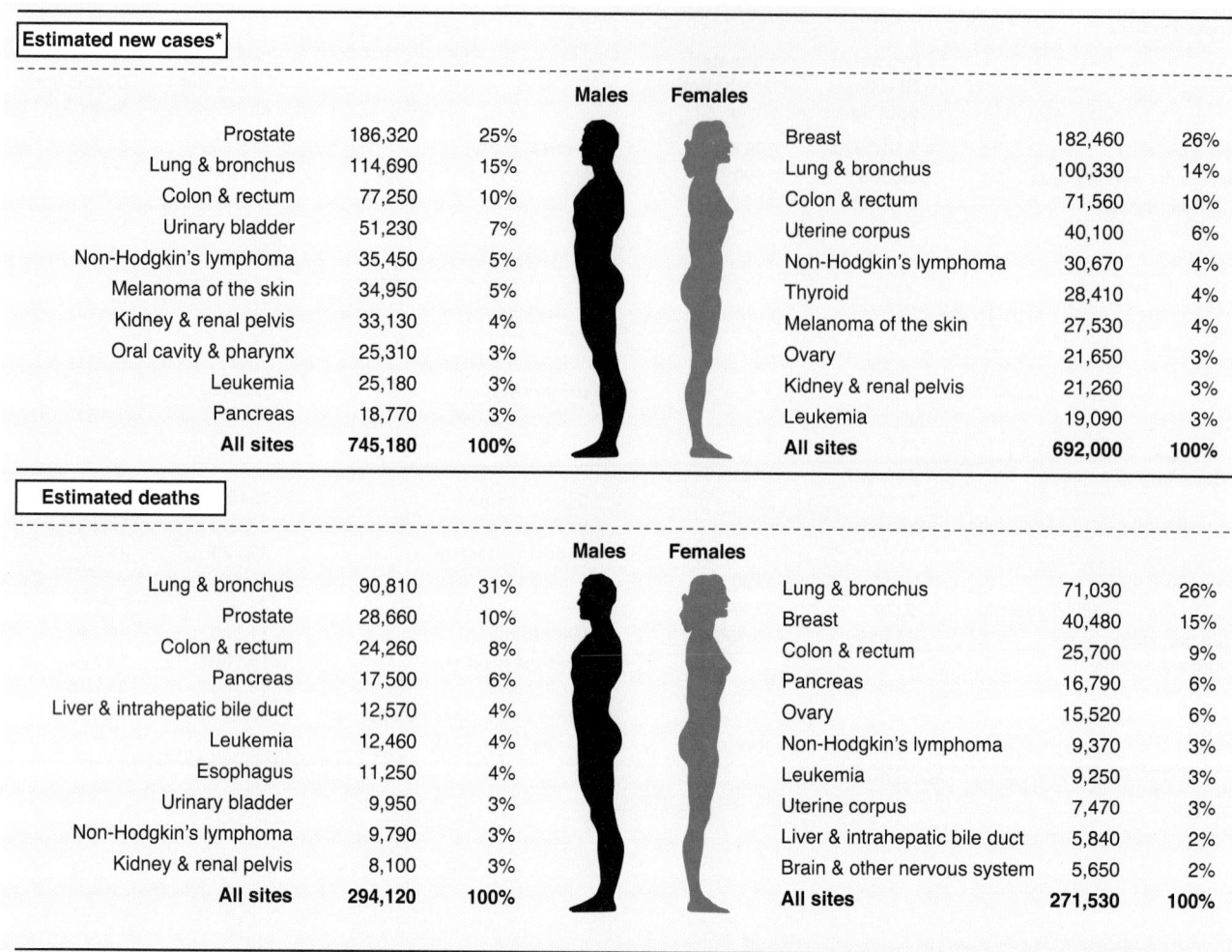

Estimated new cases*			Males	Females			
Prostate	186,320	25%		Breast	182,460	26%
Lung & bronchus	114,690	15%		Lung & bronchus	100,330	14%
Colon & rectum	77,250	10%		Colon & rectum	71,560	10%
Urinary bladder	51,230	7%		Uterine corpus	40,100	6%
Non-Hodgkin's lymphoma	35,450	5%		Non-Hodgkin's lymphoma	30,670	4%
Melanoma of the skin	34,950	5%		Thyroid	28,410	4%
Kidney & renal pelvis	33,130	4%		Melanoma of the skin	27,530	4%
Oral cavity & pharynx	25,310	3%		Ovary	21,650	3%
Leukemia	25,180	3%		Kidney & renal pelvis	21,260	3%
Pancreas	18,770	3%		Leukemia	19,090	3%
All sites	**745,180**	**100%**		**All sites**	**692,000**	**100%**

Estimated deaths			Males	Females			
Lung & bronchus	90,810	31%		Lung & bronchus	71,030	26%
Prostate	28,660	10%		Breast	40,480	15%
Colon & rectum	24,260	8%		Colon & rectum	25,700	9%
Pancreas	17,500	6%		Pancreas	16,790	6%
Liver & intrahepatic bile duct	12,570	4%		Ovary	15,520	6%
Leukemia	12,460	4%		Non-Hodgkin's lymphoma	9,370	3%
Esophagus	11,250	4%		Leukemia	9,250	3%
Urinary bladder	9,950	3%		Uterine corpus	7,470	3%
Non-Hodgkin's lymphoma	9,790	3%		Liver & intrahepatic bile duct	5,840	2%
Kidney & renal pelvis	8,100	3%		Brain & other nervous system	5,650	2%
All sites	**294,120**	**100%**		**All sites**	**271,530**	**100%**

FIG. 10-1. Ten leading cancer types with the estimated new cancer cases and deaths by sex in the United States, 2007. *Excludes basal and squamous cell skin cancers and in situ carcinomas except those of the urinary bladder. Estimates are rounded to the nearest 10. *(Modified with permission from Jemal et al.[1])*

men, 3.4 per 100,000 women) and in northern and western Africa (4.4 to 3.4 per 100,000 men, 2.5 to 3.6 per 100,000 women).[3] The difference in risk by country is presumed to be primarily due to differences in dietary factors. The risk is increased by high consumption of preserved salted foods such as meats and pickles, and decreased by high intake of fruits and vegetables.[3] There also is some international variation in the incidence of infection with *Helicobacter pylori,* which is known to play a major role in gastric cancer development.[3] Fortunately, a steady decline is being observed in the incidence and mortality rates of gastric cancer. This may be related to improvements in preservation and storage of foods as well as due to changes in the prevalence of *H. pylori.*[3]

Breast Cancer

The incidence of breast cancer is high in all of the most highly developed regions except Japan, including the United States and Canada, Australia, and Northern and Western Europe, ranging from 82.5 to 99.4 per 100,000 women per year.[3]

In comparison, the rates are relatively low (<30 per 100,000 women) in most of Africa (except South Africa) and Asia. The lowest incidence is in Central Africa (16.5 per 100,000). Although breast cancer has been linked to cancer susceptibility genes, mutations in these genes account for only 5 to 10% of breast tumors, which suggests that the wide geographic variations in breast cancer incidence are not due to geographic variations in the prevalence of these genes. Most of the differences, therefore, are attributed to differences

in reproductive factors, diet, alcohol, obesity, physical activity, and other environmental differences. Indeed, breast cancer risk increases significantly in females who have migrated from Asia to America.[3] Overall, the incidence of breast cancer is rising in most countries.

Colon and Rectal Cancer

There is a 25-fold variation in colon cancer incidence worldwide.[3] The incidence of colon and rectal cancer is higher in developed countries than in developing countries. The incidence rates are highest in North America, Australia and New Zealand, and Western Europe, and especially in Japanese men.[3] In contrast, the incidence is relatively low in North Africa, South America, and eastern, southeastern, and western Asia. These geographic differences are thought to reflect environmental exposures and are presumed to be related mainly to dietary differences in consumption of animal fat, meat, and fiber.[3]

Liver Cancer

In contrast to colon cancers, 82% of liver cancers occur in developing countries.[2] The incidence of liver cancer is especially high in China (37.9 per 100,000 men), whereas it is relatively low in North and South America and Europe (2.6 to 6.2 per 100,000 men).[2] Worldwide, the major risk factors for liver cancer are infection with hepatitis B and C viruses and consumption of foods contaminated with aflatoxin. Hepatitis B immunization in children has recently been shown to reduce the incidence of liver cancer.[3]

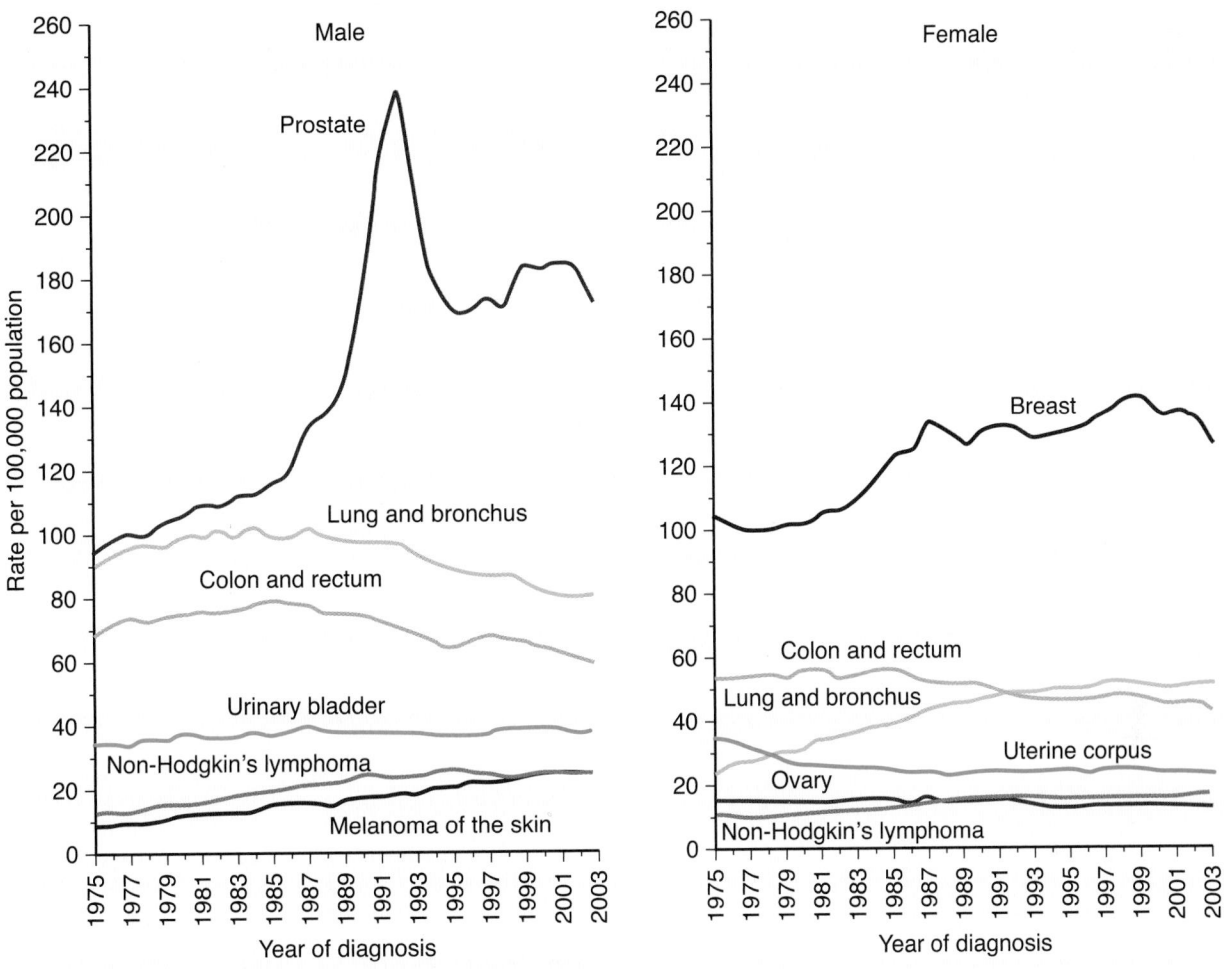

FIG. 10-2. Annual age-adjusted cancer incidence rates among males and females for selected cancer types, United States, 1975 to 2003. Rates are age adjusted to the U.S. standard population. *(Modified with permission from Jemal et al.[1])*

Prostate Cancer

The incidence of prostate cancer is dramatically higher in North America (119.9 per 100,000 men) than in China, Japan, and the rest of Asia (1.6 to 12.6 per 100,000).[3] A considerable part of the international differences in prostate cancer incidence is thought to reflect differences in diagnostic practices. As previously mentioned, the introduction of PSA screening has led to a significant increase in the diagnosis of prostate cancer in the United States (see Fig. 10-2).[1]

Global Statistics on Cancer Mortality

The mortality rates for different cancers also vary significantly among countries. This is attributable not only to variations in incidence but also to variations in survival after a cancer diagnosis. The survival rates are influenced by treatment patterns as well as by variations in cancer screening practices, which affect the stage of cancer at diagnosis. For example, the 5-year survival rate for stomach cancer is much higher in Japan, where the cancer incidence is high enough to warrant mass screening, which is presumed to lead to earlier diagnosis. In the case of prostate cancer, on the other hand, the mortality rates diverge much less than the incidence rates among countries. Survival rates for prostate cancer are much higher in North America than in developing countries.[3] It is possible that the extensive screening practices in the United States allow discovery of cancers at an earlier, more curable stage; however, it is also possible that this screening leads to discovery of more latent, less biologically aggressive cancers, which may not have caused death even if they had not been identified.

In summary, the incidence rates of many common cancers vary widely by geography. This is due in part to genetic differences, including racial and ethnic differences. It is due also in part to differences in environmental and dietary exposures, factors that can potentially be altered. Therefore, establishment of regional and international databases is critical to improving our understanding of the etiology of cancer and will ultimately assist in the initiation of targeted strategies for global cancer prevention. Furthermore, the monitoring of cancer mortality rates and 5-year cancer-specific survival rates will identify regions where there are inequities of health care, so that access to health care can be facilitated and guidelines for treatment can be established.

CANCER BIOLOGY

Hallmarks of Cancer

Although there are >100 types of cancer, it has been proposed that there are six essential alterations in cell physiology that dictate malignant growth: self-sufficiency of growth signals, insensitivity to growth-inhibitory signals, evasion of apoptosis (programmed cell death), potential for limitless replication, angiogenesis, and invasion and metastasis (Fig. 10-3).[4]

Cell Proliferation and Transformation

In normal cells, cell growth and proliferation are under strict control. In cancer cells, cells become unresponsive to normal

TABLE 10-2	Five-year relative survival rates adjusted to normal life expectancy by year of diagnosis, United States, 1975–2002

Cancer Type	Relative 5-Year Survival Rates (%)		
	1975–1977	1984–1986	1996–2002
All cancers	50	53	66
Brain	24	29	34
Breast (female)	75	79	89
Uterine cervix	70	68	73
Colon	51	59	65
Uterine corpus	87	83	84
Esophagus	5	10	16
Hodgkin's disease	73	79	86
Kidney	51	56	66
Larynx	66	66	65
Leukemia	35	42	49
Liver	4	6	10
Lung and bronchus	13	13	16
Melanoma of the skin	82	86	92
Multiple myeloma	26	29	33
Non-Hodgkin's lymphoma	48	53	63
Oral cavity	53	55	60
Ovary	37	40	45
Pancreas	2	3	5
Prostate	69	76	100
Rectum	49	57	66
Stomach	16	18	24
Testis	83	93	96
Thyroid	93	94	97
Urinary bladder	73	78	82

Source: Modified with permission from Jemal et al.[1]

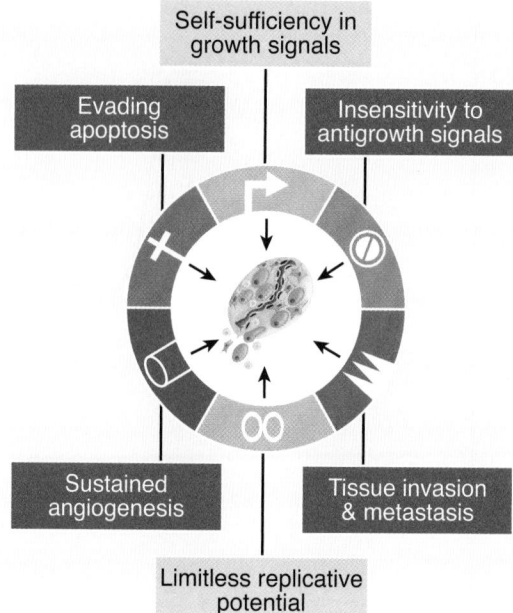

FIG. 10-3. Acquired capabilities of cancer. *(Modified with permission from Hanahan et al.[4] Copyright Elsevier.)*

growth controls, which leads to uncontrolled growth and proliferation. Human cells require several genetic changes for neoplastic transformation. Cell type–specific differences also exist for tumorigenic transformation. Abnormally proliferating, transformed cells outgrow normal cells in the culture dish (i.e., in vitro) and commonly display several abnormal characteristics.[5] These include loss of contact inhibition (i.e., cells continue to proliferate after a confluent monolayer is formed); an altered appearance and poor adherence to other cells or to the substratum; loss of anchorage dependence for growth; immortalization; and gain of tumorigenicity (i.e., the ability to give rise to tumors when injected into an appropriate host).

Cancer Initiation

Tumorigenesis is proposed to have three steps: initiation, promotion, and progression. Initiating events such as gain of function of genes known as *oncogenes* or loss of function of genes known as *tumor-suppressor genes* may lead a single cell to acquire a distinct growth advantage. Although tumors usually arise from a single cell or clone, it is thought that sometimes not a single cell but rather a large number of cells in a target organ may have undergone the initiating genetic event; thus many normal-appearing cells may have an elevated malignant potential. This is referred to as a *field effect*. The initiating events are usually genetic and occur as deletions of tumor-suppressor genes or amplification of oncogenes. Subsequent events can lead to accumulations of additional deleterious mutations in the clone.

Cancer is thought to be a disease of clonal progression as tumors arise from a single cell and accumulate mutations that confer on the tumor an increasingly aggressive behavior. Most tumors go through a progression from benign lesions to in situ tumors to invasive

cancers (e.g., atypical ductal hyperplasia to ductal carcinoma in situ to invasive ductal carcinoma of the breast). Fearon and Vogelstein proposed the model for colorectal tumorigenesis presented in Fig. 10-4.[6] Colorectal tumors arise from the mutational activation of oncogenes coupled with mutational inactivation of tumor-suppressor genes, the latter being the predominant change.[6] Mutations in at least four or five genes are required for formation of a malignant tumor, whereas fewer changes suffice for formation of a benign tumor. Although genetic mutations often occur in a preferred sequence, a tumor's biologic properties are determined by the total accumulation of its genetic changes.

Gene expression is a multistep process that starts from transcription of a gene into messenger RNA (mRNA) and then translation of this sequence into the functional protein. There are several controls at each level. In addition to alterations at the genome level (e.g., amplifications of a gene), alterations at the transcription level (e.g., methylation of the DNA leading to transcriptional silencing) or at the level of mRNA processing, mRNA stability, mRNA translation, or protein stability all can alter the levels of critical proteins and thus contribute to tumorigenesis. Alternatively, changes in the genomic sequence can lead to a mutated product with altered function.

Cell-Cycle Dysregulation in Cancer

The proliferative advantage of tumor cells is a result of their ability to bypass quiescence. Cancer cells often show alterations in signal transduction pathways that lead to proliferation in response to external signals. Mutations or alterations in the expression of cell-cycle proteins, growth factors, growth factor receptors, intracellular signal transduction proteins, and nuclear transcription factors all can lead to disturbance of the basic regulatory mechanisms that control the cell cycle, allowing unregulated cell growth and proliferation.

The cell cycle is divided into four phases (Fig. 10-5).[7] During the synthetic or S phase, the cell generates a single copy of its genetic material, whereas in the mitotic or M phase, the cellular components are partitioned between two daughter cells. The G_1 and G_2 phases represent gap phases during which the cells prepare themselves for completion of the S and M phases, respectively. When cells cease proliferation, they exit the cell cycle and enter the quiescent state referred to as G_0. In human tumor cell-cycle regulators like INK4A,

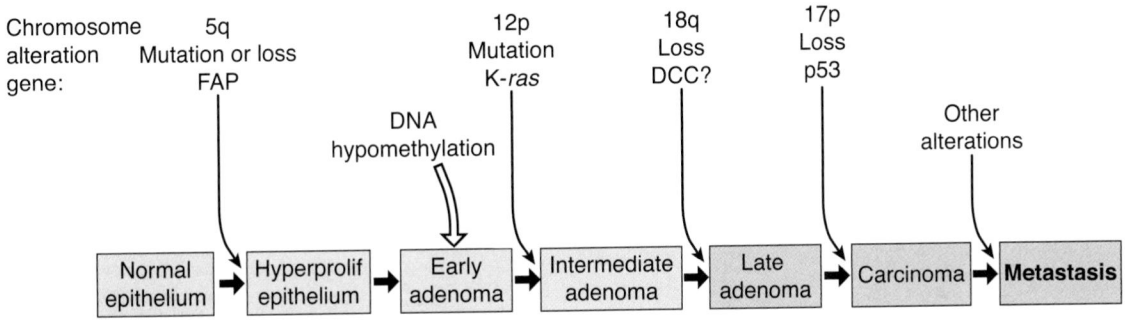

FIG. 10-4. A genetic model for colorectal tumorigenesis. Tumorigenesis proceeds through a series of genetic alterations involving oncogenes and tumor-suppressor genes. In general, the three stages of adenomas represent tumors of increasing size, dysplasia, and villous content. Individuals with familial adenomatous polyposis (FAP) inherit a mutation on chromosome arm 5q. In tumors arising in individuals without polyposis, the same region may be lost or mutated at a relatively early stage of tumorigenesis. A *ras* gene mutation (usually K-*ras*) occurs in one cell of a pre-existing small adenoma which, through clonal expansion, produces a larger and more dysplastic tumor. The chromosome arms most frequently deleted include 5q, 17p, and 18q. Allelic deletions of chromosome arms 17p and 18q usually occur at a later stage of tumorigenesis than do deletions of chromosome arm 5q or *ras* gene mutations. The order of these changes varies, however, and accumulation of these changes, rather than their order of appearance, seems most important. Tumors continue to progress once carcinomas have formed, and the accumulated chromosomal alterations correlate with the ability of the carcinomas to metastasize and cause death. DCC = deleted in colorectal cancer gene. *(Modified with permission from Fearon et al.[6] Copyright Elsevier.)*

INK4B, and KIP1 are frequently mutated or altered in expression. These alterations underscore the importance of cell-cycle regulation in the prevention of human cancers.

Oncogenes

Normal cellular genes that contribute to cancer when abnormal are called *oncogenes.* The normal counterpart of such a gene is referred to as a *proto-oncogene.* Oncogenes are usually designated by three-letter abbreviations, such as *myc* or *ras.* Oncogenes are further designated by the prefix "v-" for virus or "c-" for cell or chromosome, corresponding to the origin of the oncogene when it was first detected. Proto-oncogenes can be activated (show increased activity) or overexpressed (expressed at increased protein levels) by translo-

cation (e.g., *abl*), promoter insertion (e.g., c-*myc*), mutation (e.g., *ras*), or amplification (e.g., *HER-2/neu*). More than 100 oncogenes have been identified.

Oncogenes may be growth factors (e.g., platelet-derived growth factor), growth factor receptors (e.g., HER2), intracellular signal transduction molecules (e.g., *ras*), nuclear transcription factors (e.g., c-*myc*), or other molecules involved in the regulation of cell growth and proliferation. Growth factors are ubiquitous proteins that are produced and secreted by cells locally and that stimulate cell proliferation by binding specific cell-surface receptors on the same cells (autocrine stimulation) or on neighboring cells (paracrine stimulation). Persistent overexpression of growth factors can lead to uncontrolled autostimulation and neoplastic transformation. Alternatively, growth factor receptors can be aberrantly activated (turned on)

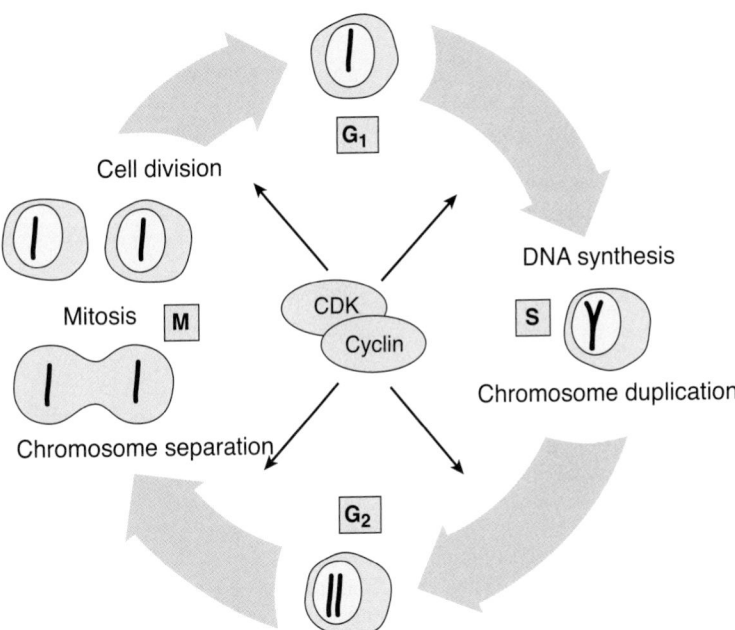

FIG. 10-5. Schematic representation of the phases of the cell cycle. Mitogenic growth factors can drive a quiescent cell from G_0 into the cell cycle. Once the cell cycle passes beyond the restriction point, mitogens are no longer required for progression into and through S phase. The DNA is replicated in S phase, and the chromosomes are condensed and segregated in mitosis. In early G_1 phase, certain signals can drive a cell to exit the cell cycle and enter a quiescent phase. Cell-cycle checkpoints have been identified in G_1, S, G_2, and M phases. CDK = cyclin-dependent kinase. *(Adapted from Kastan et al.[7])*

through mutations or overexpressed (continually presenting cells with growth-stimulatory signals, even in the absence of growth factors), which leads cells to respond as if growth factor levels are altered. The growth-stimulating effect of growth factors and other mitogens is mediated through postreceptor signal transduction molecules. These molecules mediate the passage of growth signals from the outside to the inside of the cell and then to the cell nucleus, initiating the cell cycle and DNA transcription. Aberrant activation or expression of cell-signaling molecules, cell-cycle molecules, or transcription factors may play an important role in neoplastic transformation. Two of the best-studied oncogenes, *HER2* and *ras*, are discussed here.

HER2

Protein tyrosine kinases account for a large portion of known oncogenes. HER2, also known as *neu* or c-*erb*B-2, is a member of the epidermal growth factor receptor (EGFR) family and is one of the best-characterized tyrosine kinases. Unlike other receptor tyrosine kinases, HER-2/*neu* does not have a direct soluble ligand. It plays a key role in signaling, however, because it is the preferred partner in heterodimer formation with all the other EGFR family members (EGFR/c-*erb*B-1, HER2/c-*erb*B-3, and HER3/c-*erb*B-4), which bind at least 30 ligands, including epidermal growth factor (EGF), trans-

forming growth factor α (TGFα), heparin-binding EGF-like growth factor, amphiregulin, and heregulin.[8] Heterodimerization with HER2 potentiates recycling of receptors rather than degradation, enhances signal potency and duration, increases affinity for ligands, and increases catalytic activity.[8]

HER2 can interact with different members of the HER family and activate mitogenic and antiapoptotic pathways (Fig. 10-6).[9] The specificity and potency of the intracellular signals are affected by the identity of the ligand, the composition of the receptors, and the phosphotyrosine-binding proteins associated with the erbB molecules. The Ras- and Shc-activated mitogen-activated protein kinase (MAPK) pathway is a target of all erbB ligands, which increase the transcriptional activity of early-response genes such as c-*myc*, c-*fos*, and c-*jun*.[10] MAPK-independent pathways such as the phosphoinositide-3 kinase (PI3K) pathway also are activated by most erbB dimers, although the potency and kinetics of activation may differ. Stimulation of the PI3K pathway through *HER2* signaling also can lead to activation of survival molecule Akt, which suppresses apoptosis through multiple mechanisms.

The mutant rat *neu* gene was first recognized as an oncogene in neuroblastomas from carcinogen-treated rats.[11] The *HER2* gene is frequently amplified and the protein overexpressed in many cancers, including breast, ovarian, lung, gastric, and oral cancers.

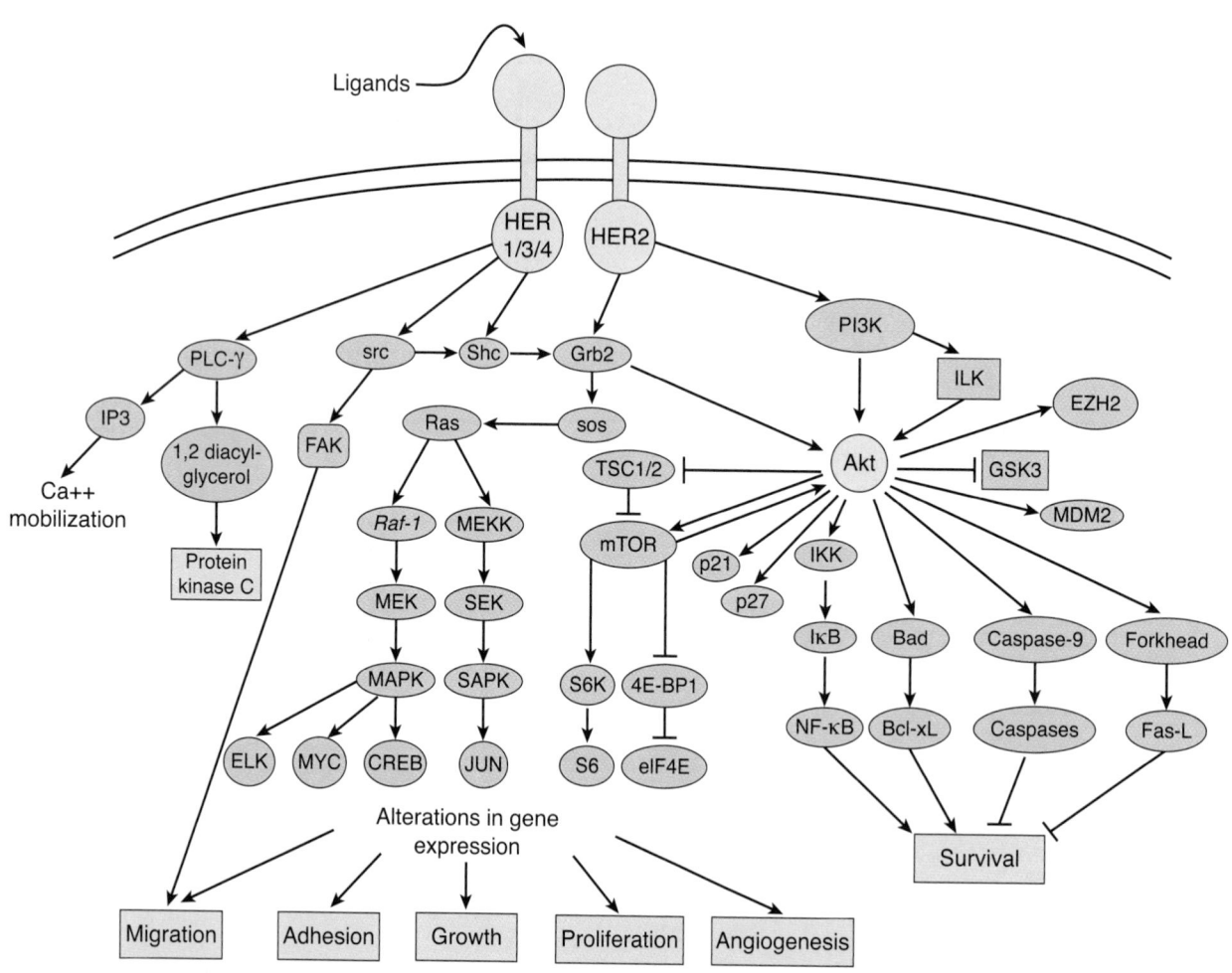

FIG. 10-6. Selected HER2 signaling pathways. HER2 can interact with different members of the HER family and activate mitogenic and antiapoptotic pathways. 4E-BP1= eIF4E binding protein 1; CREB = cyclic adenosine monophosphate element binding; eIF4E = eukaryotic initiation factor 4E; EZH = enhancer of zeste homolog; FAK = focal adhesion kinase; Fas-L = Fas ligand; GSK3 = glycogen synthase kinase-3; HER = human epidermal growth receptor; IKK = IκB kinase; ILK= integrin-linked kinase; IP3 = inositol triphosphate; IκB = inhibitor of NF-κB; MAPK = mitogen-activated protein kinase; MDM2 = mouse double minute 2 homologue; MEK = mitogen-activated protein/extracellular signal regulated kinase kinase; MEKK = MEK kinase; mTOR = mammalian target of rapamycin; NF-κB = nuclear factor κB; PI3K = phosphoinositide-3 kinase; PLC-γ= phospholipase Cγ; SAPK = stress-activated protein kinase; SEK = SAPK/extracellular signal regulated kinase kinase; TSC = tuberous sclerosis complex. *(Modified with permission from Meric-Bernstam et al.[9])*

Overexpression of HER2 results in ligand-independent activation of HER2 kinase, which leads to mitogenic signaling. HER2 overexpression is associated with increased cell proliferation and anchorage-independent growth as well as resistance to proapoptotic stimuli. Further, overexpression of HER2 increases cell migration and upregulates the activities of matrix metalloproteinases (MMPs) and in vitro invasiveness. In animal models, HER2 increases tumorigenicity, angiogenesis, and metastasis. These results all suggest that HER2 plays a key role in cancer biology.

ras

The *ras* family of genes encodes small guanosine triphosphate (GTP)–binding proteins that regulate several cellular processes. The H- and K-*ras* genes were first identified as the cellular counterparts of the oncogenes of the Harvey and Kirsten rat sarcoma viruses, whereas N-*ras* was isolated from a neuroblastoma.[12] The N-, H-, and K-*ras* genes are located on chromosomes 1, 11, and 12, respectively, and encode for 21-kDa proteins that are nearly identical in amino acid sequence but appear not to be redundant in function.[12]

ras cycles between active GTP-bound and inactive guanosine diphosphate–bound states. Various extracellular stimuli can promote ras activation, including various receptor and nonreceptor tyrosine kinases, G protein–coupled receptors, and integrins.[13] Guanine nucleotide exchange factors stimulate formation of ras-GTP. ras has an intrinsic ability to hydrolyze GTP, but this hydrolysis is slow. Guanosine triphosphatase–activating proteins (GAPs) stimulate hydrolysis of the bound GTP to return ras to its inactive form. Mutations of ras at amino acid positions 12, 13, or 61 may render ras insensitive to GAPs, which results in mutant proteins that are persistently activated. Approximately 20% of all tumors have activating mutations in one of the ras genes.[14] The frequency of ras mutations varies widely by cancer type (e.g., 90% of pancreatic cancers, but <5% of breast cancers).[12,14] Tumors that lack *ras* mutations, however, may undergo activation of the *ras* signaling pathway by other mechanisms, such as growth factor receptor activation, loss of GAP, or activation of *ras* effectors.[14]

The Ras proteins require posttranslational modification by farnesyltransferase. After association with the intracellular membrane via its farnesyl group, GTP-bound Ras then binds and activates several downstream pathways. The best-characterized downstream signaling pathway is that initiated by the serine-threonine kinase Raf. Activated Raf phosphorylates and activates MAPK1 and MAPK2 (MEK1 and MEK2).[14] MEK1 and MEK2 phosphorylate and activate the MAPKs extracellular signal regulated kinases 1 and 2 (ERK1 and ERK2). ERK phosphorylates the ETS (E26 transformation-specific) family of transcriptional factors; this leads to expression of cell-cycle regulatory proteins such as D-type cyclins, which enables the cell to progress through the G$_1$ phase of the cell cycle. Constitutive activation of Raf is common in some tumors such as non–small cell lung cancer, renal cell carcinoma, and hepatocellular cancer.[15] B-raf itself can have activating mutations in melanoma, sporadic colorectal cancer, and papillary thyroid cancer.[15] A second pathway activated by Ras is PI3K, an important mediator of the survival signaling. A third pathway is the Ras-related Ral proteins, which along with the PI3K/Akt pathway contribute to inhibition of the forkhead transcription factors that promote cell-cycle arrest by inducing p27. Further, Ras also associates with phospholipase Cε, which links Ras to activation of protein kinase C and calcium mobilization. Together, the Ras signaling pathways promote malignant transformation by increasing proliferation, which is accomplished by inducing cell-cycle regulators such as cyclin D1, which suppresses cell-cycle inhibitors like p27, and enhancing survival signaling through the PI3K/Akt pathway.

Alterations in Apoptosis in Cancer Cells

Apoptosis is a genetically regulated program to dispose of cells. Cancer cells must avoid apoptosis if tumors are to arise. The growth of a tumor mass is dependent not only on an increase in proliferation of tumor cells but also on a decrease in their apoptotic rate.

Apoptosis is distinguished from necrosis because it leads to several characteristic changes. In early apoptosis, the changes in membrane composition lead to extracellular exposure of phosphatidylserine residues, which avidly bind annexin, a characteristic that is used to discriminate apoptotic cells in laboratory studies. Late in apoptosis there are characteristic changes in nuclear morphology, such as chromatin condensation, nuclear fragmentation, and DNA laddering, as well as membrane blebbing. Apoptotic cells are then engulfed and degraded by phagocytic cells. The effectors of apoptosis are a family of proteases called *caspases* (cysteine-dependent and aspartate-directed proteases). The initiator caspases (e.g., 8, 9, and 10), which are upstream, cleave the downstream executioner caspases (e.g., 3, 6, and 7) that carry out the destructive functions of apoptosis.

Two principal molecular pathways signal apoptosis by cleaving the initiator caspases with the potential for crosstalk: the mitochondrial pathway and the death receptor pathway. In the mitochondrial (or intrinsic) pathway, death results from the release of cytochrome c from the mitochondria. Cytochrome c, procaspase 9, and apoptotic protease activating factor 1 (Apaf-1) form an enzyme complex, referred to as the *apoptosome*, that activates the effector caspases. In addition to these proteins, the mitochondria contain other proapoptotic proteins such as SMAC/DIABLO. The mitochondrial pathway can be stimulated by many factors, including DNA damage, reactive oxygen species, or the withdrawal of survival factors. The permeability of the mitochondrial membrane determines whether the apoptotic pathway will proceed. The Bcl-2 family of regulatory proteins includes proapoptotic proteins (e.g., Bax, Bad, and Bak) and antiapoptotic proteins (e.g., Bcl-2 and Bcl-xL). The activity of the Bcl-2 proteins is centered on the mitochondria, where they regulate membrane permeability. Growth factors promote survival signaling through the PI3K/Akt pathway, which phosphorylates and inactivates proapoptotic Bad. In contrast, growth factor withdrawal may promote apoptosis through signaling by unphosphorylated Bad. The heat shock proteins, including Hsp70 and Hsp27, are also involved in inhibition of downstream apoptotic pathways by blocking formation of the apoptosome complex and inhibiting release of cytochrome c from the mitochondria.[16]

The second principal apoptotic pathway is the death receptor pathway, sometimes referred to as the *extrinsic pathway*. Cell-surface death receptors include Fas/APO1/CD95, tumor necrosis factor receptor 1, and KILL-ER/DR5, which bind their ligands Fas-L, tumor necrosis factor (TNF), and TNF-related apoptosis-inducing ligand (TRAIL), respectively. When the receptors are bound by their ligands, they form a death-inducing signaling complex (DISC). At the DISC, procaspase 8 and procaspase 10 are cleaved, yielding active initiator caspases.[17] The death receptor pathway may be regulated at the cell surface by the expression of "decoy" receptors for Fas (DcR3) and TRAIL (TRID and TRUNDD). The decoy receptors are closely related to the death receptors but lack a functional death domain; therefore, they bind death ligands but do not transmit a death signal. Another regulatory group is the FADD-like interleukin-1 protease-inhibitory proteins (FLIPs). FLIPs have homology to caspase 8; they bind to the DISC and inhibit the activation of caspase 8. Finally, inhibitors of apoptosis proteins (IAPs) block caspase 3 activation and have the ability to regulate both the death receptor and the mitochondrial pathway.

In human cancers, aberrations in the apoptotic program include increased expression of Fas and TRAIL decoy receptors; increased expression of antiapoptotic Bcl-2; increased expression of the IAP-related protein survivin; increased expression of c-FLIP; mutations or downregulation of proapoptotic Bax, caspase 8, APAF1, XAF1, and death receptors CD95, TRAIL-R1, and TRAIL-R2; alterations of the p53 pathway; overexpression of growth factors and growth factor receptors; and activation of the PI3K/Akt survival pathway.[17]

Autophagy in Cancer Cells

Autophagy (self-eating) is a major cellular pathway for protein and organelle turnover. This process helps maintain a balance between anabolism and catabolism for normal cell growth and development. Inability to activate autophagy in response to nutrient deprivation, or constitutive activation of autophagy in response to stress, can lead to cell death; thus autophagy is sometimes referred to as a second form of programmed cell death. Autophagy plays an essential role during starvation, cellular differentiation, cell death, and aging. Autophagy is also involved in the elimination of cancer cells by triggering a nonapoptotic cell death program, which suggests a negative role in tumor development. Mouse models that are heterozygotes for the beclin 1 gene, an important gene for autophagy, have altered autophagic response and show a high incidence of spontaneous tumors, which establishes a role for autophagy in tumor suppression.[18] This also suggests that mutations in other genes operating in this pathway may contribute to tumor formation through deregulation of autophagy. However, autophagy also acts as a stress response mechanism to protect cancer cells from low nutrient supply or therapeutic insults. Studies on the molecular determinants of autophagy are ongoing to determine whether autophagy can be modulated for therapeutic purposes.

Cancer Invasion

A feature of malignant cells is their ability to invade the surrounding normal tissue. Tumors in which the malignant cells appear to lie exclusively above the basement membrane are referred to as *in situ cancer*, whereas tumors in which the malignant cells are demonstrated to breach the basement membrane, penetrating into surrounding stroma, are termed *invasive cancer*. The ability to invade involves changes in adhesion, initiation of motility, and proteolysis of the extracellular matrix (ECM).

Cell-to-cell adhesion in normal cells involves interactions between cell-surface proteins. Calcium adhesion molecules of the cadherin family (E-cadherin, P-cadherin, and N-cadherin) are thought to enhance the cells' ability to bind to one another and suppress invasion. Migration occurs when cancer cells penetrate and attach to the basal matrix of the tissue being invaded; this allows the cancer cell to pull itself forward within the tissue. Attachment to glycoproteins of the ECM such as fibronectin, laminin, and collagen is mediated by tumor cell integrin receptors. Integrins are a family of glycoproteins that form heterodimeric receptors for ECM molecules. The integrins can form at least 25 distinct pairings of their α and β subunits, and each pairing is specific for a unique set of ligands. In addition to regulating cell adhesion to the ECM, integrins relay molecular signals regarding the cellular environment that influence shape, survival, proliferation, gene transcription, and migration.

Factors that are thought to play a role in cancer cell motility include autocrine motility factor, autotaxin, scatter factor (also known as *hepatocyte growth factor*), TGFα, EGF, and insulin-like growth factors.

Serine, cysteine, and aspartic proteinases and MMPs have all been implicated in cancer invasion. Urokinase and tissue plasminogen activators (uPA and tPA) are serine proteases that convert plasminogen into plasmin. Plasmin, in return, can degrade several ECM components. Plasmin also may activate MMPs. uPA has been more closely correlated with tissue invasion and metastasis than tPA. Plasminogen activator inhibitors 1 and 2 (PAI-1 and PAI-2) are produced in tissues and counteract the activity of plasminogen activators.

MMPs comprise a family of metal-dependent endopeptidases. Upon activation, MMPs degrade a variety of ECM components. Although MMPs often are referred to by their common names, which reflect the ECM component for which they have specificity, a sequential numbering system has been adopted for standardization. For example, collagenase-1 is now referred to as *MMP-1*. The MMPs are further classified as secreted and membrane-type MMPs. Most of the MMPs are synthesized as inactive zymogens (pro-MMP) and are activated by proteolytic removal of the propeptide domain outside the cell by other active MMPs or serine proteinases.

MMPs are upregulated in almost every type of cancer. Some of the MMPs are expressed by cancer cells, whereas others are expressed by the tumor stromal cells. Experimental models have demonstrated that MMPs promote cancer progression by increasing cancer cell growth, migration, invasion, angiogenesis, and metastasis. MMPs exert these effects by cleaving not only structural components of the ECM but also growth factor–binding proteins, growth factor precursors, cell adhesion molecules, and other proteinases. The activity of MMPs is regulated by their endogenous inhibitors and tissue inhibitors of MMPs (TIMP-1, TIMP-2, TIMP-3, and TIMP-4).

Angiogenesis

Angiogenesis is the establishment of new blood vessels from a preexisting vascular bed. This neovascularization is essential for tumor growth and metastasis. Tumors develop an angiogenic phenotype as a result of accumulated genetic alterations and in response to local selection pressures such as hypoxia. Many of the common oncogenes and tumor-suppressor genes have been shown to play a role in inducing angiogenesis, including *ras*, HER2, and mutations in p53.

In response to the angiogenic switch, pericytes retract and the endothelium secretes several growth factors such as basic fibroblast growth factor, platelet-derived growth factor (PDGF), and insulin-like growth factor. The basement membrane and stroma around the capillary are proteolytically degraded, a process that is mediated in most part by uPA. The endothelium then migrates through the degraded matrix, initially as a solid cord and later forming lumina. Finally, sprouting tips anastomose to form a vascular network surrounded by a basement membrane.

Angiogenesis is mediated by factors produced by various cells, including tumor cells, endothelial cells, stromal cells, and inflammatory cells. The first proangiogenic factor was identified by Folkman and colleagues in 1971.[19] Since then, several other factors have been shown to be proangiogenic or antiangiogenic. Of the angiogenic stimulators, the best studied are the vascular endothelial growth factors (VEGFs). The VEGF family consists of six growth factors (VEGF-A, VEGF-B, VEGF-C, VEGF-D, VEGF-E, and placental growth factor) and three receptors (VEGFR1 or Flt-1, VEGFR2 or KDR/FLK-1, and VEGFR3 or Flt-4).[20] Neuropilin 1 and 2 also may act as receptors for VEGF.[21] VEGF is induced by hypoxia and by different growth factors and cytokines, including EGF, PDGF, TNF-α, TGFβ, and interleukin-1β. VEGF has various functions, including increasing vascular permeability, inducing endothelial cell proliferation and tube formation, and inducing endothelial cell synthesis of proteolytic enzymes such as uPA, PAI-1, urokinase plasminogen activator receptor, and MMP-1. Furthermore, VEGF may mediate blood flow by its effects on the vasodilator nitric oxide and act as an endothelial survival factor, thus protecting the integrity of the vasculature. The proliferation of new lymphatic vessels, lymphangiogenesis, is also thought to be controlled by the VEGF family. Signaling in lymphatic cells is thought to be modulated by VEGFR3.[22] Experimental studies with VEGF-C and VEGF-D have shown that they can induce tumor lymphangiogenesis and direct metastasis via the lymphatic vessels and lymph nodes.[22,23]

PDGFs A, B, C, and D also play important roles in angiogenesis. PDGFs can not only enhance endothelial cell proliferation directly but also upregulate VEGF expression in vascular smooth muscle cells, promoting endothelial cell survival via a paracrine effect.[20] The angiopoietins angiopoietin-1 and angiopoietin-2 (Ang-1 and Ang-2), in return, are thought to regulate blood vessel maturation. Ang-1 and Ang-2 both bind angiopoietin-1 receptor (also known as tyrosine-protein kinase receptor TIE-2), but only the binding of Ang-1 activates signal transduction; thus Ang-2 is an Ang-1 antagonist. Ang-1, via the Tie-2 receptor, induces remodeling and stabilization of blood vessels. Upregulation of Ang-2 by hypoxic induction of VEGF inhibits Ang-1–induced Tie-2 signaling, which results in destabilization of vessels and makes endothelial cells responsive to angiogenic signals, thus promoting angiogenesis in the presence of VEGF. Therefore the balance between these factors determines the angiogenetic capacity of a tumor.

Tumor angiogenesis is regulated by several factors in a coordinated fashion. In addition to upregulation of proangiogenic molecules, angiogenesis also can be encouraged by suppression of naturally occurring inhibitors. Such inhibitors of angiogenesis include thrombospondin 1 and angiostatin. Angiogenesis is a prerequisite not only for primary tumor growth but also for metastasis. Angiogenesis in the primary tumor, as determined by microvessel density, has been demonstrated to be an independent predictor of distant metastatic disease and survival in several cancers. Expression of angiogenic factors such as VEGFs has had prognostic value in many studies. These findings further emphasize the importance of angiogenesis in cancer biology.

Metastasis

Metastases arise from the spread of cancer cells from the primary site and the formation of new tumors in distant sites. The metastatic process consists of a series of steps that need to be completed successfully (Fig. 10-7).[24] First, the primary cancer must develop access to the circulation through either the blood circulatory system or the lymphatic system. After the cancer cells are shed into the circulation, they must survive. Next, the circulating cells lodge in a new organ and extravasate into the new tissue. Next, the cells need to initiate growth in the new tissue and eventually establish vascularization to sustain the new tumor. Overall, metastasis is an inefficient process, although the initial steps of hematogenous metastasis (the arrest of tumor cells in the organ and extravasation) are believed to be performed efficiently. Only a small subset of cancer cells is then able to initiate micrometastases, and an even smaller portion go on to grow into macrometastases.

Metastases can sometimes arise several years after the treatment of primary tumors. For example, although most breast cancer recurrences occur within the first 10 years after the initial treatment and recurrences are rare after 20 years, breast cancer recurrences have been reported decades after the original tumor. This phenomenon is referred to as *dormancy,* and it remains one of the biggest challenges in cancer biology. Persistence of solitary cancer cells in a secondary site such as the liver or bone marrow is one possible contributor to dormancy.[25] Another explanation of dormancy is that cells remain viable in a quiescent state and then become reactivated by a physiologically perturbing event. Interestingly, primary tumor removal has been proposed to be a potentially perturbing factor.[26] An alternate explanation is that cells establish preangiogenic metastases in which they continue to proliferate but that the proliferative rate is balanced by the apoptotic rate. Therefore, when these small metastases acquire the ability to become vascularized, substantial tumor growth can be achieved at the metastatic site, leading to clinical detection.

Several types of tumors metastasize in an organ-specific pattern. One explanation for this is mechanical and is based on the different circulatory drainage patterns of the tumors. When different tumor types and their preferred metastasis sites were compared, 66% of organ-specific metastases were explained on the basis of blood flow alone. The other explanation for preferential metastasis is what is referred to as the *"seed and soil" theory,* the dependence of the seed (the cancer cell) on the soil (the secondary organ). According to this theory, once cells have reached a secondary organ, their growth efficiency in that organ is based on the compatibility of the cancer cell's biology with its new microenvironment. For example, breast cancer cells may grow more efficiently in bone than in some other organs because of favorable molecular interactions that occur in the

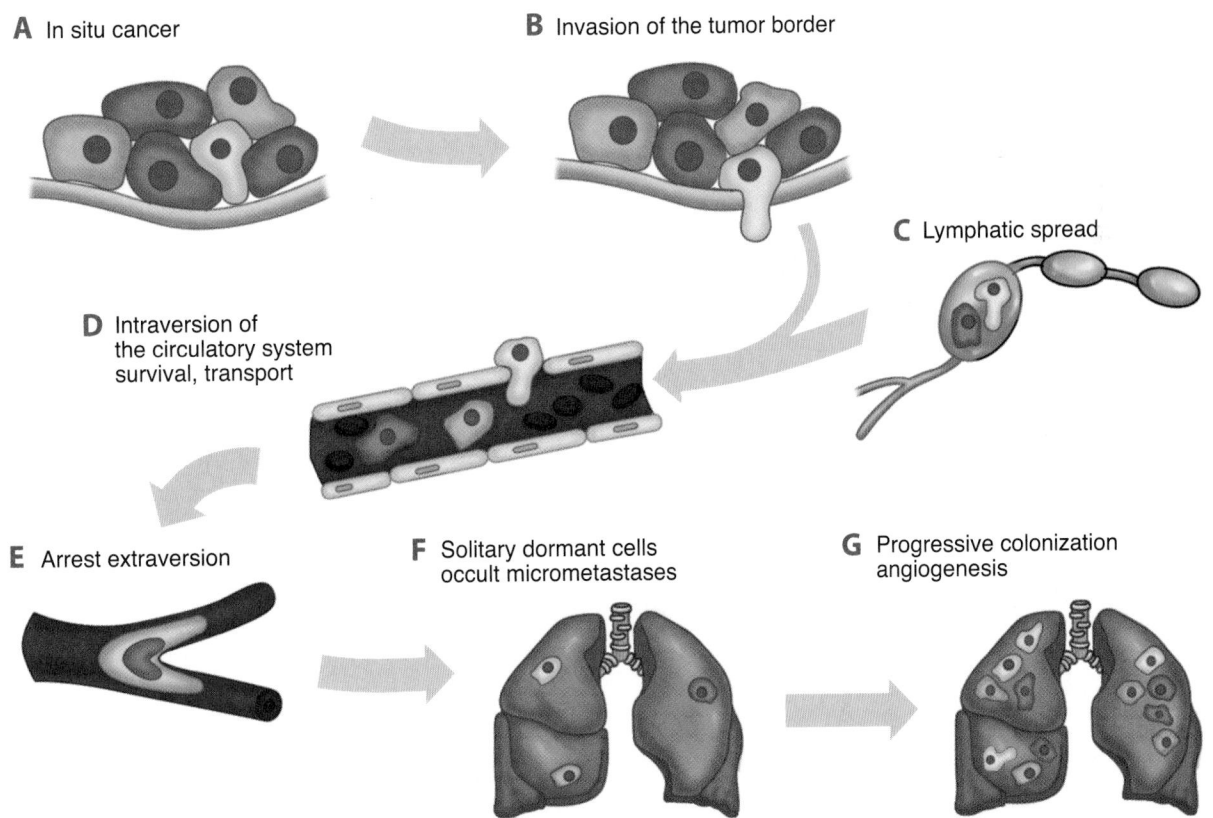

FIG. 10-7. A schematic representation of the metastatic process. **A.** The metastatic process begins with an in situ cancer surrounded by an intact basement membrane. **B.** Invasion requires reversible changes in cell-cell and cell–extracellular matrix adherence, destruction of proteins in the matrix and stroma, and motility. **C.** Metastasizing cells can enter the circulation via the lymphatics. **D.** They can also directly enter the circulation. **E.** Intravascular survival of the tumor cells and extravasation of the circulatory system follow. **F.** Metastatic single cells can colonize sites and remain dormant for years as occult micrometastases. **G.** Subsequent progression and neovascularization leads to clinically detectable metastases and progressively growing, angiogenic metastases. *(Modified with permission from Macmillan Publishers Ltd. Steeg P: Metastasis suppressors alter the signal transduction of cancer cells. Nat Rev Cancer 3:55–63. Copyright © 2003.)*

bone microenvironment. The ability of cancer cells to grow in a specific site likely depends on features inherent to the cancer cell, features inherent to the organ, and the interplay between the cancer cell and its microenvironment.[27]

Many of the oncogenes discovered to date, such as HER2 and *ras*, are thought to potentiate not only malignant transformation but also one or more of the steps required in the metastatic process. Experimental models have suggested a role for several molecules, including RhoC, osteopontin and interleukin-11, and Twist, in tumor metastasis. Metastasis also may involve the loss of metastasis-suppressor genes. Laboratory work involving cancer cell lines that have been selected to have a higher metastatic potential have led to the realization that these more highly metastatic cells have a different gene expression profile than their less metastatic parental counterparts. This in turn has led to the currently held belief that the ability of a primary tumor to metastasize may be predictable by analysis of its gene expression profile. Indeed, several studies have recently focused on identifying a gene expression profile or a "molecular signature" that is associated with metastasis. It has been shown that such a gene expression profile can be used to predict the probability that the patient will remain free of distant metastasis.[28] This suggests that the metastatic potential of a tumor is already predetermined by the genetic alterations that the cancer cells acquire early in tumorigenesis. Notably, this hypothesis differs from the multistep tumorigenesis theory in that the ability to metastasize is considered an inherent quality of the tumor from the beginning. It is assumed that metastasis develops not from a few rare cells in the primary tumor that acquire the ability to metastasize but that all cells in tumors with such molecular signatures develop the ability to metastasize. The reality probably lies in between in that some early genetic changes detectable in the entire tumor can give tumors an advantage in the metastatic process, whereas additional genetic changes can give a clone of cells additional advantages, thus allowing them to succeed in metastasis.

Cancer Stem Cells

Stem cells are cells that have the ability to perpetuate themselves through self-renewal and to generate mature cells of a particular tissue through differentiation.[29] It has recently been proposed that stem cells themselves may be the target of transformation. It was first documented for leukemia and multiple myeloma that only a small subset of cancer cells is capable of extensive proliferation. It has subsequently also been shown for many solid cancers that only a small proportion of cells is clonogenic in culture and in vivo. In leukemia and multiple myeloma only a small subset of cancer cells is capable of extensive proliferation. Similarly, in many solid tumor types only a small proportion of cells is clonogenic in culture and in vivo. If indeed tumor growth and metastasis are driven by a small population of cancer stem cells, this may alter our current approaches to cancer therapy. Currently available drugs can shrink metastatic tumors but often cannot eradicate them. The failure of these treatments usually is attributed to the acquisition of drug resistance by the cancer cells; however, the cancer stem cell hypothesis raises the possibility that existing therapies may simply fail to kill cancer stem cells effectively. Therapeutic approaches targeting stem cells specifically are under study.

CANCER ETIOLOGY

Cancer Genetics

One widely held opinion is that cancer is a genetic disease that arises from an accumulation of mutations that leads to the selection of cells with increasingly aggressive behavior. These mutations may lead either to a gain of function by oncogenes or to a loss of function by tumor-suppressor genes. Most mutations in cancer are somatic and are found only in the cancer cells. Most of our information on human cancer genes has been gained from hereditary cancers. In the case of hereditary cancers, the individual carries a particular germline mutation in every cell. In the past decade, >30 genes for autosomal

dominant hereditary cancers have been identified (Table 10-3).[30] A few of these hereditary cancer genes are oncogenes, but most are tumor-suppressor genes. Although hereditary cancer syndromes are rare, somatic mutations that occur in sporadic cancer have been found to disrupt the cellular pathways altered in hereditary cancer syndromes, which suggests that these pathways are critical to normal cell growth, cell cycle, and proliferation.

The following factors may suggest the presence of a hereditary cancer[31]:

1. Tumor development at a much younger age than usual
2. Presence of bilateral disease
3. Presence of multiple primary malignancies
4. Presentation of a cancer in the less affected sex (e.g., male breast cancer)
5. Clustering of the same cancer type in relatives
6. Occurrence of cancer in association with other conditions such as mental retardation or pathognomonic skin lesions

It is crucial that all surgeons caring for cancer patients be aware of hereditary cancer syndromes, because a patient's genetic background has significant implications for patient counseling, planning of surgical therapy, and cancer screening and prevention. Some of the more commonly encountered hereditary cancer syndromes are discussed here.

rb1 *Gene and Hereditary Retinoblastoma*

The retinoblastoma gene *rb1* was the first tumor suppressor to be cloned. The *rb1* gene product, the Rb protein, is a regulator of transcription that controls the cell cycle, differentiation, and apoptosis in normal development.[32] Retinoblastoma has long been known to occur in hereditary and nonhereditary forms. Interestingly, although most children with an affected parent develop bilateral retinoblastoma, some develop unilateral retinoblastoma. Furthermore, some children with an affected parent are not affected themselves but then have an affected child, which indicates that they are *rb1* mutation carriers. These findings led to the theory that a single mutation is not sufficient for tumorigenesis. Dr. Alfred Knudson hypothesized that hereditary retinoblastoma involves two mutations, of which one is germline and one somatic, whereas nonhereditary retinoblastoma is due to two somatic mutations (Fig. 10-8).[33] Thus both hereditary and nonhereditary forms of retinoblastoma involve the same number of mutations, a hypothesis known as *Knudson's "two-hit" hypothesis*. A "hit" may be a point mutation, a chromosomal deletion referred to as *allelic loss,* or a loss of heterozygosity, or silencing of an existing gene.

Retinoblastoma is a pediatric retinal tumor. Most of these tumors are detected within the first 7 years of life. Bilateral disease usually is diagnosed earlier, at an average age of 12 months. There is a higher incidence of second extraocular primary tumors, especially sarcomas, malignant melanomas, and malignant neoplasms of the brain and meninges in patients with germline mutations. In addition to hereditary retinoblastoma, Rb protein is commonly inactivated directly by mutation in many sporadic tumors.[34] Moreover, other molecules in the Rb pathway, such as p16 and cyclin-dependent kinases 4 and 6 (CDK4 and CDK6), have been identified in a number of sporadic tumors, which suggests that the Rb pathway is critical in malignant transformation.

p53 *and Li-Fraumeni Syndrome*

Li-Fraumeni syndrome (LFS) was first defined on the basis of observed clustering of malignancies, including early-onset breast cancer, soft tissue sarcomas, brain tumors, adrenocortical tumors, and leukemia.[35] Criteria for classic LFS in an individual (the proband) include (a) a bone or soft tissue sarcoma when younger than 45 years, (b) a first-degree relative with cancer before age 45 years, and (c) another first- or second-degree relative with either a sarcoma diagnosed at any age or any cancer diagnosed before age 45 years.[36] Approximately 70% of LFS families have been shown to have germline mutations in the tumor-suppressor gene p53.[37] Breast carcinoma, soft tissue sarcoma,

TABLE 10-3	Genes associated with hereditary cancer		
Gene	**Location**	**Syndrome**	**Cancer Sites and Associated Traits**
APC	17q21	Familial adenomatous polyposis (FAP)	Colorectal adenomas and carcinomas, duodenal and gastric tumors, desmoids, medulloblastomas, osteomas
BMPRIA	10q21-q22	Juvenile polyposis coli	Juvenile polyps of the GI tract, GI and colorectal malignancy
BRCA1	17q21	Breast-ovarian syndrome	Breast cancer, ovarian cancer, colon cancer, prostate cancer
BRCA2	13q12.3	Breast-ovarian syndrome	Breast cancer, ovarian cancer, colon cancer, prostate cancer, cancer of the gallbladder and bile duct, pancreatic cancer, gastric cancer, melanoma
p16; CDK4	9p21; 12q14	Familial melanoma	Melanoma, pancreatic cancer, dysplastic nevi, atypical moles
CDH1	16q22	Hereditary diffuse gastric cancer	Gastric cancer
hCHK2	22q12.1	Li-Fraumeni syndrome and hereditary breast cancer	Breast cancer, soft tissue sarcoma, brain tumors
hMLH1; hMSH2; hMSH6; PMS1; hPMS2	3p21; 2p22-21; 2p16; 2q31-33; 7p22	Hereditary nonpolyposis colorectal cancer	Colorectal cancer, endometrial cancer, transitional cell carcinoma of the ureter and renal pelvis, and carcinomas of the stomach, small bowel, ovary, and pancreas
MEN1	11q13	Multiple endocrine neoplasia type 1	Pancreatic islet cell cancer, parathyroid hyperplasia, pituitary adenomas
MET	7q31	Hereditary papillary renal cell carcinoma	Renal cancer
NF1	17q11	Neurofibromatosis type 1	Neurofibroma, neurofibrosarcoma, acute myelogenous leukemia, brain tumors
NF2	22q12	Neurofibromatosis type 2	Acoustic neuromas, meningiomas, gliomas, ependymomas
PTC	9q22.3	Nevoid basal cell carcinoma	Basal cell carcinoma
PTEN	10q23.3	Cowden disease	Breast cancer, thyroid cancer, endometrial cancer
rb	13q14	Retinoblastoma	Retinoblastoma, sarcomas, melanoma, and malignant neoplasms of brain and meninges
RET	10q11.2	Multiple endocrine neoplasia type 2	Medullary thyroid cancer, pheochromocytoma, parathyroid hyperplasia
SDHB; SDHC; SDHD	1p363.1-p35; 11q23; 1q21	Hereditary paraganglioma and pheochromocytoma	Paraganglioma, pheochromocytoma
SMAD4/DPC4	18q21.1	Juvenile polyposis coli	Juvenile polyps of the GI tract, GI and colorectal malignancy
STK11	19p13.3	Peutz-Jeghers syndrome	GI tract carcinoma, breast carcinoma, testicular cancer, pancreatic cancer, benign pigmentation of the skin and mucosa
p53	17p13	Li-Fraumeni syndrome	Breast cancer, soft tissue sarcoma, osteosarcoma, brain tumors, adrenocortical carcinoma, Wilms' tumor, phyllodes tumor of the breast, pancreatic cancer, leukemia, neuroblastoma
TSC1; TSC2	9q34; 16p13	Tuberous sclerosis	Multiple hamartomas, renal cell carcinoma, astrocytoma
VHL	3p25	von Hippel-Lindau disease	Renal cell carcinoma, hemangioblastomas of retina and central nervous system, pheochromocytoma
WT	11p13	Wilms' tumor	Wilms' tumor, aniridia, genitourinary abnormalities, mental retardation

Source: Modified with permission from Marsh DJ, Zori RT: Genetic insights into familial cancers – update and recent discoveries. *Cancer Lett* 181:125, 2002. Copyright Elsevier.

osteosarcoma, brain tumors, adrenocortical carcinoma, Wilms' tumor, and phyllodes tumor of the breast are strongly associated; pancreatic cancer is moderately associated; and leukemia and neuroblastoma are weakly associated with germline p53 mutations.[38] Mutations of p53 have not been detected in approximately 30% of LFS families, and it is hypothesized that genetic alterations in other proteins interacting with p53 function may play a role in these families.

Of the known genes in human cancer, p53 is the most commonly mutated. The p53 protein regulates cell-cycle progression as well as apoptotic cell death as part of stress response pathways after exposure to ionizing or ultraviolet (UV) irradiation, chemotherapy, acidosis, growth factor deprivation, or hypoxia. When cells are exposed to stressors, p53 acts as a transcription factor for genes that induce cell-cycle arrest or apoptosis. A majority of p53 mutations are found within a central DNA recognition motif and disrupt DNA binding by p53. Families with germline missense mutations in the DNA-binding domain show a more highly penetrant phenotype than families with other p53 mutations.[39] Furthermore, proband cancers are linked with significantly younger age at diagnosis in patients with missense mutations in the DNA-binding domain.[39]

hCHK2, Li-Fraumeni Syndrome, and Hereditary Breast Cancer

Germline mutations in the *hCHK2* gene have recently been identified as another susceptibility gene for LFS. The *hCHK2* gene encodes for the human homologue of the yeast Cds1 and the RAD53 G_2 checkpoint, whose activation by DNA damage prevents entry into mitosis. CHK2 directly phosphorylates p53, which suggests that CHK2 may be involved in p53 regulation after DNA damage. CHK2 also regulates *BRCA1* function after DNA damage. The protein truncation mutation *1100delC* in exon 10 identified in LFS and breast cancer abolishes the kinase function of CHK2. Another reported mutation in *hCHK2* is a missense mutation (R145W) that destabilizes the protein, shortening its half-life.[40]

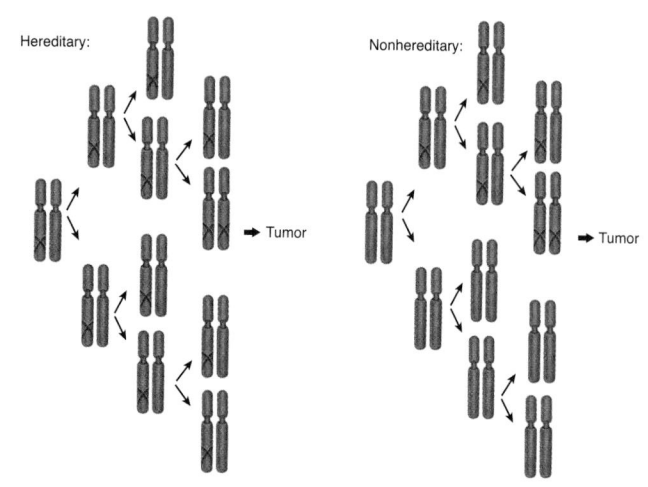

FIG. 10-8. "Two-hit" tumor formation in both hereditary and non-hereditary cancers. A "one-hit" clone is a precursor to the tumor in nonhereditary cancers, whereas all cells are one-hit clones in hereditary cancer. *(Modified with permission from Macmillan Publishers Ltd. Knudson AG: Two genetic hits (more or less) to cancer.* Nat Rev Cancer *1:157-162. Copyright © 2001.)*

Although some investigators found *hCHK2* mutations in classic LFS families, others have reported that the phenotypes of CHK2 families are not typical for LFS and involve no sarcomas or childhood cancers. The CHK2 mutation originally reported in LFS (1100delC) is found in 1.4% of population controls but is found at an increased frequency (3.1%) among breast cancer patients with a family history of the cancer.[41] Patients with bilateral breast cancers are six times more likely to have the mutation than patients with unilateral breast cancer. Thus *hCHK2* mutations may play a role in families with hereditary breast cancer as well as in families with LFS, but the extent of this is unclear. Mutations of *hCHK2* are rare in sporadic breast tumors.

BRCA1, BRCA2, *and Hereditary Breast-Ovarian Cancer Syndrome*

It is estimated that 5 to 10% of breast cancers are hereditary. Of women with early-onset breast cancer (aged 40 years or younger), nearly 10% have a germline mutation in one of the breast cancer genes *BRCA1* or *BRCA2*.[42] Mutation carriers are more prevalent among women who have a first- or second-degree relative with premenopausal breast cancer or ovarian cancer at any age. The likelihood of a *BRCA* mutation is higher in patients who belong to a population in which founder mutations may be prevalent, such as in the Ashkenazi Jewish population. For a female *BRCA1* mutation carrier, the cumulative risks of developing breast cancer and ovarian cancer by age 70 have been estimated to be 87 and 44%, respectively.[43] The cumulative risks of breast cancer and ovarian cancer by age 70 in families with *BRCA2* mutation have been estimated to be 84 and 27%, respectively.[44] Although male breast cancer can occur with either *BRCA1* or *BRCA2* mutation, the majority of families (76%) with both male and female breast cancer have mutations in *BRCA2*.[44] Besides breast and ovarian cancer, *BRCA1* and *BRCA2* mutations may be associated with increased risks for several other cancers. *BRCA1* mutations confer a fourfold increased risk for colon cancer and threefold increased risk for prostate cancer.[43] *BRCA2* mutations confer a fivefold increased risk for prostate cancer, sevenfold in men younger than 65 years.[45] Furthermore, *BRCA2* mutations confer a fivefold increased risk for gallbladder and bile duct cancers, fourfold increased risk for pancreatic cancer, and threefold increased risk for gastric cancer and malignant melanoma.[45]

BRCA1 was the first breast cancer susceptibility gene identified and has been mapped to 17q21. *BRCA2*, mapped to 13q12.3, was

reported shortly afterward. *BRCA1* and *BRCA2* encode for large nuclear proteins, 208 kDa and 384 kDa, respectively, that have been implicated in processes fundamental to all cells, including DNA repair and recombination, checkpoint control of the cell cycle, and transcription.[46] Although early studies suggested that the two proteins function together as a complex, subsequent data demonstrated that they have distinct functions.[47,48] In fact, breast cancers arising from *BRCA1* or *BRCA2* mutations are different at the molecular level and have been found to have distinct gene expression profiles.[49] *BRCA1*-associated tumors are more likely to be estrogen receptor negative, whereas *BRCA2*-associated tumors are more likely to be estrogen receptor positive. Currently, studies are ongoing to determine whether *BRCA1* and *BRCA2* status can be used to guide systemic therapy choices for breast cancer.

APC *Gene and Familial Adenomatous Polyposis*

Patients affected with familial adenomatous polyposis (FAP) characteristically develop hundreds to thousands of polyps in the colon and rectum. The polyps usually appear in adolescence and, if left untreated, progress to colorectal cancer. FAP is associated with benign extracolonic manifestations that may be useful in identifying new cases, including congenital hypertrophy of the retinal pigment epithelium, epidermoid cysts, and osteomas. In addition to colorectal cancer, patients with FAP are at risk for upper intestinal neoplasms (gastric and duodenal polyps, duodenal and periampullary cancer), hepatobiliary tumors (hepatoblastoma, pancreatic cancer, and cholangiocarcinoma), thyroid carcinomas, desmoid tumors, and medulloblastomas.

The product of the adenomatous polyposis coli tumor-suppressor gene (*APC*) is widely expressed in many tissues and plays an important role in cell-cell interactions, cell adhesion, regulation of β-catenin, and maintenance of cytoskeletal microtubules. Alterations in *APC* lead to dysregulation of several physiologic processes that govern colonic epithelial cell homeostasis, including cell-cycle progression, migration, differentiation, and apoptosis. Mutations in the *APC* gene have been identified in FAP and in 80% of sporadic colorectal cancers.[50] Furthermore, *APC* mutations are the earliest known genetic alterations in colorectal cancer progression, which emphasizes its importance in cancer initiation. The germline mutations in *APC* may arise from point mutations, insertions, or deletions that lead to a premature stop codon and a truncated, functionally inactive protein. The risk of developing specific manifestations of FAP is correlated with the position of the FAP mutations, a phenomenon referred to as *genotype-phenotype correlation*. For example, desmoids usually are associated with mutations between codons 1403 and 1578.[51,52] Mutations in the extreme 5' or 3' ends of *APC*, or in the alternatively spliced region of exon 9, are associated with an attenuated version of FAP. Better understanding of the genotype-phenotype correlations may assist in patient counseling and therapeutic planning.

Mismatch Repair Genes and Hereditary Nonpolyposis Colorectal Cancer

Hereditary nonpolyposis colorectal cancer (HNPCC), also referred to as *Lynch syndrome,* is an autosomal dominant hereditary cancer syndrome that predisposes to a wide spectrum of cancers, including colorectal cancer without polyposis. Some have proposed that HNPCC consists of at least two syndromes: Lynch syndrome 1, which entails hereditary predisposition for colorectal cancer with early age of onset (approximately age 44 years) and an excess of synchronous and metachronous colonic cancers; and Lynch syndrome 2, featuring a similar colonic phenotype accompanied by a high risk for carcinoma of the endometrium, transitional cell carcinoma of the ureter and renal pelvis, and carcinomas of the stomach, small bowel, ovary, and pancreas.[53] The diagnostic criteria for HNPCC are referred to as the *Amsterdam criteria,* or the *3-2-1-0 rule.* The classic Amsterdam criteria were revised to include other HNPCC-related cancers (Table 10-4).[54] These criteria are met when three or more family members have histologically verified, HNPCC-

| TABLE 10-4 | Revised criteria for hereditary nonpolyposis colon cancer (HNPCC) (Amsterdam criteria II) |

TABLE 10-4	Revised criteria for hereditary nonpolyposis colon cancer (HNPCC) (Amsterdam criteria II)

Three or more relatives with an HNPCC-associated cancer (colorectal cancer, endometrial cancer, cancer of the small bowel, ureter, or renal pelvis), one of whom is a first-degree relative of the other two

At least two successive generations affected

At least one case diagnosed before age 50 y

Familial adenomatous polyposis excluded

Tumors verified by pathologic examination

Source: Modified with permission from Vasen et al.[54] Copyright Elsevier.

TABLE 10-5	Cowden disease diagnostic criteria

Pathognomonic criteria

Mucocutaneous lesions

Facial trichilemmomas

Acral keratoses

Papillomatous lesions

Mucosal lesions

Major criteria

Breast cancer

Thyroid cancer, especially follicular thyroid carcinoma type

Macrocephaly (≥97th percentile)

Lhermitte-Duclos disease

Endometrial carcinoma

Minor criteria

Other thyroid lesions (e.g., goiter)

Mental retardation (intelligence quotient ≤75)

GI hamartomas

Fibrocystic disease of the breast

Lipomas

Fibromas

Genitourinary tumors (e.g., uterine fibroids) or malformation

Operational diagnosis in an individual

Mucocutaneous lesions alone if there are:

Six or more facial papules, of which three or more must be trichilemmoma, or

Cutaneous facial papules and oral mucosal papillomatosis, or

Oral mucosal papillomatosis and acral keratoses, or

Palmoplantar keratoses, six or more

Two major criteria, but one must be macrocephaly or Lhermitte-Duclos disease

One major and three minor criteria

Four minor criteria

Source: Modified with permission from Eng C: Will the real Cowden syndrome please stand up: revised diagnostic criteria. *J Med Genet* 37:828, 2000. With permission from the BMJ Publishing Group.

associated cancers (one of whom is a first-degree relative of the other two), two or more generations are involved, at least one individual was diagnosed before age 50 years, and no individuals have FAP.[54]

During DNA replication, DNA polymerases may introduce single nucleotide mismatches or small insertion or deletion loops. These errors are corrected through a process referred to as *mismatch repair*. When mismatch repair genes are inactivated, DNA mutations in other genes that are critical to cell growth and proliferation accumulate rapidly. In HNPCC, germline mutations have been identified in several genes that play a key role in DNA nucleotide mismatch repair: *hMLH1* (human mutL homologue 1), *hMSH2* (human mutS homologue 2), *hMSH6*, and *hPMS1* and *hPMS2* (human postmeiotic segregation 1 and 2), of which *hMLH1* and *hMSH2* are the most common.[55–60] The hallmark of HNPCC is microsatellite instability, which occurs on the basis of unrepaired mismatches and small insertion or deletion loops. Microsatellite instability can be tested by comparing the DNA of a patient's tumor with DNA from adjacent normal epithelium, amplifying the DNA with polymerase chain reaction (PCR) using a standard set of markers, comparing the amplified genomic DNA sequences, and classifying the degree of microsatellite instability as high, low, or stable. Such microsatellite instability testing may help select patients who are more likely to have germline mutations.

PTEN *and Cowden Disease*

Somatic deletions or mutations in the tumor-suppressor gene *PTEN* (phosphatase and tensin homologue deleted on chromosome 10) have been observed in a number of glioma and breast, prostate, and renal carcinoma cell lines and several primary tumor specimens.[61] *PTEN* also is referred to as the *gene mutated in multiple advanced cancers 1 (MMAC1)*. *PTEN* was identified as the susceptibility gene for the autosomal dominant syndrome Cowden disease (CD) or multiple hamartoma syndrome.[62] Trichilemmomas, benign tumors of the hair follicle infundibulum, and mucocutaneous papillomatosis are pathognomonic of CD. Other common features include thyroid adenomas and multinodular goiters, breast fibroadenomas, and hamartomatous GI polyps. The diagnosis of CD is made when an individual or family has a combination of pathognomonic major and/or minor criteria proposed by the International Cowden Consortium (Table 10-5).[63] CD is associated with an increased risk of breast and thyroid cancers. Breast cancer develops in 25 to 50% of affected women.[63]

PTEN encodes a 403-amino-acid protein, tyrosine phosphatase. *PTEN* negatively controls the PI3K signaling pathway for the regulation of cell growth and survival by dephosphorylating phosphoinositol 3,4,5-triphosphate; thus mutation of *PTEN* leads to constitutive activation of the PI3K/Akt signaling pathway. The "hot spot" for *PTEN* mutations has been identified in exon 5. Forty-three percent of CD mutations have been identified in this exon, which contains the tyrosine phosphatase core domain. This suggests that the *PTEN* catalytic activity is vital for its biologic function.

p16 *and Hereditary Malignant Melanoma*

The gene *P16*, also known as INK4A, CDKN1, CDKN2A, and MTS1, is a tumor suppressor that acts by binding CDK4 and CDK6 and inhibiting the catalytic activity of the CDK4-CDK6/cyclin D complex

that is required for phosphorylation of Rb and subsequent cell-cycle progression. Studies suggest that germline mutations in p16 can be found in 20% of melanoma-prone families.[64] Mutations in p16 that alter its ability to inhibit the catalytic activity of the CDK4-CDK6/cyclin D complex not only increase the risk of melanoma by 75-fold but also increase the risk of pancreatic cancer by 22-fold.[65] Interestingly, p16 mutations that do not appear to alter its function increase the risk of melanoma by 38-fold and do not increase the risk of pancreatic cancer.[65] Genetic evaluation of primary tumors has revealed that p16 is inactivated through point mutation, promoter methylation, or deletion in a significant portion of sporadic tumors, including cancers of the pancreas, esophagus, head and neck, stomach, breast, and colon, as well as melanomas.

E-Cadherin and Hereditary Diffuse Gastric Cancer

E-cadherin is a cell adhesion molecule that plays an important role in normal architecture and function of epithelial cells. The adhesive function of E-cadherin is dependent on interaction of its cytoplasmic domain with β- and γ-catenins and may be regulated by phosphorylation of β-catenin.

Hereditary diffuse gastric carcinoma is an autosomal dominant cancer syndrome that results from germline mutations in the E-cadherin gene, *CDH1*. Carriers of *CDH1* mutations have a 70 to 80% chance of developing gastric cancer.[66] Furthermore, mutations of *CDH1* have been described in sporadic cancers of the ovary, endometrium, breast, and thyroid. However, frequent mutations have been identified in only two particular tumors: diffuse gastric carcinomas and lobular breast carcinomas. Invasive lobular breast carcinomas often show inactivating mutations in combination with a loss of heterozygosity of the wild-type *CDH1* allele.[67] Interestingly, in gastric carcinomas the predominant mutations are exon skipping causing in-frame deletions, whereas most mutations identified in lobular breast cancers are premature stop codons; this suggests a genotype-phenotype correlation.

RET *Proto-Oncogene and Multiple Endocrine Neoplasia Type 2*

The *RET* (rearranged during transfection) gene encodes for a transmembrane receptor tyrosine kinase that plays a role in proliferation, migration, and differentiation of cells derived from the neural crest. Gain-of-function mutations in the *RET* gene are associated with medullary thyroid carcinoma in isolation or multiple endocrine neoplasia type 2 (MEN2) syndromes. MEN2A is associated with medullary thyroid carcinoma and pheochromocytoma (in 50%) or parathyroid adenoma (in 20%), whereas MEN2B is associated with medullary thyroid carcinoma, marfanoid habitus, mucosal neuromas, and ganglioneuromatosis.[68] *RET* mutations lead to uncontrolled growth of the thyroid C cells, and in familial medullary cancer, C-cell hyperplasia progresses to bilateral, multicentric medullary thyroid cancer. Mutations in the *RET* gene have also been identified in half of sporadic medullary thyroid cancers. The activating *RET* mutations in medullary thyroid cancer are being pursued as a therapeutic target.

Tissue Specificity of Hereditary Cancer

In spite of our increasing understanding of hereditary cancer genes, the tissue specificity of the hereditary cancers remains poorly understood. For example, although mutations in genes such as *rb* and p53 are encountered frequently in sporadic cancers arising in a variety of tissues, it is unclear why germline mutations in these genes would lead to tumors predominantly in selected tissues. However, mutations in tumor-suppressor genes alone are insufficient to produce tumors, and usually the development of cancer involves accumulation of multiple genetic alterations. The rate at which these changes occur in different tissues after inactivation of different tumor-suppressor genes may account for some of the tissue distribution seen with hereditary cancer syndromes.

Genetic Modifiers of Risk

Individuals carrying identical germline mutations vary in regard to cancer penetrance (whether cancer will develop or not) and cancer phenotype (the tissues involved). It is thought that this variability may be due to environmental influences or, if genetic, to genetic modifiers of risk. Similarly, genetic modifiers of risk also can play a role in determining whether an individual will develop cancer after exposure to carcinogens.

Chemical Carcinogens

The first report indicating that cancer could be caused by environmental factors was by John Hill, who in 1761 noted the association between nasal cancer and excessive use of tobacco snuff.[69] Currently, approximately 60 to 90% of cancers are thought to be due to environmental factors. Any agent that can contribute to tumor formation is referred to as a *carcinogen* and can be a chemical, physical, or viral agent. Chemicals are classified into three groups based on how they contribute to tumor formation. The first group of chemical agents, the genotoxins, can initiate carcinogenesis by causing a mutation. The second group, the cocarcinogens, by themselves cannot cause cancer but potentiate carcinogenesis by enhancing the potency of genotoxins. The third group, tumor promoters, enhances tumor formation when given after exposure to genotoxins.

The International Agency for Research on Cancer (IARC) maintains a registry of human carcinogens that is available through the World Wide Web (*http://www.iarc.fr*). The compounds are categorized into five groups based on an analysis of epidemiologic studies, animal models, and short-term mutagenesis tests. Group 1 contains what are considered to be proven human carcinogens, based on formal epidemiologic studies among workers who were exposed for long periods (several years) to the chemicals. Group 2A contains what are considered to be probable human carcinogens. Suggestive epidemiologic evidence exists for compounds in this group, but the data are insufficient to establish causality. There is evidence of carcinogenicity, however, from animal studies carried out under conditions relevant to human exposure. Group 2B contains what are considered to be possible carcinogens, because these substances are associated with a clear statistically and biologically significant increase in the incidence of malignant tumors in more than one animal species or strain. Group 3 agents are not classifiable as to carcinogenicity in humans. Group 4 agents are probably not carcinogenic to humans. Selected substances that have been classified as proven carcinogens (group 1) by the IARC are listed in Table 10-6.[70]

Physical Carcinogens

Physical carcinogenesis can occur through induction of inflammation and cell proliferation over a period of time or through exposure to physical agents that induce DNA damage. Foreign bodies can cause chronic irritation that can expose cells to carcinogenesis due to other environmental agents. In animal models, for example, subcutaneous implantation of a foreign body can lead to the development of tumors that have been attributed to chronic irritation from the foreign objects. In humans, clinical scenarios associated with chronic irritation and inflammation such as chronic nonhealing wounds, burns, and inflammatory bowel syndrome have all been associated with an increased risk of cancer. *H. pylori* infection is associated with

TABLE 10-6	Selected IARC group 1 chemical carcinogens[a]
Chemical	**Predominant Tumor Type[b]**
Aflatoxins	Liver cancer
Arsenic	Skin cancer
Benzene	Leukemia
Benzidine	Bladder cancer
Beryllium	Lung cancer
Cadmium	Lung cancer
Chinese-style salted fish	Nasopharyngeal carcinoma
Chlorambucil	Leukemia
Chromium [VI] compounds	Lung cancer
Coal tar	Skin cancer, scrotal cancer
Cyclophosphamide	Bladder cancer, leukemia
Diethylstilbestrol (DES)	Vaginal and cervical clear cell adenocarcinomas
Ethylene oxide	Leukemia, lymphoma
Estrogen replacement therapy	Endometrial cancer, breast cancer
Nickel	Lung cancer, nasal cancer
Tamoxifen[c]	Endometrial cancer
Vinyl chloride	Angiosarcoma of the liver, hepatocellular carcinoma, brain tumors, lung cancer, malignancies of lymphatic and hematopoietic system
TCDD (2,3,7,8-tetrachlorodibenzo-para-dioxin)	Soft tissue sarcoma
Tobacco products, smokeless	Oral cancer
Tobacco smoke	Lung cancer, oral cancer, pharyngeal cancer, laryngeal cancer, esophageal cancer (squamous cell), pancreatic cancer, bladder cancer, liver cancer, renal cell carcinoma, cervical cancer, leukemia

[a]Based on information in the IARC monographs.[70]
[b]Only tumor types for which causal relationships are established are listed. Other cancer types may be linked to the agents with a lower frequency or with insufficient data to prove causality.
[c]Tamoxifen has been shown to prevent contralateral breast cancer.
IARC = International Agency for Research on Cancer.

gastritis and gastric cancer, and thus its carcinogenicity may be considered physical carcinogenesis. Infection with the liver fluke *Opisthorchis viverrini* similarly leads to local inflammation and cholangiocarcinoma.

The induction of lung and mesothelial cancers by asbestos fibers and nonfibrous particles such as silica are other examples of foreign body–induced physical carcinogenesis.[71] Animal experiments have demonstrated that the dimensions and durability of the asbestos and other fibrous minerals are the key determinants of their carcinogenicity.[72] Short fibers can be inactivated by phagocytosis, whereas long fibers (>10 μm) are cleared less effectively and are encompassed by proliferating epithelial cells. The long fibers support cell proliferation and have been shown to preferentially induce tumors. Asbestos-associated biologic effects also may be mediated through reactive oxygen and nitrogen species. Furthermore, an interaction occurs between asbestos and silica and components of cigarette smoke. Polycyclic aromatic hydrocarbons (PAHs) in cigarette smoke are metabolized by epithelial cells and form DNA adducts. If PAH is coated on asbestos, PAH uptake is increased.[71] Both PAH and asbestos impair lung clearance, potentially increasing uptake further. Therefore, physical carcinogens may be synergistic with chemical carcinogens.

Radiation is the best-known agent of physical carcinogenesis and is classified as ionizing radiation (x-rays, gamma rays, and alpha and beta particles) or nonionizing radiation (UV). The carcinogenic potential of ionizing radiation was recognized soon after Wilhelm Conrad Roentgen's discovery of x-rays in 1895. Within the next 20 years, a large number of radiation-related skin cancers were reported. Long-term follow-up of survivors of the atomic bombing of Hiroshima and Nagasaki revealed that virtually all tissues exposed to radiation are at risk for cancer.

Radiation can induce a spectrum of DNA lesions that includes damage to the nucleotide bases and cross-linking, and DNA single- and double-strand breaks (DSBs). Misrepaired DSBs are the principal lesions of importance in the induction of chromosomal abnormalities and gene mutations. DSBs in irradiated cells are repaired primarily by a nonhomologous end-joining process, which is error prone; thus DSBs facilitate the production of chromosomal rearrangements and other large-scale changes such as chromosomal deletions. It is thought that radiation may initiate cancer by inactivating tumor-suppressor genes. Activation of oncogenes appears to play a lesser role in radiation carcinogenesis.

Although it has been assumed that the initial genetic events induced by radiation constitute direct mutagenesis from radiation, other indirect effects may contribute to carcinogenesis. For example, radiation induces genomic instability in cells that persists for at least 30 generations after irradiation. Therefore, even if cells do not acquire mutations at initial irradiation, they remain at risk for developing new mutations for several generations. Moreover, even cells that have not been directly irradiated appear to be at risk, a phenomenon referred to as the *bystander effect*.

Nonionizing UV radiation is a potent DNA-damaging agent and is known to induce skin cancer in experimental animals. Most nonmelanoma human skin cancers are thought to be induced by repeated exposure to sunlight, which leads to a series of mutations that allow the cells to escape normal growth control. Patients with inherited xeroderma pigmentosum lack one or more DNA repair pathways, which confers susceptibility to UV-induced cancers, especially on sun-exposed body parts. Patients with ataxia telangiectasia mutated syndrome also have a radiation-sensitive phenotype.

Viral Carcinogens

One of the first observations that cancer may be caused by transmissible agents was by Peyton Rous in 1910 when he demonstrated that cell-free extracts from sarcomas in chickens could transmit sarcomas to other animals injected with these extracts.[73] This was subsequently discovered to represent viral transmission of cancer by the Rous sarcoma virus. At present, several human viruses are known to have oncogenic properties, and several have been causally linked to human cancers (Table 10-7).[74] It is estimated that 15% of all human tumors worldwide are caused by viruses.[75]

Viruses may cause or increase the risk of malignancy through several mechanisms, including direct transformation, expression of oncogenes that interfere with cell-cycle checkpoints or DNA repair, expression of cytokines or other growth factors, and alteration of the immune system. Oncogenic viruses may be RNA or DNA viruses. Oncogenic RNA viruses are retroviruses and contain a reverse transcriptase. After the viral infection, the single-stranded RNA viral genome is transcribed into a double-stranded DNA copy, which is then integrated into the chromosomal DNA of the cell. Retroviral infection of the cell is permanent; thus integrated DNA sequences remain in the host chromosome. Oncogenic transforming retroviruses carry oncogenes derived from cellular genes. These cellular genes, referred to as *proto-oncogenes,* usually are involved in mitogenic signaling and growth control, and include protein kinases, G proteins, growth factors, and transcription factors (Table 10-8).[75]

Integration of the provirus upstream of a proto-oncogene may produce chimeric virus-cell transcripts and recombination during the next round of replication that could lead to incorporation of the cellular gene into the viral genome.[75] On the other hand, many retroviruses do not possess oncogenes but can cause tumors in animals regardless. This occurs by integration of the provirus near a normal cellular proto-oncogene and activation of the expression of these genes by the strong promoter and enhancer sequences in the integrated viral sequence.

Unlike the oncogenes of the RNA viruses, those of the DNA tumor viruses are viral, not cellular, in origin. These genes are required for viral replication using the host cell machinery. In permissive hosts, infection with an oncogenic DNA virus may result in a productive lytic infection, which leads to cell death and the release of newly formed viruses. In nonpermissive cells, the viral DNA can be integrated into the cellular chromosomal DNA, and some of the early viral genes can be synthesized persistently, which leads to transformation of cells to a neoplastic state. The binding of viral oncoproteins to cellular tumor-suppressor proteins p53 and Rb is fundamental to the carcinogenesis induced by most DNA viruses, although some target different cellular proteins.

Like other types of carcinogenesis, viral carcinogenesis is a multistep process. Some retroviruses contain two cellular oncogenes, rather than one, in their genome and are more rapidly tumorigenic than single-gene transforming retroviruses, which emphasizes the cooperation between transforming genes. Furthermore, some viruses encode genes that suppress or delay apoptosis.

TABLE 10-7	Selected viral carcinogens[a]
Virus	**Predominant Tumor Type[b]**
Epstein-Barr virus	Burkitt's lymphoma
	Hodgkin's disease
	Immunosuppression-related lymphoma
	Sinonasal angiocentric T-cell lymphoma
	Nasopharyngeal carcinoma
Hepatitis B virus	Hepatocellular carcinoma
Hepatitis C virus	Hepatocellular carcinoma
HIV type 1	Kaposi's sarcoma
	Non-Hodgkin's lymphoma
Human papillomavirus 16 and 18	Cervical cancer
	Anal cancer
Human T-cell lymphotropic viruses	Adult T-cell leukemia/lymphoma

[a]Based on information in the International Agency for Research on Cancer monographs.[74]
[b]Only tumor types for which causal relationships are established are listed. Other cancer types may be linked to the agents with a lower frequency or with insufficient data to prove causality.

TABLE 10-8 Cellular oncogenes in retroviruses

Oncogene	Virus Name	Origin	Protein Product
abl	Abelson murine leukemia virus	Mouse	Tyrosine kinase
fes	ST feline sarcoma virus	Cat	Tyrosine kinase
fps	Fujinami sarcoma virus	Chicken	Tyrosine kinase
src	Rous sarcoma virus	Chicken	Tyrosine kinase
erbB	Avian erythroblastosis virus	Chicken	Epidermal growth factor receptor
fms	McDonough feline sarcoma virus	Cat	Colony-stimulating factor receptor
kit	Hardy-Zuckerman 4 feline sarcoma virus	Cat	Stem cell factor receptor
mil	Avian myelocytoma virus	Chicken	Serine/threonine kinase
mos	Moloney murine sarcoma virus	Mouse	Serine/threonine kinase
raf	Murine sarcoma virus 3611	Mouse	Serine/threonine kinase
sis	Simian sarcoma virus	Monkey	Platelet-derived growth factor
H-ras	Harvey murine sarcoma virus	Rat	GDP/GTP binding
K-ras	Kirsten murine sarcoma virus	Rat	GDP/GTP binding
erbA	Avian erythroblastosis virus	Chicken	Transcription factor (thyroid hormone receptor)
ets	Avian myeloblastosis virus E26	Chicken	Transcription factor
fos	FBJ osteosarcoma virus	Mouse	Transcription factor (AP1 component)
jun	Avian sarcoma virus 17	Chicken	Transcription factor (AP1 component)
myb	Avian myeloblastosis virus	Chicken	Transcription factor
myc	MC29 myelocytoma virus	Chicken	Transcription factor (NF-κB family)

AP1 = activator protein 1; FBJ = Finkel-Biskis-Jinkins; GDP = guanosine diphosphate; GTP = guanosine triphosphate; NF-κB = nuclear factor κB.
Source: Modified with permission from Butel JS: Viral carcinogenesis: revelation of molecular mechanisms and etiology of human disease. *Carcinogenesis* 21:405, 2000. By permission of Oxford University Press.

Although immunocompromised individuals are at elevated risk, most patients infected with oncogenic viruses do not develop cancer. When cancer does develop, it usually occurs several years after the viral infection. It is estimated, for example, that the risk of hepatocellular carcinoma (HCC) among individuals infected with hepatitis C virus is 1 to 3% after 30 years.[76] There may be synergy between various environmental factors and viruses in carcinogenesis.

Recognition of a viral origin for some tumors has lead to the pursuit of vaccination as a preventive strategy. The use of childhood hepatitis B vaccination has already translated into a decrease in liver cancer incidence in the Far East.[3] Recently, vaccines against human papillomavirus have shown very promising results in preventing the development of cervical intraepithelial neoplasia and are now being pursued for primary prevention of cervical carcinoma.[77]

CANCER RISK ASSESSMENT

Cancer risk assessment is an important part of the initial evaluation of any patient. A patient's cancer risk not only is an important determinant of cancer screening recommendations but also may alter how aggressively an indeterminant finding will be pursued for diagnosis. A "probably benign" mammographic lesion, for example, defined as one with <2% probability of malignancy (American College of Radiology category III) is usually managed with a 6-month follow-up mammogram in a patient at baseline cancer risk, but obtaining a tissue diagnosis may be preferable in a patient at high risk for breast cancer.[78]

Cancer risk assessment starts with taking a complete history that includes history of environmental exposures to potential carcinogens and a detailed family history. Risk assessment for breast cancer, for example, includes obtaining a family history to determine whether another member of the family is known to carry a breast cancer susceptibility gene; whether there is familial clustering of breast cancer, ovarian cancer, thyroid cancer, sarcoma, adrenocortical carcinoma, endometrial cancer, brain tumors, dermatologic manifestations, leukemia, or lymphoma; and whether the patient is from a population at increased risk, such as individuals of Ashkenazi Jewish descent. Patients who have a family history suggestive of a cancer susceptibility syndrome such as hereditary breast-ovarian syndrome, LFS, or CD would benefit from genetic counseling and possibly genetic testing.

Patients who do not seem to have a strong hereditary component of risk can be evaluated on the basis of their age, race, personal history, and exposures. One of the most commonly used models for risk assessment in breast cancer is the Gail model.[79] Gail and colleagues analyzed the data from 2852 breast cancer cases and 3146 controls from the Breast Cancer Detection and Demonstration Project, a mammography screening project conducted in the 1970s, and developed a model for projecting breast cancer incidence. The model uses risk factors such as an individual's age, age at menarche, age at first live birth, number of first-degree relatives with breast cancer, number of previous breast biopsies, and whether the biopsy results revealed atypical ductal hyperplasia (Table 10-9).[79] This model has led to the development of a breast cancer risk assessment tool, which is available on the World Wide Web.[80] This tool incorporates the risk factors used in the Gail model, as well as race and ethnicity, and allows a health professional to project a woman's individualized estimated risk for invasive breast cancer over a 5-year period and over her lifetime (to age 90 years). Notably, these risk projections assume that the woman is undergoing regular clinical breast examinations and screening mammograms. Also of note is that this program underestimates the risk for women who have already had a diagnosis of invasive or noninvasive breast cancer and does not take into account specific genetic predispositions such as mutations in *BRCA1* or *BRCA2*. However, risk assessment tools such as this have been validated and are now in widespread clinical use. Similar models are in development or are being validated for other cancers. For example, a lung cancer risk prediction model, which includes age, sex, asbestos exposure history, and smoking history, has been found to predict risk of lung cancer.[81]

CANCER SCREENING

Early detection is the key to success in cancer therapy. Screening for common cancers using relatively noninvasive tests is expected to lead to early diagnosis, allow more conservative surgical therapies with decreased morbidity, and potentially improve surgical cure rates and overall survival rates. Key factors that influence screening guidelines are how prevalent the cancer is in the population, what risk is associated with the screening measure, and whether early diagnosis actually affects outcome. The value of a widespread screening measure is likely to go up with the prevalence of the cancer in a

TABLE 10-9 Assessment of risk for invasive breast cancer

Risk Factor	Relative Risk (%)
Age at menarche (years)	
>14	1.00
12–13	1.10
<12	1.21
Age at first live birth (years)	
Patients with no first-degree relatives with cancer	
<20	1.00
20–24	1.24
25–29 or nulliparous	1.55
≥30	1.93
Patients with one first degree-relative with cancer	
<20	1.00
20–24	2.64
25–29 or nulliparous	2.76
≥30	2.83
Patients with ≥2 first-degree relatives with cancer	
<20	6.80
20–24	5.78
25–29 or nulliparous	4.91
≥30	4.17
Breast biopsies (number)	
Patients aged <50 y at counseling	
0	1.00
1	1.70
≥2	2.88
Patients aged ≥50 y at counseling	
0	1.00
1	1.27
≥2	1.62
Atypical hyperplasia	
No biopsies	1.00
At least 1 biopsy, no atypical hyperplasia	0.93
No atypical hyperplasia, hyperplasia status unknown for at least 1 biopsy	1.00
Atypical hyperplasia in at least 1 biopsy	1.82

Source: Modified with permission from Gail MH et al: Projecting individualized probabilities of developing breast cancer for white females who are being examined annually. *J Natl Cancer Inst* 81:1879, 1989. By permission of Oxford University Press.

population, which often determines the age cutoffs for screening and explains why screening is done only for common cancers. The risks associated with the screening measure are a significant consideration, especially with more invasive screening measures such as colonoscopy. The consequences of a false-positive screening test result also need to be considered. For example, when 1000 screening mammograms are taken, only 2 to 4 new cases of cancer will be identified; this number is slightly higher (6 to 10 prevalent cancers per 1000 mammograms) for initial screening mammograms.[82] However, as many as 10% of screening mammograms may be potentially suggestive of an abnormality, which requires further imaging (i.e., a 10% recall rate). Of those women with abnormal mammogram findings, only 5 to 10% will be determined to have a breast cancer. Among women for whom biopsy is recommended, 25 to 40% will have a breast cancer. A false-positive screening result is likely to induce significant emotional distress in patients, leads to unnecessary biopsies, and has cost implications for the health care system.

The 2009 American Cancer Society guidelines for the early detection of cancer are listed in Table 10-10.[83] These guidelines are updated periodically to incorporate emerging technologies and new data on the efficacy of screening measures. Besides the American Cancer Society, several other professional bodies make recommendations for screening. Although the screening guidelines differ somewhat, most organizations do not emphasize one screening strategy as superior to another, but all emphasize the importance of age-appropriate screening.

Screening guidelines are developed for the general baseline-risk population. These guidelines need to be modified for patients who are at high risk. For example, more intensive colorectal cancer screening is recommended for individuals at increased risk because of a history of adenomatous polyps, a personal history of colorectal cancer, a family history of either colorectal cancer or colorectal adenomas diagnosed in a first-degree relative before age 60 years, a personal history of inflammatory bowel disease of significant duration, or a family history or genetic test result indicating FAP or HNPCC. For some diseases, in higher risk populations, both the screening modality and the screening intensity may be altered. For example, breast magnetic resonance imaging is recommended as an adjunct to mammography for breast cancer screening in BRCA mutation carriers, first-degree relatives of carriers, and women with a lifetime breast cancer risk of 20 to 25% or higher.[84]

CANCER DIAGNOSIS

The definitive diagnosis of solid tumors usually is obtained by performing a biopsy of the lesion. Biopsy findings determine the tumor histology and grade and thus assist in definitive therapeutic planning. When a biopsy has been performed at an outside institution, the slides should be reviewed to confirm the outside diagnosis.

Biopsy specimens of mucosal lesions usually are obtained endoscopically (e.g., via colonoscope, bronchoscope, or cystoscope). Lesions that are easily palpable, such as those of the skin, can either be excised or sampled by punch biopsy. Deep-seated lesions can be localized with computed tomographic (CT) scan or ultrasound guidance for biopsy.

A sample of a lesion can be obtained with a needle or with an open incisional or excisional biopsy. Fine-needle aspiration is easy and relatively safe, but has the disadvantage of not giving information on tissue architecture. For example, fine-needle aspiration biopsy of a breast mass can make the diagnosis of malignancy but cannot differentiate between an invasive and noninvasive tumor. Therefore core-needle biopsy is more advantageous when the histologic findings will affect the recommended therapy. Core biopsy, like fine-needle aspiration, is relatively safe and can be performed either by direct palpation (e.g., a breast mass or a soft tissue mass) or can be guided by an imaging study (e.g., stereotactic core biopsy of the breast). Core biopsies, like fine-needle aspirations, have the disadvantage of introducing sampling error. For example, 19 to 44% of patients with a diagnosis of atypical ductal hyperplasia based on core biopsy findings of a mammographic abnormality are found to have carcinoma upon excision of the lesion.[85] It is crucial to ensure that the histologic findings are consistent with the clinical scenario and to know the appropriate interpretation of each histologic finding. A needle biopsy for which the report is inconsistent with the clinical scenario should be either repeated or followed by an open biopsy.

Open biopsies have the advantage of providing more tissue for histologic evaluation and the disadvantage of being an operative procedure. Incisional biopsies are reserved for very large lesions in which a definitive diagnosis cannot be made by needle biopsy. Excisional biopsies are performed for lesions for which either core biopsy is not possible or the results are nondiagnostic. Excisional biopsies should be performed with curative intent, that is, by obtaining adequate tissue around the lesion to ensure negative surgical margins. Marking of the orientation of the margins by sutures or clips by the surgeon and inking of the specimen margins by the pathologist will allow for determination of the surgical margins and will guide surgical re-excision if one or more of the margins are positive for microscopic tumor or are close. The biopsy incision should be oriented to allow for excision of the biopsy scar if repeat operation is necessary. Furthermore, the biopsy incision should directly overlie the area to be removed rather than tunneling from another site, which runs the risk of contaminating a larger field. Finally, meticulous hemostasis during a biopsy is essential, because a hematoma can lead to contamination of the tissue planes

TABLE 10-10 American Cancer Society recommendations for early detection of cancer in average-risk, asymptomatic individuals

Cancer Site	Population	Test or Procedure	Frequency
Breast	Women aged ≥20 y	Breast self-examination	Monthly, starting at age 20
		Clinical breast examination	Every 3 y, ages 20–39
			Annual, starting at age 40
		Mammography	Annual, starting at age 40
Colorectal	Men and women aged ≥50 y	Fecal occult blood test (FOBT) or fecal immunochemical test (FIT)	Annual, starting at age 50
		or	
		Flexible sigmoidoscopy	Every 5 y, starting at age 50
		or	
		FOBT and flexible sigmoidoscopy	Annual FOBT (or FIT) and flexible sigmoidoscopy every 5 y, starting at age 50
		or	
		Double-contrast barium enema (DCBE)	DCBE every 5 y, starting at age 50
		or	
		Colonoscopy	Colonoscopy every 10 y, starting at age 50
Prostate	Men aged ≥50 y	Digital rectal examination (DRE) and prostate-specific antigen (PSA) test	Offer PSA test and DRE annually, starting at age 50, for men who have life expectancy of at least 10 y
Cervix	Women aged ≥18 y	Pap test	Cervical cancer screening beginning 3 y after first vaginal intercourse, but no later than age 21 y; screening every year with conventional Pap tests or every 2 y using liquid-based Pap tests; at or after age 30 y, women who have had three normal test results in a row may get screened every 2 to 3 y with cervical cytologic analysis alone or every 3 y with a human papillomavirus DNA test plus cervical cytologic analysis.
Endometrial	Women at menopause	—	At the time of menopause, women at average risk should be informed about the risks and symptoms of endometrial cancer and strongly encouraged to report any unexpected bleeding or spotting to their physicians.
Cancer-related checkup	Men and women aged ≥20 y	On the occasion of a periodic health examination, the cancer-related checkup should include examination of the thyroid, testicles, ovaries, lymph nodes, oral cavity, and skin, as well as health counseling about tobacco use, sun exposure, diet and nutrition, risk factors, sexual practices, and environmental and occupational exposures.	

Source: Modified with permission from Smith et al.[83]

and can make subsequent follow-up with physical examinations much more challenging.

CANCER STAGING

Cancer staging is a system used to describe the anatomic extent of a malignant process in an individual patient. Staging systems may incorporate relevant clinical prognostic factors such as tumor size, location, extent, grade, and dissemination to regional lymph nodes or distant sites. Accurate staging is essential in designing an appropriate treatment regimen for an individual patient. Staging of the lymph node basin is considered a standard part of primary surgical therapy for most surgical procedures and is discussed later in this chapter. Cancer patients who are considered to be at high risk for distant metastasis usually undergo a preoperative staging work-up. This involves a set of imaging studies of sites of preferential metastasis for a given cancer type. For example, for a patient with breast cancer, a staging work-up would include a chest radiograph, bone scan, and liver ultrasound or CT scan of the abdomen to evaluate for lung, bone, and liver metastases, respectively. A distant staging work-up usually is performed only for patients likely to have metastasis based on the characteristics of the primary tumor; for example, a staging work-up for a patient with ductal carcinoma in situ of the breast or a small invasive breast tumor is likely to be low yield and not cost effective.

Recently there also is interest in using molecular imaging with positron emission tomography (PET) scanning, or PET/CT, for cancer staging. Most commonly PET scanning is performed with fluorine 18 incorporated into fluorodeoxyglucose (FDG). FDG PET assesses the rate of glycolysis. FDG uptake is increased in most malignant tissues but also in benign pathologic conditions such as inflammatory disorders, trauma, infection, and granulomatous disease. It may be especially useful in the staging and management of lymphoma, lung cancer, and colorectal cancer. The role of PET in evaluating many other cancers is evolving, and additional molecular tracers, such as 3'-deoxy-3'-^{18}F-fluorothymidine, used to assess proliferation, are being actively pursued.

Standardization of staging systems is essential to allow comparison of results from different studies from different institutions and worldwide. The staging systems proposed by the American Joint Committee on Cancer (AJCC) and the Union Internationale Contre le Cancer (International Union Against Cancer, or UICC) are among the most widely accepted staging systems. Both the AJCC and the UICC have adopted a shared tumor, node, and metastasis (TNM) staging system that defines the cancer in terms of the anatomic extent of disease and is based on assessment of three components: the size of the primary tumor (T), the presence (or absence) and extent of nodal metastases (N), and the presence (or absence) and extent of distant metastases (M).

The TNM staging applies only to tumors that have been microscopically confirmed to be malignant. Standard TNM staging (clinical and pathologic) is completed at initial diagnosis. Clinical staging (cTNM or TNM) is based on information gained up until the initial definitive treatment. Pathologic staging (pTNM) includes clinical information and information obtained from pathologic examination of the resected primary tumor and regional lymph nodes. Other classifications, such as retreatment staging (rTNM) or autopsy staging (aTNM), should be clearly identified as such.

The clinical measurement of tumor size (T) is the one judged to be the most accurate for each individual case based on physical examination and imaging studies. For example, in breast cancer the size of the tumor could be obtained from a physical examination, mammogram, or ultrasound, and the tumor size is based only on the invasive component.

If even one lymph node is involved by tumor, the N component is at least N1. For many solid tumor types, simply the absence or presence of lymph node involvement is recorded, and the tumor is categorized either as N0 or N1. For other tumor types, the number of lymph nodes involved, the size of the lymph nodes or the lymph node metastasis, or the regional lymph node basin involved also has been shown to have prognostic value. In these cancers, the designations N1, N2, N3, and N4 suggest an increasing abnormality of lymph nodes based on size, characteristics, and location. NX indicates that the lymph nodes cannot be fully assessed.

Cases in which there is no distant metastasis are designated M0, cases in which one or more distant metastases are detected are designated M1, and cases in which the presence of distant metastasis cannot be assessed are designated MX. In clinical practice, negative findings on clinical history and examination are sufficient to designate a case as M0. However, in clinical trials, routine follow-up staging work-ups often are performed to standardize the detection of distant metastases.

The practice of dividing cancer cases into groups according to stage is based on the observation that the survival rates are higher for localized (lower-stage) tumors than for tumors that have extended beyond the organ of origin. Therefore, staging assists in selection of therapy, estimation of prognosis, evaluation of treatments, and exchange of information among treatment centers. Notably, the AJCC regularly updates its staging system to incorporate advances in prognostic technology to improve the predictive accuracy of the TNM system. Therefore it is important to know which revision of a staging system is being used when evaluating studies.

TUMOR MARKERS

Prognostic and Predictive Tissue Markers

Tumor markers are substances that can be detected in higher than normal amounts in the serum, urine, or tissues of patients with certain types of cancer. Tumors markers are produced either by the cancer cells themselves or by the body in a response to the cancer.

Over the past decade, there has been an especially high interest in identifying tissue tumor markers that can be used as prognostic or predictive markers. Although the terms *prognostic marker* and *predictive marker* are sometimes used interchangeably, the term *prognostic marker* generally is used to describe molecular markers that predict disease-free survival, disease-specific survival, and overall survival, whereas the term *predictive marker* often is used in the context of predicting response to certain therapies.

The goal is to identify prognostic markers that can give information on prognosis independent of other clinical characteristics and therefore can provide information to supplement the projections based on clinical presentation. This would allow practitioners to further classify patients as being at higher or lower risk within clinical subgroups and to identify patients who may benefit most from adjuvant therapy. For example, ideal prognostic tumor markers would be able to help determine which patients with node-negative breast cancer are at higher risk

of relapse so that adjuvant systemic therapy could be given only to that group. However, although a large number of studies have identified potential novel prognostic markers, most have not been tested with enough vigor to be shown to be of clinical utility. In the 2007 American Society of Clinical Oncology (ASCO) guidelines, it was decided that level of uPA/PAI-1 measured by enzyme-linked immunosorbent assay could be used to determine prognosis in cases of newly diagnosed node-negative breast cancer.[86] In contrast, the data for many other markers, including DNA content, proportion of tumor cells in S phase, Ki-67, cyclin E, p27, p21, thymidine kinase, topoisomerase II, HER2, p53, and cathepsin D, were felt to be insufficient to support their use in the management of breast cancer patients.[86] Similarly, in the 2006 ASCO GI tumor guidelines, the data were felt to be insufficient to recommend the routine use of p53, *ras*, thymidine synthase, dihydropyrimidine dehydrogenase, thymidine phosphorylase, microsatellite instability, 18q loss of heterozygosity, or deleted-in-colon-cancer protein in the management of patients with colorectal cancer.[87]

Predictive markers are markers that can prospectively identify patients who will benefit from a certain therapy. For example in breast cancer, estrogen receptor (ER) and HER2 assessment can identify patients who can benefit from antiestrogen therapies (e.g., tamoxifen) and anti-HER2 targeted therapies (e.g., trastuzumab), respectively, and the 2007 ASCO guidelines recommend that these markers be routinely assessed.[86] High-throughput techniques such as transcriptional profiling allow for assessment of the relative mRNA levels of thousands of genes simultaneously in a given tumor using microarray technology. With the advent of such molecular profiling technologies, researchers have focused on identifying expression profiles that are prognostic for different cancer types. For breast cancer, although many such multiparameter tests are under development, few have reached the large-scale validation stage (Table 10-11).[88] In 2007, ASCO guidelines suggested that one of these, the Onco*type* DX assay, can be used to predict recurrence in women with node-negative, ER-positive breast cancer who are treated with tamoxifen.[86] Onco*type* DX is a quantitative reverse-transcriptase polymerase chain reaction (RT-PCR) test that used paraffin-fixed tissue. A 21-gene recurrence score (RS) is generated based on the expression of 16 cancer genes and 5 reference genes. The levels of expression are used to derive an RS that ranges from 0 to 100, using a prospectively defined mathematical algorithm. This novel quantitative approach to the evaluation of the best-known molecular pathways in breast cancer has produced impressive results. Use of this multigene assay to predict recurrence was validated in the National Surgical Adjuvant Breast and Bowel Project (NSABP) B-14 trial, in which ER-positive, node-negative patients had received tamoxifen. Of the 2617 patients on the trial who had received tamoxifen, paraffin block tumor tissue samples were available for 675 of them and RT-PCR was successfully completed for 668.[89] By multivariate Cox proportional analysis, RS was found to be independently associated with recurrence risk, with a hazard ratio of 3.21 (95% confidence interval of 2.23 to 4.65, *P* <.001). The RS was indeed able to stratify patients by freedom from distant recurrence (Figs. 10-9, 10-10).[89] The ongoing Trial Assessing Individualized Options for Treatment for breast cancer (TAILORx) is

TABLE 10-11	Sensitivity and specificity of some common tumor markers		
Marker	**Cancer**	**Sensitivity (%)**	**Specificity (%)**
Prostate-specific antigen (4 μg/L)	Prostate	57–93	55–68
Carcinoembryonic antigen	Colorectal	40–47	90
	Breast	45	81
	Recurrent disease	84	100
Alpha-fetoprotein	Hepatocellular	98	65
Cancer antigen 19-9	Pancreatic	78–90	95
Cancer antigen 27-29	Breast	62	83
Cancer antigen 15-3	Breast	57	87

Source: Adapted with permission from Way et al.[88]

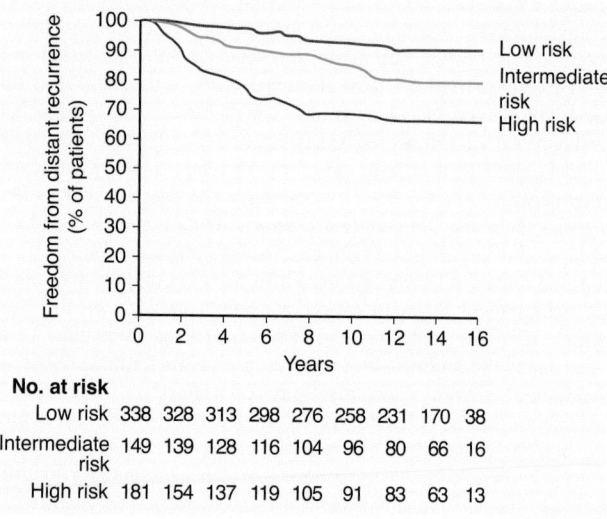

FIG. 10-9. Likelihood of distant recurrence, according to recurrence score categories. Freedom from distant recurrence according to risk group, based on recurrence scores derived from tumor levels of expression of 21 genes. (Modified with permission from Paik et al.[89] Copyright © Massachusetts Medical Society. All rights reserved.)

evaluating the utility of Oncotype DX for predicting prognosis in patients with ER-positive, node-negative tumors and will focus on women with intermediate RS scores in whom the role of chemotherapy is unclear. Several other multigene predictors for breast cancer are under development, including MammaPrint, a gene expression profiling platform assessing a 70-gene transcriptional signature.[90] This assay was approved by the Food and Drug Administration (FDA) in February 2007. The usefulness of this assay in making therapy-related decisions is being tested prospectively in a large-scale study, the Microarray in Node-Negative Disease May Avoid Chemotherapy (MINDACT) trial.

Multigene profiles to predict prognosis are in development or in validation phases for many other solid tumor types, including lung cancer, ovarian cancer, pancreatic cancer, colorectal cancer, and melanoma. Gene signatures and sequence alterations also are being studied for their ability to predict response to specific chemotherapy regimens or targeted therapies. Many of these multigene marker sets will likely be incorporated into clinical practice in the years to come.

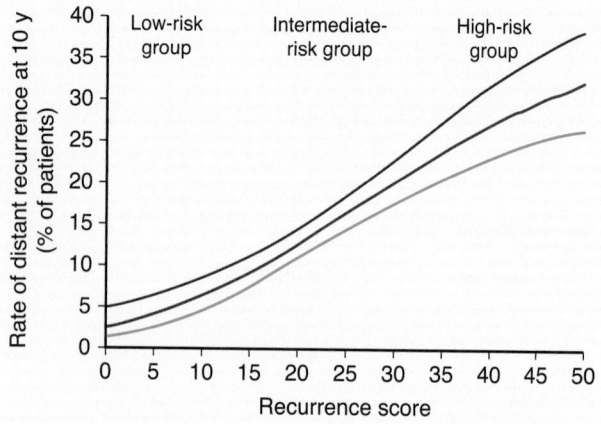

FIG. 10-10. Distant recurrence as a continuous function of the recurrence score derived from tumor levels of expression of 21 genes. (Modified with permission from Paik et al.[89] Copyright © Massachusetts Medical Society. All rights reserved.)

Serum Markers

Serum markers are under active investigation because they may allow early diagnosis of a new cancer or may be used to follow cancer response to therapy or monitor for recurrence. Unfortunately, identification of serum markers of clinical value has been challenging. Many of the tumor markers proposed so far have had low sensitivities and specificities (see Table 10-11).[88] Tumor marker levels may not be elevated in all patients with cancer, especially in the early stages, when a serum marker would be most useful for diagnosis. Therefore when a tumor marker is used to monitor recurrence, it is important to be certain that the level of the tumor marker was elevated before primary therapy. Moreover, tumor marker levels can be elevated in benign conditions. Many tumor markers are not specific for a certain type of cancer and can be elevated with more than one type of tumor. Because there may be significant laboratory variability, it is important to obtain serial results from the same laboratory. In spite of these many clinical limitations, several serum markers are in clinical use. A few of the commonly measured serum tumor markers are discussed in the following sections.

Prostate-Specific Antigen

Prostate-specific antigen (PSA) is potentially the best serum marker now available. PSA is an androgen-regulated serine protease produced by the prostate epithelium. PSA is normally present in low concentrations in the blood of all adult males. PSA levels may be elevated in the blood of men with benign prostate conditions such as prostatitis and benign prostatic hyperplasia, as well as in men with prostate cancer. PSA levels have been shown to be useful in evaluating the effectiveness of prostate cancer treatment and monitoring for recurrence after therapy. In monitoring for recurrence, a trend of increasing levels is considered more significant than a single absolute elevated value.

Although PSA is widely used for prostate cancer screening in the United States, and the American Urologic Association and the American Cancer Society both recommend yearly PSA testing for men aged 50 years and older with a life expectancy of >10 years, the specific level indicating a need to initiate a work-up, the interval at which to measure PSA levels, and the utility of PSA screening all remain controversial.[91] Therefore it is advised that before PSA screening is initiated a discussion take place with the patient about the potential benefits, limitations, and harms associated with testing. Results of a large multicenter study suggested that a total serum PSA level of 4 ng/mL should be used as a threshold for performing a prostate biopsy, but 20 to 50% of clinically significant prostate cancers occur in men with total serum PSA levels of <4 ng/mL.[92] Others have suggested that biennial PSA screening is sufficient to detect almost all prostate cancers while they are curable and that the screening interval can be altered on the basis of PSA level. Finally, although the use of serum PSA screening does lead to earlier prostate cancer detection, it remains to be demonstrated that this translates into a survival benefit. The efficacy of PSA as a screening tool is being evaluated in randomized controlled trials, and it is hoped that these will answer this question.

Carcinoembryonic Antigen

Carcinoembryonic antigen (CEA) is a glycoprotein found in the embryonic endodermal epithelium. Elevated CEA levels have been detected in patients with primary colorectal cancer as well as in patients with breast, lung, ovarian, prostate, liver, and pancreatic cancer. Levels of CEA also may be elevated in benign conditions such as diverticulitis, peptic ulcer disease, bronchitis, liver abscess, and alcoholic cirrhosis, especially in smokers and in elderly persons.

CEA measurement is most commonly used in the management of colorectal cancer. However, the appropriate use of CEA testing in patients with colorectal cancer has been debated. Use of CEA level as a screening test for colorectal cancer is not recommended. CEA levels may be useful if obtained preoperatively and postoperatively in patients with a diagnosis of colorectal cancer. Preoperative elevation of CEA level is an indicator of poor prognosis. However, the 2007 ASCO clinical practice guidelines state that the data are insufficient to support the use of CEA to determine whether to give a patient adjuvant therapy; the data are stronger for the use of CEA for monitoring for postoperative recurrence.[86] CEA measurement is the most cost-effective approach for detecting metastasis, with 64% of recurrences being detected first by an elevation in CEA level. Therefore, in cases in which the patient would be a candidate for resection of recurrent colorectal cancer or systemic therapy, the 2006 ASCO guidelines recommend that postoperative CEA testing be performed every 3 months in patients with stage II or III disease for at least 3 years.[87] CEA is the marker of choice for monitoring metastatic colorectal cancer during systemic therapy.[87]

There is also interest in using CEA levels for monitoring patients with breast cancer. However, the 2007 ASCO guidelines state that the routine use of CEA for screening, diagnosis, staging, or surveillance of breast cancer is not recommended because available data are insufficient.[86] For monitoring patients during active therapy, CEA can be used in conjunction with diagnostic imaging and history and physical examination.[86] In the absence of measurable disease, an increase in CEA level may be taken to indicate treatment failure. However, caution is advised when interpreting rising levels in the first 4 to 6 weeks of therapy.[86]

Alpha-Fetoprotein

Alpha-fetoprotein (AFP) is a glycoprotein normally produced by a developing fetus. AFP levels decrease soon after birth in healthy adults. An elevated level of AFP suggests the presence of either primary liver cancer or a germ cell tumor of the ovary or testicle. Rarely, other types of cancer such as gastric cancer are associated with an elevated AFP level. Benign conditions that can cause elevations of AFP include cirrhosis, hepatic necrosis, acute hepatitis, chronic active hepatitis, ataxia-telangiectasia, Wiskott-Aldrich syndrome, and pregnancy.[93]

The sensitivity of an elevated AFP level for detecting HCC is approximately 60%. AFP is considered to be sensitive and specific enough to be used for screening for HCC in high-risk populations. Current consensus recommendations are to screen healthy hepatitis B virus carriers with annual or semiannual measurement of AFP level and to screen carriers with cirrhosis or chronic hepatitis and patients with cirrhosis of any etiology with twice-yearly measurement of AFP level and liver ultrasonography.[94] Although AFP testing has been used widely for a long time, its efficacy in early diagnosis of HCC is limited. With improvements in imaging technology, a larger proportion of patients diagnosed with HCC are now AFP seronegative.

Cancer Antigen 19-9

Cancer antigen 19-9 (CA 19-9) is a tumor-related antigen that was originally defined by a monoclonal antibody produced by a hybridoma prepared from murine spleen cells immunized with a human colorectal cancer cell line.[87] The data are insufficient to recommend use of CA 19-9 for screening, diagnosis, surveillance, or monitoring of therapy for colon cancer.[87] Based on the 2006 ASCO guidelines, there are also insufficient data to recommend use of CA 19-9 for screening, diagnosis, or determination of the operability of pancreatic cancer.[87] However, for patients with locally advanced or metastatic cancer receiving active therapy, CA 19-9 can be measured at the start of therapy and every 1 to 3 months while therapy is given; elevations in serial CA 19-9 levels may indicate progressive disease and should be confirmed by additional studies.[87]

Cancer Antigen 15-3

Cancer antigen 15-3 (CA 15-3) is an epitope of a large membrane glycoprotein encoded by the *MUC1* gene that tumor cells shed into the bloodstream. The CA 15-3 epitope is recognized by two monoclonal antibodies in a sandwich radioimmunoassay. CA 15-3 levels are most useful in following the course of treatment in women diagnosed with advanced breast cancer. CA 15-3 levels are infrequently elevated in early breast cancer. CA 15-3 levels can be increased in benign conditions such as chronic hepatitis, tuberculosis, sarcoidosis, pelvic inflammatory disease, endometriosis, systemic lupus erythematosus, pregnancy, and lactation, and in other types of cancer such as lung, ovarian, endometrial, and GI cancers.

The sensitivity of CA 15-3 is higher for metastatic disease, and in these cases studies have shown sensitivity to be between 54 and 87%, with specificity as high as 96%. This has led to interest in using CA 15-3 for monitoring patients with advanced breast cancer for recurrence. Elevated CA 15-3 levels have been reported before relapse in 54% of patients, with a lead time of 4.2 months. Therefore, detection of elevated CA 15-3 levels during follow-up should prompt evaluation for recurrent disease. However, 6 to 8% of patients without recurrence will have elevated CA 15-3 levels that require evaluation. Moreover, monitoring with the use of CA 15-3 levels has shown no demonstrated impact on survival. Therefore, the 2007 ASCO guidelines state that the routine use of CA 15-3 for screening, diagnosis, staging, or surveillance of breast cancer is not recommended because available data are insufficient.[86] For monitoring patients during active therapy, CA 15-3 can be used in conjunction with diagnostic imaging and history and physical examination.[86] In the absence of measurable disease, an increase may be interpreted to indicate treatment failure. However, caution is advised when interpreting rising levels in the first 4 to 6 weeks of therapy.[86]

Cancer Antigen 27-29

The MUC-1 gene product in the serum may be quantitated by using radioimmunoassay with a monoclonal antibody against the cancer antigen 27-29 (CA 27-29). CA 27-29 levels can be elevated in breast cancer as well as in cancers of the colon, stomach, kidney, lung, ovary, pancreas, uterus, and liver. First-trimester pregnancy, endometriosis, benign breast disease, kidney disease, and liver disease also may be associated with elevated CA 27-29 levels.

CA 27-29 has been reported to have a sensitivity of 57%, a specificity of 98%, a positive predictive value of 83%, and a negative predictive value of 93% in detecting breast cancer recurrences.[95] Although CA 27-29 has been found to predict recurrence an average of 5.3 months before other symptoms or tests, testing of CA 27-29 levels has not been demonstrated to affect disease-free and overall survival rates.[95,96] Therefore, the 2007 ASCO guidelines state that, as with CA 15-3, the routine use of CA 27-29 for screening, diagnosis, staging, or surveillance of breast cancer is not recommended because available data are insufficient.[86] CA 27-29 levels can be used together with diagnostic imaging and history and physical examination to monitor patients during active therapy.[86] When no measurable disease is present, an increase in level may be considered to indicate treatment failure. However, rising levels in the first 4 to 6 weeks of therapy should be interpreted with caution.[86]

Circulating Tumor Cells

Circulating tumor cells (CTCs) are cells present in the blood that possess antigenic or genetic characteristics of a specific tumor type.[86] One CTC detection methodology is capture and quantitation of CTCs with immunomagnetic beads coated with antibody specific for cell-surface, epithelial, or cancer antigens. Another methodology used to detect cancer cells in the peripheral blood is RT-PCR. It has been suggested that measurement of CTCs can be an effective tool for selecting patients who have a high risk of relapse and for monitoring efficacy of cancer therapy.

CTCs have probably been most extensively studied in breast cancer, with over 400 publications to date.[86] The most promising data come from the use of CTC measures in metastatic breast cancer. In a prospective multicenter trial, the number of CTCs (≥5 CTCs vs. <5 CTCs per 7.5 mL of whole blood) before treatment of metastatic breast cancer was an independent predictor of progression-free and overall survival rates.[97] The presence of >5 CTCs after the first course of therapy predicted lack of response to treatment. This technology, known as *CellSearch,* has been approved by the FDA for clinical use. However, there are no data to prove that the use of CTC testing leads to improved survival or improved quality of life; thus the ASCO 2007 guideline update does not recommend the use of CTC measurement in any clinical setting.[86] The clinical utility of measuring CTC response to initial therapy is now being tested prospectively in a multicenter clinical trial. The use of CTC levels as a tool in treating many other types of tumor is also under active investigation, again with no level I evidence for clinical utility.

The prognostic implications of detection of CTCs by RT-PCR have been intensively studied for melanoma. In the recent multicenter Sunbelt Melanoma Trial, serial RT-PCR was performed on peripheral blood samples using four markers—tyrosinase, melanoma antigen reacting to T cell (MART-1), melanoma antigen 3 (MAGE3), and gp 100—to detect occult melanoma cells in the bloodstream.[98] Although there were no differences in survival between patients in whom at least one marker was detected and those in whom no markers were detected, the disease-free survival and distant disease-free survival were worse for patients in whom more than one marker was detected at any time during follow-up.[98] The detection of occult cancer cells with RT-PCR remains investigational, however, and is not used to direct therapy for melanoma and other cancer types at this time.

Bone Marrow Micrometastases

Micrometastatic disease in the bone marrow, also referred to as *minimal residual disease,* also is being investigated as a potential prognostic marker. Bone marrow micrometastatic disease usually is detected by staining bone marrow aspirates with monoclonal antibodies to cytokeratin, but other methodologies such as flow cytometry and RT-PCR are being explored. Breast cancer patients with bone marrow micrometastasis have larger tumors, tumors with a higher histologic grade, more lymph node metastases, and more hormone receptor–negative tumors than patients without bone marrow micrometastasis. In 4700 patients with stage I, II, or III breast cancer, micrometastasis was a significant prognostic factor associated with poor overall survival, breast cancer–specific survival, disease-free survival, and distant disease-free survival during a 10-year observation period.[99] At this time the routine use of bone marrow testing is not recommended.[86] Ongoing clinical trials are evaluating the role of routine assessment of bone marrow status in the care of patients with early and advanced breast cancer. The utility of assessment of bone marrow micrometastasis is also being evaluated in other tumor types, including gastric, esophageal, colorectal, lung, cervical, and ovarian cancer.[100]

SURGICAL APPROACHES TO CANCER THERAPY

Multidisciplinary Approach to Cancer

Although surgery is an effective therapy for most solid tumors, patients who die from cancer usually die of metastatic disease. Therefore, to improve patient survival rates, a multimodality approach including systemic therapy and radiation therapy is key for most tumors. It is important that surgeons involved in cancer care not only know the techniques for performing a cancer operation but also know the alternatives to surgery and be well versed in reconstructive options. It is also crucial that the surgeon be familiar with the indications for and complications of preoperative and postoperative chemotherapy and radiation therapy. Although the surgeon will not be delivering these other therapies, as the first physician to see a patient with a cancer diagnosis, he or she is ultimately responsible for initiating the appropriate consultations. For this reason, the surgeon often is responsible for determining the most appropriate adjuvant therapy for a given patient as well as the best sequence for therapy. In most instances, a multidisciplinary approach beginning at the patient's initial presentation is likely to yield the best result.

Surgical Management of Primary Tumors

The goal of surgical therapy for cancer is to achieve oncologic cure. A curative operation presupposes that the tumor is confined to the organ of origin or to the organ and the regional lymph node basin. Patients in whom the primary tumor is not resectable with negative surgical margins are considered to have inoperable disease. The operability of primary tumors is best determined before surgery with appropriate imaging studies that can define the extent of local-regional disease. For example, a preoperative thin-section CT scan is obtained to determine resectability of pancreatic cancer, which is based on the absence of extrapancreatic disease, the absence of tumor extension to the superior mesenteric artery and celiac axis, and a patent superior mesenteric vein–portal vein confluence.[101] Disease involving multiple distant metastases is deemed inoperable because it is usually not curable with surgery of the primary tumor. Therefore patients who are at high risk of having distant metastasis should undergo a staging work-up before surgery for the primary tumor. On occasion, primary tumors are resected in these patients for palliative reasons, such as improving the quality of life by alleviating pain, infection, or bleeding. An example of this is toilet mastectomies for large ulcerated breast tumors. Patients with limited metastases from a primary tumor on occasion are considered surgical candidates if the natural history of isolated distant metastases for that cancer type is favorable or the potential complications associated with leaving the primary tumor intact are significant.

In the past it was presumed that the more radical the surgery, the better the oncologic outcome would be. Over the past 20 years, this has been recognized as not necessarily being true, which has led to more conservative operations, with wide local excisions replacing compartmental resections of sarcomas, and partial mastectomies, skin-sparing mastectomies, and breast-conserving therapies replacing radical mastectomies for breast cancer. The uniform goal for all successful oncologic operations seems to be achieving widely negative margins with no evidence of macroscopic or microscopic tumor at the surgical margins. The importance of negative surgical margins for local tumor control and/or survival has been documented for many tumor types, including sarcoma, breast cancer, pancreatic cancer, and rectal cancer. Thus it is clear that every effort should be made to achieve microscopically negative surgical margins. Inking of the margins, orientation of the specimen by the surgeon, and immediate gross evaluation of the margins by a pathologist using frozen-section analysis when necessary may assist in achieving negative margins at the first operation. In the end, although radiation therapy and systemic therapy can assist in decreasing local recurrence rates in the setting of positive margins, adjuvant therapy cannot substitute for adequate surgery.

Although it is clear that the surgical gold standard is negative surgical margins, the appropriate surgical margins for optimal local control are controversial for many cancer types. In contrast, in melanoma the optimal margin width for any tumor depth has been defined, owing to the systematic study of this question in randomized clinical trials.[102,103] Although such randomized studies may not be possible for all tumor types, it is important to determine optimum surgical margins for each cancer type so that adjuvant radiation and systemic therapy can be offered to patients deemed to be at increased risk for local treatment failure.

Surgical Management of the Regional Lymph Node Basin

Most neoplasms have the ability to metastasize via the lymphatics. Therefore, most oncologic operations have been designed to remove the primary tumor and draining lymphatics en bloc. This type of operative approach usually is undertaken when the lymph nodes draining the primary tumor site lie adjacent to the tumor bed, as is the case for colorectal cancers and gastric cancers. For tumors in which the regional lymph node basin is not immediately adjacent to the tumor (e.g., melanomas), lymph node surgery can be performed through a separate incision. Unlike most carcinomas, soft tissue sarcomas rarely metastasize to the lymph nodes (<5%); therefore lymph node surgery usually is not necessary.

It is generally accepted that a formal lymphadenectomy is likely to minimize the risk of regional recurrence of most cancers. For example, the introduction of total mesorectal excision of rectal cancer has been associated with a large decline in local-regional recurrence, and this procedure has become the new standard of operative management.[104] On the other hand, there have been two opposing views regarding the role of lymphadenectomy in survival of cancer patients. The traditional Halsted view states that lymphadenectomy is important for staging and survival. The opposing view counters that cancer is systemic at inception and that lymphadenectomy, although useful for staging, does not affect survival. For most cancers, involvement of the lymph nodes is one of the most significant prognostic factors. Interestingly, removal of a larger number of lymph nodes has been found to be associated with an improved overall survial rate for many tumors, including breast cancer, colon cancer, and lung cancer. Although this seems to support the Halsted theory that more extensive lymphadenectomy yielding of nodes reduces the risk of regional recurrence, there may be alternative explanations for the same finding. For example, the surgeon who performs a more extensive lymphadenectomy may obtain wider margins around the tumor or even provide better overall care, such as ensuring that patients receive the appropriate adjuvant therapy or undergo a more thorough staging work-up. Alternatively, the pathologist may perform a more thorough examination, identifying more nodes and more accurately staging the nodes. The effect of appropriate staging on survival is twofold. Patients with nodal metastases may be offered adjuvant therapy, which improves their survival chances. Further, the improved staging can improve perceived survival rates through a "Will Rogers effect"; that is, identification of metastases that had formerly been silent and unidentified leads to stage migration and thus to a perceived improvement in chances of survival. Clearly the impact of lymphadenectomy on survival will not be easily resolved. Because minimizing regional recurrences as much as possible is a goal of cancer treatment, the standard of care remains lymphadenectomy for most tumors.

A relatively new development in the surgical management of the clinically negative regional lymph node basin is the introduction of lymphatic mapping technology (Fig. 10-11).[105] Lymphatic mapping and sentinel lymph node biopsy were first reported in 1977 by Cabanas for penile cancer.[106] Now, sentinel node biopsy is the standard of care for the management of melanoma and breast cancer. Moreover, the utility of sentinel node biopsy in other cancer types is being explored.

The first node to receive drainage from the tumor site is termed the sentinel node. This node is the node most likely to contain metastases, if metastases to that regional lymph node basin are present. The goal of lymphatic mapping and sentinel lymph node biopsy is to identify and remove the lymph node most likely to contain metastases in the least invasive fashion. The practice of sentinel lymph node biopsy followed by selective regional lymph node dissection for patients with a positive sentinel lymph node avoids the morbidity of lymph node dissections in patients with negative nodes. An additional advantage of the sentinel lymph node technique is that it directs attention to a single node, which allows more careful analysis of the lymph node most likely to have a positive yield and increases the accuracy of nodal staging. Two criteria are used to assess the efficacy of a sentinel lymph node biopsy: the sentinel lymph node identification rate and the false-negative rate. The sentinel lymph node identification rate is the proportion of patients in whom a sentinel lymph node was identified and removed among all patients undergoing an attempted sentinel lymph node biopsy. The false-negative rate is the proportion of patients with regional lymph node metastases in whom the sentinel lymph node was found to be negative. False-negative biopsy results may be due to identifying the wrong node or to missing the sentinel node (i.e., surgical error) or they may be due to the cancer cells' establishing metastases not in the first node encountered but in a second-echelon node (i.e., biologic variation). Alternatively, false-negative biopsy results may be due to inadequate histologic evaluation of the lymph node. The false-negative rates for sentinel lymph node biopsy in study series range between 0 and 11%. Both increases in the identification rate and decreases in the false-negative rate have been observed as surgeons gain experience with the technique.

Lymphatic mapping is performed by using isosulfan blue dye, technetium-labeled sulfur colloid or albumin, or a combination of both techniques to detect sentinel nodes. The combination of blue dye and technetium has been reported to improve the capability of detecting sentinel lymph nodes. The nodal drainage pattern usually is determined with a preoperative lymphoscintigram, and the "hot" and/or blue nodes are identified with the assistance of a gamma probe and careful nodal basin exploration. Careful manual palpation is a crucial part of the procedure to minimize the false-negative rate.

The nodes are evaluated with serial sectioning, hematoxylin and eosin staining, and immunohistochemical analysis with S-100 protein and homatropine methylbromide staining for melanoma and cytokeratin staining for breast cancer. Studies also are ongoing to evaluate the use of molecular techniques such as RT-PCR to rapidly assess the sentinel node status in the intraoperative setting. In a recent prospec-

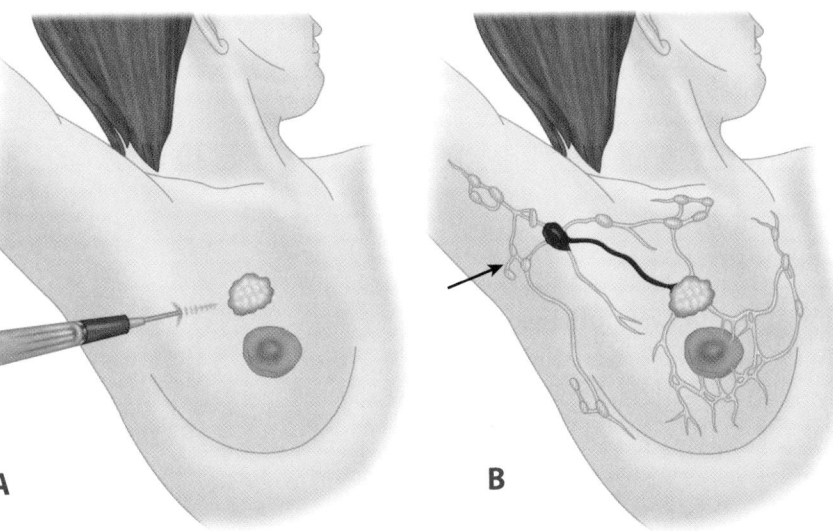

FIG. 10-11. Lymphatic mapping and sentinel lymph node biopsy for breast cancer. **A.** Peritumoral injection of blue dye. **B.** Blue dye draining into the sentinel lymph node. *[Modified with permission from Meric F, Hunt KK: Surgical options for breast cancer, in Hunt KK et al (eds): M. D. Anderson Cancer Care Series - Breast Cancer. New York: Springer-Verlag, 2001, p 187. With kind permission from Springer Science + Business Media.]*

A   **B**

tive trial, an RT-PCR assay for mammaglobin and cytokeratin 19 mRNA (GeneSearch) was found to have a sensitivity of 98.1% for detection of breast cancer metastases larger than 2 mm and 77.8% for metastases larger than 0.2 mm,[107] and it has been approved for use by the FDA. Ongoing studies are addressing how best to incorporate this and other similar technologies into clinical practice.

Another area of active investigation is the prognostic value of minimal nodal involvement. For example, in breast cancer, nodes with isolated tumor cell deposits of <0.2 mm (also called *nanometastasis*) are considered to be N0 by the sixth edition of the AJCC staging manual. However, some retrospective studies have suggested that even this amount of nodal disease burden has negative prognostic implications.[108] Molecular ultrastaging with RT-PCR for patients with node-negative disease was assessed in a prospective multicenter trial and was found not to be prognostic in malignant melanoma.[98] However, a recent meta-analysis of 22 studies enrolling 4019 patients found that PCR positivity was associated with worse overall and disease-free survival.[109] Further study of the utility of ultrastaging of nodes in breast cancer, melanoma, and several other tumor types is ongoing.

Surgical Management of Distant Metastases

The treatment of a patient with distant metastases depends on the number and sites of metastases, the cancer type, the rate of tumor growth, the previous treatments delivered and the responses to these treatments, and the patient's age, physical condition, and desires. Although once a tumor has metastasized it usually is not curable with surgical therapy, such therapy has resulted in cure in selected cases with isolated metastases to the liver, lung, or brain.

Patient selection is the key to the success of surgical therapy for distant metastases. The cancer type is a major determinant in surgical decision making. A liver metastasis from a colon cancer is more likely to be an isolated and thus resectable lesion than a liver metastasis from a pancreatic carcinoma. The growth rate of the tumor also plays an important role and can be determined in part by the disease-free interval and the time between treatment of the primary tumor and detection of the distant recurrence. Patients with longer disease-free intervals have a higher survival rate after surgical metastasectomy than those with a short disease-free interval. Similarly, patients who have synchronous metastases (metastases diagnosed at the initial cancer diagnosis) do worse after metastasectomy than patients who develop metachronous metastases (metastasis diagnosed after a disease-free interval). The natural history of metastatic disease is so poor for some tumors (e.g., pancreatic cancer) that there is no role at this time for surgical metastasectomy. In cancers with a more favorable outlook, observation for several weeks or months, potentially with initial treatment with systemic therapy, can allow the surgeon to monitor for metastases at other sites.

In curative surgery for distant metastases, as with surgery for primary tumors, the goal is to resect the metastases with negative margins. In patients with hepatic metastases that are unresectable because their location near intrahepatic blood vessels precludes a margin-negative resection, or because they are multifocal or hepatic function is inadequate, tumor ablation with cryotherapy or radiofrequency ablation is an alternative.[110,111] Curative resections or ablative procedures should be attempted only if the lesions are accessible and the procedure can be performed safely.

CHEMOTHERAPY

Clinical Use of Chemotherapy

In patients with documented distant metastatic disease, chemotherapy is usually the primary modality of therapy. The goal of therapy in this setting is to decrease the tumor burden, thus prolonging survival. It is rare to achieve cure with chemotherapy for metastatic disease for most solid tumors. Chemotherapy administered to a patient who is at high risk for distant recurrence but has no evidence of distant disease is referred to as *adjuvant chemotherapy*.

The goal of adjuvant chemotherapy is eradication of micrometastatic disease, with the intent of decreasing relapse rates and improving survival rates.

Adjuvant therapy can be administered after surgery (postoperative chemotherapy) or before surgery (preoperative chemotherapy, neoadjuvant chemotherapy, or induction therapy). A portion or all of the planned adjuvant chemotherapy can be administered before the surgical removal of the primary tumor. Preoperative chemotherapy has three potential advantages. The first is that preoperative regression of tumor can facilitate resection of tumors that were initially inoperable or allow more conservative surgery for patients whose cancer was operable to begin with. In the NSABP B-18 project, for example, women were randomly assigned to receive adjuvant doxorubicin and cyclophosphamide preoperatively or postoperatively. More patients treated before surgery than after surgery underwent breast-conserving surgery (68 vs. 60%).[112] The second advantage of preoperative chemotherapy is the treatment of micrometastases without the delay of postoperative recovery. The third advantage is the ability to assess a cancer's response to treatment clinically, after a number of courses of chemotherapy, and pathologically, after surgical resection. This is especially important if alternative treatment regimens are available to be offered to patients whose disease responded inadequately. Molecular characterization of the residual disease may also give insight into mechanisms of chemoresistance and possible therapeutic targets.

There are some potential disadvantages to preoperative chemotherapy, however. Although disease progression while the patient is receiving preoperative chemotherapy is rare in chemotherapy-sensitive tumors such as breast cancer, it is more frequent in relatively chemotherapy-resistant tumors such as sarcomas.[113] Thus, patient selection is critical to ensure that the opportunity to treat disease surgically is not lost by giving preoperative chemotherapy. Often, rates of postoperative wound infection, flap necrosis, and delays in postoperative adjuvant therapy do not differ between patients who are treated with preoperative chemotherapy and patients who are treated with surgery first. However, preoperative chemotherapy can introduce special challenges to tumor localization, margin analysis, lymphatic mapping, and pathologic staging.

Response to chemotherapy is monitored clinically with imaging studies as well as physical examinations. Response usually is defined as complete response, partial response, stable disease, or progression. Response generally is assessed using the Response Evaluation Criteria in Solid Tumors (RECIST) criteria.[114] Objective tumor response assessment is critical, because tumor response is used as a prospective endpoint in clinical trials and tumor response is a guide to clinicians regarding continuation of current therapy.

Principles of Chemotherapy

Chemotherapy destroys cells by first-order kinetics, which means that with the administration of a drug a constant percentage of cells is killed, not a constant number of cells. If a patient with 10^{12} tumor cells is treated with a dose that results in 99.9% cell kill (3-log cell kill), the tumor burden will be reduced from 10^{12} to 10^9 cells (or 1 kg to 1 g). If the patient is re-treated with the same drug, which theoretically could result in another 3-log cell kill, the cells would decrease in number from 10^9 to 10^6 (1 g to 1 mg) rather than being eliminated totally.

Chemotherapeutic agents can be classified according to the phase of the cell cycle during which they are effective. Cell-cycle phase–nonspecific agents (e.g., alkylating agents) have a linear dose-response curve, such that the fraction of cells killed increases with the dose of the drug.[115] In contrast, the cell-cycle phase–specific drugs have a plateau with respect to cell killing ability, and cell kill will not increase with further increases in drug dose.

Anticancer Agents
Alkylating Agents

Alkylating agents are cell-cycle–nonspecific agents, that is, they are able to kill cells in any phase of the cell cycle. They act by cross-linking the two strands of the DNA helix or by causing other direct damage to the DNA. The damage to the DNA prevents cell division and, if severe enough, leads to apoptosis. The alkylating agents are composed of three main subgroups: classic alkylators, nitrosoureas, and miscellaneous DNA-binding agents (Table 10-12).

Antitumor Antibiotics

Antitumor antibiotics are the products of fermentation of microbial organisms. Like the alkylating agents, these agents are cell-cycle nonspecific. Antitumor antibiotics damage the cell by interfering with DNA or RNA synthesis, although the exact mechanism of action may differ by agent.

Antimetabolites

Antimetabolites are generally cell-cycle–specific agents that have their major activity during the S phase of the cell cycle and have little effect on cells in G_0. These drugs are most effective, therefore, in tumors that have a high growth fraction. Antimetabolites are structural analogues of naturally occurring metabolites involved in DNA and RNA synthesis. Therefore, they interfere with normal synthesis of nucleic acids by substituting for purines or pyrimidines in the metabolic pathway to inhibit critical enzymes in nucleic acid synthesis. The antimetabolites include folate antagonists, purine antagonists, and pyrimidine antagonists (see Table 10-12).

Plant Alkaloids

Plant alkaloids are derived from plants such as the periwinkle plant, *Vinca rosea* (e.g., vincristine, a vinca alkaloid), or the root of American mandrake, *Podophyllum peltatum* (e.g., etoposide, a podophyllotoxin).[115] Vinca alkaloids affect the cell by binding to tubulin in the S phase. This blocks microtubule polymerization, which results in impaired mitotic spindle formation in the M phase. Taxanes such as paclitaxel, on the other hand, cause excess polymerization and stability of microtubules, which blocks the cell cycle in mitosis. The epipodophyllotoxins act to inhibit a DNA enzyme called *topoisomerase II* by stabilizing the DNA–topoisomerase II complex. This results in an inability to synthesize DNA, and thus the cell cycle is stopped in the G_1 phase.[115]

Combination Chemotherapy

Combination chemotherapy may provide greater efficacy than single-agent therapy by three mechanisms: (a) it provides maximum cell kill within the range of toxicity for each drug that can be tolerated by the host, (b) it offers a broader range of coverage of resistant cell lines in a heterogeneous population, and (c) it prevents or delays the emergence of drug-resistant cell lines.[115] When combination regimens are devised, drugs known to be active as single agents usually are selected. Drugs with different mechanisms of action are combined to allow for additive or synergistic effects. Combining cell-cycle–specific and cell-cycle–nonspecific agents may be especially advantageous. Drugs with differing dose-limiting toxic effects are combined to allow for each drug to be given at therapeutic doses. Drugs with different patterns of resistance are combined whenever possible to minimize cross-resistance. The treatment-free interval between cycles is kept to the shortest possible time that will allow for recovery of the most sensitive normal tissue.

Drug Resistance

Several tumor factors influence tumor cell kill. Tumors are heterogeneous, and, according to the Goldie-Coldman hypothesis, tumor cells are genetically unstable and tend to mutate to form different cell clones. This has been used as an argument for giving chemotherapy as soon as possible in treatment to reduce the likelihood that resistant clones will emerge. Tumor size is another important variable. The larger the tumor, the greater the heterogeneity. Moreover, according to the gompertzian model, cancer cells initially grow rapidly (exponential growth phase), then the growth slows

TABLE 10-12 Classification of chemotherapeutic agents

Alkylating agents
Classic alkylating agents
  Busulfan
  Chlorambucil
  Cyclophosphamide
  Ifosfamide
  Mechlorethamine (nitrogen mustard)
  Melphalan
  Mitomycin C
  Triethylene thiophosphoramide (thiotepa)
Nitrosoureas
  Carmustine (BCNU)
  Lomustine (CCNU)
  Semustine (MeCCNU)
  Streptozocin
Miscellaneous DNA-binding agents
  Carboplatin
  Cisplatin
  Dacarbazine (DTIC)
  Hexamethylmelamine
  Procarbazine
Antitumor antibiotics
  Bleomycin
  Dactinomycin (actinomycin D)
  Daunorubicin
  Doxorubicin
  Idarubicin
  Plicamycin (mithramycin)
Antimetabolites
Folate analogues
  Methotrexate
Purine analogues
  Azathioprine
  Mercaptopurine
  Thioguanine
  Cladribine (2-chlorodeoxyadenosine)
  Fludarabine
  Pentostatin
Pyrimidine analogues
  Capecitabine
  Cytarabine
  Floxuridine
  Gemcitabine
Ribonucleotide reductase inhibitors
  Hydroxyurea
Plant alkaloids
Vinca alkaloids
  Vinblastine
  Vincristine
  Vindesine
  Vinorelbine
Epipodophyllotoxins
  Etoposide
  Teniposide
Taxanes
  Paclitaxel
  Docetaxel
Miscellaneous agents
  Asparaginase
  Estramustine
  Mitotane

TABLE 10-13 General mechanisms of drug resistance

Cellular and biochemical mechanisms
    Decreased drug accumulation
        Decreased drug influx
        Increased drug efflux
        Altered intracellular trafficking of drug
    Decreased drug activation
    Increased inactivation of drug or toxic intermediate
    Increased repair of drug-induced damage to:
        DNA
        Protein
        Membranes
    Alteration of drug targets (quantitatively or qualitatively)
    Alteration of cofactor or metabolite levels
    Alteration of gene expression
        DNA mutation, amplification, or deletion
        Altered transcription, posttranscription processing, or translation
        Altered stability of macromolecules
Mechanisms relevant in vivo
    Pharmacologic and anatomic drug barriers (tumor sanctuaries)
    Host-drug interactions
        Increased drug inactivation by normal tissues
        Decreased drug activation by normal tissues
        Relative increase in normal tissue drug sensitivity (toxicity)
Host-tumor interactions

Source: Modified with permission from Morrow et al.[116]

down owing to hypoxia and decreased nutrient supply. Because of the larger proportion of cells dividing, smaller tumors may be more chemosensitive.

Multiple mechanisms of chemotherapy resistance have been identified (Table 10-13).[116] Cells may exhibit reduced sensitivity to drugs by virtue of their cell-cycle distribution. For example, cells in the G_0 phase are resistant to drugs active in the S phase. This phenomenon of "kinetic resistance" usually is temporary, and if the drug level can be maintained, all cells will eventually pass through the vulnerable phase of the cell cycle.[115] Alternatively, tumor cells may exhibit "pharmacologic resistance," in which the failure to kill cells is due to insufficient drug concentration. This may occur when tumor cells are located in sites where effective drug concentrations are difficult to achieve (such as the central nervous system) or can be due to enhanced metabolism of the drug after its administration, decreased conversion of the drug to its active form, or decrease in the intracellular drug level caused by increased removal of the drug from the cell associated with enhanced expression of P-glycoprotein, the protein product of multidrug resistance gene 1. Other mechanisms of resistance include decreased affinity of the target enzyme for the drug, altered amount of the target enzyme, or enhanced repair of the drug-induced defect.

For drug-sensitive cancers, another factor limiting optimal killing is improper dosing. A dose reduction of 20% because of drug toxicity can lead to a decline in the cure rate by as much as 50%.[115] On the other hand, a twofold increase in dose can be associated with a tenfold (1 log) increase in tumor cell kill.

Drug Toxicity

Tumors are more susceptible than normal tissue to chemotherapeutic agents, in part because they have a higher proportion of dividing cells. Normal tissues with a high growth fraction, such as the bone marrow, oral and intestinal mucosa, and hair follicles, are also sensitive to chemotherapeutic effects. Therefore, treatment with chemotherapeutic agents can produce toxic effects such as bone marrow suppression, stomatitis, ulceration of the GI tract, and alopecia. Toxic effects usually are graded from 0 to 4 on the basis of World Health Organization standard criteria.[117] Significant drug toxicity may necessitate a dosage reduction. A toxic effect requiring

a dose modification or change in dose intensity is referred to as a dose-limiting toxic effect. Because maintaining dose intensity is important to preserve as high a tumor cell kill as possible, several supportive strategies have been developed, such as administration of colony-stimulating factors and erythropoietin to treat poor bone marrow reserve and administration of cytoprotectants such as mesna and amifostine to prevent renal dysfunction.

Administration of Chemotherapy

Chemotherapy usually is administered systemically (IV, IM, SC, or PO). Systemic administration treats micrometastases at widespread sites and prevents systemic recurrence. However, it increases the drug's toxicity to a wide range of organs throughout the body. One method to minimize systemic toxicity while enhancing target organ delivery of chemotherapy is regional administration of chemotherapy. Many of these approaches require surgical access, such as intrahepatic delivery of chemotherapy for hepatic carcinomas or metastatic colorectal cancer using a hepatic artery infusion pump, limb perfusion for extremity melanoma and sarcoma, and intraperitoneal hyperthermic perfusion for pseudomyxoma peritonei.

HORMONAL THERAPY

Some tumors, most notably breast and prostate cancers, originate from tissues whose growth is under hormonal control. The first attempts at hormonal therapy were through surgical ablation of the organ producing the hormones involved, such as oophorectomy for breast cancer. Currently, hormonal anticancer agents include androgens, antiandrogens, antiestrogens, estrogens, glucocorticoids, gonadotropin inhibitors, progestins, aromatase inhibitors, and somatostatin analogues. Hormones or hormone-like agents can be administered to inhibit tumor growth by blocking or antagonizing the naturally occurring substance, such as with the estrogen antagonist tamoxifen. Other substances that block the synthesis of the natural hormone can be administered as alternatives. Aromatase inhibitors, for example, block the peripheral conversion of endogenous androgens to estrogens in postmenopausal women.

Hormonal therapy provides a highly tumor-specific form of therapy in sensitive tissues. In breast cancer, estrogen and progesterone receptor status is used to predict the success of hormonal therapy. Recently, several other biologic variables have been found to have an impact on the success of hormonal therapy, and these variables are likely to be incorporated into clinical practice in the near future.

TARGETED THERAPY

Over the past decade, increased understanding of cancer biology has fostered the emerging field of molecular therapeutics. The basic principle of molecular therapeutics is to exploit the molecular differences between normal cells and cancer cells to develop targeted therapies. Thus targeted therapies usually are directed at the processes involved in tumor growth rather than directly targeting the tumor cells. The ideal molecular target would be exclusively expressed in the cancer cells, be the driving force of the proliferation of the cancer cells, and be critical to their survival. A large number of molecular targets are currently being explored, both preclinically and in clinical trials. The major groups of targeted therapy agents are inhibitors of growth factor receptors, inhibitors of intracellular signal transduction, cell-cycle inhibitors, apoptosis-based therapies, and antiangiogenic compounds.

Protein kinases have come to the forefront as attractive therapeutic targets with the success of imatinib mesylate (Gleevec) in treating chronic myelogenous leukemia and GI stromal tumors, and trastuzumab (Herceptin) in treating breast cancer; these drugs work by targeting bcr-*abl*, c-*kit*, and HER2, respectively. Sequencing of the human genome has revealed approximately 500 protein kinases.

TABLE 10-14 Selected FDA-approved targeted therapies

Generic Name	Trade Name	Company	Target	FDA Approval Date	Initial Indication
Trastuzumab	Herceptin	Genentech	HER2	9/1998	Breast cancer
Imatinib	Gleevec	Novartis	c-kit, bcr-abl, PDGFR	5/2001, 12/2002	CML, GIST
Cetuximab	Erbitux	ImClone Systems	EGFR	2/2004	Colorectal cancer
Bevacizumab	Avastin	Genentech	VEGF	2/2004	Colorectal cancer, lung cancer
Erlotinib	Tarceva	Genentech, OSI Pharmaceuticals	EGFR	11/2004	Non–small cell lung cancer
Sorafenib	Nexavar	Bayer	Raf, PDGF, VEGFR, c-kit	12/2005	RCC
Sunitinib	Sutent	Pfizer	VEGFR PDGFR c-kit, Flt-3, RET	1/2006	GIST, RCC
Dasatinib	Sprycel	Bristol-Myers Squibb	bcr-abl, src family, c-kit, EPHA2, PDGFR-β	6/2006	CML
Lapatinib	Tykerb	GlaxoSmithKline	EGFR and HER2	3/2007	Breast cancer
Temsirolimus	Torisel	Wyeth	mTOR	5/2007	RCC

CML = chronic myelogenous leukemia; EGFR = epidermal growth factor receptor; EPHA2 = ephrin A2; FDA = Food and Drug Administration; Flt-3 = fms-related tyrosine kinase 3; GIST = GI stromal tumor; HER2 = human epidermal growth factor receptor 2; mTOR = mammalian target of rapamycin; PDGF = platelet-derived growth factor; PDGFR = platelet-derived growth factor receptor; RCC = renal cell carcinoma; RET = rearranged during transfection; VEGF = vascular endothelial growth factor; VEGFR = vascular endothelial growth factor receptor.

Several tyrosine kinases have been shown to have oncogenic properties (see Table 10-8), and many other protein kinases have been shown to be aberrantly activated in cancer cells.[75] Therefore, protein kinases involved in these aberrantly activated pathways are being aggressively pursued in molecular therapeutics. Potential targets like HER2 can be targeted via different strategies, such as transcriptional downregulation, targeting of mRNA, RNA inhibition, antisense strategies, direct inhibition of protein activity, and induction of immunity against the protein. Most of the compounds in development are monoclonal antibodies like trastuzumab or small-molecule kinase inhibitors like imatinib. Some of the kinases proposed as molecular targets are listed in Table 10-14. Some other agents, such as sunitinib, are multitargeted kinase inhibitors. Selected FDA-approved targeted therapies are listed in Table 10-14.

Development of molecularly targeted agents for clinical use presents several unique challenges. Once an appropriate compound is identified and confirmed to have activity in preclinical testing, predictive markers for activity in the preclinical setting must be defined. Expression of a target may not be sufficient to predict response, because the pathway of interest may not be activated or critical to the cancer's survival. Although in traditional phase I trials the goal is to identify the maximum tolerated dosage, the maximum dosage of biologic agents may not be necessary to achieve the desired biologic effect. Thus assays to verify modulation of the target need to be developed to determine at what dosage the desired effect is achieved. When phase II and III clinical trials are initiated, biomarker modulation studies should be integrated into the trial to determine whether clinical response correlates with target modulation and thus to identify additional parameters that impact response. Rational dose selection and limitation of study populations to patients most likely to respond to the molecular therapy as determined by predictive markers are most likely to lead to successful clinical translation of a product. Finally, most biologic agents are cytostatic, not cytotoxic. Thus rational combination therapy mixing new biologic agents with either established chemotherapeutic agents that have synergy or with other biologic agents is more likely to lead to cancer cures.

IMMUNOTHERAPY

The aim of immunotherapy is to induce or potentiate inherent antitumor immunity that can destroy cancer cells. Central to the process of antitumor immunity is the ability of the immune system to recognize tumor-associated antigens present on human cancers and to direct cytotoxic responses through humoral or T-cell–mediated immunity. Overall, T-cell–mediated immunity appears to have the greater potential of the two for eradicating tumor cells. T cells recognize antigens on the surfaces of target cells as small peptides presented by class I and class II MHC molecules.

Several antitumor strategies are under investigation. One approach to antitumor immunity is nonspecific immunotherapy, which stimulates the immune system as a whole through administration of bacterial agents or their products, such as bacille Calmette-Guérin. This approach is thought to activate the effectors of antitumor response such as natural killer cells and macrophages, as well as polyclonal lymphocytes.[118] Another approach to nonspecific immunotherapy is systemic administration of cytokines such as interleukin-2, interferon-α, and interferon-γ. Interleukin-2 stimulates proliferation of cytotoxic T lymphocytes and maturation of effectors such as natural killer cells into lymphokine-activated killer cells. Interferons, on the other hand, exert antitumor effects directly by inhibiting tumor cell proliferation and indirectly by activating host immune cells, including macrophages, dendritic cells, and natural killer cells, and by enhancing human leukocyte antigen (HLA) class I expression on tumor cells.[118]

Antigen-specific immunotherapy can be active, as is achieved through antitumor vaccines, or passive. In passive immunotherapy, antibodies to specific tumor-associated antigens can be produced by hybridoma technique and then administered to patients whose cancers express these antigens, inducing antibody-dependent cellular cytotoxicity.

The early attempts at vaccination against cancers used allogeneic cultured cancer cells, including irradiated cells, cell lysates, and shed antigens isolated from tissue culture supernatants. An alternate strategy is the use of autologous tumor vaccines. These have the potential advantage of being more likely to contain antigens relevant for the individual patient but have the disadvantage of requiring a large amount of tumor tissue for preparation, which restricts eligibility of patients for this modality. Strategies to enhance immunogenicity of tumor cells include the introduction of genes encoding cytokines or chemokines, and fusion of the tumor cells to allogeneic MHC class II–bearing cells.[119] Alternatively, heat shock proteins derived from a patient's tumor can be used, because heat shock protein peptide complexes are readily taken up by dendritic cells for presentation to T cells.[119]

Identification of tumor antigens has made it possible to perform antigen-specific vaccination. For example in the case of melanoma, several antigens have been identified that can be recognized by both CD8+ cytotoxic T cells and CD4+ helper T cells, including MART-1, gp 100, MAGE1, tyrosinase, TRP-1, TRP-2, and NY-ESO-1.[120] Antigens tested usually are overexpressed or mutated in cancer cells. Tissue specificity and immunogenicity are important determinants in choosing an appropriate target. Vaccines directed at defined tumor antigens aim to combine selected tumor antigens and appropriate routes for delivering these antigens to the immune system to optimize antitumor immunity.[121] Several different vaccination approaches are under study, including tumor cell–based vaccines, peptide-based vaccines, recombinant virus–based vaccines, DNA-based vaccines, and dendritic cell vaccines.

In adoptive transfer, antigen-specific effector cells (i.e., cytotoxic T lymphocytes) or antigen-nonspecific effector cells (i.e., natural killer cells) can be transferred to a patient. These effector cells can be obtained from the tumor (tumor-infiltrating lymphocytes) or the peripheral blood.

Clinical experience in patients with metastatic disease has shown objective tumor responses to a variety of immunotherapeutic modalities. It is thought, however, that the immune system is overwhelmed with the tumor burden in this setting, and thus adjuvant therapy may be preferable, with immunotherapy reserved for decreasing tumor recurrences. Trials to date suggest that immunotherapy is a potentially useful approach in the adjuvant setting. How to best select patients for this approach and how to integrate immunotherapy with other therapies are not well understood for most cancer types.

Tolerance to self-antigens expressed in tumors is a limitation in generating antitumor responses.[122] Recently, several pathways that modulate tolerance and approaches to manipulating these pathways have been identified: pathways that activate professional antigen-presenting cells such as Toll-like receptors, growth factors, and the CD40 pathway; cytokines to enhance immunoactivation; and pathways that inhibit T-cell inhibitory signals or Tregs.[122]

A new strategy being actively explored involves the use of cytotoxic T-lymphocyte antigen 4 (CTLA-4). CTLA-4 exists on the surfaces of T cells and has a homeostatic immunosuppressive function, downregulating the response of T cells to stimuli.[123] Two fully human monoclonal anti-CTLA-4 antibodies, ipilimumab and tremelimumab, are in clinical development. Anti-CTLA-4 antibodies are under study for use in melanoma as well as several other cancer types as single agents, in combination with interleukin-2, chemotherapy, or peptide vaccines.[123]

GENE THERAPY

Gene therapy is being pursued as a possible approach to modifying the genetic program of cancer cells as well as treating metabolic diseases.

The field of cancer gene therapy uses a variety of strategies, ranging from replacement of mutated or deleted tumor-suppressor genes to enhancement of immune responses to cancer cells (Fig. 10-12).[124] Indeed, in preclinical models, approaches such as replacement of tumor-suppressor genes leads to growth arrest or apoptosis. However, the translation of these findings into clinically useful tools presents special challenges.

One of the main difficulties in getting gene therapy technology from the laboratory to the clinic is the lack of a perfect delivery system. An ideal vector would be administered through a noninvasive route and would transduce all of the cancer cells and none of the normal cells. Furthermore, the ideal vector would have a high degree of activity, that is, it would produce an adequate amount of the desired gene product to achieve target cell kill. Unlike genetic diseases in which delivery of the gene of interest into only a portion of the cells may be sufficient to achieve clinical effect, cancer requires either that the therapeutic gene be delivered to all of the cancer cells or that a therapeutic effect be achieved on nontransfected cells as well as transfected cells through a bystander effect. On the other hand, treatment of a metabolic disease requires prolonged gene expression, whereas transient expression may be sufficient for cancer therapy.

Several vector systems are under study for gene therapy, however none is considered ideal. One of the promising approaches to increase the number of tumor cells transduced is the use of a replication-competent virus such as a parvovirus, human reovirus, or vesicular stomatitis virus that selectively replicates within malignant cells and lyses them more efficiently than it does normal cells. Another strategy for killing tumor cells with suicide genes exploits tumor-specific expression elements, such as the MUC-1, PSA, CEA, or VEGF promoters, that can be used to achieve tissue-specific or tumor-specific expression of the desired gene.

Because the goal in cancer therapy is to eradicate systemic disease, optimization of delivery systems is the key to success for gene therapy strategies. Gene therapy is likely to be most successful when combined with standard therapies, but it will provide the advantage of customization of therapy based on the molecular status of an individual's tumor.

RADIATION THERAPY

Physical Basis of Radiation Therapy

Ionizing radiation is energy strong enough to remove an orbital electron from an atom. This radiation can be electromagnetic, such as

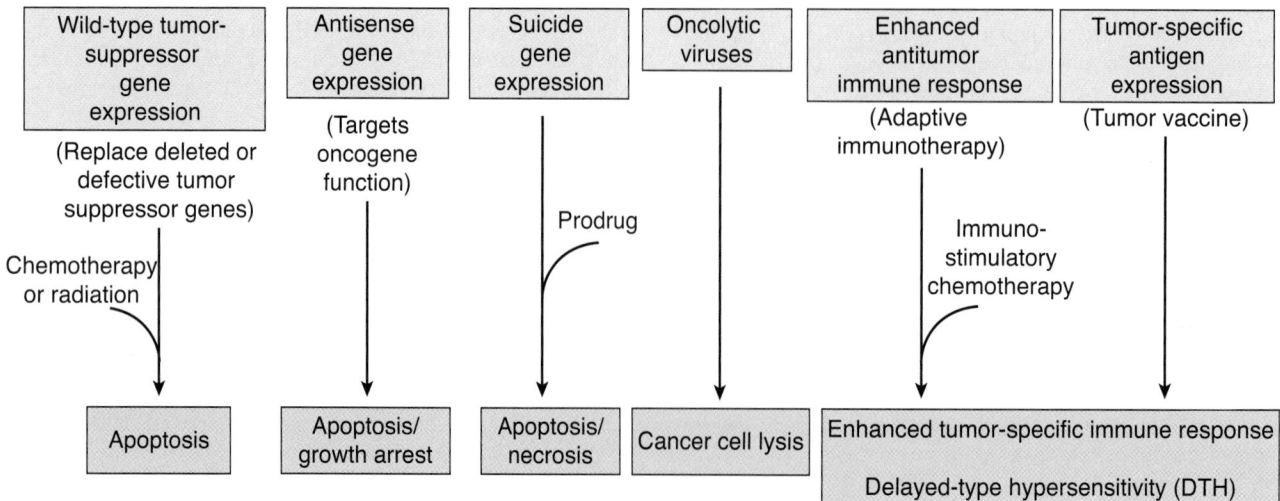

FIG. 10-12. Different strategies for gene therapy. *(Modified with permission from Cusack et al.[124] Copyright Elsevier.)*

a high-energy photon, or particulate, such as an electron, proton, neutron, or alpha particle. Radiation therapy is delivered primarily as high-energy photons (gamma rays and x-rays) and charged particles (electrons). Gamma rays are photons that are released from the nucleus of a radioactive atom. X-rays are photons that are created electronically, such as with a clinical linear accelerator. Currently, high-energy radiation is delivered to tumors primarily with linear accelerators. X-rays traverse the tissue, depositing the maximum dose beneath the surface, and thus spare the skin. Electrons are used to treat superficial skin lesions, superficial tumors, or surgical beds to a depth of 5 cm. Gamma rays typically are produced by radioactive sources used in brachytherapy.

The dose of radiation absorbed correlates with the energy of the beam. The basic unit is the amount of energy absorbed per unit of mass (joules per kilogram) and is known as a *gray (Gy)*. One gray is equivalent to 100 rads, the unit of radiation measurement used in the past.

Biologic Basis of Radiation Therapy

Radiation deposition results in DNA damage manifested by single- and double-strand breaks in the sugar phosphate backbone of the DNA molecule.[125] Cross-linking between the DNA strands and chromosomal proteins also occurs. The mechanism of DNA damage differs by the type of radiation delivered. Electromagnetic radiation is indirectly ionizing through short-lived hydroxyl radicals produced primarily by the ionization of cellular hydrogen peroxide (H_2O_2).[125] Protons and other heavy particles are directly ionizing and directly damage DNA.

Radiation damage is manifested primarily by the loss of cellular reproductive integrity. Most cell types do not show signs of radiation damage until they attempt to divide, so slowly proliferating tumors may persist for months and appear viable. Some cell types, however, undergo apoptosis.

The extent of DNA damage after radiation exposure is dependent on several factors. The most important of these is cellular oxygen. Hypoxic cells are significantly less radiosensitive than aerated cells. Because the presence of oxygen is thought to prolong the half-life of free radicals produced by the interaction of x-rays and cellular H_2O_2, indirectly ionizing radiation is less efficacious in tumors with areas of hypoxia.[125] In contrast, radiation damage from directly ionizing radiation is independent of cellular oxygen levels.

The extent of DNA damage from indirectly ionizing radiation is dependent on the phase of the cell cycle. The most radiation-sensitive phases are G_2 and M, whereas G_1 and late S phases are less sensitive. Thus irradiation of a population of tumor cells results in killing of a greater proportion of cells in G_2 and M phases. However, delivery of radiation in divided doses, a concept referred to as *fractionation*, allows the surviving G_1 and S phase cells to progress to more sensitive phases, a process referred to as *reassortment*. In contrast to DNA damage after indirectly ionizing radiation, that after exposure to directly ionizing radiation is less dependent on the cell-cycle phase.[126]

Several chemicals can modify the effects of ionizing radiation. These include hypoxic cell sensitizers such as metronidazole and misonidazole, which mimic oxygen and increase cell kill of hypoxic cells.[125] A second category of radiation sensitizers are the thymidine analogues iododeoxyuridine and bromodeoxyuridine. These molecules are incorporated into the DNA in place of thymidine and render the cells more susceptible to radiation damage; however, they are associated with considerable acute toxicity. Several other chemotherapeutic agents sensitize cells to radiation through various mechanisms, including 5-fluorouracil, actinomycin D, gemcitabine, paclitaxel, topotecan, doxorubicin, and vinorelbine.[125]

Radiation Therapy Planning

Radiation therapy is delivered in a homogeneous dose to a well-defined region that includes tumor and/or surrounding tissue at risk for subclinical disease. The first step in planning is to define the target to be irradiated as well as the dose-limiting organs in the vicinity.[127] Treatment planning includes evaluation of alternative treatment techniques, which is done through a process referred to as *simulation*. Once the beam distribution that will best achieve homogeneous delivery to the target volume and minimize the dose to the normal tissue is determined, immobilization devices and markings or tattoos on the patient's skin are used to ensure that each daily treatment is given in the same way. Conventional fractionation is 1.8 to 2 Gy/d, administered 5 days each week for 3 to 7 weeks.

Radiation therapy may be used as the primary modality for palliation in certain patients with metastatic disease, primarily patients with bony metastases. In these cases, radiation is recommended for symptomatic metastases only. However, lytic metastases in weight-bearing bones such as the femur, tibia, or humerus also are considered for irradiation. Another circumstance in which radiation therapy might be appropriate is spinal cord compression due to metastases to the vertebral body that extend posteriorly to the spinal canal.

The goal of adjuvant radiation therapy is to decrease local-regional recurrence rates. Adjuvant radiation therapy can be given before surgery, after surgery, or, in selected cases, during surgery. Preoperative radiation therapy has several advantages. It may minimize seeding of the tumor during surgery and it allows for smaller treatment fields because the operative bed has not been contaminated with tumor cells. Also, radiation therapy for inoperable tumors may achieve adequate reduction to make them operable. The disadvantages of preoperative therapy are an increased risk of postoperative wound healing problems and the difficulty in planning subsequent radiation therapy in patients who have positive surgical margins. If radiation therapy is given postoperatively, it is usually given 3 to 4 weeks after surgery to allow for wound healing. The advantage of postoperative radiation therapy is that the surgical specimen can be evaluated histologically and radiation therapy can be reserved for patients who are most likely to benefit from it. Further, the radiation therapy can be modified on the basis of margin status. The disadvantages of postoperative radiation therapy are that the volume of normal tissue requiring irradiation may be larger owing to surgical contamination of the tissue planes and that the tumor may be less sensitive to radiation owing to poor oxygenation. Postlaparotomy adhesions may decrease the mobility of the small bowel loops, increasing the risk for radiation injury in abdominal or pelvic irradiation. Given the potential advantages and disadvantages of both approaches, the roles of preoperative and postoperative radiation therapy are being actively evaluated and compared for many cancer types.

Another mode of postoperative radiation therapy is brachytherapy. In brachytherapy, unlike in external beam therapy, the radiation source is in contact with the tissue being irradiated. The radiation source may be cesium, gold, iridium, or radium. Brachytherapy is administered via temporary or permanent delivery implants such as needles, seeds, or catheters. Temporary brachytherapy catheters are placed either during open surgery or percutaneously soon after surgery. The implants are loaded interstitially, and treatment usually is given postoperatively for a short duration, such as 1 to 3 days. Although brachytherapy has the advantage of patient convenience owing to the shorter treatment duration, it has the disadvantages of leaving scars at the catheter insertion site and requiring special facilities for inpatient brachytherapy. Another short delivery approach is intraoperative radiotherapy (IORT), often used in combination with external beam therapy. The oncologic consequences of the limited treatment volume and duration associated with brachytherapy and IORT are not well understood. Accelerated partial breast irradiation with interstitial brachytherapy, intracavitary brachytherapy (MammoSite), IORT, and three-dimensional conformal external beam radiotherapy is being compared with whole breast irradiation in an intergroup phase III trial (NSABP B-39/Radiation Therapy Oncology Group 0413). Several additional studies of adjuvant IORT also are ongoing internationally.

Chemotherapy can be given before or concurrently with radiation. Chemotherapy before radiation has the advantage of reducing

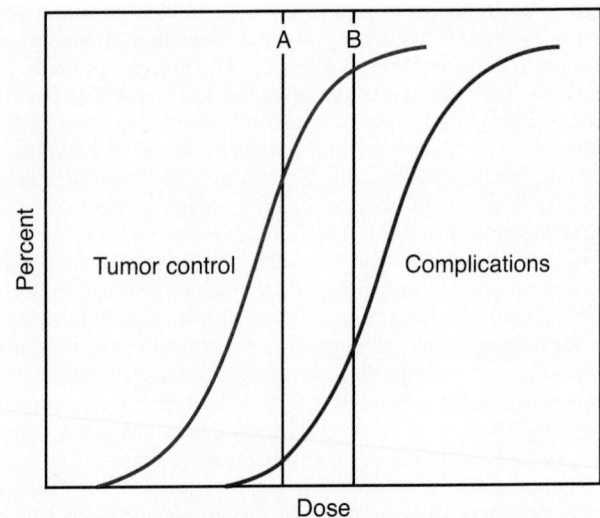

FIG. 10-13. The probability of tumor control and of complications at different radiation doses. *A.* At lower doses, the probability of complications is low, with a moderate chance of tumor control. *B.* Increasing the dose may gain a higher chance of tumor control at the price of significantly higher complication risks. *(Modified with permission from Eisbruch A, Lichter AS: What a surgeon needs to know about radiation. Ann Surg Oncol 4:516, 1997. With kind permission from Springer Science + Business Media.)*

the tumor burden, which facilitates radiation therapy. On the other hand, some chemotherapy regimens, when given concurrently with radiation, may sensitize the cells to radiation therapy.

Side Effects

Both tumor and normal tissue have radiation dose–response relationships that can be plotted as a sigmoidal curve (Fig. 10-13).[127] A minimum dose of radiation must be given before any response is seen. The response to radiation then increases slowly with an increase in dose. At a certain dose level the curves become exponential, with increases in tumor response and normal tissue toxicity with each incremental dose increase. The side effects of radiation therapy can be acute, occurring during or 2 to 3 weeks after therapy, or chronic, occurring weeks to years after therapy. The side effects depend on the tissue included in the target volume. Some of the major acute and chronic sequelae of radiation are summarized in Table 10-15.[127,128] In addition to these effects, a small increase in the risk for secondary malignancies is attributable to radiation therapy.

CANCER PREVENTION

The truth of the old axiom "An ounce of prevention is worth a pound of cure" is being increasingly recognized in oncology. Cancer prevention can be divided into three categories: (a) primary prevention (i.e., prevention of initial cancers in healthy individuals), (b) secondary prevention (i.e., prevention of cancer in individuals with premalignant conditions), and (c) tertiary prevention (i.e., prevention of second primary cancers in patients cured of their initial disease).

The systemic or local administration of therapeutic agents to prevent the development of cancer, called *chemoprevention*, is being actively explored for several cancer types. In breast cancer, the NSABP Breast Cancer Prevention Trial demonstrated that tamoxifen administration reduces the risk of breast cancer by one half and reduces the risk of estrogen receptor–positive tumors by 69% in high-risk patients.[129] Therefore, tamoxifen has been approved by the FDA for breast cancer chemoprevention. The subsequent NSABP P-2 trial demonstrated that raloxifene is as effective as tamoxifen in reducing the risk of invasive breast cancer and is associated with a lower risk of

TABLE 10-15	Local effects of radiation	
Organ	**Acute Changes**	**Chronic Changes**
Skin	Erythema, wet or dry desquamation, epilation	Telangiectasia, subcutaneous fibrosis, ulceration
GI tract	Nausea, diarrhea, edema, ulceration, hepatitis	Stricture, ulceration, perforation, hematochezia
Kidney	—	Nephropathy, renal insufficiency
Bladder	Dysuria	Hematuria, ulceration, perforation
Gonads	Sterility	Atrophy, ovarian failure
Hematopoietic tissue	Lymphopenia, neutropenia, thrombocytopenia	Pancytopenia
Bone	Epiphyseal growth arrest	Necrosis
Lung	Pneumonitis	Pulmonary fibrosis
Heart	—	Pericarditis, vascular damage
Upper aerodigestive tract	Mucositis, xerostomia, anosmia	Xerostomia, dental caries
Eye	Conjunctivitis	Cataract, keratitis, optic nerve atrophy
Nervous system	Cerebral edema	Necrosis, myelitis

Source: Modified with permission from Daly et al.[128]

thromboembolic events and cataracts but a nonstatistically significant higher risk of noninvasive breast cancer; these findings led the FDA to approve raloxifene for prevention as well. Several other agents are also under investigation.[130] Celecoxib has been shown to reduce polyp number and polyp burden in patients with familial adenomatous polyposis (FAP), which led to its approval by the FDA for these patients. In head and neck cancer, 13-*cis*-retinoic acid has been shown both to reverse oral leukoplakia and to reduce second primary tumor development.[131,132] Thus, the chemoprevention trials completed so far have demonstrated success in primary, secondary, and tertiary prevention. Although the successes of these chemoprevention studies are impressive, much remains to be done over the next few years to improve patient selection and decrease therapy-related toxic effects. It is important for surgeons to be aware of these preventive options, because they are likely to be involved in the diagnosis of premalignant and malignant conditions and will be the ones to counsel patients about their chemopreventive options.

In selected circumstances, the risk of cancer is high enough to justify surgical prevention. These high-risk settings include hereditary cancer syndromes such as hereditary breast-ovarian cancer syndrome, hereditary diffuse gastric cancer, multiple endocrine neoplasia type 2, FAP, and hereditary nonpolyposis colorectal cancer, as well as some nonhereditary conditions such as chronic ulcerative colitis. Most prophylactic surgeries are large ablative surgeries (e.g., bilateral risk-reducing mastectomy or total proctocolectomy). Therefore, it is important that the patient be completely informed about potential surgical complications as well as long-term lifestyle consequences. Further, the conservative options of close surveillance and chemoprevention need to be discussed. The patient's cancer risk needs to be assessed accurately and implications for survival discussed. Ultimately, the decision to proceed with surgical prevention should be individualized and made with caution.

TRENDS AND EVOLVING TECHNOLOGIES IN ONCOLOGY

Cancer Screening and Diagnosis

It is clear that the practice of oncology will change dramatically over the next few decades, because our understanding of the molecular basis of cancer and available technologies are evolving rapidly. One of the critical changes expected is earlier detection of cancers. With improvements in available imaging modalities and development of newer functional imaging techniques, it is likely that many tumors will be detected at earlier, more curable stages in the near future.

Another area of rapid development is the identification of serum markers. High-throughput technologies such as matrix-assisted laser desorption ionization time-of-flight mass spectroscopy and liquid chromatography ion-spray tandem mass spectroscopy have revolutionized the field of proteomics and are now being used to compare the serum protein profiles of patients with cancer with those of individuals without cancer. Identification of unique proteins as well as unique proteomic profiles for most cancer types is being pursued actively by many researchers and, if successful, could dramatically enhance our ability to detect cancers early.[133]

Surgical Therapy

The current trend in surgery is toward more conservative resections. With earlier identification of tumors, more conservative surgeries may be possible. The goal, however, is always to remove the tumor en bloc with wide negative margins. Another interesting area being explored is the destruction of tumors by techniques such as radiofrequency ablation, cryoablation, and heat-producing technologies like lasers, microwaves, or focused ultrasound. Pilot studies have demonstrated that radiofrequency ablation is effective for destruction of small primary breast cancers. Although this approach remains experimental and potentially of limited applicability because of the need for expertise in breast imaging, with the development of imaging technologies that can accurately map the extent of cancer cells, these types of noninvasive interventions are likely to come to the forefront. However, use of these techniques will be limited to treatment of cancers not involving hollow viscera.

The debate over how to manage the regional lymph node basins for certain cancer types continues. With an increasing understanding of the metastatic process, surgeons may be able to stratify patients on the basis of the likelihood that their disease will spread metastatically, based on the gene expression profile of their primary tumors, and offer regional therapy accordingly.

Systemic Therapy

The current trend in systemic therapy is toward individualized therapy. It is now presumed that all cancers of a certain cell origin are the same; thus all patients are offered the same systemic therapy. Not all patients respond to these therapies, however, which emphasizes the biologic variability within the tumor groups. Therefore, the intent is to determine the underlying biology of each tumor to tailor therapy accordingly. The transcriptional and proteomic profiling approaches are being used to identify molecular signatures that correlate with response to certain agents. It is likely that in the near future tumors can be tested and treatments individualized. Patients who will respond to conventional therapies can be treated with these regimens, whereas patients who will not respond will not, which spares them the toxicity. Instead, the latter patients can be offered novel therapies. Furthermore, with emerging biologic therapies, it is likely that patients may be given a combination of biologic therapies that specifically target the alterations in their own tumors. Patients can be genotyped for critical alleles that may affect drug metabolism and thus may influence the efficacy as well as the side effect of the drugs given. Finally, stratification of patients by gene expression profile for prognosis may assist in determining which patients are at higher risk of relapse, so that patients whose tumors have less aggressive biologic characteristics can be spared further therapy.

REFERENCES

Entries highlighted in bright blue are key references.

1. Jemal A, Siegel R, Ward E, et al: Cancer statistics, 2008. *CA Cancer J Clin* 58:71, 2008.

2. Ravdin PM, Cronin KA, Howlader N, et al: The decrease in breast-cancer incidence in 2003 in the United States. *N Engl J Med* 356:1670, 2007.

3. Parkin DM, Bray F, Ferlay J, et al: Global cancer statistics, 2002. *CA Cancer J Clin* 55:74, 2005.

4. Hanahan D, Weinberg RA: The hallmarks of cancer. *Cell* 100:57, 2000.

5. Pelengaris S, Khan M, Evan G: c-MYC: More than just a matter of life and death. *Nat Rev Cancer* 2:764, 2002.

6. Fearon ER, Vogelstein B: A genetic model for colorectal tumorigenesis. *Cell* 61:759, 1990.

7. Kastan M, Skapek S: Molecular biology of cancer: The cell cycle, in DeVita V, Hellman S, Rosenberg S (eds): *Cancer: Principles and Practice of Oncology,* 7th ed. Philadelphia: Lippincott Williams & Wilkins, 2005.

8. Eccles SA: The role of c-erbB-2/HER2/neu in breast cancer progression and metastasis. *J Mammary Gland Biol Neoplasia* 6:393, 2001.

9. Meric-Bernstam F, Hung MC: Advances in targeting human epidermal growth factor receptor-2 signaling for cancer therapy. *Clin Cancer Res* 12:6326, 2006.

10. Wang SC, Hung MC: HER2 overexpression and cancer targeting. *Semin Oncol* 28(5 Suppl 16):115, 2001.

11. Schechter AL, Stern DF, Vaidyanathan L, et al: The neu oncogene: An erb-B–related gene encoding a 185,000-Mr tumour antigen. *Nature* 312:513, 1984.

12. Malaney S, Daly RJ: The ras signaling pathway in mammary tumorigenesis and metastasis. *J Mammary Gland Biol Neoplasia* 6:101, 2001.

13. Shields JM, Pruitt K, McFall A, et al: Understanding Ras: "It ain't over 'til it's over." *Trends Cell Biol* 10:147, 2000.

14. Downward J: Targeting RAS signalling pathways in cancer therapy. *Nat Rev Cancer* 3:11, 2003.

15. Gollob JA, Wilhelm S, Carter C, et al: Role of Raf kinase in cancer: Therapeutic potential of targeting the Raf/MEK/ERK signal transduction pathway. *Semin Oncol* 33:392, 2006.

16. Kim R, Tanabe K, Uchida Y, et al: Current status of the molecular mechanisms of anticancer drug-induced apoptosis. The contribution of molecular-level analysis to cancer chemotherapy. *Cancer Chemother Pharmacol* 50:343, 2002.

17. Igney FH, Krammer PH: Death and anti-death: Tumour resistance to apoptosis. *Nat Rev Cancer* 2:277, 2002.

18. Yu EW, Koshland DE Jr.: Propagating conformational changes over long (and short) distances in proteins. *Proc Natl Acad Sci U S A* 98:9517, 2001.

19. Folkman J, Merler E, Abernathy C, et al: Isolation of a tumor factor responsible for angiogenesis. *J Exp Med* 133:275, 1971.

20. McCarty MF, Liu W, Fan F, et al: Promises and pitfalls of anti-angiogenic therapy in clinical trials. *Trends Mol Med* 9:53, 2003.

21. Soker S, Takashima S, Miao HQ, et al: Neuropilin-1 is expressed by endothelial and tumor cells as an isoform-specific receptor for vascular endothelial growth factor. *Cell* 92:735, 1998.

22. Stacker SA, Achen MG, Jussila L, et al: Lymphangiogenesis and cancer metastasis. *Nat Rev Cancer* 2:573, 2002.

23. He Y, Kozaki K, Karpanen T, et al: Suppression of tumor lymphangiogenesis and lymph node metastasis by blocking vascular endothelial growth factor receptor 3 signaling. *J Natl Cancer Inst* 94:819, 2002.

24. Steeg PS: Metastasis suppressors alter the signal transduction of cancer cells. *Nat Rev Cancer* 3:55, 2003.

25. Naumov GN, MacDonald IC, Weinmeister PM, et al: Persistence of solitary mammary carcinoma cells in a secondary site: A possible contributor to dormancy. *Cancer Res* 62:2162, 2002.

26. Demicheli R: Tumour dormancy: Findings and hypotheses from clinical research on breast cancer. *Semin Cancer Biol* 11:297, 2001.

27. Chambers AF, Groom AC, MacDonald IC: Dissemination and growth of cancer cells in metastatic sites. *Nat Rev Cancer* 2:563, 2002.

28. van de Vijver MJ, He YD, van't Veer LJ, et al: A gene-expression signature as a predictor of survival in breast cancer. *N Engl J Med* 347:1999, 2002.

29. Reya T, Morrison SJ, Clarke MF, et al: Stem cells, cancer, and cancer stem cells. *Nature* 414:105, 2001.

30. Marsh DJ, Zori RT: Genetic insights into familial cancers – update and recent discoveries. *Cancer Lett* 181:125, 2002.

31. Vahteristo P, Tamminen A, Karvinen P, et al: P53, CHK2, and CHK1 genes in Finnish families with Li-Fraumeni syndrome: Further evi-

dence of CHK2 in inherited cancer predisposition. *Cancer Res* 61:5718, 2001.

32. DiCiommo D, Gallie BL, Bremner R: Retinoblastoma: The disease, gene and protein provide critical leads to understand cancer. *Semin Cancer Biol* 10:255, 2000.

33. Knudson AG: Two genetic hits (more or less) to cancer. *Nat Rev Cancer* 1:157, 2001.

34. Harbour JW, Lai SL, Whang-Peng J, et al: Abnormalities in structure and expression of the human retinoblastoma gene in SCLC. *Science* 241:353, 1988.

35. Li FP, Fraumeni JF Jr.: Soft-tissue sarcomas, breast cancer, and other neoplasms. A familial syndrome? *Ann Intern Med* 71:747, 1969.

36. Li FP, Fraumeni JF Jr., Mulvihill JJ, et al: A cancer family syndrome in twenty-four kindreds. *Cancer Res* 48:5358, 1988.

37. Birch JM, Hartley AL, Tricker KJ, et al: Prevalence and diversity of constitutional mutations in the P53 gene among 21 Li-Fraumeni families. *Cancer Res* 54:1298, 1994.

38. Birch JM, Alston RD, McNally RJ, et al: Relative frequency and morphology of cancers in carriers of germline TP53 mutations. *Oncogene* 20:4621, 2001.

39. Birch JM, Blair V, Kelsey AM, et al: Cancer phenotype correlates with constitutional TP53 genotype in families with the Li-Fraumeni syndrome. *Oncogene* 17:1061, 1998.

40. Lee SB, Kim SH, Bell DW, et al: Destabilization of CHK2 by a missense mutation associated with Li-Fraumeni Syndrome. *Cancer Res* 61:8062, 2001.

41. Vahteristo P, Bartkova J, Eerola H, et al: A CHEK2 genetic variant contributing to a substantial fraction of familial breast cancer. *Am J Hum Genet* 71:432, 2002.

42. Loman N, Johannsson O, Kristoffersson U, et al: Family history of breast and ovarian cancers and BRCA1 and BRCA2 mutations in a population-based series of early-onset breast cancer. *J Natl Cancer Inst* 93:1215, 2001.

43. Ford D, Easton DF, Bishop DT, et al: Risks of cancer in BRCA1-mutation carriers. Breast Cancer Linkage Consortium. *Lancet* 343:692, 1994.

44. Ford D, Easton DF, Stratton M, et al: Genetic heterogeneity and penetrance analysis of the BRCA1 and BRCA2 genes in breast cancer families. The Breast Cancer Linkage Consortium. *Am J Hum Genet* 62:676, 1998.

45. Cancer risks in BRCA2 mutation carriers. The Breast Cancer Linkage Consortium. *J Natl Cancer Inst* 91:1310, 1999.

46. Venkitaraman AR: Cancer susceptibility and the functions of BRCA1 and BRCA2. *Cell* 108:171, 2002.

47. Liu Y, West SC: Distinct functions of BRCA1 and BRCA2 in double-strand break repair. *Breast Cancer Res* 4:9, 2002.

48. Venkitaraman AR: Functions of BRCA1 and BRCA2 in the biological response to DNA damage. *J Cell Sci* 114(Pt 20):3591, 2001.

49. Hedenfalk I, Duggan D, Chen Y, et al: Gene-expression profiles in hereditary breast cancer. *N Engl J Med* 344:539, 2001.

50. Sieber OM, Tomlinson IP, Lamlum H: The adenomatous polyposis coli (APC) tumour suppressor—genetics, function and disease. *Mol Med Today* 6:462, 2000.

51. Caspari R, Olschwang S, Friedl W, et al: Familial adenomatous polyposis: Desmoid tumours and lack of ophthalmic lesions (CHRPE) associated with APC mutations beyond codon 1444. *Hum Mol Genet* 4:337, 1995.

52. Davies DR, Armstrong JG, Thakker N, et al: Severe Gardner syndrome in families with mutations restricted to a specific region of the APC gene. *Am J Hum Genet* 57:1151, 1995.

53. Lynch HT, Smyrk TC, Watson P, et al: Genetics, natural history, tumor spectrum, and pathology of hereditary nonpolyposis colorectal cancer: An updated review. *Gastroenterology* 104:1535, 1993.

54. Vasen HF, Watson P, Mecklin JP, et al: New clinical criteria for hereditary nonpolyposis colorectal cancer (HNPCC, Lynch syndrome) proposed by the International Collaborative group on HNPCC. *Gastroenterology* 116:1453, 1999.

55. Leach FS, Nicolaides NC, Papadopoulos N, et al: Mutations of a mutS homolog in hereditary nonpolyposis colorectal cancer. *Cell* 75:1215, 1993.

56. Fishel R, Lescoe MK, Rao MR, et al: The human mutator gene homolog MSH2 and its association with hereditary nonpolyposis colon cancer. *Cell* 75:1027, 1993.

57. Miyaki M, Konishi M, Tanaka K, et al: Germline mutation of MSH6 as the cause of hereditary nonpolyposis colorectal cancer. *Nat Genet* 17:271, 1997.

58. Bronner CE, Baker SM, Morrison PT, et al: Mutation in the DNA mismatch repair gene homologue hMLH1 is associated with hereditary non-polyposis colon cancer. *Nature* 368:258, 1994.

59. Papadopoulos N, Nicolaides NC, Wei YF, et al: Mutation of a mutL homolog in hereditary colon cancer. *Science* 263:1625, 1994.

60. Nicolaides NC, Papadopoulos N, Liu B, et al: Mutations of two PMS homologues in hereditary nonpolyposis colon cancer. *Nature* 371:75, 1994.

61. Steck PA, Pershouse MA, Jasser SA, et al: Identification of a candidate tumour suppressor gene, MMAC1, at chromosome 10q23.3 that is mutated in multiple advanced cancers. *Nat Genet* 15:356, 1997.

62. Liaw D, Marsh DJ, Li J, et al: Germline mutations of the PTEN gene in Cowden disease, an inherited breast and thyroid cancer syndrome. *Nat Genet* 16:64, 1997.

63. Eng C: Will the real Cowden syndrome please stand up: Revised diagnostic criteria. *J Med Genet* 37:828, 2000.

64. Greene MH: The genetics of hereditary melanoma and nevi. 1998 update. *Cancer* 86(11 Suppl):2464, 1999.

65. Goldstein AM, Fraser MC, Struewing JP, et al: Increased risk of pancreatic cancer in melanoma-prone kindreds with p16INK4 mutations. *N Engl J Med* 333:970, 1995.

66. Fitzgerald RC, Caldas C: E-cadherin mutations and hereditary gastric cancer: Prevention by resection? *Dig Dis* 20:23, 2002.

67. Berx G, Van Roy F: The E-cadherin/catenin complex: An important gatekeeper in breast cancer tumorigenesis and malignant progression. *Breast Cancer Res* 3:289, 2001.

68. Alsanea O, Clark OH: Familial thyroid cancer. *Curr Opin Oncol* 13:44, 2001.

69. Redmond DE Jr.: Tobacco and cancer: The first clinical report, 1761. *N Engl J Med* 282:18, 1970.

70. *http://monographs.iarc.fr/ENG/Classification/index.php:* IARC Monographs on the Evaluation of Carcinogenic Risks to Humans, Complete List of Agents Evaluated and Their Classification, International Agency for Research on Cancer (IARC) [accessed January 16, 2008].

71. Timblin C, Jannsen-Heininger Y, Mossman B: Physical agents in human carcinogenesis, in Coleman W, Tsongalis G (eds): *The Molecular Basis of Human Cancer.* Totowa, NJ: Humana Press, 2002, p 223.

72. Stanton MF, Layard M, Tegeris A, et al: Relation of particle dimension to carcinogenicity in amphibole asbestoses and other fibrous minerals. *J Natl Cancer Inst* 67:965, 1981.

73. Rous P: A transmissible avian neoplasm. (Sarcoma of the common fowl) by Peyton Rous, M.D., *Experimental Medicine* for Sept. 1, 1910, vol. 12, pp. 696-705. *J Exp Med* 150:738, 1979.

74. *http://monographs.iarc.fr/ENG/Classification/crthgr01.php:* IARC Monographs on the Evaluation of Carcinogenic Risks to Humans, Overall Evaluations of Carcinogenicity to Humans: Group 1: Carcinogenic to Humans, International Agency for Research on Cancer (IARC) [accessed January 16, 2008].

75. Butel JS: Viral carcinogenesis: Revelation of molecular mechanisms and etiology of human disease. *Carcinogenesis* 21:405, 2000.

76. El-Serag HB: Hepatocellular carcinoma and hepatitis C in the United States. *Hepatology* 36(5 Suppl 1):S74, 2002.

77. Koutsky LA, Ault KA, Wheeler CM, et al: A controlled trial of a human papillomavirus type 16 vaccine. *N Engl J Med* 347:1645, 2002.

78. Whitman G, Stelling C: Stereotactic core needle biopsy of breast lesions: Experience at the University of Texas M. D. Anderson Cancer Center, in Singletary S (ed): *Breast Cancer.* New York: Springer-Verlag, 1999, p 4.

79. Gail MH, Brinton LA, Byar DP, et al: Projecting individualized probabilities of developing breast cancer for white females who are being examined annually. *J Natl Cancer Inst* 81:1879, 1989.

80. *http://www.cancer.gov/bcrisktool:* Breast Cancer Risk Assessment Tool, National Cancer Institute [accessed December 26, 2008].

81. Bach PB, Kattan MW, Thornquist MD, et al: Variations in lung cancer risk among smokers. *J Natl Cancer Inst* 95:470, 2003.

82. Bassett L, Hendrick R, Bassford T: Quality Determinants of Mammography. Clinical Practice Guideline No. 13, Agency for Health Care Policy and Research Publication No. 95-0632. Rockville, MD: U.S. Department of Health and Human Services, 1994.

83. Smith RA, Cokkinides V, Brawley OW. Cancer screening in the United States, 2009: a review of current American Cancer Society guidelines and issues in cancer screening. *CA Cancer J Clin* 59:27, 2009. Review.

84. Saslow D, Boetes C, Burke W, et al: American Cancer Society guidelines for breast screening with MRI as an adjunct to mammography. *CA Cancer J Clin* 57:75, 2007.

85. Jacobs TW, Connolly JL, Schnitt SJ: Nonmalignant lesions in breast core needle biopsies: To excise or not to excise? *Am J Surg Pathol* 26:1095, 2002.

86. Harris L, Fritsche H, Mennel R, et al: American Society of Clinical Oncology 2007 update of recommendations for the use of tumor markers in breast cancer. *J Clin Oncol* 25:5287, 2007.

87. Locker GY, Hamilton S, Harris J, et al: ASCO 2006 update of recommendations for the use of tumor markers in gastrointestinal cancer. *J Clin Oncol* 24:5313, 2006.

88. Way BA, Kessler G: Tumor marker overview. *Lab Med Newsl* 4:1, 1996.

89. Paik S, Shak S, Tang G, et al: A multigene assay to predict recurrence of tamoxifen-treated, node-negative breast cancer. *N Engl J Med* 351:2817, 2004.

90. van 't Veer LJ, Dai H, van de Vijver MJ, et al: Gene expression profiling predicts clinical outcome of breast cancer. *Nature* 415:530, 2002.

91. Sirovich BE, Schwartz LM, Woloshin S: Screening men for prostate and colorectal cancer in the United States: Does practice reflect the evidence? *JAMA* 289:1414, 2003.

92. Catalona WJ, Richie JP, deKernion JB, et al: Comparison of prostate specific antigen concentration versus prostate specific antigen density in the early detection of prostate cancer: Receiver operating characteristic curves. *J Urol* 152(6 Pt 1):2031, 1994.

93. *http://www.labcorp.com/datasets/labcorp/html/chapter/mono/ri000600. htm:* Alpha-Fetoprotein (AFP), Serum, Tumor Marker (Serial Monitor), Laboratory Corporation of America [accessed December 26, 2008].

94. Nguyen MH, Keeffe EB: Screening for hepatocellular carcinoma. *J Clin Gastroenterol* 35(5 Suppl 2):S86, 2002.

95. Chan DW, Beveridge RA, Muss H, et al: Use of Truquant BR radioimmunoassay for early detection of breast cancer recurrence in patients with stage II and stage III disease. *J Clin Oncol* 15:2322, 1997.

96. Outcomes of cancer treatment for technology assessment and cancer treatment guidelines. American Society of Clinical Oncology. *J Clin Oncol* 14:671, 1996.

97. Cristofanilli M, Budd GT, Ellis MJ, et al: Circulating tumor cells, disease progression, and survival in metastatic breast cancer. *N Engl J Med* 351:781, 2004.

98. Scoggins CR, Ross MI, Reintgen DS, et al: Prospective multi-institutional study of reverse transcriptase polymerase chain reaction for molecular staging of melanoma. *J Clin Oncol* 24:2849, 2006.

99. Braun S, Vogl FD, Naume B, et al: A pooled analysis of bone marrow micrometastasis in breast cancer. *N Engl J Med* 353:793, 2005.

100. Janni W, Rack B, Lindemann K, et al: Detection of micrometastatic disease in bone marrow: Is it ready for prime time? *Oncologist* 10:480, 2005.

101. Grau A, Spitz F, Bouvet M: Pancreatic adenocarcinoma, in Feig B, Berger D, Fuhrman G (eds): *The M. D. Anderson Surgical Oncology Handbook.* Philadelphia: Lippincott Williams & Wilkins, 2003, p 303.

102. Balch CM, Soong SJ, Smith T, et al: Long-term results of a prospective surgical trial comparing 2 cm vs. 4 cm excision margins for 740 patients with 1-4 mm melanomas. *Ann Surg Oncol* 8:101, 2001.

103. Moore HG, Riedel E, Minsky BD, et al: Adequacy of 1-cm distal margin after restorative rectal cancer resection with sharp mesorectal excision and preoperative combined-modality therapy. *Ann Surg Oncol* 10:80, 2003.

104. Kapiteijn E, van de Velde CJ: The role of total mesorectal excision in the management of rectal cancer. *Surg Clin North Am* 82:995, 2002.

105. Meric F, Hunt KK: Surgical options for breast cancer, in Hunt KK, Robb GL, Strom EA, et al (eds): *Breast Cancer.* New York: Springer-Verlag, 2001, p 187. MD Anderson Cancer Care Series.

106. Cabanas RM: An approach for the treatment of penile carcinoma. *Cancer* 39:456, 1977.

107. Viale G, Dell'orto P, Biasi MO, et al: Comparative evaluation of an extensive histopathologic examination and a real-time reverse-transcription-polymerase chain reaction assay for mammaglobin and cytokeratin 19 on axillary sentinel lymph nodes of breast carcinoma patients. *Ann Surg* 247:136, 2008.

108. Querzoli P, Pedriali M, Rinaldi R, et al: Axillary lymph node nanometastases are prognostic factors for disease-free survival and metastatic relapse in breast cancer patients. *Clin Cancer Res* 12:6696, 2006.

109. Mocellin S, Pilati P, Lise M, et al: Meta-analysis of hepatic arterial infusion for unresectable liver metastases from colorectal cancer: The end of an era? *J Clin Oncol* 25:5649, 2007.

110. Pearson AS, Izzo F, Fleming RY, et al: Intraoperative radiofrequency ablation or cryoablation for hepatic malignancies. *Am J Surg* 178:592, 1999.

111. Curley SA, Izzo F: Radiofrequency ablation of primary and metastatic hepatic malignancies. *Int J Clin Oncol* 7:72, 2002.

112. Fisher B, Bryant J, Wolmark N, et al: Effect of preoperative chemotherapy on the outcome of women with operable breast cancer. *J Clin Oncol* 16:2672, 1998.

113. Meric F, Hess KR, Varma DG, et al: Radiographic response to neoadjuvant chemotherapy is a predictor of local control and survival in soft tissue sarcomas. *Cancer* 95:1120, 2002.

114. Therasse P, Arbuck SG, Eisenhauer EA, et al: New guidelines to evaluate the response to treatment in solid tumors. European Organization for Research and Treatment of Cancer, National Cancer Institute of the United States, National Cancer Institute of Canada. *J Natl Cancer Inst* 92:205, 2000.

115. Page R: Principles of chemotherapy, in Pazdur R, Hoskins W, Coia L (eds): *Cancer Management: A Multidisciplinary Approach.* Melville, NY: PRR, 2001, p 21.

116. Morrow C, Cowan K: Drug resistance and its clinical circumvention, in Bast R, Kufe D, Pollock R (eds): *Cancer Medicine.* Hamilton, Ontario: BC Decker, 2000, p 539.

117. Miller AB, Hoogstraten B, Staquet M, et al: Reporting results of cancer treatment. *Cancer* 47:207, 1981.

118. Mocellin S, Rossi CR, Lise M, et al: Adjuvant immunotherapy for solid tumors: From promise to clinical application. *Cancer Immunol Immunother* 51:583, 2002.

119. Perales MA, Wolchok JD: Melanoma vaccines. *Cancer Invest* 20:1012, 2002.

120. Lizee G, Cantu MA, Hwu P: Less yin, more yang: Confronting the barriers to cancer immunotherapy. *Clin Cancer Res* 13(18 Pt 1):5250, 2007.

121. Dermime S, Armstrong A, Hawkins RE, et al: Cancer vaccines and immunotherapy. *Br Med Bull* 62:149, 2002.

122. Berinstein NL: Enhancing cancer vaccines with immunomodulators. *Vaccine* 25(Suppl 2):B72, 2007.

123. Cranmer LD, Hersh E: The role of the CTLA4 blockade in the treatment of malignant melanoma. *Cancer Invest* 25:613, 2007.

124. Cusack JC Jr., Tanabe KK: Introduction to cancer gene therapy. *Surg Oncol Clin North Am* 11:497, 2002.

125. Mundt A, Roeske J, Weichelbaum R: Principles of radiation oncology, in Bast R, Kuff D, Pollock R (eds): *Cancer Medicine.* Hamilton, Ontario: BC Decker, 2000, p 465.

126. Raju MR, Carpenter SG: A heavy particle comparative study. Part IV: Acute and late reactions. *Br J Radiol* 51:720, 1978.

127. Eisbruch A, Lichter AS: What a surgeon needs to know about radiation. *Ann Surg Oncol* 4:516, 1997.

128. Daly J, Bertagnolli M, JJ D: Oncology, in Schwartz S, Spencer F, Galloway A (eds): *Principles of Surgery.* New York: McGraw-Hill, 1999, p 297.

129. Fisher B, Costantino JP, Wickerham DL, et al: Tamoxifen for prevention of breast cancer: Report of the National Surgical Adjuvant Breast and Bowel Project P-1 Study. *J Natl Cancer Inst* 90:1371, 1998.

130. Vogel VG, Costantino JP, Wickerham DL, et al: Effects of tamoxifen vs raloxifene on the risk of developing invasive breast cancer and other disease outcomes: The NSABP Study of Tamoxifen and Raloxifene (STAR) P-2 trial. *JAMA* 295:2727, 2006.

131. Lippman SM, Batsakis JG, Toth BB, et al: Comparison of low-dose isotretinoin with beta carotene to prevent oral carcinogenesis. *N Engl J Med* 328:15, 1993.

132. Hong WK, Lippman SM, Itri LM, et al: Prevention of second primary tumors with isotretinoin in squamous-cell carcinoma of the head and neck. *N Engl J Med* 323:795, 1990.

133. Sidransky D: Emerging molecular markers of cancer. *Nat Rev Cancer* 2:210, 2002.

BACKGROUND

Although references to transplantation have existed in the scientific literature for centuries, the field of modern transplantation did not come into being until the latter half of the twentieth century. Thus, given its short history, it is truly remarkable how far this area of medicine has advanced. From an experimental procedure just 50 years ago, transplantation has evolved to become the treatment of choice for end-stage organ failure resulting from almost any of a wide variety of causes. Transplantation of the kidney, liver, pancreas, intestine, heart, and lung has now become commonplace in all parts of the world.

In fact, transplantation is now so widely accepted and successful that the main problem facing the field today is not surgical technique, rejection, or management of complications, but rather supply of organs. An increasing number of diseases and patients are now potentially treatable with transplants; however, this increase, coupled with the decrease in contraindications to transplants, has meant an increasing number of patients are now awaiting organ replacement therapy. The number of transplants performed yearly has increased over the last decade, but has not kept pace with the steadily growing waiting list. As a result, the gap is ever widening between the number of transplants performed and the number of waiting patients (Fig. 11-1).

Transplantation statistics in the United States are tracked by the United Network for Organ Sharing (UNOS). By the end of 2007, roughly 98,000 patients were awaiting a transplant, while the number of transplants performed in that year was approximately 28,000.

DEFINITIONS

Transplantation is the act of transferring an organ, tissue, or cell from one place to another. Broadly speaking, transplants are divided into three categories based on the similarity between the donor and the recipient: autotransplants, allotransplants, and xenotransplants. *Autotransplants* involve the transfer of tissue or organs from one part of an individual to another part of the same individual. They are the most common type of transplants and include skin grafts, vein grafts for bypasses, bone and cartilage transplants, and nerve trans-

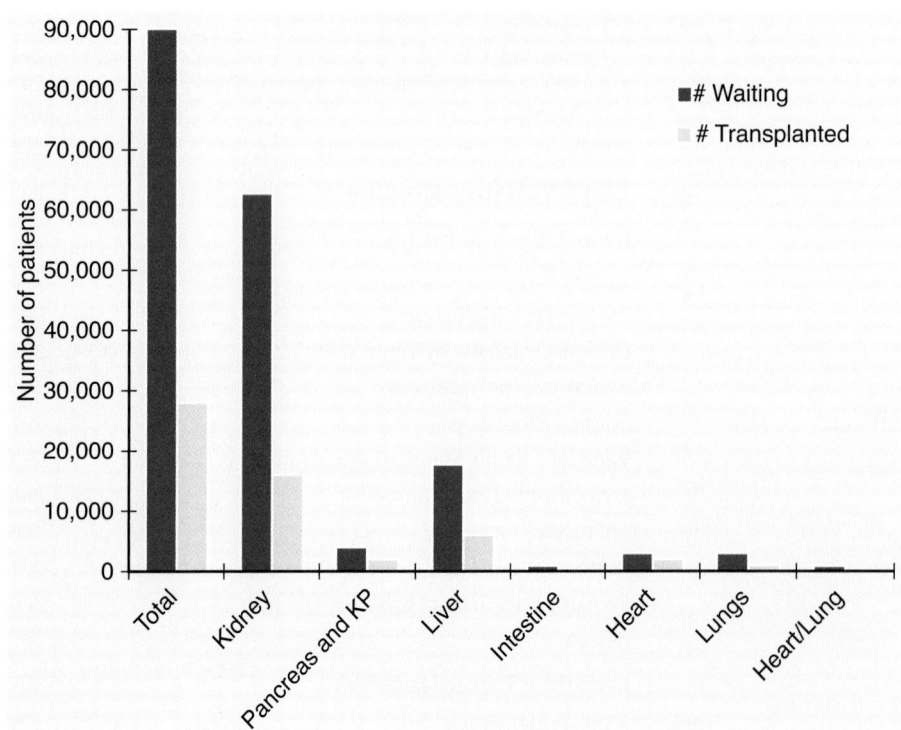

FIG. 11-1. Patients on waiting list and number of organ transplants for 2005. (U.S. data from Organ Procurement and Transplantation Network/Scientific Registry of Transplant Recipients Annual Report, *http://www.ustransplant.org*). KP = kidney and pancreas.

plants. Because the donor and the recipient are the same person and no immunologic disparity exists, no immunosuppression is required. *Allotransplants* involve transfer from one individual to a different individual of the same species—the most common scenario for most solid organ transplants performed today. Immunosuppression is required for allograft recipients to prevent rejection. Finally, *xenotransplants* involve transfer across species barriers. Currently, xenotransplants are largely relegated to the laboratory, given the complex, potent immunologic barriers to success.

This chapter deals mainly with allotransplantation. The first part discusses immunobiology, mechanisms of the rejection process, and medications currently used to achieve immunosuppression. The second part focuses on the various transplants, including kidney, pancreas, islet cell, liver, intestine, heart, and lungs. Clinical indications, surgical care, and posttransplant follow-up of these abdominal and thoracic organ recipients are described.

HISTORY

Attempts at transplantation have been documented since ancient times, but they are largely of only historic interest. They had no lasting impact on the field of modern transplantation, which did not originate until the latter half of the twentieth century. Important events in the first half of the twentieth century included the development of the surgical techniques for vascular anastomosis by Alexis Carrel; the first human-to-human kidney transplants by Yu Yu Voronoy in the 1930s (which were unsuccessful because of failure to address the immunologic barriers); and the studies of skin transplantation in animal models by Sir Peter Medawar in the 1940s.[1-3] Medawar's work was especially crucial: It provided scientific evidence for the role of the immune system in the failure of allografts to function long term, through a process later termed *rejection*. His work and observations formed the basis for modern transplant immunobiology.

The first human kidney transplant with long-term success was performed in Boston by Joseph Murray in 1954.[4] Because it was a living-donor transplant between identical twin brothers, the recipient required no immunosuppression and lived for more than 20 years, eventually dying of coronary artery disease. Soon, other centers performed similar transplants, which then led to attempts at kidney transplants between nonidentical individuals, using total body radiation and agents such as 6-mercaptopurine for immunosuppression. By the late 1950s to early 1960s, the combination of azathioprine (AZA) with corticosteroids allowed kidney allotransplantation to advance out of the realm of experimental therapy.[5,6]

Along with AZA and corticosteroids, the development of antilymphocyte serum (antibodies against human lymphoid tissue) gave clinicians reliable, adequate immunosuppression, allowing the birth of extrarenal transplants.[7] In 1963, the first liver transplant was performed by Thomas Starzl in Denver. The first pancreas transplant was performed in 1966 in Minneapolis by William Kelly and Richard Lillehei. Christiaan Barnard performed the first heart transplant in 1967 in Cape Town, South Africa. The 1970s saw other firsts with intestine, lung, and islet transplants.

Kidney transplants flourished during the 1970s, but extrarenal transplants remained largely experimental. One major reason was that rejection remained a major obstacle to the success of these transplanted organs. A dramatic change occurred, however, with the introduction in the early 1980s of cyclosporine. At that time, it was the most specific immunosuppressive agent available. It improved graft survival after kidney transplants by 30% and allowed extrarenal transplants to develop as viable therapies. Since that time, and especially in the 1990s, many new agents have been developed and approved for use in clinical transplantation; scores of others are currently being tested in clinical trials. These agents have allowed for progressively more specific targeting of the immune system pathways involved in the rejection process. As a result, rejection rates have substantially declined for all types of transplants, and graft survival rates have increased.

A large part of the recent success of transplants is due to the developments in clinical immunosuppression. But other discoveries also have played a role. More powerful immunosuppression has often meant more risk of infection with opportunistic viral, fungal, and bacterial pathogens. The development of powerful and effective antimicrobial, antifungal, and antiviral therapy (in parallel with immunosuppressive agents) has been crucial to successful solid organ transplantation.

Surgical innovations, beyond the first successful attempts at the various transplants, have continued. In the late 1980s and early 1990s, the development of deceased-donor split-liver transplant techniques and of living-donor liver transplants expanded the donor pool and helped alleviate the significant shortage of donors. The development of laparoscopic donor nephrectomy enabled faster recovery of living kidney donors, thereby increasing their numbers. The 1990s ushered in innovations with thoracic, pancreatic, and cellular transplants.

TRANSPLANT IMMUNOBIOLOGY

The technical advances and techniques that made transplants possible were described almost a hundred years ago. Yet it was only after a basic understanding of transplant immunobiology was obtained that the obstacle of rejection could be overcome, thus making clinical transplants possible. The success of transplants today is due in large part to control of the rejection process, thanks to an ever-deepening understanding of the immune process triggered by a transplant.[8]

KEY POINTS

1. The field of transplantation has made tremendous advances in the last 30 years, due mainly to refinements of surgical technique and development of effective immunosuppression medications.

2. Although immunosuppression drugs are essential for transplant, they are associated with significant short- and long-term morbidity.

3. Kidney transplantation now represents the treatment of choice for almost all patients with end-stage renal disease.

4. Liver transplantation is the viable option at present for patients with end-stage organ failure.

5. Pancreas transplantation and in the future islet cell transplantation represent the most reliable way to achieve euglycemia in the poorly controlled diabetic patient.

6. Opportunistic infections can be significantly lowered by the use of appropriate prophylaxis agents.

The immune system is important not only in graft rejection, but also in the body's defense system against viral, bacterial, fungal, and other pathogens. It also helps prevent tumor growth and helps the body respond to shock and trauma. As with the body's reaction to an infection, graft rejection is triggered when specific cells of the transplant recipient, namely T and B lymphocytes, recognize foreign antigens.

TRANSPLANT ANTIGENS

The main antigens involved in triggering rejection are coded for by a group of genes known as the *major histocompatibility complex* (MHC). These antigens, and hence genes, define the "foreign" nature of one individual to another within the same species. In humans, the MHC complex is known as the *human leukocyte antigen* (HLA) system. It comprises a series of genes located on chromosome 6. The HLA antigens are grouped into two classes, which differ in their structure and cellular distribution. Class I molecules (named HLA-A, -B, and -C) are found on the membrane of all nucleated cells. Class II molecules (named HLA-DR, -DP, and -DQ) generally are expressed by antigen-presenting cells (APCs) such as B lymphocytes, monocytes, and dendritic cells.

In a nontransplant setting, the function of the HLA gene product is to present antigens as fragments of foreign proteins that can be recognized by T lymphocytes. In the transplant setting, HLA molecules can initiate rejection and graft damage via either humoral or cellular mechanisms. Humoral rejection occurs if the recipient has circulating antibodies specific to the donor's HLA. These antibodies may be from prior exposure (i.e., blood transfusion, previous transplant, or pregnancy), or posttransplant, the recipient may develop antibodies specific to the donor's HLA. The antibodies then bind to the donor's recognized foreign antigens, activating the complement cascade and leading to cell lysis. The blood group antigens of the ABO system, although not part of the HLA system, may also trigger this form of humoral rejection.

Cellular rejection is the more common type of rejection after organ transplants. Mediated by T lymphocytes, it results from their activation and proliferation after exposure to donor MHC molecules.

ALLORECOGNITION AND DESTRUCTION

The recognition of foreign HLA antigens by the recipient T cells is referred to as *allorecognition*.[9] This process may occur by either a direct or an indirect pathway. In the direct pathway, the recipient's T cells directly interact with donor HLA molecules, leading to the generation of activated cytotoxic T cells. In the indirect pathway, the recipient's own APCs first process the donor's antigens (which may be shed from the parenchymal cells of the graft into the recipient's circulation, or alternatively may be encountered by the recipient's APCs in the graft itself); then the recipient's APCs present the donor's antigens to the recipient T cells, leading to the activation of those T cells.

Regardless of the method of presentation of foreign MHC, the subsequent steps are similar. Binding of the T cell to the foreign molecule occurs at the T-cell receptor (TCR)-CD3 complex on the surface of the lymphocyte. This binding leads to transduction of a signal to the cell, named *signal 1*. This signal by itself, however, is not sufficient to result in T-cell activation. Full activation requires transduction of a second signal that is not antigen dependent. Signal 2 is provided by the binding of accessory molecules on the T cell to corresponding molecules (ligands) on the APC. An example is CD25 on the T lymphocytes binding with its ligand B7 on the surface of the APC. Transmission of signal 1 and 2 to the cell nucleus leads to interleukin-2 (IL-2) gene expression and to production of this important cytokine. IL-2 then permits the entire cascade of T-cell activation to proceed, leading to proliferation and differentiation of these cells into cells capable of causing damage to the graft.

T-cell activation is key in initiating the rejection process, but B-cell activation and antibody production also play a role. Foreign antigens are acquired by immunoglobulin (Ig) receptors on the surface of B cells. These antigens are then processed similarly to the way that APCs process the donor's antigens. The antigen-presenting B cells can then interact with activated helper T cells. This interaction leads to B-cell proliferation, differentiation into plasma cells, and to antibody production.

CLINICAL REJECTION

Graft rejection is a complex process involving several components, including T lymphocytes, B lymphocytes, macrophages, and cytokines, with resultant local inflammatory injury and graft damage.[10-12] Rejection can be classified into four types, based on timing and pathogenesis: *hyperacute, accelerated acute, acute,* and *chronic.*

Hyperacute

This type of rejection, which usually occurs within minutes after the transplanted organ is reperfused, is due to the presence of pre-formed antibodies in the recipient, antibodies that are specific to the donor. These antibodies may be directed against the donor's HLA antigens or they may be anti-ABO blood group antibodies. Either way, they bind to the vascular endothelium in the graft and activate the complement cascade, leading to platelet activation and to diffuse intravascular coagulation. The result is a swollen, darkened graft, which undergoes ischemic necrosis. This type of rejection generally is not reversible, so prevention is key.

Prevention is best done by making sure the graft is ABO-compatible and by performing a pretransplant cross-match. The cross-match is an in vitro test that involves mixing the donor's cells with the recipient's serum to look for evidence of donor cell destruction by recipient antibodies. A positive cross-match indicates the presence of preformed antibodies in the recipient that are specific to the donor, thus a high risk of hyperacute rejection if the transplant is performed.

Accelerated Acute

This type of rejection, seen within the first few days posttransplant, involves both cellular and antibody-mediated injury. It is more common when a recipient has been sensitized by previous exposure to antigens present in the donor, resulting in an immunologic memory response.

Acute

This used to be the most common type of rejection, but with modern immunosuppression, it is becoming less and less common. Acute rejection usually is seen within days to a few months posttransplant. It is predominantly a cell-mediated process, with lymphocytes being the main cells involved. Biopsy of the affected organ demonstrates a cellular infiltrate, with membrane damage and apoptosis of graft cells. The process may be associated with systemic symptoms such as fever, chills, malaise, and arthralgias. However, with current immunosuppressive drugs, most acute rejection episodes are generally asymptomatic. They usually manifest with abnormal laboratory values (e.g., elevated creatinine in kidney transplant recipients, and elevated transaminase levels in liver transplant recipients).

Acute rejection episodes may also be mediated by a humoral, rather than cellular, immune response. B cells may generate antidonor antibodies, which can damage the graft. Establishing the diagnosis may be difficult, as biopsy may not demonstrate a significant cellular infiltrate; special immunologic stains may be necessary.

Chronic

This form of rejection occurs months to years posttransplant. Now that short-term graft survival rates have improved so markedly, chronic rejection is an increasingly common problem. Histologically, the process is characterized by atrophy, fibrosis, and arteriosclerosis. Both immune and nonimmune mechanisms are likely involved. Clinically, graft function slowly deteriorates over months to years posttransplant.

CLINICAL IMMUNOSUPPRESSION

The success of modern transplantation is in large part due to the successful development of effective immunosuppressive agents. Without these agents, only transplants between genetically identical individuals would be possible. In the 1960s, just two immunosuppressive agents were available, but more than 15 agents are now approved in the United States by the Food and Drug Administration (FDA) for clinical immunosuppression, with scores of others in various stages of clinical trials (Table 11-1). Thus the therapeutic armamentarium for transplant patients has broadened significantly, with a variety of drug combinations and protocols. Characteristics of some common immunosuppressive agents are shown in Table 11-2.

Immunosuppressive drugs generally are used in combination with others rather than alone. *Induction immunosuppression* refers to the drugs administered immediately posttransplant to induce immunosuppression. *Maintenance immunosuppression* refers to the drugs administered to maintain immunosuppression once recipients have recovered from the operative procedure.

Individual drugs can be categorized as either biologic or nonbiologic agents. *Biologic agents* consist of antibody preparations directed at various cells or receptors involved in the rejection process; they generally are used in induction (rather than maintenance) protocols. *Nonbiologic agents* form the mainstay of maintenance protocols.

Nonbiologic Agents
Corticosteroids

Historically, corticosteroids represent the first family of drugs used for clinical immunosuppression. Today steroids remain an integral component of most immunosuppressive protocols, and often are the first-line agents in the treatment of acute rejection. Despite their

TABLE 11-1 Immunosuppressive drugs by grouping

Immunophilin binders
  Calcineurin inhibitors
    Cyclosporine
    Tacrolimus
  Noninhibitors of calcineurin
    Sirolimus
Antimetabolites
  Inhibitors of de novo purine synthesis
    Azathioprine
    Mycophenolate mofetil
  Inhibitors of de novo pyrimidine synthesis
    Leflunomide
Biologic immunosuppression
  Polyclonal antibodies
    ATGAM
    Antithymocyte immunoglobulin
  Monoclonal antibodies
    Muromonab-CD3
    IL-2R (humanized)
    Belatacept
    Alemtuzumab
    Rituximab
Others
  Corticosteroids
  JAK-3 inhibitor
  Protein kinase C inhibitor (e.g., AEB)

ATGAM = antithymocyte globulin; IL-2R = interleukin-2R; JAK-3 = Janus kinase-3.

proven benefit, steroids have significant side effects, especially with long-term use. Hence, there has been considerable interest recently in withdrawing steroids from long-term maintenance protocols. The newer immunosuppressive agents may make doing so possible.

Steroids have both anti-inflammatory and immunosuppressive properties as the two are closely related. Their effects on the immune

TABLE 11-2 Summary of the main immunosuppressive drugs

Drug	Mechanism of Action	Adverse Effects	Clinical Uses	Dosage
Cyclosporine (CSA)	Binds to cyclophilin; Inhibits calcineurin and IL-2 synthesis	Nephrotoxicity; Tremor; Hypertension; Hirsutism	Improved bioavailability of microemulsion form; Used as mainstay of maintenance protocols	Oral dose is 8–10 mg/kg per day (given in two divided doses)
Tacrolimus (FK506)	Binds to FKBP; Inhibits calcineurin and IL-2 synthesis	Nephrotoxicity; Hypertension; Neurotoxicity; GI toxicity (nausea, diarrhea)	Improved patient and graft survival in (liver) primary and rescue therapy; Used as mainstay of maintenance, like CSA	IV 0.05–0.1 mg/kg per day; PO 0.15–0.3 mg/kg per day (given q12h)
Mycophenolate mofetil	Antimetabolite; Inhibits enzyme necessary for de novo purine synthesis	Leukopenia; GI toxicity	Effective for primary and rescue therapy (kidney transplants); May replace azathioprine	1 g bid PO (may need 1.5 g in black recipients)
Sirolimus	Inhibits lymphocyte effects driven by IL-2 receptor	Thrombocytopenia; Increased serum cholesterol/LDL; Vasculitis (animal studies)	May allow early withdrawal of steroids and decreased calcineurin doses	2–4 mg/d, adjusted to trough drug levels
Corticosteroids	Multiple actions; Anti-inflammatory; Inhibits lymphokine production	Cushingoid state; Glucose intolerance; Osteoporosis	Used in induction, maintenance, and treatment of acute rejection	Varies from mg to several grams/d; Maintenance doses, 5–10 mg/d
Azathioprine	Antimetabolite; Interferes with DNA and RNA synthesis	Thrombocytopenia; Neutropenia; Liver dysfunction	Used in maintenance protocols	1–3 mg/kg per day for maintenance

FKBP = FK506-binding protein; IL = interleukin; LDL = low-density lipoprotein.

system are complex. Although they have been used clinically for years, their exact mechanism of action is not fully understood. Primarily, they inhibit the production of T-cell lymphokines, which are needed to amplify macrophage and lymphocyte responses. Steroids also have a number of other immunosuppressive effects that are not as specific. For example, they cause lymphopenia secondary to the redistribution of lymphocytes from the vascular compartment back to lymphoid tissue, inhibit migration of monocytes, and function as anti-inflammatory agents by blocking various permeability-increasing agents and vasodilators.

Steroids in high doses are the first-line choice of many clinicians for the initial treatment of acute cellular rejection. Steroids also are an integral part of most maintenance immunosuppressive regimens. High-dose IV steroids usually are administered immediately posttransplant as induction therapy, followed by relatively high-dose oral steroids (e.g., prednisone at 30 mg/d in adults), tapering to the maintenance dose of 5 to 15 mg/d over 3 to 6 months.

Adverse effects of steroid therapy are numerous and contribute significantly to morbidity in transplant recipients.[13] Individual response varies markedly, but many of the side effects are dose dependent. Common side effects include mild cushingoid facies and habitus, acne, increased appetite, mood changes, hypertension, proximal muscle weakness, glucose intolerance, and impaired wound healing. Less common are posterior subcapsular cataracts, glaucoma, and aseptic necrosis of the femoral heads. High-dose steroid use, such as bolus therapy for treatment of acute rejection, increases the risk of opportunistic infections, osteoporosis, and in children, growth retardation. These serious side effects have fueled the current interest in withdrawing patients from steroids within a few months posttransplant, or avoiding steroids altogether. Promising results with steroid withdrawal and avoidance protocols have been reported with the different organ types.[14,15]

Most recent studies have concentrated on complete steroid avoidance or rapid steroid discontinuation (usually within 1 week posttransplant) rather than steroid withdrawal after 3 to 6 months posttransplant. Success rates as measured by acute rejection rates generally have been better with the former approaches. Additionally, many of the steroid-related side effects occur early, and so much of the benefit of steroid-free regimens may be lost with a withdrawal regimen. Rapid discontinuation or complete avoidance of steroids has been associated with equivalent or superior results with regard to acute rejection rates compared to steroid maintenance groups, but with significantly less steroid-related and infectious complications.

Azathioprine

An antimetabolite, AZA is a derivative of 6-mercaptopurine, the active agent. It was first introduced for clinical immunosuppression in 1962; in combination with corticosteroids, it became the standard agent worldwide for the next two decades. Until the introduction of cyclosporine, it was the most widely used immunosuppressive drug, but now has become an adjunctive component of immunosuppressive drug regimens. With the introduction of newer agents such as mycophenolate mofetil (MMF), the use of AZA has decreased significantly, and may be discontinued altogether in the near future.

AZA acts late in the immune process, affecting the cell cycle by interfering with DNA synthesis, thus suppressing proliferation of activated B and T lymphocytes. AZA is valuable in preventing the onset of acute rejection, but is not effective in the treatment of rejection episodes themselves.

The most significant side effect of AZA is bone marrow suppression. All three hematopoietic cell lines can be affected, leading to leukopenia, thrombocytopenia, and anemia. Suppression often is dose related; it usually is reversible with dose reduction or temporary cessation of the drug. Other significant side effects include hepatotoxicity, GI disturbances (nausea and vomiting), pancreatitis, and alopecia.

Cyclosporine

The introduction of cyclosporine in the early 1980s dramatically altered the field of transplantation.[16-18] It significantly improved results after kidney transplants, but its greatest impact was on extrarenal transplants. When it was introduced, cyclosporine was the most specific immunosuppressive agent available. Compared with steroids or AZA, it much more selectively inhibits the immune response. Currently, cyclosporine plays a central role in maintenance immunosuppression in many types of organ transplants.

Cyclosporine binds with its cytoplasmic receptor protein, cyclophilin, which subsequently inhibits the activity of calcineurin. Doing so impairs expression of several critical T-cell activation genes, the most important being for IL-2. As a result, T-cell activation is suppressed. The metabolism of cyclosporine is via the cytochrome P-450 system, therefore several drug interactions are possible. Inducers of P-450 such as phenytoin decrease blood levels; drugs such as erythromycin, cimetidine, ketoconazole, and fluconazole increase them.

Adverse effects of cyclosporine can be classified as renal or nonrenal. Nephrotoxicity is the most important and troubling adverse effect of cyclosporine. Cyclosporine has a vasoconstrictor effect on the renal vasculature. This vasoconstriction (likely a transient, reversible, and dose-dependent phenomenon) may cause early posttransplant graft dysfunction or may exaggerate existing poor graft function. Also, long-term cyclosporine use may result in interstitial fibrosis of the renal parenchyma, coupled with arteriolar lesions. The exact mechanism is unknown, but renal failure may eventually result.

A number of nonrenal side effects may also be seen with the use of cyclosporine. Cosmetic complications, most commonly hirsutism and gingival hyperplasia, may result in considerable distress, possibly leading to noncompliant behavior. Several neurologic complications, including headaches, tremor, and seizures, also have been reported. Other nonrenal side effects include hyperlipidemia, hepatotoxicity, and hyperuricemia.

Tacrolimus

Tacrolimus (FK506) is a metabolite of the soil fungus *Streptomyces tsukubaensis*, found in Japan. Released in the United States in April 1994 for use in liver transplantation, it is currently used in a fashion similar to cyclosporine. Tacrolimus, like cyclosporine, is a calcineurin inhibitor and has a very similar mechanism of action. Cyclosporine acts by binding cyclophilins, while tacrolimus acts by binding FK506-binding proteins (FKBPs). The tacrolimus-FKBP complex inhibits the enzyme calcineurin, which is essential for activating transcription factors in response to the rise in intracellular calcium seen with stimulation of the TCR. The net effect of tacrolimus is to inhibit T-cell function by preventing synthesis of IL-2 and other important cytokines. The main difference between tacrolimus and cyclosporine, other than the actual immunophilin each binds to, is in relative potency: Tacrolimus is 100 times more potent than cyclosporine on a molar basis. Similarly to cyclosporine, tacrolimus primarily is metabolized by the P-450 enzyme system of the liver; therefore similar drug interactions occur.

Adverse effects of tacrolimus and cyclosporine are similar. The most common problems include nephrotoxicity, neurotoxicity, impaired glucose metabolism, hypertension, infection, and GI disturbances. Nephrotoxicity is dose related and reversible with dose reduction. Neurotoxicity seen with tacrolimus ranges from mild symptoms (tremors, insomnia, and headaches) to more severe events (seizures and coma); it usually is related to high levels and resolves with dose reduction. These side effects are most common early posttransplant and subsequently tend to decrease in incidence.

The hyperglycemic effect of tacrolimus does not appear to be dose related. Its cause is unknown. However, in most studies, its incidence is significantly higher with tacrolimus than with cyclosporine. Other common side effects involve the GI tract, ranging from mild cramps to severe diarrhea. Hypertension, hypercholesterolemia, and hypomagnesemia occur with equal frequency with

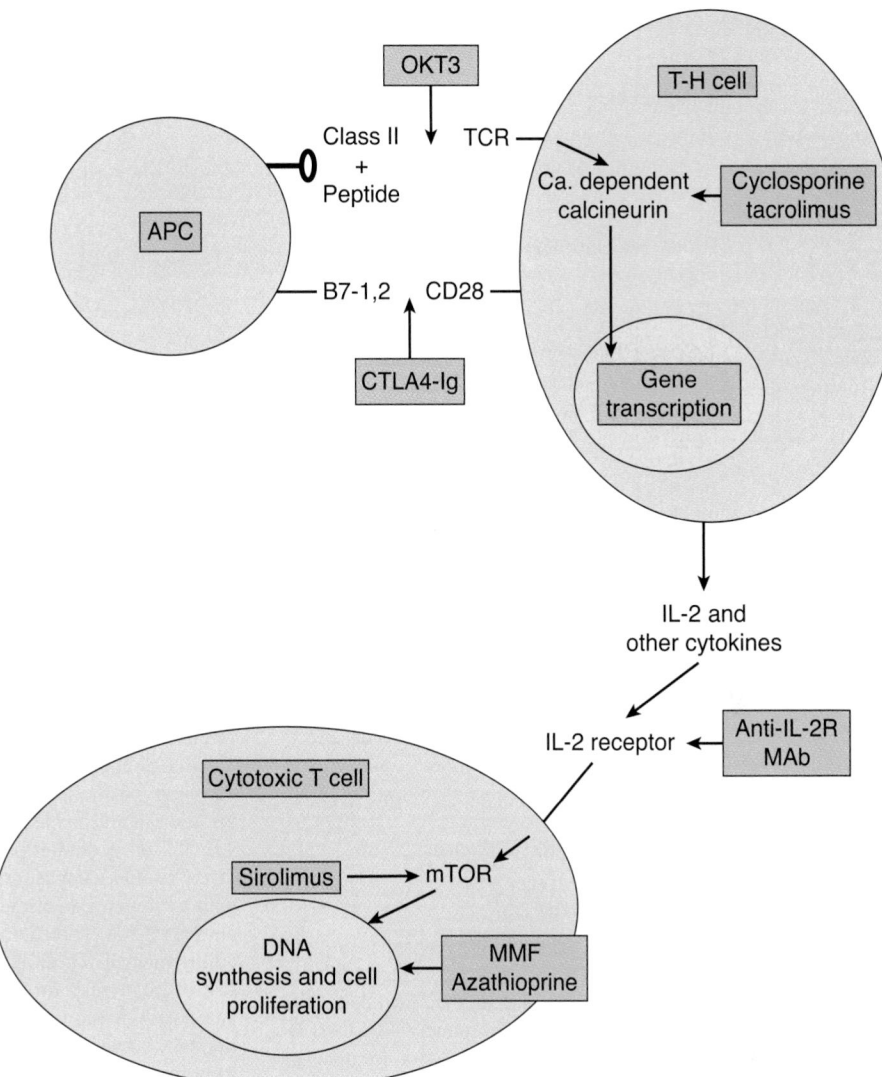

FIG. 11-2. Sites of action of immunosuppressive drugs. APC = antigen-presenting cell; CTLA4-Ig = cytotoxic T-lymphocyte-associated protein 4 immunoglobulin; IL = interleukin; MMF = mycophenolate mofetil; MAb = monoclonal antibody; mTOR = mammalian target of rapamycin; T-H Cell = helper T cell.

tacrolimus. As with other immunosuppressive drugs, infection and malignancy remain the most serious, long-term adverse events.

Sirolimus

A macrolide antibiotic derived from a soil actinomycete originally found on Easter Island (Rapa Nui), sirolimus (previously known as *rapamycin*) is structurally similar to tacrolimus and binds to the same immunophilin (FKBP). Unlike tacrolimus, it does not affect calcineurin activity, and therefore does not block the calcium-dependent activation of cytokine genes. Rather, the active complex binds so-called *target of rapamycin proteins* (Fig. 11-2), resulting in inhibition of P7056 kinase (an enzyme linked to cell division). The net result is to prevent progression from the G_1 to the S phase of the cell cycle, halting cell division.

To date, sirolimus has been used in a variety of combinations and situations. It may be used in conjunction with one of the calcineurin inhibitors. In such combinations, sirolimus usually is used to help withdraw or avoid the use of steroids completely in maintenance immunosuppressive regimens. It also has been used as an alternative to tacrolimus or cyclosporine, as part of a calcineurin-sparing protocol.[19] The advantage of this type of protocol is that it may not be associated with long-term nephrotoxicity (as may be seen with the calcineurin agents). Hence, sirolimus may prove to be better for long-term preservation of renal function in transplant recipients.

The major side effects of sirolimus include neutropenia, thrombocytopenia, and a significant elevation of the serum triglyceride and cholesterol levels. It also has been associated with impaired wound healing, leading to a higher incidence of wound-related complications.

Mycophenolate Mofetil

MMF was approved in May 1995 by the FDA for use in the prevention of acute rejection after kidney transplants. It since has been rapidly incorporated into routine clinical practice at many centers as part of maintenance regimens.[20] A semisynthetic derivative of mycophenolate acid, it is isolated from the mold *Penicillium glaucum*. It works by inhibiting inosine monophosphate dehydrogenase, which is a crucial, rate-limiting enzyme in de novo synthesis of purines. Specifically, this enzyme catalyzes the formation of guanosine nucleotides from inosine. Many cells have a salvage pathway and therefore can bypass this need for guanosine nucleotide synthesis by the de novo pathway. Activated lymphocytes, however, do not possess this salvage pathway and require de novo synthesis for clonal expansion. The net result is a selective, reversible antiproliferative effect on T and B lymphocytes.

MMF differs from cyclosporine, tacrolimus, and sirolimus in that it does not affect cytokine production or the events immediately after antigen recognition. Rather, MMF works further distally in the chain of activation events to prevent proliferation of the stimulated T cell (see Fig. 11-2). Like AZA, it is an antimetabolite; unlike AZA, its impact is selective: It only affects lymphocytes, not neutrophils or platelets. In several clinical trials, it has proven to be more effective than AZA, and has largely replaced it.

TABLE 11-3 Side effects and drug interactions of the main immunosuppressive drugs

	Common Side Effects	Other Medications That Increase Blood Levels	Other Medications That Decrease Blood Levels	Other Medications That Potentiate Toxicity
Cyclosporine (CSA)	Hypertension, nephrotoxicity, hirsutism, neurotoxicity, gingival hyperplasia	Verapamil, clarithromycin, doxycycline, azithromycin, erythromycin, fluconazole, itraconazole, ketoconazole	Isoniazid, carbamazepine, phenobarbital, phenytoin, rifampin	Nephrotoxicity: Acyclovir, ganciclovir, aminoglycosides, NSAIDs
Tacrolimus (FK506)	Hypertension, nephrotoxicity, hyperglycemia, neurotoxicity	Verapamil, clarithromycin, doxycycline, azithromycin, erythromycin, fluconazole, itraconazole, ketoconazole	Isoniazid, carbamazepine, phenobarbital, phenytoin, rifampin	Nephrotoxicity: Acyclovir, ganciclovir, aminoglycosides, NSAIDs
Sirolimus	Thrombocytopenia and nutropenia, elevated cholesterol, extremity edema, impaired wound healing	—	—	—
Mycophenolate mofetil	Leukopenia, thrombocytopenia, GI upset	—	Cholestyramine, antacids	—
Corticosteroids	Hyperglycemia, osteoporosis, cataracts, myopathy, weight gain	—	—	—
Azathioprine	Leukopenia, anemia, thrombocytopenia, GI upset	—	—	Bone marrow suppression: Allopurinol, sulfonamides

The incidence and types of adverse events with MMF are similar to those seen with AZA. Notable exceptions are GI side effects (diarrhea, gastritis, and vomiting), which are more common with MMF. Clinically, significant leukopenia also is more common, affecting about one third of recipients. Dose reduction or temporary drug cessation usually is adequate to treat leukopenia (Table 11-3).

Biologic Immunosuppression

Polyclonal antibodies directed against lymphocytes have been used in clinical transplantation since the 1960s. Monoclonal antibody (mAb) techniques were later developed and, in turn, allowed for the development of biologic agents such as muromonab-CD3 (OKT3), which were targeted to specific subsets of cells. A number of different mAbs are currently under development or have entered the phase of clinical testing for use in transplantation. Many are directed against functional secreted molecules of the immune system or their receptors, rather than against actual groups of cells.

Polyclonal Antibodies

Polyclonal antibodies are produced by immunizing animals such as horses or rabbits with human lymphoid tissue, allowing for an immune response, removing the resultant immune sera, and purifying the sera in an effort to remove unwanted antibodies. These lymphocyte-depleting antibodies are potent suppressors of the T-cell mediated immune response and selectively prevent the activation of B-cells by a range of stimuli. Polyclonal antibodies have been successfully used as induction agents to prevent rejection and to treat acute rejection episodes.

Antithymocyte Globulin Antithymocyte globulin (ATGAM) is a purified gamma globulin solution obtained by immunization of horses with human thymocytes. It contains antibodies to a wide variety of human T-cell surface antigens, including the MHC antigens. ATGAM generally must be infused via a central vein because infusion into a peripheral vein often is associated with thrombophlebitis. To avoid allergic reactions, patients should be premedicated with methylprednisolone and diphenhydramine hydrochloride. Even so, side effects may be significant because of the large amount of foreign protein. Symptoms of cytokine release syndrome include fever, chills, arthralgia, thrombocytopenia, leukopenia, and a serum sickness-like illness.

Thymoglobulin Antithymocyte immunoglobulin (Thymoglobulin) is a polyclonal antibody obtained by immunizing rabbits with human thymocytes. It has been approved by the FDA to prevent and treat rejection in solid organ transplant recipients. Multicenter randomized studies comparing antithymocyte immunoglobulin (Thymoglobulin) vs. ATGAM as induction therapy have shown that at 1-year posttransplant, there was less incidence and severity of rejection in antithymocyte immunoglobulin treated patients.[21] Five-year follow-up studies have shown that this is sustained long term. Safety profile comparison shows a higher incidence of leukopenia with antithymocyte immunoglobulin, although the rate of cytomegalovirus (CMV) infection seems to be lower. Some data suggest that antithymocyte immunoglobulin may be associated with an increased risk of posttransplant lymphoproliferative disorder (PTLD) compared with no induction, but more studies are needed for confirmation.[22] Comparison studies with muromonab-CD3 showed that muromonab-CD3 reversed a slightly higher number of rejection episodes than antithymocyte immunoglobulin in renal transplant recipients, but that both were efficient treatments; first-time use of antithymocyte immunoglobulin was associated with fewer side effects than muromonab-CD3.

Monoclonal Antibodies

mAbs have emerged as a new class of immunosuppressive agents, which appear to be effective in both the treatment and prevention of acute rejection and are well tolerated in renal transplant recipients.[23] mAbs are produced by the hybridization of murine antibody-secreting B-lymphocytes with a nonsecreting myeloma cell line. The highly specific nature of these drugs makes them less toxic than the oral, long-term maintenance agents such as corticosteroids and calcineurin inhibitors. Muromonab-CD3 remains a commonly used mAb but some of the new mAbs already have confirmed their efficacy in clinical phase III trials and are part of well-established immunosuppressive regimens. These include anti-CD25 mAbs (basiliximab and daclizumab). Other recently developed mAbs, like humanized anti-CD52 mAb alemtuzumab (Campath-1H), anti-CD20 (rituximab), anti–lymphocyte function-associated antigen-1 (anti–LFA-1), anti–intercellular adhesion molecule-1 (anti–ICAM-1) and anti–tumor necrosis factor alpha (TNF-α) (infliximab) currently are being tested and show encouraging immunosuppressive potential.

Muromonab-CD3 This MoAb is directed against the CD3 antigen complex found on all mature human T cells. The CD3 complex is an integral part of the TCR. Inactivation of CD3 by muromonab-CD3 causes the TCR to be lost from the cell surface. The T cells are then ineffective, and are rapidly cleared from the circulation and deposited into the reticuloendothelial system.

The standard dose is 5 mg/d, given IV. Smaller doses may be just as effective. Efficacy can be measured by monitoring CD3$^+$ cells in the circulation. If the drug is effective, the percentage of CD3$^+$ cells should fall to and stay below 5%. Failure to reach this level indicates an inadequate dose or the presence of antibodies directed against muromonab-CD3.

Muromonab-CD3 is highly effective and versatile. Most commonly, it is used to treat severe acute rejection episodes (i.e., those resistant to steroids). Muromonab-CD3 also has been used as prophylaxis against rejection, as induction therapy, and as primary rejection treatment.

Significant, even life-threatening adverse effects may be seen with muromonab-CD3, most commonly with the first few doses. Because muromonab-CD3 is a T-cell mitogen, most of these symptoms are thought to be mediated by T-cell release of cytokines via CD3 binding. The most common symptoms are fever, chills, and headaches. Muromonab-CD3's most serious side effect is a rapidly developing, noncardiogenic pulmonary edema. The risk of this side effect significantly increases if the patient is fluid-overloaded before beginning muromonab-CD3 treatment. Other serious side effects include encephalopathy, aseptic meningitis, and nephrotoxicity. Use of muromonab-CD3, especially multiple courses, significantly increases the risk of infection (e.g., CMV) and of neoplasms (e.g., PTLD). To reduce the side effects and the antigenicity of murine muromonab-CD3, a nonmitogenic "humanized" variant has been developed. Both in vitro and in vivo studies have found that the humanized variant of muromonab-CD3 does not activate human T cells, but retains significant immunosuppressive properties. The drug was well tolerated with minimal first-dose reactions (including lack of IL-2 release); induction of antibodies against muromonab-CD3 was not observed. Because it is less immunogenic, its half-life is much longer than that of conventional muromonab-CD3.

Anti-CD25 Monoclonal Antibodies (Basiliximab and Daclizumab)

The alpha subunit of the IL-2 receptor, also known as *Tac* or *CD25* is found exclusively on activated T cells. Blockade of this component by mAbs selectively prevents IL-2–induced T-cell activation. This selectivity makes the anti-CD25 mAbs powerful antirejection agents with no significant added risks of infection, malignancy, or other major side effects. There are two types of anti-CD25 mAbs: chimeric (approximately 75% human and 25% murine protein) and humanized (approximately 90% human and 10% murine). Basiliximab (Simulect) and daclizumab (Zenapax) are currently the two anti-CD25 mAbs approved for clinical use. They are used as part of induction immunosuppression in renal transplantation, in association with calcineurin inhibitors, corticosteroids, and MMF. A randomized, double-blind, placebo-controlled phase III trial was done comparing daclizumab vs. no induction in renal patients receiving their first cadaveric kidney transplant who received triple immunosuppression of cyclosporine, AZA, and prednisolone.[24] In the daclizumab group, fewer patients developed rejection during the first 6 months after transplantation, time to develop rejection was longer, and the numbers of rejection episodes were lower. Moreover, infusion of the antibody was not associated with any adverse reactions. There also was no difference in infection or cancer rates between the two groups. A comparable study also has been published using basiliximab in renal transplantation.[25]

Anti-CD52 Monoclonal Antibody Alemtuzumab (Campath-1H)

Alemtuzumab (Campath-1H) is a humanized rat mAb (rat Ig G2b) directed against the CD-52 antigen. It is a powerful cytolytic agent and has been used therapeutically in bone marrow transplantation, several autoimmune diseases, and organ transplantation.[26] The CD52 antigen is expressed on T and B lymphocytes, monocytes, macrophages, and eosinophils, as well as on the lining of the male reproductive tract. It is one of the most abundant antigens on the surface of lymphocytes, accounting for approximately 5% of the surface antigens. This probably explains, in part, the profound and long-lasting lymphopenia produced after the administration of one

or two doses of the antibody; these depressed lymphocyte levels may take months to years to return to normal levels. For example, two doses of alemtuzumab, 40 mg in total, given over 2 days in patients receiving a kidney transplant produce profound lymphopenia. Although B-lymphocyte counts return to normal levels within 3 to 12 months, CD4$^+$ and CD8$^+$ lymphocyte counts remain significantly depressed for as long as 3 years. After binding to its target, alemtuzumab causes cell death through several mechanisms, including complement-mediated cytolysis, antibody-mediated cytotoxicity, and apoptosis.

The most extensive experience with the use of alemtuzumab in solid organ transplantation has been in renal transplantation. It has been used in induction and maintenance therapy and treatment of acute rejection. Randomized trials comparing alemtuzumab with antithymocyte immunoglobulin found that there was no difference in patient or graft survival, acute rejection rates, or renal function; nor were there any differences in infections or incidence of diabetes or hyperlipidemia. As with all antibody treatments, there is an initial reaction with alemtuzumab administration. However, it is relatively modest and suppressed with an IV bolus injection of 1 g of methylprednisolone before administration of the antibody. Because of the long-lasting T-cell depletion, there is still concern regarding the risk of infection. An interesting observation is the occurrence of autoimmune disorders in the form of autoimmune hypothyroidism and autoimmune hemolytic anemia in rare patients treated with alemtuzumab. There is a need for large, prospective randomized control trials and long-term follow-up to establish the true role of alemtuzumab especially with respect to safety.

Anti-CD20 (Rituximab)

CD20 (human B-lymphocyte-restricted differentiation antigen, Bp35), is a protein which is located on pre-B and mature B lymphocytes. The antigen is expressed on most B-cell non-Hodgkin's lymphomas but is not found on stem cells, pro-B cells, normal plasma cells, or other normal tissues. It regulates an early step in the activation process for cell cycle initiation and differentiation, and possibly functions as a calcium ion channel. Rituximab, a chimeric murine/human mAb, approved in the United States only for the treatment of refractory or relapsed B-cell lymphomas, reacts with the CD20 antigen.[27] In transplant recipients, it is used for treatment of posttransplant lymphoproliferative disease, to anecdotally reduce preformed anti-HLA and anti-ABO antibodies, and for the prevention and treatment of acute humoral rejection. A need for controlled clinical trials clearly is needed to determine the best clinical situation in which to use this agent.

Monoclonal Antibodies to Adhesion Molecules

Adhesion molecules play a dual role in graft injury posttransplant. Initial ischemic reperfusion injury is characterized by a cellular infiltrate in the graft. This migration of cells into the graft is regulated by the endothelium, which recruits the infiltrating cells by expressing adhesion molecules on its surface. Adhesion molecules, such as the LFA-1: ICAM-1 receptor ligand pair also participate in subsequent antigen-dependent T-cell activation. When the TCR comes into contact with its target antigen, LFA-1 binds to ICAM-1 on the antigen-presenting cell (APC) surface. This binding then potentiates T-cell activation by stabilizing TCR binding to its target and transmitting amplifying signals to the cytoplasm. Therefore, mAb directed against adhesion molecules could simultaneously interrupt both the effect of ischemic injury and the alloresponse. This potential dual effect currently is being evaluated in laboratory and clinical studies.

Comparisons of the mAb directed against the alpha chain of LFA-1 (odulimomab) with antithymocyte immunoglobulin as induction therapy found, at 3 and 12 months after transplantation, similar rate and severity of rejection episodes as well as incidence of infection. An anti–LFA-1 mAb (efalizumab) was found capable of inhibiting lymphocyte adhesion, circulation, and activation. Another potential benefit of anti-LFA mAbs observed in both animal models and human beings is that they can diminish the ischemia-reperfusion injury associated with delayed graft function. The anti-CD4 mAb (priliximab) already has shown immunosuppressive potential in some therapeutic pilot studies. However, in another clinical trial, this mAb, although well tolerated, was associated with a high acute rejection rate (50% of patients developed an acute rejection episode within the first 3 months), probably because of poor drug bioavailability or possibly because of anti-murine antibody development. Due to these conflicting results, anti-CD4 mAbs are not recommended for clinical use at this time. Costimulatory blockade with anti-CD154 mAb prolongs allograft survival in nonhuman primates; but in clinical transplantation, the rejection rate has been unacceptably high and can have serious side effects, particularly thromboembolism, mediated probably by platelet activation leading to enhanced aggregation.

Belatacept: The best-characterized pathway of T-cell costimulation includes CD28, its homologue cytotoxic T-lymphocyte-associated protein 4 (CTLA4), and their ligands CD80 and CD86. CTLA4-Ig (abatacept) is a fusion protein consisting of the extra cellular domain of CTLA4 and the Fc domain of IgG. Two amino acid substitutions to this protein resulted in the development of LEA29Y or belatacept, a high-avidity molecule with slower dissociation rates.[28,29] A phase II, randomized multicenter study was done based on costimulation blockade with belatacept in renal transplantation. Renal transplant recipients were randomly assigned to receive an intensive or a less intensive regimen of belatacept or cyclosporine. All patients received induction therapy with basiliximab, MMF, and corticosteroids. The study showed that the rate of acute rejection was similar among the groups: 6% for intensive belatacept, 6% for less intensive belatacept, and 8% for cyclosporine. Subclinical rejection at routine biopsy in 6 months was more common with less intensive belatacept (20%) than with intensive belatacept (9%) or cyclosporine (11%). At 12 months, glomerular filtration rate was significantly higher with both intensive and less intensive belatacept than those treated with cyclosporine (66.3, 62.1, and 53.5 mL/min per 1.73 m^2, respectively), and chronic allograft nephropathy was less common with both regimens of belatacept than with cyclosporine (29%, 20%, and 44%, respectively). Lipid levels and blood pressure values were similar or slightly lower in the belatacept groups. The frequency of infection was similar in all three groups, around 75%. Cancers occurred in two patients treated with intensive belatacept (one breast cancer and one PTLD) and in two patients treated with cyclosporine (one skin cancer and one thyroid cancer). However, PTLD developed in two additional patients treated with the intensive regimen 2 and 13 months after replacement of belatacept with conventional immunosuppressive agents. As belatacept interacts with the CD28 pathway, there were no reports of thrombotic complications seen with intervention in the CD40: CD154 pathway. Belatacept did not appear to affect the number or activity of T regulatory cells and clinical monitoring of lymphocytes did not reveal any depleting effects. These findings suggest that belatacept acts by depleting initial T-cell activation rather than selective depletion or complement-mediated lysis. Although these results are exciting, they are preliminary, and the long-term implications can only be known with larger studies and longer-term observation.

New Agents

1. AEB: This is a new oral compound that effectively blocks early T-cell activation by selective inhibition of protein kinase C. Therefore, it has a different mechanism of action from that of calcineurin inhibitors, and early studies suggest it is not associated with the nephrotoxicity seen with calcineurin inhibitors. This agent is currently in phase II testing.
2. ISA247: This is a novel semisynthetic analogue of cyclosporine that is structurally similar to it except for a modification of a functional group. This agent has not been associated with the nephrotoxicity seen with cyclosporine and currently is in phase II testing.
3. Janus kinase-3 (JAK-3) inhibitors: JAKs are cytoplasmic tyrosine kinases that participate in the signaling of a broad range of cell surface receptors, particularly members of the cytokine receptor superfamily. JAK-3 is found primarily on hematopoietic cells and blocking this may provide a significant degree of selectivity in immunosuppression. It is currently in phase II trials.

ORGAN PROCUREMENT AND PRESERVATION

The biggest problem facing transplant centers today is the shortage of organ donors. Mechanisms that might increase the number of available organs include: (a) Optimizing the current donor pool (e.g., the use of multiple organ donors or marginal donors); (b) increasing the number of living-donor transplants (e.g., the use of living unrelated donors); (c) using unconventional and controversial donor sources (e.g., using deceased donors without cardiac activity or anencephalic donors); and (d) performing xenotransplants. The largest potential increase in the number of available organs would result from improving donation rates from suitable deceased donors. By recent estimates, over 10,000 brain-dead donors are potentially available in the United States annually. Currently, however, only about one half of them are actually used. The single most important reason for the lack of deceased-donor organ retrieval is the inability to obtain consent from the surviving next-of-kin. The need for public education is crucial, including more effective educational campaigns to increase awareness of the importance of organ transplants.

Deceased Donors

Most extrarenal transplants performed today, and roughly one half of all renal transplants, are from deceased donors. These donors are deceased individuals who meet the criteria for brain death, but whose organs are being perfused by life-support measures, allowing adequate time for referral to an organ procurement organization. A member of that organization can then ascertain whether donation is possible, and if so, approach the potential donor's family and possibly obtain consent to procure suitable organs.

Crucial to the concept of deceased-donor organ donation is the concept of brain death. Brain death means that all brain and brain stem function has irreversibly ceased, while circulatory and ventilatory functions are maintained temporarily. The clinical diagnosis of brain death rests on three criteria: (a) irreversibility of the neurologic insult; (b) absence of clinical evidence of cerebral function; and most important, (c) absence of clinical evidence of brain stem function. When testing for brain death, hypothermia, medication side effects, drug overdose, and intoxication must be excluded. Brain death can be diagnosed by routine neurologic examinations (including cold caloric and apnea testing on two separate occasions at least 6 hours apart), coupled with prior establishment of the underlying diagnosis. Confirmatory tests must verify the absence of intracranial blood flow on brain flow studies or the presence of an isoelectric electroencephalogram reading.

Once the diagnosis of brain death has been established, the process of organ donation can be initiated.[30,31] The focus then switches from the treatment of elevated intracranial pressure (ICP) to preserving organ function and optimizing peripheral oxygen delivery.[32] It is important to keep in mind that management of the deceased organ donor is an active process, requiring aggressive monitoring and intervention to ensure that perfusion to the organs of interest is not compromised. For all organ donors, core temperature, systemic arterial blood pressure, arterial oxygen saturation, and urine output must be determined routinely and frequently. Arterial blood gases, serum electrolytes, blood urea nitrogen, serum creatinine, liver enzymes, hemoglobin, and coagulation tests also need to be monitored regularly. Hemodynamic instability can be marked after brain death, with wide swings between the extremes of hypotension and hypertension. Hypotension is usually secondary to hypovolemia, due to a combination of vasomotor collapse after

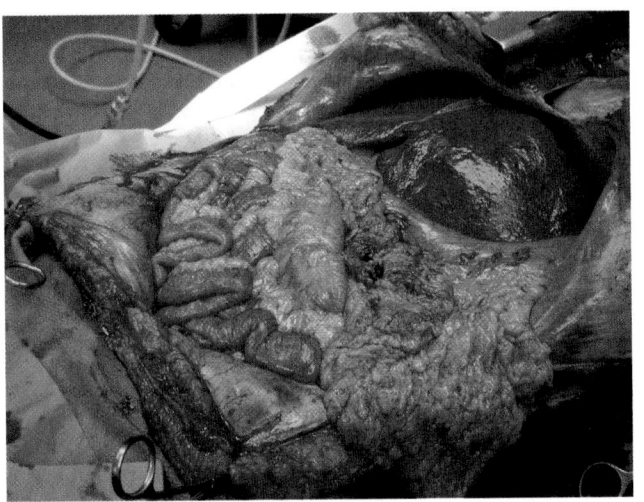

FIG. 11-3. Incision for multiorgan abdominal procurement with wide exposure of all abdominal organs.

flushing the organs with preservative solution. Other centers prefer to flush the organs early, remove the abdominal contents "en-bloc," and perform the separation and dissection of the individual organs on the back table.[34] Each technique has its potential advantages and disadvantages. Regardless of personal technique and preference, it is paramount that the transplant surgeon develops a systematic approach to safely procure the liver, pancreas, and kidneys even in the unstable donor.

The basic steps involve a long incision to provide wide exposure of all thoracic and abdominal organs (Fig. 11-3). Complete mobilization of the distal small bowel, right colon, and duodenum is performed to allow for identification of the distal aorta, iliac bifurcation, and the distal inferior vena cava (IVC). The infrarenal aorta will serve as the site for insertion of the cannula that will allow for flushing of the organs with cold preservative solution (Fig. 11-4). The supraceliac aorta is encircled followed by limited dissection of the hepatic hilum and the pancreas. The portal system can be cannulated via the inferior mesenteric vein and the organs can then be flushed with preservative solution and topically cooled with slush. The thoracic organs, liver, pancreas, and kidneys are then removed individually.

Donation after cardiac death: The non–heart-beating donor (NHBD), also referred to as the *donation after cardiac death* donor, is one type of expanded criteria donor that is increasingly being used by transplant centers to successfully boost the number of deceased donors and decrease the dire shortage of transplantable organs.[35] NHBD death is characterized by irreversible absence of circulation, in contrast to heart-beating donor death, defined by irreversible cessation of all brain functions. Organ ischemia is minimized in the brain-dead donor because circulatory arrest typically occurs concurrently with perfusion of preservation solution and rapid core cooling. NHBDs are less than ideal because the organs suffer ischemia during the prolonged periods between circulatory dysfunction, circulatory arrest, and subsequent perfusion and cooling. Furthermore, the surgical procedure for NHBD organ recovery is demanding and rushed.

brain death and the effects of treatment protocols to decrease ICP. Hypertension may also be seen, often secondary to raised ICP. It can be treated with short-acting vasodilatory agents or with rapidly reversible beta blockers.

Other key factors in donor management include respiratory maintenance, good renal perfusion with brisk urine output, and avoidance of hypothermia.

Surgical technique: The technique of multiple organ procurement (kidney, liver, pancreas, small bowel) was first described by Starzl and his colleagues in 1984.[33] Most centers have now added their own modifications to these pioneering techniques and differ primarily on their degree of in vivo dissection. Some centers perform extensive dissection of the organs to be recovered before

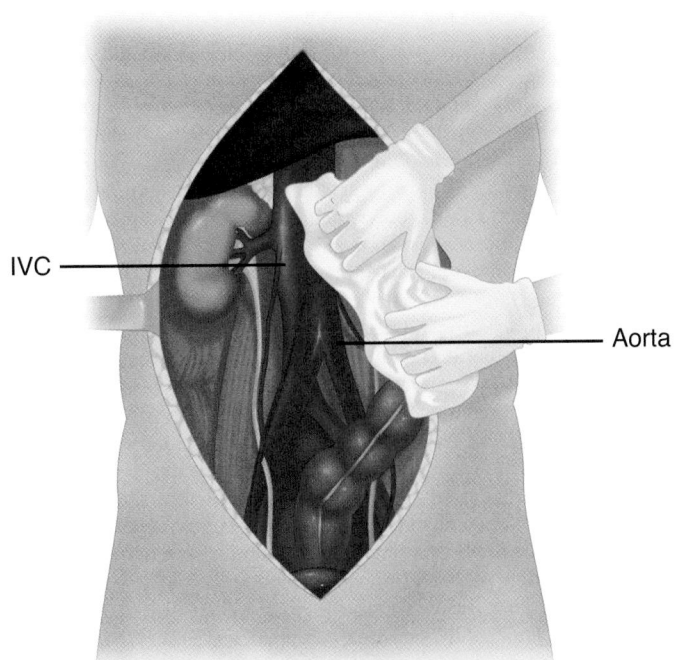

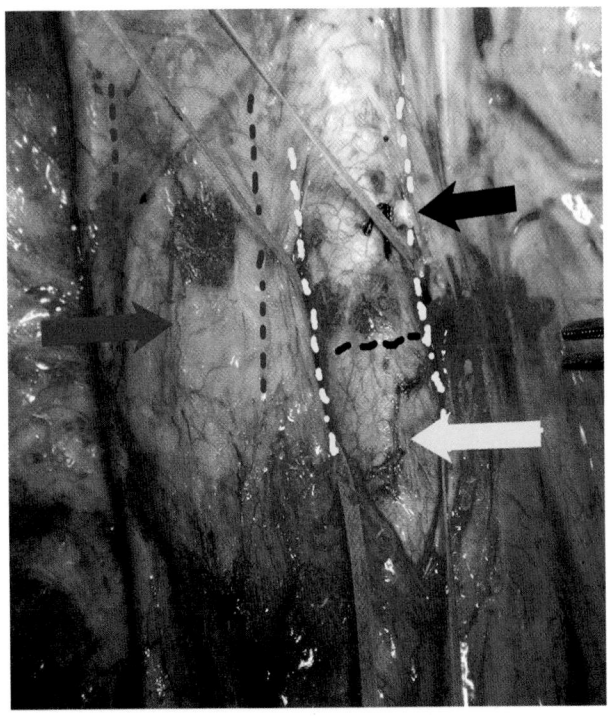

A

B

FIG. 11-4. A and **B.** With the small bowel and right colon completely mobilized, the infrarenal aorta can be isolated for insertion of the cannula that will allow the organs to be flushed with cold preservative solution. Black arrow = aorta; blue arrow = inferior vena cava (IVC); yellow arrow = cannula insertion site.

It is important to differentiate controlled from uncontrolled NHBDs. Uncontrolled NHBDs sustain circulatory arrest and either fail to respond to cardiopulmonary resuscitation and/or are declared dead on arrival to the hospital. Uncontrolled NHBD death is unplanned, so the organs suffer protracted ischemia before recovery. Although kidneys tolerate a short period of the resultant warm ischemia, transplantation of extrarenal organs from uncontrolled NHBDs carries a much greater risk. In contrast, controlled NHBDs undergo circulatory arrest following planned withdrawal of life support, most often in the operating room, with a donor surgical team readily available. Controlled NHBDs suffer terminal illness, usually a severe neurologic injury without the possibility of meaningful recovery or survival. Controlled NHBDs provide organs that are exposed to significantly less ischemic damage than those of uncontrolled NHBDs and, in general, offer superior posttransplant function when compared with uncontrolled NHBDs.

Living Donors

Living-donor transplantation is unique in that surgeons are operating on a healthy individual (i.e., a living donor) who has no medical disorders and does not require an operation. The use of living donors is an integral and important part of the field of transplantation today. The first transplants ever performed used living donors. Today, living donors are commonly used for every type of transplant except heart transplants. The number of such transplants continues to increase on a yearly basis. But living-donor transplants pose a unique set of medical, ethical, financial, and psychosocial problems that must be dealt with by the transplant team.

The use of living donors offers numerous advantages. Primary is the availability of a life-saving organ. A certain percentage of transplant candidates die while waiting for a deceased-donor organ as a direct result of a complication, or of progression of their underlying disease. For such ill candidates, the advantage of a living donor is obvious. In certain parts of the world, such as the Far East, where deceased-donor transplants are not accepted by the public, the advantage and need of the living donor is obvious. Even in countries where deceased-donor transplants are accepted, a living-donor transplant may significantly shorten the waiting time for potential recipients. A shorter waiting time generally implies a healthier candidate—one whose body has not been ravaged by prolonged end-stage organ failure. Moreover, living-donor transplants are planned (rather than emergency) procedures, allowing for better preoperative preparation of the potential recipient. Receiving an organ from a closely matched relative may also have immunologic benefits. Lastly, long-term results may be superior with living-donor transplants, which is certainly the case with kidney transplants.

The disadvantages of a living-donor transplant for the potential recipient are minimal. With some organ transplants (e.g., living-donor liver or lung), the procedure may be more technically complex, resulting in an increased incidence of surgical complications. However, this disadvantage is offset by the numerous advantages.

The major disadvantage of living-donor transplants is to the donor. Medically, there is no possibility of benefit for the donor, only potential for harm. The risk of death associated with donation depends on the organ being removed. For nephrectomy, the mortality risk is estimated to be less than 0.05%. However, for partial hepatectomy, it is about 0.5%. Risks for surgical and medical complications also depend on the procedure being performed. In addition, long-term complications or problems may be associated with partial loss of organ function through donation. The guiding principle of all living-donor transplants should be the minimization of risk to the donor. What risk there is must be carefully explained to the potential donor, and written informed consent should be obtained.

The kidney, the first organ to be used for living-donor transplants, is the most common type of organ donated by living donors today. Living-donor liver transplants are not as common, but have been performed for almost 15 years now. Initially, they involved adult donors and pediatric recipients, but now an adult donor for an adult

recipient is more common. Living-donor transplants with organs besides the kidney and liver are fairly uncommon, but are performed at various centers. Living-donor pancreas transplants involve a distal pancreatectomy, with the graft consisting of the body and tail of the pancreas; vascular inflow and outflow are provided by the splenic artery and splenic vein. Living-donor intestinal transplants usually involve removal of about 200 cm of the donor's ileum, with inflow and outflow provided by the ileocolic vessels. Living-donor lung transplants involve removal of one lobe of one lung from each of two donors; both grafts are then transplanted into the recipient.

Preservation

Organ preservation methods have played an important role in the success of cadaver-donor transplants. They have resulted in improved graft function immediately posttransplant and have diminished the incidence of primary nonfunction of organs. By prolonging the allowable cold ischemia times, they have also allowed for better organ allocation and for safer transplants.[36,37]

The most common methods involve the use of hypothermia and pharmacologic inhibition to slow down metabolic processes in the organ once it has been removed from the deceased donor. Hypothermia very effectively slows down enzymatic reactions and metabolic activity, allowing the cell to make its limited energy reserves last much longer. A temperature decrease from 37° to 4°C (98.6° to 39.2°F) (the temperature of most preservation solutions) slows metabolism about 12-fold. However, in the absence of any energy inflow into the cell, degradative reactions begin to provide the cell with an energy source. The result can be destruction of important structural elements and, eventually, structural damage to the cells and the organ. So, although hypothermia greatly slows enzymatic reactions, they continue nonetheless, leading to accumulation of potentially detrimental end products within the cell. Hypothermia also contributes to the development of cellular swelling because the membrane ion pumps are slow to function.

Cold storage solutions have been developed to improve organ preservation by ameliorating some of the detrimental effects of hypothermia alone. Essentially, these solutions suppress hypothermia-induced cellular swelling and minimize the loss of potassium from the cell. Agents that do not readily permeate the cell membrane and that have an electrolyte composition resembling the intracellular environment (low sodium, high potassium) are used, thus preventing the loss of cellular potassium.

The most commonly used fluid worldwide is the University of Wisconsin solution.[38] It contains lactobionate, raffinose, and hydroxyethyl starch. Lactobionate is impermeable and prevents intracellular swelling; it also lowers the concentration of intracellular calcineurin and free iron, which may be beneficial in reducing reperfusion injury. Hydroxyethyl starch, a synthetic colloid, may help decrease hypothermia-induced cell swelling of endothelial cells and reduce interstitial edema. Another solution that is now being used commonly is histidine-tryptophan-ketoglutarate solution.[39]

Although cold preservation has improved cadaver-donor transplant results, the amount of time that an organ can be safely preserved is limited. After that, the incidence of organ nonfunction starts to increase. With kidneys, exceeding the preservation time limit results in delayed graft function, requiring dialysis support for the recipient until function improves. With livers, the result is primary nonfunction, requiring an urgent retransplant. How long an organ can be safely preserved depends on the type of organ and on the condition of the donor. With kidneys, cold ischemic times should be kept below 36 to 40 hours; after that, delayed graft function significantly increases. With pancreata, more than 24 hours of ischemia increases problems due to pancreatitis and duodenal leaks. With livers, more than 16 hours of ischemia increases the risk for primary nonfunction and biliary complications. Hearts and lungs tolerate preservation poorly; ideally, ischemia times should be below 6 hours. With marginal donors, all of these times should be adjusted further downward.

KIDNEY TRANSPLANTATION

A kidney transplant now represents the treatment of choice for patients with end-stage renal disease (ESRD). It offers the greatest potential for restoring a healthy, productive life in most such patients. Compared with dialysis, it is associated with better patient survival and superior quality of life, and is more cost effective.[40,41] Currently, there are nearly 70,000 patients in the United States awaiting a kidney transplant. Because of the success of the procedure, the waiting list has grown dramatically since the 1990s. Unfortunately, the number of available organs has not kept pace, resulting in longer waiting times for recipients.

History

The history of kidney transplantation is in many ways the history of transplantation itself. The kidney was the first organ to be transplanted regularly, and it remains the most common organ transplanted today. The first clinical deceased-donor kidney transplant was performed in 1933 by Voronoy, a Ukrainian surgeon, with unsuccessful results secondary to rejection. In the 1950s, this immunologic barrier was circumvented by performing the kidney transplants between identical twins. The era of modern kidney transplantation began with the introduction of AZA to suppress the immune system. With the demonstration of the synergistic effect with glucocorticoids, renal transplantation was established as a viable option for the treatment of ESRD. Polyclonal antilymphocyte agents, such as antilymphocyte globulin, were soon developed, significantly contributing to the treatment of acute rejection. The introduction of cyclosporine in the 1980s significantly improved graft and patient survival rates, allowing for a dramatic increase in the number of kidney transplants.

Preoperative Evaluation

Very few absolute contraindications to kidney transplants exist. Therefore, most patients with ESRD should be considered as potential transplant candidates. However, the surgery and general anesthesia impose a significant cardiovascular stress. Subsequent lifelong immunosuppression also is associated with some risk. Pretransplant evaluation should identify any factors that would contraindicate a transplant or any risk factors that could be minimized pretransplant.[42]

The preoperative evaluation can be divided into four parts: medical, surgical, immunologic, and psychosocial. The purpose of the medical evaluation is to identify risk factors for the surgical procedure. Mortality posttransplant usually is due to underlying cardiovascular disease, so a detailed cardiac evaluation is necessary. Any history of congestive heart failure, angina, myocardial infarction, or stroke should be elicited. Patients with symptoms suggestive of cardiovascular disease or with significant risk factors (e.g., diabetes, age over 50, previous myocardial infarction) should undergo further cardiac evaluation with stress testing or angiography. Any problems identified should be treated appropriately (medically or surgically) before proceeding with the transplant.

Untreated malignancy and active infection are absolute contraindications to a transplant, because of the requisite lifelong immunosuppression. After curative treatment of malignancy, an interval of 2 to 5 years is recommended pretransplant. This recommendation is influenced by the type of malignancy, with longer observation periods for neoplasms such as melanoma or breast cancer and shorter periods for carcinoma in situ or low-grade malignancies such as basal cell carcinoma of the skin. Chronic infections such as osteomyelitis or endocarditis must be fully treated and a suitable waiting period must occur to ensure lack of recrudescence.

The medical evaluation also should concentrate on GI problems such as peptic ulcer disease, symptomatic cholelithiasis, and hepatitis. Patients who demonstrate serologic evidence of hepatitis C or B, but without evidence of active hepatic inflammation or cirrhosis, are acceptable transplant candidates. A biopsy may be helpful to determine the extent of the underlying liver disease. These patients are at increased risk for progression of their underlying liver disease after receiving immunosuppression, but exhibit excellent long-term survival rates and improved quality of life posttransplant, as compared with patients undergoing chronic dialysis.

The surgical evaluation should identify vascular or urologic abnormalities that may contraindicate or complicate a transplant. Evidence of vascular disease that is revealed by the history (claudication or rest pain) or the physical examination (diminished or absent pulse or bruit) should be evaluated further by Doppler studies or angiography. Severe aortoiliac disease may make a transplant technically impossible; an option in such patients is a revascularization procedure such as aortobifemoral graft placement pretransplant. Areas of significant arterial stenosis proximal to the planned site of implantation may need preoperative balloon angioplasty. Urologic evaluation should exclude chronic infection in the native kidney, which may require nephrectomy pretransplant. Other indications for nephrectomy include huge polycystic kidneys, significant vesicoureteral reflux, or uncontrollable renovascular hypertension. Children especially require a complete urologic examination to evaluate reflux and bladder outlet obstruction.

The immunologic evaluation involves determining blood type, tissue type (HLA-A, -B, or -DR antigens), and presence of any cytotoxic antibodies against HLA antigens (because of prior transplants, blood transfusions, or pregnancies). If a living-donor transplant is planned, a cross-match should be performed early on during the initial evaluation.

The psychosocial evaluation is necessary to ensure that transplant candidates understand the nature of the transplant procedure and its attendant risk. They must be capable of rigorously adhering to the medical regimen posttransplant. Patients who have not been compliant with their medical regimen in the past must demonstrate a willingness and capability to do so before they undergo the transplant.

Living-donor kidney transplant: One important aspect of the preoperative evaluation is the search for and evaluation of potential living donors. Living-donor kidney recipients enjoy improved long-term success, avoid a prolonged wait, and are able to plan the timing of their transplant in advance. Moreover, they have a significantly decreased incidence of acute tubular necrosis (ATN) and increased potential for HLA matching. As a result, living-donor transplants generally have better short- and long-term results, as compared with deceased-donor transplants. Of course, the risks to the living donor must be acceptably low. The donor must be fully aware of potential risks and must freely give informed consent. The search for a living donor should not be restricted to immediate family members. Results with living, unrelated donors are comparable to those with living, related (non–HLA-identical) donors.[43]

Potential living donors are first evaluated to ensure that they have normal renal function with two equally functioning kidneys and that they do not have any significant risk factors for developing renal disease (e.g., hypertension or diabetes). The anatomy of their kidneys and the vasculature can be determined by using various radiologic imaging techniques, including an IV pyelogram, arteriogram, or computed tomographic (CT) angiogram. Which kidney is removed depends on the anatomy. If there is any minor abnormality in one kidney, that kidney should be removed. If both kidneys are the same, the left kidney is preferred because of the longer left renal vein. Nephrectomy can be performed through a flank incision, by an anterior retroperitoneal approach, or by a laparoscopic technique. With the laparoscopic technique, an intraperitoneal approach is used. This involves mobilization of the colon, isolation of the ureter and renal vessels, mobilization of the kidney, division of the renal vessels, and removal of the kidney (Fig. 11-5).

Recipient Surgical Procedure

The surgical technique for kidney transplantation has changed very little from the original pelvic operation described in the 1950s. The transplanted kidney is usually placed in a heterotopic position, with

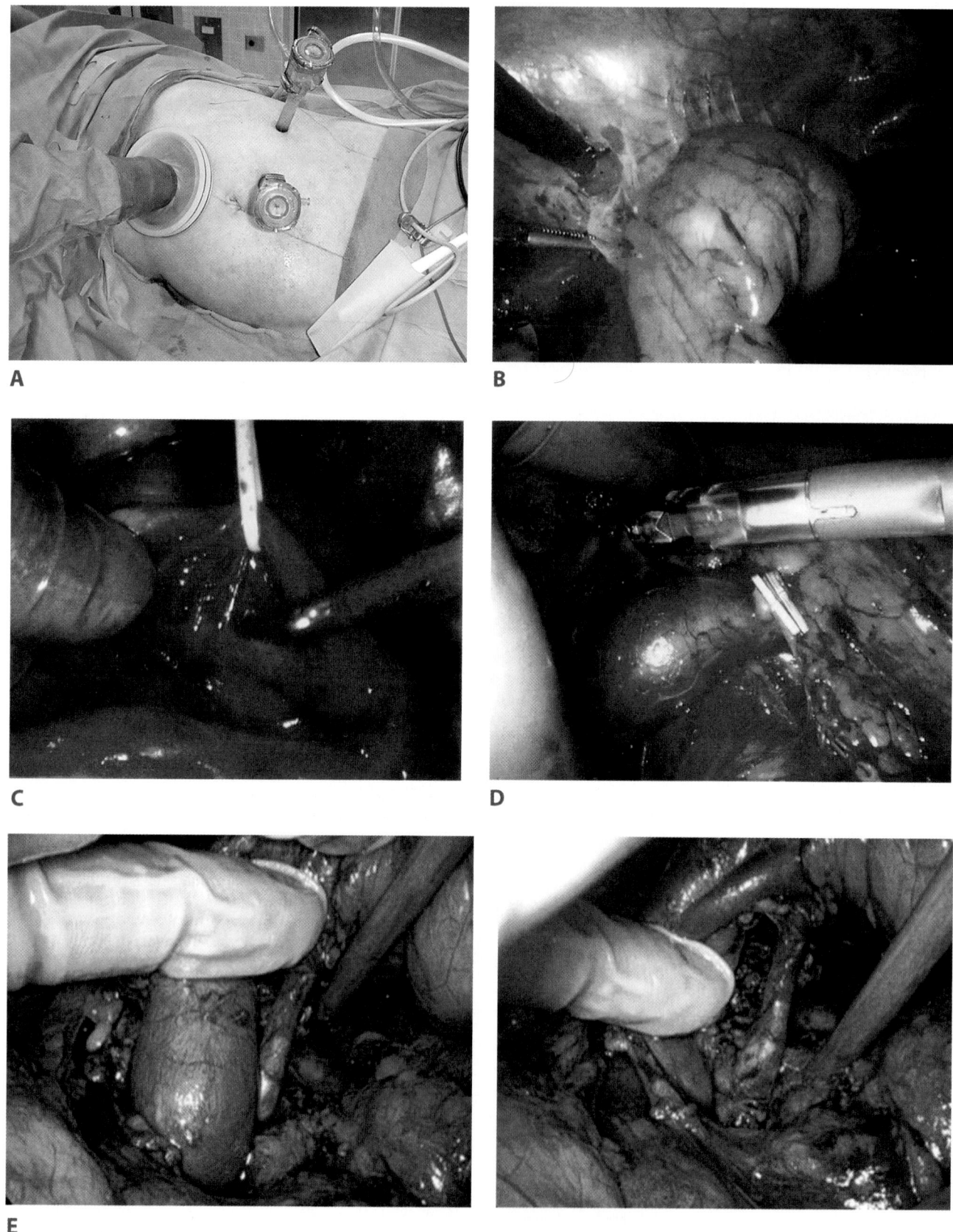

FIG. 11-5. A through **F.** Hand-assisted laparoscopic donor nephrectomy for living-donor kidney transplant. (*Continued*)

no need for native nephrectomy except in select circumstances. Retroperitoneal placement is preferred, to allow for easy access for percutaneous renal biopsy. Usually, the right iliac fossa is chosen because of the more superficial location of the iliac vein on this side

(Figs. 11-6 and 11-7). However, the left iliac fossa should be used if the recipient may be a candidate for a future pancreas transplant, if it is a second transplant, or if there is significant arterial disease on the right side.

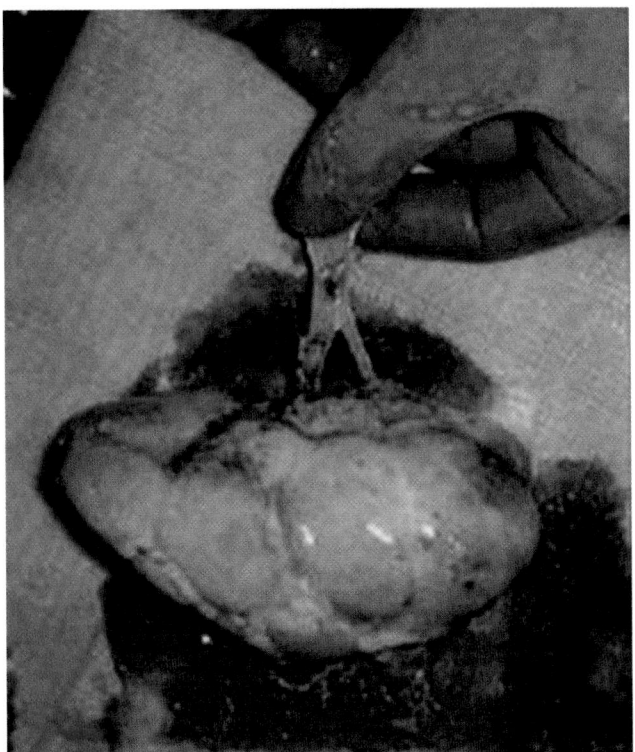

F

FIG. 11-5. (*Continued*)

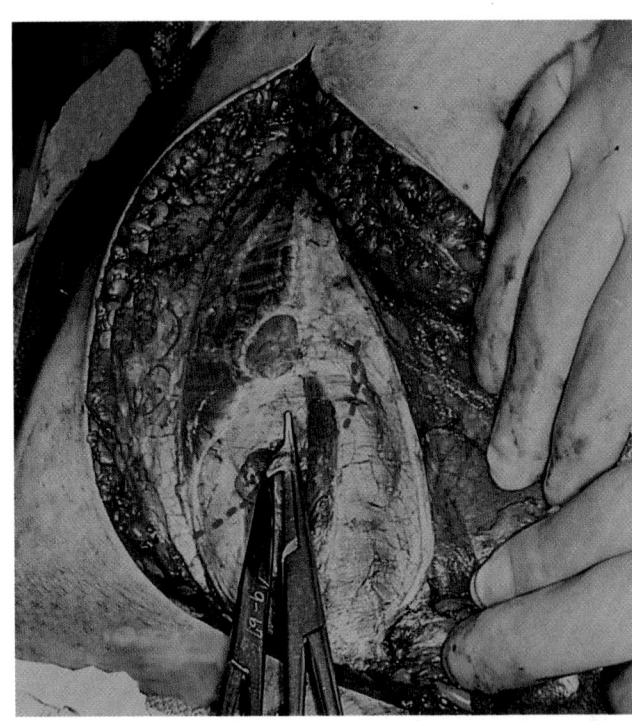

FIG. 11-7. The incision is deepened along the lateral edge of the rectus muscle, identifying and dividing the epigastric vessels.

With the standard approach, the dissection is extraperitoneal. The iliac vessels are identified and assessed for suitability for anastomosis. The internal iliac artery can be used as the inflow vessel, with an end-to-end anastomosis, or the external iliac artery can be used with an end-to-side anastomosis. To minimize the risk

of lymphocele formation after surgery, only a modest length of artery is dissected free and the lymphatics overlying the artery are ligated (Figs. 11-8 and 11-9). The donor renal vein is anastomosed end to side to the external iliac vein and the artery in a similar fashion to the iliac artery (Fig. 11-10).

After the vascular anastomosis is completed and the kidney perfused (Fig. 11-11), urinary continuity can be restored by a number of well-described techniques. The important principles are to attach the ureter to the bladder mucosa in a tension-free manner and to cover the distal 1 cm of the ureter with a submucosal tunnel, thus protecting against reflux during voiding (Figs. 11-11 and 11-12).

In approximately 10 to 15% of cases, there are multiple arteries to the kidney. Several options are possible for reconstruction in these cases, including implantation of the multiple vessels individu-

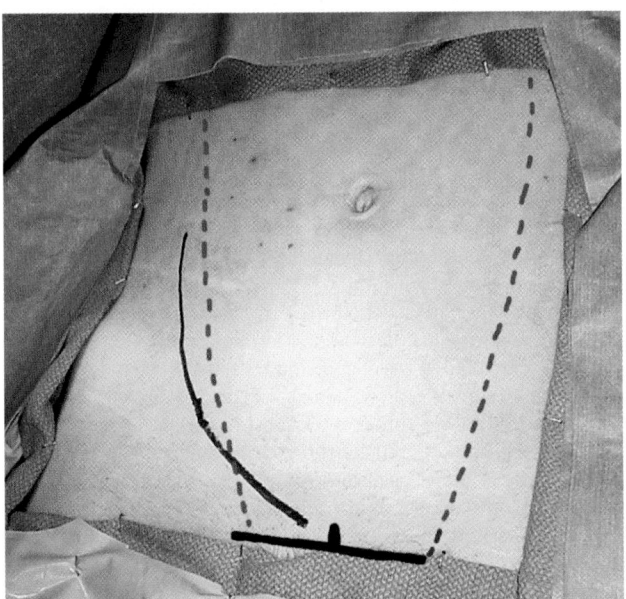

FIG. 11-6. Placement of incision for heterotopic kidney transplant in the right iliac fossa. The incision starts just above the pubic bone in the midline, curves up laterally, and then passes superiorly along the edge of the rectus muscle.

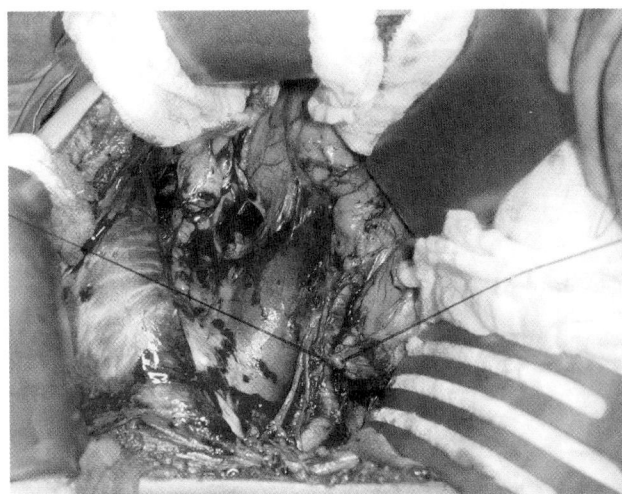

FIG. 11-8. The peritoneum is reflected medially to expose the retroperitoneal space.

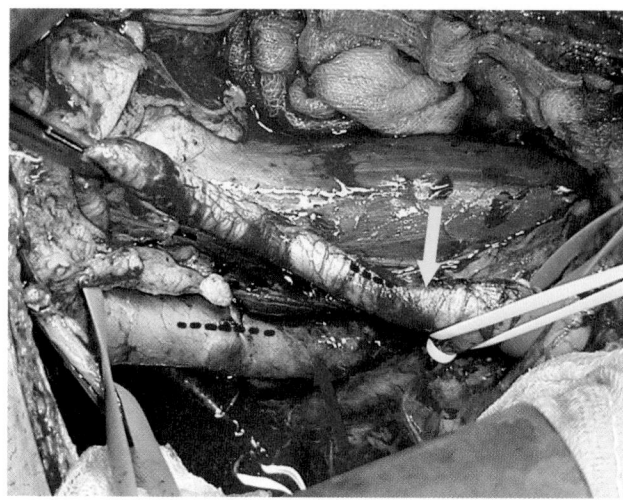

FIG. 11-9. The external iliac vessels are isolated in preparation for anastomosis to the renal vessels. Yellow arrow = external iliac artery; blue arrow = external iliac vein; dotted lines = planned site of arteriotomy and venotomy.

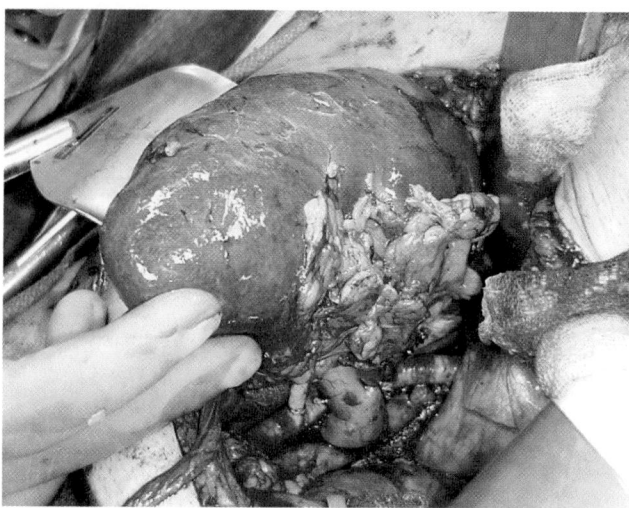

FIG. 11-11. The clamps are removed, allowing the kidney to reperfuse.

ally in the recipient (Fig. 11-13A) or back table reconstruction onto the main donor renal artery to allow for one arterial anastomosis in the recipient (Fig. 11-13B).

Intraoperative care of kidney transplant recipients is not unlike that of other patients undergoing major surgical procedures. To decrease the incidence of ATN posttransplant, a liberal hydration policy is used intraoperatively. Adequate perfusion of the transplanted kidney is important to ensure postoperative diuresis. Central venous pressure (CVP) should be maintained around 10 mmHg, and systolic blood pressure should be greater than 120 mmHg. Maintaining adequate CVP is especially important in smaller, pediatric recipients because reperfusion of an adult-sized kidney graft may divert a significant amount of their own blood volume. Administering mannitol and furosemide just before reperfusion usually is helpful in maximizing perfusion to the kidney graft.

Early Postoperative Care

The immediate postoperative care of all recipients involves (a) stabilizing the major organ systems (e.g., cardiovascular, pulmonary, and renal); (b) evaluating graft function; (c) achieving adequate immunosuppression; and (d) monitoring and treating complications directly and indirectly related to the transplant. Initially, hemodynamic stabil-

ity is assessed, as with all postsurgical patients. Blood pressure, heart rate, and urine output are measured. CVP monitoring may be useful in guiding fluid replacement therapy. Achieving hemodynamic stability is important for the recipient's overall status, but it also is necessary to optimize graft function; hemodynamically unstable recipients experience poor perfusion of their kidney graft.

Careful attention to fluid and electrolyte management is crucial. In general, recipients should be kept euvolemic or slightly hypervolemic. If initial graft function is good, fluid replacement can be regulated by hourly replacement of urine. Half-normal saline is a good solution to use for urine replacement. Aggressive replacement of electrolytes, including calcium, magnesium, and potassium, may be necessary, especially for recipients undergoing brisk diuresis. Those with ATN and fluid overload or hyperkalemia may need fluid restriction and even hemodialysis. Magnesium levels should be kept above 2 mEq/L to prevent seizures, and phosphate levels kept between 2 and 5 mEq/L for proper support of the respiratory and alimentary tracts. Marked hyperglycemia, which may be secondary to steroids, should be treated with insulin.

Hypotension is unusual early after a kidney transplant. When it occurs, it is usually related to hypovolemia. The treatment is to optimize preload and afterload and, only if necessary, to use inotropic agents such as dopamine. Systemic hypertension is more common early posttransplant. If hypertension is catecholamine-mediated or an effect of immunosuppressive agents, it usually responds well to treatment with calcium channel blockers. However, if it is secondary to fluid overload, and if the recipient has poor kidney function, dialysis may be necessary.

A critical aspect of postoperative care is the repeated evaluation of graft function, which in fact begins intraoperatively, soon after the kidney is reperfused. Signs of good kidney function include appropriate color and texture along with evidence of urine production. Postoperatively, urine output is the most readily available and easily measured indicator of graft function. Urine volume may range from none (anuria) to large quantities (polyuria). When using posttransplant urine volume to monitor graft function, the clinician should have knowledge of the recipient's pretransplant urine volume. If an individual was relatively anuric pretransplant, but then has normal urine output posttransplant, graft function is evident. However, if urine volume was significantly high pretransplant, normal urine output posttransplant does not necessarily mean good graft function; the urine may be from the native kidneys rather than from the graft. Laboratory values of obvious use in assessing graft function include serum blood urea nitrogen and creatinine levels.

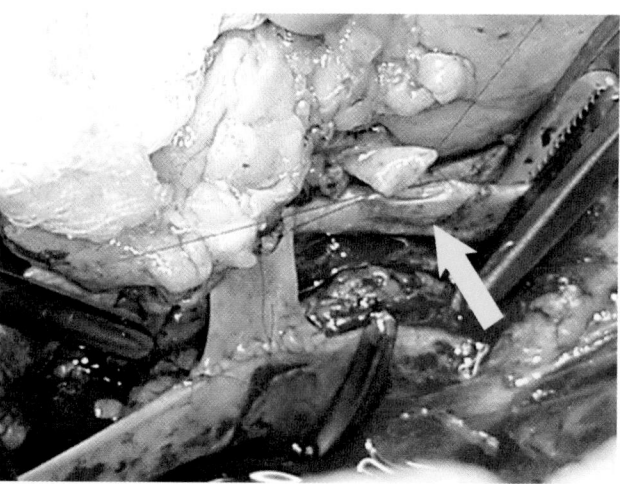

FIG. 11-10. An end-to-side anastomosis of the renal artery to the external iliac artery is performed. Yellow arrow = external iliac artery.

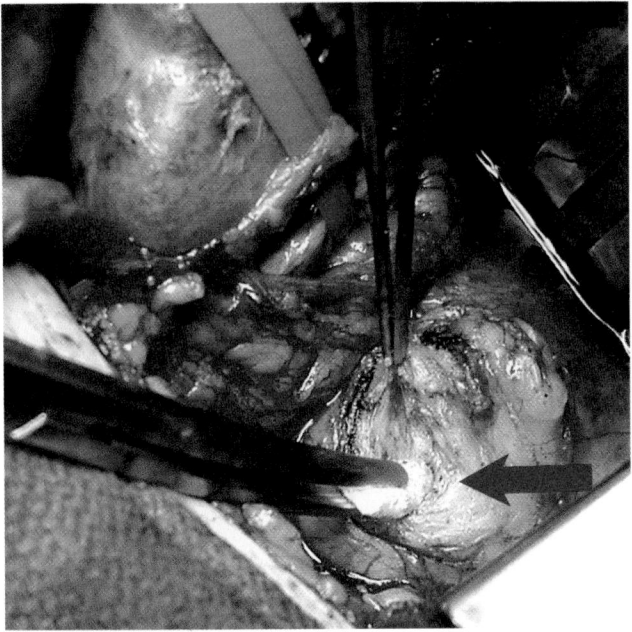

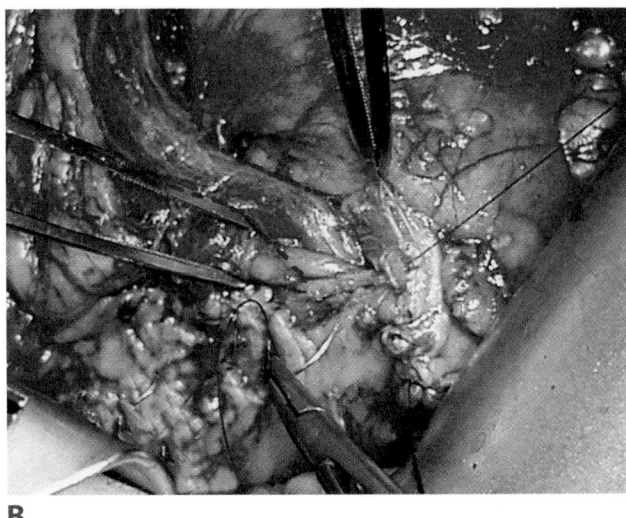

FIG. 11-12. A. Preparation of the bladder for the ureter anastomosis by division of the detrusor muscle (*arrow*). **B.** Completion of the ureter (*dashed lines*) to bladder anastomosis with closure of the detrusor muscle over the distal ureter to create an antireflux tunnel.

Recipients can be divided into three groups (by initial graft function as indicated by their urine output and serum creatinine) as those with (a) immediate graft function, characterized by a brisk diuresis posttransplant and rapidly falling serum creatinine level; (b) slow graft function, characterized by a moderate degree of kidney dysfunction posttransplant, with modest amounts of urine and a slowly falling creatinine level, but no need for dialysis at any time posttransplant; and (c) delayed graft function, which represents the far end of the spectrum of posttransplant graft dysfunction and is defined by the need for dialysis posttransplant.[44]

Decreased or minimal urine output is a frequent concern posttransplant. Most commonly, it is due to an alteration in volume status. Other causes include a blocked urinary catheter, vascular thrombosis,

a urinary leak or obstruction, early acute rejection, drug toxicity, or delayed graft function (Table 11-4). Early diagnosis is important, and begins with an assessment of the recipient's volume status. The urinary catheter is checked to exclude the presence of occlusion with clots or debris. Other diagnostic tests that may be warranted, depending on the suspected cause, include a Doppler ultrasound, nuclear medicine scan, or a biopsy.

Complications

Monitoring for potential surgical and medical complications is important. Early diagnosis and appropriate intervention can minimize the detrimental impact on the graft and recipient. Potential

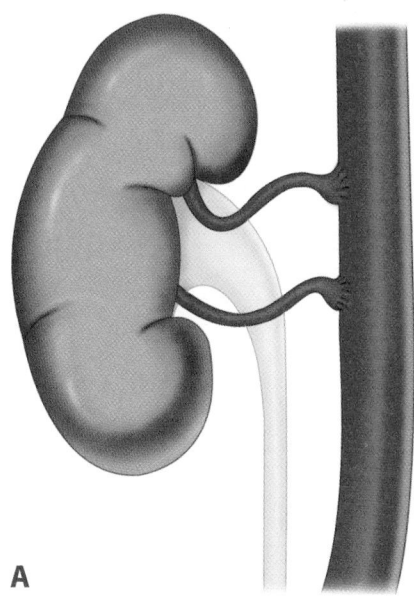

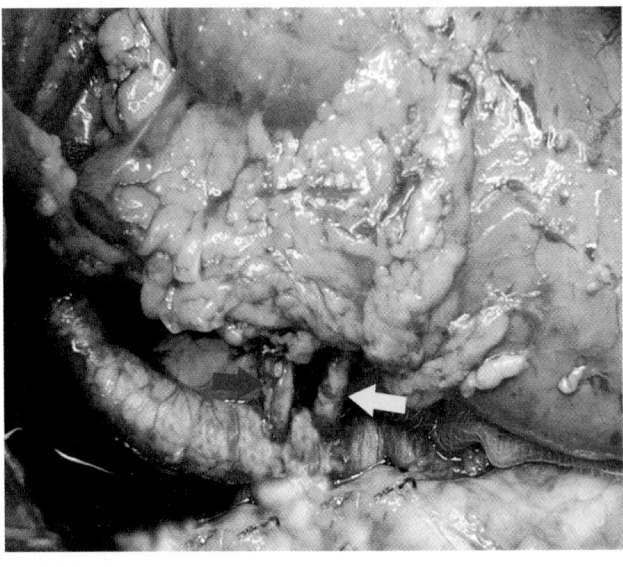

FIG. 11-13. Options for multiple renal arteries, including (**A**) implantation of both arteries separately onto recipient iliac vessel (*blue and yellow arrows*) or (**B**) bench preparation of multiple vessels with end-to-side anastomosis to main donor renal artery. (*Continued*)

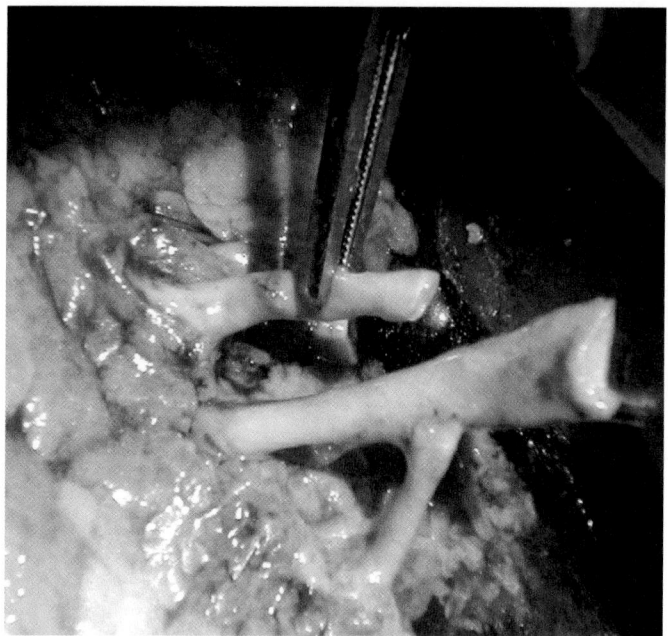 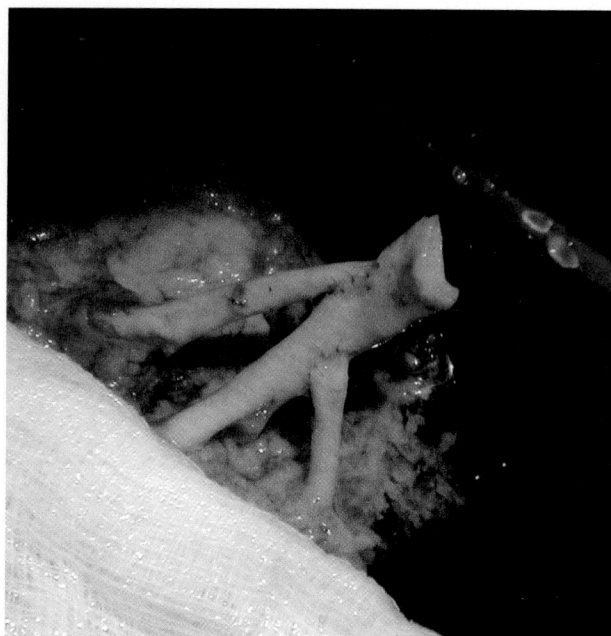

B

FIG. 11-13. (*Continued*)

complications that may occur early after surgery include hemorrhage, vascular complications, urologic complications, lymphocele, and several others.

Hemorrhage

Bleeding is uncommon after a kidney transplant; usually it occurs from unligated vessels in the graft hilum or from the retroperitoneum of the recipient. A falling hematocrit level, hypotension, or tachycardia should raise the possibility of bleeding. Surgical exploration seldom is required because bleeding often tamponades. However, ongoing transfusion requirements, hemodynamic instability, and compression of the kidney by hematoma are all indications for surgical re-exploration.

Vascular Complications

Vascular complications can involve the donor vessels (renal artery thrombosis or stenosis, renal vein thrombosis), the recipient vessels [iliac artery thrombosis, pseudoaneurysms, and deep venous thrombosis (DVT)], or both. Renal artery thrombosis usually occurs early posttransplant; it is uncommon, with an incidence of less than 1%. However, it is a devastating complication, usually resulting in graft loss. Typically, it occurs secondary to a technical problem such as intimal dissection or torsion of the vessels. Risk factors for thrombosis include hypotension, multiple renal arteries, unidentified injury to the intima of the artery, hyperacute rejection, unrelenting acute rejection, and a hypercoagulable state. Under these circumstances there is a sudden cessation of urine output. Diagnosis is made easily

---

TABLE 11-4	Causes of increased serum creatinine early after kidney transplant		
Cause	**Characteristics**	**Diagnosis**	**Treatment**
Hypovolemia	• Decreased CVP • Decreasing urine output • Low blood pressure • Low Hgb if due to bleeding	• Check Hgb and CVP	• Rehydrate with appropriate fluids
Vascular thrombosis	• Sudden drop in urine output • Dark hematuria • Tender, swollen graft	• Ultrasound with Doppler	• Re-explore for thrombectomy or nephrectomy
Bladder outlet obstruction	• Clots in urinary catheter • Sudden drop in urine output	• Distended bladder on examination or by ultrasound	• Irrigate or change bladder catheter
Ureter obstruction	—	• Euvolemic • Ultrasound showing hydroureter • Possible lymphocele on ultrasound	• Do percutaneous nephrostogram • Drainage of lymphocele (if it is the cause of ureter obstruction)
Drug toxicity	• High CSA or FK506 level	• Check drug levels	• Decrease dosage of drugs
Acute rejection	• May have risk factors such as low drug levels, high PRA	• Kidney biopsy	• Administer bolus steroid or antilymphocyte treatment • Begin plasmapheresis (and IVIG if humoral rejection)

CSA = cyclosporin A; CVP = central venous pressure; Hgb = hemoglobin; IVIG = intravenous immunoglobulin; PRA = panel reactive antibody.

with color flow Doppler studies. Urgent thrombectomy is indicated, but most such grafts cannot be salvaged and require removal. Stenosis of the renal artery is a late complication and presents with evidence of graft dysfunction or hypertension. First-line treatment is with interventional radiologic techniques; surgery is reserved for stenosis that does not respond to this therapy.

Renal vein thrombosis is not as common as its arterial counterpart, but again, graft loss is the usual end result. Causes include angulation or torsion of the vein, compression by hematomas or lymphoceles, anastomotic stenosis, and extension of an underlying DVT. Again, Doppler studies are the best diagnostic test. Urgent thrombectomy rarely is successful, and nephrectomy is usually required. Venous thromboembolic complications that affect the recipient vessels [DVT and pulmonary embolism (PE)] are not uncommon. The incidence of DVT is close to 5%; the incidence of PE 1%. Identified risk factors include recipient age over 40, hypercoagulable states, diabetes, and a history of DVT. For recipients with these risk factors, prophylaxis with low-dose heparin is recommended.

Urologic Complications

Urinary tract complications, manifesting as leakage or obstruction, generally occur in 2 to 10% of kidney recipients. The underlying cause often is related to poor blood supply and ischemia of the transplant ureter. Leakage most commonly occurs from the anastomotic site. Causes other than ischemia include undue tension created by a short ureter, and direct surgical injury. Presentation is usually early (before the fifth posttransplant week); symptoms include fever, pain, swelling at the graft site, increased creatinine level, decreased urine output, and cutaneous urinary drainage. Diagnosis can be confirmed initially with a hippurate renal scan, although a percutaneous nephrostogram is required for precise definition. Early surgical exploration with ureteral reimplantation usually is indicated, although small leaks may be managed by percutaneous nephrostomy and stent placement with good results.

Ureteral obstruction may develop early or late. Early obstruction may be due to edema, blood clots, hematomas, or torsion of the ureter. Late obstruction generally is due to scarring and fibrosis from chronic ischemia. Patients develop an elevated serum creatinine level. An ultrasound to look for hydronephrosis is a good initial test. Percutaneous transluminal dilatation, followed by placement of an internal or external stent, is a good initial treatment. If repeated dilatations and stenting are required, surgical intervention (e.g., ureteral reimplantation or ureteropyelostomy using the native ureter) should be undertaken.

Lymphocele

The reported incidence of lymphoceles (fluid collections of lymph that generally result from cut lymphatic vessels in the recipient) is 0.6 to 18%. Lymphoceles usually do not occur until at least 2 weeks posttransplant. Symptoms are generally related to the mass effect and compression of nearby structures (e.g., ureter, iliac vein, allograft renal artery), and patients develop hypertension, unilateral leg swelling on the side of the transplant, and elevated serum creatinine. Ultrasound is used to confirm a fluid collection, although percutaneous aspiration may be necessary to exclude presence of other collections such as urinomas, hematomas, or abscesses. The standard surgical treatment is creation of a peritoneal window to allow for drainage of the lymphatic fluid into the peritoneal cavity, where it can be absorbed. Either a laparoscopic or an open approach may be used. Another option is percutaneous insertion of a drainage catheter, with or without sclerotherapy; however, it is associated with some risk of recurrence or infection.

Other Complications

A wide variety of medical complications can be seen after a kidney transplant. Infections are probably the most common, but the incidence has declined significantly in recent years due to improvements in prophylaxis regimens. Common sites for infection include the

urinary tract, the pulmonary system, and the wound. Noninfectious medical complications affecting the cardiac, GI, and neurologic systems also have been well described posttransplant.[45] Such complications are often related to the administration of immunosuppressive drugs.

Late Posttransplant Care

The goal of late posttransplant care of the kidney transplant recipient is to optimize immunosuppression, carefully monitor graft function, and screen and monitor for complications that are directly or indirectly related to immunosuppressive medications. Optimizing immunosuppression entails fitting it to the individual recipient's needs. Recipients at low risk for rejection should have their immunosuppression lowered to minimize side effects and complications. Careful attention should be paid to compliance; it often is easy for recipients to become less attentive to their medications as they progress through the posttransplant period. Monitoring kidney function may help detect noncompliance, but also is important to detect late rejection episodes, recurrence of disease, or late technical problems (such as renal artery stenosis or ureteric stricture). Other potential problems in these recipients include hypercholesterolemia, hypertriglyceridemia, and increased blood pressure, which may or may not be related to the immunosuppressive drugs. Screening for malignancy (especially skin, colorectal, breast, cervical, and prostate) is important, although the incidence of many of these malignancies is equivalent to those seen in the general population. Patients should be immunized, ideally pretransplant, for *Haemophilus influenzae*, *Streptococcus pneumoniae*, and *Neisseria meningitidis*, as this is important to minimize infectious complications due to these pathogens.

Results

Posttransplant outcomes have steadily improved over the past 3 decades due to improvements in immunosuppression, organ retrieval techniques, perioperative care, and treatment of infectious posttransplant complications.[46–48] Since the late 1980s, the use of modern immunosuppressive drugs has been a primary factor, especially in those previously considered to be at high risk, such as diabetic, pediatric, and older recipients.

Most centers now report patient survival rates exceeding 95% during the first posttransplant year for all kidney recipients (Table 11-5). Living-donor transplants still have an advantage over deceased-donor transplants, but even this difference is diminishing with modern immunosuppression. The survival advantage after a transplant, as compared with dialysis, is probably greatest for

TABLE 11-5	Patient survival rates (%) after the various transplants				
Time Posttransplant	**3 Mo**	**1 Y**	**3 Y**	**5 Y**	**10 Y**
Kidney					
Deceased donor	97.9	94.7	88.1	80.7	60.7
Living donor	99.2	98.0	94.5	90.4	76.4
SPK	97.7	95.1	90.8	85.8	69.2
PAK	98.3	95.5	89.9	83.6	60.7
PTA	97.9	94.9	91.6	90.2	66.9
Liver					
Deceased donor	93.2	86.9	79.0	73.4	59.4
Living donor	95.8	91.2	82.9	76.8	76.2
Intestine	93.2	87.5	62.2	50.2	40.6
Heart	92.5	88.1	80.2	73.7	53.4
Lung	93.2	84.9	66.4	51.6	25.6
Heart-lung	77.8	66.7	53.8	43.6	27.3

PAK = pancreas after kidney; PTA = pancreas transplant alone; SPK = simultaneous pancreas-kidney.

Source: Reproduced with permission from 2006 OPTN/SRTR Annual Report, *http://www.ustransplant.org*.

TABLE 11-6	Graft survival rates (%) after the various transplants				
Time Posttransplant	**3 Mo**	**1 Y**	**3 Y**	**5 Y**	**10 Y**
Kidney					
Deceased donor	94.3	89.5	78.6	67.1	40.8
Living donor	97.2	95.1	88.4	80.3	56.5
SPK (pancreas)	89.2	85.2	79.3	71.1	54.5
PAK	86.7	78.7	67.3	56.4	27.6
PTA	87.5	72.8	58.4	53.4	25.9
Liver					
Deceased donor	89.6	82.4	73.6	67.4	53.0
Living donor	90.0	84.0	76.0	68.8	66.5
Intestine	88.3	78.5	50.6	40.1	27.9
Heart	92.0	87.5	79.4	72.6	51.5
Lung	92.5	83.3	64.4	48.9	23.4
Heart-lung	75.2	64.1	53.1	41.5	26.5

PAK = pancreas after kidney; PTA = pancreas transplant alone; SPK = simultaneous pancreas-kidney.
Source: Reproduced with permission from 2006 OPTN/SRTR Annual Report, http://www.ustransplant.org.

diabetic patients. Without a transplant, their overall survival is 26% at 5 years; with a transplant, it jumps to about 80%. The major cause of death in all kidney recipients is cardiovascular (myocardial infarction or stroke); sepsis accounts for less than 3%, while malignancy accounts for 2%.

The incidence of acute rejection has declined steadily since the early 1990s. Most centers now report acute rejection rates of 10 to 20% at 1 year posttransplant. This decline has been a major factor in the improvement in graft survival rates, which are now about 75 to 80% at 5 years and 60 to 65% at 10 years posttransplant for all kidney recipients[49] (Table 11-6). Currently, the most common cause of graft loss is recipient death (usually from cardiovascular causes) with a functioning graft. The second most common cause is chronic allograft nephropathy. Characterized by a slow, unrelenting deterioration of graft function, it likely has multiple causes (both immunologic and nonimmunologic).[50,51] The graft failure rate due to surgical technique has remained at about 2%.

PANCREAS TRANSPLANTATION

Diabetes mellitus is a very common medical condition with immense medical, social, and financial costs. In North America, it is the leading cause of kidney failure, blindness, nontraumatic amputations, and impotence. The discovery of insulin in 1922 by Banting and Best changed diabetes from a lethal disease to a chronic illness. However, even though exogenous insulin can prevent the acute metabolic complications and decrease the incidence of secondary complications associated with diabetes, it cannot provide a homeostatic environment comparable to that afforded by a functioning pancreas. Only a functioning pancreas can provide immediate insulin responses to the moment-to-moment changes in glucose levels.

A successful pancreas transplant can establish normoglycemia and insulin independence in diabetic recipients, with glucose control similar to that seen with a functioning native pancreas. A pancreas transplant also has the potential to halt progression of some secondary complications of diabetes. No current method of exogenous insulin administration can produce a euglycemic, insulin-independent state akin to that achievable with a technically successful pancreas graft. In addition to improved metabolic control and beneficial effects on secondary complications, a pancreas transplant can substantially enhance quality of life, more than that achieved by exogenous insulin administration. Indeed, the modern management of diabetes by exogenous insulin may be as burdensome as dialysis is for kidney failure, as it consists of four blood

glucose determinations daily, coupled with four insulin injections or a constantly present needle. A successful pancreas transplant obviates the need for such constant invasive monitoring.

Currently, the main drawback of a pancreas transplant is the need for immunosuppression. Pancreas transplants are now preferentially performed in diabetic patients with kidney failure who also are candidates for a kidney transplant, as they already require immunosuppression to prevent kidney rejection. However, a pancreas transplant alone (PTA) is appropriate for nonuremic diabetics if their day-to-day quality of life is so poor (e.g., labile serum glucose with ketoacidosis and/or hypoglycemic episodes, or progression of severe diabetic retinopathy, nephropathy, neuropathy, and/or enteropathy) that chronic immunosuppression is justified to achieve insulin independence.[52] As immunosuppressive agents become safer, it is likely that PTA will become increasingly common.

History

The first human pancreas transplant was performed in 1966; however, the procedure was not performed with any frequency until many years later. During the 1970s, a small number of institutions performed a few pancreas transplants, and their success rates were low, mainly because of problems with rejection. A dramatic improvement in outcome occurred in the 1980s, after advances in surgical techniques and the introduction of cyclosporine for immunosuppression. In the United States, the inception of UNOS in 1987 facilitated nationwide organ procurement and allocation. A steady growth in the application of pancreas transplants soon followed. By the mid-1990s, more than 1000 pancreas transplants were being performed annually in the United States, with improved results paralleling the introduction of even newer immunosuppressive drugs such as tacrolimus and MMF.

Results also improved because of refinements in surgical technique. By the mid-1970s, the following three techniques were in use: enteric drainage (ED), urinary drainage (first into the ureter, and later modified by direct implantation into the bladder), and duct injection. During the 1980s, bladder drainage (BD) was shown to be safe, and it became the predominant technique in all pancreas recipient categories, as it facilitated allograft monitoring via measurement of urine amylase levels. The 1990s saw a shift back to ED, especially in patients who underwent a simultaneous kidney transplant. In such recipients, the serum creatinine level could be used as a surrogate marker for pancreas rejection when both organs came from the same donor.

Preoperative Evaluation

The preoperative evaluation for pancreas transplant recipients does not differ substantially from that for diabetic kidney transplant recipients. Examination of the cardiovascular system is most important because significant coronary artery disease may be present without angina.[53] Noninvasive testing may not identify coronary artery disease, so coronary angiography is routinely performed. Detailed neurologic, ophthalmologic, metabolic, and kidney function testing may be needed to assess the degree of progression of secondary complications. Any contraindications to a transplant, such as active malignancy or infection, must be ruled out. A thorough evaluation of the peripheral vascular system is essential, given the high incidence of peripheral vascular disease in diabetics. The patency of the iliac system needs to be determined, because the iliac vessels will serve as the inflow source for the pancreas.

Once a patient is determined to be a good candidate for a pancreas transplant, with no obvious contraindications, it is important to decide which type of pancreas transplant is best for that individual. First, the degree of kidney dysfunction and the need for a kidney transplant must be determined. Patients with stable kidney function (creatinine less than 2 mg/dL and minimal protein in the urine) are candidates for a PTA. However, patients with moderate kidney insufficiency will likely require a kidney transplant as well; further deterioration of kidney function often occurs once calcineurin inhibitors are started for immunosuppression.

For patients requiring both a kidney and a pancreas transplant, various options are available. The two transplants can be performed either simultaneously or sequentially. A living donor or a deceased donor can be used, or both. Which option is best for the individual patient depends on the degree of kidney dysfunction, the availability of donors, and personal preference. The following options are currently possible:

- Deceased-donor, simultaneous pancreas-kidney transplant (SPK): The most common option worldwide, deceased-donor SPK transplants have well-documented, long-term survival results for both the kidney and the pancreas grafts. The recipient has the advantage of undergoing both transplants at the same time, and therefore may potentially become dialysis free and insulin independent at the same time. There is also an immunologic advantage, as acute rejection rates are significantly lower for SPK (vs. PTA) recipients.

- Living-donor kidney transplant, followed weeks to months later by a deceased-donor pancreas transplant [pancreas after kidney (PAK) transplant]: If a living donor is available for the kidney transplant, then this is a good option for uremic diabetic patients. It offers the possibility of performing the kidney transplant as soon as the living-donor evaluation is complete, rendering the recipient dialysis free within a short period. A living-donor (vs. deceased-donor) kidney transplant has superior long-term results. By performing the two operations sequentially instead of simultaneously, the overall surgical complication rate may be decreased, perhaps because by the time of the pancreas transplant, the effects of uremia have resolved and patients are in better metabolic and nutritional condition.[54] The disadvantage is that the long-term pancreas graft survival rates for PAK recipients are still somewhat inferior to those of individuals receiving SPK transplants.

- Simultaneous deceased-donor pancreas and living-donor kidney transplant: Candidates with a suitable living donor for the kidney transplant who have not yet progressed to dialysis can be placed on the deceased-donor pancreas transplant waiting list. When a deceased-donor pancreas becomes available, the living donor for the kidney is called in at the same time, and both procedures are performed simultaneously. Advantages include use of a living donor for the kidney, shorter waiting times, and a single operation.[55] Technically, this option may be more difficult to organize, as it requires using two full surgical teams and two full operating rooms, and at times the donor and the recipient will need to be called in from different locations. It also may create difficult timing issues for the living donor, who must come in quickly for an emergent operation.

- Living-donor, SPK transplant: If a single individual is suitable to donate both a kidney and a hemipancreas, then this may be a potential option. It is especially useful for candidates with a high level of preformed antibodies, or those who have difficulty acquiring a deceased-donor organ. The main disadvantage of this approach is to the living donor, who has to undergo a surgical procedure of substantial magnitude with its attendant risks and morbidity.

Surgical Procedure

The initial preparation of the donor pancreas is a crucial component of a successful transplant. Direct physical examination of the pancreas often is the best or only way to confirm its suitability (Fig. 11-14). If it is sclerotic, calcific, or markedly discolored, it should not be used. Before implantation, a surgical procedure is undertaken to remove the spleen and any excess duodenum, and to ligate blood vessels at the root of the mesentery (Fig. 11-15A-C). The inflow vessels to the graft are the splenic and superior mesenteric arteries; outflow is via the portal vein. Arterial reconstruction is performed before implanting the graft in the recipient. The donor superior mesenteric and splenic arteries are connected, most commonly using

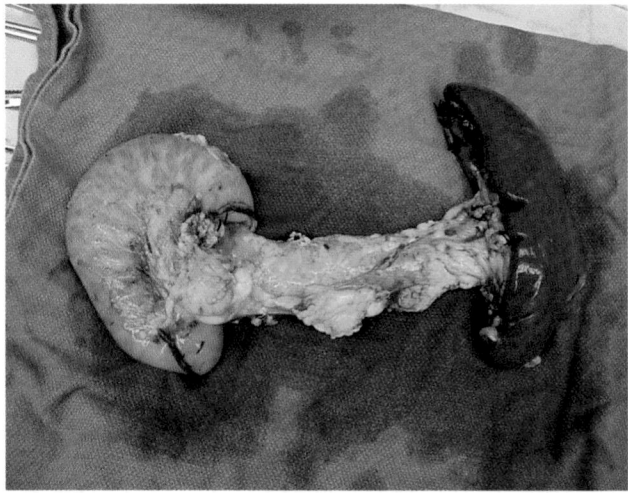

FIG. 11-14. Pancreas graft before bench preparation with spleen attached.

a reversed segment of donor iliac artery as a Y-graft (Figs. 11-15D and 11-16); doing so allows for a single arterial anastomosis in the recipient.

The pancreas graft is then implanted via an anastomosis of the aforementioned arterial graft to the recipient common iliac artery or distal aorta, and, via a venous anastomosis of the donor portal vein to the recipient iliac vein (for systemic drainage, Fig. 11-17), or to the superior mesenteric vein (for portal drainage).[56] If both a kidney and a pancreas are transplanted, they are placed in an intraperitoneal position, with the kidney usually in the left iliac fossa and the pancreas in the right iliac fossa (Fig. 11-18). If the pancreas is drained via the portal route, then it usually sits higher in the mid-abdomen (Fig. 11-19).

Once the pancreas is revascularized, a drainage procedure must be performed to handle the pancreatic exocrine secretions. Options include anastomosing the donor duodenum to the recipient bladder (Fig. 11-20) or to the small bowel, with the small bowel either in continuity or connected to a Roux-en-Y limb. Some centers always use ED, others always use BD, and others tailor the approach according to the recipient category. Both ED and BD now have a relatively low surgical risk. The main advantage of BD is the ability to directly measure enzyme activity in the pancreatic graft exocrine secretions by measuring the amount of amylase in the urine. A decrease in urine amylase is a sensitive marker for rejection, even though it is not entirely specific. Urine amylase always decreases before hyperglycemia ensues. A rise in serum amylase may precede a decrease in urine amylase, but serum amylase by itself is less sensitive (it does not always rise, but urine amylase always decreases), and is no more specific for the diagnosis of rejection. The leak rate is the same whether the pancreas is drained to the bladder or to the bowel, but the consequences of a bladder leak are much less severe than those associated with a bowel leak. The disadvantages of BD include complications such as dehydration and acidosis (from loss of alkalotic pancreatic secretions in the urine), and local problems with the bladder such as infection, hematuria, stones, and urethritis. Because of these chronic complications, between 10 and 20% of bladder-drained graft recipients are ultimately converted to ED.

ED is more physiologic and has fewer long-term complications. However, the ability to monitor for rejection is decreased, given the absence of urinary amylase. Rejection in SPK transplant recipients almost always affects both the kidney and the pancreas; therefore, the serum creatinine level can be used as a marker for rejection of the pancreas. Hence, most centers now use ED for SPK transplants. If the kidney and the pancreas are from different donors, or if a PTA is performed, then BD is preferred, so rejection of the pancreas can be detected earlier.

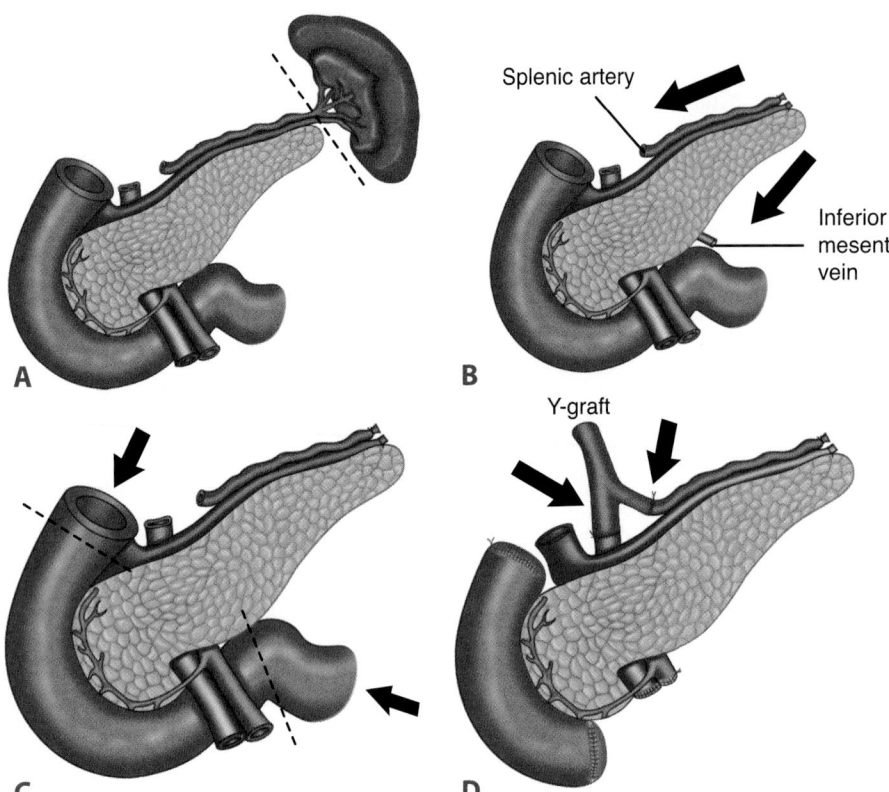

FIG. 11-15. Bench preparation of pancreas graft. Steps include (**A**) removal of the spleen; (**B**) removal of tissue along the superior and inferior aspect of the tail of the pancreas; (**C**) trimming of excess duodenum; and (**D**) ligation of vessels at the root of the mesentery and placement of arterial Y-graft.

Postoperative Care

In general, pancreas recipients do not require intensive care monitoring in the postoperative period. Laboratory values—serum glucose, hemoglobin, electrolytes, and amylase—are monitored daily. The serum glucose level is monitored even more frequently if normoglycemia is not immediately achieved. Nasogastric suction and IV fluids are continued for the first several days until bowel function returns. In the early postoperative period, regular insulin is infused to maintain plasma glucose levels less than 150 mg/dL, because chronic hyperglycemia may be detrimental to β-cells. In recipients who undergo BD, a Foley catheter is left in place for 10 to 14 days. At most centers, some form of prophylaxis is instituted against bacterial, fungal, and viral infections. In addition, many centers routinely

institute some form of prophylaxis against thrombosis of the allograft; options include low-dose heparin, low molecular weight heparin, or oral antiplatelet agents for the first week posttransplant.

Complications

One crucial aspect of posttransplant care is monitoring for rejection and complications (both surgical and medical). Rejection episodes may be identified by an increase in serum creatinine (in SPK recipients), a decrease in urinary amylase (in recipients with BD), an increase in serum amylase, or by an increase in serum glucose levels. Complications are, unfortunately, common after pancreas transplants. The pancreas graft is susceptible to a unique set of complications because of its exocrine secretions and low blood flow. However,

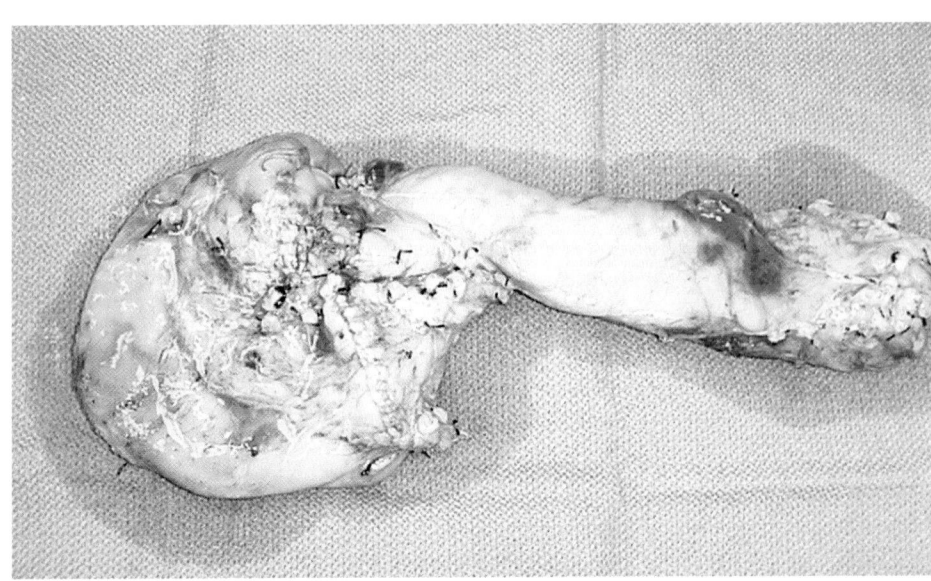

FIG. 11-16. Final appearance of benched pancreas before implantation in the recipient.

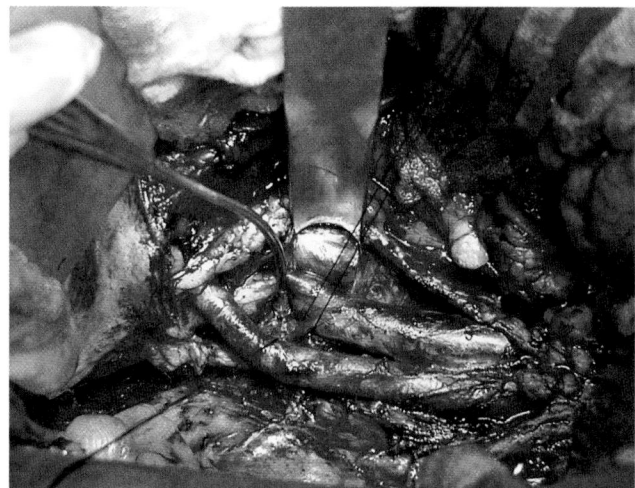

FIG. 11-17. Preparation of iliac vessels for implantation of the pancreas with ligation and division of all hypogastric veins.

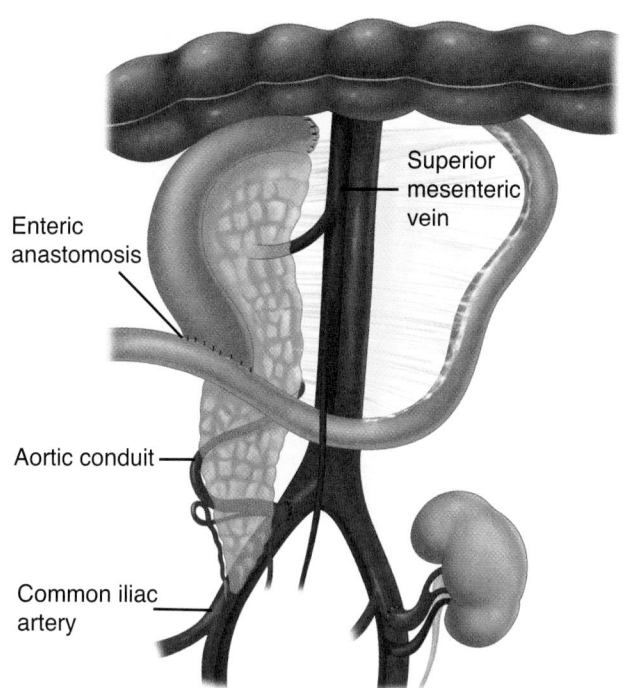

FIG. 11-19. Combined kidney and pancreas transplant with portal enteric drainage of pancreas graft. The pancreas transplant is situated higher in the abdomen and is oriented pointing toward the head of the recipient.

the incidence of graft-related complications has decreased significantly since the early 1990s due to better preservation techniques, better surgical methods, improved prophylaxis regimens, and improved immunosuppression.[57] Potential complications are described below.

Thrombosis

The incidence of thrombosis is approximately 6% for pancreas transplants reported to the UNOS registry. Low-dose heparin, dextran, or antiplatelet agents are administered routinely in the early postoperative period at many centers, although these agents slightly increase the risk of postoperative bleeding. Arterial or venous thrombosis is most common within the first several days posttransplant, heralded by an increase in blood glucose levels, an increase in insulin requirements, or a decrease in urine amylase levels. Venous thrombosis also is characteristically accompanied by hematuria, tenderness and swelling of the graft, and ipsilateral lower extremity edema. Treatment consists of graft removal.

Hemorrhage

Postoperative bleeding may be minimized by meticulous intraoperative control of bleeding sites. Hemorrhage may be exacerbated by

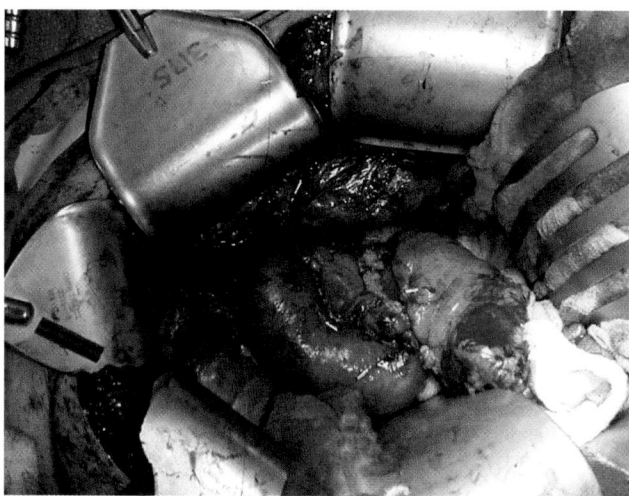

FIG. 11-18. Reperfused pancreas allograft after completion of the vascular anastomosis.

anticoagulants and antiplatelet drugs, but their benefits seem to outweigh the risks. Bleeding is a much less significant cause (<1%) of graft loss than is thrombosis, according to UNOS registry data. Significant bleeding is treated by immediate re-exploration.

Pancreatitis

Most cases of graft pancreatitis occur early, tend to be self limited, and are probably due to ischemic preservation injury. Clinical manifestations may include graft tenderness and fever, in addition to hyperamylasemia. Treatment consists of IV fluid replacement and keeping the recipient fasting. Later episodes of graft pancreatitis may be caused by reflux into the allograft duct (in recipients who undergo BD) or by cytomegalovirus (CMV) infection. Reflux is treated by urinary catheter drainage, and occasionally by conversion to ED. CMV infections are treated with appropriate antiviral agents.

Urologic Complications

Urologic complications are almost exclusively limited to recipients with BD. Hematuria is not uncommon in the first several months posttransplant, but usually it is transient and self limiting. Bladder calculi may develop because exposed sutures or staples along the duodenocystostomy serve as a nidus for stone formation. Recurrent urinary tract infections commonly occur concurrently. Treatment consists of cystoscopy with removal of the sutures or staples. Urinary leaks, most commonly from the proximal duodenal cuff or from the duodenal anastomosis to the bladder, typically occur during the first several weeks posttransplant. Small leaks can be successfully managed by prolonged (at least 2 weeks) urinary catheter drainage; larger leaks require surgical intervention.

Other urinary complications include chronic, refractory, metabolic acidosis because of bicarbonate loss, persistent and recurrent urinary tract infections, and urethritis. Along with recurrent hematuria, these complications are the major indications for converting recipients from BD to ED. Because 10 to 20% of recipients with initial BD will require conversion to ED, a recent trend has been to perform ED at the time of the transplant. ED is associated with

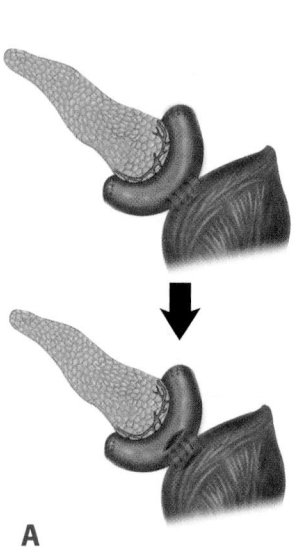

A

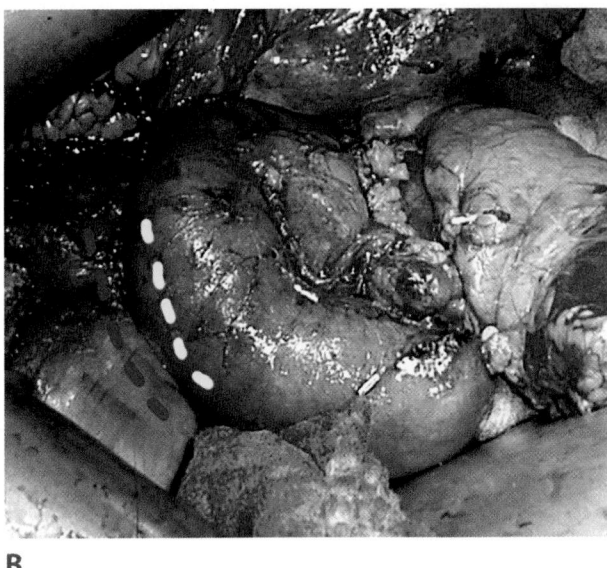

B

FIG. 11-20. A and **B.** Drainage of the exocrine secretions by anastomosis of the recipient bladder to the donor duodenum in a two-layer fashion.

significantly fewer urinary tract infections and urologic complications, but it obviates the use of urinary amylase determinations.

Infections

Infections remain a significant problem after pancreas transplants.[58] Most common are superficial wound infections and intra-abdominal infections, often related to graft complications such as leaks. Thanks to appropriate perioperative antimicrobial regimens (for prophylaxis against gram-positive bacteria, gram-negative bacteria, and yeast) the incidence of significant infections has decreased. Still, it remains about 10% and is associated with significant morbidity and mortality. Thus, if serious intra-abdominal infections occur (whether or not associated with the above complications), re-exploration and graft removal must be strongly considered, along with concurrent reduction in immunosuppression.

Results

The International Pancreas Transplant Registry (IPTR) maintains data on pancreas transplants. Analyses of IPTR data have been published yearly since the mid-1980s. The results (particularly as measured by long-term insulin independence) have continually improved over time. Patient survival rates are not significantly different between the three main recipient categories and are greater than 90% at 3 years posttransplant. Most deaths are due to pre-existing cardiovascular disease; the mortality risk of a pancreas transplant per se is extremely low (e.g., patient survival at 1 year for PTA recipients is >95%). Pancreas graft survival rates at 1 year remain higher in the SPK (~90%) than in the PAK (~85%) and PTA (~80%) categories, according to IPTR data. The differences are due in part to the decreased ability to monitor for rejection episodes in enteric-drained, solitary pancreas transplant recipients. With improving immunosuppressive protocols and the decreasing incidence of acute rejection, the difference between the three categories has been steadily decreasing since the late 1990s.[59,60]

ISLET CELL TRANSPLANTATION

The pancreas consists of two separate functional systems (endocrine and exocrine), but it is only the endocrine component that is of use in the transplant process. However, many of the complications seen with whole-organ pancreas transplants are due to the exocrine component. Therefore, the concept of transplanting simply the cells responsible for the production of insulin is very logical and attractive.

Islet cell transplantation involves extracting islets of Langerhans from a donor's pancreas and then injecting them into a diabetic recipient. These islet cells then engraft into the recipient and secrete insulin, providing excellent moment-to-moment control of blood glucose, as is seen with a whole-organ pancreas transplant. Compared with exogenous insulin injections, an islet cell transplant offers advantages similar to those of a whole-organ pancreas transplant. A successful islet transplant provides perfect glucose homeostasis, freeing the diabetic patient from the burden of frequent glucose monitoring and insulin injections. It potentially prevents secondary complications of diabetes and significantly improves quality of life.

Unlike a whole-organ pancreas transplant, an islet cell transplant is not a major surgical procedure. It generally can be performed as an outpatient procedure, with minimal recovery time for the recipient. It avoids a major surgical procedure, with its associated mortality and morbidity. Given this significantly lower surgical risk, islet cell transplants could theoretically have much wider application than whole-organ transplants.

Typically, a pancreas is procured from a suitable deceased donor. Isolating the islets is a complex process, which generally involves digesting the pancreas with a collagenase solution to separate the islet cells. The islets may then be purified (i.e., separated from the acinar cells). The purified islets can then be injected into the recipient, most commonly into the portal vein. The islet cells then engraft in the hepatic parenchyma and secrete insulin, which drains into the circulation. Potential complications associated with the injection include portal hypertension, hepatic abscesses, and bacteremia.

One major disadvantage of an islet cell transplant (similar to that of a whole-organ transplant) is the need for long-term immunosuppression. This disadvantage has limited the use of islet cell transplants to patients with kidney failure who require immunosuppression because of a kidney transplant.

This immunologic problem is compounded by the fact that islet cell rejection can be difficult to monitor and diagnose. One possible method of avoiding the need for immunosuppression is to surround the islets with a semipermeable membrane, a process called *microencapsulation*. This process would allow small molecules such as oxygen and glucose to reach the islet cells and would allow insulin to reach the systemic circulation. But microencapsulation would prevent immune cells and large molecules such as antibodies from reaching the islet cells. The islet cells would then survive and function well inside the membranes, while being protected from immunologic damage.

Islet cell transplants have been a possibility for many years, but the results have generally been poor. In 1995, a report of the International

Islet Transplant Registry indicated that of 270 recipients, only 5% were insulin independent at 1 year posttransplant. Recently, however, significantly improved results have been reported by using steroid-free immunosuppression and islet injections from multiple donors. These recent successes have stimulated a flurry of islet transplant activity at centers across the world. As results are likely to continue to improve, it is possible that islet cell transplants may come to replace whole-organ pancreas transplants.

LIVER TRANSPLANTATION

The field of liver transplantation has undergone remarkable advances in the last 2 decades. An essentially experimental procedure in the early 1980s, a liver transplant is now the treatment of choice for patients with acute and chronic liver failure. Patient survival at 1 year posttransplant has increased from 30% in the early 1980s to more than 85% at present. The major reasons for this dramatic increase include refined surgical and preservation techniques, better immunosuppressive protocols, more effective treatment of infections, and improved care during the critical perioperative period. However, a liver transplant remains a major undertaking, with the potential for complications affecting every major organ system.

History

The history of liver transplantation began with experimental transplants performed in dogs in the late 1950s. The first liver transplant attempted in humans was in 1963 by Thomas Starzl. The recipient was a 3-year-old boy with biliary atresia who unfortunately died of hemorrhage. The first successful liver transplant was in 1967, again by Starzl. Yet, for the next 10 years, liver transplants remained essentially experimental, with survival rates well below 50%. Still, advances in the surgical procedure and in anesthetic management continued to be made during that time.

The major breakthrough for the field came in the early 1980s, with the introduction and clinical use of the immunosuppressive agent cyclosporine. Patient survival dramatically improved, and liver transplantation was soon being recognized as a viable therapeutic option. Results continued to improve through the 1980s, due to ongoing improvements in immunosuppression, critical care management, surgical technique, and preservation solutions. The late 1980s and 1990s saw a dramatic increase in the number of liver transplants, and an even greater increase in the number of patients waiting for a transplant. This, in turn, increased waiting times as well as mortality rates for those waiting.

The longer waiting time and higher mortality rates for patients on the deceased-donor liver transplant waiting list led to the development of innovative surgical techniques such as split-liver transplants and living-donor liver transplants. Initially, these new techniques were mainly applied to pediatric patients because of the difficulty associated with finding appropriate size-matched organs for them. However, as the number of adults on the waiting list grew, these techniques began to be applied for adult recipients as well. The use of living-donor liver transplants progressed at an even more rapid pace in countries such as Japan, where the concept of deceased-donor organ donation was not widely accepted.

Preoperative Evaluation

A liver transplant is indicated for liver failure, whether acute or chronic. Liver failure is signaled by a number of clinical symptoms [e.g., ascites, variceal bleeding, hepatic encephalopathy (HE), and malnutrition], and by biochemical liver test results that suggest impaired hepatic synthetic function (e.g., hypoalbuminemia, hyperbilirubinemia, and coagulopathy). The cause of liver failure often influences its presentation. For example, patients with acute liver failure generally have HE and coagulopathy, whereas patients with chronic liver disease most commonly have ascites, GI bleeding, and malnutrition.

Diseases Treatable by Transplant

A host of diseases are potentially treatable by a liver transplant (Table 11-7). Broadly, they can be categorized as acute or chronic, and then subdivided by the cause of the liver disease. Chronic liver diseases account for the majority of liver transplants today. The most common cause in North America is chronic hepatitis, usually due to hepatitis C and less commonly to hepatitis B. Chronic alcohol abuse accelerates the process, especially with hepatitis C. Progression from chronic infection to cirrhosis is generally slow, usually occurring over a period of 10 to 20 years. Chronic hepatitis may also result from autoimmune causes, primarily in women. It can present either acutely over months or insidiously over years. Alcohol often plays a role in end-stage liver disease secondary to hepatitis C, but it may also lead to liver failure in the absence of viral infection. In fact, alcohol is the most common cause of end-stage liver disease in the United States. Such patients generally are suitable candidates for a transplant as long as an adequate period of sobriety can be documented.

Cholestatic disorders also account for a significant percentage of transplant candidates with chronic liver disease. In adults, the most common causes are primary biliary cirrhosis (PBC) and primary sclerosing cholangitis (PSC). PBC, a destructive disorder of interlobular bile ducts, can progress to cirrhosis and liver failure over several decades. It most commonly affects middle-aged women. PSC, a disease characterized by inflammatory injury of the bile duct, occurs mostly in young men, 70% of whom have inflammatory bowel disease. In children, biliary atresia is the most common cholestatic disorder. It is a destructive, inflammatory condition of the bile ducts, and if left untreated, it usually results in death within the first 1 to 2 years of life.

A variety of metabolic diseases can result in progressive, chronic liver injury and cirrhosis, including hereditary hemochromatosis (an autosomal recessive disorder characterized by chronic iron accumulation, which may result in cirrhosis, cardiomyopathy, and endocrine disorders including diabetes), alpha$_1$-antitrypsin deficiency (which may result in cirrhosis at any age, most commonly in the first or

TABLE 11-7	Diseases amenable to treatment by a liver transplant
Cholestatic liver diseases	
Primary biliary cirrhosis	
Primary sclerosing cholangitis	
Biliary atresia	
Alagille syndrome	
Chronic hepatitis	
Hepatitis B	
Hepatitis C	
Autoimmune hepatitis	
Alcohol liver disease	
Metabolic diseases	
Hemochromatosis	
Wilson's disease	
Alpha$_1$-antitrypsin deficiency	
Tyrosinemia	
Cystic fibrosis	
Hepatic malignancy	
Hepatocellular carcinoma	
Neuroendocrine tumor metastatic to liver	
Fulminant hepatic failure	
Others	
Cryptogenic cirrhosis	
Polycystic liver disease	
Budd-Chiari syndrome	
Amyloidosis	

second decade of life), and Wilson's disease [an autosomal recessive disorder of copper excretion, which may present as either fulminant hepatic failure (FHF) or chronic hepatitis and cirrhosis].

Hepatocellular carcinoma (HCC) may be a complication of cirrhosis from any cause, most commonly with hepatitis B, hepatitis C, hemochromatosis, and tyrosinemia. HCC patients may have stable liver disease, but are often not candidates for hepatic resection because of the underlying cirrhosis. The desire to remove the malignancy and replace the remaining liver parenchyma (both to improve liver function and remove the diseased parenchyma at risk for further carcinogenesis) led clinicians to consider the use of orthotopic liver transplantation (OLT). Long-term patient survival in early series of OLT for HCC, however, only reached 30 to 40%. It was not until patient selection strategies evolved that OLT became a more effective treatment. In a landmark 1996 study by Mazzaferro and colleagues at the University of Milan,[61] characteristics of patients with HCC that were good candidates for OLT were described. These characteristics, now commonly referred to as the *Milan criteria*, included (a) a single lesion <5 cm or 1 to 3 tumors, each <3 cm; and (b) absence of vascular or lymphatic invasion. Patients meeting these criteria achieved an impressive 85% 4-year overall patient survival, while those patients that exceeded the Milan criteria had only 50% 4-year survival. As with surgical resection, vascular invasion appears to be the most important predictor of mortality among patients undergoing OLT for HCC. Also, the fibrolamellar subtype appears to have no better prognosis than nonfibrolamellar subtypes of HCC. Liver transplantation is now a well-accepted treatment option for patients with HCC. Attention has now focused on whether there may be tumor sizes and categories that may be just outside the Milan criteria that could benefit from transplant. A host of other diseases may lead to chronic liver failure and are potentially amenable to treatment with a transplant, including Budd-Chiari syndrome (obstruction of the hepatic veins secondary to thrombus, which leads to hepatic congestion, ascites, and eventually liver damage) and polycystic liver disease (in which a large number of cysts, depending on their size, can lead to debilitating symptoms).

Acute liver disease, more commonly termed *fulminant hepatic failure*, is defined as the development of HE and profound coagulopathy shortly after the onset of symptoms, such as jaundice, in patients without pre-existing liver disease. The most common causes include acetaminophen overdose, acute hepatitis B infection, various drugs and hepatotoxins, and Wilson's disease; often, however, no cause is identified. Treatment consists of appropriate critical care support, giving patients time for spontaneous recovery. The prognosis for spontaneous recovery depends on the patient's age (those younger than 10 and older than 40 years have a poor prognosis), the underlying cause, and the severity of liver injury (as indicated by degree of HE, coagulopathy, and kidney dysfunction; Table 11-8). A subset of patients may have delayed onset of hepatic decompensation that occurs 8 weeks to 6 months after the onset of symptoms. This condition is often referred to as *subacute hepatic failure*; these patients rarely recover without a transplant.

TABLE 11-8	Indications for a liver transplant in patients with acute liver failure

Acetaminophen toxicity
   pH <7.30
   Prothrombin time >100 s (INR >6.5)
   Serum creatinine >300 μmol/L (>3.4 mg/dL)
No acetaminophen toxicity
   Prothrombin time >100 s (INR >6.5)
   age <10 or >40 y
   Non-A, non-B hepatitis
   Duration of jaundice before onset of encephalopathy >7 d
   Serum creatinine >300 μmol/L (>3.4 mg/dL)

INR = International Normalized Ratio.

Indications for Transplant

The presence of chronic liver disease alone with established cirrhosis is not an indication for a transplant. Some patients have well-compensated cirrhosis with a low expectant mortality. Patients with decompensated cirrhosis, however, have a poor prognosis without transplant. The signs and symptoms of decompensated cirrhosis include:

- HE: In its early stages, HE may begin with subtle sleep disturbances, depression, and emotional lability. Increasing severity of HE is indicated by increasing somnolence, altered speech, and in extreme cases, coma. Physical examination shows the typical flapping tremor of asterixis. Blood tests often reveal an elevated serum ammonia level. HE may occur spontaneously, but more commonly is triggered by a precipitating factor such as spontaneous bacterial peritonitis (SBP), GI bleeding, use of sedatives, constipation, or excessive dietary protein intake.

- Ascites: Ascites generally is associated with portal hypertension. The initial approach to the management of ascites is sodium restriction and diuretics. If this approach is not successful, patients may require repeated large-volume (4 to 6 L) paracentesis. A better option to diuretic-resistant ascites requiring frequent paracentesis is transjugular intrahepatic portosystemic shunting (TIPS). A potential complication of TIPS is progression of liver failure or disabling encephalopathy. Patients with signs of far-advanced liver disease, such as hyperbilirubinemia, HE, and renal dysfunction, generally are not good candidates for TIPS.

- SBP: This complication of chronic liver failure generally signals advanced disease. It often tends to be recurrent. Anaerobic gram-negative bacteria account for 60% of the cultured organisms; gram-positive cocci account for the remainder. Diagnosis is confirmed if percutaneous sampling of the abdominal fluid shows a neutrophil count of greater than 250 cells/mL. Treatment with a third-generation cephalosporin is generally effective.

- Portal hypertensive bleeding: The likelihood of patients with cirrhosis developing varices ranges from 35 to 80%. About one third of those with varices will experience bleeding. The risk of recurrent bleeding approaches 70% by 2 years after the index bleeding episode. Each episode of bleeding is associated with a 30% mortality rate. Thus, urgent treatment of the acute episode and steps to prevent rebleeding are essential. Endoscopy is indicated to diagnose and treat the acute bleed with either band ligation or sclerotherapy. Other therapies include vasoactive drugs such as octreotide or vasopressin, balloon tamponade, TIPS, and emergency surgical procedures (such as a portosystemic shunt or transection of the esophagus). Generally, patients whose endoscopic procedure fails should undergo emergency TIPS, if feasible, to control bleeding. Beta blockers have been shown to be of value in preventing the first bleeding episode in patients with varices and in preventing rebleeding.

- Hepatorenal syndrome (HRS): In patients with advanced liver disease and ascites, HRS is characterized by oliguria (<500 mL of urine/d) in association with low urine sodium (<10 mEq/L). It is a functional disorder; the kidneys have no structural abnormalities, and the urine sediment is normal. The differential diagnosis includes ATN, drug nephrotoxicity, and chronic intrinsic renal disease. HRS may be precipitated by volume depletion from diuresis, SBP, or agents such as NSAIDs. Patients may require dialysis support, but the only effective treatment is a liver transplant.

- Others: Other signs and symptoms of decompensated cirrhosis include severe weakness and fatigue, which may sometimes be the primary symptoms. Such weakness can be debilitating, leading to the inability to work or even to carry out daily functions. It may be associated with malnutrition and muscle wasting, which at times may be quite severe. Biochemical abnormalities, advanced liver disease, and loss of synthetic function are associated with a low serum albumin, a high serum bilirubin, and a rise in the serum International Normalized Ratio (INR).

Generally, FHF patients are more acutely ill than chronic liver failure patients, and thus require more intensive care pretransplant. FHF patients have more severe hepatic parenchymal dysfunction, as manifested by coagulopathy, hypoglycemia, and lactic acidosis. Infectious complications also are more common, as is the incidence of kidney failure and neurologic complications, especially cerebral edema.

Coagulopathy usually is secondary to the impaired hepatic synthesis of clotting factors. Necrosis, as a result of disseminated intravascular coagulation (DIC), may also be associated with FHF. Close attention should be given to the serum glucose level, which is more likely to be decreased in FHF patients. IV glucose should be administered at a sufficient rate to maintain euglycemia.

The prevalence of bacterial infection in FHF patients is very high, a reflection of the loss of the immunologic functions of the liver. The respiratory and urinary systems are the most common sources. In addition, almost one third of FHF patients develop some form of fungal infection, usually secondary to *Candida* species. Sepsis is generally a contraindication to a liver transplant; if it is unrecognized pretransplant, the outcome posttransplant is poor.

Multiple organ dysfunction syndrome, characterized by respiratory distress, kidney failure, increased cardiac output, and decreased systemic vascular resistance, is a well-described complication of FHF. It may be due to impaired clearance of vasoactive substances by the liver. Mechanical ventilation and dialysis support may become necessary pretransplant. Hemodynamic abnormalities may manifest as hypotension and worsening tissue oxygenation.

Cerebral edema is substantially more common in FHF patients. As many as 80% of the patients who die secondary to FHF have evidence of cerebral edema. The pathogenesis is unclear, but it may be due to potential neurotoxins that are normally cleared by the liver. Establishing the diagnosis may be problematic; patients often are sedated and ventilated, making clinical examination difficult. Radiologic imaging is neither sensitive nor specific. Several centers have tried intracranial pressure (ICP) monitoring; therapy (e.g., mannitol, hyperventilation, and thiopental) can then be directed to achieve an adequate cerebral perfusion pressure (above 50 mmHg). ICP monitoring also helps predict the likelihood of neurologic recovery posttransplant. Sustained cerebral perfusion pressures of less than 40 mmHg have been associated with postoperative neurologic death. Disadvantages of ICP monitoring include the risks of performing it in patients with severe coagulopathy; it is also a possible source of infection and may precipitate an intracranial hemorrhage.

The indications for a liver transplant are numerous (and increasing), with the number of absolute contraindications few (and decreasing with time). There are no specific age limits for recipients; their mean age is steadily increasing. Patients must have adequate cardiac and pulmonary function. Coronary artery disease is uncommon in liver transplant candidates, but those with cirrhosis may develop significant hypoxia and pulmonary hypertension. Those with severe hypoxemia or with right atrial pressures greater than 60 mmHg rarely survive a liver transplant. Other contraindications, as with other types of transplants, include uncontrolled systemic infection and malignancy. HCC patients with metastatic disease, obvious vascular invasion, or significant tumor burden are not suitable transplant candidates. Patients with other types of extrahepatic malignancy should be deferred for at least 2 years after completing curative therapy before a transplant is attempted.

Currently, the most common contraindication to a liver transplant is ongoing substance abuse. Before considering patients for a transplant, most centers require a documented period of abstinence, demonstration of compliant behavior, and willingness to pursue a chemical dependency program.

Once the indications for a transplant and the absence of contraindications have been established, a careful search for underlying medical disorders of the cardiovascular, pulmonary, neurologic,

genitourinary, and GI systems must be made. Serologic evaluation to screen for the presence of underlying viral infections is important. Unique to patients with chronic liver disease, the pretransplant evaluation must assess for any evidence of hepatopulmonary syndrome, pulmonary hypertension, and HRS.

Hepatopulmonary syndrome is characterized by impaired gas exchange, resulting from intrapulmonary arteriovenous shunts. These shunts may lead to severe hypoxemia, especially when patients are in the upright position (orthodeoxia). A transplant may be contraindicated if intrapulmonary shunting is severe, as manifested by hypoxemia that is only partially improved with high inspired oxygen concentrations.

Pulmonary hypertension is seen in a small proportion of patients with established cirrhosis. Its exact cause is unknown. Diagnosing pulmonary hypertension pretransplant is critical, because major surgical procedures in the presence of nonreversible pulmonary hypertension are associated with a very high risk of mortality.

The development of hepatorenal syndrome indicates rapid hepatic deterioration. It is a clear indication for a liver transplant. Patients with hepatorenal syndrome or with kidney failure from any cause have worse outcomes posttransplant, as compared to patients with no kidney dysfunction. Therefore, all attempts must be made to avoid or reverse any kidney dysfunction pretransplant. Once the cause of kidney dysfunction is established, appropriate therapy should be initiated, including optimization of volume status with invasive monitoring techniques, large-volume paracentesis, cessation of nephrotoxic drugs, nonpressor doses of dopamine, or judicious use of diuretics, as indicated. If such therapy is unsuccessful, dialysis support may be required until a liver transplant becomes available.

Waiting list mortality can be quite accurately predicted in chronic liver failure patients by calculating their MELD (model for end-stage liver disease)[62] score. The formula for calculation of this is:

$$\text{MELD score} = 3.8 \times \log(e)\,(\text{bilirubin mg/dL}) + 11.2 \times \log(e)\,(\text{INR}) + 9.6 \log(e)\,(\text{creatinine mg/dL})$$

A higher MELD score indicates a sicker patient, with a higher risk for mortality. In the United States, this scoring system has proven to be a useful method to determine the allocation of livers, with priority given to the sickest individuals. The calculated score does not take into account special situations such as HCC, which have a definite impact on waiting list mortality, but scoring exceptions are applied to these situations to allow for timely transplants.

Surgical Procedure

The surgical procedure is divided into three phases: preanhepatic, anhepatic, and postanhepatic. The preanhepatic phase involves mobilizing the recipient's diseased liver in preparation for its removal (Fig. 11-21). The basic steps include isolating the supra- and infrahepatic vena cava, portal vein, and hepatic artery, and dividing the bile duct (Fig. 11-22). Given existing coagulopathy and portal hypertension, the recipient hepatectomy may be the most difficult aspect of the transplant procedure. The anesthesia team must be prepared to deal with excessive blood loss.

Once the above structures have been isolated, vascular clamps are applied. The recipient's liver is removed, thus beginning the anhepatic phase. This phase is characterized by decreased venous return to the heart because of occlusion of the IVC and portal vein. Some centers routinely use a venovenous bypass (VVB) system during this time, in which blood is drawn from the lower body and bowels via a cannula in the common femoral vein and portal vein, and returned through a central venous cannula in the upper body. Potential advantages of bypass include improved hemodynamic stability, reduction of bleeding from an engorged portal system, and avoidance of elevated venous pressure in the renal veins. However, many centers do not routinely use VVB. VVB does have potential complications such as air embolism, thromboembolism, hypothermia, and trauma to vessels. Some centers use VVB selectively, reserving it for

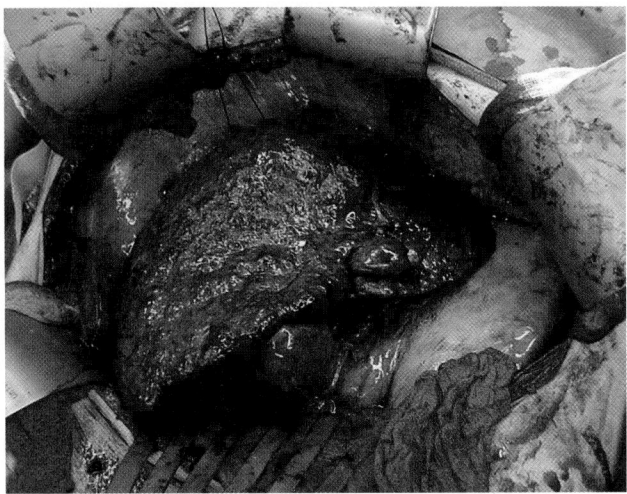

FIG. 11-21. Cirrhotic liver mobilized in preparation for complete hepatectomy.

patients who demonstrate hemodynamic instability with a trial of caval clamping. Few randomized trials have measured specific clinical outcomes with or without VVB.

With the recipient liver removed, the donor liver is anastomosed to the appropriate structures to place it in an orthotopic position. The suprahepatic caval anastomosis is performed first, followed by the infrahepatic cava and the portal vein. The portal and caval clamps may be removed at this time. The new liver is then allowed to reperfuse. Either before or after this step, the hepatic artery may be anastomosed.

With the clamps removed and the new liver reperfused, the postanhepatic phase begins, often characterized by marked changes in the recipient's status. The most dramatic changes in hemodynamic parameters usually occur on reperfusion, namely hypotension and the potential for serious cardiac arrhythmias. Severe coagulopathy may also develop because of the release of natural anticoagulants from the ischemic liver or because of active fibrinolysis. Both ε-aminocaproic acid and aprotinin have been used prophylactically to prevent fibrinolysis and decrease transfusion requirements. Electrolyte abnormalities, most commonly hyperkalemia and hypercalcemia, often are seen after reperfusion, but they usually are transient and respond well to treatment with

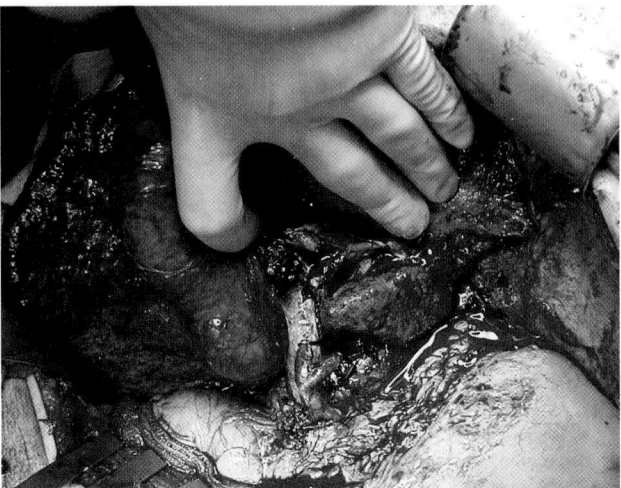

FIG. 11-22. Isolation and division of the hilar structures to diseased liver-hepatic artery, portal vein, and common bile duct.

calcium chloride and sodium bicarbonate. After reperfusion, the final anastomosis is performed, establishing biliary drainage. The recipient's remaining common bile duct (choledochoduodenostomy) or a loop of bowel (choledochojejunostomy) may be used.

Variations on the Standard Procedure

Several variations of the standard operation have been described. With the "piggyback technique," the recipient's IVC is preserved, the infrahepatic donor cava is oversewn, and the suprahepatic cava is anastomosed to the confluence of the recipient hepatic veins. Alternatively, a side-to-side caval anastomosis can be performed between the back of the donor cava and the front of the recipient cava (Fig. 11-23). With these techniques, the recipient's vena cava does not have to be completely cross-clamped during anastomosis, thus allowing blood from the lower body to return to the heart uninterrupted, without the need for VVB. The piggyback technique has many advantages, including improved hemodynamic stability, improved kidney perfusion, and avoidance of the complications possible with VVB. However, no randomized studies have demonstrated the superiority of one technique over the other.

Another important variation of the standard operation is a partial transplant, either a living-donor transplant or a deceased-donor split-liver transplant. Both have developed in response to the donor shortage and are gaining in popularity. Usually, in living-donor liver transplants for pediatric recipients, the left lateral segment or left lobe is used; for adult recipients, the right lobe is usually used. Split-liver transplants from deceased donors involve dividing the donor liver into two segments, each of which is subsequently transplanted (see Fig. 11-10).

Living-Donor Liver Transplant

Living-donor liver transplants have been performed for almost 15 years. Initially, they involved adult donors and pediatric recipients. In such cases, the left lateral segment of the donor's liver is resected (Fig. 11-24). Inflow to the graft occurs via the donor's left hepatic artery and left portal vein; outflow is via the left hepatic vein. For adult recipients, a larger piece of the liver is required; usually the right lobe is chosen (Fig. 11-25). The liver has a remarkable ability to regenerate, and the remnant piece in the donor will achieve close to the original liver volume within 4 to 6 weeks after donation. The risks for living liver donors are higher than those for living kidney donors. The risks also generally are higher for right lobe donors than for left lateral segment donors.

The greatest advantage of a living-donor liver transplant is that it avoids the often lengthy waiting period experienced with deceased-donor organ transplants. Over 17,000 people are now waiting for liver transplants in the United States, but only 5500 transplants are performed every year.[63] Roughly 15 to 25% of the candidates will die of their liver disease before having the chance to undergo a transplant. For those who do receive a transplant from a deceased donor, the waiting time can be significant, resulting in severe debilitation. With a living-donor liver transplant, this waiting time can be avoided, allowing the transplant to be performed before the recipient's health deteriorates further.

A partial hepatectomy in an otherwise healthy donor is a significant undertaking, so all potential donors must be carefully evaluated. Detailed medical screening must ensure that the donor is medically healthy; radiologic evaluation must ensure that the anatomy of the donor's liver is suitable and a psychosocial evaluation must ensure that the donor is mentally fit and not being coerced in any way. The decision to donate should be made entirely by the potential donor after careful consideration of the risks and of the potential complications.

If the recipient is a child, the lateral segment of the donor's liver (about 25% of the total liver) is removed.[64] If the recipient is an adult, a larger portion of the liver needs to be removed. Usually the right lobe of the liver, which comprises ~60% of the total liver, is used. The operative procedure involves isolating the blood vessels

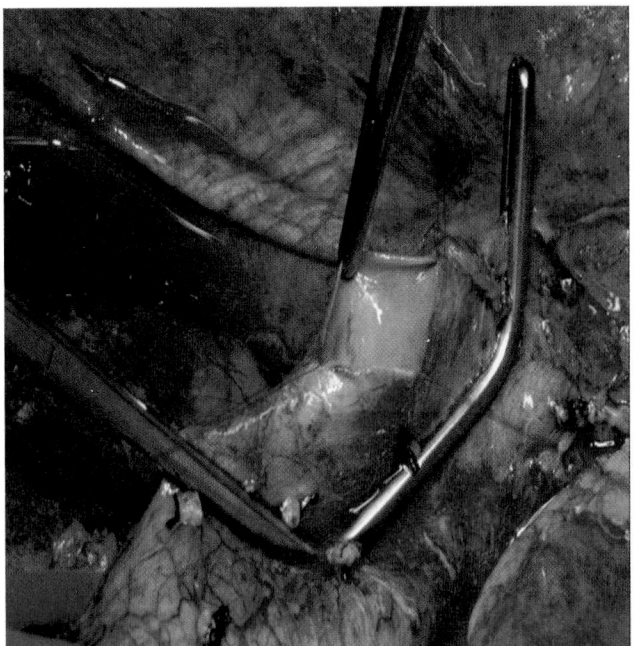

A

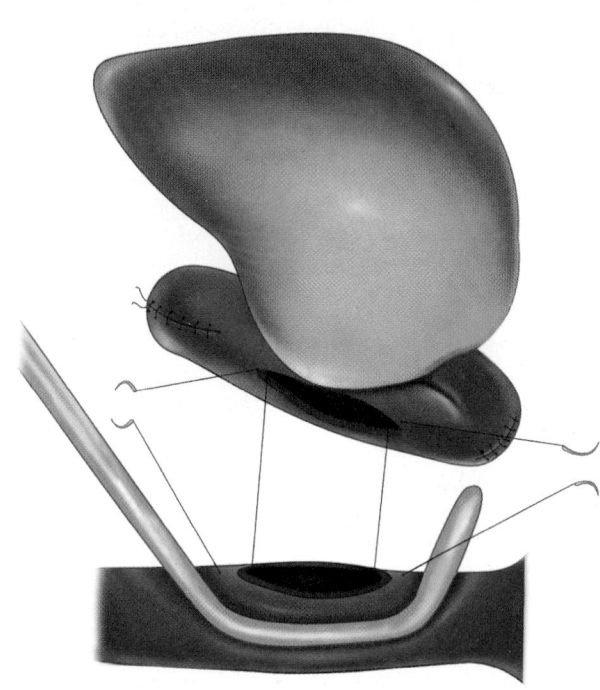

B

FIG. 11-23. A and **B.** With the native liver removed and the cava preserved, the new liver is "piggybacked" onto the cava with a side-to-side caval anastomosis.

Donor

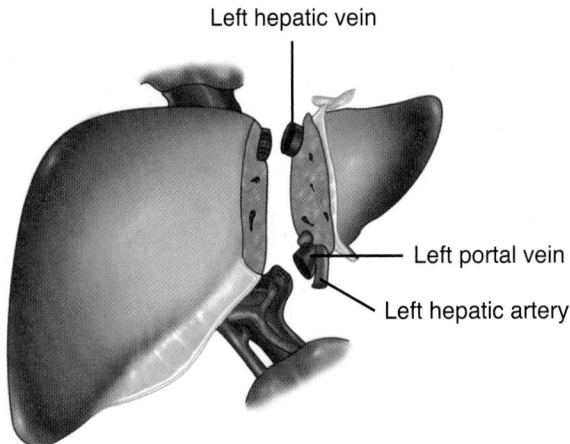

Left hepatic vein

Left portal vein

Left hepatic artery

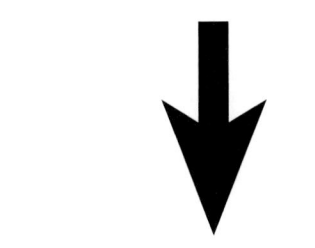

Recipient

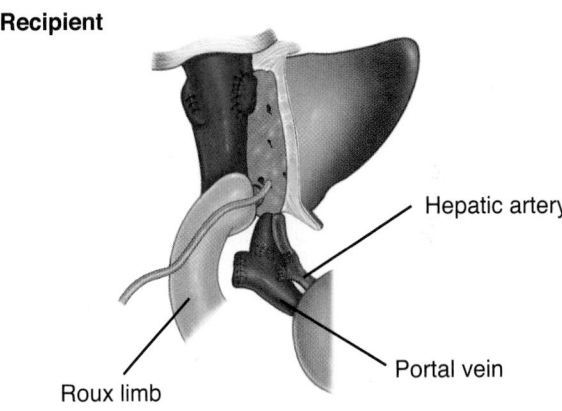

Hepatic artery

Portal vein

Roux limb

FIG. 11-24. Donor and recipient procedure for living-donor liver transplant into a pediatric recipient.

supplying the portion of the liver to be removed, transecting the hepatic parenchyma, and then removing the portion to be transplanted (Figs. 11-26, 11-27, and 11-28).

The overall incidence of complications in the donor after living-donor liver donation ranges from 20 to 30%. There is also a small risk (<0.5%) of death.[65] Bile duct problems are the most worrisome complication after donor surgery. Bile may leak from the cut surface of the liver or from the site where the bile duct is divided. That site may later become strictured. Generally, bile leaks resolve spontane-

ously with simple drainage. Strictures and sometimes bile leaks may require endoscopic retrograde cholangiopancreatography and stenting. If the above measures fail, a reoperation may be required. Intra-abdominal infections developing in donors usually are related to a biliary problem. Other complications after donor surgery may include incisional problems such as infections and hernias. The risk of deep venous thrombosis (DVT) and pulmonary embolism (PE) is the same as for other major abdominal procedures.

The recipient operation with living-donor liver transplants is not greatly different from whole-organ, deceased-donor liver transplants. The hepatectomy is performed in a similar fashion; the vena cava should be preserved in all such cases because the graft generally will only have a single hepatic vein for outflow. This is then anastomosed directly to the recipient's preserved vena cava (Fig. 11-29). Outflow problems tend to be more common with partial vs. whole transplants, especially with right lobe transplants. Various methods have been described to improve the outflow of the graft, such as including the

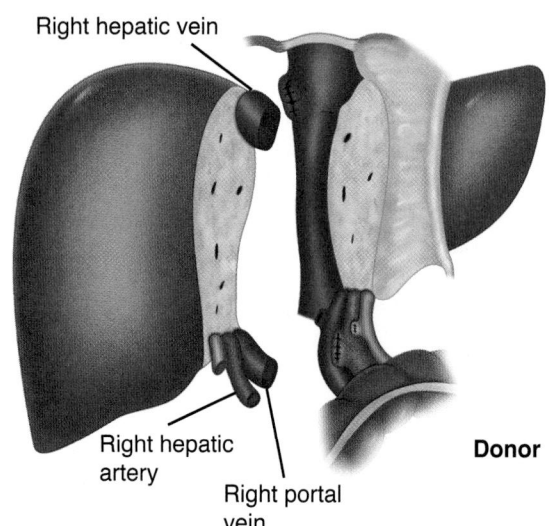

Right hepatic vein

Right hepatic artery

Right portal vein

Donor

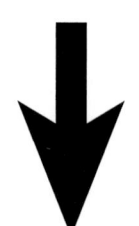

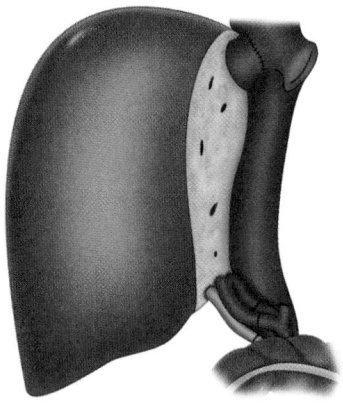

Recipient

FIG. 11-25. Donor and recipient procedure for living-donor liver transplant into an adult recipient.

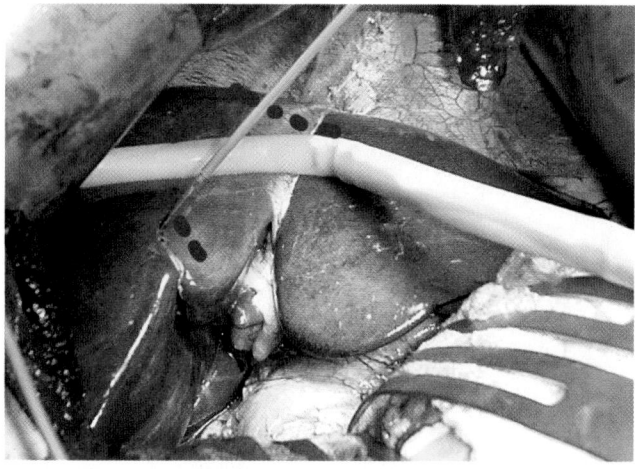

FIG. 11-26. Intraoperative ultrasound can be used to trace the course of the middle hepatic vein and choose the line of transaction, staying just to the right or the left of the vein. Dotted blue lines = middle and left hepatic veins.

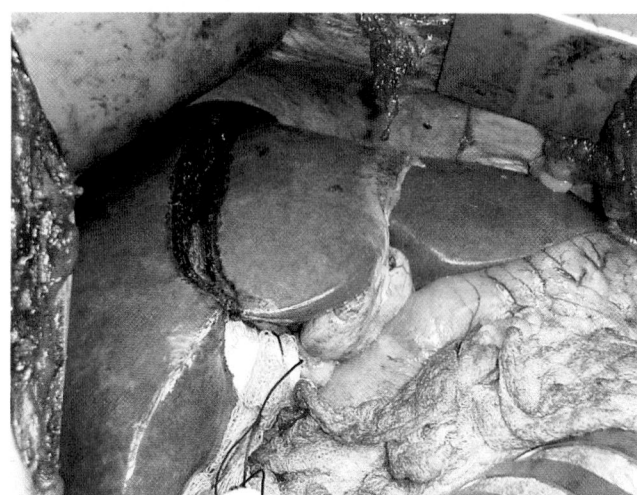

FIG. 11-27. The donor liver after completion of the parenchymal transaction and before division of the vascular structures.

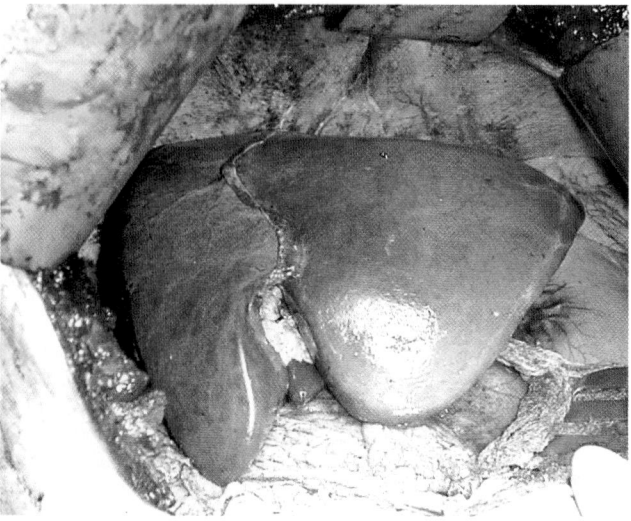

FIG. 11-28. The remnant left lobe in the donor after removal of the right lobe.

middle hepatic vein with the graft, reimplanting accessory hepatic veins, and reimplanting large tributaries that drain the right lobe into the middle hepatic vein.[66–69] Inflow to the graft can be re-established by anastomosing the donor organ hepatic artery and portal vein branch to the corresponding structures in the recipient (Fig. 11-30).

Split-Liver Transplants

Another method to increase the number of liver transplants is to split the liver from a deceased donor into two grafts, which are then transplanted into two recipients.[70] Thus, a whole adult liver from such a donor can be divided into two functioning grafts. The vast majority of split-liver transplants have been between one adult and one pediatric recipient. Usually, the liver is split into a smaller portion (the left lateral segment, which can be transplanted into a pediatric recipient) and a larger portion (the extended right lobe,

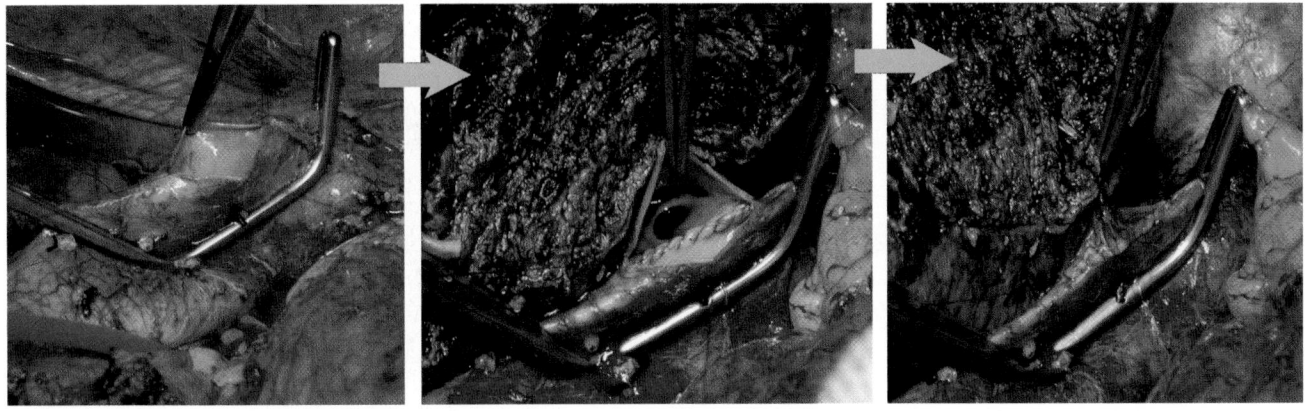

FIG. 11-29. The recipient procedure begins with completion of the outflow by anastomosis of the right hepatic vein to the recipient inferior vena cava.

which can be transplanted into a normal-sized adult recipient) (Fig. 11-31). The benefits for pediatric recipients have been tremendous, including an expansion of the donor pool and a significant decrease in waiting times and mortality rates.

Splitting the liver as described in the paragraph above has no negative impact on the adult waiting list; however, it does not improve it. Adults now account for the majority of patients awaiting a transplant, and therefore the majority of patients dying on the waiting list. So, if split-liver transplants are to have a significant impact on waiting list time and mortality, they must be performed so the resulting two grafts can be used in two adult recipients.[55,71] The concern is that the smaller of the two pieces would not be of sufficient size to sustain life in a normal-sized adult. However, with appropriate donor and recipient selection criteria, a small percentage of livers from deceased donors could be split and transplanted into two adult recipients (Fig. 11-32).

Postoperative Care

The immediate postoperative care for liver recipients involves (a) stabilizing the major organ systems (e.g., cardiovascular, pulmonary, and renal); (b) evaluating graft function and achieving adequate immunosuppression; and (c) monitoring and treating complications directly

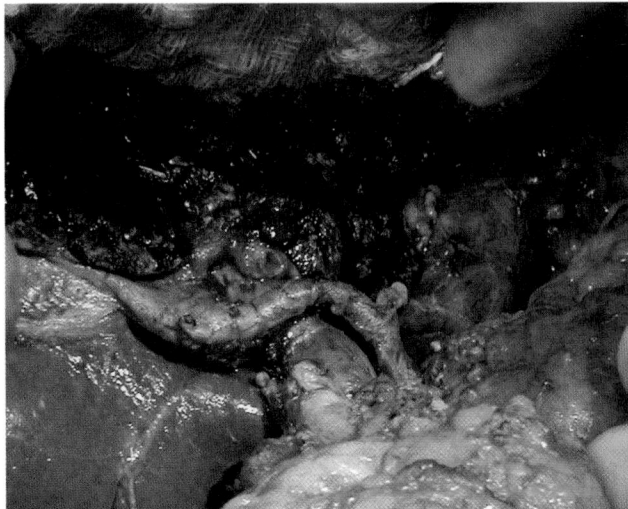

FIG. 11-30. The inflow to the right lobe graft is completed by anastomosis of the right hepatic artery and right portal vein to the corresponding structures in the recipient. Finally, the biliary system is reconstructed.

and indirectly related to the transplant.[72,73] This initial care should generally be performed in an intensive care unit (ICU) setting because recipients usually require mechanical ventilatory support for the first 12 to 24 hours. The goal is to maintain adequate oxygen saturation, acid-base equilibrium, and stable hemodynamics. Continuous hemodynamic monitoring is important to ensure adequate perfusion of the graft and vital organs. Hemodynamic instability occurring early posttransplant usually is due to fluid imbalance, but the presence of ongoing bleeding must first be excluded. Instability also may be secondary to the myocardial dysfunction that often is seen early in the reperfusion phase, but which may persist into the early postoperative period. Such dysfunction is characterized by decreased compliance and contractility of the ventricles. The usual treatment is to optimize preload and afterload, and to use inotropic agents such as dopamine or dobutamine if necessary.

Fluid management, electrolyte status, and kidney function require frequent evaluation. Most liver recipients have an increased extravascular volume but a reduced intravascular volume. Attention should be given to the potassium, calcium, magnesium, phosphate, and glucose levels. Potassium may be elevated because of poor kidney function, a residual perfusion effect, or medications. Diuretics may be required to remove excess fluid acquired intraoperatively, but they may result in hypokalemia. Magnesium levels should be kept above 2 mEq/L to prevent seizures, and phosphate levels between 2 and 5 mEq/L for proper support of the respiratory and alimentary tracts. Marked hyperglycemia, which may be secondary to steroids, should be treated with insulin. Hypoglycemia is often an indication of poor hepatic function.

A crucial aspect of postoperative care is to repeatedly evaluate graft function. In fact, doing so begins intraoperatively, soon after the liver is reperfused. Signs of hepatic function include good texture and good color of the graft, evidence of bile production, and restoration of hemodynamic stability. Postoperatively, hepatic function can be assessed using clinical signs and laboratory values. Patients who rapidly awaken from anesthesia and whose mental status progressively improves likely have a well-functioning graft. Laboratory indicators of good graft function include normalization of the coagulation profile, resolution of hypoglycemia and hyperbilirubinemia, and clearance of serum lactate. Adequate urine production and good output of bile through the biliary tube (if present) are also indicators of good graft function. Serum transaminase levels will usually rise during the first 48 to 72 hours posttransplant secondary to preservation injury, and then should fall rapidly over the next 24 to 48 hours.

Another important aspect of postoperative care is to monitor for any surgical and medical complications. The incidence of complications tends to be high after liver transplants, especially in patients who were severely debilitated pretransplant. Surgical complications

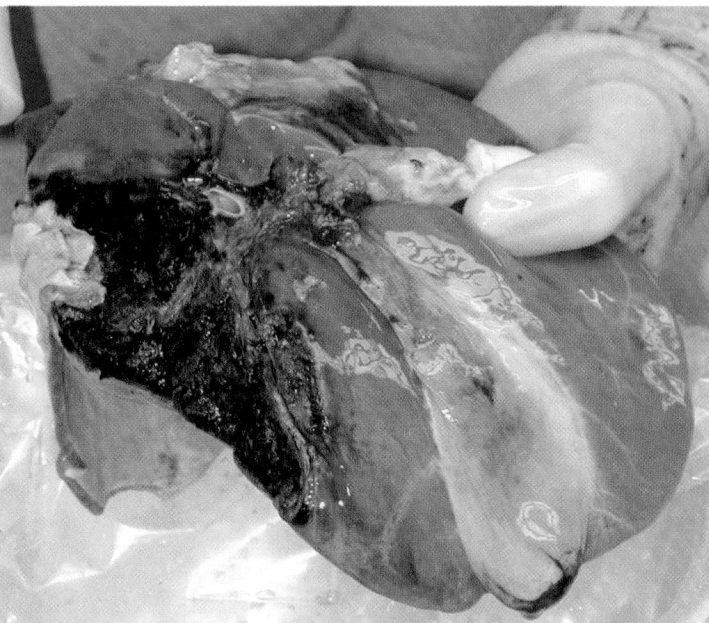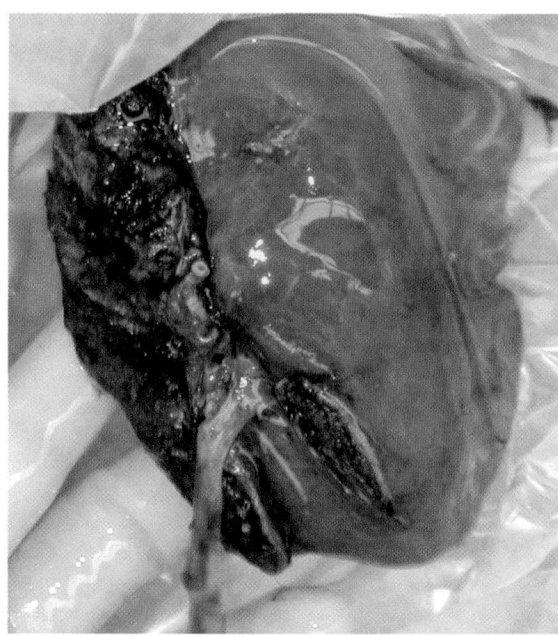

FIG. 11-31. Split liver transplant from a deceased donor for transplant into an adult and pediatric recipient.

related directly to the operation include postoperative hemorrhage and anastomotic problems.

Postoperative bleeding is common. Usually multifactorial, it may be compounded by an underlying coagulopathy resulting from deficits in coagulation, fibrinolysis, and platelet function. Blood loss should be monitored via the abdominal drains; hemoglobin levels and CVP should be measured serially. If bleeding persists despite correction of coagulation deficiencies, an exploratory laparotomy should be performed.

The incidence of vascular complications after liver transplants ranges from 8 to 12%. Thrombosis is the most common early event, with stenosis and pseudoaneurysm formation occurring later. Hepatic artery thrombosis (HAT) has a reported incidence of about 3 to 5% in adults and about 5 to 10% in children. The incidence tends to be higher in partial liver transplant recipients. After HAT, liver recipients may be asymptomatic or may develop severe liver failure secondary to extensive necrosis. Doppler ultrasound evaluation is the initial investigative method of choice, with more than 90% sensitivity and specificity. If HAT is suggested by radiologic imaging, urgent re-exploration is indicated, with thrombectomy and revision of the anastomosis. If hepatic necrosis is extensive, a retransplant is indicated. However, HAT also may present in a less dramatic fashion. Thrombosis may render the common bile duct ischemic, resulting in a localized or diffuse bile leak from the anastomosis or in a more chronic, diffuse biliary stricture.

Thrombosis of the portal vein is less common. Signs include liver dysfunction, tense ascites, and variceal bleeding. Doppler evaluation should be used to establish the diagnosis. If thrombosis is diagnosed early, operative thrombectomy and revision of the anastomosis may be successful. If thrombosis occurs late, liver function is usually preserved due to the presence of collaterals; a retransplant is then unnecessary and attention is directed toward relieving the left-sided portal hypertension.

Biliary complications remain a significant problem after liver transplants, affecting 10 to 35% of all recipients. A higher incidence generally is seen after partial liver transplants, in which bile leaks may occur from the anastomoses or from the cut surface of the liver. Biliary complications manifest either as leaks or as obstructions. Leaks tend to occur early postoperatively and often require surgical repair; obstructions usually occur later and can be managed with radiologic or endoscopic techniques. Clinical symptoms of a bile leak include fever, abdominal pain, and peritoneal irritation. Ultra-

sound may demonstrate a fluid collection; however, cholangiography is required for diagnosis. Some leaks may be successfully managed by endoscopic placement of a biliary stent. If the leak does not respond to stent placement or if the liver recipient is systemically ill, a laparotomy is warranted. Biliary strictures occur later postoperatively and manifest as cholangitis or cholestasis, or both. Initial treatment involves balloon dilatation or stent placement across the stricture site, or both. If these initial options fail, surgical revision is required.

One devastating complication posttransplant is primary nonfunction of the hepatic allograft, with an attendant mortality rate of greater than 80% without a retransplant. By definition, primary nonfunction results from poor or no hepatic function from the time of the transplant procedure. The incidence in most centers is about 3 to 5%. Factors associated with primary nonfunction include advanced donor age, increased fat content of the donor liver, prolonged donor hospitalization before organ procurement, prolonged cold ischemia time, and partial liver donation. IV prostaglandin E_1 may have some useful effects and can be administered to recipients with suspected primary nonfunction. Ultimately, however, they should be listed for an urgent retransplant.

Medical complications (both infectious and noninfectious) are common posttransplant, especially in patients who were debilitated pretransplant. Almost any organ system may be involved. The neurologic, respiratory, and renal systems are commonly affected. Neurologic complications generally manifest as a decreased level of consciousness, seizures, or focal neurologic deficits. The most common cause of a decreased level of consciousness is sedation from drugs that have accumulated in the bloodstream over a period of days. Another cause is a poorly functioning or nonfunctioning graft with resulting liver failure and hepatic encephalopathy (HE). Central pontine myelinolysis, which may result from marked fluctuations in serum sodium levels and osmolality, is an uncommon cause of a patient not regaining consciousness posttransplant. Recipients who developed FHF, especially those with severe HE and evidence of cerebral edema preoperatively, invariably have a period of diminished consciousness posttransplant. Postoperative seizures usually occur de novo and tend to be of the generalized tonic-clonic variety. Causes can include electrolyte abnormalities, effects of drugs such as cyclosporine and tacrolimus, structural abnormalities such as intracranial hemorrhage and cerebral infarctions, and infectious processes such as encephalitis or brain abscesses.

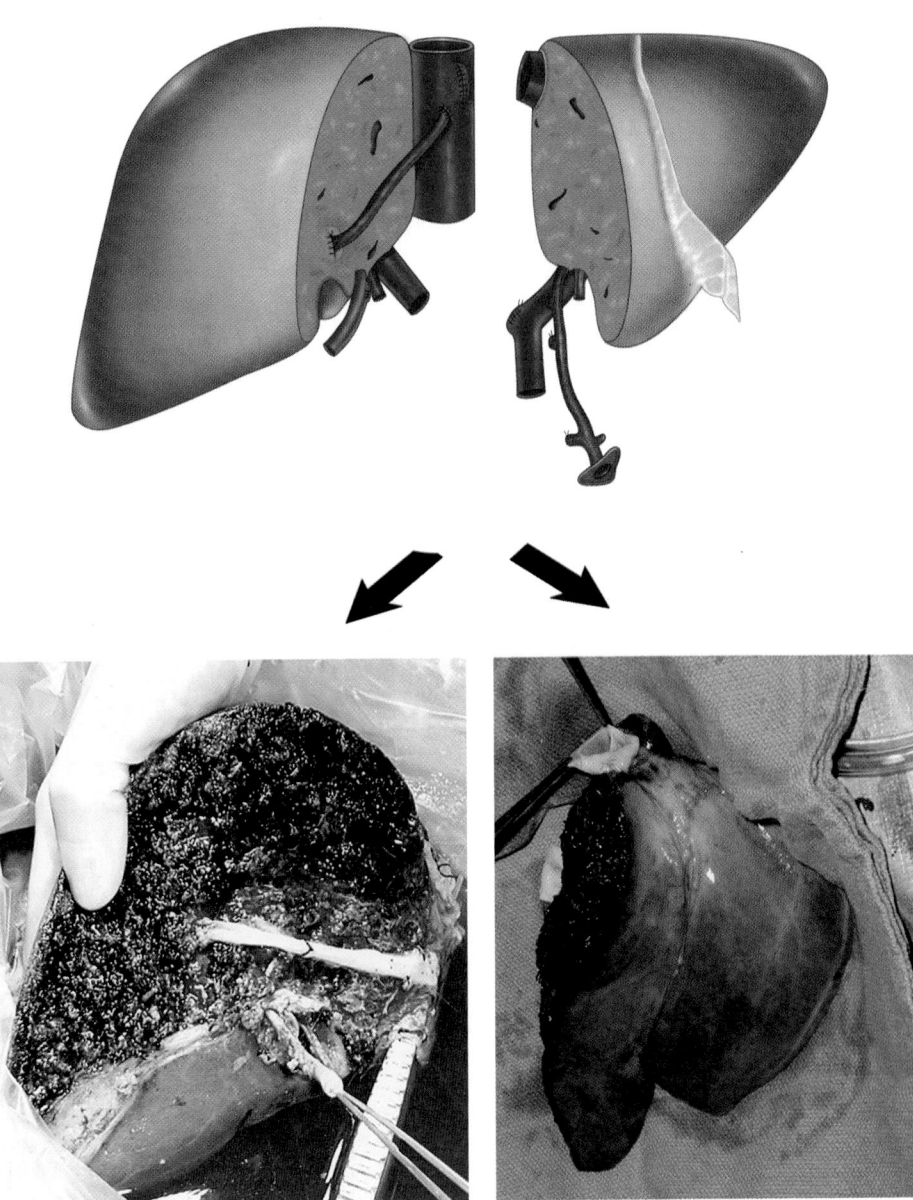

FIG. 11-32. Deceased-donor, split-liver transplant into a right lobe and left lobe for transplant into two adult recipients.

The pulmonary system is one of the most common sites of complications posttransplant. Infectious and noninfectious pulmonary complications can occur in up to 75% of liver recipients. Noninfectious complications such as pulmonary edema, pleural effusion, atelectasis, and acute respiratory distress syndrome predominate during the first week, and generally manifest with respiratory distress and hypoxemia. The lungs are a very common site of posttransplant infections, which predominate after the first posttransplant week. Organisms may be bacterial, fungal, or viral, with different pathogens predominating at different times posttransplant. Early infections posttransplant generally are secondary to gram-negative organisms or fungi. Risk factors include mechanical ventilation, atelectasis, and aspiration.

Some degree of kidney dysfunction is very common posttransplant, affecting almost all liver recipients. About 10% develop kidney failure severe enough to require dialysis. Postoperative kidney problems that may have been present pretransplant are most commonly due to HRS or ATN. Usually, such problems will improve posttransplant, but recipients with severe pretransplant kidney dysfunction are at greater risk for persistent kidney impairment posttransplant, and some patients will require renal transplantation. Other causes of postoperative renal dysfunction include systemic hypovolemia, drug nephrotoxicity, or pre-existing kidney disease.

Infectious complications after liver transplant are common and can be devastating. Early infections (within the first month posttransplant) usually are related to surgical complications, initial graft function, or pre-existing comorbid conditions. Risk factors include prolonged surgery, large-volume blood transfusions, primary nonfunction requiring a retransplant, and reoperations for bleeding or bile leaks. The most common early infections are intra-abdominal and wound infections. Intra-abdominal infections should always lead the surgeon to consider the possibility of a bile leak. If an intra-abdominal infection is suspected, a CT scan should be performed, with aspiration and culture of any fluid collections that are identified. The biliary tree should be evaluated to exclude the presence of a bile leak. Patients with FHF are at high risk for fungal infections, usually secondary to *Candida* or *Aspergillus* species. Common sites include the abdomen, lungs, and central nervous system.

Late postoperative infections (generally occurring after the first month posttransplant) are usually a reflection of the recipient's overall immunosuppressed state. Immunosuppressive drugs depress cell-mediated immunity, leading to opportunistic infections with viral, fungal, and parasitic pathogens. The risk increases with the level and length of immunosuppression, especially when acute rejection episodes are treated with bolus high-dose steroids or antilymphocyte agents. Viral infections generally are not seen until after the first month posttransplant. CMV is the most common pathogen involved. Its presentation ranges from asymptomatic infection to tissue-invasive disease. Epstein-Barr virus (EBV), another member of the herpesvirus family, also may be seen posttransplant. A wide spectrum of clinical presentations is possible, including an asymptomatic rise in antibody titers, a mononucleosis syndrome, hepatitis, and posttransplant lymphoproliferative disorder (PTLD). The most severe form of infection, PTLD can present as a localized tumor of the lymph nodes or GI tract, or rarely as a rapidly progressive, diffuse, often fatal lymphomatous infiltration.

Other aspects of postoperative care, especially in the later posttransplant period, involve careful monitoring of the recipient for any evidence of graft rejection, complications related to immunosuppression, and recurrence of the original disease.[74] After the recipient is discharged from the hospital, use of routine blood tests, including liver function tests, are important to monitor for acute rejection. The incidence of acute rejection is now about 20 to 30%; most episodes are asymptomatic and occur relatively early posttransplant. Most commonly, the serum bilirubin or transaminase levels are elevated. A percutaneous liver biopsy is then performed to confirm the diagnosis. Treatment is with high-dose corticosteroids; however, if there is no significant response, antilymphocyte therapy should be initiated. Mild acute rejection episodes often can be treated simply by temporarily increasing the baseline immunosuppression. This is especially useful in hepatitis C–positive patients in whom bolus immunosuppression represents a risk factor for recurrence of disease.

Immunosuppressive drugs are important to prevent rejection, but they are associated with a host of potential complications that recipients should be regularly evaluated for, including nephrotoxicity (especially prevalent with use of calcineurin inhibitors), cardiovascular and metabolic complications (such as hypertension, hyperlipidemia, diabetes, osteoporosis, and obesity), and malignancy (often related to long-term suppression of the immune system).

Disease recurrence is a significantly more important problem after liver transplants than with other solid organ transplants. Recurrence of hepatitis C is almost universal after transplants for this condition. Fortunately, only a minority of recipients experience aggressive recurrence leading to cirrhosis and liver failure. Ribavirin and α-interferon therapy should be considered in recipients with evidence of significant recurrence, as indicated by liver biopsy findings. Recurrence of hepatitis B has been significantly decreased by the routine use of hepatitis B immune globulin and the antiviral agent lamivudine posttransplant, but recurrence may still be seen with resistant viral strains. Other diseases that may recur posttransplant are PSC, primary hepatic malignancy, and autoimmune hepatitis.

Pediatric Liver Transplants

Liver transplants have become a well-established procedure to treat liver failure in pediatric patients. As a result of refinements in surgical technique, the advent of new immunosuppressive agents, and improvements in critical care, patient survival at 1 year has improved from 20% in the 1970s to 90% currently. In several ways, liver transplants for pediatric patients are quite similar to those for adults; however, several features make pediatric patients unique.

The clinical indications for a pediatric liver transplant are similar to those already mentioned for adults. Endpoints that require a transplant include evidence of portal hypertension as manifested by variceal bleeding and ascites, significant jaundice, intractable pruritus, encephalopathy, failing synthetic function (e.g., hypoalbuminemia or coagulopathy), poor quality of life, and failure to thrive (as manifested by poor weight gain or poor height increase).

Biliary atresia is the most common indication for a pediatric liver transplant. The incidence of biliary atresia is about one in 10,000 infant births. Once the diagnosis is established, a portoenterostomy, or Kasai procedure, is indicated to drain microscopic ducts within the porta hepatis. Successful bile flow can be achieved in 40 to 60% of patients whose Kasai procedure takes place early in their life. However, even with a Kasai procedure, 75% of children with biliary atresia eventually require a liver transplant because of progressive cholestasis followed by cirrhosis. Other cholestatic disorders that may eventually require a transplant include sclerosing cholangitis, familial cholestasis syndromes, and paucity of intrahepatic bile ducts (as seen with Alagille syndrome).

Metabolic disorders probably account for the next largest group of disorders that may require a liver transplant. Such disorders may directly result in liver failure or may have mainly extrahepatic manifestations. Alpha$_1$-antitrypsin deficiency is the most common metabolic disorder that may require a liver transplant. Such patients may present with jaundice in the neonatal period, but this usually resolves. Subsequently, they may present in late childhood or early adolescence with cirrhosis and portal hypertension. Another metabolic disorder resulting in liver failure is tyrosinemia, a hereditary disorder characterized by deficiency of an enzyme that degrades the metabolic products of tyrosine, resulting in cirrhosis and a greatly increased risk for HCC. Still another is Wilson's disease, an autosomal recessive disorder characterized by copper accumulation in the liver, central nervous system, kidneys, eyes, and other organs, that may present as fulminant, subfulminant, or chronic liver failure. Metabolic disorders that do not affect liver function, but are treatable by a liver transplant, include urea cycle defects, most commonly ornithine transcarbamoylase deficiency (which may result in profound neurologic damage if not corrected early). Primary oxalosis, which results in kidney failure due to hyperoxaluria, can be treated by a kidney transplant to correct the kidney failure and by a liver transplant to correct the enzymatic defect so renal failure does not recur.

FHF may be seen in children from similar causes as seen in adults. Of note, younger children (<10 years old) with FHF have a poor prognosis for spontaneous recovery of liver function without a transplant. Other conditions that may require a transplant include chronic hepatitis (usually due to autoimmune or viral causes), and malignancy (most commonly a hepatoblastoma).

The surgical procedure for children does not differ significantly from that used in adults. The recipient's size is a more important variable in pediatric transplants, and it has an impact on both the donor and the recipient operations. For pediatric patients (especially infants and small children), the chance of finding a size-matched graft from a deceased donor may be very small, as the vast majority of such donors are adults. With adult grafts for pediatric patients, options include reduced-size liver transplants, in which a portion of the liver, such as the right lobe or extended right lobe, is resected and discarded; split-liver transplants in which a whole liver is divided into two functional grafts; and living-donor liver transplants in which a portion, usually the left lateral segment, is resected from a living donor. Graft implantation may be more demanding in pediatric patients, given the small caliber and delicate nature of the vessels. Use of VVB usually is not technically possible because of the small size of the vessels. For that reason, and given the increasing use of partial transplants, vena cava–sparing procedures are generally performed in children.

Surgical complications, especially those related to the vascular anastomoses, tend to be more frequent in pediatric recipients. HAT is three to four times more common in children. Factors associated with this increased risk include small recipient weight (less than 10 kg), use of just the left lateral segment (rather than the whole liver), and complex arterial reconstructions.

Patient survival rates have improved dramatically for pediatric liver recipients since the early 1990s. Most centers now report patient survival of close to 90% at 1 year posttransplant. Even for small recipients, patient survival rates at 1 year are 80 to 85%. Also, pediatric recipients enjoy close to normal growth and development posttransplant. Usually, growth accelerates immediately posttransplant.

Results

Patient and graft survival rates after liver transplants have improved significantly since the mid-1990s, with most centers now reporting graft survival rates of 85 to 90% at 1 year. The main factors affecting short-term (within the first year posttransplant) patient and graft survival are the medical condition of the patient at the time of transplant and the development of early postoperative surgical complications. Severely debilitated patients with numerous comorbid conditions such as kidney dysfunction, coagulopathy, and malnutrition, have a significantly higher risk of early posttransplant mortality. Such patients are more likely to develop surgical and medical complications (especially infections) and are unable to tolerate them. The U.S. data show that for 2006, patient survival at 1 year after deceased-donor liver transplant was 87%, while graft survival was 82%.

Long-term survival rates (after the first year posttransplant) depend more on the cause of the underlying liver disease and on the presence or absence in the recipient of risk factors for other medical problems (especially cardiovascular disease). Generally, from 1 to 10 years posttransplant, survival curves decline slowly. Roughly half of the deaths in this time period are due to events not related to the underlying liver disease (e.g., myocardial infarctions, cerebrovascular accidents, and trauma). The other half of the deaths, however, are related to complications either of the underlying liver disease (e.g., recurrence) or of immunosuppression (e.g., infection or malignancy).

The original cause of liver failure has an impact on long-term survival rates as well. PBC in adults and biliary atresia in children generally are associated with a better long-term outcome, because recurrence of these diseases in the transplanted liver is rare. However, recipients with HCC or hepatitis C usually have poorer long-term outcomes, because these diseases often recur posttransplant.

INTESTINAL TRANSPLANTATION

Intestinal transplants have been performed in the laboratory for years. The first human intestinal transplant was performed in 1966, but remained essentially an experimental procedure, producing dismal results well into the 1980s. Newer immunosuppressive drugs have played a significant role in the success with the procedure since the mid-1990s. However, intestinal transplants remain the least frequently performed of all transplants, with the highest rejection rates and the lowest graft survival rates.

There are several reasons why the number of intestinal transplants has not increased dramatically. As with kidney failure patients, a medical alternative exists for patients with intestinal failure, namely, long-term total parenteral nutrition (TPN). Unlike kidney failure patients, however, patients with intestinal failure have no survival advantage with a transplant vs. medical therapy. Immunologically, the small intestine is the most difficult organ to transplant. It is populated with highly immunocompetent cells, perhaps explaining the reason for the high rejection rates and the need for higher levels of immunosuppression. Moreover, monitoring for rejection in intestinal transplant recipients is difficult, as there is no good blood or urine laboratory test to indicate it. Lastly, the intestinal lumen is filled with potential infective pathogens that can gain access to the recipient's circulation if there is any breakdown of the mucosal barrier (which can occur during an acute rejection episode).

Preoperative Evaluation

Currently an intestinal transplant is indicated for irreversible intestinal failure that is not successfully managed by TPN (because of malnutrition and failure to thrive) or that has life-threatening complications (e.g., hepatic dysfunction, repeated episodes of sepsis secondary to central access, loss of central venous access sites).[75] Currently, patients who are stable while receiving TPN without such complications generally are not considered to be suitable transplant candidates because their estimated annual survival rate is higher with TPN.

The causes of intestinal failure are different in adult than in pediatric patients. Most commonly, though, the underlying disease results in extensive resection of the small bowel with resultant short bowel syndrome.[76] The development of short bowel syndrome depends not only on the length of bowel resected, but also on the location of the resection, on the presence or absence of the ileocecal valve, and on the presence or absence of the colon. As a rough guideline, most patients can tolerate resection of 50% of their intestine with subsequent adaptation, avoiding the need for long-term parenteral nutritional support. Loss of greater than 75% of the intestine, however, usually necessitates some type of parenteral nutritional support. The most common causes of intestinal failure in children are necrotizing enterocolitis, gastroschisis, and volvulus. In adults, Crohn's disease, massive resection of ischemic bowel due to mesenteric vascular thrombosis, and trauma are the most common causes.

The pretransplant evaluation does not differ greatly from that for other transplants. Absolute contraindications such as malignancy and active infection must be ruled out, and hepatic function should be evaluated carefully. If there is evidence of significant liver dysfunction and cirrhosis, a combined liver and intestinal transplant is indicated. The serologic status of the potential recipient also should be evaluated carefully—especially regarding CMV status. Transplant candidates who are CMV-seronegative should not receive an organ from a donor who is seropositive, because of a very high incidence of highly morbid and occasionally lethal invasive CMV disease posttransplant in such recipients.

Surgical Procedure

The operative procedure varies, depending on whether or not a liver transplant also is performed.[77,78] In the case of an isolated intestinal transplant, the graft may be from a living or deceased donor. With a living donor, about 200 cm of the distal small bowel is used; inflow to the graft is via the ileocolic artery, and outflow via the ileocolic vein. With a deceased donor, the graft is based on the superior mesenteric artery for inflow and on the superior mesenteric vein for outflow. For a combined liver and intestinal transplant, the graft usually is procured intact with an aortic conduit that contains both the celiac and superior mesenteric arteries. The common bile duct can be maintained intact in the hepatoduodenal ligament along with the first part of the duodenum and a small rim of the head of the pancreas (Fig. 11-33). Doing so avoids a biliary reconstruction in the recipient.

The recipient operation varies, depending on the graft being implanted. Generally, arterial inflow to the graft is achieved using the recipient's infrarenal aorta to perform an end-to-side anastomosis. Venous drainage of the graft can be performed to the systemic or portal circulation. Systemic drainage will lead to certain metabolic abnormalities, but there is no firm evidence to suggest that such abnormalities are of any obvious detriment to the recipient. GI continuity can be achieved by a number of different methods. A stoma is useful for ready endoscopic access to the transplanted bowel to perform a biopsy, which is the only reliable method to monitor for and diagnose acute rejection.

Postoperative Care

The early posttransplant care for intestinal transplant patients is in many ways similar to that of other transplant recipients. Initial care should take place in an ICU so that fluid, electrolytes, and blood product replacement can be carefully monitored. Broad-spectrum antibiotics are routinely administered, given the high risk for infectious complications.

A number of different immunosuppressive protocols have been described. Many involve some form of induction therapy, followed by tacrolimus-based maintenance immunosuppression. Regardless of the protocol, intestinal transplants clearly have a high risk of rejection. Therefore, careful monitoring for rejection is imperative and involves endoscopy with biopsy of the graft mucosa. Acute rejection episodes often are associated with infections. Rejection

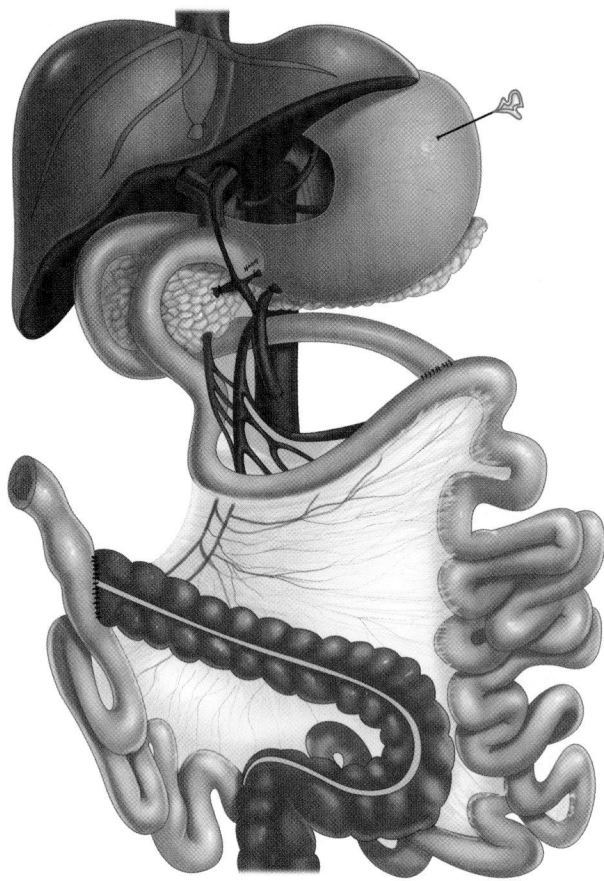

FIG. 11-33. Combined liver, pancreas, and intestine transplant.

results in damage to the intestinal mucosa, leading to impaired barrier function and bacterial translocation. Therefore, advanced rejection can be very difficult to treat as concurrent infection invariably is present.

Short-term results after intestinal transplantation have improved dramatically, mainly due to improvements in surgical technique and in immunosuppression.[79,80] Nonetheless, intestinal transplants still are associated with a high complication rate. Potential complications include enteric leaks with generalized peritonitis or localized intra-abdominal abscesses, graft thrombosis, respiratory infections, and life-threatening hemorrhage. Long-term results also have improved, but remain inferior to other types of abdominal transplants.

HEART AND LUNG TRANSPLANTATION

Heart transplantation is a well-established therapy for end-stage heart failure, and is performed in age groups from neonates to senior citizens.[81] About 3500 heart transplants are performed each year, with roughly 10% taking place in pediatric recipients. The major limitation, as with almost all other types of transplants, is the inability to meet the demand with sufficient numbers of suitable donor organs.

Lung transplantation is a newer field than heart transplantation, and far fewer lung transplants (about 1000) are performed each year. Results have improved since the early 1990s, mainly due to improvements in immunosuppression and refinements in surgical techniques, in particular with modification of the airway anastomosis.[82] A combined heart-lung transplant usually is reserved for patients who have pulmonary hypertension and obvious right-sided heart failure.[83]

Preoperative Evaluation

A heart transplant generally is indicated in the presence of end-stage heart failure. The most common cause is ischemic or dilated cardiomyopathy, followed by intractable angina, valvular disease, congenital heart disease, life-threatening recurrent ventricular arrhythmias, and isolated intracardiac tumors.

Contraindications to a heart transplant are similar to those for other types of transplants, including active malignancy or infection, numerous or advanced comorbid conditions, and obvious noncompliance with medical care recommendations. Specific to heart transplantation is the need to exclude the presence of severe, nonreversible pulmonary hypertension, which could cause acute right-sided heart failure posttransplant.

Isolated lung transplants are performed for a number of indications, including chronic obstructive pulmonary disease, idiopathic pulmonary fibrosis, cystic fibrosis, and pulmonary hypertension (without right-sided heart failure).[84–86] Patients with chronic obstructive pulmonary disease or idiopathic pulmonary fibrosis generally are treated with a single-lung transplant; those with cystic fibrosis or pulmonary hypertension (without right-sided heart failure) usually require a bilateral single-lung transplant. Patients with pulmonary hypertension with significant right-sided heart failure, or those with Eisenmenger's syndrome, usually require a combined heart-lung transplant.

Surgical Procedure
Donor Selection

As with other organ transplants, donor selection criteria are important to ensure posttransplant success. The vast majority of lung transplants are performed with organs from deceased donors. A small number of lung transplants have used living-donor organs; in such cases, two living donors each contribute a lobe of a lung, and both lobes are then implanted into the appropriate hemithorax of a single recipient.

Numerous tests can be done to try to assess the suitability of hearts and lungs from deceased donors. Ultimately, however, physical examination at the time of procurement is likely the best method. The blood group, height, and weight of the donor must be compatible with the potential recipient. A heart donor should have a normal echocardiogram and must not currently require high doses of inotropes to maintain blood pressure. The presence of significant coronary artery disease can be excluded using coronary angiography if necessary.

Lung donor criteria usually are more restrictive than heart donor criteria, but have been liberalized over the past several years. The best tests of lung donor suitability are arterial blood gas analysis, chest roentgenogram, bronchoscopy, and physical examination of the lungs at the time of procurement. Bronchoscopy is especially important, and any findings of significant secretions or evidence of bacterial or fungal infection in the donor should preclude the recovery of the lungs.

Recipient Operation

A heart transplant is an orthotopic procedure. Therefore the first step of the procedure for heart or heart-lung recipients is removal of their corresponding thoracic organs. The recipient's aorta and vena cava are cannulated, an aortic cross-clamp is applied, and the diseased heart is excised along the atrioventricular groove. The recipient is maintained on cardiopulmonary bypass during this time. The new heart is then placed in an orthotopic position, with anastomoses performed in the following order: left atrium, right atrium, pulmonary artery, and aorta. Several variations to the original technique have been described, such as performing the aortic anastomosis before the pulmonary artery anastomosis to allow reperfusion of the heart and to minimize the ischemic time. Another variation is to perform selective anastomoses of the inferior and superior vena cava (rather than just of the right atrium); doing so is believed to allow for better geometry of the right atrium and to decrease the incidence of posttransplant atrial arrhythmias.

In heart-lung transplants, the new organs are implanted en bloc. Right and left pneumonectomies are carried out, with isolation and division of the trachea just above the carina. Anastomoses are then performed between the donor and recipient trachea, right atrium, and aorta.

Single-lung transplants are performed through a standard posterolateral thoracotomy. The superior and inferior pulmonary veins, pulmonary artery, and main stem bronchus are dissected. The pulmonary artery is then clamped to assess the recipient's hemodynamic status; cardiopulmonary bypass is used if necessary, although most recipients do not require bypass support. The bronchus and appropriate vascular structures are then clamped and the pneumonectomy completed. The bronchial anastomosis is performed first, followed by the pulmonary arterial and left atrial anastomoses. A telescoped bronchial anastomosis reduces the incidence of complications, most notably leaks. A pedicle of vascularized omentum also can be wrapped around the anastomosis for further reinforcement. Bilateral single-lung transplants are performed in a similar fashion, each side sequentially.

Postoperative Care

The immediate postoperative care does not differ significantly from any other major cardiac or pulmonary procedure. However, heart or lung recipients are at greater risk for infections than their nontransplant counterparts, and require appropriate precautions and prophylaxis regimens. As with other transplant recipients, maintenance immunosuppressive therapy is started immediately posttransplant.

After heart or heart-lung transplants, cardiac output is sustained by establishing a heart rate of 90 to 110 beats per minute, using either temporary epicardial atrial pacing or low-dose isoproterenol. For recipients who may suffer transient right-sided heart failure, adequate preload is important. Use of an oximetric Swan-Ganz catheter can be helpful to monitor pulmonary artery pressure and measure cardiac output. Urine output and arterial blood gases must be carefully monitored. Hypotension and a low cardiac output usually respond to an infusion of volume and to minor adjustments in inotropic support.

Cardiac tamponade can occur in heart recipients. It should be suspected in those who become hypotensive with concurrent increases in CVP and whose mediastinal chest tube output decreases suddenly. Serious ventricular failure posttransplant is unusual and can be related to poor donor organ selection, poor graft preservation, long ischemic time, or rarely, hyperacute rejection. Inotropes and pulmonary vasodilators can be used to manage ventricular failure; if it seems likely that the graft will recover, an intra-aortic balloon pump or a ventricular assist device can be added. In the case of a very severe rejection episode, the only option is to list the recipient for a retransplant.

Lung or heart recipients are initially cared for in the ICU.[87] Attempts should be made to wean them early from the ventilator. Acute failure of a transplanted lung may be seen early posttransplant. Reasons include the inherent difficulty of lung preservation, unrecognized injury or trauma to the donor lung, and reperfusion edema. Lung graft failure can manifest as hypoxemia, infiltrates on radiographic examination, or copious secretions in the presence of reperfusion edema. Care of such recipients involves active diuresis and high levels of positive end-expiratory pressure to maintain small airway patency. They should be kept intubated as necessary and extubated as the acute injury resolves. The diagnosis of a failing lung graft should be made using transbronchial biopsy (to exclude the presence of rejection) and bronchoalveolar lavage (to exclude the presence of early infection). Extracorporeal membrane oxygenation can be used as a last resort to maintain function while a diagnosis is being established and appropriate therapy initiated.

Complications can be surgical or medical, and may occur early or late posttransplant. Many of the complications, especially those occurring late, are medical in nature and are similar to those seen after other types of transplants. Generally, they are related to the medications and to the immunosuppressed state. Examples include hypertension, hyperglycemia, osteoporosis, and malignancy. Certain complications, such as airway problems, are unique to lung and heart recipients. Rejection, both acute and chronic, can occur, but manifests in very different ways as compared with abdominal organ transplants.

Early attempts at lung transplantation were severely hampered by a high incidence of airway complications. This anastomosis is at high risk for problems because of the poor blood supply. However, increased experience and refinements in surgical technique have dramatically reduced airway complications. Nonetheless, about 10 to 15% of lung recipients develop some airway complication, often resulting in significant morbidity and occasional mortality. Airway complications can occur after heart-lung or lung transplants, but are much less common after heart-lung transplants because a good blood supply is maintained to the tracheal anastomosis. After solitary and double-lung transplants, the bronchial anastomosis is at much greater risk for partial dehiscence, airway stenosis, or both. Hypotension, poor lung preservation, rejection, and infection can compromise blood flow to the anastomoses. The result can be ischemic necrosis and poor healing of the airway, leading to partial or total dehiscence or chronic narrowing of the bronchus.

Postoperative surveillance of the bronchial anastomosis is important. In the operating room, bronchoscopy is performed to establish the baseline appearance of the anastomosis. Frequent routine bronchoscopy is useful to survey the anastomosis for early signs of dehiscence, as well as to monitor for rejection and infection. Dehiscence usually occurs within 3 to 6 weeks posttransplant. Early signs on bronchoscopy include abnormal appearance of the mucosa at the suture line, loosened sutures or knots within the airway, and herniation of tissue into the airway in case of an omental wrap. If the recipient is clinically stable and the area of dehiscence is small, conservative treatment with antibiotics and serial evaluation via bronchoscopy is appropriate. Development of a bronchopleural or bronchovascular fistula requires reoperation.

Chronic airway stenosis may develop after initial healing. It may be managed in a variety of ways, including repeated dilations of the airway with a rigid bronchoscope, use of a metallic stent, or laser photocoagulation to débride granulation tissue.

Lung or heart organ transplant recipients are susceptible to bacterial, fungal, and viral infections. Infections are particularly problematic in lung recipients, with as many as 15 to 20% likely to develop some type of significant infectious disease. Fungal infections due to *Candida* and *Aspergillus* are generally more serious than bacterial infections.[88] Most *Aspergillus* infections, which are caused by the inhalation of aerosolized fungal spores, generally occur within the first 3 months posttransplant. Among lung transplant recipients who have underlying cystic fibrosis, infections due to *Pseudomonas aeruginosa* are common. The most morbid viral infection is caused by CMV.

Rejection can be acute or chronic. Acute rejection tends to be characterized by the presence of an inflammatory infiltrate (mostly lymphocytes) in the organ parenchyma, and usually is seen early posttransplant. Chronic rejection tends to be a later phenomenon; it is characterized by obliteration of small vessels and fibrosis.[89,90] For both lung or heart recipients, rejection usually does not have clinical symptoms until the rejection episode is advanced. Therefore, routine monitoring with transbronchial biopsy (for lung recipients) and with endomyocardial biopsy (for heart recipients) is important for early diagnosis. For heart-lung recipients, rejection of the lungs may occur without rejection of the heart, so biopsy of both organs may be necessary.

Fortunately, most acute rejection episodes can be effectively reversed. Much more difficult to treat is the process of chronic rejection, which has been a major obstacle to long-term survival. In heart recipients, chronic rejection manifests as graft arteriosclerosis, which is seen in 30 to 40% of recipients by 3 years posttransplant, and in 40 to 60% of recipients by 5 years. In lung transplant recipients, chronic rejection manifests as bronchiolitis obliterans, characterized clinically by a decreased forced expiratory volume in 1 second and histologically by inflammation and fibrosis of small airways.

INFECTION AND MALIGNANCY

Immunosuppressive therapy has played an essential role in the success of clinical transplants. However, it is a double-edged sword, because suppression of the immune system prevents or decreases the risk of rejection while concomitantly predisposing the transplant recipient to a wide variety of complications, including infections and malignancies.[91] Infections in transplant recipients may be caused by so-called *opportunistic microbes*, organisms that would not be harmful to a normal, nonimmunosuppressed host, as well as more common pathogens.

Infections

Transplant recipients exhibit an increased risk for infectious complications posttransplant, which can lead to significant morbidity and mortality. Numerous risk factors include long-standing end-stage organ failure (which can lead to an immunosuppressed state even before any immunosuppressive drugs are begun), impaired tissue healing, and poor vascular flow due to coexisting illnesses such as diabetes. The transplant surgery itself, which may involve opening nonsterile viscera such as the bladder or bowel, and the posttransplant need for powerful immunosuppressive agents further increase the risk for infections.

The spectrum of possible infections in transplant recipients is wide. Infections may occur early or late posttransplant. They may be related directly to the surgical procedure, to some complication that develops afterward, or to the recipient's overall immunosuppressed state (i.e., opportunistic). Infections are classified by the type of pathogen involved into bacterial, viral, or fungal infections. However, more than one type of pathogen may be involved in several different types of infections (e.g., pneumonia may be caused by a viral, bacterial, or fungal pathogen). Moreover, a number of different pathogens may be involved in a single infection (e.g., an intra-abdominal abscess can be due to several different bacterial and fungal pathogens).

Infections also can be classified by the primary method of treatment into surgical or medical infections. Surgical infections require some surgical intervention as an integral part of their treatment. They generally occur soon after the transplant operation and usually are related directly to it, or to some complication occurring as a result of it. Surgical infections are less likely to be related to the recipient's overall immunosuppressed state, though obviously this plays some role. Typical examples of surgical infections include generalized peritonitis, intra-abdominal abscesses, and wound infections. In contrast, medical infections generally do not require an invasive intervention for treatment, but rather are primarily treated with antiviral, antibacterial, or antifungal agents. They tend to occur later posttransplant and usually are related to the recipient's overall immunosuppressive state. Typical examples of medical infections include those secondary to CMV, polyomavirus-induced nephropathy, pneumonias, and EBV-related problems.

Risk factors for posttransplant infections are classified into those present in the recipient pretransplant, those related to the donor, those related to the recipient intraoperatively, and those that occur posttransplant. Pretransplant latent infections can reactivate or worsen early posttransplant, once high-dose immunosuppression is initiated. Pretransplant immunity, or lack of immunity, to certain viral pathogens can be an especially important risk factor for posttransplant infections. For example, recipients seronegative for CMV or EBV have a high incidence of posttransplant infections with these viruses, especially if their donor was seropositive. The recipient's overall medical status may be a factor in posttransplant infections. Poor nutritional status, advanced peripheral vascular disease, frequent hospitalizations pretransplant, and recipient obesity are all well-described risk factors for posttransplant infectious complications, especially involving the wound. Donor factors may also play an important role. Although transmission of bacterial infections from the donor are uncommon, viruses such as CMV, EBV, hepatitis B or C, and HIV can certainly be transmitted to any recipient who has not had previous exposure to them.

Intraoperative risk factors for infections include a longer operative procedure with significant bleeding, prolonged cold and warm ischemia of the graft, and certain types of transplants (e.g., pancreas and intestinal transplants are associated with a significantly higher risk of infections vs. kidney transplants). Posttransplant risk factors for infection are generally related either to the development of posttransplant complications or to the level of immunosuppression. Leaks from anastomoses with spillage of contaminated fluid (e.g., bile, urine, and enteric contents) will lead to a localized and possibly generalized infection. The level of immunosuppression is an important risk factor posttransplant, especially for opportunistic infections. The higher the level of immunosuppression, the greater the risk. Long induction protocols involving powerful antilymphocyte agents or bolus antirejection treatment, particularly several treatments in sequence, have been clearly identified as risk factors for a variety of infections.

The most common surgical infections, especially in liver and pancreas transplant recipients, are intra-abdominal infections. They are also the most likely to be life threatening. They may range from diffuse peritonitis to localized abscesses. Their presentation, management, and clinical course will in part depend on their underlying cause, their location, and on the recipient's overall medical condition.

The incidence of intra-abdominal infections in transplant recipients has steadily decreased over time. Nonetheless, intra-abdominal infections continue to be a major problem. Among pancreas recipients, they are the second most common technical reason for graft loss (after vascular thrombosis). Leaks from anastomoses with spillage of contaminated fluid are probably the most significant risk factor for intra-abdominal infections. Other risk factors include increased donor age (especially in pancreas transplants), recipient obesity, donor obesity, and prolonged pretransplant dialysis, especially peritoneal dialysis.

The clinical presentation of intra-abdominal infections will depend on their severity and location. Generalized peritonitis usually is associated with some catastrophic event such as biliary disruption or graft duodenal leak with spillage of enteric contents or urine into the peritoneal cavity. It may also occur as a result of perforation of some other viscus, unrelated to the transplant (e.g., perforated gastric ulcer or perforated cecum). Generalized peritonitis is diagnosed clinically; the physical examination is the most helpful tool. Such patients appear ill, with tachycardia, elevated temperature, falling blood pressure, and diffuse tenderness with guarding on palpation of the abdomen, although immunosuppression may mask many of the usual signs and symptoms. A plain film or CT scan of the abdomen usually is not necessary, but may demonstrate free air. Treatment involves prompt return of the recipient to the operating room to determine the reason for the peritonitis; the next step often will depend on the degree of contamination.

Fortunately, most intra-abdominal infections do not fall into the generalized peritonitis category. Instead, most of them consist of localized fluid collections in and around the graft. Patients usually develop symptoms such as fever, nausea, vomiting, and abdominal distention, with localized pain and guarding over the region of the fluid collection. A CT scan with contrast is the best diagnostic tool in this clinical situation. In pancreas recipients, about one half of these localized abscesses are monomicrobial; common isolates include enterococcus, *Escherichia coli*, *Klebsiella*, and *Pseudomonas* species. The other one half of such abscesses tend to be polymicrobial, containing two or more bacteria or both bacterial and fungal species. The most common fungal species isolated is *C. albicans*, but recently *C. krusei* and *C. glabrata* have been increasing in incidence. Treatment of localized intra-abdominal infections involves adequate drainage and administration of appropriate antibacterial or antifungal agents. These infections often can be drained percutaneously under radiologic guidance, at least as an initial approach.

However, if the infected fluid is not adequately drained or if the recipient does not improve clinically, a laparotomy should be performed to achieve adequate drainage of all infected fluid.

Medical infections posttransplant tend to be more varied compared to surgical infections, and can involve bacterial, viral, or fungal pathogens. Bacterial infections primarily occur in the first few weeks posttransplant. The major sites are the incisional wound, respiratory tract, urinary tract, and bloodstream. Administration of perioperative systemic antibiotics decreases the risk and incidence of some infections. Viral infections in transplant recipients often involve the herpesvirus group; CMV is clinically the most important.[92–94] CMV establishes latent infection in its host and persists throughout life, and infection has been correlated with the overall degree of immunosuppression. CMV infection usually occurred 4 to 12 weeks posttransplant or after treatment of rejection; with routine use of antiviral prophylaxis posttransplant, however, the peak incidence of the disease has been pushed out later to 3 to 6 months posttransplant. A wide spectrum of disease manifestations may be seen during CMV infection. The infection may be subclinical, or it may present with a mild flu-like syndrome. Leukopenia, myalgia, and malaise are usual. CMV may also present as tissue-invasive disease, resulting in interstitial pneumonitis, hepatitis, or GI ulcerations. CMV-seronegative recipients of organs from CMV-seropositive donors are at highest risk. The incidence of CMV disease is reduced by use of prophylactic ganciclovir for 12 weeks posttransplant. Symptomatic disease generally is treated with IV ganciclovir or oral valganciclovir, and reduction in immunosuppression if possible.

Fungal infections are most commonly caused by *Candida* species; *Aspergillus*, *Cryptococcus*, *Blastomyces*, *Mucor*, *Rhizopus*, and other species account for a much smaller percentage of fungal infections, but are more serious.[95] Among patients who develop invasive *Candida* or *Aspergillus* infections, the mortality rate usually exceeds 20%. The standard treatment of serious posttransplant fungal infections has been with amphotericin B, along with overall reduction in immunosuppression. However, newer antifungal agents that are less toxic are showing promise.

Malignancy

Transplant recipients are at increased risk for developing certain types of de novo malignancies, including nonmelanomatous skin cancers (three- to sevenfold increased risk), lymphoproliferative disease (two- to threefold increased risk), gynecologic and urologic cancers, and Kaposi's sarcoma. The risk ranges from 1% among renal allograft recipients to approximately 5 to 6% among recipients of small bowel and multivisceral transplants.[96]

Skin Cancers

The most common malignancies in transplant recipients are skin cancers.[97] They tend to be located on sun-exposed areas and are usually squamous or basal cell carcinomas. Often they are multiple and have an increased predilection to metastasize. Human papillomavirus DNA has been detected in these tumors, suggesting that immunosuppression may have a permissive effect on viral proliferation. Diagnosis and treatment are the same as for the general population. Patients are encouraged to use sunscreen liberally and avoid significant sun exposure.

Posttransplant Lymphoproliferative Disorder

Lymphomas constitute the largest group of noncutaneous neoplasms in transplant recipients.[98–100] The vast majority (>95%) of these lymphomas consist of a spectrum of B-cell proliferation disorders associated with EBV, known collectively as *posttransplant lymphoproliferative disorder* (PTLD). Risk factors include a high degree of immunosuppression, anti–T-cell antibody therapy, and primary EBV infection posttransplant. A wide variety of clinical manifestations may be seen. Symptoms may be systemic and include fever, fatigue, weight loss, or progressive encephalopathy. Lymphadenopathy may be localized, diffuse, or absent. Intrathoracic PTLD

may present with well-circumscribed pulmonary nodules, with or without mediastinal adenopathy. Abdominal pain, rectal bleeding, or bowel perforation may occur with intra-abdominal involvement. Allograft involvement may occur and cause organ dysfunction. Central nervous system involvement is much more common (~15 to 20%), as compared with lymphomas in the nontransplant patient population.

Diagnosis is confirmed by histologic examination of tissue specimens, including in situ DNA hybridization studies to detect the EBV genome. Treatment includes reduction of immunosuppression, surgical extirpative therapy, chemotherapy, and newer agents such as monoclonal antibodies targeted to B cells (anti-CD20 mAb), the latter limited to patients whose tumors express the CD20 cell surface marker. Often a combination of these modalities is used. Mortality can exceed 50% with aggressive tumors.

Other Malignancies

A variety of other malignancies occur with increased incidence in transplant recipients. Conventional treatment is appropriate for most malignancies posttransplant. Immunosuppression should be reduced, particularly if bone marrow suppressive chemotherapeutic agents are administered. However, allograft function should be maintained for those organs that are critical to survival, such as the heart, liver, and lung. For other types of transplants with alternative therapies to fall back on if necessary (e.g., hemodialysis for kidney transplants, exogenous insulin for pancreas or islet cell transplants, and TPN for intestinal transplants), the risks of ongoing immunosuppression must be weighed against the benefits of organ function compared to the alternative therapies.

THE FUTURE OF TRANSPLANTATION

Dramatic advances have been made in the field of transplantation since the late 1970s, but it remains fraught with problems. A major disadvantage is the need for long-term, indeed lifelong, immunosuppression. Associated with immunosuppression is an increased risk for malignancies and infections, as well as a host of other potential side effects not related to the immune system. That is why tolerance, or the ability to maintain the allograft without the need for long-term immunosuppression, remains the goal for all transplant recipients. *Tolerance* is defined as a state of donor-specific hyporeactivity in the absence of immunosuppressive medications (i.e., the recipient's immune system does not attack the transplanted organ, but is intact and able to mount a response to an organ from a different donor). Many different therapeutic approaches have been tested to induce tolerance; however, none have yet shown significant promise.

Perhaps even greater than the problems of long-term immunosuppression is the significant discrepancy between the demand for, and the supply of, organs. The increase in the number of transplants being performed has not kept pace with the increase in the number of patients being placed on the waiting list. The result has been longer waiting times and sicker patients once the transplant finally takes place, if it does at all. Several methods have been proposed to increase the number of transplants being performed. The increasing use of living donors has led to an increase in the number of transplants. However, further increasing the living-donor pool by including higher-risk procedures and higher-risk donors will quickly reach a limit if donor morbidity and donor mortality increase. The use of expanded criteria donors, especially donation after cardiac death donors, has also contributed to a significant increase in the number of organs available. In the future, the use of xenografts may prove to be the solution to the organ shortage problem, but difficult immunologic hurdles remain. Mechanical devices may represent another solution and would also have the advantage of not requiring immunosuppression.[101,102] However, completely implantable, long-lasting biomechanical devices offer their own set of unique problems, which may be worse than those associated with long-term immunosuppression.

Xenotransplantation

Clinical xenotransplants (i.e., transplants of organs between different species) have offered great hope for solving the problem of the expanding waiting list, but the primary hurdle is the formidable immunologic barrier between species.[103] Other problems include the potential risk of transmission of infections (zoonoses) and the ethical problems involved with using animals for widespread human transplants.

It generally is accepted that successful xenotransplants for human beings would probably involve the use of the pig, which would likely be much more readily accepted by the general population than, for example, a primate donor.[104] Pigs also would be easier to raise on a large-scale basis and likely would be less expensive to manage, compared to primates.

The immunologic barrier in pig-to-human xenotransplants is complex, but generally involves three components. The first is hyperacute rejection (HAR), which is mediated by the presence of natural xenoantibodies in humans. These antibodies bind to antigens found mainly on vascular endothelial cells of porcine donor organs, leading to complement activation, intravascular coagulation, and rapid graft ischemia soon after the transplant. After HAR, the next barrier is delayed xenograft rejection, which occurs later than HAR, but is likely still mediated by the presence of xenoreactive antibodies combined with platelet aggregation and activation of the coagulation cascade. The third barrier is a process similar to classic T-cell–mediated acute rejection in allografts. Many different options are being tested to overcome these barriers, including the genetic engineering of pigs to express human genes, use of agents to inhibit platelet aggregation and complement activation, and administration of powerful immunosuppressive drugs.[105]

Besides the immunologic issues, the potential infectious risks also need to be more clearly defined.[106] The risks associated with the transmission of porcine viruses into human transplant recipients and then potentially into the entire human population are not fully known and must be studied in detail.

Other Therapies

Xenotransplantation is not the only therapeutic approach currently being investigated for organ replacement therapy. Other possible approaches include cellular transplants, organogenesis, and artificial and bioartificial devices.[107,108]

Cellular transplants involve the injection of cells that have the potential to replace cells in an organ that has been damaged by disease, thereby augmenting the function of that organ. An example of a cellular transplant would be the injection of stem cells or isolated hepatocytes into a failing liver. Such a procedure would most likely work best in patients with enzymatic or genetic defects. For patients with well-established chronic liver disease with cirrhosis, a cellular transplant would have limitations, because the underlying problem of portal hypertension would not be addressed. Another example of a cellular transplant would be the transplantation of stem cells or primitive muscle cells into a damaged heart. After healing, the cells could potentially function as cardiac muscle cells, thereby augmenting cardiac function. Considerable research already has been done in this area. Cellular transplants show promise, but overall have several limitations. Primary is the inability of cellular transplants to improve the function of structurally complex organs such as the kidney, which consists of several different cell types, all arranged in a specific pattern to allow for proper function.

One potential approach to overcoming this limitation is organogenesis, which essentially involves growing organs de novo from primitive cells or stem cells. However, this form of therapy is still in the theoretical phase and is unlikely to be a clinically viable option in the near future.

Much further along in the clinical realm of organ replacement therapies is the use of bioartificial and artificial mechanical devices. Considerable investigative work has been undertaken to develop a bioreactor using artificial elements and hepatocytes to treat liver failure as a bridge to liver transplantation. However, consistent results have yet to be achieved in the clinical setting. The heart model is in the most advanced stage of development. Various implantable assist devices are already in routine clinical use. Currently, these are usually temporary devices that serve as a bridge to a transplant. Several different models of a totally implantable artificial heart are also currently under development and have been used occasionally. Thromboembolic complications and infections remain the primary problems with these devices.

The future of transplantation is certainly exciting. Continued active research will focus on newer immunosuppressive drugs, tolerance, xenotransplants, cellular transplants, and artificial devices. Most transplant centers in the next decade will probably offer some combination of these new therapies to potential transplant recipients.

REFERENCES

Entries highlighted in bright blue are key references.

1. Carrel A: The transplantation of organs. *NY Med J* 99:839, 1914.
2. Guthrie CC: *Blood Vessel Surgery and Its Applications.* New York: Longmans Green, 1912.
3. Hamilton DNH, Reid WA: Yu Yu Voronoy and the first human kidney allograft. *Surg Gynecol Obstet* 159:289, 1984.
4. Merrill JP, Murray JE, Harrison JH: Successful homotransplantation of the human kidney between identical twins. *JAMA* 160:277, 1956.
5. Calne RY, Alexondre GP, Murray JE: A study of the effects of drugs in prolonged survival of homologous renal transplants in dogs. *Ann NY Acad Sci* 99:743, 1962.
6. Murray JE, Merrill JP, Harrison JH, et al: Prolonged survival of human-kidney homografts by immunosuppressive drug therapy. *N Engl J Med* 268:1315, 1963.
7. Starzl TE, Marchioro TL, Waddell WR: The reversal of rejection in human renal homografts with subsequent development of homograft tolerance. *Surg Gynecol Obstet* 117:385, 1963.
8. Valente JF, Alexander JW: Immunobiology of renal transplantation. *Surg Clin North Am* 78:1, 1998.
9. Krensky AM: Molecular basis of transplant rejection and acceptance. *Pediatr Nephrol* 5:422, 1991.
10. Ball ST, Dallman MJ: Transplantation immunology. *Curr Opin Nephrol Hypertens* 4:465, 1995.
11. Hancock WW: Current trends in transplant immunology. *Curr Opin Nephrol Hypertens* 8:317, 1999.
12. Cuturi MC, Blancho G, Josien R, et al: The biology of allograft rejection. *Curr Opin Nephrol Hypertens* 3:578, 1994.
13. Fryer JP, Granger DK, Leventhal JR, et al: Steroid-related complications in the cyclosporine era. *Clin Transplantation* 8:224, 1994.
14. Humar A, Crotteau S, Gruessner A, et al: Steroid minimization in liver transplant recipients: Impact on hepatitis C recurrence and posttransplant diabetes. *Clin Transplant* 21:526, 2007.
15. Matas AJ, Kandaswamy R, Gillingham K, et al: Prednisone free maintenance immunosuppression—a 5 year experience. *Am J Transplant* 5:2473, 2005.
16. Burke JF, Pirsch JD, Ramos EL, et al: Long-term efficacy and safety of cyclosporine in renal transplant recipients. *N Engl J Med* 331:358, 1994.
17. Calne RY, Rolles K, White DJG, et al: Cyclosporin A initially as the only immunosuppressant in 34 recipients of cadaveric organs. *Lancet* 2:1033, 1979.
18. Sweny P, Farrington K, Younis F, et al: Sixteen months experience with cyclosporin A in human kidney transplantation. *Transplant Proc* 13:365, 1981.
19. Larson TS, Dean PG, Stegall MD, et al: Complete avoidance of calcineurin inhibitors in renal transplantation: A randomized trial comparing sirolimus and tacrolimus. *Am J Transplant* 6:514, 2006.
20. Remuzzi G, Lesti M, Gotti E, et al: Mycophenolate mofetil versus azathioprine for prevention of acute rejection in renal transplantation (MYSS): A randomized trial. *Lancet* 364:503, 2004.
21. Gaber AO, First MR, Tesi RJ, et al: Results of the double-blind, randomized, multicenter, phase III clinical trial of Thymoglobulin versus ATGAM in the treatment of acute graft rejection episodes after renal transplantation. *Transplantation* 66:29, 1998.

22. Bustami RT, Ojo AO, Wolfe RA, et al: Immunosuppression and the risk of post-transplant malignancy among cadaveric first kidney transplant recipients. *Am J Transplant* 4:87, 2004.

23. Buhaescu I, Segall L, Goldsmith D, et al: New immunosuppressive therapies in renal transplantation: Monoclonal antibodies. *J Nephrol* 18:529, 2005.

24. Vincenti F, Kirkman R, Light S, et al: IL-2 receptor blockade with daclizumab to prevent acute rejection in renal transplantation. *N Engl J Med* 338:161, 1998.

25. Nashan B, Moore R, Amlot P, et al: Randomized trial of basiliximab versus placebo for control of acute cellular rejection in renal allograft recipients. *Lancet* 350:1193, 1997.

26. Morris PJ, Russell NK: Alemtuzumab (Campath-1H): A systematic review in organ transplantation. *Transplantation* 81:1361, 2006.

27. Pescovitz MD: Rituximab, an anti-CD20 MAb: History and mechanism of action. *Am J Transplant* 6:859, 2006.

28. Larsen CP, Pearson TC, Adams AB, et al: Rational development of LEA29Y (belatacept), a high-affinity variant of CTLA4-Ig with potent immunosuppressive properties. *Am J Transplant* 5:443, 2005.

29. Vincenti F, Larsen C, Durrbach A, et al: Costimulation blockade with belatacept in renal transplantation. *N Engl J Med* 353:770, 2005.

30. Van Buren CT, Barakat O: Organ donation and retrieval. *Surg Clin North Am* 74:1055, 1994.

31. Kootstra G, Kievit J, Nederstigt A: Organ donors: Heartbeating and non-heartbeating. *World J Surg* 26:181, 2002.

32. Delgado DH, Rao V, Ross HJ: Donor management in cardiac transplantation. *Can J Cardiol* 18:1217, 2002.

33. Starzl TE, Miller C, Broznick B, et al: An improved technique for multiple organ harvesting. *Surg Gynecol Obstet* 165:343, 1987.

34. Boggi U, Vistoli F, Del Chiaro M, et al: A simplified technique for the en bloc procurement of abdominal organs that is suitable for pancreas and small-bowel transplantation. *Surgery* 135:629, 2004.

35. Edwards JM, Hasz RD, Robertson VM: Non-heart-beating organ donation: Process and review. *AACN Clinical Issues* 10:293, 1999.

36. St Peter SD, Imber CJ, Friend PJ: Liver and kidney preservation by perfusion. *Lancet* 359:604, 2002.

37. Van der Werf WJ, D'Alessandro AM, Hoffmann RM, et al: Procurement, preservation, and transport of cadaver kidneys. *Surg Clin North Am* 78:41, 1998.

38. D'Alessandro AM, Southard JH, Love RB, et al: Organ preservation. *Surg Clin North Am* 74:1083, 1994.

39. Feng L, Zhao N, Yao X, et al: Histidine-tryptophan-ketoglutarate solution vs. University of Wisconsin solution for liver transplantation: A systematic review. *Liver Transpl* 13:1125, 2007.

40. Schaubel D, Desmeules M, Mao Y, et al: Survival experience among elderly end-stage renal disease patients. A controlled comparison of transplantation and dialysis. *Transplantation* 60:1389, 1995.

41. Wolfe RA, Ashby VB, Milford EL, et al: Comparison of mortality in all patients on dialysis, patients on dialysis awaiting transplantation, and recipients of a first cadaveric transplant. *N Engl J Med* 341:1725, 1990.

42. Kasiske BL, Ramos EL, Gaston RS, et al: The evaluation of renal transplant candidates: Clinical practice guidelines. *J Am Soc Nephrol* 6:1, 1995.

43. Terasaki PI, Cecka JM, Gjertson DW, et al: High survival rates of kidney transplants from spousal and living unrelated donors. *N Engl J Med* 333:333, 1995.

44. Humar A, Ramcharan T, Kandaswamy R, et al: Risk factors for slow graft function after kidney transplant: A multivariate analysis. *Clin Transplant* 16:425, 2002.

45. Sells RA: Cardiovascular complications following renal transplantation. *Transplantation Rev* 11:111, 1997.

46. Cosio F, Alamir A, Yim S, et al: Patient survival after renal transplantation: I. The impact of dialysis pretransplant. *Kidney Int* 53:767, 1998.

47. Asderakis A, Augustine T, Dyer P, et al: Pre-emptive kidney transplantation: The attractive alternative. *Nephrol Dial Transplant* 13:1799, 1998.

48. Friedman A: Strategies to improve outcomes after renal transplantation. *N Engl J Med* 346:2089, 2002.

49. Matas AJ, Humar A, Payne WD, et al: Decreased acute rejection in kidney transplant recipients is associated with decreased chronic rejection. *Ann Surg* 230:493; discussion 498, 1999.

50. Massy ZA, Guijarro C, Wiederkehr MR, et al: Chronic renal allograft rejection: Immunologic and nonimmunologic risk factors. *Kidney Int* 49:518, 1996.

51. Schweitzer EJ, Matas AJ, Gillingham K, et al: Causes of renal allograft loss: Progress in the '80s, challenges for the '90s. *Ann Surg* 214:679, 1991.

52. Sutherland DE, Gruessner RW, Najarian JS, et al: Solitary pancreas transplants: A new era. *Transplant Proc* 30:280, 1998.

53. Manske CL, Wang Y, Rector T, et al: Coronary revascularisation in insulin-dependent diabetic patients with chronic renal failure. *Lancet* 340:998, 1992.

54. Humar A, Ramcharan T, Kandaswamy R, et al: Pancreas after kidney transplant. *Am J Surg* 182:155, 2001.

55. Farney AC, Cho E, Schweitzer E, et al: Simultaneous cadaver pancreas living-donor kidney transplantation: A new approach for the type 1 diabetic uremic patient. *Ann Surg* 232:696, 2000.

56. Krishnamurthi V, Philosophe B, Bartlett ST: Pancreas transplantation: Contemporary surgical techniques. *Urol Clin North Am* 28:833, 2001.

57. Humar A, Kandaswamy R, Granger D, et al: Decreased surgical risks of pancreas transplantation in the modern era. *Ann Surg* 231:269, 2000.

58. Lumbreras C, Fernandez I, Velosa J, et al: Infectious complications following pancreatic transplantation: Incidence, microbiological and clinical characteristics, and outcome. *Clin Infect Dis* 20:514, 1995.

59. Sutherland DE, Gruessner RW, Dunn DL, et al: Lessons learned from more than 1000 pancreas transplants at a single institution. *Am Surg* 233:463, 2001.

60. McChesney LP: Advances in pancreas transplantation for the treatment of diabetes. *Dis Mon* 45:88, 1999.

61. Mazzaferro V, Regalia E, Doci R, et al: Liver transplantation for the treatment of small hepatocellular carcinomas in patients with cirrhosis. *N Engl J Med* 334:693, 1996.

62. Freeman RB Jr., Wiesner RH, Roberts JP, et al: Improving liver allocation: MELD and PELD. *Am J Transplant* 4 Suppl 9:114, 2004.

63. Pomfret EA, Fryer JP, Sima CS, et al: Liver and intestine transplantation in the United States, 1996–2005. *Am J Transplant* 7:1376, 2007.

64. Strong RW, Lynch SV, Ong TN, et al: Successful liver transplantation from a living donor to her son. *N Engl J Med* 322:1505, 1990.

65. Trotter JF, Wachs M, Everson GT, et al: Adult-to-adult transplantation of the right hepatic lobe from a living donor. *N Engl J Med* 346:1074, 2002.

66. Wachs ME, Bak TE, Karrer FM, et al: Adult living donor liver transplantation using a right hepatic lobe. *Transplantation* 66:1313, 1998.

67. Kiuchi T, Inomata Y, Uemoto S, et al: Living-donor liver transplantation in Kyoto, 1997. *Clin Transpl* 191, 1997.

68. Marcos A, Fisher RA, Ham JM, et al: Right lobe living donor liver transplantation. *Transplantation* 68:798, 1999.

69. Fan ST, Lo CM, Liu CL: Technical refinement in adult-to-adult living donor liver transplantation using right lobe graft. *Ann Surg* 231:126, 2000.

70. Rogiers X, Malago M, Gawad K, et al: In situ splitting of cadaveric livers. The ultimate expansion of a limited donor pool. *Ann Surg* 224:331, 1996.

71. Humar A, Ramcharan T, Sielaff T, et al: Split liver transplantation for 2 adult recipients: An initial experience. *Am J Transplant* 1:366, 2001.

72. Everson GT, Kam I: Immediate postoperative care, in Maddrey WC, Schiff ER, Sorrell MF (eds): *Transplantation of the Liver*. Baltimore: Lippincott Williams & Wilkins, 2001, p 131.

73. Humar A, Gruessner R: Critical care of the liver transplant recipient, in Rippe I, Fink C (eds): *Intensive Care Medicine*, 4th ed. Philadelphia: Lippincott-Raven, 1998, p 2219.

74. Brown A, Williams R: Long-term postoperative care, in Maddrey WC, Schiff ER, Sorrell MF (eds): *Transplantation of the Liver*. Baltimore: Lippincott Williams & Wilkins, 2001, p 163.

75. Buchman AL, Scolapio J, Fryer J: AGA technical review on short bowel syndrome and intestinal transplantation. *Gastroenterology* 124:1111, 2003.

76. Westergaard H: Short bowel syndrome. *Semin Gastrointest Dis* 13:210, 2002.

77. Sokal EM, Cleghorn G, Goulet O, et al: Liver and intestinal transplantation in children: Working Group Report of the First World Congress of Pediatric Gastroenterology, Hepatology, and Nutrition. *J Pediatr Gastroenterol Nutr* 35(Suppl 2):S159, 2002.

78. Kato T, Ruiz P, Thompson JF, et al: Intestinal and multivisceral transplantation. *World J Surg* 26:226, 2002.

79. Abu-Elmagd K, Bond G, Reyes J, et al: Intestinal transplantation: A coming of age. *Adv Surg* 36:65, 2002.

80. Reyes J, Mazariegos GV, Bond GM, et al: Pediatric intestinal transplantation: Historical notes, principles and controversies. *Pediatr Transplant* 6:193, 2002.

81. Miniati DN, Robbins RC: Heart transplantation: A thirty-year perspective. *Annu Rev Med* 53:189, 2002.

82. Kesten S: Advances in lung transplantation. *Dis Mon* 45:101, 1999.

83. Reichart B, Gulbins H, Meiser BM, et al: Improved results after heart-lung transplantation: A 17-year experience. *Transplantation* 75:127, 2003.

84. Cassivi SD, Meyers BF, Battafarano RJ, et al: Thirteen-year experience in lung transplantation for emphysema. *Ann Thorac Surg* 74:1663, 2002.

85. Egan TM, Detterbeck FC, Mill MR, et al: Long-term results of lung transplantation for cystic fibrosis. *Eur J Cardiothorac Surg* 22:602, 2002.

86. Egan TM, Detterbeck FC: The ABCs of LTX for BAC. *J Thorac Cardiovasc Surg* 125:20, 2003.

87. Goudarzi BM, Bonvino S: Critical care issues in lung and heart transplantation. *Crit Care Clin* 19:209, 2003.

88. Kubak BM: Fungal infection in lung transplantation. *Transpl Infect Dis* 4(Suppl 3):24, 2002.

89. Boucek RJ Jr., Boucek MM: Pediatric heart transplantation. *Curr Opin Pediatr* 14:611, 2002.

90. Marelli D, Laks H, Kobashigawa JA, et al: Seventeen-year experience with 1083 heart transplants at a single institution. *Ann Thorac Surg* 74:1558, 2002.

91. Penn I: The effect of immunosuppression on pre-existing cancers. *Transplantation* 55:742, 1993.

92. Hibberd PL, Snydman DR: Cytomegalovirus infection in organ transplant recipients. *Infect Dis Clin North Am* 9:863, 1995.

93. Kaufman DB, Leventhal JR, Gallon LG, et al: Risk factors and impact of cytomegalovirus disease in simultaneous pancreas-kidney transplantation. *Transplantation* 72:1940, 2001.

94. Dunn DL, Mayoral JL, Gillingham KJ, et al: Treatment of invasive CMV disease in solid organ transplant patients with ganciclovir. *Transplantation* 51:98, 1991.

95. Patel R, Paya CV: Infections in solid-organ transplant recipients. *Clin Microbiol Rev* 10:86, 1997.

96. Lutz J, Heemann U: Tumours after kidney transplantation. *Curr Opin Urol* 13:105, 2003.

97. Euvrard S, Kanitakis J, Claudy A: Skin cancers after organ transplantation. *N Engl J Med* 348:1681, 2003.

98. Green M: Management of Epstein-Barr virus induced post-transplant lymphoproliferative disease in recipients of solid organ transplantation. *Am J Transplant* 1:103, 2001.

99. Cockfield SM: Identifying the patient at risk for post-transplant lymphoproliferative disorder. *Transpl Infect Dis* 3:70, 2001.

100. Preiksaitis JK, Keay S: Diagnosis and management of post-transplant lymphoproliferative disorder in solid-organ transplant recipients. *Clin Infect Dis* 33(Suppl 1):S38, 2001.

101. Boehmer JP: Device therapy for heart failure. *Am J Cardiol* 91:53D, 2003.

102. Deng MC, Naka Y: Mechanical circulatory support devices—state of the art. *Heart Fail Monit* 2:120, 2002.

103. Dooldeniya MD, Warrens AN: Xenotransplantation: Where are we today? *J R Soc Med* 96:111, 2003.

104. Dorling A: Clinical xenotransplantation: Pigs might fly? *Am J Transplant* 2:695, 2002.

105. Einsiedel EF, Ross H: Animal spare parts? A Canadian public consultation on xenotransplantation. *Sci Eng Ethics* 8:579, 2002.

106. Valdes Gonzalez R: Xenotransplantation's benefits outweigh risks. *Nature* 420:268, 2002.

107. Elliott RB, Garkavenko O, Escobar L, et al: Concerns expressed about the virological risks of xenotransplantation. *Xenotransplantation* 9:422, 2002.

108. O'Connell P: Pancreatic islet xenotransplantation. *Xenotransplantation* 9:367, 2002.

Catherine L. Chen, Mark L. Shapiro,
Peter B. Angood, and Martin A. Makary

BACKGROUND

Patient harm due to medical mistakes can be catastrophic and, in some cases, result in high-profile consequences not only for the patient, but also for the surgeon and institution. A single error can even destroy a surgeon's career. Yet, medical mistakes are common to every physician, and errors themselves are unavoidably linked to human nature. Only recently has the science of the delivery of health care matured to recognize the contribution of vulnerable hospital systems in addition to individual responsibility in causing error.

Patient safety is a science that promotes the use of evidence-based medicine and commonsense improvements in an attempt to minimize the impact of human error on the routine delivery of services. Wrong-site/wrong-procedure surgeries, retained sponges, unchecked blood transfusions, mismatched organ transplants, and overlooked allergies are all examples of potentially catastrophic events that can be prevented by implementing safer hospital systems. This chapter provides an overview of the modern day field of patient safety by reviewing key measures of safety and quality, components of culture, interventions and tools, and risk management strategies in surgery.

THE SCIENCE OF PATIENT SAFETY

Medicine is considered a high-risk system with a high error rate, but these two characteristics are not always correlated. Other high-risk industries have managed to maintain an impeccably low error rate. For example, one of the highest risk systems in existence today, the U.S. Navy's nuclear submarine program, has an unmatched safety record. The nuclear fleet has achieved this safety record despite the large number of plants in operation, the added complexity of the reactors being mobile instead of fixed in one location, the secrecy of its operations, and the hazards of engaging in demanding exercises with both friendly and hostile surface ships, submarines, and aircraft.

Much of the credit is due to the culture of the nuclear submarine program, with its insistence on individual ownership, responsibility, attention to detail, professionalism, moral integrity, and mutual respect. These characteristics have created the cultural context necessary for high quality communications under high-risk and high stress conditions. Each reactor operator is aware of what is going on at all times and is responsible for understanding the implications and possible consequences of any action. Communication flows freely between crewmen and officers, and information about any mistakes that occur are dispersed rapidly through the entire system so that other workers can learn how to prevent similar mistakes in the future.[1]

High Reliability Organizations

The nuclear submarine program is an excellent example of an organization that has achieved the distinction of being considered a "high reliability organization." High reliability organization theory, which was developed by a group of social scientists at the University of California at Berkeley, recognizes that there are certain high-risk industries and organizations that have achieved very low accident and error rates compared to what would be expected given the inherent risks involved in their daily operations (Fig. 12-1). Other examples of industries or organizations that are regarded as having achieved high reliability status include aircraft carrier flight decks, nuclear power plants, and the Federal Aviation Administration's air traffic control system. In fact, one reason why nuclear power plants have such an excellent reliability record may be that their operators are often former naval submarine officers whose previous experience and training within one highly reliable organization are easily transferable to other organizations.[1]

One of the assumptions underlying the science of high reliability organizations is the following observation made by Weick in 1987: Humans who operate and manage complex systems are themselves not sufficiently complex to sense and anticipate the problems generated by the system.[2] This introduces another important idea undergirding the science of patient safety: the concept of normal accident theory. Instead of attributing accidents to individual error, this theory states that accidents are intrinsic to high-volume activities and even inevitable in some settings; that is, they are "normal" and should be expected to occur. Accidents should not be used merely to identify and punish the person at fault. As Reason states, even the "best people can make the worst errors as a result of latent conditions."[2]

Health care, naval submarines, airlines, and other industries can all be classified as "high-risk systems," which was defined by Perrow in 1984.[1] High-risk systems:

- Have the potential to create a catastrophe, loosely defined as an event leading to loss of human or animal life, despoiling of the environment, or some other situation that gives rise to the sense of "dread"
- Are complex, in that they have large numbers of highly interdependent subsystems with many possible combinations that are nonlinear and poorly understood
- Are tightly coupled, so that any perturbation in the system is transmitted rapidly between subsystems with little attenuation.

KEY POINTS

1. Patient harm due to medical mistakes can be catastrophic and, in some cases, result in high-profile consequences not only for the patient, but also for the surgeon and institution.

2. Patient safety is a science that promotes the use of evidence-based medicine and commonsense improvements in an attempt to minimize the impact of human error on the routine delivery of services.

3. The structure-process-outcome framework within the context of an organization's culture helps to clarify how risks and hazards embedded within the organization's structure may potentially lead to error and injure or harm patients.

4. Poor communication contributes to approximately 70% of the sentinel events reported to the Joint Commission on Accreditation of Healthcare Organizations.

5. Operating room briefings are team discussions of critical issues and potential hazards that can improve the safety of the operation and have been shown to improve operating room culture and decrease operating room delays.

6. National Quality Forum surgical "never events" include retained surgical items, wrong-site surgery, and death on the day of surgery of a normal healthy patient (ASA Class 1).

7. Patient rapport is the most important determinant of malpractice claims against a surgeon.

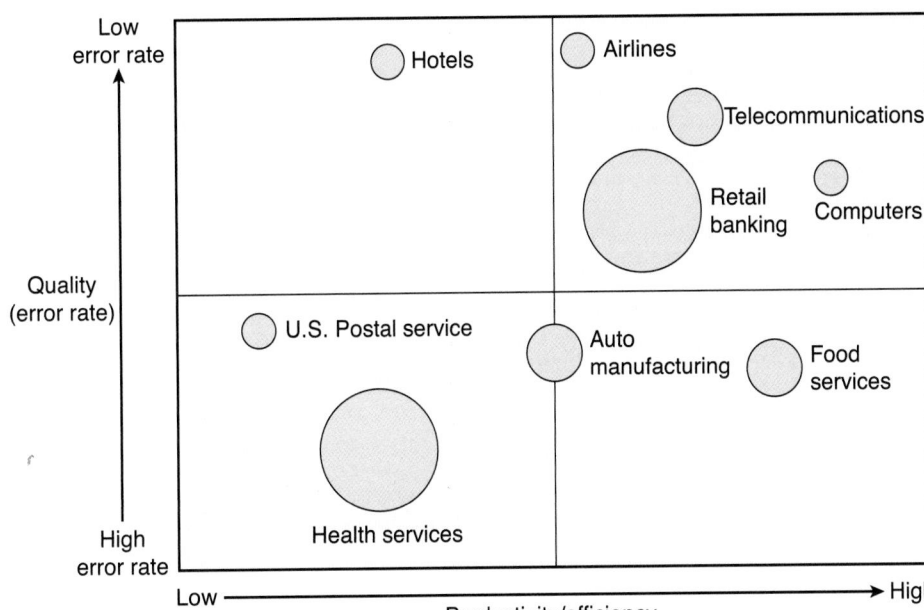

FIG. 12-1. Cross-industry comparison of size, productivity, and efficiency. *(Reproduced with permission from the Advisory Board Company, 2005.)*

However, high reliability organization theory suggests that proper oversight of people, processes, and technology can handle complex and hazardous activities and keep error rates acceptably low.[2] Studies of multiple high reliability organizations have revealed that they share the following common characteristics[2]:

- People are supportive of one another.
- People trust one another.
- People have friendly, open relationships emphasizing credibility and attentiveness.
- The work environment is resilient and emphasizes creativity and goal achievement, providing strong feelings of credibility and personal trust.

Developing these characteristics is an important step toward achieving a low error rate in any organization.

The Institute of Medicine Report

Although health care as a whole can be considered a high-risk system, the industry is far from joining the ranks of nuclear submarines and the Federal Aviation Administration as a high reliability organization. This fact was brought to light in the Institute of Medicine's report "To Err Is Human: Building a Safer Health System," which was published in 2000.[3] A landmark document in raising awareness of the magnitude of the problem of medical mistakes, the report is the most frequently cited document in the medical literature in recent years.[4] The Institute of Medicine (IOM) report shocked the health care community by concluding that between 44,000 and 98,000 deaths and over 1 million injuries occurred each year in American hospitals due to medical error. In fact, the number of deaths attributed to medical error is the aviation equivalent of one jumbo jet crash per day. As this report was disseminated, awareness about medical errors increased, and physicians and other health providers began speaking openly about mistakes and the difficulties they face when dealing with them.

The IOM report brought much-needed attention to the field of patient safety. In addition, it standardized the language used to describe errors in medicine, defining important terms for future research and quality improvement (Table 12-1). Following the publication of the IOM report, interest in patient safety research and programs increased exponentially. In an effort to improve patient safety, health services researchers began to collaborate with scientists from other disciplines, such as human factors engineering, psychology, and informatics to develop innovative solutions to longstanding safety problems. The discussion around patient safety also became more personalized by highlighting the stories of individual patients who had died from medical errors. Most importantly, the report transformed the conversation about patient safety from blaming individuals for errors to improving the systems that allow them to take place (Case 12-1).[5]

The Conceptual Model

The Donabedian model of measuring quality identifies three main types of improvements: changes to structure, process, and outcome

TABLE 12-1	Types of medical error

Adverse event
- Injury caused by medical management rather than the underlying condition of the patient
- Prolongs hospitalization, produces a disability at discharge, or both
- Classified as preventable or unpreventable

Negligence
- Care that falls below a recognized standard of care
- Standard of care is considered to be care a reasonable physician of similar knowledge, training, and experience would use in similar circumstances

Near miss
- An error that does not result in patient harm
- Analysis of near misses provides the opportunity to identify and remedy system failures before the occurrence of harm

Sentinel event
- An unexpected occurrence involving death or serious physical or psychological injury
- The injury involves loss of limb or function
- This type of event requires immediate investigation and response
- Other examples
  - Hemolytic transfusion reaction involving administration of blood or blood products having major blood group incompatibilities
  - Wrong-site, wrong-procedure, or wrong-patient surgery
  - A medication error or other treatment-related error resulting in death
  - Unintentional retention of a foreign body in a patient after surgery

From Woreta et al,[45] with permission.

CASE 12-1 Systems change resulting from medical error

Libby Zion was an 18-year-old woman who died after being admitted to the New York Hospital with fever and agitation on the evening of October 4, 1984. Her father, Sidney Zion, a lawyer and columnist for the *N.Y. Daily News*, was convinced that his daughter's death was due to inadequate staffing and overworked physicians at the hospital and was determined to bring about changes to prevent other patients from suffering as a result of the teaching hospital system. Due to his efforts to publicize the circumstances surrounding his daughter's death, Manhattan District Attorney Robert Morgenthau agreed to let a grand jury consider murder charges. Although the hospital was not indicted, in May 1986, a grand jury issued a report strongly criticizing "the supervision of interns and junior residents at a hospital in NY County."

As a result, New York State Health Commissioner David Axelrod convened a panel of experts headed by Bertrand M. Bell, a primary care physician at Albert Einstein College of Medicine who had long been critical of the lack of supervision of physicians-in-training, to evaluate the training and supervision of doctors in New York State. The Bell Commission recommended that residents work no more than 80 hours per week and no more than 24 consecutive hours per shift, and that a senior physician needed to be physically present in the hospital at all times. These recommendations were adopted by New York State in 1989. In 2003, the Accreditation Council on Graduate Medical Education followed by mandating that all residency training programs adhere to the reduced work hour schedule.

(Fig. 12-2). *Structure* refers to the physical and organizational tools, equipment, and policies that improve safety. Structural measures ask, "Do the right tools, equipment, and policies exist?" *Process* is the application of these tools, equipment, and policies/procedures to patients (good practices and evidence-based medicine). Process measures ask, "Are the right tools, policies, and equipment being used?" *Outcome* is the result on patients. Outcome measures ask, "How often are patients harmed?" In this model, structure (how care is organized) plus process (what we do) influences patient outcomes (the results achieved).[7]

The structure, process, and outcome components of quality measurement all occur within the context of an organization's overall *culture*. The local culture impacts all aspects of the delivery of care because it affects how front-line personnel understand and deliver safe patient care. In fact, culture (collective attitudes and beliefs of caregivers) is increasingly being recognized to be the fourth measurable component to the structure-process-outcome model. This recent recognition is based on growing evidence that local culture is linked to a variety of important clinical outcomes.[7] This structure-process-outcome framework within the context of an organization's culture helps to clarify how risks and hazards embedded within the organization's structure may potentially lead to error and injure or harm patients. For any new patient safety initiative to be deemed successful,

any change in structure or process must lead to a corresponding positive change in patient outcomes.[8]

CREATING A CULTURE OF SAFETY

Culture is to an organization what personality is to the individual—a hidden, yet unifying theme that provides meaning, direction, and mobilization.[2] Organizations with effective safety cultures share a constant commitment to safety as a top-level priority, a commitment that permeates the entire organization. These organizations frequently share the following characteristics[9]:

- An acknowledgment of the high-risk, error-prone nature of an organization's activities
- A nonpunitive environment where individuals are able to report errors or close calls without fear of punishment or retaliation
- An expectation of collaboration across ranks to seek solutions to vulnerabilities
- A willingness on the part of the organization to direct resources to address safety concerns

Traditional surgical culture stands almost in direct opposition to the values upheld by organizations with effective safety cultures for several reasons. Surgeons are less likely to acknowledge their propensity to make mistakes or to admit these mistakes to others.[10] Surgeons tend to minimize the effects of stress on their ability to make decisions, and often claim that their decision making is equally effective in emergency and normal situations.[11] The surgical culture, especially in the operating room (OR), is traditionally rife with hierarchy. Intimidation of other OR personal by surgeons was historically accepted as the norm. This can prevent nurses and other OR staff from pointing out potential errors or mistakes by surgeons. In the intensive care unit (ICU), when compared to physicians, nurses reported that they had more difficulty speaking up, disagreements were not appropriately resolved, and decisions were made without adequate input.[12] In addition, the field of medicine strongly values professional autonomy, which frequently promotes individualism over cooperation, often to the detriment of patient care.[13] Finally, patient safety, although often viewed as important, is seldom promoted from an organizational priority to an organizational value. Organizations often do not feel the need to devote resources to overhauling their patient safety systems as long as they perceive their existing processes to be adequate. It often takes a high-profile sentinel event to motivate leaders to commit the necessary time and resources to improving patient safety within their organization, as exemplified by the Dana-Farber Institute in the aftermath of Betsy Lehman's death (Case 12-2).

CASE 12-2 High-profile sentinel event

On December 3, 1994, Betsy Lehman, a *Boston Globe* health columnist, died as a result of receiving four times the intended dose of chemotherapy for breast cancer. Remarkably, 2 days later, Maureen Bateman, a teacher being treated for cancer, also received a chemotherapy overdose and suffered irreversible heart damage. After investigating the medication errors, the prescribing doctor, three druggists, and 15 nurses were disciplined by state regulators. The hospital was sued by the two women's families and by one of the doctors disciplined.

As a result of this widely publicized event, the Dana-Farber Cancer Institute invested more than $11 million to overhaul their safety programs, including providing new training for their employees and giving doctors more time to meet with patients. The hospital adopted a full disclosure policy so that patients would be informed anytime a mistake had affected their care. Dana-Farber also started a patient committee providing advice and feedback on ways to improve care at the hospital.

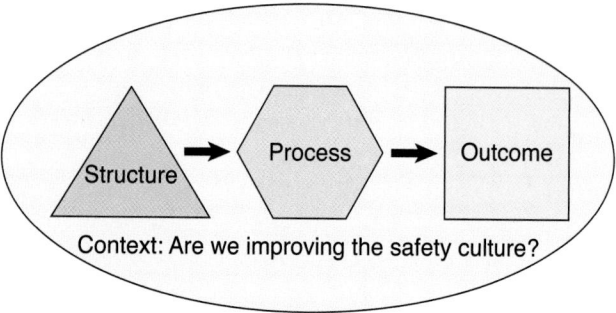

FIG. 12-2. Donebedian model for measuring quality. (*From Makary et al,[6] with permission.*)

Assessing an Organization's Safety Culture

Efforts to foster cultural change within an organization with regard to patient safety have been limited by the inability to measure the impact of any given intervention. However, previous studies have shown that employee attitudes about culture have been associated with error reduction behaviors in aviation and with patient outcomes in ICUs. The Safety Attitudes Questionnaire (SAQ) is a validated survey instrument that can be used to measure culture in a health care setting.[6] Adapted from two safety tools used in aviation, the Flight Management Attitudes Questionnaire and its predecessor, the Cockpit Management Attitudes Questionnaire, the SAQ consists of a series of questions measuring six domains: teamwork climate, safety climate, job satisfaction, perception of management, stress recognition, and working conditions.

The safety climate scale portion of the questionnaire consists of the following seven items:

- I am encouraged by my colleagues to report any patient safety concerns I may have.
- The culture in this clinical area makes it easy to learn from the mistakes of others.
- Medical errors are handled appropriately in this clinical area.
- I know the proper channels to direct questions regarding patient safety in this clinical area.
- I receive appropriate feedback about my performance.
- I would feel safe being treated here as a patient.
- In this clinical area, it is difficult to discuss mistakes.

Although perceptions of teamwork climate can differ as a function of one's role in the OR, perceptions of safety climate are relatively consistent across OR providers in a given hospital. Validated in over 500 hospitals, the SAQ is used to establish benchmark safety culture scores by health care worker type, department, and hospital. Thus, hospitals can compare their local culture between departments at their institution, among different types of health care workers within a department, and throughout the institution. Scores also are compared to national and global scores of all other participating centers seeking to compare their safety climate to national means. In addition, scores are used to evaluate the effectiveness of safety interventions by comparing the SAQ safety climate scores postimplementation to baseline scores.

Strong teamwork is at the core of any effective organization and is a key element to ensuring patient safety in the OR. Teamwork is dependent on other elements such as an organization's underlying culture and patterns of communication. The ability for junior team members and other nonsurgeon professionals, including anesthesiologists, to "speak up" about patient safety concerns is one of the most important elements in relation to creating a culture of patient safety.

TEAMWORK AND COMMUNICATION

According to the Joint Commission, communication breakdown is the most common root cause of sentinel events such as wrong-site surgery (Fig. 12-3). Poor communication contributed to nearly 70% of sentinel events reported to the Joint Commission on Accreditation of Healthcare Organizations in 2006.[14] Good communication is an essential component of teamwork and should be emphasized in any organization wishing to create a culture of patient safety. It especially is important in the OR, one of the most complex work environments in health care.

One of the best research reports ever written on the subject of breakdowns in communication was the 9/11 Commission Report.[15] The report cites Roberta Wohlsetter regarding Pearl Harbor, in which she observed that it is "much easier after the event to sort the relevant from the irrelevant signals. After the event, of course, a signal is always crystal clear; we can now see what disaster it was signaling since the disaster has occurred. But before the event it is obscure and pregnant with conflicting meanings." The circumstances leading up to 9/11 reinforce the difficulty that faces any organization charged with managing complex situations, large amounts of data, and multiple constituents. One of the criticisms of the intelligence agencies laid out in the report is that they "did not have the capability to link the collective knowledge of agents in the field to national priorities." In the same report, the authors "sympathize with the working-level officers, drowning in information and trying to decide what is important or what needs to be done when no particular action has been requested of them." In essence, much of the intelligence leading up to 9/11 could have been used to divert the attack on the United States had communications between the various agencies and individual officers clearly prioritized the threat posed by al Qaeda. In other words, the intelligence gathered actually contained the critical information needed to thwart an attack but was not prioritized sufficiently to alert the recipient of its significance until it was too late.

Similarly, within the realm of patient care, there are enormous amounts of information being exchanged between health care providers on a daily basis. Much of this information, if prioritized correctly, has the potential to prevent unintended medical errors and serious harm to patients. The importance of good communication in preventing medical error is undeniable; however, it is difficult to achieve. The traditional surgical hierarchy combined with an atmosphere of intimidation can prevent OR personnel from sharing important patient data and expressing safety concerns. Members of the team may be hesitant to raise a safety concern if they do not feel comfortable speaking up. In addition, nurses who do not feel empowered to voice their concerns have increased job dissatisfaction—a root problem in the national nursing shortage. One perioperative field study showed a 30% rate of communication

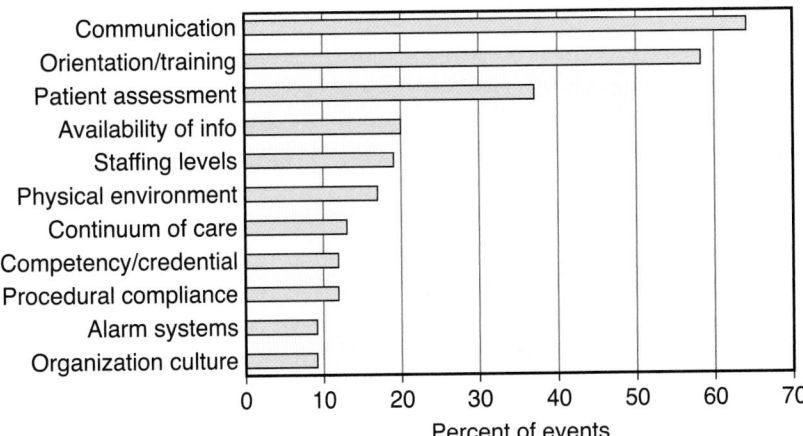

FIG. 12-3. Root causes of sentinel events 1995–2002. *(From Joint Commission.[14] © The Joint Commission, 2008. Reprinted with permission.)*

failure in the OR, with 36% of these breakdowns having a substantial impact on patient safety.[16]

In addition to overcoming the cultural barrier to better teamwork and communication in the OR, Christian and associates' prospective study of patient safety in the OR demonstrated that the standard workflow of a typical OR itself presents many opportunities for the loss or degradation of critical information.[17] Handoffs of patient care from the OR to other locations or providers are particularly prone to information loss, which has previously been demonstrated in other clinical settings. Handoffs and auxiliary tasks, such as the surgical count, frequently take place during critical portions of the case and place competing demands on provider attention from primary patient-centered activities. Communication between the surgeon and pathologist also are vulnerable, as the communication often occurs through secondary messengers such as nurses or technicians. This information loss can lead to delays, overuse of staff and resources, uncertainty in clinical decision making and planning, and oversights in patient preparation.

Measuring Teamwork

Research in commercial aviation has demonstrated a strong correlation between better teamwork and improved safety performance. Cockpit crew members' reluctance to question a captain's judgment has been identified as a root cause of aviation accidents. Attitudes about teamwork are associated with error-reduction behaviors in aviation, with patient outcomes in ICUs, and with nurse turnover in the OR. Good teamwork is associated with higher job satisfaction ratings and less sick time taken from work.

The SAQ can be used to measure teamwork, identify disconnects between or within disciplines, provide benchmarks for departments of surgery or hospitals seeking to measure their teamwork climate, and evaluate interventions aimed at improving patient safety.[18] The SAQ teamwork scores are responsive to interventions that aim to improve teamwork among operating teams, such as the implementation of ICU checklists, executive walk rounds, and preoperative briefing team discussions. The communication and collaboration sections of the SAQ reflect OR caregiver views on teamwork and can be used to distinguish meaningful interventions from impractical and ineffective programs to improve teamwork among OR professionals.

In a survey of operating room personnel across 60 hospitals, the SAQ identified substantial differences in the perception of teamwork in the OR depending on one's role. Physicians frequently rated the teamwork of others as good, while nurses at the same institutions perceived teamwork as poor (Fig. 12-4). Similar discrepancies about perceptions of collaboration between physicians and nurses have been found in ICUs. These discrepancies can be attributed to differences in the communication skills that are valued by surgeons and nurses, respectively. For example, nurses describe good collaboration as having their input respected, while physicians describe good collaboration as having nurses who can anticipate their needs and follow instructions. Efforts to improve the communication that takes place between physicians and nurses can directly improve the perception of teamwork and collaboration by the OR team (Table 12-2).

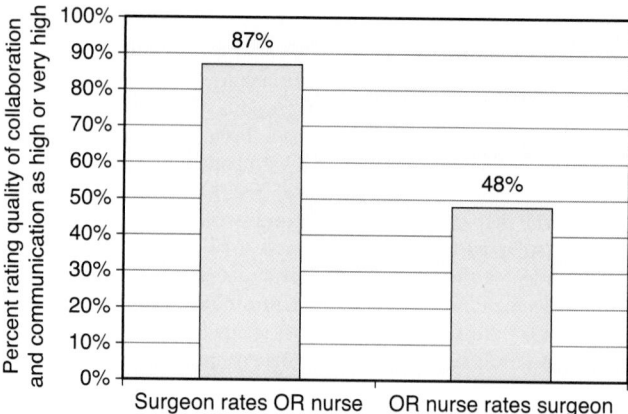

FIG. 12-4. Differences in teamwork perceptions between surgeons and operating room (OR) nurses. *(From Makary et al,[18] with permission. Copyright Elsevier.)*

Empowering well-respected surgeons to promote principles of teamwork and communication can go a long way toward transforming attitudinal and behavioral changes in fellow physicians as well as other members of the surgical team. Surgeons are increasingly encouraging the respectful and timely voicing of concerns of OR personnel related to patient safety.

COMMUNICATION TOOLS

Other high reliability organizations such as aviation frequently use tools such as prompts, checks, standard operating protocols, and communication interventions such as team briefings and debriefings. These tools identify and mitigate hazards and allow an organization to complete tasks more efficiently. They also foster a culture of open communication and speaking up if a team member senses a safety concern, a principle that has been mastered in the landmark business practices of the Toyota Production System. Safety checks and standardized team discussions serve as prompts to help "engineer out" human error, providing quality assurance and improving information flow. They also can prevent errors related to omissions, which are more likely to occur when there is information overload, multiple steps in a process, repetitions in steps, planned departures from routine processes, and when there are other interruptions and distractions present while the process is being executed. These same interventions have been shown to improve patient safety in ORs and ICUs.[19,20]

Operating Room Briefings

Preoperative briefings and checklists, when used appropriately, help to facilitate transfer of information between team members (Table 12-3). A briefing, or checklist, is any preprocedure discussion of requirements, needs, and special issues of the procedure. Briefings

TABLE 12-2	Percentage of operating room caregivers reporting a high or very high level of collaboration with other members of the operating room team			
Caregiver Position Performing Rating	**Caregiver Position Being Rated**			
	Surgeon	**Anesthesiologist**	**Nurse**	**CRNA**
Surgeon	85	84	88	87
Anesthesiologist	70	**96**	89	92
Nurse	**48**	63	81	68
CRNA	58	75	76	93

The best teamwork scores were recorded by anesthesiologists when they rated their teamwork with other anesthesiologists ("high" or "very high" 96% of the time). The lowest teamwork ratings were recorded by nurses when they rated their teamwork with surgeons ("high" or "very high" 48% of the time).
CRNA = certified registered nurse anesthetist.
From Makary et al,[18] with permission. Copyright Elsevier.

TABLE 12-3 Five-point operating room briefing

What are the **names and roles** of the team members?
Is the correct patient/procedure confirmed? [Joint Commission Universal Protocol (**TIME-OUT**)]
Have **antibiotics** been given? (if appropriate)
What are the **critical steps** of the procedure?
What are the **potential problems** for the case?

From Makary et al,[20] with permission. Copyright Elsevier.

often are locally adapted to the specific needs of the specialty (orthopaedic surgery, transplantation, etc.). They have been associated with an improved safety culture, including increased awareness of wrong-site/wrong-procedure errors, early reporting of equipment problems, and reduced operational costs. OR briefings are increasingly being used to ensure evidence-based measures, such as the appropriate administration of preoperative antibiotics and deep vein thrombosis (DVT) prophylaxis, are used. It is well recognized that a team discussion of critical issues and potential hazards improves the safety of the operation when all members of the OR team are interested in providing optimal patient care. The use of briefings also is associated with fewer unexpected delays. In one study, 30.9% of OR personnel reported a delay before the institution of OR briefings, and only 23.3% reported delays postbriefing.[21] Briefings allow personnel to discuss potential problems, before they become a "near miss" or cause actual harm, by creating an open atmosphere that empowers all team members, whether circulating nurse, medical student, or senior resident, to feel empowered to address any concerns with the attending surgeon.

The World Health Organization (WHO) has recently developed a comprehensive perioperative checklist as a primary intervention of the "Safe Surgery Saves Lives" program—an effort to reduce surgical deaths across the globe (Fig. 12-5).[22] The WHO checklist includes prompts to ensure that infection prevention measures are followed, potential airway complications are precluded (e.g., anesthesia has necessary equipment and assistance for a patient with a difficult airway), and the groundwork for effective surgical teamwork is established (e.g., proper introductions of all OR personnel). Aspects of the Joint Commission's preprocedure "Universal Protocol" (or "time-out") also are included in the checklist (e.g., checks to ensure operation performed on correct patient and correct site).

Operating Room Debriefings

Postprocedural debriefings improve patient safety by allowing for discussion and reflection on causes for errors and critical incidents that occurred during the case. The use of debriefings promotes a culture of learning from experience, and any errors or critical incidents are regarded as learning opportunities rather than cause for punishment. During the debriefing conversation, the team also can discuss what went well during the case, and designate a point person to follow up on any proposed actions that result from the discussion. In addition, most debriefings include a verification of the sponge, needle, and instrument counts, and confirm correct labeling of the surgical specimen.

Errors in surgical specimen labeling have not received as much attention as incorrect sponge or instrument counts as an indicator of the quality of communication in the OR. However, an error in verbal communication and transcription during the handoff process increases the risk of mislabeling a surgical specimen before its arrival in a pathology laboratory and can occur as a consequence of poor teamwork and communication. In one study, this type of identifica-

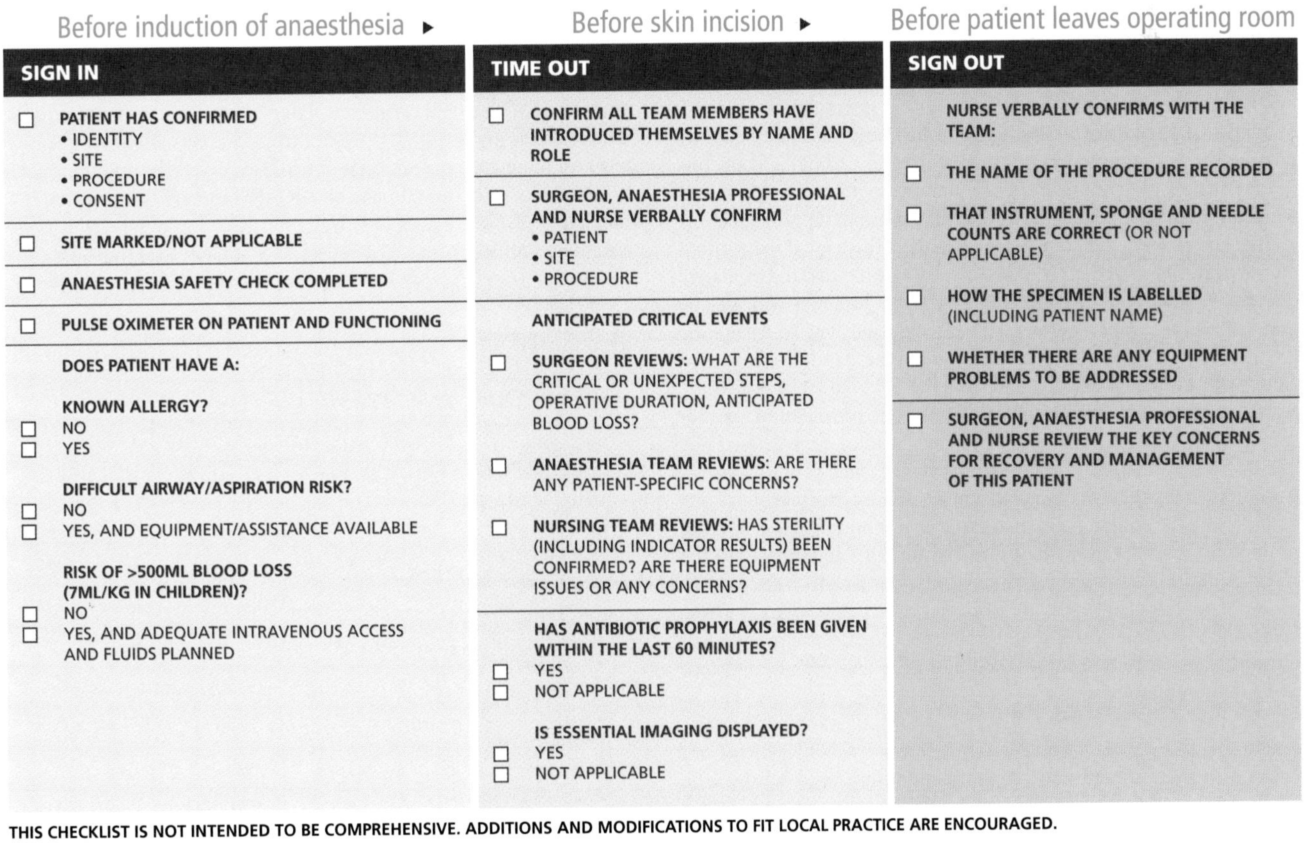

Before induction of anaesthesia ▸

SIGN IN

- ☐ PATIENT HAS CONFIRMED
  - IDENTITY
  - SITE
  - PROCEDURE
  - CONSENT
- ☐ SITE MARKED/NOT APPLICABLE
- ☐ ANAESTHESIA SAFETY CHECK COMPLETED
- ☐ PULSE OXIMETER ON PATIENT AND FUNCTIONING

DOES PATIENT HAVE A:

KNOWN ALLERGY?
- ☐ NO
- ☐ YES

DIFFICULT AIRWAY/ASPIRATION RISK?
- ☐ NO
- ☐ YES, AND EQUIPMENT/ASSISTANCE AVAILABLE

RISK OF >500ML BLOOD LOSS (7ML/KG IN CHILDREN)?
- ☐ NO
- ☐ YES, AND ADEQUATE INTRAVENOUS ACCESS AND FLUIDS PLANNED

Before skin incision ▸

TIME OUT

- ☐ CONFIRM ALL TEAM MEMBERS HAVE INTRODUCED THEMSELVES BY NAME AND ROLE
- ☐ SURGEON, ANAESTHESIA PROFESSIONAL AND NURSE VERBALLY CONFIRM
  - PATIENT
  - SITE
  - PROCEDURE

ANTICIPATED CRITICAL EVENTS
- ☐ SURGEON REVIEWS: WHAT ARE THE CRITICAL OR UNEXPECTED STEPS, OPERATIVE DURATION, ANTICIPATED BLOOD LOSS?
- ☐ ANAESTHESIA TEAM REVIEWS: ARE THERE ANY PATIENT-SPECIFIC CONCERNS?
- ☐ NURSING TEAM REVIEWS: HAS STERILITY (INCLUDING INDICATOR RESULTS) BEEN CONFIRMED? ARE THERE EQUIPMENT ISSUES OR ANY CONCERNS?

HAS ANTIBIOTIC PROPHYLAXIS BEEN GIVEN WITHIN THE LAST 60 MINUTES?
- ☐ YES
- ☐ NOT APPLICABLE

IS ESSENTIAL IMAGING DISPLAYED?
- ☐ YES
- ☐ NOT APPLICABLE

Before patient leaves operating room

SIGN OUT

NURSE VERBALLY CONFIRMS WITH THE TEAM:
- ☐ THE NAME OF THE PROCEDURE RECORDED
- ☐ THAT INSTRUMENT, SPONGE AND NEEDLE COUNTS ARE CORRECT (OR NOT APPLICABLE)
- ☐ HOW THE SPECIMEN IS LABELLED (INCLUDING PATIENT NAME)
- ☐ WHETHER THERE ARE ANY EQUIPMENT PROBLEMS TO BE ADDRESSED
- ☐ SURGEON, ANAESTHESIA PROFESSIONAL AND NURSE REVIEW THE KEY CONCERNS FOR RECOVERY AND MANAGEMENT OF THIS PATIENT

THIS CHECKLIST IS NOT INTENDED TO BE COMPREHENSIVE. ADDITIONS AND MODIFICATIONS TO FIT LOCAL PRACTICE ARE ENCOURAGED.

FIG. 12-5. World Health Organization surgical safety checklist. *[Reproduced with permission from World Health Organization Safe Surgery Saves Lives: http://www.who.int/patientsafety/safesurgery/en/ (accessed April 15, 2009).]*

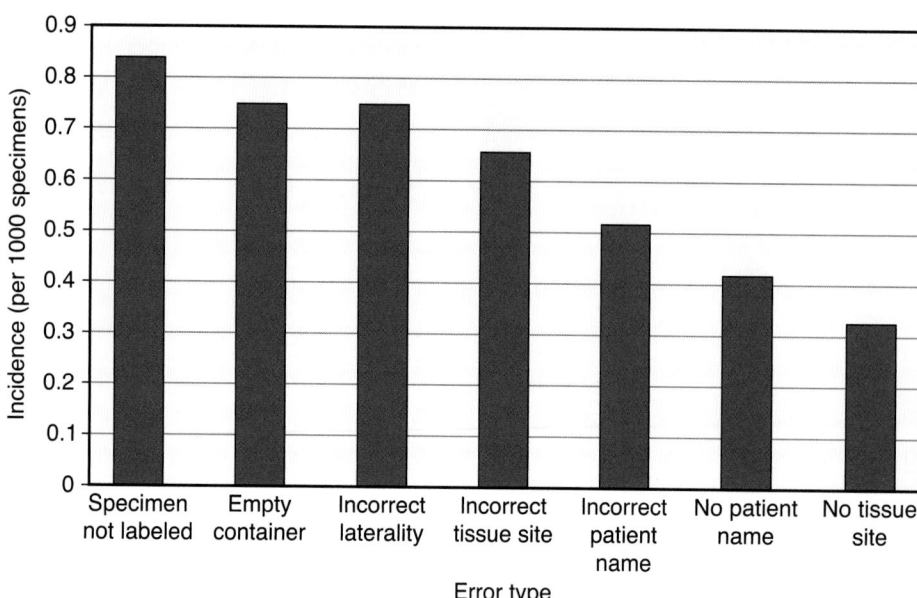

FIG. 12-6. Incidence of identification errors observed per 1000 specimens (n = 21,351). *(From Makary et al,[23] with permission. Copyright Elsevier.)*

tion error occurred in 4.3 per 1000 surgical specimens, which implies an annualized rate of occurrence of 182 mislabeled specimens per year (Fig. 12-6).[23] Errors involving specimen identification can result in delays in care, the need for an additional biopsy or therapy, failure to use appropriate therapy, or therapy administered to the wrong body site, side, or patient. These system failures can lead to significant harm to the patient, costs to the institution, and distrust by a community. Given the frequency of occurrence and the feasibility and validity of measuring them, mislabeled surgical specimens may serve as a useful indicator of patient safety in surgical patients, and should be included in any postprocedural debriefing checklist.

Sign Outs

The 9/11 Commission Report cited the lack of prioritization as the key lethal defect in communications among government agencies. Similarly, health care is another setting where information frequently passes to covering providers without prioritizing potential concerns. In other words, sign outs represent a major vulnerable process of care which, if performed inadequately, can lead to catastrophic events.

The term *sign out* can refer to either the verbal or written communication of patient information being provided to familiarize oncoming or covering physicians about the patients who will be under their care. When performed well, sign outs help to ensure the transfer of pertinent information during these handoffs in patient care, such as when taking a patient from the OR to the recovery room, or when a patient is being transferred from one physician to another during shift changes. However, previous studies have shown the handoff process to be variable, unstructured, and prone to error. Common categories of communication failure during sign outs include content omissions, such as failure to mention active medical problems or current medications and treatments, and failures in the actual communication process, such as a lack of face-to-face communication or leaving illegible or unclear notes (Case 12-3).[24] These failures led to confusion and uncertainty by the covering physician during patient care decisions, resulting in the delivery of inefficient and suboptimal care.

The use of more structured verbal communication such as the Situational Debriefing Model, otherwise known as *SBAR* (*s*ituation, *b*ackground, *a*ssessment, and *r*ecommendation), used by the U.S. Navy, can be applied to health care to improve the communication of critical information in a timely and orderly fashion.[24] In addition, all sign outs should begin with the statement "In this patient, I am most concerned about . . ." to signal to the health care provider on the receiving end the most important safety concerns regarding that specific patient.

Implementation

Tools such as checklists, sign outs, briefings, and debriefings improve communication between health care providers and create a safer patient environment (Fig. 12-7). Although their use in health care is still highly variable, specialties that have incorporated these tools, such as intensive care and anesthesia, have made impressive strides in patient safety, and the endorsement of many prominent surgeon champions is enabling the rapid diffusion of these communication tools nationally. Currently, communication breakdowns, information loss, hand off, multiple competing tasks, and high workload are considered "annoying but accepted features" of the perioperative environment by the physicians and nurses who encounter them on a daily basis.[17] As physician attitudes toward errors, stress, and teamwork in medicine become more favorable toward the common goals of reducing error and improving teamwork and communication, medicine will likely achieve many of the milestones in safety that high-reliability industries such as aviation have already accomplished.

CASE 12-3   Inadequate sign out leading to medical error

Josie King was an 18-month-old child who was admitted to Johns Hopkins Hospital in January of 2001 for first- and second-degree burns. She spent 10 days in the pediatric intensive care unit and was well on her way to recovery. She was transferred to an intermediate care floor with the expectation that she would be sent home in a few days.

The following week, her central line was removed, but nurses would not allow Josie to drink anything by mouth. Around 1 P.M. the next day, a nurse came to Josie's bedside with a syringe of methadone. Although Josie's mother told the nurse that there was no order for narcotics, the nurse insisted that the orders had been changed and administered the drug. Josie's heart stopped, and her eyes became fixed. She was moved to the pediatric intensive care unit and placed on life support. Two days later, on February 22, 2001, she died from severe dehydration.

After her death, Josie's parents, Sorrel and Jay King, were motivated to work with leaders at Johns Hopkins to ensure that no other family would have to endure the death of a child due to medical error. They later funded the Josie King Patient Safety Program and an academic scholarship in the field of safety.

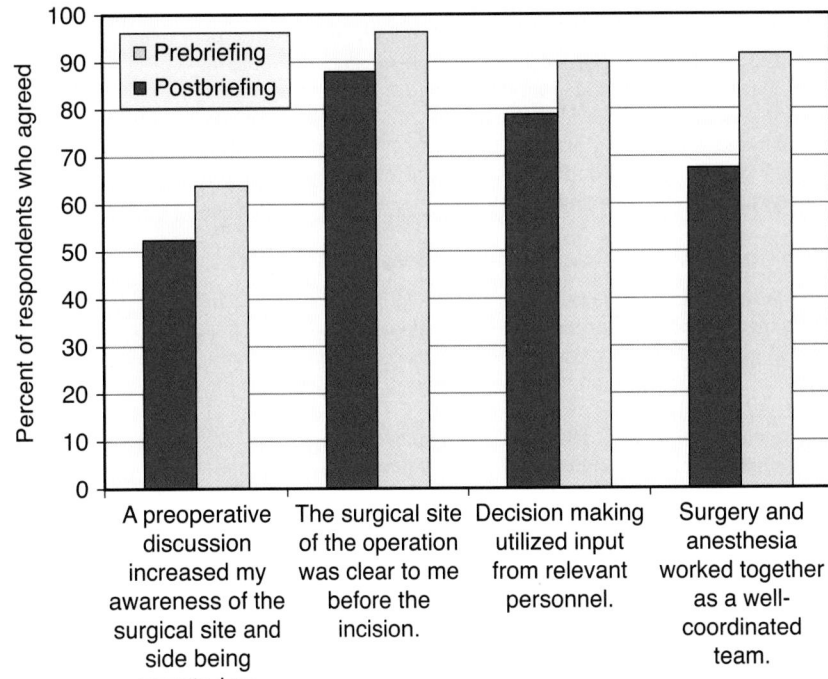

FIG. 12-7. Impact of operating room briefings on teamwork and communication. *(From Makary et al,[20] with permission. Copyright Elsevier.)*

MEASURING QUALITY IN SURGERY

Despite the newfound focus on patient safety in surgery and the number of initiatives being undertaken by many organizations to improve their safety culture, there are few tools to actually measure whether these efforts actually are effective in reducing the number of errors. Several agencies and private groups have developed criteria to evaluate quality and safety within hospitals.

Agency for Healthcare Research and Quality Patient Safety Indicators

The Agency for Healthcare Research and Quality (AHRQ) was created in 1989 as a Public Health Service agency in the Department of Health and Human Services. Its mission is to improve the quality, safety, efficiency, and effectiveness of health care for all Americans. Nearly 80% of the AHRQ's budget is awarded as grants and contracts to researchers at universities and other research institutions across the country. The AHRQ sponsors and conducts research that provides evidence-based information on health care outcomes; quality; and cost, use, and access. The information helps health care decision makers—patients and clinicians, health system leaders, purchasers, and policymakers—make more informed decisions and improve the quality of health care services.[25]

The AHRQ has advocated the use of quality indicators to measure health care quality using readily available hospital inpatient administrative data. The Patient Safety Indicators (PSIs), which were released in March 2003, are a tool to help health system leaders identify potential adverse events occurring during hospitalization. Developed after a comprehensive literature review, analysis of ICD-9-CM codes, review by a clinician panel, implementation of risk adjustment, and empirical analyses, these 27 indicators provide information on potential inhospital complications and adverse events following surgeries, procedures, and childbirth (Table 12-4).

Provider-level indicators provide a measure of the potentially preventable complication for patients who received their initial care and the complication of care within the same hospitalization, and they include only those cases where a secondary diagnosis code flags a potentially preventable complication. Area-level indicators capture all cases of the potentially preventable complication that occur

in a given area (e.g., metropolitan area or county), either during hospitalization or resulting in subsequent hospitalization.[26]

Administrative data are readily available, inexpensive, computer readable, typically continuous, and cover large populations. Their

---

TABLE 12-4 Agency for Healthcare Research and Quality patient safety indicators

Provider-level patient safety indicators
- Complications of anesthesia
- Death in low mortality diagnosis-related groups
- Decubitus ulcer
- Failure to rescue
- Foreign body left in during procedure
- Iatrogenic pneumothorax
- Selected infections due to medical care
- Postoperative hip fracture
- Postoperative hemorrhage or hematoma
- Postoperative physiologic and metabolic derangements
- Postoperative respiratory failure
- Postoperative pulmonary embolism or deep vein thrombosis
- Postoperative sepsis
- Postoperative wound dehiscence in abdominopelvic surgical patients
- Accidental puncture and laceration
- Transfusion reaction
- Birth trauma—injury to neonate
- Obstetric trauma—vaginal delivery with instrument
- Obstetric trauma—vaginal delivery without instrument
- Obstetric trauma—cesarean delivery

Area-level patient safety indicators
- Foreign body left in during procedure
- Iatrogenic pneumothorax
- Selected infections due to medical care
- Postoperative wound dehiscence in abdominopelvic surgical patients
- Accidental puncture and laceration
- Transfusion reaction
- Postoperative hemorrhage or hematoma

From Agency for Healthcare Research and Quality,[26] with permission.

potential in patient safety research is increasingly recognized. Currently, PSIs are considered indicators, not definitive measures, of patient safety concerns. They can identify potential safety problems that merit further investigation. They also can be used to better prioritize and evaluate local and national initiatives, and even as benchmarks for tracking progress in patient safety. In the future, further growth in electronic health data will make administrative data based tools like the PSIs more useful.[27]

The Surgical Care Improvement Project Measures

The Surgical Care Improvement Project (SCIP) was established in 2003 by a national partnership of organizations committed to improving surgical care by reducing the occurrence of surgical complications. The steering committee is comprised of groups such as the Centers for Medicare and Medicaid Services, the American Hospital Association, Centers for Disease Control and Prevention (CDC), Institute for Healthcare Improvement, Joint Commission on Accreditation of Healthcare Organizations, and others. The organization has a stated goal of reducing the incidence of preventable surgical complications by 25% nationally by the year 2010.[28]

The incidence of postoperative complications ranges from 6% for patients undergoing noncardiac surgery to more than 30% for patients undergoing high-risk surgery. Common postoperative complications include surgical site infections (SSIs) and postoperative sepsis, cardiovascular complications including myocardial infarction, respiratory complications including postoperative pneumonia and failure to wean, and thromboembolic complications. Patients who experience postoperative complications have increased hospital length of stay (3 to 11 days longer than those without complications), increased hospital costs (ranging from $1398 for an infectious complication to $18,310 for a thromboembolic event), and increased mortality (median patient survival decreases by 69%).[28]

Despite well-established evidence that many of these adverse events are preventable, the failure to comply with standards of care known to prevent these complications results in unnecessary harm to a large number of patients. SCIP has identified three broad areas within surgery where potential complications have a high incidence and high cost and there is a significant opportunity for prevention: SSIs, venous thromboembolism, and adverse cardiac events. The SCIP measures aim to reduce the incidence of these events during the perioperative period by advocating the use of proven process and outcome measures by participating hospitals and providers. These process and outcome measures are detailed in Table 12-5.

SSIs account for 14 to 16% of all hospital-acquired infections and are a common complication of care, occurring in 2 to 5% of patients after clean extra-abdominal operations and up to 20% of patients undergoing intra-abdominal procedures. By implementing steps to reduce SSIs, hospitals could recognize a savings of $3152 and reduction in extended length of stay by 7 days on each patient developing an infection.[29]

Adverse cardiac events occur in 2 to 5% of patients undergoing noncardiac surgery and as many as 34% of patients undergoing vascular surgery. Certain perioperative cardiac events, such as myocardial infarction, are associated with a mortality rate of 40 to 70% per event, prolonged hospitalization, and higher costs. Current studies suggest that appropriately administered beta blockers reduce perioperative ischemia, especially in patients considered to be at risk. It has been found that nearly half of the fatal cardiac events could be preventable with beta blocker therapy.[29]

DVT occurs after approximately 25% of all major surgical procedures performed without prophylaxis, and pulmonary embolism (PE) in 7% of surgeries conducted without prophylaxis. More than 50% of major orthopedic procedures are complicated by DVT, and up to 30% by PE, if prophylactic treatment is not instituted. Despite the well-established efficacy and safety of preventive measures, studies show that prophylaxis often is underused or used inappropriately. Both low-dose unfractionated heparin and low molecular weight heparin have similar efficacy in DVT and PE

TABLE 12-5	The Surgical Care Improvement Project measures

Process of care performance measures

Infection
- Prophylactic antibiotic received within 1 h before surgical incision
- Prophylactic antibiotic selection for surgical patients
- Prophylactic antibiotics discontinued within 24 h after surgery end time (48 h for cardiac patients)
- Cardiac surgery patients with controlled 6 A.M. postoperative serum glucose
- Surgery patients with appropriate hair removal
- Colorectal surgery patients with immediate postoperative normothermia

Venous thromboembolism
- Surgery patients with recommended venous thromboembolism prophylaxis ordered
- Surgery patients who received appropriate venous thromboembolism prophylaxis within 24 h before surgery to 24 h after surgery

Cardiac events
- Surgery patients on a beta blocker prior to arrival who received a beta blocker during the perioperative period

Proposed outcome measures

Infection
- Postoperative wound infection diagnosed during index hospitalization

Venous thromboembolism
- Intra- or postoperative pulmonary embolism diagnosed during index hospitalization and within 30 d of surgery
- Intra- or postoperative deep vein thrombosis diagnosed during index hospitalization and within 30 d of surgery

Cardiac events
- Intra- or postoperative acute myocardial infarction diagnosed during index hospitalization and within 30 d of surgery

Global measures
- Mortality within 30 d of surgery
- Readmission within 30 d of surgery

From Surgical Care Improvement Project,[29] with permission.

prevention. Prophylaxis using low-dose unfractionated heparin has been shown to reduce the incidence of fatal PEs by 50%.[29]

The SCIP effort provides an infrastructure and guidelines for data collection and quality improvement activities on a national scale. By achieving high levels of compliance with evidence-based practices to reduce SSIs, venous thromboembolism events, and perioperative cardiac complications, the potential number of lives saved in the Medicare patient population alone exceeds 13,000 annually.[28] Although SCIP still faces challenges with regard to implementing the proposed outcome measures at the local level, the SCIP process measures have been shown to effectively reduce perioperative complications and will continue to shape the national effort to improve the delivery of surgical care in the United States.

National Surgical Quality Improvement Program[30]

The National Surgical Quality Improvement Program (NSQIP) is a measurement program that allows hospitals to sample their rates of postoperative events and compare them to similar hospitals. Created by the Veterans Health Administration (VA) in 1991, NSQIP has been credited with measuring and improving morbidity and mortality outcomes at the VA, reducing 30-day mortality rate after major surgery by 31%, and 30-day postoperative morbidity by 45% in its first decade. Beta testing at 18 non-VA sites from 2001 to 2004 demonstrated the feasibility and utility of the program in the private sector. The program was subsequently expanded to the private sector in 2004 when the American College of Surgeons endorsed the program and encouraged hospital participation to measure and evaluate outcomes on a large scale. Currently, over 200 U.S. hospitals participate in the program.

NSQIP uses a risk-adjusted ratio of the observed to expected outcome (focusing primarily on 30-day morbidity and mortality) to compare the performance of participating hospitals with their peers. The data the program has compiled also can be used to conduct observational studies using prospectively collected information on more than 1.5 million patients and operations. The expansion of NSQIP to the private sector has helped shift the focus from merely preventing the provider errors and sentinel events highlighted by the IOM publication "To Err Is Human" to the larger goal of preventing all adverse postoperative outcomes to improve patient safety.

Several insights about patient safety have arisen as a result of NSQIP. First, safety is indistinguishable from overall quality of surgical care and should not be addressed independent of surgical quality. Defining quality in terms of keeping a patient safe from adverse outcomes allows the NSQIP data to be used to assess and improve quality of care by making improvements in patient safety. In other words, prevention of errors is synonymous with the reduction of adverse outcomes and can be used as a reliable quality measure. Second, during an episode of surgical care, adverse outcomes, and hence, patient safety, are primarily determined by the quality of the systems of care. Errors in hospitals with higher than expected observed to expected outcomes ratios are more likely to be from system errors than from provider incompetence, underscoring the importance of adequate communication, coordination, and team work in achieving quality surgical care. Finally, reliable comparative outcomes data are imperative for the identification of system problems and the assurance of patient safety from adverse outcomes. Risk-adjusted rates of adverse outcomes must be compared with similarly risk-adjusted rates at peer institutions to appreciate more subtle system errors that lead to adverse outcomes to prompt changes in the quality of an institution's processes and structures.

The Leapfrog Group

One of the largest efforts to standardize evidence-based medicine in the United States is being led by The Leapfrog Group, an alliance of large public and private health care purchasers representing more than 37 million individuals across the United States. This health care consortium was founded in 2000 with the aim to exert their combined leverage toward improving nationwide standards of health care quality, optimizing patient outcomes, and ultimately lowering health care costs. The Leapfrog Group's strategy to achieve these goals is through providing patient referral, financial incentives, and public recognition for hospitals that practice or implement evidence-based, health care standards. These include hospital use of computerized physician order entry systems, compliance with 24-hour ICU physician staffing, evaluation using a 30-point composite Leapfrog Safe Practices Score, and evidence-based hospital referral (EBHR) standards for five high-risk operations.[31]

Leapfrog encourages the use of evidence-based health care standards through the administration of an ongoing, voluntary, web-based hospital quality and safety survey. This survey is conducted in 33 regions that cover over one half of the U.S. population and 58% of all hospital beds in the country. Currently, more than 1300 hospitals participate in the survey. Leapfrog asks for information on eight high-risk conditions or procedures, including the following surgical procedures: coronary artery bypass graft, percutaneous coronary intervention, AAA repair, pancreatic resection, and esophagectomy. These procedures were chosen because evidence exists that adherence to certain process measures can dramatically improve the outcomes of these procedures. In addition, more than 100 studies also have demonstrated that better results are obtained at high-volume hospitals when undergoing cardiovascular surgery, major cancer resections, and other high-risk procedures. Hospitals fulfilling the EBHR Safety Standard are expected to meet the hospital and surgeon volume criteria shown in Table 12-6. Hospitals that do not meet these criteria but adhere to the Leapfrog-endorsed process measures for coronary artery bypass graft surgery, percutaneous coronary intervention, AAA repair, and care for high-risk neonates, receive partial

TABLE 12-6	Recommended annual volumes: hospitals and surgeons
1. Coronary artery bypass graft	≥450/100
2. Percutaneous coronary intervention	≥400/75
3. Abdominal aortic aneurysm repair	≥50/22
4. Aortic valve replacement	≥120/22
5. Pancreatic resection	≥11/2
6. Esophagectomy	≥13/2
7. Bariatric surgery	>100/20

From The Leapfrog Group,[32] with permission.

credit toward fulfilling the EBHR Safety Standard. Leapfrog purchasers work to recognize and reward hospitals that provide care for their enrollees who meet EBHR standards.[32]

In a recent study, Brooke and associates analyzed whether achieving Leapfrog's established evidence-based standards for abdominal aortic aneurysm (AAA) repair, including meeting targets for case volume and perioperative beta blocker usage, correlated with improved patient outcomes over time.[31] After controlling for differences in hospital and patient characteristics, hospitals that implemented a policy for perioperative beta blocker usage had an estimated 51% reduction in mortality following open AAA repair cases, as compared to control hospitals. Among 111 California hospitals in which endovascular AAA repair was performed, inhospital mortality was reduced by an estimated 61% over time among hospitals meeting Leapfrog case volume standards when compared to control hospitals, although this result was not statistically significant. These results suggest that hospital compliance with Leapfrog standards for elective AAA repair are an effective means to help improve inhospital mortality outcomes over time, and support further efforts aimed at standardizing patient referral to hospitals that comply with other evidence-based medicine standards for other surgical procedures.

World Health Organization "Safe Surgery Saves Lives" Initiative

In October 2004, the WHO launched a global initiative to strengthen health care safety and monitoring systems by creating the World Alliance for Patient Safety. As part of the group's efforts to improve patient safety, the alliance implemented a series of safety campaigns that brought together experts in specific problem areas through individual Global Patient Safety Challenges. The second Global Patient Safety Challenge focuses on improving the safety of surgical care. The main goal of the campaign, called *Safe Surgery Saves Lives*, is to reduce surgical deaths and complications through the universal adaptation of a comprehensive perioperative surgical safety checklist in ORs worldwide. In addition, the WHO has defined a set of uniform measures for national and international surveillance of surgical care to better assess the quantity and quality of surgical care being delivered worldwide (Table 12-7).[22] At the population level, metrics include the number of surgeon, anesthesia, and nurse providers per capita, the number of ORs per capita, and overall surgical case volumes and mortality rates. At the hospital level, metrics include

TABLE 12-7	World Health Organization basic surgical vital statistics

- Number of operating theatres per capita
- Number of trained surgeons and trained anesthesia professionals per capita
- Number of operations performed in operating theatres within per capita
- Number of deaths on the day of surgery
- Number of inhospital deaths following surgery

From World Health Organization,[22] with permission.

TABLE 12-8	Surgical "never events"

- Surgery performed on the wrong body part
- Surgery performed on the wrong patient
- Wrong surgical procedure performed on a patient
- Unintended retention of a foreign object in a patient after surgery or other procedure
- Intraoperative or immediately postoperative death in an ASA Class I patient

ASA = American Society of Anesthesiologists.
From National Quality Forum,[34] with permission.

safety improvement structures and a surgical "Apgar score," a validated method of prognosticating patient outcomes based on intraoperative events (i.e., hypotension, tachycardia, blood loss).[33]

National Quality Forum

The National Quality Forum (NQF) is a coalition of health care organizations that has worked to develop and implement a national strategy for health care quality measurement and reporting. The mission of the NQF is to improve the quality of American health care by setting national priorities and goals for performance improvement, endorsing national consensus standards for measuring and publicly reporting on performance, and promoting the attainment of national goals through education and outreach programs.

One of the major contributions of the NQF is the development of a list of Serious Reportable Events, which is frequently referred to as "*never events*."[34] According to the NQF, "never events" are errors in medical care that are clearly identifiable, preventable, and serious in their consequences for patients, and that indicate a real problem in the safety and credibility of a health care facility. Examples of "never events" include surgery performed on the wrong body part; a foreign body left in a patient after surgery; a mismatched blood transfusion; a major medication error; a severe "pressure ulcer" acquired in the hospital; and preventable postoperative deaths (Table 12-8). Criteria for inclusion as a "never event" are listed below. The event must be:

- Unambiguous (i.e., the event must be clearly identifiable and measurable, and thus feasible to include in a reporting system);
- Usually preventable, with the recognition that some events are not always avoidable, given the complexity of health care;
- Serious, resulting in death or loss of a body part, disability, or more than transient loss of a body function; and
- Any one of the following:
  - Adverse and/or,
  - Indicative of a problem in a health care facility's safety systems and/or,
  - Important for public credibility or public accountability.

These events are not a reasonable medical risk of undergoing surgery that the patient must accept, but medical errors that should never happen (Case 12-4). The occurrence of any of these events signals that an organization's patient safety culture or processes have defects that need to be evaluated and corrected to prevent the event from happening again (Table 12-9).

"NEVER EVENTS" IN SURGERY

Retained Surgical Items[35]

A retained surgical item refers to any surgical item that is found to be inside a patient after he or she has left the OR, thus requiring a second operation to remove the item. Estimates of retained foreign bodies in surgical procedures range from one case per 8000 to 18,000 operations, corresponding to one case or more each year for a typical large hospital or approximately 1500 cases per year in the United States.[36] This estimate is based on an analysis of malpractice claims and is likely to underestimate the true incidence. The risk of

CASE 12-4	Surgical "never-event"

In 2002, Mike Hurewitz, a reporter for *The Times Union* of Albany, suddenly began vomiting blood 3 days after donating part of his liver to his brother while recovering on a hospital floor in which 34 patients were being cared for by one first-year resident. He aspirated and died immediately with no other physician available to assist the overworked first-year resident.

Recognized for its advances in the field of liver transplantation, at the time, Mount Sinai Hospital was performing more adult-to-adult live-donor operations than any other hospital in the country. But the program was shut down by this event. Mount Sinai was held accountable for inadequate care and was banned from performing any live-donor adult liver transplants for more than 1 year. Of the 92 complaints investigated by the state, 75 were filed against the liver transplant unit, with 62 involving patient deaths. The state concluded that most of the 33 serious violations exhibited by the hospital occurred within the liver transplant unit.

As a result of the investigation, Mount Sinai revamped many of the procedures within its transplant unit. Among the changes, first-year residents no longer staffed the transplant service, two health care practitioners physically present in the hospital oversaw the transplant unit at all times, and any page coming from the transplant unit had to be answered within 5 minutes of the initial call. In addition, nurses monitored patients' vital signs more closely after surgery, transplant surgeons were required to make postoperative visits to both organ donor and recipient, and each registered nurse was assigned to four patients, rather than six or seven. The death also led New York to become the first state to develop guidelines for treating live organ donors. Finally, Mike Hurewitz's widow became a patient safety advocate, urging stricter controls on live donor programs.

having a retained surgical item increases during emergency surgery, when there are unplanned changes in procedure (due to new diagnoses encountered in the OR), and in patients with higher body-mass index (Table 12-10).[36]

The most common retained surgical item is a surgical sponge, but other items, such as surgical instruments and needles, can also be inadvertently left inside a patient after an operation. Retained surgical sponges are commonly discovered as an incidental finding on a routine postoperative radiograph, but also have been discovered in patients presenting with a mass or abdominal pain. Patients with sponges that were originally left in an intracavitary position (such as inside the chest or abdomen) also can present with complications such as erosion through the skin, fistula formation, bowel obstruction, hematuria, or the development of a new, tumor-like lesion.

Retained surgical needles usually are discovered incidentally, and reports of retained needles are uncommon. Retained surgical needles have not been reported to cause injury in the same way that nonsurgical needles (e.g., sewing needles, hypodermic needles) have been reported to perforate bowel or lodge in vessels and migrate. However, there have been reports of chronic pelvic pain and ocular irritation caused by retained surgical needles. A study of plain abdominal radiographs in pigs has demonstrated that medium to large size needles can easily be detected. The decision to remove these retained needles depends on whether they are symptomatic and the preference of the patient. Needles smaller than 13 mm have been found to be undetectable on plain radiograph in several studies, have not been shown to cause injury to vessels or visceral organs, and can probably be left alone.

Although the actual incidence of retained surgical instruments is unknown, they are known to be retained with far less frequency than surgical sponges. However, most of the cases that do occur are sensationalized by the lay media and draw significant attention from the general public. The initial presentation of a retained surgical instrument is pain in the surgical site or the sensation of a mass of fullness after a surgical procedure that led to the discovery of a metallic object on a radiographic study. Commonly retained

Patient	Institution	Year	Event	Root Cause	Outcome
Libby Zion	New York Hospital, New York, NY	1984	Missed allergy to Demerol	Physician fatigue	Bell Commission shortened resident work hours
Betsy Lehman	Dana-Farber Cancer Institute, Boston, MA	1994	Chemotherapy overdose	Lack of medication checks and triggers	Fired doctor, three pharmacists, 15 nurses; overhauled safety program
Josie King	Johns Hopkins Hospital, Baltimore, MD	2001	Severe dehydration	Poor communication	Increased safety research funding
Mike Hurewitz	Mt. Sinai Hospital, New York, NY	2002	Inadequate postoperative care	Inadequate supervision	Transplant program shut down until better patient safety safeguards implemented

TABLE 12-9 Four patient events that advanced the modern field of patient safety

instruments include the malleable and "FISH" instrument that are used when closing abdominal surgery.

A retained surgical foreign body should be included in the differential diagnosis of any postoperative patient who presents with pain, infection, a palpable mass, or a radiopaque structure on imaging. The diagnosis can usually be made using a computed tomographic (CT) scan, and this is often the only test that will be needed. If a retained surgical item is identified in the setting of an acute clinical presentation, the treatment usually is removal of the item. However, if the attempt to remove the retained surgical item can potentially cause more harm than the item itself, as in the case of a needle or a small part of a surgical item, then removal is occasionally not recommended. Retained surgical sponges should always be removed.

The American College of Surgeons and the Association of Perioperative Registered Nurses, in addition to the Joint Commission, have issued guidelines to try to prevent the occurrence of retained surgical items. Current recommendations include the use of standard counting procedures, performing a thorough wound exploration before closing a surgical site, and using only x-ray detectable items in the surgical wound. These organizations also strongly endorse the completion of a postoperative debriefing after every operation. An x-ray at the completion of an operation is encouraged if there is any concern for a foreign body based on any confusion regarding the counts by even a single member of the OR team, or in the presence of a risk factor.

Surgical Counts

The benefit of performing surgical counts to prevent the occurrence of retained surgical items is controversial. The increased risk of a retained surgical item during emergency surgery in the study by Gawande and colleagues appeared to be related to bypassing the surgical count in many of these cases, suggesting that the performance of a surgical count can be useful in reducing the incidence of this sentinel event.[36] However, the "falsely correct count," in which a count is performed and declared correct when it is actually incorrect, occurred in 21 to 100% of cases in which a retained surgical item was found.[35] This type of count was the most common circumstance encountered in all retained surgical item cases, which suggests that performing a surgical count in and of itself does not prevent this error from taking place. The counting protocol also imposes significant

TABLE 12-10 Risk factors for retained surgical sponges

- Emergency surgery
- Unplanned changes in procedure
- Patient with higher body-mass index
- Multiple surgeons involved in same operation
- Multiple procedures performed on same patient
- Involvement of multiple operating room nurses/staff members
- Case duration covers multiple nursing "shifts"

demands on the nursing staff and distracts them from focusing on other primarily patient-centered tasks.[17]

A retained surgical item can occur even in the presence of a known incorrect count. This event is usually a result of poor communication in which a surgeon will dismiss the incorrect count and/or fail to obtain a radiograph before the patient leaves the OR. Having stronger institutional policies in place in case of an incorrect count (such as requiring a mandatory radiograph while the patient is still in the OR) can avoid conflict among caregivers and mitigate the likelihood of a retained surgical item occurring as a result of a known incorrect count.

Although there is no single tool to prevent all errors, the development of multiple lines of defense to prevent retained surgical items and universally standardizing and adhering to OR safety protocols by all members of the surgical team will help reduce the incidence of this never event.[37] Surgeons should take the lead in the prevention of retained surgical items by avoiding the use of small or nonradiologically detectable sponges in large cavities, performing a thorough wound inspection before closing any surgical incision, and by having a vested interest in the counting procedure performed by nursing staff to keep track of sponges, needles, instruments, and any other potential retained surgical item. The value of routine radiography in the setting of emergency cases or when multiple major procedures involving multiple surgical teams are being performed to prevent a retained surgical item is becoming more apparent.

The widely accepted legal doctrine when a foreign body is erroneously left in a patient is that the mere presence of the item in the plaintiff's body indicates that the patient did not receive proper surgical care. Proof of negligence is not required in these cases because the doctrine of *Res ipsa loquitur*, or "the thing speaks for itself," applies. The characteristics of the surgeon, their style, bedside manner, honesty, and confidence demonstrated in the management of the case can go a long way in averting a lawsuit or mitigating damages.

Wrong-Site Surgery

Wrong-site surgery is any surgical procedure performed on the wrong patient, wrong body part, wrong side of the body, or wrong level of a correctly identified anatomic site. It is difficult to determine the true incidence of wrong-site surgery for several reasons. First, there is no standard definition for what constitutes wrong-site surgery among various health care organizations. Another factor is that wrong-site surgery is underreported by health care providers. Finally, the total number of potential opportunities for each type of wrong-site error is unknown. However, various studies show incidences ranging from one in 112,994 cases to one in 15,500 cases.[38] The Washington University School of Medicine suggests a rate of one in 17,000 operations, which adds up to approximately 4000 wrong-site surgeries in the United States each year. If these numbers are correct, wrong-site surgery is the third most frequent life-threatening medical error in the United States.[39]

Despite the difficulty in determining the overall incidence of wrong-site surgery, several states now require mandatory reporting of all wrong-site surgery events, including near misses. These data provide some insight into the number of actual errors compared to the number of potential opportunities to perform wrong-site surgery. Of the 427 reports of wrong-site surgery submitted from June 2004 through December 2006 to the Pennsylvania Patient Safety Reporting System, more than 40% of the errors actually reached the patient, and nearly 20% involved completion of a wrong-site procedure.[38]

The risk of performing wrong-site surgery increases when there are multiple surgeons involved in the same operation or multiple procedures are performed on the same patient, especially if the procedures are scheduled or performed on different areas of the body.[39] Time pressure, emergency surgery, abnormal patient anatomy, and morbid obesity are also thought to be risk factors.[39] Communication errors are the root cause in more than 70% of the wrong-site surgeries reported to the Joint Commission.[38] Other risk factors include receiving an incomplete preoperative assessment because documents are either unavailable or not reviewed for other reasons; having inadequate procedures in place to verify the correct surgical site; or having an organizational culture that lacks teamwork or reveres the surgeon as someone whose judgment should never be questioned.[38]

There is a one in four chance that surgeons who work on symmetric anatomic structures will be involved in a wrong-site error sometime during their careers.[39] No surgical specialty is immune. The specialties most commonly involved in reporting wrong-site surgeries according to the Joint Commission are orthopedic/podiatric surgery (41%), general surgery (20%), neurosurgery (14%), urology (11%), and maxillofacial, cardiovascular, otolaryngology, and ophthalmology (14%).[38] Most errors involved symmetric anatomic structures: lower extremities (30%), head/neck (24%), and genital/urinary/pelvic/groin (21%).[38] Although orthopedic surgery is the most frequently involved, this may be due to the higher volume of cases performed as well as the increased opportunity for lateralization errors inherent in the specialty. In addition, because the American Academy of Orthopaedic Surgeons has historically tried as a professional organization to reduce wrong-site operations, orthopedic surgeons may be more likely to report these events when they do occur.[39]

The Joint Commission Universal Protocol to Ensure Correct Surgery

The movement to eliminate wrong-site surgery began among professional orthopedic societies in the mid-1990s, when both the Canadian Orthopaedic Association and the American Academy of Orthopaedic Surgeons issued position statements and embarked on educational campaigns to prevent the occurrence of wrong-site surgery within their specialty.[39] Other organizations that issued position statements advocating for the elimination of wrong-site surgery include the North American Spine Society, the American Academy of Ophthalmology, the Association of Perioperative Registered Nurses, and the American College of Surgeons. After issuing a review of wrong-site surgery in their Sentinel Event Alert in 1998, the Joint Commission made the elimination of wrong-site surgery one of their first National Patient Safety Goals in 2003 and adopted a universal protocol for preventing wrong-site, wrong-procedure, and wrong-person surgery in 2004. The protocol has been endorsed by more than 50 professional associations and organizations.

A preoperative "time-out" or "pause for the cause" to confirm the patient, procedure, and site to be operated on before incision was recommended by the Joint Commission and is now mandatory for all ORs in the United States. Elements of the protocol include the following:

- Verifying the patient's identity
- Marking the surgical site
- Using a preoperative site verification process such as a checklist
- Confirming the availability of appropriate documents and studies before the start of a procedure
- Taking a brief time-out immediately before skin incision, in which all members of the surgical team actively communicate and provide oral verification of the patient's identity, surgical

| TABLE 12-11 | Best practices for operating room safety |

- Conduct the Joint Commission Universal Protocol ("time-out") to prevent wrong-site surgery.
- Perform an operating room briefing (checklist) to identify and mitigate hazards early.
- Promote a culture of speaking up about safety concerns.
- Use a screening x-ray to detect foreign bodies in high-risk cases.
- Begin patient sign-outs with the most likely immediate safety hazard.

From Michaels et al,[41] with permission.

site, surgical procedure, administration of preoperative medications, and presence of appropriate medical records, imaging studies, and equipment
- Monitoring compliance with protocol recommendations

Focusing on individual process components of the universal protocol, such as surgical site marking or the time-out, is not enough to prevent wrong-site surgery. Over a 30-month period in Pennsylvania, 21 wrong-side errors occurred despite the proper use of time-out procedures, with 12 of these errors resulting in complete wrong-side procedures. During the same period, correct site markings failed to prevent another 16 wrong-site surgeries, of which six were not recognized until after the procedure had been completed.[39]

Site verification begins with the initial patient encounter by the surgeon, continues throughout the preoperative verification process and during multiple critical points in the OR, and requires the active participation of the entire operating team, especially the surgeon and anesthesia provider. Based on a recent review of malpractice claims, two thirds of wrong-site operations could have been prevented by a site-verification protocol.[40]

Despite the proliferation of wrong-site protocols in the last decade, the effectiveness of surgical site verification is difficult to measure. As discussed earlier in this section, the incidence of wrong-site surgery is too rare to measure as a rate. Interestingly, the number of sentinel events reported to the Joint Commission has not changed significantly since the widespread implementation of the Universal Protocol in 2004.[39] This could be due to an increase in reporting rather than an actual increase in the incidence of wrong-site surgery. The number of sentinel events reported does not actually indicate whether or not surgical site verification protocols are effective in reducing the likelihood that a patient will be harmed when undergoing surgery.

The legal treatment of wrong-site surgery is similar to that of surgical items erroneously left in a patient: The mere fact that wrong-site surgery occurred indicates that the patient did not receive proper surgical care. Proof of negligence is not required in these cases because the doctrine of *Res ipsa loquitur*, or "the thing speaks for itself," applies. A malpractice claim may lead to a settlement or award on verdict in the 6- or 7-figure range in 2005 U.S. dollars.[39]

Ultimately, the occurrence of retained surgical items or wrong-site surgery is a reflection of the quality of professional communication between caregivers and the degree of teamwork among the members of the operating team. In addition to standardizing procedures like the surgical count, instituting mandatory postoperative radiographs in the presence of a known miscount, and reforming the processes of patient identification and site verification, to successfully minimize the risk of wrong-site surgery, organizations should also strive to create a culture of safety, create independent and redundant checks for key processes, and create a system in which caregivers can learn from their mistakes (Table 12-11).[41]

RISK MANAGEMENT

Between one half and two thirds of hospitalwide adverse events are attributable to surgical care. Most surgical errors occur in the OR and are technical in nature, including direct manual errors (such as transection of the ureter during hysterectomy) as well as judgment and knowledge errors leading to performance of an inappropriate, inadequate, or untimely procedure (i.e., performing a simple cholecystectomy for invasive adenocarcinoma of the gallbladder, or failing to intervene promptly in a patient with a leaking aortic aneurysm). Surgical complications and adverse outcomes have previously been linked to lack of surgeon specialization, low hospital volume, communication breakdowns, fatigue, surgical residents and trainees, and numerous other factors.[42]

However, poor surgical outcomes are not necessarily correlated with a surgeon's level of experience in performing a certain procedure. In one study, three fourths of the technical errors that occurred in a review of malpractice claims data involved fully trained and experienced surgeons operating within their area of expertise, and 84% occurred in routine operations that do not require advanced training beyond a standard surgical training program. Rather than surgeon expertise, these errors likely occurred due to situations complicated by patient comorbidity, complex anatomy, repeat surgery, or equipment problems (Table 12-12). Because these errors occurred during routine operations, previous suggestions to limit the performance of high-complexity operations using selective referral, regionalization, or limitation of privileging may not actually be effective in reducing the incidence of technical error among surgical patients.[42]

In any event, although there has been much emphasis on reducing the prevalence of surgical technical errors as a way of improving surgical care, the occurrence of a technical error in the OR may not be the most important indicator of whether or not a surgeon will be sued by a patient. Recent studies point to the importance of a surgeon's communication skills in averting malpractice litigation. In the American College of Surgeons' Closed Claims Study, although intraoperative organ injuries occurred in 40% of patients, reviewers felt that a surgical technical misadventure was the most deficient component of care in only 12% of patients. In fact, communication and practice pattern violations were the most common deficiency in care identified for one third of the patients in the Closed Claims Study who received the expected standard of surgical care.[43]

The Importance of Communication in Managing Risk

The manner and tone in which a physician communicates is potentially more important to avoiding a malpractice claim than the actual content of the dialogue. For example, a physician relating to a patient in a "negative" manner (e.g., using a harsh or impatient tone of voice) may trigger litigious feelings when there is a bad result, whereas a physician relating in a "positive" manner may not. Expressions of dominance, in which the voice tone is generally deep, loud, moderately fast, unaccented, and clearly articulated, may communicate a lack of empathy and understanding for the patient, whereas concern or anxiety in the surgeon's voice is often positively related to expressing concern and empathy. General and orthopedic surgeons whose tone of voice was judged to be more dominant were more likely to have been sued than those who sounded less dominant.[44]

When significant medical errors do occur, physicians have an ethical and professional responsibility to immediately disclose them

---

TABLE 12-12 Common causes of lawsuits in surgery

- Positional nerve injury
- Common bile duct injury
- Failure to diagnose or delayed diagnosis
- Failure to treat, delayed treatment, or wrong treatment
- Inadequate documentation
- Inappropriate surgical indication
- Failure to call a specialist
- Cases resulting in amputation/limb loss

---

to patients. Failure to disclose errors to patients undermines the public confidence in medicine and can create legal liability related to fraud. Physicians' fear of litigation represents a major barrier to error disclosure. However, when handled appropriately, immediate disclosure of errors frequently leads to improved patient rapport, satisfaction, and fewer malpractice claims.[45] In fact, rapport is the most important factor in determining whether a lawsuit is filed against a physician.

In 1987, the Department of Veterans Affairs Hospital in Lexington, Kentucky, implemented the nation's first formal apology and medical error full disclosure program, which called for the hospital and its doctors to work with patients and their families to settle a case. As a result, the hospital improved from having one of the highest malpractice claims totals in the VA system to being ranked among the lowest quartile of a comparative group of similar hospitals for settlement and litigation costs over a 7-year period. Its average payout in 2005 was $16,000 per settlement, vs. the national VA average of $98,000 per settlement, and only two lawsuits went to trial during a 10-year period. As a result of the success of this program, the Department of Veteran Affairs expanded the program to all VA hospitals nationwide in October 2005. This model also was replicated at the University of Michigan Health System with similar results. Its full-disclosure program cut the number of pending lawsuits by one half and reduced litigation costs per case from $65,000 to $35,000, thus saving the hospital approximately $2 million in defense litigation bills each year. In addition, University of Michigan doctors, patients, and lawyers are happier with this system. The cultural shift toward honesty and openness also has led to the improvement of systems and processes to reduce medical errors, especially repeat medical errors.[46]

With regard to risk management, the importance of good communication by surgeons and other care providers cannot be overemphasized. Whether alerting other members of the care team about a patient's needs, openly discussing any concerns the patient and/or family might have, or disclosing the cause of a medical error, open communication with all parties involved can reduce anger and mistrust of the medical system, the frequency, morbidity, and mortality of preventable adverse events, and the likelihood of litigation.

COMPLICATIONS

Despite the increased focus on improving patient safety and minimizing medical errors, it is impossible to eliminate human error entirely. Individual errors can cause minor or major complications during or after a surgical procedure. Although these types of errors may not be publicized as much as wrong-site surgery or a retained surgical item, they can still lead to surgical complications that prolong the course of illness, lengthen hospital stay, and increase morbidity and mortality rates.

Complications in Minor Procedures
Central Venous Access Catheters

Complications of central venous access catheters are common. Steps to decrease complications include the following:

- Ensure that central venous access is indicated.
- Experienced (credentialed) personnel should insert the catheter, or should supervise the insertion.
- Use proper positioning and sterile technique. Controversy exists as to whether or not placing the patient in the Trendelenburg position facilitates access.
- Central venous catheters should be exchanged only for specific indications (not as a matter of routine) and should be removed as soon as possible.

Common complications of central venous access include:

Pneumothorax Occurrence rates from both subclavian and internal jugular vein approaches are 1 to 6%. Pneumothorax rates appear to be higher among the inexperienced but occur with experienced operators as well. If the patient is stable, and the pneumothorax is small (<15%), close expectant observation may be adequate. If the patient is symptomatic, a thoracostomy tube should be placed. Occasionally, pneumothorax will occur as late as 48 to 72 hours after central venous access attempts. This usually creates sufficient compromise that a tube thoracostomy is required. Prevention requires proper positioning of the patient and correct technique. A postprocedure chest x-ray is mandatory to confirm the presence or absence of a pneumothorax, regardless of whether a pneumothorax is suspected.

Arrhythmias Arrhythmias result from myocardial irritability secondary to guidewire placement, and usually resolve when the catheter or guidewire is withdrawn from the right heart. Prevention requires electrocardiogram (EKG) monitoring whenever possible during catheter insertion.

Arterial Puncture The inadvertent puncture or laceration of an adjacent artery with bleeding can occur, but the majority will resolve with direct pressure on or near the arterial injury site. Rarely will angiography, stent placement, or surgery be required to repair the puncture site, but close observation and a chest x-ray are indicated. Prevention requires careful attention to insertion technique.

Lost Guidewire A guidewire or catheter that migrates into the vascular space completely can be readily retrieved with interventional angiography techniques. A prompt chest x-ray and close monitoring of the patient until retrieval is indicated.

Air Embolus Although estimated to occur in only 0.2 to 1% of patients, an air embolism can be dramatic and fatal. Treatment may prove futile if the air bolus is larger than 50 mL. Auscultation over the precordium may reveal a "crunching" noise, but a portable chest x-ray is required for diagnosis. If an embolus is suspected, the patient should immediately be placed into a left lateral decubitus Trendelenburg position, so the entrapped air can be stabilized within the right ventricle. Aspiration via a central venous line accessing the heart may decrease the volume of gas in the right side of the heart, and minimize the amount traversing into the pulmonary circulation. Subsequent recovery of intracardiac and intrapulmonary air may require open surgical or angiographic techniques. Prevention requires careful attention to technique.

Pulmonary Artery Rupture Flow-directed, pulmonary artery ("Swan-Ganz") catheters can cause pulmonary artery rupture due to excessive advancement of the catheter into the pulmonary circulation. There usually is a sentinel bleed noted when a pulmonary artery catheter balloon is inflated, and then the patient begins to have uncontrolled hemoptysis. Reinflation of the catheter balloon is the initial step in management, followed by immediate airway intubation with mechanical ventilation, an urgent portable chest x-ray, and notification of the OR that an emergent thoracotomy may be required. If there is no further bleeding after the balloon is reinflated, the x-ray shows no significant consolidation of lung fields from ongoing bleeding and the patient is easily ventilated, then a conservative nonoperative approach may be considered. This approach might include observation alone if the patient has no signs of bleeding or hemodynamic compromise; however, more typically a pulmonary angiogram with angioembolization or vascular stenting is required. Hemodynamically unstable patients rarely survive because of the time needed to perform the thoracotomy and identify the branch of the pulmonary artery that has ruptured.

Central Venous Line Infection The Centers for Disease Control and Prevention (CDC) reports mortality rates of 12 to 25% when a central venous line infection becomes systemic, and this carries a cost of approximately $25,000 per episode.[47–50] The CDC does not recommend routine central line changes, but when the clinical suspicion is high, the site of venous access must be changed. Additionally, nearly 15% of hospitalized patients will acquire central venous line sepsis. In many instances, once an infection is recognized as central line sepsis,

removing the line is adequate. *Staphylococcus aureus* infections, however, present a unique problem because of the potential for metastatic seeding of bacterial emboli. The required treatment is 4 to 6 weeks of tailored antibiotic therapy.

Arterial Lines

Arterial lines are placed to facilitate arterial blood gas sampling and hemodynamic monitoring. They are often left in place to make routine blood sampling easier, but this practice leads to higher complication rates.

Arterial access requires a sterile Seldinger technique, and a variety of arteries are used, such as the radial, femoral, brachial, axillary, dorsal pedis, or superficial temporal arteries. Although complications occur less than 1% of the time, they can be catastrophic. Complications include thrombosis, bleeding, hematoma, arterial spasm (nonthrombotic pulselessness), and infection. Thrombosis or embolization of an extremity arterial catheter can result in the loss of a digit, hand, or foot, and the risk is nearly the same for both femoral and radial cannulation. Thrombosis with distal tissue ischemia is treated with anticoagulation, but occasionally surgical intervention is required to re-establish adequate inflow. Pseudoaneurysms and arteriovenous fistulae can also occur.

Endoscopy and Bronchoscopy

The principal risk of GI endoscopy is perforation. Perforations occur in 1:10,000 patients with endoscopy alone, but have a higher incidence rate when biopsies are performed (up to 10%). This increased risk is due to complications of intubating a GI diverticulum (either esophageal or colonic), or from the presence of weakened or inflamed tissue in the intestinal wall (e.g., diverticulitis, glucocorticoid use, or inflammatory bowel disease).

Patients will usually complain of diffuse abdominal pain shortly after the procedure, and then will quickly progress with worsening abdominal discomfort on examination. In obtunded or elderly patients, a change in clinical status may take several hours, and occasionally as long as 24 to 48 hours, to become manifest. Radiologic studies to look for free intraperitoneal air, retroperitoneal air, or a pneumothorax are diagnostic. A delay in diagnosis results in ongoing contamination and sepsis.

Open or laparoscopic exploration locates the perforation, and allows repair and local decontamination of the surrounding tissues. The patient who may be a candidate for nonoperative management is one in which perforation arises during an elective, bowel-prepped, endoscopy, and yet the patient does not have significant pain or clinical signs of infection. The patient may be closely observed in a monitored setting, on strict dietary restriction and broad-spectrum antibiotics.

The complications of bronchoscopy include bronchial plugging, hypoxemia, pneumothorax, lobar collapse, and bleeding. When diagnosed in a timely fashion, they are rarely life threatening. Bleeding usually resolves and rarely requires surgery, but may require repeat endoscopy for thermocoagulation or fibrin glue application. The presence of a pneumothorax necessitates placement of a thoracostomy tube when significant deoxygenation occurs or the pulmonary mechanics are compromised. Lobar collapse or mucous plugging responds to aggressive pulmonary toilet, but occasionally requires repeat bronchoscopy.

Tracheostomy

Tracheostomy facilitates weaning from a ventilator, decreases length of ICU or hospital stay, and improves pulmonary toilet. Tracheostomies are now performed open, percutaneously, with or without bronchoscopy, and with or without Doppler guidance, and yet complications still arise.

Recent studies do not support obtaining a routine posttracheostomy chest x-ray after either percutaneous or open tracheostomy.[51,52] However, significant lobar collapse can occur from copious tracheal secretions or mechanical obstruction.

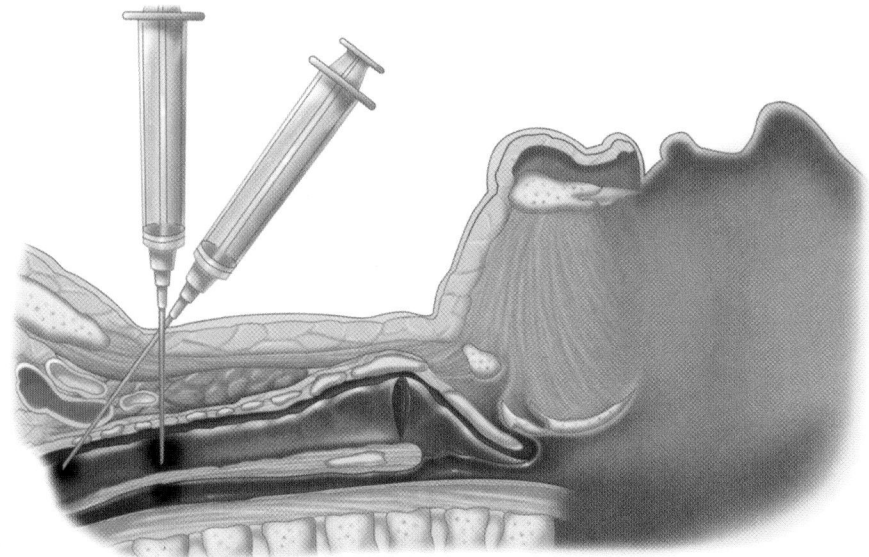

FIG. 12-8. This illustration depicts improper positioning (attitude) of the percutaneous needle. It is possible to access the innominate artery via the trachea, thus placing the patient at risk for early tracheo-innominate artery fistula.

The most dramatic complication of tracheostomy is tracheo-innominate artery fistula (TIAF) (Fig. 12-8).[53,54] This occurs rarely (~0.3%), but carries a 50 to 80% mortality rate. TIAFs can occur as early as 2 days or as late as 2 months after tracheostomy. The prototypical patient is a thin woman with a long, gracile neck. The patient may have a sentinel bleed, which occurs in 50% of TIAF cases, followed by a most spectacular bleed. Should a TIAF be suspected, the patient should be transported immediately to the OR for fiberoptic evaluation. If needed, remove the tracheostomy, and place a finger through the tracheostomy site to apply direct pressure anteriorly for compression of the innominate artery.

Percutaneous Endogastrostomy

A misplaced percutaneous endogastrostomy (PEG) may create intra-abdominal sepsis with peritonitis and/or an abdominal wall abscess with necrotizing fasciitis. As in other minor procedures, the initial placement technique must be fastidious to avoid complications. Transillumination of the abdomen may decrease the risk for error. Inadvertent colotomies, intraperitoneal leakage of tube feeds with peritonitis, and abdominal wall abscesses require surgery to correct the complications and to replace the PEG with an alternate feeding tube, usually a jejunostomy.

A dislodged or prematurely removed PEG tube must be replaced within 8 hours of dislodgment, because the gastrostomy site closes rapidly. A contrast x-ray should be performed to confirm the tube's intragastric position before feeding.

Tube Thoracostomy

Tube thoracostomy (chest tube insertion) is performed for pneumothorax, hemothorax, pleural effusions, or empyema. A chest tube can be easily placed with a combination of local analgesia and light conscious sedation. Common complications include inadequate analgesia or sedation, incomplete penetration of the pleura with formation of a subcutaneous track for the tube, lacerations to the lung or diaphragm, intraperitoneal placement of the tube through the diaphragm, and bleeding related to these various lacerations or injury to pleural adhesions. Additional problems include slippage of the tube out of position or mechanical problems related to the drainage system. All of these complications can be avoided with proper initial insertion techniques, plus a daily review of the drainage system and follow-up radiographs. Tube removal can create a residual pneumothorax if the patient does not maintain positive intrapleural pressure by Valsalva's maneuver during tube removal and dressing application.

Diagnostic Peritoneal Lavage

Diagnostic peritoneal lavage is performed in the emergent trauma setting for the hemodynamically unstable patient with neurologic impairment and an uncertain etiology for blood loss, when an abdominal trauma ultrasound is not available or is unreliable. Nasogastric and bladder catheter decompression is mandatory before diagnostic peritoneal lavage to avoid injury during the procedure (Fig. 12-9). The small or large bowel, or the major vessels of the retroperitoneum also can be punctured inadvertently, and these injuries require surgical exploration and repair.

Complications of Angiography

Intramural dissection of a cannulated artery can lead to complications such as ischemic stroke from a carotid artery dissection or occlusion, mesenteric ischemia from dissection of the superior mesenteric artery, or a more innocuous finding of "blue toe syndrome" from a dissected artery in a peripheral limb. Invasive or noninvasive imaging studies confirm the suspected problem. The severity of the ischemia and the extent of the dissection determine if anticoagulation therapy or urgent surgical exploration is indicated.

Bleeding from the vascular access site usually is obvious, but may not be visible when the blood loss is tracking into the retroperitoneal tissue planes after femoral artery cannulation. These patients can present with hemorrhagic shock; an abdominopelvic CT scan delineates the extent of bleeding into the retroperitoneum. The initial management is direct compression at the access site and clinical observation with resuscitation as indicated. Urgent surgical exploration may be required to control the bleeding site.

Renal complications of angiography occur in 1 to 2% of patients. Contrast nephropathy is a temporary and preventable complication of radiologic studies such as CT, angiography, and/or venography. Some studies suggest a benefit of N-acetylcysteine for this condition. For the patient with impaired renal function or dehydration before contrast studies, twice-daily dosing 24 hours before and on the day of the radiographic study is suggested. Nonionic contrast also may be of benefit in higher-risk patients. IV hydration before and after the procedure is the most efficient method for preventing contrast nephropathy.

Complications of Biopsies

Lymph node biopsies have direct and indirect complications that include bleeding, infection, lymph leakage, and seromas. Measures to prevent direct complications include proper surgical hemostasis, proper skin preparation, and a single preoperative dose of antibiotic

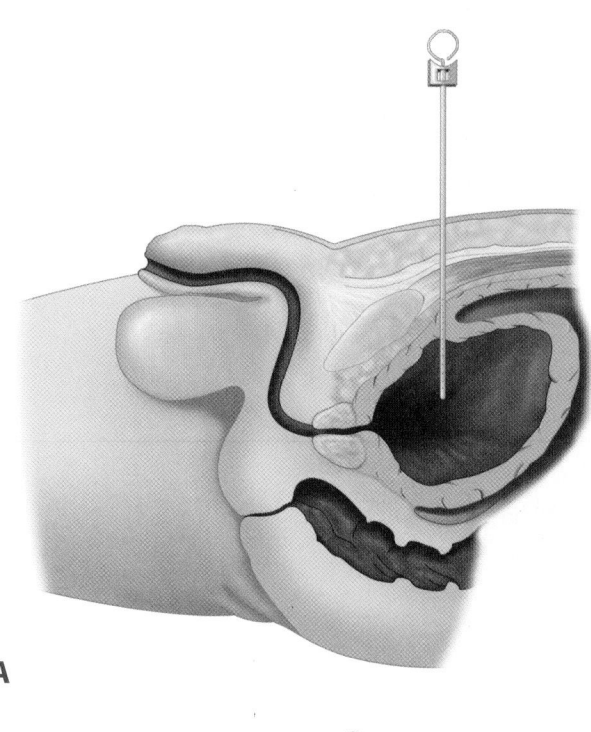

A

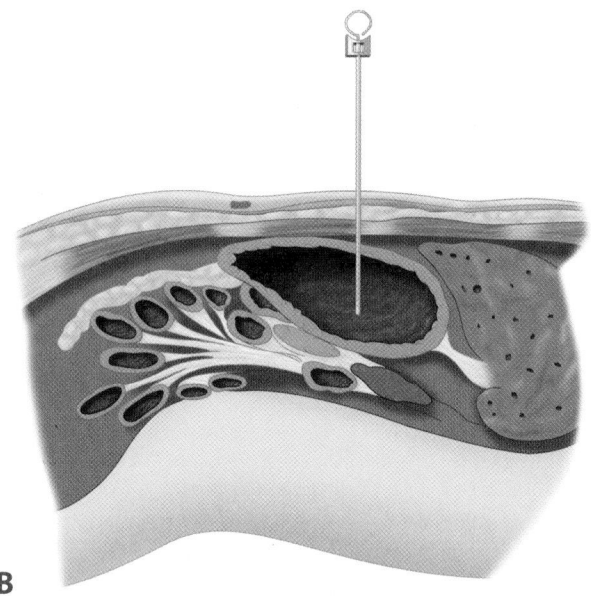

B

FIG. 12-9. The illustration depicts improper positioning of the diagnostic peritoneal lavage catheter, with overdistention of the urinary bladder (**A**) and the stomach (**B**). This error in technique clearly demonstrates the importance of decompressing hollow viscus before embarking on a diagnostic peritoneal lavage.

to cover skin flora 30 to 60 minutes before incision. Bleeding at a biopsy site usually can be controlled with direct pressure. Infection at a biopsy site will appear 5 to 10 days postoperatively, and may require opening of the wound to drain the infection. Seromas or lymphatic leaks resolve with aspiration of seromas and the application of pressure dressings, but may require repeated treatments.

Organ System Complications
Neurologic System

Neurologic complications that occur after surgery include motor or sensory deficits and mental status changes. Peripheral motor and sensory deficits are often due to neurapraxia secondary to improper positioning and/or padding during operations. Treatment is largely clinical observation, and the majority will resolve spontaneously within 1 to 3 months.

Direct injury to nerves during a surgical intervention is a well-known complication of several specific operations, including superficial parotidectomy (facial nerve), carotid endarterectomy (hypoglossal nerve), prostatectomy (nervi erigentes), and inguinal herniorrhaphy (ilioinguinal nerve). The nerve injury may simply be a stretch injury, or an unintentionally severed nerve. In addition to loss of function, severed nerves can result in a painful neuroma that may require subsequent surgery.

Mental status changes in the postoperative patient can have numerous causes (Table 12-13). Mental status changes must be carefully documented and continually assessed. CT scanning should be used early to detect intracranial causes.

Atherosclerotic disease increases the risk for intraoperative and postoperative stroke (cerebrovascular accident). Postoperatively, hypotension and hypoxemia are the most likely causes of a cerebrovascular accident. Management is largely supportive once the diagnosis is made, and includes adequate intravascular volume replacement plus optimal oxygen delivery. Neurologic consultation should be obtained so that decisions regarding thrombolysis or anticoagulation can be made in a timely fashion.

Eyes, Ears, and Nose

Corneal abrasions are unusual, but are due to inadequate protection of the eyes during anesthesia. Overlooked contact lenses in a trauma patient may cause conjunctivitis.

Persistent epistaxis can occur after nasogastric tube placement or removal, and nasal packing is the best treatment option if prolonged persistent direct pressure on the external nares fails. Anterior and posterior nasal gauze packing with balloon tamponade, angioembolization, and fibrin glue placement may be required in refractory cases. The use of antibiotics for posterior packing is controversial, but the incidence of toxic shock syndrome is documented at approximately 17:100,000 cases.

External otitis and otitis media occasionally occur postoperatively. Patients complain of ear pain or decreased hearing, and treatment includes topical antibiotics and nasal decongestion for symptomatic improvement.

TABLE 12-13	Common causes of mental status changes			
Electrolyte Imbalance	**Toxins**	**Trauma**	**Metabolic**	**Medications**
Sodium	Ethanol	Closed head injury	Thyrotoxicosis	Aspirin
Magnesium	Methanol	Pain	Adrenal insufficiency	Beta blockers
Calcium	Venoms and poisons	Shock	Hypoxemia	Narcotics
Inflammation	Ethylene glycol	Psychiatric	Acidosis	Antiemetics
Sepsis	Carbon monoxide	Dementia	Severe anemia	MAOIs
AIDS		Depression	Hyperammonemia	TCAs
Cerebral abscess		ICU psychosis	Poor glycemic control	Amphetamines
Meningitis		Schizophrenia	Hypothermia	Antiarrhythmics
Fever/hyperpyrexia			Hyperthermia	Corticosteroids, anabolic steroids

ICU = intensive care unit; MAOI = monoamine oxidase inhibitor; TCA = tricyclic antidepressant.

Ototoxicity due to aminoglycoside administration occurs in up to 10% of patients, and is often irreversible. Recent data show that iron chelating agents and alpha-tocopherol may be protective against ototoxicity. Vancomycin-related ototoxicity occurs about 3% of the time when used alone, and as often as 6% when used with other ototoxic agents, but is self limiting.[55,56]

Vascular Problems of the Neck

Complications of carotid endarterectomy include central or regional neurologic deficits or bleeding with an expanding neck hematoma. An acute change in mental status or the presence of localized neurologic deficit may require an immediate return to the OR to correct an iatrogenic occlusion. An expanding hematoma may warrant emergent airway intubation and subsequent transfer to the OR for control of hemorrhage. Intraoperative anticoagulation with heparin during carotid surgery makes bleeding a postoperative risk. Other complications can arise, such as arteriovenous fistulae, pseudoaneurysms, and infection, all of which are treated surgically.

Intraoperative hypotension during manipulation of the carotid bifurcation can occur, and is related to increased tone from baroreceptors that reflexly cause bradycardia. Should hypotension occur when manipulating the carotid bifurcation, an injection of 1% lidocaine solution around this structure should attenuate this reflexive response.

The most common late complication following carotid endarterectomy is myocardial infarction. The possibility of a postoperative myocardial infarction should be considered as a cause of labile blood pressure and arrhythmias in high-risk patients.

Thyroid and Parathyroid Glands

Surgery of the thyroid and parathyroid glands can result in hypocalcemia in the immediate postoperative period. Manifestations include EKG changes (shortened P-R interval), muscle spasm (tetany, Chvostek's sign, and Trousseau's sign), paresthesias, and laryngospasm. Treatment includes calcium gluconate infusion, and if tetany ensues, chemical paralysis with intubation. Maintenance treatment is thyroid hormone replacement (after thyroidectomy) in addition to calcium carbonate and vitamin D.

Recurrent laryngeal nerve (RLN) injury occurs in less than 5% of patients. Of those with injury, approximately 10% are permanent. As the thyroid gland is dissected from lateral to medial, the dissection near the inferior thyroid artery is a common area for RLN injury. At the conclusion of the operation, direct laryngoscopy confirms normal vocal cord apposition. The cord on the affected side will be in the paramedian position. If bilateral RLN has occurred, the chance of a successful extubation is poor. The cords are found to be in the midline, and an early sign of respiratory distress is stridor with labored breathing. If paralysis of the cords is not permanent, function may return 1 to 2 months after injury. Permanent RLN injury can be treated by various techniques to stent the cords in a position of function.

Superior laryngeal nerve injury is less debilitating, as the common symptom is loss of projection of the voice. The glottic aperture is asymmetrical on direct laryngoscopy and management is limited to clinical observation.

Respiratory System

Surgical complications that put the respiratory system in jeopardy are not always confined to technical errors. Malnutrition, inadequate pain control, inadequate mechanical ventilation, inadequate pulmonary toilet, and aspiration can cause serious pulmonary problems.

Pneumothorax can occur from central line insertion during anesthesia or from a diaphragmatic injury during an abdominal procedure. Hypotension, hypoxemia, and tracheal deviation away from the affected side may be present. A tension pneumothorax can cause complete cardiovascular collapse. Treatment is by needle thoracostomy, followed by tube thoracostomy. A large-bore needle

is placed either in the midclavicular line in the second rib interspace, or where the chest tube will be inserted, the fifth intercostal space in the anterior axillary line.

Hemothorax due to trauma or intrathoracic disease should be evacuated completely. A delay in evacuation of the hemothorax leaves the patient at risk for empyema and entrapped lung. If evacuation is incomplete with tube thoracostomy, video-assisted thoracoscopy or open evacuation and pleurodesis may be required.

Pulmonary atelectasis results in a loss of functional residual capacity (FRC) of the lung, and can predispose to pneumonia. Poor pain control in the postoperative period contributes to poor inspiratory effort and collapse of the lower lobes in particular. An increase in FRC by 700 mL or more can be accomplished by sitting patients up to greater than 45°. For mechanically ventilated patients, simply placing the head of the bed at 30 to 45° in elevation improves pulmonary outcomes. The prevention of atelectasis is facilitated by delivering adequate tidal volumes (8 to 10 mL/kg), preventing the abdominal domain from impinging on the thoracic cavity, and by sitting the patient up as much as possible. This includes having the ventilated patient out of bed and sitting in a chair if possible.

Aspiration complications include pneumonitis and pneumonia. The treatment of pneumonitis is similar to that for acute lung injury (ALI) (see below in this section), and includes oxygenation with general supportive care. Antibiotics are usually contraindicated unless known organisms are detected with bacteriologic analysis. Hospitalized patients who develop aspiration pneumonia carry a mortality rate as high as 70 to 80%. Early, aggressive, and repeated bronchoscopy for suctioning of aspirated material from the tracheobronchial tree will help to minimize the inflammatory reaction of pneumonitis and facilitate improved pulmonary toilet.

Patients with inadequate pulmonary toilet are at increased risk for bronchial plugging and lobar collapse. Patients with copious and tenacious secretions develop these plugs most often, but foreign bodies in the bronchus can be the cause of lobar collapse as well. The diagnosis of bronchial plugging is based on chest x-ray and clinical suspicion when there is acute pulmonary decompensation with increased work of breathing and hypoxemia. Fiberoptic bronchoscopy can be useful to clear mucous plugs and secretions.

Pneumonia is the second most common nosocomial infection and is the most common infection in ventilated patients. Ventilator-associated pneumonia (VAP) occurs in 15 to 40% of ventilated ICU patients, and accrues at a daily probability rate of 5% per day, up to 70% at 30 days. The 30-day mortality rate of nosocomial pneumonia can be as high as 40%, and depends on the microorganisms involved and the timeliness of initiating appropriate treatment.

Once the diagnosis of pneumonia is suspected (an abnormal chest x-ray, fever, productive cough with purulent sputum, and no other obvious fever sources), it is invariably necessary to initially begin treatment with broad-spectrum antibiotics until proper identification, colony count [≥100,000 colony-forming units (CFU)], and sensitivity of the microorganisms are determined.[57] The spectrum of antibiotic coverage should be narrowed as soon as the culture sensitivities are determined. Double-coverage antibiotic strategy for the two pathogens, *Pseudomonas* and *Acinetobacter* spp., may be appropriate if the local prevalence of these particularly virulent organisms is high. One of the most helpful tools in treating pneumonia and other infections is the tracking of a medical center's antibiogram every 6 to 12 months.[58]

Epidural analgesia decreases the risk of perioperative pneumonia. This method of pain control improves pulmonary toilet and the early return of bowel function; both have a significant impact on the potential for aspiration and for acquiring pneumonia. The routine use of epidural analgesia has a lower incidence of pneumonia than patient-controlled analgesia.[59]

ALI is a diagnosis applied to patients with similar findings to those with acute respiratory distress syndrome (ARDS). These should be considered a spectrum of the same disease process, with the difference being in the degree of oxygenation deficits of patients. The

332

TABLE 12-14	Inclusion criteria for the acute respiratory distress syndrome

Acute onset
Predisposing condition
PaO_2:FiO_2 <200 (regardless of positive end-expiratory pressure)
Bilateral infiltrates
Pulmonary artery occlusion pressure <18 mmHg
No clinical evidence of right heart failure

FiO_2 = fraction of inspired oxygen; PaO_2 = partial pressure of arterial oxygen.

CHAPTER 12

Patient Safety

pathology, pathophysiology, and the mechanism of lung injury for ALI are the same as for ARDS, except that the arterial oxygen to inspired oxygen (partial pressure of arterial oxygen:fraction of inspired oxygen) ratio is >200 for ALI and <200 for ARDS. Both types of patients will require some form of positive pressure ventilatory assistance to improve the oxygenation deficits, while simultaneously treating the primary etiology of the initiating disease.

The definition of ARDS includes five criteria (Table 12-14). The recent multicenter ARDS Research Network (ARDSnet) research trial demonstrated improved clinical outcomes for ARDS patients ventilated at tidal volumes of only 5 to 7 mL/kg.[60] It is important to note that these ventilator setting recommendations are for patients with ARDS, and not for patients requiring ventilatory support for a variety of other reasons. The beneficial effects of positive end-expiratory pressure (PEEP) for ARDS were confirmed in this study as well. The maintenance of PEEP during ventilatory support is determined based on blood gas analysis, pulmonary mechanics, and requirements for supplemental oxygen. As gas exchange improves with resolving ARDS, the initial step in decreasing ventilatory support should be to decrease the levels of supplemental oxygen first, and then to slowly bring the PEEP levels back down to minimal levels.[61] This is done to minimize the potential for recurrent alveolar collapse and a worsening gas exchange.

Not all patients can be weaned easily from mechanical ventilation. When the respiratory muscle energy demands are not balanced, or there is an ongoing active disease state external to the lungs, patients may require prolonged ventilatory support. Protocol-driven ventilator weaning strategies are successful and have become part of the standard of care. The use of a weaning protocol for patients on mechanical ventilation greater than 48 hours reduces the incidence of VAP and the overall length of time on mechanical ventilation, when compared with nonprotocol managed ventilator weaning. Unfortunately, there is still no reliable way of predicting which patient will be successfully extubated after a weaning program, and the decision for extubation is based on a combination of clinical parameters and measured pulmonary mechanics.[62] The Tobin Index (frequency:tidal volume ratio), also known as the *rapid shallow breathing index*, is perhaps the best negative predictive instrument.[63] If the result equals less than 105, then there is nearly a 70% chance the patient will pass extubation. If the score is greater than 105, the patient has an approximately 80% chance of failing extubation. Other parameters such as the negative inspiratory force, minute ventilation, and respiratory rate are used, but individually have no better predictive value than the rapid shallow breathing index.[64]

Malnutrition and poor nutritional support may adversely affect the respiratory system. The respiratory quotient (RQ), or respiratory exchange ratio, is the ratio of the rate of carbon dioxide (CO_2) produced to the rate of oxygen uptake ($RQ = \dot{V}CO_2/\dot{V}O_2$). Lipids, carbohydrates, and protein have differing effects on CO_2 production. Patients consuming a diet consisting mostly of carbohydrates would have an RQ of 1 or greater. The RQ for a diet mostly of lipids would be closer to 0.7, and that for a diet of mostly protein would be closer to 0.8. Ideally, an RQ of 0.75 to 0.85 suggests adequate balance and composition of nutrient intake. An excess of carbohydrate may negatively affect ventilator weaning because of the abnormal RQ due to higher CO_2 production and altered pulmonary gas exchange.

Although not without risk, tracheostomy will decrease the pulmonary dead space and provides for improved pulmonary toilet. When performed before the tenth day of ventilatory support, tracheostomy may decrease the incidence of VAP, the overall length of ventilator time, and the number of ICU patient days.

The occurrence of pulmonary embolism (PE) is probably underdiagnosed. Its etiology stems from DVT. The diagnosis of PE is made when a high degree of clinical suspicion for PE leads to imaging techniques such as ventilation:perfusion nuclear scans or CT pulmonary angiogram. Clinical findings include elevated central venous pressure, hypoxemia, shortness of breath, hypocarbia secondary to tachypnea, and right heart strain noted on EKG. Ventilation:perfusion nuclear scans are often indeterminate in patients who have an abnormal chest x-ray. The pulmonary angiogram remains the gold standard for diagnosing PE, but spiral CT angiogram has become an alternative method because of its relative ease of use and reasonable rates of diagnostic accuracy. For cases without clinical contraindications to therapeutic anticoagulation, patients should be empirically started on heparin infusion until the imaging studies are completed if the suspicion of a PE is strong.

Sequential compression devices on the lower extremities and low-dose subcutaneous heparin administration are routinely used to prevent DVT, and, by inference, the risk of PE. Neurosurgical and orthopedic patients have higher rates of PE, as do obese patients and those at prolonged bed rest.

When anticoagulation is contraindicated, or when a known clot exists in the inferior vena cava (IVC), therapy for PE includes insertion of an IVC filter. The Greenfield filter has been most widely studied, and it has a failure rate of less than 4%. Newer devices include those with nitinol wire that expands with body temperature and retrievable filters. Patients with spinal cord injury and multiple long-bone or pelvic fractures frequently receive IVC filters, and there appears to be a low long-term complication rate with their use.

Cardiac System

Arrhythmias are often seen preoperatively in elderly patients, but may occur postoperatively in any age group. Atrial fibrillation is the most common arrhythmia[65] and occurs between postoperative days 3 to 5 in high-risk patients. This is typically when patients begin to mobilize their interstitial fluid into the vascular fluid space. Contemporary evidence suggests that rate control is more important than rhythm control for atrial fibrillation.[66,67] The first-line treatment includes beta blockade and/or calcium channel blockade. Beta blockade must be used judiciously, because hypotension, as well as withdrawal from beta blockade with rebound hypertension, is possible. Calcium channel blockers are an option if beta blockers are not tolerated by the patient, but caution must be exercised in those with a history of congestive heart failure. Although digoxin is still a faithful standby medication, it has limitations due to the need for optimal dosing levels. Cardioversion may be required if patients become hemodynamically unstable and the rhythm cannot be controlled.

Ventricular arrhythmias and other tachyarrhythmias may occur in surgical patients as well. Similar to atrial rhythm problems, these are best controlled with beta blockade, but the use of other antiarrhythmics or cardioversion may be required if patients become hemodynamically unstable. Formal cardiac electrophysiology studies may be needed to clarify the etiology of the arrhythmias so that medical or surgical treatment can be tailored.

Cardiac ischemia is a cause of postoperative mortality. Acute myocardial infarction (AMI) can present insidiously or it can be more dramatic with the classic presentation of shortness of breath, severe angina, and sudden cardiogenic shock. The work-up to rule out an AMI includes an EKG and cardiac enzyme measurements. The patient should be transferred to a monitored (telemetry) floor as soon as a bed is available. *M*orphine, supplemental *O*xygen, *N*itroglycerine, and *A*spirin (MONA) are the initial therapeutic maneuvers for those who are being investigated for AMI.

Hypertension in the immediate postoperative period may be merely a failure of adequate pain control, but other causes include hypoxia, volume overload, and rebound hypertension from failure to resume beta blockade and/or clonidine. Perioperative hypertension carries significant morbidity and aggressive control is warranted. Twenty to 50% of patients with chronic atherosclerotic disease present with hypertension, and causes of perioperative hypertension include cerebrovascular disease, renal artery stenosis, aorto-occlusive disease, and rarely, pheochromocytoma. Routine perioperative cardiac protection with beta blockade is the standard of care for patients with a history of cardiovascular disease.

Gastrointestinal System

Surgery of the esophagus is potentially complicated because of its anatomic location and blood supply. The two primary types of esophageal resection performed are the transhiatal resection and the transthoracic (Ivor-Lewis) resection.[68] The transhiatal resection has the advantage that a formal thoracotomy incision is avoided. The dissection of the esophagus is blind, however, and an anastomotic leak occurs more than with other resections. However, when a leak does occur, simple opening of the cervical incision and draining the leak is all that is usually required.

The transthoracic Ivor-Lewis resection includes an esophageal anastomosis performed in the chest near the level of the azygos vein. These resections tend not to leak as often, but when they do, they can be difficult to control. The reported mortality is about 50% with an anastomotic leak, and the overall mortality is about 5%, which is similar to transhiatal resection. Nutritional support strategies must be considered for esophageal resection patients to maximize the potential for survival.

Nissen fundoplication is an operation that is fraught with possibilities for error. Bleeding is always a potential hazard, so dissection of the short gastric vessels must be done with care. Laparoscopic port site bleeding, injury to the aorta, and liver lacerations can also contribute to significant blood loss. The fundoplication may be too tightly wrapped or become unwrapped postoperatively. Postoperative edema and patient noncompliance will produce symptoms of odynophagia and dysphagia.

Postoperative ileus is related to dysfunction of the neural reflex axis of the intestine. Excessive narcotic use may delay return of bowel function. Epidural anesthesia results in better pain control, and there is an earlier return of bowel function, and a shorter length of hospital stay. The limited use of nasogastric tubes and the initiation of early postoperative feeding are associated with an earlier return of bowel function.

Numerous studies have shown a decreased length of stay and improved pain control when bowel surgery is performed laparoscopically. In one study, however, patients with open colon resection were fed at the same time as the laparoscopically treated patients and had no difference in hospital length of stay.[69]

Pharmacologic agents commonly used to stimulate bowel function include metoclopramide and erythromycin. Metoclopramide's action is limited to the stomach, and it may help primarily with gastroparesis. Erythromycin is a motilin agonist that works throughout the stomach and bowel. Several studies demonstrate significant benefit from the administration of erythromycin in those suffering from an ileus.[70]

Small bowel obstruction occurs in less than 1% of early postoperative patients. When it does occur, adhesions are usually the cause. Internal and external hernias, technical errors, and infections or abscesses are also causative. No one can accurately predict which patients will form obstructive postoperative adhesions, because all patients who undergo surgery form adhesions to some extent, and there is little that can limit this natural healing process. Hyaluronidase is a mucolytic enzyme that degrades connective tissue, and the use of a methylcellulose form of hyaluronidase, Seprafilm, has been shown to result in a 50% decrease in adhesion formation in some patients.[71,72] This should translate into a lower occurrence of postoperative bowel obstruction, but this has yet to be proven.

TABLE 12-15 Common causes of upper and lower gastrointestinal hemorrhage

Upper GI Bleed	Lower GI Bleed
Erosive esophagitis	Angiodysplasia
Gastric varices	Radiation proctitis
Esophageal varices	Hemangioma
Dieulafoy's lesion	Diverticulosis
Aortoduodenal fistula	Neoplastic diseases
Mallory-Weiss tear	Trauma
Peptic ulcer disease	Vasculitis
Trauma	Hemorrhoids
Neoplastic disease	Aortoenteric fistula
	Intussusception
	Ischemic colitis
	Inflammatory bowel disease
	Postprocedure bleeding

Fistulae are the abnormal communication of one structure to an adjacent structure or compartment, and are associated with extensive morbidity and mortality. Common causes for fistula formation are summarized in the pneumonic FRIENDS (Foreign body, Radiation, Ischemia/Inflammation/Infection, Epithelialization of a tract, Neoplasia, Distal obstruction, and Steroid use). The cause of the fistula must be recognized early, and treatment may include nonoperative management with observation and nutritional support, or a delayed operative management strategy that also includes nutritional support and wound care.

GI bleeding can occur perioperatively (Table 12-15). Technical errors such as a poorly tied suture, a nonhemostatic staple line, or a missed injury can all lead to postoperative intestinal bleeding.[73,74] The source of bleeding is in the upper GI tract about 85% of the time, and is usually detected and treated endoscopically. Surgical control of intestinal bleeding is required in up to 40% of patients.[75]

When patients in the ICU have a major bleed from stress gastritis, the mortality risk is as high as 50%. It is important to keep the gastric pH greater than 4 to decrease the overall risk for stress gastritis, particularly in patients mechanically ventilated for 48 hours or greater and patients who are coagulopathic.[76] Proton pump inhibitors, H_2 receptor antagonists, and intragastric antacid installation are all effective measures.

Hepatobiliary-Pancreatic System

Complications involving the hepatobiliary tree are usually due to technical errors. Laparoscopic cholecystectomy has become the standard of care for cholecystectomy, but common bile duct injury remains a nemesis of this approach. Intraoperative cholangiography has not been shown to decrease the incidence of common bile duct injuries, because the injury to the bile duct usually occurs before the cholangiogram.[77,78] Early recognition of an injury is important, because delayed bile duct leaks often require a more complex repair.

Ischemic injury due to devascularization of the common bile duct has a delayed presentation days to weeks after an operation. Endoscopic retrograde cholangiopancreatography (ERCP) demonstrates a stenotic, smooth common bile duct. Liver function studies are elevated. The recommended treatment is a Roux-en-Y hepaticojejunostomy.

A bile leak due to an unrecognized injury to the ducts may present after cholecystectomy as a biloma. These patients may present with abdominal pain and hyperbilirubinemia. The diagnosis of a biliary leak can be confirmed by CT scan, ERCP, or radionuclide scan. Once a leak is confirmed, a retrograde biliary stent and external drainage is the treatment of choice.

Hyperbilirubinemia in the surgical patient can be a complex problem. Cholestasis makes up the majority of causes for hyperbilirubinemia, but other mechanisms of hyperbilirubinemia include reabsorption of blood (e.g., hematoma from trauma), decreased bile excretion (e.g., sepsis), increased unconjugated bilirubin due to hemolysis, hyperthyroidism, and impaired excretion due to congenital abnormalities or acquired disease. Errors in surgery that cause hyperbilirubinemia largely involve missed or iatrogenic injuries.

The presence of cirrhosis predisposes to postoperative complications. Abdominal or hepatobiliary surgery is problematic in the cirrhotic patient. Ascites leak in the postoperative period can be an issue when any abdominal operation has been performed. Maintaining proper intravascular oncotic pressure in the immediate postoperative period can be difficult, and resuscitation should be maintained with crystalloid solutions. Prevention of renal failure and the management of the hepatorenal syndrome can be difficult, as the demands of fluid resuscitation and altered glomerular filtration become competitive. Spironolactone with other diuretic agents may be helpful in the postoperative care. These patients often have a labile course and bleeding complications due to coagulopathy are common. The operative mortality in cirrhotic patients is 10% for Child class A, 30% for Child class B, and 82% for Child class C patients.[79]

Pyogenic liver abscess occurs in less than 0.5% of adult admissions, due to retained necrotic liver tissue, occult intestinal perforations, benign or malignant hepatobiliary obstruction, and hepatic arterial occlusion. The treatment is long-term antibiotics with percutaneous drainage of large abscesses.

Pancreatitis can occur following injection of contrast during cholangiography and ERCP. These episodes range from a mild elevation in amylase and lipase with abdominal pain, to a fulminant course of pancreatitis with necrosis requiring surgical débridement. Traumatic injuries to the pancreas during surgical procedures on the kidneys, GI tract, or spleen comprise the most common causes. Treatment involves serial CT scans and percutaneous drainage to manage infected fluid and abscess collections. A pancreatic fistula may respond to antisecretory therapy with a somatostatin analogue, Octreotide. Management of these fistulae initially includes ERCP with or without pancreatic stenting, percutaneous drainage of any fistula fluid collections, total parenteral nutrition (TPN) with bowel rest, and repeated CT scans. The majority of pancreatic fistulae will eventually heal spontaneously.

Renal System

Renal failure can be classified as prerenal failure, intrinsic renal failure, and postrenal failure. Postrenal failure, or obstructive renal failure, should always be considered when low urine output (oliguria) or anuria occurs. The most common cause is a misplaced or clogged urinary catheter. Other, less common causes to consider are unintentional ligation or transection of ureters during a difficult surgical dissection (e.g., colon resection for diverticular disease), or a large retroperitoneal hematoma (e.g., ruptured aortic aneurysm).

Oliguria is evaluated by flushing the Foley catheter using sterile technique. When this fails to produce the desired response, it is reasonable to administer an IV fluid challenge with a crystalloid fluid bolus of 500 to 1000 mL. However, the immediate postoperative patient must be examined and have recent vital signs recorded with total intake and output tabulated, as well as urinary electrolytes measured (Table 12-16). A hemoglobin and hematocrit level should be checked immediately. Patients in compensated shock from acute blood loss may manifest anemia and end-organ malperfusion as oliguria.

Acute tubular necrosis (ATN) carries a mortality risk of 25 to 50% due to the many complications that can cause, or result from, this insult. When ATN is due to poor inflow (prerenal failure), the remedy begins with IV administration of crystalloid or colloid fluids as needed. If cardiac insufficiency is the problem, the optimization of vascular volume is achieved first, followed by inotropic agents, as needed. Intrinsic renal failure and subsequent ATN are often the result of direct renal toxins. Aminoglycosides, vancomycin, and furosemide, among other commonly used agents, contribute directly to nephrotoxicity. Contrast-induced nephropathy usually leads to a

TABLE 12-16 Urinary electrolytes associated with acute renal failure and their possible etiologies

	FE$_{Na}$	Osmolarity	UR$_{Na}$	Etiology
Prerenal	<1	>500	<20	CHF, cirrhosis
Intrinsic failure	>1	<350	>40	Sepsis, shock

CHF = congestive heart failure; FE$_{Na}$ = fractional excretion of sodium; UR$_{Na}$ = urinary excretion of sodium.

subtle or transient rise in creatinine. In patients who are volume depleted or have poor cardiac function, contrast nephropathy may permanently impair renal function.[80–83]

The treatment of renal failure due to myoglobinuria in severe trauma patients has shifted away from the use of sodium bicarbonate for alkalinizing the urine, to merely maintaining brisk urine output of 100 mL/h with crystalloid fluid infusion. Mannitol and furosemide are not recommended as long as the IV fluid achieves the goal rate of urinary output.

Musculoskeletal System

A compartment syndrome can develop in any compartment of the body. Compartment syndrome of the extremities generally occurs after a closed fracture. The injury alone may predispose the patient to compartment syndrome, but aggressive fluid resuscitation can exacerbate the problem. Pain with passive motion is the hallmark of compartment syndrome, and the anterior compartment of the leg is usually the first compartment to be involved. Confirmation of the diagnosis is obtained by direct pressure measurement of the individual compartments. If the pressures are greater than 20 to 25 mmHg in any of the compartments, then a four-compartment fasciotomy is considered. Compartment syndrome can be due to ischemia-reperfusion injury, after an ischemic time of 4 to 6 hours. Renal failure (due to myoglobinuria), foot drop, tissue loss, and a permanent loss of function are possible results of untreated compartment syndrome.

Decubitus ulcers are preventable complications of prolonged bedrest due to traumatic paralysis, dementia, chemical paralysis, or coma. Ischemic changes in the microcirculation of the skin can be significant after 2 hours of sustained pressure. Routine skin care and turning of the patient helps ensure a reduction in skin ulceration. This can be labor intensive and special mattresses and beds are available to help with this ubiquitous problem. The treatment of a decubitus ulcer in the noncoagulopathic patient is surgical débridement. Once the wound bed has a viable granulation base without an excess of fibrinous debris, a vacuum-assisted closure dressing can be applied. Wet to moist dressings with frequent dressing changes is the alternative, and is labor intensive. Expensive topical enzyme preparations are also available. If the wounds fail to respond to these measures, soft tissue coverage by flap is considered.

Contractures are the result of muscle disuse. Whether from trauma, amputation, or from vascular insufficiency, contractures can be prevented by physical therapy and splinting. If not attended to early, contractures will prolong rehabilitation and may lead to further wounds and wound healing issues. Depending on the functional status of the patient, contracture releases may be required for long-term care.

Hematologic System

The transfusion guideline of maintaining the hematocrit level in all patients at greater than 30% is no longer valid. Only those patients with symptomatic anemia, or those who have significant cardiac disease, or the critically ill patient who requires increased oxygen-carrying capacity to adequately perfuse end organs, requires higher levels of hemoglobin. Other than these select patients, the decision to transfuse should generally not occur until the hemoglobin level reaches 7 mg/dL or the hematocrit reaches 21%.

TABLE 12-17	Rate of viral transmission in blood product transfusions[a]
HIV	1:1.9 million
HBV[b]	1:137,000
HCV	1:1 million

[a]Post–nucleic acid amplification technology (1999). Earlier rates were erroneously reported higher due to lack of contemporary technology.
[b]HBV is reported with pre–nucleic acid amplification technology. Statistical information is unavailable in post–nucleic acid amplification technology at this writing. Note that bacterial transmission is 50 to 250 times higher than viral transmission per transfusion.
HBV = hepatitis B virus; HCV = hepatitis C virus.

Transfusion reactions are common complications of blood transfusion. These can be attenuated with a leukocyte filter, but not completely prevented. The manifestations of a transfusion reaction include simple fever, pruritus, chills, muscle rigidity, and renal failure due to myoglobinuria secondary to hemolysis. Discontinuing the transfusion and returning the blood products to the blood bank is an important first step, but administration of antihistamine and possibly steroids may be required to control the reaction symptoms. Severe transfusion reactions are rare but can be fatal.

Infectious complications in blood transfusion range from cytomegalovirus transmission, which is benign in the nontransplant patient, to HIV infection, to passage of the hepatitis viruses, which can lead to subsequent hepatocellular carcinoma. Although the efficiency of infectious agent screening in blood products has improved, universal precautions should be rigidly maintained for all patients (Table 12-17).

Patients on warfarin (Coumadin) who require surgery can have anticoagulation reversal by administration of fresh-frozen plasma. Each unit of fresh-frozen plasma contains 200 to 250 mL of plasma and includes one unit of coagulation factor per milliliter of plasma.

Thrombocytopenia may require platelet transfusion for a platelet count less than 20,000/mL when invasive procedures are performed, or when platelet counts are low and ongoing bleeding from raw surface areas persists. One unit of platelets will increase the platelet count by 5000 to 7500 per mL in adults. It is important to delineate the cause of the low platelet count. Usually there is a self-limiting or reversible condition such as sepsis. Rarely, it is due to heparin-induced thrombocytopenia I and II. Complications of heparin-induced thrombocytopenia II can be serious because of the diffuse thrombogenic nature of the disorder. Simple precautions to limit this hypercoagulable state include saline solution flushes instead of heparin solutions, and to limit the use of heparin-coated catheters. The treatment is anticoagulation with synthetic agents such as argatroban.

For patients with uncontrollable bleeding due to disseminated intravascular coagulopathy, an expensive but useful drug is factor VIIa.[84–86] Largely used in hepatic trauma and obstetric emergencies, this agent may mean the difference between life or death in some circumstances. The combination of ongoing, nonsurgical bleeding and renal failure can sometimes be successfully treated with desmopressin.

In addition to classic hemophilia, other inherited coagulation factor deficiencies can be difficult to manage in surgery. When required, transfusion of appropriate replacement products is coordinated with the regional blood bank center before surgery. Other blood dyscrasias seen by surgeons include hypercoagulopathic patients. Those who carry congenital anomalies such as the most common, Factor V Leiden deficiency, as well as protein C and S deficiencies, are likely to form thromboses if inadequately anticoagulated.

Abdominal Compartment Syndrome

Abdominal compartment syndrome (ACS) and intra-abdominal hypertension represent the same problem. Multisystem trauma, thermal burns, retroperitoneal injuries, and surgery related to the retroperitoneum are the major initial causative factors that may lead to ACS. Ruptured AAA, major pancreatic injury and resection, or multiple intestinal injuries are also examples of clinical situations in which a large volume of IV fluid resuscitation puts these patients at risk for intra-abdominal hypertension. Manifestations of ACS typically include progressive abdominal distention followed by increased peak airway ventilator pressures, oliguria followed by anuria, and an insidious development of intracranial hypertension.[87] These findings are related to elevation of the diaphragm and inadequate venous return from the vena cava or renal veins secondary to the transmitted pressure on the venous system.

Measurement of abdominal pressures is easily accomplished by transducing bladder pressures from the urinary catheter after instilling 100 mL of sterile saline into the urinary bladder.[88] A pressure greater than 20 mmHg constitutes intra-abdominal hypertension, but the diagnosis of ACS requires intra-abdominal pressure greater than 25 to 30 mmHg, with at least one of the following: compromised respiratory mechanics and ventilation, oliguria or anuria, or increasing intracranial pressures.[89–91]

The treatment of ACS is to open any recent abdominal incision to release the abdominal fascia, or to open the fascia directly if no abdominal incision is present. Immediate improvement in mechanical ventilation pressures, intracranial pressures, and renal output is usually noted. When expectant management for ACS is considered in the OR, the abdominal fascia should be left open and covered under sterile conditions with plans made for a second-look operation and delayed fascial closure. Patients with intra-abdominal hypertension should be monitored closely with repeated examinations and measurements of bladder pressure, so that any further deterioration is detected and operative management can be initiated. Left untreated, ACS may lead to multiple system end-organ dysfunction or failure, and has a high mortality.

Abdominal wall closure should be attempted every 48 to 72 hours until the fascia can be reapproximated. If the abdomen cannot be closed within 5 to 7 days following release of the abdominal fascia, a large incisional hernia is the net result.

Wounds, Drains, and Infection
Wound (Surgical Site) Infection

There exist no prospective, randomized, double-blind, controlled studies that demonstrate that antibiotics used beyond 24 hours in the perioperative period prevent infections. There is a general trend toward providing a single preoperative dose, as antibiotic prophylaxis may not impart any benefit at all beyond the initial dosing. Irrigation of the operative field and the surgical wound with saline solution has shown benefit in controlling wound inoculum.[92] Irrigation with an antibiotic-based solution has not demonstrated significant benefit in controlling postoperative infection.

Antibacterial-impregnated polyvinyl placed over the operative wound area for the duration of the surgical procedure has not been shown to decrease the rate of wound infection.[93–97] Although skin preparation with 70% isopropyl alcohol has the best bactericidal effect, it is flammable, and could be hazardous when electrocautery is used. The contemporary formulas of chlorhexidine gluconate with isopropyl alcohol or povidone-iodine and iodophor with alcohol are more advantageous.[98–100]

There is a difference between wound colonization and infection. Overtreating colonization is just as injurious as undertreating infection (Table 12-18). The strict definition of wound (soft tissue) infection is more than 10^5 CFU per gram of tissue. This warrants expeditious and proper antibiotic/antifungal treatment.[58,101] Often, however, clinical signs raise enough suspicion that the patient is treated before a confirmatory culture is undertaken. The clinical signs of wound infection include *rubor, tumor, calor,* and *dolor* (redness, swelling, heat, and pain), and once the diagnosis of wound infection has been established, the most definitive treatment remains open drainage of the wound to facilitate wound dressing care. The use of antibiotics for wound infection treatment should be limited.[102–105]

One type of wound dressing/drainage system that is gaining popularity is the vacuum-assisted closure dressing. The principle of

TABLE 12-18	Common causes of leukocytosis

Infection
Systemic inflammatory response syndrome
Glucocorticoid administration
Splenectomy
Leukemia
Medications
Physiologic stress
Increases in interleukin-1 and tumor necrosis factor

the system is to decrease local wound edema and to promote healing through the application of a sterile dressing that is then covered and placed under controlled suction for a period of 2 to 4 days at a time. Although costly, the benefits are frequently dramatic and may offset the costs of nursing care, frequent dressing changes, and operative wound débridement.

Drain Management

The four indications for applying a surgical drain are:

- To collapse surgical dead space in areas of redundant tissue (e.g., neck and axilla)
- To provide focused drainage of an abscess or grossly infected surgical site
- To provide early warning notice of a surgical leak (either bowel contents, secretions, urine, air, or blood)—the so-called *sentinel drain*
- To control an established fistula leak

Open drains are often used for large contaminated wounds such as perirectal or perianal fistulas and subcutaneous abscess cavities. They prevent premature closure of an abscess cavity in a contaminated wound, but do not address the fact that bacteria are free to travel in either direction along the drain tract. More commonly, surgical sites are drained by closed suction drainage systems, but data do not support closed suction drainage to "protect an anastomosis," or to "control a leak" when placed at the time of surgery. Closed suction devices can exert a negative pressure of 70 to 170 mmHg at the level of the drain, therefore the presence of this excess suction may call into question whether an anastomosis breaks down on its own, or if the drain creates a suction injury that promotes leakage (Fig. 12-10).[106]

On the other hand, CT- or ultrasound-guided placement of percutaneous drains is now the standard of care for abscesses, loculated infections, and other isolated fluid collections such as pancreatic leaks. The risk of surgery is far greater than the placement of an image-guided drain, and the risk can often be reduced in these instances by a brief course of antibiotics.

The use of antibiotics when drains are placed should be examined from a cost-benefit perspective. Antibiotics are rarely necessary when a wound is drained widely. Twenty-four to 48 hours of antibiotic use after drain placement is prophylactic, and after this period only specific treatment of positive cultures should be performed, to avoid increased drug resistance and superinfection.

Urinary Catheters

Several complications of urinary (Foley) catheters occur that lead to an increased length of hospital stay and morbidity. It is recommended that the catheter be inserted its full length up to the hub, and that urine flow is established before the balloon is inflated, because misplacement of the catheter in the urethra with premature inflation of the balloon can lead to tears and disruption of the urethra.

Enlarged prostatic tissue can make catheter insertion difficult, and a catheter coudé may be required. If this attempt is also unsuccessful, then a urologic consultation for endoscopic placement of the catheter may be required to prevent harm to the urethra. For patients with urethral strictures, filiform-tipped catheters and followers may be used, but these can potentially cause bladder injury. If endoscopic

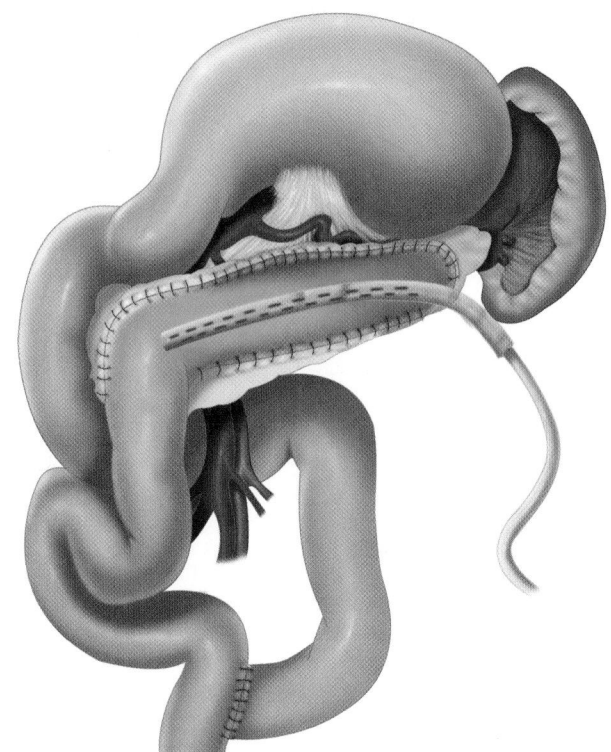

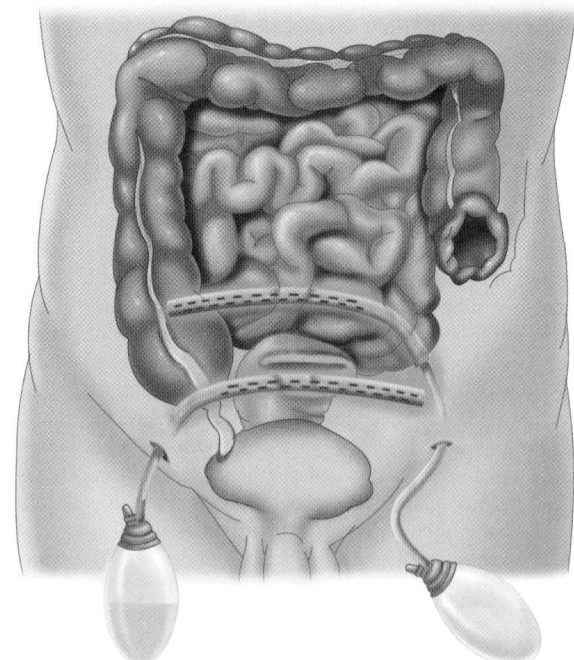

FIG. 12-10. This illustration demonstrates typical intraoperative placement of closed suction devices in pancreatic or small bowel surgery, where there may be an anastomosis. At negative pressures of 70 to 170 mmHg, these devices may actually encourage anastomotic leaks and not prevent them, or become clogged by them.

attempts fail, the patient may require a percutaneously placed suprapubic catheter to obtain decompression of the bladder. Follow-up investigations of these patients are recommended so definitive care of the urethral abnormalities can be pursued.

The most frequent nosocomial infection is urinary tract infection (UTI). These infections are classified into complicated and uncomplicated forms. The uncomplicated type is a UTI that can be treated with trimethoprim-sulfamethoxazole for 3 days. The complicated UTI usually involves the hospitalized patient with an indwelling catheter whose UTI is diagnosed as part of a fever work-up. The interpretation of urine culture results of less than 100,000 CFU/mL is controversial. Before treating such a patient, one should change the catheter and then repeat the culture to see if the catheter was simply colonized with organisms. On the other hand, an argument can be made that, until the foreign body (catheter) is removed, the bladder will continue to be the nidus of infection, and antibiotics should be started. Cultures with more than 100,000 CFU/mL should be treated with the appropriate antibiotics and the catheter removed as soon as possible. Undertreatment or misdiagnosis of a UTI can lead to urosepsis and septic shock.

Recommendations are mixed on the proper way to treat *Candida albicans* fungal bladder infections. Continuous bladder washings with fungicidal solution for 72 hours have been recommended, but this is not always effective. Replacement of the urinary catheter and a course of fluconazole are appropriate treatments, but some infectious disease specialists claim that *C. albicans* in the urine may serve as an indication of fungal infection elsewhere in the body. If this is the case, then screening cultures for other sources of fungal infection should be performed whenever a fungal UTI is found.

Empyema

One of the most debilitating infections is an empyema, or infection of the pleural space. Frequently, an overwhelming pneumonia is the source of an empyema, but a retained hemothorax, systemic sepsis, esophageal perforation from any cause, and infections with a predilection for the lung (e.g., tuberculosis) are potential etiologies as well. The diagnosis is confirmed by chest x-ray or CT scan, followed by aspiration of pleural fluid for bacteriologic analysis. Gram's stain, lactate dehydrogenase, protein, pH, and cell count are obtained, and broad-spectrum antibiotics are initiated while the laboratory studies are performed. Once the specific organisms are confirmed, anti-infective agents are tailored appropriately. Placement of a thoracostomy tube is needed to evacuate and drain the infected pleural fluid, but depending on the specific nidus of infection, video-assisted thoracoscopy may also be helpful for irrigation and drainage of the infection.

Abdominal Abscesses

Postsurgical intra-abdominal abscesses can present with vague complaints of intermittent abdominal pain, fever, leukocytosis, and a change in bowel habits. Depending on the type and timing of the original procedure, the clinical assessment of these complaints is sometimes difficult, and a CT scan is usually required. When a fluid collection within the peritoneal cavity is found on CT scan, antibiotics and percutaneous drainage of the collection is the treatment of choice. There should still be a determination as to what the cause of the infection was, so tailored antibiotic therapy can be initiated. Initial antibiotic treatment is usually with broad-spectrum antibiotics such as piperacillin-tazobactam or imipenem. Should the patient exhibit signs of peritonitis and/or have free air on x-ray or CT scan, then re-exploration should be considered.

For patients who present primarily (i.e., not postoperatively) with the clinical and radiologic findings of an abscess but are clinically stable, the etiology of the abscess must be determined. A plan for drainage of the abscess and decisions about further diagnostic studies with consideration of the timing of any definitive surgery all need to be balanced. This can be a complex set of decisions, depending on the etiology (e.g., appendicitis or diverticulitis); but if the patient exhibits signs of peritonitis, urgent surgical exploration should be performed.

Necrotizing Fasciitis

Postoperative infections that progress to the fulminant soft tissue infection known as *necrotizing fasciitis* are uncommon. Group A streptococcal (M types 1, 3, 12, and 28) soft tissue infections, as well

TABLE 12-19	Mortality associated with patients exhibiting two or more criteria for systemic inflammatory response syndrome (SIRS)
Prognosis	**Mortality (%)**
2 SIRS criteria	5
3 SIRS criteria	10
4 SIRS criteria	15–20

as infections with *Clostridium perfringens* and *C. septicum* carry a mortality of 30 to 70%. Septic shock can be present and patients can become hypotensive less than 6 hours following inoculation. Manifestations of a group A *Streptococcus pyogenes* infection in its most severe form include hypotension, renal insufficiency, coagulopathy, hepatic insufficiency, ARDS, tissue necrosis, and erythematous rash.

These findings constitute a surgical emergency and the mainstay of treatment remains wide débridement of the necrotic tissue to the level of bleeding, viable tissue. A gray serous fluid at the level of the necrotic tissue is usually noted, and as the infection spreads, thrombosed blood vessels are noted along the tissue planes involved with the infection. Typically, the patient requires serial trips to the OR for wide débridement until the infection is under control. Antibiotics are an important adjunct to surgical débridement and broad-spectrum coverage should be used because these infections may be polymicrobial (i.e., so-called *mixed-synergistic infections*). *S. pyogenes* is eradicated with penicillin, and it should still be used as the initial drug of choice.

Systemic Inflammatory Response Syndrome, Sepsis, and Multiple-Organ Dysfunction Syndrome

The systemic inflammatory response syndrome (SIRS) and the multiple organ dysfunction syndrome (MODS) carry significant mortality risks (Table 12-19). Specific criteria have been established for the diagnosis of SIRS (Table 12-20), but two criteria are not required for the diagnosis of SIRS: lowered blood pressure and blood cultures positive for infection. SIRS is the result of proinflammatory cytokines related to tissue malperfusion or injury. The dominant cytokines implicated in this process include interleukin-1, interleukin-6, and tissue necrosis factor. Other mediators include nitric oxide, inducible macrophage-type nitric oxide synthase, and prostaglandin I$_2$.

Sepsis is categorized as sepsis, severe sepsis, and septic shock. An oversimplification of sepsis would be to define it as SIRS plus infection. Severe sepsis is defined as sepsis plus signs of cellular hypoperfusion or end-organ dysfunction. Septic shock would then be sepsis associated with hypotension after adequate fluid resuscitation.

MODS is the culmination of septic shock and multiple end-organ failure.[107] Usually there is an inciting event (e.g., perforated sigmoid diverticulitis), and as the patient undergoes resuscitation, he or she develops cardiac hypokinesis and oliguric or anuric renal failure, followed by the development of ARDS and eventually septic shock with death.

Management of SIRS/MODS includes aggressive global resuscitation and support of end-organ perfusion, correction of the inciting etiology, control of infectious complications, and management of

TABLE 12-20	Inclusion criteria for the systemic inflammatory response syndrome

Temperature >38°C or <36°C (>100.4°F or <96.8°F)
Heart rate >90 beats/min
Respiratory rate >20 breaths/min or PaCO$_2$ <32 mmHg
White blood cell count <4000 or >12,000 cells/mm^3 or >10% immature forms

PaCO$_2$ = partial pressure of arterial carbon dioxide.

iatrogenic complications.[108–110] Drotrecogin α, or recombinant activated protein C, appears to specifically counteract the cytokine cascade of SIRS/MODS, but its use is still limited.[111,112] Other adjuncts for supportive therapy include tight glucose control, low tidal volumes in ARDS, vasopressin in septic shock, and steroid replacement therapy.

Nutritional and Metabolic Support Complications
Nutrition-Related Complications

A basic principle is to use enteral feeding whenever possible, but complications can intervene such as aspiration, ileus, and to a lesser extent, sinusitis. There is no difference in aspiration rates when a small-caliber feeding tube is placed transpylorically into the duodenum or if it remains in the stomach. Patients who are fed via nasogastric tubes are at risk for aspiration pneumonia, because these relatively large-bore tubes stent open the esophagus, creating the possibility of gastric reflux. The use of enteric and gastric feeding tubes obviates complications of TPN, such as pneumothorax, line sepsis, upper extremity DVT, and the related expense. There is growing evidence to support the initiation of enteral feeding in the early postoperative period, before the return of bowel function, where it is usually well tolerated.

In patients who have had any type of nasal intubation that are having high, unexplained fevers, sinusitis must be entertained as a diagnosis. CT scan of the sinuses is warranted, followed by aspiration of sinus contents so the organism(s) are appropriately treated.

Patients who have not been enterally fed for prolonged periods secondary to multiple operations, those who have had enteral feeds interrupted for any other reason, or those with poor enteral access are at risk for the refeeding syndrome, which is characterized by severe hypophosphatemia and respiratory failure. Slow progression of the enteral feeding administration rate can avoid this complication.

Common TPN problems are mostly related to electrolyte abnormalities that may develop. These electrolyte errors include deficits or excesses in sodium, potassium, calcium, magnesium, and phosphate. Acid-base abnormalities can also occur with the improper administration of acetate or bicarbonate solutions.

The most common cause for hypernatremia in hospitalized patients is underresuscitation, and conversely, hyponatremia is most often caused by fluid overload. Treatment for hyponatremia is fluid restriction in mild or moderate cases and the administration of hypertonic saline for severe cases. An overly rapid correction of the sodium abnormality may result in central pontine myelinolysis, which results in a severe neurologic deficit. Treatment for hyponatremic patients includes fluid restriction to correct the free water deficit by 50% in the first 24 hours. An overcorrection of hyponatremia can result in severe cerebral edema, a neurologic deficit, or seizures.

Glycemic Control

In 2001, Van den Berghe and colleagues demonstrated that tight glycemic control by insulin infusion is associated with a 50% reduction in mortality in the critical care setting.[113] This prospective, randomized, controlled trial of 1500 patients had two study arms: the intensive-control arm, where the serum glucose was maintained between 80 and 110 mg/dL with insulin infusion; and the control arm, where patients received an insulin infusion only if blood glucose was greater than 215 mg/dL, but serum glucose was then maintained at 180 to 200 mg/dL.

The tight glycemic control group had an average serum glucose level of 103 mg/dL, and the average glucose level in the control group was 153 mg/dL. Hypoglycemic episodes (glucose <40 mg/dL) occurred in 39 patients in the tightly controlled group, while the control group had episodes in 6 patients. The overall mortality was reduced from 8% to 4.6%, but the mortality of those patients whose ICU stay lasted longer than 5 days was reduced from 20% to 10%. Secondary findings included an improvement in overall morbidity, a decreased percentage of ventilator days, less renal impairment, and a lower incidence of bloodstream infections. These finding have been corrob-

orated by subsequent similar studies, and the principal benefit appears to be a greatly reduced incidence of nosocomial infections and sepsis. It is not known whether the benefits are due to strict euglycemia, to the anabolic properties of insulin, or both, but the maintenance of strict euglycemia appears to be a powerful therapeutic strategy.[113–115]

Metabolism-Related Complications

"Stress dose steroids" have been advocated for the perioperative treatment of patients on corticosteroid therapy, but recent studies strongly discourage the use of supraphysiologic doses of steroids when patients are on low or maintenance doses (e.g., 5 to 15 mg) of prednisone daily. Parenteral glucocorticoid treatment need only replicate physiologic replacement steroids in the perioperative period. When patients are on steroid replacement doses equal to or greater than 20 mg per day of prednisone, it may be appropriate to administer additional glucocorticoid doses for no more than two perioperative days.[116–118]

Adrenal insufficiency may be present in patients with a baseline serum cortisol less than 20 μg/dL. A rapid provocative test with synthetic adrenocorticotropic hormone may confirm the diagnosis. After a baseline serum cortisol level is drawn, 250 μg of cosyntropin is administered. At exactly 30 and 60 minutes following the dose of cosyntropin, serum cortisol levels are obtained. There should be an incremental increase in the cortisol level of between 7 and 10 μg/dL for each half hour. If the patient is below these levels, a diagnosis of adrenal insufficiency is made, and glucocorticoid and mineralocorticoid administration is then warranted. Mixed results are common, but the complication of performing major surgery on an adrenally insufficient patient is sudden or profound hypotension.[108]

Thyroid hormone abnormalities usually consist of previously undiagnosed thyroid abnormalities. Hypothyroidism and the so-called *sick-euthyroid syndrome* are more commonly recognized in the critical care setting. When surgical patients are not progressing satisfactorily in the perioperative period, screening for thyroid abnormalities should be performed. If the results show mild to moderate hypothyroidism, then thyroid replacement should begin immediately and thyroid function studies monitored closely. All patients should be reassessed after the acute illness has subsided regarding the need for chronic thyroid replacement therapy.

Problems with Thermoregulation
Hypothermia

Hypothermia is defined as a core temperature less than 35°C (95°F), and is divided into subsets of mild [35 to 32°C, (95 to 89.6°F)], moderate [32 to 28°C (89.6 to 82.4°F)], and severe [<28°C, (<82.4°F)] hypothermia. Shivering, the body's attempt to reverse the effects of hypothermia, occurs between 37 and 31°C (98.6 and 87.8°F), but ceases at temperatures below 31°C (87.8°F). Patients who are moderately hypothermic are at higher risk for complications than are those who are more profoundly hypothermic.

Hypothermia creates a coagulopathy that is related to platelet and clotting cascade enzyme dysfunction. This triad of metabolic acidosis, coagulopathy, and hypothermia is commonly found in long operative cases, and in patients with blood dyscrasias. The enzymes that contribute to the clotting cascade and platelet activity are most efficient at normal body temperatures; therefore all measures must be used to reduce heat loss intraoperatively.[119]

The most common cardiac abnormality is the development of arrhythmias when body temperature drops below 35°C (95°F). Bradycardia occurs with temperatures below 30°C (86°F). It is well known that hypothermia may induce CO_2 retention resulting in respiratory acidosis. Renal dysfunction of hypothermia manifests itself as a paradoxic polyuria, and is related to an increased glomerular filtration rate, as peripheral vascular constriction creates central shunting of blood. This is potentially perplexing in patients that are undergoing resuscitation for hemodynamic instability, because the brisk urine output provides a false sense of an adequate intravascular fluid volume.

TABLE 12-21	Common causes of elevated temperature in surgical patients

Hyperthermia	Hyperpyrexia
Environmental	Sepsis
Malignant hyperthermia	Infection
Neuroleptic malignant syndrome	Drug reaction
Thyrotoxicosis	Transfusion reaction
Pheochromocytoma	Collagen disorders
Carcinoid syndrome	Factitious syndrome
Iatrogenic	Neoplastic disorders
Central/hypothalamic responses	
Pulmonary embolism	
Adrenal insufficiency	

Neurologic dysfunction is inconsistent in hypothermia, but a deterioration in reasoning and decision-making skills progresses as body temperature falls, and profound coma (and a flat electroencephalogram) occurs as the temperature drops below 30°C (86°F). The diagnosis of hypothermia is important, so accurate measurement techniques are required to get a true core temperature.

Methods used to warm patients include warm air circulation over the patient, and heated IV fluids, and more aggressive measures such as bilateral chest tubes with warm solution lavage, intraperitoneal rewarming lavage, and extracorporeal membrane oxygenation. A rate of temperature rise of 2 to 4°C/h (3.6 to 7.2°F/h) is considered adequate, but the most common complication for nonbypass rewarming is arrhythmia with ventricular arrest.

Hyperthermia

Hyperthermia is a core temperature greater than 38.6°C (101.5°F), and has a host of etiologies (Table 12-21).[120] Hyperthermia can be environmentally induced (e.g., summer heat with inability to dissipate heat or control exposure), iatrogenically induced (e.g., heat lamps and medications), endocrine in origin (e.g., thyrotoxicosis), or neurologically induced (i.e., hypothalamic).

Malignant hyperthermia occurs after exposure to agents such as succinylcholine and some halothane-based inhalational anesthetics. The presentation is dramatic, with rapid onset of increased temperature, rigors, and myoglobinuria related to myonecrosis. Medications must be discontinued immediately and dantrolene administered (2.5 mg/kg every 5 minutes) until symptoms subside. Aggressive cooling methods are also implemented, such as an alcohol bath, or packing in ice. In cases of severe malignant hyperthermia, the mortality rate is nearly 30%.

Thyrotoxicosis can occur after surgery, due to undiagnosed Graves' disease. Hyperthermia [>40°C, (104°F)], anxiety, copious diaphoresis, congestive heart failure (present in about one fourth of episodes), tachycardia (most commonly atrial fibrillation), and hypokalemia (up to 50% of patients) are hallmarks of the disease. The treatment of thyrotoxicosis includes glucocorticoids, propylthiouracil, beta blockade, and iodide (Lugol's solution) delivered in an emergent fashion. As the name suggests, these patients are usually toxic and require supportive measures as well. Acetaminophen, cooling modalities noted in the paragraph above, and vasoactive agents often are indicated.

ISSUES IN CARING FOR OBESE PATIENTS AND PATIENTS AT THE EXTREMES OF AGE

Surgery in the obese patient has multiple risks, and it is important to optimize these patients before surgery to minimize these risks. Optimization begins preoperatively with teaching about dietary modifications, exercise, and pulmonary toilet issues. Obese patients often have eccentric left ventricular hypertrophy, right ventricular hypertrophy, and congestive heart failure. Sleep studies and patient history may also reveal significant sleep apnea and gastroesophageal reflux disease. Glycemic control is often poor and contributes significantly to infection and diabetes. The obese patient has a decrease in antithrombin III levels, and a higher risk of DVT and PE. Measures to optimize physiologic function in obese patients include keeping the head of the bed elevated at all times. This can improve the FRC of the lungs by almost a liter, thereby decreasing complications associated with atelectasis and pneumonia. Proper glycemic control via a tight insulin sliding scale is also recommended. Finally, the risk of DVT may be attenuated by immediate use of prophylactic doses of low molecular weight heparin and early ambulation.

Issues for surgery in the very young and the very old have many similarities when it comes to potential errors and complications. Perhaps the most notable similarity is the lack of physiologic reserve. The elderly may have end-organ insufficiency, while the young can have underdeveloped or anomalous organ function that may not yet have become manifest. Similarly, the immune responses at the extremes of age are often compromised. This makes diagnosing an infection difficult; elderly adults may not be capable of mounting a febrile response, and young children can often resolve fevers overnight, and the cause may remain undiagnosed.

Other alterations in these groups include the amount and distribution of total body water and total body fat. This is important to consider because some medications are predominantly distributed to fat stores, and this deposition may lead to altered drug clearance. Similarly, total body water is decreased and serum concentrations of medications may be higher than anticipated. In both groups there is a lower lean body mass, which may potentiate the adverse effects of some anesthetic agents. Metabolism of various analgesic and anesthetic agents can be protracted, leading to postoperative problems such as prolonged intubation and the need for the administration of reversal agents.

Other issues that can lead to complex decision making include those related to communication. Whether due to neurologic impairments, agitation, confusion, or an inability to comprehend a language, these factors associated with the extremes of age increase the potential for medical errors. Open and direct communication with the supporting family members is critical for optimal outcomes in these patient groups.

REFERENCES

Entries highlighted in bright blue are key references.

1. Bierly PE III, Spender JC: Culture and high reliability organizations: The case of the nuclear submarine. *Journal of Management* 21:639, 1995.
2. Ruchlin HS, Dubbs NL, Callahan MA: The role of leadership in instilling a culture of safety: Lessons from the literature. *J Healthcare Mgmt* 49:47, 2004.
3. Kohn KT, Corrigan JM, Donaldson MS: *To Err Is Human: Building a Safer Health System*. Washington, DC: National Academy Press, 1999.
4. Hindle D, Braithwaite J, Iedema R. *Patient Safety Research: A Review of the Technical Literature*. Sydney: Centre for Clinical Governance Research, University of South Wales, 2005: 8.
5. Stelfox HT, Palmisani S, Scurlock C, et al: The "To Err is Human" report and the patient safety literature. *Qual Saf Health Care* 15:174, 2006.
6. Makary MA, Sexton JB, Freischlag JA, et al: Patient safety in surgery. *Ann Surg* 243:628, 2006.
7. Berenholtz SM, Pronovost PJ: Monitoring patient safety. *Crit Care Clin* 23:659, 2007.
8. http://www.ahrq.gov/qual/medteam/medteam4.htm: Medical team training, in Baker DP, Gustafson S, Beaubien J, et al: *Medical Teamwork and Patient Safety: The Evidence-Based Relation. Literature Review*. AHRQ Publication No. 05-0053, Rockville, MD: Agency for Healthcare Research and Quality, April 2005 [accessed February 29, 2008].
9. http://www.ahrq.gov/clinic/ptsafety/chap40.htm: Pizzi LT, Goldfarb NI, Nash DB: Promoting a culture of safety, in *Making Health Care Safer: A Critical Analysis of Patient Safety Practices. Evidence Report/Technology Assessment: Number 43*. AHRQ Publication No. 01-E058, July 2001. Rockville, MD: Agency for Healthcare Research and Quality [accessed December 20, 2007].

10. Chan DK, Gallagher TH, Reznick R, et al: How surgeons disclose medical errors to patients: A study using standardized patients. *Surgery* 138:851, 2005.

11. Sexton JB, Thomas EJ, Helmreich RL: Error, stress, and teamwork in medicine and aviation: Cross sectional surveys. *BMJ* 320:745, 2000.

12. Thomas EJ, Sexton JB, Helmreich RL: Discrepant attitudes about teamwork among critical care nurses and physicians. *Crit Care Med* 31:956, 2003.

13. Amalberti R, Auroy Y, Berwick D, et al: Five system barriers to achieving ultrasafe health care. *Ann Intern Med* 142:756, 2005.

14. *http://www.jointcommission.org/SentinelEvents/Statistics*: Sentinel Event Statistics. Joint Commission website [accessed February 6, 2008].

15. *http://govinfo.library.unt.edu/911/report/index.htm*: Foresight and hindsight, in *9-11 Commission Report* [accessed February 6, 2008].

16. Lingard L, Espin S, Whyte S, et al: Communication failures in the operating room: An observational classification of recurrent types and effects. *Qual Saf Health Care* 13:330, 2004.

17. Christian CK, Gustafson ML, Roth EM, et al: A prospective study of patient safety in the operating room. *Surgery* 139:159, 2006.

18. Makary MA, Sexton JB, Freischlag JA, et al: Operating room teamwork among physicians and nurses: Teamwork in the eye of the beholder. *J Am Coll Surg* 202:746, 2006.

19. Pronovost PJ, Berenholtz SM, Goeschel CA, et al: Creating high reliability in health care organizations. *Health Services Research* 41:1599, 2006.

20. Makary MA, Mukherjee A, Sexton JB, et al: Operating room briefings and wrong-site surgery. *J Am Coll Surg* 204:236, 2007.

21. Nundy S, Mukherjee A, Sexton JB, et al: Impact of preoperative briefings on operating room delays. *Arch Surg* 143:1068, 2008.

22. World Health Organization. World Alliance for Patient Safety. *Guidelines for safe surgery* (draft). Second International Consultation. Geneva, Switzerland: January 2008.

23. Makary MA, Epstein J, Pronovost PJ, et al: Surgical specimen identification errors: A new measure of quality in surgical care. *Surgery* 141:450, 2007.

24. Arora V, Johnson J, Lovinger D, et al: Communication failures in patient sign-out and suggestions for improvement: A critical incident analysis. *Qual Saf Health Care* 14:401, 2005.

25. *http://www.ahrq.gov/about/profile.htm AHRQ Profile: Quality Research for Quality Healthcare*. AHRQ Publication No. 00-P005, March 2001. Rockville, MD: Agency for Healthcare Research and Quality [accessed February 11, 2008].

26. *http://www.qualityindicators.ahrq.gov/psi_overview.htm*: *Patient Safety Indicators Overview*. AHRQ Quality Indicators. February 2006. Rockville, MD: Agency for Healthcare Research and Quality [accessed February 11, 2008].

27. Zhan C, Miller MR: Administrative data based patient safety research: A critical review. *Qual Saf Health Care* 12:58, 2003.

28. Bratzler DW: The Surgical Infection Prevention and Surgical Care Improvement Projects: Promises and pitfalls. *Am Surg* 72:110, 2006.

29. *http://www.medqic.org/dcs/ContentServer?cid=1136495755695&pagename =Medqic%2FOtherResource%2FOtherResourcesTemplate&c=Other Resource*: SCIP Target Areas. Surgical Care Improvement Project website, January 2008 [accessed February 19, 2008].

30. Khuri SF: Safety, quality, and the National Surgical Quality Improvement Program. *Am Surg* 72:994, 2006.

31. Brooke BS, Perler BA, Dominici F, et al: California hospitals meeting Leapfrog quality standards for abdominal aortic aneurysm repair. *J Vasc Surg* 47:1155, 2008.

32. *http://www.leapfroggroup.org/media/file/Leapfrog-Evidence-Based_ Hospital_Referral_Fact_Sheet.pdf*: *Evidence-Based Hospital Referral Fact Sheet*. The Leapfrog Group website [accessed March 5, 2008].

33. Gawande AA, Kwaan MR, Regenbogen SE, et al: An Apgar score for surgery. *J Am Coll Surg* 204:201, 2007.

34. Serious Reportable Events in Healthcare 2006 Update: A Consensus Report. Washington, DC: National Quality Forum; 2007.

35. Gibbs VC, Coakley FD, Reines HD: Preventable errors in the operating room: Retained foreign bodies after surgery—Part 1. *Curr Probl Surg* 44:281, 2007.

36. Gawande AA, Studdert DM, Orav EJ, et al: Risk factors for retained instruments and sponges after surgery. *N Engl J Med* 34:229, 2003.

37. Lincourt AE, Harrell A, Cristiano J, et al: Retained foreign bodies after surgery. *J Surg Res* 138:170, 2007.

38. Doing the "right" things to correct wrong-site surgery. *Pennsylvania Patient Safety Reporting System (PA-PSRS) Patient Safety Advisory* 4:1, 2007.

39. Clarke JR, Johnston J, Finley ED: Getting surgery right. *Ann Surg* 246:395, 2007.

40. Kwaan MR, Studdert DM, Zinner MJ, et al: Incidence, patterns, and prevention of wrong-site surgery. *Arch Surg* 141:353, 2006.

41. Michaels RK, Makary MA, Dahab Y, et al: Achieving the National Quality Forum's "Never Events": Prevention of wrong site, wrong procedure, and wrong patient operations. *Ann Surg* 245:526, 2007.

42. Regenbogen SE, Greenberg CC, Studdert DM, et al: Patterns of technical error among surgical malpractice claims: An analysis of strategies to prevent injury to surgical patients. *Ann Surg* 246:705, 2007.

43. Griffen FD, Stephens LS, Alexander JB, et al: The American College of Surgeons' closed claims study: New insights for improving care. *J Am Coll Surg* 204:561, 2007.

44. Ambady N, LaPlante D, Nguyen T, et al: Surgeons' tone of voice: A clue to malpractice history. *Surgery* 132:5, 2002.

45. Woreta TA, Makary MA: Patient safety, in Makary M (ed): *General Surgery Review*. Washington, DC: Ladner-Drysdale, 2008, p 553.

46. Wojcieszak D, Banja J, Houk C: The Sorry Works! Coalition: Making the case for full disclosure. *Jt Comm J Qual Patient Saf* 32:344, 2006.

47. Kohn LT, Corrigan JM, Donaldson MS (eds): *To Err Is Human: Building a Safer Health System*. Committee on Quality of Health Care in America, Institute of Medicine, Washington, DC: National Academy Press, 2000.

48. Veenstra DL, Saint S, Sullivan SD: Cost-effectiveness of antiseptic-impregnated central venous catheters for the prevention of catheter-related bloodstream infection. *JAMA* 282:554, 1999.

49. O'Grady NP, Alexander M, Dellinger EP, et al: Guidelines for the prevention of intravascular catheter-related infections. *Am J Infect Control* 30:476, 2002.

50. Stoiser B, Kofler J, Staudinger T, et al: Contamination of central venous catheters in immunocompromised patients: A comparison between two different types of central venous catheters. *J Hosp Infect* 50:202, 2002.

51. Tyroch AH, Kaups K, Lorenzo M, et al: Routine chest radiograph is not indicated after open tracheostomy: A multicenter perspective. *Am Surg* 68:80, 2002.

52. Datta D, Onyirimba F, McNamee MJ: The utility of chest radiographs following percutaneous dilatational tracheostomy. *Chest* 123:1603, 2003.

53. Gelman JJ, Aro M, Weiss SM: Tracheo-innominate artery fistula. *J Am Coll Surg* 179:626, 1994.

54. Keceligil HT, Erk MK, Kolbakir F, et al: Tracheoinnominate artery fistula following tracheostomy. *Cardiovasc Surg* 3:509, 1995.

55. Rybak MJ, Abate BJ, Kang SL, et al: Prospective evaluation of the effect of an aminoglycoside doing regimen on rates of observed nephrotoxicity and ototoxicity. *Animicrob Agents Cheother* 43:1549, 1999.

56. Sandur S, Stoller JK: Pulmonary complications of mechanical ventilation. *Clin Chest Med* 20:223, 1999.

57. Salem M, Tainsh RE, Bromberg J, et al: Perioperative glucocorticoid coverage: A reassessment 42 years after emergence of a problem. *Ann Surg* 219:416, 1994.

58. Hughes MG, Evans HL, Chong TW, et al: Effect of an intensive care unit rotating empiric antibiotic schedule on the development of hospital-acquired infections on the non-intensive care unit ward. *Crit Care Med* 32:53, 2004.

59. Horn SD, Wright HL, Couperus JJ, et al: Association between patient-controlled analgesia pump use and postoperative surgical site infection in intestinal surgery patients. *Surg Infect (Larchmt)* 3:109, 2002.

60. The Acute Respiratory Distress Syndrome Network. Ventilation with lower tidal volumes as compared with traditional tidal volumes for acute lung injury and the acute respiratory distress syndrome. *The Acute Respiratory Distress Syndrome Network* 342:1301, 2000.

61. Valente Barbas CS: Lung recruitment maneuvers in acute respiratory distress syndrome and facilitating resolution. *Crit Care Med* 31:S265, 2003.

62. Singh JM, Stewart TE: High-frequency mechanical ventilation principles and practices in the era of lung-protective ventilation strategies. *Respir Care Clin North Am* 8:247, 2002.

63. Yang KL, Tobin MJ: A prospective study of indexes predicting the outcome of trials of weaning from mechanical ventilation. *N Engl J Med* 324:1445, 1991.

64. Epstein SK: Etiology of extubation failure and the predictive value of the rapid shallow breathing index. *Am J Respir Crit Care Med* 152:545, 1995.

65. Falk RH: Atrial fibrillation. *N Engl J Med* 344:1067, 2001.

66. Van Gelder IC, Hagens VE, Bosker HA, et al: A comparison of rate control and rhythm control in patients with recurrent persistent atrial fibrillation. *N Engl J Med* 347:1834, 2002.

67. Wyse DG, Waldo AL, DiMarco JP, et al: A comparison of rate control and rhythm control in patients with atrial fibrillation. *N Engl J Med* 347:1825, 2002.

68. Franklin RH: Ivor Lewis Lecture, 1975. The advancing frontiers of oesophageal surgery. *Ann R Coll Surg Engl* 59:284, 1977.

69. Stewart BT, Woods RJ, Collopy BT, et al: Early feeding after elective open colorectal resections: A prospective randomized trial. *Aust N Z J Surg* 68:125, 1998.

70. Asao T, Kuwano H, Nakamura J, et al: Gum chewing enhances early recovery from postoperative ileus after laparoscopic colectomy. *J Am Coll Surg* 195:30, 2002.

71. Tang CL, Seow-Choen F, Fook-Chong S, et al: Bioresorbable adhesion barrier facilitates early closure of the defunctioning ileostomy after rectal excision: A prospective, randomized trial. *Dis Colon Rectum* 46:1200, 2003.

72. Beck DE, Cohen Z, Fleshman JW, et al: A prospective, randomized, multicenter, controlled study of the safety of Seprafilm adhesion barrier in abdominopelvic surgery of the intestine. *Dis Colon Rectum* 46:1310, 2003.

73. Smoot RL, Gostout CJ, Rajan E, et al: Is early colonoscopy after admission for acute diverticular bleeding needed? *Am J Gastroenterol* 98:1996, 2003.

74. Sorbi D, Gostout CJ, Peura D, et al: An assessment of the management of acute bleeding varices: A multicenter prospective member-based study. *Am J Gastroenterol* 98:2424, 2003.

75. Domschke W, Lederer P, Lux G: The value of emergency endoscopy in upper gastrointestinal bleeding: Review and analysis of 2014 cases. *Endoscopy* 15:126, 1983.

76. Cash BD: Evidence-based medicine as it applies to acid suppression in the hospitalized patient. *Crit Care Med* 30:S373, 2002.

77. Lidwig K, Bernhardt J, Steffen H, et al: Contribution of intraoperative cholangiography to incidence and outcome of common bile duct injuries during laparoscopic cholecystectomy. *Surg Endosc* 16:1098, 2002. Epub 2002 Apr 9.

78. Flum DR, Dellinger EP, Cheadle A, et al: Intraoperative cholangiography and risk of common bile duct injury during cholecystectomy. *JAMA* 289:1639, 2003.

79. Yoon, YH, Yi Hsiao-ye, Grant BF, et al: Liver cirrhosis mortality in the United States, 1970-98. *National Institute on Alcohol Abuse and Alcoholism.* Surveillance Report No. 57, December 2001.

80. Solomon R, Werner C, Mann D, et al: Effects of saline, mannitol, and furosemide to prevent acute decreases in renal function induced by radiocontrast agents. *N Engl J Med* 331:1416, 1994.

81. Stevens MA, McCullough PA, Tobin KJ, et al: A prospective randomized trial of prevention measures in patients at high risk for contrast nephropathy: Results of the P.R.I.N.C.E. study. Prevention of radiocontrast induced nephropathy clinical evaluation. *J Am Coll Cardiol* 33:403, 1999.

82. Birck R, Krzossok S, Markowetz F, et al: Acetylcysteine for prevention of contrast nephropathy: Meta-analysis. *Lancet* 362:598, 2003.

83. Baker CS, Wragg A, Kumar S, et al: A rapid protocol for the prevention of contrast-induced renal dysfunction: The RAPPID study. *J Am Coll Cardiol* 41:2114, 2003.

84. Laffan M, O'Connell NM, Perry DJ, et al: Analysis and results of the recombinant factor VIIa extended-use registry. *Blood Coagul Fibrinolysis* 14:S35, 2003.

85. Hedner U: Dosing with recombinant factor viia based on current evidence. *Semin Hematol* 41:35, 2004.

86. Midathada MV, Mehta P, Waner M, et al: Recombinant factor VIIa in the treatment of bleeding. *Am J Clin Pathol* 121:124, 2004.

87. Bloomfield GL, Dalton JM, Sugerman HJ, et al: Treatment of increasing intracranial pressure secondary to the acute abdominal compartment syndrome in a patient with combined abdominal and head trauma. *J Trauma* 39:1168, 1995.

88. Kron I, Harman PK, Nolan SP: The measurement of intra-abdominal pressure as a criterion for abdominal re-exploration. *Ann Surg* 199:28, 1984.

89. Ivatury RR, Porter JM, Simon RJ, et al: Intra-abdominal hypertension after life-threatening penetrating abdominal trauma: Prophylaxis, incidence, and clinical relevance to gastric mucosal pH and abdominal compartment syndrome. *J Trauma* 44:1016, 1998.

90. Ivatury RR, Sugerman HJ, Peitzman AB: Abdominal compartment syndrome: Recognition and management. *Adv Surg* 35:251, 2001.

91. Saggi BH, Sugerman HJ, Ivatury RR, et al: Abdominal compartment syndrome. *J Trauma* 45:597, 1998.

92. Anglen J, Apostoles PS, Christensen G, et al: Removal of surface bacteria by irrigation. *J Orthop Res* 14:251, 1966.

93. Lewis DA, Leaper DJ, Speller DC: Prevention of bacterial colonization of wounds at operation: Comparison of iodine-impregnated ("Ioban") drapes with conventional methods. *J Hosp Infect* 5:431, 1984.

94. O'Rourke E, Runyan D, O'Leary J, et al: Contaminated iodophor in the operating room. *Am J Infect Control* 31:255, 2003.

95. Ostrander RV, Brage ME, Botte MJ: Bacterial skin contamination after surgical preparation in foot and ankle surgery. *Clin Orthop* 406:246, 2003.

96. Ghogawala Z, Furtado D: In vitro and in vivo bactericidal activities of 10%, 2.5%, and 1% povidone-iodine solution. *Am J Hosp Pharm* 47:1562, 1990.

97. Anderson RL, Vess RW, Carr JH: Investigations of intrinsic Pseudomonas cepacia contamination in commercially manufactured povidone-iodine. *Infect Control Hosp Epidemiol* 12:297, 1991.

98. Birnbach DJ, Meadows W, Stein DJ, et al: Comparison of povidone iodine and DuraPrep, an iodophor-in-isopropyl alcohol solution, for skin disinfection prior to epidural catheter insertion in parturients. *Anesthesiology* 98:164, 2003.

99. Moen MD, Noone MG, Kirson I: Povidone-iodine spray technique versus traditional scrub-paint technique for preoperative abdominal wall preparation. *Am J Obstet Gynecol* 187:1434, 2002; discussion 1436.

100. Strand CL, Wajsbort RR, Sturmann K: Effect of iodophor vs iodine tincture skin preparation on blood culture contamination rate. *JAMA* 269:1004, 1993.

101. Paterson DL, Ko WC, Von Gottberg A, et al: International prospective study of Klebsiella pneumoniae bacteremia: Implications of extended-spectrum beta-lactamase production in nosocomial infections. *Ann Intern Med* 140:26, 2004.

102. Wittmann DH, Schein M: Let us shorten antibiotic prophylaxis and therapy in surgery. *Am J Surg* 172:26S, 1966.

103. Dellinger EP: Duration of antibiotic treatment in surgical infections of the abdomen. Undesired effects of antibiotics and future studies. *Eur J Surg Suppl* 576:29, 1996; discussion 31.

104. Fry DE: Basic aspects of and general problems in surgical infections. *Surg Infect (Larchmt)* 2(Suppl 1):S3, 2001.

105. Barie PS: Modern surgical antibiotic prophylaxis and therapy—less is more. *Surg Infect (Larchmt)* 1:23, 2000.

106. Grobmyer SR, Graham D, Brennan MF, et al: High-pressure gradients generated by closed-suction surgical drainage systems. *Surg Infect (Larchmt)* 3:245, 2002.

107. Power DA, Duggan J, Brady HR: Renal-dose (low-dose) dopamine for the treatment of sepsis-related and other forms of acute renal failure: Ineffective and probably dangerous. *Clin Exp Pharmacol Physiol Suppl* 26:S23, 1999.

108. Vincent JL, Abraham, E, Annane D, et al: Reducing mortality in sepsis: New directions. *Crit Care* 6(Suppl 3):S1, 2002.

109. Malay MB, Ashton RC Jr., Landry DW, et al: Low-dose vasopressin in the treatment of vasodilatory septic shock. *J Trauma* 47:699, 1999; discussion 703.

110. Annane D, Sebille V, Charpentier C, et al: Effect of treatment with low doses of hydrocortisone and fludrocortisone on mortality in patients with septic shock. *JAMA* 288:862, 2002.

CHAPTER 12 Patient Safety

111. Dhainaut JF, Laterre PF, LaRosa SP, et al: The clinical evaluation committee in a large multicenter phase 3 trial of drotrecogin alfa (activated) in patients with severe sepsis (PROWESS): Role, methodology, and results. *Crit Care Med* 31:2291, 2003; comment, 2405.

112. Betancourt M, McKinnon PS, Massanari RM, et al: An evaluation of the cost effectiveness of drotrecogin alfa (activated) relative to the number of organ system failures. *Pharmacoeconomics* 21:1331, 2003.

113. Van den Berghe G, Wouters P, Weekers F, et al: Intensive insulin therapy in the critically ill patients. *N Engl J Med* 345:1359, 2001.

114. Finney SJ, Zekveld C, Elia A, et al: Glucose control and mortality in critically ill patients. *JAMA* 290:2041, 2003.

115. Furnary AP, Gao G, Grunkemeier GL, et al: Continuous insulin infusion reduces mortality in patients with diabetes undergoing coronary artery bypass grafting. *J Thorac Cardiovasc Surg* 125:1007, 2003.

116. La Rochelle GE Jr., La Rochelle AG, Ratner RE, et al: Recovery of the hypothalamic-pituitary-adrenal axis in patients with rheumatic diseases receiving low-dose prednisone. *Am J Med* 95:258, 1993.

117. Bromberg JS, Alfrey EJ, Barker CF, et al: Adrenal suppression and steroid supplementation in renal transplant recipients. *Transplantation* 51:385, 1991.

118. Freidman RJ, Schiff CF, Bromberg JS: Use of supplemental steroids in patients having orthopaedic operations. *J Bone Joint Surgery* 77:1801, 1995.

119. Kempainen RR, Brunette DD: The evaluation and management of accidental hypothermia. *Respir Care* 49:192, 2004.

120. O'Donnell J, Axelrod P, Fisher C, et al: Use and effectiveness of hypothermia blankets for febrile patients in the intensive care unit. *Clin Infect Dis* 24:1208, 1977.

Physiologic Monitoring of the Surgical Patient

Louis H. Alarcon

BACKGROUND

The Latin verb *monere*, which means "to warn, or advise" is the origin for the English word *monitor*. In contemporary medical practice, patients undergo monitoring to detect pathologic variations in physiologic parameters, providing advanced warning of impending deterioration in the status of one or more organ systems. The intended goal of this endeavor is that by using this knowledge, the clinician takes appropriate actions in a timely fashion to prevent or ameliorate the physiologic derangement. Furthermore, physiologic monitoring is used not only to warn, but also to titrate therapeutic interventions,

such as fluid resuscitation or the infusion of vasoactive or inotropic drugs. Monitoring tools also can be valuable for diagnostic evaluation and assessment of prognosis. The intensive care unit (ICU) and operating room are the two locations where the most advanced monitoring capabilities are routinely used in the care of critically ill patients.

In the broadest sense, physiologic monitoring encompasses a spectrum of endeavors, ranging in complexity from the routine and intermittent measurement of the classic vital signs (i.e., temperature, pulse, arterial blood pressure, and respiratory rate) to the continuous recording of the oxidation state of cytochrome oxidase, the terminal element in the mitochondrial electron transport chain. The ability to assess clinically relevant parameters of tissue and organ status and use this knowledge to improve patient outcomes represents the "holy grail" of critical care medicine. Unfortunately, consensus is often lacking regarding the most appropriate parameters to monitor to achieve this goal. Furthermore, making an inappropriate therapeutic decision due to inaccurate physiologic data or misinterpretation of good data can lead to a worse outcome than having no data at all. Of the highest importance is the integration of physiologic data obtained from monitoring into a coherent and evidenced-based treatment plan. Current technologies available to assist the clinician in this endeavor are summarized in this chapter, as well as a brief look at emerging techniques that may soon enter into clinical practice.

In essence, the goal of hemodynamic monitoring is to ensure that the flow of oxygenated blood through the microcirculation is sufficient to support aerobic metabolism at the cellular level. Mammalian cells cannot store oxygen (O_2) for subsequent use in oxidative metabolism, although a relatively tiny amount is stored in muscle tissue as oxidized myoglobin. Thus aerobic synthesis of adenosine triphosphate, the energy "currency" of cells, requires the continuous delivery of O_2 by diffusion from hemoglobin (Hgb) in red blood cells to the oxidative machinery within mitochondria. Delivery of O_2 to mitochondria may be insufficient for several reasons.

For example, cardiac output, Hgb, or the O_2 content of arterial blood can each be inadequate for independent reasons. Alternatively, despite adequate cardiac output, perfusion of capillary networks can be impaired as a consequence of dysregulation of arteriolar tone, microvascular thrombosis, or obstruction of nutritive vessels by sequestered leukocytes or platelets. Hemodynamic monitoring that does not take into account all of these factors will portray an incomplete and perhaps misleading picture of cellular physiology.

Under normal conditions when the supply of O_2 is plentiful, aerobic metabolism is determined by factors other than the availability of O_2. These factors include the hormonal milieu and mechanical workload of contractile tissue. However, in pathologic circumstances when O_2 availability is inadequate, O_2 utilization ($\dot{V}O_2$) becomes dependent upon O_2 delivery ($\dot{D}O_2$). The relationship of $\dot{V}O_2$ to $\dot{D}O_2$ over a broad range of $\dot{D}O_2$ values is commonly represented as two intersecting straight lines. In the region of higher $\dot{D}O_2$ values, the slope of the line is approximately equal to zero, indicating that $\dot{V}O_2$ is largely independent of $\dot{D}O_2$. In contrast, in the region of low $\dot{D}O_2$ values, the slope of the line is nonzero and positive, indicating that $\dot{V}O_2$ is supply dependent. The region where the two lines intersect is called the point of critical O_2 delivery ($\dot{D}O_{2crit}$), and represents the transition from supply-independent to supply-dependent O_2 uptake. Below this critical threshold of O_2 delivery (approximately 4.5 mL/kg per minute), increased O_2 extraction cannot compensate for the delivery deficit; hence, O_2

consumption begins to decrease.[1] The slope of the supply-dependent region of the plot reflects the maximal O_2 extraction capability of the vascular bed being evaluated.

The dual-line representation for depicting $\dot{D}O_2$-$\dot{V}O_2$ relationships has proven useful and informative. Nevertheless, other approaches for depicting $\dot{D}O_2$-$\dot{V}O_2$ relationships may be equally or even more relevant. For example, some investigators believe that experimentally derived $\dot{D}O_2$-$\dot{V}O_2$ data are optimally characterized by using the classic Michaelis-Menten relationship for describing the kinetics of an enzymatic reaction, a view that is prompted by the recognition that the oxygen-consuming reaction in mitochondria is catalyzed by an enzyme, cytochrome oxidase.[2]

ARTERIAL BLOOD PRESSURE

The pressure exerted by blood in the systemic arterial system, commonly referred to as *blood pressure*, is a cardinal parameter measured as part of the hemodynamic monitoring of patients. Extremes in blood pressure are either intrinsically deleterious or are indicative of a serious perturbation in normal physiology. In the past, blood pressure served as a proxy for cardiac output; the term *shock* was used more or less as a synonym for arterial hypotension. Although it is now known that arterial blood pressure is a complex function of both cardiac output and vascular input impedance, clinicians, especially inexperienced ones, tend to assume that the presence of a normal blood pressure is evidence that cardiac output and tissue perfusion are adequate. This assumption is frequently incorrect and is the reason why some critically ill patients may benefit from forms of hemodynamic monitoring in addition to measurement of arterial pressure.

Blood pressure can be determined directly by measuring the pressure within the arterial lumen or indirectly using a cuff around an extremity. When the equipment is properly set up and calibrated, direct intra-arterial monitoring of blood pressure provides accurate and continuous data. Additionally, intra-arterial catheters provide a convenient way to obtain samples of blood for measurements of arterial blood gases and other laboratory studies. Despite these advantages, intra-arterial catheters are invasive devices and occasionally are associated with serious complications. Noninvasive monitoring of blood pressure is desirable in many circumstances.

Noninvasive Measurement of Arterial Blood Pressure

Both manual and automated means for the noninvasive determination of blood pressure use an inflatable cuff to increase pressure around an extremity. If the cuff is too narrow (relative to the extremity), the measured pressure will be artifactually elevated.

KEY POINTS

1. The delivery of modern critical care is predicated on the ability to monitor a large number of physiologic variables and formulate evidenced-based therapeutic strategies to manage these variables.

2. Technologic advances in monitoring have at least a theoretical risk of exceeding our ability to understand the clinical implications of the derived information. This could result in the use of monitoring data to make inappropriate clinical decisions. Therefore, the implementation of any new monitoring technology must take into account the relevance and accuracy of the data obtained, the risks to the

patient, as well as the evidence supporting any intervention directed at correcting the detected abnormality.

3. The routine use of invasive monitoring devices, specifically the pulmonary artery catheter, must be questioned in light of the available evidence that does not demonstrate a clear benefit to its widespread use in various populations of critically ill patients.

4. The future of physiologic monitoring will be dominated by the application of noninvasive and highly accurate devices that guide evidenced-based therapy.

Therefore, the width of the cuff should be approximately 40% of its circumference.

In addition to using a cuff to cause vascular compression and thereby cessation of blood flow, noninvasive means for measuring blood pressure also require some means for detecting the presence or absence of arterial pulsations. Several methods exist for this purpose. The time-honored approach is the auscultation of the Korotkoff sounds, which are heard over an artery distal to the cuff as the cuff is deflated from a pressure higher than systolic pressure to one less than diastolic pressure. *Systolic pressure* is defined as the pressure in the cuff when tapping sounds are first audible. *Diastolic pressure* is the pressure in the cuff when audible pulsations first disappear.

Another means for pulse detection when measuring blood pressure noninvasively depends upon the detection of oscillations in the pressure within the bladder of the cuff. This approach is simple, and unlike auscultation, can be performed even in a noisy environment (e.g., a busy emergency room). Unfortunately, this approach is neither accurate nor reliable. Other methods, however, can be used to reliably detect the reappearance of a pulse distal to the cuff and thereby estimate systolic blood pressure. Two excellent and widely available approaches for pulse detection are use of a Doppler stethoscope (reappearance of the pulse produces an audible amplified signal) or a pulse oximeter (reappearance of the pulse is indicated by flashing of a light-emitting diode).

A number of automated devices are capable of repetitively measuring blood pressure noninvasively. Some of these devices measure pressure oscillations in the inflatable bladder encircling the extremity to detect arterial pulsations as pressure in the cuff is gradually lowered from greater than systolic to less than diastolic pressure.[3] Another automated noninvasive device uses a piezoelectric crystal positioned over the brachial artery as a pulse detector.[3] According to one clinical study of these approaches, the most accurate is oscillometry combined with stepped deflation of the sphygmomanometric cuff. Using this approach and comparing the results of oscillometry to those obtained by invasive intra-arterial monitoring, errors in the measurement of mean blood pressure greater than 10 or 20 mmHg occur in 0% and 8.5% of readings, respectively.[3]

Another noninvasive approach for measuring blood pressure relies on a technique called *photoplethysmography*. This method is capable of providing continuous information because systolic and diastolic blood pressures are recorded on a beat-to-beat basis. Photoplethysmography uses the transmission of infrared light to estimate the amount of Hgb (directly related to the volume of blood) in a finger placed under a servo-controlled inflatable cuff. A feedback loop controlled by a microprocessor continually adjusts the pressure in the cuff to maintain the blood volume of the finger constant. Under these conditions, the pressure in the cuff reflects the pressure in the digital artery. Although results obtained using photoplethysmography generally agree closely with those obtained by invasive monitoring of blood pressure, the difference between the two methods occasionally can be large (20 to 40 mmHg) in some patients.[4] This problem limits the usefulness of photoplethysmography as a stand-alone method for monitoring arterial blood pressure, particularly in high-risk situations. However, if initial photoplethysmographic readings are corrected by comparison with measurements obtained noninvasively by an oscillometric device, then photoplethysmography is sufficiently accurate to be used for continuous monitoring in most situations.[4]

Invasive Monitoring of Arterial Blood Pressure

Direct monitoring of arterial pressure in critically ill patients may be performed by using fluid-filled tubing to connect an intra-arterial catheter to an external strain-gauge transducer. The signal generated by the transducer is electronically amplified and displayed as a continuous waveform by an oscilloscope. Digital values for systolic and diastolic pressure also are displayed. Mean pressure, calculated by electronically averaging the amplitude of the pressure waveform, also can be displayed.

The fidelity of the catheter-tubing-transducer system is determined by numerous factors, including the compliance of the tubing, the surface area of the transducer diaphragm, and the compliance of the diaphragm. If the system is underdamped, then the inertia of the system, which is a function of the mass of the fluid in the tubing and the mass of the diaphragm, causes overshoot of the points of maximum positive and negative displacement of the diaphragm during systole and diastole, respectively. Thus in an underdamped system, systolic pressure will be overestimated and diastolic pressure will be underestimated. In an overdamped system, displacement of the diaphragm fails to track the rapidly changing pressure waveform, and systolic pressure will be underestimated and diastolic pressure will be overestimated. It is important to note that even in an underdamped or overdamped system, mean pressure will be accurately recorded, provided the system has been properly calibrated. For these reasons, when using direct measurement of intra-arterial pressure to monitor patients, clinicians should make clinical decisions based on the measured mean arterial blood pressure.

The degree of ringing (i.e., overshoot and undershoot) in a minimally damped system is determined by its resonant frequency. Ideally, the resonant frequency of the system should be at least five times greater than the highest frequency component of the pressure waveform. The resonant frequency can be too low for optimal performance if the connector tubing is too compliant or there are air bubbles in the fluid column between the arterial pressure source and the diaphragm of the transducer. For arterial pressure monitoring, the optimal resonance frequency is higher than is practically obtainable. Therefore, to prevent excessive ringing, some degree of damping is essential. To determine if the combination of resonance frequency and damping is adequate, one can pressurize the system to approximately 300 mmHg by pulling the tab that controls the valve between the monitoring system and the high-pressure bag of flush solution. When the valve is abruptly closed by allowing the tab to snap back into its normal position, a sharp pressure transient will be introduced into the system. The resulting pressure tracing can be observed on a strip chart recording. Damping is optimal if at least two oscillations are observed, and there is at least a threefold decrease in the amplitude of successive oscillations.

The radial artery at the wrist is the site most commonly used for intra-arterial pressure monitoring. It is important to recognize, however, that measured arterial pressure is determined in part by the site where the pressure is monitored. Central (i.e., aortic) and peripheral (e.g., radial artery) pressures typically are different as a result of the impedance and inductance of the arterial tree. Systolic pressures typically are higher and diastolic pressures are lower in the periphery, whereas mean pressure is approximately the same in the aorta and more distal sites.

Distal ischemia is an uncommon complication of intra-arterial catheterization. The incidence of thrombosis is increased when larger-caliber catheters are used and when catheters are left in place for an extended period of time. The incidence of thrombosis can be minimized by using a 20-gauge (or smaller) catheter in the radial artery and removing the catheter as soon as feasible. The risk of distal ischemic injury can be reduced by ensuring that adequate collateral flow is present before catheter insertion. At the wrist, adequate collateral flow can be documented by performing a modified version of the Allen test, wherein the artery to be cannulated is digitally compressed while using a Doppler stethoscope to listen for perfusion in the palmar arch vessels.

Another potential complication of intra-arterial monitoring is retrograde embolization of air bubbles or thrombi into the intracranial circulation. In order to minimize the risk of this rare but potentially devastating complication, great care should be taken to avoid flushing arterial lines when air is present in the system, and only small volumes of fluid (less than 5 mL) should be used for this purpose. Catheter-related infections can occur with any intravascular monitoring device. However, catheter-related bloodstream infection is a relatively uncommon complication of intra-arterial lines used for monitoring, occurring in 0.4 to 0.7% of catheterizations.[5] The incidence increases with longer duration of arterial catheterization.

ELECTROCARDIOGRAPHIC MONITORING

The electrocardiogram (ECG) records the electrical activity associated with cardiac contraction by detecting voltages on the body surface. A standard 3-lead ECG is obtained by placing electrodes that correspond to the left arm (LA), right arm (RA), and left leg (LL). The limb leads are defined as lead I (LA-RA), lead II (LL-RA), and lead III (LL-LA). The ECG waveforms can be continuously displayed on a monitor, and the devices can be set to sound an alarm if an abnormality of rate or rhythm is detected. Continuous ECG monitoring is widely available and applied to critically ill and perioperative patients. Monitoring of the ECG waveform is essential in patients with acute coronary syndromes or blunt myocardial injury, because dysrhythmias are the most common lethal complication. In patients with shock or sepsis, dysrhythmias can occur as a consequence of inadequate myocardial O_2 delivery or as a complication of vasoactive or inotropic drugs used to support blood pressure and cardiac output. Dysrhythmias can be detected by continuously monitoring the ECG tracing, and timely intervention may prevent serious complications. With appropriate computing hardware and software, continuous ST-segment analysis also can be performed to detect ischemia or infarction. This approach has proven useful to detect silent myocardial ischemia in patients undergoing weaning from mechanical ventilation.[6,7]

Additional information can be obtained from a 12-lead ECG, which is essential for patients with potential myocardial ischemia or to rule out cardiac complications in other acutely ill patients. Continuous monitoring of the 12-lead ECG now is available and is proving to be beneficial in certain patient populations. In a study of 185 vascular surgical patients, continuous 12-lead ECG monitoring was able to detect transient myocardial ischemic episodes in 20.5% of the patients.[7] This study demonstrated that the precordial lead V_4, which is not routinely monitored on a standard 3-lead ECG, is the most sensitive for detecting perioperative ischemia and infarction. To detect 95% of the ischemic episodes, two or more precordial leads were necessary. Thus, continuous 12-lead ECG monitoring may provide greater sensitivity than 3-lead ECG for the detection of perioperative myocardial ischemia, and is likely to become standard for monitoring high-risk surgical patients.

CARDIAC OUTPUT AND RELATED PARAMETERS

Bedside catheterization of the pulmonary artery was introduced into clinical practice in the 1970s. Although the pulmonary artery catheter (PAC) initially was used primarily to manage patients with cardiogenic shock and other acute cardiac diseases, indications for this form of invasive hemodynamic monitoring gradually expanded to encompass a wide variety of clinical conditions. Clearly, many clinicians believe that information valuable for the management of critically ill patients is afforded by having a PAC in place. However, unambiguous data in support of this view are scarce, and several studies suggest that bedside pulmonary artery catheterization may not benefit most critically ill patients, and in fact lead to some serous complications, as is discussed in Effect of Pulmonary Artery Catheterization on Outcome below.

Determinants of Cardiac Performance
Preload

Starling's law of the heart states that the force of muscle contraction depends on the initial length of the cardiac fibers. Using terminology that derives from early experiments using isolated cardiac muscle preparations, preload is the stretch of ventricular myocardial tissue just before the next contraction. Preload is determined by end-diastolic volume (EDV). For the right ventricle, central venous pressure (CVP) approximates right ventricular (RV) end-diastolic pressure (EDP). For the left ventricle, pulmonary artery occlusion pressure (PAOP), which is measured by transiently inflating a balloon at the end of a pressure monitoring catheter positioned in a small branch of the pulmonary artery, approximates left ventricular EDP. The presence of atrioventricular valvular stenosis will alter this relationship.

Clinicians frequently use EDP as a surrogate for EDV, but EDP is determined not only by volume but also by the diastolic compliance of the ventricular chamber. Ventricular compliance is altered by various pathologic conditions and pharmacologic agents. Furthermore, the relationship between EDP and true preload is not linear, but rather is exponential.

Afterload

Afterload is another term derived from in vitro experiments using isolated strips of cardiac muscle, and is defined as the force resisting fiber shortening once systole begins. Several factors comprise the in vivo correlate of ventricular afterload, including ventricular intracavitary pressure, wall thickness, chamber radius, and chamber geometry. Because these factors are difficult to assess clinically, afterload is commonly approximated by calculating systemic vascular resistance, defined as mean arterial pressure (MAP) divided by cardiac output.

Contractility

Contractility is defined as the inotropic state of the myocardium. Contractility is said to increase when the force of ventricular contraction increases at constant preload and afterload. Clinically, contractility is difficult to quantify, because virtually all of the available measures are dependent to a certain degree on preload and afterload. If pressure-volume loops are constructed for each cardiac cycle, small changes in preload and/or afterload will result in shifts of the point defining the end of diastole. These end-diastolic points on the pressure-versus-volume diagram describe a straight line, known as the *isovolumic pressure line*. A steeper slope of this line indicates greater contractility.

Placement of the Pulmonary Artery Catheter

In its simplest form, the PAC has four channels. One channel terminates in a balloon at the tip of the catheter. The proximal end of this channel is connected to a syringe to permit inflation of the balloon with air. Before insertion of the PAC, the integrity of the balloon should be verified by inflating it. To minimize the risk of vascular or ventricular perforation by the relatively inflexible catheter, it is important to verify that the inflated balloon extends just beyond the tip of the device. A second channel in the catheter contains wires that are connected to a thermistor located near the tip of the catheter. At the proximal end of the PAC, the wires terminate in a fitting that permits connection to appropriate hardware for the calculation of cardiac output using the thermodilution technique (see Measurement of Cardiac Output by Thermodilution below). The final two channels are used for pressure monitoring and the injection of the thermal indicator for determinations of cardiac output. One of these channels terminates at the tip of the catheter; the other terminates 20 cm proximal to the tip.

Placement of a PAC requires access to the central venous circulation. Such access can be obtained at a variety of sites, including the antecubital, femoral, jugular, and subclavian veins. Percutaneous placement through either the jugular or subclavian vein generally is preferred. Right internal jugular vein cannulation carries the lowest risk of complications, and the path of the catheter from this site into the right atrium is straight. In the event of inadvertent arterial puncture, local pressure is significantly more effective in controlling bleeding from the carotid artery as compared to the subclavian artery. Nevertheless, it is more difficult to keep occlusive dressings in place on the neck than in the subclavian fossa. Furthermore, the anatomic landmarks in the subclavian position are quite constant, even in patients with anasarca or massive obesity; the subclavian vein is always attached to the deep (concave) surface of the clavicle. In contrast, the appropriate landmarks to guide jugular venous cannulation are sometimes difficult to discern in obese or very edematous patients. However, ultrasonic guidance has been shown to facilitate bedside jugular venipuncture.[8]

Cannulation of the vein normally is performed percutaneously, using the Seldinger technique. A small-bore needle is inserted through the skin and subcutaneous tissue into the vein. After documenting return of venous blood, a guidewire with a flexible tip is inserted through the needle into the vein and the needle is withdrawn. A dilator/introducer sheath is passed over the wire, and the wire and the dilator are removed. The introducer sheath is equipped with a side port, which can be used for administering fluid. The introducer sheath also is equipped with a diaphragm that permits insertion of the PAC while preventing the backflow of venous blood. The proximal terminus of the distal port of the PAC is connected through low-compliance tubing to a strain-gauge transducer, and the tubing-catheter system is flushed with fluid. While constantly observing the pressure tracing on an oscilloscope, the PAC is advanced with the balloon deflated until respiratory excursions are observed. The balloon is then inflated, and the catheter advanced further, while monitoring pressures sequentially in the right atrium and right ventricle en route to the pulmonary artery. The pressure waveforms for the right atrium, right ventricle, and pulmonary artery are each characteristic and easy to recognize. The catheter is advanced out the pulmonary artery until a damped tracing indicative of the "wedged" position is obtained. The balloon is then deflated, taking care to ensure that a normal pulmonary arterial tracing is again observed on the monitor; leaving the balloon inflated can increase the risk of pulmonary infarction or perforation of the pulmonary artery. Unnecessary measurements of the PAOP are discouraged as rupture of the pulmonary artery may occur.

Hemodynamic Measurements

Even in its simplest embodiment, the PAC is capable of providing clinicians with a remarkable amount of information about the hemodynamic status of patients. Additional information may be obtained if various modifications of the standard PAC are used. By combining data obtained through use of the PAC with results obtained by other means (i.e., blood Hgb concentration and oxyhemoglobin saturation), derived estimates of systemic O_2 transport and utilization can be calculated. Direct and derived parameters obtainable by bedside pulmonary arterial catheterization are summarized in Table 13-1.

TABLE 13-1	Directly measured and derived hemodynamic data obtainable by bedside pulmonary artery catheterization	
Standard PAC	**PAC with Additional Feature(s)**	**Derived Parameters**
CVP	S$\bar{v}O_2$ (continuous)	SV (or SVI)
PAP	Q_T or Q_T* (continuous)	SVR (or SVRI)
PAOP	RVEF	PVR (or PVRI)
S$\bar{v}O_2$ (intermittent)		RVEDV
Q_T or Q_T* (intermittent)		$\dot{D}O_2$
		$\dot{V}O_2$
		ER
		Q_S/Q_T

CVP = mean central venous pressure; $\dot{D}O_2$ = systemic oxygen delivery; ER = systemic oxygen extraction ratio; PAC = pulmonary artery catheter; PAOP = pulmonary artery occlusion (wedge) pressure; PAP = pulmonary artery pressure; PVR = pulmonary vascular resistance; PVRI = pulmonary vascular resistance index; Q_S/Q_T = fractional pulmonary venous admixture (shunt fraction); Q_T = cardiac output; Q_T* = cardiac output indexed to body surface area (cardiac index); RVEDV = right ventricular end-diastolic volume; RVEF = right ventricular ejection fraction; SV = stroke volume; SVI = stroke volume index; S$\bar{v}O_2$ = fractional mixed venous (pulmonary artery) hemoglobin saturation; SVR = systemic vascular resistance; SVRI = systemic vascular resistance index; $\dot{V}O_2$ = systemic oxygen utilization.

TABLE 13-2	Formulas for calculation of hemodynamic parameters that can be derived by using data obtained by pulmonary artery catheterization

Q_T* (L·min^{-1}·m^{-2}) = Q_T/BSA, where BSA is body surface area (m^2)

SV (mL) = Q_T/HR, where HR is heart rate (min^{-1})

SVR (dyne·sec·cm^{-5}) = [(MAP − CVP) × 80]/Q_T, where MAP is mean arterial pressure (mmHg)

SVRI (dyne·sec·cm^{-5}·m^{-2}) = [(MAP − CVP) × 80]/Q_T*

PVR (dyne·sec·cm^{-5}) = [(PAP − PAOP) × 80]/QT, where PPA is mean pulmonary artery pressure

PVRI (dyne·sec·cm^{-5}·m^{-2}) = [(PAP − PAOP) × 80]/Q_T*

RVEDV (mL) = SV/RVEF

$\dot{D}O_2$ (mL·min^{-1}·m^{-2}) = Q_T* × CaO_2 × 10, where CaO_2 is arterial oxygen content (mL/dL)

$\dot{V}O_2$ (mL·min^{-1}·m^{-2}) = Q_T* × (CaO_2 − $C\bar{v}O_2$) × 10, where $C\bar{v}O_2$ is mixed venous oxygen content (mL/dL)

CaO_2 = (1.36 × Hgb × SaO_2) + (0.003 + PaO_2), where Hgb is hemoglobin concentration (g/dL), SaO_2 is fractional arterial hemoglobin saturation, and PaO_2 is the partial pressure of oxygen in arterial blood

$C\bar{v}O_2$ = (1.36 × Hgb × $S\bar{v}O_2$) + (0.003 + $P\bar{v}O_2$), where $P\bar{v}O_2$ is the partial pressure of oxygen in pulmonary arterial (mixed venous) blood

Q_S/Q_T = (CcO_2 − CaO_2)/(CcO_2 − $C\bar{v}O_2$), where CcO_2 (mL/dL) is the content of oxygen in pulmonary end capillary blood

CcO_2 = (1.36 × Hgb) + (0.003 + PAO_2), where PAO_2 is the alveolar partial pressure of oxygen

PAO_2 = [FiO_2 × (P_B − P_{H2O})] − $PaCO_2$/RQ, where FiO_2 is the fractional concentration of inspired oxygen, P_B is the barometric pressure (mmHg), P_{H2O} is the water vapor pressure (usually 47 mmHg), $PaCO_2$ is the partial pressure of carbon dioxide in arterial blood (mmHg), and RQ is respiratory quotient (usually assumed to be 0.8)

$C\bar{v}O_2$ = central venous oxygen pressure; CVP = mean central venous pressure; $\dot{D}O_2$ = systemic oxygen delivery; PAOP = pulmonary artery occlusion (wedge) pressure; PVR = pulmonary vascular resistance; PVRI = pulmonary vascular resistance index; Q_S/Q_T = fractional pulmonary venous admixture (shunt fraction); Q_T = cardiac output; Q_T* = cardiac output indexed to body surface area (cardiac index); RVEDV = right ventricular end-diastolic volume; RVEF = right ventricular ejection fraction; SV = stroke volume; SVI = stroke volume index; S$\bar{v}O_2$ = fractional mixed venous (pulmonary artery) hemoglobin saturation; SVR = systemic vascular resistance; SVRI = systemic vascular resistance index; $\dot{V}O_2$ = systemic oxygen utilization.

The equations used to calculate the derived parameters are summarized in Table 13-2. The approximate normal ranges for a number of these hemodynamic parameters (in adults) are shown in Table 13-3.

Measurement of Cardiac Output by Thermodilution

Before the development of the PAC, determining cardiac output (Q_T) at the bedside required careful measurements of O_2 consumption (Fick method) or spectrophotometric determination of indocyanine green dye dilution curves. Measurements of Q_T using the thermodilution technique are simple and reasonably accurate. The measurements can be performed repetitively, and the principle is straightforward. If a bolus of an indicator is rapidly and thoroughly mixed with a moving fluid upstream from a detector, then the concentration of the indicator at the detector will increase sharply and then exponentially diminish back to zero. The area under the resulting time-concentration curve is a function of the volume of indicator injected and the flow rate of the moving stream of fluid. Larger volumes of indicator result in greater areas under the curve, and faster flow rates of the mixing fluid result in smaller areas under the curve. When Q_T is measured by thermodilution, the indicator is heat and the detector is a temperature-sensing thermistor at the distal end of the PAC. The relationship used for calculating Q_T is called the *Stewart-Hamilton equation*:

$$Q_T = [V \times (T_B - T_I) \times K_1 \times K_2] \div \int T_B(t)dt$$

TABLE 13-3	Approximate normal ranges for selected hemodynamic parameters in adults

Parameter	Normal Range
CVP	0–6 mmHg
Right ventricular systolic pressure	20–30 mmHg
Right ventricular diastolic pressure	0–6 mmHg
PAOP	6–12 mmHg
Systolic arterial pressure	100–130 mmHg
Diastolic arterial pressure	60–90 mmHg
MAP	75–100 mmHg
Q_T	4–6 L/min
Q_T*	2.5–3.5 $L \cdot min^{-1} \cdot m^{-2}$
SV	40–80 mL
SVR	800–1400 $dyne \cdot sec \cdot cm^{-5}$
SVRI	1500–2400 $dyne \cdot sec \cdot cm^{-5} \cdot m^{-2}$
PVR	100–150 $dyne \cdot sec \cdot cm^{-5}$
PVRI	200–400 $dyne \cdot sec \cdot cm^{-5} \cdot m^{-2}$
CaO_2	16–22 mL/dL
$C\bar{v}O_2$	~15 mL/dL
$\dot{D}O_2$	400–660 $mL \cdot min^{-1} \cdot m^{-2}$
$\dot{V}O_2$	115–165 $mL \cdot min^{-1} \cdot m^{-2}$

CaO_2 = arterial oxygen content; $C\bar{v}O_2$ = central venous oxygen pressure; CVP = mean central venous pressure; $\dot{D}O_2$ = systemic oxygen delivery; MAP = mean arterial pressure; PAOP = pulmonary artery occlusion (wedge) pressure; PVR = pulmonary vascular resistance; PVRI = pulmonary vascular resistance index; Q_T = cardiac output; Q_T* = cardiac output indexed to body surface area (cardiac index); SV = stroke volume; SVI = stroke volume index; SVR = systemic vascular resistance; SVRI = systemic vascular resistance index; $\dot{V}O_2$ = systemic oxygen utilization.

where V is the volume of the indicator injected, T_B is the temperature of blood (i.e., core body temperature), T_I is the temperature of the indicator, K_1 is a constant that is the function of the specific heats of blood and the indicator, K_2 is an empirically derived constant that accounts for several factors (the dead space volume of the catheter, heat lost from the indicator as it traverses the catheter, and the injection rate of the indicator), and $\int T_B(t)dt$ is the area under the time-temperature curve. In clinical practice, the Stewart-Hamilton equation is solved by a microprocessor.

Determination of cardiac output by the thermodilution method is generally quite accurate, although it tends to systematically overestimate Q_T at low values. Changes in blood temperature and Q_T during the respiratory cycle can influence the measurement. Therefore, results generally should be recorded as the mean of two or three determinations obtained at random points in the respiratory cycle. Using cold injectate widens the difference between T_B and T_I and thereby increases signal-to-noise ratio. Nevertheless, most authorities recommend using room temperature injectate (normal saline or 5% dextrose in water) to minimize errors resulting from warming of the fluid as it transferred from its reservoir to a syringe for injection.

Technologic innovations have been introduced that permit continuous measurement of Q_T by thermodilution. In this approach, thermal transients are not generated by injecting a bolus of a cold indicator, but rather by heating the blood with a tiny filament located on the PAC upstream from the thermistor. By correlating the amount of current supplied to the heating element with the downstream temperature of the blood, it is possible to estimate the average blood flow across the filament and thereby calculate Q_T. Based upon the results of several studies, continuous determinations of Q_T using this approach agree well with data generated by conventional measurements using bolus injections of a cold indicator.[9] Information is lacking regarding the clinical value of being able to monitor Q_T continuously.

Mixed Venous Oximetry

The Fick equation can be written as $Q_T = \dot{V}O_2/(CaO_2 - C\bar{v}O_2)$, where CaO_2 is the content of O_2 in arterial blood and $C\bar{v}O_2$ is the content

of O_2 in mixed venous blood. The Fick equation can be rearranged as follows: $C\bar{v}O_2 = CaO_2 - \dot{V}O_2/Q_T$. If the small contribution of dissolved O_2 to $C\bar{v}O_2$ and CaO_2 is ignored, the rearranged equation can be rewritten as $S\bar{v}O_2 = SaO_2 - \dot{V}O_2/(Q_T \times Hgb \times 1.36)$, where $S\bar{v}O_2$ is the fractional saturation of Hgb in mixed venous blood, SaO_2 is the fractional saturation of Hgb in arterial blood, and Hgb is the concentration of Hgb in blood. Thus, it can be seen that $S\bar{v}O_2$ is a function of $\dot{V}O_2$ (i.e., metabolic rate), Q_T, SaO_2, and Hgb. Accordingly, subnormal values of $S\bar{v}O_2$ can be caused by a decrease in Q_T (due, for example, to heart failure or hypovolemia), a decrease in SaO_2 (due, for example, to intrinsic pulmonary disease), a decrease in Hgb (i.e., anemia), or an increase in metabolic rate (due, for example, to seizures or fever). With a conventional PAC, measurements of $S\bar{v}O_2$ require aspirating a sample of blood from the distal (i.e., pulmonary arterial) port of the catheter and injecting the sample into a blood gas analyzer. Therefore for practical purposes, measurements of $S\bar{v}O_2$ can be performed only intermittently.

By adding a fifth channel to the PAC, it has become possible to monitor $S\bar{v}O_2$ continuously. The fifth channel contains two fiber-optic bundles, which are used to transmit and receive light of the appropriate wavelengths to permit measurements of Hgb saturation by reflectance spectrophotometry. A clinical study of the Abbott Oximetrix PAC has documented that the device provides measurements of $S\bar{v}O_2$ that agree quite closely with those obtained by conventional analyses of blood aspirated from the pulmonary artery.[10] Despite the theoretical value of being able to monitor $S\bar{v}O_2$ continuously, data are lacking to show that this capability favorably improves outcome. Indeed, in several studies, the ability to monitor $S\bar{v}O_2$ was not shown to affect the management of critically ill patients.[11,12] Moreover, in another large study, titrating the resuscitation of critically ill patients to maintain $S\bar{v}O_2$ greater than 69% (i.e., in the normal range) failed to improve mortality or change length of ICU stay.[13] In a recent prospective, observational study of 3265 patients undergoing cardiac surgery with either a standard PAC or a PAC with continuous $S\bar{v}O_2$ monitoring, the oximetric catheter was associated with fewer arterial blood gases and thermodilution cardiac output determinations, but no difference in patient outcome.[14] Because PACs that permit continuous monitoring of $S\bar{v}O_2$ are much more expensive than conventional PACs, the routine use of these devices cannot be recommended.

The saturation of O_2 in the right atrium or superior vena cava ($ScvO_2$) correlates closely with $S\bar{v}O_2$ over a wide range of conditions,[15] although the correlation between $ScvO_2$ and $S\bar{v}O_2$ has recently been questioned.[16] Since measurement of $ScvO_2$ requires placement of a central venous catheter (CVC) rather than a PAC, it is somewhat less invasive and easier to carry out. By using a CVC equipped to permit fiber-optic monitoring of $ScvO_2$, it may be possible to titrate the resuscitation of patients with shock using a less invasive device than the PAC.[15,17]

Right Ventricular Ejection Fraction

Ejection fraction (EF) is calculated as (EDV – ESV)/EDV, where ESV is end-systolic volume. EF is an ejection-phase measure of myocardial contractility. By equipping a PAC with a thermistor with a short time constant, the thermodilution method can be used to estimate RVEF. Measurements of RVEF by thermodilution agree reasonably well with those obtained by other means, although values obtained by thermodilution typically are lower than those obtained by radionuclide cardiography.[18] Stroke volume (SV) is calculated as EDV – ESV. Left ventricular stroke volume (LVSV) also equals Q_T/HR, where HR is heart rate. Because LVSV is equal to RVSV, it is possible to estimate right ventricular end-diastolic volume by measuring RVEF, Q_T, and HR.

Several studies have attempted to assess the clinical value of RVEF measurements using these catheters. In one study, use of an RVEF catheter did not alter therapy in 93% of patients with sepsis, hemorrhagic shock, or acute respiratory distress syndrome (ARDS), but was useful in cases of abdominal compartment syndrome (ACS) with high

PAOP despite low preload.[19] In a series of 46 trauma patients who required more than 10 L of fluid in the first 24 hours of resuscitation, there was a better correlation between RV volume and Q_T than there was with PAOP.[20] However, data are lacking to show that outcomes are improved by making measurements of RVEF in addition to Q_T and other parameters measured by the conventional PAC.

Effect of Pulmonary Artery Catheterization on Outcome

In 1996, Connors and colleagues reported surprising results in a major observational study evaluating the value of pulmonary artery catheterization in critically ill patients.[21] They took advantage of an enormous data set, which had been previously (and prospectively) collected for another purpose at five major teaching hospitals in the United States. These researchers compared two groups of patients: those who did and those who did not undergo placement of a PAC during their first 24 hours of ICU care. The investigators recognized that the value of their intended analysis was completely dependent on the robustness of their methodology for case-matching, because sicker patients (i.e., those at greater risk of mortality based upon the severity of their illness) were presumably more likely to undergo pulmonary artery catheterization. Accordingly, the authors used sophisticated statistical methods for generating a cohort of study (i.e., PAC) patients, each one having a paired control matched carefully for severity of illness. A critical assessment of their published findings supports the view that the cases and their controls were indeed remarkably well matched with respect to a large number of pertinent clinical parameters. Connors and associates concluded that placement of a PAC during the first 24 hours of stay in an ICU is associated with a significant increase in the risk of mortality, even when statistical methods are used to account for severity of illness.

Although the report by Connors and coworkers generated an enormous amount of controversy in the medical community, the results reported actually confirmed the results of two prior similar observational studies. The first of these studies used as a database 3263 patients with acute myocardial infarction treated in central Massachusetts in 1975, 1978, 1981, and 1984 as part of the Worcester Heart Attack Study.[22] For all patients, hospital mortality was significantly greater for patients treated using a PAC, even when multivari-

ate statistical methods were used to control for key potential confounding factors such as age, peak circulating creatine kinase concentration, and presence or absence of new Q waves on the ECG. The second large observational study of patients with acute myocardial infarction also found that hospital mortality was significantly greater for patients managed with the assistance of a PAC, even when the presence or absence of "pump failure" was considered in the statistical analysis.[23] In neither of these reports did the authors conclude that placement of a PAC was truly the cause of worsened survival after myocardial infarction.

The available prospective, randomized controlled trials of PACization are summarized in Table 13-4. The study by Pearson and associates was underpowered with only 226 patients enrolled.[24] In addition, the attending anesthesiologists were permitted to exclude patients from the CVP group at their discretion; thus randomization was compromised. The study by Tuman and coworkers was large (1094 patients were enrolled), but different anesthesiologists were assigned to the different groups.[25] Furthermore, 39 patients in the CVP group underwent placement of a PAC because of hemodynamic complications. All of the individual single-institution studies of vascular surgery patients were relatively underpowered, and all excluded at least certain categories of patients (e.g., those with a history of recent myocardial infarction).[26,27]

In the largest randomized controlled trial of the PAC, Sandham and associates randomized 1994 American Society of Anesthesiologists class III and IV patients undergoing major thoracic, abdominal, or orthopedic surgery to placement of a PAC or CVP catheter.[28] In the patients assigned to receive a PAC, physiologic, goal-directed therapy was implemented by protocol. There were no differences in mortality at 30 days, 6 months, or 12 months between the two groups, and ICU length of stay was similar. There was a significantly higher rate of pulmonary emboli in the PAC group (0.9 vs. 0%). This study has been criticized because most of the patients enrolled were not in the highest risk category.

In the "PAC-Man" trial, a multicenter, randomized trial in 65 United Kingdom hospitals, more than 1000 ICU patients were managed with or without a PAC.[29] The specifics of the clinical management were then left up to the treating clinicians. There was no difference in hospital mortality between the two groups (with PAC 68% vs. without PAC 66%, $P = .39$). However, a 9.5% complication

---

TABLE 13-4 Summary of randomized, prospective clinical trials comparing pulmonary artery catheter with central venous pressure monitoring

Author	Study Population	Groups	Outcomes
Pearson, et al[24]	"Low-risk" patients undergoing cardiac or vascular surgery	CVP catheter (group 1); PAC (group 2); PAC with continuous $S\bar{v}O_2$, readout (group 3)	No differences among groups for mortality or length of ICU stay; significant differences in costs (group 1 < group 2 < group 3)
Tuman, et al[25]	Cardiac surgical patients	PAC; CVP	No differences between groups for mortality, length of ICU stay, or significant noncardiac complications
Bender, et al[26]	Vascular surgery patients	PAC; CVP	No differences between groups for mortality, length of ICU stay, or length of hospital stay
Valentine, et al[27]	Aortic surgery patients	PAC + hemodynamic optimization in ICU night before surgery; CVP	No difference between groups for mortality or length of ICU stay; significantly higher incidence of postoperative complications in PAC group
Sandham, et al[28]	"High-risk" major surgery	PAC; CVP	No differences between groups for mortality, length of ICU stay; increased incidence of pulmonary embolism in PAC group
Harvey, et al[29]	Medical and surgical ICU patients	PAC vs. no PAC, with option for alternative CO measuring device in non-PAC group	No difference in hospital mortality between the two groups, increased incidence of complications in the PAC group
Binanay, et al[31]	Patients with CHF	PAC vs. no PAC	No difference in hospital mortality between the two groups, increased incidence of adverse events in the PAC group
Wheeler, et al[32]	Patients with ALI	PAC vs. CVC with a fluid and inotropic management protocol	No difference in ICU or hospital mortality, or incidence of organ failure between the two groups; increased incidence of adverse events in the PAC group

ALI = acute lung injury; CHF = congestive heart failure; CO = cardiac output; CVC = central venous catheter; CVP = central venous pressure; ICU = intensive care unit; PAC = pulmonary artery catheter; $S\bar{v}O_2$ = fractional mixed venous (pulmonary artery) hemoglobin saturation.

rate was associated with the insertion or use of the PAC, although none of these complications was fatal. Clearly, these were critically ill patients, as noted by the high hospital mortality rates. Supporters of the PAC may cite methodology problems with this study, such as loose inclusion criteria and the lack of a defined treatment protocol.

A recent meta-analysis of 13 randomized studies of the PAC that included more than 5000 patients was recently published.[30] A broad spectrum of critically ill patients was included in these heterogeneous trials, and the hemodynamic goals and treatment strategies varied. Although the use of the PAC was associated with an increased use of inotropes and vasodilators, there were no differences in mortality or hospital length of stay between the patients managed with a PAC and those managed without a PAC.

Next, the ESCAPE trial (which was one of the studies included in the previous meta-analysis)[31] evaluated 433 patients with severe or recurrent congestive heart failure admitted to the ICU. Patients were randomized to management by clinical assessment and a PAC or clinical assessment without a PAC. The goal in both groups was resolution of congestive heart failure, with additional PAC targets of a pulmonary capillary occlusion pressure of 15 mmHg and a right atrial pressure of 8 mmHg. There was no formal treatment protocol, but inotropic support was discouraged. Substantial reduction in symptoms, jugular venous pressure, and edema was noted in both groups. There was no significant difference in the primary endpoint of days alive and out of the hospital during the first 6 months, or hospital mortality (PAC 10%; vs. without PAC 9%). Adverse events were more common among patients in the PAC group (21.9% vs. 11.5%; $P = .04$).

Finally, the Fluids and Catheters Treatment Trial (FACTT) conducted by the Acute Respiratory Distress Syndrome (ARDS) Clinical Trials Network was recently published.[32] The risks and benefits of PAC compared with CVCs were evaluated in 1000 patients with acute lung injury. Patients were randomly assigned to receive either a PAC or a CVC to guide management for 7 days via an explicit protocol. Patients also were randomly assigned to a conservative or liberal fluid strategy in a 2×2 factorial design (outcomes based on the fluid management strategy were published separately). Mortality during the first 60 days was similar in the PAC and CVC groups (27% and 26%; $P = .69$). The duration of mechanical ventilation and ICU length of stay also were not influenced by the type of catheter used. The type of catheter used did not affect the incidence of shock, respiratory or renal failure, ventilator settings, or requirement for hemodialysis or vasopressors. There was a 1% rate of crossover from CVC-guided therapy to PAC-guided therapy. The catheter used did not affect the administration of fluids or diuretics, and the fluid balance was similar in the two groups. The PAC group had approximately twice as many catheter-related adverse events (mainly arrhythmias).

Few subjects in critical care medicine generate more emotional responses among experts in the field than the use of the PAC. Some experts may be able to use the PAC to titrate vasoactive drugs and IV fluids for specific patients in ways that improve their outcomes. But, as these studies indicate, it is impossible to verify that use of the PAC saves lives when it is evaluated over a large population of patients. Certainly, given the current state of knowledge, routine use of the PAC cannot be justified. Whether very selective use of the device in a few relatively uncommon clinical situations is warranted or valuable remains a controversial issue. Consequently, a marked decline in the use of the PAC from 5.66 per 1000 medical admissions in 1993 to 1.99 per 1000 medical admissions in 2004 has been seen.[33] These significant reductions in the use of the PAC were noted for a variety of patients, including those admitted with myocardial infarction, surgical patients, and for patients with septicemia. Based upon the results and exclusion criteria in these prospective randomized trials, reasonable criteria for perioperative monitoring without use of a PAC are presented in Table 13-5.

One of the reasons for using a PAC to monitor critically ill patients is to optimize cardiac output and systemic O_2 delivery.

TABLE 13-5	Suggested criteria for perioperative monitoring without use of a pulmonary artery catheter in patients undergoing cardiac or major vascular surgical procedures

No anticipated need for suprarenal or supraceliac aortic cross-clamping

No history of myocardial infarction during 3 mo before operation

No history of poorly compensated congestive heart failure

No history of coronary artery bypass graft surgery during 6 wk before operation

No history of ongoing symptomatic mitral or aortic valvular heart disease

No history of ongoing unstable angina pectoris

Defining what constitutes the optimum cardiac output, however, has proven to be difficult. Based upon an extensive observational database and comparisons of the hemodynamic and O_2 transport values recorded in survivors and nonsurvivors, Bland and colleagues proposed that "goal-directed" hemodynamic resuscitation should aim to achieve a Q_T greater than 4.5 L/min per square meter and $\dot{D}O_2$ greater than 600 mL/min per square meter.[34] Prompted by these observational findings, a number of investigators have conducted randomized trials designed to evaluate the effect on outcome of goal-directed as compared to conventional hemodynamic resuscitation. Some studies provide support for the notion that interventions designed to achieve supraphysiologic goals for $\dot{D}O_2$, $\dot{V}O_2$, and Q_T improve outcome.[35-37] However, other published studies do not support this view, and a meta-analysis concluded that interventions designed to achieve supraphysiologic goals for O_2 transport do not significantly reduce mortality rates in critically ill patients.[19,38,39] At this time, supraphysiologic resuscitation of patients in shock cannot be endorsed.

There is no simple explanation for the apparent lack of effectiveness of pulmonary artery catheterization. Connors has offered several suggestions.[40] First, even though bedside pulmonary artery catheterization is quite safe, the procedure is associated with a finite incidence of serious complications, including ventricular arrhythmias, catheter-related sepsis, central venous thrombosis, pulmonary arterial perforation, and as noted above, pulmonary embolism.[28,40] The adverse effects of these complications on outcome may equal or even outweigh any benefits associated with using a PAC to guide therapy. Second, the data generated by the PAC may be inaccurate, leading to inappropriate therapeutic interventions. Third, the measurements, even if accurate, are often misinterpreted in practice. A study by Iberti and associates showed that 47% of 496 clinicians were unable to accurately interpret a straightforward recording of a tracing obtained with a PAC, and 44% could not correctly identify the determinants of systemic $\dot{D}O_2$.[41] A more recent study has confirmed that even well-trained intensivists are capable of misinterpreting results provided by pulmonary artery catheterization.[42] Furthermore, the current state of understanding is primitive when it comes to deciding what is the best management for certain hemodynamic disturbances, particularly those associated with sepsis or septic shock. Taking all of this into consideration, it may be that interventions prompted by measurements obtained with a PAC are actually harmful to patients. As a result, the marginal benefit now available by placing a PAC may be quite small. Less invasive modalities are available that can provide clinically useful hemodynamic information.

It may be true that aggressive hemodynamic resuscitation of patients, guided by various forms of monitoring, is valuable only during certain critical periods, such as the first few hours after presentation with septic shock or during surgery. For example, Rivers and colleagues reported that survival of patients with septic shock is significantly improved when resuscitation in the emergency department is guided by a protocol that seeks to keep $ScvO_2$ greater than 70%.[17] Similarly, a study using an ultrasound-based device (see Doppler Ultrasonography below) to assess cardiac filling and SV showed that maximizing SV intraoperatively results in fewer postoperative complications and shorter hospital length of stay.[43]

Minimally Invasive Alternatives to the Pulmonary Artery Catheter

Because of the cost, risks, and questionable benefit associated with bedside pulmonary artery catheterization, there has been interest for many years in the development of practical means for less invasive monitoring of hemodynamic parameters. Several approaches have been developed, which have achieved variable degrees of success. None of these methods render the standard thermodilution technique of the PAC obsolete. However, these strategies may contribute to improvements in the hemodynamic monitoring of critically ill patients.

Doppler Ultrasonography

When ultrasonic sound waves are reflected by moving erythrocytes in the bloodstream, the frequency of the reflected signal is increased or decreased, depending on whether the cells are moving toward or away from the ultrasonic source. This change in frequency is called the *Doppler shift*, and its magnitude is determined by the velocity of the moving red blood cells. Therefore, measurements of the Doppler shift can be used to calculate red blood cell velocity. With knowledge of both the cross-sectional area of a vessel and the mean red blood cell velocity of the blood flowing through it, one can calculate blood flow rate. If the vessel in question is the aorta, then Q_T can be calculated as:

$$QT = HR \times A \times \int V(t)dt$$

where A is the cross-sectional area of the aorta and $\int V(t)dt$ is the red blood cell velocity integrated over the cardiac cycle.

Two approaches have been developed for using Doppler ultrasonography to estimate Q_T. The first approach uses an ultrasonic transducer, which is manually positioned in the suprasternal notch and focused on the root of the aorta. Aortic cross-sectional area can be estimated using a nomogram, which factors in age, height, and weight, back calculated if an independent measure of Q_T is available, or by using two-dimensional transthoracic or transesophageal ultrasonography. Although this approach is completely noninvasive, it requires a highly skilled operator to obtain meaningful results, and is labor intensive. Moreover, unless Q_T measured using thermodilution is used to back-calculate aortic diameter, accuracy using the suprasternal notch approach is not acceptable.[44] Accordingly, the method is useful only for obtaining very intermittent estimates of Q_T, and has not been widely adopted by clinicians.

A more promising, albeit more invasive, approach has been introduced. In this method blood flow velocity is continuously monitored in the descending thoracic aorta using a continuous-wave Doppler transducer introduced into the esophagus in sedated or anesthetized patients. The probe is advanced into the esophagus to about 35 cm from the incisors (in adults) and connected to a monitor, which continuously displays the blood flow velocity profile in the descending aorta as well as the calculated Q_T. To maximize the accuracy of the device, the probe position must be adjusted to obtain the peak velocity in the aorta. To transform blood flow in the descending aorta into Q_T, a correction factor is applied that is based on the assumption that only 70% of the flow at the root of the aorta is still present in the descending thoracic aorta. Aortic cross-sectional area is estimated using a nomogram based on the patient's age, weight, and height. Results using these methods appear to be reasonably accurate across a broad spectrum of patients. In a multicenter study, good correlation was found between esophageal Doppler and thermodilution (r = 0.95), with a small systematic underestimation (bias 0.24 L/min) using esophageal Doppler.[45] The ultrasonic device also calculates a derived parameter termed *flow time corrected* (FTc), which is the systolic flow time in the descending aorta corrected for HR. FTc is a function of preload, contractility, and vascular input impedance. Although it is not a pure measure of preload, Doppler-based estimates of SV and FTc have been used successfully to guide volume resuscitation in high-risk surgical patients undergoing major operations.[43]

Impedance Cardiography

The impedance to flow of alternating electrical current in regions of the body is commonly called *bioimpedance*. In the thorax, changes in the volume and velocity of blood in the thoracic aorta lead to detectable changes in bioimpedance. The first derivative of the oscillating component of thoracic bioimpedance (dZ/dt) is linearly related to aortic blood flow. On the basis of this relationship, empirically derived formulas have been developed to estimate SV, and subsequently Q_T, noninvasively. This methodology is called *impedance cardiography*. The approach is attractive because it is noninvasive, provides a continuous readout of Q_T, and does not require extensive training for use. Despite these advantages, studies suggest that measurements of Q_T obtained by impedance cardiography are not sufficiently reliable to be used for clinical decision making and have poor correlation with standard methods such as thermodilution and ventricular angiography.[46,47] Impedance cardiography also has been proposed as a way to estimate LVEF, but the results obtained show poor agreement with those obtained by radionuclide ventriculography.[48,49] Based upon these data, impedance cardiography cannot be recommended at the present time for hemodynamic monitoring of critically ill patients.

Pulse Contour Analysis

Another method for determining cardiac output is an approach called *pulse contour analysis* for estimating SV on a beat-to-beat basis. The mechanical properties of the arterial tree and SV determine the shape of the arterial pulse waveform. The pulse contour method of estimating Q_T uses the arterial pressure waveform as an input for a model of the systemic circulation to determine beat-to-beat flow through the circulatory system. The parameters of resistance, compliance, and impedance are initially estimated based on the patient's age and sex, and can be subsequently refined by using a reference standard measurement of Q_T. The reference standard estimation of Q_T is obtained periodically using the indicator dilution approach by injecting the indicator into a CVC and detecting the transient increase in indicator concentration in the blood using an arterial catheter.

Measurements of Q_T based on pulse contour monitoring are comparable in accuracy to standard PAC-thermodilution methods, but it uses an approach that is less invasive since arterial and central venous, but not transcardiac, catheterization is needed.[50] Using on-line pressure waveform analysis, the computerized algorithms can calculate SV, Q_T, systemic vascular resistance, and an estimate of myocardial contractility, the rate of rise of the arterial systolic pressure (dP/dT). The use of pulse contour analysis has been applied using noninvasive photoplethysmographic measurements of arterial pressure. However, the accuracy of this technique has been questioned and its clinical use remains to be determined.[51]

Partial Carbon Dioxide Rebreathing

Partial carbon dioxide (CO_2) rebreathing uses the Fick principle to estimate Q_T noninvasively. By intermittently altering the dead space within the ventilator circuit via a rebreathing valve, changes in CO_2 production ($\dot{V}CO_2$) and end-tidal CO_2 ($ETCO_2$) are used to determine cardiac output using a modified Fick equation ($Q_T = \Delta\dot{V}CO_2 / \Delta ETCO_2$). Commercially available devices use this Fick principle to calculate Q_T using intermittent partial CO_2 rebreathing through a disposable rebreathing loop. These devices consist of a CO_2 sensor based on infrared light absorption, an airflow sensor, and a pulse oximeter. Changes in intrapulmonary shunt and hemodynamic instability impair the accuracy of Q_T estimated by partial CO_2 rebreathing. Continuous in-line pulse oximetry and inspired fraction of inspired O_2 (FiO_2) are used to estimate shunt fraction to correct Q_T.

Some studies of the partial CO_2 rebreathing approach suggest that this technique is not as accurate as thermodilution, the gold standard for measuring Q_T.[50,52] However, other studies suggest that the partial CO_2 rebreathing method for determination of Q_T compares favorably to measurements made using a PAC in critically ill patients.[53]

Transesophageal Echocardiography

Transesophageal echocardiography (TEE) has made the transition from operating room to ICU. TEE requires that the patient be sedated and usually intubated for airway protection. Using this powerful technology, global assessments of LV and RV function can be made, including determinations of ventricular volume, EF, and Q_T. Segmental wall motion abnormalities, pericardial effusions, and tamponade can be readily identified with TEE. Doppler techniques allow estimation of atrial filling pressures. The technique is somewhat cumbersome and requires considerable training and skill to obtain reliable results.

Assessing Preload Responsiveness

Although pulse contour analysis or partial CO_2 rebreathing may be able to provide estimates of SV and Q_T, these approaches alone can offer little or no information about the adequacy of preload. Thus, if Q_T is low, some other means must be used to estimate preload. Most clinicians assess the adequacy of cardiac preload by determining CVP or PAOP. However, neither CVP nor PAOP correlate well with the true parameter of interest, left ventricular end-diastolic volume (LVEDV).[54] Extremely high or low CVP or PAOP results are informative, but readings in a large middle zone (i.e., 5 to 20 mmHg) are not very useful. Furthermore, changes in CVP or PAOP fail to correlate well with changes in SV.[55] Echocardiography can be used to estimate LVEDV, but this approach is dependent on the skill and training of the individual using it, and isolated measurements of LVEDV fail to predict the hemodynamic response to alterations in preload.[56]

When intrathoracic pressure increases during the application of positive airway pressure in mechanically ventilated patients, venous return decreases, and as a consequence, LVSV also decreases. Therefore, pulse pressure variation (PPV) during a positive pressure episode can be used to predict the responsiveness of cardiac output to changes in preload.[57] PPV is defined as the difference between the maximal pulse pressure and the minimum pulse pressure divided by the average of these two pressures. This approach has been validated by comparing PPV, CVP, PAOP, and systolic pressure variation as predictors of preload responsiveness in a cohort of critically ill patients. Patients were classified as being "preload responsive" if their cardiac index increased by at least 15% after rapid infusion of a standard volume of IV fluid.[58] Receiver-operating characteristic curves demonstrated that PPV was the best predictor of preload responsiveness. Although atrial arrhythmias can interfere with the usefulness of this technique, PPV remains a useful approach for assessing preload responsiveness in most patients because of its simplicity and reliability.[56]

Tissue Capnometry

Global indices of Q_T, $\dot{D}O_2$, or $\dot{V}O_2$ provide little useful information regarding the adequacy of cellular oxygenation and mitochondrial function. On theoretical grounds, measuring tissue pH to assess the adequacy of perfusion is an attractive concept. As a consequence of the stoichiometry of the reactions responsible for the substrate level phosphorylation of adenosine diphosphate to form adenosine triphosphate, anaerobiosis is associated with the net accumulation of protons. Accordingly, knowing that tissue pH is not in the acid range should be enough information to conclude that global perfusion as well as arterial O_2 content are sufficient to meet the metabolic demands of the cells, even without knowledge of the actual values for tissue blood flow or O_2 delivery. The detection of tissue acidosis

should alert the clinician to the possibility that perfusion is inadequate. Thus, tonometric measurements of tissue P_{CO_2} in the stomach or sigmoid colon could be used to estimate mucosal pH (pH_i) and thereby monitor visceral perfusion in critically ill patients.

Unfortunately, the notion of using tonometric estimates of GI mucosal pH_i for monitoring perfusion is predicated on a number of assumptions, some of which may be partially or completely invalid. Furthermore, currently available methods for performing measurements of gastric mucosal P_{CO_2} in the clinical setting remain rather cumbersome and expensive. It is perhaps for these reasons that gastric tonometry for monitoring critically ill patients has primarily been used as a research tool.

Tonometric determination of mucosal CO_2 tension, $P_{CO_{2muc}}$, can be used to calculate pH_i by using the Henderson-Hasselbalch equation as follows:

$$pH_i = \log \left([HCO_3^-]_{muc} / 0.03 \times P_{CO_{2muc}} \right)$$

where $[HCO_3^-]_{muc}$ is the concentration of bicarbonate anion in the mucosa. Whereas $P_{CO_{2muc}}$ can be measured with reasonable accuracy and precision using tonometric methods, $[HCO_3^-]_{muc}$ cannot be measured directly, but must be estimated by assuming that the concentration of bicarbonate anion in arterial blood, $[HCO_3^-]_{art}$, is approximately equal to $[HCO_3^-]_{muc}$. Under normal conditions, the assumption that $[HCO_3^-]_{art} \cong [HCO_3^-]_{muc}$ is probably valid. Under pathologic conditions, however, the assumption that $[HCO_3^-]_{art} \cong [HCO_3^-]_{muc}$ is almost certainly invalid. For example, when blood flow to the ileal mucosa is very low, HCO_3^- in the tissue is titrated by hydrogen ions produced as a result of anaerobic metabolism, and replenishment of tissue HCO_3^- stores from arterial blood is impeded by stagnant perfusion. Thus under such conditions, $[HCO_3^-]_{muc}$ is less than $[HCO_3^-]_{art}$, and tonometric estimates of pH_i based on the Henderson-Hasselbalch equation underestimate the degree of tissue acidosis present.[59]

There is another inherent problem in using pH_i as an index of perfusion. As noted above, pH_i calculated using the Henderson-Hasselbalch equation is a function of both $P_{CO_{2muc}}$ and $[HCO_3^-]_{art}$. Under steady-state conditions, the first of these parameters, $P_{CO_{2muc}}$, reflects the balance between inflow of CO_2 into the interstitial space and outflow of CO_2 from the interstitial space. CO_2 can enter the interstitial compartment via three mechanisms: diffusion of CO_2 from arterial blood, production as a result of aerobic metabolism of carbon-containing fuels, and production as a result of titration of HCO_3^- by protons liberated during anaerobic metabolism. CO_2 leaves the interstitial compartment by diffusing into venous blood. If blood flow to the mucosa decreases, then $P_{CO_{2muc}}$ increases as a result of decreased extraction of CO_2 into venous blood. If mucosal perfusion decreases sufficiently, (i.e., to less than the anaerobic threshold for the tissue), then $P_{CO_{2muc}}$ also increases as a result of increased production due to titration of HCO_3^-.[52] Clearly, therefore, an increase in $P_{CO_{2muc}}$ *can* reflect a decrease in mucosal perfusion. However, as documented experimentally by Salzman and colleagues, an increase in $P_{CO_{2muc}}$ also can be caused by arterial hypercarbia, leading to increased diffusion of CO_2 from arterial blood into the interstitium.[60] Similarly, changes in $[HCO_3^-]_{art}$ can occur as a result of factors unrelated to either tissue perfusion or the adequacy of aerobic metabolism (e.g., diabetic ketoacidosis, iatrogenic alkalinization due to administration of sodium bicarbonate solution). For these reasons, tonometrically derived estimates of pH_i are not a reliable way to assess mucosal perfusion.

Although P_{CO_2} and pH are affected by changes in perfusion in all tissues, efforts to monitor these parameters in patients using tonometric methods have focused on the mucosa of the GI tract, particularly the stomach, for both practical and theoretical reasons. From a practical standpoint, the stomach is already commonly intubated in clinical practice for purposes of decompression and drainage or feeding. However, there are theoretical reasons why monitoring GI mucosal perfusion might be more desirable than monitoring perfusion in other sites. First, when global perfusion is compromised, blood flow to the splanchnic viscera decreases to a greater extent than does perfusion to the body as a whole.[61] Thus, the finding of compromised splanchnic perfusion may be an indicator of impending adverse changes in blood flow to other organs. Second, the gut has been hypothesized to be the "motor" of the multiple organ dysfunction syndrome (MODS), and in experimental models, intestinal mucosal acidosis, whether due to inadequate perfusion or other causes, has been associated with hyperpermeability to hydrophilic solutes.[62] Therefore, ensuring adequate splanchnic perfusion might be expected to minimize derangements in gut barrier function and, on this basis, improve outcome for patients.

The stomach, however, may not be an ideal location for monitoring tissue PCO_2. First, CO_2 can be formed in the lumen of the stomach when hydrogen ions secreted by parietal cells in the mucosa titrate luminal bicarbonate anions, which are present either as a result of backwash of duodenal secretions or secretion by gastric mucosal cells. Measurements of gastric PCO_2 and pH_i can be confounded by gastric acid secretion.[63] Consequently, accurate measurements of gastric PCO_2 and pH_i depend on pharmacologic blockade of luminal proton secretion using histamine receptor antagonists or proton pump inhibitors. The need for using pharmacologic therapy adds to the cost and complexity of the monitoring strategy. Second, enteral feeding can interfere with measurements of gastric mucosal PCO_2, necessitating temporary cessation of the administration of nutritional support or the placement of a postpyloric tube.[64]

Despite the problems noted above, measurements of gastric pH_i and/or mucosal-arterial PCO_2 gap have been proven to be a remarkably reliable predictor of outcome in a wide variety of critically ill individuals, including general medical ICU patients, victims of multiple trauma, patients with sepsis, and patients undergoing major surgical procedures.[65–67] In studies using endoscopic measurements of gastric mucosal blood flow by laser Doppler flowmetry, the development of gastric mucosal acidosis has been shown to correlate with mucosal hypoperfusion.[68] Moreover, in a landmark prospective, randomized, multicentric clinical trial of monitoring in medical ICU patients, titrating resuscitation to a gastric pH_i endpoint rather than conventional hemodynamic indices resulted in a higher 30-day survival rate.[69] In another study, trauma patients were randomized to resuscitation titrated to a gastric pH_i greater than 7.30, or to resuscitation titrated to achieve systemic $\dot{D}O_2$ or $\dot{V}O_2$ goals.[70] Although survival was not significantly different in the two arms of the study, failure to normalize gastric pH_i within 24 hours was associated with a high mortality rate (54%), whereas normalization of pH_i was associated with a significantly lower mortality rate (7%).

There is also interest in measuring tissue capnometry in less invasive sites. Results from some preliminary clinical studies support the view that the monitoring of tissue PCO_2 in the sublingual mucosa may provide valuable clinical information. Increased sublingual PCO_2 ($PslCO_2$) was associated with decreases in arterial blood pressure and Q_T in patients with shock due to hemorrhage or sepsis.[71] In a study of critically ill patients with septic or cardiogenic shock, the $PslCO_2$-$PaCO_2$ gradient was found to be a good prognostic indicator, being 9.2 ± 5.0 mmHg in the survivors and 17.8 ± 11.5 mmHg in nonsurvivors.[72] This study also demonstrated that sublingual capnography was superior to gastric tonometry in predicting patient survival. The $PslCO_2$-$PaCO_2$ gradient also correlated with the mixed venous-arterial PCO_2 gradient, but failed to correlate with blood lactate level, mixed venous O_2 saturation ($S\bar{v}O_2$), or systemic $\dot{D}O_2$. These latter findings suggest that the $PslCO_2$-$PaCO_2$ gradient may be a better marker of tissue hypoxia than are these other parameters.

Near Infrared Spectroscopic Measurement of Tissue Hemoglobin Oxygen Saturation

Near infrared spectroscopy (NIRS) allows continuous, noninvasive measurement of tissue Hgb O_2 saturation (StO_2) using near infrared wavelengths of light (700–1000 nm). This technology is based on Beer's law, which states that the transmission of light through a solution with a dissolved solute decreases exponentially as the concentration of the solute increases. In mammalian tissue, three compounds change their absorption pattern when oxygenated: cytochrome a,a_3, myoglobin, and Hgb. Because of the distinct absorption spectra of oxyhemoglobin and deoxyhemoglobin, Beer's law can be used to detect their relative concentrations within tissue. Thus, the relative concentrations of the types of Hgb can be determined by measuring the change in light intensity as it passes through the tissue. Because about 20% of blood volume is intra-arterial and the StO_2 measurements are taken without regard to systole or diastole, spectroscopic measurements are primarily indicative of the venous oxyhemoglobin concentration.

NIRS has been evaluated to assess the severity of traumatic shock in animal models and in trauma patients. Studies have shown that peripheral muscle StO_2, as determined by NIRS, is as accurate as other endpoints of resuscitation [i.e., base deficit (BD), mixed venous O_2 saturation] in a porcine model of hemorrhagic shock.[73] Continuously-measured StO_2 has been evaluated in blunt trauma patients as a predictor of the development of multiple organ dysfunction syndrome (MODS) and mortality.[74] At seven level 1 trauma centers, 383 patients were prospectively studied. StO_2 was monitored for 24 hours after admission along with vital signs and other endpoints of resuscitation such as BD. Minimum StO_2 (using a minimum $StO_2 \leq 75\%$ as a cutoff) had a similar sensitivity and specificity in predicting the development of MODS as BD ≥ 6 mEq/L. StO_2 and BD were also comparable in predicting mortality. Thus, NIRS-derived muscle StO_2 measurements perform similarly to BD in identifying poor perfusion and predicting the development of MODS or death after severe torso trauma, yet have the additional advantages of being continuous and noninvasive. Ongoing prospective studies will help determine the clinical use of continuous monitoring of StO_2 in clinical scenarios such as trauma, hemorrhagic shock, sepsis, etc.

RESPIRATORY MONITORING

The ability to monitor various parameters of respiratory function is of utmost importance in critically ill patients. Many of these patients require mechanical ventilation. Monitoring of their respiratory physiology is necessary to assess the adequacy of oxygenation and ventilation, guide weaning and liberation from mechanical ventilation, and detect adverse events associated with respiratory failure and mechanical ventilation. These parameters include gas exchange, neuromuscular activity, respiratory mechanics, and patient effort.

Arterial Blood Gases

The standard for respiratory monitoring has been to carry out intermittent measurements of arterial blood gases. Blood gas analysis provides useful information when caring for patients with respiratory failure. However, even in the absence of respiratory failure or the need for mechanical ventilation, blood gas determinations also can be valuable to detect alterations in acid-base balance due to low Q_T, sepsis, renal failure, severe trauma, medication or drug overdose, or altered mental status. Arterial blood can be analyzed for pH, PO_2, PCO_2, HCO_3^- concentration, and calculated BD. When indicated, carboxyhemoglobin and methemoglobin levels also can be measured. In recent years, efforts have been made to decrease the unnecessary use of arterial blood gas analysis. Serial arterial blood gas determinations are not necessary for routine weaning from mechanical ventilation in the majority of postoperative patients.

Most bedside blood gas analyses still involve removal of an aliquot of blood from the patient, although continuous bedside arterial blood gas determinations are now possible without sampling via an indwelling arterial catheter that contains a biosensor. In studies comparing the accuracy of continuous arterial blood gas and pH monitoring with a conventional laboratory blood gas analyzer, excellent agreement between the two methods has been demonstrated.[75] Continuous monitoring can reduce the volume of blood loss due to phlebotomy and dramatically decrease the time necessary to obtain blood gas results. Continuous monitoring, however, is expensive and is not widely used.

Determinants of Oxygen Delivery

The primary goal of the cardiovascular and respiratory systems is to deliver oxygenated blood to the tissues. $\dot{D}O_2$ is dependent to a greater degree on the O_2 saturation of Hgb in arterial blood (SaO_2) than on the partial pressure of O_2 in arterial blood (PaO_2). $\dot{D}O_2$ also is dependent on Q_T and Hgb. Dissolved O_2 in blood, which is proportional to the PaO_2, makes only a negligible contribution to $\dot{D}O_2$, as is apparent from the equation:

$$\dot{D}O_2 = Q_T \times [(Hgb \times SaO_2 \times 1.36) + (PaO_2 \times 0.0031)]$$

SaO_2 in mechanically ventilated patients depends on the mean airway pressure, the fraction of inspired O_2 (FiO_2), and $S\bar{v}O_2$. Thus, when SaO_2 is low, the clinician has only a limited number of ways to improve this parameter. The clinician can increase mean airway pressure by increasing positive end-expiratory pressure (PEEP) or inspiratory time. FiO_2 can be increased to a maximum of 1.0 by decreasing the amount of room air mixed with the O_2 supplied to the ventilator. $S\bar{v}O_2$ can be increased by increasing Hgb or Q_T or decreasing O_2 use (e.g., by administering a muscle relaxant and sedation).

Peak and Plateau Airway Pressure

Airway pressures are routinely monitored in mechanically ventilated patients. The peak airway pressure measured at the end of inspiration (P_{peak}) is a function of the tidal volume, the resistance of the airways, and lung/chest wall compliance, and peak inspiratory flow. The airway pressure measured at the end of inspiration when the inhaled volume is held in the lungs by briefly closing the expiratory valve is termed *the plateau airway pressure* ($P_{plateau}$). As a static parameter, plateau airway pressure is independent of the airway resistance and peak airway flow, and is related to the lung/chest wall compliance and delivered tidal volume. Mechanical ventilators monitor P_{peak} with each breath and can be set to trigger an alarm if the P_{peak} exceeds a predetermined threshold. $P_{plateau}$ is not measured routinely with each delivered tidal volume, but rather is measured intermittently by setting the ventilator to close the exhalation circuit briefly at the end of inspiration and record the airway pressure when airflow is zero.

If both P_{peak} and $P_{plateau}$ are increased (and tidal volume is not excessive), then the problem is a decrease in the compliance in the lung/chest wall unit. Common causes of this problem include pneumothorax, hemothorax, lobar atelectasis, pulmonary edema, pneumonia, acute respiratory distress syndrome (ARDS), active contraction of the chest wall or diaphragmatic muscles, abdominal distention, and intrinsic PEEP, such as occurs in patients with bronchospasm and insufficient expiratory times. When P_{peak} is increased but $P_{plateau}$ is relatively normal, the primary problem is an increase in airway resistance, such as occurs with bronchospasm, use of a small-caliber endotracheal tube, or kinking or obstruction of the endotracheal tube. A low P_{peak} also should trigger an alarm, as it suggests a discontinuity in the airway circuit involving the patient and the ventilator.

Ventilator-induced lung injury is now an established clinical entity of great relevance to the care of critically ill patients. Excessive airway pressure and tidal volume adversely affect pulmonary and possibly systemic responses to critical illness. Subjecting the lung parenchyma to excessive pressure, known as *barotrauma*, can result in parenchymal lung injury, diffuse alveolar damage similar to ARDS, and pneumothorax, and can impair venous return and therefore limit cardiac output. Lung-protective ventilation strategies have been developed to prevent the development of ventilator-induced lung injury and improve patient outcomes. In a large, multicenter randomized trial of patients with ARDS from a variety of etiologies, limiting plateau airway pressure to less than 30 cm H_2O and tidal volume to

less than 6 mL/kg of ideal body weight reduced 28-day mortality by 22% relative to a ventilator strategy that used a tidal volume of 12 mL/kg.[76] For this reason, monitoring of plateau pressure and using a low tidal volume strategy in patients with ARDS is now the standard of care.

Pulse Oximetry

The pulse oximeter is a microprocessor-based device that integrates oximetry and plethysmography to provide continuous noninvasive monitoring of the O_2 saturation of arterial blood (SaO_2). It is considered one of the most important and useful technologic advances in patient monitoring. Continuous, noninvasive monitoring of arterial O_2 saturation is possible using light-emitting diodes and sensors placed on the skin. Pulse oximetry uses two wavelengths of light (i.e., 660 nm and 940 nm) to analyze the pulsatile component of blood flow between the light source and sensor. Because oxyhemoglobin and deoxyhemoglobin have different absorption spectra, differential absorption of light at these two wavelengths can be used to calculate the fraction of O_2 saturation of Hgb. Under normal circumstances, the contributions of carboxyhemoglobin and methemoglobin are minimal. However, if carboxyhemoglobin levels are elevated, the pulse oximeter will incorrectly interpret carboxyhemoglobin as oxyhemoglobin and the arterial saturation displayed will be falsely elevated. When the concentration of methemoglobin is markedly increased, the SaO_2 will be displayed as 85%, regardless of the true arterial saturation.[77] The accuracy of pulse oximetry begins to decline at SaO_2 values less than 92%, and tends to be unreliable for values less than 85%.[78]

Several studies have assessed the frequency of arterial O_2 desaturation in hospitalized patients and its effect on outcome. For example, in a study of general medical patients, Bowton and associates found that patients who had an episode of hypoxemia (SaO_2 <90% for 5 minutes) in the first 24 hours of hospital admission had a mortality rate three times higher than that of patients who did not have an episode of arterial desaturation.[79] Because of its clinical relevance, ease of use, noninvasive nature, and cost-effectiveness, pulse oximetry has become a routine monitoring strategy in patients with respiratory disease, intubated patients, and those undergoing surgical intervention under sedation or general anesthesia. Pulse oximetry is especially useful in the titration of FiO_2 and PEEP for patients receiving mechanical ventilation, and during weaning from mechanical ventilation. The widespread use of pulse oximetry has decreased the need for arterial blood gas determinations in critically ill patients.

Capnometry

Capnometry is the measurement of CO_2 in the airway throughout the respiratory cycle. Capnometry is most commonly measured by infrared light absorption. CO_2 absorbs infrared light at a peak wavelength of approximately 4.27 μm. Capnometry works by passing infrared light through a sample chamber to a detector on the opposite side. More infrared light passing through the sample chamber (i.e., less CO_2) causes a larger signal in the detector relative to the infrared light passing through a reference cell. Capnometric determination of the partial pressure of CO_2 in end-tidal exhaled gas ($PETCO_2$) is used as a surrogate for the partial pressure of CO_2 in arterial blood ($PaCO_2$) during mechanical ventilation. In healthy subjects, $PETCO_2$ is about 1 to 5 mmHg less than $PaCO_2$.[80] Thus, $PETCO_2$ can be used to estimate $PaCO_2$ without the need for blood gas determination. However, changes in $PETCO_2$ may not correlate with changes in $PaCO_2$ during a number of pathologic conditions (see below).

Capnography allows the confirmation of endotracheal intubation and continuous assessment of ventilation, integrity of the airway, operation of the ventilator, and cardiopulmonary function. Capnometers are configured with either an in-line sensor or a sidestream sensor. The sidestream systems are lighter and easy to use, but the thin tubing that samples the gas from the ventilator circuit can become clogged with secretions or condensed water, preventing accurate measurements. The in-line devices are bulky and heavier, but are less likely to become clogged. Continuous monitoring with capnography has become routine during surgery under general anesthesia and for some intensive care patients. A number of situations can be promptly detected with continuous capnography. A sudden reduction in P_{ETCO_2} suggests either obstruction of the sampling tubing with water or secretions, or a catastrophic event such as loss of the airway, airway disconnection or obstruction, ventilator malfunction, or a marked decrease in Q_T. If the airway is connected and patent and the ventilator is functioning properly, then a sudden decrease in P_{ETCO_2} should prompt efforts to rule out cardiac arrest, massive pulmonary embolism, or cardiogenic shock. P_{ETCO_2} can be persistently low during hyperventilation or with an increase in dead space such as occurs with pulmonary embolization (even in the absence of a change in Q_T). Causes of an increase in P_{ETCO_2} include reduced minute ventilation or increased metabolic rate.

RENAL MONITORING

Urine Output

Bladder catheterization with an indwelling catheter allows the monitoring of urine output, usually recorded hourly by the nursing staff. With a patent Foley catheter, urine output is a gross indicator of renal perfusion. The generally accepted normal urine output is 0.5 mL/kg per hour for adults and 1 to 2 mL/kg per hour for neonates and infants. Oliguria may reflect inadequate renal artery perfusion due to hypotension, hypovolemia, or low Q_T. Low urine flow also can be a sign of intrinsic renal dysfunction. It is important to recognize that normal urine output does not exclude the possibility of impending renal failure.

Bladder Pressure

The triad of oliguria, elevated peak airway pressures, and elevated intra-abdominal pressure is known as the *abdominal compartment syndrome* (ACS). This syndrome, first described in patients after repair of ruptured abdominal aortic aneurysm, is associated with interstitial edema of the abdominal organs, resulting in elevated intra-abdominal pressure. When intra-abdominal pressure exceeds venous or capillary pressures, perfusion of the kidneys and other intra-abdominal viscera is impaired. Oliguria is a cardinal sign. Although the diagnosis of ACS is a clinical one, measuring intra-abdominal pressure is useful to confirm the diagnosis. Ideally, a catheter inserted into the peritoneal cavity could measure intra-abdominal pressure to substantiate the diagnosis. In practice, transurethral bladder pressure measurement reflects intra-abdominal pressure and is most often used to confirm the presence of ACS. After instilling 50 to 100 mL of sterile saline into the bladder via a Foley catheter, the tubing is connected to a transducing system to measure bladder pressure. Most authorities recommend that a bladder pressure greater than 20 to 25 mmHg confirms the diagnosis of ACS.[81] Less commonly, gastric or inferior vena cava pressures can be monitored with appropriate catheters to detect elevated intra-abdominal pressures.

NEUROLOGIC MONITORING

Intracranial Pressure

Because the brain is rigidly confined within the bony skull, cerebral edema or mass lesions increase intracranial pressure (ICP). Monitoring of ICP is currently recommended in patients with severe traumatic brain injury (TBI), defined as a Glasgow Coma Scale (GCS) score ≤8 with an abnormal CT scan, and in patients with severe TBI and a normal CT scan if two or more of the following are present: age greater than 40 years, unilateral or bilateral motor posturing, or systolic blood pressure less than 90 mmHg.[82] ICP monitoring also is indicated in patients with acute subarachnoid hemorrhage with coma or neurologic deterioration, intracranial hemorrhage with intraven-

tricular blood, ischemic middle cerebral artery stroke, fulminant hepatic failure with coma and cerebral edema on CT scan, and global cerebral ischemia or anoxia with cerebral edema on CT scan. The goal of ICP monitoring is to ensure that cerebral perfusion pressure (CPP) is adequate to support perfusion of the brain. CPP is equal to the difference between MAP and ICP: CPP = MAP – ICP.

One type of ICP measuring device, the ventriculostomy catheter, consists of a fluid-filled catheter inserted into a cerebral ventricle and connected to an external pressure transducer. This device permits measurement of ICP, but also allows drainage of cerebrospinal fluid (CSF) as a means to lower ICP and sample CSF for laboratory studies. Other devices locate the pressure transducer within the central nervous system and are used only to monitor ICP. These devices can be placed in the intraventricular, parenchymal, subdural, or epidural spaces. Ventriculostomy catheters are the accepted standard for monitoring ICP in patients with TBI due to their accuracy, ability to drain CSF, and low complication rate. The associated complications include infection (5%), hemorrhage (1.4%), catheter malfunction or obstruction (6.3 to 10.5%), and malposition with injury to cerebral tissue.[83]

The purpose of ICP monitoring is to detect and treat abnormal elevations of ICP that may be detrimental to cerebral perfusion and function. In TBI patients, ICP greater than 20 mmHg is associated with unfavorable outcomes.[84] However, few studies have shown that treatment of elevated ICP improves clinical outcomes in human trauma patients. In a randomized, controlled, double-blind trial, Eisenberg and colleagues demonstrated that maintaining ICP less than 25 mmHg in patients without craniectomy and less than 15 mmHg in patients with craniectomy is associated with improved outcome.[85] In patients with low CPP, therapeutic strategies to correct CPP can be directed at increasing MAP or decreasing ICP. Although it often has been recommended that CPP be maintained above 70 mmHg, the evidence to support this recommendation is not overly compelling.[86] Furthermore, a retrospective cohort study of patients with severe TBI found that ICP/CPP-targeted neurointensive care was associated with prolonged mechanical ventilation and increased therapeutic interventions, without evidence for improved outcome in patients who survive beyond 24 h.[87]

Electroencephalogram and Evoked Potentials

Electroencephalography offers the capacity to monitor global neurologic electrical activity, while evoked potential monitoring can assess pathways not detected by the conventional electroencephalogram (EEG). Continuous EEG (CEEG) monitoring in the ICU permits ongoing evaluation of cerebral cortical activity. It is especially useful in obtunded and comatose patients. CEEG also is useful for monitoring of therapy for status epilepticus and detecting early changes associated with cerebral ischemia. CEEG can be used to adjust the level of sedation, especially if high-dose barbiturate therapy is being used to manage elevated ICP. Somatosensory and brain stem evoked potentials are less affected by the administration of sedatives than is the EEG. Evoked potentials are useful for localizing brain stem lesions or proving the absence of such structural lesions in cases of metabolic or toxic coma. They also can provide prognostic data in posttraumatic coma.

A recent advance in EEG monitoring is the use of the bispectral index (BIS) to titrate the level of sedative medications. Although sedative drugs usually are titrated to the clinical neurologic examination, the BIS device has been used in the operating room to continuously monitor the depth of anesthesia. The BIS is an empiric measurement statistically derived from a database of more than 5000 EEGs.[88] The BIS is derived from bifrontal EEG recordings and analyzed for burst suppression ratio, relative alpha:beta ratio, and bicoherence. Using a multivariate regression model, a linear numeric index (BIS) is calculated, ranging from 0 (isoelectric EEG) to 100 (fully awake). Its use has been associated with lower consumption of anesthetics during surgery and earlier awakening and faster recovery from anesthesia.[89] The BIS also has been validated as a useful approach for monitoring the level of sedation for ICU patients, using the revised Sedation-Agitation Scale as a gold standard.[90]

Transcranial Doppler Ultrasonography

This modality provides a noninvasive method for evaluating cerebral hemodynamics. Transcranial Doppler (TCD) measurements of middle and anterior cerebral artery blood flow velocity are useful for the diagnosis of cerebral vasospasm after subarachnoid hemorrhage. Qureshi and associates demonstrated that an increase in the middle cerebral artery mean flow velocity as assessed by TCD is an independent predictor of symptomatic vasospasm in a prospective study of patients with aneurysmal subarachnoid hemorrhage.[91] In addition, while some have proposed using TCD to estimate ICP, studies have shown that TCD is not a reliable method for estimating ICP and CPP, and currently cannot be endorsed for this purpose.[92] TCD also is useful to confirm the clinical examination for determining brain death in patients with confounding factors such as the presence of central nervous system depressants or metabolic encephalopathy.

Jugular Venous Oximetry

When the arterial O_2 content, Hgb concentration, and the oxyhemoglobin dissociation curve are constant, changes in jugular venous O_2 saturation (SjO_2) reflect changes in the difference between cerebral O_2 delivery and demand. Generally, a decrease in SjO_2 reflects cerebral hypoperfusion, whereas an increase in SjO_2 indicates the presence of hyperemia. SjO_2 monitoring cannot detect decreases in regional cerebral blood flow if overall perfusion is normal or above normal. This technique requires the placement of a catheter in the jugular bulb, usually via the internal jugular vein. Catheters that permit intermittent aspiration of jugular venous blood for analysis or continuous oximetry catheters are available.

Low SjO_2 is associated with poor outcomes after TBI.[93] Nevertheless, the value of monitoring SjO_2 remains unproven. If it is used, it should not be the sole monitoring technique, but rather should be used in conjunction with ICP and CPP monitoring. By monitoring ICP, CPP, and SjO_2, early intervention with volume, vasopressors, and hyperventilation has been shown to prevent ischemic events in patients with TBI.[94]

Transcranial Near Infrared Spectroscopy

Transcranial NIRS is a noninvasive continuous monitoring method to determine cerebral oxygenation. It uses technology similar to that of pulse oximetry to determine the concentrations of oxy- and deoxyhemoglobin with near infrared light and sensors, and takes advantage of the relative transparency of the skull to light in the near infrared region of the spectrum. McCormick and associates demonstrated that cerebral desaturation can occur more than 2 hours before any clinical deterioration in neurologic status.[95] Nevertheless, this form of monitoring remains largely a research tool at the present time.

Brain Tissue Oxygen Tension

Although the standard of care for patients with severe TBI includes ICP and CPP monitoring, this strategy does not always prevent secondary brain injury. Growing evidence suggests that monitoring local brain tissue O_2 tension ($PbtO_2$) may be a useful adjunct to ICP monitoring in these patients. Normal values for $PbtO_2$ are 20 to 40 mmHg, and critical levels are 8 to 10 mmHg. A recent clinical study sought to determine whether the addition of a $PbtO_2$ monitor to guide therapy in severe TBI was associated with improved patient outcomes.[96] Twenty-eight patients with severe TBI (GCS score ≤8) were enrolled in an observational study at a level I trauma center. These patients received invasive ICP and $PbtO_2$ monitoring and were compared with 25 historical controls matched for age, injuries, and admission GCS score that had undergone ICP monitoring alone. Goals of therapy in both groups included maintaining an ICP <20 mmHg and a CPP >60 mmHg. Among patients with $PbtO_2$

monitoring, therapy also was directed at maintaining $PbtO_2$ >25 mmHg. The groups had similar mean daily ICP and CPP levels. The mortality rate in the historical controls treated with standard ICP and CPP management was 44%. Mortality was significantly lower in the patients who had therapy guided by $PbtO_2$ monitoring in addition to ICP and CPP (25%; P <.05). The benefits of $PbtO_2$ monitoring may include the early detection of brain tissue ischemia despite normal ICP and CPP. In addition, $PbtO_2$-guided management may reduce potential adverse effects associated with therapies to maintain ICP and CPP.

CONCLUSIONS

Modern intensive care is predicated by the need and ability to continuously monitor a wide range of physiologic parameters. This capability has dramatically improved the care of critically ill patients and advanced the development of the specialty of critical care medicine. In some cases, the technologic ability to measure such variables has surpassed our understanding of the significance or the knowledge of the appropriate intervention to ameliorate such pathophysiologic changes. In addition, the development of less invasive monitoring methods has been promoted by the recognition of complications associated with invasive monitoring devices. The future portends the continued development of noninvasive monitoring devices along with their application in an evidenced-based strategy to guide rational therapy.

REFERENCES

Entries highlighted in bright blue are key references

1. Ronco JJ, Fenwick JC, Tweeddale MG, et al: Identification of the critical oxygen delivery for anaerobic metabolism in critically ill septic and nonseptic humans. *JAMA* 270:1724, 1993.
2. Lubarsky DA, Smith LR, Sladen RN, et al: Defining the relationship of oxygen delivery and consumption: Use of biologic system models. *J Surg Res* 58:503, 1995.
3. Lehmann KG, Gelman JA, Weber MA, et al: Comparative accuracy of three automated techniques in the noninvasive estimation of central blood pressure in men. *Am J Cardiol* 81:1004, 1998.
4. Epstein RH, Bartkowski RR, Huffnagle S: Continuous noninvasive finger blood pressure during controlled hypotension. A comparison with intraarterial pressure. *Anesthesiology* 75:796, 1991.
5. Traore O, Liotier J, Souweine B: Prospective study of arterial and central venous catheter colonization and of arterial- and central venous catheter-related bacteremia in intensive care units. *Crit Care Med* 33:1276, 2005.
6. Chatila W, Ani S, Guaglianone D, et al: Cardiac ischemia during weaning from mechanical ventilation. *Chest* 109:1577, 1996.
7. Landesberg G, Mosseri M, Wolf Y, et al: Perioperative myocardial ischemia and infarction: Identification by continuous 12-lead electrocardiogram with online ST-segment monitoring. *Anesthesiology* 96:264, 2002.
8. Hayashi H, Amano M: Does ultrasound imaging before puncture facilitate internal jugular vein cannulation? Prospective randomized comparison with landmark-guided puncture in ventilated patients. *J Cardiothorac Vasc Anesth* 16:572, 2002.
9. Mihm FG, Gettinger A, Hanson CW III, et al: A multicenter evaluation of a new continuous cardiac output pulmonary artery catheter system. *Crit Care Med* 26:1346, 1998.
10. Rouby JJ, Poete P, Bodin L, et al: Three mixed venous saturation catheters in patients with circulatory shock and respiratory failure. *Chest* 98:954, 1990.
11. Jastremski MS, Chelluri L, Beney KM, et al: Analysis of the effects of continuous on-line monitoring of mixed venous oxygen saturation on patient outcome and cost-effectiveness. *Crit Care Med* 17:148, 1989.
12 Kyff JV, Vaughn S, Yang SC, et al: Continuous monitoring of mixed venous oxygen saturation in patients with acute myocardial infarction. *Chest* 95:607, 1989.
13. Gattinoni L, Brazzi L, Pelosi P, et al: A trial of goal-oriented hemodynamic therapy in critically ill patients. SVo2 Collaborative Group. *N Engl J Med* 333:1025, 1995.

14. London MJ, Moritz TE, Henderson WG, et al: Standard versus fiberoptic pulmonary artery catheterization for cardiac surgery in the Department of Veterans Affairs: A prospective, observational, multicenter analysis. *Anesthesiology* 96:860, 2002.

15. Rivers EP, Ander DS, Powell D: Central venous oxygen saturation monitoring in the critically ill patient. *Curr Opin Crit Care* 7:204, 2001.

16. Varpula M, Karlsson S, Ruokonen E, et al: Mixed venous oxygen saturation cannot be estimated by central venous oxygen saturation in septic shock. *Intensive Care Med* 32:1336, 2006.

17. Rivers E, Nguyen B, Havstad S, et al: Early goal-directed therapy in the treatment of severe sepsis and septic shock. *N Engl J Med* 345:1368, 2001.

18. Dhainaut JF, Brunet F, Monsallier JF, et al: Bedside evaluation of right ventricular performance using a rapid computerized thermodilution method. *Crit Care Med* 15:148, 1987.

19. Yu M, Takiguchi S, Takanishi D, et al: Evaluation of the clinical usefulness of thermodilution volumetric catheters. *Crit Care Med* 23:681, 1995.

20. Chang MC, Blinman TA, Rutherford EJ, et al: Preload assessment in trauma patients during large-volume shock resuscitation. *Arch Surg* 131:728, 1996.

21. Connors AF Jr., Speroff T, Dawson NV, et al: The effectiveness of right heart catheterization in the initial care of critically ill patients. SUPPORT Investigators. *JAMA* 276:889, 1996.

22. Gore JM, Goldberg RJ, Spodick DH, et al: A community-wide assessment of the use of pulmonary artery catheters in patients with acute myocardial infarction. *Chest* 92:721, 1987.

23. Zion MM, Balkin J, Rosenmann D, et al: Use of pulmonary artery catheters in patients with acute myocardial infarction. Analysis of experience in 5,841 patients in the SPRINT Registry. SPRINT Study Group. *Chest* 98:1331, 1990.

24. Pearson KS, Gomez MN, Moyers JR, et al: A cost/benefit analysis of randomized invasive monitoring for patients undergoing cardiac surgery. *Anesth Analg* 69:336, 1989.

25. Tuman KJ, McCarthy RJ, Spiess BD, et al: Effect of pulmonary artery catheterization on outcome in patients undergoing coronary artery surgery. *Anesthesiology* 70:199, 1989.

26. Bender JS, Smith-Meek MA, Jones CE: Routine pulmonary artery catheterization does not reduce morbidity and mortality of elective vascular surgery: Results of a prospective, randomized trial. *Ann Surg* 226:229, 1997.

27. Valentine RJ, Duke ML, Inman MH, et al: Effectiveness of pulmonary artery catheters in aortic surgery: A randomized trial. *J Vasc Surg* 27:203, 1998.

28. Sandham JD, Hull RD, Brant RF, et al: A randomized, controlled trial of the use of pulmonary-artery catheters in high-risk surgical patients. *N Engl J Med* 348:5, 2003.

29. Harvey S, Harrison DA, Singer M, et al: Assessment of the clinical effectiveness of pulmonary artery catheters in management of patients in intensive care (PAC-Man): A randomised controlled trial. *Lancet* 366:472, 2005.

30. Shah MR, Hasselblad V, Stevenson LW, et al: Impact of the pulmonary artery catheter in critically ill patients: Meta-analysis of randomized clinical trials. *JAMA* 294:1664, 2005.

31. Binanay C, Califf RM, Hasselblad V, et al: Evaluation study of congestive heart failure and pulmonary artery catheterization effectiveness: The ESCAPE trial. *JAMA* 294:1625, 2005.

32. Wheeler AP, Bernard GR, Thompson BT, et al: Pulmonary-artery versus central venous catheter to guide treatment of acute lung injury. *N Engl J Med* 354:2213, 2006.

33. Wiener RS, Welch HG: Trends in the use of the pulmonary artery catheter in the United States, 1993–2004. *JAMA* 298:423, 2007.

34. Bland RD, Shoemaker WC, Abraham E, et al: Hemodynamic and oxygen transport patterns in surviving and nonsurviving postoperative patients. *Crit Care Med* 13:85, 1985.

35. Shoemaker WC, Appel PL, Kram HB, et al: Prospective trial of supranormal values of survivors as therapeutic goals in high-risk surgical patients. *Chest* 94:1176, 1988.

36. Bishop MH, Shoemaker WC, Appel PL, et al: Prospective, randomized trial of survivor values of cardiac index, oxygen delivery, and oxygen consumption as resuscitation endpoints in severe trauma. *J Trauma* 38:780, 1995.

37. Yu M, Burchell S, Hasaniya NW, et al: Relationship of mortality to increasing oxygen delivery in patients > or = 50 years of age: A prospective, randomized trial. *Crit Care Med* 26:1011, 1998.

38. Heyland DK, Cook DJ, King D, et al: Maximizing oxygen delivery in critically ill patients: A methodologic appraisal of the evidence. *Crit Care Med* 24:517, 1996.

39. Alia I, Esteban A, Gordo F, et al: A randomized and controlled trial of the effect of treatment aimed at maximizing oxygen delivery in patients with severe sepsis or septic shock. *Chest* 115:453, 1999.

40. Connors AF Jr.: Right heart catheterization: Is it effective? *New Horiz* 5:195, 1997.

41. Iberti TJ, Fischer EP, Leibowitz AB, et al: A multicenter study of physicians' knowledge of the pulmonary artery catheter. Pulmonary Artery Catheter Study Group. *JAMA* 264:2928, 1990.

42. Gnaegi A, Feihl F, Perret C: Intensive care physicians' insufficient knowledge of right-heart catheterization at the bedside: Time to act? *Crit Care Med* 25:213, 1997.

43. Gan TJ, Soppitt A, Maroof M, et al: Goal-directed intraoperative fluid administration reduces length of hospital stay after major surgery. *Anesthesiology* 97:820, 2002.

44. Cerny JC, Ketslakh M, Poulos CL, et al: Evaluation of the Velcom-100 pulse Doppler cardiac output computer. *Chest* 100:143, 1991.

45. Valtier B, Cholley BP, Belot JP, et al: Noninvasive monitoring of cardiac output in critically ill patients using transesophageal Doppler. *Am J Respir Crit Care Med* 158:77, 1998.

46. Genoni M, Pelosi P, Romand JA, et al: Determination of cardiac output during mechanical ventilation by electrical bioimpedance or thermodilution in patients with acute lung injury: Effects of positive end-expiratory pressure. *Crit Care Med* 26:1441, 1998.

47. Imhoff M, Lehner JH, Lohlein D: Noninvasive whole-body electrical bioimpedance cardiac output and invasive thermodilution cardiac output in high-risk surgical patients. *Crit Care Med* 28:2812, 2000.

48. Marik PE, Pendelton JE, Smith R: A comparison of hemodynamic parameters derived from transthoracic electrical bioimpedance with those parameters obtained by thermodilution and ventricular angiography. *Crit Care Med* 25:1545, 1997.

49. Miles DS, Gotshall RW, Quinones JD, et al: Impedance cardiography fails to measure accurately left ventricular ejection fraction. *Crit Care Med* 18:221, 1990.

50. Mielck F, Buhre W, Hanekop G, et al: Comparison of continuous cardiac output measurements in patients after cardiac surgery. *J Cardiothorac Vasc Anesth* 17:211, 2003.

51. Remmen JJ, Aengevaeren WR, Verheugt FW, et al: Finapres arterial pulse wave analysis with Modelflow is not a reliable non-invasive method for assessment of cardiac output. *Clin Sci (Lond)* 103:143, 2002.

52. van Heerden PV, Baker S, Lim SI, et al: Clinical evaluation of the non-invasive cardiac output (NICO) monitor in the intensive care unit. *Anaesth Intensive Care* 28:427, 2000.

53. Odenstedt H, Stenqvist O, Lundin S: Clinical evaluation of a partial CO2 rebreathing technique for cardiac output monitoring in critically ill patients. *Acta Anaesthesiol Scand* 46:152, 2002.

54. Godje O, Peyerl M, Seebauer T, et al: Central venous pressure, pulmonary capillary wedge pressure and intrathoracic blood volumes as preload indicators in cardiac surgery patients. *Eur J Cardiothorac Surg* 13:533, 1998.

55. Lichtwarck-Aschoff M, Zeravik J, Pfeiffer UJ: Intrathoracic blood volume accurately reflects circulatory volume status in critically ill patients with mechanical ventilation. *Intensive Care Med* 18:142, 1992.

56. Gunn SR, Pinsky MR. Implications of arterial pressure variation in patients in the intensive care unit. *Curr Opin Crit Care* 7:212, 2001.

57. Michard F, Chemla D, Richard C, et al: Clinical use of respiratory changes in arterial pulse pressure to monitor the hemodynamic effects of PEEP. *Am J Respir Crit Care Med* 159:935, 1999.

58. Michard F, Boussat S, Chemla D, et al: Relation between respiratory changes in arterial pulse pressure and fluid responsiveness in septic patients with acute circulatory failure. *Am J Respir Crit Care Med* 162:134, 2000.

59. Antonsson JB, Boyle CC III, Kruithoff KL, et al: Validation of tonometric measurement of gut intramural pH during endotoxemia and mesenteric occlusion in pigs. *Am J Physiol* 259:G519, 1990.

60. Salzman AL, Strong KE, Wang H, et al: Intraluminal "balloonless" air tonometry: A new method for determination of gastrointestinal mucosal carbon dioxide tension. *Crit Care Med* 22:126, 1994.

61. Reilly PM, Wilkins KB, Fuh KC, et al: The mesenteric hemodynamic response to circulatory shock: An overview. *Shock* 15:329, 2001.

62. Fink MP: Intestinal epithelial hyperpermeability: Update on the pathogenesis of gut mucosal barrier dysfunction in critical illness. *Curr Opin Crit Care* 9:143, 2003.

63. Kolkman JJ, Groeneveld AB, Meuwissen SG: Gastric PCO_2 tonometry is independent of carbonic anhydrase inhibition. *Dig Dis Sci* 42:99, 1997.

64. Levy B, Perrigault PF, Gawalkiewicz P, et al: Gastric versus duodenal feeding and gastric tonometric measurements. *Crit Care Med* 26:1991, 1998.

65. Bjorck M, Hedberg B: Early detection of major complications after abdominal aortic surgery: Predictive value of sigmoid colon and gastric intramucosal pH monitoring. *Br J Surg* 81:25, 1994.

66. Roumen RM, Vreugde JP, Goris RJ: Gastric tonometry in multiple trauma patients. *J Trauma* 36:313, 1994.

67. Miller PR, Kincaid EH, Meredith JW, et al: Threshold values of intramucosal pH and mucosal-arterial CO_2 gap during shock resuscitation. *J Trauma* 45:868, 1998.

68. Elizalde JI, Hernandez C, Llach J, et al: Gastric intramucosal acidosis in mechanically ventilated patients: Role of mucosal blood flow. *Crit Care Med* 26:827, 1998.

69. Gutierrez G, Palizas F, Doglio G, et al: Gastric intramucosal pH as a therapeutic index of tissue oxygenation in critically ill patients. *Lancet* 339:195, 1992.

70. Ivatury RR, Simon RJ, Islam S, et al: A prospective randomized study of end points of resuscitation after major trauma: Global oxygen transport indices versus organ-specific gastric mucosal pH. *J Am Coll Surg* 183:145, 1996.

71. Weil MH, Nakagawa Y, Tang W, et al: Sublingual capnometry: A new noninvasive measurement for diagnosis and quantitation of severity of circulatory shock. *Crit Care Med* 27:1225, 1999.

72. Marik PE: Sublingual capnography: A clinical validation study. *Chest* 120:923, 2001.

73. Crookes BA, Cohn SM, Burton EA, et al: Noninvasive muscle oxygenation to guide fluid resuscitation after traumatic shock. *Surgery* 135:662, 2004.

74. Cohn SM, Nathens AB, Moore FA, et al: Tissue oxygen saturation predicts the development of organ dysfunction during traumatic shock resuscitation. *J Trauma* 62:44, 2007.

75. Haller M, Kilger E, Briegel J, et al: Continuous intra-arterial blood gas and pH monitoring in critically ill patients with severe respiratory failure: A prospective, criterion standard study. *Crit Care Med* 22:580, 1994.

76. Ventilation with lower tidal volumes as compared with traditional tidal volumes for acute lung injury and the acute respiratory distress syndrome. The Acute Respiratory Distress Syndrome Network. *N Engl J Med* 342:1301, 2000.

77. Tremper KK: Pulse oximetry. *Chest* 95:713, 1989.

78. Shoemaker WC, Belzberg H, Wo CC, et al: Multicenter study of noninvasive monitoring systems as alternatives to invasive monitoring of acutely ill emergency patients. *Chest* 114:1643, 1998.

79. Bowton DL, Scuderi PE, Haponik EF: The incidence and effect on outcome of hypoxemia in hospitalized medical patients. *Am J Med* 97:38, 1994.

80. Jubran A, Tobin MJ: Monitoring during mechanical ventilation. *Clin Chest Med* 17:453, 1996.

81. Ivatury RR, Porter JM, Simon RJ, et al: Intra-abdominal hypertension after life-threatening penetrating abdominal trauma: Prophylaxis, incidence, and clinical relevance to gastric mucosal pH and abdominal compartment syndrome. *J Trauma* 44:1016, 1998.

82. The Brain Trauma Foundation. The American Association of Neurological Surgeons. The Joint Section on Neurotrauma and Critical Care: Indications for intracranial pressure monitoring. *J Neurotrauma* 17:479, 2000.

83. The Brain Trauma Foundation. The American Association of Neurological Surgeons. The Joint Section on Neurotrauma and Critical Care: Recommendations for intracranial pressure monitoring technology. *J Neurotrauma* 17:497, 2000.

84. Juul N, Morris GF, Marshall SB, et al: Intracranial hypertension and cerebral perfusion pressure: Influence on neurological deterioration and outcome in severe head injury. The Executive Committee of the International Selfotel Trial. *J Neurosurg* 92:1, 2000.

85. Eisenberg HM, Frankowski RF, Contant CF, et al: High-dose barbiturate control of elevated intracranial pressure in patients with severe head injury. *J Neurosurg* 69:15, 1988.

86. The Brain Trauma Foundation. The American Association of Neurological Surgeons. The Joint Section on Neurotrauma and Critical Care: Guidelines for cerebral perfusion pressure. *J Neurotrauma* 17:507, 2000.

87. Cremer OL, van Dijk GW, van Wensen E, et al: Effect of intracranial pressure monitoring and targeted intensive care on functional outcome after severe head injury. *Crit Care Med* 33:2207, 2005.

88. Sigl JC, Chamoun NG: An introduction to bispectral analysis for the electroencephalogram. *J Clin Monit* 10:392, 1994.

89. Gan TJ, Glass PS, Windsor A, et al: Bispectral index monitoring allows faster emergence and improved recovery from propofol, alfentanil, and nitrous oxide anesthesia. BIS Utility Study Group. *Anesthesiology* 87:808, 1997.

90. Simmons LE, Riker RR, Prato BS, et al: Assessing sedation during intensive care unit mechanical ventilation with the Bispectral Index and the Sedation-Agitation Scale. *Crit Care Med* 27:1499, 1999.

91. Qureshi AI, Sung GY, Razumovsky AY, et al: Early identification of patients at risk for symptomatic vasospasm after aneurysmal subarachnoid hemorrhage. *Crit Care Med* 28:984, 2000.

92. Czosnyka M, Matta BF, Smielewski P, et al: Cerebral perfusion pressure in head-injured patients: A noninvasive assessment using transcranial Doppler ultrasonography. *J Neurosurg* 88:802, 1998.

93. Feldman Z, Robertson CS: Monitoring of cerebral hemodynamics with jugular bulb catheters. *Crit Care Clin* 13:51, 1997.

94. Vigue B, Ract C, Benayed M, et al: Early $SjVo_2$ monitoring in patients with severe brain trauma. *Intensive Care Med* 25:445, 1999.

95. McCormick PW, Stewart M, Goetting MG, et al: Noninvasive cerebral optical spectroscopy for monitoring cerebral oxygen delivery and hemodynamics. *Crit Care Med* 19:89, 1991.

96. Stiefel MF, Spiotta A, Gracias VH, et al: Reduced mortality rate in patients with severe traumatic brain injury treated with brain tissue oxygen monitoring. *J Neurosurg* 103:805, 2005.

Minimally Invasive Surgery, Robotics, and Natural Orifice Transluminal Endoscopic Surgery

John G. Hunter and Blair A. Jobe

INTRODUCTION

Minimally invasive surgery describes an area of surgery that crosses all traditional disciplines, from general surgery to neurosurgery. It is not a discipline unto itself, but more a philosophy of surgery, a way of thinking. Minimally invasive surgery is a means of performing major operations through small incisions, often using miniaturized, high-tech imaging systems, to minimize the trauma of surgical exposure. Some believe that the term *minimal access surgery* more accurately describes the small incisions generally necessary to gain access to surgical sites in high-tech surgery, but John Wickham's term *minimally invasive surgery* (MIS) is widely used because it describes the paradox of postmodern high-tech surgery—small holes, big operations—and the "minimalness" of the access and invasiveness of the procedures, captured in three words.

Robotic surgery today is practiced using a single platform (Intuitive, Inc., Sunnyvale, CA) and should better be termed *computer enhanced surgery* as the term *robotics* assumes autonomous action that is not a feature of the da Vinci robotic system. Instead, the da Vinci robot couples an ergonomic workstation that features stereoptic video imaging and intuitive micromanipulators (surgeon side) with a set of arms delivering specialized laparoscopic instruments enhanced with more degrees of freedom than is allowed by laparoscopic surgery alone (patient side). A computer between the surgeon side and patient side removes surgical tremor and scales motion to allow precise microsurgery, helpful for microdissection and difficult anastomoses.

Natural orifice transluminal endoscopic surgery (NOTES) is a recent extension of interventional endoscopy. Using the mouth, the anus, the vagina, and the urethra (natural orifices), flexible endoscopes are passed through the wall of the esophagus, stomach, colon, bladder, or vagina entering the mediastinum, the pleural space, or the peritoneal cavity. The advantage of this method of minimal access is principally the elimination of the scar associated with laparoscopy or thoracoscopy. Other advantages are yet to be elucidated, including pain reduction, need for hospitalization, and cost savings.

HISTORICAL BACKGROUND

Although the term *minimally invasive surgery* is relatively recent, the history of its component parts is nearly 100 years old. What is considered the newest and most popular variety of MIS, laparoscopy, is, in fact, the oldest. Primitive laparoscopy, placing a cystoscope within an inflated abdomen, was first performed by Kelling in 1901.[1] Illumination of the abdomen required hot elements at the tip of the scope and was dangerous. In the late 1950s, Hopkins described the rod lens, a method of transmitting light through a solid quartz rod with no heat and little light loss.[1] Around the same time, thin quartz fibers were discovered to be capable of trapping light internally and conducting it around corners, opening the field of fiber-optics and allowing the rapid development of flexible endoscopes.[2,3] In the 1970s, the application of flexible endoscopy grew faster than that of rigid endoscopy except in a few fields such as gynecology and orthopedics.[4] By the mid-1970s, rigid and flexible endoscopes made a rapid transition from diagnostic instruments to therapeutic ones. The explosion of video-assisted surgery in the past 20 years was a result of the development of compact, high-resolution, charge-coupled devices (CCDs) that could be mounted on the internal end of flexible endoscopes or on the external end of a Hopkins telescope. Coupled with bright light sources, fiber-optic cables, and high-resolution video monitors, the videoendoscope has changed our understanding of surgical anatomy and reshaped surgical practice.

Flexible endoscopic imaging started in the 1960s with the first bundling of many quartz fibers into bundles, one for illumination and one for imaging. The earliest upper endoscopes revolutionized the diagnosis and treatment of gastroesophageal reflux, peptic ulcer disease, and made possible early detection of upper and lower GI cancer at a stage that could be cured. The first endoscopic surgical procedure was the colonoscopic polypectomy, developed by Shinya and Wolfe, two surgeons from New York City. The percutaneous endoscopic gastrostomy (PEG) invented by Gauderer and Ponsky may have been the first NOTES procedure, reported in 1981.[5] Endoscopic pancreatic pseudocyst drainage is thought to be the next NOTES procedure developed; however, there was little energy and money put into the development of NOTES until a number of gastroenterologists claimed the ability to remove the gallbladder with a flexible endoscope, using a transgastric technique. With this pronouncement, the surgical community "woke up" and seized the momentum for NOTES research and development.

Although optical imaging produced the majority of MIS procedures, other (traditionally radiologic) imaging technologies allowed the development of innovative procedures in the 1970s. Fluoroscopic imaging allowed the adoption of percutaneous vascular procedures, the most revolutionary of which was balloon angioplasty. Balloon-based procedures spread into all fields of medicine used to open up clogged lumens with minimal access. Stents were then developed that were used in many disciplines to keep the newly ballooned segment open. The culmination of fluoroscopic balloon and stent proficiency is exemplified by the transvenous intrahepatic portosystemic shunt and by the aortic stent graft, which has nearly replaced open elective abdominal aortic aneurysm repair.

MIS procedures using ultrasound imaging have been limited to fairly crude exercises, such as fragmenting kidney stones and freezing liver tumors, because of the relatively low resolution of ultrasound devices. Newer, high-resolution ultrasound methods with high-frequency crystals may act as a guide while performing minimally invasive resections of individual layers of the intestinal wall.

Axial imaging, such as computed tomography (CT), has allowed the development of an area of MIS that often is not recognized because it requires only a CT scanner and a long needle. CT-guided drainage of abdominal fluid collections and percutaneous biopsy of abnormal tissues are minimally invasive means of performing procedures that previously required a celiotomy. CT-guided percutaneous radiofrequency (RF) ablation has emerged as a useful treatment for primary and metastatic liver tumors. This procedure also is performed laparoscopically under ultrasound guidance.[6]

A powerful, noninvasive method of imaging that will allow the development of the least invasive—and potentially noninvasive—surgery is magnetic resonance imaging (MRI).

MRI is an extremely valuable diagnostic tool, but it is only slowly coming to be of therapeutic value. One obstacle to the use of MRI for MIS is that image production and refreshment of the image as a procedure progresses are slow. Another is that all instrumentation must be nonmetallic when working with the powerful magnets of an MRI scanner. Moreover, MRI magnets are bulky and limit the surgeon's access to the patient. Open magnets have been developed that allow the surgeon to stand between two large MRI coils, obtaining access to the portion of the patient being scanned. The advantage of MRI, in addition to the superb images produced, is that there is no radiation exposure to patient or surgeon. Some neurosurgeons are accumulating experience using MRI to perform frameless stereotactic surgery.

Robotic surgery has been dreamed about for some time, and many "Rube Goldberg" devices have been developed over the years to provide mechanical assistance for the surgeon. The first computer-assisted robot, the "RoboDoc" was designed to accurately drill femoral shaft bone for wobble-free placement of hip prostheses. Although the name was appealing, the robot proved no better than a skilled orthopedic surgeon and was a good deal slower. Following this, the first and only two commercially successful robots for laparoscopic surgery were in development in California.

KEY POINTS

1. Minimally invasive surgery describes a philosophical approach to surgery in which access trauma is minimized without compromising the quality of the surgical procedure.

2. Minimally invasive surgery is dependent upon videoscopic, ultrasonographic, radiologic, and magnetic resonance imaging.

3. The carbon dioxide pneumoperitoneum used for laparoscopy induces some unique pathophysiologic consequences.

4. Training for laparoscopy requires practice outside of the operating room in a simulation laboratory and/or in animal models.

5. Laparoscopy during pregnancy is best performed in the second trimester and is safe if appropriate monitoring is performed.

6. Laparoscopic surgery for cancer is also appropriate if good tissue handling techniques are maintained.

7. Robotic surgery has been most valuable in the pelvis for performance of minimally invasive prostatectomy and gynecologic and fertility procedures.

8. Natural orifice transluminal endoscopic surgery represents a new opportunity to develop truly scar-free surgery.

Computer Motion, founded by Yulun Wang in Santa Barbara, used National Science Foundation funds to create a mechanical arm, the Aesop robot, which held and moved the laparoscope with voice, foot, or hand control. In Northern California, a master-slave system first developed for surgery on the multinational space station by Philip Green was purchased by Fred Moll and Lonnie Smith, then re-engineered with the surgeon in mind to create a remarkably intuitive computer-enhanced surgical platform. The company, Intuitive Surgical, was aptly named, and their primary product, the da Vinci robot, is the only major "robotic" surgical device currently on the market. Although eschewed by many experienced laparoscopists, the da Vinci achieved a toehold among many skilled surgeons who found that the robot could facilitate MIS procedures that were difficult with standard laparoscopic procedures.

PHYSIOLOGY AND PATHOPHYSIOLOGY OF MINIMALLY INVASIVE SURGERY

Even with the least invasive of the MIS procedures, physiologic changes occur. Many minimally invasive procedures require minimal or no sedation, and there are few adverse consequences to the cardiovascular, endocrinologic, or immunologic systems. The least invasive of such procedures include stereotactic biopsy of breast lesions and flexible GI endoscopy. Minimally invasive procedures that require general anesthesia have a greater physiologic impact because of the anesthetic agent, the incision (even if small), and the induced pneumoperitoneum.

Laparoscopy

The unique feature of laparoscopic surgery is the need to lift the abdominal wall from the abdominal organs. Two methods have been devised for achieving this.[7] The first, used by most surgeons, is a pneumoperitoneum. Throughout the early twentieth century, intraperitoneal visualization was achieved by inflating the abdominal cavity with air, using a sphygmomanometer bulb.[8] The problem with using air insufflation is that nitrogen is poorly soluble in blood and is slowly absorbed across the peritoneal surfaces. Air pneumoperitoneum was believed to be more painful than nitrous oxide (N_2O) pneumoperitoneum, but less painful than carbon dioxide (CO_2) pneumoperitoneum. Subsequently, carbon dioxide and N_2O were used for inflating the abdomen. N_2O had the advantage of being physiologically inert and rapidly absorbed. It also provided better analgesia for laparoscopy performed under local anesthesia when compared with CO_2 or air.[9] Despite initial concerns that N_2O would not suppress combustion, controlled clinical trials have established its safety within the peritoneal cavity.[10] In addition, N_2O has been shown to reduce the intraoperative end-tidal CO_2 and minute ventilation required to maintain homeostasis when compared to CO_2 pneumoperitoneum.[10] The effect of N_2O on tumor biology and the development of port site metastasis are unknown. As such, caution should be exercised when performing laparoscopic cancer surgery with this agent. Finally, the safety of N_2O pneumoperitoneum in pregnancy has yet to be elucidated.

The physiologic effects of CO_2 pneumoperitoneum can be divided into two areas: (a) gas-specific effects and (b) pressure-specific effects (Fig. 14-1). CO_2 is rapidly absorbed across the peritoneal membrane into the circulation. In the circulation, CO_2 creates a respiratory acidosis by the generation of carbonic acid.[11] Body buffers, the largest reserve of which lies in bone, absorb CO_2 (up to 120 L) and minimize the development of hypercarbia or respiratory acidosis during brief endoscopic procedures.[11] Once the body buffers are saturated, respiratory acidosis develops rapidly, and the respiratory system assumes the burden of keeping up with the absorption of CO_2 and its release from these buffers.

In patients with normal respiratory function, this is not difficult; the anesthesiologist increases the ventilatory rate or vital capacity on the ventilator. If the respiratory rate required exceeds 20 breaths per

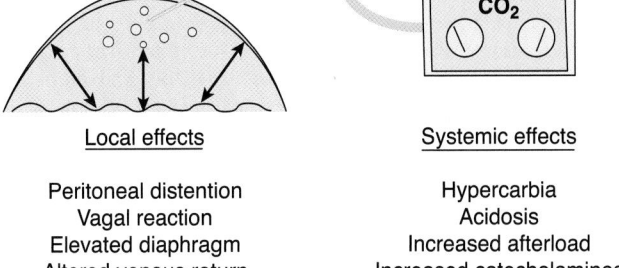

Local effects	Systemic effects
Peritoneal distention Vagal reaction Elevated diaphragm Altered venous return Pain	Hypercarbia Acidosis Increased afterload Increased catecholamines Myocardial stress

FIG. 14-1. Carbon dioxide gas insufflated into the peritoneal cavity has both local and systemic effects that cause a complex set of hemodynamic and metabolic alterations. *[Reproduced with permission from Hunter JG (ed):* Baillieres Clinical Gastroenterology Laparoscopic Surgery. *London/Philadelphia: Bailliere Tindall, 1993, p 758.]*

minute, there may be less efficient gas exchange and increasing hypercarbia.[12] Conversely, if vital capacity is increased substantially, there is a greater opportunity for barotrauma and greater respiratory motion-induced disruption of the upper abdominal operative field. In some situations, it is advisable to evacuate the pneumoperitoneum or reduce the intra-abdominal pressure to allow time for the anesthesiologist to adjust for hypercarbia.[13] Although mild respiratory acidosis probably is an insignificant problem, more severe respiratory acidosis leading to cardiac arrhythmias has been reported.[14] Hypercarbia also causes tachycardia and increased systemic vascular resistance, which elevates blood pressure and increases myocardial oxygen demand.[11,14]

The pressure effects of the pneumoperitoneum on cardiovascular physiology also have been studied. In the hypovolemic individual, excessive pressure on the inferior vena cava and a reverse Trendelenburg position with loss of lower extremity muscle tone may cause decreased venous return and decreased cardiac output.[11,15] This is not seen in the normovolemic patient. The most common arrhythmia created by laparoscopy is bradycardia. A rapid stretch of the peritoneal membrane often causes a vagovagal response with bradycardia and, occasionally, hypotension.[16] The appropriate management of this event is desufflation of the abdomen, administration of vagolytic agents (e.g., atropine), and adequate volume replacement.[17]

With the increased intra-abdominal pressure compressing the inferior vena cava, there is diminished venous return from the lower extremities. This has been well documented in the patient placed in the reverse Trendelenburg position for upper abdominal operations. Venous engorgement and decreased venous return promote venous thrombosis.[18,19] Many series of advanced laparoscopic procedures in which deep venous thrombosis (DVT) prophylaxis was not used demonstrate the frequency of pulmonary embolus. This usually is an avoidable complication with the use of sequential compression stockings, subcutaneous heparin, or low molecular weight heparin.[20] In short-duration laparoscopic procedures, such as appendectomy, hernia repair, or cholecystectomy, the risk of DVT may not be sufficient to warrant extensive DVT prophylaxis.

The increased pressure of the pneumoperitoneum is transmitted directly across the paralyzed diaphragm to the thoracic cavity, creating increased central venous pressure and increased filling pressures of the right and left sides of the heart. If the intra-abdominal pressures are kept under 20 mmHg, the cardiac output usually is well maintained.[19–21] The direct effect of the pneumoperitoneum on increasing intrathoracic pressure increases peak inspiratory pressure, pressure across the chest wall, and also, the likelihood of barotrauma. Despite these concerns, disruption of blebs and consequent pneumothoraces are rare after uncomplicated laparoscopic surgery.[21] Pneumothoraces occurring with laparoscopic esophageal surgery may be very significant. The pathophysiology and management are discussed at the end of this section. Increased intra-abdominal pressure decreases renal blood flow, glomerular filtration rate, and urine output. These effects may be mediated by direct pressure on the kidney and the renal vein.[22,23] The secondary effect of decreased renal blood flow is to increase plasma renin release, thereby increasing sodium retention. Increased circulating antidiuretic hormone levels also are found during the pneumoperitoneum, increasing free water reabsorption in the distal tubules.[24] Although the effects of the pneumoperitoneum on renal blood flow are immediately reversible, the hormonally mediated changes such as elevated antidiuretic hormone levels decrease urine output for up to 1 hour after the procedure has ended. Intraoperative oliguria is common during laparoscopy, but the urine output is not a reflection of intravascular volume status; IV fluid administration during an uncomplicated laparoscopic procedure should not be linked to urine output. Because insensible fluid losses through the open abdomen are eliminated with laparoscopy, the need for supplemental fluid during a laparoscopic surgical procedure should only keep up with venous pooling in the lower limbs, third-space losses into the bowel, and blood loss, which is generally less than occurs with an equivalent open operation.

The hemodynamic and metabolic consequences of pneumoperitoneum are well tolerated by healthy individuals for a prolonged period and by most individuals for at least a short period. Difficulties can occur when a patient with compromised cardiovascular function is subjected to a long laparoscopic procedure. It is during these procedures that alternative approaches should be considered or insufflation pressure reduced. Alternative gases that have been suggested for laparoscopy include the inert gases helium, neon, and argon. These gases are appealing because they cause no metabolic effects, but are poorly soluble in blood (unlike CO_2 and N_2O) and are prone to create gas emboli if the gas has direct access to the venous system.[19] Gas emboli are rare but serious complications of laparoscopic surgery.[20,25] They should be suspected if hypotension develops during insufflation. Diagnosis may be made by listening (with an esophageal stethoscope) for the characteristic "mill wheel" murmur. The treatment of gas embolism is to place the patient in a left lateral decubitus position with the head down to trap the gas in the apex of the right ventricle.[20] A rapidly placed central venous catheter then can be used to aspirate the gas out of the right ventricle.

In some situations, minimally invasive abdominal surgery should be performed without insufflation. This has led to the development of an abdominal lift device that can be placed through a 10- to 12-mm trocar at the umbilicus.[26] These devices have the advantage of creating little physiologic derangement, but they are bulky and intrusive. The exposure and working room offered by lift devices also are inferior to those accomplished by pneumoperitoneum. Lifting the anterior abdominal wall causes a "pinching in" of the lateral flank walls, displacing the bowel medially and anteriorly into the operative field. A pneumoperitoneum, with its well-distributed intra-abdominal pressure, provides better exposure. Abdominal lift devices also cause more postoperative pain, but they do allow the performance of MIS with standard (nonlaparoscopic) surgical instruments.

Endocrine responses to laparoscopic surgery are not always intuitive. Serum cortisol levels after laparoscopic operations are often higher than after the equivalent operation performed through an open incision.[27] The greatest difference between the endocrine response of open and laparoscopic surgery is the more rapid equilibration of most stress-mediated hormone levels after laparoscopic surgery. Immune suppression also is less after laparoscopy than after open surgery. There is a trend toward more rapid normalization of cytokine levels after a laparoscopic procedure than after the equivalent procedure performed by celiotomy.[28]

Transhiatal mobilization of the distal esophagus is commonly performed as a component of many laparoscopic upper abdominal procedures. If there is compromise of the mediastinal pleura with resultant CO_2 pneumothorax, the defect should be enlarged so as to prevent a tension pneumothorax. Even with such a strategy, tension pneumothorax may develop, as mediastinal structures may seal the hole during inspiration, allowing the chest to fill during expiration. In addition to enlargement of the hole, a thoracostomy tube (chest tube) should be placed across the breach into the abdomen with intra-abdominal pressures reduced below 8 mmHg, or a standard chest tube may be placed. When a pneumothorax occurs with laparoscopic Nissen fundoplication or Heller myotomy, it is preferable to place an 18 F red rubber catheter with multiple side holes cut out of the distal end across the defect. At the end of the procedure, the distal end of the tube is pulled out a 10-mm port site (as the port is removed), and the pneumothorax is evacuated to a primitive water seal using a bowl of sterile water or saline. During laparoscopic esophagectomy, it is preferable to leave a standard chest tube, as residual intra-abdominal fluid will tend to be siphoned through the defect postoperatively, if the tube is removed at the end of the case.

Thoracoscopy

The physiology of thoracic MIS (thoracoscopy) is different from that of laparoscopy. Because of the bony confines of the thorax, it is unnecessary to use positive pressure when working in the thorax.[29] The disadvantages of positive pressure in the chest include decreased venous return, mediastinal shift, and the need to keep a firm seal at all trocar sites. Without positive pressure, it is necessary to place a double-lumen endotracheal tube so that the ipsilateral lung can be deflated when the operation starts. By collapsing the ipsilateral lung, working space within the thorax is obtained. Because insufflation is unnecessary in thoracoscopic surgery, it can be beneficial to use standard instruments via extended port sites in conjunction with thoracoscopic instruments. This approach is particularly useful when performing advanced procedures such as thoracoscopic anatomic pulmonary resection.

Extracavitary Minimally Invasive Surgery

Many MIS procedures create working spaces in extrathoracic and extraperitoneal locations. Laparoscopic inguinal hernia repair usually is performed in the anterior extraperitoneal Retzius space.[30,31] Laparoscopic nephrectomy often is performed with retroperitoneal laparoscopy. Endoscopic retroperitoneal approaches to pancreatic necrosectomy have seen some limited use.[32] Lower extremity vascular procedures and plastic surgical endoscopic procedures require the development of working space in unconventional planes, often at the level of the fascia, sometimes below the fascia, and occasionally in nonanatomic regions.[33] Some of these techniques use insufflation of gas, but many use balloon inflation to develop the space, followed by low-pressure gas insufflation or lift devices to maintain the space (Fig. 14-2). These techniques produce fewer and less severe adverse physiologic consequences than does the pneumoperitoneum, but the insufflation of carbon dioxide into extraperitoneal locations can spread widely, causing subcutaneous emphysema and metabolic acidosis.

Anesthesia

Proper anesthesia management during laparoscopic surgery requires a thorough knowledge of the pathophysiology of the CO_2 pneumoperitoneum.[17] The laparoscopic surgeon can influence cardiovascular performance by reducing or removing the CO_2 pneumoperitoneum. Insensible fluid losses are negligible, and therefore, IV fluid administration should not exceed that necessary to maintain circulating volume. MIS procedures are often outpatient procedures, so short-acting anesthetic agents are preferable. Because the factors that require hospitalization after laparoscopic procedures include the management of nausea, pain, and urinary retention, the anesthesiologist should minimize the use of agents that provoke these conditions and maximize the use of medications that prevent such problems. Critical to the anesthesia management of these patients is the use of nonnarcotic analgesics (e.g., ketorolac) when hemostasis allows it, and the liberal use of antiemetic agents, including ondansetron and steroids.

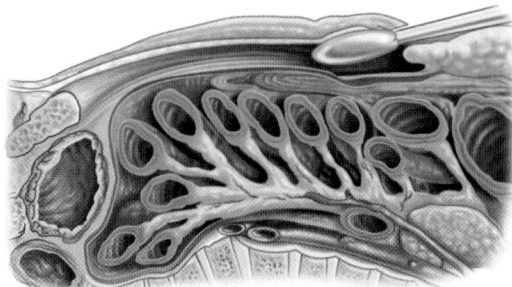

A

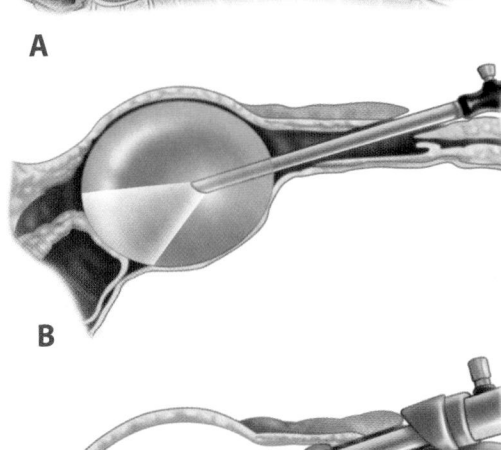

B

C

FIG. 14-2. Balloons are used to create extra-anatomic working spaces. In this example (**A** through **C**), a balloon is introduced into the space between the posterior rectus sheath and the rectus abdominal muscle. The balloon is inflated in the preperitoneal space to create working room for extraperitoneal endoscopic hernia repair.

The Minimally Invasive Team

From the beginning, the tremendous success of MIS was founded on the understanding that a team approach was necessary. The many laparoscopic procedures performed daily range from basic to advanced complexity, and require that the surgical team have an intimate understanding of the operative conduct (Table 14-1). Minimally invasive procedures require complicated and fragile equipment that demands constant maintenance. In addition, multiple intraoperative adjustments to the equipment, camera, insufflator, monitors, and patient/surgeon position are made during these procedures. As such, a coordinated team approach is mandated to ensure patient safety and excellent outcomes. More and more, flexible endoscopes are used to guide or provide quality control for laparoscopic procedures. As NOTES evolves, hybrid procedures (laparoscopy and endoscopy) and sophisticated NOTES technology will require a nursing staff capable of maintaining flexible endoscopes and understanding the operation of sophisticated endoscopic technology.

A typical MIS team may consist of a laparoscopic surgeon and an operating room (OR) nurse with an interest in laparoscopic and endoscopic surgery. Adding dedicated assistants and circulating staff with an intimate knowledge of the equipment will add to and enhance the team nucleus. Studies have demonstrated that having a

TABLE 14-1	Laparoscopic surgical procedures	
Basic	**Advanced**	
Appendectomy	Nissen fundoplication	Lymph node dissection
Cholecystectomy	Heller myotomy	Robotics
Hernia repair	Gastrectomy	Stereo imaging
	Esophagectomy	Telemedicine
	Enteral access	Laparoscopy-assisted
	Bile duct exploration	procedures
	Colectomy	Hepatectomy
	Splenectomy	Pancreatectomy
	Adrenalectomy	Prostatectomy
	Nephrectomy	Hysterectomy

designated laparoscopic team increases the efficiency and safety of laparoscopic surgery, which is translated into a benefit for patient and hospital.[34]

Room Setup and the Minimally Invasive Suite

Nearly all MIS, whether using fluoroscopic, ultrasound, or optical imaging, incorporates a video monitor as a guide. Occasionally, two images are necessary to adequately guide the operation, as in procedures such as endoscopic retrograde cholangiopancreatography, laparoscopic common bile duct exploration, and laparoscopic ultrasonography. When two images are necessary, the images should be displayed on two adjacent video monitors or projected on a single screen with a picture-in-picture effect. The video monitor(s) should be set across the operating table from the surgeon. The patient should be interposed between the surgeon and the video monitor; ideally, the operative field also lies between the surgeon and the monitor. In pelviscopic surgery it is best to place the video monitor at the patient's feet, and in laparoscopic cholecystectomy, the monitor is placed at the 10 o'clock position (relative to the patient) while the surgeon stands on the patient's left at the 4 o'clock position. The insufflating and patient-monitoring equipment ideally also is placed across the table from the surgeon, so that the insufflating pressure and the patient's vital signs and end-tidal CO_2 tension can be monitored.

The development of the minimally invasive surgical suite has been a tremendous contribution to the field of laparoscopy in that it has facilitated the performance of advanced procedures and techniques (Fig. 14-3). By having the core equipment (monitors, insufflators, and imaging equipment) located within mobile, ceiling-mounted consoles, the surgery team is able to accommodate and make small adjustments rapidly and continuously throughout the procedure. The specifically designed minimally invasive surgical suite serves to decrease equipment and cable disorganization, ease the movements of operative personnel around the room, improve ergonomics, and facilitate the use of advanced imaging equipment such as laparoscopic ultrasound.[35] Although having a minimally invasive surgical suite available is very useful, it is not essential to successfully carry out advanced laparoscopic procedures.

Patient Positioning

Patients usually are placed in the supine position for laparoscopic surgery. When the operative field is the gastroesophageal junction or the left lobe of the liver, it is easiest to operate from between the legs. The legs may be elevated in Allen stirrups or abducted on leg boards to achieve this position. When pelvic procedures are performed, it usually is necessary to place the legs in Allen stirrups to gain access to the perineum. A lateral decubitus position with the table flexed provides the best access to the retroperitoneum when performing nephrectomy or adrenalectomy. For laparoscopic splenectomy, a 45°-tilt of the patient provides excellent access to the lesser sac and the lateral peritoneal attachments to the spleen. For

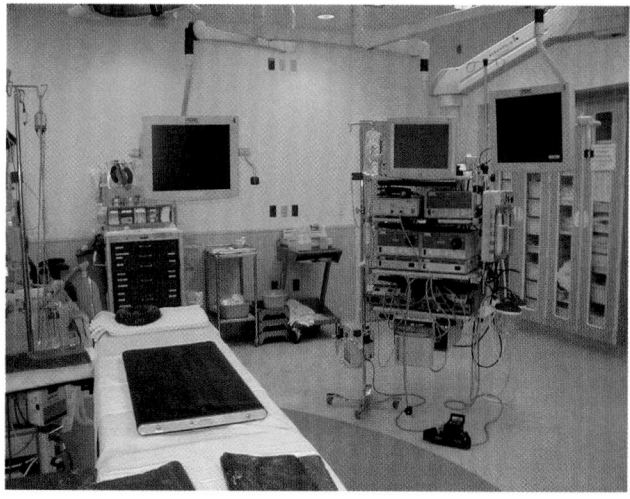

FIG. 14-3. An example of a typical minimally invasive surgery suite. All core equipment is located on easily movable consoles.

thoracoscopic surgery, the patient is placed in the lateral position with table flexion to open the intercostal spaces and the distance between the iliac crest and costal margin (Fig. 14-4).

When the patient's knees are to be bent for extended periods or the patient is going to be placed in a reverse Trendelenburg position for more than a few minutes, DVT prophylaxis should be used. Sequential compression of the lower extremities during prolonged (>90 minutes) laparoscopic procedures increases venous return and provides inhibition of thromboplastin activation.

General Principles of Access

The most natural ports of access for MIS and NOTES are the anatomic portals of entry and exit. The nares, mouth, urethra, and anus are used to access the respiratory, GI, and urinary systems. The advantage of using these points of access is that no incision is required. The disadvantages lie in the long distances between the

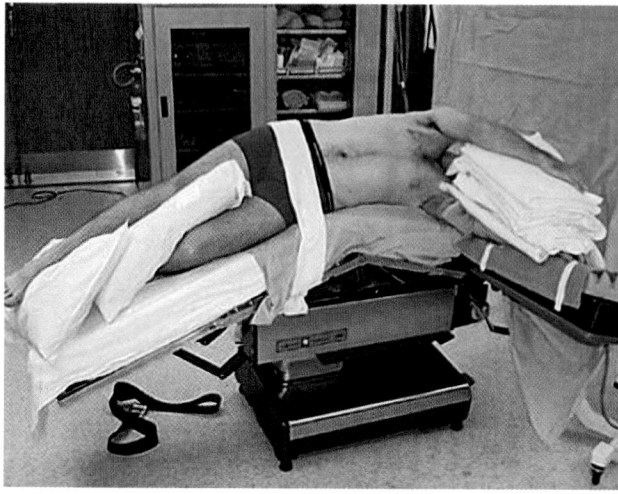

FIG. 14-4. Proper padding and protection of pressure points is an essential consideration in laparoscopic and thoracoscopic approaches. In preparation for thoracoscopy, this patient is placed in left lateral decubitus position with the table flexed, which serves to open the intercostal spaces and increase the distance between the iliac crest and the inferior costal margin.

orifice and the region of interest. For NOTES procedures, the vagina may serve as another point of access, entering the abdomen via the posterior cul–de–sac of the pelvis. Similarly, the peritoneal cavity may be reached through the side wall of the stomach or colon.

Access to the vascular system may be accomplished under local anesthesia by cutting down and exposing the desired vessel, usually in the groin. Increasingly, vascular access is obtained with percutaneous techniques using a small incision, a needle, and a guidewire, over which are passed a variety of different sized access devices. This approach, known as the *Seldinger technique*, is most frequently used by general surgeons for placement of Hickman catheters, but also is used to gain access to the arterial and venous system for performance of minimally invasive procedures. Guidewire-assisted, Seldinger-type techniques also are helpful for gaining access to the gut for procedures such as PEG, for gaining access to the biliary system through the liver, and for gaining access to the upper urinary tract.

In thoracoscopic surgery, the access technique is similar to that used for placement of a chest tube. In these procedures general anesthesia and single lung ventilation are essential. A small incision is made over the top of a rib and, under direct vision, carried down through the pleura. The lung is collapsed, and a trocar is inserted across the chest wall to allow access with a telescope. Once the lung is completely collapsed, subsequent access may be obtained with direct puncture, viewing all entry sites through the videoendoscope. Because insufflation of the chest is unnecessary, simple ports that keep the small incisions open are all that is required to allow repeated access to the thorax.

Laparoscopic Access

The requirements for laparoscopy are more involved, because the creation of a pneumoperitoneum requires that instruments of access (trocars) contain valves to maintain abdominal inflation.

Two methods are used for establishing abdominal access during laparoscopic procedures.[36,37] The first, direct puncture laparoscopy, begins with the elevation of the relaxed abdominal wall with two towel clips or a well-placed hand. A small incision is made in the umbilicus, and a specialized spring-loaded (Veress) needle is placed in the abdominal cavity (Fig. 14-5). With the Veress needle, two distinct pops are felt as the surgeon passes the needle through the abdominal wall fascia and the peritoneum. The umbilicus usually is selected as the preferred point of access because, in this location, the abdominal wall is quite thin, even in obese patients. The abdomen is inflated with a pressure-limited insufflator. CO_2 gas usually is used, with maximal pressures in the range of 14 to 15 mmHg. During the process of insufflation, it is essential that the surgeon observe the pressure and flow readings on the monitor to confirm an intraperitoneal location of the Veress needle tip (Fig. 14-6). Laparoscopic surgery can be performed under local anesthesia, but general anesthesia is preferable. Under local anesthesia, N_2O is used as the insufflating agent, and insufflation is stopped after 2 L of gas is insufflated or when a pressure of 10 mmHg is reached.

After peritoneal insufflation, direct access to the abdomen is obtained with a 5- or 10-mm trocar. The critical issues for safe direct-puncture laparoscopy include the use of a vented stylet for the trocar, or a trocar with a safety shield or dilating tip. The trocar must be pointed away from the sacral promontory and the great vessels.[38] Patient position should be surveyed before trocar placement to ensure a proper trajectory. For performance of laparoscopic cholecystectomy, the trocar is angled toward the right upper quadrant.

Occasionally, the direct peritoneal access (Hasson) technique is advisable.[39] With this technique, the surgeon makes a small incision just below the umbilicus and under direct vision locates the abdominal fascia. Two Kocher clamps are placed on the fascia, and with curved Mayo scissors, a small incision is made through the fascia and underlying peritoneum. A finger is placed into the abdomen to make sure that there is no adherent bowel. A sturdy suture is placed on each

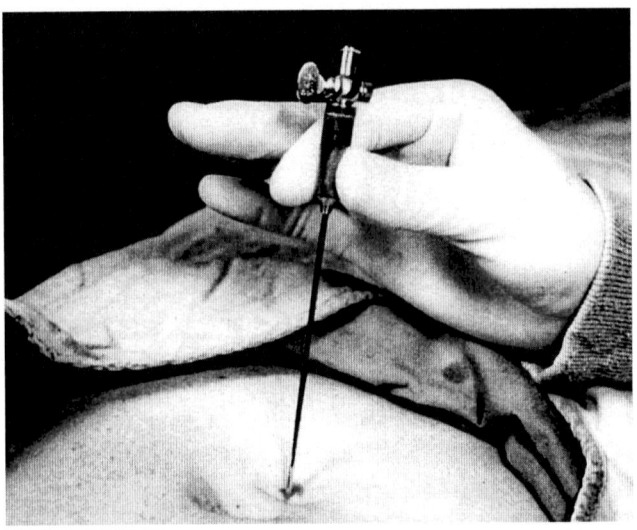
A

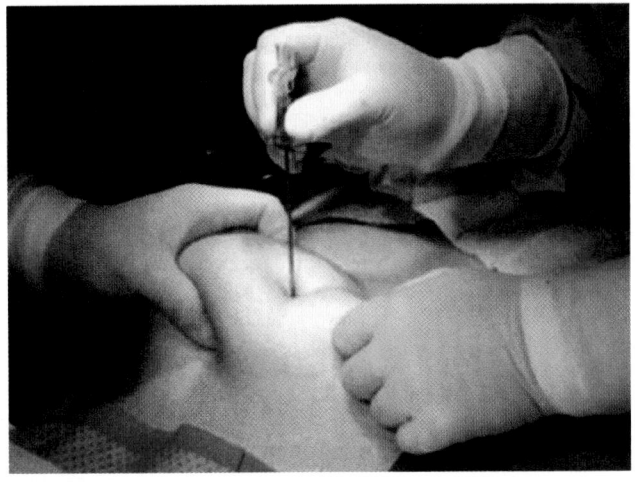
B

FIG. 14-5. A. Insufflation of the abdomen is accomplished with a Veress needle held at its serrated collar with a thumb and forefinger. **B.** Because linea alba is fused to the umbilicus, the abdominal wall is grasped with fingers or penetrating towel clip to elevate the abdominal wall away from the underlying structures.

side of the fascia and secured to the wings of a specialized trocar, which is then passed directly into the abdominal cavity (Fig. 14-7). Rapid insufflation can make up for some of the time lost with the initial dissection. This technique is preferable for the abdomen of patients who have undergone previous operations in which small bowel may be adherent to the undersurface of the abdominal wound. The close adherence of bowel to the peritoneum in the previously operated abdomen does not eliminate the possibility of intestinal injury but should make great vessel injury extremely unlikely. Because of the difficulties in visualizing the abdominal region immediately adjacent to the primary trocar, it is recommended that the telescope be passed through a secondary trocar to inspect the site of initial abdominal access.[37] Secondary punctures are made with 5- and 10-mm trocars. For safe access to the abdominal cavity, it is critical to visualize all sites of trocar entry.[38,39] At the completion of the operation, all trocars are removed under direct vision, and the insertion sites are inspected for bleeding. If bleeding occurs, direct pressure with an instrument from another trocar site or balloon tamponade

with a Foley catheter placed through the trocar site generally stops the bleeding within 3 to 5 minutes. When this is not successful, a full-thickness abdominal wall suture has been used successfully to tamponade trocar site bleeding.

It is generally agreed that 5-mm trocars need no site suturing. Ten-millimeter trocars placed off the midline and above the transverse mesocolon do not require repair. Conversely, if the fascia has been dilated to allow the passage of the gallbladder or other organ, it should be repaired at the fascial level with interrupted sutures. The port site may be closed with suture delivery systems similar to crochet needles enabling mass closure of the abdominal wall. This is especially helpful in obese patients where direct fascial closure may be challenging, through a small skin incision. Failure to close lower abdominal trocar sites that are 10 mm in diameter or larger can lead to an incarcerated hernia.

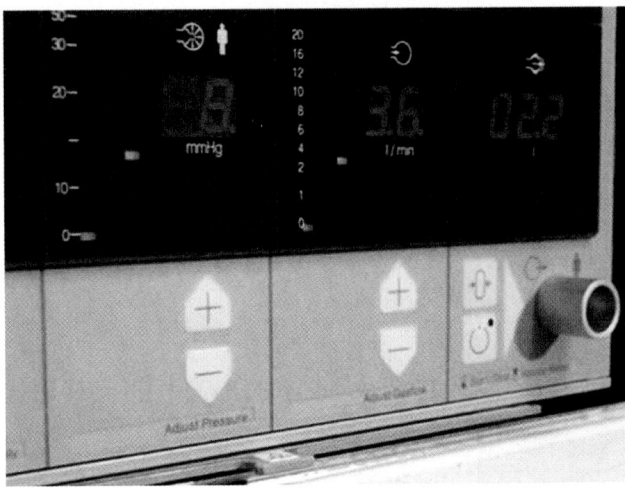

FIG. 14-6. It is essential to be able to interpret the insufflator pressure readings and flow rates. These readings indicate proper intraperitoneal placement of the Veress needle.

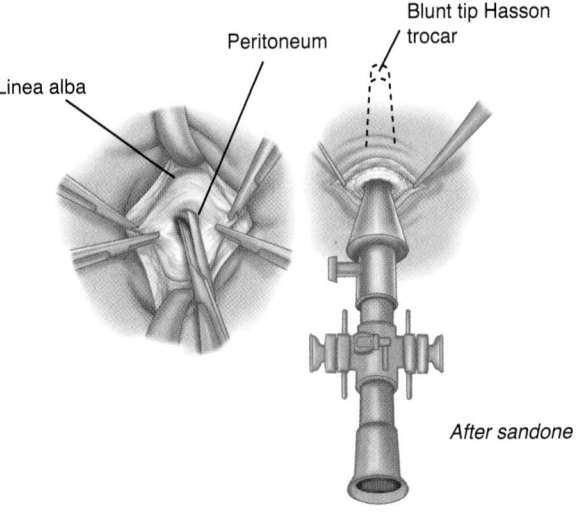

Linea alba

Peritoneum

Blunt tip Hasson trocar

After sandone

FIG. 14-7. The open laparoscopy technique involves identification and incision of the peritoneum, followed by the placement of a specialized trocar with a conical sleeve to maintain a gas seal. Specialized wings on the trocar are attached to sutures placed through the fascia to prevent loss of the gas seal.

Access for Subcutaneous and Extraperitoneal Surgery

There are two methods for gaining access to nonanatomic spaces. For retroperitoneal locations, balloon dissection is effective. This access technique is appropriate for the extraperitoneal repair of inguinal hernias and for retroperitoneal surgery for adrenalectomy, nephrectomy, lumbar discectomy, pancreatic necrosectomy, or para-aortic lymph node dissection.[40,41] The initial access to the extraperitoneal space is performed in a way similar to direct puncture laparoscopy, except that the last layer (the peritoneum) is not traversed. Once the transversalis fascia has been punctured, a specialized trocar with a balloon on the end is introduced. The balloon is inflated in the extraperitoneal space to create a working chamber. The balloon then is deflated and a Hasson trocar is placed. An insufflation pressure of 10 mmHg usually is adequate to keep the extraperitoneal space open for dissection and will limit subcutaneous emphysema. Higher gas pressures force CO_2 into the soft tissues and may contribute to hypercarbia. Extraperitoneal endosurgery provides less working space than laparoscopy but eliminates the possibility of intestinal injury, intestinal adhesion, herniation at the trocar sites, and ileus. These issues are important for laparoscopic hernia repair because extraperitoneal approaches prevent the small bowel from sticking to the prosthetic mesh.[31]

Subcutaneous surgery has been most widely used in cardiac, vascular, and plastic surgery.[33] In cardiac surgery, subcutaneous access has been used for saphenous vein harvesting, and in vascular surgery for ligation of subfascial perforating veins (Linton procedure). With minimally invasive techniques, the entire saphenous vein above the knee may be harvested through a single incision[42,43] (Fig. 14-8). Once the saphenous vein is located, a long retractor that holds a 5-mm laparoscope allows the coaxial dissection of the vein and coagulation or clipping of each side branch. A small incision above the knee also can be used to ligate perforating veins in the lower leg.

Subcutaneous access also is used for plastic surgery procedures.[43] Minimally invasive approaches are especially well suited to cosmetic surgery, in which attempts are made to hide the incision. It is easier to hide several 5-mm incisions than one long incision. The technique of blunt dissection along fascial planes combined with lighted retractors and endoscope-holding retractors is most successful for extensive subcutaneous surgery. Some prefer gas insufflation of these soft tissue planes. The primary disadvantage of soft tissue insufflation is that subcutaneous emphysema can be created.

Hand-Assisted Laparoscopic Access

Hand-assisted laparoscopic surgery is thought to combine the tactile advantages of open surgery with the minimal access of laparoscopy and thoracoscopy. This approach commonly is used to assist with difficult cases before conversion to celiotomy is necessary. Additionally, hand-assisted laparoscopic surgery is used to help surgeons negotiate the steep learning curve associated with advanced laparoscopic procedures.[44] This technology uses a "port" for the hand that preserves the pneumoperitoneum and enables endoscopic visualization in combination with the use of minimally invasive instruments (Fig. 14-9). Formal investigation of this modality has been limited primarily to case reports and small series, and has focused primarily on solid organ and colon surgery.

Intraperitoneal, intrathoracic, and retroperitoneal access for robotic surgery adheres to the principles of laparoscopic and thoracoscopic access; however, the port size for the primary puncture is 12 mm to allow placement of the stereo laparoscope.

Port Placement

Trocars for the surgeon's left and right hand should be placed at least 10 cm apart. For most operations, it is possible to orient the telescope between these two trocars and slightly back from them. The ideal trocar orientation creates an equilateral triangle between the surgeon's right hand, left hand, and the telescope, with 10 to 15

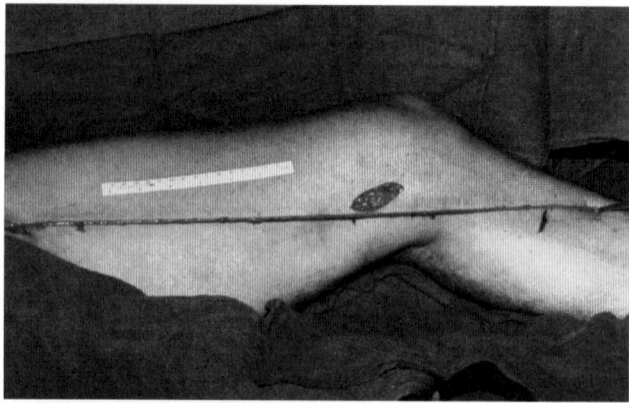

A

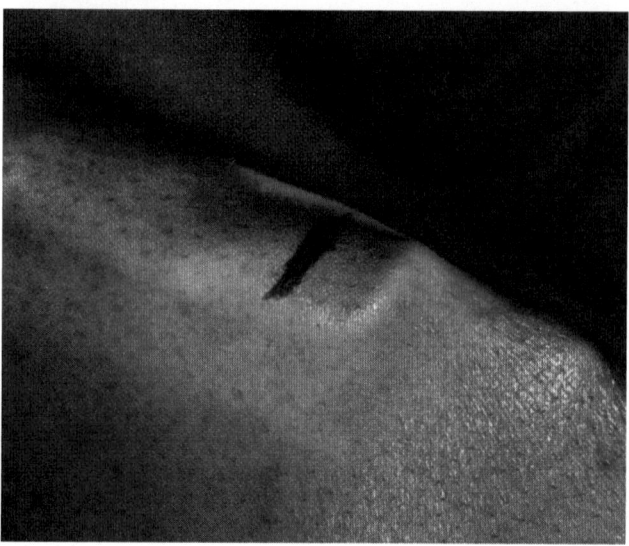

B

FIG. 14-8. A. With two small incisions, virtually the entire saphenous vein can be harvested for bypass grafting. **B.** The lighted retractor in the subcutaneous space during saphenous vein harvest is seen illuminating the skin. *[Reproduced with permission from Jones GE, Eaves FE III, Howell RL et al: Harvest of muscle, nerve, fascia, and vein, in Bostwick J III, Eaves FE III, Nahai F (eds): Endoscopic Plastic Surgery. St Louis: Quality Medical Publishing, Inc., 1995, p 542.]*

cm on each leg. If one imagines the target of the operation (e.g., the gallbladder or gastroesophageal junction) oriented at the apex of a second equilateral triangle built on the first, these four points of reference create a diamond (Fig. 14-10). The surgeon stands behind the telescope, which provides optimal ergonomic orientation but frequently requires that a camera operator (or mechanical camera holder) reach between the surgeon's hands to guide the telescope.

The position of the operating table should permit the surgeon to work with both elbows in at the sides, with arms bent 90° at the elbow.[45] It usually is necessary to alter the operating table position with left or right tilt with the patient in the Trendelenburg or reverse Trendelenburg position, depending on the operative field.[46,47]

Imaging Systems

Two methods of videoendoscopic imaging are widely used. Both methods use a camera with a CCD, which is an array of photosensitive sensor elements (pixels) that convert the incoming light intensity to an electric charge. The electric charge is subsequently converted into a black-and-white image.[48]

With videoendoscopy, the CCD chip is placed on the internal end of a long, flexible endoscope. With older flexible endoscopes,

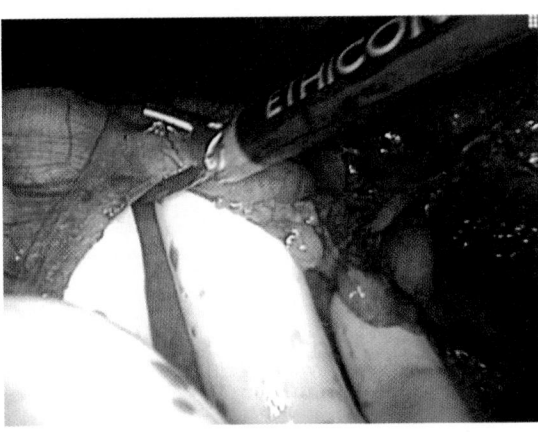

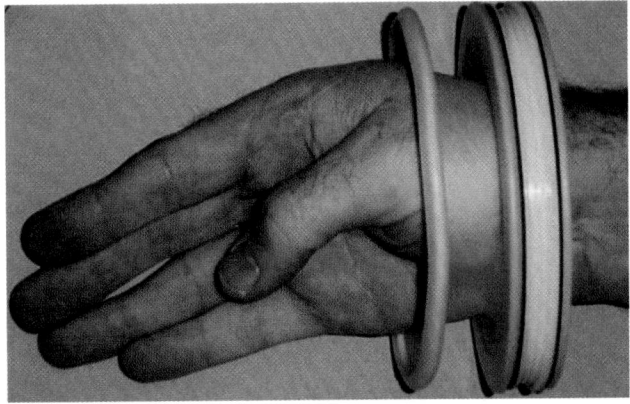

FIG. 14-9. This is an example of hand-assisted laparoscopic surgery during left colectomy. The surgeon uses a hand to provide retraction and counter tension during mobilization of the colon from its retroperitoneal attachments, as well as during division of the mesocolon. This technique is particularly useful in the region of the transverse colon.

thin quartz fibers are packed together in a bundle, and the CCD camera is mounted on the external end of the endoscope. Most standard GI endoscopes have the CCD chip at the distal end, but small, delicate choledochoscopes and nephroscopes are equipped with fiber-optic bundles.[49] Distally mounted CCD chips were developed for laparoscopy as well but have not become popular.

Video cameras come in two basic designs. Nearly all laparoscopic cameras contain a red, green, and blue input, and are identical to the color cameras used for television production.[48] An additional feature of many video cameras is digital enhancement. Digital enhancement detects edges, areas where there are drastic color or light changes between two adjacent pixels.[50] By enhancing this difference, the image appears sharper and surgical resolution is improved. New laparoscopic cameras contain a high-definition (HD) chip which increases the lines of resolution from 480 to 1080 lines. To enjoy the benefit of the clarity of HD video imaging, HD monitors also are necessary. Although this technology will inevitably replace more standard video imaging, it is not clear that the safety or efficiency of laparoscopic surgery is benefited by HD video imaging.

Priorities in a video imaging system for MIS are illumination first, resolution second, and color third. Without the first two attributes, video surgery is unsafe. Illumination and resolution are as dependent on the telescope, light source, and light cable as on the video camera used. Imaging for laparoscopy, thoracoscopy, and subcutaneous surgery uses a rigid metal telescope, usually 30 cm in length. Longer telescopes are available for obese patients and for reaching the mediastinum and deep in the pelvis from a periumbilical entry site. The standard telescope contains a series of quartz optical rods and focusing lenses.[51] Telescopes vary in size from 2 to 12 mm in diameter. Because light transmission is dependent on the cross-sectional area of the quartz rod, when the diameter of a rod/lens system is doubled, the illumination is quadrupled. Little illumination is needed in highly reflective, small spaces such as the knee, and a very small telescope will suffice. When working in the abdominal cavity, especially if blood is present, the full illumination of a 10-mm telescope usually is necessary.

Rigid telescopes may have a flat or angled end. The flat end provides a straight view (0°), and the angled end provides an oblique view (30 or 45°).[48] Angled telescopes allow greater flexibility in viewing a wider operative field through a single trocar site (Fig. 14-11); rotating an angled telescope changes the field of view. The use of an angled telescope has distinct advantages for most videoendoscopic proce-

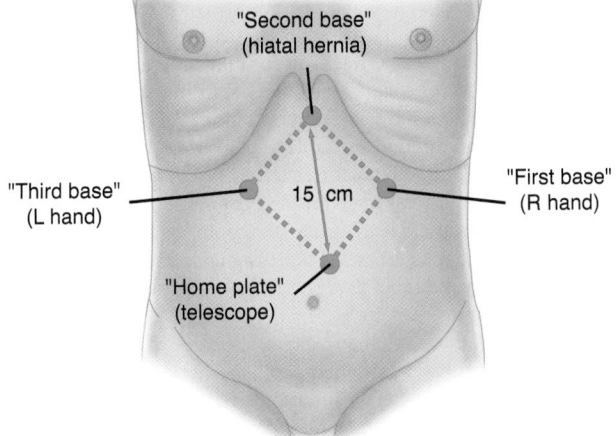

THE DIAMOND OF SUCCESS

FIG. 14-10. The diamond configuration created by placing the telescope between the left and the right hand, recessed from the target by about 15 cm. The distance between the left and the right hand is also ideally 10 to 15 cm. In this "baseball diamond" configuration, the surgical target occupies the second base position.

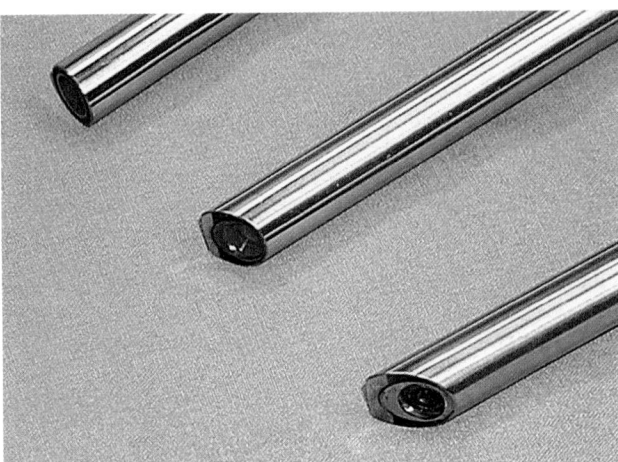

FIG. 14-11. The laparoscope tips come in a variety of angled configurations. All laparoscopes have a 70° field of view. A 30°-angled scope enables the surgeon to view this field at a 30° angle to the long axis of the scope.

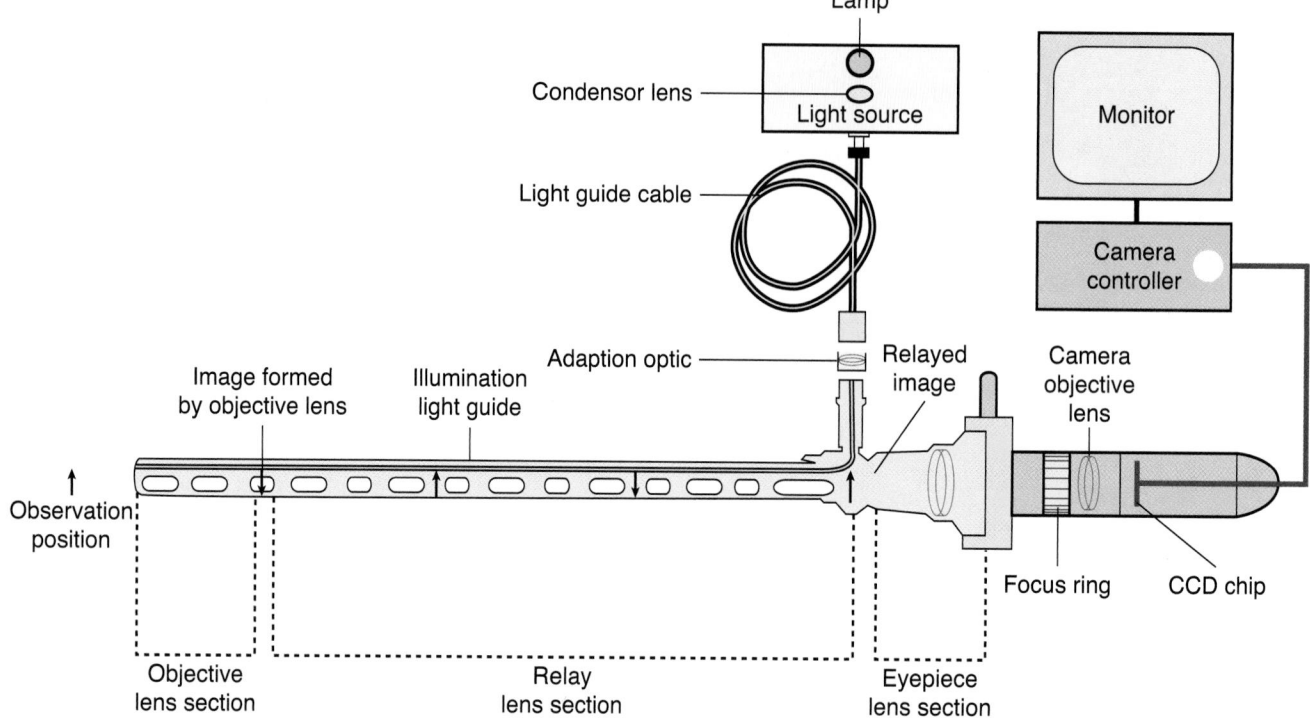

FIG. 14-12. The Hopkins rod lens telescope includes a series of optical rods that effectively transmit light to the eyepiece. The video camera is placed on the eyepiece to provide the working image. The image is only as clear as the weakest link in the image chain. CCD = charge-coupled device. (*Reproduced with permission from Prescher et al.*[48])

dures, particularly in visualizing the common bile duct during laparoscopic cholecystectomy or visualizing the posterior esophagus or the tip of the spleen during laparoscopic fundoplication.

Light is delivered to the endoscope through a fiber-optic light cable. These light cables are highly inefficient, losing >90% of the light delivered from the light source. Extremely bright light sources (300 watts) are necessary to provide adequate illumination for laparoscopic surgery.

The quality of the videoendoscopic image is only as good as the weakest component in the imaging chain (Fig. 14-12). Therefore, it is important to use a video monitor that has a resolution equal to or greater than the camera being used.[51] *Resolution* is the ability of the optical system to distinguish between line pairs. The larger the number of line pairs per millimeter, the sharper and more detailed the image. Most high-resolution monitors have up to 700 horizontal lines. High-definition television can deliver up to eight times more resolution than standard monitors; when combined with digital enhancement, a very sharp and well-defined image can be achieved.[48,51] A heads-up display is a high-resolution liquid crystal monitor that is built into eyewear worn by the surgeon.[52] This technology allows the surgeon to view the endoscopic image and operative field simultaneously. The proposed advantages of heads-up display include a high-resolution monocular image, which affords the surgeon mobility and reduces vertigo and eyestrain. However, this technology has not yet been widely adopted.

Interest in three-dimensional (3-D) laparoscopy has waxed and waned. 3-D laparoscopy provides the additional depth of field that is lost with two-dimensional endosurgery and improves performance of novice laparoscopists performing complex tasks of dexterity, including suturing and knot tying.[53] The advantages of 3-D systems are less obvious to experienced laparoscopists. Additionally, because 3-D systems require the flickering of two similar images, which are resolved with special glasses, the images' edges become fuzzy and resolution is lost. The optical accommodation necessary to rectify these slightly differing images is tiring and may

induce headaches when one uses these systems for a long period of time. The da Vinci robot uses a specialized laparoscope with two optical bundles on opposite sides of the telescope. A specialized binocular eyepiece receives input from two CCD chips, each capturing the image from one of the two quartz rod lens systems, thereby creating true 3-D imaging without using the "tricks" that have made 3-D laparoscopy so disappointing.

Energy Sources for Endoscopic and Endoluminal Surgery

Many MIS procedures use conventional energy sources, but the benefits of bloodless surgery to maintain optimal visualization has spawned new ways of applying energy. The most common energy source is RF electrosurgery using an alternating current with a frequency of 500,000 cycles/s (Hz). Tissue heating progresses through the well-known phases of coagulation [60°C (140°F)], vaporization and desiccation [100°C (212°F)], and carbonization [>200°C (392°F)].[54]

The two most common methods of delivering RF electrosurgery are with monopolar and bipolar electrodes. With monopolar electrosurgery, a remote ground plate on the patient's leg or back receives the flow of electrons that originate at a point source, the surgical electrode. A fine-tipped electrode causes a high current density at the site of application and rapid tissue heating. Monopolar electrosurgery is inexpensive and easy to modulate to achieve different tissue effects.[55] A short-duration, high-voltage discharge of current (coagulation current) provides extremely rapid tissue heating. Lower-voltage, higher-wattage current (cutting current) is better for tissue desiccation and vaporization. When the surgeon desires tissue division with the least amount of thermal injury and least coagulation necrosis, a cutting current is used.

With bipolar electrosurgery, the electrons flow between two adjacent electrodes. The tissue between the two electrodes is heated and desiccated. There is little opportunity for tissue cutting when bipolar current is used, but the ability to coapt the electrodes across

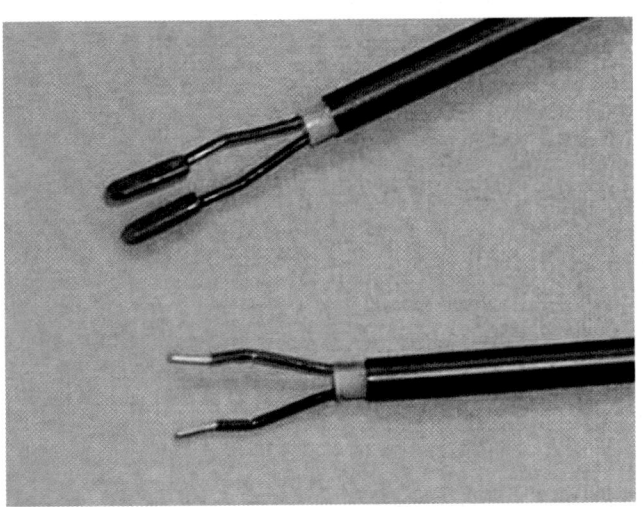

FIG. 14-13. An example of bipolar coagulation devices. The flow of electrons passes from one electrode to the other, and the intervening tissue is heated and desiccated.

a vessel provides the best method of small-vessel coagulation without thermal injury to adjacent tissues[56] (Fig. 14-13).

To avoid thermal injury to adjacent structures, the laparoscopic field of view must include all uninsulated portions of the electrosurgical electrode. In addition, the integrity of the insulation must be maintained and assured. Capacitive coupling occurs when a plastic trocar insulates the abdominal wall from the current; in turn, the current is bled off of a metal sleeve or laparoscope into the viscera[54] (Fig. 14-14A). This may result in thermal necrosis and a delayed fecal fistula. Another potential mechanism for unrecognized visceral injury may occur with the direct coupling of current to the laparoscope and adjacent bowel[54] (Fig. 14-14B).

Another method of delivering RF electrosurgery is argon beam coagulation. This is a type of monopolar electrosurgery in which a

uniform field of electrons is distributed across a tissue surface by the use of a jet of argon gas. The argon gas jet distributes electrons more evenly across the surface than does spray electrofulguration. This technology has its greatest application for coagulation of diffusely bleeding surfaces such as the cut edge of liver or spleen. It is of less value in laparoscopic procedures because the increased intra-abdominal pressures created by the argon gas jet can increase the chances of a gas embolus. It is paramount to vent the ports and closely monitor insufflation pressure when using this source of energy within the context of laparoscopy.

With endoscopic endoluminal surgery, RF alternating current in the form of a monopolar circuit represents the mainstay for procedures such as snare polypectomy, sphincterotomy, lower esophageal sphincter ablation, and "hot" biopsy.[57,58] A grounding ("return") electrode is necessary for this form of energy. Bipolar electrocoagulation is used primarily for thermal hemostasis. The electrosurgical generator is activated by a foot pedal so the endoscopist may keep both hands free during the endoscopic procedure.

Gas, liquid, and solid-state lasers have been available for medical application since the mid-1960s.[59] The CO_2 laser (wavelength 10.6 μm) is most appropriately used for cutting and superficial ablation of tissues. It is most helpful in locations unreachable with a scalpel such as excision of vocal cord granulomas. The CO_2 laser beam must be delivered with a series of mirrors and is therefore somewhat cumbersome to use. The next most popular laser is the neodymium yttrium-aluminum garnet (Nd:YAG) laser. Nd:YAG laser light is 1.064 μm (1064 nm) in wavelength. It is in the near-infrared portion of the spectrum, and, like CO_2 laser light, is invisible to the naked eye. A unique feature of the Nd:YAG laser is that 1064-nm light is poorly absorbed by most tissue pigments and therefore travels deep into tissue.[60] Deep tissue penetration provides deep tissue heating (Fig. 14-15). For this reason, the Nd:YAG laser is capable of the greatest amount of tissue destruction with a single application.[59] Such capabilities make it the ideal laser for destruction of large fungating tumors of the rectosigmoid, tracheobronchial tree, or esophagus. A disadvantage is that the deep tissue heating may cause perforation of a hollow viscus.

When it is desirable to coagulate flat lesions in the cecum, a different laser should be chosen. The frequency-doubled Nd:YAG

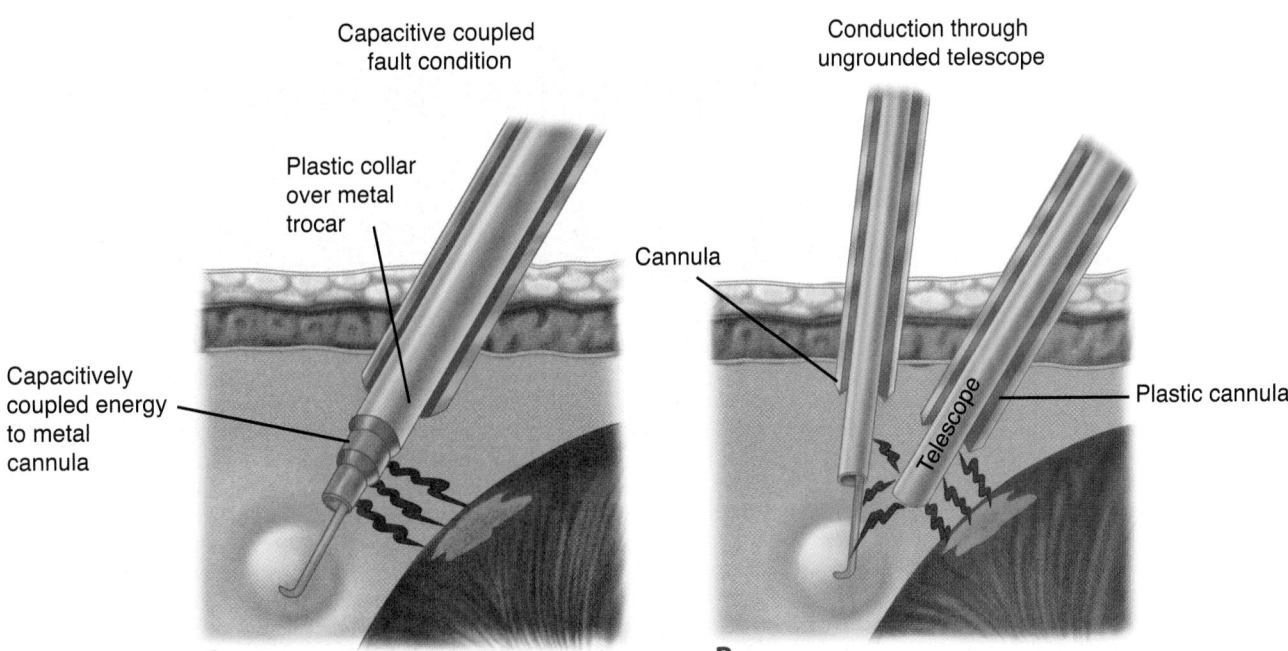

FIG. 14-14. A. Capacitive coupling occurs as a result of high current density bleeding from a port sleeve or laparoscope into adjacent bowel. **B.** Direct coupling occurs when current is transmitted directly from the electrode to a metal instrument or laparoscope, and then into adjacent tissue. *(Reproduced with permission from Odell.[54])*

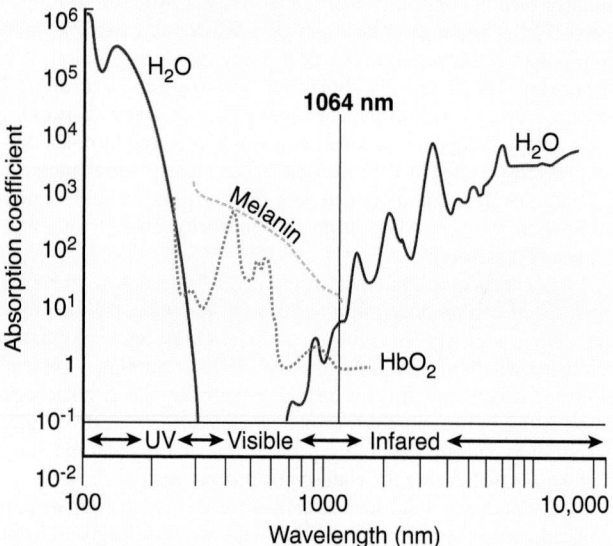

FIG. 14-15. This graph shows the absorption of light by various tissue compounds (water, melanin, and oxyhemoglobin) as a function of the wavelength of the light. The nadir of the oxyhemoglobin and melanin curves is close to 1064 nm, the wavelength of the neodymium yttrium-aluminum garnet laser. *[Reproduced with permission from Hunter JG, Sackier JM (eds): Minimally Invasive Surgery. New York: McGraw-Hill, 1993, p 28.]*

laser, also known as the *KTP laser* (potassium thionyl phosphate crystal is used to double the Nd:YAG frequency), provides 532-nm light. This is in the green portion of the spectrum, and at this wavelength, selective absorption by red pigments in tissue (such as hemangiomas and arteriovenous malformations) is optimal. The depth of tissue heating is intermediate, between those of the CO_2 and the Nd:YAG lasers. Coagulation (without vaporization) of superficial vascular lesions can be obtained without intestinal perforation.[60]

In flexible GI endoscopy, the CO_2 and Nd:YAG lasers have largely been replaced by heater probes and endoluminal stents. The heater probe is a metal ball that is heated to a temperature [60 to 100°C (140 to 212°F)] that allows coagulation of bleeding lesions without perforation.

Photodynamic therapy is a palliative treatment for obstructing cancers of the GI tract.[61] Patients are given an IV dose of porfimer sodium, which is a photosensitizing agent that is taken up by malignant cells. Two days after administration, the drug is endoscopically activated using a laser. The activated porfimer sodium generates oxygen free radicals, which kill the tumor cells. The tumor is later endoscopically débrided. The use of this modality for definitive treatment of early cancers is in experimental phases and has yet to become established.

A unique application of laser technology provides extremely rapid discharge ($<10^{-6}$ s) of large amounts of energy ($>10^3$ volts). These high-energy lasers, of which the pulsed dye laser has seen the most clinical use, allow the conversion of light energy to mechanical disruptive energy in the form of a shock wave. Such energy can be delivered through a quartz fiber, and with rapid repetitive discharges, can provide sufficient shock-wave energy to fragment kidney stones and gallstones.[62] Shock waves also may be created with miniature electric spark-plug discharge systems known as *electrohydraulic lithotriptors*. These devices also are inserted through thin probes for endoscopic application. Lasers have the advantage of pigment selectivity, but electrohydraulic lithotriptors are more popular because they are substantially less expensive and are more compact.

Methods of producing shock waves or heat with ultrasonic energy are also of interest. Extracorporeal shockwave lithotripsy

creates focused shock waves that intensify as the focal point of the discharge is approached. When the focal point is within the body, large amounts of energy are capable of fragmenting stones. Slightly different configurations of this energy can be used to provide focused internal heating of tissues. Potential applications of this technology include the ability to noninvasively produce sufficient internal heating to destroy tissue without an incision.

A third means of using ultrasonic energy is to create rapidly oscillating instruments that are capable of heating tissue with friction; this technology represents a major step forward in energy technology.[63] An example of its application is the laparoscopic coagulation shears device (Harmonic Scalpel), which is capable of coagulating and dividing blood vessels by first occluding them and then providing sufficient heat to weld the blood vessel walls together and to divide the vessel. This nonelectric method of coagulating and dividing tissue with a minimal amount of collateral damage has facilitated the performance of numerous endosurgical procedures.[64] It is especially useful in the control of bleeding from medium-sized vessels that are too big to manage with monopolar electrocautery and require bipolar desiccation followed by cutting.

Instrumentation

Hand instruments for MIS usually are duplications of conventional surgical instruments made longer, thinner, and smaller at the tip. It is important to remember that when grasping tissue with laparoscopic instruments, a greater force is applied over a smaller surface area, which increases the risk for perforation or injury.[65]

Certain conventional instruments such as scissors are easy to reproduce with a diameter of 3 to 5 mm and a length of 20 to 45 cm, but other instruments such as forceps and clamps cannot provide remote access. Different configurations of graspers were developed to replace the various configurations of surgical forceps and clamps. Standard hand instruments are 5 mm in diameter and 30 cm in length, but smaller and shorter hand instruments are now available for pediatric surgery, for microlaparoscopic surgery, and for arthroscopic procedures.[65] A unique laparoscopic hand instrument is the monopolar electrical hook. This device usually is configured with a suction and irrigation apparatus to eliminate smoke and blood from the operative field. The monopolar hook allows tenting of tissue over a bare metal wire with subsequent coagulation and division of the tissue.

Instrumentation for NOTES is still evolving, but many long micrograspers, microscissors, suturing devices, clip appliers, and visceral closure devices are evolving in design and application.

Robotic Surgery

The term *robot* defines a device that has been programmed to perform specific tasks in place of those usually performed by people. The devices that have earned the title "surgical robots" would be more aptly termed *computer-enhanced surgical devices*, as they are controlled entirely by the surgeon for the purpose of improving performance. The first computer-assisted surgical device was the laparoscopic camera holder (Aesop, Computer Motion, Goleta, Calif), which enabled the surgeon to maneuver the laparoscope either with a hand control, foot control, or voice activation (Fig. 14-16). Randomized studies with such camera holders demonstrated a reduction in operative time, steadier image, and a reduction in the number of required laparoscope cleanings.[66] This device had the advantage of eliminating the need for a human camera holder, which served to free valuable OR personnel for other duties. This technology has now been eclipsed by simpler systems using passive positioning of the camera with a mechanical arm, but the benefit of a steadier image and fewer members of the OR team remain.

The "Big Bang" in robotic surgery was the development of a *master-slave* surgical platform that returned the wrist to laparoscopic surgery and improved manual dexterity by developing an ergonomically comfortable work station, with 3-D imaging, tremor elimination, and scaling of movement (e.g., large, gross hand move-

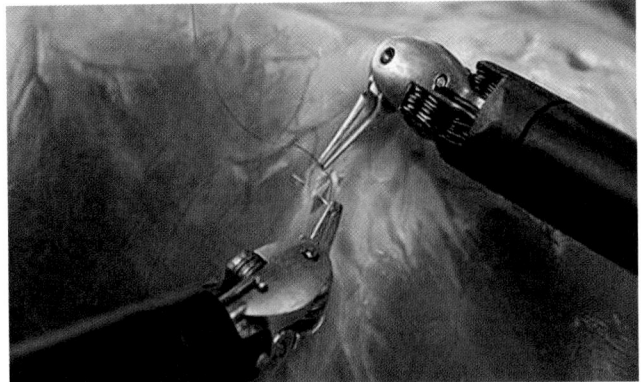

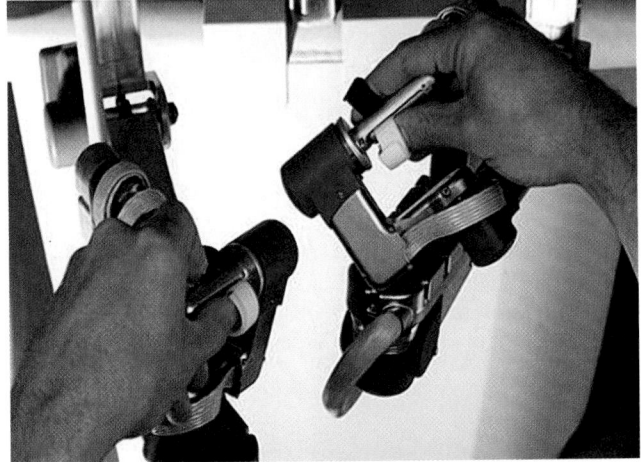

FIG. 14-16. Robotic instruments and hand controls. The surgeon is in a sitting position and the arms and wrists are in an ergonomic and relaxed position.

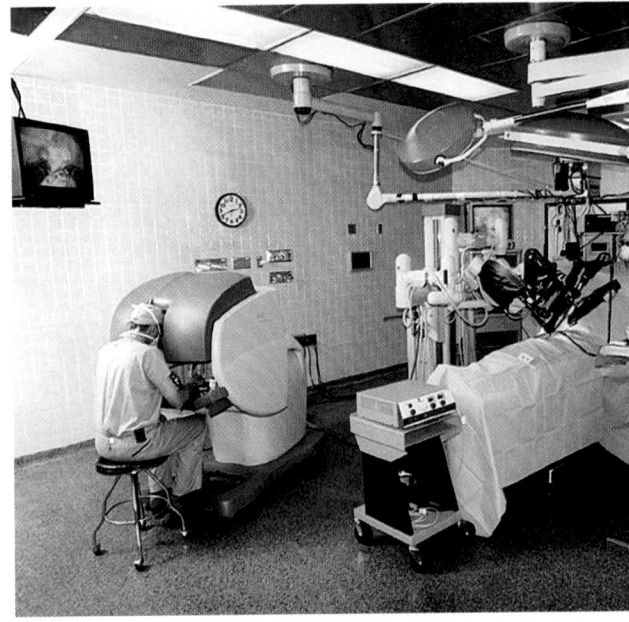

FIG. 14-17. Room setup and position of surgeon and assistant for robotic surgery.

ments can be scaled down to allow suturing with microsurgical precision) (see Fig. 14-16). The surgeon is physically separated from the operating table, and the working arms of the device are placed over the patient (Fig. 14-17). An assistant remains at the bedside and changes the instruments as needed, providing retraction as needed to facilitate the procedure. This "robotic" platform (da Vinci, Intuitive Surgical, Sunnyvale, Calif) was initially greeted with some skepticism by expert laparoscopists, as it was difficult to prove additional value for operations performed with the da Vinci robot. Not only were the operations longer, and the equipment more expensive, but additional quality could not be demonstrated. Two randomized controlled trials compared robotic and conventional laparoscopic approaches to Nissen fundoplication.[67,68] In both these trials, the operative time was longer for robotic surgery, and there was no difference in ultimate outcome. Similar results were achieved for laparoscopic cholecystectomy.[69] Nevertheless, the increased dexterity provided by the da Vinci robot convinced many surgeons and health administrators that robotic platforms were worthy of investment, for marketing purposes if for no other reason.

The success story for computer-enhanced surgery with the da Vinci started with cardiac surgery and migrated to the pelvis. Mitral valve surgery, performed with right thoracoscopic access became one of the more popular procedures performed with "the robot."[70]

The tidal wave of enthusiasm for robotic surgery came when most minimally invasive urologists declared robotic prostatectomy to be preferable to laparoscopic and open prostatectomy.[71] The great advantage—it would appear—of robotic prostatectomy is the ability to visualize and spare the pelvic nerves responsible for erectile function. In addition, the creation of the neocystourethrotomy, following prostatectomy, was greatly facilitated by needle

holders and graspers with a wrist in them. Female pelvic surgery with the "robot" also is picking up steam. The magnified imaging provided makes this approach ideal for microsurgical tasks such as reanastomosis of the Fallopian tubes.

The final frontier for computer-enhanced surgery is the promise of telesurgery, in which the surgeon is a great distance from the patient (e.g., combat or space). This application has rarely been used, as the safety provided by having the surgeon at bedside cannot be sacrificed to prove the concept. However, remote laparoscopic cholecystectomy has been performed when a team of surgeons located in New York performed a cholecystectomy on a patient located in France.[72]

Endoluminal and Endovascular Surgery

The fields of vascular surgery, interventional radiology, neuroradiology, gastroenterology, general surgery, pulmonology, and urology all encounter clinical scenarios that require the urgent restoration of luminal patency of a "biologic cylinder." Based on this need, fundamental techniques have been pioneered that are applicable to all specialties and virtually every organ system. As a result, all minimally invasive surgical procedures, from coronary artery angioplasty to palliation of pancreatic malignancy, involve the use of access devices, catheters, guidewires, balloon dilators, stents, and other devices (e.g., lasers, atherectomy catheters) that are capable of opening up the occluded biologic cylinder[73] (Table 14-2). Endoluminal balloon dilators may be inserted through an endoscope, or they may be fluoroscopically guided. Balloon dilators all have low compliance—that is, the balloons do not stretch as the pressure within the balloon is increased. The high pressures achievable in the balloon create radial expansion of the narrowed vessel or orifice, usually disrupting the atherosclerotic plaque, the fibrotic stricture, or the muscular band (e.g., esophageal achalasia).[74]

Once the dilation has been attained, it is frequently beneficial to hold the lumen open with a stent.[75] Stenting is particularly valuable in treating malignant lesions and atherosclerotic occlusions or aneurysmal disease (Fig. 14-18). Stenting is also of value to seal leaky cylinders, including aortic dissections, traumatic vascular injuries, leaking GI anastomoses, and fistulas. Stenting usually is not applicable for long-term management of benign GI strictures except in patients with limited life expectancy[75–77] (Fig. 14-19).

TABLE 14-2	Modalities and techniques of restoring luminal patency
Modality	**Technique**
Core out	Photodynamic therapy
	Laser
	Coagulation
	Endoscopic biopsy forceps
	Chemical
	Ultrasound
Fracture	Ultrasound
	Endoscopic biopsy
	Balloon
Dilate	Balloon
	Bougie
	Angioplasty
	Endoscope
Bypass	Transvenous intrahepatic portosystemic shunt
	Surgical (synthetic or autologous conduit)
Stent	Self-expanding metal stent
	Plastic stent

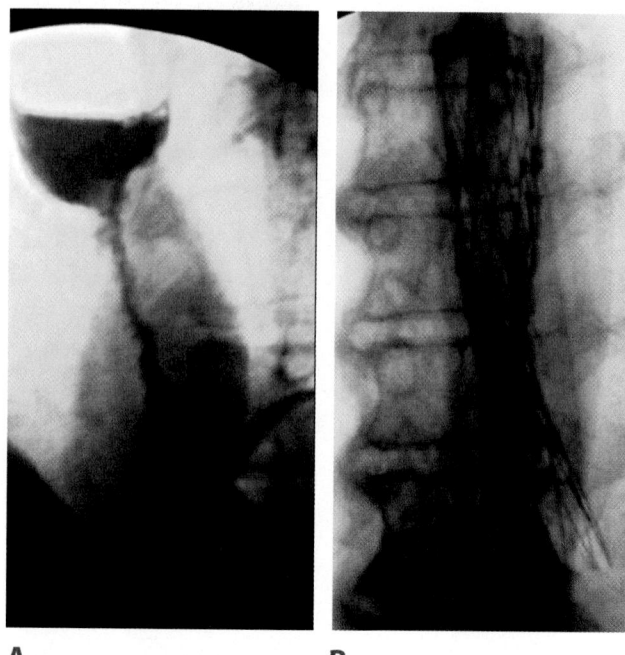

A   **B**

FIG. 14-19. This is an esophagram in a patient with severe dysphagia secondary to advanced esophageal cancer (**A**) before and (**B**) after placement of a covered self-expanding metal stent.

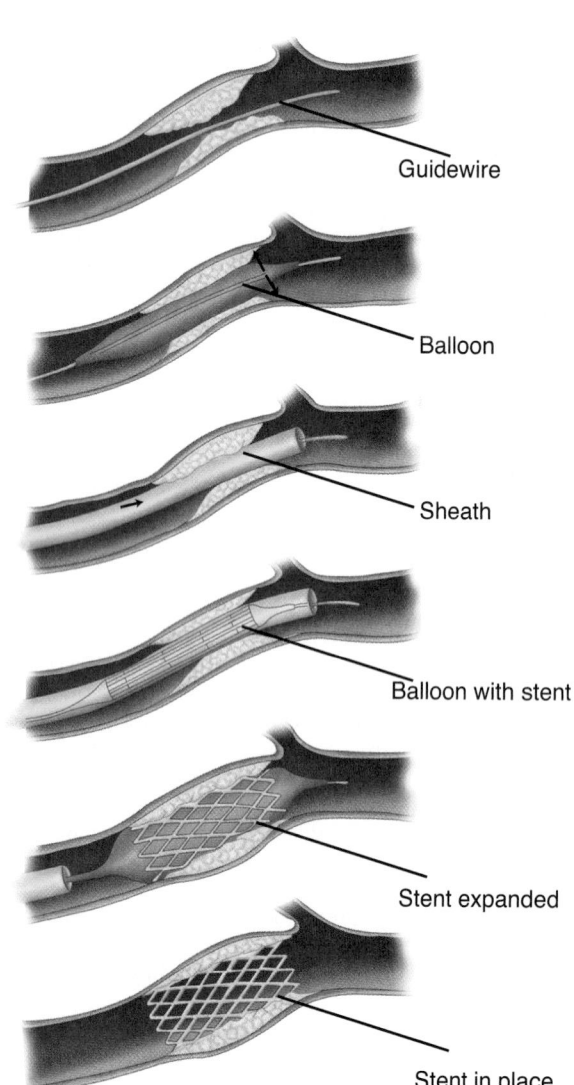

Guidewire

Balloon

Sheath

Balloon with stent

Stent expanded

Stent in place

FIG. 14-18. The deployment of a metal stent across an isolated vessel stenosis is illustrated. [Reproduced with permission from Hunter JG, Sackier JM (eds): Minimally Invasive Surgery. New York: McGraw-Hill, 1993, p 235.]

A variety of stents are available that are divided into six basic categories: plastic stents, metal stents, drug-eluting stents (to decrease fibrovascular hyperplasia), covered metal stents, anchored stent grafts, and removable covered plastic stents[76] (Fig. 14-20). Plastic stents came first and are used widely as endoprostheses for temporary bypass of obstructions in the biliary or urinary systems. Metal stents generally are delivered over a balloon and expanded with the balloon to the desired size. These metal stents usually are made of titanium or nitinol, and are still used in coronary stenting. A chemotherapeutic agent was added to coronary stents several years ago to decrease endothelial proliferation. These drug-eluting stents provide greater long-term patency but require long-term anticoagulation with antiplatelet agents to prevent thrombosis.[78] Coated metal stents are use to prevent tissue ingrowth. Ingrowth may be an advantage in preventing stent migration, but such tissue ingrowth may occlude the lumen and cause obstruction anew. This is a particular problem when stents are used for palliation of GI malignant growth, and may be a problem for the long-term use of stents in vascular disease. Filling the interstices with Silastic or other materials may prevent tumor ingrowth but also makes stent migration more likely. In an effort to minimize stent migration, stents have been incorporated with hooks and barbs at the proximal end of the stent to anchor it to the wall of the vessel. Endovascular stenting of aortic aneurysms has nearly replaced open surgery for this condition. Lastly, self-expanding plastic stents have been developed as temporary devices to be used in the GI tract to close internal fistulas and bridge leaking anastomoses.

Natural Orifice Transluminal Endoscopic Surgery

The "latest rage" in MIS is NOTES, the use of the flexible endoscope to enter the GI, urinary, or reproductive tracts, then traverse the wall of the structure to enter the peritoneal cavity, the mediastinum, or the chest. In truth, transluminal surgery has been performed in the stomach for a long time, either from the inside out (e.g. percutaneous, PEG, and transgastric pseudocyst drainage) or from the outside in (e.g., laparoscopic assisted intragastric tumor resection). The catalyzing event for NOTES was the demonstration that a porcine gall-

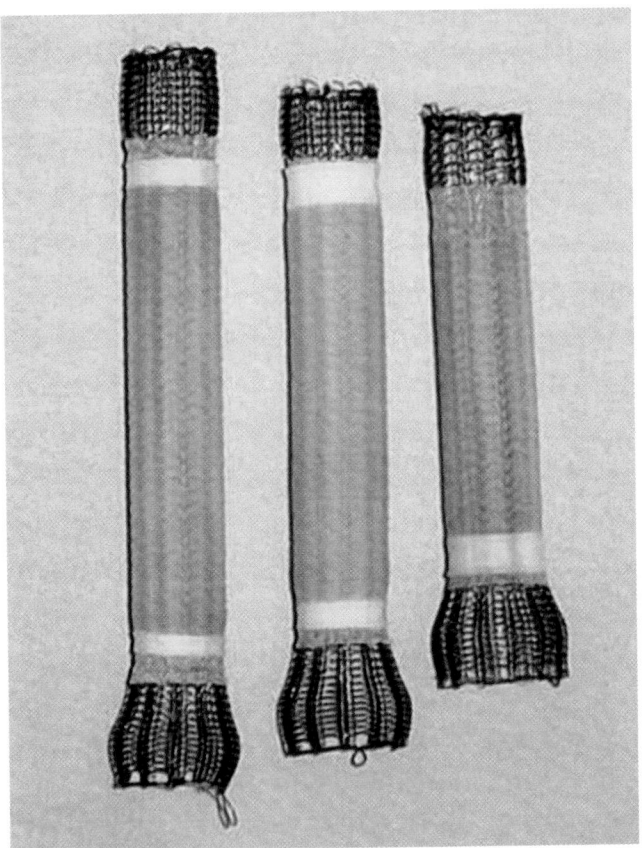

FIG. 14-20. Covered self-expanding metal stents. These devices can be placed fluoroscopically or endoscopically.

bladder could be removed with a flexible endoscope passed through the wall of the stomach, then removed through the mouth, and the demonstration in a series of 10 human cases from India of the ability to perform transgastric appendectomy. Since that time, a great deal of money has been invested by endoscopic and MIS companies to help surgeons and gastroenterologists explore this new territory. To date, the most headline-grabbing procedures have been the transvaginal and transgastric removal of the gallbladder[79–81] (Fig. 14-21). To ensure safety, all cases thus far have involved laparoscopic assistance to aid in retraction, and ensure adequate closure of the stomach. As such, the benefits of NOTES cholecystectomy have not been demonstrated convincingly, but when all laparoscopic assistance has been eliminated, this approach will surely appeal to many. Additional procedures performed with NOTES might include staging of intra-abdominal malignancy, segmental colectomy, gastrojejunostomy, and a host of other procedures capable of exciting the curious mind. In addition, the rapid growth of endoscopic technology catalyzed by NOTES has already spun off new technologies capable of performing a wide variety of endoscopic surgical procedures from endoscopic mucosal resection to ablation of Barrett's esophagus, to creation of competent antireflux valves in patients with gastroesophageal reflux disease. Although some of these applications are still considered experimental, there is little doubt that when equivalent operations can be performed with less pain, fewer scars, and less disability, patients will flock to it. Surgeons should engage only when they can perform these procedures with the safety and efficacy demanded by our profession.

SPECIAL CONSIDERATIONS

Pediatric Laparoscopy

The advantages of MIS in children may be more significant than in the adult population. MIS in the adolescent is little different from that

in the adult, and standard instrumentation and trocar positions usually can be used. However, laparoscopy in the infant and young child requires specialized instrumentation. The instruments are shorter (15 to 20 cm), and many are 3 mm in diameter rather than 5 mm. Because the abdomen of the child is much smaller than that of the adult, a 5-mm telescope provides sufficient illumination for most operations. The development of 5-mm clippers and bipolar devices has obviated the need for 10-mm trocars in pediatric laparoscopy.[82] Because the abdominal wall is much thinner in infants, a pneumoperitoneum pressure of 8 mmHg can provide adequate exposure. DVT is rare in children, so prophylaxis against thrombosis probably is unnecessary. A wide variety of pediatric surgical procedures are frequently performed with MIS access, from pull-through procedures for colonic aganglionosis (Hirschsprung's disease) to repair of congenital diaphragmatic hernias.[83]

Laparoscopy during Pregnancy

Concerns about the safety of laparoscopic cholecystectomy or appendectomy in the pregnant patient have been thoroughly investigated and are readily managed. Access to the abdomen in the pregnant patient should take into consideration the height of the uterine fundus, which reaches the umbilicus at 20 weeks. In order not to damage the uterus or its blood supply, most surgeons feel that the open (Hasson) approach should be used in favor of direct puncture laparoscopy. The patient should be positioned slightly on the left side to avoid compression of the vena cava by the uterus. Because pregnancy poses a risk for thromboembolism, sequential compression devices are essential for all procedures. Fetal acidosis induced by maternal hypercarbia also has been raised as a concern. The arterial pH of the fetus follows the pH of the mother linearly; and therefore, fetal acidosis may be prevented by avoiding a respiratory acidosis in the mother.[84] The pneumoperitoneum pressure induced by laparoscopy is not a safety issue either as it has been proved that midpregnancy uterine contractions provide a much greater pressure in utero than a pneumoperitoneum of 15 mmHg. Experience in >100 cases of laparoscopic cholecystectomy in pregnancy have been reported with uniformly good results.[85] The operation should be performed during the second trimester of pregnancy if possible. Protection of the fetus against intraoperative x-rays is imperative. Some believe it advisable to track fetal pulse rates with a transvaginal ultrasound probe; however, the significance of fetal tachycardia or bradycardia is a bit unclear in the second trimester of pregnancy. To be prudent, however, heart rate decelerations reversibly associated with pneumoperitoneum creation might signal the need to convert to open cholecystectomy or appendectomy.

Minimally Invasive Surgery and Cancer Treatment

MIS techniques have been used for many decades to provide palliation for the patient with an obstructive cancer. Laser treatment, intracavitary radiation, stenting, and dilation are outpatient techniques that can be used to re-establish the continuity of an obstructed esophagus, bile duct, ureter, or airway. MIS techniques also have been used in the staging of cancer. Mediastinoscopy is still used occasionally before thoracotomy to assess the status of the mediastinal lymph nodes. Laparoscopy also is used to assess the liver in patients being evaluated for pancreatic, gastric, or hepatic resection. New technology and greater surgical skills allow for accurate minimally invasive staging of cancer.[86] Occasionally, it is appropriate to perform palliative measures (e.g., laparoscopic gastrojejunostomy to bypass a pancreatic cancer) at the time of diagnostic laparoscopy if diagnostic findings preclude attempts at curative resection.

Initially controversial, the role of MIS to provide a safe curative treatment of cancer has proven to be no different from the principles of open surgery. All gross and microscopic tumor should be removed (an R0 resection), and an adequate lymphadenectomy should be performed to allow accurate staging. Generally, this number has been 10 to 15 lymph nodes, although there is still debate as to the value of more extensive lymphadenectomy. All of the major abdominal can-

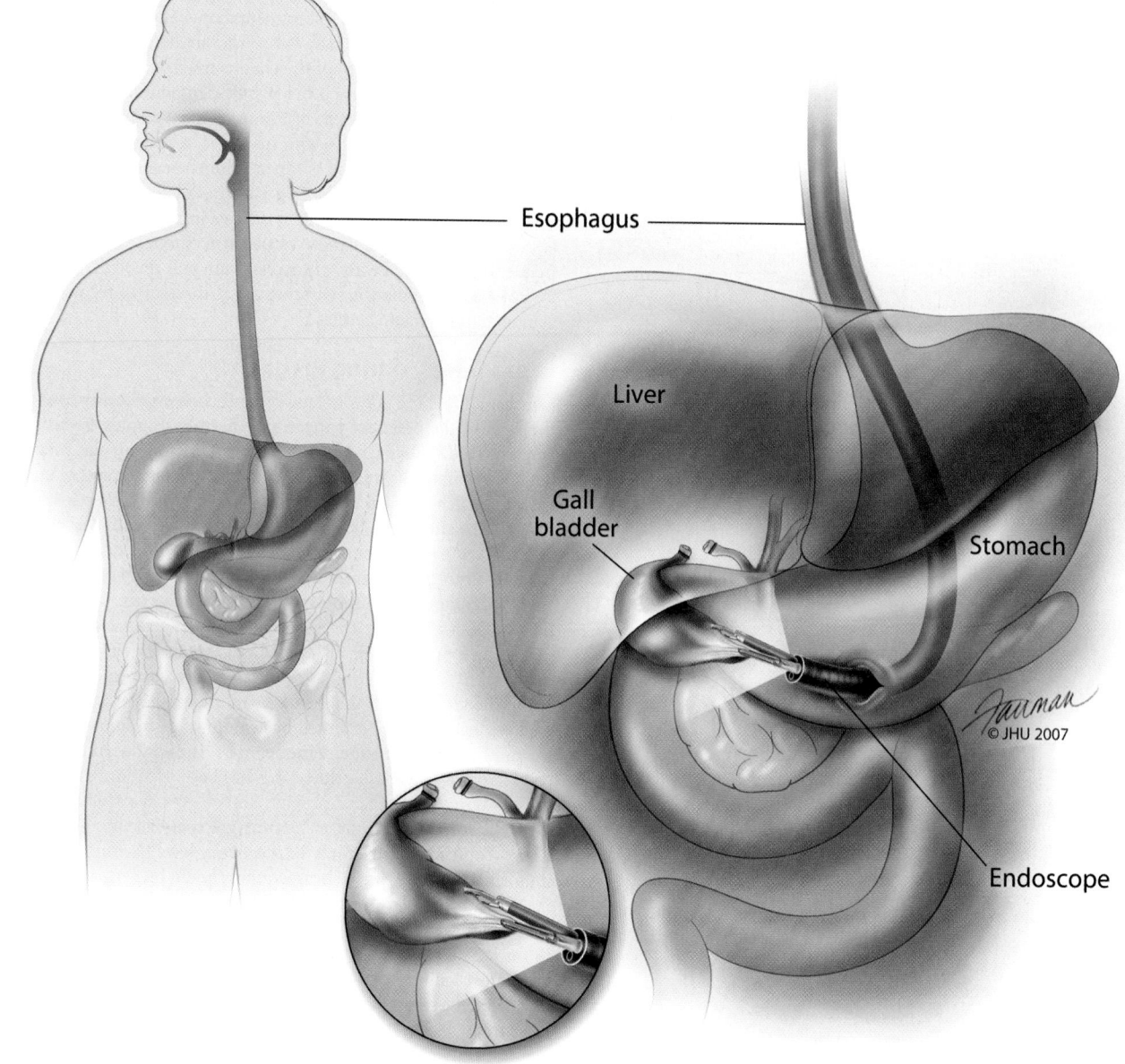

FIG. 14-21. Transgastric cholecystectomy using natural orifice transluminal endoscopic surgery technology and one to three laparoscopic ports has been performed occasionally in several locations around the world. (*Reproduced with permission from The Johns Hopkins University School of Medicine, Baltimore, Maryland.*)

cer operations have been performed with laparoscopy. Of the three major cancer resections of GI cancer (liver lobe, pancreatic head, and esophagus), only esophagectomy is routinely performed by a fair number of centers.[87,88] Laparoscopic hepatectomy has attracted a loyal following, and distal pancreatectomy frequently is performed with laparoscopic access. In Japan, laparoscopic-assisted gastrectomy has become quite popular for early gastric cancer, an epidemic in Japan far exceeding that of colon cancer in North America and Northern Europe. The most common cancer operation performed laparoscopically is segmental colectomy, which has proven itself safe and efficacious in a multicenter controlled randomized trial.[89]

Considerations in the Elderly and Infirm

Laparoscopic cholecystectomy has made possible the removal of a symptomatic gallbladder in many patients previously thought to be too elderly or too ill to undergo a laparotomy. Older patients are more likely to require conversion to celiotomy because of disease chronicity.[89]

Operations on these patients require close monitoring of anesthesia. The intraoperative management of these patients may be more difficult with laparoscopic access than with open access. The advantage of MIS lies in what happens after the operation. Much of the morbidity of surgery in the elderly is a result of impaired mobility. In addition, pulmonary complications, urinary tract sepsis, DVT, pulmonary embolism, congestive heart failure, and myocardial infarction often are the result of improper fluid management and decreased mobility. By allowing rapid and early mobilization, laparoscopic surgery has made possible the safe performance of procedures in the elderly and infirm.

Cirrhosis and Portal Hypertension

Patients with hepatic insufficiency pose a significant challenge for any type of surgical intervention.[90] The ultimate surgical outcome in this population relates directly to the degree of underlying hepatic dysfunction.[91] Often, this group of patients has minimal reserve, and the stress of an operation will trigger complete hepatic failure or hepato-renal syndrome. These patients are at risk for major hemorrhage at all levels, including trocar insertion, operative dissection in a field of dilated veins, and secondary to an underlying coagulopathy. Additionally, ascitic leak from a port site may occur, leading to bacterial peritonitis. Therefore, a watertight port site closure should be carried out in all patients.

It is essential that the surgeon be aware of the severity of hepatic cirrhosis as judged by a MELD score (Model of Endstage Liver Disease) or Child's classification. Additionally, the presence of portal hypertension is a relative contraindication to laparoscopic surgery until the portal pressures are reduced with portal decompression. For example, if a patient has an incarcerated umbilical hernia and ascites, a preoperative paracentesis or transjugular intrahepatic portosystemic shunt procedure in conjunction with aggressive diuresis may be considered. Because these patients commonly are intravascularly depleted, insufflation pressures should be reduced to prevent a decrease in cardiac output and minimal amounts of Na⁺ sparing IV fluids should be given.

Economics of Minimally Invasive Surgery

Minimally invasive surgical procedures reduce the costs of surgery most when length of hospital stay can be shortened and return to work is quickened. For example, shorter hospital stays can be demonstrated in laparoscopic cholecystectomy, Nissen fundoplication, splenectomy, and adrenalectomy. Procedures such as inguinal herniorrhaphy that are already performed as outpatient procedures are less likely to provide cost savings. Procedures that still require a 4- to 7-day hospitalization, such as laparoscopy-assisted colectomy, are less likely to deliver a lower bottom line than their open surgery counterparts. Nonetheless, with responsible use of disposable instrumentation and a commitment to the most effective use of the inpatient setting, most laparoscopic procedures can be made less expensive than their conventional equivalents.

Education and Skill Acquisition

Historically, surgeons in training (residents, registrars, and fellows) acquired their skills in minimally invasive techniques through a series of operative experiences of graded complexity. This training occurred on patients. Although such a paradigm did not compromise patient safety, learning in the OR is costly. In addition, the recent worldwide constraint placed on resident work hours makes it attractive to teach laparoscopic skills outside of the OR.

Skills labs started at nearly every surgical training center in the 1990s with a "box trainer," a rudimentary or sophisticated simulated abdominal cavity with a video camera, a monitor, trocars, laparoscopic instruments, and target models as simple as a pegboard and rubber rings, or a latex drain to practice suturing and knot tying. Virtual reality training devices present a unique opportunity to improve and enhance experiential learning in endoscopy and laparoscopy for all surgeons. This technology has the advantage of enabling objective measurement of psychomotor skills, which can be used to determine progress in skill acquisition, and ultimately, technical competency.[92] Several of these devices have been validated as a means of measuring proficiency in skill performance. More importantly, training on virtual reality platforms has proven to translate to improved operative performance in randomized trials.[93,94] In the near future, and today in some institutions, simulator training to the expert level will become a prerequisite for performance of laparoscopic procedures in the OR. The American College of Surgeons has taken a leadership position in accrediting these skills labs at American College of Surgeons–accredited educational institutes.

Telementoring

In response to the Institute of Medicine's call for the development of unique technologic solutions to deliver health care to rural and underserved areas, surgeons are beginning to explore the feasibility

of telementoring. Teleconsultation or telementoring is two-way audio and visual communication between two geographically separated providers. This communication can take place in the office setting or directly in the OR when complex scenarios are encountered. Although local communication channels may limit its performance in rural areas, the technology is available and currently is being used, especially in states and provinces with large geographically remote populations[94] (Fig. 14-22).

Innovation and Introduction of New Procedures

The revolution in minimally invasive general surgery, which occurred in 1990, created ethical challenges for the profession. The problem was this: If competence is gained from experience, how was the surgeon to climb the competence curve (otherwise known as the *learning curve*) without injuring patients? If it was indeed impossible to achieve competence without making mistakes along the way, how should one effectively communicate this to patients such that they understand the weight of their decisions? Even more fundamentally important is determining the path that should be followed before one recruits the first patient for a new procedure.

Although procedure development is fundamentally different than drug development (i.e., there is great individual variation in the performance of procedures, but no difference between one

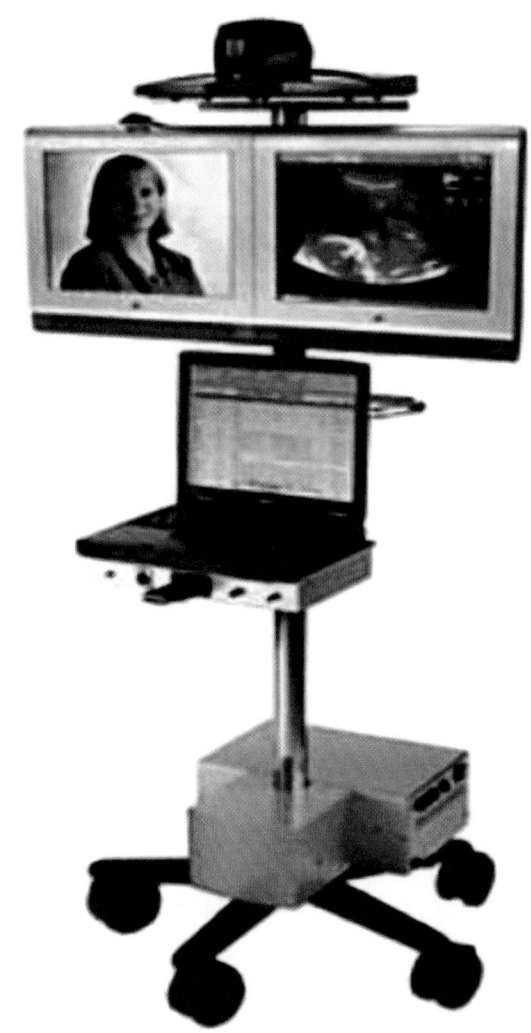

FIG. 14-22. Teleconsultation and telementoring are carried out between two providers who are geographically separated. The console has a video camera, microphone, and flat screen display that can be positioned at the operating room table or in the clinic.

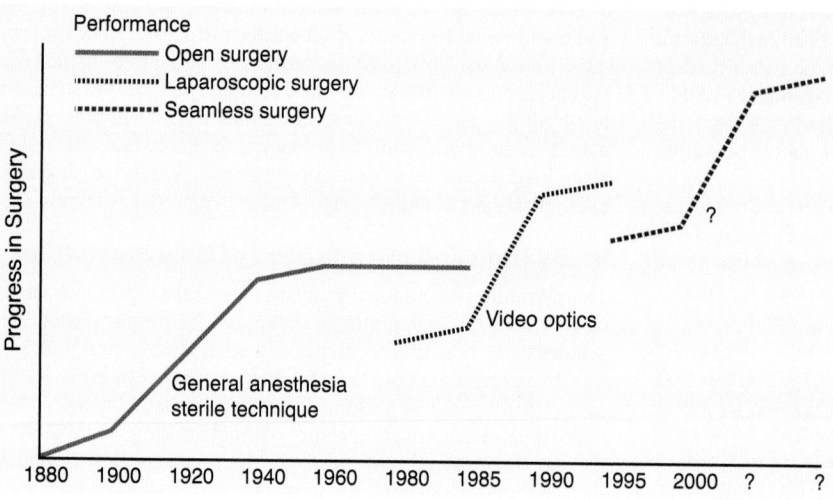

FIG. 14-23. The progress of general surgery can be reflected by a series of performance curves. General anesthesia and sterile technique allowed the development of maximally invasive open surgery over the last 125 years. Video optics allowed the development of minimally invasive surgery over the last 25 years. Noninvasive (seamless) surgery will result when a yet undiscovered transformational event allows surgery to occur without an incision, and perhaps without anesthesia.

tablet and the next), adherence to a process similar to that used to develop a new drug is a reasonable path for a surgical innovator. At the outset, the surgeon must identify the problem that is not solved with current surgical procedures. For example, although the removal of a gallbladder through a Kocher incision is certainly effective, it creates a great deal of disability, pain, and scarification. As a result of those issues, many patients with very symptomatic biliary colic delayed operation until life-threatening complications occurred. Clearly, there was a need for developing a less invasive approach (Fig. 14-23).

Once the opportunity has been established, the next step involves a search through other disciplines for technologies and techniques that might be applied. Again, this is analogous to the drug industry, where secondary drug indications have often turned out to be more therapeutically important than the primary indication for drug development. The third step is in vivo studies in the most appropriate animal model. These types of studies are controversial because of the resistance to animal experimentation, and yet without such studies, many humans would be injured or killed during the developmental phase of medical drugs, devices, and techniques. These steps often are called the *preclinical phase of procedure development*.

The decision as to when such procedures are ready to come out of the lab is a difficult one. Put simply, the procedure should be reproducible, provide the desired effect, and not have serious side effects. Once these three criteria are reached, the time for human application has arrived. Before the surgeon discusses the new procedure with patients, it is important to achieve full institutional support. Involvement of the medical board, the chief of the medical staff, and the institutional review board is essential before commencing on a new procedure. These bodies are responsible for the use of safe, high-quality medical practices within their institution, and they will demand that great caution and all possible safeguards are in place before proceeding.

The dialogue with the patient who is to be first must be thorough, brutally honest, and well documented. The psychology that allows a patient to decide to be first is quite interesting, and may, under certain circumstances, require psychiatric evaluation. Certainly if a dying cancer patient has a chance with a new drug, this makes sense. Similarly, if the standard surgical procedure has a high attendant morbidity and the new procedure offers a substantially better outcome, the decision to be first is understandable. On the other hand, when the benefits of the new approach are small and the risks are largely unknown, a more complete psychological profile may be necessary before proceeding.

For new surgical procedures, it generally is wise to assemble the best possible operative team, including a surgeon experienced with the old technique, and assistants who have participated in the earlier animal work. This initial team of experienced physicians and nurses should remain together until full competence with the procedure is attained. This may take 10 procedures, or it may take 50 procedures. The team will know that it has achieved competence when the majority of procedures take the same length of time, and the team is relaxed and sure of the flow of the operation. This will complete phase I of the procedure development.

In phase II, the efficacy of the procedure is tested in a nonrandomized fashion. Ideally, the outcome of new techniques must be as good or better than the procedure that is being replaced. This phase should occur at several medical centers to prove that good outcomes are achievable outside of the pioneering institution. These same requirements may be applied to the introduction of new technology into the OR. The value equation requires that the additional measurable procedure quality exceeds the additional measurable cost to the patient or health care system. In phase III, a randomized trial pits the new procedure against the old.

Once the competence curve has been climbed, it is appropriate for the team to engage in the education of others. During the ascension of the competence curve, other learners in the institution (i.e., surgical residents) may not have the opportunity to participate in the first case series. Although this may be difficult for them, the best interest of the patient must be put before the education of the resident.

The second stage of learning occurs when the new procedure has proven its value and a handful of experts exist, but the majority of surgeons have not been trained to perform the new procedure. In this setting, it is relatively unethical for surgeons to forge ahead with a new procedure in humans as if they had spent the same amount of time in intensive study that the first team did. The fact that one or several surgical teams were able to perform an operation does not ensure that all others with the same medical degrees can perform the operation with equal skill. It behooves the learners to contact the experts and request their assistance to ensure an optimal outcome at the new center. Although it is important that the learners contact the experts, it is equally important that the experts be willing to share their experience with their fellow professionals. As well, the experts should provide feedback to the learners as to whether they feel the learners are equipped to forge ahead on their own. If not, further observation and assistance from the experts are required. Although this approach may sound obvious, it is fraught with difficulties. In many situations ego, competitiveness, and monetary concerns have short-circuited this process and led to poor patient outcomes. To a large extent, MIS has recovered from the black eye it received early in development, when inadequately trained surgeons caused an excessive number of significant complications.

If innovative procedures and technologies are to be developed and applied without the mistakes of the past, surgeons must be honest when they answer these questions: Is this procedure safe? Would I consider undergoing this procedure if I developed a surgical indication? Is the procedure as good or better than the procedure it is replacing? Do I have the skills to apply this procedure safely and with equivalent results to the more experienced surgeon? If the answer to any of these questions is "no," or "I don't know," there is a professional obligation to seek another procedure or outside assistance before subjecting a patient to the new procedure.

REFERENCES

Entries highlighted in bright blue are key references.

1. Hopkins HH: Optical principles of the endoscope, in Berci G (ed): *Endoscopy.* New York: Appleton-Century-Crofts. 1976, p 3.
2. Katzir A: Optical fibers in medicine. *Sci Am* 260:120, 1989.
3. Hirschowitz BI: A personal history of the fiberscope. *Gastroenterology* 76:864, 1979.
4. Veritas TF: Coelioscopy: A synthesis of Georg Kelling's work with insufflation, endoscopy, and luft tamponade, in Litynski GS (ed): *Highlights in the History of Laparoscopy.* Frankfurt/Main: Barbara Bernert Verlag, 1996, p 3.
5. Ponsky JL, Gauderer MW: Percutaneous endoscopic gastrostomy: A nonoperative technique for feeding gastrostomy. *Gastroint Endosc* 27:9, 1981.
6. Wood BJ, Ramkaransingh JR, Fogo T, et al: Percutaneous tumor ablation with radiofrequency. *Cancer* 94:443, 2002.
7. Smith RS, Fry WR, Tsoi EK, et al: Gasless laparoscopy and conventional instruments: The next phase of minimally invasive surgery. *Arch Surg* 128:1102, 1993.
8. Litynski GS: *Highlights in the History of Laparoscopy.* Frankfurt/Main: Barbara Bernert Verlag, 1996, p 78.
9. Hunter JG, Staheli J, et al.: Nitrous oxide pneumoperitoneum revisited: Is there a risk of combustion? *Surg Endosc* 9:501, 1995.
10. Tsereteli Z, Terry ML, et al: Prospective randomized clinical trial comparing nitrous oxide and carbon dioxide pneumoperitoneum for laparoscopic surgery. *J Am Coll Surg* 195:173, 2002.
11. Callery MP, Soper NJ: Physiology of the pneumoperitoneum, in Hunter (ed): *Baillière's Clinical Gastroenterology: Laparoscopic Surgery.* London/Philadelphia: Baillière Tindall, 1993, p 757.
12. Ho HS, Gunther RA, et al: Intraperitoneal carbon dioxide insufflation and cardiopulmonary functions. *Arch Surg* 127:928, 1992.
13. Wittgen CM, Andrus CH, et al: Analysis of the hemodynamic and ventilatory effects of laparoscopic cholecystectomy. *Arch Surg* 126:997, 1991.
14. Cullen DJ, Eger EI: Cardiovascular effects of carbon dioxide in man. *Anesthesiol* 41:345, 1974.
15. Cunningham AJ, Turner J, et al: Transoesophageal echocardiographic assessment of haemodynamic function during laparoscopic cholecystectomy. *Br J Anaesth* 70:621, 1993.
16. Harris MNE, Plantevin OM, Crowther A, et al: Cardiac arrhythmias during anaesthesia for laparoscopy. *Br J Anaesth* 56:1213, 1984.
17. Borten M, Friedman EA: Choice of anaesthesia, in: *Laparoscopic Complications: Prevention and Management.* Toronto: BC Decker, 1986, p 173.
18. Jorgenson JO, Hanel K, Lalak NJ, et al: Thromboembolic complications of laparoscopic cholecystectomy (Letter). *Br Med J* 306:518, 1993.
19. Ho HS, Wolfe BM: The physiology and immunology of endosurgery, in Toouli JG, Gossot D, Hunter JG (eds): *Endosurgery.* New York/London: Churchill-Livingstone, 1996, p 163.
20. Sackier JM, Nibhanupudy B: The pneumoperitoneum-physiology and complications, in Toouli JG, Gossot D, Hunter JG (eds): *Endosurgery.* New York/London: Churchill-Livingstone, 1996, p 155.
21. Kashtan J, Green JF, Parsons EQ, et al: Hemodynamic effects of increased abdominal pressure. *J Surg Res* 30:249, 1981.
22. McDougall EM, Monk TG, Wolf JS Jr, et al: The effect of prolonged pneumoperitoneum on renal function in an animal model. *J Am Coll Surg* 182:317, 1996.
23. Lindberg F, Bergqvist D, Bjorck M, et al: Renal hemodynamics during carbon dioxide pneumoperitoneum: An experimental study in pigs. *Surg Endosc* 17:480, 2003.
24. Hazebroek EJ, de Vos tot Nederveen Cappel R, Gommers D, et al: Antidiuretic hormone release during laparoscopic donor nephrectomy. *Arch Surg* 137:600; discussion 605, 2002.
25. Ostman PL, Pantle-Fisher FH, Fanre EA, et al: Circulatory collapse during laparoscopy. *J Clin Anesth* 2:129, 1990.
26. Alijani A, Cuschieri A: Abdominal wall lift systems in laparoscopic surgery: Gasless and low-pressure systems. *Semin Laparosc Surg* 8:53, 2001.
27. Ozawa A, Konishi F, Nagai H, et al: Cytokine and hormonal responses in laparoscopic-assisted colectomy and conventional open colectomy. *Surg Today* 30:107, 2000.
28. Burpee SE, Kurian M, Murakame Y, et al: The metabolic and immune response to laparoscopic versus open liver resection. *Surg Endosc* 16:899, 2002.
29. Gossot D: Access modalities for thoracoscopic surgery, in Toouli JG, Gossot D, Hunter JG (eds): *Endosurgery.* New York/London: Churchill-Livingstone, 1996, p 743.
30. Memon MA, Cooper NJ, Memon B, et al: Meta-analysis of randomized clinical trials comparing open and laparoscopic inguinal hernia repair. *Br J Surg* 90:1479, 2003.
31. Himpens J: Laparoscopic preperitoneal approach to the inguinal hernia, in Toouli JG, Gossot D, Hunter JG (eds): *Endosurgery.* New York/London: Churchill-Livingstone, 1996, p 949.
32. Horvath KD, Kao LS, Wherry KL, et al: A technique for laparoscopic-assisted percutaneous drainage of infected pancreatic necrosis and pancreatic abscess. *Surg Endosc* 15:1221, 2001.
33. Eaves FF: Basics of endoscopic plastic surgery, in Bostwick J, Eaves FF, Nahai F (eds): *Endoscopic Plastic Surgery.* St Louis: Quality Medical Publishing, 1995, p 59.
34. Kenyon TA, Lenker MP, Bax TW, et al: Cost and benefit of the trained laparoscopic team. A comparative study of a designated nursing team vs a nontrained team. *Surg Endosc* 11:812, 1997.
35. Herron DM, Gagner M, Kenyon TL, et al: The minimally invasive surgical suite enters the 21st century. A discussion of critical design elements. *Surg Endosc* 15:415, 2001.
36. Byron JW, Markenson G, et al: A randomised comparison of Veress needle and direct insertion for laparoscopy. *Surg Gynecol Obstet* 177:259, 1993.
37. Fletcher DR: Laparoscopic access, in Toouli JG, Gossot D, Hunter JG (eds): *Endosurgery.* New York/London: Churchill-Livingstone, 1996, p 189.
38. Hanney RM, Alle KM, Cregan PC: Major vascular injury and laparoscopy. *Aust N Z J Surg* 65:533, 1995.
39. Catarci M, Carlini M, Gentileschi P, et al: Major and minor injuries during the creation of pneumoperitoneum. A multicenter study on 12,919 cases. *Surg Endosc* 15:566, 2001.
40. Siperstein AE, Berber E, Engle KL, et al: Laparoscopic posterior adrenalectomy: Technical considerations. *Arch Surg* 135:967, 2000.
41. Vasilev SA, McGonigle KF: Extraperitoneal laparoscopic para-aortic lymph node dissection. *Gynecol Oncol* 61:315, 1996.
42. Schurr UP, Lachat ML, Reuthebuch O, et al: Endoscopic saphenous vein harvesting for CABG—a randomized prospective trial. *Thorac Cardiovasc Surg* 50:160, 2002.
43. Lumsden AB, Eaves FF: Vein harvest, in Bostwick J, Eaves FF, Nahai F (eds): *Endoscopic Plastic Surgery.* St. Louis: Quality Medical Publishing, 1995, p 535.
44. Targarona EM, Gracia E, Rodriguez M, et al: Hand-assisted laparoscopic surgery. *Arch Surg* 138:138, 2003.
45. Berquer R, Smith WD, Davis S: An ergonomic study of the optimum operating table height for laparoscopic surgery. *Surg Endosc* 16:416, 2002.
46. Berguer R, Smith WD, Chung YH: Performing laparoscopic surgery is significantly more stressful for the surgeon than open surgery. *Surg Endosc* 15:1204, 2001.
47. Emam TA, Hanna G, Cuschieri A: Ergonomic principles of task alignment, visual display, and direction of execution of laparoscopic bowel suturing. *Surg Endosc* 16:267, 2002.
48. Prescher T: Video imaging, in Toouli JG, Gossot D, Hunter JG (eds): *Endosurgery.* New York/London: Churchill-Livingstone, 1996, p 41.
49. Margulies DR, Shabot MM: Fiberoptic imaging and measurement, in Hunter JG, Sackier JM (eds): *Minimally Invasive Surgery.* New York: McGraw-Hill, 1993, p 7.
50. Wenzl R, Lehner R, Holzer A, et al: Improved laparoscopic operating techniques using a digital enhancement video system. *J Am Assoc Gynecol Laparosc* 5:175, 1998.

51. Berci G, Paz-Partlow M: Videoendoscopic technology, in Toouli JG, Gossot D, Hunter JG (eds): *Endosurgery*. New York/London: Churchill-Livingstone, 1996, p 33.

52. Levy ML, Day JD, Albuquerque F, et al: Heads-up intraoperative endoscopic imaging: A prospective evaluation of techniques and limitations. *Neurosurgery* 40:526, 1997.

53. Taffinder N, Smith SG, Huber J, et al: The effect of a second-generation 3D endoscope on the laparoscopic precision of novices and experienced surgeons. *Surg Endosc* 13:1087, 1999.

54. Odell RC: Laparoscopic electrosurgery, in Hunter JG, Sackier JM (eds): *Minimally Invasive Surgery*. New York: McGraw-Hill, 1993, p 33.

55. Voyels CR, et al: Education and engineering solutions for potential problems with laparoscopic monopolar electrosurgery. *Am J Surg* 164:57, 1992.

56. Blanc B, d'Ercole C, Gaiato ML, et al: Cause and prevention of electrosurgical injuries in laparoscopy. *J Am Coll Surg* 179:161, 1994.

57. Tucker RD: Principles of electrosurgery, in Sivak MV (ed): *Gastroenterologic Endoscopy*, 2nd ed. Philadelphia: WB Saunders, 2000, p 125.

58. Barlow DE: Endoscopic application of electrosurgery: A review of basic principles. *Gastrointest Endosc* 28:73, 1982.

59. Trus TL, Hunter JG: Principles of laser physics and tissue interaction, in Toouli JG, Gossot D, Hunter JG (eds): *Endosurgery*. New York/London: Churchill-Livingstone, 1996, p 103.

60. Bass LS, Oz MC, Trokel SL, et al: Alternative lasers for endoscopic surgery: Comparison of pulsed thulium-holmium-chromium:YAG with continuous-wave neodymium:YAG laser for ablation of colonic mucosa. *Lasers Surg Med* 11:545, 1991.

61. Greenwald BD: Photodynamic therapy for esophageal cancer. *Chest Surg Clin North Am* 10:625, 2000.

62. Hunter JG, Bruhn E, Godman G, et al: Reflectance spectroscopy predicts safer wavelengths for pulsed laser lithotripsy of gallstones (abstract). *Gastrointest Endosc* 37:273, 1991.

63. Amaral JF, Chrostek C: Comparison of the ultrasonically activated scalpel to electrosurgery and laser for laparoscopic surgery. *Surg Endosc* 7:141, 1993.

64. Huscher CG, Liriei MM, Di Paola M, et al: Laparoscopic cholecystectomy by ultrasonic dissection without cystic duct and artery ligature. *Surg Endosc* 17:442, 2003.

65. Jobe BA, Kenyon T, Hansen PD, et al: Mini-laparoscopy: Current status, technology and future applications. *Minim Invasive Ther Allied Technol* 7:201, 1998.

66. Aiono S, Gilbert JM, Soin B, et al: Controlled trial of the introduction of a robotic camera assistant (EndoAssist) for laparoscopic cholecystectomy. *Surg Endosc* 16:1267, 2002.

67. Melvin WS, Needleman BJ, Krause KR, et al: Computer-enhanced vs. standard laparoscopic anti-reflux surgery. *J Gastrointest Surg* 6:11, 2002.

68. Costi R, Himpens J, Bruyns J, et al: Robotic fundoplication: From theoretic advantages to real problems. *J Am Coll Surg* 197:500, 2003.

69. Ruurda JP, Broeders IA, Simmermacher RP, et al: Feasibility of robot-assisted laparoscopic surgery: An evaluation of 35 robot-assisted laparoscopic cholecystectomies. *Surg Laparosc Endosc Percutan Tech* 12:41, 2002.

70. Rodriguez E, Nifong LW, Chu MW, et al: Robotic mitral valve repair for anterior leaflet and bileaflet prolapsed. *Ann Thorac Surg* 85:438; discussion 444, 2008.

71. Menon M, Tewari A, Baize B, et al: Prospective comparison of radical retropubic prostatectomy and robot-assisted anatomic prostatectomy: The Vattikuti Urology Institute experience. *Urology* 60:864, 2002.

72. Marescaux J, Leroy J, Gagner M, et al: Transatlantic robot-assisted telesurgery. *Nature* 413:379, 2001.

73. Fleischer DE: Stents, cloggology, and esophageal cancer. *Gastrointest Endosc* 43:258, 1996.

74. Foutch P, Sivak M: Therapeutic endoscopic balloon dilatation of the extrahepatic biliary ducts. *Am J Gastroenterol* 80:575, 1985.

75. Hoepffner N, Foerster EC, et al: Long-term experience in wall stent therapy for malignant choledochostenosis. *Endoscopy* 26:597, 1994.

76. Kozarek RA, Ball TJ, et al: Metallic self-expanding stent application in the upper gastrointestinal tract: Caveats and concerns. *Gastrointest Endosc* 38:1, 1992.

77. Anderson JR, Sorenson SM, Kruse A, et al: Randomized trial of endoscopic endoprosthesis versus operative bypass in malignant obstructive jaundice. *Gut* 30:1132, 1989.

78. Ruygrok PN, Sim KH, Chan C, et al: Coronary intervention with a heparin-coated stent and aspirin only. *J Invasive Cardiol* 15:439, 2003.

79. Bessler M, Stevens PD, Milone L, et al: Transvaginal laparoscopic cholecystectomy: Laparoscopically assisted. *Surg Endosc* 22:1715, 2008.

80. Marescaux J, Dallemagne B, Perretta S, et al: Surgery without scars: Report of transluminal cholecystectomy in a human being. *Arch Surg* 142:823; discussion 826, 2007.

81. Bessler M, Stevens PD, Milone L, et al: Transvaginal laparoscopic cholecystectomy: Laparoscopically assisted. *Surg Endosc* 22:1715, 2008.

82. Georgeson KE: Pediatric laparoscopy, in Toouli JG, Gossot D, Hunter JG (eds): *Endosurgery*. New York/London: Churchill-Livingstone, 1996, p 929.

83. Holcomb GW: Diagnostic laparoscopy: Equipment, technique, and special concerns in children, in Holcomb GW (ed): *Pediatric Endoscopic Surgery*. Norwalk, CT: Appleton & Lange, 1993, p 9.

84. Hunter JG, Swanstrom LL, et al: Carbon dioxide pneumoperitoneum induces fetal acidosis in a pregnant ewe model. *Surg Endosc* 9:272, 1995.

85. Morrell DG, Mullins JR, et al: Laparoscopic cholecystectomy during pregnancy in symptomatic patients. *Surgery* 112:856, 1992.

86. Callery MP, Strasberg SM, Doherty GM, et al: Staging laparoscopy with laparoscopic ultrasonography: Optimizing resectability in hepatobiliary and pancreatic malignancy. *J Am Coll Surg* 185:33, 1997.

87. Luketich JD, Alvelo-Rivera M, Buenaventura PO, et al: Minimally invasive esophagectomy: Outcomes in 222 patients. *Ann Surg* 238:486; discussion 494, 2003.

88. Fleshman J, Sargent DJ, Green E, for The Clinical Outcomes of Surgical Therapy Study Group: Laparoscopic colectomy for cancer is not inferior to open surgery based on 5-year data from the COST Study Group trial. *Ann Surg* 246:655; discussion 662, 2007.

89. Fried GM, Clas D, Meakins JL: Minimally invasive surgery in the elderly patient. *Surg Clin North Am* 74:375, 1994.

90. Borman PC, Terblanche J: Subtotal cholecystectomy: For the difficult gallbladder in portal hypertension and cholecystitis. *Surgery* 98:1, 1985.

91. Litwin DWM, Pham Q: Laparoscopic surgery in the complicated patient, in Eubanks WS, Swanstrom LJ, Soper NJ (eds): *Mastery of Endoscopic and Laparoscopic Surgery*. Philadelphia: Lippincott, Williams & Wilkins, 2000, p 57.

92. Gallagher AG, Smith CD, Bowers SP, et al: Psychomotor skills assessment in practicing surgeons experienced in performing advanced laparoscopic procedures. *J Am Coll Surg* 197:479, 2003.

93. Seymour NE, Gallagher AG, Roman SA, et al: Virtual reality training improves operating room performance: Results of a randomized, double-blinded study. *Ann Surg* 236:458; discussion 463, 2002.

94. Anvari M: Telesurgery: Remote knowledge translation in clinical surgery. *World J Surg* 31:1545, 2007.

Molecular and Genomic Surgery

Xin-Hua Feng, Xia Lin, and F. Charles Brunicardi

OVERVIEW OF MOLECULAR CELL BIOLOGY

One of the goals of modern biology is to analyze the molecular structure and gain a fuller understanding of how cells, tissues, organs, and entire organisms function, both in a normal state and under pathologic conditions. Significant progress has been made in molecular studies of metabolism pathways, gene expression, cellular signaling, and organ development in human beings. The advent of recombinant DNA technology, polymerase chain reaction (PCR) techniques, and completion of the Human Genome Project are positively affecting human society by not only broadening our knowledge and understanding of disease development but also by bringing about necessary changes in disease treatment.

Today's practicing surgeons are becoming increasingly aware that many modern surgical procedures rely on the information gained through molecular research. Genomic information, such as BRCA and *RET* proto-oncogene, is being used to help direct prophylactic

procedures to remove potentially harmful tissues before they do damage to patients. Molecular engineering has led to cancer-specific gene therapy that could serve in the near future as a more effective adjunct to surgical debulking of tumors than radiation or chemotherapy, so surgeons will benefit from a clear introduction to how basic biochemical and biologic principles relate to the developing area of molecular biology.

This chapter reviews the current information on modern molecular biology for the surgical community. It is written with the intent of serving two functions. The first is to introduce or update the readers about the general concepts of molecular cell biology, which are essential for comprehending the real power and potential of modern molecular technology. The second aim is to inform the reader about the modern molecular techniques that are commonly used for surgical research and to provide a fundamental introduction on the background of how these techniques are developed and applied to benefit patients.

Basic Concepts of Molecular Research

The modern era of molecular biology, which has been mainly concerned with how genes govern cell activity, began in 1953 when James D. Watson and Francis H. C. Crick made one of the greatest scientific discoveries by deducing the double-helical structure of deoxyribonucleic acid, or DNA.[1,2] The year 2003 marked the fiftieth anniversary of this great discovery. Before 1953, one of the most mysterious aspects of biology was how genetic material was precisely duplicated from one generation to the next. Although DNA had been implicated as genetic material, it was the base-paired structure of DNA that provided a logical interpretation of how a double helix could "unzip" to make copies of itself. This DNA synthesis, termed *replication*, immediately gave rise to the notion that a template was involved in the transfer of information between generations, and thus confirmed the suspicion that DNA carried an organism's hereditary information.

Within cells, DNA is packed into chromosomes. One important feature of DNA as genetic material is its ability to encode important information for all of a cell's functions (Fig. 15-1). Based on the principles of base complementarity, scientists also discovered how information in DNA is accurately transferred into the protein structure. DNA serves as a template for RNA synthesis, termed *transcription*, including messenger RNA (mRNA, or the protein-encoding RNA), ribosomal RNA (rRNA), and transfer RNA (tRNA). mRNA carries the information from DNA to make proteins, termed *translation*, with the assistance of rRNA and tRNA. Each of these steps is precisely controlled in such a way that genes are properly expressed in each cell at a specific time and location. In recent years, new classes of noncoding RNAs, for example, microRNA (or miRNA) and Piwi-interacting RNA (or piRNA), have been identified that regulate gene expression through mRNA degradation. Consequently, the differential gene activity in a cell determines its actions, properties, and functions.

Molecular Approaches to Surgical Research

Rapid advances in molecular and cellular biology over the past half century have revolutionized the understanding of disease and will radically transform the practice of surgery. In the future, molecular techniques will be increasingly applied to surgical disease and will lead to new strategies for the selection and implementation of operative therapy. Surgeons should be familiar with the fundamental principles of molecular and cellular biology so that emerging scientific breakthroughs can be translated into improved care of the surgical patient.

The greatest advances in the field of molecular biology have been in the areas of analysis and manipulation of DNA.[1] Since Watson and Crick's discovery of DNA structure, an intensive effort has been made to unlock the deepest biologic secrets of DNA. Among the

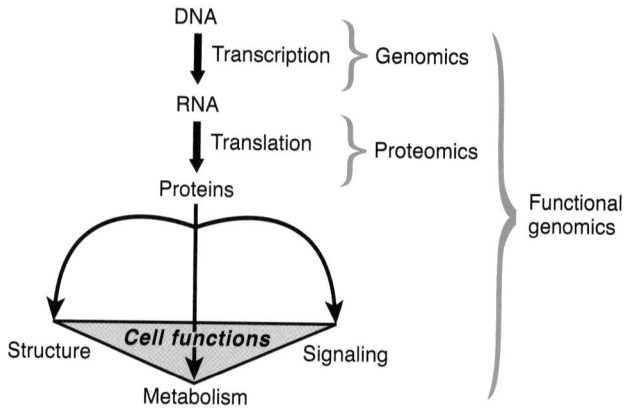

FIG. 15-1. The flow of genetic information from DNA to protein to cell functions. The process of transmission of genetic information from DNA to RNA is called *transcription*, and the process of transmission from RNA to protein is called *translation*. Proteins are the essential controlling components for cell structure, cell signaling, and metabolism. *Genomics* and *proteomics* are the study of the genetic composition of a living organism at the DNA and protein level, respectively. The study of the relationship between genes and their cellular functions is called *functional genomics*.

avalanche of technical advances, one discovery in particular has drastically changed the world of molecular biology: the uncovering of the enzymatic and microbiologic techniques that produce recombinant DNA. Recombinant DNA technology involves the enzymatic manipulation of DNA and, subsequently, the cloning of DNA. DNA molecules are cloned for a variety of purposes including safeguarding DNA samples, facilitating sequencing, generating probes, and expressing recombinant proteins in one or more host organisms. DNA can be produced by a number of means, including restricted digestion of an existing vector, PCR, and cDNA synthesis. As DNA cloning techniques have developed over the last quarter century, researchers have moved from studying DNA to studying the functions of proteins, and from cell and animal models to molecular therapies in humans. Expression of recombinant proteins provides a method for analyzing gene regulation, structure, and function. In recent years the uses for recombinant proteins have expanded to include a variety of new applications, including gene therapy and biopharmaceuticals. The basic molecular approaches for modern

KEY POINTS

1. The advent of recombinant DNA technology, polymerase chain reaction techniques, and completion of the human genome have revolutionized the understanding of disease development and also radically transformed the practice of medicine and surgery.

2. Genes govern cell activity in different cell types, which ultimately leads to the health of the human organism. The cellular diversity is controlled by the *genome* and accomplished by tight regulation of gene expression in a given cell at a given time.

3. Human diseases arise from improper changes in the genome. The continuous understanding of how the genome functions will make it possible to tailor medicine on an individual basis. The goal of personalized genomic medicine is to attack the disease by choosing personalized treatments that work with the individual's genomic profile. Personalized genomic medicine will undoubtedly revolutionize the practice of modern medicine.

4. Improving the outlook for human diseases can only come from a better understanding of the molecular signaling mechanisms that cause these diseases and subsequent successful therapeutic regimens.

surgical research include DNA cloning, cell manipulation, disease modeling in animals, and clinical trials in human patients.

FUNDAMENTALS OF MOLECULAR AND CELL BIOLOGY

DNA and Heredity

DNA forms a right-handed, double-helical structure that is composed of two antiparallel strands of unbranched polymeric deoxyribonucleotides linked by phosphodiester bonds between the 5' carbon of one deoxyribose moiety to the 3' carbon of the next (Fig. 15-2). DNA is composed of four types of deoxyribonucleotides: adenine (A), cytosine (C), guanine (G), and thymine (T). The nucleotides are joined together by phosphodiester bonds. In the double-helical structure deduced by Watson and Crick, the two strands of DNA are complementary to each other. Because of size, shape, and chemical composition, A always pairs with T, and C with G, through the formation of hydrogen bonds between complementary bases that stabilize the double helix.

Recognition of the hereditary transmission of genetic information is attributed to the Austrian monk, Gregor Mendel. His seminal work, ignored upon publication until its rediscovery in 1900, established the laws of segregation and of independent assortment. These two principles established the existence of paired elementary units of heredity and defined the statistical laws that govern them.[3] DNA was isolated in 1869, and a number of important observations of the inherited basis of certain diseases were made in the early part of the twentieth century. Although today it appears easy to understand how DNA replicates, before the 1950s, the idea of DNA as the primary genetic material was not appreciated. The modern era of molecular biology began in 1944 with the demonstration that DNA was the substance that carried genetic information. The first experimental evidence that DNA was genetic material came from simple transformation experiments conducted in the 1940s using *Streptococcus pneumoniae*. One strain of the bacteria could be converted into another by incubating it with DNA from the other, just as the treatment of the DNA with deoxyribonuclease would inactivate the transforming activity of the DNA. Similarly, in the early 1950s, before the discovery of the double-helical structure of DNA, the entry of viral DNA and not the protein into the host bacterium was believed to be necessary to initiate infection by the bacterial virus or bacteriophage. Key historical events concerning genetics are outlined in Table 15-1.

Building blocks of DNA

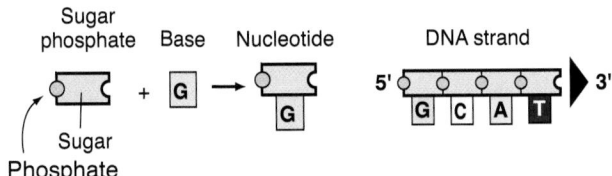

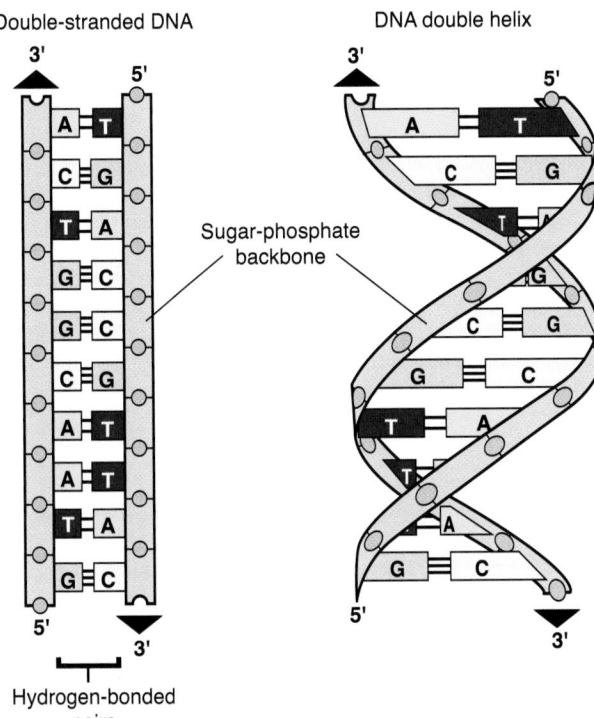

FIG. 15-2. Schematic representation of a DNA molecule forming a double helix. DNA is made of four types of nucleotides, which are linked covalently into a DNA strand. A DNA molecule is composed of two DNA strands held together by hydrogen bonds between the pair bases. The arrowheads at the ends of the DNA strands indicate the polarities of the two strands, which run antiparallel to each other in the DNA molecule. The diagram at the bottom left of the figure shows the DNA molecule straightened out. In reality, the DNA molecule is twisted into a double helix, of which each turn of DNA is made up of 10.4 nucleotide pairs, as shown on the right. (*From Alberts et al,[1] with permission.*)

TABLE 15-1 Historical events in genetics and molecular biology

Year	Investigator	Event
1865	Mendel	Laws of genetics established
1869	Miescher	DNA isolated
1905	Garrod	Human inborn errors of metabolism
1913	Sturtevant	Linear map of genes
1927	Muller	X-rays cause inheritable genetic damage
1928	Griffith	Transformation discovered
1941	Beadle and Tatum	"One gene, one enzyme" concept
1944	Avery, MacLeod, McCarty	DNA as material of heredity
1950	McKlintock	Existence of transposons confirmed
1953	Watson and Crick	Double-helical structure of DNA
1957	Benzer and Kornberg	Recombination and DNA polymerase
1966	Nirenberg, Khorana, Holley	Genetic code determined
1970	Temin and Baltimore	Reverse transcriptase
1972	Cohen, Boyer, Berg	Recombinant DNA technology
1975	Southern	Transfer of DNA fragments from sizing gel to nitrocellulose (Southern blot)
1977	Sanger, Maxim, Gilbert	DNA sequencing methods
1982	—	GenBank database established
1985	Mullis	Polymerase chain reaction
1986	—	Automated DNA sequencing
1989	Collins	Cystic fibrosis gene identified by positional cloning and linkage analysis
1990	—	Human Genome Project initiated
1997	Roslin Institute	Mammalian cloning (Dolly)
2001	IHGSC and Celera Genomics	Draft versions of human genome sequence published
2003	—	Human Genome Project completed

IHGSC = International Human Genome Sequencing Consortium.

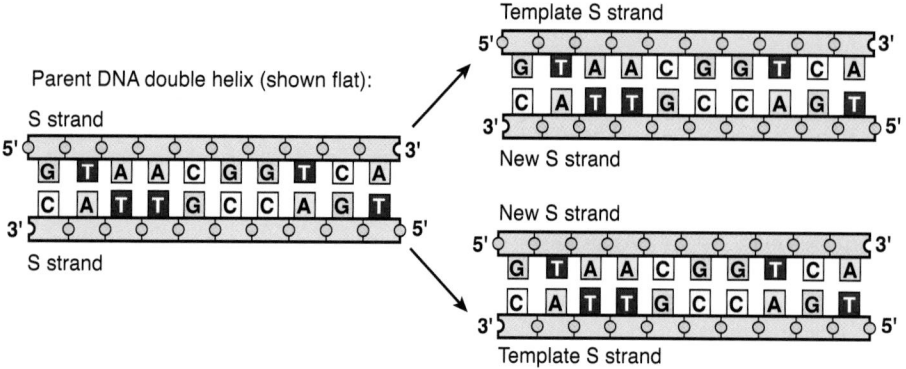

DNA is a template for its own duplication

FIG. 15-3. DNA replication. As the nucleotide A only pairs with T, and G with C, each strand of DNA can determine the nucleotide sequence in its complementary strand. In this way, double-helical DNA can be copied precisely. *(From Alberts et al,¹ with permission.)*

For cells to pass on the genetic material (DNA) to each progeny, the amount of DNA must be doubled. Watson and Crick recognized that the complementary base-pair structure of DNA implied the existence of a template-like mechanism for the copying of genetic material.² The transfer of DNA material from the mother cell to daughter cells takes place during somatic cell division (also called *mitosis*). Before a cell divides, DNA must be precisely duplicated. During replication, the two strands of DNA separate and each strand creates a new complementary strand by precise base-pair matching (Fig. 15-3). The two, new, double-stranded DNAs carry the same genetic information, which can then be passed on to two daughter cells. Proofreading mechanisms ensure that the replication process occurs in a highly accurate manner. The fidelity of DNA replication is absolutely crucial to maintaining the integrity of the genome from generation to generation. However, mistakes can still occur during this process, resulting in *mutations*, which may lead to a change of the DNA's encoded protein and, consequently, a change of the cell's behavior. The reliable dependence of many features of modern organisms on subtle changes in genome is linked to Mendelian inheritance and also contributes to the processes of Darwinian evolution. In addition, massive changes, so-called *genetic instability*, can occur in the genome of somatic cells such as cancer cells.

Gene Regulation

Living cells have the necessary machinery to enzymatically transcribe DNA into RNA and translate the mRNA into protein. This machinery accomplishes the two major steps required for gene expression in all organisms: transcription and translation (Fig. 15-4). However, gene regulation is far more complex, particularly in eukaryotic organisms. For example, many gene transcripts must be spliced to remove the intervening sequences. The sequences that are spliced off are called *introns*, which appear to be useless, but in fact may carry some regulatory information. The sequences that are joined together, and are eventually translated into protein, are called *exons*. Additional regulation of gene expression includes modification of mRNA, control of mRNA stability, and its nuclear export into cytoplasm (where it is assembled into ribosomes for translation). After mRNA is translated into protein, the levels and functions of the proteins can be further regulated posttranslationally. However, the following sections will mainly focus on gene regulation at transcriptional and translational levels.

Transcription

Transcription is the enzymatic process of RNA synthesis from DNA.⁴ In bacteria, a single RNA polymerase carries out all RNA synthesis, including that of mRNA, rRNA, and tRNA. Transcription often is coupled with translation in such a way that an mRNA molecule is completely accessible to ribosomes, and bacterial protein synthesis begins on an mRNA molecule even while it is still being synthesized. Therefore, a discussion of gene regulation with a look at the simpler prokaryotic system precedes that of the more complex transcription and posttranscriptional regulation of eukaryotic genes.

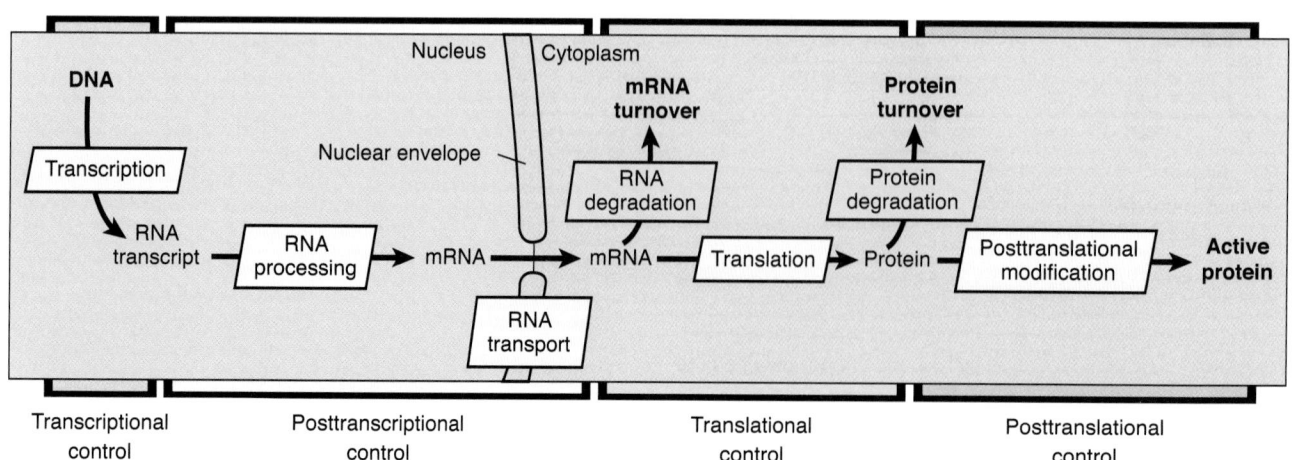

FIG. 15-4. Four major steps in the control of eukaryotic gene expression. Transcriptional and posttranscriptional control determine the level of messenger RNA (mRNA) that is available to make a protein, while translational and posttranslational control determine the final outcome of functional proteins. Note that posttranscriptional and posttranslational controls consist of several steps.

Transcription in Bacteria Initiation of transcription in prokaryotes begins with the recognition of DNA sequences by RNA polymerase. First, the bacterial RNA polymerase catalyzes RNA synthesis through loose binding to any region in the double-stranded DNA and then through specific binding to the *promoter* region with the assistance of accessory proteins called σ factors (sigma factors). A promoter region is the DNA region upstream of the transcription initiation site. RNA polymerase binds tightly at the promoter sites and causes the double-stranded DNA structure to unwind. Consequently, few nucleotides can be base-paired with the DNA template to begin transcription. Once transcription begins, the σ factor is released. The growing RNA chain may begin to peel off as the chain elongates. This occurs in such a way that there are always about 10 to 12 nucleotides of the growing RNA chains that are base-paired with the DNA template.

The bacterial promoter contains a region of about 40 bases that include two conserved elements called *–35 region* and *–10 region*. The numbering system begins at the initiation site, which is designated +1 position, and counts backward (in negative numbers) on the promoter and forward on the transcribed region. Although both regions on different promoters are not the same sequences, they are fairly conserved and very similar. This conservation provides the accurate and rapid initiation of transcription for most bacterial genes. It is also common in bacteria that one promoter serves to transcribe a series of clustered genes, called an *operon*. A single transcribed mRNA contains a series of coding regions, each of which is later independently translated. In this way, the protein products are synthesized in a coordinated manner. Most of the time these proteins are involved in the same metabolic pathway, thus demonstrating that the control by one operon is an efficient system. After initiation of transcription, the polymerase moves along the DNA to elongate the chain of RNA, although at a certain point, it will stop. Each step of RNA synthesis, including initiation, elongation, and termination, will require the integral functions of RNA polymerase as well as the interactions of the polymerase with regulatory proteins.

Transcription in Eukaryotes Transcription mechanisms in eukaryotes differ from those in prokaryotes. The unique features of eukaryotic transcription are as follows: (a) Three separate RNA polymerases are involved in eukaryotes: RNA polymerase I transcribes the precursor of 5.8S, 18S, and 28S rRNAs; RNA polymerase II synthesizes the precursors of mRNA as well as microRNA; RNA polymerase III makes tRNAs and 5S rRNAs. (b) In eukaryotes, the initial transcript is often the precursor to final mRNAs, tRNAs, and rRNAs. The precursor is then modified and/or processed into its final functional form. RNA splicing is one type of processing to remove the noncoding introns (the region between coding exons) on an mRNA. (c) In contrast to bacterial DNA, eukaryotic DNA often is packaged with histone and nonhistone proteins into chromatins. Transcription will only occur when the chromatin structure changes in such a way that DNA is accessible to the polymerase. (d) RNA is made in the nucleus and transported into cytoplasm, where translation occurs. Therefore, unlike bacteria, eukaryotes undergo uncoupled transcription and translation.

Eukaryotic gene transcription also involves the recognition and binding of RNA polymerase to the promoter DNA. However, the interaction between the polymerase and DNA is far more complex in eukaryotes than in prokaryotes. Because the majority of studies have been focused on the regulation and functions of proteins, this chapter primarily focuses on how protein-encoding mRNA is made by RNA polymerase II.

Translation

DNA directs the synthesis of RNA; RNA in turn directs the synthesis of proteins. Proteins are variable-length polypeptide polymers composed of various combinations of 20 different amino acids and are the working molecules of the cell. The process of decoding information on mRNA to synthesize proteins is called *translation* (see Fig. 15-1). Translation takes place in ribosomes composed of rRNA and ribosomal proteins. The numerous discoveries made during the 1950s made it easy to understand how DNA replication and transcription involves base-pairing between DNA and DNA, or DNA and RNA. However, at that time it was still impossible to comprehend how mRNA transfers the information to the protein-synthesizing machinery. The genetic information on mRNA is composed of arranged sequences of four bases that are transferred to the linear arrangement of 20 amino acids on a protein. Amino acids are characterized by a central carbon unit linked to four side chains: an amino group ($-NH_2$), a carboxy group ($-COOH$), a hydrogen, and a variable ($-R$) group. The amino acid chain is assembled via peptide bonds between the amino group of one amino acid and the carboxy group of the next. Because of this decoding, the information carried on mRNA relies on tRNA. Translation involves all three RNAs. The precise transfer of information from mRNA to protein is governed by *genetic code*, the set of rules by which codons are translated into an amino acid (Table 15-2). A *codon*, a

TABLE 15-2 The genetic code

		Second Base in Codon													
		U			C			A			G				
First Base in Codon	U	UUU	Phe	[F]	UCU	Ser	[S]	UAU	Tyr	[Y]	UGU	Cys	[C]	U	Third Base in Codon
		UUC	Phe	[F]	UCC	Ser	[S]	UAC	Tyr	[Y]	UGC	Cys	[C]	C	
		UUA	Leu	[L]	UCA	Ser	[S]	UAA	*STOP*	—	UGA	*STOP*	—	A	
		UUG	Leu	[L]	UCG	Ser	[S]	UAG	*STOP*	—	UGG	Trp	[W]	G	
	C	CUU	Leu	[L]	CCU	Pro	[P]	CAU	His	[H]	CGU	Arg	[R]	U	
		CUC	Leu	[L]	CCC	Pro	[P]	CAC	His	[H]	CGC	Arg	[R]	C	
		CUA	Leu	[L]	CCA	Pro	[P]	CAA	Gln	[Q]	CGA	Arg	[R]	A	
		CUG	Leu	[L]	CCG	Pro	[P]	CAG	Gln	[Q]	CGG	Arg	[R]	G	
	A	AUU	Ile	[I]	ACU	Thr	[T]	AAU	Asn	[N]	AGU	Ser	[S]	U	
		AUC	Ile	[I]	ACC	Thr	[T]	AAC	Asn	[N]	AGC	Ser	[S]	C	
		AUA	Ile	[I]	ACA	Thr	[T]	AAA	Lys	[K]	AGA	Arg	[R]	A	
		AUG	Met	[M]	ACG	Thr	[T]	AAG	Lys	[K]	AGG	Arg	[R]	G	
	G	GUU	Val	[V]	GCU	Ala	[A]	GAU	Asp	[D]	GGU	Gly	[G]	U	
		GUC	Val	[V]	GCC	Ala	[A]	GAC	Asp	[D]	GGC	Gly	[G]	C	
		GUA	Val	[V]	GCA	Ala	[A]	GAA	Glu	[E]	GGA	Gly	[G]	A	
		GUG	Val	[V]	GCG	Ala	[A]	GAG	Glu	[E]	GGG	Gly	[G]	G	

A = adenine; C = cytosine; G = guanine; U = uracil; Ala = alanine; Arg = arginine; Asn = asparagine; Asp = aspartic acid; Cys = cysteine; Glu = glutamic acid; Gln = glutamine; Gly = glycine; His = histidine; Ile = isoleucine; Leu = leucine; Lys = lysine; Met = methionine; Phe = phenylalanine; Pro = proline; Ser = serine; Thr = threonine; Trp = tryptophan; Tyr = tyrosine; Val = valine. Letter in [ ] indicates single lettercode for amino acid.

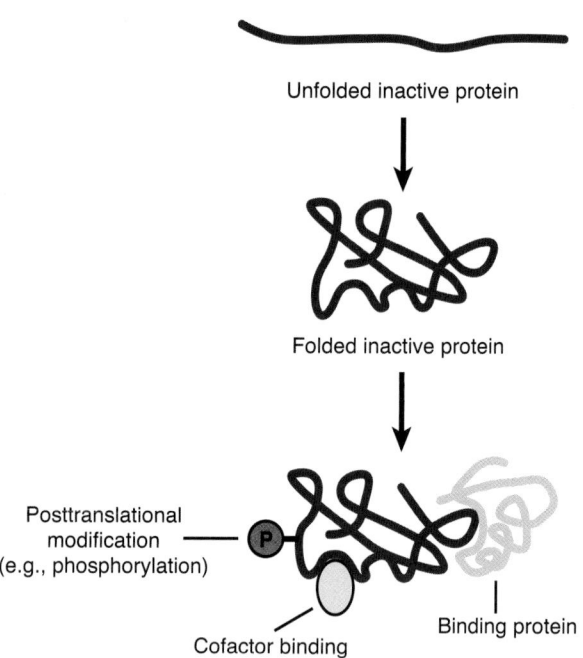

Unfolded inactive protein

Folded inactive protein

Posttranslational modification (e.g., phosphorylation)

Cofactor binding

Binding protein

Mature inactive protein

FIG. 15-5. Maturation of a functional protein. Although the linear amino acid sequence of a protein often is shown, the function of a protein also is controlled by its correctly folded three-dimensional structure. In addition, many proteins also have covalent posttranslational modifications such as phosphorylation or noncovalent binding to a small molecule or a protein.

triplet of three bases, codes for one amino acid. In this case, random combinations of the four bases form $4 \times 4 \times 4$, or 64 codes. Because 64 codes are more than enough for 20 amino acids, most amino acids are coded by more than one codon. The start codon is AUG, which also corresponds to methionine; therefore, almost all proteins begin with this amino acid. The sequence of nucleotide triplets that follows the start codon signal is termed the *reading frame*. The codons on mRNA are sequentially recognized by tRNA adaptor proteins. Specific enzymes termed *aminoacyl-tRNA synthetases* link a specific amino acid to a specific tRNA. The translation of mRNA to protein requires the ribosomal complex to move stepwise along the mRNA until the initiator methionine sequence is identified. In concert with various protein initiator factors, the methionyl-tRNA is positioned on the mRNA and protein synthesis begins. Each new amino acid is added sequentially by the appropriate tRNA in conjunction with proteins called *elongation factors*. Protein synthesis proceeds in the amino-to-carboxy-terminus direction.

The biologic versatility of proteins is astounding. Among many other functions, proteins serve as enzymes that catalyze critical biochemical reactions, carry signals to and from the extracellular environment, and mediate diverse signaling and regulatory functions in the intracellular environment. They also transport ions and various small molecules across plasma membranes. Proteins make up the key structural components of cells and the extracellular matrix and are responsible for cell motility. The unique functional properties of proteins are largely determined by their structure (Fig. 15-5).

Regulation of Gene Expression

The human organism is made up of a myriad of different cell types that, despite their vastly different characteristics, contain the same genetic material. This cellular diversity is controlled by the *genome* and accomplished by tight regulation of gene expression. This leads to the synthesis and accumulation of different complements of RNA

and, ultimately, to the proteins found in different cell types. For example, muscle and bone express different genes or the same genes at different times. Moreover, the choice of which genes are expressed in a given cell at a given time depends on signals received from its environment. There are multiple levels at which gene expression can be controlled along the pathway from DNA to RNA to protein (see Fig. 15-4). *Transcriptional control* refers to the mechanism for regulating when and how often a gene is transcribed. Splicing of the primary RNA transcript (*RNA processing control*) and selection of completed mRNAs for nuclear export (*RNA transport control*) represent additional potential regulatory steps. The mRNAs in the cytoplasm can be selectively translated by ribosomes (*translational control*), or selectively stabilized or degraded (*mRNA degradation control*). Finally, the resulting proteins can undergo selective activation, inactivation, or compartmentalization (*protein activity control*).

Because a large number of genes are regulated at the transcriptional level, regulation of gene transcripts (i.e., mRNA) often is referred to as *gene regulation* in a narrow definition. Each of the steps during transcription is properly regulated in eukaryotic cells. Because genes are differentially regulated from one another, one gene can be differentially regulated in different cell types or at different developmental stages. Therefore, gene regulation at the level of transcription is largely context dependent. However, there is a common scheme that applies to transcription at the molecular level (Fig. 15-6). Each gene promoter possesses unique sequences called *TATA boxes* that can be recognized and bound by a large complex containing RNA polymerase II, forming the basal transcription machinery. Usually located upstream of the TATA box (but sometimes longer distances) are a number of regulatory sequences referred to as *enhancers* that are recognized by regulatory proteins called *transcription factors*. These transcription factors specifically bind to the enhancers, often in response to environmental or developmental cues, and cooperate with each other and with basal transcription factors to initiate transcription. Regulatory sequences that negatively regulate the initiation of transcription also are present on the promoter DNA. The transcription factors that bind to these sites are called *repressors*, in contrast to the *activators* that activate transcription. The molecular interactions between transcription factors and promoter DNA, as well as between the cooperative transcription factors, are highly regulated and context-dependent. Specifically, the recruitment of transcription factors to the promoter DNA occurs in response to physiologic signals. A number of structural motifs in these DNA-binding transcription factors facilitate this recognition and interaction. These include the helix-turn-helix, the homeodomain motif, the zinc finger, the leucine zipper, and the helix-loop-helix motifs.

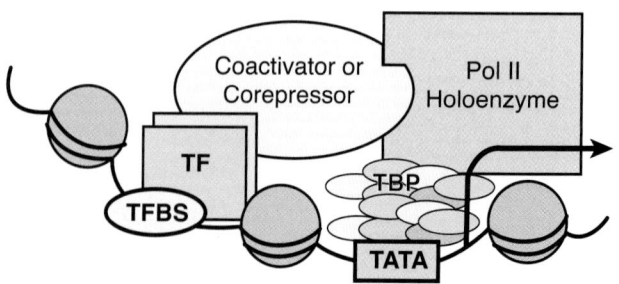

Coactivator or Corepressor

Pol II Holoenzyme

TF

TFBS

TBP

TATA

FIG. 15-6. Transcriptional control by RNA polymerase. DNA is packaged into a chromatin structure. TATA = the common sequence on the promoter recognized by TBP and polymerase II holoenzyme; TBP = TATA-binding protein and associated factors; TF = hypothetical transcription factor; TFBS = transcription factor binding site; ball-shaped structures = nucleosomes. Coactivator or corepressor are factors linking the TF with the Pol II complex.

Human Genome

Genome is a collective term for all genes present in one organism. The human genome contains DNA sequences of 3 billion base-pairs, carried by 23 pairs of chromosomes. The human genome has an estimated 25,000 to 30,000 genes, and overall it is 99.9% identical in all people.[5,6] Approximately 3 million locations where single-base DNA differences exist have been identified and termed *single nucleotide polymorphisms*. Single nucleotide polymorphisms may be critical determinants of human variation in disease susceptibility and responses to environmental factors.

The completion of the human genome sequence in 2003 represented another great milestone in modern science. The human genome project created the field of *genomics*, which is the study of genetic material in detail (see Fig. 15-1). The medical field is building upon the knowledge, resources, and technologies emanating from the human genome to further the understanding of the relationship of the genes and their mutations to human health and disease. This expansion of genomics into human health applications resulted in the field of genomic medicine.

The emergence of genomics as a science will transform the practice of medicine and surgery in this century. This breakthrough has allowed scientists the opportunity to gain remarkable insights into the lives of humans. Ultimately, the goal is to use this information to develop new ways to treat, cure, or even prevent the thousands of diseases that afflict humankind. In the twenty-first century, work will begin to incorporate the information embedded in the human genome sequence into surgical practices. By doing so, the genomic information can be used for diagnosing and predicting disease and disease susceptibility. Diagnostic tests can be designed to detect errant genes in patients suspected of having particular diseases or of being at risk for developing them. Furthermore, exploration into the function of each human gene is now possible, which will shed light on how faulty genes play a role in disease causation. This knowledge also makes possible the development of a new generation of therapeutics based on genes. Drug design is being revolutionized as researchers create new classes of medicines based on a reasoned approach to the use of information on gene sequence and protein structure function rather than the traditional trial-and-error method. Drugs targeted to specific sites in the body promise to have fewer side effects than many of today's medicines. Finally, other applications of genomics will involve the transfer of genes to replace defective versions or the use of gene therapy to enhance normal functions such as immunity.

Proteomics refers to the study of the structure and expression of proteins as well as the interactions among proteins encoded by a human genome (see Fig. 15-1).[7] A number of Internet-based repositories for protein sequences exist, including Swiss-Prot (*http://www.expasy.ch*). These databases allow comparisons of newly identified proteins with previously characterized sequences to allow prediction of similarities, identification of splice variants, and prediction of membrane topology and posttranslational modifications. Tools for proteomic profiling include two-dimensional gel electrophoresis, time-of-flight mass spectrometry, matrix-assisted laser desorption/ionization, and protein microarrays. *Structural proteomics* aims to describe the three-dimensional structure of proteins that is critical to understanding function. *Functional genomics* seeks to assign a biochemical, physiologic, cell biologic, and/or developmental function to each predicted gene. An ever-increasing arsenal of approaches, including transgenic animals, RNA interference (RNAi), and various systematic mutational strategies, will allow dissection of functions associated with newly discovered genes. Although the potential of this field of study is vast, it is in its early stages.

It is anticipated that a genomic and proteomic approach to human disease will lead to a new understanding of pathogenesis that will aid in the development of effective strategies for early diagnosis and treatment.[8] For example, identification of altered protein expression in organs, cells, subcellular structures, or protein complexes may lead to development of new biomarkers for disease detection. Moreover, improved understanding of how protein structure determines function will allow rational identification of therapeutic targets, and thereby not only accelerate drug development, but also lead to new strategies to evaluate therapeutic efficacy and potential toxicity.[7]

Cell Cycle and Apoptosis

Every organism has many different cell types. Many cells grow, while some cells such as nerve cells and striated muscle cells do not. All growing cells have the ability to duplicate their genomic DNA and pass along identical copies of this genetic information to every daughter cell. Thus, the cell cycle is the fundamental mechanism to maintain tissue homeostasis. A cell cycle comprises four periods: G_1 (first gap phase before DNA synthesis), S (synthesis phase when DNA replication occurs), G_2 (the gap phase before mitosis), and M (mitosis, the phase when two daughter cells with identical DNA are generated) (Fig. 15-7). After a full cycle, the daughter cells enter G_1 again, and when they receive appropriate signals, undergo another cycle, and so on. The machinery that drives cell cycle progression is made up of a group of enzymes called *cyclin-dependent kinases* (CDK). Cyclin expression fluctuates during the cell cycle, and cyclins are essential for CDK activities and form complexes with CDK. The cyclin A/CDK1 and cyclin B/CDK1 drive the progression for the M phase, while cyclin A/CDK2 is the primary S phase complex. Early G_1 cyclin D/CDK4/6 or late G_1 cyclin E/CDK2 controls the G_1-S transition. There also are negative regulators for CDK termed *CDK inhibitors*, which inhibit the assembly or activity of the cyclin-CDK complex. Expression of cyclins and CDK inhibitors often are regulated by developmental and environmental factors.

The cell cycle is connected with signal transduction pathways as well as gene expression. While the S and M phases rarely are subjected to changes imposed by extracellular signals, the G_1 and G_2 phases are the primary periods when cells decide whether to move on to the next phase or not. During the G_1 phase, cells receive green- or red-light signals, S phase entry or G_1 arrest, respectively. Growing cells proliferate only when supplied with appropriate mitogenic growth factors. Cells become committed to entry of the cell cycle only toward the end of G_1. Mitogenic signals stimulate the activity of early G_1 CDKs (e.g., cyclin D/CDK4) that inhibit the activity of pRb protein and activate the transcription factor called *E2F* to induce the expression of batteries of genes essential for G_1-S progression. Meanwhile, cells also receive antiproliferative signals such as those from tumor suppressors. These antiproliferative signals also act in the G_1 phase to stop cells' progress into the S phase by inducing CKI production. For example, when DNA is damaged, cells will repair the damage before entering the S phase. Therefore, G_1 contains one of the most important checkpoints for cell cycle progression. If the analogy is made that CDK is to a cell as an engine is to a car, then cyclins and CKI are the gas pedal and brake, respectively. Accelerated proliferation or improper cell cycle progression with damaged DNA would be disastrous. Genetic gain-of-function mutations in oncogenes (that often promote expression or activity of the cyclin/CDK complex) or loss-of-function mutations in tumor suppressor (that stimulate production of CKI) are causal factors for malignant transformation.

In addition to cell cycle control, cells use genetically programmed mechanisms to kill cells. This cellular process, called *apoptosis* or *programmed cell death*, is essential for the maintenance of tissue homeostasis (Fig. 15-8).

Normal tissues undergo proper apoptosis to remove unwanted cells, those that have completed their jobs or have been damaged or improperly proliferated. Apoptosis can be activated by many physiologic stimuli such as death receptor signals (e.g., Fas or cytokine tumor necrosis factor), growth factor deprivation, DNA damage, and stress signals. Two major pathways control the biochemical mechanisms governing apoptosis: the death receptor and mitochondrial. However, recent advances in apoptosis research suggest an interconnection of the two pathways. What is central to the apoptotic machinery is the activation of a cascade of proteinases called caspases. Similarly to CDK in the cell cycle, activities and

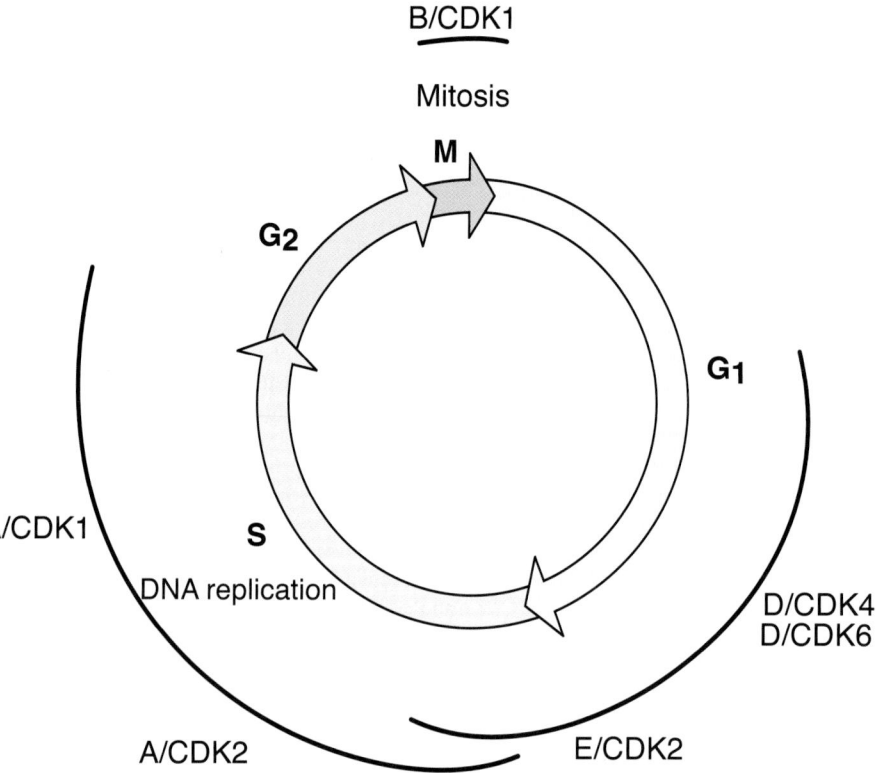

FIG. 15-7. The cell cycle and its control system. M is the mitosis phase, when the nucleus and the cytoplasm divide; S is the phase when DNA is duplicated; G_1 is the gap between M and S; G_2 is the gap between S and M. A complex of cyclin and cyclin-dependent kinase (CDK) controls specific events of each phase. Without cyclin, CDK is inactive. Different cyclin/CDK complexes are shown around the cell cycle. A, B, D, and E stand for cyclin A, cyclin B, cyclin D, and cyclin E, respectively.

expression of caspases are well controlled by positive and negative regulators. The complex machinery of apoptosis must be tightly controlled. Perturbations of this process can cause neoplastic transformation or other diseases.

Signal Transduction Pathways

Gene expression in a genome is controlled in a temporal and spatial manner, at least in part by signaling pathways.[9] A signaling pathway generally begins at the cell surface and, after a signaling relay by a cascade of intracellular effectors, ends up in the nucleus (Fig. 15-9). All cells have the ability to sense changes in their external environment. The bioactive substances to which cells can respond are many and include proteins, short peptides, amino acids, nucleotides/nucleosides, steroids, retinoids, fatty acids, and dissolved gases. Some of these substances are lipophilic and thereby can cross the plasma membrane by diffusion to bind to a specific target protein within the cytoplasm (intracellular receptor). Other substances bind directly

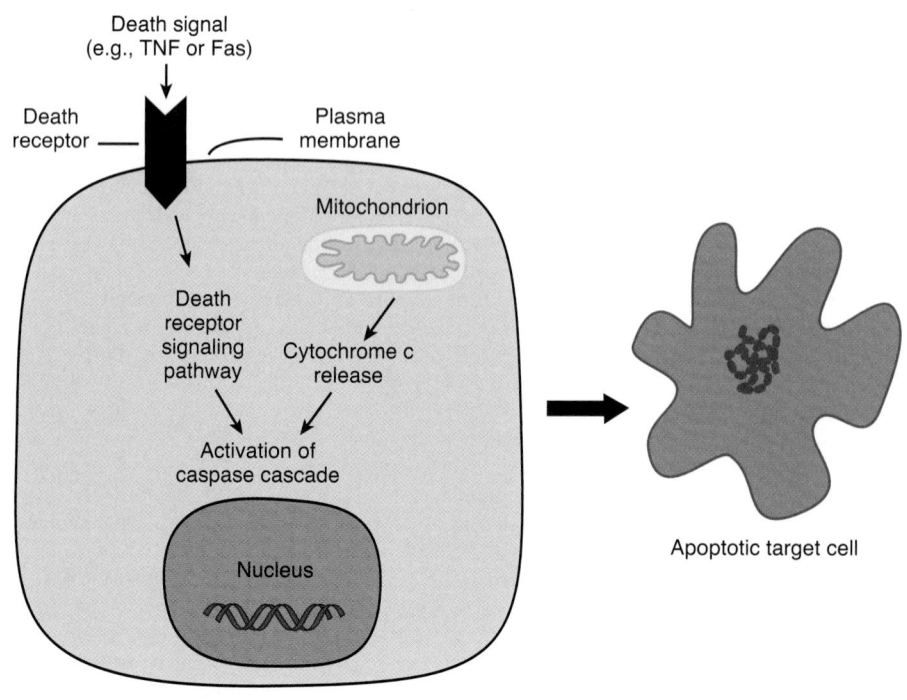

FIG. 15-8. A simplified view of the apoptosis pathways. Extracellular death receptor pathways include the activation of Fas and tumor necrosis factor (TNF) receptors, and consequent activation of the caspase pathway. Intracellular death pathway indicates the release of cytochrome c from mitochondria, which also triggers the activation of the caspase cascade. During apoptosis, cells undergo DNA fragmentation, nuclear and cell membrane breakdown, and are eventually digested by other cells.

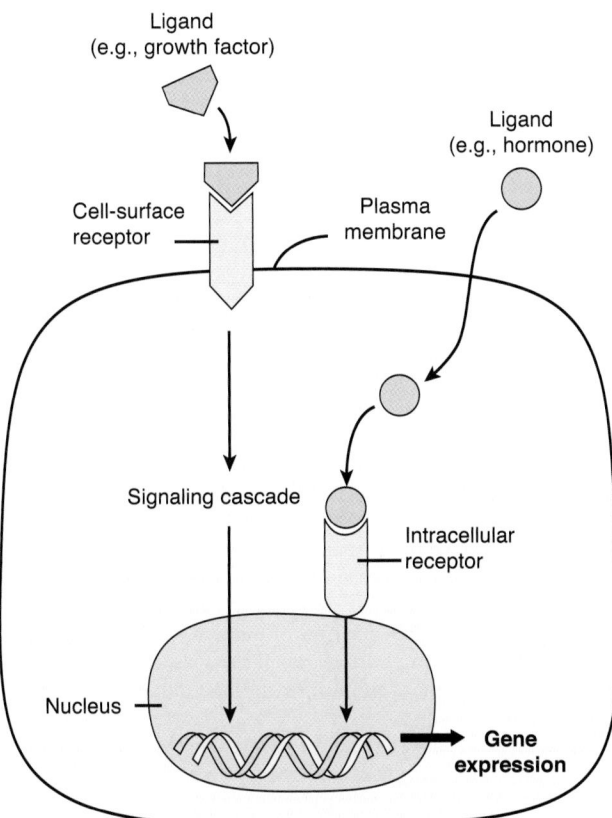

FIG. 15-9. Cell-surface and intracellular receptor pathways. Extracellular signaling pathway: Most growth factors and other hydrophilic signaling molecules are unable to move across the plasma membrane and directly activate cell-surface receptors such as G-protein coupled receptors and enzyme-linked receptors. The receptor serves as the receiver, and in turn activates the downstream signals in the cell. Intracellular signaling pathway: Hormones or other diffusible molecules enter the cell and bind to the intracellular receptor in the cytoplasm or in the nucleus. Either extracellular or intracellular signals often reach the nucleus to control gene expression.

continually are subject to multiple input signals that simultaneously and sequentially activate multiple receptor and non–receptor-mediated signal transduction pathways, which form a signaling network. Although the regulators responsible for cell behavior are rapidly identified as a result of genomic and proteomic techniques, the specific functions of the individual proteins, how they assemble, and the networks that control cellular behavior remain to be defined. An increased understanding of cell regulatory pathways—and how they are disrupted in disease—will likely reveal common themes based on protein interaction domains that direct associations of proteins with other polypeptides, phospholipids, nucleic acids, and other regulatory molecules. Advances in the understanding of signaling networks will require methods of investigation that move beyond traditional "linear" approaches into medical informatics and computational biology. The bewildering biocomplexity of such networks mandates multidisciplinary and transdisciplinary research collaboration. The vast amount of information that is rapidly emerging from genomic and proteomic data mining will require the development of new modeling methodologies within the emerging disciplines of medical mathematics and physics.

Signaling pathways often are grouped according to the properties of signaling receptors. Many hydrophobic signaling molecules are able to diffuse across plasma membranes and directly reach specific cytoplasmic targets. Steroid hormones, thyroid hormones, retinoids, and vitamin D are examples that exert their activity upon binding to structurally related receptor proteins that are members of the *nuclear hormone receptor superfamily*. Ligand binding induces a conformational change that enhances transcriptional activity of these receptors. Most extracellular signaling molecules interact with transmembrane protein receptors that couple ligand binding to intracellular signals, leading to biologic actions.

There are three major classes of cell-surface receptors: *transmitter-gated ion channels*, *seven-transmembrane G-protein coupled receptors (GPCRs)*, and *enzyme-linked receptors*. The superfamily of GPCRs is one of the largest families of proteins, representing over 800 genes of the human genome. Members of this superfamily share a characteristic seven-transmembrane configuration. The ligands for these receptors are diverse and include hormones, chemokines, neurotransmitters, proteinases, inflammatory mediators, and even sensory signals such as odorants and photons. Most GPCRs signal through *heterotrimeric G proteins*, which are guanine-nucleotide regulatory complexes. Thus the receptor serves as the receiver, the G protein serves as the transducer, and the enzyme serves as the effector arm. *Enzyme-linked receptors* possess an extracellular ligand-recognition domain and a cytosolic domain that either has intrinsic enzymatic activity or directly links with an enzyme. Structurally, these receptors usually have only one transmembrane-spanning domain. Of at least five forms of enzyme-linked receptors classified by the nature of the enzyme activity to which they are coupled, the growth factor receptors such as tyrosine kinase receptor or serine/threonine kinase receptors mediate diverse cellular events including cell growth, differentiation, metabolism, and survival/apoptosis. Dysregulation (particularly mutations) of these receptors is thought to underlie conditions of abnormal cellular proliferation in the context of cancer. The following sections will further review two examples of growth factor signaling pathways and their connection with human diseases.

Insulin Pathway and Diabetes[11]

The discovery of insulin in the early 1920s is one of the most dramatic events in the treatment of human disease. *Insulin* is a peptide hormone that is secreted by the β-cell of the pancreas. Insulin is required for the growth and metabolism of most mammalian cells, which contain cell-surface insulin receptors (InsR). Insulin binding to InsR activates the kinase activity of InsR. InsR then adds phosphoryl groups, a process referred to as *phosphorylation*, and subsequently activates its immediate intracellular effector, called *insulin receptor substrate* (IRS). IRS plays a central role in coordinating the signaling

with a transmembrane protein (cell-surface receptor). Binding of ligand to receptor initiates a series of biochemical reactions (*signal transduction*) typically involving protein-protein interactions and the transfer of high-energy phosphate groups, leading to various cellular end responses.

Control and specificity through simple protein-protein interactions—referred to as *adhesive interactions*—is a common feature of signal transduction pathways in cells.[10] Signaling also involves catalytic activities of signaling molecules, such as protein kinases/phosphatases, that modify the structures of key signaling proteins. Upon binding and/or modification by upstream signaling molecules, downstream effectors undergo a conformational (allosteric) change and, consequently, a change in function. The signal that originates at the cell surface and is relayed by the cytoplasmic proteins often ultimately reaches the transcriptional apparatus in the nucleus. It alters the DNA binding and activities of transcription factors that directly turn genes on or off in response to the stimuli. Abnormal alterations in signaling activities and capacities in otherwise normal cells can lead to diseases such as cancer.

Advances in biology in the last two decades have dramatically expanded the view on how cells are wired with signaling pathways. In a given cell, many signaling pathways operate simultaneously and crosstalk with one another. A cell generally may react to a hormonal signal in a variety of ways: (a) by changing its metabolite or protein, (b) by generating an electric current, or (c) by contracting. Cells

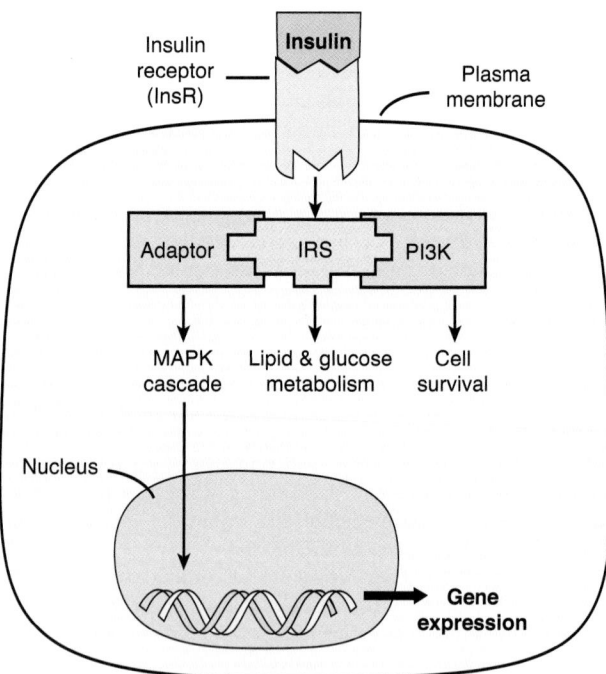

FIG. 15-10. Insulin-signaling pathway. Insulin is a peptide growth factor that binds to and activates the heterotetrameric receptor complex (InsR). InsR possesses protein tyrosine kinase activity and is able to phosphorylate the downstream insulin receptor substrate (IRS). Phosphorylated IRS serves as a scaffold and controls the activation of multiple downstream pathways for gene expression, cell survival, and glucose metabolism. Inactivation of the insulin pathway can lead to type 2 diabetes.

of insulin by activating distinct signaling pathways, the PI3K-Akt pathway and MAPK pathway, both of which possess multiple protein kinases that can control transcription, protein synthesis, and glycolysis (Fig. 15-10).

The primary physiologic role of insulin is in glucose homeostasis, which is accomplished through the stimulation of glucose uptake into insulin-sensitive tissues such as fat and skeletal muscle. Defects in insulin synthesis/secretion and/or responsiveness are major causal factors in diabetes, one of the leading causes of death and disability in the United States, affecting an estimated 16 million Americans. Type 2 diabetes accounts for about 90% of all cases of diabetes. Clustering of type 2 diabetes in certain families and ethnic populations points to a strong genetic background for the disease. More than 90% of affected individuals have insulin resistance, which develops when the body is no longer able to respond correctly to insulin circulating in the blood. Although relatively little is known about the biochemical basis of this metabolic disorder, it is clear that the insulin-signaling pathways malfunction in this disease. It is also known that genetic mutations in the InsR or IRS cause type 2 diabetes, although which one is not certain. The majority of type 2 diabetes cases may result from defects in downstream-signaling components in the insulin-signaling pathway. Type 2 diabetes also is associated with declining β-cell function, resulting in reduced insulin secretion; these pathways are under intense study. A full understanding of the basis of insulin resistance is crucial for the development of new therapies for type 2 diabetes. Furthermore, apart from type 2 diabetes, insulin resistance is a central feature of several other common human disorders, including atherosclerosis and coronary artery disease, hypertension, and obesity.

Transforming Growth Factor β (TGFβ) Pathway and Cancers[12]

Growth factor signaling controls cell growth, differentiation, and apoptosis. Although insulin and many mitogenic growth factors

promote cell proliferation, some growth factors and hormones inhibit cell proliferation. Transforming growth factor β (TGFβ) is one of them. The balance between mitogens and TGFβ plays an important role in controlling the proper pace of cell cycle progression. The growth inhibition function of TGFβ signaling in epithelial cells plays a major role in maintaining tissue homeostasis.

The TGFβ superfamily comprises a large number of structurally related growth and differentiation factors that act through a receptor complex at the cell surface (Fig. 15-11). The complex consists of transmembrane serine/threonine kinases. The receptor signals through activation of heterotrimeric complexes of intracellular effectors called SMADs (which are contracted from homologous *Caenorhabditis elegans* Sma and *Drosophila* Mad, two evolutionarily conserved genes for TGFβ signaling). Upon phosphorylation by the receptors, SMAD complexes translocate into the nucleus, where they bind to gene promoters and cooperate with specific transcription factors to regulate the expression of genes that control cell proliferation and differentiation. For example, TGFβ strongly induces the transcription of a gene called $p15^{INK4B}$ (a type of CKI) and, at the same time, reduces the expression of many oncogenes such as *c-Myc*. The outcome of the altered gene expression leads to the inhibition of cell cycle progression. Meanwhile, the strength and duration of TGFβ signaling is fine-tuned by a variety of positive or negative modulators, including protein phosphatases. Therefore, controlled activation of TGFβ signaling is an intrinsic mechanism for cells to ensure controlled proliferation.

Resistance to TGFβ's anticancer action is one hallmark of human cancer cells. TGFβ receptors and SMADs are identified as tumor suppressors. The TGFβ signaling circuit can be disrupted in a variety of ways and in different types of human tumors. Some lose TGFβ responsiveness through downregulation or mutations of their TGFβ

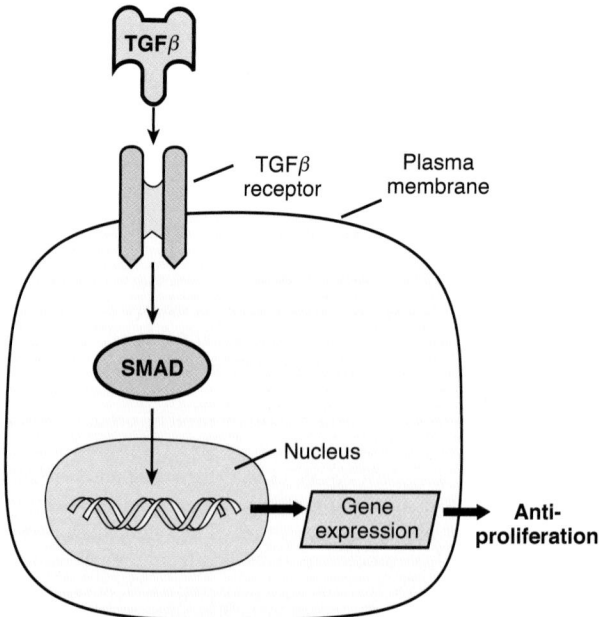

FIG. 15-11. TGFβ signaling pathway. The TGFβ family has at least 29 members encoded in the human genome. They are also peptide growth factors. Each member binds to a heterotetrameric complex consisting of a distinct set of type I and type II receptors. TGFβ receptors are protein serine/threonine kinases and can phosphorylate the downstream substrates called *SMAD proteins*. Phosphorylated SMADs are directly transported into the nucleus, where they bind to the DNA and regulate gene expression that is responsible for inhibition of cell proliferation. Inactivation of the TGFβ pathway through genetic mutations in the TGFβ receptors or SMADs is frequent in human cancer, leading to the uncontrolled proliferation of cancer cells.

receptors. The cytoplasmic SMAD4 protein, which transduces signals from ligand-activated TGFβ receptors to downstream targets, may be eliminated through mutation of its encoding gene. The locus encoding cell cycle inhibitor p15^{INK4B} may be deleted. Alternatively, the immediate downstream target of its actions, cyclin-dependent kinase 4 (CDK4), may become unresponsive to the inhibitory actions of p15^{INK4B} because of mutations that block p15^{INK4B} binding. The resulting cyclin D/CDK4 complexes constitutively inactivate tumor suppressor pRb by hyperphosphorylation. Finally, functional pRb, the end target of this pathway, may be lost through mutation of its gene. For example, in pancreatic and colorectal cancers, 100% of cells derived from these cancers carry genetic defects in the TGFβ signaling pathway. Therefore, the antiproliferative pathway converging onto pRb and the cell division cycle is, in one way or another, disrupted in a majority of human cancer cells. Besides cancer, dysregulation of TGFβ signaling also has been associated with other human diseases such as Marfan syndrome and thoracic aortic aneurysm.

Gene Therapy and Molecular Drugs in Cancer

Modern advances in the use of molecular biology to manipulate genomes have greatly contributed to the understanding of the molecular basis for how cells live, die, or differentiate. Given the fact that human diseases arise from improper changes in the genome, the continuous understanding of how the genome functions will make it possible to tailor medicine on an individual basis. Although significant hurdles remain, the course toward therapeutic application of molecular biology already has been mapped out by many proof-of-principle studies in the literature. In this section, cancer is used as an example to elaborate some therapeutic applications of molecular biology. Modern molecular medicine includes gene therapy and molecular drugs that target genes or gene products that wire human cells.

Cancer is a complex disease, involving uncontrolled growth and spread of tumor cells (Fig. 15-12). Cancer development depends on the acquisition and selection of specific characteristics that set the tumor cell apart from normal somatic cells. Cancer cells have defects in regulatory circuits that govern normal cell proliferation and homeostasis. Many lines of evidence indicate that tumorigenesis in humans is a multistep process and that these steps reflect genetic alterations that drive the progressive transformation of normal human cells into highly malignant derivatives. The genomes of tumor cells are invariably altered at multiple sites, having suffered disruption through lesions as subtle as point mutations and as obvious as changes in chromosome complement. A succession of genetic changes, each conferring one or another type of growth advantage, leads to the progressive conversion of normal human cells into cancer cells.

Cancer research in the past 20 years has generated a rich and complex body of knowledge, revealing cancer to be a disease involving dynamic changes in the genome. The causes of cancer include genetic predisposition, environmental influences, infectious agents, and aging. These transform normal cells into cancerous ones by derailing a wide spectrum of regulatory pathways including signal transduction pathways, cell cycle machinery, or apoptotic pathways.[13] The early notion that cancer was caused by mutations in genes critical for the control of cell growth implied that genome stability is important for preventing oncogenesis. There are two classes of cancer genes in which alteration has been identified in human and animal cancer cells: oncogenes, with dominant gain-of-function mutations, and tumor suppressor genes, with recessive loss-of-function mutations. In normal cells, oncogenes promote cell growth by activating cell cycle progression, while tumor suppressors counteract oncogenes' functions. Therefore, the balance between oncogenes and tumor suppressors maintains a well-controlled state of cell growth.

During the development of most types of human cancer, cancer cells can break away from primary tumor masses, invade adjacent

CHAPTER 15 Molecular and Genomic Surgery

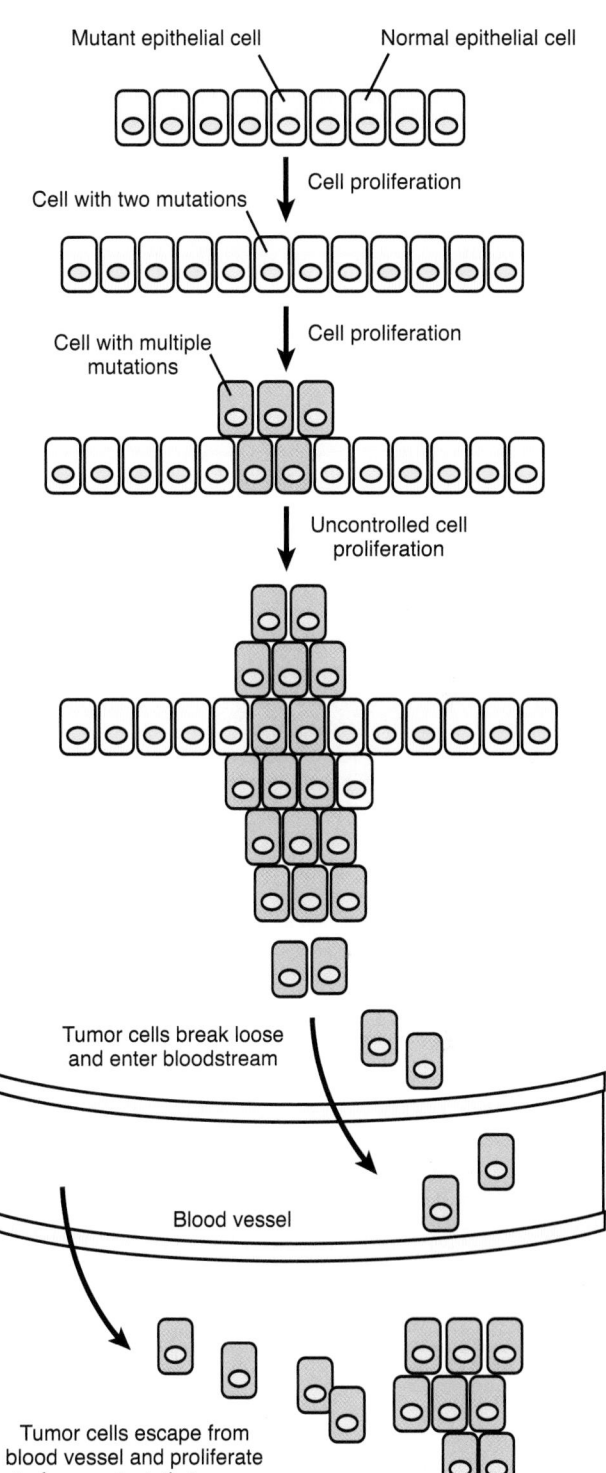

FIG. 15-12. Tumor clonal evolution and metastasis. A tumor develops from mutant cells with multiple genetic mutations. Through repeated alterations in the genome, mutant epithelial cells are able to develop into a cluster of cells (called a *tumor clone*) that proliferates in an uncontrollable fashion. Further changes in the tumor cells can transform the tumor cells into a population of cells that can enter the blood vessels and repopulate in a new location.

tissues, and hence travel to distant sites where they form new colonies. This spreading process of tumor cells, called *metastasis*, is the cause of 90% of human cancer deaths. Metastatic cancer cells that enter the bloodstream can reach virtually all tissues of the body. Bones are one of the most common places for these cells to settle and start growing again. Bone metastasis is one of the most frequent causes of pain in people with cancer. It also can cause bones to break and create other symptoms and problems for patients.

The progression in the knowledge of cancer biology has been accelerating in recent years. All of the scientific knowledge acquired through hard work and discovery has made it possible for cancer treatment and prevention. As a result of explosive new discoveries, some modern treatments were developed. The success of these therapies, together with traditional treatments such as surgical procedures, is further underscored by the fact that in 2002 the cancer rate was reduced in the United States. Current approaches to the treatment of cancer involve killing cancer cells with toxic chemicals, radiation, or surgery. Alternatively, several new biologic- and gene-based therapies are aimed at enhancing the body's natural defenses against invading cancers. Understanding the biology of cancer cells has led to the development of designer therapies for cancer prevention and treatment. Gene therapy, immune system modulation, genetically engineered antibodies, and molecularly designed chemical drugs are all promising fronts in the war against cancer.

Immunotherapy

The growth of the body is controlled by many natural signals through complex signaling pathways. Some of these natural agents have been used in cancer treatment and have been proven effective for fighting several cancers through the clinical trial process. These naturally occurring biologic agents, such as interferons, interleukins, and other cytokines, can now be produced in the laboratory. These agents, as well as the synthetic agents that mimic the natural signals, are given to patients to influence the natural immune response agents either by directly altering the cancer cell growth, or by acting indirectly to help healthy cells control the cancer. One of the most exciting applications of immunotherapy has come from the identification of certain tumor targets called *antigens* and the aiming of an antibody at these targets. This was first used as a means of localizing tumors in the body for diagnosis, and was more recently used to attack cancer cells. Trastuzumab (Herceptin) is an example of such a drug.[14] Trastuzumab is a monoclonal antibody that neutralizes the mitogenic activity of cell-surface growth factor receptor HER-2. Approximately 25% of breast cancers overexpress HER-2. These tumors tend to grow faster and generally are more likely to recur than tumors that do not overproduce HER-2. Trastuzumab is designed to attack cancer cells that overexpress HER-2. Trastuzumab slows or stops the growth of these cells and increases the survival of HER-2–positive breast cancer patients. Another significant example is the administration of interleukin-2 (IL-2) to patients with metastatic melanoma or kidney cancer, which has been shown to mediate the durable regression of metastatic cancer. IL-2, a cytokine produced by human helper T lymphocytes, has a wide range of immune regulatory effects, includ-

ing the expansion of lymphocytes following activation by a specific antigen. IL-2 has no direct impact on cancer cells. The impact of IL-2 on cancers in vivo derives from its ability to expand lymphocytes with antitumor activity. The expanded lymphocytes somehow recognize the antigen on cancer cells. Thus, the molecular identification of cancer antigens has opened new possibilities for the development of effective immunotherapies for patients with cancer. Clinical studies using immunization with peptides derived from cancer antigens have shown that high levels of lymphocytes with antitumor activity can be produced in cancer-bearing patients. Highly avid antitumor lymphocytes can be isolated from immunized patients and grown in vitro for use in cell-transfer therapies.

Chemotherapy

The primary function of anticancer chemicals is to block different steps involved in cell growth and replication. These chemicals often block a critical chemical reaction in a signal transduction pathway or during DNA replication or gene expression. For example, STI571, also known as *Gleevec*, is one of the first molecularly targeted drugs based on the changes that cancer causes in cells.[15] STI571 offers promise for the treatment of chronic myeloid leukemia (CML) and may soon surpass interferon-γ as the standard treatment for the disease. In CML, STI571 is targeted at the Bcr-Abl kinase, an activated oncogene product in CML (Fig. 15-13). Bcr-Abl is an overly activated protein kinase resulting from a specific genetic abnormality generated by chromosomal translocation that is found in the cells of patients with CML. STI571-mediated inhibition of Bcr-Abl-kinase activity not only prevents cell growth of Bcr-Abl–transformed leukemic cells, but also induces apoptosis. Clinically, the drug quickly corrects the blood cell abnormalities caused by the leukemia in a majority of patients, achieving a complete disappearance of the leukemic blood cells and the return of normal blood cells. Additionally, the drug appears to have some effect on other cancers including certain brain tumors and GI stromal tumors, a very rare type of stomach cancer.

Gene Therapy

Gene therapy is an experimental treatment that involves genetically altering a patient's own tumor cells or lymphocytes (cells of the immune system, some of which can attack cancer cells). For years, the concept of gene therapy has held promise as a new, potentially potent weapon to attack cancer. Although a rapid progression in the understanding of the molecular and clinical aspects of gene therapy has been witnessed in the past decade, gene therapy treatment has not yet been shown to be superior to standard treatments in humans.

Several problems must be resolved to transform it into a clinically relevant form of therapy. The major issues that limit its translation to the clinic are improving the selectivity of tumor targeting, im-

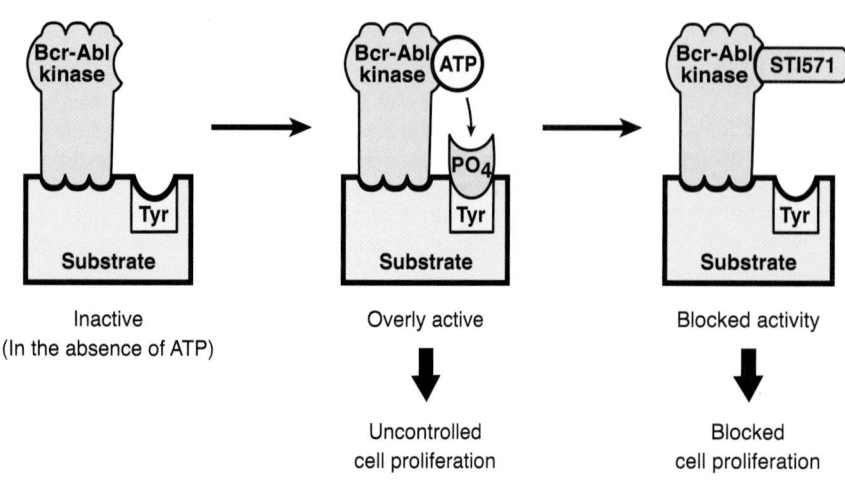

FIG. 15-13. Mechanism of STI571 as a molecular drug. Bcr-Abl is an overly activated oncogene product resulting from a specific genetic abnormality generated by chromosomal translocation that is found in cells of patients with chronic myeloid leukemia. Bcr-Abl is an activated protein kinase and thus requires adenosine triphosphate (ATP) to phosphorylate substrates, which in turn promote cell proliferation. STI571 is a small molecule that competes with the ATP-binding site and thus blocks the transfer of phosphoryl group to substrate. PO_4 = phosphate; Tyr = tyrosine.

proving the delivery to the tumor, and the enhancement of the transduction rate of the cells of interest. In most gene therapy trials for malignant diseases, tumors can be accessed and directly injected (in situ gene therapy). The in situ gene therapy also offers a better distribution of the vector virus throughout the tumor. Finally, a combination of gene therapy strategies will be more effective than the use of a single gene therapy system. An important aspect of effective gene therapy involves the choice of appropriate genes for manipulation. Genes that promote the production of messenger chemicals or other immune-active substances can be transferred into the patient's cells. These include genes that inhibit cell cycle progression, induce apoptosis, enhance host immunity against cancer cells, block the ability of cancer cells to metastasize, and cause tumor cells to undergo suicide. Recent development of RNAi technology, which uses a loss-of-function approach to block gene functions, ensures a new wave of hopes for gene therapy. Nonetheless, gene therapy is still experimental and is being studied in clinical trials for many different types of cancer. The mapping of genes responsible for human cancer is likely to provide new targets for gene therapy in the future. The preliminary results of gene therapy for cancer are encouraging, and as advancements are made in the understanding of the molecular biology of human cancer, the future of this rapidly developing field holds great potential for treating cancer.

It is noteworthy that the use of multiple therapeutic methods has proven more powerful than a single method. The use of chemotherapy after surgery to destroy the few remaining cancerous cells in the body is called *adjuvant* therapy. Adjuvant therapy was first tested and found to be effective in breast cancer. It was later adopted for use in other cancers. A major discovery in chemotherapy is the advantage of multiple chemotherapeutic agents (known as *combination* or *cocktail chemotherapy*) over single agents. Some types of fast-growing leukemias and lymphomas (tumors involving the cells of the bone marrow and lymph nodes) responded extremely well to combination chemotherapy, and clinical trials led to gradual improvement of the drug combinations used. Many of these tumors can be cured today by combination chemotherapy. As cancer cells carry multiple genetic defects, the use of combination chemotherapy, immunotherapy, and gene therapies may be more effective in treating cancers.

Stem Cell Research

Stem cell biology represents a cutting-edge scientific research field with potential clinical applications.[16] It may have an enormous impact on human health by offering hope for curing human diseases such as diabetes mellitus, Parkinson's disease, neurologic degeneration, and congenital heart disease. Stem cells are endowed with two remarkable properties (Fig. 15-14). First, stem cells can proliferate in an undifferentiated but pluripotent state, and as a result can self-

renew. Second, they have the ability to differentiate into many specialized cell types. There are two groups of stem cells: embryonic stem (ES) cells and adult stem cells. Human ES cells are derived from early preimplantation embryos called *blastocysts* (5 days postfertilization), and are capable of generating all differentiated cell types in the body. Adult stem cells are present in and can be isolated from adult tissues. They often are tissue specific and only can generate the cell types comprising a particular tissue in the body; however, in some cases they can transdifferentiate into cell types found in other tissues. Hematopoietic stem cells are adult stem cells. They reside in bone marrow and are capable of generating all cell types of the blood and immune system.

Stem cells can be grown in culture and be induced to differentiate into a particular cell type, either in vitro or in vivo. With the recent and continually increasing improvement in culturing stem cells, scientists are beginning to understand the molecular mechanisms of stem cell self-renewal and differentiation in response to environmental cues. It is believed that discovery of the signals that control self-renewal vs. differentiation will be extremely important for the therapeutic use of stem cells in treating disease. It is possible that success in the study of the changes in signal transduction pathways in stem cells will lead to the development of therapies to specifically differentiate stem cells into a particular cell type to replace diseased or damaged cells in the body. Recently, stem cell research has been transformed by the discovery from the Shinya Yamanaka group and the James Thomsen group, who have found that a simple genetic manipulation can reprogram adult differentiated cells into pluripotent cells.[17] This exciting discovery not only bypasses the ethical issues of using early embryos to generate ES cells, but also ensures a potentially limitless source of patient-specific stem cells for tissue engineering and transplantation medicine.

Personalized Genomic Medicine

Genes determine our susceptibility to diseases and direct our body's response to medicine. Because an individual's genes differ from those of another, the determination of each individual's genome has the potential to improve the predication, prevention, and treatment of disease. Sequencing of individual genomes holds the key to realize this revolution called *personalized genomic medicine*. Next generation sequencing such as 454 Life Sciences technology is promising to reduce the time and cost so that genome sequencing can be affordable in the health care system. The goal of personalized genomic medicine is to spot the gene variations in each individual and to attack the disease by choosing personalized treatments that work with the individual's genomic profile. Personalized genomic medicine will undoubtedly revolutionize the practice of modern medicine.

TECHNOLOGIES OF MOLECULAR AND CELL BIOLOGY

DNA Cloning

Since the advent of recombinant DNA technology three decades ago, hundreds of thousands of genes have been identified. Recombinant DNA technology is the technology that uses advanced enzymatic and microbiologic techniques to manipulate DNA.[18] Pure pieces of any DNA can be inserted into bacteriophage DNA or other carrier DNA such as plasmids to produce recombinant DNA in bacteria. In this way, DNA can be reconstructed, amplified, and used to manipulate the functions of individual cells or even organisms. This technology, often referred to as *DNA cloning*, is the basis of all other DNA analysis methods. It is only with the awesome power of recombinant DNA technology that the completion of the Human Genome Project was possible. It also has led to the identification of the entire gene complements of organisms such as viruses, bacteria, worms, flies, and plants.

Molecular cloning refers to the process of cloning a DNA fragment of interest into a DNA vector that ultimately is delivered

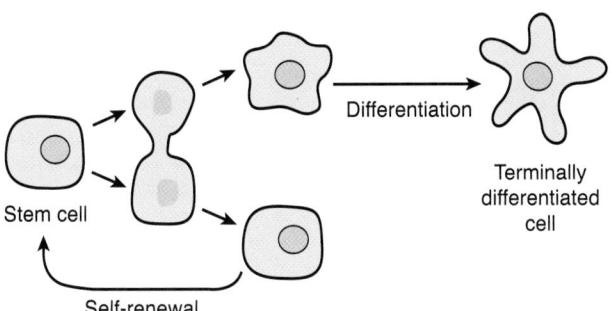

FIG. 15-14. Stem cells. A stem cell is capable of self-renewal (unlimited cell cycle) and differentiation (becoming nondividing cells with specialized functions). Differentiating stem cells often undergo additional cell divisions before they become fully mature cells that carry out specific tissue functions.

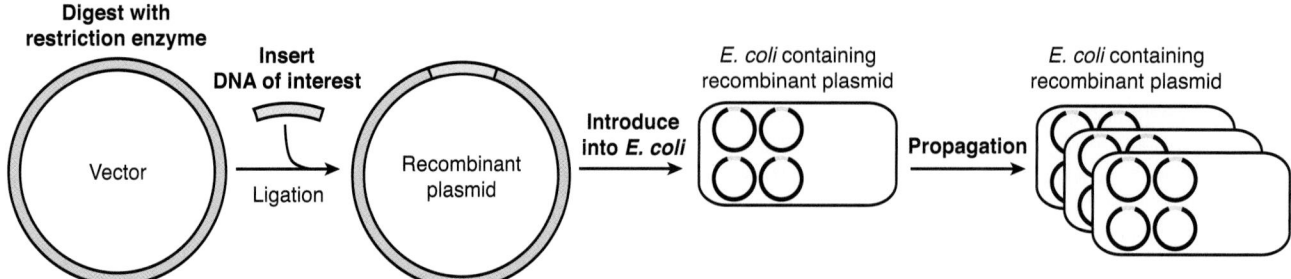

FIG. 15-15. Generation of recombinant DNA. The vector is a circular DNA molecule that is capable of replicating in *Escherichia coli* cells. Insert DNA (often your favorite gene) is ligated to the vector after ends of both DNA are properly treated with restriction enzymes. Ligated DNA (i.e., the recombinant plasmid DNA) is then transformed into *E. coli* cells, where it replicates to produce recombinant progenies. *E. coli* cells carrying the recombinant plasmid can be propagated to yield large quantities of plasmid DNA.

into bacterial or mammalian cells or tissues[19,20] (Fig. 15-15). This represents a very basic technique that is widely used in almost all areas of biomedical research. DNA vectors often are called *plasmids*, which are extrachromosomal molecules of DNA that vary in size and can replicate and be transmitted from bacterial cell to cell. Plasmids can be propagated either in the cytoplasm, or after insertion, as part of the bacterial chromosome in *Escherichia coli*. The process of molecular cloning involves several steps of manipulation of DNA. First, the vector plasmid DNA is cleaved with a restriction enzyme to create compatible ends with the foreign DNA fragment to be cloned. The vector and the DNA fragment are then joined in vitro by a DNA ligase. Alternatively, DNA cloning can be simply done through the so-called *Gateway Technology* that allows for the rapid and efficient transfer of DNA fragments between different cloning vectors while maintaining reading frame and orientation, without the use of restriction endonucleases and DNA ligase. The technology, which is based on the site-specific recombination system of bacteriophage l, is simple, fast, robust and automatable, thus compatible for high-throughput DNA cloning.

Finally, the ligation product or the Gateway reaction product is introduced into competent host bacteria; this procedure is called *transformation*, which can be done by either calcium/heat shock or electroporation. Precautions must be taken in every step of cloning to generate the desired DNA construct. The vector must be correctly prepared to maximize the creation of recombinants; for example, it must be enzymatically treated to prevent self-ligation. Host bacteria must be made sufficiently competent to permit the entry of recombinant plasmids into cells. The selection of desired recombinant plasmid-bearing *E. coli* normally is achieved by the property of drug resistance conferred by the plasmid vectors. The plasmids encoding markers provide specific resistance to (i.e., the ability to grow in the presence of) antibiotics such as ampicillin, kanamycin, and tetracycline. The foreign component in the plasmid vector can be a mammalian expression cassette, which can direct expression of foreign genes in mammalian cells. The resulting plasmid vector can be amplified in *E. coli* to prepare large quantities of DNA for its subsequent applications such as transfection, gene therapy, transgenics, and knockout mice.

Detection of Nucleic Acids and Proteins
Southern Blot Hybridization

Southern blotting refers to the technique of transferring DNA fragments from an electrophoresis gel to a membrane support, and the subsequent analysis of the fragments by hybridization with a radioactively labeled probe (Fig. 15-16).[21] Southern blotting is named after E. M. Southern, who in 1975 first described the technique of DNA analysis. It enables reliable and efficient analysis of size-fractionated DNA fragments in an immobilized membrane support. Southern blotting is composed of several steps. It normally begins with the digestion of the DNA samples with appropriate restriction enzymes

and the separation of DNA samples in an agarose gel with appropriate DNA size markers. The DNA gel is stained with ethidium bromide and photographed with a ruler laid alongside the gel so that band positions can later be identified on the membrane. The DNA gel then is treated so the DNA fragments are denatured (i.e., strand separation). The DNA then is transferred onto a nitrocellulose membrane by capillary diffusion or under electricity. After immobiliza-

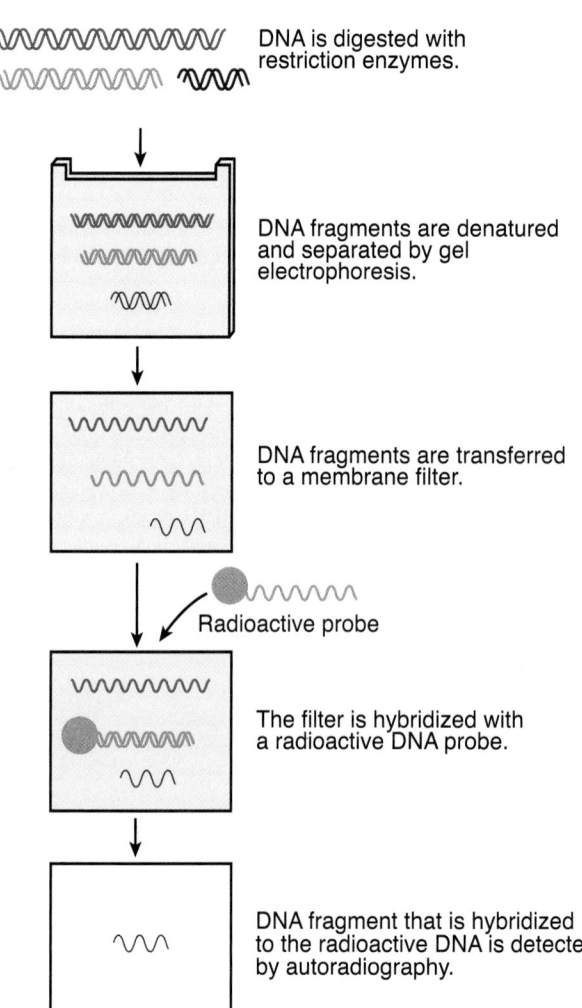

DNA is digested with restriction enzymes.

DNA fragments are denatured and separated by gel electrophoresis.

DNA fragments are transferred to a membrane filter.

Radioactive probe

The filter is hybridized with a radioactive DNA probe.

DNA fragment that is hybridized to the radioactive DNA is detected by autoradiography.

FIG. 15-16. Southern blotting. Restriction enzymatic fragments of DNA are separated by agarose gel electrophoresis, transferred to a membrane filter, and then hybridized to a radioactive probe.

tion, the DNA can be subjected to hybridization analysis, enabling bands with sequence similarity to a radioactively labeled probe to be identified.

The development of Southern transfer and the associated hybridization techniques made it possible for the first time to obtain information about the physical organization of single and multicopy sequences in complex genomes. The later application of Southern blotting hybridization to the study of restriction fragment length polymorphisms opened up new possibilities such as genetic fingerprinting and prenatal diagnosis of genetic diseases.

Northern Blot Hybridization

Northern blotting refers to the technique of size fractionation of RNA in a gel and the transferring of an RNA sample to a solid support (membrane) in such a manner that the relative positions of the RNA molecules are maintained. The resulting membrane then is hybridized with a labeled probe complementary to the mRNA of interest. Signals generated from detection of the membrane can be used to determine the size and abundance of the target RNA. In principle, Northern blot hybridization is similar to Southern blot hybridization (and hence its name), with the exception that RNA, not DNA, is on the membrane. Although reverse-transcriptase polymerase chain reaction has been used in many applications (described in Polymerase Chain Reaction below), Northern analysis is the only method that provides information regarding mRNA size and has remained a standard method for detection and quantitation of mRNA. The process of Northern hybridization involves several steps, as does Southern hybridization, including electrophoresis of RNA samples in an agarose-formaldehyde gel, transfer to a membrane support, and hybridization to a radioactively labeled DNA probe. Data from hybridization allow quantification of steady-state mRNA levels, and at the same time, provide information related to the presence, size, and integrity of discrete mRNA species. Thus, Northern blot analysis, also termed *RNA gel blot analysis*, commonly is used in molecular biology studies relating to gene expression.

Polymerase Chain Reaction

PCR is an in vitro method for the polymerase-directed amplification of specific DNA sequences using two oligonucleotide primers that hybridize to opposite strands and flank the region of interest in the target DNA (Fig. 15-17).[22] One cycle of PCR reaction involves template denaturation, primer annealing, and the extension of the annealed primers by DNA polymerase. Because the primer extension products synthesized in one cycle can serve as a template in the next, the number of target DNA copies nearly doubles at each cycle. Thus, a repeated series of cycles result in the exponential accumulation of a specific fragment in which the termini are sharply defined by the 5' ends of the primers. The introduction of the thermostable DNA polymerase (e.g., Taq polymerase) transforms the PCR into a simple and robust reaction. The reaction components (e.g., template, primers, Taq polymerase, 2'-deoxynucleoside 5'-triphosphates, and buffer) could all be assembled and the amplification reaction carried out by simply cycling the temperatures within the reaction tube. The specificity and yield in amplifying a particular DNA fragment by PCR reaction is affected by the proper setting of the reaction parameters (e.g., enzyme, primer, and Mg^{2+} concentration, as well as the temperature cycling profile). Modifying various PCR parameters to optimize the specificity of amplification yields more homogenous products, even in rare template reactions.

The emergence of the PCR technique has dramatically altered the approach to both fundamental and applied biologic problems. The capability of amplifying a specific DNA fragment from a gene or the whole genome greatly advances the study of the gene and its function. It is simple, yet robust, speedy, and most of all, flexible. As a recombinant DNA tool, it underlies almost all of molecular biology. This revolutionary technique enabled the modern methods for the isolation of genes, construction of a DNA vector, introduction of alterations into DNA, and quantitation of gene expression, making it a fundamental cornerstone of genetic and molecular analysis.

Immunoblotting and Immunoprecipitation

Analyses of proteins are primarily carried out by antibody-directed immunologic techniques. For example, Western blotting, also called *immunoblotting*, is performed to detect protein levels in a population of cells or tissues, whereas immunoprecipitation is used to concentrate proteins from a larger pool. Using specific antibodies, microscopic analysis called *immunofluorescence* and *immunohistochemistry* is possible for the subcellular localization and expression of proteins in cells or tissues, respectively.

Immunoblotting refers to the process of identifying a protein from a mixture of proteins (Fig. 15-18). It consists of five steps: (a) sample preparation; (b) electrophoresis (separation of a protein mixture by sodium dodecyl sulfate-polyacrylamide gel electrophoresis); (c) transfer (the electrophoretic transfer of proteins from gel onto membrane support, (e.g., nitrocellulose, nylon, or polyvinylidene difluoride); (d) staining (the subsequent immunodetection of target proteins with specific antibody); and (e) development (colorimetric or chemiluminescent visualization of the antibody-recognized protein). Thus, immunoblotting combines the resolution of gel electrophoresis with the specificity of immunochemical detection. Immunoblotting is a powerful tool used to determine a number of important characteristics of proteins. For example, immunoblotting analysis will determine the presence and the quantity of a protein in a given cellular condition and its relative molecular weight. Immunoblotting also can be used to determine whether posttranslational modification such as phosphorylation has occurred on a protein. Importantly, through immunoblotting analysis, a comparison of the protein levels and modification states in normal vs. diseased tissues is possible.

Immunoprecipitation, another widely used immunochemical technique, is a method that uses antibody to enrich a protein of interest and any other proteins that are associated with it (Fig. 15-19). The principle of the technique lies in the property of a strong and specific affinity between antibodies and their antigens to locate and pull down target proteins in solution. Once the antibody-antigen (target protein) complexes are formed in the solution, they are collected and purified using small agarose beads with covalently attached protein A or protein G. Both protein A and protein G specifically interact with the antibodies, thus forming a large immobilized complex of antibody-antigen bound to beads. The purified protein can then be analyzed by a number of biochemical methods. When immunoprecipitation is combined with immunoblotting, it can be used for the sensitive detection of proteins in low concentrations, which would otherwise be difficult to detect. Moreover, combined immunoprecipitation and immunoblotting analysis is very efficient in analyzing the protein-protein interactions or determining the posttranslational modifications of proteins. In addition, immunoprecipitated proteins can be used as preparative steps for assays such as intrinsic or associated enzymatic activities. The success of immunoprecipitation is influenced by two major factors: (a) the abundance of the protein in the original preparation and (b) the specificity and affinity of the antibody for this protein.

DNA Microarray

Now that the human genome sequence is completed, the primary focus of biologists is rapidly shifting toward gaining an understanding of how genes function. One of the interesting findings about the human genome is that there are only approximately 25,000 to 30,000 protein-encoding genes. However, it is known that genes and their products function in a complicated and yet orchestrated fashion and that the surprisingly small number of genes from the genome sequence is sufficient to make a human being. Nonetheless, with the tens of thousands of genes present in the genome, traditional methods in molecular biology, which generally work on a one-gene-in-one-experiment basis, cannot generate the whole picture of ge-

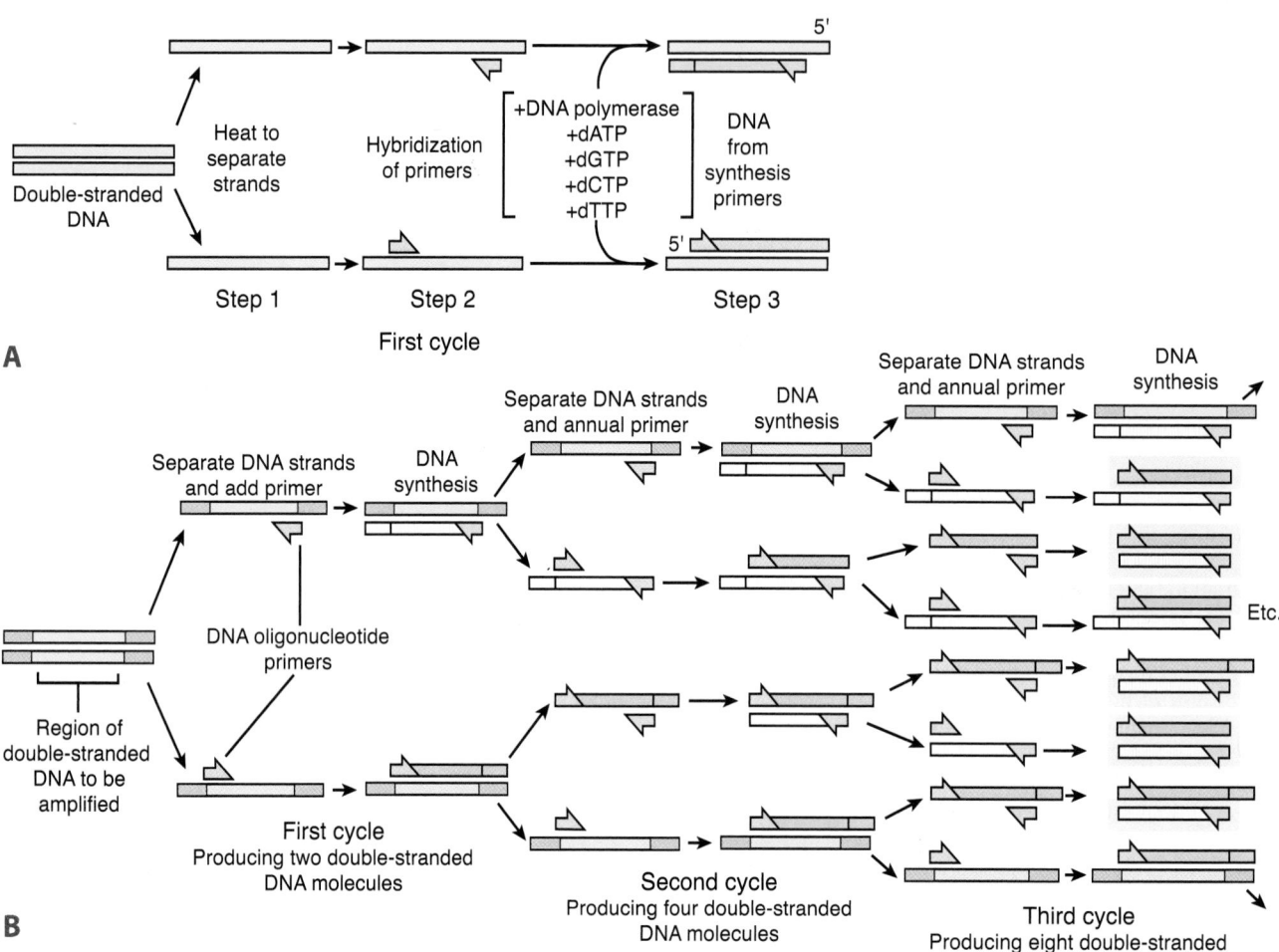

FIG. 15-17. Amplification of DNA using the polymerase chain reaction technique. Knowledge of the DNA sequence to be amplified is used to design two synthetic DNA oligonucleotides, each complementary to the sequence on one strand of the DNA double helix at opposite ends of the region to be amplified. These oligonucleotides serve as primers for in vitro DNA synthesis, which is performed by a DNA polymerase, and they determine the segment of the DNA that is amplified. **A.** PCR starts with a double-stranded DNA, and each cycle of the reaction begins with a brief heat treatment to separate the two strands (*Step 1*). After strand separation, cooling of the DNA in the presence of a large excess of the two primer DNA oligonucleotides allows these primers to hybridize to complementary sequences in the two DNA strands (*Step 2*). This mixture is then incubated with DNA polymerase and the four deoxyribonucleoside triphosphates so that DNA is synthesized, starting from the two primers (*Step 3*). The entire cycle is then begun again by a heat treatment to separate the newly synthesized DNA strands. **B.** As the procedure is performed over and over again, the newly synthesized fragments serve as templates in their turn, and, within a few cycles, the predominant DNA is identical to the sequence bracketed by and including the two primers in the original template. Of the DNA put into the original reaction, only the sequence bracketed by the two primers is amplified because there are no primers attached anywhere else. In the example illustrated in **B**, three cycles of reaction produce 16 DNA chains, eight of which (*boxed in brown*) are the same length as and correspond exactly to one or the other strand of the original bracketed sequence shown at the far left; the other strands contain extra DNA downstream of the original sequence, which is replicated in the first few cycles. After three more cycles, 240 of the 256 DNA chains correspond exactly to the original bracketed sequence, and after several more cycles, essentially all of the DNA strands have this unique length. (*From Alberts et al,[1] with permission.*)

nome function. In the past several years, a new technology called *DNA microarray* has attracted tremendous interest among biologists as well as clinicians. This technology promises to monitor the whole genome on a single chip so researchers can have a better picture of the interactions among thousands of genes simultaneously.

DNA microarray, also called *gene chip*, *DNA chip*, and *gene array*, refers to large sets of probes of known sequences orderly arranged on a small chip, enabling many hybridization reactions to be carried out in parallel in a small device (Fig. 15-20).[23] Like Southern and Northern hybridization, the underlying principle of this technology is the remarkable ability of nucleic acids to form a duplex between two strands with complementary base sequences. DNA microarray provides a medium for matching known and unknown DNA samples based on base-pairing rules, and automating the process of

identifying the unknowns. Microarrays require specialized robotics and imaging equipment that spot the samples on a glass or nylon substrate, carry out the hybridization, and analyze the data generated. DNA microarrays containing different sets of genes from a variety of organisms are now commercially available, allowing biologists to simply purchase the chips and perform hybridization and data collection. The massive scale of microarray experiments requires the aid of computers. They are used during the capturing of the image of the hybridized target, the conversion of the image into usable measures of the extent of hybridization, and the interpretation of the extent of hybridization into a meaningful measure of the amount of the complementary sequence in the target. Some data-analysis packages are available commercially or can be found in the core facility of certain institutions.

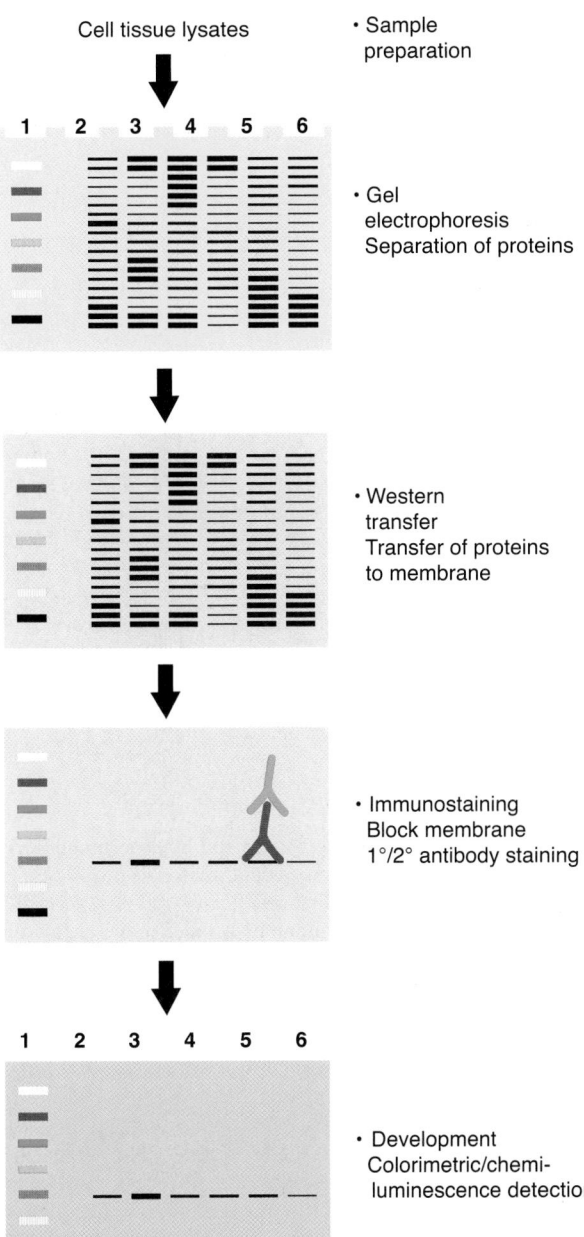

Cell tissue lysates

- Sample preparation

- Gel electrophoresis Separation of proteins

- Western transfer Transfer of proteins to membrane

- Immunostaining Block membrane 1°/2° antibody staining

- Development Colorimetric/chemiluminescence detection

FIG. 15-18. Immunoblotting. Proteins are prepared from cells or tissues, separated according to size by sodium dodecyl sulfatepolyacrylamide gel electrophoresis, and transferred to a membrane filter. Detection of a protein of interest can be done by sequential incubation with a primary antibody directed against the protein, and then with an enzyme-conjugated secondary antibody that recognizes the primary antibody. Visualization of the protein is carried out by using colorimetric or luminescent substrates for the conjugated enzyme.

DNA microarray technology has produced many significant results in quite different areas of application. There are two major application forms for the technology: identification of sequence (gene/gene mutation) and determination of expression level (abundance) of genes. For example, analysis of genomic DNA detects amplifications and deletions found in human tumors. Differential gene expression analysis also has uncovered networks of genes differentially present in cancers that cannot be distinguished by conventional means. Significantly, recent advancements in next generation sequencing (e.g., Solexa and 454 technology) have dem-

onstrated the precision and speed to analyze gene expression in any genome.

Cell Manipulations
Cell Culture

Cell culture has become one of the most powerful techniques, as cultured cells are being used in a diversity of biologic fields ranging from biochemistry to molecular and cellular biology.[24] Through their ability to be maintained in vitro, cells can be manipulated by the introduction of genes of interest (cell transfection) and be transferred into in vivo biologic receivers (cell transplantation) to study the biologic effect of the interested genes (Fig. 15-21). In general, cell culture procedures are simple and straightforward. In the laboratory, cells are cultured either as a monolayer (in which cells grow as one layer on culture dishes) or in suspension.

It is important to know the wealth of information concerning cell culturing before attempting the procedure. For example, conditions of culture will depend on the cell types to be cultured (e.g., origins of the cells such as epithelial or fibroblasts, or primary vs. immortalized/transformed cells). It also is necessary to use special culture medium that has been used to establish the cell line (if it is a cell line), including the type and concentration of serum used to maintain the growth of cells in vitro. If primary cells are derived from human patients or animals, some commercial resources have a variety of culture media available for testing. Generally, cells are manipulated in a sterile hood and the working surfaces are wiped with 80% ethyl alcohol solution. Cultured cells are maintained in a humidified carbon dioxide incubator at 37°C (98.6°F), and need to be examined daily under an inverted microscope to check for possible contamination and confluency (the area cells occupy on the dish). As a general rule, cells should be fed with fresh medium every 2 to 3 days and split when they reach confluency. Depending upon the growth rate of cells, the actual time and number of plates required to split cells in two varies from cell line to cell line. Splitting a monolayer requires the detachment of cells from plates by using a trypsin treatment, of which concentration and time period vary depending on cell lines. If cultured cells grow continuously in suspension, they are split or subcultured by dilution.

Because cell lines may change their properties when cultured, it is not possible to maintain cell lines in culture indefinitely. Therefore, it is essential to store cells at various time passages for future use. The common procedure is to use cryopreservation. The solution for cryopreservation is fetal calf serum containing 10% dimethyl sulfoxide or glycerol, stored in liquid nitrogen [−196°C (−320.8°F)]. Cells can be stored for many years using this method.

Cell Transfection

Cells are cultured for two reasons: to maintain and to manipulate them (see Fig. 15-21). The transfer of foreign macromolecules, such as nucleic acid, into living cells provides an efficient method for studying a variety of cellular processes and functions at the molecular level. DNA transfection has become an important tool for studying the regulation and function of genes. The cDNA to be expressed should be in a plasmid vector, behind an appropriate promoter working in mammalian cells (e.g., the constitutively active cytomegalovirus promoter or inducible promoter). Depending on the cell type, many ways of introducing DNA into mammalian cells have been developed. Commonly used approaches include calcium phosphate, electroporation, liposome-mediated transfection, the nonliposomal formulation, and the use of viral vectors. These methods have shown variable success when attempting to transfect a wide variety of cells. Transfection can be performed in the presence or absence of serum. It is suggested to test the transfection efficiency of cell lines of interest by comparing transfection with several different approaches. For a detailed transfection protocol, it is best to follow the manufacturer's instructions for the particular reagent. General considerations for a successful transfection depend on several parameters, such as the quality and quantity of DNA and cell culture (type of cell and

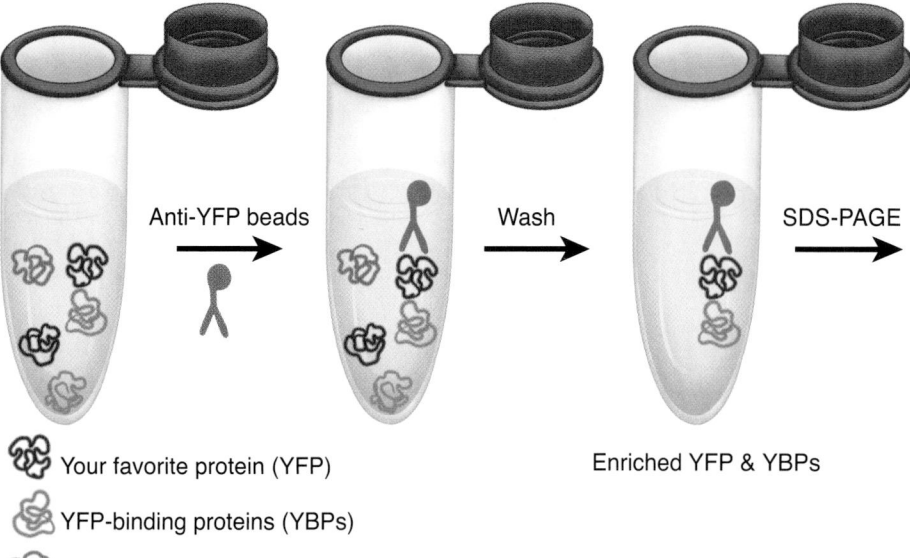

Your favorite protein (YFP)

YFP-binding proteins (YBPs)

Junk proteins

Anti-YFP conjugated to beads

Enriched YFP & YBPs

FIG. 15-19. Immunoprecipitation. Proteins prepared from cells or tissues can be enriched using an antibody directed against them. The antibody is first conjugated to agarose beads and then incubated with protein mixture. Owing to the specific high-affinity interaction between antibody and its antigen (the protein), the antigen-antibody complex can be collected on beads by centrifugation. The immunoprecipitated protein can then be analyzed by immunoblotting. Alternatively, if proteins are radiolabeled in cells or tissues, detection of immunoprecipitated proteins can be achieved by simple sodium dodecyl sulfate-polyacrylamide gel electrophoresis followed by autoradiography.

growth phase). To minimize variations in both of these in transfection experiments, it is best to use cells that are healthy, proliferate well, and are plated at a constant density. After DNA is introduced into the cells, it is normally maintained epitopically in cells and will be diluted while host cells undergo cell division. Therefore, functional assays should be performed 24 to 72 hours after transfection, also termed *transient transfection*. In many applications, it is important to study the long-term effects of DNA in cells by stable transfection. Stable cell clones can be selected for DNA integration into the host cell genome, when plasmids carry an antibiotic-resistant marker. In the presence of antibiotics, only those cells that continuously carry the antibiotic-resistant marker (after generations of cell division) can survive. One application of stable transfection is the generation of transgenic or knockout mouse models, in which the transgene has to be integrated in the mouse genome. Stable cells also can be transplanted into host organs.

Genetic Manipulations

Understanding how genes control the growth and differentiation of the mammalian organism has been the most challenging topic of modern research. It is essential for us to understand how genetic mutations and chemicals lead to the pathologic condition of human bodies. The knowledge and ability to change the genetic program will inevitably make a great impact on society and have far-reaching effects on how we think of ourselves.

The mouse has become firmly established as the primary experimental model for studying how genes control mammalian development. Genetically altered mice are powerful model systems in which to study the function and regulation of genes.[25] The gene function can be studied by creating mutant mice through homologous recombination (gene knockout). A gene of interest also can be introduced into the mouse (transgenic mouse) to study its effect on development or diseases. As mouse models do not precisely represent human biology, genetic manipulations of human somatic or ES cells provide a great means for the understanding of the molecular networks in human cells. In all cases, the gene to be manipulated must first be cloned. Gene cloning has been made easy by recombinant DNA technology and the availability of human and mouse genomes (see the Human Genome section). The following section briefly describes the technologies and the principles behind them.

Transgenic Mice

During the past 20 years, DNA cloning and other techniques have allowed the introduction of new genetic material into the mouse germline. As early as 1980, the first genetic material was successfully introduced into the mouse germline by using pronuclear microinjection of DNA (Fig. 15-22). These animals, called *transgenic*, contain foreign DNA within their genomes. In simple terms, a transgenic mouse is created by the microinjection of DNA into the one-celled mouse embryo, allowing the efficient introduction of cloned genes into the developing mouse somatic tissues, as well as into the germline.

Designs of a Transgene The transgenic technique has proven to be extremely important for basic investigations of gene regulation, creation of animal models of human disease, and genetic engineering of livestock. The design of a transgene construct is a simple task. Like constructs used in cell transfection, a simple transgene construct consists of a protein-encoding gene and a promoter that precedes it. The most common applications for the use of transgenic mice are similar to those in the cell culture system: (a) to study the functions of proteins encoded by the transgene and (b) to analyze the tissue-specific and developmental-stage–specific activity of a gene promoter. Examples of the first application include overexpression of oncogenes, growth factors, hormones, and other key regulatory genes, as well as genes of viral origins. Overexpression of the transgene normally represents gain-of-function mutations. The tissue distribution or expression of a transgene is determined primarily by *cis*-acting promoter enhancer elements within or in the immediate vicinity of the genes themselves. Thus, controlled expression of the transgene can be made possible by using an inducible or tissue-specific promoter. Furthermore, transgenic mice carrying dominant negative mutations of a regulatory gene also have been generated. For example, a truncated growth factor receptor that can bind to the ligand, but loses its catalytic activity when expressed in mice, can block the growth factor binding to the endogenous protein. In this way, the transgenic mice exhibit a loss of function of phenotype, possibly resembling the knockout of the endogenous gene. The second application of the transgenic expression is to analyze the gene promoter of interest. The gene promoter of interest normally is fused to a reporter gene that encodes β-galactosidase (also called *LacZ*),

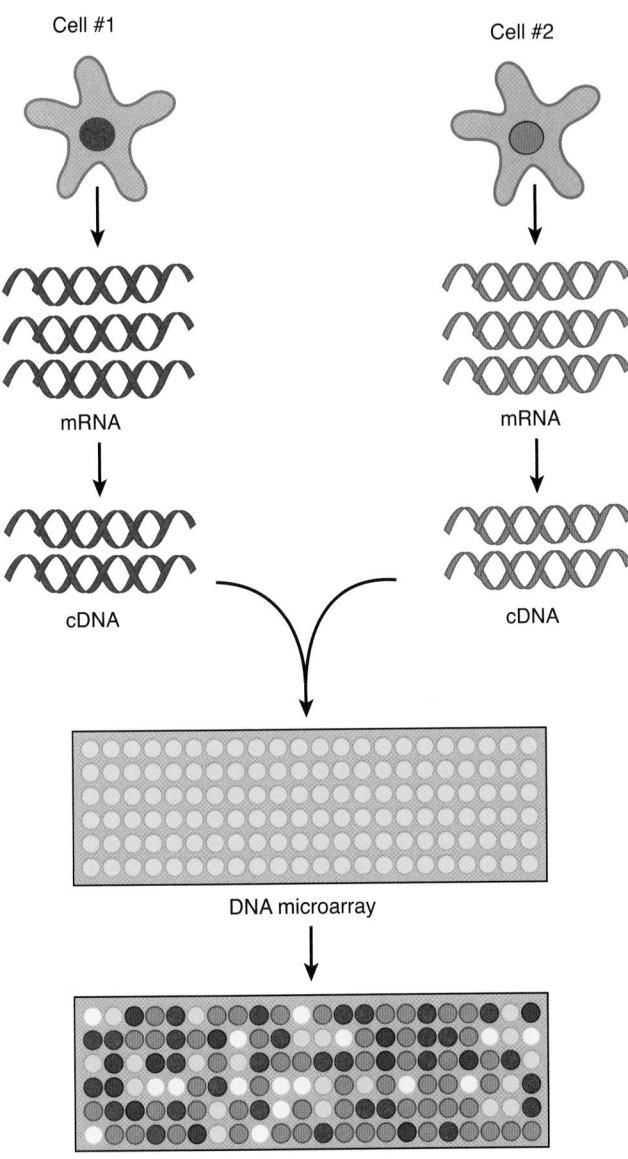

Cell #1
Cell #2

mRNA
mRNA

cDNA
cDNA

DNA microarray

DNA microarray data

FIG. 15-20. DNA microarrays. DNA microarrays, also referred to as *gene chips*, have arrayed oligonucleotides or complementary DNAs (cDNAs) corresponding to tens or hundreds of distinct genes. DNA microarray is used to comparatively analyze gene expression in different cells or tissues. Messenger RNAs (mRNAs) extracted from different sources are converted into cDNAs, which are then labeled with different fluorescent dyes. The two fluorescent cDNA probes are mixed and hybridized to the same DNA microarrays. The ratio of dark brown to light brown fluorescence at each spot on the chip represents the relative expression of levels of that gene between two different cells. In the example shown in the figure, cDNA from cell #1 is labeled with dark brown fluorescence and the cell #2 light brown fluorescence. On the microarray, dark brown spots demonstrate that the gene in cell sample #1 is expressed at a higher level than the corresponding gene in cell sample #2. The light brown spots indicate that the gene in cell sample #1 also is expressed at a higher level than the corresponding gene in cell sample #2. Beige spots represent equal expression of the gene in both cell samples.

luciferase, or green fluorescence protein. Chemical staining of LacZ activity or detection of chemiluminescence/fluorescence can easily visualize the expression of the reporter gene. The amount of the reporter gene activity represents the activity of the promoter, and

thus, reporter activities are tightly correlated to expression of the gene in which the promoter is used to drive the reporter gene expression.

Production of Transgenic Mice The success of generating transgenic mice is largely dependent upon the proper quality and concentration of the DNA supplied for microinjection. For DNA to be microinjected into mouse embryos, it should be linearized by restriction digestion to increase the chance of proper transgene integration. Concentration of DNA should be accurately determined. Mice that develop from injected eggs often are termed *founder* mice.

Genotyping of Transgenic Mice The screening of founder mice and the transgenic lines derived from the founders is accomplished by determining the integration of the injected gene into the genome. This normally is achieved by performing PCR or Southern blot analysis with a small amount of DNA extracted from the mouse tail. Once a given founder mouse is identified to be transgenic, it will be mated to begin establishing a transgenic line.

Analysis of Phenotype of Transgenic Mice Phenotypes of transgenic mice are dictated by both the expression pattern and biologic functions of the transgene. Depending on the promoter and the transgene, phenotypes can be predictable or unpredictable. Elucidation of the functions of the transgene-encoded protein in vitro often offers some clue to what the protein might do in vivo. When a constitutively active promoter is used to drive the expression of transgenes, mice should express the gene in every tissue; however, this mouse model may not allow the identification and study of the earliest events in disease pathogenesis. Ideally, the use of tissue-specific or inducible promoter allows one to determine if the pathogenic protein leads to a reversible or irreversible disease process. For example, rat insulin promoter can target transgene expression exclusively in the β-cells of pancreatic islets. The phenotype of insulin promoter-mediated transgenic mice is projected to affect the function of human β-cells.

Gene Knockout in Mice

The isolation and genetic manipulation of ES cells represents one of the most important milestones for modern genetic technologies. Several unique properties of these ES cells, such as the pluripotency to differentiate into different tissues in an embryo, make them an efficient vehicle for introducing genetic alterations into this species. Thus, this technology provides an important breakthrough, making it possible to genetically manipulate ES cells in a controlled way in the culture dish and then introduce the mutation into the germline (Fig. 15-23). This not only makes mouse genetics a powerful approach for addressing important gene functions but also identifies the mouse as a great system to model human disease.

Targeting Vector The basic concept in building a target vector to knock out a gene is to use two segments of homologous sequence to a gene of interest that flank a part of the gene essential for functions (e.g., the coding region). In the target vector, a positive selectable marker (e.g., the *neo* gene) is placed between the homology arms. Upon the homologous recombination between the arms of the vector and the corresponding genomic regions of the gene of interest in ES cells, the positive selectable marker will replace the essential segment of the target gene, thus creating a null allele. In addition, a negative selectable marker also can be used alone or in combination with the positive selectable marker, but must be placed outside of the homologous arms to enrich for homologous recombination. To create a conditional knockout (i.e., gene knockout in a spatiotemporal fashion), site-specific recombinases such as the popular cre-loxP system are used. If the consensus loxP sequences that are recognized by cre recombinases are properly designed into targeting loci, controlled expression of the recombinase as a transgene can result in the site-specific recombination at the right time and in the right place (i.e., cell type or tissue). This method is markedly useful to prevent developmental compensations and to introduce null mutations in the adult mouse that would otherwise

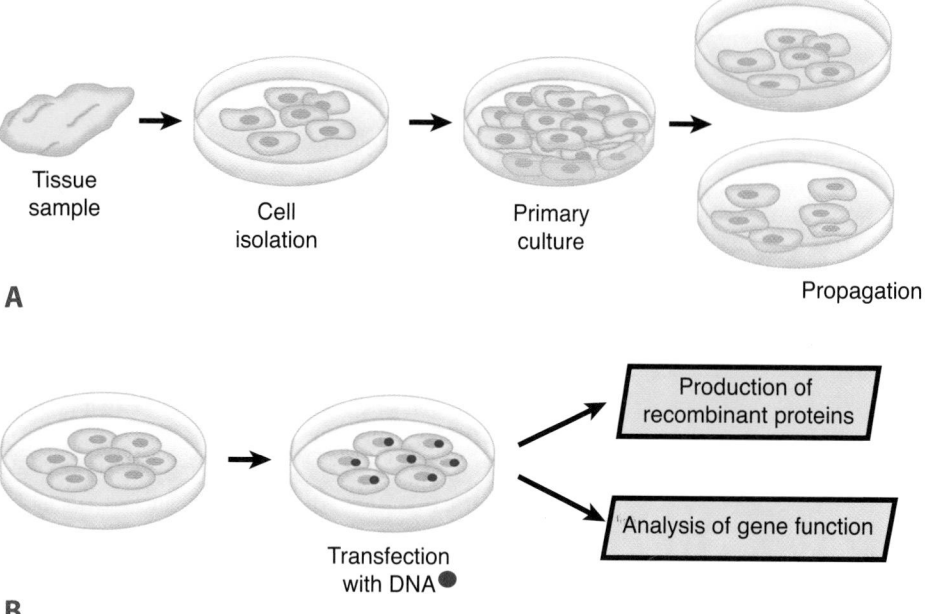

A

B

Transfection
with DNA●

FIG. 15-21. Cell culture and transfection. **A.** Primary cells can be isolated from tissues and cultured in medium for a limited period of time. After genetic manipulations to overcome the cell aging process, primary cells can be immortalized into cell lines for long-term culture. **B.** DNA can be introduced into cells to produce recombinant gene products or to analyze the biologic functions of the gene.

be lethal. Overall, this cre-loxP system allows for spatial and temporal control over transgene expression and takes advantage of inducers with minimal pleiotropic effects.

Introduction of the Targeting Vector into ES Cells ES cell lines can be obtained from other investigators, commercial sources, or established from blastocyst-stage embryos. To maintain ES cells at their full developmental potential, optimal growth conditions should be provided in culture. If culture conditions are inappropriate or inadequate, ES cells may acquire genetic lesions or alter their gene expression patterns, and consequently decrease their pluripotency. Excellent protocols are available in public domains or in mouse facilities in most institutions.

To alter the genome of ES cells, the targeting vector DNA then is transfected into ES cells. Electroporation is the most widely used and the most efficient transfection method for ES cells. Similar procedures for stable cell transfection are used for selecting ES cells that carry the targeting vector. High-quality, targeting-vector DNA free of contaminating chemicals is first linearized and then electroporated into ES cells. Stable ES cells are selected in the presence of a positive selectable antibiotic drug. After a certain period of time and depending on the type of antibiotics, all sensitive cells die and the resistant cells grow into individual colonies of the appropriate size for subcloning by picking. It is extremely important to mini-

mize the time during which ES cells are in culture between selection and injection into blastocysts. Before injecting the ES cells, DNA is prepared from ES colonies to screen for positive ES cells that exhibit the correct integration or homologous recombination of the targeting vector. Positive ES colonies are then expanded and used for creation of chimeras.

Creation of the Chimera A chimeric organism is one in which cells originate from more than one embryo. Here, chimeric mice are denoted as those that contain some tissues from the ES cells with an altered genome. When these ES cells give rise to the lineage of the germ layer, the germ cells carrying the altered genome can be passed on to the offspring, thus creating the germline transmission from ES cells. There are two methods for introducing ES cells into preimplantation-stage embryos: injection and aggregation. The injection of embryonic cells directly into the cavity of blastocysts is one of the fundamental methods for generating chimeras, but aggregation chimeras also have become an important alternative for transmitting the ES cell genome into mice. The mixture of recognizable markers (e.g., coat color) that are specific for the donor mouse and ES cells can be used to identify chimeric mice. However, most experimenters probably use existing mouse core facilities already established in some institutions, or contract a commercial vendor for the creation of a chimera.

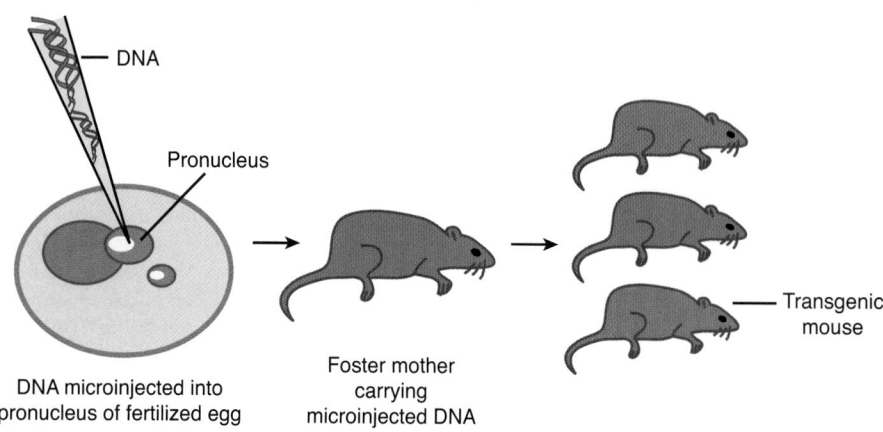

DNA microinjected into
pronucleus of fertilized egg

Foster mother
carrying
microinjected DNA

Transgenic
mouse

FIG. 15-22. Transgenic mouse technology. DNA is microinjected into a pronucleus of a fertilized egg, which is then transplanted into a foster mother. The microinjected egg develops offspring mice. Incorporation of the injected DNA into offspring is indicated by the different coat color of offspring mice.

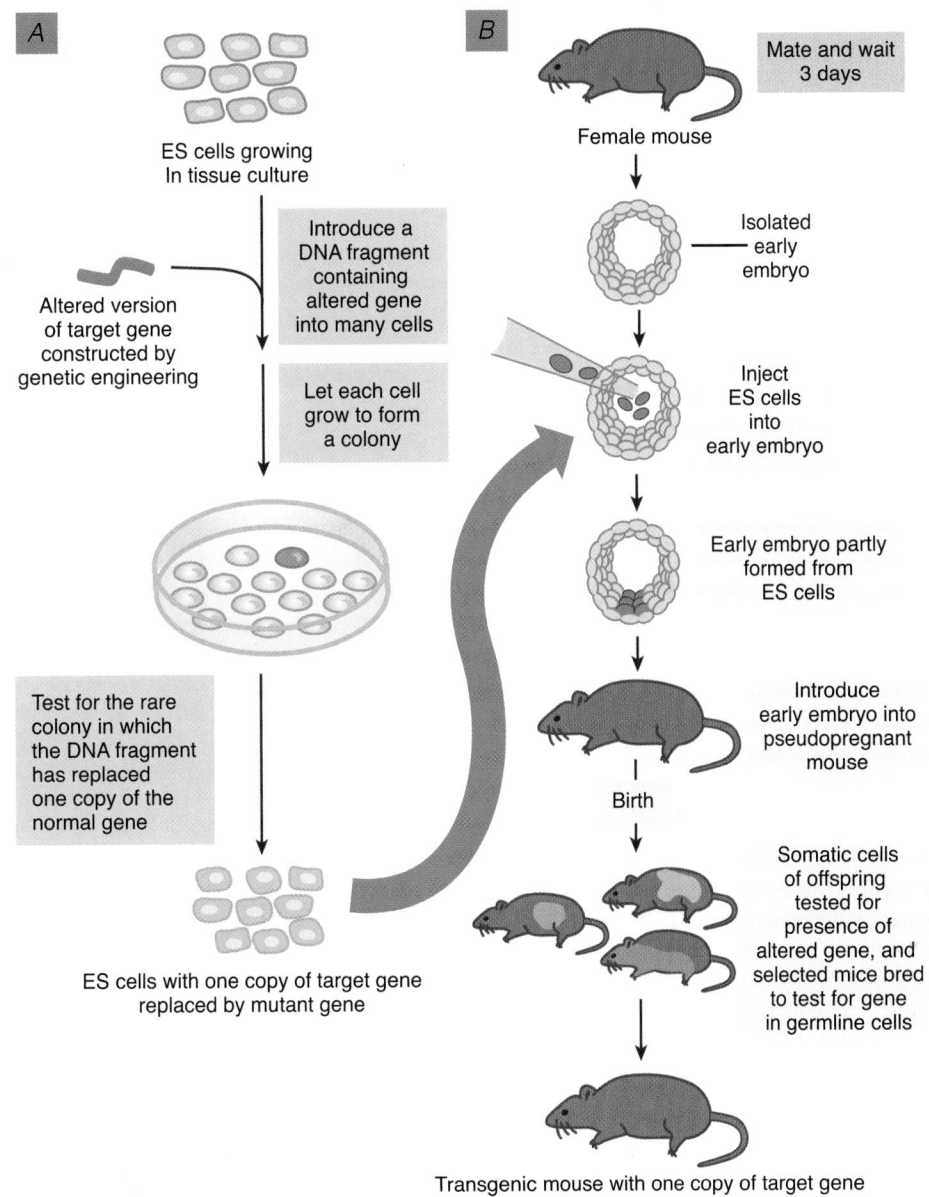

FIG. 15-23. Knockout mouse technology. Summary of the procedures used for making gene replacements in mice. In the first step (**A**), an altered version of the gene is introduced into cultured embryonic stem (ES) cells. Only a few rare ES cells will have their corresponding normal genes replaced by the altered gene through a homologous recombination event. Although the procedure is often laborious, these rare cells can be identified and cultured to produce many descendants, each of which carries an altered gene in place of one of its two normal corresponding genes. In the next step of the procedure (**B**), these altered ES cells are injected into a very early mouse embryo; the cells are incorporated into the growing embryo, and a mouse produced by such an embryo will contain some somatic cells that carry the altered gene. Some of these mice also will contain germline cells that contain the altered gene. When bred with a normal mouse, some of the progeny of these mice will contain the altered gene in all of their cells. If two such mice are in turn bred (not shown), some of the progeny will contain two altered genes (one on each chromosome) in all of their cells. If the original gene alteration completely inactivates the function of the gene, these mice are known as *knockout mice*. When such mice are missing genes that function during development, they often die with specific defects long before they reach adulthood. These defects are carefully analyzed to help decipher the normal function of the missing gene. *(From Alberts et al,[1] with permission.)*

Genotyping and Phenotyping of Knockout Animals The next step is to analyze whether germline transmission of targeted mutation occurs in mice. DNA from a small amount of tissue from offspring of the chimera is extracted and subjected to genomic PCR or Southern blot DNA hybridization. Positive mice (i.e., those with properly integrated targeting vector into the genome) will be used for the propagation of more knockout mice for phenotype analysis. When the knockout genes are crucial for early embryogenesis, mice often die in utero, an occurrence called *embryonic lethality*. When

this happens, only the phenotype of the homozygous (both alleles ablated) knockout mouse embryos and the phenotype of the heterozygous (only one allele ablated) adult mice can be studied. Because most are interested in the phenotype of adult mice, in particular when using mice as disease models, it is recommended to create the conditional knockout using the cre-loxP system so that the gene of interest can be knocked out at will.

To date, more than 5000 genes have been disrupted by homologous recombination and transmitted through the germline. The phenotypic studies of these mice provide ample information on the functions of these genes in growth and differentiation of organisms, and during development of human diseases.

RNA Interference

Although gene ablation in animal models provides an important means to understand the in vivo functions of genes of interest, animal models may not adequately represent human biology. Alternatively, gene targeting can be used to knock out genes in human cells, including human ES cells. A number of recent advances have made gene targeting in somatic cells as easy as in murine ES cells.[25] However, gene targeting (knocking out both alleles) in somatic cells is a time-consuming process.

Development of RNAi technology in the past few years has provided a more promising approach to understanding the biologic functions of human genes in human cells.[26] RNAi is an ancient natural mechanism by which small, double-stranded RNA (dsRNA) acts as a guide for an enzyme complex that destroys complementary RNA and downregulates gene expression in a sequence-specific manner. Although the mechanism by which dsRNA suppresses gene expression is not entirely understood, experimental data provide important insights. In nonmammalian systems such as *Drosophila*, it appears that longer dsRNA is processed into 21–23 nt dsRNA (called *small interfering RNA* or *siRNA*) by an enzyme called *Dicer* containing RNase III motifs. The siRNA apparently then acts as a guide sequence within a multicomponent nuclease complex to target complementary mRNA for degradation. Because long dsRNA induces a potent antiviral response pathway in mammalian cells, short siRNAs are used to perform gene silencing experiments in mammalian cells (Fig. 15-24).

For siRNA studies in mammalian cells, researchers have used two 21-mer RNAs with 19 complementary nucleotides and 3' terminal noncomplementary dimers of thymidine or uridine. The antisense siRNA strand is fully complementary to the mRNA target sequence. Target sequences for an siRNA are identified visually or by software.

The target 19 nucleotides should be compared to an appropriate genome database to eliminate any sequences with significant homology to other genes. Those sequences that appear to be specific to the gene of interest are the potential siRNA target sites. A few of these target sites are selected for siRNA design. The antisense siRNA strand

is the reverse complement of the target sequence. The sense strand of the siRNA is the same sequence as the target mRNA sequence. A deoxythymidine dimer is routinely incorporated at the 3' end of the sense strand siRNA, although it is unknown whether this noncomplementary dinucleotide is important for the activity of siRNAs.

There are two ways to introduce siRNA to knock down gene expression in human cells:

1. RNA transfection: siRNA can be made chemically or using an in vitro transcription method. Like DNA oligos, chemically synthesized siRNA oligos can be commercially ordered. However, synthetic siRNA is expensive and several siRNAs may have to be tried before a particular gene is successfully silenced. In vitro transcription provides a more economic approach. Both short and long RNA can be synthesized using bacteriophage RNA polymerase T7, T3, or SP6. In the case of long dsRNAs, RNase such as recombinant Dicers will be used to process the long dsRNA into a mixture of 21–23 nt siRNA. siRNA oligos or mixtures can be transfected into a few characterized cell lines such as HeLa (human cervical carcinoma) and 293T cells (human kidney carcinoma). Transfection of siRNA directly into primary cells may be difficult.

2. DNA transfection: Expression vectors for expressing siRNA have been made using RNA polymerase III promoters such as U6 and H1. These promoters precisely transcribe a hairpin structure of dsRNA, which will be processed into siRNA in the cell (see Fig. 15-24). Therefore, properly-designed DNA oligos corresponding to the desired siRNA will be inserted downstream of the U6 or H1 promoter. There are two advantages of the siRNA expression vectors over siRNA oligos. First, it is easier to transfect DNA into cells. Second, stable populations of cells can be generated that maintain the long-term silencing of target genes. Furthermore, the siRNA expression cassette can be incorporated into a retroviral or adenoviral vector to provide a wide spectrum of applications in gene therapy.

There has been a fast and fruitful development of RNAi tools for in vitro and in vivo use in mammals. These novel approaches, together with future developments, will be crucial to put RNAi technology to use for effective disease therapy or to exert the awesome power of mammalian genetics. Therefore, the applications of RNAi to

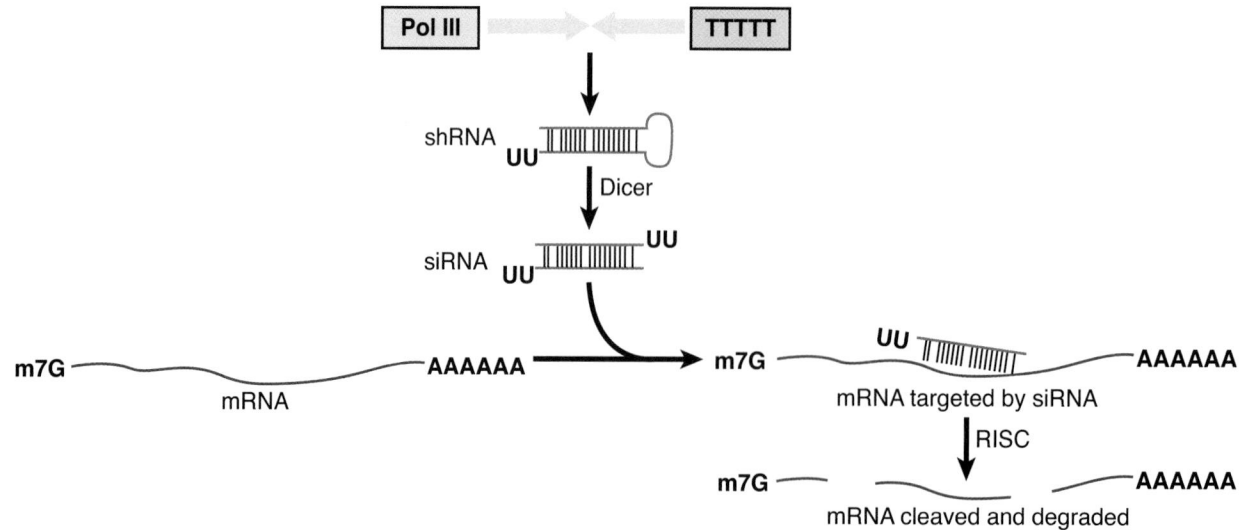

FIG. 15-24. RNA inference in mammalian cells. Small interfering RNA (siRNA) can be produced from a polymerase III–driven expression vector. Such a vector first synthesizes a 19–29 nt double-stranded (ds)RNA stem and a loop (labeled as *shRNA* in the figure), and then the RNase complex called *Dicer* processes the hairpin RNA into a small dsRNA (labeled as *siRNA* in the figure). siRNA can be chemically synthesized and directly introduced into the target cell. In the cell, through RNA-induced silencing complex (RISC), siRNA recognizes and degrades target messenger RNAs (mRNAs).

human health are enormous. siRNA can be applied as a new tool for sequence-specific regulation of gene expression in functional genomics and biomedical studies. With the availability of the human genome sequences, RNAi approaches hold tremendous promise for unleashing the dormant potential of sequenced genomes.

Practical applications of RNAi will possibly result in new therapeutic interventions. In 2002, the concept of using siRNA in battling infectious diseases and carcinogenesis was proven effective. These include notable successes in blocking replication of viruses, such as HIV, hepatitis B virus, and hepatitis C virus, in cultured cells using siRNA targeted at the viral genome or the human gene encoding viral receptors. RNAi has been shown to antagonize the effects of hepatitis C virus in mouse models. In cancers, silencing of oncogenes such as *c-Myc* or *Ras* can slow down the proliferation rate of cancer cells. Finally, siRNA also has potential applications for some dominant genetic disorders.

The twenty-first century, already heralded as the "century of the gene," carries great promise for alleviating suffering from disease and improving human health. On the whole, completion of the human genome blueprint, the promise of gene therapy, and the existence of stem cells has captured the imagination of the public and the biomedical community for good reason. Aside from their potential in curing human diseases, these emerging technologies also have provoked many political, economic, religious, and ethical discussions. As more is discerned about the technologic advances, more attention must also be paid to concerns for their inherent risks and social implications. Surgeons must take the opportunity to collaborate with basic scientists to develop the field of personalized genomic surgery this century.

REFERENCES

Entries highlighted in bright blue are key references.

1. Alberts B, Johnson A, Lewis J, et al: *Molecular Biology of the Cell*, 4th ed. New York: Garland Science, 2002.
2. Watson JD, Crick FH: Molecular structure of nucleic acids; a structure for deoxyribose nucleic acid. *Nature* 171:737, 1953.
3. Mendel G: Versuche über Planzen-Hybriden. *Verhandlungen des naturforschenden Vereines, Abhandlungen.* Brünn: 4, 3, 1866.
4. Carey M, Smale ST: *Transcriptional Regulation in Eukaryotes.* New York: Cold Spring Harbor Laboratory Press, 2000.
5. Wolfsberg TG, Wetterstrand KA, Guyer MS, et al: A user's guide to the human genome. *Nature Genetics* Supplement, 2002. (Also see the Nature website: *http://www.nature.com/nature/supplements/collections/humangenome/.*)
6. U.S. Department of Energy: Genomics and its impact on science and society: The human genome project and beyond. Published online by Human Genome Management Information System (HGMIS): *http://www.ornl.gov/hgmis/publicat/primer*, March 2003.
7. Simpson RJ: *Protein and Proteomics.* New York: Cold Spring Harbor Laboratory Press, 2003.
8. Hanash S: Disease proteomics. *Nature* 422:226, 2003.
9. Ptashne M, Gann A: *Genes & Signals.* New York: Cold Spring Harbor Laboratory Press, 2002.
10. Pawson T, Nash P: Assembly of cell regulatory systems through protein interaction domains. *Science* 300:445, 2003.
11. Lizcano JM, Alessi DR: The insulin signalling pathway. *Curr Biol* 12:R236, 2002.
12. Feng XH, Derynck R: Specificity and versatility in TGF-beta signaling through Smads. *Annu Rev Cell Dev Biol* 21:659, 2005.
13. Hanahan D, Weinberg RA: The hallmarks of cancer. *Cell* 100:57, 2000.
14. McNeil C: Heceptin raises its sights beyond advanced breast cancer. *J Natl Cancer Inst* 90:882, 1998.
15. Druker BJ, Tamura S, Buchdunger E, et al: Effects of a selective inhibitor of the Abl tyrosine kinase on the growth of Bcr-Abl positive cells. *Nat Med* 2:561, 1996.
16. Kiessling AA, Anderson SC: *Human Embryonic Stem Cells: An Introduction to the Science and Therapeutic Potential.* Boston: Jones & Bartlett Pub, 2003.
17. Vogel G: Breakthrough of the year: Reprogramming cells. *Science* 322:1766, 2008.
18. Cohen SN, Chang AC, Boyer HW, et al: Construction of biologically functional bacterial plasmids in vitro. *Proc Natl Acad Sci U S A* 70:3240, 1973.
19. Sambrook J: *Molecular Cloning, A Laboratory Manual*, 3rd ed. New York: Cold Spring Harbor Laboratory Press, 2001.
20. Ausubel FM, Brent R, Kingston RE, et al: *Current Protocols in Molecular Biology.* New York: John Wiley & Sons, 2003.
21. Southern EM: Detection of specific sequences among DNA fragments separated by gel electrophoresis. *J Mol Biol* 98:503, 1975.
22. Mullis K, Faloona F, Scharf S, et al: Specific enzymatic amplification of DNA in vitro: The polymerase chain reaction. *Cold Spring Harb Symp Quant Biol* 51:263, 1986.
23. Bowtell D, Sambrook J: *DNA Microarrays, A Molecular Cloning Manual.* New York: Cold Spring Harbor Laboratory Press, 2003.
24. Bonifacino JS, Dasso M, Harford JB, et al: *Current Protocols in Cell Biology.* New York: John Wiley & Sons, 2003.
25. Nagy A, Gertsenstein M, Vintersten K, et al: *Manipulating The Mouse Embryo, A Laboratory Manual*, 3rd ed. New York: Cold Spring Harbor Laboratory Press, 2003.
26. Hannon GJ: *RNAi, A Guide To Gene Silencing.* New York: Cold Spring Harbor Laboratory Press, 2003.

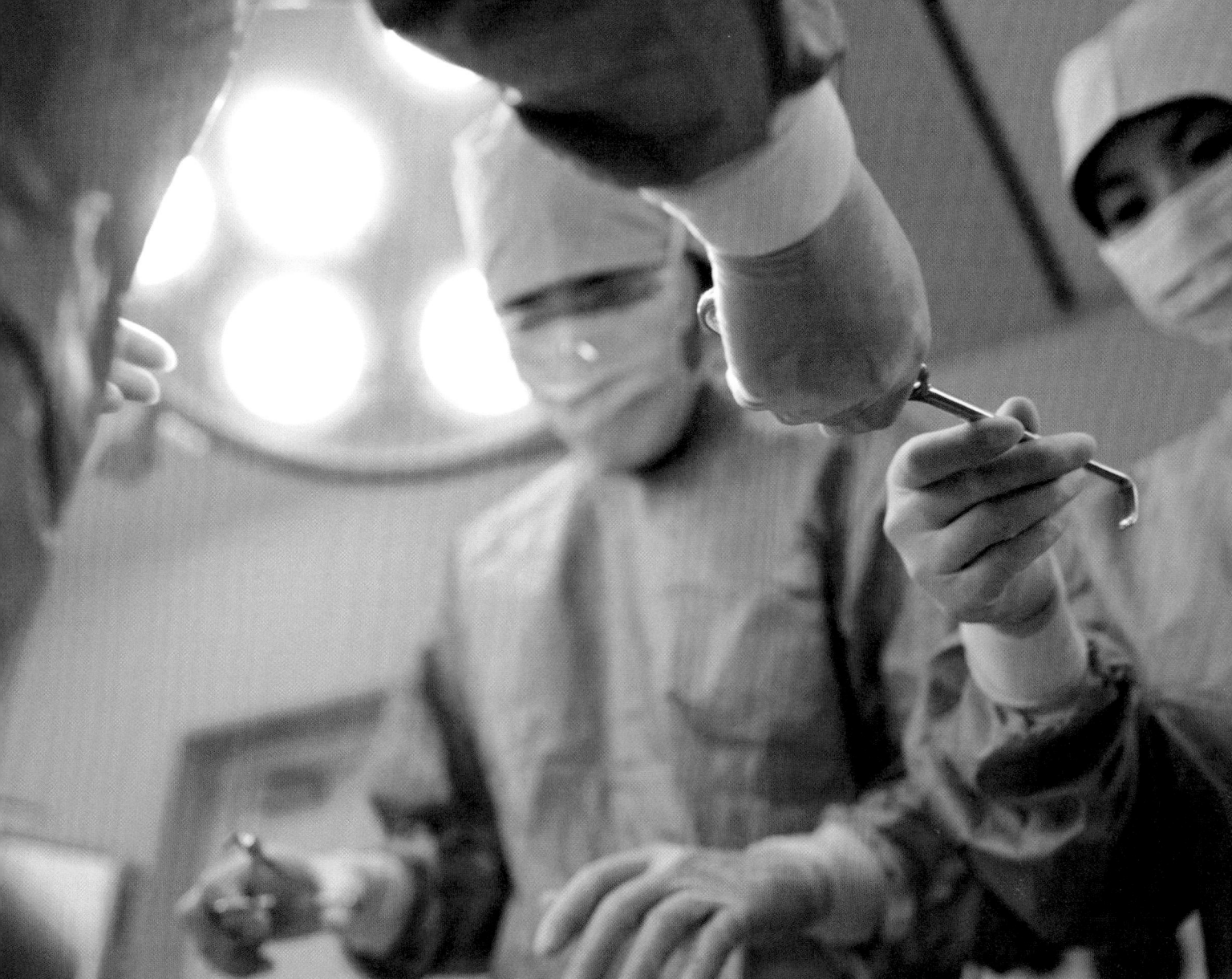

PART II
Specific Considerations

CHAPTER 16

The Skin and Subcutaneous Tissue

Patrick Cole, Lior Heller, Jamal Bullocks,
Larry H. Hollier, and Samuel Stal

BACKGROUND

As the largest human organ, the skin is one of the most complex and physiologically underappreciated elements of our bodies. Beneath its uniform appearance, the skin demonstrates profound regional variation due to the highly structured organization of many different cell types and dermal elements. Although primarily valued as a protective barrier allowing interface with our surroundings, the structure and physiology of the skin is complex and fascinating. As an environmental buffer, the skin protects against a vast array of destructive forces: The structural integrity of the epidermis creates a semipermeable barrier to chemical absorption, prevents fluid loss, protects against penetration of solar radiation, rebuffs infectious agents, and dermal durability resists physical forces. In addition, the skin's ability to regulate body heat makes it the body's primary thermoregulatory organ. The relative ease of analyzing skin specimens has made the skin one of the best-studied tissues of the human body. Not only does this fascinating organ form the primary focus of the subspecialties of plastic surgery and dermatology, but it also has driven research in a broad number of fields, including immunology, transplantation, and would healing.

ANATOMY AND PHYSIOLOGY OF THE SKIN

Anatomically, the skin may be divided into three layers: the epidermis, basement membrane, and dermis.[1-3] With very little extracellular matrix (ECM), the epidermis is composed primarily of specialized cells that perform vital functions. Sandwiched between epidermal and dermal structures, the basement membrane anchors these layers together.[1-3] This membrane fulfills many biologic functions, including tissue organization, growth factor reservoir, support of cell monolayers during tissue development, and semipermeable selective barrier. In addition to its role in providing soft-tissue durability, the dermis is primarily composed of a dense ECM that provides support for a complex network of nerves, vasculature, and adnexal structures.[3,4] The ECM is a collection of fibrous proteins and associated glycoproteins embedded in a hydrated ground substance of glycosaminoglycans and proteoglycans. These distinct molecules are organized into a highly ordered network that is closely associated with the cells that produce them. In addition to providing the architectural framework that imparts mechanical support and viscoelasticity, the ECM can regulate the neighboring cells, including their ability to migrate, proliferate, and survive injury.[2,4,5]

The Epidermis

Composed primarily of keratinocytes, the epidermis is a dynamic, multilayered composite of maturing cells. From internal to external-most layer, the epidermis is composed of the (a) stratum germina-tum, (b) stratum spinosum, (c) stratum granulosum, (d) stratum lucidum, and finally, (e) the stratum corneum. Basal cells are a mitotically active, single-cell layer of the least-differentiated keratinocytes at the base of epidermal structure.[2,6] As basal cells multiply, they leave the basal lamina to begin their differentiation and upward migration. In the spinous layer, keratinocytes are linked together by tonofibrils and produce keratin. As these cells drift upward, they lose their mitotic ability. With entry into the granular layer, cells accumulate keratohyalin granules.[1,4,6] In the horny layer, keratinocytes age, lose their intercellular connections, and shed. From basal layer exit to shedding, keratinocyte transit time approximates 40 to 56 days.[2,3]

Melanocytes and other cellular components within the skin deter absorption of harmful radiation. Initially derived from precursor cells of the neural crest, melanocytes extend dendritic processes upward into epidermal tissues from their position beneath the basal cell layer.[5,7] They number approximately one for every 35 keratinocytes, and produce melanin from tyrosine and cysteine. Once the pigment is packaged into melanosomes within the melanocyte cell body, these pigment molecules are transported into the epidermis via dendritic processes.[6,7] As dendritic processes (apocopation) are sheared off, melanin is transferred to keratinocytes via phagocytosis. Despite differences in skin tone, the density of melanocytes is constant among individuals. It is the rate of melanin production, transfer to keratinocytes, and melanosome degradation that determine the degree of skin pigmentation.[5,6] Whereas people of North European ancestry have melanocytes that release relatively low amounts of melanin, those of African descent demonstrate the same overall quantity of melanocytes, but with much higher melanin production. Genetically activated factors as well as ultraviolet (UV) radiation, hormones such as estrogen, adrenocorticotropic hormone, and melanocyte-stimulating hormone, increase melanin production.[6,7]

Cutaneous melanocytes play a critical role in neutralizing the sun's harmful rays. UV-induced damage affects the function of tumor suppressor genes, directly causes cell death, and facilitates neoplastic transformation.[2-5] Although a majority of solar radiation that reaches the Earth is UVA (315 to 400 nm), the majority of skin damage is caused by UVB (240 to 315 nm). UVB is the major factor in sunburn injury, and is a known risk factor in the development of melanoma. Although UVB causes considerable DNA damage in the skin, UVA has only recently has been shown to damage DNA, proteins, and lipids.[8-11] In addition, UV-related damage can either be potentiated by or contribute to effects of other harmful agents such as ionizing radiation, viruses, or chemical carcinogens.[3-6]

As a durable barrier against external forces, the skin relies on a complex network of filaments to maintain cellular integrity. Intermediate filaments, called *keratins*, are found within the spindle layer and provide flexible scaffolding that enables the keratinocyte to resist external stress.[4,6] Various keratins are expressed according to keratinocyte maturation phase, and mitotically active keratinocytes mainly

KEY POINTS

1. The epidermis consists of five layers. The two most superficial layers (the stratum corneum and lucidum) contain nonviable keratinocytes.

2. Collagen III provides tensile strength to the dermis and epidermis.

3. Adult dermis contains a 4:1 ratio of type I:type III collagen.

4. Of the congenital skin disorders, only pseudoxanthoma elasticum and cutis laxia are responsive to surgical rejuvenation.

5. Hemangioma is the most common cutaneous lesion of infancy and a large majority spontaneously involute (resolve) past the first year of patient age.

6. Basal cell carcinoma (BCC) is the most common form of skin cancer and nodular BCC is the most frequent form of this tumor.

7. Breslow thickness is the most important prognostic variable predicting survival in those with cutaneous melanoma.

express keratins 5 and 14.[6,7] Point mutations affecting these genes may result in blistering diseases, such as epidermolysis bullosa, associated with spontaneous release of dermal-epidermal attachments.[4,7]

In addition to its role in resisting radiation, toxin absorption, and deforming forces, the skin is a critically immunoreactive barrier.[4,6] Following migration into epidermal structure from the bone marrow, Langerhans' cells act as the skin's macrophages. This specialized cell type expresses class II major histocompatibility antigens, and has antigen-presenting capabilities.[4,7] In addition to initiating rejection of foreign bodies, Langerhans' cells play a crucial role in immunosurveillance against viral infections and neoplasms of the skin.[2,7]

The Dermis

The dermis is mostly comprised of structural proteins, and to a smaller degree, cellular components.[2,4–6] Collagen, the main functional protein within the dermis, constitutes 70% of dermal dry weight and is responsible for its remarkable tensile strength.[4,5] Tropocollagen, a collagen precursor, consists of three polypeptide chains (hydroxyproline, hydroxylysine, and glycine) wrapped in a helix.[2,6] These long molecules are then cross-linked to one another to form collagen fibers. Of the seven structurally distinct collagens, the skin primarily contains type I. Fetal dermis contains mostly type III (reticulin fibers) collagen, but this only remains in the basement membrane zone and perivascular regions during postnatal development.[6,7] Elastic fibers are highly branched proteins capable of stretching to twice their resting length. In addition to resisting stretch forces, these fibers allow a return to baseline form after the skin responds to deforming stress.[4,6] Ground substance, consisting of various polysaccharide–polypeptide (glycosaminoglycans) complexes, is an amorphous material that occupies the remaining spaces. These glycosaminoglycans, secreted by fibroblasts, can hold up to 1000 times their own volume in water and constitute most of dermal volume.[6,7]

The blood supply to the dermis is based on an intricate network of blood vessels which provide vascular inflow to superficial structures, as well as regulate body temperature.[3–7] This is achieved with the help of vertical vascular channels that interconnect two horizontal plexuses, one within the papillary dermis, and the other at the dermal–subcutaneous junction.[4,6] Glomus bodies are tortuous arteriovenous shunts that allow a substantial increase in superficial blood flow when stimulated to open.[3,5]

Cutaneous sensation is achieved via activation of a complicated plexus of dermal autonomic fibers synapsed to sweat glands, erector pili, and vasculature control points.[6,7] These fibers also connect to corpuscular receptors that relay information from the skin back to the central nervous system. Meissner's, Ruffini's, and Pacini's corpuscles transmit information on local pressure, vibration, and touch.[4,6] In addition, "unspecialized" free nerve endings report temperature, touch, pain, and itch sensations.[4,6]

Cutaneous Adnexal Structures

The skin has three main adnexal structures: eccrine glands, pilosebaceous units, and apocrine glands.[4–7] The sweat-producing eccrine glands are located over the entire body but are concentrated on the palms, soles, axillae, and forehead.[3,4] Although pheromone-producing apocrine glands play a distinct role in lower mammalian life, these structures have not been shown to demonstrate significant activity in human populations.[5,7] However, large populations of apocrine glands are primarily found in the human axillae and anogenital region. It is these structures that predispose both regions to suppurative hydroadenitis.[4,6] Hair follicles are mitotically active germinal centers that produce hair, a cylinder of tightly packed cornified epithelial cells. Together with oil-secreting sebaceous glands, these two structures form a pilosebaceous unit.[3,4,7] In addition to the production of hair, hair follicles perform several vital functions. The hair follicle contains a reservoir of pluripotential stem cells critical in epidermal reproductivity.[2,7] These cells are capable of near limitless expansion to replace lost or injured cells, as well as restore epidermal continuity after wounding. For example,

in skin graft harvest, residual hair follicles supply new keratinocytes to regenerate the epidermis and restore skin integrity.[3,5]

INJURIES TO THE SKIN AND SUBCUTANEOUS TISSUE

Each day, the skin and subcutaneous tissue face an endless supply of stimuli that threaten to break tissue integrity. Such lapses in continuity provide entry of microorganisms, allow injury to deeper tissue layers, and prompt local tissue inflammation. In addition to penetrating trauma, the environment offers a host of potentially injurious elements, such as caustic substances, extreme temperatures, prolonged or excessive pressure, and radiation.

Traumatic Injuries

Traumatic wounds may be caused by penetrating, blunt, and shear force, bite, and degloving injuries. Although clean lacerations may be closed primarily after irrigation, débridement, and careful evaluation, contaminated or infected wounds should be allowed to heal by secondary intention or delayed primary closure.[8–10] Débridement of nonviable tissue and aggressive irrigation of the wound are principles guiding the management of more complex wounds. Tangential abrasions should be approached similarly to second-degree burns, and degloving injuries considered third-degree or full-thickness burns.[8–10] Degloved skin may be partially salvaged by placing it back on the wound like a skin graft. In addition, replacement of clean, avulsed tissue can effectively provide wound coverage as a biologic dressing.[8–10] As the injured tissues declare their viability throughout the post-injury period, necrotic debris is removed. Areas of uncovered wound bed undergo delayed primary closure, are allowed to granulate in, or undergo definitive reconstruction.[8–10]

Bite wounds account for 4.5 million injuries each year, and prompt 2% of all emergency rooms visits.[8–10] These small puncture wounds may initially seem innocuous, but the impregnation of oral bacteria into deep, contained tissue layers can lead to significant morbidity if unrecognized (Fig. 16-1). The most common infectious organisms found with human bites are *Viridans streptococci*, *Staphylococcus aureus*, *Eikenella corrodens*, *Haemophilus influenzae*, and beta-lactamase-producing bacteria.[8–10] Dog bites account for the most frequent animal-related wound. Because the canine jaw can exert over 450 pounds of pressure per square inch,[9,10] dog bites often add a crushing element in addition to penetrating injury as well as an avulsion element. Although the dog bite injury may contaminate tissues with both aerobic and anaerobic organisms, the most commonly cultured bacteria include *Pasteurella multocida*, *Staphylococcus* species, alpha-hemolytic streptococci, *E. corrodens*, *Actinomyces*, and *Fusobacterium*.[8–10] The bite wound, whether from human or animal, is a contaminated wound and should not be closed primarily. Selected facial wounds may be closed primarily after very thorough cleansing and initiation of antibiotic therapy. Although there remains a potential risk of serious infection, this risk may be low enough on the face to weigh in favor of the improved long-term wound appearance after primary closure. The great majority of bite wounds should be approached via drainage, copious irrigation, débridement of necrotic material, antibiotic therapy, extremity immobilization, and elevation.[8–10]

Exposure to Caustic Substances

Injuries secondary to caustic substance exposure may be categorized as resulting from either acidic or alkali solutions. The effect of acid exposure on the skin is determined by the concentration, duration of contact, amount, and penetrability.[11–13] Deep tissue *coagulative* injury may result, damaging nerves, blood vessels, tendons, and bone.[12–15] The initial treatment should include copious skin irrigation for at least 30 minutes with either saline or water.[11–15] This dilutes active acid solution and helps return the skin to normal pH. Injuries associated with hydrofluoric acid present an additional treatment

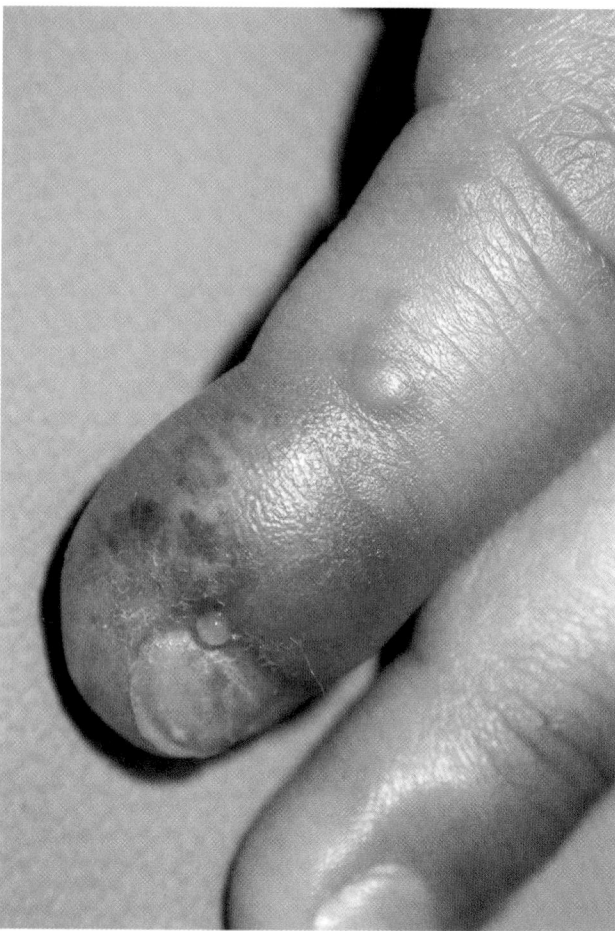

FIG. 16-1. Digital infection following puncture or bite wounds often contain a variety of bacteria, and rapid spread of infection is possible in the absence of antibiotic therapy.

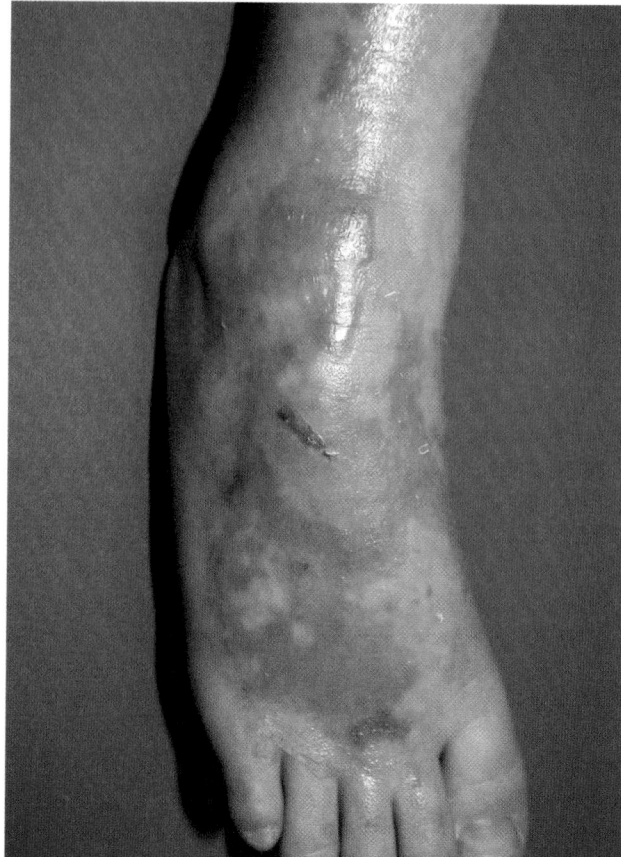

FIG. 16-2. Infiltration of IV fluid may produce significant soft-tissue injury. However, a great majority of these wounds respond well to conservative management, including frequent dressing change and continued wound care.

challenge. Fluoride ions continue to injure underlying tissue until they are neutralized with calcium, and absorb the body's calcium supply, which may prompt cardiac arrythmia.[12,14,15] Topical quaternary ammonium compounds are widely used, and topical calcium carbonate gel also effectively detoxifies fluoride ions.[14,15]

Alkaline agents often used as household cleaning agents are responsible for more than 15,000 skin burns in the United States annually.[12,13] After penetrating the skin, alkaline substances cause fat saponification that facilitates tissue penetration and increases tissue damage. In addition, the *liquefactive* injury produced by alkali burns provides a longer, more sustained period of injury.[12,13] Immediate irrigation of the affected area with continuous water flow should be maintained for at least 2 hours, or until symptomatic relief is achieved.

Intravenous fluid (IVF) extravasation—leakage of injectable fluids into interstitial space—is considered a chemical burn (Fig. 16-2). In contrast to many cutaneous injuries, this type of insult occurs from underneath the skin surface and is actually a deep injury. Extravasation produces injury via chemical toxicity, osmotic toxicity, or from pressure effects in a closed environment.[12,13] This displacement may be the result of IV catheter movement or increased vascular permeability. The most common substances associated with these injuries are cationic solutions (e.g., potassium ion, calcium ion, bicarbonate), osmotically active chemicals (e.g., total parenteral nutrition or hypertonic dextrose solutions), and antibiotics or cytotoxic drugs.[12,13] The dorsum of the hand is the most common site of extravasation in the adult, which may result in extensor tendon exposure.

Patients undergoing chemotherapy have a 4.7% risk for developing extravasation, and children present an incidence as high as 58%.[16,17] Newborn babies are at particular risk due to the fragility and small caliber of their veins, their poor ability to verbalize pain, and the frequent use of pressurized IVF pumps used in their care. The most common IVF extravasations causing necrosis in the infant are high-concentration dextrose solutions, calcium, bicarbonate, and parenteral nutrition.[16,17] In the adult population, commonly extravasated drugs are chemotherapeutic agents, such as doxorubicin (Adriamycin) and paclitaxel.[18] The direct toxic effects of doxorubicin causes cellular death that is perpetuated by release of doxorubicin-DNA complexes from dead cells. This cellular death prevents release of cytokines and growth factors, which may ultimately result in wound healing failure.[18] Following extravasation, edema, erythema, and induration usually are present. Injury to underlying nerves, muscles, tendons, and blood vessels must be taken into account. Although a majority of such injuries are successfully managed through a conservative approach, many treatment options are available.[16–18] In the severe infusion injury, vigorous liposuction with a small cannula may be used to introduce saline flush into the injured area. The flush is then allowed to egress via the small liposuction wounds.[16–18] Although patients more than 24 hours after extravasation injury have shown no benefit from flushout, this technique has proved useful in the acute setting. Surgery should be limited to patients with necrotic tissue, pain, or damage of underlying structures.[16–18]

Hyper- and Hypothermic Injury

Skin exposed to temperature extremes is at significant risk of hypo- or hyperthermic injury. Depending upon the temperature, period, and method of exposure, hyperthermic burns may cause varying degrees of tissue injury affecting the skin at different levels of depth.[19] The central area of injury, the zone of coagulation, is exposed to the most direct heat transfer and typically becomes necrotic.[20,21] Surrounding the zone of coagulation is the zone of stasis, which has marginal tissue perfusion and questionable viability. The outermost area, the zone of hyperemia, is most similar to uninjured tissue and demonstrates increased blood flow due to the body's response to injury.[20,21] A more detailed discussion of burn wounds may be found in Chap. 8. Hypothermic injury (frostbite) results in the acute freezing of tissues and is the product of two factors: (a) duration of exposure, and (b) the temperature gradient at the skin surface.[22,23] Severe hypothermia primarily exerts its damaging effect by causing direct cellular injury to blood vessel walls and microvascular thrombosis. In addition, the skin's tensile strength decreases by 20% in a cold environment [12°C, (53.6°F)].[22,23] The treatment protocol for frostbite includes rapid rewarming, close observation, elevation and splinting, daily hydrotherapy, and serial débridements.[22,23]

Pressure Injury

Prolonged, excessive pressure often results in pressure ulcer formation. As pressure is applied to overlying tissues, cutaneous vascular flow is decreased, rendering local tissues functionally ischemic.[23–25] As little as 1 hour of 60 mmHg pressure produces histologically identifiable venous thrombosis, muscle degeneration, and tissue necrosis.[23–25] Although normal arteriole, capillary, and venule pressures are 32, 20, and 12 mmHg, respectively, sitting can produce pressures as high 300 mmHg at the ischial tuberosities.[23–25] Healthy individuals regularly shift their body weight, even while asleep. However, sacral pressure can build to 150 mmHg when lying on a standard hospital mattress.[24,25] Patients unable to sense pain or shift their body weight, such as paraplegics or bedridden individuals, may develop prolonged elevated tissue pressures and local necrosis. Because muscle tissue is more sensitive to ischemia than skin, necrosis usually extends to a deeper area than that apparent on superficial inspection.[24,25] The elements of pressure sore treatment include relief of pressure, wound care, and systemic enhancement, such as optimization of nutrition. Air flotation mattresses and gel seat cushions redistribute pressure, decrease the incidence of pressure ulcers, and are cost-effective in the care of patients at high risk.[24,25] In addition, many institutions provide nutritional support services to facilitate proper dietary intake. Surgical management should include débridement of all necrotic tissue followed by thorough irrigation. Shallow ulcers may be allowed to close by secondary intention, but deeper wounds with involvement of the underlying bone require surgical débridement and coverage.[24,25]

Radiation Exposure

Radiation injuries are frequently produced by a wide range of environmental elements, such as solar (UV) exposure, iatrogenic management, and industrial/occupational applications.[26,27] Solar or UV radiation is the most common form of radiation exposure. The UV spectrum is divided into UVA (400 to 315 nm), UVB (315 to 290 nm), and UVC (290 to 200 nm).[27–29] With regard to skin damage and development of skin cancers, significant wavelengths are in the UV spectrum. The ozone layer absorbs UVC wavelengths below 290 nm, allowing only UVA and UVB to reach the earth.[50,52] UVB is responsible for the acute sunburns and for the chronic skin damage leading to malignant degeneration, although it makes up less than 5% of the solar UV radiation that hits the earth.[27–29]

Ionizing radiation effectively blocks mitosis in rapidly dividing cell types,[26,28,29] and has become a mainstay in the treatment of various malignancies. The extent of cellular damage is dependent on radiation dose, exposure period, and the cell type being treated.[27–29] Acute radiation changes include erythema and basal epithelial cellular death in the area of direct application. With cellular repair, permanent hyperpigmentation is observed in healing areas. Four to 6

months following radiation application, chronic radiation changes are characterized by a loss of capillaries via thrombosis and fibrinoid necrosis of vessel walls.[27,29] Progressive fibrosis and hypovascularity may eventually lead to ulceration when poor vascular inflow results in poor tissue perfusion that progresses as the skin ages.[27–29]

INFECTIONS OF THE SKIN AND SUBCUTANEOUS TISSUE

Heralded by erythema, warmth, tenderness, and edema, cellulitis is a superficial, spreading infection of the skin and subcutaneous tissue. The most common organisms associated with cellulitis are group A streptococci and *S. aureus*.[30] Unless associated with significant patient morbidities, uncomplicated cellulitis usually can be managed with oral antibiotics on an outpatient basis.

Folliculitis, Furuncles, and Carbuncles

Folliculitis is an infection of the hair follicle. The causative organism is usually *Staphylococcus*, but gram-negative organisms may cause follicular inflammation as well. A furuncle (boil) begins as folliculitis, but may eventually progress to form a fluctuant nodule.[30,31] Whereas folliculitis usually resolves with adequate hygiene, soaking the furuncle in warm water hastens liquefaction and hastens spontaneous rupture. More involved, deep-seated infections that result in multiple draining cutaneous sinuses are called carbuncles. Along with furuncles, these lesions often require incision and drainage before healing can be initiated.[30,31]

Necrotizing Soft-Tissue Infections

Although many soft-tissue infections remain localized, some result in rapid, necrotizing spread and septic shock. The most common sites are the external genitalia, perineum, or abdominal wall (*Fournier gangrene*).[30–32] Currently, classification of these infections is based on (a) the tissue plane affected and extent of invasion, (b) the anatomic site, and (c) the causative pathogen(s).[30–32] Deep soft-tissue infections are classified as either necrotizing fasciitis or necrotizing myositis. Necrotizing fasciitis represents a rapid, extensive infection of the fascia deep to the adipose tissue. Necrotizing myositis primarily involves the muscles but typically spreads to adjacent soft tissues.[30–32] The most common organisms isolated from patients presenting with necrotizing soft-tissue infections include the gram-positive organisms: group A streptococci, enterococci, coagulase-negative staphylococci, *S. aureus*, *S. epidermidis*, and *Clostridium* species.[30–32] Gram-negative species frequently associated with necrotizing infections include *Escherichia coli*, *Enterobacter*, *Pseudomonas* species, *Proteus* species, *Serratia* species, and bacteroides.[30–32] Polymicrobial infections tend to be more common than single organism disease in these cases.[31,32]

Clinical risk factors for necrotizing soft-tissue infection include diabetes mellitus, malnutrition, obesity, chronic alcoholism, peripheral vascular disease, chronic lymphocytic leukemia, steroid use, renal failure, cirrhosis, and autoimmune deficiency syndrome.[30–32] Appropriate management starts with prompt recognition, broad-spectrum IV antibiotics, aggressive surgical débridement, and intensive care unit support.[30–32] Débridement must be extensive, including all skin, subcutaneous tissue, and muscle, until there is no further evidence of infected tissue. Initial resection is followed by frequent returns to the operating room for additional débridement as required.[31,32] In addition, aggressive fluid replacement is typically needed to offset acute renal failure from ongoing sepsis.[31,32]

Hidradenitis Suppurativa

Hidradenitis suppurativa is a defect of the terminal follicular epithelium.[33,34] Because the follicular defect results in apocrine gland blockage, obstructed infection leads to abscess formation throughout affected axillary, inguinal, and perianal regions. Following spontaneous rupture of these localized collections, foul-smelling sinuses form and repeated infections create a wide area of inflamed, painful tissue.[33,34] Treatment of acute infections includes application of warm compresses, antibiotics, and open drainage. In cases of chronic hidradenitis, wide excision is required and closure may be achieved via skin graft or local flap placement.[33,34]

Actinomycosis

Actinomycosis is a granulomatous suppurative bacterial disease caused by *Actinomyces*. In addition to *Nocardia, Actinomadura*, and *Streptomyces, Actinomyces* infections may produce deep cutaneous infections that present as nodules and spread to form draining tracts within surrounding soft tissue.[35,36] Forty to 60% of the actinomycotic infections occur within the face or head.[35,36] Actinomycotic infection usually results following tooth extraction, odontogenic infection, or facial trauma.[35,36] Accurate diagnosis depends on careful histologic analysis, and the presence of sulfur granules within purulent specimen is pathognomonic.[35] Penicillin and sulfonamides are typically effective against these infections. However, areas of deep-seated infection, abscess, or chronic scarring may require surgical therapy.[35,36]

VIRAL INFECTIONS OF THE SKIN AND SUBCUTANEOUS TISSUE

Human Papillomavirus

Warts are epidermal growths resulting from human papillomavirus (HPV) infection. Different morphologic types have a tendency to occur at different areas of the body. The common wart (verruca vulgaris) is found on the fingers and toes and is rough and bulbous (Fig. 16-3). Plantar warts (verruca plantaris) occur on the soles and palms, and may resemble a common callus. Flat warts (verruca plana) are slightly raised and flat. This particular subtype tends to appear on the face, legs, and hands.[37–39] Venereal warts (condylomata acuminata) grow in the moist areas around the vulva, anus, and scrotum. Histologic examination demonstrates hyperkeratosis (hypertrophy of the horny layer), acanthosis (hypertrophy of the spinous layer), and papillomatosis.[37–39] A multitude of various therapies have been created to eradicate the papillomatous growth. Warts may be removed via application of chemicals, such as formalin, podophyllum, and phenol-nitric acid.[37–39] Curettage with electrodesiccation also can be used for scattered lesions. Treatment of extensive areas of skin requires surgical excision under general anesthesia.[37–39] Because of the infectious etiology, recurrences are

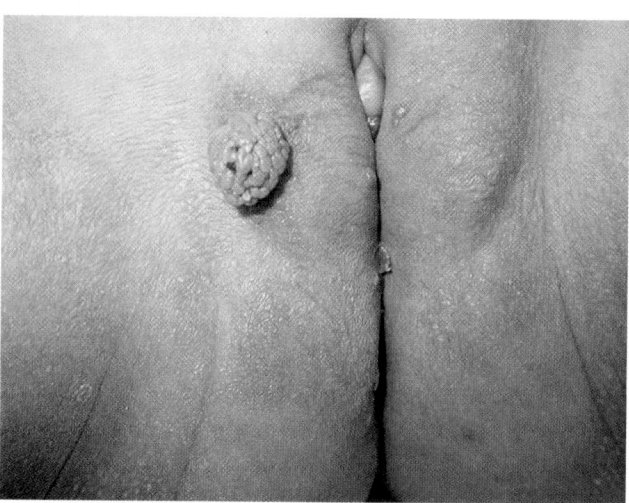

FIG. 16-4. Human papillomavirus affecting digital and genitourinary sites often proves most problematic for the patient.

common, and repeated excisions are often necessary. Some warts (especially HPV types 5, 8, and 10) are associated with squamous cell cancers, therefore lesions that grow rapidly, atypically, or ulcerate should be biopsied.[38,39]

Condylomata acuminata is one of the most common sexually transmitted diseases, and largely results from HPV types 6 and 11 (Fig. 16-4).[37–39] Extensive growths, facilitated by concomitant HIV infection, are often multiple and can grow large in size (Buschke-Löwenstein tumor). In addition to local destruction or excision, adjuvant therapy with interferon, isotretinoin, or autologous tumor vaccine decreases recurrence rates.[38,39] Immune response modifiers, such as imiquimod, may also optimize long-term eradication of HPV-induced anogenital lesions.[37–39] Because larger lesions have a significant risk of malignant transformation, close observation of lesion return or atypical presentation should be advised.

Human Immunodeficiency Virus

Patients with HIV commonly display a variety of skin manifestations. As a result of intrinsic wound-healing deficiencies and much lower resilience, these patients frequently develop chronic wounds.[40–42] In addition, the risk of postoperative soft-tissue complications directly increases with disease progression. The cause for delayed wound healing is unknown but is thought to be secondary to: (a) decreasing T-cell CD4$^+$ count, (b) opportunistic infection, (c) low serum albumin, and (d) poor nutrition.[40–42] Overall, these effects are thought to result in poor collagen cross-linking and deposition producing a profound compromise in wound healing.[40–42]

INFLAMMATORY DISEASES OF THE SKIN AND SUBCUTANEOUS SOFT TISSUE

Pyoderma Gangrenosum

Pyoderma gangrenosum is a relatively uncommon destructive cutaneous lesion. Clinically, a rapidly enlarging, necrotic lesion with undermined border and surrounding erythema characterize this disease.[43–45] Linked to underlying systemic disease in 50% of cases, these lesions are commonly associated with inflammatory bowel disease, rheumatoid arthritis, hematologic malignancy, and monoclonal immunoglobulin A gammapathy.[43–45] Recognition of the underlying disease is of paramount importance. Management of pyoderma gangrenosum ulcerations without correction of underlying systemic disorders is fraught with complication. A majority of patients receive systemic steroids or cyclosporine.[43–45] Although medical management alone may slowly result in wound healing,

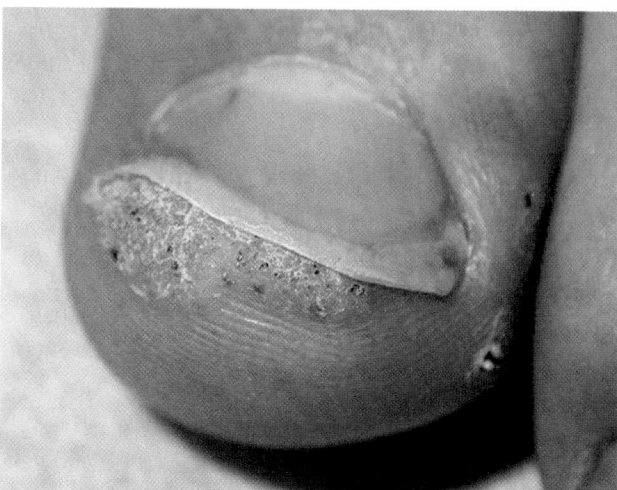

FIG. 16-3. The common wart, caused by cutaneous infection with human papillomavirus, may affect all areas covered by epidermal tissues.

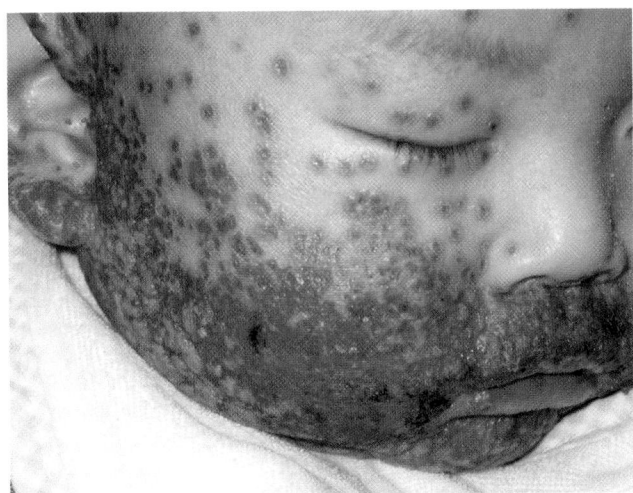

FIG. 16-5. Staphylococcal scalded skin syndrome is associated with retained foreign objects colonized with toxin-secreting staphylococcus strains.

many physicians advocate chemotherapy with aggressive wound care and skin graft coverage.[43-45]

Staphylococcal Scalded Skin Syndrome and Toxic Epidermal Necrolysis

Staphylococcal scalded skin syndrome (SSSS) and toxic epidermal necrolysis (TEN) create a similar clinical picture including skin erythema, bullae formation, and wide areas of tissue loss (Fig. 16-5).[46,47] SSSS is caused by an exotoxin produced during staphylococcal infection of the nasopharynx or middle ear.[46,47] TEN is an immune response to certain drugs such as sulfonamides, phenytoin, barbiturates, and tetracycline.[46,47] Diagnosis is made via skin biopsy. Histologic analysis of SSSS reveals a cleavage plane in the granular layer of the epidermis.[46,47] In contrast, TEN results in structural defects at the dermoepidermal junction and is similar to a second-degree burn.[46,47] Treatment involves fluid and electrolyte replacement, as well as wound care similar to burn therapy. Whereas those with more than 30% of total body surface area involvement are classified as TEN, patients with less than 10% of epidermal detachment are categorized as Stevens-Johnson syndrome.[46,47] In Stevens-Johnson syndrome, respiratory and alimentary tract epithelial sloughing may result in intestinal malabsorption and pulmonary failure. Patients with significant soft-tissue loss should be treated in burn units with specially trained staff and critical equipment.[46,47] Although corticosteroid therapy has not been efficacious, temporary coverage via cadaveric, porcine skin, or semisynthetic biologic dressings (Biobrane) allows the underlying epidermis to regenerate spontaneously.[46,47]

BENIGN TUMORS OF THE SKIN AND SUBCUTANEOUS TISSUE

Cysts (Epidermal, Dermoid, Trichilemmal)

Cutaneous cysts are categorized as either epidermal, dermoid, or trichilemmal.[48,49] Although surgeons often refer to cutaneous cysts as sebaceous cysts because they appear to contain sebum, this is a misnomer and the substance is actually keratin.[48,49] Epidermal cysts are the most common type of cutaneous cyst, and may present as a single, firm nodule anywhere on the body. Dermoid cysts are congenital lesions that result when epithelium is trapped during fetal midline closure.[48,49] Although the eyebrow is the most frequent site of presentation, dermoid cysts are common anywhere from the nasal tip to the forehead.[48,49] Trichilemmal (pilar) cysts, the second

most common cutaneous cyst, occur more often on the scalp of females.[48,49] When ruptured, these cysts have an intense, characteristic odor.

On clinical examination, it is difficult to distinguish one type of cyst from another: Each cyst presents as a subcutaneous, thinwalled nodule containing a white, creamy material.[48,49] Histologic examination reveals several key features. Cyst walls consist of an epidermal layer oriented with the basal layer superficial, and the more mature layers deep (i.e., with the epidermis growing into the center of the cyst).[48,49] The desquamated cells (keratin) collect in the center to form the cyst. Epidermal cysts have a mature epidermis complete with granular layer.[48,49] Dermoid cysts demonstrate squamous epithelium, eccrine glands, and pilosebaceous units. In addition, these particular cysts may develop bone, tooth, or nerve tissue on occasion.[48,49] Trichilemmal cyst walls do not contain a granular layer; however, these cysts contain a distinctive outer layer resembling the root sheath of a hair follicle (trichilemmoma).[48-50] Each of these cysts typically remain unnoticed and asymptomatic until they rupture, cause local inflammation, or become infected. Once infected, these cysts behave similar to abscesses, and incision and drainage is recommended. After resolution of inflammation, the cyst wall must be removed in its entirety or the cyst will recur.[48-50]

Keratoses (Seborrheic, Solar)

Seborrheic keratoses arise in sun-exposed areas of the body such as the face, forearms, and back of the hands.[51-53] Most notable in the older age groups, lesions appear light brown or yellow and have a velvety, greasy texture. Seborrheic keratoses are considered premalignant lesions, and squamous cell carcinoma (SCC) may develop over time.[52,53] Interestingly, sudden eruptions of multiple lesions may be associated with internal malignancies.[50,52] However, seborrheic keratoses are rarely mistaken for other lesions, so biopsy and treatment are seldom required.[50,52] Histologically, these lesions contain atypical-appearing keratinocytes and evidence of dermal solar damage.[50,52] Although malignancies that do develop rarely metastasize, lesion destruction is the treatment of choice. Treatments often include application of topical 5-fluorouracil, surgical excision, electrodesiccation, and dermabrasion.[50,52]

Nevi (Acquired and Congenital)

Depending on the location of nevus cells, acquired melanocytic nevi are classified as junctional, compound, or dermal.[54-57] This classification does not represent different types of nevi, but rather different stages in nevus maturation. Initially, nevus cells accumulate in the epidermis (junctional).[55-57] As they mature, nevus cells migrate partially into the dermis (compound) and finally rest completely within dermal tissues (dermal). Eventually most lesions undergo involution. Congenital nevi are relatively rare, and may be found in less than 1% of neonates.[54,56,57] These lesions are larger and often contain hair. Histologically, congenital and acquired nevi appear similar. Giant congenital lesions (giant hairy nevi) most often occur in a swim trunk distribution, chest, or back (Fig. 16-6).[54-57] Not only are these lesions cosmetically unpleasant, but congenital nevi may develop into malignant melanoma in 1 to 5% of cases.[54-57] Total excision of the nevus is the treatment of choice; however, the lesion is often so large that inadequate tissue for wound closure precludes complete resection. Instead, serial excisions with local tissue expansion/advancement are frequently required over several years.[54-57]

Vascular Tumors of the Skin and Subcutaneous Tissue

Hemangiomas are benign vascular neoplasms that present soon after birth (Fig. 16-7). They initially undergo rapid cellular proliferation over the first year of life, then undergo slow involution throughout childhood.[58-60] Histologically, hemangiomas are composed of mitotically active endothelial cells surroundings several, confluent blood-filled spaces. Although these lesions may enlarge

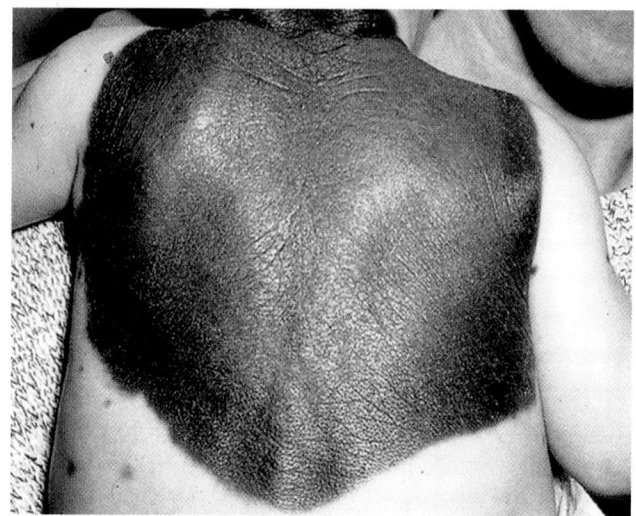

FIG. 16-6. Although the giant nevus may be aesthetically concerning, these lesions present a roughly 5% risk of malignant transformation over one's lifetime.

systemic prednisone or interferon alpha-2a treatment use.[58–60] In the absence of acute surgical indications or significant patient/parent concern, many lesions are allowed to spontaneously involute. However, hemangiomata that remain into adolescence or involute to leave an unsightly telangiectasia typically require surgical excision for optimal resolution.[58–60]

In contrast to neoplasms, vascular malformations are a result of structural abnormalities formed during fetal development.[61,62] Unlike hemangiomas, vascular malformations grow in proportion to the body and never involute. Histologically, they contain enlarged vascular spaces lined by nonproliferating endothelium.[61,62] Arteriovenous malformations are high-flow lesions that often present as subcutaneous masses associated with locally elevated temperature, dermal stain, thrill, and bruit. In addition, overlying ischemic ulcers, adjacent bone destruction, or local hypertrophy may occur.[61,62] Very large malformations may cause cardiac enlargement and congestive heart failure. Complications of arteriovenous malformations, such as pain, hemorrhage, ulceration, cardiac effects, or local tissue destruction, should prompt attempts at lesion destruction.[61,62] Therapy consists of surgical resection. Even when complete lesion resection is not possible, significant debulking may greatly diminish symptomatology. In addition, angiography with selective embolization just before surgery greatly facilitates operative removal.[61,62]

The capillary malformation, or port-wine stain, is a flat, dull-red lesion often located on the trigeminal (cranial nerve V) distribution on the face, trunk, or extremities (Fig. 16-8).[61,62] Presentation within the V1 or V2 facial regions should prompt concern of a possible link to more systemic syndromes such as Sturge-Weber syndrome (leptomeningeal angiomatosis, epilepsy, and glaucoma).[61,62] Histologically, these nevi are composed of ectatic capillaries lined by

significantly in the first year of life, approximately 90% involute over time.[58–60] Acute treatment is limited to hemangiomata that interfere with function, such as airway, vision, and feeding. In addition, lesions resulting in systemic problems, such as thrombocytopenia or high-output cardiac failure, should prompt resection. The growth of rapidly enlarging lesions also can be halted with

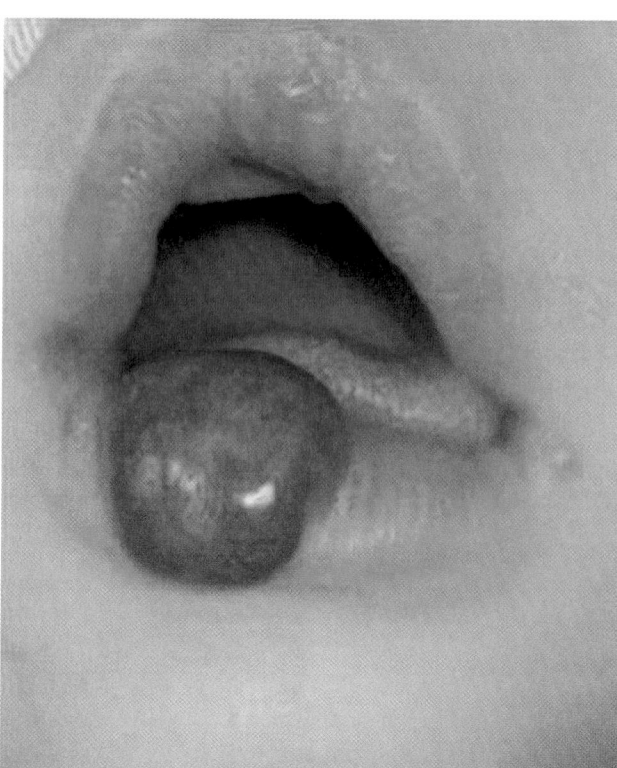

FIG. 16-7. Hemangiomas most often present at approximately 2 to 4 weeks after birth, rapidly proliferate during infancy, reach a plateau phase, then involute over several years. Unless the hemangiomatous mass obstructs the airway, visual axis, or imposes psychological harm to a preschool age child, these tumors typically are allowed to spontaneously involute.

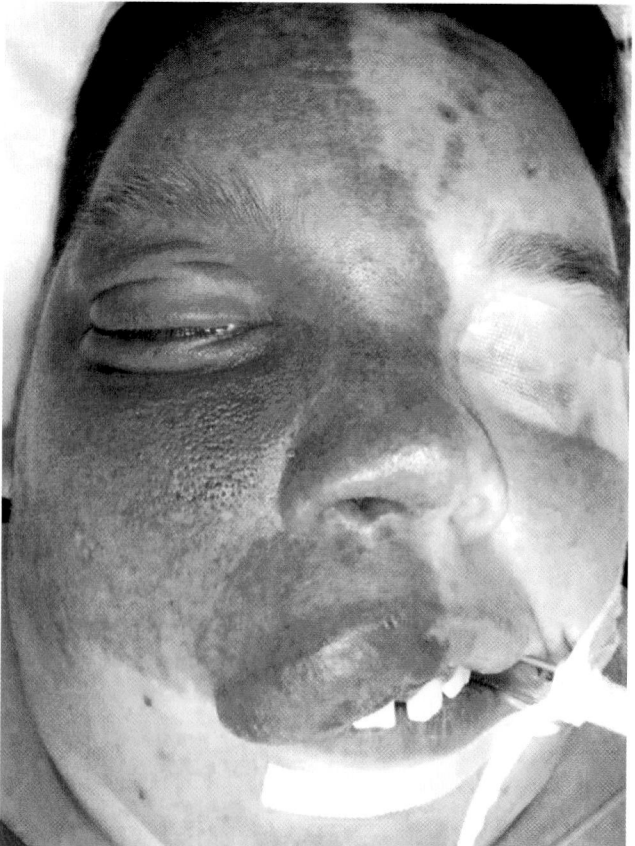

FIG. 16-8. A capillary hemangioma (also known as a *port-wine stain*) present upon the midface may signify Churg-Strauss syndrome, and computed tomography of the brain is appropriate to rule out intracranial berry aneurysms.

mature endothelium. Unsightly lesions may be treated with pulsed dye laser, covered with cosmetics, or surgically excised.[61,62]

Glomus tumor is an uncommon, benign neoplasm of the extremity. Representing less than 1.5% of all benign, soft-tissue extremity tumors, these lesions arise from dermal neuromyoarterial apparatus (glomus bodies).[63,64] Glomus tumor more commonly affects the hand, and presentation within the subungual region of the toe is rare. Diagnosis of these lesions is traditionally delayed, and atypical presentation on the foot or toes often leads to even greater diagnostic challenges. In addition to the severe pain, point tenderness and cold sensitivity are associated with these lesions and subungual glomus tumors typically appear as blue, subungual discolorations of 1 to 2 mm. Tumor excision is the treatment of choice.[63,64]

Soft-Tissue Tumors (Acrochordons, Dermatofibromas, Lipomas)

Lipomas are the most common subcutaneous neoplasm.[64] Although they are found most frequently on the trunk, these lesions may appear anywhere. Typically soft and fleshy on palpation, lipomas may grow to a large size and become substantially deforming. Histologic examination reveals a lobulated tumor composed of normal fat cells.[64] Although fears of malignant degeneration have prompted resection in the past, no report of such malignancy has been substantiated. To date, the lipoma is widely viewed as benign with essentially no risk of malignant devolvement.[64] Although observation is an option, surgical excision is required for tumor removal. Acrochordons (skin tags) are fleshy, pedunculated masses located on the preauricular areas, axillae, trunk, and eyelids.[65-67] They are composed of hyperplastic epidermis over a fibrous connective tissue stalk. These lesions are usually small, and are frequently treated via "tying off" or with resection in the clinic.[65-67] Dermatofibromas are solitary, soft-tissue nodules usually approximating 1 to 2 cm in diameter, and are found primarily on the legs and flanks. Histologically, these lesions are composed of unencapsulated connective tissue whorls containing fibroblasts.[65-67] Although a majority of dermatofibromas can be diagnosed clinically, atypical presentation or course should prompt excisional biopsy to assess for malignancy. Although these tumors may be managed conservatively, operative removal is the treatment of choice.[66-68]

Neural Tumors (Neurofibromas, Neurilemomas, Granular Cell Tumors)

Benign, cutaneous neural tumors such as neurofibromas, neurilemomas, and granular cell tumors primarily arise from the nerve sheath.[65,68] Neurofibromas can be sporadic and solitary. However, a majority are associated with café au lait spots, Lisch nodules, and an autosomal dominant inheritance (von Recklinghausen's disease).[65,66] These lesions are firm, discrete nodules attached to a nerve. Histologically, proliferation of perineurial and endoneurial fibroblasts with Schwann cells embedded in collagen are noted. In contrast to direct nerve attachment as seen with neurofibromas, neurilemomas are solitary tumors arising from cells of the peripheral nerve sheath.[65,66] These lesions are discrete nodules that may induce local or radiating pain along the distribution of the nerve. Microscopically, the tumor contains Schwann cells with nuclei packed in palisading rows. Surgical resection is the management option of choice. Granular cell tumors are usually solitary lesions of the skin or, more commonly, the tongue.[65,66] They consist of granular cells derived from Schwann cells that often infiltrate the surrounding striated muscle. Based on the severity of symptomatology, operative resection is the primary therapy of choice.[65-68]

MALIGNANT TUMORS OF THE SKIN

Although malignancies arising from cells of the dermis or adnexal structures are relatively uncommon, the skin is frequently subject to epidermal tumors, such as basal cell carcinoma (BCC), SCC, and melanoma.[69-72] Each of these tumors has received exhaustive study, and several key factors associated with their development have been identified. Perhaps of greatest significance is that increased exposure to UV radiation is associated with an increased development of all skin cancer.[69-72] Clinical studies reveal that persons with outdoor occupations are at greater risk, as are those with fair complexions and people living in regions receiving higher per capita sunlight. In addition, albino individuals of dark-skinned races are prone to develop cutaneous neoplasms that are typically rare in nonalbino members of the same group. This observation suggests that melanin, and its ability to limit UV radiation tissue penetration, plays a large role in carcinogenesis protection.[69-72]

Skin cancer development also has been strongly linked to chemical carcinogens such as tar, arsenic, and nitrogen mustard. Radiation therapy directed at skin lesions increases the risk for local BCC and SCC.[69-72] As an ongoing area of intense research interest, certain subtypes of HPV have been linked to SCC.[69-72] Additionally, chronically irritated or nonhealing areas such as burn scars, sites of repeated bullous skin sloughing, and decubitus ulcers present an elevated risk of developing SCC.[69-72] Systemic immunologic dysfunction is also related to an increase in cutaneous malignancies. Immunosuppressed patients receiving chemotherapy, those with advanced HIV/AIDS, and immunosuppressed transplant recipients have an increased incidence of BCC, SCC, and melanoma.[69-72]

Basal Cell Carcinoma

Arising from the basal layer of the epidermis, BCC is the most common type of skin cancer. Based on gross and histologic morphology, BCC has been divided into several subtypes: nodular, superficial spreading, micronodular, infiltrative, pigmented, and morpheaform.[69-72]

Nodulocystic or noduloulcerative type accounts for 70% of BCC tumors. Waxy and frequently cream colored, these lesions present with rolled, pearly borders surrounding a central ulcer. Although superficial basal cell tumors commonly occur on the trunk and form a red, scaling lesion, pigmented BCC lesions are tan to black in color. Morpheaform BCC often appears as a flat, plaque-like lesion.[69-72] This particular variant is considered relatively aggressive and should prompt early excision. A rare form of BCC is the basosquamous type, which contains elements of both basal cell and squamous cell cancer. These lesions may metastasize similar to SCC, and should be treated aggressively.[69-72]

BCCs are slow growing, and metastasis is extremely rare.[69-72] Due to this slow developmental progression, patients often neglect these lesions for years and presentation with extensive local tissue destruction is common. The majority of small (less than 2 mm), nodular lesions may be treated via curettage, electrodesiccation, or laser vaporization.[69-72]

Although effective, these techniques destroy any potential tissue sample for confirmatory pathology diagnosis and tumor margin analysis. Surgical excision may be used to both effect complete tumor removal as well as allow proper laboratory evaluation. Basal cell tumors located at areas of great aesthetic value, such as the cheek, nose, or lip, may be best approached with Mohs' surgery.[69-72] Typically completed by specialized dermatology surgeons, Mohs' surgery uses minimal tissue resection and immediate microscopic analysis to confirm appropriate resection. Large tumors, those that invade surrounding structures, and aggressive histologic types (morpheaform, infiltrative, and basosquamous) are best treated by surgical excision with 0.5-cm to 1-cm margins.[69-72]

Squamous Cell Carcinoma

SCCs arise from epidermal keratinocytes (Fig. 16-9). While less common than BCC, SCC is more devastating due to an increased invasiveness and tendency to metastasize.[69-72] Before local invasion, in situ SCC lesions are termed *Bowen's disease*. In situ SCC tumors specific to the penis are referred to as *erythroplasia of Queyrat*.[67,68] Following tissue invasion, tumor thickness correlates well with malignant behav-

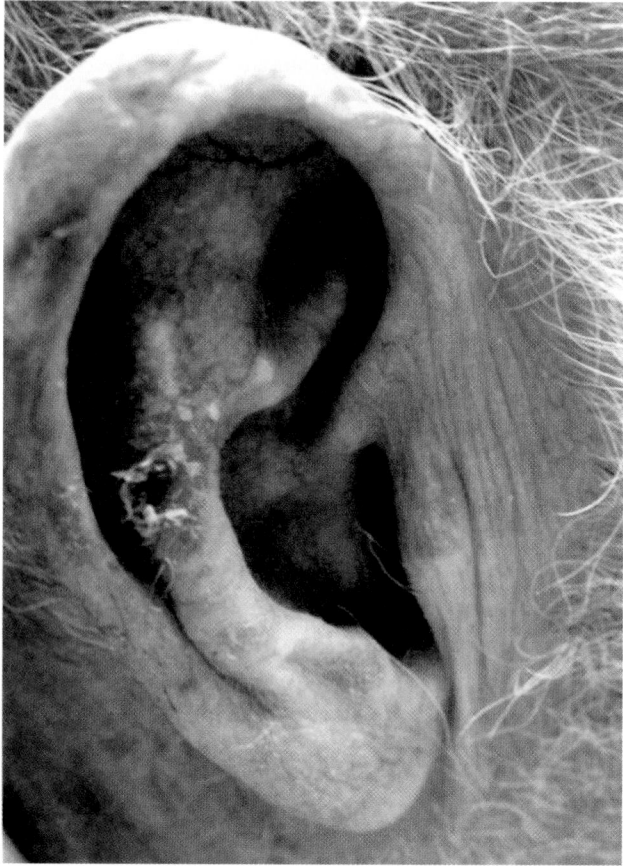

FIG. 16-9. Although basal cell carcinoma is the most common tumor involving the head and neck, squamous cell carcinoma (pictured here) occurs with high frequency on the nose, ears, and lower lip.

ior. Tumor recurrence is more prevalent once SCC tumors grow more than 4 mm in thickness, and lesions that metastasize are typically at least 10 mm in diameter.[69–72] Tumor location is also of great prognostic importance. Although SCC tumors in areas with cumulative solar damage are less aggressive, and respond well to local excision, lesions arising in burn scars (Marjolin's ulcer), areas of chronic osteomyelitis, and areas of previous injury metastasize early.[69–72]

Although small lesions can be treated with curettage and electrodesiccation, most surgeons recommend surgical excision. Lesions should be excised with a 1-cm margin, and histologic confirmation of tumor-free borders is mandatory.[69–72] Tumors within areas of great aesthetic value, such as the cheek, nose, or lip, may be best approached with Mohs' surgery. This precise, specialized surgical technique uses minimal tissue resection and immediate microscopic analysis to confirm appropriate resection yet limit removal of valuable anatomy. The need for lymph node (LN) dissection in the setting of SCC remains a topic of debate. Regional LN excision is indicated for clinically palpable nodes.[69–72] However, SCC lesions arising in chronic wounds are more aggressive and regional lymph node metastases are observed more frequently. In this instance, lymphadenectomy before development of palpable nodes (prophylactic LN dissection) is indicated. Metastatic disease is a poor prognostic sign, and only 13% of patients typically survive 10 years.[69–72]

Mohs' Surgery for Squamous and Basal Cell Carcinomas

Basal and squamous cell lesions often present on sun-exposed portions of the body such as the head and face. Unfortunately, these areas are of great aesthetic value and significant tissue loss may significantly alter facial symmetry, contour, and continuity. Developed in 1936, Mohs' technique uses serial excision in small increments coupled with immediate microscopic analysis to ensure tumor removal, yet limit resection of aesthetically valuable tissue.[70–72] One distinct advantage of Mohs' technique is that all specimen margins are evaluated. In contrast, traditional histologic examination surveys selected portions on surgical margin. The major benefit of Mohs' technique is the ability to remove a tumor with minimal sacrifice of uninvolved tissue.[70–72] Although this procedure is of particular value when managing tumors of the eyelid, nose, or cheek, one major drawback is procedure length. Total lesion excision may require multiple attempts at resection, and many procedures may be carried out over several days. Recurrence and metastases rates are comparable to those of wide local excision.[70–72]

Malignant Melanoma

The increasing rate of melanoma diagnoses is the highest of any cancer in the United States. The age-adjusted incidence of invasive melanoma in the United States increased from approximately 4 to 18 per 100,000 white males between 1973 and 1998.[73] With this increasing prevalence, it is critical that physicians recognize and appropriately manage these lesions early.

The pathogenesis of melanoma is complex and remains poorly understood to date. Melanoma may arise from transformed melanocytes anywhere that these cells have migrated during normal embryogenesis (Fig. 16-10).[73–76] Although nevi (freckles) are benign melanocytic neoplasms found on the skin of many people, dysplastic nevi contain a histologically identifiable focus of atypical melanocytes. These lesions are thought to represent an intermediate stage between benign nevus and true malignant melanoma.[73–76] Studies demonstrate increased relative risk of melanoma development based on increasing numbers of dysplastic nevi found on the patient. In addition, a strong genetic component has been described.[73–76] Up to 14% of malignant melanomas occur in a familial pattern, and family members of those with either dysplastic nevi or melanoma are at increased risk for tumor development.[73–76]

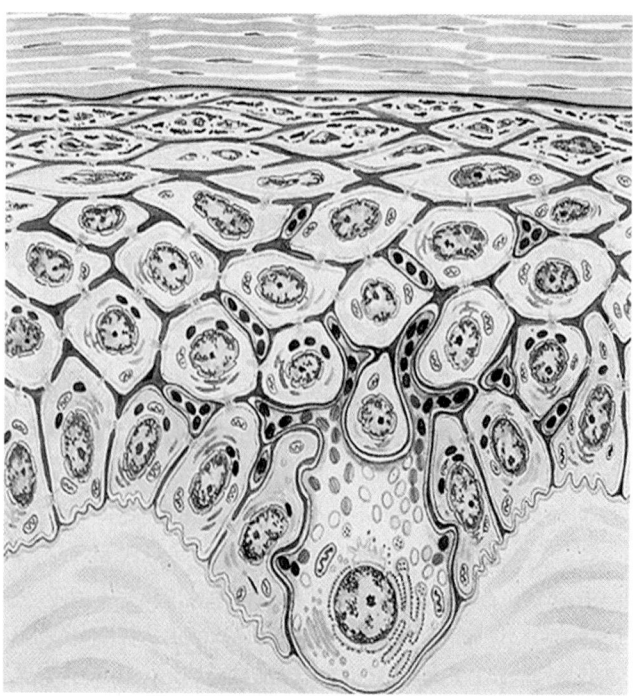

FIG. 16-10. Following malignant transformation, invasive melanoma cells replicate, penetrate surrounding epidermal layers, and migrate to more distant tissues.

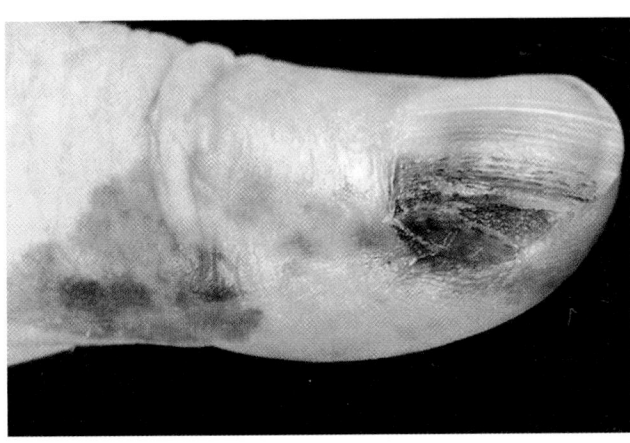

FIG. 16-11. Lateral view of a subungual melanoma demonstrating apparent proximal digital extension.

Once the melanocyte has transformed into the malignant phenotype, tumor growth occurs radially in the epidermal plane.[73-76] Even though microinvasion of the dermis may have occurred, metastases do not occur until these melanocytes form dermal nests. During the subsequent vertical growth phase, cells develop different cell-surface antigens and their malignant behavior becomes much more aggressive.[73-76] Study of these cell populations in culture medium demonstrates substantially lengthened cellular life span and increased malignant growth despite significantly poor nutrient medium.[73-76]

Although the eye and anus are notable sites, over 90% of melanomas are found on the skin (Fig. 16-11).[73-76] In addition, 4% of tumors are discovered as metastases without any identifiable primary site. Suspicious features suggestive of melanoma include any pigmented lesion with an irregular border, darkening coloration, ulceration, and raised surface.[73-76] Although many benign lesions may fit these descriptors, it is perhaps most critical to note recent changes in nevus appearance that may denote malignant transformation. In addition, approximately 5 to 10% of melanomas are nonpigmented.[73-76]

In order of decreasing frequency, the four types of melanoma are superficial spreading, nodular, lentigo maligna, and acral lentiginous.[73-76] The most common type, superficial spreading, accounts for up to 70% of melanomas. These lesions occur anywhere on the skin except the hands and feet. They are typically flat and measure 1 to 2 cm in diameter at diagnosis.[73-76] Before vertical extension, a prolonged radial growth phase is characteristic of these lesions. Typically of darker coloration and often raised, the nodular type accounts for 15 to 30% of melanomas.[73-76] These lesions are noted for their lack of radial growth; hence, all nodular melanomas are in the vertical growth phase at diagnosis. Although considered a more aggressive lesion, the prognosis for patients with nodular-type melanomas is similar to that for a patient with a superficial spreading lesion of the same depth. Lentigo maligna accounts for 4 to 15% of melanomas, and occurs most frequently on the neck, face, and hands of the elderly.[73-76] Although they tend to be quite large at diagnosis, these lesions have the best prognosis because invasive growth occurs late. Less than 5% of lentigo maligna are estimated to evolve into melanoma.[74,75] Acral lentiginous melanoma is the least common subtype, and constitutes only 2 to 8% of melanomas in white populations. Although acral lentiginous melanoma among dark-skinned people is relatively rare, this type accounts for 29 to 72% of all melanomas in dark-skinned people (African Americans, Asians, and Hispanics).[74,75] Acral lentiginous melanoma most frequently is encountered on the palms, soles, and subungual regions. Most common on the great toe or thumb, subungual lesions appear as blue-black discolorations of the posterior nail fold. The additional presence of pigmentation in the proximal or lateral nail folds (Hutchinson's sign) is diagnostic of subungual melanoma.[73-76]

Several clinical features of melanoma have been identified as significant prognostic indicators. Independent of histologic type and depth of invasion, those with lesions of the extremities have a better prognosis than patients with melanomas of the head, neck, or trunk (10-year survival rate of 82% for localized disease of the extremity compared to a 68% survival rate with a lesion of the face).[73-76] Lesion ulceration carries a worse prognosis. The 10-year survival rate for patients with local disease (stage I) and an ulcerated melanoma was 50% compared to 78% for the same stage lesion without ulceration.[73-76] Early studies identified that the incidence of ulceration increases with increasing thickness, from 12.5% in melanomas less than 0.75 mm to 72.5% in melanomas greater than 4.0 mm.[74,76] Recent evidence suggests that tumors ulcerate as the result of increased angiogenesis.[73-76] Gender is also a substantial prognostic indicator. Numerous studies demonstrate that females have an improved survival compared to males.[74,75] Women tend to acquire melanomas in more favorable anatomic sites, and these lesions are less likely to contain ulceration. After correcting for thickness, age, and location, females continue to have a higher survival rate than men (10-year survival rate of 80% for women vs. 61% for men with stage I disease).[74-76] In general, there is no significant difference between different histologic tumor types in terms of prognosis, when matched for tumor thickness, gender, age, or other. Nodular melanomas have the same prognosis as superficial spreading types when lesions are matched for depth of invasion. Lentigo maligna types, however, have a better prognosis even after correcting for thickness, and acral lentiginous lesions have a worse prognosis. Even though the various types of melanoma have similar prognoses when controlled for the other prognostic factors, acral lentiginous melanoma has a shorter interval to recurrence.[74-76]

The most current staging system, from the American Joint Committee on Cancer (AJCC), contains the best method of interpreting clinical information in regard to prognosis of this disease (Fig. 16-12).[74-76] Historically, the vertical thickness of the primary tumor (Breslow thickness) and the anatomic depth of invasion (Clark level) have represented the dominant factors in the T classification. The T classification of lesions comes from the original observation by Clark that prognosis is directly related to the level of invasion of the skin by the melanoma. Whereas Clark used the histologic level [I, superficial to basement membrane (in situ); II, papillary dermis; III, papillary/reticular dermal junction; IV, reticular dermis; and V, subcutaneous fat], Breslow modified the approach to obtain a more reproducible measure of invasion by the use of an ocular micrometer. The lesions were measured from the granular layer of the epidermis or the base of the ulcer to the greatest depth of the tumor (I, 0.75 mm or less; II, 0.76 to 1.5 mm; III, 1.51 to 4.0 mm; IV, 4.0 mm or more).[74-76] These levels of invasion have been subsequently modified and incorporated in the AJCC staging system. The new staging system has largely replaced the Clark level with another histologic feature, ulceration, based on analysis of large databases available to the AJCC Melanoma Committee.[75,76]

Evidence of tumor in regional LNs is a poor prognostic sign associated with a precipitous drop in survival at 15-year follow-up.[77-81] Based on the tumor, node, and metastasis tumor staging system, this finding advances any classification from stage I or II to stage III. Identification of distant metastasis is the worst prognostic sign and is classified as stage IV disease. Although occasional survival for several years has been noted, median survival ranges from 2 to 7 months depending on the number and site of metastases.[77-81]

Diagnosis of melanoma typically requires excisional biopsy (Fig. 16-13). A 1-mm margin of normal skin is taken if the wound can be closed primarily.[73-76] If removal of the entire lesion creates too large a defect, then an incisional biopsy of a representative part is recommended. Biopsy incisions should be made with the expectation that a subsequent wide excision of the biopsy site may be done.

With diagnosis made, treatment of melanoma may range from simple excision to more complex lymphadenectomy or immunotherapy (see Fig. 16-13). Regardless of tumor depth or extension, surgical excision is the management of choice. Lesions 1 mm or less

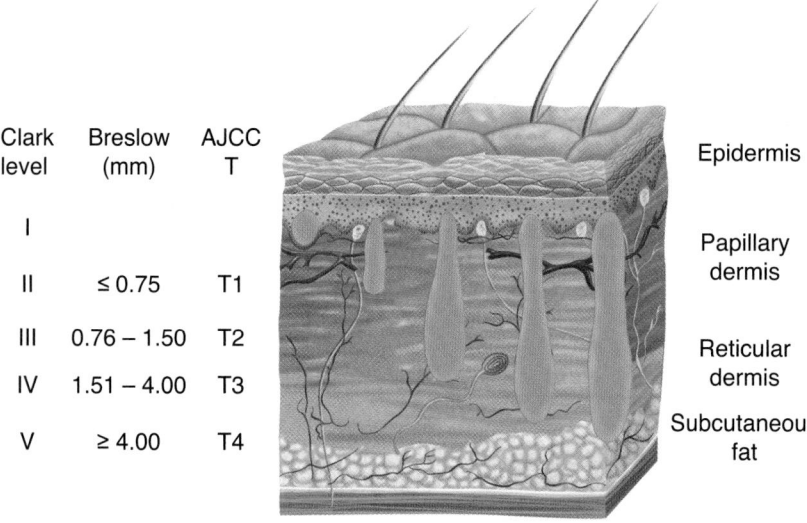

Clark level	Breslow (mm)	AJCC T
I		
II	≤ 0.75	T1
III	0.76 – 1.50	T2
IV	1.51 – 4.00	T3
V	≥ 4.00	T4

Epidermis

Papillary dermis

Reticular dermis

Subcutaneous fat

FIG. 16-12. Although Breslow's thickness has traditionally been used to anticipate clinical outcomes based on the depth of melanoma invasion, more recent staging criteria advanced by the American Joint Committee on Cancer (AJCC) are today's standard of care.

in thickness can be treated with a 1-cm margin.[73-76] For lesions 1 mm to 4 mm thick, a 2-cm margin is recommended. Lesions of greater than 4 mm may be treated with 3-cm margins.[73-76] The surrounding tissue should be removed down to the fascia to remove all lymphatic channels. If the deep fascia is not involved by the tumor, removing it does not affect recurrence or survival rates, so the fascia is left intact.[73-76]

Treatment of regional LNs that do not obviously contain tumor in patients without evidence of metastasis is an area of continued debate. In patients with thin lesions (less than 1 mm), the tumor cells are still localized in the surrounding tissue, and the cure rate is excellent with wide excision of the primary lesion; therefore treatment of regional LNs is not beneficial (Fig. 16-14).[73-76] With lesions deeper than 4 mm, it is highly likely that the tumor cells already have spread to the regional LNs and distant sites. Removal of the melanomatous LNs has no effect on survival.[73-76] Most of these patients die of metastatic disease before developing problems in regional nodes.

In patients with intermediate-thickness tumors (T2 and T3, 1 to 4.0 mm) and no clinical evidence of nodal or metastatic disease, the use of prophylactic dissection (elective LN dissection on clinically negative nodes) is controversial. To date, no prospective, randomized studies have demonstrated that elective LN dissection improves survival in patients with intermediate-thickness melanomas. However, 25 to 50% of LN specimens contain micrometastases in these cases and recurrence may be decreased with LN dissection.[77-81]

Sentinel lymphadenectomy for malignant melanoma is gaining acceptance (Fig. 16-15). The sentinel node may be preoperatively located with the use of a gamma camera, which identifies the radioisotope injected into the primary lesion.[77-81] Whereas preoperative identification may provide the surgeon greater reliability in localizing the LN, intraoperative mapping with 1% isosulfan blue dye injection may be equally effective.[77-81] Both techniques identify the lymphatic drainage from the primary lesion, and determine the first (sentinel) LN draining the tumor area.[77-81] If micrometastasis is identified in the removed node by frozen-section examination, a complete LN dissection is performed.[77-81] This method may be used to identify patients who would benefit from LN dissection, while sparing others an unnecessary operation.

All microscopically or clinically positive LNs should be removed by regional nodal dissection.[77-81] When groin LNs are removed, the deep (iliac) nodes must be removed along with the superficial (inguinal) nodes, or disease will recur in that region. For axillary dissections, the nodes medial to the pectoralis minor muscle also must be resected.[77-81] For lesions on the face, anterior scalp, and ear, a superficial parotidectomy to remove parotid nodes and a modified neck dissection is recommended.[77-81]

Once melanoma has spread to a distant site, median survival is 7 to 8 months and the 5-year survival rate is less than 5%.[77-81] Solitary lesions in the brain, GI tract, or skin that are symptomatic should be excised when possible. Although cure is extremely rare, the degree of palliation can be high and asymptomatic survival prolonged.[77-81]

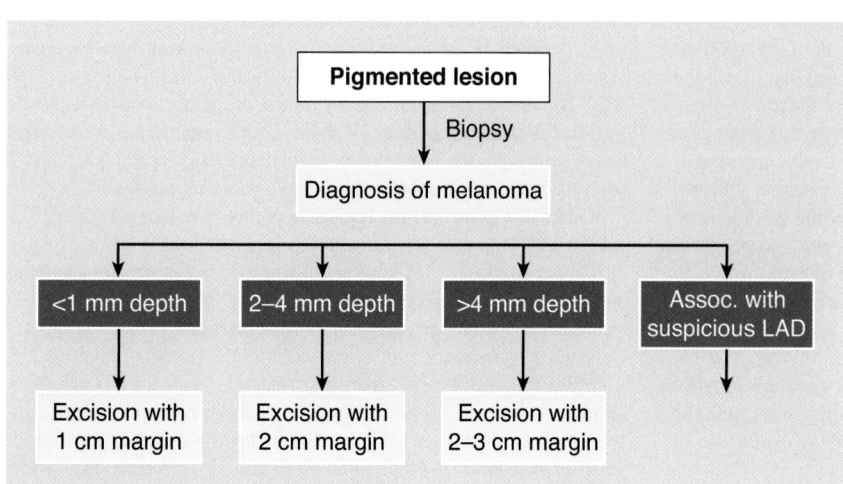

FIG. 16-13. The diagnosis of melanoma should be made via excisional biopsy. Based on tumor depth, appropriate margins may be planned. Indications for lymph node evaluation continue to advance as our understanding of tumor behavior improves and outcome data become available. LAD = lymphadenopathy.

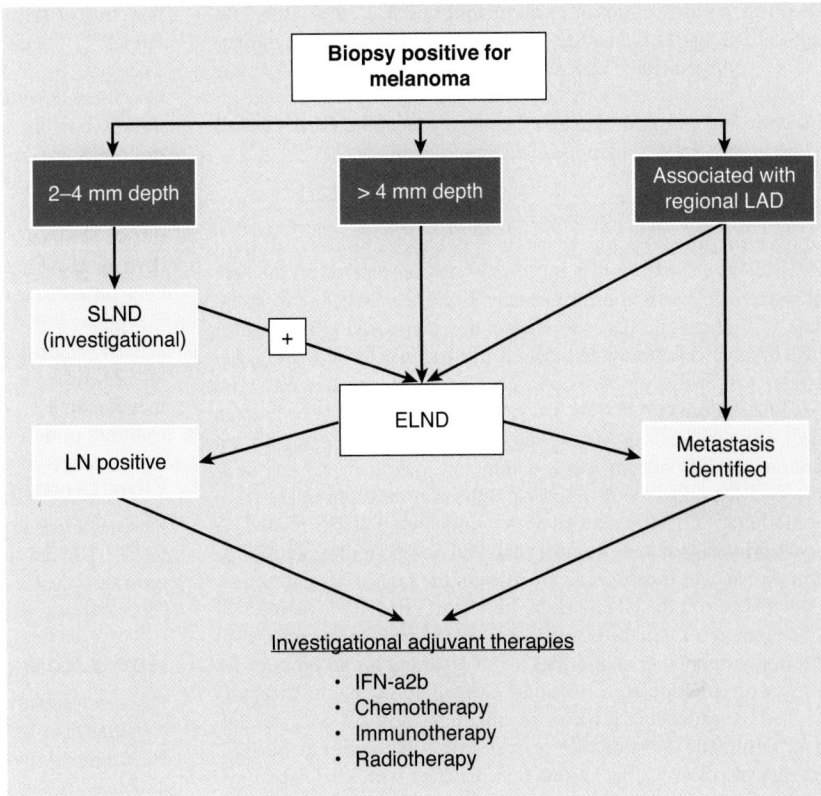

FIG. 16-14. Melanoma treatment algorithm. The algorithmic approach to melanoma has taken many forms throughout the last several decades. However, as our diagnostic technology, therapeutic approaches, and ability to assess outcome improves, the current algorithm incorporates these advances. ELND = elective lymph node dissection; IFN-a2b = interferon alfa-2b; LAD = lymphadenopathy; LN = lymph node; SLND = sentinel lymph node dissection.

A decision to operate on metastatic lesions must be made after careful deliberation with the patient and the treating oncologist.

Locally recurrent, lymphatic-invading, or tumors unamenable to surgical excision present a significant management challenge. In-transit disease (local disease in lymphatics) develops in 5 to 8% of melanoma patients with a high-risk primary melanoma (>1.5 mm).[77-81] Hyperthermic regional perfusion with a chemotherapeutic agent (e.g., melphalan) is presently the treatment of choice. The goal of regional perfusion therapy is to increase the dosage of the chemotherapeutic agent to maximize tumor response while limiting systemic toxic effects.[77-81] Melphalan generally is heated to an elevated temperature [up to 41.5°C, (106.7°F)] and perfused for 60 to 90 minutes. Although difficult to perform and associated with complications (neutropenia, amputation, death), it does produce a high response rate (greater than 50%).[74,77-79] The introduction of tumor necrosis factor alpha or interferon-γ with melphalan results in the regression of more than 90% of cutaneous in-transit metastases.[75-77]

Although initially thought to be ineffective in the treatment of melanoma, the use of radiation therapy, regional and systemic chemotherapy, and immunotherapy are all under investigation. High-dose-per-fraction radiation produces a better response rate than low-dose large-fraction therapy.[79-81] As the treatment of choice for patients with symptomatic multiple brain metastases, radiation therapy produced measurable improvement in tumor size, symptomatology, or performance status in 70% of treated patients.[79-81]

Another promising area of nonsurgical melanoma treatment is the use of immunologic manipulation. Interferon alfa-2b is the only Food and Drug Administration–approved adjuvant treatment for AJCC stages IIB/III melanoma.[80,81] In these patients, both the relapse-free interval and overall survival were improved with use of INF-α.[80,81] Side effects were common and frequently severe; the majority of the patients required modification of the initial dosage and 24% discontinued treatment.[80,81] Immunotherapy also continues to be a field of great promise. Vaccines have been developed with the hope of stimulating the body's own immune system against the tumor. Melanoma cells contain a number of distinctly different cell-surface antigens, and monoclonal antibodies have been raised against these antigens.[80,81] These antibodies have been used alone or linked to a radioisotope or cytotoxic agent in an effort to selectively kill tumor cells. All treatments are currently investigational. One defined-antigen vaccine has entered clinical testing; the ganglioside G_{M2}. Gangliosides are carbohydrate antigens found on the surface of melanomas as well as many other tumors.[80,81]

ADDITIONAL MALIGNANCIES OF THE SKIN

Merkel Cell Carcinoma (Primary Neuroendocrine Carcinoma of the Skin)

Once thought to be a variant of SCC, Merkel cell carcinomas are actually of neuroepithelial differentiation.[82,83] These tumors are asso-

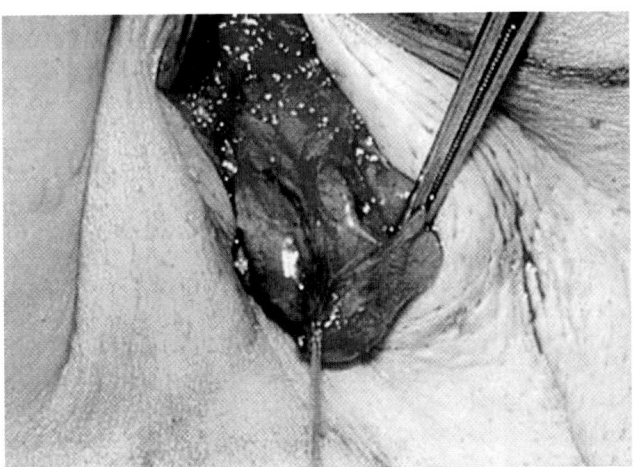

FIG. 16-15. Intraoperative view of sentinel lymph node identification during distal melanoma excision.

ciated with a synchronous or metasynchronous SCC 25% of the time. Due to their aggressive nature, wide local resection with 3-cm margins is recommended.[82,83] Local recurrence rates are high, and distant metastases occur in one third of patients. Prophylactic regional LN dissection and adjuvant radiation therapy are recommended. Overall, the prognosis is worse than for malignant melanoma.[82,83]

Kaposi's Sarcoma

Kaposi's sarcoma (KS) appears as rubbery bluish nodules that occur primarily on the extremities but may appear anywhere on the skin and viscera. These lesions are usually multifocal rather than metastatic.[84–88] Histologically, the lesions are composed of capillaries lined by atypical endothelial cells. Early lesions may resemble hemangiomas, while older lesions contain more spindle cells and resemble sarcomas.[84–86] Classically, KS is seen in people of Eastern Europe or sub-Saharan Africa. The lesions are locally aggressive but undergo periods of remission. A different variety of KS has been described for people with AIDS or with immunosuppression from chemotherapy.[84–86] For reasons not yet understood, AIDS-related KS occurs primarily in male homosexuals and not in IV drug abusers or hemophiliacs. In this form of the disease, the lesions spread rapidly to the nodes, and the GI and respiratory tract often are involved.[84–86] Development of AIDS-related KS is associated with concurrent infection with a herpes-like virus.[84–86] Treatment for all types of KS consists of radiation to the lesions. Combination chemotherapy is effective in controlling the disease, although most patients develop an opportunistic infection during or shortly after treatment. Surgical treatment is reserved for lesions that interfere with vital functions, such as bowel obstruction or airway compromise.[84–86]

Extramammary Paget's Disease

This tumor is histologically similar to the mammary type. It is a cutaneous lesion that appears as a pruritic red patch that does not resolve.[85] Biopsy demonstrates classic Paget's cells. Paget's disease is thought to be a cutaneous extension of an underlying adenocarcinoma, although an associated tumor cannot always be demonstrated.[85]

Angiosarcoma

Angiosarcomas may arise spontaneously, mostly on the scalp, face, and neck. They usually appear as a bruise that spontaneously bleeds or enlarges without trauma.[87,88] Tumors also may arise in areas of prior radiation therapy or in the setting of chronic lymphedema of the arm, such as after mastectomy (Stewart-Treves syndrome).[87,88] The angiosarcomas that arise in these areas of chronic change occur decades later. The tumors consist of anaplastic endothelial cells surrounding vascular channels. Although total excision of early lesions can provide occasional cure, the prognosis usually is poor, with 5-year survival rates of less than 20%. Chemotherapy and radiation therapy are used for palliation.[87,88]

Dermatofibrosarcoma Protuberans

Dermatofibrosarcoma protuberans (DFSP) accounts for 1 to 2% of all soft-tissue sarcomas, occurs most frequently in persons aged 20 to 50 years, and is more common in males.[88,89] The most common presenting location is on the trunk (50 to 60%), although the proximal extremities (20 to 30% of cases), as well as head and neck also are frequently affected (10 to 15%).[88,89] DFSP often appears as a pink, nodular lesion that may ulcerate and become infected. Histologically, the lesions contain atypical spindle cells, probably of fibroblast origin, located around a core of collagen tissue. Despite what appears to be complete lesion excision, local recurrence remains frequent and mortality associated with metastasis relatively high.[88,89] To date, the minimum resection margin needed to achieve local control remains undefined. Local recurrence rates of up to 50% have been reported after simple excision, and wide local excision with 3-cm margins is linked to a 20% recurrence rate. Most authorities seem to advocate a three-dimensional margin of 2 to 3 cm with

resection of skin, subcutaneous tissue, and the underlying investing fascia.[88,89] The periosteum and a portion of the bone may also need to be resected to achieve negative deep surgical margins. In addition to achieving wide macroscopic resection, conformation of negative microscopic margins is especially critical. DFSP is considered to be a radiosensitive tumor, and radiotherapy following wide local excision has reached local control rates approximating 95% at 10 years.[88,89] Continued study of chemotherapy efficacy on DFSP also has produced optimistic results. Imatinib, a selective inhibitor of platelet-derived growth factor (PDGF) β-chain alpha and PDGF receptor beta protein-tyrosine kinase activity, alters the biologic effects of deregulated PDGF receptor signaling. Clinical trials have shown activity against localized and metastatic DFSP containing the t(17:22) translocation, suggesting that targeting the PDGF receptors may become a new therapeutic option for DFSP. Phase II clinical trials are underway.[88,89]

Fibrosarcoma

Fibrosarcomas are hard, irregular masses found in the subcutaneous fat.[88,89] The fibroblasts appear markedly anaplastic with disorganized growth. If they are not excised completely, metastases usually develop. The 5-year survival rate after excision is approximately 60%.[88,89]

Liposarcoma

Liposarcomas arise in the deep muscle planes, and, rarely, from the subcutaneous tissue.[88,89] They occur most commonly on the thigh. An enlarging lipoma should be excised and inspected to distinguish it from a liposarcoma. Wide excision is the treatment of choice, with radiation therapy reserved for metastatic disease.[88,89]

SYNDROMIC SKIN MALIGNANCIES

Several genetic syndromes are associated with an increased incidence of skin malignancy. Although many are related to development of a specific lesion, others appear to produce a more generic prevalence for neoplastic formation. Based on their respective genetic defects, syndromes associated with BCC, SCC, and melanoma have all been identified and well described. Diseases linked with BCC include the basal cell nevus (Gorlin's) syndrome and nevus sebaceus of Jadassohn.[90–92] Basal cell nevus syndrome is an autosomal dominant disorder characterized by the growth of hundreds of BCCs during young adulthood. Palmar and plantar pits are a common physical finding and represent foci of neoplasms.[90–92] Treatment is limited to excision of only aggressive and symptomatic lesions. Nevus sebaceus of Jadassohn is a lesion containing several cutaneous tissue elements that develops during childhood.[90–92] This lesion is associated with a variety of neoplasms of the epidermis, but most commonly BCC. Diseases associated with SCC may have a causative role in the development of carcinoma. Skin diseases that cause chronic wounds, such as epidermolysis bullosus and lupus erythematosus, are associated with a high incidence of SCC.[90–92] Epidermodysplasia verruciformis is a rare autosomal recessive disease associated with infection with HPV. Large verrucous lesions develop early in life and often progress to invasive SCC in middle age.[90–92] Xeroderma pigmentosum is an autosomal recessive disease associated with a defect in cellular repair of DNA damage. The inability of the skin to correct DNA damage from UV radiation leaves these patients prone to cutaneous malignancies.[90–92] SCCs are most frequent, but BCCs, melanomas, and even acute leukemias are seen. Dysplastic nevi are considered precursors to melanoma. Familial dysplastic nevus syndrome is an autosomal dominant disorder.[90–92] Patients develop multiple dysplastic nevi, and longitudinal studies have demonstrated an almost 100% incidence of melanoma. Gene mapping of the defects found in familial dysplastic nevus syndrome has identified several candidate "melanoma" genes.[90–94] It remains to be determined whether these germline mutations also are found in sporadic cases of melanoma. Much like other familial malignancy syndromes, genetic analysis of the hereditary defect may shed much needed light on the molecular mechanisms that lead to malignant transformation. Much like familial polyposis coli and the association with colon cancer, familial dysplastic nevus syndrome is treated by close surveillance and frequent biopsy of all suspicious lesions. Similarly, the development of colon cancer can be arrested with total proctocolectomy; unfortunately, a similar solution is not possible in patients with familial dysplastic nevi.[90–94]

FUTURE DEVELOPMENTS IN SKIN SURGERY

The last decade has seen unprecedented advances in our understanding of the skin and its pathology as well as our ability to protect and replace it. Autologous skin grafts remain the best method to cover skin defects, but donor-site problems and limited availability of autologous skin remain problematic.[95–98] Tissue expansion with subcutaneous balloon implants produces new epidermis, and mobilization achieved via expansion remains a highly effective approach to wound coverage.[95–98] Still, optimal wound coverage lies in the development of engineered skin replacements. Current research is directed at identifying different materials and cells that can be used to replace both epidermis and dermis.

Several dermal replacements based on synthetic materials or cadaveric sources are in clinical use (Fig. 16-16). A bovine-collagen and shark-proteoglycan–based dermis (Integra) has been used primarily in burn patients for more than a decade.[95–98] This prosthetic dermis, available in ready-to-use form, can cover large surface areas. Vascularization of this dermis takes 2 to 3 weeks, and final epidermal coverage of the wound requires a thin skin graft.[95–98] The final result is functionally and aesthetically good, but the high cost has been problematic. Cadaveric dermis, with all of the cellular elements removed, is not antigenic and is not rejected by the recipient patient.[95–98] This human dermal matrix is commercially-available (AlloDerm) and functions much like Integra, with similar limitations of engraftment and high cost. Both forms of dermal replacements are more frequently used in delayed reconstruction of burn patients than in the acute setting.[95–98]

Another issue confounding surgeons is the lack of means to quickly provide numerous autologous skin cells for permanent skin replacement. The expansion of epidermis by the growth and maturation of keratinocytes in culture is readily performed.[95–98] A small skin biopsy specimen can produce enough autologous epithelium to cover the entire body surface. However, on the body, the cultured epidermis often blisters and sloughs as a consequence of slow restoration of the basement membrane. Improving the durability of

these cells may one day negate autologous skin grafting technique or the requirement for cadaveric soft tissues. In addition, as more is learned about the protein factors that control wound healing and tissue growth, the replacement for damaged skin will eventually come from complete organogenesis of tissue.[95–98] Characterization of these growth factors on a structural and functional level is progressing rapidly. Factors have been isolated that cause specific mesenchymal cells to proliferate, migrate, and organize into structures such as capillaries or even rudimentary organoid tissue.[95–98]

CONCLUSION

Anatomically, the epidermal, basement membrane, and dermal layers of the skin each play a vital role in maintaining dermal/epidermal integrity. Multiple, complex mechanisms within these soft tissues protect us from injury as well as relay external information along a vast neural network. In addition to penetrating trauma, the environment offers a host of potentially injurious elements such as caustic substances, extreme temperatures, prolonged or excessive pressure, and radiation. Infections ranging from simple bacterial to necrotizing, life-threatening disease may also affect the skin and subcutaneous tissues. Perhaps of greatest public concern, a multitude of benign and malignant tumors threaten to disrupt, disfigure, and invade normal skin structure. Although the risks associated with many of these lesions are great, a broad variety of medical and surgical management options currently exist. Although contemporary medicine may not have an optimal answer for each threat the skin may face, continued research, advances in our understanding, and technical improvements in the field promise to enhance our ability to replace and protect the skin well into the future.

REFERENCES

Entries highlighted in bright blue are key references

1. Byrne C, Hardman M, Nield K: Covering the limb—Formation of the integument. *J Anat* 202:113, 2003.
2. Ballantyne D, Converse J: *Experimental Skin Grafts and Transplantation Immunity*. New York: Springer-Verlag, 1979.
3. Nemes Z, Steinert PM: Bricks and mortar of the epidermal barrier. *Exp Mol Med* 31:5, 1999.
4. Flaxman BA, Sosio AC, Van Scott EJ: Changes in melanosome distribution in Caucasoid skin following topical application of N-mustard. *J Invest Dermatol* 60:321, 1973.
5. Halaban R: The regulation of normal melanocyte proliferation. *Pigment Cell Res* 13:4, 2000.
6. Fuchs E, Cleveland DW: A structural scaffolding of intermediate filaments in health and disease. *Science* 279:514, 1998.
7. Meigel WN, Gay S, Weber L: Dermal architecture and collagen type distribution. *Arch Dermatol Res* 259:1, 1977.
8. Madoff LC: Infectious complications of bites and burns, in Braunwald E, Fauci AS, Kasper DL, et al (eds): *Harrison's Principles of Internal Medicine*, 15th ed. New York: McGraw Hill, 2001, p 817.
9. Presutti RJ: Bite wounds: Early treatment and prophylaxis against infectious complications. *Postgrad Med* 101:243, 1997.
10. Halikis MN, Taleisnik J: Soft-tissue injuries of the wrist. *Clin Sports Med* 15:235, 1996.
11. Leonard LG, Scheulen JJ, Munster AM: Chemical burns: Effect of prompt first aid. *J Trauma* 22:420, 1982.
12. Herbert K, Lawrence JC: Chemical burns. *Burns* 15:381, 1989.
13. Andrews K, Mowlavi A, Milner SM: The treatment of alkaline burns of the skin by neutralization. *Plast Reconstr Surg* 111:1618, 2003.
14. Matsuno K: The treatment of hydrofluoric acid burns. *Occup Med* 46:313, 1996.
15. Anderson WJ, Anderson JR: Hydrofluoric acid burns of the hand: Mechanism of injury and treatment. *J Hand Surg* 13:52, 1988.
16. Khan MS, Holmes JD: Reducing the morbidity from extravasation injuries. *Ann Plast Surg* 48:628, 2002.
17. Kumar RJ, Pegg SP, Kimble RM: Management of extravasation injuries. *ANZ J Surg* 71:285, 2001.

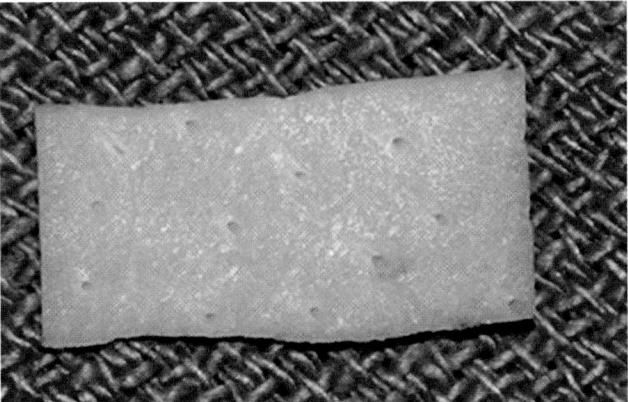

FIG. 16-16. The most recent generation of dermal matrix replacement tissues includes both cadaveric and xenographic materials. AlloDerm (pictured here) may be placed over various deeper tissues to provide a dermal scaffold onto which autologous skin may be grafted.

18. Goolsby TV, Lombardo FA: Extravasation of chemotherapeutic agents: prevention and treatment. *Semin Oncol* 33:139, 2006.

19. Sakallioglu AE, Haberal M: Current approach to burn critical care. *Minerva Med* 98:569, 2007.

20. Pereira C, Gold W, Herndon D: Review paper: Burn coverage technologies: Current concepts and future directions. *J Biomater Appl* 22:101, 2007.

21. Biem J, Koehncke N, Classen D, et al: Out of the cold: Management of hypothermia and frostbite. *CMAJ* 168:305, 2003.

22. Murphy JV, Banwell PE, Roberts AHN, et al: Frostbite: Pathogenesis and treatment. *J Trauma* 48:171, 2000.

23. Nola GT, Vistnes LM: Differential response of skin and muscle in the experimental production of pressure sores. *Plast Reconstr Surg* 66:728, 1980.

24. Thomas DR: Pressure ulcers, in Cassel CK, Cohen HJ, Larson EB, et al (eds): *Geriatric Medicine*, 3rd ed. New York: Springer, 1997, p 767.

25. Goode PS, Allman RM: Pressure ulcers, in Duthie EH Jr., Katz PR (eds): *Practice of Geriatrics*, 3rd ed. Philadelphia: WB Saunders, 1998, p 228.

26. Gottlober P, Steinert M, Weiss M, et al: The outcome of local radiation injuries: 14 years of follow-up after the Chernobyl accident. *Radiat Res* 155:409, 2001.

27. Poh-Fitzpatrick MB: The biologic actions of solar radiation on skin, with a note on sunscreens. *J Dermatol Surg* 3:169, 1977.

28. Mao J, Fatunase OA, Marks LB: Cytoprotection for radiation-associated normal tissue injury. *Cancer Treat Res* 139:307, 2008.

29. Smart RC: Radiation protection in Australia: A thirty year perspective. *Australas Phys Eng Sci Med* 30:155, 2007.

30. Cunningham JD, Silver L, Rudikoff D: Necrotizing fasciitis: A plea for early diagnosis and treatment. *Mt Sinai J Med* 68:253, 2001.

31. Yuen KY, Ma L, Wong SSY, et al: Fatal necrotizing fasciitis due to *Vibrio damsela*. *Scand J Infect Dis* 25:659, 1993.

32. Cainzos M, Gonzalez-Rodriguez FJ: Necrotizing soft tissue infections. *Curr Opin Crit Care* 13:433, 2007.

33. Brown TJ, Rosen T, Orengo IF: Hidradenitis suppurativa. *South Med J* 91:1107, 1998.

34. Slade DE, Powell BW, Mortimer PS: Hidradenitis suppurativa: Pathogenesis and management. *Br J Plast Surg* 56:451, 2003.

35. Miller M, Haddad AJ: Cervicofacial actinomycosis. *Oral Surg Oral Med Oral Pathol Oral Radiol Endod* 83:496, 1998.

36. Nielsen PM, Novak A: Acute cervicofacial actinomycosis. *Int J Oral Maxillofac Surg* 16:440, 1987.

37. Brentjens MH, Yeung-Yue KA, Lee PC, et al: Human papillomavirus: A review. *Dermatol Clin* 20:315, 2002.

38. Welch JL, Edison KE: Treatment options for the common wart. *Mo Med* 104:502, 2007.

39. Davis PA, Corless DJ, Gazzard BG, et al: Increased risk of wound complications and poor wound healing following laparotomy in HIV-seropositive and AIDS patients. *Dis Surg* 16:60, 1999.

40. Eriguchi M, Takeda Y, Yoshizaki I, et al: Surgery in patients with HIV infection: Indications and outcome. *Biomed Pharmacother* 51:474, 1997.

41. Luck JV Jr.: Orthopaedic surgery on the HIV-positive patient: Complications and outcome. *Instr Course Lect* 43:543, 1994.

42. Davis PA, Wastell C: A comparison of biomechanical properties of excised mature scars from HIV patients and non-HIV controls. *Am J Surg* 180:217, 2000.

43. Brunsting LA, Goeckerman WH, O'Leary PA: Pyoderma (ecthyma) gangrenosum—clinical and experimental observations in five cases occurring in adults. *Arch Dermatol* 22:655, 1930.

44. Von Den Driesch P: Pyoderma gangrenosum: A report of 44 cases with follow-up. *Br J Dermatol* 137:1000, 1997.

45. Wollina U: Clinical management of pyoderma gangrenosum. *Am J Clin Dermatol* 3:149, 2002.

46. Patel GK, Finlay AY: Staphylococcal scalded skin syndrome: Diagnosis and management. *Am J Clin Dermatol* 4:165, 2003.

47. Atiyeh BS, Dham R, Yassin MF, et al: Treatment of toxic epidermal necrolysis with moisture-retentive ointment: A case report and review of the literature. *Dermatol Surg* 29:185, 2003.

48. Mackie RM: Epidermoid cyst, in Champion RH, Burton JL, Burns DA, et al (eds): *Rook/Wilkinson/Ebling Textbook of Dermatology*, vol. 2, 6th ed. Oxford: Blackwell Science, 1998, p 1666.

49. Szeremeta W, Parikh TD, Widelitz JS: Congenital nasal malformations. *Otolaryngol Clin North Am.* 40:97, 2007.

50. Satyaprakash AK, Sheehan DJ, Sangüeza OP: Proliferating trichilemmal tumors: A review of the literature. *Dermatol Surg* 33:1102, 2007.

51. Braun RP, Rabinovitz H, Oliviero M, et al: Dermoscopic diagnosis of seborrheic keratosis. *Clin Dermatol* 20:270, 2002.

52. Fu W, Cockerell CJ: The actinic (solar) keratosis. *Arch Dermatol* 139:66, 2003.

53. Robins P, Gupta AK: The use of topical fluorouracil to treat actinic keratosis. *Cutis* 70:4, 2002.

54. Castilla EE, DaGraca-Dutra M, Orioli-Parreiras IM: Epidemiology of congenital pigmented nevi: I. Incidence rates and relative frequencies. *Br J Dermatol* 104:307, 1981.

55. Rhodes AR, Melsk JW: Small congenital nevocellular nevi and the risk of cutaneous melanoma. *J Pediatr* 100:216, 1982.

56. Schaffer JV. Pigmented lesions in children: When to worry. *Curr Opin Pediatr* 16:430, 2007.

57. Krengel S, Hauschild A, Schäfer T: Melanoma risk in congenital melanocytic naevi: A systematic review. *Br J Dermatol* 155:1, 2006.

58. Fishman SJ, Mulliken JB: Hemangiomas and vascular malformations of infancy and childhood. *Pediatr Clin North Am* 40:1177, 1993.

59. Sadan N, Wolach B: Treatment of hemangiomas of infants with high doses of prednisone. *J Pediatr* 128:141, 1996.

60. Marler JJ, Mulliken JB: Vascular anomalies: Classification, diagnosis, and natural history. *Facial Plast Surg Clin North Am* 9:495, 2001.

61. Garzon MC, Huang JT, Enjolras O, et al: Vascular malformations: Part I. *J Am Acad Dermatol* 56:353, 2007.

62. Legiehn GM, Heran MK: Classification, diagnosis, and interventional radiologic management of vascular malformations. *Orthop Clin North Am* 37:435, 2006.

63. McDermott EM, Weiss AP: Glomus tumors. *J Hand Surg [Am]* 31:1397, 2006.

64. Mentzel T: Cutaneous lipomatous neoplasms. *Semin Diagn Pathol* 18:250, 2001.

65. Marks R, Kopf AW: Cancer of the skin in the next century. *Int J Dermatol* 34:445, 1995.

66. Luce EA: Oncologic considerations in nonmelanotic skin cancer. *Clin Plast Surg* 22:39, 1995.

67. Epstein JH: Photocarcinogenesis, skin cancer, and aging. *J Am Acad Dermatol* 9:487, 1983.

68. Sober AJ, Burstein JM: Precursors to skin cancer. *Cancer* 75:645, 1995.

69. Gallagher RP, Hill GB, Bajdik CD, et al: Sunlight exposure, pigmentation factors, and risk of nonmelanocytic skin cancer: II. Squamous cell carcinoma. *Arch Dermatol* 131:164, 1995.

70. Fleming ID, Amonette R, Monaghan T, et al: Principles of management of basal and squamous cell carcinoma of the skin. *Cancer* 75(Suppl 2):699, 1995.

71. Friedman HI, Cooper PH, Wanebo HJ: Prognostic and therapeutic use of microstaging of cutaneous squamous cell carcinomas of the trunk and extremities. *Cancer* 56:109, 1985.

72. Mohs FE: *Chemosurgery, Microscopically Controlled Surgery for Skin Cancer*. Springfield: Charles C Thomas, 1978.

73. Desmond RA, Soong S-J: Epidemiology of malignant melanoma. *Surg Clin North Am* 83:1, 2003.

74. Balch CM, Buzaid AC, Soong SJ, et al: Final version of the American Joint Committee on Cancer staging system for cutaneous melanoma. *J Clin Oncol* 16:3635, 2001.

75. Balch CM, Soong SJ, Gershenwald JE, et al: Prognostic factors analysis of 17,600 melanoma patients: Validation of the American Joint Committee on Cancer melanoma staging system. *J Clin Oncol* 16:3622, 2001.

76. Essner R: Surgical treatment of malignant melanoma. *Surg Clin North Am* 83:109, 2003.

77. Leong SPL: Selective lymphadenectomy for malignant melanoma. *Surg Clin North Am* 83:157, 2003.

78. Lee ML, Tomsu K, Von Eschen KB: Duration of survival for disseminated malignant melanoma: Results of a meta-analysis. *Melanoma Res* 10:81, 2000.

79. Karakousis CP, Velez A, Driscoll DL, et al: Metastasectomy in malignant melanoma. *Surgery* 115:295, 1994.

80. Kirkwood JM, Strawderman MH, Ernstoff MS, et al: Interferon alfa-2b adjuvant therapy of high-risk resected cutaneous melanoma: The Eastern Cooperative Oncology Group trial EST 1684. *J Clin Oncol* 14:7, 1996.

81. Kadison AS, Morton DL: Immunotherapy of malignant melanoma. *Surg Clin North Am* 83:343, 2003.

82. O'Connor WJ, Brodland DG: Merkel cell carcinoma. *Dermatol Surg* 22:262, 1996.

83. Chanda JJ: Extramammary Paget's disease: Prognosis and relationship to internal malignancy. *J Am Acad Dermatol* 13:1009, 1985.

84. Noel JC, Hermans P: Herpes virus-like DNA sequence and Kaposi's sarcoma: Relationship with epidemiology, clinical spectrum, and histologic features. *Cancer* 77:2132, 1996.

85. Szajerka T, Jablecki JL: Kaposi's sarcoma revisited. *AIDS Rev* 9:230, 2007.

86. Angeletti PC, Zhang L, Wood C: The viral etiology of AIDS-associated malignancies. *Adv Pharmacol* 56:509, 2008.

87. Skubitz KM, D'Adamo DR: Sarcoma. *Mayo Clin Proc* 82:1409, 2007.

88. McArthur G: Dermatofibrosarcoma protuberans: Recent clinical progress. *Ann Surg Oncol* 14:2876, 2007.

89. Korkolis DP, Liapakis IE, Vassilopoulos PP: Dermatofibrosarcoma protuberans: Clinicopathological aspects of an unusual cutaneous tumor. *Anticancer Res* 27:1631, 2007.

90. Miettinen M: From morphological to molecular diagnosis of soft tissue tumors. *Adv Exp Med Biol* 587:99, 2006.

91. Wolf K, Friedl P: Molecular mechanisms of cancer cell invasion and plasticity. *Br J Dermatol* 154(Suppl 1):11, 2006.

92. Barbagallo JS, Kolodzieh MS, Silverberg NB, et al: Neurocutaneous disorders. *Dermatol Clin* 20:547, 2002.

93. Goyal JL, Rao VA, Srinivasan R, et al: Oculocutaneous manifestations in xeroderma pigmentosa. *Br J Ophthalmol* 78:295, 1994.

94. Somoano B, Tsao H: Genodermatoses with cutaneous tumors and internal malignancies. *Dermatol Clin.* 26:69, 2008.

95. Ryan CM, Schoenfeld DA, Malloy M, et al: Use of Integra artificial skin is associated with decreased length of stay for severely injured adult burn survivors. *J Burn Care Rehabil* 23:311, 2002.

96. Terino EO: AlloDerm acellular dermal graft: Applications in aesthetic soft-tissue augmentation. *Clin Plast Surg* 28:83, 2001.

97. Klein MB, Chang J, Young DM: Update on skin replacements, in Habal M (ed): *Advances in Plastic and Reconstructive Surgery*. New York: Mosby, 1998, p 223.

98. Nunez-Gutierrez H, Castro-Munozledo F, Kuri-Harcuch W: Combined use of allograft and autograft epidermal cultures in therapy of burns. *Plast Reconstr Surg* 98:929, 1996.

The Breast

Kelly K. Hunt, Lisa A. Newman,
Edward M. Copeland III, and Kirby I. Bland

A BRIEF HISTORY OF BREAST CANCER THERAPY

Breast cancer, with its uncertain cause, has captured the attention of surgeons throughout the ages. Despite centuries of theoretical meandering and scientific inquiry, breast cancer remains one of the most dreaded of human diseases.[1–12] The story of efforts to cope with breast cancer is complex, and there is no successful conclusion as in diseases for which cause and cure are known. However, progress has been made in lessening the horrors that formerly devastated the body and psyche. Currently, 50% of American women will consult a surgeon regarding breast disease, 25% will undergo breast biopsy, and 12% will develop some variant of breast cancer.

The Smith Surgical Papyrus (3000–2500 B.C.) is the earliest known document to refer to breast cancer. The cancer was in a man, but the description encompassed most of the common clinical features. In reference to this cancer, the author concluded, "There is no treatment."[1] There were few other historical references to breast cancer until the first century. In *De Medicina,* Celsus commented on the value of operations for early breast cancer: "None of these may be removed but the cacoethes (early cancer), the rest are irritated by every method of cure. The more violent the operations are, the more angry they grow."[2] In the second century, Galen inscribed his classical clinical observation: "We have often seen in the breast a tumor exactly resembling the animal the crab. Just as the crab has legs on both sides of his body, so in this disease the veins extending out from the unnatural growth take the shape of a crab's legs. We have often cured this disease in its early stages, but after it has reached a large size, no one has cured it. In all operations we attempt to excise the tumor in a circle where it borders on the healthy tissue."[3]

The galenic system of medicine ascribed cancers to an excess of black bile and concluded that excision of a local bodily outbreak could not cure the systemic imbalance. Theories espoused by Galen dominated medicine until the Renaissance. The majority of respected surgeons considered operative intervention to be a futile and ill-advised endeavor. However, beginning with Morgagni, surgical resections were more frequently undertaken, including some early attempts at mastectomy and axillary dissection. Le Dran repudiated Galen's humoral theory in the eighteenth century and stated that breast cancer was a local disease that spread by way of lymph vessels to axillary lymph nodes. When operating on a woman with breast cancer, he routinely removed any enlarged axillary lymph nodes.[5]

In the nineteenth century, Moore, of the Middlesex Hospital, London, emphasized complete resection of the breast for cancer and stated that palpable axillary lymph nodes also should be removed.[11] In a presentation before the British Medical Association in 1877, Banks supported Moore's concepts and advocated the resection of axillary lymph nodes even when palpable lymphadenopathy was not evident, recognizing that occult involvement of axillary lymph nodes was frequently present. In 1894, Halsted and Meyer reported their operations for treatment of breast cancer.[4] By demonstrating superior local-regional control rates after radical resection, these surgeons established radical mastectomy as state-of-the-art treatment for that era. Both Halsted and Meyer advocated complete dissection of axillary lymph node levels I to III. Both routinely resected the long thoracic nerve and the thoracodorsal neurovascular bundle with the axillary contents.

In 1943, Haagensen and Stout described the grave signs of breast cancer, which included (a) edema of the skin of the breast, (b) skin ulceration, (c) chest wall fixation, (d) an axillary lymph node >2.5 cm in diameter, and (e) fixed axillary lymph nodes. Women with two or more signs had a 42% local recurrence rate and only a 2% 5-year disease-free survival rate.[6] Based on these findings, they declared that women with grave signs were beyond cure by radical surgery. Approximately 25% of women were excluded from surgery based on these criteria of inoperability. Today, with comprehensive mammography screening, only 10% of women are found to have such advanced breast cancers. In 1948, Patey and Dyson of the Middlesex Hospital, London, advocated a modified radical mastectomy for the management of advanced operable breast cancer, explaining, "Until an effective general agent for treatment of carcinoma of the breast is developed, a high proportion of these cases are doomed to die."[12] Their technique included removal of the breast and axillary lymph nodes with preservation of the pectoralis major muscle. They showed that removal of the pectoralis minor muscle allowed access to and clearance of axillary lymph node levels I to III. Subsequently, Madden advocated a modified radical mastectomy that preserved both the pectoralis major and pectoralis minor muscles, even though this approach prevented complete dissection of the apical (level III) axillary lymph nodes.[7]

In the 1970s, there was a transition from the Halsted radical mastectomy to the modified radical mastectomy as the surgical procedure most frequently used by American surgeons to treat breast cancer. This transition acknowledged that (a) extirpation of the pectoralis major muscle was not essential for local-regional control in stage I and stage II breast cancer, and (b) neither the modified radical mastectomy nor the Halsted radical mastectomy consistently achieved local-regional control of stage III breast cancer. The National Surgical Adjuvant Breast and Bowel Project (NSABP) B-04 trial conducted by Fisher and colleagues compared local and regional treatments of breast cancer. Life table estimates were obtained for 1665 women enrolled and followed for a mean of 120 months (Fig. 17-1). This study randomly divided clinically node-negative women into three treatment groups: (a) Halsted radical mastectomy; (b) total mastectomy plus radiation therapy; and (c) total mastectomy alone. Clinically node-positive women were treated with Halsted radical mastectomy or total mastectomy plus radiation therapy. This trial accrued patients between 1971 and 1974, an era that predated widespread availability of effective systemic therapy for breast cancer. Outcomes from this trial therefore reflect survival associated with local-regional therapy only. There were no differences in survival between the three groups of node-negative women or between the two groups of node-positive women (see Fig. 17-1A). Correspondingly, there were no differences in survival during the

CHAPTER 17 The Breast

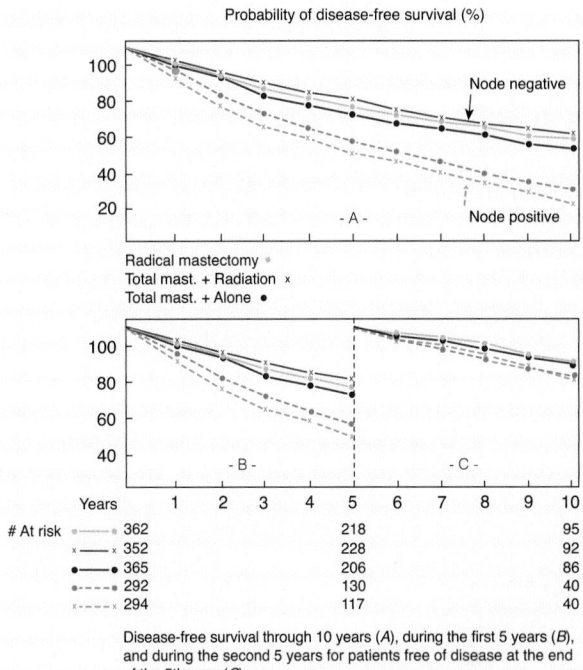

FIG. 17-1. Results of the National Surgical Adjuvant Breast and Bowel Project B-04 trial. Disease-free survival for women treated by radical mastectomy (*orange circles*), total mastectomy plus radiation (*x's*), or total mastectomy alone (*blue circles*). (*Reproduced with permission from Fisher B, et al: Ten-year results of a randomized clinical trial comparing radical mastectomy and total mastectomy with or without radiation.* N Engl J Med 312:674, 1985. Copyright © Massachusetts Medical Society. All rights reserved.)

KEY POINTS

1. The breast receives its principal blood supply from perforating branches of the internal mammary artery, lateral branches of the posterior intercostal arteries, and branches from the axillary artery, including the highest thoracic, lateral thoracic, and pectoral branches of the thoracoacromial artery.

2. The axillary lymph nodes usually receive >75% of the lymph drainage from the breast, and the rest flows through the lymph vessels that accompany the perforating branches of the internal mammary artery and enters the parasternal (internal mammary) group of lymph nodes.

3. Breast development and function are initiated by a variety of hormonal stimuli, with the major trophic effects being modulated by estrogen, progesterone, and prolactin.

4. Benign breast disorders and diseases are related to the normal processes of reproductive life and to involution, and there is a spectrum of breast conditions that ranges from normal to disorder to disease (aberrations of normal development and involution classification).

5. To calculate breast cancer risk using the Gail model, a woman's risk factors are translated into an overall risk score by multiplying her relative risks from several categories. This risk score is then compared with an adjusted population risk of breast cancer to determine the woman's individual risk. This model is not appropriate for use in women with a known *BRCA1* or *BRCA2* mutation or women with lobular or ductal carcinoma in situ.

6. Routine use of screening mammography in women ≥50 years of age reduces mortality from breast cancer by 33%.

7. Core-needle biopsy is the preferred method for diagnosis of palpable or nonpalpable breast abnormalities.

8. When a diagnosis of breast cancer is made, the surgeon should determine the clinical stage, histologic characteristics, and appropriate biomarker levels before initiating local therapy.

9. Sentinel node dissection is the preferred method for staging of the regional lymph nodes in women with clinically node-negative invasive breast cancer.

10. Local-regional and systemic therapy decisions for an individual patient with breast cancer are best made using a multidisciplinary treatment approach.

first and second 5-year follow-up periods (see Fig. 17-1B and 17-1C). These overall survival equivalence patterns have persisted at 25 years of follow-up.[13]

Other prospective clinical trials that compared the Halsted radical mastectomy to the modified radical mastectomy were the Manchester trial, reported by Turner and colleagues, and the University of Alabama trial, reported by Maddox and colleagues.[8,9] In both studies, the type of surgical procedure did not influence recurrence rates for patients with stage I and stage II breast cancer. The criterion for accrual to the Alabama Breast Cancer Project (1975 to 1978) was a T1 to T3 breast cancer with no apparent distant metastases. Patients received a radical or a modified radical mastectomy. Node-positive patients received adjuvant cyclophosphamide (Cytoxan), methotrexate, and 5-fluorouracil chemotherapy or adjuvant melphalan. After a median follow-up period of 15 years, neither type of surgery nor type of chemotherapy was shown to affect local-regional, disease-free, or overall survival.[8] Since the 1970s, considerable progress has been made in the integration of surgery, radiation therapy, and chemotherapy to control local-regional disease, enhance survival, and increase the possibility of breast conservation. Local-regional control is achieved for nearly 80% of women with advanced breast cancers.

EMBRYOLOGY AND FUNCTIONAL ANATOMY OF THE BREAST

Embryology

At the fifth or sixth week of fetal development, two ventral bands of thickened ectoderm (mammary ridges, milk lines) are evident in the embryo.[14] In most mammals, paired breasts develop along these ridges, which extend from the base of the forelimb (future axilla) to the region of the hind limb (inguinal area). These ridges are not prominent in the human embryo and disappear after a short time, except for small portions that may persist in the pectoral region. Accessory breasts (*polymastia*) or accessory nipples (*polythelia*) may occur along the milk line (Fig. 17-2) when normal regression fails. Each breast develops when an ingrowth of ectoderm forms a primary tissue bud in the mesenchyme. The primary bud, in turn, initiates the development of 15 to 20 secondary buds. Epithelial cords develop from the secondary buds and extend into the surrounding mesenchyme. Major (lactiferous) ducts develop, which open into a shallow mammary pit. During infancy, a proliferation of mesenchyme transforms the mammary pit into a nipple. If there is failure of a pit to elevate above skin level, an inverted nipple results. This congenital malformation occurs in 4% of infants. At birth, the breasts are identical in males and females, demonstrating only the presence of major ducts. Enlargement of the breast may be evident and a secretion, referred to as *witch's milk,* may be produced. These transitory events occur in response to maternal hormones that cross the placenta.

The breast remains undeveloped in the female until puberty, when it enlarges in response to ovarian estrogen and progesterone, which initiate proliferation of the epithelial and connective tissue elements. However, the breasts remain incompletely developed until pregnancy occurs. Absence of the breast (*amastia*) is rare and results from an arrest in mammary ridge development that occurs during the sixth fetal week. Poland's syndrome consists of hypoplasia or complete absence of the breast, costal cartilage and rib defects, hypoplasia of the subcutaneous tissues of the chest wall, and brachysyndactyly. Breast hypoplasia also may be iatrogenically induced before puberty by trauma, infection, or radiation therapy. *Symmastia* is a rare anomaly recognized as webbing between the breasts across the midline. Accessory nipples (polythelia) occur in <1% of infants and may be associated with abnormalities of the urinary tract (renal agenesis and cancer), abnormalities of the cardiovascular system (conduction disturbances, hypertension, congenital heart anomalies), and other conditions (pyloric stenosis, epilepsy, ear

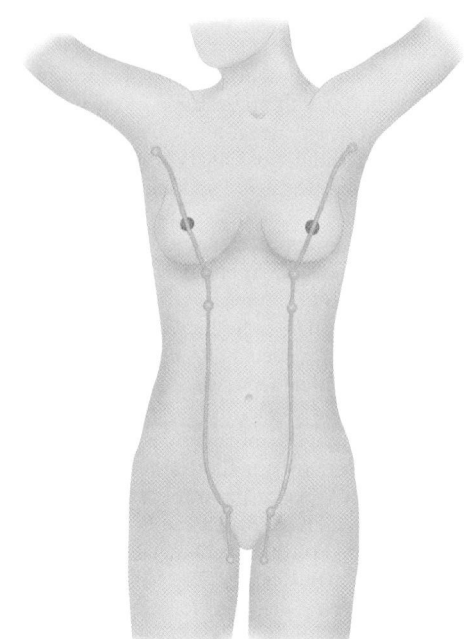

FIG. 17-2. The mammary milk line. *(Reproduced with permission from Bland et al,[14] p 214. Copyright Elsevier.)*

abnormalities, arthrogryposis). Supernumerary breasts may occur in any configuration along the mammary milk line but most frequently occur between the normal nipple location and the symphysis pubis. Turner's syndrome (ovarian agenesis and dysgenesis) and Fleischer's syndrome (displacement of the nipples and bilateral renal hypoplasia) may have polymastia as a component. Accessory axillary breast tissue is uncommon and usually is bilateral.

Functional Anatomy

The breast is composed of 15 to 20 lobes (Fig. 17-3), which are each composed of several lobules.[15] Fibrous bands of connective tissue travel through the breast (Cooper's suspensory ligaments), insert perpendicularly into the dermis, and provide structural support. The mature female breast extends from the level of the second or third rib to the inframammary fold at the sixth or seventh rib. It extends transversely from the lateral border of the sternum to the anterior axillary line. The deep or posterior surface of the breast rests on the fascia of the pectoralis major, serratus anterior, and external oblique abdominal muscles, and the upper extent of the rectus sheath. The retromammary bursa may be identified on the posterior aspect of the breast between the investing fascia of the breast and the fascia of the pectoralis major muscles. The axillary tail of Spence extends laterally across the anterior axillary fold. The upper outer quadrant of the breast contains a greater volume of tissue than do the other quadrants. The breast has a protuberant conical form. The base of the cone is roughly circular, measuring 10 to 12 cm in diameter. Considerable variations in the size, contour, and density of the breast are evident among individuals. The nulliparous breast has a hemispheric configuration with distinct flattening above the nipple. With the hormonal stimulation that accompanies pregnancy and lactation, the breast becomes larger and increases in volume and density, whereas with senescence, it assumes a flattened, flaccid, and more pendulous configuration with decreased volume.

Nipple-Areola Complex

The epidermis of the nipple-areola complex is pigmented and is variably corrugated. During puberty, the pigment becomes darker and the nipple assumes an elevated configuration. During pregnancy, the areola enlarges and pigmentation is further enhanced. The areola

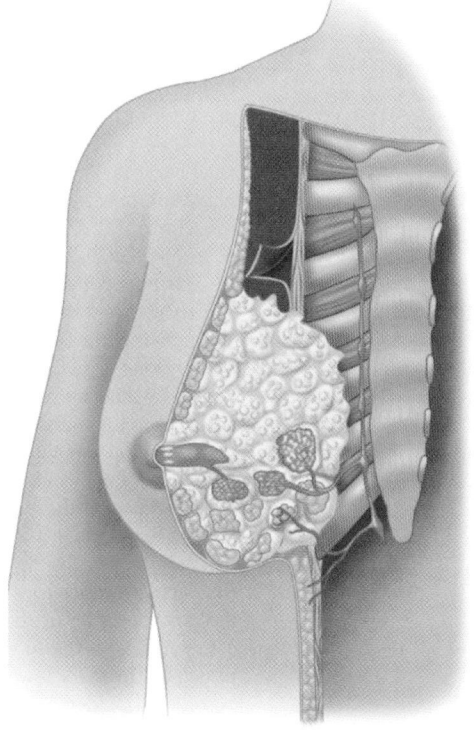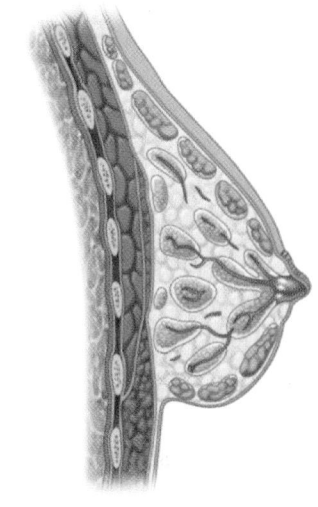

FIG. 17-3. Anatomy of the breast. Tangential and cross-sectional (sagittal) views of the breast and associated chest wall. *(Reproduced with permission from Romrell et al,[15] p 20. Copyright Elsevier.)*

contains sebaceous glands, sweat glands, and accessory glands, which produce small elevations on the surface of the areola (Montgomery's tubercles). Smooth muscle bundle fibers, which lie circumferentially in the dense connective tissue and longitudinally along the major ducts, extend upward into the nipple, where they are responsible for the nipple erection that occurs with various sensory stimuli. The dermal papilla at the tip of the nipple contains numerous sensory nerve endings and Meissner's corpuscles. This rich sensory innervation is of functional importance, because the sucking of the infant initiates a chain of neurohumoral events that results in milk letdown.

Inactive and Active Breast

Each lobe of the breast terminates in a major (lactiferous) duct (2 to 4 mm in diameter), which opens through a constricted orifice (0.4 to 0.7 mm in diameter) into the ampulla of the nipple (see Fig. 17-3). Immediately below the nipple-areola complex, each major duct has a dilated portion (lactiferous sinus), which is lined with stratified squamous epithelium. Major ducts are lined with two layers of cuboidal cells, whereas minor ducts are lined with a single layer of columnar or cuboidal cells. Myoepithelial cells of ectodermal origin reside between the epithelial cells in the basal lamina and contain myofibrils. In the inactive breast, the epithelium is sparse and consists primarily of ductal epithelium (Fig. 17-4). In the early phase of the menstrual cycle, minor ducts are cord-like with small lumina. With estrogen stimulation at the time of ovulation, alveolar epithelium increases in height, duct lumina become more prominent, and some secretions accumulate. When the hormonal stimulation decreases, the alveolar epithelium regresses.

With pregnancy, the breast undergoes proliferative and developmental maturation. As the breast enlarges in response to hormonal stimulation, lymphocytes, plasma cells, and eosinophils accumulate within the connective tissues. The minor ducts branch and alveoli develop. Development of the alveoli is asymmetric, and variations in the degree of development may occur within a single lobule (Fig. 17-5). With parturition, enlargement of the breasts occurs via hypertrophy of alveolar epithelium and accumulation of secretory products in the lumina of the minor ducts. Alveolar epithelium contains

abundant endoplasmic reticulum, large mitochondria, Golgi complexes, and dense lysosomes. Two distinct substances are produced by the alveolar epithelium: (a) the protein component of milk, which is synthesized in the endoplasmic reticulum (merocrine secretion); and (b) the lipid component of milk (apocrine secretion), which forms as free lipid droplets in the cytoplasm. Milk released in the first few days after parturition is called *colostrum* and has low lipid content but contains considerable quantities of antibodies. The lymphocytes and plasma cells that accumulate within the connective tissues of the breast are the source of the antibody component. With subsequent reduction in the number of these cells, the production of colostrum decreases and lipid-rich milk is released.

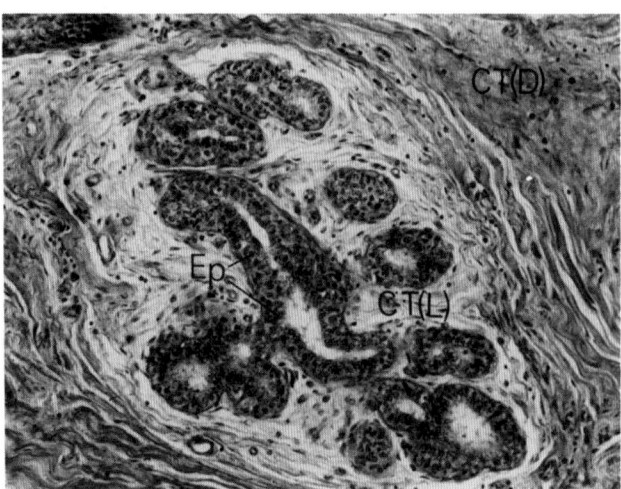

FIG. 17-4. Inactive human breast (×160). The epithelium (*Ep*), which is primarily ductal, is embedded in loose connective tissue [*CT(L)*]. Dense connective tissue [*CT(D)*] surrounds the lobule. *(Reproduced with permission from Romrell et al,[15] p 22. Copyright Elsevier.)*

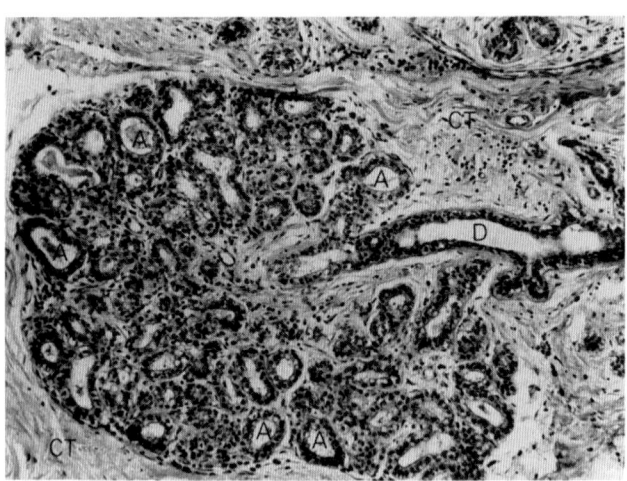

FIG. 17-5. Active human breast: pregnancy and lactation (×160). The alveolar epithelium becomes conspicuous during the early proliferative period. An alveolus (*A*) and a duct (*D*) are shown. The alveolus is surrounded by cellular connective tissue (*CT*). *(Reproduced with permission from Romrell et al,[15] p 23. Copyright Elsevier.)*

Blood Supply, Innervation, and Lymphatics

The breast receives its principal blood supply from (a) perforating branches of the internal mammary artery; (b) lateral branches of the posterior intercostal arteries; and (c) branches from the axillary artery, including the highest thoracic, lateral thoracic, and pectoral branches of the thoracoacromial artery (Fig. 17-6). The second, third, and fourth anterior intercostal perforators and branches of the internal mammary artery arborize in the breast as the medial mammary arteries. The lateral thoracic artery gives off branches to the serratus anterior, pectoralis major and pectoralis minor, and subscapularis muscles. It also gives rise to lateral mammary branches. The veins of the breast and chest wall follow the course of the arteries, with venous drainage being toward the axilla. The three principal groups of veins are (a) perforating branches of the internal thoracic vein, (b) perforating branches of the posterior intercostal veins, and (c) tributaries of the axillary vein. Batson's vertebral venous plexus, which invests the vertebrae and extends from the base of the skull to the sacrum, may provide a route for breast cancer metastases to the vertebrae, skull, pelvic bones, and central nervous system. Lymph vessels generally parallel the course of blood vessels.

Lateral cutaneous branches of the third through sixth intercostal nerves provide sensory innervation of the breast (lateral mammary branches) and of the anterolateral chest wall. These branches exit the intercostal spaces between slips of the serratus anterior muscle. Cutaneous branches that arise from the cervical plexus, specifically the anterior branches of the supraclavicular nerve, supply a limited area of skin over the upper portion of the breast. The intercostobrachial nerve is the lateral cutaneous branch of the second intercostal nerve and may be visualized during surgical dissection of the axilla. Resection of the intercostobrachial nerve causes loss of sensation over the medial aspect of the upper arm.

The boundaries for lymph drainage of the axilla are not well demarcated, and there is considerable variation in the position of the axillary lymph nodes. The six axillary lymph node groups recognized by surgeons (Figs. 17-7 and 17-8) are (a) the axillary vein group (lateral), which consists of four to six lymph nodes that lie medial or posterior to the vein and receive most of the lymph drainage from the upper extremity; (b) the external mammary group (anterior or pectoral group), which consists of five or six lymph nodes that lie along the lower border of the pectoralis minor muscle contiguous with the lateral thoracic vessels and receive most of the lymph drainage from the lateral aspect of the breast; (c) the scapular group (posterior or subscapular), which consists of five to seven lymph nodes that lie along the posterior wall of the axilla at the lateral border of the scapula contiguous with the subscapular vessels and receive lymph drainage principally from the lower posterior neck, the posterior trunk, and the posterior shoulder; (d) the central group, which consists of three or four sets of lymph nodes that are embedded in the fat of the axilla lying immediately posterior to the pectoralis minor muscle and receive lymph drainage both from the axillary vein, external mammary, and scapular groups of lymph nodes, and directly from the breast; (e) the subclavicular group (apical), which consists of six to twelve sets of lymph nodes that lie posterior and superior to the upper border of the pectoralis minor muscle and receive lymph drainage from all of the other groups of axillary lymph nodes; and (f) the interpectoral group (Rotter's nodes), which consists of one to four lymph nodes that are interposed between the pectoralis major and pectoralis minor muscles and receive lymph drainage directly from the breast. The lymph fluid that passes through the interpectoral group of lymph nodes passes directly into the central and subclavicular groups.

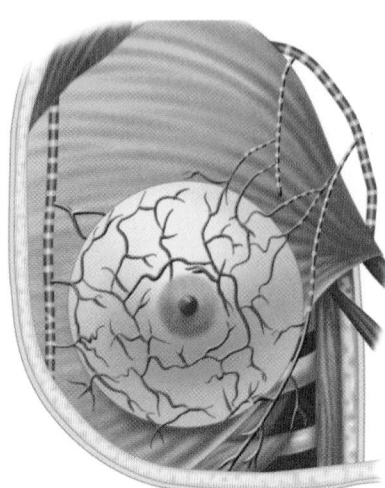

FIG. 17-6. Arterial supply to the breast, axilla, and chest wall. *(Reproduced with permission from Romrell et al,[15] p 28. Copyright Elsevier.)*

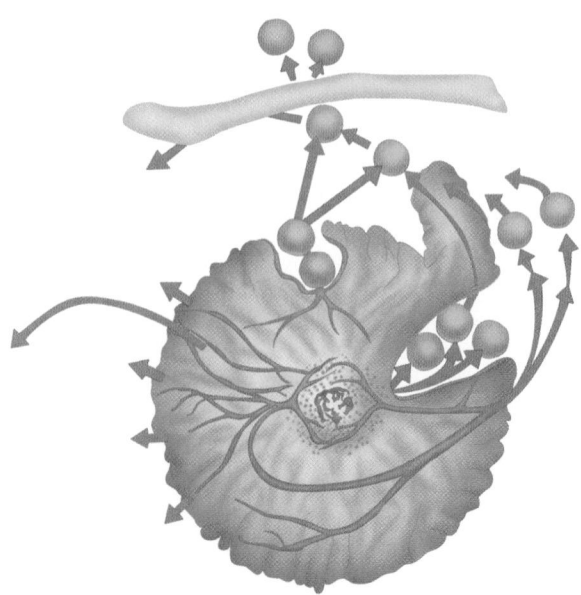

FIG. 17-7. Lymphatic pathways of the breast. *Arrows* indicate the direction of lymph flow. *(Reproduced with permission from Romrell et al,[15] p 30. Copyright Elsevier.)*

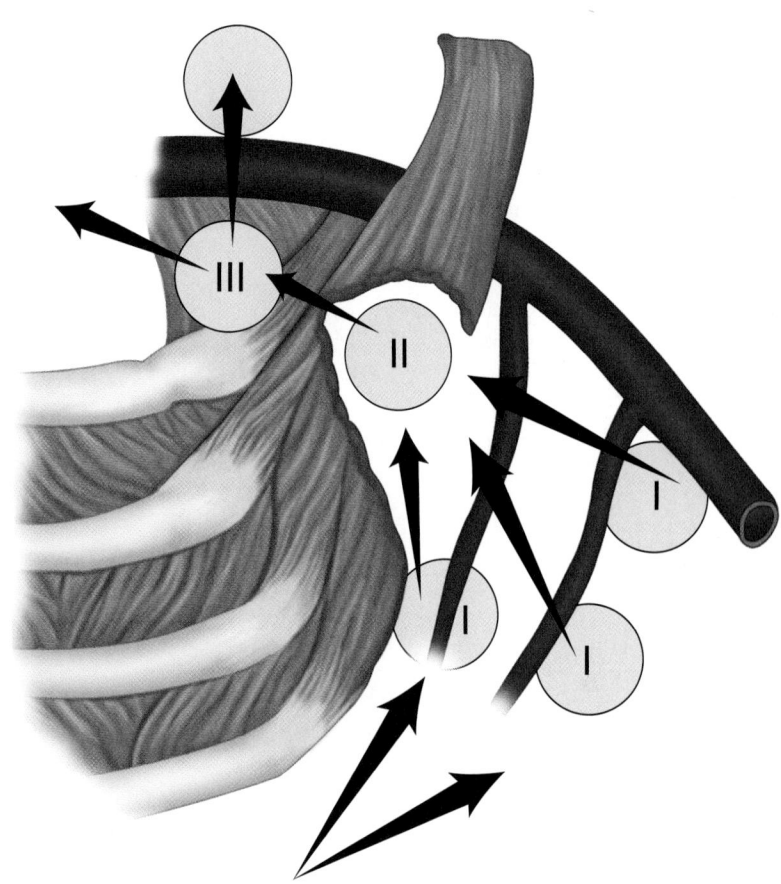

FIG. 17-8. Axillary lymph node groups. Level I includes lymph nodes located lateral to the pectoralis minor muscle (PM); level II includes lymph nodes located deep to the PM; and level III includes lymph nodes located medial to the PM. *Arrows* indicate the direction of lymph flow. The axillary vein with its major tributaries and the supraclavicular lymph node group are also illustrated. *(Reproduced with permission from Romrell et al,[15] p 32. Copyright Elsevier.)*

As indicated in Fig. 17-8, the lymph node groups are assigned levels according to their anatomic relationship to the pectoralis minor muscle. Lymph nodes located lateral to or below the lower border of the pectoralis minor muscle are referred to as *level I lymph nodes,* which include the axillary vein, external mammary, and scapular groups. Lymph nodes located superficial or deep to the pectoralis minor muscle are referred to as *level II lymph nodes,* which include the central and interpectoral groups. Lymph nodes located medial to or above the upper border of the pectoralis minor muscle are referred to as *level III lymph nodes,* which consist of the subclavicular group. The plexus of lymph vessels in the breast arises in the interlobular connective tissue and in the walls of the lactiferous ducts and communicates with the subareolar plexus of lymph vessels. Efferent lymph vessels from the breast pass around the lateral edge of the pectoralis major muscle and pierce the clavipectoral fascia, ending in the external mammary (anterior, pectoral) group of lymph nodes. Some lymph vessels may travel directly to the subscapular (posterior, scapular) group of lymph nodes. From the upper part of the breast, a few lymph vessels pass directly to the subclavicular (apical) group of lymph nodes. The axillary lymph nodes usually receive >75% of the lymph drainage from the breast. The rest is derived primarily from the medial aspect of the breast, flows through the lymph vessels that accompany the perforating branches of the internal mammary artery, and enters the parasternal (internal mammary) group of lymph nodes.

PHYSIOLOGY OF THE BREAST

Breast Development and Function

Breast development and function are initiated by a variety of hormonal stimuli, including estrogen, progesterone, prolactin, oxytocin, thyroid hormone, cortisol, and growth hormone.[16,17] Estro-

gen, progesterone, and prolactin especially have profound trophic effects that are essential to normal breast development and function. Estrogen initiates ductal development, whereas progesterone is responsible for differentiation of epithelium and for lobular development. Prolactin is the primary hormonal stimulus for lactogenesis in late pregnancy and the postpartum period. It upregulates hormone receptors and stimulates epithelial development. Figure 17-9 depicts the secretion of neurotrophic hormones from the hypothalamus, which is responsible for regulation of the secretion of the hormones that affect the breast tissues. The gonadotropins luteinizing hormone (LH) and follicle-stimulating hormone (FSH) regulate the release of estrogen and progesterone from the ovaries. In turn, the release of LH and FSH from the basophilic cells of the anterior pituitary is regulated by the secretion of gonadotropin-releasing hormone (GnRH) from the hypothalamus. Positive and negative feedback effects of circulating estrogen and progesterone regulate the secretion of LH, FSH, and GnRH. These hormones are responsible for the development, function, and maintenance of breast tissues (Fig. 17-10). In the female neonate, circulating estrogen and progesterone levels decrease after birth and remain low throughout childhood because of the sensitivity of the hypothalamic-pituitary axis to negative feedback from these hormones. With the onset of puberty, there is a decrease in the sensitivity of the hypothalamic-pituitary axis to negative feedback and an increase in its sensitivity to positive feedback from estrogen. These physiologic events initiate an increase in GnRH, FSH, and LH secretion and ultimately an increase in estrogen and progesterone secretion by the ovaries, which leads to establishment of the menstrual cycle. At the beginning of the menstrual cycle, there is an increase in the size and density of the breasts, which is followed by engorgement of the breast tissues and epithelial proliferation. With the onset of menstruation, the breast engorgement subsides and epithelial proliferation decreases.

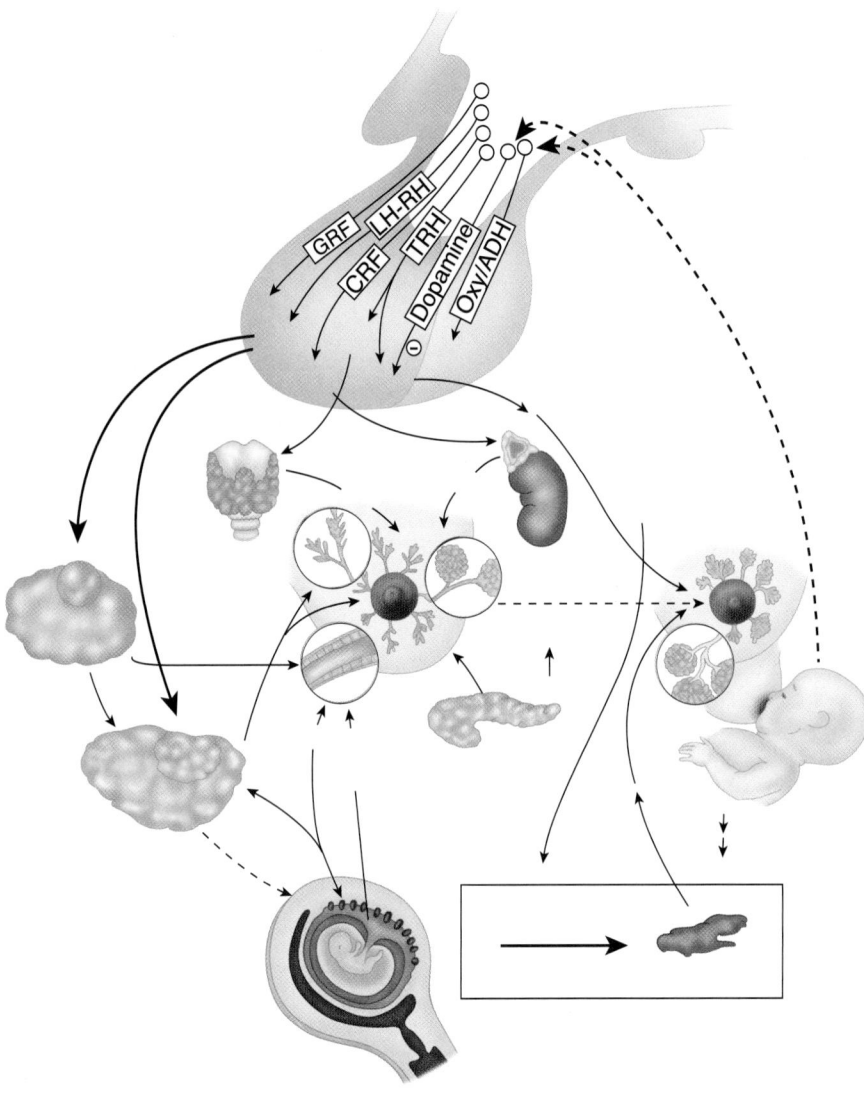

FIG. 17-9. Overview of the neuroendocrine control of breast development and function. ADH = antidiuretic hormone; CRF = corticotropin-releasing factor; GRF = growth hormone releasing factor; LH-RH = luteinizing hormone–releasing hormone; Oxy = oxytocin; TRH = thyrotropin-releasing hormone. *[Reproduced with permission from Kass R et al.: Breast physiology: normal and abnormal development and function, in: Bland and Copeland (eds): The Breast: Comprehensive Management of Benign and Malignant Disorders. Philadelphia: Saunders, 2004, p 54. Copyright Elsevier.]*

Pregnancy, Lactation, and Senescence

A dramatic increase in circulating ovarian and placental estrogens and progestins is evident during pregnancy, which initiates striking alterations in the form and substance of the breast (see Fig. 17-10B).[16–18] The breast enlarges as the ductal and lobular epithelium proliferates, the areolar skin darkens, and the accessory areolar glands (Montgomery's glands) become prominent. In the first and second trimesters, the minor ducts branch and develop. During the third trimester, fat droplets accumulate in the alveolar epithelium and colostrum fills the alveolar and ductal spaces. In late pregnancy, prolactin stimulates the synthesis of milk fats and proteins.

After delivery of the placenta, circulating progesterone and estrogen levels decrease, which permits full expression of the lactogenic action of prolactin. Milk production and release are controlled by neural reflex arcs that originate in nerve endings of the nipple-areola complex. Maintenance of lactation requires regular stimulation of these neural reflexes, which results in prolactin secretion and milk letdown. Oxytocin release results from the auditory, visual, and olfactory stimuli associated with nursing. Oxytocin initiates contraction of the myoepithelial cells, which results in compression of alveoli and expulsion of milk into the lactiferous sinuses. After weaning of the infant, prolactin and oxytocin release decreases. Dormant milk causes increased pressure within the ducts and alveoli, which results in atrophy of the epithelium (Fig. 17-10C). With menopause there is a decrease in the secretion of estrogen and progesterone by the ovaries and involution of the ducts and alveoli of the breast. The surrounding fibrous connective tissue increases in density, and breast tissues are replaced by adipose tissues (Fig. 17-10D).

Gynecomastia

Gynecomastia refers to an enlarged breast in the male.[19] Physiologic gynecomastia usually occurs during three phases of life: the neonatal period, adolescence, and senescence. Common to each of these phases is an excess of circulating estrogens in relation to circulating testosterone. Neonatal gynecomastia is caused by the action of placental estrogens on neonatal breast tissues, whereas in adolescence, there is an excess of estradiol relative to testosterone, and with senescence, the circulating testosterone level falls, which results in relative hyperestrinism. In gynecomastia, the ductal structures of the male breast enlarge, elongate, and branch with a concomitant increase in epithelium. During puberty, the condition often is unilateral and typically occurs between ages 12 and 15 years. In contrast, senescent gynecomastia is usually bilateral. In the nonobese male, breast tissue measuring at least 2 cm in diameter must be present before a diagnosis of gynecomastia may be made. Mammography and ultrasonography are used to differentiate breast tissues. Dominant masses or areas of firmness, irregularity, and asymmetry suggest the possibility of a breast cancer, particularly in the older male. Gynecomastia generally does not predispose the male breast to cancer. However, the hypoandrogenic state of Klinefelter's syndrome (XXY),

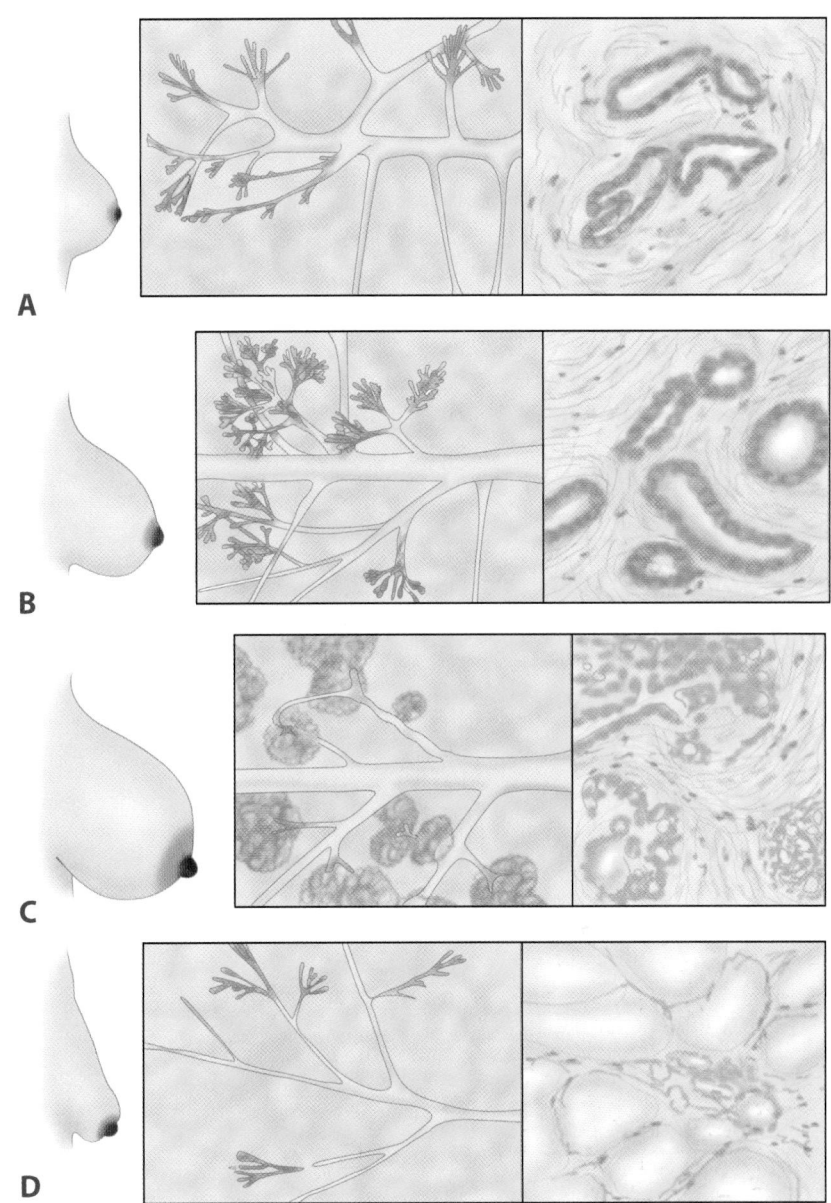

FIG. 17-10. The breast at different physiologic stages. The central column contains three-dimensional depictions of microscopic structures. **A.** Adolescence. **B.** Pregnancy. **C.** Lactation. **D.** Senescence.

in which gynecomastia is usually evident, is associated with an increased risk of breast cancer. Table 17-1 presents a clinical classification of gynecomastia.

Table 17-2 identifies the pathophysiologic mechanisms that may initiate gynecomastia. Estrogen excess results from an increase in the secretion of estradiol by the testicles or by nontesticular tumors, nutritional alterations such as protein and fat deprivation, endocrine disorders (hyperthyroidism, hypothyroidism), and hepatic disease

(nonalcoholic and alcoholic cirrhosis). Refeeding gynecomastia is related to the resumption of pituitary gonadotropin secretion after pituitary shutdown. Androgen deficiency may initiate gynecomastia. Concurrently occurring with decreased circulating testosterone levels is an elevated level of circulating testosterone-binding globulin, which results in a reduction of free testosterone. This senescent gynecomastia usually occurs in men aged 50 to 70 years. Klinefelter's syndrome (XXY) is manifested by gynecomastia, hypergonadotropic hypogonadism, and azoospermia. Primary testicular failure also may be caused by adrenocorticotropic hormone deficiency, hereditary defects of androgen synthesis, and congenital anorchia (eunuchoidal males). Secondary testicular failure may result from trauma, orchitis, and cryptorchidism. Renal failure, regardless of cause, also may initiate gynecomastia. Drugs with estrogenic activity (digitalis, estrogens, anabolic steroids, marijuana) or drugs that enhance estrogen synthesis (human chorionic gonadotropin) may cause gynecomastia. Drugs that inhibit the action or synthesis of testosterone (cimetidine, ketoconazole, phenytoin, spironolactone, antineoplastic agents, diazepam) also have been implicated. Drugs such as reserpine, theophylline, verapamil, tricyclic antidepressants, and furosemide induce

TABLE 17-1	Clinical classification of gynecomastia
Grade I	Mild breast enlargement without skin redundancy
Grade IIa	Moderate breast enlargement without skin redundancy
Grade IIb	Moderate breast enlargement with skin redundancy
Grade III	Marked breast enlargement with skin redundancy and ptosis, which simulates a female breast

Source: Modified with permission from Simon BE: Classification and surgical correction of gynecomastia. *Plas Reconstr Surg* 51:48, 1973, Wolters Kluwer Health.

TABLE 17-2 Pathophysiologic mechanisms of gynecomastia

I. Estrogen excess states
  A. Gonadal origin
    1. True hermaphroditism
    2. Gonadal stromal (nongerminal) neoplasms of the testis
      a. Leydig cell (interstitial)
      b. Sertoli cell
      c. Granulosa-theca cell
    3. Germ cell tumors
      a. Choriocarcinoma
      b. Seminoma, teratoma
      c. Embryonal carcinoma
  B. Nontesticular tumors
    1. Adrenal cortical neoplasms
    2. Lung carcinoma
    3. Hepatocellular carcinoma
  C. Endocrine disorders
  D. Diseases of the liver—nonalcoholic and alcoholic cirrhosis
  E. Nutrition alteration states
II. Androgen deficiency states
  A. Senescence
  B. Hypoandrogenic states (hypogonadism)
    1. Primary testicular failure
      a. Klinefelter's syndrome (XXY)
      b. Reifenstein's syndrome
      c. Rosewater-Gwinup-Hamwi familial gynecomastia
      d. Kallmann syndrome
      e. Kennedy's disease with associated gynecomastia
      f. Eunuchoidal state (congenital anorchia)
      g. Hereditary defects of androgen biosynthesis
      h. Adrenocorticotropic hormone deficiency
    2. Secondary testicular failure
      a. Trauma
      b. Orchitis
      c. Cryptorchidism
      d. Irradiation
  C. Renal failure
III. Drug effects
IV. Systemic diseases with idiopathic mechanisms

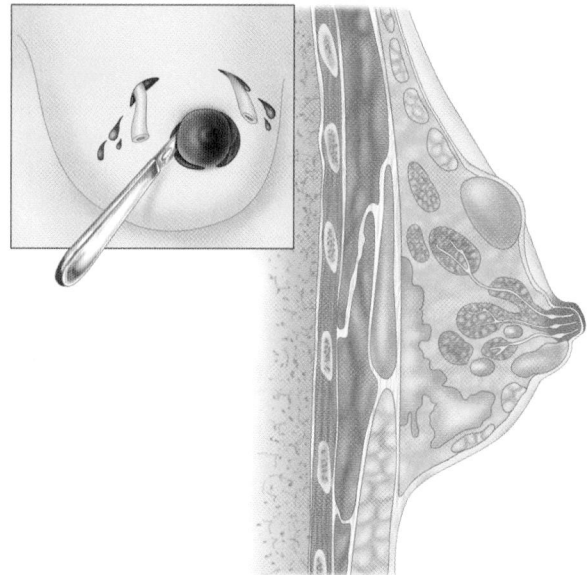

FIG. 17-11. Breast abscesses. Sagittal view of the breast with sites of potential abscess formation. Deep abscesses may be multilocular and may communicate with subcutaneous or subareolar sites. *Insert* depicts drainage of a multilocular breast abscess through circumareolar incisions and other incisions that parallel Langer's lines.

gynecomastia through idiopathic mechanisms. When gynecomastia is caused by androgen deficiency, then testosterone administration may cause regression. When it is caused by medications, then these are discontinued if possible. When endocrine defects are responsible, then these receive specific therapy. When gynecomastia is progressive and does not respond to other treatments, surgical therapy is considered. Attempts to reverse gynecomastia with danazol have been successful, but the androgenic side effects of the drug are considerable.

INFECTIOUS AND INFLAMMATORY DISORDERS OF THE BREAST

Except during the postpartum period, infections of the breast are rare and are classified as intrinsic (secondary to abnormalities in the breast) or extrinsic (secondary to an infection in an adjacent structure, e.g., skin, thoracic cavity).

Bacterial Infection

Staphylococcus aureus and *Streptococcus* species are the organisms most frequently recovered from nipple discharge from an infected breast.[16] Breast abscesses are typically seen in staphylococcal infections and present with point tenderness, erythema, and hyperther-

mia. These abscesses are related to lactation and occur within the first few weeks of breastfeeding. Figure 17-11 depicts the progression of a staphylococcal infection, which may result in subcutaneous, subareolar, interlobular (periductal), and retromammary abscesses (unicentric or multicentric), necessitating operative drainage of fluctuant areas. Preoperative ultrasonography is effective in delineating the required extent of the drainage procedure, which is best accomplished via circumareolar incisions or incisions paralleling Langer's lines. Although staphylococcal infections tend to be more localized and may be situated deep in the breast tissues, streptococcal infections usually present with diffuse superficial involvement. They are treated with local wound care, including application of warm compresses, and the administration of IV antibiotics (penicillins or cephalosporins). Breast infections may be chronic, possibly with recurrent abscess formation. In this situation, cultures are performed to identify acid-fast bacilli, anaerobic and aerobic bacteria, and fungi. Uncommon organisms may be encountered, and long-term antibiotic therapy may be required.

Biopsy of the abscess cavity wall is generally recommended at the time of incision and drainage to rule out underlying or coexisting breast cancer with necrotic tumor.

Hospital-acquired puerperal infections of the breast are much less common nowadays, but nursing women who present with milk stasis or noninfectious inflammation may still develop this problem. Epidemic puerperal mastitis is initiated by highly virulent strains of methicillin-resistant *S. aureus* that are transmitted via the suckling neonate and may result in substantial morbidity and occasional mortality. Purulent fluid may be expressed from the nipple. In this circumstance, breastfeeding is stopped, antibiotics are started, and surgical therapy is initiated. *Nonepidemic (sporadic) puerperal mastitis* refers to involvement of the interlobular connective tissue of the breast by an infectious process. The patient develops nipple fissuring and milk stasis, which initiate a retrograde bacterial infection. Emptying of the breast using breast suction pumps shortens the duration of symptoms and reduces the incidence of recurrences. The addition of antibiotic therapy results in a satisfactory outcome in >95% of cases.

Zuska's disease, also called *recurrent periductal mastitis,* is a condition of recurrent retroareolar infections and abscesses.[21,22] This syndrome is managed symptomatically, by antibiotics coupled with incision and drainage as necessary. Attempts to obtain durable long-term control by wide débridement of chronically infected tissue and/or terminal duct resection are frequently frustrated by postoperative infections. Smoking has been implicated as a risk factor for this condition.

Mycotic Infections

Fungal infections of the breast are rare and usually involve blasto-mycosis or sporotrichosis.[20] Intraoral fungi that are inoculated into the breast tissue by the suckling infant initiate these infections, which present as mammary abscesses in close proximity to the nipple-areola complex. Pus mixed with blood may be expressed from sinus tracts. Antifungal agents can be administered for the treatment of systemic (noncutaneous) infections. This therapy generally eliminates the necessity of surgical intervention, but occasionally drainage of an abscess, or even partial mastectomy, may be necessary to eradicate a persistent fungal infection. *Candida albicans* affecting the skin of the breast presents as erythematous, scaly lesions of the inframammary or axillary folds. Scrapings from the lesions demonstrate fungal elements (filaments and binding cells). Therapy involves the removal of predisposing factors such as maceration and the topical application of nystatin.

Hidradenitis Suppurativa

Hidradenitis suppurativa of the nipple-areola complex or axilla is a chronic inflammatory condition that originates within the accessory areolar glands of Montgomery or within the axillary sebaceous glands.[20] Women with chronic acne are predisposed to developing hidradenitis. When located in and about the nipple-areola complex, this disease may mimic other chronic inflammatory states, Paget's disease of the nipple, or invasive breast cancer. Involvement of the axillary skin is often multifocal and contiguous. Antibiotic therapy with incision and drainage of fluctuant areas is appropriate treatment. Excision of the involved areas may be required. Large areas of skin loss may necessitate coverage with advancement flaps or split-thickness skin grafts.

Mondor's Disease

Mondor's disease is a variant of thrombophlebitis that involves the superficial veins of the anterior chest wall and breast.[23] In 1939, Mondor described the condition as "string phlebitis," a thrombosed vein presenting as a tender, cord-like structure.[24] Frequently involved veins include the lateral thoracic vein, the thoracoepigastric vein, and, less commonly, the superficial epigastric vein. Typically, a woman presents with acute pain in the lateral aspect of the breast or the anterior chest wall. A tender, firm cord is found to follow the distribution of one of the major superficial veins. Rarely, the presentation is bilateral, and most women have no evidence of thrombophlebitis in other anatomic sites. This benign, self-limited disorder is not indicative of a cancer. When the diagnosis is uncertain, or when a mass is present near the tender cord, biopsy is indicated. Therapy for Mondor's disease includes the liberal use of anti-inflammatory medications and application of warm compresses along the symptomatic vein. Restriction of motion of the ipsilateral extremity and shoulder as well as brassiere support of the breast are important. The process usually resolves within 4 to 6 weeks. When symptoms persist or are refractory to therapy, excision of the involved vein segment is appropriate.

COMMON BENIGN DISORDERS AND DISEASES OF THE BREAST

Benign breast disorders and diseases encompass a wide range of clinical and pathologic entities. Surgeons require an in-depth understanding of benign breast disorders and diseases so that clear explanations may be given to affected women, appropriate treatment instituted, and unnecessary long-term follow up avoided.

Aberrations of Normal Development and Involution

The basic principles underlying the aberrations of normal development and involution (ANDI) classification of benign breast conditions are the following: (a) benign breast disorders and diseases are related to the normal processes of reproductive life and to involution; (b) there is a spectrum of breast conditions that ranges from normal to disorder to disease; and (c) the ANDI classification encompasses all aspects of the breast condition, including pathogenesis and the degree of abnormality.[25] The horizontal component of Table 17-3 defines ANDI along a spectrum from normal, to mild abnormality (disorder), to severe abnormality (disease). The vertical component indicates the period during which the condition develops.

Early Reproductive Years

Fibroadenomas are seen predominantly in younger women aged 15 to 25 years (Fig. 17-12).[26] Fibroadenomas usually grow to 1 or 2 cm in diameter and then are stable but may grow to a larger size. Small

TABLE 17-3 ANDI classification of benign breast disorders

	Normal	Disorder	Disease
Early reproductive years (age 15–25 y)	Lobular development	Fibroadenoma	Giant fibroadenoma
	Stromal development	Adolescent hypertrophy	Gigantomastia
	Nipple eversion	Nipple inversion	Subareolar abscess
			Mammary duct fistula
Later reproductive years (age 25–40 y)	Cyclical changes of menstruation	Cyclical mastalgia	Incapacitating mastalgia
		Nodularity	
	Epithelial hyperplasia of pregnancy	Bloody nipple discharge	
Involution (age 35–55 y)	Lobular involution	Macrocysts	—
		Sclerosing lesions	
	Duct involution		
	Dilatation	Duct ectasia	Periductal mastitis
	Sclerosis	Nipple retraction	—
	Epithelial turnover	Epithelial hyperplasia	Epithelial hyperplasia with atypia

ANDI = aberrations of normal development and involution.
Source: Modified with permission from Hughes LE: Aberrations of normal development and involution (ANDI): A concept of benign breast disorders based on pathogenesis, in Hughes LE, et al (eds): *Benign Disorders and Diseases of the Breast: Concepts and Clinical Management.* London: WB Saunders, 2000, p 23. Copyright Elsevier.

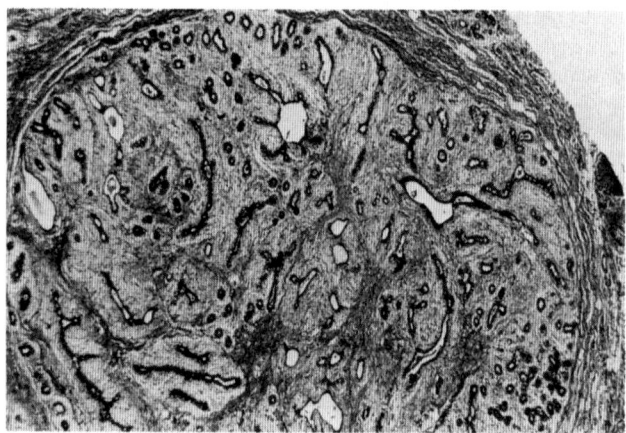

FIG. 17-12. Fibroadenoma (×10). *(Courtesy of Dr. R. L. Hackett.)*

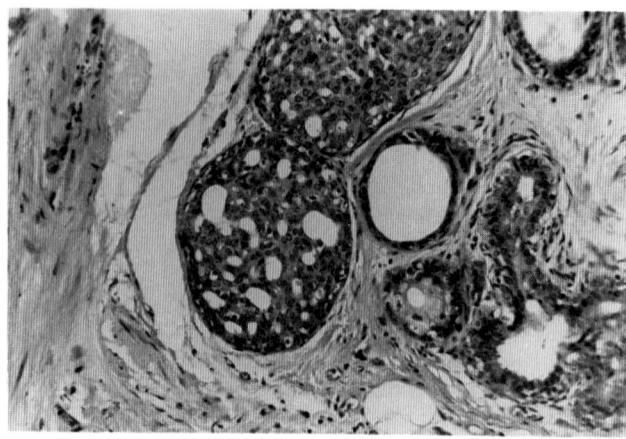

A

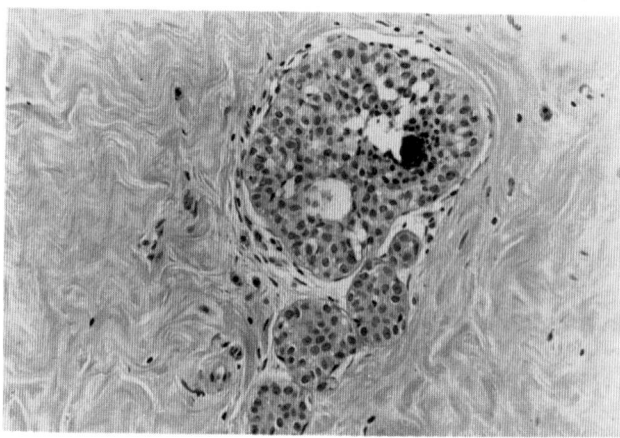

B

FIG. 17-13. A. Ductal epithelial hyperplasia. The irregular intracellular spaces and variable cell nuclei distinguish this process from carcinoma in situ. **B.** Lobular hyperplasia. The presence of alveolar lumina and incomplete distention distinguish this process from carcinoma in situ. *(Courtesy of Dr. R. L. Hackett.)*

fibroadenomas (≤1 cm in size) are considered normal, whereas larger fibroadenomas (≤3 cm) are disorders and giant fibroadenomas (>3 cm) are disease. Similarly, multiple fibroadenomas (more than five lesions in one breast) are very uncommon and are considered disease. The precise etiology of adolescent breast hypertrophy is unknown. A spectrum of changes from limited to massive stromal hyperplasia (gigantomastia) is seen. Nipple inversion is a disorder of development of the major ducts, which prevents normal protrusion of the nipple. Mammary duct fistulas arise when nipple inversion predisposes to major duct obstruction, leading to recurrent subareolar abscess and mammary duct fistula.

Later Reproductive Years

Cyclical mastalgia and nodularity usually are associated with premenstrual enlargement of the breast and are regarded as normal. Cyclical pronounced mastalgia and severe painful nodularity are viewed differently than are physiologic discomfort and lumpiness. Painful nodularity that persists for >1 week of the menstrual cycle is considered a disorder. In epithelial hyperplasia of pregnancy, papillary projections sometimes give rise to bilateral bloody nipple discharge.

Involution

Involution of lobular epithelium is dependent on the specialized stroma around it. However, an integrated involution of breast stroma and epithelium is not always seen, and disorders of the process are common. When the stroma involutes too quickly, alveoli remain and form microcysts, which are precursors of macrocysts. Macrocysts are common, are often subclinical, and do not require specific treatment. Sclerosing adenosis is considered a disorder of both the proliferative and the involutional phases of the breast cycle. Duct ectasia (dilated ducts) and periductal mastitis are other important components of the ANDI classification. Periductal fibrosis is a sequela of periductal mastitis and may result in nipple retraction. Sixty percent of women ≥70 years of age exhibit some degree of epithelial hyperplasia (Fig. 17-13). Atypical proliferative diseases include ductal and lobular hyperplasia, both of which display some features of carcinoma in situ. Women with atypical ductal or lobular hyperplasia have a fourfold increase in breast cancer risk (Table 17-4).

Pathology of Nonproliferative Disorders

Of paramount importance for the optimal management of benign breast disorders and diseases is the histologic differentiation of benign, atypical, and malignant changes.[27,28] Determining the clinical significance of these changes is a problem that is compounded by inconsistent nomenclature. The classification system originally developed by Page separates the various types of benign breast disorders and diseases into three clinically relevant groups: nonpro-

liferative disorders, proliferative disorders without atypia, and proliferative disorders with atypia (Table 17-5). Nonproliferative disorders of the breast account for 70% of benign breast conditions and carry no increased risk for the development of breast cancer. This category includes cysts, duct ectasia, periductal mastitis, calcifications, fibroadenomas, and related disorders.

TABLE 17-4	Cancer risk associated with benign breast disorders and in situ carcinoma of the breast
Abnormality	**Relative Risk**
Nonproliferative lesions of the breast	No increased risk
Sclerosing adenosis	No increased risk
Intraductal papilloma	No increased risk
Florid hyperplasia	1.5 to 2-fold
Atypical lobular hyperplasia	4-fold
Atypical ductal hyperplasia	4-fold
Ductal involvement by cells of atypical ductal hyperplasia	7-fold
Lobular carcinoma in situ	10-fold
Ductal carcinoma in situ	10-fold

Source: Modified from Dupont WD, et al: Risk factors for breast cancer in women with proliferative breast disease. *N Engl J Med* 312:146, 1985.

TABLE 17-5 Classification of benign breast disorders

Nonproliferative disorders of the breast
  Cysts and apocrine metaplasia
  Duct ectasia
  Mild ductal epithelial hyperplasia
  Calcifications
  Fibroadenoma and related lesions
Proliferative breast disorders without atypia
  Sclerosing adenosis
  Radial and complex sclerosing lesions
  Ductal epithelial hyperplasia
  Intraductal papillomas
Atypical proliferative lesions
  Atypical lobular hyperplasia
  Atypical ductal hyperplasia

Source: Modified from Consensus Meeting[29] with permission. Copyright © American Medical Association.

Breast macrocysts are an involutional disorder, have a high frequency of occurrence, and are often multiple. Duct ectasia is a clinical syndrome characterized by dilated subareolar ducts that are palpable and often associated with thick nipple discharge. Haagensen regarded duct ectasia as a primary event that led to stagnation of secretions, epithelial ulceration, and leakage of duct secretions (containing chemically irritating fatty acids) into periductal tissue.[30] This sequence was thought to produce a local inflammatory process with periductal fibrosis and subsequent nipple retraction. An alternative theory considers periductal mastitis to be the primary process, which leads to weakening of the ducts and secondary dilatation. It is possible that both processes occur and together explain the wide spectrum of problems seen, which include nipple discharge, nipple retraction, inflammatory masses, and abscesses.

Calcium deposits are frequently encountered in the breast. Most are benign and are caused by cellular secretions and debris or by trauma and inflammation. Calcifications that are associated with cancer include microcalcifications, which vary in shape and density and are <0.5 mm in size, and fine, linear calcifications, which may show branching. Fibroadenomas have abundant stroma with histologically normal cellular elements. They show hormonal dependence similar to that of normal breast lobules in that they lactate during pregnancy and involute in the postmenopausal period. Adenomas of the breast are well circumscribed and are composed of benign epithelium with sparse stroma, which is the histologic feature that differentiates them from fibroadenomas. They may be divided into tubular adenomas and lactating adenomas. Tubular adenomas are seen in young nonpregnant women, whereas lactating adenomas are seen during pregnancy or during the postpartum period. Hamartomas are discrete breast tumors that are usually 2 to 4 cm in diameter, firm, and sharply circumscribed. Adenolipomas consist of sharply circumscribed nodules of fatty tissue that contain normal breast lobules and ducts.

Fibrocystic Disease

The term *fibrocystic disease* is nonspecific. Too frequently, it is used as a diagnostic term to describe symptoms, to rationalize the need for breast biopsy, and to explain biopsy results. Synonyms include fibrocystic changes, cystic mastopathy, chronic cystic disease, chronic cystic mastitis, Schimmelbusch's disease, mazoplasia, Cooper's disease, Reclus' disease, and fibroadenomatosis. *Fibrocystic disease* refers to a spectrum of histopathologic changes that are best diagnosed and treated specifically.

Pathology of Proliferative Disorders without Atypia

Proliferative breast disorders without atypia include sclerosing adenosis, radial scars, complex sclerosing lesions, ductal epithelial hyperplasia, and intraductal papillomas.[27,28] Sclerosing adenosis is prevalent during the childbearing and perimenopausal years and has no malignant potential. Histologic changes are both proliferative (ductal proliferation) and involutional (stromal fibrosis, epithelial regression). Sclerosing adenosis is characterized by distorted breast lobules and usually occurs in the context of multiple microcysts, but occasionally presents as a palpable mass. Benign calcifications are often associated with this disorder. Central sclerosis and varying degrees of epithelial proliferation, apocrine metaplasia, and papilloma formation characterize radial scars and complex sclerosing lesions of the breast. Lesions up to 1 cm in diameter are called *radial scars,* whereas larger lesions are called *complex sclerosing lesions.* Radial scars originate at sites of terminal duct branching where the characteristic histologic changes radiate from a central area of fibrosis. All of the histologic features of a radial scar are seen in the larger complex sclerosing lesions, but there is a greater disturbance of structure with papilloma formation, apocrine metaplasia, and occasionally sclerosing adenosis.

Mild ductal hyperplasia is characterized by the presence of three or four cell layers above the basement membrane. Moderate ductal hyperplasia is characterized by the presence of five or more cell layers above the basement membrane. Florid ductal epithelial hyperplasia occupies at least 70% of a minor duct lumen. It is found in >20% of breast tissue specimens, is either solid or papillary, and is associated with an increased cancer risk (see Table 17-4). Intraductal papillomas arise in the major ducts, usually in premenopausal women. They generally are <0.5 cm in diameter but may be as large as 5 cm. A common presenting symptom is nipple discharge, which may be serous or bloody. Grossly, intraductal papillomas are pinkish tan, friable, and usually attached to the wall of the involved duct by a stalk. They rarely undergo malignant transformation, and their presence does not increase a woman's risk of developing breast cancer (unless accompanied by atypia). However, multiple intraductal papillomas, which occur in younger women and are less frequently associated with nipple discharge, are susceptible to malignant transformation.

Pathology of Atypical Proliferative Diseases

The atypical proliferative diseases have some of the features of carcinoma in situ but either lack a major defining feature of carcinoma in situ or have the features in less than fully developed form.[30] In 1978, Haagensen and colleagues described lobular neoplasia, a spectrum of disorders ranging from atypical lobular hyperplasia to lobular carcinoma in situ (LCIS).[31]

Treatment of Selected Benign Breast Disorders and Diseases

Cysts

Because needle biopsy of breast masses may produce artifacts that make mammography assessment more difficult, many radiologists prefer to image breast masses before performing needle biopsy.[32,33] In practice, however, the first investigation of palpable breast masses is frequently needle biopsy, which allows for the early diagnosis of cysts. A 21-gauge needle attached to a 10-mL syringe is placed directly into the mass, which is fixed by fingers of the nondominant hand. The volume of a typical cyst is 5 to 10 mL but it may be 75 mL or more. If the fluid that is aspirated is not bloodstained, then the cyst is aspirated to dryness, the needle is removed, and the fluid is discarded, because cytologic examination of such fluid is not cost effective. After aspiration, the breast is carefully palpated to exclude a residual mass. If one exists, ultrasound examination is performed to exclude a persistent cyst, which is reaspirated if present. If the mass is solid, a tissue specimen is obtained. When cystic fluid is bloodstained, 2 mL of fluid is taken for cytologic examination. The mass is then imaged with ultrasound and any solid area on the cyst wall is sampled by needle biopsy. The presence of blood is usually obvious, but in cysts with dark fluid, an occult blood test or microscopic examination will eliminate any doubt. The two cardinal rules of safe cyst aspiration are that (a) the mass must disappear completely after aspiration, and (b) the fluid must not be blood-stained. If either of these conditions is not met, then ultrasound with needle biopsy or pneumocystography can be performed. A simple cyst is rarely of concern, but a complex cyst may be the result of an underlying malignancy. A pneumocystogram is obtained by injecting air into the cyst and then obtaining a repeat mammogram. When this technique is used, the wall of the cyst cavity can be more carefully assessed for any irregularities.

Fibroadenomas

Removal of all fibroadenomas has been advocated irrespective of patient age or other considerations, and solitary fibroadenomas in young women are frequently removed to alleviate patient concern. Yet most fibroadenomas are self-limiting and many go undiagnosed, so a more conservative approach is reasonable. Careful ultrasound examination with core-needle biopsy will provide for an accurate diagnosis. Ultrasonography may reveal specific features that are pathognomonic for fibroadenoma. In this situation a core-needle biopsy may not be necessary. Subsequently, the patient is counseled concerning the ultrasound and biopsy results, and excision of the fibroadenoma may be avoided. Cryoablation is an approved treatment for fibroadenomas of the breast. With short-term follow-up a significant percentage of fibroadenomas will decrease in size and will no longer be palpable.[34] However, many will remain palpable, especially those larger than 2 cm. Therefore, women should be counseled that the options for treatment include surgical removal, cryoablation, or observation.

Sclerosing Disorders

The clinical significance of sclerosing adenosis lies in its mimicry of cancer. It may be confused with cancer on physical examination, by mammography, and at gross pathologic examination. Excisional biopsy and histologic examination are frequently necessary to exclude the diagnosis of cancer. The diagnostic work-up for radial scars and complex sclerosing lesions frequently involves stereoscopic biopsy. It usually is not possible to differentiate these lesions with certainty from cancer by mammographic features, so biopsy is recommended. The mammographic appearance of a radial scar or sclerosing adenosis (mass density with spiculated margins) will usually lead to an assessment that the results of a core-needle biopsy showing benign disease are discordant with the radiographic findings. Breast radiologists will therefore often forego image-guided needle biopsy of a lesion suspicious for radial scar and refer the case directly to a surgeon for wire localized excisional biopsy.

Periductal Mastitis

Painful and tender masses behind the nipple-areola complex are aspirated with a 21-gauge needle attached to a 10-mL syringe. Any fluid obtained is submitted for cytologic examination and for culture using a transport medium appropriate for the detection of anaerobic organisms. In the absence of pus, women are started on a combination of metronidazole and dicloxacillin while awaiting the results of culture. Antibiotics are then continued based on sensitivity tests. Many cases respond satisfactorily, but when considerable purulent material is present, surgical treatment is recommended. Unlike puerperal abscesses, a subareolar abscess is usually unilocular and often is associated with a single duct system. Preoperative ultrasound will accurately delineate its extent. The surgeon may either undertake simple drainage with a view toward formal surgery, should the problem recur, or proceed with definitive surgery. In a woman of childbearing age, simple drainage is preferred, but if there is an anaerobic infection, recurrent infection frequently develops. Recurrent abscess with fistula is a difficult problem and may be treated by fistulectomy or by major duct excision, depending on the circumstances (Table 17-6). When a localized periareolar abscess recurs at the previous site and a fistula is present, the preferred

TABLE 17-6	Treatment of recurrent subareolar sepsis	
Suitable for Fistulectomy	**Suitable for Total Duct Excision**
Small abscess localized to one segment	Large abscess affecting >50% of the areolar circumference
Recurrence involving the same segment	Recurrence involving a different segment
Mild or no nipple inversion	Marked nipple inversion
Patient unconcerned about nipple inversion	Patient requests correction of nipple inversion
Younger patient	Older patient
No discharge from other ducts	Purulent discharge from other ducts
No prior fistulectomy	Recurrence after fistulectomy

Source: Modified with permission from Hughes LE: The duct ectasia/periductal mastitis complex, in Hughes LE, et al (eds): *Benign Disorders and Diseases of the Breast: Concepts and Clinical Management.* London: WB Saunders, 2000, p 162. Copyright © Elsevier.

operation is fistulectomy, which has minimal complications and a high degree of success. However, when subareolar sepsis is diffuse rather than localized to one segment or when more than one fistula is present, total duct excision is the most expeditious approach. The first circumstance is seen in young women with squamous metaplasia of a single duct, whereas the latter circumstance is seen in older women with multiple ectatic ducts. Age is not always a reliable guide, however, and fistula excision is the preferred initial procedure for localized sepsis irrespective of age. Antibiotic therapy is useful for recurrent infection after fistula excision, and a 2- to 4-week course is recommended before total duct excision.

Nipple Inversion

More women request correction of congenital nipple inversion than request correction for the nipple inversion that occurs secondary to duct ectasia. Although the results are usually satisfactory, women seeking correction for cosmetic reasons should always be made aware of the surgical complications of altered nipple sensation, nipple necrosis, and postoperative fibrosis with nipple retraction. Because nipple inversion is a result of shortening of the subareolar ducts, a complete division of these ducts is necessary for permanent correction of the disorder.

RISK FACTORS FOR BREAST CANCER

Hormonal and Nonhormonal Risk Factors

Increased exposure to estrogen is associated with an increased risk for developing breast cancer, whereas reducing exposure is thought to be protective.[35–41] Correspondingly, factors that increase the number of menstrual cycles, such as early menarche, nulliparity, and late menopause, are associated with increased risk. Moderate levels of exercise and a longer lactation period, factors that decrease the total number of menstrual cycles, are protective. The terminal differentiation of breast epithelium associated with a full-term pregnancy is also protective, so older age at first live birth is associated with an increased risk of breast cancer. Finally, there is an association between obesity and increased breast cancer risk. Because the major source of estrogen in postmenopausal women is the conversion of androstenedione to estrone by adipose tissue, obesity is associated with a long-term increase in estrogen exposure.

Nonhormonal risk factors include radiation exposure. Young women who receive mantle radiation therapy for Hodgkin's lymphoma have a breast cancer risk that is 75 times greater than that of age-matched control subjects. Survivors of the atomic bomb blasts in Japan during World War II have a very high incidence of breast cancer, likely because of somatic mutations induced by the radiation exposure. In both circumstances, radiation exposure during adolescence, a period of active breast development, magnifies the deleterious effect. Studies also suggest that the risk of breast cancer increases as the amount of alcohol a woman consumes increases. Alcohol consumption is known to increase serum levels of estradiol. Finally, evidence suggests that long-term consumption of foods with a high fat content contributes to an increased risk of breast cancer by increasing serum estrogen levels.

Risk Assessment Models

The average lifetime risk of breast cancer for newborn U.S. females is 12%.[42,43] The longer a woman lives without cancer, the lower her risk of developing breast cancer. Thus, a woman aged 50 years has an 11% lifetime risk of developing breast cancer, and a woman aged 70 years has a 7% lifetime risk of developing breast cancer. Because risk factors for breast cancer interact, evaluating the risk conferred by combinations of risk factors is difficult. Two risk assessment models are currently used to predict the risk of breast cancer. From the Breast Cancer Detection Demonstration Project, a mammography screening program conducted in the 1970s, Gail and colleagues developed the most frequently used model, which incorporates age at menarche, the number of breast biopsies, age at first live birth, and the number of first-degree relatives with breast cancer. It predicts the cumulative risk of breast cancer according to decade of life. To calculate breast cancer risk using the Gail model, a woman's risk factors are translated into an overall risk score by multiplying her relative risks from several categories (Table 17-7). This risk score is then compared to an adjusted population risk of breast cancer to determine a woman's individual risk. A software program incorporating the Gail model is available from the National Cancer Institute at *http://bcra.nci.nih.gov/brc*. This model was recently modified to more accurately assess risk in African American women.[45,46]

Claus and colleagues, using data from the Cancer and Steroid Hormone Study, a case-control study of breast cancer, developed the other frequently used risk assessment model, which is based on assumptions about the prevalence of high-penetrance breast cancer susceptibility genes.[47] Compared with the Gail model, the Claus model incorporates more information about family history but excludes other risk factors. The Claus model provides individual estimates of breast cancer risk according to decade of life based on presence of first- and second-degree relatives with breast cancer and their age at diagnosis. Risk factors that are less consistently associated with breast cancer (diet, use of oral contraceptives, lactation) or are rare in the general population (radiation exposure) are not included in either the Gail or Claus risk assessment model. Other models have been proposed that account for mammographic breast density in assessing breast cancer risk.[48,49] None of these models accounts for the risk associated with mutations in the breast cancer susceptibility genes *BRCA1* and *BRCA2*.

Risk Management

Several important medical decisions may be affected by a woman's underlying risk of developing breast cancer.[50-58] These decisions include when to use postmenopausal hormone replacement therapy, at what age to begin mammography screening, when to use tamoxifen to prevent breast cancer, and when to perform prophylactic mastectomy to prevent breast cancer. Postmenopausal hormone replacement therapy was widely prescribed in the 1980s and 1990s because of its effectiveness in controlling the symptoms of estrogen deficiency; namely, vasomotor symptoms such as hot flashes, night sweats and their associated sleep deprivation, osteoporosis, and cognitive changes. Furthermore, these hormone supplements were thought to reduce coronary artery disease as well. Use of combined estrogen and progesterone became standard for women who had not undergone hysterectomy, because unopposed estrogen increases the risk of uterine cancer. Concerns of prolonging a woman's lifetime exposure to estrogen, coupled with conflicting data regarding the impact of these hormones on cardiovascular health, motivated the implementation of large-scale phase III clinical trials to definitively evaluate the risks vs. benefits of postmenopausal hormone replacement therapy. The Women's Health

TABLE 17-7 Relative risk estimates for the Gail model	
Variable	**Relative Risk**
Age at menarche (years)	
≥14	1.00
12–13	1.10
<12	1.21
Number of biopsies/history of benign breast disease, age <50 y	
0	1.00
1	1.70
≥2	2.88
Number of biopsies/history of benign breast disease, age ≥50 y	
0	1.02
1	1.27
≥2	1.62
Age at first live birth (years)	
<20 y	
Number of first-degree relatives with history of breast cancer	
0	1.00
1	2.61
≥2	6.80
20–24 y	
Number of first-degree relatives with history of breast cancer	
0	1.24
1	2.68
≥2	5.78
25–29 y	
Number of first-degree relatives with history of breast cancer	
0	1.55
1	2.76
≥2	4.91
≥30 y	
Number of first-degree relatives with history of breast cancer	
0	1.93
1	2.83
≥2	4.17

Source: Modified with permission from Armstrong K, et al: Primary care: Assessing the risk of breast cancer. *N Engl J Med* 342:564, 2000. Copyright © Massachusetts Medical Society. All rights reserved.

Initiative was therefore designed by the National Institutes of Health as a series of clinical trials to study the effects of diet, nutritional supplements, and hormones on the risk of cancer, cardiovascular disease, and bone health in postmenopausal women. Findings from primary studies of postmenopausal hormone replacement therapy were released in 2002, demonstrating conclusively that breast cancer risk is threefold to fourfold higher after >4 years of use and there is no significant reduction in coronary artery or cerebrovascular risks.

Routine use of screening mammography in women ≥50 years of age reduces mortality from breast cancer by 33%. This reduction comes without substantial risks and at an acceptable economic cost. However, the use of screening mammography in women <50 years of age is more controversial for several reasons: (a) breast density is greater and screening mammography is less likely to detect early breast cancer; (b) screening mammography results in more false-positive test findings, which results in unnecessary biopsies; and (c) younger women are less likely to have breast cancer, so fewer young women will benefit from screening. On a population basis, however, the benefits of screening mammography in women between the ages of 40 and 49 years still appear to outweigh the risks. Targeting mammography to women at higher risk of breast cancer may also improve the balance of risks and benefits. In one study of women aged 40 to 49 years, an abnormal mammography finding was three times more likely to be cancer in a woman with a family history of breast cancer than in a woman without such a history. Furthermore, as noted previously in the section Risk Assessment Models, mounting data regarding mammographic breast density demonstrate an independent correlation with breast cancer risk. Incorporation of breast density measurements into breast cancer risk assessment models appears to be a promising strategy for increasing the accuracy of these tools. Unfortunately, widespread application of these modified models is hampered by inconsistencies in the reporting of mammographic density. Current recommendations are that women undergo baseline mammography at age 35 and then have annual mammographic screening beginning at age 40.

Tamoxifen, a selective estrogen receptor modulator, was the first drug shown to reduce the incidence of breast cancer in healthy women. The Breast Cancer Prevention Trial (NSABP P-01) randomly assigned >13,000 women with a 5-year Gail relative risk of breast cancer of 1.70 or higher to receive tamoxifen or placebo. After a mean follow-up period of 4 years, the incidence of breast cancer was reduced by 49% in the group receiving tamoxifen.[50] Tamoxifen therapy currently is recommended only for women who have a Gail relative risk of 1.70 or higher. In addition, deep vein thrombosis occurs 1.6 times as often, pulmonary emboli 3.0 times as often, and endometrial cancer 2.5 times as often in women taking tamoxifen. The increased risk for endometrial cancer is restricted to early-stage cancers in postmenopausal women. Cataract surgery is required almost twice as often among women taking tamoxifen. Gail and colleagues subsequently developed a model that accounts for underlying risk of breast cancer as well as comorbidities to determine the net risk-benefit ratio of tamoxifen use for chemoprevention.[59] Most recently, the NSABP completed its second chemoprevention trial, designed to compare tamoxifen and raloxifene for breast cancer risk reduction in high-risk postmenopausal women. Raloxifene, another selective estrogen receptor modulator, was selected for the experimental arm in this follow-up prevention trial because its use in managing postmenopausal osteoporosis suggested that it might be even more effective at breast cancer risk reduction, but without the adverse effects of tamoxifen on the uterus. The P-2 trial, the Study of Tamoxifen and Raloxifene (known as the *STAR trial*), randomly assigned 19,000 postmenopausal women at high-risk for breast cancer to receive either tamoxifen or raloxifene. At a median follow-up of 5 years, the two agents were found to be nearly identical in their ability to reduce breast cancer risk, but raloxifene was associated with a more favorable adverse event profile.[60] Of note, both drugs reduce the risk of developing breast cancer by approximately 50%. Although tamoxifen has been shown to reduce the incidence of LCIS and ductal carcinoma in situ (DCIS), raloxifene did not have an effect on the frequency of these diagnoses.

A retrospective study of women at high risk for breast cancer found that prophylactic mastectomy reduced their risk by >90%.[52] However, the effects of prophylactic mastectomy on the long-term quality of life are poorly quantified. A study involving women who were carriers of a breast cancer susceptibility gene (BRCA) mutation found that the benefit of prophylactic mastectomy differed substantially according to the breast cancer risk conferred by the mutations. For women with an estimated lifetime risk of 40%, prophylactic mastectomy added almost 3 years of life, whereas for women with an estimated lifetime risk of 85%, prophylactic mastectomy added >5 years of life.[56]

BRCA Mutations
BRCA1

Five to 10% of breast cancers are caused by inheritance of germline mutations such as *BRCA1* and *BRCA2*, which are inherited in an autosomal dominant fashion with varying penetrance (Table 17-8).[61–67] *BRCA1* is located on chromosome arm 17q, spans a genomic region of approximately 100 kilobases (kb) of DNA, and contains 22 coding

TABLE 17-8	Incidence of sporadic, familial, and hereditary breast cancer
Sporadic breast cancer	65–75%
Familial breast cancer	20–30%
Hereditary breast cancer	5–10%
BRCA1[a]	45%
BRCA2	35%
p53[a] (Li-Fraumeni syndrome)	1%
STK11/LKB1[a] (Peutz-Jeghers syndrome)	<1%
PTEN[a] (Cowden disease)	<1%
MSH2/MLH1[a] (Muir-Torre syndrome)	<1%
ATM[a] (Ataxia-telangiectasia)	<1%
Unknown	20%

[a]Affected gene.
Source: Adapted from Martin.[54]

protein of 1863 amino acids. Both *BRCA1* and *BRCA2* function as tumor-suppressor genes, and for each gene, loss of both alleles is required for the initiation of cancer. Data accumulated since the isolation of the *BRCA1* gene suggest a role in transcription, cell-cycle control, and DNA damage repair pathways. More than 500 sequence variations in *BRCA1* have been identified. It now is known that germline mutations in *BRCA1* represent a predisposing genetic factor in as many as 45% of hereditary breast cancers and in at least 80% of hereditary ovarian cancers. Female mutation carriers have up to a 90% lifetime risk for developing breast cancer and up to a 40% lifetime risk for developing ovarian cancer. Breast cancer susceptibility in these families appears as an autosomal dominant trait with high penetrance. Approximately 50% of children of carriers inherit the trait. In general, *BRCA1*-associated breast cancers are invasive ductal carcinomas, are poorly differentiated, and are hormone receptor negative. *BRCA1*-associated breast cancers have a number of distinguishing clinical features, such as an early age of onset compared with sporadic cases; a higher prevalence of bilateral breast cancer; and the presence of associated cancers in some affected individuals, specifically ovarian cancer and possibly colon and prostate cancers.

Several founder mutations have been identified in *BRCA1*. The two most common mutations are 185delAG and 5382insC, which account for 10% of all the mutations seen in *BRCA1*. These two mutations occur at a 10-fold higher frequency in the Ashkenazi Jewish population than in non-Jewish whites. The carrier frequency of the 185delAG mutation in the Ashkenazi Jewish population is 1% and, along with the 5382insC mutation, accounts for almost all *BRCA1* mutations in this population. Analysis of germline mutations in Jewish and non-Jewish women with early-onset breast cancer indicates that 20% of Jewish women who develop breast cancer before age 40 years carry the 185delAG mutation.

BRCA2

BRCA2 is located on chromosome arm 13q and spans a genomic region of approximately 70 kb of DNA. The 11.2-kb coding region contains 26 coding exons.[61–67] It encodes a protein of 3418 amino acids. The *BRCA2* gene bears no homology to any previously described gene, and the protein contains no previously defined functional domains. The biologic function of *BRCA2* is not well defined, but like *BRCA1*, it is postulated to play a role in DNA damage response pathways. *BRCA2* messenger RNA also is expressed at high levels in the late G_1 and S phases of the cell cycle. The kinetics of *BRCA2* protein regulation in the cell cycle is similar to that of *BRCA1* protein, which suggests that these genes are coregulated. The mutational spectrum of *BRCA2* is not as well established as that of *BRCA1*. To date, >250 mutations have been found. The breast cancer risk for *BRCA2* mutation carriers is close to 85%, and the lifetime ovarian cancer risk, while lower than for *BRCA1*, is still estimated to be close to 20%. Breast cancer susceptibility in *BRCA2* families is an autosomal dominant trait and has a high penetrance. Approximately 50% of children of carriers inherit the trait. Unlike male carriers of *BRCA1* mutations, men with germline mutations in *BRCA2* have an estimated breast cancer risk of 6%, which represents a 100-fold increase over the risk in the general male population. *BRCA2*-associated breast cancers are invasive ductal carcinomas, which are more likely to be well differentiated and to express hormone receptors than are *BRCA1*-associated breast cancers. *BRCA2*-associated breast cancer has a number of distinguishing clinical features, such as an early age of onset compared with sporadic cases, a higher prevalence of bilateral breast cancer, and the presence of associated cancers in some affected individuals, specifically ovarian, colon, prostate, pancreatic, gallbladder, bile duct, and stomach cancers, as well as melanoma. A number of founder mutations have been identified in *BRCA2*. The 6174delT mutation is found in Ashkenazi Jews with a prevalence of 1.2%. Another *BRCA2* founder mutation, 999del5, is observed in Icelandic and Finnish populations.

Identification of BRCA Mutation Carriers

Identifying hereditary risk for breast cancer is a four-step process that includes (a) obtaining a complete, multigenerational family history, (b) assessing the appropriateness of genetic testing for a particular patient, (c) counseling the patient, and (d) interpreting the results of testing.[68] Genetic testing should not be offered in isolation, but only in conjunction with patient education and counseling, including referral to a genetic counselor. Initial determinations include whether the individual is an appropriate candidate for genetic testing and whether genetic testing will be informative for personal and clinical decision making. A thorough and accurate family history is essential to this process, and the maternal and paternal sides of the family are both assessed, because 50% of the women with a *BRCA* mutation have inherited the mutation from their fathers. To help surgeons advise women about testing, statistically based models that determine the probability that an individual carries a *BRCA* mutation have been developed. A hereditary risk of breast cancer is considered if a family includes two or more women who developed ovarian cancer or breast cancer before age 50 years. Any woman diagnosed with breast cancer before age 50 years or with ovarian cancer at any age is asked about first-, second-, and third-degree relatives on either side of the family with either of these diagnoses. Breast and ovarian cancer in the same individual, and male breast cancer at any age, also suggest the possibility of hereditary breast and ovarian cancer. The threshold for genetic testing is lower in individuals who are members of ethnic groups in whom the mutation prevalence is increased. For instance, the possibility of hereditary cancer is considered for any Ashkenazi Jewish woman with early-onset breast cancer.

BRCA Mutation Testing

Appropriate counseling for the individual being tested for *BRCA* mutation is strongly recommended, and documentation of informed consent is required.[68-69] The test that is clinically available for analyzing *BRCA* mutation is gene sequence analysis. In a family with a history suggestive of hereditary breast cancer and no previously tested member, the most informative strategy is first to test an affected family member. This person undergoes complete sequence analysis of both the *BRCA1* and *BRCA2* genes. If a mutation is identified, relatives are usually tested only for that specific mutation. An individual of Ashkenazi Jewish ancestry is tested initially for the three specific mutations that account for hereditary breast and ovarian cancer in that population. If results of that test are negative, it may then be appropriate to fully analyze the *BRCA1* and *BRCA2* genes.

A positive test result is one that discloses the presence of a *BRCA* mutation that interferes with translation or function of the *BRCA* protein. A woman who carries a deleterious mutation has a breast cancer risk of up to 85% as well as a greatly increased risk of ovarian cancer. A negative test result is interpreted according to the individual's personal and family history, especially whether a mutation has been previously identified in the family, in which case the woman is generally tested only for that specific mutation. If the mutation is not present, the woman's risk of breast or ovarian cancer may be no greater than that of the general population. In addition, no *BRCA* mutation can be passed on to the woman's children. In the absence of a previously identified mutation, a negative test result in an affected individual generally indicates that a *BRCA* mutation is not responsible for the familial cancer. However, the possibility remains of an unusual abnormality in one of these genes that cannot yet be identified through clinical testing. It also is possible that the familial cancer is indeed caused by an identifiable *BRCA* mutation but that the individual tested had sporadic cancer, a situation known as *phenocopy*. This is especially possible if the individual tested developed breast cancer close to the age of onset of the general population (age 60 years or older) rather than before age 50 years, as is characteristic of *BRCA* mutation carriers. Overall, the false-negative rate for *BRCA* mutation testing is <5%. Some test results, especially when a single base-pair change (missense mutation) is identified, may be difficult to interpret. This is because single base-pair changes do not always result in a nonfunctional protein. Thus, missense mutations not located within critical functional domains, or those that cause only minimal changes in protein structure, may not be disease associated and are usually reported as indeterminate results. In communicating indeterminate results to women, care must be taken to relay the uncertain cancer risk associated with this type of mutation and to emphasize that ongoing research might clarify its meaning. In addition, testing other family members with breast cancer to determine if a genetic variant tracks with their breast cancer may provide clarification as to its significance. Indeterminate genetic variance currently accounts for 12% of the test results.

Concern has been expressed that the identification of hereditary risk for breast cancer may interfere with access to affordable health insurance. This concern refers to discrimination directed against an individual or family based solely on an apparent or perceived genetic variation from the normal human genotype. The Health Insurance Portability and Accountability Act of 1996 (HIPAA) made it illegal in the United States for group health plans to consider genetic information as a pre-existing condition or to use it to deny or limit coverage. Most states also have passed laws that prevent genetic discrimination in the provision of health insurance. In addition, individuals applying for health insurance are not required to report whether relatives have undergone genetic testing for cancer risk, only whether those relatives have actually been diagnosed with cancer. Currently there is little documented evidence of genetic discrimination resulting from findings of available genetic tests.

Cancer Prevention for BRCA Mutation Carriers

Risk management strategies for *BRCA1* and *BRCA2* mutation carriers include the following:

1. Prophylactic mastectomy and reconstruction
2. Prophylactic oophorectomy and hormone replacement therapy
3. Intensive surveillance for breast and ovarian cancer
4. Chemoprevention

Although removal of breast tissue reduces the likelihood that *BRCA1* and *BRCA2* mutation carriers will develop breast cancer, mastectomy does not remove all breast tissue and women continue to be at risk because a germline mutation is present in any remaining breast tissue. For postmenopausal *BRCA1* and *BRCA2* mutation carriers who have not had a mastectomy, it may be advisable to avoid hormone replacement therapy, because no data exist regarding the effect of the therapy on the penetrance of breast cancer susceptibility genes. Because breast cancers in *BRCA* mutation carriers have the same mammographic appearance as breast cancers in noncarriers, a screening mammogram is likely to be effective in *BRCA* mutation carriers, provided it is performed and interpreted by an experienced radiologist with a high level of suspicion. Present screening recommendations for *BRCA* mutation carriers who do not undergo prophylactic mastectomy include clinical breast examination every 6 months and mammography every 12 months beginning at age 25 years, because the risk of breast cancer in *BRCA* mutation carriers increases after age 30 years. Recent attention has been focused on the use of magnetic resonance imaging (MRI) for breast cancer screening in high-risk individuals and known *BRCA* mutation carriers. MRI appears to be more sensitive at detecting breast cancer in younger women with dense breasts.[70] However, MRI does lead to the detection of benign breast lesions that cannot easily be distinguished from malignancy, and these false-positive events can result in more interventions, including biopsies. The current recommendations from the American Cancer Society are for annual MRI in women with a 20 to 25% or greater lifetime risk of developing breast cancer, including women with a strong family history of breast or ovarian cancer and women who were treated for Hodgkin's disease in their teens or early twenties.[71] Despite a 49% reduction in the incidence of breast cancer in high-risk women taking tamoxifen, it is too early to recommend the use of tamoxifen uniformly for *BRCA* mutation carriers. Cancers arising in *BRCA1* mutation carriers are usually high grade and are most often hormone receptor negative. Approximately 66% of *BRCA1*-associated DCIS lesions are estrogen receptor negative, which suggests early acquisition of the hormone-independent phenotype. Tamoxifen appears to be more effective at preventing estrogen receptor–positive breast cancers.

The risk of ovarian cancer in *BRCA1* and *BRCA2* mutation carriers ranges from 20 to 40%, which is 10 times higher than that in the general population. Prophylactic oophorectomy is a reasonable prevention option in mutation carriers. The American College of Obstetrics and Gynecology recommends that women with a documented *BRCA1* or *BRCA2* mutation consider prophylactic oophorectomy at the comple-

tion of childbearing or at the time of menopause. Hormone replacement therapy is discussed with the patient at the time of oophorectomy. The Cancer Genetics Studies Consortium recommends yearly transvaginal ultrasound timed to avoid ovulation and annual measurement of serum cancer antigen 125 levels beginning at age 25 years as the best screening modalities for ovarian carcinoma in *BRCA* mutation carriers who have opted to defer prophylactic oophorectomy.

Other hereditary syndromes associated with an increased risk of breast cancer include Cowden disease (*PTEN* mutations, in which cancers of the thyroid, GI tract, and benign skin and subcutaneous nodules are also seen), Li-Fraumeni syndrome (p53 mutations, also associated with sarcomas, lymphomas, and adrenocortical tumors), and syndromes of breast and melanoma.

EPIDEMIOLOGY AND NATURAL HISTORY OF BREAST CANCER

Epidemiology

Breast cancer is the most common site-specific cancer in women and is the leading cause of death from cancer for women aged 20 to 59 years.[72-73] It accounts for 26% of all newly diagnosed cancers in females and is responsible for 15% of the cancer-related deaths in women.[73] It was predicted that approximately 182,460 invasive breast cancers would be diagnosed in women in the United States in 2008 and that 40,480 would die from breast cancer.[74] Breast cancer was the leading cause of cancer-related mortality in women until 1987, when it was surpassed by lung cancer (Fig. 17-14). In the 1970s, the

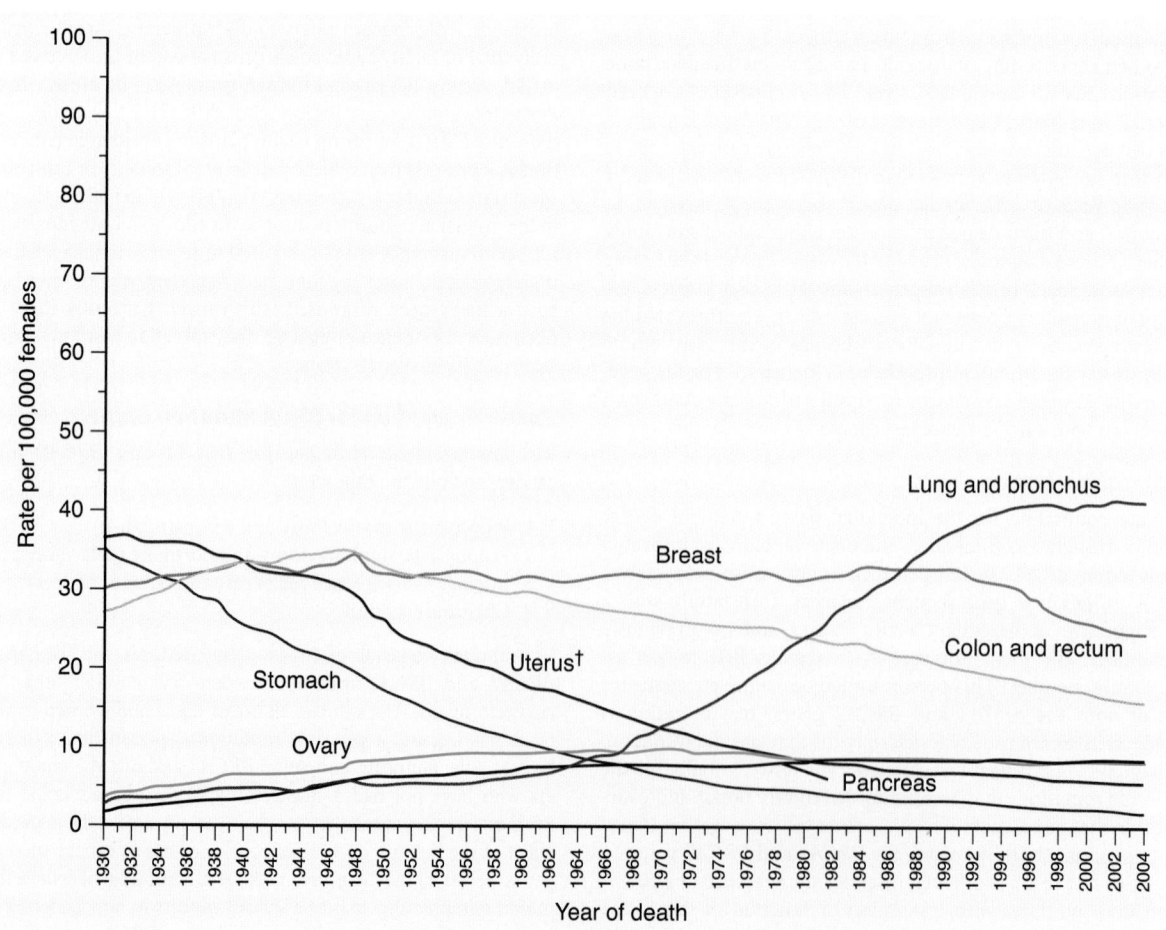

FIG. 17-14. Death rates for cancer at selected organ sites in U.S. females. These are age-adjusted rates per 100,000 population. †The uterine cancer death rate is derived by combining the cervical and corpus death rates. Note the steep rise in the lung cancer death rate after 1960. *(Reproduced with permission from Jemal A, et al: Cancer statistics, 2008. CA Cancer J Clin 58:71, 2008.)*

probability that a woman in the United States would develop breast cancer was estimated at 1 in 13; in 1980 it was 1 in 11; and in 2004 it was 1 in 8. Cancer registries in Connecticut and upper New York State document that the age-adjusted incidence of new breast cancer cases had steadily increased since the mid-1940s. The incidence in the United States, based on data from nine Surveillance, Epidemiology, and End Results (SEER) registries, has been decreasing by 23% per year since 2000. The increase had been approximately 1% per year from 1973 to 1980, and there was an additional increase in incidence of 4% between 1980 and 1987, which was characterized by frequent detection of small primary cancers. The increase in breast cancer incidence occurred primarily in women ≥55 years and paralleled a marked increase in the percentage of older women who had mammograms taken. At the same time, incidence rates for regional metastatic disease dropped and breast cancer mortality declined. From 1960 to 1963, 5-year overall survival rates for breast cancer were 63 and 46% in white and African American women, respectively, whereas the rates for 1981 to 1983 were 78 and 64%, respectively. For 1987 to 1989 rates were 85 and 71%, respectively.

There is a 10-fold variation in breast cancer incidence among different countries worldwide. Cyprus and Malta have the highest age-adjusted mortality for breast cancer (29.6 per 100,000 population), whereas Haiti has the lowest (2.0 deaths per 100,000 population). The United States has an age-adjusted mortality for breast cancer of 19.0 cases per 100,000 population. Women living in less-industrialized nations tend to have a lower incidence of breast cancer than women living in industrialized countries, although Japan is an exception. In the United States, Mormons, Seventh Day Adventists, American Indians, Alaska natives, Hispanic/Latina Americans, and Japanese and Filipino women living in Hawaii have a below-average incidence of breast cancer, whereas nuns (due to nulliparity) and Ashkenazi Jewish women have an above-average incidence.

The incidence rates of breast cancer increased in most countries through the 1990s. Since the estimates for 1990, there was an overall increase in incidence rates of approximately 0.5% annually. It was predicted that there would be approximately 1.4 million new cases in 2010. The cancer registries in China have noted annual increases in incidence of up to 3 to 4%, and in eastern Asia, increases are similar.

Recent data from the SEER program reveal declines in breast cancer incidence over the past decade, and this is widely attributed to decreased use of hormone replacement therapy as a consequence of the Women's Health Initiative reports.[75]

Breast cancer burden has well-defined variations by geography (Fig. 17-15), regional lifestyle, and racial or ethnic background.[76] In general, both breast cancer incidence and mortality are relatively lower among the female populations of Asia and Africa, relatively underdeveloped nations, and nations that have not adopted the Westernized reproductive and dietary patterns. In contrast, European and North American women and women from heavily industrialized or westernized countries have a substantially higher breast cancer burden. These international patterns are mirrored in breast cancer incidence and mortality rates observed for the racially, ethnically, and culturally diverse population of the United States (Fig. 17-16).[77]

Although often related, the factors that influence breast cancer incidence may differ from those that affect mortality. Incidence rates are lower among populations that are heavily weighted with women

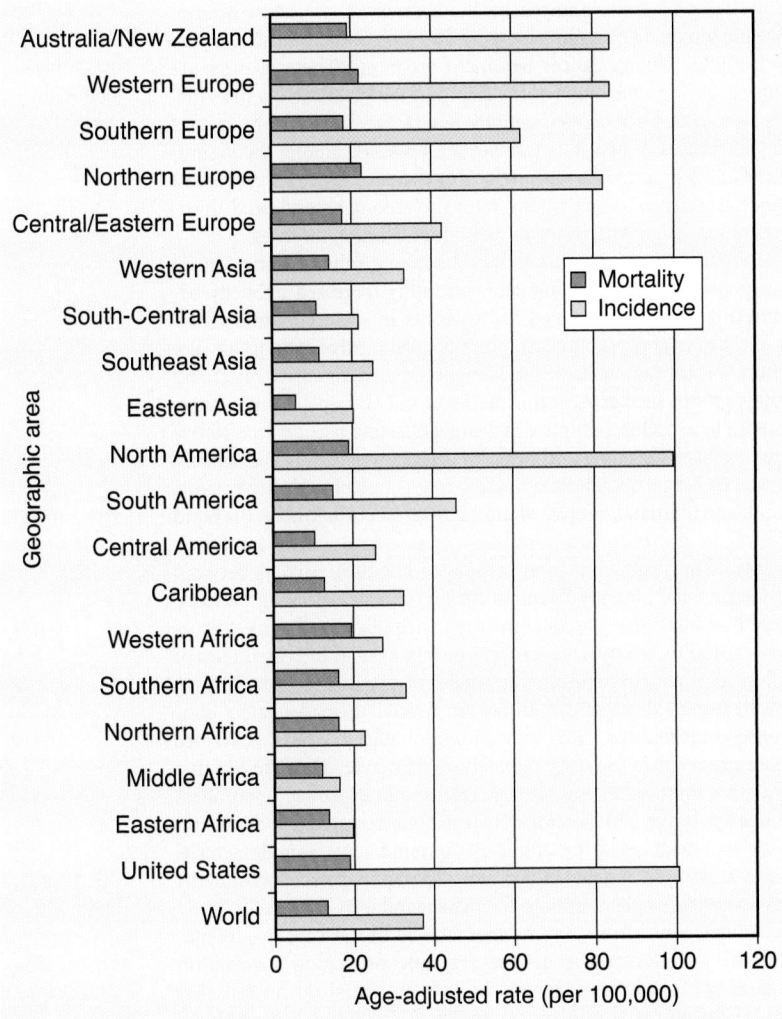

FIG. 17-15. International variation in breast cancer incidence and mortality. *(Reproduced with permission from Ferlay et al.[76])*

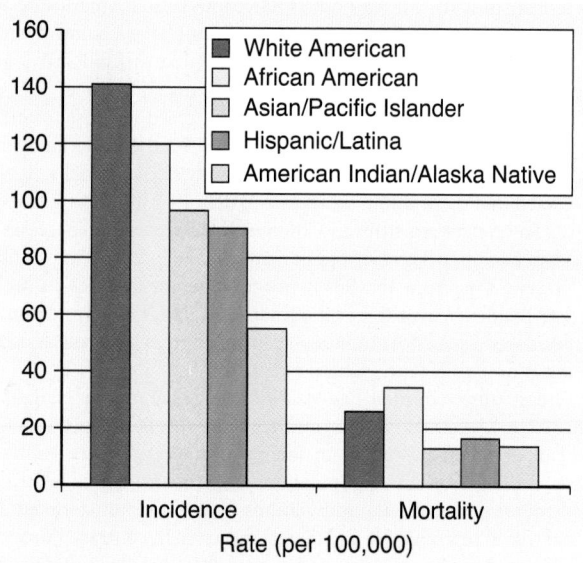

FIG. 17-16. Breast cancer incidence and mortality rates in the United States, 1998 to 2002, by ethnic background. *(Reproduced from Ries.[77])*

who begin childbearing at young ages and who have multiple full-term pregnancies followed by prolonged lactation. These are features that characterize many underdeveloped nations and also many eastern nations. Breast cancer mortality rates should be lower in populations that have a lower incidence, but the mortality burden will simultaneously be adversely affected by the absence of effective mammographic screening programs for early detection and diminished access to multidisciplinary cancer treatment programs. These features are likely to account for much of the disproportionate mortality risks that are seen in underdeveloped nations. Similar factors probably account for differences in breast cancer burden observed among the various racial and ethnic groups within the United States. Interestingly, breast cancer incidence and mortality rates rise among second- and third-generation Asian Americans as they adopt Western lifestyles.

Disparities in breast cancer survival among subsets of the American population are appropriately generating increased publicity because they are closely linked to disparities in socioeconomic status. Poverty rates and proportions of the population that lack health care insurance are two to three times higher among minority racial and ethnic groups such as African Americans and Hispanic/Latino Americans. These socioeconomic disadvantages create barriers to effective breast cancer screening and result in delayed breast cancer diagnosis, advanced stage distribution, inadequacies in comprehensive treatment, and ultimately increased mortality rates. Furthermore, the rapid growth in the Hispanic population is accompanied by increasing problems in health education because of linguistic barriers between physicians and recently immigrated, non-English-speaking patients. Recent studies also are documenting inequities in the treatments delivered to minority breast cancer patients, such as increased rates of failure to provide systemic therapy and breast reconstruction. Some of the treatment delivery disparities are related to inadequately controlled comorbidities (such as hypertension and diabetes), which are more prevalent in minority populations. However, some studies that adjust for these factors report persistent and unexplained unevenness in treatment recommendations. It is clear that breast cancer disparities associated with racial or ethnic background have a multifactorial cause, and improvements in outcome will require correction of many public health problems at both the patient and provider levels.

Advances in the ability to characterize breast cancer subtypes and the genetics of the disease are now provoking speculation regarding possible hereditary influences on breast cancer risk that are related to racial or ethnic ancestry.[78] These questions become

particularly compelling when one looks at disparities in breast cancer burden between African Americans and white Americans. Lifetime risk of breast cancer is lower for African Americans, yet a paradoxically increased breast cancer mortality risk also is seen. African Americans also have a younger age distribution for breast cancer; among women <45 years of age, breast cancer incidence is highest among African Americans compared to other subsets of the American population. Lastly and most provocatively, African American women of all ages have notably higher incidence rates for estrogen receptor–negative tumors. These same patterns of disease are seen in contemporary female populations of western, sub-Saharan Africa, who are likely to share ancestry with African American women as a consequence of the Colonial-era slave trade. Interestingly, male breast cancer also is seen with increased frequency among both African Americans and Africans.

Natural History

Bloom and colleagues described the natural history of breast cancer based on the records of 250 women with untreated breast cancers who were cared for on charity wards in the Middlesex Hospital, London, between 1805 and 1933. The median survival of this population was 2.7 years after initial diagnosis (Fig. 17-17).[79] The 5- and 10-year survival rates for these women were 18.0 and 3.6%, respectively. Only 0.8% survived for 15 years or longer. Autopsy data confirmed that 95% of these women died of breast cancer, whereas the remaining 5% died of other causes. Almost 75% of the women developed ulceration of the breast during the course of the disease. The longest surviving patient died in the nineteenth year after diagnosis.

Primary Breast Cancer

More than 80% of breast cancers show productive fibrosis that involves the epithelial and stromal tissues. With growth of the cancer and invasion of the surrounding breast tissues, the accompanying desmoplastic response entraps and shortens Cooper's suspensory ligaments to produce a characteristic skin retraction. Localized edema (peau d'orange) develops when drainage of lymph fluid from the skin

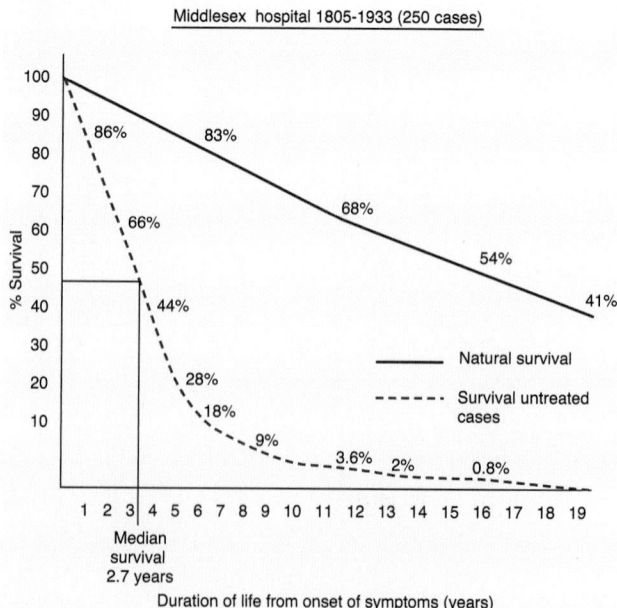

FIG. 17-17. Survival of women with untreated breast cancer compared with natural survival. *[Reproduced with permission from Bloom HJG, Richardson WW, Harries EJ: Natural history of untreated breast cancer (1803–1933): Comparison of untreated and treated cases according to histological grade of malignancy. Br Med J 2:213, 1962. With permission from the BMJ Publishing Group.]*

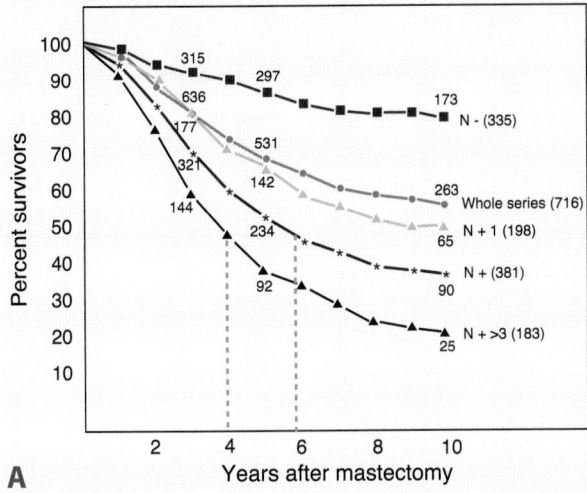

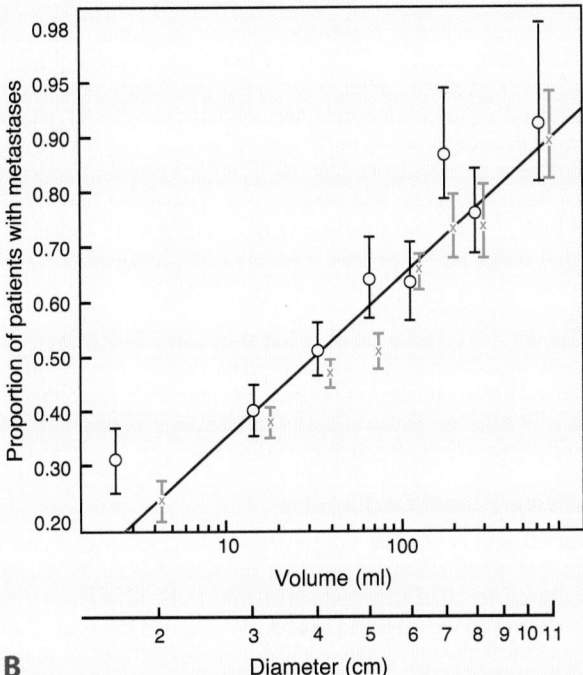

FIG. 17-18. A. Overall survival for women with breast cancer according to axillary lymph node status. The time periods are years after radical mastectomy. *(Reproduced with permission from Valagussa P, et al: Patterns of relapse and survival following radical mastectomy. Analysis of 716 consecutive patients. Cancer 41:1170, 1978. Copyright © American Cancer Society. This material is reproduced with permission of Wiley-Liss, Inc., a subsidiary of John Wiley & Sons, Inc.)* **B.** Risk of metastases according to breast cancer volume and diameter. *(Reproduced with permission from Koscielny S et al: Breast cancer: Relationship between the size of the primary tumour and the probability of metastatic dissemination. Br J Cancer 49:709, 1984.)*

is disrupted. With continued growth, cancer cells invade the skin, and eventually ulceration occurs. As new areas of skin are invaded, small satellite nodules appear near the primary ulceration. The size of the primary breast cancer correlates with disease-free and overall survival, but there is a close association between cancer size and axillary lymph node involvement (Fig. 17-18). In general, up to 20% of breast cancer recurrences are local-regional, >60% are distant, and 20% are both local-regional and distant.

Axillary Lymph Node Metastases

As the size of the primary breast cancer increases, some cancer cells are shed into cellular spaces and transported via the lymphatic network of the breast to the regional lymph nodes, especially the axillary lymph nodes. Lymph nodes that contain metastatic cancer are at first ill defined and soft but become firm or hard with continued growth of the metastatic cancer. Eventually the lymph nodes adhere to each other and form a conglomerate mass. Cancer cells may grow through the lymph node capsule and fix to contiguous structures in the axilla, including the chest wall. Typically, axillary lymph nodes are involved sequentially from the low (level I) to the central (level II) to the apical (level III) lymph node groups. Although >95% of the women who die of breast cancer have distant metastases, the most important prognostic correlate of disease-free and overall survival is axillary lymph node status (see Fig. 17-18A). Women with node-negative disease have less than a 30% risk of recurrence, compared with as much as a 75% risk for women with node-positive disease.

Distant Metastases

At approximately the twentieth cell doubling, breast cancers acquire their own blood supply (neovascularization). Thereafter, cancer cells may be shed directly into the systemic venous blood to seed the pulmonary circulation via the axillary and intercostal veins or the vertebral column via Batson's plexus of veins, which courses the length of the vertebral column. These cells are scavenged by natural killer lymphocytes and macrophages. Successful implantation of metastatic foci from breast cancer predictably occurs after the primary cancer exceeds 0.5 cm in diameter, which corresponds to the twenty-seventh cell doubling. For 10 years after initial treatment, distant metastases are the most common cause of death in breast cancer patients. For this reason, conclusive results cannot be derived from breast cancer trials until at least 5 to 10 years have elapsed. Although 60% of the women who develop distant metastases will do so within 24 months of treatment, metastases may become evident as late as 20 to 30 years after treatment of the primary cancer. Common sites of involvement, in order of frequency, are bone, lung, pleura, soft tissues, and liver.

HISTOPATHOLOGY OF BREAST CANCER

Carcinoma In Situ

Cancer cells are in situ or invasive depending on whether or not they invade through the basement membrane.[80,81] Broders's original description of in situ breast cancer stressed the absence of invasion of cells into the surrounding stroma and their confinement within natural ductal and alveolar boundaries.[80] Because areas of invasion may be minute, the accurate diagnosis of in situ cancer necessitates the analysis of multiple microscopic sections to exclude invasion. In 1941, Foote and Stewart published a landmark description of LCIS, which distinguished it from DCIS.[81] In the late 1960s, Gallagher and Martin published their study of whole-breast sections and described a stepwise progression from benign breast tissue to in situ cancer and subsequently to invasive cancer. They coined the term *minimal breast cancer* (LCIS, DCIS, and invasive cancers smaller than 0.5 cm in size) and stressed the importance of early detection.[85] It is now recognized that each type of minimal breast cancer has a distinct clinical and biologic behavior. Before the widespread use of mammography, diagnosis of breast cancer was by physical examination. At that time, in situ cancers constituted <6% of all breast cancers, and LCIS was more frequently diagnosed than DCIS by a ratio of >2:1. However, when screening mammography became popular, a 14-fold increase in the incidence of in situ cancer (45%) was demonstrated, and DCIS was more frequently diagnosed than LCIS by a ratio of >2:1. Table 17-9 lists the clinical and pathologic characteristics of DCIS and LCIS. *Multicentricity* refers to the occurrence of a second breast cancer outside the breast quadrant of the primary cancer (or at least 4 cm away), whereas *multifocality* refers to the occurrence of a second

TABLE 17-9	Salient characteristics of in situ ductal (DCIS) and lobular (LCIS) carcinoma of the breast	
	LCIS	DCIS
Age (years)	44–47	54–58
Incidence[a]	2–5%	5–10%
Clinical signs	None	Mass, pain, nipple discharge
Mammographic signs	None	Microcalcifications
Premenopausal	2/3	1/3
Incidence of synchronous invasive carcinoma	5%	2–46%
Multicentricity	60–90%	40–80%
Bilaterality	50–70%	10–20%
Axillary metastasis	1%	1–2%
Subsequent carcinomas:		
Incidence	25–35%	25–70%
Laterality	Bilateral	Ipsilateral
Interval to diagnosis	15–20 y	5–10 y
Histologic type	Ductal	Ductal

[a]In biopsy specimens of mammographically detected breast lesions.
Source: Reproduced with permission from Frykberg ER, et al: Current concepts on the biology and management of in situ (Tis, stage 0) breast carcinoma, in Bland KI, et al (eds): *The Breast: Comprehensive Management of Benign and Malignant Diseases.* Philadelphia: WB Saunders, 1998, p 1020. Copyright Elsevier.

TABLE 17-10	Classification of breast ductal carcinoma in situ (DCIS)		
Histologic Subtype	Determining Characteristics		
	Nuclear Grade	Necrosis	DCIS Grade
Comedo	High	Extensive	High
Intermediate[a]	Intermediate	Focal or absent	Intermediate
Noncomedo[b]	Low	Absent	Low

[a]Often a mixture of noncomedo patterns.
[b]Solid, cribriform, papillary, or focal micropapillary.
Source: Adapted with permission from Connolly JL, et al: Ductal carcinoma in situ of the breast: Histologic subtyping and clinical significance. *PPO Updates* 10:1, 1996.

cancer within the same breast quadrant as the primary cancer (or within 4 cm of it). Multicentricity occurs in 60 to 90% of women with LCIS, whereas the rate of multicentricity for DCIS is 40 to 80%. LCIS occurs bilaterally in 50 to 70% of cases, whereas DCIS occurs bilaterally in 10 to 20% of cases.

Lobular Carcinoma In Situ

LCIS originates from the terminal duct lobular units and develops only in the female breast. It is characterized by distention and distortion of the terminal duct lobular units by cancer cells, which are large but maintain a normal nuclear:cytoplasmic ratio. Cytoplasmic mucoid globules are a distinctive cellular feature. LCIS may be observed in breast tissues that contain microcalcifications, but the calcifications associated with LCIS typically occur in adjacent tissues. This neighborhood calcification is a feature that is unique to LCIS and contributes to its diagnosis. The frequency of LCIS in the general population cannot be reliably determined because it usually presents as an incidental finding. The average age at diagnosis is 44 to 47 years, which is approximately 15 to 25 years younger than the age at diagnosis for invasive breast cancer. LCIS has a distinct racial predilection, occurring 12 times more frequently in white women than in African American women. Invasive breast cancer develops in 25 to 35% of women with LCIS. Invasive cancer may develop in either breast, regardless of which breast harbored the initial focus of LCIS, and is detected synchronously with LCIS in 5% of cases. In women with a history of LCIS, up to 65% of subsequent invasive cancers are ductal, not lobular, in origin. For these reasons, LCIS is regarded as a marker of increased risk for invasive breast cancer rather than as an anatomic precursor.

Ductal Carcinoma In Situ

Although DCIS is predominantly seen in the female breast, it accounts for 5% of male breast cancers. Published series suggest a detection frequency of 7% in all biopsy tissue specimens. The term *intraductal carcinoma* is frequently applied to DCIS, which carries a high risk for progression to an invasive cancer. Histologically, DCIS is characterized by a proliferation of the epithelium that lines the minor ducts, resulting in papillary growths within the duct lumina. Early in their development, the cancer cells do not show pleomorphism, mitoses, or atypia, which leads to difficulty in distinguishing

early DCIS from benign hyperplasia. The papillary growths (papillary growth pattern) eventually coalesce and fill the duct lumina so that only scattered, rounded spaces remain between the clumps of atypical cancer cells, which show hyperchromasia and loss of polarity (cribriform growth pattern). Eventually pleomorphic cancer cells with frequent mitotic figures obliterate the lumina and distend the ducts (solid growth pattern). With continued growth, these cells outstrip their blood supply and become necrotic (comedo growth pattern). Calcium deposition occurs in the areas of necrosis and is a common feature seen on mammography. DCIS is now frequently classified based on nuclear grade and the presence of necrosis (Table 17-10). Based on multiple consensus meetings, grading of DCIS has been recommended. Although there is no universal agreement on classification, most systems endorse the use of cytologic grade and presence or absence of necrosis.[82]

The risk for invasive breast cancer is increased nearly fivefold in women with DCIS.[83] The invasive cancers are observed in the ipsilateral breast, usually in the same quadrant as the DCIS that was originally detected, which suggests that DCIS is an anatomic precursor of invasive ductal carcinoma (Fig. 17-19).

Invasive Breast Carcinoma

Invasive breast cancers have been described as lobular or ductal in origin.[84–87] Early classifications used the term *lobular* to describe invasive cancers that were associated with LCIS, whereas all other invasive cancers were referred to as *ductal*. Current histologic classifications recognize special types of breast cancers (10% of total cases), which are defined by specific histologic features. To qualify as a special-type cancer, at least 90% of the cancer must contain the defining histologic features. Eighty percent of invasive breast cancers are described as invasive ductal carcinoma of no special type (NST). These cancers generally have a worse prognosis than special-type cancers. Foote and Stewart originally proposed the following classification for invasive breast cancer[81]:

1. Paget's disease of the nipple
2. Invasive ductal carcinoma
3. Adenocarcinoma with productive fibrosis (scirrhous, simplex, NST), 80%
4. Medullary carcinoma, 4%
5. Mucinous (colloid) carcinoma, 2%
6. Papillary carcinoma, 2%
7. Tubular carcinoma, 2%
8. Invasive lobular carcinoma, 10%
9. Rare cancers (adenoid cystic, squamous cell, apocrine)

Paget's disease of the nipple was described in 1874. It frequently presents as a chronic, eczematous eruption of the nipple, which may be subtle but may progress to an ulcerated, weeping lesion. Paget's disease usually is associated with extensive DCIS and may be associated with an invasive cancer. A palpable mass may or may not be present. A nipple biopsy specimen will show a population of cells

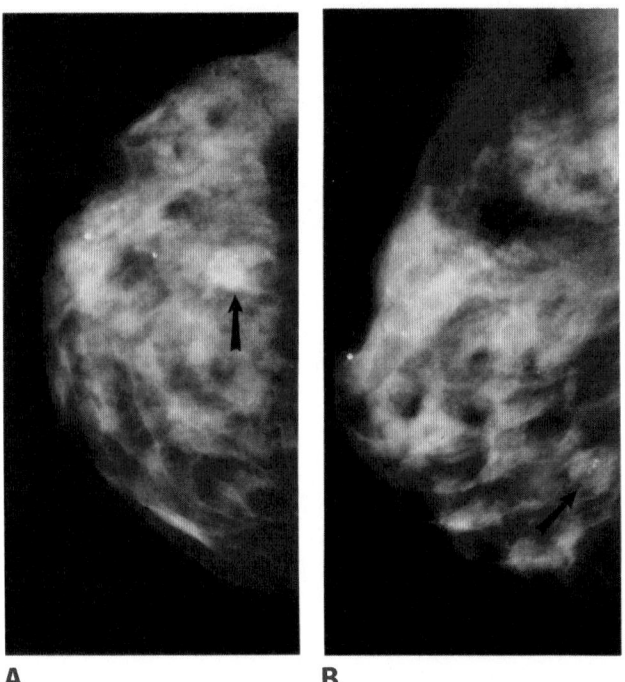

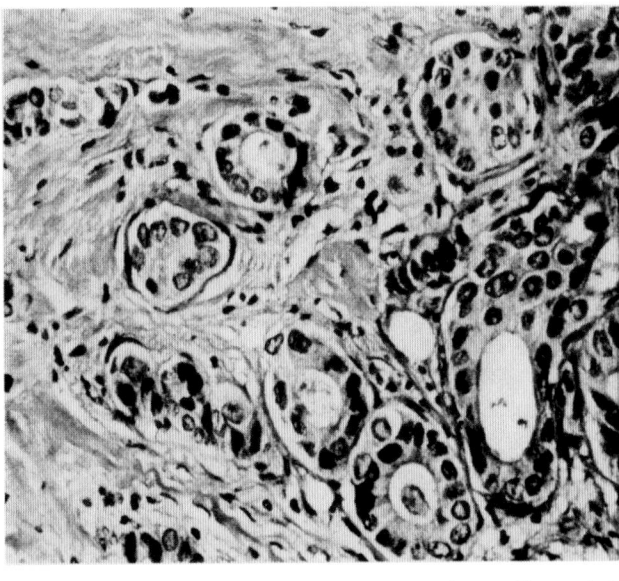

FIG. 17-20. Invasive ductal carcinoma with productive fibrosis (scirrhous, simplex, no special type) (×62.5). *(Courtesy of Dr. R. L. Hackett.)*

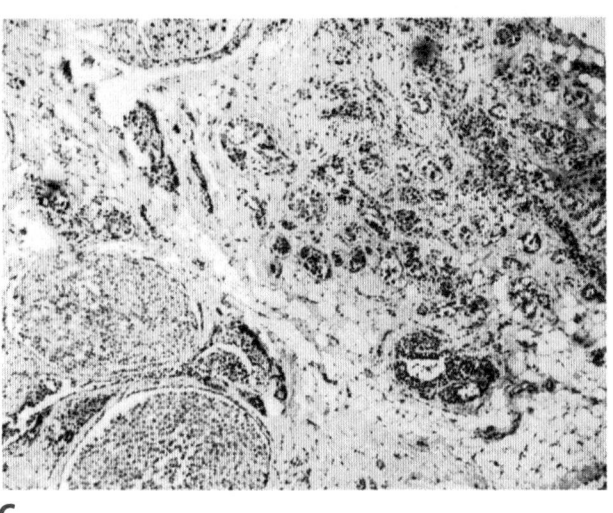

FIG. 17-19. Ductal carcinoma in situ (DCIS). Craniocaudal (**A**) and mediolateral oblique (**B**) mammographic views show a poorly defined 1.2-cm mass (*arrow*) containing microcalcifications. Histopathologic preparation of the surgical specimen (**C**) confirms DCIS with areas of invasion (hematoxylin and eosin stain, ×32).

that are identical to the underlying DCIS cells (pagetoid features or pagetoid change). Pathognomonic of this cancer is the presence of large, pale, vacuolated cells (Paget cells) in the rete pegs of the epithelium. Paget's disease may be confused with superficial spreading melanoma. Differentiation from pagetoid intraepithelial melanoma is based on the presence of S-100 antigen immunostaining in melanoma and carcinoembryonic antigen immunostaining in Paget's disease. Surgical therapy for Paget's disease may involve lumpectomy, mastectomy, or modified radical mastectomy, depending on the extent of involvement and the presence of invasive cancer.

Invasive ductal carcinoma of the breast with productive fibrosis (scirrhous, simplex, NST) accounts for 80% of breast cancers and presents with macroscopic or microscopic axillary lymph node metastases in up to 60% of cases. This cancer usually occurs in perimenopausal or postmenopausal women in the fifth to sixth decades of life as a solitary, firm mass. It has poorly defined margins and its cut surfaces show a central stellate configuration with chalky white or yellow streaks extending into surrounding breast tissues. The cancer cells often are arranged in small clusters, and there is a broad spectrum of histologic types with variable cellular and nuclear grades (Fig. 17-20).

Medullary carcinoma is a special-type breast cancer; it accounts for 4% of all invasive breast cancers and is a frequent phenotype of *BRCA1* hereditary breast cancer. Grossly, the cancer is soft and hemorrhagic. A rapid increase in size may occur secondary to necrosis and hemorrhage. On physical examination, it is bulky and often positioned deep within the breast. Bilaterality is reported in 20% of cases. Medullary carcinoma is characterized microscopically by (a) a dense lymphoreticular infiltrate composed predominantly of lymphocytes and plasma cells; (b) large pleomorphic nuclei that are poorly differentiated and show active mitosis; and (c) a sheet-like growth pattern with minimal or absent ductal or alveolar differentiation (Fig. 17-21). Approximately 50% of these cancers are associated with DCIS, which characteristically is present at the periphery of the cancer, and <10% demonstrate hormone receptors. In rare circumstances, mesenchymal metaplasia or anaplasia is noted. Because of the intense lymphocyte response associated with the cancer, benign or hyperplastic enlargement of the lymph nodes of the axilla may contribute to erroneous clinical staging. Women with this cancer have a better 5-year survival rate than those with NST or invasive lobular carcinoma.

Mucinous carcinoma (colloid carcinoma), another special-type breast cancer, accounts for 2% of all invasive breast cancers and typically presents in the elderly population as a bulky tumor. This cancer is defined by extracellular pools of mucin, which surround aggregates of low-grade cancer cells. The cut surface of this cancer is glistening and gelatinous in quality. Fibrosis is variable, and when abundant it imparts a firm consistency to the cancer. Approximately 66% of mucinous carcinomas display hormone receptors. Lymph node metastases occur in 33% of cases, and 5- and 10-year survival rates are 73 and 59%, respectively. Because of the mucinous component, cancer cells may not be evident in all microscopic sections, and analysis of multiple sections is essential to confirm the diagnosis of a mucinous carcinoma.

Papillary carcinoma is a special-type cancer of the breast that accounts for 2% of all invasive breast cancers. It generally presents in

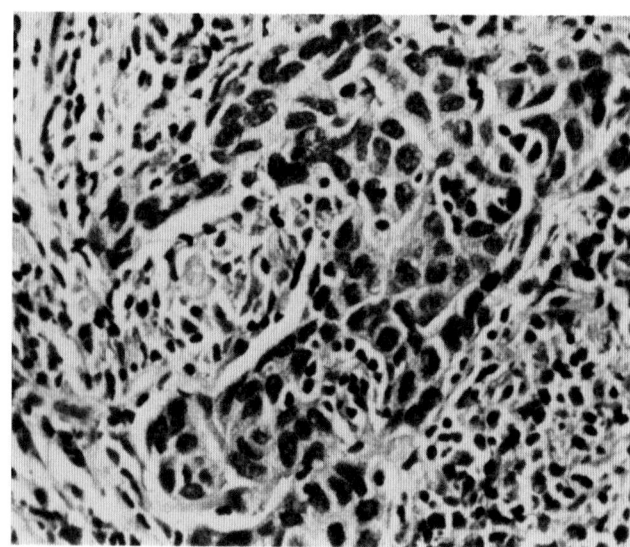

FIG. 17-21. Medullary breast carcinoma (×250). *(Reproduced with permission from Simpson et al,[87] p 285. Copyright Elsevier.)*

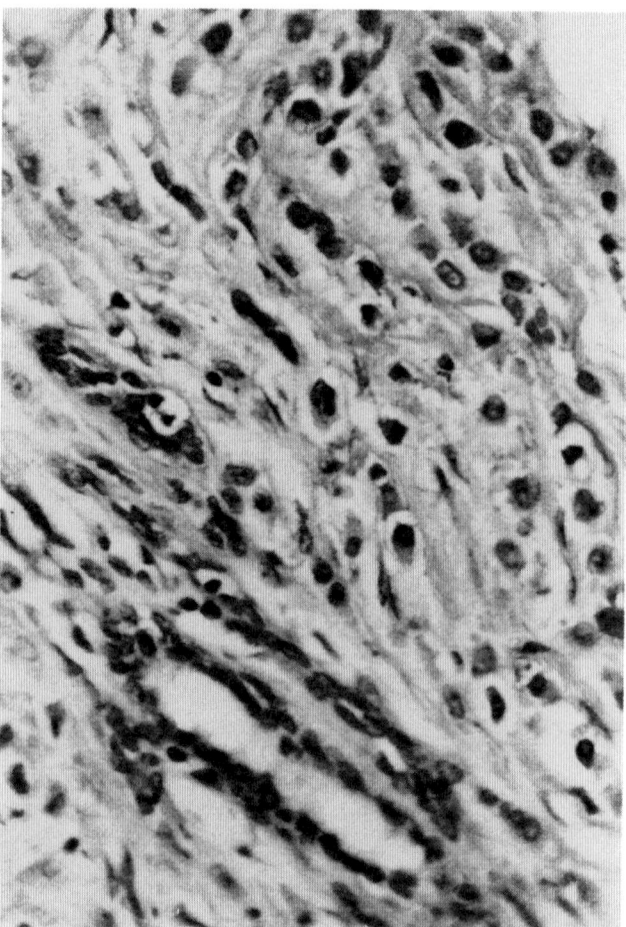

FIG. 17-22. Lobular carcinoma (×250). Uniform, relatively small lobular carcinoma cells are seen arranged in a single-file orientation ("Indian file"). *(Reproduced with permission from Simpson et al,[87] p 285. Copyright Elsevier.)*

the seventh decade of life and occurs in a disproportionate number of nonwhite women. Typically, papillary carcinomas are small and rarely attain a size of 3 cm in diameter. These cancers are defined by papillae with fibrovascular stalks and multilayered epithelium. McDivitt and colleagues noted that these tumors showed a low frequency of axillary lymph node metastases and had 5- and 10-year survival rates similar to those for mucinous and tubular carcinoma.[88]

Tubular carcinoma is another special-type breast cancer and accounts for 2% of all invasive breast cancers. It is reported in as many as 20% of women whose cancers are diagnosed by mammographic screening and usually is diagnosed in the perimenopausal or early menopausal periods. Under low-power magnification, a haphazard array of small, randomly arranged tubular elements is seen. Approximately 10% of women with tubular carcinoma or with invasive cribriform carcinoma, a special-type cancer closely related to tubular carcinoma, will develop axillary lymph node metastases, which are usually confined to the lowest axillary lymph nodes (level I). However, the presence of metastatic disease in one or two axillary lymph nodes does not adversely affect survival. Distant metastases are rare in tubular carcinoma and invasive cribriform carcinoma. Long-term survival approaches 100%.

Invasive lobular carcinoma accounts for 10% of breast cancers. The histopathologic features of this cancer include small cells with rounded nuclei, inconspicuous nucleoli, and scant cytoplasm (Fig. 17-22). Special stains may confirm the presence of intracytoplasmic mucin, which may displace the nucleus (signet-ring cell carcinoma). At presentation, invasive lobular carcinoma varies from clinically inapparent cancers to those that replace the entire breast with a poorly defined mass. It is frequently multifocal, multicentric, and bilateral. Because of its insidious growth pattern and subtle mammographic features, invasive lobular carcinoma may be difficult to detect.

DIAGNOSIS OF BREAST CANCER

In 33% of breast cancer cases, the woman discovers a lump in her breast. Other less frequent presenting signs and symptoms of breast cancer include (a) breast enlargement or asymmetry; (b) nipple changes, retraction, or discharge; (c) ulceration or erythema of the skin of the breast; (d) an axillary mass; and (e) musculoskeletal discomfort. However, up to 50% of women presenting with breast complaints have no physical signs of breast pathology. Breast pain usually is associated with benign disease.

Misdiagnosed breast cancer accounts for the greatest number of malpractice claims for errors in diagnosis and for the largest number of paid claims. Litigation often involves younger women, whose physical examination and mammogram may be misleading. If a young woman (≤45 years) presents with a palpable breast mass and equivocal mammographic findings, ultrasound examination and biopsy are used to avoid a delay in diagnosis.

Examination
Inspection

The surgeon inspects the woman's breast with her arms by her side (Fig. 17-23A), with her arms straight up in the air (Fig. 17-23B), and with her hands on her hips (with and without pectoral muscle contraction).[89,90] Symmetry, size, and shape of the breast are recorded, as well as any evidence of edema (peau d'orange), nipple or skin retraction, or erythema. With the arms extended forward and in a sitting position, the woman leans forward to accentuate any skin retraction.

Palpation

As part of the physical examination, the breast is carefully palpated. Examination of the patient in the supine position (see Fig. 17-23C) is best performed with a pillow supporting the ipsilateral hemithorax. The surgeon gently palpates the breast from the ipsilateral side, making certain to examine all quadrants of the breast from the sternum laterally to the latissimus dorsi muscle and from the clavicle inferiorly to the upper rectus sheath. The surgeon performs the examination with the palmar aspects of the fingers, avoiding a

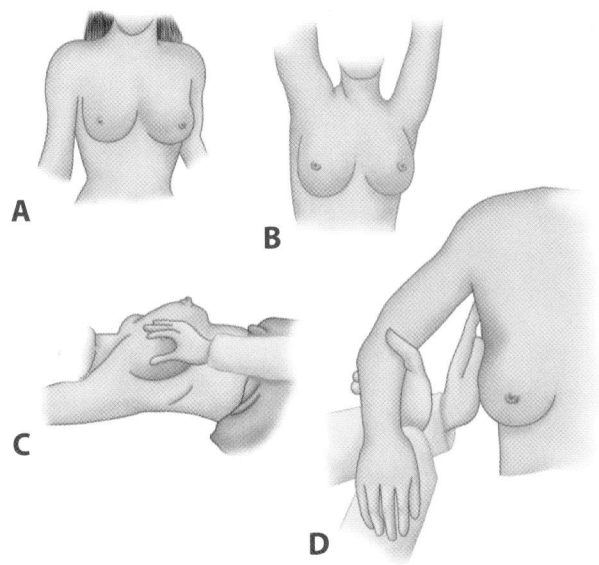

FIG. 17-23. Examination of the breast. **A.** Inspection of the breast with arms at sides. **B.** Inspection of the breast with arms raised. **C.** Palpation of the breast with the patient supine. **D.** Palpation of the axilla.

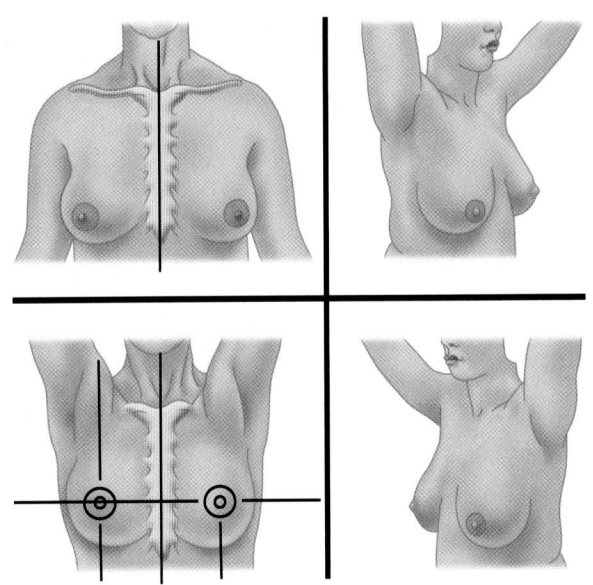

FIG. 17-24. A breast examination record. *(Reproduced with permission from Cliggott Publishing Co.)*

grasping or pinching motion. The breast may be cupped or molded in the surgeon's hands to check for retraction. A systematic search for lymphadenopathy then is performed. Figure 17-23D shows the position of the patient for examination of the axilla. By supporting the upper arm and elbow, the surgeon stabilizes the shoulder girdle. Using gentle palpation, the surgeon assesses all three levels of possible axillary lymphadenopathy. Careful palpation of supraclavicular and parasternal sites also is performed. A diagram of the chest and contiguous lymph node sites is useful for recording location, size, consistency, shape, mobility, fixation, and other characteristics of any palpable breast mass or lymphadenopathy (Fig. 17-24).

Imaging Techniques

Mammography

Mammography has been used in North America since the 1960s, and the techniques used continue to be modified and improved to enhance image quality (Fig. 17-25A and C).[91-94] Conventional mammography delivers a radiation dose of 0.1 cGy per study. By comparison, chest radiography delivers 25% of this dose. However, there is no increased breast cancer risk associated with the radiation dose delivered with screening mammography. Screening mammography is used to detect unexpected breast cancer in asymptomatic women. In this regard, it supplements history taking and physical examination. With screening mammography, two views of the breast are obtained, the craniocaudal (CC) view (Fig. 17-25D) and the mediolateral oblique (MLO) view (Fig. 17-25E). The MLO view images the greatest volume of breast tissue, including the upper outer quadrant and the axillary tail of Spence. Compared with the MLO view, the CC view provides better visualization of the medial aspect of the breast and permits greater breast compression. Diagnostic mammography is used to evaluate women with abnormal findings such as a breast mass or nipple discharge. In addition to the MLO and CC views, a diagnostic examination may use views that better define the nature of any abnormalities, such as the 90-degree lateral and spot compression views. The 90-degree lateral view is used along with the CC view to triangulate the exact location of an abnormality. Spot compression

may be done in any projection by using a small compression device, which is placed directly over a mammographic abnormality that is obscured by overlying tissues (Fig. 17-25F). The compression device minimizes motion artifact, improves definition, separates overlying tissues, and decreases the radiation dose needed to penetrate the breast. Magnification techniques (×1.5) often are combined with spot compression to better resolve calcifications and the margins of masses. Mammography also is used to guide interventional procedures, including needle localization and needle biopsy.

An experienced radiologist can detect breast cancer with a false-positive rate of 10% and a false-negative rate of 7%. Specific mammographic features that suggest a diagnosis of breast cancer include a solid mass with or without stellate features, asymmetric thickening of breast tissues, and clustered microcalcifications. The presence of fine, stippled calcium in and around a suspicious lesion is suggestive of breast cancer and occurs in as many as 50% of nonpalpable cancers. These microcalcifications are an especially important sign of cancer in younger women, in whom it may be the only mammographic abnormality. The clinical impetus for screening mammography came from the Health Insurance Plan study and the Breast Cancer Detection Demonstration Project, which demonstrated a 33% reduction in mortality for women after screening mammography. Mammography was more accurate than clinical examination for the detection of early breast cancers, providing a true-positive rate of 90%. Only 20% of women with nonpalpable cancers had axillary lymph node metastases, compared with 50% of women with palpable cancers.[95] Current guidelines of the National Comprehensive Cancer Network suggest that normal-risk women ≥20 years of age should have a breast examination at least every 3 years. Starting at age 40 years, breast examinations should be performed yearly and a yearly mammogram should be taken. Prospective randomized studies of mammography screening confirm a 40% reduction in stage II, III, and IV cancer in the screened population, with a 30% increase in overall survival.

Xeromammography techniques are identical to those of mammography with the exception that the image is recorded on a xerography plate, which provides a positive rather than a negative image

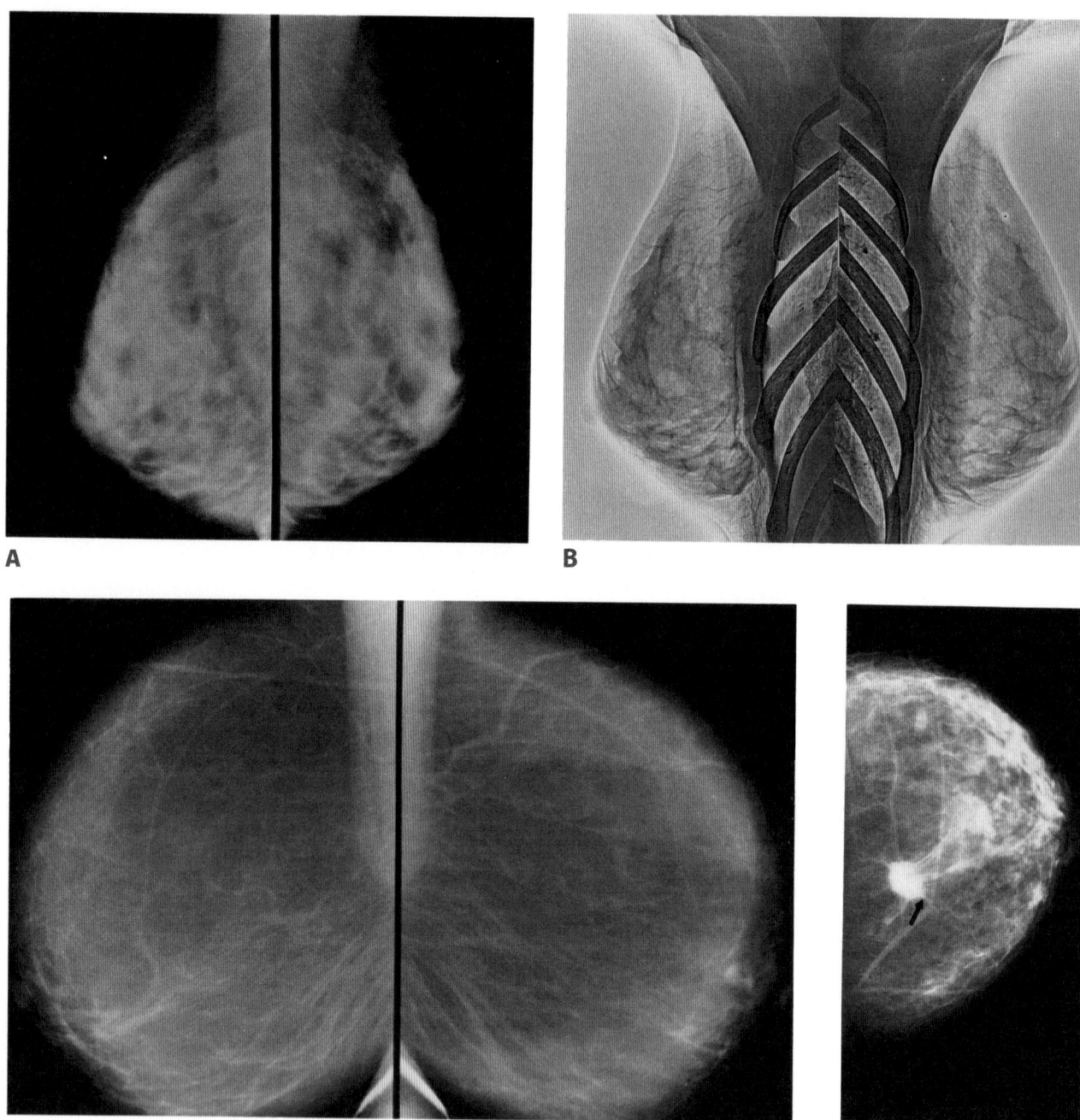

FIG. 17-25. Mammography and xeromammography. **A.** Mammogram of a premenopausal breast with a dense fibroglandular pattern. **B.** Xeromammogram of the breast shown in **A**. Xeromammography allows visualization from the nipple to the ribs, whereas mammography permits better visualization of the axillary tail of Spence. **C.** Mammogram of a postmenopausal breast with a sparse fibroglandular pattern. **D.** Invasive breast cancer (*arrow*) shown in the craniocaudal mammography view. *(Continued)*

(see Fig. 17-25B). Details of the entire breast and the soft tissues of the chest wall may be recorded with one exposure. Screen film mammography has replaced xeromammography because it requires a lower dose of radiation and provides similar image quality. Digital mammography was developed to allow the observer to manipulate the degree of contrast in the image. This is especially useful in women with dense breasts and women <50 years of age. Recently, investigators directly compared digital vs. screen film mammography in a prospective trial enrolling over 42,000 women.[96] They found that digital and screen film mammography had similar accuracy; however, digital mammography was more accurate in women <50 years of age,

women with mammographically dense breasts, and premenopausal or perimenopausal women.

Ductography

The primary indication for ductography is nipple discharge, particularly when the fluid contains blood. Radiopaque contrast media is injected into one or more of the major ducts and mammography is performed. A duct is gently enlarged with a dilator and then a small, blunt cannula is inserted under sterile conditions into the nipple ampulla. With the patient in a supine position, 0.1 to 0.2 mL of dilute contrast media is injected and CC and MLO mammographic views are

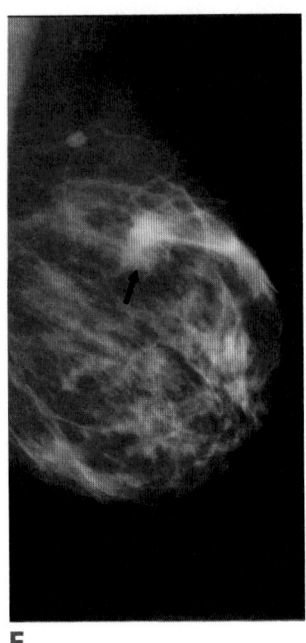

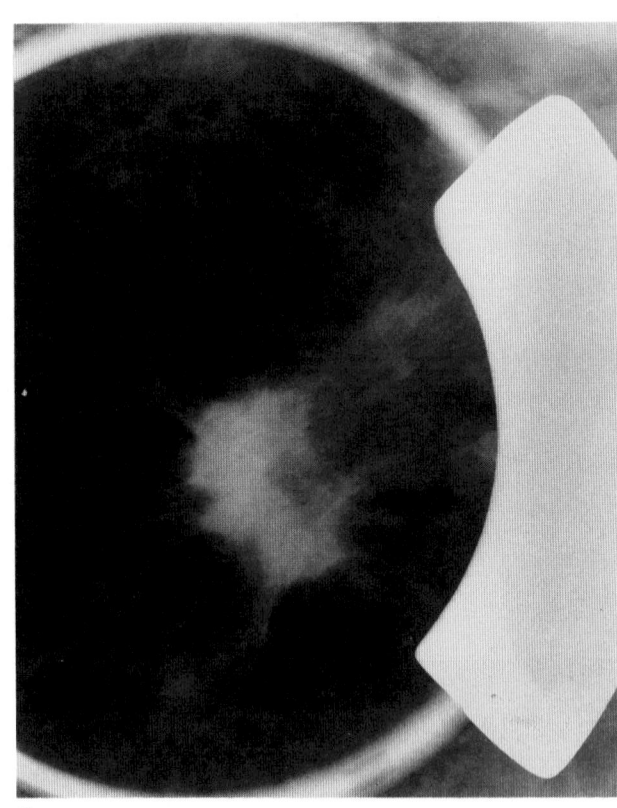

FIG. 17-25. *(Continued)* **E.** Invasive breast cancer *(arrow)* shown in the mediolateral oblique mammography view. **F.** Cone-compression mammography view of the cancer seen in **D** and **E**. Note that the speculated margins of the cancer are accentuated by cone compression. *(Courtesy of Dr. B. Steinbach.)*

E

F

obtained without compression. Intraductal papillomas are seen as small filling defects surrounded by contrast media (Fig. 17-26). Cancers may appear as irregular masses or as multiple intraluminal filling defects.

Ultrasonography

Second only to mammography in frequency of use for breast imaging, ultrasonography is an important method of resolving equivocal mammographic findings, defining cystic masses, and demonstrating the echogenic qualities of specific solid abnormalities. On ultrasound examination, breast cysts are well circumscribed, with smooth margins and an echo-free center (Fig. 17-27). Benign breast masses usually show smooth contours, round or oval shapes, weak internal echoes, and well-defined anterior and posterior margins. Breast cancer characteristically has irregular walls (Fig. 17-28) but may have

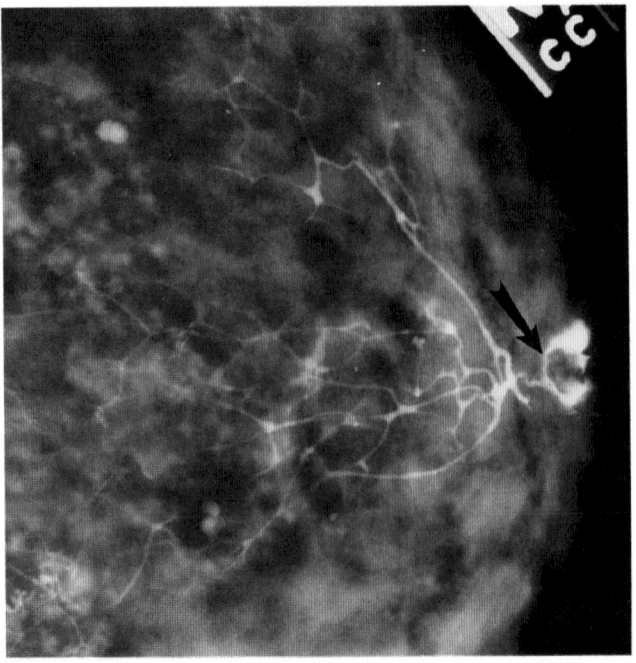

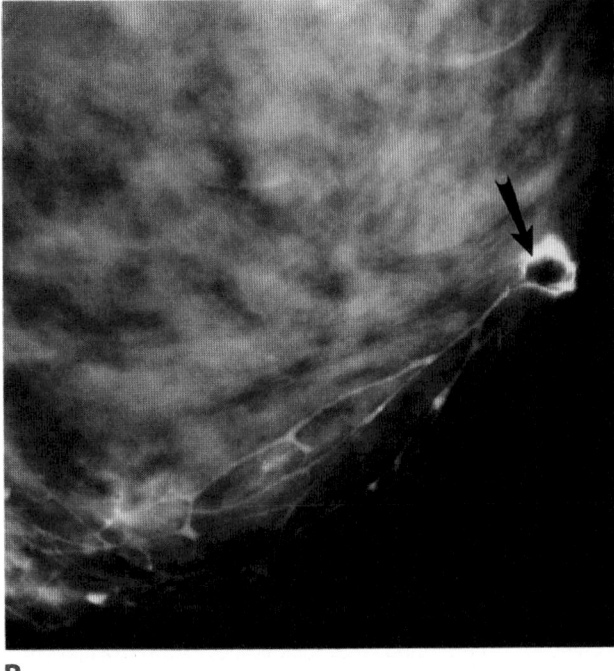

A

B

FIG. 17-26. Ductogram. Craniocaudal (**A**) and mediolateral oblique (**B**) mammographic views demonstrate a mass *(arrows)* posterior to the nipple and outlined by contrast, which also fills the proximal ductal structures. *(Courtesy of Dr. B. Steinbach.)*

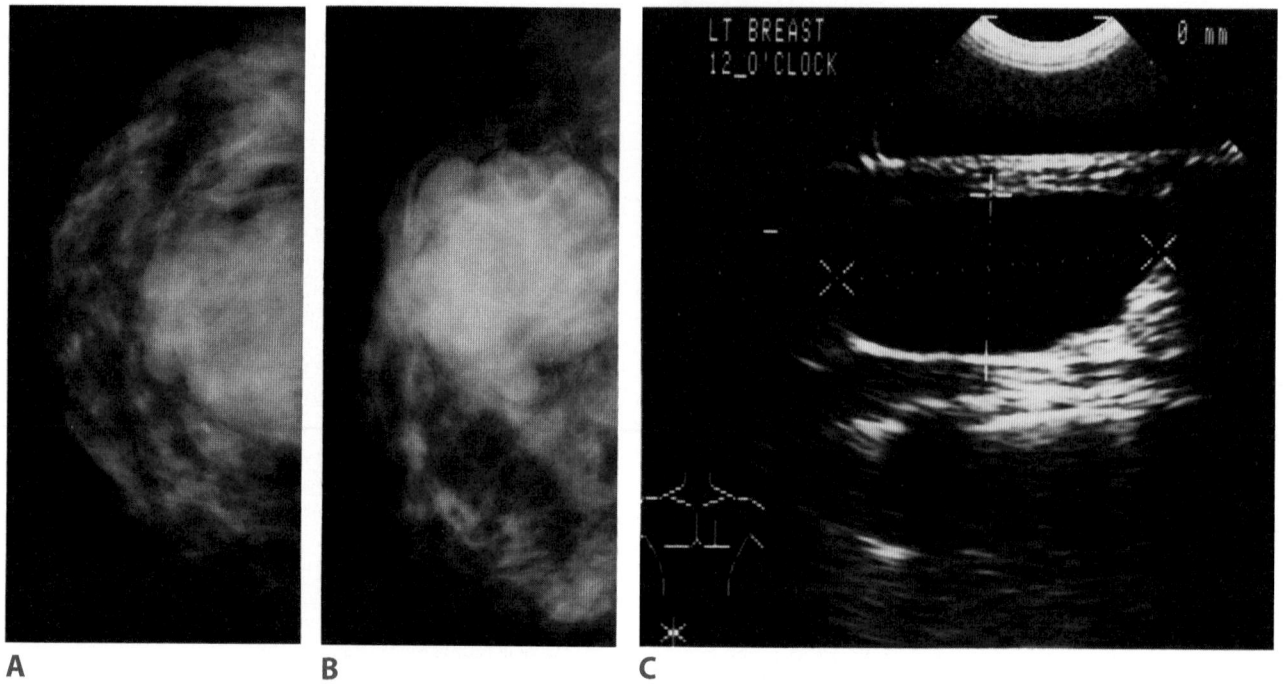

FIG. 17-27. Breast cyst. Craniocaudal (**A**) and mediolateral oblique (**B**) mammographic views show a large lobulated mass. Ultrasound image of the mass (**C**) shows it to be anechoic with a well-defined back wall, characteristic of a cyst. *(Courtesy of Dr. B. Steinbach.)*

smooth margins with acoustic enhancement. Ultrasonography is used to guide fine-needle aspiration biopsy, core-needle biopsy, and needle localization of breast lesions. Its findings are highly reproducible and it has a high patient acceptance rate, but it does not reliably detect lesions that are ≤1 cm in diameter.

Magnetic Resonance Imaging

In the process of evaluating MRI as a means of characterizing mammographic abnormalities, additional breast lesions have been detected. However, in the circumstance of negative findings on both mammography and physical examination, the probability of a breast cancer being diagnosed by MRI is extremely low. There is current interest in the use of MRI to screen the breasts of high-risk women and of women with a newly diagnosed breast cancer. In the first case, women who have a strong family history of breast cancer or who carry known genetic mutations require screening at an early age, but mammographic evaluation is limited because of the increased breast density in younger women. In the second case, an MRI study of the contralateral breast in women with a known breast cancer has shown a contralateral breast cancer in 5.7% of these women.

Breast Biopsy
Nonpalpable Lesions

Image-guided breast biopsies are frequently required to diagnose nonpalpable lesions.[97] Ultrasound localization techniques are used when a mass is present, whereas stereotactic techniques are used when no mass is present (microcalcifications only). The combination of diagnostic mammography, ultrasound or stereotactic localization, and fine-needle aspiration (FNA) biopsy achieves almost 100% accuracy in the diagnosis of breast cancer. However, although FNA biopsy permits cytologic evaluation, core-needle or open biopsy also permits the analysis of breast tissue architecture and allows the pathologist to determine whether invasive cancer is present. This permits the surgeon and patient to discuss the specific management of a breast cancer before therapy begins. Core-needle biopsy is preferred over open biopsy for nonpalpable breast lesions because a single surgical procedure can be planned based on the results of the

core biopsy. The advantages of core-needle biopsy include a low complication rate, avoidance of scarring, and a lower cost.

Palpable Lesions

FNA biopsy of a palpable breast mass can easily proceed in an outpatient setting.[98] A 1.5-in, 22-gauge needle attached to a 10-mL syringe is used. Use of a syringe holder enables the surgeon performing the FNA biopsy to control the syringe and needle with one hand while positioning the breast mass with the opposite hand. After the needle is placed in the mass, suction is applied while the needle is moved back and forth within the mass. Once cellular material is seen at the hub of the needle, the suction is released and the needle is withdrawn. The cellular material is then expressed onto microscope slides. Both air-dried and 95% ethanol–fixed microscopic sections are prepared for analysis. When a breast mass is clinically and mammographically suspicious, the sensitivity and specificity of FNA biopsy approaches 100%. Core-needle biopsy of palpable breast masses is performed using a 14-gauge needle, such as the Tru-Cut needle. Automated devices also are available. Tissue specimens are placed in formalin and then processed to paraffin blocks. Although the false-negative rate for core-needle biopsy specimens is very low, a tissue specimen that does not show breast cancer cannot conclusively rule out that diagnosis because a sampling error may have occurred. The clinical, radiographic, and pathologic findings should be in concordance. If the biopsy findings do not concur with the clinical and radiographic findings, the clinician should proceed with an image-guided or open biopsy to be certain that the target lesion has been adequately sampled for diagnosis.

BREAST CANCER STAGING AND BIOMARKERS

Breast Cancer Staging

The clinical stage of breast cancer is determined primarily through physical examination of the skin, breast tissue, and regional lymph nodes (axillary, supraclavicular, and cervical).[99] However, clinical determination of axillary lymph node metastases has an accuracy of

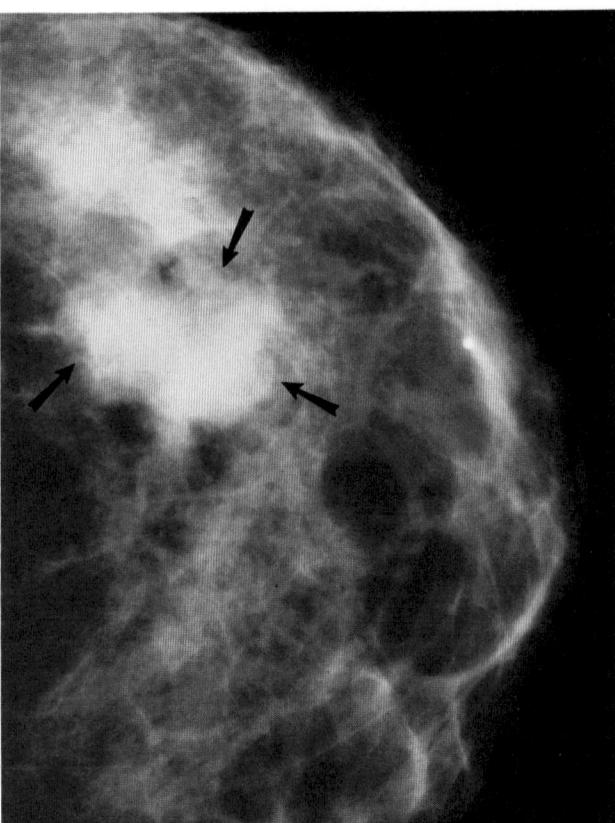

A

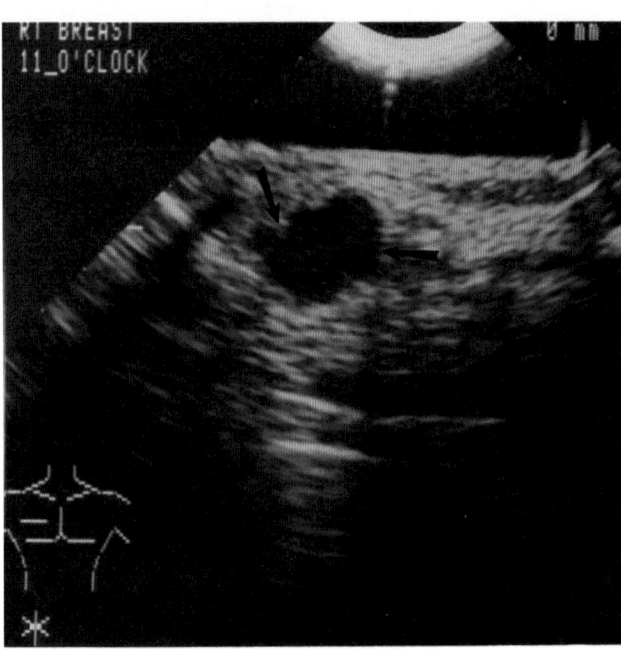

B

FIG. 17-28. Breast cancer. **A.** Craniocaudal mammographic view of a palpable mass (*arrows*). **B.** Ultrasound image demonstrating a solid mass with irregular borders (*arrows*) consistent with cancer.

only 33%. Mammography, chest radiography, and intraoperative findings (primary tumor size, chest wall invasion) also provide necessary staging information. Pathologic stage combines the findings from pathologic examination of the resected primary breast cancer and axillary or other regional lymph nodes. Fisher and colleagues found that accurate predictions regarding the occurrence of

distant metastases were possible after resection and pathologic analysis of 10 or more level I and II axillary lymph nodes.[100] A frequently used staging system is the TNM (tumor, nodes, and metastasis) system. The American Joint Committee on Cancer (AJCC) has modified the TNM system for breast cancer (Tables 17-11 and 17-12). Koscielny and colleagues demonstrated that tumor size correlates with the presence of axillary lymph node metastases (see Fig. 17-18B). Others have shown an association between tumor size, axillary lymph node metastases, and disease-free survival. The single most important predictor of 10- and 20-year survival rates in breast cancer is the number of axillary lymph nodes involved with metastatic disease. Routine biopsy of internal mammary lymph nodes is not generally performed; however, with the advent of sentinel lymph node dissection and the use of preoperative lymphoscintigraphy for localization of the sentinel nodes, surgeons have begun to biopsy the internal mammary nodes in some cases. The sixth edition of the AJCC staging system does allow for staging based on findings from the internal mammary sentinel nodes.[99] Drainage to the internal mammary nodes is more frequent with central and medial quadrant cancers. Clinical or pathologic evidence of metastatic spread to supraclavicular lymph nodes is no longer considered systemic or stage IV disease, but routine scalene or supraclavicular lymph node biopsy is not indicated.

Biomarkers

Breast cancer biomarkers are of several types. Risk factor biomarkers are those associated with increased cancer risk.[101–105] These include familial clustering and inherited germline abnormalities, proliferative breast disease with atypia, and mammographic densities. Exposure biomarkers are a subset of risk factors that include measures of carcinogen exposure such as DNA adducts. Surrogate endpoint biomarkers are biologic alterations in tissue that occur between cancer initiation and development. These biomarkers are used as endpoints in short-term chemoprevention trials and include histologic changes, indices of proliferation, and genetic alterations leading to cancer. Prognostic biomarkers provide information regarding cancer outcome irrespective of therapy, whereas predictive biomarkers provide information regarding response to therapy. Candidate prognostic and predictive biomarkers and biologic targets for breast cancer include (a) indices of proliferation such as proliferating cell nuclear antigen (PCNA) and Ki-67; (b) indices of apoptosis and apoptosis modulators such as bcl-2 and the bax:bcl-2 ratio; (c) indices of angiogenesis such as vascular endothelial growth factor (VEGF) and the angiogenesis index; (d) growth factors and growth factor receptors such as human epidermal growth factor receptor 2 (HER-2)/*neu*, epidermal growth factor receptor (EGFr), transforming growth factor, platelet-derived growth factor, and the insulin-like growth factor family; (e) the steroid hormone receptor pathway; (f) the cell cycle, cyclins, and cyclin-dependent kinases; (g) the proteasome; (h) the COX-2 enzyme; (i) the peroxisome proliferator-activated receptors (PPARs); (j) tumor-suppressor genes such as p53; and (k) the mammalian target of rapamycin (mTOR) signaling pathway.

Indices of Proliferation

PCNA is a nuclear protein associated with a DNA polymerase whose expression increases in phase G_1 of the cell cycle, reaches its maximum at the G_1/S interface, and then decreases through G_2.[106–109] Immunohistochemical staining for PCNA outlines the proliferating compartments in breast tissue. Good correlation is noted between PCNA expression and (a) cell-cycle distributions seen on flow cytometry based on DNA content, and (b) uptake of bromodeoxyuridine and the proliferation-associated Ki-67 antigen. Individual proliferation markers are associated with slightly different phases of the cell cycle and are not equivalent. PCNA and Ki-67 expression are positively correlated with p53 overexpression, high S-phase fraction, aneuploidy, high mitotic index, and high histologic grade in human breast cancer specimens, and are negatively correlated with estrogen receptor content.

CHAPTER 17

The Breast

TABLE 17-11 TNM staging system for breast cancer

Primary tumor (T) Definitions for classifying the primary tumor (T) are the same for clinical and for pathologic classification. If the measurement is made by physical examination, the examiner will use the major headings (T1, T2, or T3); if other measurements, such as mammographic or pathologic measurements, are used, the subsets of T1 can be used. Tumors should be measured to the nearest 0.1-cm increment.

TX	Primary tumor cannot be assessed
T0	No evidence of primary tumor
Tis	Carcinoma in situ
Tis (DCIS)	Ductal carcinoma in situ
Tis (LCIS)	Lobular carcinoma in situ
Tis (Paget's)	Paget's disease of the nipple with no tumor (NOTE: Paget's disease associated with a tumor is classified according to the size of the tumor)
T1	Tumor ≤2 cm in greatest dimension
T1mic	Microinvasion ≤0.1 cm or less in greatest dimension
T1a	Tumor >0.1 cm but not >0.5 cm in greatest dimension
T1b	Tumor >0.5 cm but not >1 cm in greatest dimension
T1c	Tumor >1 cm but not >2 cm in greatest dimension
T2	Tumor >2 cm but not >5 cm in greatest dimension
T3	Tumor >5 cm in greatest dimension
T4	Tumor of any size with direct extension to (a) chest wall or (b) skin, only as described below
T4a	Extension to chest wall, not including pectoralis muscle
T4b	Edema (including peau d'orange), or ulceration of the skin of the breast, or satellite skin nodules confined to the same breast
T4c	Both T4a and T4b
T4d	Inflammatory carcinoma

Regional lymph nodes—Clinical (N)

NX	Regional lymph nodes cannot be assessed (e.g., previously removed)
N0	No regional lymph node metastasis
N1	Metastasis to movable ipsilateral axillary lymph node(s)
N2	Metastases in ipsilateral axillary lymph nodes fixed or matted, or in clinically apparent[a] ipsilateral internal mammary nodes in the absence of clinically evident axillary lymph node metastasis
N2a	Metastasis in ipsilateral axillary lymph nodes fixed to one another (matted) or to other structures
N3	Metastasis only in clinically apparent[a] ipsilateral internal mammary nodes and in the absence of clinically evident axillary lymph node metastasis; metastasis in ipsilateral infraclavicular lymph node(s) with or without axillary lymph node involvement, or in clinically apparent[a] ipsilateral internal mammary lymph node(s) and in the presence of clinically evident axillary lymph node metastasis; or metastasis in ipsilateral supraclavicular lymph node(s) with or without axillary or internal mammary lymph node involvement
N3a	Metastasis in ipsilateral infraclavicular lymph node(s)
N3b	Metastasis in ipsilateral internal mammary lymph nodes(s) and axillary lymph node(s)
N3c	Metastasis in ipsilateral supraclavicular lymph node(s)

Regional lymph nodes—Pathologic (pN)

pNX	Regional lymph nodes cannot be assessed (e.g., previously removed, or not removed for pathologic study)
pN0[b]	No regional lymph node metastasis histologically, no additional examination for isolated tumor cells [NOTE: Isolated tumor cells (ITC) are defined as single tumor cells or small cell clusters not >0.2 mm, which are usually detected only by immunohistochemical (IHC) or molecular methods but which may be verified on hematoxylin and eosin stains; ITCs do not usually show evidence of malignant activity (e.g., proliferation or stromal reaction)]
pN0(i−)	No regional lymph node metastasis histologically, negative IHC results
pN0(i+)	No regional lymph node metastasis histologically, positive IHC results, no IHC cluster >0.2 mm
pN0(mol−)	No regional lymph node metastasis histologically, negative molecular findings [reverse-transcriptase polymerase chain reaction (RT-PCR)]
pN0(mol+)	No regional lymph node metastasis histologically, positive molecular findings (RT-PCR)
pN1	Metastasis in 1 to 3 axillary lymph nodes, and/or in internal mammary nodes with microscopic disease detected by sentinel lymph nodes dissection, not clinically apparent[c]
pN1mi	Micrometastasis (>0.2 mm, none >2.0 mm)
pN1a	Metastasis in 1 to 3 axillary lymph nodes
pN1b	Metastasis in internal mammary nodes with microscopic disease detected by sentinel lymph node dissection, not clinically apparent[c]
pN1c	Metastasis in 1 to 3 axillary lymph nodes and in internal mammary lymph nodes with microscopic disease detected by sentinel lymph node dissection but not clinically apparent[c] (if associated with >3 positive axillary lymph nodes, the internal mammary nodes are classified as pN3b to reflect increased tumor burden)
pN2	Metastasis in 4 to 9 axillary lymph nodes, or in clinically apparent[a] internal mammary lymph nodes in the absence of axillary lymph node metastasis
pN2a	Metastasis in 4 to 9 axillary lymph nodes (at least one tumor deposit >2.0 mm)
pN2b	Metastasis in clinically apparent[a] internal mammary lymph nodes in the absence of axillary lymph node metastasis
pN3	Metastasis in ≥10 axillary lymph nodes, or in infraclavicular lymph nodes, or in clinically apparent[a] ipsilateral internal mammary lymph nodes in the presence of 1 or more positive axillary lymph nodes; or in >3 axillary lymph nodes with clinically negative microscopic metastasis in internal mammary lymph nodes; or in ipsilateral supraclavicular lymph nodes
pN3a	Metastasis in ≥10 axillary lymph nodes (at lease one tumor deposit >2.0 mm), or metastasis to the infraclavicular lymph nodes
pN3b	Metastasis in clinically apparent[a] ipsilateral internal mammary lymph nodes in the presence of ≥1 positive axillary lymph nodes; or in >3 axillary lymph nodes and in internal mammary lymph nodes with microscopic disease detected by sentinel lymph node dissection, not clinically apparent[c]
pN3c	Metastasis in ipsilateral supraclavicular lymph nodes

Distant metastasis (M)

MX	Distant metastasis cannot be assessed
M0	No distant metastasis
M1	Distant metastasis

[a]*Clinically apparent* is defined as detected by imaging studies (excluding lymphoscintigraphy) or by clinical examination or grossly visible pathologically.

[b]Classification is based on axillary lymph node dissection with or without sentinel lymph node dissection. Classification based solely on sentinel lymph node dissection without subsequent axillary lymph node dissection is designated (sn) for "sentinel node" e.g., pN−(l+) (sn).

[c]*Not clinically apparent* is defined as not detected by imaging studies (excluding lymphoscintigraphy) or by clinical examination.

Source: Reprinted with permission from American Joint Committee on Cancer: *AJCC Cancer Staging Manual*, 6th ed. New York: Springer, 2002, p 227–228. Used with permission of the American Joint Committee on Cancer (AJCC), Chicago, Illinois. The original source of the material is the AJCC Cancer Staging Manual, Sixth Edition (2002) published by Springer Science and Business Media LLC, *www.springerlink.com*.

TABLE 17-12 TNM stage groupings

Stage 0	Tis	N0	M0
Stage I	T1[a]	N0	M0
Stage IIA	T0	N1	M0
	T1[a]	N1	M0
	T2	N0	M0
Stage IIB	T2	N1	M0
	T3	N0	M0
Stage IIIA	T0	N2	M0
	T1[a]	N2	M0
	T2	N2	M0
	T3	N1	M0
	T3	N2	M0
Stage IIIB	T4	N0	M0
	T4	N1	M0
	T4	N2	M0
Stage IIIC	Any T	N3	M0
Stage IV	Any T	Any N	M1

[a]T1 includes T1mic.

Source: Reprinted with permission from American Joint Committee on Cancer: *AJCC Cancer Staging Manual*, 6th ed. New York: Springer, 2002, pp 228. Used with permission of the American Joint Committee on Cancer (AJCC), Chicago, Illinois. The original source of the material is the AJCC Cancer Staging Manual, Sixth Edition (2002) published by Springer Science and Business Media LLC, *www.springerlink.com*.

Indices of Apoptosis

Alterations in programmed cell death (apoptosis), which may be triggered by p53-dependent or p53-independent factors, may be important prognostic and predictive biomarkers in breast cancer.[110–112] Bcl-2 family proteins appear to regulate a step in the evolutionarily conserved pathway for apoptosis, with some members functioning as inhibitors of apoptosis and others as promoters of apoptosis. *BCL2* is the only oncogene that acts by inhibiting apoptosis rather than by directly increasing cellular proliferation. The death-signal protein bax is induced by genotoxic stress and growth factor deprivation in the presence of wild-type (normal) p53 and/or AP-1/fos. The bax:bcl-2 ratio and the resulting formation of either bax-bax homodimers, which stimulate apoptosis, or bax–bcl-2 heterodimers, which inhibit apoptosis, represent an intracellular regulatory mechanism with prognostic and predictive implications. In breast cancer, overexpression of bcl-2 and a decrease in the bax:bcl-2 ratio correlate with high histologic grade, the presence of axillary lymph node metastases, and reduced disease-free and overall survival rates. Similarly, decreased bax expression correlates with axillary lymph node metastases, a poor response to chemotherapy, and decreased overall survival.

Indices of Angiogenesis

Angiogenesis is necessary for the growth and invasiveness of breast cancer and promotes cancer progression through several different mechanisms, including delivery of oxygen and nutrients and the secretion of growth-promoting cytokines by endothelial cells.[113,114] VEGF induces its effect by binding to transmembrane tyrosine kinase receptors. Overexpression of VEGF in invasive breast cancer is correlated with increased microvessel density and recurrence in node-negative breast cancer. An angiogenesis index has been developed in which microvessel density (CD31 expression) is combined with expression of thrombospondin (a negative modulator of angiogenesis) and p53 expression. Both VEGF expression and the angiogenesis index may have prognostic and predictive significance in breast cancer. Antiangiogenesis breast cancer therapy is now being studied in human trials. The use of bevacizumab (a monoclonal antibody to VEGF) was recently approved by the U.S. Food and Drug Administration (FDA) for use in metastatic breast cancer in combination with paclitaxel chemotherapy. This approval was based on results from a phase III trial by the Eastern Cooperative Oncology Group. The group's E2100 trial showed that when bevacizumab was added to paclitaxel chemotherapy, median progression-free survival increased to 11.3 months from the 5.8 months seen in patients who received paclitaxel alone.[115]

Growth Factor Receptors and Growth Factors

Overexpression of EGFr in breast cancer correlates with estrogen receptor–negative status and with p53 overexpression.[116–118] Similarly, increased immunohistochemical membrane staining for the HER-2/*neu* growth factor receptor in breast cancer is associated with mutated p53 Ki-67 overexpression and estrogen receptor–negative status. HER-2/*neu* is a member of the EGFr family of growth factor receptors in which ligand binding results in receptor homodimerization and tyrosine phosphorylation by tyrosine kinase domains within the receptor. Tyrosine phosphorylation is followed by signal transduction, which results in changes in cell behavior. An important property of this family of receptors is that ligand binding to one receptor type also may result in heterodimerization between two different receptor types that are coexpressed; this leads to transphosphorylation and transactivation of both receptors in the complex (transmodulation). In this context, the lack of a specific ligand for the HER-2/*neu* receptor suggests that HER-2/*neu* may function solely as a coreceptor, modulating signaling by other EGFr family members. HER-2/*neu* is both an important prognostic factor and a predictive factor in breast cancer.[119] When overexpressed in breast cancer, HER-2/*neu* promotes enhanced growth and proliferation, and increases invasive and metastatic capabilities. Clinical studies have shown that patients with HER-2/*neu*–overexpressing breast cancer have poorly differentiated tumors with high proliferation rates, positive lymph nodes, decreased hormone receptor expression, and an increased risk of recurrence and death due to breast cancer.[119–123] Routine testing of the primary tumor specimen for HER-2/*neu* expression should be performed on all invasive breast cancers. This can be done with immunohistochemical analysis to evaluate for overexpression of the cell-surface receptor at the protein level or by using fluorescent in situ hybridization to evaluate for gene amplification. Patients whose tumors overexpress HER-2/*neu* are candidates for anti–HER-2/*neu* therapy. Trastuzumab (Herceptin) is a recombinant humanized monoclonal antibody directed against HER-2/*neu*. Randomized clinical trials have demonstrated that single-agent trastuzumab therapy is an active and well-tolerated option for first-line treatment of women with HER-2/*neu*–overexpressing metastatic breast cancer. More recently, adjuvant trials demonstrated that trastuzumab also was highly effective in the treatment of women with early-stage breast cancer when used in combination with chemotherapy. Patients who received trastuzumab in combination with chemotherapy had a 52% reduction in the risk of breast cancer recurrence compared with those who received chemotherapy alone.[124]

Steroid Hormone Receptor Pathway

Hormones play an important role in the development and progression of breast cancer. Estrogens, estrogen metabolites, and other steroid hormones such as progesterone all have been shown to have an effect. Breast cancer risk is related to estrogen exposure over time. In postmenopausal women, hormone replacement therapy consisting of estrogen plus progesterone increases the risk of breast cancer by 26% compared to placebo.[125] Patients with hormone receptor–positive tumors survive two to three times longer after a diagnosis of metastatic disease than do patients with hormone receptor–negative tumors. Patients with tumors negative for both estrogen receptors and progesterone receptors are not considered candidates for hormonal therapy. Tumors positive for estrogen or progesterone receptors have a higher response rate to endocrine therapy than tumors that do not express estrogen or progesterone receptors. Tumors positive for both receptors have a response rate of >50%, tumors negative for both receptors have a response rate of <10%, and tumors positive for one receptor but not the other have an intermediate response rate of 33%. The determination of estrogen and progesterone receptor status used to require biochemical evaluation of fresh tumor tissue. Today, however, estrogen and progesterone receptor status can be measured in archived tissue using immunohistochemical techniques. Hormone receptor status also can be measured in specimens obtained with fine-needle aspiration biopsy or core-needle biopsy, and this can help guide treatment planning. Testing for estrogen and progesterone receptors should be performed on all primary invasive breast cancer specimens. The tumor hormone receptor status should be ascertained for both premenopausal and postmenopausal patients to identify patients who are most likely to benefit from endocrine therapy.

The remaining biomarkers and biologic targets listed earlier are still in preclinical and clinical trials evaluating their importance in breast cancer for both prognostic and predictive purposes.

Coexpression of Biomarkers

Selection of optimal therapy for breast cancer requires both an accurate assessment of prognosis and an accurate prediction of response to therapy. The breast cancer markers that are most important in determining therapy are estrogen receptor, progesterone receptor, and HER-2/*neu*. Clinicians evaluate clinical and pathologic staging and the expression of estrogen receptor, progesterone receptor, and HER-2/*neu* in the primary tumor to assess prognosis and assign therapy. Adjuvant! Online (*http://www.adjuvantonline.com*) is a program available to clinicians that incorporates clinical and pathologic factors for an individual patient and calculates risk of recurrence and death due to breast cancer and then provides an assessment of the reduction in risk of recurrence that would be expected with the use of combination chemotherapy, endocrine therapy, or both of these. Adjuvant! Online was developed using information from the SEER database, the Early Breast Cancer Trialists' Collaborative Group overview analyses, and results from other individual published trials.[126] The website is updated and modified as new information becomes available. Clinicopathologic factors are used to separate breast cancer patients into broad prognostic groups, and treatment decisions are made on this basis (Table 17-13). When this approach is used, up to 70% of early breast cancer patients receive adjuvant chemotherapy that is either unnecessary or ineffective. As described earlier, a wide variety of biomarkers have been shown to individually predict prognosis and response to therapy, but they do not improve the accuracy of either the assessment of prognosis or the prediction of response to therapy.

As knowledge regarding cellular, biochemical, and molecular biomarkers for breast cancer increases, prognostic indices are being developed that combine the predictive power of several individual biomarkers with the relevant clinicopathologic factors.

Most recently, technologic advances have led to the ability to measure the expression of multiple genes in a tumor sample simultaneously. This gene expression profiling can provide information about tumor behavior that can be used in determining prognosis and therapy.[127] These high-throughput analyses require bioinformatics support that can categorize and analyze the immense amount of data that are generated. This allows for a detailed stratification of breast cancer patients for assessment of prognosis and for prediction of response to therapy. The Onco*type* DX is a 21-gene assay that has been validated in newly diagnosed patients with node-negative, estrogen receptor–positive breast cancer.[128] A recurrence score is generated, and those patients with high recurrence scores are found to benefit the most from chemotherapy, whereas those with low recurrence scores benefit most from tamoxifen and may not require chemotherapy. There is currently an ongoing clinical trial, the Trial Assessing Individualized Options for Treatment for breast cancer (TAILORx), that randomly assigns patients with an intermediate recurrence score to hormonal therapy alone or to chemotherapy followed by hormonal therapy. The MammaPrint test was recently approved by the FDA for use in patients with newly diagnosed, node-negative breast cancer. The MammaPrint test is based on a 70-gene profile, and fresh tissue is required to perform the assay. The Onco*type* DX assay is performed using paraffin-embedded tumor tissue and therefore can be carried out on archived samples.

OVERVIEW OF BREAST CANCER THERAPY

Before diagnostic biopsy, the surgeon must discuss with the patient the possibility that a suspicious mass or mammographic finding may be a breast cancer. Once a diagnosis of breast cancer is made, the type of therapy offered to a breast cancer patient is determined by the stage of the disease. Laboratory tests and imaging studies are performed based on the initial stage as presented in Table 17-14. Before therapy is initiated, the patient and the surgeon must share a clear perspective on the planned course of treatment.

In Situ Breast Cancer (Stage 0)

Both LCIS and DCIS may be difficult to distinguish from atypical hyperplasia or from cancers with early invasion.[50,129–134] Expert pathologic review is required in all cases. Bilateral mammography is performed to determine the extent of the in situ cancer and to exclude a second cancer. Because LCIS is considered a marker for increased risk rather than an inevitable precursor of invasive disease, the current treatment options for LCIS include observation, chemoprevention with tamoxifen, and bilateral total mastectomy. The goal of treatment is to prevent or detect at an early stage the invasive

---

TABLE 17-13 Traditional prognostic and predictive factors for invasive breast cancer

Tumor Factors	Host Factors
Nodal status	Age
Tumor size	Menopausal status
Histologic/nuclear grade	Family history
Lymphatic/vascular invasion	Previous breast cancer
Pathologic stage	Immunosuppression
Hormone receptor status	Nutrition
DNA content (ploidy, S-phase fraction)	Prior chemotherapy
Extent of intraductal component	Prior radiation therapy
HER-2/*neu* expression	

Source: Modified with permission from Beenken SW, et al: Breast cancer genetics, in Ellis N (ed): *Inherited Cancer Syndromes.* New York: Springer-Verlag, 2003, p 112. With kind permission of Springer Science + Business Media.

TABLE 17-14 Diagnostic studies for breast cancer patients

	Cancer Stage				
	0	**I**	**II**	**III**	**IV**
History & physical	X	X	X	X	X
Complete blood count, platelet count		X	X	X	X
Liver function tests and alkaline phosphatase level		X	X	X	X
Chest radiograph		X	X	X	X
Bilateral diagnostic mammograms, ultrasound as indicated	X	X	X	X	X
Hormone receptor status		X	X	X	X
HER-2/*neu* expression	X	X	X	X	X
Bone scan[a]			X	X	X
Abdominal (without or without pelvis) computed tomographic scan or ultrasound or magnetic resonance imaging			X	X	X

[a]Bone scan performed for stage II only if localized symptoms are present or serum alkaline phosphatase level is elevated.
Abdominal imaging and bone scanning are indicated for evaluation of symptoms or abnormal laboratory test results at any presenting stage.
Source: Adapted with permission from Carlson RW, et al: Breast cancer, in *NCCN Practice Guidelines in Oncology.* Fort Washington, Penn: National Comprehensive Cancer Network, 2006.

cancer that subsequently develops in 25 to 35% of these women. There is no benefit to excising LCIS, because the disease diffusely involves both breasts in many cases and the risk of invasive cancer is equal for both breasts. The use of tamoxifen as a risk reduction strategy should be considered in women with a diagnosis of LCIS.

Women with DCIS and evidence of extensive disease (>4 cm of disease or disease in more than one quadrant) usually require mastectomy. For women with limited disease, lumpectomy and radiation therapy are recommended. Low-grade DCIS of the solid, cribriform, or papillary subtype that is <0.5 cm in diameter may be managed by lumpectomy alone without radiation if the margins of resection are widely free of disease. For nonpalpable DCIS, needle localization techniques are used to guide the surgical resection. Specimen mammography is performed to ensure that all visible evidence of cancer is excised. Adjuvant tamoxifen therapy is considered for DCIS patients. The gold standard against which breast conservation therapy for DCIS is evaluated is mastectomy. Women treated with mastectomy have local recurrence and mortality rates of <2%. Women treated with lumpectomy and adjuvant radiation therapy have a similar mortality rate, but the local recurrence rate increases to 9%. Forty-five percent of these recurrences will be invasive cancer when radiation therapy is not used. The use of radiation therapy markedly decreases the risk of in-breast recurrence and significantly reduces the risk that any recurrence will be invasive disease. Both Lagios and Gump noted that recurrence of DCIS was greatest when the cancers were >2.5 cm in size, the criteria for histologic confirmation of clear margins were not rigorously applied, and the DCIS was of the comedo type. They noted that recurrences frequently occurred within the original surgery site, which indicates that inadequate clearance of DCIS, rather than the biology of the cancer, was responsible.[135]

Early Invasive Breast Cancer (Stage I, IIA, or IIB)

NSABP B-06 compared total mastectomy to lumpectomy with or without radiation therapy in the treatment of women with stage I and II breast cancer.[136–143] After 5- and 8-year follow-up periods, the disease-free, distant disease-free, and overall survival rates for lumpectomy with or without radiation therapy were similar to those observed after total mastectomy. However, the incidence of ipsilat-

eral breast cancer recurrence (in-breast recurrence) was higher in the lumpectomy group not receiving radiation therapy. These findings supported the use of lumpectomy and radiation therapy in the treatment of stage I and II breast cancer. Reanalysis of the study results was undertaken after 20 years of follow-up. The reanalysis confirmed that there was no difference in disease-free survival rates after total mastectomy or after lumpectomy with or without adjuvant radiation therapy. The in-breast recurrence rate was higher in the lumpectomy alone group (39.2%) than in the lumpectomy plus adjuvant radiation therapy group (14.3%). These findings are detailed in Fig. 17-29.

Currently, mastectomy with assessment of axillary lymph node status and breast conserving surgery with assessment of axillary lymph node status and radiation therapy are considered equivalent treatments for patients with stage I and II breast cancer. Axillary lymphadenopathy confirmed to be metastatic disease or metastatic disease in a sentinel lymph node (see later) necessitates an axillary lymph node dissection. Breast conservation is considered for all patients because of the important cosmetic advantages. Relative contraindications to breast conservation therapy include (a) prior radiation therapy to the breast or chest wall, (b) involved surgical margins or unknown margin status after re-excision, (c) multicentric disease, and (d) scleroderma or lupus erythematosus.

Traditionally, dissection of the level I and II axillary lymph nodes has been performed in early invasive breast cancer. Sentinel lymph node dissection is now considered the standard for evaluation of the axillary lymph node status in women who have clinically negative lymph nodes. Candidates for this procedure have clinically uninvolved axillary lymph nodes with a T1 or T2 primary breast cancer. Controversy remains about the suitability of sentinel node dissection in women with larger primary tumors (T3) and those treated with neoadjuvant chemotherapy.[144] If the sentinel lymph node cannot be identified or is found to harbor metastatic disease, then an axillary lymph node dissection should be performed.

Adjuvant chemotherapy for patients with early invasive breast cancer is considered for all patients with node-positive cancers, all patients with cancers that are >1 cm, and patients with node-negative cancers of >0.5 cm when adverse prognostic features are present. Adverse prognostic factors include blood vessel or lymph vessel invasion, high nuclear grade, high histologic grade, HER-2/*neu* over-

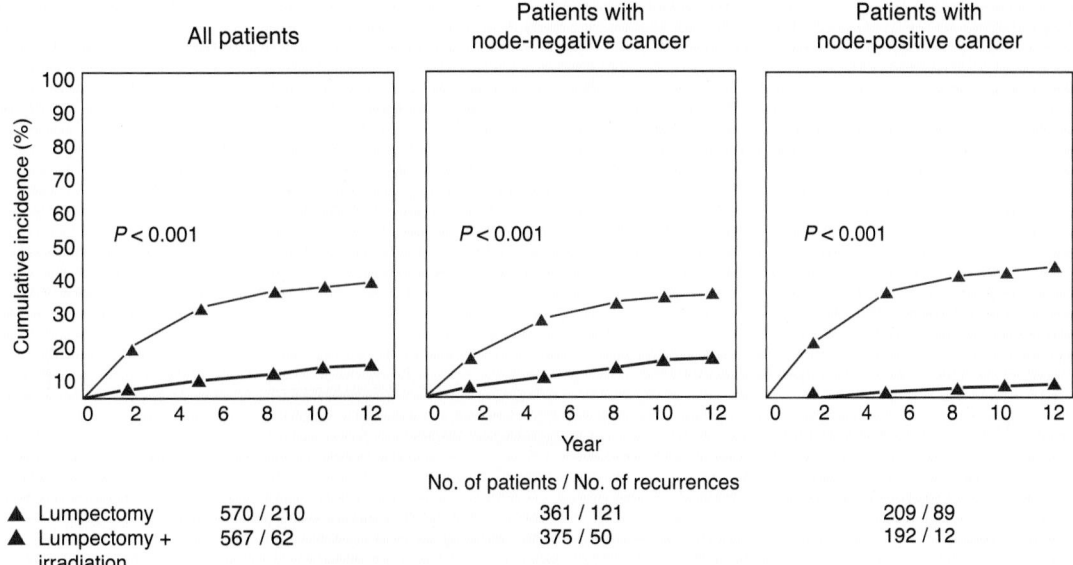

FIG. 17-29. Results of the National Surgical Adjuvant Breast and Bowel Project B-06 trial. Life-table analysis showing the incidence of recurrent cancer in the ipsilateral breast after lumpectomy or lumpectomy with adjuvant radiation therapy in 1137 patients with clear surgical margins. (*Reproduced with permission from Fisher B, Anderson S: Reanalysis and results after 12 years of follow-up in a randomized clinical trial comparing total mastectomy with lumpectomy with or without irradiation in the treatment of breast cancer. N Engl J Med 333:1456, 1995. Copyright © Massachusetts Medical Society. All rights reserved.*)

expression, and negative hormone receptor status. Tamoxifen therapy is considered for women with hormone receptor–positive cancers that are >1 cm. HER-2/*neu* expression is determined for all patients with newly diagnosed breast cancer and may be used to provide prognostic information in patients with node-negative breast cancer and predict the relative efficacy of various chemotherapy regimens. Trastuzumab is the only HER-2/*neu*–targeted agent that is currently approved for use in the metastatic and the adjuvant setting. The FDA approved trastuzumab in November 2006 for use as part of a treatment regimen containing doxorubicin, cyclophosphamide, and paclitaxel for treatment of HER-2/*neu*–positive, node-positive breast cancer.

Advanced Local-Regional Breast Cancer (Stage IIIA or IIIB)

Women with stage IIIA and IIIB breast cancer have advanced local-regional breast cancer but have no clinically detected distant metastases.[145] In an effort to provide optimal local-regional disease-free survival as well as distant disease-free survival for these women, surgery is integrated with radiation therapy and chemotherapy (Fig. 17-30). Neoadjuvant chemotherapy should be considered in the initial management of all patients with locally advanced stage III breast cancer. Surgical therapy for women with stage III disease is usually a modified radical mastectomy, followed by adjuvant radiation therapy. Chemotherapy is used to maximize distant disease-free survival, whereas radiation therapy is used to maximize local-regional disease-free survival. In selected patients with stage IIIA cancer, neoadjuvant (preoperative) chemotherapy can reduce the size of the primary cancer and permit breast-conserving surgery. Investigators from the M. D. Anderson Cancer Center reported that low local-regional failure rates could be achieved in selected patients with stage III disease treated with neoadjuvant chemotherapy followed by breast-conserving surgery and radiation.[146] The 5-year actuarial ipsilateral breast tumor recurrence–free survival rates in this study were 95%. They noted that the ipsilateral breast tumor recurrence rates increased when patients had clinical N2 or N3 disease, >2 cm of residual disease in the breast at surgery, a pattern of multifocal residual disease in the breast at surgery, and lymphovascular space invasion in the primary tumor. This study and others demonstrate that breast-conserving surgery can be used for appropriately selected patients with locally advanced breast cancer who achieve a good response with neoadjuvant chemotherapy. For patients with stage IIIA disease who experience minimal response to chemotherapy and for patients with stage IIIB breast cancer, neoadjuvant chemotherapy can decrease the local-regional cancer burden enough to permit subsequent modified radical mastectomy to establish local-regional control. In both stage IIIA and IIIB disease, surgery is followed by adjuvant radiation therapy.

Internal Mammary Lymph Nodes

Metastatic disease to internal mammary lymph nodes may be occult, may be evident on chest radiograph or CT scan, or may present as a painless parasternal mass with or without skin involvement. There is no consensus regarding the need for internal mammary lymph node radiation therapy in women who are at increased risk for occult involvement (cancers involving the medial aspect of the breast, axillary lymph node involvement) but who show no signs of internal mammary lymph node involvement. Systemic chemotherapy and radiation therapy are indicated in the treatment of grossly involved internal mammary lymph nodes.

Distant Metastases (Stage IV)

Treatment for stage IV breast cancer is not curative but may prolong survival and enhance a woman's quality of life.[147] Hormonal therapies that are associated with minimal toxicity are preferred to cytotoxic chemotherapy. Appropriate candidates for initial hormonal therapy include women with hormone receptor–positive cancers; women with bone or soft tissue metastases only; and women

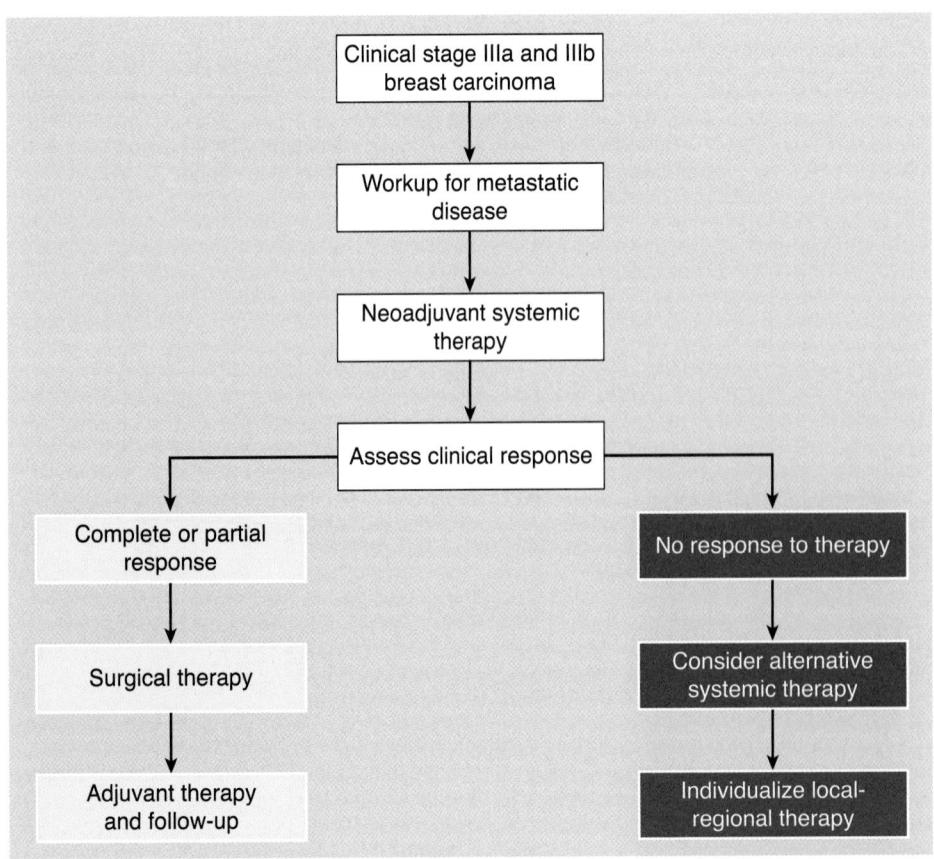

FIG. 17-30. Treatment pathways for stage IIIA and stage IIIB breast cancer.

with limited and asymptomatic visceral metastases. Systemic chemotherapy is indicated for women with hormone receptor–negative cancers, symptomatic visceral metastases, and hormone-refractory metastases. Women with stage IV breast cancer may develop anatomically localized problems that will benefit from individualized surgical treatment, such as brain metastases, pleural effusion, pericardial effusion, biliary obstruction, ureteral obstruction, impending or existing pathologic fracture of a long bone, spinal cord compression, and painful bone or soft tissue metastases. Bisphosphonates, which may be given in addition to chemotherapy or hormone therapy, should be considered in women with bone metastases. Whether to perform surgical resection of the local-regional disease in women with stage IV breast cancer has recently been debated after several reports have suggested that women who undergo resection of the primary disease have improved survival over those who do not. Khan and associates used the National Cancer Data Base to identify patterns of treatment in women with metastatic breast cancer and found that those who had surgical resection with negative margins had a better prognosis than those women who did not have surgical therapy.[148] Gnerlich and colleagues reported similar findings using the SEER database, and there have been several reports subsequent to this study from single institutions that have confirmed these findings.[149] Some have suggested that the findings of improved survival are due to selection bias and that local therapy should be reserved for palliation of symptoms. A proposal has recently gone forward to study this question in a randomized fashion through the Breast Cancer Intergroup of North America. In the meantime, surgical management of patients with stage IV disease should be addressed by obtaining multidisciplinary input and by considering the treatment goals of each individual patient and the patient's treating physicians.

Local-Regional Recurrence

Women with local-regional recurrence of breast cancer may be separated into two groups: those who have had mastectomy and those who have had lumpectomy. Women treated previously with mastectomy undergo surgical resection of the local-regional recurrence and appropriate reconstruction. Chemotherapy and antiestrogen therapy are considered, and adjuvant radiation therapy is given if the chest wall has not previously received radiation therapy. Women treated previously with a breast conservation procedure undergo a mastectomy and appropriate reconstruction. Chemotherapy and antiestrogen therapy are considered.

Breast Cancer Prognosis

Survival rates for women diagnosed with breast cancer between 1983 and 1987 have been calculated based on SEER program data. The 5-year survival rate for patients with stage I disease is 94%; for patients with stage IIA disease, 85%; and for patients with stage IIB tumors, 70%. For patients with stage IIIA disease the 5-year survival rate is 52%; for patients with stage IIIB cancers, 48%; and for patients with stage IV tumors, 18%. Breast cancer survival has significantly increased over the past 2 decades due to improvements in screening and local and systemic therapies. Data from the American College of Surgeons National Cancer Data Base indicate the 5-year survival for patients with stage I cancer to be 100%; for those with stage IIA tumors, 92%; for those with stage IIB disease, 81%; for patients with stage IIIA cancers, 67%; and for those with stage IIIB disease, 54%.[150]

SURGICAL TECHNIQUES IN BREAST CANCER THERAPY

Excisional Biopsy with Needle Localization

Excisional biopsy implies complete removal of a breast lesion with a margin of normal-appearing breast tissue. In the past, surgeons would obtain prior consent from the patient allowing mastectomy if the initial biopsy results confirmed cancer. Today it is important to consider the options for local therapy (lumpectomy vs. mastectomy with or without reconstruction) and the need for nodal assessment with sentinel node dissection. Figure 17-31 illustrates methods of obtaining a cosmetically acceptable breast scar. Excellent scars generally result from circumareolar incisions through which subareolar and centrally located breast lesions may be approached. Elsewhere, incisions that parallel Langer's lines, which are lines of tension in the skin that are generally concentric with the nipple-areola complex, result in acceptable scars except in the lower half of the breast, where the use of radial incisions typically provides the best outcome. Whenever possible, the surgeon should consider keeping the biopsy incision within the boundaries of the skin excision that may be required as part of a subsequent mastectomy (Fig. 17-32). When the tumor is quite distant from the central breast, the biopsy incision can be excised separately from the primary mastectomy incision, should a mastectomy be required. Radial incisions in the upper half of the breast are not recommended because of possible scar contracture resulting in displacement of the ipsilateral nipple-areola complex.

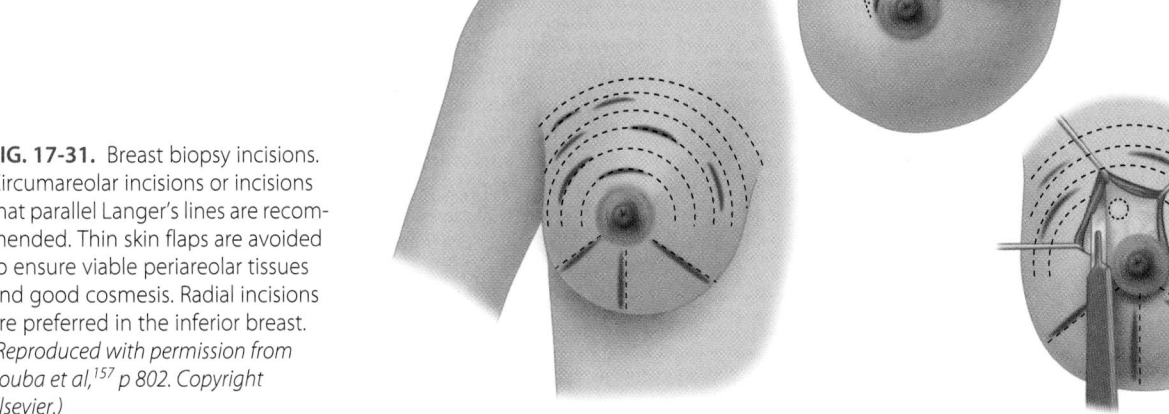

FIG. 17-31. Breast biopsy incisions. Circumareolar incisions or incisions that parallel Langer's lines are recommended. Thin skin flaps are avoided to ensure viable periareolar tissues and good cosmesis. Radial incisions are preferred in the inferior breast. *(Reproduced with permission from Souba et al,[157] p 802. Copyright Elsevier.)*

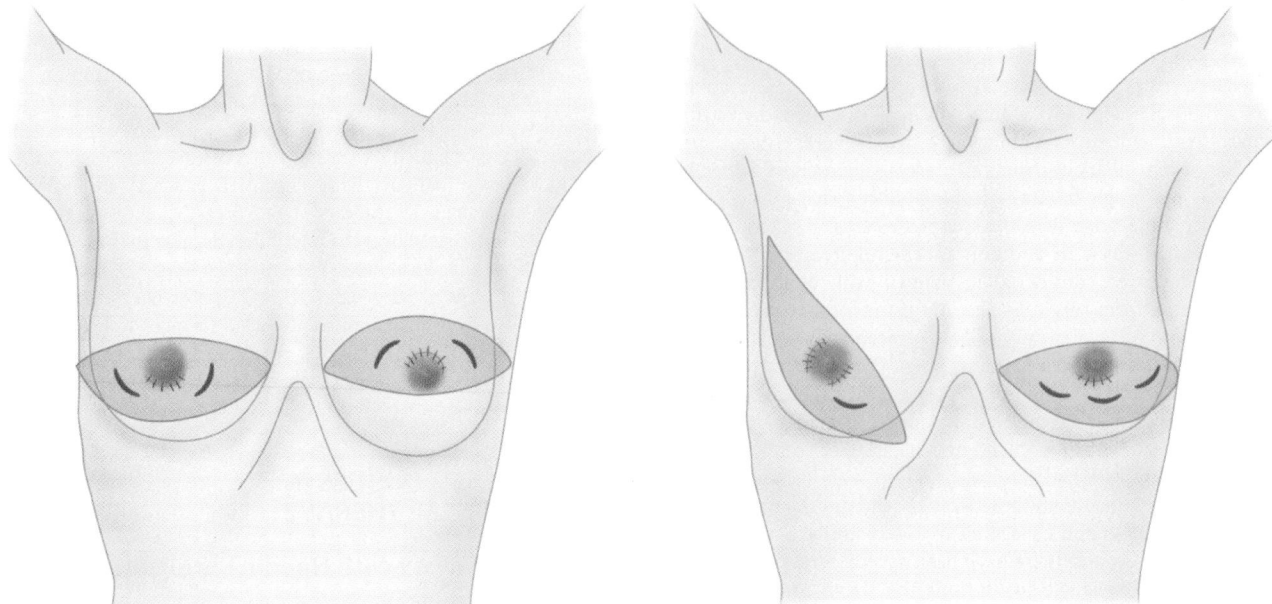

FIG. 17-32. Placement of breast biopsy incisions. Breast biopsy incisions are positioned within the boundaries of subsequent mastectomy skin incisions, and their placement allows for 1-cm or larger margins around the biopsy scar. *(Reproduced with permission from Souba et al,[157] p 802. Copyright Elsevier.)*

Similarly, curvilinear incisions in the lower half of the breast may displace the nipple-areolar complex downward.

After excision of a suspicious breast lesion, the biopsy tissue specimen is orientated for the pathologist using sutures, clips, or dyes. Additional margins (superior, inferior, medial, lateral, superficial, and deep) may be taken from the surgical bed to confirm complete excision of the suspicious lesion. Electrocautery or absorbable ligatures are used to achieve wound hemostasis. Although approximation of the breast tissues in the excision bed is usually not necessary, cosmesis may occasionally be facilitated by approximation of the surgical defect using 3-0 absorbable sutures. A running subcuticular closure of the skin using 4-0 or 5-0 absorbable monofilament sutures is performed, followed by approximation of the skin edges with adhesive skin closure strips (Steri-Strips). Wound drainage is avoided.

Excisional biopsy with needle localization requires a preoperative visit to the mammography suite for placement of a localization wire. The lesion can also be targeted by sonography in the imaging suite or in the operating room. The lesion to be excised is accurately localized by mammography, and the tip of a thin wire hook is positioned close to the lesion (Fig. 17-33). Using the wire hook as a guide, the surgeon subsequently excises the suspicious breast lesion while removing a margin of normal-appearing breast tissue. Before the patient leaves the operating room, specimen radiography is performed to confirm complete excision of the suspicious lesion (Fig. 17-34).

Sentinel Lymph Node Dissection

Sentinel lymph node dissection is primarily used to assess the regional lymph nodes in women with early breast cancers who are clinically node negative by physical examination and imaging studies.[151-159] This method also is accurate in women with larger tumors (T3 N0), but nearly 75% of these women will prove to have axillary lymph node metastases on histologic examination. A recent publication of the American Society of Clinical Oncology made recommendations for the use of sentinel lymph node dissection in patients with early-stage breast cancer.[144] To develop practice guidelines analysts used data from one prospective randomized trial comparing sentinel node dissection with axillary node dissection, four

meta-analyses, and published results from 69 single-institution and multicenter trials in which sentinel node dissection test performance was evaluated along with axillary node dissection. The American Society of Clinical Oncology guidelines did not recommend using sentinel node dissection in patients with T3, T4, or inflammatory breast cancers because the current level of evidence was felt to be insufficient. Other clinical situations in which the guidelines recommended against the use of sentinel node dissection included cases involving palpable axillary lymphadenopathy, pregnancy, DCIS without mastectomy, prior axillary surgery, or prior nononcologic breast surgery, and after preoperative chemotherapy. Although limited data are available, it was felt that sentinel node dissection was acceptable under the circumstances of multicentric tumors, DCIS with mastectomy, older age, obesity, male breast cancer, need for evaluation of internal mammary lymph nodes, and prior diagnostic or excisional biopsy, and before the use of preoperative systemic chemotherapy.

Evidence from large prospective studies suggests that the combination of intraoperative gamma probe detection of radioactive colloid and intraoperative visualization of isosulfan blue dye (Lymphazurin) is more accurate for identification of sentinel nodes than the use of either agent alone. Some surgeons use preoperative lymphoscintigraphy, although it is not required for identification of the sentinel nodes. On the day before surgery, or the day of surgery, the radioactive colloid is injected either in the breast parenchyma around the primary tumor or prior biopsy site or into the subareolar region or subdermally in proximity to the primary tumor site. With a 25-gauge needle, 0.5 mCi of 0.2-μm technetium 99m–labeled sulfur colloid is injected for same-day surgery or a higher dose of 2.5 mCi of technetium-labeled sulfur colloid is administered when the isotope is to be injected on the day before surgery. Subdermal injections are given in proximity to the cancer site or in the subareolar location. Later, in the operating room, 3 to 5 mL of isosulfan blue dye is injected either in the breast parenchyma or in the subareolar location. It is not recommended that the blue dye be used in a subdermal injection because this can result in tattooing of the skin. For nonpalpable cancers, the injection of the technetium-labeled sulfur colloid solution can be guided by either intraoperative ultrasound or by a localization wire that is placed preoperatively

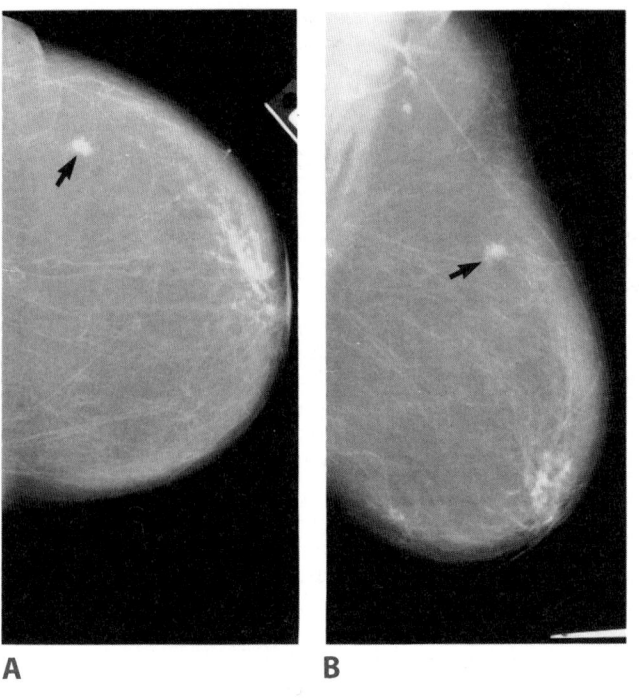
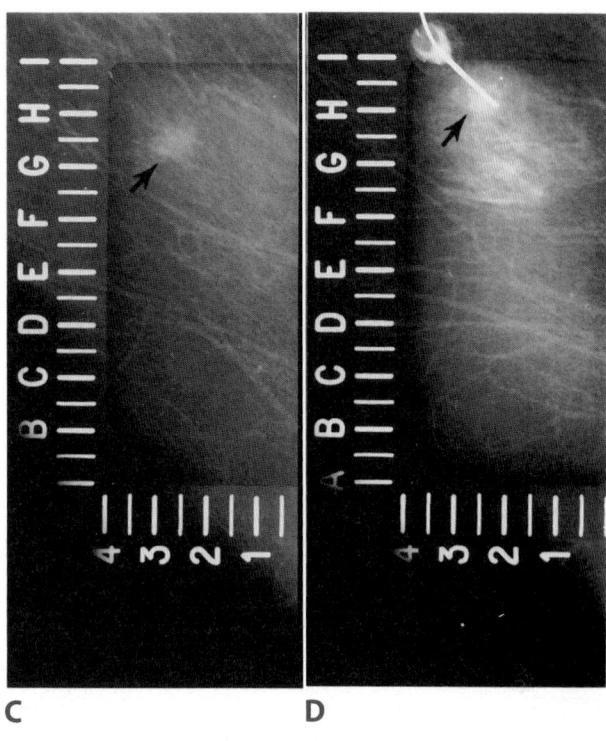

FIG. 17-33. Nonpalpable breast cancer. **A** and **B.** Craniocaudal (**A**) and mediolateral oblique (**B**) mammography views of the breast demonstrate an 8-mm spiculated mass (*arrows*) subsequently shown to be a cancer. **C** and **D.** Method of needle localization. The numbers and letters of the localization plate allow biplanar positioning of the guidewire (*arrows*). (*Courtesy of Dr. B. Steinbach.*)

under ultrasound or stereotactic guidance. It is helpful for the radiologist to mark the skin overlying the breast cancer at the time of needle localization using an indelible marker. In women who have undergone previous excisional biopsy, the injections are made in the breast parenchyma around the biopsy cavity but not into the cavity itself. Women are told preoperatively that the isosulfan blue dye injection will cause a change in the color of their urine and that there is a very small risk of allergic reaction to the dye (1 in 10,000). Anaphylactic reactions have been documented. The use of radioactive colloid is safe, and radiation exposure is very low.

A hand-held gamma counter is used to transcutaneously identify the location of the sentinel lymph node. This can help to guide placement of the incision. A 3- to 4-cm incision is made in line with that used for an axillary dissection, which is a curved transverse incision in the lower axilla just below the hairline. After dissecting through the subcutaneous tissue, the surgeon dissects through the axillary fascia, being mindful to identify blue lymphatic channels. Following these channels can lead directly to the sentinel node and limit the amount of dissection through the axillary tissues. The gamma counter is used to facilitate the dissection and to pinpoint the location of the sentinel lymph node. As the dissection continues, the signal from the probe increases in intensity as the sentinel lymph node is approached. The sentinel lymph node also is identified by visualization of isosulfan blue dye in the afferent lymph vessel and in the lymph node itself. Before the sentinel lymph node is removed, a 10-second in vivo radioactivity count is obtained. After removal of the sentinel lymph node, a 10-second ex vivo radioactive count is obtained, and the lymph node is then sent to the pathology laboratory for either permanent- or frozen-section analysis. The lowest false-negative rates for sentinel lymph node dissection have been obtained when all blue lymph nodes and all lymph nodes with radiation counts >10% of the 10-second ex vivo count of the sentinel lymph node are harvested (10% rule). Based on this, the gamma counter is used before closing the axillary wound to measure residual radioactivity in the surgical bed. A search is made for additional sentinel lymph nodes. This

procedure is repeated until residual radioactivity in the surgical bed is less than 10% of the 10-second ex vivo count of the most radioactive sentinel lymph node and all blue nodes have been removed.

Results from the NSABP B-32 randomized trial on the technical aspects of sentinel node surgery were recently published.[160] This trial compared sentinel node dissection alone with sentinel node dissection plus immediate axillary dissection in women with early-stage breast cancer. The overall success rate for identification of a sentinel node was 97.2%. The false-negative rate was reported to be 9.8% and was influenced by tumor location, type of diagnostic biopsy, and number of sentinel nodes removed at surgery. The authors reported that tumors located in the lateral breast were more likely to have a false-negative sentinel node. This may be explained by difficulty in discriminating the hot spot in the axilla when the radioisotope has been injected at the primary tumor site in the lateral breast. Those patients who had undergone an excisional biopsy before the sentinel node procedure were significantly more likely to have a false-negative sentinel node. This report further confirms that surgeons should use needle biopsy for diagnosis whenever possible and reserve excisional biopsy for the rare situations in which needle biopsy findings are nondiagnostic. Finally, removal of a larger number of sentinel nodes at surgery appears to reduce the false-negative rate. In the NSABP B-32 trial, the false-negative rate was reduced from 17.7 to 10% when two sentinel nodes were recovered and to 6.9% when three sentinel nodes were removed. Yi and associates recently reported that the number of sentinel nodes that need to be removed for accurate staging is influenced by individual patient and primary tumor factors.[161]

Investigators in the NSABP B-32 trial reported finding sentinel nodes outside of the level I and II axillary nodes in 1.4% of cases. This finding was significantly influenced by the site of radioisotope injection. When a subareolar or periareolar injection site was used, there were no instances of sentinel nodes identified outside of the level I or II axilla, compared with a rate of 20% when a peritumoral injection was used. This supports the overall concept that the

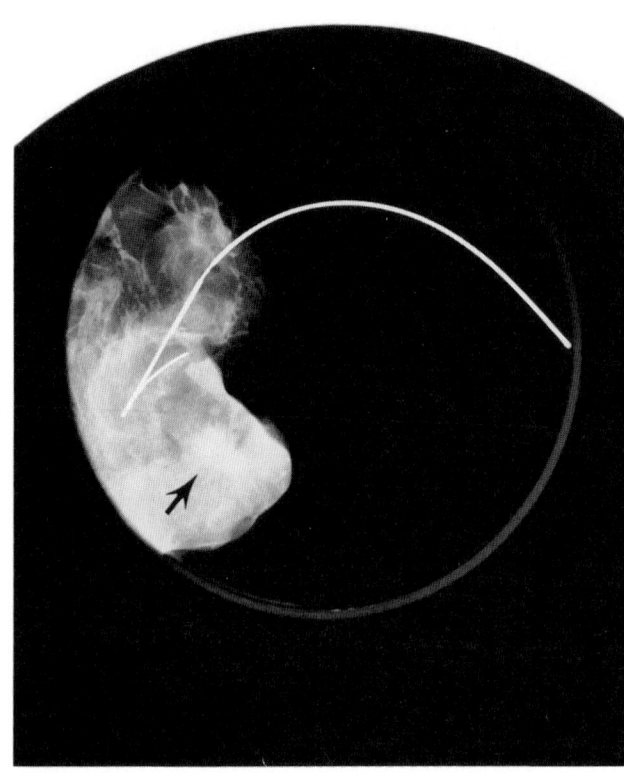

FIG. 17-34. Specimen mammography. The specimen mammogram contains the suspicious mass (*arrow*) seen on preoperative imaging. *(Courtesy of Dr. B. Steinbach.)*

sentinel node is the first site of drainage from the lymphatic vessels of the primary tumor. Although many patients will have similar drainage patterns from injections given at the primary tumor site and at the subareolar plexus, some patients will have extra-axillary drainage, either alone or in combination with axillary node drainage, and this is best assessed with a peritumoral injection of the radioisotope.

The morbidity of sentinel node dissection alone vs. sentinel node dissection with a completion axillary node dissection has been reported by investigators from the American College of Surgeons Oncology Group Z0010 and Z0011 trials.[162,163] Immediate effects of sentinel node dissection alone in the Z0010 trial included wound infection in 1%, axillary seroma in 7.1%, and axillary hematoma in 1.4%.[162] At 6 months after surgery, axillary paresthesias were reported in 8.6% of patients, decreased range of motion in the upper extremity was present in 3.8%, and 6.9% had a change in arm circumference of >2 cm on the affected side, which was reported as lymphedema. Younger patients were more likely to experience paresthesias, whereas increasing age and body mass index were more predictive of lymphedema. When adverse surgical effects were examined in the Z0011 trial, patients who underwent sentinel node dissection with axillary dissection had more wound infections, seromas, and paresthesias than those patients who underwent sentinel node dissection alone. Lymphedema at 1 year after surgery was reported by 13% of patients in the sentinel node plus axillary dissection group but by only 2% in the sentinel node alone group. Arm circumference measurements were greater at 1 year in the group undergoing sentinel node plus axillary dissection, but the difference between the two groups was not statistically significant.[163]

The initial publications from the NSABP and American College of Surgeons Oncology Group multicenter trials provide important information to clinicians regarding the use of sentinel node dissection in early-stage breast cancer patients. Information on recurrence patterns, survival differences, and the impact of micrometastases in the sentinel nodes on outcomes requires further maturation of the

data. These trials do not address the use of sentinel node dissection in other patient populations, such as patients with DCIS, patients receiving preoperative chemotherapy, and patients with prior breast or axillary surgery.

Another area of sentinel node technology that requires standardization is the pathologic processing of the sentinel nodes. Most pathology laboratories perform a more detailed analysis of the sentinel nodes than is routinely done for axillary nodes recovered from a level I and II axillary node dissection. This can include examining thin sections of the node with step sectioning at multiple levels through the paraffin blocks or performing immunohistochemical staining of the sentinel node for cytokeratin or a combination of these techniques. Intraoperative assessment of sentinel nodes also varies for different clinicians and pathology laboratories. Some centers prefer to use touch preparation cytologic analysis of the sentinel nodes, whereas others use frozen-section analysis, and the sensitivity and specificity of these assays vary considerably. The GeneSearch Breast Lymph Node Assay is a real-time reverse-transcriptase polymerase chain reaction assay that detects breast tumor cell metastasis in lymph nodes through the identification of the gene expression markers mammaglobin and cytokeratin 19. These markers are present in higher levels in breast tissue and not in nodal tissue (cell type–specific messenger RNA). The GeneSearch assay generates expression data for genes of interest, which are then evaluated against predetermined criteria to provide a qualitative (positive/negative) result. The assay is designed to detect foci that correspond to metastases which are seen with examination by standard hematoxylin and eosin staining and measure >0.2 mm. The GeneSearch assay results have been compared with permanent-section histologic analysis and frozen-section analysis of sentinel nodes in a prospective trial, and the assay was recently approved by the FDA for the intraoperative assessment of sentinel nodes.[164] When a positive node is identified intraoperatively by touch preparation, frozen-section analysis, or GeneSearch assay, the surgeon can proceed with immediate completion of axillary node dissection. Although there are a number of nomograms and predictive models designed to determine which patients with a positive sentinel node are at risk for harboring additional positive nonsentinel nodes in the axilla, completion axillary dissection remains the standard practice.[165]

Breast Conservation

Breast conservation involves resection of the primary breast cancer with a margin of normal-appearing breast tissue, adjuvant radiation therapy, and assessment of regional lymph node status.[166,167] Resection of the primary breast cancer is alternatively called *segmental mastectomy, lumpectomy, partial mastectomy, wide local excision,* and *tylectomy.* For many women with stage I or II breast cancer, breast-conserving therapy (BCT) is preferable to total mastectomy because BCT produces survival rates equivalent to those after total mastectomy while preserving the breast.[168] Six prospective randomized trials have shown that overall and disease-free survival rates are similar with BCT and mastectomy. Three of the studies showed higher local-regional failure rates in patients undergoing BCT; however, in two of these studies, there were no clear criteria for histologically negative margins.[166-169] Recent data from the Early Breast Cancer Trialists' Collaborative Group revealed that avoiding local recurrence translates into a survival advantage.[169] When all of this information is taken together, BCT is considered to be oncologically equivalent to mastectomy.

In addition to being equivalent to mastectomy in terms of oncologic safety, BCT appears to offer advantages over mastectomy with regard to quality of life and aesthetic outcomes. BCT allows for preservation of breast shape and skin as well as preservation of sensation, and provides an overall psychologic advantage associated with breast preservation.

Breast conservation surgery is currently the standard treatment for women with stage 0, I, or II invasive breast cancer. Women with DCIS require only resection of the primary cancer and adjuvant radiation therapy without assessment of regional lymph nodes. When a lumpectomy is performed, a curvilinear incision lying concentric to the nipple-areola complex is made in the skin overlying the breast cancer when the tumor is in the upper aspect of the breast. Radial incisions are preferred when the tumor is in the lower aspect of the breast. Skin encompassing any prior biopsy site generally is excised, but skin excision is not otherwise necessary unless there is direct involvement of the overlying skin by the primary tumor. The breast cancer is removed with an envelope of normal-appearing breast tissue that is adequate to achieve at least a 2-mm cancer-free margin. Specimen orientation is performed by the surgeon. Additional margins from the surgical bed are taken as needed to provide a histologically negative margin. Requests for determination of hormone receptor status and HER-2/*neu* expression are conveyed to the pathologist.

Sentinel lymph node dissection is now the preferred staging procedure with a clinically node-negative axilla. When the procedures are sequenced in the operating room, the sentinel node procedure usually is performed before removal of the primary breast tumor. When indicated, intraoperative assessment of the sentinel node can proceed while the segmental mastectomy is being performed. When the sentinel lymph node does not contain metastatic disease, axillary lymph node dissection is avoided. It is the surgeon's responsibility to ensure complete removal of cancer in the breast. Ensuring surgical margins that are free of breast cancer will minimize the chances of local recurrence and will enhance cure rates. Local recurrence of breast cancer after conservation surgery is determined primarily by the adequacy of surgical margins. Cancer size and the extent of skin excision are not significant factors in this regard. It is the practice of many North American and European surgeons to undertake re-excision when residual cancer within 2 mm of a surgical margin is determined by histopathologic examination. If clear margins are not obtainable with re-excision, mastectomy is required.

The use of oncoplastic surgery can be entertained at the time of segmental mastectomy or at a later time to improve the overall aesthetic outcome. Oncoplastic techniques range from a simple reshaping of breast tissue to local tissue rearrangement to the use of pedicled flaps or breast reduction techniques. The overall goal is to achieve the best possible aesthetic result. In determining which patients are candidates for oncoplastic breast surgery, several factors should be considered, including the extent of the resection of breast tissue necessary to achieve negative margins, the location of the primary tumor within the breast, and the size of the patient's breast and body habitus. Oncoplastic techniques are of prime consideration when (a) a significant area of breast skin will need to be resected with the specimen to achieve negative margins; (b) a large volume of breast parenchyma will be resected resulting in a significant defect; (c) the tumor is located between the nipple and the inframammary fold, an area often associated with unfavorable cosmetic outcomes; or (d) excision of the tumor and closure of the breast may result in malpositioning of the nipple.

Mastectomy and Axillary Dissection

A skin-sparing mastectomy removes all breast tissue, the nipple-areola complex, and scars from any prior biopsy procedures.[170,171] There is a recurrence rate of less than 6 to 8%, comparable to the long-term recurrence rates reported with standard mastectomy, when skin-sparing mastectomy is used for patients with T1 to T3 cancers. A total (simple) mastectomy without skin sparing removes all breast tissue, the nipple-areola complex, and skin. An extended simple mastectomy removes all breast tissue, the nipple-areola complex, skin, and the level I axillary lymph nodes. A modified radical mastectomy removes all breast tissue, the nipple-areola complex, skin, and the level I and level II axillary lymph nodes. The Halsted radical mastectomy removes all breast tissue and skin, the nipple-areola complex, the pectoralis major and pectoralis minor muscles, and the level I, II, and III axillary lymph nodes. The use of systemic chemotherapy and hormonal therapy as well as adjuvant

radiation therapy for breast cancer have nearly eliminated the need for the radical mastectomy.

For a variety of biologic, economic, and psychosocial reasons, some women desire mastectomy rather than breast conservation. Women who are less concerned about cosmesis may view mastectomy as the most expeditious and desirable therapeutic option because it avoids the cost and inconvenience of radiation therapy. Women whose primary breast cancers cannot be excised with a reasonable cosmetic result or those who have extensive microcalcifications are best treated with mastectomy. Women with large cancers that occupy the subareolar and central portions of the breast and women with multicentric primary cancers also undergo mastectomy.

Modified Radical Mastectomy

A modified radical mastectomy preserves both the pectoralis major and pectoralis minor muscles, allowing removal of level I and level II axillary lymph nodes but not the level III (apical) axillary lymph nodes (Figs. 17-35 and 17-36).[170] The Patey modification removes the pectoralis minor muscle and allows complete dissection of the level III axillary lymph nodes (Figs. 17-37 and 17-38). A modified radical mastectomy permits preservation of the medial (anterior thoracic) pectoral nerve, which courses in the lateral neurovascular bundle of the axilla and usually penetrates the pectoralis minor to supply the lateral border of the pectoralis major. Anatomic boundaries of the modified radical mastectomy are the anterior margin of the latissimus dorsi muscle laterally, the midline of the sternum medially, the subclavius muscle superiorly, and the caudal extension of the breast 2 to 3 cm inferior to the inframammary fold inferiorly (see Fig. 17-35 *inset*). Skin-flap thickness varies with body habitus but ideally is 7 to 8 mm inclusive of skin and tela subcutanea. Once the skin flaps are fully developed, the fascia of the pectoralis major muscle and the overlying breast tissue are elevated off the underlying musculature, which allows for the complete removal of the breast.

Subsequently, an axillary lymph node dissection is performed. The most lateral extent of the axillary vein is identified and the areolar tissue of the lateral axillary space is elevated as the vein is cleared on its anterior and inferior surfaces. The areolar tissues at the junction of the axillary vein and the anterior edge of the latissimus dorsi muscle, which include the lateral and subscapular lymph node groups (level I), are cleared in an inferomedial direction. Care is taken to preserve the thoracodorsal neurovascular bundle. The dissection then continues medially with clearance of the central axillary lymph node group (level II). The long thoracic nerve of Bell is identified and preserved as it travels in the investing fascia of the serratus anterior muscle. Every effort is made to preserve this nerve, because permanent disability with a winged scapula and shoulder weakness will follow denervation of the serratus anterior muscle. If there is palpable lymphadenopathy at the apex of the axilla, the tendinous portion of the pectoralis minor muscle is divided near its insertion onto the coracoid process (see Fig. 17-37 *inset*), which allows dissection of the axillary vein medially to the costoclavicular (Halsted's) ligament. Finally, the breast and axillary contents are removed from the surgical bed and are sent for pathologic assessment. The Patey modification originally involved removal of the pectoralis muscle (see Fig. 17-38). However, some surgeons now divide only the tendon of the pectoralis minor muscle at its insertion onto the coracoid process while leaving the rest of the muscle intact.

Seromas beneath the skin flaps or in the axilla represent the most frequent complication of mastectomy and axillary lymph node dissection, reportedly occurring in as many as 30% of cases. The use of closed-system suction drainage reduces the incidence of this complication. Catheters are retained in the wound until drainage diminishes to <30 mL per day. Wound infections occur infrequently after a mastectomy and the majority are a result of skin-flap necrosis. Cultures of specimens taken from the infected wound for aerobic and anaerobic organisms, débridement, and antibiotic therapy are effective management. Moderate or severe hemorrhage in the postopera-

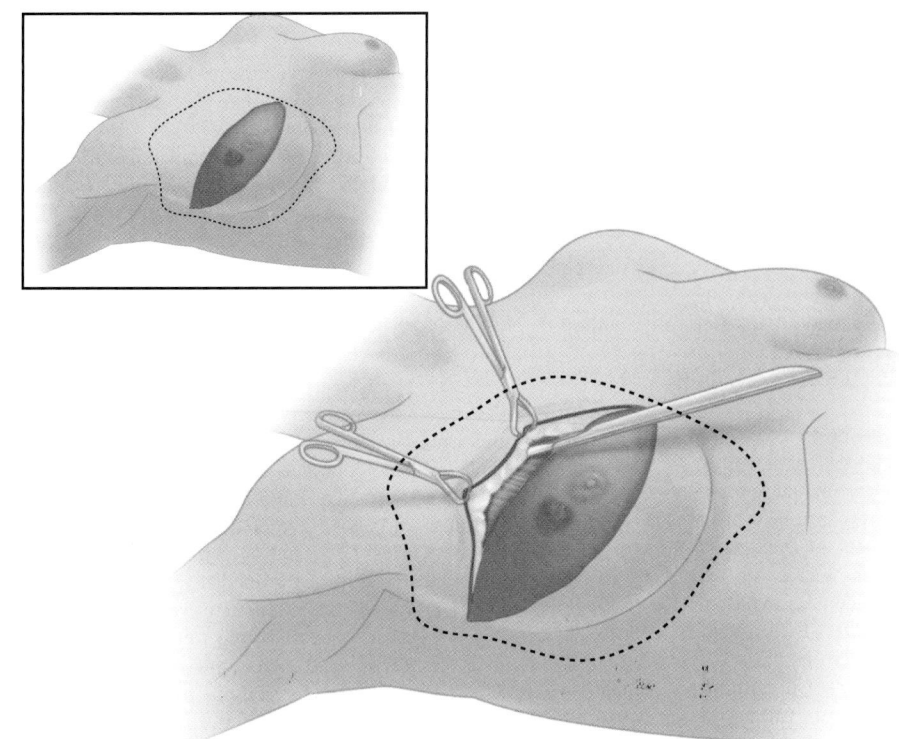

FIG. 17-35. Modified radical mastectomy: elevation of skin flaps. Skin flaps are 7 to 8 mm in thickness, inclusive of the skin and tela subcutanea. *Inset* depicts the limits of the modified radical mastectomy. *(Reproduced with permission from Bland et al,[170] p 905. Copyright Elsevier.)*

tive period is rare and is best managed with early wound exploration for control of hemorrhage and re-establishment of closed-system suction drainage. The incidence of functionally significant lymphedema after a modified radical mastectomy is 10 to 20%. Extensive axillary lymph node dissection, the delivery of radiation therapy, the presence of pathologic lymph nodes, and obesity are predisposing factors. The use of individually fitted compressive sleeves and intermittent compression devices may be necessary.

Reconstruction of the Breast and Chest Wall

The goals of reconstructive surgery after a mastectomy for breast cancer are wound closure and breast reconstruction, which is either immediate or delayed.[172] For most women, wound closure after mastectomy is accomplished with simple approximation of the wound edges. However, if a more radical removal of skin and subcutaneous tissue is necessary, a pedicled myocutaneous flap from the latissimus dorsi muscle is generally the best approach for wound coverage. A skin graft provides functional coverage that will tolerate adjuvant radiation therapy; however, this is not preferred, because poor graft adherence may delay delivery of radiation therapy. Breast reconstruction after prophylactic mastectomy or after mastectomy for early invasive breast cancer is performed at the same time as the mastectomy. This allows for a skin-sparing mastectomy to be performed, which offers the best overall cosmetic outcomes. Reconstruction can proceed with an expander/implant reconstruction or with

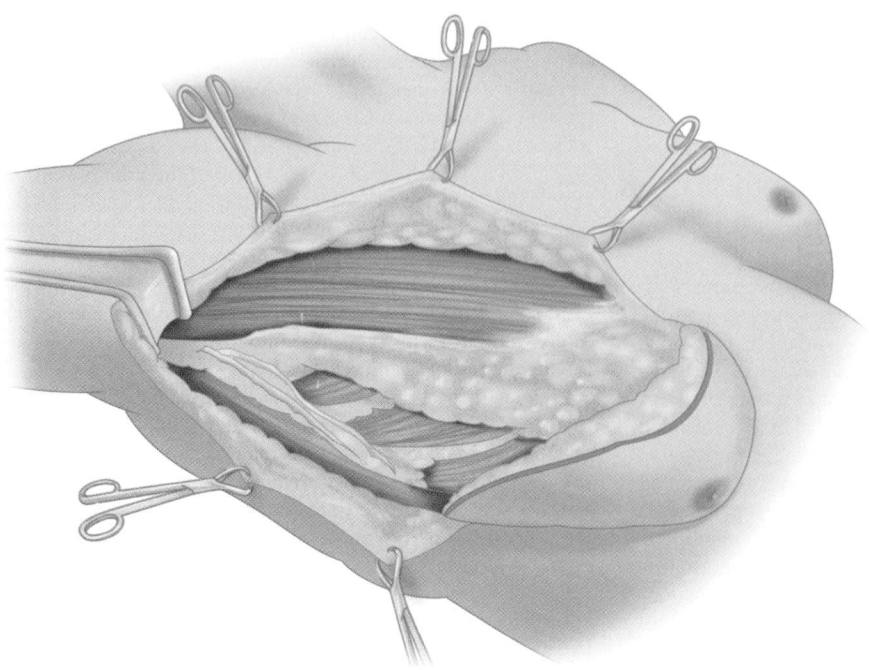

FIG. 17-36. Modified radical mastectomy: resection of breast tissue. The pectoralis major muscle is cleared of its fascia as the overlying breast is elevated. The latissimus dorsi muscle is the lateral boundary of the dissection. *(Reproduced with permission from Bland et al,[170] p 906. Copyright Elsevier.)*

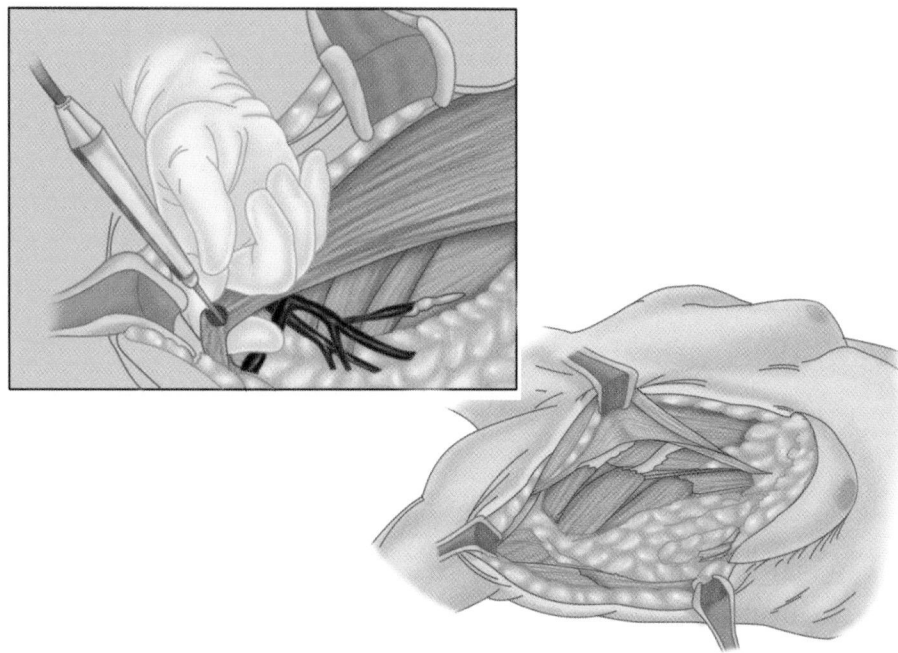

FIG. 17-37. Modified radical mastectomy (Patey): axillary lymph node dissection. The dissection proceeds from lateral to medial, with complete visualization of the anterior and inferior aspects of the axillary vein. Loose areolar tissue at the junction of the axillary vein and the anterior margin of the latissimus dorsi muscle is swept inferomedially inclusive of the lateral (axillary) lymph node group (level I). Care is taken to preserve the thoracodorsal artery, vein, and nerve in the deep axillary space. The lateral lymph node group is resected in continuity with the subscapular lymph node group (level I) and the external mammary lymph node group (level I). Dissection anterior to the axillary vein allows removal of the central lymph node group (level II) and the apical (subclavicular) lymph node group (level III). The superomedial limit of this dissection is the clavipectoral fascia (Halsted's ligament). *Inset* depicts division of the insertion of the pectoralis minor muscle at the coracoid process. The surgeon's finger shields the underlying brachial plexus. *(Reproduced with permission from Bland et al,[170] p 908.)*

autologous tissue such as a pedicled myocutaneous flap or a free flap using microvascular techniques. In patients with advanced breast cancer reconstruction is delayed until after completion of adjuvant radiation therapy to ensure that local-regional control of disease is obtained. If chest wall coverage is needed to replace a large skin or soft tissue defect, many different types of myocutaneous flaps are employed, but the latissimus dorsi and the rectus abdominus myocutaneous flaps are most frequently used. The latissimus dorsi myocutaneous flap consists of a skin paddle based on the underlying latissimus dorsi muscle, which is supplied by the thoracodorsal artery with contributions from the posterior intercostal arteries. A transverse rectus abdominis myocutaneous (TRAM) flap consists of a skin paddle based on the underlying rectus abdominis muscle, which is supplied by vessels from the deep inferior epigastric artery. The free TRAM flap uses microvascular anastomoses to establish blood supply to the flap. When the bony chest wall is involved with cancer, resection of a portion of the bony chest wall is indicated. If only one or two ribs are resected and soft tissue coverage is provided, reconstruction of the bony defect is usually not necessary, because scar tissue will stabilize the chest wall. If more than two ribs are sacrificed, it is advisable to stabilize the chest wall with prosthetic material, which is then covered with soft tissue by using a latissimus dorsi or TRAM flap.

NONSURGICAL BREAST CANCER THERAPIES

Radiation Therapy

Radiation therapy is used for all stages of breast cancer depending on whether the patient is undergoing BCT or mastectomy.[173–179] For women with limited DCIS (stage 0) in whom negative margins are achieved by segmental mastectomy, adjuvant radiation therapy is

given to reduce the risk of local recurrence. Low-grade DCIS of the solid, cribriform, or papillary subtypes that is <0.5 cm in diameter and is excised with widely negative margins may be managed by excision alone. For women with stage I, IIA, or IIB breast cancer in which negative margins are achieved by segmental mastectomy, adjuvant radiation therapy is given to reduce the risk of local recurrence. Those women treated with mastectomy who have cancer at the surgical margins are at sufficiently high risk for local recurrence to warrant the use of adjuvant radiation therapy to the chest wall and supraclavicular lymph nodes. Women with metastatic disease involving four or more axillary lymph nodes and premenopausal women with metastatic disease involving one to three lymph nodes also are at increased risk for recurrence and are candidates for the use of chest wall and supraclavicular lymph node radiation therapy. In advanced local-regional breast cancer (stage IIIA or IIIB), women are at high risk for recurrent disease after surgical therapy, and adjuvant radiation therapy is used to reduce the recurrence rates (Fig. 17-39). Current recommendations for stages IIIA and IIIB breast cancer are (a) adjuvant radiation therapy to the breast and supraclavicular lymph nodes after neoadjuvant chemotherapy and segmental mastectomy with or without axillary lymph node dissection, (b) adjuvant radiation therapy to the chest wall and supraclavicular lymph nodes after neoadjuvant chemotherapy and mastectomy with or without axillary lymph node dissection, and (c) adjuvant radiation therapy to the chest wall and supraclavicular lymph nodes after segmental mastectomy or mastectomy with axillary lymph node dissection and adjuvant chemotherapy.

The use of partial breast irradiation (PBI) for patients treated with breast-conserving surgery is currently being compared with whole-breast irradiation in a phase III randomized trial. PBI can be delivered via brachytherapy, external beam radiation therapy using three-dimensional conformal radiation, or intensity-modulated ra-

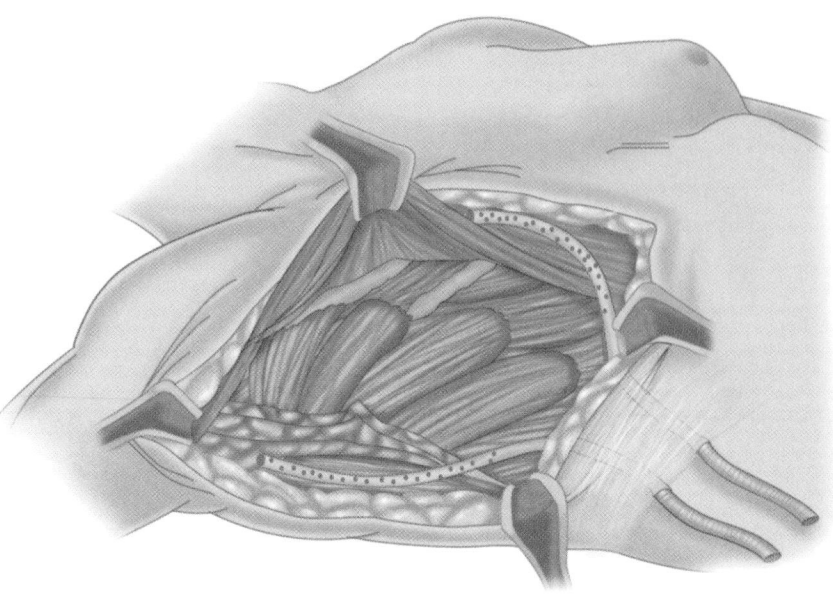

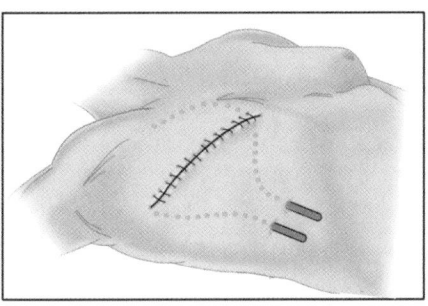

FIG. 17-38. Modified radical mastectomy (Patey): completed dissection. The completed dissection includes the pectoralis minor muscle from its insertion to its origin from the second to fifth ribs. Rotter's lymph nodes (level I) are left attached to the pectoralis minor muscle as it is removed. Both medial and lateral pectoral nerves are preserved to ensure innervation of the lateral and medial heads (respectively) of the pectoralis major muscle. *Inset* depicts the positioning of closed-suction catheters, which are brought out through the inferior flap. The lateral catheter is placed 2 cm inferior to the axillary vein. The medial catheter is positioned anterior to the pectoralis major muscle. *(Reproduced with permission from Bland et al,[170] p 909. Copyright Elsevier.)*

diation therapy. Although initial results are promising in highly selected low-risk populations, PBI should be used in the clinical setting only as part of a prospective trial.

Chemotherapy

Adjuvant Chemotherapy

The Early Breast Cancer Trialists' Collaborative Group overview analysis of adjuvant chemotherapy demonstrated reductions in the odds of recurrence and of death in women ≤70 years of age with stage I, IIA, or IIB breast cancer.[180–185] For those ≥70 years of age, the lack of definitive clinical trial data regarding adjuvant chemotherapy prevented definitive recommendations. Adjuvant chemotherapy is of minimal benefit to women with negative nodes and cancers ≤0.5 cm in size and is not recommended. Women with negative nodes and cancers 0.6 to 1.0 cm are divided into those with a low risk of recurrence and those with unfavorable prognostic features that portend a higher risk of recurrence and a need for adjuvant chemotherapy. Adverse prognostic factors include blood vessel or lymph vessel invasion, high nuclear grade, high histologic grade, HER-2/*neu* overexpression, and negative hormone receptor status. Adjuvant chemotherapy is recommended for women with these unfavorable prognostic features. Table 17-15 lists the frequently used chemotherapy regimens for breast cancer.

For women with hormone receptor–negative cancers that are >1 cm in size, adjuvant chemotherapy is appropriate. However, women with node-negative hormone receptor–positive cancers and T1 tumors are candidates for antiestrogen therapy with or without chemotherapy. For special-type cancers (tubular, mucinous, medullary, etc), adjuvant chemotherapy or antiestrogen therapy for cancers <3 cm in size is controversial. For women with node-positive tumors or with a special-type cancer that is >3 cm, the use of chemotherapy is appropriate. Those with hormone receptor–positive tumors should receive

antiestrogen therapy as well. Current treatment recommendations for stage IIIA breast cancer include preoperative chemotherapy with a doxorubicin (Adriamycin)-containing regimen followed by either a modified radical mastectomy or segmental mastectomy with axillary dissection followed by adjuvant radiation therapy. These recommendations are based in part on the results of the NSABP B-15 trial. In this study, women with node-positive, tamoxifen-nonresponsive cancers who were ≤59 years of age were randomly assigned to receive either 2 months of therapy with doxorubicin and cyclophosphamide or 6 months of cyclophosphamide, methotrexate, and cyclophosphamide, methotrexate, 5-fluorouracil. There was no difference in relapse-free survival or overall survival rates, and women preferred the shorter regimen.[186]

Neoadjuvant (Preoperative) Chemotherapy

In the early 1970s, the National Cancer Institute in Milan, Italy, initiated two prospective randomized multimodality clinical trials for women with T3 or T4 breast cancer.[187] The best results were achieved when surgery was interposed between chemotherapy courses, with 82% local-regional control and 25% 5-year disease-free survival. The NSABP B-18 trial evaluated the role of neoadjuvant chemotherapy in women with operable stage II and III breast cancer.[188] Women entered into this study were randomly assigned to receive either surgery followed by chemotherapy or neoadjuvant chemotherapy followed by surgery. There was no difference in the 5-year disease-free survival rates for the two groups, but after neoadjuvant chemotherapy there was an increase in the number of lumpectomies performed and a decreased incidence of node positivity. It was suggested that neoadjuvant chemotherapy be considered for the initial management of breast cancers judged too large for initial lumpectomy.

The use of neoadjuvant chemotherapy has expanded from its initial use in the setting of large and locally advanced breast cancers

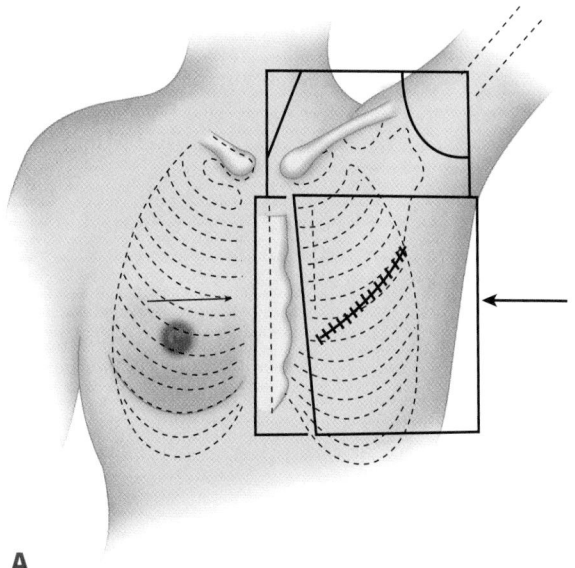

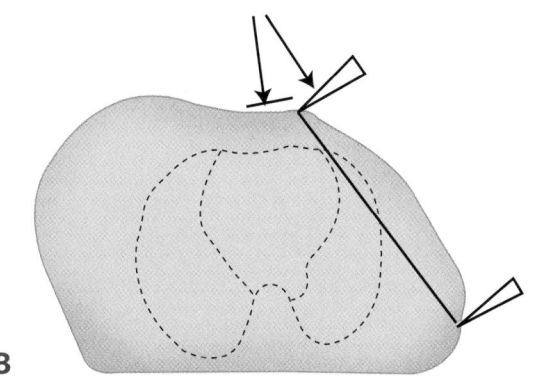

FIG. 17-39. Radiation therapy for stage IIIA and stage IIIB breast cancer. **A.** Comprehensive chest wall and regional lymph node radiation therapy. **B.** Cross-sectional view showing the tangential field. *[Reproduced with permission from Beenken SW, et al: Radiation therapy for stage IIIA and stage IIIB breast cancer, in Bland KI (ed): The Practice of General Surgery. Philadelphia: WB Saunders, 2002, p 983. Copyright © Elsevier.]*

TABLE 17-15	Adjuvant chemotherapy regimens for breast cancer

HER-2/*neu* Negative (Non–Trastuzumab-Containing Regimens)	HER-2/*neu* Positive (Trastuzumab-Containing Regimens)
FAC/CAF	AC → T + concurrent trastuzumab (T = paclitaxel)
FEC/CEF	Docetaxel + trastuzumab → FEC
AC or EC	TCH (docetaxel, carboplatin, trastuzumab)
TAC (T = docetaxel)	Chemotherapy followed by trastuzumab sequentially
A → CMF	AC → docetaxel + trastuzumab
E → CMF	
CMF	
AC × 4	
A → T → C (T = paclitaxel)	
FEC → T (T = docetaxel)	
TC (T = docetaxel)	

A = Adriamycin (doxorubicin); C = cyclophosphamide; E = epirubicin; F = 5-fluorouracil; M = methotrexate; T = Taxane (docetaxel or paclitaxel); → = followed by.
Source: Adapted with permission from Carlson RW, et al: Breast cancer, in *NCCN Practice Guidelines in Oncology*. Fort Washington, Penn: National Comprehensive Cancer Network, 2006.

mastectomy or lumpectomy with axillary lymph node dissection if necessary, followed by adjuvant radiation therapy. For inoperable stage IIIA and for stage IIIB breast cancer, neoadjuvant chemotherapy is used to decrease the local-regional cancer burden. This may then permit subsequent modified radical or radical mastectomy, which is followed by adjuvant radiation therapy.

Nodal Evaluation in Patients Receiving Neoadjuvant Chemotherapy The management of the axilla after neoadjuvant chemotherapy has not been specifically addressed in randomized trials. Standard practice has been to perform an axillary lymph node dissection after chemotherapy or to perform a sentinel lymph node dissection before chemotherapy for nodal staging before chemotherapy is initiated. A number of small single-institution studies, one multicenter study, and a recent meta-analysis have explored the use of sentinel lymph node dissection at the completion of chemotherapy. The published results from these studies have demonstrated the feasibility of sentinel lymph node dissection in breast cancer patients after neoadjuvant chemotherapy and have suggested that the procedure is accurate for nodal staging in this patient population.[191,192] Although the issue has not been specifically addressed in the published trials, the presence of suspected or documented axillary metastases at initial presentation generally is considered a relative contraindication to sentinel lymph node dissection after neoadjuvant chemotherapy, and these patients usually undergo axillary lymph node dissection after completion of chemotherapy.

Neoadjuvant Endocrine Therapy

Neoadjuvant endocrine therapy has most commonly been used in elderly women who were deemed poor candidates for surgery or cytotoxic chemotherapy. However, as clinicians have gained experience with neoadjuvant treatment strategies, it is now clear from examination of predictors of complete pathologic response that estrogen receptor–positive tumors do not shrink in response to chemotherapy as readily as estrogen receptor–negative tumors.[193] Fisher and colleagues examined the results of the NSABP B-14 and B-20 trials and found that, as age increased, women obtained less benefit from chemotherapy. They recommended that factors[194] including tumor estrogen receptor concentration, nuclear grade, histologic grade, tumor type, and markers of proliferation should be considered in these patients before choosing between the use of chemotherapy and hormonal therapy. If in fact the tumor is estrogen receptor rich, these patients may benefit more from endocrine therapy in the neoadjuvant setting than they might if they received

to use in any patient who is deemed to be a candidate for systemic chemotherapy based on primary tumor factors or nodal staging. The use of neoadjuvant chemotherapy offers the opportunity to observe the response of the intact primary tumor and any regional nodal metastases to a specific chemotherapy regimen.[189] For patients whose tumors remain stable in size or even progress with the initial neoadjuvant chemotherapy regimen, a new regimen can be instituted that uses another class of agents.

After treatment with neoadjuvant chemotherapy, patients are assessed for clinical and pathologic response to the regimen. Patients whose tumors achieve a pathologic complete response to neoadjuvant chemotherapy have been shown to have survival outcomes far superior to those of patients whose tumors demonstrate only a partial response or remain stable. Patients who experience progression of disease during neoadjuvant chemotherapy have the poorest survival.[190]

Current recommendations for treatment of operable advanced local-regional breast cancer are neoadjuvant chemotherapy with a doxorubicin-containing or taxane-containing regimen, followed by standard chemotherapy. Neoadjuvant endocrine therapy has been shown to shrink tumors, enabling breast-conserving surgery in women with hormone receptor–positive disease who otherwise would have to be treated with mastectomy.

With the use of neoadjuvant chemotherapy or endocrine therapy, observation of the response of the intact tumor and/or nodal metastases to a specific regimen could ultimately help to define which patients will benefit from specific therapies in the adjuvant setting. In adjuvant trials the primary endpoint is typically survival, whereas in neoadjuvant trials the endpoints are more often clinical or pathologic response rates. There are a number of clinical trials underway comparing neoadjuvant chemotherapy and endocrine therapy regimens with pretreatment and posttreatment biopsy samples obtained from the primary tumors in all of the participants. These samples are being subjected to intensive genomic and proteomic analyses that may help to define a more personalized or individualized approach to breast cancer treatment in the future.

For women with stage IV breast cancer, an antiestrogen (tamoxifen for premenopausal women or an aromatase inhibitor for postmenopausal women) is the preferred therapy. However, women with hormone receptor–negative cancers with symptomatic visceral metastasis or with hormone-refractory cancer may receive systemic chemotherapy. Pamidronate may be given to women with osteolytic bone metastases in addition to hormonal therapy or standard chemotherapy.[195] Women with metastatic breast cancer also may be enrolled into clinical trials exploring novel biologic therapies alone or in combination with chemotherapeutics.

Antiestrogen Therapy

Within the cytosol of breast cancer cells are specific proteins (receptors) that bind and transfer steroid moieties into the cell nucleus to exert specific hormonal effects.[184,196–200] The most widely studied hormone receptors are the estrogen receptor and progesterone receptor. Hormone receptors are detectable in >90% of well-differentiated ductal and lobular invasive cancers. Sequential studies of hormone receptor status reveal no differences between the primary cancer and metastatic disease in the same patient.

After binding to estrogen receptors in the cytosol, tamoxifen blocks the uptake of estrogen by breast tissue. Clinical responses to antiestrogen are evident in >60% of women with hormone receptor–positive breast cancers but in <10% of women with hormone receptor–negative breast cancers. An overview analysis by the Early Breast Cancer Trialists' Collaborative Group showed that adjuvant therapy with tamoxifen produced a 25% reduction in the annual risk of breast cancer recurrence and a 7% reduction in annual breast cancer mortality.[201] The analysis also showed a 39% reduction in the risk of cancer in the contralateral breast. The antiestrogens do have defined toxicity, including bone pain, hot flashes, nausea, vomiting, and fluid retention. Thrombotic events occur in <3% of treated women. Cataract surgery is more frequently performed in patients receiving tamoxifen. A long-term risk of tamoxifen use is endometrial cancer, although it occurs rarely. Tamoxifen therapy usually is discontinued after 5 years. In postmenopausal women, aromatase inhibitors are now considered as first-line therapy in the adjuvant setting or as a secondary agent after 1 to 2 years of adjuvant tamoxifen therapy. The aromatase inhibitors are less likely to cause endometrial cancer but do lead to changes in bone mineral density that may result in osteoporosis and an increased rate of fractures in postmenopausal women.

The NSABP P-1 trial was the first large-scale U.S. breast cancer prevention trial, and it demonstrated a 49% reduction in the incidence of invasive breast cancer in high-risk women who were treated with tamoxifen.[50] This reduction was demonstrated for all age groups treated, for all projected levels of risk, and for women with a prior history of either LCIS or atypical ductal hyperplasia. The reduction was demonstrable within the first year of follow-up and continued through a 6-year follow-up period. This led to approval of tamoxifen as a chemopreventive agent for women with a Gail relative risk of 1.70 or greater. Treatment consists of tamox-

ifen (20 mg/d) for up to 5 years to reduce the risk of breast cancer. The NSABP P-2 prevention trial compared the use of raloxifene, a selective estrogen receptor modulator used to prevent osteoporosis in postmenopausal women, with the use of tamoxifen in postmenopausal women at increased risk for breast cancer (Study of Tamoxifen and Raloxifene, or STAR trial). In the STAR trial, 19,747 postmenopausal women were randomly assigned to receive tamoxifen (20 mg daily) or raloxifene (60 mg daily) for 5 years. The initial results revealed 163 invasive breast cancers in the tamoxifen group and 168 invasive breast cancers in the raloxifene group.[60] Fewer noninvasive cancers were diagnosed in the tamoxifen group. An important outcome was the finding of 36% fewer cases of uterine cancer in the raloxifene group. Overall there were no differences between tamoxifen and raloxifene with respect to the risks of other invasive cancers, ischemic heart disease events, numbers of stroke, or osteoporotic fractures reported. The number of thromboembolic events and incidence of cataracts were lower in the raloxifene group. Overall, the STAR trial revealed that raloxifene is as effective as tamoxifen for reducing the risk of invasive breast cancer in high-risk women. There was a difference in favor of tamoxifen with respect to number of noninvasive breast cancers, but this was not statistically significant. Perhaps most importantly when a chemoprevention regimen is considered, raloxifene appears to have a better toxicity profile than tamoxifen, including both a lower risk of thromboembolic events and a lower risk of cataracts.

Tamoxifen therapy is also considered for women with DCIS that is found to be estrogen receptor positive on immunohistochemical studies. The goals of such therapy are to decrease the risk of an ipsilateral recurrence after breast conservation therapy for DCIS and to decrease the risk of a primary invasive breast cancer or a contralateral breast cancer event.

Node-negative women with hormone receptor–positive breast cancers that are 1 to 3 cm in size are candidates for adjuvant endocrine therapy with or without chemotherapy. For node-positive women and for all women with a cancer that is >3 cm in size, the use of endocrine therapy in addition to adjuvant chemotherapy is appropriate. Women with hormone receptor–positive cancers achieve significant reduction in risk of recurrence and mortality due to breast cancer through the use of endocrine therapies. For women with stage IV breast cancer, an antiestrogen is the preferred initial therapy. For women with prior antiestrogen exposure, recommended second-line hormonal therapies include aromatase inhibitors in postmenopausal women and progestins, androgens, high-dose estrogen, or oophorectomy (medical, surgical, or radioablative) in premenopausal women. Women who respond to hormonal therapy with either shrinkage of their breast cancer or long-term stabilization of disease receive additional hormonal therapy at the time of progression. Women with hormone receptor–negative cancers, with symptomatic visceral metastasis, or with hormone-refractory disease receive systemic chemotherapy rather than hormone therapy.

Ablative Endocrine Therapy

In the past, oophorectomy, adrenalectomy, and/or hypophysectomy were the primary endocrine modalities used to treat metastatic breast cancer, but today they are rarely used. Oophorectomy was used in premenopausal breast cancer patients who presented with skin or bony metastases after a disease-free interval that exceeded 18 months. In contrast, pharmacologic doses of exogenous estrogens were given to postmenopausal women with similar recurrences. For both groups, the response rates were nearly 30%. Adrenalectomy and hypophysectomy were effective in individuals who had previously responded to either oophorectomy or exogenous estrogen therapy, and the response to these additional procedures was nearly 30%. Visceral metastases (lung, liver) responded infrequently to any form of hormonal manipulation. Aminoglutethimide blocks enzymatic conversion of cholesterol to γ-5-pregnenolone and inhibits the conversion of androstenedione to estrogen in peripheral tissues. Dose-dependent and transient side effects include ataxia, dizziness, and lethargy. After treatment with this agent (medical adrenalectomy), adrenal suppression necessitates glucocorticoid therapy. Neither permanent adrenal insufficiency nor acute crises have been observed. Because the adrenal glands are the major site for production of endogenous estrogens after menopause, treatment with aminoglutethimide has been compared prospectively with surgical adrenalectomy and hypophysectomy in postmenopausal women and is equally efficacious.

Anti–HER-2/*neu* Antibody Therapy

The determination of tumor HER-2/*neu* expression for all newly diagnosed patients with breast cancer is now recommended.[201–204] It is used for prognostic purposes in node-negative patients to assist in the selection of adjuvant chemotherapy because response rates appear to be better with doxorubicin-based adjuvant chemotherapy in patients with tumors that overexpress HER-2/*neu*, and as baseline information in case the patient develops recurrent disease that may benefit from anti–HER-2/*neu* therapy (trastuzumab). Patients with tumors that overexpress HER-2/*neu* may benefit if trastuzumab is added to paclitaxel chemotherapy. Cardiotoxicity may develop if trastuzumab is delivered concurrently with doxorubicin-based chemotherapy.

Trastuzumab was initially approved for the treatment of HER-2/*neu*–positive breast cancer in patients with metastatic disease. Once efficacy was demonstrated for patients with metastatic disease, the NSABP and the North Central Cancer Treatment Group conducted phase III trials evaluating the impact of adjuvant trastuzumab therapy in patients with early-stage breast cancer. After approval from the FDA, these groups amended their adjuvant trastuzumab trials (B-31 and N9831, respectively), to provide for a joint efficacy analysis. The first joint interim efficacy analysis demonstrated an improvement in 3-year disease-free survival from 75% in the control arm to 87% in the trastuzumab arm (hazard ratio = 0.48, P <.0001). There was an accompanying 33% reduction in mortality in the patients who received trastuzumab (hazard ratio = 0.67, P = .015). The magnitude of reduction in hazard for disease-free survival events crossed prespecified early reporting boundaries, so the data-monitoring committees for both groups recommended that randomized accrual to the trials be ended, and the results were subsequently published.[124]

Buzdar and colleagues at the M. D. Anderson Cancer Center reported the results of a randomized phase II neoadjuvant trial of trastuzumab in combination with sequential paclitaxel followed by FEC-75 (5-fluorouracil, epirubicin, cyclophosphamide) vs. the same chemotherapy regimen without trastuzumab in 42 women with early-stage operable breast cancer. The pathologic complete response rates in this trial increased from 25 to 66.7% when chemotherapy was given concurrently with trastuzumab. None of the patients receiving the concurrent trastuzumab and FEC regimen developed symptoms of congestive heart failure. However, given the small sample size in this report, the 95% confidence interval for developing heart failure was 0 to 14.8%.[205] A subsequent report which included additional patients treated with concurrent chemotherapy and trastuzumab further confirmed the high pathologic complete response rates and continued to show that cardiac function was preserved.[206] This regimen is currently being tested in a phase III multicenter trial sponsored by the American College of Surgeons Oncology Group.

SPECIAL CLINICAL SITUATIONS

Nipple Discharge
Unilateral Nipple Discharge

Nipple discharge is a finding that can be seen in a number of clinical situations. It may be suggestive of cancer if it is spontaneous, unilateral, localized to a single duct, present in women ≥40 years of age, bloody, or associated with a mass. A trigger point on the breast may be present so that pressure around the nipple-areolar complex

induces discharge from a single duct. In this circumstance, mammography and ultrasound are indicated for further evaluation. A ductogram also can be useful and is performed by cannulating a single discharging duct with a small nylon catheter or needle and injecting 1.0 mL of water-soluble contrast solution. Nipple discharge associated with a cancer may be clear, bloody, or serous. Testing for the presence of hemoglobin is helpful, but hemoglobin may also be detected when nipple discharge is secondary to an intraductal papilloma or duct ectasia. Definitive diagnosis depends on excisional biopsy of the offending duct and any associated mass lesion. A 3.0 lacrimal duct probe can be used to identify the duct that requires excision. Another approach is to inject methylene blue dye within the duct after ductography. The nipple must be sealed with collodion or a similar material so that the blue dye does not discharge through the nipple but remains within the distended duct facilitating its localization. Needle localization biopsy is performed when there is an associated mass that lies >2.0 to 3.0 cm from the nipple.

Bilateral Nipple Discharge

Nipple discharge is suggestive of a benign condition if it is bilateral and multiductal in origin, occurs in women ≤39 years of age, or is milky or blue-green. Prolactin-secreting pituitary adenomas are responsible for bilateral nipple discharge in <2% of cases. If serum prolactin levels are repeatedly elevated, plain radiographs of the sella turcica are indicated and thin section CT scan is required. Optical nerve compression, visual field loss, and infertility are associated with large pituitary adenomas.

Axillary Lymph Node Metastases in the Setting of an Unknown Primary Cancer

A woman who presents with an axillary lymph node metastasis that is consistent with a breast cancer metastasis has a 90% probability of harboring an occult breast cancer.[207] However, axillary lymphadenopathy is the initial presenting sign in only 1% of breast cancer patients. Fine-needle aspiration biopsy, core-needle biopsy, or open biopsy of an enlarged axillary lymph node is performed to confirm metastatic disease. When metastatic cancer is found, immunohistochemical analysis may classify the cancer as epithelial, melanocytic, or lymphoid in origin. The presence of hormone receptors (estrogen or progesterone receptors) suggests metastasis from a breast cancer but is not diagnostic. The search for a primary cancer includes careful examination of the thyroid, breast, and pelvis, including the rectum. The breast should be examined with diagnostic mammography, ultrasonography, and MRI to evaluate for an occult primary lesion. Further radiologic and laboratory studies should include chest radiography and liver function studies. Chest, abdominal, and pelvic CT scans also are indicated, as is a bone scan to rule out distant metastasis. Suspicious findings on mammography, ultrasonography, or MRI necessitate breast biopsy. When a breast cancer is found, treatment consists of an axillary lymph node dissection with a mastectomy or preservation of the breast followed by whole-breast radiation therapy. Chemotherapy and endocrine therapy should be considered.

Breast Cancer during Pregnancy

Breast cancer occurs in 1 of every 3000 pregnant women, and axillary lymph node metastases are present in up to 75% of these women.[208] The average age of the pregnant woman with breast cancer is 34 years. Fewer than 25% of the breast nodules developing during pregnancy and lactation will be cancerous. Ultrasonography and needle biopsy are used in the diagnosis of these nodules. Open biopsy may be required. Mammography is rarely indicated because of its decreased sensitivity during pregnancy and lactation; however, the fetus can be shielded if mammography is needed. Approximately 30% of the benign conditions encountered will be unique to pregnancy and lactation (galactoceles, lobular hyperplasia, lactating adenoma, and mastitis or abscess). Once a breast cancer is diagnosed, complete blood count, chest radiography (with shielding of the abdomen), and liver function studies are performed.

Because of the potential deleterious effects of radiation therapy on the fetus, radiation cannot be considered until the fetus is delivered. A modified radical mastectomy can be performed during the first and second trimesters of pregnancy, even though there is an increased risk of spontaneous abortion after first-trimester anesthesia. During the third trimester, lumpectomy with axillary node dissection can be considered if adjuvant radiation therapy is deferred until after delivery. Lactation is suppressed. Chemotherapy administered during the first trimester carries a risk of spontaneous abortion and a 12% risk of birth defects. There is no evidence of teratogenicity resulting from administration of chemotherapeutic agents in the second and third trimesters. For this reason, many clinicians now consider the optimal strategy to be delivery of chemotherapy in the second and third trimesters as a neoadjuvant approach, which allows local therapy decisions to be made after the delivery of the baby. Pregnant women with breast cancer often present at a later stage of disease because breast tissue changes that occur in the hormone-rich environment of pregnancy obscure early cancers. However, pregnant women with breast cancer have a prognosis, stage by stage, that is similar to that of nonpregnant women with breast cancer.

Male Breast Cancer

Fewer than 1% of all breast cancers occur in men.[209,210] The incidence appears to be highest among North Americans and the British, in whom breast cancer constitutes as much as 1.5% of all male cancers. Jewish and African American males have the highest incidence. Male breast cancer is preceded by gynecomastia in 20% of men. It is associated with radiation exposure, estrogen therapy, testicular feminizing syndromes, and Klinefelter's syndrome (XXY). Breast cancer is rarely seen in young males and has a peak incidence in the sixth decade of life. A firm, nontender mass in the male breast requires investigation. Skin or chest wall fixation is particularly worrisome.

DCIS makes up <15% of male breast cancer, whereas infiltrating ductal carcinoma makes up >85%. Special-type cancers, including infiltrating lobular carcinoma, have occasionally been reported. Male breast cancer is staged in the same way as female breast cancer, and stage by stage, men with breast cancer have the same survival rate as women. Overall, men do worse because of the advanced stage of their cancer (stage III or IV) at the time of diagnosis. The treatment of male breast cancer is surgical, with the most common procedure being a modified radical mastectomy. Sentinel node dissection has been shown to be feasible and accurate for nodal assessment in men presenting with a clinically node-negative axillary nodal basin. Adjuvant radiation therapy is appropriate in cases in which there is a high risk for local-regional recurrence. Eighty percent of male breast cancers are hormone receptor positive, and adjuvant tamoxifen is considered. Systemic chemotherapy is considered for men with hormone receptor–negative cancers and for men with large primary tumors, multiple positive nodes, and locally advanced disease.

Phyllodes Tumors

The nomenclature, presentation, and diagnosis of phyllodes tumors (including cystosarcoma phyllodes) have posed many problems for surgeons.[211] These tumors are classified as benign, borderline, or malignant. Borderline tumors have a greater potential for local recurrence. Mammographic evidence of calcifications and morphologic evidence of necrosis do not distinguish between benign, borderline, and malignant phyllodes tumors. Consequently, it is difficult to differentiate benign phyllodes tumors from the malignant variant and from fibroadenomas. Phyllodes tumors are usually sharply demarcated from the surrounding breast tissue, which is compressed and distorted. Connective tissue composes the bulk of these tumors, which have mixed gelatinous, solid, and cystic areas. Cystic areas represent sites of infarction and necrosis. These gross alterations give the gross cut tumor surface its classical leaf-like (phyllodes) appearance. The stroma of a phyllodes tumor generally

has greater cellular activity than that of a fibroadenoma. After microdissection to harvest clusters of stromal cells from fibroadenomas and from phyllodes tumors, molecular biology techniques have shown the stromal cells of fibroadenomas to be either polyclonal or monoclonal (derived from a single progenitor cell), whereas those of phyllodes tumors are always monoclonal.

Most malignant phyllodes tumors (Fig. 17-40) contain liposarcomatous or rhabdomyosarcomatous elements rather than fibrosarcomatous elements. Evaluation of the number of mitoses and the presence or absence of invasive foci at the tumor margins may help to identify a malignant tumor. Small phyllodes tumors are excised with a margin of normal-appearing breast tissue. When the diagnosis of a phyllodes tumor with suspicious malignant elements is made, re-excision of the biopsy site to ensure complete excision of the tumor with a 1-cm margin of normal-appearing breast tissue is indicated. Large phyllodes tumors may require mastectomy. Axillary dissection is not recommended because axillary lymph node metastases rarely occur.

Inflammatory Breast Carcinoma

Inflammatory breast carcinoma (stage IIIB) accounts for <3% of breast cancers. This cancer is characterized by the skin changes of

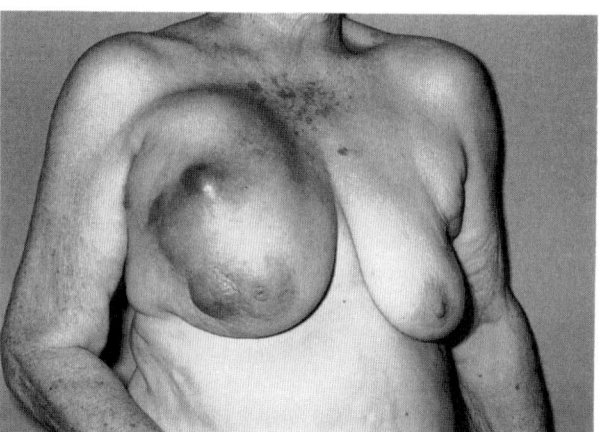

A

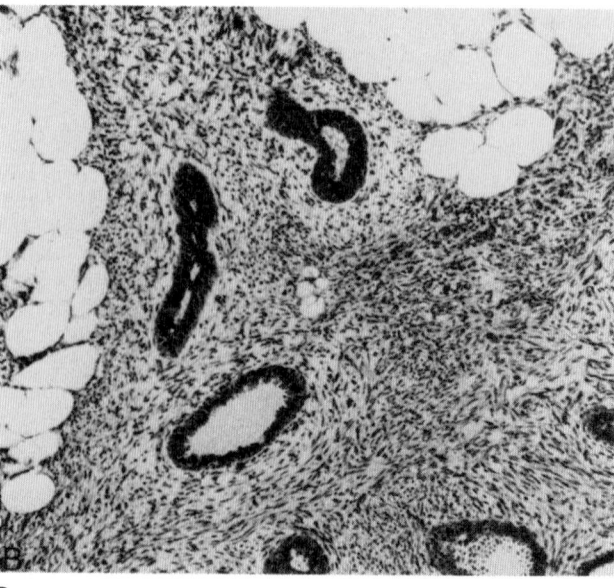

B

FIG. 17-40. A. Malignant phyllodes tumor (cystosarcoma phyllodes). **B.** Histologic features of a malignant phyllodes tumor (hematoxylin and eosin stain, ×100).

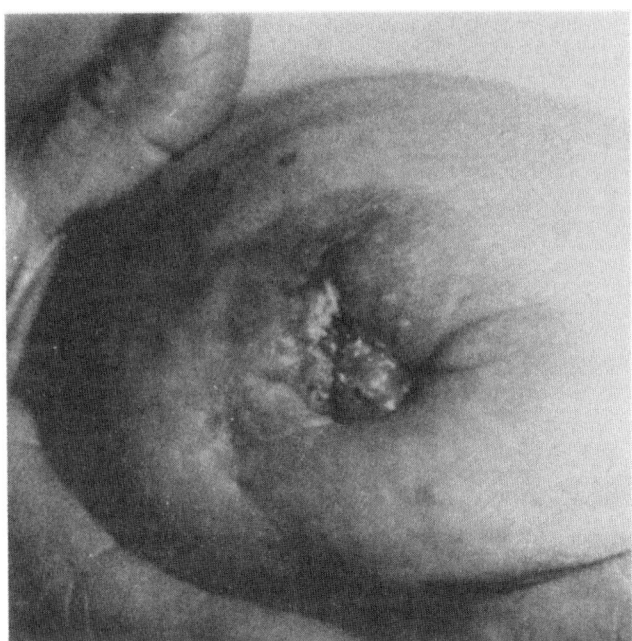

FIG. 17-41. Inflammatory breast carcinoma. Stage IIIB cancer of the breast with erythema, skin edema (peau d'orange), nipple retraction, and satellite skin nodules.

brawny induration, erythema with a raised edge, and edema (peau d'orange).[212] Permeation of the dermal lymph vessels by cancer cells is seen in skin biopsy specimens. There may be an associated breast mass (Fig. 17-41). The clinical differentiation of inflammatory breast cancer may be extremely difficult, especially when a locally advanced scirrhous carcinoma invades dermal lymph vessels in the skin to produce peau d'orange and lymphangitis (Table 17-16). Inflammatory breast cancer also may be mistaken for a bacterial infection of the breast. More than 75% of women who have inflammatory breast cancer present with palpable axillary lymphadenopathy, and distant metastases also are frequently present. A report of the SEER program described distant metastases at diagnosis in 25% of white women with inflammatory breast carcinoma.

Surgery alone and surgery with adjuvant radiation therapy have produced disappointing results in women with inflammatory breast cancer. However, neoadjuvant chemotherapy with a doxorubicin-

TABLE 17-16	Inflammatory vs. noninflammatory breast cancer
Inflammatory	**Noninflammatory**
Dermal lymph vessel invasion is present with or without inflammatory changes.	Inflammatory changes are present without dermal lymph vessel invasion.
Cancer is not sharply delineated.	Cancer is better delineated.
Erythema and edema frequently involve >33% of the skin over the breast.	Erythema is usually confined to the lesion, and edema is less extensive.
Lymph node involvement is present in >75% of cases.	Lymph nodes are involved in approximately 50% of the cases.
Distant metastases are present in 25% of cases.	Distant metastases are less common at presentation.
Distant metastases are more common at initial presentation.	

Source: Modified with permission from Chittoor SR, et al: Locally advanced breast cancer: Role of medical oncology, in Bland KI, et al (eds): *The Breast: Comprehensive Management of Benign and Malignant Diseases.* Philadelphia: WB Saunders, 1998, p 1281. Copyright Elsevier.

containing regimen may effect dramatic regressions in up to 75% of cases. In this setting, modified radical mastectomy is performed to remove residual cancer from the chest wall and axilla. Adjuvant chemotherapy may be indicated depending on final pathologic assessment of the breast and regional nodes. Finally, the chest wall and the supraclavicular, internal mammary, and axillary lymph node basins receive adjuvant radiation therapy. This multimodal approach results in 5-year survival rates that approach 30%.

Rare Breast Cancers

Squamous Cell (Epidermoid) Carcinoma

Squamous cell (epidermoid) carcinoma is a rare cancer that arises from metaplasia within the duct system and generally is devoid of distinctive clinical or radiographic characteristics.[213] Regional metastases occur in 25% of patients, whereas distant metastases are rare.

Adenoid Cystic Carcinoma

Adenoid cystic carcinoma is very rare, accounting for <0.1% of all breast cancers. It is typically indistinguishable from adenoid cystic carcinoma arising in salivary tissues. These cancers are generally 1 to 3 cm in diameter at presentation and are well circumscribed. Axillary lymph node metastases are rare, but deaths from pulmonary metastases have been reported.

Apocrine Carcinoma

Apocrine carcinomas are well-differentiated cancers that have rounded vesicular nuclei and prominent nucleoli. There is a very low mitotic rate and little variation in cellular features. However, apocrine carcinomas may display an aggressive growth pattern.

Sarcomas

Sarcomas of the breast are histologically similar to soft tissue sarcomas at other anatomic sites. This diverse group includes fibrosarcoma, malignant fibrous histiocytoma, liposarcoma, leiomyosarcoma, malignant schwannoma, rhabdomyosarcoma, osteogenic sarcoma, and chondrosarcoma. The clinical presentation is typically that of a large, painless breast mass with rapid growth. Diagnosis is by core-needle biopsy or by open incisional biopsy. Sarcomas are graded based on cellularity, degree of differentiation, nuclear atypia, and mitotic activity. Primary treatment is wide local excision, which may necessitate mastectomy. Axillary dissection is not indicated unless there is palpable lymphadenopathy. Angiosarcomas are classified as de novo, as postradiation, or as arising in association with postmastectomy lymphedema. In 1948, Stewart and Treves described lymphangiosarcoma of the upper extremity in women with ipsilateral lymphedema after radical mastectomy.[214] *Angiosarcoma* is now the preferred name. The average interval between modified radical or radical mastectomy and the development of an angiosarcoma is 10.5 years. Sixty percent of women developing this cancer have a history of adjuvant radiation therapy. Forequarter amputation may be necessary to palliate the ulcerative complications and advanced lymphedema.

Lymphomas

Primary lymphomas of the breast are rare, and there are two distinct clinicopathologic variants. One type occurs in women ≤39 years of age, is frequently bilateral, and has the histologic features of Burkitt's lymphoma. The second type is seen in women ≥40 years of age and is usually of the B-cell type. Breast involvement by Hodgkin's lymphoma has been reported. An occult breast lymphoma may be diagnosed after detection of palpable axillary lymphadenopathy. Treatment depends on the stage of disease. Lumpectomy or mastectomy may be required. Axillary dissection for staging and for clearance of palpable disease is appropriate. Recurrent or progressive local-regional disease is best managed by chemotherapy and radiation therapy. The prognosis is favorable, with 5- and 10-year survival rates of 74 and 51%, respectively.

REFERENCES

Entries highlighted in bright blue are key references.

1. Breasted JH: *The Edwin Smith Surgical Papyrus.* Chicago: University of Chicago Press, 1930, p 405. Classics of Medicine Library, vol. III.

2. Celsus AC: De Medicina, Vol II. *Loeb Classical Library Ed,* Book V. Cambridge: Harvard University Press, 1935, p. 131.

3. Beenken SW, et al: History of the therapy of breast cancer, in Bland and Copeland (eds): *The Breast: Comprehensive Management of Benign and Malignant Disorders.* Philadelphia: Saunders, 2004, p 5.

4. Halsted WS: I. The results of operations for the cure of cancer of the breast performed at the Johns Hopkins Hospital from June, 1889, to January, 1894. *Ann Surg* 20:497, 1894.

5. Le Dran F: Mémoire avec une précis de plusieurs observations sur le cancer. *Mem Acad Roy Chir Paris* 3:1, 1757.

6. Haagensen CD, Stout AP: Carcinoma of the breast (II. Criteria of Operability). *Ann Surg* 118:859, 1943.

7. Madden JL: Modified radical mastectomy. *Surg Gynecol Obstet* 121:1221, 1965.

8. Maddox WA, et al: A randomized prospective trial of radical (Halsted) mastectomy versus modified radical mastectomy in 311 breast cancer patients. *Ann Surg* 198:207, 1983.

9. Turner L, et al: Radical versus modified radical mastectomy for breast cancer. *Ann R Col Surg Engl* 63:239, 1981.

10. Meyer W: An improved method of the radical operation for carcinoma of the breast. *Med Rec* 46:746, 1894.

11. Moore C: On the influence of inadequate operations on the theory of cancer. *R Med Chir Soc* 1:244, 1867.

12. Patey DH, Dyson WH: The prognosis of carcinoma of the breast in relation to the type of operation performed. *Br J Cancer* 2:7, 1948.

13. Fisher B, et al: Twenty-five-year follow-up of a randomized trial comparing radical mastectomy, total mastectomy, and total mastectomy followed by irradiation. *N Engl J Med* 347:567, 2002.

14. Bland KI, Romrell LJ: Congenital and acquired disturbances of breast development and growth, in Bland KI, Copeland EM III (eds): *The Breast: Comprehensive Management of Benign and Malignant Diseases.* Philadelphia: WB Saunders, 1998, p 214.

15. Romrell LJ, Bland KI: Anatomy of the breast, axilla, chest wall, and related metastatic sites, in Bland KI, Copeland EM III (eds): *The Breast: Comprehensive Management of Benign and Malignant Diseases.* Philadelphia: WB Saunders, 1998, p 19.

16. Lonnerdal B: Nutritional and physiologic significance of human milk proteins. *Am J Clin Nutr* 77:1537S, 2003.

17. Rosenbloom AL: Breast physiology: Normal and abnormal development and function, in Bland KI, Copeland EM III (eds): *The Breast: Comprehensive Management of Benign and Malignant Diseases.* Philadelphia: WB Saunders, 1998, p 38.

18. Van de Perre P: Transfer of antibody via mother's milk. *Vaccine* 21:3374, 2003.

19. Bland KI, Graves TA: Gynecomastia, in Bland KI, Copeland EM III (eds): *The Breast: Comprehensive Management of Benign and Malignant Diseases.* Philadelphia: WB Saunders, 1998, p 153.

20. Bland KI: Inflammatory, infectious, and metabolic disorders of the breast, in Bland KI, Copeland EM III (eds): *The Breast: Comprehensive Management of Benign and Malignant Diseases.* Philadelphia: WB Saunders, 1998, p 75.

21. Furlong AJ, et al: Periductal inflammation and cigarette smoke. *J Am Coll Surg* 179:417, 1994.

22. Zuska J, Crile G Jr., Ayres WW: Fistulas of lactiferous ducts. *Am J Surg* 81:312, 1951.

23. Camiel MR: Mondor's disease in the breast. *Am J Obstet Gynecol* 152(7 Pt 1):879, 1985.

24. Mondor H: Tronculite sous-cutanée subaiguë de la paroi thoracique antero-latérale. *Mem Acad Chir Paris* 65:1271, 1939.

25. Hughes LE, Mansel RE, Webster DJ: Aberrations of normal development and involution (ANDI): A new perspective on pathogenesis and nomenclature of benign breast disorders. *Lancet* 2:1316, 1987.

26. Archer F, Omar M: The fine structure of fibro-adenoma of the human breast. *J Pathol* 99:113, 1969.

27. Page DL, Anderson TJ: *Diagnostic Histopathology of the Breast.* Edinburgh: Churchill Livingstone, 1987.

28. Page DL, Simpson JF: Benign, high-risk, and premalignant lesions of the breast, in Bland KI, Copeland EM III (eds): *The Breast: Comprehensive Management of Benign and Malignant Diseases.* Philadelphia: WB Saunders, 1998, p 191.

29. Consensus Meeting: Is "fibrocystic disease" of the breast precancerous? *Arch Pathol Lab Med* 110:171, 1986.

30. Haagensen CD: *Diseases of the Breast,* 3rd ed. Philadelphia: WB Saunders, 1986.

31. Haagensen CD, et al: Lobular neoplasia (so-called lobular carcinoma in situ) of the breast. *Cancer* 42:737, 1978.

32. Gadd MA, Souba WW: Evaluation and treatment of benign breast disorders, in Bland KI, Copeland EM III (eds): *The Breast: Comprehensive Management of Benign and Malignant Diseases.* Philadelphia: WB Saunders, 1998, p 233.

33. Marchant DJ: Benign breast disease. *Obstet Gynecol Clin North Am* 29:1, 2002.

34. Nurko J, et al: Interim results from the FibroAdenoma Cryoablation Treatment Registry. *Am J Surg* 190:647; discussion 651, 2005.

35. Bernstein L, et al: Physical exercise and reduced risk of breast cancer in young women. *J Natl Cancer Inst* 86:1403, 1994.

36. Blackburn GL, et al: Diet and breast cancer. *J Womens Health (Larchmt)* 12:183, 2003.

37. Goss PE, Sierra S: Current perspectives on radiation-induced breast cancer. *J Clin Oncol* 16:338, 1998.

38. Hulka BS: Epidemiologic analysis of breast and gynecologic cancers. *Prog Clin Biol Res* 396:17, 1997.

39. Pujol P, Galtier-Dereure F, Bringer J: Obesity and breast cancer risk. *Hum Reprod* 12 Suppl 1:116, 1997.

40. Singletary SE: Rating the risk factors for breast cancer. *Ann Surg* 237:474, 2003.

41. Wynder EL, et al: Breast cancer: Weighing the evidence for a promoting role of dietary fat. *J Natl Cancer Inst* 89:766, 1997.

42. Claus EB, Risch N, Thompson WD: Autosomal dominant inheritance of early-onset breast cancer. Implications for risk prediction. *Cancer* 73:643, 1994.

43. Domchek SM, et al: Application of breast cancer risk prediction models in clinical practice. *J Clin Oncol* 21:593, 2003.

44. Gail MH, et al: Projecting individualized probabilities of developing breast cancer for white females who are being examined annually. *J Natl Cancer Inst* 81:1879, 1989.

45. Gail MH, et al: Projecting individualized absolute invasive breast cancer risk in African American women. *J Natl Cancer Inst* 99:1782, 2007.

46. Edwards BK, et al: Annual report to the nation on the status of cancer, 1975–2002, featuring population-based trends in cancer treatment. *J Natl Cancer Inst* 97:1407, 2005.

47. Claus EB, et al: The calculation of breast cancer risk for women with a first degree family history of ovarian cancer. *Breast Cancer Res Treat* 28:115, 1993.

48. Chen J, et al: Projecting absolute invasive breast cancer risk in white women with a model that includes mammographic density. *J Natl Cancer Inst* 98:1215, 2006.

49. Kerlikowske K, et al: Longitudinal measurement of clinical mammographic breast density to improve estimation of breast cancer risk. *J Natl Cancer Inst* 99:386, 2007.

50. Fisher B, et al: Tamoxifen for prevention of breast cancer: Report of the National Surgical Adjuvant Breast and Bowel Project P-1 Study. *J Natl Cancer Inst* 90:1371, 1998.

51. Grodstein F, et al: Postmenopausal hormone therapy and mortality. *N Engl J Med* 336:1769, 1997.

52. Hartmann LC, et al: Efficacy of bilateral prophylactic mastectomy in women with a family history of breast cancer. *N Engl J Med* 340:77, 1999.

53. Kerlikowske K, et al: Efficacy of screening mammography. A meta-analysis. *JAMA* 273:149, 1995.

54. Rowe TC, et al: DNA damage by antitumor acridines mediated by mammalian DNA topoisomerase II. *Cancer Res* 46:2021, 1986.

55. Sakorafas GH: The management of women at high risk for the development of breast cancer: Risk estimation and preventative strategies. *Cancer Treat Rev* 29:79, 2003.

56. Schrag D, et al: Decision analysis—effects of prophylactic mastectomy and oophorectomy on life expectancy among women with BRCA1 or BRCA2 mutations. *N Engl J Med* 336:1465, 1997.

57. Vogel VG: Management of the high-risk patient. *Surg Clin North Am* 83:733, 2003.

58. Wu K, Brown P: Is low-dose tamoxifen useful for the treatment and prevention of breast cancer? *J Natl Cancer Inst* 95:766, 2003.

59. Gail MH, et al: Weighing the risks and benefits of tamoxifen treatment for preventing breast cancer. *J Natl Cancer Inst* 91:1829, 1999.

60. Vogel VG, et al: Effects of tamoxifen vs raloxifene on the risk of developing invasive breast cancer and other disease outcomes: The NSABP Study of Tamoxifen and Raloxifene (STAR) P-2 trial. *JAMA* 295:2727, 2006.

61. Ford D, et al: Genetic heterogeneity and penetrance analysis of the BRCA1 and BRCA2 genes in breast cancer families. The Breast Cancer Linkage Consortium. *Am J Hum Genet* 62:676, 1998.

62. Gowen LC, et al: BRCA1 required for transcription-coupled repair of oxidative DNA damage. *Science* 281:1009, 1998.

63. Martin AM, Weber BL: Genetic and hormonal risk factors in breast cancer. *J Natl Cancer Inst* 92:1126, 2000.

64. Oddoux C, et al: The carrier frequency of the BRCA2 6174delT mutation among Ashkenazi Jewish individuals is approximately 1%. *Nat Genet* 14:188, 1996.

65. Roa BB, et al: Ashkenazi Jewish population frequencies for common mutations in BRCA1 and BRCA2. *Nat Genet* 14:185, 1996.

66. Rosen EM, et al: BRCA1 gene in breast cancer. *J Cell Physiol* 196:19, 2003.

67. Wooster R, Weber BL: Breast and ovarian cancer. *N Engl J Med* 348:2339, 2003.

68. Warner E, et al: Prevalence and penetrance of BRCA1 and BRCA2 gene mutations in unselected Ashkenazi Jewish women with breast cancer. *J Natl Cancer Inst* 91:1241, 1999.

69. Schneider KA: Genetic counseling for BRCA1/BRCA2 testing. *Genet Test* 1:91, 1997.

70. Kriege M, et al: Efficacy of MRI and mammography for breast-cancer screening in women with a familial or genetic predisposition. *N Engl J Med* 351:427, 2004.

71. Saslow D, et al: American Cancer Society guidelines for breast screening with MRI as an adjunct to mammography. *CA Cancer J Clin* 57:75, 2007.

72. Guinee VF: Epidemiology of breast cancer, in Bland KI, Copeland EM III (eds): *The Breast: Comprehensive Management of Benign and Malignant Diseases.* Philadelphia: WB Saunders, 1998, p 339.

73. Jemal A, et al: Cancer statistics 2008. *CA Cancer J Clin* 58:71, 2008.

74. American Cancer Society: *Cancer Facts and Figures 2008.* Atlanta: American Cancer Society, 2008. *Available at http://www.cancer.org/downloads/STT/2008CAFFfinalsecured.pdf* [accessed January 29, 2009].

75. Clarke CA, et al: Recent declines in hormone therapy utilization and breast cancer incidence: Clinical and population-based evidence. *J Clin Oncol* 24:e49, 2006.

76. Ferlay J, et al: *Globocan 2002: Cancer Incidence, Mortality and Prevalence Worldwide.* Lyon, France: IARC Press, 2004. IARC Cancer Base No. 5, Version 2.0.

77. Ries LAG, et al: SEER Cancer Statistics Review, 1975-2002, National Cancer Institute. Bethesda, MD, *http://seer.cancer.gov/csr/1975_2002/* [accessed January 29, 2009].

78. Fregene A, Newman LA: Breast cancer in sub-Saharan Africa: How does it relate to breast cancer in African-American women? *Cancer* 103:1540, 2005.

79. Bloom HJ, Richardson WW, Harries EJ: Natural history of untreated breast cancer (1805–1933). Comparison of untreated and treated cases according to histological grade of malignancy. *Br Med J* 2:213, 1962.

80. Broders AC: Carcinoma in situ contrasted with benign penetrating epithelium. *JAMA* 99:1670, 1932.

81. Foote FWJ, Stewart FW: Lobular carcinoma in situ: A rare form of mammary carcinoma. *Am J Pathol* 17:491, 1941.

82. Consensus conference on the classification of ductal carcinoma in situ. *Hum Pathol* 28:1221, 1997.

83. Recht A, et al: The fourth EORTC DCIS Consensus meeting (Chateau Marquette, Heemskerk, The Netherlands, 23–24 January 1998)—conference report. *Eur J Cancer* 34:1664, 1998.

84. Devitt JE, Barr JR: The clinical recognition of cystic carcinoma of the breast. *Surg Gynecol Obstet* 159:130, 1984.

85. Gallager HS, Martin JE: The study of mammary carcinoma by mammography and whole organ sectioning. Early observations. *Cancer* 23:855, 1969.

86. Seth A, et al: Gene expression profiling of ductal carcinomas in situ and invasive breast tumors. *Anticancer Res* 23:2043, 2003.

87. Simpson JF, Wilkinson EJ: Malignant neoplasia of the breast: Infiltrating carcinomas, in Bland KI, Copeland EM III (eds): *The Breast: Comprehensive Management of Benign and Malignant Diseases.* Philadelphia: WB Saunders, 1998, p 285.

88. McDivitt RW, et al.: Tubular carcinoma of the breast: Clinical and pathological observations concerning 135 cases. *Am J Surg Pathol* 6:401, 1982.

89. Jatoi I: Screening clinical breast examination. *Surg Clin North Am* 83:789, 2003.

90. Rosato FE, Rosato EL: Examination techniques: Roles of the physician and patient in evaluating breast diseases, in Bland KI, Copeland EM III (eds): *The Breast: Comprehensive Management of Benign and Malignant Diseases.* Philadelphia: WB Saunders, 1998, p 615.

91. Bassett LW: Breast imaging, in Bland KI, Copeland EM III (eds): *The Breast: Comprehensive Management of Benign and Malignant Diseases.* Philadelphia: WB Saunders, 1998, p 648.

92. Fletcher SW, Elmore JG: Clinical practice. Mammographic screening for breast cancer. *N Engl J Med* 348:1672, 2003.

93. Miller AB: Screening and detection, in Bland KI, Copeland EM III (eds): *The Breast: Comprehensive Management of Benign and Malignant Diseases.* Philadelphia: WB Saunders, 1998, p 625.

94. Schnall MD: Breast MR imaging. *Radiol Clin North Am* 41:43, 2003.

95. Seidman H, et al.: Survival experience in the Breast Cancer Detection Demonstration Project. *CA Cancer J Clin* 37:258, 1987.

96. Pisano ED, et al: Diagnostic performance of digital versus film mammography for breast-cancer screening. *N Engl J Med* 353:1773, 2005.

97. Robinson DS, Sundaram M: Stereotactic imaging and breast biopsy, in Bland KI, Copeland EM III (eds): *The Breast: Comprehensive Management of Benign and Malignant Diseases.* Philadelphia: WB Saunders, 1998, p 698.

98. Wilkinson EJ, Masood S: Cytologic needle samplings of the breast: Techniques and end results, in Bland KI, Copeland EM III (eds): *The Breast: Comprehensive Management of Benign and Malignant Diseases.* Philadelphia: WB Saunders, 1998, p 705.

99. Breast, in Greene FL, et al (eds): *AJCC Cancer Staging Manual,* 6th ed. New York: Springer-Verlag, 2002, p 223.

100. Fisher B, Slack NH: Number of lymph nodes examined and the prognosis of breast carcinoma. *Surg Gynecol Obstet* 131:79, 1970.

101. Dillon DA: Molecular markers in the diagnosis and staging of breast cancer. *Semin Radiat Oncol* 12:305, 2002.

102. Esteva FJ, et al: Molecular prognostic factors for breast cancer metastasis and survival. *Semin Radiat Oncol* 12:319, 2002.

103. Haffty BG: Molecular and genetic markers in the local-regional management of breast cancer. *Semin Radiat Oncol* 12:329, 2002.

104. Morabito A, et al: Prognostic and predictive indicators in operable breast cancer. *Clin Breast Cancer* 3:381, 2003.

105. Rogers CE, et al: Molecular prognostic indicators in breast cancer. *Eur J Surg Oncol* 28:467, 2002.

106. Monaghan P, et al: Growth factor stimulation of proliferating cell nuclear antigen (PCNA) in human breast epithelium in organ culture. *Cell Biol Int Rep* 15:561, 1991.

107. Siitonen SM, et al: Intratumor variation in cell proliferation in breast carcinoma as determined by antiproliferating cell nuclear antigen monoclonal antibody and automated image analysis. *Am J Clin Pathol* 99:226, 1993.

108. Tuccari G, et al: PCNA/cyclin expression in breast carcinomas: Its relationships with Ki-67, ER, PgR immunostainings and clinico-pathologic aspects. *Pathologica* 85:47, 1993.

109. van Dierendonck JH, et al: Cell-cycle–related staining patterns of antiproliferating cell nuclear antigen monoclonal antibodies. Comparison with BrdUrd labeling and Ki-67 staining. *Am J Pathol* 138:1165, 1991.

110. Allan DJ, et al: Reduction in apoptosis relative to mitosis in histologically normal epithelium accompanies fibrocystic change and carcinoma of the premenopausal human breast. *J Pathol* 167:25, 1992.

111. Bargou RC, et al: Expression of the bcl-2 gene family in normal and malignant breast tissue: Low bax-alpha expression in tumor cells correlates with resistance towards apoptosis. *Int J Cancer* 60:854, 1995.

112. Binder C, et al: Expression of Bax in relation to Bcl-2 and other predictive parameters in breast cancer. *Ann Oncol* 7:129, 1996.

113. Brown LF, et al: Expression of vascular permeability factor (vascular endothelial growth factor) and its receptors in breast cancer. *Hum Pathol* 26:86, 1995.

114. Gasparini G, et al: Prognostic significance of vascular endothelial growth factor protein in node-negative breast carcinoma. *J Natl Cancer Inst* 89:139, 1997.

115. Miller K, et al: Paclitaxel plus bevacizumab versus paclitaxel alone for metastatic breast cancer. *N Engl J Med* 357:2666, 2007.

116. Athanassiadou PP, et al: Presence of epidermal growth factor receptor in breast smears of cyst fluids: Relationship to electrolyte ratios and pH concentration. *Cancer Detect Prev* 16:113, 1992.

117. Tsutsumi Y, et al: neu oncogene protein and epidermal growth factor receptor are independently expressed in benign and malignant breast tissues. *Hum Pathol* 21:750, 1990.

118. van de Vijver MJ, et al: Neu-protein overexpression in breast cancer. Association with comedo-type ductal carcinoma in situ and limited prognostic value in stage II breast cancer. *N Engl J Med* 319:1239, 1989.

119. Slamon DJ, et al: Human breast cancer: Correlation of relapse and survival with amplification of the HER-2/neu oncogene. *Science* 235:177, 1987.

120. Gusterson BA, et al: Prognostic importance of c-erbB-2 expression in breast cancer. International (Ludwig) Breast Cancer Study Group. *J Clin Oncol* 10:1049, 1992.

121. McCann AH, et al: Prognostic significance of c-erbB-2 and estrogen receptor status in human breast cancer. *Cancer Res* 51:3296, 1991.

122. Slamon DJ, et al: Studies of the HER-2/neu proto-oncogene in human breast and ovarian cancer. *Science* 244:707, 1989.

123. Wright C, et al: Expression of c-erbB-2 oncoprotein: A prognostic indicator in human breast cancer. *Cancer Res* 49:2087, 1989.

124. Romond EH, et al: Trastuzumab plus adjuvant chemotherapy for operable HER2-positive breast cancer. *N Engl J Med* 353:1673, 2005.

125. Chlebowski RT, et al: Influence of estrogen plus progestin on breast cancer and mammography in healthy postmenopausal women: The Women's Health Initiative Randomized Trial. *JAMA* 289:3243, 2003.

126. Ravdin PM, et al: Computer program to assist in making decisions about adjuvant therapy for women with early breast cancer. *J Clin Oncol* 19:980, 2001.

127. Perou CM, et al: Distinctive gene expression patterns in human mammary epithelial cells and breast cancers. *Proc Natl Acad Sci U S A* 96:9212, 1999.

128. Paik S, et al: A multigene assay to predict recurrence of tamoxifen-treated, node-negative breast cancer. *N Engl J Med* 351:2817, 2004.

129. Julien JP, et al: Radiotherapy in breast-conserving treatment for ductal carcinoma in situ: First results of the EORTC randomised phase III trial 10853. EORTC Breast Cancer Cooperative Group and EORTC Radiotherapy Group. *Lancet* 355:528, 2000.

130. Lagios MD, et al: Mammographically detected duct carcinoma in situ. Frequency of local recurrence following tylectomy and prognostic effect of nuclear grade on local recurrence. *Cancer* 63:618, 1989.

131. Rosai J: Borderline epithelial lesions of the breast. *Am J Surg Pathol* 15:209, 1991.

132. Schnitt SJ, et al: Interobserver reproducibility in the diagnosis of ductal proliferative breast lesions using standardized criteria. *Am J Surg Pathol* 16:1133, 1992.

133. Silverstein MJ, et al: The influence of margin width on local control of ductal carcinoma in situ of the breast. *N Engl J Med* 340:1455, 1999.

134. Tan-Chiu E, et al: The effect of tamoxifen on benign breast disease: Findings from the National Surgical Adjuvant Breast and Bowel Project (NSABP) breast cancer prevention trial (BCPT) [abstract 7]. *Breast Cancer Res Treat* 69:210, 2001.

135. Lagios MD: Duct carcinoma in situ: Biological implications for clinical practice. *Semin Oncol* 23:6, 1996

136. Effects of radiotherapy and surgery in early breast cancer. An overview of the randomized trials. Early Breast Cancer Trialists' Collaborative Group. *N Engl J Med* 333:1444, 1995.

137. Arriagada R, et al: Conservative treatment versus mastectomy in early breast cancer: Patterns of failure with 15 years of follow-up data. Institut Gustave-Roussy Breast Cancer Group. *J Clin Oncol* 14:1558, 1996.

138. Cooke T, et al: HER2 as a prognostic and predictive marker for breast cancer. *Ann Oncol* 12 Suppl 1:S23, 2001.

139. Fisher B, et al: Twenty-year follow-up of a randomized trial comparing total mastectomy, lumpectomy, and lumpectomy plus irradiation for the treatment of invasive breast cancer. *N Engl J Med* 347:1233, 2002.

140. Fisher B, et al: Reanalysis and results after 12 years of follow-up in a randomized clinical trial comparing total mastectomy with lumpectomy with or without irradiation in the treatment of breast cancer. *N Engl J Med* 333:1456, 1995.

141. Gump FE, Jicha DL, Ozello L: Ductal carcinoma in situ (DCIS): A revised concept. *Surgery* 102:790, 1987.

142. Paik S, et al: HER2 and choice of adjuvant chemotherapy for invasive breast cancer: National Surgical Adjuvant Breast and Bowel Project Protocol B-15. *J Natl Cancer Inst* 92:1991, 2000.

143. Veronesi U, et al: Twenty-year follow-up of a randomized study comparing breast-conserving surgery with radical mastectomy for early breast cancer. *N Engl J Med* 347:1227, 2002.

144. Lyman GH, et al: American Society of Clinical Oncology guideline recommendations for sentinel lymph node biopsy in early-stage breast cancer. *J Clin Oncol* 23:7703, 2005.

145. Hortobagyi GN, Singletary SE, et al: Treatment of locally advanced and inflammatory breast cancer, in Harris JR, et al (eds): *Diseases of the Breast.* Philadelphia: Lippincott Williams & Wilkins, 2000, p 645.

146. Chen AM, et al: Breast conservation after neoadjuvant chemotherapy: The MD Anderson Cancer Center experience. *J Clin Oncol* 22:2303, 2004.

147. Favret AM, et al: Locally advanced breast cancer: Is surgery necessary? *Breast J* 7:131, 2001.

148. Khan SA, Stewart AK, Morrow M: Does aggressive local therapy improve survival in metastatic breast cancer? *Surgery* 132:620; discussion 626, 2002.

149. Gnerlich J, et al: Surgical removal of the primary tumor increases overall survival in patients with metastatic breast cancer: Analysis of the 1988–2003 SEER data. *Ann Surg Oncol* 14:2187, 2007.

150. *http://www.facs.org/cancer/ncdb:* National Cancer Data Base (NCDB), 2002–2008, American College of Surgeons, Commission on Cancer [accessed January 29, 2009].

151. Bass SS, et al: Lymphatic mapping and sentinel lymph node biopsy. *Breast J* 5:288, 1999.

152. Cox CE, et al: Importance of lymphatic mapping in ductal carcinoma in situ (DCIS): Why map DCIS? *Am Surg* 67:513; discussion 519, 2001.

153. Dupont E, et al: Learning curves and breast cancer lymphatic mapping: Institutional volume index. *J Surg Res* 97:92, 2001.

154. Krag D, et al: The sentinel node in breast cancer—a multicenter validation study. *N Engl J Med* 339:941, 1998.

155. McMasters KM, et al: Sentinel-lymph-node biopsy for breast cancer—not yet the standard of care. *N Engl J Med* 339:990, 1998.

156. O'Hea BJ, et al: Sentinel lymph node biopsy in breast cancer: Initial experience at Memorial Sloan-Kettering Cancer Center. *J Am Coll Surg* 186:423, 1998.

157. Souba WW, Bland KI: Indications and techniques for biopsy, in Bland KI, Copeland EM III (eds): *The Breast: Comprehensive Management of Benign and Malignant Diseases.* Philadelphia: WB Saunders, 1998, p 802.

158. Veronesi U, et al: Sentinel-node biopsy to avoid axillary dissection in breast cancer with clinically negative lymph-nodes. *Lancet* 349:1864, 1997.

159. Wilke LG, Giuliano A: Sentinel lymph node biopsy in patients with early-stage breast cancer: Status of the National Clinical Trials. *Surg Clin North Am* 83:901, 2003.

160. Krag DN, et al: Technical outcomes of sentinel-lymph-node resection and conventional axillary-lymph-node dissection in patients with clinically node-negative breast cancer: Results from the NSABP B-32 randomised phase III trial. *Lancet Oncol* 8:881, 2007.

161. Yi M, et al: How many sentinel lymph nodes are enough during sentinel lymph node dissection for breast cancer? *Cancer* 113:30, 2008.

162. Wilke LG, et al: Surgical complications associated with sentinel lymph node biopsy: Results from a prospective international cooperative group trial. *Ann Surg Oncol* 13:491, 2006.

163. Lucci A, et al: Surgical complications associated with sentinel lymph node dissection (SLND) plus axillary lymph node dissection compared with SLND alone in the American College of Surgeons Oncology Group Trial Z0011. *J Clin Oncol* 25:3657, 2007.

164. Julian TB, et al: Novel intraoperative molecular test for sentinel lymph node metastases in patients with early-stage breast cancer. *J Clin Oncol* 26:3338, 2008.

165. Van Zee KJ, et al: A nomogram for predicting the likelihood of additional nodal metastases in breast cancer patients with a positive sentinel node biopsy. *Ann Surg Oncol* 10:1140, 2003.

166. Fisher B: Lumpectomy (segmental mastectomy and axillary dissection), in Bland KI, Copeland EM III (eds): *The Breast: Comprehensive Management of Benign and Malignant Diseases*. Philadelphia: WB Saunders, 1998, p 917.

167. Newman LA, Washington TA: New trends in breast conservation therapy. *Surg Clin North Am* 83:841, 2003.

168. NIH consensus conference. Treatment of early-stage breast cancer. *JAMA* 265:391, 1991.

169. Clarke M, et al: Effects of radiotherapy and of differences in the extent of surgery for early breast cancer on local recurrence and 15-year survival: An overview of the randomised trials. *Lancet* 366:2087, 2005.

170. Bland KI, Chang HR, et al: Modified radical mastectomy and total (simple) mastectomy, in Bland KI, Copeland EM III (eds): *The Breast: Comprehensive Management of Benign and Malignant Diseases*. Philadelphia: WB Saunders, 1998, p 881.

171. Simmons RM, Adamovich TL: Skin-sparing mastectomy. *Surg Clin North Am* 83:885, 2003.

172. McCraw JB, Papp C, et al: Breast reconstruction following mastectomy, in Bland KI, Copeland EM III (eds): *The Breast: Comprehensive Management of Benign and Malignant Diseases*. Philadelphia: WB Saunders, 1998, p 962.

173. Fortin A, et al: Impact of locoregional radiotherapy in node-positive patients treated by breast-conservative treatment. *Int J Radiat Oncol Biol Phys* 56:1013, 2003.

174. Hellman S: Stopping metastases at their source. *N Engl J Med* 337:996, 1997.

175. Overgaard M, et al: Postoperative radiotherapy in high risk premenopausal women with breast cancer who receive adjuvant chemotherapy. *N Engl J Med* 337:949, 1997.

176. Overgaard M, et al: Postoperative radiotherapy in high-risk postmenopausal breast-cancer patients given adjuvant tamoxifen: Danish Breast Cancer Cooperative Group DBCG 82c randomised trial. *Lancet* 353:1641, 1999.

177. Ragaz J, et al: Adjuvant radiotherapy and chemotherapy in node-positive premenopausal women with breast cancer. *N Engl J Med* 337:956, 1997.

178. Recht A, Edge SB: Evidence-based indications for postmastectomy irradiation. *Surg Clin North Am* 83:995, 2003.

179. Recht A, et al: Postmastectomy radiotherapy: Clinical practice guidelines of the American Society of Clinical Oncology. *J Clin Oncol* 19:1539, 2001.

180. Tamoxifen for early breast cancer: An overview of the randomised trials. Early Breast Cancer Trialists' Collaborative Group. *Lancet* 351:1451, 1998.

181. Polychemotherapy for early breast cancer: An overview of the randomised trials. Early Breast Cancer Trialists' Collaborative Group. *Lancet* 352:930, 1998.

182. Fisher B, et al: Two months of doxorubicin-cyclophosphamide with and without interval reinduction therapy compared with 6 months of cyclophosphamide, methotrexate, and fluorouracil in positive-node breast cancer patients with tamoxifen-nonresponsive tumors: Results from the National Surgical Adjuvant Breast and Bowel Project B-15. *J Clin Oncol* 8:1483, 1990.

183. Kelleher M, Miles D: 21. The adjuvant treatment of breast cancer. *Int J Clin Pract* 57:195, 2003.

184. Loprinzi CL, Thome SD: Understanding the utility of adjuvant systemic therapy for primary breast cancer. *J Clin Oncol* 19:972, 2001.

185. Wood WC, et al: Dose and dose intensity of adjuvant chemotherapy for stage II, node-positive breast carcinoma. *N Engl J Med* 330:1253, 1994.

186. Fisher B, et al.: Two months of doxorubicin-cyclophosphamide with and without interval reinduction therapy compared with 6 months of cyclophosphamide, methotrexate, and fluorouracil in positive-node breast cancer patients with tamoxifen-nonresponsive tumors: Results from the National Surgical Adjuvant Breast and Bowel Project B-15. *J Clin Oncol* 8:1483, 1990.

187. Bonadonna G, et al: New adjuvant trials for resectable breast cancer at the Istituto Nazionale Tumori of Milan. *Recent Results Cancer Res* 91:210, 1984.

188. Fisher B, et al: Effect of preoperative chemotherapy on the outcome of women with operable breast cancer. *J Clin Oncol* 16:2672, 1998.

189. Buchholz TA, et al: Neoadjuvant chemotherapy for breast carcinoma: Multidisciplinary considerations of benefits and risks. *Cancer* 98:1150, 2003.

190. Kuerer HM, et al: Clinical course of breast cancer patients with complete pathologic primary tumor and axillary lymph node response to doxorubicin-based neoadjuvant chemotherapy. *J Clin Oncol* 17:460, 1999.

191. Mamounas EP, et al: Sentinel node biopsy after neoadjuvant chemotherapy in breast cancer: Results from National Surgical Adjuvant Breast and Bowel Project Protocol B-27. *J Clin Oncol* 23:2694, 2005.

192. Xing Y, et al: Meta-analysis of sentinel lymph node biopsy after preoperative chemotherapy in patients with breast cancer. *Br J Surg* 93:539, 2006.

193. Guarneri V, et al: Prognostic value of pathologic complete response after primary chemotherapy in relation to hormone receptor status and other factors. *J Clin Oncol* 24:1037, 2006.

194. Fisher B, et al: Treatment of lymph-node-negative, oestrogen-receptor-positive breast cancer: Long-term findings from National Surgical Adjuvant Breast and Bowel Project randomised clinical trials. *Lancet* 364:858, 2004.

195. Conte PF, et al: Delay in progression of bone metastases in breast cancer patients treated with intravenous pamidronate: Results from a multinational randomized controlled trial. The Aredia Multinational Cooperative Group. *J Clin Oncol* 14:2552, 1996.

196. Baum M, Buzdar A: The current status of aromatase inhibitors in the management of breast cancer. *Surg Clin North Am* 83:973, 2003.

197. Bonneterre J, et al: Anastrozole versus tamoxifen as first-line therapy for advanced breast cancer in 668 postmenopausal women: Results of the Tamoxifen or Arimidex Randomized Group Efficacy and Tolerability study. *J Clin Oncol* 18:3748, 2000.

198. Buzdar A, et al: Phase III, multicenter, double-blind, randomized study of letrozole, an aromatase inhibitor, for advanced breast cancer versus megestrol acetate. *J Clin Oncol* 19:3357, 2001.

199. Buzdar AU, et al: Anastrozole versus megestrol acetate in the treatment of postmenopausal women with advanced breast carcinoma: Results of a survival update based on a combined analysis of data from two mature phase III trials. Arimidex Study Group. *Cancer* 83:1142, 1998.

200. Campos SM, Winer EP: Hormonal therapy in postmenopausal women with breast cancer. *Oncology* 64:289, 2003.

201. Effects of chemotherapy and hormonal therapy for early breast cancer on recurrence and 15-year survival: An overview of the randomised trials. *Lancet* 365:1687, 2005.

202. Paik S, et al: Real-world performance of HER2 testing—National Surgical Adjuvant Breast and Bowel Project experience. *J Natl Cancer Inst* 94:852, 2002.

203. Press MF, et al: Evaluation of HER-2/neu gene amplification and overexpression: Comparison of frequently used assay methods in a molecularly characterized cohort of breast cancer specimens. *J Clin Oncol* 20:3095, 2002.

204. Volpi A, et al: Prognostic significance of biologic markers in node-negative breast cancer patients: A prospective study. *Breast Cancer Res Treat* 63:181, 2000.

205. Buzdar AU, et al: Significantly higher pathologic complete remission rate after neoadjuvant therapy with trastuzumab, paclitaxel, and epirubicin chemotherapy: Results of a randomized trial in human epidermal growth factor receptor 2–positive operable breast cancer. *J Clin Oncol* 23:3676, 2005.

206. Buzdar AU, et al: Neoadjuvant therapy with paclitaxel followed by 5-fluorouracil, epirubicin, and cyclophosphamide chemotherapy and concurrent trastuzumab in human epidermal growth factor receptor 2–positive operable breast cancer: An update of the initial randomized study population and data of additional patients treated with the same regimen. *Clin Cancer Res* 13:228, 2007.

207. Tench DW, Page DL: The unknown primary presenting with axillary lymphadenopathy, in Bland KI, Copeland EM III (eds): *The Breast: Comprehensive Management of Benign and Malignant Diseases*. Philadelphia: WB Saunders, 1998, p 1447.

208. Robinson DS, Sundaram M, et al: Carcinoma of the breast in pregnancy and lactation, in Bland KI, Copeland EM III (eds): *The Breast: Comprehensive Management of Benign and Malignant Diseases*. Philadelphia: WB Saunders, 1998, p 1433.

209. Giordano SH, Buzdar AU, Hortobagyi GN: Breast cancer in men. *Ann Intern Med* 137:678, 2002.

210. Wilhelm MC, Langenburg SE, et al: Cancer of the male breast, in Bland KI, Copeland EM III (eds): *The Breast: Comprehensive Management of Benign and Malignant Diseases*. Philadelphia: WB Saunders, 1998, p 1416.

211. Khan SA, Badve S: Phyllodes tumors of the breast. *Curr Treat Options Oncol* 2:139, 2001.

212. Chittoor SR, Swain SM: Locally advanced breast cancer: Role of medical oncology, in Bland KI, Copeland EM III (eds): *The Breast: Comprehensive Management of Benign and Malignant Diseases*. Philadelphia: WB Saunders, 1998, p 1403.

213. Mies C: Mammary sarcoma and lymphoma, in Bland KI, Copeland EM III (eds): *The Breast: Comprehensive Management of Benign and Malignant Diseases*. Philadelphia: WB Saunders, 1998, p 307.

214. Stewart FW, Treves N: Lymphangiosarcoma in postmastectomy lymphedema: A report of six cases in elephantiasis chirurgica. *Cancer* 1:64, 1948.

CHAPTER 18

Disorders of the Head and Neck

Richard O. Wein, Rakesh K. Chandra,
and Randal S. Weber

A COMPLEX REGION

The head and neck constitute a complex anatomic region where different pathologies may affect an individual's ability to see, smell, hear, speak, obtain nutrition and hydration, or breathe. The use of a multidisciplinary approach to many of the disorders in this region is essential in an attempt to achieve the best functional results with care. This chapter reviews many of the common diagnoses encountered in the field of otolaryngology-head and neck surgery and aims to provide an overview that clinicians can use as a foundation for understanding of this region. As is the case with every field of surgery, care for patients with disorders of the head and neck is constantly changing as issues of quality of life and the economics of medicine continue to evolve.

BENIGN CONDITIONS OF THE HEAD AND NECK

Ear Infections

Infections may involve the external, middle, and/or internal ear. In each of these scenarios, the infection may follow an acute or chronic course and may be associated with both otologic and intracranial complications. Otitis externa typically refers to infection of the skin of the external auditory canal (EAC).[1] Acute otitis externa is commonly known as *swimmer's ear*, because moisture that persists within the canal after swimming often initiates the process and leads to skin maceration and itching. Typically, the patient subsequently traumatizes the canal skin by scratching (i.e., with a cotton swab or fingernail), thus eroding the normally protective skin/cerumen barrier. Because the environment within the external ear canal is already dark, warm, and humid, it then becomes susceptible to rapid microbial proliferation and tissue cellulitis. The most common organism responsible is *Pseudomonas aeruginosa*, although other bacteria and fungi may also be implicated. Table 18-1 summarizes the microbiology of common otolaryngologic conditions. Symptoms and signs of otitis externa include itching during the initial phases and pain with swelling of the canal soft tissues as the infection progresses. Infected,

desquamated debris accumulates within the canal. In the chronic inflammatory stage of the infection, the pain subsides, but profound itching occurs for prolonged periods with gradual thickening of the external canal skin. Standard treatment requires removal of debris under otomicroscopy and application of appropriate topical antimicrobials such as neomycin/polymyxin or quinolone-containing eardrops, which often include topical steroid such as hydrocortisone or dexamethasone to nonspecifically decrease pain and swelling. Recent studies have demonstrated superiority of quinolone-containing preparations in achieving faster clinical resolution.[1] Nonantibiotic antimicrobial preparations, such as 2% acetic acid, may also have a role, particularly for mixed bacterial/fungal infections. The patient should also be instructed to keep the ear dry. Systemic antibiotics are reserved for those with severe infections, diabetics, and immunosuppressed patients.

Diabetic, elderly, and immunodeficient patients are susceptible to a condition called *malignant otitis externa*, a fulminant necrotizing infection of the otologic soft tissues combined with osteomyelitis of the temporal bone. In addition to the above findings, cranial neuropathies may be observed. The classic physical finding is granulation tissue along the floor of the EAC. Symptoms include persistent otalgia for longer than 1 month and purulent otorrhea for several weeks. These patients require aggressive medical therapy, including IV antibiotics covering *Pseudomonas*.[2] Other gram-negative bacteria and fungi are occasionally implicated, necessitating culture-directed therapy in those cases. Patients who do not respond to medical management require surgical débridement. This condition may progress to involvement of the adjacent skull base and soft tissues, meningitis, brain abscess, and death.

In its acute phase, otitis media typically implies a bacterial infection of the middle ear. This diagnosis accounts for 25% of pediatric antibiotic prescriptions and is the most common bacterial infection of childhood. Most cases occur before 2 years of age and are secondary to immaturity of the eustachian tube. Contributing factors include upper respiratory viral infection and day-care attendance, as well as craniofacial conditions affecting eustachian tube function, such as cleft palate. It is also possible that social factors such as day-care attendance and the overprescription of antibiotics has led to antibiotic resistance.

Classification of the infection as acute is based upon the duration of the process being less than 3 weeks. In this phase, otalgia and fever are the most common symptoms and physical exam reveals a bulging, opaque tympanic membrane (Fig. 18-1). The most common organ-

TABLE 18-1	Microbiology of common otolaryngologic infections
Condition	**Microbiology**
Otitis externa and malignant otitis externa	*Pseudomonas aeruginosa*, fungi (*Aspergillus* most common)
Acute otitis media	*Streptococcus pneumoniae, Haemophilus influenzae, Moraxella catarrhalis*
Chronic otitis media	Above bacteria, staphylococci, other streptococci; may be polymicrobial; exact role of bacteria unclear
Acute sinusitis	Viral upper respiratory infection, *S. pneumoniae, H. influenzae, M. catarrhalis*
Chronic sinusitis	Above bacteria, staphylococci, other streptococci; may be polymicrobial; exact role of bacteria unclear; may represent immune response to fungi
Pharyngitis	Viral, streptococci (usually pyogenes)

KEY POINTS

1. Disorders of the head and neck can cause significant cosmetic and functional impairment. The practitioner must be empathetic to the effect of these morbidities on quality of life.

2. Infectious conditions of the head and neck may present with life-threatening sequelae such as loss of airway or intracranial extension.

3. Patients with obstructive sleep apnea require evaluation to determine the specific anatomic site(s) of involvement. Long-term cardiovascular problems are a significant concern in these patients.

4. Repair of traumatic soft-tissue injuries requires precise realignment of anatomic landmarks such as the gray line and vermilion border.

5. The key principle in the surgical repair of facial fractures is immobilization, which may require plates, screws, wires, and/or intermaxillary fixation.

6. Concurrent abuse of tobacco and alcohol are synergistic in increasing the risk of developing head and neck cancer.

7. Hoarseness, a nonhealing oral ulcer, or cervical lymphadenopathy of greater than 2 weeks duration requires evaluation.

8. Monomodality therapy (surgery or radiation) is used for early stage (I/II) head and neck cancer, whereas combination surgery and chemoradiation is used with advanced stage (III/IV) malignancies.

9. The most significant recent advance in the treatment of head and neck cancer is the use of epidermal growth factor receptor inhibitor-based chemotherapy.

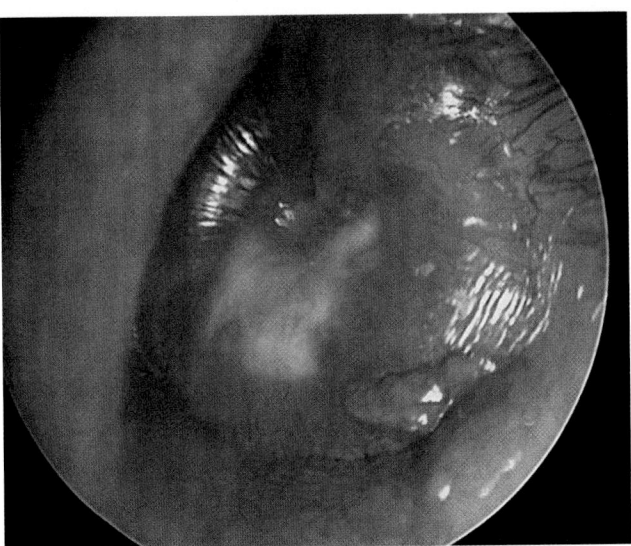

FIG. 18-1. Acute otitis media.

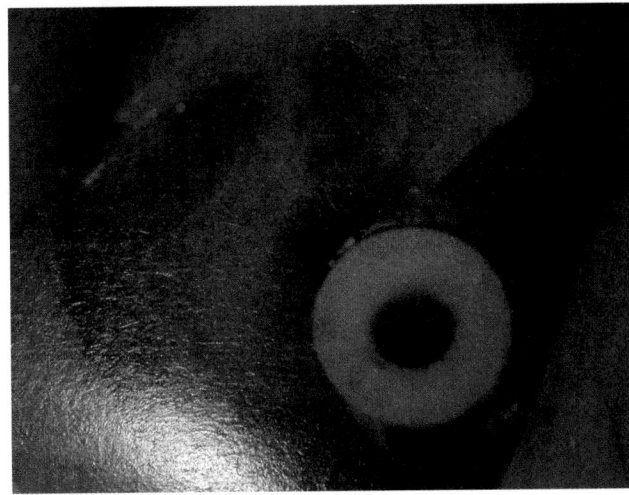

FIG. 18-2. Myringotomy and tube.

isms responsible are *Streptococcus pneumoniae, Haemophilus influenzae,* and *Moraxella catarrhalis.* If the process lasts 3 to 8 weeks, it is deemed subacute. Chronic otitis media, lasting more than 8 weeks, usually results from an unresolved acute otitis media. Twenty percent of patients demonstrate a persistent middle ear effusion 8 weeks after resolution of the acute phase. Rather than a purely infectious process, however, it represents chronic inflammation and hypersecretion by the middle ear mucosa associated with eustachian tube dysfunction, viruses, allergy, ciliary dysfunction, and other factors. The bacteriology is variable, but often includes those found in acute otitis media and may be polymicrobial. The exact role of bacteria in the pathophysiology is controversial. The patient experiences otalgia, ear fullness, and conductive hearing loss. Physical examination reveals a retracted tympanic membrane that may exhibit an opaque character or an air-fluid level. Bubbles may be seen behind the retracted membrane.

Treatment for uncomplicated otitis media is oral antibiotic therapy. However, penicillin resistance of the commonly implicated organisms is rising such that almost 100% of *Moraxella,* 50 to 70% of *Haemophilus,* and up to 40% of pneumococcal strains are resistant.[3] Beta-lactamase-resistant combinations, cephalosporins, and macrolides are often required, although amoxicillin and sulfas are still considered first-line drugs. Chronic otitis media is frequently treated with myringotomy and tube placement (Fig. 18-2). This is indicated for frequent acute episodes, chronic effusions persisting beyond 3 months, and those associated with significant conductive hearing loss. The purpose of this procedure is to remove the effusion and provide a route for middle ear ventilation. Tympanic membrane perforation during acute otitis media frequently results in resolution of severe pain and provides for drainage of purulent fluid and middle ear ventilation. These perforations will heal spontaneously after the infection has resolved in the majority of cases. Chronic otitis media, however, may be associated with nonhealing tympanic membrane perforations. Patients may have persistent otorrhea, which is treated with topical drops. Preparations containing aminoglycoside are avoided, because this class of drugs is toxic to the inner ear. Solutions containing alcohol or acetic acid may be irritative or caustic to the middle ear, and are also avoided in the setting of a perforation.

Nonhealing perforation requires surgical closure (tympanoplasty) after medical treatment of any residual acute infection. Chronic inflammation may also be associated with erosion of the ossicular chain, which can be reconstructed with various prostheses or autologous ossicular replacement techniques. Cholesteatoma is an epidermoid cyst of the middle ear and/or mastoid, which causes bone destruction secondary to its expansile nature and through enzymatic destruction. Cholesteatoma develops as a consequence of eustachian tube dysfunction and chronic otitis media secondary to retraction of squamous elements of the tympanic membrane into the middle ear space. Squamous epithelium may also migrate into the middle ear via a perforation. Chronic mastoiditis that fails medical management or is associated with cholesteatoma is treated by mastoidectomy.

Complications of otitis media may be grouped into two categories: intratemporal (otologic) and intracranial.[4] Fortunately, complications are rare in the antibiotic era, but mounting antibiotic resistance necessitates an increased awareness of these conditions. Intratemporal complications include acute coalescent mastoiditis, petrositis, facial nerve paralysis, and labyrinthitis. In acute coalescing mastoiditis, destruction of the bony lamellae by an acute purulent process results in severe pain, fever, and swelling behind the ear. The mastoid air cells coalesce into one common space filled with pus. Mastoid infection may also spread to the petrous apex, causing retro-orbital pain and sixth-nerve palsy. These diagnoses are confirmed by computed tomographic (CT) scan.

Facial nerve paralysis may also occur secondary to an acute inflammatory process in the middle ear or mastoid.[5] Intratemporal complications are managed by myringotomy tube placement in addition to appropriate IV antibiotics. In acute coalescent mastoiditis, and petrositis, mastoidectomy is also performed as necessary to drain purulent foci. Labyrinthitis refers to inflammation of the inner ear. Most cases are idiopathic or are secondary to viral infections of the endolymphatic space. The patient experiences vertigo with sensorineural hearing loss, and symptoms may smolder over several weeks. Labyrinthitis associated with middle ear infection may be serous or suppurative. In the former case, bacterial products and/or inflammatory mediators transudate into the inner ear via the round window membrane, establishing an inflammatory process therein. Total recovery is eventually possible after the middle ear is adequately treated. Suppurative labyrinthitis, however, is a much more toxic condition in which the acute purulent bacterial infection extends into the inner ear and causes marked destruction of the sensory hair cells and neurons of the eighth-nerve ganglion. This condition may hallmark impending meningitis and must be treated rapidly. The goal of management of inner ear infection, which occurs secondary to middle ear infection, is to "sterilize" the middle ear space with antibiotics and the placement of a myringotomy tube.

Meningitis is the most common intracranial complication. Otologic meningitis in children is most commonly associated with a *H. influenzae* type B infection. Other intracranial complications include epidural abscess, subdural abscess, brain abscess, otitic hydrocephalus (pseudotumor), and sigmoid sinus thrombophlebitis. In these cases, the otogenic source must be urgently treated with antibiotics and myringotomy tube placement. Mastoidectomy and neurosurgical consultation may be necessary.

Bell's palsy, or idiopathic facial paralysis, may be considered within the spectrum of otologic disease given the facial nerve's course through the temporal bone. This entity is the most common etiology of facial nerve paralysis and is clinically distinct from that occurring as a complication of otitis media in that the otologic exam is normal. Historically, Bell's palsy was synonymous with "idiopathic" facial paralysis. It is now accepted, however, that the majority of these cases represent a viral neuropathy caused by herpes simplex. Treatment includes oral steroids plus antiviral therapy (i.e., acyclovir). Complete recovery is the norm, but does not occur universally, and selected cases may benefit from surgical decompression of the nerve within its bony canal. Electrophysiologic testing has been used to identify those patients in whom surgery might be indicated.[6] The procedure involves decompression of the nerve via exposure in the middle cranial fossa. Varicella zoster virus may also cause facial nerve paralysis when the virus reactivates from dormancy in the nerve. This condition, known as *Ramsay Hunt syndrome*, is characterized by severe otalgia followed by the eruption of vesicles of the external ear. Treatment is similar to Bell's palsy, but full recovery is only seen in approximately two thirds of cases.

Traumatic facial nerve injuries may occur secondary to accidental trauma or surgical injury. The former is detailed in Sinus Inflammatory Disease below. Iatrogenic facial nerve trauma most often occurs during mastoidectomy.[7] When the facial nerve is injured intraoperatively, it is explored. Injury to greater than 50% of the neural diameter of the facial nerve is addressed either with primary reanastomosis or reconstructed with the use a nerve graft. Complete recovery of nerve function is uncommon in these cases.

Sinus Inflammatory Disease

Sinusitis is a clinical diagnosis based on patient signs and symptoms.[8] The Task Force on Rhinosinusitis (sponsored by the American Academy of Otolaryngology–Head and Neck Surgery) has established criteria to define "a history consistent with sinusitis" (Table 18-2). To qualify for the diagnosis, the patient must exhibit at least two major factors or one major and two minor factors. The classification of sinusitis as acute vs. subacute or chronic is primarily based on the time course over which those criteria have been met. If signs and symptoms are present for at least 7 to 10 days, but for less than 4 weeks, the process is designated acute sinusitis. Subacute sinusitis is present for 4 to 12 weeks and chronic sinusitis is diagnosed when the patient has had signs and symptoms for at least 12 weeks. In addition, the diagnosis of chronic sinusitis requires some objective demonstration of mucosal inflammatory disease. This may be accomplished by endoscopic examination or radiologically (i.e., CT scan).

TABLE 18-2	Factors associated with a history of rhinosinusitis[a]

Major Factors	Minor Factors
Facial congestion/fullness	Headache
Facial pain/pressure	Maxillary dental pain
Nasal drainage/discharge	Cough
Postnasal drip	Halitosis (bad breath)
Nasal obstruction/blockage	Fatigue
Hyposmia/anosmia (decreased or absent sense of smell)	Ear pain, pressure, or fullness
Fever (acute sinusitis only)	Fever
Purulence on nasal endoscopy (diagnostic by itself)	

[a]Either two major factors or one major and two minor factors are required. Purulence on nasal endoscopy is diagnostic. Fever is a major factor only in the acute stage.

Acute sinusitis typically follows a viral upper respiratory infection whereby sinonasal mucosal inflammation results in closure of the sinus ostium. This results in stasis of secretions, tissue hypoxia, and ciliary dysfunction. These conditions promote bacterial proliferation and acute inflammation. The mainstay of treatment is the use of antibiotics that are empirically directed toward the three most common organisms *S. pneumoniae*, *H. influenzae*, and *M. catarrhalis*. As with otitis media, antibiotic resistance is a mounting concern. Nosocomial acute sinusitis frequently involves *Pseudomonas* or *S. aureus*, both of which may also exhibit significant antibiotic resistance. Other treatments include topical and systemic decongestants, nasal saline spray, topical nasal steroids, and oral steroids in selected cases. In the acute setting, surgery is reserved for complications or pending complications, which may include extension to the eye (orbital cellulitis or abscess) or the intracranial space (meningitis, intracranial abscess). It should also be noted that, strictly speaking, a viral upper respiratory infection (common cold) is a form of acute sinusitis. The working definition outlined above, however, attempts to exclude these cases by requiring that symptoms be present for at least 7 to 10 days, by which time the common cold should be in a resolution phase. Use of this working definition strives to avoid unnecessary antibiotic prescriptions and further promotion of resistance.

Chronic sinusitis represents a heterogeneous group of patients with multifactorial etiologies contributing to ostial obstruction, ciliary dysfunction, and inflammation. Components of genetic predisposition, allergy, anatomic obstruction, bacteria, fungi, and environmental factors play varying roles, depending on the individual patient. As of yet, no immunologic "final common pathway" has been defined, but the clinical picture is well described. Diagnosis is suspected according to the criteria in Table 18-2, with clinical signs and symptoms persisting for at least 12 weeks. Chronic sinusitis may also be associated with the presence of nasal polyps. Chronic sinusitis with and without polyposis is thought to reflect an immunologically distinct disease process.[8] Mucosal inflammation in nonpolypoid chronic sinusitis is predominantly mediated by neutrophils, consistent with immune response to bacterial infection. In contrast, inflammatory infiltrates observed in polypoid chronic sinusitis are typically eosinophilic. Multiple theories have been proposed for the latter condition, and recent investigation has suggested that patients with polyposis may mount abnormal immunologic reactions toward fungi that colonize the sinonasal tract or to staphylococcal enterotoxin.[8] Regardless of pathophysiology, polyps themselves may further block sinus outflow, resulting in further stasis of secretions and bacterial proliferation.

Nasal endoscopy is a critical element of the diagnosis of chronic sinusitis. Anatomic abnormalities, such as septal deviation, nasal polyps, and purulence may be observed (Figs. 18-3 and 18-4). The finding of purulence or polypoid change by nasal endoscopy is supportive of the diagnosis of chronic sinusitis, if symptoms persist for at least 12 weeks. In this setting, purulence may represent an acute exacerbation of chronic sinusitis. Pus found on endoscopic exam may be cultured, and subsequent antibiotic therapy can be directed accordingly. The spectrum of bacteria found in chronic sinusitis is highly variable and includes higher prevalences of polymicrobial infections and antibiotic-resistant organisms. Overall, *S. aureus*, coagulase-negative staphylococci, gram-negative bacilli, and streptococci are isolated, in addition to the typical pathogens of acute sinusitis. The increased prevalence of community acquired methicillin resistant *S. aureus* is a mounting concern.[9]

The diagnosis of chronic sinusitis can be confirmed by CT scan, which demonstrates mucosal thickening and/or sinus opacification. It should be underscored, however, that CT scan is probably not the diagnostic gold standard because many asymptomatic patients will demonstrate findings on sinus CT scan. Also, patients with positive findings on nasal endoscopy may have normal CT scans. Overall, the decision to treat medically should be based upon patient history and nasal endoscopy, rather than results of the CT scan. Furthermore, over 75% of patients with normal findings on nasal endoscopy will

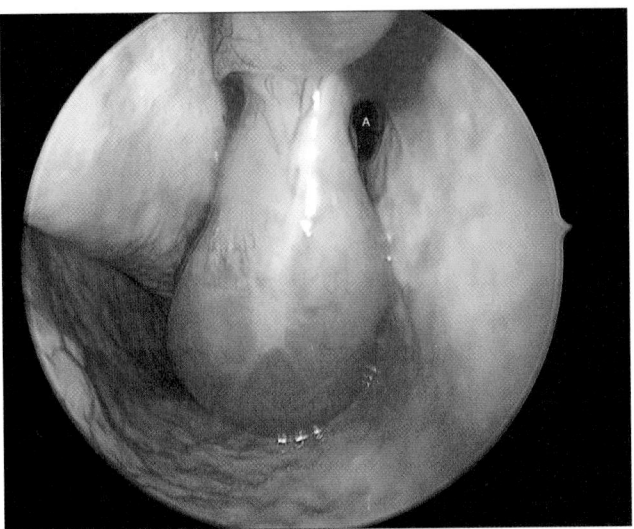

FIG. 18-3. Endoscopic view of nasal polyp obstructing the posterior nasal airway. A small residual air passage (A) is seen between the polyp and the nasal septum.

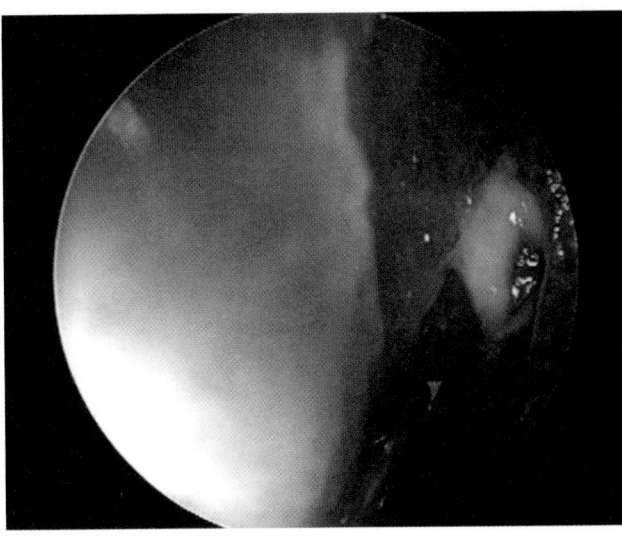

FIG. 18-4. Endoscopic view of pus in the middle meatus admixed with polypoid change. This can be swabbed for culture, as shown, in the outpatient setting under endoscopic guidance.

have normal CT scans, underscoring the importance of endoscopy in the decision-to-treat process. Although acute sinusitis often is treated empirically by the primary care practitioner, when clinical criteria for chronic sinusitis are met, this typically prompts otolaryngology referral for nasal endoscopy, aggressive medical therapy, and possibly surgery. When surgery is used, the CT scan, if acquired with the appropriate protocol, can also be used for stereotactic intraoperative navigation to confirm relationships between the disease process, medial orbital wall, and skull base during surgery (Fig. 18-5).

Medical management of chronic sinusitis includes a prolonged course of oral antibiotics for 3 to 6 weeks, nasal and/or oral steroids, and nasal irrigations with saline or antibiotic solutions.[8] Underlying allergic disease may be managed with antihistamines and possible allergy immunotherapy. Although the role of these treatments in resolving chronic sinusitis remains questionable, they may be considered in patients with comorbid allergic rhinitis or as part of empiric management before consideration of surgery. The use of oral steroids may also be selected empirically, particularly in patients with comor-

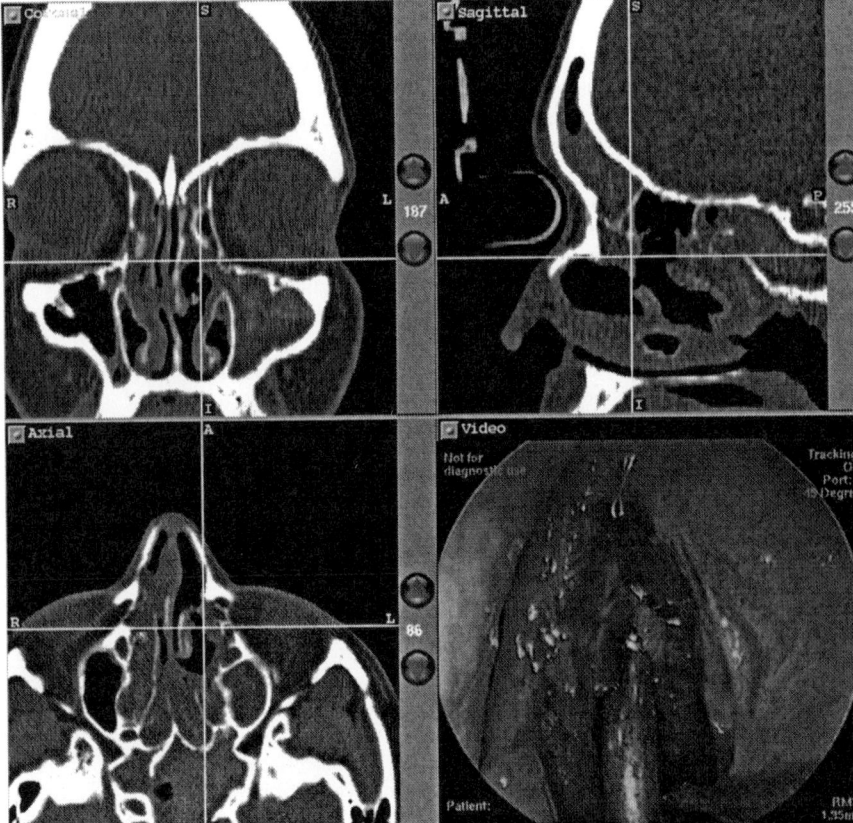

FIG. 18-5. Triplanar computed tomographic reconstructions as used for intraoperative stereotactic navigation. The coronal (upper left), axial (lower left), and sagittal (upper right) planes are seen, with the cross hairs localizing the anatomic position indicated in the endoscopic view (lower left). This particular patient has classic allergic fungal sinusitis, which has the radiologic hallmark of whitish hyperdense foci with areas of gray sinus opacification, as is seen in the maxillary sinus on the coronal image and in the sphenoid on the sagittal view.

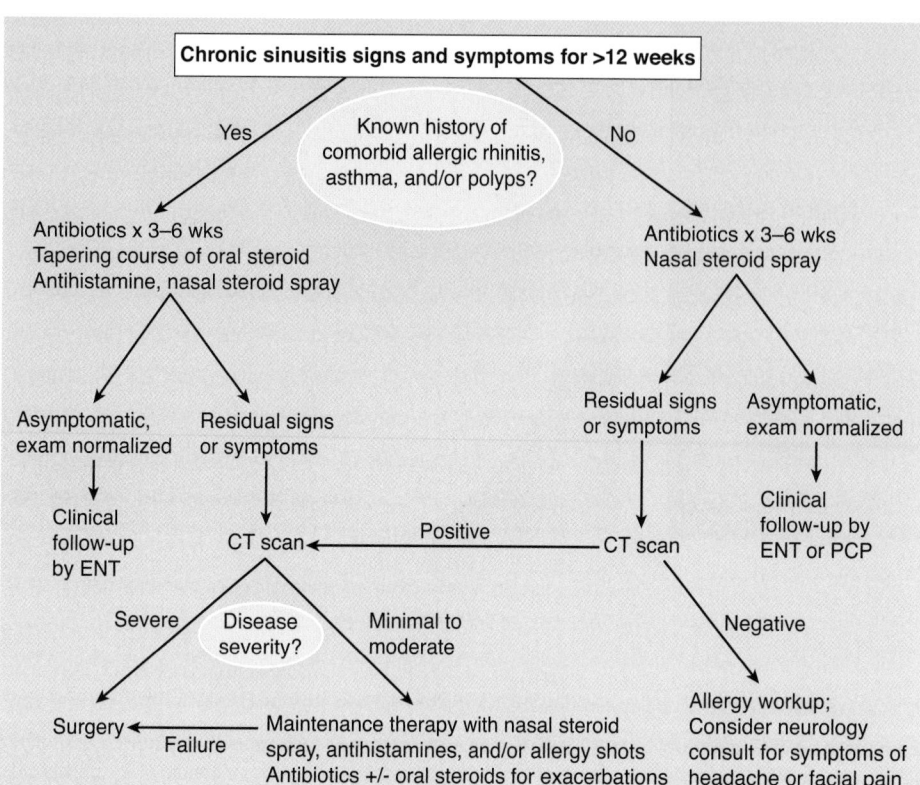

FIG. 18-6. Algorithm of chronic sinusitis signs and symptoms for 12 weeks. CT = computed tomography; ENT = ear, nose, and throat; PCP = primary care physician.

bid chronic airway inflammatory diseases such as nasal polyps, allergic rhinitis, or asthma.[10] The decision to use oral steroids must be individualized with consideration of the risks and side effects of these medications. As yet, there is no consensus regarding what constitutes a "maximum" course of medical therapy that should be attempted before consideration of surgery for chronic sinusitis. A proposed therapeutic algorithm is outlined (Fig. 18-6). It should be noted that unless there is suspicion of neoplasm or pending complication of sinusitis, the decision to proceed with surgery is highly individualized. This is because surgery for uncomplicated chronic sinusitis is elective, and patients who "fail" medical management will exhibit significant variability in symptoms, physical signs, and CT findings. More aggressive medical and surgical management may be necessary in patients with comorbid chronic inflammatory disease of the airways such as allergic rhinitis, nasal polyposis, and asthma. Surgery is typically preformed endoscopically where the goals are to remove polyps, enlarge the natural sinus ostia (see Fig. 18-5, Fig. 18-7), and to remove chronically infected bone to promote both ventilation and drainage of the sinus cavities. Inspissated mucin or pus is drained and cultured. Eventual resolution of the chronic inflammatory process can be attained with a combination of meticulous surgery and directed medical therapy, although the patient must understand that surgery may not alter the underlying immunologic pathophysiology.

The role of fungi in sinusitis is an area of active investigation. Fungal sinusitis may take on both noninvasive and invasive forms. The noninvasive form includes the presence of a fungal ball and allergic fungal sinusitis, both of which occur in immunocompetent patients.

A fungal ball is typically seen in individuals with chronic (or recurrent acute) symptoms that are often subtle and limited to a single sinus. Patients may complain about the perception of a foul odor and occasionally report expelling fungal debris upon nose blowing. A fungal ball (Fig. 18-8) consisting of *Aspergillus fumigatus* usually is found in the maxillary sinus, with scant inflammatory cell infiltration. Surgery to remove the fungal ball and re-establish sinus ventilation is almost always curative. This can be accomplished endoscopically.

Classic allergic fungal sinusitis is thought to involve direct stimulation of eosinophils by a subset of helper T cells (T_H2) primed by fungal antigens. This results in vigorous inflammation and polyp growth, and some have proposed that other forms of chronic sinusitis may represent more subtle manifestations of this pathophysiology.[11] Patients often present with chronic sinusitis that has been especially refractory to medical management. CT scan has characteristic features, and endoscopic evaluation reveals florid polyposis and inspissated mucin containing fungal debris and products of eosinophil breakdown. The implicated organisms are usually those of the Dematiaceae family, but *Aspergillus* species are also seen. Treatment includes systemic steroids, surgery, and nasal irrigations. Oral antifungal therapy is sometimes indicated as well.

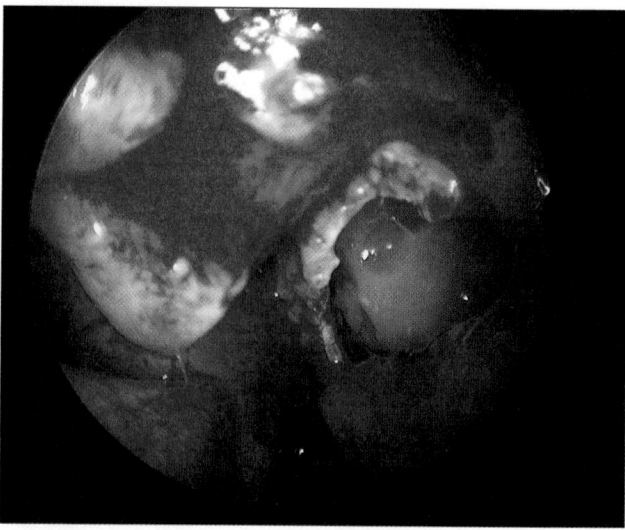

FIG. 18-7. Endoscopic surgical enlargement of the left maxillary sinus and view of pus within the sinus lumen.

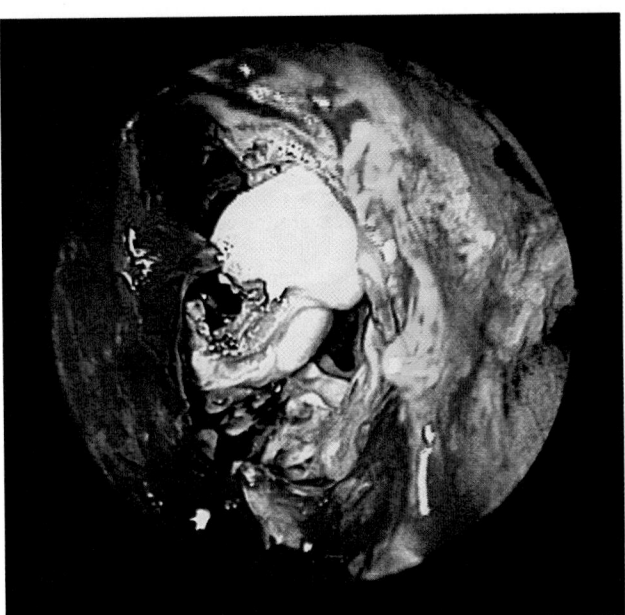

FIG. 18-8. Sinus fungal ball.

Immunocompetent patients may occasionally develop an indolent form of invasive fungal sinusitis, but more commonly, invasive fungal sinusitis affects immunocompromised patients, diabetics, or the elderly.[11] Fungal invasion of the microvasculature causes ischemic necrosis and black eschar of the sinonasal mucosa. Aspergillus and fungi of the Mucoraceae family are often implicated with the latter more common in diabetic patients. Treatment requires aggressive surgical débridement and IV antifungals, but the prognosis is dismal.

Pharyngeal and Adenotonsillar Disease

The pharyngeal mucosa contains significant concentrations of lymphoid tissue, predisposing this area to reactive inflammatory changes. Lymphoid tissue of various pharyngeal subsites forms the so-called *Waldeyer's tonsillar ring*, consisting of the palatine tonsils ("the tonsils"), lingual tonsil (lymphoid tissue accumulation within the tongue base), and adenoid. The mucosa of the posterior and lateral pharyngeal walls is also rich with lymphoid cells. Infection, immune-mediated inflammatory disease, or local stressors, such as radiation or acid reflux, may initiate lymphoid reactivity and associated symptoms. Chronic or recurrent adenotonsillitis and adenotonsillar hypertrophy are the most common disorders affecting these structures.

In the vast majority of cases, infectious pharyngitis is viral rather than bacterial in origin. Most cases resolve without complication from supportive care and possibly antibiotics. Patients with tonsillitis typically present with sore throat, dysphagia, and fever. The mucosa is inflamed. Tonsillar exudates and cervical adenitis may be seen when the etiology is bacterial. If adenoiditis is present, the symptoms may be similar to those of sinusitis, but visual evaluation of the adenoid, at least in children, requires endoscopy and/or radiographic imaging (lateral neck soft-tissue x-ray). Tonsillitis and adenoiditis may follow acute, recurrent acute, and chronic temporal patterns.

It should be noted, however, that clinical diagnosis often is inaccurate for determining whether the process is bacterially induced. When the patient also has hoarseness, rhinorrhea, cough, and no evidence of exudates or adenitis, an upper respiratory viral infection can be presumed. When a bacterial cause is suspected,[12] antibiotics should be initiated to cover the usual organisms: group A beta-hemolytic streptococci (*Streptococcus pyogenes*), *S. pneumoniae*, and group C and G streptococci. *H. influenzae* and anaerobes

also have been implicated. It is particularly important to identify group A beta-hemolytic streptococci in pediatric patients to initiate timely antibiotic therapy, given the risk of rheumatic fever, which may occur in up to 3% of cases if antibiotics are not used. Historically, if bacterial pharyngitis was suspected in a child, oropharyngeal swab with culture was performed to identify group A beta-hemolytic streptococci. Currently, rapid antigen assays are available with sensitivity and specificity of approximately 85% and 90%, respectively. Some authors advocate culture only when these are negative. Unnecessary antibiotic therapy for patients who are unlikely to have a bacterial etiology should be avoided, given the already mounting antibiotic resistance problem. When suspicion for a bacterial process is high, or with positive culture/antigen assay results, treatment may include penicillins, cephalosporins, or macrolides in penicillin-allergic patients.

Complications of *S. pyogenes* pharyngitis may be systemic, including rheumatic fever, poststreptococcal glomerulonephritis, and scarlet fever. The incidence of glomerulonephritis is not influenced by antibiotic therapy. Scarlet fever results from production of erythrogenic toxins by streptococci. This causes a punctate rash, first appearing on the trunk and then spreading distally, sparing the palms and soles. The so-called *strawberry tongue* also is seen. Locoregional complications include peritonsillar abscess and, rarely, deep-neck space abscess. Peritonsillar abscess is typically drained transorally under local anesthesia, as is the authors' practice, but some suggest that needle aspiration without incision is sufficient.[13] Deep neck space abscess, which more commonly is odontogenic in origin, usually requires operative incision and drainage via a transcervical approach.

Atypical cases of pharyngitis may be caused by *Corynebacterium diphtheriae*, *Bordetella pertussis* (whooping cough), syphilis, *Neisseria gonorrhoeae*, and fungi. Diphtheria is a potentially fatal condition associated with toxin-mediated tissue necrosis and a gray membrane on the mucosal surface. Cardiorespiratory collapse may ensue from systemic circulation of the toxin. Treatment includes the use of antitoxin. Fortunately, diphtheria is rare in developed countries as a consequence of childhood vaccinations. Childhood vaccination also has almost eliminated whooping cough in developed nations. This entity follows a protracted, but usually self-limiting course. During the secondary phase of syphilis, ulcerations with raised red margins (resembling the chancre lesion) may be observed on the pharyngotonsillar mucosa. Identification of these less typical organisms requires a high index of suspicion and application of appropriate culture techniques and/or serologic tests. *Candida albicans* is the most common fungal organism to cause pharyngitis. This organism is a normal component of the oral flora, but under conditions of immunosuppression, broad-spectrum antibacterial therapy, poor oral hygiene, or vitamin deficiency, it may become pathogenic. Whitish-cheesy or creamy mucosal patches are observed with underlying erythema, and diagnosis is easily established by Gram's stain of this material, revealing budding yeast and pseudohyphae. Oral and topical antifungals are usually effective, and immunosuppressed patients may require prophylactic therapy.

In addition to viral upper respiratory viruses, herpes simplex virus, Epstein-Barr virus (EBV), cytomegalovirus, and HIV are associated with pharyngitis. Systemic EBV infection represents clinical mononucleosis, although syphilis, cytomegalovirus, and HIV are known to cause mononucleosis-like syndromes. These conditions, particularly EBV, may exhibit an exudative pharyngotonsillitis that may be confused with a bacterial etiology. Progression of the clinical picture reveals lymphadenopathy, splenomegaly, and hepatitis. Diagnosis is established based on the detection of heterophile antibodies or atypical lymphocytes in the peripheral blood. Occasionally, pharyngeal biopsy or cervical lymph node biopsy is required to establish the diagnosis.

Noninfectious causes of pharyngitis must also be considered. These include mucositis from chemoradiation therapy, which may be associated with fungal superinfection. Pharyngitis may also be seen in immune-mediated conditions such as erythema multiforme, bullous pemphigoid, and pemphigus vulgaris. In addition, reflux is being increasingly identified as a cause of both laryngitis and pharyngitis, particularly when the symptoms are chronic. A 24-hour pH probe is the gold standard diagnostic test, and treatment is usually successful with lifestyle modification, although proton pump inhibitors are often prescribed.[14]

Obstructive adenotonsillar hyperplasia may present with nasal obstruction, rhinorrhea, voice changes, dysphagia, and sleep-disordered breathing or OSA, depending on the particular foci of lymphoid tissue involved.

Tonsillectomy and adenoidectomy are indicated for chronic or recurrent acute infection and for obstructive hypertrophy.[15] The American Academy of Otolaryngology–Head and Neck Surgery Clinical Indicators Compendium suggests tonsillectomy after three or more infections per year despite adequate medical therapy. Some feel that tonsillectomy is indicated in children who miss 2 or more weeks of school annually secondary to tonsil infections. Multiple techniques have been described, including electrocautery, sharp dissection, laser, and radiofrequency ablation. There is no consensus as to the best method. In cases of chronic or recurrent infection, surgery is considered only after failure of medical therapy. Patients with recurrent peritonsillar abscess should undergo tonsillectomy when the acute inflammatory changes have resolved. Selected cases, however, require tonsillectomy in the acute setting for the management of severe inflammation, systemic toxicity, or impending airway compromise. Adenoidectomy, in conjunction with myringotomy and tube placement, may be beneficial for children with chronic or recurrent otitis media.[16] This is because the adenoid appears to function as a bacterial reservoir that seeds the middle ear via the eustachian tube. Adenoidectomy is also the first line of surgical management for children with chronic sinusitis. In addition to acting as a bacterial reservoir, an obstructive adenoid impairs mucociliary clearance from the sinonasal tract into the pharynx.

The primary complications of tonsillectomy[17] include bleeding, airway obstruction, death, and readmission for dehydration secondary to postoperative dysphagia. Complications of adenoidectomy also include hemorrhage, as well as nasopharyngeal stenosis and velopharyngeal insufficiency. In the latter condition, nasal regurgitation of liquids and hypernasal speech are experienced. Patients with significant airway obstruction secondary to adenotonsillar hypertrophy are also at risk for postobstructive pulmonary edema syndrome, once the obstruction is relieved by adenotonsillectomy. Overall, bleeding is the most significant risk and may require a return trip to the operating room for control. With the exception of bleeding, which is observed in 3 to 5% of patients, most of these complications are rare or self limiting. It deserves special notation that adenotonsillectomy in a child with Down syndrome requires attention to the cervical spine. Patients with this syndrome may exhibit atlantoaxial instability, resulting in cervical spine injury if the neck is extended for the procedure. Baseline radiographs, with appropriate orthopedic or neurosurgical consultation, are indicated preoperatively. Surgery for adenotonsillar hypertrophy may be indicated when the patient exhibits sleep-disordered breathing.

Sleep disorders represent a continuum from simple snoring to upper airway resistance syndrome to obstructive sleep apnea (OSA).[18] Upper airway resistance syndrome and OSA are associated with snoring, excessive daytime somnolence, fatigue, and frequent sleep arousals. In OSA, polysomnogram demonstrates at least 10 episodes of apnea or hypopnea per hour of sleep. The average number of apneas and hypopneas per hour can be used to calculate a respiratory disturbance index, which, along with oxygen saturation, can be used to grade the severity of OSA. These episodes occur as a result of collapse of the pharyngeal soft tissues during sleep. In adults, it should be noted that in addition to tonsil size, factors such as tongue size and body mass index (especially >35 kg/m^2) are significant predictors of OSA. Other anatomic findings associated with OSA include obese neck, retrognathia, low hyoid bone, and enlarged soft palate. Surgery should be considered after failure of more conservative measures,

such as weight loss, elimination of alcohol use, use of oral appliances to open the airway during sleep, and continuous positive airway pressure. Selection of surgical procedure should be tailored to the particular patient's pattern of obstruction. In children, surgical management typically involves tonsillectomy and/or adenoidectomy, because the disorder is usually caused, at least in part, by hypertrophy or collapse of these structures. In any individual patient, the anatomy must be carefully evaluated to determine whether the site of airway collapse is in the retropalatal region, retrolingual area, or both. A therapeutic algorithm for adults is proposed (Fig. 18-9), based on site of obstruction and severity of disease. In adults, uvulopalatoplasty is frequently performed to alleviate soft-palate collapse and is the most common operation performed for sleep-disordered breathing. The goal of this procedure is to remove redundant tissue from the uvula and soft palate, along with obstructive tonsillar tissue. This can be accomplished with cold steel, laser, and/or cautery. Adults with significant nasal obstruction may benefit from septoplasty, reduction in size of the inferior turbinates, and possibly external nasal surgery. Patients with a significant component of retrolingual obstruction may be candidates for tongue base reduction, tongue base advancement, or hyoid suspension. Additionally, a variety of maxillomandibular advancement procedures also have been described to enlarge the anterior-posterior dimension of the retrolingual airway. Patients with moderate to severe sleep apnea frequently manifest involvement of the tongue base. However, management of this subgroup may be difficult, as procedures addressing the retrolingual airway can involve difficult recovery, significant morbidity, and limited success. These patients often continue to require continuous positive airway pressure despite performance of multilevel surgical procedures. Patients with severe OSA (respiratory disturbance index >40, lowest nocturnal oxygen saturation <70%) and unfavorable anatomy or comorbid cardiopulmonary disease may require tracheotomy,[19] which is the only surgical "cure" for OSA. Tracheotomy should be offered in patients with evidence of right heart failure (cor pulmonale), which is a potential sequela of severe OSA or undertreated cases of moderate OSA.

On the opposite end of the spectrum, many patients present with snoring but fail to exhibit OSA according to polysomnographic criteria. These "social snorers" may pursue elective procedures that stiffen the uvula and soft palate. This may be accomplished by the application of radiofrequency energy or cautery to induce submucosal scar, or by palatal implants. Elective uvulopharyngoplasty may also be a consideration in this population.

Benign Conditions of the Larynx

Disorders of voice may affect a wide array of patients with respect to age, gender, and socioeconomic status. The principal symptom of these disorders, at least when a mass lesion is present, is hoarseness. Other vocal manifestations include hypophonia or aphonia, breathiness, and pitch breaks. Benign laryngeal disorders may also be associated with airway obstruction, dysphagia, and reflux.[20] Smoking may also be a risk factor for benign disease, but this element of the history should raise the index of suspicion for malignancy.

Recurrent respiratory papillomatosis (RRP) reflects involvement of human papillomavirus (HPV) within the mucosal epithelium of the upper aerodigestive tract. The larynx is the most frequently involved site, and subtypes 6 and 11 are the most often implicated. The disorder typically presents in early childhood, secondary to viral acquisition during vaginal delivery. Many cases resolve after puberty, but the disorder may progress into adulthood. Adult-onset RRP typically occurs in the third or fourth decade of life, is usually less severe, and is more likely to involve extralaryngeal sites of the upper aerodigestive tract. With laryngeal involvement, RRP is most likely to present with hoarseness, although airway compromise may be observed. The diagnosis can be established with office endoscopy. Currently, there is no "cure" for RRP. Treatment involves operative microlaryngoscopy with excision or laser ablation, and

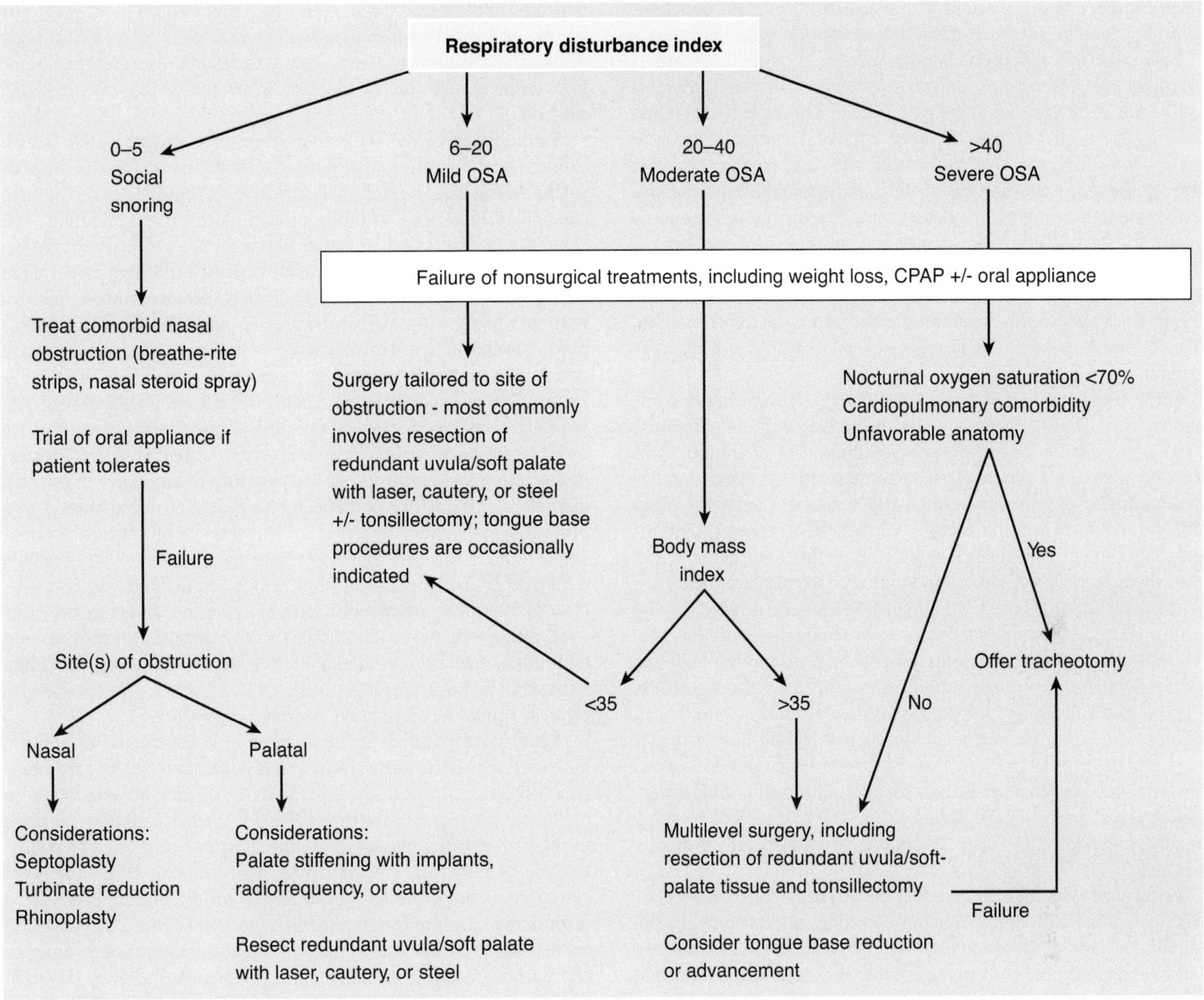

Respiratory disturbance index

0–5
Social
snoring

6–20
Mild OSA

20–40
Moderate OSA

>40
Severe OSA

Failure of nonsurgical treatments, including weight loss, CPAP +/- oral appliance

Treat comorbid nasal
obstruction (breathe-rite
strips, nasal steroid spray)

Trial of oral appliance if
patient tolerates

Failure

Surgery tailored to site of
obstruction - most commonly
involves resection of
redundant uvula/soft palate
with laser, cautery, or steel
+/- tonsillectomy; tongue base
procedures are occasionally
indicated

Body mass
index

Nocturnal oxygen saturation <70%
Cardiopulmonary comorbidity
Unfavorable anatomy

Yes

Offer tracheotomy

Site(s) of obstruction

<35   >35

No

Nasal   Palatal

Considerations:
Septoplasty
Turbinate reduction
Rhinoplasty

Considerations:
Palate stiffening with implants,
radiofrequency, or cautery

Resect redundant uvula/soft palate
with laser, cautery, or steel

Multilevel surgery, including
resection of redundant uvula/soft-
palate tissue and tonsillectomy

Consider tongue base reduction
or advancement

Failure

FIG. 18-9. Algorithm of respiratory disturbance index. CPAP = continuous positive airway pressure; OSA = obstructive sleep apnea.

the natural history is eventual recurrence. Therefore, surgery has an ongoing role for palliation of the disease. Multiple procedures are typically required over the patient's lifetime. Several medical therapies, including intralesional cidofovir injection and oral indole-3-carbinol, are being investigated to determine their abilities to retard recurrence. Additionally, the advent of HPV vaccines has suggested a role for this therapy in prevention of RRP.[21]

Laryngeal granulomas typically occur in the posterior larynx on the arytenoid mucosa (Fig. 18-10). These lesions develop secondary to multiple factors,[22] including reflux, voice abuse, chronic throat clearing, endotracheal intubation, and vocal fold paralysis. Effective management requires identification of the underlying cause(s). Patients report pain (often with swallowing) more commonly than vocal changes. In addition to fiber-optic laryngoscopy, work-up may include voice analysis, laryngeal electromyography (EMG), and pH probe testing.[23] Treatment is individualized, depending on the contributing factors identified. First-line modalities that may be used include voice rest, voice retraining therapy, and antireflux therapy. The management of vocal cord paresis/paralysis is discussed later in this section. It is notable that the majority of cases demonstrate a component of reflux and when maximal medical therapy has failed, fundoplication may be indicated. The role of surgical excision is somewhat controversial, because it does not address the underlying etiology and is frequently associated with recurrence. Nonetheless, excision is indicated when carcinoma is suspected or when the patient has airway obstruction. Surgery may also be indicated in

selected cases when a granuloma has matured into a fibroepithelial polyp, or when the patient (e.g., a performing artist) requires prompt removal for voice restoration. Surgical excision is optimally performed under jet ventilation so as to avoid endotracheal intubation.

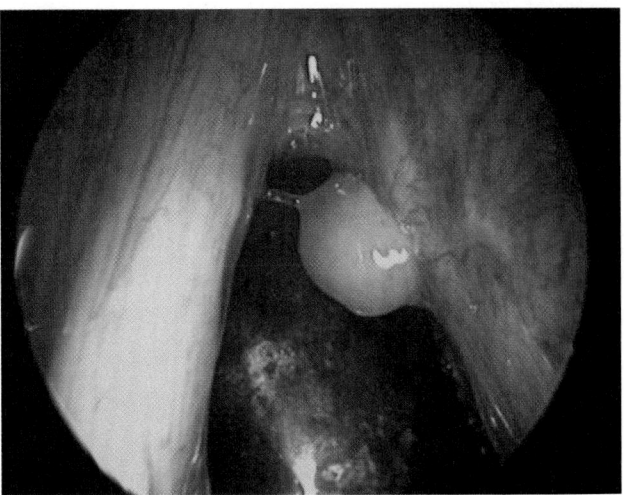

FIG. 18-10. Laryngeal granuloma.

During surgery, it is important to preserve the arytenoid perichondrium to promote epithelialization postoperatively.

Edema in the superficial lamina propria of the vocal cord is known as *polypoid corditis, polypoid laryngitis, polypoid degeneration of the vocal cord,* or *Reinke's edema.*[24] The superficial lamina propria just underlies the vibratory epithelial surface. Edema is thought to arise from injury to the capillaries that exist in this layer, with subsequent extravasation of fluid. Patients report progressive development of a rough, low-pitched voice. Females more commonly present for medical attention because the lowered vocal frequency is more evident, given the higher fundamental frequency of the female voice. The etiology is also multifactorial and may involve smoking, laryngopharyngeal reflux, hypothyroidism, and vocal hyperfunction. Most of these patients are heavy smokers. Findings are typically bilateral.

Focal, unilateral hemorrhagic vocal cord polyps are more common in men. These occur secondary to capillary rupture within the mucosa by shearing forces during voice abuse. Use of anticoagulant or antiplatelet drugs may be a risk factor. As with laryngeal granulomas, treatment of polypoid corditis and vocal cord polyps requires addressing the underlying factors. Conservative management includes absolute discontinuance of smoking, reflux management, and voice therapy. Notably, topical and systemic steroids are ineffective for these conditions. For polypoid corditis, elective surgery may be performed under microlaryngoscopy to evacuate the gelatinous matrix within the superficial lamina propria and trim excess mucosa. Focal polyps may be excised superficially under microlaryngoscopy. Surgery, particularly for polypoid corditis, will be less effective in patients who continue to smoke, although it should be noted that because of their heavy smoking history, surgery might be necessary to rule out occult malignancy. Surgery for polypoid corditis and hemorrhagic polyps may be accomplished either with cold steel or by using the carbon dioxide (CO_2) laser. Postoperative voice therapy is usually indicated.

Vocal cord cysts may occur under the laryngeal mucosa, particularly in regions containing mucous-secreting glands, such as the supraglottic larynx. Occasionally, they derive from minor salivary glands, and congenital cysts may persist as remnants of the branchial arch. Cysts may present in a variety of ways depending on the size and site of origin (Fig. 18-11). Cysts of the vocal cord may be difficult to distinguish from vocal polyps, and video stroboscopic laryngoscopy may be necessary to help establish the diagnosis. Cysts observed in children can be quite large, thus compromising the airway. Lesions of the true vocal cord usually present with hoarseness. Treatment again

depends on the size and site of the cyst. Large cysts of the supraglottic larynx are treated by marsupialization with cold steel or a CO_2 laser. Those of the vocal cord itself require careful microsurgical technique for complete removal of the cyst while preserving the overlying mucosa.

Leukoplakia of the vocal fold represents a white patch (which cannot be wiped off) on the mucosal surface, usually on the superior surface of the true vocal cord. Rather than a diagnosis per se, the term *leukoplakia* describes a finding on laryngoscopic examination. The significance of this finding is that it may represent squamous hyperplasia, dysplasia, and/or carcinoma. Lesions exhibiting hyperplasia have a 1 to 3% risk of progression to malignancy. In contrast, that risk is 10 to 30% for those demonstrating dysplasia. Furthermore, leukoplakia may be observed in association with inflammatory and reactive pathologies, including polyps, nodules, cysts, granulomas, and papillomas. The wide, differential diagnosis for leukoplakia necessitates sound clinical judgment when selecting lesions that require operative direct laryngoscopy with biopsy for histopathologic analysis. Features of ulceration and erythroplasia are particularly suggestive of possible malignancy. A history of smoking and alcohol abuse should also prompt a malignancy work-up. In the absence of suspected malignancy, conservative measures are used for 1 month. These include reduction of caffeine and alcohol, which are dehydrating and promote laryngopharyngeal reflux, proper hydration, and elimination of vocal abuse behaviors. Antireflux therapy, including proton pump inhibitors, may be prescribed. Investigational therapies, including retinoids, also have been attempted. Any lesions that progress, persist, or recur should be considered for excisional biopsy.

Vocal cord paralysis most commonly is iatrogenic in origin,[25] following surgery to the thyroid, parathyroid, carotid, or cardiothoracic structures. Vocal cord paralysis may also be secondary to malignant processes in the lungs, thoracic cavity, skull base, or neck. In the pediatric population up to one fourth of cases may be neurologic in origin, with Arnold-Chiari malformation being the most common. Overall, the left vocal cord is more commonly involved secondary to the longer course of the recurrent laryngeal nerve (RLN) on that side, which extends into the thoracic cavity. When anterior approaches to the cervical spine are performed, however, the right RLN is at an increased risk, because it courses more laterally to the tracheoesophageal complex. Neurotoxic medications, trauma, intubation injury, and atypical infections are less common causes of vocal cord paralysis. The cause remains idiopathic in up to 20% of adults and 35% of children. These cases should prompt an imaging work-up to examine the course of the vagal/RLN in question: from the skull base to the aortic arch on the left, and from skull base to the subclavian on the right.

"Idiopathic" left true vocal cord paralysis may be a presenting sign of malignancy involving the lung, thyroid, or esophagus. Adults typically present with hoarseness and the voice may be breathy if the contralateral vocal cord has not compensated to close the glottic valve. If the proximal vagus nerve or the superior laryngeal nerve is involved, the patient may demonstrate aspiration secondary to diminished supraglottic sensation. Stridor, weak cry, and respiratory distress are seen in children, but adults typically do not exhibit signs of airway compromise unless paralysis is bilateral. Flexible fiberoptic laryngoscopy usually confirms the diagnosis, but laryngeal EMG may be necessary to distinguish vocal cord paralysis from mechanical fixation secondary to scar tissue or cricoarytenoid joint fixation. The position of the paralyzed fold depends on the residual innervation, pattern of reinnervation, and the degrees of atrophy and fibrosis of the laryngeal musculature. In bilateral vocal cord paralysis, the cords are often paralyzed in a paramedian position, creating airway compromise that necessitates tracheotomy. Once an airway is secure, vocal cord lateralization or arytenoidectomy may be performed electively to provide an adequate airway. Treatment of unilateral vocal cord paralysis includes speech therapy, which promotes glottic closure to optimize the voice and prevent aspiration. Some patients do well with this modality alone.

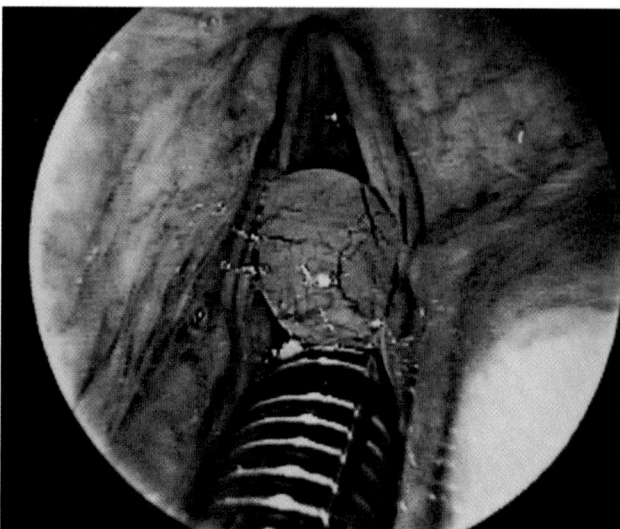

FIG. 18-11. Large cyst of vocal cord.

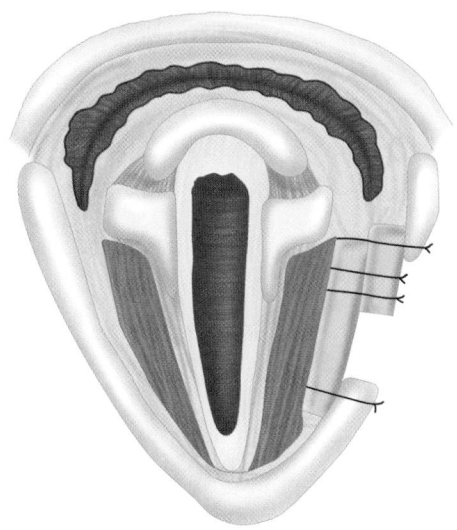

FIG. 18-12. Cross-section of the larynx demonstrating the principle of medialization laryngoplasty. An implant is used to push the paralyzed vocal cord toward the midline.

Surgical treatment to augment or medialize the paralyzed vocal fold is performed to provide a surface against which the contralateral normal fold may make contact. Injection laryngoplasty may be performed under office or operative laryngoscopy with a variety of autologous (fat, collagen) or alloplastic (hydroxylapatite, silicone, Teflon) compounds. Autologous materials are preferred. Teflon injection is of historical significance only secondary to the incidence of severe foreign body inflammatory reactions. Injection of the vocal fold increases its bulk to optimize closure with the contralateral normal fold. This technique also is useful for vocal cord atrophy, which may occur with aging. Recent trends include the use of micronized human collagen for this purpose, which has shown promising results. Laryngeal framework surgery involves the implantation of cartilage, hydroxylapatite, Gore-Tex, or silicone under the musculomembranous fold via an external approach through a window in the thyroid cartilage (Fig. 18-12).[26] This may be combined with procedures to adduct the vocal process of the arytenoids. Laryngeal reinnervation (with ansa cervicalis to RLN transfer) and pacing have also been attempted with varying success.

Vascular Lesions

Vascular lesions can be broadly classified into two groups: hemangiomas and vascular malformations.[27] Hemangiomas are the most common vascular lesions present in infancy and childhood. These lesions are present at birth in up to 30% of cases, but usually become apparent in the first few weeks of life. The lesions proliferate in size over the first year before beginning involution, which subsequently occurs over the next 2 to 12 years. Forty percent of cases will resolve completely, while the remainder require intervention. Once the proliferative phase has ended, the lesion should be observed every 3 months for involution, and surgery should be considered for those that have not significantly involuted by 3 to 4 years of age. Surgical treatment of proliferating hemangiomas is reserved for lesions associated with severe functional or cosmetic problems, such as those involving the nasal tip or periorbital region. Treatment is performed with either the flashlamp-pumped pulsed-dye laser (FPDL), the potassium titanyl phosphate (KTP) laser, or the neodymium yttrium-aluminum garnet (Nd:YAG) laser, repeated every 4 to 6 weeks until the lesion disappears. Systemic steroids may be used to arrest rapidly proliferating lesions until the child reaches 12 to 18 months, after which growth should stabilize or involution begin. Subcutaneous interferon alfa-2a may also be used for this purpose. This treatment, however, is associated with neurologic side effects

and should be used with caution.[27,28] Vascular malformations, in contrast, are almost always present at birth and slowly enlarge without proliferation.[29] These may arise from capillaries, venules, veins, arteriovenous channels, and/or lymphatics. Capillary malformations usually involve the midline neck or forehead, and may fade with age. Venular malformations are also known as *port-wine stains*. These lesions often follow facial dermatomes and usually thicken with age. Venous malformations are composed of ectatic veins within the lips, tongue, or buccal area. These may present as purple masses or subcutaneous/submucosal nodules. Arteriovenous malformations are rare malformations of arteriovenous channels that failed to regress during development.

Lymphatic malformations or lymphangiomas of the head and neck usually involve the cervical area, in which case they are more commonly macrocystic and well demarcated. Those arising above the hyoid bone tend to be microcystic and have an infiltrative quality. Lymphangiomas may become secondarily infected and may rapidly enlarge, causing airway compromise. These lesions may also be associated with feeding difficulties and failure to thrive.

Capillary hemangiomas and superficial port-wine stains are effectively treated by FPDL. The KTP or Nd:YAG laser is used for deeper port-wine stains. Venous malformations may be treated with laser, sclerotherapy, and/or surgical excision, depending on the depth, size, and location. Superficial lesions are treated with the Nd:YAG laser, which has deeper penetration than either the FPDL or KTP laser. Deeper venous malformations may benefit from Nd:YAG therapy of the superficial component followed by meticulous surgical excision of the deeper component. Sclerotherapy should be undertaken with extreme caution in the head and neck, because the valveless quality of the veins in this region introduces significant risk of cavernous sinus thrombosis. Arteriovenous malformations require formal surgical resection with negative margins. Preoperative angiographic embolization is frequently used to facilitate surgery. Microvascular reconstruction may be necessary, depending on the extent of the resection required. Surgical excision is also required for lymphatic malformations, although superficial lesions are sometimes treatable with the CO_2 laser. This often is difficult for microcystic cases given the infiltrative nature. Sclerotherapy with OK-432 is effective in macrocystic lymphangiomas, and multiple other sclerosing agents, including bleomycin, have been explored.[30]

TRAUMA OF THE HEAD AND NECK

Management of soft-tissue trauma in the head and neck has several salient features. Skin injuries may be classified as abrasions, contusions, or lacerations. Abrasions represent superficial epidermal injury and are treated with cleansing, saline irrigation, and removal of dirt or other foreign bodies. The latter step is important because retained materials may form a nidus for infection or foreign-body reaction and may cause tattooing of the skin after healing. Topical antibiotic dressing is applied until re-epithelialization is complete. The patient is instructed to avoid sunlight, because this can cause pigmentary abnormalities during the healing process, which matures over a 6- to 12-month period. Contusions may include ecchymosis and/or frank hematoma. Treatment includes head-of-bed elevation to decrease tissue edema, application of ice, and drainage of hematoma. Lacerations must also be cleansed and irrigated, with removal of any associated dirt or foreign bodies. Most lacerations without significant tissue loss can be closed primarily, and primary closure is preferred when possible. Closure of trapdoor lacerations requires conservative undermining of surrounding tissue and good approximation of subdermal levels before epidermal closure. A pressure dressing is also applied. These measures are used to avoid a pincushion deformity (Fig. 18-13).

Typically, subdermal layers are approximated with an absorbable 3-0 or 4-0 suture such as Vicryl or polydioxanone, and the skin is closed using 5-0 or 6-0 monofilament nylon or Prolene. Sutures

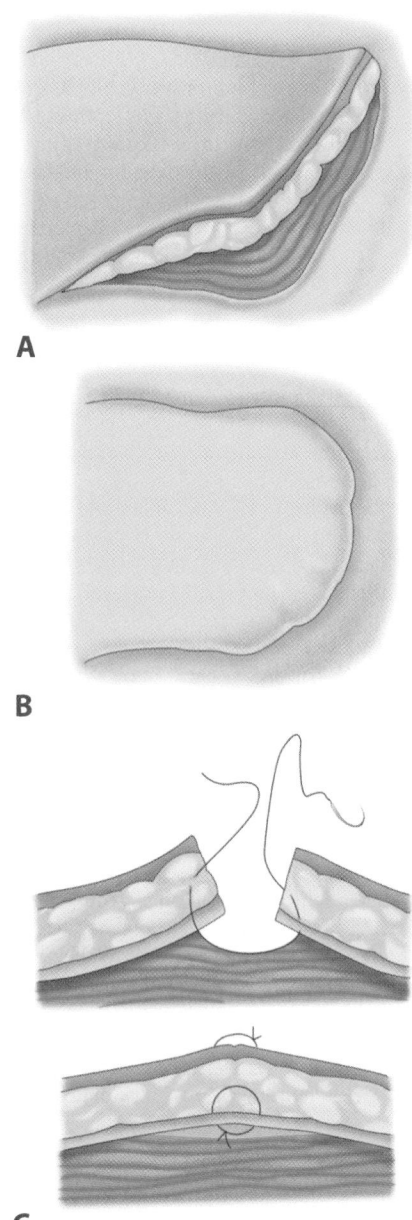

FIG. 18-13. Trap door laceration (**A**) healed with a "pin cushion" deformity (**B**). Soft-tissue layers must be meticulously approximated (**C**) to avoid this complication.

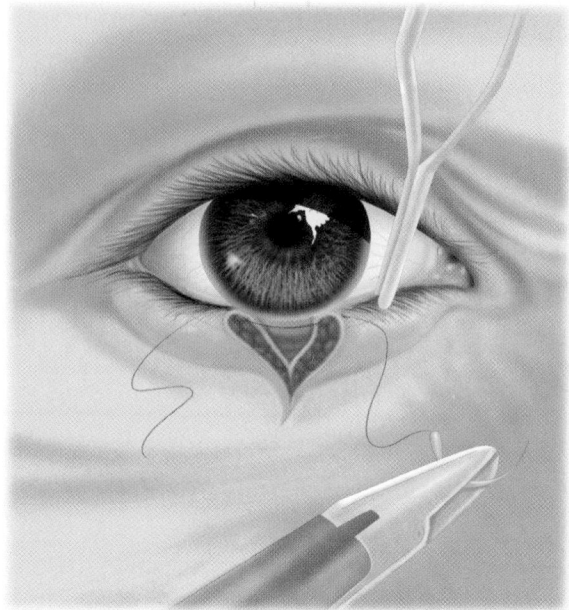

FIG. 18-14. Alignment of the gray line is the key step in the repair of eyelid lacerations.

procedures may be required. With laceration of the auricle, key structures such as the helical rim and antihelix must be carefully aligned. These injuries must be repaired so that the cartilage is covered. The principles of auricular repair are predicated on the fact that the cartilage has no intrinsic blood supply and is thus susceptible to ischemic necrosis following trauma. The suture should be

are removed after 4 to 5 days, but may be removed earlier in thin-skinned areas. The wound is treated with antibiotic ointments. Systemic antibiotics are indicated for through-and-through mucosal lacerations, contaminated wounds, bite injuries, and when delayed closure is performed (>72 hours). The chosen antibiotic should cover *S. aureus.* In many such wounds, healing by secondary intention may be preferable.

Wound closure must be understood in the context of the cosmetic and functional anatomic landmarks of the head and neck. Management of injuries to the eyelid requires identification of the orbicularis oculi, which is closed in a separate layer. The gray line (conjunctival margin; Fig. 18-14) must be carefully approximated to avoid lid notching or height mismatch. Management of lip injuries follows the same principle. The orbicularis oris must be closed, and the vermilion border carefully approximated (Fig. 18-15). Injuries involving one fourth the width of the eyelid or one third the width of the lip may be closed primarily; otherwise, flap or grafting

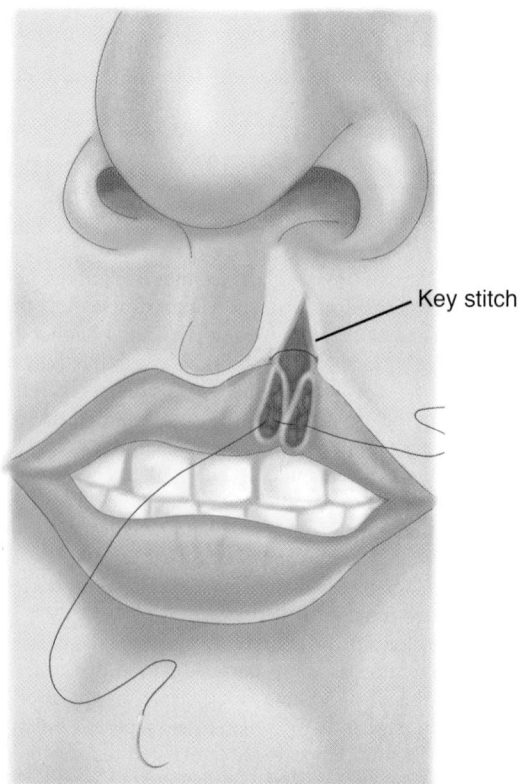

Key stitch

FIG. 18-15. Approximation of the vermilion border is the key step in the repair of lip lacerations.

passed through the perichondrium, while placement through the cartilage itself should be avoided.

Auricular hematomas should be drained promptly, with placement of a bolster as a pressure dressing. A pressure dressing is frequently advocated after closure of an ear laceration. It also deserves note that the surgeon must avoid the temptation to perform aggressive débridement after injuries to the eyelid or auricle. Given the rich vascular supply to the face and neck, many soft-tissue components that appear devitalized will indeed survive.

Most traumatic facial nerve injuries are secondary to temporal bone trauma, which is discussed below in this section. Soft-tissue injuries occurring in the misfile may involve distal facial nerve branches. Those injured anterior to a vertical line dropped from the lateral cantus do not require repair secondary to collateral innervation in the anterior midface. Posterior to this line, the nerve should be repaired, primarily if possible, using 8-0 to 10-0 monofilament suture to approximate the epineurium under microscopic visualization. If neural segments are missing, cable grafting is performed using either the greater auricular (provides 7 to 8 cm) or sural nerve (up to 30 cm) as a donor. Injuries to the buccal branch should alert the examiner to a possible parotid duct injury. This structure lies along an imaginary line drawn from the tragus to the midline upper lip, running along with the buccal branch of the facial nerve. The duct should be repaired over a 22-gauge stent or marsupialized into the oral cavity.

Facial bone fractures most commonly involve the mandible. Fractures most often involve the angle, body, or condyle, and in most cases, two or more sites are almost always involved (Fig. 18-16). Fractures are described as either favorable or unfavorable, depending on whether or not the masticatory musculature tends to pull the fracture into reduction or distraction. Vertically favorable fractures are brought into reduction by the masseter, while horizontally favorable fractures are brought into reduction by the pterygoid musculature. The fracture is usually evaluated radiographically using a Panorex, but specialized plain film views, and occasionally CT scan, are necessary in selected cases. Classical management of mandible fractures dictated closed reduction and a 6-week period of intermaxillary fixation (IMF) with arch bars applied via circumdental wiring. Comminuted, displaced, or unfavorable fractures underwent open reduction and wire fixation in addition to IMF. Currently, arch bars and IMF are performed to establish occlusion. The fracture is then exposed and reduced, using transoral approaches where possible.

Transcervical approaches are required to address fractures of the ramus or posterior body, with careful attention given to preserving the marginal mandibular branch of the facial nerve. Rigid fixation is then accomplished by the application of plates and screws. Selected fractures, such as those of the body, benefit from dynamic compression plating, which applies pressure toward the fracture line. With rigid fixation, IMF is required to establish occlusion intraoperatively, and is not necessarily continued for a full 6 weeks postoperatively. This is preferable because IMF is associated with gingival and dental disease, as well as with significant weight loss and malnutrition, during the fixation period. New techniques have included the 4-point fixation technique, where the maxilla and mandible are held in occlusion by wires attached to intraoral cortical bone screws, with two screws above and below the occlusal line anteriorly. In edentulous patients, determining the baseline occlusion is of less significance because dentures may be refashioned once healing is complete. If IMF is required to aid in immobilization of the fracture in an edentulous patient, interosseous wiring and/or the fabrication of custom-made splints is required.

Midface fractures are classically described in three patterns: Le Fort I, II, and III. A full understanding of midface structure is first necessary (Fig. 18-17). Three vertical buttresses support the midface: the nasofrontal-maxillary, the frontozygomaticomaxillary, and pterygomaxillary.[31] The five weaker, horizontal buttresses include the frontal bone, nasal bones, upper alveolus, zygomatic arches, and the infraorbital region. Classical signs of midface fractures in general include subconjunctival hemorrhage; malocclusion; midface numbness or hypesthesia (maxillary division of the trigeminal nerve); facial ecchymoses/hematoma; ocular signs/symptoms; and mobility of the maxillary complex.

Le Fort I fractures occur transversely across the alveolus, above the level of the teeth apices. In a pure Le Fort I fracture, the palatal vault is mobile while the nasal pyramid and orbital rims are stable. The Le Fort II fracture extends through the nasofrontal buttress, medial wall of the orbit, across the infraorbital rim, and through the zygomaticomaxillary articulation. The nasal dorsum, palate, and medial part of the infraorbital rim are mobile. The Le Fort III fracture is also known as *craniofacial disjunction*. The frontozygomaticomaxillary, frontomaxillary, and frontonasal suture lines are disrupted. The entire face is mobile from the cranium. It is convenient to conceptualize complex midface fractures according to these patterns (Fig. 18-18); however, in reality, fractures reflect a combination of these three types. Also, the fracture pattern may vary between the left and right sides of the midface. Lateral blows to the cheek may be associated

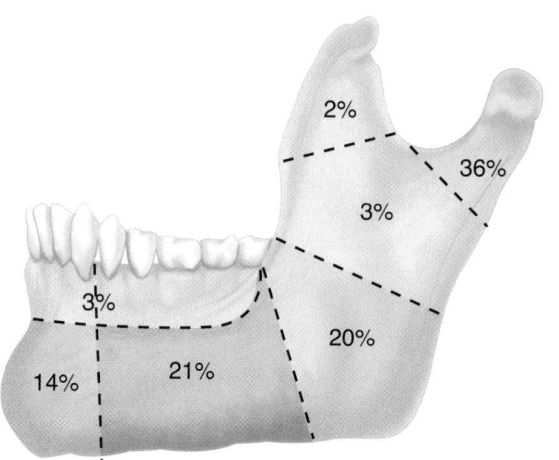

FIG. 18-16. Sites of common mandible fractures.

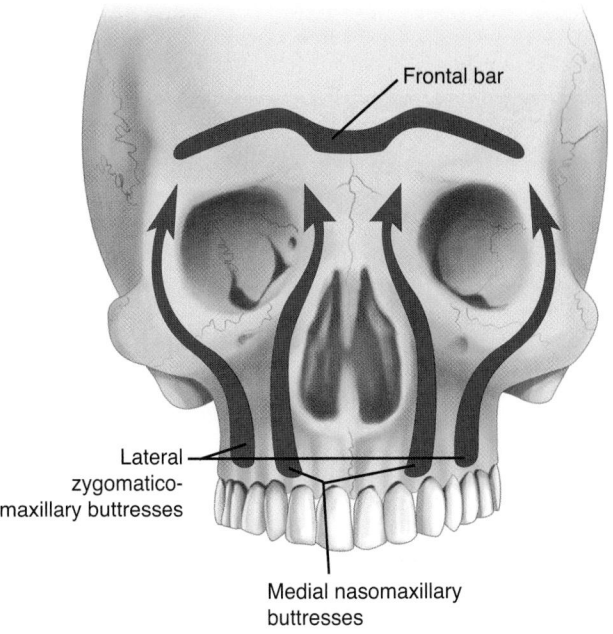

FIG. 18-17. Major buttresses of the midface.

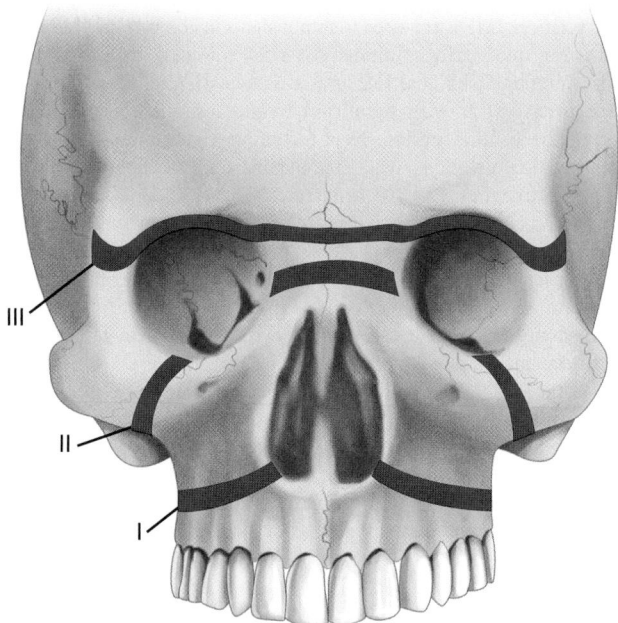

FIG. 18-18. Classic Le Fort fracture patterns.

with isolated zygoma fractures. The zygoma is typically displaced inferiorly and medially with disruption of the suture lines between the temporal, frontal, and maxillary bones and the zygoma. Disruption of the latter articulation may be associated with depression into the maxillary sinus and blood in the sinus cavity. Fractures of the midface and/or zygoma may be associated with an orbital blowout, whereas the orbital floor is disrupted and orbital soft tissues subsequently herniate into the maxillary sinus (Fig. 18-19). The mechanism of orbital blowout may involve propagation of adjacent fracture lines or may be the result of a sudden increase in intraorbital pressure during the injury. This may be associated with enophthalmos or entrapment of the inferior oblique muscle. The latter results in diplopia upon upward gaze. Entrapment is confirmed by forced duction testing, where, under topical or general anesthesia, the muscular attachment of the inferior oblique is grasped with forceps and manipulated to determine passive ocular mobility. Fractures of

the midface, zygoma, and orbital floor are best evaluated using CT scan, and repair requires a combination of transoral and external approaches to achieve at least two points of fixation for each fractured segment.[32] Significant areas of bone loss can be reconstructed with commercially available hydroxyapatite bone cements, an osteoconductive calcium-phosphate matrix. Blowout fractures demonstrating significant entrapment or enophthalmos are treated by orbital exploration and reinforcement of the floor with mesh or bone grafting.

Temporal bone fractures occur in approximately one fifth of skull fractures. As with fractures of the mandible and midface, blunt trauma (from motor vehicle accident or assault) usually is implicated. Unfortunately, the incidence of temporal bone fracture from gunshot wounds to the head is rising. Fractures are divided into two patterns (Fig. 18-20), longitudinal and transverse, based on the clinical picture and CT imaging. In practice, most fractures are oblique. By classical descriptions, longitudinal fractures constitute 80% and are associated with lateral skull trauma. Signs and symptoms include conductive hearing loss, ossicular injury, bloody otorrhea, and labyrinthine concussion. The facial nerve is injured in approximately 20% of cases. In contrast, the transverse pattern constitute only 20% of temporal bone fractures and occurs secondary to fronto-occipital trauma. The facial nerve is injured in 50% of cases. These injuries frequently involve the otic capsule to cause sensorineural hearing loss and loss of vestibular function. Hemotympanum may be observed. A cerebrospinal fluid (CSF) leak must be suspected in temporal bone trauma. This resolves with conservative measures in most cases. The most significant consideration in the management of temporal bone injuries is the status of the facial nerve. Delayed or partial paralysis will almost always resolve with conservative management. However, immediate paralysis that does not recover within 1 week should be considered for nerve decompression. Electroneurography and EMG have been used to help

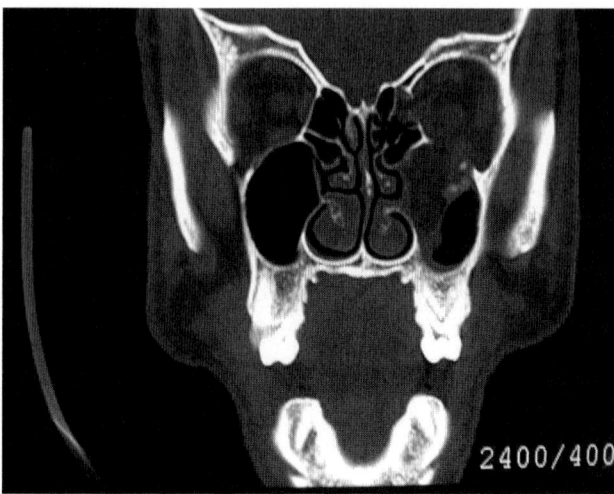

FIG. 18-19. Coronal computed tomography demonstrating an orbital blowout fracture with herniation of orbital contents into the maxillary sinus.

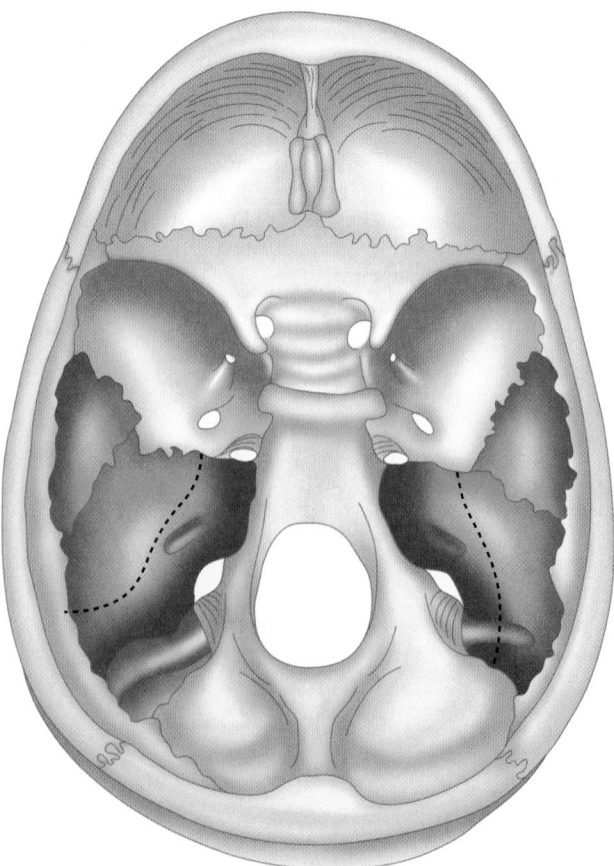

FIG. 18-20. View of cranial surface of skull base. Longitudinal (*left*) and transverse (*right*) temporal bone fractures.

determine which patients with delayed-onset complete paralysis will benefit from surgical decompression. The finding of greater than 90% degeneration more than 72 hours after the onset of complete paralysis is considered an indication for surgery.[33] Multiple approaches have been described for facial nerve decompression, some of which sacrifice hearing. These patients may have severe intracranial or vascular injuries such that the decision to operate must also be made in the context of the patient's overall medical stability. It is of paramount importance to protect the eye in patients with facial nerve paralysis of any etiology, because absence of an intact blink reflex will predispose to corneal drying and abrasion. This requires the placement of artificial tears throughout the day with lubricant ointment, eye taping, and/or a humidity chamber at night.[34,35]

TUMORS OF THE HEAD AND NECK

When a discussion of neoplasms of the head and neck is initiated, the conversation frequently focuses on squamous cell carcinoma. This is because the majority of malignancies of this region are represented by this pathology. The diagnosis and treatment of lesions spanning from the lips and oral cavity to the larynx and hypopharynx requires a similar methodic approach.

The selection of treatment protocols varies for each site within the upper aerodigestive tract. The importance of multidisciplinary management cannot be underestimated. Presentation of cases before a tumor board allowing review of a patient's history, physical examination findings, imaging, and prior pathology specimens allows for confirmation of the patient's status. Additionally, it should encourage discussion from multiple points of view concerning the most appropriate treatment options available. Participation in the discussion with representatives of radiation oncology, medical oncology, surgical oncology, oral maxillofacial surgery/dental medicine, along with radiologists and pathologists specializing in upper aerodigestive tract disorders benefits not only the patient but also represents an excellent teaching opportunity for all disciplines.

The development of organ preservation protocol and the evolution of free tissue reconstructive techniques are some of the most significant advances made within the field during the last two decades. The future of the treatment of head and neck cancer lies within the field of molecular biology. As more is understood about the genetics of cancer, tailoring treatment options to a particular tumor mutation has the capacity to maximize survival while achieving the highest quality of life.

Etiology and Epidemiology

It should come as no surprise that abuse of tobacco and alcohol are the most common preventable risk factors associated with the development of head and neck cancers. This relationship is synergistic rather than additive. Smoking confers a 1.9-fold increased risk to males and a threefold increased risk to females for developing a head and neck carcinoma, when compared to nonsmokers. The risk increases as the number of years smoking and number of cigarettes smoked per day increases. Alcohol alone confers a 1.7-fold increased risk to males drinking one to two drinks per day, when compared to nondrinkers. This increased risk rises to greater than threefold for heavy drinkers. Individuals who both smoke (two packs per day) and drink (four units of alcohol per day) had an odds ratio of 35 for the development of a carcinoma when compared to controls.[36] Users of smokeless tobacco have a four times increased risk of oral cavity carcinoma when compared to nonusers.

Tobacco is the leading preventable cause of death in the United States and is responsible for one of every five deaths.[37] Approximately one fourth of U.S. adults habitually use tobacco products, with recent trends demonstrating an increase in the use of tobacco products by women. The evidence supporting the need for head and neck cancer patients to pursue smoking cessation after treatment is compelling. In a study by Moore,[38] 40% of patients who continued to smoke after definitive treatment for an oral cavity malignancy went on to recur or develop a second head and neck malignancy. For patients who stopped smoking after treatment, only 6% went on to develop a recurrence. Induction of specific p53 mutations within upper aerodigestive tract tumors has been noted in patients with histories of tobacco and alcohol use.[39,40]

When smokers who develop head and neck squamous cell carcinomas are compared to nonsmokers, differences between the two populations emerge. Koch and associates[41] noted that nonsmokers were represented by a disproportionate number of women and were more frequently at the extremes of age (<30 or >85 years of age). Tumors from nonsmokers presented more frequently in the oral cavity, specifically within the oral tongue, buccal mucosa, and alveolar ridge. Smokers presented more frequently with tumors of the larynx, hypopharynx, and floor of mouth. Former smokers, defined as those individuals who had quit greater than 10 years prior, demonstrated a profile more consistent with nonsmokers.

In India and Southeast Asia, the product of the areca catechu tree, known as a betel nut, is chewed in a habitual manner and acts as a mild stimulant similar to that of coffee. The nut is chewed in combination with lime and cured tobacco as a mixture known as a quid. The long-term use of the betel nut quid can be destructive to oral mucosa and dentition and is highly carcinogenic.[42] Another habit associated with oral malignancy is that of reverse smoking, where the lighted portion of the tobacco product is within the mouth during inhalation. The risk of hard palate carcinoma is 47 times greater in reverse smokers when compared to nonsmokers.

HPV is an epitheliotropic virus that has been detected to varying degrees within samples of oral cavity squamous cell carcinoma. Infection alone is not considered sufficient for malignant conversion; however, results of multiple studies suggest a role of HPV in a subset of head and neck squamous cell carcinoma. Approximately 40% of tonsillar carcinomas demonstrate evidence of HPV types 16 and 18.

Environmental ultraviolet light exposure has been associated with the development of lip cancer. The projection of the lower lip, as it relates to this solar exposure, has been used to explain why the majority of squamous cell carcinomas arise along the vermilion border of the lower lip. In addition, pipe smoking also has been associated with the development of lip carcinoma. Factors such as mechanical irritation, thermal injury, and chemical exposure have been described as an explanation for this finding.

Other entities associated with oral malignancy include Plummer-Vinson syndrome (achlorhydria, iron-deficiency anemia, mucosal atrophy of mouth, pharynx, and esophagus), chronic infection with syphilis, and immunocompromised status (30-fold increase with renal transplant).

Although evidence linking HIV infection to squamous cell carcinoma of the head and neck is lacking, several AIDS-defining malignancies, including Kaposi's sarcoma, and non-Hodgkin's lymphoma may require the care of an otolaryngologist.

Anatomy and Histopathology

The upper aerodigestive tract is divided into several distinct sites that include the oral cavity, pharynx, larynx, and nasal cavity/paranasal sinuses. Within these sites are individual subsites with specific anatomic relationships that affect diagnosis, tumor spread, and selection of treatment options. The spread of a tumor from one site to another is determined by the course of the nerves, blood vessels, lymphatic pathways, and fascial planes. The fascial planes serve as barriers to the direct invasion of tumor and facilitate the pattern of spread to regional lymph nodes.

The oral cavity extends from the vermilion border of the lip to the hard-palate/soft-palate junction superiorly, to circumvallate papillae inferiorly, and to the anterior tonsillar pillars laterally (Fig. 18-21). It is divided into seven subsites: lips, alveolar ridges, oral tongue, retromolar trigone, floor of mouth, buccal mucosa, and hard palate. Advanced oral cavity lesions may present with mandibular and/or maxillary involvement requiring special consideration

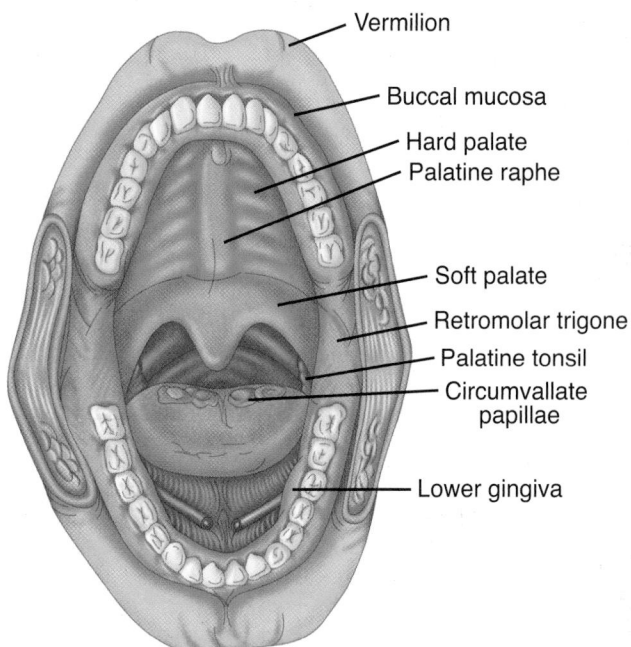

- Vermilion
- Buccal mucosa
- Hard palate
- Palatine raphe
- Soft palate
- Retromolar trigone
- Palatine tonsil
- Circumvallate papillae
- Lower gingiva

FIG. 18-21. Oral cavity landmarks.

at the time of resection and reconstruction. Regional metastatic spread of lesions of the oral cavity is to the lymphatics of the submandibular and the upper jugular region (levels I, II, and III).

The pharynx is divided into three regions: nasopharynx, oropharynx, and hypopharynx. The nasopharynx extends from the posterior nasal septum and choana to the skull base and includes the fossa of Rosenmüller and torus tubarius of the eustachian tubes laterally. The inferior margin of the nasopharynx is the superior surface of the soft palate. The adenoids, typically involuted in adults, are located with the posterior aspect of this site. Given the midline location of the nasopharynx, bilateral regional metastatic spread is common in these lesions. Lymphadenopathy of the posterior triangle (level V) of the neck should provoke consideration for a nasopharyngeal primary.

The major sites within the oropharynx are the tonsillar region, base of tongue, soft palate, and posterolateral pharyngeal walls. Regional lymphatic drainage for oropharyngeal lesions frequently occurs to the upper and lower cervical lymphatics (levels II, III, IV). Retropharyngeal metastatic lymphatic spread may occur with oropharyngeal lesions.

The hypopharynx extends from the vallecula to the lower border of the cricoid posterior and lateral to the larynx. The subsites of this region include the pyriform fossa, the postcricoid space, and posterior pharyngeal wall. Regional lymphatic spread is frequently bilateral and to the mid- and lower cervical lymph nodes (levels III, IV).

The larynx is divided into three regions: the supraglottis, glottis, and subglottis. The supraglottic larynx includes the epiglottis, false vocal cords, medial surface of the aryepiglottic folds, and the roof of the laryngeal ventricles. The glottis includes the true vocal cords, anterior and posterior commissure, and the floor of the laryngeal ventricle. The subglottis extends from below the true vocal cords to the cephalic border of the cricoid within the airway. The supraglottis has a rich lymphatic network, which accounts for the high rate of bilateral spread of metastatic disease that is not typically seen with the glottis. Glottic and subglottic lesions, in addition to potential spread to the cervical chain lymph nodes, may also spread to the paralaryngeal and paratracheal lymphatics and require attention to prevent lower central neck recurrence.

Carcinogenesis

Development of a tumor represents the loss of cellular signaling mechanisms involved in the regulation of growth. Following malig-

nant transformation, the processes of replication (mitosis), programmed cell death (apoptosis), and the interaction of a cell with its surrounding environment are altered. Advances in molecular biology have allowed for the identification of many of the mutations associated with this transformation.

Overexpression of mutant p53 is associated with carcinogenesis at multiple sites within the body. Point mutations in p53 have been reported in up to 45% of head and neck carcinomas. Koch and associates[41] noted that p53 mutation is a key event in the malignant transformation of greater than 50% of head and neck squamous cell carcinomas in smokers.

Carcinogenesis has long been explained as a two-hit process, involving DNA damage and the progression of mutated cells through the cell cycle. These two events also are known as *initiation* and *promotion*. It has been proposed that up to six to 10 independent genetic mutations are required for the development of a malignancy. Overexpression of mitogenic receptors, loss of tumor-suppressor proteins, expression of oncogene-derived proteins that inhibit apoptosis, and overexpression of proteins that drive the cell cycle can allow for unregulated cell growth.

Genetic mutations may occur as a result of environmental exposure (e.g., radiation or carcinogen exposure), viral infection, or spontaneous mutation (deletions, translocations, frame shifts). Common genetic alterations, such as loss of heterozygosity at 3p, 4q, and 11q13, and the overall number of chromosomal microsatellite losses are found more frequently in the tumors of smokers than in the tumors of nonsmokers.[41]

Second Primary Tumors in the Head and Neck

Patients diagnosed with a head and neck cancer are predisposed to the development of a second tumor within the aerodigestive tract. The overall rate of second primary tumors is approximately 14%. A second primary tumor detected within 6 months of the diagnosis of the initial primary lesion is defined as a synchronous neoplasm. The prevalence of synchronous tumors is approximately 3 to 4%. The detection of a second primary lesion more than 6 months after the initial diagnosis is referred to as metachronous tumor. Eighty percent of second primaries are metachronous and at least half of these lesions develop within 2 years of the diagnosis of the original primary. The incidence and site of the second primary tumor vary and depend on the site and the inciting factors associated with the initial primary tumor. The importance of advocating smoking cessation and addressing alcoholism in these patients cannot be overemphasized.

Patients with a primary malignancy of the oral cavity or pharynx are most likely to develop a second lesion within the cervical esophagus, whereas patients with a carcinoma of the larynx are at risk for developing a neoplasm in the lung. As such, the presentation of a new-onset dysphagia, unexplained weight loss, or chronic cough/hemoptysis must be assessed thoroughly in patients with a history of prior treatment for a head and neck cancer.

A staging examination is recommended at the initial evaluation of all patients with primary cancers of the upper aerodigestive tract. This may involve a direct laryngoscopy, rigid/flexible esophagoscopy, and rigid/flexible bronchoscopy also known as "panendoscopy." Some surgeons argue against the use of bronchoscopy because of the low yield of the examination in asymptomatic patients with a normal chest x-ray. Additionally, some surgeons prefer to use a barium swallow instead of esophagoscopy as a preoperative evaluation. Despite the different practices concerning pretreatment evaluation of asymptomatic patients, it should be noted that patients with symptoms potentially representing those of metastatic spread of disease require a work-up greater than a screening evaluation.

Staging

Staging for upper aerodigestive tract malignancies is defined by the American Joint Committee on Cancer[43] and follows the TNM (primary tumor, regional nodal metastases, distant metastasis) staging format. The T staging criteria for each site varies depending

TABLE 18-3 TNM staging for oral cavity carcinoma

Primary tumor

TX	Unable to assess primary tumor
T0	No evidence of primary tumor
Tis	Carcinoma in situ
T1	Tumor is <2 cm in greatest dimension
T2	Tumor >2 cm and <4 cm in greatest dimension
T3	Tumor >4 cm in greatest dimension
T4 (lip)	Primary tumor invading cortical bone, inferior alveolar nerve, floor of mouth, or skin of face (e.g., nose or chin)
T4a (oral)	Tumor invades adjacent structures (e.g., cortical bone, into deep tongue musculature, maxillary sinus) or skin of face
T4b (oral)	Tumor invades masticator space, pterygoid plates, or skull base and/or encases the internal carotid artery

Regional lymphadenopathy

NX	Unable to assess regional lymph nodes
N0	No evidence of regional metastasis
N1	Metastasis in a single ipsilateral lymph node, 3 cm or less in greatest dimension
N2a	Metastasis in single ipsilateral lymph node, >3 cm and <6 cm
N2b	Metastasis in multiple ipsilateral lymph nodes, all nodes <6 cm
N2c	Metastasis in bilateral or contralateral lymph nodes, all nodes <6 cm
N3	Metastasis in a lymph node >6 cm in greatest dimension

Distant metastases

MX	Unable to assess for distant metastases
M0	No distant metastases
M1	Distant metastases

TNM staging

Stage 0	Tis	N0	M0
Stage I	T1	N0	M0
Stage II	T2	N0	M0
Stage III	T3	N0	M0
	T1–3	N1	M0
Stage IVa	T4a	N0	M0
	T4a	N1	M0
	T1–4a	N2	M0
Stage IVb	Any T	N3	M0
	T4b	Any N	M0
Stage IVc	Any T	Any N	M1

TNM = tumor, nodes, and metastasis.
Source: Used with the permission of the American Joint Committee on Cancer (AJCC), Chicago, Illinois. The original source for this material is the AJCC Cancer Staging Manual, Sixth Edition (2002) published by Springer Science and Business Media LLC, www.springerlink.com.

upon the relevant anatomy (e.g., vocal cord immobility is typical of T3 lesions). Table 18-3 demonstrates TNM staging for oral cavity lesions. The N classification system is uniform for all head and neck sites except for the nasopharynx.

Upper Aerodigestive Tract
Lip

The lips represent a transition from external skin to internal mucous membrane that occurs at the vermilion border. The underlying musculature of the orbicularis oris creates a circumferential ring that allows the mouth to have a sphincter-like function. Cancer of the lip is most commonly seen in white men from the ages of 50 to 70 years, but can be seen in younger patients, particularly those with fair complexions. Risk factors include prolonged exposure to sunlight, fair complexion, immunosuppression, and tobacco use.

The majority of lip malignancies present on the lower lip (88 to 98%), followed by the upper lip (2 to 7%) and oral commissure (1%). The histology of lip cancers is predominantly squamous cell carci-

noma; however, other tumors, such as keratoacanthoma, verrucous carcinoma, basal cell carcinoma, malignant melanoma, minor salivary gland malignancies, and tumors of mesenchymal origin (e.g., malignant fibrous histiocytoma, leiomyosarcoma, and rhabdomyosarcoma), may also present in this location. Basal cell carcinoma presents more frequently on the upper lip than lower.

Clinical findings in lip cancer include an ulcerated lesion on the vermilion or cutaneous surface. Careful palpation is important in determining the actual size and extent of these lesions. The presence of paresthesia in the area adjacent to the lesion may indicate mental nerve involvement.

Characteristics of lip primaries that negatively affect prognosis include perineural invasion, involvement of the underlying maxilla/mandible, presentation on the upper lip or commissure, regional lymphatic metastasis, and age younger than 40 years at onset. Lip cancer results in fewer than 200 patient deaths annually and is stage dependent. Early diagnosis coupled with adequate treatment results in a high likelihood of disease control.

The treatment for lip cancer is determined by the overall health of the patient, size of the primary lesion, and the presence of regional metastases. Small primary lesions may be treated with surgery or radiation with equal success and acceptable cosmetic results. However, surgical excision with histologic confirmation of tumor-free margins is the preferred treatment modality. Lymph node metastasis occurs in fewer than 10% of patients with lip cancer (Fig. 18-22). The primary echelon of nodes at risk is in the submandibular and submental regions. In the presence of clinically evident neck metastasis, neck dissection is indicated. The overall 5-year cure rate of lip cancer approximates 90% and drops to 50% in the presence of neck metastases.[44] Postoperative radiation is administered to the primary site and neck for patients with close or positive margins, lymph node metastases, or perineural invasion.

The reconstruction of lip defects after tumor excision requires innovative techniques to provide oral competence, maintenance of dynamic function, and acceptable cosmesis. The typical lip length is 6 to 7 cm. This simple fact is important because the reconstructive algorithms available to the head and neck surgeon are based on the proportion of lip resected. Realignment of the vermilion border during the reconstruction and preservation of the oral commissure (when possible) are important principles in attempting to attain an

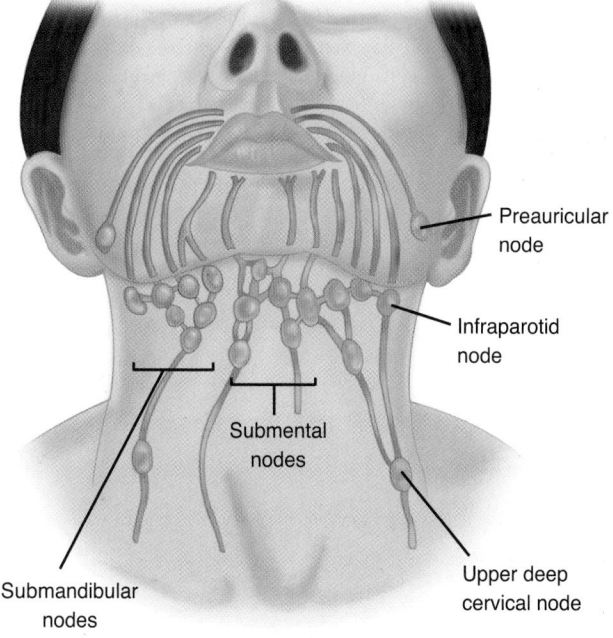

FIG. 18-22. Lymphatics of the lip.

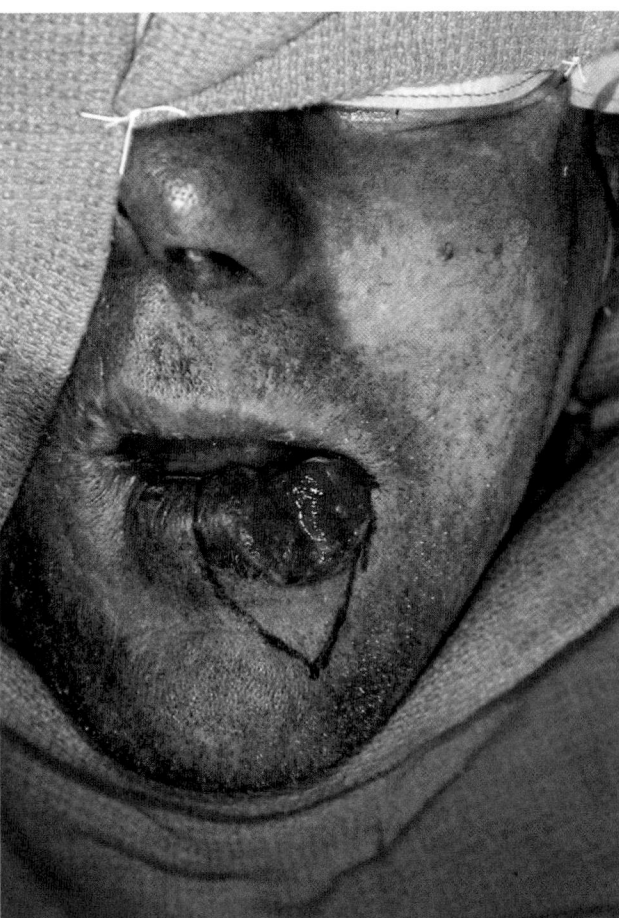

FIG. 18-23. Wedge resection of lower lip squamous cell carcinoma.

have also been described.[46] Details regarding specific techniques of reconstruction are not discussed in this chapter.[45]

Oral Cavity

As previously mentioned in Anatomy and Histopathology, the oral cavity is composed of several sites with different anatomic relationships. The majority of tumors in the oral cavity are squamous cell carcinomas (>90%). Each site is briefly reviewed with emphasis placed on anatomy, diagnosis, and treatment options.

Oral Tongue

The oral tongue is a muscular structure with overlying nonkeratinizing squamous epithelium. The posterior limit of the oral tongue is the circumvallate papillae, whereas its ventral portion is contiguous with the anterior floor of mouth. The tongue is composed of four intrinsic and four extrinsic muscles separated at the midline by the median fibrous septum. Tumors of the tongue begin in the stratified epithelium of the surface and eventually invade into the deeper muscular structures. The tumors may present as ulcerations or as exophytic masses (Fig. 18-25).[47] The regional lymphatics of the oral cavity are to the submandibular space and the upper cervical lymph nodes (Fig. 18-26). The lingual nerve and the hypoglossal nerve may be directly invaded by locally extensive tumors (Fig. 18-27). Involvement results in ipsilateral paresthesias and deviation of the tongue on protrusion with fasciculations and eventual atrophy. Tumors on the tongue may occur on any surface, but are most commonly seen on the lateral and ventral surfaces.[48] Primary tumors of the mesenchymal components of the tongue include leiomyomas, leiomyosarcomas, rhabdomyosarcomas, and neurofibromas.

Surgical treatment of small (T1–T2) primary tumors is wide local excision with either primary closure or healing by secondary intention. The CO_2 laser may be used for excision of early tongue cancers or for ablation of premalignant lesions. A partial glossectomy, which removes a significant portion of the lateral oral tongue, still permits reasonably effective postoperative function. Resection of larger tumors of the tongue that invade deeply can result in significant functional impairment. If lingual contact with the palate, lip and teeth is decreased, it will result in impaired articulation. The use of soft, pliable fasciocutaneous free flaps can provide intraoral bulk and preservation of tongue mobility. Prosthetic augmentation can allow for contact between the remaining tongue tissue and the palate, improving a patient's ability to speak and swallow. Treatment of the regional lymphatics is typically performed with the same modality used to address the primary site. When the primary site is addressed surgically, modified radical neck dissection (MRND) or selective neck dissection (SND) is performed. Depth of invasion of the primary tumor can direct the need for elective lymph node dissection with early stage lesions.[49]

Floor of Mouth

The floor of mouth is the mucosally covered semilunar area that extends from the anterior tonsillar pillar posteriorly to the frenulum

acceptable cosmetic result. Resection with primary closure is possible with a defect of up to one third of the lip (Fig. 18-23). When the resection includes one third to one half of the lip, rectangular excisions can be closed using Burow's triangles in combination with advancement flaps and releasing incisions in the mental crease.[44,45] Borrowing tissue from the upper lip can repair other medium-size defects. For larger defects of up to 75%, the Karapandzic flap uses a sensate, neuromuscular flap that includes the remaining orbicularis oris muscle, conserving its blood supply from branches of the labial artery (Fig. 18-24). The lip-switch (Abbe-Estlander) flap or a stair-step advancement technique can be used to repair defects of either the upper or lower lip. Microstomia is a potential complication with these types of lip reconstruction. For very large defects, Webster or Bernard types of repair using lateral nasolabial flaps with buccal advancement

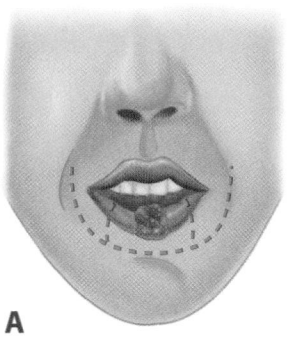
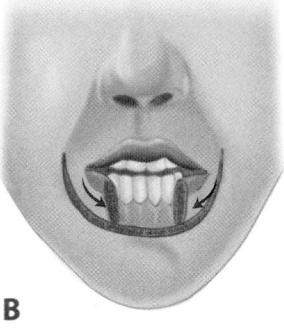
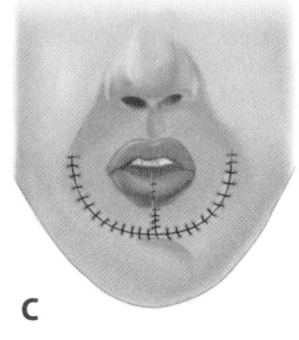

A **B** **C**

FIG. 18-24. A through **C.** Karapandzic labioplasty for lower lip carcinoma.

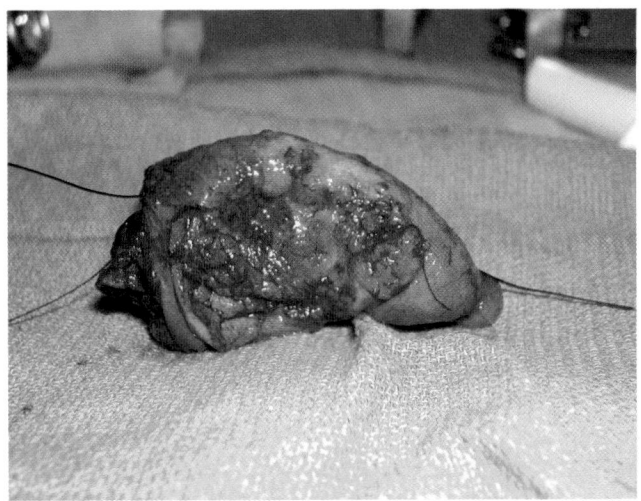

FIG. 18-25. Oral tongue squamous cell carcinoma.

anteriorly, and from the inner surface of the mandible to the ventral surface of the oral tongue. The ostia of the submaxillary and sublingual glands are contained in the anterior floor of mouth. The muscular floor of mouth is composed of the sling-like genioglossus, mylohyoid, and hyoglossus muscles, which serve as a barrier to spread of disease. Invasion into these muscles can result in decreased tongue mobility and poor articulation. Another pathway for spread of tumor is along the salivary ducts, which can result in direct extension into the sublingual space.

Anterior or lateral extension to the mandibular periosteum is of primary importance in the preoperative assessment for these lesions. Imaging studies of the mandible, including CT scan, magnetic resonance imaging (MRI), and Panorex radiography, are helpful for ascertaining bone invasion. A careful clinical evaluation, which includes bimanual palpation to assess adherence or fixation to adjacent bone, is also essential (Fig. 18-28). The absence of fixation of the lesion to the inner mandibular cortex indicates that a mandible-sparing procedure is feasible.[50] Deep invasion into the intrinsic musculature of the tongue causes fixation and mandates a partial glossectomy in conjunction with resection of the floor of mouth. Lesions in the anterior floor of mouth may invade the sublingual gland or submandibular duct and require resection of either of these structures in continuity with the primary lesion. Direct extension of tumors into or through the sublingual space and into the submaxillary space may necessitate the need for removal of the primary tumor with the neck dissection specimen in continuity.

The resection of large tumors of the floor of mouth may require a lip-splitting incision (Fig. 18-29) and immediate reconstruction. The goals are to obtain watertight closure to avoid a salivary fistula and to avoid tongue tethering to maximize mobility. For small mucosal lesions, wide local excision can be followed by placement of a split-thickness skin graft over the muscular bed. Larger defects that require marginal or segmental mandibulectomy require complex reconstruction with a fasciocutaneous or a vascularized osseous free flap.

Alveolus/Gingiva

The alveolar mucosa overlies the bone of the mandible and maxilla. It extends from the gingivobuccal sulcus to the mucosa of the floor of mouth and hard palate. The posterior limits are the pterygopalatine arch and the ascending portion of the ramus of the mandible. Because of the tight attachment of the alveolar mucosa to the mandibular and

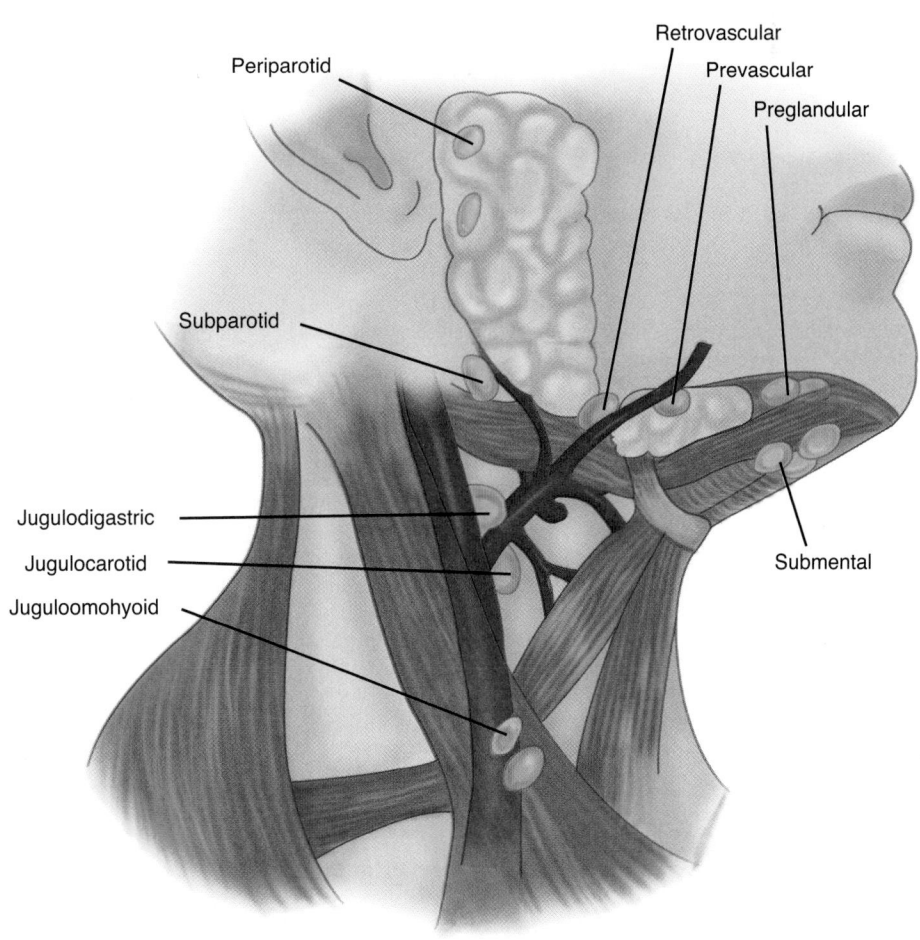

FIG. 18-26. Primary lymphatics for oral cavity lesions.

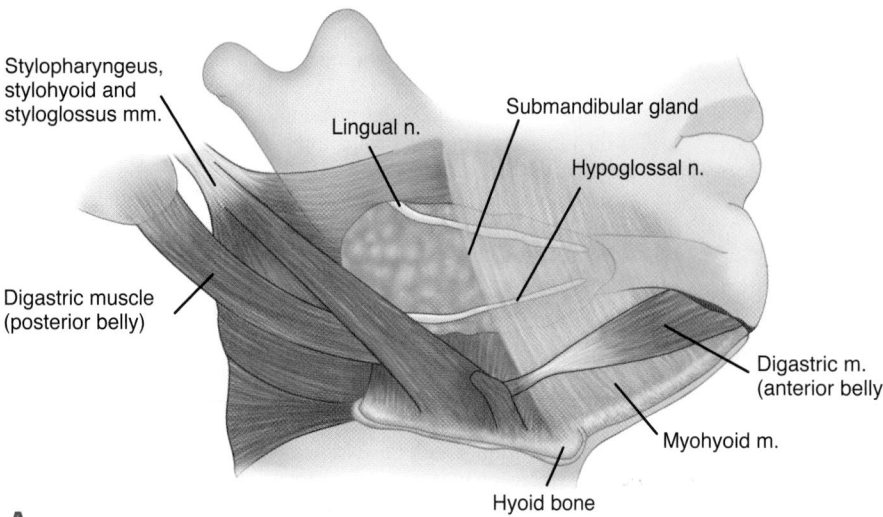

A

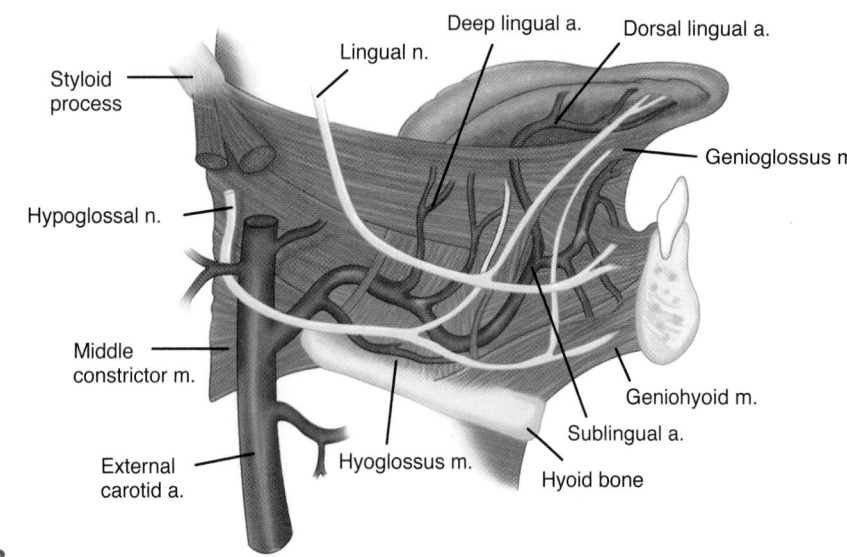

B

FIG. 18-27. **A** and **B.** Anatomy of the floor of mouth and submandibular space. a. = artery; m. = muscle; n. = nerve.

maxillary periosteum, treatment of lesions of the alveolar mucosa frequently requires resection of the underlying bone.

Marginal resection of the mandible can be performed for tumors of the alveolar surface that present with minimal bone invasion. Although access for such a procedure can be performed by using an anterior mandibulotomy (Fig. 18-30), use of transoral and pull-through procedures is preferred if a coronal or sagittal marginal mandibulotomy is performed. For more extensive tumors that invade into the medullary cavity, segmental mandibulectomy is necessary. Preoperative radiographic evaluation of the mandible plays an important role in determining the type of bone resection required. For radiographic evaluation of the mandible, Panorex views demonstrate gross cortical invasion. MRI is the best modality for demonstrating invasion of the medullary cavity of the mandible. Sectional CT scanning with bone settings is the optimum modality for imaging subtle cortical invasion. Gross bony invasion involvement at the mandibular symphysis negatively impacts locoregional control.[51]

Retromolar Trigone

The retromolar trigone is represented by tissue posterior to the posterior inferior alveolar ridge and ascends over the inner surface of the ramus of the mandible. Similar to alveolar lesions, early involve-

ment of the mandible is common because of the lack of intervening soft tissue in the region. The clinical presentation of trismus represents involvement of the muscles of mastication and may indicate spread to the skull base. Tumors of the region may extend posteriorly into the oropharyngeal anatomy or laterally to invade the mandible. As a result, resection of retromolar trigone tumors usually requires a marginal or segmental mandibulectomy with a soft-tissue and/or osseous reconstruction to maximize a patient's postoperative ability for speech and swallowing. Ipsilateral neck dissection is performed because of the risk of metastasis to the regional lymphatics. Huang and associates demonstrated a 5-year, disease-free survival rate for T1 lesions of 76%, which declined to 54% for T4 disease. Patients with N0 disease had a 5-year survival rate of 69%.[52]

Buccal Mucosa

The buccal mucosa includes all of the mucosal lining from the inner surface of the lips to the line of attachment of mucosa of the alveolar ridges and pterygomandibular raphe. The etiologies of malignancies in the buccal area include lichen planus, chronic dental trauma, and the habitual use of tobacco and alcohol. Tumors in this area have a propensity to spread locally and to metastasize to regional lymphatics. Local intraoral spread may necessitate resection of the

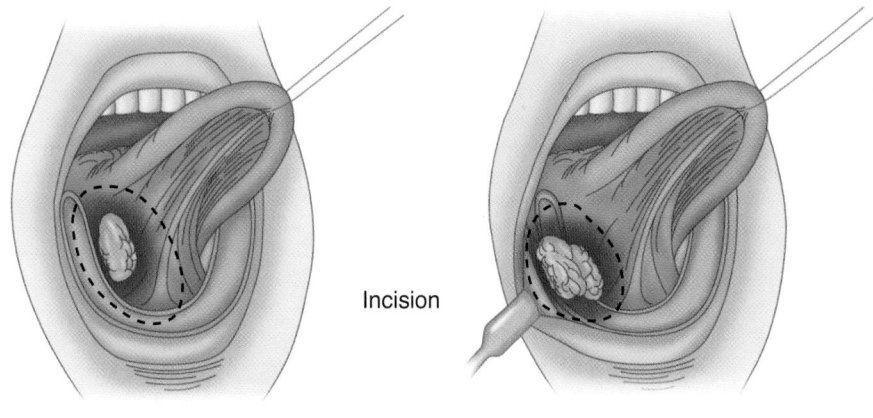

Incision

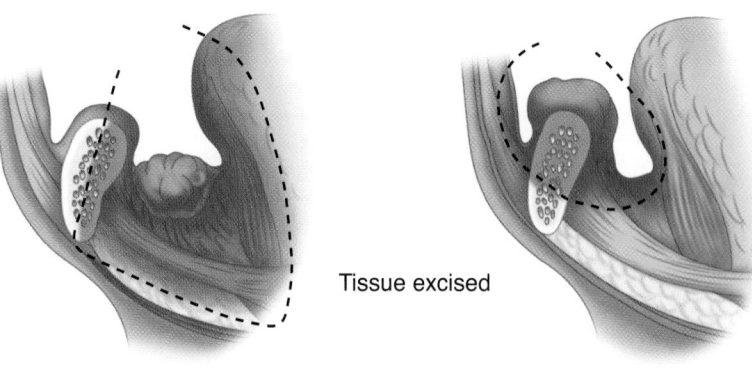

Tissue excised

FIG. 18-28. A and **B.** Differences in the transoral resection of a floor of mouth and alveolar ridge lesion.

A

B

alveolar ridge of the mandible or maxilla. Lymphatic drainage is to the facial and the submandibular nodes (level I). Small lesions can be excised surgically, but more advanced tumors require combined surgery and postoperative radiation.[53] Deep invasion into the cheek may require through-and-through resection. Reconstruction aimed at providing both internal and external lining may be accomplished

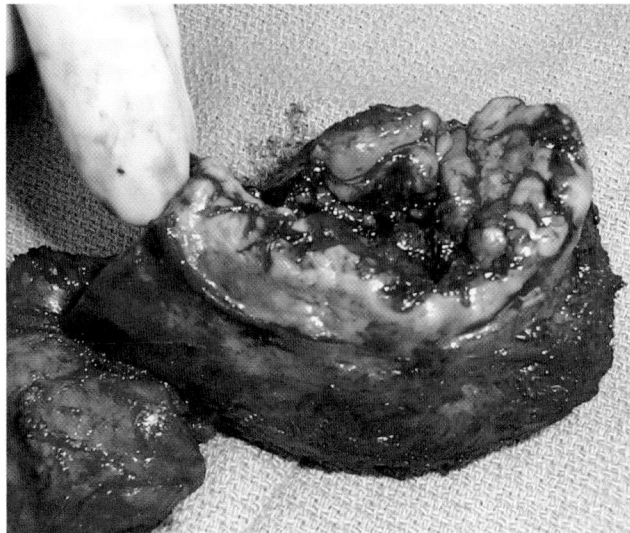

FIG. 18-29. Composite resection specimen of a T4 floor of mouth squamous cell.

with a folded fasciocutaneous free flap or a combination of pedicled and free tissue techniques.

Palate

The hard palate is defined as the semilunar area between the upper alveolar ridge and the mucous membrane covering the palatine process of the maxillary palatine bones. It extends from the inner surface of the superior alveolar ridge to the posterior edge of the palatine bone. Most squamous cell carcinomas of the hard palate are caused by habitual tobacco and alcohol use. Chronic irritation from ill-fitting dentures also may play a causal role. Inflammatory lesions arising on the palate may mimic malignancy and can be differentiated by biopsy. Necrotizing sialometaplasia appears on the palate as a butterfly-shaped ulcer that clinically appears similar to a neoplasm. Treatment is symptomatic and biopsy confirms its benign nature. Torus palatini are bony outgrowths of the midline palate and do not specifically require surgical treatment unless symptomatic.

Squamous cell carcinoma and minor salivary gland tumors are the most common malignancies of the palate.[54] The latter include adenoid cystic carcinoma, mucoepidermoid carcinoma, adenocarcinoma, and polymorphous low-grade adenocarcinoma. Mucosal melanoma may occur on the palate and presents as a nonulcerated, pigmented plaque. Kaposi's sarcoma of the palate is the most common intraoral site for this tumor. Tumors may present as either an ulcerative, exophytic, or submucosal mass. Minor salivary gland tumors tend to arise at the junction of the hard and soft palate. Direct infiltration of bone leads to extension into the floor of the nasal cavity and/or maxillary sinus. Squamous cell carcinoma of the hard palate is treated surgically. Adjuvant radiation is indicated for advanced staged tumors. Because the periosteum of the palate can act as a barrier to spread of tumor, mucosal excision may be adequate for very superfi-

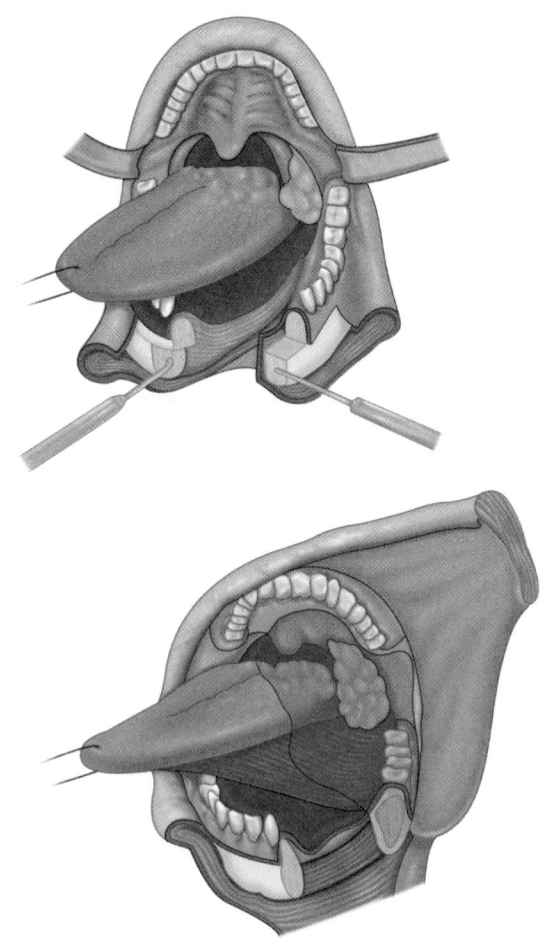

FIG. 18-30. Anterior mandibulotomy with mandibular swing to approach a posterior lesion.

cial lesions. Involvement of the periosteum requires removal of a portion of the bony palate. Partial palatectomy of infrastructure maxillectomy may be required for larger lesions involving the palate or maxillary antrum. Malignancies may extend along the greater palatine nerve making biopsy important for identifying neurotropic spread. Through-and-through defects of the palate require a dental prosthesis for rehabilitation of swallowing and speech.

Oropharynx

The oropharynx extends from the soft palate to the superior surface of the hyoid bone (or floor of the vallecula) and includes the base of tongue, the inferior surface of the soft palate and uvula, the anterior and posterior tonsillar pillars, the glossotonsillar sulci, tonsils, and the lateral and posterior pharyngeal walls. Laterally, the borders of this region are the pharyngeal constrictors and the medial aspect of the mandible. Direct extension of tumors from the oropharynx into these lateral tissues may involve spread into the parapharyngeal space. The ascending ramus of the mandible can be involved when tumors invade the medial pterygoid muscle.

As was true of the oral cavity, the histology of the majority of tumors in this region is squamous cell carcinoma. Although less common, minor salivary gland tumors may present as submucosal masses in the tongue base and soft palate. Additionally, the tonsils and tongue base may be the presenting site for a lymphoma noted clinically as asymmetrical enlargement.

Oropharyngeal cancer may present as an ulcerative lesion or an exophytic mass. Tumor fetor from necrosis is common. A muffled or "hot potato" voice is seen with large tongue base tumors. Dysphagia

and weight loss are common symptoms. Referred otalgia, mediated by the tympanic branches of cranial nerve (CN) IX and CN X, is a common complaint. Trismus may indicate advanced disease and usually results from involvement of the pterygoid musculature. The incidence of regional metastases from cancers of the oropharynx is high. Consequently, ipsilateral or bilateral nontender cervical lymphadenopathy is a common presenting sign.

Imaging studies are important for adequate staging and should assess for extension to the larynx, parapharyngeal space, pterygoid musculature, mandible, and nasopharynx. Lymph node metastasis from oropharyngeal cancer most commonly occurs in the subdigastric area of level II. Metastases also are found in levels III, IV, and V, in addition to the retropharyngeal and parapharyngeal lymph nodes. Approximately one half of patients have metastases at the time of presentation. Bilateral metastases are common from tumors arising in the tongue base and soft palate.[55]

The treatment goals for patients with oropharyngeal cancer include maximizing survival and preserving function. Management of squamous cell cancers of this region includes surgery alone, primary radiation alone, surgery with postoperative radiation, and combined chemotherapy with radiation therapy.[56] Tumors of the oropharynx tend to be radiosensitive.[57] Patients with early stage lesions may be candidates for monomodality radiation alone. Adequate treatment of the neck is important with oropharyngeal squamous cancer because of the high risk of regional metastasis. Concomitant chemoradiation is used in patients with advanced stage (III, IV) oropharyngeal carcinoma.[58] This approach has been effectively demonstrated to preserve function and is associated with survivorship comparable to surgery with postoperative radiation.

Tumors of the soft palate and tonsil extending to the tongue base are associated with poor survival. Extensive oropharyngeal cancers may require surgical resection and postoperative radiotherapy.[59] Lesions that involve the mandible require composite resections, such as the classic jaw-neck resection or "commando" procedure. Surgical management of the tongue base may require total glossectomy for extensive lesions crossing the anatomic midline. The potential need for synchronous performance of total laryngectomy at the time of tongue base resection should be explained to the patient. Preservation of the larynx after total glossectomy is associated with a significant risk of postoperative dysphagia and aspiration.[60]

Swallowing rehabilitation in patients with oropharyngeal carcinoma is an important aspect of posttreatment care. For soft palate defects, palatal obturators may assist in providing a seal between the nasopharynx and the posterior pharyngeal wall.[61] Nasal regurgitation of air and liquids can be decreased with use. Close cooperation between the head and neck surgeon and the maxillofacial prosthodontist is essential to provide patients with the optimum prosthetic rehabilitation. Preoperative planning can result in the creation of a defect that better tolerates obturation. For patients with postglossectomy defects, palatal augmentation prostheses can provide bulk extending inferiorly from the palate. The prosthesis decreases the volume of the oral cavity and allows the remaining tongue or soft tissue to articulate with the palate. It also facilitates posterior projection of the food bolus during the oral and pharyngeal phases of swallowing.

Hypopharynx and Cervical Esophagus

The hypopharynx extends from the vallecula to the lower border of the cricoid cartilage and includes the pyriform sinuses, the lateral and posterior pharyngeal walls, and the postcricoid region (Fig. 18-31). Squamous cancers of the hypopharynx frequently present at an advanced stage. Clinical findings are similar to those of lower oropharyngeal lesions and include a neck mass, muffled or hoarse voice, referred otalgia, dysphagia, and weight loss. A common symptom is dysphagia, starting with solids and progressing to liquids, leaving patients malnourished at the time of presentation. Invasion of the larynx by direct extension can result in vocal cord paralysis and may lead to airway compromise.

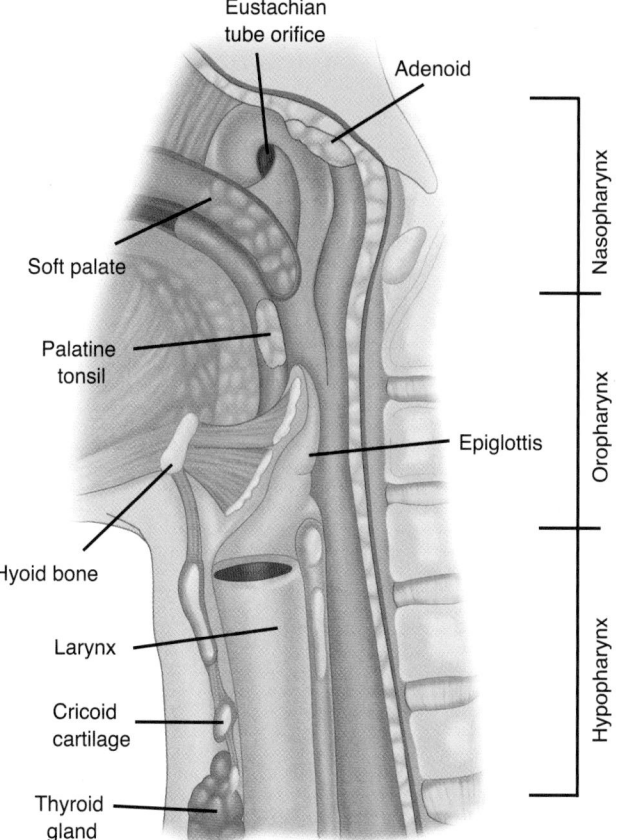

FIG. 18-31. Relationship of nasopharynx, oropharynx, and hypopharynx.

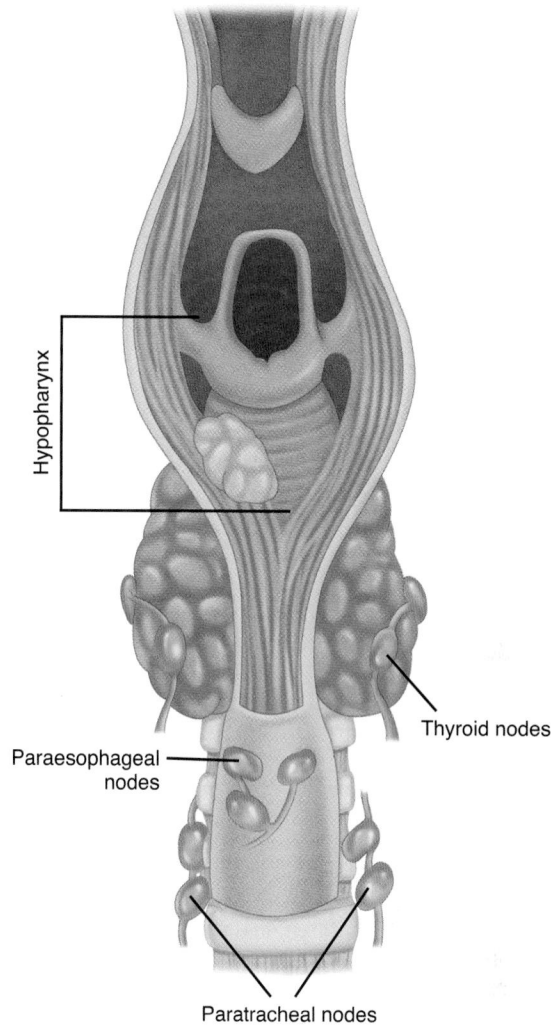

FIG. 18-32. View of the hypopharynx demonstrating the potential pathways of spread of tumor and pertinent anatomy.

Routine office examination should include flexible fiber-optic laryngoscopy to properly assess the extent of tumor. During examination, the patient should be instructed to perform a Valsalva's maneuver, which will result in passive opening of the pyriform sinuses and postcricoid regions, providing improved visualization. Decreased laryngeal mobility or fixation may indicate invasion of the prevertebral fascia and unresectability. Barium swallow can provide information regarding postcricoid and upper esophageal extension, potential multifocality within the esophagus, and document the presence of aspiration. CT and/or MRI imaging should be obtained through the neck and upper chest to assess for invasion of the laryngeal framework and to identify for regional metastases, with special attention given to the paratracheal and upper mediastinal lymph nodes (Fig. 18-32). Bilateral metastatic adenopathy in the paratracheal chain is common and the majority of patients present with nodal disease at the time of diagnosis.

Tumors of the hypopharynx and cervical esophagus are associated with poorer survival rates than are other sites in the head and neck because of advanced stage and lymph node metastasis at presentation. Surgery with postoperative radiation therapy improves locoregional control compared to single-modality therapy in the treatment of advanced stage tumors.[62] Definitive radiation therapy may be effective for limited T1 tumors, whereas concomitant chemoradiation is generally used for T2 and T3 tumors.[63] Surgical salvage after radiation failure has a success rate of less than 50% and can be associated with significant wound-healing complications.

Larynx-preserving surgical procedures for tumors of the hypopharynx are possible for only a limited number of lesions. Tumors of the medial pyriform wall or pharyngoepiglottic fold may be resected with partial laryngopharyngectomy. In this circumstance, the tumor must not involve the apex of the pyriform sinus, vocal cord mobility must be unimpaired, and the patient must have adequate pulmonary reserve. Given the increased risk for postoperative aspiration associated with various forms of partial laryngectomy, a history significant for pulmonary disease is a contraindication for performing the procedures. Because the majority of patients with tumors of the hypopharynx present with large lesions with significant submucosal spread, total laryngectomy often is required to achieve negative resection margins. Resection of the primary tumor and surrounding pharyngeal tissue is performed en bloc. Bilateral neck dissection is frequently indicated given the elevated risk of nodal metastases found with these lesions.

When laryngopharyngectomy is performed for hypopharyngeal tumors the surgical defect is repaired by primary closure when possible. Generally, 4 cm or more of pharyngeal mucosa is necessary for primary closure to provide an adequate lumen for swallowing and to minimize the risk of stricture formation. Larger surgical defects require closure with the aid of pedicled myocutaneous flaps or microvascular reconstruction with radial forearm or jejunal free flap. When total laryngopharyngoesophagectomy is necessary, gastric pull-up is performed.

Cervical esophageal cancer may be managed surgically or by concomitant chemoradiation. Preservation of the larynx is possible if the cricopharyngeus muscle demonstrates limited involvement. Unfortunately, this is not often the case and many patients with cervical esophageal cancer require laryngectomy. Total esophagectomy is performed because of the tendency for multiple primary tumors and skip lesions seen with esophageal cancers.

Despite aggressive treatment strategies, the 5-year survival rate for cervical esophageal cancer is less than 20%. Given the presence of paratracheal lymphatic spread, surgical treatment for tumors of this area must include paratracheal lymph node dissection, in addition to treatment of the lateral cervical lymphatics.

Larynx

Laryngeal carcinoma is a diagnosis typically entertained in individuals with prominent smoking histories and the complaint of a change in vocal quality (Fig. 18-33). The borders of the larynx span from the epiglottis superiorly to the cricoid cartilage inferiorly. The lateral limits of the larynx are the aryepiglottic folds. The larynx is composed of three regions: the supraglottis, the glottis, and the subglottis (Fig. 18-34).

The supraglottis includes the epiglottis, aryepiglottic folds, arytenoids, and ventricular bands (false vocal folds). The inferior boundary of the supraglottis is a horizontal plane passing through the lateral margin of the ventricle. The glottis is composed of the true vocal cords (superior and inferior surfaces) and includes the anterior and posterior commissures. The subglottis extends from the inferior surface of the glottis to the lower margin of the cricoid cartilage. The soft-tissue compartments of the larynx are separated by fibroelastic membranes, which can act as barriers to the spread of cancer. These membranes thicken medially to form the false vocal fold and the vocal ligament (the true vocal cord).

The supraglottic larynx contains pseudostratified, ciliated respiratory epithelium that covers the false vocal cords. The epiglottis and the vocal cords are lined by stratified, nonkeratinizing squamous epithelium. The subglottic mucosa is pseudostratified, ciliated respiratory epithelium. Minor salivary glands are also found in the supraglottis and subglottis. Tumor types that arise in the larynx are primarily squamous cell carcinoma but also include tumors of neuroendocrine origin, squamous papillomas, granular cell tumors, and tumors of salivary origin. Several histologic variants of squamous cell carcinoma exist and include verrucous, basaloid squamous cell, adenosquamous, and spindle cell carcinoma. Tumors of the laryngeal framework include synovial sarcoma, chondroma, and chondrosarcoma.

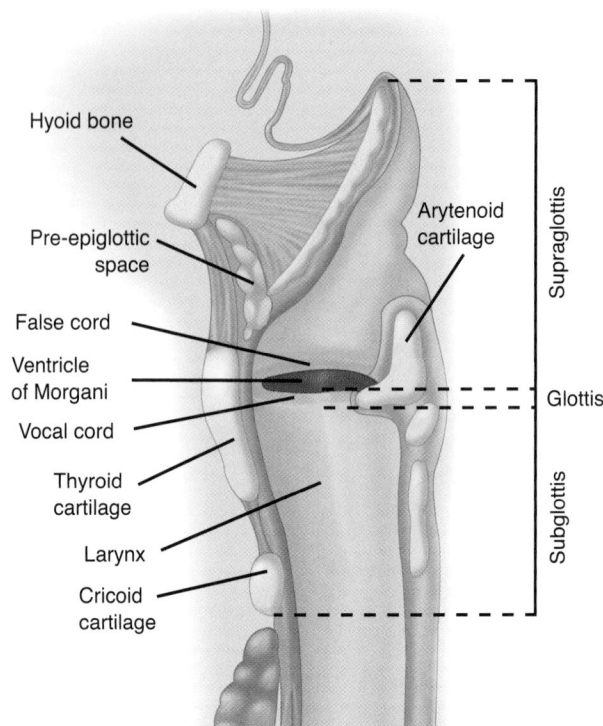

FIG. 18-34. Sagittal view of the larynx with the divisions of the supraglottis, glottis, and subglottis demonstrated.

The normal functions of the larynx are airway patency, protection of the tracheobronchial tree during swallowing, and phonation. Patients with tumors of the supraglottic larynx may present with symptoms of chronic sore throat, dysphonia ("hot potato" voice), dysphagia, or a neck mass secondary to regional metastasis. Supraglottic tumors may cause vocal cord fixation by inferior extension in the paraglottic space or direct invasion of the cricoarytenoid joint. Anterior extension of tumors arising on the laryngeal surface of the epiglottis into the pre-epiglottic space produces a muffled quality to the voice. Referred otalgia or odynophagia is encountered with advanced supraglottic cancers. Bulky tumors of the supraglottis may result in airway compromise. In contrast to most supraglottic lesions, hoarseness is an early symptom in patients with tumors of the glottis.[64] Airway obstruction from a glottic tumor is usually a late symptom and is the result of tumor bulk or impaired vocal cord mobility. Decreased vocal cord mobility may be caused by direct muscle invasion or involvement of the RLN. Fixation of the vocal cord indicates invasion into the vocalis muscle, paraglottic space, or cricoarytenoid joint. Superficial tumors that are bulky may appear to cause cord fixation through mass effect. Subglottic cancers are relatively uncommon and typically present with vocal cord paralysis (usually unilateral) and/or airway compromise.

The staging classification for squamous cell cancers of the larynx includes assessment of vocal cord mobility as well as local tumor extension. Accurate clinical staging of laryngeal tumors requires flexible fiber-optic endoscopy in the office and direct microlaryngoscopy under general anesthesia. Direct laryngoscopy, used to assess the extent of local spread, may be combined with esophagoscopy or bronchoscopy to adequately stage the primary tumor and to exclude the presence of a synchronous lesion. Key areas to note for tumor extension in supraglottic tumors are the vallecula, base of tongue, ventricle, arytenoid, and anterior commissure. For glottic cancers, it is important to determine extension to the false cords, anterior commissure, arytenoid, and subglottis.

Radiographic imaging by CT and/or MRI provides important staging information and is crucial for identifying cartilage erosion or

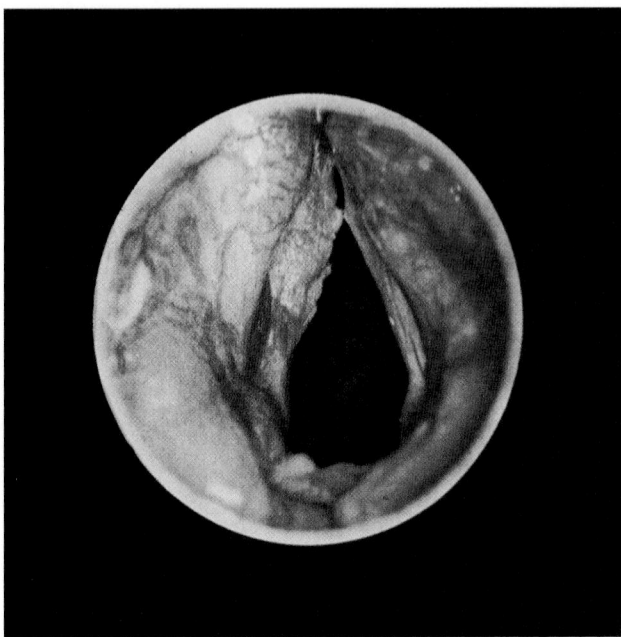

FIG. 18-33. Endoscopic view of a laryngeal squamous carcinoma.

invasion and extension into the pre-epiglottic or paraglottic spaces. High quality, thin-section images through the larynx should be obtained in patients with laryngeal tumors and used with clinical assessment to arrive at a final disease pretreatment staging. Lymph node metastasis may be defined more readily with the use of imaging studies.

Lymphatic drainage of the larynx is distinct for each subsite. Two major groups of laryngeal lymphatic pathways exist: those that drain areas superior to the ventricle, and those that drain areas inferior to it. Supraglottic drainage routes pierce the thyrohyoid membrane with the superior laryngeal artery, vein, and nerve, and drain mainly to the subdigastric and superior jugular nodes.[64] Those from the glottic and subglottic areas exit via the cricothyroid ligament and end in the prelaryngeal node (the Delphian node), the paratracheal nodes, and the deep cervical nodes along the inferior thyroid artery. Limited glottic cancers typically do not spread to regional lymphatics (1 to 4%). However, there is a high incidence of lymphatic spread from supraglottic (30 to 50%) and subglottic cancers (40%).

When considering treatment for laryngeal tumors, it is useful to categorize them as a continuum from early tumors (those with a small area of involvement resulting in minimal functional impairment) to advanced tumors (those with significant airway compromise and local extension). For example, severe dysplasia and carcinoma in situ often can be treated successfully with CO_2 laser resection or conservative surgical approaches. In contrast, more advanced tumors may require partial laryngectomy[65] (Fig. 18-35) or even total laryngectomy (Fig. 18-36). Further complicating the treatment paradigm is the role of radiotherapy, with or without chemotherapy, with the goal of laryngeal preservation.[66]

Prognostic factors for patients with cancer of the larynx are tumor size, nodal metastasis, perineural invasion, and extracapsular spread of disease in cervical lymph nodes. Patient comorbidities are important to consider when arriving at a treatment plan for patients with laryngeal cancer.

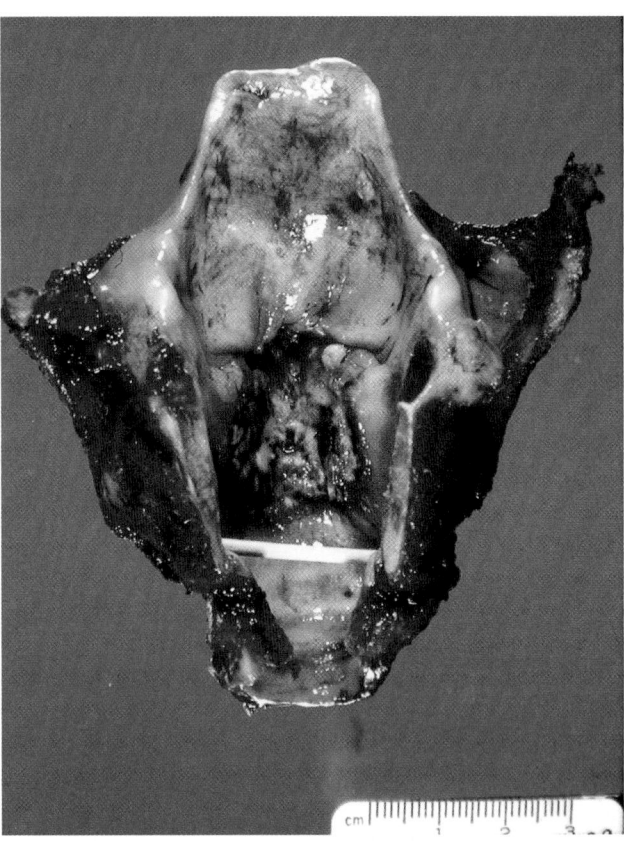

FIG. 18-36. Total laryngectomy specimen featuring a glottic squamous carcinoma.

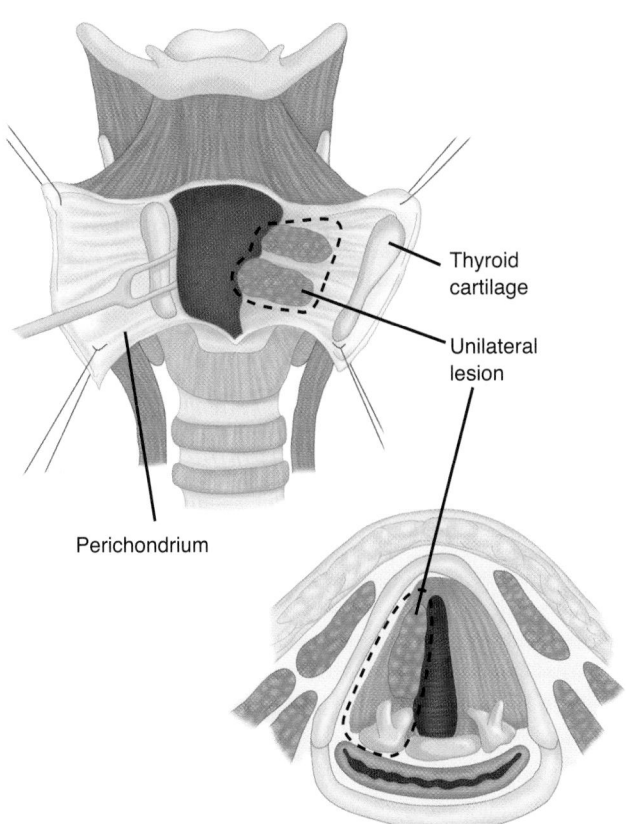

FIG. 18-35. Example of the resection of a vertical partial laryngectomy for an early stage glottic carcinoma.

For severe dysplasia or carcinoma in situ of the vocal cord, complete removal of the involved mucosa with microlaryngoscopy is an effective treatment. Patients with limited involvement of the arytenoid or anterior commissure are the best candidates for a good posttreatment vocal quality result with this approach. Multiple procedures may be necessary to control the disease and to prevent progression to an invasive cancer. Close follow-up examinations and smoking cessation are mandatory adjuncts of therapy. For early stage cancers of the glottis and the supraglottis, radiation therapy is equally as effective as surgery in controlling disease.

Critical factors in determining the appropriate treatment modality are comorbid conditions (chronic obstructive pulmonary disease, cardiovascular, and renal disease) and tumor extension. Voice preservation and maintenance of quality of life are key issues and significantly impact therapeutic decisions. The use of radiation therapy for early stage disease of the glottis and supraglottis provides excellent disease control with reasonable, if not excellent, preservation of vocal quality. Partial laryngectomy for small glottic cancers provides excellent tumor control, but vocal quality can vary. For supraglottic cancers without arytenoid or vocal cord extension, standard supraglottic laryngectomy results in excellent disease control with good voice function. For advanced tumors with extension beyond the endolarynx or with cartilage destruction, total laryngectomy followed by postoperative radiation is still considered the standard of care.[67] In this setting, reconstruction by means of a pectoralis major flap (Fig. 18-37) or free flap reconstruction is required for lesions with pharyngeal extension.

Subglottic cancers, constituting only 1% of laryngeal tumors, are typically treated with total laryngectomy. Because these tumors present with adenopathy in 40% of patients, special attention must be given to the treatment of paratracheal lymph nodes.[68]

Laryngeal Preservation Techniques

Superficial cancers confined to the true vocal cord can be treated with a variety of surgical options. These include endoscopic vocal

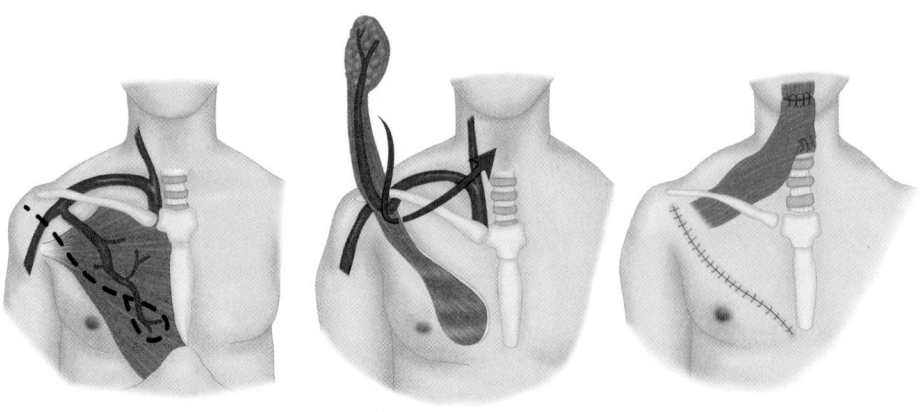

FIG. 18-37. Pectoralis flap reconstruction of a laryngectomy patient requires soft-tissue augmentation for pharynx closure.

cord stripping, microflap dissection, partial cordectomy, and CO_2 laser resection. Although using a CO_2 laser can provide excellent hemostasis and minimize damage to the adjacent uninvolved tissue, scarring associated with its use is considered more significant than with conventional "cold" techniques. Microflap dissection, using a subepithelial infusion of a saline-epinephrine solution into Reinke's space, allows for assessment of depth of invasion and the ability to resect the lesion as a single unit. Use of an operative microscope aids the precision of such dissections. Open laryngofissure and cordectomy may be reserved for more invasive tumors.

For larger tumors of the glottis with impaired vocal cord mobility, a variety of partial resections exist that permit preservation of reasonable vocal quality. For lesions involving the anterior commissure with limited subglottic extension, an anterofrontal partial laryngectomy is indicated. For lateralized T2 or T3 glottic tumors without cartilage destruction, a vertical partial laryngectomy is feasible. In this circumstance, reconstruction is accomplished by means of a false vocal cord imbrication to simulate a true vocal cord on the side of the resection.

For T3 glottic lesions not involving the pre-epiglottic space or cricoarytenoid joint, a supracricoid laryngectomy with cricohyoidopexy or cricohyoidoepiglottopexy (CHEP) are options.[65] The supracricoid laryngectomy technique uses the remaining arytenoids as the phonatory structures, which come into apposition with epiglottic remnant in the CHEP, or with the tongue base in the cricohyoidopexy. Oncologic advantages of this procedure include the complete removal of the paraglottic spaces and thyroid cartilage. The supracricoid laryngectomy with CHEP is associated with excellent disease control and a high rate of tracheostomy decannulation. Favorable deglutition rates and a breathy vocal quality are seen postoperatively with this procedure. For lesions with involvement of the cricoarytenoid joint and/or extension to the level of the cricoid, total laryngectomy is required.

The risk for aspiration is high following certain partial laryngectomies. Patient selection is vital to successful application of these techniques. Presurgical pulmonary assessment may be necessary. One simple measurement of functional reserve is to have the patient climb two flights of stairs. Those able to do so without stopping are more likely to be candidates for conservation surgical procedures. For patients that are not candidates for partial laryngectomy, total laryngectomy is considered the best surgical option for locoregional control. Total laryngectomy may also be the preferred treatment for those patients who are noncompliant, given the importance of postoperative follow-up and monitoring for recurrence.

The approach to the treatment for patients with advanced tumors of the larynx and hypopharynx has evolved over time. Chemoradiation has demonstrated the ability for comparable locoregional disease control and overall survival similar to open surgical approaches. The Radiation Therapy Oncology Group 91-11 trial demonstrated a higher laryngeal preservation rate among patients receiving concomitant chemotherapy and radiotherapy than in those patients receiving radiation alone or sequential chemotherapy followed by radiation therapy.[69] A randomized laryngeal preservation trial of neoadjuvant induction chemotherapy followed by radiation therapy has yielded survival rates similar to those of laryngectomy, with the benefit of preservation of the larynx in 65% of patients.[66] Surgical salvage is available in cases of treatment failure or recurrent disease.

Speech and Swallowing Rehabilitation

Involvement of a speech and swallowing therapist is critical in the preoperative counseling and postoperative rehabilitation of patients with laryngeal cancer. Speech rehabilitation options after total laryngectomy include esophageal speech, tracheoesophageal puncture, and use of an electrolarynx. Esophageal speech is produced by actively swallowing and releasing air from the esophagus resulting in vibrations of the esophageal walls and pharynx. The sounds produced can be articulated into words. The ability to create esophageal speech depends on the motivation of patients and their ability to control the upper esophageal sphincter, allowing injection and expulsion of air in a controlled fashion. Unfortunately, less than 20% of postlaryngectomy patients develop fluent esophageal speech.

A tracheoesophageal puncture is a fistula created between the trachea and esophagus that permits placement of a one-way valve that allows air from the trachea to enter the upper esophagus. The valve prevents retrograde passage of food or saliva into the trachea. Patients that undergo placement of a tracheoesophageal puncture have a success rate of greater than 80% in achieving functional speech.

For patients unable to develop esophageal speech, the electrolarynx creates vibratory sound waves when held against the neck or cheek. The vibrations create sound waves that the patient articulates into words. A disadvantage of the electrolarynx is the mechanical quality of the sound produced. This device is most useful in the postoperative period before training for esophageal speech.

Postoperative swallowing rehabilitation is another important task performed by the speech and swallowing team. Patient instruction in various swallowing techniques and evaluation for the appropriate diet consistency allow a patient to initiate oral intake of nutrition while minimizing the risk of aspirating. Flexible fiberoptic laryngoscopy can be performed transnasally and provides valuable information to assist in the assessment of dysphagia. The oral intake of various consistencies of liquids and solids can be observed with endoscopic assessment of laryngeal penetrance. A similar assessment may be performed with a modified barium swallow allowing the analysis of the various phases of swallowing.

Unknown Primary Tumors

When patients present with cervical nodal metastases without clinical or radiologic evidence of an upper aerodigestive tract primary tumor, they are referred to as having an unknown primary. Given the difficulty in performing a detailed examination in the clinical setting of the base of tongue, the tonsillar fossa, and the nasopharynx, examination under anesthesia with directed tissue biopsies has been advocated. Ipsilateral tonsillectomy, direct laryngoscopy with base of tongue and pyriform biopsies, examination of the nasopharynx, and bimanual examination can allow for identification of a primary site in a portion of patients previously considered to have an unknown primary. In those individuals in whom a primary site cannot be ascertained, empiric treatment of the mucosal sources of the upper aerodigestive tract at risk (from nasopharynx to hypopharynx) and the cervical lymphatics with concomitant chemoradiation is advocated. For patients with advanced neck disease (N2a or greater) or with persistent lymphadenopathy after radiation, a postradiation neck dissection may be necessary. For patients in whom the primary lesion is identified, a more limited radiation treatment field may be used.

Nose and Paranasal Sinuses

The nose and paranasal sinuses are the sites of a great deal of infectious and inflammatory pathology. The diagnosis of tumors within this region is frequently made after a patient has been unsuccessfully treated for recurrent sinusitis and undergoes diagnostic imaging. Symptoms associated with sinonasal tumors are subtle and insidious. They include chronic nasal obstruction, facial pain, headache, epistaxis, and facial numbness. As such, tumors of the paranasal sinuses frequently present at an advanced stage. Orbital invasion can result in proptosis, diplopia, epiphora, and vision loss. Paresthesia within the distribution of CN V2 is suggestive of pterygopalatine fossa or skull base invasion and is generally a poor prognostic factor. Maxillary sinus tumors can present with loose dentition indicating erosion of the alveolar and/or palatal bones. Tumors found to arise posterior to Ohngren's line are associated with a worse prognosis than are more anteriorly based lesions (Fig. 18-38).[70]

A variety of benign tumors arise in the nasal cavity and paranasal sinuses and include inverted papillomas, hemangiomas, hemangiopericytomas, angiofibromas, minor salivary tumors, and benign fibrous histiocytomas. Fibro-osseous and osseous lesions, such as fibrous dysplasias, ossifying fibromas, osteomas, and myxomas, can also arise in this region. Additionally, herniation of intracranial con-

tents into the nasal cavity can occur with the erosion of the anterior skull base with the resultant presentation of a sinonasal mass on clinical examination.

Malignant tumors of the sinuses are predominantly squamous cell carcinomas. Sinonasal undifferentiated carcinoma,[71] adenocarcinoma, mucosal melanoma, lymphoma, olfactory neuroblastoma, rhabdomyosarcoma, and angiosarcoma are some of the other malignancies that have been described. Metastases from the kidney, breast, lung, and thyroid may also present as an intranasal mass. Regional metastasis is uncommon with tumors of the paranasal sinuses (14 to 16%) and occurs in the parapharyngeal, retropharyngeal, and subdigastric nodes of the jugular chain.

The diagnosis of an intranasal mass is made with the assistance of a headlight and nasal speculum or nasal endoscopy. The site of origin, involved bony structures, and the presence of vascularity should be assessed. For paranasal sinus tumors, MRI and CT scanning often are complementary studies in determining orbital and intracranial extension.[72] Benign processes frequently present as slow-growing expansile tumors with limited erosion of surrounding bone, as compared to the lytic destruction typically associated with malignancies. Skull base foramen should be closely examined for enlargement that may be suggestive of perineural invasion. Examination for cavernous sinus extension, cribriform plate erosion, and dural enhancement is necessary to assess for resectability and the type of surgical approach that is possible. A meningocele or encephalocele will present as a unilateral pulsatile mass. Biopsy of a unilateral nasal mass should be deferred until imaging studies are obtained. Untimely biopsy can result in a CSF leak. If hypervascularity is suspected, biopsy should be performed under controlled conditions in the operating room.

The standard treatment for malignant tumors of the paranasal sinuses is surgical resection with postoperative radiation therapy. Tumors arising along the medial wall of the maxillary sinus may be treated by means of a medial maxillectomy. The treatment of advanced tumors of the paranasal sinuses frequently involves a multispecialty approach. Members of this team include the head and neck surgeon, neurosurgeon, prosthodontist, ophthalmologist, and reconstructive surgeon. Each team member is necessary to facilitate the goal of safe and complete tumor removal. For vascular tumors, preoperative embolization performed within 24 hours of the planned surgical resection may reduce intraoperative hemorrhage.

Prognosis is dependent on tumor location and extension to the surrounding anatomy. Infrastructure maxillectomy, which includes removal of the hard palate and the lower maxillary sinus, is necessary for inferiorly based tumors of the maxillary sinus. For tumors in the upper portion of the maxillary sinus, complete maxillectomy (including removal of the orbital floor) is performed. If there is invasion of the orbital fat, exenteration of the orbital contents is required. Removal of the bony floor of the orbit and preservation of the globe are possible where there is absence of invasion through the orbital periosteum. However, reconstruction of the orbital floor to recreate a stable support for the orbital contents is essential. Removal of anterior cheek skin is indicated when there is tumor extension into the overlying subcutaneous fat and dermis.

For tumors involving the ethmoid sinuses, the integrity of the cribriform plate is assessed with preoperative imaging. Complete sphenoethmoidectomy or medial maxillectomy may suffice if the tumor is localized to the lateral nasal wall. Endoscopic resection with the assistance of image-guidance technology is gaining increasing acceptance for low-grade resectable lesions such as inverted papilloma.

If erosion of the cribriform has occurred, an anterior craniofacial resection is the standard operative approach. The head and neck surgeon and neurosurgeon work in concert to perform this procedure. The neurosurgeon performs a frontal craniotomy for exposure of the anterior cranial fossa floor, whereas the head and neck surgeon proceeds through a transfacial or endoscopic approach to resect the inferior bony attachments. Paranasal sinus malignancies that are deemed unresectable are those with bilateral optic nerve

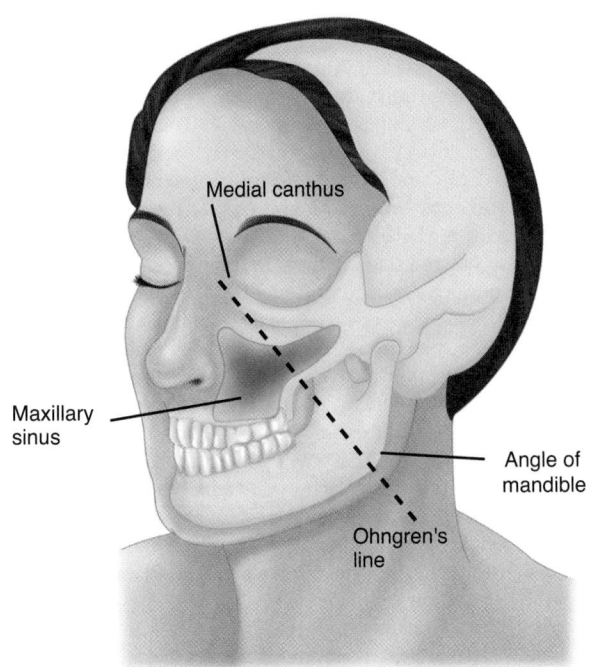

FIG. 18-38. Example of the Ohngren's line and the relationship to the maxilla.

Medial canthus

Maxillary sinus

Angle of mandible

Ohngren's line

involvement, massive brain invasion, or carotid encasement.[73] Post-operative rehabilitation after orbital exenteration is accomplished by soft-tissue reconstruction and placement of a maxillofacial prosthesis. Combined treatment with surgery and postoperative radiotherapy for squamous cell carcinoma of the sinuses results in survival superior to either radiation or surgery alone. Chemotherapy has a limited application and may be used for specific indications. Rhabdomyosarcoma is primarily treated with chemotherapy followed by radiation therapy. Surgery is reserved for persistent disease after chemoradiation. Sinonasal undifferentiated carcinoma is highly aggressive and typically is not adequately controlled with standard therapy. Chemotherapy in this setting may help to reduce the tumor bulk and allow for orbital preservation.

Nasopharynx

The nasopharynx extends in a plane superior to the hard palate from the choana, to the posterior nasal cavity, to the posterior pharyngeal wall. It includes the fossa of Rosenmüller, the eustachian tube orifices (torus tubarius), and the site of the adenoid pad. Tumors arising in the nasopharynx are usually of squamous cell origin and range from lymphoepithelioma to well-differentiated carcinoma. However, the differential diagnosis for nasopharyngeal tumors is broad and also includes lymphoma, chordoma, chondroma, nasopharyngeal cyst (Tornwaldt's cyst), angiofibroma, minor salivary gland tumor, paraganglioma, rhabdomyosarcoma, extramedullary plasmacytoma, and sarcoma.

Risk factors for nasopharyngeal carcinoma include area of habitation, ethnicity, and tobacco use. There is an increased incidence of nasopharyngeal cancer in southern China, Africa, Alaska, and in Greenland Eskimos. A strong correlation exists between nasopharyngeal cancer and the presence of EBV infection, such that EBV titers may be used as a means to follow a patient's response to treatment.

Symptoms associated with nasopharyngeal tumors include nasal obstruction, posterior (level V) neck mass, epistaxis, headache, serous otitis media with hearing loss, and otalgia. Cranial nerve involvement is indicative of skull base extension and advanced disease. Lymphatic spread occurs to the posterior cervical, upper jugular, and retropharyngeal nodes. Bilateral regional metastatic spread is common. Distant metastasis is present in 5% of patients at presentation.

Examination of the nasopharynx is facilitated by the use of the flexible or rigid fiber-optic endoscope. Evaluation with imaging studies is important for staging and treatment planning. CT with contrast is used for determining bone destruction, while MRI is used to assess for intracranial and soft-tissue extension. Erosion or enlargement of neural foramina (on CT imaging) or enhancement of cranial nerves (on MRI) is indicative of perineural spread of disease and portends a worse prognosis. The status of the cavernous sinus and optic chiasm should also be assessed. The standard treatment for nasopharyngeal carcinoma is chemoradiation. Combination therapy produces superior survival rates for nasopharyngeal carcinoma in comparison to radiation alone.[74] Intracavitary radiation boost with implants to the tumor may be included as an adjunct to external beam radiotherapy to improve local control of advanced tumors. Surgical treatment for nasopharyngeal carcinoma is rarely feasible, but may be considered in selected cases as salvage therapy for patients with localized recurrences.

For minor salivary gland and low-grade tumors of the nasopharynx, resection can be performed via a variety of approaches. Lateral rhinotomy or midface degloving approaches can provide good access for removal of tumors in the posterior nasal cavity extending into the nasopharynx. Endoscopic removal is also possible in selected cases. A variety of surgical approaches also exist for more posteriorly located tumors extending to the sphenoid and clivus. Transpalatal approaches used in combination with transmaxillary and transcervical routes can provide good surgical access in addition to providing adequate control of the carotid artery. The emergence of endoscopic techniques has provided a significant advancement in the surgical management of lesions in these two sites.

Ear and Temporal Bone

Tumors of the ear and temporal bone are uncommon and account for less than 1% of all head and neck malignancies. Primary sites include the external ear (pinna), EAC, middle ear, mastoid, or petrous portion of the temporal bone. The most common histology is squamous cell carcinoma. Minor salivary gland tumors, including adenoid cystic carcinoma and adenocarcinoma, may also present in this region. The pinna, because of its exposure to ultraviolet light, is a common site for basal cell and squamous cell carcinoma to arise. Direct extension of tumors from the parotid gland and periauricular skin may occur in this region. Metastases from distant sites occur primarily to the petrous bone and arise in the breast, kidney, lung, and prostate. In the pediatric population, tumors of the temporal bone are most commonly soft-tissue sarcomas. For advanced stage tumors with extensive temporal bone extension, the complex anatomy of the temporal bone makes removal of tumors with functional preservation challenging.

The diagnosis of tumors of the ear and temporal bone is frequently delayed because the initial presentation of these patients is mistaken for benign infectious disease. When patients fail to improve with conservative care and symptoms evolve to potentially include facial nerve paralysis or worsening hearing loss, the need for imaging and biopsy become obvious. Granulation tissue in the EAC or middle ear should be biopsied in patients with atypical presentations or histories consistent with chronic otologic disease.[75] The complexity of the temporal bone anatomy makes the use of imaging studies of paramount importance in the staging and treatment of tumors in this region.

Small skin cancers on the helix of the ear can be readily treated with simple excision and primary closure. Mohs' microsurgery with frozen section margin control also can be used for cancer of the external ear. In lesions that are recurrent or invade the underlying perichondrium and cartilage, rapid spread through tissue planes can occur. Tumors may extend from the cartilaginous external canal to the bony canal and invade the parotid, temporomandibular joint, and skull base. For extensive, pinna-based lesions, procedures such as auriculectomy may be required. Postoperative radiation therapy may be required for advanced skin cancer with positive margins, perineural spread, or multiple involved lymph nodes.

Tumors involving the EAC and middle ear may present with persistent otorrhea, otalgia, EAC or periauricular mass, hearing loss, and facial nerve weakness or paralysis. The patient resembles the presentation of an external otitis unresponsive to standard medical therapy. Sleeve resections are reserved for small superficial tumors involving the cartilaginous external canal. Tumors involving the petrous apex or intracranial structures may present with headache and palsies of CN V and VI. The optimal treatment for tumors of the middle ear and bony external canal is en bloc resection followed by radiation therapy. Management of the regional lymphatics is determined by the site and stage of the tumor at presentation. Temporal bone resections are classified as lateral or subtotal (Fig. 18-39). The lateral temporal bone resection removes the bony and cartilaginous canal, tympanic membrane, and ossicles. The subtotal temporal bone resection includes the removal of the ear canal, middle ear, inner ear, and facial nerve. It is indicated for malignant tumors extending into the middle ear.

Postoperative radiation therapy in the treatment of malignancies of the temporal bone usually is indicated and improves local control over surgery alone. Five-year survival rates are approximately 50% for patients with tumors confined to the external canal and decrease with medial tumor extension. Prognosis is poor when tumor involves the petrous apex.[76]

The purpose of reconstruction after temporal bone resection is to provide vascularized tissue and bulk to the site of resection. Prevention of CSF leak by watertight dural closure and prevention of meningitis are important goals of repair. Additionally, the reconstruction enables protection of vascular structures and the surrounding bone to prepare the patient for postoperative radiation

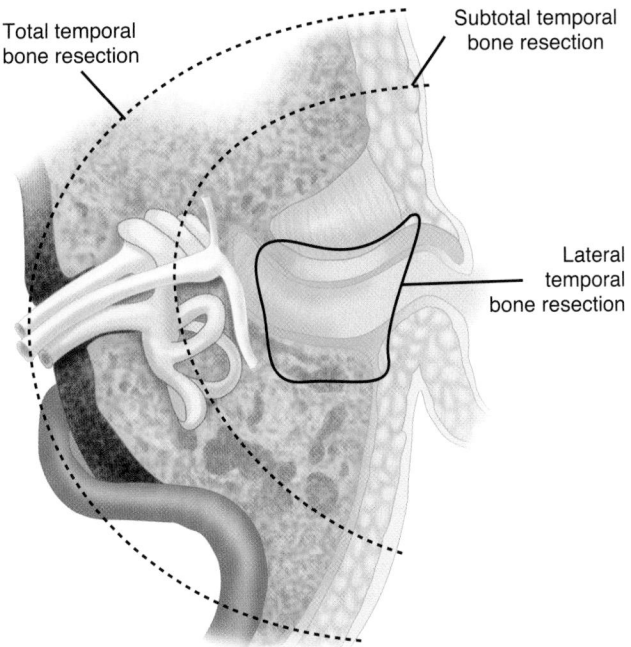

FIG. 18-39. Examples of resection specimens for lateral temporal bone resection, subtotal temporal bone resection, and total temporal bone resection.

therapy. Commonly used reconstruction methods are regional pedicle myocutaneous flaps (e.g., pectoralis major) and free flaps (rectus abdominis, radial forearm, or latissimus dorsi). The loss of the pinna produces significant external deformity; however, a prosthetic ear may produce acceptable rehabilitation. When the facial nerve is sacrificed, rehabilitation is necessary and includes the use of interposition nerve grafts, hypoglossal to facial nerve anastomosis, and static or dynamic sling techniques. In patients with poor eye closure, taping of the eyelids and the liberal use of eye lubrication can prevent exposure keratitis. Additionally, tarsorrhaphy, lid-shortening procedures, and the use of gold weight implants can provide upper eyelid closure and protect the cornea.

Neck

The diagnostic evaluation of a neck mass requires a planned approach that does not compromise the effectiveness of future treatment options. A neck mass in a 50-year-old smoker/drinker with a synchronous oral ulcer is different from cystic neck mass in an 18-year-old that enlarges with an upper respiratory infection. As with all diagnoses, a complete history with full head and neck exam, including flexible laryngoscopy, are critical to complete evaluation. The differential diagnosis of a neck mass is dependent on its location and the patient's age. In children, most neck masses are inflammatory or congenital. However, in the adult population, a neck mass greater than 2 cm in diameter has a greater than 80% probability of being malignant. Once the physician has developed a differential diagnosis, interventions to confirm or dispute diagnoses are initiated. Fine-needle aspiration (FNA), with or without the assistance of ultrasound or CT guidance, can provide valuable information for early treatment planning. The use of imaging (CT and/or MRI) is dictated by the patient's clinical presentation. Imaging enables the physician to evaluate the anatomic relationships of the mass to the surrounding anatomy of the neck and sharpen the differential. A cystic lesion may represent benign pathology such as a branchial cleft cyst; however, it may also represent a regional metastasis of a tonsil/base of tongue squamous cell carcinoma or a papillary thyroid carcinoma. In this circumstance, evaluation of these potential primary sites can alter the planned operative intervention.

If a variety of diagnoses are still being entertained after FNA and imaging, an open biopsy may be necessary. For patients with the potential diagnosis of lymphoma, a biopsy sacrificing normal anatomical structures is not necessary. Ensuring appropriate processing of biopsied materials, sent in saline or in formalin, and sparing undue trauma to tissues can decrease the need for rebiopsy. Appropriate placement of the incision for an open biopsy should be considered if the need for neck dissection or composite resection is later required.

Patterns of Lymph Node Metastasis

The regional lymphatic drainage of the neck is divided into seven levels. These levels allow for a standardized format for radiologists, surgeons, pathologists, and radiation oncologists to communicate concerning specific sites within the neck (Fig. 18-40). The levels are defined as the following:

Level I—the submental and submandibular nodes
Level Ia—the submental nodes; medial to the anterior belly of the digastric muscle bilaterally, symphysis of mandible superiorly, and hyoid inferiorly
Level Ib—the submandibular nodes and gland; posterior to the anterior belly of digastric, anterior to the posterior belly of digastric, and inferior to the body of the mandible
Level II—upper jugular chain nodes
Level IIa—jugulodigastric nodes; deep to sternocleidomastoid (SCM) muscle, anterior to the posterior border of the muscle, posterior to the posterior aspect of the posterior belly of digastric, superior to the level of the hyoid, inferior to spinal accessory nerve (CN XI)
Level IIb—submuscular recess; superior to spinal accessory nerve to the level of the skull base
Level III—middle jugular chain nodes; inferior to the hyoid, superior to the level of the cricoid, deep to SCM muscle from posterior border of the muscle to the strap muscles medially
Level IV—lower jugular chain nodes; inferior to the level of the cricoid, superior to the clavicle, deep to SCM muscle from posterior border of the muscle to the strap muscles medially
Level V—posterior triangle nodes
Level Va—lateral to the posterior aspect of the SCM muscle, inferior and medial to splenius capitis and trapezius, superior to the spinal accessory nerve

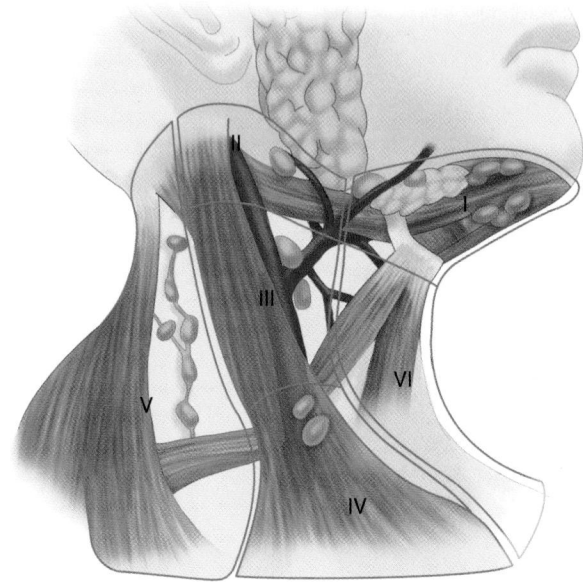

FIG. 18-40. Levels of the neck denoting lymph node bearing regions.

Level Vb—lateral to the posterior aspect of SCM muscle, medial to trapezius, inferior to the spinal accessory nerve, superior to the clavicle

Level VI—anterior compartment nodes; inferior to the hyoid, superior to suprasternal notch, medial to the lateral extent of the strap muscles bilaterally

Level VII—paratracheal nodes; inferior to the suprasternal notch in the upper mediastinum

Patterns of spread from primary tumor sites in the head and neck to cervical lymphatics are well described.[77] The location and incidence of metastasis vary according to the primary site. Primary tumors within the oral cavity and lip metastasize to the nodes in levels I, II, and III. Skip metastases may occur with oral tongue cancers such that involvement of nodes in level III or IV may occur without involvement of higher echelon nodes (levels I & II). Tumors arising in the oropharynx, hypopharynx, and larynx most commonly spread to the lymph nodes of the lateral neck in levels II, III, and IV. Isolated level V lymphadenopathy is uncommon with oral cavity, pharyngeal, and laryngeal primaries. Malignancies of the nasopharynx and thyroid commonly spread to level V nodes in addition to the jugular chain nodes. Retropharyngeal lymph nodes are sites for metastasis from tumors of the nasopharynx, soft palate, and lateral and posterior walls of the oropharynx and hypopharynx. Tumors of the hypopharynx, cervical esophagus, and thyroid frequently involve the paratracheal nodal compartment, and may extend to the lymphatics in the upper mediastinum (level VII). The Delphian node, a pretracheal lymph node, may become involved by advanced tumors of the glottis with subglottic spread.

The philosophy for the treatment of the cervical lymphatics in head and neck cancer has evolved significantly since the mid-1970s. The presence of cervical metastasis decreases the 5-year survival rate in patients with upper aerodigestive malignancies by approximately 50%. As such, adequate treatment of the N_0 and N_+ neck in these patients has always been viewed as a priority in an effort to increase disease-free survival rates. Traditionally, the gold standard for control of cervical metastasis has been the radical neck dissection (RND) first described by Crile. The classic RND removes levels I to V of the cervical lymphatics in addition to the SCM, internal jugular vein, and the spinal accessory nerve (CN XI). Any modification of the RND that preserves nonlymphatic structures (i.e., CN XI, SCM muscle, or internal jugular vein) is defined as a *modified radical neck dissection* (MRND). A neck dissection that preserves lymphatic compartments normally removed as part of a classic RND is termed a *selective neck dissection* (SND). Bocca[78] and colleagues demonstrated that the MRND, or "functional neck dissection," was equally effective in controlling regional metastasis as the RND, in addition to noting that the functional results in patients were superior. With outcome data supporting the use of SND and MRND, these procedures have become the preferred alternative for the treatment of cervical metastases when indicated.[79,80]

SND options have become increasingly popular given the benefits of improved shoulder function and cosmetic impact on neck contour when compared to MRND. The principle behind preservation of certain nodal groups is that specific primary sites preferentially drain their lymphatics in a predictable pattern. Types of SND include the supraomohyoid neck dissection, the lateral neck dissection, and the posterolateral neck dissection.[81] The supraomohyoid dissection, typically used with oral cavity malignancies, removes lymph nodes in levels I to III (Fig. 18-41). The lateral neck dissection, frequently used for laryngeal malignancies, removes those nodes in levels II through IV (Fig. 18-42). The posterolateral neck dissection, used with thyroid cancer, removes the lymphatics in levels II to V (Fig. 18-43). In the clinically negative neck (N_0), if the risk for occult metastasis is greater than 20%, elective treatment of the nodes at risk is generally advocated. This may be in the form of elective neck irradiation or elective neck dissection. An additional role of SND is as a staging tool to determine the need for postoperative radiation therapy. Regional control after selective dissection has been shown to be as effective for controlling regional disease as the MRND in the N_0 patient. Aware-

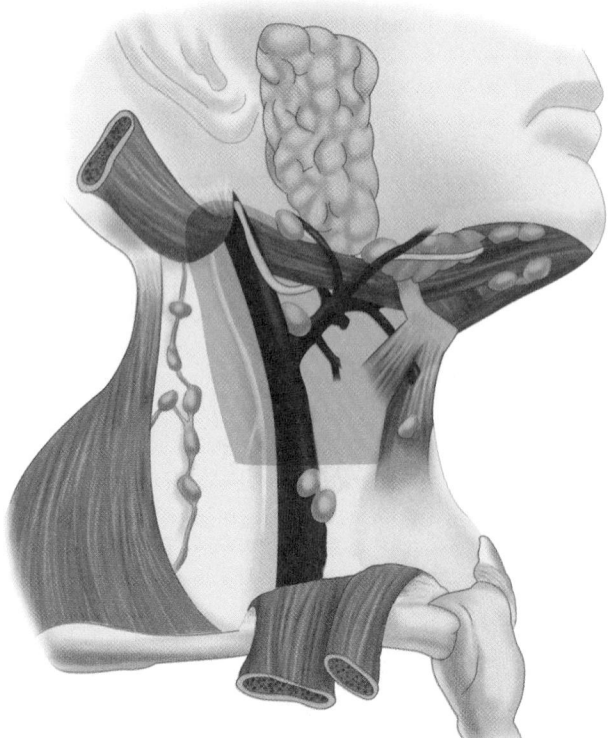

FIG. 18-41. Shaded region indicates the region included in a supraomohyoid neck dissection.

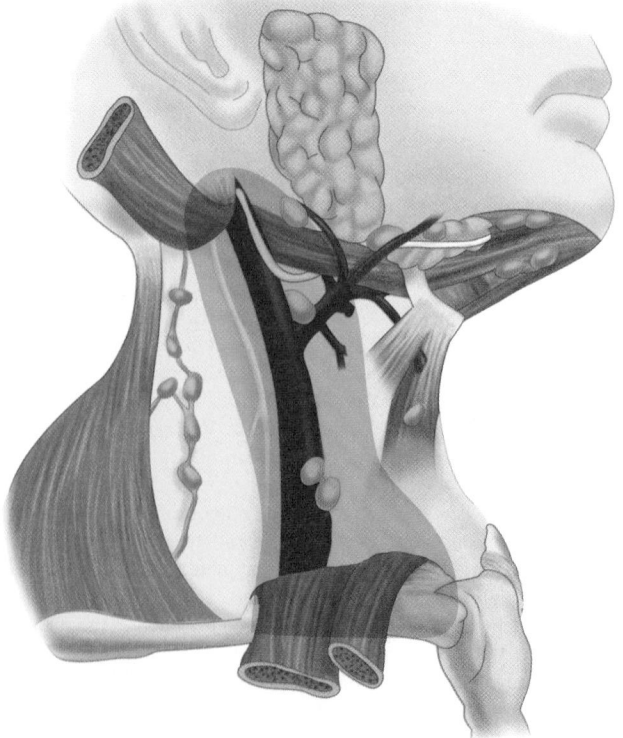

FIG. 18-42. Shaded region indicates the region included in a lateral neck dissection.

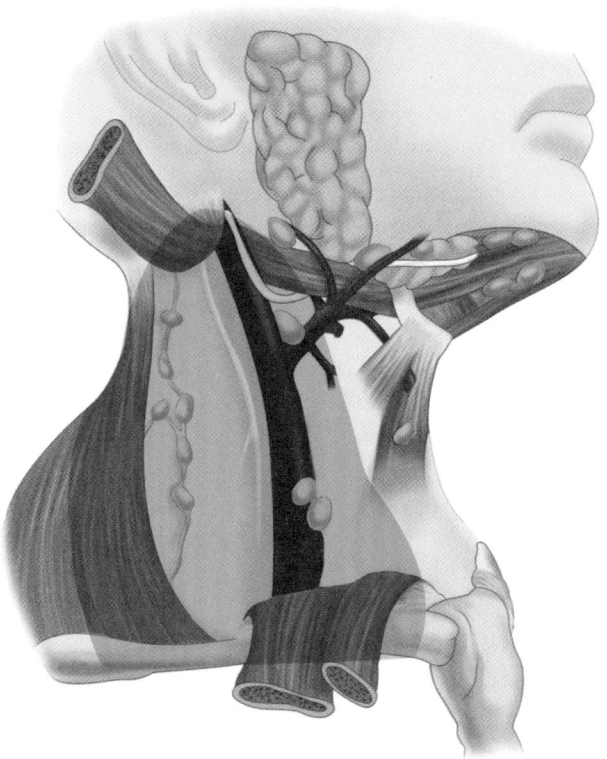

FIG. 18-43. Shaded region indicates the region included in a posterolateral neck dissection.

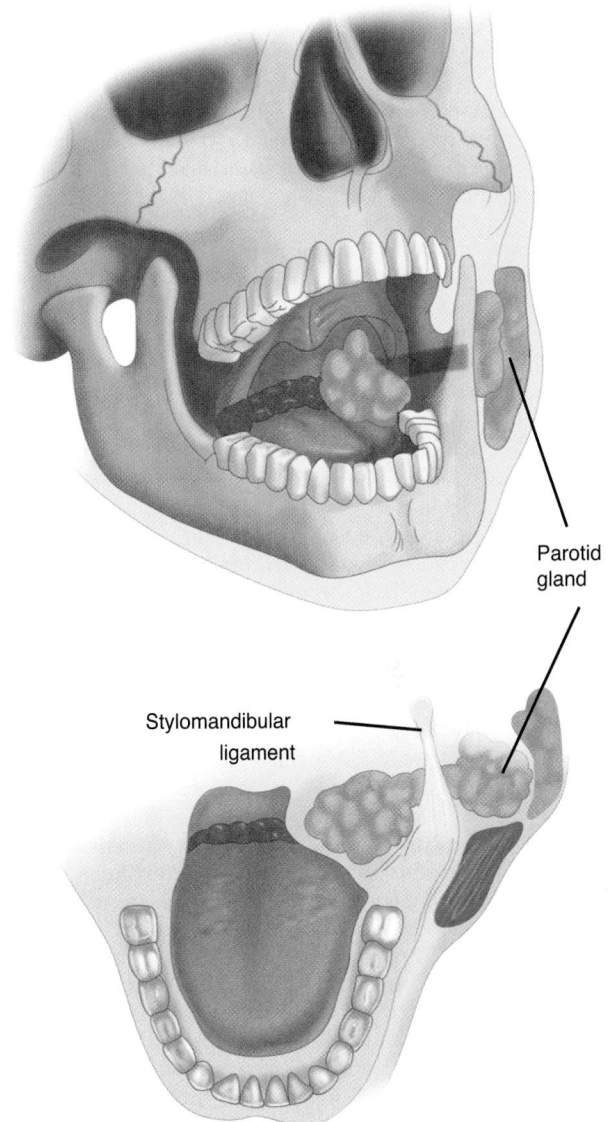

Parotid gland

Stylomandibular ligament

FIG. 18-44. Parapharyngeal mass—prestyloid with prominent oropharyngeal presentation typical of a dumbbell tumor.

ness of the potential for "skip metastases," in particular with lateral oral tongue lesions, may require extension of a standard SND to include additional levels for selected lesions.[82] The treatment option selected for the primary site cancer is a significant factor in determining which therapeutic modality will be selected for the treatment of the regional lymphatics.

For clinically N$_+$ necks, frequently the surgical treatment of choice is the MRND or RND. SND options have been advocated by some authors for treatment of limited N1 disease, however, they do not have a role in the treatment of advanced N stage disease. When extracapsular spread, perineural invasion, vascular invasion, and the presence of multiple involved lymph nodes are noted, surgical management of the neck alone is not adequate.[83] Adjuvant radiation therapy, and possibly chemoradiation, is indicated in these cases.

A planned postradiation neck dissection for patients undergoing radiation as a primary therapy is another indication for the use of neck dissection. In patients with existing advanced N stage disease (N2a or greater) or in patients with a partial response in the neck to therapy, neck dissection is performed 6 to 8 weeks after completion of radiation.

Regional metastases that encase the carotid artery or that demonstrate fixation of nodes to surrounding structures (e.g., prevertebral muscles) decrease 5-year survival rates significantly, to the range of 15 to 22%. The associated morbidity is high with procedures involving carotid resection (cerebrovascular accident and death) and must be weighed carefully when deciding if surgery is to be pursued. Surgically debulking metastatic disease does not improve survival and is not advocated. Recurrent neck metastasis after comprehensive neck dissection or radiation is associated with very poor survival.

Parapharyngeal Space Masses

The parapharyngeal space is a potential space, shaped like an inverted pyramid spanning the skull base to the hyoid. The boundaries of the space are separated by the styloid process and its associated fascial attachments into the "prestyloid" and "poststyloid" compartments.[84] The contents of the prestyloid space are the parotid, fat, and lymph nodes. The poststyloid compartment is composed of CNs IX to XII, the carotid space contents, cervical sympathetic chain, fat, and lymph nodes. Tumors in this space can produce displacement of the lateral pharyngeal wall medially into the oropharynx (Fig. 18-44), dysphagia, cranial nerve dysfunction, Horner's syndrome, or vascular compression.

Of the masses found in the parapharyngeal space, 40 to 50% of the tumors are of salivary gland origin. Tumors of neurogenic origin such as paragangliomas (glomus vagale, carotid body tumor), schwannomas, and neurofibromas are responsible for 20 to 25% of parapharyngeal masses. Lymph node metastases and primary lymphoma represent 15% of lesions. With this in mind, when reviewing preoperative imaging, one can assume that tumors arising anterior to the styloid process are most likely of salivary gland origin, whereas those of the poststyloid compartment are vascular or neurogenic. This is helpful in that angiography is not as necessary for prestyloid lesions as it may be for vascular poststyloid tumors. If a paraganglioma is suspected, a 24-hour urinary catecholamine collection should be obtained to allow for optimal premedication for patients with functional tumors. Embolization may be considered for vascular tumors before surgery in an attempt to decrease intraoperative blood loss.

Surgical access to these tumors may require a transmandibular and/or lateral cervical approach. It is inadvisable to approach parapharyngeal space tumors transorally without having the necessary exposure and control of the associated vasculature that is afforded by these approaches. Some tumors of the parapharyngeal space (e.g., dumbbell tumors of deep parotid origin) are amenable to removal by a combined transparotid and transcervical approach while allowing for dissection and displacement of the facial nerve to assist removal of tumor.

Benign Neck Masses

A number of benign masses of the neck occur that require surgical management. Many of these masses are seen in the pediatric population. The differential diagnosis includes thyroglossal duct cyst, branchial cleft cyst, lymphangioma (cystic hygroma), hemangioma, and dermoid cyst.

Thyroglossal duct cysts represent the vestigial remainder of the tract of the descending thyroid gland from the foramen cecum, at the tongue base, into the lower anterior neck during fetal development. They present as a midline or paramedian cystic mass adjacent to the hyoid bone. After an upper respiratory infection, the cyst may enlarge or become infected. Surgical management of a thyroglossal duct cyst requires removal of the cyst, the tract, and the central portion of the hyoid bone (Sistrunk procedure), as well as a portion of the tongue base up to the foramen cecum. Before excision of a thyroglossal duct cyst, an imaging study such as ultrasound is performed to identify if normal thyroid tissue exists in the lower neck, and lab assay is performed to assess if the patient is euthyroid.

Congenital branchial cleft remnants are derived from the branchial cleft apparatus that persists after fetal development. There are several types, numbered according to their corresponding embryologic branchial cleft. First branchial cleft cysts and sinuses are associated intimately with the EAC and the parotid gland. Second and third branchial cleft cysts are found along the anterior border of the SCM muscle and can produce drainage via a sinus tract to the neck skin (Fig. 18-45). Secondary infections can occur, producing enlargement, cellulitis, and neck abscess that requires operative drainage. The removal of branchial cleft cysts and fistula requires removal of the fistula tract to the point of origin to decrease the risk of recurrence. The second branchial cleft remnant tract courses between the internal and external carotid arteries and proceeds into the tonsillar fossa. The third branchial cleft remnant courses posterior to the common carotid artery, ending in the pyriform sinus region. Cystic metastasis from squamous cell carcinoma of the tonsil or tongue base to a cervical lymph node can be confused for a branchial cleft cyst in an otherwise asymptomatic patient. Dermoid cysts tend to present as midline masses and represent trapped epithelium originating from the embryonic closure of the midline.

Lymphatic malformations such as lymphangiomas and cystic hygromas can be difficult management problems. They typically present as mobile, fluid-filled masses. Because of their predisposition to track extensively into the surrounding soft tissues, complete removal of these lesions can be challenging. Recurrence and regrowth occur with incomplete removal. Cosmetic deformity and/or nerve injury can result when extensive surgical dissection is performed for large lesions. In newborns and infants, there is higher associated morbidity when cystic hygromas and lymphangiomas become massive, require tracheostomy, and involve the deep neck and mediastinum.

Deep-Neck Fascial Planes

The fascial planes of the neck provide boundaries that are clinically applicable because they determine the pathway of spread of an infection. The deep cervical fascia is composed of three layers. These are the investing (superficial deep), pretracheal, and the prevertebral fascias. The superficial layer of the deep cervical fascia forms a cone around the neck and spans from skull base and mandible to the clavicle and manubrium. This layer surrounds the SCM muscle and covers the anterior and posterior triangles of the neck. The pretracheal fascia is found within the anterior compartment, deep to the strap muscles and surrounds the thyroid gland, trachea, and esophagus. This fascia blends laterally to the carotid sheath. Infections in this region may track along the trachea or esophagus into the mediastinum. The prevertebral fascia extends from the skull base to the thoracic vertebra and covers the prevertebral musculature and cervical spine. If an infection were to communicate anteriorly through the prevertebral fascia, it would enter the retropharyngeal

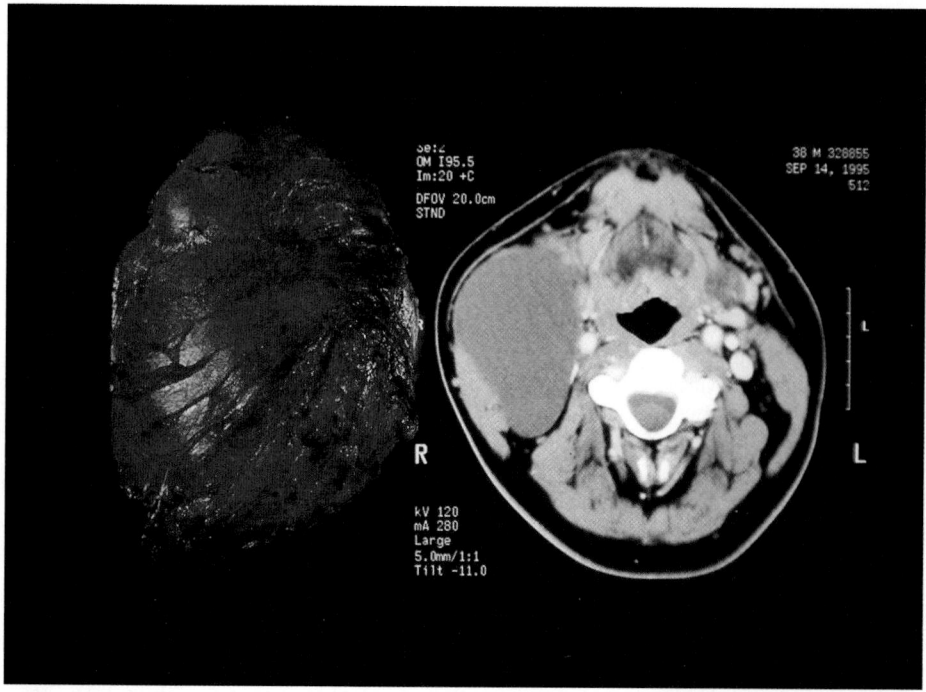

FIG. 18-45. CT scan demonstrating a branchial cleft cyst with operative specimen.

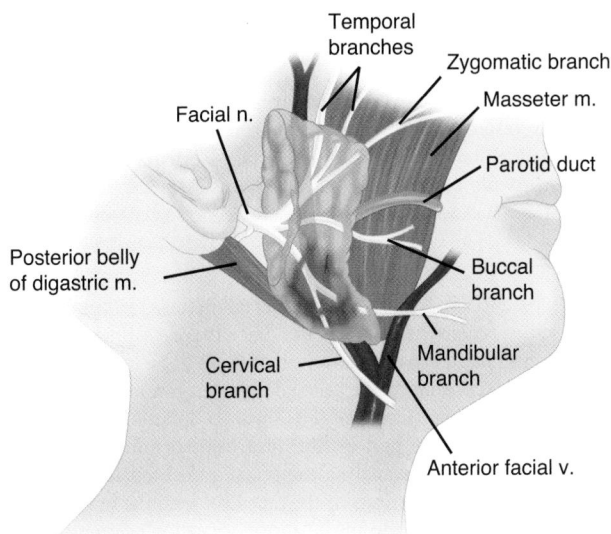

FIG. 18-46. Example of a tumor in the parotid with the pattern of the facial nerve and associated anatomy. m. = muscle; n. = nerve; v. = vein.

space. Infectious extension into this space is complicated by the fact that this region, located posterior to the buccopharyngeal fascia, extends from the skull base to the mediastinum.

Salivary Gland Tumors

Tumors of the salivary gland are relatively uncommon and represent less than 2% of all head and neck neoplasms. The major salivary glands are the parotid, submandibular, and sublingual glands. Minor salivary glands are found throughout the submucosa of the upper aerodigestive tract with the highest density found within the palate. Eighty-five percent of salivary gland neoplasms arise within the parotid gland (Fig. 18-46). The majority of these neoplasms are benign, with the most common histology being pleomorphic adenoma (benign mixed tumor). In contrast, approximately 50% of tumors arising in the submandibular and sublingual glands are malignant. Tumors arising from minor salivary gland tissue carry an even higher risk for malignancy (75%).

Salivary gland tumors are usually slow growing and well circumscribed. Patients with a mass and findings of rapid growth, pain, paresthesias, and facial nerve weakness are at increased risk of harboring a malignancy. The facial nerve, which separates the superficial and deep lobes of the parotid, may be directly involved by tumors in 10 to 15% of patients. Additional findings ominous for malignancy include skin invasion and fixation to the mastoid tip. Trismus suggests invasion of the masseter or pterygoid muscles.[85]

Submandibular and sublingual gland tumors present as a neck mass or floor of mouth swelling, respectively. Malignant tumors of the sublingual or submandibular gland may invade the lingual or hypoglossal nerves, causing paresthesias or paralysis.[86] Bimanual examination is important for determining the size of the tumor and possible fixation to the mandible or involvement of the tongue.

Minor salivary gland tumors present as painless submucosal masses and are most frequently seen at the junction of the hard and soft palate. Minor salivary gland tumors arising in the prestyloid parapharyngeal space may produce medial displacement of the lateral oropharyngeal wall and tonsil.

The incidence of metastatic spread to cervical lymphatics is variable and depends on the histology, primary site, and stage of the tumor. Parotid gland malignancies can metastasize to the intra- and periglandular nodes. The next echelon of lymphatics for the parotid is the upper jugular nodal chain. Although the risk of lymphatic

metastasis is low for most salivary gland malignancies, lesions that are considered high grade or that demonstrate perineural invasion have a higher propensity for regional spread. Tumors arising in patients of advanced age also tend to have more aggressive behavior. Initial nodal drainage for the submandibular gland is the level Ia and Ib lymph nodes and submental nodes followed by the upper and midjugular nodes. Extraglandular extension of tumor and lymph node metastases are adverse prognostic factors for submandibular gland tumors.

Diagnostic imaging is standard for the evaluation of salivary gland tumors. MRI is the most sensitive study to determine soft-tissue extension and involvement of adjacent structures. Unfortunately, imaging studies lack the specificity for differentiating benign and malignant neoplasms. Diagnosis of salivary gland tumors is frequently aided by the use of FNA. In the hands of an experienced cytologist familiar with salivary gland pathology, FNA can provide an accurate preoperative diagnosis in 70 to 80% of cases. This can help the operative surgeon with treatment planning and patient counseling, but should be viewed in the context that a more extensive procedure may be ultimately required. The final histopathologic diagnosis is confirmed by surgical excision.

Benign and malignant tumors of the salivary glands are divided into epithelial, nonepithelial, and metastatic neoplasms. Benign epithelial tumors include pleomorphic adenoma (80%), monomorphic adenoma, Warthin's tumor, oncocytoma, or sebaceous neoplasm. Nonepithelial benign lesions include hemangioma, neural sheath tumor, and lipoma. Treatment of benign neoplasms is surgical excision of the affected gland or, in the case of the parotid, excision of the superficial lobe with facial nerve dissection and preservation. The minimal surgical procedure for neoplasms of the parotid is superficial parotidectomy with preservation of the facial nerve. Enucleation of the tumor mass is not recommended because of the risk of incomplete excision and tumor spillage. Tumor spillage of a pleomorphic adenoma during removal can lead to problematic recurrences.

Malignant epithelial tumors range in aggressiveness from low to high grade. Their behavior depends on tumor histology, degree of invasiveness, and the presence of regional metastasis. The most common malignant epithelial neoplasm of the salivary glands is mucoepidermoid carcinoma. The low-grade mucoepidermoid carcinoma is composed of largely mucin-secreting cells, whereas in high-grade tumors, the epidermoid cells predominate. High-grade mucoepidermoid carcinomas resemble nonkeratinizing squamous cell carcinoma in their histologic features and clinical behavior. Adenoid cystic carcinoma, which has a propensity for neural invasion, is the second most common malignancy in adults. Skip lesions along nerves are common and can lead to treatment failures because of the difficulty in treating the full extent of invasion. Adenoid cystic carcinomas have a high incidence of distant metastasis, but display indolent growth. It is not uncommon for patients to experience lengthy survival despite the presence of disseminated disease. The most common malignancies in the pediatric population are mucoepidermoid carcinoma and acinic cell carcinoma. For minor salivary glands, the most common malignancies are adenoid cystic carcinoma, mucoepidermoid carcinoma, and low-grade polymorphous adenocarcinoma. Carcinoma ex pleomorphic adenoma is an aggressive malignancy that arises from a pre-existing benign mixed tumor.

The primary treatment of salivary malignancies is surgical excision. In this setting, basic surgical principles include the en bloc removal of the involved gland with preservation of all nerves unless directly invaded by tumor. For parotid tumors that arise in the lateral lobe, superficial parotidectomy with preservation of CN VII is indicated. If the tumor extends into the deep lobe of the parotid, a total parotidectomy with nerve preservation is performed. Although malignant tumors may abut the facial nerve, if a plane of dissection can be developed without leaving gross tumor, it is preferable to preserve the nerve. If the nerve is encased by tumor (or is noted to be nonfunctional preoperatively) and preservation would result leaving gross residual disease, nerve sacrifice should be considered.

The removal of submandibular malignancies includes en bloc resection of the gland and submental and submandibular lymph nodes. Radical resection is indicated with tumors that invade the mandible, tongue, or floor of mouth. Therapeutic removal of the regional lymphatics is indicated for clinical adenopathy or when the risk of occult regional metastasis exceeds 20%. High-grade mucoepidermoid carcinomas, for example, have a high risk of regional disease and require elective treatment of the regional lymphatics. When gross nerve invasion is found (lingual or hypoglossal), sacrifice of the nerve is indicated with retrograde frozen section biopsies to determine the extent of involvement. If the nerve is invaded at the level of the skull base foramina, a surgical clip may be left in place to mark the area for inclusion in postoperative radiation fields. The presence of skip metastases in the nerve with adenoid cystic carcinoma makes recurrence common with this pathology.

Postoperative radiation treatment plays an important role in the treatment of salivary malignancies. The presence of extraglandular disease, perineural invasion, direct invasion of regional structures, regional metastasis, and high-grade histology are all indications for radiation treatment.

RECONSTRUCTION IN HEAD AND NECK SURGERY

Defects of soft tissue and bony anatomy of the head and neck can occur after oncologic resection. Tumor surgery frequently necessitates removal of structures related to speech and swallowing. Loss of sensation and motor function can produce dysphagia through impairment of food bolus formation, manipulation, and propulsion. Removal of laryngeal, tongue base, and hypopharyngeal tumors can lead to impairment in airway protective reflexes and predispose to aspiration. Cosmetic deformities that result from surgery can also significantly impact the quality of life of a patient. Current surgical management of head and neck tumors requires restoration of form and function through application of contemporary reconstruction techniques.

Basic principles of reconstruction include attempting to replace resected tissue components (bone, skin, soft tissue) with tissue with similar qualities. However, restoring a patient's functional capacity does not always require strict observation of this rule. The head and neck reconstructive surgeon must consider a patient's preoperative comorbidities and anatomy when constructing a care plan.

A stepladder analogy has been used to describe the escalation in complexity of reconstructive options in the repair of head and neck defects. It is important to remember that the most complex procedure is not always the most appropriate. Progression for closure by secondary intention, primary closure, skin grafts, local flaps, regional flaps, and free-tissue transfer flaps (free flaps) run the gamut of options available. The most appropriate reconstructive technique used is based on the medical condition of the patient, the location and size of the defect to be repaired, and the functional impairment associated with the defect.

Small defects of the skin of the medial canthus, scalp, and nose may be allowed to heal by secondary intention with excellent cosmetic and functional results. When considering primary closure, the excision should be placed in the lines of relaxed skin tension and should attempt to not distort surrounding anatomy such as the hairline, eyelids, or lips.

Skin Grafts

Split and full-thickness skin grafts are used in the head and neck for a variety of defects. Following oral cavity resections, split-thickness grafts can provide adequate reconstruction of the mucosal surface if an adequate vascular tissue bed is available to support the blood supply needed for graft survival. These grafts start to incorporate into the recipient site in approximately 5 days and do not provide replacement of absent soft-tissue bulk; however, they are a simple low morbidity technique for covering mucosal defects that allow for monitoring for local recurrence. Full-thickness grafts are used on the face when local rotational flaps are not available. These grafts have less contracture over time than split-thickness grafts. Grafts can be harvested from the postauricular or supraclavicular areas to maximize the match of skin characteristics. Dermal grafts have been used to provide coverage for exposed vessels in the neck, reconstruct mucosal defects, and assist in providing soft-tissue bulk.

Local Flaps

Local flaps encompass a large number of mainly random-pattern flaps used to reconstruct defects in adjacent areas. It is beyond the scope of this chapter to enumerate all of these flaps, but they should be designed according to the relaxed skin tension lines of the face and neck skin. These lines are tension lines inherent in the facial regions and caused in part by the insertions of muscles of facial animation. Incisions paralleling the relaxed skin tension lines that respect the aesthetic subunits of the face heal with the least amount of tension and camouflage into a more appealing cosmetic result. Poorly designed incisions or flaps result in widened scars and distortion of important aesthetic units.

Regional Flaps

Regional flaps are those that are available as pedicled transfer of soft tissue from areas adjacent to the defect. These flaps have an axial blood supply that traverses the flap longitudinally from proximal to distal between the fascia and subcutaneous tissue. Single-stage reconstruction is possible, and harvest may occur simultaneously with the resection of primary disease resulting in a decrease in overall operative time.

The deltopectoral fasciocutaneous flap is a medially based flap from the anterior chest wall reliant on the perforators of the internal mammary artery. Its pliability permits folding, making it capable for use with reconstruction of pharyngoesophageal defects. A disadvantage is that use of the flap requires a second stage detaching the proximal chest component and completion of insetting approximately 3-4 weeks after the original procedure.

Several myocutaneous flaps exist for head and neck reconstruction. The vascular pedicle of these flaps permits a wide arc of rotation, making them ideal for a variety of different reconstructive needs. The trapezius muscle provides a number of soft-tissue flaps that can be rotated to reconstruct a number of defects in the head and neck. The superior trapezius flap is based on paraspinous perforators and is ideal for lateral neck defects. The lateral island trapezius flap, based on the transverse cervical and dorsal scapular vessels, allows for harvest of a soft-tissue paddle below the inferior border of the scapula. This flap is ideal for reconstruction of scalp and lateral skull base defects.

The pectoralis myocutaneous flap is based on the pectoral branch of the thoracoacromial artery (medial) and the lateral thoracic artery (lateral). The latter vessel may be sacrificed to increase the arc of rotation. This workhorse flap includes the pectoralis major muscle, either alone or with overlying anterior chest skin. The pectoralis myocutaneous flap has enjoyed tremendous popularity because of its ease of harvest, the ability to tailor its thickness to the defect, and limited donor site morbidity. It can be used for reconstruction of the oropharynx, oral cavity, and the hypopharynx and in some cases can be tubed to replace cervical esophageal defects. Bulk associated with this flap may make certain applications less practical, and this problem is exacerbated in obese patients. The arc of rotation limits the superior extent of this flap to the zygomatic arch externally and the superior pole of the tonsil internally.

The latissimus dorsi flap provides a large source of soft tissue and has a wide arc of rotation. The flap is based on the thoracodorsal vasculature. This flap can be used as a regional rotational flap or as a free flap. Lateral decubitus positioning is typically required for harvesting this flap, making it less attractive for simultaneous cancer ablation and reconstruction.

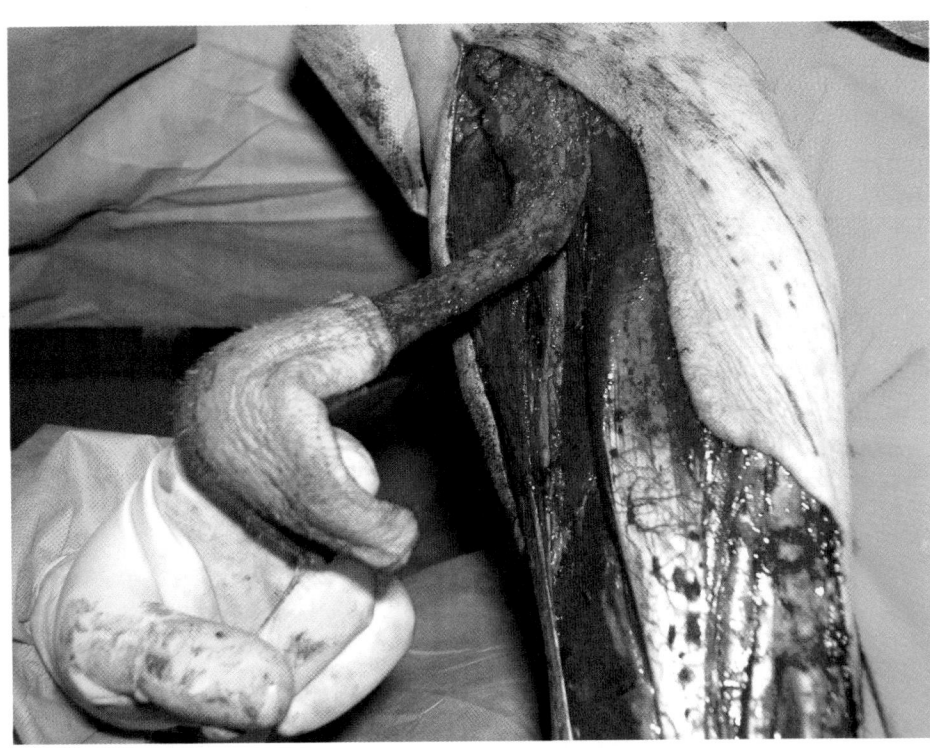

FIG. 18-47. Radial forearm free flap before harvest from the arm.

Free-Tissue Transfer

Free-tissue transfer with microvascular anastomosis affords the reconstructive surgeon unparalleled ability to replace tissue loss with tissues of similar characteristics. There are a number of donor sites available for various types of flaps, including osteomyocutaneous, myocutaneous, fasciocutaneous, fascial, and myoosseous flaps. The flaps most popular in head and neck reconstructive armamentarium are those with ease of harvest from a standpoint of patient positioning and those that allow for a two-teamed approach for simultaneous flap harvesting and oncologic resection.[87]

The radial forearm fasciocutaneous flap (Fig. 18-47) is a hardy flap with constant vascular anatomy and a long vascular pedicle, allowing for ease of insetting and choice in anastomotic vascular recipient sites. It is pliable and can be reinnervated as a sensate flap, making it ideal for repair of oral cavity and oropharyngeal defects. It can be tubed to repair hypopharyngeal and upper esophageal defects.[88,89]

The anterolateral thigh flap, based on the descending branch of the lateral circumflex femoral artery, has the capacity for a large pliable skin paddle with muscle that is capable of being tubed and is used to reconstruct similar defects as that of the radial forearm flap while providing more tissue bulk.

The fibular osteocutaneous or osteomyocutaneous flap allows for one-stage reconstruction of resected mandible. In the adult, up to 20 cm of bone can be harvested with a cuff of soleus and flexor hallucis longus muscle for additional soft-tissue bulk. The donor site defect is well tolerated as long as approximately 7 cm of bone are retained proximally and distally for knee and ankle stability.[90]

Iliac crest osteocutaneous flaps are also used for the reconstruction of mandible defects. The natural shape of this donor site bone is similar to the mandibular angle. The thick stock of bone provided by the iliac crest allows for better vertical reconstruction of the mandible while spanning a segmental defect. However, for lengthy mandibular defects (greater than 10 cm), the fibular flap usually is chosen. Additionally, for shorter mandible defects, other free flaps, including osseous components such as scapular and radial forearm flaps, can be used. The scapular flap can provide approximately 12 cm of scapula bone and is based on the circumflex scapular artery. This flap can be combined with parascapular and scapular skin islands and portions of latissimus dorsi and serratus anterior mus-

cle. The radial forearm osteocutaneous flap can provide a limited quantity of bone with the soft-tissue component of the flap but is associated with an increased risk of donor site fracture.

Large soft-tissue defects can result from trauma, excision of skull base tumors, and tumors involving large segments of skin. Furthermore, after extensive skull base resections in the anterior and lateral skull base, the need for separation of the oropharyngeal and sinonasal tracts from the dura requires soft-tissue interposition between the dura and the contaminated upper aerodigestive tract. The rectus abdominis flap, based on the deep inferior epigastric vessels, provides a large amount of soft tissue and is ideal for closure of wounds of the lateral skull base and dura.

For reconstruction of defects of the hypopharynx and cervical esophagus, both free flaps and regional pedicled flaps are available. The free transfer of a jejunal segment can be performed based on branches of the superior mesenteric artery. Other free flaps used in this area include fasciocutaneous flaps, such as tubed radial forearm flap. The gastric pull-up is a regional flap that is also in use for reconstruction of cervical esophageal defects. The stomach is mobilized and pedicled on the right gastric and gastroepiploic vessels into the defect via tunneling through the thoracic cavity.

TRACHEOSTOMY

Tracheostomy is indicated in the management of patients who require prolonged intubation, access for frequent pulmonary suctioning, and in those patients with neurologic deficits that impair protective airway reflexes. Its use in head and neck surgery is often for the temporary management of the airway in the perioperative period. After surgical resection of oral cavity and oropharyngeal cancers, edema of the upper aerodigestive tract occurs necessitating perioperative tracheostomy to prevent loss of the airway.

The avoidance of prolonged orotracheal and nasotracheal intubation decreases the risk of laryngeal and subglottic injury and potential stenosis, facilitates oral and pulmonary suctioning, and decreases patient discomfort. When the tracheostomy is no longer needed, the tube is removed and closure of the opening usually occurs spontaneously over a 2-week period. Complications of tracheostomy include pneumothorax, RLN injury, tracheal stenosis, wound infection with large-vessel erosion, and failure to close after decannulation. The use of cricothyroidotomy as an alternative to tracheostomy for patients who require prolonged intubation is associated with a higher incidence of vocal cord dysfunction and subglottic stenosis. When cricothyroidotomy is used in the setting of establishing an emergency airway, conversion to a standard tracheostomy should be considered if decannulation is not anticipated within 5 to 7 days.

Placement of a tracheostomy does not obligate a patient to loss of speech. When a large cuffed tracheostomy tube is in place, expecting a patient to be capable of normal speech is impractical. However, after a patient is downsized to an uncuffed tracheostomy tube, intermittent finger occlusion or Passy-Muir valve placement will allow a patient to communicate while still using the tracheostomy to bypass the upper airway. When a patient no longer has the original indication for the tracheostomy and can tolerate capping of the tracheal tube for greater than 24 hours, decannulation is considered safe. If an upper airway mass or tissue reconstruction was the indication for the tracheostomy, pre-decannulation flexible laryngoscopic examination of the airway is recommended.[91]

LONG-TERM MANAGEMENT AND REHABILITATION

Palliative Care

For patients with unresectable disease or distant metastases, palliative care options exist. Palliative treatment is aimed at improving a patient's symptoms and may include radiation, chemotherapy, or consultation with a pain specialist. The head and neck surgeon has the options of tracheostomy and gastrostomy tube placement for patients progressing with worsening airway compromise and dysphagia, respectively. Hospice is also an option for patients with a limited short-term outlook; hospice allows a patient to retain dignity at the time of greatest adversity.

Follow-Up Care

Patients diagnosed and treated for a head and neck tumor require follow-up care aimed at monitoring for recurrence and the side effects of therapy. For malignancies of the upper aerodigestive tract, the American Head and Neck Society offers a formula for follow-up appointments (Table 18-4).[92]

In addition to a formal head and neck examination, patients should be questioned about any emerging symptoms related to their primary tumor. New-onset pain, otalgia, hoarseness, and dysphagia are some of the problems that may indicate the need to evaluate further for recurrence. Worsening dysphagia may also be a presenting symptom for a patient developing a pharyngeal stricture. Such a patient may require dilatation and/or placement of a gastrostomy tube for nutrition. Additionally, a number of patients who undergo head and neck radiation will develop hypothyroidism years after treatment. Patients with shoulder dysfunction after surgery should be considered for physical therapy consultation to minimize the long-term effects of their surgical care. Patients with chronic pain-related issues can benefit from consultation with a pain specialist to construct a treatment regimen to provide adequate control of long-term discomfort. Long-term follow-up with a dentist experienced in caring for patients with a history of therapeutic radiation therapy is vital if prevention of osteoradionecrosis is to be achieved.

REFERENCES

Entries highlighted in bright blue are key references.

1. Senturia BA, Marcus MD, Lucente FE: *Diseases of the External Ear*, 2nd ed. New York: Grune and Stratton, 1980.
2. Kimmelman CP, Lucente FE: Use of ceftazidime for malignant external otitis. *Ann Otol Rhinol Laryngol* 98:721, 1989.
3. Sutton D, Derkay CS, Darrow DH, et al: Resistant bacteria in the middle ear fluid at the time of tympanostomy tube surgery. *Ann Otol Rhinol Laryngol* 109:24, 2000.
4. Nissen AJ, Bui H: Complications of chronic otitis media. *Ear Nose Throat J* 75:284, 1996.
5. Antonelli PJ, Garside JA, Mancuso AA, et al: Computed tomography and the diagnosis of coalescent mastoiditis. *Otolaryngol Head Neck Surg* 120:350, 1999.
6. Gantz BJ, Rubinstein JT, Gidley P, et al: Surgical management of Bell's palsy. *Laryngoscope* 109:1177, 1999.
7. Green JD, Shelton C, Brackman DE: Surgical management of iatrogenic facial nerve injuries. *Otolaryngol Head Neck Surg* 111:606, 1994.
8. Lanza DC, Kennedy DW: Adult rhinosinusitis defined. *Otolaryngol Head Neck Surg* 117:S1, 1997.
9. Brook I: Microbiology and management of sinusitis. *J Otolaryngol* 25:249, 1996.
10. Benninger MS, Anon J, Mabry RL: The medical management of rhinosinusitis. *Otolaryngol Head Neck Surg* 117:S41, 1997.
11. Cody DT, Neel HB, Ferrerio JA, et al: Allergic fungal sinusitis: The Mayo Clinic experience. *Laryngoscope* 104:1074, 1994.
12. deShazo RD, O'Brien M, Chapin K, et al: A new classification and diagnostic criteria for invasive fungal sinusitis. *Arch Otolaryngol Head Neck Surg* 123:1181, 1997.
13. Bisno AL, Gerber MA, Gwaltney JM, et al: Diagnosis and management of group A streptococcal pharyngitis: A practice guideline. *Clin Infect Dis* 25:574, 1997.
14. Thompson LDR, Wenig BM, Kornblut BM: Pharyngitis, in Bailey BJ, Calhoun KH, Derkay CS, et al (eds): *Head and Neck Surgery—Otolaryngology*, 3rd ed. Philadelphia: Lippincott Williams and Wilkins, 2001, p 543.
15. Paradise J, Bluestone C, Bachman R, et al: Efficacy of tonsillectomy in recurrent throat infections in severely affected children. *N Engl J Med* 310:674, 1984.
16. Gates G, Cooper J, Avery C, et al: Chronic secretory otitis media: Effects of surgical management. *Ann Otol Rhinol Laryngol Suppl* 98:2, 1989.
17. Gerber ME, O'Connor DM, Adler E, et al: Selected risk factors in pediatric adenotonsillectomy. *Arch Otolaryngol Head Neck Surg* 122:811, 1996.
18. Friedman M, Tanyeri H, La Rossa M, et al: Clinical predictors of obstructive sleep apnea. *Laryngoscope* 109:1901, 1999.
19. Standards of Practice Committee of the American Sleep Disorders Association: Practice parameters for the use of laser assisted uvuloplasty. *Sleep* 17:744, 1994.
20. Zeitels SM, Casiano RR, Gardner GM, et al: Management of common voice problems: Committee report. *Otolaryngol Head Neck Surg* 126:333, 2002.
21. Rosen CA, Woodson GE, Thompson JW, et al: Preliminary results of the use of indole 3-carbinol for recurrent respiratory papillomatosis. *Otolaryngol Head Neck Surg* 118:810, 1998.
22. Gray S, Hammond E, Hanson DF: Benign pathologic responses of the larynx. *Ann Otol Rhinol Laryngol* 104:13, 1995.
23. Koufman JA: The otolaryngologic manifestations of gastroesophageal reflux disease (GERD). *Laryngoscope* 53(Suppl):1, 1991.
24. Nasri S, Sercarz JA, McAlpin T, et al: Treatment of vocal fold granuloma using botulism toxin type A. *Laryngoscope* 105:585, 1995.
25. Benninger MS, Crumley RL, Ford CN, et al: Evaluation and treatment of the unilateral paralyzed vocal fold. *Otolaryngol Head Neck Surg* 111:497, 1994.
26. Ishiki N: Vocal mechanics and the basis for phonosurgery. *Laryngoscope* 108:1761, 1998.

TABLE 18-4 American Head and Neck Society follow-up appointment formula

Posttreatment	Follow-Up Period
1st y	Every 1–3 mo
2nd y	Every 2–4 mo
3rd y	Every 3–6 mo
4th y	Every 4–6 mo
5th y and after	Every 12 mo

27. Hochman M, Vural E, Suen J, et al: Contemporary management of vascular lesions of the head and neck. *Curr Opin Otolaryngol Head Neck Surg* 7:161, 1999.

28. Waner M: The treatment of vascular lesions. *Facial Plast Surg Clin North Am* 4:275, 1996.

29. Kohut MP, Hansen M, Pribaz JJ, et al: Arteriovenous malformations of the head and neck: Natural history and management. *Plast Reconstr Surg* 102:643, 1998.

30. Giguere CM, Bauman NM, Smith RJH: New treatment options for lymphangioma in infants and children. *Ann Otol Rhinol Laryngol* 111:1066, 2002.

31. Gruss JS, Macinnon SE: Complex midface fractures: Role of buttress reconstruction and immediate bone grafts. *Plast Reconstr Surg* 78:9, 1988.

32. Shumrick K, Kersten R, Kulwin D, et al: Extended access/internal approaches for the management of facial trauma. *Arch Otolaryngol Head Neck Surg* 118:1105, 1992.

33. Coker NJ: Facial electroneurography: Analysis of techniques and correlation with degenerating motor neurons. *Laryngoscope* 102:747, 1992.

34. Brodie HA, Thompson TC: Management of complications from 820 temporal bone fractures. *Am J Otol* 18:188, 1997.

35. Darrouzet V, Duclos J, Liguoro D: Management of facial paralysis resulting from temporal bone fractures: Our experience in 115 cases. *Otolaryngol Head Neck Surg* 125:787, 2001.

36. Blot WJ, McLaughlin JK, Winn DM, et al: Smoking and drinking in relation to oral and pharyngeal cancer. *Cancer Res* 48:3282, 1988.

37. Rigotti NA: Treatment of tobacco use and dependence. *N Engl J Med* 346:506, 2002.

38. Moore C: Cigarette smoking and cancer of the mouth, pharynx and larynx. *JAMA* 218:553, 1971.

39. Brennan JA, Boyle JO, Koch WM, et al: Association between cigarette smoking and mutation of the p53 gene in squamous cell carcinoma of the head and neck. *N Engl J Med* 332:712, 1995.

40. Boyle JO, Koch W, Hrubin PA, et al: The incidence of P53 mutations increase with progression of head and neck cancer. *Cancer Res* 53:4477, 1993.

41. Koch WM, Lango M, Sewell D, et al: Head and neck cancer in nonsmokers: A distinct clinical and molecular entity. *Laryngoscope* 109:1544, 1999.

42. Jusawalla DJ, Despandi VA: Evaluation of cancer risk in tobacco chewers and smokers. An epidemiologic assessment. *Cancer* 28:244, 1971.

43. Joint Committee on Cancer: *American Joint Committee on Cancer Staging Manual*, 6th ed. Chicago: American, 2002.

44. Zitsch RP, Park CW, Renner FJ, et al: Outcome analysis for lip carcinoma. *Otolaryngol Head Neck Surg* 113:589, 1995.

45. Calhoun K: Reconstruction of small- and medium-sized defects of the lower lip. *Am J Otolaryngol* 13:16, 1992.

46. Conley JJ, Donovan DT: A new technique for total reconstruction of the lower lip in a patient with malignant melanoma. *Otolaryngol Head Neck Surg* 94:393, 1986.

47. Franceschi D, Gupta R, Spiro RH, et al: Improved survival in the treatment of squamous carcinoma of the oral tongue. *Am J Surg* 166:360, 1993.

48. Lydiatt DD, Robbins KT, Byers RM, et al: Treatment of stage I and II oral cancer. *Head Neck* 15:308, 1993.

49. Spiro RH, Huvos AG, Wong GY, et al: Predictive value of tumor thickness in squamous carcinoma confined to the tongue and floor of mouth. *Am J Surg* 152:345, 1986.

50. Rodgers LW Jr., Stringer SP, Mendenhall WM, et al: Management of squamous cell carcinoma of the floor of mouth. *Head Neck* 15:16, 1993.

51. Overholt SM, Eicher SA, Wolf P, et al: Prognostic factors affecting outcome in lower gingival carcinoma. *Laryngoscope* 106:1335, 1996.

52. Huang CJ, Chao KSC, Tsai J, et al: Cancer of retromolar trigone: Long-term radiation therapy outcome. *Head Neck* 23:758, 2001.

53. Bloom ND, Spiro RH: Carcinoma of the cheek mucosa: A retrospective analysis. *Am J Surg* 154:411, 1987.

54. Beckhardt RN, Weber RS, Zane R, et al: Minor salivary gland tumors of the palate: Clinical and pathologic correlates of outcome. *Laryngoscope* 11:1155, 1995.

55. Bradford CR, Futran N, Peters G: Management of tonsil cancer. *Head Neck* 21:657, 1999.

56. Lee, HJ, Zelefsky MJ, Kraus DH, et al: Long-term regional control after radiation therapy and neck dissection for base of tongue carcinoma. *Int J Rad Oncology Biol Phys* 38:995, 1997.

57. Peters LJ, Weber RS, Morrison WH, et al: Neck surgery in patients with primary oropharyngeal cancer treated by radiotherapy. *Head Neck* 18:552, 1996.

58. Ang KK, Peters LJ, Weber RS, et al: Concomitant boost radiotherapy schedules in the treatment of carcinoma of the oropharynx and nasopharynx. *Int J Radiat Oncol Biol Phys* 19:1339, 1990.

59. Weber RS, Gidley P, Morrison WH, et al: Treatment selection for carcinoma of the base of tongue. *Am J Surg* 160:415, 1990.

60. Weber RS, Ohlms L, Bowman J, et al: Functional results after total or near total glossectomy with laryngeal preservation. *Arch Otolaryngol Head Neck Surg* 117:512, 1991.

61. Weber RS, Peters LJ, Wolf P, et al: Squamous cell carcinoma of the soft palate, uvula, and anterior faucial pillar. *Otolaryngol Head Neck Surg* 99:16, 1988.

62. Frank J, Garb J, Kay S, et al: Postoperative radiotherapy improves survival in squamous cell carcinoma of the hypopharynx. *Am J Surg* 168:476, 1994.

63. Lefebve JL, Chevalier D, Luboinski B, et al: Larynx preservation in piriform sinus cancer: Preliminary results of a European organization for research and treatment of cancer phase III trial. *J Natl Cancer Inst* 88:890, 1996.

64. Hartig G, Truelson J, Weinstein GS. Supraglottic cancer. *Head Neck* 22:426, 2000.

65. Laccourreye H, Laccourreye O, Weinstein GS, et al: Supracricoid laryngectomy with cricohyoidoepiglottopexy: A partial laryngeal procedure for selected glottic carcinomas. *Ann Otol Rhinol Laryngol* 99:421, 1990.

66. Wolf GT, Hong WK, Fischer SG, et al: Induction chemotherapy plus radiation compared with surgery plus radiation in patients with advanced laryngeal cancer. *N Engl J Med* 324:1685, 1991.

67. Medina JE, Khafif A: Early oral feeding following total laryngectomy. *Laryngoscope* 111:368, 2001.

68. Weber RS, Marvel J, Smith P, et al: Paratracheal lymph node dissection for carcinoma of the larynx, hypopharynx, and cervical esophagus. *Otolaryngol Head Neck Surg* 108:11, 1993.

69. Weber RS, Berket BA, Forastiere A, et al: Outcome of salvage total laryngectomy following organ preservation therapy: The Radiation Therapy Oncology Group trial 91-11. *Arch Otolaryngol Head Neck Surg* 129:44, 2003.

70. Osguthorpe JD: Sinus neoplasia. *Arch Otolaryngol Head Neck Surg* 120:19, 1994.

71. Levine PA, Frierson HF, Mills SE, et al: Sinonasal undifferentiated carcinoma: A distinctive and highly aggressive neoplasm. *Laryngoscope* 97:905, 1987.

72. Senior BA, Lanza DC, Kennedy DW, et al: Computer-assisted resection of benign sinonasal tumors with skull base and orbital extension. *Arch Otolaryngol Head Neck Surg* 123:706, 1997.

73. Isaacs RS, Donald PJ: Sphenoid and sellar tumors. *Otolaryngol Clin North Am* 28:1191, 1995.

74. Al-Sarraf M, LeBlanc M, Giri PG, et al: Chemoradiotherapy versus radiotherapy in patients with advanced nasopharyngeal cancer: Phase III randomized intergroup 0099. *J Clin Oncol* 16:1310, 1998.

75. Kuhel W, Hume CR, Selesnick SH: Cancer of the external auditory canal and temporal bone. *Otolaryngol Clin North Am* 29:827, 1996.

76. Prasad S, Janecka IP: Efficacy of surgical treatments for squamous cell carcinoma of the temporal bone: A literature review. *Otolaryngol Head Neck Surg* 110:270, 1994.

77. Shah JP: Patterns of cervical lymph node metastasis from squamous carcinomas of the upper aerodigestive tract. *Am J Surg* 160:405, 1990.

78. Bocca E, Pignataro O, Oldino C: Functional neck dissection: An evaluation and review of 843 cases. *Laryngoscope* 94:942, 1984.

79. Medina JE, Byers RM: Supraomohyoid neck dissection: Rationale, indications and surgical technique. *Head Neck* 11:111, 1989.

80. Eicher SA, Weber RS: Surgical management of cervical lymph node metastases. *Curr Opin Oncol* 8:215, 1996.

81. Robbins KT, Atkinson JLD, Byers RM, et al: The use and misuse of neck dissection for head and neck cancer. *J Am Coll Surg* 193:91, 2001.

82. Byers RM, Weber RS, Andrews T, et al: Frequency and therapeutic implications of "skip metastases" in the neck from squamous carcinoma of the oral tongue. *Head Neck* 19:14, 1997.

83. Myers EN, Fagan JJ: Treatment of the N+ neck in squamous cell carcinoma of the upper aerodigestive tract. *Otolaryngol Clin North Am* 31:671, 1998.

84. Eisele DE, Netterville J, Hoffman H, et al: Parapharyngeal space masses. *Head Neck* 21:154, 1999.

85. Frankenthaler RA, Luna MA, Lee S, et al: Prognostic variables in parotid gland cancer. *Arch Otol Head Neck Surg* 117:1251, 1991.

86. Weber RS, Byers RM, Petit B, et al: Submandibular gland tumors: Adverse histologic factors and therapeutic implications. *Arch Otolaryngol Head Neck Surg* 116:1055, 1990.

87. Blackwell KE, Buchbinder D, Biller HF: Reconstruction of massive defects in the head and neck: The role of simultaneous distant and regional flaps. *Head Neck* 19:620, 1997.

88. Anthony JP, Neligan PC, Rotstein LE, et al: Reconstruction of partial laryngopharyngectomy defects. *Head Neck* 19:541, 1997.

89. Schusterman M, Shestak K, de Vries EL, et al: Reconstruction of the cervical esophagus: Free jejunal transfer versus gastric pull-up. *Plast Reconstr Surg* 85:16, 1990.

90. Urken ML, Buchbinder D, Costantino PD, et al: Oromandibular reconstruction using microvascular composite flaps: Report of 210 cases. *Arch Otolaryngol Head Neck Surg* 124:46, 1998.

91. Wenig BL, Applebaum EL: Indications for and technique for tracheostomy. *Clin Chest Med* 1293:545, 1991.

92. The American Society for Head and Neck Surgery and the Society of Head and Neck Surgeons: *Clinical Practice Guidelines for the Diagnosis and Management of Cancer of the Head and Neck.* 1996. Also see *http://www.headandneckcancer.org/clinicalresources/docs/oralcavity.php.*

Chest Wall, Lung, Mediastinum, and Pleura

Katie S. Nason, Michael A. Maddaus, and James D. Luketich

TRACHEA

Anatomy

An understanding of the relevant anatomy of the trachea is essential for surgeons of all specialties (Fig. 19-1).[1] The trachea is composed of cartilaginous and membranous portions, beginning with the cricoid cartilage, the first complete cartilaginous ring of the airway. The cricoid cartilage consists of an anterior arch and a posterior broad-based plate. Articulating with the posterior cricoid plate are the arytenoid cartilages. The vocal cords originate from the arytenoid cartilages and then attach to the thyroid cartilage. The subglottic space, the narrowest part of the trachea with an internal diameter of approximately 2 cm, begins at the inferior surface of the vocal cords and extends to the first tracheal ring. The remainder of the distal trachea is 10.0 to 13.0 cm long, consists of 18 to 22 rings, and has an internal diameter of 2.3 cm.

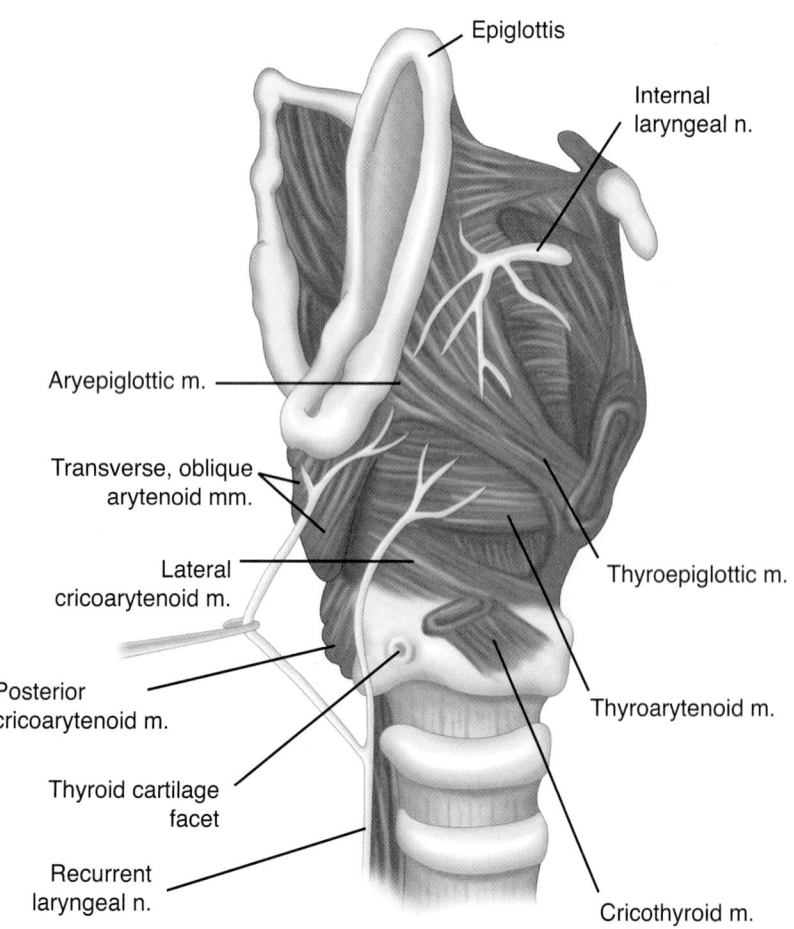

FIG. 19-1. Anatomy of the larynx and upper trachea. m. = muscle; n. = nerve.

The tracheal blood supply enters the airway near the junction of the membranous and cartilaginous portions of the airway (Fig. 19-2). It is segmental, which means that each entering small branch supplies a segment of 1.0 to 2.0 cm, which limits circumferential mobilization to that same distance. The arteries supplying the trachea include the inferior thyroid, subclavian, supreme intercostal, internal thoracic, innominate, and superior and middle bronchial arteries. The vessels are interconnected along the lateral surface of the trachea by an important longitudinal vascular anastomosis that feeds transverse segmental vessels to the soft tissues between the cartilages.

KEY POINTS

1. Lung cancer continues to be a highly lethal and extremely common cancer, with 5-year survival of 15%. Lung cancer incidence is second only to the incidence of prostate cancer in men and breast cancer in women. Squamous cell carcinoma and adenocarcinoma of the lung are the most common subtypes and are rarely found in the absence of a smoking history. Nonsmokers who live with smokers have a 24% increased risk of lung cancer compared to nonsmokers who do not live with smokers.

2. Endoscopic bronchial ultrasound is a valuable new tool that can enhance the accuracy and safety of transbronchial biopsies of both the primary tumor (when it abuts the central airways) and the mediastinal lymph nodes and should become part of the surgeon's armamentarium for the diagnosis and treatment of lung cancer.

3. The assessment of patient risk before thoracic resection is based on clinical judgment and data.

4. Impaired exchange of carbon monoxide is associated with a significant increase in the risk of postoperative pulmonary complications, independent of the patient's smoking history. In patients undergoing pulmonary resection, the risk of any pulmonary complication increases by 42% for every 10% decline in the percent carbon monoxide diffusion capacity (%DLCO), and this measure may be a useful parameter in risk stratification of patients for surgery.

5. Maximum oxygen consumption ($\dot{V}O_2$max) values provide important additional information in those patients with severely impaired DLCO and forced expiratory volume in 1 second. Values of <10 mL/kg per minute generally prohibit any major pulmonary resection, because the mortality in patients with these levels is 26% compared with only 8.3% in patients whose $\dot{V}O_2$max is ≥10 mL/kg per minute; values of >15 mL/kg per minute generally indicate the patient's ability to tolerate pneumonectomy.

6. Major changes in the tumor, node, and metastasis (TNM) staging system for lung cancer have been proposed. Tumor stage will be further subdivided into T1a and T1b, T2a and T2b, T3, and T4. Satellite nodules in the same lobe will be considered T3 and malignant pleural and pericardial effusions will be considered metastatic disease rather than T4 disease.

7. Increasing evidence suggests a significant role for gastroesophageal reflux disease in the pathogenesis of chronic lung diseases such as bronchiectasis and idiopathic pulmonary fibrosis, and it may also contribute to bronchiolitis obliterans syndrome in lung transplant patients.

8. Multidrug-resistant tuberculosis (MDRTB) organisms are present in approximately 10% of new tuberculosis cases and 40% of recurrent cases. Another rare disease variant termed *extensively drug-resistant tuberculosis* has also been identified. The causative organisms are resistant not only to isoniazid and rifampin, as are the MDRTB organisms, but also to at least one of the injectable second-line drugs such as capreomycin, amikacin, and kanamycin.

9. Treatment of pulmonary aspergilloma is individualized. Asymptomatic patients can be observed without any additional therapy. Similarly, mild hemoptysis, which is not life-threatening, can be managed with medical therapy, including antifungals and cough suppressant. Amphotericin B is the drug of choice, although voriconazole has recently been used for treatment of aspergillosis, with fewer side effects and equivalent efficacy. Massive hemoptysis had traditionally been an indication for urgent or emergent operative intervention. However, with the advancement of endovascular techniques, bronchial artery embolization in select centers with experience in these techniques has been effective.

10. Treatment for candidal infection, like that for other fungal infections, has changed dramatically in the past decade. The availability of multiple effective therapies allows for specific tailoring of treatment, including combination regimens, based on the patient's ability to tolerate associated toxicities, the microbiologic information for the specific candidal species, and the route of administration. Although their demonstrated efficacy is similar to that of other classes of antifungal drugs, the triazoles and echinocandins appear to have fewer side effects and are better tolerated than these other drug classes.

11. In patients with malignant pleural effusion, poor expansion of the lung (because of entrapment by tumor or adhesions) generally predicts a poor result with pleurodesis and is the primary indication for placement of indwelling pleural catheters. These catheters have dramatically changed the management of end-stage cancer treatment, because they substantially shorten the amount of time patients spend in the hospital during their final weeks of life.

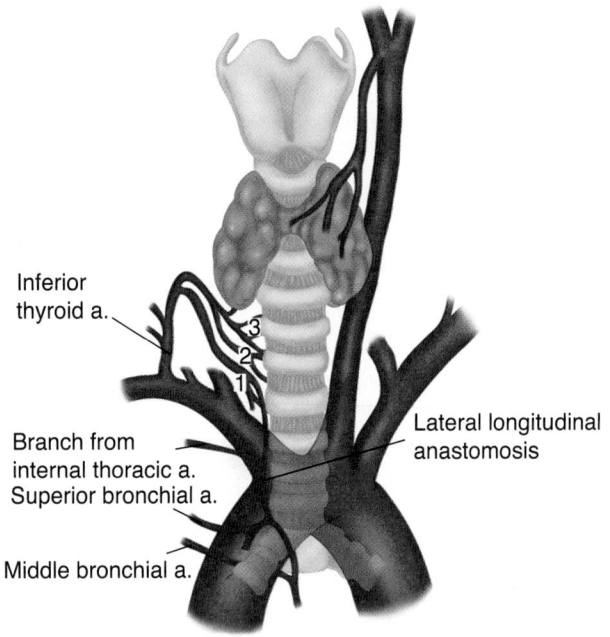

FIG. 19-2. Arterial blood supply to the larynx and upper trachea. a. = artery.

Inferior thyroid a.

Branch from internal thoracic a.
Superior bronchial a.

Middle bronchial a.

Lateral longitudinal anastomosis

Tracheal Injury

Injury secondary to endotracheal intubation is most commonly the result of overinflation of the cuff. Although high-volume/low-pressure cuffs are now ubiquitous, they can easily be overinflated, and pressures can be generated that are high enough to cause ischemia of the contiguous airway wall. In some patients, periods of ischemia as short as 4 hours may be all that is required to induce an ischemic event significant enough to lead to scarring and stricture. With prolonged overinflation and consequent full-thickness destruction of the airway,

fistula development between the innominate artery and esophagus may ensue. For these reasons, it is good practice in all intubations, no matter how brief, to inflate the cuff only to the level necessary to prevent air leakage around the cuff. In circumstances of prolonged ventilatory support and high airway pressures, cuff pressure monitoring (to maintain pressures below 20 mmHg) is advisable.

Tracheal stenosis is nearly always iatrogenic. It is secondary to either endotracheal intubation or tracheostomy. Collectively, such tracheal injuries are referred to as *postintubation injuries*. Clinically significant tracheal stenosis is common after tracheostomy due to scarring and local injury, and occurs in 3 to 12% of cases.[2] Factors associated with an increased risk of tracheal stenosis include incorrect placement of the tracheostomy through the first tracheal ring or the cricothyroid membrane where the airway is narrowest, use of a large tracheostomy tube, and transverse incision on the trachea. However, even a properly placed tracheostomy can lead to tracheal stenosis secondary to scarring and local injury, and mild ulceration and stenosis frequently are seen after tracheostomy removal. The rate of stomal stenosis can be minimized by using the smallest tracheostomy tube possible and downsizing as soon as the patient will tolerate it, and by using a vertical tracheal incision without removing cartilage.

Clinically, stridor and dyspnea on exertion are the primary symptoms of tracheal stenosis. The length of time to onset of symptoms after extubation or after tracheostomy decannulation varies, usually ranging from 2 to 12 weeks; however, symptoms can appear immediately or as long as 1 to 2 years later. Frequently, patients are misdiagnosed as having asthma or bronchitis, and treatment for such illnesses can persist for some time before the correct diagnosis is discovered. Generally, the intensity of symptoms experienced is related to the degree of stenosis and to the patient's underlying pulmonary disease.

Acute Management

The treatment of tracheal stenosis is resection and primary anastomosis. In nearly all postintubation injuries the injury is transmural, and significant portions of the cartilaginous structural support are destroyed (Fig. 19-3). Measures such as laser ablation are temporizing. In the early phase of evaluating patients, dilation using a rigid broncho-

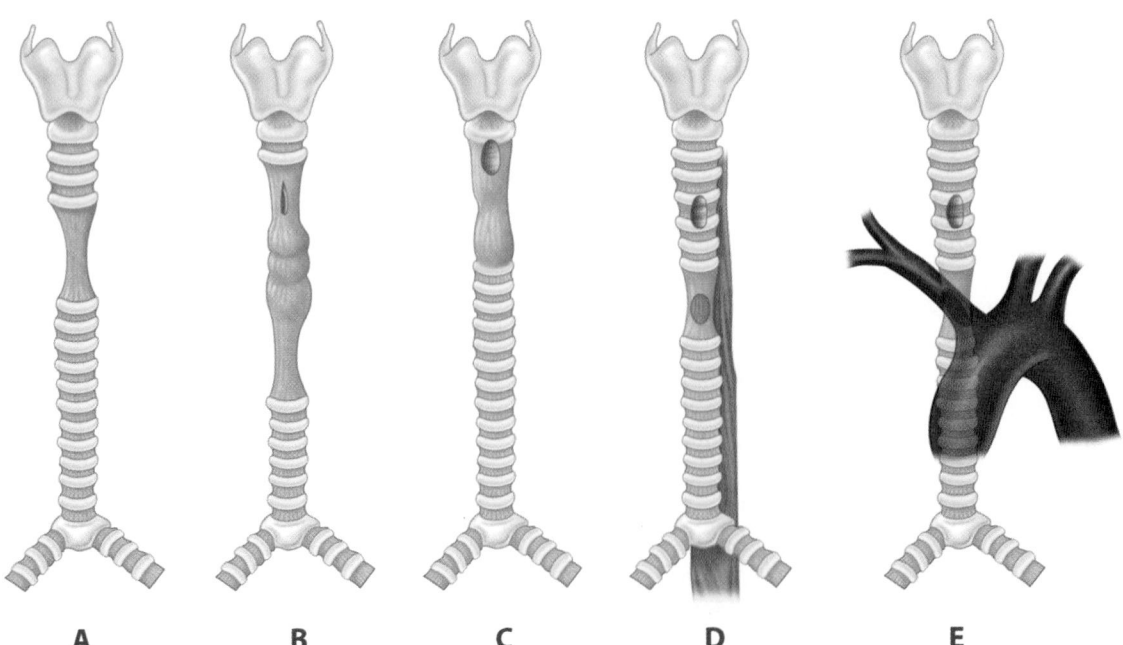

A   B   C   D   E

FIG. 19-3. Diagram of the principal postintubation lesions. **A.** A circumferential lesion at the cuff site after the use of an endotracheal tube. **B.** Potential lesions after the use of tracheostomy tubes. Anterolateral stenosis can be seen at the stomal level. Circumferential stenosis can be seen at the cuff level (lower than with an endotracheal tube). The segment in between is often inflamed and malacic. **C.** Damage to the subglottic larynx. **D.** Tracheoesophageal fistula occurring at the level of the tracheostomy cuff. Circumferential damage is usual at this level. **E.** Tracheoinnominate artery fistula. *(Adapted with permission from Grillo.[2])*

scope is useful to gain immediate relief of dyspnea and to allow full assessment of the lesion. It is important to carefully document the length and position of the stenosis as well as the location in relation to the vocal cords. Rarely, if ever, is a tracheostomy necessary. For patients who are not operative candidates due to associated comorbidities, internal stents, typically silicone T tubes, are useful. Wire mesh stents should not be used, given their known propensity to erode through the wall of the airway. The use of balloon dilation and tracheoplasty also has been described, although their efficacy is marginal. Efforts focused on tissue engineering may provide suitable material for tracheal replacement in long-segment tracheal stenosis in the future.

Most intubation injuries are located in the upper third of the trachea, so tracheal resection usually is done through a collar incision. Resection typically involves 2 to 4 cm of trachea for benign stenosis. However, a primary anastomosis can still be performed without undue tension, even if up to one half of the trachea needs to be resected.[2] When resection for a postintubation injury is performed, it is critical to fully resect all inflamed and scarred tissue. Tracheostomies and stents are not required postoperatively, and the patient often is extubated in the operating room or shortly thereafter.

Tracheal Fistulas
Tracheoinnominate Artery Fistula

Tracheoinnominate artery fistula has two causes: too low a placement of the tracheostomy and hyperinflation of the tracheal cuff.

When performing a tracheostomy, the surgeon must be diligent about proper identification of the tracheal rings. Tracheostomies should be placed through the second to fourth tracheal rings without reference to the location of the sternal notch. When they are placed below the fourth tracheal ring, the inner curve of the tracheostomy cannula will be positioned to exert pressure on the upper surface of the innominate artery, which will lead to arterial erosion. Similarly, the tracheal cuff, when hyperinflated, will cause ischemic injury to the airway and subsequent erosion into the artery and fistula development. Most cuff-induced fistulas develop within 2 weeks after placement of the tracheostomy.

Clinically, tracheoinnominate artery fistulas present with bleeding. A premonitory hemorrhage often occurs, and although it usually is not massive, it must not be ignored or simply attributed to general airway irritation or wound bleeding. With significant bleeding, the tracheostomy cuff can be hyperinflated to temporarily occlude the arterial injury. If such an effort is unsuccessful, the tracheostomy incision should immediately be opened widely and a finger inserted to compress the artery against the manubrium (Fig. 19-4). The patient can then be orally intubated, and the airway suctioned free of blood. Emergent surgical resection of the involved segment of artery is performed, usually without reconstruction.

Tracheoesophageal Fistula

Tracheoesophageal fistulas (TEFs) occur primarily in patients with an indwelling nasogastric tube who are also receiving prolonged me-

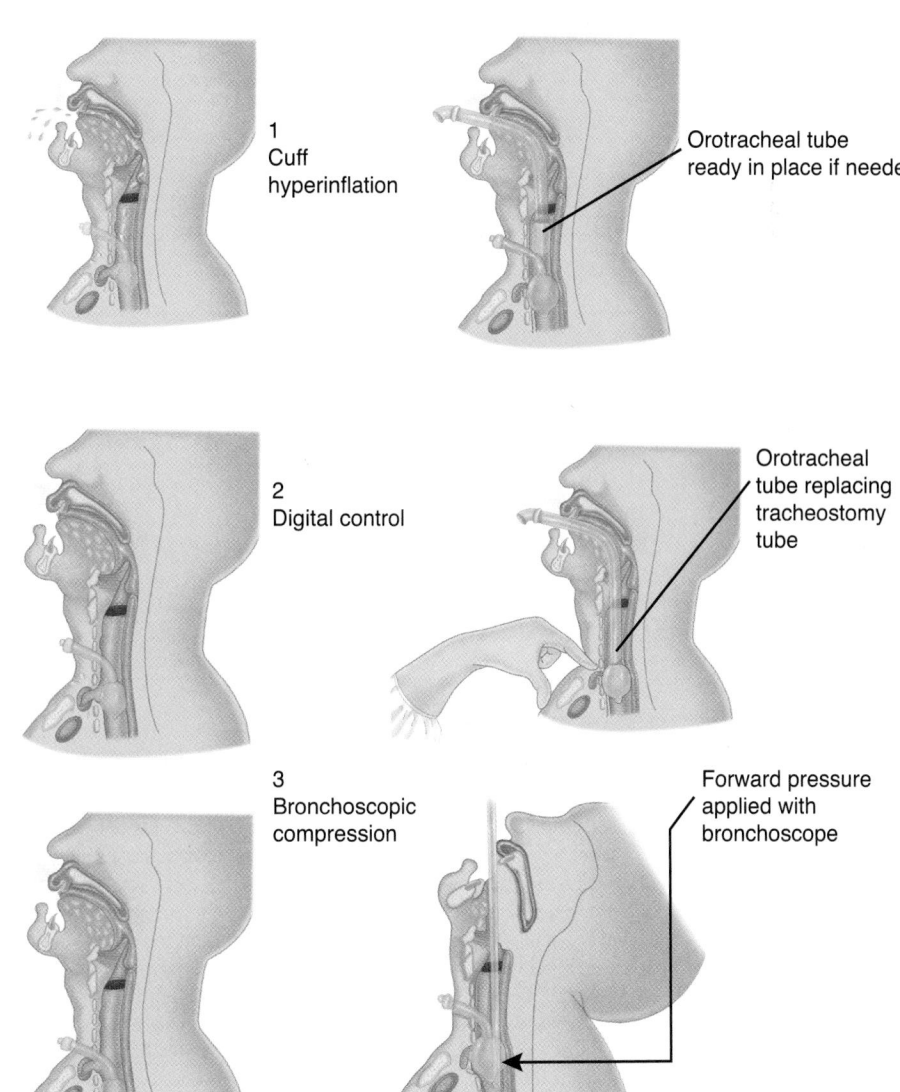

1 Cuff hyperinflation

Orotracheal tube ready in place if needed

2 Digital control

Orotracheal tube replacing tracheostomy tube

3 Bronchoscopic compression

Forward pressure applied with bronchoscope

FIG. 19-4. Steps in the emergency management of a tracheoinnominate artery fistula.

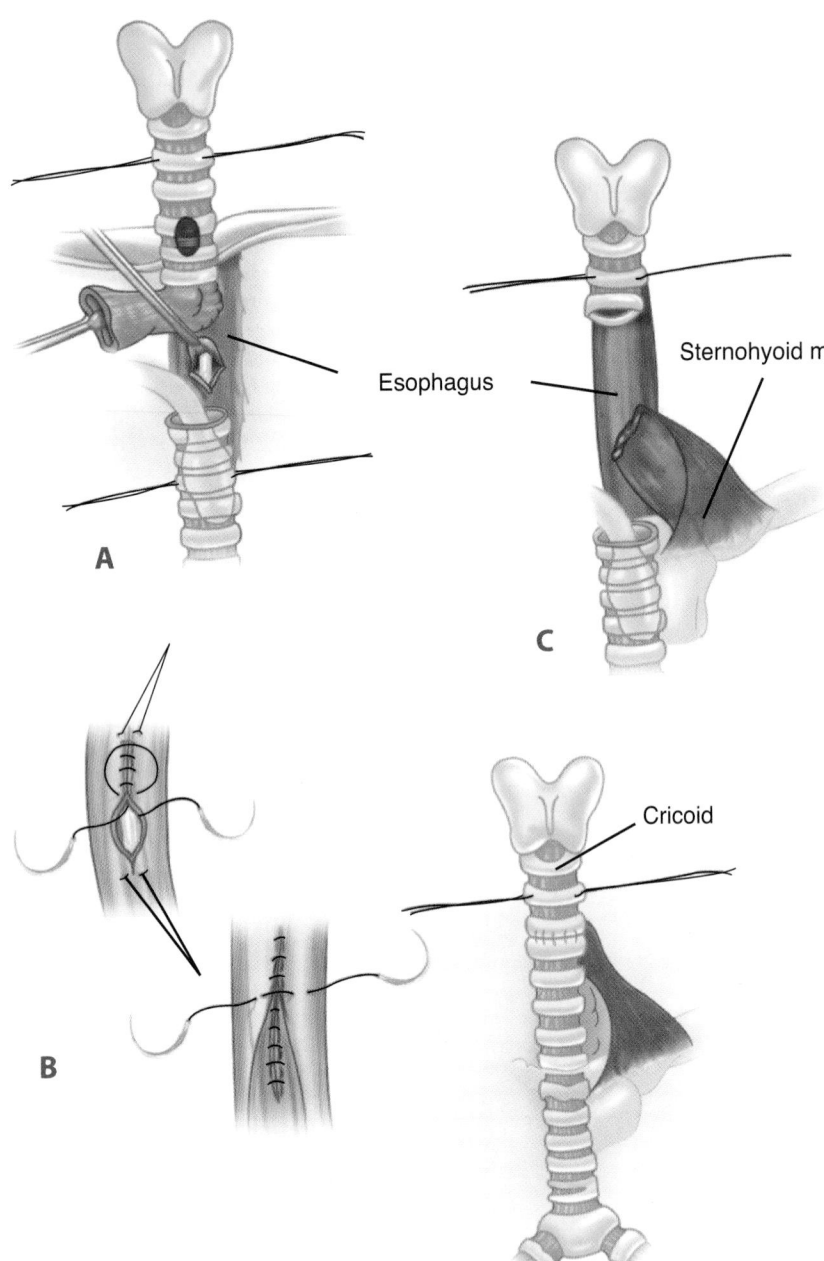

FIG. 19-5. Single-stage operation for closure of a tracheoesophageal fistula and tracheal resection. **A.** The fistula is divided and the trachea is transected below the level of damage. **B.** The fistula is closed on the tracheal side in a single layer and on the esophageal side in a double layer. **C.** The damaged trachea segment is resected. **D.** View of completed tracheal anastomosis. m. = muscle.

chanical ventilatory support.[3] Cuff compression of the membranous trachea against the nasogastric tube leads to airway and esophageal injury and fistula development. Clinically, saliva, gastric contents, or tube feeding contents are noted in the material suctioned from the airway. Distention of the stomach secondary to positive pressure ventilation can occur. Diagnosis of a suspected TEF is by bronchoscopy. Withdrawal of the endotracheal tube with the bronchoscope inserted allows the fistula at the cuff site to be seen. Alternatively, esophagoscopy will enable visualization of the cuff of the endotracheal tube in the esophagus.

First and foremost, treatment of a TEF requires weaning the patient from the ventilator and then extubating as soon as possible. During the weaning period, the nasogastric tube should be removed, with attention given to ensuring that the cuff of the endotracheal tube is placed below the fistula and that it is not overinflated. Then a gastrostomy tube should be placed for aspiration (to prevent reflux) and a jejunostomy tube for feeding. If aspiration is relentless and is not managed by the aforementioned steps, esophageal diversion with esophagostomy can be performed. Once the patient is weaned from the ventilator, a single-

stage operation should be done, consisting of tracheal resection and primary anastomosis, repair of the esophageal defect, and interposition of a muscle flap between the trachea and esophagus (Fig. 19-5).[4]

Tracheal Neoplasms

Primary tracheal neoplasms are exceedingly rare, and the diagnosis frequently is delayed. The most common primary tracheal neoplasms are squamous cell carcinomas (related to smoking) and adenoid cystic carcinomas. Clinically, tracheal tumors present with cough, dyspnea, hemoptysis, stridor, or symptoms of invasion of contiguous structures (such as the recurrent laryngeal nerve or the esophagus). The most common radiologic finding of tracheal malignancy is tracheal stenosis, but it is seen in only 50% of cases. With tumors other than squamous cell carcinomas, symptoms may persist for months because of slow tumor growth rates. Stage of presentation is advanced, with approximately 50% of patients presenting with stage IV disease. Overall 5-year survival for patients with tracheal neoplasms is 40%, but survival falls to 15% for those with stage IV disease.[5]

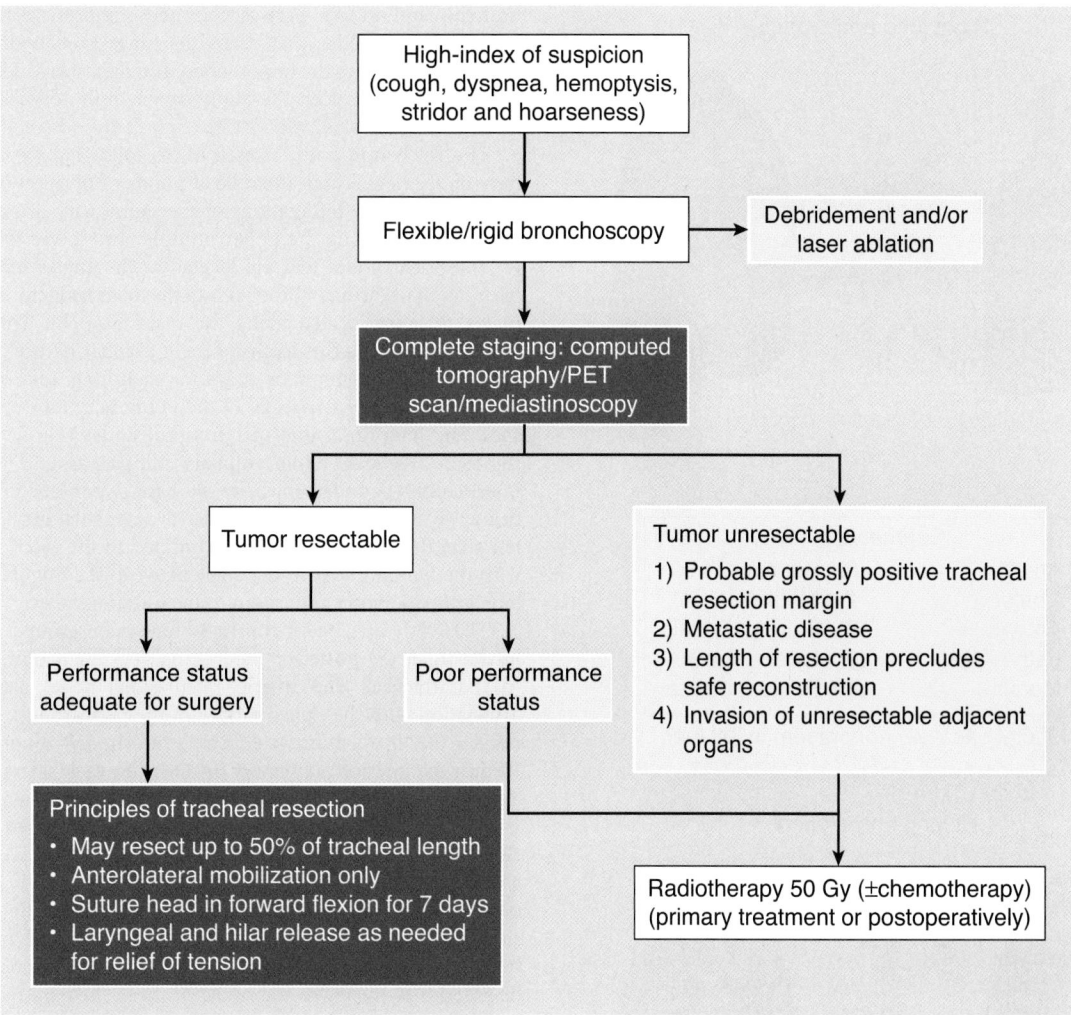

FIG. 19-6. Algorithm for evaluation and treatment of tracheal neoplasm. PET = positron emission tomography.

Squamous cell carcinomas often present with regional lymph node metastases and are frequently not resectable at the time of presentation. Their biologic behavior is similar to that of squamous cell carcinomas of the lung. Adenoid cystic carcinomas, which are a type of salivary gland tumor, are generally slow growing, spread submucosally, and tend to infiltrate along nerve sheaths and within the tracheal wall. Spread to regional lymph nodes can occur. Although indolent in nature, adenoid cystic carcinomas are malignant and can spread to the lungs and bones. Squamous cell carcinomas and adenoid cystic carcinomas represent approximately 65% of all tracheal neoplasms. The remaining 35% is composed of small cell carcinomas, mucoepidermoid carcinomas, adenocarcinomas, lymphomas, and others.[6]

Therapy

A treatment algorithm for tracheal neoplasms is presented in Fig. 19-6. Evaluation and treatment of patients with tracheal tumors should include neck and chest computed tomography (CT) and rigid bronchoscopy. Rigid bronchoscopy permits general assessment of the airway and tumor; it also allows débridement or laser ablation of the tumor to provide relief of dyspnea. If the tumor is judged to be completely resectable, primary resection and anastomosis is the treatment of choice.[7]

The length limit of tracheal resection is roughly 50% of the trachea. To prevent tension on the anastomosis postoperatively, specialized maneuvers are necessary, such as anterolateral tracheal mobilization, suturing of the chin to the sternum with the head flexed forward for 7 days, laryngeal release, and right hilar release.

For most tracheal resections (which involve much less than 50% of the airway), anterolateral tracheal mobilization and suturing of the chin to the sternum for 7 days are done routinely. Use of laryngeal and hilar release is determined at the time of surgery, based on the surgeon's judgment of the degree of tension present.

Radiotherapy is frequently given postoperatively after resection of both adenoid cystic carcinomas and squamous cell carcinomas, due to their radiosensitivity.[8] A dose of 50 Gy or higher is usual. For patients with unresectable tumors, radiation may be given as the primary therapy with the expectation of temporary local control, but it is rarely curative. For recurrent airway compromise, stenting or laser therapies should be considered part of the treatment algorithm.

LUNG

Anatomy
Segmental Anatomy

The segmental anatomy of the lungs and bronchial tree is illustrated in Fig. 19-7.[9] Note the continuity of the pulmonary parenchyma between adjacent segments of each lobe. In contrast, separation of the bronchial and vascular stalks allows subsegmental and segmental resections, if the clinical situation requires it or if lung tissue can be preserved.

Lymphatic Drainage

Many lymphatic vessels are located beneath the visceral pleura of each lung, in the interlobular septa, in the submucosa of the

Right lung and bronchi

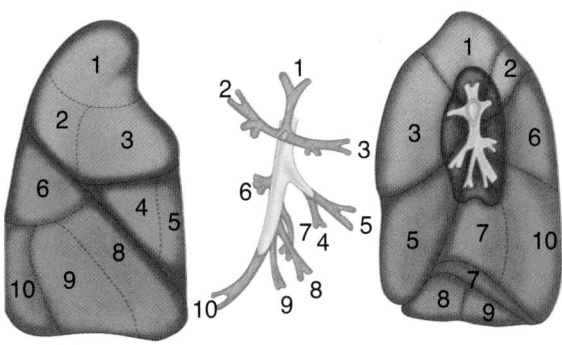

Segments	
1. Apical	6. Superior
2. Posterior	7. Medial Basal *
3. Anterior	8. Anterior Basal
4. Lateral	9. Lateral Basal
5. Medial	10. Posterior Basal

* Medial basal (7) not present in left lung

Left lung and bronchi

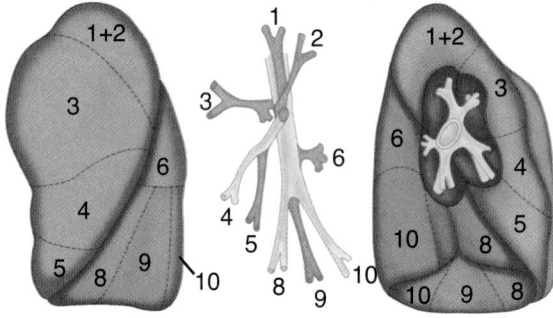

FIG. 19-7. Segmental anatomy of the lungs and bronchi.

bronchi, and in the perivascular and peribronchial connective tissue. Lymph nodes that drain the lungs are divided into two groups according to the tumor, node, and metastasis (TNM) staging system for lung cancer: the pulmonary lymph nodes, N1; and the mediastinal nodes, N2 (Fig. 19-8).

The N1 lymph nodes consist of the following: (a) intrapulmonary or segmental nodes that lie at points of division of segmental bronchi or in the bifurcations of the pulmonary artery; (b) lobar nodes that lie along the upper, middle, and lower lobe bronchi; (c) interlobar nodes that are located in the angles formed by the bifurcation of the main bronchi into the lobar bronchi; and (d) hilar nodes that are located along the main bronchi. The interlobar lymph nodes lie in the depths of the interlobar fissure on each side and constitute a lymphatic sump for each lung, referred to as the *lymphatic sump of Borrie*; all of the pulmonary lobes of the corresponding lung drain into this group of nodes (Fig. 19-9). On the right side, the nodes of the lymphatic sump lie around the bronchus intermedius (bounded above by the right upper lobe bronchus and below by the middle lobe and superior segmental bronchi). On the left side, the lymphatic sump is confined to the interlobar fissure, with the lymph nodes in the angle between the lingular and lower lobe bronchi and in apposition to the pulmonary artery branches.

The N2 lymph nodes consist of four main groups: (a) anterior mediastinal, (b) posterior mediastinal, (c) tracheobronchial, and (d) paratracheal. The anterior mediastinal nodes are located in association with the upper surface of the pericardium, the phrenic nerves, the ligamentum arteriosum, and the left innominate vein. Within the inferior pulmonary ligament on each side are the paraesophageal lymph nodes, which are part of the posterior mediastinal group. Additional paraesophageal nodes can be located more superiorly, between the esophagus and trachea near the arch of the azygos vein. The tracheobronchial lymph nodes are made up of three subgroups that are located near the bifurcation of the trachea: the subcarinal nodes, the lymph nodes that lie in the obtuse angle between the trachea and each main stem bronchus, and nodes that lie anterior to the lower end of the trachea. The paratracheal lymph nodes are located in proximity to the trachea in the superior mediastinum. Those on the right side form a chain with the tracheobronchial nodes inferiorly and with some of the deep cervical nodes above (scalene lymph nodes). Lymphatic drainage of the right lung is ipsilateral, except for occasional bilateral drainage to the superior mediastinum. Ipsilateral and contralateral drainage from the left lung, particularly the left lower lobe, to the superior mediastinum occur with the same frequency.

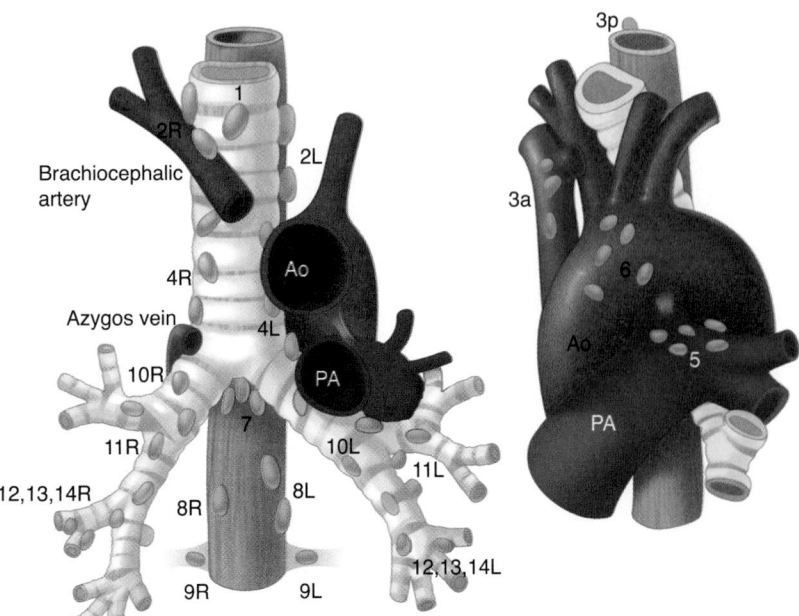

FIG. 19-8. The location of regional lymph node stations for lung cancer staging. Station, Description: 1, highest mediastinal lymph nodes; 2, upper paratracheal nodes; 3, prevascular, precarinal and retrotracheal nodes; 4, lower paratracheal nodes; 5, aorto-pulmonary nodes; 6, pre-aortic nodes; 7, subcarnal nodes; 8, paraesophageal nodes; 9, pulmonary ligament nodes; 10, tracheobronchial nodes; 11, interlobular nodes; 12, lobar bronchial nodes; 13, segmental nodes; 14, subsegmental nodes. Note: Stations 12, 13, and 14 are not shown in their entirety. *(Reproduced with permission from Ferguson, MK: Thoracic Surgery Atlas. W.B. Saunders, Inc., Philadelphia, PA, 2007. Copyright Elsevier.)*

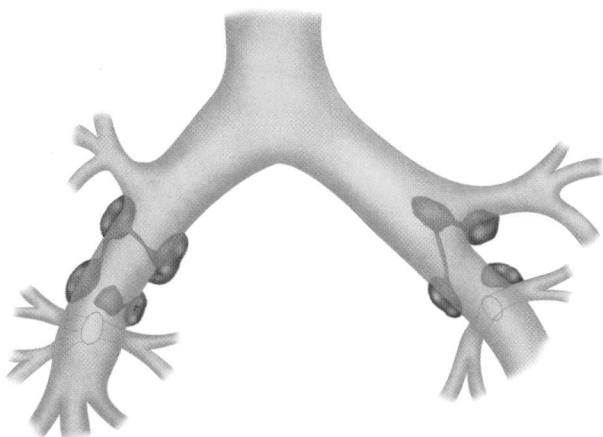

FIG. 19-9. The lymphatic sump of Borrie includes the groups of lymph nodes that receive lymphatic drainage from all pulmonary lobes of the corresponding lung.

Computed Tomography

Spiral (helical) CT allows continuous scanning as the patient is moved through a scanning gantry so that an x-ray beam can trace a

helical curve in relation to the patient's position. The entire thorax can be imaged during a solitary breath hold, so motion artifacts are eliminated, which results in superior image quality (compared with conventional CT scanning), particularly in the detection of pulmonary nodules and central airway abnormalities.[10] The shorter acquisition time of spiral CT allows for consistent contrast filling of the great vessels, which results in markedly improved visualization of pathologic states and anatomic variation contiguous to vascular structures. In addition, three-dimensional spiral CT images can be reconstructed for enhanced visualization of spatial anatomic relationships.[11]

In general, slice thickness is proportional to image resolution; as slice thickness increases, volume averaging increases, which results in a decline in image resolution. Slice thickness is determined by the structure being imaged as well as by the indication for the study. Thin sections (1- to 2-mm collimation) at 1-cm intervals should be used to evaluate pulmonary parenchyma and peripheral bronchi. If the goal is to find any pulmonary metastases, thin sections at intervals of 5- to 7-mm collimation are recommended. For assessing the trachea and central bronchi, collimation of 3 to 5 mm is recommended. Virtually all institutions have protocols for spiral CT scanning. Providing accurate clinical history and data is of paramount importance to obtaining appropriate imaging. In addition, the astute clinician must be well versed in normal thoracic anatomy to appreciate pathologic changes and management strategies (Fig. 19-10).

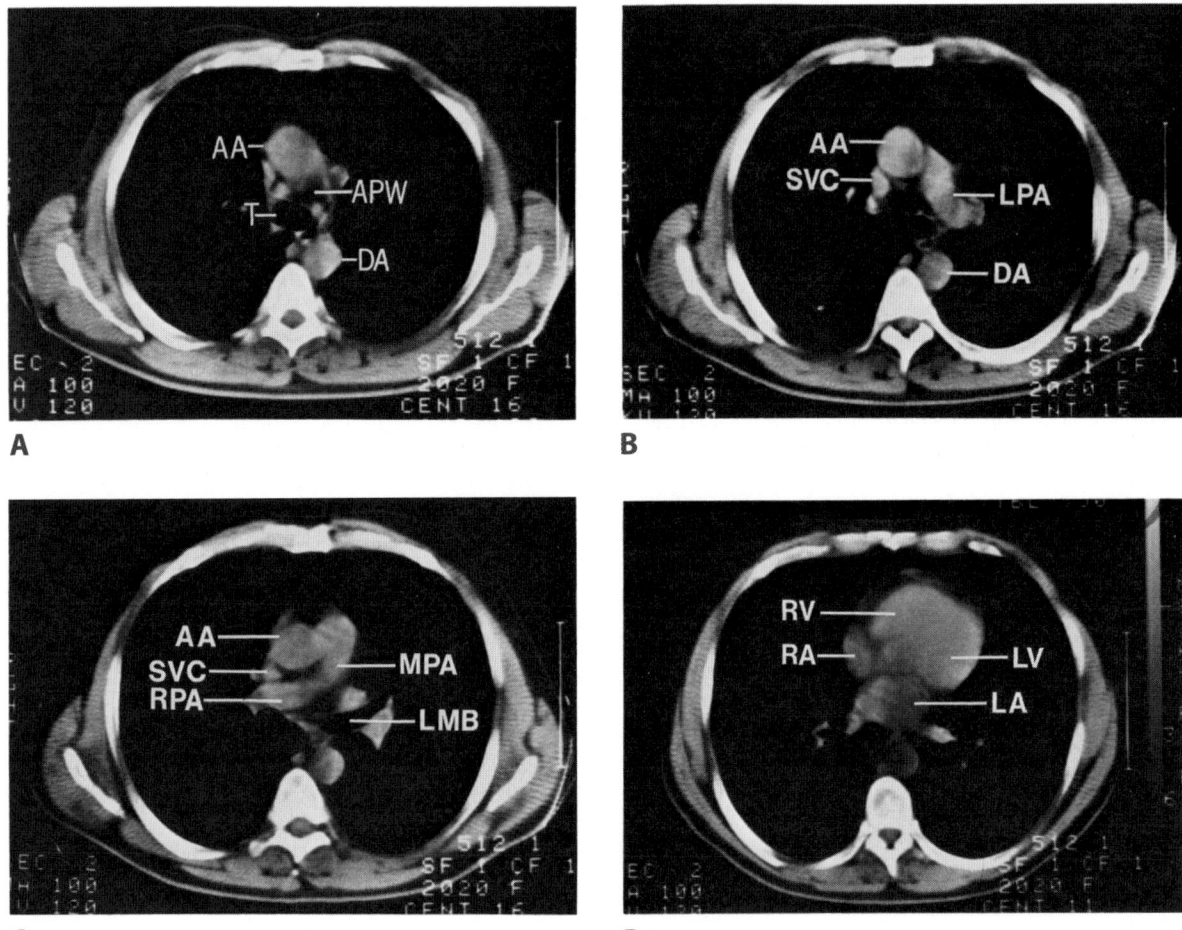

FIG. 19-10. Spiral computed tomographic scan showing normal transverse chest anatomy at four levels. **A.** At the level of the tracheal bifurcation, the aorticopulmonary window (APW) can be seen. **B.** The origin of the left pulmonary artery (LPA) can be seen at a level 1 cm inferior to **A. C.** The origin and course of the right pulmonary artery (RPA) can be seen at this next most cephalad level. The left upper lobe bronchus can be seen at its origin from the left main bronchus (LMB). **D.** Cardiac chambers and pulmonary veins are seen in the lower thorax. AA = ascending aorta; DA = descending aorta; LA = left atrium; LV = left ventricle; MPA = main pulmonary artery; RA = right atrium; RV = right ventricle; SVC = superior vena cava; T = trachea.

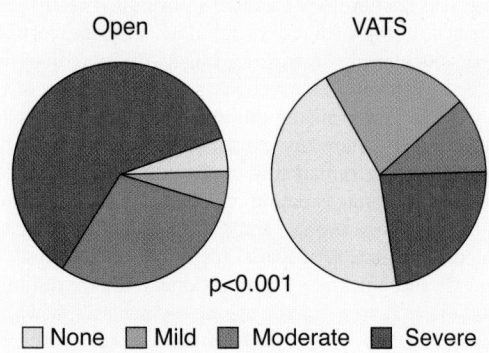

FIG. 19-11. Pie chart comparison of pain control at 3 weeks after lobectomy by standard thoracotomy or video-assisted thoracic surgery (VATS). The pie charts show that patients undergoing VATS have significantly less pain ($P < .01$) as measured by the most potent analgesic still required: severe—schedule II narcotic; moderate—schedule III or lower narcotic; mild—NSAID or acetaminophen. (Reproduced with permission from Demmy TL, et al: Is video-assisted thoracic surgery lobectomy better? Quality of life considerations. Ann Thorac Surg 85:S719, 2008. Copyright © Elsevier.)

Thoracic Surgical Approaches

Thoracic surgical approaches have changed over recent years with advancements in minimally invasive approaches. A surgeon trained in advanced minimally invasive techniques can now perform sympathectomy, segmental lung resections, lobectomies, and mediastinal resections through multiple thoracoscopic ports and small access incisions without the need for a substantial, rib-spreading incision. Although there has not been a documented change in mortality using these approaches, subjective measures of quality of life after video-assisted thoracic surgery (VATS), such as pain level (Fig. 19-11) and perceived functional recovery, consistently and reproducibly favor VATS over thoracotomy. Objective measures such as functional status as measured by 6-minute walk, return to work, and ability to tolerate chemotherapy also favor VATS over thoracotomy. Finally, recovery of respiratory function occurs earlier in patients undergoing VATS. These findings are pronounced in patients with chronic obstructive pulmonary disease (COPD) and in the elderly, populations whose quality of life can be dramatically impacted by changes in their respiratory symptoms and function, thoracic pain, and physical performance.[12] Table 19-1 provides a summary of populations that may benefit from VATS approaches.

Mediastinoscopy is generally used for diagnostic assessment of mediastinal lymphadenopathy and staging of lung cancer. Mediastinoscopy is performed via a transverse 2- to 3-cm incision approximately 1 cm above the suprasternal notch. The incision is carried through the platysma. The midline of the strap muscles is identified and dissected laterally. Care is taken to avoid any venous structures that may overlie these muscles, which are highly variable in size and position. The pretracheal fascia is incised. Blunt dissection along the anterior trachea is performed to the level of the carina with careful note of the position of the innominate artery. The innominate artery can be located close to the suprasternal notch, particularly in women; therefore, blind use of electrocautery is to be avoided. The mediastinoscope is inserted, and anatomic definition of the trachea, carina, and lateral aspect of both proximal bronchi is achieved with blunt dissection using a long suction catheter. Long biopsy forceps can be inserted through the scope for sampling. The standard staging procedure for lung cancer includes biopsies of the paratracheal (stations 4R and 4L) and subcarinal lymph nodes (station 7).

Before the widespread use of VATS and CT-guided biopsy, a modified Chamberlain procedure was used for evaluation of aortopulmonary window lymph nodes. In this procedure a 4- to 5-cm

TABLE 19-1	Special circumstances under which lobectomy by video-assisted thoracic surgery may be preferable
Condition	**Examples**
Pulmonary compromise	Poor FEV_1/D_{LCO}, heavy smoking, sleep apnea, recent pneumonia
Cardiac dysfunction	Congestive heart failure, severe coronary artery disease, recent myocardial infarction, valvular disease
Extrathoracic malignancy	Solitary brain metastasis from lung cancer, deep pulmonary metastases requiring lobectomy
Poor physical performance	Performance status equivalent to a Zubrod score of 2 or 3, morbid obesity
Rheumatologic/orthopedic condition	Spinal disease, severe rheumatoid arthritis, severe kyphosis, lupus erythematosus, osteomyelitis
Advanced age	Age >70 y
Vascular problems	Aneurysm, severe peripheral vascular disease
Recent or impending major operation	Urgent abdominal operation, joint replacement requiring use of crutches, need for contralateral thoracotomy
Psychologic/neurologic conditions	Substance abuse, poor command following, pain syndromes
Immunosuppression/impaired wound healing	Recent transplantation, diabetes

D_{LCO} = carbon monoxide diffusion capacity; FEV_1 = forced expiratory volume in 1 s.
Source: Reproduced with permission from Demmy TL, et al: Is video-assisted thoracic surgery lobectomy better? Quality of life considerations. Ann Thorac Surg 85:S719, 2008. Copyright © Elsevier.

incision is made over the left second costal cartilage, which, on occasion, is excised. The internal mammary vessels may be ligated or preserved. The dissection proceeds into the mediastinum along the aortic arch. Biopsy of the aortopulmonary window lymph nodes and anterior mediastinal lymphomas just beneath the second and third costal cartilage can then be performed. Improved techniques in CT-guided biopsy, positron emission tomography (PET), and VATS have significantly reduced the need for this operative approach.

The most frequently used incision for an open procedure in thoracic surgery is the posterolateral thoracotomy. The posterolateral thoracotomy incision can be used for most pulmonary resections, for esophageal operations, and for the approach to the posterior mediastinum and vertebral column (Fig. 19-12). The patient is placed in the lateral decubitus position. A pitfall of thoracic incisions in a lateral decubitus position is the potential for injury to the brachial plexus and axillary vascular structures secondary to displacement of the shoulder. Therefore careful attention must be paid to positioning the patient on the operating table after anesthesia has been induced. The skin incision typically starts at the anterior axillary line just below the nipple level and extends posteriorly below the tip of the scapula. The incision then proceeds in a cranial direction halfway between the vertebral border of the scapula and the spinous processes of the vertebrae. The latissimus dorsi is divided and the serratus anterior is retracted. Before entering the pleural space, the surgeon confirms that the anesthesiologist has excluded ventilation to the operative lung by clamping the proper lumen of a double-lumen endotracheal tube. The pleural space is then entered at the fifth interspace by dividing the intercostal muscles with electrocautery above the sixth rib. A rib spreader is placed into the thoracic cavity and minimally opened. The division of the intercostal muscles anteriorly (to the level of the internal mammary artery) and posteriorly (to the level of the paraspinous tendons) is continued using electrocautery from the inside of the thoracic cavity as an internal thoracotomy. The internal thoracotomy will prevent rib fracture during subsequent spreading of the retractor. If necessary, a portion of rib can be removed posteriorly to improve visibility and prevent injury to a rib,

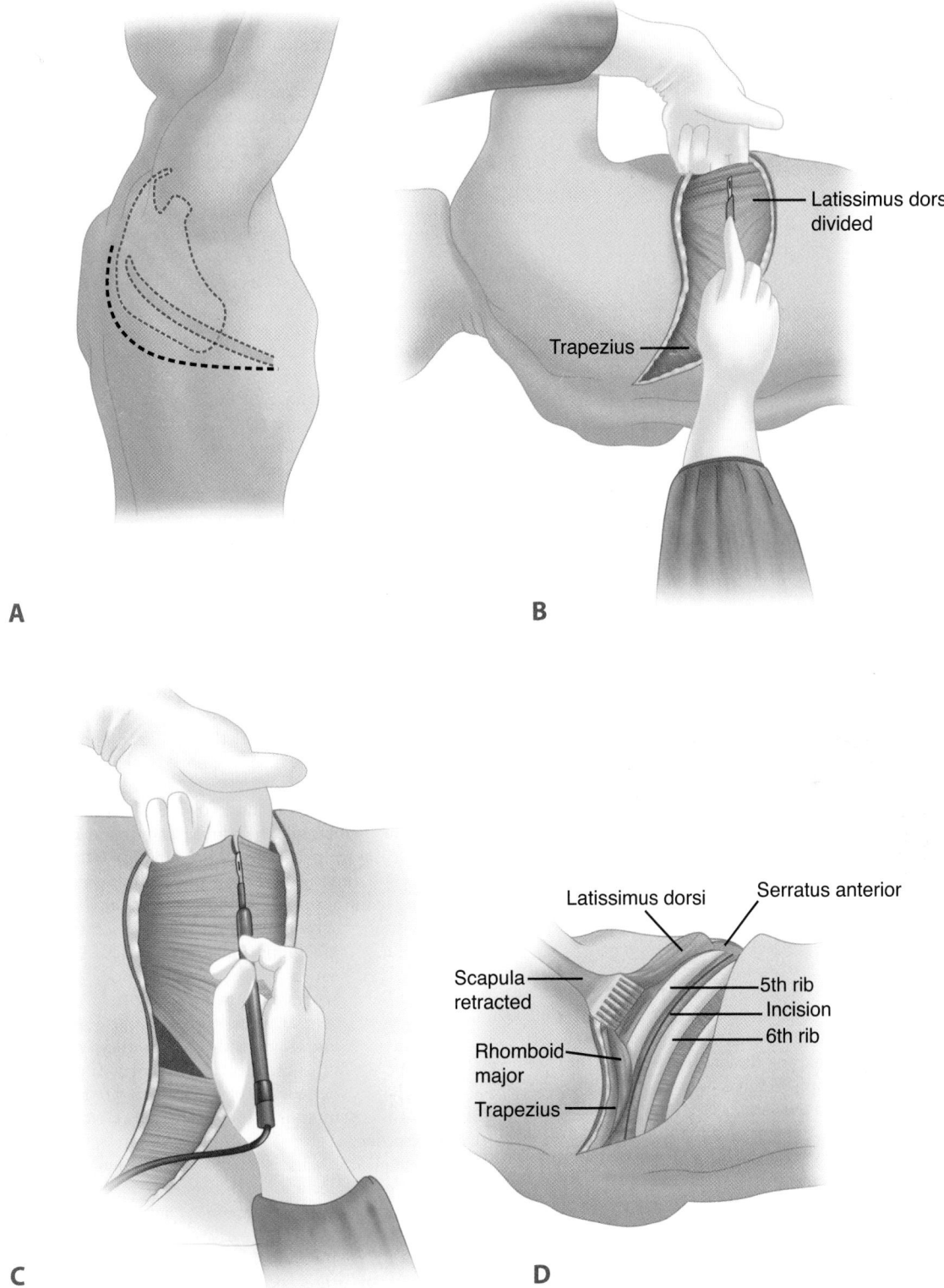

A

B

Latissimus dorsi
divided

Trapezius

C

D

Latissimus dorsi   Serratus anterior

Scapula
retracted

5th rib
Incision
6th rib

Rhomboid
major

Trapezius

FIG. 19-12. The posterolateral thoracotomy incision. **A.** Skin incision from the anterior axillary line to the lower extent of the scapula tip. **B** and **C.** Division of the latissimus dorsi and shoulder girdle musculature. **D.** The pleural cavity is entered after dividing the intercostal muscles along the lower margin of the interspace, with care taken not to injure the neurovascular bundle lying below each rib.

which can lead to increased postoperative pain and prolong restricted motion of the rib cage. Should a rib fracture occur, resection of any broken edges is recommended to help reduce postoperative pain.

The anterolateral thoracotomy has traditionally been used in trauma victims. This approach allows quick entry into the chest with the patient supine. When hemodynamic instability is present, the

lateral decubitus position significantly compromises control over the patient's cardiopulmonary system and resuscitation efforts, whereas the supine position allows the anesthesiologist full access to the patient. The incision is submammary, beginning at the sternal border overlying the fourth intercostal space and extending to the midaxillary line. The pectoralis major muscle and some of the pectoralis

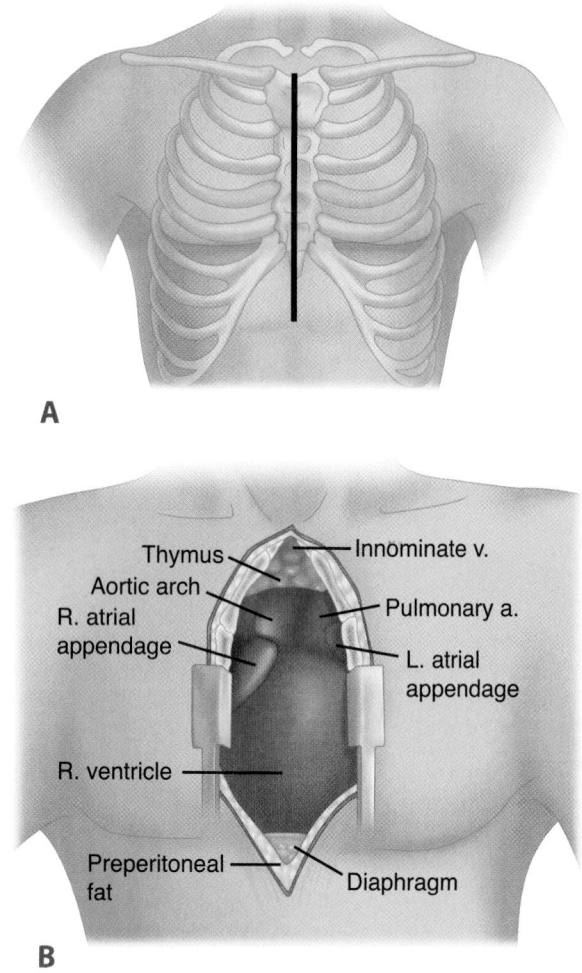

FIG. 19-13. The median sternotomy incision. **A.** Skin incision from the suprasternal notch to the xiphoid process. **B.** Exposure of the pleural space. a. = artery; v. = vein.

minor are divided, and the incision is carried through the serratus anterior muscle. The intercostal muscles are divided with cautery over the top of the subjacent rib. Should more exposure be necessary, the sternum can be transected and the incision carried to the contralateral thoracic cavity ("clamshell" thoracotomy). A bilateral anterior thoracotomy incision with a transverse sternotomy (clamshell thoracotomy) is a standard operative approach to the heart and mediastinum in certain elective circumstances. It is the preferred incision for double-lung transplantation. A partial median sternotomy also can be added to an anterior thoracotomy ("trap door" or "hemiclam" thoracotomy) for access to mediastinal structures. A hypesthetic nipple is a frequent complication of this approach.

The median sternotomy incision allows exposure of anterior mediastinal structures and is principally used for cardiac operations. The surgeon has access to both pleural cavities and can avoid incision into the pleural cavity if it is unnecessary. The skin incision extends from the suprasternal notch to the xiphoid process (Fig. 19-13). A sternal saw is used to split the sternum. Advantages of this approach include decreased postoperative pain and less compromise of pulmonary function than with a lateral thoracotomy. Disadvantages of the incision include an increased risk of infection if a tracheostomy is needed concomitantly or before the sternotomy is completely healed.

Video-Assisted Thoracoscopic Surgery

VATS has become an accepted approach for diagnosis and treatment of pleural effusions and recurrent pneumothorax, and for lung biopsy, lobectomy or segmental resection, resection of bronchogenic and mediastinal cysts, esophageal myotomy, and intrathoracic esophageal mobilization for esophagectomy.[13] VATS is performed via two to four incisions measuring 0.5 to 1.2 cm in length to allow insertion of the thoracoscope and instruments. The incision location varies according to the procedure. For VATS lobectomy, port placement varies according to the lobe being resected and is highly variable among surgeons.[14] The basic principle is to position the ports high enough on the thoracic cage to have access to the hilar structures (Fig. 19-14). Endoscopic staplers are used to divide the major vascular structures and bronchus.

At the conclusion of a thoracic operation, the pleural cavity typically is drained with one or more chest tubes. Each chest tube is brought out through a separate stab incision in the chest wall below the level of the thoracotomy or through a VATS port site. If the visceral pleura has not been violated and there is no concern of pneumothorax or hemothorax (i.e., after VATS sympathectomies), a chest tube is unnecessary. The lung is then ventilated and placed under positive pressure ventilation to assist with re-expansion of atelectatic segments. Thoracic incisions should be closed in layers: the intercostal space with three to four interrupted sutures, two running sutures for musculofascial layers, and a running subcuticular suture or staples for the skin closure.

Postoperative Care
Chest Tube Management

Chest tubes are routinely placed into the pleural space at the conclusion of all operations involving resection or manipulation of lung tissue. The reason for pleural tube placement is twofold: first, the tube allows evacuation of air if an air leak is present. Second, blood and pleural fluid can be drained, which prevents accumulations within the pleural space that would compromise the patient's respiratory status. The tube is removed when the air leak is resolved and when the volume of drainage decreases below an acceptable level over 24 hours. The ideal volume of drainage over a 24-hour period that predicts safe chest tube removal is unknown. The ability of the pleural lymphatics to absorb fluid is substantial. It can be as high as 0.40 mL/kg per hour in a healthy individual, possibly resulting in the absorption of up to 500 mL of fluid over a 24-hour period. The capacity of the pleural space to manage and absorb fluid is high if the pleural lining and lymphatics are healthy.

In the past, many surgeons required a drainage volume of <150 mL over 24 hours before removing a chest tube. Recently, however, it has been shown that pleural tubes can be removed after VATS lobectomy or thoracotomy with 24-hour drainage volumes as high as 400 mL without subsequent development of pleural effusions.[15] Currently, it is the practice of these authors to remove chest tubes when 24-hour output is ≤400 mL after lobectomy or lesser pulmonary resections.

If the pleural space is altered (e.g., malignant pleural effusion, pleural space infections or inflammation, or pleurodesis), strict adherence to a volume requirement before tube removal is appropriate (typically 100 to 150 mL over 24 hours). Such circumstances alter normal pleural fluid dynamics.

The use of suction and the management of air leaks vary. Suction levels of –20 cm H_2O have been routinely used after pulmonary surgery in an effort to eradicate residual air spaces and to control postoperative parenchymal air leaks. However, it has been shown that the routine use of a water seal (with the patient off suction) actually promotes more rapid healing of parenchymal air leaks.[16] The main factors guiding the use of a water seal are the degree of air leakage and the degree of expansion of the remaining lung. If the leak is significant enough to induce atelectasis or collapse of the lung during use of a water seal (off suction), suction should be used to achieve lung re-expansion.

A systematic approach to the evaluation of an air leak and/or incompletely drained pneumothorax with associated pulmonary collapse is important. The chest tube and its attached tubing should be

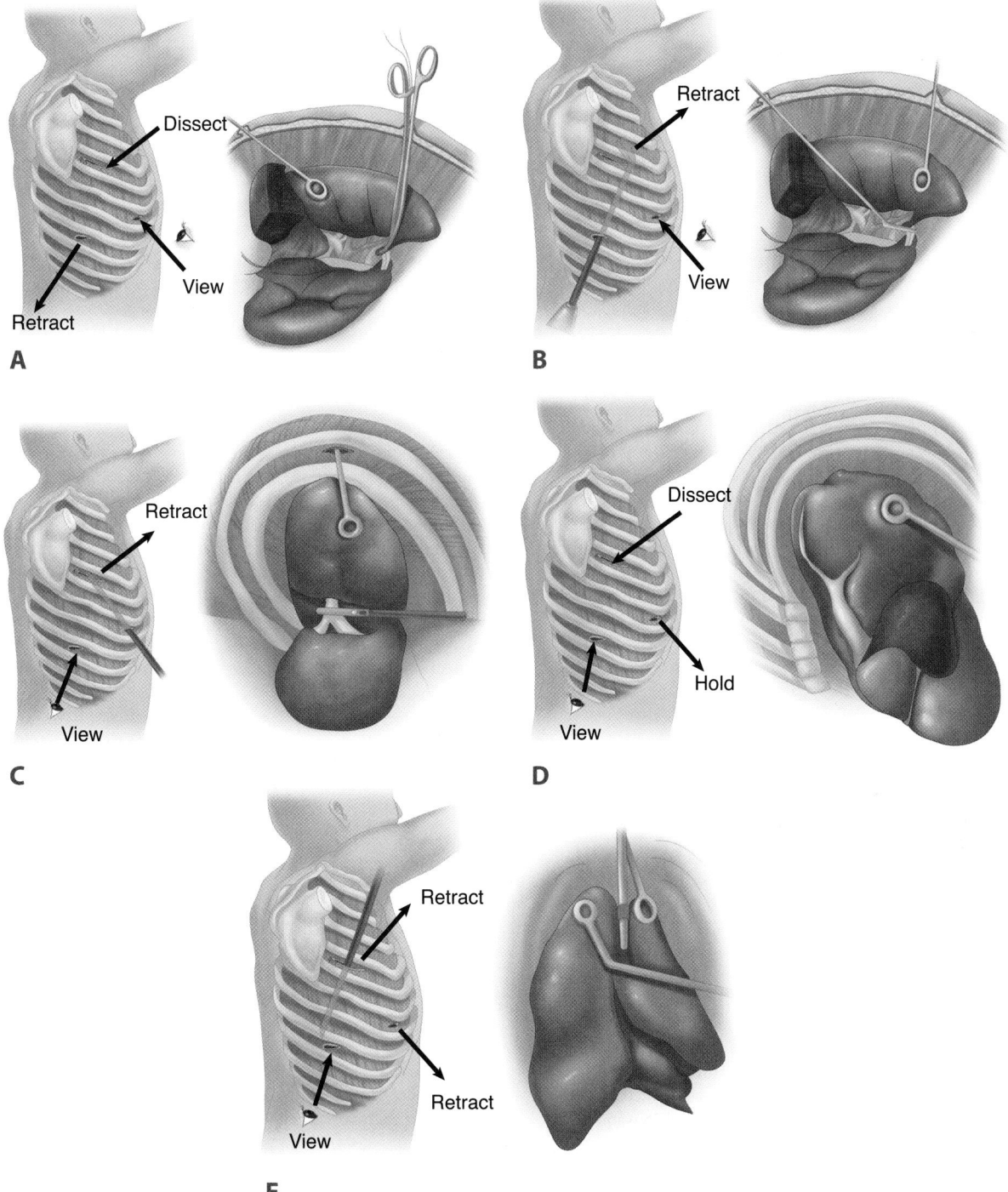

FIG. 19-14. Selected video-assisted thoracic surgery lobectomy maneuvers. All the maneuvers are shown with the patient positioned in the left lateral decubitus position. The same maneuvers can be performed in mirror image for left-sided work. **A.** Medial viewing and inferior holding of lung to allow dissection through the access incision. Example shows dissection of the apical hilum. **B.** Medial viewing and access holding of lung to allow stapling of hilar structures from below. Example shows division of the apical pulmonary artery trunk to the right upper lobe (upper lobe branch of vein divided and reflected away). **C.** Standard viewing and use of working port to dissect and divide structures while lung is retracted through access incision. Example shows use of stapler to divide pulmonary artery to right lower lobe. **D.** Standard viewing and use of working port to retract lung and access incision to dissect structures. This method is commonly used to dissect the pulmonary artery in the major fissure. Example shows inferior pulmonary vein after the pulmonary ligament was divided using this maneuver. **E.** Standard viewing and use of access incision to deliver stapler to divide fissures. Example shows division of the posterior fissure between the right lower lobe and the upper lobe. *(Reproduced with permission from Demmy et al.[14] Copyright Elsevier.)*

examined to ensure that the chest tube is patent and that the attached tubing is not kinked or mechanically obstructed, such as occurs when the patient is lying on the tube. Once the surgeon has confirmed that the chest tube is patent, the patient is asked to voluntarily cough or perform Valsalva's maneuver. This maneuver increases the intrathoracic pressure and will push air contained in the hemithorax out of the chest tube. During the cough, the water seal chamber is observed. If bubbles pass through the water seal chamber, an air leak is presumed. Occasionally, if the chest tube is not secured snugly at the skin surface, air can enter into the hemithorax around the tube with respiration; thus an air leak will be present, although not emanating from the lung itself. During the voluntary cough, the fluid level in the water seal chamber should move up and down with the cough and with deep respiration, reflecting the pleural pressure changes occurring with these maneuvers. A stationary fluid level implies a mechanical blockage, either due to external tube compression or to a clot or debris within the tube.

Pain Control

Good pain control after posterolateral thoracotomy is critical. It permits the patient to actively participate in breathing maneuvers designed to clear and manage secretions, and promotes ambulation and a feeling of well-being. The most common routes for pain medication are epidural, paravertebral, and IV. To maximize efficacy, epidural catheters should be inserted at about the T6 level, roughly at the level of the scapular tip. Lower placement risks inadequate pain control, and higher placement may provoke hand and arm numbness. Typically, a combination of fentanyl at 0.3 μg/mL and either bupivacaine (0.125%) or ropivacaine (0.1%) is used. Ropivacaine has less cardiotoxicity than bupivacaine; thus, in the event of inadvertent IV injection, the potential for refractory complete heart block as is seen with bupivacaine is significantly less. Paravertebral anesthesia can be initiated using the same epidural catheter kit with placement 2.5 cm lateral to the spinous process at T4 to T6. Combinations of narcotics and topical analgesics are then infused as with epidural catheters.

When the catheter is properly placed, well-managed epidural anesthesia can provide outstanding pain control without significant systemic sedation.[17] Urinary retention is a frequent side effect, particularly in males, who require an indwelling urinary catheter. In addition, the use of local anesthetics may cause sympathetic outflow blockade, leading to vasodilation and hypotension that often require IV administration of vasoconstrictors (an alpha agonist such as phenylephrine) and/or fluid administration. In such circumstances, fluid administration for hypotension may be undesirable in pulmonary surgery patients, particularly after pneumonectomy. Paravertebral anesthesia provides equivalent pain control with less effect on hemodynamics.[18]

Alternatively, IV narcotics delivered via a patient-controlled analgesia device can be used, often in conjunction with ketorolac. Titration of basal and intermittent dosing often is necessary to balance the degree of pain relief with the degree of sedation. Oversedation and narcotization of patients is as undesirable as failure to provide adequate pain control, because of the significant risk of secretion retention and development of atelectasis or pneumonia. Proper pain control with IV narcotics is a balance of pain relief and sedation.

Whether receiving pain control medication via the epidural, paravertebral, or IV route, the patient typically is transitioned to oral pain medication on the third or fourth postoperative day. During both the parenteral and oral phase of pain management, use of a standardized regimen of stool softeners and laxatives is advisable to prevent severe constipation.

Respiratory Care

Good respiratory care is the result of a commitment by the surgeon and by all other health care professionals involved. The team should be educated about the techniques of good respiratory care. The best respiratory care is achieved when the patient is able to deliver an effective cough to clear secretions. The process ideally begins preoperatively, with clear instructions on using pillows (or other support devices) over the wound and then applying pressure. Postoperatively, proper pain control without oversedation (as outlined earlier) is essential. Multiple studies have shown that a variety of adjunct respiratory care techniques (e.g., intermittent positive pressure breathing and incentive spirometry) may not be of benefit. These findings are consistent with the impression of these authors

that routine respiratory care is best accomplished by a dedicated team and educated patients.

In patients whose pulmonary function is significantly impaired preoperatively, generating an effective cough postoperatively may be nearly impossible. In this setting, routine nasotracheal suctioning can be used but is uncomfortable for the patient. A better alternative is placement of a percutaneous transtracheal suction catheter at the time of surgery. This catheter is comfortable for the patient and allows regular and convenient suctioning.

Postoperative Complications

Postpneumonectomy pulmonary edema occurs in 1 to 5% of patients undergoing pneumonectomy, with a higher incidence after right pneumonectomy. Clinically, symptoms of respiratory distress manifest hours to days after surgery. Radiographically, diffuse interstitial infiltration or frank alveolar edema is seen. The pathophysiologic causes remain poorly understood but are related to factors that increase permeability and filtration pressure and decrease lymphatic drainage from the affected lung. The syndrome reportedly is associated with a nearly 100% mortality rate even with aggressive therapy. Treatment consists of ventilatory support, fluid restriction, and diuretics.

Other postoperative complications include air leak and bronchopleural fistula. Although these are two very different problems, distinguishing between them may be difficult. Postoperative air leaks are common after pulmonary resection, particularly in patients with emphysematous changes, because the fibrotic changes and destroyed blood supply impair healing of surface injuries. Prolonged air leaks—that is, those lasting over 5 days—may be treated by diminishing or discontinuing suction (if used), by continuing chest drainage, or by instilling a pleurodesic agent, usually talcum powder.

If the leak is moderate to large, a high index of suspicion should be maintained for bronchopleural fistula from the resected bronchial stump, particularly if the patient is immunocompromised or received induction chemotherapy and/or radiation therapy. If a bronchopleural fistula is suspected, flexible bronchoscopy is performed. Management options include continued prolonged chest tube drainage, reoperation and reclosure (with stump reinforcement with intercostals or a serratus muscle pedicle flap), or, for fistulas <4 mm, bronchoscopic fibrin glue application. Patients often have concomitant empyemas, and open drainage may be necessary.

Solitary Pulmonary Nodule

A solitary pulmonary nodule is typically described as a single, well-circumscribed, spherical lesion. It is ≤3 cm in diameter and is completely surrounded by normal aerated lung parenchyma.[19] There are no associated changes of atelectasis, hilar enlargement, or pleural effusion. The American College of Chest Physicians discourages use of the term *coin lesion* because these lesions are spherical. The majority are detected incidentally on chest radiographs or CT scans obtained for some other purpose. Originally defined by findings on chest radiographs, solitary pulmonary nodules were identified on 0.09 to 0.2% of all chest radiographs in large screening studies as early as 1950.[20,21] With the advent of low-dose screening CT, however, many of these lesions are ultimately found to be associated with multiple (one to six) other, usually subcentimeter, nodules. In the Early Lung Cancer Action project, 23% (233/1000) of healthy volunteers were found to have between 1 to 6 nodules on screening CT. Notably, 12% (27/233) had nodule-associated malignant disease.[22] Approximately 150,000 solitary nodules are found incidentally each year. The clinical significance of such a lesion depends on whether or not it represents a malignancy.

Differential Diagnosis

The differential diagnosis of a solitary pulmonary nodule can be distilled down to a differentiation between malignancy and other numerous benign conditions. Ideally, diagnostic approaches would provide a clear distinction between the two, so that definitive surgical resection could be reserved for the malignant nodule and resection avoided when the nodule is benign. In unselected patient populations, a new solitary pulmonary nodule observed on a chest radiograph has a 20 to 40% likelihood of being malignant, with the risk approximately 50% or higher in smokers. Factors influencing the probability of cancer in a solitary pulmonary nodule include evidence for growth over time, density of the lesion on CT scan (with 40 to 50% of partial solid nodules cancerous compared with only 15% of solid nodules <1 cm and nonsolid nodules), associated symptoms, patient age, sex, cigarette smoking history, occupational history, and the prevalence of endemic granulomatous disease.

Infectious granulomas arising in response to a variety of organisms comprise 70 to 80% of this type of benign solitary nodule; hamartomas are the next most common single cause, accounting for approximately 10%. The differential diagnosis of a solitary pulmonary nodule should include a broad variety of congenital, neoplastic, inflammatory, vascular, and traumatic disorders.

Imaging

Chest thin section CT scanning is critical in characterizing nodule location, size, margin morphology, calcification pattern, and growth rate.[23] Because of the increased sensitivity of CT (compared with radiography) for detection of small nodules, CT often reveals more than a single pulmonary nodule; up to 50% of patients thought to have a single lesion based on chest radiograph are proven to harbor multiple nodules when examined by CT. Beyond a certain number, multiple nodules more likely represent metastases or granulomatous disease, which alters work-up. Lesions >3 cm are regarded as masses and are more likely malignant. Irregular, lobulated, or spiculated edges strongly suggest malignancy. The corona radiata sign (consisting of fine linear strands extending 4 to 5 mm outward and appearing spiculated on radiographs) is highly cancer specific (Fig. 19-15).

Calcification within a nodule suggests a benign lesion. Four patterns of benign calcification are common: diffuse, solid, central, and laminated or "popcorn." Granulomatous infections such as tuberculosis can demonstrate the first three patterns, whereas the popcorn pattern is most common in hamartomas.

Calcification that is stippled, amorphous, or eccentric usually is associated with cancer. Characteristically neoplasms grow, and several studies have confirmed that lung cancers have volume-doubling times of 20 to 400 days.[24] Lesions with shorter doubling times are likely due to infection, and longer doubling times suggest benign tumors but can indicate slower-growing lung cancer. Traditionally, size stability over 2 years on chest radiographs has been considered a sign of a benign tumor. However, this long-held notion has been challenged by recent investigations, which demonstrated only a 65% positive predictive value for chest radiographs.[25] Thus size stability of a pulmonary mass on chest films is a relatively unreliable indicator of a benign lesion that must be interpreted with caution.

PET scanning takes advantage of another biologic property of neoplasms: increased glucose uptake commensurate with increased metabolic activity. ^{18}F-fluorodeoxyglucose (FDG) is used to measure glucose metabolism in cells imaged by PET. Most lung tumors have increased signatures of glucose uptake, compared with healthy tissues. PET is becoming widely used to help differentiate benign from malignant nodules.[26] One meta-analysis estimated its sensitivity for identifying neoplasms as 97% and its specificity as 78%.[27] False-negative results can occur (especially in patients who have bronchoalveolar carcinomas (BACs), carcinoids, and tumors <1 cm in diameter), as can false-positive results (because of confusion with other infectious or inflammatory processes).

Biopsy vs. Resection

The surgeon must have an evidence-based algorithm for approaching the diagnosis and treatment of a pulmonary nodule. Guidelines have been developed based on a systematic literature review and consensus of clinical experts in the field[19] (Fig. 19-16). Only through biopsy can

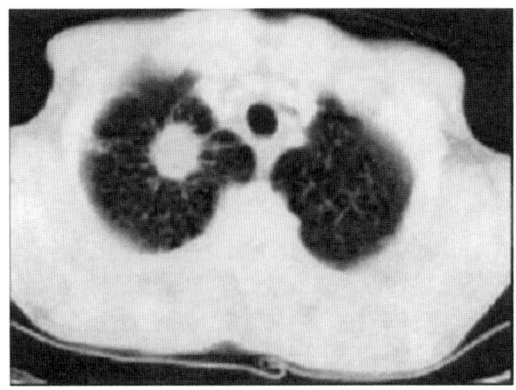

A

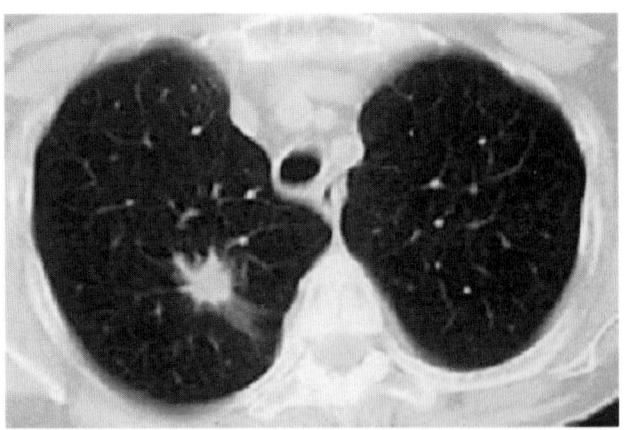

B

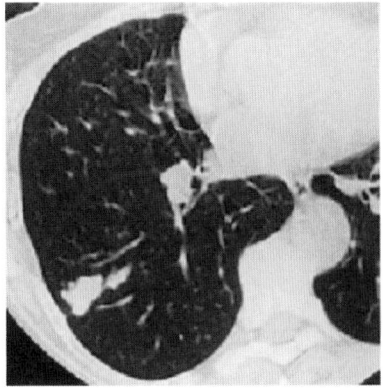

C

FIG. 19-15. Computed tomographic scan images of solitary pulmonary nodules. **A.** The corona radiata sign demonstrated by a solitary nodule. Multiple fine striations extend perpendicularly from the surface of the nodule like the spokes of a wheel. **B.** A biopsy-proven adenocarcinoma demonstrating spiculation. **C.** A lesion with a scalloped border, an indeterminate finding suggesting an intermediate probability of malignancy.

a pulmonary nodule be definitively diagnosed. Bronchoscopy has a 20 to 80% sensitivity for detecting a neoplastic process within a solitary pulmonary nodule, depending on the nodule size, its proximity to the bronchial tree, and the prevalence of cancer in the population being sampled. Transthoracic fine-needle aspiration (FNA) biopsy can accurately identify the status of peripheral pulmonary lesions in up to 95% of patients; the false-negative rate ranges from 3 to 29%.[28] Complications may occur at a relatively high rate (e.g., a

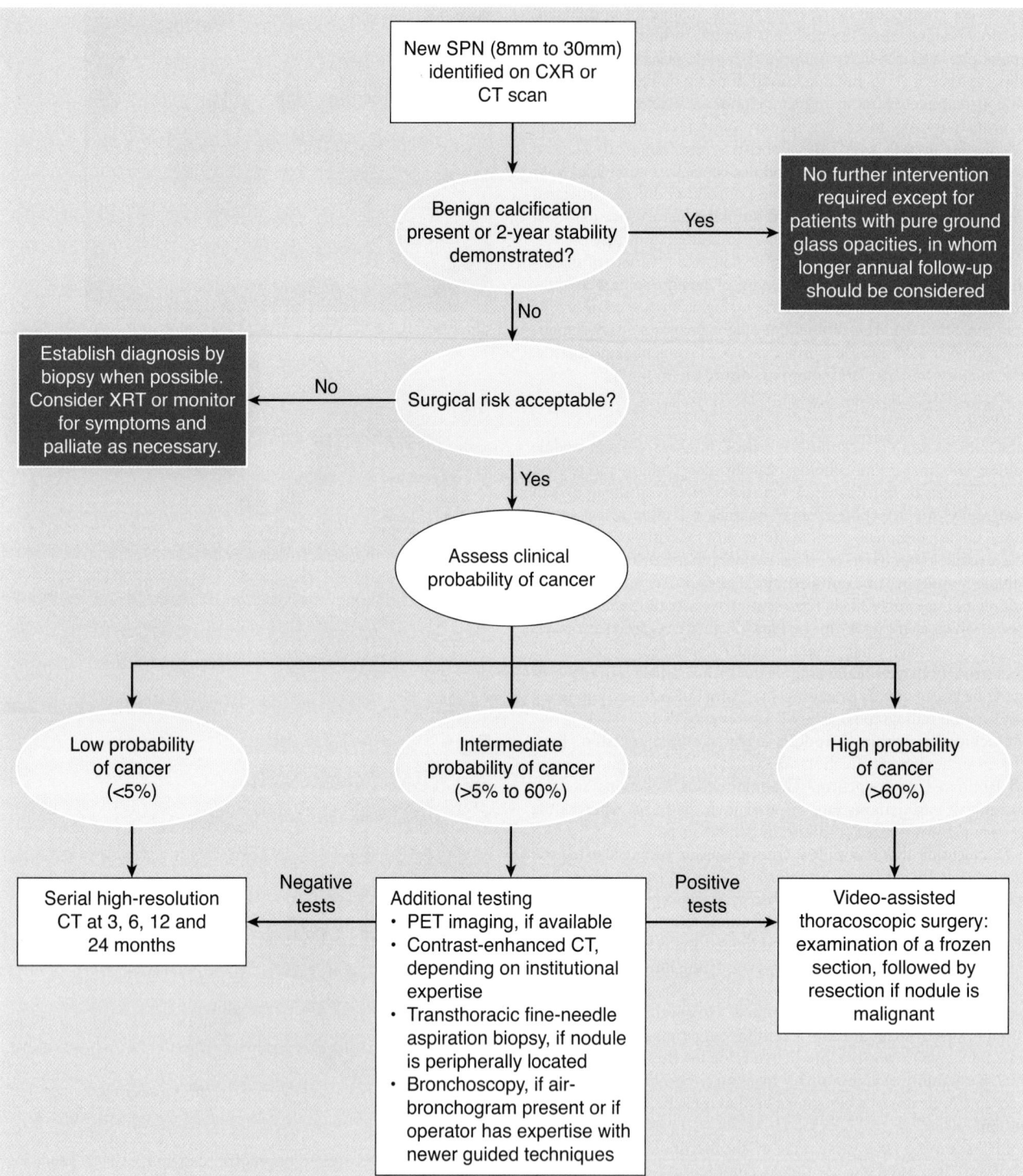

FIG. 19-16. Recommended management algorithm for patients with solitary pulmonary nodules (SPNs) measuring 8 mm to 30 mm in diameter. CT = computed tomography; CXR = chest radiograph; PET = positron emission tomography; XRT; radiotherapy. *(Reproduced with permission from Gould.[19])*

30% rate of pneumothorax). VATS often is used for excising and diagnosing indeterminate pulmonary nodules. Lesions most suitable for VATS are those that are located in the outer one third of the lung and those that are <3 cm in diameter. Certain principles must be followed when excising potentially malignant lesions via VATS. The nodule must not be directly manipulated with instruments, the visceral pleura overlying the nodule must not be violated, and the excised nodule must be extracted from the chest within a bag to prevent seeding of the chest wall. Some groups advocate proceeding directly to VATS in the work-up of a solitary pulmonary nodule in

appropriate clinical circumstances, citing superior diagnostic accuracy and low surgical risks.[29]

Lung Neoplasms

Lung cancer is the leading cancer killer in the United States. Every year, it accounts for 30% of all cancer deaths—more than cancers of the breast, prostate, and ovary combined. It is the second most frequently diagnosed cancer in the United States, behind prostate cancer in men and breast cancer in women (Fig. 19-17). In the annual

Estimated new cases*

			Males	Females			
Prostate	186,320	25%		Breast	182,460	26%
Lung & bronchus	114,690	15%		Lung & bronchus	100,330	14%
Colon & rectum	77,250	10%		Colon & rectum	71,560	10%
Urinary bladder	51,230	7%		Uterine corpus	40,100	6%
Non-Hodgkin lymphoma	35,450	5%		Non-Hodgkin lymphoma	30,670	4%
Melanoma of the skin	34,950	5%		Thyroid	28,410	4%
Kidney & renal pelvis	33,130	4%		Melanoma of the skin	27,530	4%
Oral cavity & pharynx	25,310	3%		Ovary	21,650	3%
Leukemia	25,180	3%		Kidney & renal pelvis	21,260	3%
Pancreas	18,770	3%		Leukemia	19,090	3%
All sites	**745,180**	**100%**		**All sites**	**692,000**	**100%**

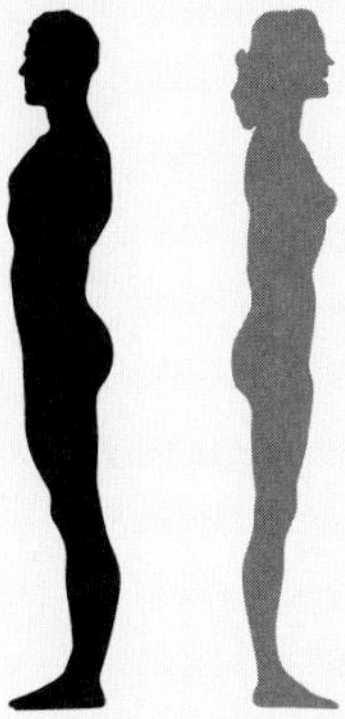

Estimated deaths

			Males	Females			
Lung & bronchus	90,810	31%		Lung & bronchus	71,030	26%
Prostate	28,660	10%		Breast	40,480	15%
Colon & rectum	24,260	8%		Colon & rectum	25,700	9%
Pancreas	17,500	6%		Pancreas	16,790	6%
Liver & intrahepatic bile duct	12,570	4%		Ovary	15,520	6%
Leukemia	12,460	4%		Non-Hodgkin lymphoma	9,370	3%
Esophagus	11,250	4%		Leukemia	9,250	3%
Urinary bladder	9,950	3%		Uterine corpus	7,470	3%
Non-Hodgkin lymphoma	9,790	3%		Liver & intrahepatic bile duct	5,840	2%
Kidney & renal pelvis	8,100	3%		Brain & other nervous system	5,650	2%
All sites	**294,120**	**100%**		**All sites**	**271,530**	**100%**

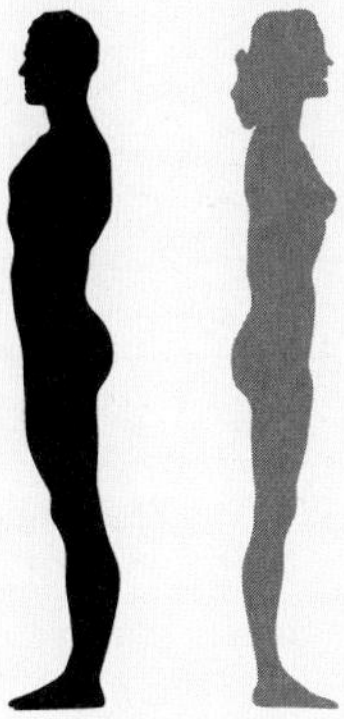

FIG. 19-17. Ten leading cancer types among estimated new cancer cases and cancer-related deaths by sex in the United States, 2008. *Excludes basal and squamous cell skin cancers and in situ carcinomas except those of the urinary bladder. *(Reproduced with permission from Jemal A, et al: Cancer statistics, 2008. CA Cancer J Clin 58:71, 2008. © 2008 American Cancer Society.)*

report to the nation on the status of cancer in 2007, it was noted that the incidence of lung cancer in men has begun to decrease, while incidence has remained stable in women. Annual death rates for men also have declined. Annual death rates for women continue to increase, although at a significantly slower pace than noted in previous reports.[30] Most patients are diagnosed at an advanced stage of disease, so therapy is rarely curative. The overall 5-year survival for all patients with lung cancer is 15%, which makes lung cancer the most lethal of the leading four cancers (Fig. 19-18).

Survival of patients with lung cancer varies according to several demographic and social factors. Positive survival factors are female sex (5-year survival of 18.3% for women vs. 13.8% for men), younger age (5-year survival of 22.8% for those <45 years vs. 13.7% for those >65 years), and white race (5-year survival of 16.1% for whites vs. 12.2% for African Americans). When access to advanced medical care is unrestricted, as for the military population, the racial difference in survival disappears, which suggests that these differences in survival may be explained, at least in part, by less access to advanced medical care and later diagnosis for African Americans.[31]

Epidemiology

Cigarette smoking is the primary cause of lung cancer, with smoking-related cancers accounting for approximately 75% of all lung cancers worldwide in 2007. Two lung cancer types, squamous cell carcinoma and small cell carcinoma, are extraordinarily rare in the absence of cigarette smoking. The risk of developing lung cancer escalates with the number of cigarettes smoked and the number of years of smoking, and is higher when unfiltered cigarettes are used. Conversely, the risk of lung cancer declines with smoking cessation (Table 19-2).[32] Even after smoking cessation, however, the risk never drops to that of people who never smoked, regardless of the length of abstinence. Approximately 25% of all lung cancers worldwide and 53% of cancers in women are not related to smoking, and the majority of these (62%) are adenocarcinomas. Table 19-3 summarizes the existing data regarding the etiology of lung cancer in nonsmokers.[33]

Secondhand (or passive) smoke exposure has been shown to confer an excess risk of developing lung cancer of 24% when a nonsmoker lives with a smoker.[34] Pre-existing lung disease confers an increased risk of lung cancer—up to 13%—for individuals who have never smoked. This increase is thought to be related to poor clearance of inhaled carcinogens and/or to the effects of chronic inflammation.

Other causes of lung cancer include exposure to a number of industrial compounds, including asbestos, arsenic, and chromium compounds. Of particular note is the ominous combination of asbestos exposure and cigarette smoking, which together have a multiplicative effect on risk, as opposed to an additive effect. Patients with COPD are at higher risk for lung cancer than would be predicted based on smoking risk alone. A previous history of tuberculosis with secondary scar formation also leads to a higher risk of primary lung carcinoma.

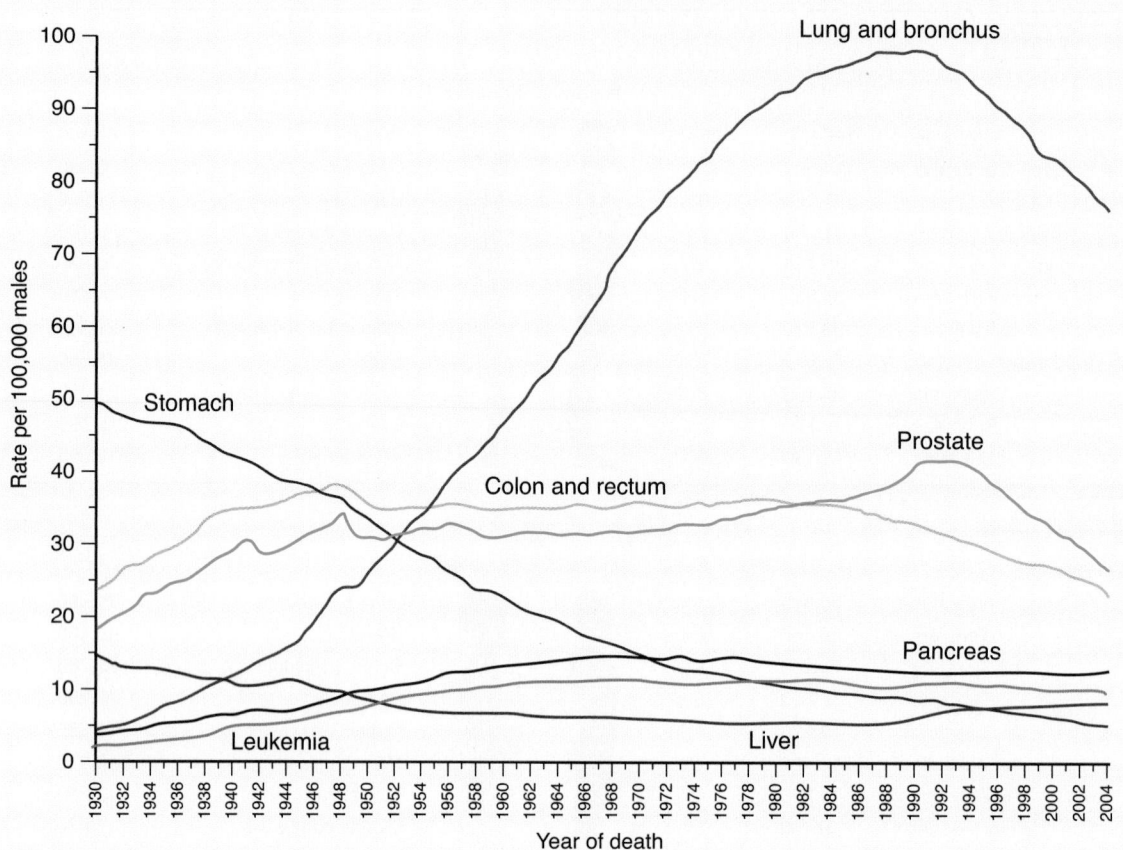

FIG. 19-18. Age-adjusted cancer-related mortality rates in men for selected cancers in the United States, 1930 to 2004. Rates are age adjusted to the 2000 U.S. standard population. *(Reproduced with permission from Jemal A, et al: Cancer statistics, 2008. CA Cancer J Clin 58:71, 2008. © 2008 American Cancer Society.)*

Over 3000 chemicals have been identified in tobacco smoke, but the main chemical carcinogens are polycyclic aromatic hydrocarbons. Once inhaled and absorbed, these compounds become mutagenic through their activation by specific enzymes, binding to macromolecules such as DNA and then inducing mutations.

In treating any patient with a history of smoking, it is important to remember that field cancerization of the entire aerodigestive tract has likely occurred. The patient's risk is increased for cancers of the oral cavity, pharynx, larynx, tracheobronchial tree and lung, and esophagus. In examining such patients, a detailed history must be taken and physical examination of these organ systems performed.

Normal Lung Histology

The lung can be conveniently viewed as two linked components: the tracheobronchial tree (or conducting airways component) and the alveolar spaces (or gas exchange component). The tracheobronchial tree consists of approximately 23 airway divisions to the level of the alveoli. It includes the main bronchi, lobar bronchi, segmental bronchi (to designated bronchopulmonary segments), and terminal bronchioles (i.e., the smallest airway vessels, which lack alveoli and are lined by bronchial epithelium). The tracheobronchial tree is normally lined by pseudostratified ciliated columnar cells and mucous (or goblet) cells, both of which derive from basal cells (Fig. 19-19). Ciliated cells predominate. Goblet cells, which release mucus, can significantly increase in number in acute bronchial injury, such as exposure to cigarette smoke. The normal bronchial epithelium also contains bronchial submucosal glands, which are mixed salivary-type glands containing mucous cells, serous cells, and Kulchitsky cells. Kulchitsky cells are neuroendocrine cells; they also are found within the surface epithelium (see Fig. 19-19). The bronchial submucosal glands can give rise to salivary gland–type tumors (previously referred to as *bronchial gland tumors*), including mucoepidermoid carcinomas and adenoid cystic carcinomas.

The alveolar spaces or alveoli have two primary cell types, referred to as *type I and II pneumocytes*. Type I pneumocytes cover 95% of the surface area of the alveolar wall but constitute only 40% of the total number of alveolar epithelial cells. These cells are not capable of regeneration because they have no mitotic potential. Type II pneumocytes cover only 3% of the alveolar surface but constitute 60% of the alveolar epithelial cells. In addition, clusters of neuroendocrine cells are seen in the alveolar spaces.

Preinvasive Lesions

As with epithelial tumors in other organs, precancerous changes can be seen in the respiratory tract. Three precancerous lesions are currently recognized: squamous dysplasia and carcinoma in situ,

TABLE 19-2	Relative risk of lung cancer in smokers
Smoking Category	**Relative Risk**
Never smoked	1.0
Currently smoke	15.8–16.3
Formerly smoked	
Years of abstinence	
1–9	5.9–19.5
10–19	2.0–6.1
>20	1.9–3.7

Source: Adapted from Samet,[32] p 673.

TABLE 19-3 Summary of selected studies of risk factors for lung cancer in individuals who never smoked

Risk Factor	Risk Estimate (95% CI)	Comments	Reference
Environmental tobacco smoke	1.19 (90% CI: 1.04–1.35)	Meta-analysis of 11 U.S. studies of spousal exposure (females only)	225
	1.21 (1.13–1.30)	Meta-analysis of 44 case-control studies worldwide of spousal exposure	226
	1.22 (1.13–1.33)	Meta-analysis of 25 studies worldwide of workplace exposure	226
	1.24 (1.18–1.29)	Meta-analysis of 22 studies worldwide of workplace exposure	227
Residential radon	8.4% (3.0–15.8%) per 100 Bq m³ increase in measured radon	Meta-analysis of 13 European studies	228
	11% (0–28%) per 100 Bq m³	Meta-analysis of 7 North American studies	229
Cooking oil vapors	2.12 (1.81–2.47)	Meta-analysis of 7 studies from China and Taiwan (females who never smoked)	230
Indoor coal and wood burning	2.66 (1.39–5.07)	Meta-analysis of 7 studies from China and Taiwan (both sexes)	230
	1.22 (1.04–1.44)	Large case-control study (2861 cases and 3118 controls) from Eastern and Central Europe (both sexes)	231
	2.5 (1.5–3.6)	Large case-control study (1205 cases and 1541 controls) from Canada (significant for women only)	232
Genetic factors: family history, CYP1A1 Ile462Val polymorphism, *XRCC1* variants	1.51 (1.11–2.06)	Meta-analysis of 28 case-control, 17 cohort, and 7 twin studies	233
	2.99 (1.51–5.91)	Meta-analysis of 14 case-control studies of Caucasian never smokers	234
	2.04 (1.17–3.54)	Meta-analysis of 21 case-control studies of Caucasian and Asian never smokers (significant for Caucasians only)	235
	No association	Meta-analysis of 13 case-control studies	236
	No association overall; reduced risk 0.65 (0.46–0.83) with Arg194Trp polymorphism and 0.56 (0.36–0.86) with Arg280His for heavy smokers	Large case-control study from Europe (2188 cases and 2198 controls)	237
	Increased risk for never smokers 1.3 (1.0–1.8) and decreased risk for heavy smokers 0.5 (0.3–1.0) with Arg299Gln	Large case-control study from the United States (1091 cases and 1240 controls)	238
Viral factors: HPV 16 and 18	10.12 (3.88–26.4) for never smoking women >60 y	Case-control study (141 cases, 60 controls) from Taiwan of never smoking women	239

Bq = becquerels; CI = confidence interval; CYP1A1 = cytochrome P-450 enzyme 1A1; HPV = human papilloma virus.
Source: Reprinted by permission from Macmillan Publishers Ltd. Sun S, Schiller JH, Gazdar AF: Lung cancer in never smokers–a different disease. *Nature Rev Cancer* 7:778 Copyright © 2007.

atypical adenomatous hyperplasia, and diffuse idiopathic pulmonary neuroendocrine cell hyperplasia. The term *precancerous* does not mean that an inevitable progression to invasive carcinoma will occur, but such lesions, particularly those with high-grade dysplasia,[35,36] do constitute a clear marker of the potential for later development of invasive cancer.

Squamous Dysplasia and Carcinoma In Situ Cigarette smoke can induce a metaplastic change of the tracheobronchial pseudostratified epithelium to squamous mucosa, which is a normal response to injury. With the development of cellular abnormalities in the metaplastic squamous mucosa, squamous dysplasia evolves. It involves increased cell size, an increased number of cell layers, an increased nucleus:cytoplasm ratio, increased mitoses, and changes in cellular polarity. Gradations are considered mild, moderate, or severe. Carcinoma in situ represents carcinoma still confined by the basement membrane. Once the in situ tumor invades beyond the basement membrane, invasive squamous cell carcinoma is present.

Atypical Adenomatous Hyperplasia Atypical adenomatous hyperplasia is defined as a lesion <5.0 mm consisting of epithelial cells lining the alveoli that are similar to type II pneumocytes. Histologically, atypical adenomatous hyperplasia is similar to BAC. It represents the beginning stage of a stepwise evolution to BAC and then to adenocarcinoma.

Diffuse Idiopathic Pulmonary Neuroendocrine Cell Hyperplasia Diffuse idiopathic pulmonary neuroendocrine cell hyperplasia is a rare lesion representing a diffuse proliferation of neuroendocrine cells but without invasion of the basement membrane. It can exist as a diffuse increase in the number of single neuroendocrine cells or as small lesions <5.0 mm in diameter. Lesions that are >5.0 mm in size or that breach the basement membrane are carcinoid tumors.

Invasive or Malignant Lesions

The term *bronchial carcinoma* is synonymous with lung cancer in general. Both terms refer to any epithelial carcinoma occurring in the bronchopulmonary tree. Currently, the pathologic diagnosis of lung cancer is based on light microscopic criteria, and cancers are broadly divided into two main groups: non–small cell lung carcinomas and neuroendocrine tumors (typical carcinoid, atypical carcinoid, large cell neuroendocrine carcinoma, and small cell carcinoma).[37] Immunohistochemical staining and electron microscopy are used as adjuncts in diagnosis, particularly in the assessment of potential neuroendocrine tumors.

Non–Small Cell Lung Carcinoma The term *non–small cell lung carcinoma (NSCLC)* encompasses many tumor cell types, including large cell carcinoma, squamous cell carcinoma, adenocarcinoma, and BAC, and is used to distinguish these tumors from small cell carcinoma. Although they differ in appearance histologically, their clinical behavior and treatment options are similar. Because of this, they are usually thought of as a uniform group. Each type, however, has unique features that affect its clinical presentation and findings.

Squamous Cell Carcinoma Squamous cell carcinomas account for 30 to 40% of lung cancers. Squamous cell carcinoma is the cancer most frequently found in men and is highly correlated with cigarette smoking. Histologically, cells develop a pattern of clusters with intracellular bridges and keratin pearls. Importantly, squamous cell carcinoma is primarily located centrally and arises in the major bronchi, often causing the typical symptoms of centrally located tumors, such as hemoptysis, bronchial obstruction with atelectasis, dyspnea, and pneumonia. Occasionally a more peripherally based squamous cell carcinoma will develop in a tuberculosis scar or in the wall of a bronchiectatic cavity. Central necrosis is frequent and

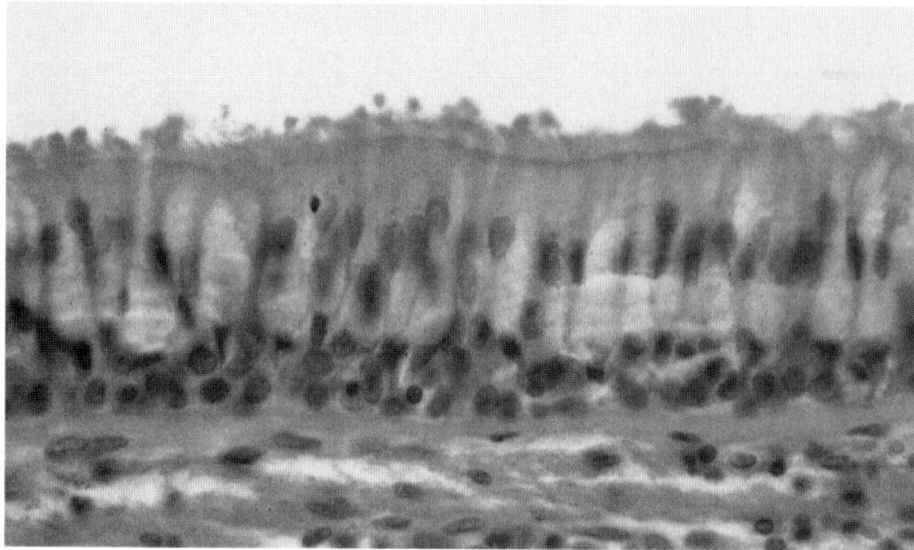

A

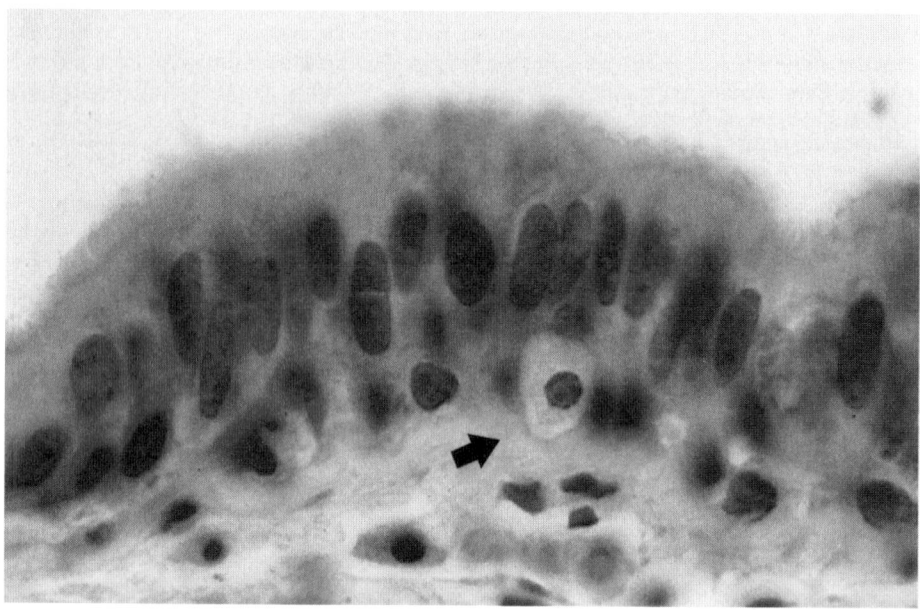

B

FIG. 19-19. Normal lung histology. **A.** Pseudostratified ciliated columnar cells and mucous cells normally line the tracheobronchial tree. **B.** A Kulchitsky cell is depicted (*arrow*).

may lead to the radiographic findings of a cavity (possibly with an air-fluid level). Such cavities may become infected, with resultant abscess formation.

Adenocarcinoma The incidence of adenocarcinoma has increased over the last several decades, and adenocarcinomas now account for 25 to 40% of all lung cancers. Adenocarcinoma is the most frequent histologic type found in women and occurs more frequently in females than in males.[38] Unlike squamous cell carcinoma, adenocarcinoma is most often a peripherally based tumor; thus it frequently is discovered incidentally on routine chest radiographs. Symptoms of chest wall invasion or malignant pleural effusions dominate. Histologically, adenocarcinoma is composed of glands with or without mucin production, combined with destruction of contiguous lung architecture.

Bronchoalveolar Carcinoma BAC is a relatively unusual (5% of all lung cancers) subtype of adenocarcinoma. BAC has a unique growth pattern and differs from adenocarcinoma in that, rather than invading and destroying contiguous lung parenchyma, tumor

cells multiply and fill the alveolar spaces. For a tumor to be classified as a pure BAC, there can be no evidence of destruction of surrounding lung parenchyma. When sites of classic BAC are demonstrated within glandular destruction of contiguous lung architecture, the tumor is classified as adenocarcinoma with BAC features.

Because of their growth within alveoli, BAC tumor cells from one site can aerogenously seed other parts of the same lobe or lung, or the contralateral lung. This growth pattern and tendency to seed can produce three radiographic presentations: a single nodule, multiple nodules (in single or multiple lobes), or a diffuse form with an appearance mimicking that of a lobar pneumonia. Because tumor cells fill the alveolar spaces and envelop small airways rather than destroying them, air bronchograms can be seen, unlike with other carcinomas.

Large Cell Carcinoma Large cell carcinomas account for 10 to 20% of lung cancers and may be located centrally or peripherally. As implied by the name, the cells are large, with diameters of 30 to 50 μm. They are often admixed with other cell types such as squamous cells or adenocarcinoma. Large cell carcinoma can be confused with a large cell variant of neuroendocrine carcinoma, with immunohistochemical staining usually allowing diagnostic distinction between the two.

Neuroendocrine Neoplasms Neuroendocrine tumors of the lung have been plagued by a confusing array of differing classifications. Over the last decade, progress in immunohistochemical and electron microscopic techniques have significantly improved the understanding and classification of these tumors.[39] In particular, immunohistochemical staining for neuroendocrine markers (including chromogranins, synaptophysin, CD57, and neuron-specific enolase) is essential to accurate diagnosis of most tumors.

Recently, neuroendocrine lung tumors have been reclassified into neuroendocrine hyperplasia and three separate grades of neuroendocrine carcinoma (NEC).[39] Listed below is the grading system now applied to NEC (left column), with the previously used common name (right column):

Grade I NEC	Classic or typical carcinoid
Grade II NEC	Atypical carcinoid
Grade III NEC	Large cell type
	Small cell type

Grade I NEC (classic or typical carcinoid) is a low-grade NEC. An epithelial tumor, it arises primarily in the central airways, although 20% of the time it occurs peripherally. It occurs primarily in younger patients. Because of the central location, it classically presents with hemoptysis, with or without airway obstruction and pneumonia. Histologically, tumor cells are arranged in cords and clusters with a rich vascular stroma. This vascularity can lead to life-threatening hemorrhage with even simple bronchoscopic biopsy maneuvers. Regional lymph node metastases are seen in 15% of patients but rarely spread systemically or cause death.

Grade II NEC (atypical carcinoid) comprises a group of tumors with a degree of aggressive clinical behavior. Unlike Grade I NEC, these tumors are etiologically linked to cigarette smoking and are more likely to be peripherally located. Histologic findings may include areas of necrosis, nuclear pleomorphism, and higher mitotic rates. These tumors have a much higher malignant potential. Lymph node metastases are found in 30 to 50% of patients. At the time of their diagnosis, 25% of patients already have remote metastases.

Grade III NEC large cell–type tumors occur primarily in heavy smokers. These tumors tend to be found in the middle to peripheral lung fields. They are often large with central necrosis and a high mitotic rate. Their neuroendocrine nature is revealed by positive immunohistochemical staining for at least one neuroendocrine marker.

Grade III NEC small cell type [small cell lung carcinoma (SCLC)] is the most malignant NEC and accounts for 25% of all lung cancers. These tumors are centrally located and consist of smaller cells with a diameter of 10 to 20 μm that have little cytoplasm and very dark nuclei. The tumors also have a high mitotic rate and areas of extensive necrosis. Multiple mitoses are easily seen. Importantly, examination of very small bronchoscopic biopsy specimens can distinguish NSCLC from SCLC, but crush artifact may make NSCLC appear similar to SCLC. If uncertainty exists, special immunohistochemical staining or rebiopsy (or both) are necessary. These tumors are the leading producer of paraneoplastic syndromes.

Salivary Gland–Type Neoplasms The tracheobronchial tree has salivary-type submucosal bronchial glands interspersed throughout. These glands can give rise to tumors that are histologically identical to those seen in the salivary glands. The two most common are adenoid cystic carcinoma and mucoepidermoid carcinoma. Both tumors occur centrally due to their site of origin. Adenoid cystic carcinoma is a slow-growing tumor that is locally and systemically invasive. It tends to grow submucosally and infiltrate along perineural sheaths. Mucoepidermoid carcinoma consists of squamous and mu-

cous cells and is graded as low or high grade, depending on the mitotic rate and degree of necrosis.

Clinical Presentation

Lung cancer displays one of the most diverse presentation patterns of all human maladies (Table 19-4). The wide range of symptoms and signs is related to (a) histologic features, which often help determine the anatomic site of origin in the lung; (b) the specific tumor location in the lung and its relationship to surrounding structures; (c) biologic features, and the production of a variety of paraneoplastic syndromes; and (d) the presence or absence of metastatic disease.

Tumor Histology

Squamous cell and small cell carcinomas frequently arise in main, lobar, or first segmental bronchi, which are collectively referred to as the *central airways*. Symptoms of airway irritation or obstruction are common and include cough, hemoptysis, wheezing (due to high-grade airway obstruction), dyspnea (due to bronchial obstruction with or without postobstructive atelectasis), and pneumonia (caused by airway obstruction with secretion retention and atelectasis).

In contrast, adenocarcinomas often are located peripherally. For this reason, they are often discovered incidentally as an asymptomatic peripheral lesion on chest radiograph. When symptoms occur, they are due to pleural or chest wall invasion (pleuritic or chest wall pain) or pleural seeding with malignant pleural effusion.

BAC (a variant of adenocarcinoma) may present as a solitary nodule, as multifocal nodules, or as a diffuse infiltrate mimicking an infectious pneumonia (pneumonic form). In the pneumonic form, severe dyspnea and hypoxia may occur, sometimes with expectoration of large volumes (over 1 L/d) of light tan fluid, with resultant dehydration and electrolyte imbalance. Because BAC tends to fill the alveolar spaces as it grows (as opposed to the typical invasion, destruction, and compression of lung architecture seen with other cell types), air bronchograms may be seen radiographically within the tumor.

Tumor Location

Symptoms related to the local intrathoracic effect of the primary tumor can be conveniently divided into two groups: pulmonary and nonpulmonary thoracic symptoms.

TABLE 19-4 Clinical presentation of lung cancer

Category	Symptom	Cause
Pulmonary symptoms	Cough	Bronchus irritation or compression
	Dyspnea	Airway obstruction or compression
	Wheezing	>50% airway obstruction
	Hemoptysis	Tumor erosion or irritation
	Pneumonia	Airway obstruction
Nonpulmonary thoracic symptoms	Pleuritic pain	Parietal pleural irritation or invasion
	Local chest wall pain	Rib and/or muscle involvement
	Radicular chest pain	Intercostal nerve involvement
	Pancoast's syndrome	Stellate ganglion, chest wall, brachial plexus involvement
	Hoarseness	Recurrent laryngeal nerve involvement
	Swelling of head and arms	Bulky involved mediastinal lymph nodes Medially based right upper lobe tumor

Pulmonary Symptoms Pulmonary symptoms result from the direct effect of the tumor on the bronchus or lung tissue. Symptoms (in order of frequency) include cough (secondary to irritation or compression of a bronchus), dyspnea (usually due to central airway obstruction or compression, with or without atelectasis), wheezing (with narrowing of a central airway by >50%), hemoptysis (typically, blood streaking of mucus that rarely is massive and indicates a central airway location), pneumonia (usually due to airway obstruction by the tumor), and lung abscess (due to necrosis and cavitation, with subsequent infection).

Nonpulmonary Thoracic Symptoms Nonpulmonary thoracic symptoms result from invasion of the primary tumor directly into a contiguous structure (e.g., chest wall, diaphragm, pericardium, phrenic nerve, recurrent laryngeal nerve, superior vena cava, and esophagus) or from mechanical compression of a structure (e.g., esophagus or superior vena cava) by enlarged tumor-bearing lymph nodes.

Peripherally located tumors (often adenocarcinomas) extending through the visceral pleura lead to irritation or growth into the parietal pleura and potentially to continued growth into the chest wall structures. Three types of symptoms are possible, depending on the extent of chest wall involvement: (a) pleuritic pain, from noninvasive contact of the parietal pleura with inflammatory irritation and from direct parietal pleural invasion; (b) localized chest wall pain, with deeper invasion and involvement of the rib and/or intercostal muscles; and (c) radicular pain, from involvement of the intercostal nerve(s). Radicular pain may be mistaken for renal colic in the case of lower lobe tumors that invade the posterior chest wall.

Tumors (usually adenocarcinomas) originating in the posterior apex of the chest, referred to as *superior sulcus tumors,* may produce Pancoast's syndrome. Depending on the exact tumor location, symptoms can include apical chest wall and/or shoulder pain (from involvement of the first rib and chest wall), Horner syndrome (unilateral enophthalmos, ptosis, miosis, and facial anhidrosis from invasion of the stellate sympathetic ganglion), and radicular arm pain (from invasion of T1, and occasionally C8, brachial plexus nerve roots).

Invasion of the primary tumor into the mediastinum may lead to involvement of the phrenic or recurrent laryngeal nerves. The phrenic nerve traverses the thoracic cavity along the superior vena cava and anterior to the pulmonary hilum. Direct invasion of the nerve occurs with tumors of the medial surface of the lung or with anterior hilar tumors. Symptoms may include shoulder pain (referred), hiccups, and dyspnea with exertion because of diaphragm paralysis. Radiographically, the diagnosis is suggested by unilateral diaphragm elevation on chest radiograph and can be confirmed by fluoroscopic examination of the diaphragm with breathing and sniffing (the sniff test).

Recurrent laryngeal nerve involvement most commonly occurs on the left side, given the hilar location of the left recurrent laryngeal nerve as it passes under the aortic arch. Paralysis may occur from invasion of the vagus nerve above the aortic arch by a medially based left upper lobe tumor, from invasion of the recurrent laryngeal nerve directly by a hilar tumor, or from invasion by hilar or aortopulmonary lymph nodes involved with metastatic tumor. Symptoms include voice change, often referred to as *hoarseness* but more typically a loss of tone associated with a breathy quality, and coughing, particularly when drinking liquids.

Superior vena caval syndrome most frequently occurs with small cell carcinoma, with bulky enlargement of involved mediastinal lymph nodes and compression of the superior vena cava. Occasionally, a medially based right upper lobe tumor can produce the syndrome with direct invasion. Symptoms include variable degrees of swelling of the head, neck, and arms; headache; and conjunctival edema. Pericardial invasion may lead to pericardial effusions (benign or malignant), associated with increasing levels`of dyspnea and/or arrhythmias, and with the potential to develop pericardial tamponade. Diagnosis requires a high index of suspicion in the

setting of a medially based tumor with symptoms of dyspnea and is confirmed by CT scan or echocardiography.

Direct invasion of a vertebral body produces symptoms of back pain, which is often localized and severe. If the neural foramina are involved, radicular pain may also be present. Involvement of the esophagus is usually secondary to external compression by enlarged lymph nodes involved with metastatic disease, usually with lower lobe tumors. Finally, invasion of the diaphragm by a tumor at the base of a lower lobe may produce dyspnea, pleural effusion, or referred shoulder pain.

Tumor Biology

Lung cancers, both non–small cell and small cell, are capable of producing a variety of paraneoplastic syndromes, most often from tumor production and release of biologically active materials systemically (Table 19-5). The majority of such syndromes are caused by small cell carcinomas, including many endocrinopathies. Para-

---

TABLE 19-5 Paraneoplastic syndromes in patients with lung cancer

Endocrine
Hypercalcemia (ectopic parathyroid hormone)
Cushing's syndrome
Syndrome of inappropriate secretion of antidiuretic hormone
Carcinoid syndrome
Gynecomastia
Hypercalcitoninemia
Elevated growth hormone level
Elevated levels of prolactin, follicle-stimulating hormone, luteinizing hormone
Hypoglycemia
Hyperthyroidism

Neurologic
Encephalopathy
Subacute cerebellar degeneration
Progressive multifocal leukoencephalopathy
Peripheral neuropathy
Polymyositis
Autonomic neuropathy
Eaton-Lambert syndrome
Optic neuritis

Skeletal
Clubbing
Pulmonary hypertrophic osteoarthropathy

Hematologic
Anemia
Leukemoid reactions
Thrombocytosis
Thrombocytopenia
Eosinophilia
Pure red cell aplasia
Leukoerythroblastosis
Disseminated intravascular coagulation

Cutaneous
Hyperkeratosis
Dermatomyositis
Acanthosis nigricans
Hyperpigmentation
Erythema gyratum repens
Hypertrichosis lanuginosa acquista

Other
Nephrotic syndrome
Hypouricemia
Secretion of vasoactive intestinal peptide with diarrhea
Hyperamylasemia
Anorexia or cachexia

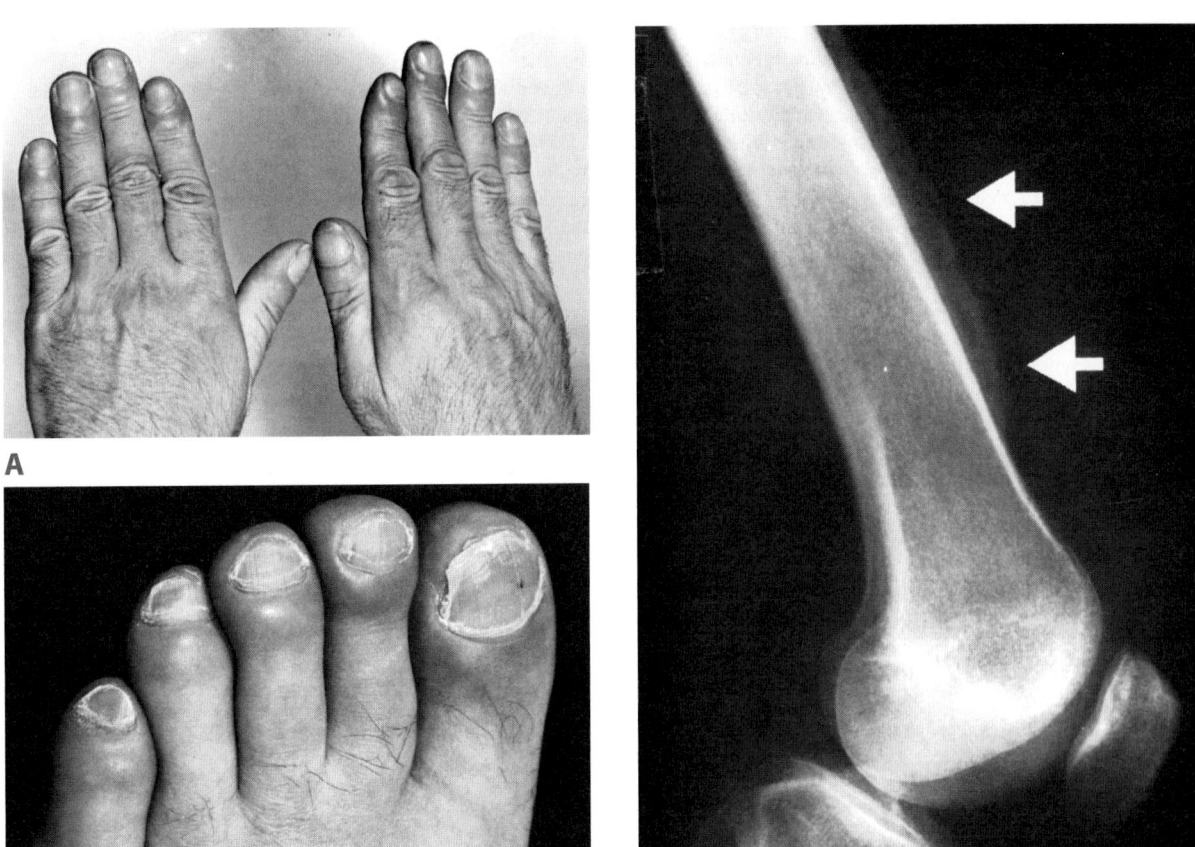

FIG. 19-20. Pulmonary hypertrophic osteoarthropathy associated with small cell carcinoma. **A.** Painful clubbing of the fingers. **B.** Painful clubbing of the toes (close-up). **C.** The *arrows* point to new bone formation on the femur.

neoplastic syndromes may produce symptoms even before symptoms are produced by the primary tumor, thereby leading to early diagnosis. Their presence does not influence resectability or the potential to successfully treat the tumor. Symptoms of the syndrome often will abate with successful treatment, and recurrence may be heralded by recurrent paraneoplastic symptoms. Many of the symptoms induced by these syndromes mimic those of the generalized debility caused by metastatic disease.

One of the more common paraneoplastic syndromes in patients with SCLC is hypertrophic pulmonary osteoarthropathy (HPO). Clinically, the syndrome is characterized by tenderness and swelling of the ankles, feet, forearms, and hands. It is due to periostitis of the fibula, tibia, radius, metacarpals, and metatarsals. Symptoms may be severe and debilitating. Clubbing of the digits occurs with or independently of HPO in up to 30% of patients with SCLC (Fig. 19-20). Symptoms of HPO may antedate the diagnosis of cancer by months. Radiographically, plain films of the affected areas show periosteal inflammation and elevation. A bone scan demonstrates intense but symmetric uptake of radiotracer in the long bones. Relief is afforded by treatment with aspirin or NSAIDs and by successful surgical or medical eradication of the tumor.

Hypercalcemia occurs in up to 10% of patients with lung cancer and is most often due to metastatic disease. However, 15% of cases are caused by secretion of ectopic parathyroid hormone–related peptide, most often with squamous cell carcinoma. A diagnosis of ectopic parathyroid hormone secretion can be made by measurement of elevated serum levels of parathyroid hormone; however, the clinician must also rule out concurrent metastatic bone disease by a bone scan. Symptoms of hypercalcemia include lethargy, depressed level of consciousness, nausea, vomiting, and dehydration. Most

patients have resectable tumors, and after complete resection the calcium level will normalize. Unfortunately, tumor recurrence is extremely common and may manifest as recurrent hypercalcemia.

Endocrinopathies are caused by the release of hormones or hormone analogues into the systemic circulation. Most occur with SCLCs. The syndrome of inappropriate secretion of antidiuretic hormone occurs in 10 to 45% of patients with SCLC. Characterized by confusion, lethargy, and possible seizures, it is diagnosed by the presence of hyponatremia, low serum osmolality, and high urinary sodium and osmolality. Another cause of hyponatremia can be the ectopic secretion of atrial natriuretic peptide.

Cushing's syndrome is due to production of an adrenocorticotropic hormone (ACTH)–like molecule and occurs principally in patients with SCLC. ACTH production is autonomous and not suppressible by dexamethasone. Immunoreactive ACTH is present in nearly all extracts of SCLC. A high percentage of patients with SCLC have elevated ACTH levels by radioimmunoassay, yet <5% have symptoms of Cushing's syndrome. Because the serum elevation of ACTH is rapid, appearance of the physical signs of Cushing's syndrome (e.g., truncal obesity, buffalo hump, striae) is unusual. Symptoms are primarily related to the metabolic consequences of severe hypokalemia, metabolic alkalosis, and hyperglycemia. Diagnosis is made by demonstrating hypokalemia (potassium level of <3.0 mmol/L), nonsuppressible elevated plasma levels of cortisol that lack the normal diurnal variation, elevated blood ACTH levels, or elevated urinary levels of 17-hydroxycorticosteroids, all of which are not suppressible by administration of exogenous dexamethasone.

Peripheral and central neuropathies are among the most common paraneoplastic syndromes in lung cancer, particularly in SCLC and squamous cell carcinoma. Unlike other paraneoplastic syndromes, which are usually due to ectopic secretion of an active substance, these syndromes are felt to be immune mediated. Antigens normally expressed only by the nervous system are believed to be aberrantly expressed by the cancer cells, generating antibodies leading either to interference with neurologic function or to immune neurologic destruction. Up to 16% of patients with lung cancer have evidence of neuromuscular disability, and of these patients, half have small cell carcinomas and 25% have squamous cell carcinomas. In patients with neurologic or muscular symptoms, central nervous system (CNS) metastases must be ruled out with CT or magnetic resonance imaging (MRI) of the head. Other metastatic disease leading to disability must also be excluded.

Lambert-Eaton syndrome is a myasthenia-like syndrome usually seen in patients with SCLC. It is caused by a neuromuscular conduction defect. Gait abnormalities are due to proximal muscle weakness and fatigability, and particularly affect the thighs. Symptoms can occur before symptoms of the primary tumor and may actually precede radiographic evidence of the tumor. The syndrome is produced by immunoglobulin G antibodies targeting voltage-gated calcium channels, which function in the release of acetylcholine from presynaptic sites at the motor end plate. Therapy is directed at the primary tumor with resection, radiation, and/or chemotherapy. Many patients have dramatic improvement after resection or successful medical therapy. For patients with refractory symptoms, treatment consists of administration of guanidine hydrochloride, immunosuppressive agents such as prednisone and azathioprine, and occasionally plasma exchange. Unlike in myasthenia gravis patients, neostigmine is usually ineffective.

Metastatic Symptoms

Lung cancer metastases occur most commonly to the CNS, vertebral bodies, bone, liver, adrenal glands, lungs, skin, and soft tissues. At diagnosis, 10% of patients with primary lung cancer have CNS metastases; another 10 to 15% will go on to develop CNS metastases after diagnosis. Focal symptoms are most common and include headache, nausea and vomiting, seizures, hemiplegia, and speech difficulty. Lung cancer is the most common cause of spinal cord compression, which may occur by invasion of an intervertebral foramen from a primary tumor contiguous with the spine or from direct extension of a vertebral metastasis. Bony metastases, such as to the vertebral bodies or ribs, are identified in 25% of all patients with lung cancer. They are primarily lytic and produce pain locally; thus any new and localized skeletal symptoms must be evaluated

radiographically. Liver metastases are most often an incidental finding on CT scan. Adrenal metastases are also typically asymptomatic and are usually discovered by routine CT scan. They may lead to adrenal hypofunction. Skin and soft tissue metastases occur in 8% of patients dying of lung cancer and generally present as painless subcutaneous or intramuscular masses. Occasionally, the tumor erodes through the overlying skin, with necrosis and creation of a chronic wound. Excision may then be necessary for both mental and physical palliation.

Nonspecific Symptoms

Lung cancer often produces a variety of nonspecific symptoms such as anorexia, weight loss, fatigue, and malaise. The cause of these symptoms is often unclear, but their presence should raise concern about possible metastatic disease.

Diagnosis, Evaluation, and Staging

In a patient with either a histologically confirmed lung cancer or a pulmonary lesion suspected to be a lung cancer, assessment encompasses three areas: the primary tumor, presence of metastatic disease, and functional status (the patient's ability to tolerate a pulmonary resection). A discrete approach to each of these three areas allows the surgeon to systematically evaluate the patient, perform accurate clinical stage assignment, and assess the patient's functional suitability for pulmonary resection (Table 19-6).

Assessment of the Primary Tumor Assessment of the primary tumor begins with the history and directed questions regarding the presence or absence of pulmonary, nonpulmonary, thoracic, and paraneoplastic symptoms. Because patients often come to the surgeon with a chest radiograph or CT scan demonstrating the lesion, the location of the tumor can help direct the clinician in taking the history and performing the physical examination.

If the patient does not already have a chest CT scan, CT should be performed expeditiously as the next stage in evaluating a new patient. Routine chest CT should include IV administration of a contrast agent to enable delineation of mediastinal lymph nodes relative to normal mediastinal structures. Chest CT allows assessment of the primary tumor and its relationship to surrounding and contiguous structures. It also indicates whether invasion of contiguous structures has occurred. Recommendations for treatment and options for obtaining a tissue diagnosis require a thorough assessment of these CT findings.

TABLE 19-6   Evaluation of patients with lung cancer

	Primary Tumor	Metastatic Disease	Functional Assessment
History	Pulmonary Nonpulmonary thoracic Paraneoplastic	Weight loss Malaise New bone pain Neurologic signs or symptoms Skin lesions	Ability to walk up two flights of stairs Ability to walk on a flat surface indefinitely
Physical examination	Voice	Supraclavicular node palpation Skin examination Neurologic examination	Accessory muscle usage Air flow by auscultation Force of cough
Radiographic examination	Chest CT	Chest CT, PET	Chest CT: tumor anatomy, atelectasis
Tissue analysis	Bronchoscopy Transthoracic needle aspiration and biopsy	Bone scan, head MRI, abdominal CT Bronchoscopic lymph node FNA Endoscopic ultrasound Mediastinoscopy Biopsy of suspected metastasis	Quantitative perfusion scan
Other	Thoracoscopy	—	Pulmonary function tests (FEV$_1$, D$_{LCO}$, O$_2$ consumption)

CT = computed tomography; D$_{LCO}$ = carbon monoxide diffusion capacity; FEV$_1$ = forced expiratory volume in 1 s; FNA = fine-needle aspiration; MRI = magnetic resonance imaging; PET = positron emission tomography.

The determination of invasion often is made from the patient's history and the location of the primary tumor. For example, a tumor abutting the chest wall with underlying rib destruction provides clear evidence of local invasion. It is common to see the primary tumor abutting the chest wall without evidence of rib destruction. In this circumstance, a history of the presence or absence of pain in the area is an accurate guide to the likelihood of parietal pleural, rib, or intercostal nerve involvement. Similar observations apply to tumors abutting the recurrent laryngeal nerve, phrenic nerve, diaphragm, vertebral bodies, and chest apex. Thoracotomy should not be denied because of presumptive evidence of invasion of the chest wall, vertebral body, or mediastinal structures; proof of invasion may require thoracoscopy or even thoracotomy.

MRI of pulmonary lesions and mediastinal nodes has been disappointing; overall, it offers no real improvement over CT scanning. There may be an important role for MRI, however, in defining a tumor's relationship to a major vessel due to its excellent imaging of vascular structures. This is especially true if the use of a contrast agent is contraindicated. Thus routine use of MRI in lung cancer patients is reserved for those with allergies to contrast agents or with suspected mediastinal, vascular, or vertebral body invasion.

Tissue diagnosis of the primary tumor can be made from specimens obtained through bronchoscopy or needle biopsy. Bronchoscopy provides additional useful information regarding tumor location within the airway and may guide operative planning. It is particularly useful for centrally located tumors, which have a higher probability of being visualized and being within reach of endobronchial biopsy forceps. In addition, bronchoscopy enables visualization of the entire tracheobronchial tree and thus allows the surgeon to identify the presence of additional unsuspected endobronchial lesions.

Diagnostic tissue can be obtained from bronchoscopy by one of four methods: (a) brushings and washings for cytologic analysis, (b) direct forceps biopsy of a visualized lesion, (c) fine-needle aspiration (FNA) with a Wang needle of an externally compressing lesion without a visualized endobronchial tumor, and (d) transbronchial biopsy with the use of forceps guided to the lesion by fluoroscopy. For peripheral lesions (roughly the outer half of the lung), transbronchial fluoroscopic biopsy often is performed first, followed by collection of brushings and washings. The intent is to improve the yield of the biopsy by picking up additional cells after disruption of the lesion by the biopsy forceps. For central lesions, direct forceps biopsy by bronchoscopic visualization often is possible, and again is followed by collection of brushings and washings. For central lesions with external airway compression but no visible endobronchial lesions, Wang needle FNA through the bronchoscope is performed. Endoscopic bronchial ultrasound (EBUS) is a valuable new tool that can facilitate the accuracy and safety of these transbronchial biopsies of both the primary tumor (when it abuts the central airways) and the mediastinal lymph nodes,[40] and should become part of the surgeon's armamentarium for the diagnosis and treatment of lung cancer.

Transthoracic needle aspiration is ideally suited for peripheral lesions not easily accessible by bronchoscopy. Under imaging guidance (fluoroscopy or CT), either an FNA or core-needle biopsy is performed. The primary complication is pneumothorax (occurring in up to 50% of patients), which is usually minor and requires no treatment. Three biopsy results are possible: malignancy, a specific benign process, or indeterminate findings. The overall false-negative rate is 20 to 30%; therefore, unless a specific benign diagnosis (such as granulomatous inflammation or hamartoma) is made, malignancy is not ruled out and further efforts at diagnosis are warranted.

Thoracoscopy is a valuable staging tool for assessing the primary tumor's relationship to other intrathoracic structures, because it is frequently difficult to discern whether the primary tumor has invaded a contiguous structure (such as the chest wall or mediastinum). It is also useful for obtaining tissue diagnoses for tumors that are inaccessible by imaging-guided procedures or for which the biopsy results were indeterminate. Peripheral lesions are readily accessible by thora-

coscopic wedge excision of the lesion, and if the patient's pulmonary reserve is adequate, the surgeon can then proceed to lobectomy (either VATS or open) after frozen-section diagnosis.

A thoracotomy is occasionally necessary to diagnose and stage a primary tumor. Although this occurs in <5% of patients, two circumstances may require such an approach: (a) the presence of a deep-seated lesion that yielded an indeterminate needle biopsy result or that could not be biopsied for technical reasons, or (b) inability to determine invasion of a mediastinal structure by any method short of palpation. In the case of a deep-seated lesion without a diagnosis, FNA, biopsy using a core needle, or preferably an excisional biopsy can be performed with frozen-section analysis. If the biopsy result is indeterminate, a lobectomy may instead be necessary. When a pneumonectomy is required, a tissue diagnosis of cancer must be made before proceeding.

Assessment of Metastatic Disease Distant metastases are found in approximately 40% of patients with newly diagnosed lung cancer. The presence of lymph node or systemic metastases may imply inoperability. A patient's risk of harboring metastatic disease must be carefully considered by the surgeon.

As with assessment of the primary tumor, assessment for the presence of metastatic disease should begin with the history taking and physical examination, with a focus on the presence or absence of new bone pain, neurologic symptoms, and new skin lesions. In addition, constitutional symptoms (e.g., anorexia, malaise, and unintentional weight loss of >5% of body weight) suggest either a large tumor burden or the presence of metastases. Physical examination should focus on the patient's overall appearance, and any evidence of weight loss such as redundant skin or muscle wasting should be noted. A complete examination of the head and neck, including evaluation of cervical and supraclavicular lymph nodes and the oropharynx, should be performed because of the strong association of oropharyngeal primary tumors and lung cancer. This is particularly true for patients with a significant history of tobacco use. The skin should be thoroughly examined. Routine laboratory studies include serum levels of hepatic enzymes (e.g., serum glutamic oxaloacetic transaminase and alkaline phosphatase), as well as serum calcium level (to detect bone metastases or the ectopic parathyroid syndrome). Elevation of either hepatic enzyme levels or serum calcium levels typically occurs with extensive metastases.

Mediastinal Lymph Nodes Chest CT scanning permits assessment of possible metastatic spread to the mediastinal lymph nodes. It continues to be the most effective noninvasive method available to assess the mediastinal and hilar nodes for enlargement. However, a positive CT finding (i.e., nodal diameter >1.0 cm) predicts actual metastatic involvement in only approximately 70% of lung cancer patients. Thus even when enlarged mediastinal lymph nodes are noted on CT scan, up to 30% of such nodes are enlarged due to noncancerous reactive causes such as inflammation related to atelectasis or pneumonia secondary to the tumor. Therefore, no patient should be denied an attempt at curative resection just because of a positive CT finding of mediastinal lymph node enlargement. Any CT finding of metastatic nodal involvement must be confirmed histologically. The negative predictive value of normal-appearing lymph nodes by CT (lymph nodes <1.0 cm) is better than the positive predictive value of a suspicious-appearing lymph node, particularly with small squamous cell tumors. With normal-size lymph nodes and a T1 tumor, the false-negative rate is <10%, which leads many surgeons to omit mediastinoscopy. However, the false-negative rate increases to nearly 30% with centrally located and T3 tumors. In this situation, mediastinoscopy is routinely recommended, because it has been demonstrated that T3 adenocarcinomas or large cell carcinomas have a higher rate of early micrometastasis. Therefore, all such patients should undergo mediastinoscopy.

PET scanning for metastatic disease is based on the detection of positrons emitted by FDG, a D-glucose analogue labeled with positron-emitting fluorine. After cellular uptake and phosphorylation, FDG is not metabolized further, which leads to intracellular accumulation. This accumulation, combined with a cancer's intrinsically higher rate of glucose metabolism, results in accumulation and potential visualization. A significant advantage of PET scanning is the ability to image the whole body after a single FDG injection, which allows simultaneous evaluation of the primary lung lesion, mediastinal lymph nodes, and distant organs.

Mediastinal lymph node staging by PET scanning appears to have greater accuracy than staging by CT scanning. PET staging of mediastinal lymph nodes has been evaluated in two meta-analyses. The overall sensitivity of PET for detection of mediastinal lymph node metastases was 0.79 [95% confidence interval (CI) = 0.76 to 0.82], with a specificity of 0.91 (95% CI = 0.89 to 0.93), and an accuracy of 0.92 (95% CI = 0.90 to 0.94).[41,42]

When results of PET and CT scans were compared in patients who also underwent lymph node biopsies, PET had a sensitivity of 88% and a specificity of 91%, whereas CT scanning had a sensitivity of 63% and a specificity of 76%. Combining CT and PET scanning may lead to even greater accuracy.[43] In one study of CT, PET, and mediastinoscopy in 68 patients with potentially operable, non–small cell lung carcinoma (NSCLC), CT correctly identified the nodal stage in 40 patients (59%). It understaged the tumor in 12 patients and overstaged it in 16. PET correctly identified the nodal stage in 59 patients (87%). It understaged the tumor in five patients and overstaged it in four. For detecting N2 and N3 disease, the combination of PET and CT scanning yielded a sensitivity, specificity, and accuracy of 93%, 95%, and 94%, respectively. The values for CT scan alone were 75%, 63%, and 68%, respectively. With the recent development of combined PET-CT scanners, continued improvement in accuracy may be anticipated. However, with mediastinal lymph nodes, mediastinoscopy is recommended for histologic verification of disease in nodes determined to be cancerous by PET.

Endoesophageal ultrasound (EUS) has recently emerged as a method of staging in NSCLC. EUS can accurately visualize mediastinal paratracheal lymph nodes (stations 4R, 7, and 4L) and other lymph node stations (stations 8 and 9). It is able to visualize primary lung lesions contiguous with or near the esophagus (see Fig. 19-8). Using FNA techniques and, more recently, core-needle biopsy, samples of lymph nodes or primary lesions can be obtained. Diagnostic yield is improved with intraoperative cytologic evaluation, which can be performed with the cytopathologist in the operating room. Limitations of EUS include the inability to visualize the anterior (pretracheal) mediastinum, and thus it does not replace mediastinoscopy for complete mediastinal nodal staging. However, it may not be necessary to perform mediastinoscopy if findings on EUS are positive for N2 nodal disease, particularly if more than one station is found to harbor metastases.

Bronchoscopic FNA of paratracheal lymph nodes (primarily stations 4R, 7, and 4L) also can be performed. A significant disadvantage is the relatively blind nature of the aspiration. Station 7 can be reliably accessed, but other paratracheal lymph node locations must be estimated and aspiration attempted; therefore bronchoscopic FNA has limited usefulness. Both EUS and bronchoscopic FNA lack the ability for complete staging afforded by mediastinoscopy, which enables sampling of all upper mediastinal nodal stations and determination of the degree of lymph node involvement (from microscopic to complete nodal replacement). The addition of EBUS-guided lymph node FNA is currently under study at many institutions. Because the biopsy is image guided and the biopsy needed is directed at an angle from the scope, the limitations of the transbronchial biopsy are overcome. Using this technology, it is possible to obtain FNA cytologic samples from level 4, level 7, level 10, and level 11 lymph nodes. Accuracy of the technique compared to the gold standard of mediastinoscopy is still being determined. Like mediastinoscopy, it does not allow assessment of level 3, 5, or 6 nodal stations. With this additional modality, it may be possible to use a combination of EUS and EBUS to determine clinical stage, with mediastinoscopy reserved for restaging after induction chemo-

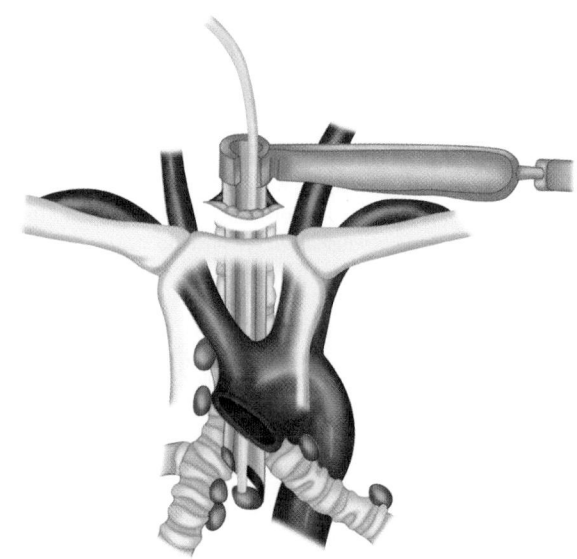

FIG. 19-21. Cervical mediastinoscopy. Paratracheal and subcarinal lymph node tissues (within the pretracheal space) can be sampled using a mediastinoscope introduced through a suprasternal skin incision.

therapy and/or radiation therapy. Further studies are needed, including determination of appropriate training and credentialing for those performing the procedure, before this approach can be considered a replacement for mediastinoscopy. For the foreseeable future, therefore, mediastinoscopy remains the standard method of tissue staging of the mediastinum.

Cervical mediastinoscopy has several advantages over other techniques of mediastinal lymph node staging (Fig. 19-21). It can provide a tissue diagnosis, allows sampling of all paratracheal and subcarinal lymph nodes, and permits visual determination of the presence of extracapsular extension of nodal metastases. With complex hilar or right paratracheal primary tumors, it allows direct biopsies and assessment of invasion into the mediastinum.

An absolute indication for obtaining a tissue diagnosis is mediastinal lymph node enlargement of >1.0 cm by CT scan. As stated earlier, EUS, EBUS, or transbronchial biopsy all can be used for this diagnosis. If the results are negative from these less invasive means, mediastinoscopy is mandatory, because the rates of false-negative biopsy results in this setting are high and the likelihood of metastatic disease is significant. When the size of mediastinal lymph nodes is normal, mediastinoscopy generally is recommended for centrally located tumors, for T2 and T3 primary tumors, and occasionally for T1 adenocarcinomas or large cell carcinomas (due to their higher rate of metastatic spread). Some surgeons perform mediastinoscopy in all lung cancer patients because of the poor survival associated with surgical resection of N2 disease.

Patients with left upper lobe tumors may have localized regional spread to station 5 and 6 lymph nodes, without mediastinal paratracheal involvement (see Fig. 19-8). Traditionally, such patients have undergone left anterior mediastinotomy (Chamberlain procedure). A left parasternal transverse incision is made with reflection of the mediastinal pleura laterally. The anterior mediastinal tissue is entered, which allows biopsy of station 5 and 6 lymph nodes and of primary tumors of the left hilum. More recently, left thoracoscopic (VATS) biopsy of these nodal stations is performed, particularly in centers experienced with VATS lobectomy. If there is a low index of suspicion, the patient can be scheduled for VATS biopsy and lobectomy under the same anesthesia if the nodes are negative. If the index of suspicion is high, the VATS biopsy is performed as a separate procedure. Cervical mediastinoscopy should precede both

TABLE 19-7	Indications for prethoracotomy biopsy of station 5 and 6 lymph nodes

1. Enrollment criteria for induction therapy protocol require pathologic confirmation of N2 disease.
2. Computed tomographic scan shows evidence of bulky nodal metastases or extracapsular spread that could prevent complete resection.
3. Tissue diagnosis of a hilar mass or of lymph nodes causing recurrent laryngeal nerve paralysis is needed.

anterior mediastinotomy and VATS biopsy, even if the patient has normal paratracheal lymph nodes. Additional diagnostic evaluation of the lymph nodes in station 5 and 6 may be unnecessary if the cervical lymph nodes are proven to be benign via biopsy during cervical mediastinoscopy and the preoperative CT scan suggests complete resectability of the tumor and potentially involved mediastinal lymphadenopathy. There are, however, several indications for prethoracotomy biopsy of station 5 and 6 lymph nodes, which are listed in Table 19-7. It is particularly important to prove pathologically that mediastinal lymph nodes are involved before deciding that the patient is *not* a candidate for resection.

Pleural Effusion A pleural effusion found on a CT scan (or chest radiograph) is not automatically a malignant effusion. Malignant pleural effusion can be diagnosed only by finding malignant cells in a sample of pleural fluid examined microscopically. Pleural effusion is often secondary to the atelectasis or consolidation seen with central tumors, or it can be reactive or secondary to cardiac dysfunction. However, pleural effusion associated with a peripherally based tumor, particularly one that abuts the visceral or parietal pleural surface, does have a higher probability of being malignant. Regardless, no pleural effusion should be assumed to be malignant. Cytologic proof of the presence of malignant cells is required. Thoracoscopy may be indicated to rule out pleural metastases in selected patients. It can be performed as part of a separate staging procedure, often with mediastinoscopy, or immediately before a planned thoracotomy.

Distant Metastases Until recently, detection of distant metastases outside the thorax was performed with a combination of chest CT scan and multiorgan scanning (e.g., brain CT or MRI, abdominal CT, and bone scan). Chest CT scans always include the upper abdomen and allow visualization of the liver and adrenal glands. Liver abnormalities that are not clearly simple cysts or hemangiomas need to be further evaluated, typically by MRI scanning. Adrenal enlargement, nodules, or masses also should be further evaluated by MRI and occasionally by needle biopsy. It must be remembered that adrenal adenomas, which are found in 2% of the general population and in up to 8% of patients with hypertension, may be mistakenly assumed to represent metastases. Adrenal adenomas have a high lipid content (secondary to steroid production), but metastases and most primary adrenal malignancies contain little if any lipid; thus MRI usually is able to distinguish the two.

In the absence of neurologic symptoms or signs, the probability of negative results on a CT scan of the head is 95%. Bone scans are notorious for their high sensitivity but low specificity and have a known overall false-positive rate of 40%. False-positive findings for any organ often lead to further noninvasive and invasive evaluation, and may even lead to denial of surgical resection. For these reasons, routine preoperative multiorgan scanning is not recommended for patients with a negative clinical evaluation and clinical stage I disease. However, it is recommended for patients with regionally advanced (clinical stage II, IIIA, and IIIB) disease. Any patient with a clinical evaluation suggestive of metastases, regardless of clinical stage, should undergo radiographic evaluation for metastatic disease.

PET scanning has supplanted multiorgan scanning in the search for distant metastases to the liver, adrenal glands, and bones. Currently, chest CT and PET are routine in the evaluation of patients with lung cancer. Brain MRI should be performed when the suspicion

or risk of brain metastases is increased. Several reports have shown that PET scanning appears to detect an additional 10 to 15% of distant metastases not detected by routine chest or abdominal CT and bone scans.[44–46] The PET finding of FDG uptake at a distant site must be proven not to be a metastasis. This often is accomplished with MRI and/or biopsies.

Integrated PET-CT scanners recently have become available. Early reports have demonstrated better accuracy in detection and localization of lymph node and distant metastases than with independently performed PET and CT scans (Fig. 19-22). This technology appears to overcome the problem of imprecise information on the exact location of focal abnormalities seen on PET scans and will likely become the standard imaging modality for lung cancer.

With any radiologic assessment for cancer, a common problem faced by surgeons is whether the results are true-positive or false-positive. Because a false-positive result can have a dramatic impact on the therapeutic course for a patient, the accuracy of a given scan must be ensured. The patient must be given the benefit of any doubt about the accuracy of a scan; the result must be proven, most often by a biopsy, to be true-positive.

Assessment of Functional Status For patients with a potentially resectable primary tumor, the patient's functional status and ability to tolerate either lobectomy or pneumonectomy needs to be carefully assessed. The surgeon should first estimate the likelihood of pneumonectomy, lobectomy, or possibly sleeve resection, given the CT scan results (see discussion of surgical resection in "Treatment"). A sequential process of evaluation then unfolds.

A patient's history is the most important tool for gauging risk. It must be emphasized that numbers alone [e.g., forced expiratory volume in 1 second (FEV_1) and carbon monoxide diffusion capacity (D_{LCO})] do not supplant the clinician's assessment. The clinical assessment entails the observation of the patient's general vigor and attitude. The late Dr. Robert Ginsberg best summarized the impact of a patient's vigor and attitude:

> Other factors that may predict a poor outcome from surgical intervention are difficult to classify. It has been my distinct impression that the patient's attitude toward the disease, the desire to have a favorable outcome, and confidence in the doctor is predictive of success. A prospective analysis of quality of life following lung cancer treatment, performed by the Lung Cancer Study Group, confirmed that the patient's attitude toward the disease was the best indicator of long-term survival. Except in life-threatening situations, patients should never be cajoled or forced into accepting surgery. In most cases, this led to disastrous results. At times, it is best to defer surgical intervention to the patient with a significant negative outlook, especially if other curative options (e.g., radiotherapy for cancer) are available. [Personal communication to author (JDL).]

When obtaining the patient's history, specific questions should be routinely asked that help determine the amount of lung that the patient will likely tolerate having resected. Can the patient walk on a flat surface indefinitely, without oxygen and without having to stop and rest secondary to dyspnea? If so, the patient will be very likely to tolerate thoracotomy and lobectomy. Can the patient walk up two flights of stairs (up two standard levels), without having to stop and rest secondary to dyspnea? If so, the patient will likely tolerate pneumonectomy. Finally, nearly all patients, except those who show carbon dioxide retention on arterial blood gas analysis, will be able to tolerate periods of single-lung ventilation and wedge resection.

Other pertinent elements of the history are current smoking status and sputum production. Current smokers have a significantly increased risk of postoperative pulmonary complications, defined as respiratory failure requiring intensive care unit care or reintubation, pneumonia, atelectasis requiring bronchoscopy, pulmonary embolism, and need for oxygen supplementation at the time of hospital discharge (Fig. 19-23).[38] Patients with more than a 60 pack-

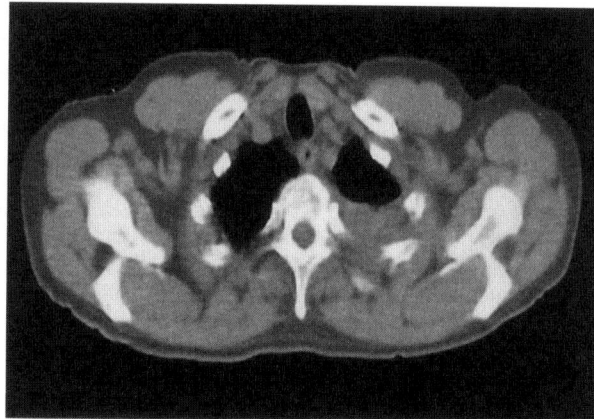

A

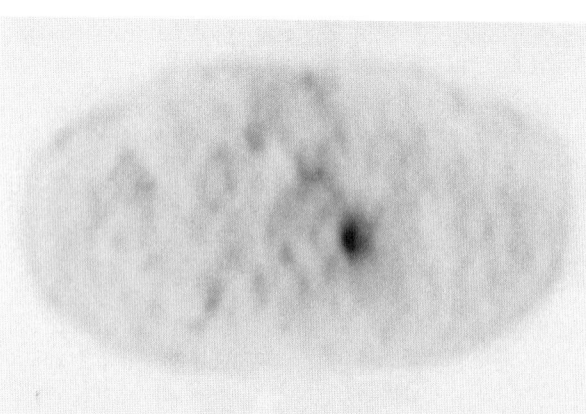

B

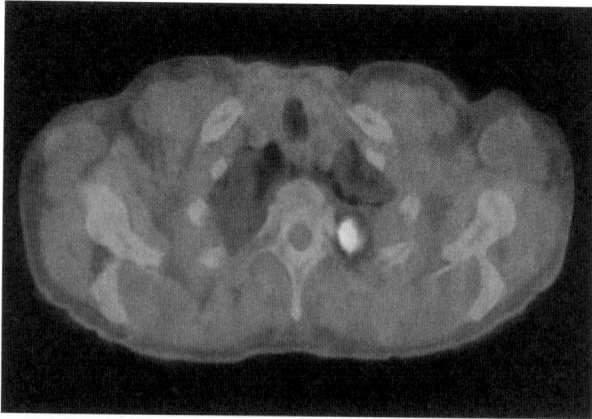

C

FIG. 19-22. Imaging of non–small cell lung cancer by integrated positron emission tomography–computed tomography (PET-CT) scan. **A.** CT scan of the chest showing a tumor in the left upper lobe. **B.** PET scan of the chest at the identical cross-sectional level. **C.** Coregistered PET-CT scan clearly showing tumor invasion (confirmed intraoperatively). *(Adapted with permission from Lardinois D, et al: Staging of non–small cell lung cancer with integrated positron-emission tomography and computed tomography. N Engl J Med 348:2504. Copyright © Massachusetts Medical Society. All rights reserved.)*

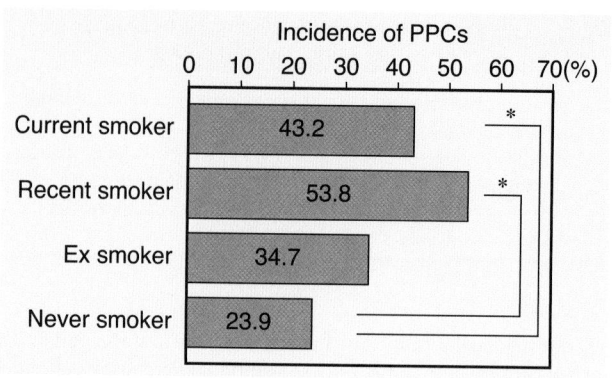

FIG. 19-23. The incidence of postoperative pulmonary complications (PPCs) in patients who underwent pulmonary surgery stratified by timing of smoking cessation in comparison to incidence in patients who never smoked. *P <.05. *(Reproduced with permission from Nakagawa et al.[36])*

impaired exchange of carbon dioxide was predictive of increased risk, independent of the smoking history. For every 10% decline in percent DLCO the risk of any pulmonary complication (as estimated by the odds ratio) increased by 42% (odds ratio = 1.42; 95% CI = 1.16 to 1.75; P = .008).[38] To diminish the risk significantly requires cessation of smoking at least 8 weeks preoperatively, a requirement that often is not feasible for a cancer patient. Nevertheless, efforts to abstain should be encouraged, ideally for 2 weeks before surgery. Smoking cessation on the day of surgery leads to increased sputum production and potential secretion retention postoperatively, and some authors have reported increased rates of pulmonary complications in this group.[47]

Patients with chronic daily sputum production will have more problems postoperatively with retention and atelectasis; they are also at higher risk for pneumonia. Sputum culture, antibiotic administration, and bronchodilators may be warranted preoperatively.

The physical examination should focus on the following signs of chronic obstructive pulmonary disease (COPD) or airflow limitation: cyanosis, peripheral edema from right heart failure, mild post-cough shortness of breath, use of accessory muscles for breathing, decreased air entry, wheezes or crackles, and a "wet" cough. The combination of the patient's answers to the questions on exercise tolerance presented earlier and results of the cough test allow the experienced thoracic surgeon to gauge operative risk remarkably well.

Pulmonary function studies are routinely performed when any resection greater than a wedge resection will be performed. Of all the measurements available, the two most valuable are FEV_1 and DLCO.

General guidelines for the use of FEV_1 in assessing the patient's ability to tolerate pulmonary resection are as follows: patients with an FEV_1 of >2.0 L can tolerate pneumonectomy, and those with an FEV_1 of >1.5 L can tolerate lobectomy. It must be emphasized that these are guidelines only. It is also important to note that the raw value is often imprecise, because normal values are reported as "percent predicted" based on corrections made for age, height, and gender. For example, a raw FEV_1 value of 1.3 L in a 62-year-old, 75-in male has a percent predicted value of 30% (because the normal expected value is 4.31 L); in a 62-year-old, 62-in female, the percent predicted value is 59% (normal expected value of 2.21 L). The male patient falls into the high-risk group for lobectomy, whereas the female could potentially tolerate pneumonectomy.

The percent predicted value for both FEV_1 and DLCO correlates with the risk of development of complications postoperatively, particularly pulmonary complications. Complication rates are significantly higher among patients with percent predicted values of <50%, with the risk of complications increasing in a stepwise fashion for each 10% decline. Figure 19-24 shows the relationship between predicted postoperative DLCO and estimated operative mortality.

year history of smoking are 2.5 times more likely to develop any pulmonary complication and three times more likely to develop pneumonia than patients with a history of 60 or fewer pack-years (odds ratio = 2.54; 95% CI = 1.28 to 5.04; P = .0008). In addition,

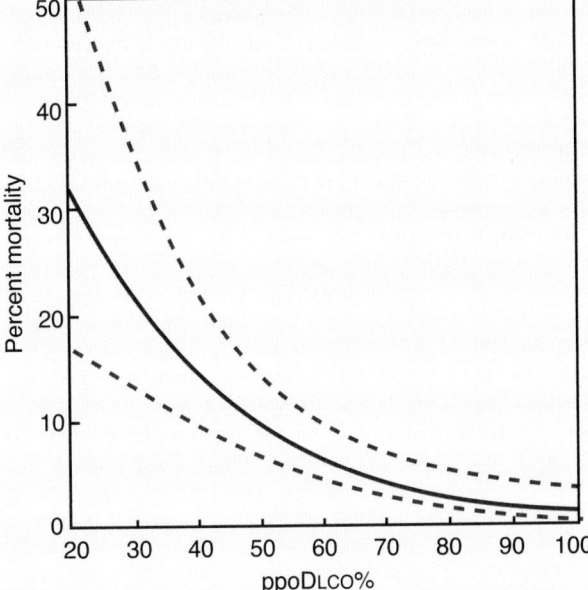

FIG. 19-24. Operative mortality after major pulmonary resection for non–small cell lung cancer (334 patients) as a function of the percent predicted postoperative carbon monoxide diffusion capacity (ppoDLCO%). *Solid line* is the logistic regression model; *dashed lines* represent the 95% confidence limits. *(Adapted with permission from Wang J, et al: Diffusing capacity predicts operative mortality but not long-term survival after resection for lung cancer.* J Thorac Cardiovasc Surg *117:582, 1999. Copyright Elsevier.)*

To calculate the predicted postoperative value for FEV_1 or DLCO, the percent predicted value of FEV_1 or DLCO is multiplied by the fraction of remaining lung after the proposed surgery. For example, in a planned right upper lobectomy, a total of three segments will be removed. Therefore, removing 3 of a total of 20 segments will leave the patient with $(20 - 3/20) \times 100 = 85\%$ of original lung capacity.

Of the two patients mentioned earlier, the man will have a postoperative percent predicted FEV_1 of $30\% \times 0.85 = 25\%$, whereas the woman will have a postoperative percent predicted FEV_1 of 50%.

The effect of the primary tumor on lung function must also be considered. Figure 19-25 shows a tumor with significant right main stem airway obstruction with associated atelectasis and volume loss of the right lung. At presentation, the patient was dyspneic with ambulation and the FEV_1 was 1.38 L. The referring physician told the patient that surgery was not feasible because he would require pneumonectomy, which he would not be able to tolerate. This case history illustrates a common pitfall for clinicians: failure to determine a patient's functional status before the development of the tumor. Six months earlier, this patient could walk up two flights of stairs without dyspnea. Similarly, if a patient with limited pulmonary function experiences complete collapse of a lobe (e.g., right upper lobe) and has only a mild decline in functional status, the surgeon can anticipate that the patient will tolerate lobectomy because the lobe already is not functioning and in fact may be contributing to a shunt.

Quantitative perfusion scanning is used in select circumstances to help estimate the functional contribution of a lobe or whole lung. Such perfusion scanning is most useful when the impact of a tumor on pulmonary physiology is difficult to discern. With complete collapse of a lobe or whole lung, the impact is apparent, and perfusion scanning is usually unnecessary. However, with centrally located tumors associated with partial obstruction of a lobar or main bronchus or of the pulmonary artery, perfusion scanning may be valuable in predicting the postoperative result of resection. For example, if the quantitative perfusion to the right lung is measured to be 21% (normal is 55%) and the patient's percent predicted FEV_1 is 60%, the predicted postoperative FEV_1 after a right pneumonectomy would be $60\% \times 0.79 = 47\%$, which indicates the ability to tolerate pneumonectomy. If the perfusion value is 55%, the predicted postoperative value would be 27%, and pneumonectomy would pose a significantly higher risk.

Exercise testing that yields maximum oxygen consumption ($\dot{V}O_2max$) has emerged as a valuable decision-making technique to help in evaluation of patients with abnormal FEV_1 and DLCO. Table 19-8 provides a summary of the existing data regarding the relationship between $\dot{V}O_2max$ and postoperative mortality risk. It is not uncommon to encounter patients with significant reductions in percent predicted FEV_1 and DLCO whose history shows a functional

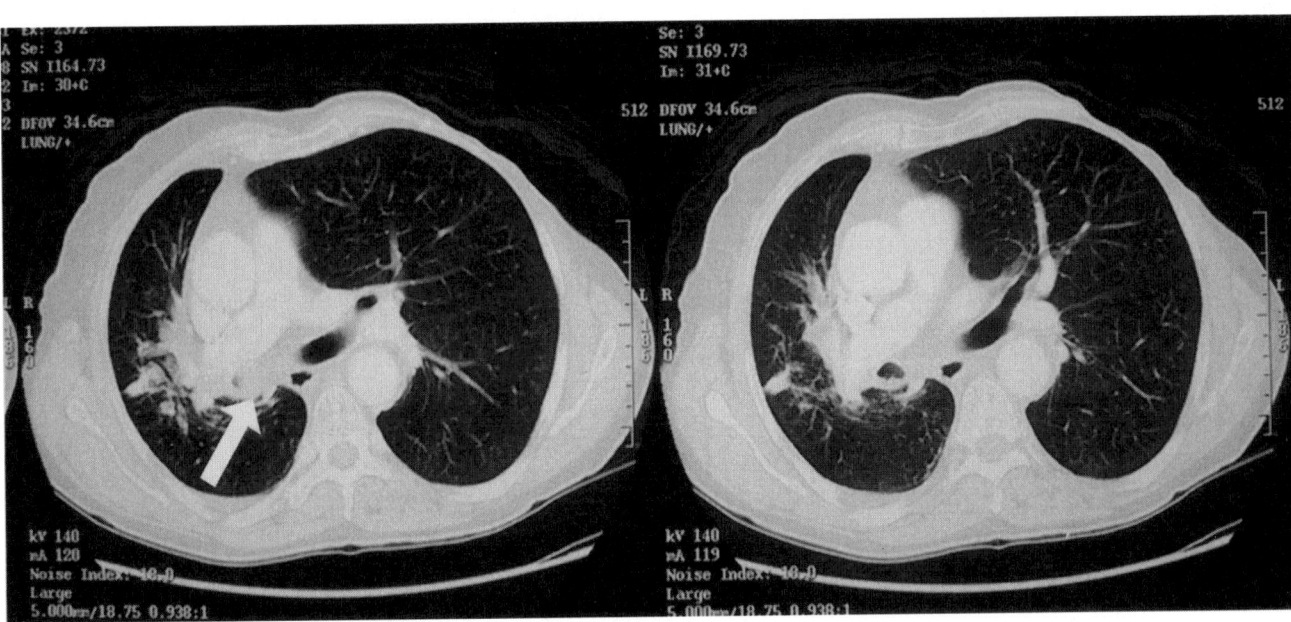

FIG. 19-25. Chest computed tomographic scan of an obstructing right main stem lung tumor. *Arrow* indicates location of right main bronchus. The right lung volume is much less than the left lung volume.

TABLE 19-8 Relation between maximum oxygen consumption ($\dot{V}O_2$max) as determined by preoperative exercise testing and perioperative mortality

Study	Deaths/Total
$\dot{V}O_2$max 10–15 mL/kg per minute	
Smith et al[196]	1/6 (33%)
Bechard and Wetstein[197]	0/15 (0%)
Olsen et al[198]	1/14 (7.1%)
Walsh et al[199]	1/5 (20%)
Bolliger et al[200]	2/17 (11.7%)
Markos et al[201]	1/11 (9.1%)
Wang et al[202]	0/12 (0%)
Win et al[203]	2/16 (12.5%)
Total	8/96 (8.3%)
$\dot{V}O_2$max <10 mL/kg per minute	
Bechard and Wetstein[197]	2/7 (29%)
Olsen et al[198]	3/11 (27%)
Holden et al[204]	2/4 (50%)
Markos et al[201]	0/5 (0%)
Total	7/27 (26%)

Source: Reproduced with permission from Colice et al.[48]

status that is inconsistent with the pulmonary function test results. In these circumstances, and in other situations in which decision making is difficult, the $\dot{V}O_2$max should be measured. Values of <10 mL/kg per minute generally prohibit any major pulmonary resection, because the mortality associated with this level is 26%, compared with only 8.3% for $\dot{V}O_2$max levels of ≥10 mL/kg per minute; $\dot{V}O_2$max levels >15 mL/kg per minute generally indicate the patient's ability to tolerate pneumonectomy.

The risk assessment for a patient is based on a combination of clinical judgment and data. Commonly, there are gray areas in which data such as those described earlier can enable more accurate determination of the risk. This risk assessment must be integrated with the experienced clinician's sense of the patient and with the patient's attitude toward the disease and toward life. Figure 19-26 provides a useful algorithm for determining suitability for lung resection.[48]

Lung Cancer Staging Systems

The staging of any tumor is an attempt to measure or estimate the extent of disease present and in turn use that information to help determine the patient's prognosis. The staging of solid epithelial tumors is based on the tumor, node, and metastasis (TNM) staging system. The T status provides information about the primary tumor itself, such as its size and relationship to surrounding structures; the N status provides information about regional lymph nodes; and the M status provides information about the presence or absence of metastatic disease. Table 19-9 lists the TNM descriptors that have been developed for use in NSCLC. These recommendations have been in place since 1997 and are in the process of revision for the next edition of the Union Internationale Contre le Cancer staging system. The proposed changes are discussed at length in the following paragraphs.[49–54]

The designation of lymph nodes as N1, N2, or N3 requires familiarity with the lymph node map devised by Naruke and colleagues in 1978,[55] which was subsequently modified by the American Thoracic Society in 1983 and by Mountain and Dresler in 1997[56,57] (see Fig. 19-8). Because the mapping system is based on clearly delineated anatomic boundaries, accurate and reproducible localization of thoracic lymph nodes is possible, which allows detailed nodal staging for individual patients and facilitates standardization of nodal assessment among surgeons.

A tumor in a given patient is typically classified into a clinical stage and a pathologic stage. The clinical stage (cTNM) is derived from an assessment of all data short of surgical resection of the primary tumor and lymph nodes. Thus clinical staging information includes the history and physical examination, radiographic test results, and diagnostic biopsy information. A therapeutic plan is then generated based on the clinical stage. After surgical resection of the tumor and lymph nodes, a postoperative pathologic stage (pTNM) is determined, providing further prognostic information.

In 1986, an international staging system for lung cancer was developed by Mountain and applied to a database of >3000 patients from the M. D. Anderson Hospital in Houston, Texas, and the Lung Cancer Study Group.[58] In 1997, Mountain reviewed the survival data from an additional 1524 patients beyond the original database. Taking into account the combined total of 5319 patients, he revised the staging system.[59] These changes were subsequently adopted by the American Joint Committee on Cancer. The 1997 version of the international staging system, which is still in use, is shown in Table 19-9.

Significant variation in survival is seen within stage groupings, however (Table 19-10), which has prompted a critical evaluation of the variables that predict poor long-term survival. For example, a tumor that is ≤1.0 cm in diameter has a significantly better prognosis than tumors 2.0 to 3.0 cm in diameter. The wide range of postoperative 5-year survival rates (5 to 25%) after surgical resection of patients with N2 nodal involvement demonstrates the effect of the number and location of involved nodal stations and of the presence of extracapsular nodal extension.

To address the wide variability in survival within stages, the International Association for the Study of Lung Cancer Staging Committee was created in 1999. A database encompassing over 100,000 patients worldwide has been created and intensively examined for important determinants of survival by tumor, node, and metastasis staging.[51–54] The results of this analysis, as well as recommended changes to the TNM staging system, have been recently published after vigorous analysis of multinational data.[50–53] These changes were validated in 23,583 patients and shown to predict survival better than the current staging system.[31,54] Proposed changes to the TNM staging are outlined in Tables 19-11 and 19-12.

Treatment

Early-Stage Disease Early-stage disease typically is defined as stages I and II. In this group are T1 and T2 tumors (with or without local N1 nodal involvement) and T3 tumors (without N1 nodal involvement). This group represents a small, but increasing, proportion of the total number of patients diagnosed with lung cancer each year (approximately 20% of 101,844 patients from 1989 to 2003).[49]

The current standard of treatment is surgical resection, accomplished by lobectomy or pneumonectomy, depending on the tumor location. Despite use of the term *early stage,* 5-year survival is suboptimal, and the results of surgery as a single treatment modality remain disappointing. Patients with stage IA non–small cell lung cancer (NSCLC) who were offered resection but refused any treatment, including chemotherapy and radiation, were recently reported to have a median survival of 14 months and a 5-year survival rate of 22%.[60] For tumors evaluated postoperatively as pathologic stage IA disease, 5-year survival is better after surgical resection than with no treatment, but still only 67%, as reported in 1997 by Mountain.[59] The figures decline with higher-stage disease. Advanced age at diagnosis, male sex, low socioeconomic status, nonsurgical treatment, and poor histologic grade are associated with increased mortality risk on multivariate analysis.[49] The overall 5-year survival rate for stage I tumors as a group is approximately 65%; for stage II disease it is approximately 41%.

Appropriate surgical procedures for patients with early-stage disease include lobectomy, sleeve lobectomy, and occasionally pneumonectomy with mediastinal lymph node dissection or sampling. Sleeve resection is performed for tumors located at airway bifurcations when an adequate bronchial margin cannot be obtained by

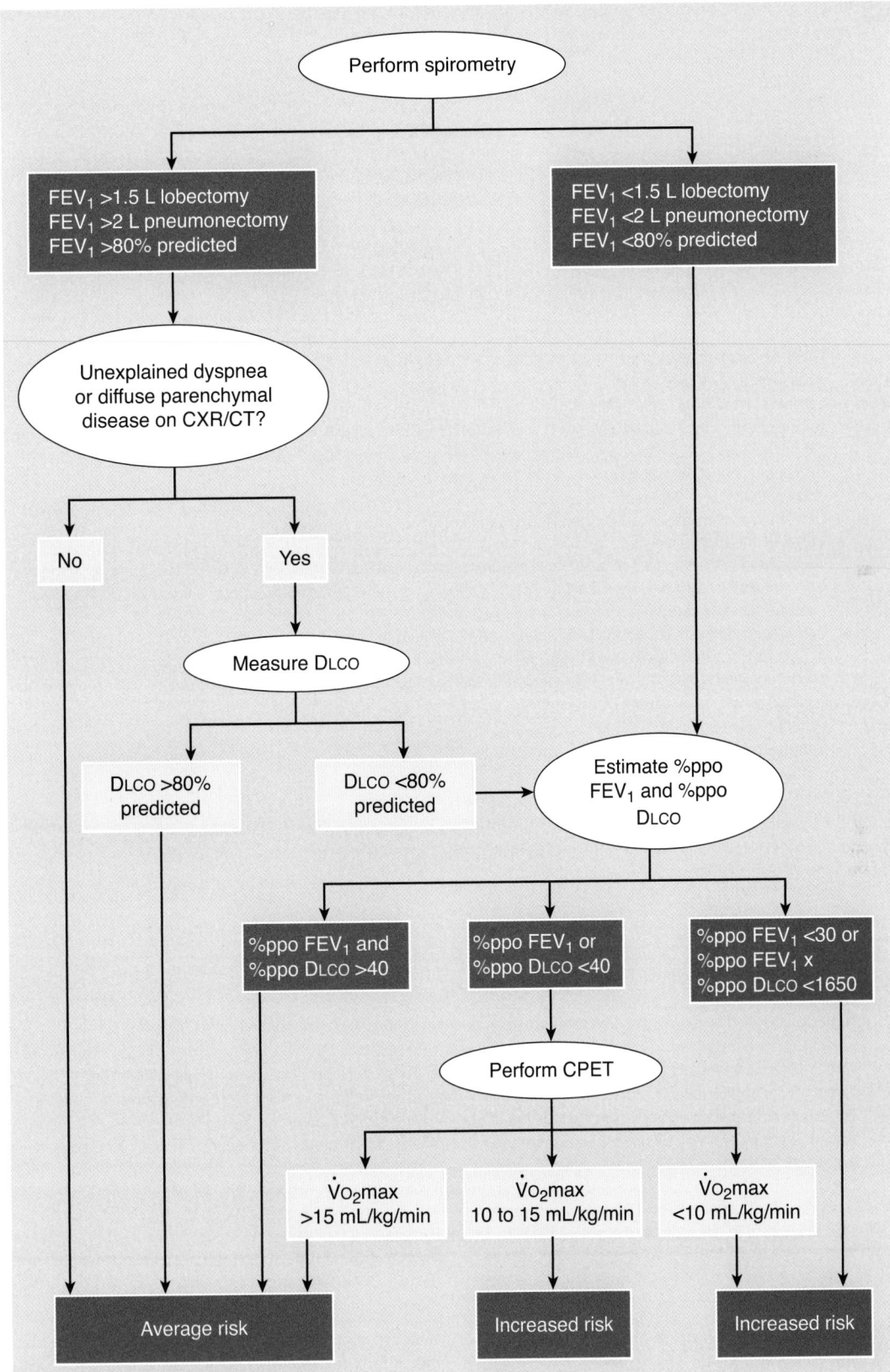

FIG. 19-26. Algorithm for preoperative evaluation of pulmonary function and reserve before resectional lung surgery. CPET = cardiopulmonary exercise test; CT = computed tomographic scan; CXR = chest radiograph; D$_{LCO}$ = carbon monoxide diffusion capacity; FEV$_1$ = forced expiratory volume in 1 second; %ppo = percent predicted postoperative lung function; V̇o$_2$max = maximum oxygen consumption. *(Reproduced with permission from Colice et al.[48])*

TABLE 19-9	American Joint Committee on Cancer staging system for lung cancer

Stage	TNM
IA	T1 N0 M0
IB	T2 N0 M0
IIA	T1 N1 M0
IIB	T2 N1 M0
	T3 N0 M0
IIIA	T3 N1 M0
	T1–3 N2 M0
IIIB	T4 Any N M0
	Any T N3 M0
IV	Any T Any N M1

TNM definitions

T	**TX**	Positive malignant cell, but primary tumor not visualized by imaging or bronchoscopy
	T0	No evidence of primary tumor
	Tis	Carcinoma in situ
	T1	Tumor ≤3 cm, surrounded by lung or visceral pleura, without bronchoscopic evidence of invasion more proximal than the lobar bronchus
	T2	Tumor with any of the following features of size or extent: • >3 cm in greatest dimension • Involves main bronchus, ≥2 cm distal to the carina • Invades the visceral pleura • Associated with atelectasis or obstructive pneumonitis that extends to the hilar region but does not involve the entire lung
	T3	Tumor of any size that directly invades any of the following: chest wall (including superior sulcus tumors), diaphragm, mediastinal pleura, parietal pericardium; or tumor in the main bronchus <2 cm distal to the carina, but without involvement of the carina; or associated atelectasis or obstructive pneumonitis of the entire lung
	T4	Tumor of any size that invades any of the following: mediastinum, heart, great vessels, trachea, esophagus, vertebral body, carina; or tumor with a malignant pleural or pericardial effusion, or with satellite tumor nodule(s) within the ipsilateral primary-tumor lobe of the lung
N	**NX**	Regional lymph nodes cannot be assessed
	N0	No regional lymph node metastasis
	N1	Metastasis to ipsilateral peribronchial and/or ipsilateral hilar lymph nodes, and intrapulmonary nodes involved by direct extension of the primary tumor
	N2	Metastasis to ipsilateral mediastinal and/or subcarinal lymph node(s)
	N3	Metastasis to contralateral mediastinal, contralateral hilar, ipsilateral or contralateral scalene, or supraclavicular lymph node(s)
M	**MX**	Presence of distant metastasis cannot be assessed
	M0	No distant metastasis
	M1	Distant metastasis present [including metastatic tumor nodule(s) in the ipsilateral nonprimary tumor lobe(s) of the lung]

Summary of staging definitions

Occult stage	Microscopically identified cancer cells in lung secretions on multiple occasions (or multiple daily collections); no discernible primary cancer in the lung
Stage 0	Carcinoma in situ
Stage IA	Tumor surrounded by lung or visceral pleura ≤3 cm arising more than 2 cm distal to the carina (T1 N0)
Stage IB	Tumor surrounded by lung >3 cm, or tumor of any size with visceral pleura involved arising more than 2 cm distal to the carina (T2 N0)
Stage IIA	Tumor ≤3 cm not extended to adjacent organs, with ipsilateral peribronchial and hilar lymph node involvement (T1 N1)
Stage IIB	Tumor >3 cm not extended to adjacent organs, with ipsilateral peribronchial and hilar lymph node involvement (T2 N1) Tumor invading chest wall, pleura, or pericardium but not involving carina, nodes negative (T3 N0)
Stage IIIA	Tumor invading chest wall, pleura, or pericardium and nodes in hilum or ipsilateral mediastinum (T3, N1–2) or tumor of any size invading ipsilateral mediastinal or subcarinal nodes (T1–3, N2)
Stage IIIB	Direct extension to adjacent organs (esophagus, aorta, heart, cava, diaphragm, or spine); satellite nodule same lobe, or any tumor associated with contralateral mediastinal or supraclavicular lymph node involvement (T4 or N3)
Stage IV	Separate nodule in different lobes or any tumor with distant metastases (M1)

TABLE 19-10	Cumulative percentage of survival by stage after treatment for lung cancer

Pathologic Stage	Time after Treatment	
	24 mo (%)	**60 mo (%)**
pT1 N0 M0 ($n = 511$)	86	67
pT2 N0 M0 ($n = 549$)	76	57
pT1 N1 M0 ($n = 76$)	70	55
pT2 N1 M0 ($n = 288$)	56	39
pT3 N0 M0 ($n = 87$)	55	38

Source: Modified from Mountain.[59]

standard lobectomy. Pneumonectomy rarely is performed; primary indications for pneumonectomy in early-stage disease include the presence of large central tumors involving the distal main stem bronchus and inability to completely resect involved N1 lymph nodes. The latter circumstance occurs with bulky adenopathy or with extracapsular nodal spread. Carcinoma arising in the extreme apex of the chest with associated arm and shoulder pain, atrophy of the muscles of the hand, and Horner syndrome was first described by Henry Pancoast in 1932.[61] Any tumor of the superior sulcus, including tumors without evidence of involvement of the neurovascular bundle, is now commonly known as *Pancoast's tumor*. The designation should be reserved for those tumors involving the parietal pleura

TABLE 19-11 Summary of proposed lung cancer staging revisions

Current TNM Staging		Proposed (IASLC) TNM Staging

Tumor Stage

T1 (up to 3 cm) ⟶ T1a ≤2 cm / T1b >2 cm to ≤3 cm

T2 (>3 cm) ⟶ T2a >3 cm to ≤5 cm / T2b >5 cm to ≤7 cm / T3 >7 cm

T ⟶ Mediastinal invasion ⟶ Remain T4

Satellite nodules ⟶ Downstage to T3

Malignant pleural or pericardial effusion ⟶ Malignant pleural effusion M1a / Malignant pericardial effusion M1b*

Metastasis Stage

M1a (ipsilateral intrapulmonary nodules ⟶ Downstage to T4

*Additional recommendation after further validation that was not in the proposal for changes to the TNM system by Goldstraw et al.[51]

IASLC = International Association for the Study of Lung Cancer; TNM = tumor, nodes, and metastasis.

or deeper structures overlying the first rib. Chest wall involvement at or below the second rib should not be considered Pancoast's tumor.[62] Treatment involves a multidisciplinary approach. Goals of operative treatment obviously include curative resection; however, due to the location of the tumor and involvement of the neurovascular bundle that supplies the ipsilateral extremity, preserving postoperative function of the extremity also is critical. The recommendation for resection of Pancoast's tumors (apical tumors) depends on the results of mediastinal lymph node analysis. Survival of those with N2 nodal spread in this setting is poor, and in part because of the risk of morbidity and mortality, surgical resection has no role. For this reason, resection should always be preceded by mediastinoscopy.

Historically, Pancoast's tumors have been difficult to treat, with high rates of local recurrence and poor 5-year survival with radiation and/or surgical resection. Tumor invasion into surrounding structures prompted investigations into modalities such as induction radiation and, more recently, concomitant radiation and chemotherapy, to improve rates of complete resection. The Southwest Oncology Group formally studied the use of induction chemoradiotherapy followed by surgery, and long-term results are now available. The treatment regimen was well tolerated, with 95% of patients completing induction treatment. Complete resection was achieved in 76%. Five-year survival was 44% overall and 54% when complete resection was achieved. Disease progression with this regimen was predomi-

nantly at distant sites, with the brain being the most common.[63] A treatment algorithm for Pancoast's tumors is presented in Fig. 19-27.

Surgical excision is performed via thoracotomy with en bloc resection of the chest wall, vascular structures, and anatomic lobectomy. A portion of the lower trunk of the brachial plexus and the stellate ganglion are also typically resected. With chest wall involvement, en bloc chest wall resection, along with lobectomy, is performed, with or without chest wall reconstruction. For small rib resections or those posterior to the scapula, chest wall reconstruction is usually unnecessary. Larger defects (two rib segments or more) usually are reconstructed with polytetrafluoroethylene (Gore-Tex) material to provide chest wall contour and stability.

En bloc resection also is used for other locally advanced tumors (T3) with direct invasion of the adjacent chest wall, diaphragm, or pericardium. If a large portion of the pericardium is removed, reconstruction with thin Gore-Tex membrane will be required to prevent cardiac herniation and venous obstruction.

If a patient is deemed medically unfit for major pulmonary resection due to inadequate pulmonary reserve or other medical conditions, then options include limited surgical resection and radiotherapy. Limited resection, defined as segmentectomy or wedge resection, can be used only for more peripheral T1 or T2 tumors. A randomized trial of lobectomy vs. limited resection for stage I NSCLC conducted by the Lung Cancer Study group con-

TABLE 19-12 International Association for the Study of Lung Cancer proposed changes to the tumor, nodes, and metastasis (TNM) staging system for 2009

Sixth Edition T/M Descriptor	Proposed T/M	N0	N1	N2	N3
T1 (≤2 cm)	T1a	IA	IIA	IIIA	IIIB
T1 (>2 to 3 cm)	T1b	IA	IIA	IIIA	IIIB
T2 (≤5 cm)	T2a	IB	**IIA**	IIIA	IIIB
T2 (>5 to 7 cm)	T2b	**IIA**	IIB	IIIA	IIIB
T2 (>7 cm)	T3	**IIB**	**IIIA**	IIIA	IIIB
T3 invasion	—	IIB	IIIA	IIIA	IIIB
T4 (same-lobe nodules)	—	**IIB**	**IIIA**	**IIIA**	IIIB
T4 (extension)	T4	**IIIA**	**IIIA**	IIIB	IIIB
M1 (ipsilateral lung)	—	**IIIA**	**IIIA**	**IIIB**	**IIIB**
T4 (pleural effusion)	M1a	**IV**	**IV**	**IV**	**IV**
M1 (contralateral lung)	—	IV	IV	IV	IV
M1 (distant)	M1b	IV	IV	IV	IV

Cells in bold represent a change from the sixth edition for a particular TNM category.

Source: Reproduced with permission from Goldstraw et al.[51]

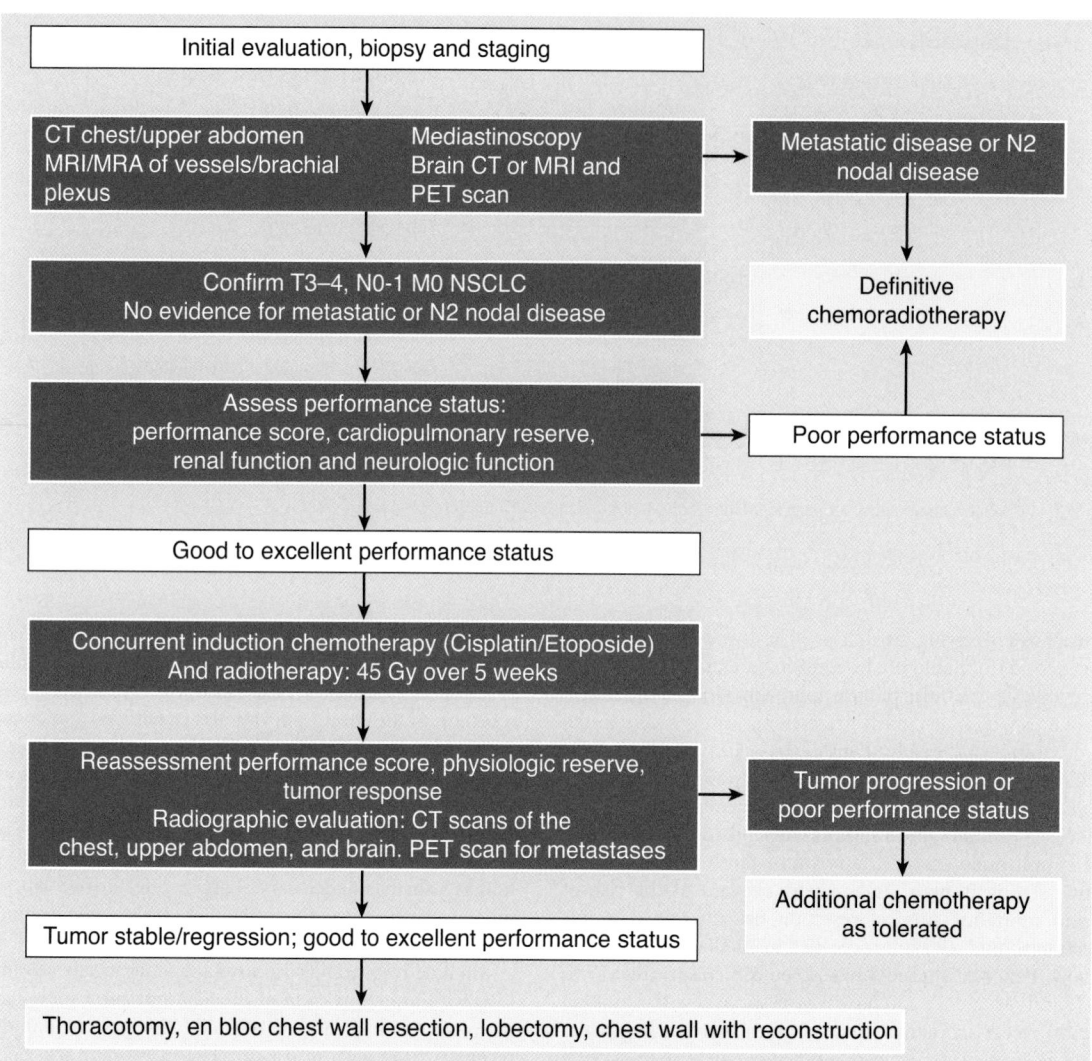

FIG. 19-27. Treatment algorithm for Pancoast's tumors. CT = computed tomography; MRA = magnetic resonance angiography; MRI = magnetic resonance imaging; NSCLC = non–small cell lung cancer; PET = positron emission tomography.

firmed an increased risk of local recurrence, found a slight trend toward decreased overall survival, and concluded that limited resection, even for small, localized tumors, should not be the only therapy.[64,65] Other studies suggest decreased long-term survival rate for tumor size >3 cm but not for smaller tumors, probably due to incomplete resection of occult intrapulmonary lymphatic tumor metastasis.[66] Table 19-13 shows the findings of a meta-analysis by Nakamura and colleagues comparing the mortality and morbidity outcomes for segmental resection and lobectomy. With the increasing prevalence of screening CT in high-risk populations, this topic is again the subject of intensive review. Studies are ongoing to evaluate the role of limited resection, including limited resection with and without brachytherapy in high-risk operative candidates. In addition, the Cancer and Leukemia Group B has initiated a randomized trial of lobectomy vs. sublobar resection (CALGB 140503) that will address the question of whether sublobar resection is equivalent to lobectomy for tumors ≤2 cm in size with no evidence of nodal involvement. At this time, however, for patients who will tolerate lobectomy, complete resection remains the standard of care.

Another option for patients who are poor operative candidates is definitive radiotherapy. Traditional external beam radiation is used to deliver a total dose of 60 to 65 Gy, producing 5-year survival rates of approximately 30% in patients with stage I disease. Significant advances have been made in the focused delivery of radiation

for definitive treatment of early-stage lung cancer, including tomotherapy and robotic radiosurgery (CyberKnife) therapy. These treatments deliver high doses of radiation in several sessions directly to the tumor rather than to the tumor and surrounding normal lung. This minimizes the toxicity of the treatment to surrounding lung parenchyma. Preservation of normal lung is critical for patients with limited pulmonary reserve. Excellent 5-year survival and low recurrence rates are being reported. In addition, the therapy is well tolerated, with minimal side effects.

The role of chemotherapy in early-stage NSCLC is evolving. Postoperative adjuvant chemotherapy previously was found to be of no benefit in multiple prospective randomized trials; however, newer, more effective agents have been of benefit, although the final results of current trials are pending. Similarly, prospective phase II studies have shown a potential benefit for preoperative (or induction) chemotherapy.[67,68] There are concerns that induction chemotherapy may result in increased perioperative morbidity or mortality; however, except in patients undergoing right-sided pneumonectomy after induction chemotherapy, the incidence of perioperative morbidity and mortality is not different for the two groups.[69]

Locoregional Advanced Disease Surgical resection as sole therapy has a limited role in treatment of stage III disease.[70] T3 N1 tumors can be treated with surgery alone, and a 5-year survival rate of approximately 25% is seen with such therapy. Patients with N2

| TABLE 19-13 | Summary of studies comparing limited resection and lobectomy |

Study	Study Design	Stage	No. of Limited Resections	No. of Lobectomies	Reasons for Limited Resection	Survival Difference
Hoffman and Ransdell (1980)[205]	RS	IA	33 (W)	40[g]	Poor cardiopulmonary function and smaller lesions	NS
Read et al (1990)[206]	RS	IA	113 (107 S + 6 W)	131	ND	NS (CSS)
Date et al (1994)[207]	MPS	IA	16 (6 S + 10 W)	16	Poor pulmonary function	Lobectomy better
Warren and Faber (1994)[66]	RS	IA + IB	66 (S)	103	Poor cardiopulmonary function and smaller lesions	Lobectomy better
Harpole et al (1995)[208]	RS	IA + IB	75 (W)	193	Poor cardiopulmonary function and smaller lesions	NS (CSS)
LCSG (1996)[64,209]	RCT	IA	122 (82 S + 40 W)	125	Randomization	NS
Kodama et al (1997)[210]	RS	IA	46[b] (W)	77	Intentional resection for small lesions	NS
Landreneau et al (1997)[211]	RS	IA	102 (W)	117	Poor cardiopulmonary function	NS
Pastorino et al (1997)[212]	RS	IA + IB	53 (S + W)	367	ND	NS
Kwiatkowski et al (1998)[213]	RS	IA + IB	58 (S + W)	186[c]	ND	Lobectomy better
Okada et al (2001)[214]	RS	IA ≤2 cm	70 (S)	139	Intentional resection for small lesions ≤2 cm	NS
Koike et al (2003)[215]	RS	IA ≤2 cm	74 (60 S + 14 W)	159	Intentional resection for small lesions ≤2 cm	NS
Campione et al (2004)[216]	RS	IA	21 (S)	100	Poor cardiopulmonary function	NS
Keenan et al (2004)[217]	RS	IA + IB	54 (S)	147	Poor pulmonary function	NS

[a]Tumors peripherally located.
[b]Only intentional resection.
[c]Including 13 pneumonectomies.
CSS = cancer-specific survival; LCSG = Lung Cancer Study Group; MPS = matched-pair study; ND = not described; NS = not significant; RCT = randomized controlled trial; RS = retrospective study; S = segmentectomy; W = wedge resection.
Source: Reprinted by permission from Macmillan Publishers Ltd. Nakamura H, et al: Survival following lobectomy vs. limited resection for stage I lung cancer: A meta-analysis. *Br J Cancer* 92:1033, Copyright © 2005.

disease are a heterogeneous group. Patients with clinically evident N2 disease (i.e., bulky adenopathy on CT scan or mediastinoscopy, with lymph nodes often replaced by tumor) have a 5-year survival rate of 5 to 10% with surgery alone. In contrast, patients with microscopic N2 disease discovered incidentally in one lymph node station after surgical resection have a 5-year survival rate that may be as high as 30%. Surgery is occasionally appropriate for select patients with T4, N0 or N1, M0 primary tumors (e.g., tumors invading the superior vena caval, carinal or vertebral body involvement, or satellite nodules in the same lobe); surgery generally does *not* have a role in the care of patients with a tumor of any size and N3 disease or with T4 tumors and N2 disease. Survival rates remain low for these patients.

Definitive radiotherapy is predominantly used for palliation of symptoms in patients with poor performance status, because the cure rate of radiotherapy as a single modality in patients with N2 or N3 disease is <7%. Recently improvement has been seen with three-dimensional conformal radiotherapy and altered fractionation. Such poor results for patients with stage IIIA lung cancer reflect the limitations of locoregional therapy in treating a disease process that results in death because of systemic metastatic spread.

Definitive treatment of stage III disease (when surgery is not felt to be feasible at any time) is usually a combination of chemotherapy and radiotherapy. Two strategies for delivery are available. Sequential chemoradiation involves full-dose systemic chemotherapy (i.e., cisplatin combined with a second agent) followed by standard radiotherapy (approximately 60 Gy). The combination of chemotherapy followed by radiation has been shown to improve the 5-year survival rate to 17%, compared with 6% with radiotherapy alone.[71]

An alternative approach, referred to as *concurrent chemoradiation,* is to administer chemotherapy and radiotherapy at the same time. When certain chemotherapeutic agents are given at the same time as radiotherapy, tumor cells become sensitized to the radiation, which enhances the radiation effect. The advantages of this approach are improved local control of the primary tumor and associated nodal disease and a lack of delay in administering radiotherapy. A

disadvantage, however, is the necessary reduction in chemotherapy dosage to diminish overlapping toxicities, which can potentially lead to undertreatment of systemic micrometastases. Randomized trials have shown a modest 5-year survival benefit compared with chemotherapy alone.

Preoperative (Induction) Chemotherapy for Non–Small Cell Lung Cancer The use of chemotherapy before possible surgical resection has a number of potential advantages:

1. The tumor's blood supply is still intact, which allows better chemotherapy delivery and avoids tumor cell hypoxia (in any residual microscopic tumor remaining postoperatively), which would increase radioresistance.
2. The primary tumor may be downstaged with enhanced resectability.
3. Patients are better able to tolerate chemotherapy before surgery and are more likely to complete the prescribed regimen than when chemotherapy is given after surgery.
4. Preoperative chemotherapy functions as an in vivo test of the primary tumor's sensitivity to chemotherapy.
5. Response to chemotherapy can be monitored and used to guide decisions about additional therapy.
6. Systemic micrometastases are treated.
7. Patients who have progressive disease (non-responders) are identified and spared a pulmonary resection.

Potential disadvantages include the following:

1. In theory the perioperative complication rate may increase (predominantly in patients requiring right pneumonectomy after induction chemotherapy).
2. While the patient is receiving chemotherapy, potentially curative resection is delayed; if the patient does not respond, this delay could result in tumor spread.

In stage IIIA N2 disease, the response rates to such chemotherapy are high—in the range of 70%. The treatment is generally safe,

TABLE 19-14 Selected randomized trials of neoadjuvant chemotherapy for stage III non–small cell lung cancer

Trial (Reference)	No. of Patients (Stage III)	Chemotherapy	Response Rate (%)	pCR (%)	Complete Resection	PFS	OS	5-y Survival
Rosell et al[71]	60 (60)	Mitomycin Ifosfamide Cisplatin	60	4	85%	12 vs. 5 mo (DFS; $P = .006$)	22 vs. 10 mo ($P = .005$)	16% vs. 0%
Roth et al[73]	60 (60)	Cyclophosphamide Etoposide Cisplatin	35	NR	39% vs. 31%	Not reached vs. 9 mo ($P = .006$)	64 vs. 11 mo ($P = .008$)	56% vs. 15%[a]
Pass et al[218]	27 (27)	Etoposide Cisplatin	62	8	85% vs. 86%	12.7 vs. 5.8 mo ($P = .083$)	28.7 vs. 15.6 mo ($P = .095$)	NR
Nagai et al[219]	62 (62)	Cisplatin Vindesine	28	0	65% vs. 77%	NR	17 vs. 16 mo ($P = .5274$)	10% vs. 22%
Gilligan et al[220]	519 (80)	Platinum based[b]	49	4	82% vs. 80%	NR	54 vs. 55 mo ($P = .86$)	44% vs. 45%
Depierre et al[221]	355 (167)	Mitomycin Ifosfamide Cisplatin	64	11	92% vs. 86%	26.7 vs. 12.9 mo ($P = .033$)	37 vs. 26 mo ($P = .15$)	43.9% vs. 35.3%[c]
Pisters et al[222]	354 (113)[d]	Carboplatin Paclitaxel	41	NR	94% vs. 89%	33 vs. 21 mo ($P = .07$)	75 vs. 46 mo ($P = .19$)	50% vs. 43%
Sorensen et al[223]	90 (NR)	Paclitaxel Carboplatin	46	0	79% vs. 70%	NR	34.4 vs. 22.5 mo (NS)	36% vs. 24% (NS)
Mattson et al[224]	274 (274)	Docetaxel	28	NR	77% vs. 76%[e]	9 vs. 7.6 mo (NS)	14.8 vs. 12.6 mo (NS)	NR

[a]3-y survival.

[b]Options included MVP (mitomycin C, vindesine, and platinum), MIC (mitomycin, ifosfamide, and cisplatin), NP (cisplatin and vinorelbine), PacCarbo (paclitaxel and carboplatin), GemCis (gemcitabine and cisplatin), and DocCarbo (docetaxel and carboplatin).

[c]4-y survival.

[d]113 patients (32%) were reported to have stage IIB or IIIA disease.

[e]22 patients in the chemotherapy arm and 29 patients in the control arm had resectable disease.

DFS = disease-free survival; NR = not recorded; NS = not significant; OS = overall survival; pCR = pathologic complete response; PFS = progression-free survival.

Source: Reproduced with permission from The Journal of the National Comprehensive Cancer Network. Allen J, Jahanzeb M. Neoadjuvant chemotherapy in stage III NSCLC. *J Natl Compr Canc Netw* 6:285, 2008, Table 2 © 2008 National Comprehensive Cancer Network, Inc.

because it does not cause a significant increase in perioperative morbidity. Two randomized trials have now compared surgery alone for patients with N2 disease to preoperative chemotherapy followed by surgery.[68,70] Both trials were stopped before complete accrual because of a significant increase in survival in the chemotherapy arm. The initially observed survival differences have been maintained up to 3 years and beyond (Table 19-14). Given these results, induction chemotherapy with cisplatin-based regimens (two to three cycles) has become standard for patients with N2 disease.

The role of surgery in Stage IIIA NSCLC is still the subject of intense debate. Many surgeons and oncologists differentiate between microscopic and bulky N2 lymphadenopathy and the number of involved N2 nodal stations in determining whether to proceed with resection after induction therapy. Although randomized trials specifically investigating resection after induction therapy in patients with single-station microscopic disease have not yet been performed, proceeding to resection is thought to be appropriate by many surgeons. Furthermore, histologic confirmation of N2 nodal metastases is imperative; false-positive findings on PET scan are unacceptably high, and reliance on this modality will lead to significant undertreatment of patients with earlier-stage cancers. This is particularly true in regions with a high incidence of granulomatous diseases. Patients should not be denied surgical resection after induction chemotherapy unless they have proven N2 disease, because the survival of patients with early-stage NSCLC is significantly better with resection than with chemotherapy alone.

The use of induction chemotherapy in patients with stage I and II disease is undergoing investigation. Table 19-15 summarizes the findings of a systematic review and meta-analysis reporting stage-specific 5-year survival benefit after induction chemotherapy followed by surgical resection. As shown in Table 19-15, an absolute survival benefit of 4 to 7% can be realized using induction chemotherapy for all stages of lung cancer.

Surgery in Stage IV Disease The treatment of patients with stage IV disease is chemotherapy. However, on occasion, patients with a single site of metastasis are encountered, particularly patients with adenocarcinomas who have a solitary brain metastasis. In this highly select group, 5-year survival rates of 10 to 15% can be achieved with surgical excision of the brain metastasis and the primary tumor, provided it is early stage.

Small Cell Lung Carcinoma Small cell lung carcinoma (SCLC) accounts for approximately 20% of primary lung cancers and generally is not treated surgically. These aggressive neoplasms have early,

TABLE 19-15 Five-year stage-specific survival after induction chemotherapy followed by surgery

Stage	5-y Survival (%)	Absolute Benefit (%)	New 5-y Survival (%)
IA	75	4	79
IB	55	6	61
IIA	50	7	57
IIB	40	7	47
IIIA	15–35	6–7	21–42
IIIB	5–10	3–5	8–15

Source: Reproduced with permission from Burdett SS, Stewart LA, Rydzewska L. Chemotherapy and surgery versus surgery alone in non-small cell lung cancer. Cochrane Database Syst Rev 2007:CD006157. John Wiley & Sons, Ltd. Copyright Cochrane Collaboration.

widespread metastases. Histologically, they can be difficult to distinguish from lymphoproliferative lesions and atypical carcinoid tumors. Therefore, a definitive diagnosis must be established with adequate tissue samples. Three groups of SCLC are recognized: pure small cell carcinoma (sometimes referred to as *oat cell carcinoma*), small cell carcinoma with a large cell component, and combined (mixed) tumors.

Unlike with NSCLC, the clinical stage of SCLC is defined broadly by the presence of either local "limited" or distant "disseminated" disease. SCLC presenting with bulky locoregional disease but no evidence for distant metastatic disease is termed *limited* SCLC. Most often, the primary tumor is large and associated with bulky mediastinal adenopathy, which may lead to obstruction of the superior vena cava. SCLC falling into the other clinical stage, termed *disseminated,* usually presents with metastatic disease throughout the patient's body. Regardless of the stage of presentation, treatment is primarily chemotherapy and radiation. Surgery is appropriate for the rare patient with an incidentally discovered peripheral nodule that is found to be SCLC. If a stage I SCLC is identified after resection, postoperative chemotherapy usually is given.

Metastatic Lesions to the Lung The cause of one or more new pulmonary nodules in a patient with a previous malignancy can be difficult to discern.[72] Features suggestive of metastatic disease are multiplicity; smooth, round borders on CT scan; and temporal proximity to the original primary lesion. One must always entertain the possibility that a single new lesion is a primary lung cancer. The probability of a new primary cancer vs. a metastasis in patients presenting with solitary lesions depends on the type of initial neoplasm. The likelihood of a new primary lung cancer is highest in patients with a history of uterine carcinoma (74%), bladder carcinoma (89%), lung carcinoma (92%), and head and neck carcinoma (94%).[73]

Surgical resection of pulmonary metastases has a role in properly selected patients.[74] Resection of pulmonary metastases is associated with modest survival benefits in a very select group of patients. The general principles of patient selection for metastasis resection are listed in Table 19-16.

The technical aim of pulmonary metastasis resections is complete resection of all macroscopic tumors. In addition, any adjacent structure involved should be resected en bloc (i.e., chest wall, diaphragm, and pericardium). Multiple lesions and/or hilar lesions may require lobectomy. Pneumonectomy rarely is justified or used.

Pulmonary metastasis resection can be carried out via thoracotomy or VATS techniques. McCormack and colleagues reported their experience at Memorial Sloan-Kettering in a prospective study of 18 patients who had no more than two pulmonary metastatic lesions and underwent VATS resection.[75] A thoracotomy was performed during the same operation; if palpation identified any additional lesions, they were resected. The study concluded that the probability that a metastatic lesion will be missed by VATS excision is 56%. The patients in that study were evaluated by standard chest CT scan, because spiral CT scanning was not yet available. It remains controversial whether metastasis resection should be performed via thoracotomy or VATS. Proponents of an open approach

TABLE 19-17	Actuarial survival data from the International Registry of Lung Metastases	
Survival	**Complete Resection (%)**	**Incomplete Resection (%)**
5 y	36	13
10 y	26	7
15 y	22	—

refer to the above-referenced study. Proponents of VATS techniques argue that the resolution of spiral CT scanning is so far superior to that of conventional CT that any data collected using old standard CT scans are no longer applicable; they also point to the significantly reduced pain and faster recovery when VATS is used. To date, no prospective study using spiral CT scanning has been performed to resolve this clinical dilemma.

The best data regarding outcomes after resection of pulmonary metastases come from the International Registry of Lung Metastases. The registry was established in 1991 by 18 thoracic surgery departments in Europe, the United States, and Canada, and included data on 5206 patients. Approximately 88% of patients underwent complete resection. An analysis of survival at 5, 10, and 15 years (with grouping of all primary tumor types) was performed (Table 19-17). Multivariate analysis showed a better prognosis for patients with germ cell tumors, osteosarcomas, a disease-free interval of >36 months, and a single metastasis.[76]

Pulmonary Infections
Lung Abscess

A *lung abscess* is a localized area of pulmonary parenchymal necrosis caused by an infectious organism. Tissue destruction results in a solitary or dominant cavity measuring at least 2 cm in diameter. Less often, there may be multiple, smaller cavities (<2 cm). In that case, the infection typically is referred to as *necrotizing pneumonia*. An abscess that is present for >6 weeks is considered chronic.

Based on the etiology (Table 19-18), lung abscesses are further classified as primary or secondary. A primary lung abscess occurs, for example, in immunocompromised patients (as a result of malignancy, chemotherapy, organ transplantation, etc), in patients in whom highly virulent organisms incite a necrotizing pulmonary infection, and in patients who have a predisposition to aspirate oropharyngeal or GI secretions. A secondary lung abscess occurs in patients with an underlying condition such as a partial bronchial obstruction, a lung infarct, or adjacent suppurative infections (subphrenic or hepatic abscesses).[77]

The incidence of bacterial lung abscess in the United States has declined significantly over the past 50 years, with a concomitant decrease in the mortality rate from between 30 and 40% to between 5 and 10%. This decrease has been attributed to the development of bactericidal antibiotics. Factors associated with a worse outcome include advanced patient age, prolonged symptoms, comorbid disease, nosocomial infection, and perhaps larger cavity size. More recently, a greater proportion of lung abscesses have been associated with pulmonary malignancies or immunosuppression, which has resulted in an increase in lung abscesses caused by unusual or opportunistic organisms.

Pathogenesis Lung abscess is the result of a lower respiratory tract infection only by organisms that cause necrosis. Microorganisms gain access to the respiratory tract via inhalation of aerosolized particles, aspiration of oropharyngeal secretions, or hematogenous spread from distant sites. Direct extension from a contiguous site is less frequent. Most primary lung abscesses are suppurative bacterial infections secondary to aspiration. Risk factors for increased aspiration include impaired consciousness, suppressed cough reflex, dysfunctional esophageal motility, laryngopharyngeal reflux disease, and centrally acting neurologic diseases (e.g., stroke). At the time of

TABLE 19-16	General principles governing appropriate selection of patients for pulmonary metastasectomy

1. Primary tumor must already be controlled.
2. Patient must be able to tolerate general anesthesia, potential single-lung ventilation, and the planned pulmonary resection.
3. Metastases must be completely resectable based on computed tomographic imaging.
4. There is no evidence of extrapulmonary tumor burden.
5. Alternative superior therapy must not be available.

TABLE 19-18 Causes of lung abscess

I. Primary
   A. Necrotizing pneumonia
      1. *Staphylococcus aureus, Klebsiella, Pseudomonas, Mycobacterium*
      2. *Bacteroides, Fusobacterium, Actinomyces*
      3. *Entamoeba, Echinococcus*
   B. Aspiration pneumonia
      1. Anesthesia
      2. Stroke
      3. Drugs or alcohol
   C. Esophageal disease
      1. Achalasia, Zenker's diverticulum, gastroesophageal reflux
   D. Immunodeficiency
      1. Cancer (and chemotherapy)
      2. Diabetes
      3. Organ transplantation
      4. Steroid therapy
      5. Malnutrition
II. Secondary
   A. Bronchial obstruction
      1. Neoplasm
      2. Foreign body
   B. Systemic sepsis
      1. Septic pulmonary emboli
      2. Seeding of pulmonary infarct
   C. Complication of pulmonary trauma
      1. Infection of hematoma or contusion
      2. Contaminated foreign body or penetrating injury
   D. Direct extension from extraparenchymal infection
      1. Pleural empyema
      2. Mediastinal, hepatic, subphrenic abscess

Source: Adapted with permission from Rusch VW, et al: Chest wall, pleura, and mediastinum, in Schwartz SI, et al (eds): *Principles of Surgery*, 7th ed. New York: McGraw-Hill, 1999, p 735.

aspiration, the composition of the oropharyngeal flora determines the etiologic organisms; those organisms that are most numerous or virulent proliferate and emerge as single or predominant pathogens. With increasing use of proton pump inhibitors to suppress acid secretion in the stomach, the oropharyngeal flora has shifted, and risk of aspiration-associated bacterial infections has increased.[78] Secondary lung abscesses occur most often distal to an obstructing bronchial carcinoma. Infected cysts or bullae are not considered true abscesses.

The characteristic pathologic features of aspiration pneumonia include alveolar edema and infiltration with inflammatory cells. Because of the effect of gravity, foci of infection tend to develop in the subpleural regions of the superior segments of the lower lobes and in the posterior segments of the upper lobes. The right lung is involved more frequently, presumably because of the less acute angle of the right main bronchus. Thus, the right upper and lower lobes are most commonly affected, followed by the left lower lobe and right middle lobe.

Microbiology In community-acquired pneumonia, the causative bacteria are predominantly gram positive; in hospital-acquired pneumonia, 60 to 70% of the organisms are gram negative. Gram-negative bacteria associated with nosocomial pneumonia include *Klebsiella pneumoniae, Haemophilus influenzae, Proteus* species, *Pseudomonas aeruginosa, Escherichia coli, Enterobacter cloacae,* and *Eikenella corrodens.* Immunosuppressed patients may develop abscesses caused by the usual pathogens as well as less virulent and opportunistic organisms such as *Salmonella* species, *Legionella* species, *Pneumocystis jiroveci,* atypical mycobacteria, and fungi.

Normal oropharyngeal secretions contain many more *Streptococcus* species and more anaerobes (approximately 1×10^8 organisms/

mL) than aerobes (approximately 1×10^7 organisms/mL). Pneumonia that follows from aspiration, with or without abscess development, is typically polymicrobial. An average of two to four isolates present in large numbers have been cultured from lung abscesses sampled percutaneously. Overall, at least 50% of these infections are caused by purely anaerobic bacteria, 25% are caused by mixed aerobes and anaerobes, and 25% or fewer are caused by aerobes only.

Clinical Features and Diagnosis The typical presentation may include productive cough, fever [>38.9°C (102°F)], chills, leukocytosis (>15,000 cells/mm³), weight loss, fatigue, malaise, pleuritic chest pain, and dyspnea. Lung abscesses also may present in a more indolent fashion, with weeks to months of cough, malaise, weight loss, low-grade fever, night sweats, leukocytosis, and anemia. After aspiration pneumonia, 1 to 2 weeks typically elapse before cavitation occurs; 40 to 75% of such patients produce a putrid, foul-smelling sputum. Severe complications such as massive hemoptysis, endobronchial spread to other portions of the lungs, rupture into the pleural space and development of pyopneumothorax, or septic shock and respiratory failure are rare in the modern antibiotic era. The mortality rate is approximately 5 to 10% except in immunosuppressed patients, in whom rates range from 9 to 28%.

The chest radiograph is the primary tool for diagnosing a lung abscess (Fig. 19-28). Its distinguishing characteristic is a density or mass with a relatively thin-walled cavity. Frequently, an air-fluid level is observed within the abscess, indicating a communication with the tracheobronchial tree. CT scan of the chest is useful to clarify the diagnosis when the chest radiograph is equivocal, assess for endobronchial obstruction and/or an associated mass, and evaluate other pathologic anomalies. A cavitating lung carcinoma frequently is mistaken for a lung abscess. Other possible differential diagnoses include loculated or interlobar empyema, infected lung cysts or bullae, tuberculosis, bronchiectasis, fungal infections, and noninfectious inflammatory conditions (e.g., Wegener's granulomatosis).

Identification of the specific etiologic organism should ideally occur before antibiotic administration. Attempts should be made to obtain an adequate specimen for culture analysis to appropriately direct antibiotic therapy and minimize the risk of promoting drug-resistant bacterial speciation. Unfortunately, routine sputum cultures are often of limited usefulness because of contamination with upper respiratory tract flora. Bronchoscopy, which is essential to rule out endobronchial obstruction due to tumor or foreign body, is ideal for obtaining uncontaminated cultures using bronchoalveolar lavage. Culture samples also can be obtained by percutaneous transthoracic FNA under ultrasound or CT guidance.

Management Systemic antibiotics directed against the causative organism represent the mainstay of therapy. For community-acquired infections secondary to aspiration, likely pathogens are oropharyngeal streptococci and anaerobes. Penicillin G, ampicillin, and amoxicillin are the main therapeutic agents, but a beta-lactamase inhibitor or metronidazole should be added because of the increasing prevalence of gram-negative anaerobes that produce beta-lactamase. Clindamycin is also a primary therapeutic agent. For hospital-acquired infections, frequently encountered causative agents include *Staphylococcus aureus* and aerobic gram-negative bacilli, common organisms of the oropharyngeal flora. Piperacillin or ticarcillin with a beta-lactamase inhibitor (or equivalent alternatives) provides better coverage of likely pathogens. The duration of antimicrobial therapy is variable: 1 to 2 weeks for simple aspiration pneumonia and 3 to 12 weeks for necrotizing pneumonia and lung abscess. It is probably best to treat until the cavity is resolved or until serial radiographs show significant improvement. Parenteral therapy generally is used until the patient is afebrile and able to demonstrate consistent enteral intake. Oral therapy can then be used to complete the course of therapy.

Surgical drainage of lung abscesses is uncommon, because drainage usually occurs spontaneously via the tracheobronchial tree. Indications for intervention are listed in Table 19-19.

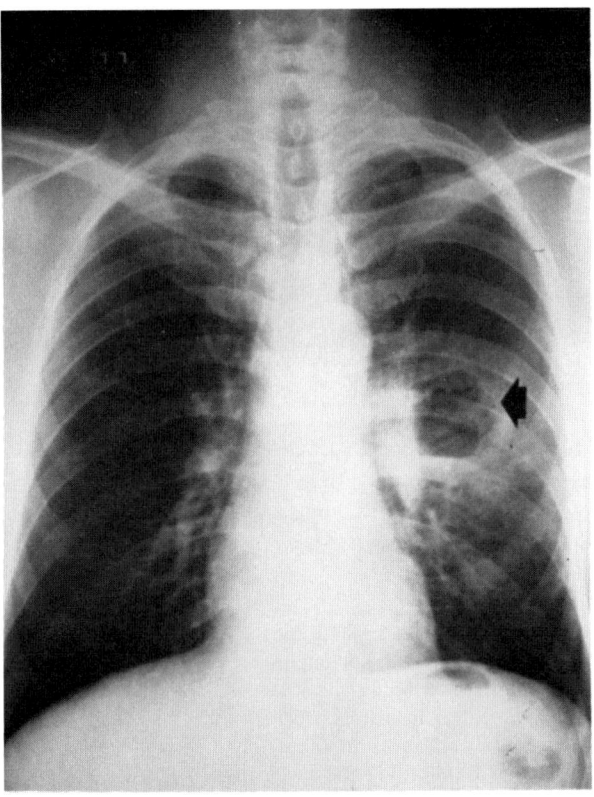

A

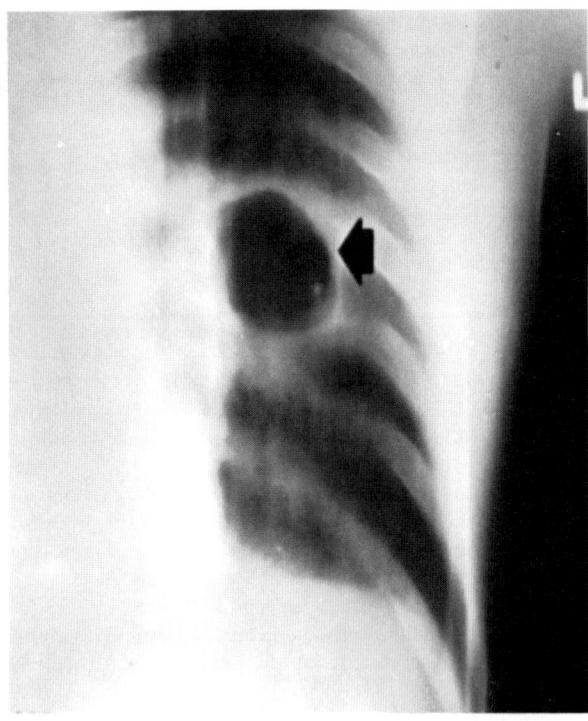

B

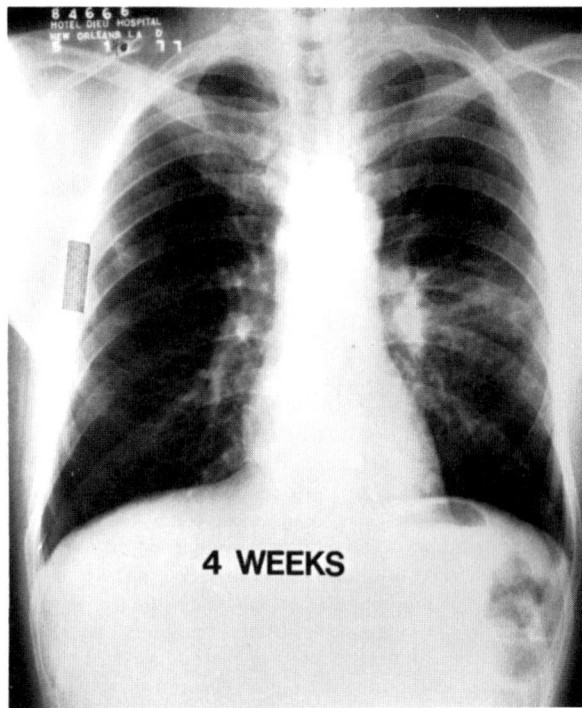

4 WEEKS

C

FIG. 19-28. Lung abscess resulting from emesis and aspiration after an alcoholic binge. **A.** Chest radiograph showing an abscess cavity in the left upper lobe (*arrow*). **B.** Coronal tomogram highlighting the thin wall of the abscess (*arrow*). **C.** Healing of the abscess cavity after 4 weeks of antibiotic therapy and postural drainage.

External drainage may be accomplished with tube thoracostomy, percutaneous drainage, or surgical cavernostomy. The choice between thoracostomy placement and radiologic placement of a drainage catheter depends on the treating physician's preference and the availability of interventional radiology. Surgical resection is required in <10% of lung abscess patients. Lobectomy is the preferred intervention for bleeding from a lung abscess or pyopneumothorax. An important intraoperative consideration is to protect the contralateral lung with a double-lumen tube, bronchial blocker, or contralateral main stem intubation. Surgical treatment has a 90% success rate, with an associated mortality of 1 to 13%.

Bronchiectasis

Bronchiectasis is defined as a pathologic and permanent dilation of bronchi with bronchial wall thickening. This condition may be localized to certain bronchial segments or it may be diffuse throughout the bronchial tree, typically affecting the medium-sized airways. Overall, this is a rare clinical entity in the United States with a prevalence of <1 in 10,000.

Pathogenesis Development of bronchiectasis can be attributed to either congenital or acquired causes. The principal congenital diseases that lead to bronchiectasis include cystic fibrosis, primary

TABLE 19-19	Indications for surgical drainage procedures for lung abscesses

1. Failure of medical therapy
2. Abscess under tension
3. Abscess increasing in size during appropriate treatment
4. Contralateral lung contamination
5. Abscess >4–6 cm in diameter
6. Necrotizing infection with multiple abscesses, hemoptysis, abscess rupture, or pyopneumothorax
7. Inability to exclude a cavitating carcinoma

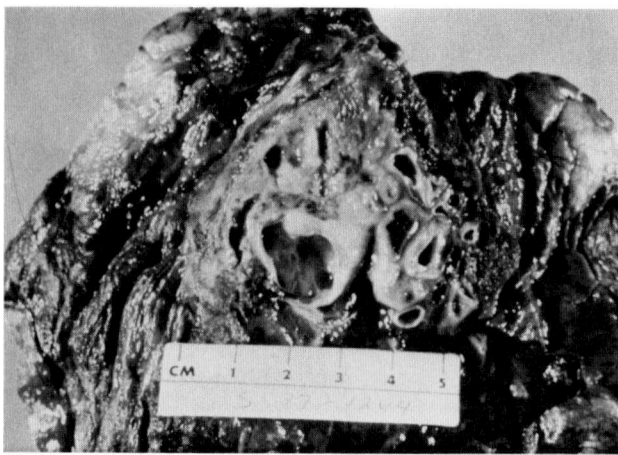

FIG. 19-29. Multiple cystic-type bronchiectatic cavities can be seen on a cut section of the right lower lobe of the lung.

ciliary dyskinesia, and immunoglobulin deficiencies (e.g., selective immunoglobulin A deficiency). Congenital causes tend to produce a diffuse pattern of bronchial involvement.

Acquired causes are categorized broadly as infectious and inflammatory. Adenoviruses and influenza viruses are the predominant childhood viral infections associated with the development of bronchiectasis. Chronic infection with tuberculosis remains an important worldwide cause of bronchiectasis.

More significant in the United States are nontuberculous mycobacterial (NTM) infections that cause bronchiectasis, particularly infection by *Mycobacterium avium-intracellulare* complex. Recently, several studies have suggested an association between chronic gastroesophageal reflux disease, acid suppression, and NTM infection with bronchiectasis.[79,80] This interaction is thought to be related to chronic aspiration of colonized gastric secretions in the setting of acid suppression. Although a causative relationship has not been proven, these findings suggest a role for gastroesophageal reflux disease in the pathogenesis of this disease process.

Noninfectious causes of bronchiectasis include inhalation of toxic gases such as ammonia, which results in severe and destructive airway inflammatory responses. Allergic bronchopulmonary aspergillosis, Sjögren's syndrome, and alpha$_1$-antitrypsin deficiency are some additional examples of presumed immunologic disorders that may be accompanied by bronchiectasis.

The common pathway shared by all of these causes of bronchiectasis is impairment of airway defenses or deficits in immunologic mechanisms that permit bacterial colonization and establishment of chronic infection. Common causative organisms include *Haemophilus* species (55%), *Pseudomonas* species (26%), and *Streptococcus pneumoniae* (12%).[81] Both the bacterial organisms and the inflammatory cells recruited to thwart the bacteria elaborate proteolytic and oxidative molecules, which progressively destroy the muscular and elastic components of the airway walls; those components are then replaced by fibrous tissue. Thus chronic airway inflammation is the essential pathologic feature of bronchiectasis. The dilated airways usually are filled with thick purulent material; more distal airways are often occluded by secretions or obliterated by fibrous tissue. The vascularity of affected bronchial walls increases, bronchial arteries become hypertrophied, and abnormal anastomoses form between the bronchial and pulmonary arterial circulation.

There are three principal types of bronchiectasis, based on pathologic morphology: cylindrical—uniformly dilated bronchi; varicose—an irregular or beaded pattern of dilated bronchi; and saccular (cystic)—peripheral balloon-type bronchial dilation (Fig. 19-29). The saccular type is the most common after bronchial obstruction or infection.

Clinical Manifestations and Diagnosis A daily persistent cough and purulent sputum production are the typical symptoms of bronchiectasis. The quantity of daily sputum production (10 mL to >150 mL) tends to correlate with disease extent and severity. Often, patients with bronchiectasis may appear asymptomatic or have a dry, nonproductive cough ("dry bronchiectasis"). These patients are likely to have involvement of the upper lobes. The clinical course is characterized by progressive symptoms and respiratory impair-

ment. Increasing resting and exertional dyspnea are the result of progressive airway obstruction. Acute exacerbations may be triggered by viral or bacterial pathogens. Hemoptysis may become more frequent as the disease progresses, and bleeding is attributable to chronically inflamed, friable airway mucosa. In more advanced stages, massive bleeding may result from erosions of the hypertrophied bronchial arteries.

The current gold standard of diagnosis is chest CT scanning, which affords a highly detailed cross-sectional view of bronchial architecture. Both mild and severe forms of bronchiectasis are readily demonstrated with this imaging modality. A chest radiograph, although less sensitive, may reveal characteristic signs of bronchiectasis such as lung hyperinflation, bronchiectatic cysts, and dilated, thick-walled bronchi forming train track–like patterns radiating from the lung hila. Sputum culture may identify characteristic pathogens, including *H. influenzae, S. pneumoniae,* and *P. aeruginosa.* Acid-fast bacillus smears and cultures of sputum should be performed to evaluate for the presence of NTM, which are common in this setting. The severity of airway obstruction should be determined by spirometry, which also can evaluate the course of disease.

Management Standard therapy includes optimizing clearance of secretions from the tracheobronchial tree, using bronchodilators to reverse any airflow limitation, and correcting reversible underlying causes whenever possible.[82] Chest physiotherapy based on vibration, percussion, and postural drainage is widely accepted as the basis for therapy, although randomized trials demonstrating efficacy are lacking. Acute exacerbations should be treated with courses of broad-spectrum antibiotics tailored to culture and sensitivity profiles. Usually, a 2- to 3-week course of IV antibiotics, followed by an oral regimen, will result in a longer-lasting remission. Hyperosmolar agents such as 7% normal saline and dry mannitol also have been suggested as reasonable adjuncts to maintain quality of life and decrease exacerbations by reducing sputum volume, improving mucociliary clearance, and slowing the decline in lung function, although adequately powered randomized trials of these therapies have not been performed.

Over the past decade, investigations into the use of inhaled antibiotics such as tobramycin and colistin have suggested that they improve resolution of bacterial infection and slow the decline in pulmonary function associated with bronchiectasis, but large, randomized trials showing overall clinical benefit have not yet been published.[83,84] Macrolide antibiotics have also generated significant interest, for both their antibacterial and nonantibacterial properties. Macrolide antibiotics have been shown to decrease sputum production, inhibit cytokine release, and inhibit neutrophil adhesion and formation of reactive oxygen species. They also inhibit migration of

Pseudomonas, disrupt biofilm, and prevent release of virulence factors.[85] Although macrolide therapy does appear to be efficacious, it is important to remember that macrolides have significant activity against NTM, and widespread prophylactic use in patients with bronchiectasis may lead to the emergence of multidrug-resistant NTM species.

Surgical resection of a localized bronchiectatic segment or lobe may benefit patients with refractory symptoms who are receiving maximal medical therapy. Multifocal disease must be excluded before any surgery is attempted; any uncorrectable predisposing factor (e.g., ciliary dyskinesia) also must be excluded. An important surgical tenet is to preserve as much normal parenchyma as possible. Patients with end-stage lung disease from bronchiectasis may be potential candidates for bilateral lung transplantation. Surgical resection also is indicated in patients with large hemoptysis secondary to hypertrophied bronchial arteries. Because resection may not always be clinically practical, bronchial artery embolization is an alternative.

Mycobacterial Infections

Epidemiology Tuberculosis is a widespread problem that affects nearly one third of the world's population. Currently, approximately 9 million new cases of tuberculosis are reported annually worldwide and almost 2 million tuberculosis-related deaths occur—more than for any other single infectious disease. In 2007, it was the leading killer of persons infected with HIV.[86] In the United States, infection with mycobacteria is also a significant health problem, with an estimated 3 to 4% of infected individuals developing active disease within the first year, and 5 to 15% of all patients thereafter. During the 1980s a resurgence of tuberculosis occurred, related primarily to the emergence of AIDS. More than 20,000 new cases of tuberculosis are now reported annually in the United States, although there has been a sharp decline in the incidence of new cases among U.S.-born citizens since 1993 (2.1 per 100,000, which represents a decrease of 71% since 1993). This is partly attributable to renewed public and federal interest in eliminating tuberculosis from the United States.[87]

The elderly, minorities, and recent immigrants are the populations that most commonly show clinical manifestations of infection, yet no age group, sex, or race is exempt from infection. In most large urban centers, reported cases of tuberculosis are more numerous among the homeless, prisoners, and drug-addicted populations. Tuberculosis in immunocompromised patients also contributes to the increased incidence, and such patients often develop unusual systemic as well as pulmonary manifestations.[88] In comparison with past decades, surgical intervention now is required more frequently in patients with multidrug-resistant tuberculosis (MDRTB) who do not respond to medical treatment and in selected patients with NTM infections.

Microbiology Mycobacterial species are obligate aerobes. They are primarily intracellular parasites with slow rates of growth. Their defining characteristic is the property of acid-fastness, which is the ability to withstand decolorization by an acid-alcohol mixture after being stained.

Mycobacterium tuberculosis is the highly virulent bacillus of this species that produces invasive infection among humans, principally pulmonary tuberculosis. Because of improper application of antimycobacterial drugs and multifactorial interactions, MDRTB organisms have emerged that are defined by their resistance to at least two of the first-line antimycobacterial drugs (isoniazid and rifampin). Approximately 10% of new tuberculosis cases and 40% of recurrent cases are attributed to MDRTB organisms. In addition, there is another rare variant termed *extensively drug-resistant tuberculosis,* which is caused by organisms resistant to isoniazid and rifampin, all fluoroquinolones, and at least one of the injectable second-line drugs (capreomycin, amikacin, kanamycin).[89]

The more important NTM organisms include *Mycobacterium kansasii, M. avium, M. avium-intracellulare* complex (MAC), and *M. fortuitum.* The highest incidence of *M. kansasii* infection is in midwestern U.S. cities among middle-aged males in good socioeconomic environments. MAC organisms are important agents of infection in elderly and immunocompromised patient groups. *M. fortuitum* infections are common complications of underlying severe debilitating disease. None of these organisms is as contagious as *M. tuberculosis.*

Pathogenesis and Pathology The main route of transmission is via airborne inhalation of viable mycobacteria. Three stages of primary infection have been described. In the first stage, alveolar macrophages become infected through ingestion of the bacilli. These infected macrophages then release chemoattractants to recruit additional macrophages. In the second stage, from days 7 to 21, the patient typically remains asymptomatic while the bacteria multiply within the infected macrophages. The third stage is characterized by the onset of cell-mediated immunity (CD4+ helper T cells) and delayed-type hypersensitivity. Activated macrophages acquire an increased capacity for bacterial killing. Macrophage death increases, which results in the formation of a granuloma, the characteristic lesion found on pathologic examination.

Tuberculous granulomas are composed of blood-derived macrophages, degenerating macrophages or epithelioid cells, and multinucleated giant cells (fused macrophages with nuclei around the periphery, also known as *Langerhans cells*). T lymphocytes are found at the periphery of granulomas. The low oxygen content of this environment inhibits macrophage function and bacillary growth, with subsequent central caseation as macrophage death occurs. A Ghon complex is a single small lung lesion that often is the only remaining trace of a primary infection. The primary infection usually is located in the peripheral portion of the middle zone of the lungs. Reactivation of tuberculosis infection may occur after hydrolytic enzymes liquify the caseum. Typically, the apical and posterior segments of the upper lobes and the superior segments of the lower lobes are involved. Edema, hemorrhage, and mononuclear cell infiltration also are present. The tuberculous cavity may become secondarily infected with other bacteria, fungi, or yeasts, all of which may contribute to enhanced tissue destruction.

The pathologic changes caused by NTM organisms are similar to those produced by *M. tuberculosis.* MAC infections commonly occur not only in immunocompromised patients but also in patients with previously damaged lungs. Caseous necrosis is uncommon, and the infection is characterized by clusters of tissue macrophages filled with mycobacteria. There is a poor granulomatous response, and immune cell infiltration is confined to the interstitium and alveolar walls. Cavitary disease is infrequent, although nodules may be noted.

Clinical Presentation and Diagnosis The clinical course of infection and the presentation of symptoms are influenced by many factors, including the site of primary infection, the stage of disease, and the degree of cell-mediated immunity. Approximately 80 to 90% of tuberculosis patients present with clinical disease in the lungs. In 85 to 90% of these patients, involution and healing occur, which leads to a dormant phase that may last a lifetime. The only evidence of tuberculosis infection may be a positive skin reaction to tuberculin challenge or a Ghon complex observed on chest radiograph. Within the first 2 years of primary infection, reactivation may occur in up to 10 to 15% of infected patients. In 80%, reactivation occurs in the lungs; other reactivation sites include the lymph nodes, pleura, and musculoskeletal system.

After primary infection, pulmonary tuberculosis frequently is asymptomatic. Systemic symptoms of low-grade fever, malaise, and weight loss are subtle and may go unnoticed. A productive cough may develop, usually after tubercle cavitation. Many radiographic patterns can be identified at this stage, including local exudative lesions, local fibrotic lesions, cavitation, bronchial wall involvement, acute tuberculous pneumonia, bronchiectasis, bronchostenosis, and tuberculous granulomas. Hemoptysis often develops from complications of disease such as bronchiectasis or erosion into vascular malformations associated with cavitation. Extrapulmonary involvement is due to hematogenous or lymphatic spread from pulmonary lesions. Virtually any organ can become infected, which gives rise to the protean manifestations of tuberculosis. Of note to the thoracic surgeon, the pleura, chest wall, and mediastinal organs may all be involved. More than one third of immunocompromised patients have disseminated disease, with hepatomegaly, diarrhea, splenomegaly, and abdominal pain.

A definitive diagnosis of tuberculosis requires identification of the mycobacterium in a patient's bodily fluids or involved tissues. Skin testing using purified protein derivative is important for epidemiologic purposes and can help exclude infection in uncomplicated cases. For pulmonary tuberculosis, sputum examination is inexpensive and has a high diagnostic yield. Bronchoscopy with alveolar lavage also may be a useful diagnostic adjunct and has high diagnostic accuracy. Chest CT scan can delineate the extent of parenchymal disease.

Management Medical therapy is the primary mode of treatment of pulmonary tuberculosis and often is initiated before a mycobacterial pathogen is definitively identified. Combinations of two or more drugs are routinely used to minimize resistance, which inevitably develops with only single-agent therapy. A current treatment algorithm is outlined in Fig. 19-30. First-line drugs include isonicotinic acid hydrazine (isoniazid), ethambutol, rifampin, and pyrazinamide. Second-line drugs include cycloserine, ethionamide, kanamycin, ciprofloxacin, and amikacin, among others. In the case of MDRTB organisms, four or more antimycobacterial drugs often are used, generally for 18 to 24 months. Rifampin and isoniazid augmented with one or more second-line drugs are most commonly used to treat NTM infections. Generally, therapy lasts approximately 18 months. The overall response is satisfactory in 70 to 80% of patients with *M. kansasii* infection. Surgical intervention rarely is required in those 20 to 30% who do not respond to medical therapy. In contrast, pulmonary MAC infections respond poorly, even to combinations of four or more drugs, and most patients eventually require surgical intervention. Overall, sputum conversion is achieved in only 50 to 80% of those with NTM infections, and relapses occur in up to 20% of patients.

In the United States, surgical intervention is most often required to treat patients infected with MDRTB organisms whose lungs have been destroyed and who have persistent thick-walled cavitation.[90] The indications for surgery related to mycobacterial pulmonary infections are presented in Table 19-20.

The governing principle of mycobacterial surgery is to remove all gross disease while preserving any uninvolved lung tissue. Scattered

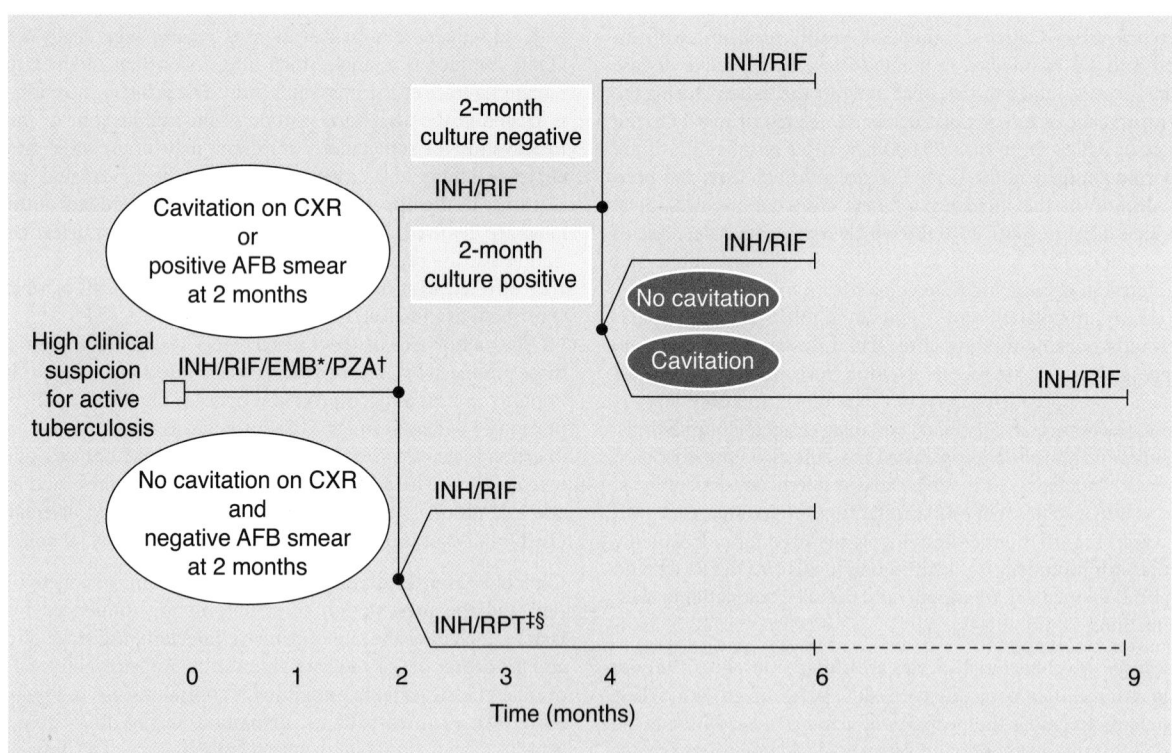

FIG. 19-30. Treatment algorithm for tuberculosis. Patients in whom tuberculosis is proven or strongly suspected should have treatment initiated with isoniazid (INH), rifampin (RIF), pyrazinamide (PZA), and ethambutol (EMB) for the initial 2 months. A repeat smear and culture should be performed when 2 months of treatment has been completed. If cavities were seen on the initial chest radiograph (CXR) or the acid-fast bacillus (AFB) smear results are positive at completion of 2 months of treatment, the continuation phase of treatment should consist of INH and RIF daily or twice daily for 4 months to complete a total of 6 months of treatment. If cavitation was present on the initial CXR and the culture results at the time of completion of 2 months of therapy are positive, the continuation phase should be lengthened to 7 months (total of 9 months of treatment). If the patient has HIV infection and the CD4+ cell count is <100/μL, the continuation phase should consist of daily or three times weekly INH and RIF. In HIV-uninfected patients with no cavitation on CXR and negative results on AFB smears at completion of 2 months of treatment, the continuation phase may consist of either once weekly INH and rifapentine (RPT) or daily or twice weekly INH and RIF to complete a total of 6 months of treatment (*bottom*). For patients receiving INH and RPT whose 2-month culture results are positive, treatment should be extended by an additional 3 months (total of 9 months). *EMB may be discontinued when results of drug susceptibility testing indicate no drug resistance. †PZA may be discontinued after it has been taken for 2 months (56 doses). ‡RPT should not be used in HIV-infected patients with tuberculosis or in patients with extrapulmonary tuberculosis. §Therapy should be extended to 9 months if results of 2-month culture are positive. (*Reproduced with permission from Blumberg HM, et al: American Thoracic Society/Centers for Disease Control and Prevention/Infectious Diseases Society of America: Treatment of tuberculosis. Am J Respir Crit Care Med 167:603, 2003. Official Journal of the American Thoracic Society. Copyright © American Thoracic Society.*)

TABLE 19-20	Indications for surgery to treat mycobacterial pulmonary infections

1. Complications resulting from previous thoracic surgery to treat tuberculosis
2. Failure of optimized medical therapy (e.g., progressive disease, lung gangrene, or intracavitary aspergillosis superinfection)
3. Need for tissue acquisition for definitive diagnosis
4. Complications of pulmonary scarring (e.g., massive hemoptysis, cavernomas, bronchiectasis, or bronchostenosis)
5. Extrapulmonary thoracic involvement
6. Pleural tuberculosis
7. Nontuberculous mycobacterial infection

nodular disease may be left intact, given its low mycobacterial burden. Antimycobacterial medications should be given preoperatively (for approximately 3 months) and continued postoperatively for 12 to 24 months. Overall, >90% of patients who were deemed good surgical candidates are cured when appropriate medical and surgical therapy is used.

Actinomycetic Infections

Actinomycosis Members of the families Actinomycetaceae and Nocardiaceae were once considered fungi but are now classified as bacteria. Actinomycosis is a chronic disease usually caused by *Actinomyces israelii*. It is characterized by chronic suppuration, sinus formation, and discharge of purulent material containing yellow-brown sulfur granules.[90] Approximately 15% of infections involve the thorax; organisms enter the lungs via the oral cavity (where they normally reside). Because the disease is uncommon, making the correct diagnosis can be challenging,[92] and the clinician must first suspect the disease and then perform appropriate culture analysis under anaerobic conditions. Lung involvement can present with progressive pulmonary fibrosis in the periphery. Pleural and chest wall involvement (periostitis of the ribs) is an associated finding. Treatment consists of prolonged high-dose penicillin, which is very effective. Because of the intense fibrotic reaction surrounding affected parenchyma, surgery is seldom possible.

Nocardiosis *Nocardia asteroides* is an aerobic, acid-fast, gram-positive organism that usually causes nocardiosis, a disease similar to actinomycosis with additional CNS involvement. In addition, hematogenous dissemination from a pulmonary focus may lead to generalized systemic infection. The disease process ranges from benign, self-limited suppuration of skin and subcutaneous tissues to pulmonary (extensive parenchymal necrosis and abscesses) and systemic (e.g., CNS) manifestations. In immunosuppressed patients, pulmonary cavitation or hematogenous dissemination may be accelerated. Prolonged treatment (2 to 3 months) with sulfadiazine, minocycline, or trimethoprim-sulfamethoxazole is typically required. Surgery to drain abscesses and empyema is indicated.

Pulmonary Mycoses

An important differential diagnosis to consider in thoracic pathology in general is a mycotic lung infection, which can mimic a bronchial carcinoma or tuberculosis. Most fungi are secondary or opportunistic pathogens that cause pulmonary and systemic infections in humans only when natural host resistance is impaired. Clinically significant examples include species of *Aspergillus, Cryptococcus, Candida,* and *Mucor.* However, some fungi are primary or true pathogens, able to cause infections in otherwise healthy patients. Some examples endemic in the United States are species of *Histoplasma, Coccidioides,* and *Blastomyces.*[93]

The incidence of fungal infections has increased significantly, with many new opportunistic fungi emerging. This increase is attributed to the growing population of immunocompromised patients (i.e., organ transplant recipients, cancer patients under-going chemotherapy, HIV-infected patients, and young and elderly patients), who are more likely to become infected with fungi.[94] Other at-risk patient populations include those who are malnourished, severely debilitated, or diabetic, or who have hematologic disorders. Patients receiving high-dose, intensive antibiotic therapies are also susceptible. Definitive diagnosis of a fungal infection is achieved by directly identifying the organism in body exudates or tissues, preferably by growing in culture. Serologic testing to identify mycotic-specific antibodies also may be a useful diagnostic tool. Although these infections were previously difficult to treat, several new classes of antifungal agents are now available that are effective against many life-threatening fungi and are less toxic than older agents. In addition, thoracic surgery may be a useful therapeutic adjunct for patients with pulmonary mycoses.

Aspergillosis The genus *Aspergillus* comprises over 350 species, three of which are most commonly responsible for clinical disease: *A. fumigatus, A. flavus,* and *A. niger. Aspergillus* is a saprophytic, filamentous fungus with septate hyphae. Spores (2.5 to 3 μm in diameter) are released and easily inhaled by susceptible patients; because the spores are microns in size, they are able to reach the distal bronchi and alveoli.

Aspergillosis can manifest as one of three clinical syndromes: *Aspergillus* hypersensitivity lung disease, aspergilloma, or invasive pulmonary aspergillosis. Overlap occurs between these syndromes, depending on the patient's immune status.[95] Hypersensitivity results in productive cough, fever, wheezing, pulmonary infiltrates, eosinophilia, and elevated levels of immunoglobulin E antibodies to *Aspergillus.*

Aspergilloma (fungus ball) is a matted sphere of hyphae, fibrin, and inflammatory cells that tends to colonize pre-existing intrapulmonary cavities. Grossly, it appears as a round or oval, friable, gray (or red, brown, or even yellow), necrotic-looking mass (Fig. 19-31). This form is the most common presentation of noninvasive pulmonary aspergillosis. Although some aspergillomas are found incidentally during radiographic evaluation for other reasons, they most commonly present with hemoptysis. Other common complaints include chronic and productive cough, clubbing, malaise, or weight loss. Chest radiography can suggest the diagnosis by the finding of a crescentic radiolucency above a rounded radiopaque lesion (Monad sign).

Treatment of pulmonary aspergilloma is individualized. Asymptomatic patients can be observed without any additional therapy. Similarly, mild hemoptysis that is not life-threatening can be managed with medical therapy, including antifungals and cough suppressants. Amphotericin B is the drug of choice, although voriconazole recently has been used for treatment of aspergillosis, with fewer side effects and equivalent efficacy.

Massive hemoptysis had traditionally been an indication for urgent or emergent operative intervention. However, with the advancement of endovascular techniques, bronchial artery embolization in select centers with experience in these techniques has been effective. Patients can now be successfully stabilized with endovascular embolization and may, in many cases, require no further intervention. This approach is particularly important to consider in patients with severely impaired pulmonary function who may not have sufficient reserve to tolerate even a very small pulmonary resection. Other indications for surgical intervention include recurrent hemoptysis, particularly after bronchial artery embolization[96]; chronic cough with systemic symptoms; progressive infiltrate around the mycetoma; and a pulmonary mass of unknown cause.

When operative intervention is indicated, the surgeon must remain cognizant of the goals of the procedure. Because this disease typically occurs in patients with significantly impaired pulmonary function, attempts should be made to excise all diseased tissue with as limited a resection as possible. Once resection is completed, the postresection space in the hemithorax should be obliterated with a pleural tent, pneumoperitoneum, pulmonary decortications, intrathoracic rotation of a muscle, or omental flap or thoracoplasty.

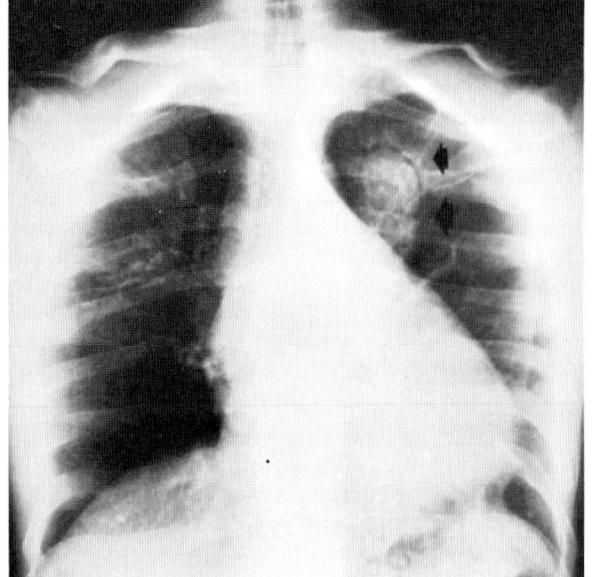

A

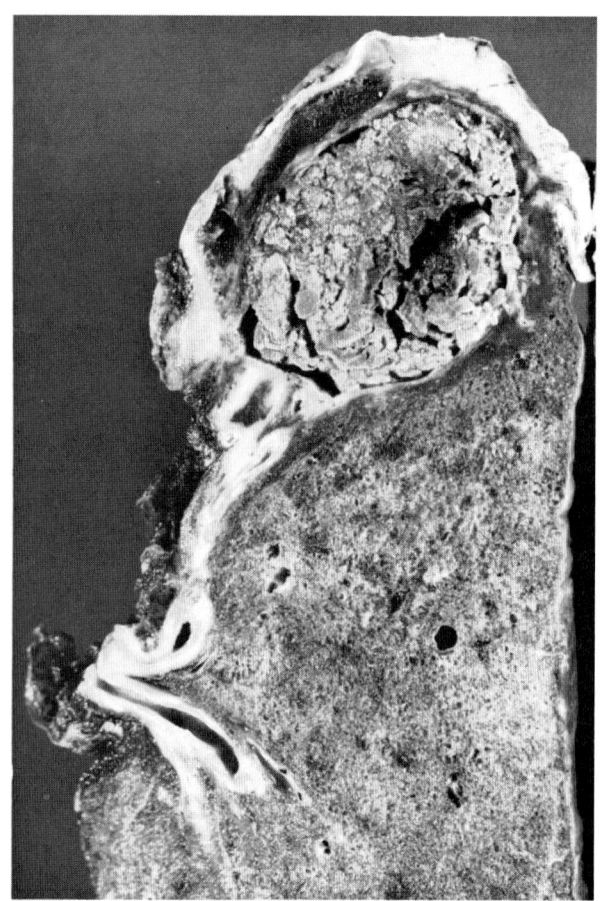

B

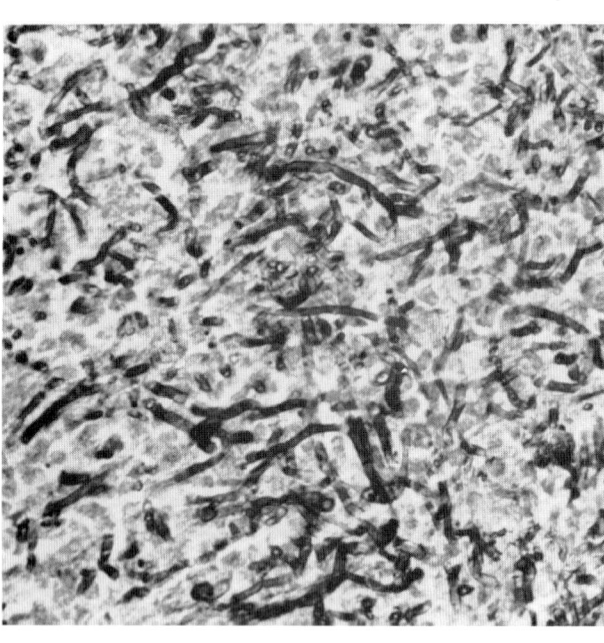

C

FIG. 19-31. Pulmonary aspergilloma. **A.** The chest radiograph shows a solid mass within a cavity surrounded by a rim of air between the mass and cavity wall (Monad sign, *arrows*). **B.** A cut section shows the fungus ball occupying an old, fibrotic cavity. **C.** Histologic stain reveals characteristic *Aspergillus* hyphae invading the wall of the cavity.

Long-term follow-up is necessary, given that the recurrence rate after surgery is approximately 7%.

Invasive pulmonary aspergillosis typically affects immunocompromised patients who have dysfunctional cellular immunity, namely, defective polymorphonuclear leukocytes. Invasion of pulmonary parenchyma and blood vessels by a necrotizing bronchopneumonia may be complicated by thrombosis, hemorrhage, and then dissemination. Patients present with fever that is nonresponsive to antibiotic therapy in the setting of neutropenia. They may also have pleuritic chest pain, cough, dyspnea, or hemoptysis. Chest CT scanning, in addition to routine radiography, may reveal finer details of the infective process and characteristic signs (e.g., halo sign and cavitary lesions). Treatment of invasive pulmonary aspergillosis has been revolutionized in the past decade, with a randomized trial demonstrating a significant survival benefit with voriconazole over amphotericin B.[97] The mortality rate is high, ranging from 93 to 100% in bone marrow transplant recipients to approximately 38% in kidney transplant recipients, although this is

improved to approximately 60% at 12 weeks with voriconazole therapy. Several other advances in diagnosis and treatment, including CT scanning in high-risk populations and development of additional triazoles and echinocandins, have improved early identification and response to therapy in this patient population. Serologic tests have been developed, but their accuracy is limited at this time. Additional treatment considerations include the use of hematopoietic growth factors to minimize the neutropenic period, which contributes to uncontrolled disease. Surgical removal of the infectious nidus is advocated by some groups because medical treatment is associated with such poor outcomes.

Cryptococcosis Cryptococcosis is a subacute or chronic infection caused by *Cryptococcus neoformans*, a round, budding yeast (5 to 20 μm in diameter) that is sometimes surrounded by a characteristic wide gelatinous capsule. Cryptococci typically are present in soil and dust contaminated by pigeon droppings. When inhaled, such droppings can cause a nonfatal disease primarily affecting the pulmonary and central nervous systems. At present, cryptococcosis is the fourth most common opportunistic infection in patients with HIV infection, affecting 6 to 10% of that population. Four basic pathologic patterns are seen in the lungs of infected patients: granulomas, granulomatous pneumonia, diffuse alveolar or interstitial involvement, and proliferation of fungi in alveoli and lung vasculature. Symptoms are nonspecific, as are the radiographic findings. *Cryptococcus* may be isolated from sputum, bronchial washings, samples obtained by percutaneous needle aspiration of the lung, or cerebrospinal fluid. Multiple antifungal agents are effective against *C. neoformans,* including amphotericin B and the azoles.

Candidiasis *Candida* organisms are oval, budding cells (with or without mycelial elements) that colonize the oropharynx of many healthy individuals. The fungi of this genus are common hospital and laboratory contaminants. Usually, *C. albicans* causes disease in the oral or bronchial mucosa, among other anatomic sites. Other potentially pathogenic *Candida* species include *C. tropicalis, C. glabrata,* and *C. krusei.* Historically, *C. albicans* was the pathogen that most commonly caused invasive candidal infection. However, more recent reports suggest the other *Candida* species, particularly *C. glabrata* and *C. krusei,* are becoming more prevalent. These species are relatively resistant to fluconazole, and the shift is likely related to the widespread use of this antifungal agent.[98]

Candida infections have increased in incidence and are no longer confined to immunocompromised patients. Rising incidence of infection has been seen in patients with any of the following risk factors: critical illness of long duration; long-term use of antibiotics, particularly multiple drugs; indwelling urinary or vascular catheter; and GI perforation or burn wounds.[99] With respect to the thorax, such patients commonly have candidal pneumonia, pulmonary abscess, esophagitis, and mediastinitis. Pulmonary candidal infections typically result in an acute or chronic granulomatous reaction. Because *Candida* can invade blood vessel walls and a variety of tissues, systemic or disseminated infections can occur, but are less common.

Treatment of candidal infection, similar to that of other fungal infections, has changed dramatically in the past decade. Amphotericin B, often in combination with 5-fluorocytosine, is a proven therapeutic treatment for *Candida* tissue infections. Newer classes of antifungals have been developed. The fungicidal medications include polyenes (amphotericin B deoxycholate and various lipid-associated amphotericin B preparations) and the echinocandins (caspofungin, micafungin, and anidulafungin). Fungistatic drugs include the triazoles (fluconazole, itraconazole, voriconazole, and posaconazole).[98] The availability of multiple effective therapies allows for specific tailoring of treatment, including the use of combination regimens, based on the patient's ability to tolerate associated toxicities, the microbiologic information for the specific candidal species, and the route of administration. Although their demonstrated efficacy is similar, the triazoles and echinocandins appear to have fewer side effects and are better tolerated than the other classes of antifungal drugs. For patients with *Candida* mediastinitis (which has a mortality rate of over 50%), surgical intervention to débride all infected tissues is required, in addition to prolonged administration of antifungal drugs.

Mucormycosis The *Mucor* species, rare members of the class Zygomycetes, are responsible for rapidly fatal disease in immunocompromised patients. Other disease-causing species of the class Zygomycetes include *Absidia, Rhizopus,* and *Mortierella.*[100] These fungi are characterized by nonseptate, branching hyphae and are difficult to culture. Infection occurs via inhalation of spores. Neutropenia, acidosis, diabetes, and hematologic malignancy all predispose patients to clinical susceptibility. In the lungs, disease consists of blood vessel invasion, thrombosis, and infarction of infected organs. Tissue destruction is significant, along with cavitation and abscess formation. Initial treatment is to correct underlying risk factors and administer antifungal therapies, although the optimal duration and optimal total dose are unknown. Surgical resection of

any localized disease should be performed after initial medical treatment attempts fail.

Primary Fungal Pathogens *Histoplasma capsulatum* is a dimorphic fungus existing in mycelial form in soil contaminated by fowl or bat excreta, and in yeast form in human hosts. Histoplasmosis primarily affects the respiratory system after spores are inhaled. It is the most common of all fungal pulmonary infections. In the United States, this disease is endemic in the Midwest and Mississippi River Valley, where approximately 500,000 new cases arise each year. Active, symptomatic disease is uncommon. Acute forms of the disease present as primary or disseminated pulmonary histoplasmosis; chronic forms present as pulmonary granulomas (histoplasmomas), chronic cavitary histoplasmosis, mediastinal granulomas, fibrosing mediastinitis, or broncholithiasis. In immunocompromised patients, the infection becomes systemic and more virulent; because cell-mediated immunity is impaired, uninhibited fungal proliferation occurs within pulmonary macrophages and then spreads. Histoplasmosis is definitively diagnosed by fungal smear, culture, direct biopsy of infected tissues, or serologic testing.

The clinical presentation depends on the inoculum size and on host factors. Patients with acute pulmonary histoplasmosis commonly present with fever, chills, headache, chest pain, musculoskeletal pain, and nonproductive cough. Chest radiographs may be normal or may show mediastinal lymphadenopathy and patchy parenchymal infiltrates. Most patients improve in a few weeks and do not require antifungal therapy. Amphotericin B is the treatment of choice if moderate symptoms persist for 2 to 4 weeks; if the illness is extensive, including dyspnea and hypoxia; and if patients are immunosuppressed.[101]

As the pulmonary infiltrates from acute histoplasmosis heal, consolidation into a solitary nodule or histoplasmoma may occur. This condition is asymptomatic and usually is seen incidentally on radiographs as a coin-shaped lesion. Central calcification may occur; if so, no further treatment is required. Noncalcified lesions require further diagnostic work-up including chest CT scan, needle biopsy, or surgical excision to rule out a malignancy. Figure 19-32 shows the differences in pathologic findings between infections in normal and in immunocompromised hosts.[102]

When lymph nodes and pulmonary granulomas calcify over time, pressure atrophy on the bronchial wall may result in erosion and migration of the granulomatous mass into the bronchus, causing broncholithiasis. Typical symptoms include cough, hemoptysis, and dyspnea. Life-threatening complications include massive hemoptysis or bronchoesophageal fistula. In addition to radiography, bronchoscopy should be performed to aid in diagnosis. Definitive treatment is surgical; the bronchial mass should be removed and any associated complications repaired. Endobronchial débridement is not advised, because this can result in massive, fatal bleeding.

Chronic cavitary histoplasmosis occurs in approximately 10% of patients who become symptomatic after infection. Most such patients have pre-existing lung pathology such as COPD or emphysema. The disease begins with colonization of diseased lung spaces, development of ongoing pneumonitis and necrosis, cavity enlargement, new cavity formation, and eventual spread to other areas of lung. Nonspecific symptoms, such as cough, sputum production, fever, weight loss, weakness, and hemoptysis are common. Chest radiography may reveal intrapulmonary cavitation and scarring. Occasionally, partial resolution of the inflammatory changes may be observed. Triazole therapy (such as itraconazole or ketoconazole) provides effective therapy. Occasionally, combination therapy or the use of polyenes (such as lipid-associated amphotericin B) or echinocandins is necessary for management of more severe infections. In patients with adequate pulmonary reserve and localized, thick-walled cavities that have been unresponsive to antifungal therapy, surgical excision should be considered.

Disseminated histoplasmosis occurs most frequently in patients who are severely immunocompromised, such as posttransplantation

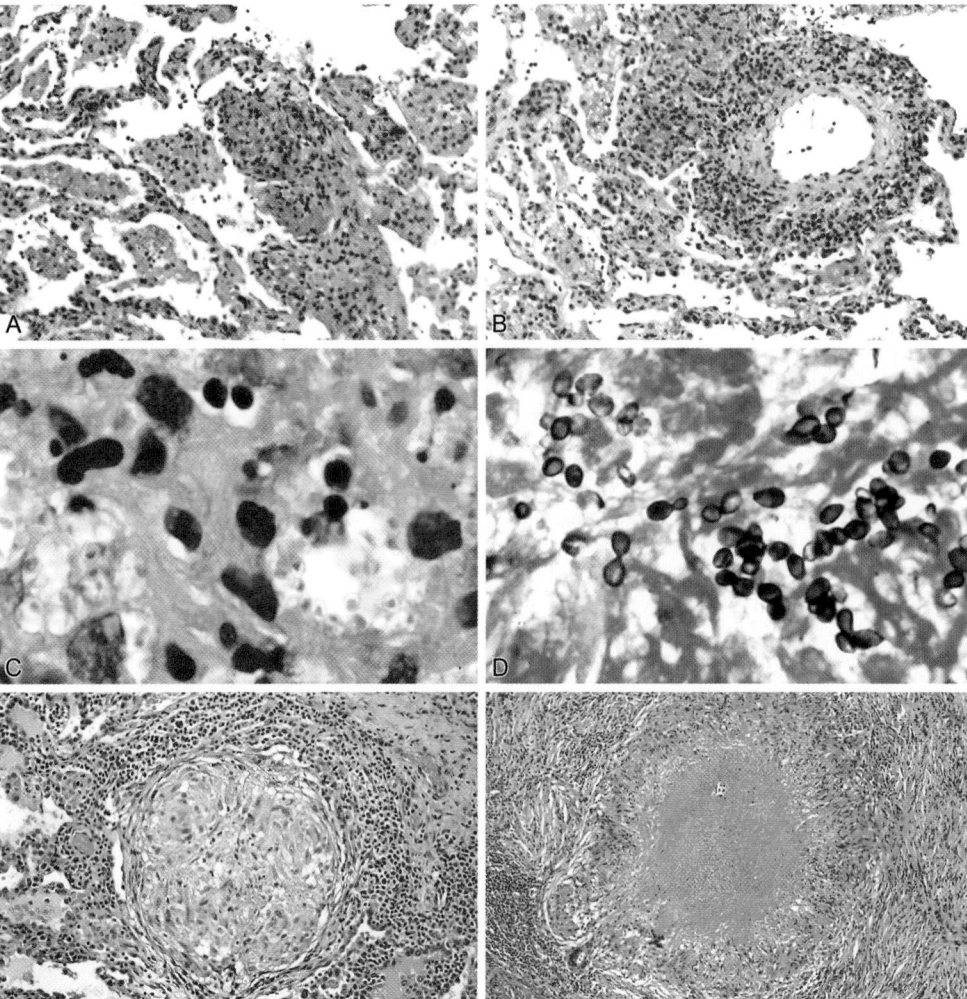

FIG. 19-32. Pathologic findings of infection in normal and immunocompromised hosts. Histopathologic preparations are shown contrasting acute diffuse pulmonary involvement in a lung segment of a normal host with a probable primary infection (**A** through **D**) with pulmonary granulomas from an immunocompromised patient who had an opportunistic reinfection with *Histoplasma capsulatum* (**E, F**). **A.** Diffuse interstitial pneumonitis in an adult (normal host) with recent heavy environmental exposure and subsequent development of progressive pulmonary disease. There is an inflammatory cell infiltrate primarily involving the interalveolar interstitial spaces but present within many alveolar spaces as well. The exudate consists mostly of mononuclear phagocytes, lymphocytes, and occasional plasma cells. Many of the alveolar walls are markedly thickened [hematoxylin and eosin stain (H&E), ×50]. **B.** Another area from the same lung as in **A** showing focal vasculitis with an infiltrate of lymphocytes and macrophages (H&E, ×25). **C.** Relatively large alveolar macrophages packed with single and budding yeasts 2 to 4 μm in diameter (same lung as in **A** and **B**). The basophilic cytoplasm of these yeasts is retracted from their thin outer cell walls, leaving halo-like clear areas that can be confused with capsules (H&E, ×500). **D.** Intracellular and extracellular yeasts, 2 to 4 μm in diameter, some of which are single, budding, or in short chains (Gomori methenamine silver stain, ×500). **E.** Nonnecrotizing (sometimes called *epithelioid cell* or *noncaseating*) granuloma from a patient who had recently received chemotherapy for a germ cell tumor (different patient than in **A** through **D**). This lesion consists of a focal collection of macrophages (sometimes referred to as *histiocytes* or *epithelioid cells*) plus lymphocytes and occasional plasma cells. A few multinucleated macrophages are present. A thin layer of fibroblasts circumscribes the lesion. Yeasts of *H. capsulatum,* probably present within macrophages of this lesion at an earlier stage, were not identified in this granuloma or in any of several other nonnecrotizing granulomas within the specimen. Lesions of this type often undergo necrosis to become necrotizing granulomas (H&E, ×50). **F.** Necrotizing (sometimes referred to as *caseating*) granuloma from the same lung as in **E**. This lesion has a necrotic center surrounded by macrophages, encapsulating fibroblasts, fibrous connective tissue in the periphery, and scattered lymphocytes. A prominent giant cell is present in the lower left of the granuloma (at approximately 8 o'clock). Micro-organisms are usually present only in relatively small numbers in these types of lesions. They are most frequently detected within the most central necrotic material in these granulomas (H&E, ×25). *(Reproduced with permission from Hage et al.[102])*

patients, HIV-infected patients, and patients using immunosuppressive medications. The presentation is a spectrum of illness, ranging from nonspecific signs of fever, weight loss, and malaise to shock, respiratory distress, and multiorgan failure. Diagnosis can be made with a combination of *Histoplasma* urine antigen testing, serologic assay, and fungal culture and should be suspected in patients with the aforementioned symptoms in any endemic area, particularly if the

patient is immunosuppressed. Any of the antifungal therapies can be used in the treatment of disseminated histoplasmosis.[103] Use of amphotericin B has decreased the mortality rate to <25% in this type of serious infection.

Coccidioides immitis is an endemic fungus found in the soil and dust of the southwestern United States. The major risk factors for symptomatic infection are related to occupation, host factors, and exposure to the fungus in endemic areas. Those in occupations that involve significant exposure to soil, such as agricultural workers and military personnel, especially in endemic areas, are at substantial risk. Those with immunosuppression due to medications or illness (such as AIDS) are also at risk.[104] The infection results from inhalation of spores (arthroconidia), which individually swell into spherules that later subdivide into endospores. Positive results from cultures of sputum, other body fluid, or tissue are necessary for a definitive diagnosis. Of patients who develop symptomatic disease, 95% have pulmonary involvement, which can be divided into three main categories, depending on the associated signs and symptoms: primary, complicated, and residual pulmonary coccidioidomycosis. Primary pulmonary coccidioidomycosis occurs in approximately 40% of people who inhale spores. The other 60% will remain asymptomatic and develop lifelong immunity. The symptoms of coccidioidomycosis, known as *valley fever,* consist of fever, chills, headache, erythema multiforme, erythema nodosum, polyarthralgias, nonproductive cough, and chest pain. Chest radiographic findings of hilar and paratracheal adenopathy and the aforementioned constellation of atypical symptoms are suggestive of pulmonary coccidioidomycosis. When symptoms and radiographic findings persist for longer than 6 to 8 weeks, the disease is considered to be persistent coccidioidal pneumonia, which occurs in approximately 1% of patients. Progression to caseous nodules, cavities, and calcified, fibrotic, or ossified lesions indicates complicated or residual stages of the disease.

There are several relative indications for surgery in pulmonary coccidioidomycosis. A rapidly expanding (>4 cm) cavity that is close to the visceral pleura presents a high risk for rupture into the pleural space and subsequent empyema. Life-threatening hemoptysis or hemoptysis that is persistent despite medical therapy, symptomatic fungus ball, and bronchopleural fistula are also indications for operative intervention. Long-standing cavities with sputum persistently positive for the fungus and pulmonary nodules that degenerate over time should also be resected. Finally, any nodule that causes concern for malignancy must be biopsied and/or resected to determine the underlying cause.

Diagnosis of coccidioidomycosis is confirmed by histopathologic, mycologic, and serologic evaluation. In a small minority of infected patients (0.5%) extrapulmonary disease may develop, with involvement of the meninges, bones, joints, skin, or soft tissues. Immunocompromised patients are especially susceptible to disseminated coccidioidomycosis, which carries a mortality rate of >40%. Treatment options for this disease vary depending on the severity of the disease as well as the stage. Amphotericin B deoxycholate or the triazoles continue to be the primary antifungal medications. Treatment of primary pulmonary coccidioidomycosis remains controversial, because in most patients the infection will resolve without further intervention. Itraconazole and fluconazole are effective treatments for patients with mild to moderate disease with evidence of pulmonary cavitation or progressive chronic pulmonary lesions. Amphotericin B is warranted for patients with severe pulmonary or disseminated disease and for immunocompromised patients.

Blastomyces dermatitidis is a round, single-budding yeast with a characteristic thick, refractile cell wall. It resides in the soil as a nonmotile spore called a *conidia.* Exposure occurs when contaminated soil is disturbed and the conidia are aerosolized. The spore is inhaled and transforms into a yeast phase at body temperature.[105] The majority of exposed persons develop a self-limited infection. A small minority of patients develop chronic pulmonary infection or disseminated disease, including cutaneous, osteoarticular, or genitourinary involvement.

B. dermatitidis has a worldwide distribution. In the United States it is endemic in the central states.[106] In the chronic infection, the organism induces a granulomatous and pyogenic reaction with microabscesses and giant cells; caseation, cavitation, and fibrosis may also occur. Symptoms are nonspecific and consistent with chronic pneumonia in 60 to 90% of patients. They include cough, mucoid sputum production, chest pain, fever, malaise, weight loss,

and, uncommonly, hemoptysis. In acute disease, radiographs are either completely negative or have nonspecific findings; in chronic disease, fibronodular lesions (with or without cavitation) similar to those of tuberculosis are noted. Pulmonary parenchymal abnormalities in the upper lobe(s) may be noted. Mass lesions similar to carcinoma are common, and lung biopsy is frequently performed. Over 50% of patients with chronic blastomycosis also have extrapulmonary manifestations, but <10% of patients present with severe clinical manifestations.[105]

Once a patient manifests symptoms of chronic blastomycosis, antifungal treatment is required to achieve resolution. If the disease is untreated, mortality approaches 60%.[105] While controversial, many support a short course of triazole therapy (oral itraconazole 200 mg daily) for 6 months as the treatment of choice for most patients with mild to moderate forms of the disease. Itraconazole has poor CNS penetration. The most common site of recurrence after apparently successful therapy is in the CNS. In the absence of therapy, close follow-up is warranted for evidence of progression to chronic or extrapulmonary disease. Amphotericin B is indicated for patients with severe or life-threatening disease, CNS involvement, disseminated disease, or extensive lung involvement, and for immunocompromised patients. After adequate drug therapy, surgical resection of known cavitary lesions should be considered, because viable organisms are known to persist in such lesions.

Antifungals Limitations still exist in the treatment of fungal pneumonias. The major classes of antifungal therapies now include the polyenes (amphotericin and lipid-associated amphotericin), the triazoles (fluconazole, voriconazole, itraconazole), and the echinocandins (caspofungin, micafungin, and anidulafungin). These agents differ in terms of their side-effect profiles, efficacy against various fungi, and fungicidal vs. fungistatic characteristics. The important disease-specific characteristics of these agents have been detailed earlier. Amphotericin B, a by-product of the actinomycete *Streptomyces nodosus,* has served as the mainstay for deep, systemic fungal infections. A complex lipophilic organic compound or polyene, amphotericin B binds to ergosterol in the cell membranes of fungi, causing disruption and ion leakage. However, nephrotoxicity limits its usefulness and applicability. Three lipid-based formulations of amphotericin B have now shown decreased nephrotoxicity and higher drug-dose delivery. Higher costs and limited data concerning greater efficacy have tempered widespread adoption of these three drugs as first-line antifungal therapy. Susceptible fungi convert 5-fluorocytosine (flucytosine) to 5-fluorouracil, which inhibits DNA and RNA synthesis. Flucytosine is commonly used in combination with amphotericin B in patients with cryptococcal or candidal infections to decrease the amount of amphotericin B necessary. The azole compounds include miconazole, ketoconazole, fluconazole, itraconazole, and voriconazole.[107] This class of drugs inhibits the enzyme cytochrome P-450, thereby interfering with fungal cell membrane synthesis; in the presence of these drugs, lanosterol is not converted to ergosterol, a necessary fungal component.

Echinocandins are a new class of antifungals that inhibit cell wall synthesis by interfering with glucan synthesis. Caspofungin was the first echinocandin to be approved by the U.S. Food and Drug Administration for the treatment of invasive pulmonary aspergillosis that is refractory to first-line agents. The most common associated side effects are headache, transient elevation of transaminase levels, and infusion-related venous effects.[108] This class of antifungals has become an integral part of the management of candidiasis.

Massive Hemoptysis

Massive hemoptysis generally is defined as expectoration of >600 mL of blood within a 24-hour period. It is a medical emergency associated with a mortality rate of 30 to 50%. Most clinicians would agree that losing over a liter of blood via the airway within 1 day is significant, yet use of an absolute volume criterion presents difficulties. First, it is difficult for the patient or caregivers to quantify the volume of blood being lost. Second, and most relevant, the rate of bleeding necessary to produce respiratory compromise is highly dependent on the individual's prior respiratory status. For example, the loss of 100 mL of blood over 24 hours in a 40-year-old male with normal pulmonary function would be of little immediate consequence, because his normal cough would ensure his ability to clear the blood and secretions. In contrast, the same amount of bleeding in a 69-year-old male with severe COPD, chronic bronchitis, and an FEV_1 of 1.1 L may be life-threatening.

Anatomy

The lungs have two sources of blood supply: the pulmonary and bronchial arterial systems. The pulmonary system is a high-compliance, low-pressure system, and the walls of the pulmonary arteries are very thin and delicate. The bronchial arteries, part of the systemic circulation, have systemic pressures and thick walls; most branches originate from the proximal thoracic aorta. Most cases of massive hemoptysis involve bleeding from the bronchial artery circulation or from the pulmonary circulation pathologically exposed to the high pressures of the bronchial circulation. In many cases of hemoptysis, particularly those due to inflammatory disorders, the bronchial arterial tree becomes hyperplastic and tortuous. The systemic pressures within these arteries, combined with a disease process within the airway and erosion, lead to bleeding.

Causes

Significant hemoptysis has many causes, which can broadly be categorized into pulmonary, extrapulmonary, and iatrogenic causes. Table 19-21 summarizes the most common causes of hemoptysis.[109] Most are secondary to inflammatory processes. An acute necrotizing pneumonic infection can lead to destruction and erosion of vascular structures and bleeding. Chronic inflammatory disorders (e.g., bronchiectasis, cystic fibrosis, tuberculosis) lead to localized bronchial arterial proliferation, and with erosion, bleeding of these hypervascular areas occurs.

Tuberculosis also can cause hemoptysis by erosion of a broncholith (a calcified tuberculous lymph node) into a vessel or, when a tuberculous cavity is present, by erosion of a blood vessel within

TABLE 19-21 Pulmonary and extrapulmonary causes of massive hemoptysis

Pulmonary	Extrapulmonary	Iatrogenic
Pulmonary parenchymal disease	Congestive heart failure	Intrapulmonary catheter
Bronchitis	Coagulopathy	
Bronchiectasis	Mitral stenosis	
Tuberculosis	Medications	
Lung abscess		
Pneumonia		
Cavitary fungal infection (e.g., aspergilloma)		
Lung parasitic infection (ascariasis, schistosomiasis, paragonimiasis)		
Pulmonary neoplasm		
Pulmonary infarction or embolism		
Trauma		
Arteriovenous malformation		
Pulmonary vasculitis		
Pulmonary endometriosis		
Wegener's granulomatosis		
Cystic fibrosis		
Pulmonary hemosiderosis		

TABLE 19-22 Treatment priorities in the management of massive hemoptysis

1. Achieve respiratory stabilization and prevent asphyxiation.
2. Localize the bleeding site.
3. Control the hemorrhage.
4. Determine the cause.
5. Definitively prevent recurrence.

the cavity. Within such cavities, aneurysms of the pulmonary artery (referred to as *Rasmussen aneurysms*) can develop that are accompanied by subsequent erosion and massive bleeding.

Hemoptysis due to lung cancer is usually mild, resulting in blood-streaked sputum. Massive hemoptysis in patients with lung cancer typically is caused by malignant invasion of pulmonary artery vessels by large central tumors. Although rare, it is often a terminal event.

Management

The treatment of patients with life-threatening hemoptysis is best carried out by a multidisciplinary team of intensive care physicians, interventional radiologists, and thoracic surgeons. Table 19-22 provides an algorithm for management of patients with massive hemoptysis.

The pragmatic clinical definition of *massive hemoptysis* is a degree of bleeding that threatens respiratory stability. Therefore clinical judgment of the risk of respiratory compromise is the first step in evaluating a patient.[110,111] Two scenarios are possible: (a) bleeding is significant and persistent, but its rate allows a rapid but sequential diagnostic and therapeutic approach, and (b) bleeding is so rapid that emergency airway control and therapy are necessary.

Scenario 1: Significant, Persistent, but Nonmassive Bleeding
Although bleeding is brisk in scenario 1, the patient may be able to maintain clearance of the blood and secretions with his or her own respiratory reflexes. Immediate measures are admission to an intensive care unit, strict bedrest, Trendelenburg positioning with the affected side down (if known), administration of humidified oxygen, monitoring of oxygen saturation and arterial blood gas levels, and insertion of large-bore IV catheters. Strict bedrest with sedation may lead to slowing or cessation of bleeding, and the judicious use of IV narcotics or other relaxants to mildly sedate the patient and diminish some of the reflexive airway activity is often necessary. Also recommended are administration of aerosolized adrenaline, IV antibiotic therapy if needed, and correction of abnormal blood coagulation. Finally, unless contraindicated, IV vasopressin (20 units over 15 minutes, followed by an infusion of 0.2 unit/min) can be given.

A chest radiograph is the first test and often proves to be the most revealing. Localized lesions may be seen, but the effects of blood soiling of other areas of the lungs may predominate, obscuring the area of pathology. Chest CT scanning provides more detail and is nearly always performed if the patient is stable. Pathologic areas may be obscured by blood soiling.

Flexible bronchoscopy is the next step in evaluating the patient's condition. Some clinicians argue that rigid bronchoscopy should always be performed. However, if the patient is clinically stable and the ongoing bleeding is not imminently threatening, flexible bronchoscopy is appropriate. It allows diagnosis of airway abnormalities and will usually permit localization of the bleeding site to a lobe or even a segment. The person performing the bronchoscopy must be prepared with excellent suction and must be able to perform saline lavage with a dilute solution of epinephrine.

Most cases of massive hemoptysis arise from the bronchial arterial tree; therefore, the next therapeutic option frequently is selective bronchial arteriography and embolization. Prearteriogram bronchoscopy is extremely useful to direct the angiographer. However, if bronchoscopy fails to localize the bleeding site, then bilateral bronchial arteriography can be performed. Typically, the abnormal vascularity is visualized, rather than extravasation of the contrast dye. Embolization will acutely arrest the bleeding in 80 to 90% of patients. However, 30 to 60% of patients will have recurrences. Therefore, embolization should be viewed as an immediate but probably temporizing measure to acutely control bleeding. Subsequently, definitive treatment of the underlying pathologic process is appropriate. If bleeding persists after embolization, a pulmonary artery source should be suspected and pulmonary angiography performed.

If respiratory compromise is impending, orotracheal intubation should be performed. After intubation, flexible bronchoscopy should be performed to clear blood and secretions and to attempt localization of the bleeding site. Depending on the possible causes of the bleeding, bronchial artery embolization or (if appropriate) surgery can be considered.

Scenario 2: Significant, Persistent, and Massive Bleeding Life-threatening bleeding requires emergency airway control and preparation for potential surgery. Such patients are best cared for in an operating room equipped with rigid bronchoscopy equipment. Immediate orotracheal intubation may be necessary to gain control of ventilation and suctioning. However, rapid transport to the operating room and rigid bronchoscopy should be facilitated. Rigid bronchoscopy allows adequate suctioning of bleeding with visualization of the bleeding site; the nonbleeding side can be cannulated with the rigid scope and the patient ventilated. After stabilization, ice-saline lavage of the bleeding site can then be performed (up to 1 L in 50-mL aliquots); bleeding stops in up to 90% of patients.[112]

Alternatively, blockade of the main stem bronchus of the affected side can be accomplished with a double-lumen endotracheal tube, with a bronchial blocker, or by intubation of the nonaffected side using an uncut standard endotracheal tube. Placement of a double-lumen endotracheal tube is challenging in these circumstances, given the bleeding and secretions. Proper placement and suctioning may be difficult, and attempts could compromise the patient's ventilation. The best option is to place a bronchial blocker in the affected bronchus with inflation. The blocker is left in place for 24 hours and the area is then re-examined bronchoscopically. After this 24-hour period, bronchial artery embolization can be performed.

Surgical Intervention In most patients, bleeding can be stopped, recovery can occur, and plans can be made to definitively treat the underlying cause. In scenario 1 (significant, persistent, but nonmassive bleeding), the patient may undergo further evaluation as an inpatient or outpatient. Chest CT scanning and pulmonary function studies should be performed preoperatively. In scenario 2 (significant, persistent, and massive bleeding), surgery, if appropriate, usually will be performed during the same hospitalization in which the rigid bronchoscopy or main stem bronchus blockade is carried out. In <10% of patients, emergency surgery will be necessary, delayed only by efforts to localize the bleeding site by rigid bronchoscopy.

Surgical treatment is individualized according to the source of bleeding and the patient's medical condition, prognosis, and pulmonary reserve. General indications for urgent surgery are presented in Table 19-23. In patients with significant cavitary disease or fungus balls, the walls of the cavities are eroded and necrotic; rebleeding will likely ensue. In addition, bleeding from cavitary lesions may be due to pulmonary artery erosion, which requires surgery for control.

End-Stage Lung Disease
Lung Volume Reduction Surgery

Lung volume reduction surgery (LVRS) was originally described by Brantigan in the late 1950s, and the procedure was resurrected and refined by Cooper and associates in the early 1990's.[113–115] As described by Cooper, the ideal patient for LVRS has heterogeneous emphysema with apical predominance; that is, the worst emphysematous changes are in the apex of both lungs (as seen on chest CT scan). The physiologic lack of function of these areas is demonstrated

TABLE 19-23	General indications for urgent operative intervention for massive hemoptysis

1. Presence of a fungus ball
2. Presence of a lung abscess
3. Presence of significant cavitary disease
4. Failure to control the bleeding

by quantitative perfusion scan, which shows minimal or no perfusion. When these nonfunctional areas are surgically excised, the volume of the lung is reduced, which theoretically restores respiratory mechanics. Diaphragm position and function are improved, and there may be an improvement in the dynamic small airway collapse in the remaining lung. After favorable outcomes were reported for LVRS in studies at the Barnes-Jewish Hospital and in other various smaller trials, application of LVRS rapidly escalated.

In the mid-1990s, analysis of Medicare claims for LVRS revealed an operative mortality of 16.9% and a 1-year mortality of 23%. In 1997 the National Emphysema Treatment Trial conducted a randomized study involving 1218 patients that used a noncrossover design to compare medical and surgical management after a 10-week pretreatment pulmonary rehabilitation program. Subgroup analysis demonstrated that in patients with the anatomic changes delineated by Cooper and colleagues, LVRS significantly improved exercise capacity, lung function, quality of life, and dyspnea compared with medical therapy. After 2 years, functional improvements began to decline toward baseline. In medically treated patients, similar parameters steadily declined below baseline. LVRS was associated with increased short-term morbidity and mortality and did not confer a survival benefit over medical therapy.[116]

Lung Transplantation

Cooper and associates at the University of Toronto performed the first successful single-lung transplant in 1983.[117] Pasque and colleagues introduced the modern technique of bilateral sequential lung (BSL) transplant in 1990.[118]

Today, the most common indications for referral for a lung transplantation are COPD and idiopathic pulmonary fibrosis (IPF). Most patients with IPF and older patients with COPD are offered a single-lung transplant. Younger COPD patients and patients with alpha$_1$-antitrypsin deficiency and severe hyperinflation of the native lungs are offered BSL transplantation. Most patients with primary pulmonary hypertension and almost all patients with cystic fibrosis are treated with BSL transplantation. Heart-lung transplantation is reserved for patients with irreversible ventricular failure or uncorrectable congenital cardiac disease.

Patients with COPD are considered for placement on the transplant waiting list when their FEV$_1$ has fallen to below 25% of its predicted value. Patients with significant pulmonary hypertension should be listed earlier. IPF patients should be referred when their forced vital capacity has fallen to <60% or their carbon monoxide diffusion capacity (D$_{LCO}$) is <50% of the predicted value.

In the past, patients with primary pulmonary hypertension and New York Heart Association class III or IV symptoms were listed for a lung transplant. However, treatment of such patients with IV prostacyclin and other pulmonary vasodilators has now markedly altered that strategy. Virtually all patients with primary pulmonary hypertension are now treated with IV epoprostenol. Some of these patients have experienced a marked improvement in their symptoms associated with a decrease in their pulmonary arterial pressures and an increase in exercise capacity. Listing of these patients is deferred until they develop New York Heart Association class III or IV symptoms or until their mean pulmonary artery pressure rises above 75 mmHg. Medium-term and bronchiolitis obliterans syndrome–free survival rates of patients who underwent a lung transplantation at the University of Minnesota during a recent 5-year

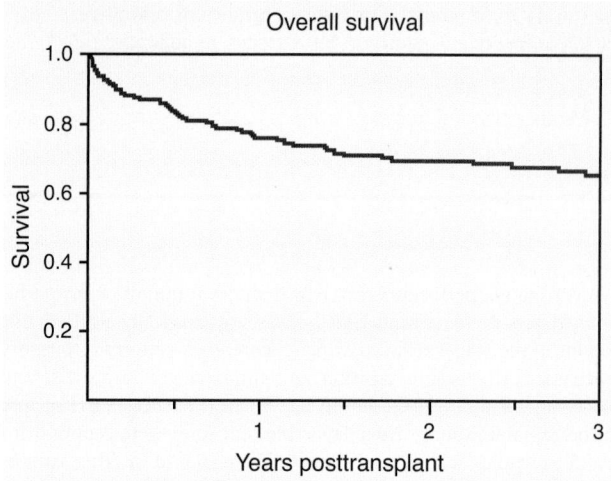

FIG. 19-33. Overall survival rate after lung transplantation at the University of Minnesota.

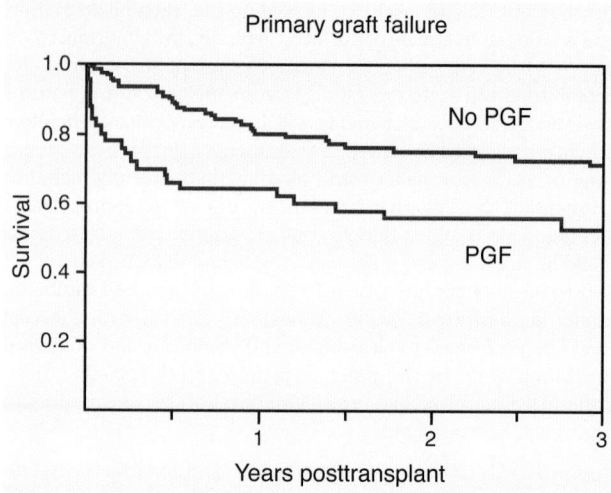

FIG. 19-35. Survival rate after lung transplantation at the University of Minnesota for patients with and without primary graft failure (PGF).

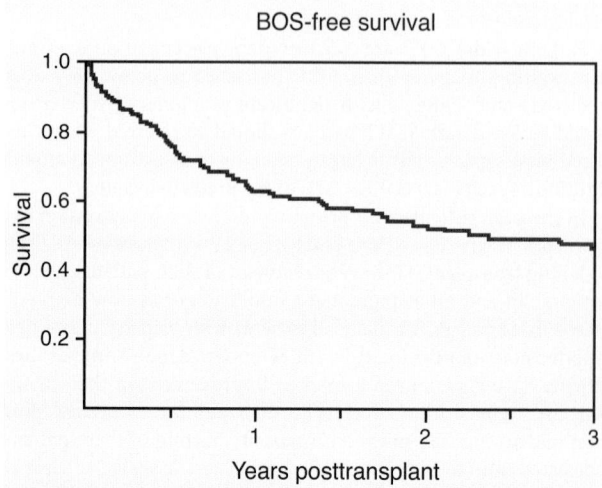

FIG. 19-34. Survival rate after lung transplantation in the absence of bronchiolitis obliterans syndrome (BOS) at the University of Minnesota.

period are shown in Figs. 19-33 and 19-34.[119] The mortality of patients while awaiting transplantation is approximately 10%. In an effort to expand the number of lung donors, many transplant groups have liberalized their criteria for donor selection. Still, the partial pressure of arterial oxygen should be >300 mmHg on a fraction of inspired oxygen of 100%. In special circumstances, lungs may be used from donors with a smoking history; from donors >50 years of age; and from donors with positive Gram's stains or infiltrates on chest radiograph.[120–123] The use of two living donors, each donating a single lower lobe, is another strategy for increasing the donor pool. Recipient outcomes are similar to outcomes of those with cadaver donors in carefully selected patients.

Most of the early mortality after lung transplantation is related to primary graft failure resulting from a severe ischemia-reperfusion injury to the lung(s) (Fig. 19-35). Reperfusion injury is characterized radiographically by interstitial and alveolar edema, and clinically by hypoxia and ventilation-perfusion mismatch. Donor neutrophils and recipient lymphocytes probably play an important role in the pathogenesis of reperfusion injury. The most important impediment to longer-term survival after lung transplantation is the development of bronchiolitis obliterans syndrome, a manifestation

of chronic rejection. Episodes of acute rejection are the major risk factors for developing bronchiolitis obliterans syndrome. Other injuries to the lung (including early reperfusion injury and injury from chronic gastroesophageal reflux disease) may also adversely affect long-term outcomes of patients.[119,124]

Spontaneous Pneumothorax

Spontaneous pneumothorax is secondary to intrinsic abnormalities of the lung, and the most common cause is rupture of an apical subpleural bleb. The cause of these blebs is unknown, but they occur more frequently in smokers and males, and they tend to be seen predominately in young postadolescent males with a tall, thin body habitus. Treatment is generally insertion of a chest tube with water seal. If a leak is present and it persists for >3 days, thoracoscopic management (i.e., bleb resection with pleurodesis by talc or pleural abrasion) is performed. Recurrences or complete lung collapse with the first episode are generally indications for thoracoscopic intervention.[125] Additional indications for intervention on the first episode include exposure to occupational hazards such as air travel, deep sea diving, or travel to remote locations. CT findings of multiple small bullae or a large bleb are associated with an increased risk of recurrent pneumothorax.[126] Many surgeons are now using screening CT to recommend VATS bleb resection with pleurodesis for first-episode spontaneous pneumothorax.

Other causes of spontaneous pneumothorax are emphysema (rupture of a bleb or bulla), cystic fibrosis, AIDS, metastatic cancer (especially sarcoma), asthma, lung abscess, and occasionally lung cancer. Catamenial pneumothorax, a rare but interesting type of spontaneous pneumothorax in women in their second and third decades, occurs within 72 hours of the onset of menses and is possibly related to endometriosis. Management of pneumothorax in these circumstances often is tied to treatment of the specific disease process and may involve tumor resection, thoracoscopic pleurectomy, or talc pleurodesis.

CHEST WALL

Chest Wall Mass
Clinical Approach

Surgeons confronted with a patient with a chest wall mass must be aware that their approach to diagnosis and treatment has significant impact on the patient's chances for long-term survival. All chest wall tumors should be considered malignant until proven otherwise. It is critically important that the surgeon(s) be mindful of this

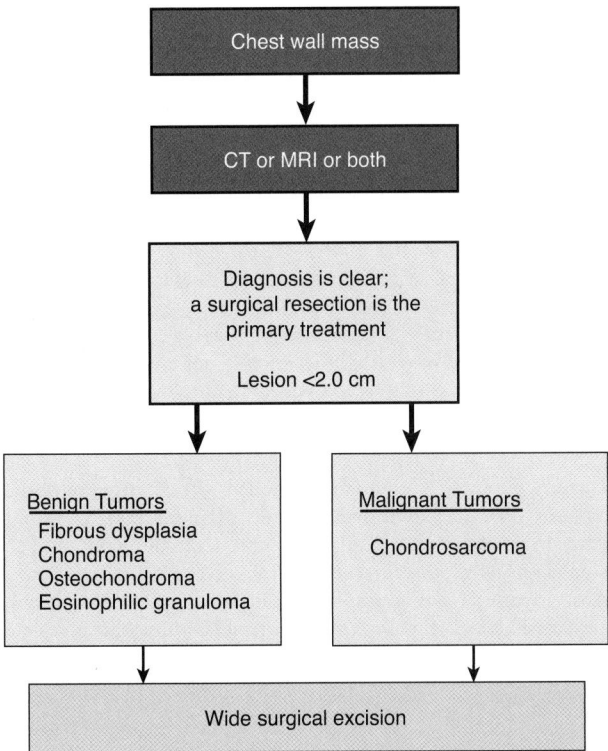

FIG. 19-36. Systematic approach for evaluating a chest wall mass when the clinical scenario is uncomplicated and initial imaging studies suggest a clear diagnosis. CT = computed tomography; MRI = magnetic resonance imaging.

tenet and well versed in the diagnostic and treatment principles for chest wall malignancies. These tenets must be applied starting with the initial biopsy, because the placement of the incision can significantly affect success in achieving complete resection and reconstructing the chest wall. Complete resection is imperative if there is any hope for cure and/or long-term survival. A general approach is outlined in Figs. 19-36 and 19-37.

Patients with either a benign or malignant chest wall tumor typically present with complaints of a slowly enlarging palpable mass (50 to 70%), chest wall pain (25 to 50%), or both. The interval from the time the patient first notices the mass until the time the patient is seen by medical providers often can be months. Interestingly, masses often are not noticed by patients until they experience a trauma to the area.

Pain from a chest wall mass is typically localized to the area of the tumor. Pain is more often present (and more intense) with malignant tumors, but it also can be present with up to one third of benign tumors. With Ewing's sarcoma, fever and malaise may also be present. Age can provide guidance regarding the possibility of malignancy. Patients with benign chest wall tumors are on average 26 years old; the average age for patients with malignant tumors is 40 years. Overall, the probability that a chest wall tumor is malignant is 50 to 80%.

Evaluation and Management

Laboratory evaluations are usually of little help in assessing chest wall masses. In plasmacytoma, there may be monoclonality of one of the immunoglobulins with normal levels of other immunoglobulins. Another exception is osteosarcoma, in which alkaline phosphatase levels may be elevated. Still another exception is Ewing's sarcoma, in which the erythrocyte sedimentation rate may be elevated.

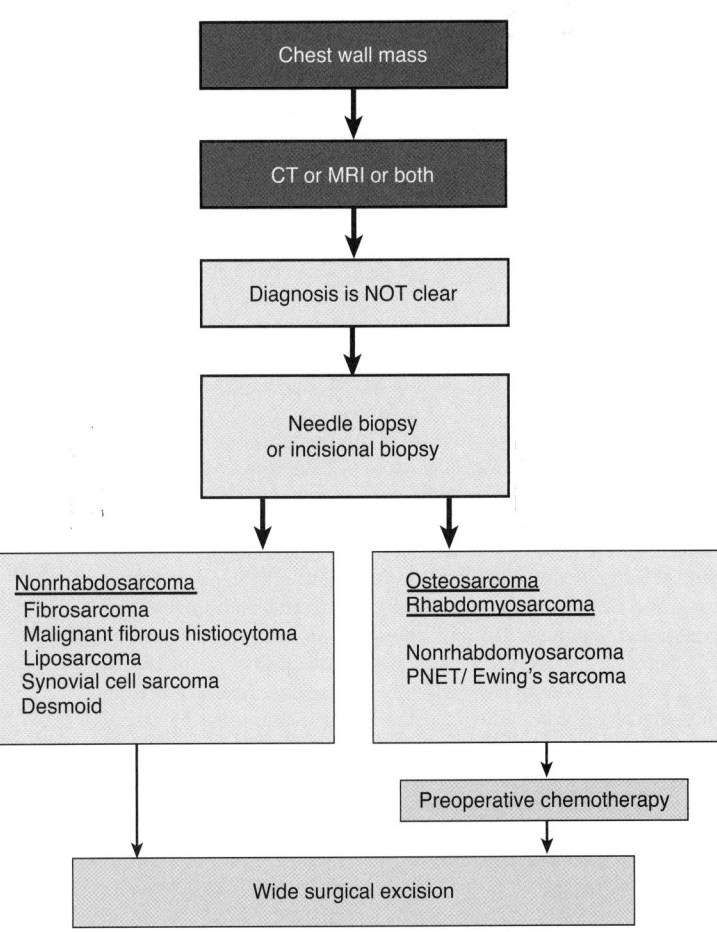

FIG. 19-37. Systematic approach for evaluating a chest wall mass for which the diagnosis is not unequivocal. A tissue diagnosis is critical for effective management of chest wall masses. CT = computed tomography; MRI = magnetic resonance imaging; PNET = primitive neuroectodermal tumor.

Radiography Radiographic evaluation begins with a chest radiograph, which may reveal evidence of rib destruction and calcification within the lesion, and, if old films are available, provide a clue to growth rate. CT scanning should be done in all patients to evaluate the nature of the primary lesion, to determine its relationship to contiguous structures (e.g., mediastinum, lung, soft tissues, and other skeletal elements), and to search for possible pulmonary metastases. Importantly, contiguous involvement of underlying lung or other soft tissues or the presence of pulmonary metastases does not preclude successful surgery. CT also is valuable in assessing for the presence of extraosseous bone formation and bone destruction, both typically seen with osteosarcoma.

MRI has a number of advantages in the radiographic evaluation of chest wall masses, particularly those that may be malignant. Multiple planes of imaging (coronal, sagittal, and oblique) are possible. MRI also may better define the relationship between tumor and muscle. For tumors contiguous to or near neurovascular structures or the spine, MRI and magnetic resonance angiography with multiple planes of imaging provide invaluable information about the tumor. Thus they greatly facilitate preoperative planning and may further delineate tissue abnormalities, potentially enhancing the ability to distinguish benign from malignant sarcomas.

Biopsy The first step in the management of all chest wall tumors is to obtain a tissue diagnosis. Inappropriate or misguided attempts at tissue diagnosis through casual open biopsy techniques have the potential (if the lesion is a sarcoma) to seed surrounding tissues and contiguous body cavities (e.g., the pleural space) with tumor cells, potentially compromising local tumor control and patient survival. Accurate typing of chest wall sarcomas has a profound impact on their management.

Tissue diagnosis can be made by one of three methods: a needle biopsy (typically CT guided, FNA, or core biopsy), an incisional biopsy, or an excisional biopsy. Until recently, the thoracic surgery literature has been dogmatic in advocating only an excisional biopsy.[127] Reasons for insisting on this technique were that (a) the entire mass is removed, which allows 100% accurate sampling and diagnosis; (b) unlike with incisional biopsy, the potential problem of seeding the surrounding soft tissues with tumor cells does not exist; and (c) adjuvant chemotherapy can be administered.

Management of extremity sarcomas has changed dramatically in the last decade, however. Neoadjuvant therapy is now the standard of care for certain sarcomas. Because sarcomas of the thorax are the same as sarcomas of the extremities, management principles for both should be parallel, whenever technically and medically possible.

An excisional biopsy should still be performed when the initial diagnosis (based on radiographic evaluation) indicates that the lesion is benign or when the lesion has the classic appearance of a chondrosarcoma (in which case definitive surgical resection can be undertaken). Any lesion of <2.0 cm can be excised as long as the resulting wound is small enough to close primarily.

When the diagnosis cannot be made by radiographic evaluation, a needle biopsy (FNA or core) should be performed. Pathologists experienced with sarcomas can accurately diagnose approximately 90% of patients using FNA techniques. A needle biopsy (FNA or core) has the advantage of avoiding wound and body cavity contamination (a potential complication with an incisional biopsy).

If results of a needle biopsy are nondiagnostic, an incisional biopsy may be performed, with the following caveats. When an incisional biopsy is performed, the skin incision must be placed directly over the mass and oriented to allow subsequent excision of the scar. Development of skin flaps must be avoided, and in general no drains are used. A drain may be placed if a hematoma is likely to develop, because this can potentially limit soft tissue contamination by tumor cells. Subsequently, if definitive surgical resection is undertaken, the entire area of the biopsy (including skin and the drain track) must be excised en bloc with the tumor.

Chest Wall Neoplasms

Benign Tumors

Chondroma Chondromas are one of the more common benign tumors of the chest wall. They are primarily seen in children and young adults. Chondromas usually occur at the costochondral junction anteriorly. Given their typical location and the young age of most patients, chondromas may be confused with costochondritis. Clinically, a mass (usually without pain) is present in the case of chondromas. Radiographically, the lesion is lobulated and radiodense; it may have diffuse or focal calcifications and may displace the bony cortex without penetration. Chondromas may grow to huge sizes if left untreated. Treatment is surgical resection with a 2-cm margin. One must be certain, however, that the lesion is not a well-differentiated chondrosarcoma. In this case, a wider 4-cm margin is required to prevent local recurrence. Therefore, large chondromas should be treated surgically as low-grade chondrosarcomas.[128]

Fibrous Dysplasia The ribs are a frequent site of origin of fibrous dysplasia. As with chondromas, fibrous dysplasia most frequently occurs in young adults. Pain is an infrequent complaint, and the lesion is typically located in the posterolateral aspect of the rib cage. Fibrous dysplasia may be associated with trauma. Radiographically, an expansile mass is present, with cortical thinning and no calcification. Local excision with a 2-cm margin is curative.

Osteochondroma Osteochondromas are the most common benign bone tumor. Many are detected as incidental radiographic findings. Most are solitary. If a patient has multiple osteochondromas, the surgeon must have a high index of suspicion for malignancy, because the incidence of chondrosarcoma is significantly higher in this population.

Osteochondromas occur in the first 2 decades of life, and they arise at or near the growth plate of bones. The lesions are benign during youth or adolescence. Osteochondromas that enlarge after completion of skeletal growth have the potential to develop into chondrosarcomas.

Osteochondromas in the thorax arise from the rib cortex. They are one of several components of the autosomal dominant syndrome known as *hereditary multiple exostoses*. When part of this syndrome, osteochondromas have a high rate of degeneration into chondrosarcomas. Any patient with hereditary multiple exostoses syndrome who develops new pain at the site of an osteochondroma or who notes gradual growth in the mass over time should be carefully evaluated for osteosarcoma. Local excision of a benign osteochondroma is sufficient treatment. If malignancy is determined, wide excision is performed, with a 4-cm margin.

Eosinophilic Granuloma Eosinophilic granulomas are benign osteolytic lesions. They were originally thought to be destructive lesions with large numbers of eosinophilic cells. Yet eosinophilic granulomas of the ribs also can occur as solitary lesions or as part of a more generalized disease process of the lymphoreticular system termed *Langerhans cell histiocytosis (LCH)*. In LCH, the involved tissue is infiltrated with large numbers of histiocytes (similar to Langerhans cells seen in skin and other epithelia), which are often organized as granulomas. The cause is unknown. Of all LCH bone lesions, 79% are solitary eosinophilic granulomas, 7% involve multiple eosinophilic granulomas, and 14% belong to other forms of more systemic LCH.

Isolated single eosinophilic granulomas can occur in the ribs, skull, pelvis, mandible, humerus, and other sites. They are diagnosed primarily in children between the ages of 5 and 15 years. Because of the associated pain and tenderness, they may be confused with Ewing's sarcoma or with an inflammatory process such as osteomyelitis. Healing may occur spontaneously, but the typical treatment is limited surgical resection with a 2-cm margin.

Desmoid Tumors Desmoid tumors are unusual soft tissue neoplasms that arise from fascial or musculoaponeurotic structures. Histologically, they consist of proliferations of benign-appearing fibroblastic cells, abundant collagen, and few mitoses. Accordingly, some authorities consider desmoid tumors to be a form of fibrosarcoma.

Desmoid tumors have recently been shown to possess alterations in the adenomatous polyposis coli/β-catenin pathway, and cyclin D1 dysregulation is thought to play a significant role in their pathogenesis.[129] Associations with other diseases and conditions are well documented, especially those with similar alterations in the adenomatous polyposis coli pathway, such as familial adenomatous polyposis (Gardner's syndrome). Other conditions with increased risk of desmoid tumor formation include states of increased estrogen levels (pregnancy) and trauma. Surgical incisions (abdominal and thoracic) have been the site of desmoid development, either in or near the scar.

Clinically, patients are usually in the third to fourth decade of life and have pain, a chest wall mass, or both. The tumor usually is fixed to the chest wall but not to the overlying skin. No radiographic findings are typical, but MRI may delineate muscle or soft tissue infiltration. Histologic diagnosis may not be possible by a needle biopsy because of low cellularity. An open incisional biopsy often is necessary for lesions over 3 to 4 cm, with attention to the caveats listed earlier (see "Biopsy").

Desmoid tumors do not metastasize, but they have a strong propensity to recur locally, with local recurrence rates as high as 5 to 50%, sometimes despite complete initial resection with histologically negative margins.[130] Such locally aggressive behavior is secondary to microscopic tumor infiltration of muscle and surrounding soft tissues.

Surgery consists of wide local excision with a margin of 2 to 4 cm and with intraoperative assessment of resection margins by frozen-section analysis. Typically, a rib is removed above and below the tumor with a 4- to 5-cm margin of rib. A margin of <1 cm results in much higher local recurrence rates.[131] If a major neurovascular structure would have to be sacrificed, which would lead to high morbidity, then a margin of <1 cm would have to suffice. Survival after wide local excision with negative margins is 90% at 10 years.

Primary Malignant Chest Wall Tumors

A malignant tumor of the chest wall is either a metastatic lesion from another primary tumor or a sarcoma. Although many different cell types are seen in sarcomas, the primary features affecting prognosis are histologic grade and responsiveness to chemotherapy.

Sarcomas can be divided into two broad groups according to potential responsiveness to chemotherapy (Table 19-24). Preoperative (neoadjuvant) chemotherapy offers the ability to (a) assess tumor chemosensitivity by the degree of tumor size reduction and microscopic necrosis, (b) determine to which chemotherapeutic agents the tumor is sensitive, and (c) lessen the extent of surgical resection by reducing tumor size. Patients whose tumors are responsive to preoperative chemotherapy (as judged by the reduction in the size of the primary tumor and/or by the degree of necrosis seen histologically after resection) have a much better prognosis than those whose tumors show a poor response.

Information about the tumor's propensity to respond to chemotherapy, the patient's physiologic state and capacity to receive treatment, and the presence or absence of metastatic disease can then be used to determine optimal therapy. The following guidelines, based on tumor type and assuming fitness for therapy, can be used to direct therapy. Based on the tumor's known potential response to chemotherapy or the presence of metastatic disease, the initial treatment is either (a) preoperative chemotherapy [for patients with osteosarcoma, rhabdomyosarcoma, primitive neuroectodermal tumor (PNET), or Ewing's sarcoma] followed by surgery and postoperative chemotherapy, (b) primary surgical resection and reconstruction (for patients with nonmetastatic malignant fibrous histiocytoma, fibrosarcoma, liposarcoma, or synovial sarcoma), or (c) neoadjuvant chemotherapy followed by surgical resection if indicated in patients with metastatic soft tissue sarcomas. Exceptions to these guidelines may apply at specific centers at which the impact of neoadjuvant chemotherapy on soft tissue sarcomas is under investigation. Typically such exceptions

TABLE 19-24 Classification of sarcomas by therapeutic response

Tumor Type	Chemotherapy Sensitivity
Osteosarcoma	+
Rhabdomyosarcoma	+
Primitive neuroectodermal tumor	+
Ewing's sarcoma	+
Malignant fibrous histiocytoma	±
Fibrosarcoma	±
Liposarcoma	±
Synovial sarcoma	±

apply to pediatric patients and to adult patients who have deep, high-grade, nonmetastatic tumors >10 cm in diameter.

Malignant Chest Wall Bone Tumors

Chondrosarcoma Chondrosarcomas are the most common primary chest wall malignancies. As with chondromas, they usually arise anteriorly from the costochondral arches. These slowly enlarging, often painful masses of the anterior chest wall can reach massive proportions.[128] CT scan shows a radiolucent lesion, often with stippled calcifications pathognomonic for chondrosarcomas (Fig. 19-38). The involved bony structures also are destroyed. Metastatic disease to the lungs or bones should be ruled out by CT and bone scan.

Most chondrosarcomas are slow-growing, low-grade tumors. For this reason, any lesion in the anterior chest wall likely to be a low-grade chondrosarcoma should be treated with wide (4-cm) resection. Chondrosarcomas are not sensitive to chemotherapy or radiation therapy. Prognosis is determined by tumor grade and extent of resection. With a low-grade tumor and wide resection, patient survival at 5 to 10 years can be as high as 60 to 80%.

Osteosarcoma Osteosarcomas are the most common bone malignancy, but they are an uncommon malignancy of the chest wall, representing only 10% of all malignant chest wall tumors.[132] They present as rapidly enlarging, painful masses. Although they primarily occur in young adults, osteosarcomas can occur in patients >40 years of age, sometimes in association with previous radiation therapy, Paget's disease, or chemotherapy.

Radiographically, the typical appearance consists of spicules of new periosteal bone formation producing a sunburst appearance. As with chondrosarcomas, careful CT assessment of the pulmonary parenchyma for metastasis is necessary. Osteosarcomas have a propensity to spread to the lungs. Up to one third of patients present with metastatic disease.

Osteosarcomas are potentially sensitive to chemotherapy. Currently, administration of chemotherapy before surgical resection is common. After chemotherapy, complete resection is performed with wide (4-cm) margins, followed by reconstruction. In patients presenting with lung metastases that are potentially amenable to surgical resection, induction chemotherapy may be given, followed by surgical resection of the primary tumor and of the pulmonary metastases. After surgical treatment of known disease, additional maintenance chemotherapy usually is recommended.

Other Tumors *Primitive Neuroectodermal Tumors* PNETs derive from primordial neural crest cells that migrate from the mantle layer of the developing spinal cord. This group of tumors includes neuroblastomas, ganglioneuroblastomas, and ganglioneuromas. Ewing's sarcomas and Askin's tumors are closely related to PNETs. Askin's tumor was originally described by Askin in 1979 as a "malignant, small cell tumor of the thoracopulmonary region," and is now known to be a member of the Ewing's sarcoma/PNET family.[132,133] Histologically, Ewing's sarcomas and PNETs are small round cell tumors; both possess a translocation between the long arms of chromosomes 11 and 22 within their genetic makeup. They also share a consistent

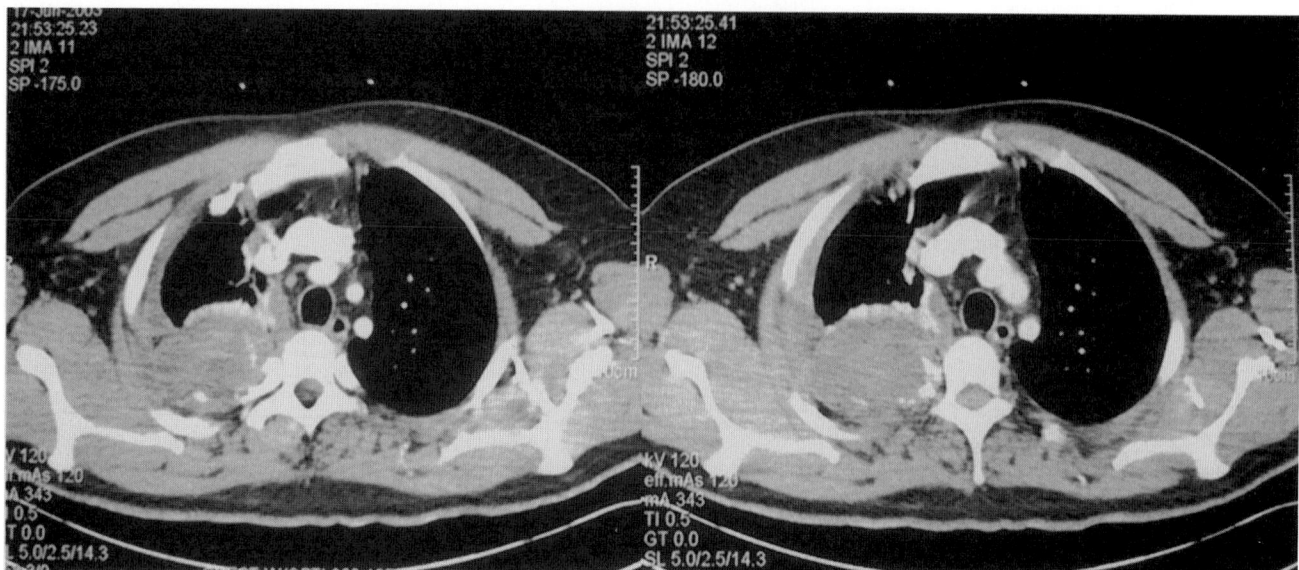

FIG. 19-38. Chest computed tomographic scan showing a right posterior lung tumor. In the appropriate clinical setting, stippled calcifications (white streaks in right lung mass) are highly indicative of chondrosarcomas.

pattern of proto-oncogene expression and have been found to express the product of the *MIC2* gene.

Ewing's Sarcoma Ewing's sarcoma occurs in adolescents and young adults, who present with progressive chest wall pain but without a mass. Systemic symptoms of malaise and fever are often present. Laboratory studies reveal an elevated erythrocyte sedimentation rate and mild elevation of white blood cell count.

Radiographically, the characteristic onion peel appearance is produced by multiple layers of periosteum in the bone formation. Evidence of bony destruction is also common. The diagnosis can be made by a percutaneous needle biopsy or an incisional biopsy.

These tumors have a strong propensity to spread to the lungs and skeleton. Due to their clinically aggressive behavior, patient survival rates are only ≤50% at 3 years. Increasing tumor size is associated with decreasing survival. Treatment has improved significantly and now consists of multiagent chemotherapy, radiation therapy, and surgery. Patients are typically treated preoperatively with chemotherapy and re-evaluated with radiographic imaging. When residual disease is identified, surgical resection and reconstruction are performed, followed by maintenance chemotherapy.

Plasmacytoma Solitary plasmacytomas of the chest wall are very rare, and only 25 to 30 cases are seen annually in the United States.[132] The typical presentation is pain without a palpable mass. Radiographs show an osteolytic lesion. As with other chest wall tumors, a needle biopsy is performed under CT guidance for diagnosis. Histologically, the lesion is identical to that of multiple myeloma, with sheets of plasma cells. It occurs at an average age of 55 years. Evaluation for systemic myeloma is performed with bone marrow aspiration, testing of calcium levels, and measurement of urinary Bence Jones protein levels. If the results of these studies are negative, then a solitary plasmacytoma is diagnosed. Surgery is usually limited to a biopsy only, which may be excisional. Treatment consists of irradiation with doses of 4000 to 5000 cGy. Up to 75% of patients go on to develop systemic multiple myeloma. Patient survival at 10 years is approximately 20%.

Malignant Chest Soft Tissue Sarcomas

Soft tissue sarcomas of the chest wall are uncommon (Fig. 19-39). They include fibrosarcomas, liposarcomas, malignant fibrous histiocytomas, rhabdomyosarcomas, angiosarcomas, and other extremely rare lesions. Leiomyosarcoma and GI stromal tumors are the most common, representing approximately 65% of the total. Localized disease is present in 55 to 60% of cases; the remaining approximately 40% of cases show an even split between regional and distant spread.[134] Despite the prevalence of localized disease, soft tissue sarcomas of the chest wall are associated with significantly worse survival than are similar tumors located on the extremities or in the head and neck region. The factors affecting risk of death from soft tissue sarcomas are presented in Table 19-25.

Patients receiving surgical intervention have significantly better overall survival. Median survival with surgical resection is 25 months compared to 8 months without resection. Additional prognostic variables that are important for long-term survival include tumor size, grade, and stage, and achievement of a negative resection margin.[134] With the exception of rhabdomyosarcomas, the primary treatment of these lesions is wide surgical resection with 4-cm margins and reconstruction.[135] Rhabdomyosarcomas are sensitive to chemotherapy and often are treated with preoperative chemotherapy. As with all sarcomas, soft tissue sarcomas of the chest wall have a propensity to spread to the lungs.

Malignant Fibrous Histiocytoma Malignant fibrous histiocytomas were originally thought to derive from histiocytes because of the microscopic appearance of cultured tumor cells. Subsequently it was shown that their likely origin is the fibroblast. Malignant fibrous histiocytomas are generally the most common soft tissue sarcoma of late adult life, although they very rarely occur on the chest wall. The typical age at presentation is between 50 and 70 years. These tumors are rare in those <20 years of age. They present with pain, with or without a palpable mass. Radiographically, a mass is usually evident, with destruction of surrounding tissue and bone. Treatment is wide resection with a margin of ≥4 cm and reconstruction. Over two thirds of patients develop distant metastasis or local recurrence.

Liposarcoma Liposarcomas make up 15% of chest wall sarcomas. Most liposarcomas are low-grade tumors that have a propensity to recur locally, given their infiltrative nature. Clinically, they present most often as painless masses. Treatment is wide resection and reconstruction. Intraoperative margins should be evaluated (as with all sarcomas) and resection continued, if feasible, until margins are negative. Local recurrence can be treated with re-excision, and radiotherapy is occasionally used.

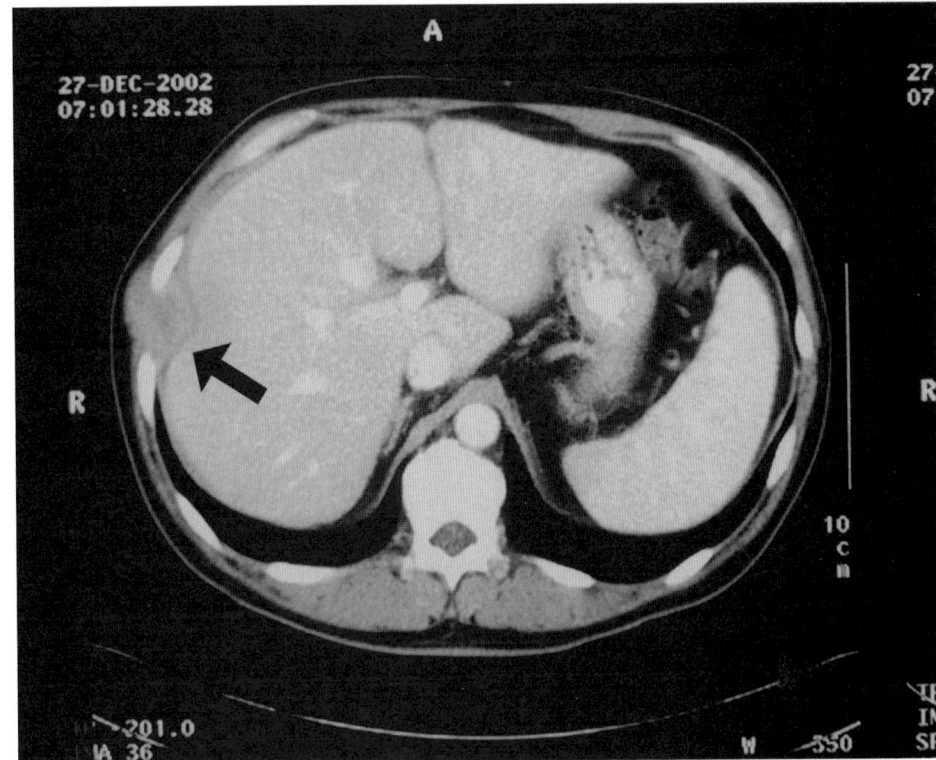

FIG. 19-39. Chest computed tomographic scan showing a right chest wall tumor (*arrow*). Tissue diagnosis revealed that this mass was a leiomyosarcoma.

TABLE 19-25	Cox proportional hazards model for risk of death from soft tissue sarcoma			
	n	**Hazard Ratio**	**95% CI**	***P* Value**
Gender				
Male	3937	Reference group	Reference group	Reference group
Female	4113	0.897	0.843–0.955	.001
Age				
50 y	1837	Reference group	Reference group	Reference group
51–70 y	3099	1.131	1.026–1.247	.013
>70 y	3114	1.538	1.395–1.697	<.001
Race				
Caucasian	7152	Reference group	Reference group	Reference group
Non-Caucasian	898	1.212	1.093–1.344	<.001
Histologic type				
Fibrosarcoma	489	Reference group	Reference group	Reference group
MFH	2529	1.281	1.097–1.495	.002
Liposarcoma	1534	0.894	0.759–1.054	.182
LMS/GIST	3498	1.204	1.033–1.403	.018
Location				
Head and neck	576	Reference group	Reference group	Reference group
Trunk	4054	1.255	1.096–1.438	.001
Extremity	2474	1.003	0.875–1.151	.960
Retroperitoneum	946	1.276	1.093–1.489	.002
Stage				
Localized	5006	Reference group	Reference group	Reference group
Regional	1724	1.575	1.458–1.702	<.001
Distant	1320	2.897	2.660–3.155	<.001
Surgical treatment				
Yes	6754	Reference group	Reference group	Reference group
No	1296	1.562	1.443–1.691	<.001
Radiation therapy				
Yes	2175	Reference group	Reference group	Reference group
No	5875	1.151	1.070–1.239	<.001
Chemotherapy				
Yes	1062	Reference group	Reference group	Reference group
No	6988	0.909	0.829–0.996	.041

CI = confidence interval; GIST = gastrointestinal stromal tumor; LMS = leiomyosarcoma; MFH = malignant fibrous histiocytoma.
Source: Reproduced with permission from Gutierrez et al.[134] Copyright Elsevier.

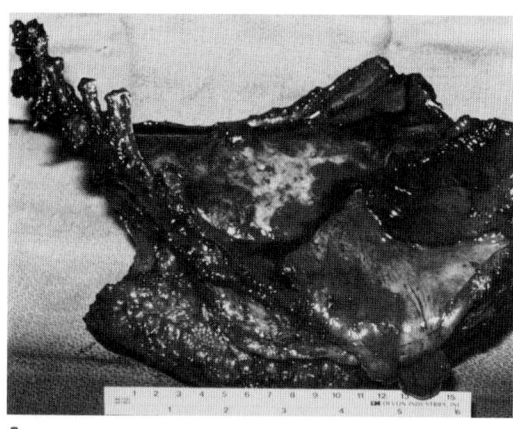

A

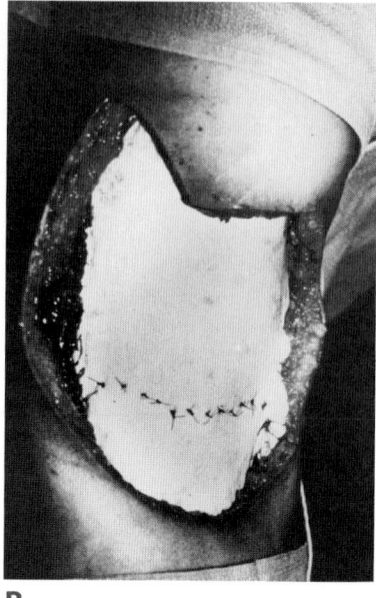

B

FIG. 19-40. Principles of reconstruction after resection of a chest wall tumor (osteogenic sarcoma) are illustrated. **A.** En bloc resection of the involved chest wall, including normal ribs above and below the tumor as well as pulmonary parenchyma, must be performed. The resected specimen is shown. **B.** A prosthesis has been sewn in place. In the lower third of the prosthesis, the line of diaphragm reattachment is seen. The skin defect was closed with a myocutaneous flap from the ipsilateral rectus muscle.

Fibrosarcoma Fibrosarcomas often present as large painful masses. Radiographically, a mass is seen with surrounding tissue destruction. Treatment is wide local excision with intraoperative frozen-section analysis of margins, followed by reconstruction. Local and systemic recurrence is frequent. Patient survival at 5 years is approximately 50 to 60%.

Rhabdomyosarcoma Rhabdomyosarcomas are rare tumors of the chest wall. Microscopically, they are a spindle cell tumor. The diagnosis often depends on immunohistochemical staining for muscle markers. Rhabdomyosarcomas are sensitive to chemotherapy. Treatment consists of preoperative chemotherapy with subsequent surgical resection.

Chest Wall Reconstruction

The status of the margins after resection of chest wall tumors is the primary determinant of long-term freedom from recurrence and overall survival. As a result, adequate margins of normal tissue must be included in the en bloc resection. En bloc resection should include involved ribs, sternum, superior sulcus, or spine if necessary, and invasion of these structures should not be considered a contraindication to surgery in an otherwise fit patient. The principles of surgery for any malignant chest wall tumor are to strategically plan the anatomy of resection and to carefully assess what structures will need to be sacrificed to obtain a 4-cm margin. Reconstruction at the same operation can be accomplished using prosthetic materials and myocutaneous flaps.[136] An acceptable cosmetic result is possible with creative use of myocutaneous flaps, even when the defect is large.

Because of the high rate of malignancy of chest wall neoplasms, any mass that likely represents a primary tumor must be aggressively managed. When malignancy is suspected, preliminary plans must be made for chest wall reconstruction that will allow resection of a generous margin of normal tissue around the neoplasm. The resection should include at least one normal adjacent rib above and below the tumor, with all intervening intercostal muscles and pleura. In addition, an en bloc resection of overlying chest wall muscles such as the pectoralis minor or major, serratus anterior, or latissimus dorsi muscle often is necessary. When the periphery of the lung is involved with the neoplasm, it is appropriate to resect the adjacent part of the pulmonary lobe in continuity (Fig. 19-40). Involvement of the sternum by a malignant tumor requires total resection of the sternum with the adjacent cartilage. Techniques for postoperative respiratory support are now good enough that resection should not be compromised because of any concern about the patient's ability to be adequately ventilated in the early postoperative period.

The extent of resection depends on the tumor's location and on any involvement of contiguous structures. Laterally based lesions often require simple wide excision, with resection of any contiguously involved lung, pleura, muscle, or skin. Anteriorly based lesions contiguous with the sternum require partial sternectomy. Primary malignant tumors of the sternum may require complete sternectomy. Posterior lesions involving the rib heads over their articulations with the vertebral bodies may, depending on the extent of rib involvement, require partial en bloc vertebrectomy.

Reconstruction of a large defect in the chest wall requires the use of some type of material to prevent lung herniation and to provide stability for the chest wall (see Fig. 19-40). Mild degrees of paradoxical motion are often well tolerated if the area of instability is relatively small. Several authors, notably Pairolero and Arnold from the Mayo Clinic, have reported extensive experience with chest wall reconstruction after removal of significant portions of the bony thorax.[137] Historically, a wide variety of materials have been used to re-establish chest wall stability, including rib autografts, steel struts, acrylic plates, and numerous synthetic meshes. The current preference is either a 2-mm polytetrafluoroethylene (Gore-Tex) patch or a double-layer polypropylene (Marlex) mesh sandwiched with methyl methacrylate. Several properties make Gore-Tex an excellent material for use in chest wall reconstruction. It is impervious to fluid, which prevents pleural fluid from entering the chest wall. This quality minimizes the formation of seromas, which can compromise viability of the myocutaneous flap and provide a nidus for infection. In addition, it provides excellent rigidity and stability when secured taut to the surrounding bony structure and, as a result, provides a firm platform for myocutaneous flap reconstruction.

Except for smaller lesions, tissue coverage requires the use of myocutaneous flaps (latissimus dorsi, serratus anterior, rectus abdominis, or pectoralis major muscle).[138–140] Optimal management of larger tumors includes careful preoperative planning and execution of the surgery by the thoracic surgeon and an experienced plastic surgeon to ensure optimal physiologic and cosmetic results.

MEDIASTINUM

General Concepts
Anatomy and Pathologic Entities

The mediastinum, the central part of the thoracic cavity, can be divided into compartments for classification of anatomic components and disease processes. Although there is substantial overlap,

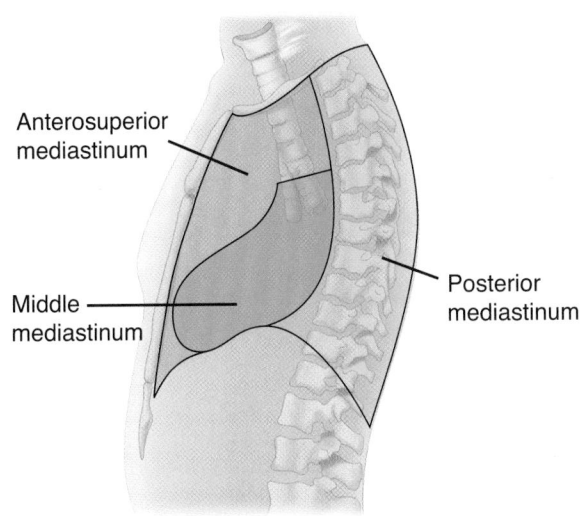

FIG. 19-41. Anatomic division of the mediastinum.

islands of thymic cellular components (Fig. 19-43). The middle mediastinal compartment contains the pericardium and its contents, the ascending and transverse aorta, the superior and inferior venae cavae, the brachiocephalic artery and vein, the phrenic nerves, the upper vagus nerve trunks, the trachea, the main bronchi and their associated lymph nodes, and the central portions of the pulmonary arteries and veins. The posterior compartment contains the descending aorta, esophagus, thoracic duct, azygos and hemiazygos veins, and lymph nodes. Numerous pathologic variants may be present in the various compartments, with much overlap. Table 19-26 includes the most common pathologic entities, listed by compartment.[141,142]

History and Physical Examination

The type of mediastinal pathology encountered varies significantly by age of the patient. In adults, the most common tumors include neurogenic tumors of the posterior compartment, benign cysts occurring in any compartment, and thymomas of the anterior mediastinum (Table 19-27). In children, neurogenic tumors of the posterior mediastinum are also common. Lymphoma is the second most common mediastinal tumor, usually located in the anterior or middle compartment, and thymoma is rare (Table 19-28). In both age groups, approximately 25% of mediastinal tumors are malignant. Pediatric tumors are discussed in Chap. 39.

In most recent series, up to two thirds of mediastinal tumors in adults are discovered as asymptomatic abnormalities on radiologic studies ordered to investigate other problems. When symptomatic, these tumors are significantly more likely to be malignant. Characteristics such as size, location, rate of growth, and associated inflammation are important factors that correlate with symptoms. Large, bulky tumors, expanding cysts, and teratomas can cause compression of mediastinal structures, in particular the trachea, and lead to cough, dyspnea on exertion, or stridor. Chest pain or dyspnea may be reported secondary to associated pleural effusions, cardiac tamponade, or phrenic nerve involvement. Occasionally, a mediastinal mass near the aortopulmonary window may be identified in a work-up for hoarseness because of left recurrent laryngeal nerve involvement (Fig. 19-44). The patient whose CT scan is shown in Fig. 19-44 presented with hoarseness and was found to have a primary lung cancer with metastases to the level 5 and 6 lymph nodes in the region of the aortopulmonary window. Her hoarseness was due to nodal compres-

this compartmentalization facilitates understanding of general concepts of surgical interest. Several classification schemes exist, but for the purposes of this chapter, the three-compartment model is used (Fig. 19-41). This model includes the anterior compartment (often referred to as *anterosuperior*), the visceral compartment (middle), and the paravertebral sulci bilaterally (posterior compartment). The anterior compartment lies between the sternum and the anterior surface of the heart and great vessels. The visceral or middle compartment is located between the great vessels and the trachea. Posterior to these two compartments lies the paravertebral sulci bilaterally and the periesophageal area.

The normal content of the anterior compartment includes the thymus gland or its remnant, the internal mammary artery and vein, lymph nodes, and fat. During childhood, the size of the thymus gland is impressive, and it occupies the entire anterior mediastinum (Fig. 19-42). After adolescence, the thymus gland decreases in both thickness and length and takes on a more fatty content, with only residual

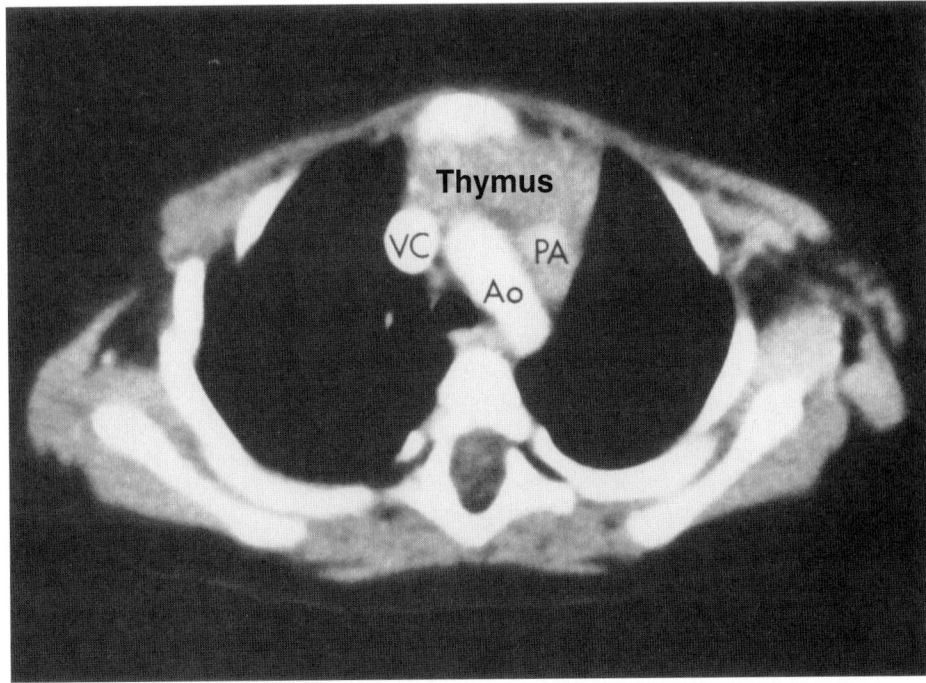

FIG. 19-42. Normal appearance of the thymus gland in childhood. Ao = aorta; PA = pulmonary artery; VC = vena cava.

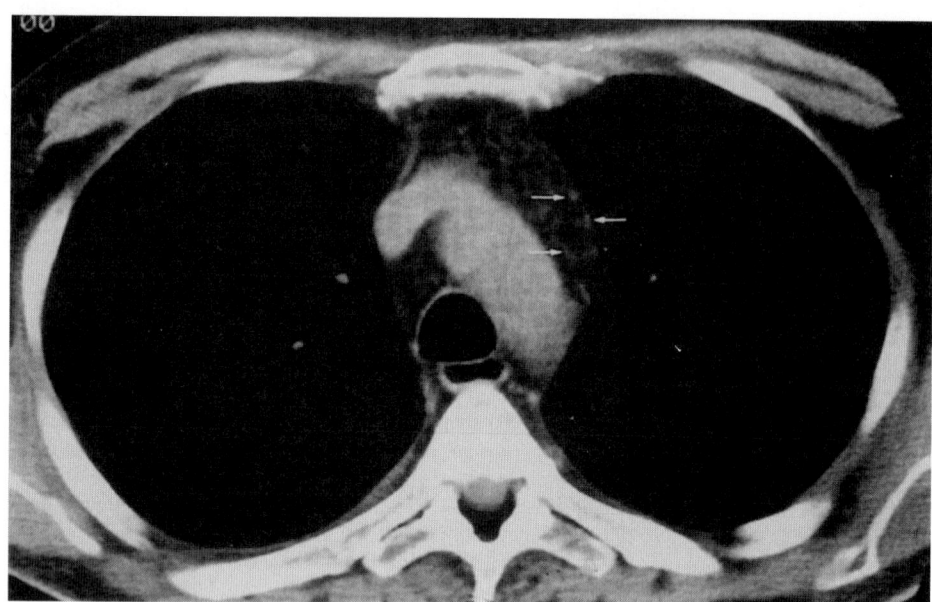

FIG. 19-43. Computed tomographic scan showing the normal appearance of an involuted thymus gland in an adult. Note the near-total fatty appearance of the gland with only tiny islands of soft tissue scattered within it (*small arrows*).

sion of the left recurrent laryngeal nerve. In the era of screening CT examinations, a higher percentage of malignant tumors of the mediastinum are being discovered as asymptomatic, incidental masses.

The history and physical examination in conjunction with the imaging findings may suggest a specific diagnosis (Table 19-29). In one recent series, systemic symptoms were present in 50% of patients with a mediastinal mass and a lymphoproliferative disorder, compared with only 29% of patients with other masses (such as thymic or neurogenic lesions). Laboratory signs of inflammation were also noted: The erythrocyte sedimentation rate and C-reactive protein levels were elevated and leukocytosis was present in 86% of patients with a lymphoproliferative disorder, compared with only 58% of patients with other types of mediastinal masses.

Diagnostic Evaluation
Imaging and Serum Markers

A number of asymptomatic mediastinal masses are suggested by chest radiographs but are generally poorly defined by this study. CT has become the most common imaging modality for evaluation of mediastinal masses.[143] Contrast-enhanced CT scans for clear delineation of anatomy are preferred. MRI may be indicated in the workup of a mediastinal mass, particularly in patients contemplating

surgical resection. Specifically, MRI is more accurate than CT in determining if there is invasion of vascular structures or spinal involvement.

Several other imaging modalities are available to evaluate mediastinal masses of suspected endocrine origin (Table 19-30). Single-photon emission computed tomography (SPECT) technology may be used to improve image contrast and give information on three-dimensional localization of some tumors of endocrine origin. SPECT has largely replaced conventional two-dimensional nuclear imaging. If a thyroid origin is suspected, a thyroid scan using iodine 131 or iodine 123 can identify most intrathoracic goiters and define the extent of functioning thyroid tissue. If a thyroid scan is indicated, it should precede other scans requiring iodine-containing

TABLE 19-27   Mediastinal tumors in adults

Tumor Type	Percentage of Total	Location
Neurogenic tumors	21	Posterior
Cysts	20	All
Thymomas	19	Anterior
Lymphomas	13	Anterior/middle
Germ cell tumors	11	Anterior
Mesenchymal tumors	7	All
Endocrine tumors	6	Anterior/middle

Source: Reproduced from Shields TW: Primary lesions of the mediastinum and their investigation and treatment, in Shields TW (ed): *General Thoracic Surgery*, 4th ed. Baltimore: Lippincott Williams & Wilkins, 1994, p 1731.

TABLE 19-26   Usual location of the common primary tumors and cysts of the mediastinum

Anterior Compartment	Visceral Compartment	Paravertebral Sulci
Thymoma	Enterogenous cyst	Neurilemoma-schwannoma
Germ cell tumor	Lymphoma	Neurofibroma
Lymphoma	Pleuropericardial cyst	Malignant schwannoma
Lymphangioma	Mediastinal granuloma	Ganglioneuroma
Hemangioma	Lymphoid hamartoma	Ganglioneuroblastoma
Lipoma	Mesothelial cyst	Neuroblastoma
Fibroma	Neuroenteric cyst	Paraganglioma
Fibrosarcoma	Paraganglioma	Pheochromocytoma
Thymic cyst	Pheochromocytoma	Fibrosarcoma
Parathyroid adenoma	Thoracic duct cyst	Lymphoma

Source: Reproduced with permission from Shields TW: The mediastinum and its compartments, in Shields TW (ed): *Mediastinal Surgery*. Philadelphia: Lea & Febiger, 1991, p 5.

TABLE 19-28   Mediastinal tumors in children

Tumor Type	Percentage of Total	Location
Neurogenic tumors	40	Posterior
Lymphomas	18	Anterior/middle
Cysts	18	All
Germ cell tumors	11	Anterior
Mesenchymal tumors	9	All
Thymomas	Rare	Anterior

Source: Reproduced with permission from Silverman NA, et al: Mediastinal masses. *Surg Clin North Am* 60:760, 1980. Copyright Elsevier.

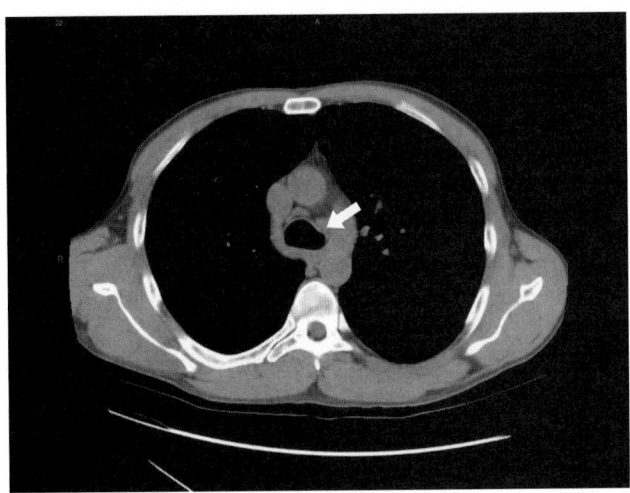

FIG. 19-44. Computed tomographic scan of a patient who presented with hoarseness due to compression of the left recurrent laryngeal nerve caused by mediastinal lymph node metastases to the aortopulmonary window area (*arrow*) from a primary lung cancer.

contrast agents, because these would interfere with subsequent iodine tracer uptake by thyroid tissue and scanning. If a pheochromocytoma or neuroblastoma is suspected, octreotide scans or *m*-iodobenzylguanidine (iobenguane I 123, or MIBG) scans are helpful in diagnosis and localization. A sestamibi scan may be useful for diagnosing and localizing a mediastinal parathyroid gland.

PET scanning has improved the noninvasive staging of lung cancer and esophageal cancer. The utility of PET in staging the mediastinum for NSCLC is reviewed in "Mediastinal Lymph Nodes" earlier in this chapter. The value of PET in staging other tumors of the mediastinum is not as clear. It is useful for distinguishing malignant from benign tumors. It may help detect distant metastases in some patients. For example, in patients with esophageal cancer, up to 10% of those with negative results on a metastatic survey by conventional imaging, including CT scan, will have a positive finding on PET scan for distant metastases.[144] The role of routine PET imaging in staging surgically resectable lesions of the mediastinum has not been established.

The use of serum markers to evaluate a mediastinal mass can be invaluable in some patients. For example, seminomatous and non-

TABLE 19-30   Nuclear imaging relevant to the mediastinum

Radiopharmaceutical, Radionuclide, or Radiochemical	Label	Disease of Interest
Iodine	^{131}I, ^{123}I	Retrosternal goiter, thyroid cancer
Monoclonal antibodies	^{111}In, ^{99m}Tc	NSCLC, colon and breast cancer, prostate cancer metastases
Octreotide	^{111}In	Amine precursor uptake decarboxylation tumors: carcinoid, gastrinoma, insulinoma, small cell lung cancer, pheochromocytoma, glucagonoma, medullary thyroid carcinoma, paraganglioma
Gallium	^{67}Ga	Lymphoma, NSCLC, melanoma
Sestamibi	^{99m}Tc	Medullary thyroid carcinoma, nonfunctional papillary or follicular thyroid carcinoma, Hürthle cell thyroid carcinoma, parathyroid adenoma or carcinoma
Thallium	^{201}Tl	See sestamibi
MIBG	^{131}I, ^{123}I	Pheochromocytoma, neuroblastoma; see also octreotide
Fluorodeoxyglucose	^{18}F	General oncologic imaging, breast and colon cancer, melanoma

MIGB = *m*-iodobenzylguanidine; NSCLC = non–small cell lung cancer.
Source: Reproduced with permission from McGinnis KM, et al: Markers of the mediastinum, in Pearson FG, et al (eds): *Thoracic Surgery*, 2nd ed. New York: Churchill Livingstone, 2002, p 1675. Copyright Elsevier.

seminomatous germ cell tumors can frequently be diagnosed and often distinguished from one another by the levels of alpha-fetoprotein (AFP) and human chorionic gonadotropin (hCG). In over 90% of nonseminomatous germ cell tumors, either the AFP or the hCG level will be elevated. Results are close to 100% specific if the level of either AFP or hCG is >500 ng/mL. Some centers initiate chemotherapy based on this result alone, without a biopsy. In contrast, the AFP level is always normal in patients with mediastinal seminomas; only 10% will have an elevated hCG level, which usually is <100 ng/mL. Other serum markers, such as intact parathyroid hormone level for ectopic parathyroid adenomas, may be useful for diagnosis and also for intraoperative confirmation of complete resection. After successful resection of a parathyroid adenoma, the level of this hormone should rapidly normalize.

Diagnostic Nonsurgical Biopsy of the Mediastinum

The indications and decision-making steps for performing a diagnostic biopsy of a mediastinal mass remain somewhat controversial. In some patients, given the results of noninvasive imaging and the history, surgical removal may be the obvious choice; preoperative biopsy may be unnecessary and even hazardous. In other patients whose primary treatment is likely to be nonsurgical, a biopsy is essential. Even when biopsy appears to be a reasonable goal, needle aspiration of the mediastinal mass may be considered hazardous or of low diagnostic yield.

Percutaneous biopsy may be technically difficult because of the overlying bony thoracic cavity and the proximity to lung tissue, the heart, and great vessels. FNA biopsy minimizes some of these potential hazards and may be effective in diagnosing mediastinal thyroid tissue, cancers, carcinomas, seminomas, inflammatory processes, and cysts.[145] Other noncarcinomatous malignancies such as

TABLE 19-29   Signs and symptoms suggestive of various diagnoses in the setting of a mediastinal mass

Diagnosis	History and Physical Findings	Compartment Location of Mass
Lymphoma	Night sweats, weight loss, fatigue, extrathoracic adenopathy, elevated erythrocyte sedimentation rate or C-reactive protein level, leukocytosis	Any compartment
Thymoma with myasthenia gravis	Fluctuating weakness, early fatigue, ptosis, diplopia	Anterior
Mediastinal granuloma	Dyspnea, wheezing, hemoptysis	Visceral (middle)
Germ cell tumor	Male gender, young age, testicular mass, elevated levels of human chorionic gonadotropin and/or alpha-fetoprotein	Anterior

lymphoproliferative disorders, thymomas, and benign tumors may require larger pieces of tissue. Such biopsy specimens may be obtained by a core-needle technique (which may not be safe depending on the location of the mass) or by surgery. In light of the issues cited, it is not surprising that the approach to biopsy of mediastinal masses may be different from center to center. Significant controversy exists in the literature regarding this topic. However, the treatment of up to 60% of patients with anterior mediastinal masses is ultimately nonsurgical, so it is essential to understand all options for obtaining adequate tissue for a definitive diagnosis using the least invasive approach. In one recent study, the authors used the medical history, physical examination, laboratory findings (erythrocyte sedimentation rate, C-reactive protein level, and presence of leukocytosis), and CT scan to assign patients to a possible lymphoproliferative diagnosis or a possible nonlymphoproliferative diagnosis. The authors concluded that if features suggest one of the lymphoproliferative group of mediastinal masses, the patient should undergo a surgical biopsy, because larger pieces of tissues were required to make the diagnosis in their series. However, if a nonlymphoproliferative diagnosis was suggested, they recommended FNA before a potential surgical resection, because the yield of accurate diagnoses by FNA was higher in that group.[146]

In 1989, the American Thoracic Society published a position statement declaring that "cutting needles should not be used to biopsy diffuse infiltrative lung diseases or lesions in or adjacent to the mediastinum or hilar areas."[147] Since that time, however, institutions with significant interventional expertise have challenged that statement. In one series of 142 patients with mediastinal masses, CT-guided transthoracic core-needle biopsies were performed using 14- to 22-gauge needles. The sensitivity of the procedure was 98.9% and the specificity was 100%. Inadequate material was obtained from only 0.7% of patients, with no pneumothoraces or bleeding complications reported.[147] The diagnostic yield is lower in series including a higher number of patients with lymphoproliferative disorders. Other series also reported a higher complication rate of 8 to 23% for pneumothorax and up to 10% for hemoptysis. In describing another series of anterior mediastinal masses, Herman and colleagues reported that needle biopsy was >90% specific in diagnosing most carcinomatous tumors, but its accuracy for diagnosing lymphomas was <50%.[148]

Similar controversy exists regarding the yield of needle biopsies for definitively diagnosing germ cell tumors and thymomas. Knapp described 56 patients with malignant germ cell tumors of the mediastinum. Various combinations of germ cell elements were present in 34% of tumors, so open biopsies with multiple tissue sections were seen as advisable. For another series of 79 patients with mediastinal masses suspected to be malignant, Larsen reported that endoscopic ultrasound-guided FNA had a sensitivity of 92% and a specificity of 100%.[145,149]

In the authors' experience, CT-guided needle biopsy has proven most useful for investigating tumors that are clearly unresectable or for assessing suspected carcinomatous tumors. For mediastinal masses suggestive of a lymphoma, obtaining larger pieces of tissue by mediastinoscopy to sample paratracheal adenopathy is preferred. Thoracoscopic biopsies are preferred for other locations. If an anterior mediastinal mass appears localized and is consistent with a thymoma, surgical resection is performed. For most localized tumors of the posterior mediastinum suspected to be neurogenic in origin, surgical resection without biopsy also is the preference of these authors. FNA guided by endoscopic ultrasound and endobronchial ultrasound and even core biopsy (guided by endoscopic ultrasound) are increasingly used for cytologic and tissue diagnosis of mediastinal masses and lymphadenopathy. Demonstration of the safety of the use of Tru-Cut core-needle biopsy (TCB) is a significant advance in the minimally invasive evaluation of mediastinal lymphadenopathy and periesophageal tumors, because the yield and accuracy are significantly improved with this procedure. When FNA and TCB were combined, the accuracy was 98%, compared with 79% for each modality independently. In addition, the results of the TCB changed the diagnosis in nine cases that had been missed by FNA due to inadequacy of the specimens. Finally, TCB was better at diagnosis of benign diseases than was FNA. Accessible nodal stations include subcarinal (level 7), aortopulmonary (level 5), periesophageal (level 8), inferior pulmonary ligament (level 9), and peritracheal (level 4) stations.[150] Technical expertise in these modalities should be pursued by thoracic and general surgeons.

Surgical Biopsy and Resection of Mediastinal Masses

For tumors of the mediastinum that are not amenable to an endoscopic or CT-guided needle biopsy or that do not yield sufficient tissue for diagnosis, a surgical biopsy is indicated. The definitive approach to a surgical biopsy of the anterior mediastinum is through a median sternotomy. At the time of sternotomy, if the lesion is easily resectable, it should be completely removed. Given the invasiveness of the procedure and the inability in some patients to obtain a definitive diagnosis by frozen-section analysis, less invasive procedures are preferable if the lesion is large or if the CT scan or history suggests that surgery is not the best definitive treatment. Masses in the paratracheal region are easily biopsied by mediastinoscopy. For tumors of the anterior or posterior mediastinum, a left or right VATS approach often allows safe and adequate surgical biopsy. In some patients, an anterior mediastinotomy (i.e., Chamberlain procedure) may be ideal for an anterior tumor or a tumor with significant parasternal extension. Before a surgical biopsy is pursued, a discussion should be held with the pathologist regarding routine histologic assessment, special stains and markers, and requirements for lymphoma work-up.

The gold standard for the resection of most mediastinal masses is through a median sternotomy or lateral thoracotomy. In some cases, a lateral thoracotomy with sternal extension (hemiclamshell) provides excellent exposure for extensive mediastinal tumors that have a lateral component. This standard has been successfully challenged for some anterior mediastinal lesions. For example, good results have been reported using a cervical incision with a sternal retractor for thymus removal. The upward lift allows the surgeon reasonable access to the anterior mediastinum and has proven adequate in some centers for definitive resection of the thymus gland for myasthenia gravis.[151] Similarly, several large series have now shown that a right or left VATS approach can be successful for removal of the thymus gland and for resection of small (1 to 2 cm) encapsulated thymomas.[152,153] Most would agree that if a larger anterior mediastinal tumor is seen or malignancy is suspected, a median sternotomy with a more radical resection should be performed.

Neoplasms

Thymus

Thymic Hyperplasia Diffuse thymic hyperplasia was first described in children after successful chemotherapy for lymphoma. It has now been described in adults and is referred to as *rebound thymic hyperplasia.*[154] It is most frequently reported after chemotherapy for lymphoma or germ cell tumors. Initially, atrophy of the thymic gland is seen; later, on follow-up scans, the patient is noted to have thymic gland enlargement, which can be dramatic. The usual time course for thymic hyperplasia to develop is approximately 9 months after cessation of chemotherapy, but it has been reported anywhere from 2 weeks to 12 months after chemotherapy. Benign hyperplasia must be clearly distinguished from recurrent lymphoma or germ cell tumors. Doing so may be difficult, because thymic hyperplasia is dramatic in some patients, requiring careful follow-up and, at a minimum, serial CT scans. PET scanning may be helpful; a low standardized uptake value of tracer on PET scan suggests a benign tumor, but little has been published on this topic. Biopsies may be required if the clinical index of suspicion is high.

Thymic Tumors *Thymoma* Thymoma is the most frequently encountered neoplasm of the anterior mediastinum in adults (seen most frequently between 40 and 60 years of age). They are rare in children. Most patients with thymomas are asymptomatic, but depending on the institutional referral patterns, between 10 and 50% have symptoms suggestive of myasthenia gravis or have circulating antibodies to acetylcholine receptor. However, <10% of patients with myasthenia gravis are found to have a thymoma on CT. Thymectomy leads to improvement or resolution of symptoms of myasthenia gravis in only approximately 25% of patients with thymomas. In contrast, in patients with myasthenia gravis and no thymoma, thymectomy results are superior: up to 50% of patients have a complete remission and 90% improve. In 5% of patients with thymomas, other paraneoplastic syndromes, including red cell aplasia, hypogammaglobulinemia, systemic lupus erythematosus, Cushing's syndrome, or syndrome of inappropriate secretion of antidiuretic hormone may be present. Large thymic tumors may present with symptoms related to a mass effect, which may include cough, chest pain, dyspnea, or superior vena caval syndrome.

The diagnosis may be suspected based on CT scan and history, but imaging alone is not diagnostic. In most centers, the diagnosis is made after surgical resection because of the relative difficulty of performing a needle biopsy and the likelihood that removal will ultimately be recommended. However, CT-guided FNA biopsy has been reported to have a diagnostic sensitivity of 87% and a specificity of 95% in specialized centers. Cytokeratin is the marker that best distinguishes thymomas from lymphomas. In most patients, the distinction between lymphoma and thymoma can be made on CT scan, because most lymphomas are associated with marked lymphadenopathy and thymomas most frequently appear as a solitary encapsulated mass. PET may have a role in differentiating thymic cancer from thymoma, because thymic cancer tends to be very FDG avid.[155]

The most commonly accepted staging system for thymomas is that of Masaoka.[156] It is based on the presence or absence of gross or microscopic invasion of the capsule and surrounding structures, as well as on the presence or absence of metastases (Table 19-31).

Histologically, thymomas generally are characterized by a mixture of epithelial cells and mature lymphocytes. Grossly, many thymomas remain well-encapsulated. Even those with capsular invasion often lack histologic features of malignancy; they appear cytologically benign and identical to early-stage tumors. This lack of classic cellular features of malignancy is the reason that most pathologists use the term *thymoma* or *invasive thymoma* rather than *malignant thymoma*. Thymic tumors with malignant cytologic features are classified separately and referred to as *thymic carcinomas*.

The definitive treatment for thymomas is complete surgical removal of all resectable tumors. Local recurrence rates and survival vary according to stage (Fig. 19-45). Resection generally is accomplished by median sternotomy with extension to hemiclamshell in more advanced cases. In centers with significant experience with VATS procedures, thymoma is not a contraindication to a VATS approach, provided the principles of resection are adhered to, such as a complete resection without disruption of the capsule. Even advanced tumors with local invasion of resectable structures such as the pericardium, superior vena cava, or innominate vessels should be considered for resection with reconstruction. The role of adjuvant or

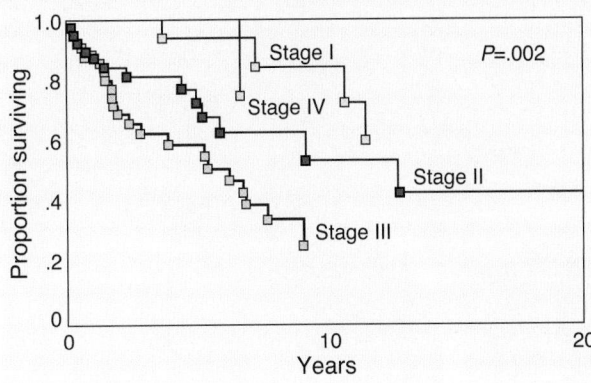

FIG. 19-45. Stage-specific survival for thymomas.

neoadjuvant therapies for advanced-stage tumors remains unclear. Traditionally, stage II thymomas have been treated by complete surgical resection followed by mediastinal irradiation, but due to the relatively small number of cases, randomized trials have not been done. A recent retrospective review of a single-institution series of stage II thymoma patients showed no difference in survival or local recurrence after complete surgical resection alone, compared with surgical resection with radiotherapy.[157] Advanced thymomas have been shown to respond to platinum-based chemotherapy and to corticosteroids.[158] One summary of chemotherapy trials showed an overall response rate of approximately 70%.[159] Combining radiotherapy and chemotherapy for local progression also has been successful in some small series; the combination appears to prolong survival, although most advanced-stage, unresectable thymomas will recur.[160] Therefore, it is imperative that all patients with thymomas undergo a thorough evaluation for potential resection.

Thymic Carcinoma Thymic carcinomas are unlike encapsulated or invasive thymomas in that they are unequivocally malignant at the microscopic level. Suster and Rosai classified thymic carcinomas into low-grade and high-grade tumors.[161] Low-grade tumors are well differentiated with squamous cell, mucoepidermoid, or basaloid features. High-grade thymic carcinomas include those with lymphoepithelial, small cell neuroendocrine, sarcomatoid, clear cell, and undifferentiated or anaplastic features. Compared with thymomas, they are a more heterogeneous group of malignancies with a propensity for early local invasion and widespread metastases. Complete resection is occasionally curative, but most thymic carcinomas will recur and are refractory to chemotherapy.[158] The prognosis of patients with such tumors remains poor.

Thymolipoma Thymolipomas are rare benign tumors that may grow to a very large size before being diagnosed. On CT scan, their appearance can be dramatic, with a characteristic fat density dotted by isolated areas of soft tissue density representing islands of thymic tissue (Fig. 19-46). Thymolipomas are generally well-encapsulated, soft, and pliable masses that do not invade surrounding structures. Resection is recommended for large masses.

Neurogenic Tumors

Most neurogenic tumors of the mediastinum arise from the cells of the nerve sheath, from ganglion cells, or from the paraganglionic system (Table 19-32). The incidence, cell types, and risk of malignancy strongly correlate with patient age. Tumors of nerve sheath origin predominate in adults. Most present as asymptomatic incidental findings and most are benign. In children and young adults, tumors of the autonomic ganglia predominate, with up to two thirds being malignant.[162]

Nerve Sheath Tumors Nerve sheath tumors account for 20% of all mediastinal tumors. More than 95% of nerve sheath tumors are

TABLE 19-31	Masaoka staging system for thymoma
Stage I	Encapsulated tumor with no gross or microscopic evidence of capsular invasion
Stage II	Gross capsular invasion or invasion into the mediastinal fat or pleura or microscopic capsular invasion
Stage III	Gross invasion into the pericardium, great vessels, or lung
Stage IVA	Pleural or pericardial dissemination
Stage IVB	Lymphogenous or hematogenous metastasis

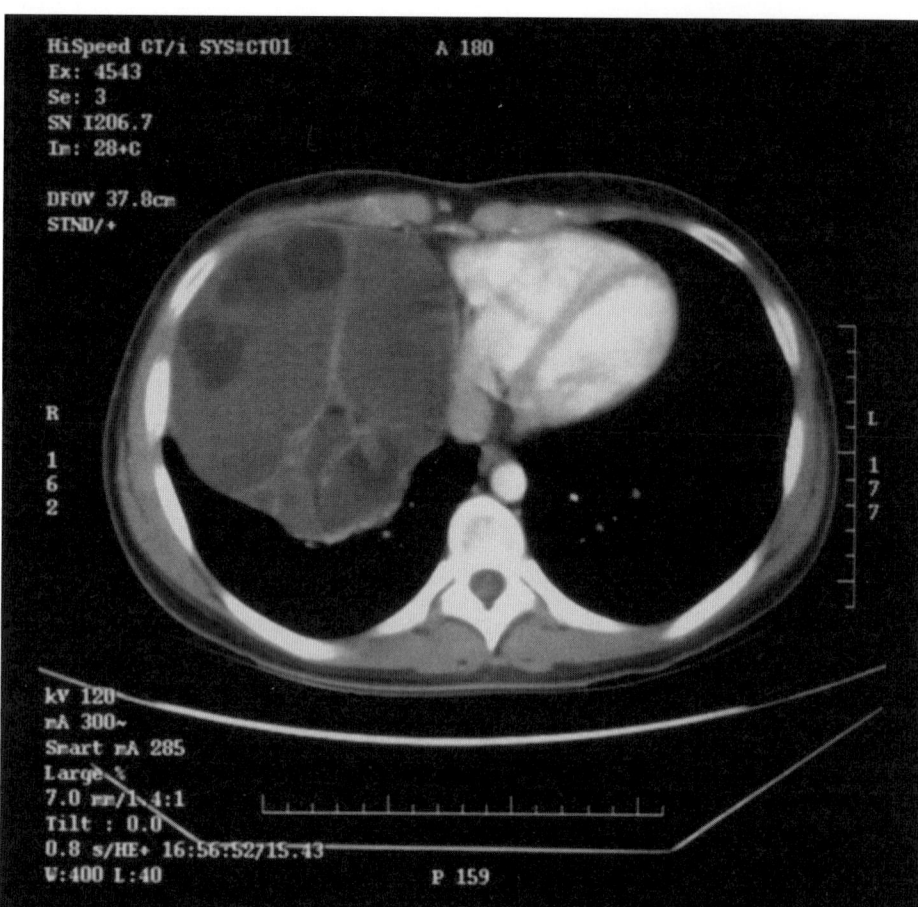

FIG. 19-46. Massive thymolipoma, which was asymptomatic, in an 18-year-old woman.

benign neurilemomas or neurofibromas. Malignant neurosarcomas are much less common.

Neurilemoma Neurilemomas, also called *schwannomas,* arise from Schwann cells in intercostal nerves. They are firm, well encapsulated, and generally benign. Two characteristic histologic components of benign neurilemomas exist and are referred to as Antoni type A and Antoni type B regions. Antoni type A regions contain compact spindle cells with twisted nuclei and nuclear palisading. Antoni type B regions contain loose and myxoid connective tissue with a haphazard cellular arrangement. These characteristics allow them to be distinguished from malignant, fibrosarcomatous tumors, which lack encapsulation and have no Antoni features. If routine CT scan suggests extension of a neurilemoma into the intervertebral foramen, MRI is suggested to evaluate the extent of this dumbbell configuration (Fig. 19-47). Such a configuration may lead to cord compression and paralysis, and re-

quires a more complex surgical approach. It is recommended that most nerve sheath tumors be resected. Traditionally, this has been performed by open thoracotomy, but a VATS approach has been established as safe and effective for simple surgeries and, in experienced centers, even the more complex operations.[163] It is reasonable to follow small, asymptomatic paravertebral tumors in older patients or in patients for whom surgery presents a high risk. In children, ganglioneuroblastomas or neuroblastomas are more common; therefore, all neurogenic tumors should be completely resected.

Neurofibroma Neurofibromas have components of both nerve sheaths and nerve cells and account for up to 25% of nerve sheath tumors. Up to 40% of patients with mediastinal fibromas have generalized neurofibromatosis (von Recklinghausen's disease). Approximately 70% of neurofibromas are benign. Malignant degeneration to a neurofibrosarcoma may occur in 25 to 30% of patients.[164] The risk of malignant degeneration is increased in those of advanced age, those with von Recklinghausen's disease, and those with previous exposure to radiation. Neurofibrosarcomas carry a poor prognosis because of rapid growth and aggressive local invasion along nerve bundles. Complete surgical resection is the mainstay of treatment. Adjuvant radiotherapy or chemotherapy does not confer a significant benefit but may be added if complete resection is not possible.[165] The 5-year survival rate is 53% but drops to 16% in patients who have neurofibromatosis or large tumors (>5 cm).

Ganglion Cell Tumors Ganglion cell tumors arise from the sympathetic chain or from the adrenal medulla. Histologic cell types include ganglioneuromas, ganglioneuroblastomas, and neuroblastomas.

Ganglioneuroma Ganglioneuromas are well-differentiated, benign tumors that are characterized histologically by well-differentiated ganglion cells with a background of Schwann cells. They tend to occur in young adults and to be asymptomatic, although diarrhea

TABLE 19-32	Classification of neurogenic tumors of the mediastinum	
Tumor Origin	**Benign**	**Malignant**
Nerve sheath	Neurilemoma, neurofibroma, melanotic schwannoma, granular cell tumor	Neurofibrosarcoma
Ganglion cell	Ganglioneuroma	Ganglioneuroblastoma, neuroblastoma
Paraganglionic cell	Chemodectoma, pheochromocytoma	Malignant chemodectoma, malignant pheochromocytoma

Source: Reproduced with permission from Bousamra.[162] Copyright Elsevier.

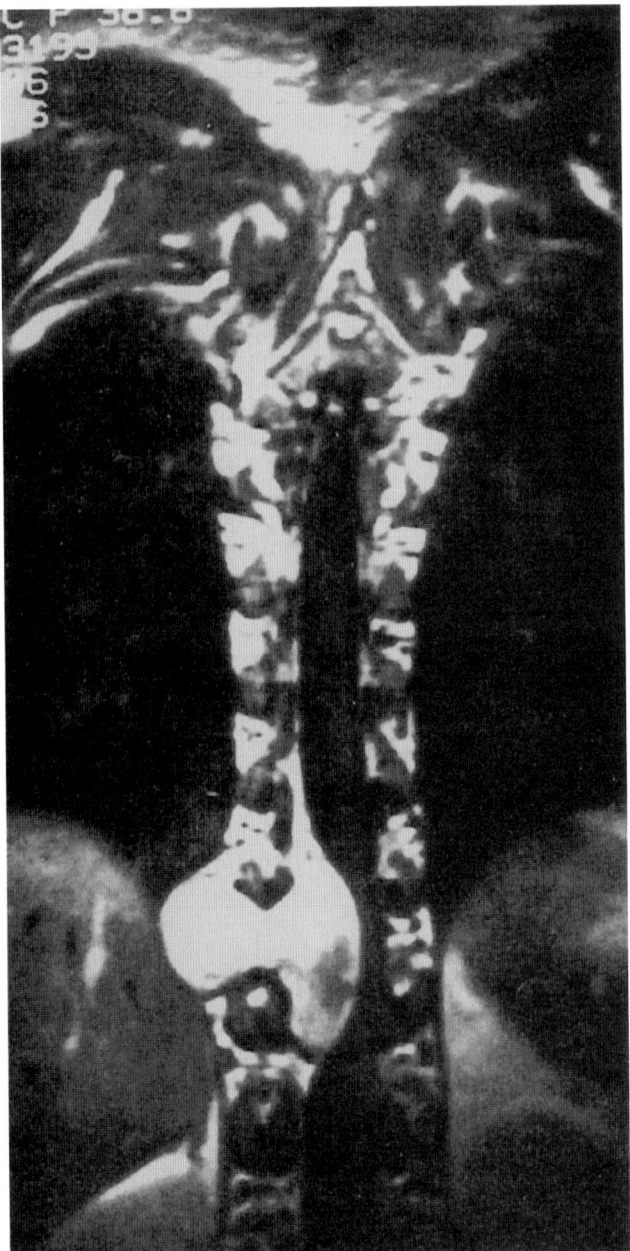

FIG. 19-47. Magnetic resonance image of a neurogenic tumor with extension into the spinal canal via the foramen, which gives a typical dumbbell appearance.

the most common intrathoracic malignancy of childhood. The adrenal gland is a common primary site, but 14% of all neuroblastomas arise in the thorax, where the tumors are commonly associated with extension into the spinal canal and osseous invasion. These thoracic tumors are not as recalcitrant to chemotherapy and surgical resection as are other chest malignancies; they are more likely to be resectable, with less invasion of surrounding organs. More than half occur in children <2 years of age; 90% arise within the first decade of life. These tumors are therefore discussed in more detail in Chap. 39 on pediatric surgery.

Paraganglionic Tumors Paraganglionic tumors arising in the thoracic cavity include chemodectomas and pheochromocytomas. Only 10% of all pheochromocytomas are located in an extra-adrenal site. Intrathoracic pheochromocytomas are one of the rarest tumors. Approximately 10% of thoracic pheochromocytomas are malignant, a rate similar to that of adrenal tumors. The most common thoracic location is within the costovertebral sulcus, but paraganglionic tumors also arise within the visceral compartment of the mediastinum. These catecholamine-producing lesions can lead to life-threatening hemodynamic problems, so complete removal is important. Diagnosis generally is confirmed by the measurement of elevated levels of urinary catecholamines and their metabolites. Localization is by CT scan, aided by MIBG scintigraphy. Preoperative care includes alpha- and beta-adrenergic blockade to prevent intraoperative malignant hypertension and arrhythmias. These tumors tend to be highly vascular and should be approached with care. Chemodectomas are rare tumors that may be located around the aortic arch, vagus nerves, or aorticosympathetics. They rarely secrete catecholamines and are malignant in up to 30% of patients.

Lymphoma

Overall, lymphomas are the most common malignancy of the mediastinum. In approximately 50% of patients who have both Hodgkin's and non-Hodgkin's lymphoma, the mediastinum is the primary site. The anterior compartment is most commonly involved, with occasional involvement of the middle compartment and hilar nodes. The posterior compartment is rarely involved. Chemotherapy and/or radiotherapy results in a cure rate of up to 90% for early-stage Hodgkin's disease and up to 60% for more advanced stages.

Mediastinal Germ Cell Tumors

Germ cell tumors are uncommon neoplasms, with only approximately 7000 diagnosed each year. However, they are the most common malignancy in young men between the ages of 15 and 35 years. Most germ cell tumors are gonadal in origin. Those with the mediastinum as the primary site are rare, constituting <5% of all germ cell tumors, and <1% of all mediastinal tumors (usually occurring in the anterior compartment). If a malignant mediastinal germ cell tumor is found, it is important to exclude a gonadal primary tumor. Primary mediastinal germ cell tumors (including teratomas, seminomas, and nonseminomatous malignant germ cell tumors) are a heterogeneous group of benign and malignant neoplasms thought to originate from primitive pluripotent germ cells "misplaced" in the mediastinum during embryonic development. Previously, most mediastinal germ cell tumors were thought to be metastatic. However, two lines of evidence suggest that many mediastinal germ cell tumors are primary, developing from pluripotent primordial germ cells in the mediastinum: (a) several autopsy series showed that patients with germ cell tumors in extragonadal sites, presumed previously to have originated from the gonads, had no evidence of an occult primary tumor or of any residual scar of the gonads, even after an exhaustive search; and (b) patients treated by surgery or radiation for their mediastinal germ cell tumors had long-term survival with no late testicular recurrences.[166]

About one third of all primary mediastinal germ cell tumors are seminomatous. Two thirds are nonseminomatous tumors or teratomas. Treatment and prognosis vary considerably within these two groups. Mature teratomas are benign and can generally be diagnosed by the characteristic CT findings of a multilocular cystic tumor,

related to secretion of vasoactive intestinal peptide has been described. These tumors have a propensity for intraspinal canal extension, although they remain well encapsulated. Complete resection is curative, and the risk of local recurrence is low.

Ganglioneuroblastoma Ganglioneuroblastomas contain a mixture of benign ganglion cells and malignant neuroblasts. The distribution of these cells within the tumor is predictive of the clinical course. The nodular pattern is associated with a high incidence of metastatic disease; tumors with the diffuse pattern rarely metastasize. On gross examination, these tumors often remain encapsulated; histologically, there are focal calcifications around regions of neuroblasts. Ganglioneuroblastomas arise most frequently in infants and children <3 years of age. The majority of tumors are resectable, and the 5-year survival rate is 80%.

Neuroblastoma Neuroblastomas are highly malignant. They are the most common extracranial solid malignancy in pediatric patients and encapsulated with combinations of fluid, soft tissue, calcium, and/or fat attenuation in the anterior compartment. FNA biopsy alone may be diagnostic for seminomas, and usually levels of serum markers, including hCG and AFP, are normal. In 10% of seminomas, hCG levels are slightly elevated. FNA findings, along with high hCG and AFP levels, can accurately diagnose nonseminomatous tumors. If the diagnosis remains uncertain after assessment of FNA findings and serum marker levels, then core-needle biopsy or surgical biopsy may be required. An anterior mediastinotomy (Chamberlain procedure) or thoracoscopy is the most frequent diagnostic surgical approach.

Teratoma Teratomas are the most common type of mediastinal germ cell tumors, accounting for 60 to 70% of such tumors. They contain two or three embryonic layers that may include teeth, skin, hair (ectodermal), cartilage and bone (mesodermal), or bronchial, intestinal, or pancreatic tissue (endodermal). Therapy for mature, benign teratomas is surgical resection, which confers an excellent prognosis.

Rarely, teratomas may contain a focus of carcinoma. These malignant teratomas (or teratocarcinomas) are locally aggressive. Often diagnosed at an unresectable stage, they respond poorly to chemotherapy and in a limited manner to radiotherapy; the prognosis is uniformly poor.

Seminoma Most patients with seminomas have advanced disease at the time of diagnosis and present with symptoms of local compression, including superior vena caval syndrome, dyspnea, or chest discomfort. With advanced disease, the preferred treatments are combination cisplatin-based chemotherapy regimens with bleomycin and either etoposide or vinblastine. Complete responses have been reported in over 75% of patients treated with these regimens. Surgical resection may be curative for small asymptomatic seminomas that are found incidentally on screening CT scans. Surgical resection of residual masses after chemotherapy may be indicated.

Nonseminomatous Germ Cell Tumors Nonseminomatous germ cell tumors include embryonal cell carcinomas, choriocarcinomas, endodermal sinus tumors, and mixed types. They are often bulky, irregular tumors of the anterior mediastinum with areas of low attenuation on CT scan because of necrosis, hemorrhage, or cyst formation. Frequently, adjacent structures have become involved, with metastases to regional lymph nodes, pleura, and lungs. Lactate dehydrogenase (LDH), AFP, and hCG levels are frequently elevated. Chemotherapy is the preferred treatment and includes combination therapy with cisplatin, bleomycin, and etoposide. With this regimen, survival is 67% at 2 years and 60% at 5 years. Surgical resection of residual masses is indicated, because it may guide further therapy. Up to 20% of residual masses contain additional tumors; in another 40%, mature teratomas; and the remaining 40%, fibrotic tissue.

Mediastinal Cysts
Primary Mediastinal Cyst

Benign cysts account for up to 25% of mediastinal masses. Most are located in the middle compartment, and they are the most frequent type of mass occurring in this compartment. A CT scan showing characteristic features of near-water density in a typical location is virtually 100% diagnostic.[167]

Pericardial Cyst

Pericardial cysts, the most common type of mediastinal cysts, are usually asymptomatic and detected incidentally. Typically they contain a clear fluid and appear in the right costophrenic angle. The cyst wall lining is a single layer of mesothelial cells. For most simple, asymptomatic pericardial cysts, observation alone is recommended. Surgical resection or aspiration may be indicated for complex cysts or large symptomatic cysts.

Bronchogenic Cyst

Bronchogenic cysts are developmental anomalies that occur during embryogenesis and manifest as an abnormal budding of the foregut or tracheobronchial tree. Most frequently they arise in the mediastinum, but approximately 15% occur within the pulmonary parenchyma. The most frequent mediastinal location is just posterior to the carina or main stem bronchus. Thin walled and lined with respiratory epithelium, they contain a protein-rich mucoid material and varying amounts of seromucous glands, smooth muscle, and cartilage. They may communicate with the tracheobronchial tree.

The management of bronchogenic cysts remains controversial. In children, most such cysts are symptomatic. Resection generally is recommended, because serious complications may ensue if the cyst becomes larger or infected. Complications include airway obstruction, infection, rupture, and, rarely, malignant transformation.[168,169]

In adults, over half of all bronchogenic cysts are found incidentally during work-up for an unrelated problem or during screening. The natural history of an incidentally diagnosed, asymptomatic bronchogenic cyst is unknown, but it is clear that many such cysts do not lead to clinical problems. In one study of young military personnel, 78% of all bronchogenic cysts found on routine chest radiographs were asymptomatic.[170] However, in other reports with more comprehensive follow-up, up to 67% of adults with incidentally found bronchogenic cysts eventually became symptomatic.[171] Symptoms include chest pain, cough, dyspnea, and fever. Serious complications are less common and include hemodynamic compromise, airway obstruction, pulmonary artery obstruction, hemoptysis, and malignant degeneration. Symptomatic bronchogenic cysts should be removed. Traditionally, removal has been via posterolateral thoracotomy.[171] Resection of infected cysts may be quite difficult because of the presence of dense adhesions; elective removal often is recommended before infection has a chance to occur. Thoracoscopic exploration and resection are possible for small cysts with minimal adhesions. The goal of minimally invasive or open surgery should be complete removal of the cyst wall.

Enteric Cyst

Most clinicians agree that in contrast to bronchogenic cysts, esophageal cysts should be removed, regardless of the presence or absence of symptoms. Esophageal cysts have a propensity for serious complications secondary to enlargement, which leads to hemorrhage, infection, or perforation. Thus, surgical resection is the treatment of choice for both adults and children.

Thymic Cyst

Thymic cysts generally are asymptomatic and are discovered incidentally during radiographic work-up for an unrelated problem. Simple cysts are of no consequence; however, the occasional cystic neoplasm must be ruled out. Cystic components occasionally are seen in patients with thymoma and Hodgkin's disease.

Ectopic Endocrine Glands

Up to 5% of all mediastinal masses are estimated to be of thyroid origin. However, most of these masses are simple extensions of thyroid masses. They usually are nontoxic, and over 95% of such masses can be completely resected through a cervical approach. True ectopic thyroid tissue in the mediastinum is rare. Ten to 20% of abnormal parathyroid glands are found in the mediastinum; most can be removed during exploration from a cervical incision. In cases of true mediastinal parathyroid glands, thoracoscopic or open resection may be indicated. Location generally can be pinpointed by a combination of CT and sestamibi scanning.

Mediastinitis
Acute Mediastinitis

Acute mediastinitis is a fulminant infectious process that spreads along the fascial planes of the mediastinum. Infections originate most commonly from esophageal perforations, sternal infections, and oropharyngeal or neck infections, but a number of less common etiologic factors can lead to this deadly process (Table 19-33).

TABLE 19-33	Etiologic factors in acute mediastinitis

Esophageal perforation
  Iatrogenic
    Balloon dilatation (for achalasia)
    Bougienage (for peptic stricture)
    Esophagoscopy
    Sclerotherapy (for variceal bleeding)
  Spontaneous
    Postemetic (Boerhaave's syndrome)
    Straining during:
      Elimination
      Weight lifting
    Seizure
    Pregnancy
    Childbirth
  Ingestion of foreign bodies
  Trauma
    Blunt
    Penetrating
  Postsurgical
    Infection
    Anastomotic leak
  Erosion by cancer
Deep sternotomy wound infection
Oropharynx and neck infections
Ludwig's angina
Quinsy
Retropharyngeal abscess
Cellulitis and suppurative lymphadenitis of the neck
Infections of the lung and pleura
Subphrenic abscess
Rib or vertebral osteomyelitis
Hematogenous or metastatic abscess

Source: Reproduced with permission from Razzuk MA, et al: Infections of the mediastinum, in Pearson FG, et al (eds): *Thoracic Surgery*, 2nd ed. New York: Churchill Livingstone, 2002, p 1604. Copyright Elsevier.

As infections from any of these sources enter the mediastinum, spread may be rapid along the continuous fascial planes connecting the cervical and mediastinal compartments. Clinical signs and symptoms include fever, chest pain, dysphagia, respiratory distress, and cervical and upper thoracic subcutaneous crepitus. In severe cases, the clinical course can rapidly deteriorate to florid sepsis, hemodynamic instability, and death. Thus, a high index of suspicion is required in the context of any infection with access to the mediastinal compartments.

A chest CT scan can be particularly helpful in determining the extent of spread and the best approach to surgical drainage. Acute mediastinitis is a true surgical emergency, and treatment must be instituted immediately and must be aimed at correcting the primary problem, such as the esophageal perforation or oropharyngeal abscess. Another major concern is débridement and drainage of the spreading infectious process within the mediastinum, neck, pleura, and other tissue planes. Antibiotic administration, fluid resuscitation, and other supportive measures are important, but surgical correction of the problem at its source and open débridement of infected areas are critical measures. Surgical débridement may need to be repeated and other planes and cavities explored depending on the patient's clinical status. Blood cell counts and serial CT scans also may be required. Persistent sepsis or collections on CT scan may require further radical surgical débridement.

Chronic Mediastinitis

Sclerosing or fibrosing mediastinitis is a result of chronic inflammation of the mediastinum, most frequently as a result of granulomatous infections such as histoplasmosis or tuberculosis. The process begins in lymph nodes and continues as a chronic, low-grade inflammation leading to fibrosis and scarring. In many patients, the clinical manifestations are silent. However, if the fibrosis is progressive and severe, it may lead to encasement of the mediastinal structures, causing entrapment and compression of the low-pressure veins (including the superior vena cava and innominate and azygos veins). This fibrotic process can compromise other structures such as the esophagus and pulmonary arteries. There is no definitive treatment. Surgery is indicated only for diagnosis or in specific patients to relieve airway or esophageal obstruction or to achieve vascular reconstruction. Reports of palliative success with less invasive procedures (such as dilation and stenting of airways, the esophagus, or the superior vena cava) are promising. In one series of 22 patients, ketoconazole was effective in controlling progression.[172] In another series of 71 patients, 30% died during long-term follow-up. Chronic mediastinitis is similar to the fibrotic changes that occur in other sites, including retroperitoneal fibrosis, sclerosing cholangitis, and Riedel's thyroiditis.

PLEURA AND PLEURAL SPACE

Anatomy

The parietal pleura is a mesothelial lining of each hemithorax that invaginates at the hilum of each lung and continues on to cover each lung as the visceral pleura. Between these two surfaces is the potential pleural space, which is normally occupied only by a thin layer of lubricating pleural fluid. Two physiologic processes hold the visceral pleura of the lung in close apposition to the parietal pleura of the chest wall: those mechanisms that constantly remove pleural fluid and those that prevent an accumulation of free gas in the pleural space. A network of somatic, sympathetic, and parasympathetic fibers innervates the parietal pleura. Irritation of the parietal surface by inflammation, tumor invasion, trauma, and other processes can lead to a sensation of chest wall pain. The visceral pleura have no somatic innervation.[173,174]

Pleural Effusion

Pleural effusion refers to any significant collection of fluid within the pleural space. Normally, there is an ongoing balance between the flow of lubricating fluid into the pleural space and its continuous absorption. Between 5 and 10 L of fluid normally enters the pleural space daily by filtration through microvessels supplying the parietal pleura (located mainly in the less dependent regions of the cavity). The net balance of pressures in these capillaries leads to fluid flow from the parietal pleural surface into the pleural space, and the net balance of forces in the pulmonary circulation leads to absorption through the visceral pleura. Normally, 15 to 20 mL of pleural fluid is present at any given time. Any disturbance in these forces can lead to imbalance and accumulation of pleural fluid. Common pathologic conditions in North America that lead to pleural effusion include congestive heart failure, bacterial pneumonia, malignancy, and pulmonary emboli (Table 19-34).[175]

Diagnostic Work-Up

The initial diagnostic work-up for pleural effusion is guided in large part by the patient's history and findings of the physical examination. Bilateral pleural effusions are due to congestive heart failure in over 80% of patients. If the clinical history suggests this diagnosis, a trial of diuresis (rather than thoracentesis) may be indicated. Up to 75% of effusions due to congestive heart failure resolve within 48 hours with diuresis alone.

A patient presenting with cough, fever, leukocytosis, and unilateral infiltrate and effusion is likely to have a parapneumonic process. If the effusion is small and the patient responds to antibiotic therapy, a diagnostic thoracentesis may be unnecessary. However, a patient who has an obvious pneumonia and a large pleural effusion that is purulent and foul smelling has an empyema. Aggressive drainage

TABLE 19-34 Leading causes of pleural effusion in the United States, based on data from patients undergoing thoracentesis

Cause	Annual Incidence	Transudate	Exudate
Congestive heart failure	500,000	Yes	No
Pneumonia	300,000	No	Yes
Cancer	200,000	No	Yes
Pulmonary embolus	150,000	Sometimes	Sometimes
Viral disease	100,000	No	Yes
Coronary artery bypass surgery	60,000	No	Yes
Cirrhosis with ascites	50,000	Yes	No

with chest tubes is required, possibly with surgical intervention. Outside of the setting of congestive heart failure or small effusions associated with an improving pneumonia, most patients with pleural effusions of unknown cause should undergo thoracentesis.

A general classification of pleural fluid collections into transudates and exudates is helpful in understanding the various causes (Table 19-35). Transudates are protein-poor ultrafiltrates of plasma that form because of alterations in systemic hydrostatic pressures or colloid osmotic pressures (e.g., with congestive heart failure or cirrhosis). On gross visual inspection, a transudative effusion is generally clear or straw colored. Exudates are protein-rich pleural fluid collections that generally occur because of inflammation or invasion of the pleura by tumors. Grossly, they are often turbid, bloody, or purulent. Grossly bloody effusions in the absence of

trauma are frequently malignant but also may occur in the setting of a pulmonary embolism or pneumonia. Several criteria have traditionally been used to differentiate transudates from exudates. An effusion is considered exudative if the ratio of pleural fluid protein to serum protein is >0.5 and the LDH ratio is >0.6 or the absolute pleural LDH level is more than two thirds of the normal upper limit for serum. If these criteria suggest a transudate, the patient should be carefully evaluated for congestive heart failure, cirrhosis, and other conditions associated with transudative effusion.

If an exudative effusion is suggested, further diagnostic studies may be helpful. If total and differential cell counts reveal a predominance of neutrophils (>50% of cells), the effusion is likely to be associated with an acute inflammatory process (such as a parapneumonic effusion or empyema, pulmonary embolus, or pancreatitis). A predominance of mononuclear cells suggests a more chronic inflammatory process (such as cancer or tuberculosis). Gram's staining and culture should be performed, if possible with inoculation of fluid specimens into culture bottles at the bedside. Pleural fluid glucose levels are frequently decreased (<60 mg/dL) with complex parapneumonic effusions or malignant effusions. Cytologic testing should be done on exudative effusions to rule out an associated malignancy. Cytologic analysis is accurate in diagnosing >70% of malignant effusions associated with adenocarcinomas but is less sensitive for those associated with mesotheliomas (<10%), squamous cell carcinomas (20%), or lymphomas (25 to 50%). If the diagnosis remains uncertain after drainage and fluid analysis, thoracoscopy and direct biopsy are indicated. Tuberculous effusions can now be diagnosed accurately by measurement of increased levels of adenosine deaminase (>40 units/L) in the pleural fluid.[176,177] Pulmonary embolism should be suspected in a patient with a pleural effusion occurring in association with pleuritic chest pain, hemoptysis, or dyspnea out of proportion to the size of the effusion. These effusions may be transudative, but if an associated infarct occurs near the pleural

TABLE 19-35 Differential diagnosis of pleural effusions

I. Transudative pleural effusions
  A. Congestive heart failure
  B. Cirrhosis
  C. Nephrotic syndrome
  D. Superior vena caval obstruction
  E. Fontan procedure
  F. Urinothorax
  G. Peritoneal dialysis
  H. Glomerulonephritis
  I. Myxedema
  J. Cerebrospinal fluid leaks to pleura
  K. Hypoalbuminemia
  L. Pulmonary emboli
  M. Sarcoidosis
II. Exudative pleural effusions
  A. Neoplastic diseases
    1. Metastatic disease
    2. Mesothelioma
    3. Body cavity lymphoma
    4. Pyothorax-associated lymphoma
  B. Infectious diseases
    1. Tuberculosis
    2. Other bacterial infections
    3. Fungal infections
    4. Parasitic infections
    5. Viral infections
  C. Pulmonary embolization
  D. Gastrointestinal disease
    1. Pancreatic disease

    2. Subphrenic abscess
    3. Intrahepatic abscess
    4. Intrasplenic abscess
    5. Esophageal perforation
    6. After abdominal surgery
    7. Diaphragmatic hernia
    8. Endoscopic variceal sclerosis
    9. After liver transplantation
  E. Heart diseases
    1. After coronary artery bypass graft surgery
    2. Post–cardiac injury (Dressler's) syndrome
    3. Pericardial disease
  F. Obstetric and gynecologic diseases
    1. Ovarian hyperstimulation syndrome
    2. Fetal pleural effusion
    3. Postpartum pleural effusion
    4. Megis' syndrome
    5. Endometriosis
  G. Collagen vascular diseases
    1. Rheumatoid pleuritis
    2. Systemic lupus erythematosus
    3. Drug-induced lupus
    4. Immunoblastic lymphadenopathy
    5. Sjögren's syndrome
    6. Familial Mediterranean fever
    7. Churg-Strauss syndrome
    8. Wegeners granulomatosis
  H. Drug-induced pleural disease
    1. Nitrofurantoin

    2. Dantrolene
    3. Methysergide
    4. Ergot alkaloids
    5. Amiodarone
    6. Interleukin-2
    7. Procarbazine
    8. Methotrexate
    9. Clozapine
  I. Miscellaneous diseases and conditions
    1. Asbestos exposure
    2. After lung transplantation
    3. After bone marrow transplantation
    4. Yellow nail syndrome
    5. Sarcoidosis
    6. Uremia
    7. Trapped lung
    8. Therapeutic radiation exposure
    9. Drowning
    10. Amyloidosis
    11. Milk of calcium pleural effusion
    12. Electrical burns
    13. Extramedullary hematopoiesis
    14. Rupture of mediastinal cyst
    15. Acute respiratory distress syndrome
    16. Whipple's disease
    17. Iatrogenic pleural effusions
  J. Hemothorax
  K. Chylothorax

TABLE 19-36 Primary organ site or neoplasm type in male patients with malignant pleural effusions

Primary Site or Tumor Type	No. of Male Patients	Percentage of Male Patients
Lung	140	49.1
Lymphoma/leukemia	60	21.1
Gastrointestinal tract	20	7.0
Genitourinary tract	17	6.0
Melanoma	4	1.4
Miscellaneous less common tumors	10	3.5
Primary site unknown	31	10.9
Total	285	100

Source: Reproduced with permission from Johnston WW: The malignant pleural effusion: A review of cytopathologic diagnoses of 584 specimens from 472 consecutive patients. *Cancer* 56:905, 1985.

TABLE 19-37 Primary organ site or neoplasm type in female patients with malignant pleural effusions

Primary Site or Tumor Type	No. of Female Patients	Percentage of Female Patients
Breast	70	37.4
Female genital tract	38	20.3
Lung	28	15.0
Lymphoma	14	8.0
Gastrointestinal tract	8	4.3
Melanoma	6	3.2
Urinary tract	2	1.1
Miscellaneous less common tumors	3	1.6
Primary site unknown	17	9.1
Total	187	100.0

Source: Reproduced with permission from Johnston WW: The malignant pleural effusion: A review of cytopathologic diagnoses of 584 specimens from 472 consecutive patients. *Cancer* 56:905, 1985.

surface, an exudate may be seen. If a pulmonary embolism is suspected in a postoperative patient, most clinicians would obtain a spiral CT scan. Alternatively, duplex ultrasonography of the lower extremities may yield a diagnosis of deep vein thrombosis, which calls for anticoagulant therapy and precludes the need for a specific diagnosis of pulmonary embolism. In some patients, a blood test for levels of D-dimer may be helpful; if results of a sensitive D-dimer blood test are negative, pulmonary embolism may be ruled out.

Malignant Pleural Effusion

Malignant pleural effusions may occur in association with a number of different malignancies, most commonly lung cancer, breast cancer, and lymphomas, depending on the patient's age and gender (Tables 19-36 and 19-37).[178] Malignant effusions are exudative and often tinged with blood. An effusion in the setting of a malignancy means a more advanced stage of disease and generally indicates an unresectable tumor. Mean survival in such cases is 3 to 11 months. Occasionally, benign pleural effusions may be associated with a bronchogenic NSCLC, and surgical resection may still be indicated if the results of cytologic testing of the effusion is negative for malignancy. An important issue is the size of the effusion and the degree of dyspnea that results. Symptomatic, moderate to large effusions should be drained by chest tube, pigtail catheter, or VATS, followed by instillation of a sclerosing agent. Before the pleural cavity is sclerosed, whether by chest tube or VATS, the lung should be nearly fully expanded. Poor expansion of the lung (because of entrapment by tumor or adhesions) generally predicts a poor result with pleurodesis and is the primary indication for placement of indwelling pleural catheters. These catheters have dramatically changed the management of end-stage cancer treatment because they substantially shorten the amount of time patients spend in the hospital during their final weeks of life.[179] The choices for sclerosing agent include talc, bleomycin, and doxycycline. Success rates for controlling the effusion range from 60 to 90%, depending on the exact scope of the clinical study, the degree of lung expansion after the pleural fluid is drained, and the care with which the outcomes were reported. Figure 19-48 presents a decision algorithm for the management of malignant pleural effusion.

Empyema

Thoracic empyema is defined by a purulent pleural effusion. The most common causes are parapneumonic, but postsurgical or posttraumatic empyema also is common (Table 19-38). The finding of grossly purulent, foul-smelling pleural fluid makes the diagnosis of empyema obvious on visual examination at the bedside. In the early stage, small to moderate turbid pleural effusions in the setting of a pneumonic process may require further pleural fluid analysis. Close clinical follow-up also is imperative to determine if progression to empyema is occurring. A deteriorating clinical course or a

pleural pH of <7.20 and a glucose level of <40 mg/dL indicates the need to drain the fluid.

Patients of all ages can develop empyema, but the frequency is increased in older or debilitated patients. Common associated conditions include a pneumonic process in patients with pulmonary disorders and neoplasms, cardiac problems, diabetes mellitus, drug and alcohol abuse, neurologic impairments, postthoracotomy problems, and immunologic impairments. The mortality rate for empyema frequently depends on the degree of severity of the comorbidity; it may range from as low as 1% to >40% in immunocompromised patients.

Pathophysiology

The spectrum of organisms involved in pneumonic processes that progress to empyema is changing. Pneumococci and staphylococci continue to be the most common, but gram-negative aerobic bacteria and anaerobes are becoming more prevalent. Cases involving mycobacteria or fungi are rare. Multiple organisms may be isolated in up to 50% of patients, but cultures may be sterile if antibiotic therapy was initiated before specimens were obtained for culture or if the culture process was not efficient. Therefore, it is imperative that the choice of antibiotics be guided by the clinical scenario and not just the organisms found on culture. Broad-spectrum coverage may still be required even when cultures have failed to grow out an organism or when a single organism is grown but the clinical picture is more consistent with a multiorganism process. Commonly identified gram-negative organisms include *E. coli*, *Klebsiella* and *Pseudomonas* species, and Enterobacteriaceae. Anaerobic organisms may be fastidious and difficult to document by culture and are associated with infections in patients with periodontal diseases, aspiration syndromes, alcoholism or drug abuse, or gastroesophageal reflux as well as patients undergoing general anesthesia.

The route of organism entry into the pleural cavity may be by contiguous spread from pneumonia, lung abscess, liver abscess, or another infectious process with contact with the pleural space. Organisms also may enter the pleural cavity by direct contamination from thoracentesis, thoracic surgical procedures, esophageal injuries, or trauma.

As organisms enter the pleural space, an influx of polymorphonuclear cells occurs, with a subsequent release of inflammatory mediators and toxic oxygen radicals. In attempting to control the invading organisms, these mechanisms lead to variable degrees of endothelial injury and capillary instability. An influx of fluid into the pleural space then occurs, followed by a process that overwhelms the normal exit avenues of the pleural lymphatic network.

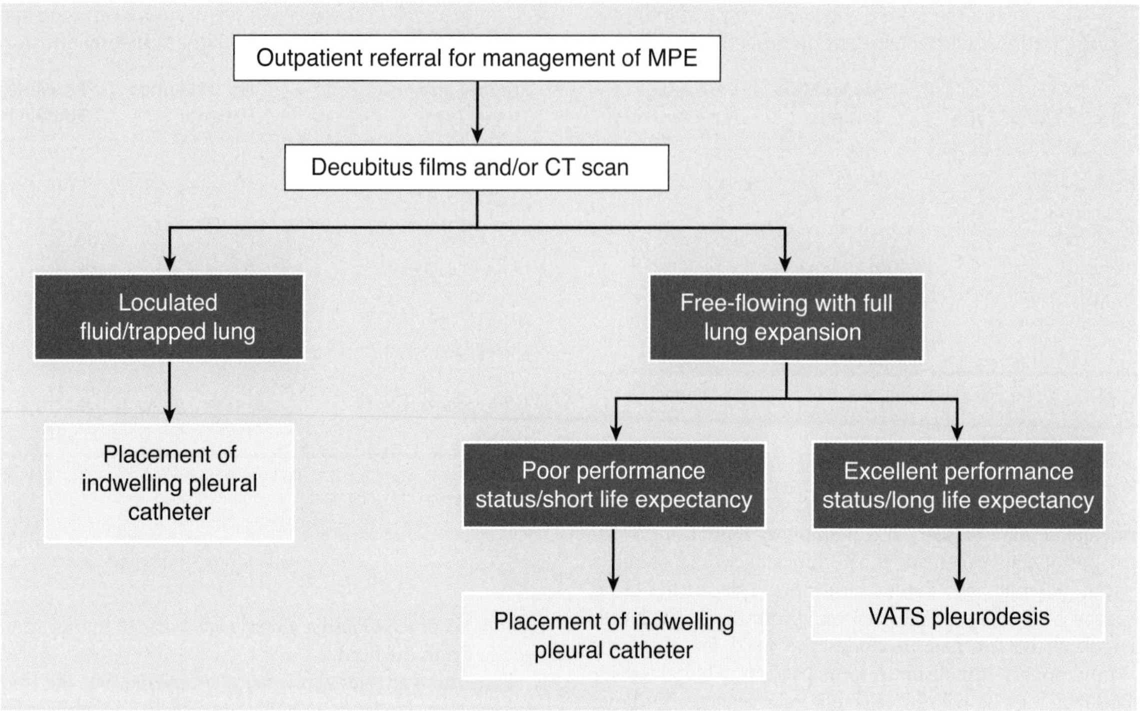

FIG. 19-48. Treatment decision algorithm for the management of malignant pleural effusion (MPE). CT = computed tomography; VATS = video-assisted thoracic surgery.

This early effusion is watery and free flowing in the pleural cavity. Thoracentesis at this stage yields fluid with a pH typically >7.3, a glucose level of >60 mg/dL, and a low LDH level (<500 units/L). At this stage, the decision to use antibiotics alone or to perform a repeat thoracentesis, chest tube drainage, thoracoscopy, or open thoracotomy depends on the amount of pleural fluid, its consistency, the clinical status of the patient, the degree of expansion of the lung after drainage, and the presence of loculated fluid in the pleural space (vs. free-flowing purulent fluid). If relatively thin, purulent pleural fluid is found early in the setting of a pneumonic process, the fluid often can be completely drained with simple large-bore thoracentesis. If complete lung expansion is obtained and the pneumonic process is responding to antibiotics, no further drainage may be necessary. A finding of pleural fluid with a pH <7.2 and with a low glucose level means that a more aggressive approach to drainage should be pursued.

The pleural fluid may become thick and loculated over the course of hours to days and may be associated with fibrinous adhesions (the fibrinopurulent stage). At this stage, chest tube insertion with closed-system drainage or drainage with thoracoscopy may be necessary to remove the fluid and adhesions and to allow complete lung expansion.[180] Further progression of the inflammatory process leads to the formation of a pleural peel, which may be flimsy and easy to remove early on. As the process progresses, however, a thick pleural rind may develop, leaving a trapped lung. Complete lung decortication by thoracotomy or, in some patients, thoracoscopy would then be necessary.

Management

If there is a residual space, persistent pleural infection is likely to occur. A persistent pleural space may be secondary to contracted, but intact, underlying lung; or it may be secondary to surgical lung resection. If the space is small and well drained by chest tubes, a conservative approach may be possible. This requires leaving the chest tubes in place and attached to closed-system drainage until symphysis of the visceral and parietal surfaces takes place. At this point, the chest tubes can be removed from suction. If the residual pleural space remains stable, the tubes can be cut and advanced out of the chest over the course of several weeks. If the patient's condition is stable, tube removal frequently can be done in the outpatient setting, guided by the degree of drainage and the size of the residual space visualized on serial CT scans. The presence of larger spaces may require open thoracotomy and decortication in an attempt to re-expand the lung to fill this residual space. If re-expansion fails or appears to carry too high a risk, then open drainage, rib resection, and prolonged packing may be required, with delayed closure with muscle flaps or thoracoplasty.[181] Most chronic pleural space problems can be avoided by early specialized thoracic surgical consultation and complete drainage of empyemas, which allows space obliteration by the reinflated lung.

Chylothorax

Chylothorax develops most commonly after surgical trauma to the thoracic duct or a major branch but may also be associated with a number of other conditions (Table 19-39).[182] It generally is unilateral; for example, it may occur on the right after esophagectomy, in which

| TABLE 19-38 | Pathogenesis of empyema |

Contamination from a source contiguous to the pleural space (50–60%)
　Lung
　Mediastinum
　Deep cervical area
　Chest wall and spine
　Subphrenic area
Direct inoculation of the pleural space (30–40%)
　Minor thoracic interventions
　Postoperative infections
　Penetrating chest injuries
Hematogenous infection of the pleural space from a distant site (<1%)

Source: Reproduced with permission from Paris F, et al: Empyema and bronchopleural fistula, in Pearson FG, et al (eds): *Thoracic Surgery*, 2nd ed. New York: Churchill Livingstone, 2002, p 1177. Copyright Elsevier.

TABLE 19-39 Etiology of chylothorax

Congenital
  Atresia of thoracic duct
  Thoracic duct–pleural space fistula
  Birth trauma
Traumatic and/or iatrogenic
  Blunt injury
  Penetrating injury
  Surgery
    Cervical
      Excision of lymph nodes
      Radical neck dissection
    Thoracic
      Correction of patent ductus arteriosus
      Correction of coarctation of the aorta
      Vascular procedure involving the origin of the left subclavian
        artery
      Esophagectomy
      Sympathectomy
      Resection of thoracic aneurysm
      Resection of mediastinal tumors
      Left pneumonectomy
    Abdominal
      Sympathectomy
      Radical lymph node dissection
    Diagnostic procedures
      Translumbar arteriography
      Subclavian vein catheterization
      Left-sided heart catheterization
Neoplasms
Infections
  Tuberculous lymphadenitis
  Nonspecific mediastinitis
  Ascending lymphangitis
  Filariasis
Miscellaneous
  Venous thrombosis
    Left subclavian-jugular vein
    Superior vena cava
  Pulmonary lymphangiomatosis

Source: Reproduced with permission from Cohen RG, et al: The pleura, in Sabiston DC, et al (eds): *Surgery of the Chest*, 6th ed. Philadelphia: Elsevier, 1995. Copyright Elsevier.

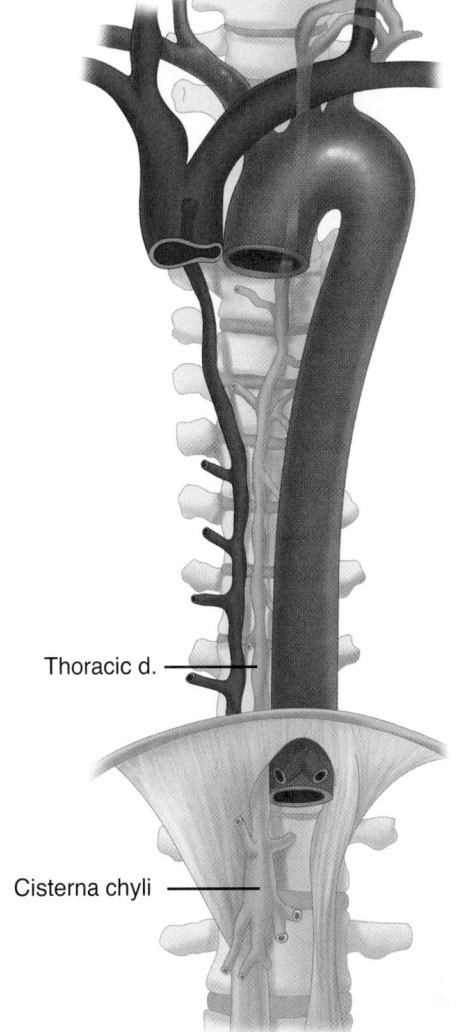

FIG. 19-49. Normal thoracic duct anatomy. The esophagus comes into close proximity to the thoracic duct (d.) as it enters the chest from its origin in the abdomen at the cisterna chyli.

the duct is most frequently injured during dissection of the distal esophagus. The esophagus comes into close proximity to the thoracic duct as it enters the chest from its origin in the abdomen at the cisterna chyli (Fig. 19-49). If the mediastinal pleura is disrupted on both sides, bilateral chylothoraces may occur. Left-sided chylothorax may develop after a left-sided neck dissection, especially in the region of the confluence of the subclavian and internal jugular veins. Chylothorax also may follow nonsurgical trauma, including penetrating or blunt injuries to the chest or neck area, central line placements, and other surgical misadventures. It is also seen in neonates, probably secondary to birth trauma. It may be seen in association with a variety of benign and malignant diseases that generally involve the lymphatic system of the mediastinum or neck. Given the significant variability of the course of the thoracic duct within the chest, some injuries are inevitable. The direct relationship of chylothorax to a surgical procedure, traumatic event, or neoplastic process may not always be obvious. Understanding the anatomy and course of the thoracic duct and some of its more common variants is helpful.

Pathophysiology

Most commonly, the thoracic duct originates in the abdomen from the cisterna chyli, which is located in the midline, near the level of the second lumbar vertebra. From this origin, the thoracic duct ascends into the chest through the aortic hiatus at the level of T10 to T12 and courses just to the right of the aorta (see Fig. 19-49). As the thoracic duct courses cephalad above the diaphragm, it most commonly remains in the right chest, lying just behind the esophagus, between the aorta and azygos vein. The duct continues superiorly, lying just to the right of the vertebral column. Then, at about the level of the fifth or sixth thoracic vertebra, it crosses behind the aorta and the aortic arch into the left posterior mediastinum. From this location, it again courses superiorly, staying near the esophagus and mediastinal pleura as it exits the thoracic inlet. As it exits the thoracic inlet, it passes just to the left, just behind the carotid sheath and anterior to the inferior thyroid and vertebral bodies. Just medial to the anterior scalene muscle, it courses inferiorly and drains into the union of the internal jugular and subclavian veins. Given the extreme variability in the position of the main duct and its branches, accumulation of chyle in the chest or flow from penetrating wounds may be seen in association with a variety of traumatic events and medical conditions.[183]

The main function of the duct is to transport fat absorbed from the digestive system. The composition of normal chyle is fat, with variable amounts of protein and lymphatic material (Table 19-40). Given the high volumes of chyle that flow through the thoracic duct,

TABLE 19-40 Composition of chyle

Component	Amount (per 100 mL)
Total fat	0.4–5 g
Total cholesterol	65–220 mg
Total protein	2.21–5.9 g
Albumin	1.1–4.1 g
Globulin	1.1–3.1 g
Fibrinogen	16–24 g
Sugars	48–200 g
Electrolytes	Similar to levels in plasma
Cellular elements	
Lymphocytes	400–6800/mm³
Erythrocytes	50–600/mm³
Antithrombin globulin	>25% of plasma concentration
Prothrombin	>25% of plasma concentration
Fibrinogen	>25% of plasma concentration

Source: Reproduced with permission from Miller.[182] Copyright Elsevier.

significant injuries can cause leaks in excess of 2 L/d. If this leakage is left untreated, protein, volume, and lymphocyte depletion can lead to serious metabolic effects and death. The diagnosis generally requires thoracentesis, the results of which may be grossly suggestive; often the pleural fluid is milky and nonpurulent. However, if the patient is under *nil per os* (nothing by mouth, or NPO) orders, the pleural fluid may not be grossly abnormal. Laboratory analysis of the pleural fluid shows a high lymphocyte count and high triglyceride levels. If the triglyceride level is >110 mg/100 mL, a chylothorax is almost certainly present (99% accuracy rate). If the triglyceride level is <50 mg/100 mL, there is only a 5% chance of chylothorax. In many clinical situations, the accumulation of chyle may be slow because minimal digestive fat is flowing through the GI tract after major trauma or surgery, so the diagnosis may be more difficult to establish.

Management

The treatment plan for any chylothorax depends on its cause, the amount of drainage, and the clinical status of the patient (Fig. 19-50). In general, the treatment for most patients is a short period of chest tube drainage, NPO orders, TPN, and observation. Chest cavity drainage must be adequate to allow complete lung re-expansion. The use of somatostatin has been advocated by some authors, with variable results.[184] If significant chyle drainage (>500 mL/d in an adult, >100 mL/d in an infant) continues despite TPN and good lung expansion, early surgical ligation of the duct is recommended. Ligation can be approached best by right thoracotomy and, in some experienced centers, by right VATS. Chylothoraces due to malignant conditions often respond to radiotherapy and/or chemotherapy and less commonly require surgical ligation. Untreated chylothoraces are associated with significant nutritional and immunologic depletion that leads to significant mortality. Before the introduction of surgical ligation of the thoracic duct, the mortality rate from chylothorax exceeded 50%. With the availability of TPN for nutritional supplementation and surgical ligation for persistent leaks, the mortality rate of chylothorax is <10%.

Access and Drainage of Pleural Fluid Collections
Approaches and Techniques

Once the decision is made to invasively access a pleural effusion, the next step is to determine if a sample of the fluid is required or if complete drainage of the pleural space is desired. This step is influenced by the clinical history, the type and amount of fluid present, the nature of the collection (such as free flowing or loculated), the cause, and the likelihood of recurrence. For small, free-flowing effusions, outpatient thoracentesis with a relatively small-bore needle or catheter (14- to 16-gauge) can be performed (Fig. 19-51). This approach

can be used to sample fluid or to completely drain free-flowing pleural effusions. Fluid should be grossly examined as it is drained. Clear straw-colored fluid is often transudative; turbid or bloody fluid is often exudative.

The site of entry for drainage of a pleural effusion or pneumothorax may be based on the chest radiograph alone if the effusion is demonstrated to be free flowing. For large, free-flowing effusions, a low posterolateral approach at the eighth or ninth intercostal space affords good access. If the effusion is more complex with loculations, an approach guided by CT scan or ultrasound may be indicated. If complete drainage is the goal and the fluid is nonbloody and nonviscous, a small-bore (14- to 16-gauge) pigtail catheter is inserted and connected to a closed drainage system with applied suction (typically –20 cm H_2O) or water seal. If the fluid is bloody or turbid, a larger-diameter drainage tube (such as a 28F chest tube) may be required. In general, the smallest-bore drainage catheter that will effectively drain the pleural space should be chosen. The use of smaller-diameter catheters significantly decreases the pain associated with the placement of chest tubes.[185,186] For clinical situations requiring biopsy or for potential interventions such as adhesiolysis or pleurodesis, minimally invasive surgery using a VATS approach may be indicated.

Complications of Pleural Drainage

The most common complication of invasive procedures to access the pleural space is inadvertent access to another cavity or organ. Examples include puncture of the underlying lung, with air leakage and pneumothorax; subdiaphragmatic entry, with damage to the liver, spleen, or other intra-abdominal viscera; bleeding secondary to intercostal vessel injury or, most commonly, larger vessel injury; and even cardiac puncture. Sometimes bleeding may be the result of an underlying coagulopathy or anticoagulant therapy. Other technical complications include loss of a catheter, guidewire, or fragment in the pleural space, and infections. Occasionally, rapid drainage of a large effusion can be followed by shortness of breath, clinical instability, and a phenomenon referred to as *postexpansion pulmonary edema*. For this reason, it is recommended to drain only up to 1 L initially. Most complications can be avoided by consulting with a clinician experienced in pleural drainage techniques.

Tumors of the Pleura
Malignant Mesothelioma

Malignant mesothelioma is the most common type of tumor of the pleura. The annual incidence in the United States is approximately 3000 cases. Other tumors of the pleura are much less common and include benign and malignant fibrous tumors of the pleura, lipomas, and cysts. In 20% of malignant mesotheliomas, the tumor arises from the peritoneum. Exposure to asbestos is the major known risk factor and can be established in over 50% of patients. Geographic areas of increased incidence are frequently the sites of industries using asbestos in the manufacturing process, such as shipbuilding. The risk extends beyond the worker directly exposed to the asbestos; family members exposed to the dust from clothing or the work environment are also at risk. Other risk factors have been identified, including exposure to fibers with physical properties similar to those of amphibole and exposure to radiation. Cigarette smoking does not appear to increase the risk of malignant mesothelioma, even though asbestos exposure and smoking synergistically increase the risk for lung cancer. Malignant mesotheliomas have a male predominance of 2:1 and are most common after the age of 40.

Pathophysiology The exact etiologic role of asbestos fibers has not been elucidated; however, the physical characteristics of specific fibers (referred to as *serpentine* or *amphibole*) have been shown to be important. The serpentine fibers are large and curly and generally are not able to travel beyond larger airways. However, the narrow, straight amphibole fibers, in particular the crocidolite fibers, may navigate distally into the pulmonary parenchyma and are most clearly associated with mesotheliomas. The latency period between asbestos

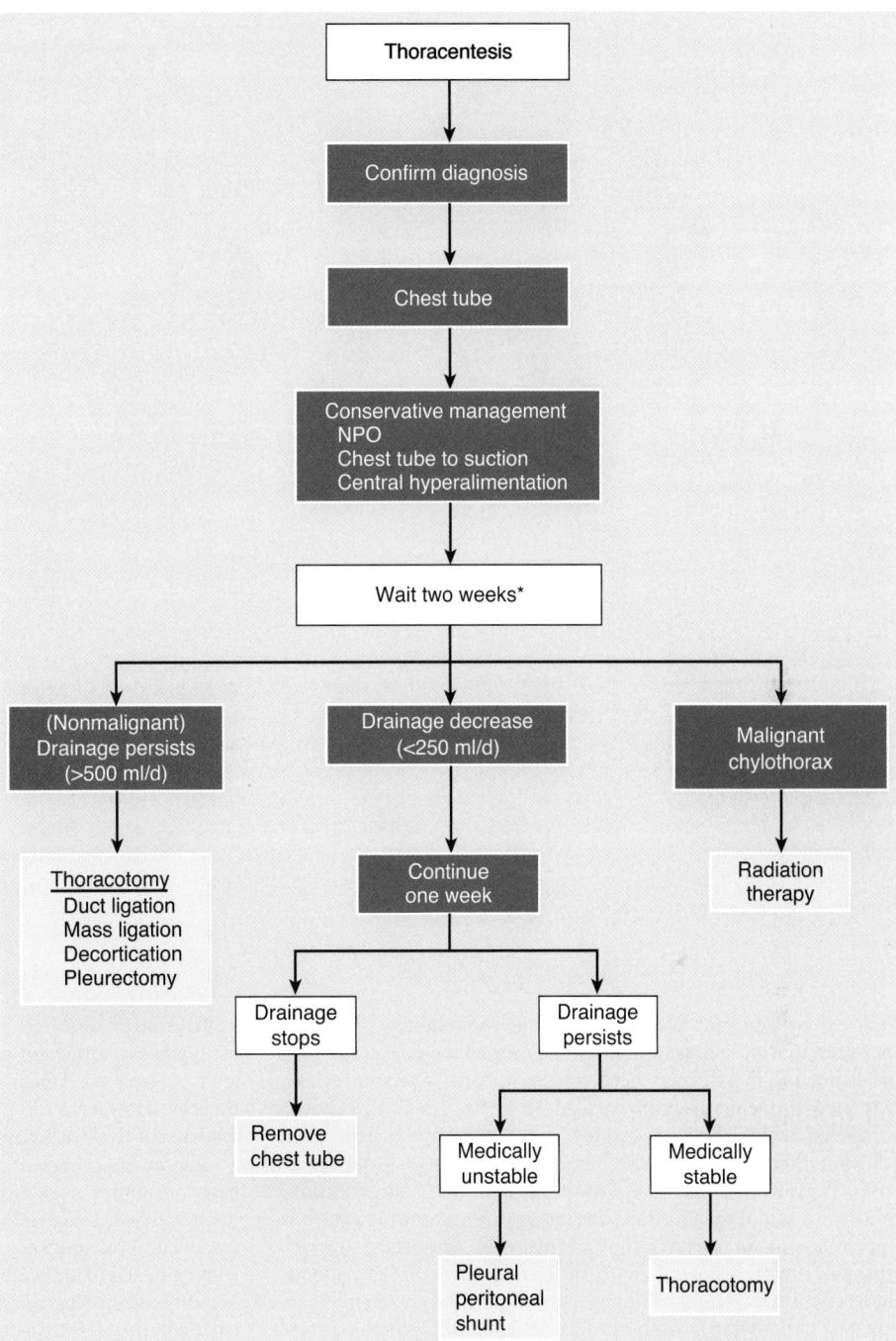

FIG. 19-50. Algorithm for the management of chylothorax. *If high output persists (>50 mL/d), early surgical ligation of the thoracic duct may be considered. NPO = nothing by mouth.

exposure and the development of mesothelioma is at least 20 years. The tumor generally is multicentric, with multiple pleura-based nodules coalescing to form sheets of tumor. This process initially involves the parietal pleura, generally with early spread to the visceral surfaces and with a variable degree of invasion of surrounding structures. Autopsy studies have shown that most patients have distant metastases, but the natural history of the disease in untreated patients culminates in death due to local extension.

Clinical Presentation Most patients present with dyspnea and chest pain. Over 90% have a pleural effusion. Results of thoracentesis are diagnostic in <10% of patients. Frequently, thoracoscopy or open pleural biopsy with special staining of tumor samples is required to differentiate mesotheliomas from adenocarcinomas (Table 19-41). Once the diagnosis is confirmed, cell types can be distinguished (e.g., epithelial, sarcomatous, and mixed). Epithelial types are associated with a more favorable prognosis, and in some

patients long-term survival may be seen with no treatment. Sarcomatous and mixed tumors share a more aggressive course.

Management The treatment of malignant mesotheliomas remains controversial. It has been the subject of a number of recent clinical trials, the vast majority showing limited success.[187] A new staging system has been devised that has clearly shown prognostic value (Table 19-42).[188] However, although prognosis does depend on the stage of the disease, the problem is that many patients present with advanced local or distant disease beyond curative potential. Treatment options include supportive care only, surgical resection, and multimodality approaches (using a combination of surgery, chemotherapy, and radiation therapy).

Surgical options include palliative approaches such as pleurectomy or talc pleurodesis. Palliative approaches may lead to local control and a modest improvement in short-term survival. More radical surgical approaches (such as extrapleural pneumonectomy

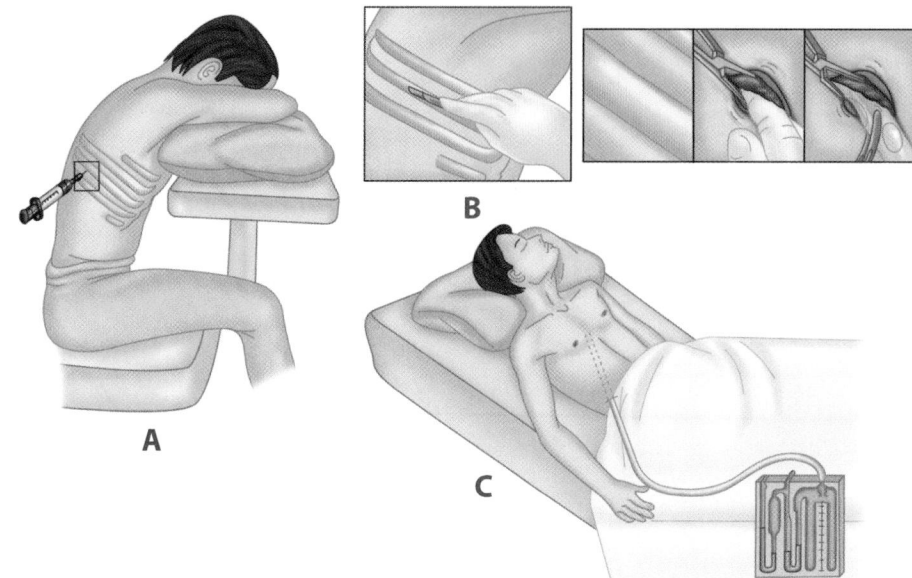

FIG. 19-51. Techniques for aspiration and drainage of a pleural effusion. **A.** Needle aspiration. With careful appraisal of the radiographic findings, the best interspace is selected, and fluid is aspirated with a needle and syringe. Large volumes of fluid can be removed with a little patience and a large-bore needle. **B.** Chest tube insertion. After careful skin preparation, draping, and administration of local anesthesia, a short skin incision is made over the correct interspace. The incision is deepened into the intercostal muscles, and the pleura is penetrated (usually with a clamp). When any doubt exists about the status of the pleural space at the site of puncture, the wound is enlarged bluntly to admit a finger, which can be swept around the immediately adjacent pleural space to assess the situation and break down any adhesions. The tube is inserted, with the tip directed toward the optimal position suggested by the chest radiographs. In general, a high anterior tube is best for air (pneumothorax) and a low posterior tube is best for fluid. A 28 to 32F tube is adequate for most situations. A 36F tube is preferred for hemothorax or for a viscous empyema. Many surgeons prefer a very small tube (16F to 20F) for drainage of simple pneumothorax. **C.** The tube is connected to a water-seal drainage system. Suction is added, if necessary, to expand the lung. Suction usually will be required in a patient with a substantial air leak (bronchopleural fistula).

followed by adjuvant chemotherapy and radiotherapy) have an increased morbidity rate; moreover, the mortality rate exceeds 10% in all but the most experienced centers. In one Japanese review, extrapleural pneumonectomy yielded no improvement in survival compared with debulking surgery and showed no benefit over adjuvant therapy: the overall 5-year survival in all groups was <10%.[189] However, several reports of trials of radical surgery combined with multimodality adjuvant therapy have shown reasonable improvements in survival for patients with early-stage tumors (compared with historical controls). In one series of 183 patients undergoing extrapleural pneumonectomy and adjuvant chemotherapy and radiotherapy, a subset of 31 patients had favorable prognostic features (i.e., tumors of the epithelial cell type, negative resection margins, and negative extrapleural node status). This patient subset with favorable indicators had a 5-year survival rate of 46%, compared with 15% for the entire group.[190]

In another series, 88 patients with mesotheliomas were studied prospectively. Adjuvant radiation therapy was given to 54 patients after extrapleural pneumonectomy; the median survival was 17 months. However, for patients with stage I and II disease, the median survival was significantly longer at 33.0 months.[191]

The authors' current approach to malignant mesotheliomas is based on tumor stage and pulmonary performance status. For patients with early-stage mesotheliomas and good pulmonary function, extrapleural pneumonectomy is recommended, especially for those with epithelial mesotheliomas. Patients are referred for clinical trials of multimodality therapy, if available. If disease is more advanced, or if patients have less than optimal pulmonary function or performance status, talc pleurodesis or supportive therapy is recommended.

Intrapleural therapy has been explored to improve the locoregional control of malignant mesotheliomas. In a phase II trial, 37 patients underwent pleurectomy with decortication, followed by intrapleural and systemic therapy with cisplatin and mitomycin C. Their median survival was 17 months, with a locoregional recurrence rate of 80%.[192] According to another study, the addition of hyperthermic intrapleural perfusion seems to be pharmacokinetically advantageous; of seven patients, three underwent pleurectomy with decortication and received hyperthermic cisplatin. Systemic drug concentrations were greater after pleurectomy with decortication than after pleuropneumonectomy. The ratio of local tissue platinum concentration to perfusate platinum concentration tended to be higher after hyperthermic perfusion than after normothermic perfusion.[193]

Another promising alternative to enhance the local efficacy of chemotherapy against malignant mesotheliomas is L-NDDP (cis-bis-neodecanoato-trans-R,R-1,2-diaminocyclohexane platinum), a new lipophilic cisplatin analogue produced by the University of Texas M. D. Anderson Cancer Center in Houston, Texas. A phase

TABLE 19-41	Differentiation of mesothelioma from adenocarcinoma	
	Mesothelioma	**Adenocarcinoma**
Immunohistochemical results		
Carcinoembryonic antigen	Negative	Positive
Vimentin	Positive	Negative
Low molecular weight cytokeratins	Positive	Negative
Electron microscopic features	Long, sinuous villi	Short, straight villi with fuzzy glycocalyx

TABLE 19-42 International Mesothelioma Interest Group staging system for diffuse malignant pleural mesothelioma

T Tumor

T1	T1a	Tumor limited to the ipsilateral parietal ± mediastinal ± diaphragmatic pleura	
		No involvement of the visceral pleura	
	T1b	Tumor involving the ipsilateral parietal ± mediastinal ± diaphragmatic pleura	
		Tumor also involving the visceral pleura	

T2   Tumor involving each of the ipsilateral pleural surfaces (parietal, mediastinal, diaphragmatic, and visceral pleurae) with at least one of the following features:
> Involvement of diaphragmatic muscle
> Extension of tumor from visceral pleura into the underlying pulmonary parenchyma

T3   Describes locally advanced but potentially resectable tumor
Tumor involving all of the ipsilateral pleural surfaces (parietal, mediastinal, diaphragmatic, and visceral pleurae) with at least one of the following features:
> Involvement of the endothoracic fascia
> Extension into the mediastinal fat
> Solitary, completely resectable focus of tumor extending into the soft tissues of the chest wall
> Nontransmural involvement of the pericardium

T4   Describes locally advanced technically unresectable tumor
Tumor involving all of the ipsilateral pleural surfaces (parietal, mediastinal, diaphragmatic, and visceral pleurae) with at least one of the following features:
> Diffuse extension or multifocal masses of tumor in the chest wall, with or without associated rib destruction
> Direct transdiaphragmatic extension of tumor to the peritoneum
> Direct extension of tumor to the contralateral pleura
> Direct extension of tumor to mediastinal organs
> Direct extension of tumor into the spine
> Tumor extending through to the internal surface of the pericardium with or without a pericardial effusion; or tumor involving the myocardium

N Lymph Nodes

NX	Regional lymph nodes cannot be assessed
N0	No regional lymph node metastasis
N1	Metastases in the ipsilateral bronchopulmonary or hilar lymph nodes
N2	Metastases in the subcarinal or the ipsilateral mediastinal lymph nodes including the ipsilateral internal mammary nodes
N3	Metastases in the contralateral mediastinal, contralateral internal mammary, or ipsilateral or contralateral supraclavicular lymph nodes

M Metastases

MX	Presence of distant metastases cannot be assessed
M0	No distant metastases
M1	Distant metastases present

Staging

Stage I			
IA	T1a	N0	M0
IB	T1b	N0	M0
Stage II	T2	N0	M0
Stage III	Any T3	Any N1	M0
		Any N2	
Stage IV	Any T4	Any N3	Any M1

Source: Reproduced with permission from International Mesothelioma Interest Group: A proposed new international TNM staging system for malignant pleural mesothelioma. *Chest* 108:1122, 1995.

II trial of L-NDDP enrolled 38 patients to receive a thoracoscopic biopsy and cytologic examination before and after treatment. Of the 33 patients who received treatment, 14 (42%) had a complete pathologic response; of the patients with positive cytologic results, 18 (78%) had a complete cytologic response.[194]

Fibrous Tumors of the Pleura

Fibrous tumors of the pleura are unrelated to asbestos exposure or malignant mesotheliomas. They generally occur as a single pedunculated mass arising from the visceral pleura. Frequently, they are discovered incidentally on routine chest radiographs without an associated pleural effusion. Fibrous tumors of the pleura may be benign or malignant. Symptoms such as cough, chest pain, and dyspnea occur in 30 to 40% of patients. Less common are fever, hypertrophic pulmonary osteoarthropathy, hemoptysis, and hy-poglycemia. Hypoglycemia occurs in only approximately 4% of patients and resolves with surgical resection, as do the other symptoms. Given the localized, pedunculated nature of both benign and malignant fibrous tumors of the pleura, most are cured by complete surgical resection. Incompletely resected malignant tumors may recur locally or metastasize; frequently, they are fatal within 2 to 5 years.[195]

ACKNOWLEDGMENT

The authors wish to thank Shannon Wyszomierski and Holly Rorabaugh for their invaluable help in compiling this chapter for the ninth edition. The authors also express appreciation to their spouses, Chris and Lee.

REFERENCES

Entries highlighted in bright blue are key references.

1. Cusimano RJ, Pearson FG: Anatomy, physiology, and embryology of the upper airway, in Pearson FG, et al (ed): *Thoracic Surgery*, 2nd ed. New York: Churchill Livingstone, 2002, p 215.

2. Grillo HC: Surgical treatment of postintubation tracheal injuries. *J Thorac Cardiovasc Surg* 8:860, 1979.

3. Couraud L, Ballester MJ, Delaisement C: Acquired tracheoesophageal fistula and its management. *Semin Thorac Cardiovasc Surg* 8:392, 1996.

4. Mathisen DJ, Grillo HC, Wain JC, et al: Management of acquired nonmalignant tracheoesophageal fistula. *Ann Thorac Surg* 52:759, 1991.

5. Bhattacharyya N: Contemporary staging and prognosis for primary tracheal malignancies: A population-based analysis. *Otolaryngol Head Neck Surg* 131:639, 2004.

6. Gaissert HA, Grillo HC, Shadmehr MB, et al: Uncommon primary tracheal tumors. *Ann Thorac Surg* 82:268, 2006.

7. Regnard JF, Fourquier P, Levasseur P: Results and prognostic factors in resections of primary tracheal tumors: A multicenter retrospective study. The French Society of Cardiovascular Surgery. *J Thorac Cardiovasc Surg* 111:808; discussion 813, 1996.

8. Chow DC, Komaki R, Libshitz HI, et al: Treatment of primary neoplasms of the trachea. The role of radiation therapy. *Cancer* 71:2946, 1993.

9. Rice TW: Anatomy of the lung, in Pearson FG, et al (ed): *Thoracic Surgery,* 2nd ed. New York: Churchill Livingstone, 2002, p 427.

10. Remy-Jardin M, Remy J, Giraud F, et al: Pulmonary nodules: Detection with thick-section spiral CT versus conventional CT. *Radiology* 187:513, 1993.

11. Naidich DP: Helical computed tomography of the thorax: Clinical applications. *Radiol Clin North Am* 32:759, 1994.

12. Kent MS, Schuchert M, Fernando H, et al: Minimally invasive esophagectomy: State of the art. *Dis Esophagus* 19:137, 2006.

13. Swanson SJ, Herndon JE 2nd, D'Amico TA, et al: Video-assisted thoracic surgery lobectomy: Report of CALGB 39802—a prospective, multi-institution feasibility study. *J Clin Oncol* 25:4993, 2007.

14. Demmy TL, James TA, Swanson SJ, et al: Troubleshooting video-assisted thoracic surgery lobectomy. *Ann Thorac Surg* 79:1744; discussion 1753, 2005.

15. Cerfolio RJ, Bryant AS: Results of a prospective algorithm to remove chest tubes after pulmonary resection with high output. *J Thorac Cardiovasc Surg* 135:269, 2008.

16. Cerfolio RJ, Bass C, Katholi CR: Prospective randomized trial compares suction versus water seal for air leaks. *Ann Thorac Surg* 71:1613, 2001.

17. Bauer C, Hentz JG, Ducrocq X, et al: Lung function after lobectomy: A randomized, double-blinded trial comparing thoracic epidural ropivacaine/sufentanil and intravenous morphine for patient-controlled analgesia. *Anesth Analg* 105:238, 2007.

18. Casati A, Alessandrini P, Nuzzi M, et al: A prospective, randomized, blinded comparison between continuous thoracic paravertebral and epidural infusion of 0.2% ropivacaine after lung resection surgery. *Eur J Anaesthesiol* 23:999, 2006.

19. Gould MK, Fletcher J, Iannettoni MD, et al: Evaluation of patients with pulmonary nodules: When is it lung cancer? ACCP evidence-based clinical practice guidelines (2nd edition). *Chest* 132(3 Suppl):108S, 2007.

20. Comstock GW, Vaughan RH, Montgomery G: Outcome of solitary pulmonary nodules discovered in an x-ray screening program. *N Engl J Med* 254:1018, 1956.

21. Good CA, Wilson TW: The solitary circumscribed pulmonary nodule; study of seven hundred five cases encountered roentgenologically in a period of three and one-half years. *J Am Med Assoc* 166:210, 1958.

22. Henschke CI, McCauley DI, Yankelevitz DF, et al: Early Lung Cancer Action Project: Overall design and findings from baseline screening. *Lancet* 354:99, 1999.

23. Marten K, Grabbe E: The challenge of the solitary pulmonary nodule: Diagnostic assessment with multislice spiral CT. *Clin Imaging* 27:156, 2003.

24. Detterbeck FC, Gibson CJ: Turning gray: The natural history of lung cancer over time. *J Thorac Oncol* 3:781, 2008.

25. Yankelevitz DF, Henschke CI: Does 2-year stability imply that pulmonary nodules are benign? *AJR Am J Roentgenol* 168:325, 1997.

26. Stroobants S, Verschakelen J, Vansteenkiste J: Value of FDG-PET in the management of non-small cell lung cancer. *Eur J Radiol* 45:49, 2003.

27. Gould MK, Maclean CC, Kuschner WG, et al: Accuracy of positron emission tomography for diagnosis of pulmonary nodules and mass lesions: A meta-analysis. *JAMA* 285:914, 2001.

28. Ost D, Fein AM, Feinsilver SH: Clinical practice. The solitary pulmonary nodule. *N Engl J Med* 348:2535, 2003.

29. Cardillo G, Regal M, Sera F, et al: Videothoracoscopic management of the solitary pulmonary nodule: a single-institution study on 429 cases. *Ann Thorac Surg* 75:1607, 2003.

30. Espey DK, Wu XC, Swan J, et al: Annual report to the nation on the status of cancer, 1975–2004, featuring cancer in American Indians and Alaska Natives. *Cancer* 110:2119, 2007.

31. Mulligan CR, Meram AD, Proctor CD, et al: Unlimited access to care: Effect on racial disparity and prognostic factors in lung cancer. *Cancer Epidemiol Biomarkers Prev* 15:25, 2006.

32. Samet JM: Health benefits of smoking cessation. *Clin Chest Med* 12:669, 1991.

33. Sun S, Schiller JH, Gazdar AF: Lung cancer in never smokers—a different disease. *Nat Rev Cancer* 7:778, 2007.

34. Hackshaw AK, Law MR, Wald NJ: The accumulated evidence on lung cancer and environmental tobacco smoke. *BMJ* 315:980, 1997.

35. Jeremy George P, Banerjee AK, et al: Surveillance for the detection of early lung cancer in patients with bronchial dysplasia. *Thorax* 62:43, 2007.

36. Wang GF, Lai MD, Yang RR, et al: Histological types and significance of bronchial epithelial dysplasia. *Mod Pathol* 19:429, 2006.

37. Gould VE, Warren WH: Epithelial tumors of the lung. *Chest Surg Clin N Am* 10:709, 2000.

38. Barrera R, Shi W, Amar D, et al: Smoking and timing of cessation: Impact on pulmonary complications after thoracotomy. *Chest* 127:1977, 2005.

39. Cerilli LA, Ritter JH, Mills SE, et al: Neuroendocrine neoplasms of the lung. *Am J Clin Pathol* 116 Suppl:S65, 2001.

40. Rivera MP, Mehta AC: Initial diagnosis of lung cancer: ACCP evidence-based clinical practice guidelines (2nd edition). *Chest* 132(3 Suppl):131S, 2007.

41. Dwamena BA, Sonnad SS, Angobaldo JO, et al: Metastases from non-small cell lung cancer: Mediastinal staging in the 1990s—meta-analytic comparison of PET and CT. *Radiology* 213:530, 1999.

42. Toloza EM, Harpole L, McCrory DC: Noninvasive staging of non-small cell lung cancer: A review of the current evidence. *Chest* 123(1Suppl):137S, 2003.

43. Goldberg M, Unger M: Lung cancer. Diagnostic tools. *Chest Surg Clin N Am* 10:763, 2000.

44. Saunders CA, Dussek JE, O'Doherty MJ, et al: Evaluation of fluorine-18-fluorodeoxyglucose whole body positron emission tomography imaging in the staging of lung cancer. *Ann Thorac Surg* 67:790, 1999.

45. Weder W, Schmid RA, Bruchhaus H, et al: Detection of extrathoracic metastases by positron emission tomography in lung cancer. *Ann Thorac Surg* 66:886, 1998.

46. Rao J, Abella-Columna E, Pounds TR, et al: Prevalence of metastatic disease and impact of PET on management in staging lung cancer: a clinical series of 400 patients. *J Nucl Med* 41 Suppl:75P, 2000.

47. Nakagawa M, Tanaka H, Tsukuma H, et al: Relationship between the duration of the preoperative smoke-free period and the incidence of postoperative pulmonary complications after pulmonary surgery. *Chest* 120:705, 2001.

48. Colice GL, Shafazand S, Griffin JP, et al: Physiologic evaluation of the patient with lung cancer being considered for resectional surgery: ACCP evidenced-based clinical practice guidelines (2nd edition). *Chest* 132(3 Suppl):161S, 2007.

49. Ou SH, Zell JA, Ziogas A, et al: Prognostic factors for survival of stage I nonsmall cell lung cancer patients: A population-based analysis of 19,702 stage I patients in the California Cancer Registry from 1989 to 2003. *Cancer* 110:1532, 2007.

50. Ou SH, Zell JA, Ziogas A, et al: Prognostic significance of the non-size-based AJCC T2 descriptors: Visceral pleura invasion, hilar atelectasis, or obstructive pneumonitis in stage IB non-small cell lung cancer is dependent on tumor size. *Chest* 133:662, 2008.

51. Goldstraw P, Crowley J, Chansky K, et al: The IASLC Lung Cancer Staging Project: Proposals for the revision of the TNM stage groupings in the forthcoming (seventh) edition of the TNM classification of malignant tumours. *J Thorac Oncol* 2:706, 2007.

52. Groome PA, Bolejack V, Crowley JJ, et al: The IASLC Lung Cancer Staging Project: Validation of the proposals for revision of the T, N, and M descriptors and consequent stage groupings in the forthcoming (seventh) edition of the TNM classification of malignant tumours. *J Thorac Oncol* 2:694, 2007.

53. Shepherd FA, Crowley J, Van Houtte P, et al: The International Association for the Study of Lung Cancer lung cancer staging project: Proposals regarding the clinical staging of small cell lung cancer in the forthcoming (seventh) edition of the tumor, node, metastasis classification for lung cancer. *J Thorac Oncol* 2:1067, 2007.

54. Zell JA, Ignatius Ou SH, Ziogas A, et al: Validation of the proposed International Association for the Study of Lung Cancer non–small cell lung cancer staging system revisions for advanced bronchioloalveolar carcinoma using data from the California Cancer Registry. *J Thorac Oncol* 2:1078, 2007.

55. Naruke T, Suemasu K, Ishikawa S: Lymph node mapping and curability at various levels of metastasis in resected lung cancer. *J Thorac Cardiovasc Surg* 76:832, 1978.

56. Mountain CF, Dresler CM: Regional lymph node classification for lung cancer staging. *Chest* 111:1718, 1997.

57. American Thoracic Society. Medical section of the American Lung Association. Clinical staging of primary lung cancer. *Am Rev Respir Dis* 127:659, 1983.

58. Mountain CF: A new international staging system for lung cancer. *Chest* 89(4 Suppl):225S, 1986.

59. Mountain CF: Revisions in the International System for Staging Lung Cancer. *Chest* 111:1710, 1997.

60. Raz DJ, Zell JA, Ou SH, et al: Natural history of stage I non–small cell lung cancer: Implications for early detection. *Chest* 132:193, 2007.

61. Pancoast HK: Superior pulmonary sulcus tumor: Tumor characterized by pain, Horner's syndrome, destruction of bone and atrophy of hand muscles. *JAMA* 99:1391, 1932.

62. Rusch VW: Management of Pancoast tumours. *Lancet Oncol* 7:997, 2006.

63. Rusch VW, Giroux DJ, Kraut MJ, et al: Induction chemoradiation and surgical resection for superior sulcus non–small-cell lung carcinomas: Long-term results of Southwest Oncology Group Trial 9416 (Intergroup Trial 0160). *J Clin Oncol* 25:313, 2007.

64. Ginsberg RJ, Rubinstein LV: Randomized trial of lobectomy versus limited resection for T1 N0 non–small cell lung cancer. Lung Cancer Study Group. *Ann Thorac Surg* 60:615, 1995.

65. Nakamura H, Kazuyuki S, Kawasaki N, et al: History of limited resection for non–small cell lung cancer. *Ann Thorac Cardiovasc Surg* 11:356, 2005.

66. Warren WH, Faber LP: Segmentectomy versus lobectomy in patients with stage I pulmonary carcinoma. Five-year survival and patterns of intrathoracic recurrence. *J Thorac Cardiovasc Surg* 107:1087; discussion 1093, 1994.

67. Pisters KM, Ginsberg RJ, Giroux DJ, et al: Induction chemotherapy before surgery for early-stage lung cancer: A novel approach. Bimodality Lung Oncology Team. *J Thorac Cardiovasc Surg* 119:429, 2000.

68. Rosell R, Gomez-Codina J, Camps C, et al: A randomized trial comparing preoperative chemotherapy plus surgery with surgery alone in patients with non–small-cell lung cancer. *N Engl J Med* 330:153, 1994.

69. Brouchet L, Bauvin E, Marcheix B, et al: Impact of induction treatment on postoperative complications in the treatment of non–small cell lung cancer. *J Thorac Oncol* 2:626, 2007.

70. Roth JA, Atkinson EN, Fossella F, et al: Long-term follow-up of patients enrolled in a randomized trial comparing perioperative chemotherapy and surgery with surgery alone in resectable stage IIIA non–small-cell lung cancer. *Lung Cancer* 21:1, 1998.

71. Dillman RO, Herndon J, Seagren SL, et al: Improved survival in stage III non–small-cell lung cancer: Seven-year follow-up of cancer and leukemia group B (CALGB) 8433 trial. *J Natl Cancer Inst* 88:1210, 1996.

72. Cahan WG, Shah JP, Castro EB: Benign solitary lung lesions in patients with cancer. *Ann Surg* 187:241, 1978.

73. Pastorino U, Pezzella F: Lung metastases and second lung cancer: role of surgery. In: Brambilla C, Brambilla E (eds): *Lung Tumors: Fundamental Biology and Clinical Management.* New York: M. Dekker, 1999, p 679.

74. Davidson RS, Nwogu CE, Brentjens MJ, et al: The surgical management of pulmonary metastasis: Current concepts. *Surg Oncol* 10:35, 2001.

75. McCormack PM, Bains MS, Begg CB, et al: Role of video-assisted thoracic surgery in the treatment of pulmonary metastases: Results of a prospective trial. *Ann Thorac Surg* 62:213; discussion 216, 1996.

76. Pastorino U, Buyse M, Friedel G, et al: Long-term results of lung metastasectomy: Prognostic analyses based on 5206 cases. *J Thorac Cardiovasc Surg* 113:37, 1997.

77. Mansharamani N, Balachandran D, Delaney D, et al: Lung abscess in adults: Clinical comparison of immunocompromised to non-immunocompromised patients. *Respir Med* 96:178, 2002.

78. Laheij RJ, Sturkenboom MC, Hassing RJ, et al: Risk of community-acquired pneumonia and use of gastric acid-suppressive drugs. *JAMA* 292:1955, 2004.

79. Thomson RM, Armstrong JG, Looke DF: Gastroesophageal reflux disease, acid suppression, and *Mycobacterium avium* complex pulmonary disease. *Chest* 131:1166, 2007.

80. Koh WJ, Lee JH, Kwon YS, et al: Prevalence of gastroesophageal reflux disease in patients with nontuberculous mycobacterial lung disease. *Chest* 131:1825, 2007.

81. Angrill J, Agusti C, de Celis R, et al: Bacterial colonisation in patients with bronchiectasis: Microbiological pattern and risk factors. *Thorax* 57:15, 2002.

82. Barker AF: Bronchiectasis. *N Engl J Med* 346:1383, 2002.

83. Bilton D, Henig N, Morrissey B, et al: Addition of inhaled tobramycin to ciprofloxacin for acute exacerbations of *Pseudomonas aeruginosa* infection in adult bronchiectasis. *Chest* 130:1503, 2006.

84. Steinfort DP, Steinfort C: Effect of long-term nebulized colistin on lung function and quality of life in patients with chronic bronchial sepsis. *Intern Med J* 37:495, 2007.

85. Ilowite J, Spiegler P, Chawla S: Bronchiectasis: New findings in the pathogenesis and treatment of this disease. *Curr Opin Infect Dis* 21:163, 2008.

86. http://www.cdc.gov/tb/WorldTBDay/resources_global.htm: Fact Sheets: A Global Perspective on Tuberculosis, 2008, Centers for Disease Control and Prevention [accessed April 1, 2008].

87. Taylor Z, Nolan CM, Blumberg HM: Controlling tuberculosis in the United States. Recommendations from the American Thoracic Society, CDC, and the Infectious Diseases Society of America. *MMWR Recomm Rep* 54(RR-12):1, 2005.

88. Frieden TR, Sterling TR, Munsiff SS, et al: Tuberculosis. *Lancet* 362:887, 2003.

89. http://www.cdc.gov/tb/pubs/tbfactsheets/mdrtb.htm: Fact Sheet: Multi-drug-Resistant Tuberculosis (MDR TB), 2008, Centers for Disease Control and Prevention [accessed April 1, 2008].

90. Iseman MD: Treatment of multidrug-resistant tuberculosis. *N Engl J Med* 329:784, 1993.

91. Conant EF, Wechsler RJ: Actinomycosis and nocardiosis of the lung. *J Thorac Imaging* 7:75, 1992.

92. Mabeza GF, Macfarlane J: Pulmonary actinomycosis. *Eur Respir J* 21:545, 2003.

93. Wheat LJ, Goldman M, Sarosi G: State-of-the-art review of pulmonary fungal infections. *Semin Respir Infect* 17:158, 2002.

94. Kubak BM: Fungal infection in lung transplantation. *Transpl Infect Dis* 4(Suppl 3):24, 2002.

95. Marr KA, Patterson T, Denning D: Aspergillosis. Pathogenesis, clinical manifestations, and therapy. *Infect Dis Clin North Am* 16:875, 2002.

96. Corr P: Management of severe hemoptysis from pulmonary aspergilloma using endovascular embolization. *Cardiovasc Intervent Radiol* 9:807, 2006.

97. Herbrecht R, Denning DW, Patterson TF, et al: Voriconazole versus amphotericin B for primary therapy of invasive aspergillosis. *N Engl J Med* 347:408, 2002.

98. Playford EG, Sorrell TC: Optimizing therapy for *Candida* infections. *Semin Respir Crit Care Med* 28:678, 2007.

99. Ostrosky-Zeichner L, Rex JH, Bennett J, et al: Deeply invasive candidiasis. *Infect Dis Clin North Am* 16:821, 2002.

100. Gonzalez CE, Rinaldi MG, Sugar AM: Zygomycosis. *Infect Dis Clin North Am* 16:895, 2002.

101. Wheat LJ, Kauffman CA: Histoplasmosis. *Infect Dis Clin North Am* 17:1, 2003.

102. Hage CA, Wheat LJ, Loyd J, et al: Pulmonary histoplasmosis. *Semin Respir Crit Care Med* 29:151, 2008.

103. Assi MA, Sandid MS, Baddour LM, et al: Systemic histoplasmosis: A 15-year retrospective institutional review of 111 patients. *Medicine (Baltimore)* 86:162, 2007.

104. Spinello IM, Munoz A, Johnson RH: Pulmonary coccidioidomycosis. *Semin Respir Crit Care Med* 29:166, 2008.

105. Pappas PG: Blastomycosis. *Semin Respir Crit Care Med* 25:113, 2004.

106. Bradsher RW, Chapman SW, Pappas PG: Blastomycosis. *Infect Dis Clin North Am* 17:21, 2003.

107. Pound MW, Drew RH, Perfect JR: Recent advances in the epidemiology, prevention, diagnosis, and treatment of fungal pneumonia. *Curr Opin Infect Dis* 15:183, 2002.

108. Playford EG, Sorrell TC: Optimizing therapy for *Candida* infections. *Semin Respir Crit Care Med* 28:678, 2007.

109. Corder R: Hemoptysis. *Emerg Med Clin North Am* 21:421, 2003.

110. Conlan AA: Massive hemoptysis—diagnostic and therapeutic implications. *Surg Annu* 17:337, 1985.

111. Cahill BC, Ingbar DH: Massive hemoptysis. Assessment and management. *Clin Chest Med* 15:147, 1994.

112. Conlan AA, Hurwitz SS: Management of massive haemoptysis with the rigid bronchoscope and cold saline lavage. *Thorax* 35:901, 1980.

113. Brantigan OC, Mueller E, Kress MB: A surgical approach to pulmonary emphysema. *Am Rev Respir Dis* 80:194, 1959.

114. Cooper JD, Patterson GA: Lung-volume reduction surgery for severe emphysema. *Chest Surg Clin N Am* 5:815, 1995.

115. Cooper JD, Trulock EP, Triantafillou AN, et al: Bilateral pneumectomy (volume reduction) for chronic obstructive pulmonary disease. *J Thorac Cardiovasc Surg* 109:106, 1995

116. Russi EW, Bloch KE, Weder W: Lung volume reduction surgery: What can we learn from the National Emphysema Treatment Trial? *Eur Respir J* 22:571, 2003.

117. Cooper JD, Pearson FG, Patterson GA, et al: Technique of successful lung transplantation in humans. *J Thorac Cardiovasc Surg* 93:173, 1987.

118. Pasque MK, Cooper JD, Kaiser LR, et al: Improved technique for bilateral lung transplantation: Rationale and initial clinical experience. *Ann Thorac Surg* 49:785, 1990.

119. Dahlberg PS, Prekker ME, Hertz M, et al: Recent trends in lung transplantation: the University of Minnesota experience. *Clin Transpl,* p 243, 2002.

120. Bhorade SM, Vigneswaran W, McCabe MA, et al: Liberalization of donor criteria may expand the donor pool without adverse consequence in lung transplantation. *J Heart Lung Transplant* 19:1199, 2000.

121. Kron IL, Tribble CG, Kern JA, et al: Successful transplantation of marginally acceptable thoracic organs. *Ann Surg* 217:518; discussion 522, 1993.

122. Pierre AF, Sekine Y, Hutcheon MA, et al: Marginal donor lungs: A reassessment. *J Thorac Cardiovasc Surg* 123:421; discussion 427, 2002.

123. Sundaresan S, Semenkovich J, Ochoa L, et al: Successful outcome of lung transplantation is not compromised by the use of marginal donor lungs. *J Thorac Cardiovasc Surg* 109:1075; discussion 1079, 1995.

124. Palmer SM, Miralles AP, Howell DN, et al: Gastroesophageal reflux as a reversible cause of allograft dysfunction after lung transplantation. *Chest* 118:1214, 2000.

125. Inderbitzi RG, Leiser A, Furrer M, et al: Three years' experience in video-assisted thoracic surgery (VATS) for spontaneous pneumothorax. *J Thorac Cardiovasc Surg* 107:1410, 1994.

126. Warner BW, Bailey WW, Shipley RT: Value of computed tomography of the lung in the management of primary spontaneous pneumothorax. *Am J Surg* 162:39, 1991.

127. Cavanaugh DG, Cabellon S Jr., Peake JB: A logical approach to chest wall neoplasms. *Ann Thorac Surg* 41:436, 1986.

128. Somers J, Faber LP: Chondroma and chondrosarcoma. *Semin Thorac Cardiovasc Surg* 11:270, 1999.

129. Andino L, Cagle PT, Murer B, et al: Pleuropulmonary desmoid tumors: Immunohistochemical comparison with solitary fibrous tumors and assessment of beta-catenin and cyclin D1 expression. *Arch Pathol Lab Med* 130:1503, 2006.

130. Baliski CR, Temple WJ, Arthur K, et al: Desmoid tumors: A novel approach for local control. *J Surg Oncol* 80:96, 2002.

131. Abbas AE, Deschamps C, Cassivi SD, et al: Chest-wall desmoid tumors: Results of surgical intervention. *Ann Thorac Surg* 78:1219; discussion 1219, 2004.

132. Liptay MJ, Fry WA: Malignant bone tumors of the chest wall. *Semin Thorac Cardiovasc Surg* 11:278, 1999.

133. Askin FB, Rosai J, Sibley RK, Dehner LP, et al: Malignant small cell tumor of the thoracopulmonary region in childhood: A distinctive clinicopathologic entity of uncertain histogenesis. *Cancer* 43:2438, 1979.

134. Gutierrez JC, Perez EA, Franceschi D, et al: Outcomes for soft-tissue sarcoma in 8249 cases from a large state cancer registry. *J Surg Res* 141:105, 2007.

135. Walsh GL, Davis BM, Swisher SG, et al: A single-institutional, multidisciplinary approach to primary sarcomas involving the chest wall requiring full-thickness resections. *J Thorac Cardiovasc Surg* 121:48, 2001.

136. Incarbone M, Pastorino U: Surgical treatment of chest wall tumors. *World J Surg* 25:218, 2001.

137. Arnold PG, Pairolero PC: Chest-wall reconstruction: an account of 500 consecutive patients. *Plast Reconstr Surg* 98:804, 1996.

138. Mansour KA, Thourani VH, Losken A, et al: Chest wall resections and reconstruction: A 25-year experience. *Ann Thorac Surg* 73:1720; discussion 1725, 2002.

139. Deschamps C, Tirnaksiz BM, Darbandi R, et al: Early and long-term results of prosthetic chest wall reconstruction. *J Thorac Cardiovasc Surg* 117:588; discussion 591, 1999.

140. Graeber GM: Chest wall resection and reconstruction. *Semin Thorac Cardiovasc Surg* 11:251, 1999.

141. Kirschner PA: Anatomy and surgical access of the mediastinum, in Pearson FG, et al (ed): *Thoracic Surgery,* 2nd ed. New York: Churchill Livingstone, 2002, p 1563.

142. Strollo DC, Rosado-de-Christenson ML, Jett JR: Primary mediastinal tumors. Part II: Tumors of the middle and posterior mediastinum. *Chest* 112:1344, 1997.

143. Baron RL, Levitt RG, Sagel SS, et al: Computed tomography in the evaluation of mediastinal widening. *Radiology* 138:107, 1981.

144. Luketich JD, Friedman DM, Weigel TL, et al: Evaluation of distant metastases in esophageal cancer: 100 consecutive positron emission tomography scans. *Ann Thorac Surg* 68:1133; discussion 1136, 1999.

145. Larsen SS, Krasnik M, Vilmann P, et al: Endoscopic ultrasound guided biopsy of mediastinal lesions has a major impact on patient management. *Thorax* 57:98, 2002.

146. Hoerbelt R, Keunecke L, Grimm H, et al: The value of a noninvasive diagnostic approach to mediastinal masses. *Ann Thorac Surg* 75:1086, 2003.

147. Sokolowski JW, Jr., Burgher LW, Jones FL, Jr., Patterson JR, et al: Guidelines for percutaneous transthoracic needle biopsy. This position paper of the American Thoracic Society was adopted by the ATS Board of Directors, June 1988. *Am Rev Respir Dis* 140:255, 1989.

148. Herman SJ, Holub RV, Weisbrod GL, et al: Anterior mediastinal masses: Utility of transthoracic needle biopsy. *Radiology* 180:167, 1991.

149. Knapp RH, Hurt RD, Payne WS, et al: Malignant germ cell tumors of the mediastinum. *J Thorac Cardiovasc Surg* 89:82, 1985.

150. Storch I, Shah M, Thurer R, et al: Endoscopic ultrasound-guided fine-needle aspiration and Tru-Cut biopsy in thoracic lesions: When tissue is the issue. *Surg Endosc J* 22:86, 2008.

151. Meyers BF, Cooper JD: Transcervical thymectomy for myasthenia gravis. *Chest Surg Clin N Am* 11:363, 2001.

152. Yim AP, Kay RL, Izzat MB, et al: Video-assisted thoracoscopic thymectomy for myasthenia gravis. *Semin Thorac Cardiovasc Surg* 11:65, 1999.

153. Yim AP: Video-assisted thoracoscopic resection of anterior mediastinal masses. *Int J Surg* 81:350, 1996.

154. Small EJ, Venook AP, Damon LE: Gallium-avid thymic hyperplasia in an adult after chemotherapy for Hodgkin disease. *Cancer* 72:905, 1993.

155. Quint LE: PET: Other thoracic malignancies. *Cancer Imaging* 6:S82, 2006.

156. Masaoka A, Monden Y, Nakahara K, et al: Follow-up study of thymomas with special reference to their clinical stages. *Cancer* 48:2485, 1981.

157. Mangi AA, Wright CD, Allan JS, et al: Adjuvant radiation therapy for stage II thymoma. *Ann Thorac Surg* 74:1033, 2002.

158. Chahinian AP: Chemotherapy of thymomas and thymic carcinomas. *Chest Surg Clin N Am* 11:447, 2001.

159. Loehrer PJ, Sr., Perez CA, Roth LM, et al: Chemotherapy for advanced thymoma. Preliminary results of an intergroup study. *Ann Intern Med* 113(7):520, 1990.

160. Blumberg D, Port JL, Weksler B, et al: Thymoma: A multivariate analysis of factors predicting survival. *Ann Thorac Surg* 60:908; discussion 914, 1995.

161. Suster S, Rosai J: Thymic carcinoma. A clinicopathologic study of 60 cases. *Cancer* 67:1025, 1991.

162. Bousamra M: Neurogenic tumors of the mediastinum, in Pearson FG, et al (ed): *Thoracic Surgery,* 2nd ed. New York: Churchill Livingstone, 2002, p 1732.

163. Venissac N, Leo F, Hofman P, et al: Mediastinal neurogenic tumors and video-assisted thoracoscopy: Always the right choice? *Surg Laparosc Endosc Percutan Tech* 14:20, 2004.

164. Coleman BG, Arger PH, Dalinka MK, et al: CT of sarcomatous degeneration in neurofibromatosis. *AJR Am J Roentgenol* 140:383, 1983.

165. Ducatman BS, Scheithauer BW, Piepgras DG, et al: Malignant peripheral nerve sheath tumors. A clinicopathologic study of 120 cases. *Cancer* 57:2006, 1986.

166. Nichols CR, Saxman S, Williams SD, et al: Primary mediastinal nonseminomatous germ cell tumors. A modern single institution experience. *Cancer* 65:1641, 1990.

167. Rice TW: Benign neoplasms and cysts of the mediastinum. *Semin Thorac Cardiovasc Surg* 4:25, 1992.

168. Di Lorenzo M, Collin PP, Vaillancourt R, et al: Bronchogenic cysts. *J Pediatr Surg* 24:988, 1989.

169. Ribet ME, Copin MC, Gosselin B: Bronchogenic cysts of the mediastinum. *J Thorac Cardiovasc Surg* 109:1003, 1995.

170. Fontenelle LJ, Armstrong RG, Stanford W, et al: The asymptomatic mediastinal mass. *Arch Surg* 102:98, 1971.

171. St-Georges R, Deslauriers J, Duranceau A, et al: Clinical spectrum of bronchogenic cysts of the mediastinum and lung in the adult. *Ann Thorac Surg* 52:6, 1991.

172. Urschel HC, Jr., Razzuk MA, Netto GJ, et al: Sclerosing mediastinitis: improved management with histoplasmosis titer and ketoconazole. *Ann Thorac Surg* 50:215, 1990.

173. Agostoni E: Mechanics of the pleural space, in Fisherman AP, Macklem PT, Mead J et al (eds): Mechanics of breathing, in *Handbook of Physiology*, vol 3. Bethesda, Md: American Physiological Society, 1986.

174. Lawrence GH: Considerations of the anatomy and physiology of the pleural space, in Lawrence GH (ed): *Problems of the Pleural Space.* Philadelphia: WB Saunders, 1983.

175. Rusch VW: Pleural effusion: Benign and malignant, in Pearson FG, et al (ed): *Thoracic Surgery,* 2nd ed. New York: Churchill Livingstone, 2002, p 1157.

176. Ocana I, Martinez-Vazquez JM, Segura RM, et al: Adenosine deaminase in pleural fluids. Test for diagnosis of tuberculous pleural effusion. *Chest* 84:51, 1983.

177. Lee YC, Rogers JT, Rodriguez RM, et al: Adenosine deaminase levels in nontuberculous lymphocytic pleural effusions. *Chest* 120:356, 2001.

178. Johnston WW: The malignant pleural effusion. A review of cytopathologic diagnoses of 584 specimens from 472 consecutive patients. *Cancer* 56:905, 1985.

179. Tremblay A, Michaud G: Single-center experience with 250 tunnelled pleural catheter insertions for malignant pleural effusion. *Chest* 129:362, 2006.

180. Light RW: Parapneumonic effusions and empyema. *Clin Chest Med* 6:55, 1985.

181. Miller JI Jr.: The history of surgery of empyema, thoracoplasty, Eloesser flap, and muscle flap transposition. *Chest Surg Clin N Am* 10:45, 2000.

182. Miller JI Jr.: Diagnosis and management of chylothorax. *Chest Surg Clin N Am* 6:139, 1996.

183. Malthaner RA, Inculet RI: The thoracic duct and chylothorax, in Pearson FG, et al (ed): *Thoracic Surgery,* 2nd ed. New York: Churchill Livingstone, 2002, p 1228.

184. Roehr CC, Jung A, Proquitte H, et al: Somatostatin or octreotide as treatment options for chylothorax in young children: a systematic review. *Intensive Care Med* 32:650, 2006.

185. Gammie JS, Banks MC, Fuhrman CR, et al: The pigtail catheter for pleural drainage: A less invasive alternative to tube thoracostomy. *JSLS* 3:57, 1999.

186. Luketich JD, Kiss M, Hershey J, et al: Chest tube insertion: A prospective evaluation of pain management. *Clin J Pain* 14:152, 1998.

187. Khalil MY, Mapa M, Shin HJ, et al: Advances in the management of malignant mesothelioma. *Curr Oncol Rep* 5:334, 2003.

188. Rusch VW: A proposed new international TNM staging system for malignant pleural mesothelioma. From the International Mesothelioma Interest Group. *Chest* 108:1122, 1995.

189. Takagi K, Tsuchiya R, Watanabe Y: Surgical approach to pleural diffuse mesothelioma in Japan. *Lung Cancer* 31:57, 2001.

190. Sugarbaker DJ, Flores RM, Jaklitsch MT, et al: Resection margins, extrapleural nodal status, and cell type determine postoperative long-term survival in trimodality therapy of malignant pleural mesothelioma: Results in 183 patients. *J Thorac Cardiovasc Surg* 117:54; discussion 63, 1999.

191. Rusch VW, Rosenzweig K, Venkatraman E, et al: A phase II trial of surgical resection and adjuvant high-dose hemithoracic radiation for malignant pleural mesothelioma. *J Thorac Cardiovasc Surg* 122:788, 2001.

192. Rusch V, Saltz L, Venkatraman E, et al: A phase II trial of pleurectomy/decortication followed by intrapleural and systemic chemotherapy for malignant pleural mesothelioma. *J Clin Oncol* 12:1156, 1994.

193. Ratto GB, Civalleri D, Esposito M, et al: Pleural space perfusion with cisplatin in the multimodality treatment of malignant mesothelioma: A feasibility and pharmacokinetic study. *J Thorac Cardiovasc Surg* 117:759, 1999.

194. Lu C, Perez-Soler R, Piperdi B, et al: Phase II study of a liposome-entrapped cisplatin analog (L-NDDP) administered intrapleurally and pathologic response rates in patients with malignant pleural mesothelioma. *J Clin Oncol* 23:3495, 2005.

195. England DM, Hochholzer L, McCarthy MJ: Localized benign and malignant fibrous tumors of the pleura. A clinicopathologic review of 223 cases. *Am J Surg Pathol* 13:640, 1989.

196. Smith TP, Kinasewitz GT, Tucker WY, et al: Exercise capacity as a predictor of post-thoracotomy morbidity. *Am Rev Respir Dis* 129:730, 1984.

197. Bechard D, Wetstein L: Assessment of exercise oxygen consumption as preoperative criterion for lung resection. *Ann Thorac Surg* 44:344, 1987.

198. Olsen GN, Weiman DS, Bolton JW, et al: Submaximal invasive exercise testing and quantitative lung scanning in the evaluation for tolerance of lung resection. *Chest* 95:267, 1989.

199. Walsh GL, Morice RC, Putnam JB, Jr., et al: Resection of lung cancer is justified in high-risk patients selected by exercise oxygen consumption. *Ann Thorac Surg* 58:704, 1994.

200. Bolliger CT, Jordan P, Soler M, et al: Exercise capacity as a predictor of postoperative complications in lung resection candidates. *Am J Respir Crit Care Med* 151:1472, 1995.

201. Markos J, Mullan BP, Hillman DR, et al: Preoperative assessment as a predictor of mortality and morbidity after lung resection. *Am Rev Respir Dis* 139:902, 1989.

202. Wang J, Olak J, Ultmann RE, et al: Assessment of pulmonary complications after lung resection. *Ann Thorac Surg* 67:1444, 1999.

203. Win T, Jackson A, Sharples L, et al: Cardiopulmonary exercise tests and lung cancer surgical outcome. *Chest* 127:1159, 2005.

204. Holden DA, Rice TW, Stelmach K, et al: Exercise testing, 6-min walk, and stair climb in the evaluation of patients at high risk for pulmonary resection. *Chest* 102:1774, 1992.

205. Hoffmann TH, Ransdell HT: Comparison of lobectomy and wedge resection for carcinoma of the lung. *J Thorac Cardiovasc Surg* 79:211, 1980.

206. Read RC, Yoder G, Schaeffer RC: Survival after conservative resection for T1 N0 M0 non-small cell lung cancer. *Ann Thorac Surg* 49:391, 1990.

207. Date H, Andou A, Shimizu N: The value of limited resection for "clinical" stage I peripheral non-small cell lung cancer in poor-risk patients: comparison of limited resection and lobectomy by a computer-assisted matched study. *Tumori* 80:422, 1994.

208. Harpole DH, Jr., Herndon JE, 2nd, Young WG, Jr., et al: Stage I nonsmall cell lung cancer. A multivariate analysis of treatment methods and patterns of recurrence. *Cancer* 76:787, 1995.

209. Lederle FA: Lobectomy versus limited resection in T1 N0 lung cancer. *Ann Thorac Surg* 62:1249, 1996.

210. Kodama K, Doi O, Higashiyama M, et al: Intentional limited resection for selected patients with T1 N0 M0 non-small-cell lung cancer: A single-institution study. *J Thorac Cardiovasc Surg* 114:347, 1997.

211. Landreneau RJ, Sugarbaker DJ, Mack MJ, et al: Wedge resection versus lobectomy for stage I (T1 N0 M0) non-small-cell lung cancer. *J Thorac Cardiovasc Surg* 113:691, 1997.

212. Pastorino U, Andreola S, Tagliabue E, et al: Immunocytochemical markers in stage I lung cancer: relevance to prognosis. *J Clin Oncol* 15:2858, 1997.

213. Kwiatkowski DJ, Harpole DH, Jr., Godleski J, et al: Molecular pathologic substaging in 244 stage I non-small-cell lung cancer patients: Clinical implications. *J Clin Oncol* 16:2468,1998.

214. Okada M, Yoshikawa K, Hatta T, et al: Is segmentectomy with lymph node assessment an alternative to lobectomy for non-small cell lung cancer of 2 cm or smaller? *Ann Thorac Surg* 71:956, 2001.

215. Koike T, Yamato Y, Yoshiya K, et al: Intentional limited pulmonary resection for peripheral T1 N0 M0 small-sized lung cancer. *J Thorac Cardiovasc Surg* 125:924, 2003.

216. Campione A, Ligabue T, Luzzi L, et al: Comparison between segmentectomy and larger resection of stage IA non-small cell lung carcinoma. *J Cardiovasc Surg (Torino)* 45:67, 2004.

217. Keenan RJ, Landreneau RJ, Maley RH, Jr., et al: Segmental resection spares pulmonary function in patients with stage I lung cancer. *Ann Thorac Surg* 78:228. 2004.

218. Pass HI, Pogrebniak HW, Steinberg SM, et al: Randomized trial of neoadjuvant therapy for lung cancer: interim analysis. *Ann Thorac Surg* 53:992, 1992.

219. Nagai K, Tsuchiya R, Mori T, et al: A randomized trial comparing induction chemotherapy followed by surgery with surgery alone for patients with stage IIIA N2 non-small cell lung cancer (JCOG 9209). *J Thorac Cardiovasc Surg* 125:254, 2003.

220. Gilligan D, Nicolson M, Smith I, et al: Preoperative chemotherapy in patients with resectable non-small cell lung cancer: results of the MRC LU22/NVALT 2/EORTC 08012 multicentre randomised trial and update of systematic review. *Lancet* 369:1929, 2007.

221. Depierre A, Milleron B, Moro-Sibilot D, et al: Preoperative chemotherapy followed by surgery compared with primary surgery in resectable stage I (except T1N0), II, and IIIa non-small-cell lung cancer. *J Clin Oncol* 20:247, 2002.

222. Pisters K, Vallieres E, Bunn PA, Jr., et al: S9900: Surgery alone or surgery plus induction (ind) paclitaxel/carboplatin (PC) chemotherapy in early stage non-small cell lung cancer (NSCLC): Follow-up on a phase III trial. *J Clin Oncol* 25:7520, 2007.

223. Sorensen JB, Riska H, Ravn J, et al: Scandinavian phase III trial of neoadjuvant chemotherapy in NSCLC stages IB-IIIA/T3. *ASCO Meeting Abstracts* 23:7146, 2005.

224. Mattson KV, Abratt RP, ten Velde G, et al: Docetaxel as neoadjuvant therapy for radically treatable stage III non-small-cell lung cancer: A multinational randomised phase III study. *Ann Oncol* 14:116, 2003.

225. Population Risk of Lung Cancer from Passive Smoking, in: *Respiratory health effects of passive smoking: lung cancer and other disorders.* Washington, D.C.: Office of Health and Environmental Assessment, Office of Research and Development, U.S. Environmental Protection Agency, 1992.

226. Public Health Service. Office of the Surgeon General, United States. Office on Smoking and Health. *The health consequences of involuntary exposure to tobacco smoke: a report of the Surgeon General.* Rockville,

MD; Washington, DC: U.S. Dept. of Health and Human Services, Public Health Service for sale by the Supt. of Documents, U.S. G.P.O.; 2006.

227. Stayner L, Bena J, Sasco AJ, et al: Lung cancer risk and workplace exposure to environmental tobacco smoke. *Am J Public Health* 97:545, 2007.

228. Darby S, Hill D, Auvinen A, et al: Radon in homes and risk of lung cancer: collaborative analysis of individual data from 13 European case-control studies. *BMJ* 330:223, 2005.

229. Krewski D, Lubin JH, Zielinski JM, et al: A combined analysis of North American case-control studies of residential radon and lung cancer. *J Toxicol Environ Health A* 69:533, 2006.

230. Zhao Y, Wang S, Aunan K, et al: Air pollution and lung cancer risks in China—a meta-analysis. *Sci Total Environ* 366:500, 2006.

231. Lissowska J, Bardin-Mikolajczak A, Fletcher T, et al: Lung cancer and indoor pollution from heating and cooking with solid fuels: the IARC international multicentre case-control study in Eastern/Central Europe and the United Kingdom. *Am J Epidemiol* 162:326, 2005.

232. Ramanakumar AV, Parent ME, Siemiatycki J: Risk of lung cancer from residential heating and cooking fuels in Montreal, Canada. *Am J Epidemiol* 165:634, 2007.

233. Matakidou A, Eisen T, Houlston RS: Systematic review of the relationship between family history and lung cancer risk. *Br J Cancer* 93:825, 2005.

234. Hung RJ, Boffetta P, Brockmoller J, et al: CYP1A1 and GSTM1 genetic polymorphisms and lung cancer risk in Caucasian non-smokers: a pooled analysis. *Carcinogenesis* 24:875, 2003.

235. Raimondi S, Boffetta P, Anttila S, et al: Metabolic gene polymorphisms and lung cancer risk in non-smokers. An update of the GSEC study. *Mutat Res* 592:45, 2005.

236. Hung RJ, Hall J, Brennan P, et al: Genetic polymorphisms in the base excision repair pathway and cancer risk: a HuGE review. *Am J Epidemiol* 162:925, 2005.

237. Hung RJ, Brennan P, Canzian F, et al: Large-scale investigation of base excision repair genetic polymorphisms and lung cancer risk in a multicenter study. *J Natl Cancer Inst* 97:567, 2005.

238. Zhou W, Liu G, Miller DP, et al. Polymorphisms in the DNA repair genes XRCC1 and ERCC2, smoking, and lung cancer risk. *Cancer Epidemiol Biomarkers Prev* 12:359, 2003.

239. Cheng YW, Chiou HL, Sheu GT, et al. The association of human papillomavirus 16/18 infection with lung cancer among nonsmoking Taiwanese women. *Cancer Res* 61:2799, 2001.

CHAPTER 20

Congenital Heart Disease

Tara B. Karamlou, Karl F. Welke,
and Ross M. Ungerleider

PARADIGM SHIFT

Congenital heart surgery is a constantly evolving field. The last 20 years have brought about rapid developments in the technologic realm as well as a more thorough understanding of both the anatomy and pathophysiology of congenital heart disease (CHD), leading to the improved care of patients with this challenging disease.[1,2]

These new advancements created a paradigm shift in the field of pediatric heart surgery. The traditional strategy of initial palliation followed by definitive correction at a later age, which had pervaded the thinking of most surgeons, began to evolve to one emphasizing early repair, even in the tiniest patients.[2] Furthermore, some of the defects that were virtually uniformly fatal [such as hypoplastic left-heart syndrome (HLHS)] now can be successfully treated with aggressive forms of palliation using cardiopulmonary bypass (CPB), resulting in outstanding survival for many of these children.

Because the goal in most cases of CHD is now early repair, as opposed to subdividing lesions into cyanotic or noncyanotic lesions, a more appropriate classification scheme divides particular defects into three categories based on the feasibility of achieving this goal: (a) defects that have no reasonable palliation and for which repair is the only option; (b) defects for which repair is not possible and for which palliation is the only option; and (c) defects that can either be repaired or palliated in infancy.[3] It bears mentioning that all defects in the second category are those in which the appropriate anatomic components either are not present, as in HLHS, or cannot be created from existing structures.

DEFECTS WHERE REPAIR IS THE ONLY OR BEST OPTION

Atrial Septal Defect

An atrial septal defect (ASD) is defined as an opening in the interatrial septum that enables the mixing of blood from the systemic venous and pulmonary venous circulations.

Embryology

The atrial and ventricular septa form between the third and sixth weeks of fetal development. After the paired heart tubes fuse into a single tube folded onto itself, the distal portion of the tube causes an indentation to form in the roof of the common atrium. Near this portion of the roof, the septum primum arises and extends into a crescentic formation toward the atrioventricular (AV) junction. The gap remaining between the septum primum and the developing tissues of the AV junction is called the *ostium primum*. Before the septum primum fuses completely with the endocardial cushions, a series of fenestrations appear in the septum primum that coalesce into the ostium secundum. During this coalescence, the septum

secundum grows downward from the roof of the atrium, parallel to and to the right of the septum primum. The septum primum does not fuse, but creates an oblique pathway, called the *foramen ovale*, within the interatrial septum. After birth, the increase in left atrial (LA) pressure normally closes this pathway, obliterating the interatrial connection.[4]

Anatomy

ASDs can be classified into three different types: (a) sinus venosus defects, comprising approximately 5 to 10% of all ASDs; (b) ostium primum defects, which are more correctly described as partial AV canal defects; and (c) ostium secundum defects, which are the most prevalent subtype, comprising 80% of all ASDs (Fig. 20-1).[5]

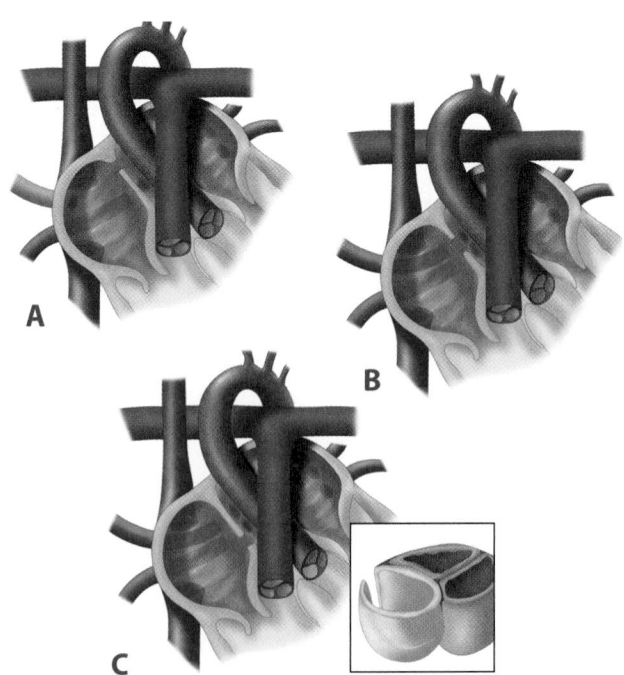

FIG. 20-1. The anatomy of atrial septal defects. In the sinus venosus type (**A**), the right upper and middle pulmonary veins frequently drain to the superior vena cava or right atrium. **B.** Secundum defects generally occur as isolated lesions. **C.** Primum defects are part of a more complex lesion and are best considered as incomplete atrioventricular septal defects. *[Reproduced with permission from Greenfield LJ, Mulholland MW, Oldham KT, et al (eds):* Surgery: Scientific Principles and Practice, *3rd ed. Philadelphia: Lippincott Williams & Wilkins, 2001, p 1444.]*

Pathophysiology

ASDs result in an increase in pulmonary blood flow secondary to left-to-right shunting through the defect. The direction of the intracardiac shunt is predominantly determined by the compliance of the respective ventricles. In utero, the distensibility, or compliance, of the right and left ventricles (LVs) is equal, but postnatally the LV becomes less compliant than the right ventricle (RV). This shift occurs because the resistance of the downstream vascular beds changes after birth. The pulmonary vascular resistance (PVR) falls with the infant's first breath, decreasing RV pressure, whereas the systemic vascular resistance rises dramatically, increasing LV pressure. The increased LV pressure creates a thicker muscle mass, which offers a greater resistance to diastolic filling than does the RV; thus, the majority of flow through the ASD occurs from left to right. The greater volume of blood returning to the right atrium causes volume overload in the RV, but because of its lower muscle mass and low-resistance output, it easily distends to accommodate this load.[5,6]

The long-term consequences of RV volume overload include hypertrophy with elevated RV end-diastolic pressure and a relative pulmonary stenosis across the pulmonary valve, because it cannot accommodate the increased RV flow. The resistance at the level of the pulmonary valve then contributes a further pressure load on the RV, which accelerates RV hypertrophy. Compliance gradually decreases as the right ventricular pressure approaches systemic pressure, and the size of the left-to-right shunt decreases. Patients at this stage have a balanced circulation and may deceptively appear less symptomatic.

A minority of patients with ASDs develop progressive pulmonary vascular changes as a result of chronic overcirculation. The increased PVR in these patients leads to an equalization of left and right ventricular pressures, and their ratio of pulmonary (Qp) to systemic flow (Qs), Qp:Qs, will approach 1.[5,7] This does not mean, however, that there is no intracardiac shunting, only that the ratio between the left-to-right component and the right-to-left component is equal.

The ability of the RV to recover normal function is related to the duration of chronic overload, because those undergoing ASD closure before age 10 years have a better likelihood of achieving normal RV function in the postoperative period.[3]

The physiology of sinus venosus ASDs is similar to that discussed above for simple ASDs except that these are frequently accompanied by anomalous pulmonary venous drainage. This often results in significant hemodynamic derangements that accelerate the clinical course of these infants.

The same increase in symptoms is true for those with ostium primum defects because the associated mitral insufficiency from the "cleft" mitral valve can lead to more atrial volume load and increased atrial level shunting.

Diagnosis

Patients with ASDs may present with few physical findings. Auscultation may reveal prominence of the first heart sound with fixed splitting of the second heart sound. This results from the relatively fixed left-to-right shunt throughout all phases of the cardiac cycle. A diastolic flow murmur indicating increased flow across the tricuspid valve may be discerned, and, frequently, an ejection flow murmur can be heard across the pulmonary valve. A right ventricular heave and increased intensity of the pulmonary component of the second heart sound indicates pulmonary hypertension and possible unrepairability.

Chest radiographs in the patient with an ASD may show evidence of increased pulmonary vascularity, with prominent hilar markings and cardiomegaly. The electrocardiogram (ECG) shows right axis deviation with an incomplete bundle-branch block. When right bundle-branch block is associated with a leftward or superior axis, an AV canal defect should be strongly suspected.[8]

Diagnosis is clarified by two-dimensional echocardiography, and use of color flow mapping facilitates an understanding of the physiologic derangements created by the defects.[9] Older children and adults with unrepaired ASDs may present with stroke or systemic embolism from paradoxical embolism or atrial arrhythmias from dilation of the right atrium.

Echocardiography also enables the clinician to estimate the amount of intracardiac shunting, can demonstrate the degree of mitral regurgitation in patients with ostium primum defects, and with the addition of microcavitation, can assist in the detection of sinus venosus defects.[5]

The advent of two-dimensional echocardiography with color flow Doppler has largely obviated the need for cardiac catheterization because the exact nature of the ASD can be precisely defined by echo alone. However, in cases where the patient is older than age 40 years, catheterization can quantify the degree of pulmonary hypertension present, because those with a fixed PVR greater than 12 U/mL are considered inoperable.[10] Cardiac catheterization also can be useful in that it provides data that enable the calculation of Qp and Qs so that the magnitude of the intracardiac shunt can be determined. The ratio (Qp:Qs) can then be used to determine whether closure is indicated in equivocal cases, because a Qp:Qs greater than

---

KEY POINTS

1. Congenital heart disease comprises a wide morphologic spectrum. In general, lesions can be conceptualized as those which can be completely repaired, those that should be palliated, and those that can be either repaired or palliated depending on particular patient and institutional characteristics.

2. Percutaneous therapies for congenital heart disease are quickly becoming important adjuncts, and in some cases, alternatives, to standard surgical therapy. Important examples include percutaneous closure of atrial and ventricular septal defects, the hybrid approach to hypoplastic left heart syndrome, radiofrequency perforation of the pulmonary valve, and percutaneous pulmonary valve placement. Further studies are necessary to establish criteria and

current benchmarks for the safe integration of these novel approaches into the care of patients with congenital heart surgery.

3. Outcomes have improved substantially over time in congenital heart surgery, and most complex lesions can be operated in early infancy. Neurologic protection, however, remains a key issue in the care of neonates undergoing surgery with cardiopulmonary bypass and deep hypothermic circulatory arrest. New monitoring devices and perioperative strategies are currently under investigation. Attention in the field has shifted currently from analyses of perioperative mortality, which for most lesions is under 10%, to longer-term outcomes, including quality of life and neurologic function.

1.5:1 is generally accepted as the threshold for surgical intervention. Finally, in patients older than age 40 years, cardiac catheterization can be important to disclose the presence of coronary artery disease.

In general, ASDs are closed when patients are between 4 and 5 years of age. Children of this size can usually be operated on without the use of blood transfusion and generally have excellent outcomes. Patients who are symptomatic may require repair earlier, even in infancy. Some surgeons, however, advocate routine repair in infants and children, as even smaller defects are associated with the risk of paradoxical embolism, particularly during pregnancy. In a review by Reddy and colleagues, 116 neonates weighing less than 2500 g who underwent repair of simple and complex cardiac defects with the use of CPB were found to have no intracerebral hemorrhages, no long-term neurologic sequelae, and a low operative-mortality rate (10%). These results correlated with the length of CPB and the complexity of repair.[11] These investigators also found an 80% actuarial survival at 1 year, and, more important, that growth following complete repair was equivalent to weight-matched neonates free from cardiac defects.[11]

Treatment

ASDs can be repaired in a facile manner using standard CPB techniques through a midline sternotomy approach.[7] The details of the repair itself are generally straightforward. An oblique atriotomy is made, the position of the coronary sinus and all systemic and pulmonary veins are determined, and the rim of the defect is completely visualized. Closure of ostium secundum defects is accomplished either by primary repair or by insertion of a patch that is sutured to the rim of the defect. The decision about whether patch closure is necessary can be determined by the size and shape of the defect as well as by the quality of the edges.

The type of repair used for sinus venosus ASDs associated with partial anomalous pulmonary venous connection is dictated by the location of the anomalous pulmonary veins. If the anomalous veins connect to the atria or to the superior vena cava (SVC) caudal to where the cava is crossed by the right pulmonary artery (RPA), the ASD can be repaired by inserting a patch, with redirection of the pulmonary veins behind the patch to the left atrium. Care must be taken with this approach to avoid obstruction of the pulmonary veins or the SVC, although usually the SVC is dilated and provides ample room for patch insertion. If the anomalous vein connects to the SVC cranial to the RPA an alternative technique, the Warden procedure, may be necessary. In this operation, the SVC is transected cranial to the connection of the anomalous vein (usually the right superior pulmonary vein). The caudal end of the transected cava is oversewn. The cranial end of the transected cava is anastomosed to the auricle of the right atrium. Inside the atrium, a patch is used to redirect pulmonary venous blood flow to the left atrium. In contrast to the repair for a defect where the pulmonary veins enter the right atrium or the SVC below the right PA, the patch covers the superior vena caval right atrial junction so that blood from the anomalous pulmonary vein that enters the cava is directed to the left atrium. Blood returning from the upper body enters the right atrium via the anastomosis between the SVC and the right auricle.

These operative strategies have been well established, with a low complication rate and a mortality rate approaching zero. As such, attention has shifted to improving the cosmetic result and minimizing hospital stay and convalescence. Multiple new strategies have been described to achieve these aims, including the right submammary incision with anterior thoracotomy, limited bilateral submammary incision with partial sternal split, transxiphoid window, and limited midline incision with partial sternal split.[4,12–14] Some centers use video-assisted thoracic surgery in the submammary and transxiphoid approaches to facilitate closure within a constricted operative field. The morbidity and mortality of all of these approaches are comparable to those of the traditional median sternotomy; however, each has technical drawbacks. The main concern is that operative precision be maintained with limited exposure. Luo and associates described a prospective randomized study compar-

ing ministernotomy (division of the upper sternum for aortic and pulmonary lesions, and the lower sternum for septal lesions) to full sternotomy in 100 consecutive patients undergoing repair of septal lesions.[14] The patients in the ministernotomy group had longer procedure times (by 15 to 20 minutes), less bleeding, and shorter hospital stays. These results have been echoed by other investigators from Boston who maintain that ministernotomy provides a cosmetically acceptable scar without compromising aortic cannulation or limiting the exposure of crucial mediastinal structures.[12] This approach also can be easily extended to a full sternotomy should difficulty or unexpected anomalies be encountered.[13]

First performed in 1976, transcatheter closure of ASDs with the use of various occlusion devices is gaining widespread acceptance.[15] Certain types of ASDs, including patent foramen ovale (PFO), secundum defects, and some fenestrated secundum defects, are amenable to device closure, as long as particular anatomic criteria (e.g., an adequate superior and inferior rim for device seating and distance from the AV valve) are met. Since the introduction of percutaneous closure (PC), there has been a dramatic rise in device closure prevalence to the point where device closure has supplanted surgical therapy as the dominant treatment modality for secundum ASD.[16] A study from the author's group[16] recently found that ASD/PFO closures per capita increased dramatically from 1.08 per 100,000 population in 1988 to 2.59 per 100,000 population in 2005, an increase of 139%. When analyzed by closure type, surgical closure increased by only 24% (from 0.86 per 100,000 population in 1988 to 1.07 per 100,000 in 2005) whereas PC increased by 3475% (from 0.04 per 100,000 population in 1988 to 1.43 per 100,000 in 2005). Importantly, this study determined that the paradigm shift favoring PC has occurred mainly due to increased prevalence of closure in adults over age 40 years rather than an increase in closure in infants or children. Complications reported to occur with transcatheter closure include air embolism (1 to 3%); thromboembolism from the device (1 to 2%); disturbed AV valve function (1 to 2%); systemic/pulmonary venous obstruction (PVO) (1%); perforation of the atrium or aorta with hemopericardium (1 to 2%); atrial arrhythmias (1 to 3%); and malpositioning/embolization of the device requiring intervention (2 to 15%).[4,17] Thus, although percutaneous approaches are cosmetic and often translate into shorter periods of convalescence, their attendant risks are not trivial, especially because their use may not result in complete closure of the septal defect.

Results

Surgical repair of ASDs is associated with a mortality rate near zero.[4,5,7,8,11] Early repairs in neonates weighing less than 1000 g have been increasingly reported with excellent results.[11] Uncommonly, atrial arrhythmias or significant LA hypertension may occur soon after repair. The latter is caused by the noncompliant small, LA chamber and generally resolves rapidly.

Aortic Stenosis

Anatomy and Classification

The spectrum of aortic valve abnormality represents the most common form of CHD, with the great majority of patients being asymptomatic until midlife. Obstruction of the left ventricular outflow tract (LVOT) occurs at multiple levels: subvalvular, valvular, and supravalvular (Fig. 20-2). The critically stenotic aortic valve in the neonate or infant is commonly unicommissural or bicommissural, with thickened, dysmorphic, and myxomatous leaflet tissue and a reduced cross-sectional area at the valve level. Associated left-sided lesions are often present. In a review of 32 cases from the Children's Hospital in Boston, 59% had unicommissural valves and 40% had bicommissural valves.[18] Associated lesions were frequent, occurring in 88% of patients, most commonly patent ductus arteriosus (PDA), mitral regurgitation, and hypoplastic LV. Endocardial fibroelastosis also is common among infants with critical aortic stenosis (AS).[19] In this condition, the LV is largely nonfunctional, and these patients are not

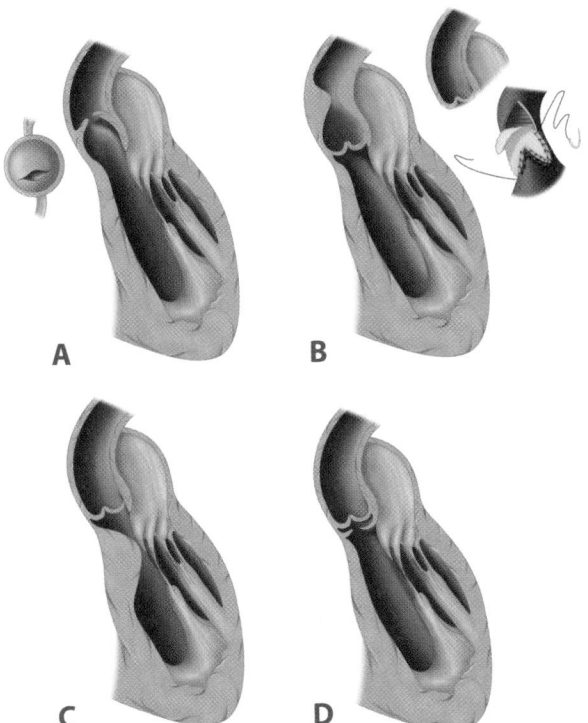

FIG. 20-2. The anatomy of the types of congenital aortic stenosis. **A.** Valvar aortic stenosis. **B.** Supravalvar aortic stenosis and its repair (*insert*). **C.** Tunnel-type subvalvar aortic stenosis. **D.** Membranous subvalvar aortic stenosis. *[Reproduced with permission from Greenfield LJ, Mulholland MW, Oldham KT, et al (eds): Surgery: Scientific Principles and Practice, 3rd ed. Philadelphia: Lippincott Williams & Wilkins, 2001, p 1448.]*

candidates for balloon valvotomy, simple valve replacement, or repair, because the LV is incapable of supporting the systemic circulation. Often, the LV is markedly hypertrophic with a reduced cavity size, but on rare occasion, a dilated LV, reminiscent of overt heart failure, is encountered.[20]

Pathophysiology

The unique intracardiac and extracardiac shunts present in fetal life allow even neonates with critical AS to survive. In utero, left ventricular hypertrophy and ischemia cause LA hypertension, which reduces the right-to-left flow across the foramen ovale. In severe cases, a reversal of flow may occur, causing right ventricular volume loading. The RV then provides the entire systemic output via the PDA (ductal-dependent systemic blood flow). Although cardiac output is maintained, the LV suffers continued damage as the intracavitary pressure precludes adequate coronary perfusion, resulting in LV infarction and subendocardial fibroelastosis. The presentation of the neonate with critical AS is then determined by both the morphology of the LV and other left-sided heart structures, the degree of left ventricular dysfunction, and the completeness of the transition from a parallel circulation to an in-series circulation (i.e., on closure of the foramen ovale and the ductus arteriosus). Those infants with mild-to-moderate AS in which LV function is preserved are asymptomatic at birth. The only abnormalities may be a systolic ejection murmur and ECG evidence of left ventricular hypertrophy. However, those neonates with severe AS and compromised LV function are unable to provide adequate cardiac output at birth, and will present in circulatory collapse once the ductus closes, with dyspnea, tachypnea, irritability, narrowed pulse pressure, oliguria, and profound metabolic acidosis.[7,21] If ductal patency is maintained, systemic perfusion will be provided by the RV via ductal flow, and cyanosis may be the only finding.

Diagnosis

Neonates and infants with severe valvular AS may have a relatively nonspecific history of irritability and failure to thrive. Angina, if present, is usually manifested by episodic, inconsolable crying that coincides with feeding. As discussed previously, evidence of poor peripheral perfusion, such as extreme pallor, indicates severe left ventricular outflow tract obstruction (LVOTO). Differential cyanosis is an uncommon finding, but is present when enough antegrade flow occurs only to maintain normal upper body perfusion, while a large PDA produces blue discoloration of the abdomen and legs.

Physical findings include a systolic ejection murmur, although a quiet murmur may paradoxically indicate a more severe condition with reduced cardiac output. A systolic click correlates with a valvular etiology of obstruction. As LV dysfunction progresses, evidence of congestive heart failure (CHF) occurs.

The chest radiograph is variable, but may show dilatation of the aortic root, and the ECG often demonstrates LV hypertrophy. Echocardiography with Doppler flow is extremely useful in establishing the diagnosis, as well as quantifying the transvalvular gradient.[22] Furthermore, echocardiography can facilitate evaluation for the several associated defects that can be present in critical neonatal AS, including mitral stenosis, LV hypoplasia, LV endocardial fibroelastosis, subaortic stenosis, ventricular septal defect (VSD), or coarctation. The presence of any or several of these defects has important implications related to treatment options for these patients. Although cardiac catheterization is not routinely performed for diagnostic purposes, it can be invaluable as part of the treatment algorithm if the lesion is amenable to balloon valvotomy.

Treatment

The first decision that must be made in the neonate with critical LVOTO is whether the patient is a candidate for biventricular or univentricular repair. Central to this decision is assessment of the degree of hypoplasia of the LV and other left-sided structures. Alsoufi and colleagues[23] recently described a rational approach to the neonate with critical LVOTO (Fig. 20-3). The infant with severe AS requires urgent intervention. Preoperative stabilization, however, has dramatically altered the clinical algorithm and outcomes for this patient population.[19,21] The preoperative strategy begins with endotracheal intubation and inotropic support. Prostaglandin infusion is initiated to maintain ductal patency, and confirmatory studies are performed before operative intervention.

Therapy is generally indicated in the presence of a transvalvular gradient of 50 mmHg with associated symptoms including syncope, CHF, or angina, or if a gradient of 50 to 75 mmHg exists with concomitant ECG evidence of LV strain or ischemia. In the critically ill neonate, there may be little gradient across the aortic valve because of poor LV function. These patients depend on patency of the ductus arteriosus to provide systemic perfusion from the RV, and all ductal-dependent patients with critical AS require treatment. However, the decision regarding treatment options must be based on a complete understanding of associated defects. For example, in the presence of a hypoplastic LV (left ventricular end-diastolic volume <20 mL/m^2), or a markedly abnormal mitral valve, isolated aortic valvotomy should not be performed because studies have demonstrated high mortality in this population following isolated valvotomy.[24]

Patients who have a LV capable of providing systemic output are candidates for intervention to relieve AS, generally through balloon valvotomy. Very rarely, if catheter-based therapy is not an option, relief of valvular AS in infants and children can be accomplished with surgical valvotomy using standard techniques of CPB and direct exposure to the aortic valve. A transverse incision is made in the ascending aorta (AA) above the sinus of Valsalva, extending close to, but not into, the noncoronary sinus. Exposure is attained with placement of a retractor into the right coronary sinus. After inspection of the valve, the chosen commissure is incised to within 1 to 2 mm of the aortic wall (Fig. 20-4).

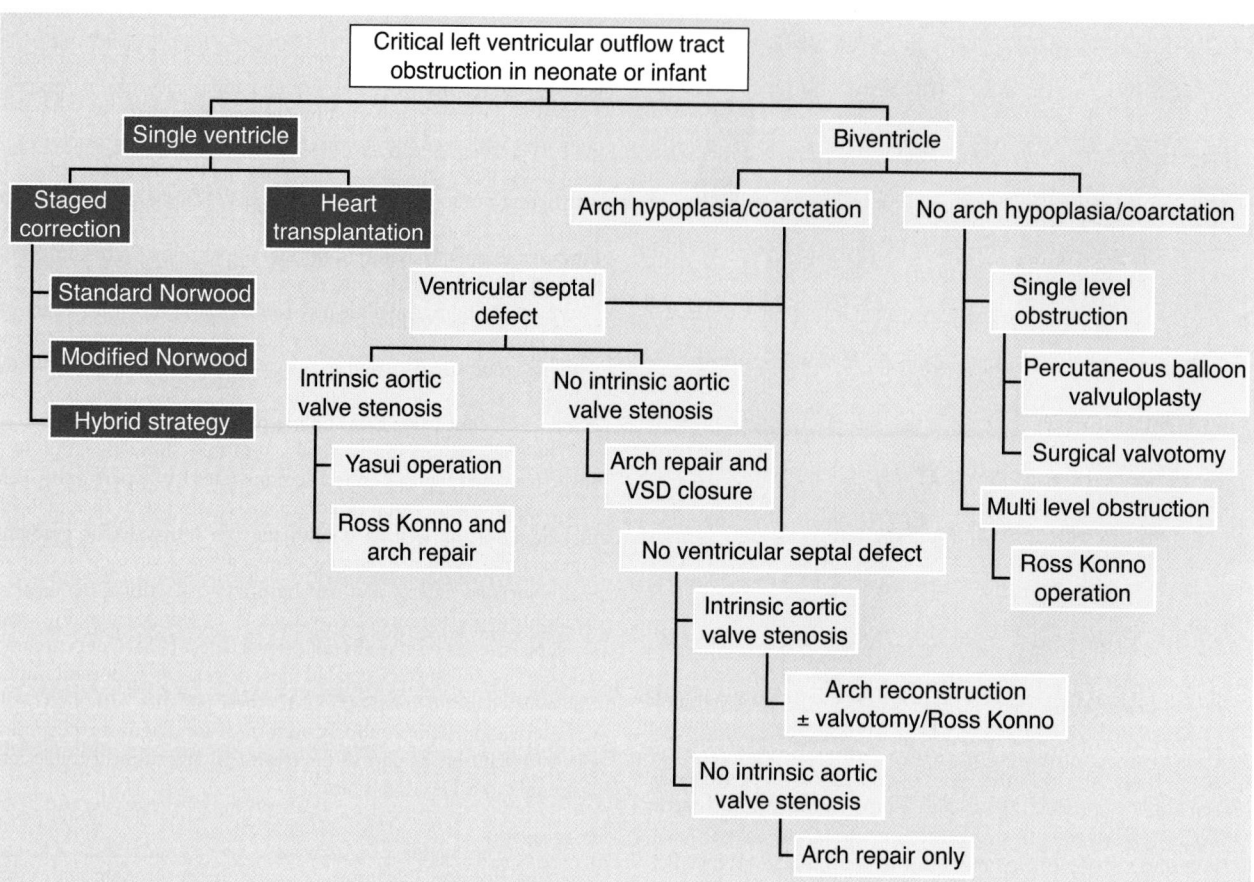

FIG. 20-3. Treatment algorithm for neonates and infants with critical left ventricular outflow tract obstruction. Patients can be initially triaged to either a single or a biventricular approach depending on presenting morphologic, demographic, and institutional factors. VSD = ventricular septal defect. *(From Alsoufi et al,[23] Fig. 1, with permission. Copyright Elsevier.)*

Balloon valvotomy performed in the catheterization lab is the procedure of choice for reduction of transvalvular gradients in symptomatic infants and children. This procedure is an ideal palliative option because mortality from surgical valvotomy can be high due to the critical nature of these patients' condition. Furthermore, balloon valvotomy provides relief of the valvular gradient and allows future surgical intervention (which is generally required in most patients when a larger prosthesis can be implanted) to be performed on an unscarred chest. An important issue when planning aortic valvotomy, whether percutaneously or via open surgical technique, is the risk of inducing hemodynamically significant aortic regurgitation. Induction of more than moderate aortic regurgitation is poorly tolerated in the infant with critical AS, and may require an urgent procedure to replace or repair the aortic valve.

In general, catheter-based balloon valvotomy has supplanted open surgical valvotomy. The decision regarding the most appropriate method to use depends on several factors including the available medical expertise, the patient's overall status and hemodynamics, and the presence of associated cardiac defects requiring repair.[25] Although evidence is emerging to the contrary, simple valvotomy, whether performed using percutaneous or open technique, is generally considered a palliative procedure. The goal is to relieve LVOTO without producing clinically significant regurgitation, to allow sufficient annular growth for eventual aortic valve replacement. The majority of infants who undergo aortic valvotomy will require further intervention on the aortic valve within 10 years following initial intervention.[26]

Valvotomy may result in aortic insufficiency that, although not important enough to require intervention in infancy, alone or in combination with AS may result in the need for an aortic valve

replacement. Neonates with severely hypoplastic LVs or significant LV endocardial fibroelastosis may not be candidates for two-ventricle repair and are treated the same as infants with the HLHS, which is discussed later (see Hypoplastic Left-Heart Syndrome below).

Many surgeons previously avoided aortic valve replacement for AS in early childhood because the more commonly used mechanical valves would be outgrown and require replacement later, and the obligatory anticoagulation for mechanical valves resulted in a substantial risk for complications. In addition, mechanical valves had an important incidence of bacterial endocarditis or perivalvular leak requiring reintervention.

The use of allografts and the advent of the Ross procedure have largely obviated these issues and made early definitive correction of critical AS a viable option.[19,27,28] Donald Ross first described transposition of the pulmonary valve into the aortic position with allograft reconstruction of the pulmonary outflow tract in 1967.[27] The result of this operation is a normal trileaflet semilunar valve made of a patient's native tissue with the potential for growth to adult size in the aortic position in place of the damaged aortic valve (Fig. 20-5). The Ross procedure has become a useful option for aortic valve replacement in children, because it has improved durability and can be performed with acceptable morbidity and mortality rates. The placement of a pulmonary conduit, which does not grow and becomes calcified and stenotic over time, does obligate the patient to reoperation to replace the right-ventricle to PA conduit. Karamlou and colleagues[29] reviewed the outcomes and associated risk factors for aortic valve replacement in 160 children from the Hospital for Sick Children in Toronto. They found that younger age, lower operative weight, concomitant performance of aortic root replacement or reconstruction, and use of prosthesis type other than a pulmonary

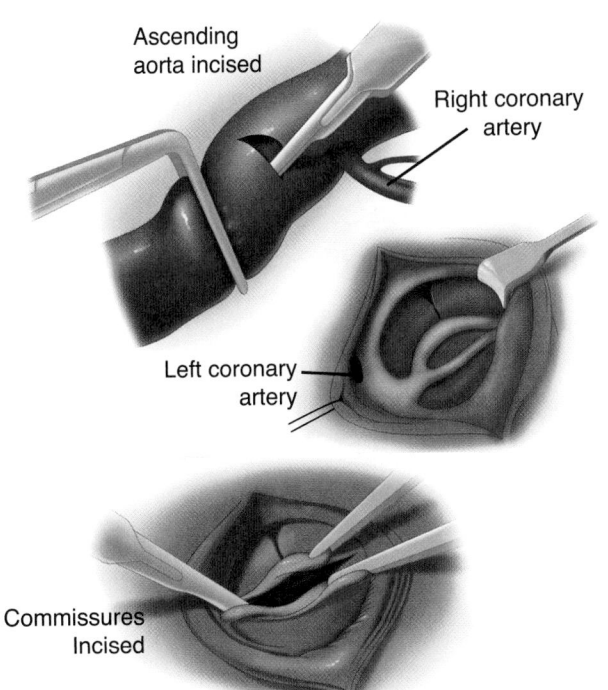

FIG. 20-4. Aortic valvotomy with cardiopulmonary bypass. A transverse incision is made in the ascending aorta above the sinuses of Valsalva, extending close to, but not into, the noncoronary sinus. Exposure is accomplished with placement of a retractor into the right coronary sinus. After inspection of the valve, the chosen commissure is incised to within 1 to 2 mm of the aortic wall. *(Reproduced with permission from Doty DB:* Cardiac Surgery: A Looseleaf Workbook and Update Service. *Chicago: Year Book, 1986.)*

Labels in figure: Ascending aorta incised; Right coronary artery; Left coronary artery; Commissures Incised

autograft were significant predictors of death, while the use of a bioprosthetic or allograft valve type and earlier year of operation were identified as significant risk factors for repeated aortic valve replacement. Autograft use was associated with a blunted progression of the peak prosthetic valve gradient and a rapid decrease in the left ventricular end-diastolic dimension (Fig. 20-6). In agreement with these findings, Lupinetti and Jones compared allograft aortic valve replacement with the Ross procedure and found a more significant transvalvular gradient reduction and regression of left ventricular hypertrophy in those patients who underwent the Ross procedure.[30] In some cases, the pulmonary valve may not be usable because of associated defects or congenital absence. These children are not candidates for the Ross procedure and are now most frequently treated with cryopreserved allografts (cadaveric human aortic valves). At times, there may be a size discrepancy between the right ventricular outflow tract (RVOT) and the LVOT, especially in cases of severe critical AS in infancy. For these cases, the pulmonary autograft is placed in a manner that also provides enlargement of the aortic annulus (Ross/Konno) (Fig. 20-7).

Subvalvular AS occurs beneath the aortic valve and may be classified as discrete or tunnel-like (diffuse). A thin, fibromuscular diaphragm immediately proximal to the aortic valve characterizes discrete subaortic stenosis. This diaphragm typically extends for 180° or more in a crescentic or circular fashion, often attaching to the mitral valve as well as the interventricular septum.[21] The aortic valve itself is usually normal in this condition, although the turbulence imparted by the subvalvular stenosis may affect leaflet morphology and valve competence.

Diffuse subvalvular AS results in a long, tunnel-like obstruction that may extend to the left ventricular apex. In some individuals, there may be difficulty in distinguishing between hypertrophic cardiomyopathy and diffuse subaortic stenosis. Operation for subvalvu-

lar AS is indicated with a gradient exceeding 30 mmHg, the presence of aortic valve insufficiency, or when symptoms indicating LVOTO are present.[30] Given that repair of isolated, discrete, subaortic stenosis can be done with low rates of morbidity and mortality, some surgeons advocate repair in all cases of discrete AS, to avoid progression of the stenosis and the development of aortic insufficiency, although more recent data demonstrate that subaortic resection should be delayed until the LV gradient exceeds 30 mmHg because most children with an initial LV gradient less than 30 mmHg have quiescent disease.[31] Diffuse AS is a more complex lesion and often requires aortoventriculoplasty as described in the previous paragraph. Results are generally excellent, with operative mortality less than 5%.[32]

Supravalvular AS occurs more rarely, and also can be classified into a discrete type, which produces an hourglass deformity of the aorta, and a diffuse form that can involve the entire arch and brachiocephalic arteries. The aortic valve leaflets are usually normal, but in some cases, the leaflets may adhere to the supravalvular stenosis, thereby narrowing the sinuses of Valsalva in diastole and restricting coronary artery perfusion. In addition, accelerated intimal hyperplastic changes in the coronary arteries can be demonstrated in these patients because the proximal position of the coronary arteries subjects them to abnormally high perfusion pressures.

The signs and symptoms of supravalvular AS are similar to other forms of LVOTO. An asymptomatic murmur is the presenting manifestation in approximately one half of these patients. Syncope, poor exercise tolerance, and angina may all occur with nearly equal frequency. Supravalvar AS is associated with Williams syndrome, a constellation of elfin facies, mental retardation, and hypercalcemia.[33] Following routine evaluation, cardiac catheterization should be performed to delineate coronary anatomy, as well as to delineate the degree of obstruction. A gradient of 50 mmHg or greater is an indication for operation. However, the clinician must be cognizant of any coexistent lesions, most commonly pulmonic stenosis, which may add complexity to the repair.

The localized form of supravalvular AS is treated by creating an inverted Y-shaped aortotomy across the area of stenosis, straddling the right coronary artery. The obstructing shelf is then excised and a pantaloon-shaped patch is used to close the incision.[21]

The diffuse form of supravalvular stenosis is more variable, and the particular operative approach must be tailored to each specific patient's anatomy. In general, either an aortic endarterectomy with patch augmentation can be performed, or if the narrowing extends past the aorta arch, a prosthetic graft can be placed between the ascending and descending aorta. Operative results for discrete supravalvular AS are generally good, with a hospital mortality of less than 1% and an actuarial survival rate exceeding 90% at 20 years.[34] In contrast, however, the diffuse form is more hazardous to repair, and carried a mortality of 15% in a series.[34,35]

Patent Ductus Arteriosus

Anatomy

The ductus arteriosus is derived from the sixth aortic arch and normally extends from the main or left PA to the upper descending thoracic aorta, distal to the left subclavian artery. In the normal fetal cardiovascular system, ductal flow is considerable (approximately 60% of the combined ventricular output), and is directed exclusively from the PA to the aorta.[36] In infancy, the length of the ductus may vary from 2 to 8 mm, with a diameter of 4 to 12 mm.

Locally produced and circulating prostaglandin E_2 (PGE_2) and PGI_2 induce active relaxation of the ductal musculature, maintaining maximal patency during the fetal period.[37] At birth, increased pulmonary blood flow metabolizes these prostaglandin products, and absence of the placenta removes an important source of them, resulting in a marked decrease in these ductal-relaxing substances. In addition, release of histamines, catecholamines, bradykinin, and acetylcholine all promote ductal contraction. Despite all of these complex interactions, the rising oxygen tension in the fetal blood is the main stimulus causing smooth muscle contraction and ductal

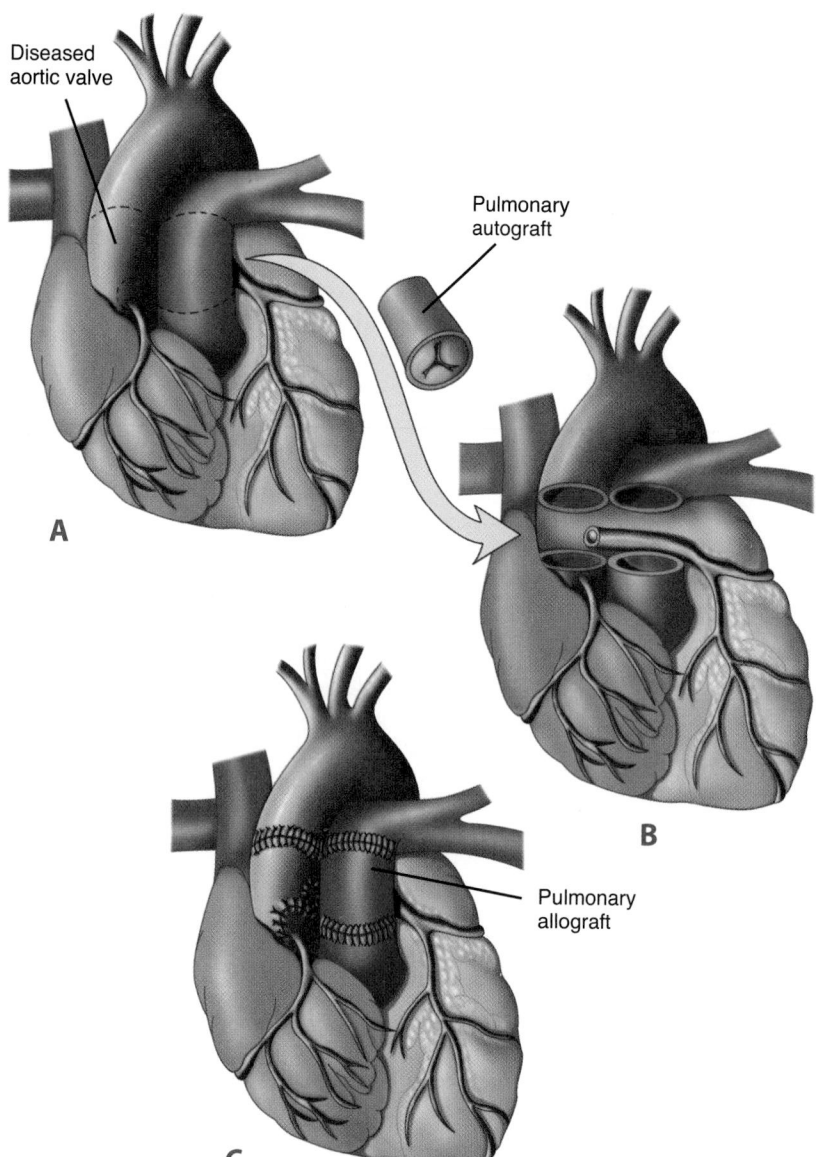

FIG. 20-5. A through **C.** The pulmonary autograft for aortic valve replacement. The aortic valve and adjacent aorta are excised, preserving buttons of aortic tissue around the coronary ostia. The pulmonary valve and main pulmonary artery are excised and transferred to the aortic position. The coronary buttons are then attached to the neoaortic root. A pulmonary allograft is inserted to re-establish the right ventricular outflow tract. *(From Koucho-kos NT, Davila-Roman VG, Spray TL, et al: Replacement of the aortic root with a pulmonary autograft in children and young adults with aortic-valve disease. N Engl J Med 330:1, 1994. Copyright © Massachusetts Medical Society. All rights reserved.)*

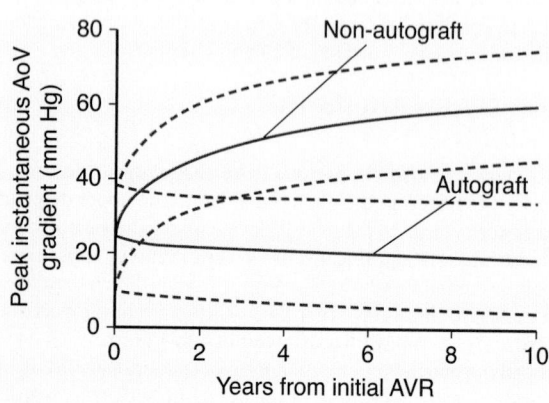

FIG. 20-6. Predicted progression of the peak instantaneous prosthetic valve gradient after initial aortic valve replacement (AVR) stratified by prosthesis type (autograft vs. nonautograft) for a hypothetical patient of 3 years undergoing AVR in 1990. Solid lines represent point estimates from a mixed linear regression model (surrounded by their 90% confidence intervals in dashed lines). AoV = aortic valve. *(From Karamlou et al,[29] with permission.)*

closure within 10 to 15 hours postnatally.[38] Anatomic closure by fibrosis produces the ligamentum arteriosum connecting the PA to the aorta.

Delayed closure of the ductus is termed *prolonged patency*, whereas failure of closure causes *persistent patency*, which may occur as an isolated lesion or in association with more complex congenital heart defects. In many of these infants with more complex congenital heart defects, either pulmonary or systemic perfusion may depend on ductal flow, and these infants may decompensate if exogenous PGE is not administered to maintain ductal patency.

Natural History

The incidence of PDA is approximately 1 in every 2000 births; however, it increases dramatically with increasing prematurity.[39] In some series, PDAs have been noted in 75% of infants of 28 to 30 weeks gestation. Persistent patency occurs more commonly in females, with a 2:1 ratio.[39]

PDA is not a benign entity, although prolonged survival has been reported. The estimated death rate for infants with isolated, untreated PDA is approximately 30%.[40] The leading cause of death is CHF, with respiratory infection as a secondary cause. Endocarditis is more likely to occur with a small ductus and is rarely fatal if aggressive antibiotic therapy is initiated early.

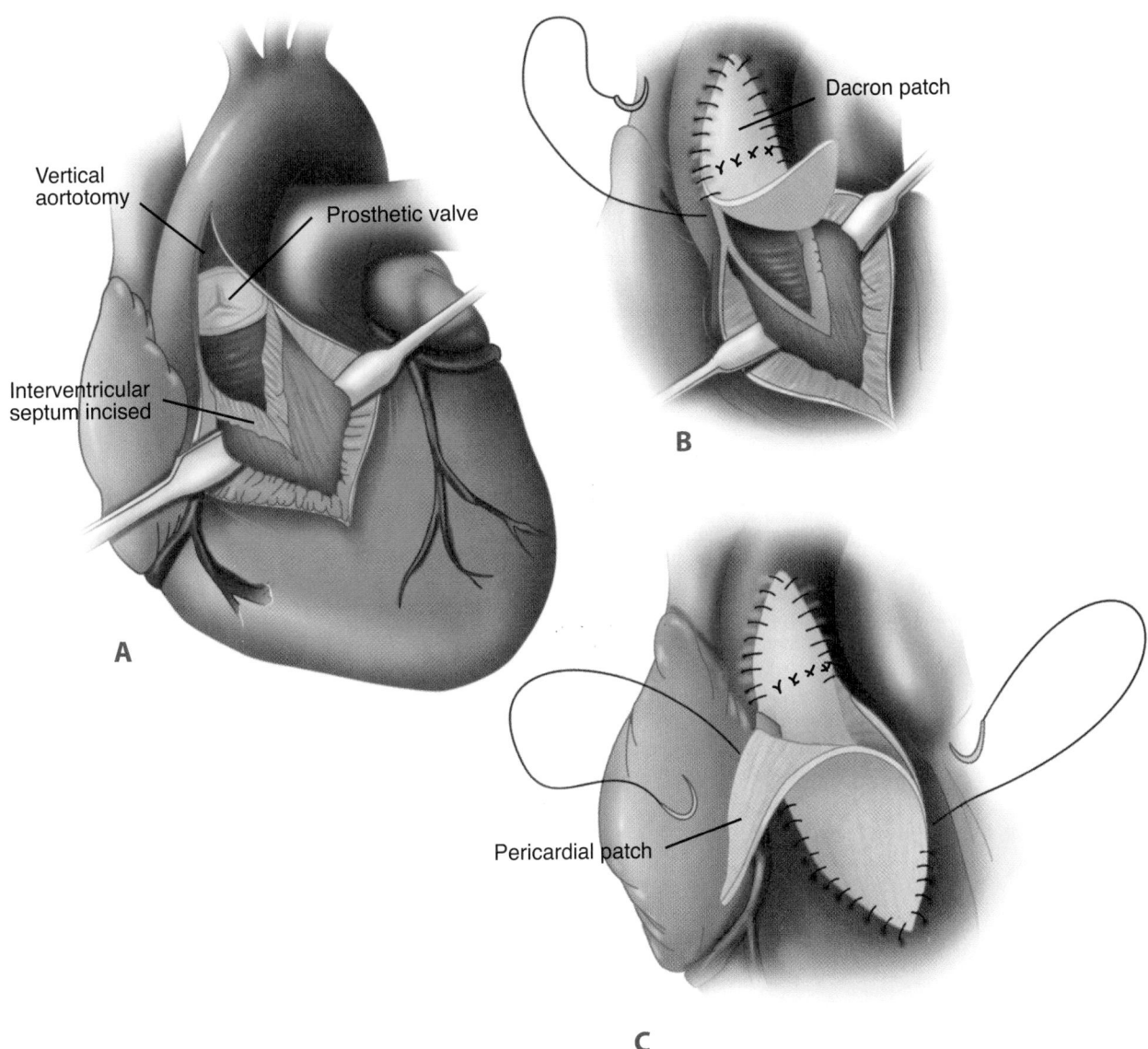

FIG. 20-7. The Konno-Rastan aortoventriculoplasty permits significant enlargement of the aortic annulus and subaortic region. **A.** A vertical aortotomy is made to the left of the right coronary artery and extended into the right ventricular outflow tract. After excising the aortic valve the interventricular septum is incised and an aortic valve prosthesis is secured within the enlarged annulus. **B.** A Dacron patch that is attached to the sewing ring of the prosthesis closes the interventricular septum and the aortotomy. **C.** A separate pericardial patch closes the right ventriculotomy. *(Reproduced with permission from Misbach GA, Turley K, Ullyot DJ, et al: Left ventricular outflow enlargement by the Konno procedure. J Thorac Cardiovasc Surg 84:696, 1982. Copyright Elsevier.)*

Clinical Manifestations and Diagnosis

After birth, in an otherwise normal cardiovascular system, a PDA results in a left-to-right shunt that depends on both the size of the ductal lumen and its total length. As the PVR falls 16 to 18 weeks postnatally, the shunt will increase, and its flow will ultimately be determined by the relative resistances of the pulmonary and systemic circulations.

The hemodynamic consequences of an unrestrictive ductal shunt are left ventricular volume overload with increased LA and PA pressures, and right ventricular strain from the augmented afterload. These changes result in increased sympathetic discharge, tachycardia, tachypnea, and ventricular hypertrophy. The diastolic shunt results in lower aortic diastolic pressure and increases the potential for myocardial ischemia and underperfusion of other systemic organs, while the increased pulmonary flow leads to increased work of breathing and decreased gas exchange. Unrestrictive ductal flow may lead to pulmonary hypertension within the first year of life. These changes will be

significantly attenuated if the size of the ductus is only moderate, and completely absent if the ductus is small.

Physical examination of the afflicted infant will reveal evidence of a hyperdynamic circulation with a widened pulse pressure and a hyperactive precordium. Auscultation demonstrates a systolic or continuous murmur, often termed a *machinery murmur.* Cyanosis is not present in uncomplicated isolated PDA.

The chest radiograph may reveal increased pulmonary vascularity or cardiomegaly, and the ECG may show LV strain, LA enlargement, and possibly RV hypertrophy. Echocardiogram with color mapping reliably demonstrates the patency of the ductus as well as estimates the shunt size. Cardiac catheterization is necessary only when pulmonary hypertension is suspected.

Therapy

The presence of a persistent PDA is sufficient indication for closure because of the increased mortality and risk of endocarditis.[2,4] In older patients with pulmonary hypertension, closure may not improve symptoms and is associated with much higher mortality.

In premature infants, aggressive intervention with indomethacin or ibuprofen to achieve early closure of the PDA is beneficial unless contraindications such as necrotizing enterocolitis or renal insufficiency are present.[41] Term infants, however, are generally unresponsive to pharmacologic therapy with indomethacin, so mechanical closure must be undertaken once the diagnosis is established. This can be accomplished either surgically or with catheter-based therapy.[12,42,43] Currently, transluminal placement of various occlusive devices, such as the Rashkind double-umbrella device or embolization with Gianturco coils, is in widespread use.[42] However, there are a number of complications inherent with the use of percutaneous devices, such as thromboembolism, endocarditis, incomplete occlusion, vascular injury, and hemorrhage secondary to perforation.[43] In addition, these techniques may not be applicable in very young infants, as the peripheral vessels do not provide adequate access for the delivery devices.

Surgical closure can be achieved via either open or video-assisted approaches. The open approach uses a posterior lateral thoracotomy in the fourth or fifth intercostal space on the side of the aorta (generally the left). The lung is then retracted anteriorly. In the neonate, the PDA is singly ligated with a surgical clip or permanent suture. In older patients the PDA is triply ligated. Care must be taken to avoid the recurrent laryngeal nerve that courses around the PDA. The PDA also can be ligated via a median sternotomy; however, this approach generally is reserved for patients who have additional cardiac or great vessel lesions requiring repair. Occasionally, a short, broad ductus, in which the dimension of its width approaches that of its length, will be encountered. In this case, division between vascular clamps with oversewing of both ends is advisable (Fig. 20-8). In

extreme cases, the use of CPB to decompress the large ductus during ligation is an option.

Video-assisted thoracoscopic occlusion, using metal clips, also has been described, although it offers few advantages over the standard surgical approach.[12] Preterm newborns and children may do well with the thoracoscopic technique, while older patients (older than age 5 years) and those with smaller ducts (<3 mm) do well with coil occlusion. In fact, Moore and colleagues concluded from their series that coil occlusion is the procedure of choice for ducts smaller than 4 mm.[44] Complete closure rates using catheter-based techniques have steadily improved. Comparative studies of cost and outcome between open surgery and transcatheter duct closure, however, have shown no overwhelming choice between the two modalities.[12] Burke prospectively reviewed coil occlusion and video-assisted thoracic surgery at Miami Children's Hospital, and found both options to be effective and less morbid than traditional thoracotomy.[12]

Outcomes

In premature infants, the surgical mortality is very low, although the overall hospital death rate is significant as a consequence of other complications of prematurity. In older infants and children, mortality is less than 1%. Bleeding, chylothorax, vocal cord paralysis, and the need for reoperation occur infrequently. With the advent of muscle-sparing thoracotomy, the risk of subsequent arm dysfunction or breast abnormalities is virtually eliminated.[45]

Aortic Coarctation
Anatomy

Coarctation of the aorta (COA) is defined as a luminal narrowing in the aorta that causes an obstruction to blood flow. This narrowing

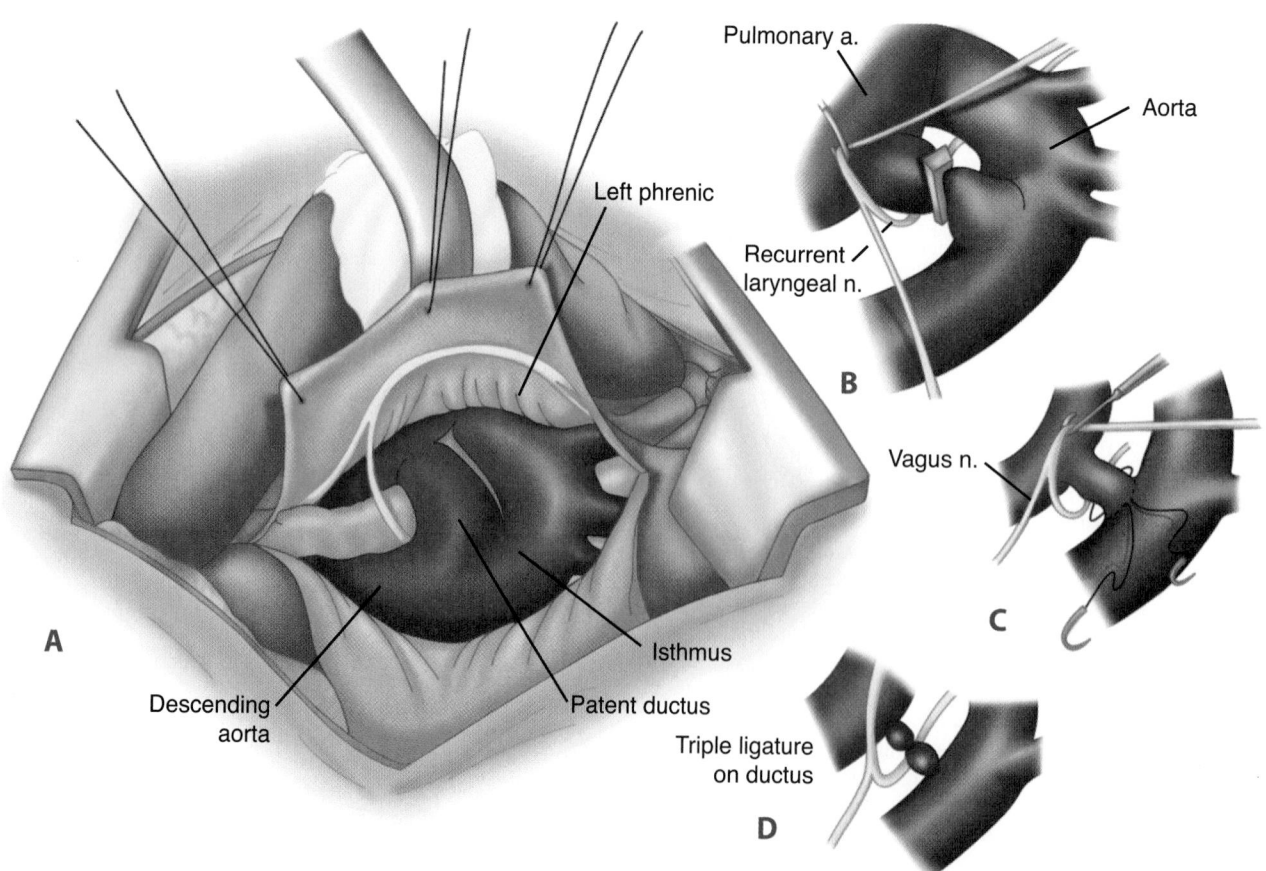

FIG. 20-8. A. Surgeon's perspective of infant patent ductus arteriosus exposed via a left thoracotomy. **B.** The pleura over the aortic isthmus is incised and mobilized. **C** and **D.** Technique of triple ligation. a. = artery; n. = nerve. (*From Castaneda et al,[7] p 208, with permission. Copyright Elsevier.*)

is most commonly located distal to the left subclavian artery. The embryologic origin of COA is a subject of some controversy. One theory holds that the obstructing shelf, which is largely composed of tissue found within the ductus, forms as the ductus involutes.[46] The other theory holds that a diminished aortic isthmus develops secondary to decreased aortic flow in infants with enhanced ductal circulation.

Extensive collateral circulation develops, predominantly involving the intercostals and mammary arteries as a direct result of aortic flow obstruction. This translates into the well-known finding of "rib-notching" on chest radiograph, as well as a prominent pulsation underneath the ribs.

Other associated anomalies, such as VSD, PDA, and ASD, may be seen with COA, but the most common is that of a bicuspid aortic valve, which can be demonstrated in 25 to 42% of cases.[47]

Pathophysiology

Infants with COA develop symptoms consistent with left ventricular outflow obstruction, including pulmonary overcirculation and, later, biventricular failure. In addition, proximal systemic hypertension develops as a result of mechanical obstruction to ventricular ejection, as well as hypoperfusion-induced activation of the renin–angiotensin–aldosterone system. Interestingly, hypertension is often persistent after surgical correction despite complete amelioration of the mechanical obstruction and pressure gradient.[48] It has been shown that early surgical correction may prevent the development of long-term hypertension, which undoubtedly contributes to many of the adverse sequelae of COA, including the development of circle of Willis aneurysms, aortic dissection and rupture, and an increased incidence of coronary arteriopathy with resulting myocardial infarction.[49]

Diagnosis

COA is likely to become symptomatic either in the newborn period if other anomalies are present or in the late adolescent period with the onset of left ventricular failure. Physical examination will demonstrate a hyperdynamic precordium with a harsh murmur localized to the left chest and back. Femoral pulses will be dramatically decreased when compared to upper extremity pulses, and differential cyanosis may be apparent until ductal closure.

Echocardiography will reliably demonstrate the narrowed aortic segment, as well as define the pressure gradient across the stenotic segment. In addition, detailed information regarding other associated anomalies can be gleaned. Aortography is reserved for those cases in which the echocardiographic findings are equivocal.

Therapy

The routine management of hemodynamically significant COA in all age groups has traditionally been surgical. Transcatheter repairs are used with increasing frequency in older patients and those with recoarctation following surgical repair. Balloon dilatation of native coarctation in neonates has been used with poor results. The most common surgical techniques in current use are resection with end-to-end anastomosis or extended end-to-end anastomosis, taking care to remove all residual ductal tissue.[50,51] Extended end-to-end anastomosis may also allow the surgeon to treat transverse arch hypoplasia which is commonly encountered in infants with aortic coarctation.[52,53] The subclavian flap aortoplasty is another repair, although it is used less frequently in the modern era because of the risk of late aneurysm formation and possible underdevelopment of the left upper extremity or ischemia.[51] In this method, the left subclavian artery is transected and brought down over the coarcted segment as a vascularized patch. The main benefit of these techniques is that they do not involve the use of prosthetic materials, and evidence suggests that extended end-to-end anastomosis may promote arch growth, especially in infants with the smallest initial aortic arch diameters.[52]

Despite the benefits, however, extended end-to-end anastomosis may not be feasible when there is a long segment of coarctation or in the presence of previous surgery, because sufficient mobilization of the aorta above and below the lesion may not be possible. In this instance, prosthetic materials, such as a patch aortoplasty, in which a prosthetic patch is used to enlarge the coarcted segment, or an interposition tube graft must be used.

The most common complications after COA repair are late restenosis and aneurysm formation at the repair site.[54–56] Aneurysm formation is particularly common after patch aortoplasty when using Dacron material. In a large series of 891 patients, aneurysms occurred in 5.4% of the total, with 89% occurring in the group who received Dacron-patch aortoplasty, and only 8% in those who received resection with primary end-to-end anastomosis.[54] A further complication, although uncommon, is lower-body paralysis resulting from ischemic spinal cord injury during the repair. This dreaded outcome complicates 0.5% of all surgical repairs, but its incidence can be lessened with the use of some form of distal perfusion, preferably left heart bypass with the use of femoral arterial or distal thoracic aorta for arterial inflow and the femoral vein or left atrium for venous return.[50] These techniques are generally reserved for older patients with complex coarctations that may need prolonged aortic cross-clamp times for repair, often in the setting of large collateral vessels and/or previous surgery.

Hypertension is also well recognized following repair of COA. Bouchart and colleagues reported that in a cohort of 35 hypertensive adults (mean age 28 years) undergoing repair, despite a satisfactory anatomic outcome, only 23 patients were normotensive at a mean follow-up period of 165 months.[55] Likewise, Bhat and associates reported that in a series of 84 patients (mean age at repair was 29 years), 31% remained hypertensive at a mean follow-up of 5 years following surgery.[56]

Although operative repair is still the gold standard, treatment of COA by catheter-based intervention has become more widespread. Both balloon dilatation and primary stent implantation have been used successfully. The most extensive study of the results of balloon angioplasty reported on 970 procedures: 422 native and 548 recurrent COAs. Mean gradient reduction was 74 ± 24% for native and 70 ± 31% for recurrent COA.[57] This demonstrated that catheter-based therapy could produce equally effective results both in recurrent and in primary COA, a finding with far-reaching implications in the new paradigm of multidisciplinary treatment algorithms for CHD. In the valvuloplasty and angioplasty of congenital anomalies report, higher preangioplasty gradient, earlier procedure date, older patient age, and the presence of recurrent COA were independent risk factors for suboptimal procedural outcome.[57]

The gradient after balloon dilatation in most series is generally acceptable. However, there is a significant minority (0 to 26%) for whom the procedural outcome is suboptimal, with a postprocedure gradient of 20 mmHg or greater. These patients may be ideal candidates for primary stent placement. Restenosis is much less common in children, presumably reflecting the influence of vessel wall scarring and growth in the pediatric age group.

Deaths from the procedure also are infrequent (less than 1% of cases), and the main major complication is aneurysm formation, which occurs in 7% of patients.[50] With stent implantation, many authors have demonstrated improved resolution of stenosis compared with balloon dilatation alone, yet the long-term complications on vessel wall compliance remain largely unknown because only midterm data are widely available.

In summary, children younger than age 6 months with native COA should be treated with surgical repair, while those requiring intervention at later ages may be ideal candidates for balloon dilatation or primary stent implantation.[50] Additionally, catheter-based therapy should be used for those cases of restenosis following either surgical or primary endovascular management.

Truncus Arteriosus
Anatomy

Truncus arteriosus is a rare anomaly, comprising between 1 and 4% of all cases of CHD.[58] It is characterized by a single great artery that

Collett & Edwards

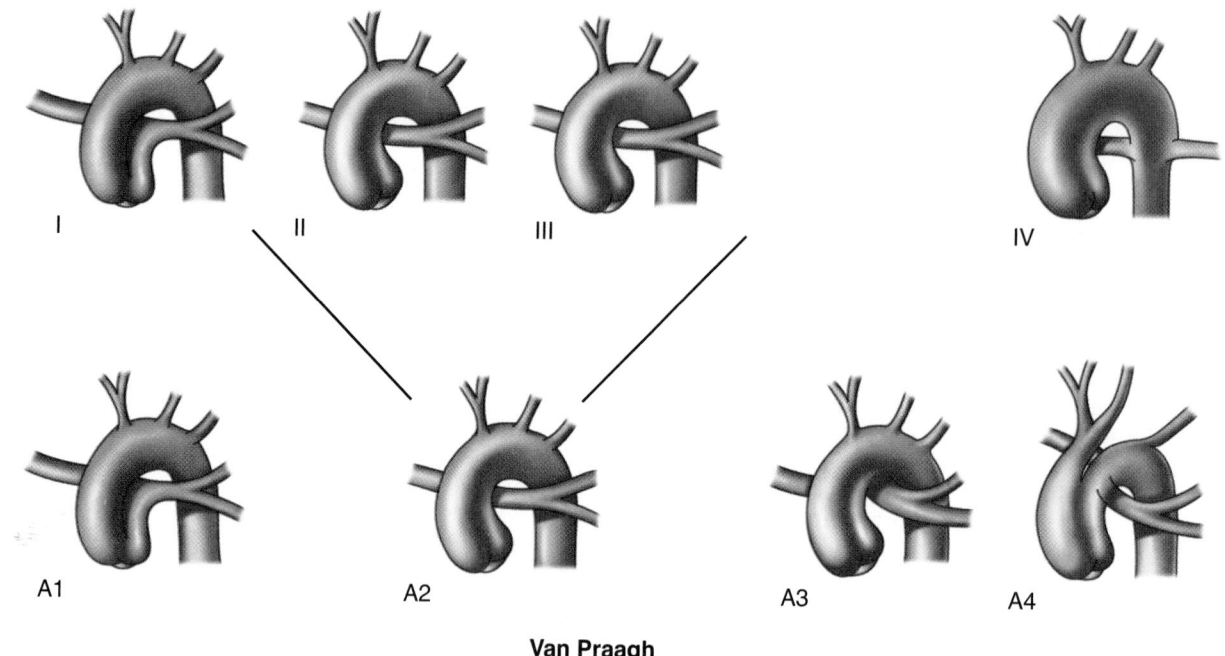

Van Praagh

FIG. 20-9. There are similarities between the Collett and Edwards and the Van Praagh classifications of truncus arteriosus. Type I is the same as A1. Types II and III are grouped as a single type A2 because they are not significantly distinct embryologically or therapeutically. Type A3 denotes unilateral pulmonary artery with collateral supply to the contralateral lung (hemitruncus). Type A4 is truncus associated with interrupted aortic arch (13% of all cases of truncus arteriosus). *[Reproduced with permission from Fyler DC: Truncus arteriosus, in Fyler DC (ed): Nadas' Pediatric Cardiology. Philadelphia: Hanley & Belfus, 1992, p 676. Copyright Elsevier. As adapted with permission from Hernanz-Schulman M, Fellows KE: Persistent truncus arteriosus: Pathologic, diagnostic and therapeutic considerations. Semin Roentgenol 20:121, 1985. Copyright Elsevier.]*

arises from the heart, overrides the ventricular septum, and supplies the pulmonary, systemic, and coronary circulations.

The two major classification systems are those of Collett and Edwards, described in 1949, and Van Praagh and Van Praagh, described in 1965 (Fig. 20-9).[59,60] The Collett and Edwards classification focuses mainly on the origin of the pulmonary arteries from the common arterial trunk, whereas the Van Praagh system is based on the presence or absence of a VSD, the degree of formation of the aorticopulmonary septum, and the status of the aortic arch.

During embryonic life, the truncus arteriosus normally begins to separate and spiral into a distinguishable anterior PA and posterior aorta. Persistent truncus, therefore, represents an arrest in embryologic development at this stage.[61] Other implicated events include twisting of the dividing truncus because of ventricular looping, subinfundibular atresia, and abnormal location of the semilunar valve anlages.[62]

The neural crest may also play a crucial role in the normal formation of the great vessels, as experimental studies in chick embryos have shown that ablation of the neural crest results in persistent truncus arteriosus.[63] The neural crest also develops into the pharyngeal pouches that give rise to the thymus and parathyroids, which likely explains the prevalent association of truncus arteriosus and DiGeorge syndrome.[64]

The annulus of the truncal valve usually straddles the ventricular septum in a "balanced" fashion; however, it is not unusual for it to be positioned predominantly over the RV, which increases the potential for LVOT obstruction following surgical repair. In the great majority of cases, the leaflets are thickened and deformed, which leads to valvular insufficiency. There are usually three leaflets (60%), but occasionally a bicuspid (50%), or even a quadricuspid valve (25%), is present.[65]

In truncus arteriosus, the pulmonary trunk bifurcates, with the left and right pulmonary arteries forming posteriorly and to the left

in most cases. The caliber of the pulmonary arterial branches is usually normal, with stenosis or diffuse hypoplasia occurring in rare instances.

The coronary arteries may be normal; however, anomalies are not unusual and occur in 50% of cases.[65,66] Many of these are relatively minor, although two variations are of particular importance, because they have implications in the conduct of operative repair. The first is that the left coronary ostium may arise high in the sinus of Valsalva or even from the truncal tissue at the margin of the PA tissue. This coronary artery can be injured during repair when the pulmonary arteries are removed from the trunk or when the resulting truncal defect is closed. The second is that the right coronary artery can give rise to an important accessory anterior descending artery, which often passes across the RV in the exact location where the right ventriculotomy is commonly performed during repair.[65,66]

Physiology and Diagnosis

The main pathophysiologic consequences of truncus arteriosus are (a) the obligatory mixing of systemic and pulmonary venous blood at the level of the VSD and truncal valve, which leads to arterial saturations near 85%, and (b) the presence of a nonrestrictive left-to-right shunt, which occurs during both systole and diastole, the volume of which is determined by the relative resistances of the pulmonary and systemic circulations.[65] Additionally, truncal valve stenosis or regurgitation, the presence of important LVOTO, and stenosis of PA branches can further contribute to both pressure- and volume loading of the ventricles. The presence of these lesions often results in severe heart failure and cardiovascular instability early in life. PVR may develop as early as 6 months of age, leading to poor results with late surgical correction.

Patients with truncus arteriosus usually present in the neonatal period, with signs and symptoms of CHF and mild to moderate cyanosis. A pan-systolic murmur may be noted at the left sternal border, and occasionally a diastolic murmur may be heard in the presence of truncal regurgitation.

Chest radiography will be consistent with pulmonary overcirculation, and a right aortic arch can be appreciated 35% of the time. The ECG is usually nonspecific, demonstrating normal sinus rhythm with biventricular hypertrophy.

Echocardiography with Doppler color flow or pulsed Doppler is diagnostic, and usually provides sufficient information to determine the type of truncus arteriosus, the origin of the coronary arteries, and their proximity to the pulmonary trunk, the character of the truncal valves, and the extent of truncal insufficiency.[65] Cardiac catheterization can be helpful in cases where pulmonary hypertension is suspected, or to further delineate coronary artery anomalies before repair.

The presence of truncus is an indication for surgery. Repair should be undertaken in the neonatal period, or as soon as the diagnosis is established. Eisenmenger's physiology, which is found primarily in older children, is the only absolute contraindication to correction.

Repair

Truncus arteriosus was first managed with PA banding as described by Armer and colleagues in 1961.[67] However, this technique led to only marginal improvements in 1-year survival rates because ventricular failure inevitably occurred. In 1967, however, complete repair was accomplished by McGoon and his associates based on the experimental work of Rastelli, who introduced the idea that an extracardiac valved conduit could be used to restore ventricular-to-PA continuity.[68] Over the next 20 years, improved survival rates led to uniform adoption of complete repair even in the youngest and smallest infants.[58,65,69]

Surgical correction entails the use of CPB. Repair is completed by separation of the pulmonary arteries from the aorta, closure of the aortic defect (occasionally with a patch) to minimize coronary flow complications, placement of a valved cryopreserved allograft or jugular venous valved conduit (Contegra) to reconstruct the RVOT, and ventricular septal defect closure. Important branch pulmonary arterial stenosis should be repaired at the time of complete repair, and can usually be accomplished with longitudinal allograft patch arterioplasty. Severe truncal valve insufficiency occasionally requires truncal valve replacement, which can be accomplished with a cryopreserved allograft.[70]

Results

The results of complete repair of truncus have steadily improved. Ebert reported a 91% survival rate in his series of 77 patients who were younger than 6 months of age; later reports by others confirmed these findings and demonstrated that excellent results could be achieved in even smaller infants with complex-associated defects.[11,69]

Newer extracardiac conduits also have been developed and used with success, which has widened the repertoire of the modern congenital heart surgeon and improved outcomes.[71] Severe truncal regurgitation, interrupted aortic arch (IAA), coexistent coronary anomalies, chromosomal or genetic anomalies, and age younger than 100 days are risk factors associated with perioperative death and poor outcome.

Total Anomalous Pulmonary Venous Connection

Total anomalous pulmonary venous connection (TAPVC) occurs in 1 to 2% of all cardiac malformations and is characterized by abnormal drainage of the pulmonary veins into the right heart, whether through connections into the right atrium or into its tributaries.[72] Accordingly, the only mechanism by which oxygenated blood can return to the left heart is through an ASD, which is almost uniformly present with TAPVC.

Unique to this lesion is the absence of a definitive form of palliation. Thus, TAPVC with concomitant obstruction represents one of the only true surgical emergencies across the entire spectrum of congenital heart surgery.

Anatomy and Embryology

The lungs develop from an outpouching of the foregut, and their venous plexus arises as part of the splanchnic venous system. TAPVC arises when the pulmonary vein evagination from the posterior surface of the left atrium fails to fuse with the pulmonary venous plexus surrounding the lung buds. In place of the usual connection to the left atrium, at least one connection of the pulmonary plexus to the splanchnic plexus persists. Accordingly, the pulmonary veins drain to the heart through a systemic vein (Fig. 20-10).

Darling and colleagues classified TAPVC according to the site or level of connection of the pulmonary veins to the systemic venous system[73]: type I (45%), anomalous connection at the supracardiac level; type II (25%), anomalous connection at the cardiac level; type III (25%), anomalous connection at the infracardiac level; and type

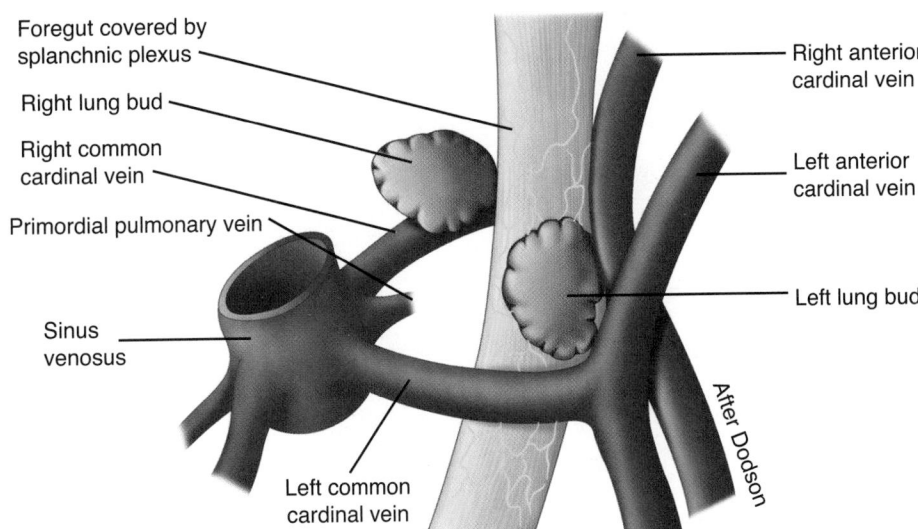

FIG. 20-10. Total anomalous pulmonary venous connection results when the primordial pulmonary vein fails to unite with the plexus of veins that surround the lung buds and is derived from the splanchnic venous plexus, including the cardinal veins and umbilicovitelline veins. *(From Castaneda et al,[7] p 158, with permission. Copyright Elsevier.)*

Foregut covered by splanchnic plexus

Right lung bud

Right common cardinal vein

Primordial pulmonary vein

Sinus venosus

Left common cardinal vein

Right anterior cardinal vein

Left anterior cardinal vein

Left lung bud

After Dodson

IV (5%), anomalous connection at multiple levels.[74] Within each category, further subdivisions can be implemented, depending on whether PVO exists. Obstruction to pulmonary venous drainage is a powerful predictor of adverse natural outcome and occurs most frequently with the infracardiac type, especially when the pattern of infracardiac connection prevents the ductus venosus from bypassing the liver.[75]

Pathophysiology and Diagnosis

Because both pulmonary and systemic venous blood return to the right atrium in all forms of TAPVC, a right-to-left intracardiac shunt must be present for the afflicted infant to survive. This invariably occurs via a nonrestrictive PFO. Because of this obligatory mixing, cyanosis is usually present, and its degree depends on the ratio of pulmonary to systemic blood flow. Decreased pulmonary blood flow is a consequence of PVO, the presence of which is unlikely if the right ventricular pressure is less than 85% of systemic pressure.[76]

The child with TAPVC may present with severe cyanosis and respiratory distress necessitating urgent surgical intervention if a severe degree of PVO is present. However, in cases where there is no obstructive component, the clinical picture is usually one of pulmonary overcirculation, hepatomegaly, tachycardia, and tachypnea with feeding. In a child with serious obstruction, arterial blood gas analysis reveals severe hypoxemia (PO_2 less than 20 mmHg), with metabolic acidosis.[77]

Chest radiography will show normal heart size with generalized pulmonary edema. Two-dimensional echocardiography is very useful in establishing the diagnosis, and also can assess ventricular septal position, which may be leftward secondary to small left ventricular volumes, as well as estimate the right ventricular pressure based on the height of the tricuspid regurgitant jet. Echocardiography can usually identify the pulmonary venous connections (types I–IV), and it is rarely necessary to perform other diagnostic tests.

Cardiac catheterization is not recommended in these patients because the osmotic load from the IV contrast can exacerbate the degree of pulmonary edema.[78] When cardiac catheterization is performed, equalization of oxygen saturations in all four heart chambers is a hallmark finding in this disease because the mixed blood returned to the right atrium gets distributed throughout the heart.

Therapy

Operative correction of TAPVC requires anastomosis of the common pulmonary venous channel to the left atrium, obliteration of the anomalous venous connection, and closure of the ASD.[77,79]

All types of TAPVC are approached through a median sternotomy, and many surgeons use deep hypothermic circulatory arrest to achieve an accurate and widely patent anastomosis. The technique for supracardiac TAPVC includes early division of the vertical vein, retraction of the aorta and the SVC laterally to expose the posterior aspect of the left atrium and the pulmonary venous confluence, and a side-to-side anastomosis between a long, horizontal biatrial incision and a longitudinal incision within the pulmonary venous confluence. The ASD can then be closed with an autologous pericardial or synthetic patch.

In patients with TAPVC to the coronary sinus without obstruction, a simple unroofing of the coronary sinus can be performed through a single right atriotomy with concomitant closure of the ASD. If PVO is present, the repair should include generous resection of roof of the coronary sinus.[77]

Repair of infracardiac TAPVC entails ligation of the vertical vein at the diaphragm, followed by construction of a proximal, patulous longitudinal venotomy. This repair is usually performed by "rolling" the heart toward the left, thus exposing the left atrium where it usually overlies the descending vertical vein (Fig. 20-11).

The perioperative care of these infants is crucial because episodes of pulmonary hypertension can occur within the first 48 hours, which contribute significantly to mortality following repair.[6,78,79] Muscle relaxants and narcotics should be administered during this period to maintain a constant state of anesthesia. Arterial partial pressure of carbon dioxide should be maintained at

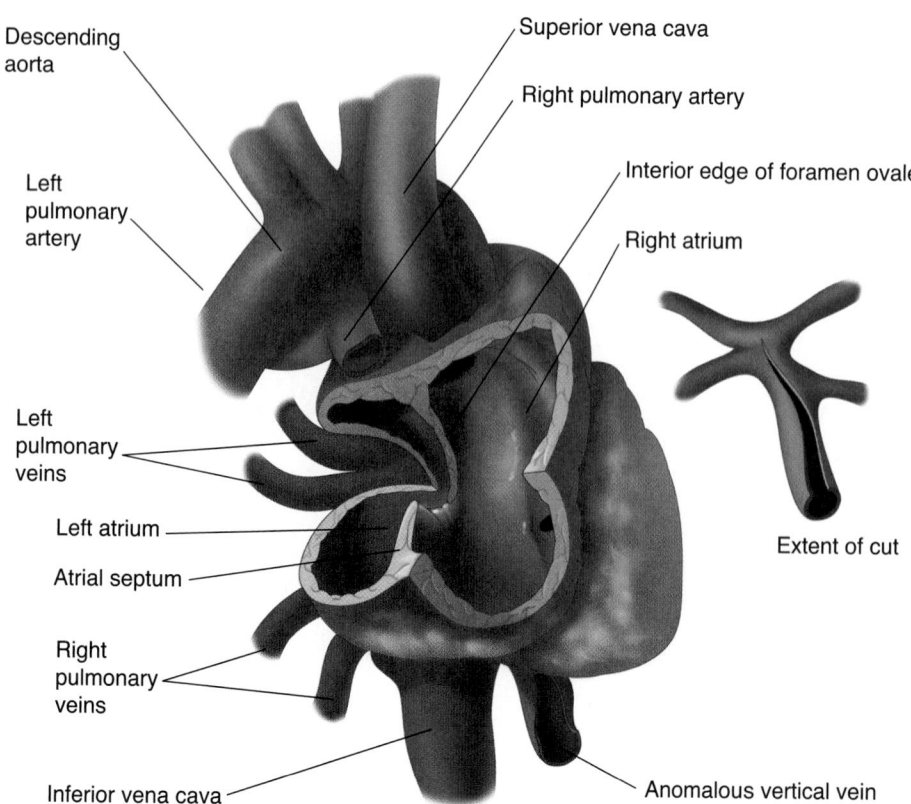

FIG. 20-11. Operative exposure obtained with infradiaphragmatic total anomalous pulmonary venous connection, using an approach from the right. *(From Castaneda et al,[7] p 161, with permission. Copyright Elsevier.)*

30 mmHg with use of a volume ventilator and the fraction of inspired oxygen should be increased to keep the pulmonary arterial pressure at less than two thirds of the systemic pressure.

Results

Results of TAPVC in infancy have markedly improved, with an operative mortality of 5% or less in some series.[77–80] This improvement is probably multifactorial, mainly as a consequence of early noninvasive diagnosis and aggressive perioperative management. The routine use of echocardiography; improvements in myocardial protection with specific attention to the RV; creation of a large, tension-free anastomosis with maximal use of the venous confluence and atrial tissue; careful geometric alignment of the pulmonary venous sinus with the body of the left atrium avoiding tension and rotation of the pulmonary veins; and prevention of pulmonary hypertensive events have likely played a major role in reducing operative mortality. The importance of risk factors for early mortality, such as venous obstruction at presentation, urgency of operative repair, and infradiaphragmatic anatomic type, has been debated.[79,81]

Bando and colleagues[82] made the controversial statement that both preoperative PVO and anatomic type had been neutralized as potential risk factors beyond calendar year 1991. Hyde and associates[80] similarly reported that connection type was not related to outcome. However, a recent, large, single institution report of 377 children with TAPVC by the author from the Hospital for Sick Children in Toronto[83] found that, although outcomes had improved over time, patient anatomic factors were still important determinants of both survival and the need for subsequent reoperation. Risk factors for postrepair death were earlier operation year, younger age at repair, cardiac connection type, and postoperative PVO. Risk-adjusted estimated 1-year survival for a patient repaired at birth with unfavorable morphology in 2006 is 37% (95% confidence intervals: 8 to 80%) compared to 96% (95% confidence intervals: 91 to 99%) for a patient with favorable morphology repaired at age 1 year. Freedom from reoperation was 82% ± 6% at 11 years postrepair, with increased risk associated with mixed connection and postoperative PVO. (Fig. 20-12).

The most significant postoperative complication of TAPVC repair is PVO, which occurs 9 to 11% of the time, regardless of the surgical technique used. Mortality varies between 30 and 45% and alternative catheter interventions do not offer definitive solutions.[78] Recurrent PVO can be localized at the site of the pulmonary venous anastomosis (extrinsic), which can usually be cured with patch enlargement or balloon dilatation, or it may be secondary to endocardial thickening of the pulmonary venous ostia frequently resulting in diffuse pulmonary venous sclerosis (intrinsic), which carries a 66% mortality rate because few good solutions exist.[75] More commonly, postrepair left ventricular dysfunction can occur as the noncompliant LV suddenly is required to handle an increased volume load from redirected pulmonary venous return. This can manifest as an increase in PA pressure but is distinguishable from primary pulmonary hypertension (another possible postoperative complication following repair of TAPVC) from the elevated LA pressure and LV dysfunction along with echocardiographic evidence of poor LV contractility. In pulmonary hypertension, the LA pressure may be low, the LV may appear "underfilled" (by echocardiography), and the RV may appear dilated. In either case, postoperative support for a few days with extracorporeal membrane oxygenation may be lifesaving, and TAPVC should be repaired in centers that have this capacity.

Some investigators have speculated that preoperative PVO is associated with increased medial thickness within the pulmonary vasculature, which may predispose these infants to intrinsic pulmonary venous stenosis despite adequate pulmonary venous decompression.[80] The majority of studies demonstrating that preoperative PVO is a predictor of subsequent need for reoperation to correct recurrent PVO lend credence to this notion. Another complication following repair of TAPVC is the development of atrial arrhythmias secondary to altered atrial geometry and LA enlargement procedures. These arrhythmias may be asymptomatic, and certain sur-

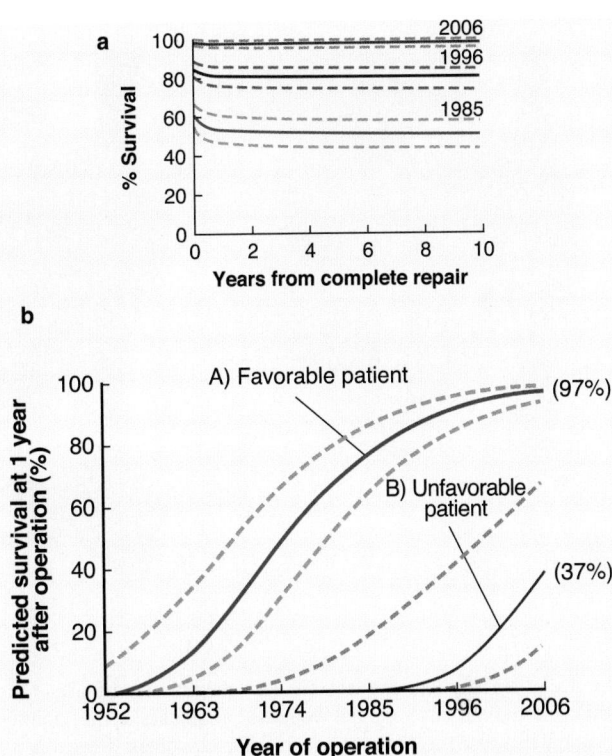

FIG. 20-12. a. Risk-adjusted survival from repair improved significantly with increasing year of operation, indicating a strong era effect. Solid lines are continuous point estimates enclosed by dashed 95% confidence limits showing three different solutions to the multivariable equation for death after repair. All other predictors have been set to mean values to illustrate the favorable influence of later operation year on survival after repair. **b.** Risk-adjusted nomograms show 1-year survival after repair expressed as a function of increasing year of operation for two different patients. The top line (*A*) shows the multivariable solution for a patient with favorable anatomic characteristics (noncardiac connection without pulmonary venous obstruction) undergoing repair at 1 year of age; the bottom line (*B*) shows the solution for a patient with unfavorable characteristics (cardiac connection with pulmonary venous obstruction) undergoing operation at birth. The nomograms show that the more recent era has improved survival in all patients, especially within the last few decades. However, unfavorable anatomic characteristics have not been neutralized as important determinants of postrepair survival despite improvements in perioperative care. Numbers in parentheses represent parametric estimates of median survival at 1 year after repair in 2005. [*From Karamlou et al,[83] (Fig. 2), with permission.*]

geons therefore advocate routine long-term follow-up with 24-hour ECG monitoring to facilitate their detection and treatment.[81]

Cor Triatriatum

Anatomy

Cor triatriatum is a rare CHD characterized by the presence of a fibromuscular diaphragm that partitions the left atrium into two chambers: a superior chamber that receives drainage from the pulmonary veins, and an inferior chamber that communicates with the mitral valve and the LV (Fig. 20-13). An ASD frequently exists between the superior chamber and the right atrium, or, more rarely, between the right atrium and the inferior chamber.[84]

Pathophysiology and Diagnosis

Cor triatriatum results in obstruction of pulmonary venous return to the left atrium. The degree of obstruction is variable and depends on

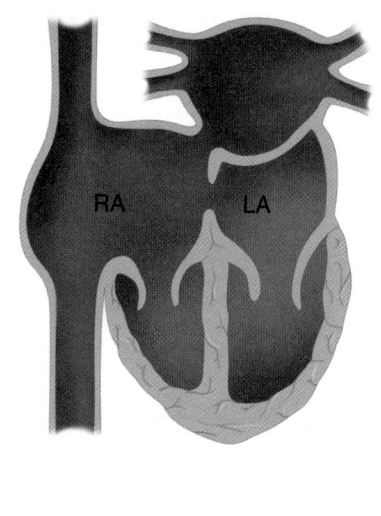
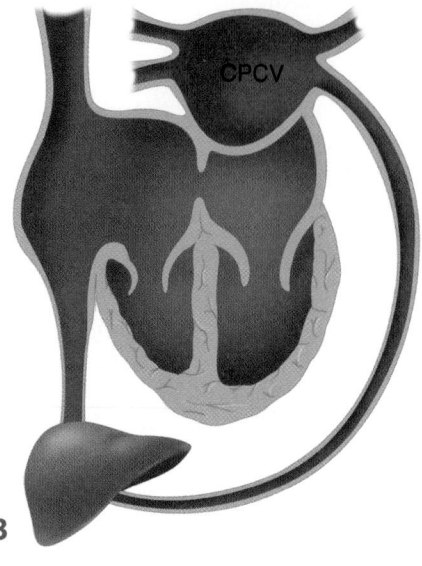

FIG. 20-13. Variants of cor triatriatum with imperforate membrane between common pulmonary venous chamber (*CPVC*) and left atrium (*LA*). **A.** Common chamber draining to right atrium directly. **B.** Common chamber draining into systemic venous circulation via anomalous vein. RA = right atrium. *[Adapted with permission from Lucas RV: Anomalous venous connections, pulmonary and systemic, in Adams FH, Emmanouilides GC (eds):* Moss' Heart Disease in Infants, Children, and Adolescents, *3rd ed. Baltimore: Lippincott Williams & Wilkins, 1983.]*

the size of fenestrations present in the LA membrane, the size of the ASD, and the existence of other associated anomalies. If the communication between the superior and inferior chambers is less than 3 mm, patients usually are symptomatic during the first year of life. The afflicted infant will present with the stigmata of low cardiac output and pulmonary venous hypertension, as well as CHF and poor feeding.

Physical examination may demonstrate a loud pulmonary S_2 sound and a right ventricular heave, as well as jugular venous distention and hepatomegaly. Chest radiography will show cardiomegaly and pulmonary vascular prominence, and the ECG will suggest right ventricular hypertrophy. Two-dimensional echocardiography provides a definitive diagnosis in most cases, with catheterization necessary only when echocardiographic evaluation is equivocal.

Therapy

Operative treatment for cor triatriatum is fairly simple. CPB and cardioplegic arrest are used. A right atriotomy usually allows access to the LA membrane through the existing ASD, because it is dilated secondary to communication with the pulmonary venous chamber. The membrane is then excised, taking care not to injure the mitral valve or the interatrial septum, and the ASD is closed with a patch. Alternatively, if the right atrium is small, the membrane can be exposed through an incision directly into the superior LA chamber, just anterior to the right pulmonary veins.[7,82] Surgical results are uniformly excellent for this defect, with survival approaching 100%.

The use of catheter-based intervention for this diagnosis remains controversial, although there have been two recent reports of successful balloon dilatation.[83]

Aortopulmonary Window
Embryology and Anatomy

Aortopulmonary window (APW) is a rare congenital lesion, occurring in about 0.2% of patients, characterized by incomplete development of the septum that normally divides the truncus into the aorta and the PA.[85]

In the vast majority of cases, APW occurs as a single defect of minimal length, which begins a few millimeters above the semilunar valves on the left lateral wall of the aorta (Fig. 20-14). Coronary artery anomalies, such as aberrant origin of the right or left coronary artery from the main PA, are occasionally present.

Pathophysiology and Diagnosis

The dominant pathophysiology of APW is that of a large left-to-right shunt with increased pulmonary flow and the early develop-

ment of CHF. Like other lesions with left-to-right flow, the magnitude of the shunt is determined by the size of the defect, as well as the PVR.

Infants with APW present with frequent respiratory tract infections, tachypnea with feeding, and failure to thrive. Cyanosis is usually absent because these infants deteriorate before the onset of significant pulmonary hypertension. The rapid decline with this defect occurs because shunt flow continues during both phases of the cardiac cycle, which limits systemic perfusion and increases ventricular work.[86]

The diagnosis of APW begins with the physical examination, which may demonstrate a systolic flow murmur, a hyperdynamic precordium, and bounding peripheral pulses. The chest radiograph will show pulmonary overcirculation and cardiomegaly, and the ECG will usually demonstrate either left ventricular hypertrophy or biventricular hypertrophy. Echocardiography can detect the defect and also provide information about associated anomalies. Retrograde aortography will confirm the diagnosis, but is rarely necessary.

Therapy

All infants with APW require surgical correction once the diagnosis is made. Repair is undertaken through a median sternotomy and the use of CPB. The pulmonary arteries are occluded once the distal aorta is cannulated, and a transaortic repair using a prosthetic patch for PA closure is then carried out. The coronary ostia must be carefully visualized and included on the aortic side of the patch. Alternatively, a two-patch technique can be used, which may eliminate recurrent

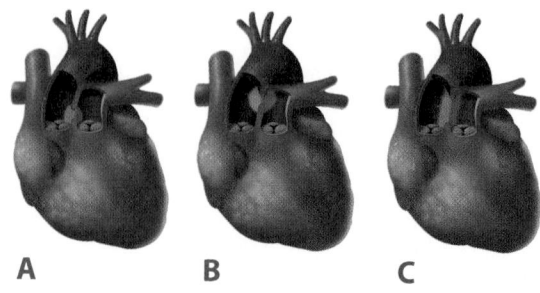

FIG. 20-14. A through **C.** Classification of aortopulmonary window. *(Reproduced with permission from Mori K, Ando M, Takao A: Distal type of aortopulmonary window: report of 4 cases. Br Heart J 40:681, 1978. With permission from the BMJ Publishing Group.)*

FIG. 20-15. Two-patch repair of aortopulmonary window. **A.** The aorta and right atrium are cannulated through a median sternotomy and, once the patient is on cardiopulmonary bypass, the right and left pulmonary arteries are occluded with snares. The ducts arteriosus (when present) can be ligated. The aorta is cross-clamped and the heart arrested with cardioplegia. The aortopulmonary window is then divided, with the left coronary ostia being carefully protected. **B.** A piece of previously prepared pulmonary homograft material is used to patch the aortic defect. In older children polytetrafluoroethylene material can be safely used. **C.** Once the aortic portion of the defect has been safely repaired, the aortic cross-clamp may be removed to restore perfusion to the heart. During rewarming the pulmonary portion of the defect is repaired using a similar piece of homograft or polytetrafluoroethylene. **D.** At the completion of repair, the patient is easily weaned from cardiopulmonary bypass, and the cannulas are removed. This type of repair restores normal anatomy, with a reduced likelihood of long-term fistula formation. *(From Gaynor et al,[87] with permission.)*

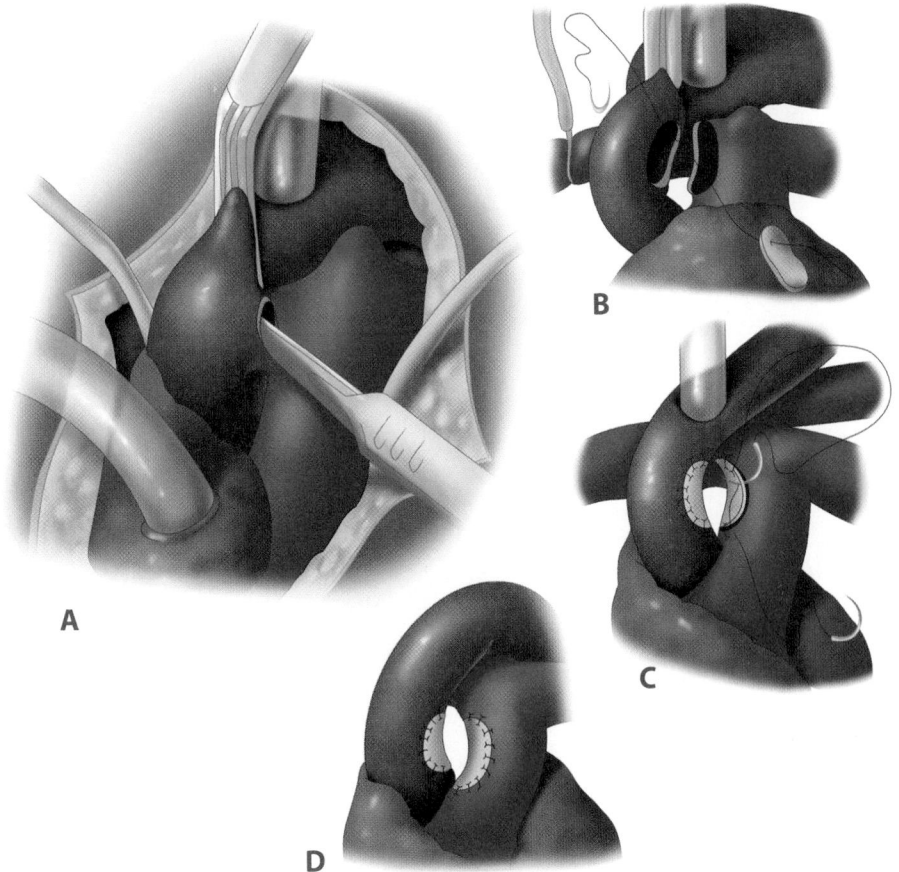

fistulas from suture line leaks that occasionally occur with the single-patch method (Fig. 20-15).[85]

Results

Results are generally excellent, with an operative mortality in most large series of less than 5%.[85]

DEFECTS REQUIRING PALLIATION

Tricuspid Atresia

Tricuspid atresia occurs in 2 to 3% of patients with CHD and is characterized by atresia of the tricuspid valve. This results in discontinuity between the right atrium and RV. The RV is generally hypoplastic, and left-heart filling is dependent on an ASD. Tricuspid atresia is the most common form of the single-ventricle complex, indicating that there is functionally only one ventricular chamber.

Anatomy

As mentioned, tricuspid atresia results in a lack of communication between the right atrium and the RV, and in the majority of patients there is no identifiable valve tissue or remnant.[88] The right atrium is generally enlarged and muscular, with a fibrofatty floor. An unrestrictive ASD is usually present. The LV is often enlarged as it receives both systemic and pulmonary blood flow, but the left AV valve usually is normal.

The RV, however, usually is severely hypoplastic, and there is sometimes a ventricular septal defect in its trabeculated or infundibular portion. In many cases, the interventricular communication is a site of obstruction to pulmonary blood flow, but obstruction may also occur at the level of the outlet valve or in the subvalvular infundibulum.[87] In most cases, pulmonary blood flow is dependent on the presence of a PDA, and there may be no flow into the pulmonary circulation except for this PDA.

Tricuspid atresia is classified according to the relationship of the great vessels and by the degree of obstruction to pulmonary blood flow (Fig. 20-16). Because of the rarity of tricuspid atresia with transposed great arteries, this chapter will focus solely on tricuspid atresia with normally related great vessels.

Pathophysiology

The main pathophysiology in tricuspid atresia is that of a univentricular heart of left ventricular morphology. That is, the LV must receive systemic blood via the interatrial communication, and then distribute it to both the pulmonary circulation and the systemic circulation. Unless there is a VSD (as is found in some cases), pulmonary flow is dependent upon the presence of a PDA. As the ductus begins to close shortly after birth, infants become intensely cyanotic. Re-establishing ductal patency (with PGE_1) restores pulmonary blood flow and stabilizes patients for surgical intervention. Pulmonary hypertension is unusual in tricuspid atresia. However, occasional patients have a large VSD between the LV and the infundibular portion of the RV (just below the pulmonary valve). If there is no obstruction at the level of this VSD or at the valve, these infants may actually present with heart failure from excessive pulmonary blood flow. Regardless of whether these infants are "ductal-dependent" for pulmonary blood flow or have pulmonary blood flow provided across a VSD, they will be cyanotic because the obligatory right-to-left shunt at the atrial level will provide complete mixing of systemic and pulmonary venous return so that the LV ejects a hypoxemic mixture into the aorta.

Diagnosis

The signs and symptoms of tricuspid atresia are dependent on the underlying anatomic variant, but most infants are cyanotic and hypoxic as a result of decreased pulmonary blood flow and the

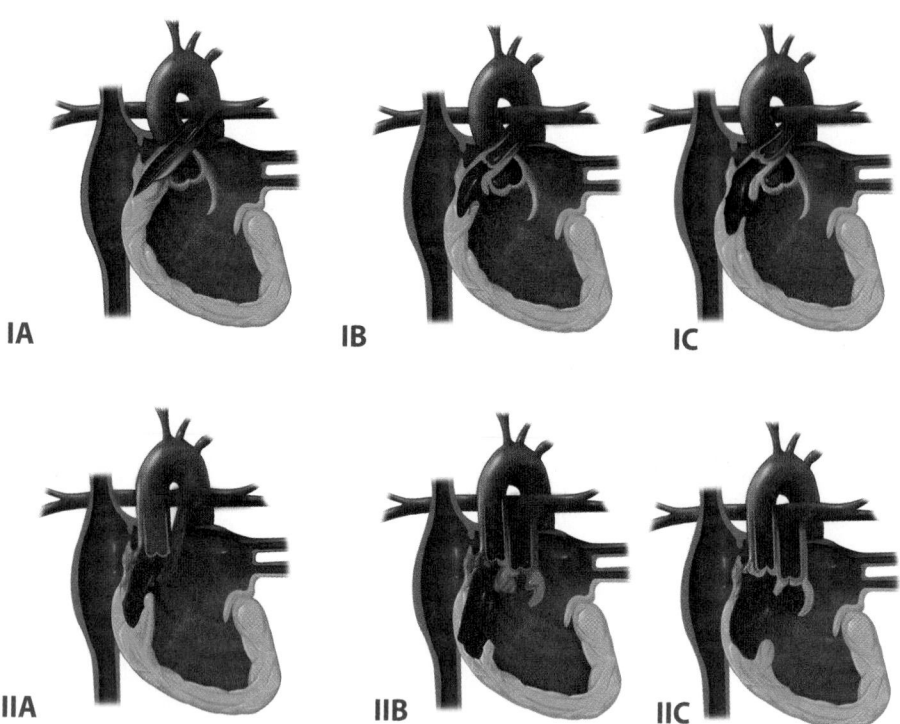

FIG. 20-16. Classification of tricuspid atresia. Type I, normally related great arteries with: **IA,** pulmonary atresia with virtual absence of right ventricle; **IB,** pulmonary stenosis with small ventricular septal defect; **IC,** normal pulmonary valve, large ventricular septal defect. Type II, transposed great arteries with: **IIA,** pulmonary atresia; **IIB,** pulmonary or subpulmonary stenosis; **IIC,** normal or enlarged pulmonary valve and artery without subpulmonary stenosis. [*Reproduced with permission from Tricuspid atresia, in Mavroudis C and Backer CL (eds):* Pediatric Cardiac Surgery, *2nd ed. St. Louis: Mosby, 1994, p 381.*]

complete mixing at the atrial level. When pulmonary blood flow is provided through a VSD, there may be a prominent systolic murmur. Tricuspid atresia with pulmonary blood flow from a PDA may present with the soft, continuous murmur of a PDA in conjunction with cyanosis.

In the minority of patients with tricuspid atresia, symptoms of CHF will predominate. This is often related to excessive flow across a VSD. The natural history of the muscular VSDs in these infants is that they will close and the CHF will dissipate and transform into cyanosis with reduced pulmonary blood flow. Chest radiography will show decreased pulmonary vascularity. The ECG is strongly suggestive, because uncharacteristic left axis deviation will be present, owing to underdevelopment of the RV. Two-dimensional echocardiography readily confirms the diagnosis and the anatomic subtype.

Treatment

The treatment for tricuspid atresia in the earlier era of palliation was aimed at correcting the defect in the pulmonary circulation. That is, patients with too much pulmonary flow received a pulmonary band, and those with insufficient flow received a systemic-to-PA shunt. Systemic-to-PA shunts, or Blalock-Taussig (B-T) shunts, were first applied to patients with tricuspid atresia in the 1940s and 1950s.[89] Likewise PA banding was applied to patients with tricuspid atresia and congestive failure in 1957. However, despite the initial relief of either cyanosis or CHF, long-term mortality was high, as the single ventricle was left unprotected from either volume or pressure overload.[90]

Recognizing the inadequacies of the initial repairs, Glenn described the first successful cavopulmonary anastomosis, an end-to-side RPA-to-SVC shunt in 1958, and later modified this to allow flow to both pulmonary arteries.[91] This end-to-side RPA-to-SVC anastomosis was known as the *bidirectional Glenn*, and is the first stage to final Fontan repair in widespread use today (Fig. 20-17). The Fontan repair was a major advancement in the treatment of CHD, as it essentially bypassed the right heart, and allowed separation of the pulmonary and systemic circulations. It was first performed by Fontan in 1971, and consisted of a classic Glenn anastomosis, ASD closure, and direct connection of the right atrium to the proximal end of the left PA using an aortic homograft.[92] The main PA was ligated, and a homograft valve was inserted into the orifice of the IVC.

Multiple modifications of this initial repair were performed over the next 20 years. One of the most important was the description by deLeval and colleagues of the creation of an interatrial lateral tunnel that allowed the inferior vena caval blood to be channeled exclusively to the SVC.[93] A total cavopulmonary connection could then be accomplished by dividing the SVC and suturing the superior portion to the upper side of the RPA and the inferior end to the augmented undersurface of the RPA. Pulmonary flow then occurs passively, in a laminar fashion, driven by the central venous pressure. This repair became known as the *modified Fontan operation*.

Another important modification, the fenestrated Fontan repair, was introduced in 1988.[94-96] In this procedure, a residual 20 to 30% right-to-left shunt is either created or left unrepaired at the time of cavopulmonary connection to help sustain systemic output in the face of transient elevations in the PVR postoperatively (Fig. 20-18).[94]

The last notable variation on the original Fontan repair uses an extracardiac prosthetic tube graft, usually 20 mm in diameter, as the conduit directing IVC blood to the pulmonary arteries.[95] This technique has the advantages of decreasing atrial geometric alterations by avoiding intra-atrial suture lines, and improving flow dynamics in the systemic venous pathway by maximizing laminar flow. Several investigators have shown a decrease in supraventricular arrhythmias, as well as an improvement in ventricular function, which may be secondary to decreased atrial tension and alleviation of chronic elevations in coronary sinus pressure.[95,96] The extracardiac Fontan operation can be completed without the use of CPB in selected cases, which may further improve outcomes.[97]

One potential disadvantage of the extracardiac Fontan is that it delays performance of the Fontan to allow placement of a conduit of sufficient size. Despite these innovative approaches, the current strategy for operative management still relies on the idea of palliation. Patients are approached in a staged manner, to maximize their physiologic state so that they will survive to undergo a Fontan operation. The therapeutic strategy must begin in the neonatal period and should be directed toward reducing the patient's subsequent risk factors for a Fontan procedure. Accordingly, small systemic pulmonary shunts, which are usually performed through a median sternotomy, should be constructed for palliation of ductus-dependent univentricular physiology. This can easily be replaced with a bidirec-

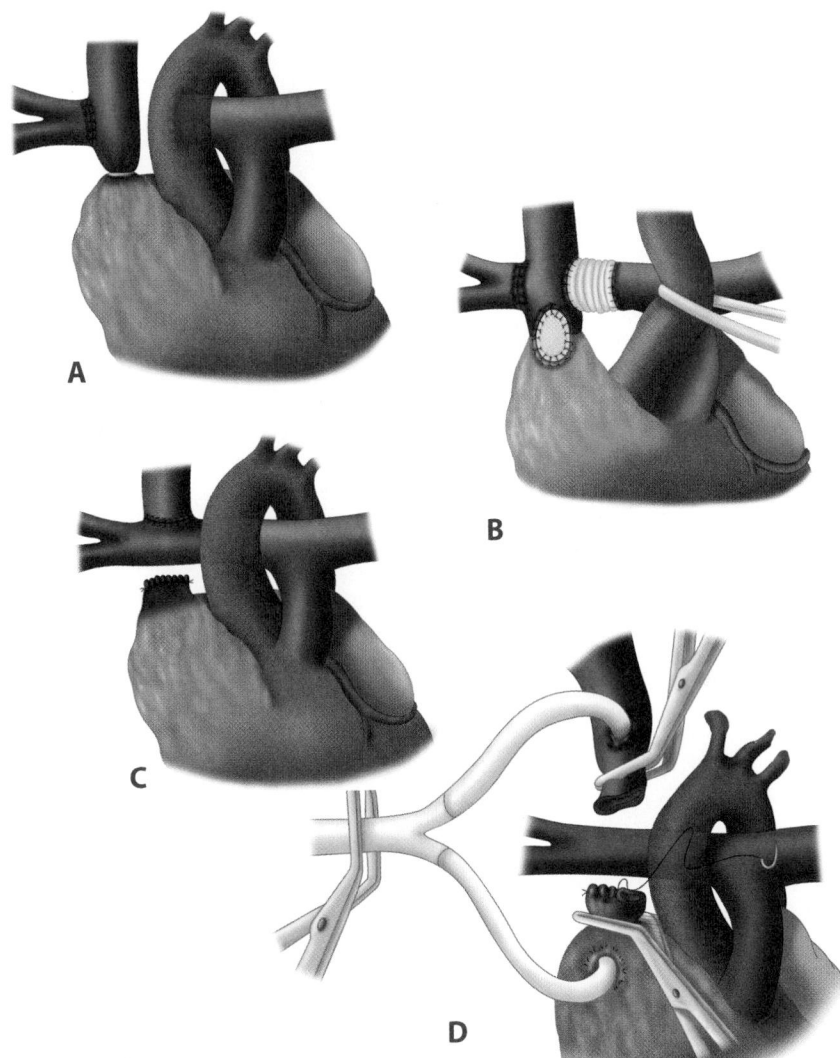

FIG. 20-17. Superior vena cava–pulmonary artery shunts. **A.** Classic Glenn shunt. End-to-side right pulmonary artery (RPA)-to-superior vena cava (SVC) anastomosis with ligation of SVC–right atrial junction. **B.** Method of takedown of classic Glenn shunt and creation of total cavopulmonary anastomosis during Fontan operation. **C.** Bidirectional Glenn shunt (bidirectional SVC–pulmonary artery shunt), end-to-side SVC-to-RPA anastomosis. **D.** Method of construction of bidirectional Glenn shunt, one cannula in the high SVC or innominate vein and another cannula in the right atrium connected to a Y-connector. *[Reproduced with permission from Tricuspid atresia, in Mavroudis C, Backer CL (eds):* Pediatric Cardiac Surgery, *2nd ed. St. Louis: Mosby, 1994, p 383.]*

tional Glenn shunt or hemi-Fontan operation at 6 months of life. In non–ductus-dependent univentricular physiology, the infant can be managed medically until primary construction of a bidirectional cavopulmonary anastomosis becomes feasible. This is possible in the majority of cases because the physiologically elevated PVR prevents pulmonary overcirculation during the neonatal period.

Occasionally, if a previous B-T shunt was performed, arterio-plasty of the RPA may be required to ensure adequate size and unobstructed bilateral flow.[2] The bidirectional Glenn shunt or hemi-Fontan operation effectively avoids recirculation of both systemic and pulmonary venous return, thus preventing volume overload of the single ventricle and its attendant sequelae.[95] PA banding is necessary in 10 to 15% of patients with markedly increased pulmonary blood flow and florid CHF.

The Fontan is usually performed when the child is between 2 and 4 years of age, and it is generally successful if the infant was staged properly, with a protected single ventricle, and there is adequate PA growth. The PVR should be below 4 Wood's units, and the ejection fraction should be more than 45% to ensure success.[98] In patients with high PA pressure, fenestration of the atrial baffle may be helpful because their PVR may preclude adequate cardiac output postoperatively.[92,96]

Results

Reports of the Fontan procedure for tricuspid atresia have been encouraging, with an overall survival of 86% and an operative

mortality of 2%.[8,99] The main complications following repair are atrial arrhythmias, particularly atrial flutter; conduit obstruction requiring reoperation; protein-losing enteropathy; and decreased exercise tolerance.

A prospective multi-institutional study from the Congenital Heart Surgeons' Society reported the outcomes of 150 neonates with tricuspid atresia and normally related great vessels.[99] Five-year survival was 86%, and by the age of 2 years, 89% had undergone cavopulmonary anastomosis, and 75% of those surviving cavopulmonary anastomosis underwent a Fontan operation within 3 years. Competing risks methodology was used in this study to determine the rates of transition to end states and their associated determinants (Fig. 20-19). Risk factors for death without cavopulmonary anastomosis in this study included the presence of mitral regurgitation and palliation with systemic-to-pulmonary artery shunts not originating from the innominate artery. Factors associated with decreased transition rate to cavopulmonary anastomosis included patient variables (younger age at admission to a participating institution and noncardiac anomalies) and procedural variables (larger systemic-to-pulmonary arterial shunt diameter and previous palliation).[99]

Hypoplastic Left-Heart Syndrome

HLHS comprises a wide spectrum of cardiac malformations, including hypoplasia or atresia of the aortic and mitral valves and hypoplasia of the LV and AA.[100] HLHS has a reported prevalence of 0.2 per 1000 live births and occurs twice as often in boys as in girls.

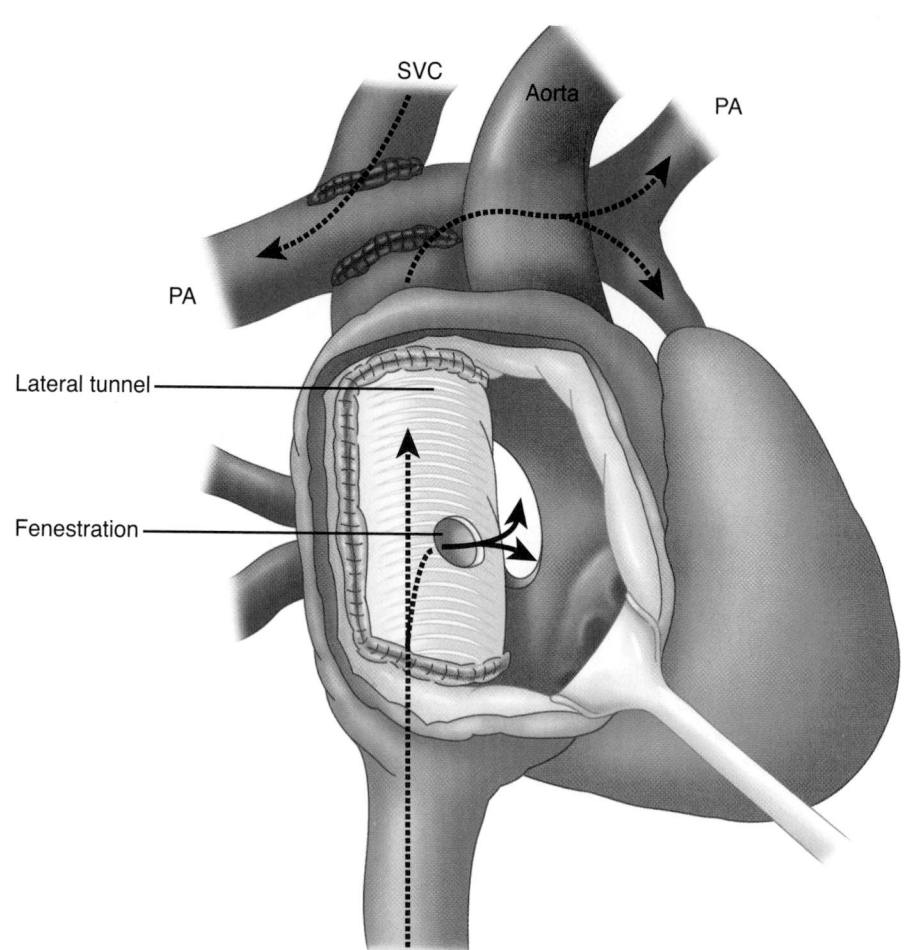

FIG. 20-18. The fenestrated Fontan procedure. Using a polytetrafluoroethylene patch, a tunnel is created in the lateral wall of the right atrium to direct inferior vena cava (IVC) flow to the superior vena cava (SVC) that is anastomosed to the pulmonary artery (PA). A 4- to 5-mm fenestration in the baffle diminishes systemic venous pressure and improves cardiac output at the expense of a small decrease in systemic arterial oxygen saturation. *(Reproduced with permission from Kopf GS, Kleinman CS, Hijazi ZM, et al: Fenestrated Fontan operation with delayed transcatheter closure of atrial septal defect: Improved results in high-risk patients. J Thorac Cardiovasc Surg 103:1039, 1992. Copyright Elsevier.)*

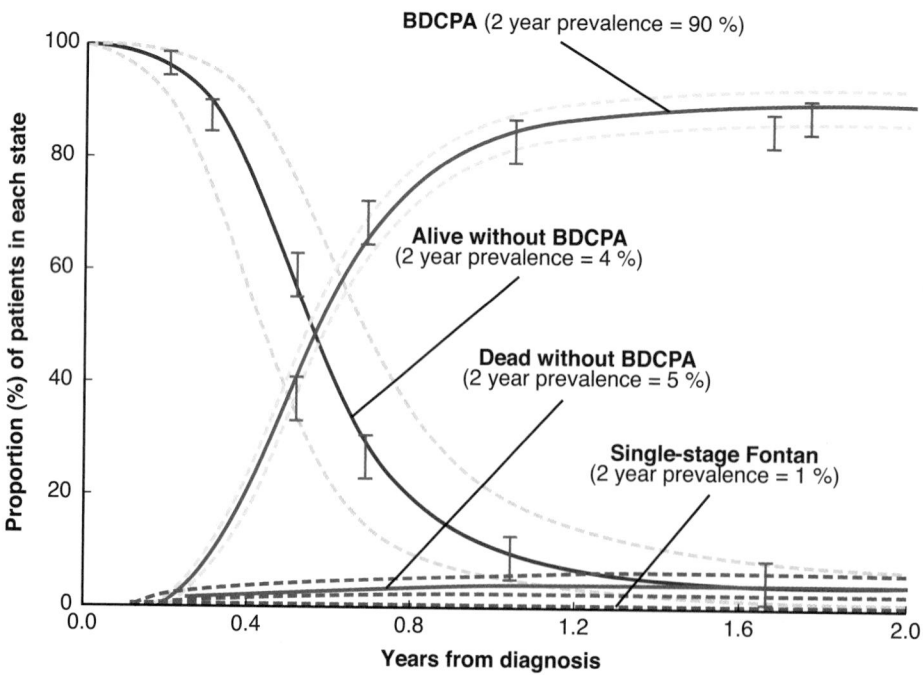

FIG. 20-19. Competing risks depiction of events after diagnosis in 150 patients with tricuspid atresia. All patients began alive and thereafter migrated to one of four mutually exclusive end states [death, bidirectional cavopulmonary anastomosis (BDCPA), single-stage Fontan completion, or remaining alive without BDCPA] at time-dependent rates defined by the underlying hazard functions. At any point in time, the sum of proportions of children in each state is 100%. For example, estimated prevalences after 2 years from diagnosis are as follows: 89% BDCPA, 6% dead without BDCPA, 4% alive without BDCPA, and 1% single-stage Fontan completion. Solid lines represent parametric point estimates; dashed lines enclose 70% confidence intervals; circles with error bars represent nonparametric estimates; numbers in parentheses indicate the estimated proportion of patients in each state at 2 years from diagnosis. *(From Karamlou et al,[99] Fig. 1, with permission. Copyright Elsevier.)*

Left untreated, HLHS is invariably fatal and is responsible for 25% of early cardiac deaths in neonates.[101] However, the evolution of palliative surgical procedures has dramatically improved the outlook for patients with HLHS, and an improved understanding of anatomic and physiologic alterations have spurred advances in parallel arenas such as intrauterine diagnosis and fetal intervention, echocardiographic imaging, and neonatal critical care.

Anatomy

As implied by its name, HLHS involves varying degrees of underdevelopment of left-sided structures, including the LV and the aortic and mitral valves. Thus, HLHS can be classified into four anatomic subtypes based on the valvular morphology: (a) aortic and mitral stenosis; (b) aortic and mitral atresia; (c) aortic atresia and mitral stenosis; and (d) AS and mitral atresia. Aortic atresia tends to be associated with more severe degrees of hypoplasia of the AA than does AS.

Even in cases without frank aortic atresia, however, the aortic arch is generally hypoplastic and, in severe cases, may even be interrupted. There is an associated coarctation shelf in 80% of patients with HLHS, and the ductus itself is usually quite large, as is the main PA.[7] The segmental pulmonary arteries, however, are small, secondary to reduced intrauterine pulmonary blood flow, which is itself a consequence of the left-sided outflow obstruction. The LA cavity is generally smaller than normal, and is accentuated because of the leftward displacement of the septum primum. There is almost always an interatrial communication via the foramen ovale, which can be large, but more commonly restricts right-to-left flow. In rare cases, there is no atrial-level communication, which can be lethal for these infants because there is no way for pulmonary venous return to cross over to the RV.

Associated defects can occur with HLHS, and many of them have importance with respect to operative repair. For example, if a ventricular septal defect is present, the LV can retain its normal size during development even in the presence of mitral atresia. This is because a right-to-left shunt through the defect impels growth of the LV.[102] This introduces the feasibility of biventricular repair for this subset of patients.

Although HLHS undoubtedly results from a complex interplay of developmental errors in the early stages of cardiogenesis, many investigators have hypothesized that the altered blood flow is responsible for the structural underdevelopment that characterizes HLHS. In other words, if the stimulus for normal development of the AA from the primordial aortic sac is high-pressure systemic blood flow from the LV through the aortic valve, then an atretic or stenotic aortic valve, which impedes flow and leads to only low-pressure diastolic retrograde flow via the ductus, will change the developmental signals and result in hypoplasia of the downstream structures. Normal growth and development of the LV and mitral valve can be secondarily affected, resulting in hypoplasia or atresia of these structures.[100]

Pathophysiology and Diagnosis

In HLHS, pulmonary venous blood enters the left atrium, but atrial systole cannot propel blood across the stenotic or atretic mitral valve into the LV. Thus, the blood is shunted across the foramen ovale into the right atrium, where it contributes to volume loading of the RV. The end result is pulmonary venous hypertension from outflow obstruction at the level of the left atrium, as well as pulmonary overcirculation and right ventricular failure. As the PVR falls postnatally, the condition is exacerbated because right ventricular output is preferentially directed away from the systemic circulation, resulting in profound underperfusion of the coronary arteries and the vital organs. Closure of the ductus is incompatible with life in these neonates.

Neonates with severe HLHS receive all pulmonary, systemic, and coronary blood flow from the RV. Generally, a child with HLHS will present with respiratory distress within the first day of life, and mild cyanosis may be noted. These infants must be rapidly triaged to a tertiary center, and echocardiography should be performed to confirm the diagnosis. PGE$_1$ must be administered to maintain ductal patency, and the ventilatory settings adjusted to avoid excessive oxygenation and increase carbon dioxide tension. These maneuvers will maintain PVR and promote improved systemic perfusion.[2,7,100] Cardiac catheterization generally should be avoided because it is not usually helpful and might result in injury to the ductus and compromised renal function secondary to the osmotic dye load.

Treatment

In 1983, Norwood and colleagues described a two-stage palliative surgical procedure for relief of HLHS[103] that was later modified to the currently used three-stage method of palliation.[104] Stage 1 palliation, also known as the *modified Norwood procedure*, bypasses the LV by creating a single outflow vessel, the neoaorta, which arises from the RV.[105]

The current technique of arch reconstruction involves completion of a connection between the pulmonary root, the native AA, and a piece of pulmonary homograft used to augment the diminutive native aorta. There are several modifications of this anastomosis, most notably the Damus-Kaye-Stansel (DKS) anastomosis, which involves dividing both the aorta and the PA at the sinotubular junction. The proximal aorta is anastomosed to the proximal PA creating a "double-barreled" outlet from the heart. This outlet is anastomosed to the distal aorta, which can be augmented with homograft material if there is an associated coarctation. At the completion of arch reconstruction, a 3.5- or 4-mm shunt is placed from the innominate artery to the right PA. The interatrial septum is then widely excised, thereby creating a large interatrial communication and preventing pulmonary venous hypertension (Fig. 20-20).

The DKS connection, as described in the previous paragraph, might avoid postoperative distortion of the tripartite connection in the neoaorta, and thus decrease the risk of coronary insufficiency.[105,106] It can be used when the aorta is 4 mm or larger. Unfortunately, in many infants with HLHS, especially if there is aortic atresia, the aorta is diminutive and often less than 2 mm in diameter.

The postoperative management of infants following stage 1 palliation is complex because favorable outcomes depend on establishing a delicate balance between pulmonary and systemic perfusion. Literature suggests that these infants require adequate postoperative cardiac output to supply both the pulmonary and the systemic circulations and that the use of oximetric catheters to monitor S$\bar{v}$O$_2$ aids clinicians in both the selection of inotropic agents and in ventilatory management.[106,107] The introduction of a modification that includes arch reconstruction and placement of the shunt between the RV and the PA (Sano shunt) diminishes the diastolic flow created by the classical aortopulmonary shunt and may augment coronary perfusion, resulting in improved postoperative cardiac function. A current prospective, randomized, multi-institutional trial sponsored by the National Institutes of Health, the systemic ventricle reconstruction trial, is currently evaluating the outcomes of neonates having either a modified B-T shunt or a Sano shunt.[107,108]

Although surgical palliation with the Norwood procedure is still the mainstay of therapy for infants with HLHS, a combined surgical and percutaneous option (hybrid procedure), which consists of bilateral PA banding and placement of a ductal stent, has emerged as a promising alternative that obviates the need for CPB in the fragile neonatal period.[109,110] The hybrid procedure can also be used as a bridge to heart transplantation in those infants with severe AV valve regurgitation or otherwise unsuitable single-ventricle anatomy.

Following stage 1 palliation, the second surgical procedure is the creation of a bidirectional cavopulmonary shunt or hemi-Fontan, generally at 3 to 6 months of life when the PVR has decreased to normal levels. This is the first step in separating the pulmonary and systemic circulations, and it decreases the volume load on the single ventricle. The existing innominate artery-to-pulmonary shunt (or RV-pulmonary shunt) is eliminated during the same operation (Fig. 20-21).

The third stage of surgical palliation, known as the *modified Fontan procedure*, completes the separation of the systemic and pulmonary circulations and is performed between 18 months and 3 years of age, or when the patient experiences increased cyanosis

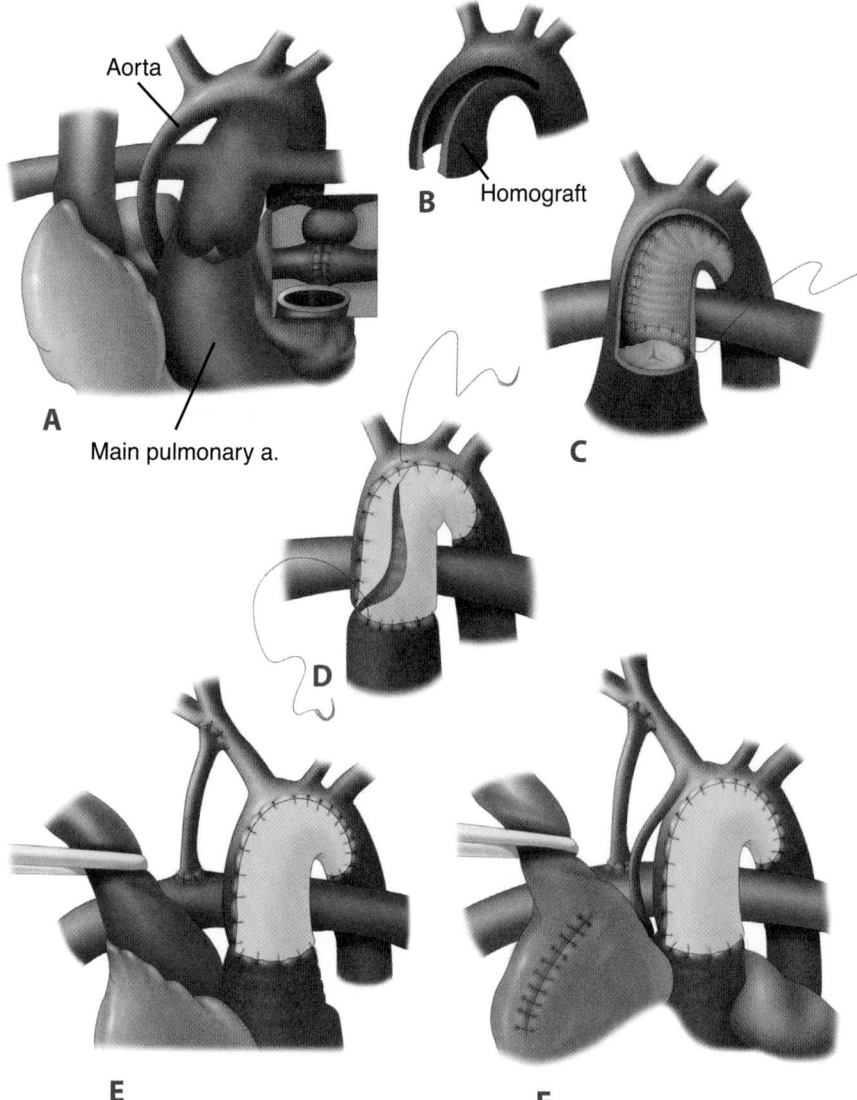

FIG. 20-20. Current techniques for first-stage palliation of the hypoplastic left-heart syndrome. **A.** Incisions used for the procedure, incorporating a cuff of arterial wall allograft. The distal divided main pulmonary artery may be closed by direct suture or with a patch. **B.** Dimensions of the cuff of the arterial wall allograft. **C.** The arterial wall allograft is used to supplement the anastomosis between the proximal divided main pulmonary artery and the ascending aorta, aortic arch, and proximal descending aorta. **D** and **E.** The procedure is completed by atrial septectomy and a 3- to 5-mm modified right Blalock shunt. **F.** When the ascending aorta is particularly small, an alternative procedure involves placement of a complete tube of arterial allograft. The tiny ascending aorta may be left in situ, as indicated, or implanted into the side of the neoaorta. a. = artery. *(From Castaneda et al,[7] p 371, with permission. Copyright Elsevier.)*

(i.e., has outgrown the capacity to perfuse the systemic circulation with adequately oxygenated blood). This has traditionally required a lateral tunnel within the right atrium to direct blood from the IVC to the PA, allowing further relief of the volume load on the RV, and providing increased pulmonary blood flow to alleviate cyanosis. More recently, many favor using an extracardiac conduit (e.g., 20-mm tube graft) to connect the IVC to the PA.

Not all patients with HLHS require this three-stage palliative repair. Some infants afflicted with a milder form of HLHS, recently described as *hypoplastic left-heart complex*, have aortic or mitral hypoplasia without intrinsic valve stenosis and antegrade flow in the AA. In this group, a two-ventricle repair can be achieved with a reasonable outcome. Tchervenkov recently published the results of 12 patients with hypoplastic left-heart complex who underwent biventricular repair at a mean age of 7 days.[107] The operative technique consisted of a pulmonary homograft patch aortoplasty of the aortic arch and AA and closure of the interatrial and interventricular communications.[110,111] The left heart was capable of sustaining systemic perfusion in 92% of patients, and early mortality was 15.4%. Four patients required reoperations to relieve LVOTO, most commonly between 12 and 39 months following repair.

Although the Norwood procedure is the most widely performed initial operation for HLHS, transplantation can be used as a first-line therapy and may be preferred when anatomic or physiologic considerations exist that preclude a favorable outcome with palliative repair. Significant tricuspid regurgitation, intractable PA hy-

pertension, or progressive right ventricular failure, are cases where cardiac replacement may be advantageous. Widespread adaptation of transplantation as first-line treatment for HLHS has been limited by improved Norwood survival rates as the operation and pre- and postoperative management of the patient have evolved, as well as limited organ availability. Organ availability should be considered before electing transplantation, as 24% of infants died awaiting transplantation in the largest series to date.[111,112]

Results

Outcomes for HLHS are still significantly worse than those for other complex cardiac defects. However, with improvements in perioperative care and modifications in surgical technique, the survival following the Norwood procedure now exceeds 80% in experienced centers.[100,106,108,110] The outcome for low-birth-weight infants has improved, but low weight still remains a major predictor of adverse survival, especially when accompanied by additional cardiac defects, such as systemic outflow obstruction, or extracardiac anomalies.[110]

DEFECTS THAT MAY BE PALLIATED OR REPAIRED

Ebstein's Anomaly
Anatomy

Ebstein's anomaly is a rare defect, occurring in less than 1% of CHD patients. The predominant maldevelopment in this lesion is the

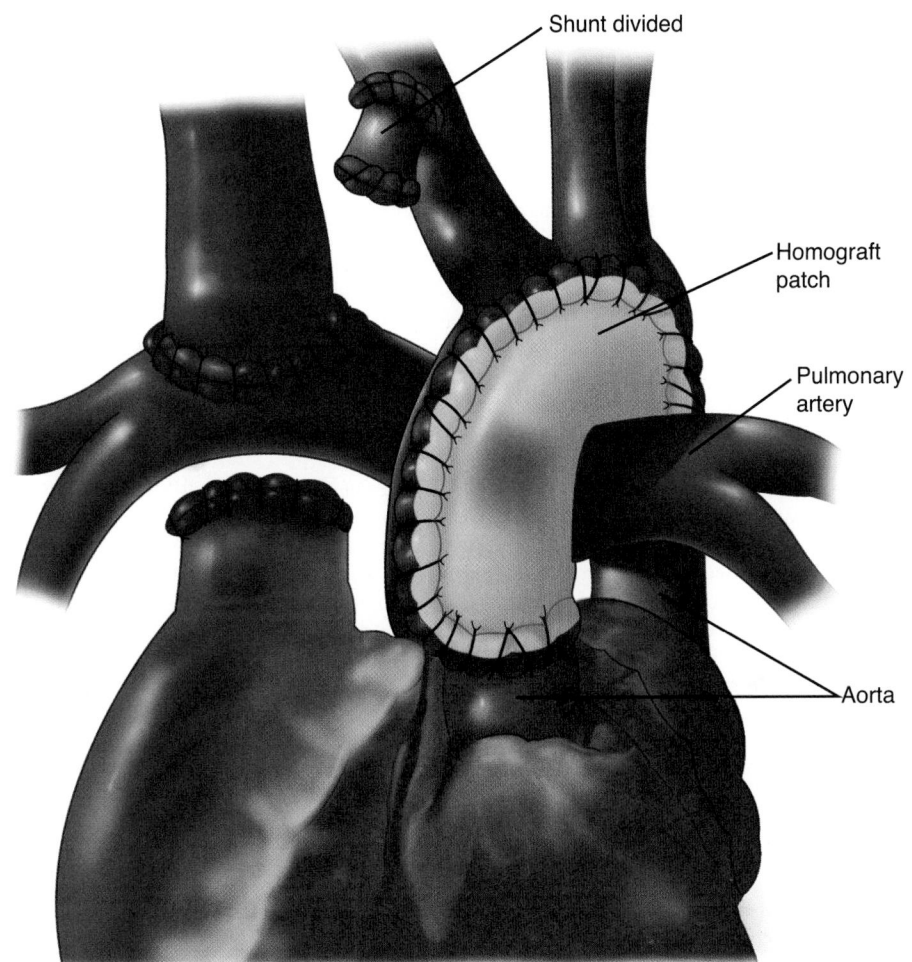

FIG. 20-21. Technique of a bidirectional Glenn shunt. The divided right superior vena cava has been anastomosed at the previous site of the distal anastomosis of the modified right Blalock shunt. The cardiac end of the divided superior vena cava may also be anastomosed to the right pulmonary artery, with the internal orifice being closed with a Gore-Tex patch. *(From Castaneda et al,[7] p 376, with permission. Copyright Elsevier.)*

inferior displacement of the tricuspid valve into the RV, although Bove and others[113] have emphasized that Ebstein's anomaly is primarily a defect in right ventricular morphology rather than an isolated defect in the tricuspid valve. The anterior leaflet is usually attached in its normal position to the annulus, but the septal and posterior leaflets are displaced toward the ventricle. This effectively divides the RV into two parts: the inlet portion (atrialized RV) and the outlet portion (true or trabeculated RV). The atrialized RV is usually thin and dilated. Similarly, the tricuspid annulus and the right atrium are extremely dilated, and the tricuspid valve is usually regurgitant with a "sail-like" leaflet. There is commonly an ASD present, which results in a right-to-left shunt at the atrial level. Occasionally, there is true anatomic pulmonary atresia or milder forms of RVOT obstruction. A Wolff-Parkinson-White (WPW) syndrome type of accessory pathway with associated pre-excitation is present in 15% of patients.[109,110]

Pathophysiology

Right ventricular dysfunction occurs in patients with Ebstein's anomaly because of two basic mechanisms: the inflow obstruction at the level of the atrialized ventricle, which produces ineffective RV filling and contractile dysfunction. Inflow obstruction and tricuspid regurgitation, which is exacerbated by progressive annular dilatation, both produce ineffective RV filling. Contractile dysfunction of the RV is a result of a decrease in the number of myocardial fibers, as well as the discordant contraction of the large atrialized portion.

The lack of forward flow at the right ventricular level may lead to physiologic or functional pulmonary atresia, and the infant is dependent on ductal patency for survival. All systemic venous return must be directed through an ASD to the left atrium, where it

can be shunted through the ductus for gas exchange. However, the left ventricular function is usually compromised in infants with severe Ebstein's anomaly as well, because the enormous RV and the to-and-fro flow within the atrialized RV prevent adequate intracardiac mixing. Left ventricular function may also be severely compromised in Ebstein's anomaly because the large RV causes left ventricular compression.

Diagnosis

There is a spectrum of clinical presentation in the infants with Ebstein's anomaly that mirrors the anatomic spectrum of this anomaly. Some infants with less severe forms may present with a mild degree of cyanosis, whereas the onset of clinical symptoms in patients' surviving childhood is gradual, with the average age of diagnosis in the mid-teens.

However, the infant with severe atrialization and pulmonary stenosis will be both cyanotic and acidotic at birth. The chest radiograph may demonstrate the classic appearance, which consists of a globular "wall-to-wall" heart, similar to that seen with pericardial effusion. The ECG may show right bundle-branch block and right axis deviation. WPW syndrome, as mentioned above in Anatomy under Ebstein's Anomaly, is a common finding in these patients. Echocardiography will confirm the diagnosis, as well as provide critical information, including tricuspid valvular function, size of the atrialized portion of the RV, degree of pulmonary stenosis, and the atrial size.[6,113,114]

The Great Ormond Street Score,[115] which consists of the area of the right atrium plus the area of the atrialized portion of the RV divided by the diastolic area of the remaining cardiac chambers, has been proposed as a useful prognostic tool to stratify neonates with

Ebstein's. A score greater than unity is essentially 100% mortality. Electrophysiology study with radiofrequency ablation is indicated in patients with evidence of WPW syndrome, or in children with a history of supraventricular tachycardia, undefined wide-complex tachycardia, or syncope.

Treatment

Surgery is indicated for symptomatic infants and for older children and adults with arrhythmias, progressive cyanosis, or New York Heart Association class III or IV. However, the operative repair may be different, depending on the patient's age, because older children usually are candidates for a biventricular or one-and-a-half ventricle repair, whereas moderate survival has been reported for neonates, using a procedure that converts the anatomy to a single ventricle physiology, as described by Starnes and coworkers.[115,116]

The surgical approach in widespread use today for patients surviving infancy was described by Danielson and colleagues in 1992.[6,114,117] This procedure entails excision of redundant right atrial tissue and patch closure of any associated ASD, plication of the atrialized portion of the ventricle with obliteration of the aneurysmal cavity, posterior tricuspid annuloplasty to narrow the tricuspid annulus, reconstruction of the tricuspid valve if the anterior leaflet is satisfactory, or replacement of the tricuspid valve if necessary.[117] If the tricuspid valve is not amenable to reconstruction, valve replacement should be considered. Care must be taken when performing the posterior annuloplasty, or during the conduct of tricuspid valve replacement, to avoid the conduction system, because complete heart block can complicate this procedure. In addition, patients who demonstrated preoperative evidence of pre-excitation should undergo electrophysiologic mapping and ablation.

Neonatal Ebstein's anomaly is a separate entity. Results with surgical correction have been poor, and many neonates are not candidates for operative repair as described in the paragraph above. Surgical options for the symptomatic neonate include palliative procedures, the one-and-a-half ventricle repair, or conversion to single-ventricle physiology.[1,7,118] Arguably, the most favorable outcomes in symptomatic neonatal Ebstein's or repair in slightly older infants has been using the right ventricular exclusion premise. This technique, known as the *Starnes procedure*,[116] uses a fenestrated patch to close the tricuspid valve orifice coupled with systemic-to-pulmonary artery shunt. The patch must be fenestrated to allow decompression of the RV in instances of anatomic pulmonary atresia. Although Knott-Craig and colleagues[118,119] have described tricuspid valve repair for the full spectrum of neonates and infants with excellent short- and midterm results, these have not been reproduced in other institutions. The one-and-a-half ventricle repair was first described by Billingsly and coworkers as an attempt to achieve a more physiologic "pulsatile" pulmonary circulation in those patients with a hypoplastic or dysplastic RV.[120] This is accomplished by diverting the superior vena caval blood directly into the pulmonary arterial system by a bidirectional cavopulmonary shunt while recruiting the RV to propel the inferior vena caval blood directly to the pulmonary arteries via the RVOT. Thus, the hemodynamics of the one-and-a-half ventricle repair are characterized by separate systemic and pulmonary circulations in series. The systemic circulation is fully supported by a systemic ventricle, and the pulmonary circulation is supported by both the bidirectional Glenn shunt and the hypoplastic (pulmonary) ventricle. Proponents of this approach report a decreased right atrial pressure and a decrease in IVC hypertension, which is theorized to be responsible for many of the dreaded complications of the Fontan circulation, including protein-losing encephalopathy, hepatic congestion, atrial arrhythmias, and systemic ventricular failure. In addition, the maintenance of pulsatile pulmonary blood flow, as opposed to continuous laminar flow as in the Fontan circulation, may be advantageous to the pulmonary microcirculation, although it has not been proven in any studies thus far.[120,121] Certain criteria, most notably an adequate tricuspid valve Z score, as well as the absence of severe pulmonary hypertension or

concomitant defects requiring intricate intracardiac repair, should be satisfied before electing the one-and-a-half ventricle approach.[121,122] Patients who do not fulfill these criteria may be approached with a two-ventricle repair and atrial fenestration, or a Fontan repair.

In the infant with severe Ebstein's anomaly, initial stabilization with prostaglandin to maintain ductal patency, mechanical ventilation, and correction of cyanosis is mandatory. Metabolic acidosis, if present from compromised systemic perfusion, must be aggressively treated with afterload reduction. Many of these infants will improve over 1 to 2 weeks as PVR falls and they are able to improve antegrade flow into the pulmonary circulation through their abnormal RV and tricuspid valve. When stabilization and medical palliation fails, surgical management remains an option, although its success depends on numerous anatomic factors (e.g., adequacy of the tricuspid valve, RV, and pulmonary outflow tract), and surgery for symptomatic neonates with Ebstein's anomaly carries a high risk. Knott-Craig and associates reported three cases where two-ventricle repair was undertaken by subtotal closure of the ASD, extensive resection of the right atrium, and vertical plication of the atrialized chamber.[117,118] Five-year follow-up revealed all patients to be asymptomatic and in sinus rhythm without medications.

Results

In the neonatal period, the most common postoperative problem, whether after a simple palliative procedure such as a B-T shunt or following a more extensive procedure such as attempted exclusion of the RV, has been low cardiac output. Supraventricular tachycardia also has been problematic postoperatively. Complete heart blockage necessitating pacemaker implantation should be uncommon if the techniques described to avoid suturing between the coronary sinus and the tricuspid annulus are used.

There are few published reports of outcomes, owing to the rarity of this defect. However, based on the natural history of this condition, which is remarkably benign for the majority of older patients, the outlook should be excellent for patients who have survived ASD closure, plication, and tricuspid annuloplasty.[7,113,117,118]

Transposition of the Great Arteries

Anatomy

Complete transposition is characterized by connection of the atria to their appropriate ventricles with inappropriate ventriculoarterial connections. Thus, the aorta arises anteriorly from the RV, while the PA arises posteriorly from the LV. Van Praagh and coworkers introduced the term *D-transposition of the great arteries* (D-TGA) to describe this defect, while L-TGA describes a form of corrected transposition where there is concomitant AV discordance.[123,124]

D-TGA requires an obligatory intracardiac mixing of blood, which usually occurs at both the atrial and the ventricular levels or via a patent ductus. Significant coronary anomalies occur frequently in patients with D-TGA.[7] The most common pattern, occurring in 68% of cases, is characterized by the left main coronary artery arising from the leftward coronary sinus, giving rise to the left anterior descending and circumflex arteries. The most common variant is for the circumflex coronary artery to arise as a branch from the right coronary artery instead of from the left coronary artery.

Pathophysiology

D-TGA results in parallel pulmonary and systemic circulations, with patient survival dependent on intracardiac mixing of blood. After birth, both ventricles are relatively noncompliant, and thus, infants initially have higher pulmonary flow owing to the decreased downstream resistance. This causes LA enlargement and a left-to-right shunt via the PFO.

Postnatally, the LV does not hypertrophy because it is not subjected to systemic afterload. The lack of normal extrauterine left ventricular maturation has important implications for the timing of surgical repair because the LV must be converted to the systemic ventricle and be able to function against systemic vascular resistance. If complete repair is done within the first few weeks of life the LV usually adapts easily to systemic resistance since it is conditioned to high intrauterine PVR. After a few weeks of life, the LV that is conditioned to the decrease in pulmonary resistance that occurs when the lungs inflate after birth may have difficulty adapting to systemic vascular resistance without preoperative preparation or postoperative support. Novel techniques of LV "preparation" using a pulmonary arterial band have been used in cases where complete repair has been delayed.

Clinical Manifestations and Diagnosis

Infants with D-TGA and an intact ventricular septum are usually cyanotic at birth, with an arterial PO_2 between 25 and 40 mmHg. If ductal patency is not maintained, deterioration will be rapid with ensuing metabolic acidosis and death. Conversely, those infants with a coexisting VSD may be only mildly hypoxemic and may come to medical attention after 2 to 3 weeks, when the falling PVR leads to symptoms of CHF.

The ECG will reveal right ventricular hypertrophy, and the chest radiograph will reveal the classic egg-shaped configuration. Definitive diagnosis is made by echocardiography, which reliably demonstrates ventriculoarterial discordance and any associated lesions. Cardiac catheterization is rarely necessary, except in those infants requiring surgery after the neonatal period to assess the suitability of the LV to support the systemic circulation. Limited catheterization, however, is useful for performance of atrial septostomy in those neonates with inadequate intracardiac mixing.

Surgical Repair

Blalock and Hanlon introduced the first operative intervention for D-TGA with the creation of an atrial septectomy to enhance intracardiac mixing.[125] This initial procedure was feasible in the precardiopulmonary bypass era, but carried a high mortality rate. Later, Rashkind and Cuaso developed a catheter-based balloon septostomy, which largely obviated the need for open septectomy.[42]

These early palliative maneuvers, however, met with limited success, and it was not until the late 1950s, when Senning and Mustard developed the first "atrial repair," that outcomes improved. The Senning operation consisted of rerouting venous flow at the atrial level by incising and realigning the atrial septum over the pulmonary veins and using the right atrial free wall to create a pulmonary venous baffle (Fig. 20-22).[126] Although the Mustard repair was similar, it made use of either autologous pericardium or synthetic material to create the interatrial baffle.[118] These atrial switch procedures resulted in a physiologic correction, but not an anatomic one, as the systemic circulation is still based on the RV. Still, survival rose to 95% in most centers by using an early balloon septostomy followed by an atrial switch procedure at 3 to 8 months of age.[126,127]

Despite the improved early survival rates, long-term problems, such as SVC or PVO, baffle leak, arrhythmias, tricuspid valve regurgitation, and right ventricular failure, prompted the development of the arterial switch procedure by Jatene in 1975.[128] The arterial switch procedure involves the division of the aorta and the PA, posterior translocation of the aorta (Lecompte maneuver), mobilization of the coronary arteries, placement of a pantaloon-shaped pericardial patch, and proper alignment of the coronary arteries on the neoaorta (Fig. 20-23).

The most important consideration is the timing of surgical repair, because arterial switch should be performed within 2 weeks after birth, before the LV loses its ability to pump against systemic afterload.[2,4,7] In patients presenting later than 2 weeks, the LV can be retrained with preliminary PA banding and aortopulmonary shunt followed by definitive repair. Alternatively, the unprepared LV can be supported following arterial switch with a mechanical assist device for a few days while it recovers ability to manage systemic pressures. Echocardiography can be used to assess left

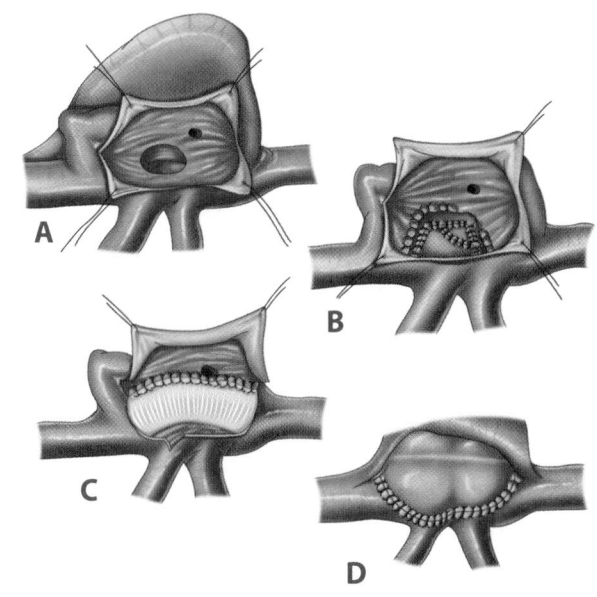

FIG. 20-22. The Senning operation. **A.** The atrial septum is cut near the tricuspid valve, creating a flap attached posteriorly between the caval veins. **B.** The flap of atrial septum is sutured to the anterior lip of the orifices of the left pulmonary veins, effectively separating the pulmonary and systemic venous channels. **C.** The posterior edge of the right atrial incision is sutured to the remnant of the atrial septum, diverting the systemic venous channel to the mitral valve. **D.** The anterior edge of the right atrial incision (lengthened by short incisions at each corner) is sutured around the cava above and below to the lateral edge of the LA incision, completing the pulmonary channel and diversion of pulmonary venous blood to the tricuspid valve area. *[Reproduced with permission from D-Transposition of the great arteries, in Mavroudis C, Backer CL (eds):* Pediatric Cardiac Surgery, *2nd ed. St. Louis: Mosby, 1994, p 345.]*

ventricular performance and guide operative planning in these circumstances.

The subset of patients who present with D-TGA complicated by LVOTO and VSD may not be suitable for an arterial switch operation. The Rastelli operation, first performed in 1968, uses placement of an intracardiac baffle to direct left ventricular blood to the aorta and an extracardiac valved conduit to establish continuity between the RV and the PA, which has led to successful outcomes in these complex patients.[129]

Results

For patients with D-TGA, intact ventricular septum, and VSD, the arterial switch operation provides excellent long-term results with a mortality rate of less than 5%. Operative risk is increased when unfavorable coronary anatomic configurations are present, or when augmentation of the aortic arch is required. The most common complication is supravalvular pulmonary stenosis, occurring 10% of the time, which may require reoperation.[4,7,130]

Results of the Rastelli operation have improved substantially, with an early mortality rate of 5% in a review.[131] Late mortality rate results were less favorable because conduit failure requiring reoperation, pacemaker insertion, or relief of LVOTO as frequent.

Double-Outlet Right Ventricle
Anatomy

Double-outlet right ventricle (DORV) accounts for 5% of CHD and exists when both the aorta and PA arise wholly, or in large part, from the RV. DORV encompasses a spectrum of malformations, because the incomplete shift of the aorta toward the LV is often

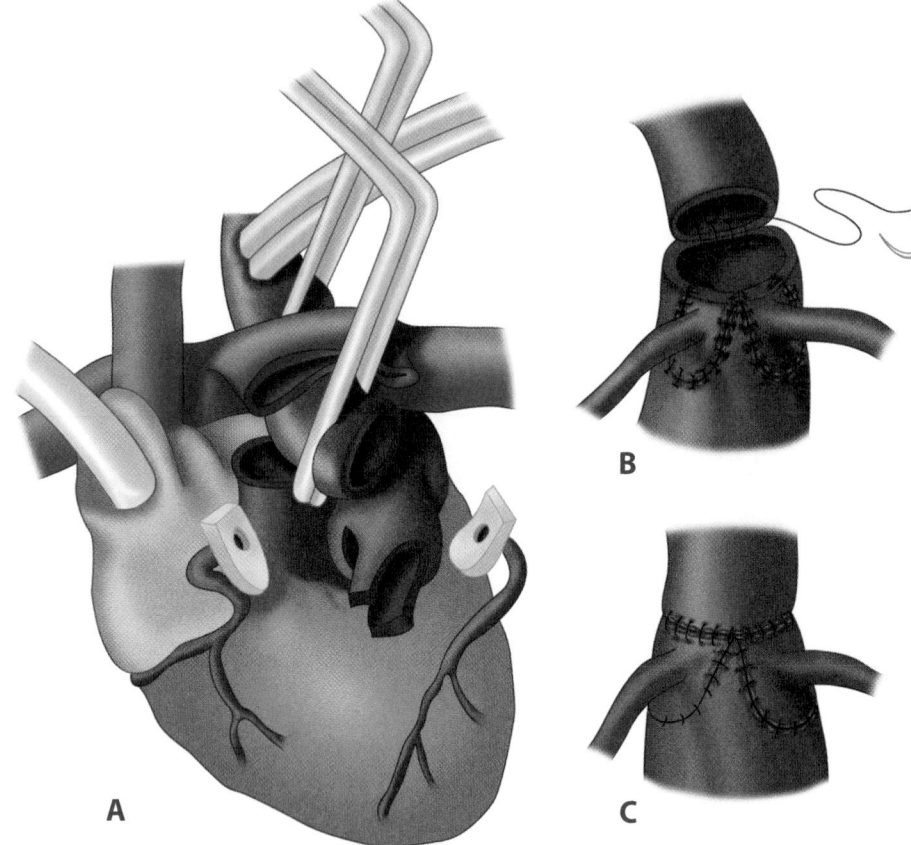

FIG. 20-23. A. The maneuver of Lecompte (positioning the pulmonary artery anterior to the aorta) is shown with aortic cross-clamp repositioning to retract the pulmonary artery during the neoaortic reconstruction. **A** and **B.** After the coronary patches are rotated for an optimal lie, they are sutured to the linearly incised sinuses of Valsalva at the old pulmonary artery (neoaorta) (**C**). *[Reproduced with permission from Backer CL, Idriss FS, Mavroudis C: Surgical techniques and intraoperative judgments to facilitate the arterial switch operation in transposition with intact ventricular septum, in Mavroudis C, Backer CL (eds): Arterial Switch.* Cardiac Surgery: State of the Art Review, *Vol. 5, no. 1. Philadelphia: Hanley & Belfus, 1991, p 108. Copyright Elsevier.]*

associated with other abnormalities of cardiac development, such as ventricular looping and infundibular-truncal spiraling.[132] The vast majority of hearts exhibiting DORV have a concomitant VSD, which varies in its size and spatial association with the great vessels. The VSD is usually nonrestrictive and represents the only outflow for the LV; its location relative to the great vessels dictates the dominant physiology of DORV, which can be analogous to that of a large isolated VSD, tetralogy of Fallot, or D-TGA. In 1972, Lev[133] suggested considering DORV as a spectrum of hearts that "pass imperceptibly from tetralogy with VSD with overriding aorta into DORV with subaortic VSD." Thus, Lev and colleagues described a classification scheme for DORV based on the "commitment" of the VSD to either or both great arteries.[7,133] The VSD can be subaortic, doubly committed, noncommitted, or subpulmonic.

The subaortic type is the most common (50%) and occurs when the VSD is located directly beneath the aortic annulus. Doubly committed VSD (10%) is present when the VSD lies beneath both the aorta and the PA, which are usually side by side in this lesion. The noncommitted VSD (10 to 20%) exists when the VSD is remote from the great vessels. The subset of DORV hearts with the VSD located beneath the pulmonary valve also are classified as the Taussig-Bing syndrome.[134] This occurs in 30% of cases of DORV with VSD, and it occurs when the aorta rotates more anteriorly, with the PA rotated more posteriorly (Fig. 20-24).

Clinical Manifestations and Diagnosis

Patients with DORV typically present with one of the following three scenarios: (a) those with doubly committed or subaortic VSD present with CHF and a high propensity for pulmonary hypertension, much like those infants with a large single VSD; (b) those with a subaortic VSD and pulmonary stenosis present with cyanosis and hypoxia, much like those infants with tetralogy of Fallot; and (c) those with subpulmonic VSD present with cyanosis much like those with D-TGA, because streaming directs desaturated systemic venous blood to the aorta and oxygenated blood to the PA.[132] Thus,

the three critical factors influencing the clinical presentation and subsequent management of infants with DORV are the size and location of the VSD, the presence or absence of important RVOT obstruction, and the presence of other anomalies (especially associated hypoplasia of left-sided structures sometimes seen with subpulmonary VSD).

Echocardiography is the mainstay of diagnosis, and can also provide valuable information regarding the feasibility of biventricular repair. Specific anatomic questions that should be resolved to assist in surgical planning in addition to those mentioned above include the coronary anatomy (presence of a conal branch or left anterior descending from the right coronary coursing across the conus), the presence of additional muscular VSDs remote from either great vessel, and the distance between the tricuspid and pulmonary valve. Cardiac catheterization is rarely necessary in neonates or infants, except to determine the degree of pulmonary hypertension and to determine the effects of previous palliative procedures on the pulmonary arterial anatomy.

Therapy

The goals of corrective surgery are to relieve pulmonary stenosis, to provide separate and unobstructed outflow pathways from each ventricle to the correct great vessel, and to achieve separation of the systemic and pulmonary circulations.

Double-Outlet Right Ventricle with Noncommitted Ventricular Septal Defect

The repair of hearts with DORV and noncommitted VSD can be accomplished by constructing an intraventricular tunnel connecting the VSD to the aorta, closing the PA, and placing a valved extracardiac conduit from the RV to the PA. In those patients without pulmonary stenosis who have intractable congestive failure, a PA band can be placed in the first 6 months to control PA overcirculation and prevent the development of pulmonary hypertension.

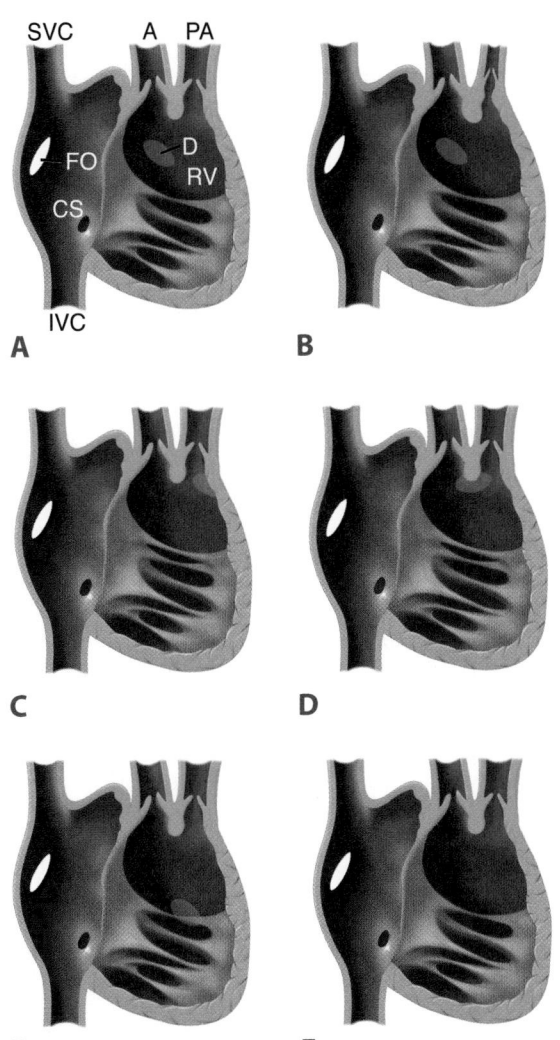

FIG. 20-24. The relationship of the ventricular septal defect (VSD) to the great arteries in double-outlet right ventricle (DORV). **A.** Subaortic VSD without pulmonary stenosis. **B.** Subaortic VSD with pulmonary stenosis. **C.** Subpulmonary VSD (Taussig-Bing malformation). **D.** Doubly committed VSD. **E.** Noncommitted (remote) VSD. **F.** Intact interventricular septum. A = aorta; CS = coronary sinus; D = ventricular septal defect; FO = foramen ovale; IVC = inferior vena cava; PA = pulmonary artery; RV = right ventricle; SVC = superior vena cava. *(Adapted with permission from Zamora R, Moller JH, and Edwards JE: Double-outlet right ventricle. Chest 68:672, 1975.)*

Those infants with pulmonary stenosis can be managed with a systemic-to-pulmonary shunt followed by biventricular repair as described by Belli and colleagues in 1999, or with a modified Fontan.[135] There is no consensus on the timing of repair, but literature suggests that repair within the first 6 months is associated with better outcome. However, in cases where an extracardiac valved conduit is necessary, it is better to delay definitive repair until the child is 2 to 3 years of age, because this allows placement of a larger conduit and possibly reduces the number of future obligatory conduit replacements.[7,132]

Double-Outlet Right Ventricle with Subaortic or Doubly Committed Ventricular Septal Defect without Pulmonary Stenosis

Patients with CORV with subaortic or doubly committed VSD without pulmonary stenosis can be treated by creating an intracardiac baffle that directs blood from the LV into the aorta. Enlargement of

the VSD may be necessary to allow ample room for the baffle; this should be done anterosuperiorly to avoid injury to the conduction system that normally lies inferoposteriorly along the border of the VSD. In addition, other important considerations in constructing the LV outflow tunnel include the prominence of the conal septum, the attachments of the tricuspid valve to the conal septum, and the distance between the tricuspid and pulmonary valves. In some instances, unfavorable anatomy may preclude placement of an adequate intracardiac baffle, necessitating single ventricle repair.

Double-Outlet Right Ventricle with Subaortic or Doubly Committed Ventricular Septal Defect with Pulmonary Stenosis

Repair of DORV with subaortic or doubly committed VSD with pulmonary stenosis is similar to Double-Outlet Right Ventricle with Subaortic or Doubly Committed Ventricular Septal Defect without Pulmonary Stenosis described above except that concomitant RVOT reconstruction must be performed in addition to the intracardiac tunnel. The RVOT augmentation can be accomplished with the placement of a transannular patch or with placement of an extracardiac valved conduit when an anomalous left anterior descending artery precludes use of a patch.

Taussig-Bing Syndrome without Pulmonary Stenosis

Infants with Taussig-Bing syndrome without pulmonary stenosis are best treated with a balloon septostomy during the neonatal period to improve mixing, followed by VSD closure baffling LV egress to the PA and an arterial switch operation. The Kawashima procedure,[136] in which an intraventricular tunnel is used to baffle LV egress directly to the aorta, may alternatively be used when the aorta is more posterior or when there is associated pulmonary stenosis.

Taussig-Bing Syndrome with Pulmonary Stenosis

Taussig-Bing syndrome with pulmonary stenosis may be treated with a variety of techniques, depending on the specific anatomic details and the expertise of the treatment team. A Rastelli-type repair, which involves construction of an intraventricular tunnel through the existing VSD that connects the LV to both great vessels, followed by division of the PA at its origin and insertion of a valved conduit from the RV to the distal PA, can be performed.[137] Alternatively, a Yasui procedure, which involves baffling the VSD to the PA, creation of a DKS anastomosis between the PA and the aorta with patch augmentation can be accomplished concomitant with placement of a RV-PA conduit.[138]

Results

The results of DORV repairs are generally favorable, especially for the tetralogy-type DORV with subaortic VSD.[139,140] However, more complex types of DORV, including noncommitted VSD and Taussig-Bing type, still carry important morbidity and mortality.[125,139,140] Furthermore, repeated interventions for RVOT reconstruction or staged operations for patients triaged to single ventricle pathways pose late hazards for patients surviving initial repair. A recent single institution series evaluated 393 patients with DORV.[139] The authors found that the need for reintervention approached 37% at 15 years following repair. Arterial switch operation, as opposed to Rastelli-type repair, was associated with an increased risk of early postrepair mortality, but mitigated against the risk of late death. Patients with hypoplastic left-sided structures and a nonsubaortic VSD may fare better with a single-ventricle repair.

Tetralogy of Fallot
Anatomy

The original description of TOF by Ettienne Louis Fallot,[141] as the name implies, included four abnormalities: a large perimembra-

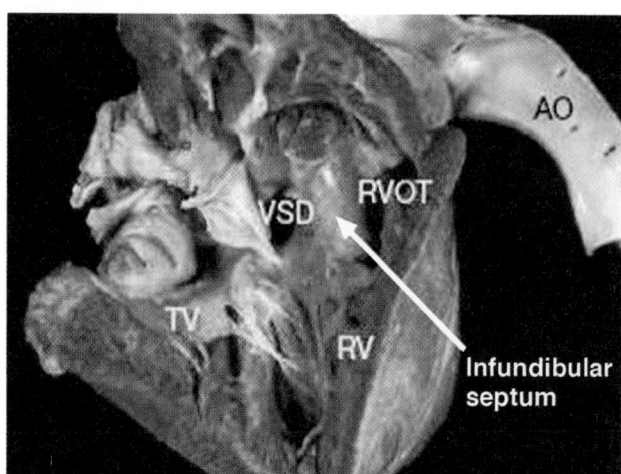

FIG. 20-25. Pathologic specimen of the heart in a patient with tetralogy of Fallot. The four anatomic components comprising tetralogy of Fallot can be conceptualized as a *monology of Fallot*, because they can be explained by malposition of the interventricular septum. AO = aorta; RV = right ventricle; RVOT = right ventricular outflow tract; TV = tricuspid valve; VSD = ventricular septal defect. *(From Van Praagh et al,[142] with permission. © Elsevier Ltd.)*

nous VSD adjacent to the tricuspid valve; an overriding aorta; a variable degree of RVOT obstruction, which might include hypoplasia and dysplasia of the pulmonary valve as well as obstruction at the subvalvular and PA level; and right ventricular hypertrophy. More recently, Van Praagh and colleagues[142] pointed out that TOF could be more correctly termed *monology of Fallot*, because the four components are explained by the malposition of the infundibular septum. When the infundibular septum is displaced anteriorly and leftward, the RVOT is narrowed and its anterior displacement results in failure of fusion of the ventricular septum between the arms of the trabecula-septomarginalis (Fig. 20-25).

The morphology of TOF is markedly heterogeneous and includes an absent pulmonary valve, concomitant AV septal defects, and pulmonary atresia with major aortopulmonary collaterals. The present discussion will focus only on the so-called *classic presentation of TOF* without coexisting intracardiac defects.

Anomalous coronary artery patterns, related to either origin or distribution, have been described in TOF.[143] However, the most surgically important coronary anomaly occurs when the left anterior descending artery arises as a branch of the right coronary artery. This occurs in approximately 3% of cases of TOF and may preclude placement of a transannular patch, as the left anterior descending coronary artery crosses the RVOT at varying distances from the pulmonary valve annulus.[144]

Pathophysiology and Clinical Presentation

The initial presentation of a child afflicted with TOF depends on the degree of RVOT obstruction. Those children with cyanosis at birth usually have severe pulmonary annular hypoplasia with concomitant hypoplasia of the peripheral pulmonary arteries. Most children, however, present with mild cyanosis at birth, which then progresses as the right ventricular hypertrophy further compromises the RVOT. Cyanosis usually becomes significant within the first 6 to 12 months of life, and the child may develop characteristic "tet" spells, which are periods of extreme hypoxemia. These spells are characterized by decreased pulmonary blood flow and an increase in aortic flow. They can be triggered by any stimulus that decreases systemic vascular resistance, such as fever or vigorous physical activity. Cyanotic spells increase in severity and frequency as the child grows, and older patients with uncorrected TOF may often squat,

which increases peripheral vascular resistance and relieves the cyanosis.

Physical examination in the older patient with TOF may demonstrate clubbing, polycythemia, or brain abscesses. Chest radiography will demonstrate a boot-shaped heart, and ECG will show the normal pattern of right ventricular hypertrophy. Echocardiography confirms the diagnosis because it demonstrates the position and nature of the VSD, defines the character of the RVOT obstruction, and often visualizes the branch pulmonary arteries and the proximal coronary arteries. Cardiac catheterization is rarely necessary and is actually risky in TOF because it can create spasm of the RVOT muscle and result in a hypercyanotic episode (tet spell). Occasionally, aortography is necessary to delineate the coronary artery anatomy.

Treatment

John Deanfield[145] said ". . . long follow-up inevitably means surgery in an earlier era: More recent surgery, at a younger age, with better preoperative, operative, and postoperative care, will improve long-term results. Data from the former (earlier) era will be overly pessimistic." This statement is particularly pertinent as surgical correction of TOF has evolved from a staged approach of antecedent palliation in infancy followed by intracardiac repair to primary repair during the first few months of life without prior palliative surgery.

However, systemic-to-pulmonary shunts, generally a B-T shunt, may still be preferred with an unstable neonate younger than 6 months of age, when an extracardiac conduit is required because of an anomalous left anterior descending coronary artery, or when pulmonary atresia, significant branch PA hypoplasia, or severe noncardiac anomalies coexist with TOF.

Traditionally, TOF was repaired through a right ventriculotomy, providing excellent exposure for closure of the VSD and relief of the RVOT obstruction, but concerns that the resultant scar would significantly impair right ventricular function or lead to lethal arrhythmias led to the development of a transatrial approach. Transatrial repair, except in cases when the presence of diffuse RVOT hypoplasia requires insertion of a transannular patch, is now being increasingly advocated by many, although its superiority has not been conclusively demonstrated.[146]

The operative technique involves the use of CPB. All existing systemic-to-pulmonary arterial shunts, as well as the ductus arteriosus, are ligated. A right atriotomy is then made, and the anatomy of the VSD and the RVOT are assessed by retracting the tricuspid valve (Fig. 20-26). The outflow tract obstruction is relieved by resecting the offending portion of the infundibular septum as well as any muscle trabeculations. If necessary, a pulmonary valvotomy or, alternatively, a longitudinal incision in the main PA can be performed to improve exposure. The diameter of the pulmonary valve annulus is assessed by inserting Hegar dilators across the outflow tract; if the PA/AA diameter is less than 0.5, or the estimated RV/LV pressure is greater than 0.7, a transannular patch is inserted.[21,147] Patch closure of the VSD is then accomplished, taking care when placing sutures along the posteroinferior portion to avoid the conduction system.

Results

Operative mortality for primary repair of TOF in infancy is less than 5% in most series.[4,7,146,148] Previously reported risk factors such as transannular patch insertion or younger age at time of repair have been eliminated secondary to improved intraoperative and postoperative care.

A major complication of repaired TOF is the development of pulmonary insufficiency, which subjects the RV to the adverse effects of acute and chronic volume overload. This is especially problematic if residual lesions such as a VSD or peripheral pulmonary stenosis exist. Pulmonary valve regurgitation after repair of TOF is relatively well tolerated in the short term, partly because the hypertrophied RV usually adapts to the altered hemodynamic load.[139,149] The detrimental effects of chronic pulmonary valve regur-

FIG. 20-26. The anatomy from the perspective of the right atrial (RA) approach, shown as if the right atrial free wall and tricuspid valve were translucent. The free edge of the tricuspid leaflets is shown by dashed lines. **A.** The difference from the right ventricular (RV) perspective is in the apparent position of the parietal extension. From the RA perspective the surgeon looks *beneath* this, as the parietal extension arches *over* the right ventricular outflow tract. **B.** The same perspective without the outline of the tricuspid valve leaflets. The parietal extension is transected at its origin from the infundibular septum, dissected up toward the free wall, and amputated at the free wall. **C.** A pledgetted mattress suture is placed from the RA side through the base of the commissural tissue between septal and tricuspid leaflets and through the patch. **D.** The suturing is continued onto the parietal extension and infundibular septum, visualizing and staying close to the aortic valve leaflets to avoid leaving a hole between muscular bands. When working from the RA, it is particularly important to stay close to the aortic valve leaflets in the direction of the septum to avoid narrowing the RV outflow tract. **E.** The repair of the ventricular septal defect is completed. Note that the suture line is away from the bundle of His and its branches, except where it crosses the right bundle branch anteroinferiorly. ant. = anterior; ML = mitral leaflet; post. = posterior; TV = tricuspid valve. *(Reproduced with permission from Kirklin JW, Barratt-Boyes BG: Cardiac Surgery, 2nd ed. New York: Churchill Livingstone, 1993, p 863. Copyright © Elsevier.)*

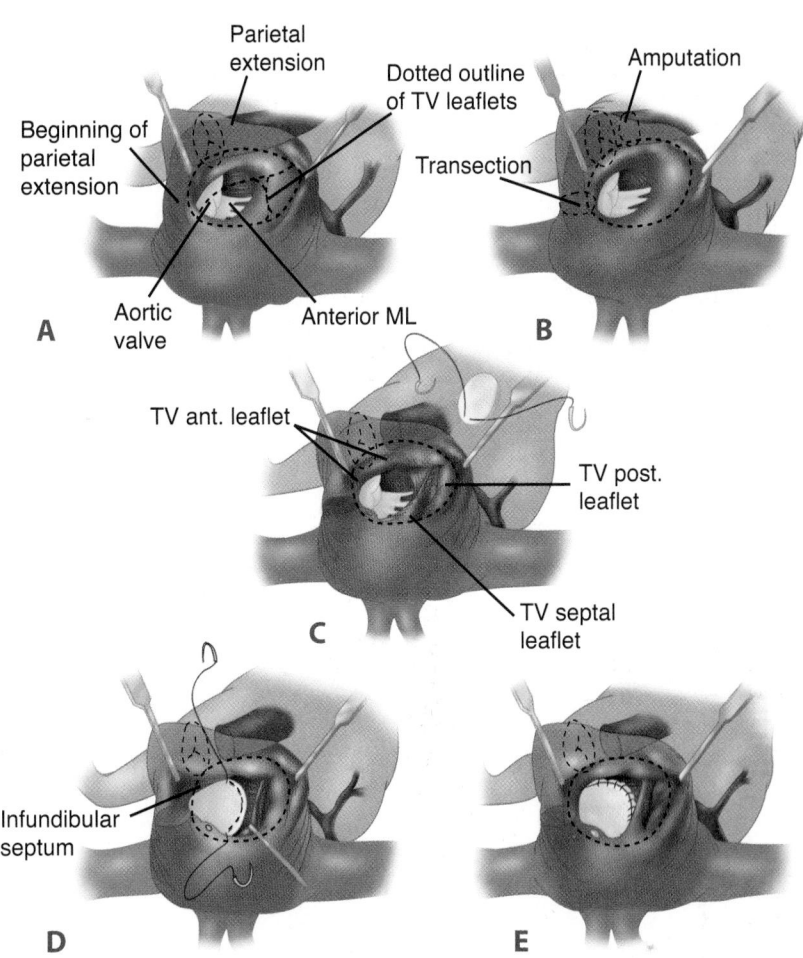

gitation are, however, numerous, and include progressive right ventricular dilatation and failure, tricuspid valve regurgitation, exercise intolerance, arrhythmia, and sudden death. Mechanoelectrical interaction, by which a dilatated RV provides the substrate for electrical instability, might underlie the propensity toward ventricular arrhythmia.[150] In support of this contention, Gatzoulis and colleagues [140,150] found that the risk of symptomatic arrhythmia was high in patients with marked right ventricular enlargement and QRS prolongation on resting ECG of more than 180 milliseconds. Karamlou and associates have shown that similar structural and hemodynamic abnormalities, including a larger right atrial volume and right ventricular chamber size, are also related to atrial arrhythmias in patients following TOF repair.[151] The authors found that prolongation of the QRS duration, beyond a threshold of 160 milliseconds, increased the risk of atrial arrhythmias.[151] Together, these data show that a similar mechanism could be responsible for both atrial and ventricular arrhythmias after repair in TOF patients.

When significant deterioration of ventricular function occurs, insertion of a pulmonary valve may be required, although this is rarely necessary in infants. Unfortunately, there are no universal criteria establishing the timing of pulmonary valve replacement, though dilation of the RV, prolongation of the QRS duration beyond 180 milliseconds, important atrial arrhythmias, or impaired ventricular function are widely used.

Arrhythmias are potentially the most serious late complication following TOF repair. In a multicenter cohort of 793 patients studied by Gatzoulis and colleagues,[150] a steady increase was documented in the prevalence of ventricular and atrial tachyarrhythmia and sudden cardiac death in the first 5 to 10 years following intracardiac repair. Clinical events were reported in 12% of patients at 35 years after repair. Prevalence of atrial arrhythmias from other studies, however, ranges from 1 to 11%,[140,150] which is a reflection of the strong time dependence of arrhythmia onset.

Underlying causes of arrhythmia following repair are complex and multifactorial, resulting in poorly defined optimum screening and treatment algorithms. Older repair age has been associated with an increased frequency of both atrial and ventricular arrhythmias. Impaired ventricular function secondary to a protracted period of cyanosis before repair might contribute to the propensity for arrhythmia in older patients.

Ventricular Septal Defect
Anatomy

VSD refers to a hole between the LVs and RVs. These defects are common, comprising 20 to 30% of all cases of CHD, and may occur as an isolated lesion or as part of a more complex malformation.[152] VSDs vary in size from 3 to 4 mm to more than 3 cm, and are classified into four types based on their location in the ventricular septum: perimembranous, AV canal, outlet or supracristal, and muscular (Fig. 20-27).

Perimembranous VSDs are the most common type requiring surgical intervention, constituting approximately 80% of cases.[153] These defects involve the membranous septum and include the malalignment defects seen in TOF. In rare instances, the anterior and septal leaflets of the tricuspid valve adhere to the edges of the perimembranous defect, forming a channel between the LV and the right atrium. These defects result in a large left-to-right shunt owing to the large pressure differential between the two chambers.

AV canal defects, also known as *inlet defects*, occur when part or all of the septum of the AV canal is absent. The VSD lies beneath the tricuspid valve and is limited upstream by the tricuspid annulus, without intervening muscle.

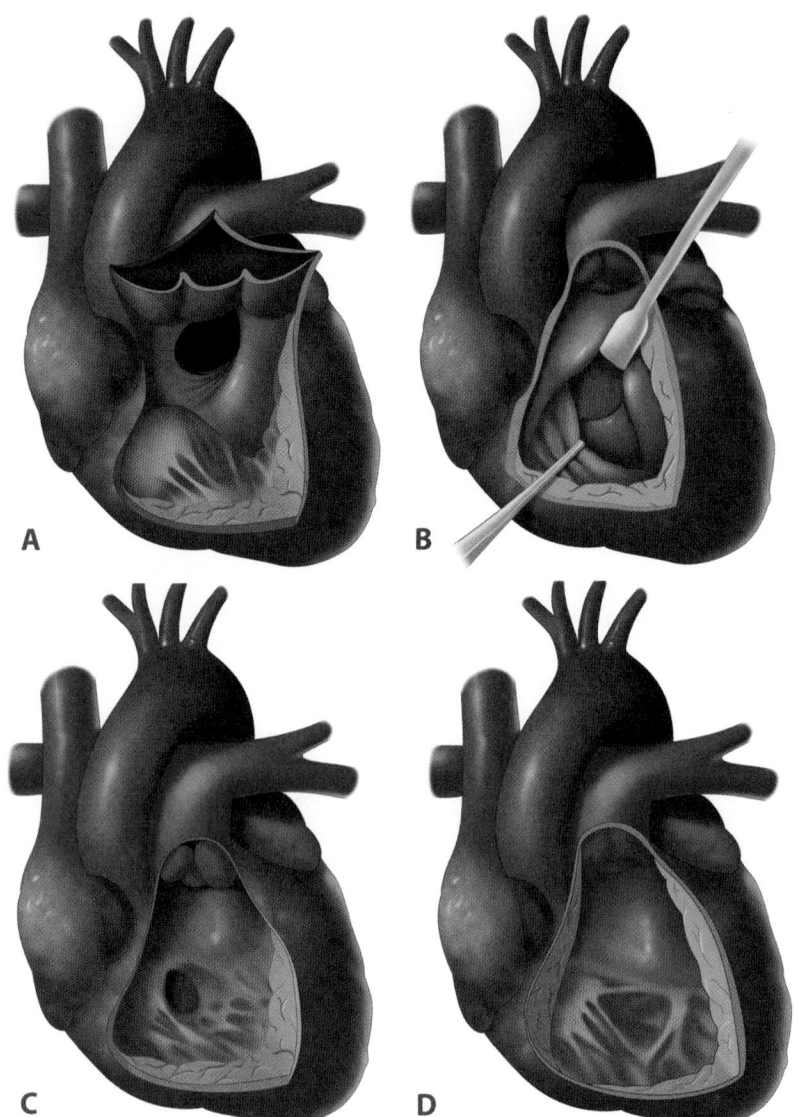

FIG. 20-27. Classic anatomic types of ventricular septal defect (VSD). **A.** Type I (conal, infundibular, supracristal, subarterial) VSD. **B.** Type II or perimembranous VSD. **C.** Type III VSD (atrioventricular canal type or inlet septum type). **D.** Type IV VSD (single or multiple). *[Reproduced with permission from Ventricular septal defect, in Mavroudis C, Backer CL (eds): Pediatric Cardiac Surgery, 2nd ed. St. Louis: Mosby, 1994, p 70. Copyright Elsevier.]*

The supracristal or outlet VSD results from a defect within the conal septum. Characteristically, these defects are limited upstream by the pulmonary valve and are otherwise surrounded by the muscle of the infundibular septum.

Muscular VSDs are the most common type, and may lie in four locations: anterior, midventricular, posterior, or apical. These are surrounded by muscle, and can occur anywhere along the trabecular portion of the septum. The rare "Swiss-cheese" type of muscular VSD consists of multiple communications between the right and LVs, complicating operative repair.

Pathophysiology and Clinical Presentation

The size of the VSD determines the initial pathophysiology of the disease. Large VSDs are classified as nonrestrictive, and are at least equal in diameter to the aortic annulus. These defects allow free flow of blood from the LV to the RV, elevating right ventricular pressures to the same level as systemic pressure. Consequently, the pulmonary-to-systemic flow ratio (Qp:Qs) is inversely dependent on the ratio of PVR to systemic vascular resistance. Nonrestrictive VSDs produce a large increase in pulmonary blood flow, and the afflicted infant will present with symptoms of CHF. However, if untreated, these defects will cause pulmonary hypertension with a corresponding increase in PVR. This will lead to a reversal of flow (a right-to-left shunt), which is known as Eisenmenger's syndrome.

Small restrictive VSDs offer significant resistance to the passage of blood across the defect, and therefore, right ventricular pressure is either normal or only minimally elevated and Qp:Qs rarely exceeds 1.5.[4,7] These defects are generally asymptomatic because there are few physiologic consequences. However, there is a long-term risk of endocarditis, because endocardial damage from the jet of blood through the defect may serve as a possible nidus for colonization.

Diagnosis

The child with a large VSD will present with severe CHF and frequent respiratory tract infections. Those children with Eisenmenger's syndrome may be deceptively asymptomatic until frank cyanosis develops.

The chest radiograph will show cardiomegaly and pulmonary overcirculation and the ECG will show signs of left ventricular or biventricular hypertrophy. Echocardiography provides definitive diagnosis, and can estimate the degree of shunting as well as pulmonary arterial pressures. Cardiac catheterization has largely been supplanted by echocardiography, except in older children where measurement of pulmonary resistance is necessary before recommending closure of the defect.

Treatment

VSDs may close or narrow spontaneously, and the probability of closure is inversely related to the age at which the defect is observed.

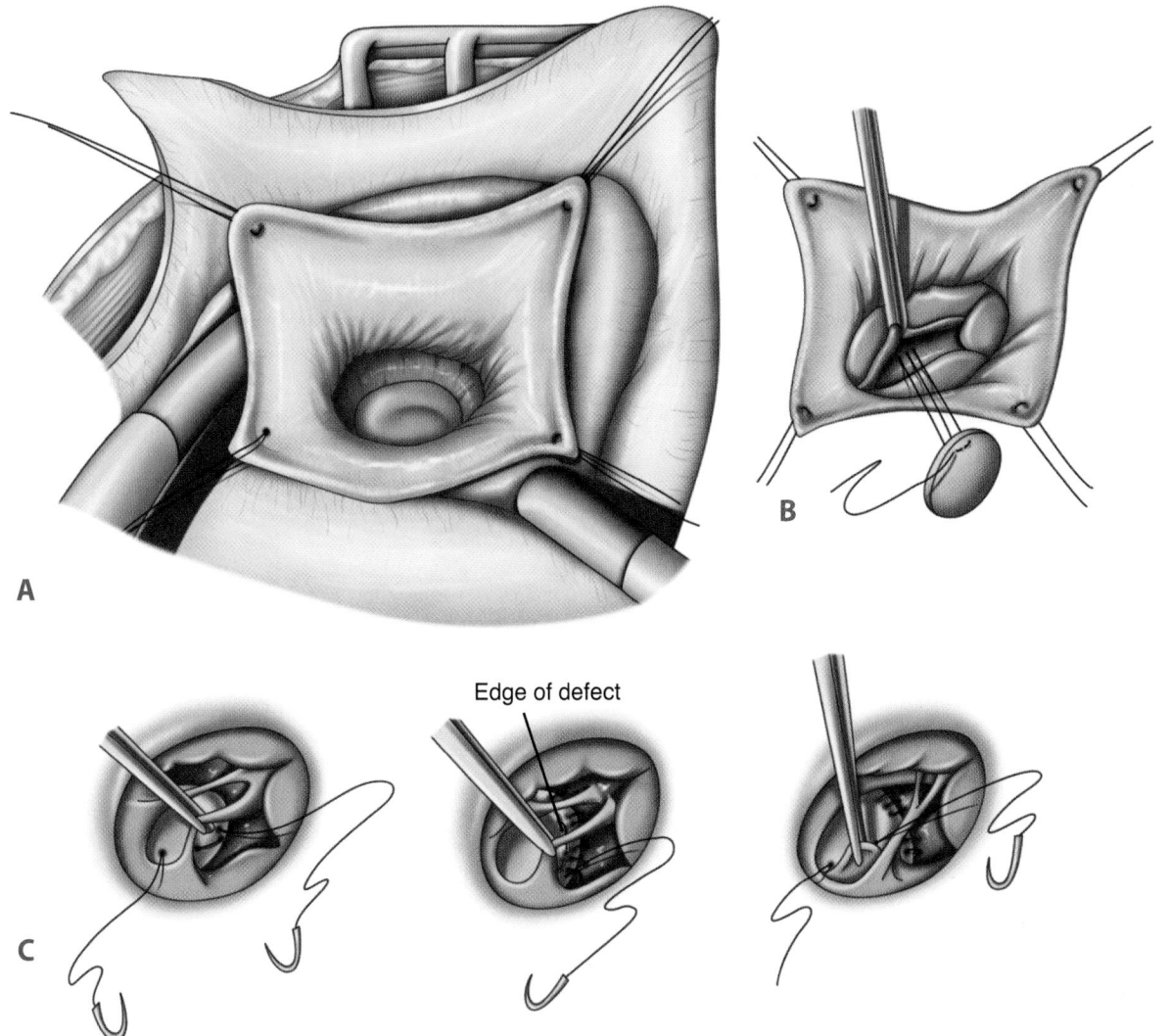

FIG. 20-28. A. Right atrial incision and exposure of perimembranous ventricular septal defect (VSD) in the region of the tricuspid anteroseptal commissure. Stay sutures have been placed to slightly evert the atrial wall. Note that initially, the superior edge of this typical perimembranous defect is not visible. The atrioventricular node is in the muscular portion of the atrioventricular septum, just on the atrial side of the commissure between the tricuspid septal and anterior leaflets. The bundle of His thus penetrates at the posterior angle of the VSD, where it is vulnerable to injury. **B** and **C.** The repair of the perimembranous VSD is completed with use of a slightly oversized Dacron patch, taking care to place stitches 3 to 5 mm away from the edge of the defect itself to avoid injury to the conduction system. *[Reproduced with permission from Walters HL, Pacifico AD, Kirklin JK: Ventricular septal defects, in Sabiston DC, Lyerly HK (eds): Textbook of Surgery: The Biologic Basis of Modern Surgical Practice. Philadelphia: W.B. Saunders, 1997, p 2014. Copyright Elsevier.]*

Thus, infants at 1 month of age have an 80% incidence of spontaneous closure, whereas a child at 12 months of age has only a 25% chance of closure.[153] This has an important impact on operative decision making, because a small or moderate-size VSD may be observed for a period of time in the absence of symptoms. Large defects and those in severely symptomatic neonates should be repaired during infancy to relieve symptoms and because irreversible changes in PVR may develop during the first year of life.

Repair of isolated VSDs requires the use of CPB with moderate hypothermia and cardioplegic arrest. The right atrial approach is preferable for most defects, except apical muscular defects, which often require a left ventriculotomy for adequate exposure. Supracristal defects may alternatively be exposed via a longitudinal incision in the right ventricular outflow tract, below the pulmonary valve. Regardless of the type of defect present, a right atrial approach can be used initially to inspect the anatomy, as this may be abandoned should it offer inadequate exposure for repair. After careful inspection of the heart for any associated malformations, a patch repair is used, taking care to avoid the conduction system (Fig. 20-28).

Routine use of intraoperative transesophageal echocardiography should be used to assess for any residual defects.

Successful percutaneous device closure of VSDs using the Amplatzer muscular VSD has been described.[154] The device has demonstrated a 100% closure rate in a small series of patients with isolated or residual VSDs, or as a collaborative treatment strategy for the VSD component in more complex congenital lesions. Proponents of device closure argue that their use can decrease the complexity of surgical repair, avoid reoperation for a small residual lesion, or avoid the need for a ventriculotomy.

Multiple or "Swiss-cheese" VSDs represent a special case, and many cannot be repaired during infancy. In those patients in whom definitive VSD closure cannot be accomplished, temporary placement of a PA band can be used to control pulmonary flow. This allows time for spontaneous closure of many of the smaller defects, thus simplifying surgical repair.

Some centers, however, have advocated early definitive repair of the Swiss-cheese septum, by using oversize patches, fibrin glue, and combined intraoperative device closure, as well as techniques to complete the repair transatrially.[155] At the University of California, San Francisco, 69% of patients with multiple VSDs underwent single-stage correction, and the repaired group had improved outcome as compared to the palliated group.[154]

Results

Even in very small infants, closure of VSDs can be safely performed with hospital mortality near 0%.[4,7,155,156] The main risk factor remains the presence of other associated lesions, especially when present in symptomatic neonates with large VSDs.

Atrioventricular Canal Defects
Anatomy

AV canal defects result from failure of fusion of the endocardial cushions in the central portion of the heart, causing a lesion that involves the atrial and the ventricular septum, as well as the anterior mitral and septal tricuspid valve leaflets. Defects involving primarily the atrial septum are known as *partial AV canal defects* and frequently occur in conjunction with a cleft anterior mitral leaflet. Complete AV canal defects have a combined deficiency of the atrial and ventricular septum associated with a common AV orifice rather than separate tricuspid and mitral valves. The common AV valve generally has five leaflets: three lateral (free wall) and two bridging (septal) leaflets. The defect in the ventricular septum can lie either between the two bridging leaflets, or beneath them. The relationship between the septal defect and the anterior bridging leaflet forms the basis of the Rastelli classification for complete AV canal defects (Fig. 20-29).[157]

Pathophysiology and Diagnosis

Partial AV canal defects, in the absence of AV valvular regurgitation, frequently resemble isolated ASDs. Left-to-right shunting predominates as long as PVR remains low. However, 40% of patients with partial AV canal defects have moderate-to-severe valve incompetence, and progressive heart failure occurs early in this patient population.[158] Complete AV canal defects produce more severe pathophysiologic changes, because the large intracardiac communication and signifi-

cant AV valve regurgitation contribute to ventricular volume loading and pulmonary hypertension. Children with complete AV canal defects develop signs of CHF within the first few months of life.

Physical examination may reveal a right ventricular heave and a systolic murmur. Children may also present with endocarditis or paradoxical emboli as a result of the intracardiac communication. Chest radiography will be consistent with CHF, and the ECG demonstrates right ventricular hypertrophy with a prolonged PR interval.

Two-dimensional echocardiography with color-flow mapping is confirmatory, but cardiac catheterization can be used to define the status of the pulmonary vasculature, with a PVR greater than 12 Woods units indicating inoperability.[158]

Treatment

The management of patients with AV canal defects can be especially challenging. Timing of operation is individualized. Those patients with partial defects can be electively repaired between 2 and 5 years of age, whereas complete AV canal defects should be repaired within the first year of life to prevent irreversible changes in the pulmonary circulation. Complete repair in infancy should be accomplished, with palliative procedures such as PA banding reserved for only those infants with other complex lesions, or who are too ill to tolerate CPB.

The operative technique requires the use of either continuous hypothermic CPB or, for small infants, deep hypothermic circulatory arrest. The heart is initially approached through an oblique right atriotomy, and the anatomy is carefully observed. In the case of a partial AV canal, the cleft in the mitral valve is repaired with interrupted sutures and the ASD is closed with a pericardial patch.[159] Complete AV canal defects are repaired by patch closure of the VSD, separating the common AV valve into tricuspid and mitral components and suspending the neovalves from the top of the VSD patch, and closing the ASD.

Results

Partial AV canal defects have an excellent outcome, with a mortality rate of 0 to 2% in most series.[157] Complete AV canal defects are

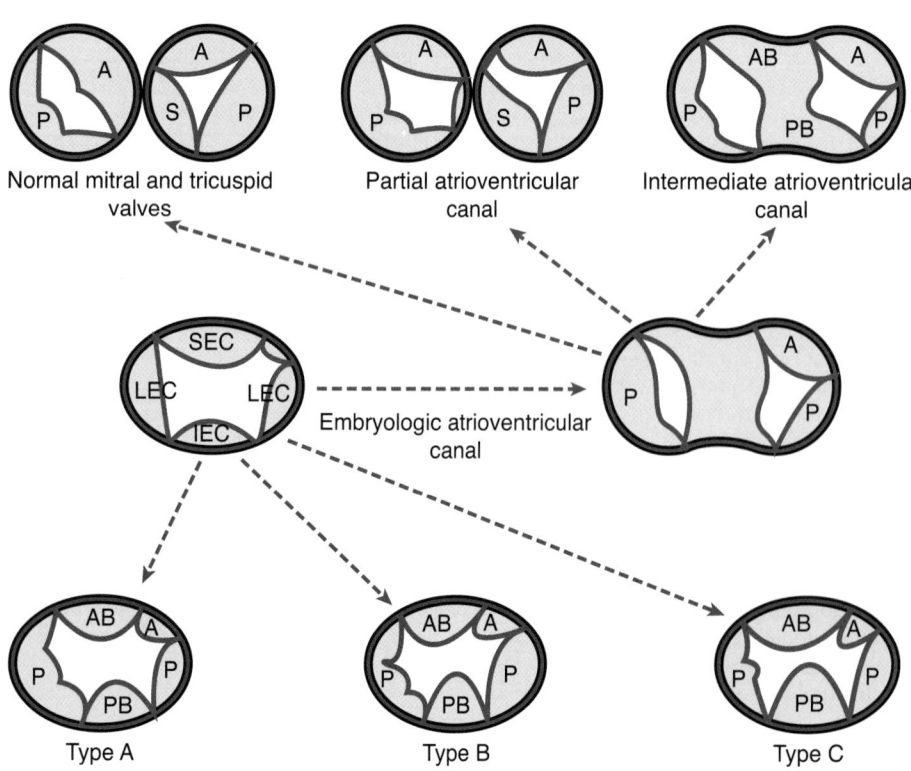

Normal mitral and tricuspid valves

Partial atrioventricular canal

Intermediate atrioventricular canal

Embryologic atrioventricular canal

Type A

Type B

Type C

Complete atrioventricular canal

FIG. 20-29. Formation of mitral and tricuspid leaflets and probable embryogenesis of partial, intermediate, and complete forms of atrioventricular canal defects. A = anterior; AB = anterior bridging leaflet; IEC = inferior endocardial cushion; LEC = lateral endocardial cushion; P = posterior; PB = posterior bridging leaflet; S = septal; SEC = superior endocardial cushion. [*Reproduced from Feldt RH, Porter CJ, Edwards WD, et al: Defects of the atrial septum and the atrioventricular canal, in Adams FH, Emmanouilides GC (eds): Moss' Heart Disease in Infants, Children, and Adolescents, 4th ed. Baltimore: Lippincott Williams & Wilkins, 1989. © Mayo Clinic ID #: CP1214116B-2.*]

associated with a poorer prognosis, with an operative mortality of 3 to 13%.

The most frequently encountered postoperative problems are complete heart block (1 to 2%), right bundle-branch block (22%), arrhythmias (11%), RVOT obstruction (11%), and severe mitral regurgitation (13 to 24%).[157] The increasing use of intraoperative transesophageal echocardiography may positively influence outcomes, as the adequacy of repair can be assessed and treated without need for subsequent reoperation.[157,158]

Interrupted Aortic Arch

Anatomy

IAA is a rare defect, comprising approximately 1% of all cases of CHD.[7,159] It is defined as an absence of luminal continuity between the ascending and descending aorta, and does not occur as an isolated defect in most cases, because a VSD or PDA is usually present. IAA is classified based on the location of the interruption (Fig. 20-30).

Clinical Manifestations and Diagnosis

Infants with IAA have ductal-dependent systemic blood flow and will develop profound metabolic acidosis and hemodynamic collapse upon ductal closure. In the rare instance of failed ductal closure, the diagnosis may be missed during infancy, and the child will present with symptoms of CHF from a persistent left-to-right shunt.

Once definitive diagnosis is made in infants, usually with echocardiography, preparations are made for operative intervention, and PGE$_1$ is infused to maintain ductal patency and correct acidosis. The infant's hemodynamic status should be optimized with mechanical ventilation and inotropic support. An effort should be made to increase PVR by decreasing the fractional inspired oxygen and avoiding hyperventilation, because this will preferentially direct blood into the systemic circulation.

Treatment

Initial strategies for the management of IAA involved palliation though a left thoracotomy by using one of the arch vessels as a conduit to restore aortic continuity. PA banding can be simultaneously performed to limit left-to-right shunting, because it is not feasible to repair the VSD or other intracardiac communications with this approach.

However, complete surgical repair in infants with IAA is now preferable. The operative technique involves use of a median sternotomy and CPB with short periods of circulatory arrest. Aortic arch reconstruction can be accomplished with either direct anastomosis or patch aortoplasty followed by closure of the VSD.[159]

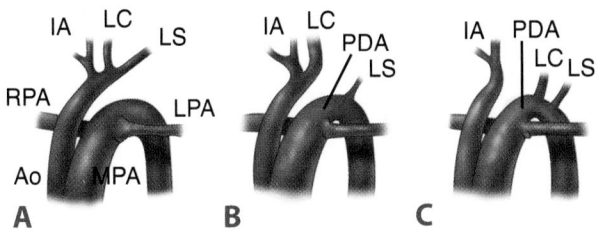

FIG. 20-30. Anatomic types of interrupted aortic arch. **A.** Interruption distal to the left subclavian artery. **B.** Interruption between the left subclavian and left carotid arteries. **C.** Interruption between the left carotid and innominate arteries. Ao = aorta; IA = innominate artery; LPA, MPA, RPA = left, main, and right pulmonary arteries; LC = left carotid artery; LS = left subclavian artery; PDA = patent ductus arteriosus. *[Reproduced with permission from Jonas RA: Interrupted aortic arch, in Mavroudis C, Backer CL (eds):* Pediatric Cardiac Surgery, *2nd ed. St. Louis: Mosby, 1994, p 184. Copyright Elsevier.]*

In certain cases, the defect will involve hypoplasia of the left heart, precluding attempts at definitive repair. These infants should be managed with a Norwood procedure followed by a Fontan repair.

Results

Outcomes in infants with IAA have improved substantially over the last decades as a result of improved perioperative care. Operative mortality is now less than 10% in most series.[157] Some authors advocate the use of patch augmentation of the aorta to ensure adequate relief of LVOTO and to diminish anastomotic tension, thus reducing the subsequent risk of restenosis and tracheobronchial compression.[7,157,160]

REFERENCES

Entries highlighted in bright blue are key references.

1. Ohye RG, Edward LB: Advances in congenital heart surgery. *Curr Opin Pediatr* 13:473, 2001.
2. Kouchoukos NT, Blackstone EH, Doty DB, et al: Atrial septal defect and partial anomalous pulmonary venous connection, in Kouchoukos NT, Blackstone EH, Doty DB, et al (eds): *Kirklin/Barrat-Boyes Cardiac Surgery*, 3rd ed. Philadelphia: Churchill Livingstone, 2003, p 716.
3. Liberthson RR, Boucher CA, Strauss HW, et al: Right ventricular function in adult atrial septal defect. *Am J Cardiol* 47:56, 1981.
4. Mosca RS, Hirsch JC, Bove EL: Congenital heart disease and cardiac tumors, in Greenfield LJ, Mulholland MW, Oldham KT, et al (eds): *Surgery: Scientific Principles and Practice*, 3rd ed. Philadelphia: Lippincott Williams and Wilkins, 2001, p 1443.
5. Ungerleider RM: Atrial septal defects, ostium primum defects, and atrioventricular canals, in Sabiston DC, Lyerly HK (eds): *Surgery. The Biological Basis of Modern Surgical Practice*, 15th ed. Philadelphia: W.B. Saunders, 1997, p 1980.
6. Wenn S, Qayyum SR, Anderson RH, et al: Septation and separation within the outflow tract of the developing heart. *J Anat* 202:327, 2003.
7. Castaneda AR, Jonas RA, Mayer JE, et al: *Cardiac Surgery of the Neonate and Infant*. Philadelphia: W.B. Saunders, 1994.
8. Kirklin JW, Pacifico AD, Kirklin JK: The surgical treatment of atrioventricular canal defects, in Arciniegas E (ed): *Pediatric Cardiac Surgery*. Chicago: Yearbook Medical, 1985, p 2398.
9. Peterson GE, Brickner ME, Reimold SC: Transesophageal echocardiography: Clinical indications and applications. *Circulation* 107:2398, 2003.
10. Kouchoukos NT, Blackstone EH, Doty DB, et al: Atrial septal defect and partial anomalous pulmonary venous connection, in Kouchoukos NT, Blackstone EH, Doty DB, et al (eds): *Kirklin/Barrat-Boyes Cardiac Surgery*, 3rd ed. Philadelphia: Churchill Livingstone, 2003, p 740.
11. Reddy VM: Cardiac surgery for premature and low birth weight neonates. *Semin Thorac Cardiovasc Surg Pediatr Card Surg Annu* 4:271, 2001.
12. Burke RP: Reducing the trauma of congenital heart surgery. *Semin Thorac Cardiovasc Surg Pediatr Card Surg Annu* 4:216, 2001.
13. Khan JH, McElhinney DB, Reddy M, et al: Repair of secundum atrial septal defect: Limiting the incision without sacrificing exposure. *Ann Thorac Surg* 66:1433, 1998.
14. Luo W, Chang C, Chen S: Ministernotomy versus full sternotomy in congenital heart defects: A prospective randomized study. *Ann Thorac Surg* 71:473, 2001.
15. King TD, Mills NL: Secundum atrial septal defects: Nonoperative closure during cardiac catheterization. *JAMA* 235:2506, 1976.
16. Karamlou T, Diggs BS, McCrindle BW, et al: The rush to atrial septal defect closure: Is the introduction of percutaneous closure driving utilization? *Ann Thorac Surg* 86:1584, 2008.
17. Rigby ML: The era of transcatheter closure of atrial septal defects [editorial]. *Heart* 81:227, 1999.
18. Zeevi B, Keane JF, Castaneda AR, et al: Neonatal critical valvular aortic stenosis. A comparison of surgical and balloon dilatation therapy. *Circulation* 80:831, 1989.
19. Brown JW, Stevens LS, Holly S, et al: Surgical spectrum of aortic stenosis in children: A thirty-year experience with 257 children. *Ann Thorac Surg* 45:393, 1988.
20. Kouchoukos NT, Blackstone EH, Doty DB, et al: Congenital aortic stenosis, in Kouchoukos NT, Blackstone EH, Doty DB, et al (eds):

Kirklin/Barrat-Boyes Cardiac Surgery, 3rd ed. Philadelphia: Churchill Livingstone, 2003, p 1269.

21. Lupinetti FM, Bove EL: Left ventricular outflow tract obstruction, in Mavroudis C, Backer CL (eds): *Pediatric Cardiac Surgery*, 2nd ed. St. Louis: Mosby, 1994, p 435.

22. Gupta ML, Lantin-Hermoso MR, Rao PS: What's new in pediatric cardiology. *Indian J Pediatr* 70:41, 2003.

23. Alsoufi B, Karamlou T, McCrindle BW, et al: Management options in neonates and infants with critical left ventricular outflow tract obstruction. *Eur J Cardiothorac Surg* 31:1013, 2007.

24. Hammon JW Jr., Lupinetti FM, Maples MD, et al: Predictors of operative mortality in critical aortic stenosis presenting in infancy. *Ann Thorac Surg* 45:537, 1988.

25. Mosca RS, Iannettoni MD, Schwartz SM, et al: Critical aortic stenosis in the neonate: A comparison of balloon valvuloplasty and transventricular dilatation. *J Thorac Cardiovasc Surg* 109:147, 1995.

26. Moore P, Egito E, Mowrey H, et al: Midterm results of balloon dilatation of congenital aortic stenosis: Predictors of success. *J Am Coll Cardiol* 27:1257, 1996.

27. Ross DN: Replacement of aortic and mitral valves with a pulmonary autograft. *Lancet* 57:956, 1967.

28. Jones TK, Lupinetti FM: Comparison of Ross procedures and aortic valve allografts in children. *Ann Thorac Surg* 66:S170, 1998.

29. Karamlou T, Jang K, Williams WG, et al: Outcomes and associated risk factors for aortic valve replacement in 160 children: A competing risks analysis. *Circulation* 29:3462, 2005.

30. Marasini M, Zannini L, Ussia GP, et al: Discrete subaortic stenosis: Incidence, morphology, and surgical impact of associated subaortic anomalies. *Ann Thorac Surg* 75:1763, 2003.

31. Karamlou T, Gurofsky R, Bojcevski A, et al: Prevalence and associated risk factors for intervention in 313 children with subaortic stenosis. *Ann Thorac Surg* 84:900, 2007.

32. Somerville J, Stone S, Ross D: Fate of patients with fixed subaortic stenosis after surgical removal. *Br Heart J* 43:629, 1980.

33. Williams JC, Barratt-Boyes BG, Lowe JB: Supravalvular aortic stenosis. *Circulation* 24:1311, 1961.

34. van Son JM, Danielson GK, Puga FJ, et al: Supravalvular aortic stenosis: Long-term results of surgical treatment. *J Thorac Cardiovasc Surg* 107:103, 1994.

35. Sharma BK, Fujiwara H, Hallman GL, et al: Supravalvular aortic stenosis: A 29-year review of surgical experience. *Ann Thorac Surg* 51:1031, 1991.

36. McElhinney DB, Petrossian E, Tworetzky W, et al: Issues and outcomes in the management of supravalvular aortic stenosis. *Ann Thorac Surg* 69:562, 2000.

37. Clyman RI, Mauray F, Roman C, et al: Circulating PGE_2 concentration and patent ductus arteriosus in fetal and neonatal lambs. *J Pediatr* 97:455, 1982.

38. McMurphy DM, Heymann MA, Rudolph AM, et al: Developmental change in constriction of the ductus arteriosus: Response to oxygen and vasoactive substances in the isolated ductus arteriosus of the fetal lamb. *Periatr Res* 6:231, 1972.

39. Mitchell SC, Korones SB, Berendes HW: Congenital heart disease in 56,109 births. Incidence and natural history. *Circulation* 43:323, 1971.

40. Campbell M: Natural history of persistent ductus arteriosus. *Br Heart J* 30:4, 1968.

41. Itabashi K, Ohno T, Nishida H: Indomethacin responsiveness of patent ductus arteriosus and renal abnormalities in preterm infants treated with indomethacin. *J Pediatr* 143:203, 2003.

42. Rashkind WJ, Cuaso CC: Transcatheter closure of patent ductus arteriosus. *Pediatr Cardiol* 1:3, 1979.

43. Moore JW, Schneider DJ, Dimeglio D: The duct-occlud device: Design, clinical results, and future directions. *J Interv Cardiol* 14:231, 2001.

44. Moore P, Egito E, Mowrey H, et al: Midterm results of balloon dilation of congenital aortic stenosis: Predictors of success. *J Am Coll Cardiol* 27:1257, 1996.

45. Mavroudis C, Backer CL, Gevitz M: Forty-six years of patent ductus arteriosus division at Children's Memorial Hospital of Chicago. Standards for comparison. *Ann Thorac Surg* 220:402, 1994.

46. Elzenga NJ, Gittenberger-de Groot AC, Oppenheimer-Dekker A: Coarctation and other obstructive arch anomalies: Their relationship to the ductus arteriosus. *Int J Cardiol* 13:289, 1986.

47. Locher JP, Kron IL: Coarctation of the aorta, in Mavroudis C, Backer CL (eds): *Pediatric Cardiac Surgery*. St. Louis: Mosby, 1994, p 167.

48. Presbitero P, Demaie D, Villani M, et al: Long-term results (15–30 years) of surgical repair of coarctation. *Br Heart J* 57:462, 1987.

49. Cohen M, Fuster V, Steele PM, et al: Coarctation of the aorta: Long-term follow-up and prediction of outcome after surgical correction. *Circulation* 80:840, 1989.

50. Hornung TS, Benson LN, McLaughlin PR: Interventions for aortic coarctation. *Cardiol Rev* 10:139, 2002.

51. Waldhausen JA, Nahrwold DL: Repair of coarctation of the aorta with a subclavian flap. *J Thorac Cardiovasc Surg* 51:532, 1966.

52. Karamlou T, Bernasconi A, Jaeggi E, et al: Factors associated with arch reintervention and growth of the aortic arch after coarctation repair in neonates weighing less than 2.5 kg. *J Thorac Cardiovasc Surg*, 2009 (in press).

53. van Heurn LW, Wong CM, Speigelhalter DJ, et al: Surgical treatment of aortic coarctation in infants younger than 3 months: 1985–1990. Success of extended end-to-end arch aortoplasty. *Journal Thorac Cardiovasc Surg* 107:74, 1994.

54. Knyshov GV, Sitar LL, Glagola MD, et al: Aortic aneurysms at the site of the repair of coarctation of the aorta: A review of 48 patients. *Ann Thorac Surg* 61:935, 1996.

55. Bouchart F, Dubar A, Tabley A, et al: Coarctation of the aorta in adults: Surgical results and long-term follow-up. *Ann Thorac Surg* 70:1483, 2000.

56. Bhat MA, Neelakhandran KS, Unnikriahnan M, et al: Fate of hypertension after repair of coarctation of the aorta in adults. *Br J Surg* 88:536, 2001.

57. McCrindle BW, Jones TK, Morrow WR, et al: Acute results of balloon angioplasty of native coarctation versus recurrent aortic obstruction are equivalent. Valvuloplasty and Angioplasty of Congenital Anomalies (VACA) Registry Investigators. *J Am Coll Cardiol* 28:1810, 1996.

58. Hopkins RA, Wallace RB: Truncus arteriosus, in Sabiston DC, Lyerly HK (eds): *Textbook of Surgery: The Biologic Basis of Modern Surgical Practice*, 15th ed. Philadelphia: W.B. Saunders, 1997, p 2052.

59. Collett RW, Edwards JE: Persistent truncus arteriosus: A classification according to anatomic subtypes. *Surg Clin North Am* 29:1245, 1949.

60. Van Praagh R, Van Praagh S: The anatomy of common aorticopulmonary trunk (truncus arteriosus communis) and its embryologic implications: A study of 57 necroscopy cases. *Am J Cardiol* 16:406, 1965.

61. De la Cruz MV, Pio da Rocha J: An ontogenic theory for the explanation of congenital malformations involving the truncus and conus. *Am Heart J* 51:782, 1976.

62. Manner J: Cardiac looping in the chick embryo: A morphologic review with special reference to terminological and biomechanical aspects of the looping process. *Anat Rec* 259:242, 2000.

63. Hutson MR, Kirby ML: Neural crest and cardiovascular development: A 20-year perspective. *Birth Defects Res Part C Embryo Today* 69:2, 2003.

64. Kouchoukos NT, Blackstone EH, Doty DB, et al: Truncus arteriosus, in Kouchoukos NT, Blackstone EH, Doty DB, et al (eds): *Kirklin/Barrat-Boyes Cardiac Surgery*, 3rd ed. Philadelphia: Churchill Livingstone, 2003, p 1201.

65. Mavroudis C, Backer CL: Truncus arteriosus, in Mavroudis C, Backer CL (eds): *Pediatric Cardiac Surgery*, 2nd ed. St. Louis: Mosby, 1994, p 237.

66. Chiu IS, Wu SJ, Chen MR, et al: Anatomic relationship of the coronary orifice and truncal valve in truncus arteriosus and their surgical implication. *J Thorac Cardiovasc Surg* 123:350, 2002.

67. Armer RM, De Oliveira PF, Lurie PR: True truncus arteriosus. Review of 17 cases and report of surgery in 7 patients. *Circulation* 24:878, 1961.

68. McGoon DC, Rastelli GC, Ongley PA: An operation for the correction of truncus arteriosus. *JAMA* 205:69, 1968.

69. Ebert PA: Truncus arteriosus, in Glenn WWL, Baue AE, Geha AS (eds): *Thoracic and Cardiovascular Surgery*, 4th ed. Norwalk: Appleton-Century-Crofts, 1983, p 731.

70. Forbess JM, Shah AS, St Louis JD, et al: Cryopreserved homografts in the pulmonary position: Determinants of durability. *Ann Thorac Surg* 71:54, 2001.

71. Aupecle B, Serraf A, Belli E, et al: Intermediate follow-up of a composite stentless porcine valved conduit of bovine pericardium in the pulmonary circulation. *Ann Thorac Surg* 74:127, 2002.

72. Kouchoukos NT, Blackstone EH, Doty DB, et al: Total anomalous pulmonary venous connection, in Kouchoukos NT, Blackstone EH, Doty DB, et al (eds): *Kirklin/Barrat-Boyes Cardiac Surgery*, 3rd ed. Philadelphia: Churchill Livingstone, 2003, p 758.

73. Darling RC, Rothney WB, Craij JM: Total pulmonary venous drainage into the right side of the heart. *Lab Invest* 6:44, 1957.

74. Delisle G, Ando M, Calder AL, et al: Total anomalous pulmonary venous connection: Report of 93 autopsied cases with emphasis on diagnostic and surgical considerations. *Am Heart J* 91:99, 1976.

75. Michielon G, Di Donato RM, Pasquini L, et al: Total anomalous pulmonary venous connection: Long-term appraisal with evolving technical solutions. *Eur J Cardiothorac Surg* 22:184, 2002.

76. Jonas RA, Smolinsky A, Mayer JE, et al: Obstructed pulmonary venous drainage with total anomalous pulmonary venous connection to the coronary sinus. *Am J Cardiol* 59:431, 1987.

77. Austin EH: Disorders of pulmonary venous return, in Sabiston DC, Lyerly HK (eds): *Textbook of Surgery: The Biological Basis of Modern Surgical Practice*, 15th ed. Philadelphia: W.B. Saunders, 1997, p 2001.

78. Ricci M, Elliott M, Cohen GA, et al: Management of pulmonary venous obstruction after correction of TAPVC: Risk factors for adverse outcome. *Eur J Cardiothorac Surg* 24:28, 2003.

79. Serraf A, Bruniaux J, Lacour-Gayet F, et al: Obstructed total anomalous pulmonary venous return. Toward neutralization of a major risk factor. *J Thorac Cardiovasc Surg* 101:601, 1991.

80. Hyde JAJ, Stumper O, Barth MJ, et al: Total anomalous pulmonary venous connection: Outcome of surgical correction and management of recurrent venous obstruction. *Eur J Cardiothorac Surg* 15:735, 1999.

81. Korbmacher B, Buttgen S, Schulte HD, et al: Long-term results after repair of total anomalous pulmonary venous connection. *Thorac Cardiovasc Surg* 49:101, 2001.

82. Bando K, Turrentine MW, Ensing GJ, et al: Surgical management of total anomalous pulmonary venous connection. Thirty-year trends. *Circulation* 94:II12, 1996.

83. Karamlou T, Gurofsky R, Al Sukhni E, et al: Factors associated with mortality and reoperation in 377 children with total anomalous pulmonary venous connection. *Circulation* 115:1591, 2007.

84. Salomone G, Tiraboschi R, Bianchi T, et al: Cor triatriatum: Clinical presentation and operative results. *J Thorac Cardiovasc Surg* 101:1088, 1991.

85. Cooley DA, McNamara DG, Latson JR: Aorticopulmonary septal defect: Diagnosis and surgical treatment. *Surgery* 42:101, 1957.

86. Huang TC, Lee CL, Lin CC, et al: Use of an Inoue balloon dilatation method for treatment of cor triatriatum stenosis in a child. *Catheter Cardiovasc Interv* 57:252, 2002.

87. Gaynor JW, Ungerleider RM: Aortopulmonary window, in Mavroudis C, Backer CL (eds): *Pediatric Cardiac Surgery*, 2nd ed. St. Louis: Mosby, 1994, p 250.

88. Ohtake S, Mault JR, Lilly MK, et al: Effect of a systemic-pulmonary artery shunt on myocardial function and perfusion in a piglet model. *Surg Forum* 42:200, 1991.

89. Scalia D, Russo P, Anderson RH, et al: The surgical anatomy of hearts with no direct communication between the right atrium and the ventricular mass—so-called tricuspid atresia. *J Thorac Cardiovasc Surg* 87:743, 1984.

90. Cheung HC, Lincoln C, Anderson RH, et al: Options for surgical repair in hearts with univentricular atrioventricular connection and subaortic stenosis. *J Thorac Cardiovasc Surg* 100:672, 1990.

91. Trusler GA, Williams WG: Long-term results of shunt procedures for tricuspid atresia. *Ann Thorac Surg* 29:312, 1980.

92. Dick M, Gyler DC, Nadas AS: Tricuspid atresia: Clinical course in 101 patients. *Am J Cardiol* 36:327, 1975.

93. Glenn WWL, Patino JF: Circulatory by-pass of the right heart. Preliminary observations on the direct delivery of vena caval blood into the pulmonary arterial circulation. Azygous vein-pulmonary artery shunt. *Yale J Biol Med* 27:147, 1954.

94. Fontan F, Baudet E: Surgical repair of tricuspid atresia. *Thorax* 26:240, 1971.

95. deLeval MR, Kilner P, Gerwillig M, et al: Total cavopulmonary connection: A logical alternative to atriopulmonary connection for complex Fontan operations. *J Thorac Cardiovasc Surg* 96:682, 1988.

96. Laks H, Haas GS, Pearl JM, et al: The use of an adjustable interatrial communication in patients undergoing the Fontan and definitive heart procedures [abstract]. *Circulation* 78:357, 1988.

97. Haas GS, Hess H, Black M, et al: Extracardiac conduit Fontan procedure: Early and intermediate results. *Eur J Cardiothorac Surg* 17:648, 2000.

98. Tokunaga S, Kado H, Imoto Y, et al: Total cavopulmonary connection with an extracardiac conduit: Experience with 100 patients. *Ann Thorac Surg* 73:76, 2002.

99. Karamlou T, Ashburn DA, Caldarone CA, et al: Matching procedure to morphology improves outcome in neonates with tricuspid atresia. *J Thorac Cardiovasc Surg* 130:1503, 2005.

100. Bardo DME, Frankel DG, Applegate KE, et al: Hypoplastic left heart syndrome. *Radiographics* 21:706, 2001.

101. Norwood WI: Hypoplastic left heart syndrome. *Ann Thorac Surg* 52:688, 1991.

102. Bronshtein M, Zimmer EZ: Early sonographic diagnosis of fetal small left heart ventricle with a normal proximal outlet tract: A medical dilemma. *Prenat Diagn* 17:249, 1997.

103. Norwood WI, Lang P, Hansen DD: Physiologic repair of aortic atresia-hypoplastic left heart syndrome. *N Engl J Med* 308:23, 1983.

104. Norwood WI: Hypoplastic left heart syndrome. *Ann Thorac Surg* 52:688, 1991.

105. Tweddell JS, Hoffman GM, Mussatto KA, et al: Improved survival of patients undergoing palliation of hypoplastic left heart syndrome: Lessons learned from 115 consecutive patients. *Circulation* 106:I82, 2002.

106. Tweddell JS, Hoffan GM, Ghanayem NS, et al: Ventilatory control of pulmonary vascular resistance is not necessary to achieve a balanced circulation in the postoperative Norwood patient. *Circulation* 100:I671, 1999.

107. Tchervenkov CI: Two-ventricle repair for hypoplastic left heart syndrome. *Semin Thorac Cardiovasc Surg Pediatr Card Surg Annu* 4:89, 2001.

108. http://www.clinicaltrials.gov: Single Ventricle Reconstruction Trial NCT00115934. [accessed June 21, 2008].

109. Akinturerk H, Michel-Behnke I, Valeske K, et al: Stenting of the arterial duct and banding of the pulmonary arteries: Basis for combined Norwood stage I and II repair in hypoplastic left heart. *Circulation* 105:1099, 2002.

110. Caldarone CA, Benson L, Holtby H, et al: Initial experience with hybrid palliation for neonates with single ventricle physiology. *Ann Thorac Surg* 84:1294, 2007.

111. Bailey LL, Gundry SR, Razzouk AJ, et al: Bless the babies: 115 late survivors of heart transplantation during the first year of life. The Loma Linda University Pediatric Heart Transplant Group. *J Thorac Cardiovas Surg* 105:805, 1993.

112. Gaynor JW, Mahle WT, Cohen MI, et al: Risk factors for mortality after the Norwood procedure. *Eur J Cardiothorac Surg* 22:88, 2002.

113. Bove EL: How I Manage Neonatal Ebstein's (abstract). 88th Annual Meeting of the American Association of Thoracic Surgery, San Diego, CA, May 10, 2008.

114. Matthew ST, Federico GF, Singh BK: Ebstein's anomaly presenting as Wolff-Parkinson-White syndrome in a postpartum patient. *Cardiol Rev* 11:208, 2003.

115. Celermajer DS, Cullen S, Sullivan ID, et al: Outcome in neonates with Ebstein's anomaly. *J Am Coll Cardiol* 19:1041, 1992.

116. Starnes VA, Pitlick PT, Bernstein D, et al: Ebstein's anomaly appearing in the neonate. *J Thorac Cardiovasc Surg* 101:1082, 1991.

117. Danielson GK, Driscoll DJ, Mair DD, et al: Operative treatment of Ebstein's anomaly. *J Thorac Cardiovasc Surg* 104:1195, 1992.

118. Knott-Craig CJ, Overholt ED, Ward KE, et al: Neonatal repair of Ebstein's anomaly: Indications, surgical technique, and medium-term follow-up. *Ann Thorac Surg* 69:1505, 2000.

119. Yetman AT, Freedom RM, McCrindle BW: Outcome in cyanotic neonates with Ebstein's anomaly. *Am J Cardiol* 81:749, 1998.

120. Billingsly AM, Laks H, Boyce SW, et al: Definitive repair in patients with pulmonary atresia and intact ventricular septum. *J Thorac Cardiovasc Surg* 97:746, 1989.

121. Stellin G, Vida VL, Milanesi O, et al: Surgical treatment of complex cardiac anomalies: The "one and one half ventricle repair." *Eur J Cardiothorac Surg* 22:435, 2002.

122. Chowdhury UK, Airan B, Sharma R, et al: One and a half ventricle repair with pulsatile Glenn: Results and guidelines for patient selection. *Ann Thorac Surg* 71:2000, 2001.

123. Van Praagh R, Van Praagh S, Vlad P: Anatomic subtypes of congenital dextrocardia: Diagnostic and embryologic implications. *Am J Cardiol* 13:510, 1964.

124. Van Praagh R, Van Praagh S: Isolated ventricular inversion: A consideration of the morphogenesis, definition, and diagnosis of nontransposed and transposed great arteries. *Am J Cardiol* 17:395, 1966.

125. Blalock A, Hanlon CR: The surgical treatment of complete transposition of the aorta and the pulmonary artery. *Surg Gynecol Obstet* 90:1, 1950.

126. Senning A: Surgical correction of transposition of the great vessel. *Surgery* 45:966, 1959.

127. Mustard WT, Chute AL, Keith JD: A surgical approach to transposition of the great vessels with extracorporeal circuit. *Surgery* 36:39, 1954.

128. Jatene AD, Fontes VF, Paulista PP, et al: Successful anatomic correction of transposition of the great vessels: A preliminary report. *Arq Bras Cardiol* 28:461, 1975.

129. Rastelli GC: A new approach to the "anatomic" repair of transposition of the great arteries. *Mayo Clin Proc* 44:1, 1969.

130. Culbert EL, Ashburn DA, Cullen-Dean G, et al: Quality of life after repair of transposition of the great arteries. *Circulation* 108:857, 2003.

131. Dearani JA, Danielson GK, Puga FJ, et al: Late results of the Rastelli operation for transposition of the great arteries. *Semin Thorac Cardiovasc Surg Pediatr Card Surg Annu* 4:3, 2001.

132. Freedom RM, Yoo SJ: Double-outlet right ventricle: Pathology and angiocardiography. *Semin Thorac Cardiovasc Surg Pediatr Card Surg Annu* 3:3, 2000.

133. Lev M, Bharati S, Meng CCL, et al: A concept of double outlet right ventricle. *J Thorac Cardiovasc Surg* 64:271, 1972.

134. Taussig HB, Bing RJ: Complete transposition of the aorta and a levoposition of the pulmonary artery. *Am Heart J* 37:551, 1949.

135. Belli E, Serraf A, Lacour-Gayet F, et al: Double-outlet right ventricle with non-committed ventricular septal defect. *Eur J Cardiothorac Surg* 15:747, 1999.

136. Kawashima Y, Matsuda H. Yagihara T, et al: Intraventricular repair for Taussig-Bing anomaly. *J Thorac Cardiovasc Surg* 105:591, 1993.

137. Rastelli GC, McGoon DC, Wallace RB: Anatomic correction of transposition of the great arteries with ventricular septal defect and subpulmonic stenosis. *J Thorac Cardiovasc Surg* 58:545, 1969.

138. Yasui H, Kado H, Nakano E et al: Primary repair of interrupted aortic arch with severe stenosis in neonates. *J Thorac Cardiovasc Surg* 93:539, 1987.

139. Bradley TJ, Karamlou T, Kulik A, et al. Determinants of repair type, reintervention, and mortality in 393 children with double-outlet right ventricle. *J Thorac Cardiovasc Surg* 134:967, 2007.

140. Brown JW, Ruzmetov M, Okada Y, et al: Surgical results in patients with double outlet right ventricle: A 20-year experience. *Ann Thorac Surg* 72:1630, 2001.

141. Fallot A: Contribution a l'anatomie pathologique de la maladie bleue (cyanose cardiaque) [French]. *Marseille Med* 25:77, 1888.

142. Van Praagh R, et al: Tetralogy of Fallot: Underdevelopment of the pulmonary infundibulum and its sequelae. *Am J Cardiol* 26:25, 1970.

143. Need LR, Powell AJ, del Nido P, et al: Coronary echocardiography in tetralogy of Fallot: Diagnostic accuracy, resource utilization, and surgical implications over 13 years. *J Am Coll Cardiol* 36:1371, 2000.

144. Mahle WT, McBride MG, Paridon SM: Exercise performance in tetralogy of Fallot: The impact of primary complete repair in infancy. *Pediatr Cardiol* 23:224, 2002.

145. Deanfield JE: Adult congenital heart disease with special reference to the data on long-term follow-up of patients surviving to adulthood with or without surgical correction. *Eur Heart J* 13:111, 1992.

146. Alexiou C, Chen Q, Galogavrou M, et al: Repair of tetralogy of Fallot in infancy with a transventricular or a transatrial approach. *Eur J Cardiothorac Surg* 22:174, 2002.

147. Walsh EP, Rockenmacher S, Keane JF, et al: Late results in patients with tetralogy of Fallot repaired during infancy. *Circulation* 77:1062, 1988.

148. Karamlou T, McCrindle BW, Williams WG: Surgery insight: Late complications following repair of tetralogy of Fallot and related surgical strategies for management. *Nature Cardiovasc Med* 3:611, 2006.

149. Kouchoukos NT, Blackstone EH, Doty DB, et al: Ventricular septal defect, in Kouchoukos NT, Blackstone EH, Doty DB, et al (eds): *Kirklin/Barrat-Boyes Cardiac Surgery*, 3rd ed. Philadelphia: Churchill Livingstone, 2003, p 851.

150. Gatzoulis MA, et al: Mechanoelectrical interaction in tetralogy of Fallot. QRS prolongation relates to right ventricular size and predicts malignant ventricular arrhythmias and sudden death. *Circulation* 92:231, 1995.

151. Karamlou T, et al: Outcomes after late reoperation in patients with repaired tetralogy of Fallot: The impact of arrhythmia and arrhythmia surgery. *Ann Thorac Surg* 81:1786, 2006.

152. Turner SW, Hornung T, Hunter S: Closure of ventricular septal defects: A study of factors influencing spontaneous and surgical closure. *Cardiol Young* 12:357, 2002.

153. Waight DJ, Bacha EA, Khahana M, et al: Catheter therapy of Swiss cheese ventricular septal defects using the Amplatzer muscular VSD occluder. *Catheter Cardiovasc Interv* 55:360, 2002.

154. Seddio F, Reddy VM, McElhinney DB, et al: Multiple ventricular septal defects: How and when should they be repaired? *J Thorac Cardiovasc Surg* 117:134, 1999.

155. Rastelli G, Kirklin JW, Titus JL: Anatomic observations on complete form of persistent common atrioventricular canal with special reference to atrioventricular valves. *Mayo Clin Proc* 41:296, 1966.

156. Tsang VT, Hsia TY, Yates RW, et al: Surgical repair of supposedly multiple defects within the apical part of the muscular ventricular septum. *Ann Thorac Surg* 73:58, 2002.

157. Ungerleider RM: Atrial septal defects, ostium primum defects, and atrioventricular canals, in Sabiston DC, Lyerly HK (eds): *Textbook of Surgery: The Biologic Basis of Modern Surgical Practice*. Philadelphia: W.B. Saunders, 1997, p 1993.

158. Kouchoukos NT, Blackstone EH, Doty DB, et al: Coarctation of the aorta and interrupted aortic arch, in Kouchoukos NT, Blackstone EH, Doty DB, et al (eds): *Kirklin/Barrat-Boyes Cardiac Surgery*, 3rd ed. Philadelphia: Churchill Livingstone, 2003, p 1353.

159. Ungerleider RM, Kisslo JA, Greeley WJ, et al: Intraoperative prebypass and postbypass epicardial color flow imaging in the repair of atrioventricular septal defects. *J Thorac Cardiovasc Surg* 98:1146, 1989.

160. Roussin R, Belli E, Lacour-Gayet F, et al: Aortic arch reconstruction with pulmonary autograft patch aortoplasty. *J Thorac Cardiovasc Surg* 123:443, 2002.

Acquired Heart Disease

Charles F. Schwartz, Gregory A. Crooke,
Eugene A. Grossi, and Aubrey C. Galloway

CARDIAC ASSESSMENT

Clinical Evaluation

The importance of the history and physical examination when evaluating a patient with acquired heart disease for potential surgery cannot be overemphasized. It is imperative that the surgeon be well aware of the functional status of the patient and the clinical relevance of each symptom, because surgical decisions depend upon the accurate assessment of the significance of a particular pathologic finding. Likewise, as the number of diagnostic tests continues to increase, appropriate sequencing of the diagnostic work-up requires a clinical perspective that is obtained through the history and physical examination. Associated risk factors and coexisting conditions must be identified, as they significantly influence a patient's operative risk for cardiac or noncardiac surgery. Furthermore, the operative strategy is affected by specific physical findings and important history, such as previous cardiac or thoracic surgery, peripheral vascular occlusive disease, or prior saphenous vein stripping. The safe surgeon is one who can integrate clinical evidence and diagnostic information to establish a scientifically based operative plan.

Symptoms

The classic symptoms of heart disease are fatigue, angina, dyspnea, edema, hemoptysis, palpitations, and syncope, as outlined by Braunwald.[1] When a patient describes or complains of any of these symptoms, the clinical scenario leading to it must be explored in detail, including symptom intensity, duration, provocation, and conditions that lead to relief. The initial goal is to determine whether a symptom is cardiac or noncardiac in origin, as well as to determine the clinical significance of the complaint. An important feature of cardiac disease is that myocardial function or coronary blood supply that may be adequate at rest may become completely inadequate with exercise or exertion. Thus, chest pain or dyspnea that occurs primarily during exertion is frequently cardiac in origin, while symptoms that occur at rest often are not.

In addition to evaluating the patient's primary symptoms, the history should include a family history, past medical history [prior surgery or myocardial infarction (MI), concomitant hypertension, diabetes, and other associated diseases], personal habits (smoking, alcohol or drug use), functional capacity, and a detailed review of systems. After a careful assessment of a patient's symptoms, appropriate diagnostic studies are ordered and interpreted. The classic symptoms are reviewed in detail below.

Easy fatigability is a frequent but nonspecific symptom of cardiac disease that can arise from many causes. In some patients, this symptom reflects a generalized decrease in cardiac output or low-grade heart failure. The significance of subjective easy fatigability is vague and nonspecific.

Angina pectoris is the hallmark of myocardial ischemia secondary to coronary artery disease (CAD), although a variety of other conditions can produce chest pain, and the clinician must determine if chest pain is of cardiac or noncardiac origin. Classic angina is precordial pain described as squeezing, heavy, or burning in nature, lasting from 2 to 10 minutes. The pain is usually substernal, radiating into the left shoulder and arm, but occasionally occurs in the midepigastrium, jaw, right arm, or midscapular region. Angina usually is provoked by exercise, emotion, sexual activity, or eating, and is relieved by rest or nitroglycerin. Angina is present in its classic form in 75% of patients with coronary disease, while atypical symptoms occur in 25% of patients and more frequently in women. A small but significant number of patients have "silent" ischemia, typically occurring in diabetics. Angina also is a classic symptom of aortic stenosis, occurring secondary to a combination of left ventricular (LV) hypertrophy, increased intracardiac pressure, increased ventricular wall tension (leading to higher oxygen requirements), and decreased cardiac output. This combination results in a myocardial oxygen supply-demand mismatch with resultant ischemia and angina.

Noncardiac causes of chest pain that may be confused with angina include gastroesophageal reflux disease, esophageal spasm, musculoskeletal pain, peptic ulcer disease, pulmonary embolus, costochondritis (Tietze's syndrome), biliary tract disease, pleuritis, pulmonary hypertension, pericarditis, and aortic dissection.

The physiologic change in most patients with heart failure is a rise in LV end-diastolic pressure, followed by cardiac enlargement. While Starling's law describes the compensatory mechanism of the heart of increased work in response to increased diastolic fiber length, symptoms develop as this compensatory mechanism fails, resulting in a progressive rise in LV end-diastolic pressure. Because this development is eventually damaging to the myocardial muscle and may ultimately result in a dilated cardiomyopathy, data suggest that surgery should be considered for many patients before the development of dyspnea or congestive heart failure (CHF). Nevertheless, exertional dyspnea is often the first sign of LV dysfunction, and should prompt an evaluation for an underlying cardiac cause.

Dyspnea may appear as an early sign in patients with mitral stenosis due to restriction of flow from the left atrium into the left ventricle. However, with other forms of heart disease, dyspnea is a late sign, as it develops only after the left ventricle has failed and the end-diastolic pressure rises significantly. Dyspnea associated with mitral insufficiency, aortic valve disease, or coronary disease represents relatively advanced pathophysiology.

A number of other respiratory symptoms represent different degrees of pulmonary congestion. These include orthopnea, paroxysmal nocturnal dyspnea, cough, hemoptysis, and pulmonary edema. Occasionally, dyspnea represents an "angina equivalent," occurring secondary to ischemia-related LV dysfunction. This finding is more common in women and in diabetic patients.

Left-sided heart failure may result in fluid retention and pulmonary congestion, subsequently leading to pulmonary hypertension and progressive right-sided heart failure. A history of exertional dyspnea with associated edema is frequently due to heart failure. In contrast, primary right heart failure may result from right ventricular injury and dysfunction or from primary tricuspid valve (TV) disease. Right atrial pressure, normally <5 to 8 mmHg, may be elevated to 15 to 30 mmHg or higher. Retention of >7 to 10 lb of fluid results in visible lower extremity edema, usually equal bilaterally. Additionally, jugular venous distention and hepatomegaly develop with severe right heart failure. In chronic, severe heart failure, generalized fluid retention may be quite severe, accompanied by ascites and massive hepatomegaly.

Palpitations are secondary to rapid, forceful, ectopic, or irregular heartbeats. Palpitations frequently are innocuous, but occasionally represent significant or potentially life-threatening arrhythmias. The underlying cardiac arrhythmia may range from premature atrial or ventricular contractions to atrial fibrillation, atrial flutter, paroxysmal atrial or junctional tachycardia, or sustained ventricular tachycardia.

Atrial fibrillation is one of the most common causes of palpitations. It is a common arrhythmia in patients with mitral stenosis, and results from left atrial enlargement that evolves from sustained elevation in left atrial pressure. With other forms of heart disease, arrhythmias are less common and occur sporadically. In general, arrhythmias are more frequent in older patients, resulting from intrinsic disease in sinus node (sick sinus syndrome) or disease of the atrioventricular (AV) conduction mechanism resulting in complete or intermittent heart block.

Severe, life-threatening forms of ventricular tachycardia or ventricular fibrillation may occur in any patient with ischemic disease, either from ongoing ischemia or from prior infarction and myocardial scarring.

Syncope, or sudden loss of consciousness, is usually a result of sudden decreased perfusion of the brain. The differential diagnosis includes: (a) third-degree heart block with bradycardia or asystole, (b) malignant ventricular tachyarrhythmias or ventricular fibrillation, (c) aortic stenosis, (d) hypertrophic cardiomyopathy, (e) carotid artery disease, (f) seizure disorders, and (g) vasovagal reaction. Any episode of syncope must be evaluated thoroughly, as many of these conditions can result in sudden death.

Functional Disability and Angina

An important part of the history is the assessment of the patient's overall cardiac functional disability, which is a good approximation of the severity of the patient's underlying disease. The New York Heart Association (NYHA) has developed a classification of patients with heart disease based on symptoms and functional disability (Table 21-1). The NYHA classification has been extremely useful in evaluating a patient's severity of disability, in comparing treatment regimens, and in predicting operative risk.

The NYHA functional classification system is widely used and adequate for the majority of patients. However, when a more precise functional analysis is necessary, the specific activity scale proposed

---

TABLE 21-1 New York Heart Association functional classification

Class I: Patients with cardiac disease but without resulting limitation of physical activity. Ordinary physical activity does not cause undue fatigue, palpitation, dyspnea, or angina pain.

Class II: Patients with cardiac disease resulting in slight limitation of physical activity. They are comfortable at rest. Ordinary physical activity results in fatigue, palpitation, dyspnea, or angina pain.

Class III: Patients with cardiac disease resulting in marked limitation of physical activity. They are comfortable at rest. Less than ordinary physical activity causes fatigue, palpitation, dyspnea, or anginal pain.

Class IV: Patients with cardiac disease resulting in an inability to carry on any physical activity without discomfort. Symptoms of cardiac insufficiency or of the anginal syndrome may be present even at rest. If any physical activity is undertaken, discomfort is increased.

---

by Goldman and based upon the estimated metabolic cost of various activities is used. A different grading system for patients with ischemic disease, developed by the Canadian Cardiovascular Society (CCS), is used to assess the severity of angina (Table 21-2).

Cardiac Risk Assessment in General Surgery Patients

Cardiac risk stratification for patients undergoing noncardiac surgery is a critical part of the preoperative evaluation of the general surgery patient. The joint American College of Cardiology/American Heart Association task force, chaired by Eagle, recently reported guidelines and recommendations, which are summarized in this section. In general, the preoperative cardiovascular evaluation involves an assessment of clinical markers, the patient's underlying functional capacity, and various surgery-specific risk factors.

TABLE 21-2 Canadian Cardiovascular Society angina classification

Class I: Ordinary physical activity, such as walking or climbing stairs, does not cause angina. Angina may occur with strenuous or rapid or prolonged exertion at work or recreation.

Class II: There is slight limitation of ordinary activity. Angina may occur with walking or climbing stairs rapidly, walking uphill, walking or stair climbing after meals or in the cold, in the wind, or under emotional stress, or walking more than two blocks on the level, or climbing more than one flight of stairs under normal conditions at a normal pace.

Class III: There is marked limitation of ordinary physical activity. Angina may occur after walking one or more blocks on the level or climbing one flight of stairs under normal conditions at a normal pace.

Class IV: There is inability to carry on any physical activity without discomfort; angina may be present at rest.

KEY POINTS

1. The long-term outcomes of coronary artery bypass graft surgery remain superior to coronary stenting for patients with left main disease and multivessel coronary artery disease in diabetic patients.

2. Congestive heart failure is reaching epidemic proportions. Effective surgical strategies exist for these patients, ranging from valve repair to ventricular assist devices.

3. Mitral valve repair rather than replacement affords superior long-term benefits to patients with degenerative mitral valve disease.

4. Aortic valve replacement is routinely and safely performed in patients over 80 years old.

The *clinical markers* that predict an increased risk of a cardiac event during noncardiac surgery are divided into three grades. *Major* predictors include unstable coronary syndromes, including acute or recent MI and unstable angina (CCS class III or IV), decompensated heart failure (NYHA class IV), and significant arrhythmias and severe valvular disease. *Intermediate* predictors are mild angina (CCS class I or II), old MI, compensated heart failure (NYHA class II and III), diabetes, and renal insufficiency. *Mild* predictors are advanced age, uncontrolled systemic hypertension, irregular rhythm, prior stroke, abnormal electrocardiogram (ECG), and mild functional disability.

Specific *surgical risk factors or procedures* expose the patient to greater or lesser risk of a cardiovascular event. *High-risk* procedures include emergent, major procedures in the elderly; major vascular procedures (e.g., thoracic, abdominal aortic, or peripheral vascular); and long general surgical procedures with anticipated large fluid shifts and/or blood loss (e.g., pancreatectomy, hepatic resection, or abdominoperineal resection). *Intermediate-risk* procedures include any intraperitoneal or intrathoracic operation, carotid endarterectomy, and orthopedic, prostate, and head and neck procedures. *Low-risk* procedures include endoscopic, breast, cataract, and superficial operations.

Based upon the clinical markers, the functional class of the patient, and the proposed surgical procedure, the patient is assigned a high, intermediate, or low cardiac risk, and then managed appropriately. In some patients, further risk stratification is required, such as patients with intermediate cardiac risk factors who are undergoing a high-risk surgical procedure. These patients should undergo exercise stress testing or provocative testing (dipyridamole thallium or dobutamine stress echocardiography) before an operation. In patients who are considered high cardiac risk due to clinical markers or by virtue of noninvasive testing, coronary angiography may be recommended before surgery. CAD is then managed according to the classic indications. In patients who are thought to be low or moderate cardiac risk, medical management alone is sufficient.

Due to the common atherosclerotic etiology and the close association between clinically relevant CAD and peripheral vascular disease (PVD), patients undergoing major vascular surgery should be screened closely, either by history or provocative stress testing. Those patients with symptoms suggestive of ischemia, with a decreased ejection fraction due to prior MI, or with provocative stress testing suggestive of ischemia should undergo coronary angiography or a newer cardiac computed tomography (CT) modality before vascular surgery. Any significant underlying coronary disease should be aggressively treated, either with intensive perioperative management or with coronary revascularization before surgery, using standard indications. This aggressive screening approach, followed by appropriate intervention in patients with significant CAD, has greatly lowered the operative risk of patients undergoing major vascular surgery.

Diagnostic Studies

Electrocardiogram and Chest X-Ray

ECG and the chest x-ray are two classic diagnostic studies. The ECG is used to detect rhythm disturbances, heart block, atrial or ventricular hypertrophy, ventricular strain, myocardial ischemia, and MI. Standard posterior-anterior and lateral chest x-rays are excellent for determining cardiac enlargement and pulmonary congestion, as well as for assessing associated pulmonary pathology.

Echocardiography

Echocardiography has become the most widely used cardiac diagnostic study. This test incorporates the use of ultrasound and reflected acoustic waves for cardiac imaging. Blood flow velocities are assigned colors to help visually evaluate them. This information is superimposed onto the two-dimensional image, giving a graphic illustration of the directional intracardiac flow pattern and an assessment of valvular insufficiency.

Standard transthoracic echocardiography has become an excellent noninvasive screening test to evaluate cardiac size, wall motion, and valvular pathology. Corrective operation for valvular disease is now frequently performed on younger patients based on this study alone.

Transesophageal echocardiography (TEE), performed by the placement of a two-dimensional transducer in a flexible endoscope, improves the image quality by minimizing scatter from the chest wall. This test, although invasive, is particularly useful in the evaluation of valvular disease, and may elucidate exact leaflet pathology. Additionally, atherosclerotic disease of the aortic arch and descending aorta can be accurately assessed with this study. Moreover, TEE studies are used when more precise imaging is required or when the diagnosis is uncertain after a transthoracic study.

Dobutamine stress echocardiography has evolved as an important noninvasive provocative study. This study is used to assess cardiac wall motion in response to inotropic stimulation, as wall motion abnormalities reflect underlying ischemia. Several reports have documented the accuracy of dobutamine stress echocardiography in identifying patients with significant CAD. The predictive value of a positive test for MI or death after noncardiac surgery is approximately 10%, while 20 to 40% will have some cardiac event. A negative test is 93 to 100% predictive that no cardiac event will occur.

Radionuclide Studies

Currently the most widely used myocardial perfusion screening study is the thallium scan, which uses the nuclide thallium-201. Initial uptake of thallium-201 into myocardial cells is dependent upon myocardial perfusion, while delayed uptake depends on myocardial viability. Thus, reversible defects occur in underperfused, ischemic, but viable zones, while fixed defects occur in areas of infarction. Fixed defects on the thallium scan suggest nonviable myocardium and may be of prognostic value.

The exercise thallium test is widely used to identify inducible areas of ischemia and is 95% sensitive in detecting multivessel coronary disease. This is the best overall test to detect myocardial ischemia, but requires the patient to exercise on the treadmill. The study also gives excellent, specific information about the patient's cardiac functional status.

The dipyridamole thallium study is a provocative study using IV dipyridamole, which induces vasodilation and consequently unmasks myocardial ischemia in response to stress. This is the most widely used provocative study for risk stratification for patients who cannot exercise. In patients undergoing noncardiac surgery, the predictive value of a positive dipyridamole thallium study is 5 to 20% for MI or death, while a negative study is 99 to 100% predictive that a cardiac event will not occur. It is, therefore, a very effective screening study for moderate- to high-risk patients who require a general surgery procedure.

Global myocardial function is frequently evaluated by a gated blood pool scan (equilibrium radionuclide angiocardiography) using technetium-99m. This study can detect areas of hypokinesis and measure left ventricular ejection fraction (LVEF), end-systolic volume, and end-diastolic volume. An exercise-gated blood pool scan is an excellent method to assess a patient's global cardiac response to stress. Normally, the ejection fraction will increase with exercise, but with significant CAD or valvular disease, the ejection fraction may remain unchanged or even decrease. The resting-gated blood pool scan determines the degree of prior cardiac injury and assesses baseline cardiac function, whereas the exercise-gated blood pool scan assesses the functional response to stress.

Positron Emission Tomography Scan

The positron emission tomography (PET) scan is a radionuclide imaging technique used to assess myocardial viability in underperfused areas of the heart. The technique may be more sensitive than the thallium scan for this purpose.[2] The PET scan is based on the myocardial metabolism of glucose or other compounds tagged with positron-emitting isotopes. PET allows the noninvasive functional assessment of perfusion, substrate metabolism, and cardiac innervation in vivo. The PET scan may be most useful in determining whether an area of apparently infarcted myocardium may, in fact, be hibernating and capable of responding to revascularization. These data can be used to determine whether patients with CHF might improve with operative revascularization.

Magnetic Resonance Imaging Viability Studies

Magnetic resonance imaging (MRI) may be used to delineate the transmural extent of MI and to distinguish between reversible and irreversible myocardial ischemic injury.[3] This test has proven to be useful in the assessment of patients with myocardial scarring and ventricular aneurysms, when ventricular remodeling surgery is an option.

Cardiac Catheterization

The cardiac catheterization study remains an important part of cardiac diagnosis. Complete cardiac catheterization includes the measurement of intracardiac pressures and cardiac output, localization and quantification of intracardiac shunts, determination of internal cardiac anatomy and ventricular wall motion by cineradiography, and determination of coronary anatomy by coronary angiography. However, most cardiac catheterizations today are focused studies (e.g., coronary angiography alone), because echocardiography and other noninvasive studies can accurately evaluate valvular pathology and cardiac function.

During cardiac catheterization the cardiac output can be calculated using the Fick oxygen method, where cardiac index (1/min per square meter) = oxygen consumption (mL/min per square meter) arteriovenous oxygen content difference (mL/min). For determining the arteriovenous oxygen difference, the oxygen content is calculated separately in the arterial and venous circulations by the formula:

$$\text{Oxygen content (mL oxygen/L blood)} =$$
$$\text{hemoglobin (g/100 mL)} \times \text{percent hemoglobin saturation} \times$$
$$1.36 \text{ (mL oxygen/g hemoglobin)} \times 10.$$

Calculation of systemic vascular resistance (SVR) is by the formula:

$$\text{SVR} = \text{(mean systemic arterial pressure} -$$
$$\text{mean right atrial pressure)} \times 80/\text{systemic blood flow}$$
(cardiac output). The normal SVR is 1200 dynes•sec•cm^{-5}.

The pulmonary vascular resistance (PVR) is calculated by the formula:

$$\text{PVR} = \text{(mean pulmonary artery pressure} -$$
$$\text{mean left atrial pressure)} \times 80/\text{pulmonary blood flow}$$
(equal to the cardiac output when no shunt is present).
The normal PVR is 70 to 80 dynes•sec•cm^{-5}.

The area of a cardiac valve can be determined from measured cardiac output and intracardiac pressures using Gorlin's formula. This formula relates valve area to the flow across the valve divided by the square root of the transvalvular pressure gradient. The Gorlin formula indicates that a relatively small transvalvular pressure gradient may actually represent severe valvular stenosis when the patient's cardiac output is low, demonstrating the danger of basing a surgical decision on the transvalvular gradient alone. The significance of valvular stenosis should be based on the calculated valve area [the normal mitral valve (MV) area is 4 to 6 cm^2 and the normal aortic valve area is 2.5 to 3.5 cm^2 in adults].

Coronary angiography remains the primary diagnostic procedure for determining the degree of CAD (Fig. 21-1). The left coronary system supplies the major portion of the LV myocardium through the left main, left anterior descending, and circumflex coronary arteries. The right coronary artery supplies the right ventricle, and the posterior descending artery supplies the inferior wall of the left ventricle. The AV nodal artery arises from the right coronary artery in 80 to

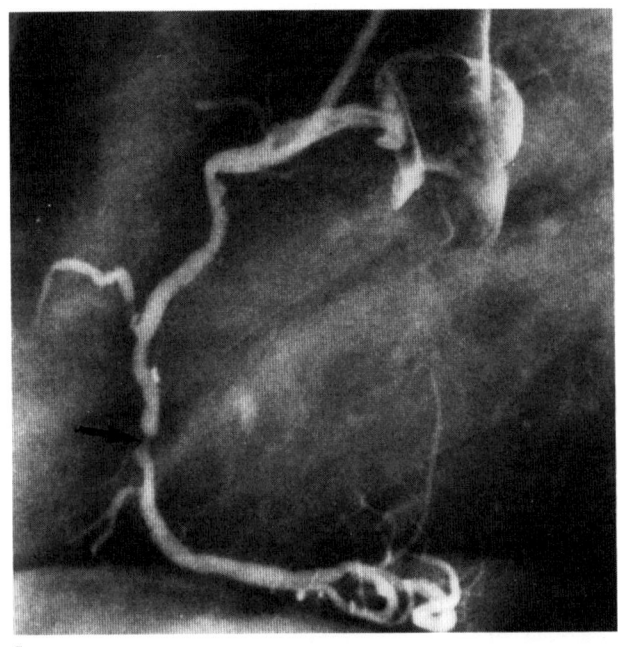

A

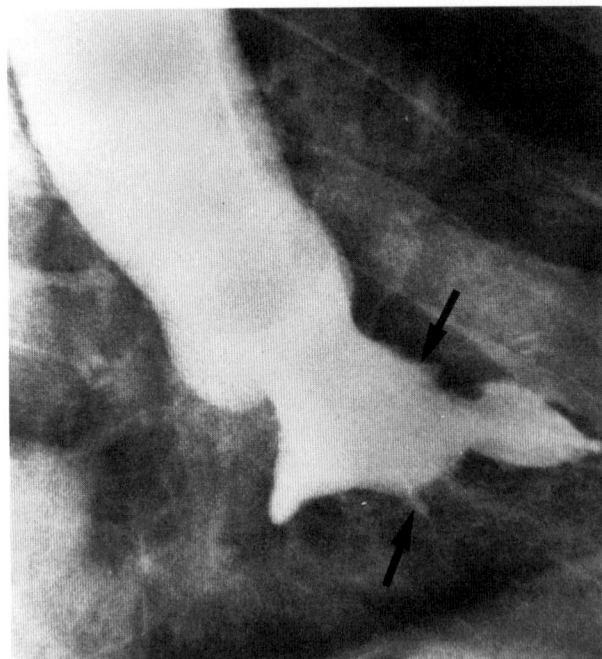

B

FIG. 21-1. Cardiac catheterization. **A.** Coronary angiogram demonstrating a severely stenotic atherosclerotic lesion in the right coronary artery. **B.** A systolic left ventriculogram of a patient with a normal ejection fraction (*arrows* indicate normal systolic contraction of LV walls).

85% of patients, termed *right dominant circulation*. In 15 to 20% of cases, the circumflex branch of the left coronary system supplies the posterior descending branch and the AV nodal artery, termed *left dominant*, while 5% are codominant.

Computed Tomography Coronary Angiography

Technologic advances in CT now allow less invasive imaging of the coronary anatomy. Newer rapid CT coronary angiography has been shown to be extremely sensitive in detecting coronary stenoses. These tests initially assess luminal calcium and a "calcium score" is derived. CT angiography has provided comparable results to traditional angiography in some recent studies.[4]

Extracorporeal Perfusion

History

With initial intracardiac surgical procedures being performed by brief asystole and systemic hypothermia or cross-perfusion from a parent, reliable cardiopulmonary support of the patient became a necessary development.

The pioneering efforts of Gibbon were largely responsible for such a development of the extracorporeal circulation circuit (cardiopulmonary bypass or CPB). Starting in 1932, Gibbon's laboratory investigations continued until, in 1953, he performed the first successful open heart operation in a human supported by a CPB machine.[5] Intrinsic to this device was the capacity for gas exchange with oxygenation and carbon dioxide (CO_2) removal. Subsequently, refinements in the circuit led to the development of bubble oxygenators and the now widely used membrane oxygenators which use a hollow fiber membrane for the blood-gas interface.

In recent years, the focus of perfusion technology has been on the development of perfusion systems that inflict less trauma on the patient's blood. One such advance was the introduction of biocompatible circuits to perfusion technology. This concept involves coating the plastic circuits with biocompatible materials that result in less activation of complement and other inflammatory cytokines during extracorporeal perfusion.

Technique

Heparin is the most important medication used during CPB; it allows the blood to transverse the CPB circuit without clotting. Typically, 3 to 4 mg/kg of heparin is given to elevate activated clotting time (ACT) above 500 seconds. In a typical modern circuit, vacuum-assisted venous drainage removes blood from a patient and a pump then pushes it thru a membrane oxygenator and filter before returning it to the patient. Traditionally, venous blood was drained from the right atrium by gravity through large bore cannulas, but more recently, vacuum-assisted venous drainage has been increasingly used, which allows use of smaller-diameter venous drainage cannulas. Systemic flow rates during extracorporeal perfusion depend on the body oxygen consumption requirements of the patient, which are dependent upon the patient's body temperature. Normothermic perfusion is done at a flow rate of about 2.5 to 3.5 L/min per square meter, which is the normal cardiac index. Because hypothermia decreases the metabolic rate [approximately 50% for each 7°C (12.6°F)], the necessary flow rates can be diminished as the patient is cooled. Safe bypass flow rates for 30°C (86°F) are 1.8 to 2.3 L/min per square meter, for 25°C (77°F) 1.5 to 1.8 L/min per square meter, and for 20°C (68°F) 1.2 to 1.5 L/min per square meter.

Gas flow through the oxygenator is adjusted to produce an arterial oxygen tension above 150 mmHg and the CO_2 tension 35 to 45 mmHg. Systemic temperature is controlled with a heat exchanger in the circuit; the temperature is usually lowered to 25 to 32°C (77° to 89.6°F), although colder temperatures are occasionally necessary for some complicated procedures. Free intrapericardial or intracardiac blood is aspirated with a suction apparatus, filtered, and returned to the pump circuit's reservoir. A cell-saving device is likewise used to reprocess spilled blood before and after the heparinization of CPB. This technique washes the blood and extracts the red blood cells for transfusion back to the patient.

Venous blood returning to the heart-lung machine will usually have an oxygen saturation >60%. With adequate flow rates and oxygen saturations, metabolic acidosis of a significant degree does not occur. Patients are constantly monitored for signs of underoxygenation. Heparin is gradually metabolized by the body, and so additional heparin is given to keep the ACT above 500 to 600 seconds.

Once the operation is completed and the patient is systemically rewarmed to normothermic levels, the perfusion is slowed and then stopped as the patient's blood is returned from the pump reservoir to the patient. Before discontinuing bypass, the surgeon checks several important variables: ECG (for rate, rhythm, and ST-segment changes), potassium level, hematocrit, myocardial contractility, and hemostasis of the suture lines. Both visual inspection and TEE are used to assess contractility. Postbypass, the patient's blood pressure and cardiac function are monitored closely. A Swan-Ganz catheter can measure the cardiac output and the pulmonary capillary wedge pressure to provide a guide to left atrial preload. If the cardiac output and blood pressure are inadequate despite an adequate preload, inotropic support is initiated. Hypotension from a low peripheral vascular resistance and normal myocardial contractility is treated with vasoconstrictors.

Once hemodynamic stability is achieved, heparin is neutralized with protamine. If a coagulopathy is present, the ACT may not return to prebypass levels, indicating the need for coagulation products, such as fresh-frozen plasma, platelets, or clotting factor concentrates. Although this is infrequent, it does occur in complex operations and longer pump runs.

Systemic Response

Systemic responses to extracorporeal perfusion mainly involve platelet dysfunction and a generalized systemic inflammatory response syndrome. This is apparently due to the activation of complement and other acute-phase inflammatory components by blood contact with the extracorporeal circuit. The severity of the inflammatory response and the level of subsequent end-organ dysfunction are related to the length of the pump time, with complement and cytokine activation leading to an upregulation of white blood cell adhesion molecules and the ability of white blood cells to release superoxide. White blood cell upregulation or "priming" produced by extracorporeal circulation results in increased capillary permeability throughout the body, with the "primed" white blood cells placing the patient in a potentially vulnerable state for 24 to 48 hours, during which any secondary insult may result in various levels of multiorgan dysfunction. Other effects may include mental confusion, renal insufficiency, decreased oxygen exchange (pulmonary dysfunction), transient hepatic dysfunction, and hyperamylasemia. Low levels of a consumptive coagulopathy and hyperfibrinolysis from plasmin activation may also be present. Current research is focused on minimizing the body's systemic inflammatory response during extracorporeal circulation by coating circuits with biocompatible materials or by blockading specific cytokines. Aprotinin and steroids may attenuate the inflammatory response to bypass, while aprotinin and ε-aminocaproic acid diminish coagulopathy. There remains controversy as to the risk-benefit ratio of aprotinin, with concerns about renal and neurologic adverse events. Zero-balance ultrafiltration (Z-BUF) is a method of ultrafiltration during CPB. This technique removes significant amounts of inflammatory mediators associated with CPB and potentially attenuates the adverse effects of bypass while maintaining the patient's volume status. Recent studies have shown that Z-BUF reduces pulmonary edema and protects against lung injury.[6] Additionally, the use of Z-BUF has been shown to decrease the concentrations of interleukin-6 and interleukin-8 that are markers of systemic inflammation associated with CPB.

Myocardial Protection

Cardioplegia was developed as a protective solution to induce both cardiac asystole and protect the myocardium from ischemic injury. When infused through the coronary circulation, cold high-potassium cardioplegic solution produces diastolic arrest and slows the metabolic activity, protecting the heart from ischemia. The arrested heart allows the surgeon to work precisely on the heart in a motionless, bloodless field. With current cardioplegic techniques the heart can be stopped and protected for 2 to 3 hours quite safely, allowing time for complicated procedures to be performed with good recovery of cardiac function.

Both crystalloid and blood cardioplegic solutions are widely used, with the exact composition of the cardioplegic mixture varying among different institutions. With periods of cardiac arrest up to 90 minutes, there is little measurable difference in the two techniques, although blood cardioplegia may allow the heart to be safely arrested for longer periods.

CORONARY ARTERY DISEASE

History

In the 1930s, investigators attempted to increase the blood supply to the ischemic heart by developing collateral circulation with vascular adhesions. Beck, the leading investigator, tried different methods for many years, but ultimately failed. An ingenious concept arose in 1946, when Vineberg developed the technique of implantation of the internal mammary artery (IMA) into a tunnel in the myocardium. This was applied clinically by Vineberg and Miller in 1951 and continued for many years. Interestingly, the artery remained patent in >90% of patients, but the amount of flow through the artery was small, and the procedure was subsequently abandoned. Coronary artery endarterectomy for coronary revascularization was attempted by Longmire in 1956 with short-term success. Late results were poor, however, due to progressive restenosis and occlusion. Shortly thereafter, CPB was used to facilitate coronary revascularization, and Senning reported vein patch graft arterioplasty in 1961.

The development of the coronary artery bypass operation in the 1960s was a dramatic medical milestone. In the United States, the principal credit belongs to Favalaro and Effler from the Cleveland Clinic. In 1967, they began the first series of coronary bypass grafts with saphenous vein grafts using CPB. This launched the modern era of coronary bypass surgery. An additional breakthrough came in 1968 when Green and colleagues performed the first left IMA to left anterior descending artery (LAD) bypass, using CPB and an operative microscope. Kolessov had independently performed IMA to left coronary artery bypass grafting (CABG) on the beating heart in Russia in 1964, although his work was largely unknown for many years. Subsequently, coronary artery bypass surgery became one of the most widely applied surgical procedures in the United States and throughout the world.

Etiology and Pathogenesis

The etiology of CAD is primarily atherosclerosis. The disease is multifactorial, with the primary risk factors being hyperlipidemia, smoking, diabetes, hypertension, obesity, sedentary lifestyle, and male gender. Newly identified risk factors include elevated levels of C-reactive protein, lipoprotein (a), and homocysteine. The atherosclerotic process results in the formation of obstructive lesions in the aorta, the peripheral vessels, and the coronary arteries. Atherosclerosis is the leading cause of death in the Western world, and acute MI alone accounts for 25% of the deaths in the United States each year. The most important factor in the long-term treatment of coronary disease is modification of risk factors, including the immediate cessation of smoking, control of hypertension, weight loss, exercise, and reduction of serum cholesterol. If dietary control of cholesterol cannot be achieved in patients with coronary disease, evidence suggests that the early use of medications (such as statins) to lower cholesterol can significantly reduce cardiovascular risk.

The basic lesion is a segmental plaque within the coronary artery. Involvement of small distal vessels is usually less extensive, while arterioles and intramyocardial vessels are usually free of disease. This segmental localization makes CABG possible. Among the three major coronary arteries, the proximal LAD is frequently stenosed or occluded, with the distal half of the artery remaining patent. The right coronary artery is often stenotic or occluded throughout its course, but the posterior descending and left AV groove branches are almost always patent. The circumflex artery is often diseased proximally, but one or more distal marginal branches

are usually patent. With progressive disease, platelet aggregation in the narrowed lumen or plaque hemorrhage or rupture may lead to unstable symptoms or to acute thrombosis and MI.

Clinical Manifestations

Myocardial ischemia from CAD may result in angina pectoris, MI, CHF, cardiac arrhythmias, and sudden death. Angina is the most frequent symptom, but MI may appear without prior warning. CHF usually results as a sequela of MI, with significant muscular injury resulting in an ischemic myopathy. Myocardial injury and scarring can then lead to serious ventricular arrhythmias that may result in sudden death.

Angina pectoris, the most common manifestation, manifests by periodic chest discomfort, usually substernal, and typically appears with exertion. These symptoms usually subside within 3 to 5 minutes and are relieved by sublingual nitroglycerin. In 20 to 25% of patients, the pain may be atypical and radiate to the jaw, shoulder, or epigastrium. Some patients, especially women or diabetics, have no symptoms of angina and experience primarily exertional dyspnea. Establishing a diagnosis of myocardial ischemia in these patients is difficult and perhaps impossible without provocative diagnostic studies. The differential diagnosis in patients with atypical symptoms includes aortic stenosis, hypertrophic cardiomyopathy, musculoskeletal disorders, pulmonary disease, gastritis or peptic ulcer disease, gastroesophageal reflux, diffuse esophageal spasm, and anxiety.

MI is the most common serious complication of CAD, with 1.1 million infarcts occurring in the United States annually. Modern therapy, which involves early reperfusion with either thrombolytic therapy or emergent angioplasty, has lowered the mortality to <5%. MI may result in acute cardiac failure and cardiogenic shock, or in mechanical rupture of infarcted zones of the heart.

In a certain number of patients who have MI, CHF develops, resulting from significant loss of LV function. When areas of salvageable myocardium are still present, angina is associated with heart failure, and significant improvement can be obtained with CABG. In contrast, with patients with late-stage chronic congestive failure due to diffuse myocardial scarring, the outlook is ominous. Bypass grafting may not be beneficial in these patients unless viable myocardium is present with reversible ischemia. Surgical ventricular remodeling, long-term support with a ventricular assist device, or cardiac transplantation become the only options in such patients.

Preoperative Evaluation

A complete history and physical examination should be performed in every patient with suspected CAD, along with a chest x-ray, ECG, and baseline echocardiogram. In patients with atypical symptoms, provocative stress tests, such as adenosine thallium or dobutamine echocardiography, may be beneficial in deciding if a cardiac catheterization is indicated. CT angiography is now used to evaluate intraluminal calcium and also is accurate in the assessment of previous bypass grafts. However, cardiac catheterization remains the gold standard of evaluation, as it outlines the location and severity of the coronary disease and accurately assesses cardiac function. "Angiographically significant" coronary stenosis is considered to be present when the diameter is reduced by >50%, corresponding to a reduction in cross-sectional area >75%. Furthermore, the number, location, and severity of the coronary stenoses are used to determine the appropriate method of revascularization.

Ventricular function is expressed as the LVEF, with 0.55 to 0.70 considered as normal, 0.40 to 0.55 as mildly depressed, <0.40 as moderately depressed, and <0.25 as severely depressed. An ejection fraction <0.25 is usually associated with severe heart failure. The LVEF is used to determine operative risk and long-term prognosis. Regional wall motion may also be analyzed, either by cardiac catheterization or echocardiography.

Studies such as the PET scan, thallium scan, dobutamine echocardiogram, or MRI viability scan may be used to determine myocardial viability and the reversibility of ischemia in areas of the heart that might benefit from revascularization. A patient is not "inoperable" simply because the LV function is severely depressed, if a significant amount of myocardium has reversible ischemia and is thought to be viable but hibernating.

Coronary Artery Bypass Grafting

Indications

CABG may be indicated in patients with chronic angina, unstable angina, or postinfarction angina, and in asymptomatic patients with severe proximal lesions or patients with atypical symptoms who have easily provoked ischemia during stress testing.

Chronic Angina In some patients with chronic angina, CABG is associated with improved survival and improved complication-free survival when compared to medical management. In general, patients with more severe angina (CCS class III or IV symptoms) are most likely to benefit from bypass. For patients with less severe angina (CCS class I or II), other factors, such as the anatomic distribution of disease (left main coronary disease or triple-vessel) and the degree of LV dysfunction, are used to determine which patients will most benefit from surgical revascularization.

Three historic randomized trials were conducted to determine which patients with mild degrees of chronic angina would have improved survival from coronary bypass surgery. These studies provided the initial background data to support the widespread use of CABG.

The Veterans Administration Cooperative Study. This study involved 668 males with mild to moderate angina, treated between 1972 and 1974, and demonstrated improved long-term survival in patients with left main disease treated with surgical therapy.[7] Largely based on this trial, surgery has been recommended for virtually all patients with significant left main arterial disease. Subsequent studies have shown that patients with left main arterial disease treated with surgery have a median survival of 13.3 years, vs. 6.6 years in those treated medically.[8]

The European Coronary Surgery Study Group. This study, done between 1973 and 1976, randomized male patients with mild to moderate angina into medical or surgical therapy.[9] Surgery was found to be associated with improved survival in patients with triple-vessel disease and in patients with double-vessel disease with proximal left anterior descending and circumflex artery lesions.

Coronary Artery Surgery Study. This multicenter study performed between 1975 and 1979 randomized patients with mild angina (class I or II) into medical or surgical therapy. Late results demonstrated improved survival with surgery in patients with triple-vessel disease and depressed cardiac function.

Other nonrandomized trials and studies involving the overall Coronary Artery Surgery Study registry (of both randomized and nonrandomized patients) have suggested that surgical intervention might improve survival and event-free intervals in other patients with triple-vessel disease. A study by Jones and colleagues from Duke University evaluated the long-term benefits of bypass surgery and angioplasty vs. medical therapy in 9263 patients with documented CAD treated between 1984 and 1990.[10] Treatment was nonrandomized, with 2449 patients receiving medical therapy, 3890 patients receiving bypass surgery, and 2924 patients receiving angioplasty. Both the surgery and angioplasty treatment groups had better long-term survival than medical therapy for all levels of disease severity, with surgery having the best survival benefit in patients with triple-vessel disease and in patients with double-vessel disease with proximal LAD stenosis.

To summarize, although medical therapy may be appropriate for many patients with chronic stable angina, bypass surgery is indicated for most patients with multivessel disease and CCS class III or IV symptoms. In patients with milder (CCS class I or II) symptoms, surgery results in improved survival in those with left main stenosis and those with triple-vessel disease and depressed LV function or diabetes. Certain other anatomic or physiologic subsets of patients,

such as those with multivessel disease and tight proximal left anterior descending stenosis or easily provoked ischemia during stress testing, are also likely to have a survival benefit with surgery.

Unstable Angina Unstable angina exists when angina is persistent or rapidly progressive despite optimal medical therapy. This occurs from severe ischemia and represents an unstable clinical situation, usually leading to MI. It commonly represents plaque rupture or hemorrhage, often with local thrombus and spasm, resulting in a sudden decrease in regional blood flow. Patients with unstable angina should be promptly hospitalized for intensive medical therapy and undergo prompt cardiac catheterization. Most patients with unstable angina will require urgent revascularization with either percutaneous coronary intervention (PCI) or CABG.

Acute Myocardial Infarction CABG generally does not have a primary role in the treatment of uncomplicated acute MI, as PCI or thrombolysis is the preferred method of emergent revascularization in these patients. However, patients with subendocardial MI and underlying left main disease or postinfarction angina and multivessel involvement may require surgery.

The primary indication for surgery after acute transmural MI is in patients who develop mechanical complications, such as postinfarction ventricular septal defect (VSD), papillary muscle rupture with mitral insufficiency, or LV rupture. Postinfarction VSD typically occurs 4 to 5 days after MI, occurring in approximately 1% of patients. These patients usually present with CHF and pulmonary edema, and a new systolic murmur.[11] Once recognized, patients with a postinfarction VSD should have an intra-aortic balloon pump (IABP) placed and undergo emergent repair. The operative mortality ranges from 10 to 20%. Another mechanical complication of acute MI is papillary muscle rupture with acute mitral insufficiency. These patients also typically present 4 to 5 days postinfarction with heart failure and a new murmur. Prompt valve repair or replacement offers the only meaningful chance for survival. Operative risk is 10 to 20%. The third mechanical complication of MI is LV free wall rupture. These patients present with cardiogenic shock, often with acute tamponade. Emergent surgery has a success rate of approximately 50%.

Percutaneous Coronary Intervention vs. Coronary Artery Bypass Grafting

PCI, or angioplasty, was developed by Gruentzig in 1977 and has significantly changed the treatment of patients with CAD.[12] Over 750,000 PCIs are now performed in the United States each year. The indications for PCI have continually expanded as this technology has advanced. A number of large, randomized studies have compared outcomes of patients with coronary disease treated with PCI and CABG. These studies have attempted to identify the optimal therapy for patients with coronary disease, based on their anatomy and risk stratification. Three large, representative studies are summarized here.

The Bypass Angioplasty Revascularization Investigation Trial. This trial, sponsored by the National Institutes of Health, randomized 1792 patients with multivessel coronary disease to either coronary bypass (*n* = 914) or PCI (*n* = 915).[13] Inhospital event rates for CABG and PCI were 1.3 and 1.1% for mortality, 4.6 and 2.1% for MI, and 0.8 and 0.2% for stroke. There was no significant difference in 5-year survival—89.3% for CABG and 86.3% for PCI. However, the PCI group required more repeat interventions, with 54% within 5 years vs. only 8% for CABG. In diabetic patients with triple-vessel disease, CABG offered a clear survival advantage at 5 years, 80.6 vs. 65.5% with PCI (*P* = .003).

Arterial Revascularization Therapies Study Group. This large trial compared outcomes in 1205 patients randomly assigned to CABG (*n* = 605) or PCI (*n* = 600).[14] Unlike the *Bypass Angioplasty Revascularization Investigation* trial, PCI patients in this trial received coronary stents. At 1 year, death, stroke, and MI rates were similar, although PCI patients had more recurrent symptoms, 16.8

635

vs. 3.5% in CABG patients. The 1-year event-free survival rate was 73.8% with PCI compared with 87.8% with CABG.

Most recently, stents coated with pharmacologic agents (such as paclitaxel or sirolimus) aimed at reducing instent restenosis have been introduced.[15] These stents are in wide use presently, however, long-term results remain unknown.[16]

New York State Study Group. This patient cohort includes greater than 59,000 patients in New York receiving either coronary stenting or CABG with 3-year follow-up. Propensity analysis was used to adjust for varying clinical cofactors. Long-term patient survival was superior with CABG rather than stenting in patients with two or more diseased coronary arteries.[17]

Summary

When comparing CABG to PCI for the treatment of patients with CAD, results demonstrate that with appropriate patient selection both procedures are safe and effective, with little difference in mortality. PCI is associated with less short-term morbidity, decreased cost, and shorter hospital stay, but requires more late reinterventions. CABG provides more complete relief of angina, requires fewer reinterventions, and is more durable. Additionally, CABG appears to offer a survival advantage in diabetic patients with multivessel disease.

Operative Techniques and Results

Conventional Coronary Artery Bypass Grafting Conventional CABG is performed through a median sternotomy incision (Fig. 21-2), using CPB for extracorporeal perfusion and cardioplegia for intraoperative myocardial protection of the heart.

In the vast majority of patients the left IMA is used as the primary conduit for bypassing the LAD, which is the most important vessel in the heart (Fig. 21-3). The IMA is harvested from the chest wall and usually is used as an in situ graft, remaining connected proximally to the native left subclavian artery. As such, the IMA remains metabolically active and enlarges over time in response to demand. The IMA

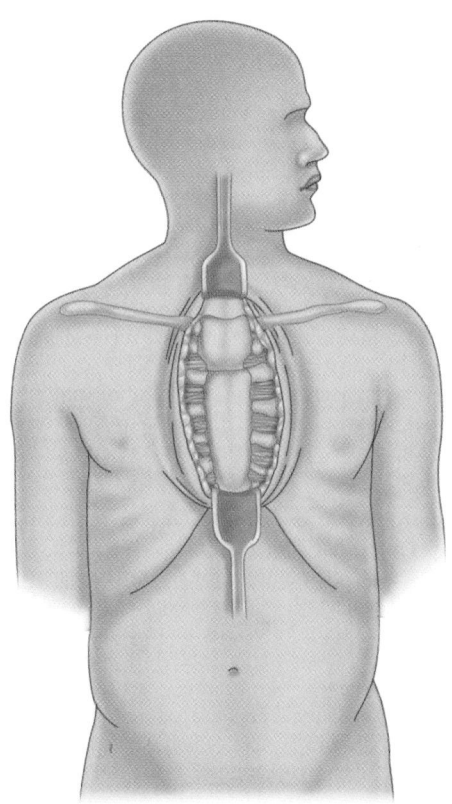

FIG. 21-2. Median sternotomy incision. *(Illustration courtesy of Heartport, Inc., Redwood City, CA.)*

CHAPTER 21 Acquired Heart Disease

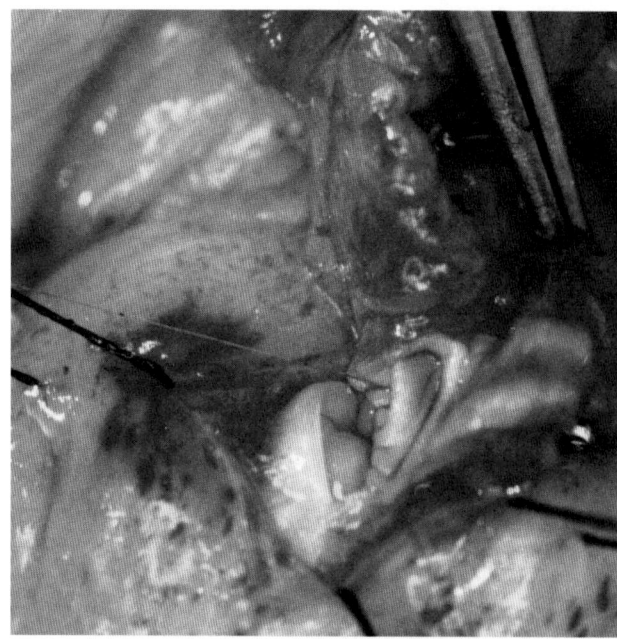

A

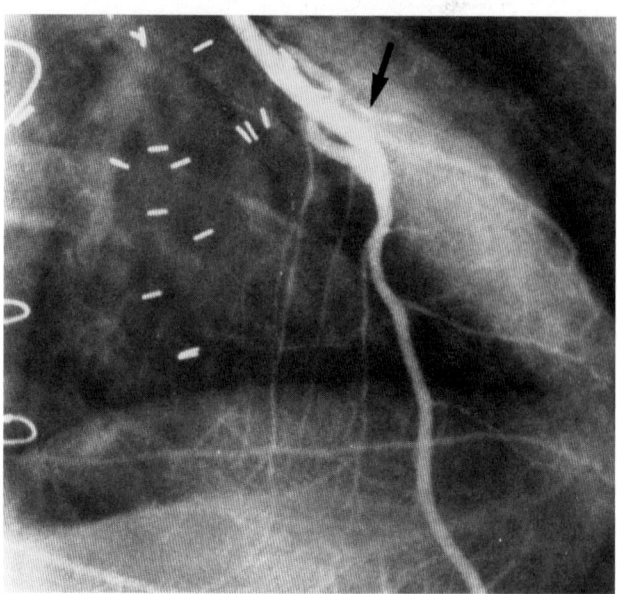

B

FIG. 21-3. Coronary artery bypass grafting. **A.** Operative photograph of anastomosis between the left internal mammary artery and the left anterior descending artery. The anastomosis was completed using optical magnification, microvascular technique, and a continuous 8-0 suture. **B.** Fifteen-year follow-up coronary angiogram demonstrating a widely patent left internal mammary artery–left anterior descending artery bypass graft. The *arrow* demonstrates the anastomotic site. The mammary artery is virtually free of graft atherosclerosis.

is resistant to intrinsic atherosclerotic disease and its patency is rarely compromised by luminal stenosis. After CPB is initiated and the heart is arrested, the IMA to left anterior descending anastomosis is constructed end-to-side with fine sutures.

Loop reported a series of 2306 internal mammary grafts and 3625 vein grafts, demonstrating that use of an IMA graft significantly improved survival at 10 years. Patients who had IMA grafts also had fewer late complications with a decreased risk of MI and reoperation. The left IMA has a 10-year patency rate of approximately 95% when used as an in situ graft to the LAD.

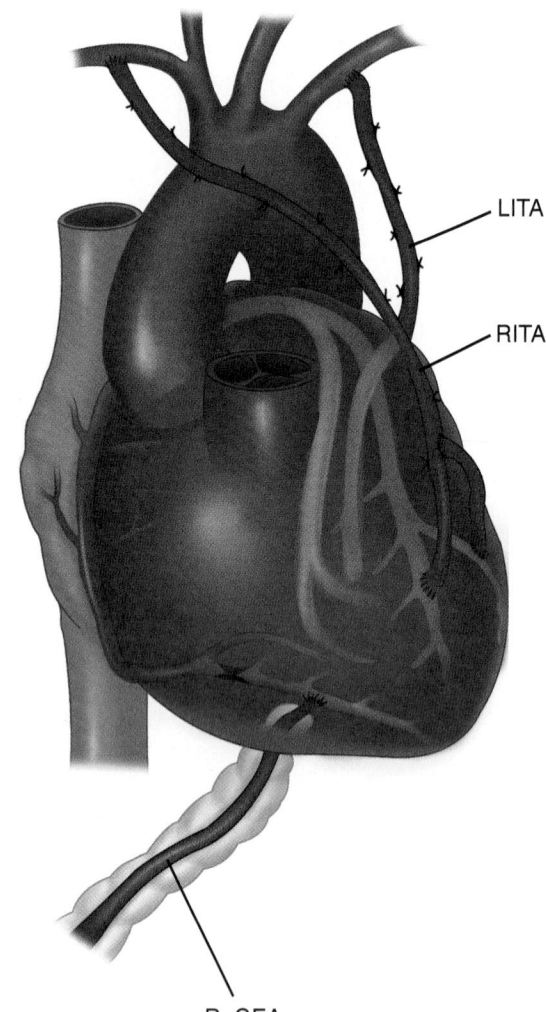

FIG. 21-4. Arterial revascularization. Schematic of arterial conduits used in coronary artery bypass grafting, showing left internal mammary (or thoracic) artery (LITA), right internal mammary (or thoracic) artery (RITA), and composite graft using radial and gastroepiploic arteries (R+GEA). *(Reproduced with permission from Pevni D, Kramer A, Paz Y, et al: Composite arterial grafting with double skeletonized internal thoracic arteries. Eur J Cardiothorac Surg 20:299, 2001. Copyright Elsevier.)*

The excellent results obtained with in situ left IMA grafts prompted many other centers to use the right IMA in coronary revascularization. The right IMA may be used to provide a second arterial conduit as either an in situ or a free graft (Fig. 21-4). Dion reported 400 consecutive patients in whom both left and right IMAs were used, and found equivalent patency with the left and the right IMA.[18] Lytle and colleagues showed excellent late results and no increase in perioperative risk in >500 cases in which both IMAs were used.[19] Even when the IMA is used as a "free" graft, patency rates are approximately 70 to 80% at 10 years.

Saphenous vein grafts, which were initially the primary conduits used for CABG, continue to be used widely, usually for grafting secondary targets on the lateral and posterior walls of the heart. Once CPB has been established and the heart arrested, a small arteriotomy is performed in the coronary artery, and the distal anastomosis is performed between the saphenous vein and the coronary artery. The proximal anastomosis then connects each vein graft to the ascending aorta. The 10-year patency of saphenous vein grafts is only approximately 65%, however, and patency is limited by the development of progressive intimal hyperplasia and late vein graft atherosclerosis.

In an attempt to achieve better long-term patency than that obtainable with saphenous vein grafts and encouraged by the excellent late patency of internal mammary arterial grafts, surgeons have explored the use of other arterial conduits. The most widely used has been the radial artery graft. After an Allen test has been performed to assure adequate blood flow to the hand, the radial artery can be harvested and used as a free graft. Reports have demonstrated excellent early and midterm patency rates with radial artery grafts. Other alternative arterial grafts include the right gastroepiploic artery, usually used as an in situ pedicled graft, and the inferior epigastric artery, which is used as a free graft. Reports are mixed regarding late patency rates of the gastroepiploic and inferior epigastric arteries, however. Although the expanded use of arterial grafts is appealing, a significant improvement in patency rates of arterial conduits other than the IMA compared to vein grafts has yet to be verified.

Results The operative mortality for coronary artery bypass is 1 to 3%, depending on the number of risk factors present. Both the Society of Thoracic Surgeons (STS) and New York state have established large databases to establish risk factors and report outcomes. Variables that have been identified as influencing operative risk according to STS risk modeling include: female gender, age, race, body surface area, NYHA class IV status, low ejection fraction, hypertension, PVD, prior stroke, diabetes, renal failure, chronic obstructive pulmonary disease, immunosuppressive therapy, prior cardiac surgery, recent MI, urgent or emergent presentation, cardiogenic shock, left main coronary disease, and concomitant valvular disease. Perioperative complications include MI, bleeding, stroke, arrhythmias, tamponade, wound infection, aortic dissection, pneumonia, respiratory failure, renal failure, GI complications, and multiorgan failure.

Late results demonstrate that relief of angina is striking after CABG. Angina is completely relieved or markedly decreased in >98% of patients, and recurrent angina is rare in the first 5 to 7 years. Reintervention is required in <10% of patients within 5 years. Symptoms begin to recur more frequently between 8 and 15 years due to progression of disease or late graft occlusion. However, tight control of risk factors can minimize the risk of recurrence. Cessation of smoking and control of hypercholesterolemia are especially important, as late graft occlusion is five to seven times higher in patients who continue to smoke or have persistent hypercholesterolemia. If recurrent angina develops, angiography should be performed promptly, followed by repeat revascularization as indicated.

Exercise capacity generally improves significantly after CABG, with most patients demonstrating a markedly improved functional response to exercise secondary to improved blood flow. This functional improvement lasts up to 10 years, with longer improvement in patients receiving IMA grafts.

Late survival is similarly excellent after CABG, with a 5-year survival of >90% and a 10-year survival of 75 to 90%, depending on the number of comorbidities present. Late survival is influenced by age, diabetes, LV function, NYHA class, CHF, associated valvular insufficiency, completeness of revascularization, and the nonuse of an IMA graft. Intense medical therapy for control of diabetes, hypercholesterolemia, and hypertension, and cessation of smoking significantly improve late survival.

Off-Pump Coronary Artery Bypass One of the most significant developments in cardiac surgery in the last 15 to 20 years has been the introduction of off-pump coronary artery bypass (OPCAB). This involves performing coronary bypass surgery on a beating heart, without the use of CPB. The main concept in this surgical approach is the elimination of the deleterious consequences of CPB.

The initial experiences with beating heart techniques took place in Argentina under Benetti. This procedure is performed with the assistance of stabilization devices, which allow precise anastomoses while the heart remains beating. During OPCAB surgery, the coronary artery is temporarily snared or occluded to provide a relatively bloodless field for the creation of the anastomosis. Because this interval of regional ischemia may produce a critical

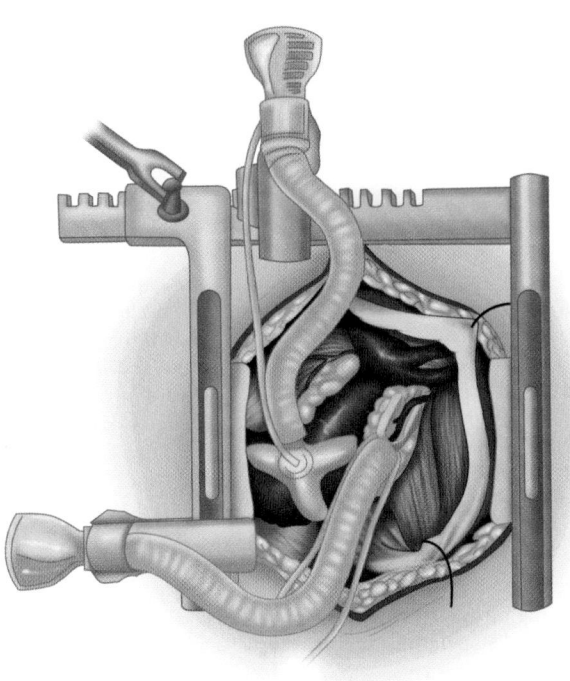

FIG. 21-5. Off-pump coronary artery bypass technique. Illustration demonstrating setup for off-pump coronary artery bypass graft. Shown are a retractor, a stabilizing device, and a displacement device. (*Illustration courtesy of Medtronic, Inc., Minneapolis, MN.*)

reduction in cardiac function or arrhythmias, several methods such as intracoronary shunts or preischemic conditioning have been developed to minimize the risks of temporary coronary occlusion during construction of the anastomosis.

The temporary displacement of the heart while performing posterior and inferior wall grafts may lead to a reduction in cardiac output and subsequent hemodynamic instability. Many intraoperative maneuvers have been proposed to minimize these effects (Fig. 21-5). These include use of the right lateral decubitus and Trendelenburg ("head down") positions, administration of fluids, opening the right pleural cavity to minimize the compression of the right heart by the pericardium, and the use of pericardial sutures to aid in tilting the heart. Additionally, suction devices are used to position the apex of the heart. These devices limit the compression of the left ventricle and therefore assist in maintaining hemodynamic stability.

Results The OPCAB technique has been extensively studied and results compared to conventional surgery. Initial attention was given to assessing the accuracy of graft placement with the OPCAB approach, which required grafting onto the beating heart. Puskas and associates assessed 421 grafts in 167 patients and found an overall early graft patency of 98.8%, with 100% patency of 163 IMA grafts.[20] These results were equivalent to those published for conventional CABG. Similarly, when evaluating patients receiving multiple arterial grafts, Kim and colleagues found no difference in the 1-year patency of arterial grafts performed with OPCAB compared with traditional methods.[21]

Sabik and coworkers compared overall results in 406 OPCAB patients with 406 conventional CABG patients.[22] The operative mortality and the risks of stroke, MI, and reoperation for bleeding were similar, while OPCAB patients had less risk of encephalopathy, sternal infection, blood transfusion, and renal failure. A prospective randomized comparison between OPCAB and conventional CABG reported by Puskas demonstrated equivalent operative mortality and risk of stroke in each group, but less myocardial injury, fewer blood transfusions, earlier postoperative extubation, and earlier hospital discharge in OPCAB patients.

A study performed by Grossi at New York University in high-risk patients with severe atheromatous aortic arch disease who required CABG compared outcomes in 245 OPCAB patients with outcomes in 245 conventional patients, using propensity case-matching methodology. In this high-risk patient population, OPCAB was associated with a decreased risk of death (6.5 vs. 11.4%), stroke (1.6 vs. 5.7%), and all perioperative complications. Others have similarly shown significant reductions in both mortality and major neurologic events with the OPCAB technique.[23,24]

Minimally Invasive Direct Coronary Artery Bypass An even less invasive off-pump approach for CABG, termed *minimally invasive direct coronary artery bypass*, or MIDCAB, uses a small left anterior minithoracotomy incision to perform bypass grafting on the beating heart, without CPB. The technique uses a mechanical stabilizer to isolate the coronary artery and facilitate the anastomosis and an in situ left IMA graft. The technique is mainly useful in performing bypasses to the anterior wall of the heart, primarily to the LAD or to the diagonal branches.

Results The operative mortality for MIDCAB has been <2%, and the patency rate of the IMA graft has been approximately 98%.[25] Because both the use of CPB and the need for sternotomy are eliminated, MIDCAB patients have less pain and blood loss, fewer perioperative complications, and a shorter recovery time than conventional CABG patients. This technique is generally only applicable to patients with single-vessel disease, and therefore, outcomes after MIDCAB are probably best compared with PCI. Diegeler and associates reported a prospective, randomized trial that compared results of MIDCAB and PCI for treatment of isolated, proximal LAD stenosis.[26] This study found that the combined perioperative risks of death and MI were equivalent, but the MIDCAB patients had better relief of angina and required fewer subsequent reinterventions. Similarly, a prospective, randomized study reported by Drenth and colleagues compared MIDCAB with PCI and stenting in patients with isolated high-grade LAD stenosis. At 6 months, quantitative coronary angiography showed anastomotic stenosis in 4% after MIDCAB, but restenosis at the intervention site in 29% after PCI (P <.001).[27] Thus, the late results with MIDCAB for revascularization of the LAD appear to be significantly more durable than those achieved with PCI.

New Developments

Total Endoscopic Coronary Artery Bypass Minimal access coronary artery bypass performed using endoscopic instrumentation is facilitated with the latest generation of surgical robotic technology. Made possible by advancements in articulation of robotic instruments to more closely approximate the movement of human hands, total endoscopic coronary artery bypass has been reported on both the arrested and beating heart.[28] Robotic instrumentation also has been described to perform IMA harvests as part of the MIDCAB technique. Although early results are promising, larger series with long-term data are necessary before total endoscopic coronary artery bypass moves out of the experimental phase.

Transmyocardial Laser Revascularization Transmyocardial laser revascularization (TMR) uses a high-powered CO_2 laser or holmium:yttrium-aluminum-garnet laser to drill multiple holes (1 cm²) through the myocardium into the ventricular cavity. The procedure is performed on the beating heart with the laser pulses gated to the R wave on the ECG. The TMR procedure has been used primarily for patients with refractory angina who are unsuitable candidates for standard CABG due to poor distal coronary artery anatomy. The mechanism of benefit of TMR remains uncertain. It has been demonstrated that the transmyocardial laser channels are rapidly occluded and do not allow a direct flow from the ventricle to the myocardium. The most likely possibility is that TMR works by stimulating angiogenesis in the area of injury.

Burkhoff and coworkers reported the results of a large, randomized, multicenter trial with TMR in 182 patients with CCS angina class III or IV, reversible ischemia, and incomplete response to other therapies. They found TMR to be associated with significant increases in exercise tolerance, reduction in angina score, and improvements in quality of life.[29] Despite subjective reports of improvement, however, the results of objective cardiac perfusion measurements after TMR have been inconclusive, and multiple randomized trials have failed to demonstrate any survival benefit with the procedure. Thus, the exact role of TMR and its relationship to medical therapeutic angiogenesis remains to be determined.

Biomolecular Therapy and Tissue Engineering Tissue engineering and biomolecular or gene therapy may be possible in the near future to replace the dysfunctional tissue or to improve organ function with an assembly that contains specific populations of living cells. Significant progress has been made in understanding the cellular and molecular mechanisms of cardiovascular disease, leading to new forms of molecular-genetic therapy. These innovations are currently being tried experimentally for genetically engineered or modified veins and arteries, engineered heart valves, stem cell or progenitor cell cardiomyocyte restoration therapy, and therapeutic angiogenesis. Much of this work has focused on vascular mitogens, on intracellular signaling pathways, and on the underlying genetic functions that control the cellular response.

In the field of CAD, several gene therapy protocols are now under active investigation. These include: (a) genetic engineering of vein grafts that are resistant to atherosclerosis or restenosis; (b) gene therapy for coronary arteries to prevent restenosis after angioplasty or surgical endarterectomy; (c) genetic manipulation of the coronary and peripheral vascular system in an attempt to prevent lipid accumulation and progression of atherosclerosis; (d) the biomolecular delivery of growth factors or genetic material into the coronary system or myocardium to promote therapeutic angiogenesis; and (e) the total bioengineering of blood vessels using cell seeding techniques and a biodegradable scaffold. Although these innovations are currently experimental, biomolecular adjuvant therapy offers great promise for the future.

Anastomotic Devices Significant technologic progress has led to the development of devices that mechanically construct proximal and distal vascular anastomoses, without the need for sutures or knot tying. The goals for these devices are to provide safe, rapid, and reproducible anastomoses; reduce operative time; limit anastomotic variability between surgeons; and improve graft patency. If perfected, such devices may facilitate newer minimally invasive endoscopic or robotic surgical techniques by eliminating the difficulties associated with suturing and knot tying in small spaces. Proximal anastomotic devices, some in early clinical trials, are designed to create aortosaphenous anastomoses without the need for aortic cross-clamping. This may have particular significance in patients with severe atherosclerotic aortic disease in whom prevention of aortic manipulation is crucial in preventing embolic complications. Distal anastomotic devices are also in experimental use, and may facilitate off-pump or minimally invasive CABG.

VALVULAR HEART DISEASE

General Principles

The surgical treatment of valve disease has increased significantly in recent years. According to the STS database, valve operations accounted for 14% of all classified procedures performed in 1996. By 2002, that percentage had increased to 20% of all classified procedures. Due to increased PCI and better medical management of coronary disease, CABG volume declined by 15% between 1996 and 1999. However, during this same period, aortic valve replacements increased by 12% and MV operations increased by 58%.

Valvular heart disease can result in a *pressure load* (valvular stenosis), a *volume load* (valvular insufficiency), or both (mixed stenosis and insufficiency). Aortic stenosis increases the afterload of the left ventricle, resulting in LV hypertrophy, while both aortic and mitral insufficiency result in a significant volume overload of the left ventricle, producing cardiac dilatation. Although the heart can effectively compensate for these hemodynamic changes for some time, progressive deterioration in cardiac function develops, leading to valvular cardiomyopathy. The decision to proceed with surgical intervention is based on the patient's history, symptoms, physical findings, and the results of diagnostic studies, including echocardiography, cardiac catheterization, and radionuclide tests. Demonstration of a decreased ejection fraction at rest (or a rise in the end-systolic volume by echocardiography) or a fall in ejection fraction during exercise are probably the most accurate signs that the systolic function of the heart is beginning to deteriorate and that surgery should be performed promptly. As surgeons have gained experience and as new technologies have been advanced, surgical risk has been reduced and long-term results have improved. Therefore, surgical therapy is now recommended at a much earlier stage of the disease process in an attempt to maintain normal cardiac function long after valve surgery. Studies have proven earlier intervention in mitral disease has clearly shown long-term benefit.[30] Survival after cardiac valve replacement is strongly influenced by the myocardial function at the time of operation. For example, Chaliki and associates reported that the operative risk for aortic valve replacement for aortic insufficiency in patients with a low ejection fraction was 14%, compared to 3.7% in patients with preserved LV function.[31] At 10 years, only 41 ± 9% of those patients with reduced ejection fraction had survived, compared with 70 ± 3% of those with normal ventricular function. Postoperative cardiac function generally returns to normal if the operation is performed at an early phase of ventricular dysfunction. Even with impaired LV function, NYHA class IV disability, and pulmonary hypertension, patients with valvular heart disease are rarely inoperable. After the hemodynamic burden on the ventricle has been removed with corrective surgery, the patient is treated with an aggressive medical heart failure regimen (digitalis, diuretics, afterload reduction, and beta blockers when indicated), usually with significant improvement. Additionally, aortic valve replacement in high risk, elderly patients can be performed with excellent results.[32] Except in the rare case of advanced cardiomyopathy combined with other systemic disease, surgery should not be denied to most elderly or high-risk patients. The typical valve-related complications from valvular surgery include thromboembolic events, anticoagulant-related hemorrhage, prosthetic valve failure, endocarditis, prosthetic paravalvular leakage, and failure of valve repair.

Surgical Options

Valve replacement can be performed with either mechanical or tissue valves. Current mechanical valves include tilting disk and older ball-in-cage designs. Tissue for valve replacement can be xenograft (porcine valves, bovine or equine pericardium), homograft (human cadaver donor), or autograft (translocation of pulmonic valve). Valve repair is increasingly an option, as opposed to valve replacement, especially for patients with mitral or TV insufficiency. The recommendations for valve repair or replacement, type of prosthesis, and operative approach are based on multiple factors, such as the patient's age, lifestyle, associated medical conditions, access to follow-up health care, desire for future pregnancy, and experience of the surgeon. The risks, benefits, and options should be discussed in detail with the patient before arriving at a joint decision. General considerations regarding these choices are discussed in the following paragraphs.

Mechanical prostheses are highly durable but require permanent anticoagulation therapy to minimize the risk of valve thrombosis and thromboembolic complications. Such lifelong anticoagulation therapy carries the risk of hemorrhagic complications and may dictate lifestyle changes. For some patients, the typical mechanical valve closing sound adversely affects quality of life. Mechanical prostheses are usually preferable in patients with a long life expectancy who want to minimize the risk of reoperation and are suitable candidates for anticoagulation.[33]

Tissue valves are naturally less thrombogenic, and generally do not require anticoagulation therapy. Consequently, tissue valves have lower risks of thromboembolic and anticoagulant-related complications, with the total yearly risk of all valve-related complications being considerably less than with mechanical valves. Unfortunately, tissue valves are more prone to structural failure due to late calcification of the xenograft tissue. However, because of improved methods of valve preservation and chemical impregnation to slow calcification of the tissue, the currently available tissue valves are becoming increasingly durable, and it is anticipated that it may take 15 to 20 years before structural failure will occur in these prostheses.

For aortic valve replacement, a mechanical prosthesis, a newer-generation tissue valve (either stented or nonstented), a homograft, or a pulmonary autograft (Ross procedure) may be recommended, depending on the patient's lifestyle and desire to avoid anticoagulation therapy. Some type of tissue valve is usually recommended for patients >65 years of age because anticoagulation therapy may be hazardous and valve durability is better in older patients. For patients >65 years of age, Jamieson and colleagues demonstrated a risk of tissue valve structural deterioration of <10% at 15 years.[34]

Valve repair can be performed in the vast majority of patients with mitral insufficiency as discussed later in this chapter. In certain patients, valve replacement may still be indicated, particularly with rheumatic disease and valvular stenosis. When valve replacement is necessary, a tissue valve is an appropriate choice in women planning pregnancy or in patients >60 to 65 years of age. A mechanical prosthesis is recommended for younger patients, especially if the patient is in atrial fibrillation, because anticoagulation therapy is already required in this group.

Mechanical Valves

A common mechanical valve used in the United States is the St. Jude Medical bileaflet prosthesis (Fig. 21-6). Mechanical (disk) valves have excellent flow characteristics, an acceptably low risk of late valve-related complications, and an extremely low risk of mechanical valve

failure. With proper anticoagulation and keeping the International Normalized Ratio (INR) at two to three times the normal for mechanical aortic valves and 2.5 to 3.5 times the normal for mechanical MVs, the incidence of thromboembolism is approximately 1 to 2% per patient per year, and the risk of anticoagulant-related hemorrhage is 0.5 to 2% per patient per year. Careful monitoring of the INR reduces the risk of thromboembolic events, minimizes anticoagulation-related complications, and improves survival.[35]

Tissue Valves

Several types of xenograft tissue valves are available and widely used (Fig. 21-7). The stented valves are most common (either porcine or bovine pericardial), while stentless valves are being increasingly used by some groups. Again, the chief advantage of tissue valves is the low incidence of thromboembolism and the absence of the need for anticoagulation therapy. Stented tissue valves have the drawback of having higher gradients across the valve, particularly in smaller sizes (indexed prosthetic valve area <0.85 cm² valve area per square meter body surface area). Therefore, this group of patients may have less symptomatic improvement and a suboptimal hemodynamic response to exercise.[36] However, most patients experience excellent symptomatic improvement and have a normal response to exercise after stented tissue valve replacement.

Nevertheless, the limitations in flow characteristics observed in small sizes of stented tissue valves led to the development of stentless valves in an attempt to maximize the effective valve orifice area by eliminating the profile of the stent, and to take advantage of the natural dynamic nature of the aortic annulus. Since the first clinical report of a stentless porcine valve in 1990 by David and associates,[37] several stentless aortic bioprostheses have been introduced (Fig. 21-8). The technique of implantation varies (subcoronary or miniroot), but the results have been excellent in most series. Patients undergoing stentless valve replacement have been found to have a significant reduction

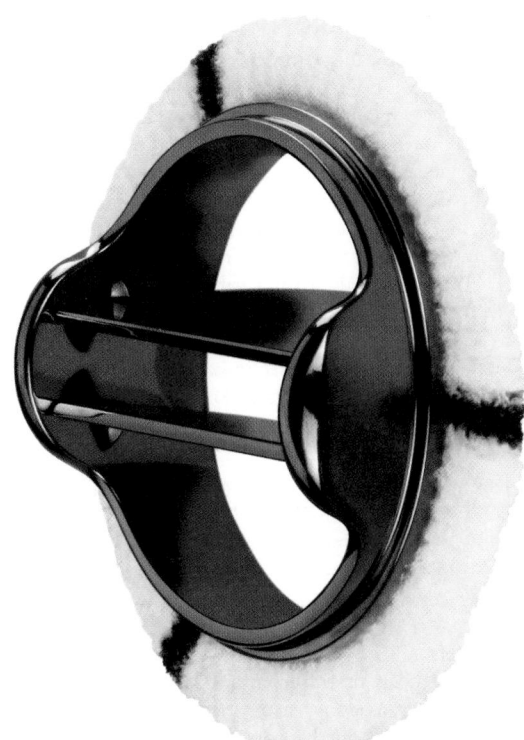

FIG. 21-6. Mechanical valve. St. Jude Medical bileaflet prosthesis. *(Photo courtesy of St. Jude Medical, Inc., St. Paul, MN. All rights reserved.)*

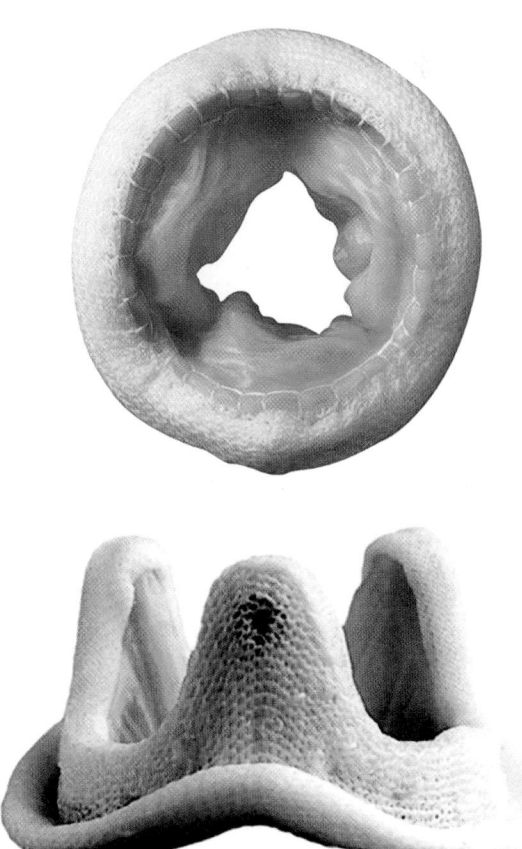

FIG. 21-7. Bioprosthetic valves. *(Photos courtesy of Medtronic, Inc., Minneapolis, MN.)*

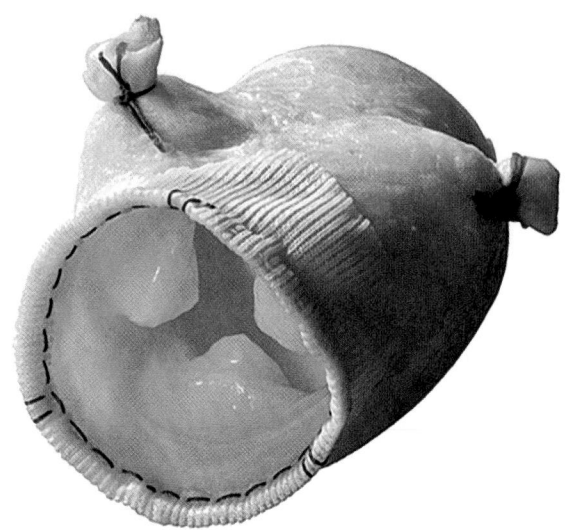

FIG. 21-8. Freestyle xenograft root and valve prosthesis. *(Photo courtesy of Medtronic, Inc., Minneapolis, MN.)*

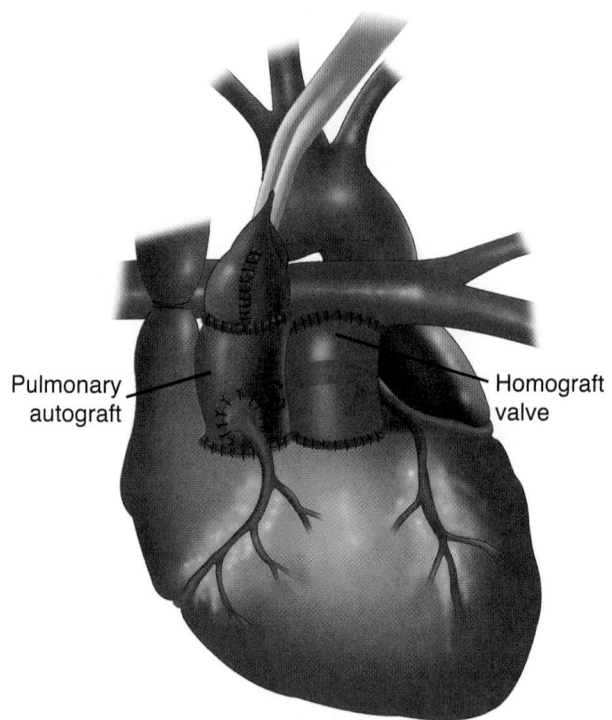

FIG. 21-9. Diagram of a completed Ross procedure. The aortic valve has been replaced with the patient's own pulmonary valve (pulmonary autograft), and the coronary arteries have been reimplanted. The pulmonary valve has been replaced with a homograft valve (aortic or pulmonary) obtained from a cadaver. *(Reproduced with permission from Oury JH: Clinical aspects of the Ross procedure: Indications and contraindications. Semin Thorac Cardiovasc Surg 8:328, 1996. Copyright Elsevier.)*

in transvalvular gradient, both at rest and with exercise. Although the long-term durability of stentless valves has not yet been established, these valves offer excellent hemodynamics, and durability is anticipated to be similar to that achieved with stented xenografts.

Homografts

Surgical alternatives to prosthetic valve replacement have been developed in an attempt to use the body's natural tissue and lower the incidence of valve-related complications. In the 1960s, Ross in England and Barrett-Boyes in New Zealand described a procedure for aortic valve replacement using antibiotic-preserved aortic homograft (allograft) valves.[38,39] Since this time, homografts have been used more frequently for aortic and pulmonary valve replacements. Similarly to patients receiving xenografts, the rate of thromboembolic complications is low, and long-term anticoagulation therapy is not required. In addition, homografts have much lower transvalvular pressure gradients than stented tissue valves. Although homografts are attractive options in many instances, there are some limitations to their widespread use. During the first year of implantation, homograft valves rapidly lose their original cellular components and normal tissue architecture. Newer methods of homograft preservation that result in significant retention of cellular viability are possible using cryopreservation techniques, widening the availability of homografts and potentially improving the long-term results. The main disadvantage of a homograft valve is its uncertain durability, especially in young patients, as structural degeneration of the valve tissue leads to graft dysfunction and valve failure. The 15-year durability is approximately that of a xenograft.

Autografts

Ross described a potentially durable but more complicated alternative for aortic valve replacement with natural autologous tissue, using the patient's native pulmonary valve as an autograft for aortic valve replacement and replacing the pulmonary valve with a homograft (Fig. 21-9). This operation, referred to as the Ross procedure, has the advantage of placing an autologous valve into the aortic position, which functions physiologically and does not require anticoagulation therapy. Results have shown minimal-to-absent transvalvular gradients, with improvement in LV function both at rest and during exercise. Ross reported late follow-up of 339 autograft patients with a rate of freedom from autograft replacement of 85% at 20 years, and a rate of freedom from all valve-related events of 70% at 20 years. Others have reported less durable results, with a combined failure rate of the autograft or pulmonary homograft of 30 to 40% at 12 to 15 years. The Ross procedure may be indicated for younger patients who require aortic valve replacement and want to avoid the need for anticoagulation.

Valve Repair

Valve repair has become the procedure of choice for most patients with MV insufficiency, while repair of the aortic valve is feasible in certain situations. In the 1960s McGoon, Kay, and Reed each developed separate plication techniques for reconstruction of the MV for mitral insufficiency. However, the primary advance in MV repair resulted from work by Carpentier in the 1970s. Valve repair has subsequently proved to be highly reproducible for correction of mitral insufficiency, with excellent durability and freedom from late valve-related complications. The 15-year freedom from valve repair failure is >90% in patients with degenerative mitral insufficiency. Valve repair offers significant advantages over valve replacement, primarily lower risks of thromboembolic- and anticoagulant-related complications. Survival may also be improved in certain groups of patients after valve repair.

Mitral Valve Disease

In the 1920s the first attempts to surgically correct mitral stenosis via a closed atrial approach demonstrated the feasibility of mitral valve surgery. Now, with good preoperative pathophysiologic evaluation and precise surgical technique, mitral valve surgery has become one of the most successful procedures performed by cardiac surgeons.

Mitral Stenosis

Etiology MV stenosis or mixed mitral stenosis and insufficiency almost always are caused by rheumatic heart disease, although a definite clinical history can be obtained in only 50% of patients. Congenital mitral stenosis is rarely seen in adults. Occasionally, intracardiac tumors such as a left atrial myxoma may obstruct the mitral orifice and cause symptoms that mimic mitral stenosis.

Pathology Although the rheumatic inflammatory process is associated with some degree of pancarditis involving the endocardium, myocardium, and pericardium, permanent injury results predominantly from the endocarditis, with progressive fibrosis of the valves. Rheumatic valvulitis produces three distinct degrees of pathologic change: fusion of the commissures alone, commissural fusion plus subvalvular shortening of the chordae tendineae, and extensive fixation of the valve and subvalvular apparatus with calcification and scarring of both leaflets and chordae (Fig. 21-10). The degree of pathology present should be determined preoperatively, as this predicts the suitability of balloon valvuloplasty, surgical commissurotomy, or valve replacement.

Pathophysiology Mitral stenosis usually has a prolonged course after the initial rheumatic infection, and symptoms may not appear for 10 to 20 years. The progression to valvular fibrosis and calcification may be related to repeated episodes of rheumatic fever, or may result from scarring produced by inflammation and turbulent blood flow.

Mitral stenosis leads to a progressive decrease in the MV area, which results in a transvalvular gradient across the stenotic valve during diastole. The normal cross-sectional area of the MV is 4 to 6 cm^2. Symptoms may progressively develop with moderate stenosis, defined as a cross-sectional area of 1.0 to 1.5 cm^2. Severe symptomatic stenosis occurs when the MV area is <0.8 to 1.0 cm^2.

The pathophysiology associated with mitral stenosis results from an elevation in left atrial pressure, producing pulmonary venous congestion and pulmonary hypertension. As the left atrium dilates, atrial fibrillation may develop, exacerbating the patient's symptoms and resulting in an increased likelihood of clot formation and embolization. The LV function usually remains normal because the ventricle is protected by the stenotic valve.

Clinical Manifestations The main symptoms of mitral stenosis are exertional dyspnea and decreased exercise capacity. Dyspnea occurs when the left atrial pressure becomes elevated due to the stenotic

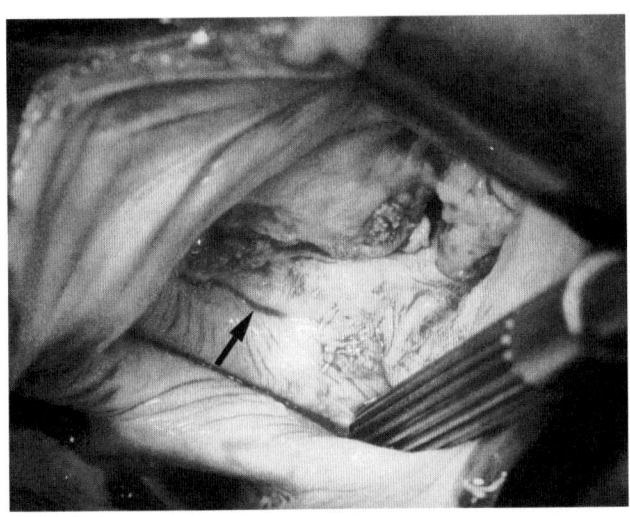

A

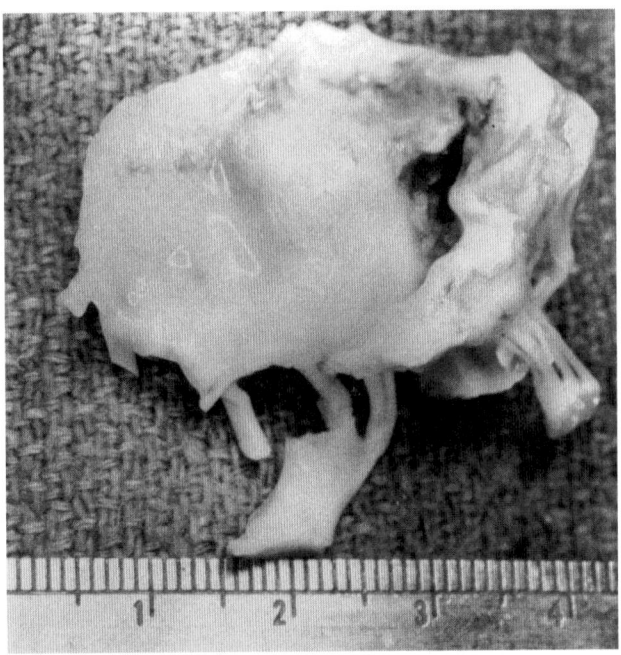

B

FIG. 21-10. Mitral replacement. **A.** Operative photograph of rheumatic mitral valve with calcific mitral stenosis, viewed through a left atriotomy incision. *Arrow* points to "bar" of heavily calcified posterior annulus. **B.** Excised calcified mitral valve with fibrotic, shortened chordae tendineae. **C.** St. Jude mechanical mitral valve visualized through the open left atrium. Pledget reinforced sutures were used to secure the valve into the native annulus.

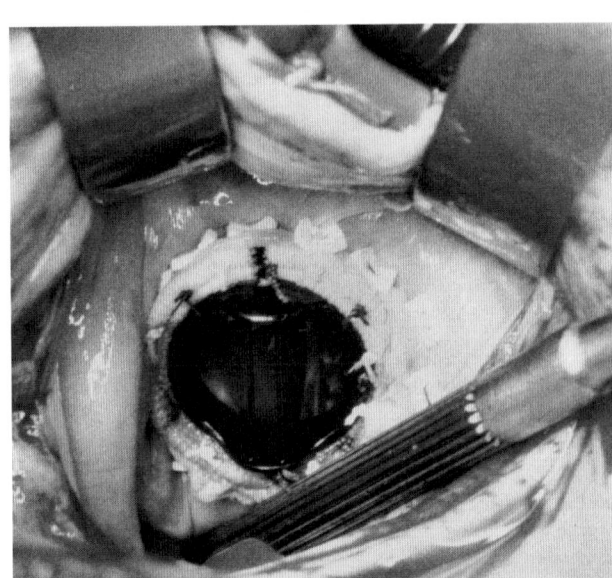

C

valve, resulting in pulmonary congestion. Orthopnea and paroxysmal nocturnal dyspnea may also occur, or in advanced cases, hemoptysis. The most serious development is pulmonary edema. When the stenosis is chronic, with pulmonary hypertension, the patient may develop right-sided heart failure, which manifests as jugular venous distention, hepatomegaly, ascites, or ankle edema.

Atrial fibrillation develops in a significant number of patients with chronic mitral stenosis, and in some patients, arterial embolization is the initial presenting symptom. Atrial thrombi result from dilation of the left atrium, with stasis of blood. The left atrial appendage becomes especially susceptible to clot formation. Angina is a rare symptom that may result from coronary embolization.

The characteristic auscultatory findings of mitral stenosis, called the *auscultatory triad*, are an increased first heart sound, an opening snap, and an apical diastolic rumble. A loud pansystolic murmur transmitted to the axilla usually indicates associated mitral insufficiency. A systolic murmur along the left lower sternal border, loudest near the xiphoid process, commonly occurs with associated tricuspid insufficiency.

Diagnostic Studies The ECG may show atrial fibrillation, left atrial enlargement (P mitrale), and right-axis deviation, or it may be normal. On chest x-ray, enlargement of the left atrium is typically seen on the posteroanterior film as a double contour visible behind the right atrial shadow. The overall cardiac size may be normal, but enlargement of the left atrium and the pulmonary artery (PA) may obliterate the normal concavity between the aorta and the left ventricle, producing a "straight" left border of the heart. Calcifications of the MV also may be seen. In the lung fields, the typical abnormalities consistent with pulmonary congestion may be present.

The Doppler echocardiogram is diagnostic. TEE is a particularly useful test because it provides enhanced resolution and unobstructed visualization of the MV and the posterior cardiac structures, including the left atrium and the atrial appendage. Echocardiography gives a very accurate measurement of the transvalvular gradient and the cross-sectional area of the MV, and allows assessment of the degree of leaflet mobility, calcification, and subvalvular fusion, each of which may be important in predicting the feasibility of valve repair.

Cardiac angiography should be performed in patients in whom concomitant CAD is likely, based on the patient's history or risk factors, and in most patients >55 years of age. Right heart catheterization may be valuable in patients with pulmonary hypertension, although a reliable estimate of the PA pressures can usually be determined from Doppler echocardiography.

Indications for Valvuloplasty or Commissurotomy Although percutaneous balloon valvuloplasty has become an acceptable alternative for many patients with uncomplicated mitral stenosis, open mitral commissurotomy remains an extremely reproducible and durable option. Commissurotomy has the advantage of allowing the surgeon to address nonpliable or calcified MVs, mobilize fused papillary muscles to correct subvalvular restrictive disease, effectively repair patients with mixed stenosis and insufficiency, and remove left atrial clot. Either balloon valvuloplasty or open surgical commissurotomy is indicated for symptomatic patients with moderate (MV area <1.5 cm^2) or severe (MV area <1.0 cm^2) mitral stenosis. Similarly, the development of pulmonary hypertension or embolic events in the presence of mitral stenosis is considered a relative indication for treatment. If the need for surgery is uncertain, exercise echocardiography may be useful, with a significant increase in the transvalvular gradient and a rise in PA pressure being indications for intervention.

Mitral Insufficiency

Etiology Degenerative disease is the most common cause of mitral insufficiency in the United States, accounting for 50 to 60% of the patients requiring surgery. Other causes include rheumatic fever (15 to 20%), ischemic disease (15 to 20%), endocarditis, congenital abnormalities, and cardiomyopathy.

Pathology The major structural components of the MV are the annulus, the leaflets, the chordae tendinae, and the papillary muscles. A defect in any of these components may create mitral insufficiency. A functional classification for mitral insufficiency was proposed by Carpentier,[40] who characterized three basic types of functionally diseased valves. Type I insufficiency occurs from annular dilatation or leaflet perforation with normal leaflet motion. Type II occurs from leaflet prolapse or ruptured chordae tendinae with increased leaflet motion, typically occurring in patients with degenerative disease. Degenerative causes include myxomatous degeneration and fibroelastic deficiency. With myxomatous degeneration, thickened excessive leaflet tissue is present, with leaflet prolapse occurring from chordal elongation or chordal rupture. The valve usually has a billowing appearance (Barlow's syndrome). By contrast, patients with fibroelastic deficiency have thinned leaflets and chordae, with chordal elongation or rupture. In both types, the mitral annulus is invariably dilated. Type III insufficiency occurs from restricted leaflet motion, with the leaflets not reaching the proper plane of closure during systole. Type III insufficiency typically occurs in rheumatic patients and in patients with chronic ischemic insufficiency.

In patients with rheumatic disease, the chordae tendinae are thickened and foreshortened, producing restrictive leaflet motion. Posterior dilatation of the mitral annulus also usually is present. With ischemic insufficiency, ventricular injury results in tethering of the mitral leaflets, producing restrictive leaflet motion, and central insufficiency, often with secondary annular dilation.

Pathophysiology The basic physiologic abnormality in patients with mitral insufficiency is regurgitation of a portion of the LV stroke volume into the left atrium. This results in decreased forward blood flow and an elevated left atrial pressure, producing pulmonary congestion and volume overload of the left ventricle.

As mitral insufficiency progresses, there is a corresponding increase in the size of the left atrium, and eventually, atrial fibrillation results. Concurrently, the left ventricle dilates. Initially the LV stroke volume increases by Starling's law, but eventually, this compensatory mechanism fails, and the ejection fraction decreases. However, decreased systolic function of the heart is a relatively late finding, because the ventricle is "unloaded" as a result of the valvular insufficiency. Once LV dysfunction and heart failure develop, the left ventricle usually has been significantly and often irreversibly injured.

Clinical Manifestations In patients with acute mitral regurgitation (MR), CHF develops suddenly, while in patients with chronic mitral insufficiency, the left atrium and ventricle become compliant, and symptoms do not develop until later in the course of the disease when the ventricle eventually fails, resulting in exertional dyspnea, decreased exercise capacity, and orthopnea. As LV dysfunction progresses, symptoms of pulmonary congestion become more prominent, ultimately resulting in pulmonary hypertension and right-sided heart failure.

On physical examination, the characteristic findings of mitral insufficiency are an apical holosystolic murmur and a forceful apical impulse. The apical murmur usually is harsh and transmitted to the axilla (in cases of anterior leaflet pathology), or to the left sternal border (typically in cases of posterior leaflet pathology), although this is variable. However, the severity of the insufficiency may not correlate with the intensity of the murmur.

Diagnostic Studies The severity of mitral insufficiency can be determined accurately with echocardiography, along with the site of valvular prolapse or restriction, and the level of LV function. An important measurement is the size of the cardiac chambers. The size of the left atrium reflects the chronicity and severity of the insufficiency. With severe, chronic mitral insufficiency, dilatation of the left atrium to 5 to 6 cm or greater is common. This is important because the propensity for atrial fibrillation is greatly increased when the left atrial size is >4.5 to 5 cm. The LV diastolic dimensions become enlarged relatively early because of volume overload, but

LV systolic function is usually well maintained early in the course of the disease. Once the echocardiogram demonstrates a decrease in LV systolic function, manifested as a rise in the end-systolic dimension of the heart and a drop in the ejection fraction, this is an indication that the left ventricle is beginning to decompensate. If there is uncertainty about the physiologic significance of mitral insufficiency, exercise stress-echocardiography may be used. Normally the ejection fraction rises with exercise, but a fall in ejection fraction with exercise is an early sign of LV systolic dysfunction.

Indications for Operation Delaying an operation until the patient is severely symptomatic and the heart is markedly dilated often results in a certain degree of irreversible ventricular injury. According to the American College of Cardiology/American Heart Association guidelines, MV repair or replacement is recommended in any symptomatic patient with mitral insufficiency, even with normal LV function (defined as ejection fraction >60% and end-systolic dimension <45 mm).[41] Surgery also is currently recommended in asymptomatic patients with severe mitral insufficiency if there are signs of LV systolic dysfunction (increased end-systolic dimension or decreased ejection fraction). Recent onset of atrial fibrillation, pulmonary hypertension, or an abnormal response to exercise testing are considered relative indications for surgery.

MV surgery should be strongly considered in most patients while they remain asymptomatic, before significant LV dysfunction.[42] A retrospective study by David and associates compared 289 symptomatic with 199 asymptomatic patients undergoing MV repair for degenerative disease.[43] Survival at 15 years was 76% for asymptomatic patients, identical to that for the general population matched for age and sex, compared to a survival of 53% for symptomatic patients.

Operative Techniques

The traditional approach for MV surgery is through a median sternotomy incision with CPB and cardioplegic arrest. The MV is exposed through a left atrial incision, made posterior and parallel to the intra-atrial groove. After the left atrial incision is made, self-retaining retractor blades are inserted to expose the MV. In certain patients, exposure through the posterior left atrial approach may not be optimal. This is particularly true in patients with a small left atrium, a deep chest, or an aortic prosthesis in place, and in reoperations in which the tissue is fixed and nonelastic. Alternative incisions for exposing the difficult MV include a right atriotomy with transseptal incision, a superior approach through the dome of the atrium, and a biatrial transseptal approach.

Commissurotomy Once CPB has been established and the heart has been arrested, the left atrium is opened and the MV is visualized. Initially, the atrial cavity is examined for thrombi, especially within the atrial appendage. The MV is assessed by evaluating leaflet mobility, commissural fusion, and the degree of fibrosis in the subvalvular apparatus. A right-angle clamp often is placed beneath the commissures, gently applying horizontal tension to evaluate commissural fusion.

Once the commissure has been accurately identified and the chordae noted, a right-angle clamp is introduced beneath the fused commissure, stretching the adjacent chordae and leaflets, after which the commissure is carefully incised. The incision is made 2 to 3 mm at a time, serially confirming that the separated margins of the commissural leaflet remain attached to chordae tendineae. The usual commissurotomy curves slightly anteriorly and does not go directly laterally. The incision should stop 1 to 2 mm from the valve annulus where the leaflet tissue becomes thin, indicating the transition from the fused commissure to the normal commissural leaflet of the MV. Once the commissurotomy is completed, any fused papillary muscle is incised as necessary to minimize restriction and improve mobility of the attached leaflet.

After separation of the commissure and mobilization of the underlying chordae tendineae and papillary muscle, leaflet mobility is assessed visually. The anterior leaflet is grasped with a forceps and

moved throughout the entire range of motion, looking for subvalvular restriction or leaflet rigidity. In some patients, restricted motion may be further improved by dividing secondary chordae or by the selective débridement of calcium. Extremely thickened chordae can be mobilized by excision of a triangular portion of the fused cords. If extensive débridement and mobilization of the chordal structures are necessary, valve replacement usually is more appropriate. At least 30% of patients undergoing commissurotomy require more than simple incision of the commissure to produce an adequate mitral orifice and to restore mobility to the valve. Competence of the valve is assessed by injection of cold saline into the ventricle.

If the patient is in atrial fibrillation, the atrial appendage is closed with a continuous suture of 3-0 polypropylene to minimize the subsequent risk of emboli. Recently, intraoperative radiofrequency ablation procedures of the left atrium combined with MV surgery have become widely used in an attempt to convert these patients to sinus rhythm.

Mitral Valve Replacement MV replacement is necessary when the extent of disease precludes commissurotomy or valve reconstruction. Valve replacement is most likely in patients with long-standing rheumatic disease. Once the valve is exposed and the need for valve replacement is determined, an incision is made in the anterior mitral leaflet, usually starting at the 12 o'clock position, and most of the anterior leaflet is resected. The posterior leaflet is preserved whenever possible, and the chordal attachments to both leaflets are preserved or reattached to the annulus, as this has been shown to improve LV function and lower the risk of posterior LV free wall rupture, a potentially lethal complication of valve replacement. However, chordal preservation is not always possible in patients with extensive rheumatic disease, because of extensive valvular thickening and calcification.

When the MV is excised, an appropriate-sized replacement valve is selected. This valve usually is attached with 12 to 16 mattress sutures. A pledgeted mattress suture technique is recommended because it minimizes the risk of perivalvular leakage. The sutures may be inserted from the atrial to the ventricular side, everting the annulus and seating the valve intra-annularly, or from the ventricular side to the atrial side, resulting in supra-annular positioning of the prosthetic valve. Care is taken to insert the sutures precisely into the annular tissue because excessively deep insertion of sutures may injure critical structures, including the circumflex coronary artery posterolaterally (from the surgeon's perspective, at 7 to 8 o'clock), the AV node anteromedially (at 1 to 2 o'clock), or the aortic valve anterolaterally (at 10 to 12 o'clock). Once the sutures are placed through the mitral annulus, they are placed through the valve sewing ring. The valve is then lowered onto the annulus and the sutures are tied and cut. The atriotomy incision is closed, and after air is removed from the cardiac chambers, the aortic cross-clamp is removed and the heart is reperfused.

Mitral Valve Reconstruction The basic techniques of MV reconstruction include resection of the posterior leaflet, chordal shortening, chordal transposition, artificial chordal replacement, and triangular resection for repair of the anterior leaflet disease. An annuloplasty to correct associated annular dilation also is recommended in most cases.

The intraoperative assessment of the valvular pathology is an important step in valve reconstruction. A localized roughened area of atrial endocardium, termed a *jet lesion*, may be present from regurgitant blood striking the endocardium, providing a guide to the location of the insufficiency. Subsequently, the commissures are examined, noting whether these are prolapsed, fused, or malformed. The closing plane of the leaflets in the area supported by commissural chordae is determined next, and the anterior and posterior leaflets are then examined, noting areas of prolapse or restriction. Such abnormalities as perforation, fibrosis, calcification, or leaflet clefts also must be recognized. Finally, the degree of annular enlargement is assessed.

Proper evaluation of the degree of leaflet prolapse is critical. The "billowing" MV originally described by Barlow has excessive leaflet tissue, but may remain competent if the chordae are not elongated. In such cases, the rough free edge of the leaflet closes at the proper level, even though the midportion of the leaflet may contain excessive tissue. The anterolateral commissural chordae are seldom elongated, so elevating the commissural leaflet with a nerve hook provides a valuable reference point from which the degree of elongation of other chordae may be determined. Chordal rupture or total lack of structural support leads to prolapse and a completely flail leaflet.

Posterior Leaflet Procedures Quadrangular resection of the posterior leaflet has become the mainstay of MV reconstruction (Figs. 21-11 and 21-12). A rectangular excision is performed, cutting directly down to, but not through, the mitral annulus. Diseased tissue in the posterior leaflet is excised with a quadrangular excision, usually removing 1 to 2 cm of tissue. Strong chordae of proper length are identified on each side of the excised leaflet and encircled with retraction sutures.

Once the quadrangular excision has been performed, the annulus of the excised segment of leaflet is corrected either by simple annular plication, folding plasty, or sliding plasty. The simple annular plication is performed with several interrupted sutures placed about 5 mm apart. These are started centrally and extended to include a few millimeters of annulus adjacent to the remaining leaflets. When these annular sutures are tied, the leaflet margins are automatically brought into apposition without any tension. If there were tension on the leaflet tissues, there would be a serious possibility of dehiscence of the subsequent leaflet repair. Once the annular sutures have been tied, the leaflet margins are approximated with simple or figure-of-eight sutures, usually 4-0 or 5-0 polypropylene, depending on the thickness of the leaflets.

The folding plasty technique, described by the group from New York University (NYU), involves folding down the cut vertical edges of the posterior leaflet to the annulus and closing the ensuing cleft.[44] With this technique the central height of the posterior leaflet is reduced, the edge of leaflet coaptation is moved posteriorly, and annular plication is either eliminated or reduced. This elimination of annular plication avoids the serious complication of circumflex artery kinking, which may occur in the setting of left dominant coronary artery circulation and a large posterior leaflet resection. The sliding plasty technique reported by Carpentier and associates also is successful in reducing posterior leaflet height and moving the edge of leaflet coaptation posteriorly.

Often, the valve appears quite competent after the leaflet repair has been completed. Gently injecting saline into the ventricle with a bulb syringe and noting both the mobility of the leaflets and their apposition is an excellent visual guide for assessing competency. If localized insufficiency remains in other areas, additional procedures can be performed.

Anterior Leaflet Procedures Four primary techniques are used for anterior leaflet reconstruction: chordal shortening, chordal transposition, artificial chordal replacement, and triangular resection of anterior leaflet tissue with primary repair. With chordal shortening, the elongated chord is imbricated either onto the free edge of the leaflet or onto the papillary muscle. In contrast, the chordal transposition technique uses a segment of structurally intact posterior leaflet directly opposite the prolapsed anterior leaflet. A small quadrangular excision of the posterior leaflet with the attached chordae is performed, and the mobilized leaflet and chordae are then transposed onto the anterior leaflet to provide structural support. The defect created in the posterior leaflet is then repaired in the manner described in the Posterior Leaflet Procedures section. Artificial chordae replacement has been used by some groups as an alternative for anterior leaflet repair, using polytetrafluoroethylene sutures that are attached to both the papillary muscle and the free edge of the prolapsing leaflet to re-establish structural support. Finally, triangular resection and primary repair has been increasingly used at NYU for treatment of anterior leaflet prolapse (Fig. 21-13). The adjacent intact chordae are identified, and triangular resection is performed to remove the prolapsing segment of the leaflet and any ruptured chordae. The technique is particularly helpful when a large amount of redundant anterior leaflet tissue is present, as in patients with myxomatous degeneration and Barlow's syndrome. Additionally, Gortex neochordae have shown excellent results for the treatment of prolapsing leaflet segments.[45]

Repair of Leaflet Perforation Leaflet perforations can be repaired by primary suture closure or by closure with a pericardial patch. Extensive leaflet destruction is best managed with MV replacement.

Annuloplasty Use of a MV annuloplasty device (ring or partial band) to correct annular dilation during valve repair decreases the risk of late repair failure.[46] The primary purpose of an annuloplasty device is to correct the associated annular dilation that invariably occurs in patients with chronic mitral insufficiency, regardless of etiology, and results in worsening central insufficiency due to lack of leaflet coaptation. Various types of annuloplasty devices are available, including rigid or semirigid rings that geometrically remodel the annulus, flexible rings or bands that provide no geometric remodeling but restrict annular dilation while maintaining physiologic sphincter motion of the annulus, and semirigid bands that provide both annular remodeling and physiologic annular sphincter motion (Fig. 21-14). The relative advantages of the different types of devices remain under investigation, but it is widely accepted that use

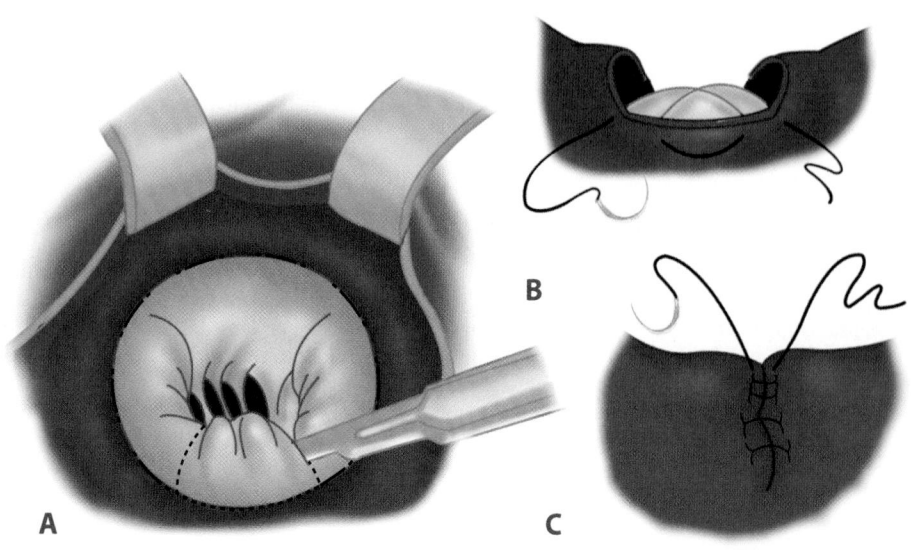

FIG. 21-11. A through **C.** Repair of posterior prolapse. Illustration of rectangular resection and repair for correction of posterior leaflet prolapse. *(Reproduced with permission from Galloway AC, Colvin SB, Baumann SG, et al: Current concepts of mitral valve reconstruction for mitral insufficiency. Circulation 78:1087, 1988.)*

A

B

C

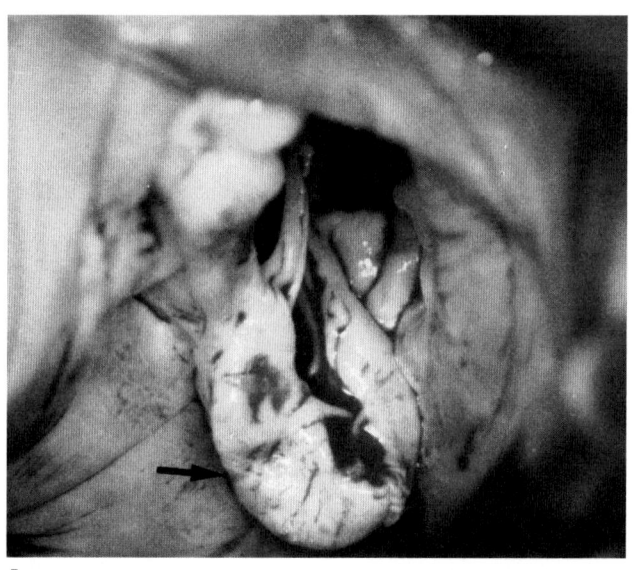

A

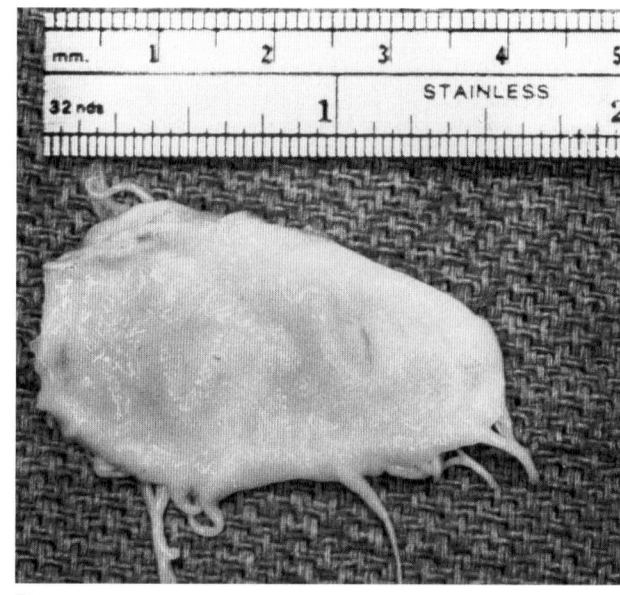

B

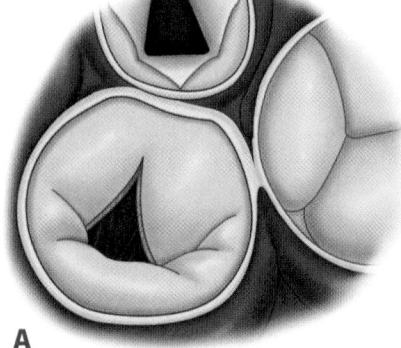

C

FIG. 21-12. Mitral repair operation. **A.** Operative photograph demonstrating myxomatous mitral valve with massive prolapse and a flail posterior leaflet (indicated by the *arrow*). **B.** Specimen of resected mitral valve posterior leaflet. **C.** Operative photograph of completed Carpentier-type mitral valve reconstruction. The *narrow arrow* indicates the posterior leaflet repair, while the *wide arrow* demonstrates the ring annuloplasty. Note the total correction of leaflet prolapse and annular dilation.

FIG. 21-13. Repair of anterior leaflet prolapse. **A.** Illustration of triangular resection of the anterior mitral leaflet. **B.** Suture repair of the defect.

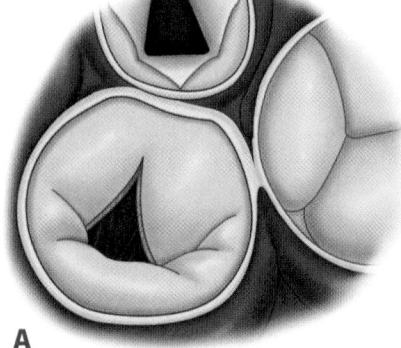

A

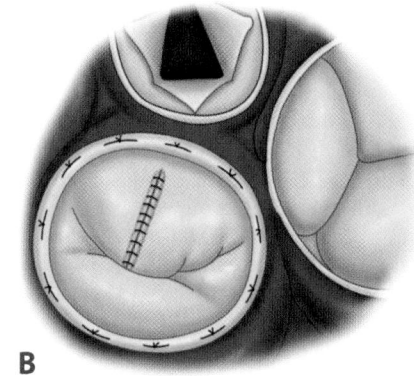

B

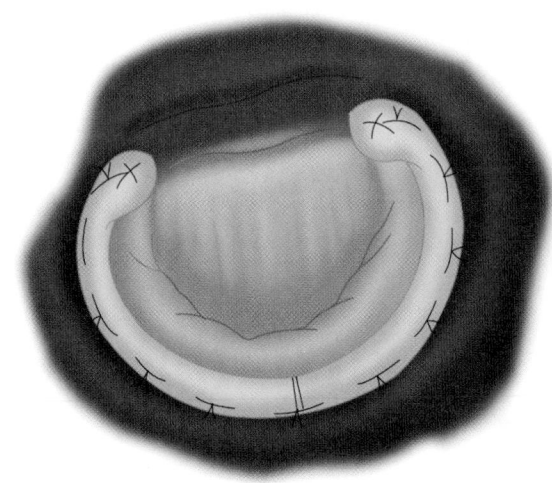

FIG. 21-14. Annuloplasty device. Illustration of Colvin-Galloway Future Band Annuloplasty sewn into mitral valve annulus. Annuloplasty device corrects annular dilatation and restores appropriate geometric configuration to the annulus. *(Illustration courtesy of Medtronic, Inc., Minneapolis, MN.)*

of an annuloplasty device to correct annular dilation improves long-term repair durability.

Results

Commissurotomy The operative risk for open mitral commissurotomy is <1%, and long-term results have been excellent. Choudhary and associates reported a 10-year freedom from MV failure after open commissurotomy of 87 ± 3.5%.[47] The incidence of thromboembolism was only 0.5% per patient-year. Antunes and colleagues reported favorable long-term results after open commissurotomy in 100 patients with a mean follow-up of 8.5 years.[48] The 9-year actuarial freedom from reoperation was 98%, and 93% were in NYHA functional class I or II. Open mitral commissurotomy is a well-established procedure, allowing effective correction of mitral stenosis.

Balloon Valvuloplasty Percutaneous mitral balloon valvuloplasty has recently been developed as an alternative treatment for mitral stenosis. The choice between surgical commissurotomy and balloon valvuloplasty varies widely among centers. The main advantages of commissurotomy over balloon valvuloplasty are that, during surgery, the fused chordae can be surgically divided and mobility restored.

A prospective and randomized study has suggested that percutaneous balloon valvuloplasty and surgical commissurotomy result in comparable clinical improvement in selected patients with mitral stenosis.[49] MV areas were larger early after surgical commissurotomy, but were similar after 24 months. Patients receiving balloon valvuloplasty require more rigid selection criteria, as the procedure becomes less effective if the patient has significant calcification of the valve or fusion of the subvalvular apparatus.

Valve Replacement The operative mortality rate for MV replacement is 2 to 6%, depending on the number of comorbidities present. The major predictors of increased operative risk after MV replacement are age, LV function, emergency operation, NYHA functional status, previous cardiac surgery, associated CAD, and concomitant disease in another valve. Mohty and associates reported late survival rates after MV replacement of 71 ± 3%, 49 ± 3%, and 29 ± 4% at 5, 10, and 15 years, respectively.[50] The major factors influencing long-term survival are age, urgency of operation, NYHA functional status, mitral insufficiency (vs. stenosis), ischemic etiology, pulmonary hypertension, and the need for concomitant coronary bypass or procedures on another valve.

Improved engineering of mechanical prostheses has produced valves with lower intrinsic thrombogenicity and better durability, resulting in fewer late valve-related complications. Khan and co-workers compared late results in 513 patients receiving mechanical valves with 402 patients receiving tissue valves.[51] There was no difference in survival or in thromboembolic or anticoagulation-related complications between the groups. However, freedom from reoperation at 15 years was 98% with mechanical valves and 79% with tissue valves. Thus, while mechanical valves and tissue valves result in similar long-term survival, there is an increased risk of late reoperation in patients receiving tissue valves.

Valve Repair The operative risk for MV repair is <1 to 2%, and late results have demonstrated that, compared to replacement, repair is associated with improved survival and better freedom from valve-related complications. A report on 1195 patients undergoing valve repair and ring annuloplasty demonstrated that the actuarial freedoms from complications at 5 and 10 years, respectively, were as follows: thromboembolic, 92 and 88%; anticoagulant-related complications, 98 and 96%; endocarditis, 97 and 96%; and reoperation, 91 and 84%.[52] The need for anterior leaflet repair (as compared to posterior leaflet repair or annuloplasty alone) did not compromise the 5-year results in terms of patient survival, risk of reoperation, or freedom from valve-related complications. The freedom from reoperation, however, has been shown to be significantly better in nonrheumatic patients (93% at 5 years, 88% at 10 years) than in rheumatic patients (86% at 5 years, 73% at 10 years; P <.005).

Braunberger and associates reported long-term (20-year) results after mitral repair in 162 patients with nonrheumatic MV insufficiency.[53] The 20-year Kaplan-Meier survival rate was 48%, which is similar to the normal age-matched population. Freedom from cardiac death was 92 and 81% at 10 and 20 years, respectively. The linearized risk of reoperation rate was 0.4% per patient-year, although the need for anterior leaflet repair did decrease late repair durability. Repair of posterior leaflet prolapse resulted in a 98.5% freedom from reoperation at 10 years, while anterior leaflet repair had an 86.2% freedom from reoperation at 10 years (P <.03).

Mohty and associates reported the results of 679 MV repairs and 238 valve replacements performed at the Mayo Clinic between 1980 and 1995.[50] Survival after valve repair was better than after valve replacement (68 ± 2% vs. 49 ± 3% at 10 years, and 37 ± 5% vs. 29 ± 4% at 15 years), with an adjusted odds ratio for death of 0.68 for repair vs. replacement (P <.002). The overall late risk of reoperation after valve repair was only 16% at 15 years.

Minimally Invasive Mitral Valve Surgery Newer techniques that allow MV repair or replacement to be performed with a minimally invasive incision have been increasingly used over the last decade. Most techniques employ either minithoracotomy or a partial sternotomy incision. At NYU, minimally invasive MV surgery has been performed through a small right anterior thoracotomy incision, entering the chest through the third or fourth intercostal space (Fig. 21-15). Others have used partial upper sternotomy, partial lower sternotomy, or parasternal incisions. The ascending aorta may be directly cannulated for perfusion, or cannulation may be performed through the femoral artery, while venous drainage for CPB may be achieved either directly from the right atrium or percutaneously from the femoral vein. Similar to traditional surgery, the operation is performed with moderate systemic hypothermia [28 to 30°C (82.4 to 86°F)] and cardioplegia is used for myocardial protection. The aorta may be directly occluded with a flexible or special long cross-clamp or occluded internally with a balloon catheter. Long instruments are required, but standard valve techniques are used.

Grossi and associates analyzed the initial NYU minimally invasive MV experience in 714 patients operated on between 1996 and 2001. Hospital mortality was 1.1% for isolated MV repair and 5.8% for isolated valve replacement. The risk of complications was similar to that reported with conventional surgery, although minimally invasive

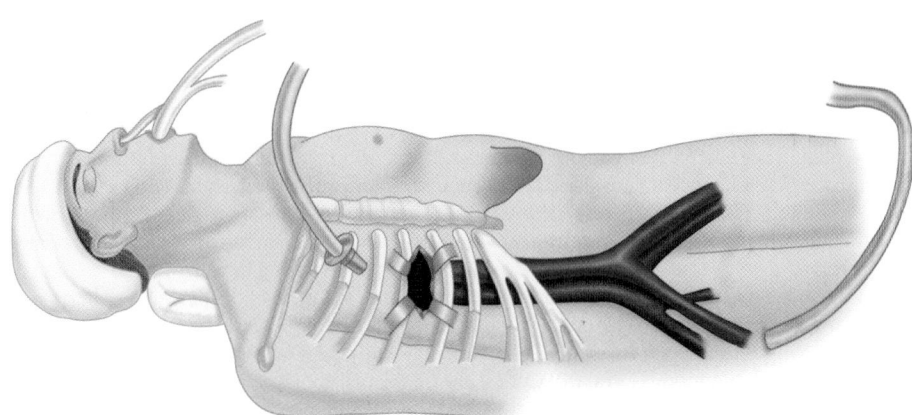

FIG. 21-15. Minimally invasive valve operation. Schematic diagram demonstrating operative approach for minimally invasive mitral valve surgery. A fourth interspace anterolateral minithoracotomy is shown, with direct aortic cannulation through a separate second interspace incision and venous cannulation via the right femoral vein. *(Reproduced with permission from Sharony R, Grossi EA, Saunders PC, et al: Repair of tricuspid regurgitation: the posterior annuloplasty technique.* Operative Techniques in Thoracic and Cardiovascular Surgery: A Comparative Atlas. *8(4):177–183, 2003.)*

patients needed less blood and had less pain, fewer infections, a shorter hospital stay, and a quicker overall recovery.[54,55] Galloway and colleagues reported late results after minimally invasive valve repair, demonstrating that repair durability, freedom from valve-related complications, and survival were equivalent to results achieved with the traditional sternotomy approach. Thus, the results after minimally invasive valve surgery are encouraging, and more widespread use of minimally invasive techniques is likely in the future.

New Developments

Edge-to-Edge Repair In 1995, Alfieri described the "double-orifice" or "edge-to-edge" repair as an alternative technique for repair for mitral insufficiency.[56] With this technique, the free edge of the anterior leaflet is sutured to the opposing free edge of the posterior leaflet, converting the valve into a double-orifice "bow tie." The edge-to-edge technique has been used for anterior leaflet pathology, ischemic insufficiency, endocarditis, and dilated cardiomyopathy. This method may be used as a primary repair technique or as an alternative after incomplete correction with other methods. However, the late results after edge-to-edge repair are not well established, and some reports suggest that the edge-to-edge technique may negatively influence late repair durability.[57]

Robotic Mitral Valve Surgery Recent technologic achievements in optics and computerized telemanipulation have enabled robotically assisted MV operations. Chitwood and associates[58] and Mohr and associates[59] have reported encouraging results with robotically and videoscopically assisted MV repair, with femoral perfusion and a transthoracic aortic cross-clamp. The da Vinci robot is currently available for surgical use. It is a master-slave (console-effector) telemanipulation system equipped with a three-dimensional camera. It has been reported that the articulated wrist-like instruments and three-dimensional visualization of the da Vinci surgical system enable precise tissue telemanipulation. These systems still have significant limitations, however, and may not be readily adaptable to performing the multiple complex tasks necessary for valve surgery.[60] The large nationwide trial of the da Vinci robot for MV repair has reported good results, but a disappointingly high early valve repair failure rate.

Aortic Valve Disease

Effective surgical treatment of aortic valve disease became possible in 1960 with the development of satisfactory prosthetic valves by Starr and Edwards and by Harken and associates.

Aortic Stenosis

Etiology In the adult North American population, the primary causes of aortic stenosis include acquired calcific disease, bicuspid aortic valve, and rheumatic disease. Acquired calcific aortic stenosis typically occurs in the seventh or eighth decade of life, and is the most frequent etiology, accounting for over half of the cases. Acquired calcific stenosis, also termed *degenerative aortic stenosis* or *senile aortic stenosis*, appears to be related to the aging process, with progressive degeneration leading to valve damage and calcification, although a causative role of lipids has been demonstrated recently. Lipid-lowering drugs seem to slow the progression of acquired calcific stenosis.

Bicuspid aortic valve accounts for approximately one third of the cases of aortic stenosis in adults, typically presenting in the fourth or fifth decade of life, after years of turbulent flow through the bicuspid valve result in damage and calcification.

The third major cause of aortic stenosis, rheumatic heart disease, accounts for approximately 10 to 15% of patients in North America, but is more common in underdeveloped countries. With rheumatic disease, the degree of stenosis progresses with time. Concomitant MV disease almost always is present, although not always clinically significant.

Pathophysiology Generally, the aortic valve must be reduced to one third its normal cross-sectional area before significant hemodynamic changes occur. A normal aortic valve has a cross-sectional area of 2.5 to 3.5 cm^2. Moderate aortic stenosis is defined as an aortic valve area between 1.0 and 1.5 cm^2, while severe stenosis is defined as a valve area <1.0 cm^2.[41] Patients with severe stenosis typically have a mean transvalvular pressure gradient >50 mmHg, although the gradient is dependent on both the valve area and the cardiac output, and therefore, may not be severely elevated if the cardiac output is low. Once the valve area is <0.5 cm^2, with a transvalvular gradient of 100 mmHg or greater, the degree of stenosis is considered critical.

Aortic stenosis results in increased myocardial work and progressive concentric LV hypertrophy with little ventricular dilatation. This results in a thick, noncompliant ventricle, leading to early diastolic dysfunction. The significance of diastolic dysfunction has been intensively studied and has been implicated as a major cause of CHF in patients with aortic stenosis. The systolic function of the ventricle usually remains well preserved for many years, but eventually deteriorates due to long-standing increased afterload.

Myocardial ischemia develops in some patients with severe aortic stenosis, usually in response to exercise. The LV mass and LV systolic wall tension are increased, resulting in increased oxygen demand. Simultaneously, the cardiac output often is low and does not increase in response to exercise. The end-diastolic pressure of the ventricle becomes progressively elevated during exercise, resulting in increased demand, but with poor perfusion of the subendocardium.

Clinical Manifestations The classic symptoms of aortic stenosis include exertional dyspnea, decreased exercise capacity, heart failure, angina, and syncope. Once the patient becomes symptomatic, prompt operation is indicated. If heart failure, angina, or syncope is present, the need for surgery is more urgent, as the risk of death exceeds 30 to 50% over the next 5 years. Sudden death, which accounts for a significant number of fatalities from aortic stenosis, possibly due to arrhythmias, becomes a more likely threat once the patient becomes severely symptomatic.

The most common symptoms are exertional dyspnea and decreased exercise capacity (NYHA class II or III), which are indicative of progressive LV decompensation. The presence of NYHA class IV symptoms, manifest as CHF, orthopnea, pulmonary edema, and right-sided heart dysfunction, is a more ominous finding. Once CHF is present, the mortality approaches 40% over 2 to 3 years.

Angina pectoris, which may develop in patients with advanced disease, is a manifestation of increased LV mass and increased myocardial strain, resulting in subendocardial ischemia. Subclinical ischemic episodes may be associated with silent myocardial necrosis, and patients with little history and few prior symptoms may present with markedly depressed LV function, with large amounts of myocardium replaced by scar tissue.

Syncope may develop in patients with severe aortic stenosis secondary to the severe flow limitations imposed by the tightly stenotic valve and decreased cerebral blood flow. Syncope typically develops in response to exercise but may occur when patients vasodilate from any cause after minimal effort and with little warning. In a small proportion of patients, syncope results from heart block. The average life expectancy once angina or syncope has appeared is 3 to 5 years.

With auscultation, the principal finding is a harsh, diamond-shaped (crescendo-decrescendo) systolic murmur at the base of the heart (right second intercostal space) with radiation to the carotid arteries. The two components of the S_2 may become synchronous, or aortic valve closure may even follow pulmonic valve closure, causing paradoxical splitting of the S_2. An S_4 gallop at the apex reflects the presence of LV hypertrophy or heart failure. The apical impulse has been described as a "prolonged heave," while the pulse pressure in the peripheral circulation is usually narrow and sustained (pulsus parvus et tardus).

Diagnostic Studies On x-ray the heart size may be either normal or enlarged due to LV hypertrophy. Calcification of the valve often is visible in older patients. The ECG may demonstrate LV hypertrophy but may also be normal. Conduction abnormalities are common, apparently from spicules of calcium projecting into the conduction bundle located at the base of the commissure between the right cusp and noncoronary cusp, and some patients may develop complete heart block. Atrial fibrillation generally indicates the presence of advanced disease with a prolonged elevation of intracardiac pressures.

The diagnosis of aortic stenosis is now most frequently made by echocardiography, which provides an accurate estimate of the peak and mean systolic transvalvular gradients, which allows calculation of the aortic valve area. Because the Doppler echocardiogram measures flow velocity, the peak instantaneous pressure gradient may overestimate the true peak gradient, and the mean gradient is usually more accurate. The echocardiogram also can demonstrate the amount of calcium in the leaflets, the degree of leaflet immobility, the left atrial size, the degree of LV hypertrophy, the end-systolic and end-diastolic dimensions of the left ventricle, and the LV function. Finally, the echocardiogram is important for identifying any occult subvalvular stenosis and for differentiating valvular stenosis from idiopathic hypertrophic subaortic stenosis (IHSS).

Cardiac catheterization readily confirms the diagnosis by measuring the aortic transvalvular gradient and permitting calculation of the cross-sectional area of the valve, but is often unnecessary for this purpose in the current era due to the accuracy of echocardiography. However, coronary angiography should be performed in patients >55 years of age and in patients at high risk for CAD. The degree of pulmonary hypertension also should be measured in patients with severe CHF and NYHA class IV symptoms.

Operative Indications Patients with aortic stenosis typically respond well to aortic valve replacement, which immediately relieves the increased afterload. A special subgroup of patients includes those with critical aortic stenosis and advanced LV systolic dysfunction. These patients have an increased operative risk, but may still have significant improvement after valve replacement as long as the ventricle is not irreversibly damaged.[61] Echocardiographic signs of LV dysfunction must be carefully assessed even in asymptomatic patients, because it is well documented that once ventricular systolic dysfunction occurs, symptoms progressively develop within 1 to 2 years, with CHF and ventricular damage progressing thereafter.

Aortic valve replacement is indicated for virtually all symptomatic patients with aortic stenosis. Even in patients with NYHA class IV symptoms and poor ventricular function, surgery has been found to improve both functional status and survival. In asymptomatic patients with moderate to severe stenosis, periodic echocardiographic studies are performed to assess the transvalvular gradient, valve area, LV size, and LV function. Surgery is indicated with the first sign of LV systolic dysfunction, manifest on echocardiography as either a rise in the LV end-systolic size or a drop in the LVEF. Surgery also may be recommended for asymptomatic patients with aortic stenosis who have a progressive increase in the transvalvular gradient on serial echocardiographic studies, a rapid rise in diastolic dimensions, a valve area <0.80 cm^2, progressive pulmonary hypertension, or right ventricular dysfunction during exercise testing.

Aortic Insufficiency

Etiology and Pathology A variety of diseases can produce aortic valve insufficiency, including degenerative diseases, inflammatory or infectious diseases (endocarditis, rheumatic fever), congenital diseases, aortoannular ectasia or aneurysm of the aortic root, and aortic dissection. Mixed valvular stenosis and insufficiency can develop in any patient with aortic stenosis, regardless of etiology.

Degenerative valvular disease is a manifestation of fibroelastic deficiency or myxomatous degeneration that produces thin and elongated valvular tissue. The aortic valve leaflets sag into the ventricular lumen, often with no other tissue abnormality, producing central aortic insufficiency. The gross and histologic appearances suggest that this is a variant of the more common MV prolapse.

Infectious and inflammatory etiologies of aortic insufficiency include bacterial endocarditis and rheumatic fever. Streptococci, staphylococci, or enterococci are the most common bacteria involved, in decreasing order of frequency. Syphilis is increasingly rare. Rheumatic fever often produces mixed stenosis and insufficiency but may produce aortic insufficiency alone. Concomitant MV disease is invariably present.

Patients who have a congenitally bicuspid aortic valve rarely become symptomatic during childhood, but prolonged turbulence may lead to aortic stenosis, mixed stenosis and insufficiency, or pure insufficiency later in life. Congenital causes of aortic insufficiency account for 10 to 15% of the patients operated on for aortic insufficiency as adults. Congenital aortic insufficiency may also occur secondary to subaortic VSD, with valvular insufficiency developing from a Venturi effect that results in prolapse of the aortic valve leaflet into the septal defect.

Aneurysmal dilation of the aortic root is thought to be secondary to idiopathic or known connective tissue disorders, with the idiopathic variety seen with increasing frequency as the average age of the population increases. In the less severe forms of degenerative diseases of the aorta, such as idiopathic cystic medial necrosis, there may be a localized aneurysm in the ascending aorta or aortic root, with or without associated aortic valve insufficiency, depending on the degree of distortion of the sinotubular junction. Aortoannular ectasia with aneurysm of the aortic root occurs in its most extreme form in patients with Marfan syndrome or Ehlers-Danlos syndrome. These connective tissue disorders involve defective genes coding for fibrillin cross-linkage or collagen synthesis, resulting in extensive weakness within the aortic wall with frequent involvement of the aortic root. A common presentation is aneurysmal dilation of the entire aortic root with concomitant aortic valve insufficiency. These patients also have an increased risk of aneurysmal disease elsewhere in the aorta, a high incidence of MV prolapse, and a greatly increased risk of aortic dissection. Typically, the aortic root gradually enlarges, starting in the sinuses of Valsalva and progressing until the entire root is involved. Valvular insufficiency results from dilatation of both the aortic sinotubular junction and the aortic valve annulus. The size and shape of the aneurysm is characteristic, resembling an inverted, truncated cone, with the narrow apex in the mid-to-distal ascending aorta and a large dilated aortic root.

Acute aortic dissection may produce aortic valve insufficiency by detachment of the commissures and prolapse of the valve cusps, usually involving the noncoronary cusp and the commissure between the left and right cusps. In patients with chronic dissection, the sinotubular junction is usually dilated and distorted, producing leaflet prolapse and valvular insufficiency. Both the aortic root and ascending aorta may be aneurysmal secondary to the chronic dissection.

Pathophysiology With aortic valve insufficiency, blood regurgitates into the left ventricle during diastole, producing LV volume overload (increased preload). The ventricle compensates by the Starling mechanism and increases the LV stroke volume during systole. A widened pulse pressure and low diastolic pressure result in diminished coronary perfusion, while oxygen demand is increased secondary to the large stroke volume and increased cardiac work. Progressive valvular insufficiency results in ventricular dilation and eccentric LV hypertrophy, with the heart initially compensating to maintain a normal ratio of wall thickness to cavity size. Because ventricular compliance is normal, the LV diastolic pressure does not increase initially, and the patient usually remains asymptomatic for a long period of time despite significant diastolic volume overload. As the heart continues to dilate, however, the ventricular muscle can no longer compensate and the ratio of wall thickness to cavity size decreases. The systolic wall tension required for ejection eventually exceeds the ability of the ventricular muscle to contract, resulting in "afterload mismatch" and progressive systolic dysfunction. Further progression leads to LV failure and pulmonary hypertension. In the advanced stages, fibrosis develops within the myocardium, which further contributes to systolic dysfunction, ultimately resulting in a dilated myopathic ventricle.

Clinical Manifestations Symptoms develop at variable rates in patients with aortic insufficiency, depending on the acuity and severity of the insufficiency and the compliance and strength of the heart muscle. Frequently, the patient who gradually develops moderate to severe insufficiency remains asymptomatic for many years, often 10 or more. Once symptoms appear, however, ventricular function usually is significantly depressed and rapid clinical deterioration occurs over the next 4 to 5 years. The terminal illness usually is progressive heart failure and arrhythmias.

The most common symptoms are dyspnea on exertion and decreased exercise capacity. These symptoms gradually increase in severity as the ventricle deteriorates. Palpitations are also common, apparently arising from forceful contraction of the dilated left ventricle. NYHA class IV symptoms, angina, and right heart failure occur with advanced disease or with severe incompetence in which the regurgitant flow exceeds 50% of forward flow.

Palpation reveals an enlarged heart and a prominent cardiac impulse described as a *forceful thrust*, with the point of maximal impact displaced inferiorly and leftward. The hallmark of aortic insufficiency is a high-pitched decrescendo diastolic murmur heard best in the left third intercostal space with the patient erect and leaning forward. The length of the murmur may correspond with the severity of the insufficiency, but the intensity does not. If the murmur is loudest to the right of the sternum, aortoannular ectasia is likely. A light systolic ejection murmur due to increased flow across the aortic valve may also be present. An S_3 gallop, if present, is indicative of heart failure. A middiastolic rumble at the apex that simulates mitral stenosis has been described, the Austin Flint murmur. This murmur is produced by the aortic insufficiency impeding the opening of the MV during diastole.

Examination of the peripheral arterial circulation may reveal several abnormalities. The pulse pressure is widened, partly from an increase in systolic pressure, but principally from a decrease in diastolic pressure, which may be in the range of 30 to 40 mmHg. The true diastolic pressure, measured by direct arterial puncture, is never <30 to 35 mmHg, even though, on auscultation, a diastolic pressure of zero may be obtained in some patients. Peripheral pulses usually are forceful, bounding, and quickly collapsing, termed *Corrigan's* or *water-hammer pulses*. "Pistol shot" sounds may be heard with the stethoscope over peripheral arteries. A wide variety of other auscultatory phenomena have been described, some over a century ago, all indicating vasodilatation and a hyperdynamic peripheral circulation.

Diagnostic Studies The chest x-ray usually shows impressive cardiac enlargement, with the apex displaced downward and to the left and a markedly enlarged cardiac-thoracic ratio. The ECG is normal early in the disease, but with cardiac enlargement, signs of LV hypertrophy become prominent. Sinus rhythm usually is present initially, although atrial fibrillation is common later in the course of the disease.

Echocardiography, which measures the degree of valvular insufficiency, the LV end-diastolic and end-systolic dimensions, the left atrial size, and the LV function, is the primary diagnostic tool. The echocardiogram also is used to assess the degree of mitral or tricuspid insufficiency and estimate the PA pressure.

The classic finding on cardiac catheterization is the reflux of contrast material from the aortic root into the ventricle with aortic root angiography, graded from 1+ to 4+. However, due to the accuracy of current echocardiography, angiographic studies to diagnose aortic insufficiency are no longer necessary in most cases. Aortic root angiography or MRI studies may be performed if aneurysmal disease is suspected. If surgery is planned, coronary angiography should be performed to rule out CAD in patients with appropriate risk factors. In patients with heart failure the LV end-diastolic pressure may be elevated to 15 to 20 mmHg and sometimes higher, with an associated rise in the PA pressure.

Operative Indications The development of symptoms is an absolute indication for surgery in patients with aortic insufficiency. It has long been recognized, however, that postponing surgery until the patient becomes severely symptomatic is potentially dangerous, as many patients will have already developed substantial ventricular enlargement and cardiac dysfunction by that time. Therefore, echocardiographic studies are routinely used to determine the appropriate timing for surgical intervention, which should be performed before the development of symptoms and before the ventricular function severely deteriorates. Asymptomatic patients with severe aortic insufficiency should be referred for surgery at the first sign of deteriorating LV systolic function on echocardiography, which manifests as a rise in the end-systolic dimension of the ventricle or by a drop in the ejection fraction. Operative results indicate that cardiac function will return to normal and long-term survival will be improved significantly if an operation is done at this stage.

In the authors' experience, valve replacement should be performed even in patients with low ejection fractions and advanced NYHA class IV symptoms, especially if recruitable ventricular wall motion is present with inotropic stimuli. Most class IV patients will improve significantly after surgery, although the degree of improvement may be uncertain for 6 to 12 months. Intensive postoperative medical therapy with a heart failure regimen that includes afterload reduction, low-dose beta blockers, and diuretics is beneficial in this group of patients to help remodel the left ventricle. Because ventricular arrhythmias are a common cause of death in patients with markedly depressed LV function, evidence supports routine electrophysiologic testing and implantation of an automatic internal cardiac defibrillator (ICD) if inducible arrhythmias are present.

Operative Techniques

Aortic Valve Replacement Aortic valve replacement has traditionally been performed through a median sternotomy incision, and this approach remains the standard in most cardiac centers. CPB with moderate systemic hypothermia is used, the aorta is cross-clamped, and the heart is protected by cardioplegia delivered antegrade into the aortic root directly into the coronary ostia by hand-held cannulas, or retrograde through the coronary sinus. Typically, a LV vent is inserted through the right superior pulmonary vein to keep the field free of blood during the procedure and to aid in deairing after blood flow is re-established to the heart.

After the heart has been arrested, an oblique or hockey-stick–shaped aortotomy incision is made, beginning approximately 1 cm above the right coronary artery and extending medially toward the PA and inferiorly into the noncoronary sinus. The aortic valve is excised totally (Fig. 21-16), removing all leaflets and any fragments of calcium present in the annulus. A gauze pack may be placed in the ventricle before removal of the valve to minimize the risk of calcium spillage and embolization. Serial irrigations of the ventricle are performed after removal of the valve and débridement of calcium.

At NYU, pledgeted horizontal mattress sutures are routinely used, as this technique is thought to minimize the risk of paravalvular leakage. Other suturing techniques for placement of the valve include simple interrupted sutures, figure-of-eight sutures, and continuous sutures. Care is taken to avoid damage to the coronary ostia, to the conduction bundle adjacent to the membranous septum between the right and the noncoronary valve cusps, and to the MV posteriorly. The valve may be seated on the annulus in either of

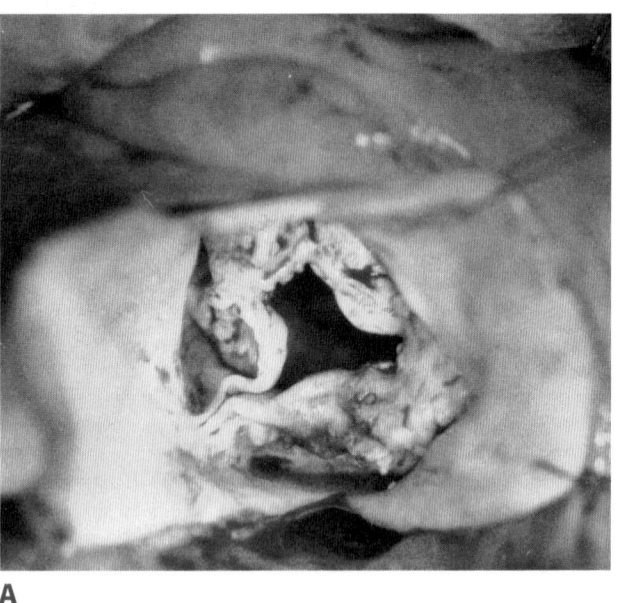 **A**
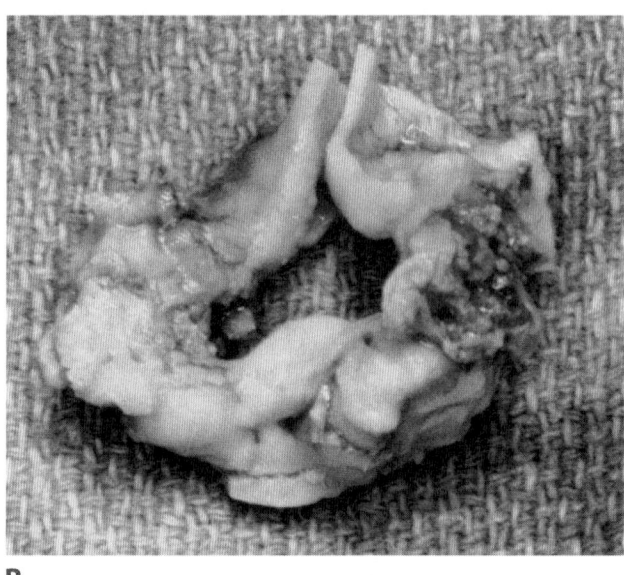 **B**
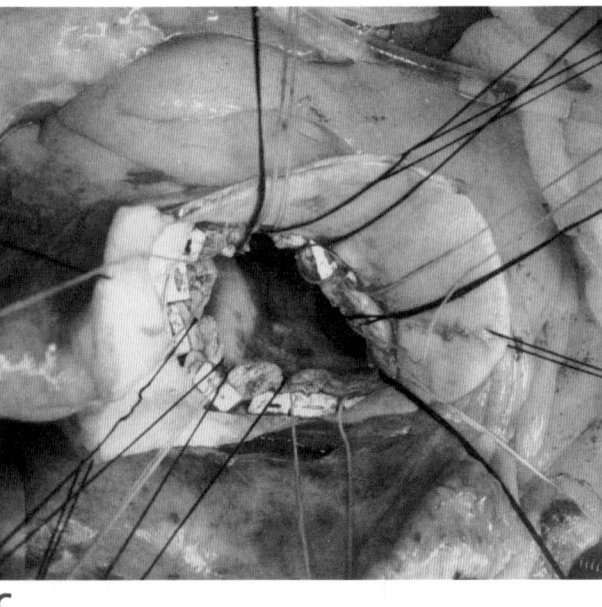 **C**
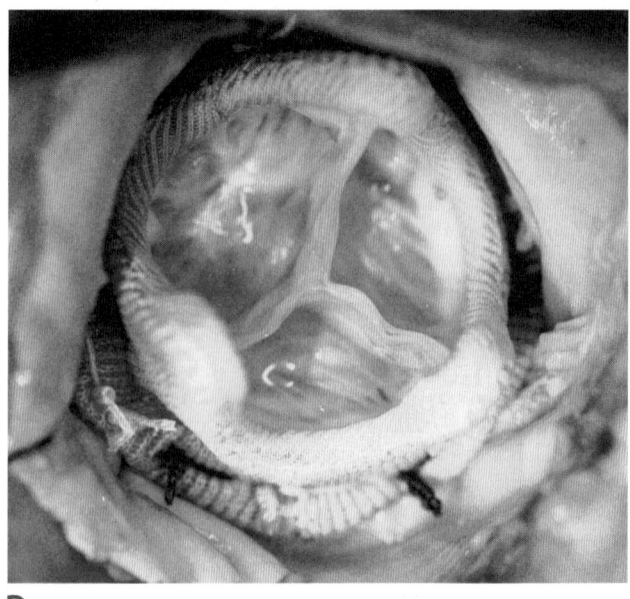 **D**

FIG. 21-16. Operation for calcific aortic stenosis. **A.** Operative photograph of calcific aortic stenosis seen through an oblique aortotomy incision. **B.** Excised aortic valve. The valve leaflets were completely immobile and fixed in the midposition, producing a mixture of aortic stenosis and aortic insufficiency. **C.** After excising the valve, pledget reinforced mattress sutures have been placed into the aortic valve annulus. The sutures will be subsequently placed through the sewing ring of the prosthetic valve. **D.** Porcine valve in the aortic position before closure of the aortotomy incision.

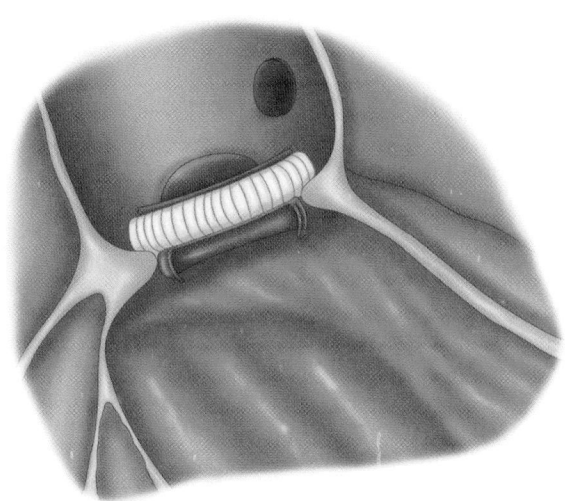

FIG. 21-17. Aortic valve replacement. Supra-annular placement of a St. Jude Hemodynamic Plus valve in the aortic position. *(Illustration courtesy of St. Jude Medical, Inc., St. Paul, MN. All rights reserved.)*

two ways. For supra-annular placement (Fig. 21-17), the sutures are placed from below the annulus in an upward direction, through the annulus, and then through the valve sewing ring. For intra-annular placement, the sutures are placed from above the annulus downward and then back up through the sewing ring, which results in the valve resting completely within the annulus.

Mechanical valves are widely used in younger patients. Two configurations are available, a single tilting disk and a bileaflet disk. The flow characteristics are extremely good with all current mechanical valves, and even better in newer designs that allow supra-annular valve placement and therefore increase the effective orifice size that can be implanted for a particular sized annulus. The flow characteristics of the valve become important when the aortic annulus is small to minimize the postoperative gradient across the smaller prosthesis. Patients with mechanical valves routinely require lifelong anticoagulation with warfarin to minimize the risk of thromboembolic complications.

Tissue valves are most commonly used in older patients, although they now are increasingly used in younger patients who want to avoid the need for long-term anticoagulation therapy. Tissue valves may be either stented or stentless, with the traditional stented valves being easier to implant, and the stentless valves having better flow characteristics, particularly in smaller valve sizes. Current tissue valves have a projected durability of 15 years or longer and do not require long-term anticoagulation.

However, a small aortic root may be a particularly difficult problem when tissue valves are placed, as the stented tissue valves have relatively poor flow characteristics in smaller sizes. This can potentially result in patient-prosthesis mismatch, which may occur if the implanted prosthesis is equal to or <19 mm and the patient's body surface area is >1.7 m^2, or when the prosthetic valve area is <0.85 cm^2/m^2. Controversy exists regarding the impact of small prosthetic valves on late survival, although avoiding patient-prosthesis mismatch clearly results in better postoperative LV mass regression. Surgical options to avoid patient-prosthesis mismatch include use of valves that have better flow characteristics in small sizes, such as supra-annular mechanical valves, stentless tissue valves, or homografts. Alternately, a larger size stented tissue valve can be placed using procedures to enlarge the aortic annulus.

Results The operative risk for aortic valve replacement is 1 to 5% for most patients, but may be considerably higher in elderly patients with multiple comorbidities and in patients with severely depressed LV function. Chaliki and associates[31] reported that aortic valve replacement in patients with aortic insufficiency and poor LV function (ejection fraction <35%) resulted in increased operative risk, 14% compared to 3.7% in patients with ejection fractions >50%. Ten-year survival was 70% in patients with good ventricular function, but only 42% in patients with ejection fractions <35%.

The STS National Database lists the clinical variables affecting the operative risk associated with valve surgery. The major risk factors are age, body surface area, diabetes, renal failure, hypertension, chronic lung disease, PVD, cerebrovascular accident, infectious endocarditis, prior cardiac operation, MI, cardiogenic shock, NYHA functional status, and elevated PA mean pressure. The overall incidence of perioperative stroke is 2.8 to 4.8%.

The 10-year survival after aortic valve replacement in patients <65 years of age exceeds 80% but may be significantly worse in patients with severely impaired ventricular function. The factors affecting late survival are age, NYHA functional status, ventricular function, concomitant CAD, concomitant disease in another valve and diabetes, previous MI, CHF, and urgent or emergent surgery.

Postoperative Care Postoperative care is usually uneventful after aortic valve replacement in patients with normal LV function. However, patients with significantly reduced LV function may have a complicated postoperative course. Arrhythmias are relatively common, and continuous ECG monitoring is required for the first 48 hours. Anticoagulation therapy is started 1 day after mechanical valve replacement, targeting an INR of 2.5 to 3 times normal. Antiplatelet therapy with aspirin is used in patients with tissue valves, homografts, or autografts. The postoperative hospital stay is usually approximately 5 days, depending on the patient's age and overall physical condition. Early cardiac rehabilitation is particularly helpful in elderly patients.

Except for patients with severe ventricular dysfunction, most patients become asymptomatic and regain a normal range of physical activity within 1 to 2 months after operation. Periodic medical evaluations should be instituted for all patients because of the problems inherent with use of any prosthetic valve. The patient should have long-term monitoring for proper anticoagulation therapy (with the INR followed in patients on warfarin), and the valve function should be periodically assessed by echocardiography. Thromboembolism, anticoagulant-related hemorrhage, endocarditis, and prosthetic valve failure are the principal late complications. Both thromboembolism and anticoagulant-related hemorrhage occur with incidences of 1 to 2% per year after mechanical valve replacement, despite careful anticoagulation therapy and monitoring. Patients with tissue valves have a risk of thromboembolism of 0.5 to 1% per year, but anticoagulant-related hemorrhage is less common because warfarin is not required. Endocarditis remains an infrequent but serious late hazard after valve replacement, and routine antibiotic prophylaxis is recommended lifelong for any invasive procedure that might produce a transient bacteremia.

Aortic Valve Repair Aortic valve repair rarely has been used as the primary treatment for aortic insufficiency because of the high risk of late repair failure. Recently, however, David, Yacoub, and Casselman independently described different techniques for valve repair in patients with aortic insufficiency, with encouraging results.[62–64]

David's approach is based on the principle that aortic insufficiency in patients with aortoannular ectasia is secondary to annular dilatation and distortion of the sinotubular junction. David's approach involved excising the aneurysmal portion of the aortic root and reimplanting the aortic valve inside a tubular Dacron graft, using a technique similar to homograft implantation, with reimplantation of the coronary arteries. Late results were reported in 230 patients who underwent aortic valve-sparing operations for aortic insufficiency. The 8-year survival was 83% and the 8-year freedom from reoperation was 99%.

Yacoub reported a similar valve-sparing technique for patients with annuloaortic ectasia. With Yacoub's technique the aortic wall and sinuses of Valsalva are excised down to the anatomic annulus. The Dacron graft is sutured to the annulus, the valve is resuspended, and the coronary buttons are reimplanted.

The technique described by Casselman and associates for repair of aortic insufficiency in patients with bicuspid aortic valves involves triangular resection of the redundant segment of the involved valve cusp in an attempt to achieve cusp symmetry, followed by annular plication of one or both commissures. Results were reported after repair in 94 patients. The freedom from reoperation was 95%, 87%, and 84% at 1, 5, and 7 years, respectively.

Ross Procedure The Ross procedure involves replacement of the aortic valve with an autograft from the patient's native pulmonary valve. The resected pulmonary valve is then replaced with a pulmonary homograft. Variations of the technique of implantation of the autograft for the aortic valve replacement include free-hand replacement with resuspension of the valve commissures, and cylinder root replacement with reimplantation of the coronary artery ostia (see Fig. 21-9).

The cylinder root replacement technique is the most reproducible. With this method, the native aorta is transected 5 mm above the sinotubular ridge. The aortic valve leaflets and the aortic tissue in the sinuses of Valsalva are totally removed, preserving the left main and right coronary arteries on buttons of aortic tissue. The main PA is transected at the bifurcation, and a separate incision is made below the pulmonary valve in the right ventricular outflow tract. The pulmonary valve and artery are enucleated en bloc from the outflow tract bed, with care being taken to avoid injury to the first septal perforator as the valve is removed from the septum medially. The pulmonary autograft annulus is sutured to the aortic annulus with continuous or interrupted sutures, and the coronary arteries are reimplanted into the autograft. The pulmonary valve and right ventricular outflow are reconstructed in standard fashion with a homograft.

The Ross procedure has risks similar to those associated with standard aortic valve replacement, although the risk of bleeding may be slightly higher. The primary benefit is that patients do not require long-term anticoagulation and the risk of thromboembolism is negligible. Midterm durability of both the autograft and the pulmonary homograft has been good at 7 to 12 years postoperatively. Paparella and associates reported results in 155 patients, with an 86% 7-year period of freedom from severe recurrent insufficiency. However, progressive late aortic insufficiency has been described in a number of patients, along with calcification of the pulmonary homograft and pulmonary stenosis.[65] The risk of late reoperation ranges from 30 to 50% at 15 to 20 years.

Minimally Invasive Aortic Valve Surgery Minimally invasive approaches for aortic valve surgery have recently become an acceptable alternative to conventional median sternotomy. Both ministernotomy and minithoracotomy approaches have been used with excellent success.[66,67] Although the proposed benefits of minimally invasive aortic valve replacement remain controversial, several centers have reported results that are at least comparable to standard surgery, but with less need for blood transfusions and shorter hospital stays.[68,69] Recent review of the extensive NYU experience demonstrated a survival advantage for this minimally invasive approach for high-risk patients requiring aortic valve surgery over the last decade.[32]

At NYU, minimally invasive aortic valve replacement is performed through a right anterior minithoracotomy incision, with central aortic cannulation and vacuum-assisted venous drainage. An external cross-clamp is applied directly to the aorta, and the heart is protected with traditional cardioplegic methods. This approach has now been used in >1000 patients. A report by Grossi and colleagues demonstrated that patients treated with the minimally invasive approach had less need for blood transfusions, fewer infections, and a shorter hospital stay than matched patients receiving traditional surgery.[54] Sharony and coworkers reported results in elderly patients, demonstrating shorter hospital stay and rehabilitation time.[67] Thus, minimally invasive approaches for aortic valve replacement appear promising and deserve further investigation.

Idiopathic Hypertrophic Subaortic Stenosis

Patients with hypertrophic cardiomyopathy or IHSS have varying degrees of subaortic LV outflow tract obstruction, usually associated with systolic anterior motion of the MV. Systolic anterior motion of the valve has been explained by the presence of Venturi forces created by the high-velocity flow in the narrowed outflow tract, which pulls the adjacent anterior leaflet of the MV into the outflow tract, worsening outflow obstruction. The subaortic obstruction may have a dynamic component and can usually be provoked with volume depletion, vasodilators, or inotropes. The intracavitary pressure of the left ventricle is usually markedly elevated, and the ventricle is hypercontractile with impaired diastolic relaxation. The degree of LV outflow tract obstruction at rest is a strong predictor of progression to severe symptoms of heart failure and death. However, most patients with hypertrophic cardiomyopathy and subaortic obstruction will respond to medical therapy, and only a minority will require surgical intervention.

Operative Techniques

Surgical septal myotomy and myectomy, developed by Morrow, has shown consistent results and remains the primary technique for treatment of IHSS.[70] This approach requires resection of a trough of muscle from the subaortic outflow tract. Typically, the resection is 1 cm wide and 1 cm deep, and extends the length of the septum to below the lower edge of the anterior leaflet of the MV. The resected trough should remain leftward of the right coronary ostium to avoid heart block but should routinely produce a left bundle-branch block. A modification of the Morrow myectomy, termed extended myectomy, involves mobilization and partial excision of the papillary muscles. The extended approach has been suggested to resect the deeper portion of the septal bulge and redirect the flow medially and anteriorly away from the MV, abolishing systolic anterior motion. However, there are few data to suggest that the extended myectomy procedure improves late outcomes.

Tricuspid Stenosis and Insufficiency

Acquired TV disease can be classified as organic or functional. Organic disease is almost always a result of either rheumatic fever or endocarditis. In patients with rheumatic disease, tricuspid stenosis or insufficiency virtually never occurs as an isolated lesion, but only in association with extensive disease of the MV. With mitral disease, the frequency of associated tricuspid disease is 10 to 15%, although an incidence as high as 30% has been reported. Rarely, blunt trauma produces rupture of a papillary muscle or chordae tendineae with resultant tricuspid insufficiency.

Functional tricuspid regurgitation is much more common than insufficiency from organic disease. Functional tricuspid regurgitation develops from dilatation of the tricuspid annulus and right ventricle as a result of pulmonary hypertension and right ventricular failure. These abnormalities usually result from MV disease or from other conditions that result in LV failure and pulmonary hypertension.

With tricuspid stenosis, the pathologic changes are similar to those found with the more familiar mitral stenosis, with fusion of the commissures. Because right atrial pressure is normally only 4 to 5 mmHg, significant tricuspid stenosis may be present with a valve orifice considerably larger than that seen with mitral stenosis. With rheumatic disease, mixed tricuspid stenosis and insufficiency or pure insufficiency may result from fibrosis and contraction of the valve leaflets, often in association with shortening and fusion of chordae tendineae. Calcification is rare.

Functional dilatation of the tricuspid annulus results in tricuspid insufficiency. The valve leaflets appear stretched, but otherwise are pliable and seemingly normal, even though serious regurgitation is present. The dilatation and deformity of the annulus are irreversible. Valves with severe functional insufficiency and a markedly dilated annulus usually do not regain competency, even after the MV disease is corrected and PA systolic pressure returns to normal.

Pathophysiology

With tricuspid stenosis or severe insufficiency, the mean right atrial pressure becomes elevated to 10 to 20 mmHg or higher. The higher pressures are found with a TV orifice <1.5 cm^2 and a mean diastolic gradient between the atrium and ventricle of 5 to 15 mmHg or in patients with pulmonary hypertension and severe insufficiency. When the mean right atrial pressure remains >15 mmHg, hepatomegaly, ascites, and leg edema usually appear.

Clinical Manifestations

The symptoms and signs of TV disease are similar to those of right heart failure resulting from MV disease. They result from chronic elevation of right atrial pressure above the range of 15 to 20 mmHg. Clinical manifestations include jugulovenous distention, hepatomegaly, pedal edema, and ascites. With long-standing severe tricuspid insufficiency, hepatic dysfunction and clotting abnormalities may develop.

The characteristic murmur of tricuspid stenosis is best heard as a diastolic murmur at the lower end of the sternum. It is a low-pitched murmur of medium intensity and can easily be overlooked because it is well localized at the lower end of the sternum. During inspiration, the intensity of the murmur increases as the volume of blood returning to the heart is temporarily raised by an increase in intrathoracic negative pressure. Tricuspid insufficiency produces a prominent systolic murmur heard best at the left lower sternal border. The murmur often is found in association with an enlarged, pulsating liver and prominent and engorged jugular veins. A prominent jugular venous pulsation, especially when the cardiac rhythm is sinus, may be the best clue to unsuspected tricuspid disease. A hepatojugular reflex also may be noted.

Diagnostic Studies

The x-ray shows enlargement of the right atrium and right ventricle. Echocardiography confirms the diagnosis and differentiates stenosis from insufficiency. Cardiac catheterization is no longer necessary in most cases.

Indications for Surgery

Indications for surgery are based primarily on clinical findings, which are correlated with echocardiographic findings and hemodynamics. Severe insufficiency is indicated by echocardiography when the area of the regurgitant jet occupies a large part of the atrium, the effective regurgitant orifice is >40 mm^2, or the width of the vena contracta (narrowest flow) is >6.5 mm.[71] Severe tricuspid regurgitation should clearly be repaired because it has been widely demonstrated that annuloplasty provides excellent late results with little added morbidity. Mild degrees of tricuspid insufficiency are usually left alone, especially in the absence of pulmonary hypertension, while repair of moderate insufficiency requires further consideration of the clinical findings and symptoms present. However, effective TV repair minimizes the risk of late right-sided heart failure and reoperation.

Operative Techniques

In the small minority of patients whose tricuspid stenosis is secondary to pure commissural fusion, a commissurotomy may be performed, usually combined with an annuloplasty. More commonly, valve replacement is necessary when significant tricuspid stenosis is present because the entire valve and subvalvular apparatus are damaged. When a prosthetic valve is inserted, care is required in suture placement along the septal leaflet where the conduction bundle is located, and sutures should be placed more superficially in this area.

In patients with functional tricuspid insufficiency, the annulus is markedly dilated while the leaflets appear entirely normal. Virtually all such patients can be treated by annuloplasty. The suture annuloplasty techniques proposed by Kay and Boyd and the De Vega annuloplasty technique have been highly reliable. Alternatively, a flexible or rigid annuloplasty device may be used.

Results

Data on more than 300 patients from the authors' institution show that the suture annuloplasty repair for functional tricuspid insufficiency is reproducible in the absence of significant intrinsic leaflet disease. Valve repair using a posterior suture annuloplasty technique was 98% durable at 7 years. Similar results have been reported with the De Vega annuloplasty.[72] Other centers prefer the use of rigid or flexible annuloplasty devices for correction of tricuspid insufficiency, especially if the right heart pressures are expected to remain chronically elevated.

When TV replacement is required, the options include use of either a tissue valve or a mechanical valve. Carrier and associates reported follow-up on 97 patients who underwent TV replacement with either tissue valves ($n = 82$) or mechanical valves ($n = 15$).[73] The 5-year freedom from reoperation was 92% in patients with mechanical valves and 97% in patients with tissue valves ($P = .2$). Data suggest that the risk of valve thrombosis is increased in mechanical valves placed in the tricuspid position, as emphasized in a report by Kawano and colleagues that demonstrated a 30% risk of mechanical valve thrombosis in the tricuspid position over 15 years, with a linearized rate of 2.9% per patient-year.[74] Bioprostheses are therefore preferred for most patients requiring TV replacement.

Multivalve Disease

Disease involving multiple valves is relatively common, particularly in patients with rheumatic disease. Prominent signs in one valve can readily mask disease in others. With aortic valve disease, functional mitral insufficiency can result from a progressive rise in the LV end-diastolic pressure and volume. Similarly, MV disease may result in pulmonary hypertension, right heart failure, and functional tricuspid insufficiency. Often these secondary functional changes resolve without treatment if the primary pathology is corrected in a timely fashion. Certainly, multiple-valve surgery has a higher operative risk than single-valve procedures, in part because the condition often represents more advanced disease and is associated with significant cardiac dysfunction.

In a 1992 report by Galloway and colleagues, 513 patients with multiple-valve disease treated surgically between 1976 and 1985 were studied to assess factors influencing operative risk and long-term survival.[75] Three groups accounted for the majority of the cases: 58% had aortic valve and MV disease, 29% had MV and TV disease, and 12% had triple-valve disease (aortic, MV, and TV). Preoperative CHF was present in 91%, 41% were NYHA class III, and 54% were NYHA class IV. The average PA systolic pressure was 60 mmHg. Despite chronic symptoms and severe disease, the overall operative mortality rate was 12.5% and the 5-year survival rate was 67%. The variables predicting decreased survival time were systolic PA pressure, age, triple-valve procedures, concomitant coronary bypass grafting, previous heart surgery, and diabetes. After operation, 80% of the patients improved to NYHA class I or II, demonstrating that most patients will have significant clinical improvement despite advanced symptoms preoperatively. The 5-year freedom from late cardiac-related death or complications was 82%.

Aortic and Mitral Valve Disease

Nine combinations of valvular pathology can produce aortic and MV disease because each valve can be stenotic, insufficient, or both. Stenosis in both valves may lead to underestimation of the degree of aortic stenosis, because return of blood to the left ventricle is limited as a result of mitral stenosis. Aortic insufficiency, which produces the Austin Flint murmur, might overshadow and mask true mitral stenosis. With functional mitral insufficiency resulting from severe aortic disease, aortic valve replacement can lead to resolution of insufficiency in some patients, but patients with more severe mitral insufficiency may require mitral repair or replacement. Patients presenting with aortic valve and MV disease should be examined closely for these and other considerations.

Mitral and Tricuspid Valve Disease

Multiple combinations of valvular pathology are possible with mitral and tricuspid disease, but mitral disease with functional tricuspid insufficiency is the most common scenario, resulting from chronic pulmonary hypertension and right heart failure. The presence of associated tricuspid insufficiency increases the operative risk for patients undergoing MV surgery. The risk for isolated MV and TV disease is approximately 6%.

Triple-Valve Disease

Triple-valve surgery can be challenging because the clinical condition usually is a result of chronic aortic and mitral disease with severe pulmonary hypertension, biventricular failure, and functional tricuspid insufficiency. Occasionally, rheumatic disease affects all three valves. The degree of pulmonary hypertension is the most significant predictor of survival in patients with triple-valve disease. The operative morality for 61 triple-valve procedures in an NYU report was only 5.6% when the PA systolic pressure was <60 mmHg, but >25% when the PA pressures were above 60 mmHg and the patients were >70 years of age.[75] This emphasizes the value of an early operation, before the development of irreversible ventricular dysfunction and chronic pulmonary hypertension.

SURGICAL THERAPY FOR THE FAILING HEART

Epidemiology of Congestive Heart Failure

CHF affects 5.2 million people in the United States with >500,000 new cases per year. Patients with NYHA IV CHF from CAD have an extremely poor outlook, with 43% and 18% survival at 1 and 3 years, respectively, and the risk of sudden cardiac death is higher, being 6 to 9 times greater than the general population. In the United States, there were >1 million hospital discharges for CHF in 2005 and >3.4 million outpatient visits. The estimated cost of care in 2008 was $3.48 billion.

Etiology and Pathophysiology

The causes of heart failure differ widely. It can be broken down to idiopathic or secondary causes. Causes include hypertension, CAD, structural valve disease, and other miscellaneous causes such as postviral, postpartum, and hypertrophic.

Often, the inciting event is an injury. This can be regional or global. In the case of MI, after a heart attack, the affected region becomes akinetic with the ingrowth of scar tissue. This area no longer contracts. If the area is large enough, the remaining walls have to compensate. This sometimes requires enlargement of the ventricle to maintain adequate cardiac output. An additional effect is the change in the normal elliptical shape of the ventricle. Additional adverse side effects include elevated left atrial pressures, ventricular and atrial dysrhythmias, LV dyssynchrony, and geometric distortion of the MV apparatus. This process is referred to as *remodeling*.

Surgery for Cardiomyopathy and Congestive Heart Failure

Heart transplant remains the gold standard for the surgical treatment of end-stage heart disease. Late- and end-stage heart disease, also known as *cardiomyopathy*, often is accompanied by symptoms of CHF. The increasing incidence of heart failure combined with new surgical modalities, improved safety of conventional surgery, and better understanding of the natural history of heart failure, has pushed surgery for CHF into the mainstream of cardiac surgery. There is an increased demand for patients with late-stage or end-stage heart disease to be considered for surgical therapies.[76]

The goals of surgical therapy include improving survival, improving symptoms or the quality of life, or preventing further ongoing insults. Although ideal, a survival benefit in the short or intermediate term is not always possible, and certainly, by the time CHF has presented, surgical therapy is palliative in most cases.

Dobutamine echocardiography is a valuable diagnostic test in patients with cardiomyopathy. This test provides the usual two-dimensional pictures of regional cardiac function. Improved segmental contractility at low doses (5 mcg/kg per minute) and worsening function higher doses indicate both viability and predict functional recovery after revascularization. Cardiac MRI has become a preferred diagnostic test, providing the surgeon with the three-dimensional shape and function of the heart. Wall thinness and lack of myocardial thickening are good indicators of chronic scaring. Gadolinium hyperenhancement quantifies the amount of scar tissues in the segments of heart and its absence is highly predictive of recovery of function after revascularization. Finally, cardiopulmonary exercise testing is used to measure the degree of cardiac dysfunction as it pertains to a heart's ability to support metabolism. In patients with severe heart failure, it allows interpretation of symptoms and determination of prognosis. It also can be used to determine whether a patient is potentially best suited for cardiac transplantation.

Ischemic Cardiomyopathy

Surgical coronary revascularization is one of the most commonly performed procedures for CHF. Coronary bypass grafting is the primary strategy of treatment for ischemic cardiomyopathy.

Good target vessels are essential to successful revascularization in ischemic cardiomyopathy. Old age and poor quality of distal coronary vessels were the significant risk factors for successful outcome after surgical revascularization, with completely poor distal vessels having a 100% predictive value of hospital death and, thus, should be considered a strong contraindication.[77]

Myocardial viability is the pivotal variable in the assessment of these patients. Ongoing angina is often a sufficient indicator to proceed to surgery. In the patient with ischemic cardiomyopathy and CHF symptoms alone that are not related to acute ischemia, viability testing is used to determine whether surgery will improve outcomes. Patients with viability have significantly improved hospital survival and 2-year outcomes compared to those without, whereas patients with no viability show no benefit from surgical revascularization. In fact, patients with viable myocardium who did not undergo revascularization had double the mortality rate of all patients without viability and five times the mortality rate of those who underwent revascularization.[78] This underscores both the importance of viable myocardium as well as the adverse consequences of not offering a patient with viability surgical intervention.

Other risk factors for short and intermediate term outcomes include LV size and LV dyssynchrony. A LV end-systolic dimension >100mL/m^2 carries an adverse prognosis. Short-term and long-term survival after CABG were significantly reduced in those patients whose preoperative LV dimensions exceeded this threshold, 85 vs. 53% at 5 years (P <.05). Similarly, freedom from recurrent CHF was 85 vs. 31% at 5 years (P <.01).[79] LV dyssynchrony held a much higher predictive value than even viability in moderate to high-risk revascularization. Hospital mortality was 2.9 vs. 27.3% (P <.001), with an ongoing effect over the next 2 years.[80]

Functional Mitral Regurgitation

Functional mitral regurgitation (FMR) is defined as MR secondary to ventricular dysfunction with structurally normal valve leaflets and subvalvular apparatus. In these cases, there is a failure of the valve leaflets to adequately coapt, causing the valve to leak. Structural problems in the geometry, size, and function of the left ventricle are responsible for the mitral dysfunction. There are several components of LV abnormalities that contribute to the pathology. First is LV dyssynchrony. Poor coordination of the contraction of the septum and lateral walls can cause MR that varies in intensity during the cardiac cycle, and can sometime be severe. The classic Carpentier classification system refers to functional regurgitation as a I/IIIb type of lesion. Annular dilatation (type I) and LV distortion (type IIIB) both play roles. FMR can further be classified. Ischemic functional mitral regurgitation (IMR) is a consequence of myocardial ischemia and almost always infarction. Pure FMR is associated with dilated cardiomyopathies. There are many differences and similarities between these subsets.

As the ventricular geometry and function of the left ventricle deteriorate, there is enlargement of the septal lateral dimension of the mitral annulus, reducing the coaptation length on the edges of the MV. Additionally, and more importantly, as the left ventricle enlarges, the papillary muscles are pulled down away from the mitral annulus and outward. This prevents the leaflets of the MV from coming back to the annular plane and further impairs the coaptation. In dilated (nonischemic) cardiomyopathy, this tends to be a symmetric event. In ischemic MR, the area of LV dysfunction most often correlates with the area of MI and secondary remodeling, usually in the inferior and posterior segments of the left ventricle. This correlated with coronary events in the inferior and terminal circumflex coronary distributions. The result is usually a more heterogeneous pathologic process with annular enlargement in the P3 area, and disproportional displacement of the posterior medical papillary muscle. Usually, there is significant decrease in the overall LVEF. LV remodeling leads to an enlarged ventricle with a less elliptical shape, and more MR. This increased regurgitation leads to increased preload, increased wall tension, and increased LV work load, all of which contribute to further LV dysfunction and to progressive heart failure.

The impact of IMR/FMR on long-term survival is significant. The presence of MR is a marker of the severity of disease. After MI, the presence of any MR reduced the 5-year survival from 61 to 38% (P <.001). Patients with moderate or greater MR had only a 29% 5-year survival compared to those with milder MR who had 47% 5-year survival (P <.0001).[81] Medical therapy and PCI have not reduced the impact of IMR on late mortality after MI.[82]

Many patients with IMR come to the operating room with indications for coronary revascularization in the setting of reduced ventricular function. Some patients present with primary CHF and valve indications for surgery. Current recommendations are to surgically address the MV if the MR is severe or if the MR is moderate and symptoms of CHF are present. A growing number of centers will address moderate MR in those patients who are at otherwise low risk for CABG.

MV repair is the procedure of choice. Currently, the recommendations are to use a complete semirigid or rigid ring and to downsize the mitral annulus by two full ring sizes. This seems to provide the greatest success in a competent MV, and seems to promote reverse remodeling and more effectively guard against recurrence. MV replacement, with sparing of the subvalvar apparatus, is indicated when there are complicated issues such as severe tethering of the leaflets, massive LV dilation, or NYHA class 4 symptoms.

Outcomes from surgery are heterogeneous and correlate to the severity of the case mix. Operative mortality runs from <1 to 9% in contemporary series and is related to the severity of LV dysfunction, acuity of presentation, severity of MR, severity of heart failure, and medical comorbidities. It is currently believed at most large centers that the addition of a MV procedure has little impact on short-term mortality in the majority of patients. Revascularization improves survival of patients with ischemic MR. It is unclear whether the addition of a MV procedure further improves survival.[83] Adherence to a strict downsizing strategy of the mitral ring appears to mitigate against recurrence and allow for some reverse remodeling.[84]

In a 2006 FDA trial study, isolated MV repairs in a predominately nonischemic cardiomyopathy population had a surprisingly low surgical mortality of 1.6% with a 2-year survival of 85%.[85] In addition, there was improvement in NYHA class and quality of life, and echocardiographic evidence of improved cardiac performance.

Left Ventricular Aneurysmorrhaphy and Surgical Ventricular Reconstruction

The third clinical component of ischemic cardiomyopathy is the postinfarction ventricular aneurysm or postinfarction areas of akinesia associated with significant LV enlargement. Similar to the previously discussed pathologies of ischemic cardiomyopathy and functional mitral regurgitation, this is a heterogeneous group of patients with differing amounts of coronary disease and viable myocardium.

Approximately 5 to 10% of transmural MIs result in LV aneurysms, which develop 4 to 8 weeks following transmural infarct as necrotic myocardium is replaced by fibrous tissue. Collateral coronary circulation in the area of the infarct and reperfusion of the infarct vessel probably limits aneurysm formation in many patients by maintaining partial myocardial viability.

The classic aneurysm is an avascular thin scar, 4 to 6 mm thick, which bulges outward (paradoxical motion) when the remaining LV muscle contracts in systole (Fig. 21-18). More than 80% of aneurysms are in the anteroseptal and apical portions of the left ventricle, resulting from occlusions of the left anterior descending coronary artery. Patients with anteroapical aneurysms usually also have significant aneurysmal dilation of the upper part of the ventricular septum. Posterior ventricular aneurysms are less common (15 to 20%), and lateral wall aneurysms are rare. Mural thrombus can be found attached to the ventricular surface of the aneurysm in more than one half of patients.

As the aneurysm enlarges, it is associated with a progressive deterioration of LV function due to the LV remodeling. As stated in the Functional MR section, remodeling consists of increasing LV volume, a more spherical LV shape, and worsening efficiency and energetics of the remaining remote myocardium, all leading to globally decreased LV performance. The LV end-diastolic and end-systolic volumes both increase, and the LV end-diastolic pressure is usually elevated. The combination of elevated intracavitary pressure and radius results in a significant elevation in wall tension, according to Laplace's law, and oxygen requirements are increased. The increased wall tension and oxygen consumption may result in angina, which may be worsened by accompanying coronary disease in noninfarcted areas of the heart. Areas of scar tissue around the edge of the aneurysm frequently serve as foci for ventricular arrhythmias, which are prominent in 15 to 20% of patients with LV aneurysms. Symptoms of LV aneurysms include angina, CHF, ventricular arrhythmias, rare embolic phenomenon, and, almost never, rupture.

Diagnostic Evaluation

Diagnostic evaluation is most often for CAD, then to identify those patients who may benefit from surgical ventricular reconstruction. Evidence of a large prior anterior wall MI or a total LAD occlusion should prompt an investigation of the left ventricle size and shape by right anterior oblique or biplane ventriculogram. Transthoracic echocardiography gives important information regarding LV function, size, and MV function, and also can suggest apical LV dyskinesis or thrombus. It is now accepted that cardiac MRI is now the best diagnostic modality, accurately identifying areas of viability by localizing thinned and scarred areas of the myocardium.

Indications for Surgery

Many patients come to surgery for standard coronary bypass indications. The rest present during evaluation for CHF or arrhythmias. CHF or advanced NYHA functional class is not a prerequisite for surgery. Although not absolute, the indications for this procedure mandate an

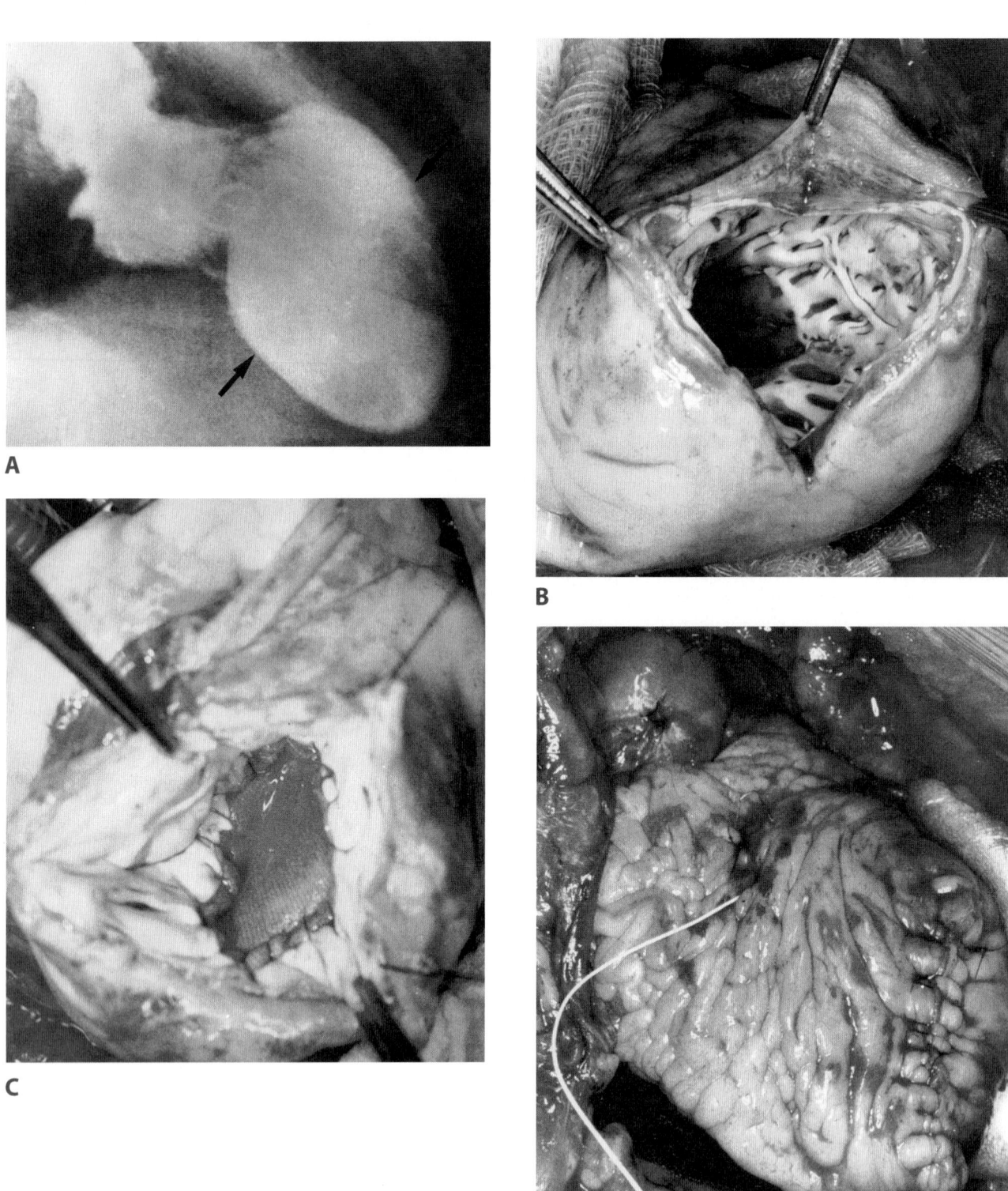

A

B

C

D

FIG. 21-18. Left ventricular aneurysm. **A.** A left ventriculogram demonstrating a large left ventricular aneurysm. *Arrows* point to outline of aneurysm cavity distal to the normal ventricle. Note the contrast to the normal left ventriculogram demonstrated in Fig. 21-1B. **B.** Operative photograph of open left ventricular aneurysm. Aneurysmal involvement of the ventricular septum was present, and significant subendocardial scar is seen. **C.** Aneurysm repair using a Dacron patch and the endoaneurysmorrhaphy technique, which excludes the aneurysm and the aneurysmal septum from the normal part of the left ventricular cavity. **D.** The wall of the aneurysm has been closed over the Dacron patch, completing the endoaneurysmorrhaphy technique.

enlarged left ventricle, left ventricular end-diastolic volume index >110 mL/m² or left ventricular end-systolic volume index >80 mL/m², and an anterior septal MI with an area of akinetic or dyskinetic wall with thinned myocardium subtending about 30% of the total circumference of the heart. There has to be good basilar heart function and reasonable distal coronary targets for those patients with ischemic myocardium that requires revascularization. Relative contraindications include the absence of thinned myocardium, poor distal coronary artery targets, poor basilar heart function, poor right ventricular function, and severe pulmonary hypertension without significant MR.

Surgery

Like ischemic MR, the primary therapy for a left ventricular aneurysm is surgical revascularization. Operative principles stress complete revascularization, including the LAD if possible. The classic repair was performed by excision of the aneurysm and linear closure of the ventricle. Disadvantages of this linear closure technique included not addressing the thinned, aneurysmal septum, and the possible undesirable geometry of the remaining left ventricle. Therefore, more physiologic techniques of ventricular reconstruction have evolved in the hands of Jatene, Cooley, and Dor. These intracavitary repair techniques all share the principle of downsizing the left ventricle, and excluding the infarct area high up on the anterior septum to achieve a more physiologic size and shape ventricle.[86-88]

Results

As a proof of concept, a large international study (RESTORE) investigated outcomes after surgical anterior ventricular endocardial restoration in 439 patients with ischemic cardiomyopathy as a result of anterior infarction. They found an overall hospital mortality of 6.6%, with an increase in ejection fraction from 29.7 to 40% and a 3-year survival rate approaching 90%. These encouraging results suggest the benefit that patients with ischemic cardiomyopathy may gain from ventricular remodeling procedures.[89]

The operative mortality for surgical ventricular restoration is 4.9%. Significant MR increases the operative risk to 13%.[90] LV performance improved, with the ejection fraction increasing from 33 to 40%, left ventricular end-diastolic volume decreasing from 211 to 142 mL, and left ventricular end-systolic volume from 145 to 88 mL. NYHA class decreased from 2.7 + 0.9 to 1.6 + 0.7 late after surgery and 10-year survival was 63%. Risk factors for poor outcomes included MR >2+, advanced NYHA class, and diastolic dysfunction. Other benefits included documentation of improved remote regional wall motion, improvements in ventricular synchrony, and improvements in the neurohumoral profile of heart failure patients.

Cardiac Restraint Devices

Another attempt at halting ventricular remodeling and inducing "reverse remodeling" is the use of external restraint devices. The Acorn CorCap Cardiac Restraint Device is an external mesh that is applied to myopathic ventricles either at the time of MV surgery or as a stand-alone procedure. As an adjunct to MV remodeling annuloplasty the cardiac restraint device added a significant but probably clinically unimportant additional reduction in ventricular size and return to a more elliptical shape. In stand-alone patients, there was improved freedom from adverse cardiac events and improvements in quality of life as well as reduction in LV volumes and sphericity.[85] The Myocor Coapsys device is another external restraint system that also addresses ventricular shape. This device consists of a set of pads external to the LV connected by a intracavitary suture. The suture is tightened to both reshape the LV and treat FMR.[91] Both of the above devices are under clinical investigation.

Mechanical Circulatory Support

Intra-Aortic Balloon Pump

The IABP is the first line and most common technique for mechanical circulatory support. It is easily deployable in the catheterization laboratory, operating room, or at the bedside. A balloon catheter is inserted through the femoral artery and advanced into the thoracic aorta. With electronic synchronization, the balloon is inflated during diastole and deflated during systole. Coronary blood flow is increased by improved diastolic perfusion, and afterload is reduced. The cardiac index typically improves after insertion, and the preload decreases. Total myocardial oxygen consumption is diminished by approximately 15%.

The most frequent indications for use of IABP are to provide hemodynamic support during or after cardiac catheterization, cardiogenic shock, weaning from CPB, and for preoperative use in high-risk patients and refractory unstable angina. The use of a preoperative IABP in patients with severe LV dysfunction or unstable angina with critical coronary anatomy has resulted in improved outcomes. Kang reported significantly lower risk-adjusted mortality in high-risk patients requiring CABG if a preoperative IABP was used.[92]

Generally, the IABP is used for a few days with minimal morbidity. Analysis of 911 patients undergoing CABG who received IABP revealed that the duration of IABP therapy ranged from 20 hours to 21 days (mean 3.8 days). Major complications occurred in 5.9% of the patients, and minor complications in 5.8%. Ischemia of the limb requiring thromboembolectomy developed in 2.7%.[93] Limb ischemia on the side of insertion is the most serious complication, and the extremity must be examined frequently for viability.

Ventricular Assist Devices

Indications for ventricular assist device (VAD) support are anytime the heart can no longer support the oxygen delivery demands of the body. Patients can have pre-existing chronic heart failure or acute heart failure after MI, viral illness, or after unsuccessful surgery or intervention. Indications include cardiac index <2 L/min per square meter, systolic blood pressure <90 mmHg, pulmonary capillary wedge pressure or CVP >18, SVR >2100, low urine output, metabolic acidosis, and decreased mental status. Contraindications are relative but include sepsis, severe PVD, as well as end-stage renal disease, malignancy, central nervous system injury or irreversible dysfunction, severe hepatic disease, and severe chronic pulmonary disease. These contraindications need to be weighed individually according to the type and goals of support.

The goals of therapy are the preservation of end-organ perfusion and function. Goals can further be divided into short-term or long-term support. In general, one thinks of VADs as used for support while the heart recovers (bridge to recovery), support while the patient waits for a heart transplant (bridge to transplant), or as the final option in a nonheart transplant candidate with chronic heart failure (destination therapy). Patient selection, including contraindications, as well as device selection, takes into account both the etiology goals of therapy.

Cannulation Strategies

Support of the left ventricle is accomplished by draining blood away from the left ventricle and pumping it into the aorta. Cannulas can be inserted into the LV apex, or the left atrium for inflow to the pump. Return is through an arterial cannula or graft to the ascending or descending aorta. Right-sided devices most often drain the right ventricle by a cannula in the right atrium. Blood is returned to the patient via a cannula or graft in the PA or right ventricular outflow tract.

Pulsatile VADs almost always work in asynchrony to the native heart. Although they are a parallel circuit, almost all of the cardiac output is derived from the VAD, and often, the aortic valve does not open. Pulsatile devices approved by the Food and Drug Administration (FDA) include the Abiomed BVS5000 and AB5000, HeartMate XVE, Novacor (recently withdrawn from the market by the manufacturer), and the Thoratec PVAD and IVAD devices. Newer, nonpulsatile devices provide assistance to the native left ventricle, often with a dramatic reduction in systemic pulsatile flow. Second generation axial flow pumps include the HeartMate II with imminent FDA approval for bridge to transplant, the DeBakey MicroMed, and the Jarvik 2000. The recent pivotal trial comparing the nonpulsatile HeartMate II to the HeartMate XVE showed a dramatic reduction in complications with the newer generation axial flow device.[94] The so-called third generation pumps include smaller centrifugal pumps with either fluid film or magnetic levitation impeller support to further reduce blood trauma and improve durability.

Right Ventricular and Biventricular Assist Devices

The majority of patients with chronic heart failure require left ventricular assist device (LVAD) support. Usually a moderate amount of RV dysfunction can be managed by perioperative inotropes and pulmonary vasodilators such as milrinone and nitric oxide. Some LVAD patients need temporary mechanical RV support that can then be weaned. Isolated right ventricular assist devices are unusual. Biventricular support is used for acute cardiogenic shock after an MI or post–open heart surgery. Chronic biventricular failure in some cases can be managed as a bridge to transplant with an implantable biventricular assist device (BiVAD) with either the Thoratec devices or the CardioWest Total Artificial Heart. Although the patients with a Thoratec BiVAD can be discharged home on support, there is no destination therapy option for biventricular failure.

Bridge to Recovery The most common scenarios for this type of support is after a MI and after open heart surgery when ventricular performance is inadequate to allow weaning from CPB or to support the individual while the heart recovers. MI is most commonly treated with PCI or thrombolytic therapy. Patients who are in shock and continue to be despite opening the culprit vessel are candidates for mechanical support. The IABP is the standard of care, along with inotropes and vasopressors. For those patients who are still in cardiogenic shock, a quick progression to assist device support can be life saving. Those patients in post-MI shock with either unreconstructable coronary disease or what is predicted to be unsalvageable LV function can be implanted with a long-term device as a bridge to transplant. After open heart surgery, patients who continue to be in cardiogenic shock despite IABP and inotropic support have an extremely high mortality. Samuels reviewed 3400 open heart surgery patients and found patients requiring two and three high-dose inotropes had a hospital mortality of 42 and 80% respectively, thus providing a "rule of thumb" guide for consideration of assist device support.[95] Using this as a guide for early post-cardiotomy VAD support their group was able to wean 62% and discharge 28% of patients with severe, refractory postcardiac surgery acute heart failure.

Bridge to Transplant LVAD as a bridge to transplant was first performed at Stanford in 1984. LVAD as a bridge to transplant is indicated in patients on the transplant waiting list with severe refractory heart failure. These patients are candidates for heart transplant, but are not predicted to survive the waiting list period secondary to sequelae of cardiac failure including worsening end-organ function, rising PA pressures, or those with refractory cardiogenic shock on escalating inotropes, and those with malignant ventricular arrhythmias or sudden death. The incidence of patients on mechanical circulatory support at the time of cardiac transplant has increased to 28%. There is equivalent posttransplant survival in patients coming to transplant on continuous inotropic support or on LVAD support. Survival to transplant is about 70%. Complications include infections of the drive line, pocket, and device itself, device malfunction, sepsis, multisystem organ failure, right heart failure, stroke, bleeding, and pulmonary complications. The most common cause of death is multisystem organ failure, with advanced age >60 and the need for right ventricular assist device support being the biggest operative risk factors.

Destination Therapy This is a relatively new concept where the assist device is implanted as a permanent solution to end-stage heart disease. Initially, this has been reserved for patients with extremely limited life expectancy who were not candidates for heart transplant.[96] The REMATCH trial showed a 48% reduction in mortality for the LVAD group as compared to optimal medical management. The survival for the LVAD group was 52 and 23% compared to the optimal medical management, which was 25 and 8% at 1 and 2 years, respectively. Current indications include: (a) NYHA IV symptoms for >60 days, (b) LVEF <25%, (c) peak oxygen consumption <12 mL/kg per minute or inability to wean from inotropic support, and (d) contraindications to heart transplant. Currently, the HeartMate XVE is the only device approved for destination therapy in the United States, though several others are in clinical trials. Limitations include medical comorbidities complicating the insertion, size requirements, and device longevity, morbidity, and limitations on activities. Early post-REMATCH registration data now show a modest improvement to 63% 1-year survival. Patient selection plays an important role in the outcomes of destination therapy.[94] High-risk patients have an 11 to 28% 1-year survival while those with lower preoperative risk profiles have a 62 to 81% 1-year survival. The most significant indicator of outcomes is the 90-day mortality. Technical improvements and patient selection have tremendous impact. With a fixed number of heart transplants being performed, interest in applications is quickly widening and there are many devices in the development and testing phases. As devices improve in the future, it is expected that the indications for destination therapy and the demand will grow to help meet the growing number of patients with end-stage heart disease.

Total Artificial Heart A total artificial heart (TAH) will be the conceptual end solution for cardiac replacement of the failing heart. This technology has moved in a vastly different direction than VADs. Assist devices work in parallel to the left ventricle, and are becoming simpler, smaller, and valveless, in contrast to the TAH, which displaces the heart and retains pulsatile flow. The original Jarvik TAH is still in use as the CardioWest BiVAD and is used as a bridge to transplant. More recently, the AbioCor TAH has been implanted as part of an FDA trial and recently obtained FDA Humanitarian Device Exemption approval in 2006. Despite tremendous improvements in design and technology, limitations and complications include mobility, stroke, infection, and space limitations in the recipient chest. Current indications include patients <75 years of age with severe irreversible biventricular failure or end-stage heart disease who are not transplant or LVAD candidates, and cannot be weaned from multiple inotropic support or mechanical biventricular support. Total cardiac replacement with an artificial heart, however, is still in the experimental arena. Long-term risks include thromboembolic complications, the risk of infection, and trauma to blood elements.

SURGERY FOR ARRHYTHMIAS

History

Cardiac surgery for arrhythmias began with the treatment of Wolff-Parkinson-White syndrome (ventricular pre-excitation and tachycardia) by surgical division. Subsequently, the surgical treatment of medically refractory AV node re-entrant tachycardia was performed. Subsequently, the development and efficacy of catheter-based endovascular techniques supplanted these more invasive surgical procedures.

Surgery for Atrial Fibrillation

Starting in the 1980s, a series of surgical procedures were developed to address atrial fibrillation. James Cox first developed an "atrial isolation" procedure, followed by Guiraudon's "corridor procedure." A fuller understanding of the electrophysiologic basis of atrial tachyarrhythmias as well as the goals of intact sinus mechanism, AV synchrony, and atrial transport led to the development of the Cox Maze procedures.[97] This operation, in its current form, consists of a series of surgical incisions and reconstruction of the atria such that the sinus mechanism is preserved and macroreentrant circuits necessary for atrial fibrillation to form are prevented. This procedure has a 98% success rate, an extremely low follow-up neurologic event rate, and is the gold standard for the nonmedical treatment of refractory atrial fibrillation.[98]

In 1998, Haissaguerre demonstrated that paroxysmal atrial fibrillation is initiated by ectopic beats in the pulmonary veins.[99] This led to successful catheter-based ablation of the pulmonary vein ostia for paroxysmal atrial fibrillation, with satisfactory results. This has led to the successful addition of "pulmonary vein ablation" to such surgical procedures as MV reconstruction. Although these procedures are less successful, they are much less complicated to perform and have been performed with low morbidity. Likewise, recently, a series of "lesser invasive" surgical procedures have been designed to electrically exclude the pulmonary veins as well as create other "lines" of ablation that block conduction to treat atrial tachyarrhythmias. These procedures use various thermal energy sources (radio frequency energy, microwave, high intensity focused ultrasound, cryo energy) to creates various lesion sets from outside the atria via a minimally invasive approach. It is known, however, that with chronic atrial fibrillation, there is modification of the atrial substrate such that the tissue permanently fibrillates without the need for an instigating stimulus. The learned adage is that atrial fibrillation begets atrial fibrillation. It is not yet clear if and where these procedures will be most successful and beneficial for which subtypes of atrial fibrillation.

Pacemakers

Pacemakers were first developed in the 1950s. A lead was fixed to the surface of the heart (epicardial lead), the pacemaker was AC powered, and the patient was limited by the tether of the power cord. Soon these devices became miniaturized and battery driven so they could be externally worn. In 1960 the first totally implantable pacemaker was placed in a patient; the battery had a life of about 12 to 18 months. It is sobering to remember that before pacemakers, the mean life expectancy of a patient with symptomatic complete heart block was 6 months.

Currently, pacemakers are implanted with transvenous leads that require only a subcutaneous access procedure and fluoroscopic control. The pacemaker system typically consists of transvenous leads introduced into the subclavian veins and a "generator," which is a small sealed unit that contains both the controlling electronics and the battery. These units typically last 8 to 10 years, after which the leads are disconnected and reconnected to a new generator. External pacing generators are still used when only temporary pacing is needed, as in postcardiac surgical patients.

Pacemakers not only treat bradyarrhythmias, but also synchronize atrial and ventricular contractions. Epicardial lead systems are reserved today for small infants and patients without direct access to the endocardium of the right ventricle (patients status post-Fontan procedure or TV replacement). Additionally, epicardial leads are used for "dyssynchrony pacing" in patients with heart failure. These patients with impaired ventricular function can benefit from both left- and right-sided pacing if a significant intraventricular conduction defect exists.[100]

Defibrillators

In the 1990s, a new class of implantable devices was created—ICDs. Although these devices all had basic bradycardiac pacemaker capability, they also had the capacity to detect and treat ventricular tachyarrhythmias. When a persistent ventricular tachycardia is detected, the ICD battery charges a capacitor for several seconds and treats the arrhythmia by delivering upward of 30 joules of energy (at approximately 750 volts) across the myocardium. While these devices at first required a thoracotomy or sternotomy to implant them, transvenous lead access is now routine. Implantation was first reserved for sudden death survivors (due to ventricular tachycardia) or those high-risk patients with inducible arrhythmias. The high success rates of this therapy lead to the MADIT and SCDHFT trials.[101] These studies demonstrated a survival advantage to empiric ICD implantation in patients with both ischemic and nonischemic cardiomyopathy.

SURGERY FOR PERICARDIAL DISEASE

Acute Pericarditis

Acute pericarditis results from acute inflammation of the pericardial space, and may result in substernal chest pain or ECG changes. A pericardial friction rub may be heard on physical examination. The pain often is inspiratory, worsened in the supine position, and relieved by leaning forward. The associated ECG changes commonly include sinus tachycardia with concave upward ST-segment elevation throughout the precordium. The ECG typically progresses to T-wave inversion, followed by the total resolution of all changes. The causes of acute pericarditis are variable, including infection, MI, trauma, neoplasm, radiation, autoimmune diseases, drugs, nonspecific causes, and others. Untreated pericarditis may result in progressive development of a pericardial effusion with subsequent cardiac tamponade. Infectious causes may result in septic complications. Chronic constrictive pericarditis may develop after resolution of the acute process.

Diagnosis

The diagnostic work-up should attempt to determine the underlying cause of the pericarditis. Blood tests should include erythrocyte sedimentation rate, hematocrit level, white blood cell count, bacterial cultures, viral titers, blood urea nitrogen, T_3, T_4, thyroid-stimulating hormone, antinuclear antibody, rheumatoid factor, and myocardial enzyme levels. The ECG may be typical or nonspecific. The chest x-ray may be normal or may demonstrate an enlarged cardiac silhouette or a pleural effusion. An echocardiogram to evaluate the degree of pericardial effusion is essential. A pericardiocentesis or pericardial biopsy may be necessary when the diagnosis or etiology is uncertain.

Treatment

The preferred treatment depends on the underlying cause. Purulent pyogenic pericarditis requires drainage and prolonged IV antibiotic therapy. Postpericardiotomy syndrome, post-MI syndrome, viral pericarditis, and idiopathic pericarditis often are self-limiting, but can require a short course of treatment with NSAIDs. If a significant pericardial effusion is present, drainage is indicated if tamponade occurs or if resolution is not prompt with anti-inflammatory agents. A 5- to 7-day course of steroids is occasionally necessary. Follow-up studies should be done to document resolution of pericardial effusion or to assess for late constrictive pericarditis.

Chronic Constrictive Pericarditis

Etiology

In the majority of patients, the cause of chronic constrictive pericarditis is unknown and probably is the end stage of an undiagnosed viral pericarditis. Tuberculosis is a rarity. Intensive radiation is a significant cause in some series. Constrictive pericarditis may develop after an open-heart operation. Previous cardiac surgery was reported to be the cause in 39% of the patients treated surgically for constrictive pericarditis at the authors' institution.

Pathology and Pathophysiology

The pericardial cavity is obliterated by fusion of the parietal pericardium to the epicardium, forming dense scar tissue that encases and constricts the heart. In chronic cases, areas of calcification develop, adding an additional element of constriction. The ultimate form of this process is "coeur de stein" in which the entire visceral surface of the heart is covered with an armor-like calcification.

The pathophysiology of this disease remains the limitation of diastolic filling of the ventricles. This results in a decrease in cardiac output from a decrease in stroke volume. The right ventricular diastolic pressure is increased, with a corresponding increase in right atrial and central venous pressure ranging from 10 to 30 mmHg. This venous hypertension may produce hepatomegaly, ascites, peripheral edema, and a generalized increase in blood volume. The disease is slowly progressive with increasing ascites and edema. Fatigability and dyspnea on exertion are common, but dyspnea at rest is unusual. The ascites often is severe, and the diagnosis is easily confused with cirrhosis. Hepatomegaly and ascites often are the most prominent physical abnormalities. Peripheral edema is moderate in some patients, but severe in others. These findings are manifestations of advanced congestive failure from any form of heart disease. With constrictive pericarditis, however, the usual cardiac findings are a heart of normal size without murmurs or abnormal sounds. Atrial fibrillation is present in about one third of the patients, and a pleural effusion is common in more severe cases. A paradoxical pulse is found in a small proportion of patients.

Laboratory Findings

Venous pressure is elevated, often to 15 to 20 mmHg or higher. The ECG, though not diagnostic, usually is abnormal with a low voltage and inverted T waves. The chest x-ray usually shows a heart of normal size, but pericardial calcification may be seen in a significant proportion of cases and often is the first clue to the diagnosis. Echocardiogram, MRI, or CT scan may demonstrate a thickened pericardium.

Findings on cardiac catheterization are highly characteristic. There is elevation of the right ventricular diastolic pressure with a change in contour, showing an early filling with a subsequent plateau, called the *square root sign*. There also is "equalization" of pressures in the different cardiac chambers, because right atrial pressure, right ventricular diastolic pressure, PA diastolic pressure, pulmonary wedge pressure, and left atrial pressure are similar. The one condition that cannot be excluded without myocardial biopsy is a restrictive cardiomyopathy, and this disease process is often misdiagnosed as "constrictive" pericarditis. Echocardiographic features have been used in an attempt to distinguish between these two processes.

Treatment

A pericardiectomy should be done promptly in symptomatic patients. An operation can be done through a sternotomy incision or a long left anterolateral thoracotomy. The constricting pericardium should be removed from all surfaces of the ventricle, mobilizing the heart so it can be held freely upward in the hand. Removal of the pericardium over the atria and the venae cavae is considered optional, although this usually is done as well. CPB is not usually necessary, but may be needed in the event of significant hemorrhage. The pericardium is removed anteriorly from the pulmonary veins on the right to the pulmonary veins on the left. Both phrenic nerves are identified, mobilized, and protected. Particular care is taken to remove pericardial tissue over the PA, where residual constriction can seriously impair the operative results.

As the constricting scar develops from organization of an exudate between the pericardium and the epicardium, the plane of dissection may be external to the epicardium, which will greatly decrease operative hemorrhage. If the epicardium is thickened, it must be removed from the underlying myocardium, although this is tedious and results in diffuse bleeding.

Intracardiac pressures may be measured before and after pericardiectomy. Often with a complete pericardiectomy the characteristic pressure abnormalities are eliminated or greatly improved. If significant abnormalities remain, the operative field should be carefully checked for any residual sites of constriction. In the past, slow recovery over many months probably was a result of inadequate pericardiectomy, not underlying ventricular atrophy.

Results

After a radical pericardiectomy that corrects the hemodynamic abnormalities, patients improve promptly with a massive diuresis. If a prompt diuresis does not occur, the original diagnosis should be questioned. The risk of an operation varies with the age of the patient and the severity of the disease; the mortality rate usually is <5%. A good result can be anticipated for >95% of the patients. The authors have previously reported surgical treatment for chronic constrictive pericarditis with total pericardiectomy, with an operative mortality rate of 3%. After the operation hemodynamic abnormalities were promptly corrected, ascites and peripheral edema resolved, and functional status improved dramatically.

CARDIAC NEOPLASMS

Overview

Primary cardiac neoplasms are rare, reported to occur with incidences ranging from 0.001 to 0.3% in autopsy series. Benign tumors account for 75% of primary neoplasms and malignant tumors account for 25%. The most frequent primary cardiac neoplasm is myxoma, comprising 30 to 50%. Other benign neoplasms, in decreasing order of occurrence, include lipoma, papillary fibroelastoma, rhabdomyoma, fibroma, hemangioma, teratoma, lymphangioma, and others. Most primary malignant neoplasms are sarcomas (angiosarcoma, rhabdomyosarcoma, fibrosarcoma, leiomyosarcoma, and liposarcoma), with malignant lymphomas accounting for 1 to 2%.

Metastatic cardiac neoplasms are more common than primary neoplasms, occurring in 4 to 12% of patients dying of cancer. Symptoms include dyspnea, fever, malaise, weight loss, arthralgias, and dizziness. Clinical findings may include murmurs of mitral stenosis or insufficiency, heart failure, pulmonary hypertension, and systemic embolization. Usually, the diagnosis is readily established by two-dimensional echocardiography. TEE may be useful when transthoracic findings are equivocal or confusing. MRI has been of value in diagnosis, providing excellent cardiac definition. Cardiac catheterization is not necessary in the majority of cases, but may be necessary when other cardiac disease is suspected or if other diagnostic studies are equivocal.

Excision is the treatment of choice for most benign tumors. Care is taken to avoid deformity or destruction of adjacent cardiac structures, and reconstruction of the involved cardiac chamber is sometimes necessary. Total excision of metastatic or primary malignant neoplasms is less frequently possible but should be attempted. Otherwise incisional diagnostic biopsy is performed. Multimodality therapy with excision, chemotherapy, and radiotherapy is indicated for most malignant cardiac neoplasms.

Myxomas

Sixty to 75% of cardiac myxomas develop in the left atrium, almost always from the atrial septum near the fossa ovalis. Most other myxomas develop in the right atrium; <20 have been reported in the right or left ventricle. The predilection for a myxoma to develop from the rim of the fossa ovalis in the left atrium has been studied, but no satisfactory explanation has been found.

Myxomas are true neoplasms, although their similarity to an organized atrial thrombus has led to considerable debate. The occurrence of myxomas in the absence of other organic heart disease, histochemical studies of myxomas demonstrating mucopolysaccharide and glycoprotein, and a distinct histologic appearance indicate that myxomas are true neoplasms. Although they can recur locally, they do not invade or metastasize and are considered benign.

Pathology

The tumors usually are polypoid, projecting into the atrial cavity from a 1- to 2-cm stalk attached to the atrial septum. The size ranges from 0.5 to >10 cm. Only the superficial layer of the septum is involved; invasion of the septum does not occur. Some myxomas grow slowly; a few patients have symptoms for many years. There is no tendency to invade other areas of the heart, and distant metastases are rarely reported. The friable consistency of a myxoma is of particular significance because frequently, the first presentation is that of an embolic event.

Histologically, a myxoma is covered with endothelium and composed of a myxomatous stroma with large stellate cells mixed with fusiform or multinucleated cells. Mitoses are infrequent. Lymphocytes and plasmacytes are regularly found. Hemosiderin, a result of hemorrhage into the tumor, is commonly present. Myxoma cells usually express interleukin-6, and some tumors have abnormal cellular DNA content.

Sporadic myxomas usually present in the fifth or sixth decade of life but have been described in younger and older patients. Familial myxomas (autosomal dominant) can occur, usually presenting at <30 years of age. The familial myxoma syndrome includes myxomas, freckles, pigmented nevi, nodular adrenal cortical disease, and mammary myomatous fibroadenomas. Testicular tumors and pituitary adenomas with two or more components are required for diagnosis.

Pathophysiology

A myxoma may be completely asymptomatic until it grows large enough to obstruct the MV or TV or fragments to produce emboli. Embolization has been estimated to occur in 40 to 50% of patients. A pedunculated myxoma may be quite mobile, moving through the cardiac chamber with each contraction. Intermittent acute obstruction of the mitral orifice has been reported to produce syncope and even sudden death (Fig. 21-19). In a series of 49 patients, it has been reported that most myxomas originated from the left atrium (87.7%), but also much less frequently from the MV (6.1%), from the right atrium (4.1%), and from the left and right atria (2%). These myxomas prolapsed into the left ventricle in 40.8% of the patients, creating mitral stenosis in 10.2%, and even LV outflow tract obstruction in 2%.[102] Some myxomas produce generalized symptoms resembling an autoimmune disorder, including fever, weight loss, digital clubbing, myalgia, and arthralgia. These patients may have an immune reaction to the neoplasm, as elevated levels of interleukin-6 and elevated levels of antimyocardial antibodies have been described.

Clinical Manifestations

Symptoms may include those of MV obstruction that resemble mitral stenosis; peripheral embolization; or generalized autoimmune symptoms. The diagnosis often is made after an embolic episode from histologic examination of the surgically removed embolus, or as a result of subsequent diagnostic studies to determine the reason for embolism. The precision and reliability of two-dimensional echocardiography has greatly simplified diagnosis. Angiography is optional unless additional disease is suspected. CT scan has been reported to be helpful with small tumors, but MRI is more definitive.

Treatment

Surgery should be performed as soon as possible after the diagnosis has been established due to the inherent risk of a disabling or fatal cerebral embolus. Either a sternotomy or a minimally invasive approach can be used. Once extracorporeal circulation has been established, the aorta is clamped to avoid embolism. Palpation is avoided. The right atrium is opened, and the fossa ovalis incised to expose the stalk of the myxoma. The left atrium is then opened in the interatrial groove. With the tumor visualized, the segment of atrial septum from which the tumor arises is excised, after which the tumor is removed through the left atrium. The defect in the atrial septum is closed primarily or with a small patch. This technique is simple and allows exploration of atria and ventricles.

A few cases of recurrent myxoma have been reported, some of which have been re-excised successfully. Although thought to result from inadequate excision of the site of origin, some have recurred at more remote sites in the atrium, indicating the multipotential source of these unusual neoplasms. Periodic echocardiography should be routinely performed for several years after an operation.

Keeling and associates described their experience with a series of 49 patients with cardiac myxomas over 20 years. Cardiac myxomas represented 86% of all surgically treated cardiac tumors. The early mortality rate was 2%, while the rate of reoperation was 2% after 24 years.[102]

Metastatic Neoplasms

Cardiac metastases have been found in 4 to 12% of autopsies performed for neoplastic disease. Although they have occurred from primary neoplasms developing in almost every known site of the body, the most common have been carcinoma of the lung or breast, melanoma, and lymphoma. Cardiac metastases involving only the heart are very unusual. Similarly, a solitary cardiac metastasis is rare; usually there are multiple areas of involvement. Cardiac involvement is common with leukemia or lymphoma, developing in 25 to 40% of patients.[103] All areas of the heart are involved with equal frequency except the cardiac valves, perhaps because lymphatics are absent in valvular tissue.

The diagnosis of a primary cardiac malignant tumor may be suspected in a patient in whom an unexplained hemorrhagic pericar-

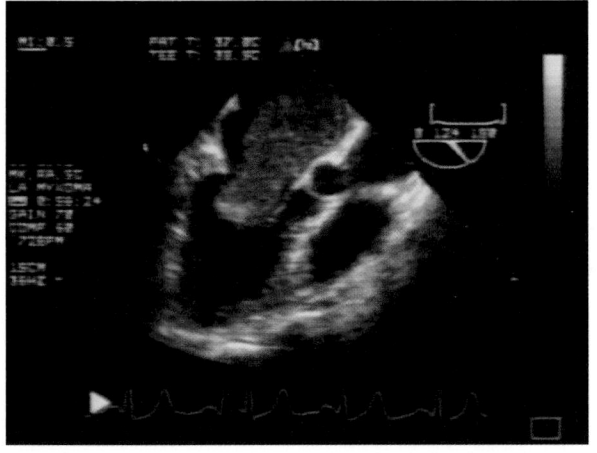
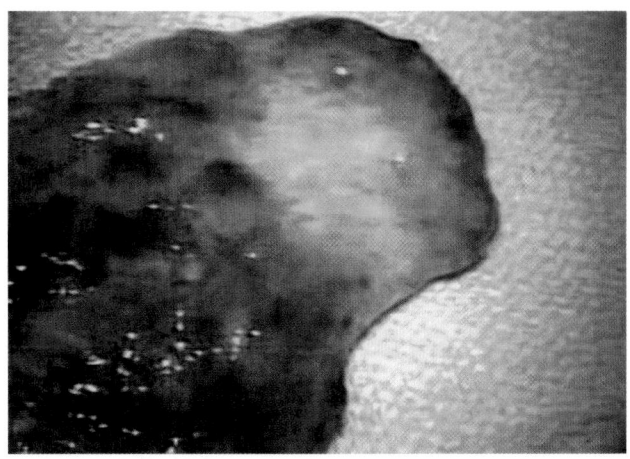

A **B**

FIG. 21-19. Massive left atrial myxoma. **A.** Intraoperative echocardiogram of a large left atrial mass, diagnosed preoperatively as a left atrial myxoma. The mass can be seen prolapsing through the mitral valve orifice causing intermittent symptoms of mitral stenosis. **B.** The resected specimen. The neck of the mass that was obstructing the mitral orifice is clearly delineated.

dial effusion develops, especially in association with a bizarre cardiac shadow on the radiograph. Echocardiography should confirm the presence of an abnormal cardiac mass. Thoracotomy or sternotomy usually is required to establish the diagnosis. Combined chemotherapy and radiation is indicated, but only rarely is effective therapy possible.

Miscellaneous Neoplasms

Unusual benign lesions of the heart include fibromas, lipomas, angiomas, teratomas, and cysts. Fewer than 50 of each of these types of lesion have been reported. Fibromas have been found most frequently in the left ventricle, often as 2- to 5-cm nodules within the muscle. Sudden death, probably from a cardiac arrhythmia, has been reported with these tumors.

Lipomas are rare asymptomatic tumors found projecting from the epicardial or endocardial surface of the heart in older patients. Angiomas are small, focal, vascular malformations of no clinical significance, although they may be associated with heart block. Pericardial teratomas and bronchogenic cysts are rare lesions that can cause symptoms from compression of the right atrium with obstruction of venous return. Most of these occur in children and can be up to 10 cm in diameter. Myxomas are by far the most common benign tumor in adults; they are seldom found in children except as part of the familial syndrome described in the Pathology section.

Renal cell carcinoma, Wilms' tumor, uterine tumors, and adrenal tumors may have direct intracardiac extension. Excision of these infradiaphragmatic tumors by radical surgery associated with cavoatrial thrombectomy has been suggested, and extracorporeal circulation and deep circulatory arrest provide an optimal technique for removing the tumor thrombus, even in the presence of metastatic disease, and have good early and long-term results.

REFERENCES

Entries highlighted in bright blue are key references.

1. Libby P. *Braunwald's Heart Disease: A Textbook of Cardiovascular Medicine*, 8th ed. Philadelphia: Saunders Elsevier, 2007.
2. Slart RH, Bax JJ, van Veldhuisen DJ, et al: Imaging techniques in nuclear cardiology for the assessment of myocardial viability. *Int J Cardiovasc Imaging* 22:63, 2006.
3. Treede H, Becker C, Reichenspurner H, et al: Multidetector computed tomography (MDCT) in coronary surgery: First experiences with a new tool for diagnosis of coronary artery disease. *Ann Thorac Surg* 74:S1398, 2002.
4. Nieman K, Oudkerk M, Rensing BJ, et al: Coronary angiography with multi-slice computed tomography. *Lancet* 357:599, 2001.
5. Gibbon JH Jr. Application of a mechanical heart and lung apparatus to cardiac surgery. *Minn Med* 37:171, 1954.
6. Liu J, Ji B, Long C, et al: Comparative effectiveness of methylprednisolone and zero-balance ultrafiltration on inflammatory response after pediatric cardiopulmonary bypass. *Artif Organs* 31:571, 2007.
7. Eleven-year survival in the Veterans Administration randomized trial of coronary bypass surgery for stable angina. The Veterans Administration Coronary Artery Bypass Surgery Cooperative Study Group. *N Engl J Med* 311:1333, 1984.
8. Caracciolo EA, Davis KB, Sopko G, et al: Comparison of surgical and medical group survival in patients with left main equivalent coronary artery disease. Long-term CASS experience. *Circulation* 91:2335, 1995.
9. Varnauskas E: Twelve-year follow-up of survival in the randomized European Coronary Surgery Study. *N Engl J Med* 319:332, 1988.
10. Jones RH, Kesler K, Phillips HR 3rd, et al: Long-term survival benefits of coronary artery bypass grafting and percutaneous transluminal angioplasty in patients with coronary artery disease. *J Thorac Cardiovasc Surg* 111:1013, 1996.
11. Chaux A, Blanche C, Matloff JM, et al: Postinfarction ventricular septal defect. *Semin Thorac Cardiovasc Surg* 10:93, 1998.
12. Gruentzig AR: Percutaneous transluminal coronary angioplasty. *Semin Roentgenol* 16:152, 1981.
13. Comparison of coronary bypass surgery with angioplasty in patients with multivessel disease. The Bypass Angioplasty Revascularization Investigation (BARI) Investigators. *N Engl J Med* 335:217, 1996.
14. Abizaid A, Costa MA, Centemero M, et al: Clinical and economic impact of diabetes mellitus on percutaneous and surgical treatment of multivessel coronary disease patients: Insights from the Arterial Revascularization Therapy Study (ARTS) trial. *Circulation* 104:533, 2001.
15. Morice MC, Serruys PW, Sousa JE, et al: A randomized comparison of a sirolimus-eluting stent with a standard stent for coronary revascularization. *N Engl J Med* 346:1773, 2002.
16. Stettler C, Wandel S, Allemann S, et al: Outcomes associated with drug-eluting and bare-metal stents: A collaborative network meta-analysis. *Lancet* 370:937, 2007.
17. Hannan EL, Racz MJ, Walford G, et al: Long-term outcomes of coronary-artery bypass grafting versus stent implantation. *N Engl J Med* 352:2174, 2005.
18. Dion R, Etienne PY, Verhelst R, et al: Bilateral mammary grafting. Clinical, functional and angiographic assessment in 400 consecutive patients. *Eur J Cardiothorac Surg* 7:287; discussion 94, 1993.
19. Lytle BW, Cosgrove DM, Loop FD, et al: Perioperative risk of bilateral internal mammary artery grafting: analysis of 500 cases from 1971 to 1984. *Circulation* 74:III37, 1986.
20. Puskas JD, Thourani VH, Marshall JJ, et al: Clinical outcomes, angiographic patency, and resource utilization in 200 consecutive off-pump coronary bypass patients. *Ann Thorac Surg* 71:1477; discussion 83, 2001.
21. Kim KB, Lim C, Lee C, et al: Off-pump coronary artery bypass may decrease the patency of saphenous vein grafts. *Ann Thorac Surg* 72:S1033, 2001.
22. Sabik JF, Gillinov AM, Blackstone EH, et al: Does off-pump coronary surgery reduce morbidity and mortality? *J Thorac Cardiovasc Surg* 124:698, 2002.
23. Patel NC, Pullan DM, Fabri BM: Does off-pump total arterial revascularization without aortic manipulation influence neurological outcome? A study of 226 consecutive, unselected cases. *Heart Surg Forum* 5:28, 2002.
24. Calafiore AM, Di Mauro M, Canosa C, et al: Early and late outcome of myocardial revascularization with and without cardiopulmonary bypass in high risk patients (EuroSCORE > or = 6). *Eur J Cardiothorac Surg* 23:360, 2003.
25. Oliveira SA, Lisboa LA, Dallan LA, et al: Minimally invasive single-vessel coronary artery bypass with the internal thoracic artery and early postoperative angiography: Midterm results of a prospective study in 120 consecutive patients. *Ann Thorac Surg* 73:505, 2002.
26. Diegeler A, Thiele H, Falk V, et al: Comparison of stenting with minimally invasive bypass surgery for stenosis of the left anterior descending coronary artery. *N Engl J Med* 347:561, 2002.
27. Drenth DJ, Winter JB, Veeger NJ, et al: Minimally invasive coronary artery bypass grafting versus percutaneous transluminal coronary angioplasty with stenting in isolated high-grade stenosis of the proximal left anterior descending coronary artery: Six months' angiographic and clinical follow-up of a prospective randomized study. *J Thorac Cardiovasc Surg* 124:130, 2002.
28. Falk V, Walther T, Autschbach R, et al: Robot-assisted minimally invasive solo mitral valve operation. *J Thorac Cardiovasc Surg* 115:470, 1998.
29. Burkhoff D, Schmidt S, Schulman SP, et al: Transmyocardial laser revascularisation compared with continued medical therapy for treatment of refractory angina pectoris: A prospective randomised trial. ATLANTIC Investigators. Angina Treatments-Lasers and Normal Therapies in Comparison. *Lancet* 354:885, 1999.
30. Enriquez-Sarano M, Avierinos JF, Messika-Zeitoun D, et al: Quantitative determinants of the outcome of asymptomatic mitral regurgitation. *N Engl J Med* 352:875, 2005.
31. Chaliki HP, Mohty D, Avierinos JF, et al: Outcomes after aortic valve replacement in patients with severe aortic regurgitation and markedly reduced left ventricular function. *Circulation* 106:2687, 2002.
32. Grossi EA, Schwartz CF, Yu PJ, et al: High-risk aortic valve replacement: are the outcomes as bad as predicted? *Ann Thorac Surg* 85:102; discussion 7, 2008.
33. Jamieson WR, von Lipinski O, Miyagishima RT, et al: Performance of bioprostheses and mechanical prostheses assessed by composites of valve-related complications to 15 years after mitral valve replacement. *J Thorac Cardiovasc Surg* 129:1301, 2005.
34. Jamieson WR, David TE, Feindel CM, et al: Performance of the Carpentier-Edwards SAV and Hancock-II porcine bioprostheses in aortic valve replacement. *J Heart Valve Dis* 11:424, 2002.

35. Butchart EG, Payne N, Li HH, et al: Better anticoagulation control improves survival after valve replacement. *J Thorac Cardiovasc Surg* 123:715, 2002.

36. Pibarot P, Dumesnil JG, Jobin J, et al: Hemodynamic and physical performance during maximal exercise in patients with an aortic bioprosthetic valve: comparison of stentless versus stented bioprostheses. *J Am Coll Cardiol* 34:1609, 1999.

37. David TE, Pollick C, Bos J: Aortic valve replacement with stentless porcine aortic bioprosthesis. *J Thorac Cardiovasc Surg* 99:113, 1990.

38. Ross DN: Homograft replacement of the aortic valve. *Lancet* 2:487, 1962.

39. Barratt-Boyes BG: Homograft aortic valve replacement in aortic incompetence and stenosis. *Thorax* 19:131, 1964.

40. Carpentier A. Cardiac valve surgery—the "French correction." *J Thorac Cardiovasc Surg* 86:323, 1983.

41. Bonow RO, Carabello BA, Kanu C, et al: ACC/AHA 2006 guidelines for the management of patients with valvular heart disease: A report of the American College of Cardiology/American Heart Association Task Force on Practice Guidelines (writing committee to revise the 1998 Guidelines for the Management of Patients With Valvular Heart Disease): Developed in collaboration with the Society of Cardiovascular Anesthesiologists: Endorsed by the Society for Cardiovascular Angiography and Interventions and the Society of Thoracic Surgeons. *Circulation* 114:e84, 2006.

42. Enriquez-Sarano M: Timing of mitral valve surgery. *Heart* 87:79, 2002.

43. David TE, Ivanov J, Armstrong S, et al: Late outcomes of mitral valve repair for floppy valves: Implications for asymptomatic patients. *J Thorac Cardiovasc Surg* 125:1143, 2003.

44. Grossi EA, Galloway AC, Kallenbach K, et al: Early results of posterior leaflet folding plasty for mitral valve reconstruction. *Ann Thorac Surg* 65:1057, 1998.

45. David TE: Artificial chordae. *Semin Thorac Cardiovasc Surg* 16:161, 2004.

46. Gillinov AM, Cosgrove DM: Mitral valve repair for degenerative disease. *J Heart Valve Dis* 11:S15, 2002.

47. Choudhary SK, Dhareshwar J, Govil A, et al: Open mitral commissurotomy in the current era: Indications, technique, and results. *Ann Thorac Surg* 75:41, 2003.

48. Antunes MJ, Vieira H, Ferrao de Oliveira J: Open mitral commissurotomy: The 'golden standard.' *J Heart Valve Dis* 9:472, 2000.

49. Cardoso LF, Grinberg M, Rati MA, et al: Comparison between percutaneous balloon valvuloplasty and open commissurotomy for mitral stenosis. A prospective and randomized study. *Cardiology* 98:186, 2002.

50. Mohty D, Orszulak TA, Schaff HV, et al: Very long-term survival and durability of mitral valve repair for mitral valve prolapse. *Circulation* 104:I1, 2001.

51. Khan SS, Trento A, DeRobertis M, et al: Twenty-year comparison of tissue and mechanical valve replacement. *J Thorac Cardiovasc Surg* 122:257, 2001.

52. Galloway AC, Grossi EA, Bizekis CS, et al: Evolving techniques for mitral valve reconstruction. *Ann Surg* 236:288; discussion 93, 2002.

53. Braunberger E, Deloche A, Berrebi A, et al: Very long-term results (more than 20 years) of valve repair with carpentier's techniques in nonrheumatic mitral valve insufficiency. *Circulation* 104:I8, 2001.

54. Grossi EA, Galloway AC, Ribakove GH, et al: Impact of minimally invasive valvular heart surgery: A case-control study. *Ann Thorac Surg* 71:807, 2001.

55. Grossi EA, Zakow PK, Ribakove G, et al: Comparison of post-operative pain, stress response, and quality of life in port access vs. standard sternotomy coronary bypass patients. *Eur J Cardiothorac Surg* 16:S39, 1999.

56. Fucci C, Sandrelli L, Pardini A, et al: Improved results with mitral valve repair using new surgical techniques. *Eur J Cardiothorac Surg* 9:621; discussion 6, 1995.

57. Lorusso R, Fucci C, Pentiricci S, et al: "Double-orifice" technique to repair extensive mitral valve excision following acute endocarditis. *J Cardiac Surg* 13:24, 1998.

58. Chitwood WR Jr., Elbeery JR, Chapman WH, et al: Video-assisted minimally invasive mitral valve surgery: The "micro-mitral" operation. *J Thorac Cardiovasc Surg* 113:413, 1997.

59. Mohr FW, Falk V, Diegeler A, et al: Minimally invasive port-access mitral valve surgery. *J Thorac Cardiovasc Surg* 115:567; discussion 74, 1998.

60. Nifong LW, Chu VF, Bailey BM, et al: Robotic mitral valve repair: Experience with the da Vinci system. *Ann Thorac Surg* 75:438; discussion 43, 2003.

61. Green GR, Miller DC: Continuing dilemmas concerning aortic valve replacement in patients with advanced left ventricular systolic dysfunction. *J Heart Valve Dis* 6:562, 1997.

62. David TE, Feindel CM: An aortic valve-sparing operation for patients with aortic incompetence and aneurysm of the ascending aorta. *J Thorac Cardiovasc Surg* 103:617; discussion 22, 1992.

63. Sarsam MA, Yacoub M: Remodeling of the aortic valve anulus. *J Thorac Cardiovasc Surg* 105:435, 1993.

64. Casselman FP, Gillinov AM, Akhrass R, et al: Intermediate-term durability of bicuspid aortic valve repair for prolapsing leaflet. *Eur J Cardiothorac Surg* 15:302, 1999.

65. Paparella D, David TE, Armstrong S, et al: Mid-term results of the Ross procedure. *J Cardiac Surg* 16:338, 2001.

66. Gundry SR, Shattuck OH, Razzouk AJ, et al: Facile minimally invasive cardiac surgery via ministernotomy. *Ann Thorac Surg* 65:1100, 1998.

67. Sharony R, Grossi EA, Saunders PC, et al: Minimally invasive aortic valve surgery in the elderly: A case-control study. *Circulation* 108:II43, 2003.

68. Cosgrove DM 3rd, Sabik JF, Navia JL: Minimally invasive valve operations. *Ann Thorac Surg* 65:1535; discussion 8, 1998.

69. Byrne JG, Aranki SF, Couper GS, et al: Reoperative aortic valve replacement: partial upper hemisternotomy versus conventional full sternotomy. *J Thorac Cardiovasc Surg* 118:991, 1999.

70. Morrow AG, Fogarty TJ, Hannah H 3rd, et al: Operative treatment in idiopathic hypertrophic subaortic stenosis. Techniques, and the results of preoperative and postoperative clinical and hemodynamic assessments. *Circulation* 37:589, 1968.

71. Tribouilloy CM, Enriquez-Sarano M, Bailey KR, et al: Quantification of tricuspid regurgitation by measuring the width of the vena contracta with Doppler color flow imaging: A clinical study. *J Am Coll Cardiol* 36:472, 2000.

72. De Vega NG. [Selective, adjustable and permanent annuloplasty. An original technic for the treatment of tricuspid insufficiency]. *Rev Esp Cardiol* 25:555, 1972.

73. Carrier M, Hebert Y, Pellerin M, et al: Tricuspid valve replacement: An analysis of 25 years of experience at a single center. *Ann Thorac Surg* 75:47, 2003.

74. Kawano H, Oda T, Fukunaga S, et al: Tricuspid valve replacement with the St. Jude Medical valve: 19 years of experience. *Eur J Cardiothorac Surg* 18:565, 2000.

75. Galloway AC, Grossi EA, Baumann FG, et al: Multiple valve operation for advanced valvular heart disease: Results and risk factors in 513 patients. *J Am Coll Cardiol* 19:725, 1992.

76. Cowie MR, Mosterd A, Wood DA, et al: The epidemiology of heart failure. *Eur Heart J* 18:208, 1997.

77. Langenburg SE, Buchanan SA, Blackbourne LH, et al: Predicting survival after coronary revascularization for ischemic cardiomyopathy. *Ann Thorac Surg* 60:1193; discussion 6, 1995.

78. Chareonthaitawee P, Gersh BJ, Araoz PA, et al: Revascularization in severe left ventricular dysfunction: The role of viability testing. *J Am Coll Cardiol* 46:567, 2005.

79. Yamaguchi A, Ino T, Adachi H, et al: Left ventricular volume predicts postoperative course in patients with ischemic cardiomyopathy. *Ann Thorac Surg* 65:434, 1998.

80. Penicka M, Bartunek J, Lang O, et al: Severe left ventricular dyssynchrony is associated with poor prognosis in patients with moderate systolic heart failure undergoing coronary artery bypass grafting. *J Am Coll Cardiol* 50:1315, 2007.

81. Grigioni F, Enriquez-Sarano M, Zehr KJ, et al: Ischemic mitral regurgitation: Long-term outcome and prognostic implications with quantitative Doppler assessment. *Circulation* 103:1759, 2001.

82. Ellis SG, Whitlow PL, Raymond RE, et al: Impact of mitral regurgitation on long-term survival after percutaneous coronary intervention. *Am J Cardiol* 89:315, 2002.

83. Trichon BH, Glower DD, Shaw LK, et al: Survival after coronary revascularization, with and without mitral valve surgery, in patients with ischemic mitral regurgitation. *Circulation* 108:II103, 2003.

84. Bax JJ, Braun J, Somer ST, et al: Restrictive annuloplasty and coronary revascularization in ischemic mitral regurgitation results in reverse left ventricular remodeling. *Circulation* 110:II103, 2004.

85. Acker MA, Bolling S, Shemin R, et al: Mitral valve surgery in heart failure: Insights from the Acorn Clinical Trial. *J Thorac Cardiovasc Surg* 132:568, 577.e1, 2006.

86. Jatene AD: Left ventricular aneurysmectomy. Resection or reconstruction. *J Thorac Cardiovasc Surg* 89:321, 1985.

87. Cooley DA: Ventricular endoaneurysmorrhaphy: A simplified repair for extensive postinfarction aneurysm. *J Cardiac Surg* 4:200, 1989.

88. Dor V, Saab M, Coste P, et al: Left ventricular aneurysm: A new surgical approach. *Thorac Cardiovasc Surg* 37:11, 1989.

89. Athanasuleas CL, Stanley AW Jr., Buckberg GD, et al: Surgical anterior ventricular endocardial restoration (SAVER) in the dilated remodeled ventricle after anterior myocardial infarction. RESTORE group. Reconstructive Endoventricular Surgery, returning Torsion Original Radius Elliptical Shape to the LV. *J Am Coll Cardiol* 37:1199, 2001.

90. Menicanti L, Castelvecchio S, Ranucci M, et al: Surgical therapy for ischemic heart failure: Single-center experience with surgical anterior ventricular restoration. *J Thorac Cardiovasc Surg* 134:433, 2007.

91. Grossi EA, Woo YJ, Schwartz CF, et al: Comparison of Coapsys annuloplasty and internal reduction mitral annuloplasty in the randomized treatment of functional ischemic mitral regurgitation: Impact on the left ventricle. *J Thorac Cardiovasc Surg* 131:1095, 2006.

92. Kang N, Edwards M, Larbalestier R: Preoperative intraaortic balloon pumps in high-risk patients undergoing open heart surgery. *Ann Thorac Surg* 72:54, 2001.

93. Meharwal ZS, Trehan N: Vascular complications of intra-aortic balloon insertion in patients undergoing coronary reavscularization: Analysis of 911 cases. *Eur J Cardiothorac Surg* 21:741, 2002.

94. Lietz K, Long JW, Kfoury AG, et al: Outcomes of left ventricular assist device implantation as destination therapy in the post-REMATCH era: Implications for patient selection. *Circulation* 116:497, 2007.

95. Samuels LE, Kaufman MS, Thomas MP, et al: Pharmacological criteria for ventricular assist device insertion following postcardiotomy shock: Experience with the Abiomed BVS system. *J Cardiac Surg* 14:288, 1999.

96. Rose EA, Gelijns AC, Moskowitz AJ, et al: Long-term mechanical left ventricular assistance for end-stage heart failure. *N Engl J Med* 345:1435, 2001.

97. Cox JL, Jaquiss RD, Schuessler RB, et al: Modification of the maze procedure for atrial flutter and atrial fibrillation. II. Surgical technique of the maze III procedure. *J Thorac Cardiovasc Surg* 110:485, 1995.

98. Cox JL, Ad N, Palazzo T: Impact of the maze procedure on the stroke rate in patients with atrial fibrillation. *J Thorac Cardiovasc Surg* 118:833, 1999.

99. Haissaguerre M, Jais P, Shah DC, et al: Spontaneous initiation of atrial fibrillation by ectopic beats originating in the pulmonary veins. *N Engl J Med* 339:659, 1998.

100. Pires LA, Abraham WT, Young JB, et al: Clinical predictors and timing of New York Heart Association class improvement with cardiac resynchronization therapy in patients with advanced chronic heart failure: Results from the Multicenter InSync Randomized Clinical Evaluation (MIRACLE) and Multicenter InSync ICD Randomized Clinical Evaluation (MIRACLE-ICD) trials. *Am Heart J* 151:837, 2006.

101. Klein H, Auricchio A, Reek S, et al: New primary prevention trials of sudden cardiac death in patients with left ventricular dysfunction: SCD-HEFT and MADIT-II. *Am J Cardiol* 83:91D, 1999.

102. Keeling IM, Oberwalder P, Anelli-Monti M, et al: Cardiac myxomas: 24 years of experience in 49 patients. *Eur J Cardiothorac Surg* 22:971, 2002.

103. Neragi-Miandoab S, Kim J, Vlahakes GJ: Malignant tumours of the heart: A review of tumour type, diagnosis and therapy. *Clin Oncol (R Coll Radiol)* 19:748, 2007.

CHAPTER 22

Thoracic Aneurysms and Aortic Dissection

Scott A. LeMaire, Kapil Sharma,
and Joseph S. Coselli

ANATOMY OF THE AORTA

The aorta consists of two major segments—the proximal aorta and the distal aorta—whose anatomic characteristics affect both the clinical manifestations of disease in these segments and the selection of treatment strategies for such disease (Fig. 22-1). The proximal aortic segment includes the ascending aorta and the transverse aortic arch. The ascending aorta begins at the aortic valve and ends at the origin of the innominate artery. The first portion of the ascending aorta is the aortic root, which includes the aortic valve annulus and the three sinuses of Valsalva; the coronary arteries originate from two of these sinuses. The aortic root joins the tubular portion of the ascending aorta at the sinotubular ridge. The transverse aortic arch is the area from which the brachiocephalic branches arise. The distal aortic segment includes the descending thoracic aorta and the abdominal aorta. The descending thoracic

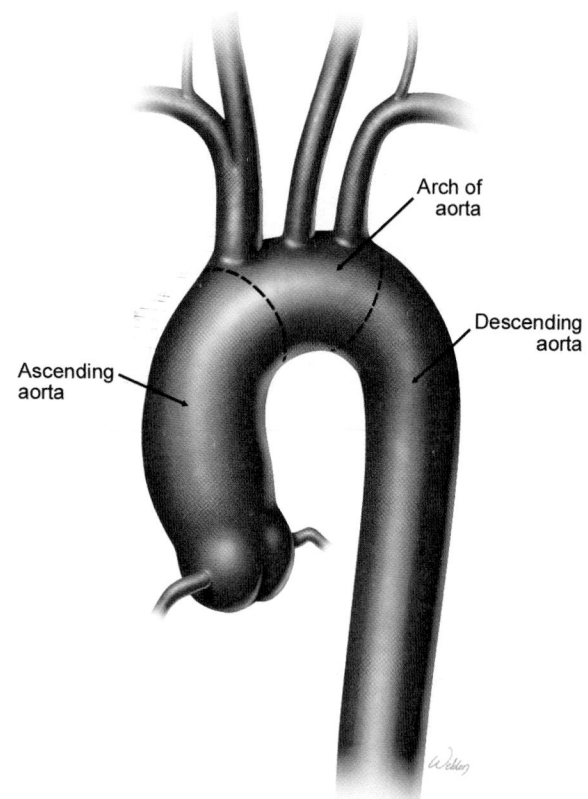

FIG. 22-1. Illustration of normal thoracic aortic anatomy. The brachiocephalic vessels arise from the transverse aortic arch and are used as anatomic landmarks to define the aortic regions. The ascending aorta is proximal to the innominate artery, whereas the descending aorta is distal to the left subclavian artery.

aorta begins distal to the origin of the left subclavian artery and extends to the diaphragmatic hiatus, where it joins the abdominal aorta. The descending thoracic aorta gives rise to multiple bronchial and esophageal branches, as well as to the segmental intercostal arteries, which provide circulation to the spinal cord.

The volume of blood that flows through the thoracic aorta at high pressure is far greater than that found in any other vascular structure. For this reason, any condition that disrupts the integrity of the thoracic aorta, such as aortic dissection, aneurysm rupture, or traumatic injury, can have catastrophic consequences.

Historically, open surgical repair of such conditions has been an intimidating undertaking associated with significant morbidity and mortality. Strategies for protecting the brain and spinal cord during such repairs have become critical in preventing devastating complications. In recent years, endovascular therapy for thoracic aortic disease in selected patients has become accepted practice, producing fewer adverse outcomes than traditional approaches do.

THORACIC AORTIC ANEURYSMS

Aortic aneurysm is defined as a permanent, localized dilatation of the aorta to a diameter that is at least 50% greater than is normal at that anatomic level.[1] The annual incidence of thoracic aortic aneurysms is estimated to be 5.9 per 100,000 persons.[2] The clinical manifestations, methods of treatment, and treatment results in patients with aortic aneurysms vary according to the cause and the aortic segment involved. Causes of thoracic aortic aneurysms include degenerative disease of the aortic wall, aortic dissection, aortitis, infection, and trauma. Aneurysms can be localized to a single aortic segment, or they can involve multiple segments. Thoracoabdominal aortic aneurysms, for example, involve both the descending thoracic aorta and the abdominal aorta. In the most extreme cases, the entire aorta is aneurysmal; this condition is often called *mega-aorta*.

Aortic aneurysms can be either "true" or "false." True aneurysms can take two forms: fusiform and saccular. Fusiform aneurysms are more common and can be described as symmetrical dilatations of the aorta. Saccular aneurysms are localized outpouchings of the aorta. False aneurysms, also called *pseudoaneurysms*, are leaks in the aortic wall that cause blood to collect in pouches of scar tissue on the exterior of the aorta.

Aneurysms of the thoracic aorta consistently increase in size and eventually progress to cause serious complications. These include rupture, which is usually a fatal event. Therefore, aggressive treatment is indicated in all but the poorest surgical candidates. Small, asymptomatic thoracic aortic aneurysms can be followed, especially in high-surgical-risk patients, and can be treated surgically later if symptoms or complications develop, or if progressive enlargement occurs.

KEY POINTS

1. Assessing urgency of repair for an aortic aneurysm is essential to developing an appropriate management plan. Although emergent repair carries greater operative risk than does elective repair, any inappropriate delay of repair risks death.

2. Surgical repair of an aortic aneurysm requires the development of a patient-tailored plan based on careful preoperative medical evaluation. When possible, optimization of a patient's health status to mitigate existing comorbidities is essential before surgical intervention.

3. Ascending aortic aneurysms that are symptomatic or >5.5 cm should be repaired.

4. Ascending aortic dissection is a life-threatening condition, and immediate operative repair is indicated.

5. The natural progression of an aortic aneurysm is continued expansion and eventual rupture. Hence, regular noninvasive imaging studies, as part of a lifelong surveillance plan, are necessary to ensure long-term patient health. Even small asymptomatic aneurysms are routinely imaged to assess overall growth and yearly rate of expansion.

6. Although endovascular devices are approved for use in repairing simple descending thoracic aortic aneurysms, the long-term durability of this type of aortic repair has yet to be clearly established.

7. The development and use of surgical adjuncts like antegrade selective cerebral perfusion and cerebrospinal fluid drainage have significantly reduced morbidity rates associated with complex aortic repair.

Meticulous control of hypertension is the primary medical treatment for patients with small, asymptomatic aneurysms.

Elective resection with graft replacement is indicated in asymptomatic patients with an aortic diameter of at least twice normal in the involved segment (5 to 6 cm in most thoracic segments). Elective repair is contraindicated by extreme operative risk due to severe coexisting cardiac or pulmonary disease and by other conditions that limit life expectancy, such as malignancy. An emergency operation is performed for any patient in whom a ruptured aneurysm is suspected.

Patients with thoracic aortic aneurysm often have coexisting aneurysms of other aortic segments. A common cause of death after repair of a thoracic aortic aneurysm is rupture of a different aortic aneurysm. Therefore, staged repair of multiple aortic segments often is necessary. As with any major operation, careful preoperative evaluation for coexisting disease and subsequent medical optimization are essential for successful surgical treatment.

An alternative to traditional open repair of a descending thoracic aortic aneurysm is endovascular stent grafting. Certain anatomic criteria must be satisfied for this treatment option to be considered, including the presence of at least a 2-cm landing zone of healthy aortic tissue proximally and distally to the aneurysm to be excluded. Although data on long-term outcomes are still lacking, endovascular repair of descending thoracic aortic aneurysm has become an accepted practice that produces excellent midterm results.

Etiology and Pathogenesis
General Considerations

The normal aorta derives its elasticity and tensile strength from the medial layer, which contains approximately 45 to 55 lamellae of elastin, collagen, smooth muscle cells, and ground substance. Elastin content is highest within the ascending aorta, as would be expected because of its compliant nature, and decreases distally into the descending and abdominal aorta. Maintenance of the aortic matrix involves complex interactions among smooth muscle cells, macrophages, proteases, and protease inhibitors. Any alteration in this delicate balance can lead to aortic disease.

Thoracic aortic aneurysms have a variety of causes (Table 22-1). Although these disparate pathologic processes differ in biochemical and histologic terms, they share the final common pathway of progressive aortic expansion and eventual rupture.

Hemodynamic factors clearly contribute to the process of aortic dilatation. The vicious cycle of increasing diameter and increasing wall tension, as characterized by Laplace's law (tension = pressure × radius), is well established. Turbulent blood flow is also recognized as a factor. Poststenotic aortic dilatation, for example, occurs in some patients with aortic valve stenosis or coarctation of the descending thoracic aorta. Hemodynamic derangements, however, are only one piece of a complex puzzle.

TABLE 22-1 Causes of thoracic aortic aneurysms

Nonspecific medial degeneration
Aortic dissection
Genetic disorders
    Marfan syndrome
    Loeys-Dietz syndrome
    Ehlers-Danlos syndrome
    Familial aortic aneurysms
    Congenital bicuspid aortic valve
Poststenotic dilatation
Infection
Aortitis
    Takayasu's arteritis
    Giant cell arteritis
    Rheumatoid aortitis
Trauma

Atherosclerosis is commonly cited as a cause of thoracic aortic aneurysms. However, although atherosclerotic disease often is found in conjunction with aortic aneurysms, the notion that atherosclerosis is a distinct cause of aneurysm formation has been challenged. In thoracic aortic aneurysms, atherosclerosis appears to be a coexisting process, rather than the underlying cause.

Research into the pathogenesis of abdominal aortic aneurysms has focused on the molecular mechanisms of aortic wall degeneration and dilatation. For example, imbalances between proteolytic enzymes (e.g., matrix metalloproteinases) and their inhibitors contribute to abdominal aortic aneurysm formation. Building on these advances, current investigations are attempting to determine whether similar inflammatory and proteolytic mechanisms are involved in thoracic aortic disease, in hope of identifying potential molecular targets for pharmacologic therapy.

Nonspecific Medial Degeneration

Nonspecific medial degeneration is the most common cause of thoracic aortic disease. Histologic findings of mild medial degeneration, including fragmentation of elastic fibers and loss of smooth muscle cells, are expected in the aging aorta. However, an advanced, accelerated form of medial degeneration leads to progressive weakening of the aortic wall, aneurysm formation, and eventual dissection, rupture, or both. The underlying causes of medial degenerative disease remain unknown.

Aortic Dissection

An aortic dissection usually begins as a tear in the inner aortic wall, which initiates a progressive separation of the medial layers and creates two channels within the aorta. This event profoundly weakens the outer wall. As the most common catastrophe involving the aorta, dissection represents a major, distinct cause of thoracic aortic aneurysms and is discussed in detail in the second half of this chapter.

Genetic Disorders

Marfan Syndrome Marfan syndrome is an autosomal dominant genetic disorder characterized by a specific connective tissue defect that leads to aneurysm formation. The phenotype of patients with Marfan syndrome typically includes a tall stature, high palate, joint hypermobility, eye lens disorders, mitral valve prolapse, and aortic aneurysms. The aortic wall is weakened by fragmentation of elastic fibers and deposition of extensive amounts of mucopolysaccharides (a process previously called *cystic medial degeneration*). Patients with Marfan syndrome have a mutation in the fibrillin gene located on the long arm of chromosome 15. The traditionally held view is that abnormal fibrillin in the extracellular matrix decreases connective tissue strength in the aortic wall and produces abnormal elasticity, which predisposes the aorta to dilatation from wall tension caused by left ventricular ejection impulses.[3] More recent evidence, however, shows that the abnormal fibrillin causes degeneration of the aortic wall matrix by increasing the activity of transforming growth factor beta (TGF-β).[4] Between 75 and 85% of patients with Marfan syndrome have dilatation of the ascending aorta and annuloaortic ectasia (dilatation of the aortic sinuses and annulus).[5] Such aortic abnormalities are the most common cause of death among patients with Marfan syndrome.[6] Marfan syndrome also is frequently associated with aortic dissection.

Ehlers-Danlos Syndrome Ehlers-Danlos syndrome includes a spectrum of inherited connective tissue disorders of collagen synthesis. The subtypes represent differing defective steps of collagen production. Vascular type Ehlers-Danlos syndrome is characterized by an autosomal dominant defect in type III collagen synthesis, which can have life-threatening cardiovascular manifestations. Spontaneous arterial rupture, usually involving the mesenteric vessels, is the most common cause of death in these patients. Thoracic aortic aneurysms and dissections are less commonly associated with Ehlers-Danlos syndrome, but when they do occur, they pose a particularly challenging surgical problem because of the reduced integrity of the aortic tissue in patients with Ehlers-Danlos syndrome.

Loeys-Dietz Syndrome Recently described, Loeys-Dietz syndrome is phenotypically distinct from Marfan syndrome. It is characterized as an aneurysmal syndrome with widespread systemic involvement. Loeys-Dietz syndrome is an aggressive, autosomal dominant condition that is distinguished by the triad of arterial tortuosity and aneurysms, hypertelorism (widely spaced eyes), and bifid uvula or cleft palate. It is caused by heterozygous mutations in the genes encoding TGF-β receptors, rather than fibrillin 1.[7,8]

Familial Aortic Aneurysms Families without the heritable connective tissue disorders described earlier also can be affected by genetic conditions that cause thoracic aortic aneurysms. In fact, it is estimated that at least 20% of patients with thoracic aortic aneurysms and dissections have a genetic predisposition to them. The involved mutations are characterized by autosomal dominant inheritance with decreased penetrance and variable expression. Thus far, mutations involving the genes for TGF-β receptor 2 (*TGFβR2*), β-myosin heavy chain (*MYH11*), and α-smooth muscle cell actin (*ACTA2*) have been identified as causes of familial thoracic aortic aneurysms and dissection. Two other loci—on chromosomes 5 and 11—also have been associated with this condition, but the responsible genes have not yet been clearly identified.[9]

Congenital Bicuspid Aortic Valve Bicuspid aortic valve is the most common congenital malformation of the heart or great vessels, affecting up to 2% of Americans.[10] Compared to patients with normal, trileaflet aortic valves, patients with bicuspid aortic valves have an increased incidence of ascending aortic aneurysm formation and, often, a more rapid rate of aortic enlargement.[11] Fifty percent to 70% of adults with bicuspid aortic valve, but without significant valve dysfunction, have echocardiographically detectable aortic dilatation.[12,13] This dilatation usually is limited to the ascending aorta and root.[14] Dilation occasionally is found in the arch and only rarely in the descending or abdominal aorta. In addition, aortic dissection occurs 10 times more often in patients with bicuspid valves than in the general population.[15] Recent findings suggest that aneurysms associated with bicuspid aortic valves have a fundamentally different pathobiologic cause than aneurysms that occur in patients with trileaflet valves.[16]

The exact mechanism responsible for aneurysm formation in patients with bicuspid aortic valves remains controversial. The two most popular theories posit that the dilatation is caused by (a) a congenital defect involving the aortic wall matrix that results in progressive degeneration, or (b) ongoing hemodynamic stress caused by turbulent flow through the diseased valve. It is likely that both proposed mechanisms are involved: patients with bicuspid aortic valves may have a congenital connective tissue abnormality that predisposes the aorta to aneurysm formation, especially in the presence of chronic turbulent flow through a deformed valve.

In support of the theory that aneurysms result from vascular matrix remodeling that causes structural weakness of the aortic wall, evidence suggests that fibrillin 1 content is significantly lower and matrix metalloproteinase activity is significantly higher in the aortic media in patients with bicuspid aortic valves than in persons with normal tricuspid aortic valves.[16–18] In recent years, clinical studies have increasingly supported the theory that aortic wall fragility, not turbulent flow, is the main mechanism of dilatation in these patients. For example, one study showed that the aorta progressively dilates when the bicuspid valve is replaced with a prosthesis, despite the elimination of the hemodynamic lesion.[19] In addition, several studies have found evidence of a genetic predisposition to this condition.[20–22]

Infection

Primary infection of the aortic wall resulting in aneurysm formation is rare. Although these lesions are termed *mycotic aneurysms*, the responsible pathogens usually are bacteria rather than fungi. Bacterial

invasion of the aortic wall may result from bacterial endocarditis, endothelial trauma caused by an aortic jet lesion, or extension from an infected laminar clot within a pre-existing aneurysm. The most common causative organisms are *Staphylococcus aureus, Staphylococcus epidermidis, Salmonella,* and *Streptococcus.*[23,24] Unlike most other causes of thoracic aortic aneurysms, which generally produce fusiform aneurysms, infection often produces saccular aneurysms located in areas of aortic tissue destroyed by the infectious process.

Although syphilis was once the most common cause of ascending aortic aneurysms, the advent of effective antibiotic therapy has made syphilitic aneurysms a rarity in developed nations. In other parts of the world, however, syphilitic aneurysms remain a major cause of morbidity and mortality. The spirochete *Treponema pallidum* causes an obliterative endarteritis of the vasa vasorum that results in medial ischemia and loss of the elastic and muscular elements of the aortic wall. The ascending aorta and arch are the most commonly involved areas. The emergence of HIV infection in the 1980s was associated with a substantial increase in the incidence of syphilis in both HIV-positive and HIV-negative patients. Because syphilitic aortitis often presents 10 to 30 years after the primary infection, the incidence of associated aneurysms may increase in the near future.

Aortitis

In patients with pre-existing degenerative thoracic aortic aneurysms, localized transmural inflammation and subsequent fibrosis can develop. The dense aortic infiltrate responsible for the fibrosis consists of lymphocytes, plasma cells, and giant cells. The cause of the intense inflammatory reaction is unknown. Although the severe inflammation is a superimposed problem rather than a primary cause, its onset within an aneurysm can further weaken the aortic wall and precipitate expansion.

Systemic autoimmune disorders also cause thoracic aortitis. Aortic Takayasu's arteritis generally produces obstructive lesions related to severe intimal thickening, but associated medial necrosis can lead to aneurysm formation. In patients with giant cell arteritis (temporal arteritis), granulomatous inflammation may develop that involves the entire thickness of the aortic wall, causing intimal thickening and medial destruction. Rheumatoid aortitis is an uncommon systemic disease that is associated with rheumatoid arthritis and ankylosing spondylitis. The resulting medial inflammation and fibrosis can affect the aortic root, causing annular dilatation, aortic valve regurgitation, and ascending aortic aneurysm formation.

Pseudoaneurysms

Pseudoaneurysms of the thoracic aorta usually represent chronic leaks that are contained by surrounding tissue and fibrosis. By definition, the wall of a pseudoaneurysm is not formed by intact aortic tissue; rather, the wall develops from organized thrombus and associated fibrosis. Pseudoaneurysms can arise from primary defects in the aortic wall (e.g., after trauma or contained aneurysm rupture) or from anastomotic leaks that occur after cardiovascular surgery. Anastomotic pseudoaneurysms can be caused by technical problems or by deterioration of the native aortic tissue, graft material, or suture. Tissue deterioration usually is related to either progressive degenerative disease or infection. Improvements in sutures, graft materials, and surgical techniques have decreased the incidence of thoracic aortic pseudoaneurysms.

Natural History

Treatment decisions in cases of thoracic aortic aneurysm are guided by our current understanding of the natural history of these aneurysms, which classically is characterized as progressive aortic dilatation and eventual dissection, rupture, or both. An analysis by Elefteriades of data from 1600 patients with thoracic aortic disease has helped quantify these well-recognized risks.[25] Average expansion rates were 0.07 cm/y in ascending aortic aneurysms and 0.19 cm/y in descending thoracic aortic aneurysms. As expected, aortic diameter was a strong predictor of rupture, dissection, and mortality. For thoracic aortic aneurysms >6 cm in diameter, annual rates of catastrophic complications were 3.6% for rupture, 3.7% for dissection, and 10.8% for death. Critical diameters, at which the incidence of expected complications significantly increased, were 6.0 cm for aneurysms of the ascending aorta and 7.0 cm for aneurysms of the descending thoracic aorta; the corresponding risks of rupture after reaching these diameters were 31 and 43%, respectively.[26]

Certain types of aneurysms have an increased propensity for expansion and rupture. For example, aneurysms in patients with Marfan syndrome dilate at an accelerated rate and rupture or dissect at smaller diameters than non–Marfan-related aneurysms. Before the era of surgical treatment for aortic aneurysms, this aggressive form of aortic disease resulted in an average life expectancy of 32 years for Marfan patients; aortic root complications caused the majority of deaths.[27] Saccular aneurysms, which commonly are associated with aortic infection and typically affect only a discrete small section of the aorta, tend to grow more rapidly than fusiform aneurysms, which are associated with more widespread degenerative changes and generally affect a larger section of the aorta.

One common clinical scenario deserves special attention. A moderately dilated ascending aorta (i.e., 4 to 5 cm) often is encountered during aortic valve replacement or coronary artery bypass operations. The natural history of these ectatic ascending aortas has been defined by several studies. Michel and colleagues[28] studied patients whose ascending aortic diameters were >4 cm at the time of aortic valve replacement; 25% of these patients required reoperation for ascending aortic replacement. Prenger and colleagues[29] reported that aortic dissection occurred in 27% of patients who had aortic diameters of >5 cm at the time of aortic valve replacement.

Clinical Manifestations

In many patients with thoracic aortic aneurysms, the aneurysm is discovered incidentally when imaging studies are performed for unrelated reasons. Therefore, patients often are asymptomatic at the time of diagnosis. However, thoracic aortic aneurysms that initially go undetected eventually create symptoms and signs that correspond with the segment of aorta that is involved. These aneurysms have a wide variety of manifestations, including compression or erosion of adjacent structures, aortic valve regurgitation, distal embolism, and rupture.

Local Compression and Erosion

Initially, aneurysmal expansion and impingement on adjacent structures causes mild, chronic pain. The most common symptom in patients with ascending aortic aneurysms is anterior chest discomfort; the pain is frequently precordial in location but may radiate to the neck and jaw, mimicking angina. Aneurysms of the ascending aorta and transverse aortic arch can cause symptoms related to compression of the superior vena cava, the pulmonary artery, the airway, or the sternum. Rarely, these aneurysms erode into the superior vena cava or right atrium, causing acute high-output failure. Expansion of the distal aortic arch can stretch the recurrent laryngeal nerve, which results in left vocal cord paralysis and hoarseness. Descending thoracic and thoracoabdominal aneurysms frequently cause back pain localized between the scapulae. When the aneurysm is largest in the region of the aortic hiatus, it may cause middle back and epigastric pain. Thoracic or lumbar vertebral body erosion typically causes severe, chronic back pain; extreme cases can present with spinal instability and neurologic deficits from spinal cord compression. Although mycotic aneurysms have a peculiar propensity to destroy vertebral bodies, spinal erosion also occurs with degenerative aneurysms. Descending thoracic aortic aneurysms may cause varying degrees of airway obstruction, manifesting as cough, wheezing, stridor, or pneumonitis. Pulmonary or airway erosion presents as hemoptysis. Compression and erosion of the esophagus cause dysphagia and hematemesis, respectively. Thoracoabdominal aortic aneurysms can cause duodenal obstruction or, if they erode through the bowel wall, GI bleeding. Jaundice due to compression of the liver

or porta hepatis is uncommon. Erosion into the inferior vena cava or iliac vein presents with an abdominal bruit, widened pulse pressure, edema, and heart failure.

Aortic Valve Regurgitation

Ascending aortic aneurysms can cause displacement of the aortic valve commissures and annular dilatation. The resulting deformation of the aortic valve leads to progressively worsening aortic valve regurgitation. In response to the volume overload, the heart remodels and becomes increasingly dilated. Patients with this condition may present with progressive heart failure, a widened pulse pressure, and a diastolic murmur.

Distal Embolization

Thoracic aortic aneurysms—particularly those involving the descending and thoracoabdominal aorta—are commonly lined with friable, atheromatous plaque and mural thrombus. This debris may embolize distally, causing occlusion and thrombosis of the visceral, renal, or lower-extremity branches.

Rupture

Patients with ruptured thoracic aortic aneurysms often experience sudden, severe pain in the anterior chest (ascending aorta), upper back or left chest (descending thoracic aorta), or left flank or abdomen (thoracoabdominal aorta). When ascending aortic aneurysms rupture, they usually bleed into the pericardial space, producing acute cardiac tamponade and death. Descending thoracic aortic aneurysms rupture into the pleural cavity, producing a combination of severe hemorrhagic shock and respiratory compromise. External rupture is extremely rare; saccular syphilitic aneurysms have been observed to rupture externally after eroding through the sternum.

Diagnostic Evaluation

Although certain constellations of symptoms and signs are highly suggestive of thoracic aortic aneurysm, diagnosing and characterizing these aneurysms requires imaging studies. In addition to establishing the diagnosis, imaging studies provide critical information that guides the selection of treatment options. Optimal imaging techniques for the thoracic and thoracoabdominal aorta are somewhat institution-specific, varying with the availability of imaging equipment and expertise.

Plain Radiography

Plain radiographs of the chest, abdomen, or spine often provide enough information to support the initial diagnosis of thoracic aortic aneurysm. Ascending aortic aneurysms produce a convex shadow to the right of the cardiac silhouette. The anterior projection of an ascending aneurysm results in the loss of the retrosternal space in the lateral view. An aneurysm may be indistinguishable from elongation and tortuosity.[30] It is important to recognize that chest radiographs (CXRs) often appear normal in patients with thoracic aortic disease and thus cannot exclude the diagnosis of aortic aneurysm. Aortic root aneurysms, for example, often are hidden within the cardiac silhouette. Plain CXRs may reveal convexity in the right superior mediastinum, loss of the retrosternal space, or widening of the descending thoracic aortic shadow, which may be highlighted by a rim of calcification outlining the dilated aneurysmal aortic wall. Aortic calcification also may be seen in the upper abdomen on a standard radiograph made in the anteroposterior or lateral projection (Fig. 22-2). Once a thoracic aortic aneurysm is detected on plain radiographs, additional studies are required to define the extent of aortic involvement.

Ultrasonography

Although useful in evaluating infrarenal abdominal aortic aneurysms, standard transabdominal ultrasonography does not allow visualization of the thoracic aorta. During ultrasound evaluation of a suspected infrarenal abdominal aortic aneurysm, if a definitive

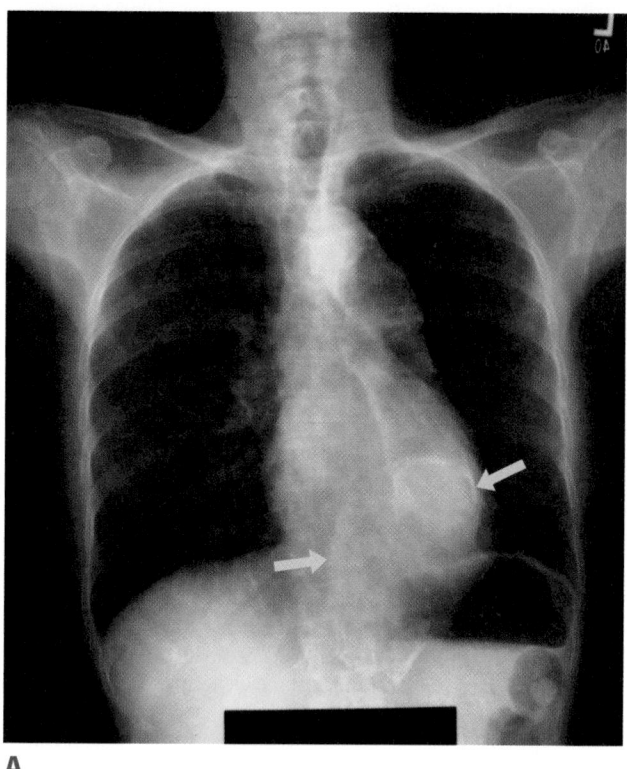

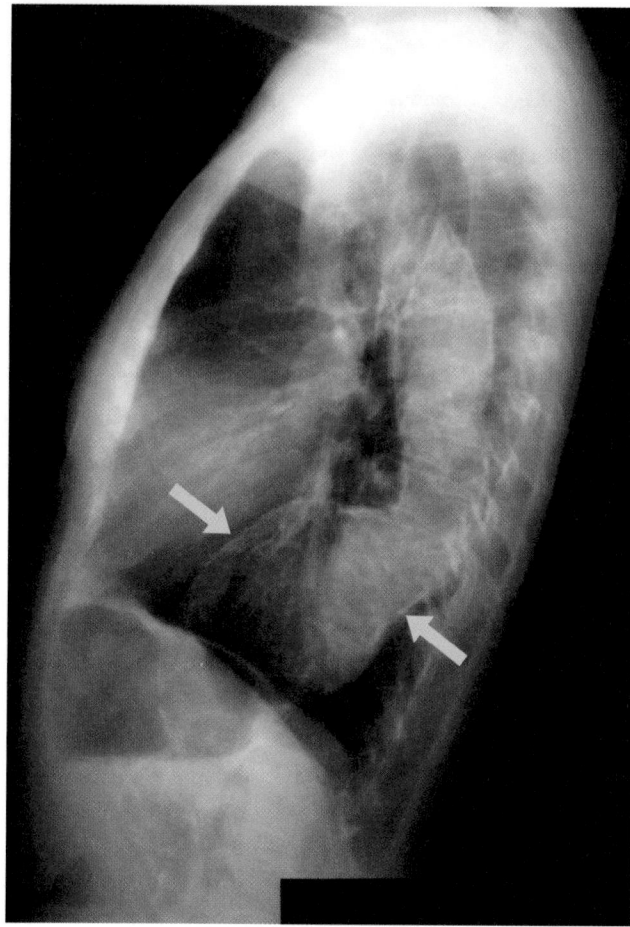

FIG. 22-2. Chest radiographs showing a calcified rim (*arrows*) in the aortic wall of a thoracoabdominal aortic aneurysm. **A.** Anteroposterior view. **B.** Lateral view.

neck cannot be identified at the level of the renal arteries, the possibility of thoracoabdominal aortic involvement should be suspected and investigated by using other imaging modalities.

Echocardiography

Ascending aortic aneurysms are commonly discovered during echocardiography in patients presenting with symptoms or signs of aortic valve regurgitation. Both transthoracic and transesophageal echocardiography provide excellent visualization of the ascending aorta, including the aortic root.[31] Transesophageal echocardiography (TEE) also allows visualization of the descending thoracic aorta but is not ideal for evaluating the transverse aortic arch (which is obscured by air in the tracheobronchial tree) or the upper abdominal aorta. Effective echocardiography requires considerable technical skill, both in obtaining adequate images and in interpreting them. This imaging modality has the added benefit of assessing cardiac function and revealing any other abnormalities that may be present.

Computed Tomography

Computed tomographic (CT) scanning is widely available and provides visualization of the entire thoracic and abdominal aorta. Consequently, CT is the most common—and arguably the most useful—imaging modality for evaluating thoracic aortic aneurysms.[32] Systems capable of constructing multiplanar images and performing three-dimensional aortic reconstructions are widely available. In addition to establishing the diagnosis, CT provides information about an aneurysm's location, extent, anatomic anomalies, and relationship to major branch vessels. CT is particularly useful in determining the absolute diameter of the aorta, especially in the presence of laminated clot. Contrast-enhanced CT provides information about the aortic lumen and can detect mural thrombus, aortic dissection, inflamma-

tory periaortic fibrosis, and mediastinal or retroperitoneal hematoma due to contained aortic rupture. The major disadvantage of contrast-enhanced CT scanning is the possibility of contrast-induced acute renal failure in patients who are at risk (e.g., patients with pre-existing renal disease or diabetes).[33] If possible, surgery is performed ≥1 day after contrast administration to allow time to observe renal function and to permit diuresis of the contrast agent. If renal insufficiency occurs or is worsened, elective surgery is postponed until renal function returns to normal or stabilizes.

Magnetic Resonance Angiography

Magnetic resonance angiography (MRA) is becoming widely available and has the ability to facilitate visualization of the entire aorta. This modality produces aortic images comparable to those produced by contrast-enhanced CT but does not necessitate exposure to ionizing radiation. In addition, MRA offers excellent visualization of branch vessel details, and it is useful in detecting branch vessel stenosis.[34] Current limitations of MRA include high expense and a susceptibility to artifacts created by ferromagnetic materials. Also, a few recent studies have suggested that gadolinium—the contrast agent for MRA—may be linked to nephrogenic systemic fibrosis and acute renal failure in patients with advanced renal insufficiency.[35] Furthermore, the MRA environment is not appropriate for many critically ill patients.

Aortography and Cardiac Catheterization

Although diagnostic aortography was, until recently, considered the gold standard for evaluating thoracic aortic disease, CT and MRA have largely replaced this modality. Technologic improvements have enabled CT and MRA to provide excellent aortic imaging while causing less morbidity than catheter-based studies do, so CT and

MRA should now be considered the gold standard. Therefore, the role of diagnostic angiography in patients with thoracic aortic disease is currently limited. However, the advent of endovascular therapies has given catheter-based angiography a new role, because intraprocedural angiography is an essential component of endovascular procedures.

In selected cases, aortography is used to gain important information when other types of studies are contraindicated or have not provided satisfactory results. For example, information about obstructive lesions of the brachiocephalic, visceral, renal, or iliac arteries is useful when surgical treatment is being planned; if other imaging studies have not provided adequate detail, aortograms can be obtained in patients with suspected branch vessel occlusive disease.

Unlike standard aortography, cardiac catheterization continues to play a major role in diagnosis and preoperative planning, especially in patients with ascending aortic involvement. Proximal aortography can reveal not only the status of the coronary arteries and left ventricular function but also the degree of aortic valve regurgitation, the extent of aortic root involvement, coronary ostial displacement, and the relationship of the aneurysm to the arch vessels.

The value of the information one can obtain from catheter-based diagnostic studies should be weighed against the established limitations and potential complications of such studies. A key limitation of aortography is that it images only the lumen and may therefore underrepresent the size of large aneurysms that contain laminated thrombus. Manipulation of intraluminal catheters can result in embolization of laminated thrombus or atheromatous debris. Proximal aortography carries a 0.6 to 1.2% risk of stroke. Other risks include allergic reaction to contrast agent, iatrogenic aortic dissection, and bleeding at the arterial access site. In addition, the volumes of contrast agent required to adequately fill large aneurysms can cause significant renal toxicity. To minimize the risk of contrast nephropathy, patients receive periprocedural IV fluids for hydration, mannitol for diuresis, and acetylcysteine.[36,37] As with contrast-enhanced CT, surgery is performed ≥1 day after angiography whenever possible to ensure that renal function has stabilized or returned to baseline.

Treatment

Determination of the Appropriate Treatment

Once a thoracic aortic aneurysm is detected, management begins with patient education, particularly if the patient is asymptomatic. A detailed medical history is collected, a physical examination is performed, and a systematic review of medical records is carried out to clearly assess the presence or absence of pertinent symptoms and signs, despite any initial denial of symptoms by the patient. Signs of genetic diseases such as Marfan syndrome are thoroughly reviewed. If clinical criteria are met for such a genetic condition, confirmatory laboratory tests are conducted. Patients with such genetic diseases are best treated in a dedicated aortic clinic where they can be appropriately followed. Surveillance CT scans and aggressive blood pressure control are the mainstays of initial management for asymptomatic patients. When patients become symptomatic or their aneurysms grow to meet certain size criteria, the patients become surgical candidates.

Since the last edition of this textbook was published, endovascular therapy has become an accepted treatment for thoracic aortic aneurysms. Although its role in treating proximal aortic disease and thoracoabdominal aortic aneurysms remains experimental, endoluminal stenting is approved by the Food and Drug Administration for the treatment of isolated descending thoracic aortic aneurysms. For aneurysms with proximal aortic involvement and for thoracoabdominal aortic aneurysms, open procedures remain the gold standard and preferred approach.

Determination of the Extent and Severity of Disease

Serial CT scans are critical when one is evaluating a thoracic aneurysm, determining treatment strategy, and planning necessary procedures. Note that, commonly, patients with a thoracic aortic aneurysm

also have a remote aneurysm.[2] In such cases, the more threatening lesion usually is addressed first. In many patients, staged operative procedures are necessary for complete repair of extensive aneurysms involving the ascending aorta, transverse arch, and descending thoracic or thoracoabdominal aorta.[38] When the descending segment is not disproportionately large (compared with the proximal aorta) and is not causing symptoms, the proximal aortic repair is carried out first. An important benefit of this approach is that it allows treatment of valvular and coronary artery occlusive disease at the first operation.

Proximal aneurysms (proximal to the left subclavian artery) usually are addressed via a sternotomy approach. Left thoracotomy incisions are used for open repairs of aneurysms involving the descending thoracic aorta, unless the aneurysm fulfills certain endovascular criteria. A CT scan can reveal detailed information about aortic calcification and luminal thrombus. These details are important in preventing embolization during surgical manipulation.

Indications for Operation Thoracic aortic aneurysms are repaired to prevent fatal rupture. Therefore, on the basis of the natural history studies discussed earlier, elective operation is recommended when the diameter of an ascending aortic aneurysm is >5.5 cm, when the diameter of a descending thoracic aortic aneurysm is >6.5 cm, or when the rate of dilatation is >1 cm/y.[25,39] In patients with connective tissue disorders, such as Marfan and Loeys-Dietz syndromes, the threshold for operation is lower with regard to both absolute size (5.0 cm for the ascending aorta and 6.0 cm for the descending thoracic aorta) and rate of growth. Smaller ascending aortic aneurysms (4.0 to 5.5 cm) also are considered for repair when they are associated with significant aortic valve regurgitation.

The acuity of presentation is a major factor in decisions about the timing of surgical intervention. Many patients are asymptomatic at the time of presentation, so there is time for thorough preoperative evaluation and improvement of their current health status, such as through smoking cessation and other optimization programs. In contrast, patients who present with symptoms may need urgent operation. Symptomatic patients are at increased risk of rupture and warrant expeditious evaluation. The onset of new pain in patients with known aneurysms is especially concerning, because it may herald significant expansion, leakage, or impending rupture. Because emergent interventions produce worse outcomes than elective procedures do, emergent intervention is reserved for patients who present with rupture or superimposed acute dissection.[40]

Open Repair vs. Endovascular Repair As noted earlier, endovascular repair of thoracic aortic aneurysms has become an accepted treatment option in selected patients, particularly patients with isolated degenerative descending thoracic aortic aneurysms. For endovascular repairs to produce optimal outcomes, several anatomic criteria must be met. For one, the proximal and distal neck diameters should fall within a range that will allow proper sealing. Also, the proximal and distal necks should be at least 20 mm long so that an appropriate landing-zone seal can be made. Note that the limiting structures proximally and distally are the brachiocephalic vessels and celiac axis, respectively. Another anatomic limitation for this therapy relates to vascular access: The femoral and iliac arteries have to be wide enough to accommodate the large sheaths necessary to deploy the stent grafts. Occasionally, a "side graft" must be anastomosed to the iliac artery through a retroperitoneal incision because of poor distal access. When any of these anatomic criteria is not met, an open approach is preferable to an endovascular approach. Of note, attempts have been made to extend the use of endovascular therapy to aortic arch aneurysms and thoracoabdominal aortic aneurysms. Reports of these types of purely endovascular repair are limited. Still experimental, hybrid approaches involve debranching the aortic arch or the visceral vessels of the abdominal aorta followed by endovascular exclusion of the aneurysm. Figure 22-3 provides an algorithm for the management of descending thoracic aortic aneurysm.

The patients who benefit more from an endovascular approach than from traditional open techniques are those who are of ad-

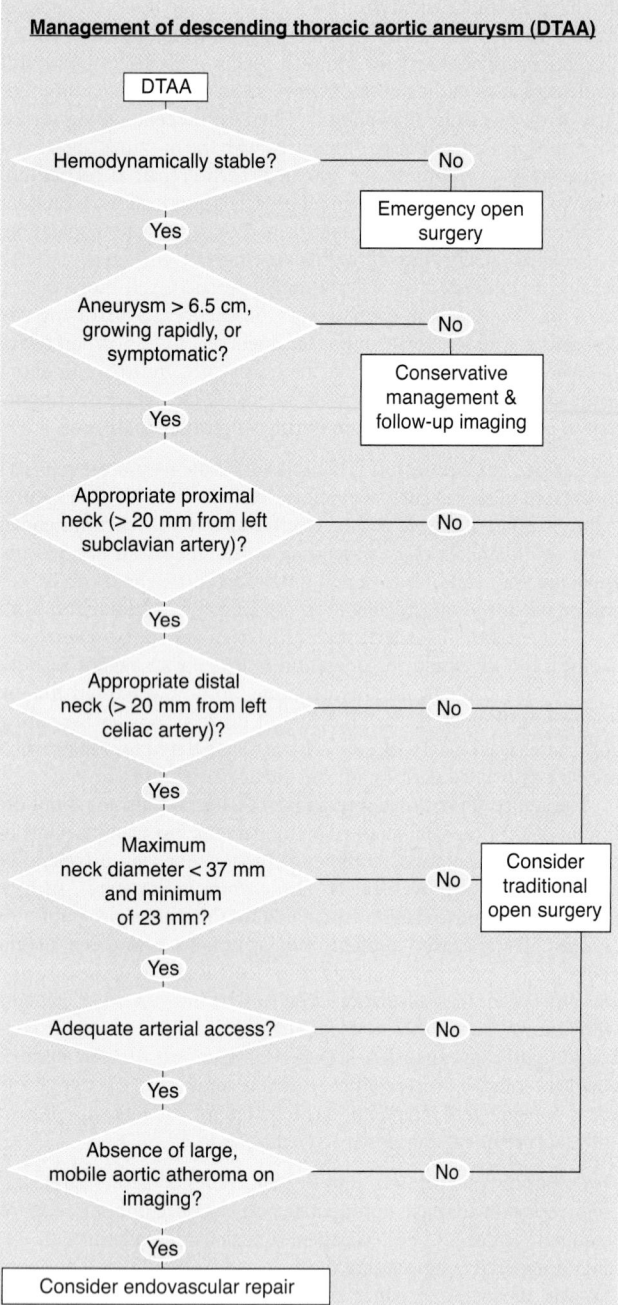

Management of descending thoracic aortic aneurysm (DTAA)

DTAA

Hemodynamically stable? — No → Emergency open surgery

Yes

Aneurysm > 6.5 cm, growing rapidly, or symptomatic? — No → Conservative management & follow-up imaging

Yes

Appropriate proximal neck (> 20 mm from left subclavian artery)? — No

Yes

Appropriate distal neck (> 20 mm from left celiac artery)? — No

Yes

Maximum neck diameter < 37 mm and minimum of 23 mm? — No → Consider traditional open surgery

Yes

Adequate arterial access? — No

Yes

Absence of large, mobile aortic atheroma on imaging? — No

Yes

Consider endovascular repair

FIG. 22-3. Algorithm for the management of descending thoracic aortic aneurysm as used to facilitate decisions regarding treatment.

vanced age or have significant comorbidities. The open repair of a descending thoracic aortic aneurysm can result in significant pulmonary morbidity. Therefore, patients with borderline pulmonary reserve may be best suited for an endovascular or hybrid procedure. In contrast, patients with significant intraluminal atheroma are best served by an open approach because of the risk of embolization and stroke posed by catheter manipulations. Similarly, patients with connective tissue disease should undergo an open procedure and generally are not considered candidates for endovascular repair. Endovascular repair in the setting of connective tissue disorders has been met with poor results, which are mainly due to progressive dilatation, stent graft migration, and endoleak.

Preoperative Assessment and Preparation

Given the impact of comorbid conditions on perioperative complications, a careful preoperative assessment of physiologic reserve is

critical in assessing operative risk. Therefore, most patients undergo a thorough evaluation—with emphasis on cardiac, pulmonary, and renal function—before undergoing elective surgery.[41,42]

Cardiac Evaluation Coronary artery disease is common in patients with thoracic aortic aneurysms and is responsible for a substantial proportion of early and late postoperative deaths in such patients. Similarly, valvular disease and myocardial dysfunction have important implications when one is planning anesthetic management and surgical approaches for aortic repair. Transthoracic echocardiography is a satisfactory noninvasive method for evaluating both valvular and biventricular function. Dipyridamole-thallium myocardial scanning identifies regions of myocardium that have reversible ischemia, and this test is more practical than exercise testing in older patients with concomitant lower-extremity peripheral vascular disease. Cardiac catheterization and coronary arteriography are performed in patients who have evidence of coronary disease—as indicated by either the patient's history or the results of noninvasive studies—or who have a left ventricular ejection fraction of ≤30%. If significant valvular or coronary artery disease is identified before a proximal aortic operation, the disease can be addressed directly during the procedure. Patients who have asymptomatic distal aortic aneurysms and severe coronary occlusive disease undergo percutaneous transluminal angioplasty or surgical revascularization before the aneurysmal aortic segment is replaced.

Pulmonary Evaluation Pulmonary function screening with arterial blood gas measurement and spirometry is routinely performed before thoracic aortic operations. Patients with a forced expiratory volume in 1 second of >1.0 L and a partial pressure of carbon dioxide of <45 mmHg are considered surgical candidates. In suitable patients, borderline pulmonary function can be improved by implementing a regimen that includes smoking cessation, weight loss, exercise, and treatment of bronchitis for a period of 1 to 3 months before surgery. Although surgery is not withheld from patients with symptomatic aortic aneurysms and poor pulmonary function, adjustments in operative technique should be made to maximize these patients' chances of recovery. In such patients, preserving the left recurrent laryngeal nerve, the phrenic nerves, and diaphragmatic function is particularly important.

Renal Evaluation Renal function is assessed preoperatively by measuring serum electrolyte, blood urea nitrogen, and creatinine levels. Information about kidney size and perfusion can be obtained from the CT scan or aortogram used to evaluate the aorta.

Accurate information about baseline renal function has important therapeutic and prognostic implications. For example, perfusion strategies and perioperative medications are adjusted according to renal function. Patients with severely impaired renal function frequently require at least temporary hemodialysis after surgery. These patients also have a mortality rate that is significantly higher than normal. Patients with thoracoabdominal aortic aneurysms and poor renal function secondary to severe proximal renal occlusive disease undergo renal artery endarterectomy, stenting, or bypass grafting during the aortic repair.

Operative Repair

Proximal Thoracic Aortic Aneurysms *Open Repair* Operations to repair proximal aortic aneurysms—which involve the ascending aorta, transverse aortic arch, or both—are performed through a midsternal incision and require cardiopulmonary bypass. The best choice of aortic replacement technique varies depending on the extent of the aneurysm and the condition of the aortic valve. The spectrum of operations ranges from simple graft replacement of the tubular portion of the ascending aorta (Fig. 22-4) to graft replacement of the entire proximal aorta, including the aortic root, and reattachment of the coronary arteries and brachiocephalic branches. The options for treating aortic valve disease, repairing aortic aneurysms, and maintaining perfusion during repair procedures each deserve detailed consideration (Table 22-2).

TABLE 22-2 Options for open surgical repair of proximal aortic aneurysms

Options for treating aortic valve disease
    Aortic valve annuloplasty (annular plication)
    Aortic valve replacement with mechanical or biologic prosthesis
    Aortic root replacement
        Composite valve graft
        Aortic homograft
        Stentless porcine root
        Pulmonary autograft (Ross procedure)
        Valve-sparing techniques
Options for graft repair of the aortic aneurysm
    Patch aortoplasty
    Ascending replacement only
    Beveled hemiarch replacement
    Total arch replacement with reattachment of brachiocephalic branches
    Total arch replacement with bypass grafts to the brachiocephalic branches
    Elephant trunk technique
Perfusion options
    Standard cardiopulmonary bypass
    Hypothermic circulatory arrest without adjuncts
    Hypothermic circulatory arrest with adjuncts
        Retrograde cerebral perfusion
        Selective antegrade cerebral perfusion
            Balloon perfusion catheters
            Right axillary artery cannulation
        Combined antegrade and retrograde cerebral perfusion

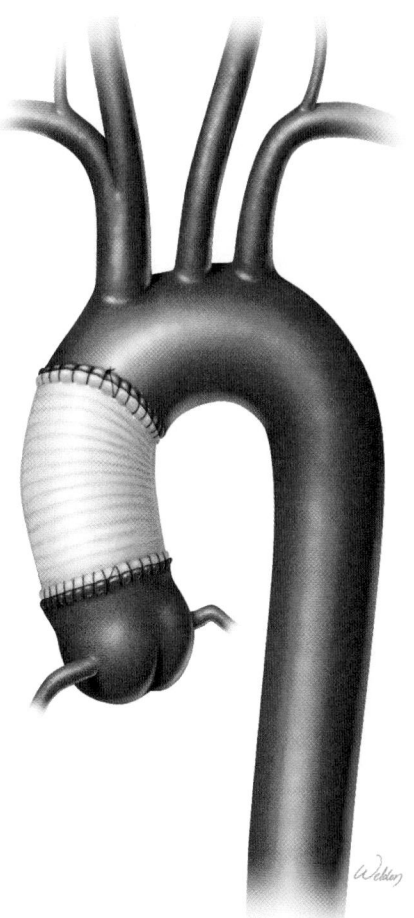

FIG. 22-4. Illustration of an ascending aortic repair. The tubular portion of the ascending aorta has been replaced by a graft, and the native aortic root and arch are left intact.

Aortic Valve Disease and Root Aneurysms Many patients undergoing proximal aortic operations have aortic valve disease that requires concomitant surgical correction. When such disease is present and the sinus segment is normal, separate repair or replacement of the aortic valve and graft replacement of the tubular segment of the ascending aorta are carried out. Mild to moderate valve regurgitation with annular dilatation in this setting can be addressed by plicating the annulus with mattress sutures placed below each commissure. The valve is replaced with a stented biologic or mechanical prosthesis in patients with more severe valvular regurgitation or with valvular stenosis. Separate replacement of the aortic valve and ascending aorta is not performed in patients with Marfan syndrome, because progressive dilatation of the remaining sinus segment eventually leads to complications that necessitate reoperation. Therefore, patients with Marfan syndrome or annuloaortic ectasia require some form of aortic root replacement.[43]

In most cases, the aortic root is replaced with a mechanical or biologic graft that has both a valve and an aortic conduit. Currently, three graft options are commercially available: composite valve grafts, which consist of a bileaflet mechanical valve attached to a polyester tube graft; aortic root homografts, which are harvested from cadavers and cryopreserved; and stentless porcine aortic root grafts.[44,45]

Another option for selected patients is the Ross procedure, in which the patient's pulmonary artery root is excised and placed in the aortic position. The right ventricular outflow tract is reconstructed by using a cryopreserved pulmonary homograft. This option is rarely used, largely because of its technical demands and because of concerns about the potential for autograft dilatation in patients with connective tissue disorders.[46] An additional option is valve-sparing

aortic root replacement, which has evolved substantially during the past decade.[47] The valve-sparing technique that is currently favored is called *aortic root reimplantation* and involves excising the aortic sinuses, attaching a prosthetic graft to the patient's annulus, and resuspending the native aortic valve inside the graft. The superior hemodynamics of the native valve and the avoidance of anticoagulation are major advantages of the valve-sparing approach. Long-term results in carefully selected patients have been excellent.[48] The durability of this procedure in patients with either Marfan syndrome or bicuspid aortic valves has been the subject of controversy. Recently, in appropriately experienced centers, this technique has shown encouraging long-term durability for patients with Marfan syndrome.[49,50] Also, there is evidence that valve-sparing techniques can produce acceptable outcomes in patients with bicuspid aortic valves.[51]

Regardless of the type of conduit used, aortic root replacement requires reattaching the coronary arteries to openings in the graft. In the original procedure described by Bentall and De Bono,[52] this was accomplished by suturing the intact aortic wall surrounding each coronary artery to the openings in the graft. The aortic wall was then wrapped around the graft to establish hemostasis. However, this technique frequently produced leaks at the coronary reattachment sites that eventually led to pseudoaneurysm formation. Cabrol's modification, in which a separate, small tube graft is sutured to the coronary ostia and the main aortic graft, achieves tension-free coronary anastomoses and reduces the risk of pseudoaneurysm formation.[53] Kouchoukos's button modification of the Bentall procedure is currently the most widely used technique.[54] The aneurysmal aorta is excised, and buttons of aortic wall are left surrounding both coronary arteries, which are then mobilized and sutured to the aortic graft (Fig. 22-5). The coronary suture lines may be reinforced with polytetrafluoroethylene felt or pericardium to enhance hemostasis. When the coronary arteries cannot be mobilized adequately because of extremely large aneurysms or scarring from previous surgery, the Cabrol technique can be used. Another option, originally described by Zubiate and Kay,[55] is the construction of bypass grafts by using interposition saphenous vein or synthetic grafts.

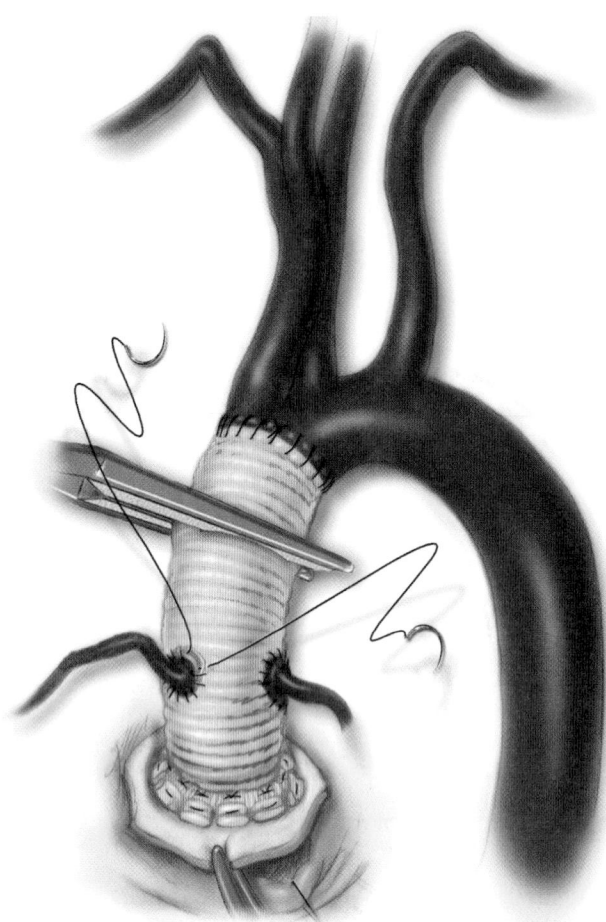

FIG. 22-5. Illustration of the modified Bentall procedure for replacing the aortic root and ascending aorta. The aortic valve and entire ascending aorta, including the sinuses of Valsalva, have been replaced by a mechanical composite valve graft. The coronary arteries with buttons of surrounding aortic tissue have been mobilized and are being reattached to openings in the aortic graft.

Aortic Arch Aneurysms Several options are also available for handling aneurysms that extend into the transverse aortic arch. The surgical approach depends on the extent of involvement and the need for cardiac and cerebral protection. Saccular aneurysms that arise from the lesser curvature of the distal transverse arch and that encompass <50% of the aortic circumference are treated by patch graft aortoplasty. For fusiform aneurysms, when the distal portion of the arch is a reasonable size, a single, beveled replacement of the lower curvature (hemiarch) is performed. More extensive arch aneurysms require total replacement involving a distal anastomosis to the proximal descending thoracic aorta and separate reattachment of the brachiocephalic branches. The brachiocephalic vessels are reattached to one or more openings made in the graft, or if these vessels are aneurysmal, they are replaced with separate, smaller grafts. In the most extreme cases, the aneurysm involves the entire arch and extends into the descending thoracic aorta. Such aneurysms are approached by using Borst's elephant trunk technique of staged total arch replacement (Fig. 22-6).[57] The distal anastomosis is constructed so that a portion of the graft is left suspended within the proximal descending thoracic aorta. During a subsequent operation, this "trunk" is used to facilitate repair of the descending thoracic aorta through a thoracotomy incision. This technique permits access to the distal portion of the graft at the second operation without the need for dissection around the distal transverse aortic arch; this reduces the risk of injuring the left recurrent laryngeal nerve, esophagus, and pulmonary artery if an open approach is used at the second stage. As

described in the section on hybrid repair of arch aneurysms (see later), the elephant trunk can be completed by using a hybrid endovascular approach in certain settings.

Cardiopulmonary Bypass Perfusion Strategies Like the operations themselves, perfusion strategies used during proximal aortic surgery depend on the extent of the repair. Aneurysms that are isolated to the ascending segment can be replaced by using standard cardiopulmonary bypass and distal ascending aortic clamping. This provides constant perfusion of the brain and other vital organs during the repair. Aneurysms involving the transverse aortic arch, however, cannot be clamped during the repair, which necessitates the temporary withdrawal of cardiopulmonary bypass support; this is called *circulatory arrest*. To protect the brain and other vital organs during the circulatory arrest period, profound cooling must be initiated before pump flow is stopped. An electroencephalogram is monitored during cooling. Once electrocerebral silence is achieved—indicating cessation of brain activity and minimization of metabolic requirements—the pump flow is stopped, and the arch is repaired. Electrocerebral silence usually occurs when the patient's nasopharyngeal temperature falls below 18°C (64.4°F). Although brief periods of circulatory arrest generally are well tolerated, this technique does have substantial limitations. The well-recognized risks of brain injury and death increase dramatically as the duration of circulatory arrest increases. Techniques for monitoring the brain during circulatory arrest have proven benefits in pediatric patients.[58] Whether transcranial Doppler ultrasonography and near-infrared spectroscopy are of any benefit in adult patients remains to be determined.

Two perfusion strategies have been developed to reduce the risks that circulatory arrest entails: retrograde cerebral perfusion and selective antegrade cerebral perfusion. Retrograde cerebral perfusion delivers cold, oxygenated blood from the pump into a cannula placed in the superior vena cava (Fig. 22-7A). This technique was introduced in the hope that the retrograde delivery of blood would provide oxygen to the brain; however, accumulating evidence suggests that it does not.[59-62] The apparent benefits of this technique are more likely due to maintenance of cerebral hypothermia and retrograde flushing of air and debris.

Selective antegrade cerebral perfusion delivers blood directly into the brachiocephalic arteries while circulatory arrest is maintained in the rest of the body.[63] This technique originally required cumbersome bypass grafts and cannulas and consequently fell out of favor. However, recent technologic improvements and new strategies for delivery have resulted in a resurgence of interest in this technique, which should now be considered a standard adjunct for cerebral protection during hypothermic circulatory arrest. One common way of delivering antegrade cerebral perfusion involves the insertion of small, flexible balloon perfusion catheters into one or more of the branch arteries (Fig. 22-7B). Another method, which is rapidly gaining popularity because of its relative simplicity, involves cannulating the right axillary artery (Fig. 22-8).[64] After circulatory arrest is induced and the proximal innominate artery is occluded, the axillary artery cannula delivers blood into the cerebral circulation via the right common carotid artery. Note that, with this technique, blood flow to the left side of the brain requires an intact circle of Willis. Antegrade cerebral perfusion via the right axillary artery has become our standard adjunct for cerebral perfusion during circulatory arrest.

Several reports have noted the safety of using only deep to moderate hypothermia [25° to 30°C (77° to 86°F)] when antegrade cerebral perfusion is used during circulatory arrest.[65,66] The advantages of moderate hypothermia relate mainly to avoiding the severe coagulopathy that develops with deep hypothermia. Some authors have raised concerns that reducing the degree of hypothermia narrows the safety margin that profound hypothermia provides, because it increases the risk of ischemic complications involving the spinal cord, kidneys, and other organs that are left unprotected while the brain receives antegrade cerebral perfusion.[67] To address this issue, some groups have devised perfusion strategies that provide flow to the descending aorta during arch repair.[68,69]

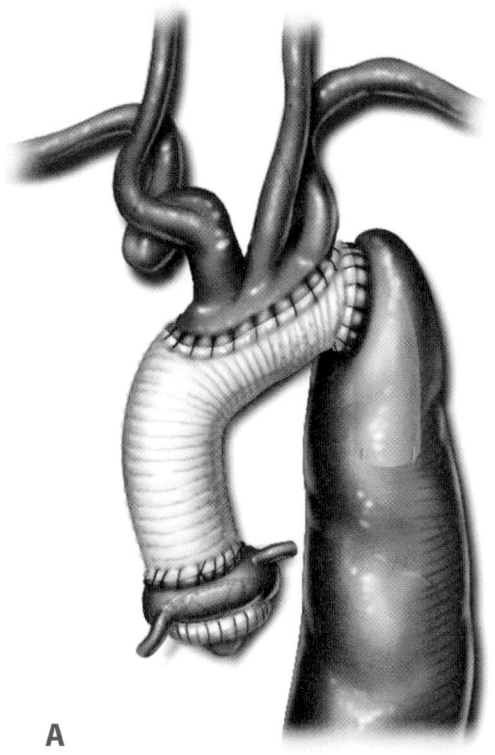

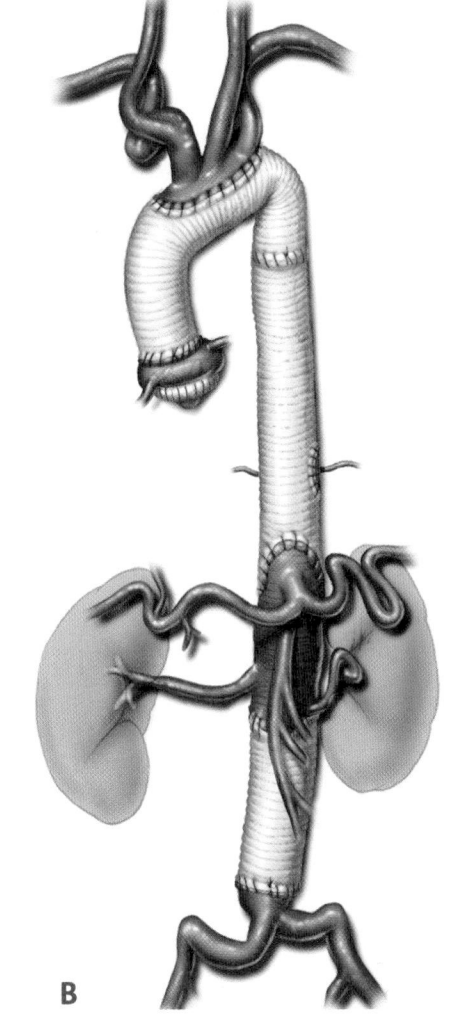

FIG. 22-6. Illustration of Borst's elephant trunk technique. **A.** Stage 1: The proximal repair includes replacement of the ascending aorta and entire arch, with island reattachment of the brachiocephalic vessels. The distal anastomosis is constructed such that a section of the graft is left suspended within the proximal descending thoracic aorta. **B.** Stage 2: The distal repair uses the floating "trunk" for the proximal anastomosis. *(Reproduced with permission from LeMaire et al.[56] Copyright Elsevier.)*

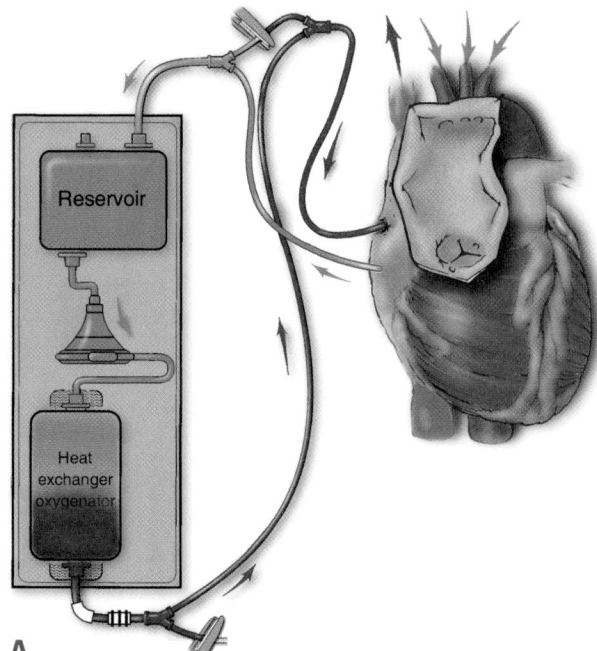

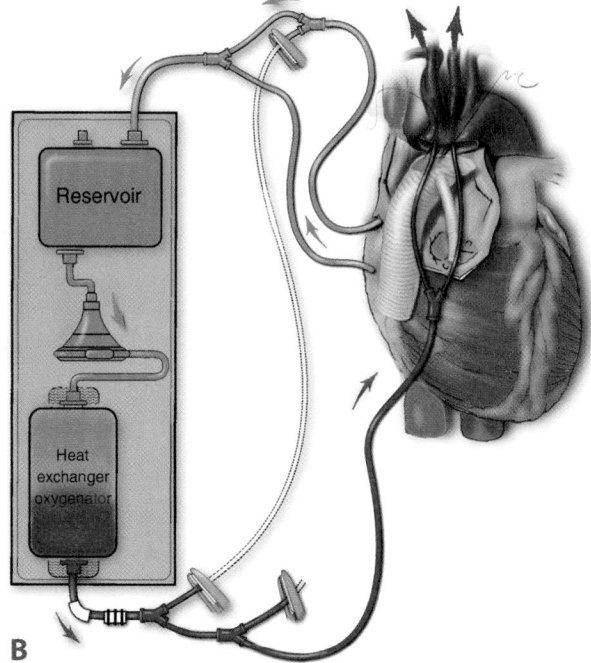

FIG. 22-7. Illustration of perfusion strategies used during aortic arch aneurysm repair performed under hypothermic circulatory arrest. **A.** Retrograde cerebral perfusion. Oxygenated blood is delivered through a cannula placed in the superior vena cava. **B.** Antegrade cerebral perfusion. Oxygenated blood is delivered through balloon perfusion catheters inserted into the innominate and left common carotid arteries. *[Images adapted from Gravlee GP, Davis RF, Kurusz M, et al (eds):* Cardiopulmonary Bypass: Principles and Practice, *2nd ed. Philadelphia: Lippincott Williams & Wilkins, 2000, Chap. 34, Fig. 34.3B.]*

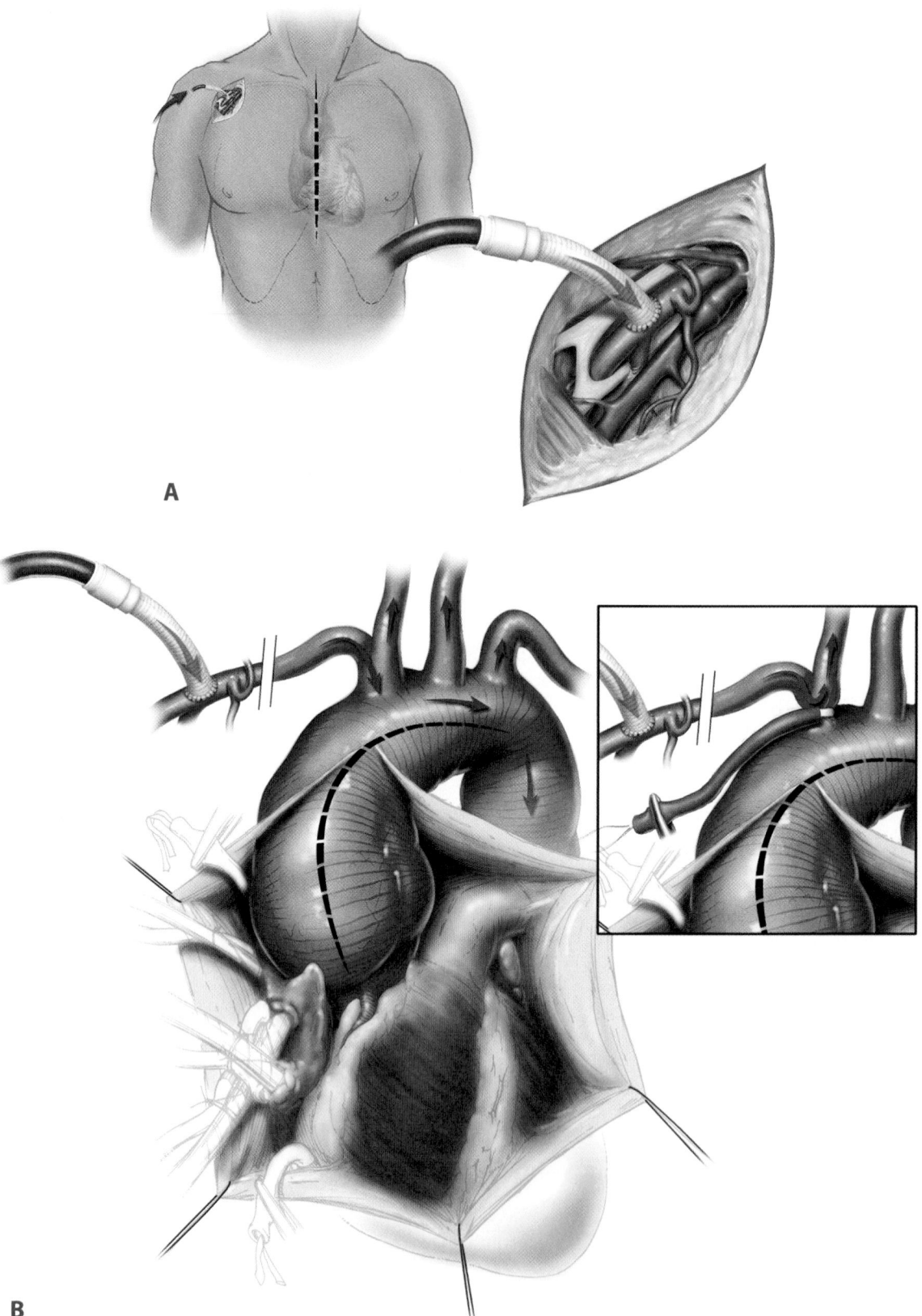

A

B

FIG. 22-8. Illustration of an alternative technique for delivering antegrade cerebral perfusion during aortic arch repairs. **A.** A graft sewn to the right axillary artery is used to return oxygenated blood from the cardiopulmonary bypass circuit. **B.** After adequate hypothermia is established, the innominate artery is occluded with a tourniquet (*inset*) so that flow is diverted to the right common carotid artery, which maintains cerebral circulation. [*Images adapted from Gravlee GP, Davis RF, Stammers AH, et al (eds):* Cardiopulmonary Bypass: Principles and Practice, 3rd ed. *Philadelphia: Lippincott Williams & Wilkins, 2008, Chap. 32, Fig. 1A and 1B.*]

Endovascular Repair Experience with purely endovascular treatment of proximal aortic disease remains limited and only investigational. The unique anatomy of the aortic arch and the need for uninterrupted cerebral perfusion pose difficult challenges. There are reports of the use of "homemade" grafts to exclude arch aneurysms; however, these grafts are highly experimental at this time. For example, in 1999, Inoue and colleagues[70] reported placing a triple-branched stent graft in a patient with an aneurysm of the aortic arch. The three brachiocephalic branches were positioned by placing percutaneous wires in the right brachial, left carotid, and left brachial arteries. The patient underwent two subsequent procedures: surgical repair of a right brachial pseudoaneurysm and placement of a distal stent graft extension to control a major perigraft leak. Since then, efforts to employ endovascular techniques in the treatment of the proximal aorta have been essentially limited to the use of approved devices for off-label indications, such as the exclusion of pseudoaneurysms in the ascending aorta.

Hybrid Repair Unlike purely endovascular approaches, hybrid repairs of the aortic arch have entered the mainstream clinical arena, although they remain controversial. Hybrid arch repairs involve some form of "debranching" of the brachiocephalic vessels, followed by endovascular exclusion of some or all of the aortic arch (Fig. 22-9). Although this technique has many variants, they often involve sewing a branched graft to the proximal ascending aorta with the use of a partial aortic clamp. The branches of the graft are then sewn to the arch vessels. Once the arch is "debranched," the arch aneurysm can be excluded with an endograft. The arguments for using a hybrid approach to treat aortic arch aneurysms include the elimination of cardiopulmonary bypass, circulatory arrest, and cardiac ischemia.

It is not yet clear whether hybrid repairs are as durable as traditional ones.[71] Also, there is a risk of embolization and stroke due to wire and device manipulation within the aortic arch. There are no large-scale studies comparing hybrid and traditional repairs. In a recent expert consensus document, the recommendation was to limit direct stenting of the aortic arch to patients who fall into the high surgical risk category. These are patients with significant comorbidities such as chronic pulmonary disease.[72]

Distal Thoracic Aortic Aneurysms *Open Repair* In patients with descending thoracic or thoracoabdominal aortic aneurysms, several aspects of treatment—including preoperative risk assessment, anesthetic management, choice of incision, and use of protective adjuncts—are dictated by the overall extent of aortic involvement. By definition, descending thoracic aortic aneurysms involve the portion

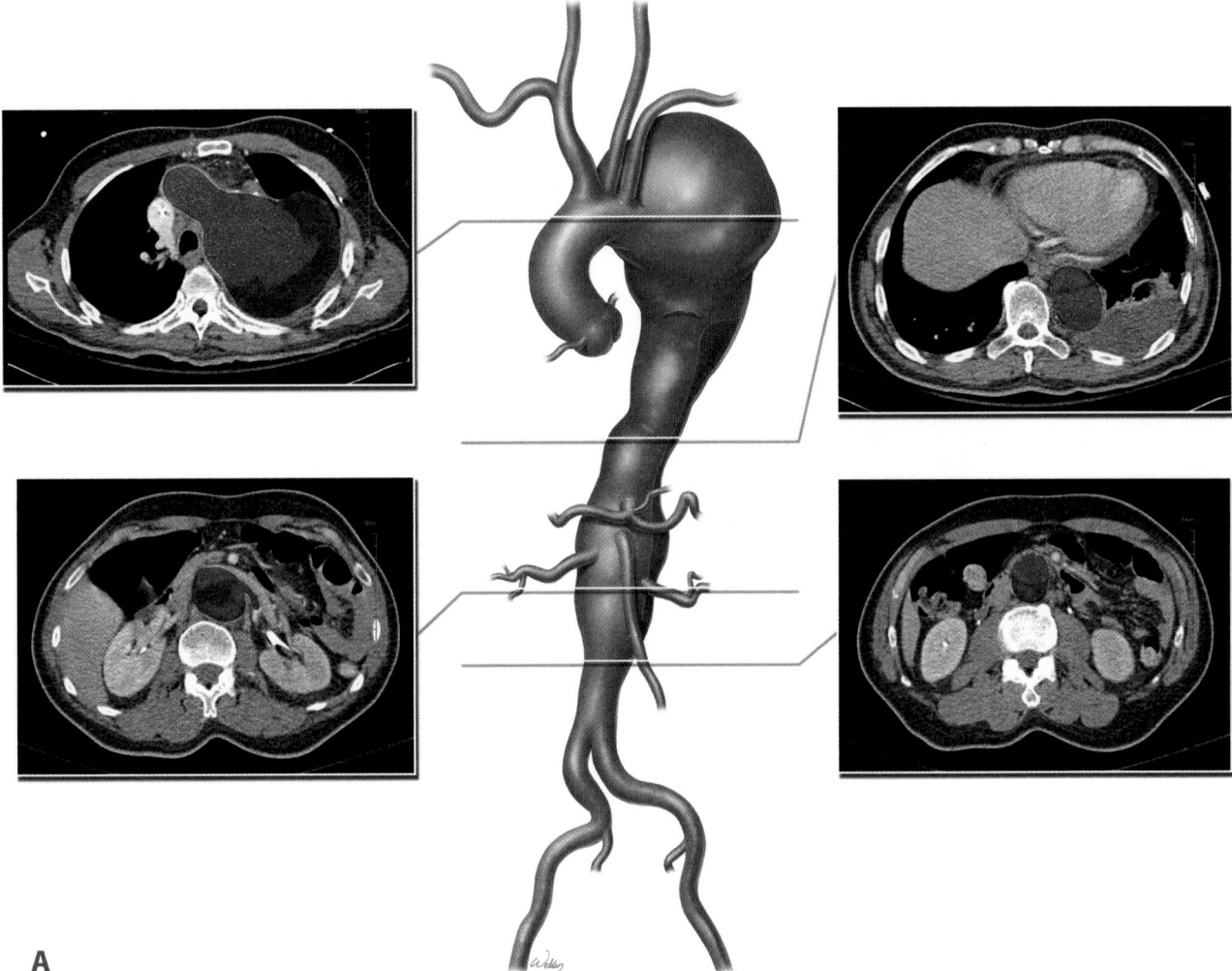

A

FIG. 22-9. Illustration of a hybrid approach—which combines open and endovascular techniques—for repair of an extensive aortic aneurysm. **A.** Preoperative computed tomographic images detail an enormous aneurysm involving the aortic arch and entire thoracoabdominal aorta. (*Continued*)

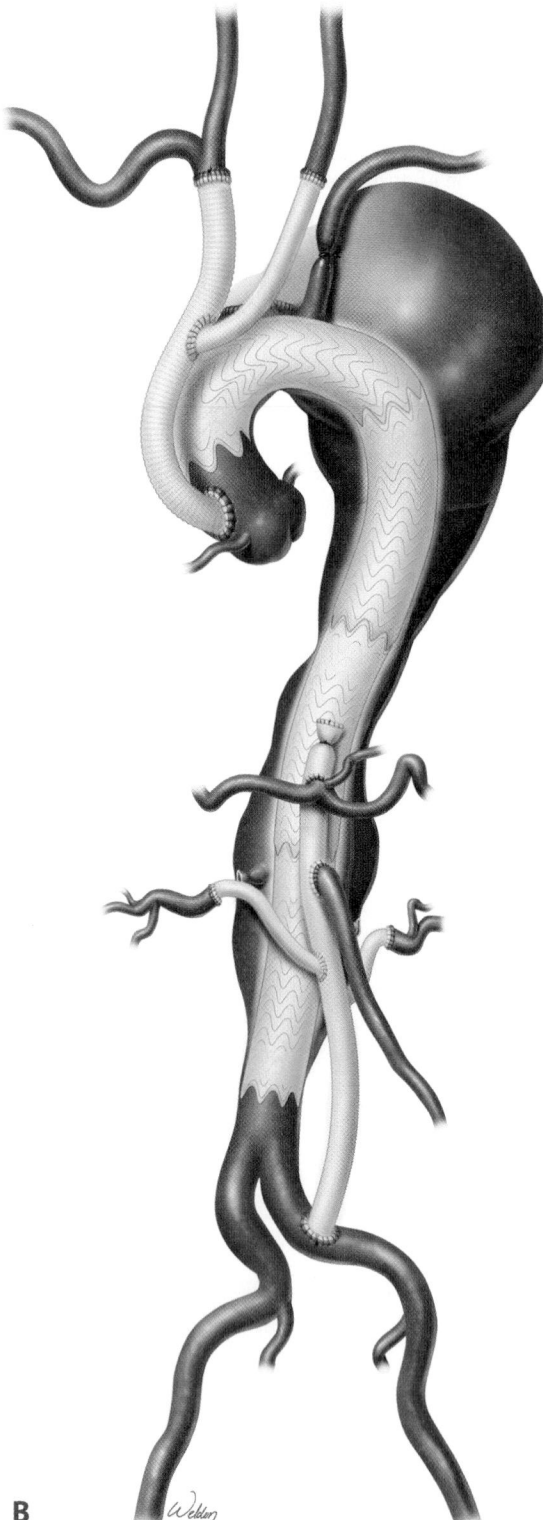

B

Weldon

FIG. 22-9. *(Continued)* **B.** Debranching the arch and thoracoabdominal segments allows the use of a series of endovascular stent grafts to exclude the entire aneurysm.

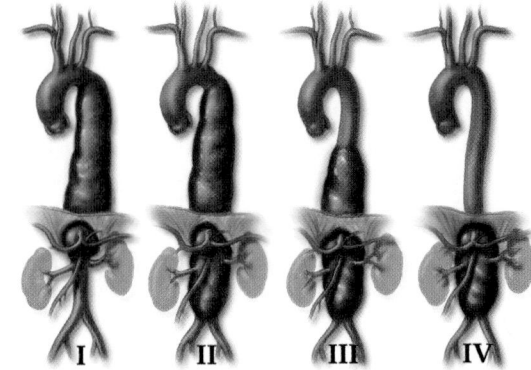

FIG. 22-10. Illustration of the Crawford classification of thoracoabdominal aortic aneurysms based on the extent of aortic involvement. *[Reproduced with permission from Coselli JS, LeMaire SA: Descending and Thoracoabdominal Aortic Aneurysms, in Cohn LH (ed): Cardiac Surgery in the Adult, 3rd ed. New York: McGraw-Hill, Inc., 2008, Chap. 54, Fig. 54-5.]*

beginning near the left subclavian artery, and extend down to encompass the aorta at the origins of the celiac axis and superior mesenteric arteries. The renal arteries also may be involved. Extent II aneurysms also arise near the left subclavian artery but extend distally into the infrarenal abdominal aorta, and they often reach the aortic bifurcation. Extent III aneurysms originate in the lower descending thoracic aorta (below the sixth rib) and extend into the abdomen. Extent IV aneurysms begin within the diaphragmatic hiatus and often involve the entire abdominal aorta.

Descending thoracic aortic aneurysms are repaired through a left thoracotomy. In patients with thoracoabdominal aortic aneurysms, the thoracotomy is extended across the costal margin and into the abdomen. Use of a double-lumen endobronchial tube allows selective ventilation of the right lung and deflation of the left lung. Transperitoneal exposure of the thoracoabdominal aorta is achieved by performing medial visceral rotation and circumferential division of the diaphragm. During a period of aortic clamping, the diseased segment is replaced with a polyester tube graft. Important branch arteries—including intercostal arteries and the celiac, superior mesenteric, and renal arteries—are reattached to openings made in the side of the graft. Visceral and renal artery occlusive disease is commonly encountered during aneurysm repair; options for correcting branch vessel stenosis include endarterectomy, direct arterial stenting, and bypass grafting.

Clamping the descending thoracic aorta causes ischemia of the spinal cord and abdominal viscera. Clinically significant manifestations of hepatic, pancreatic, and bowel ischemia are relatively uncommon. However, both acute renal failure and spinal cord injury resulting in paraplegia or paraparesis remain major causes of morbidity and mortality after these operations. Therefore, several aspects of the operation are devoted to minimizing spinal and renal ischemia (Table 22-3). Our multimodal approach to spinal cord protection includes expeditious repair to minimize aortic clamping time, moderate systemic heparinization (1.0 mg/kg) to prevent small-vessel thrombosis, mild permissive hypothermia [32° to 34°C (89.6° to 93.2°F)] nasopharyngeal temperature], and reattachment of segmental intercostal and lumbar arteries. As the aorta is replaced from proximal to distal, the aortic clamp is moved sequentially to lower positions along the graft to restore perfusion to newly reattached branch vessels. During extensive thoracoabdominal aortic repairs (i.e., Crawford extent I and II aneurysms), cerebrospinal fluid drainage is used. The benefits of this adjunct, which improves spinal perfusion by reducing cerebrospinal fluid pressure, have been confirmed in a prospective, randomized trial performed by our group.[73] Motor

of the aorta between the left subclavian artery and the diaphragm. Thoracoabdominal aneurysms can involve the entire thoracoabdominal aorta, from the origin of the left subclavian artery to the aortic bifurcation, and are categorized according to the Crawford classification scheme (Fig. 22-10). Extent I thoracoabdominal aortic aneurysms involve most of the descending thoracic aorta, usually

TABLE 22-3	Current strategy for spinal cord and visceral protection during repair of distal thoracic aortic aneurysms

All extents
- Permissive mild hypothermia [32–34°C (89.6–93.2°F), nasopharyngeal]
- Moderate heparinization (1 mg/kg)
- Aggressive reattachment of segmental arteries, especially between T8 and L1
- Sequential aortic clamping when possible
- Perfusion of renal arteries with 4°C (39.2°F) crystalloid solution when possible

Crawford extent I and II thoracoabdominal repairs
- Cerebrospinal fluid drainage
- Left heart bypass during proximal anastomosis
- Selective perfusion of celiac axis and superior mesenteric artery during intercostal and visceral anastomoses

evoked potentials often are used to monitor the spinal cord throughout the operation.[74,75] Left heart bypass, which provides perfusion of the distal aorta and its branches during the clamping period, is also used during extensive thoracoabdominal aortic repairs.[76–78] Because left heart bypass unloads the heart, it is also useful in patients with poor cardiac reserve. Balloon perfusion cannulas connected to the left heart bypass circuit can be used to deliver blood directly to the celiac axis and superior mesenteric artery during their reattachment. The potential benefits of reducing hepatic and bowel ischemia include reduced risks of postoperative coagulopathy and bacterial translocation, respectively. Whenever possible, renal protection is achieved by perfusing the kidneys with cold [4°C (39.2°F)] crystalloid. In a randomized clinical trial, reduced kidney temperature was found to be associated with renal protection, and the use of cold crystalloid independently predicted preserved renal function.[79]

In certain cases, hypothermic circulatory arrest is required for descending thoracic or thoracoabdominal aortic repairs.[80] The primary indication for this approach is the inability to clamp the aorta because of rupture, extremely large aneurysm size, or extension of the aneurysm into the distal transverse aortic arch.

As discussed earlier, complete repair of extensive aneurysms involving the ascending aorta, transverse arch, and descending thoracic aorta generally requires staged operations. In such procedures, when the descending or thoracoabdominal component is symptomatic (e.g., causes back pain or has ruptured) or is disproportionately large (compared with the ascending aorta), the distal segment is treated during the initial operation, and repair of the ascending aorta and transverse aortic arch is performed as a second procedure. A reversed elephant trunk repair, in which a portion of the proximal end of the aortic graft is inverted down into the lumen, can be performed during the first operation; this technique facilitates the second-stage repair of the ascending aorta and transverse aortic arch (Fig. 22-11).[81]

Although spinal cord ischemia and renal failure receive the most attention, several other complications warrant consideration. The most common complication of extensive repairs is pulmonary dysfunction. With aneurysms adjacent to the left subclavian artery, the vagus and left recurrent laryngeal nerves are often adherent to the aortic wall and thus are susceptible to injury. Vocal cord paralysis should be suspected in patients who have postoperative hoarseness, and the presence of nerve damage should be confirmed by endoscopic examination. Vocal cord paralysis can be treated effectively by direct cord medialization (type 1 thyroplasty). Injury to the esophagus during the proximal anastomosis can have catastrophic consequences. Carefully separating the proximal descending thoracic aorta from the underlying esophagus before performing the proximal anastomosis minimizes the risk of a secondary aortoesophageal fis-

tula. In patients who have previously undergone coronary artery bypass with a left internal thoracic artery graft, clamping proximal to the left subclavian artery can precipitate severe myocardial ischemia and cardiac arrest. When the need to clamp at this location is anticipated in these patients, a left common carotid to subclavian bypass is performed to prevent cardiac complications.

Endovascular Repair *Descending Thoracic Aortic Aneurysms* Stent graft repair of descending thoracic aortic aneurysms has become an accepted treatment option for selected patients.[72] In 1991, Parodi and associates[82] reported using endovascular stent grafting to repair abdominal aortic aneurysms. Only 3 years after this seminal report was published, Dake and colleagues[83] reported performing endovascular descending thoracic aortic repair with "homemade" stent grafts in 13 patients.

At this time, endografting is primarily used to treat degenerative descending thoracic aortic aneurysms. However, many authors have reported using this new, less invasive option in patients with aortic dissection or with traumatic, mycotic, or ruptured aneurysms of the descending thoracic aorta.

In elderly patients with severe comorbidity and patients who have undergone previous complex thoracic aortic procedures, endovascular repair is a particularly attractive alternative to standard surgical procedures. As mentioned previously, appropriate patient selection depends on specific measurements taken from preoperative CT angiograms.

To protect patients against spinal cord ischemia during these endovascular repairs, many surgeons use cerebrospinal fluid drainage. Fluid is drained to maintain a cerebrospinal fluid pressure of approximately 12 to 14 mmHg. The first step in the repair procedure is to obtain appropriate vascular access for the insertion of the thoracic stent graft. If the femoral artery will not accommodate the necessary sheath, then an iliac artery is exposed. A graft can be sewn to the iliac artery in an end-to-side fashion to facilitate the deployment of the endograft. After 5000 to 10,000 units of heparin are administered, a guidewire and the delivery sheath are inserted into the access artery under fluoroscopic guidance. The endograft is then advanced into the aorta and suitably positioned. Note that when a C-arm is used, the best view of the distal arch and descending thoracic aorta is usually in the left anterior oblique position at an angle of approximately 40 to 50 degrees. The device is then deployed, and the proximal and distal ends are expanded by using a balloon catheter, which optimizes the seal between the device and the aortic wall at this landing zone. An aortogram is then taken to rule out any endoleak, and protamine is administered.

It is common to cover the left subclavian artery with the endograft to lengthen the proximal landing zone.[84] However, recent findings suggest that the risk of spinal cord complications is heightened when the subclavian artery is covered and not revascularized, presumably because of a loss of collateral circulation to the spinal cord.[85] To prevent this complication, a carotid to subclavian bypass can be easily constructed to maintain vertebral artery blood flow and minimize neurologic injury (Fig. 22-12).[86,87] In addition, new generations of stent grafts are being designed with side branches that can be placed within the left subclavian artery. This feature is particularly attractive if the proximal neck is short or if the patient has a patent left internal thoracic artery to left anterior descending coronary artery bypass.

Elephant Trunk Completion The advent of endograft stenting has provided surgeons with an excellent method of completing elephant trunk repairs endovascularly, rather than taking the open approach through a thoracotomy.[88] Recall that an elephant trunk is used when an aortic aneurysm extends from the distal arch to the descending thoracic aorta. An endograft can be deployed at the time of elephant trunk construction or during a separate, subsequent procedure.[89] When the stent is deployed in a retrograde manner in such a second-stage procedure, the procedure is facilitated by placing radiopaque markers at the end of the elephant trunk during the first-stage

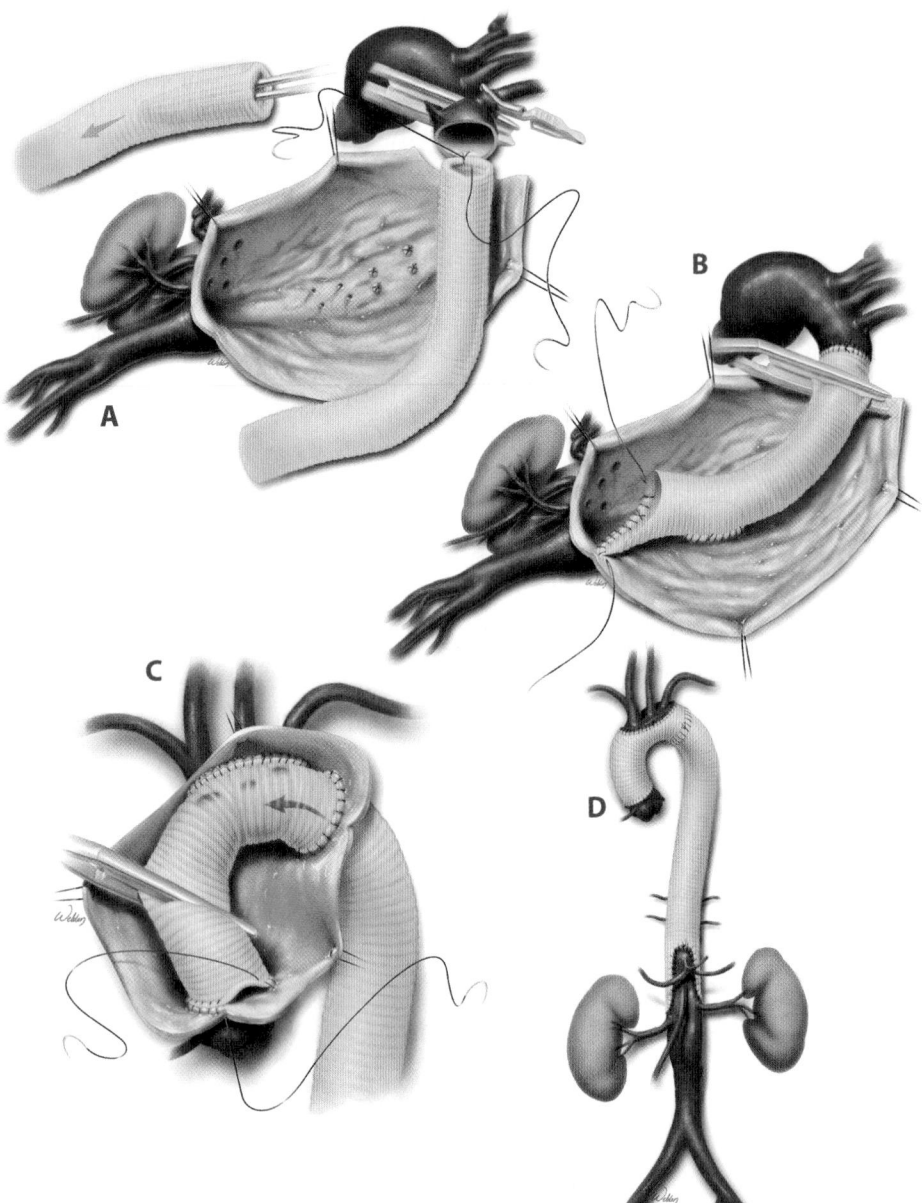

FIG. 22-11. Illustration of the reversed elephant trunk technique. **A.** Stage 1: The distal aorta is repaired through a left thoracoabdominal approach. The aneurysm is opened after the aorta is clamped between the left common carotid artery and the left subclavian artery, which is also clamped. Before the proximal anastomosis is performed, the end of the graft is partly invaginated to leave a "trunk" for the subsequent repair. Proximal intercostal arteries are oversewn. **B.** After the proximal suture line is completed, the clamps are repositioned to restore blood flow to the left subclavian artery. The repair is completed by reattaching patent intercostal arteries to an opening in the side of the graft and creating a beveled distal anastomosis at the level of the visceral branches. **C.** Stage 2: The proximal aorta is repaired through a median sternotomy. The aortic arch is opened under hypothermic circulatory arrest. The "trunk" is pulled out and used to replace the aortic arch and ascending aorta. This eliminates the need for a new distal anastomosis and simplifies the procedure. Circulatory arrest and operative time, along with their attendant risks, are reduced. **D.** The completed two-stage repair of the entire thoracic aorta. *(Reproduced with permission from Coselli JS, LeMaire SA, Carter SA, et al: The reversed elephant trunk technique used for treatment of complex aneurysms of the entire thoracic aorta. Ann Thorac Surg 80:2166, 2005, Figs. 2, 3, 7, and 8. Copyright Elsevier.)*

procedure. This allows the distal end of the trunk to be identified via fluoroscopy. A guidewire can then be manipulated into the trunk and advanced into the ascending aorta to stabilize it during stent deployment. Note that advancing a wire in retrograde fashion from the femoral artery into the elephant trunk can be challenging. Occasionally, the wire must be advanced in an antegrade fashion from a brachial artery.

Thoracoabdominal Aortic Aneurysms Like the endovascular repair of proximal aortic disease, endovascular thoracoabdominal aortic aneurysm repair remains experimental. However, such repairs have been shown to be feasible in a handful of specialized centers. Endovascular thoracoabdominal aortic aneurysm repairs are quite complex, because at least one of the visceral arteries must be incorporated into the repair. The number of visceral branches that need to be addressed varies with the extent of aortic coverage.[90] The types of stent grafts used include fenestrated grafts, reinforced fenestrated grafts, and branched grafts, as well as modular combinations of grafts. Graft fenestrations and branch vessels are typically aligned by using inflatable angioplasty balloons. Procedure time is not insignificant, nor is

the amount of contrast medium required to obtain the highly detailed images needed to plan these procedures. In addition, some of the stent grafts used in endovascular thoracoabdominal aortic aneurysm repair are custom-made in advance and thus may take several weeks to obtain; therefore, their use is limited to cases of elective repair.[91]

It should be noted that, like open thoracoabdominal aortic aneurysm repair, endovascular repair carries risks of paraplegia, renal failure, stroke, and death, despite the apparent benefits of its being a less invasive procedure. Until prospective studies demonstrate consistent and favorable results, endovascular thoracoabdominal aortic aneurysm repair must be considered purely investigational.

Hybrid Repair As discussed previously, hybrid repairs can be performed in patients with aortic arch aneurysms that extend into the descending thoracic aorta. For example, the arch can be replaced by using the elephant trunk technique (see Fig. 22-6A), after which the descending thoracic aorta can be excluded endovascularly by using the elephant trunk as the proximal landing zone. When the descending thoracic aortic aneurysm only extends into the distal arch (Fig. 22-13), the arch can be debranched by constructing

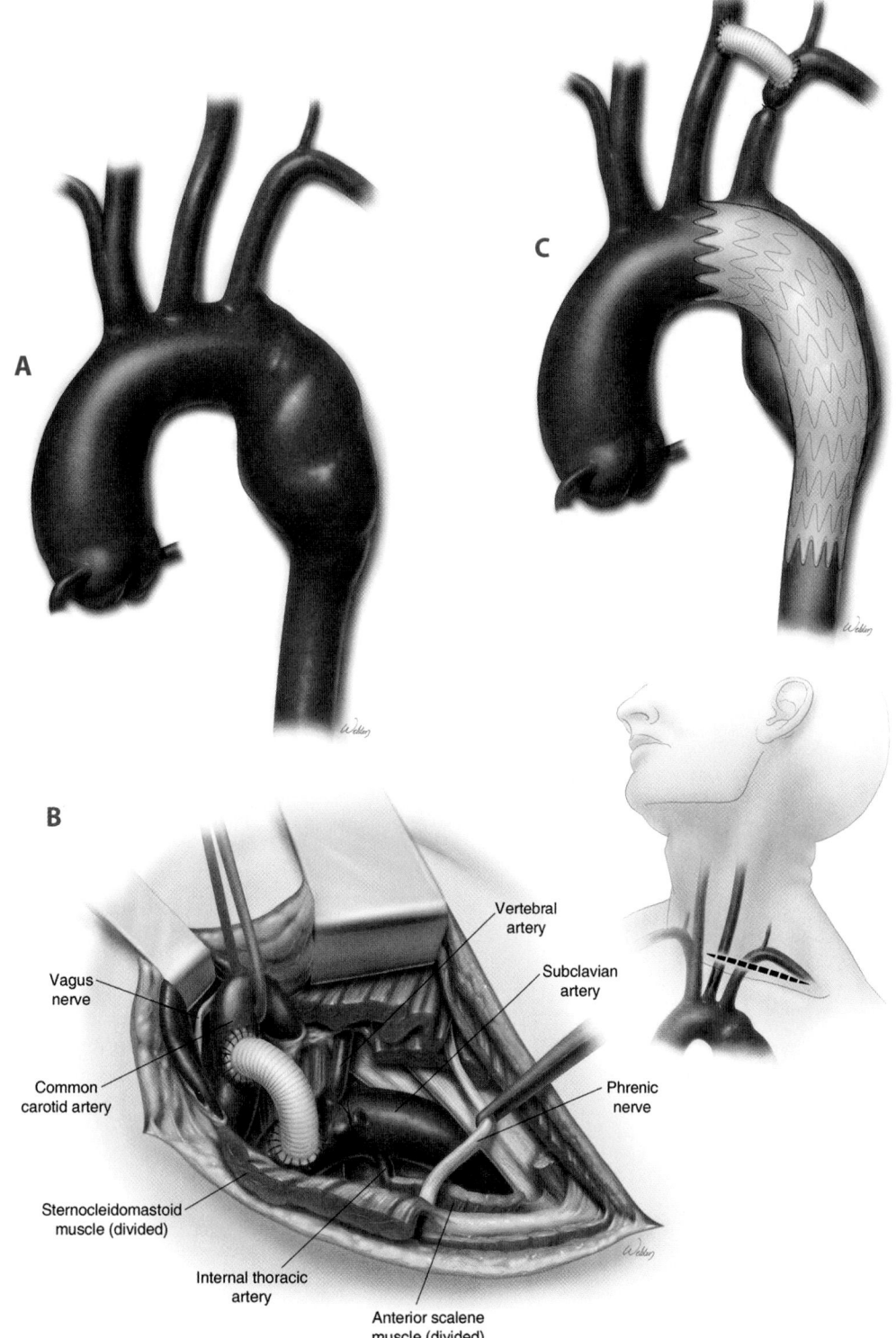

FIG. 22-12. Illustration of a hybrid repair of the proximal descending thoracic aorta. **A.** The preoperative representation of the aneurysm shows that establishing a 2-cm proximal landing zone for a stent graft will require covering the origin of the left subclavian artery. **B.** Through a supraclavicular approach, a bypass from the left common carotid artery to the left subclavian artery is performed to reroute circulation and create a landing zone for the stent graft. After the bypass is completed, the left subclavian artery is ligated proximal to the graft. **C.** In the completed hybrid repair, the aneurysm has been excluded successfully by a stent graft that covers the origin of the left subclavian artery, and blood flow to the left vertebral artery and arm is preserved by the bypass graft. *(Reproduced with permission from Bozinovski et al,[86] Figs. 9, 10, and 11. Copyright © Elsevier.)*

bypass grafts off of the ascending aorta, then placing stent grafts across the arch and descending thoracic aorta.[86]

There have been several reports of hybrid thoracoabdominal aortic aneurysm repair.[92,93] This approach is gaining momentum, especially in patient-tailored interventions for patients at high surgical risk, such as those who have limited physiologic reserve, are of advanced age, or have significant comorbidities. Hybrid procedures use open surgical techniques to reroute blood supply to the visceral arteries so that their

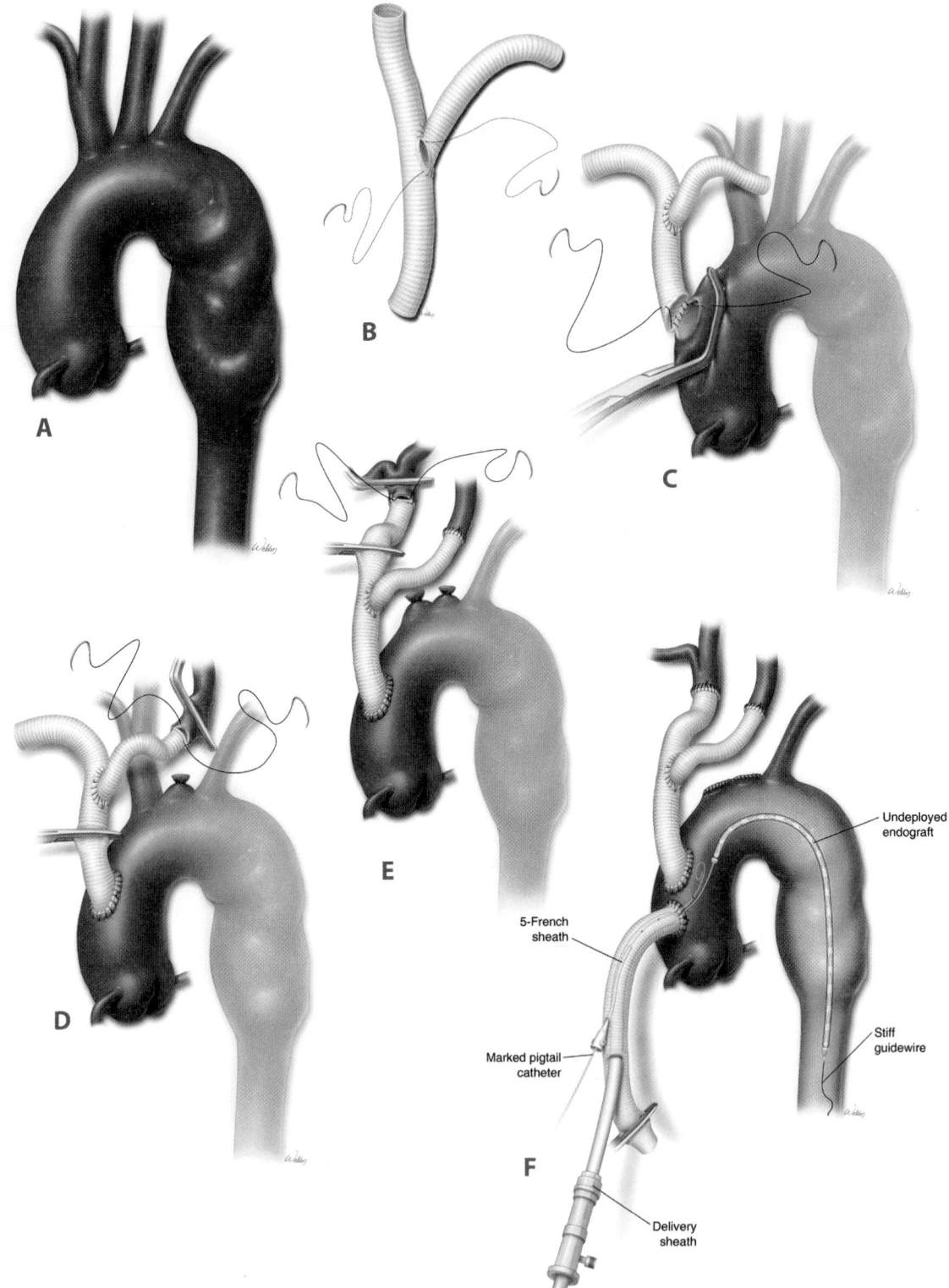

FIG. 22-13. Illustration of a hybrid repair of the distal aortic arch and proximal descending thoracic aorta. **A.** Preoperative representation of the aneurysm shows dilatation of the distal aortic arch, which makes the arch an unsuitable landing zone. **B.** A Y graft is created from 8- and 10-mm grafts. This graft will be used to debranch the arch. **C.** After sternotomy, a small section of the ascending aorta is excluded by a side-biting clamp. The beveled end of the Y graft is sutured to an opening in the aorta. **D.** The 8-mm end of the Y graft is used to bypass the left common carotid artery. **E.** The 10-mm end is used to bypass the innominate artery. **F.** Antegrade deployment of the stent graft can be performed through a conduit graft sewn to the ascending aorta below the Y graft. (*Continued*)

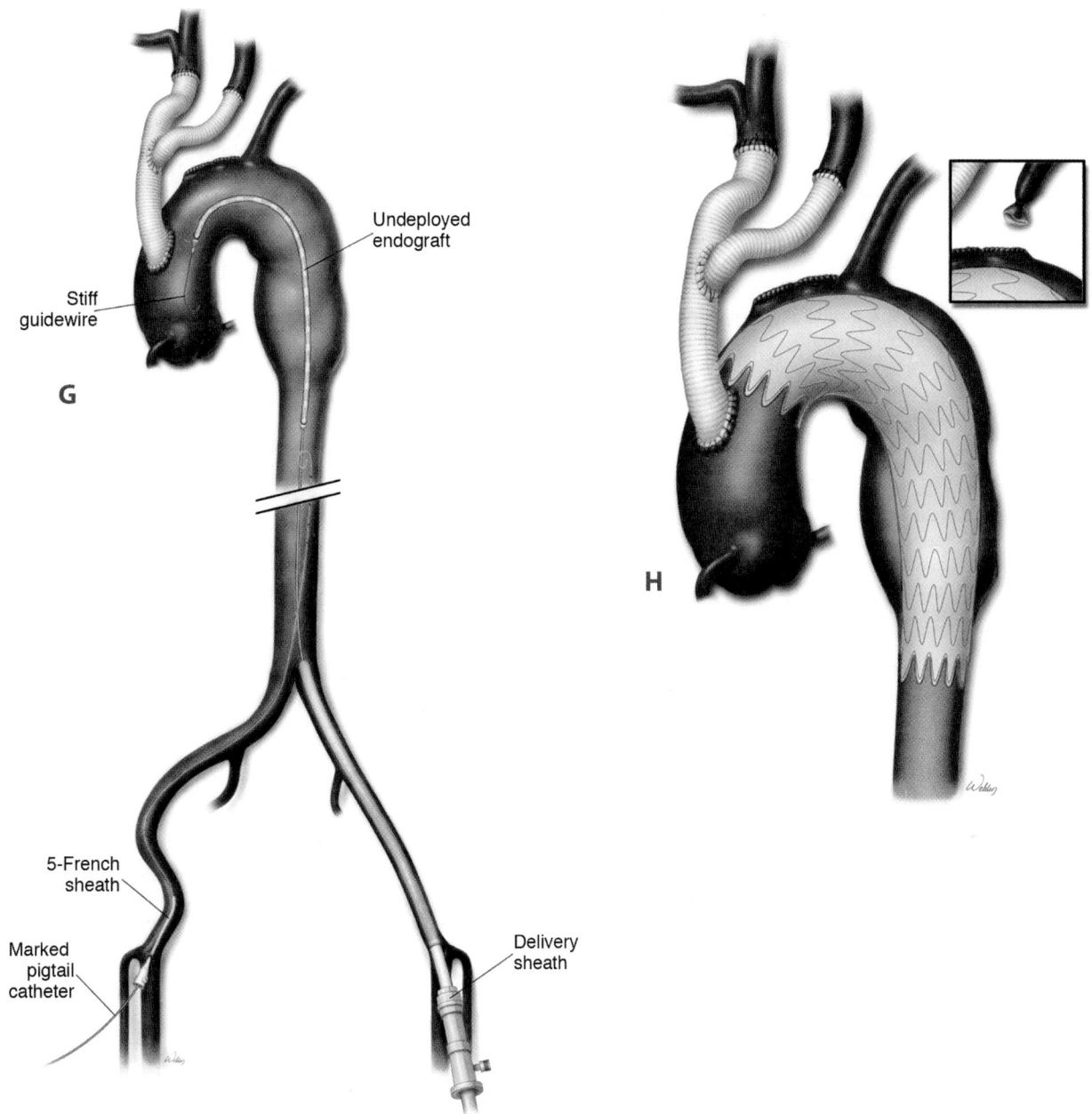

FIG. 22-13. *(Continued)* **G.** Alternatively, retrograde deployment of the stent graft can be performed via the femoral artery. **H.** In the completed hybrid repair, the endovascular graft is properly seated, and the bypass grafts ensure blood flow into the innominate and left common carotid arteries. The left subclavian artery can often be fully occluded by the stent graft without complication. The inset figure depicts an alternate approach in which the left subclavian artery has been ligated to prevent back-bleeding and type II endoleak. *(Reproduced with permission from Bozinovski et al,[86] Figs. 1–8. Copyright © Elsevier.)*

aortic origins can be covered by stent grafts without causing visceral ischemia (see Fig. 22-9). Endovascular methods are then used (either as part of the same procedure or at a later stage) to repair the aortic aneurysm, often with a simple tube stent graft, which is more readily available than the customized, modular stent grafts deployed in strictly endovascular repairs. Several reports of small series suggest that these hybrid repairs produce acceptable outcomes among patients with elevated surgical risk.[92,93] For low-risk surgical patients, it is likely that open surgical repair will remain the gold standard until the durability of hybrid repairs has been established.

Postoperative Considerations

Open Procedures Aortic anastomoses are often extremely fragile during the early postoperative period. Even brief episodes of postoperative hypertension can disrupt suture lines and precipitate severe bleeding or pseudoaneurysm formation. Therefore, during the initial 24 to 48 hours, meticulous blood pressure control is maintained to protect the integrity of the anastomoses. Generally, we liberally use nitroprusside and IV beta antagonists to keep the mean arterial blood pressure between 80 and 90 mmHg. In patients with extremely friable aortic tissue, such as those with Marfan syndrome, we lower the target range to 70 to 80 mmHg. It is a delicate balancing act, as one must be mindful of spinal cord perfusion and avoid periods of relative hypotension while maintaining these low pressures.

A second threat to anastomotic integrity is graft infection. To reduce the risk of this complication, IV antibiotics are continued throughout the postoperative course until all drains, chest tubes, and central venous lines are removed.

Endovascular Procedures As experience with descending thoracic aortic stent grafts continues to accumulate, so too do reports of complications specifically related to device deployment. Many of these complications are directly related to manipulation of the delivery system within the iliac arteries and aorta.[94] Patients with small, calcified, tortuous iliofemoral arteries are at particularly high risk for life-threatening iliac artery rupture. The potential for aortic injury precipitating immediate operation is well described in the abdominal aortic stent graft literature; however, thus far, there are few reports of thoracic aortic rupture during stent graft procedures. A more common and equally deadly complication is acute iatrogenic retrograde dissection into the aortic arch and ascending aorta. There are already several reports of this complication, most involving new-generation devices and requiring emergency repair of the ascending aorta and aortic arch via sternotomy and cardiopulmonary bypass.[95,96] Such a dissection converts a localized descending thoracic aortic aneurysm into an acute problem involving the entire thoracic aorta.

Another significant complication of descending thoracic aortic stent grafting is endoleak. First-generation stents were associated with an incidence of endoleak of up to 46%; however, this percentage is declining as stent graft technology continues to evolve.[97,98] An endoleak occurs when there is a persistent flow of blood (visible on radiologic imaging) into the aneurysm sac. These occurrences are not benign, because they lead to continual pressurization of the sac, which can cause expansion or even rupture. This complication is categorized according to the cause of the leak. Type I endoleaks, which result from an incomplete seal between the graft and aorta at attachment sites, are the most unstable and can precipitate aortic rupture. Therefore, aggressive intervention is warranted as soon as such leaks are identified. Type II endoleaks occur when the sac is filled by collateral arteries, such as patent intercostal arteries. These leaks are more benign than type I leaks and can simply be monitored with regular imaging. If the aneurysm sac expands or the leak persists, the collateral arteries can occasionally be occluded by using percutaneous interventions. Type III endoleaks are caused by either a tear in the graft fabric or an incomplete seal between two devices. This variety of endoleak is rare and should be treated aggressively. Typically, another endograft can be used to cover and seal the leak. Type IV endoleaks are extremely rare and were seen more often with earlier devices made of porous materials through which blood could leak. Type V endoleaks are characterized by endotension, in which there is evidence of aneurysm expansion even though the leak has no identifiable source. Type IV and V endoleaks can be treated by overstenting the existing graft with another stent graft.

Other device-related problems include stent graft misdeployment, device migration, and endograft kinking. Although not all complications related to stent grafts are fatal, endovascular repairs should be performed by expert teams qualified to address the variety of problems that may arise. Also, because late graft-related complications are common, regularly scheduled radiologic imaging surveillance is of the utmost importance.

AORTIC DISSECTION

Pathology and Classification

Aortic dissection, the most common catastrophic event involving the aorta, is a progressive separation of the aortic wall layers that usually occurs after a tear forms in the intima and inner media. As the separation of the layers of the media propagates, at least two channels form (Fig. 22-14): the original lumen, which remains lined by the intima and which is called the *true lumen*, and the newly formed channel within the layers of the media, which is called the *false lumen*. The dissecting membrane separates the true and false lumens. Additional tears in the dissecting membrane that allow communication between the two channels are called *re-entry sites*. Although the separation of layers primarily progresses distally along the length of the aorta, it can also proceed in a proximal direction; this process often is referred to as *proximal extension* or *retrograde dissection*.

The extensive disruption of the aortic wall has severe anatomic consequences (Fig. 22-15). First, the outer wall of the false lumen is extremely thin, inflamed, and fragile, which makes it prone to expansion or rupture in the face of ongoing hemodynamic stress. Second, the expanding false lumen can compress the true lumen and cause *malperfusion syndrome* by interfering with blood flow in the aorta or any of its branch vessels, including the coronary, carotid, intercostal, visceral, renal, and iliac arteries. Finally, when the separation of layers occurs within the aortic root, the aortic valve commissures can become unhinged, which results in acute valvular regurgitation. The clinical consequences of each of these sequelae are addressed in detail in the section on clinical manifestations later.

Dissection vs. Aneurysm

The relationship between dissection and aneurysmal disease requires clarification. Dissection and aneurysm are separate entities, although they often coexist and are mutual risk factors. In most cases, dissection occurs in patients without aneurysms. The subsequent progressive dilatation of the weakened outer aortic wall results in an aneurysm. On the other hand, in patients with degenerative aneurysms, the ongoing deterioration of the aortic wall can lead to a superimposed dissection. The overused term *dissecting aneurysm* should be reserved for this specific situation.

Classification

For management purposes, aortic dissections are classified according to their location and chronicity. Improvements in imaging have increasingly revealed variants of aortic dissection that probably represent different forms along the spectrum of this condition.

Location Dissections are categorized according to their anatomic location and extent to guide treatment. The two traditional classification schemes that remain in common use are the DeBakey and

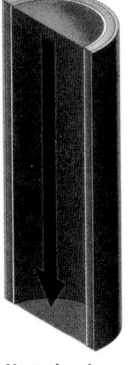 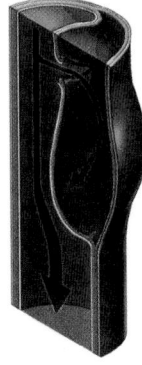 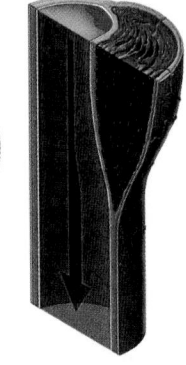 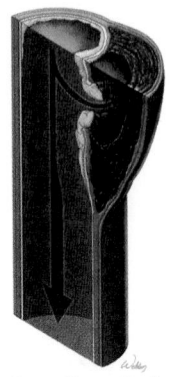

Normal aorta **Aortic dissection** **Intramural hematoma** **Penetrating aortic ulcer**

FIG. 22-14. Illustration of longitudinal sections of the aortic wall and lumen. Blood flows freely downstream in normal aortic tissue. In classic aortic dissection, blood entering the media through a tear creates a false channel in the wall. Intramural hematomas arise when hemorrhage from the vasa vasorum causes blood to collect within the media; the intima is intact. Penetrating aortic ulcers are deep atherosclerotic lesions that burrow into the aortic wall and allow blood to enter the media. In each of these conditions, the outer aortic wall is severely weakened and prone to rupture.

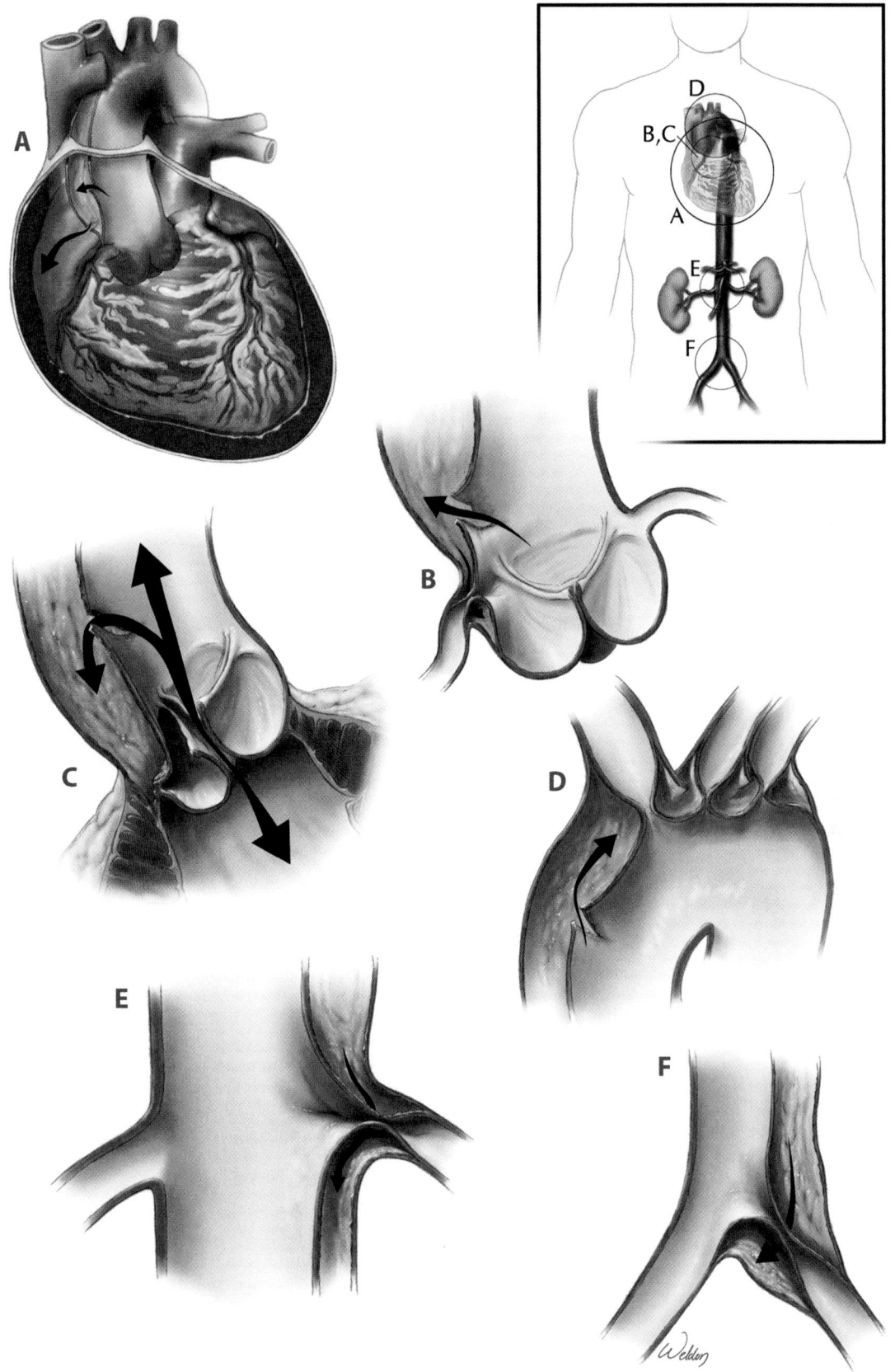

FIG. 22-15. Illustration of the potential anatomic consequences of aortic dissection, with a mapped diagram of affected regions (*inset*).
A. Ascending aortic rupture and cardiac tamponade. **B.** Disruption of coronary blood flow. **C.** Injury to the aortic valve causing regurgitation.
D, E, and **F.** Compromised blood flow to branch vessels causing ischemic complications. *[Images adapted from Creager MA, Dzau VS, Loscalzo J (eds): Vascular Medicine. Philadelphia: WB Saunders, 2006, Fig. 35-1.]*

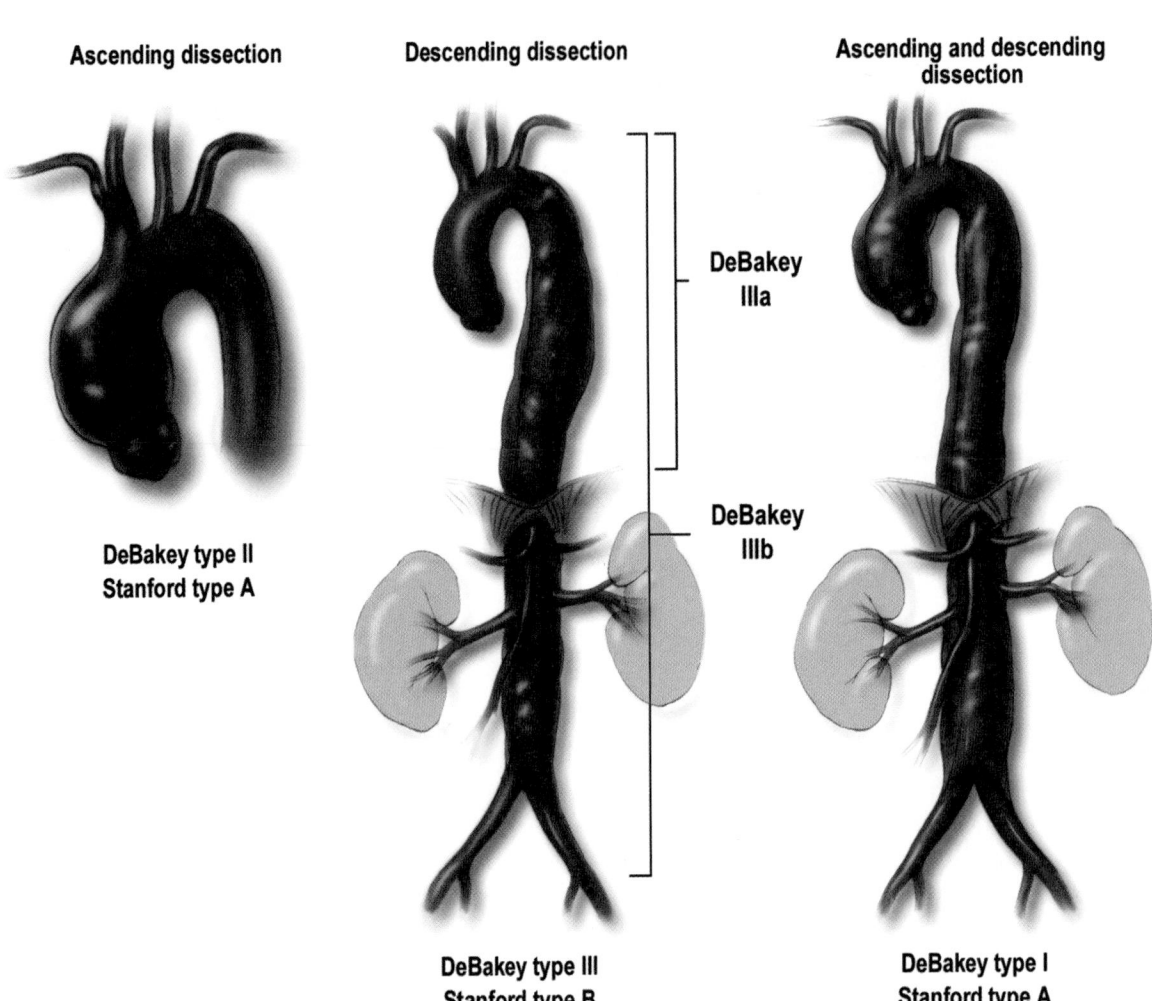

Ascending dissection

DeBakey type II
Stanford type A

Descending dissection

DeBakey
IIIa

DeBakey
IIIb

DeBakey type III
Stanford type B

Ascending and descending dissection

DeBakey type I
Stanford type A

FIG. 22-16. Illustration of the classification schemes for aortic dissection based on which portions of the aorta are involved. Dissection can be confined to the ascending aorta (*left*) or descending aorta (*middle*), or it can involve the entire aorta (*right*). [*Reproduced with permission from Creager MA, Dzau VS, Loscalzo J (eds):* Vascular Medicine. *Philadelphia: WB Saunders, 2006. Copyright © Saunders/Elsevier, 2006, Fig. 35-2.*]

the Stanford classification systems (Fig. 22-16).[99,100] In their current forms, both of these schemes describe the segments of aorta that are involved in the dissection, rather than the site of the initial intimal tear. The main drawback of the Stanford classification system is that it does not distinguish between patients with isolated ascending aortic dissection and patients with dissection involving the entire aorta. Both types of patients would be classified as having type A dissections, despite the fact that their treatment, follow-up, and prognosis are substantially different. Borst and associates[101] devised a different system of classifying aortic dissections that they contended was simpler and more descriptive than the traditional DeBakey and Stanford schemes. In this system, the ascending aorta and descending aorta are considered independently. This is useful because treatment strategies are chosen according to which segments are involved. For example, patients with isolated ascending aortic dissections often undergo emergent operation. In contrast, when only the descending and thoracoabdominal portions are involved, the initial treatment is usually medical; surgery is reserved for patients in whom complications develop. Patients with dissections that involve both the ascending and descending aorta often undergo surgical repair of the ascending dissection, followed by aggressive medical treatment of the descending dissection.

Chronicity Aortic dissection also is categorized according to the time elapsed since the initial tear. Dissection is considered acute within the first 14 days after the initial tear; after 14 days, the dissection is considered chronic. Although arbitrary, the distinction between acute and chronic dissections has important implications,

not only for decision-making about perioperative management strategies and operative techniques, but also for evaluating surgical results. Figure 22-17 provides an algorithm for the management of acute aortic dissection. In light of the importance of acuity, Borst and associates[101] have proposed a third phase—termed *subacute*—to describe the transition between the acute and chronic phases. The subacute period encompasses days 15 through 60 after the initial tear. Although this is past the traditional 14-day acute phase, patients with subacute dissection continue to have extremely fragile aortic tissue, which may complicate operative treatment and increase the risks associated with surgery.

Variants As noted earlier, advancements in noninvasive imaging of the aorta have revealed variants of aortic dissection (see Fig. 22-14). The recently introduced term *acute aortic syndrome* encompasses classic aortic dissection and its variants. Other aortic syndromes, which were once thought to be rare, include *intramural hematoma (IMH)* and *penetrating aortic ulcer (PAU)*. Although the issue is somewhat controversial, the current consensus is that, in most cases, these variants of dissection should be treated identically to classic dissection.

An IMH is a collection of blood within the aortic wall, without an intimal tear, that is believed to be due to rupture of the vasa vasorum within the media. The accumulation of blood can result in a secondary intimal tear that ultimately leads to a dissection.[102] Because IMH and aortic dissection represent a continuum, it is possible that IMH is seen less frequently than aortic dissection because IMH rapidly progresses to true dissection. The prevalence of IMH among

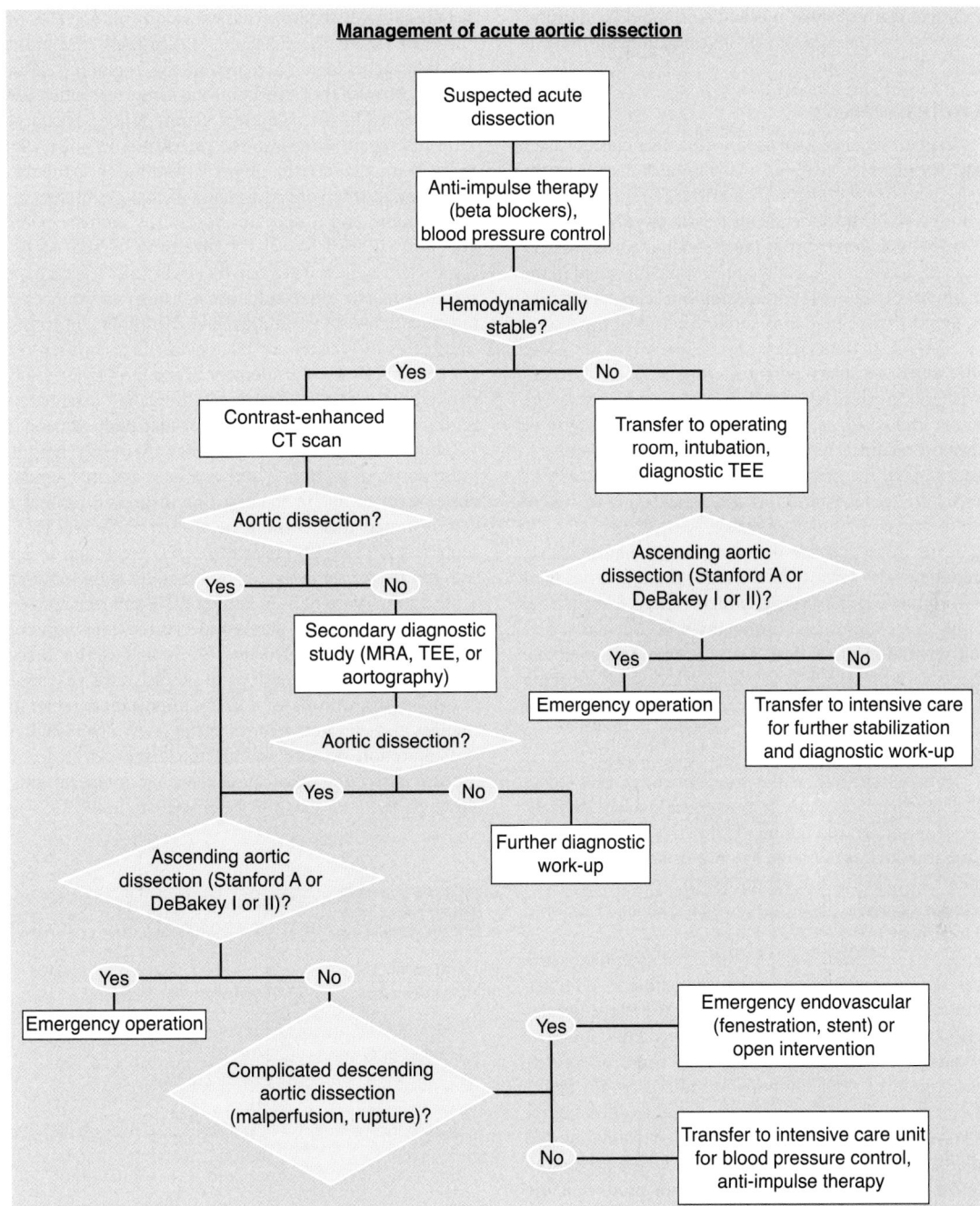

FIG. 22-17. Algorithm used to facilitate decisions regarding treatment of acute aortic dissection. CT = computed tomography; MRA = magnetic resonance angiography; TEE = transesophageal echocardiography.

patients with acute aortic syndromes is approximately 6%, with 16% progressing to full dissection.[103] An IMH can be classified according to its location (i.e., ascending or descending) and should be treated analogously to classic dissection.[104]

A PAU is essentially a disrupted atherosclerotic plaque that projects into the aortic wall and is associated with surrounding hematoma. Eventually, the ulcer can penetrate the aortic wall, which leads to dissection or rupture. The rate of disease progression is higher than that of IMH alone.[105]

Etiology and Natural History

Aortic dissection is a lethal condition with a reported incidence of 3.5 per 100,000 in the United States.[106] Without appropriate mod-

ern medical or surgical treatment, most patients (approximately 90%) die within 3 months of dissection, mostly from rupture.[107,108]

Although several risk factors for aortic dissection have been identified, the specific causes remain unknown. Ultimately, any condition that weakens the aortic wall increases the risk of aortic dissection. Common general cardiovascular risk factors, such as smoking, hypertension, atherosclerosis, and hypercholesterolemia, are associated with aortic dissection. Patients with connective tissue disorders, aortitis, bicuspid aortic valve, or pre-existing medial degenerative disease are at risk for dissection, especially if they already have a thoracic aortic aneurysm.[15] Aortic injury during cardiac catheterization or surgery is a common cause of iatrogenic dissection. Other situations that are associated with aortic dissection include cocaine abuse and amphetamine abuse.[109] Advances in the understanding of the molecular mechanisms behind abdominal aortic aneurysms have prompted similar investigations of thoracic aortic dissection.[110,111]

Clinical Manifestations

The onset of dissection often is associated with severe chest or back pain, classically described as "tearing," that migrates distally as the dissection progresses along the length of the aorta. The location of the pain often indicates which aortic segments are involved. Pain in the anterior chest suggests involvement of the ascending aorta, whereas pain in the back and abdomen generally indicates involvement of the descending and thoracoabdominal aorta. Additional clinical sequelae of acute aortic dissection are best considered in terms of the dissection's potential anatomic manifestations at each level of the aorta (see Fig. 22-15 and Table 22-4). Thus, potential complications of dissection of the aorta (and involved secondary arteries) are highly varied, including, but not limited to, cardiac ischemia (coronary artery) or tamponade, stroke (brachiocephalic arteries), paraplegia or paraparesis (intercostal arteries), mesenteric ischemia (superior mesenteric artery), kidney failure (renal arteries), and limb ischemia or loss of motor function (brachial or femoral arteries).

Ascending aortic dissection can directly injure the aortic valve, causing regurgitation. The severity of the regurgitation varies with the degree of commissural disruption, which ranges from partial separation of only one commissure, producing mild valvular regurgitation, to full separation of all three commissures and complete prolapse of the valve into the left ventricle, producing severe acute heart failure. Patients with acute aortic valve regurgitation may report worsening dyspnea.

Ascending dissections also can extend into the coronary arteries or shear the coronary ostia off of the true lumen, causing acute coronary occlusion; when this occurs, it most often involves the right coronary artery. The sudden disruption of coronary blood flow can cause a myocardial infarction. Because symptoms and signs consistent with myocardial ischemia are produced, this presentation can mask the presence of aortic dissection, which results in delayed diagnosis and treatment.

The thin and inflamed outer wall of a dissected ascending aorta often produces a serosanguineous pericardial effusion that can accumulate and cause tamponade. Suggestive signs include jugular venous distention, muffled heart tones, pulsus paradoxus, and low-voltage electrocardiogram (ECG) tracings. Free rupture into the pericardial space produces rapid tamponade and is generally fatal.

As the dissection progresses, any branch vessel from the aorta can become involved, which results in compromised blood flow and ischemic complications (i.e., *malperfusion*). Therefore, depending on which arteries are involved, the dissection can produce acute stroke, paraplegia, hepatic failure, bowel infarction, renal failure, or a threatened ischemic limb.

Diagnostic Evaluation

Because of the variations in severity and the wide variety of potential clinical manifestations, the diagnosis of acute aortic dissection can be challenging.[112–114] Only 3 out of every 100,000 patients who present to an emergency department with acute chest, back, or abdominal pain are eventually diagnosed with aortic dissection. Not surprisingly, diagnostic delays are common; delays beyond 24 hours after hospitalization occur in up to 39% of cases. Unfortunately, delays in diagnosis lead to delays in treatment, which can have disastrous consequences. The European Society of Cardiology Task Force on Aortic Dissection stated, "The main challenge in managing acute aortic dissection is to suspect and thus diagnose the disease as early as possible."[112] A high index of suspicion is critical, particularly in younger, atypical patients, who may have connective tissue disorders or other, less common risk factors.

Most patients with acute aortic dissection (80 to 90%) experience severe pain in the chest, back, or abdomen.[112–114] The pain usually occurs suddenly, has a sharp or tearing quality, and often migrates

distally as the dissection progresses along the aorta. For classification purposes (acute vs. subacute vs. chronic), the onset of pain is generally considered to represent the beginning of the dissection process. Most of the other common symptoms either are nonspecific or are caused by the secondary manifestations of dissection.

A discrepancy between the extremities in pulse, blood pressure, or both is the classic physical finding in patients with aortic dissection. It often occurs because of changes in flow in the true and false lumens, and it does not necessarily indicate extension into an extremity branch vessel. Involvement of the aortic arch often creates differences between the right and left arms, whereas descending aortic dissection often causes differences between the upper and lower extremities. Like symptoms, most of the physical signs after dissection are related to the secondary manifestations and therefore vary considerably (Table 22-4). For example, signs of stroke or a threatened ischemic limb may dominate the physical findings in patients with carotid or iliac malperfusion, respectively.

Unfortunately, laboratory studies are of little help in diagnosing acute aortic dissection. There has been recent interest in using D-dimer level to aid in making this diagnosis. Several reports have demonstrated that D-dimer is an extremely sensitive indicator of acute aortic dissection; elevated levels are found in approximately 97% of affected patients.[115] Tests that are commonly used to detect acute coronary events—including ECG and tests for serum markers of myocardial injury—deserve special consideration and need to be interpreted carefully. Normal ECGs and serum marker levels in patients with acute chest pain should raise suspicion about the possibility of aortic dissection. It is important to remember that ECG changes and elevated serum marker levels associated with myocardial infarction do not exclude the diagnosis of aortic dissection, because dissection can cause coronary malperfusion. Ultimately, although the issue has not been well studied, ECGs seem to have

TABLE 22-4	Anatomic complications of aortic dissection and their associated symptoms and signs
Anatomic Manifestation	**Symptoms and Signs**
Aortic valve insufficiency	Dyspnea
	Murmur
	Pulmonary rales
	Shock
Coronary malperfusion	Chest pain with characteristics of angina
	Nausea, vomiting
	Shock
	Ischemic changes on electrocardiogram
	Elevated levels of cardiac enzymes
Pericardial tamponade	Dyspnea
	Jugular venous distention
	Pulsus paradoxus
	Muffled cardiac tones
	Shock
	Low-voltage electrocardiogram
Subclavian or iliofemoral artery malperfusion	Cold, painful extremity
	Extremity sensory and motor deficits
	Peripheral pulse deficit
Carotid artery malperfusion	Syncope
	Focal neurologic deficit (transient or persistent)
	Carotid pulse deficit
	Coma
Spinal malperfusion	Paraplegia
	Incontinence
Mesenteric malperfusion	Nausea, vomiting
	Abdominal pain
Renal malperfusion	Oliguria or anuria
	Hematuria

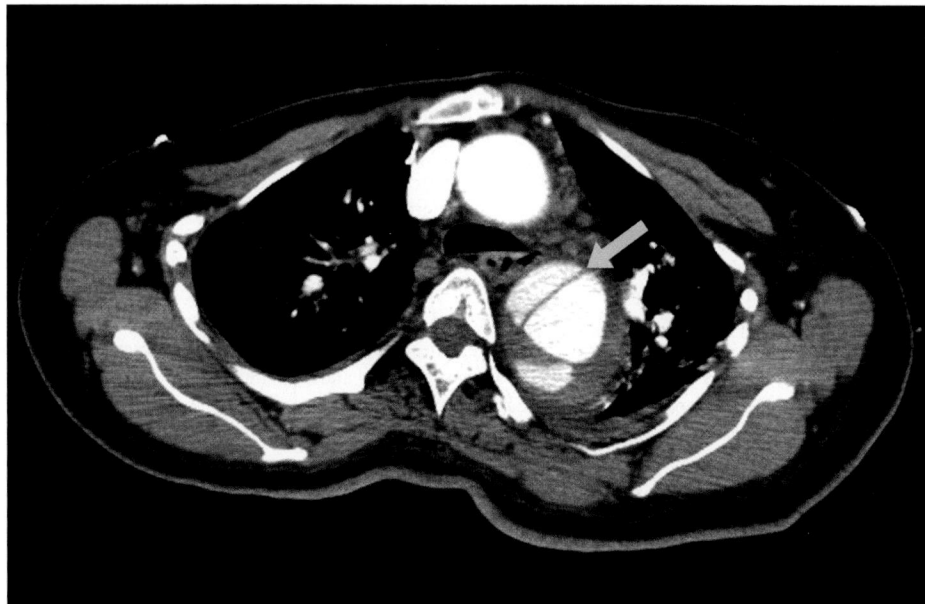

FIG. 22-18. Computed tomographic scan showing chronic aortic dissection in the distal aorta. The dissecting membrane (*arrow*) has separated the aorta into two channels—the true and false lumens.

little utility for detecting or ruling out dissection. Similarly, although chest x-rays (CXRs) may show a widened mediastinum or abnormal aortic contour, up to 16% of patients with dissection have a normal-appearing CXR.[114] The value of the CXR for detecting aortic dissection is limited, with a sensitivity of 67% and a specificity of 86%.[116]

Once the diagnosis of dissection is considered, the thoracic aorta should be imaged with CT, MRA, or echocardiography. The accuracy of these noninvasive imaging tests has all but eliminated the need for diagnostic aortography in most patients with suspected aortic dissection. Currently, the diagnosis usually is established with contrast-enhanced CT. The classic diagnostic feature is a double-lumen aorta (Fig. 22-18). In addition, CT scans provide essential information about the segments of the aorta involved; the acuity of the dissection; aortic dilatation, including the presence of pre-existing degenerative aneurysms; and the development of threatening sequelae, including pericardial effusion, early aortic rupture, and branch vessel compromise. Although MRA also provides excellent imaging, the MR suite is not well suited for critically ill patients. In patients who cannot undergo contrast-enhanced CT or MRA, transthoracic echocardiography can be used to establish the diagnosis. Transesophageal echocardiography (TEE) is excellent for determining the presence of dissection, aneurysm, and IMH in the ascending aorta.

Contrast-enhanced CT has a sensitivity of 98% and a specificity of 87% for diagnosis of aortic dissection. Although MRA is now considered the gold standard, with both a sensitivity and a specificity of 98%, CT scanning is the preferred imaging modality in the emergency department, mainly because of its swift image acquisition.[117] In appropriate hands, TEE has a demonstrated sensitivity and specificity as high as 98 and 95%, respectively.[118] Furthermore, TEE offers important information about ventricular function and aortic valve competency. Finally, TEE is the diagnostic modality of choice for hemodynamically unstable patients in whom the diagnosis of ascending dissection is suspected; ideally, these patients should be taken to the operating room, where the TEE can be performed and, if the TEE is confirmatory, surgery can be started immediately.

In selected patients with ascending aortic dissection (i.e., those who have evidence of pre-existing coronary artery disease), coronary angiography is performed before surgery. Specific relative indications in these patients include a history of angina or myocardial infarction, a recent myocardial perfusion study with abnormal results, previous coronary artery bypass or angioplasty, and acute ischemic changes on ECG. Contraindications include hemodynamic instability, aortic rupture, and pericardial effusion.[119] In our practice, patients with acute aortic dissections rarely undergo coronary angiography. However, all patients presenting for elective repair of chronic ascending dissections have diagnostic coronary angiograms taken.

Of note, when malperfusion of the renal, visceral, or lower extremity arteries develops, the patient is usually treated in an angiography suite or hybrid operating room. Although the dissection usually is diagnosed on CT scan, these patients undergo aortography, during which the mechanism of the malperfusion is ascertained and, if possible, corrected. Hence, aortography may be obsolete as a diagnostic test for dissection, but it is beneficial for patients with malperfusion.

Treatment

Initial Assessment and Management

Regardless of the location of the dissection, the initial treatment is the same for all patients with suspected or confirmed acute aortic dissection (see Fig. 22-17). Furthermore, because of the potential for rupture before the diagnosis is confirmed, aggressive pharmacologic management is started once there is clinical suspicion of dissection, and this treatment is continued during the diagnostic evaluation. The goals of pharmacologic treatment are to stabilize the dissection and prevent rupture.

Patients are monitored closely in an intensive care unit. Indwelling radial arterial catheters are used to monitor blood pressure and optimize titration of antihypertensive agents. Blood pressures in a malperfused limb can underrepresent the central aortic pressure; therefore, blood pressure is measured in the arm with the best pulse. Central venous catheters assure reliable IV access for delivering vasoactive medications. Pulmonary artery catheters are reserved for patients with severe cardiopulmonary dysfunction.

In addition to confirming the diagnosis of dissection and defining its acuity and extent, the initial evaluation focuses on determining whether any of several life-threatening complications are present. Particular attention is paid to changes in neurologic status, peripheral pulses, and urine output. Serial laboratory studies—including arterial blood gas concentrations, complete blood cell count, prothrombin and partial thromboplastin times, and serum levels of electrolytes, creatinine, blood urea nitrogen, and liver enzymes—are useful for detecting organ ischemia and optimizing management.

The initial management strategy, commonly described as *antihypertensive therapy* or *blood pressure control,* focuses on reducing aortic wall stress, the force of left ventricular ejection, chronotropy, and the rate of change in blood pressure (dP/dT). Reductions in dP/dT are achieved by lowering both cardiac contractility and blood pressure. The drugs initially used to accomplish these goals include IV beta-adrenergic blockers, direct vasodilators, calcium channel blockers, and angiotensin-converting enzyme inhibitors. These agents are used to achieve a heart rate between 60 and 80 bpm, a systolic blood pressure between 100 and 110 mmHg, and a mean arterial blood pressure between 60 and 75 mmHg. These hemodynamic targets are maintained as long as urine output remains adequate and neurologic function is not impaired. Achieving adequate pain control with IV opiates, such as morphine and fentanyl, is important for maintaining acceptable blood pressure control.

Beta antagonists are administered to all patients with acute aortic dissections unless there are strong contraindications, such as severe heart failure, bradyarrhythmia, high-grade atrioventricular conduction block, or bronchospastic disease. Esmolol can be useful in patients with bronchospastic disease because it is a cardioselective, ultra-fast-acting agent with a short half-life. Labetalol, which causes both nonselective beta blockade and postsynaptic alpha$_1$-blockade, reduces systemic vascular resistance without impairing cardiac output. Doses of beta antagonists are titrated to achieve a heart rate of 60 to 80 bpm. In patients who cannot receive beta antagonists, calcium channel blockers such as diltiazem are an effective alternative. Nitroprusside, a direct vasodilator, can be administered once beta blockade is adequate. When used alone, however, nitroprusside can cause reflex increases in heart rate and contractility, elevated dP/dT, and progression of aortic dissection. Enalapril and other angiotensin-converting enzyme inhibitors are useful in patients with renal malperfusion. These drugs inhibit renin release, which may improve renal blood flow.

Treatment of Ascending Aortic Dissection

Acute Ascending Dissection Ascending aortic repairs performed in the chronic phase of dissection uniformly have better outcomes than repairs performed in the acute phase. Unfortunately, the risk of a fatal complication, such as aortic rupture, during medical management outweighs the risk associated with early operation. Therefore, acute ascending aortic dissection has traditionally been considered an absolute indication for emergency surgical repair. However, specific patient groups may benefit from nonoperative management or delayed operation.[120] Delayed repair should be considered for patients who (a) present with acute stroke or mesenteric ischemia, (b) are elderly and have substantial comorbidity, (c) are in stable condition and may benefit from transfer to specialized centers, or (d) have undergone a cardiac operation in the remote past. Regarding the last group, it is important that the previous operation not be too recent; dissections that occur during the first 3 weeks after cardiac surgery pose a high risk of rupture and tamponade, and such dissections warrant early operation.[121]

In the absence of the circumstances listed earlier, most patients with acute ascending aortic dissection undergo emergent graft replacement of the ascending aorta. The operation is conducted in a manner similar to that described for aneurysms of the transverse aortic arch in the previous section. Immediately before the operation begins, intraoperative TEE is commonly performed to further assess baseline myocardial and valvular function and, if necessary, to confirm the diagnosis. The operation is performed via a median sternotomy with cardiopulmonary bypass and hypothermic circulatory arrest (Fig. 22-19). In preparation for circulatory arrest, cannulas are placed in the right axillary artery (to provide arterial inflow) and the right atrium (to provide venous drainage).[96,122] If profound hypothermic circulatory arrest is used, the patient traditionally is cooled until electroencephalographic monitoring shows electrocere-

bral silence; this generally occurs at nasopharyngeal temperatures of <18°C (64.4°F).[123] Alternatively, if antegrade cerebral perfusion can be reliably established, the arch repair can be conducted under deep hypothermia [23° to 25°C (73.4° to 77°F)]. After an appropriate level of cooling has been achieved, cardiopulmonary bypass is stopped, and the ascending aorta is opened. The innominate artery is then occluded with a clamp or snare, and flow from the axillary artery cannula is used to provide selective antegrade cerebral perfusion. A separate perfusion catheter can be placed in the left common carotid artery to ensure perfusion of the left side of the brain. This strategy of performing the distal anastomosis during circulatory arrest, often termed *open distal anastomosis*, obviates the need to place a clamp across the fragile aorta, avoiding further aortic damage. Also, it allows the surgeon to carefully inspect the aortic arch for intimal tears. The entire arch is replaced only if a primary intimal tear is located in the arch or if the arch is aneurysmal; in most acute cases, a less extensive, beveled "hemiarch" repair is adequate.[124] The distal aortic cuff is prepared by tacking the inner and outer walls together and using surgical adhesive to obliterate the false lumen and strengthen the tissue. A polyester tube graft is sutured to the distal aortic cuff. The anastomosis between the graft and the aorta is fashioned so that blood flow will be directed into the true lumen; this often alleviates any distal malperfusion problems that were present preoperatively. After the distal anastomosis is reinforced with additional adhesive, the graft is deaired and clamped, full cardiopulmonary bypass is resumed, rewarming is initiated, and the proximal portion of the repair is started. In the absence of annuloaortic ectasia or Marfan syndrome—which generally necessitate aortic root replacement—aortic valve regurgitation can be corrected by resuspending the commissures onto the outer aortic wall.[125] The proximal aortic cuff is prepared with tacking sutures and surgical adhesive before the proximal aortic anastomosis is performed.

In the majority of patients who undergo surgical repair of acute ascending dissection, the dissection persists distal to the site of the operative repair. Extensive dilatation of the descending aorta develops in approximately 25% of the survivors, and rupture of the dilated distal aorta is the most common cause of late death in these patients. Freedom from distal reoperation is reported as 88% at 5 years and 76% at 10 years.[126] Therefore, after ascending aortic repair, most of these patients require aggressive treatment of the remaining acute descending aortic dissection, as described in detail later.

Chronic Ascending Dissection Occasionally, patients with ascending aortic dissection present for repair in the chronic phase. In most respects, the operation is similar to that for acute dissection repair. The greater tissue strength in the chronic setting, which makes suturing safer, is a notable difference. In addition, the false lumen is not obliterated at the distal anastomosis; instead, the dissecting membrane is fenestrated into the arch to assure perfusion of both lumens and to prevent postoperative malperfusion complications. Unlike operations for acute dissection, operations for chronic dissection are often aggressive repairs that extend into the arch and root, because the tissues are much less fragile.

Treatment of Descending Aortic Dissection

Nonoperative Management Nonoperative, pharmacologic management of acute descending aortic dissection results in lower morbidity and mortality rates than surgical treatment does.[114] The most common causes of death during nonoperative treatment are aortic rupture and end-organ malperfusion. Therefore, patients are continually reassessed for new complications. At least two serial CT scans—usually obtained on day 2 or 3 and on day 8 or 9 of treatment—are compared with the initial scan to rule out significant aortic expansion.

Once the patient's condition has been stabilized, pharmacologic management is gradually shifted from IV to oral medications. Oral therapy, usually including a beta antagonist, is initiated when systolic pressure is consistently between 100 and 110 mmHg and

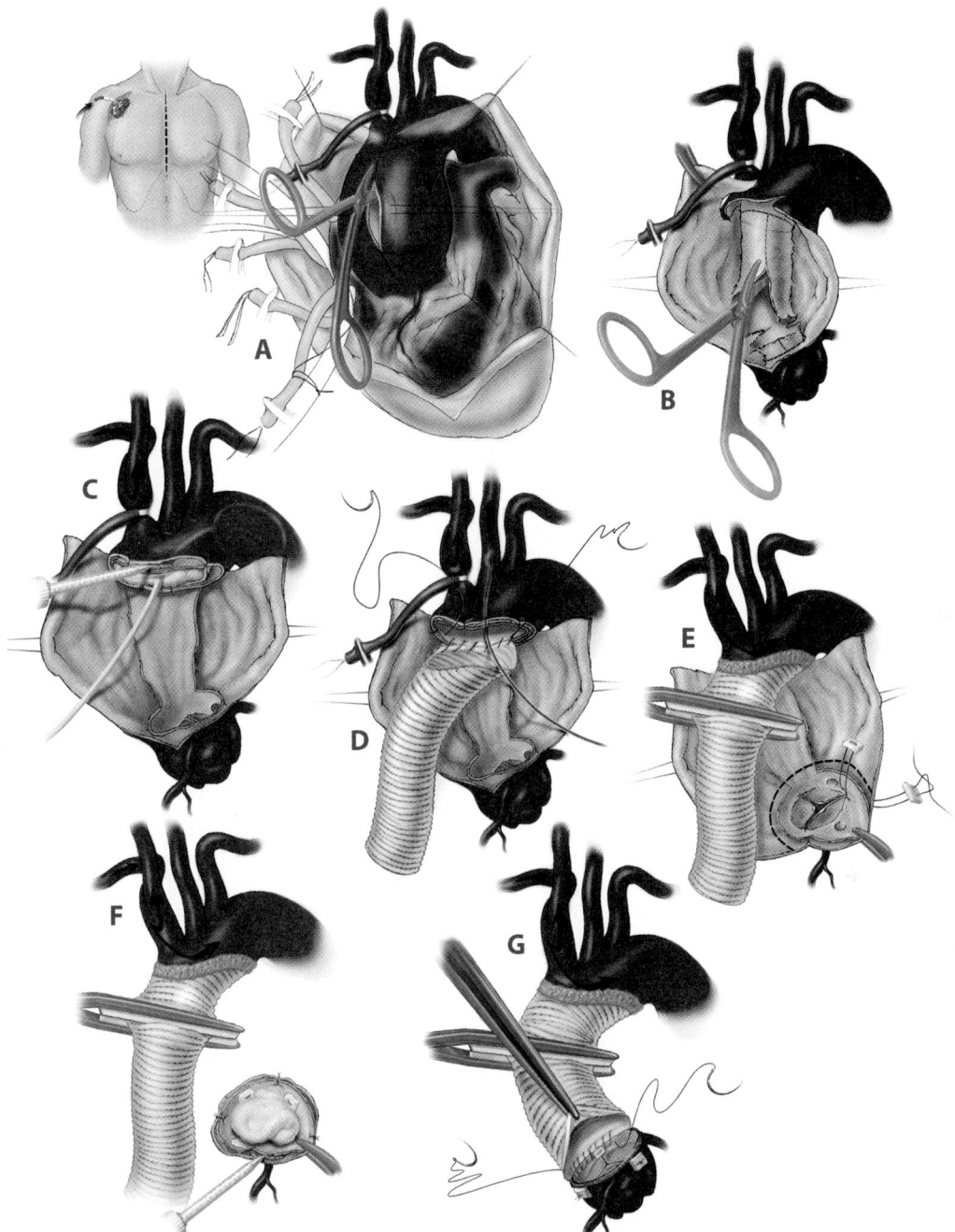

FIG. 22-19. Illustration of proximal aortic repair for acute ascending aortic dissection. **A.** This repair requires a median sternotomy and cardiopulmonary bypass. The ascending aorta is opened during hypothermic circulatory arrest, while antegrade cerebral perfusion is delivered via an axillary artery graft (see Fig. 22-8). **B.** The dissecting membrane is removed to expose the true lumen. **C.** Surgical adhesive is used to obliterate the false lumen and strengthen the aorta for the distal anastomosis. A 30-mL balloon catheter is placed in the true lumen to compress the distal false lumen; this helps keep the adhesive within the proximal false lumen, which maximizes the strength of the repair and prevents distal embolization of the adhesive through re-entry sites. A moist gauze sponge is placed in the true lumen to prevent the adhesive from running into the brachiocephalic vessels. **D.** An open distal anastomosis prevents clamp injury of the arch tissue and allows inspection of the arch lumen. A balloon perfusion catheter in the left common carotid artery ensures antegrade perfusion of the left cerebral circulation. If the origin of the dissection (i.e., intimal tear or disruption) does not extensively involve the greater curvature of the aortic arch, and if there is no evidence of a pre-existing arch aneurysm, a beveled, hemi-arch repair is carried out, preserving most of the greater curvature of the arch. The aorta is transected, beginning at the greater curvature immediately proximal to the origin of the innominate artery and extending distally toward the lesser curvature to the level of the left subclavian artery. Consequently, most of the transverse aortic arch, except for the dorsal segment containing the brachiocephalic arteries, is removed. An appropriately sized, sealed (with collagen or gelatin) Dacron tube graft is selected, and the beveled distal anastomosis is made with continuous 3-0 or 4-0 monofilament suture. **E.** After the anastomosis is covered with additional adhesive and cardiopulmonary bypass is resumed, the aortic valve is assessed. Disrupted commissures are resuspended with pledgeted mattress sutures to restore valvular competence. **F.** The aorta is generally transected at the sinotubular junction, and adhesive is used to obliterate the false lumen within the proximal aortic stump. A moist gauze sponge is placed within the true lumen to prevent the adhesive from injuring the aortic valve leaflets or entering the coronary artery ostia. **G.** After the adhesive has set, the proximal anastomosis is carried out at the sinotubular junction, incorporating the distal margin of the commissures. *[Reproduced with permission from Creager MA, Dzau VS, Loscalzo J (eds): Vascular Medicine. Philadelphia: WB Saunders, 2006. Copyright © Saunders/Elsevier, 2006, Fig. 35-3A–G.]*

the neurologic, renal, and cardiovascular systems are stable. Many patients can be discharged after their blood pressure is well controlled with oral agents and after serial CT scans confirm the absence of aortic expansion.

Long-term pharmacologic therapy is important for patients with chronic aortic dissection. Beta blockers remain the drugs of choice.[127] In a 20-year follow-up study, DeBakey and colleagues[128] found that inadequate blood pressure control was associated with late aneurysm formation. Aneurysms developed in only 17% of patients with "good" blood pressure control, compared with 45% of patients with "poor" control.

Aggressive imaging follow-up is recommended for all patients with chronic aortic dissection.[129] Both contrast-enhanced CT and MRA scans provide excellent aortic imaging and facilitate serial comparisons to detect progressive aortic expansion. The first surveillance scan is obtained approximately 6 weeks after the onset of dissection. Subsequent scans are obtained at least every 3 months for the first year, every 6 months for the second year, and annually thereafter. Scans are obtained more frequently in high-risk patients, such as those with Marfan syndrome, and in those in whom significant aortic expansion is detected. For patients who have undergone graft repair of descending aortic dissection, annual CT or MRA scans are also obtained to detect false aneurysm formation or dilatation of unrepaired segments of aorta. Early detection of worrisome changes allows timely, elective intervention before rupture or other complications develop. The importance of careful follow-up was illustrated by Glower and associates,[130] who reported long-term outcomes in patients who had undergone repair of chronic aortic dissection. Nearly 20% of late deaths were caused by aortic rupture, and 25% of patients required additional surgical repair during the follow-up period.

Indications for Surgery Surgery is typically reserved for patients who experience complications.[131] In general terms, surgical intervention for acute descending aortic dissection is intended to prevent or repair ruptures and relieve ischemic manifestations.

During the acute phase of a dissection, the specific indications for operative intervention include aortic rupture, increasing periaortic or pleural fluid volume, rapidly expanding aortic diameter, uncontrolled hypertension, and persistent pain despite adequate medical therapy. Acute dissection superimposed on a pre-existing aneurysm is considered a life-threatening condition and is therefore another indication for operation. Finally, patients who have a history of noncompliance with medical therapy may ultimately benefit more from surgical treatment if they are otherwise reasonable operative candidates.

Acute malperfusion syndromes also warrant intervention. In the recent past, visceral and renal malperfusion were considered indications for operation. Percutaneous interventions, however, have largely replaced open surgery for treatment of these complications. When the endovascular approach is unavailable or unsuccessful, surgical options can be used.

In the chronic phase, the indications for operative intervention for aortic dissections are similar to those for degenerative thoracic aortic aneurysms. These indications include rapid expansion of the aneurysm and other factors that increase the likelihood of rupture. Elective operation is considered when the affected segment has reached a diameter of 6.0 to 6.5 cm or when an aneurysm has enlarged by >1 cm during a 1-year period. A lower threshold often is used for patients with Marfan syndrome.

Endovascular Treatment *Malperfusion Syndrome* Endovascular therapy is routinely used in patients with descending aortic dissection complicated by visceral malperfusion.[132] Abdominal malperfusion syndrome often is fatal; prompt identification of visceral ischemia and expedited treatment to restore hepatic, GI, and renal perfusion are imperative for a positive outcome. As described in a later section, several open surgical techniques can be used to re-establish blood flow to compromised organs. However,

in the acute setting, open surgery is associated with poor outcomes. Therefore, endovascular intervention is the preferred initial approach in this setting. In one endovascular technique known as *endovascular fenestration*, a balloon is used to create a tear in the dissection flap, which allows blood to flow in both the true and false lumens. This technique can be used when a visceral branch is being supplied by an underperfused true or false lumen. Placement of a stent graft in the true lumen of the aorta can resolve a "dynamic" malperfusion. Occasionally, a small stent must be placed directly in the lumen of a visceral or renal artery because the dissection has propagated into the branch, creating "static" malperfusion at the origin.

Iliofemoral malperfusion causing limb-threatening leg ischemia also can be treated via an endovascular approach. However, direct surgical revascularization—usually by placing a femoral-to-femoral arterial bypass graft—is a better option whenever the endovascular procedure cannot be performed expeditiously.

Acute Dissection There is considerable interest in using endovascular stent grafts to treat uncomplicated acute descending dissection. The goal of this treatment strategy is to use the stent graft to cover the intimal tear, seal the entry site of the dissection, and eventually cause thrombosis of the false lumen. However, whether this approach is more effective than conventional nonoperative management has not been established; therefore, at this time, the use of endografts in patients with classic dissection remains investigational.[133] Such procedures take place in a hybrid operating room, where access to the true lumen is gained from the femoral arteries. An aortogram is taken, and the intimal tear is identified. Note that the diameter of the true lumen is measured on both the aortogram and a preoperative contrast-enhanced CT scan. A stent graft approximately 10% wider in diameter than the true lumen is selected for these cases. Unlike stents deployed in treating most descending thoracic aortic aneurysms, stents deployed in treating descending aortic dissections must *not* be ballooned, because ballooning can cause a new intimal tear, retrograde dissection into the ascending aorta, or even aortic rupture.

Chronic Dissection Endovascular treatment of chronic descending aortic dissection also is currently under investigation.[134] These dissections are particularly challenging, because the relative rigidity of the dissecting membrane and the presence of multiple re-entry sites make it difficult to exclude the false lumen. Furthermore, interfering with false lumen perfusion may cause ischemic complications, such as bowel infarction or renal failure. Until the safety and effectiveness of endovascular repair for this condition have been demonstrated, patients with chronic descending aortic dissection should be treated with conventional nonoperative management until indications for open surgical repair develop.

Penetrating Aortic Ulcer Unlike patients with classic descending aortic dissection, those with PAUs appear to be very well suited for endovascular intervention. Covering the focal ulceration with a stent graft has been shown to be an effective treatment.[135]

Open Repair *Acute Dissection* In patients with acute aortic dissection, surgical repair of the descending thoracic or thoracoabdominal aorta is associated with high morbidity and mortality.[114] Therefore, the primary goals of surgery are to prevent fatal rupture and to restore branch vessel perfusion.[131] A limited graft repair of the life-threatening aortic lesion achieves these goals while minimizing risks. Because the most common site of rupture in descending aortic dissection is in the proximal third of the descending thoracic aorta, the upper half of the descending thoracic aorta is usually repaired. The distal half also may be replaced if it exceeds 4 cm in diameter. Graft replacement of the entire thoracoabdominal aorta is not attempted in this setting unless a large coexisting aneurysm mandates this radical approach. Similarly, the repair is not extended into the aortic arch unless the arch is aneurysmal, even if the primary tear is located there. Patients with chronic dissection who require emergency repair because of acute pain or rupture also undergo limited graft replacement of the symptomatic segment.

Because repairing acute dissections entails an increased risk of paraplegia, adjuncts that provide spinal cord protection, such as cerebrospinal fluid drainage and left heart bypass, are used liberally during such repairs,[136] even if the repair is confined to the upper descending thoracic aorta. Proximal control usually is obtained between the left common carotid and left subclavian arteries; any mediastinal hematoma near the proximal descending thoracic aorta is avoided until proximal control is established. After the aorta is opened, the dissecting membrane is excised from the section undergoing graft replacement. The proximal and distal anastomoses use all layers of the aortic wall, thereby excluding the false lumen in the suture lines and directing all blood flow into the true lumen. Although the relative lack of mural thrombus assures the presence of multiple patent intercostal arteries, extreme tissue fragility may preclude their reattachment.

Malperfusion Syndrome Lower-extremity ischemia is commonly addressed with surgical extra-anatomic revascularization techniques, such as femoral-to-femoral bypass grafting. In patients with abdominal organ ischemia, flow to the compromised bed must be reestablished swiftly. When an endovascular approach is unavailable or unsuccessful, open surgery is necessary. Although they are considered second-line therapies, multiple techniques are available, including graft replacement of the aorta (with flow redirected into the true lumen), open aortic fenestration, and visceral or renal artery bypass.

Chronic Dissection A more aggressive replacement usually is performed during elective aortic repairs in patients with chronic dissection. In many regards, the operative approach used in these patients is identical to that used for descending thoracic and thoracoabdominal aortic aneurysms, as described in the first half of this chapter (Fig. 22-20). One key difference is the need to excise as

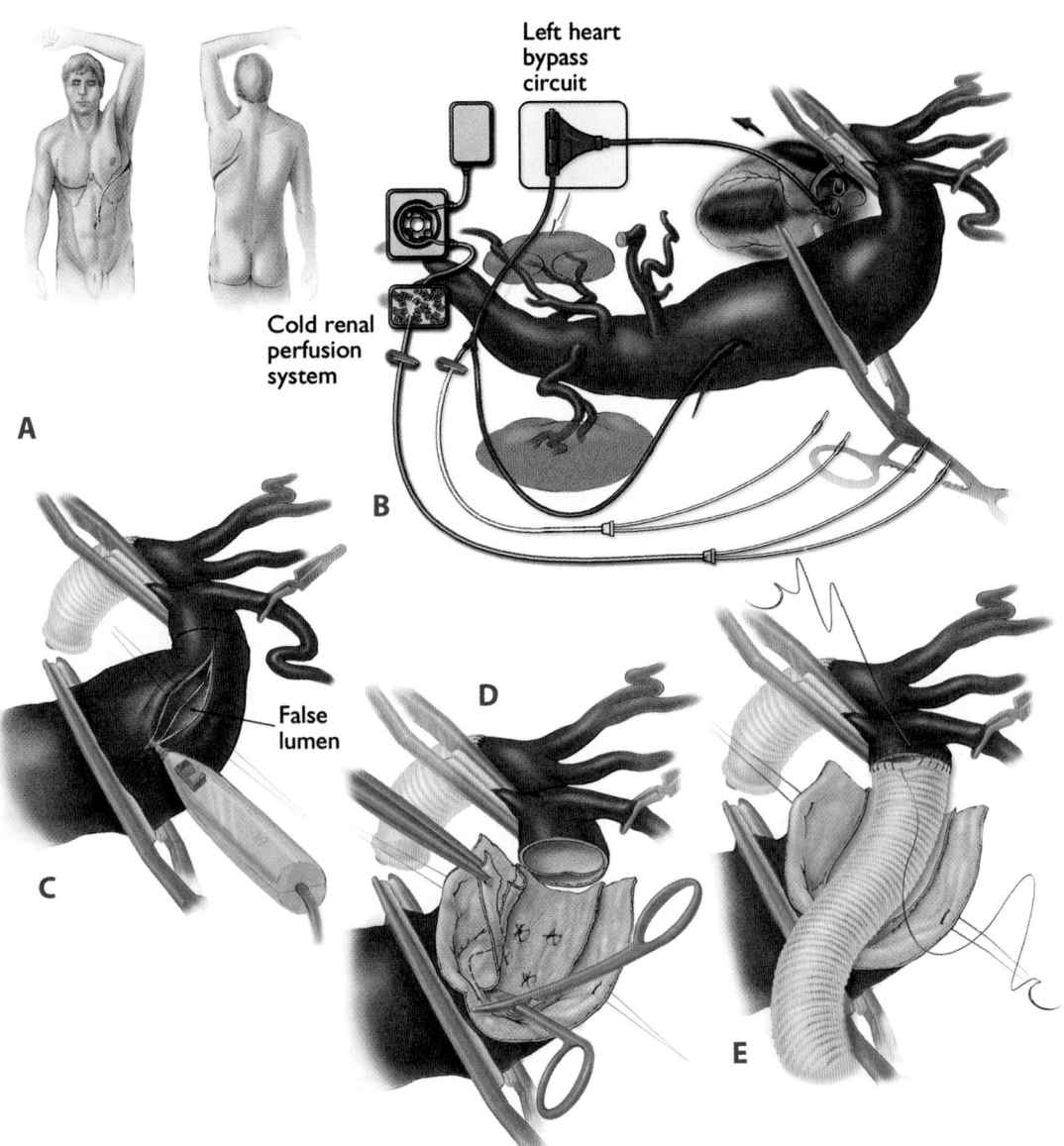

FIG. 22-20. Illustration of distal aortic repair of a chronic dissection. **A.** Thoracoabdominal incision. **B.** Extent II thoracoabdominal aortic aneurysm resulting from chronic aortic dissection. The patient has previously undergone composite valve graft replacement of the aortic root and ascending aorta. After left heart bypass is initiated, the proximal portion of the aneurysm is isolated by placing clamps on the left subclavian artery, between the left common carotid and left subclavian arteries, and across the middle descending thoracic aorta. **C.** The isolated segment of aorta is opened by using electrocautery. **D.** The dissecting membrane is excised, and bleeding intercostal arteries are oversewn. The aorta is prepared for proximal anastomosis by transecting it distal to the proximal clamp and separating this portion from the esophagus (not shown). **E.** The proximal anastomosis between the aorta and an appropriately sized Dacron graft is completed with continuous polypropylene suture. (*Continued*)

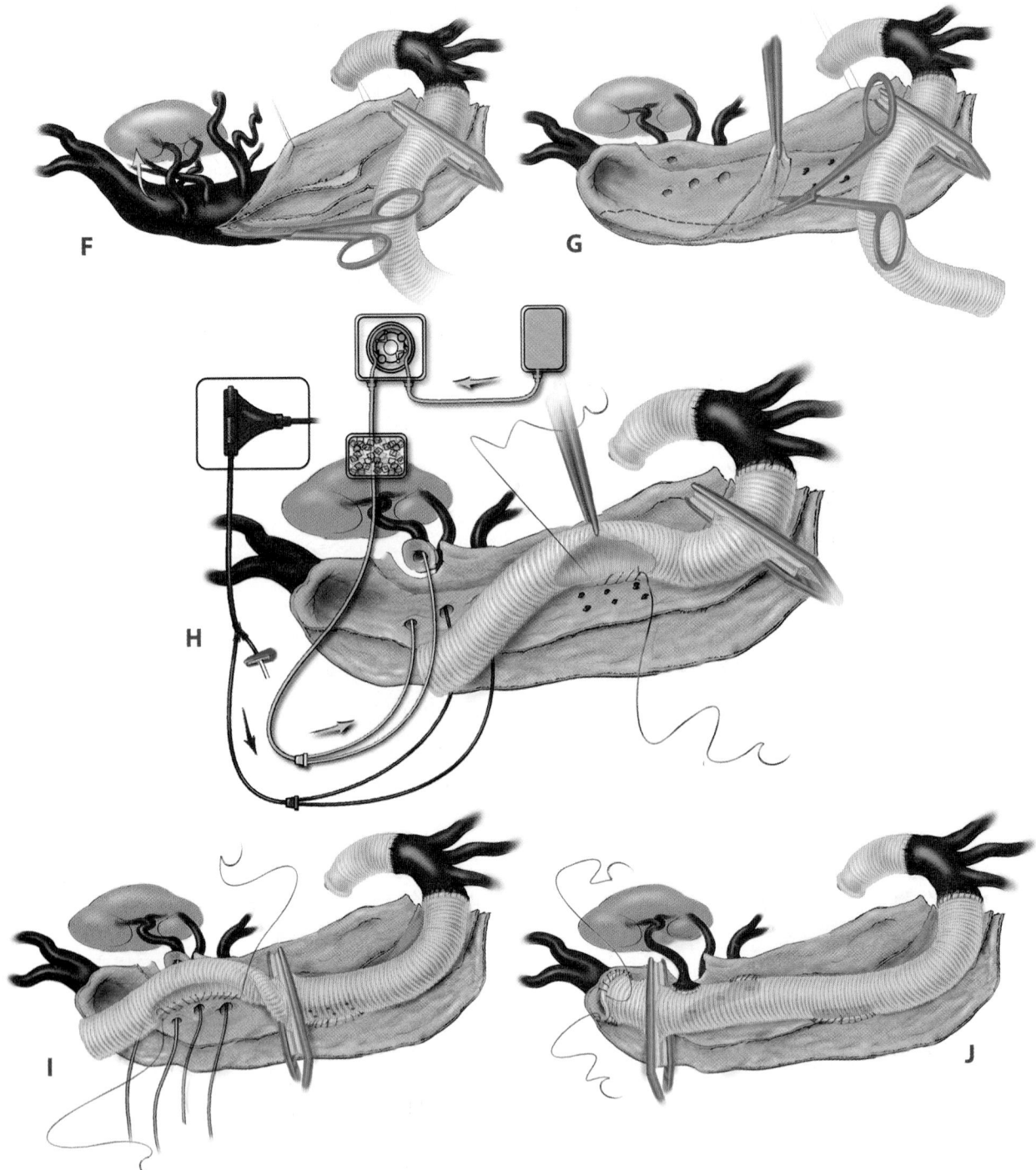

FIG. 22-20. *(Continued)* **F.** After left heart bypass has been stopped and the distal aortic cannula has been removed, the proximal clamp is repositioned onto the graft, the other two clamps are removed, and the remainder of the aneurysm is opened. **G.** The rest of the dissecting membrane is excised, and the openings to the celiac, superior mesenteric, and renal arteries are identified. **H.** Selective visceral perfusion with oxygenated blood from the bypass circuit is delivered through balloon perfusion catheters placed in the celiac and superior mesenteric arterial ostia. Cold crystalloid is delivered to the renal arteries. The critical intercostal arteries are reattached to an opening cut in the graft. **I.** To minimize spinal cord ischemia, the proximal clamp is repositioned distal to the intercostal reattachment site. A second oval opening is fashioned in the graft adjacent to the visceral vessels. Selective perfusion of the visceral arteries continues during their reattachment to the graft. A separate anastomosis is often required to reattach the left renal artery. **J.** After the balloon perfusion catheters are removed and the visceral anastomosis is completed, the clamp is again moved distally, restoring blood flow to the celiac, renal, and superior mesenteric arteries. The final anastomosis is created between the graft and the distal aorta. *[Reproduced with permission from Creager MA, Dzau VS, Loscalzo J (eds): Vascular Medicine. Philadelphia: WB Saunders, 2006. Copyright © Saunders/Elsevier, 2006, Fig. 35-8A–J.]*

much dissecting membrane as possible to clearly identify the true and false lumens and to locate all important branch vessels. When the dissection extends into the visceral or renal arteries, the membrane can be fenestrated, or the false lumen can be obliterated with sutures or intraluminal stents. Asymmetric expansion of the false lumen can create wide separation of the renal arteries. This problem is addressed by reattaching the mobilized left renal artery to a separate opening in the graft or by performing a left renal artery bypass with a side graft. Wedges of dissecting membrane also are excised from the aorta adjacent to the proximal and distal anastomoses, which allows blood to flow through both true and false lumens. When placing the proximal clamp is not technically feasible, hypothermic circulatory arrest can be used to facilitate the proximal portion of the repair.

OUTCOMES

Improvements in anesthesia, surgical techniques, and perioperative care have led to substantial improvements in outcome after thoracic aortic aneurysm repair. When performed in specialized centers, these operations are associated with excellent survival rates and acceptable morbidity rates. The interpretation of outcomes data is complicated by site-specific variables, such as the number of years reported and whether data are taken from single-practice centers or from pooled, multi-center, or national registries, and by patient-specific variables, such as type of enrollment, urgency and extent of repair, concomitant procedures performed, and the presence of pre-existing risk factors such as advanced age, previous cardiovascular repair, disease of any system or organ, or connective tissue disorder.

Repair of Proximal Aortic Aneurysms

Risks associated with the open repair of the proximal aorta vary by extent of repair and are greatest for repairs involving total arch replacement. All varieties of aortic root replacement have shown acceptable early mortality rates and few complications. Two groups with 20 and 27 years' experience with composite valve graft replacement reported early mortality rates of 5.6% and 1.9%, respectively, with the more recent repairs having better outcomes.[137,138] Early mortality rates for stentless porcine tissue root replacements are also low, ranging from 3.6 to 6.0%.[139–143]

Repairs incorporating the ascending aorta and aortic arch have acceptable outcomes, with risk increasing as larger sections of the aortic arch are incorporated into the repair.[144,145] Reported early mortality rates after stage 1 elephant trunk repairs range from 2.3 to 13.9%.[56,71,146–148]

The risk of operative death and stroke in these repairs is additionally increased by severe atherosclerosis of the ascending aorta, and a revised surgical strategy is often needed to avoid clamping this section of the aorta. In a review of literature accompanying Zingone and colleagues' own data for 36 such patients, pooled early death rates averaged 9.0% (ranged from 3.7 to 25.0%) and pooled stroke rates averaged 5.3% (ranged from 0 to 17.6%).[149] Their revised patient strategy included the use of hypothermic circulatory arrest in most patients (94%) and resulted in two early deaths (6%), one stroke (3%), and five patients with neurocognitive disturbances (14%). Other studies indicate that the enhanced risk of neurocognitive disturbances in ascending repairs using circulatory arrest are not offset by lower rates of early mortality.[150,151]

In a report by Kazui and Bashar[152] covering 20 years of experience and 472 consecutive patients who underwent aortic arch repair with selective antegrade cerebral perfusion, early mortality was 9.3% for all repairs and 4.1% for more recent repairs. The stroke rate was 3.2% for permanent deficits and 4.7% for temporary deficits. Recent innovations in aortic arch replacement, such as the use of extra-anatomic grafts and moderate hypothermia, have also produced good results, including early mortality rates ranging from 0 to 4.7%, permanent stroke rates ranging from 0 to 4.0%, and rates of transient neurologic dysfunction ranging from 0 to 4.9%.[153–155]

Treatment of Acute Ascending Aortic Dissection

The International Registry of Acute Aortic Dissection (IRAD) provides the most comprehensive data on contemporary outcomes in patients with acute aortic dissection. This registry was established in 1996 and has accumulated data from >1600 patients treated for acute aortic dissection at 22 centers in 11 countries. A recent IRAD analysis of data for 682 patients who underwent surgical repair of acute ascending aortic dissection revealed an inhospital mortality rate of 23.9%. The investigators identified several preoperative predictors of early mortality, including age >70 years, previous cardiac surgery, hypotension or shock at presentation, migrating pain, cardiac tamponade, pulse deficit, and evidence of myocardial ischemia or infarction on ECG.[156]

Repair of Distal Aortic Aneurysms

Endovascular Repair of Descending Thoracic Aortic Aneurysms

In the earliest series of endovascular repairs of descending thoracic aortic aneurysms, mortality and morbidity were difficult to assess. Most of the reported series were small and contained a large proportion of high-risk patients with substantial comorbidity. For example, in the Stanford experience with "first-generation" stent grafts in 103 patients with descending thoracic aortic aneurysms, the operative mortality rate was 9%, the stroke rate was 7%, the paraplegia/paraparesis rate was 3%, and actuarial survival was only 73 ± 5% at 2 years. However, 62 patients (60%) were not considered candidates for thoracotomy and open surgical repair; as expected, this group experienced the majority of the morbidity and mortality.[97] In a follow-up series, the Stanford group reported survival rates of 74% at 1 year and 31% at 5 years after stent grafting in patients who were deemed not to be surgical candidates; in contrast, survival rates were 93% at 1 year and 78% at 5 years (P <.001) after stent grafting in patients who were deemed reasonable candidates for conventional open repair.[157] This study also found a 30% incidence of late aortic complications, which stresses the necessity for appropriate follow-up. A recent prospective, nonrandomized, multicenter trial compared 140 patients who underwent endograft exclusion with 94 historical or concurrent patients who underwent open repair. The stent graft group had significantly less morbidity and early mortality than the open repair group, although no significant between-group difference was observed in the rate of stroke (3.6% and 4.3%, respectively).[158] At 5 years, the two groups differed significantly in their aneurysm-related mortality rates (2.8% for endovascular patients and 11.7% for open repair patients) but not in their rates of all-cause mortality (which were 32% and 31%, respectively).[159]

The efficacy of endovascular treatment of chronic descending thoracic aortic dissection has not been established. Small series have demonstrated the feasibility of this type of repair.[117,160] For example, in a recent study of six patients who had undergone such repairs, Czerny and colleagues[160] found no evidence of complication or aneurysmal expansion in any patient during the period between 4 months and 25 months after the procedure. The INSTEAD trial (INvestigation of STEnt grafts in patients with type B Aortic Dissection) involving 136 patients with uncomplicated chronic descending aortic dissection is being conducted to determine whether stent grafting improves all-cause mortality at 1 year when used as an adjunct to medical antihypertensive therapy.[134] Early results of this randomized trial, which completed enrollment in 2005, already appear to show increased mortality in the stent recipients.[161] Thus, at present, the use of stent grafts to treat chronic descending aortic dissection should be considered experimental.

Open Repair of Descending Thoracic and Thoracoabdominal Aortic Aneurysms

Contemporary results of open repairs of descending thoracic aortic aneurysms indicate that early mortality rates range from 4.4 to 8.0% and paraplegia rates range from 2.3 to 5.7%; stroke rates are generally lower, ranging from 1.8 to 2.1%.[162–164] In our series, although the risk of paraplegia increased with the extent of repair, the risk of mortality was greatest for those undergoing repair of the proximal two thirds of the descending aorta.[162] As expected, stroke rates after distal aortic repairs were highest when the clamp site was near the left subclavian artery.

Several studies have compared endovascular and surgical approaches to descending thoracic aortic repair. Some studies found no significant differences in rates of early death, stroke, and paraplegia,[165-167] whereas others found that surgical patients had higher rates of early mortality (27%)[168] and paraplegia (14%).[158]

Contemporary series of open thoracoabdominal aortic repairs show acceptable survival. Reported outcome rates range from 5 to 12% for early mortality, 4 to 9.5% for paraplegia, 1.7 to 5.2% for stroke, and 6 to 12% for renal complications. These series reports generally summarize 10 to 20 years of surgical experience.[163,169-171] Even for complex thoracoabdominal aortic repairs, such as stage 2 elephant trunk repairs, several centers report acceptable early mortality rates ranging from 0 to 10%.[56,71,146-148] Worse outcomes are also documented, as in a statewide, nonfederal analysis of 1010 patients in which the early mortality rate was 25%. Of note, 40% of these patients were treated at centers averaging only one thoracoabdominal aortic aneurysm repair per year.[172] Cowan and colleagues,[173] who examined the influence of familiarity with the procedure on rates of mortality and morbidity after thoracoabdominal aortic aneurysm repair, reported that patients treated at low-volume centers fared less well. Replacing the entire thoracoabdominal aorta (i.e., performing an extent II repair) carries the highest risk of death, bleeding, renal failure, and paraplegia.[78,163,169]

Treatment of Acute Descending Aortic Dissection
Nonoperative Management

The inhospital mortality rate for patients with acute descending aortic dissection who receive nonoperative treatment is nearly 10%.[114,174] The primary causes of death during nonoperative management are rupture, malperfusion, and cardiac failure. Risk factors associated with treatment failure—defined as death or need for surgery—include an enlarged aorta, persistent hypertension despite maximal treatment, oliguria, and peripheral ischemia. Among patients who receive nonoperative treatment for descending aortic dissection and who survive the acute period, approximately 90% remain alive 1 year later and approximately 76% are alive 3 years later.[175]

Endovascular Treatment

For malperfusion of the visceral or renal arteries, an endovascular approach is ideal. The Stanford group reported a 93% technical success rate for endovascular reperfusion of an ischemic bed.[176] Their experience with the use of first-generation stents to treat acute complicated descending dissections was also encouraging: Complete thrombosis of the false lumen occurred in 79% of patients. The early mortality rate was 16%, comparable to that associated with open techniques.[177] A recent meta-analysis of observational studies of endovascular stenting, which included 248 patients with acute descending aortic dissection, found a 30-day mortality rate of 9.8%. When compared with mortality rates obtained from IRAD data, this rate is substantially lower than the rate associated with open surgical treatment, but similar to the rate achieved with nonoperative management.[178]

Open Repair

We recently reported our 16-year experience with 76 patients with acute descending aortic dissection. Complexities included emergent (86%) or urgent (14%) repair, rupture (22%), pain (53%), and aneurysm superimposed on the dissection (96%). The 30-day mortality rate was 15%, and the inhospital mortality rate was 22%.[179] There were 5 cases of paraplegia (7%), five strokes (7%), and 15 cases of renal failure (20%). In a recent multicenter study, the IRAD investigators found a 33% inhospital mortality rate among 52 patients with acute dissection who underwent open surgical re-

placement of the descending thoracic aorta.[180] Another study found that, of patients who survive surgical treatment of acute descending aortic dissection, approximately 96% were alive at 1 year and approximately 83% were alive at 3 years after the procedure.[175]

ACKNOWLEDGMENTS

The authors wish to thank Susan Y. Green, MPH, Stephen N. Palmer, PhD, ELS, and Angela T. Odensky, MA, for editorial assistance, and Scott A. Weldon, MA, CMI, and Carol P. Larson, CMI, for creating the illustrations.

REFERENCES

Entries highlighted in bright blue are key references.

1. Johnston KW, Rutherford RB, Tilson MD, et al: Suggested standards for reporting on arterial aneurysms. Subcommittee on Reporting Standards for Arterial Aneurysms, Ad Hoc Committee on Reporting Standards, Society for Vascular Surgery and North American Chapter, International Society for Cardiovascular Surgery. *J Vasc Surg* 13:452, 1991.
2. Bickerstaff LK, Pairolero PC, Hollier LH, et al: Thoracic aortic aneurysms: A population-based study. *Surgery* 92:1103, 1982.
3. Segura AM, Luna RE, Horiba K, et al: Immunohistochemistry of matrix metalloproteinases and their inhibitors in thoracic aortic aneurysms and aortic valves of patients with Marfan's syndrome. *Circulation* 98(19 Suppl):II331, 1998.
4. Neptune ER, Frischmeyer PA, Arking DE, et al: Dysregulation of TGF-β activation contributes to pathogenesis in Marfan syndrome. *Nat Genet* 33:407, 2003.
5. Marsalese DL, Moodie DS, Vacante M, et al: Marfan's syndrome: Natural history and long-term follow-up of cardiovascular involvement. *J Am Coll Cardiol* 14:422, 1989.
6. Adams JN, Trent RJ: Aortic complications of Marfan's syndrome. *Lancet* 352:1722, 1998.
7. Loeys BL, Schwarze U, Holm T, et al: Aneurysm syndromes caused by mutations in the TGF-β receptor. *N Engl J Med* 355:788, 2006.
8. LeMaire SA, Pannu H, Tran-Fadulu V, et al: Severe aortic and arterial aneurysms associated with a TGFBR2 mutation. *Nat Clin Pract Cardiovasc Med* 4:167, 2007.
9. Pannu H, Avidan N, Tran-Fadulu V, et al: Genetic basis of thoracic aortic aneurysms and dissections: Potential relevance to abdominal aortic aneurysms. *Ann N Y Acad Sci* 1085:242, 2006.
10. Hoffman JI, Kaplan S: The incidence of congenital heart disease. *J Am Coll Cardiol* 39:1890, 2002.
11. Keane MG, Wiegers SE, Plappert T, et al: Bicuspid aortic valves are associated with aortic dilatation out of proportion to coexistent valvular lesions. *Circulation* 102(19 Suppl 3):III35, 2000.
12. Nistri S, Sorbo MD, Marin M, et al: Aortic root dilatation in young men with normally functioning bicuspid aortic valves. *Heart* 82:19, 1999.
13. Cecconi M, Manfrin M, Moraca A, et al: Aortic dimensions in patients with bicuspid aortic valve without significant valve dysfunction. *Am J Cardiol* 95:292, 2005.
14. Sabet HY, Edwards WD, Tazelaar HD, et al: Congenitally bicuspid aortic valves: A surgical pathology study of 542 cases (1991 through 1996) and a literature review of 2,715 additional cases. *Mayo Clin Proc* 74:14, 1999.
15. Larson EW, Edwards WD: Risk factors for aortic dissection: A necropsy study of 161 cases. *Am J Cardiol* 53:849, 1984.
16. LeMaire SA, Wang X, Wilks JA, et al: Matrix metalloproteinases in ascending aortic aneurysms: Bicuspid versus trileaflet aortic valves. *J Surg Res* 123:40, 2005.
17. Fedak PW, de Sa MP, Verma S, et al: Vascular matrix remodeling in patients with bicuspid aortic valve malformations: Implications for aortic dilatation. *J Thorac Cardiovasc Surg* 126:797, 2003.
18. Koullias GJ, Korkolis DP, Ravichandran P, et al: Tissue microarray detection of matrix metalloproteinases, in diseased tricuspid and bicuspid aortic valves with or without pathology of the ascending aorta. *Eur J Cardiothorac Surg* 26:1098, 2004.
19. Yasuda H, Nakatani S, Stugaard M, et al: Failure to prevent progressive dilation of ascending aorta by aortic valve replacement in patients with

bicuspid aortic valve: Comparison with tricuspid aortic valve. *Circulation* 108 Suppl 1:II291, 2003.

20. Martin LJ, Ramachandran V, Cripe LH, et al: Evidence in favor of linkage to human chromosomal regions 18q, 5q and 13q for bicuspid aortic valve and associated cardiovascular malformations. *Hum Genet* 121:275, 2007.

21. Wessels MW, Berger RM, Frohn-Mulder IM, et al: Autosomal dominant inheritance of left ventricular outflow tract obstruction. *Am J Med Genet* 134A:171, 2005.

22. McKellar SH, Tester DJ, Yagubyan M, et al: Novel NOTCH1 mutations in patients with bicuspid aortic valve disease and thoracic aortic aneurysms. *J Thorac Cardiovasc Surg* 134:290, 2007.

23. Johnson JR, Ledgerwood AM, Lucas CE: Mycotic aneurysm: New concepts in therapy. *Arch Surg* 118:577, 1983.

24. Brown SL, Busuttil RW, Baker JD, et al: Bacteriologic and surgical determinants of survival in patients with mycotic aneurysms. *J Vasc Surg* 1:541, 1984.

25. Elefteriades JA: Natural history of thoracic aortic aneurysms: Indications for surgery, and surgical versus nonsurgical risks. *Ann Thorac Surg* 74:S1877, 2002.

26. Davies RR, Goldstein LJ, Coady MA, et al: Yearly rupture or dissection rates for thoracic aortic aneurysms: Simple prediction based on size. *Ann Thorac Surg* 73:17, 2002.

27. Murdoch JL, Walker BA, Halpern BL, et al: Life expectancy and causes of death in the Marfan syndrome. *N Engl J Med* 286:804, 1972.

28. Michel PL, Acar J, Chomette G, et al: Degenerative aortic regurgitation. *Eur Heart J* 12:875, 1991.

29. Prenger K, Pieters F, Cheriex E: Aortic dissection after aortic valve replacement: Incidence and consequences for strategy. *J Card Surg* 9:495, 1994.

30. Isselbacher EM: Thoracic and abdominal aortic aneurysms. *Circulation* 111:816, 2005.

31. Wiet SP, Pearce WH, McCarthy WJ, et al: Utility of transesophageal echocardiography in the diagnosis of disease of the thoracic aorta. *J Vasc Surg* 20:613, 1994.

32. Fillinger MF: Imaging of the thoracic and thoracoabdominal aorta. *Semin Vasc Surg* 13:247, 2000.

33. Weisbord SD, Palevsky PM: Radiocontrast-induced acute renal failure. *J Intensive Care Med* 20:63, 2005.

34. Danias P, Eldeman R, Manning W: Magnetic resonance angiography of the great vessels and the coronary arteries, in Pohost GM (ed): *Imaging in Cardiovascular Disease*. Philadelphia: Lippincott Williams & Wilkins, 2000, p 449.

35. Ergun I, Keven K, Uruc I, et al: The safety of gadolinium in patients with stage 3 and 4 renal failure. *Nephrol Dial Transplant* 21:697, 2006.

36. Tepel M, van der Giet M, Schwarzfeld C, et al: Prevention of radiographic-contrast-agent-induced reductions in renal function by acetylcysteine. *N Engl J Med* 343:180, 2000.

37. Merten GJ, Burgess WP, Gray LV, et al: Prevention of contrast-induced nephropathy with sodium bicarbonate: A randomized controlled trial. *JAMA* 291:2328, 2004.

38. Coselli JS, LeMaire SA, Buket S: Marfan syndrome: The variability and outcome of operative management. *J Vasc Surg* 21:432, 1995.

39. Coady MA, Rizzo JA, Elefteriades JA: Developing surgical intervention criteria for thoracic aortic aneurysms. *Cardiol Clin* 17:827, 1999.

40. LeMaire SA, Rice DC, Schmittling ZC, et al: Emergency surgery for thoracoabdominal aortic aneurysms with acute presentation. *J Vasc Surg* 35:1171, 2002.

41. LeMaire SA, Miller CC III, Conklin LD, et al: A new predictive model for adverse outcomes after elective thoracoabdominal aortic aneurysm repair. *Ann Thorac Surg* 71:1233, 2001.

42. LeMaire SA, Miller CC III, Conklin LD, et al: Estimating group mortality and paraplegia rates after thoracoabdominal aortic aneurysm repair. *Ann Thorac Surg* 75:508, 2003.

43. Gott VL, Cameron DE, Alejo DE, et al: Aortic root replacement in 271 Marfan patients: A 24-year experience. *Ann Thorac Surg* 73:438, 2002.

44. Deleuze PH, Fromes Y, Khoury W, et al: Eight-year results of Freestyle stentless bioprosthesis in the aortic position: A single-center study of 500 patients. *J Heart Valve Dis* 15:247, 2006.

45. Carrel TP, Berdat P, Englberger L, et al: Aortic root replacement with a new stentless aortic valve xenograft conduit: Preliminary hemodynamic and clinical results. *J Heart Valve Dis* 12:752, 2003.

46. Oury JH: Clinical aspects of the Ross procedure: Indications and contraindications. *Semin Thorac Cardiovasc Surg* 8:328, 1996.

47. Fazel SS, David TE: Aortic valve-sparing operations for aortic root and ascending aortic aneurysms. *Curr Opin Cardiol* 22:497, 2007.

48. David TE, Ivanov J, Armstrong S, et al: Aortic valve-sparing operations in patients with aneurysms of the aortic root or ascending aorta. *Ann Thorac Surg* 74:S1758, 2002.

49. David TE, Feindel CM, Webb GD, et al: Aortic valve preservation in patients with aortic root aneurysm: Results of the reimplantation technique. *Ann Thorac Surg* 83:S732, 2007.

50. Kallenbach K, Baraki H, Khaladj N, et al: Aortic valve-sparing operation in Marfan syndrome: What do we know after a decade? *Ann Thorac Surg* 83:S764, 2007.

51. El Khoury G, Vanoverschelde JL, Glineur D, et al: Repair of bicuspid aortic valves in patients with aortic regurgitation. *Circulation* 114(1 Suppl):I610, 2006.

52. Bentall H, De Bono A: A technique for complete replacement of the ascending aorta. *Thorax* 23:338, 1968.

53. Cabrol C, Pavie A, Gandjbakhch I, et al: Complete replacement of the ascending aorta with reimplantation of the coronary arteries: New surgical approach. *J Thorac Cardiovasc Surg* 81:309, 1981.

54. Kouchoukos NT, Wareing TH, Murphy SF, et al: Sixteen-year experience with aortic root replacement: Results of 172 operations. *Ann Surg* 214:308, 1991.

55. Zubiate P, Kay JH: Surgical treatment of aneurysm of the ascending aorta with aortic insufficiency and marked displacement of the coronary ostia. *J Thorac Cardiovasc Surg* 71:415, 1976.

56. LeMaire SA, Carter SA, Coselli JS: The elephant trunk technique for staged repair of complex aneurysms of the entire thoracic aorta. *Ann Thorac Surg* 81:1561, 2006.

57. Borst HG, Frank G, Schaps D: Treatment of extensive aortic aneurysms by a new multiple-stage approach. *J Thorac Cardiovasc Surg* 95:11, 1988.

58. Nelson DP, Andropoulos DB, Fraser CD Jr.: Perioperative neuroprotective strategies. *Semin Thorac Cardiovasc Surg Pediatr Card Surg Annu*, p 49, 2008.

59. Wong CH, Bonser RS: Retrograde cerebral perfusion: Clinical and experimental aspects. *Perfusion* 14:247, 1999.

60. Coselli JS, LeMaire SA: Experience with retrograde cerebral perfusion during proximal aortic surgery in 290 patients. *J Card Surg* 12(2 Suppl):322, 1997.

61. Matalanis G, Hata M, Buxton BF: A retrospective comparative study of deep hypothermic circulatory arrest, retrograde, and antegrade cerebral perfusion in aortic arch surgery. *Ann Thorac Cardiovasc Surg* 9:174, 2003.

62. Okita Y, Minatoya K, Tagusari O, et al: Prospective comparative study of brain protection in total aortic arch replacement: Deep hypothermic circulatory arrest with retrograde cerebral perfusion or selective antegrade cerebral perfusion. *Ann Thorac Surg* 72:72, 2001.

63. Kazui T, Inoue N, Yamada O, et al: Selective cerebral perfusion during operation for aneurysms of the aortic arch: A reassessment. *Ann Thorac Surg* 53:109, 1992.

64. Sinclair MC, Singer RL, Manley NJ, et al: Cannulation of the axillary artery for cardiopulmonary bypass: Safeguards and pitfalls. *Ann Thorac Surg* 75:931, 2003.

65. Pacini D, Leone A, Di Marco L, et al: Antegrade selective cerebral perfusion in thoracic aorta surgery: Safety of moderate hypothermia. *Eur J Cardiothorac Surg* 31:618, 2007.

66. Zierer A, Aybek T, Risteski P, et al: Moderate hypothermia (30 °C) for surgery of acute type A aortic dissection. *Thorac Cardiovasc Surg* 53:74, 2005.

67. Svensson LG: Antegrade perfusion during suspended animation? *J Thorac Cardiovasc Surg* 124:1068, 2002.

68. Panos A, Myers PO, Kalangos A: Novel technique for aortic arch surgery under mild hypothermia. *Ann Thorac Surg* 85:347, 2008.

69. Della Corte A, Scardone M, Romano G, et al: Aortic arch surgery: Thoracoabdominal perfusion during antegrade cerebral perfusion may reduce postoperative morbidity. *Ann Thorac Surg* 81:1358, 2006.

70. Inoue K, Hosokawa H, Iwase T, et al: Aortic arch reconstruction by transluminally placed endovascular branched stent graft. *Circulation* 100(19 Suppl):II316, 1999.

71. Svensson LG, Kim KH, Blackstone EH, et al: Elephant trunk procedure: Newer indications and uses. *Ann Thorac Surg* 78:109, 2004.

72. Svensson LG, Kouchoukos NT, Miller DC, et al: Expert consensus document on the treatment of descending thoracic aortic disease using endovascular stent-grafts. *Ann Thorac Surg* 85(1 Suppl):S1, 2008.

73. Coselli JS, LeMaire SA, Köksoy C, et al: Cerebrospinal fluid drainage reduces paraplegia after thoracoabdominal aortic aneurysm repair: Results of a randomized clinical trial. *J Vasc Surg* 35:631, 2002.

74. Jacobs MJ, Mess W, Mochtar B, et al: The value of motor evoked potentials in reducing paraplegia during thoracoabdominal aneurysm repair. *J Vasc Surg* 43:239, 2006.

75. van Dongen EP, Schepens MA, Morshuis WJ, et al: Thoracic and thoracoabdominal aortic aneurysm repair: Use of evoked potential monitoring in 118 patients. *J Vasc Surg* 34:1035, 2001.

76. Coselli JS: The use of left heart bypass in the repair of thoracoabdominal aortic aneurysms: Current techniques and results. *Semin Thorac Cardiovasc Surg* 15:326, 2003.

77. Coselli JS, LeMaire SA: Left heart bypass reduces paraplegia rates after thoracoabdominal aortic aneurysm repair. *Ann Thorac Surg* 67:1931, 1999.

78. Safi HJ, Miller CC III, Huynh TT, et al: Distal aortic perfusion and cerebrospinal fluid drainage for thoracoabdominal and descending thoracic aortic repair: Ten years of organ protection. *Ann Surg* 238:372, 2003.

79. Köksoy C, LeMaire SA, Curling PE, et al: Renal perfusion during thoracoabdominal aortic operations: Cold crystalloid is superior to normothermic blood. *Ann Thorac Surg* 73:730, 2002.

80. Kouchoukos NT, Masetti P, Rokkas CK, et al: Hypothermic cardiopulmonary bypass and circulatory arrest for operations on the descending thoracic and thoracoabdominal aorta. *Ann Thorac Surg* 74:S1885, 2002.

81. Coselli JS, Oberwalder P: Successful repair of mega aorta using reversed elephant trunk procedure. *J Vasc Surg* 27:183, 1998.

82. Parodi JC, Palmaz JC, Barone HD: Transfemoral intraluminal graft implantation for abdominal aortic aneurysms. *Ann Vasc Surg* 5:491, 1991.

83. Dake MD, Miller DC, Semba CP, et al: Transluminal placement of endovascular stent-grafts for the treatment of descending thoracic aortic aneurysms. *N Engl J Med* 331:1729, 1994.

84. Riesenman PJ, Farber MA, Mendes RR, et al: Coverage of the left subclavian artery during thoracic endovascular aortic repair. *J Vasc Surg* 45:90, 2007.

85. Buth J, Harris PL, Hobo R, et al: Neurologic complications associated with endovascular repair of thoracic aortic pathology: Incidence and risk factors. A study from the European Collaborators on Stent/Graft Techniques for Aortic Aneurysm Repair (EUROSTAR) registry. *J Vasc Surg* 46:1103, 2007.

86. Bozinovski J, LeMaire SA, Weldon SA, et al: Hybrid repairs of the distal aortic arch and proximal descending thoracic aorta. *Op Tech Thorac Cardiovasc Surg* 12:167, 2007.

87. Woo EY, Bavaria JE, Pochettino A, et al: Techniques for preserving vertebral artery perfusion during thoracic aortic stent grafting requiring aortic arch landing. *Vasc Endovascular Surg* 40:367, 2006.

88. Fann JI, Dake MD, Semba CP, et al: Endovascular stent-grafting after arch aneurysm repair using the "elephant trunk." *Ann Thorac Surg* 60:1102, 1995.

89. Lin PH, Dardik A, Coselli JS: A simple technique to facilitate antegrade thoracic endograft deployment using a hybrid elephant trunk procedure under hypothermic circulatory arrest. *J Endovasc Ther* 14:669, 2007.

90. Greenberg RK, West K, Pfaff K, et al: Beyond the aortic bifurcation: Branched endovascular grafts for thoracoabdominal and aortoiliac aneurysms. *J Vasc Surg* 43:879, 2006.

91. Anderson JL, Adam DJ, Berce M, et al: Repair of thoracoabdominal aortic aneurysms with fenestrated and branched endovascular stent grafts. *J Vasc Surg* 42:600, 2005.

92. Black SA, Wolfe JH, Clark M, et al: Complex thoracoabdominal aortic aneurysms: Endovascular exclusion with visceral revascularization. *J Vasc Surg* 43:1081, 2006.

93. Zhou W, Reardon M, Peden EK, et al: Hybrid approach to complex thoracic aortic aneurysms in high-risk patients: Surgical challenges and clinical outcomes. *J Vasc Surg* 44:688, 2006.

94. Modine T, Lions C, Destrieux-Garnier L, et al: Iatrogenic iliac artery rupture and type A dissection after endovascular repair of type B aortic dissection. *Ann Thorac Surg* 77:317, 2004.

95. Bethuyne N, Bove T, Van den Brande P, et al: Acute retrograde aortic dissection during endovascular repair of a thoracic aortic aneurysm. *Ann Thorac Surg* 75:1967, 2003.

96. Pasic M, Schubel J, Bauer M, et al: Cannulation of the right axillary artery for surgery of acute type A aortic dissection. *Eur J Cardiothorac Surg* 24:231, 2003.

97. Dake MD, Miller DC, Mitchell RS, et al: The "first generation" of endovascular stent-grafts for patients with aneurysms of the descending thoracic aorta. *J Thorac Cardiovasc Surg* 116:689, 1998.

98. Appoo JJ, Moser WG, Fairman RM, et al: Thoracic aortic stent grafting: Improving results with newer generation investigational devices. *J Thorac Cardiovasc Surg* 131:1087, 2006.

99. DeBakey ME, Henly WS, Cooley DA, et al: Surgical management of dissecting aneurysms of the aorta. *J Thorac Cardiovasc Surg* 49:130, 1965.

100. Daily PO, Trueblood HW, Stinson EB, et al: Management of acute aortic dissections. *Ann Thorac Surg* 10:237, 1970.

101. Borst HG, Heinemann MK, Stone CD: *Surgical Treatment of Aortic Dissection.* New York: Churchill Livingstone, 1996.

102. Nienaber CA, Sievers HH: Intramural hematoma in acute aortic syndrome: More than one variant of dissection? *Circulation* 106:284, 2002.

103. Evangelista A, Mukherjee D, Mehta RH, et al: Acute intramural hematoma of the aorta: A mystery in evolution. *Circulation* 111:1063, 2005.

104. Maraj R, Rerkpattanapipat P, Jacobs LE, et al: Meta-analysis of 143 reported cases of aortic intramural hematoma. *Am J Cardiol* 86:664, 2000.

105. Ganaha F, Miller DC, Sugimoto K, et al: Prognosis of aortic intramural hematoma with and without penetrating atherosclerotic ulcer: A clinical and radiological analysis. *Circulation* 106:342, 2002.

106. Clouse WD, Hallett JW Jr., Schaff HV, et al: Acute aortic dissection: Population-based incidence compared with degenerative aortic aneurysm rupture. *Mayo Clin Proc* 79:176, 2004.

107. Hirst AE Jr., Johns VJ Jr., Kime SW Jr.: Dissecting aneurysm of the aorta: A review of 505 cases. *Medicine (Baltimore)* 37:217, 1958.

108. Anagnostopoulos CE, Prabhakar MJ, Kittle CF: Aortic dissections and dissecting aneurysms. *Am J Cardiol* 30:263, 1972.

109. Daniel JC, Huynh TT, Zhou W, et al: Acute aortic dissection associated with use of cocaine. *J Vasc Surg* 46:427, 2007.

110. Wang X, LeMaire SA, Chen L, et al: Increased collagen deposition and elevated expression of connective tissue growth factor in human thoracic aortic dissection. *Circulation* 114(1 Suppl):I200, 2006.

111. Wang X, LeMaire SA, Chen L, et al: Decreased expression of fibulin-5 correlates with reduced elastin in thoracic aortic dissection. *Surgery* 138:352, 2005.

112. Erbel R, Alfonso F, Boileau C, et al: Diagnosis and management of aortic dissection. *Eur Heart J* 22:1642, 2001.

113. Klompas M: Does this patient have an acute thoracic aortic dissection? *JAMA* 287:2262, 2002.

114. Hagan PG, Nienaber CA, Isselbacher EM, et al: The International Registry of Acute Aortic Dissection (IRAD): New insights into an old disease. *JAMA* 283:897, 2000.

115. Sodeck G, Domanovits H, Schillinger M, et al: D-dimer in ruling out acute aortic dissection: A systematic review and prospective cohort study. *Eur Heart J* 28:3067, 2007.

116. von Kodolitsch Y, Nienaber CA, Dieckmann C, et al: Chest radiography for the diagnosis of acute aortic syndrome. *Am J Med* 116:73, 2004.

117. Nienaber CA, von Kodolitsch Y, Nicolas V, et al: The diagnosis of thoracic aortic dissection by noninvasive imaging procedures. *N Engl J Med* 328:1, 1993.

118. Keren A, Kim CB, Hu BS, et al: Accuracy of biplane and multiplane transesophageal echocardiography in diagnosis of typical acute aortic dissection and intramural hematoma. *J Am Coll Cardiol* 28:627, 1996.

119. Miller JS, LeMaire SA, Coselli JS: Evaluating aortic dissection: When is coronary angiography indicated? *Heart* 83:615, 2000.

120. Scholl FG, Coady MA, Davies R, et al: Interval or permanent nonoperative management of acute type A aortic dissection. *Arch Surg* 134:402, 1999.

121. Gillinov AM, Lytle BW, Kaplon RJ, et al: Dissection of the ascending aorta after previous cardiac surgery: Differences in presentation and management. *J Thorac Cardiovasc Surg* 117:252, 1999.

122. Yavuz S, Goncu MT, Turk T: Axillary artery cannulation for arterial inflow in patients with acute dissection of the ascending aorta. *Eur J Cardiothorac Surg* 22:313, 2002.

123. Coselli JS, Crawford ES, Beall AC Jr., et al: Determination of brain temperatures for safe circulatory arrest during cardiovascular operation. *Ann Thorac Surg* 45:638, 1988.

124. Kirsch M, Soustelle C, Houel R, et al: Risk factor analysis for proximal and distal reoperations after surgery for acute type A aortic dissection. *J Thorac Cardiovasc Surg* 123:318, 2002.

125. Westaby S, Saito S, Katsumata T: Acute type A dissection: Conservative methods provide consistently low mortality. *Ann Thorac Surg* 73:707, 2002.

126. Geirsson A, Bavaria JE, Swarr D, et al: Fate of the residual distal and proximal aorta after acute type A dissection repair using a contemporary surgical reconstruction algorithm. *Ann Thorac Surg* 84:1955, 2007.

127. Genoni M, Paul M, Jenni R, et al: Chronic beta-blocker therapy improves outcome and reduces treatment costs in chronic type B aortic dissection. *Eur J Cardiothorac Surg* 19:606, 2001.

128. DeBakey ME, McCollum CH, Crawford ES, et al: Dissection and dissecting aneurysms of the aorta: Twenty-year follow-up of five hundred twenty-seven patients treated surgically. *Surgery* 92:1118, 1982.

129. Fann JI, Smith JA, Miller DC, et al: Surgical management of aortic dissection during a 30-year period. *Circulation* 92(9 Suppl):II113, 1995.

130. Glower DD, Speier RH, White WD, et al: Management and long-term outcome of aortic dissection. *Ann Surg* 214:31, 1991.

131. Elefteriades JA, Hartleroad J, Gusberg RJ, et al: Long-term experience with descending aortic dissection: The complication-specific approach. *Ann Thorac Surg* 53:11, 1992.

132. Barnes DM, Williams DM, Dasika NL, et al: A single-center experience treating renal malperfusion after aortic dissection with central aortic fenestration and renal artery stenting. *J Vasc Surg* 47:903, 2008.

133. Kusagawa H, Shimono T, Ishida M, et al: Changes in false lumen after transluminal stent-graft placement in aortic dissections: Six years' experience. *Circulation* 111:2951, 2005.

134. Nienaber CA, Zannetti S, Barbieri B, et al: INvestigation of STEnt grafts in patients with type B Aortic Dissection: Design of the INSTEAD trial—a prospective, multicenter, European randomized trial. *Am Heart J* 149:592, 2005.

135. Demers P, Miller DC, Mitchell RS, et al: Stent-graft repair of penetrating atherosclerotic ulcers in the descending thoracic aorta: Mid-term results. *Ann Thorac Surg* 77:81, 2004.

136. Coselli JS, LeMaire SA, de Figueiredo LP, et al: Paraplegia after thoracoabdominal aortic aneurysm repair: Is dissection a risk factor? *Ann Thorac Surg* 63:28, 1997.

137. Aomi S, Nakajima M, Nonoyama M, et al: Aortic root replacement using composite valve graft in patients with aortic valve disease and aneurysm of the ascending aorta: Twenty years' experience of late results. *Artif Organs* 26:467, 2002.

138. Kindo M, Billaud P, Gerelli S, et al: Twenty-seven-year experience with composite valve graft replacement of the aortic root. *J Heart Valve Dis* 16:370, 2007.

139. Kon ND, Cordell AR, Adair SM, et al: Aortic root replacement with the freestyle stentless porcine aortic root bioprosthesis. *Ann Thorac Surg* 67:1609, 1999.

140. David TE, Mohr FW, Bavaria JE, et al: Initial experience with the Toronto Root bioprosthesis. *J Heart Valve Dis* 13:248, 2004.

141. Melina G, De Robertis F, Gaer JA, et al: Mid-term pattern of survival, hemodynamic performance and rate of complications after Medtronic Freestyle versus homograft full aortic root replacement: Results from a prospective randomized trial. *J Heart Valve Dis* 13:972, 2004.

142. Gleason TG, David TE, Coselli JS, et al: St. Jude Medical Toronto biologic aortic root prosthesis: Early FDA phase II IDE study results. *Ann Thorac Surg* 78:786, 2004.

143. Kincaid EH, Cordell AR, Hammon JW, et al: Coronary insufficiency after stentless aortic root replacement: Risk factors and solutions. *Ann Thorac Surg* 83:964, 2007.

144. Achneck HE, Rizzo JA, Tranquilli M, et al: Safety of thoracic aortic surgery in the present era. *Ann Thorac Surg* 84:1180, 2007.

145. Estrera AL, Miller CC III, Madisetty J, et al: Ascending and transverse aortic arch repair: The impact of glomerular filtration rate on mortality. *Ann Surg* 247:524, 2008.

146. Heinemann MK, Buehner B, Jurmann MJ, et al: Use of the "elephant trunk technique" in aortic surgery. *Ann Thorac Surg* 60:2, 1995.

147. Safi HJ, Miller CC III, Estrera AL, et al: Staged repair of extensive aortic aneurysms: Long-term experience with the elephant trunk technique. *Ann Surg* 240:677, 2004.

148. Sundt TM, Moon MR, DeOliviera N, et al: Contemporary results of total aortic arch replacement. *J Card Surg* 19:235, 2004.

149. Zingone B, Rauber E, Gatti G, et al: Diagnosis and management of severe atherosclerosis of the ascending aorta and aortic arch during cardiac surgery: Focus on aortic replacement. *Eur J Cardiothorac Surg* 31:990, 2007.

150. Immer FF, Barmettler H, Berdat PA, et al: Effects of deep hypothermic circulatory arrest on outcome after resection of ascending aortic aneurysm. *Ann Thorac Surg* 74:422, 2002.

151. Fleck TM, Czerny M, Hutschala D, et al: The incidence of transient neurologic dysfunction after ascending aortic replacement with circulatory arrest. *Ann Thorac Surg* 76:1198, 2003.

152. Kazui T, Bashar AH: Aortic arch replacement using a trifurcated graft. *Ann Thorac Surg* 81:1552, 2006.

153. Suzuki K, Kazui T, Bashar AH, et al: Total aortic arch replacement in patients with arch vessel anomalies. *Ann Thorac Surg* 81:2079, 2006.

154. Spielvogel D, Etz CD, Silovitz D, et al: Aortic arch replacement with a trifurcated graft. *Ann Thorac Surg* 83:S791, 2007.

155. Kamiya H, Hagl C, Kropivnitskaya I, et al: Quick proximal arch replacement with moderate hypothermic circulatory arrest. *Ann Thorac Surg* 83:1055, 2007.

156. Rampoldi V, Trimarchi S, Eagle KA, et al: Simple risk models to predict surgical mortality in acute type A aortic dissection: The International Registry of Acute Aortic Dissection score. *Ann Thorac Surg* 83:55, 2007.

157. Demers P, Miller DC, Mitchell RS, et al: Midterm results of endovascular repair of descending thoracic aortic aneurysms with first-generation stent grafts. *J Thorac Cardiovasc Surg* 127:664, 2004.

158. Bavaria JE, Appoo JJ, Makaroun MS, et al: Endovascular stent grafting versus open surgical repair of descending thoracic aortic aneurysms in low-risk patients: A multicenter comparative trial. *J Thorac Cardiovasc Surg* 133:369, 2007.

159. Makaroun MS, Dillavou ED, Wheatley GH, et al: Five-year results of endovascular treatment with the Gore TAG device compared with open repair of thoracic aortic aneurysms. *J Vasc Surg* 47:912, 2008.

160. Czerny M, Zimpfer D, Rodler S, et al: Endovascular stent-graft placement of aneurysms involving the descending aorta originating from chronic type B dissections. *Ann Thorac Surg* 83:1635, 2007.

161. Nienaber CA: Results from the INSTEAD trial. Paper presented at: Sixth Annual International Symposium on Advances in Understanding Aortic Diseases; September 30–October 1, 2005; Berlin, Germany.

162. Coselli JS, LeMaire SA, Conklin LD, et al: Left heart bypass during descending thoracic aortic aneurysm repair does not reduce the incidence of paraplegia. *Ann Thorac Surg* 77:1298, 2004.

163. Chiesa R, Melissano G, Civilini E, et al: Ten years' experience of thoracic and thoracoabdominal aortic aneurysm surgical repair: Lessons learned. *Ann Vasc Surg* 18:514, 2004.

164. Estrera AL, Miller CC III, Chen EP, et al: Descending thoracic aortic aneurysm repair: 12-year experience using distal aortic perfusion and cerebrospinal fluid drainage. *Ann Thorac Surg* 80:1290, 2005.

165. Stone DH, Brewster DC, Kwolek CJ, et al: Stent-graft versus open-surgical repair of the thoracic aorta: Mid-term results. *J Vasc Surg* 44:1188, 2006.

166. Matsumura JS, Cambria RP, Dake MD, et al: International controlled clinical trial of thoracic endovascular aneurysm repair with the Zenith TX2 endovascular graft: 1-year results. *J Vasc Surg* 47:247, 2008.

167. Dick F, Hinder D, Immer FF, et al: Outcome and quality of life after surgical and endovascular treatment of descending aortic lesions. *Ann Thorac Surg* 85:1605, 2008.

168. Brandt M, Hussel K, Walluscheck KP, et al: Stent-graft repair versus open surgery for the descending aorta: A case-control study. *J Endovasc Ther* 11:535, 2004.

169. Coselli JS, Bozinovski J, LeMaire SA: Open surgical repair of 2286 thoracoabdominal aortic aneurysms. *Ann Thorac Surg* 83:S862, 2007.

170. Schepens MA, Kelder JC, Morshuis WJ, et al: Long-term follow-up after thoracoabdominal aortic aneurysm repair. *Ann Thorac Surg* 83:S851, 2007.

171. Conrad MF, Crawford RS, Davison JK, et al: Thoracoabdominal aneurysm repair: A 20-year perspective. *Ann Thorac Surg* 83:S856, 2007.

172. Rigberg DA, McGory ML, Zingmond DS, et al: Thirty-day mortality statistics underestimate the risk of repair of thoracoabdominal aortic aneurysms: A statewide experience. *J Vasc Surg* 43:217, 2006.

173. Cowan JA Jr., Dimick JB, Henke PK, et al: Surgical treatment of intact thoracoabdominal aortic aneurysms in the United States: Hospital and surgeon volume-related outcomes. *J Vasc Surg* 37:1169, 2003.

174. Suzuki T, Mehta RH, Ince H, et al: Clinical profiles and outcomes of acute type B aortic dissection in the current era: Lessons from the International Registry of Acute Aortic Dissection (IRAD). *Circulation* 108 Suppl 1:II312, 2003.

175. Tsai TT, Fattori R, Trimarchi S, et al: Long-term survival in patients presenting with type B acute aortic dissection: Insights from the International Registry of Acute Aortic Dissection. *Circulation* 114:2226, 2006.

176. Slonim SM, Miller DC, Mitchell RS, et al: Percutaneous balloon fenestration and stenting for life-threatening ischemic complications in patients with acute aortic dissection. *J Thorac Cardiovasc Surg* 117:1118, 1999.

177. Dake MD, Kato N, Mitchell RS, et al: Endovascular stent-graft placement for the treatment of acute aortic dissection. *N Engl J Med* 340:1546, 1999.

178. Eggebrecht H, Nienaber CA, Neuhauser M, et al: Endovascular stent-graft placement in aortic dissection: A meta-analysis. *Eur Heart J* 27:489, 2006.

179. Bozinovski J, Coselli JS: Outcomes and survival in surgical treatment of descending thoracic aorta with acute dissection. *Ann Thorac Surg* 85:965, 2008.

180. Trimarchi S, Nienaber CA, Rampoldi V, et al: Role and results of surgery in acute type B aortic dissection: Insights from the International Registry of Acute Aortic Dissection (IRAD). *Circulation* 114(1 Suppl):I357, 2006.

Arterial Disease

Peter H. Lin, Panagiotis Kougias,
Carlos Bechara, Catherine Cagiannos,
Tam T. Huynh, and Changyi J. Chen

GENERAL APPROACH TO THE VASCULAR PATIENT

Because the vascular system involves every organ system in our body, the symptoms of vascular disease are as varied as those encountered in any medical specialty. Lack of adequate blood supply to target organs typically presents with pain; for example, calf pain with lower extremity (LE) claudication, postprandial abdominal pain from mesenteric ischemia, and arm pain with axillosubclavian arterial occlusion. In contrast, stroke and transient ischemic attack (TIA) are the presenting symptoms from middle cerebral embolization as a consequence of a stenosed internal carotid artery (ICA). The pain syndrome of arterial disease usually is divided clinically into acute and chronic types, with all shades of severity between the two extremes. Sudden onset of pain can indicate complete occlusion of a critical vessel, leading to more severe pain and critical ischemia in the target organ, resulting in lower limb gangrene or intestinal infarction. Chronic pain results from a slower, more progressive atherosclerotic occlusion, which can be totally or partially compensated by developing collateral vessels. Acute on chronic is another pain pattern in which a patient most likely has an underlying arterial stenosis that suddenly occludes; for example, the patient with a history of calf claudication who now presents with sudden, severe acute limb-threatening ischemia. The clinician should always try to understand and relate the clinical manifestations to the underlying pathologic process.

Vascular History

Appropriate history should be focused on the presenting symptoms related to the vascular system (Table 23-1). Of particular importance in the previous medical history is noting prior vascular interventions (endovascular or open surgical), and all vascular patients should have inquiry made about their prior cardiac history and current cardiac symptoms. Approximately 30% of vascular patients will be diabetic. A history of prior and current smoking status should be noted.

TABLE 23-1 Pertinent elements in vascular history
• History of stroke or transient ischemic attack
• History of coronary artery disease, including previous myocardial infarction and angina
• History of peripheral arterial disease
• History of diabetes
• History of hypertension
• History of tobacco use
• History of hyperlipidemia

The patient with carotid disease in most cases is completely asymptomatic, having been referred based on the finding of a cervical bruit or duplex finding of stenosis. Symptoms of carotid territory TIAs include transient monocular blindness (amaurosis), contralateral weakness or numbness, and dysphasia. Symptoms persisting longer than 24 hours constitute a stroke. In contrast, the patient with chronic mesenteric ischemia is likely to present with postprandial abdominal pain and weight loss. The patient fears eating because of the pain, avoids food, and loses weight. It is very unlikely that a patient with abdominal pain who has not lost weight has chronic mesenteric ischemia.

The patient with LE pain on ambulation has intermittent claudication that occurs in certain muscle groups; for example, calf pain upon exercise usually reflects superficial femoral artery (SFA) disease, while pain in the buttocks reflects iliac disease. In most cases, the pain manifests in one muscle group below the level of the affected artery, occurs only with exercise, and is relieved with rest only to recur at the same location, hence the term *window gazers disease*. Rest pain (a manifestation of severe underlying occlusive disease) is constant and occurs in the foot (not the muscle groups), typically at the metatarsophalangeal junction, and is relieved by dependency. Often, the patient is prompted to sleep with their foot hanging off one side of the bed to increase the hydrostatic pressure.

KEY POINTS

1. Carotid intervention as a preventive strategy should be performed in patients with 50% or greater symptomatic internal carotid artery stenosis, and those with 80% or greater asymptomatic internal carotid artery stenosis. Carotid intervention for asymptomatic stenosis between 60% and 79% remains controversial, and is a function of an operator's stroke rate. The choice of intervention—carotid endarterectomy vs. carotid stenting—remains controversial; currently, carotid endarterectomy appears to be associated with lower stroke rate, whereas carotid stenting is more suitable under certain anatomic or physiologic conditions.

2. Abdominal aortic aneurysms should be repaired when the risk of rupture, determined mainly by aneurysm size, exceeds the risk of death due to perioperative complications or concurrent illness. Endovascular repair is associated with less perioperative morbidity and mortality compared to open reconstruction, and is preferred for high-risk patients who meet specific anatomic criteria.

3. Symptomatic mesenteric ischemia should be treated to improve quality of life and prevent bowel infarction. Operative treatment—bypass—is superior to endovascular intervention, although changes in wire and stent technology have improved the results of mesenteric stenting in recent series.

4. Aortoiliac occlusive disease can be treated with either endovascular means or open reconstruction, depending on patient risk stratification, occlusion characteristics, and symptomatology.

5. Claudication is a marker of extensive atherosclerosis, and is mainly managed with risk factor modification and pharmacotherapy. Only 5% of claudicants will need intervention because of disabling extremity pain. The five-year mortality of a patient with claudication approaches 30%. Patients with rest pain or tissue loss need expeditious evaluation and vascular reconstruction to ameliorate the severe extremity pain and prevent limb loss.

6. For infrainguinal occlusive disease, open revascularization is more durable than endovascular treatment. The latter, however, is associated with significantly less morbidity, may represent the procedure of choice in high-risk patients, and can provide adequate inflow to treat limited areas of tissue loss.

Vascular Physical Examination

Specific vascular examination should include abdominal aortic palpation, carotid artery examination, and pulse examination of the LE (femoral, popliteal, posterior tibial, and dorsalis pedis arteries). The abdomen should be palpated for an abdominal aortic aneurysm (AAA), detected as an expansile pulse above the level of the umbilicus. It also should be examined for the presence of bruits. Because the aorta typically divides at the level of the umbilicus, an aortic aneurysm is most frequently palpable in the epigastrium. In thin individuals, a normal aortic pulsation is palpable, while in obese patients even large aortic aneurysms may not be detectable. Suspicion of a clinically enlarged aorta should lead to the performance of an ultrasound scan for a more accurate definition of aortic diameter.

The carotids should be auscultated for the presence of bruits, although there is a higher correlation with coronary artery disease (CAD) than underlying carotid stenosis. A bruit at the angle of the mandible is a significant finding, leading to follow-up duplex scanning. The differential diagnosis is a transmitted murmur from a sclerotic or stenotic aortic valve. The carotid is palpable deep to the sternocleidomastoid muscle in the neck. Palpation, however, should be gentle and rarely yields clinically useful information.

Upper extremity examination is necessary when an arteriovenous graft is to be inserted in patients who have symptoms of arm pain with exercise. Thoracic outlet syndrome can result in occlusion or aneurysm formation of the subclavian artery. Distal embolization is a manifestation of thoracic outlet syndrome; consequently, the fingers should be examined for signs of ischemia and ulceration. The axillary artery enters the limb below the middle of the clavicle, where it can be palpated in thin patients. It usually is easily palpable in the axilla and medial upper arm. The brachial artery is most easily located at the antecubital fossa immediately medial to the biceps tendon. The radial artery is palpable at the wrist anterior to the radius.

For LE vascular examination, the femoral pulse usually is palpable midway between the anterior superior iliac spine and the pubic tubercle. The popliteal artery is palpated in the popliteal fossa with the knee flexed to 45° and the foot supported on the examination table to relax the calf muscles. Palpation of the popliteal artery is a bimanual technique. Both thumbs are placed on the tibial tuberosity anteriorly and the fingers are placed into the popliteal fossa between the two heads of the gastrocnemius muscle. The popliteal artery is palpated by compressing it against the posterior aspect of the tibia just below the knee. The posterior tibial pulse is detected by palpation 2 cm posterior to the medial malleolus. The dorsalis pedis is detected 1 cm lateral to the hallucis longus extensor tendon, which dorsiflexes the great toe and is clearly visible on the dorsum of the foot. Pulses can be graded using either the traditional four-point scale or the basic two-point scale system (Table 23-2). The foot also should be carefully examined for pallor on elevation and rubor on dependency, as these findings are indicative of chronic ischemia. Note should also be made of nail changes and loss of hair. Ulceration and other findings specific to disease states are described in relevant sections below.

After reconstructive vascular surgery, the graft may be available for examination, depending on its type and course. The in situ LE graft runs in the subcutaneous fat and can be palpated along most of its length. A change in pulse quality, aneurysmal enlargement, or a new bruit should be carefully noted. Axillofemoral grafts, femoral-to-femoral grafts, and arteriovenous access grafts usually can be easily palpated as well.

Noninvasive Diagnostic Evaluation of the Vascular Patient

Ankle-Brachial Index

There is increasing interest in the use of the ankle-brachial index (ABI) to evaluate patients at risk for cardiovascular events. An ABI <0.9 correlates with increased risk of myocardial infarction and

TABLE 23-2 Grading scales for peripheral pulses

Traditional Scale		Basic Scale	
4+	Normal	2+	Normal
3+	Slightly reduced	1+	Diminished
2+	Markedly reduced	0	Absent
1+	Barely palpable	—	—
0	Absent	—	—

indicates significant, although perhaps asymptomatic, underlying peripheral vascular disease. The ABI is determined in the following ways. Blood pressure (BP) is measured in both upper extremities using the highest systolic BP as the denominator for the ABI. The ankle pressure is determined by placing a BP cuff above the ankle and measuring the return to flow of the posterior tibial and dorsalis pedis arteries using a pencil Doppler probe over each artery. The ratio of the systolic pressure in each vessel divided by the highest arm systolic pressure can be used to express the ABI in both the posterior tibial and dorsalis pedis arteries (Fig. 23-1). Normal is more than 1. Patients with claudication typically have an ABI in the 0.5 to 0.7 range, and those with rest pain are in the 0.3 to 0.5 range. Those with gangrene have an ABI of <0.3. These ranges can vary depending on the degree of compressibility of the vessel. The test is less reliable in patients with heavily calcified vessels. Due to noncompressibility, some patients such as diabetics and those with end-stage renal disease may have an ABI of 1.40 or greater and require additional noninvasive diagnostic testing to evaluate for peripheral arterial disease (PAD). Alternative tests include toe-brachial pressures, pulse volume recordings, transcutaneous oxygen measurements, or vascular imaging (duplex ultrasound).

Segmental Limb Pressures

By placing serial BP cuffs down the LE and then measuring the pressure with a Doppler probe as flow returns to the artery below the cuff, it is possible to determine segmental pressures down the leg. These data can then be used to infer the level of the occlusion. The systolic pressure at each level is expressed as a ratio, with the highest systolic pressure in the upper extremities as the denominator. Normal segmental pressures commonly show high thigh pressures 20 mmHg or greater in comparison to the brachial artery pressures. The low thigh pressure should be equivalent to brachial pressures. Subsequent pressures should fall by no more than 10 mmHg at each level. A pressure gradient of 20 mmHg between two subsequent levels is usually indicative of occlusive disease at that level. The most frequently used index is the ratio of the ankle pressure to the brachial pressure, the ABI. Normally the ABI is >1.0, and a value <0.9 indicates some degree of arterial obstruction and has been shown to be correlated with an increased risk of coronary heart disease.[1] Limitations of relying on segmental limb pressures include: (a) missing isolated moderate stenoses (usually iliac) that produce little or no pressure gradient at rest; (b) falsely elevated pressures in patients with diabetes and end-stage renal disease; and (c) the inability to differentiate between stenosis and occlusion.[2] Patients with diabetes and end-stage renal disease have calcified vessels that are difficult to compress, thus rendering this method inaccurate, due to recording of falsely elevated pressure readings. Noncompressible arteries yield ankle systolic pressures of 250 mmHg or greater and an ABI of >1.40. In this situation, absolute toe and ankle pressures can be measured to gauge critical limb ischemia. Ankle pressures <50 mmHg or toe pressures <30 mmHg are indicative of critical limb ischemia. The toe pressure is normally 30 mmHg less than the ankle pressure, and a toe-brachial index of <0.70 is abnormal. False-positive results with the toe-brachial index are unusual. The main limitation of this technique is that it may be impossible to measure pressures in the first and second toes due to pre-existing ulceration.

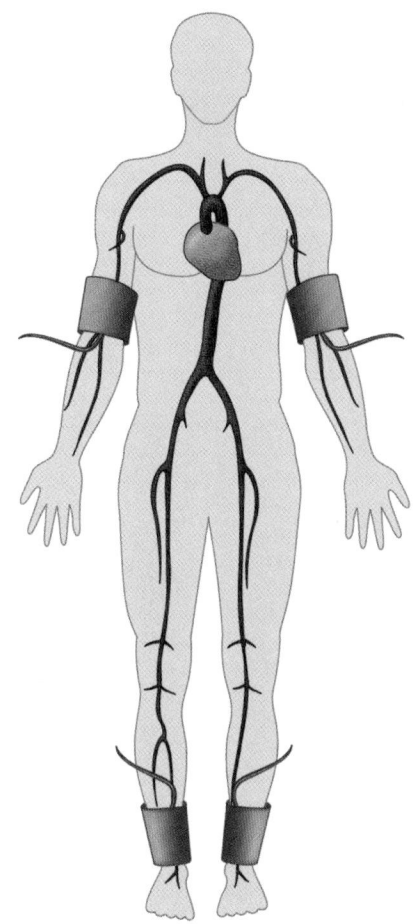

Right ABI = ratio of

Higher of the right ankle systolic pressures (posterior tibial or dorsalis pedis)

Higher arm systolic pressure (left or right arm)

Left ABI = ratio of

Higher of the left ankle systolic pressures (posterior tibial or dorsalis pedis)

FIG. 23-1. Calculating the ankle-brachial index.

Higher arm systolic pressure (left or right arm)

Pulse Volume Recording

In patients with noncompressible vessels, segmental plethysmography can be used to determine underlying arterial occlusive disease. Cuffs placed at different levels on the leg detect changes in leg volume and produce a pulse volume recording (PVR) when connected to a plethysmograph (Fig. 23-2). To obtain accurate PVR waveforms the cuff is inflated to 60 to 65 mmHg to detect volume changes without causing arterial occlusion. Pulse volume tracings are suggestive of proximal disease if the upstroke of the pulse is not brisk, the peak of the wave tracing is rounded, and there is disappearance of the dicrotic notch.

Although isolated segmental limb pressures and PVR measurements are 85% accurate when compared with angiography in detecting and localizing significant atherosclerotic lesions, when used in combination, accuracy approaches 95%.[3] For this reason, it is suggested that these two diagnostic modalities be used in combination when evaluating PAD.

Radiological Evaluation of the Vascular Patient

Ultrasound

Ultrasound examinations are relatively time consuming, require experienced technicians, and may not visualize all arterial segments. Dop-

pler waveform analysis can suggest atherosclerotic occlusive disease if the waveforms in the insonated arteries are biphasic, monophasic, or asymmetrical. B-mode ultrasonography provides black and white, real-time images. B-mode ultrasonography does not evaluate blood flow; thus, it cannot differentiate between fresh thrombus and flowing blood, which have the same echogenicity. Calcification in atherosclerotic plaques will cause acoustic shadowing. B-mode ultrasound probes cannot be sterilized. Use of the B-mode probe intraoperatively requires a sterile covering and gel to maintain an acoustic interface. Experience is needed to obtain and interpret images accurately. Duplex ultrasonography entails performance of B-mode imaging, spectral Doppler scanning, and color flow duplex scanning. The caveat to performance of duplex ultrasonography is meticulous technique by a certified vascular ultrasound technician, so that the appropriate 60° Doppler angle is maintained during insonation with the ultrasound probe. Alteration of this angle can markedly alter waveform appearance and subsequent interpretation of velocity measurements. Direct imaging of intra-abdominal vessels with duplex ultrasound is less reliable because of the difficulty in visualizing the vessels through overlying bowel. These disadvantages currently limit the applicability of duplex scanning in the evaluation of aortoiliac and infrapopliteal disease. In a recent study, duplex ultrasonography had lower sensitiv-

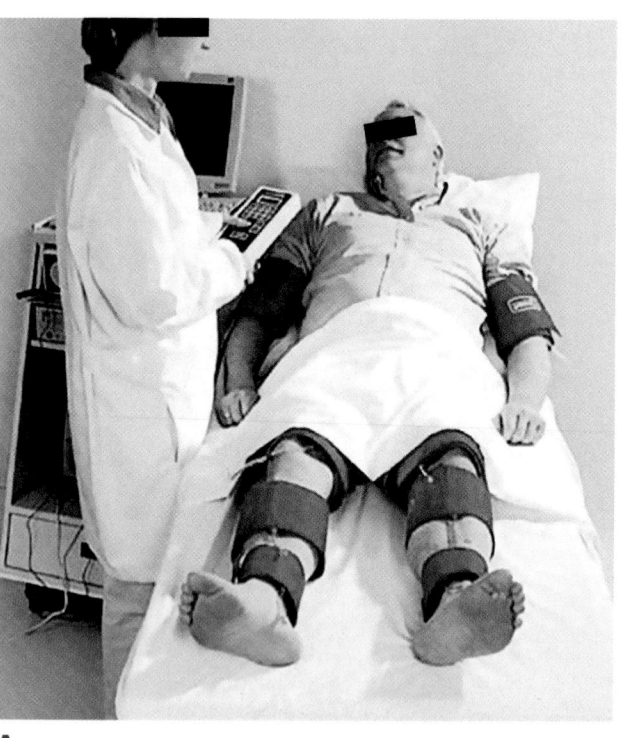

A

FIG. 23-2. A. Pulse volume recording is done by connecting blood pressure cuffs and plethysmograph to various levels of the leg. **B.** Typical report of peripheral vascular study with arterial segmental pressure measurement plus Doppler evaluation of the lower extremity.

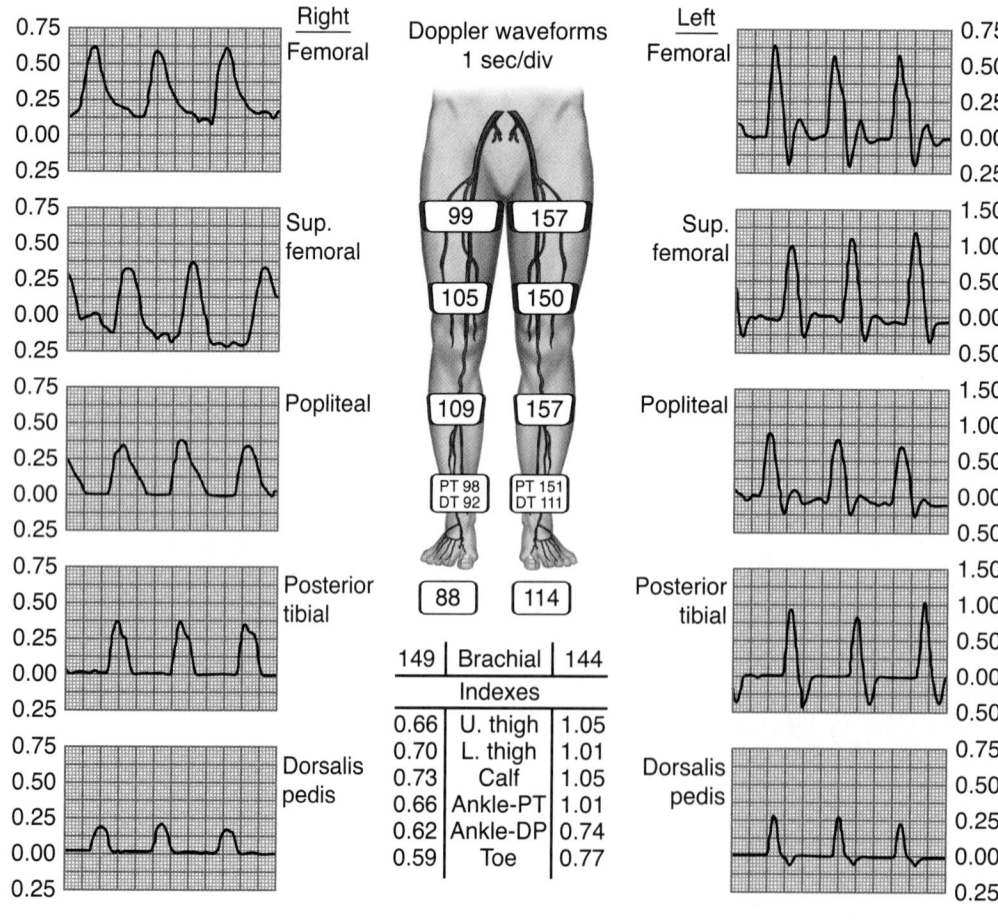

B

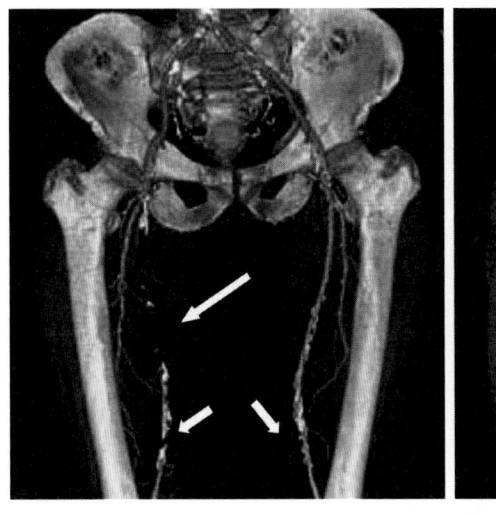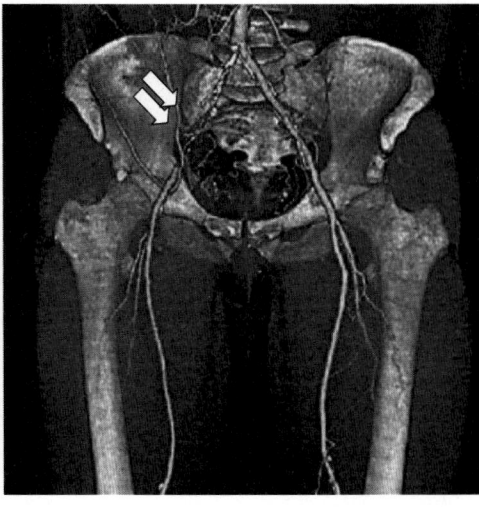

FIG. 23-3. A multidetector computed tomographic angiogram with three-dimensional reconstruction of the iliofemoral arterial circulation in two patients with lower leg claudication. **A.** A 50-year-old man with an occluded right superficial femoral artery (*single long arrow*) with reconstituted superficial femoral artery at the level of midthigh. Arterial calcifications (*short arrows*) in the bilateral distal superficial femoral arteries. **B.** A 53-year-old man with occluded right common iliac artery (*double arrows*).

A   **B**

ity in the calculation of infrapopliteal vessel stenosis in comparison to conventional digital subtraction or computer tomography angiography.[4] Few surgeons rely solely on duplex ultrasonography for preoperative planning in LE revascularizations. However, in the hands of experienced ultrasonographers, LE arteries can be assessed accurately by determining the significance of velocity criteria across the arterial stenosis. Duplex scanning is unable to evaluate recently implanted polytetrafluoroethylene (PTFE) and polyester (Dacron) grafts because they contain air, which prevents ultrasound penetration.

Computed Tomography Angiography

Computed tomography angiography (CTA) is a noninvasive, contrast-dependent method for imaging the arterial system. It depends on IV infusion of iodine-based contrast agents. The patient is advanced through a rotating gantry, which images serial transverse slices. The contrast-filled vessels can be extracted from the slices and rendered in three-dimensional format (Fig. 23-3). The extracted images can also be rotated and viewed from several different directions during postacquisition image processing. This technology has been advanced as a consequence of aortic endografting. CTA provides images for postprocessing that can be used to display the aneurysm in a format that demonstrates thrombus, calcium, lumen, and the outer wall, and allows "fitting" of a proposed endograft into the aneurysm (Fig. 23-4). CTA is increasingly being used to image the carotid bifurcation, and as computing power increases, the speed of image acquisition and resolution will continue to increase. The major limitations of multidetector CTA are use of contrast and

presence of artifacts caused by calcification and stents. CTA can overestimate the degree of instent stenosis, while heavy calcification can limit the diagnostic accuracy of the method by causing a "blooming artifact."[5] The artifacts can be overcome with alteration in image acquisition technique. There are no randomized trials to document the superiority of multidetector CTA over traditional angiography, but there is emerging evidence to support the claim that multidetector CTA has sensitivity, specificity, and accuracy that rival invasive angiography.[5]

Magnetic Resonance Angiography

Magnetic resonance angiography (MRA) has the advantage of not requiring iodinated contrast agents to provide vessel opacification (Fig. 23-5). Gadolinium is used as a contrast agent for MRA studies, and as it is generally not nephrotoxic, it can be used in patients with elevated creatinine. MRA is contraindicated in patients with pacemakers, defibrillators, spinal cord stimulators, intracerebral shunts, cochlear implants, and cranial clips. Patients with claustrophobia may require sedation to be able to complete the test. The presence of metallic stents causes artifacts and signal dropout; however, these can be dealt with using alternations in image acquisition and processing. Nitinol stents produce minimal artifact.[6] Compared to other modalities, MRA is relatively slow and expensive. However, due to its noninvasive nature and decreased nephrotoxicity, MRA is being used more frequently for imaging vasculature in various anatomic distributions.

Diagnostic Angiography

Diagnostic angiography is considered the gold standard in vascular imaging. In many centers, its use is rapidly decreasing due to the development of noninvasive imaging modalities such as duplex arterial mapping, CTA, and MRA. Nevertheless, contrast angiography still remains in widespread use. The essential aspects of angiography are vascular access and catheter placement in the vascular bed that requires examination. The imaging system and the contrast agent are used to opacify the target vessel. Although in the past this function has largely been delegated to the interventional radiology service, an increasing number of surgeons are performing this procedure and following the diagnostic imaging with immediate surgical or endovascular intervention. There are several considerations when relying on angiography for imaging.

Approximately 70% of atherosclerotic plaques occur in an eccentric location within the blood vessel; therefore, images can be misleading when trying to evaluate stenoses because angiography is limited to a uniplanar "lumenogram." With increased use of intra-

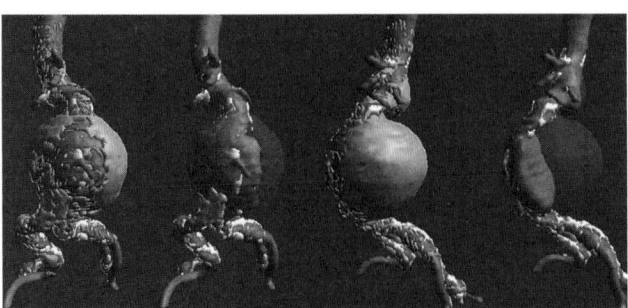

FIG. 23-4. Three-dimensional computed tomographic angiogram of an abdominal aortic aneurysm that displays various aneurysm components, including thrombus, aortic calcification, blood circulation, and aneurysm wall.

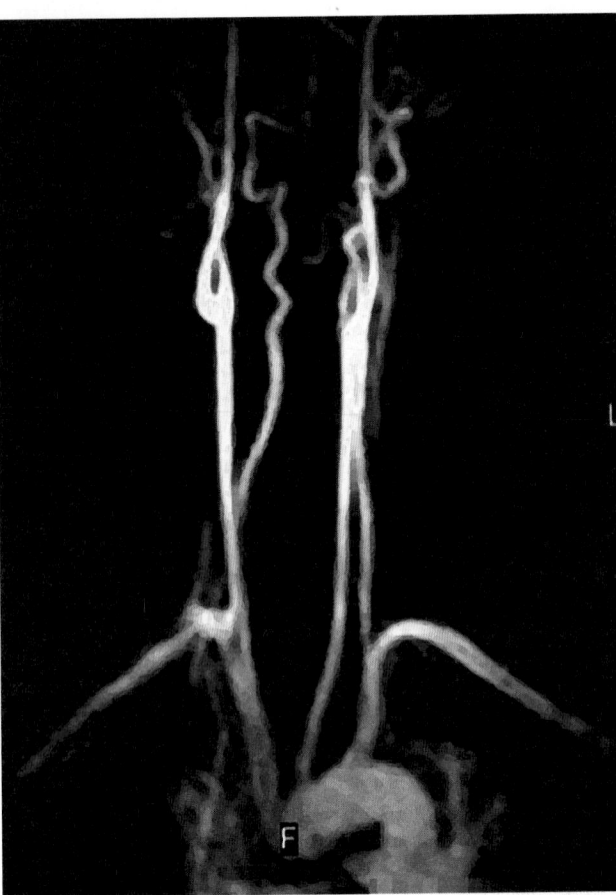

FIG. 23-5. Magnetic resonance angiogram of aortic arch and carotid arteries. This study can provide a three-dimensional analysis of vascular structures such as aortic arch branches, as well as carotid and vertebral arteries.

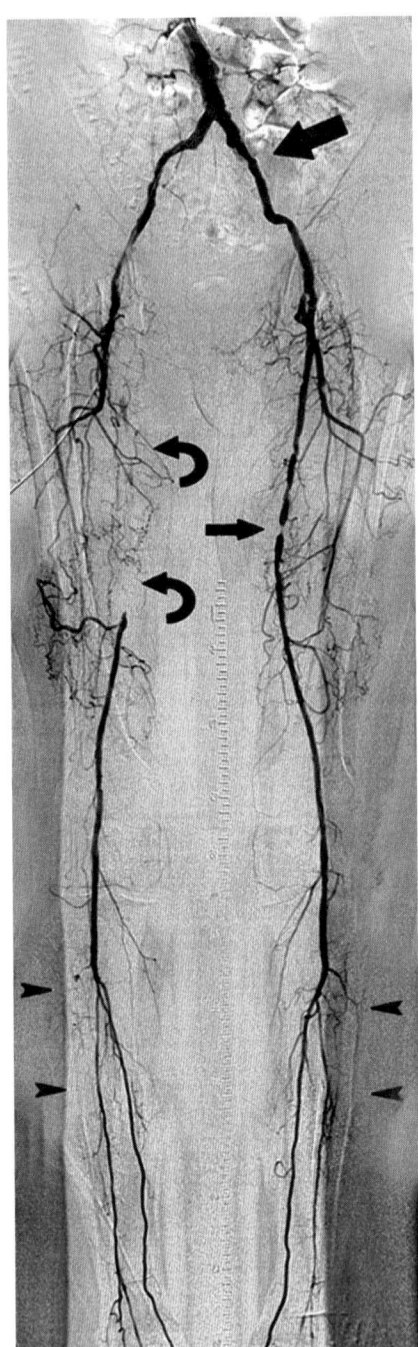

FIG. 23-6. Digital subtraction angiography provides excellent visualization of intravascular circulation with intra-arterial contrast administration. As depicted in this digital subtraction angiography study, multilevel lesions are demonstrated that include a focal left iliac artery stenosis (*large arrow*), right superficial femoral occlusion (*curved arrows*), left superficial femoral stenosis (*small arrow*), and multiple tibial artery stenoses (*arrowheads*).

vascular stent deployment, it has been also noted that assessment of stent apposition and stent position in relation to surrounding branches may be inaccurate. Furthermore, angiography exposes the patient to the risks of both ionizing radiation and intravascular contrast. Nevertheless, contrast angiography remains the most common invasive method of vascular investigation for both diagnostic and therapeutic intervention. The angiogram usually provides the final information needed to decide whether or not to proceed with operation or endovascular interventions.

Digital subtraction angiography (DSA) offers some advantages over conventional cut-film angiography, such as excellent visualization despite use of lower volumes of contrast media. In particular when multilevel occlusive lesions limit the amount of contrast reaching distal vessels, supplemental use of digital subtraction angiographic techniques may enhance visualization and definition of anatomy. Intra-arterial DSA uses a portable, axially rotatable imaging device that can obtain views from different angles. DSA also allows for real-time video replay (Fig. 23-6). An entire extremity can be filmed with DSA, using repeated injections of small amounts of contrast agent to obtain sequential angiographic images, the so-called *pulse-chase technique.*

Preoperative Cardiac Evaluation

The most important and controversial aspect of preoperative evaluation in patients with atherosclerotic disease requiring surgical intervention is the detection and subsequent management of associated CAD.[7] Several studies have documented the existence of significant CAD in 40 to 50% or more of patients requiring peripheral vascular reconstructive procedures, 10 to 20% of whom may be relatively asymptomatic largely because of their inability to exercise.[8] Myocardial infarction is responsible for the majority of both early and late postoperative deaths. Most available screening methods lack sensitivity and specificity to predict postoperative cardiac complications. There have been conflicting reports regarding the utility of preoperative dipyridamole-thallium nuclear imaging or dobutamine-echocardiography to stratify vascular patients in terms of perioperative cardiac morbidity and mortality. In nearly one half of patients, thallium imaging proves to be unnecessary because cardiac risk can be predicted by clinical information alone.[7] Even with coronary angiography, it is difficult to relate anatomic findings to functional significance, and hence, surgical risk. There are no data confirming that percutaneous coronary interventions or surgical revascularization before vascular surgical procedures impacts mortality or incidence of myocardial infarctions. In fact, coronary angiography is associated with its own inherent risks, and patients undergoing coronary artery bypass grafting or coronary percutaneous transluminal angioplasty (PTA) before needed aortoiliac reconstructions are subjected to the risks and complications of both procedures.

The Coronary Artery Revascularization Prophylaxis trial showed that coronary revascularization in patients with peripheral vascular disease and significant CAD, who are considered high risk for perioperative complications, did not reduce overall mortality or perioperative myocardial infarction.[9] Additionally, patients who underwent prophylactic coronary revascularization had significant delays before undergoing their vascular procedure and increased limb morbidity compared to patients who did not. Studies do support improvement in cardiovascular and overall prognosis with medical optimization of patients. Therefore, use of perioperative beta blockade, as well as use of antiplatelet medication, statins, and angiotensin-converting enzyme (ACE) inhibitors is encouraged in vascular patients.[10,11]

BASIC PRINCIPLES OF ENDOVASCULAR THERAPY

Cardiovascular disease remains a major cause of mortality in the developed world since the beginning of the twenty-first century. Although surgical revascularization has played a predominant role in the management of patients with vascular disease, the modern treatment paradigms have evolved significantly with increased emphasis of catheter-based percutaneous interventions over the past two decades. The increasing role of this minimally invasive vascular intervention is fueled by various factors, including rapid advances in imaging technology and reduced morbidity and mortality in endovascular interventions, as well as faster convalescence following percutaneous therapy when compared to traditional operations. There is little doubt that, with continued device development and refined image-guided technology, endovascular intervention will provide improved clinical outcomes and play an even greater role in the treatment of vascular disease.

The technique of percutaneous access for both the diagnostic and therapeutic management of vascular disease has resulted in tremendous changes in the practice of several subspecialties, including interventional radiology, invasive cardiology, and vascular surgery. The development of catheter and endoscopic instrumentation allows the vascular surgeon to operate via an intra- or extraluminal route. Endovascular techniques are now able to treat the full spectrum of vascular pathology, including stenoses and occlusions resulting from several etiologies, aneurysmal pathology, and traumatic lesions. Many of these procedures have only recently been developed, and, as such, have not been investigated in a manner that would enable an accurate comparison with the more traditional methods of open surgical intervention. Long-term follow-up for these procedures is frequently lacking. However, because of the potential to treat patients with decreased mortality and morbidity, endovascular skills and techniques are being adopted into mainstream vascular surgery.

Needles and Access

Needles are used to achieve percutaneous vascular access. The size of the needle will be dictated by the diameter of the guidewire used. Most often, an 18-gauge needle is used, as it will accept a 0.035-in guidewire. A 21-gauge micropuncture needle will accept a 0.018-in guidewire. The most popular access needle is the Seldinger needle, which can be used for single- and double-wall puncture techniques.

Femoral arterial puncture is the most common site for access. The common femoral artery (CFA) is punctured over the medial third of the femoral head, which is landmarked using fluoroscopy. The single-wall puncture technique requires a sharp, beveled needle tip and no central stylet. The anterior wall of the vessel is punctured with the bevel of the needle pointing up and pulsatile back-bleeding indicates an intraluminal position. This method is most useful for graft punctures, patients with abnormal clotting profiles, or if thrombolytic therapy is anticipated. Once the needle assumes an intraluminal position, verified by pulsatile back-bleeding, the guidewire may be advanced. This is always passed gently and under fluoroscopic guidance to avoid subintimal dissection or plaque disruption. Double-wall puncture techniques are performed with a blunt needle that has a removable inner cannula. The introducer needle punctures both walls of the artery and is withdrawn until bleeding is obtained to confirm intraluminal position before advancing a guidewire. There can be troublesome bleeding from the posterior arterial wall puncture; therefore, single puncture techniques are preferred.

Retrograde femoral access is the most common arterial access technique (Fig. 23-7). The advantages of this technique include the size and fixed position of the CFA, as well as the relative ease of compression against the femoral head at the end of the procedure. Care should be taken to avoid puncturing the external iliac artery (EIA) above the inguinal ligament because this can result in retroperitoneal hemorrhage secondary to ineffective compression of the puncture site. Likewise, puncturing too low, at or below the CFA bifurcation can result in thrombosis or pseudoaneurysm formation of the SFA or profunda femoris artery (PFA). Antegrade femoral access is more difficult than retrograde femoral access and there is a greater tendency to puncture the SFA, but it is invaluable when the aortic bifurcation cannot be traversed or when devices are not long enough to reach a lesion from a contralateral femoral access approach. Occasionally, when the distal aorta or bilateral iliac arteries are inaccessible because of the extent of atherosclerotic lesions, scarring, or presence of bypass conduits, the brachial artery must be used to obtain access for diagnostic and therapeutic interventions. The left brachial artery is punctured, as this avoids the origin of the carotid artery and thus decreases the risk of catheter-related emboli to the brain. The artery is accessed with a micropuncture needle just proximal to the antecubital crease. The use of brachial access is associated with a higher risk of thrombosis and nerve injuries than femoral access.

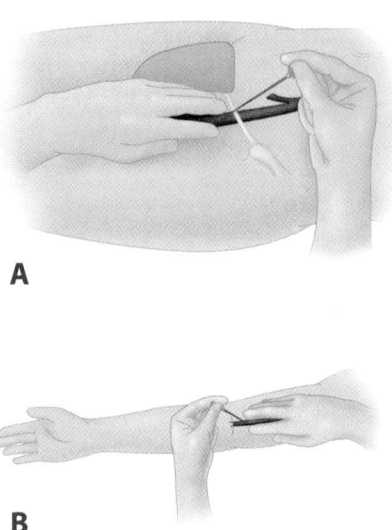

A

B

FIG. 23-7. A. Antegrade femoral artery access. The needle is inserted just below the inguinal ligament in the common femoral artery whereby the guidewire is inserted in the ipsilateral superficial femoral artery. **B.** Brachial artery approach. The needle is inserted in a retrograde fashion in the brachial artery just above the antecubital fossa, whereby the guidewire is next inserted in the brachial artery.

Guidewires

Guidewires are used to introduce, position, and exchange catheters. A guidewire generally has a flexible and stiff end. In general, only the flexible end of the guidewire is placed in the vessel. All guidewires are composed of a stiff inner core and an outer tightly coiled spring that allows a catheter to track over the guidewire. There are five essential characteristics of guidewires: size, length, stiffness, coating, and tip configuration.

Guidewires come in different maximum transverse diameters ranging from 0.011 to 0.038 in. For most aortoiliac procedures, a 0.03-in wire is most commonly used while the smaller diameter 0.018-in guidewires are reserved for selective small vessel angiography, such as infrageniculate or carotid lesions. In addition to diameter size, guidewires come in varying lengths usually ranging from 180 to 260 cm in length. Increasing the length of the wire always makes it more difficult to handle and increases the risk of contamination. While performing a procedure, it is important to maintain the guidewire across the lesion until the completion arteriogram has been satisfactorily completed.

The stiffness of the guidewire is also an important characteristic. Stiff wires allow for passage of large aortic stent graft devices without kinking. They are also useful when trying to perform sheath or catheter exchanges around a tortuous artery. An example of a stiff guidewire is the Amplatz wire. Hydrophilic coated guidewires, such as the Glidewire, have become invaluable tools for assisting in difficult catheterizations. The coating is primed by bathing the guidewire in saline solution. The slippery nature of this guidewire along with its torque capability significantly facilitates passage of this guidewire in difficult catheterizations. Guidewires also come in various tip configurations. Angled tip wires like the angled Glidewire can be steered to manipulate a catheter across a tight stenosis or to select a specific branch of a vessel. The Rosen wire has a soft curled end that makes it ideal for renal artery stenting. The soft curl of this wire prevents it from perforating small renal branch vessels.

Hemostatic Sheaths

The hemostatic sheath is a device through which endovascular procedures are performed. The sheath acts to protect the vessel from injury as wires and catheters are introduced (Fig. 23-8). A one-way valve prevents bleeding through the sheath, and a side port allows contrast or heparin flushes to be administered during the procedure. Sheaths are sized by their inner diameter. The most commonly used sheaths for percutaneous access have a 5Fr to 9Fr inner diameter, but with open surgical exposure of the CFA, sheaths as large as 26Fr can be introduced. Sheaths also vary in length and long sheaths are available so that interventions remote from the site of arterial access can be performed.

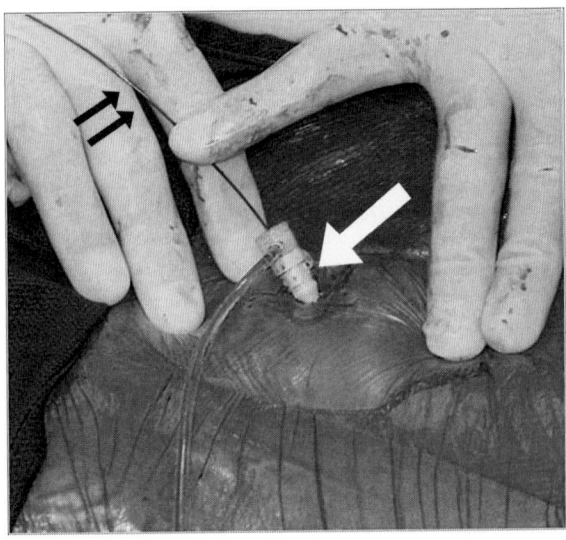

FIG. 23-8. All percutaneous endovascular procedures are performed through an introducer sheath (*large arrow*), which provides an access conduit from skin to intravascular compartment. The sheath also acts to protect the vessel from injury as guidewires (*small arrows*) and catheters are introduced.

Catheters

A wide variety of catheters exist that differ primarily in the configuration of the tip. The multiple shapes permit access to vessels of varying dimensions and angulations. Catheters are used to perform angiography, protect the passage of balloons and stents, and can be used to direct the guidewire through tight stenoses or tortuous vessels.

Angioplasty Balloons

Angioplasty balloons differ primarily in their length and diameter, as well as the length of the catheter shaft. As balloon technology has advanced, lower profiles have been manufactured (i.e., the size that the balloon assumes upon deflation). Balloons are used to perform angioplasty on vascular stenoses, to deploy stents, and to assist with additional expansion after insertion of self-expanding stents (Fig. 23-9). Besides length and diameter, operators need to be familiar with several other balloon characteristics. Noncompliant and low-compliance balloons tend to be inflated to their preset diameter and offer greater dilating force at the site of stenosis. Low-compliance

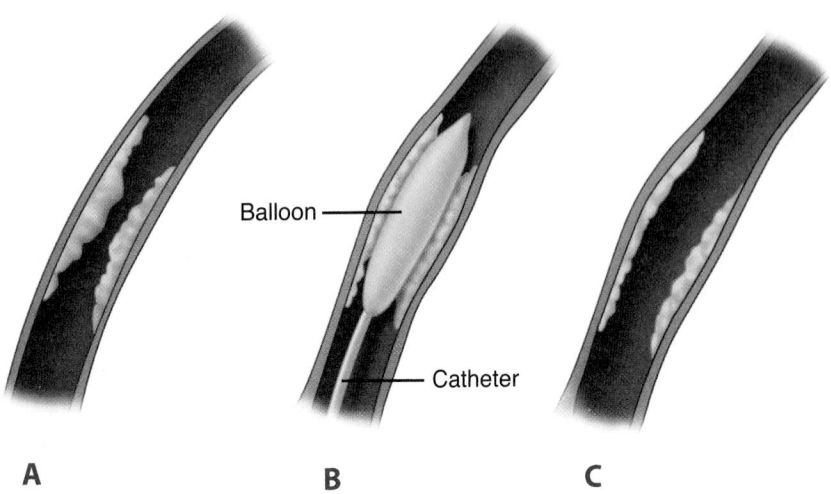

Balloon

Catheter

A **B** **C**

FIG. 23-9. A. An artery with luminal narrowing caused by plaque. **B.** A balloon angioplasty catheter is positioned within the diseased artery, which is inflated to enlarge the intravascular channel. **C.** The plaque is compressed with widened flow lumen as the result of balloon angioplasty.

balloons are the mainstay for peripheral intervention. Lower profile balloons are less likely to get caught during passage through stents and are easier to pull out of sheaths. Under fluoroscopic guidance, balloon inflation is performed until the waist of the atherosclerotic lesion disappears and the balloon is at the full profile. The duration of balloon inflation and pressures used for the angioplasty depend on the indication for the intervention as well as the location and characteristics of the lesion being treated. Frequently, several inflations are required to achieve a full profile of the balloon. Occasionally, a lower profile balloon is needed to predilate the tight stenosis so that the selected balloon catheter can cross the lesion. After inflation, most balloons do not regain their preinflation diameter and assume a larger profile. Trackability, pushability, and crossability of the balloon should all be considered when choosing a particular balloon. Lastly, shoulder length is an important characteristic to consider when selecting a balloon because of the potential to cause injury during performance of PTA in adjacent arterial segments. There is always risk of causing dissection or rupture during PTA, thus a completion angiogram is performed while the wire is still in place. Leaving the wire in place provides access for repeating the procedure, or placing a stent or stent graft if warranted.

Stents

Vascular stents are commonly used after an inadequate angioplasty with dissection or elastic recoil of an arterial stenosis. They serve to buttress collapsible vessels and help prevent atherosclerotic restenosis. Appropriate indications for primary stenting of a lesion without an initial trial of angioplasty alone are evolving in manners that are dependent on the extent and site of the lesion. Stents are manufactured from a variety of metals, including stainless steel, tantalum, cobalt-based alloy, and nitinol. Vascular stents are classified into two basic categories: balloon-expandable stents and self-expanding stents.

Self-expanding stents (Fig. 23-10) are deployed by retracting a restraining sheath. They usually consist of Elgiloy (a cobalt, chromium, nickel alloy) or nitinol (a shape memory alloy composed of nickel and titanium), the latter of which will contract and assume a heat-treated shape above a transition temperature that depends upon the composition of the alloy. Self-expanding stents will expand to a final diameter that is determined by stent geometry, hoop strength, and vessel size. The self-expanding stent is mounted on a central shaft and is placed inside an outer sheath. It relies on a mechanical spring-like action to achieve expansion. With deployment of these stents, there is some degree of foreshortening that has to be taken into account when choosing the area of deployment. In this way, self-expanding stents are more difficult to place with absolute precision. There are several advantages related to self-expanding stents. Self-expanding stents generally come in longer lengths than balloon-expandable stents and are therefore used to treat long and tortuous lesions. Their ability to continually expand after delivery allows them to accommodate adjacent vessels of different size. This makes these stents ideal for placement in the ICA. These stents are always oversized by 1 to 2 mm relative to the largest diameter of normal vessel adjacent to the lesion to prevent immediate migration.

Balloon-expandable stents are usually composed of stainless steel, mounted on an angioplasty balloon, and deployed by balloon inflation (Fig. 23-11). They can be manually placed on a chosen balloon catheter or obtained premounted on a balloon catheter. The capacity of a balloon-expandable stent to shorten in length during deployment depends on both stent geometry and the final diameter to which the balloon is expanded. These stents are more rigid and are associated with a shorter time to complete endothelialization. They are often of limited flexibility and have a higher degree of crush resistance when compared to self-expanding. This makes them ideal for short-segment lesions, especially those that involve the ostia, such as proximal common iliac or renal artery stenosis.

The most exciting area of development in stents is the evolution of drug-eluting stents (DES). These stents are usually composed of

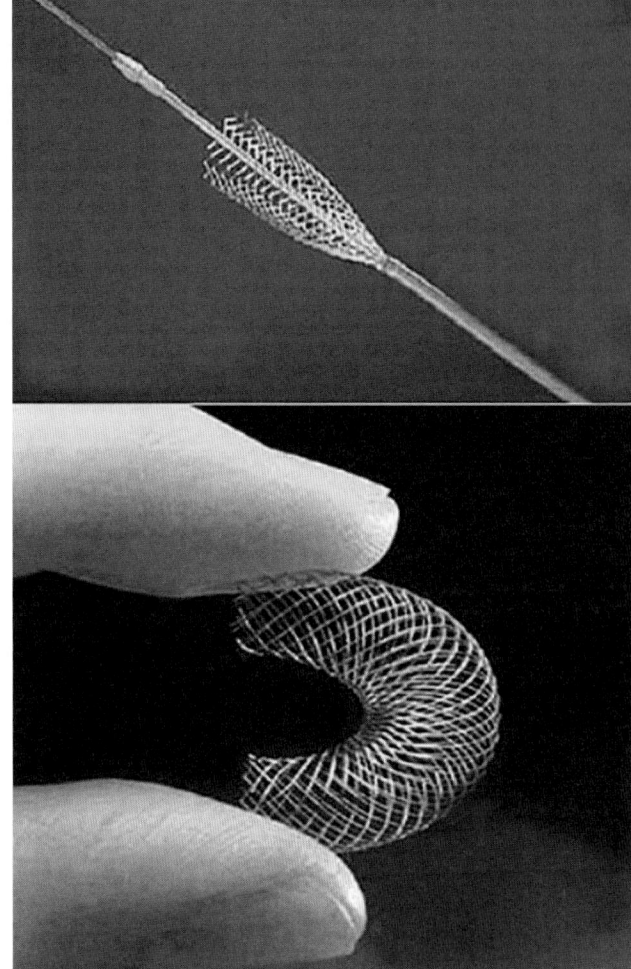

FIG. 23-10. Self-expanding stents are made of tempered stainless steel or nitinol, an alloy of nickel and titanium, and are restrained when folded inside a delivery catheter. After release from the restraining catheter, the self-expanding stents will expand to a final diameter that is determined by stent geometry, hoop strength, and vessel size.

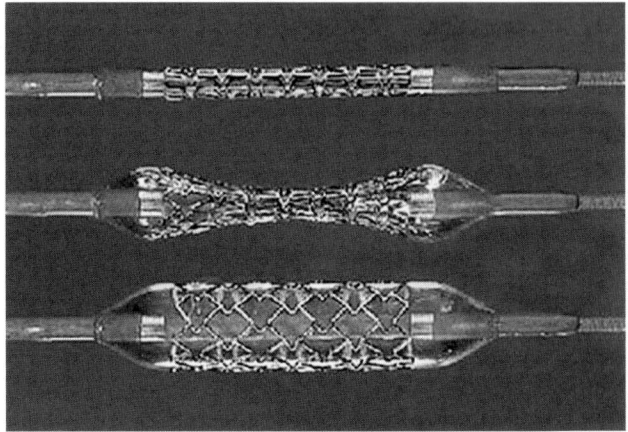

FIG. 23-11. In a balloon-expandable stent, the stent is premounted on a balloon catheter. The balloon stretches the stent members beyond their elastic limit. The stent is deployed by full balloon expansion. This type of stent has a higher degree of crush resistance when compared to self-expanding. This makes them ideal for short-segment calcified ostial lesions.

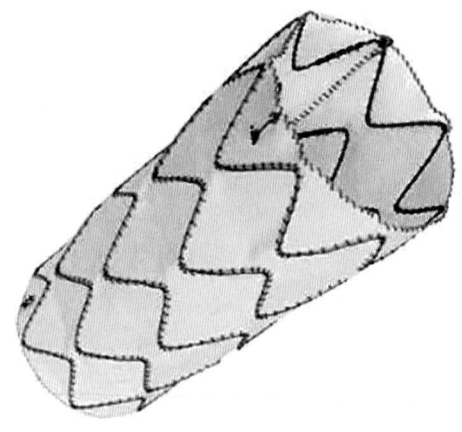
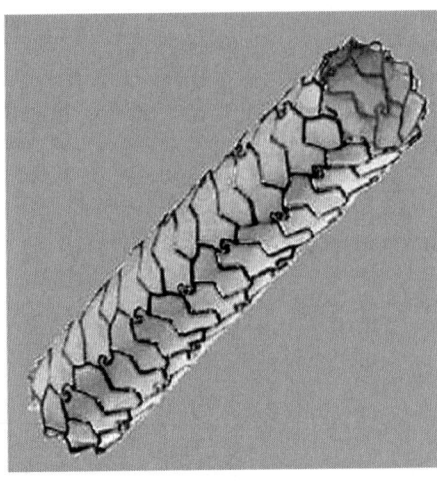

FIG. 23-12. A stent graft is a combination of a metal stent covered with fabric that is commonly used for aneurysm exclusion.

nitinol and have various anti-inflammatory drugs bonded to them. Over time, the stents release the drug into the surrounding arterial wall and help prevent restenosis. Numerous randomized controlled trials have proven their benefit in coronary arteries.[12] Clinical studies have similarly proved early efficacy of DES in the treatment of PAD.

Stent Grafts

The combination of a metal stent covered with fabric gave birth to the first stent grafts. Covered stents have been designed with either a surrounding PTFE or polyester fabric and have been used predominantly for treatment of traumatic vascular lesions, including arterial disruption and arteriovenous fistulas (Fig. 23-12). However, these devices may well find a growing role in treatment of iliac or femoral arterial occlusive disease as well as popliteal aneurysms.

Endovascular aneurysm repair using the concept of stent grafts was initiated by Parodi in 1991.[13] Since that time, a large number of endografts have been inserted under the auspices of clinical trials at first and now as Food and Drug Administration (FDA)-approved devices. Current FDA-approved devices include (a) AneuRx device (Medtronic/AVE, Santa Rosa, Calif), (b) Gore Excluder device (WL Gore & Associates, Flagstaff, Ariz), (c) Endologix Powerlink device (Endologix Inc., Irvine, Calif), (d) Zenith device (Cook Inc., Bloomington, Ind), and (e) Talent device (Medtronic/AVE, Santa Rosa, Calif). All of these devices require that patients have an infrarenal aneurysm with at least a 15-mm proximal aortic neck below the renal arteries, and not >60° of angulation. For those patients with associated common iliac artery (CIA) aneurysmal disease, endovascular treatment can be achieved by initial coil embolization of the ipsilateral hypogastric artery with extension of the endovascular device into the EIA. Clinical trials are underway with devices that will expand indications to aneurysms involving the visceral segment of the abdominal aorta. The FDA has similarly approved several thoracic endografts for the treatment of descending thoracic aortic aneurysm. Early studies have demonstrated short-term efficacy of thoracic aortic devices in the treatment of traumatic aortic transections, and aortic dissections.[14-16] A larger experience with these devices exists in both Europe and Asia, and trials are underway in the United States with several devices.

CAROTID ARTERY DISEASE

Atherosclerotic occlusive plaque is by far the most common pathology seen in the carotid artery bifurcation. Thirty to 60% of all ischemic strokes are related to atherosclerotic carotid bifurcation occlusive disease. In the following section, discussion will be focused on clinical presentation, diagnosis, and management, including medical therapy, surgical carotid endarterectomy, and stenting of atherosclerotic carotid occlusive disease. In the second part of the section, a brief review will be focused on other less common non-atherosclerotic diseases involving the extracranial carotid artery, including kink and coil, fibromuscular dysplasia (FMD), arterial dissection, aneurysm, radiation arteritis, Takayasu's arteritis, and carotid body tumor.

Epidemiology and Etiology of Carotid Occlusive Disease

Approximately 700,000 Americans suffer a new or recurrent stroke each year.[17] Eighty-five percent of all strokes are ischemic and 15% are hemorrhagic. Hemorrhagic strokes are caused by head trauma or spontaneous disruption of intracerebral blood vessels. Ischemic strokes are due to hypoperfusion from arterial occlusion, or less commonly due to decreased flow resulting from proximal arterial stenosis and poor collateral network. Common causes of ischemic strokes are cardiogenic emboli (35%), carotid artery disease (30%), lacunar (10%), miscellaneous (10%), and idiopathic (15%).[17] The term *cerebrovascular accident* (CVA) often is used interchangeably to refer to an ischemic stroke. A *transient ischemic attack* (TIA) is defined as a temporary focal cerebral or retinal hypoperfusion state that resolves spontaneously within 24 hours after its onset. However, the majority of TIAs resolve within minutes, and longer lasting neurologic deficits more likely represent a stroke. Recently, the term *brain attack* has been coined to refer to an acute stroke or TIA, denoting the condition as a medical emergency requiring immediate attention, similar to a heart attack.

Stroke due to carotid bifurcation occlusive disease usually is caused by atheroemboli (Fig. 23-13). The carotid bifurcation is an area of low-flow velocity and low-shear stress. As the blood circulates through the carotid bifurcation, there is separation of flow into the low-resistance ICA, and the high-resistance external carotid artery. Characteristically, atherosclerotic plaque forms in the outer wall opposite to the flow divider (Fig. 23-14). Atherosclerotic plaque formation is complex, beginning with intimal injury, platelet deposition, smooth muscle cell proliferation, and fibroplasia, and leading to subsequent luminal narrowing. With increasing degree of stenosis in the ICA, flow becomes more turbulent, and the risk of atheroembolization escalates. The severity of stenosis is commonly divided into three categories according to the luminal diameter reduction: mild (less than 50%), moderate (50 to 69%), and severe (70 to 99%). Severe carotid stenosis is a strong predictor for stroke.[18] In turn, a prior history of neurologic symptoms (TIA or stroke) is an important determinant for recurrent ipsilateral stroke. The risk factors for the development of carotid artery bifurcation disease are similar to those causing atherosclerotic occlusive disease in other vascular beds. Increasing age, male gender, hypertension, tobacco

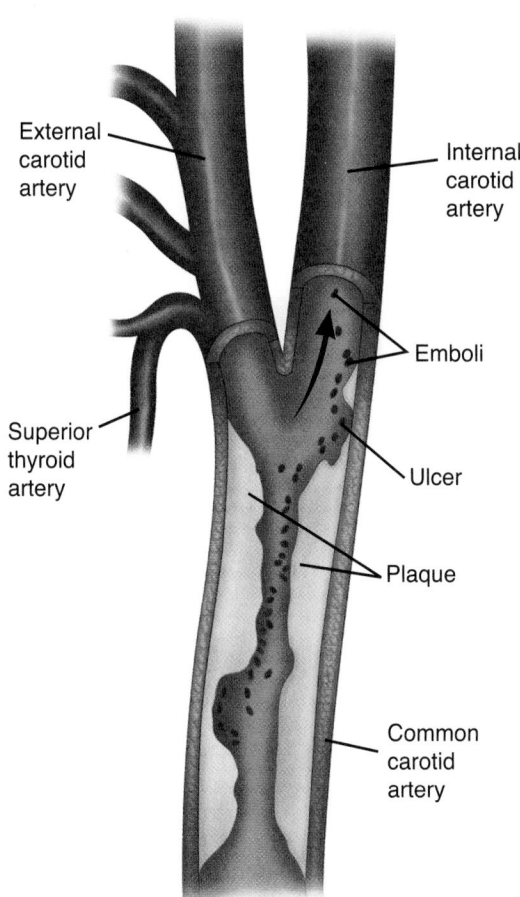

FIG. 23-13. Stroke due to carotid bifurcation occlusive disease is usually caused by atheroemboli arising from the internal carotid artery, which provides the majority of blood flow to the cerebral hemisphere. With increasing degree of stenosis in the carotid artery, flow becomes more turbulent, and the risk of atheroembolization escalates.

smoking, diabetes mellitus, homocysteinemia, and hyperlipidemia are well-known predisposing factors for the development of atherosclerotic occlusive disease.

Clinical Manifestations of Cerebral Ischemia

TIA is a focal loss of neurologic function, lasting for <24 hours. *Crescendo TIAs* refer to a syndrome comprising repeated TIAs within a short period of time that is characterized by complete neurologic recovery in between. At a minimum the term should probably be reserved either for those with daily events or multiple resolving attacks within 24 hours. Hemodynamic TIAs represent focal cerebral events that are aggravated by exercise or hemodynamic stress and typically occur after short bursts of physical activity, postprandially or after getting out of a hot bath. It is implied that these are due to severe extracranial disease and poor intracranial collateral recruitment. *Reversible ischemic neurologic deficits* refer to ischemic focal neurologic symptoms lasting longer than 24 hours but resolving within 3 weeks. When a neurologic deficit lasts longer than 3 weeks, it is considered a *completed stroke*. *Stroke in evolution* refers to progressive worsening of the neurologic deficit, either linearly over a 24-hour period, or interspersed with transient periods of stabilization and/or partial clinical improvement.

The patients who suffer CVAs typically present with three categories of symptoms, including ocular symptoms, sensory/motor deficit, and/or higher cortical dysfunction. The common ocular symptoms associated with extracranial carotid artery occlusive disease include amaurosis fugax and presence of Hollenhorst plaques. Amaurosis fugax, commonly referred to as *transient monocular blindness*, is a temporary loss of vision in one eye that patients typically describe as a window shutter coming down or gray shedding of the vision. This partial blindness usually lasts for a few minutes and then resolves. Most of these phenomena (>90%) are due to embolic occlusion of the main artery or the upper or lower divisions. Monocular blindness progressing over a 20-minute period suggests a migrainous etiology. Occasionally, the patient will recall no visual symptoms while the optician notes a yellowish plaque within the retinal vessels, which is also known as the *Hollenhorst plaque*. These are frequently derived from cholesterol embolization

FIG. 23-14. A. The carotid bifurcation is an area of low-flow velocity and low-shear stress. As the blood circulates through the carotid bifurcation, there is separation of flow into the low-resistance internal carotid artery and the high-resistance external carotid artery. **B.** The carotid atherosclerotic plaque typically forms in the outer wall opposite to the flow divider due in part to the effect of the low-shear stress region, which also creates a transient reversal of flow during cardiac cycle.

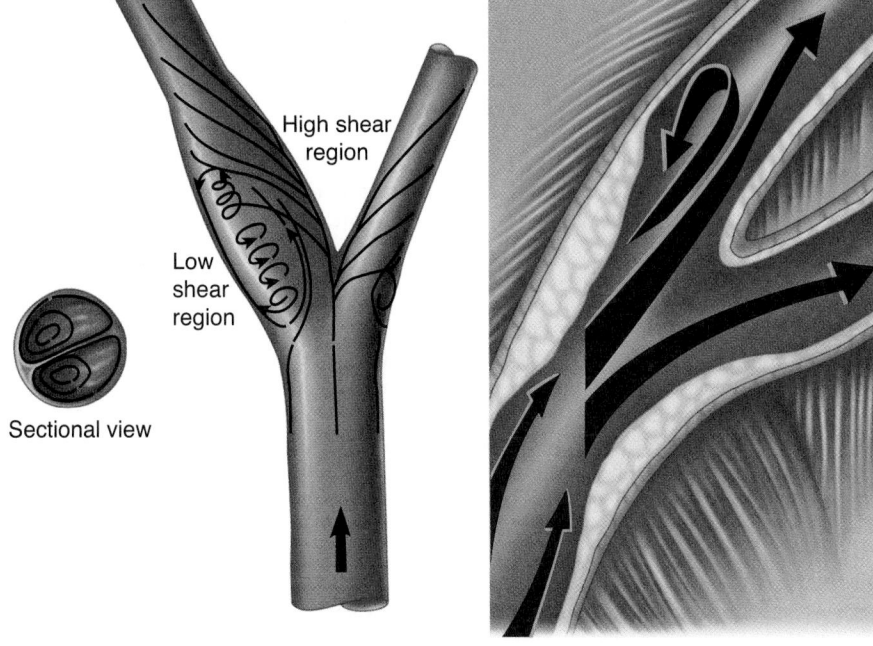

Sectional view

High shear region

Low shear region

A

B

from the carotid bifurcation and warrant further investigation. Additionally, several ocular symptoms may be caused by microembolization from the extracranial carotid diseases, including monocular vision loss due to retinal artery or optic nerve ischemia, the ocular ischemia syndrome, and visual field deficits secondary to cortical infarction and ischemia of the optic tracts. Typical motor and/or sensory symptoms associated with CVAs are located in either an ipsilateral or contralateral neurologic deficit. Ischemic events tend to have an abrupt onset, with the severity of the insult being apparent from the onset and not usually associated with seizures or paraesthesia. In contrast, they represent loss or diminution of neurologic function. Furthermore, motor or sensory deficits can be unilateral or bilateral, with the upper and lower limbs being variably affected depending on the site of the cerebral lesion.

The combination of a motor and sensory deficit in the same body territory is suggestive of a cortical thromboembolic event as opposed to lacunar lesions secondary to small vessel disease of the penetrating arterioles. However, a small proportion of the latter may present with a sensorimotor stroke secondary to small vessel occlusion within the posterior limb of the internal capsule. Pure sensory and pure motor strokes and those strokes where the weakness affects one limb only or does not involve the face are more typically seen with lacunar as opposed to cortical infarction. A number of higher cortical functions, including speech and language disturbances, can be affected by thromboembolic phenomena from the carotid artery with the most important clinical example for the dominant hemisphere being dysphasia or aphasia, and visuospatial neglect being an example of nondominant hemisphere injury.

Diagnostic Evaluation

Duplex ultrasonography is the most widely used screening tool to evaluate for atherosclerotic plaque and stenosis of the extracranial carotid artery. It is also commonly used to monitor patients serially for progression of disease, or after intervention (carotid endarterectomy or angioplasty). Duplex ultrasound of the carotid artery combines B-mode gray-scale imaging and Doppler waveform analysis. Characterization of the carotid plaque on gray-scale imaging provides useful information about its composition. However, there are currently no universal recommendations that can be made based solely on the sonographic appearance of the plaque. On the other hand, criteria have been developed and well refined for grading the degree of carotid stenosis based primarily on Doppler-derived velocity waveforms.

The external carotid artery has a high-resistance flow pattern with a sharp systolic peak and a small amount of flow in diastole. In contrast, a normal ICA will have a low-resistance flow pattern with a broad systolic peak and a large amount of flow during diastole. The flow pattern in the common carotid artery (CCA) resembles that in the ICA, as 80% of the flow is directed to the ICA, with waveforms that have broad systolic peaks and a moderate amount of flow during diastole. Conventionally, velocity measurements are recorded in the common, external carotid bulb, and the proximal, mid-, and distal portions of the ICA. Characteristically, the peak systolic velocity is increased at the site of the vessel stenosis. The end-diastolic velocity is increased with a greater degree of stenosis. In addition, stenosis of the ICA can lead to color shifts with color mosaics indicating a poststenotic turbulence. Dampening of the Doppler velocity waveforms are typically seen in areas distal to severe carotid stenosis where blood flow is reduced. It is well known that occlusion of the ipsilateral ICA can lead to a "falsely" elevated velocity on the contralateral side due to an increase in compensatory blood flow. In the presence of a high-grade stenosis or occlusion of the ICA, the ipsilateral CCA displays high flow resistance waveforms, similar to that seen in the external carotid artery. If there is a significant stenosis in the proximal CCA, its waveforms may be dampened with low velocities.

The Doppler grading systems of carotid stenosis were initially established by comparison to angiographic findings of disease.

TABLE 23-3	Carotid duplex ultrasound criteria for grading internal carotid artery stenosis			
Degree of Stenosis (%)	ICA PSV (cm/s)	ICA/CCA PSV Ratio	ICA EDV (cm/s)	Plaque Estimate (%)[a]
Normal	<125	<2.0	<40	None
<50	<125	<2.0	<40	<50
50–69	125–230	2.0–4.0	40–100	≥50
≥70 to less than near occlusion	>230	>4.0	>100	≥50
Near occlusion	High, low, or not detected	Variable	Variable	Visible
Total occlusion	Not detected	Not applicable	Not detected	Visible, no lumen

[a]Plaque estimate (diameter reduction) with gray-scale and color Doppler ultrasound. ICA = internal carotid artery; CCA = common carotid artery; PSV = peak systolic velocity; EDV = end-diastolic velocity.

Studies have shown variability in the measurements of the duplex properties by different laboratories, as well as heterogeneity in the patient population, study design, and techniques. One of the most commonly used classifications was established at the University of Washington School of Medicine in Seattle. Diameter reduction of 50 to 79% is defined by peak systolic velocity >125 cm/sec with extensive spectral broadening. For stenosis in the range of 80 to 99%, the peak systolic velocity is >125 cm/sec and peak diastolic velocity is >140 cm/sec. The ratio of internal carotid to common carotid artery (ICA/CCA) peak systolic velocity has also been part of various ultrasound diagnostic classifications. A ratio >4 is a great predictor of angiographic stenosis of 70 to 99%. A multispecialty consensus panel has developed a set of criteria for grading carotid stenosis by duplex examination (Table 23-3).[19]

MRA is increasingly being used to evaluate for atherosclerotic carotid occlusive disease and intracranial circulation. MRA is noninvasive and does not require iodinated contrast agents. MRA uses phase contrast or time-of-flight, with either two-dimensional or three-dimensional data sets for greater accuracy. Three-dimensional, contrast-enhanced MRA allows data to be obtained in coronal and sagittal planes with improved image qualities due to shorter study time. In addition, the new MRA techniques allow for better reformation of images in various planes to allow better grading of stenosis. There have been numerous studies comparing the sensitivity and specificity of MRA imaging for carotid disease to duplex and selective contrast angiography.[20] Magnetic resonance imaging (MRI) of the brain is essential in the assessment of acute stroke patients. MRI with diffusion-weighted imaging can differentiate areas of acute ischemia, areas still at risk for ischemia (penumbra), and chronic cerebral ischemic changes. However, computed tomographic (CT) imaging remains the most expeditious test in the evaluation of acute stroke patients to rule out intracerebral hemorrhage. Recently, multidetector CTA has gained increasing popularity in the evaluation of carotid disease.[21] This imaging modality can provide volume rendering, which allows rotation of the object with accurate anatomic structures from all angles (Fig. 23-15). The advantages of CTA over MRA include faster data acquisition time and better spatial resolution. However, grading of carotid stenosis by CTA requires further validation at the time of this writing before it can be widely applied.

Historically, DSA has been the gold standard test to evaluate the extra- and intracranial circulation (Fig. 23-16). This is an invasive procedure, typically performed via a transfemoral puncture, and involves selective imaging of the carotid and vertebral arteries using iodinated contrast. The risk of stroke during cerebral angiography is generally reported at approximately 1%, and is typically due to

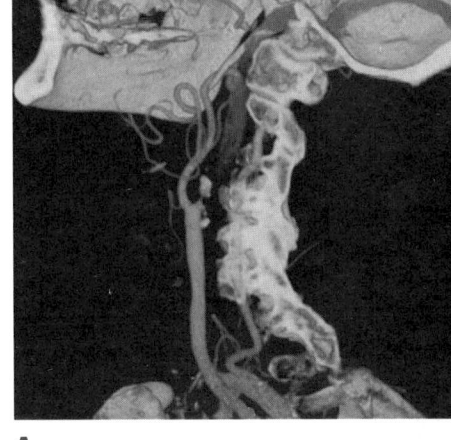
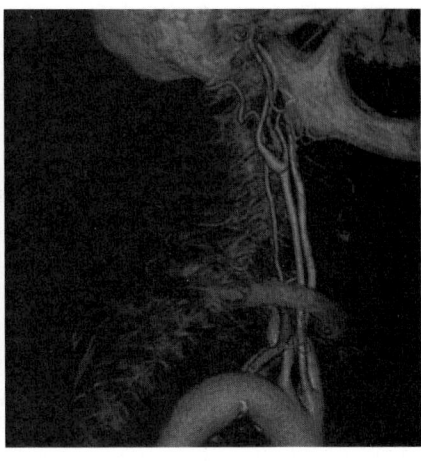

FIG. 23-15. A. Carotid computed tomography angiography is a valuable imaging modality that can provide a three-dimensional image reconstruction with high image resolution. A carotid artery occlusion is noted in the internal carotid artery. **B.** The entire segment of extracranial carotid artery is visualized from the thoracic compartment to the base of skull. **A** **B**

atheroembolization related to wire and catheter manipulation in the arch aorta or proximal branch vessels. Over the past decades, however, the incidence of neurologic complications following angiography has been reduced, due to the use of improved guidewires and catheters, better resolution digital imaging, and increased experience. Local access complications of angiography are infrequent and include development of hematoma, pseudoaneurysm, distal embolization, or acute vessel thrombosis. Currently, selective angiography is particularly used for patients with suspected intracranial disease and for patients in whom percutaneous revascularization is considered. The techniques of carotid angioplasty and stenting for carotid bifurcation occlusive disease are described in the "Techniques of Carotid Angioplasty and Stenting" section. Preoperative CTA or MRA is routinely utilized to get information about the aortic arch anatomy and pres-

ence of concomitant intracranial disease and collateral pathway in planning our strategy for carotid stenting or endarterectomy.

Treatment of Carotid Occlusive Disease

Conventionally, patients with carotid bifurcation occlusive disease are divided into two broad categories: patients without prior history of ipsilateral stroke or TIA (asymptomatic) and those with prior or current ipsilateral neurologic symptoms (symptomatic). It is estimated that 15% of all strokes are preceded by a TIA. The 90-day risk of a stroke in a patient presenting with a TIA is 3 to 17%.[17] According to the Cardiovascular Health Study, a longitudinal, population-based study of CAD and stroke in men and women, the prevalence of TIA in men was 2.7% between the ages of 65 to 69 and 3.6% for ages 75 to 79; the prevalence in women was 1.4% and 4.1%, respectively.[22] There have been several studies reporting on the effectiveness of stroke prevention with medical treatment and carotid endarterectomy for symptomatic patients with moderate to severe carotid stenosis. Early and chronic aspirin therapy has been shown to reduce stroke recurrence rate in several large clinical trials.[23]

Symptomatic Carotid Stenosis

Currently, most stroke neurologists prescribe both aspirin and clopidogrel for secondary stroke prevention in patients who had experienced a TIA or stroke.[17] In patients with symptomatic carotid stenosis, the degree of stenosis appears to be the most important predictor in determining risk for an ipsilateral stroke. The risk of a recurrent ipsilateral stroke in patients with severe carotid stenosis approaches 40%. Two large multicenter randomized clinical trials, the European Carotid Surgery Trial and the North American Symptomatic Carotid Endarterectomy Trial, have both shown a significant risk reduction in stroke for patients with symptomatic high-grade stenosis (70 to 99%) undergoing carotid endarterectomy when compared to medical therapy alone.[24,25] There has been much discussion regarding the different methodology used in the measurement of carotid stenosis and calculation of the life-table data between the two studies, which still led to similar results.[26] Findings of these two landmark trials have also been reanalyzed in many subsequent publications. The main conclusions of the trials remain validated and widely acknowledged. Briefly, the North American Symptomatic Carotid Endarterectomy Trial study showed that, for high-grade carotid stenosis, the cumulative risk of ipsilateral stroke was 26% in the medically treated group and 9% in the surgically treated group at 2 years. For patients with moderate carotid artery stenosis (50 to 69%), the benefit of carotid endarterectomy is less but still favorable when compared to medical treatment alone; the 5-year fatal or nonfatal ipsilateral stroke rate was 16% in the surgically treated group vs. 22% in the medically treated group.[27] The risk of stroke was

FIG. 23-16. A carotid angiogram reveals an ulcerated carotid plaque (*arrow*) in the proximal internal carotid artery, which also resulted in a high-grade, internal, carotid artery stenosis.

similar for the remaining group of symptomatic patients with less than 50% carotid stenosis, whether they had endarterectomy or medical treatment alone. The European Carotid Surgery Trial reported similar stroke risk reduction for patients with severe symptomatic carotid stenosis and no benefit in patients with mild stenosis, when carotid endarterectomy was performed vs. medical therapy.[25]

The optimal timing of carotid intervention after acute stroke, however, remains debatable. Earlier studies showed an increased rate of postoperative stroke exacerbation and conversion of a bland to hemorrhagic infarction when carotid endarterectomy was carried out within 5 to 6 weeks after acute stroke. The dismal outcome reported in the early experience was likely related to poor patient selection. The rate of stroke recurrence is not insignificant during the interval period and may be reduced with early intervention for symptomatic carotid stenosis. Contemporary series have demonstrated acceptable low rates of perioperative complications in patients undergoing carotid endarterectomy within 4 weeks after acute stroke.[27] In a recent retrospective series, carotid artery stenting, when performed early (<2 weeks) after the acute stroke, was associated with higher mortality than when delayed (>2 weeks).[28]

Asymptomatic Carotid Stenosis

Whereas there is universal agreement that carotid revascularization (endarterectomy or stenting) is effective in secondary stroke prevention for patients with symptomatic moderate and severe carotid stenosis, the management of asymptomatic patients remains an important controversy to be resolved. Generally, the detection of carotid stenosis in asymptomatic patients is related to the presence of a cervical bruit or based on screening duplex ultrasound findings. In one of the earlier observational studies, the authors showed that the annual rate of occurrence of neurologic symptoms was 4% in a cohort of 167 patients with asymptomatic cervical bruits followed prospectively by serial carotid duplex scan.[29] The mean annual rate of carotid stenosis progression to a greater than 50% stenosis was 8%. The presence of or progression to a greater than 80% stenosis correlated highly with either the development of a total occlusion of the ICA or new symptoms. The major risk factors associated with disease progression were cigarette smoking, diabetes mellitus, and age. This study supported the contention that it is prudent to follow a conservative course in the management of asymptomatic patients presenting with a cervical bruit.

One of the first randomized clinical trials on the treatment of asymptomatic carotid artery stenosis was the Asymptomatic Carotid Atherosclerosis Study, which evaluated the benefits of medical management with antiplatelet therapy vs. carotid endarterectomy.[30] Over a 5-year period, the risk of ipsilateral stroke in individuals with a carotid artery stenosis greater than 60% was 5.1% in the surgical arm. On the other hand, the risk of ipsilateral stroke in patients treated with medical management was 11%. Carotid endarterectomy produced a relative risk reduction of 53% over medical management alone. The results of a larger randomized trial from Europe, The Asymptomatic Carotid Surgery Trial, confirmed similar beneficial stroke risk reduction for patients with asymptomatic greater than 70% carotid stenosis undergoing endarterectomy compared to medical therapy.[31] An important point derived from this latter trial was that even with improved medical therapy, including the addition of statin drugs and clopidogrel, medical therapy was still inferior to endarterectomy in the primary stroke prevention for patients with high-grade carotid artery stenosis. It is generally agreed that asymptomatic patients with severe carotid stenosis (80 to 99%) are at significantly increased risk for stroke and stand to benefit from either surgical or endovascular revascularization. However, revascularization for asymptomatic patients with a less severe degree of stenosis (60 to 79%) remains controversial.

Carotid Endarterectomy vs. Angioplasty and Stenting

Currently, the argument is no longer that medical therapy alone is inferior to surgical endarterectomy in stroke prevention for severe

TABLE 23-4	Conditions qualifying patients as "high surgical risk" for carotid endarterectomy
Anatomical Factors	**Physiological Factors**
• High carotid bifurcation (above C2 vertebral body)	• Age ≥80 y
• Low common carotid artery (below clavicle)	• Left ventricular ejection fraction ≤30%
• Contralateral carotid occlusion	• New York Heart Association Class III/IV congestive heart failure
• Restenosis of ipsilateral prior carotid endarterectomy	• Unstable angina: Canadian Cardiovascular Society Class III/IV angina pectoris
• Previous neck irradiation	• Recent myocardial infarction
• Prior radical neck dissection	• Clinically significant cardiac disease (congestive heart failure, abnormal stress test, or need for coronary revascularization)
• Contralateral laryngeal nerve palsy	• Severe chronic obstructive pulmonary disease
• Presence of tracheostomy	• End-stage renal disease on dialysis

carotid stenosis. Rather, the debate now revolves around whether carotid angioplasty and stenting produces the same benefit that has been demonstrated by carotid endarterectomy. Since carotid artery stenting was approved by the FDA in 2004 for clinical application, this percutaneous procedure has become a treatment alternative in patients who are deemed "high-risk" for endarterectomy (Table 23-4). In contrast to many endovascular peripheral arterial interventions, percutaneous carotid stenting represents a much greater challenging procedure, because it requires complex, catheter-based skills using the 0.014-in guidewire system and distal protection device. Moreover, current carotid stent devices predominantly use the monorail guidewire system that requires more technical agility, in contrast to the over-the-wire catheter system that is routinely used in peripheral interventions. This percutaneous intervention often requires balloon angioplasty and stent placement through a long carotid guiding sheath via a groin approach. Poor technical skills can result in devastating treatment complications such as stroke, which can occur due in part to plaque embolization during the balloon angioplasty and stenting of the carotid artery. Because of these various procedural components that require high technical proficiency, many early clinical investigations of carotid artery stenting, which included physicians with little or no carotid stenting experience, resulted in alarmingly poor clinical outcomes. A recent Cochrane review noted that, before 2006, a total of 1269 patients had been studied in five randomized controlled trials comparing percutaneous carotid intervention and surgical carotid reconstruction.[32] Taken together, these trials revealed that carotid artery stenting had a greater procedural risk of stroke and death when compared to carotid endarterectomy (odds ratio 1.33; 95% CI 0.86–2.04). Additionally, greater incidence of carotid restenosis was noted in the stenting group than the endarterectomy cohorts. However, the constant improvement of endovascular devices, procedural techniques, and adjunctive pharmacologic therapy will likely improve the treatment success of percutaneous carotid intervention. Critical appraisals of these trials comparing the efficacy of carotid stenting vs. endarterectomy are available for review.[33] Several ongoing clinical trials will undoubtedly provide more insights on the efficacy of carotid stenting in the near future.

Surgical Techniques of Carotid Endarterectomy

Although carotid endarterectomy is one of the earliest vascular operations ever described and its techniques have been perfected in the last two decades, surgeons continue to debate many aspects of this procedure. For instance, there is no universal agreement with regard to the best anesthetic of choice, the best intraoperative cerebral monitoring, whether to "routinely" shunt, open vs. eversion endarterectomy, and patch vs. primary closure. Various anesthetic options are available for a patient undergoing carotid endarterectomy including general, local, and regional anesthesia. Typically, the anesthesia of choice depends on the preference of the surgeon, anesthesiologist, and patient. However, depending on the anesthetic given, the surgeon must decide whether intraoperative cerebral monitoring is necessary or intra-arterial carotid shunting will be used. In general, if the patient is awake, then his or her abilities to respond to commands during carotid clamp period determine the adequacy of collateral flow to the ipsilateral hemisphere. On the other hand, intraoperative electroencephalogram or transcranial power Doppler (TCD) has been used to monitor for adequacy of cerebral perfusion during the clamp period for patients undergoing surgery under general anesthesia. Focal ipsilateral decreases in amplitudes and slowing of electroencephalogram waves are indicative of cerebral ischemia. Similarly, a decrease to less than 50% of baseline velocity in the ipsilateral middle cerebral artery is a sign of cerebral ischemia. For patients with poor collateral flow exhibiting signs of cerebral ischemia, intra-arterial carotid shunting with removal of the clamp will restore cerebral flow for the remaining part of the surgery. Stump pressures have been used to determine the need for intra-arterial carotid shunting. Some surgeons prefer to shunt all patients on a routine basis and do not use intraoperative cerebral monitoring.

The patient's neck is slightly hyperextended and turned to the contralateral side, with a roll placed between the shoulder blades. An oblique incision is made along the anterior border of the sternocleidomastoid muscle centered on top of the carotid bifurcation (Fig. 23-17). The platysma is divided completely. Typically, tributaries of the anterior jugular vein are ligated and divided. The dissection is carried medial to the sternocleidomastoid. The superior belly of the omohyoid muscle is usually encountered just anterior to the CCA. This muscle can be divided. The carotid fascia is incised and the CCA is exposed. The CCA is mobilized cephalad toward the bifurcation. The dissection of the carotid bifurcation can cause reactive bradycardia related to stimulation of the carotid body. This reflex can be blunted with injection of lidocaine 1% into the carotid body or reversed with administration of IV atropine. A useful landmark in the dissection of the carotid bifurcation is the common facial vein. This vein can be ligated and divided. Frequently, the twelfth cranial nerve (hypoglossal nerve) traverses the carotid bifurcation just behind the common facial vein. The external carotid artery is mobilized just enough to get a clamp across. Often, a branch of the external carotid artery crossing to the sternocleidomastoid can be divided to allow further cephalad mobilization of the ICA. For high bifurcation, division of the posterior belly of the digastric muscle is helpful in establishing distal exposure of the ICA.

IV heparin sulfate (1 mg/kg) is routinely administered just before carotid clamping. The ICA is clamped first using a soft, noncrushing vascular clamp to prevent distal embolization. The external and common carotid arteries are clamped subsequently. A longitudinal arteriotomy is made in the distal CCA and extended into the bulb and past the occlusive plaque into the normal part of the ICA. Endarterectomy is carried out to remove the occlusive plaque (Fig. 23-18). If necessary, a temporary shunt can be inserted from the CCA to the ICA to maintain continuous antegrade cerebral blood flow (Fig. 23-19). Typically, a plane is teased out from the vessel wall, and the entire plaque is elevated and removed. The distal transition line in the ICA where the plaque had been removed must be examined carefully and should be smooth. Tacking sutures are placed when an intimal flap remains in this transition to ensure no obstruction to flow (Fig. 23-20). The occlusive plaque is usually removed from the origin of the external carotid artery using the eversion technique. The endarterectomized surface is then irrigated and any debris removed. A patch (autogenous saphenous vein, synthetic such as polyester, PTFE, or biologic material) is sewn to close the arteriotomy (Fig. 23-21). Whether patch closure is necessary in all patients and which patch is the best remain controversial. However, most surgeons agree that patch closure is indicated particularly for the small vessel (<7 mm). The eversion technique also has been advocated for removing the plaque from the ICA. In the eversion technique, the ICA is transected at the bulb, the edges of the divided vessel are everted, and the occluding plaque is "peeled" off the vessel wall. The purported advantages of the eversion technique are no need for patch closure and a clear visualization of the distal transition area. Reported series

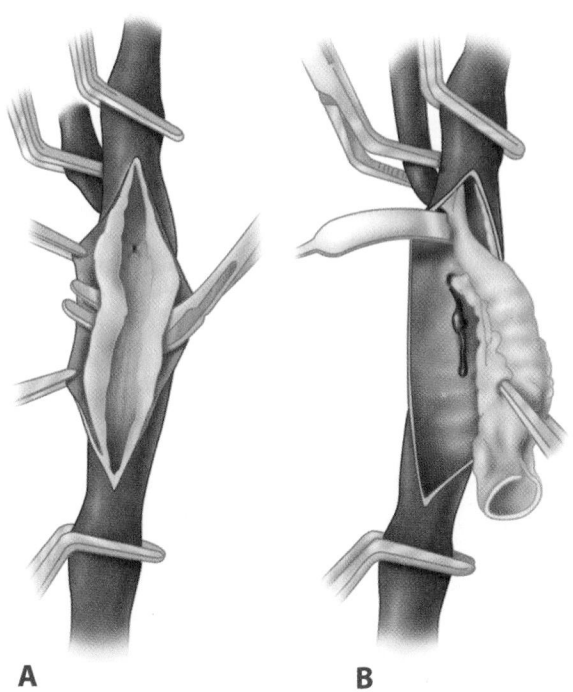

FIG. 23-18. A. During carotid endarterectomy, vascular clamps are applied in common carotid, external carotid, and internal carotid arteries. Carotid plaque is elevated from the carotid lumen. **B.** Carotid plaque is removed and the arteriotomy is closed either primarily or with a patch angioplasty.

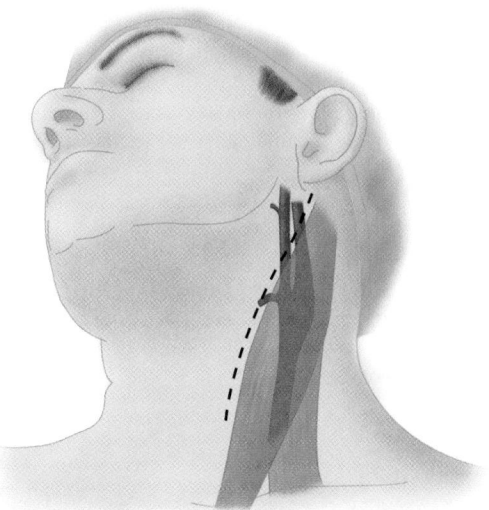

FIG. 23-17. To perform carotid endarterectomy, the patient's neck is slightly hyperextended and turned to the contralateral side. An oblique incision is made along the anterior border of the sternocleidomastoid muscle centered on top of the carotid bifurcation.

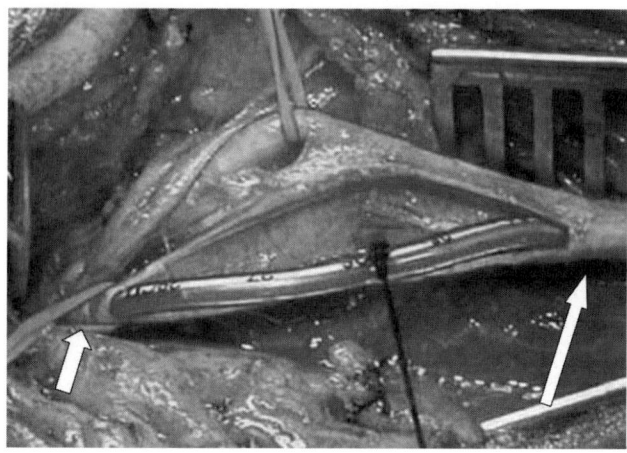

FIG. 23-19. A temporary carotid shunt is inserted from the common carotid artery (*long arrow*) to the internal carotid artery (*short arrow*) during carotid endarterectomy to provide continuous antegrade cerebral blood flow.

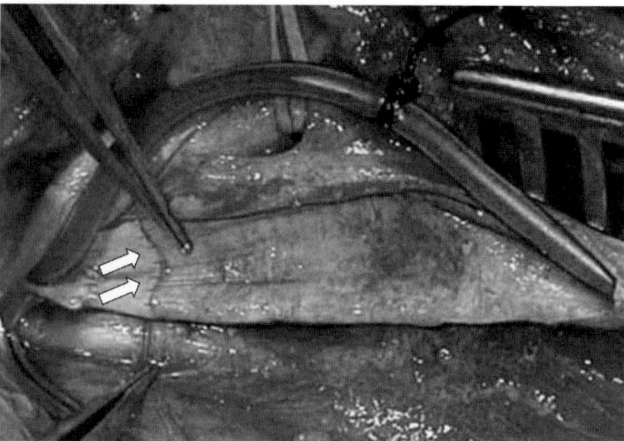

FIG. 23-20. The distal transition line (left side of the picture) in the internal carotid artery where the plaque had been removed must be examined carefully and should be smooth. Tacking sutures (*arrows*) are placed when an intimal flap remains in this transition to ensure no obstruction to flow.

have not shown a clear superiority of one technique over the others.[34] Surgeons will likely continue to use the technique of their choice. Just before completion of the anastomosis to close the arteriotomy, it is prudent to flush the vessels of any potential debris. When the arteriotomy is closed, flow is restored to the external carotid artery first and to the ICA second. IV protamine sulfate can be given to reverse the effect of heparin anticoagulation following carotid endarterectomy. The wound is closed in layers. After surgery, the patient's neurologic condition is assessed in the operating room (OR) before transfer to the recovery area.

Complications of Carotid Endarterectomy

Most patients tolerate carotid endarterectomy very well and typically are discharged home within 24 hours after surgery. Complications after endarterectomy are infrequent but can be potentially life threatening or disabling. Acute ipsilateral stroke is a dreaded complication following carotid endarterectomy. Cerebral ischemia can be due to either intraoperative or postoperative events. Embolizations from the occlusive plaque or prolonged cerebral ischemia are potential causes of intraoperative stroke. The most common cause of postoperative stroke is due to embolization. Less frequently, acute carotid artery occlusion can cause acute postoperative stroke. This is usually due to carotid artery thrombosis related to closure of the arteriotomy, an occluding intimal flap, or distal carotid dissection. When patients experience acute symptoms of neurologic ischemia after endarterectomy, immediate intervention may be indicated. Carotid duplex scan can be done expeditiously to assess

patency of the extracranial ICA. Re-exploration is mandated for acute carotid artery occlusion. Cerebral angiography can be useful if intracranial revascularization is considered.

Local complications related to surgery include excessive bleeding and cranial nerve palsies. Postoperative hematoma in the neck after carotid endarterectomy can lead to devastating airway compromise. Any expanding hematoma should be evacuated and active bleeding stopped. Securing an airway is critical and can be extremely difficult in patients with large postoperative neck hematomas. The reported incidence of postoperative cranial nerve palsies after carotid endarterectomy varies from 1 to 30%.[35] Well-recognized injuries involve the marginal mandibular, vagus, hypoglossal, superior laryngeal, and recurrent laryngeal nerves. Often these are traction injuries but can also be due to severance of the respective nerves.

Techniques of Carotid Angioplasty and Stenting

Percutaneous carotid artery stenting has become an accepted alternative treatment in the management of patients with carotid bifurcation disease (Fig. 23-22). The perceived advantages of percutaneous carotid revascularization are related to the minimal invasiveness of the procedure compared to surgery. There are anatomical conditions based on angiographic evaluation in which carotid artery stenting should be avoided due to increased procedural-related risks (Table 23-5). In preparation for carotid stenting, the patient should be given oral clopidogrel 3 days before the intervention if the patient was not already taking the drug. The procedure is done in either the OR with angiographic capabilities or in a dedicated angiography room. The

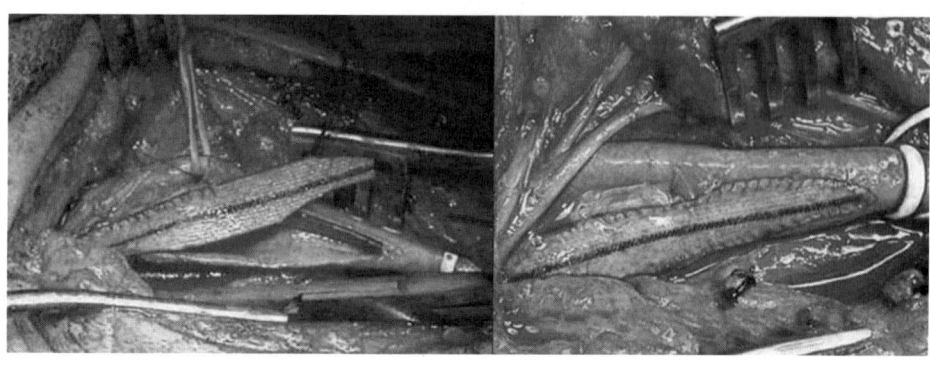

A **B**

FIG. 23-21. A. An autologous or synthetic patch can be used to close the carotid arteriotomy incision, which maintains the luminal patency. **B.** A completion closure of carotid endarterectomy incision using a synthetic patch.

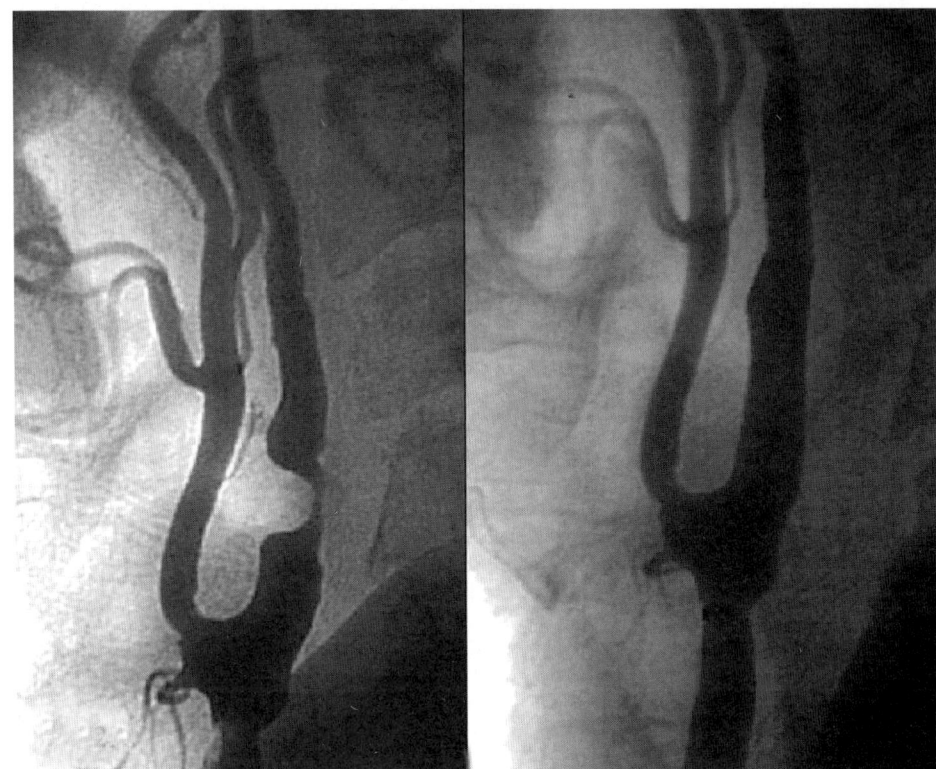

FIG. 23-22. A. Carotid angiogram demonstrated a high-grade stenosis of the left internal carotid artery. **B.** Completion angiogram demonstrating a satisfactory result following a carotid stent placement.

A   **B**

patient is placed in the supine position. The patient's BP and cardiac rhythm are closely monitored.

To gain access to the carotid artery, a retrograde transfemoral approach is most commonly used as the access site for carotid intervention. Using the Seldinger technique, a diagnostic 5F or 6F sheath is inserted in the CFA. A diagnostic arch aortogram is obtained. The carotid artery to be treated is then selected using a 5F diagnostic catheter, and contrast is injected to show the carotid anatomy. It is important to assess the contralateral carotid artery, vertebrobasilar, and intracranial circulation if these are not known based on the preoperative, noninvasive studies. Once the decision is made to proceed with carotid artery stenting, with the tip of the diagnostic catheter still in the CCA, a 0.035-in, 260-cm long stiff glide wire is placed in the ipsilateral external carotid artery. Anticoagulation with IV bivalirudin bolus (0.75mg/kg) followed by an infusion rate of 2.5 mg/kg per hour for the remainder of the procedure is routinely administered. Next, the diagnostic catheter is withdrawn and a 90-cm 6F guiding sheath is advanced into the CCA over the stiff glide wire. It is critical not to advance the sheath beyond the occlusive plaque in the carotid bulb. The stiff wire is then removed and preparation is made to deploy the distal embolic protection device (EPD). Several distal EPDs are available (Table 23-6). The EPD device is carefully deployed beyond the target lesion. With regard to the carotid stents, there are several stents that have received approval from the FDA and are commercially available for carotid revascularization (Table 23-7). All current carotid stents use the rapid-exchange monorail 0.014-in platform. The size selection is typically based on the size of CCA. Predilatation using a 4-mm balloon may be necessary to allow passage of the stent delivery catheter. Once the stent is deployed across the occlusive plaque, postdilatation is usually performed using a 5.5-mm or less balloon. It's noteworthy that balloon dilation of the carotid bulb may lead to immediate bradycardia due to stimulation of the glossopharyngeal nerve. The EPD is then retrieved and the procedure is completed with removal of the sheath from the femoral artery. The puncture site is closed using an available closure device or with manual compression. Throughout the procedure, the patient's neurologic function is closely monitored. The bivalirudin infusion is stopped, and the patient is kept on clopidogrel (75 mg daily) for at least 1 month and aspirin indefinitely.

TABLE 23-5	Unfavorable carotid angiographic appearance in which carotid stenting should be avoided

- Extensive carotid calcification
- Polypoid or globular carotid lesions
- Severe tortuosity of the common carotid artery
- Long segment stenoses (>2 cm in length)
- Carotid artery occlusion
- Severe intraluminal thrombus (angiographic defects)
- Extensive middle cerebral artery atherosclerosis

TABLE 23-6	Commonly used embolic protection devices (EPDs)

Mechanism	Name of EPD	Pore Size (micrometers)
Distal balloon occlusion	PercuSurge Guard Wire, Export catheter (Medtronic)	N/A
Distal filter	Angioguard (Cordis)	100
	Accunet (Abbott)	150
	Emboshield (Abbott)	140
	FilterWire (Boston Scientific)	110
	SpiderRx (EV3)	<100
Flow reversal[a]	Parodi Neuro Protection (Gore)	N/A

N/A = not applicable.
[a]Currently in clinical trial (EMPIRE) in United States.

TABLE 23-7	Currently approved carotid stents in the United States			
Name of Stent	Manufacturer	Cell Design	Tapered Stent	Delivery System Size (F)
Acculink	Abbott	Open	Yes	6
Exact	Abbott	Closed	Yes	6
NexStent	Boston Scientific	Closed	Self-tapering	5
Protégé RX	EV3	Open	Yes	6
Precise RX	Cordis	Open	No	6
Exponent	Medtronic	Open	No	6

Complications of Carotid Stenting

Although there have been no randomized trials comparing carotid stenting with and without EPD, the availability of EPDs appears to have reduced the risk of distal embolization and stroke. The results of the various clinical trials and registries of carotid stenting have been reported and compared. It is well known that distal embolization as detected by TCD is much more frequent with carotid stenting, even with EPD, when compared to carotid endarterectomy. However, the clinical significance of the distal embolization detected by TCD is not clear, as most are asymptomatic. Acute carotid stent thrombosis is rare. The incidence of instent carotid restenosis is not well known but is estimated at 10 to 30%. Duplex surveillance shows elevated peak systolic velocities within the stent after carotid stenting can occur frequently. However, velocity criteria are being formulated to determine the severity of instent restenosis after carotid stenting by ultrasound duplex.[36] It appears that systolic velocities exceeding 300 to 400 cm/s would represent greater than 70 to 80% restenosis. Bradycardia and hypotension occurs in up to 20% of patients undergoing carotid stenting.[37] Systemic administration of atropine is usually effective in reversing the bradycardia. Other technical complications of carotid stenting are infrequent and include carotid artery dissection, and access site complications such as groin hematoma, femoral artery pseudoaneurysm, distal embolization, and acute femoral artery thrombosis.

Non-Atherosclerotic Disease of the Carotid Artery
Carotid Coil and Kink

A carotid coil consists of an excessive elongation of the ICA producing tortuosity of the vessel (Fig. 23-23). Embryologically, the carotid artery is derived from the third aortic arch and dorsal aortic root, and is uncoiled as the heart and great vessels descend into the mediastinum. In children, carotid coils appear to be congenital in origin. In contrast, elongation and kinking of the carotid artery in adults is associated with the loss of elasticity and an abrupt angulation of the vessel. Kinking is more common in women than men. Cerebral ischemic symptoms caused by kinks of the carotid artery are similar to those from atherosclerotic carotid lesions, but are more likely due to cerebral hypoperfusion than embolic episodes. Classically, sudden head rotation, flexion, or extension can accentuate the kink and provoke ischemic symptoms. Most carotid kinks and coils are found incidentally on carotid duplex scan. However, interpretation of the Doppler frequency shifts and spectral analysis in tortuous carotid arteries can be difficult because of the uncertain angle of insonation. Cerebral angiography, with multiple views taken in neck flexion, extension, and rotation, is useful in the determination of the clinical significance of kinks and coils.

Fibromuscular Dysplasia

FMD usually involves medium-sized arteries that are long and have few branches (Fig. 23-24). Women in the fourth or fifth decade of life are more commonly affected than men. Hormonal effects on the

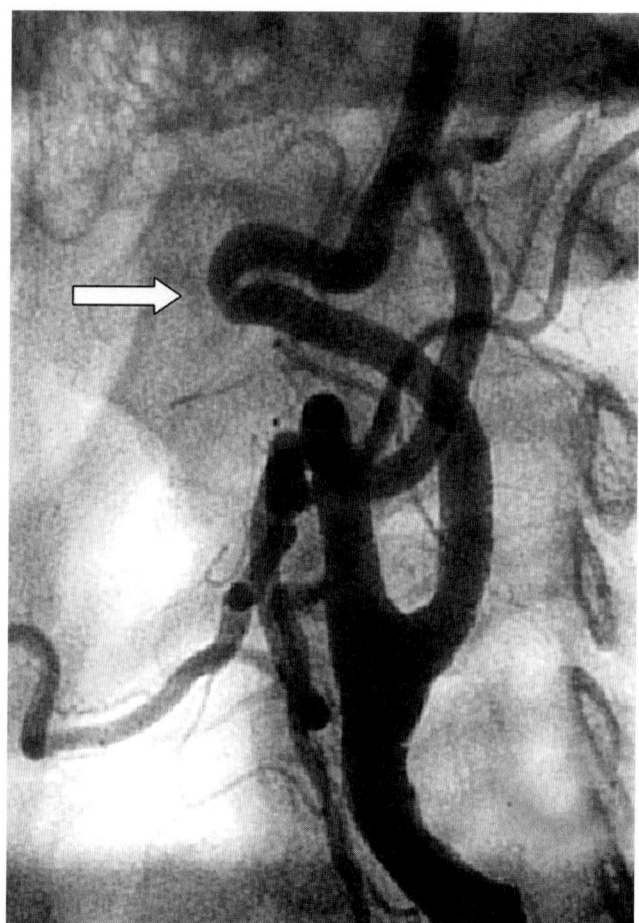

FIG. 23-23. Excessive elongation of the carotid artery can result in carotid kinking (*arrow*), which can compromise cerebral blood flow and lead to cerebral ischemia.

vessel wall are thought to play a role in the pathogenesis of FMD. FMD of the carotid artery is commonly bilateral, and in about 20% of patients, the vertebral artery also is involved.[38] An intracranial saccular aneurysm of the carotid siphon or middle cerebral artery can be identified in up to 50% of the patients with FMD. Four histological types of FMD have been described in the literature. The most common type is medial fibroplasia, which may present as a focal stenosis or multiple lesions with intervening aneurysmal outpouchings. The disease involves the media with the smooth muscle being replaced by fibrous connective tissue. Commonly, mural dilations and microaneurysms can be seen with this type of FMD. Medial hyperplasia is a rare type of FMD, with the media demonstrating excessive amounts of smooth muscle. Intimal fibroplasia accounts for 5% of all cases and occurs equally in both sexes. The media and adventitia remain normal, and there is accumulation of subendothelial mesenchymal cells with a loose matrix of connective tissue causing a focal stenosis in adults. Finally, premedial dysplasia represents a type of FMD with elastic tissue accumulating between the media and adventitia. FMD also can involve the renal and the external iliac arteries. It is estimated that approximately 40% of patients with FMD present with a TIA due to embolization of platelet aggregates.[38] DSA demonstrates the characteristic "string of beads" pattern, which represents alternating segments of stenosis and dilatation. The string of beads can also be shown noninvasively by CTA or MRA. FMD should be suspected when an increased velocity is detected across a stenotic segment without associated atherosclerotic changes on carotid duplex ultrasound. Antiplatelet medication is the generally accepted therapy for asymptomatic

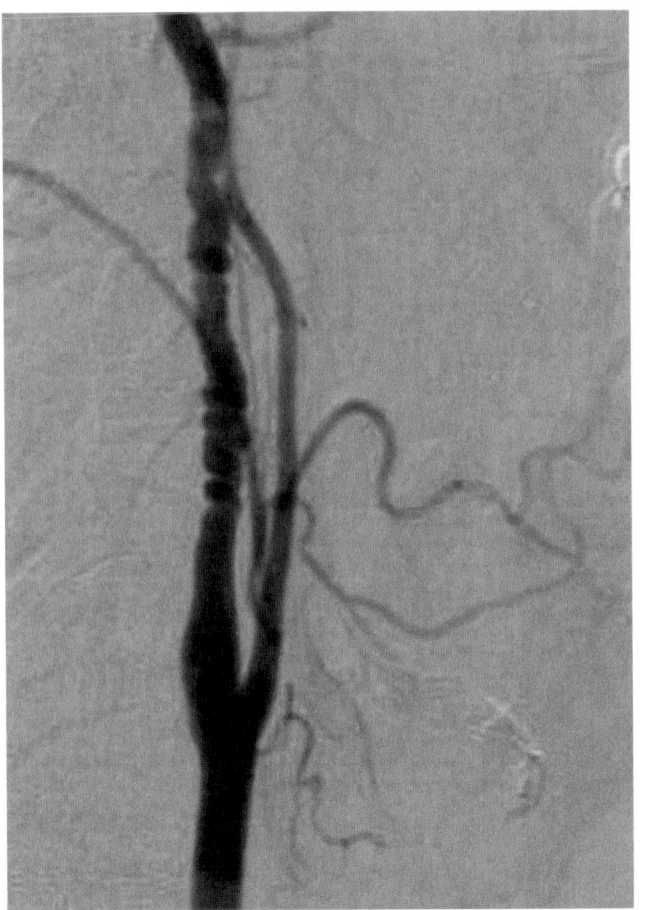

FIG. 23-24. A carotid fibromuscular dysplasia with typical characteristics of multiple stenosis with intervening aneurysmal outpouching dilatations. The disease involves the media, with the smooth muscle being replaced by fibrous connective tissue.

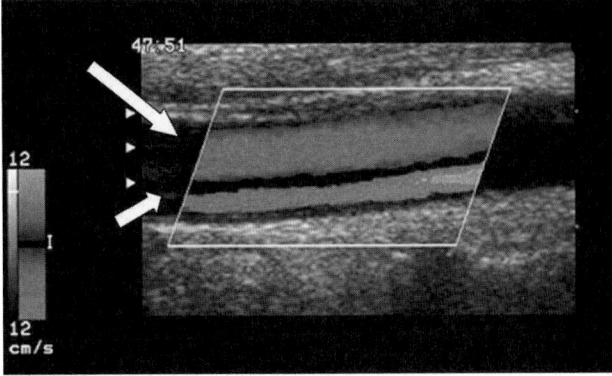

FIG. 23-25. Carotid ultrasound reveals a patient with a carotid artery dissection in which carotid flow is separated in the true flow lumen (*long arrow*) from the false lumen (*short arrow*).

lesions. Endovascular treatment is recommended for patients with documented lateralizing symptoms. Surgical correction is rarely indicated.

Carotid Artery Dissection

Dissection of the carotid artery accounts for approximately 20% of strokes in patients younger than 45 years of age. The etiology and pathogenesis of spontaneous carotid artery dissection remains incompletely understood. Arterial dissection involves hemorrhage within the media, which can extend into the subadventitial and subintimal layers. When the dissection extends into the subadventitial space, there is an increased risk of aneurysm formation. Subintimal dissections can lead to intramural clot or thrombosis. Traumatic dissection is typically a result of hyperextension of the neck during blunt trauma, neck manipulation, strangulation, or penetrating injuries to the neck. Even in supposedly spontaneous cases, a history of preceding unrecognized minor neck trauma is not uncommon. Connective disorders such as Ehlers-Danlos syndrome, Marfan syndrome, alpha$_1$-antitrypsin deficiency, or FMD may predispose to carotid artery dissection. Iatrogenic dissections also can occur due to catheter manipulation or balloon angioplasty.

Typical clinical features of carotid artery dissection include unilateral neck pain, headache, and ipsilateral Horner's syndrome in up to 50% of patients, followed by manifestations of the cerebral or ocular ischemia and cranial nerve palsies. Neurologic deficits can result either because of hemodynamic failure (caused by luminal stenosis) or by an artery to artery thromboembolism. The ischemia may cause TIAs or infarctions, or both. Catheter angiography has

been the method of choice to diagnose arterial dissections, but with the advent of duplex ultrasonography, MRI/MRA, and CTA, most dissections can now be diagnosed using noninvasive imaging modalities (Fig. 23-25). The dissection typically starts in the ICA distal to the bulb. Uncommonly, the dissection can start in the CCA, or is an extension of a more proximal aortic dissection. Medical therapy has been the accepted primary treatment of symptomatic carotid artery dissection. Anticoagulation (heparin and warfarin) and antiplatelet therapy have been commonly used, although there have not been any randomized studies to evaluate their effectiveness. The prognosis depends on the severity of neurologic deficit but is generally good in extracranial dissections. The recurrence rate is low. Therapeutic interventions have been reserved for recurrent TIAs or strokes, or failure of medical treatment. Endovascular options include intra-arterial stenting, coiling of associated pseudoaneurysms, or more recently, deployment of covered stents.

Carotid Artery Aneurysms

Carotid artery aneurysms are rare, encountered in less than 1% of all carotid operations (Fig. 23-26). The true carotid artery aneurysm generally is due to atherosclerosis or medial degeneration. The carotid bulb is involved in most carotid aneurysms, and bilaterality is present in 12% of the patients. Patients typically present with a pulsatile neck mass. The available data suggest that, untreated, these aneurysms lead to neurologic symptoms from embolization. Thrombosis and rupture of the carotid aneurysm is rare. Pseudoaneurysms of the carotid artery can result from injury or infection. Mycotic aneurysms often involve syphilis in the past, but are now more commonly associated with peritonsillar abscesses caused by *Staphylococcus aureus* infection. FMD and spontaneous dissection of the carotid artery can lead to the formation of true aneurysms or pseudoaneurysms. Whereas conventional surgery has been the primary mode of treatment in the past, carotid aneurysms are currently being treated more commonly using endovascular approaches.[39]

Carotid Body Tumor

The carotid body originates from the third branchial arch and from neuroectodermal-derived neural crest lineage. The normal carotid body is located in the adventitia or periadventitial tissue at the bifurcation of the CCA (Fig. 23-27). The gland is innervated by the glossopharyngeal nerve. Its blood supply is derived predominantly from the external carotid artery, but also can come from the vertebral artery. Carotid body tumor is a rare lesion of the neuroendocrine system. Other glands of neural crest origin are seen in the neck, parapharyngeal spaces, mediastinum, retroperitoneum, and adrenal medulla. Tumors involving these structures have been referred to as *paraganglioma*, *glomus tumor*, or *chemodectoma*.

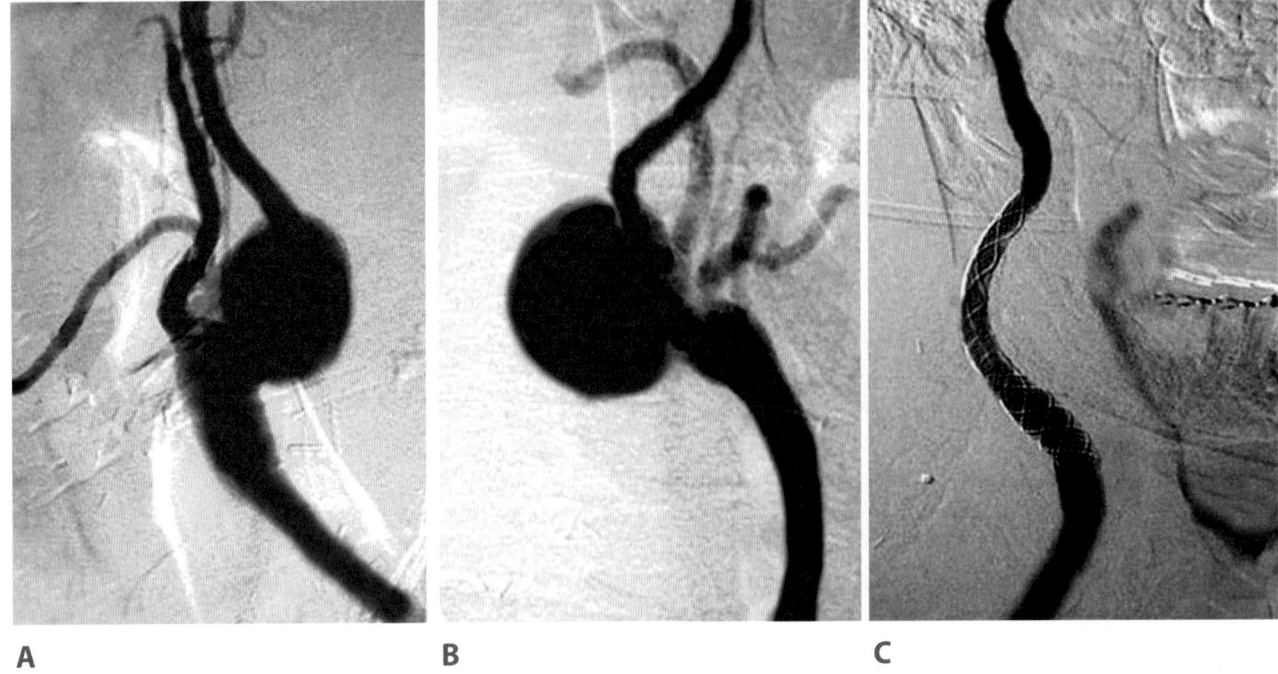

FIG. 23-26. A. An anteroposterior angiogram of the neck revealing a carotid artery aneurysm. **B.** A lateral projection of the carotid artery aneurysm. **C.** Following endovascular placement, the carotid artery aneurysm is successfully excluded.

Approximately 5 to 7% of carotid body tumors are malignant. Although chronic hypoxemia has been invoked as a stimulus for hyperplasia of carotid body, approximately 35% of carotid body tumors are hereditary. The risk of malignancy is greatest in young patients with familial tumors.

Symptoms related to the endocrine products of the carotid body tumor are rare. Patients usually present between the fifth and seventh decade of life with an asymptomatic lateral neck mass. The diagnosis of carotid body tumor requires confirmation on imaging studies. Carotid duplex scan can localize the tumor to the carotid bifurcation, but CT or MR imaging usually is required to further delineate the relationship of the tumor to the adjacent structures. Classically, a carotid body tumor will widen the carotid bifurcation. The Shamblin classification describes the tumor extent: I. tumor is <5 cm and relatively free of vessel involvement; II. tumor is intimately involved but does not encase the vessel wall; and III. tumor is intramural and encases the carotid vessels and adjacent nerves.[40] With good resolution CT and MR imaging, arteriography usually is not required. However, arteriography can provide an assessment of the vessel invasion and intracranial circulation, and

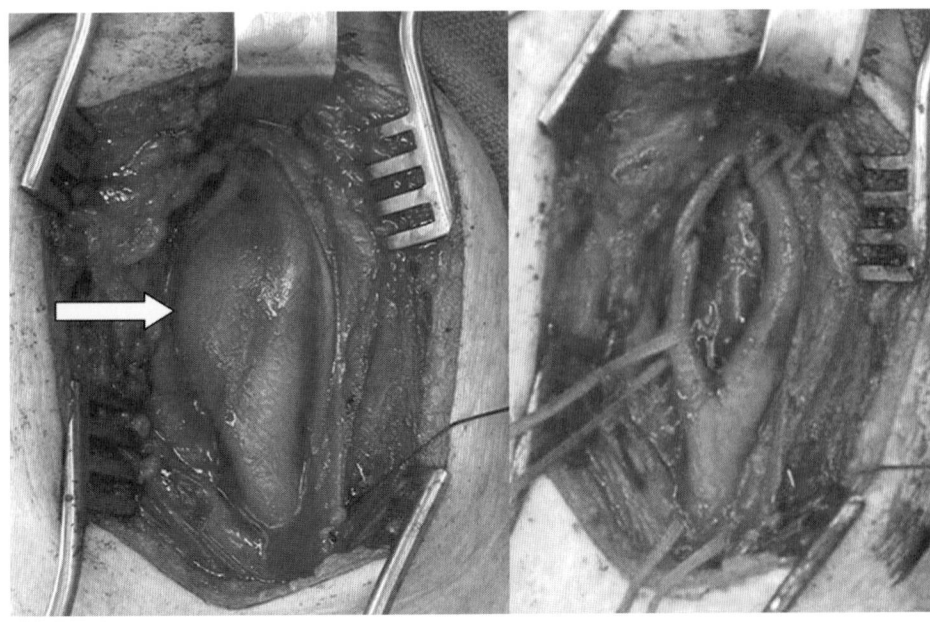

FIG. 23-27. A. A carotid body tumor (*arrow*) located adjacent to the carotid bulb. **B.** Following peri-adventitial dissection, the carotid body tumor is removed.

allows for preoperative embolization of the feeder vessels, which has been reported to reduce intraoperative blood loss. Surgical resection is the recommended treatment for suspected carotid body tumor.

Carotid Trauma

Blunt or penetrating trauma to the neck can cause injury to the carotid artery. Notwithstanding the massive bleeding from carotid artery transection, injury to the carotid artery can result in carotid dissection, thrombosis, or pseudoaneurysm formation. Carotid duplex ultrasound can be useful to locate the site of injury in the cervical segment of the carotid artery. Spiral CTA has become the modality of choice to detect extracranial carotid artery injury. Confirmation of carotid injury by contrast cerebral angiography remains the gold standard diagnostic test. Injuries to the cervical segment of the common and internal carotid arteries can be repaired surgically. Acute carotid artery thrombosis usually is treated medically with anticoagulation if the patient is asymptomatic. Revascularization should be considered for patients presenting with ongoing cerebral ischemia related to carotid artery thrombosis. Traumatic carotid artery dissection can cause cerebral ischemia due to thromboembolization, decreased flow, or thrombosis. Commonly, the dissection involves the distal portion of the cervical and petrous segment of the ICA. Medical management with antiplatelet or anticoagulation usually is adequate for uncomplicated traumatic carotid dissection. In patients with pseudoaneurysms of the carotid artery that are located in a segment that is out of surgical reach, the use of selective coil embolization of the pseudoaneurysm or exclusion of the pseudoaneurysm by a covered stent graft has been reported. Bare metal stent has been used with success in the treatment of traumatic carotid artery dissection.

ABDOMINAL AORTIC ANEURYSM

In spite of more than 50,000 patients undergoing elective repair of abdominal aortic aneurysm (AAA) each year in the United States, approximately 15,000 patients die annually as a result of ruptured aneurysm, making it the tenth leading cause of death in men in this country.[41] The incidence appears to be increasing, and this is due in part to improvements in diagnostic imaging and, more importantly, is a result of a growing elderly population. With early diagnosis and timely intervention, aneurysm rupture–related death is largely preventable. Conventional treatment of an AAA involves replacing the aneurysmal segment of the aorta with a prosthetic graft, with the operation performed through a large abdominal incision. Techniques for this open abdominal surgery have been refined, adapted, and extensively studied by vascular surgeons over the past four decades. Despite a well-documented, low perioperative mortality rate of 2 to 3% in large academic institutions, the thought of undergoing an open abdominal aortic operation often provokes a sense of anxiety in many patients due in part to the postoperative pain associated with the large abdominal incision as well as the long recovery time needed before the patient can return to normal physical activity.

The most common location of aortic aneurysms is the infrarenal aorta. Endovascular stent graft placement represents a revolutionary and minimally invasive treatment for infrarenal AAAs that only requires 1 to 2 days of hospitalization, and the patient can return to normal physical activity within 1 week. The concept of using an endoluminal device in the management of vascular disease was first proposed by Dotter and colleagues, who successfully treated a patient with iliac occlusion using transluminal angioplasty in 1964.[42] Nearly three decades later, Parodi and colleagues reported the first successful endovascular repair of AAA using a stent graft device.[13] Since then, a variety of stent graft technologies have been developed to treat the AAA. The rapid innovation of this new treatment modality has undoubtedly captured the attention of patients with aortic aneurysms as well as physicians who practice endovascular therapy. Physicians in general should be knowledgeable regarding available treatment options to provide adequate evaluation and education to patients and their families. The following discussion is to outline the treatment options for AAAs, including conventional repair and endovascular approach. Advantages and potential complications of these treatments also will be addressed.

Natural History of Aortic Aneurysm

The natural history of an AAA is to expand and rupture. AAA exhibits a "staccato" pattern of growth, where periods of relative quiescence may alternate with expansion. Therefore, although an individual pattern of growth cannot be predicted, average aggregate growth is approximately 3 to 4 mm/y. There is some evidence to suggest that larger aneurysms may expand faster than smaller aneurysms, but there is significant overlap between the ranges of growth rates at each strata of size.

Rupture risk appears to be directly related to aneurysm size as predicted by Laplace's law. Although more sophisticated methods of assessing rupture risk based on finite element analysis of wall stress is under active investigation, maximum transverse diameter remains the standard method of risk assessment for aneurysm rupture. In the past, AAA rupture risk has been overestimated. More recently, two landmark studies have served to better define the natural history of AAA.[43,44] Based on best available evidence, the annualized risk of rupture is given in Table 23-8. The rupture risk is quite low for aneurysms <5.5 cm and begins to rise exponentially thereafter. This size can serve as an appropriate threshold for recommending elective repair provided one's surgical mortality is below 5%. For each size strata, however, women appear to be at higher risk for rupture than men, and a lower threshold of 4.5 to 5.0 cm may be reasonable in good-risk patients. Although data are less compelling, a pattern of rapid expansion of >0.5 cm within 6 months can be considered a relative indication for elective repair. Aneurysms that fall below these indications may safely be followed with CT or ultrasound at 6-month intervals, with long-term outcomes equivalent to earlier surgical repair. Interestingly, in the ADAM study, 80% of all patients with AAA who were followed in this manner eventually came to repair within 5 years.[44]

Unless symptomatic or ruptured, AAA repair is a prophylactic repair. The rationale for recommending repair is predicated on the assumption that the risk of aneurysm rupture exceeds the combined risk of death from all other causes such as cardiopulmonary disease and cancer. On the other hand, our limitation in predicting timing and cause of death is underscored by the observation that over 25% of patients who were deemed unfit for surgical repair because of their comorbidities died from rupture of their aneurysms within 5 years.

Clinical Manifestations

Most AAAs are asymptomatic, and they are usually found incidentally during work-up for chronic back pain or kidney stones. Physical

TABLE 23-8	Annualized risk of rupture of abdominal aortic aneurysm (AAA) based on size		
Description	**Diameter of Aorta (cm)**	**Estimated Annual Risk of Rupture (%)**	**Estimated 5-y Risk of Rupture (%)**[a]
Normal aorta	2–3	0	0 (unless AAA develops)
Small AAA	4–5	1	5–10
Moderate AAA	5–6	2–5	30–40
Large AAA	6–7	3–10	>50
Very large AAA	>7	>10	Approaching 100

[a]The estimated 5-y risk is more than five times the estimated annual risk because over that 5 y, the AAA, if left untreated, will continue to grow in size.

examination is neither sensitive nor specific except in thin patients. Large aneurysms may be missed in the obese, while normal aortic pulsations may be mistaken for an aneurysm in thin individuals. Rarely, patients present with back pain and/or abdominal pain with a tender pulsatile mass. Patients with these symptoms must be treated as if they had a rupture until proven otherwise. If the patient is hemodynamically stable and the aneurysm is intact on a CT scan, the patient is admitted for BP control with IV antihypertensive agents and repaired usually within 12 to 24 hours or at least during the same hospitalization. In contrast, patients who are hemodynamically unstable with a history of acute back pain and/or syncope, and a known unrepaired AAA or a pulsatile abdominal mass should be immediately taken to the OR with a presumed diagnosis of a ruptured AAA.

Overall mortality of AAA rupture is 71 to 77%, which includes all out-of-hospital and inhospital deaths, as compared to 2 to 6% for elective open surgical repair.[45] Nearly one half of all patients with ruptured AAA will die before reaching the hospital. For the remainder, surgical mortality is 45 to 50% and has not substantially changed in the last 30 years.

Relevant Anatomy

An AAA is defined as a pathologic focal dilation of the aorta that is >30 mm or 1.5 times the adjacent diameter of the normal aorta (Fig. 23-28). Male aortas tend to be larger than female, and there is generalized growth of the aortic diameter with each decade of life. Ninety percent of AAA are infrarenal in location and have a fusiform morphology. There is a higher predilection for juxtarenal and suprarenal AAA in women as compared to men. Concomitant common iliac and/or hypogastric artery aneurysms can be found in 20 to 25% of patients. Although the etiology of most aortic aneurysms is atherosclerotic, clinically significant peripheral occlusive disease is unusual and present in less than 10% of all cases.

Although extravascular anatomy is important for open surgical repair of AAA, intravascular anatomy and aortoiliac morphology are important for endovascular repair. Pertinent anatomic dimensions include the diameter of the proximal, nondilated, infrarenal aortic neck, which can range from 18 to 30 mm, CIA, from 8 to 16 mm, and external iliac arteries, 6 to 10 mm. Morphologically, the aortic neck can manifest complex angulation above and below the renal arteries due to a combination of elongation and anterolateral displacement by the posterior bulge of the aneurysmal aorta. Furthermore, the shape of the proximal neck is rarely tubular, but often is conical, reverse conical, or barrel shaped. Distally, the iliac arteries can have severe tortuosity with multiple compound turns. Although not significant from a hemodynamic standpoint, severe iliac calcifications combined with extreme tortuosity can pose a formidable challenge during endovascular repair.

Diagnostic Evaluation

Preoperative evaluation should include routine history and physical examination with particular attention to (a) any symptoms referable to the aneurysm, which may impact the timing of repair, (b) a history of pelvic surgery or radiation, in the event retroperitoneal exposure is required or interruption of hypogastric circulation is planned, (c) claudication suggestive of significant iliac occlusive disease, (d) LE bypass or other femoral reconstructive procedures, and (e) chronic renal insufficiency or contrast allergy.

Cross-sectional imaging is required for definitive evaluation of AAA. Although ultrasound is safe, widely available, relatively accurate, and inexpensive, and, therefore, is the screening modality of choice, the CT scan remains the gold standard for determination of anatomic eligibility for endovascular repair. Size of AAA may differ up to 1 cm between CT and ultrasound, and, during longitudinal follow-up, comparisons should be made between identical modalities. With modern multirow detector scanners, a timed-bolus IV contrast enhanced, 2.5 to 3.0-mm slice spiral CT of the chest, abdomen, and pelvis can be performed in <30 seconds with a single breath hold. Extremely high-resolution images are obtained with submillimeter spatial resolution (Fig. 23-29). Proper window level and width (brightness and contrast) is important for discrimination among aortic wall, calcific plaque, thrombus, and lumen. The only major drawback to CT is the risk of contrast nephropathy in diabetics and in patients with renal insufficiency.

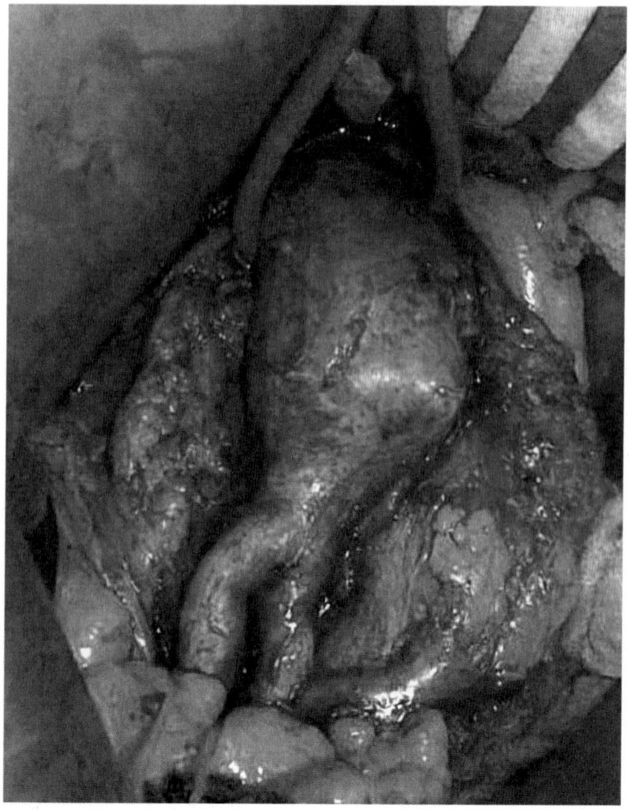

FIG. 23-28. An operative view of an infrarenal aortic aneurysm.

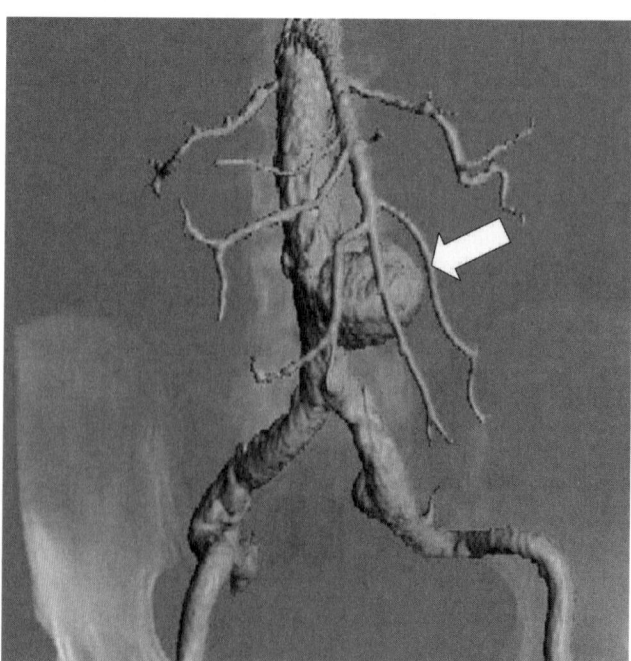

FIG. 23-29. High resolution of image displaying an aortic aneurysm (*arrow*) can be achieved with multidetector computed tomographic angiography.

The spiral technique further affords the ability for three-dimensional reconstruction. Three-dimensional reconstructions can yield important morphologic information that is critical to endovascular therapy. Using third-party software, these images can be viewed and manipulated on a desktop computer and so-called "center-line" (transverse slices perpendicular to the central flow-lumen of the aorta) diameter and length measurements obtained. Conventional angiography has a minimal role in the current management of AAA. Angiography is invasive with an increased risk of complications. Indications for angiography are isolated to concomitant iliac occlusive disease (present in less than 10% of patients with AAA) and unusual renovascular anatomy.

Surgical Repair of Abdominal Aortic Aneurysm

General anesthesia is necessary when performing a conventional open AAA repair. Although a retroperitoneal incision is a well-accepted surgical approach, a midline transabdominal incision remains the more common approach for open aortic aneurysm operation. Because the abdominal incision can lead to significant pain and discomfort, an epidural catheter can be placed before the operation for postoperative analgesic infusion to provide pain control. Once the abdominal cavity is opened, the small intestines and transverse colon are retracted to expose the retroperitoneum overlying the AAA. The retroperitoneum is next divided, followed by isolation of both proximal and distal segments of the AAA. IV heparin (100 IU/kg) is given, followed by clamping of the proximal and distal segments of the aneurysm. The aneurysm sac is opened next, and a prosthetic graft is used to reconstruct the aorta. If the aneurysm only involved the abdominal aorta, a tube graft can be used to replace the aorta (Fig. 23-30). If the aneurysm extends distally to the iliac arteries, a prosthetic bifurcated graft is used for either an aortobi-iliac or aortobifemoral bypass reconstruction (Fig. 23-31). The overlying aneurysm sac and the retroperitoneum are closed to cover the prosthetic bypass graft to minimize potential bowel contact to the graft. Small and large intestines are returned to the abdominal cavity followed by the closure of the abdominal fascia and skin.

Advantages and Risks of Open Abdominal Aortic Aneurysm Repair

The main advantage of a conventional open repair is that the AAA is permanently eliminated because it is entirely replaced by a prosthetic aortic graft. The risk of aneurysm recurrence or delayed rupture no longer exists. As a result, long-term imaging surveillance is not needed with these patients. In contrast, the long-term efficacy of endovascular repair remains unclear. Consequently, long-term imaging surveillance is critical to ensure that the aortic aneurysm remains properly sealed by the stent graft. Other potential advantages of open repair include direct assessment of the circulatory integrity of the colon. If signs of colonic ischemia become evident after aortic bypass grafting, a concomitant mesenteric artery bypass can be performed to revascularize the colonic circulation. In addition, open repair permits the surgeons to explore for other abdominal pathologies such as GI tumors, liver mass, or cholelithiasis.

As for the risks associated with open repair, cardiac complications, in the form of either myocardial infarction or arrhythmias, remain the most common morbidity, with an incidence between 2 and 6%.[46] Another significant complication is renal failure or transient renal insufficiency as a result of perioperative hypotension, atheromatous embolization, inadvertent injury to the ureter, preoperative contrast-induced nephropathy, or suprarenal aortic clamp-

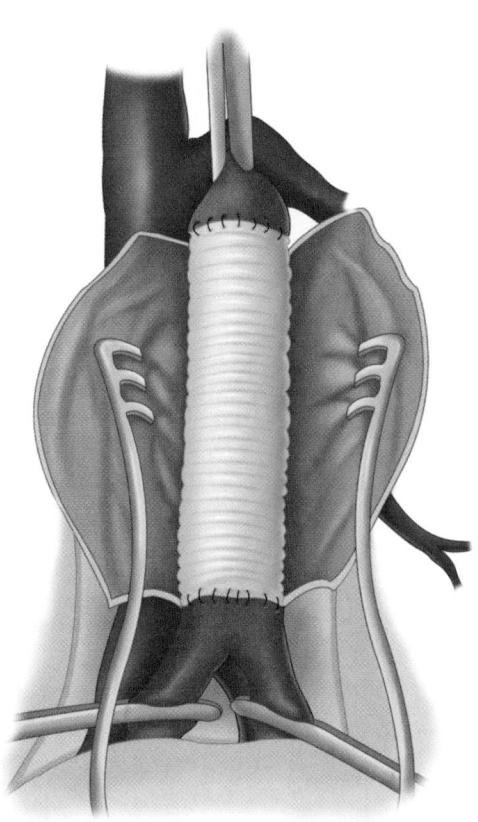

A

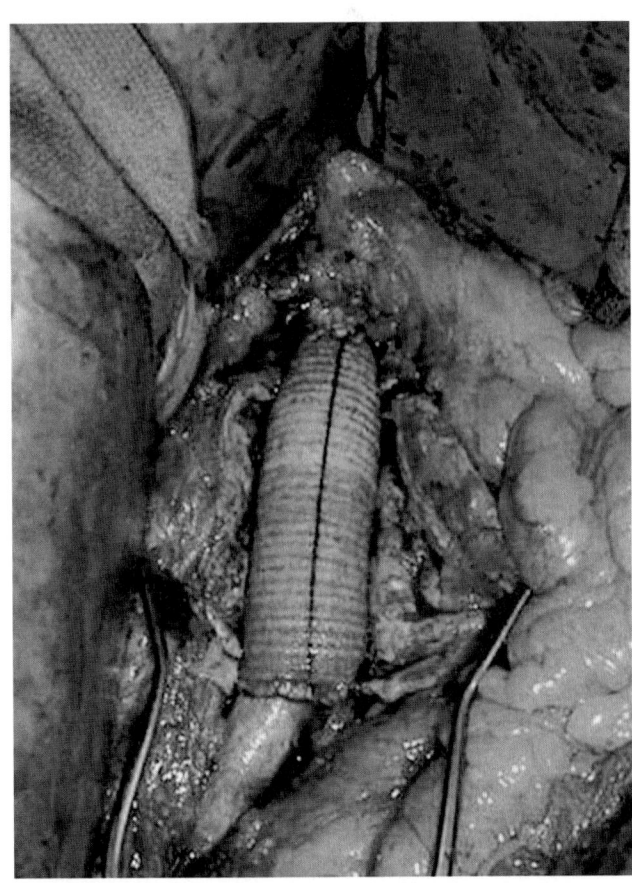

B

FIG. 23-30. A. Schematic depiction of an aortic tube graft used to repair an aortic aneurysm. **B.** Intraoperative image of an aortic tube graft reconstruction.

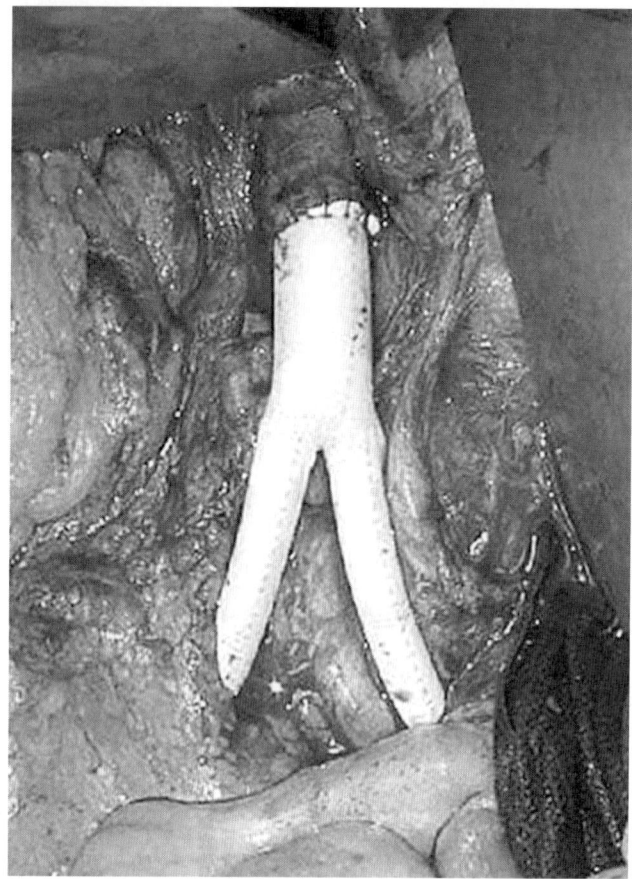

FIG. 23-31. Intraoperative view of a bifurcated graft used to repair an aortic aneurysm.

ing. Although the incidence of renal failure is less than 2% in elective aneurysm repair, it can occur in more than 20% of patients after repair of a ruptured AAA.[46]

Ischemic colitis is a devastating potential complication after open repair. The likelihood of such a complication is highest in those who had a prior colon resection and undergo repair of a ruptured AAA, due to the loss of collateral blood supply to the rectosigmoid colon. It is estimated that 5% of patients who undergo elective aneurysm repair will develop partial-thickness ischemic colitis but without significant clinical sequelae.[47] However, if the partial-thickness ischemia progresses to full-thickness gangrene and peritonitis, mortality can be as high as 90%.[47]

The incidence of prosthetic graft infection ranges between 1 and 4% after open repair.[47] It is more common in those who undergo repair of a ruptured AAA. If the prosthetic graft is not fully covered by the aneurysm sac or retroperitoneum, intestinal adhesion with subsequent bowel erosion may occur, resulting in an aortoenteric fistula. The predominant sign of such a complication is massive hematemesis, and it typically occurs years after the operation. Despite these potential complications, however, the majority of patients who undergo successful elective open repair have an uneventful recovery.

Endovascular Repair of Abdominal Aortic Aneurysm

More than a decade has passed since the first report of human implantation of a homemade stent graft for endovascular repair of an AAA by Parodi in 1991.[3] Several prospective clinical trials across different devices and analysis of large Medicare administrative databases and meta-analyses of published literature have consistently demonstrated significantly decreased operative time, blood loss, hospital length of stay, and overall perioperative morbidity and mortality of endovascular repair as compared to open surgical repair. For patients who are at increased risk for surgery because of age or comorbidity, endovascular repair is a superior, minimally invasive alternative.

The principle of endovascular repair of AAA involves the implantation of an aortic stent graft that is fixed proximally and distally to the nonaneurysmal aortoiliac segment, and thereby endoluminally excludes the aneurysm from the aortic circulation (Fig. 23-32). Unlike open surgical repair, endovascular treatment does not remove or eliminate the aneurysm sac, which therefore is subjected to potential aneurysm expansion or even rupture as persistent aneurysm sac pressurization may occur following endograft implantation. Importantly, aortic branches such as lumbar arteries or the inferior mesenteric artery (IMA) are ligated, which can lead to persistent aneurysm pressurization and aneurysm expansion. Currently, five devices are available for elective repair of

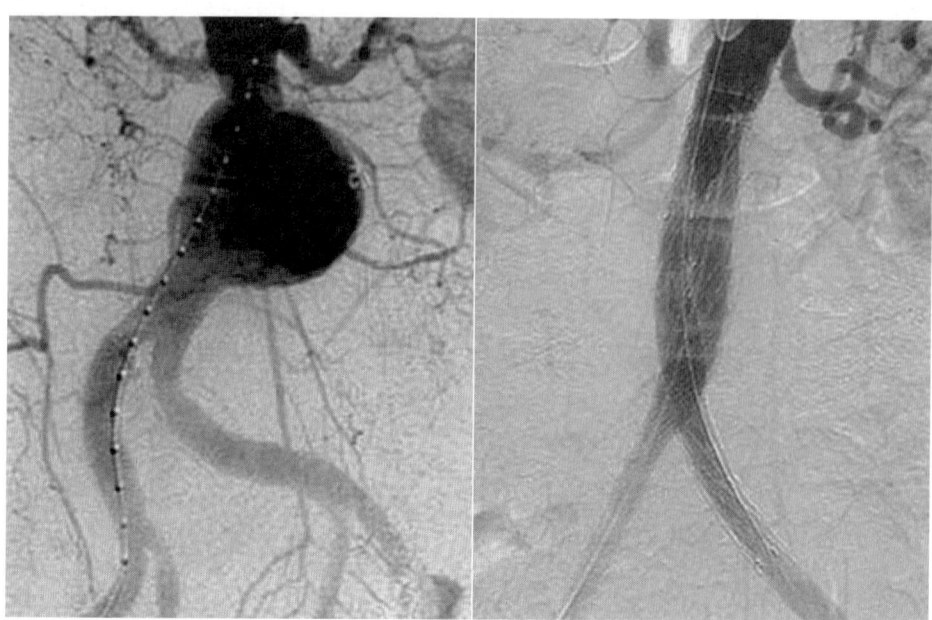

A   **B**

FIG. 23-32. A. An aortogram demonstrating a large, infrarenal, abdominal aortic aneurysm. **B.** Following endovascular stent graft implantation, the aortic aneurysm is successfully excluded.

intact infrarenal AAA: (a) AneuRx device (Medtronic/AVE, Santa Rosa, Calif), (b) Gore Excluder device (WL Gore & Associates, Flagstaff, Ariz), (c) Endologix Powerlink device (Endologix Inc., Irvine, Calif), (d) Zenith device (Cook Inc., Bloomington, Ind), and (e) Talent device (Medtronic/AVE, Santa Rosa, Calif). Despite some differences in physical appearance, mechanical properties, and materials, they will be discussed collectively in this chapter. They are all modular devices consisting of a primary device or main body and one or two iliac limbs that insert into the main body to complete the repair. Depending on the device, there are varying degrees of flexibility in the choice of iliac limbs that can be matched to the main body, which can impact the customizability for a particular anatomy.

Patient Selection for Endovascular Aortic Aneurysm Repair

Anatomic eligibility for endovascular repair is mainly based on three areas: the proximal aortic neck, CIAs, and the external iliac and common femoral arteries, which relate to the proximal and distal landing zones or fixation sites and the access vessels, respectively. The requirements for the proximal aortic neck are a diameter of 18 to 28 mm and a minimum length of 15 mm (Table 23-9). Usually, multiple measurements of the diameter are taken along the length of the neck to assess its shape. All diameter measurements are midwall to midwall of the vessel. Secondary considerations include mural calcifications (<50% circumference), luminal thrombus (<50% circumference), and angulation (<45°). Presence of a significant amount of any one of these secondary features in combination with a relatively short proximal neck may compromise successful short- and long-term fixation of the stent graft and exclusion of the aneurysm. The usual distal landing zone is the CIA. The EIA may serve as an alternate site when the ipsilateral CIA is aneurysmal or ectatic. The treatable diameters of CIAs range from 8 to 20 mm, and there should be at least 20 mm of patent artery of uniform diameter to allow adequate fixation. And finally, at least one of two common femoral and external iliac arteries must be at least 7 mm in diameter to safely introduce the main delivery sheath. Slightly smaller iliac diameters may be tolerated depending on the specific device and in the absence of severe tortuosity and calcific disease. Difficult access is one of the main causes of increased procedural times and intraoperative complications. Using these criteria, approximately 60% of all AAA are anatomic candidates for endovascular repair.

The next step in the preoperative planning is device selection. Typically, the proximal diameter of the main device is oversized by 10 to 20% of the nominal diameter of the aortic neck. Distally, the iliac limbs are oversized by 1 to 4 mm depending on the individual device's instructions for use. The biggest challenge to proper device selection remains determining the optimal length from the renal arteries to the hypogastric arteries. Despite availability of sophisticated three-dimensional reconstructions, the exact path that a device will take from the proximal aortic neck to the distal iliac arteries is difficult to predict. It is dependent on a host of factors related to the mechanical properties of the stent graft and the morphology of the aortoiliac flow lumen. "Plumb-line" measurements of axial CT images can be quite inaccurate, typically grossly underestimating the length, while center-line measurements usually overestimate the length. Angiographic measurements using a marker catheter are invasive, require contrast and radiation exposure, and also are inaccurate because the marker catheter fails to take into account the stiffness of the stent graft. The consequences of not choosing the correct length of the device include inadvertent coverage of the hypogastric artery if too long and the need for additional devices if too short.

Advantages and Risks of Endovascular Repair

The obvious advantage of an endovascular AAA repair is its minimally invasive nature. Typically, patients who undergo this procedure stay in the hospital for only 1 to 3 days, in contrast to the 5- to 10-day stay required after conventional open surgical repair. In most clinical practices, patients who have had an endovascular repair are routinely transferred to a general vascular ward from the postanesthesia recovery unit, avoiding admission to a more costly intensive care unit (ICU).

Because an abdominal incision is not necessary in endovascular repair, the procedure is particularly beneficial in patients with severe pulmonary disease such as chronic obstructive pulmonary disease or emphysema. Patients can sustain adequate breathing in the postoperative period, thereby avoiding respiratory complications or prolonged mechanical ventilation. Because the abdominal cavity has not been entered, the risk of GI complications such as ileus, ventral hernia, or bowel obstruction due to intestinal adhesion also is greatly reduced. Moreover, regional or epidural anesthesia can be used, avoiding the risks associated with general anesthesia in patients with severe cardiopulmonary dysfunction.

Despite its many advantages, endovascular repair does have potential complications. Because the stent graft device is attached endoluminally within the abdominal aorta, an endoleak due to incomplete stent graft exclusion of the aneurysm can occur. With this type of leak, blood flow persists outside the lumen of the endoluminal graft but within an aneurysm sac. A meta-analysis of 1118 patients who underwent successful endovascular repair found an endoleak incidence of 24%.[48] Although a small endoleak usually poses little clinical significance because it will typically become thrombosed spontaneously, a large or persistent endoleak may lead to continuous aneurysm perfusion and ultimately to aneurysm rupture. The rupture rate following an endovascular AAA repair has been reported to be <0.8%.[49]

Stent graft iliac limb dysfunction resulting in thrombosis has been reported following endovascular repair.[16,48] One possible cause is aneurysm remodeling, resulting in a shortening in the aortic length, which can cause the stent graft to kink. Alternatively, progression of an underlying iliac atherosclerotic lesion may cause compression of the iliac limb and ultimately result in graft-limb occlusion. Treatment options include thrombolysis or graft thrombectomy to determine the underlying cause and possibly additional stent graft placement. Renal artery occlusion may occur due to improper stent graft positioning or migration.[16,46,48] Graft limb separation or dislocation also has been reported.[16,46,48]

In patients with AAA and concurrent iliac artery aneurysms who undergo preoperative coil embolization of the internal iliac artery, 20 to 45% experience symptoms of pelvic ischemia.[50] These symptoms may include buttock claudication, impotence, gluteal skin sloughing, and colonic ischemia. Other complications pertaining to endovascular repair relate to the access site and include groin hematoma and wound infection. Occasionally, the stent graft device can malfunction by either failing to deploy or dislodging during the deployment procedure.[16,49] If the device cannot be salvaged or rescued endoluminally, open surgical repair of the aneurysm may be necessary.

Technical Considerations of Endovascular Aortic Aneurysm Repair

Although endovascular AAA repair may be performed in any venue with appropriate digital fluoroscopic imaging capability, due to the

TABLE 23-9	Ideal characteristics of an aneurysm for endovascular abdominal aortic aneurysm repair
Neck length (mm)	>15
Neck diameter (mm)	>18, <32
Aortic neck angle (°)	<60
Neck mural calcification (% circumference)	<50
Neck luminal thrombus (% circumference)	<50
Common iliac artery diameter (mm)	between 8–20
Common iliac artery length (mm)	>20
External iliac artery diameter (mm)	>7

need for absolute sterility and aseptic technique, it is most safely performed in a surgical suite. The patient is prepped and draped just as in open AAA repair. Patients with renal insufficiency should be started on perioperative oral *N*-acetylcysteine and sodium bicarbonate infusion to reduce the risk of contrast nephropathy. A variety of anesthetic options may be used. Regional anesthesia may be appropriate for patients with pulmonary disease. There are reports of success with local anesthetics alone, as the incisions are typically smaller than a typical open inguinal hernia repair.[51]

Bilateral transverse oblique incisions are made just below the inguinal ligament to expose approximately 2 to 3 cm of common femoral arteries and obtain proximal control. Special attention is paid to avoid the groin crease to decrease the risk of wound complications. Some have advocated a completely percutaneous access using the "pre-close" technique with the Perclose suture-mediated vascular closure device (Abbott Perclose, Redwood City, Calif). Review of reported series on this technique suggest a technical success rate of 95% for medium size sheaths ranging from 12F to 16F, and 75% success for 18F to 24F sizes.

Transfemoral access is obtained using standard Seldinger technique. Initial soft-tipped starter guidewires are exchanged for stiff guidewires that are advanced to the thoracic arch. IV heparin at 80 IU/kg is administered and the activated clotting time is maintained at 200 to 250 seconds. These guidewires provide the necessary support for the subsequent introduction of the large-diameter delivery catheters and devices. In the absence of special anatomic considerations, the primary device is inserted through the right side and the contralateral iliac limb is inserted through the left side. After administration of heparin, the delivery catheter or the introducer sheath is advanced to the L1–L2 vertebral space, which typically marks the location of the renal arteries. An angiographic catheter is advanced from the contralateral femoral artery to the same level.

A road-mapping aortogram is obtained to localize the renal arteries. The primary device is rotated to the desired orientation and deployed immediately below the lowest renal artery (Fig. 23-33). The angiographic catheter is replaced with a directional catheter and an angled guidewire, and the opening for the contralateral limb on the main device is cannulated. Intrastent passage of the guidewire is confirmed, and the angled guidewire is replaced with a stiff guidewire. The contralateral iliac limb is inserted into the docking opening of the primary device and deployed. A completion angiogram is performed looking for patency of the renal and hypogastric arteries, the device limbs, proximal and distal fixation, and endoleak. Adjunctive interventions, including additional devices, balloons, bare stents, etc., are performed as needed. The procedure is concluded with routine repairs of the femoral arteries and closure of the groin incisions. The patients are recovered in the recovery room for 2 to 4 hours and admitted to the general care floor. Although in the past, patients were admitted to the ICU, this is rarely needed. Most patients can be started on a regular diet that evening and discharged the next morning.

Surveillance following Endovascular Aortic Aneurysm Repair

Lifelong follow-up is essential to the long-term success after endovascular AAA repair. Indeed, one may go so far as to say that absence of appropriate follow-up is tantamount to not having had a repair at all. A triple-phase (noncontrast, contrast, delayed) spiral CT scan and a four-view (anteroposterior, lateral, and two obliques) abdominal x-ray should be obtained within the first month. Subsequent imaging can be obtained at 6-month intervals in the first 1 to 2 years and yearly thereafter. After the first 6 months, patients who cannot travel easily may obtain their studies locally and submit them for review. The CT scan is for detection of endoleaks, subtle proximal migrations, and changes in aneurysm size. The abdominal x-ray gives a "bird's-eye" view of the overall morphology of the stent graft. Subtle changes in conformation of the iliac limbs relative to each other and/or the spine can provide early signs of impending

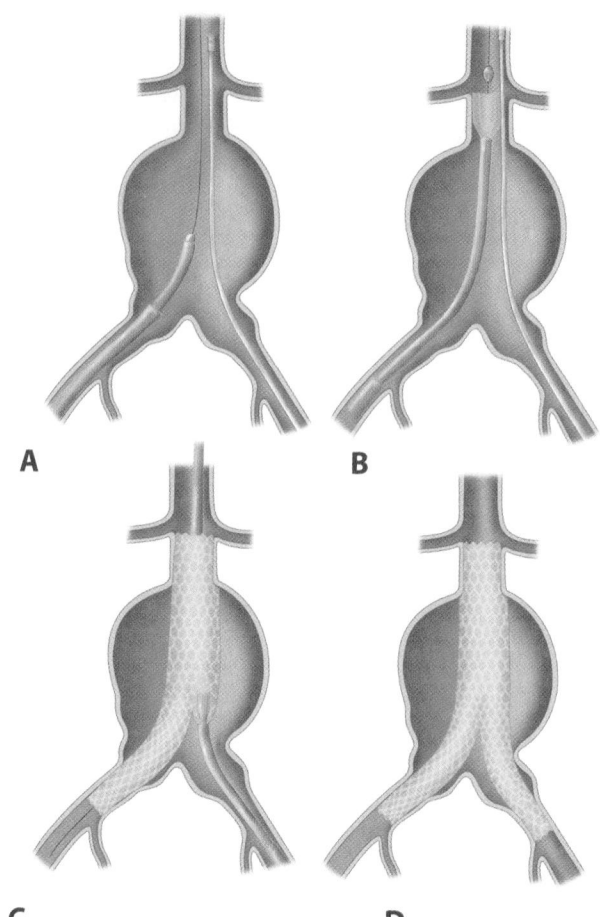

FIG. 23-33. A. During an endovascular aortic aneurysm repair, the main endograft device is inserted through a femoral artery approach. **B.** The device is deployed in the aorta just below the renal arteries. **C.** A contralateral iliac endograft device is inserted through a contralateral gate opening that is next deployed. **D.** Completion deployment of the endograft device should fully exclude an aortic aneurysm while arterial flow to the renal and hypogastric arteries should remain patent.

component separation or loss of fixation. Further, stent fractures and/or suture breaks that can compromise long-term device integrity sometimes only can be detected on a plain film and not on a CT scan.

Results from Clinical Studies Comparing Endovascular vs. Open Repair

The primary success rate after endovascular repair of AAA has been reported to be as high as 95%.[16,45] The less invasive nature of this procedure is appealing to many physicians and patients. In addition, virtually all reports indicate decreased blood loss, transfusion requirements, and length of ICU and hospital stay for endovascular repair of AAAs when compared to the standard surgical approach.[16,45,52] With the advent of bifurcated grafts and improved delivery systems in the future, the only real limitation will be cost. When evaluating the literature for results from clinical series, it is important to look at a comparison of endoluminal vs. open repair, device specific outcome, and cost analysis studies.

Early reports on results with endovascular repair were often flawed due to selection biases. This is because from its inception, endovascular repair has been used mostly in patients who are at higher risk for open repair. At the same time, only patients with favorable anatomy including less tortuosity and the presence of a suitable infrarenal neck were considered for endovascular repair. Randomization is also difficult because most patients who anatomically qualify for endovascular repair would withdraw from the study if randomized to open repair. Consequently, there are very few randomized, controlled trials that have compared outcomes in patients with similar risk factors and anatomy that are eligible for both types of repair. Two such European trials have published short-term outcome data that are unbiased in design.

The DREAM trial is a multicenter randomized trial that compared open vs. endovascular repair among a group of 345 patients at 28 European centers using multiple different devices including: Gore, AneuRx, and Zenith.[53] Patients were included only if they were considered to be candidates for both types of repairs. The operative mortality rate was 4.6% in the operative group vs. 1.2% in the endoluminal group at 30 days. When looking at the combined rate of operative mortality and severe complications, there was an incidence of 9.8% in the open-repair vs. 4.7% in the endoluminal group. The difference here was largely due to the higher frequency of pulmonary complications seen in the open group. There was a higher incidence of graft-related complications in the endoluminal group. There was no difference in the nonvascular-local complication rate among the two groups.

The EVAR-1 trial is also a multicenter randomized trial that compared open to endoluminal repair.[52] This study was conducted on 1082 patients at 34 centers in the United Kingdom using all available devices. Short-term mortality at 30 days was 4.7% in the open and 1.7% in the endoluminal group. The inhospital mortality rate was also increased in the open when compared to the endoluminal group (6.2 to 2.1%). As expected, the secondary-intervention rate was higher in the endoluminal group (9.8 to 5.8%). Complication rates were not reported with the EVAR-1 trial. There are criticisms that can be applied to both of these trials. Patients had to be eligible for either type of repair to be included in the study. Consequently, these findings cannot be generalized for patients who are too sick to undergo open surgery or in those patients whose anatomy precludes them from undergoing endovascular repair.

Device-Specific Outcome

Matsmura and associates compared endoluminal to open repair using the Excluder device.[54] In their review, they demonstrated a 30-day mortality rate of 1% along with an endoleak rate of 17 and 20% at 1 and 2-year intervals.[54] The limb narrowing, limb migration, and trunk migration were all 1% at 2 years. There were no deployment failures or early conversions. There was an annual 7% reintervention rate. Aneurysm growth was demonstrated in 14% of patients at 2 years. The Zenith device by Cook has been studied by Greenberg and associates, who compared standard surgical repair to endoluminal repair in low-risk patients as well as endoluminal repair in high-risk patients.[55] They reported a 30-day mortality rate

of 3.5% that was equal to the open group. The rate of endoleak was 7.4 and 5.4% at 1 and 2-year intervals. There was a 5.3% migration of 5 mm after 1 year. Freedom from rupture was 100% in the low-risk and 98.9% in the high-risk endoluminal group at 2 years. Experience with the AneuRx device has been reported by Zarins and associates.[56] In their 4-year review, they found a 30-day mortality rate of 2.8%. Endoleak rate at 4 years was 13.9%, aneurysm enlargement was 11.5%, and stent graft migration was 9.5%. Freedom from rupture was noted to be 98.4% at 4 years. Criado and associates have reported on their 1-year experience with the Talent LPS device by Medtronic.[57] They report a 30-day mortality rate of 0.8%. Endoleak rate was 10%. Three deployment failures were noted, and freedom from rupture was 100%. Aneurysm growth and migration rates were divided into three different neck-size groups. Patients with a wide neck (>26 mm) had a 3% growth and migration rate. Narrow-neck patients (<26 mm) had a 1% growth rate and a 2% migration rate. Interestingly, short-neck patients (<15 mm) had no aneurysm growths and a 2% migration rate.

Cost Analysis

The current climate of cost containment and limited reimbursement for heath care services mandates a critical analysis of the economic impact of any new medical technology on the market. The inhospital costs for both endovascular and open repair include graft cost, OR fees, radiology, pharmacy, ancillary care, ICU charges, and floor charges. Despite the improved morbidity and mortality rates, several early studies have reported no cost benefit with the application of endovascular repair.[58,59] The limiting factor appears to be the cost of the device. Despite commercialization of endovascular repair, the device costs are still in the range of $5000 to $6000 with no signs of abating. A recent report by Angle and associates further corroborates previous studies.[60] In their review, despite decreased hospital and ICU stays and use of pharmacy and respiratory services, cost of endovascular repair was 1.74 times greater than the standard surgical approach. In addition, these cost analysis studies are centered on inhospital costs and do not even begin to address secondary costs such as postoperative surveillance that is required with endovascular repair.

Classification and Management of Endoleak

An endoleak is an extravasation of contrast outside the stent graft and within the aneurysm sac (Fig. 23-34). It can be present in up to 20 to 30% of all endovascular AAA repairs in the early postoperative period.[61] In general, over one half of these endoleaks will resolve spontaneously during the first 6 months, resulting in a 10% incidence of chronic endoleaks in all cases beyond the first year of follow-up. Endoleaks can be detected using conventional angiography, contrast CT (Fig. 23-35), MRA (magnetic resonance angiography), and color flow duplex ultrasound. Although there is no

FIG. 23-34. Four types of endoleak that include: type I endoleak = attachment site leak; type II endoleak = side branch leak caused by lumbar or side branches; type III endoleak = endograft junctional leak due to overlapping device components; type IV endoleak = endograft fabric or porosity leak.

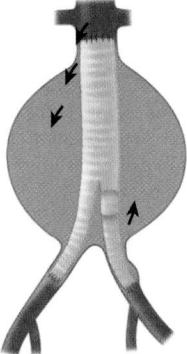
Type I endoleak

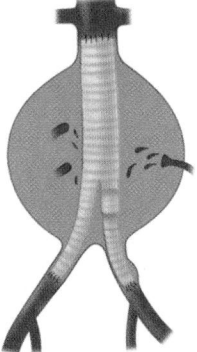
Type II endoleak

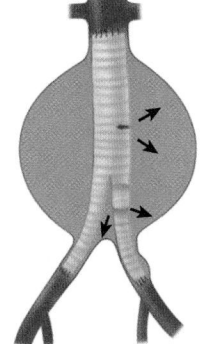
Type III endoleak

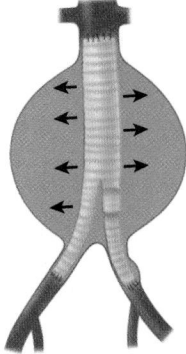
Type IV endoleak

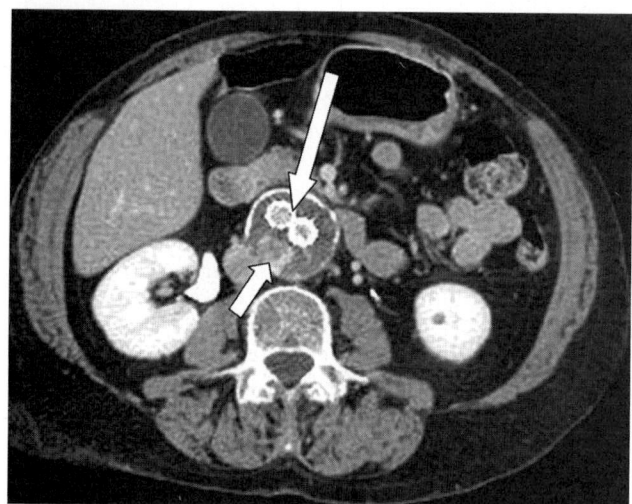

FIG. 23-35. A computed tomographic scan demonstrating an endoleak (*small arrow*) as evidenced by contrast flow outside the aortic endograft (*long arrow*).

recognized gold standard, in practice, angiography is considered the least sensitive but most specific for characterizing the source of the endoleak, while the CT scan is the most sensitive but least specific. Widespread availability and reliability that is relatively independent of technique have made the CT scan the de facto standard imaging modality for postoperative surveillance. Conversely, routine use of duplex ultrasound and MRA has been limited by the lack of proper equipment and local expertise. On the other hand, investigational techniques such as time-resolved MRA may provide greater sensitivity and specificity than either angiography or CT in the future.

Four types of endoleaks have been described (Table 23-10). *Type I endoleak* refers to fixation-related leaks that occur at the proximal or distal attachment sites. These represent less than 5% of all endoleaks and are seen as an early blush of contrast into the aneurysm sac from the proximal or distal ends of the device during completion angiography.[61,62] Although seen as a marker of poor patient selection or inadequate repair, over 80% of these leaks spontaneously seal in the first 6 months. Persistent type I endoleaks, on the other hand, require prompt treatment. *Type II endoleak* refers to retrograde flow originating from a lumbar, inferior mesenteric, accessory renal, or hypogastric artery. They are the most common type of endoleak, accounting for 20 to 30% of all cases, and about one half resolve spontaneously. On angiography, they are seen as a late filling of the aneurysm sac from a branch vessel(s). Type II endoleaks carry a relatively benign natural history and do not merit intervention unless associated with aneurysm growth. *Type III endoleaks* refer to a failure of device integrity or component separation from modular systems. If detected intraoperatively or in the early perioperative period, it is usually from inadequate overlap between two stent grafts, while in the late period, it may be from a fabric tear or junctional separation from conformational changes of

the aneurysm. Regardless of the etiology or timing, these should be promptly repaired. And lastly, *type IV endoleak* refers to the diffuse, early blush seen during completion angiography due to graft porosity and/or suture holes of some Dacron-based devices. It does not have any clinical significance and usually cannot be seen after 48 hours and heparin reversal. Endoleaks that have initially been considered type IV that persist become type III endoleaks by definition, as it indicates a more significant material defect than simple porosity or a suture hole.

Endotension following Endovascular Aortic Aneurysm Repair

In approximately 5% of cases after an apparently successful endovascular repair, the aneurysm continues to grow without any demonstrable endoleak.[63] This phenomenon has been described as *endotension*. Although it was initially thought that an endoleak was really present but simply not detected, cases have been reported where the aneurysm has been surgically opened and the contents were completely devoid of any blood and no extravasation could be found. The mechanism of continued pressurization of the aneurysm sac following successful exclusion from the arterial circulation remains unsolved at this time. One putative mechanism has been linked to a transudative process related to certain expanded PTFE graft materials.[64] More importantly, however, the natural history of these enlarging aneurysms without endoleaks is unknown, but to date there has been no evidence to suggest that they carry an increased risk of rupture. Conservatively speaking, until further, long-term data become available, if the patient is a suitable surgical risk, elective open conversion should be considered.

Secondary Interventions following Endovascular Aortic Aneurysm Repair

There is approximately a 10 to 15% per year risk of secondary interventions following endovascular AAA repair.[16,55,65] These procedures are critical in the long-term success of the primary procedure in prevention of aneurysm rupture and aneurysm-related death. These secondary procedures, in order of frequency, include proximal or distal extender placement for migrations, highly-selective or translumbar embolization for type II endoleaks, direct surgical or laparoscopic branch vessel ligations, bridging cuffs for component separations, and late open surgical conversions.

Multiple large series have reported an annual rupture rate of approximately 1 to 1.5% per year after endovascular repair.[16,55,65] The EUROSTAR registry reports a rupture rate of 2.3% over a 15-month period in patients with an endoleak, compared with 0.3% in those without.[66] Various causes of late ruptures have been reported in the literature, although presence of a persistent endoleak with aneurysm enlargement remains a common culprit for this complication. It has been shown that even successfully excluded aneurysm can lead to the development of attachment-site leaks and device failure, caused in part by aneurysm remodeling resulting in stent migration or kinking.[67]

Treatment of rupture may be open conversion or endovascular stent graft placement. May and associates reported a mortality rate of 43% in those patients who underwent open conversion.[68] Emergent endovascular repair should be considered in these patients because it is potentially much faster and incurs less physiologic stress than open conversion. Several reports have shown that endovascular repair can be performed successfully in patients previously treated with endoluminal prostheses.[69,70]

MESENTERIC ARTERY DISEASE

Vascular occlusive disease of the mesenteric vessels is a relatively uncommon but potentially devastating condition that generally presents in patients more than 60 years of age, is three times more frequent in women, and has been recognized as an entity since

TABLE 23-10	Endoleak classification
Classification	**Description**
Type I endoleak	Attachment site leak
Type II endoleak	Side branch leak caused by lumbar or inferior mesenteric artery
Type III endoleak	Junctional leak (of overlapping endograft components)
Type IV endoleak	Endograft fabric or porosity leak

1936.[71] The incidence of such a disease is low and represents 2% of the revascularization operations for atheromatous lesions. The most common cause of mesenteric ischemia is atherosclerotic vascular disease. Autopsy studies have demonstrated splanchnic atherosclerosis in 35 to 70% of cases.[72] Other etiologies exist and include FMD, panarteritis nodosa, arteritis, and celiac artery (CA) compression from a median arcuate ligament, but they are unusual and have an incidence of one in nine compared to that of atherosclerosis.

Chronic mesenteric ischemia is related to a lack of blood supply in the splanchnic region and is caused by disease in one or more visceral arteries: the celiac trunk, the SMA, and the IMA. Mesenteric ischemia is thought to occur when two of the three visceral vessels are affected with severe stenosis or occlusion; however, in as many as 9% of cases, only a single vessel is involved [superior mesenteric artery (SMA) in 5% and celiac trunk in 4% of cases].[73] This disease process may evolve in a chronic fashion, as in the case of progressive luminal obliteration due to atherosclerosis. On the other hand, mesenteric ischemia can occur suddenly, as in the case of thromboembolism. Despite recent progress in perioperative management and better understanding in pathophysiology, mesenteric ischemia is considered one of the most catastrophic vascular disorders, with mortality rates ranging from 50 to 75%. Delay in diagnosis and treatment are the main contributing factors in its high mortality. It is estimated that mesenteric ischemia accounts for one in every 1000 hospital admissions in this country. The prevalence is rising due in part to the increased awareness of this disease, the advanced age of the population, and the significant comorbidity of these elderly patients. Early recognition and prompt treatment before the onset of irreversible intestinal ischemia are essential to improve the outcome.

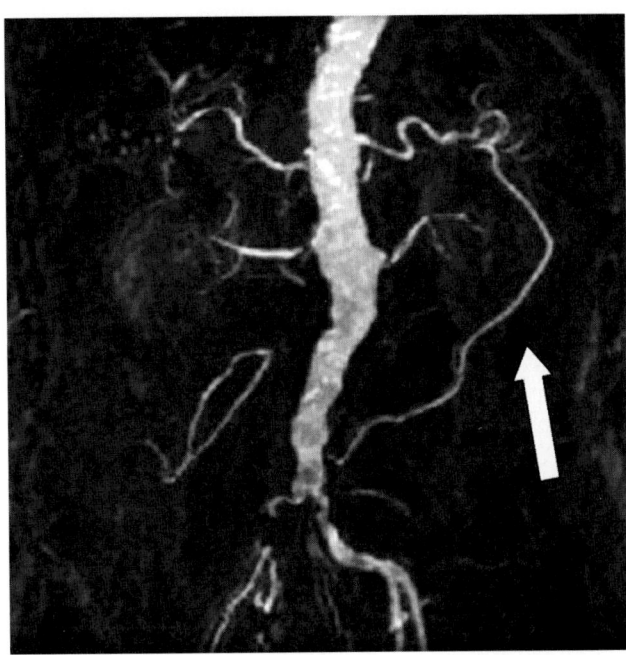

FIG. 23-36. An aortogram showing a prominent collateral vessel that is the arc of Riolan (*arrow*) in a patient with an inferior mesenteric artery occlusion. This vessel network provides collateral flow between the superior mesenteric artery and inferior mesenteric artery.

Anatomy and Pathophysiology

Mesenteric arterial circulation is remarkable for its rich collateral network. Three main mesenteric arteries provide the arterial perfusion to the GI system: the CA, SMA, and IMA. In general, the CA provides arterial circulation to the foregut (distal esophagus to duodenum), hepatobiliary system, and spleen; the SMA supplies the midgut (jejunum to midcolon); and the IMA supplies the hindgut (midcolon to rectum). The CA and SMA arise from the ventral surface of the infradiaphragmatic suprarenal abdominal aorta, while the IMA originates from the left lateral portion of the infrarenal aorta. These anatomic origins in relation to the aorta are important when a mesenteric angiogram is performed to determine the luminal patency. To fully visualize the origins of the CA and SMA, it is necessary to perform both an anteroposterior and a lateral projection of the aorta because most arterial occlusive lesions occur in the proximal segments of these mesenteric trunks.

Because of the abundant collateral flow between these mesenteric arteries, progressive diminution of flow in one or even two of the main mesenteric trunks is usually tolerated, provided that uninvolved mesenteric branches can enlarge over time to provide sufficient compensatory collateral flow. In contrast, acute occlusion of a main mesenteric trunk may result in profound ischemia due to lack of sufficient collateral flow. Collateral network between the CA and the SMA exist primarily through the superior and inferior pancreaticoduodenal arteries. The IMA may provide collateral arterial flow to the SMA through the marginal artery of Drummond, the arc of Riolan, and other unnamed retroperitoneal collateral vessels termed *meandering mesenteric arteries* (Fig. 23-36). Lastly, collateral visceral vessels may provide important arterial flow to the IMA and the hindgut through the hypogastric arteries and the hemorrhoidal arterial network.

Regulation of mesenteric blood flow is largely modulated by both hormonal and neural stimuli, which characteristically regulate systemic blood flow. In addition, the mesenteric circulation responds to the GI contents. Hormonal regulation is mediated by splanchnic vasodilators such as nitric oxide, glucagon, and vasoactive intestinal peptide. Certain intrinsic vasoconstrictors such as

vasopressin can diminish the mesenteric blood flow. On the other hand, neural regulation is provided by the extensive visceral autonomic innervation.

Clinical manifestation of mesenteric ischemia is predominantly postprandial abdominal pain, which signifies that the increased oxygen demand of digestion is not met by the GI collateral circulation. The postprandial pain frequently occurs in the midabdomen, suggesting that the diversion of blood flow from the SMA to supply the stomach impairs perfusion to the small bowel. This leads to transient anaerobic metabolism and acidosis. Persistent or profound mesenteric ischemia will lead to mucosal compromise with release of intracellular contents and by-products of anaerobic metabolism to the splanchnic and systemic circulation. Injured bowel mucosa allows unimpeded influx of toxic substances from the bowel lumen with systemic consequences. If full-thickness necrosis occurs in the bowel wall, intestinal perforation ensues, which will lead to peritonitis. Concomitant atherosclerotic disease in cardiac or systemic circulation frequently compounds the diagnostic and therapeutic complexity of mesenteric ischemia.

Types of Mesenteric Artery Occlusive Disease

There are three major mechanisms of visceral ischemia involving the mesenteric arteries, which include: (a) acute mesenteric ischemia, which can be either embolic or thrombotic in origin; (b) chronic mesenteric ischemia; and (c) nonocclusive mesenteric ischemia. Despite the variability of these syndromes, a common anatomic pathology is involved in these processes. The SMA is the most commonly involved vessel in acute mesenteric ischemia. Acute thrombosis occurs in patients with underlying mesenteric atherosclerosis, which typically involves the origin of the mesenteric arteries while sparing the collateral branches. In acute embolic mesenteric ischemia, the emboli typically originate from a cardiac source and frequently occur in patients with atrial fibrillation or following myocardial infarction (Figs. 23-37 and 23-38). Nonocclusive mesenteric ischemia is characterized by a low flow state in otherwise normal mesenteric arteries, and most frequently occurs in critically

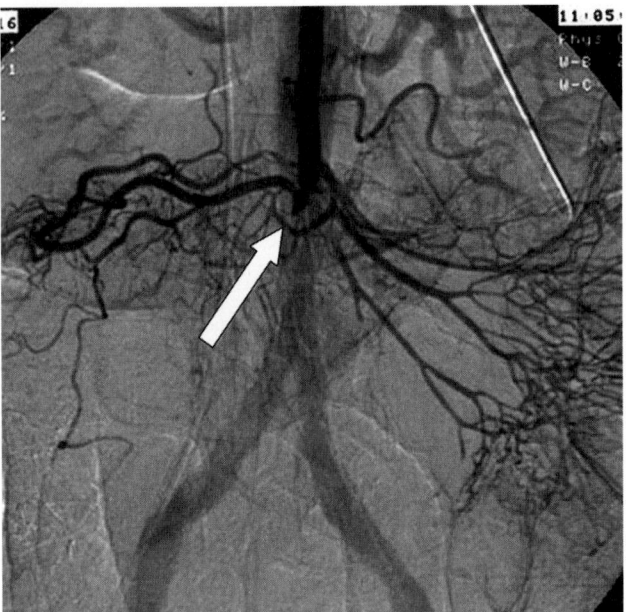

FIG. 23-37. An anteroposterior view of a selective superior mesenteric artery angiogram showed an abrupt cutoff of the middle colic artery, which was caused by emboli (*arrow*) due to atrial fibrillation.

ill patients on vasopressors. Finally, chronic mesenteric ischemia is a functional consequence of a long-standing atherosclerotic process that typically involves at least two of the three main mesenteric vessels. The gradual development of the occlusive process allows the development of collateral vessels that prevent the manifestations of acute ischemia, but are not sufficient to meet the high postprandial intestinal oxygen requirements, giving rise to the classical symptoms of postprandial abdominal pain and the resultant food fear.

Several less common syndromes of visceral ischemia involving the mesenteric arteries can also cause serious debilitation. Chronic mesenteric ischemic symptoms can occur due to extrinsic compression of the CA by the diaphragm, which is termed the *median arcuate ligament syndrome*, or *celiac artery compression syndrome*. Acute visceral ischemia may occur following an aortic operation,

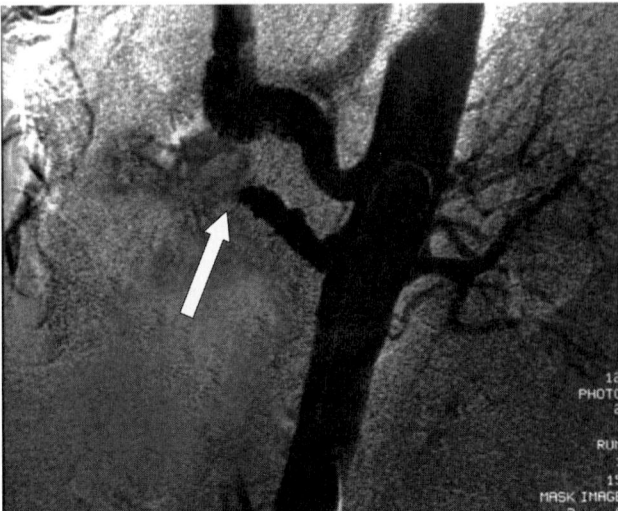

FIG. 23-38. A lateral mesenteric angiogram showing an abrupt cutoff of the proximal superior mesenteric artery, which is consistent with superior mesenteric artery embolism (*arrow*).

due to ligation of the IMA in the absence of adequate collateral vessels. Furthermore, acute visceral ischemia may develop in aortic dissection that involves the mesenteric arteries, or after coarctation repair. Finally, other unusual causes of ischemia include mesenteric arteritis, radiation arteritis, and cholesterol emboli.

Clinical Manifestations

Abdominal pain out of proportion to physical findings is the classic presentation in patients with acute mesenteric ischemia and occurs following an embolic or thrombotic ischemic event of the SMA. Other manifestations include sudden onset of abdominal cramps in patients with underlying cardiac or atherosclerotic disease, often associated with bloody diarrhea, as a result of mucosal sloughing secondary to ischemia. Fever, nausea, vomiting, and abdominal distention are some common but nonspecific manifestations. Diffuse abdominal tenderness, rebound, and rigidity are late signs and usually indicate bowel infarction and necrosis.

Clinical manifestations of chronic mesenteric ischemia are more subtle owing to the extensive collateral development. However, when intestinal blood flow is unable to meet the physiologic GI demands, mesenteric insufficiency ensues. The classic symptoms include postprandial abdominal pain, "food fear," and weight loss. Persistent nausea, and occasionally diarrhea, may coexist. Diagnosis remains challenging, and most of the patients will undergo an extensive and expensive GI tract work-up for the above symptoms before referral to a vascular service.

The typical patients who develop nonocclusive mesenteric ischemia are elderly patients. Comorbidities include congestive heart failure, acute myocardial infarction with cardiogenic shock, hypovolemic or hemorrhagic shock, sepsis, pancreatitis, and administration of digitalis or vasoconstrictor agents such as epinephrine. Abdominal pain is only present in approximately 70% of these patients. When present, the pain is usually severe but may vary in location, character, and intensity. In the absence of abdominal pain, progressive abdominal distention with acidosis may be an early sign of ischemia and impending bowel infarction.

Abdominal pain due to narrowing of the origin of the CA may occur as a result of extrinsic compression or impingement by the median arcuate ligament (Fig. 23-39). This condition is known as *celiac artery compression syndrome* or *median arcuate ligament syndrome*. Angiographically, there is CA compression that augments with deep expiration, and poststenotic dilatation. The CA compression syndrome has been implicated in some variants of chronic mesenteric ischemia. Most patients are young females between 20 and 40 years of age. Abdominal symptom is nonspecific, but the pain is localized in the upper abdomen, which may be precipitated by meals.

Diagnostic Evaluation

The differential diagnosis of acute mesenteric ischemia includes other causes of severe abdominal pain of acute onset, such as perforated viscus, intestinal obstruction, pancreatitis, cholecystitis, and nephrolithiasis. Laboratory evaluation is neither sensitive nor specific in distinguishing these various diagnoses. In the setting of mesenteric ischemia, complete blood count may reveal hemoconcentration and leukocytosis. Metabolic acidosis develops as a result of anaerobic metabolism. Elevated serum amylase may indicate a diagnosis of pancreatitis, but is also common in the setting of intestinal infarction. Finally, increased lactate levels, hyperkalemia, and azotemia may occur in the late stages of mesenteric ischemia.

Plain abdominal radiographs may provide helpful information to exclude other causes of abdominal pain such as intestinal obstruction, perforation, or volvulus, which may exhibit symptoms mimicking intestinal ischemia. Pneumoperitoneum, pneumatosis intestinalis, and gas in the portal vein may indicate infarcted bowel. In contrast, radiographic appearance of an adynamic ileus with a gasless abdomen is the most common finding in patients with acute mesenteric ischemia.

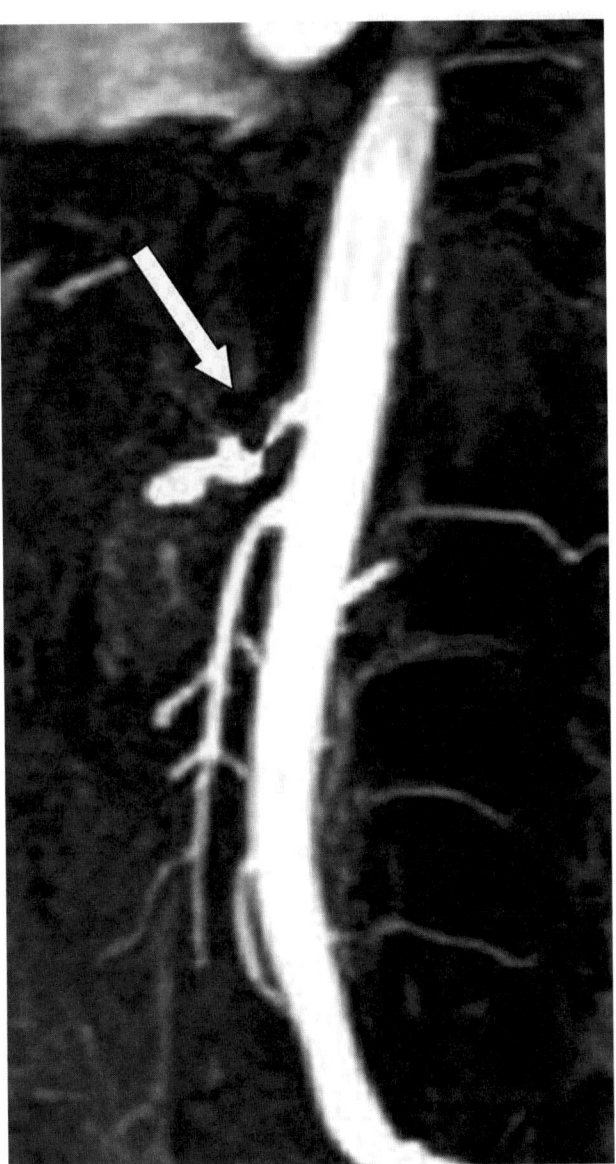

FIG. 23-39. A lateral projection of the magnetic resonance angiography of the aorta showing a chronic compression of the celiac artery (*arrow*) by the median arcuate ligament.

Upper endoscopy, colonoscopy, or barium radiography does not provide any useful information when evaluating acute mesenteric ischemia. Moreover, barium enema is contraindicated if the diagnosis of mesenteric ischemia is being considered. The intraluminal barium can obscure accurate visualization of mesenteric circulation during angiography. In addition, intraperitoneal leakage of barium can occur in the setting of intestinal perforation, which can lead to added therapeutic challenges during mesenteric revascularization.

Diagnosis of chronic mesenteric ischemia can be more challenging. Usually, before the evaluation by a vascular service, the patients have undergone an extensive work-up for the symptoms of chronic abdominal pain, weight loss, and anorexia. Rarely, the vascular surgeon is the first to encounter a patient with the above symptoms. In this situation, it is advisable to keep in mind that mesenteric ischemia is a rare entity, and that a full diagnostic work-up that should include CT scan of the abdomen and evaluation by a gastroenterologist should be performed. Mesenteric occlusive disease may coexist with malignancy, and symptoms of mesenteric vessel stenosis may be the result of extrinsic compression by a tumor.

Duplex ultrasonography is a valuable noninvasive means of assessing the patency of the mesenteric vessels. Moneta and associ-

ates evaluated the use of duplex ultrasound in the diagnosis of mesenteric occlusive disease in a blinded prospective study.[74,75] A peak systolic velocity in the SMA >275 cm/s demonstrated a sensitivity of 92%, specificity of 96%, and an overall accuracy of 96% for detecting more than 70% stenosis. The same authors found sensitivity and specificity of 87% and 82%, respectively, with an accuracy of 82% in predicting more than 70% celiac trunk stenosis. Duplex has been successfully used for follow-up after open surgical reconstruction or endovascular treatment of the mesenteric vessels to assess recurrence of the disease. Finally, spiral computed tomography with three-dimensional reconstruction (Fig. 23-40) as well as MRA (Fig. 23-41) have been promising in providing clear radiographic assessment of the mesenteric vessels.

The definitive diagnosis of mesenteric vascular disease is made by biplanar mesenteric arteriography, which should be performed promptly in any patient with suspected mesenteric occlusion. It typically shows occlusion or near-occlusion of the CA and SMA at or near their origins from the aorta. In most cases, the IMA has been previously occluded secondary to diffuse infrarenal aortic atherosclerosis. The differentiation of the different types of mesenteric arterial occlusion may be suggested with biplanar mesenteric arteriogram. Mesenteric emboli typically lodge at the orifice of the middle colic artery, which creates a "meniscus sign" with an abrupt cutoff of a normal proximal SMA several centimeters from its origin on the aorta. Mesenteric thrombosis, in contrast, occurs at the most proximal SMA, which tapers off at 1 to 2 cm from its origin. In the case of chronic mesenteric occlusion, the appearance of collateral circulation is typically present. Nonocclusive mesenteric ischemia produces an arteriographic image of segmental mesenteric vasospasm with a relatively normal appearing main SMA trunk (Fig. 23-42).

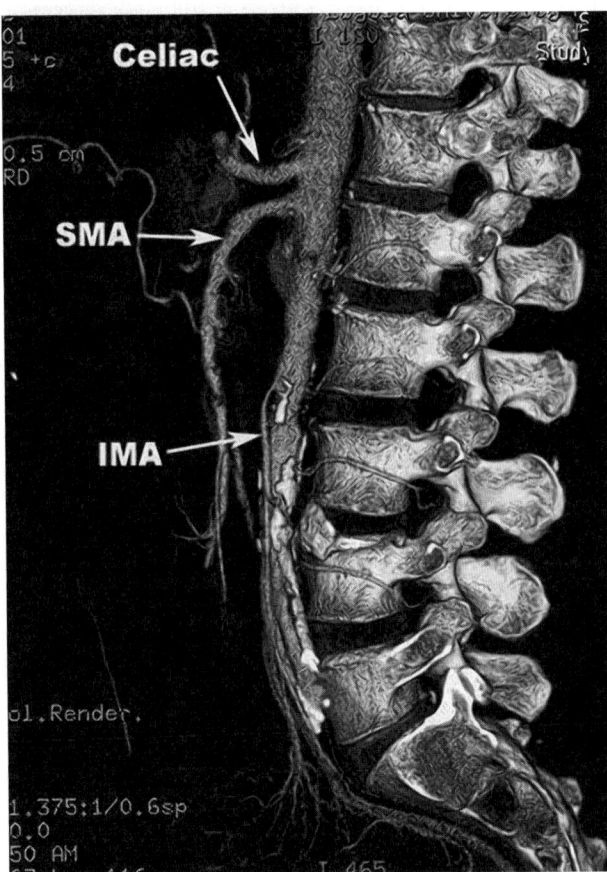

FIG. 23-40. Computed tomographic angiogram of the abdomen with three-dimensional reconstruction provides a clear view of the celiac artery, superior mesenteric artery (SMA), and inferior mesenteric artery (IMA).

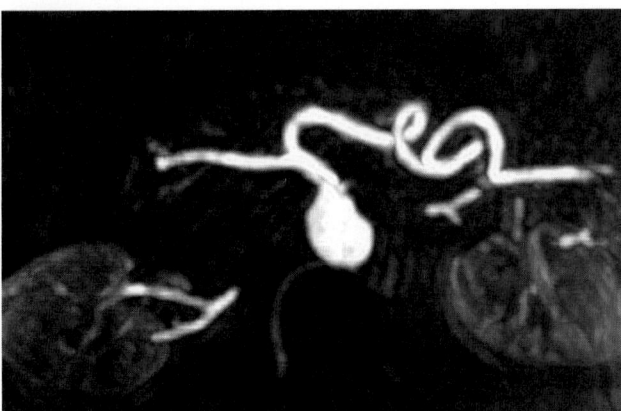

FIG. 23-41. A cross-sectional view of a magnetic resonance angiography provides a clear view of the luminal patency of the superior mesenteric artery.

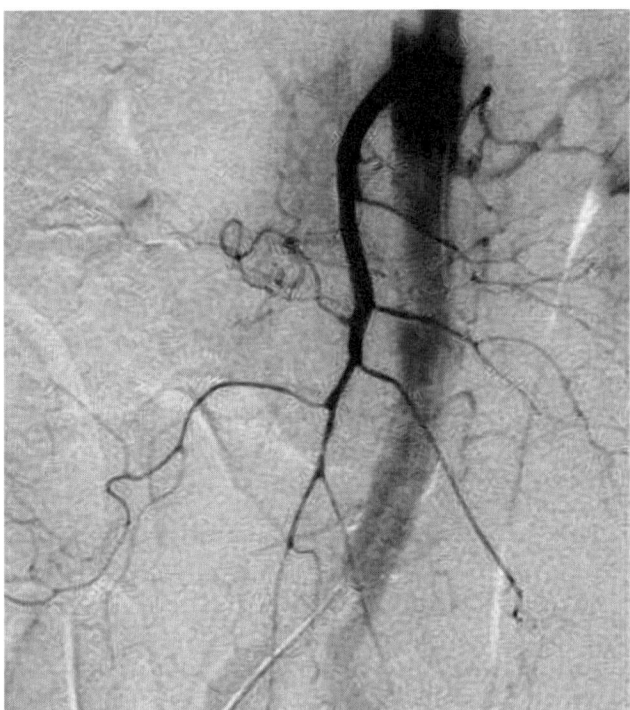

FIG. 23-42. Mesenteric arteriogram showing nonocclusive mesenteric ischemia as evidenced by diffuse spasm of intestinal arcades with poor filling of intramural vessels.

Mesenteric arteriography also can play a therapeutic role. Once the diagnosis of nonocclusive mesenteric ischemia is made on the arteriogram, an infusion catheter can be placed at the SMA orifice and vasodilating agents such as papaverine can be administered intra-arterially. The papaverine infusion may be continued postoperatively to treat persistent vasospasm, a common occurrence following mesenteric reperfusion. Transcatheter thrombolytic therapy has little role in the management of thrombotic mesenteric occlusion. Although thrombolytic agents may transiently recannulate the occluded vessels, the underlying occlusive lesions require definitive treatment. Furthermore, thrombolytic therapy typically requires a prolonged period of time to restore perfusion, during which the intestinal viability will be difficult to assess.

A word of caution would be appropriate here regarding patients with typical history of chronic intestinal angina who present with an acute abdomen and classical findings of peritoneal irritation. Arteriography is the gold standard for the diagnosis of mesenteric occlusive disease; however, it can be a time-consuming diagnostic modality. In this group of patients, immediate exploration for assessment of intestinal viability and vascular reconstruction is the best choice.

Surgical Repair
Acute Embolic Mesenteric Ischemia

Initial management of patients with acute mesenteric ischemia includes fluid resuscitation and systemic anticoagulation with heparin to prevent further thrombus propagation. Significant metabolic acidosis not responding to fluid resuscitation should be corrected with sodium bicarbonate. A central venous catheter, peripheral arterial catheter, and a Foley catheter should be placed for hemodynamic status monitoring. Appropriate antibiotics are given before surgical exploration. The operative management of acute mesenteric ischemia is dictated by the cause of the occlusion. It is helpful to obtain a preoperative mesenteric arteriogram to confirm the diagnosis and to plan appropriate treatment options. However, the diagnosis of mesenteric ischemia frequently cannot be established before surgical exploration; and therefore, patients in a moribund condition with acute abdominal symptoms should undergo immediate surgical exploration, avoiding the delay required to perform an arteriogram.

The primary goal of surgical treatment in embolic mesenteric ischemia is to restore arterial perfusion with removal of the embolus from the vessel. The abdomen is explored through a midline incision, which often reveals variable degrees of intestinal ischemia from the midjejunum to the ascending or transverse colon. The transverse colon is lifted superiorly, and the small intestine is reflected toward the right upper quadrant. The SMA is approached at the root of the small bowel mesentery, usually as it emerges from beneath the pancreas to cross over the junction of the third and fourth portions of the duodenum. Alternatively, the SMA can be approached by incising the retroperitoneum lateral to the fourth portion of the duodenum, which is rotated medially to expose the SMA. Once the proximal SMA is identified and controlled with vascular clamps, a transverse arteriotomy is made to extract the embolus, using standard balloon embolectomy catheters. In the event the embolus has lodged more distally, exposure of the distal SMA may be obtained in the root of the small bowel mesentery by isolating individual jejunal and ileal branches to allow a more comprehensive thromboembolectomy. Following the restoration of SMA flow, an assessment of intestinal viability must be made, and nonviable bowel must be resected. Several methods have been described to evaluate the viability of the intestine, which include intraoperative IV fluorescein injection and inspection with a Wood's lamp, and Doppler assessment of antimesenteric intestinal arterial pulsations. A second-look procedure should be considered in many patients, and is performed 24 to 48 hours following embolectomy. The goal of the procedure is reassessment of the extent of bowel viability, which may not be obvious immediately following the initial embolectomy. If nonviable intestine is evident in the second-look procedure, additional bowel resections should be performed at that time.

Acute Thrombotic Mesenteric Ischemia

Thrombotic mesenteric ischemia usually involves a severely atherosclerotic vessel, typically the proximal CA and SMA. Therefore, these patients require a reconstructive procedure to the SMA to bypass the proximal occlusive lesion and restore adequate mesenteric flow. The saphenous vein is the graft material of choice, and prosthetic materials should be avoided in patients with nonviable bowel, due to the risk of bacterial contamination if resection of necrotic intestine is performed. The bypass graft may originate from either the aorta or iliac artery. Advantages from using the supraceliac infradiaphragmatic aorta as opposed to the infrarenal aorta as the inflow vessel include a more smooth graft configuration with less chance of kinking, and the absence of atherosclerotic disease in the supraceliac aortic segment. Exposure of the supraceliac aorta is technically more challenging and time consuming than that of the iliac artery, which, unless calcified, is an appropriate inflow. Patency rates are similar regardless of inflow vessel choice.[76]

Chronic Mesenteric Ischemia

The therapeutic goal in patients with chronic mesenteric ischemia is to revascularize mesenteric circulation and prevent the development of bowel infarction. Mesenteric occlusive disease can be treated successfully by either transaortic endarterectomy or mesenteric artery bypass. Transaortic endarterectomy is indicated for ostial lesions of patent CA and SMA. A left medial rotation is performed, and the aorta and the mesenteric branches are exposed. A lateral aortotomy is performed, encompassing both the CA and SMA orifices. The visceral arteries must be adequately mobilized so that the termination site of endarterectomy can be visualized. Otherwise, an intimal flap may develop, which can lead to early thrombosis or distal embolization.

For occlusive lesions located 1 to 2 cm distal to the mesenteric origin, mesenteric artery bypass should be performed. Multiple mesenteric arteries are typically involved in chronic mesenteric ischemia, and both the CA and SMA should be revascularized whenever possible. In general, bypass grafting may be performed either antegrade from the supraceliac aorta or retrograde from either the infrarenal aorta or iliac artery. Both autogenous saphenous vein grafts and prosthetic grafts have been used with satisfactory and equivalent success. An antegrade bypass also can be performed using a small-caliber bifurcated graft from the supraceliac aorta to both the CA and SMA, which yields an excellent long-term result.[76]

Celiac Artery Compression Syndrome

The decision to intervene in patients with CA compression syndrome should be based on both an appropriate symptom complex and the finding of CA compression in the absence of other findings to explain the symptoms. The treatment goal is to release the ligamentous structure that compresses the proximal CA and to correct any persistent stricture by bypass grafting. The patient should be cautioned that relief of the celiac compression cannot be guaranteed to relieve the symptoms. In a number of reports on endovascular management of chronic mesenteric ischemia, the presence of CA compression syndrome has been identified as a major factor of technical failure and recurrence. Therefore, angioplasty and stenting should not be undertaken if extrinsic compression of the CA by the median arcuate ligament is suspected based on preoperative imaging studies. Open surgical treatment should be performed instead.[77,78]

Endovascular Treatment

Chronic Mesenteric Ischemia

Endovascular treatment of mesenteric artery stenosis or short segment occlusion by balloon dilatation or stent placement represents a less invasive therapeutic alternative to open surgical intervention, particularly in patients whose medical comorbidities place them in a high operative risk category. Endovascular therapy is also suited to patients with recurrent disease or anastomotic stenosis following previous open mesenteric revascularization. Prophylactic mesenteric revascularization is rarely performed in the asymptomatic patient undergoing an aortic procedure for other indications.[79] However, the natural history of untreated chronic mesenteric ischemia may justify revascularization in some minimally symptomatic or asymptomatic patients if the operative risks are acceptable, because the first clinical presentation may be acute intestinal ischemia in as many as 50% of the patients, with a mortality rate that ranges from 15 to 70%.[79] This is particularly true when the SMA is involved. Mesenteric angioplasty and stenting is particularly suitable for this patient subgroup given its low morbidity and mortality. Because of the limited experience with stent use in mesenteric vessels, appropriate indications for primary stent placement have

not been clearly defined. Guidelines generally include calcified ostial stenoses, high-grade eccentric stenoses, chronic occlusions, and significant residual stenosis greater than 30% or the presence of dissection after angioplasty. Restenosis after PTA is also an indication for stent placement.[80]

Acute Mesenteric Ischemia

Catheter-directed thrombolytic therapy is a potentially useful treatment modality for acute mesenteric ischemia, which can be initiated with intra-arterial delivery of thrombolytic agent into the mesenteric thrombus at the time of diagnostic angiography. Various thrombolytic medications, including urokinase (Abbokinase, Abbott Laboratory, North Chicago, Ill) or recombinant tissue plasminogen activator (Activase, Genentech, South San Francisco, Calif), have been reported to be successful in a small series of case reports. Catheter-directed thrombolytic therapy has a higher probability of restoring mesenteric blood flow success when performed within 12 hours of symptom onset. Successful resolution of a mesenteric thrombus will facilitate the identification of the underlying mesenteric occlusive disease process. As a result, subsequent operative mesenteric revascularization or mesenteric balloon angioplasty and stenting may be performed electively to correct the mesenteric stenosis. There are two main drawbacks with regard to thrombolytic therapy in mesenteric ischemia. Percutaneous, catheter-directed thrombolysis (CDT) does not allow the possibility to inspect the potentially ischemic intestine following restoration of the mesenteric flow. Additionally, a prolonged period of time may be necessary to achieve successful CDT, due in part to serial angiographic surveillance to document thrombus resolution. An incomplete or unsuccessful thrombolysis may lead to delayed operative revascularization, which may further necessitate bowel resection for irreversible intestinal necrosis. Therefore, catheter-directed thrombolytic therapy for acute mesenteric ischemia should only be considered in selected patients under a closely scrutinized clinical protocol.

Nonocclusive Mesenteric Ischemia

The treatment of nonocclusive mesenteric ischemia is primarily pharmacologic with selective mesenteric arterial catheterization followed by infusion of vasodilatory agents such as tolazoline or papaverine. Once the diagnosis is made on the mesenteric arteriography (see Fig. 23-42), intra-arterial papaverine is given at a dose of 30 to 60 mg/h. This must be coupled with the cessation of other vasoconstricting agents. Concomitant IV heparin should be administered to prevent thrombosis in the cannulated vessels. Treatment strategy thereafter is dependent on the patient's clinical response to the vasodilator therapy. If abdominal symptoms improve, mesenteric arteriography should be repeated to document the resolution of vasospasm. The patient's hemodynamic status must be carefully monitored during papaverine infusion, as significant hypotension can develop in the event that the infusion catheter migrates into the aorta, which can lead to systemic circulation of papaverine. Surgical exploration is indicated if the patient develops signs of continued bowel ischemia or infarction as evidenced by rebound tenderness or involuntary guarding. In these circumstances, papaverine infusion should be continued intraoperatively and postoperatively. The OR should be kept as warm as possible, and warm irrigation fluid and laparotomy pads should be used to prevent further intestinal vasoconstriction during exploration.

Techniques of Endovascular Interventions

To perform endovascular mesenteric revascularization, intraluminal access is performed via a femoral or brachial artery approach. Once an introducer sheath is placed in the femoral artery, an anteroposterior and lateral aortogram just below the level of the diaphragm is obtained with a pigtail catheter to identify the origin of the CA and SMA. Initial catheterization of the mesenteric artery can be performed using a variety of selective angled catheters, which include the RDC, Cobra-2, Simmons I (Boston Scientific/Meditech,

Natick, Mass), or SOS Omni catheter (AngioDynamics, Queensbury, NY). Once the mesenteric artery is cannulated, systemic heparin (5000 IU) is administered IV. A selective mesenteric angiogram is then performed to identify the diseased segment, which is followed by the placement of a 0.035-in or less traumatic 0.014- to 0.018-in guidewire to cross the stenotic lesion. Once the guidewire is placed across the stenosis, the catheter is carefully advanced over the guidewire across the lesion. In the event that the mesenteric artery is severely angulated as it arises from the aorta, a second stiffer guidewire (Amplatz or Rosen Guidewire, Boston Scientific) may be exchanged through the catheter to facilitate the placement of a 6F guiding sheath (Pinnacle, Boston Scientific).

With the image intensifier angled in a lateral position to fully visualize the proximal mesenteric segment, a balloon angioplasty is advanced over the guidewire through the guiding sheath and positioned across the stenosis. The balloon diameter should be chosen based on the vessel size of the adjacent normal mesenteric vessel. Once balloon angioplasty is completed, a postangioplasty angiogram is necessary to document the procedural result. Radiographic evidence of either residual stenosis or mesenteric artery dissection constitutes suboptimal angioplasty results that warrant mesenteric stent placement. Moreover, atherosclerotic involvement of the proximal mesenteric artery or vessel orifice should be treated with a balloon-expandable stent placement. These stents can be placed over a low profile 0.014- or 0.018-in guidewire system. It is preferable to deliver the balloon-mounted stent through a guiding sheath, which is positioned just proximal to the mesenteric orifice while the balloon-mounted stent is advanced across the stenosis. The stent is next deployed by expanding the angioplasty balloon to its designated inflation pressure. The balloon is then deflated and carefully withdrawn through the guiding sheath.

Completion angiogram is performed by hand injecting a small volume of contrast though the guiding sheath. It is critical to maintain the guidewire access until a satisfactory completion angiogram is obtained. If the completion angiogram reveals suboptimal radiographic results, such as residual stenosis or dissection, additional catheter-based intervention can be performed through the same guidewire. These interventions may include repeat balloon angioplasty for residual stenosis or additional stent placement for mesenteric artery dissection. During the procedure, intra-arterial infusion of papaverine or nitroglycerine can be used to decrease vasospasm. Administration of antiplatelet agents is also recommended, for at least 6 months or even indefinitely if other risk factors of cardiovascular disease are present.

Complications of Endovascular Treatment

Complications are not common and rarely become life threatening. These include access site thrombosis, hematomas, and infection. Dissection can occur during PTA and is managed with placement of a stent. Balloon-mounted stents are preferred over the self-expanding ones because of the higher radial force and the more precise placement. Distal embolization has also been reported but it never resulted in acute intestinal ischemia, likely due to the rich network of collaterals already developed.[81]

Clinical Results of Interventions for Mesenteric Ischemia

The first successful percutaneous angioplasty of the SMA was reported in 1980.[82] Since 1995, 11 series and multiple scattered case reports have reported results from endovascular management of mesenteric occlusive disease.[76,81] In a literature review, Aburhama and associates showed that endovascular intervention had an overall technical success rate of 91%, early and late pain relief of 84 and 71%, respectively, and 30-day morbidity and mortality rates of 16.4 and 4.3, respectively. The average patency was 63% during an average 26-month follow-up.[81]

In a recent review of the literature from published series since 1995, restenosis was developed in 22% of patients during 24.5

months of average follow-up.[76] The long-term clinical relief without reintervention was 82%. Among the patients that had a technical failure, 15 were ultimately diagnosed with median arcuate ligament syndrome and underwent successful surgical treatment, an observation that emphasizes the need for careful patient selection. Interestingly, the addition of selective stenting after PTA that was started in 1998 slightly increases the technical success rate, but is not correlated with any substantial overall clinical benefit or improved, long-term patency rates.

In contrast to the endovascular treatment, open surgical techniques have achieved an immediate clinical success that approaches 100%, a surgical mortality rate from 0 to 17%, and an operative morbidity rate that ranges from 19 to 54% in a number of different series.[76,78,79] AbuRahma and colleagues reported their experience of endovascular interventions of 22 patients with symptomatic mesenteric ischemia due to either SMA or CA stenosis.[81] They noted excellent initial technical and clinical success rates, which were 96% (23/24) and 95% (21/22), respectively, with no perioperative mortality or major morbidity. During a mean follow-up of 26 months (range 1 to 54 months), the primary late clinical success rate was 61% and freedom from recurrent stenosis was 30%. The freedom from recurrent stenosis rates at 1, 2, 3, and 4 years were 65%, 47%, 39%, and 13%, respectively. The authors concluded that mesenteric stenting, which provides excellent early results, is associated with a relatively high incidence of late restenosis.[81]

Several studies have attempted to compare the endovascular to standard open surgical approach.[83,84] The results of the open surgery appear to be more durable, but tend to be associated with higher morbidity and mortality rates and an overall longer hospital stay. In one study that compared the clinical outcome of open revascularization with percutaneous stenting for patients with chronic mesenteric ischemia, 28 patients underwent endovascular treatment and 85 patients underwent open mesenteric bypass grafting.[84] Both patient cohorts had similar baseline comorbidities and symptom duration, so there was no difference in early inhospital complication or mortality rates. Moreover, both groups had similar 3-year cumulative recurrent stenosis and mortality rates. However, patients treated with mesenteric stenting had a significantly higher incidence of recurrent symptoms. The authors concluded that operative mesenteric revascularization should be offered to patients with low surgical risk.[84]

Based on the above results one could argue that mesenteric angioplasty and stenting demonstrate an inferior technical and clinical success rate. Long-term patency rates appear to also be superior with the open technique. There is a general consensus, however, that the endovascular approach is associated with lower morbidity and mortality rates and is therefore more suitable for high-risk patients. One should also keep in mind that practices representing standard of care for stent placement today were absent in the early era of endovascular experience. These include perioperative heparinization and short-term antiplatelet therapy, use of stents with higher radial force, routine use of postoperative surveillance with arterial duplex and early reintervention to prevent a high-grade stenosis to progress to occlusion, and placement of drug-eluting stents (DES).

RENAL ARTERY DISEASE

Obstructive lesions of the renal artery can produce hypertension, resulting in a condition known as *renovascular hypertension*, which is the most common form of hypertension amenable to therapeutic intervention, and affects 5 to 10% of all hypertensive patients in the United States.[85] Patients with renovascular hypertension are at an increased risk for irreversible end-organ dysfunction, including permanent kidney damage, if inadequate pharmacologic therapies are used to control the BP. The majority of patients with renal artery obstructive disease have vascular lesions of either atherosclerotic disease or fibrodysplasia involving the renal arteries. The proximal portion of the renal artery represents the most common location for the development of atherosclerotic disease. It is well established that renal artery intervention, either by surgical or endovascular revascularization, provides an effective treatment for controlling renovascular hypertension as well as preserving renal function. The decision for intervention is complex, and needs to take into consideration a variety of anatomic, physiologic, and clinical features, unique for the individual patient.

Etiology

Approximately 80% of all renal artery occlusive lesions are caused by atherosclerosis, which typically involves a short segment of the renal artery ostia, and represents spillover disease from a severely atheromatous aorta (Fig. 23-43).[86] Atherosclerotic lesions are bilateral in two thirds of patients. Individuals with this disease commonly present during the sixth decade of life. Men are affected twice as frequently as women. Atherosclerotic lesions in other territories such as the coronary, mesenteric, cerebrovascular, and peripheral arterial circulation are common. When a unilateral lesion is present, the disease process equally affects the right and left renal artery.[87]

The second most common cause of renal artery stenosis is FMD, which accounts for 20% of cases, and is most frequently encountered in young, often multiparous women.[88] FMD of the renal artery represents a heterogeneous group of lesions that can produce histopathologic changes in the intima, media, or adventitia. The most common variety consists of medial fibroplasia, in which thickened fibromuscular ridges alternate with attenuated media producing the classic angiographic "string of beads" appearance (Figs. 23-44 and 23-45). The cause of medial fibroplasia remains unclear. Most common theories involve a modification of arterial smooth muscle cells in response to estrogenic stimuli during the reproductive years, unusual traction forces on affected vessels, and mural ischemia from impairment of vasa vasorum blood flow.[88] Fibromuscular hyperplasia usually affects the distal two thirds of the main renal artery, and the right renal artery is affected more frequently than the left. Other less common causes of renal artery stenosis include renal artery aneurysm (compressing the adjacent normal renal artery), arteriovenous malformations, neurofibromatosis, renal artery dissections, renal artery trauma, Takayasu's arteritis, and renal arteriovenous fistula.

Clinical Manifestations

Renovascular hypertension is the most common sequelae of renal artery occlusive disease. Its prevalence varies from 2% in patients

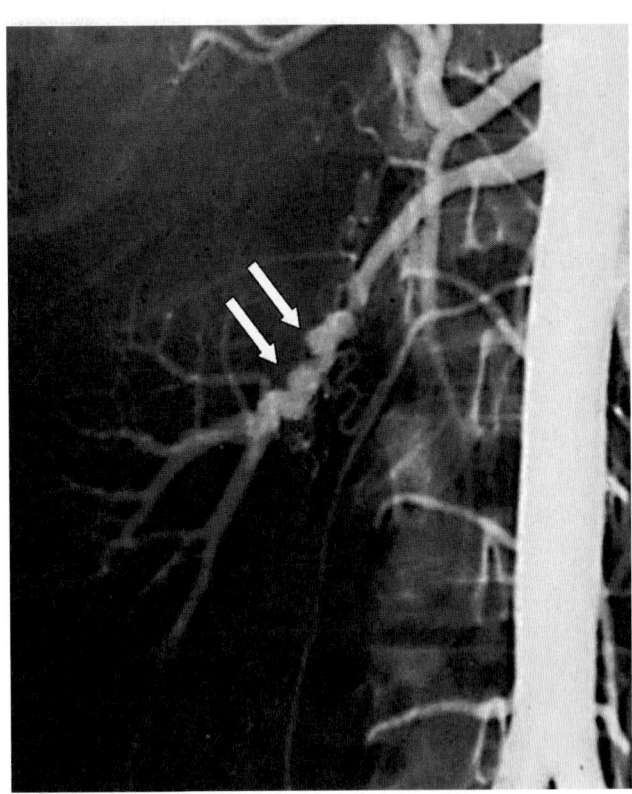

FIG. 23-44. Abdominal aortogram revealed a left renal artery fibromuscular dysplasia (*arrows*) with a characteristic "string of beads" appearance.

with diastolic BP >100 mmHg, to almost 30% in those with diastolic BP over 125 mmHg.[86] Clinical features that may indicate the presence of renovascular hypertension include the following: (a) systolic and diastolic upper abdominal bruits, (b) diastolic hypertension of >115 mmHg, (c) rapid onset of hypertension after the age of 50 years, (d) a sudden worsening of mild to moderate essential hypertension, (e) hypertension that is difficult to control with three or more antihypertensives, (f) development of renal insufficiency after ACE inhibitors, and (g) development of hypertension during childhood.

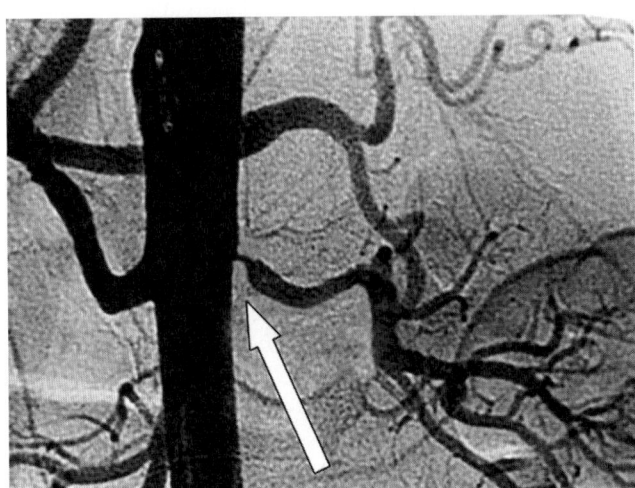

FIG. 23-43. Occlusive disease of the renal artery typically involves the renal ostium (*arrow*) as a spillover plaque extension from aortic atherosclerosis.

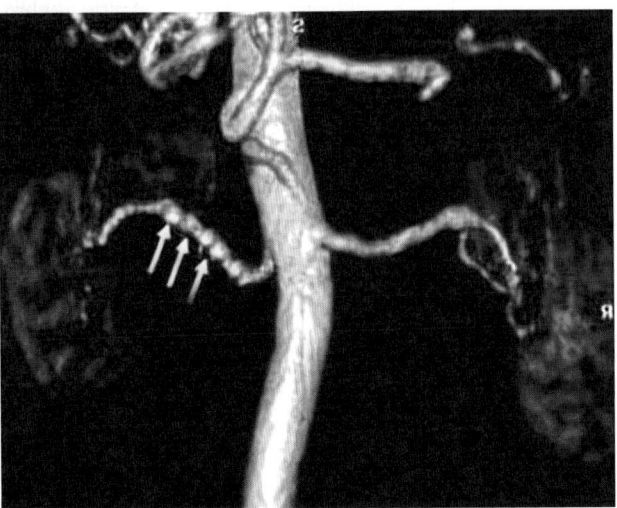

FIG. 23-45. Magnetic resonance angiography of the abdominal aorta revealed the presence of a left renal artery fibromuscular dysplasia (*arrows*).

All patients with significant hypertension, especially elevated diastolic BP, must be considered as suspect for renovascular disease. Young adults with hypertension have a great deal to gain by avoiding lifelong treatment if renovascular hypertension is diagnosed and corrected. Appropriate diagnostic studies and intervention must be timely instituted to detect the possibility of renovascular hypertension in patients with primary hypertension who present for clinical evaluation.

Diagnostic Evaluation

The diagnostic requisites for renovascular hypertension include both hypertension and renal artery stenosis. Impairment of the renal function may coexist, although the occurrence of renal insufficiency before the development of hypertension is uncommon. Nearly all diagnostic studies for renovascular hypertension evaluate either the anatomic stenosis or renal parenchymal dysfunction attributed to the stenosis. This section provides an overview of the strengths and limitations of the most common tests used in the diagnostic evaluation of the patient with suspected renovascular hypertension before intervention.

Captopril renal scanning is a functional study that assesses renal perfusion before and after administration of the ACE inhibitor captopril. Captopril inhibits the secretion of angiotensin II. Through this mechanism it reduces the efferent arteriole vasoconstriction and, as a result, the glomerular filtration rate (GFR). The test consists of a baseline renal scan, and a second renal scan after captopril administration. Positive result indicates that captopril administration (a) increases the time to peak activity to more than 11 minutes or (b) the GFR ratio between sides increases to greater than 1.5:1 compared to a normal baseline scan. Significant parenchymal disease limits the reliability of this study.

Renal artery duplex ultrasonography is a noninvasive test of assessing renal artery stenosis both by visualization of the vessel and measurement of the effect of stenosis on blood flow velocity and waveforms. The presence of a severe renal artery stenosis correlates with peak systolic velocities of >180 cm/s and the ratio of these velocities to those in the aorta of >3.5 (Table 23-11). Renal artery duplex is a technically demanding examination, requiring a substantial amount of operator expertise. In addition, the presence of bowel gas and obesity make the exam difficult to perform and interpret. However, in experienced hands and with appropriate patient selection, it can be a high-yield examination and is typically the initial screening test for patients with suspected renal artery occlusive disease.

Selective catheterization of the renal vein via a femoral vein approach for assessing renin activity is a more invasive test of detecting the physiologic sequelae of renal artery stenosis. If unilateral disease is present the affected kidney should secrete high levels of renin while the contralateral kidney should have low renin production. A ratio between the two kidneys, or the renal vein renin ratio, of >1.5 is indicative of functionally important renovascular hypertension, and it also predicts a favorable response from renovascular revascularization. Because this study assesses the ratio between the two kidneys, it is not useful in patients with bilateral disease because both kidneys may secrete abnormally elevated renin levels.

The renal:systemic renin index (RSRI) is calculated by subtracting systemic renin activity from individual renal vein renin activity and dividing the remainder by systemic renin activity. This value represents the contribution of each kidney to renin production. In the absence of renal artery stenosis, the renal vein renin activity from each kidney is typically 24% or 0.24 higher than the systemic level. As the result, the total of both kidneys' renin activity is usually 48% greater than the systemic activity, a value that represents a steady state of renal renin activity. The RSRI of the affected kidney in patients with renovascular hypertension is >0.24. In the case of unilateral renal artery stenosis with normal contralateral kidney, the increase in ipsilateral renin release is normally balanced by suppression of the contralateral kidney renin production, which results in a drop in its RSRI to <0.24. Bilateral renal artery disease may negate the contralateral compensatory response, and the autonomous release of renin from both diseased kidneys may result in the sum of the individual RSRIs being considerably >0.48. The prognostic value of RSRI remains limited in that approximately 10% of patients with favorable clinical response following renovascular revascularization do not exhibit contralateral renin suppression. As a result, the use of RSRI must be applied with caution in the management of patients with renovascular hypertension.

MRA with IV gadolinium contrast enhancement has been increasingly used for renal artery imaging because of its ability to provide high-resolution images (Figs. 23-46 and 23-47) while using a minimally nephrotoxic agent. Flow void may be inaccurately interpreted as occlusion or stenosis in MRA. Therefore, unless the quality of the image analysis software is superior, MRA should be interpreted with caution and used in conjunction with other modalities before making plans for operative or endovascular treatment.

DSA remains the gold standard to assess renal artery occlusive disease. A flush aortogram is performed first so that any accessory renal arteries can be detected and the origins of all the renal arteries are adequately displayed. The presence of collateral vessels circumventing a renal artery stenosis strongly supports the hemodynamic importance of the stenosis. A pressure gradient of 10 mmHg or greater is necessary for collateral vessel development, which also is associated with activation of the renin-angiotensin cascade.

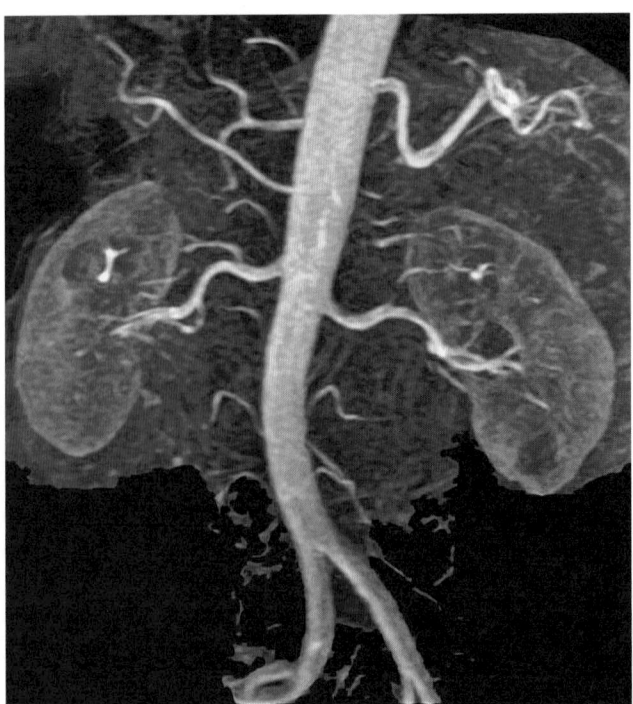

FIG. 23-46. Magnetic resonance angiography of the abdominal aorta revealed bilateral normal renal arteries.

TABLE 23-11	Renal duplex diagnostic criteria	
Renal Artery Diameter Reduction	**Renal Artery PSV**	**RAR**
Normal	<180 cm/s	<3.5
<60%	≥180 cm/s	<3.5
≥60%	≥180 cm/s	≥3.5
Occlusion	No signal	No signal

PSV = peak systolic velocity; RAR = renal-to-aortic ratio.

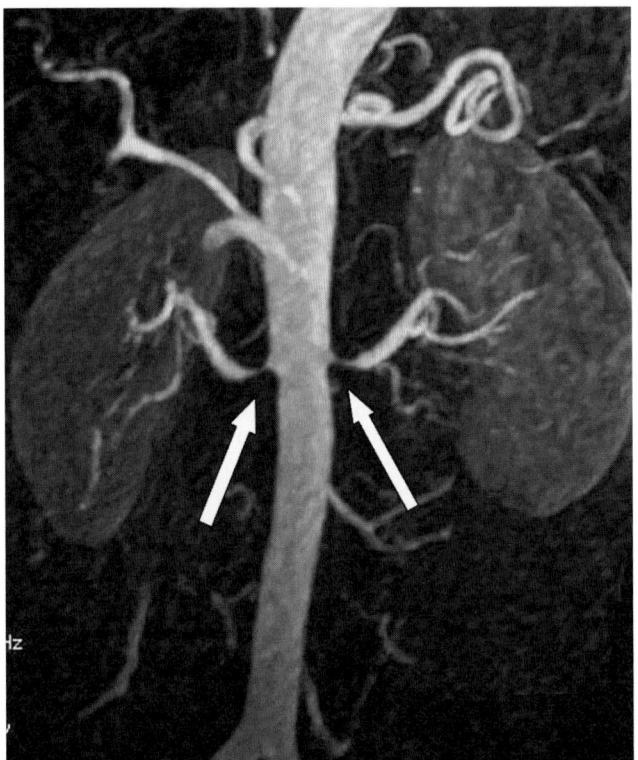

FIG. 23-47. Magnetic resonance angiography of the abdominal aorta revealed bilateral ostial renal artery stenosis (*arrows*).

TABLE 23-12 Indications for renal artery revascularization

Angiography criteria
- Fibromuscular dysplasia lesion
- Pressure gradient >20 mmHg
- Affected/unaffected kidney renin ratio >1.5:1

Clinical criteria
- Refractory or rapidly progressive hypertension
- Hypertension associated with flash pulmonary edema without coronary artery disease
- Rapidly progressive deterioration in renal function
- Intolerance to antihypertensive medications
- Chronic renal insufficiency related to bilateral renal artery occlusive disease or stenosis to a solitary functioning kidney
- Dialysis-dependent renal failure in a patient with renal artery stenosis but without another definite cause of end-stage renal disease
- Recurrent congestive heart failure or flash pulmonary edema not attributable to active coronary ischemia

Treatment Indications

The therapeutic goals in patients with renovascular disease include: (a) improved BP control to prevent end-organ damage on systems such as the cerebral, coronary, pulmonary, and peripheral circulations; and (b) preservation and possibly improvement of the renal function (Table 23-12).

The indications for endovascular treatment for renal artery occlusive disease include 70% or greater stenosis of one or both renal arteries and at least one of the following clinical criteria:

- Inability to adequately control hypertension despite appropriate antihypertensive regimen.
- Chronic renal insufficiency related to bilateral renal artery occlusive disease or stenosis to a solitary functioning kidney.
- Dialysis-dependent renal failure in a patient with renal artery stenosis but without another definite cause of end-stage renal disease.
- Recurrent congestive heart failure or flash pulmonary edema not attributable to active coronary ischemia.

Before 1990, the most common treatment modality in patients with renal artery occlusive disease was surgical revascularization, with either renal artery bypass grafting or renal artery endarterectomy. The advancement of endovascular therapy in the past decade has led to various minimally invasive treatment strategies such as renal artery balloon angioplasty or stenting to control hypertension or to preserve renal function.

Surgical Reconstruction

The typical approach for surgical renal artery revascularization involves a midline xiphoid-to-pubis incision. The posterior peritoneum is incised, and the duodenum is mobilized to the right, starting at the ligament of Treitz. The left renal hilum can be exposed by extending the retroperitoneal dissection to the left along the avascular plane along the inferior border of the pancreas.

Mobilization of the left renal vein is essential in these cases and can be achieved by dividing the gonadal, iliolumbar, and adrenal veins. The proximal portion of the right renal artery can be exposed through the base of the mesentery by retraction of the left renal vein cephalad and the vena cava to the right. Accessing the most distal portion of the right renal artery requires a Kocher maneuver and duodenal mobilization. Another approach useful for treating bilateral renal artery lesions involves mobilization of the entire small bowel and the right colon, with a dissection that starts at the ligament of Treitz, and proceeds toward the cecum and then along the line of Todd in the right paracolic gutter. Simultaneous dissection along the inferior border of the pancreas provides additional visualization of the left renal artery. Finally, division of the diaphragmatic crura that encircle the suprarenal aorta may sometimes be necessary to achieve suprarenal clamping.

Types of Surgical Reconstruction

Aortorenal bypass is the most frequently performed reconstruction of ostial occlusive renal artery disease. After proximal and distal control is obtained, an elliptical segment of the aorta is excised, and the proximal anastomosis is performed in end-to-side fashion. Autologous vein is the preferred conduit. If the vein is not suitable, then prosthetic material can be used. An end-to-end anastomosis is then performed between the conduit of choice and the renal artery using either a 6-0 or 7-0 polypropylene suture. The length of the arteriotomy needs to be at least three times the diameter of the renal artery to prevent anastomotic restenosis. If the surgeon plans to perform a side-to-side anastomosis between the conduit and the renal artery, then it is performed first, and the aortic anastomosis follows.

Endarterectomy, either transrenal or transaortic, is an alternative to bypass for short ostial lesions, or in patients with multiple renal arteries. The transrenal endarterectomy is performed with a transverse longitudinal incision on the aorta that extends into the diseased renal artery. After the plaque removal, the arteriotomy is closed with a prosthetic patch. Transaortic endarterectomy is well suited for patients with multiple renal arteries and short ostial lesions. The aorta is opened longitudinally and aortic sleeve endarterectomy is performed, followed by eversion endarterectomy of the renal arteries. Adequate mobilization of the renal arteries is essential for a safe and complete endarterectomy.

Hepatorenal and splenorenal bypass are alternative options of revascularizations for patients who might not tolerate aortic clamping, or for those with calcified aorta that precludes adequate control. For hepatorenal bypass, a right subcostal incision is used, and the hepatic artery is exposed with an incision in the lesser omentum. A Kocher maneuver is performed, the right renal vein is identified and mobilized, and the right renal artery is identified and controlled posteriorly to the vein. The greater saphenous vein is the conduit of choice. The anastomosis is performed end to side with the common hepatic artery, and end to end with the renal artery anterior to the inferior vena cava. The splenorenal bypass is performed via a left subcostal incision. The splenic artery is mobilized from the lesser sac, brought through a retropancreatic plane, and anastomosed end to end to the renal artery.

Reimplantation of the renal artery is an attractive option of reconstruction in children, or in adults with ostial lesions. A redundant renal artery is a prerequisite for the procedure. After mobilization, the artery is transected and spatulated, eversion endarterectomy is performed, if necessary, and an end-to-side anastomosis with the aorta is created.

Clinical Results of Surgical Repair

Results reflect the need for performance of renal artery bypass in high-volume and experienced centers. In a review from a large tertiary center, 92% of the patients with non-atherosclerotic vascular disease had good response to hypertension, but only 43% were completely cured and were taken off antihypertensives.[89] Patients younger than 45 years old fare better with a cure rate of 68% and an improvement rate of 32%. In patients with atherosclerotic renal artery disease, the cure rate was even smaller (12%), and the overall response to hypertension rate was 85%. The operative mortality was 3.1% and 0% in the atherosclerotic and non-atherosclerotic groups, respectively.

Renal function improvement occurs within the first week of the operation in approximately two thirds of the patients. A progressive decrease in the GFR is seen after this initial improvement, but the rate of decrease is less compared to the group of patients who did not respond at all to operative intervention. Up to three fourths of patients were permanently removed from dialysis in a large series.[90] Favorable response of renal function to revascularization improves overall survival.

Endovascular Treatment

Endovascular treatment of renal artery occlusive disease was first introduced by Grüntzig who successfully dilated a renal artery stenosis using a balloon catheter technique. This technique requires passage of a guidewire under fluoroscopic control typically from a femoral artery approach to across the stenosis in the renal artery. A balloon-dilating catheter is passed over the guidewire and positioned within the area of stenosis and inflated to produce a controlled disruption of the arterial wall. Alternatively, a balloon-mounted, expandable stent can be used to primarily dilate the renal artery stenosis. Completion angiography usually is performed to assess the immediate results. The technical aspect of an endovascular renal artery revascularization is discussed in Techniques of Renal Artery Angioplasty and Stenting below.

Techniques of Renal Artery Angioplasty and Stenting

Access to the renal artery for endovascular intervention is typically performed via a femoral artery approach, although a brachial artery approach can be considered in the event of severe aortoiliac occlusive disease, aortoiliac aneurysm, or severe caudal renal artery angulation. Once an introducer sheath is placed in the femoral artery, an aortogram is performed with a pigtail catheter placed in the suprarenal aorta. Additional oblique views are frequently necessary to more precisely visualize the orifice of the stenosed renal artery and thoroughly assess the presence of accessory renal arteries. Noniodinated contrast agents such as carbon dioxide and gadolinium can be used in endovascular renal intervention in patients with renal dysfunction or history of allergic reaction.

After systemic heparinization, catheterization of the renal artery can be performed using a variety of selective angled catheters including the RDC, Cobra-2, Simmons I, or SOS Omni catheter (Boston Scientific/Meditech, Natick, Mass; Cook, Bloomington, Ind; Medtronic, Santa Rosa, Calif; Cordis, Warren, NJ; or AngioDynam-

ics, Queensbury, NY). A selective renal angiogram is then performed to confirm position, and the lesion is crossed with either a 0.035-in or a 0.018- to 0.014-in guidewire. It is important to maintain the distal wire position without movement in the tertiary renal branches while guiding sheath placement to reduce the possibility of parenchymal perforation and spasm. A guiding sheath or a guiding catheter is then advanced at the orifice of the renal artery to provide a secure access for balloon and stent deployment.

Balloon angioplasty is performed with a balloon sized to the diameter of the normal renal artery adjacent to the stenosis. Choosing a balloon with a 4-mm diameter is a reasonable first choice. The luminal diameter of the renal artery can be further assessed by comparing it to the fully inflated balloon. Such a comparison may provide a reference guide to determine whether renal artery dilatation with a larger diameter angioplasty balloon is necessary.

Once balloon angioplasty of the renal artery is completed, an angiogram is performed to document the procedural result. Radiographic evidence of either residual stenosis or renal artery dissection constitutes suboptimal angioplasty results, which warrants an immediate renal artery stent placement. Moreover, atherosclerotic involvement of the very proximal renal artery that involves the vessel orifice typically requires stent placement. A balloon-expandable stent is typically used, and is positioned in such a way so that it protrudes into the aorta by 1 to 2 mm. The size of the stent is determined by the size of the renal artery, taking into account a desirable 10 to 20% oversizing. After the stent deployment, the angiogram is repeated and, upon a satisfactory result, the devices are withdrawn. It is critical to maintain the guidewire access across the renal lesion until satisfactory completion angiogram is obtained. Spasm of the branches of the renal artery will usually respond to nitroglycerin 100 to 200 mcg administered through the guiding sheath directly into the renal artery.

While endovascular therapy of renal artery occlusive disease is considerably less invasive than conventional renal artery bypass operation, complications relating to this treatment modality can occur. In a study in which Guzman and colleagues compared the complications following renal artery angioplasty and surgical revascularization, the authors noted that major complication rates following endovascular and surgical treatment were 17% and 31%, respectively. In contrast, significantly greater minor complications were associated with the endovascular cohort, which was 48%, in contrast to 7% in the surgical group.[91] In a prospective randomized study that compared the clinical outcome of renal artery balloon angioplasty vs. stenting for renal ostial atherosclerotic lesion, comparable complications rates were found in the two groups, which were 39% and 43%, respectively. However, the incidence of restenosis rate at 6 months was significantly higher in the balloon angioplasty cohort than the stenting group, which was 48% in contrast to 14% at 6 months. This study underscores the clinical superiority of renal stenting compared to renal balloon angioplasty alone in patients with ostial stenosis.[92]

Deterioration in renal function, albeit transient, is a common complication following endovascular renal artery intervention. This is most likely the combined result of the use of iodinated contrast, and the occurrence of renal parenchymal embolism due to wire and catheter manipulation. In most cases, this is a temporary problem, as supportive care with adequate fluid hydration is sufficient to reverse the renal dysfunction. However, transient hemodialysis may become necessary in approximately 1% of patients. Other complications include vascular access complications (bleeding, hematoma, femoral nerve injury, arteriovenous fistula, and pseudoaneurysm), target vessel dissection, perinephric hematoma, early postoperative renal artery thrombosis, and extremity atheroembolism from thrombus in the aorta or the iliac arteries.

Clinical Results of Endovascular Interventions

Percutaneous Transluminal Balloon Angioplasty

FMD of the renal artery is the most common treatment indication for percutaneous, transluminal balloon angioplasty. Patients with symptomatic FM, such as hypertension or renal insufficiency, usually respond well to renal artery balloon angioplasty alone.[93] In contrast, balloon angioplasty generally is not an effective treatment for patients with renal artery stenosis or proximal occlusive disease of the renal artery, due to the high incidence of restenosis with balloon angioplasty alone. In the latter group of patients, primary stent placement is the preferred endovascular treatment. The long-term benefit of renal artery balloon angioplasty in patients with FMD was reported by Surowiec and colleagues.[93] They followed 14 patients who underwent 19 interventions on 18 renal artery segments. The technical success rate of balloon angioplasty for FMD was 95%. Primary patency rates were 81%, 69%, 69%, and 69% at 2, 4, 6, and 8 years, respectively. Assisted primary patency rates were 87%, 87%, 87%, and 87% at 2, 4, 6, and 8 years, respectively. The restenosis rate was 25% at 8 years. Clinical benefit, as defined by either improved or cured hypertension, was found in 79% of patients overall, with two thirds of patients having maintained this benefit at 8 years. The authors concluded that balloon angioplasty is highly effective in symptomatic FMD with excellent durable functional benefits.[93]

The utility of balloon angioplasty alone in the treatment of renovascular hypertension appears to be limited. Van Jaarsveld and associates performed a prospective study in which patients with renal artery stenosis were randomized to either drug therapy or balloon angioplasty treatment.[94] A total of 106 patients with 50% diameter stenosis or greater plus hypertension or renal insufficiency were randomized in the study. At 3 months, there was no difference in the degree to which BP was controlled between the two groups. However, the degree and dose of antihypertensive medications was slightly lowered in the balloon angioplasty group. The above advantage of the angioplasty group completely disappeared at 12 months, making the authors conclude that, in the treatment of patients with hypertension and renal artery stenosis, percutaneous transluminal balloon angioplasty alone offers minimal advantage over antihypertensive drug therapy.

Renal Artery Stenting

Endovascular stent placement is the treatment of choice for patients with symptomatic or high-grade renal artery occlusive disease (Fig. 23-48). This is due in part to the high incidence of restenosis with balloon angioplasty alone, particularly in the setting of ostial stenosis. Renal artery stenting is also indicated for renal artery dissection caused by balloon angioplasty or other catheter-based interventions. Numerous studies have clearly demonstrated the clinical efficacy of renal artery stenting when compared to balloon angioplasty alone in patients with high-grade renal artery stenosis.

White and colleagues conducted a study to evaluate the role of renal artery stenting in patients with poorly controlled hypertension and renal artery lesions that did not respond well to balloon angioplasty alone.[95] The technical success of the procedure was 99%. The mean BP values were 173 ± 25/88 ± 17 mmHg before stent implantation and 146 ± 20/77 ± 12 mmHg 6 months after renal artery stenting (P <.01). Angiographic follow-up with 67 patients (mean 8.7 ± 5 months) demonstrated restenosis, as defined by 50% or greater luminal narrowing, occurred in 15 patients (19%). The study concluded that renal artery stenting is a highly effective treatment for renovascular hypertension, with a low angiographic restenosis rate. In another similar study, Blum and colleagues prospectively performed renal artery stenting in 68 patients (74 lesions) with ostial renal artery stenosis and suboptimal balloon angioplasty.[96] Patients were followed for a mean of 27 months with measurements of BP and serum creatinine (Scr), duplex sonography, and intra-arterial angiography. Five-year patency was 84.5% (mean follow-up was 27 months). Restenosis occurred in eight of 74 arteries (11%), but, after reintervention, the secondary, 5-year patency rate was 92.4%. BP was cured or improved in 78% of patients. The authors concluded that primary stent placement is an effective treatment for renal artery stenosis involving the ostium.

The clinical utility of renal artery stenting in renal function preservation was analyzed by several studies, which measured serial Scr levels to determine the response of renal function following endovascular intervention.[97] In a study reported by Harden and colleagues, who performed 33 renal artery stentings in 32 patients with renal insufficiency, they noted that renal function improved or stabilized in 22 patients (69%).[98] In a similar study, Watson and associates evaluated the effect of renal artery stenting on renal function by comparing the slopes of the regression lines derived from the reciprocal of Scr vs. time.[97] With a total of 61 renal stentings performed in 33 patients, the authors found that after stent placement, the slopes of the reciprocal of the serum creatinine (1/Scr) were positive in 18 patients and less negative in seven patients. The study concludes that in patients with chronic renal insufficiency due to obstructive renal artery stenosis, renal artery stenting is effective in improving or stabilizing renal function.

The clinical outcome of several large clinical studies of renal artery stenting in the treatment of renovascular hypertension or chronic renal insufficiency is shown in Table 23-13.[95,96,98–104] These studies uniformly demonstrated an excellent technical success rate with low incidence of restenosis or procedural-related complications. A similar analysis was reported by Leertouwer and colleagues who performed a meta-analysis of 14 studies comparing patients with renal arterial stent placement to those who underwent balloon angioplasty alone for renal arterial stenosis.[105] The study found that stent placement proved highly successful, with an initial technical success of 98%. The

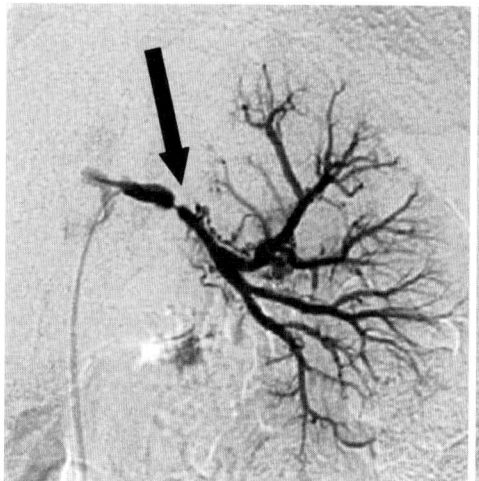
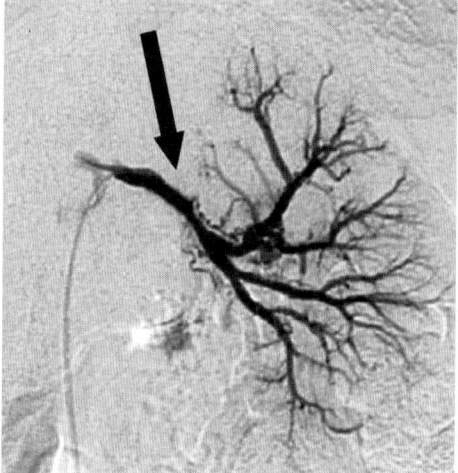

FIG. 23-48. Renal artery stenting. **A.** Focal lesion in the renal artery (*arrow*). **B.** Poststenting angiogram reveals a satisfactory result following a renal artery stenting placement (*arrow*).

A   **B**

| TABLE 23-13 | Clinical outcome of renal artery stent placement in the treatment of renovascular hypertension and renal insufficiency |

Author	Year	Patient No.	Technical Success (%)	Follow-Up (mo) (%)	Renal Insufficiency (%)		Renovascular Hypertension (%)		Complications (%)	Restenosis (%)
					Stable	Improved	Cured	Improved		
Iannone[102]	1996	63	99	10	45	36	4	35	13	14
Harden[98]	1997	32	100	6	34	34	N/A	N/A	3	13
Blum[96]	1997	68	100	27	N/A	N/A	16	62	0	11
White[95]	1997	100	99	6	N/A	20	N/A	N/A	2	19
Shannon[104]	1998	21	100	9	29	43	N/A	N/A	9	0
Rundback[103]	1998	45	94	17	N/A	N/A	N/A	N/A	9	25
Dorros[100]	1998	163	100	48	N/A	N/A	3	51	11	N/A
Henry[101]	1999	210	99	25	N/A	29	19	61	3	9
Bush[99]	2001	73	89	20	21	38	13	61	12	16

N/A = not available.

overall cure rate for hypertension was 20%, whereas hypertension was improved in 49%. Renal function improved in 30% and stabilized in 38% of patients. The restenosis rate at follow-up of 6 to 29 months was 17%. Renal stenting resulted in a higher technical success rate and a lower restenosis rate when compared to balloon angioplasty alone.

AORTOILIAC OCCLUSIVE DISEASE

The distal abdominal aorta and the iliac arteries are common sites affected by atherosclerosis. The symptoms and natural history of the atherosclerotic process affecting the aortoiliac arterial segment are influenced by the disease distribution and extent. Atherosclerotic plaques may cause clinical symptoms by restricting blood flow due to luminal obstruction or by embolizing atherosclerotic debris to the LE circulation. If the aortoiliac plaques reach sufficient mass that impinge on the arterial lumen, obstruction of blood flow to lower extremities occurs. Various risk factors exist that can lead to the development of aortoiliac occlusive disease. Recognition of these factors and understanding this disease entity will enable physicians to prescribe the appropriate treatment strategy that may alleviate symptoms and improve quality of life.

Diagnostic Evaluation

On clinical examination, patients often have weakened femoral pulses and a reduced ABI. Verification of iliac occlusive disease is usually made by color duplex scanning that reveals either a peak systolic velocity ratio of 2.5 or greater at the site of stenosis and/or a monophasic waveform. Noninvasive tests such as pulse volume recording (PVR) of the LE with estimation of the thigh-brachial pressure index may be suggestive of aortoiliac disease. MRA and multidetector CTA are increasingly being used to determine the extent and type of obstruction. DSA offers the interventionalist the benefit of making a diagnosis and the option of performing an endovascular treatment in a single session. Angiography provides important information regarding distal arterial runoff vessels as well as the patency of the profunda femoris artery (PFA). Presence of pelvic and groin collaterals is important in providing crucial collateral flow in maintaining lower limb viability. It must be emphasized, however, that patients should be subjected to angiography only if their symptoms warrant surgical intervention.

Differential Diagnosis

Degenerative hip or spine disease, lumbar disc herniation, spinal stenosis, diabetic neuropathy, and other neuromuscular problems can produce symptoms that may be mistaken for vascular claudication. Such cases can be distinguished from true claudication by the fact that the discomfort from neuromuscular problems often is relieved by sitting or lying down, as opposed to cessation of

ambulation. In addition, complaints that are experienced upon standing suggest nonvascular causes. When confusion persists, the use of noninvasive vascular laboratory testing modalities, including treadmill exercise, can help establish the diagnosis.

Collateral Arterial Network

The principal collateral pathways in severe aortoiliac artery occlusive disease or chronic aortic occlusion that may provide blood flow distal to the aortoiliac lesion include: (a) the SMA to the distal IMA via its superior hemorrhoidal branch to the middle and inferior hemorrhoidals to the internal iliac artery (39%); (b) the lumbar arteries to the superior gluteal artery to the internal iliac system (37%); (c) the lumbar arteries to the lateral and deep circumflex arteries to the common femoral artery (CFA) (12%); and (d) Winslow's pathway from the subclavian to the superior epigastric artery to the inferior epigastric artery to the external iliac arteries at the groin (Fig. 23-49). In general, treatment indications for aortoiliac artery occlusive disease include

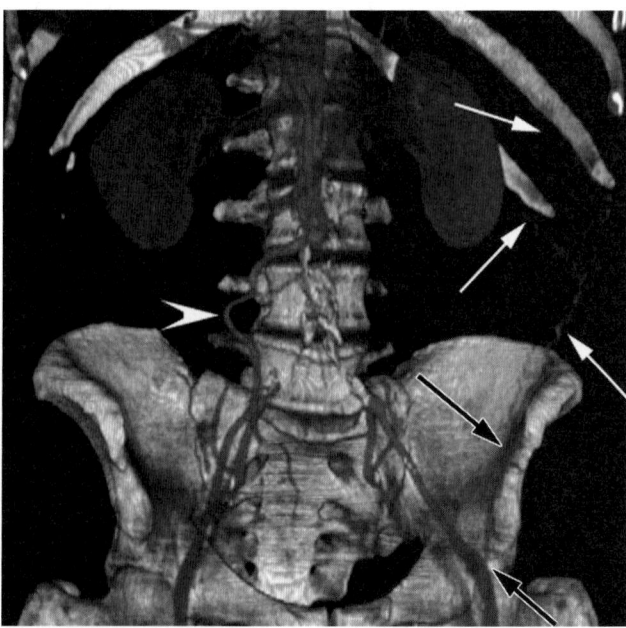

FIG. 23-49. Pertinent collateral pathways are developed in the event of chronic severe aortoiliac occlusive disease. As illustrated in this multidetector computed tomography angiography, these collaterals include epigastric arteries (*large white arrows*), an enlarged inferior mesenteric artery (*white arrowhead*), and enlarged lumbar arteries (*black arrows*).

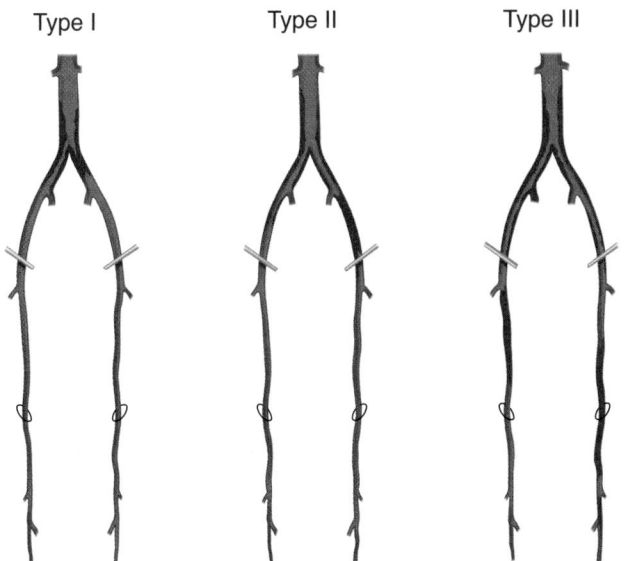

Type I   Type II   Type III

FIG. 23-50. Aortoiliac disease can be classified into three types. Type I represents focal disease affecting the distal aorta and proximal common iliac artery. Type II represents diffuse aortoiliac disease above the inguinal ligament. Type III represents multisegment occlusive disease involving aortoiliac and infrainguinal arterial vessels.

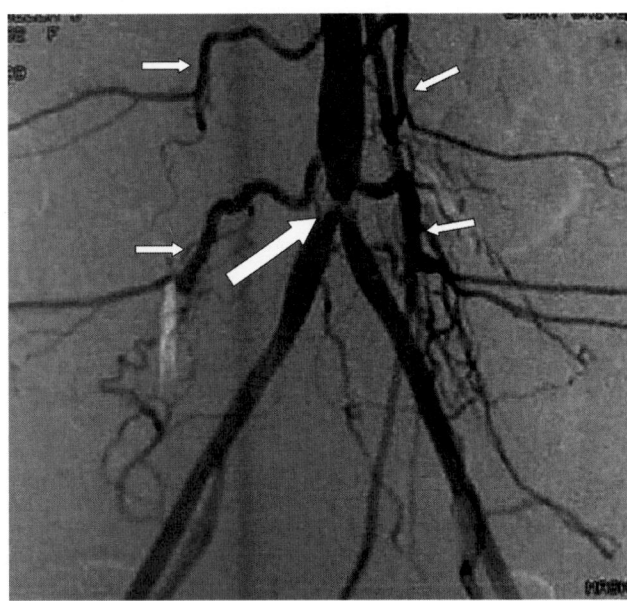

FIG. 23-51. Type I aortoiliac disease is confined to the distal abdominal aorta (*long arrow*) or proximal common iliac arteries. Due to the localized nature of this type of aortic obstruction and formation of collateral blood flow around the occluded segment (*short arrows*), limb-threatening symptoms are rare in the absence of more distal disease.

disabling claudication, ischemic rest pain, nonhealing LE tissue wound, and LE microembolization that arise from aortoiliac lesions.

Disease Classification

Based on the atherosclerotic disease pattern, aortoiliac occlusive disease can be classified into three various types (Fig. 23-50). Type

I aortoiliac disease, which occurs in 5 to 10% of patients, is confined to the distal abdominal aorta and common iliac vessels (Fig. 23-51). Due to the localized nature of this type of aortic obstruction and formation of collateral blood flow around the occluded segment, limb-threatening symptoms are rare in the absence of more distal disease (Fig. 23-52). This type of aortoiliac occlusive disease occurs in a relatively younger group of patients (aged in their mid-50s),

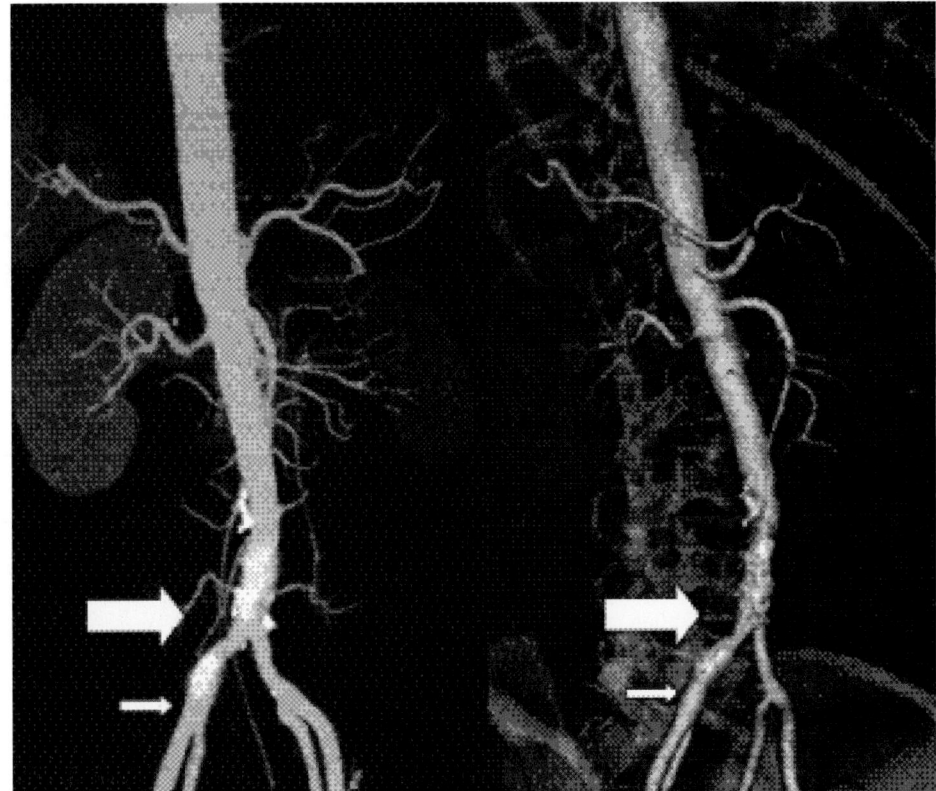

FIG. 23-52. Multidetector computed tomography angiography of the aortoiliac artery circulation in a 63-year-old man with buttock claudication. Three-dimensional image reconstruction showing intra-arterial calcification of the aorta (*large arrows*) and right common iliac artery (*small arrows*). This is consistent with a type I aortoiliac occlusive disease.

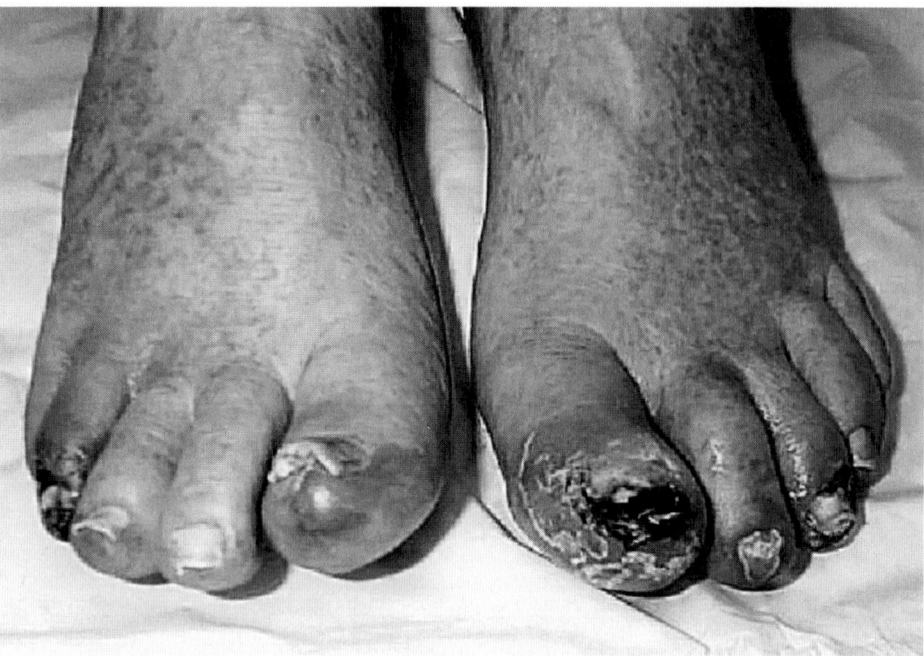

FIG. 23-53. Atherosclerotic disease involving the aortoiliac segment can result in microembolization of the lower leg circulation, resulting in trash foot or digital gangrene of toes.

compared with patients who have more femoropopliteal disease. Patients with a type I disease pattern have a lower incidence of hypertension and diabetes, but a significant frequency of abnormal blood lipid levels, particularly type IV hyperlipoproteinemia. Symptoms typically consist of bilateral thigh or buttock claudication and fatigue. Men report diminished penile tumescence and may have complete loss of erectile function. These symptoms in the absence of femoral pulses constitute Leriche's syndrome. Rest pain is unusual with isolated aortoiliac disease unless distal disease coexists. Occasionally patients report a prolonged history of thigh and buttock claudication that recently has become more severe. It is likely that this group has underlying aortoiliac disease that has progressed to acute occlusion of the terminal aorta. Others may present with "trash foot" that represents microembolization into the distal vascular bed (Fig. 23-53).

Type II aortoiliac disease represents a more diffuse atherosclerotic progression that involves predominately the abdominal aorta with disease extension into the CIA. This disease pattern affects approximately 25% of patients with aortoiliac occlusive disease. Type III aortoiliac occlusive disease, which affects approximately 65% of patients with aortoiliac occlusive disease, is widespread disease that is seen above and below the inguinal ligament (Fig. 23-54). Patients with "multilevel" disease are older, more commonly male (with a male-to-female ratio of 6:1), and much more likely to have diabetes, hypertension, and associated atherosclerotic disease involving cerebral, coronary, and visceral arteries. Progression of the occlusive process is more likely in these patients than in those with localized aortoiliac disease. For these reasons, most patients with a type III pattern tend to present with symptoms of advanced ischemia and require revascularization for limb salvage rather than for claudication. These patients have a decreased 10-year life expectancy when compared to patients with localized aortoiliac disease.

The most commonly used classification system of iliac lesions has been set forth by the TASC II group with recommended treatment options. This lesion classification categorizes the extent of atherosclerosis and has suggested a therapeutic approach based on this classification (Table 23-14 and Fig. 23-55).[2] According to this consensus document, endovascular therapy is the treatment of choice for type A lesions, and surgery is the treatment of choice for type D lesions. Endovascular treatment is the preferred treatment for type B lesions, and surgery is the preferred treatment for good-risk patients

with type C lesions. In comparison to the 2000 TASC II document, the commission has not only made allowances for treatment of more extensive lesions, but also took into account the continuing evolution of endovascular technology and the skills of individual interventionalists when stating that the patient's comorbidities, fully informed patient preference, and the local operator's long-term

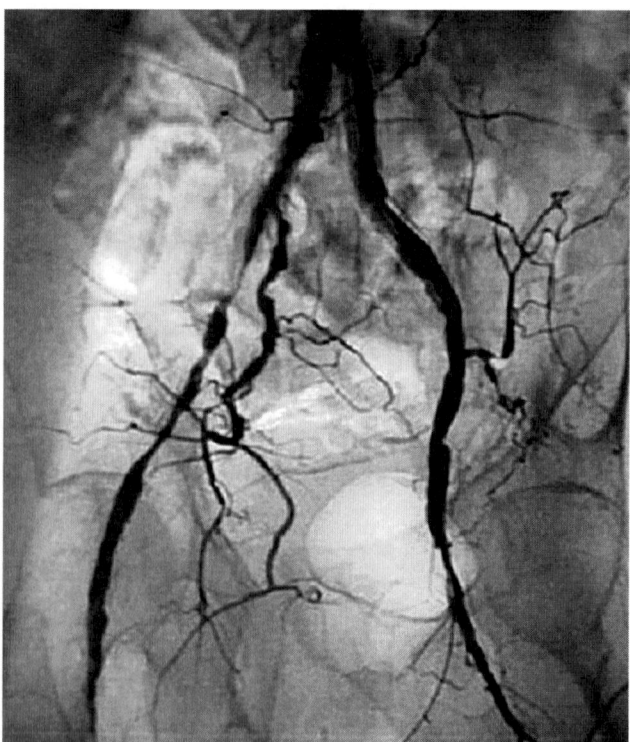

FIG. 23-54. Type III aortoiliac occlusive disease is a multilevel disease pattern that affects the aortoiliac segment as well as infrainguinal femoropopliteal vessels. Most patients with this disease pattern tend to present with symptoms of advanced ischemia and require revascularization for limb salvage rather than for claudication.

TABLE 23-14 TASC II classification of aortoiliac occlusive lesions

Type A lesions
- Unilateral or bilateral stenoses of CIA
- Unilateral or bilateral single short (≤3 cm) stenosis of EIA

Type B lesions
- Short (≤3 cm) stenosis of infrarenal aorta
- Unilateral CIA occlusion
- Single or multiple stenosis totaling 3–10 cm involving the EIA not extending into the CFA
- Unilateral EIA occlusion not involving the origins of internal iliac or CFA

Type C lesions
- Bilateral CIA occlusions
- Bilateral EIA stenoses 3–10 cm long not extending into the CFA
- Unilateral EIA stenosis extending into the CFA
- Unilateral EIA occlusion that involves the origins of internal iliac and/or CFA
- Heavily calcified unilateral EIA occlusion with or without involvement of origins of internal iliac and/or CFA

Type D lesions
- Infrarenal aortoiliac occlusion
- Diffuse disease involving the aorta and both iliac arteries requiring treatment
- Diffuse multiple stenoses involving the unilateral CIA, EIA, and CFA
- Unilateral occlusions of both CIA and EIA
- Bilateral occlusions of EIA
- Iliac stenoses in patients with AAA requiring treatment and not amenable to endograft placement or other lesions requiring open aortic or iliac surgery

AAA = abdominal aortic aneurysm; CFA = common femoral artery; CIA = common iliac artery; EIA = external iliac artery; TASC II = Trans-Atlantic Inter-Society Consensus.

success rates must be considered when making treatment decisions for type B and type C lesions.[2,106]

General Treatment Considerations

There is no effective medical therapy for the management of aortoiliac disease, but control of risk factors may help slow progression of atherosclerosis. Patients should have hypertension, hyperlipidemia, and diabetes mellitus controlled. They should be advised to stop smoking.

severe pulmonary disease. Further propose retroperitoneal approach include less GI third-space fluid losses, and ease with whi be accessed. There are randomized rep and refute the superiority of this a nated, knitted Dacron graft is used anastomosis, which can then be end-to-side fashion using 3–0 anastomosis should be made to decrease the incidenc atherosclerotic occlusiv

An end-to-end pro patients with an a extending up to t the end-to-end chance of co have not b ency bet for an of ba

condition or

In most cases, ABI disease in both iliac systems. severely affected than the other, progression eral bypass does not complicate the procedure of physiologic stress of the operation. ABF reliably relieves sympto has excellent long-term patency (approximately 70 to 75% at 10 years), and can be completed with a tolerable perioperative mortality (2 to 3%).[107]

Technical Considerations for Aortobifemoral Bypass

Both femoral arteries are initially exposed to ensure that they are adequate for the distal anastomoses. The abdomen is then opened in the midline, the small intestine is retracted to the right, and the posterior peritoneum overlying the aorta is incised. A retroperitoneal approach may be selected as an alternative in certain situations. This approach involves making a left flank incision and displacing the peritoneum and its contents to the right. Such an approach is contraindicated if the right renal artery is acutely occluded, because visualization from the left flank is very poor. Tunneling of a graft to the right femoral artery also is more difficult from a retroperitoneal approach, but can be achieved. The retroperitoneal approach has been reputed to be better tolerated than midline laparotomy for patients with multiple previous abdominal operations and with

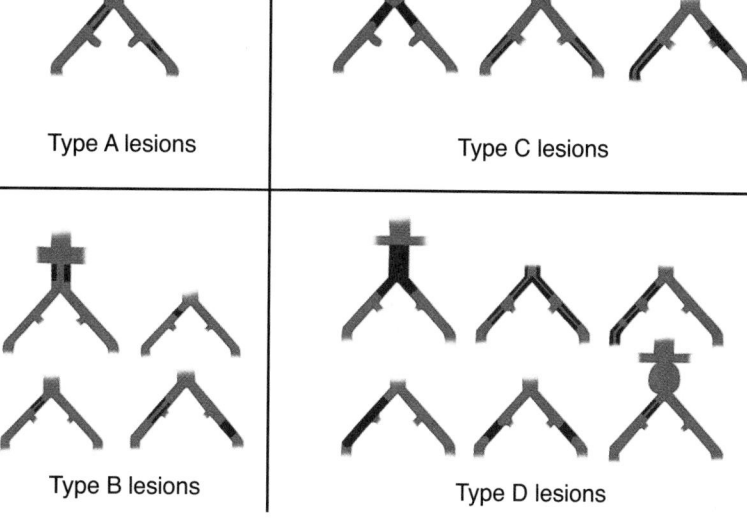

FIG. 23-55. Schematic depiction of Trans-Atlantic Inter-Society Consensus classification of aortoiliac occlusive lesions.

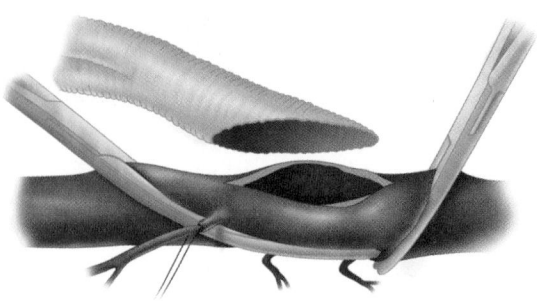

FIG. 23-57. In an end-to-side aortic anastomosis, the end of a prosthetic graft is connected to the side of an aortic incision.

d advantages of the
disturbance, decreased
the pararenal aorta can
orts, however, that support
pproach. A collagen-impreg-
to perform the proximal aortic
made in either an end-to-end or
polypropylene suture. The proximal
as close as possible to the renal arteries
of restenosis from progression of the
process in the future.

ximal aortic anastomosis is necessary in those
ortic aneurysm or complete aortic occlusion
he renal arteries (Fig. 23-56). Although in theory,
configuration allows for less turbulence and less
mpetitive flow with still patent host iliac vessels, there
een consistent results to substantiate differences in pat-
veen end-to-end and end-to-side grafts. Relative indications
end-to-side proximal aortic anastomosis include the presence
rge aberrant renal arteries, an unusually large IMA with poor
ck-bleeding, suggesting inadequate collateralization, and/or occlusive disease involving bilateral external iliac arteries. Under such
circumstances, end-to-end bypass from the proximal aorta to the
femoral level devascularizes the pelvic region because there is no
antegrade or retrograde flow in the occluded external iliac arteries to
supply the hypogastric arteries. As a result of the pelvic devascularization, there is an increased incidence of impotence, postoperative
colon ischemia, buttock ischemia, and paraplegia secondary to
spinal cord ischemia, despite the presence of excellent femoral and
distal pulses.

An end-to-side proximal aortic anastomosis can be associated
with certain disadvantages, which include the potential for distal
embolization when applying a partially occlusive aortic clamp (Fig.
23-57). Furthermore, the distal aorta often proceeds to total occlusion after an end-to-side anastomosis. There may also be a higher
incidence of aortoenteric fistula following construction of end-to-
side proximal anastomoses because the anterior projection makes
subsequent tissue coverage and reperitonealization of the graft
more difficult. The limbs of the graft are tunneled through the
retroperitoneum to the groin, where an end-to-side anastomosis is
fashioned between the graft and the bifurcation of the CFA using
5-0 polypropylene suture. Endarterectomy or patch angioplasty of
the profunda femoris may be required concurrently. Once the
anastomoses have been fashioned and the graft thoroughly flushed,
the clamps are removed and the surgeon carefully controls the
degree of aortic occlusion until full flow is re-established. During
this period the patient must be carefully monitored for hypotension.
Declamping hypotension is a complication of sudden restoration of
aortic flow, particularly following prolonged occlusion. Once flow
has been re-established, the peritoneum is carefully reapproximated
over the prosthesis to prevent fistulization into the intestine.

Despite the presence of multilevel disease in most patients, a
properly performed aortobifemoral operation can provide arterial
inflow and alleviate claudication symptoms in 70 to 80% of patients;
however, 10 to 15% of patients will require simultaneous outflow
reconstruction to address distal ischemia and facilitate limb salvage.
The advantage of concomitant distal revascularization is avoidance
of reoperation in a scarred groin. As a rule, if the profunda femoris
can accept a 4-mm probe and if a No. 3 Fogarty embolectomy
catheter can be passed distally for 20 cm or more, the PFA will be
sufficient for outflow and concomitant distal revascularization is
not necessary.

Aortic Endarterectomy

Aortoiliac endarterectomy is rarely performed, as it is associated with
greater blood loss, greater sexual dysfunction, and is more difficult to
perform. Long-term patency is comparable with aortobifemoral
grafting, and thus it remains a reasonable option in cases in which the
risk of infection of a graft is excessive, because it involves no prosthetic tissue. Aortoiliac endarterectomy was useful when disease was
localized to either the aorta or CIAs; however, at present, aortoiliac
PTA, stents, and other catheter-based therapies have become first-
line treatments in this scenario. Endarterectomy should not be performed if the aorta is aneurysmal because of continued aneurysmal
degeneration of the endarterectomized segment. If there is total
occlusion of the aorta to the level of the renal arteries, aortic transection several centimeters below the renal arteries with thrombectomy
of the aortic cuff followed by graft insertion is easier and more
expeditious when compared to endarterectomy. Involvement of the
EIA makes aortic endarterectomy more difficult to complete because
of decreased vessel diameter, increased length, and exposure issues.
The ability to establish an appropriate endarterectomy plane is compromised due to the muscular and inherently adherent nature of the
media in this location. There is a higher incidence of early thrombosis
and late failure with extended aortoiliofemoral endarterectomy when
compared to bypass grafting as a result of recurrent stenosis.

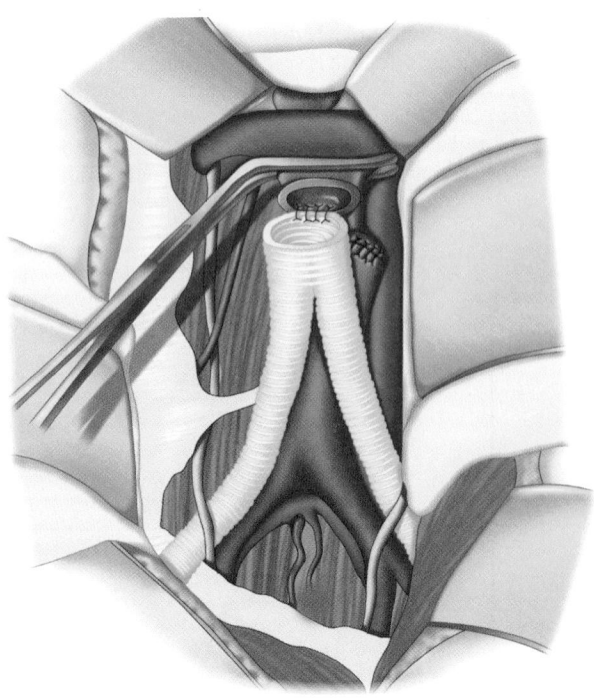

FIG. 23-56. In an end-to-end proximal aortic anastomosis, the aorta is divided in half. The proximal end of the aorta is anastomosed to the end of a prosthetic graft while the distal divided aortic stump is oversewn.

Axillofemoral Bypass

An axillofemoral bypass is an extra-anatomic reconstruction that derives arterial inflow from the axillary artery to the femoral artery. This is a treatment option for those patients with medical comorbidities that prohibit an abdominal vascular reconstruction. It may be performed under local anesthesia and is used for limb salvage. Extra-anatomic bypasses have lower patency when compared to aorto-bifemoral, and therefore, are seldom recommended for claudication. Before performing this operation, the surgeon should check pulses and BP in both arms to ensure that there is no obvious disease affecting flow through the axillary system. Angiography of the axillo-subclavian vasculature is not necessary, but can be helpful if performed at the time of aortography. The axillary artery is exposed below the clavicle, and a 6- to 8-mm externally reinforced PTFE graft is tunneled subcutaneously down the lateral chest wall and lateral abdomen to the groin. It is anastomosed to the ipsilateral distal at the CFA bifurcation into the superficial femoral and profunda femoris arteries. A femorofemoral crossover graft using a 6- to 8-mm externally reinforced PTFE graft is then used to revascularize the opposite extremity if necessary. Reported patency rates over 5 years vary from 30 to 80%.[108] Paradoxically, although it is a less complex procedure than aortofemoral grafting, the mortality rate is higher (10%), reflecting the compromised medical status of these patients.[108]

Iliofemoral Bypass

One option for patients with unilateral occlusion of the distal common iliac or external iliac arteries is iliofemoral grafting (Fig. 23-58). Long-term patency is comparable to aortounifemoral bypass and because the procedure can be performed using a retroperitoneal approach without clamping the aorta, the perioperative mortality is less.[108]

Femorofemoral Bypass

A femorofemoral bypass is another option for patients with unilateral stenosis or occlusion of the common or EIA who have rest pain, tissue loss, or intractable claudication. The primary (assisted) patency at 5 years is reported to be 60 to 70%, and, although this is inferior when compared to aortofemoral bypass, there are physiologic benefits, especially for patients with multiple comorbidities, because it is not necessary to cross-clamp the aorta.[109] There are no studies supporting the superiority of unsupported or externally supported PTFE over Dacron for choice of conduit. The fear of the recipient extremity stealing blood from the extremity ipsilateral to the donor limb is not realized unless the donor iliac artery and donor outflow arteries are diseased.[109] Depending on the skills of the interventionalist/surgeon, many iliac lesions classified as TASC II B, C, or D can now be addressed using an endovascular approach, thus obviating the need to perform a femorofemoral bypass. Additionally, femorofemoral bypass can be used as an adjuvant procedure after iliac inflow has been optimized with endovascular methods.

Obturator Bypass

An obturator bypass is used to reconstruct arterial anatomy in patients with groin sepsis resulting from prior prosthetic grafting, intra-arterial drug abuse, groin neoplasm, or damage from prior groin irradiation. This bypass can originate from the CIA, EIA, or uninvolved limb of an ABF. A conduit of Dacron, PTFE, or autologous vein is tunneled through the anteromedial portion of the obturator membrane to the distal superficial femoral or popliteal artery. The obturator membrane must be divided sharply so as to avoid injury to adjacent structures, and care must be taken to identify the obturator artery and nerve that pass posterolaterally. After the bypass is completed and the wounds isolated, the infected area is entered, the involved arteries are débrided to healthy tissue, and vascularized muscle flaps are mobilized to cover the ligated ends.[110] There have been varied results in terms of patency and limb salvage for obturator bypass. Some authors have reported 57% 5-year patency and 77% 5-year limb salvage rates, whereas others have shown a high rate of reinfection and low patency requiring reintervention.[110,111]

Thoracofemoral Bypass

The indications for thoracofemoral bypass are (a) multiple prior surgeries with a failed infrarenal aortic reconstruction and (b) infected aortic prosthesis. This procedure is more physiologically demanding than other extra-anatomic reconstructions because the patient must not only tolerate clamping the descending thoracic aorta but also performance of a left thoracotomy. The graft is tunneled to the left CFA from the left thorax posterior to the left

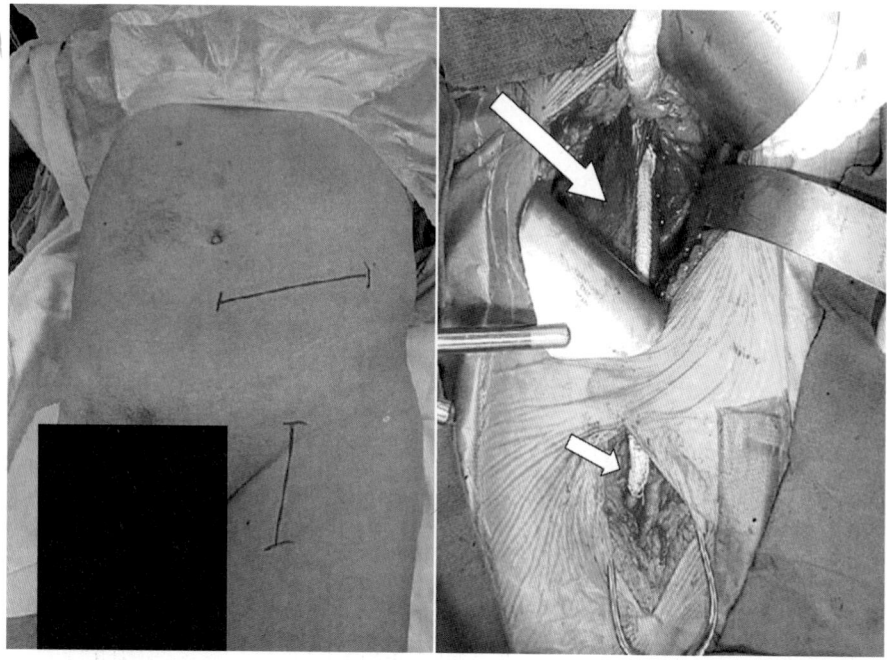

FIG. 23-58. A. Skin markings showing the incisions of an iliofemoral bypass. **B.** A prosthetic bypass graft is used for an iliofemoral artery bypass in which the proximal anastomosis is connected to the common iliac artery (*long arrow*) while the distal anastomosis is connected to the common femoral artery (*short arrow*).

A   **B**

kidney in the anterior axillary line using a small incision in the periphery of the diaphragm and an incision in the left inguinal ligament to gain access to the extraperitoneal space from below. The right limb is tunneled in the space of Retzius in an attempt to decrease kinking that is more likely to occur with subcutaneous, suprapubic tunneling. Thoracofemoral bypass has long-term patency comparable to aortofemoral bypass.

Complications of Surgical Aortoiliac Reconstruction

With current surgical techniques and conduits, early postoperative hemorrhage is unusual and occurs in 1 to 2% of cases. It is usually the result of technical oversight or coagulation abnormality.[112] Acute limb ischemia (ALI) occurring after aortoiliac surgery may be the result of acute thrombosis or distal thromboembolism. The surgeon can prevent thromboembolic events by (a) avoiding excessive manipulation of the aorta, (b) ensuring adequate systemic heparinization, (c) judicious placement of vascular clamps, and (d) thorough flushing before restoring blood flow. Acute thrombosis of an aortofemoral graft limb in the early perioperative period occurs in 1 to 3% of patients.[112] Thrombectomy of the graft limb is performed through a transverse opening in the hood of the graft at the femoral anastomosis. With this approach, it is possible to inspect the interior of the anastomosis and pass embolectomy catheters distally to clear the superficial femoral and profunda arteries. Various complications may be encountered following aortoiliac or aortobifemoral reconstruction (Table 23-15).

Intestinal ischemia following aortic reconstruction occurs in approximately 2% of cases; however, with colonoscopy, mucosal ischemia, which is a milder form, is seen more frequently. The surgeon can identify patients who require concomitant revascularization of the IMA, hypogastric arteries, or mesenteric arteries by examining the preoperative arteriogram for the presence of associated occlusive lesions in the celiac axis, the superior mesenteric arteries, or both. Likewise patients with patent and enlarged IMA or a history of prior colonic resections will benefit from IMA reimplantation.

In a comprehensive review of 747 patients who had aortoiliac operations for occlusive disease, secondary operations for late complications such as reocclusion, pseudoaneurysms, and infection were necessary in 21% of cases over a 22-year period.[113] The most frequent late complication is graft thrombosis. Limb occlusion occurs in 5 to 10% of patients within 5 years of the index operation and in 15 to 30% of patients 10 years or more after the index operation.[112,113] Anastomotic pseudoaneurysms occur in 1 to 5% of femoral anastomoses in patients with aortofemoral grafts.[114] Predisposing factors to pseudoaneurysm formation include progression of degenerative changes within the host artery, excessive tension at the anastomosis, and infection.[114] Due to the associated risks of thrombosis, distal embolization, infection, and rupture, anastomotic aneurysms should be repaired expeditiously.

Infection following aortoiliac reconstruction is a devastating complication that occurs in 1% of cases. Femoral anastomoses of aortofemoral reconstructions and axillofemoral bypasses are prone to infection.[113,114] Use of prophylactic antibiotics and meticulous surgical technique are vital in preventing contamination of the graft at the time of implantation. If infection appears to be localized to a single groin, one may consider the treatment strategies of graft preservation, aggressive local wound débridement, antibiotic solution irrigation, and soft tissue coverage with rotational muscle flaps. This nonexcisional treatment approach may be useful in selective cases of localized femoral graft infection. Most patients with infected aortoiliofemoral reconstructions usually require graft excision and revascularization via remote uncontaminated routes or the use of in situ replacement to clear the infective process and maintain limb viability. Aortoenteric fistula and associated GI hemorrhage are devastating complications, with a 50% incidence of death or limb loss. The incidence of aortoenteric fistula formation appears to be higher after an end-to-side proximal anastomosis, because it is more difficult to cover the prosthesis with viable tissue and avoid contact with the GI tract with this configuration.[113,114] Treatment of aortoenteric fistula requires resection of all prosthetic material, closure of the infrarenal abdominal aorta, repair of the GI tract, and revascularization by means of an extra-anatomic graft.

Endovascular Treatment for Aortic Disease

Although aortofemoral bypass surgery has excellent long-term patency and can be performed with low mortality rates, there are patients who are unable to withstand the physiologic stress of longer open procedures performed under general anesthesia, which require aortic cross-clamping, and which are associated with greater blood loss. These patients are more suited to endovascular interventions despite the decreased durability and requirement for more frequent reinterventions.

Focal Aortic Stenosis

The endovascular technique used to treat infrarenal aortic stenoses is similar to that used for iliac artery disease. Bilateral CFA access is established followed by insertion of a 10F sheath. The lesion is crossed using a hydrophilic wire and a supporting selective catheter and then changed for a stiffer guidewire. A self-expanding nitinol stent or a balloon-expandable stent mounted on a larger caliber angioplasty balloon is implanted followed by adequate postdilation. At the physician's discretion, "kissing" stents, simultaneous bilateral proximal iliac stents, are deployed if the lesion is in the distal aorta in the proximity of the aortic bifurcation. The role of covered stents such as cuffs made for endoluminal abdominal aortic aneurysm (AAA) repair has not been rigorously studied. The aortic diameter should be sized with a calibrated catheter during the angiography or by preintervention CT scanning to avoid undersizing. Balloon size will range from 12 to 18 mm in most cases. A single stent generally is sufficient in most cases. Large Palmaz-type stents mounted on XXL balloons (Meditech, Westwood, Mass) have been successfully used and may be inflated up to 25 mm in diameter if needed. Newer self-expanding stents also have been used. Concentric aortic stenosis may encroach upon the IMA and coverage of this vessel may be unavoidable. Care should be taken to use low inflation pressures (5 mmHg) to minimize the risk of

---

TABLE 23-15 Perioperative complications of aortobifemoral bypass grafting

Medical complications
- Perioperative myocardial infarction
- Respiratory failure
- Ischemia-induced renal failure
- Bleeding from IV heparinization
- Stroke

Procedure-related complications

Early
- Declamping shock
- Graft thrombosis
- Retroperitoneal bleeding
- Groin hematoma
- Bowel ischemia/infarction
- Peripheral embolization
- Erectile dysfunction
- Lymphatic leak
- Chylous ascites
- Paraplegia

Late
- Graft infection
- Anastomotic pseudoaneurysm
- Aortoenteric fistula
- Aortourinary fistula
- Graft thrombosis

aortic rupture. Patient complaints of back or abdominal pain during balloon inflation should be taken seriously, as they may suggest impending rupture. In case of a calcified small caliber, hypoplastic aorta (≤12 mm, typically in female patients), it is recommended to use smaller diameter stents. To achieve clinical improvement, these patients can be recanalized to an aortic diameter of 8 or 9 mm. Distal embolization is one of the potential complications of endovascular treatment for aortic stenoses. Full heparinization, meticulous technique during wire and catheter manipulations, and primary stenting reduce the risk of this complication. Because calcified aortic stenoses are prone to rupture during dilation, it is recommended that the extent of the calcification should be determined beforehand with preoperative CT scans. In case of aortic rupture, as long as wire access has been maintained, an occlusion balloon can be inflated proximal to the disrupted segment to achieve hemostasis and the rupture can be covered with a stent graft or repaired with open surgery.

Occlusive Lesions of the Aortic Bifurcation

Occlusive lesions are treated with the kissing balloon technique to avoid dislodging aortic plaque. Two angioplasty balloons of equal size are positioned across the ostia of the CIAs, using a retrograde approach, and inflated. Simultaneous balloon dilatation at the origins of both CIAs is advocated, even in the presence of a unilateral lesion, to protect the contralateral CIA from dissection or plaque embolization. Calcified lesions, which typically occur at the aortic bifurcation, are not amenable to balloon dilatation, and frequently require that a distal aortic reconstruction be performed using "kissing stents." Fears that the proximal ends of the stents that extend into the distal aorta will become a nidus for thrombus formation, or cause hemolysis have not been realized. The results are difficult to interpret because these bifurcation lesions are usually included in studies with iliac artery lesions. Patency rates for aortic bifurcation PTA range from 76 to 92% at 3 years.[115] The largest series reported to date includes 79 patients with aortic bifurcation lesions. The cumulative clinical success rate at a mean of 4 years was 93%.[116] In more recent years, stents have been used to reconstruct the aortic bifurcation.[117] The kissing stent technique is well suited for orificial lesions. Technical success with kissing stents at the aortic bifurcation has been reported to be 95 to 100%.[117] In the largest series reported, the primary patency at 3 years was 79%.[118]

Endovascular Treatment for Iliac Artery Disease

Percutaneous Transluminal Angioplasty

PTA is most useful in the treatment of isolated iliac stenoses of <4 cm in length. When used for stenoses rather than occlusion, a 2-year patency of 86% can be achieved.[119] The complication rate is approximately 2%, consisting of distal embolization, medial dissection, and acute thrombosis.

Technical Considerations for Iliac Interventions

Crossing a high-grade stenosis or occlusion can be challenging in the iliac arteries. It is vital to image the lesion well because multiple views and use of the image intensifier will frequently uncover the anatomic reason for the difficulty. Frequently, the difficulty is the result of vessel tortuosity that cannot be appreciated on the original view. Use of an angled hydrophilic guidewire and an angled catheter can provide steering and add extra support for the wire trying to cross the lesion. Patience, persistence, and periodic reimaging will facilitate the crossing of a lesion in the great majority of cases. Guidewire traversal must be achieved for performance of endovascular iliac intervention. Over 90% of iliac occlusions can be passed with simple guidewire techniques.

The preferred approach for recanalizing a CIA occlusion is retrograde passage of devices from an ipsilateral CFA puncture because, in this manner, distance to the lesion is short and access is straighter. A stenosis is normally crossed using a combination of a soft-tip 0.035-in guidewire (i.e., Bentson type wire) or hydrophilic wire and a 5 F straight or selective catheter. One of the hazards of retrograde recanalization is that the guidewire stays in a subintimal location, and cannot be redirected into the true lumen at the aortic bifurcation. There are several approaches that can be used to achieve re-entry of total chronic occlusions. Specialized catheters allow passage of a needle and guidewire across the intima distal to the occlusion. Intravascular ultrasound can be used for true lumen re-entry under fluoroscopic guidance. Another method of achieving true lumen re-entry involves performing the recanalization from an antegrade contralateral CFA approach. A 4 F Berenstein catheter (Cordis Corp., Miami Lakes, FL) is used to probe the occlusion. The lesion can be crossed in most instances (5 to 20% failure rate) with a hydrophilic guidewire or, occasionally, with its stiffer back end. As soon as the guidewire crosses the obstruction and lies within the ipsilateral EIA lumen, it is snared and partially pulled out of the ipsilateral CFA. A short catheter is then inserted in a retrograde fashion over the wire end into the abdominal aorta proximal to the lesion. The hydrophilic guidewire is then exchanged for a stiffer Amplatz (Boston Scientific, Natick, MA) guidewire to facilitate iliac stenting.

Obtaining arterial access when there are absent femoral pulsations is aided by the use of ultrasound guidance and "road-map" imaging software that is available on modern angiographic equipment. When the lesion is successfully crossed, balloons of an appropriate size and length are selected for the angioplasty. Most CIAs will accommodate 8- to 10-mm diameter balloons, while most EIAs will accommodate 6- to 8-mm diameter balloons. Inflation is performed with caution, especially if there is heavy calcification, and should be guided by patient discomfort, pressure gauge readings, and changes in balloon outline.

If guidewire traversal is straightforward, consideration should be given to the presence of an acute thrombosis that may benefit from CDT. If guidewire traversal is challenging, it is unlikely that CDT will be beneficial. Investigators have found that routine thrombolysis and balloon dilation of occluded arteries before stent placement is associated with an increased incidence of distal embolic events.[120] Stents should be placed after inadequate angioplasty. Stents are warranted when there is a greater than 30% residual stenosis, when there is a flow-limiting dissection, or when there is a pressure gradient of 5 mmHg or greater across the treated segment.[121] Placement of stents can precipitate distal embolization in up to 10%, especially if lesions are friable and vulnerable to manipulation. Routine primary stent placement is not recommended because it has not been found to be superior to selective stenting in terms of outcomes or cost.[122]

Primary Stenting vs. Selective Stenting in Iliac Arteries

Primary stenting rather than selective stenting should be considered for longer iliac lesions and for all TASC II C and D lesions. The primary patency rates at 1, 2, and 3 years were 96%, 90%, and 72% for longer lesions (>5 cm) that were primarily stented vs. 46%, 46%, and 28% with selective stenting.[122] Primary stenting generally is advocated for chronic iliac artery occlusions, recurrent stenosis after previous iliac PTA, and for complex stenoses with eccentric, calcified, ulcerated plaques, or plaques with spontaneous dissection. All these lesions are prone to distal embolization during manipulation of wires and angioplasty balloons. Distal embolization with isolated PTA is not common for uncomplicated lesions, but can occur in up to 24% of cases, when treating ulcerated plaques, aortoiliac bifurcation lesions, or iliac occlusions.[122] It is believed that direct stent placement without predilation significantly reduces the risk of distal embolization by trapping potentially emboligenic material between the arterial wall and the stent mesh. Although PTA has demonstrated excellent results in focal stenoses of the abdominal aorta and iliacs, primary stenting in these locations is safe, improves patency rates, reduces the degree of restenosis when compared with PTA alone, and also decreases the risk of distal embolization. Additional potential advantages of direct stenting include shorter procedural time and less radiation exposure. The Dutch Iliac Stent Trial has provided evidence that refutes the superiority of primary stenting over angioplasty alone.[123] Most interventionalists continue to perform angioplasty first and stent selectively for inadequate results. The approach to aortoiliac stenting is intuitive. Individual judgment and experience are important in the decision-making process, and there are lesions with unstable morphology such as long occlusions, ulceration, and dissection that warrant primary stenting.

Stent Graft Placement for Aortoiliac Interventions

Stent grafts have been used to treat complex iliac lesions in an attempt to exclude these sources of embolization. A recent report suggested that the use of stent grafts was beneficial for TASC II C and D lesions.[124] Bosiers and colleagues published a series involving 91 limbs with diseased iliacs that they treated with 107 stent grafts. They reported successful deployment in all patients without distal embolization or vessel rupture and a primary patency rate of 91.1% at 1-year follow-up.[125] The authors commented about their concerns of causing embolization during placement of the stent grafts and recommended that, once an occlusion was traversed with the guidewire, to gently predilate with a 5-mm balloon, followed by smooth stent graft insertion into the newly created channel. The role of stent grafts in aortoiliac occlusive disease has not been fully elucidated yet.

Complications of Endovascular Aortoiliac Interventions

Iliac artery angioplasty is associated with a 2 to 4% major complication rate and 4 to 15% minor complication rate. Many of these minor complications are related to the arterial puncture site. The most frequent complications relate to access site cannulation. Hemorrhage can range from the more common access site hematoma to the rarer retroperitoneal and intraperitoneal hemorrhage. Distal embolization occurs in 2 to 10% of iliac PTA and stenting procedures.[112] Percutaneous catheter aspiration should be the initial treatment for calf vessel embolization, but, for larger emboli such as those that lodge in the profunda femoris or common femoral arteries, surgical embolectomy may be required because the embolic material contains atherosclerotic plaque, which is not amenable to transcatheter aspiration or CDT. The incidence of pseudoaneurysm formation at the puncture site is 0.5%. The treatment of choice for pseudoaneurysms >2 cm in diameter is percutaneous thrombin injection under ultrasound guidance. Arterial rupture may complicate the procedure in 0.3% of cases. Tamponade of the ruptured artery with an occlusion balloon should be performed, and a covered stent should be placed. In case of failure, surgical treatment is required.

Clinical Results Comparing Surgical and Endovascular Treatment of Aortoiliac Disease

The mortality risk for ABF in patients with isolated, localized aortoiliac disease is relatively low, whereas, for patients with concomitant atherosclerosis in coronary, carotid, and visceral vessels, mortality and morbidity are higher. For this reason, the cumulative long-term survival rate for patients having aortoiliac reconstruction remains 10 to 15 years less than anticipated for a normal age- and sex-matched population. Twenty-five to 30% of patients with concomitant atherosclerosis in other vascular distributions are dead within 5 years, and 50 to 60% will have died by 10 years.[114]

Compared with conventional ABF, common iliac angioplasty was shown to have a 10 to 20% lower overall patency rate. It should be noted that these results were reported in early trials that used older generations of endovascular equipment. With continued progress and newer angioplasty balloons and stenting practices, more comparable outcomes are being reported. Review of the literature confirms that there is an 85 to 90% graft patency rate at 5 years and 70 to 75% at 10 years after aortobifemoral reconstruction.[126] Due in part to factors including continued refinements in anesthetic management, intraoperative monitoring, and postoperative intensive care, low perioperative mortality rates for ABF can be achieved commonly in today's clinical practice.

Despite its lower long-term success, common iliac angioplasty is a useful procedure in patients with focal disease and mild symptoms in whom a major surgical revascularization is not justified. Angioplasty of the iliac vessels can be a useful adjunct to distal surgical bypass as well, increasing the success of distal revascularization and eliminating the risks associated with aortoiliac bypass. Thus, with long-term patency less than, but comparable to, open surgical bypass, and with more favorable morbidity rates, iliac angioplasty has become a well-accepted modality of treatment for iliac occlusive disease. Ideal iliac angioplasty lesions are nonocclusive and short. Patency after intervention is better when lesions occur in larger diameter vessels, when stenoses rather than occlusions are treated, when runoff vessels are patent, and when the indication for intervention is lifestyle-limiting claudication rather than critical limb ischemia.

Becker and associates estimated a 5-year patency rate of 72% in an analysis of 2697 cases of iliac angioplasty and noted a better patency (79%) in claudicants.[127] Less favorable results are obtained with long stenoses, external iliac stenoses, and tandem lesions. The reported technical and initial clinical success of balloon angioplasty in iliac artery stenoses exceeds 90% in most series and the 5-year patency rates range between 54 and 92%.[128] The reported technical and initial clinical success of balloon angioplasty in iliac artery occlusions ranges between 78 and 98% and the 3-year patency rates range between 48 and 85%.[128]

Factors reported to affect the patency of aortoiliac endovascular interventions adversely include quality of runoff vessels, severity of ischemia, and length of diseased segments treated. Likewise, as vessel diameter and flow rates change, so do success rates after angioplasty. It was reported in the literature that location of the lesion at the EIA adversely affects both primary and assisted-primary patency. Following angioplasty of the CIA, patency rates were 81 and 52% at 1 and 6 years, whereas, after EIA angioplasty, they were 74 and 48% at 1 and 4 years.[129] Although there is literature that supports location of the lesion in the EIA as a factor that adversely affects both primary and assisted-primary patency, this has not been a universal finding.[129] Female patients are also reported to have lower patency rates than males following iliac PTA, with or without stent placement in the EIA.[130]

Stenting of the iliac arteries provides a durable and curative treatment, with a 3-year patency rate of 41 to 92% for stenoses and a 3-year patency rate of 64 to 85% and 4-year patency rate of 54 to 78% for occlusions.[128] A meta-analysis of 2116 patients by Bosch and Hunink showed that aortoiliac PTA resulted in a 39% improvement in long-term patency compared to balloon angioplasty, despite the fact that complication rates and 30-day mortality rates did not differ significantly.[131] Park and colleagues presented long-term follow-up results in a cohort of patients with all four TASC II types of iliac lesions. The authors presented primary patency rates of 87%, 83%, 61%, and 49% at 3, 5, 7, and 10 years, respectively, after the index intervention.[132] Leville and associates achieved primary and secondary patency rates of 76 and 90%, respectively, after 3 years, in a cohort of patients that they stented for iliac occlusions. The authors postulated that endovascular treatment for iliac occlusive disease should be extended to type C and D lesions, because they observed no detectable differences between the four TASC II classifications in terms of primary and secondary patency rates.[133] They concluded that presence of TASC II C and D lesions should not preclude endovascular treatment and believe that endovascular attempts should be exhausted before open surgical repair of iliac occlusions is attempted because of the decreased perioperative morbidity and good midterm durability.

Not all results have been in favor of stenting, and, at present, universal primary stenting cannot be recommended. Although stents are often used to improve the outcome of PTA, there is no general consensus that stenting should be mandatory in all iliac lesions. Complex, ulcerated iliac lesions with high embologenic potential or recanalized chronic iliac occlusions may be an exception. In the Dutch Iliac Trial, primary stenting did not prove to be superior to iliac angioplasty and selective stenting. The researchers in this prospective, randomized, multicenter study concluded that balloon angioplasty with selective stenting had comparable 2-year patency rates with primary stenting; 77 and 78%, respectively. It must be noted, however, that it was necessary to stent 43% of the patients in the PTA treatment group due to unsatisfactory angioplasty results.[123] The 5-year outcomes between the two groups were also similar, with 82 and 80% of the treated iliac segments remaining free of the need for new revascularization procedures after a mean follow-up of 5.6 ± 1.3 years.[123]

LOWER EXTREMITY ARTERIAL OCCLUSIVE DISEASE

The symptoms of LE occlusive disease are classified into two large categories: ALI and chronic limb ischemia (CLI). Ninety percent (90%) of acute ischemias are either thrombotic or embolic. Frequently, sudden onset of limb-threatening ischemia may be the result of acute exacerbation of the pre-existing atherosclerotic disease. Chronic ischemia is largely due to atherosclerotic changes of the LE that manifest from asymptomatic to limb-threatening gangrene. As the population ages, the prevalence of chronic occlusive disease of the LE is increasing and it significantly influences lifestyle, morbidity, and mortality. In addition, multiple comorbid conditions increase risks of surgical procedures. Endovascular interventions become an important alternative in treating LE occlusive disease. However, despite rapid evolving endovascular technology, LE endovascular intervention continues to be one of the most controversial areas of endovascular therapy.

Epidemiology

In a detailed review of the literature, McDaniel and Cronenwett concluded that claudication occurred in 1.8% of patients under 60 years of age, 3.7% of patients between 60 and 70 years of age, and 5.2% of patients over 70 years of age.[134] Leng and his colleagues scanned 784 subjects using ultrasound in a random sample of men and women ages 56 to 77 years. Of the subjects that were scanned, 64% demonstrated atherosclerotic plaque.[135] However, a large number of patients had occlusive disease without significant symptoms. In a study by Schroll and Munck, only 19% of the patients with peripheral vascular disease were symptomatic.[136] Using ankle-brachial indices (ABIs), Stoffers and colleagues scanned 3171 individuals between the ages of 45 and 75 and identified 6.9% of patients who had ABIs <0.95, only 22% of whom had symptoms.[137] In addition, they demonstrate that the concomitant cardiovascular and cerebrovascular diseases were three to four times higher among the group with asymptomatic peripheral vascular diseases than those without peripheral vascular disease. Furthermore, they confirm that 68% of all peripheral arterial obstructive diseases were unknown to the primary care physician and this group mainly represented less advanced cases of atherosclerosis. However, among patients with an ABI ratio <0.75, 42% were unknown to the primary physicians.

Diagnostic Evaluation

The diagnosis of LE occlusive disease often is made based upon a focused history and physical examination, and confirmed by the imaging studies. A well-performed physical examination often reveals the site of lesions by detecting changes in pulses, temperature, and appearances. The bedside ABIs using BP cuff also aid in diagnosis. Various clinical signs and symptoms are useful to differentiate conditions of viable, threatened, and irreversible limb ischemia caused by arterial insufficiency (Table 23-16).

Noninvasive studies are important in documenting the severity of occlusive disease objectively. Ultrasound Dopplers measuring ABIs and segmental pressures are widely used in North America and Europe. Normal ABI is >1.0. In patients with claudication, ABIs decrease to 0.5 to 0.9 and to even lower levels in patients with rest pain or tissue loss.[138] Segmental pressures are helpful in identifying

TABLE 23-16 Signs and symptoms of acute limb ischemia

Description	Category		
	Viable	**Threatened**	**Irreversible**
Clinical description	Not immediately threatened	Salvageable if promptly treated	Major tissue loss, amputation unavoidable
Capillary return	Intact	Intact, slow	Absent (marbling)
Muscle weakness	None	Mild, partial	Profound, paralysis (rigor)
Sensory loss	None	Mild, incomplete	Profound anesthetic
Arteriovenous Doppler finding	Audible	Inaudible or audible	Inaudible

the level of involvement. Decrease in segmental pressure between two segments indicates significant disease. Ultrasound duplex scans are used to identify the site of lesion by revealing flow disturbance and velocity changes. A meta-analysis of 71 studies by Koelemay and associates confirmed that duplex scanning is accurate for assessing arterial occlusive disease in patients suffering from claudication or critical ischemia, with an accumulative sensitivity of 80% and specificity of over 95%.[139] Adding an ultrasound contrast agent further increases sensitivity and specificity to ultrasound technology.[140] Other noninvasive imaging technologies such as MRA and CTA are rapidly evolving and gaining popularity in the diagnosis of LE occlusive disease (Figs. 23-59 and 23-60).

Contrast angiography remains the gold standard in imaging study. Using contrast angiography, interventionists can locate and size the anatomic significant lesions and measure the pressure gradient across the lesion, as well as plan for potential intervention. Angiography is, however, semi-invasive and should be confined to patients for whom surgical or percutaneous intervention is contemplated. Patients with borderline renal function may need to have alternate contrast agents such as gadolinium or carbon dioxide to avoid contrast-induced nephrotoxicity.

Differential Diagnosis

Arterial insufficiency frequently leads to muscle ischemic pain involving the LE muscularly, particularly during exercise. Intermittent claudication is pain affecting the calf, and, less commonly, the thigh and buttock, which is induced by exercise and relieved by rest. Symptom severity varies from mild to severe. Intermittent claudication occurs as a result of muscle ischemia during exercise caused by obstruction to arterial flow. For differential diagnosis of intermittent claudication, there are a variety of neurologic, musculoskeletal, and venous conditions that may produce symptoms of calf pain (Table 23-17). Additionally, various non-atherosclerotic conditions also can cause symptoms consistent with intermittent LE claudication (Table 23-18). Nocturnal calf muscle spasms or night cramps are not indicative of arterial disease. They are common but are difficult to diagnose with certainty. Foot ulceration is not always the result of arterial insufficiency. Ischemic ulcers occur on the toes or lateral side of the foot and are painful. By comparison, venous ulcers, which also are common, occur above the medial malleolus. These venous stasis ulcers are typically surrounded by a peripheral area of darkened skin discoloration that is also known as *lipodermatosclerosis.* Neuropathic ulcers usually are found on weight-bearing surfaces, have thick calluses, and are pain free. Ulcers may be the result of more than one etiology. Rest pain must be distinguished from peripheral neuropathy, which is prevalent in diabetic patients. Patients with diabetic neuropathy tend to have decreased vibration and position sense and decreased reflexes. Spinal stenosis causes pain that is exacerbated with standing and back extension.

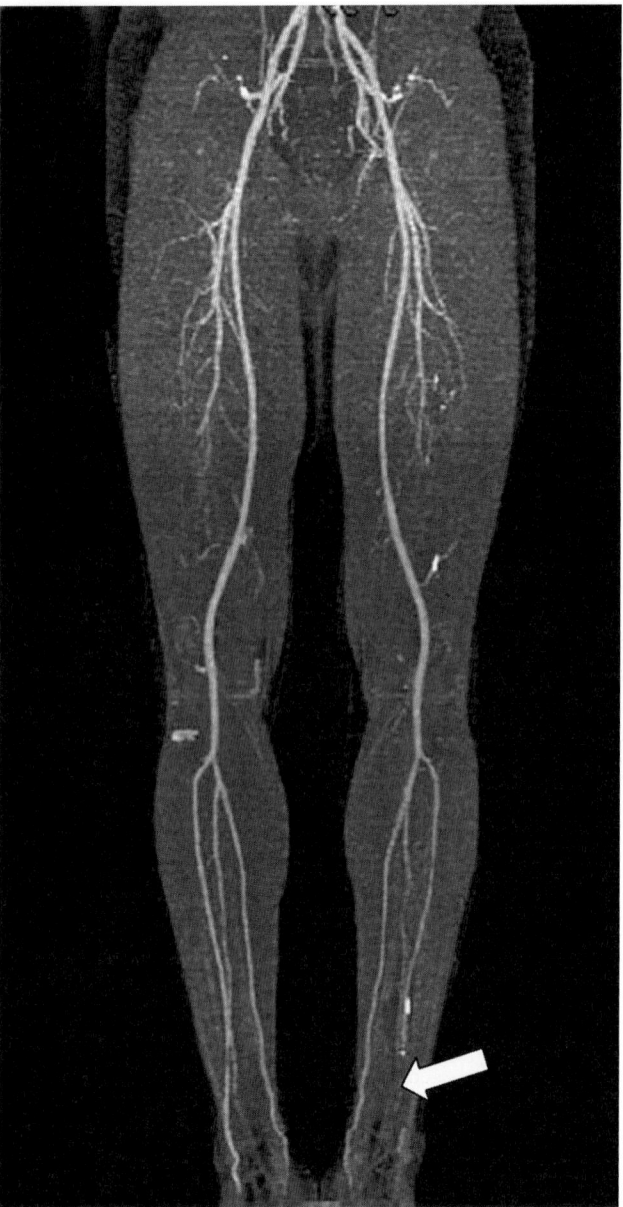

FIG. 23-59. A high-resolution computed tomography angiography of a patient with normal right lower extremity arterial circulation. Distal occlusive disease is noted in the left tibial arteries (*arrow*).

Lower Extremity Occlusive Disease Classification

LE occlusive disease may range from exhibiting no symptoms to limb-threatening gangrene. There are two major classifications based on the clinical presentations.

The Fontaine classification uses four stages: Fontaine I is the stage when patients are asymptomatic; Fontaine II is when they have mild (IIa) or severe (IIb) claudication; Fontaine III is when they have ischemic rest pain; and Fontaine IV is when patients suffer tissue loss such as ulceration or gangrene (Table 23-19).[141]

The Rutherford classification has four grades (0–III) and seven categories (0–6). Asymptomatic patients are classified into category 0; claudicants are stratified into grade I and divided into three categories based on the severity of the symptoms; patients with rest pain belong to grade II and category 4; patients with tissue loss are classified into grade III and categories 5 and 6, based on the significance of the tissue loss.[2] These clinical classifications help to establish uniform standards in evaluating and reporting the results of diagnostic measurements and therapeutic interventions (see Table 23-19).

The most clinically useful classification of LE atherosclerotic disease should be based on morphologic characters of the lesions. The TASC II task force published a guideline separating LE arterial diseases into femoropopliteal and infrapopliteal lesions (Table 23-20). This guideline is particularly useful in determining intervention strategies based on the disease classifications. Based on the guideline, femoropopliteal lesions are divided into four types: A, B, C, and D. Type A lesions are single focal lesions <3 cm in length that did not involve the origins of the superficial femoral artery (SFA) or the distal popliteal artery; Type B lesions are single lesions 3 to 5 cm in length not involving the distal popliteal artery or multiple or heavily calcified lesions <3 cm in length; Type C lesions are multiple stenoses or occlusions >15 cm in length, or recurrent stenoses or occlusions that need treatment after two endovascular interventions. Type D lesions were those with complete occlusion of CFA, SFA, or popliteal artery.[2]

In a similar fashion, infrapopliteal arterial diseases are classified into four types based on TASC II guideline (Fig. 23-61). Type A lesions are single lesions <1 cm in length not involving the trifurcation; Type B lesions are multiple lesions <1 cm in length or single lesions shorter than 1 cm involving the trifurcation; Type C lesions are those lesions extensively involving trifurcation or those that are 1- to 4-cm stenotic or 1- to 2-cm occlusive lesions; Type D lesions are occlusions longer than 2 cm or diffuse diseases.[2]

Etiology of Acute Limb Ischemia

ALI is defined as *sudden loss of limb perfusion* and the term is applicable up to 2 weeks after an initiating event. Although the instances of acute leg ischemia caused by emboli have decreased due to more effective treatment of rheumatic fever and atrial fibrillation, the incidence of thrombotic acute leg ischemia has increased. Even with the extensive use of newer endovascular techniques including thrombolysis, most published series report a 10 to 30% 30-day amputation rate.[2] The short-term mortality of patients presenting with acute ischemia is 15 to 20%. The most common etiologies of ALI include embolism, native vessel thrombosis, reconstruction thrombosis, trauma, and complications of peripheral aneurysm. Most cases of acute LE ischemia are the result of thrombosis of a prosthetic conduit. This stems from increased use of prosthetic conduits to address CLI.

Presenting symptoms in ALI are pain and loss of sensory or motor function. The abruptness and time of onset of the pain, its location and intensity, as well as change in severity over time, should all be taken into consideration. The duration and intensity of the pain and presence of motor or sensory changes are very important in clinical decision making and urgency of revascularization. Thrombolysis may be less effective for thrombosis of a 2-week or longer duration compared with acute thrombosis.[142]

Arterial Embolism

The heart is the most common source of distal emboli, which account for more than 90% of peripheral arterial embolic events. Atrial fibrillation is the most common source. Sudden cardioversion results in the dilated noncontractile atrial appendage regaining contractile activity, which can dislodge the contained thrombus. Other cardiac sources include mural thrombus overlying a myocardial infarction, or thrombus forming within a dilated left ventricular aneurysm. Mural thrombi also can develop within a ventricle dilated by cardiomyopathy. Emboli that arise from a ventricular aneurysm or from a dilated cardiomyopathy can be very large and can lodge at the aortic bifurcation (saddle embolus), thus rendering both legs ischemic. Diseased valves are another source of distal embolization. Historically, this occurred as a result of rheumatic heart disease. Currently, subacute and acute bacterial endocarditis are the more common causes. Infected emboli can seed the recipient vessel wall, creating mycotic aneurysms.

An electrocardiogram will diagnose atrial fibrillation. A transthoracic or transesophageal echocardiogram should be performed to look for a cardiac source. It is important to seek other sources of

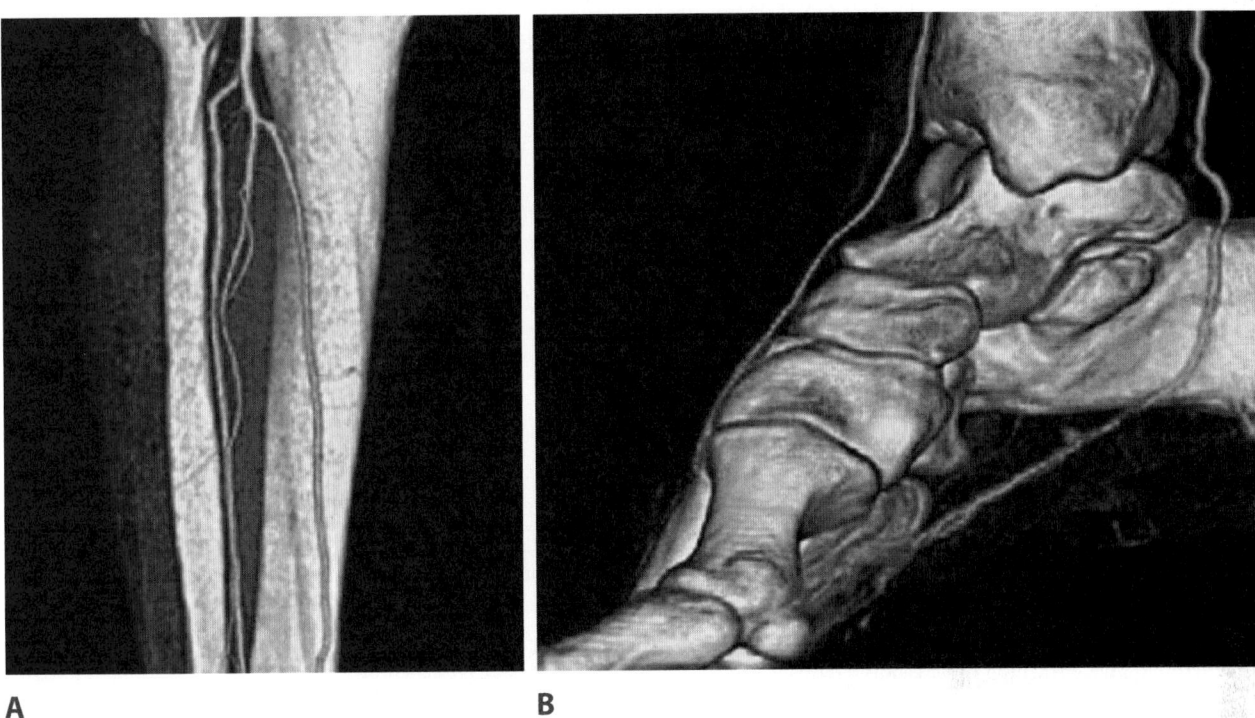

A   **B**

FIG. 23-60. A. A multidetector computed tomographic angiography of a patient with an infrapopliteal arterial circulation. **B.** Pedal arterial circulation. The high spatial resolution and image quality of these images show three patent infrapopliteal runoff vessels and patent pedal vessels at the foot level.

TABLE 23-17   Differential diagnosis of intermittent claudication

Condition	Location of Pain or Discomfort	Characteristic Discomfort	Onset Relative to Exercise	Effect of Rest	Effect of Body Position	Other Characteristics
Intermittent claudication (calf)	Calf muscles	Cramping pain	After same degree of exercise	Quickly relieved	None	Reproducible
Chronic compartment syndrome	Calf muscles	Tight, bursting pain	After much exercise (e.g., jogging)	Subsides very slowly	Relief speeded by elevation	Typically heavy-muscled athletes
Venous claudication	Entire leg, but usually worse in thigh and groin	Tight, bursting pain	After walking	Subsides slowly	Relief speeded by elevation	History of iliofemoral deep venous thrombosis, signs of venous congestion, edema
Nerve root compression (e.g., herniated disk)	Radiates down leg, usually posteriorly	Sharp lancinating pain	Soon, if not immediately after onset	Not quickly relieved (also often present at rest)	Relief may be aided by adjusting back position	History of back problems
Symptomatic Baker's cyst	Behind knee, down calf	Swelling, soreness, tenderness	With exercise	Present at rest	None	Not intermittent
Intermittent claudication (hip, thigh, buttock)	Hip, thigh, buttocks	Aching discomfort, weakness	After same degree of exercise	Quickly relieved	None	Reproducible
Hip arthritis	Hip, thigh, buttocks	Aching discomfort	After variable degree of exercise	Not quickly relieved (and may be present at rest)	More comfortable sitting, weight taken off legs	Variable, may relate to activity level, weather changes
Spinal cord compression	Hip, thigh, buttocks (follows dermatome)	Weakness more than pain	After walking or standing for same length of time	Relieved by stopping only if position changed	Relief by lumbar spine flexion (sitting or stooping forward)	Frequent history of back problems, provoked by increased intra-abdominal pressure
Intermittent claudication (foot)	Foot, arch	Severe deep pain and numbness	After same degree of exercise	Quickly relieved	None	Reproducible
Arthritic, inflammatory process	Foot, arch	Aching pain	After variable degree of exercise	Not quickly relieved (and may be present at rest)	May be relieved by not bearing weight	Variable, may relate to activity level

TABLE 23-18	Non-atherosclerotic causes of intermittent claudication

- Aortic coarctation
- Arterial fibrodysplasia
- Iliac syndrome of the cyclist
- Peripheral emboli
- Persistent sciatic artery
- Popliteal aneurysm
- Popliteal cyst
- Popliteal entrapment
- Primary vascular tumors
- Pseudoxanthoma elasticum
- Remote trauma or radiation injury
- Takayasu's disease
- Thromboangiitis obliterans

the embolus using CT scanning of the descending thoracic and abdominal aorta. More unusual sources include mural thrombus from an aortic aneurysm and, occasionally, idiopathic arterial-to-arterial thrombus occurs, usually from a thrombus that has formed in an atherosclerotic aortic arch or descending thoracic aorta. The presence of mobile plaque on transesophageal echocardiography is suggestive of this source.

Paradoxical embolus occurs when a patient has a patent foramen ovale and an embolus from a deep venous thrombosis which embolizes across the atrial defect into the left side of the heart and passes into the peripheral circulation. This is diagnosed using a bubble echocardiography, in which air bubbles introduced into the venous circulation can be seen traversing the septal defect.

Arterial Thrombosis

Thrombosis can occur in native arteries and in arterial reconstructions. Patients with thrombosed arterial segments often have an underlying atherosclerotic lesion at the site of thrombosis, or aneurysmal degeneration with mural thrombosis. It is important to obtain a history, determine risk factors for atherosclerosis and hypercoagulable status, and examine the contralateral extremity for circulatory problems. Patients with thrombosis of prior arterial reconstructions have limb incisions from previous surgery, and graft occlusion can be confirmed with duplex imaging.

Clinical Manifestations of Acute Limb Ischemia

Acute LE ischemia manifests with the "five Ps": *p*ain, *p*allor, *p*aresthesias, *p*aralysis, and *p*ulselessness, to which some add a sixth "P"—

TABLE 23-19	Classification of peripheral arterial disease based on the Fontaine and Rutherford classifications

Fontaine Classification		Rutherford Classification		
Stage	**Clinical**	**Grade**	**Category**	**Clinical**
I	Asymptomatic	0	0	Asymptomatic
IIa	Mild claudication	I	1	Mild claudication
IIb	Moderate to severe claudication	I	2	Moderate claudication
		I	3	Severe claudication
III	Ischemic rest pain	II	4	Ischemic rest pain
IV	Ulceration or gangrene	III	5	Minor tissue loss
		III	6	Major tissue loss

TABLE 23-20	TASC II classification of femoral popliteal occlusive lesions

Type A lesions
- Single stenosis ≤10 cm in length
- Single occlusion ≤5 cm in length

Type B lesions
- Multiple lesions (stenoses or occlusions), each ≤5 cm
- Single stenosis or occlusion ≤15 cm not involving the infra geniculate popliteal artery
- Single or multiple lesions in the absence of continuous tibial vessels to improve inflow for a distal bypass
- Heavily calcified occlusion ≤5 cm in length
- Single popliteal stenosis

Type C lesions
- Multiple stenoses or occlusions totaling >15 cm with or without heavy calcification
- Recurrent stenoses or occlusions that need treatment after two endovascular interventions

Type D lesions
- Chronic total occlusions of CFA or SFA (>20 cm, involving the popliteal artery)
- Chronic total occlusion of popliteal artery and proximal trifurcation vessels

CFA = common femoral artery; SFA = superficial femoral artery; TASC II = Trans-Atlantic Inter-Society Consensus.

*p*oikilothermia or "*p*erishing cold." Pain is the usual symptom that causes a patient to present to the emergency room. The most common location for an embolus to lodge in the leg is at the common femoral bifurcation. Typically a patient will complain of foot and calf pain. Pulses are absent and there may be diminution of sensation. Inability to move the affected muscle group is a sign of very severe ischemia and necessitates urgent revascularization. During evaluation of the affected extremity, it is important to compare findings with the contralateral limb. Clinical evaluation is extremely important in determining the etiology and location of the obstruction. One of the most important pieces of information to

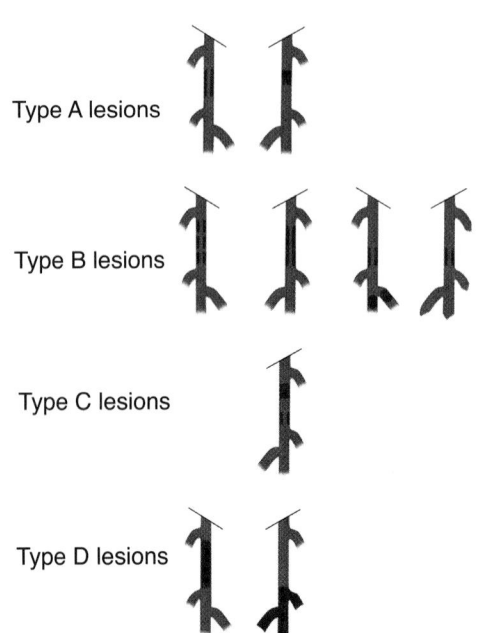

FIG. 23-61. Schematic depiction of Trans-Atlantic Inter-Society Consensus classification of femoral popliteal occlusive lesions.

obtain is whether the patient has had prior vascular procedures or if there is a history of LE claudication. Either of these features suggests pre-existing vascular disease, renders revascularization more complicated, and usually mandates angiography to permit surgical planning. On the contrary, in a patient with no history suggestive of prior vascular disease, the etiology is most likely embolic and simple thrombectomy is more likely to be successful.

Absent bilateral femoral pulses in a patient with bilateral LE ischemia are most likely due to saddle embolus to the aortic bifurcation. A palpable femoral pulse and absent popliteal and distal pulses may either be due to distal common femoral embolus (the pulse being palpable above the level of occlusion) or embolus to the superficial femoral or popliteal arteries. Typically, emboli lodge at arterial bifurcations where they are trapped due to sudden reductions in arterial diameter. A popliteal trifurcation embolus will present with calf ischemia and absent pedal pulses, possibly with a popliteal pulse present. The finding of palpable contralateral pulses and the absence of ipsilateral pulses in the acutely ischemic leg is suggestive of an embolus, irrespective of presence of Doppler signals. Arteriography is not mandatory in patients without antecedent history suggestive of vascular disease; nevertheless, all patients should be positioned on the OR table in such a way that fluoroscopic access to the entire inflow and outflow tract is possible, if necessary.

The main question to be answered by the history and physical examination is the severity of the ALI, which is the major consideration in early management decisions. Patients with ALI should be evaluated in a fashion that takes into consideration the severity and duration of ischemia at the time of presentation. Ideally, all patients with acute ischemia should be investigated with imaging, especially if there is an antecedent vascular reconstruction; however, the clinical condition and access to resources must guide further investigations.[2] Unnecessary delays can result in amputation. Arteriography, if it can be performed in a timely fashion, is an excellent modality for localizing obstructions and deciding which type of intervention (endovascular, embolectomy, or bypass) patients will benefit more from. One of the goals of treatment for ALI is to prevent thrombus propagation; therefore, expedient anticoagulation with heparin is indicated as soon as the diagnosis is suspected.

Treatment Considerations for Acute Limb Ischemia

In the absence of any significant contraindication, the patient with an ischemic LE should be immediately anticoagulated. This will prevent propagation of the clot into unaffected vascular beds. IV fluid should be started and a Foley catheter inserted to monitor urine output. Baseline labs should be obtained and creatinine levels noted. A hypercoagulable work-up should be performed before initiation of heparin if there is sufficient suspicion. According to results from randomized trials, there is no clear superiority for thrombolysis over surgery in terms of 30-day limb salvage or mortality. Access to each treatment option is a major issue in the decision-making process, as time is often critical. National registry data from the United States reveal that surgery is used three- to fivefold more frequently than thrombolysis. Three randomized studies have investigated the role of catheter-directed thrombolytic therapy in the treatment of ALI.[143]

Endovascular Treatment

The potential to reduce mortality and morbidity while achieving limb salvage is the impetus that makes thrombolysis preferable to open surgery as first-line treatment in patients with ALI (class I and IIa). Advantages of thrombolytic therapy over balloon embolectomy include the reduced endothelial trauma and potential for more gradual and complete clot lysis in branch vessels usually too small to access by embolectomy balloons. It is hoped that the more gradual clot dissolution with thrombolysis may decrease the incidence of reperfusion injury that is encountered after open surgical procedures where rapid return of blood flow may precipitate compartment syndrome. Skeletal muscle tissue appears to be most vulnerable to ischemia. Pathophysiologic studies reveal that irreversible damage to muscle tissue starts after 3 hours of ischemia and is nearly complete at 6 hours. Progressive microvascular damage appears to follow rather than precede skeletal muscle tissue damage. The more severe the cellular damage, the greater the microvascular changes. When the musculature and microvasculature are severely damaged, amputation rather than attempts at revascularization may be the most prudent course to prevent washout of toxic by-product from the ischemic limb into the systemic circulation. The mortality rate associated with reperfusion syndrome is high, because of the development of concomitant adult respiratory distress syndrome, shock, disseminated intravascular coagulation, and renal failure.

Patients with small-vessel occlusion are poor candidates for surgery because they lack distal target vessels to use for bypass. These patients should be offered a trial of thrombolysis unless they have contraindications to thrombolysis or their ischemia is so severe that the time needed to achieve adequate lysis is considered too long. The major contraindications of thrombolysis are recent stroke, intracranial primary malignancy, brain metastases, or intracranial surgical intervention. Relative contraindications for performance of thrombolysis include renal insufficiency, allergy to contrast material, cardiac thrombus, diabetic retinopathy, coagulopathy, and recent arterial puncture or surgery (Table 23-21).

Advances in clot removal techniques with percutaneous mechanical thrombectomy and thromboaspiration may extend the applicability of this intervention to patients with more advanced degrees of ALI (class IIb) and contraindications to thrombolysis. Several thrombectomy devices have received FDA approval for acute LE arterial thrombosis. The utility of these thrombectomy devices is that they can be used as stand-alone therapy when there are contraindications for thrombolytic therapy. Additionally, these thrombectomy devices can be used in conjunction with thrombolytic agents, for pharmacomechanical thrombectomy, to enhance clot lysis, and to limit the doses and time required for thrombolysis.[144,145]

Surgical Treatment
Embolectomy

When a decision is made to proceed with open surgical intervention, the abdomen, contralateral groin, and entire LE are prepped in the field. The groin is opened through a vertical incision, exposing the CFA and its bifurcation. Frequently, the location of the embolus at the

TABLE 23-21	Contraindications to thrombolytic therapy

Absolute contraindications

Established cerebrovascular events (including transient ischemic attack) within last 2 mo
Active bleeding diathesis
Recent (<10 d) GI bleeding
Neurosurgery (intracranial or spinal) within last 3 mo
Intracranial trauma within last 3 mo
Intracranial malignancy or metastasis

Relative major contraindications

Cardiopulmonary resuscitation within last 10 d
Major nonvascular surgery or trauma within last 10 d
Uncontrolled hypertension (>180 mmHg systolic or >110 mmHg diastolic)
Puncture of noncompressible vessel
Intracranial tumor
Recent eye surgery

Minor contraindications

Hepatic failure, particularly with coagulopathy
Bacterial endocarditis
Pregnancy
Diabetic hemorrhagic retinopathy

femoral bifurcation is readily apparent by the presence of a palpable proximal femoral pulse, which disappears distally. The artery is clamped and opened transversely over the bifurcation. Thrombus is extracted by passing a Fogarty balloon embolectomy catheter. Good back-bleeding and antegrade bleeding suggest that the entire clot has been removed. Embolic material often forms a cast of the vessel and is sent for culture and histologic examination. Completion angiography is advisable to ascertain the adequacy of clot removal. The artery is then closed and the patient fully anticoagulated.

When an embolus lodges in the popliteal artery, in most cases it can be extracted via a femoral incision using a balloon embolectomy catheter approach. A femoral approach is preferred because the larger diameter of the femoral artery results in decreased likelihood of arterial compromise when the arteriotomy is closed. The disadvantage with using the femoral approach for embolectomy is the greater difficulty involved in directing the embolectomy catheter into each of the infrapopliteal arteries. Use of fluoroscopic imaging and an over-the-wire thrombectomy catheter can overcome this problem. Alternatively, use of a separate incision to expose the popliteal bifurcation may be necessary to achieve a complete thrombectomy.

A more complex situation arises when a patient has antecedent peripheral vascular disease and in situ thrombosis develops on top of pre-existing atheroma because, frequently, embolectomy catheters will not pass through these occlusions. Similarly, when a bypass graft fails, it is usually due to progression of atheroma proximal or distal to the graft anastomoses, or to intrinsic stenoses that develop within a vein graft. In these scenarios, expeditious angiography is useful, to determine the extent of the occlusion, to search for inflow and distal outflow vessels, and to decide whether thrombolysis or surgery will be the better intervention. Although the surgeon's preference tends to dictate the approach selected, the decision is based on the presence or absence of good target vessels and availability of a suitable bypass conduit. If there are good distal vessels and the saphenous vein is suitable, surgical bypass is recommended, as it is fast, durable, and reliable. In the absence of a good distal target and saphenous vein, or in a patient at high risk for surgery, lysis is recommended.

Bypass Graft Thrombectomy

Bypass thrombectomy is more likely to succeed with prosthetic bypasses. Bypass graft revision or replacement is more appropriate for acute vein graft failures as they are less likely to respond to thrombolysis and require some type of revision such as valve lysis, interposition, or extension. Thrombectomy of autogenous grafts is prone to failure unless an anatomic cause for failure such as a retained valve or unligated side branch is found and corrected. The performance of a fasciotomy to circumvent reperfusion injury/compartment syndrome is an important consideration.

Complications Related to Treatment for Acute Limb Ischemia

Adverse events related to CDT are primarily related to bleeding complications. The overall risk of hemorrhagic stroke from a thrombolysis procedure has been reported to be 1 to 2.3%, with 50% of hemorrhagic complications occurring during the thrombolytic procedure.[146] Hematoma at the vascular puncture site has been reported in 12 to 17% of cases. GI bleeding is reported in 5 to 10% of cases. Hematuria following thrombolysis is uncommon and should prompt a search for urinary tumors. Hemorrhage requiring transfusion can occur in approximately 25% of patients undergoing thrombolysis.[138,143] Lytic agents are absolutely contraindicated in patients with intracranial surgery, intracranial hemorrhage within the last 3 months, or in the presence of any active bleeding. Most bleeding complications occur at the arterial puncture sites, but concealed retroperitoneal bleeding is possible. The most feared complication that patients can sustain is intracerebral hemorrhage. Older patients may be more susceptible to this complication and

TABLE 23-22	Complications of arterial revascularization
Compartment syndrome	
Ischemic neuropathy	
Muscle necrosis	
Recurrent thrombosis	
Lower leg swelling	
Reperfusion syndrome	
Hypotension	
Hyperkalemia	
Myoglobinuria	
Renal failure	

thus many interventionalists are extremely reticent to use thrombolysis in patients older than 80 years of age.

Patients who are treated for acute ischemia are susceptible to two major complications following revascularization, which include reperfusion and compartment syndromes. Other procedure-related complications can include arterial rethrombosis, recurrent embolization, and arterial injuries secondary to the balloon catheter manipulations.

Reperfusion of the ischemic limb is variable in its physiologic effects and directly relates to the severity and extent of the ischemia. Patients with a saddle embolus of the aortic bifurcation and severely ischemic limbs may develop the full-blown "reperfusion syndrome," whereas patients with minimal muscle ischemia who are reperfused in a timely fashion essentially develop no effects. Many patients with ALI have severe underlying cardiac disease and are unable to tolerate even short ischemic periods. Complications occurring after revascularization of the LE and causes of recurrent thrombosis are listed in Table 23-22.

Compartment syndrome occurs after prolonged ischemia is followed by reperfusion. The capillaries leak fluid into the interstitial space in the muscles, which are enclosed within a nondistensible fascial envelope. When the pressure inside the compartment exceeds the capillary perfusion pressure, nutrient flow ceases and progressive ischemia occurs, even in the presence of peripheral pulses. Consequently, every patient who has sustained an ischemic event and is reperfused is monitored for compartment syndrome, which is characterized by excessive pain in the compartment, pain on passive stretching of the compartment, and sensory loss due to nerve compression of the nerves coursing though the compartment (Table 23-23 and Fig. 23-62). The most commonly affected compartment is the anterior compartment in the leg. Numbness in the web space between the first and second toes is diagnostic due to compression of the deep peroneal nerve. Compartment pressure is measured by inserting an arterial line into the compartment and recording the pressure. Although controversial, pressures >20 mmHg are an indication for fasciotomy. Compartment pressures are relieved in the leg by medial and lateral incisions. Through the medial incision, long openings are then made in the fascia of the superficial and deep posterior compartments. Through the lateral incision, the anterior and peroneal compartments are opened. Both skin and fascial incisions should be of adequate length to ensure full compartment decompression. Laboratory evidence of rhabdomyolysis is seen in 20%. The myoglobin from damaged muscle precipitates in kidney tubules and causes acute tubular necrosis. Alkalinization of urine increases the solubility of myoglobin, thus preventing it from crystallizing in the tubules. In addition to alkalinization, therapy consists of forced saline diuresis and removal of the source of dead muscle that is releasing the myoglobin.

Clinical Manifestations of Chronic Limb Ischemia

The term *chronic limb ischemia* is reserved for patients with objectively proven arterial occlusive disease and symptoms lasting for more than 2 weeks. Symptoms include rest pain and tissue loss such

TABLE 23-23 Fascial compartments of the lower leg

	Anterior Compartment	Lateral Compartment	Superficial Posterior Compartment	Deep Posterior Compartment
Muscles	Tibialis anterior Extensor digitorum longus Peroneus tertius Extensor hallucis longus Extensor digitorum brevis Extensor hallucis brevis	Peroneus longus Peroneus brevis	Gastrocnemius Plantaris Soleus	Tibialis posterior Flexor digitorum longus Flexor hallucis longus
Artery	Anterior tibial artery	Anterior and posterior tibial branches of the popliteal artery	—	Posterior tibial artery Peroneal artery
Nerve	Deep peroneal nerve	Superficial peroneal nerve	—	Tibial nerve

as ulceration or gangrene (Table 23-24). The diagnosis should be corroborated with noninvasive diagnostic tests such as the ABI, toe pressures, and transcutaneous oxygen measurements. Ischemic rest pain most commonly occurs below an ankle pressure of 50 mmHg or a toe pressure <30 mmHg.[2] Ulcers are not always of an ischemic etiology (Table 23-25). In many instances, there are other etiologic factors (traumatic, venous, or neuropathic) that are contributory, but it is underlying peripheral arterial disease (PAD) that may be responsible for delayed or absent healing (Fig. 23-63). Healing of ulcers requires an inflammatory response and greater perfusion than is required to support intact skin and underlying tissues. As a result, the ankle and toe pressure levels needed for healing are higher than the pressures seen with ischemic rest pain. For patients with ulcers or gangrene, the presence of CLI is suggested by an ankle pressure <70 mmHg or a toe systolic pressure <50 mmHg.[2] It is important to understand that there is no definite consensus regarding the vascular hemodynamic parameters required to make the diagnosis of CLI.

One of the most common sites for occlusive disease is in the distal SFA as it passes deep through the adductor canal. It may be

that the entrapment by the adductor hiatus prevents the compensatory dilation that occurs in atherosclerotic vessels. Stenoses, which develop here, progress to occlusion of the distal third of the SFA (Fig. 23-64). When distal SFA occlusion develops slowly, it may be totally asymptomatic because of development of collaterals from the proximal SFA or the profunda femoris artery (PFA) can bypass the occlusion and reconstitute the popliteal artery. Symptom development is a function of the extent of occlusion, adequacy of collaterals, and also the activity level of the patients.

Presenting symptoms of femoropopliteal occlusive disease are broadly classified into two types: limb-threatening and non–limb-threatening ischemia. Claudication is non–limb-threatening, while rest pain, ulceration, and gangrene are limb-threatening and warrant urgent intervention. Occlusive disease of the femoral artery may be isolated or occur in conjunction with multilevel disease that involves both the aortoiliac segment and the tibial vessels. Symptoms in patients with multilevel disease are more severe than in those with single-level disease. Pain from isolated SFA and popliteal occlusion typically manifests as calf claudication. Cramping pain develops in

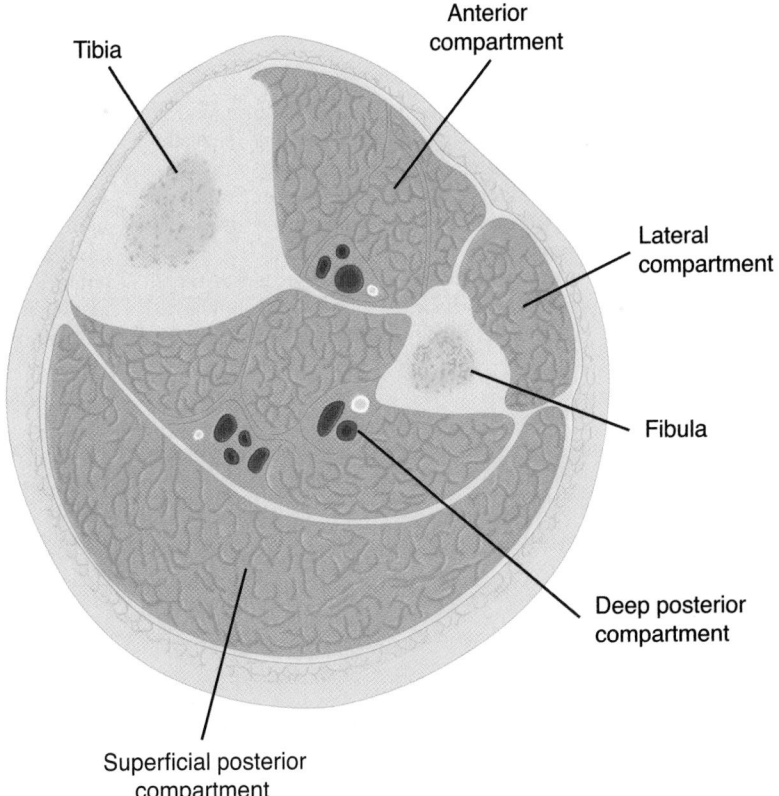

FIG. 23-62. Schematic illustration of fascial compartments of the lower extremity.

TABLE 23-24 Clinical categories of chronic limb ischemia

Grade	Category	Clinical Description	Objective Criteria
0	0	Asymptomatic—no hemodynamically significant occlusive disease	Normal treadmill or reactive hyperemia test
	1	Mild claudication	Able to complete treadmill exercise[a]; AP after exercise >50 mmHg but at least 20 mmHg lower than resting value
I	2	Moderate claudication	Between categories 1 and 3
	3	Severe claudication	Cannot complete standard treadmill exercise[a] and AP after exercise <50 mmHg
II[b]	4	Ischemic rest pain	Resting AP <40 mmHg, flat or barely pulsatile ankle or metatarsal PVR; TP <30 mmHg
III[b]	5	Minor tissue loss—nonhealing ulcer, focal gangrene with diffuse pedal ischemia	Resting AP <60 mmHg, ankle or metatarsal PVR flat or barely pulsatile; TP <40 mmHg
	6	Major tissue loss—extending above TM level, functional foot no longer salvageable	Same as category 5

[a]5 minutes at 2 miles per hour on a 12% incline of treadmill exercise.
[b]Grades II and III, categories 4, 5, and 6, are encompassed by the term *chronic critical ischemia*.
AP = ankle pressure; PVR = pulse volume recording; TM = transmetatarsal; TP = toe pressure.

TABLE 23-25 Symptoms and signs of neuropathic ulcer versus ischemic ulcer

Neuropathic Ulcer	Ischemic Ulcer
Painless	Painful
Normal pulses	Absent pulses
Regular margins, typically punched-out appearance	Irregular margin
Often located on plantar surface of foot	Commonly located on toes, glabrous margins
Presence of calluses	Calluses absent or infrequent
Loss of sensation, reflexes, and vibration	Variable sensory findings
Increased in blood flow (atrioventricular shunting)	Decreased in blood flow
Dilated veins	Collapsed veins
Dry, warm foot	Cold foot
Bony deformities	No bony deformities
Red or hyperemic in appearance	Pale and cyanotic in appearance

factors. In comparison, rest pain is constant, and usually occurs in the forefoot across the metatarsophalangeal joint. It is worse at night and requires placing the foot in a dependent position to improve symptoms. Patients may report that they either sleep in a chair or hang the foot off the side of the bed. The pain is severe and relentless, even with narcotics. Ischemic ulceration most commonly involves the toes. Any toe can be affected. Occasionally, ulcers develop on the dorsum of the foot. Ulceration can occur in atypical positions in an ischemic foot from trauma such as friction from poorly fitting shoes. Injury to a foot with borderline ischemia can convert an otherwise stable situation into one that is limb-threatening. The initial development of gangrene commonly involves the digits. As with all vascular patients, it is important to evaluate their risk factors, intercurrent cardiac diseases, and any prior vascular interventions.

Treatment Considerations for Chronic Limb Ischemia

Patients with vascular diseases frequently have complicated medical comorbidities. Careful patient evaluation and selection should be performed for any peripheral arterial vascular procedure. The fundamental principle is to assess not only the surgical risk from the peripheral arterial system but also the global nature of the atherosclerotic process. Full cardiac evaluations are often necessary due to the high incidence of concomitant atherosclerotic coronary arteries disease, resulting in a high risk for ischemic events. Hertzer and associates reviewed coronary angiographies on 1000 patients undergoing elective vascular procedures and identified 25% of concomitant correctable CAD, including 21% in patients undergoing elective peripheral vascular intervention.[8] Conte and associates analyzed their 20-year experience in a tertiary practice setting in 1642 open LE reconstructive surgeries and concluded that pa-

the calf on ambulation, occurs at a reproducible distance, and is relieved by rest. Activities such as climbing stairs or going uphill also exacerbate the pain. Many patients report worsening symptoms during cold weather. It is important to evaluate whether the symptoms are progressive or static. In >70% of patients, the disease is stable, particularly with risk factor modification.

Progression of the underlying atherosclerotic process is more likely to occur in patients with diabetes, those who continue to smoke, and those who fail to modify their atherosclerotic risk

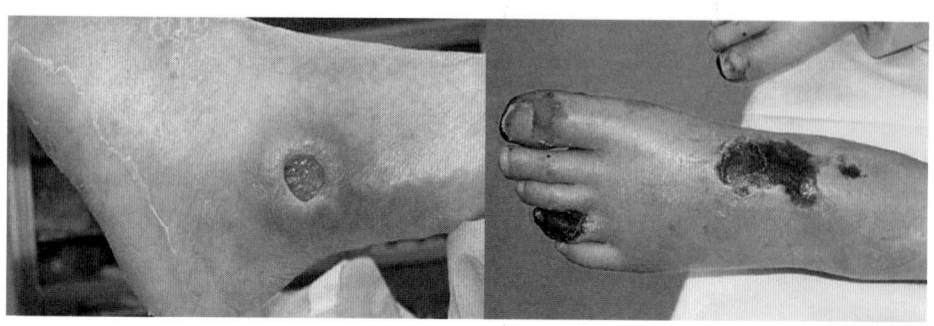

A   **B**

FIG. 23-63. A. A neuropathic ulcer is characterized by a punched-out appearance with loss of sensation in the surrounding skin. The foot may be warm to touch, and pulses may be present in the distal pedal arteries. **B.** An ischemic ulcer is characterized by a gangrenous skin change in the foot or toes. The foot is usually cold to touch with absent pedal pulses. The foot is painful to touch with decreased distal capillary refills.

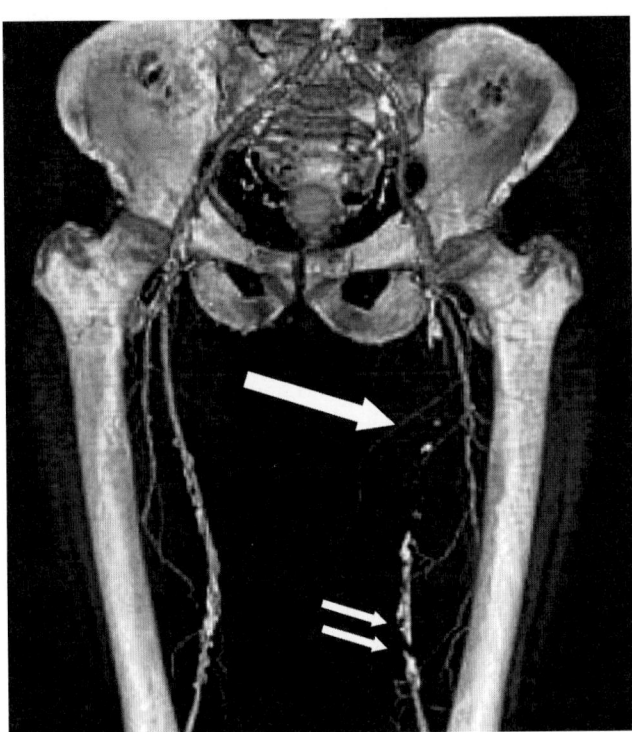

FIG. 23-64. Computed tomography angiogram of a patient with an occluded left superficial femoral artery (*single long arrow*) with reconstituted superficial femoral artery at the level of midthigh. Diffuse arterial calcifications (*double small arrows*) are noted in the mid and distal left superficial femoral arteries.

cular procedures should be performed by a competent vascular interventionist who understands the vascular disease process and is familiar with a variety of endovascular techniques. In addition, certain lesions such as long segment occlusion, heavily calcified lesion, orifice lesion, or lesions that can be not be traversed by a guidewire may not be amendable to endovascular treatment or may be associated with poor outcomes. A proper selection of patients and techniques is critical in achieving a good long-term outcome.

Endovascular intervention for LE occlusive disease is continuously evolving. Success and patency rates of endovascular intervention are closely related to the anatomic and morphologic characters of the treated lesions. The TASC II work group made recommendations on the intervention strategies of LE arterial diseases based on the morphologic characters. Based on the TASC II guidelines, endovascular treatment is recommended for type A lesions, open surgery is recommended for Type D lesions, and no recommendations were made for Types B and C lesions. However, with rapid advancement in endovascular technologies, there are increased numbers of lesions amendable to endovascular interventions.

There is less literature support on infrapopliteal endovascular intervention due to higher complication and lower success rates. The treatment is restricted to patients with limb-threatening ischemia who lack surgical alternatives. However, with further advancement of endovascular technology and the development of new devices, endovascular intervention will become an integral part of treatment (Table 23-26). By itself or combined with open technique, percutaneous intervention plays an important role in therapeutic options for LE occlusive disease. As described by the TASC II guidelines, four criteria should be measured to evaluate the clinical success of the treatment: improvement in walking distance, symptomatic improvement, quality of life, and overall graft patency. These criteria should all be carefully weighed and evaluated for each individual before endovascular therapy.

Endovascular Treatment
Technical Considerations

A sterile field is required in either an OR or an angiography suite with image capability. The most common and safest access site is the CFA via either a retrograde or antegrade approach. For diagnostic angiography, arterial access should be contralateral to the symptomatic sides. For therapeutic procedures, location of the lesion and the anatomic structures of the arterial tree determine the puncture site. To avoid puncturing the iliac artery or SFA, the femoral head is

tients requiring LE reconstruction presented an increasingly complex medical and surgical challenge compared with the previous decade.[147] With aging of the population, there are a growing number of vascular patients who have prohibitive medical comorbidities that are deemed high-risk for open surgical repair. Endovascular intervention provides an attractive alternative.

As for open surgical repair, the clinical indications for endovascular intervention of LE PADs include lifestyle-limiting claudication, ischemic rest pain, and tissue loss or gangrene. Importantly, endovas-

TABLE 23-26	Summary of endovascular treatment strategies using device-based infrapopliteal intervention

Intervention	Advantages	Disadvantages
Angioplasty	• Easy to use • Broad range of applications	• Failure in long lesions, calcified lesions, and disease at multiple levels
Balloon-expandable stent	• Overcomes arterial recoil from angioplasty • Useful in treatment of flow-limiting dissection	• Crushability can lead to restenosis • Poor distal runoff can result in stent thrombosis; limited data
Self-expanding stent	• Vessel conformability and wall apposition prevents kinking and crushing of stent	• Limited sizes; limited data; multicenter trials under way
Bioabsorbable stent	• Overcomes arterial recoil from angioplasty • Absorbed long-term to prevent risk of stent thrombosis	• Limited data; multicenter trials under way
Cryoplasty	• Reduces the risk of flow-limiting dissection, therefore reducing the need for stent implantation	• Short-term results of a multicenter trial are promising; however, long-term data are limited
Cutting balloon	• Useful in anastomotic segments of bypass grafts and instent restenosis where "watermelon seeding" can prevent adequate expansion of plaque	• Limited data
Mechanical atherectomy	• Allows for debulking of plaque without the need for stent implantation in most cases • Allows for removal of plaque for histologic analysis	• Limited use in areas of heavy calcification • No large, randomized, prospective trial comparing this technique to angioplasty and stenting
Laser	• Useful in acute thrombotic and chronic total occlusions	• Minimal data in infrapopliteal arteries • Need adjunctive treatment with angioplasty, stenting, or atherectomy

located under the fluoroscopy and used as the guide for the level of needle entry. In addition, there are several useful techniques in helping access a pulseless CFA, including puncturing guided by ultrasound, using a micropuncture kit, and targeting calcification in a calcified vessel. An antegrade approach may be challenging, particularly in obese patients. Meticulous technique is crucial in preventing complications, and a bony landmark can be used as guidance to ensure CFA puncture.

Traversing the lesion with a wire is the most critical part of the procedure. Typically, 0.035-in guidewires are used for femoropopliteal lesions and 0.014- or 0.018-in guidewires are used for infrapopliteal access. Hydrophilic-coated wires, such as Glide wires, are useful in navigating through tight stenosis or occlusion. An angled-tip wire with a torque device may be helpful in crossing an eccentric lesion, and a shaped selective catheter is frequently used in helping manipulate the wire across the lesion. The soft and floppy end of the wire is carefully advanced, crossing the lesion under fluoroscopy, and gentle force is applied while manipulating the wire. Once the lesion has been traversed, one needs to pay particular attention to the tip of the wire to ensure a secure wire access and avoid vessel wall perforation or dissection.

Once the access to the diseased vessel is secured and the wire has successfully traversed the lesion, several treatment modalities can be used either used alone or in conjunction with others, including angioplasty, stent or stent graft placement, and atherectomy. The available angioplasty techniques are balloon angioplasty, cryoplasty, subintimal angioplasty (SA), and cutting balloon. The most commonly used atherectomy techniques include percutaneous atherectomy catheter and laser atherectomy device.

Systemic anticoagulation should be maintained routinely during LE arterial interventions to minimize the risk of pericatheter thrombosis. Unfractionated heparin is the most commonly used agent, given on a weight-based formula. It is a common clinical practice to use a 80 to 100 mg/kg initial bolus for a therapeutic procedure to achieve the activated clotting time above 250 seconds on the catheter insertion and subsequently 1000 units for each additional hour of the procedure. Newer agents such as low molecular weight heparin, platelet IIb/IIIa inhibitor, direct thrombin inhibitor, or recombinant hirudin have been available and can be used either alone or in conjunction with heparin, particularly in patients sensitive to unfractionated heparin. After procedures, all patients are placed on antiplatelet therapy such as aspirin. Additional antiplatelet agents such as clopidogrel (Plavix) are given to selected patients with stent placement for at least 6 weeks after LE interventions, unless otherwise contraindicated.

Percutaneous Transluminal Balloon Angioplasty

After the lesion is crossed with a wire, an appropriate balloon angioplasty catheter is selected and tracked along the wire to traverse the lesion. The length of the selected catheter should be slightly longer than the lesion and the diameter should be equal to the adjacent normal vessel. The balloon tends to be approximately 10 to 20% oversized. The radiopaque markers of the balloon catheter are placed so that they will straddle the lesion. Then, the balloon is inflated with saline and contrast mixture to allow visualization of the insufflation process under the fluoroscopy (Fig. 23-65). The patient may experience mild pain, which is not uncommon. However, severe pain can be indicative of vessel rupture, dissection, or other complications. An angiography is crucial in confirming the intraluminal location of the catheter and absence of contrast extravasation. The inflation is continued until the waist of the atherosclerotic lesion disappears and the balloon is at full profile. Frequently, several inflations are required to achieve full profile of the balloon (Fig. 23-66). Occasionally, a lower profile balloon is needed to predilate the tight stenosis so that the selected balloon catheter can cross the lesion.

Besides length and diameter, the operators need to be familiar with several balloon characters. Noncompliant and low-compliant balloons tend to be inflated to their preset diameter and offer greater dilating force at the site of stenosis. Low-compliant balloons are the mainstay for peripheral intervention. A balloon with a low profile is used to minimize complication at the entry site and for crossing the tight lesions. Upon inflation, most balloons do not rewrap to their preinflation diameter and assume a larger profile. Furthermore, trackability, pushability, and crossability of the balloon should be considered when choosing a particular type. Lastly, shoulder length is an important characteristic when performing PTA to avoid injury to the adjacent arterial segments. After PTA, a completion angiogram is performed while the wire is still in place. Leaving the wire in place provides access for repeating the procedure if the result is unsatisfactory.

PTA is an established and effective therapy for select patients with LE occlusive diseases. Studies have shown that PTA of the femoropopliteal segment achieved over a 90% technical success rate

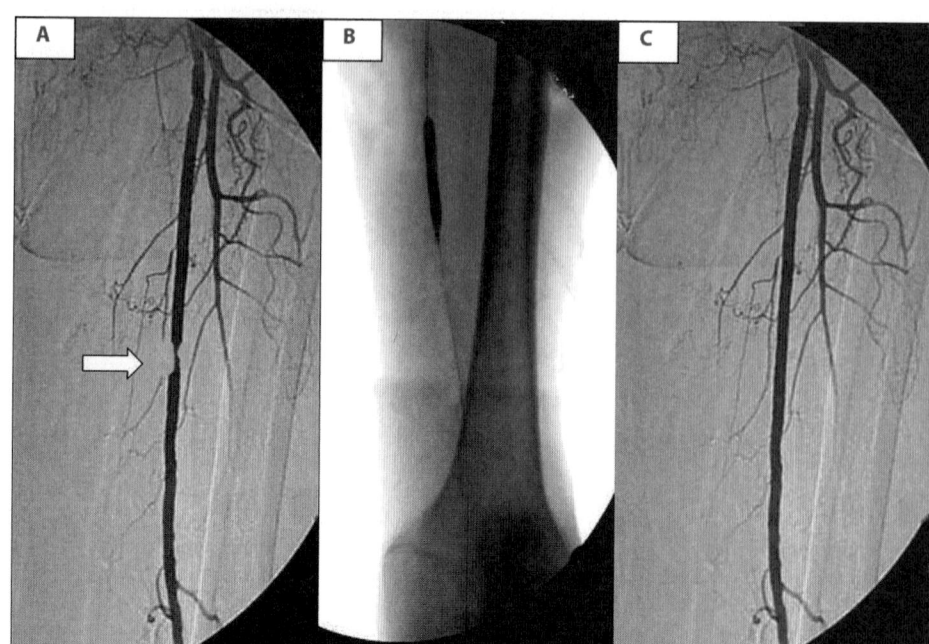

FIG. 23-65. A. Angiogram demonstrating a focal stenosis in the superficial femoral artery (*arrow*). **B.** This lesion was treated with a balloon angioplasty catheter that inflated a dilating balloon and expanded the flow lumen. **C.** Completion angiogram demonstrating satisfactory radiographic result.

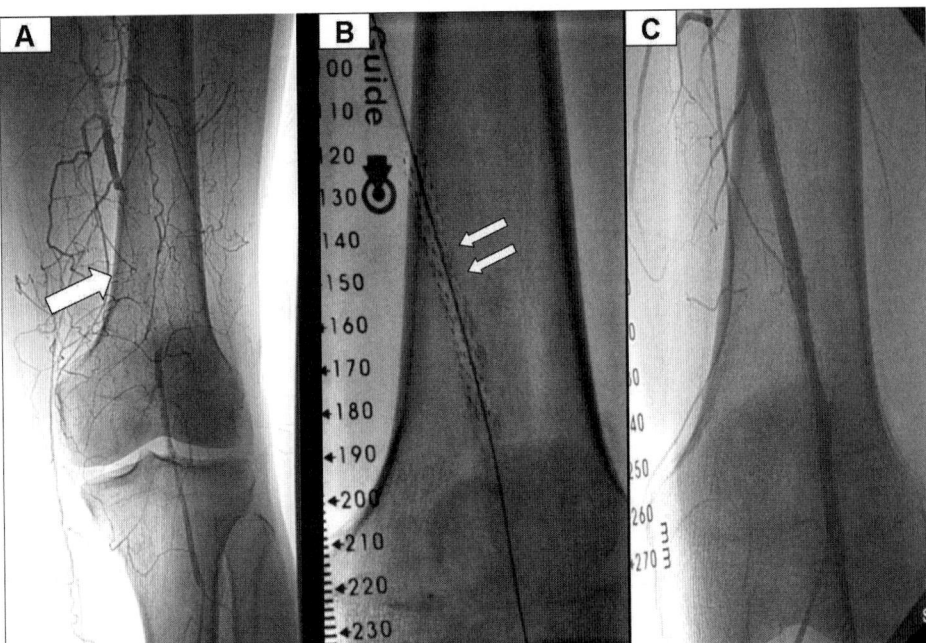

FIG. 23-66. A. Angiogram demonstrating a segmental occlusion in the distal superficial femoral artery (*single arrow*). **B.** This lesion was treated with cryoplasty, which lowered the balloon catheter temperature to a temporary freezing state during the balloon angioplasty procedure (*double arrows*). **C.** Completion angiogram demonstrated satisfactory result with no evidence of vessel dissection.

and a 38 to 58% 5-year primary patency rate.[148–150] However, efficacy of PTA is highly dependent upon anatomic selection and patient condition.[106] PTA of lesions longer than 7 to 10 cm offer limited patency, while PTA of shorter lesions, such as those that are <3 cm, have fairly good results. Lofberg and associates performed 127 femoropopliteal PTA procedures and reported a primary 5-year success rate of 12% in limbs with an occlusion longer than 5 cm vs. 32% in limbs with an occlusion <5 cm in length.[151] Occlusive lesions have much worse initial technical success rates than stenotic lesions. Concentric lesions respond better to PTA than eccentric lesions, and heavy calcifications have a negative impact on success rates. A meta-analysis by Hunink and associates showed that adjusted 5-year primary patencies after angioplasty of femoropopliteal lesions varied from 12 to 68%, the best results being for patients with claudication and stenotic lesions.[150] Distal runoff is another powerful predictor of long-term success. Johnston analyzed 254 consecutive patients who underwent femoral and popliteal PTA and reported that 5-year patency rates of 53% for stenotic lesions and 36% for occlusive lesions in patients with good runoffs vs. a 5-year patency of 31% for stenotic lesions and 16% for occlusive lesions in patients with poor runoff.[149] Literature reviews showed that 5-year patency rates varied from 27 to 67% based on the runoff statuses.[150]

Due to limited success with infrapopliteal PTA, the indication for infrapopliteal artery PTA is stringent, reserved for limb salvage. Current patency rates from infrapopliteal PTA can be improved further by proper patient selection, ensuring straight-line flow to the foot in at least one tibial vessel, and close patient surveillance for early reintervention. Possible future advances including the use of drug-eluting stents (DES), cutting balloons, and atherectomy devices are being investigated to improve clinical outcomes following endovascular interventions on the tibial arteries. Varty and associates reported a 1-year limb salvage rate of 77% in patients with critical ischemia who underwent infrapopliteal PTA.[152] In patients with favorable anatomies, a 2-year limb salvage rate after infrapopliteal artery PTA is expected to exceed 80%.

Subintimal Angioplasty

The technique of SA was first described in 1987 when successful establishment of flow was made by accidental creation of a subintimal channel during treatment of a long popliteal artery occlusion. SA is recommended for chronic occlusion, long segments of lesion, and heavily calcified lesions. In addition, this technique is applicable for vessels with diffuse diseases and for vessels that had previously failed an intraluminal approach because it is difficult to negotiate the wire across the entire diseased segment without dissection.

The principle of this technique is to bypass the occlusion by deliberately creating a subintimal dissection plan commencing proximal to the lesion and continuing in the subintimal space before breaking back into the true lumen distal to the lesion. The occluded lumen is recanalized through the subintimal plan. SA can be performed through either ipsilateral antegrade or contralateral retrograde using the CFA approach. If selecting contralateral CFA puncture, a long guiding sheath is placed across the aortic bifurcation to provide access for the femoropopliteal and infrapopliteal vessels. The subintimal dissection is initiated at the origin of an occlusion by directing the tip of an angled guidewire, usually an angled hydrophilic wire such as Glidewire. A supporting catheter is used to guide the tip of the guidewire away from the important collaterals. When the wire is advanced, a loop is naturally formed at the tip of the guidewire. Once the subintimal plan is entered, the wire tends to move freely in the dissection space. Subintimal location of the wire and the catheter can be confirmed by injecting a small amount of diluted contrast. At this point, the wire and the catheter are then advanced along the subintimal plan until the occlusion segment is passed. A loss of resistance is often encountered as the guidewire re-enters the true lumen distal to the occlusion. Recanalization is confirmed by advancing the catheter over the guidewire beyond the point of re-entry and obtaining an angiogram. This is followed by a balloon angioplasty. To confirm the patency following balloon dilatation, a completion angiogram is performed before withdrawing the catheter and wire. If flow is impaired, repeat balloon dilatation may be necessary. Frequently, a stent is required to maintain a patent lumen and treat residual stenosis if more than a 30% luminal reduction is confirmed on completion angiogram.

Multiple studies have demonstrated the efficacy of SA. Bolia and his colleagues and London and his colleagues reported their extensive experiences on SA for treating long segment occlusions of infrainguinal vessels.[153,154] They achieved a technical success rate of over 80% for both femoropopliteal and tibial arteries. One-year patency rates varied from 53% for infrapopliteal vessels to 71% for femoropopliteal segments. Limb salvage rates reached over 80% at 12 months. They also reported that the factors influencing patency are smoking, number of runoff vessels, and occlusion length. Studies by other groups showed similar results.[155,156] Treiman and colleagues treated 25 patients with 6- to 18-cm femoropopliteal occlusion and achieved a technical success rate of 92% and a 12-month primary patency rate of 92%,[156] while Lipsitz and associates reported a technical success rate of 87% in treating 39 patients and achieved a 12-month cumulative patency rate of 74%.[155] Additionally, Ingle and associates reported a technical success rate of 87% on 67 patients with femoropopliteal lesions and a 36-month limb salvage rate of 94%.[157] As demonstrated herein, although technical success rates are similar in most series, the patency rates vary widely in different studies. Patient selection, anatomic character, and lesion locations may account for the wide range of outcomes.

Stent Placement

Although suggested by Dotter during the late 1960s, the use of an endoluminal stent was not pursued until the limitations of PTA were widely recognized. There are several situations where stent placement is appealing. The primary indication is the potential salvage of an unacceptable angioplasty result. Stent placement is typically used when residual stenosis after PTA is 30% or greater. An endoluminal stent is also used for dissection, perforation, and other PTA complications. Primary stent placement has become a viable alternative for treating ulcerative lesions that may potentially be the source for embolization. Primary stent is also used to treat occlusive lesions that have a tendency of reocclusion and distal embolization after PTA. In addition, an endoluminal stent is potentially beneficial for early restenosis post-PTA. DESs are currently under investigation in the United States and may be promising in decreasing restenotic rates.

Even though technical success rates are high, a published series on femoropopliteal artery stents show that patency rates are comparable to PTA alone with primary patency rates varying from 18 to 72% at 3 years.[106,158] Gray and associates stented 58 limbs after suboptimal PTA for long SFA lesions and demonstrated a 1-year primary patency rate of 22%.[159] However, Mewissen treated 137 limbs using self-expanding SMART nitinol stents in patients with TASC II A, B, and C femoropopliteal lesions and reported a 1-year primary patency rate of 76% and a 24-month primary patency rate of 60%.[160] Appropriate patient selection and the anatomic characteristics of the lesions are crucial in the success of treatment outcomes. Additionally, stent characteristics may contribute to the patency rate.

Several clinical studies have demonstrated the significant improvements of the new generation of nitinol stents for the SFA lesions: the German Multicenter Experience, the Mewissen trial, the BLASTER Trial, and the SIROCCO trials.[161] The German Multicenter Experience was a retrospective review of 111 SFA stenting procedures and found the 6-month patency rates for Smart stents and Wall stents were 82% and 37%, respectively. The BLASTER (Bilateral Lower Arterial Stenting Employing Reopro) Trial evaluated the feasibility of using nitinol stents with and without IV abciximab for the treatment of femoral artery disease. Preliminary results showed a 1-year clinical patency rate of 83%.[162]

Furthermore, DESs, which proved effective at decreasing restenosis in coronary intervention, may offer another promising alternative in LE diseases. The drug, released over a period of time, interferes with smooth muscle cell proliferation, the main cellular element and source of extracellular-matrix–producing restenosis. The first DES clinical trial used Cordis Cypher SMART stents coated with sirolimus (SIROCCO trial).[163] The SIROCCO results showed binary inlesion restenosis rates of 0% in the sirolimus-eluting group vs. 23.5% in the noneluting group at 6-month follow-up angiography.

Stent Graft

The concept of endobypass using stent graft in treating atherosclerotic SFA disease has been entertained. A stent graft is placed percutaneously across a long segment or multiple segments of lesions and is used to create a femoropopliteal bypass. Theoretically, endobypass has the potential of being as successful as surgical bypass graft by relining the vessel wall in its anatomical position without the negative impact of anastomosis. Stent grafts can be divided into two categories: unsupported and fully supported. The unsupported grafts consist of segments of bypass graft, such as PTFE, with an expandable stent at one or both ends. The unsupported grafts are flexible with a low profile, but prone to external compression. The supported stent grafts consist of a metallic skeleton covered with graft fabric. The presence of a dense metal skeleton promotes an extensive inflammatory response and increases the risk of thrombosis. There is no FDA-approved stent graft for peripheral intervention. However, Viabahn (WL Gore, Calif) is the most commonly used device in the United States, composed of an ultrathin PTFE graft externally supported by a self-expanding nitinol meshwork. The Viabahn device has a specific delivery mechanism—pulling back the attached string—which results in a proximal-to-distal delivery of the endoprosthesis.

Although it is an intriguing concept, data on endobypass results are limited and the graft thrombosis rate is high. Additionally, covering major collateral vessels can potentially jeopardize the viability of the limb if stent graft occlusion occurs. Bauermeister treated 35 patients with Hemobahn and reported a 28.6% occlusion rate on an average 7-month follow-up.[164] Kedora and colleagues recently conducted a prospective, randomized study comparing covered PTFE/nitinol self-expanding stent grafts with prosthetic above-the-knee femoropopliteal bypass. Fifty limbs were randomized into each group. Primary patency at 1-year was approximately 74% for both cohorts, with a mean follow-up of 18 months. The covered nitinol PTFE stent graft in the SFA had a 1-year patency rate comparable to surgical bypass, with a significantly shorter hospital stay (0.9 vs. 3.1 days).[165]

Atherectomy

The basic principle of atherectomy is to remove the atheroma from obstructed arterial vessels. There are currently five atherectomy devices approved by the FDA: Simpson AtheroCath (DVI, Redwood City, Calif), Transluminal Extraction Catheter (Interventional Technologies, San Diego, Calif), Theratec recanalization arterial catheter (Trac-Wright), Auth Rotablator (Heart Technologies, Redmond, Wash), and SilverHawk system (FoxHollow Technologies, Redwood City, Calif). These devices either cut and remove or pulverize the atheroma plaques.

The Simpson AtheroCath has a directional cutting element that is exposed to one third of the circumference of the arterial wall. The atheroma protruding into the window is excised and pushed into the collection chamber. The Transluminal Extraction Catheter has an over-the-wire, nondirectional cutter mounted on the distal end of a torque tube. The excised atheroma is simultaneously removed by aspiration through the torque tube. The Theratec recanalization arterial catheter is a nondirectional, noncoaxial, atheroablative device. The rotating cam tip pulverizes the atheromatous lesion into minute particles. The Auth Rotablator is a nondirectional, coaxial, atheroablative device with a metal burr embedded with fine diamond chips. Lastly, the SilverHawk device, approved by the FDA for peripheral use in 2003, is a monorail catheter designed to overcome the drawback of direction atherectomy catheter, such as the Simpson AtheroCath. The working end consists of a hinged housing unit containing a carbide cutting blade. The blade is activated from the motor drive unit and the catheter is then advanced through the length of the lesion. Once each pass is completed, the cutter then packs the tissue into the distal end of the nosecone to maximize collection capacity. The SilverHawk can then either be removed or torqued to treat a different quadrant in the same lesion or other lesions.

Despite the promising early technical and clinical success, the mid- and long-term results have been disappointing due to a high incidence of restenosis. However, a multicenter clinical registry of plaque atherectomy in patients with femoropopliteal occlusive disease showed potential clinical efficacy of this technology as the 6- and 12-month rates of survival free of target lesion revascularization were 90 and 80%, respectively.[166] Importantly, nearly three fourths (73%) of patients treated with plaque excision modality did not require adjunctive endovascular therapy as infrainguinal stenting was necessary in only 6.3% of lesions. Results from the TALON registry support the role of plaque excision in selective patients with LE arterial disease.[166]

Laser Atherectomy

Since laser atherectomy was reported in the 1960s, a variety of innovative approaches have been developed in an effort to overcome the limitation of laser angioplasty. Recent developments in excimer laser technology have led to increased optimism regarding the ability to safely deliver laser energy. Excimer laser atherectomy approved by the FDA for peripheral artery intervention uses precision laser energy control (shallow tissue penetration) and safer wavelengths (ultraviolet as opposed to the infrared spectra in older laser technology), which decreases perforation and thermal injury to the treated vessels.

A laser atherectomy catheter, with diameters varying from 0.9 mm to 2.5 mm, is tracked over the guidewire to the desired target. Once activated, the excimer laser uses ultraviolet energy to ablate the lesion and create a nonthrombogenic arterial lumen. This lumen is further dilated by an angioplasty balloon. Because the excimer laser can potentially reduce the rate of distal embolization by evaporating the lesion, it may be used as an adjunct tool for ostial lesions and lesions that can be traversed by a wire but not an angioplasty balloon catheter.

Several studies regarding the use of excimer laser atherectomy combined with balloon angioplasty on LE occlusive disease have shown promising clinical outcomes.[167,168] Peripheral excimer laser angioplasty trials involved 318 patients with chronic SFA occlusion. They achieved a technical success rate of 83.2%, a 1-year primary patency rate of 33.6%, and an assisted primary patency rate of 65%.[168] Steinkamp and his colleagues treated 127 patients with long-segment of popliteal artery occlusion using laser atherectomy followed by balloon angioplasty and reported a 3-year primary patency rate of 22%.[169] The multicenter clinical trial evaluating the use of laser angioplasty for critical limb ischemia supports the efficacy of this treatment modality in selective patients as the 6-month primary patency rate and clinical improvement were 33 and 89%, respectively.[167]

Complications of Endovascular Interventions
Angioplasty-Related Complications

Complications related to PTA vary widely, including dissection, rupture, embolization, pseudoaneurysms, restenosis, hematoma, and acute occlusion secondary to thrombosis, vasospasm, or intimal injury. Clark and associates analyzed the data from 205 patients in the SCVIR Transluminal Angioplasty and Revascularization registry and reported a complication rate of 7.3% for patients undergoing femoropopliteal angioplasty.[170] Minor complications accounted for 75% of the cases, including distal emboli (41.7%), puncture site hematomas (41.7%), contained vessel rupture (8.3%), and vagal reactions (8.3%). In another study, Axisa and colleagues reported an overall rate of significant complications for patients undergoing PTA of the lower extremities as 4.2%, including retroperitoneal bleeding (0.2%), false aneurysm (0.2%), ALI (1.5%), and vessel perforation (1.7%).[171]

Complications limiting the application of SA are parallel to those of PTA. A study investigating the use of SA in 65 patients with SFA occlusion found that complications developed in 15% of patients.[172] These complications included significant stenosis (44%), SFA rupture (6%), distal embolization (3%), retroperitoneal hemorrhage (1.5%), and pseudoaneurysm (1.5%). Additional complications reported consist of perforation, thrombosis, dissection, and extensions beyond the planned re-entry site.[173] Importantly, damage to significant collateral vessels may occur in 1 to 1.5% of patient who undergo SA. If a successful channel is not achieved in this situation, the patient may have a compromised distal circulation that necessitates distal bypass. Cryoplasty is a modified form of angioplasty, and long-term results on LE intervention are not yet available. Fava and associates treated

15 patients with femoropopliteal disease and had a 13% complication rate involving guidewire dissection and PTA-induced dissection of a tandem lesion remote to the cryoplasty zone.[174]

Endoluminal Stent and Stent Graft–Related Complications

In addition to the aforementioned complications with angioplasty, endoluminal stents are associated with the risk of stent fraction and deformity. The adductor canal has nonlaminar flow dynamics, especially with walking. The forces exerted on the SFA include torsion, compression, extension, and flexion. These forces exert significant stress on the SFA and stents. In addition, the LE is subject to external trauma, which further increases the risk of stent deformity and fracture (Fig. 23-67). The SIROCCO study showed that stent fracture, although not associated with clinical symptoms, occurs in 18.2% of the procedures involving both the DES and control stent.[163]

Stent grafts may present an additional complication of covering important collaterals, which results in compromised distal circula-

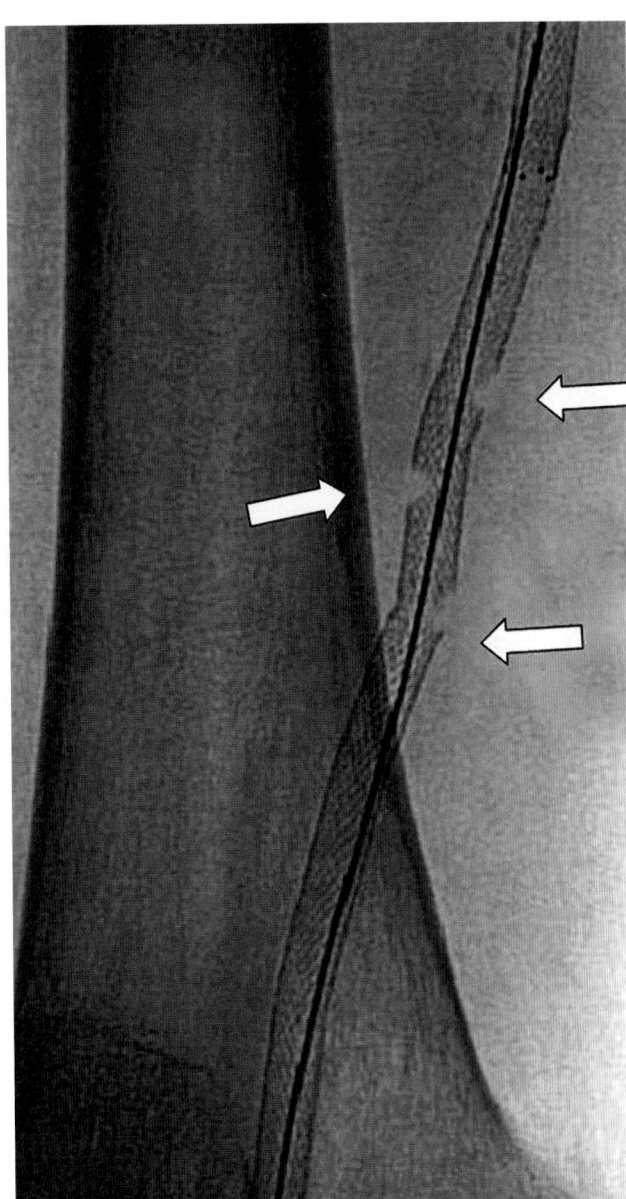

FIG. 23-67. Due to various geometric forces, including torsion, compression, extension, and flexion, which exert on the superficial femoral artery, stent fracture (*arrows*) is a known complication following superficial femoral artery stent placement.

tion. A prospective study evaluating Hemobahn stent grafts in the treatment of femoropopliteal arterial occlusions demonstrated a 23% immediate complication rate, including distal embolization (7.7%), groin hematoma (13.5%), and arteriovenous fistula (1.9%).[175]

Atherectomy-Related Complications

Overall complication rates associated with atherectomy range from 15.4 to 42.8% and include spasm, thrombosis, dissection, perforation, distal emboli, no reflow, and hematoma.[176,177] Jahnke and associates conducted a prospective study evaluating high-speed, rotational atherectomy in 15 patients with infrapopliteal occlusive disease. They yielded a 94% technical success rate, which was complicated by vessel rupture (5%), distal embolization (5%), and arterial spasm (5%).[175] Although the excimer laser atherectomy reduces embolic events by evaporating the lesion, embolization still remains a problematic complication. Studies show that distal embolic events occur in 3 to 4% of procedures, and perforation in 2.2 to 4.3% of cases.[168,169] Other complications compromising laser atherectomy therapy include acute reocclusion, vasospasm, direct vessel injury, and dissection.

Surgical Treatment for Chronic Limb Ischemia Due to Femoropopliteal Disease

Endarterectomy

Endarterectomy has a limited, albeit important, role in LE occlusive disease. It is most frequently used when there is disease in the CFA or involving the PFA. In this procedure, the surgeon opens the diseased segment longitudinally and develops a cleavage plane within the media that is developed proximally and distally. This permits the inner layer containing the atheroma to be excised. Great care must be taken at the distal end of the endarterectomy to ensure either a smooth transition or to tack down the distal endpoint to prevent the flow from elevating a potentially occlusive atheromatous flap. Currently, there is essentially no role for long open endarterectomy in the treatment of SFA stenoses or occlusions. The high incidence of restenosis is what limits use of endarterectomy in this location. Short-segment stenoses are more appropriately treated with balloon angioplasty. Endarterectomy using a catheter-based approach (e.g., Moll endarterectomy device) supplemented with stent grafting or stenting across the endpoint of the endarterectomy is currently being re-evaluated; however, no long-term data are available.

Bypass Grafting

Bypass grafting remains the primary intervention for LE occlusive disease. The type of bypass and conduit are important variables to consider. Patients with occlusive disease limited to the SFA, who have at least 4 cm (ideally 10 cm) of normal popliteal artery reconstituted above the knee joint and at least one continuous vessel to the foot, can be treated with an above-knee (AK) femoropopliteal bypass graft. Despite the fact that in this above-knee location, the differential patencies between prosthetic (PTFE) and vein graft are comparable; undoubtedly, it remains ideal to use a saphenous vein as the bypass conduit, if possible. Saving the vein for future coronary artery bypass or distal leg bypass grafting has been shown to be a flawed argument. One must also take into consideration that the consequences to the vascular outflow after a thrombosed prosthetic are worse than after a thrombosed vein graft.

When the disease extends to involve the popliteal artery or the tibial vessels, the surgeon must select an appropriate outflow vessel to perform a bypass. Suitable outflow vessels are defined as uninterrupted flow channels beyond the anastomosis into the foot. In order of descending preference, they are: AK popliteal artery, below-knee (BK) popliteal artery, posterior tibial artery, anterior tibial artery, and peroneal artery. In patients with diabetes, it is frequently the peroneal artery that is spared. Although the peroneal artery has no direct flow into the foot, collateralization to the posterior tibial and anterior tibial arteries makes it an appropriate outflow vessel. There

is no objective evidence to preferentially select tibial over peroneal arteries if they are vessels of equal caliber and quality. The dorsalis pedis, which is the continuation of the anterior tibial in the foot, is frequently spared from atherosclerotic disease and can be used as a target for distal bypasses. Patency is affected by the length of the bypass (longer bypasses have reduced patency), quality of the recipient artery, extent of runoff to the foot, and quality of the conduit (saphenous vein/graft). Five-year assisted patency rates for infrapopliteal venous bypasses are 60%. Venous conduits also have been shown to be suitable for bypasses to plantar arteries. In this location, venous conduits have a 3-year limb salvage of 84% and a 3-year secondary patency of 74%.[2] A meta-analysis suggests unsatisfactory results when PTFE-coated grafts are used to bypass to infrapopliteal arteries. In this location, prosthetic grafts have a 5-year primary patency rate of 30.5%.[178] Additionally, due to distal embolization and compromise of outflow vessels, prosthetic graft occlusion may have more severe consequences than vein graft occlusion.[178]

Two techniques are used for distal bypass grafting: reversed saphenous vein grafting and in situ saphenous vein grafting. There is no difference in outcomes (patency or limb salvage) between these techniques.[2] In the former, the vein is excised in its entirety from the leg using open or endoscopic vein harvest, reversed to render the valves nonfunctional, and tunneled from the CFA inflow to the distal target vessels. End-to-side anastomoses are then created.

Several adjunctive techniques have been tried to improve the patency of bypass grafts to tibial arteries. Creation of an arteriovenous fistula at the distal anastomosis is one option, but it has not been shown to improve patency.[179] Another method involves creating various configurations of vein cuffs or patches at the distal anastomosis in an attempt to streamline the flow and to reduce the likelihood of neointimal hyperplasia. Results with this approach are more promising, especially when done to improve patency of a below-the-knee prosthetic; however, there are no definitive comparative trials that support the superiority of one configuration over another.

Amputation

Primary amputation is defined as an amputation that is performed without a prior attempt at surgical or endovascular revascularization. It is rarely necessary in patients who, as a result of neglect, present with class III ALI. Primary amputation may play a role in patients with critical limb ischemia who are deemed nonambulatory because of knee contractures, debilitating strokes, or dementia.

Complications of Surgical Reconstruction

Vein Graft Stenoses

Fifteen percent of vein grafts will develop intrinsic stenoses within the first 18 months following implantation. Consequently, patients with a vein graft were entered into duplex surveillance protocols (scans every 3 months) to detect elevated (>300 cm/s) or abnormally low (<45 cm/s) graft velocities early. Stenoses greater than 50%, especially if associated with changes in ABI, should be repaired to prevent graft thrombosis. Repair usually entails patch angioplasty or short-segment venous interposition, but PTA/stenting is an option for short, focal lesions. Grafts with stenoses that are identified and repaired before thrombosis have assisted primary patency identical to primary patency, whereas a thrombosed autogenous bypass has limited longevity, resulting from ischemic injury to the vein wall. Secondary patency is markedly inferior to primary assisted patency. The recommendation for routine duplex ultrasound surveillance of autogenous infrainguinal bypasses was recently brought into question by a randomized, controlled trial that demonstrated no cost benefit or quality-of-life improvement after 18 months in patients with femoropopliteal venous bypasses.[180] Many surgeons continue with programs of vein graft surveillance, as has been suggested in older trials, awaiting further confirmation of the findings from the more recent study. When intervening on a failing infrainguinal bypass, the original indication for surgery is an important consideration. Limb salvage rates for occluded grafts are better if the indication for the original bypass was claudication rather than rest pain or tissue loss. An acutely occluded infrainguinal graft (≤30 postoperative days) has a 25% limb salvage rate.[181]

Limb Swelling

Limb swelling is common following revascularization and usually returns to baseline within 2 to 3 months. The etiology is multifactorial, with lymphatic interruption, interstitial edema, and disruption of venous drainage all contributing. Limb swelling tends to worsen with repeat revascularization (see Table 23-22).

Wound Infection

Because the most common inflow vessel for distal bypass is the CFA, groin infection is common and occurs in 7% of cases.[182] When an autogenous conduit such as a saphenous vein is used, most infection can be managed with local wound care because it involves the subcutaneous tissue or skin rather than infection of the actual vein. When a prosthetic graft has been used, management of graft infection is a major undertaking. Infection of a LE prosthetic bypass graft is associated with a significant amputation rate because of the tendency for graft thrombosis and anastomotic disruption. Prosthetic graft infections cannot be eradicated with antibiotics, and they mandate graft excision and complex revascularization using a vein, if available.

Choice of Conduit for Infrainguinal Bypass Grafting

Autogenous Vein

Autogenous vein is superior to prosthetic conduits for all infrainguinal bypasses, even in the AK position. This preference is applicable not only for the initial bypass but also for reoperative cases. For long bypasses, ipsilateral great saphenous vein (GSV), contralateral GSV, small saphenous vein, arm vein, and spliced vein are used, in decreasing order of preference. If only a short segment of vein is missing, the SFA can be endarterectomized and the proximal anastomosis performed distally to decrease the length of the conduit and to avoid harvesting and splicing additional vein. When GSV is not available and a relatively short bypass is necessary, arm vein or small saphenous vein is effective. Small saphenous vein is of particular use when a posterior approach is used. If a longer bypass with vein is necessary, arm vein is preferable because it is less awkward to harvest. Another conduit alternative is to harvest the upper arm basilic, median cubital, and cephalic veins in continuity, while incising valves in the basilic segment and using the cephalic segment in reversed configuration to provide a relatively long, unspliced autogenous conduit.[183]

Cryopreserved Grafts

Cryopreserved grafts are usually cadaveric arteries or veins that have been subjected to rate-controlled freezing with dimethyl sulfoxide and other cryopreservants. Cryopreserved vein grafts are more expensive than prosthetic grafts and are more prone to failure. The endothelial lining is lost as part of the freezing process, making these grafts prone to early thrombosis. Cryopreserved grafts also are prone to aneurysmal degeneration. Despite the fact that these grafts have not performed as well as prosthetic bypasses and autogenous vein in clinical practice, they can still play a role when revascularization is required following removal of infected prosthetic bypass grafts, especially when autogenous vein is unavailable to create a new bypass through clean tissue planes.[184]

Human Umbilical Vein

Human umbilical vein (HUV) is less commonly used than PTFE, because it is thicker and more cumbersome to handle and because of concerns about aneurysmal degeneration. HUV allografts are stabilized with glutaraldehyde and do not have viable cells or antigenic reactivity. These grafts have poor handling characteristics and require extra care when suturing because of an outer Dacron mesh wrapping, which is used to decrease aneurysmal degeneration. Dardik and colleagues have reported favorable results after using HUV and an adjunctive distal arteriovenous fistula.[185] One trial comparing HUV with PTFE and saphenous vein showed that HUV was better than PTFE but worse than saphenous vein in terms of 5-year patency in the AK location.[186] In a systematic review, HUV appears to perform better than cryopreserved veins.[187]

Prosthetic Conduits and Adjunctive Modifications

If vein is truly unavailable, PTFE or Dacron is the best option for AK bypass. The addition of rings to PTFE did not confer benefit in a single prospective, randomized clinical trial.[188] For infrageniculate prosthetic bypasses, use of a vein patch, cuff, or other venous anastomotic modification can improve patency (52% patency at 2 years for PTFE with vein cuff vs. 29% for PTFE with no cuff) and also improve limb salvage (84% vs. 62%).[189]

Although prosthetic grafts are readily available, easy to handle, and do not require extensive dissection to harvest, their propensity to undergo thrombosis and develop neointimal hyperplasia makes them a less favorable alternative when compared to vein. In a recent review of vein and prosthetic AK femoropopliteal bypasses, the 5-year primary patency rates were reported to be 74 and 39%, respectively.[190] Outcomes were even worse for BK prosthetic bypasses. Unfortunately, the use of autologous venous conduits is not possible in as many as 30% of patients. The GSV may be unsuitable because of small size and poor quality or unavailable due to prior harvest.

Methods to improve prosthetic graft performance have consisted of altering the geometry at the distal anastomosis to get the benefit obtained with vein cuffs (Distaflo, Bard Peripheral Vascular, Tempe, Ariz) and covalently bonding agents onto the luminal surface with anticoagulant, anti-inflammatory and antiproliferative characteristics (Propaten, Gore, Flagstaff, Ariz). One randomized trial that compared precuffed PTFE and PTFE with a vein cuff enrolled 104 patients at 10 centers. Eighty-nine patients were randomized to 47 precuffed PTFE bypasses and 44 bypasses with a vein cuff. At 1 and 2 years, primary patency rates were 52 and 49% for the precuffed group and 62 and 44% for the vein cuffed group, respectively. At 1 year and 2 years, the limb salvage rate was 72 and 65% for the precuffed group and 75 and 62% in the vein cuffed group, respectively. Although numbers are small and follow-up short, the midterm analysis revealed that Distaflo precuffed grafts and PTFE grafts with vein cuff had similar results. The authors concluded that a precuffed graft was a reasonable alternative for infragenicular reconstruction in the absence of saphenous vein.[191] Other authors have been less optimistic and question if there is any benefit derived from geometrically altering prosthetic conduits.[192]

Another approach for improving outcomes when using prosthetic for bypass grafts involves bonding anticoagulants to the conduit. The Gore Propaten graft has heparin bonded onto the luminal surface of the PTFE graft using Carmeda BioActive Surface technology, which immobilizes the heparin molecule with a single covalent bond that does not alter its anticoagulant properties.[193] The heparin binding does not alter the microstructure and handling characteristics of the PTFE. A prospective, randomized trial by Devine and associates suggested that heparin-bonded Dacron or PTFE was superior to plain PTFE for AK popliteal bypasses. The 3-year primary patency for the heparin-bonded grafts was 55% compared with 42% for PTFE ($P < .044$). Both of these patency rates are inferior to GSV; however, if the improved results with heparin bonding continue to be substantiated, then heparin-bonded prosthetic grafts will become the preferred conduit for AK bypass in the absence of suitable vein.[194] A recent review of available studies with this graft showed an 80% 1-year patency for BK bypasses.[195] Randomized, controlled clinical trials with more patients and longer follow-up are necessary to validate whether the PROPATEN vascular graft is superior to other prosthetics, and if, indeed, it is comparable to autogenous vein for BK interventions.

Clinical Results of Surgical and Endovascular Interventions for Femoropopliteal Occlusive Disease

Balloon angioplasty of the femoropopliteal vessels has not enjoyed the degree of success seen with iliac angioplasty. Patency in this region is dependent upon whether the patient presents with claudication vs. limb-threatening ischemia, the status of the distal runoff vessels, and lesion morphology.[2] Initial technical success for femoropopliteal angioplasty is seen in 80 to 90% of cases, with failures to cross a lesion occurring in 7% of stenoses and 18% of occlusive lesions. Studies have shown that PTA of the femoropopliteal segment achieved greater than a 90% technical success rate and had a 59% primary patency rate at 5-years.[148,149] PTA of lesions longer than 7 to 10 cm results in compromised patency, while PTA of shorter lesions (<3 cm) gives fairly good results. Lofberg and associates performed 127 femoropopliteal PTA procedures and reported a primary patency rate at 5-year follow-up of 12% in limbs with occlusion longer than 5 cm vs. 32% in limbs with occlusion <5 cm in length.[151] Occlusive lesions have much worse initial technical success rates than stenotic lesions. Concentric lesions respond better to PTA than eccentric lesions, and heavy calcifications have a negative impact on success rates. Distal runoff is another powerful predictor of long-term success.

Johnston and associates analyzed 254 consecutive patients who underwent femoropopliteal PTA and reported a 5-year patency rate of 53% for stenotic lesions and 36% for occlusive lesions in patients with good runoff vs. 5-year patency of 31% for stenotic lesions and 16% for occlusive lesions in patients with poor runoff.[149] A meta-analysis by Hunink and colleagues showed that adjusted 5-year primary patencies after angioplasty of femoropopliteal lesions varied from 12 to 68%, the best results occurring in patients with claudication and stenotic lesions.[150] Although the initial technical success is better for stenoses than occlusions, long-term patency rates for stenoses and short occlusions have been variable and there have been conflicting results regarding the efficacy of stent use. Early published series that examined efficacy of femoropopliteal artery stents showed patency rates that were comparable to stand-alone PTA with primary patency rates varying from 18 to 72% at 3 years.[158] Patient selection and the anatomic character of the lesions may play important roles in the outcomes. Additionally, stent characteristics may contribute to the patency rate. Several clinical studies have demonstrated significant improvements in patency when the newer generations of nitinol stents are used to treat SFA lesions.[160,196]

Mewissen treated 137 lower limbs in 122 patients with CLI, secondary to TASC II A (n = 12) or TASC II B or C (n = 125) lesions in the SFA. Patients were treated with Cordis SMART self-expanding nitinol stents. Binary restenosis (>50%) was measured by standard duplex velocity criteria at various postintervention intervals. Primary stent patency, defined as absence of binary restenosis in this study, was calculated by life table methods from the time of intervention. The mean lesion length was 12.2 cm (range, 4 to 28 cm). The technical success was 98%. Mean follow-up was 302 days. The primary stent patency rates were 92%, 76%, 66%, and 60% at 6, 12, 18, and 24-months, respectively.[160] Fereira and associates treated 59 patients who had 74 femoropopliteal lesions (60% TASC II D) with Zilver nitinol self-expanding stents (COOK, Bloomington, Ind). Mean recanalization length was 19 cm (range 3 to 53 cm). Mean follow-up time was 2.4 years (range 3 days to 4.8 years). Kaplan-Meier estimates for primary patency rates were 90%, 78%, 74%, 69%, and 69% at 1, 2, 3, 4, and 4.8 years, respectively.[197]

There is general agreement that for suboptimal PTA of an SFA lesion, stent placement is indicated, but a recent randomized trial by Schillinger and associates suggests that primary stenting results in lower restenosis rates than PTA and selective stenting. Restenosis rates at 2 years were 45.7% vs. 69.2% in favor of primary stenting compared with PTA and optional secondary stenting using an intention-to-treat analysis (P = .031). Consistently, stenting, both primary and selective, was superior to stand-alone PTA with respect to the occurrence of restenosis (49.2% vs. 74.3%; P = .028) by a treatment-received analysis.[198]

Nitinol bare metal stents that are designed specifically for BK interventions are showing very encouraging results. Bosiers and colleagues reported their 12-month results using the commercially available non–drug-eluting Xpert (Abbott Vascular, Santa Clara, Calif) nitinol stent system in BK arterial interventions.[199] They had a 12-month primary patency rate of 76.3%, and a limb salvage rate of 95.9%. They followed patients to 12 months and performed angiography with quantitative vessel analysis on the 73% of patients available. Angiography revealed a binary restenosis rate (>50%) of only 20.5%, which is comparable to well-accepted coronary DES study outcomes. The authors attributed this optimal performance to the maintenance of flow dynamics because the stent was specifically designed for use in small vessels.[199] Kickuth and colleagues also have obtained good results using the Xpert stent. After stent placement, the primary cumulative patency rate at 6 months for the study group of 35 patients was 82%. The sustained clinical improvement rate as evidenced by improved ABI was 80%, and freedom from major amputation was 100% at the 6-month follow-up. The rate of major complications was 17%.[200]

Wolf and associates published a multicenter, prospective randomized trial comparing PTA with bypass in 263 men who had iliac, femoral, or popliteal artery obstruction.[201] In 56 patients, cumulative 1-year primary patency after PTA was 43% and, after bypass surgery, was 82%, demonstrating that for long SFA stenoses or occlusions, surgery is better than PTA. Another recent randomized study (BASIL trial) of 452 patients with CLI demonstrated no difference in amputation-free survival at 6 months between surgery and PTA/stenting. The authors commented that surgery was somewhat more expensive and recommended that endovascular intervention should be used as first-line therapy, especially in medically unfit patients. They did conclude that at 2-year follow-up, healthy patients without medical comorbidities derived greater benefit from surgery because it was associated with decreased need for reintervention and had a decreased hazard ratio in terms of all-cause mortality.[202] Using the 2000 TASC II definitions and a Markov state transition model decision analysis, Nolan and colleagues showed that PTA/stenting surpasses bypass efficacy for TASC II C lesions if PTA/stenting primary patency is greater than 32% at 5 years, patient age is >80 years, and/or GSV bypass operative mortality is greater than 6%.[106,203]

NON-ATHEROSCLEROTIC DISORDERS OF BLOOD VESSELS

The majority of cases of peripheral vascular disease that are seen by vascular surgeons are attributable to underlying atherosclerosis. Non-atherosclerotic disease states that result in arterial pathology are less commonly encountered, but are nonetheless important, as they are potentially treatable lesions that may mimic atherosclerotic lesions and result in vascular insufficiency (see Table 23-18). A thorough knowledge of these rare disease states is important for the practicing vascular surgeon to make medical recommendations and provide appropriate surgical treatment.

Giant Cell Arteritis (Temporal Arteritis)

Giant cell arteritis is also known as *temporal arteritis*, which is a systemic chronic inflammatory vascular disease with many characteristics similar to those of Takayasu's disease. The histologic and pathologic changes as well as laboratory findings are similar. Patients tend to be white women over the age of 50 years old, with a high incidence in Scandinavia and among women of Northern European descent. Genetic factors may play a role in disease pathogenesis, with a human leukocyte antigen (HLA) variant having been identified. Differences exist between Takayasu's and giant cell arteritis in terms of presentation, disease location, and therapeutic efficacy. The inflammatory process typically involves the aorta and its extracranial branches, of which the superficial temporal artery is specifically affected.

The clinical syndrome begins with a prodromal phase of constitutional symptoms, including headache, fever, malaise, and myalgia. The patients may be initially diagnosed with coexisting polymyalgia rheumatica; an HLA-related association may exist between the two diseases. As a result of vascular narrowing and end-organ ischemia, complications may occur such as visual alterations, including blindness and mural weakness, resulting in acute aortic dissection that may be devastating. Ischemic optic neuritis resulting in partial or complete blindness occurs in up to 40% of patients and is considered a medical emergency. Cerebral symptoms occur when the disease process extends to the carotid arteries. Jaw claudication and temporal artery tenderness may be experienced. Aortic lesions usually are asymptomatic until later stages and consist of thoracic aneurysms and aortic dissections.

The diagnostic gold standard is a temporal artery biopsy, which will show the classic histologic findings of multinucleated giant cells with a dense perivascular inflammatory infiltrate. Treatment regimens are centered on corticosteroids, and giant cell arteritis tends to rapidly respond. Remission rates are high, and treatment tends to have a beneficial and preventative effect on the development of subsequent vascular complications.

Takayasu's Arteritis

Takayasu's arteritis is a rare but well-recognized chronic inflammatory arteritis affecting large vessels, predominantly the aorta and its main branches (Table 23-27).[204] Chronic vessel inflammation leads to wall thickening, fibrosis, stenosis, and thrombus formation. Symptoms are related to end-organ ischemia. The acute inflammation can destroy the arterial media and lead to aneurysm formation. This rare autoimmune disease occurs predominantly in women between the ages of 10 and 40 years old who are of Asian descent. Genetic studies have demonstrated a high frequency of HLA haplotypes in patients from Japan and Mexico, suggesting increased susceptibility to developing the disease in patients with certain alleles. However, these associations have not been seen in North America. Vascular inflammation leads to arterial wall thickening, stenosis, and eventually, fibrosis and thrombus formation. The pathologic changes produce stenosis, dilation, aneurysm formation, and/or occlusion.

The clinical course of Takayasu's arteritis begins with a "prepulseless" phase in which the patient demonstrates constitutional symptoms. These include fever, anorexia, weight loss, general malaise, arthralgias, and malnutrition. As the inflammation progresses and stenoses develop, more characteristic features of the disease become evident. During the chronic phase, the disease is inactive or "burned out." It is during this latter stage that patients most frequently present with bruits and vascular insufficiency according to the arterial bed involved. Laboratory data may show elevations in erythrocyte sedimentation rate, C-reactive protein, white blood cell count, or con-

versely, anemia may predominate. Characteristic clinical features during the second phase vary according to the involved vascular bed and include hypertension reflecting renal artery stenosis, retinopathy, aortic regurgitation, cerebrovascular symptoms, angina and congestive heart failure, abdominal pain or GI bleeding, pulmonary hypertension, or extremity claudication.

The gold standard for diagnosis remains angiography showing narrowing or occlusion of the entire aorta or its primary branches, or focal or segmental changes in large arteries in the upper or lower extremities. Six types of Takayasu's arteritis exist and are graded in terms of severity: type I, affecting the aorta and arch vessels; type IIa, affecting the ascending aorta, aortic arch, and branches; type IIb, affecting the ascending aorta, aortic arch and branches, and thoracic descending aorta; type III, affecting the thoracic descending aorta, abdominal aorta, and/or renal arteries; type IV, affecting the abdominal aorta and/or renal arteries; and type V, with combined features of types IIb and IV.[204]

Treatment consists of steroid therapy initially, with cytotoxic agents used in patients who do not achieve remission. Surgical treatment is performed only in advanced stages, and bypass needs to be delayed during active phases of inflammation. There is no role for endarterectomy, and synthetic or autogenous bypass grafts need to be placed onto disease-free segments of vessels. For focal lesions, there have been reports of success with angioplasty.[205–207]

Ehlers-Danlos Syndrome

Ehlers-Danlos syndrome is one of the more significant inheritable disorders affecting the connective tissue, along with Marfan syndrome. This syndrome represents a heterogeneous group of connective tissue disorders (types I through IV) that were first described in 1682 by van Meekeren.[208] It is an autosomal dominant disorder affecting approximately one in 5000 persons that is characterized by skin elasticity, joint hypermobility, tissue fragility, multiple ecchymoses, and subcutaneous pseudotumors. Ehlers-Danlos syndrome is a disorder of fibrillar collagen metabolism with identifiable, specific defects that have been found in the collagen biosynthetic pathway that produce clinically distinct forms of this disease. Ten different phenotypes have been described, each with variable modes of inheritance and biochemical defects. Of the four basic types of collagen found in the body, the predominant type in blood vessels is type III. Within the vessel wall, type III collagen contributes to structural integrity and tensile strength, as well as playing a role in platelet aggregation and thrombus formation.

Of the three types of Ehlers-Danlos syndrome that have arterial complications, type IV represents 5% of cases and is the one most likely to be seen by a vascular surgeon. These patients synthesize abnormal type III collagen (mutation COL3A1), and represent 5% of all cases.[208] Affected individuals do not show the typical skin and joint manifestations, and thus typically present for diagnosis when a major vascular catastrophe occurs. In a review of 36 patients with this disorder, Cikrit and colleagues reported a 44% mortality rate from major hemorrhage before any surgical intervention.[209] In the 20 patients who underwent 29 vascular procedures, there was a 29% mortality rate. Arterial rupture, aneurysm formation, and acute aortic dissection may occur in any major artery, with the most frequent site of rupture being the abdominal cavity. Repair is problematic, as the vessel wall is soft and sutures pull through the fragile tissue. Ligation may be the only option in many circumstances.

Marfan Syndrome

Another heterogeneous heritable disorder of connective tissue, Marfan syndrome is characterized by abnormal musculoskeletal, ocular, and cardiovascular features first described by Antoine Marfan in 1896.[210] The inborn error of metabolism in this syndrome has been localized to the long arm of chromosome 15 (15q21.3). Defects occur in fibrillin, a basic protein in the microfibrillar apparatus that serves as a backbone for elastin, which is one of the main extracellular structural proteins in blood vessels. This is an autoso-

	TABLE 23-27	Angiographic classification of Takayasu's arteritis

Type	Vessel Involvement
I	Branches from the aortic arch
IIa	Ascending aorta, aortic arch and its branches
IIb	Ascending aorta, aortic arch and its branches, thoracic descending aorta
III	Thoracic descending aorta, abdominal aorta, and/or renal arteries
IV	Abdominal aorta and/or renal arteries
V	Combined features of types IIb and IV

Involvement of the coronary or pulmonary arteries are designated as C (+) or P (+), respectively.

mal dominant gene with high penetrance; however, approximately 15 to 20% of cases are secondary to new spontaneous mutations.[210]

Classic recognizable features of Marfan syndrome include tall stature, long limbs (dolichostenomelia), long fingers (arachnodactyly), joint hyperextensibility, chest wall deformities, and scoliosis. Ocular manifestations are flattened corneas, lens subluxation, and myopia. Ninety-five percent of patients have cardiovascular involvement, which may include ascending aortic dilatation, mitral valve prolapse, valvular regurgitation, and aortic dissection. Skin, central nervous system, and pulmonary features may be present as well. Aortic root dilatation will generally occur in all patients. This may not be evident on standard chest radiograph until dilatation has resulted in an ascending aortic aneurysm, aortic valve regurgitation, or dissection. Left untreated, the cardiovascular complications are devastating and reduce the life expectancy to about 40 years for men and slightly higher for women. Death is usually attributable to life-threatening complications of aortic regurgitation, dissection, and rupture after the ascending aorta has dilated to 6 cm or more.

Aggressive medical management with beta-adrenergic blocking agents and other BP lowering regimens is crucial to treatment. Surgical intervention entails replacement of the aortic root with a composite valve graft (e.g., Bentall procedure).[205] Prophylactic operative repair is indicated for an aneurysm >5.5 cm, with an acceptable perioperative mortality of less than 5%.

Pseudoxanthoma Elasticum

Pseudoxanthoma elasticum is a rare inherited disorder of connective tissue that is characterized by an unbalanced elastic fiber metabolism and synthesis, resulting in fragmentation and calcification of the fibers. Clinical manifestations occur in the skin, ocular, GI, and cardiovascular systems.[206] Characteristic skin lesions are seen in the axilla, antecubital and popliteal fossae, and groin. The yellow, xanthoma-like papules occur in redundant folds of skin and are said to resemble plucked chicken skin. The inheritance pattern includes both autosomal dominant and recessive types and has a prevalence of one in 160,000 individuals.[183] The ATP-binding cassette subfamily C member 6 (ABCC6) gene has been demonstrated to be responsible, and 43 mutations have been identified, all of which lead to calcification of the internal elastic laminae of medium-sized vessel walls.[206]

Cardiovascular features are common and include premature CAD, cerebrovascular disease, renovascular hypertension, diminished peripheral pulses, and restrictive cardiomyopathy. Symptom onset typically occurs in the second decade of life, with onset at an average age of 13 years. Patients should be counseled to reduce potential contributing factors for atherosclerosis such as tobacco use and high cholesterol levels. Calcium intake should be restricted in adolescents, as a positive correlation has been found between disease severity and calcium intake.[206] Surgical management involves standard vascular techniques, with the exception that arterial conduits should not be used in cardiac bypass.

Kawasaki Disease

Kawasaki disease was first described in 1967, as a mucocutaneous lymph node syndrome occurring in young children. In most studies, more than one half of the patients are younger than 2 years of age, with a higher prevalence in boys.[207] Although originally described in Japan, the disease is found worldwide. An infectious agent may be causative; however, no specific agent has been identified. Immune activation with the contribution of cytokines, elastases, growth factors, and metalloproteinases is believed to be a mechanism for inflammation and aneurysm formation. Coronary artery aneurysms, the hallmark of the disease, histologically demonstrate a panarteritis with fibrinoid necrosis. Coronary arteriography may show occlusions, recanalization, and localized stenosis, in addition to multiple aneurysms. A variety of constitutional symptoms and signs resulting from systemic vasculitis are present in the acute phase of the illness.[207]

Medical therapy for Kawasaki disease clearly decreases the manifestations of coronary artery involvement. IV gamma globulin and aspirin therapy are most successful if begun within the first 10 days of illness. Up to 20% of untreated patients will develop coronary arterial lesions.[207] A long-term, low-dose aspirin therapy regimen usually is recommended.

Inflammatory Arteritis and Vasculitis

Chronic inflammatory arteritis and vasculitis (i.e., inflammatory changes within veins as well as arteries) include a spectrum of disease processes caused by immunologic mechanisms. These terms signify a necrotizing transmural inflammation of the vessel wall associated with antigen-antibody immune complex deposition within the endothelium. These conditions show pronounced cellular infiltration in the adventitia, thickened intimal fibrosis, and organized thrombus.[204] These disease processes may clinically mimic atherosclerosis, and most are treated by corticosteroid therapy or chemotherapeutic agents. Even so, it is important to recognize distinguishing characteristics of each disease to establish the course of treatment and long-term prognosis. A classification system of systemic vasculitis by vessel size is shown in Table 23-28.

Behçet's Disease

Behçet's disease is a rare syndrome characterized by oral and genital ulcerations and ocular inflammation, affecting males in Japan and the Mediterranean. An HLA linkage has been found, indicating a genetic component to the etiology. Vascular involvement is seen in 7 to 38% of patients, and is localized to the abdominal aorta, femoral artery, and pulmonary artery.[211] Vascular lesions also may include venous complications such as deep venous thrombosis or superficial thrombophlebitis. Arterial aneurysmal degeneration can occur; however, this is an uncommon, albeit potentially devastating, complication. Multiple true aneurysms and pseudoaneurysms may develop, and rupture of an aortic aneurysm is the major cause of death in patients with Behçet's disease.[212]

Histologically, degeneration of the vasa vasorum with surrounding perivascular lymphocyte infiltration is seen, along with thickening of the elastic laminae around the tunica media.[213] Aneurysm formation is believed to be associated with a loss of the nutrient flow and elastic component of the vessels, leading to progressive dilatation. Multiple aneurysms are relatively common, with a reported occurrence of 36% in affected Japanese patients.[212] Furthermore, pseudoaneurysm formation after surgical bypass is common at anastomotic suture lines due to the vascular wall fragility and medial destruction. Systemic therapy with corticosteroids and immunosuppressive agents may diminish symptoms related to the inflammatory process; however, they have no effect on the rate of disease progression and arterial degeneration.[212]

Polyarteritis Nodosa

Polyarteritis nodosa (PAN) is another systemic inflammatory disease process, which is characterized by a necrotizing inflammation of medium-sized or small arteries that spares the smallest blood vessels

TABLE 23-28	Classification of vasculitis based on vessel involvement
Large vessel vasculitis	
Takayasu's arteritis	
Giant cell arteritis	
Behçet's disease	
Medium-sized vessel vasculitis	
Polyarteritis nodosa	
Kawasaki disease	
Buerger's disease	
Small vessel vasculitis	
Hypersensitivity angiitis	

(i.e., arterioles and capillaries). This disease predominantly affects men more than women by a 2:1 ratio. PAN develops subacutely, with constitutional symptoms that last for weeks to months. Intermittent, low-grade fever, malaise, weight loss, and myalgia are common presenting symptoms. As medium-sized vessels lie within the deep dermis, cutaneous manifestations occur in the form of livedo reticularis, nodules, ulcerations, and digital ischemia.[214] Skin biopsies of these lesions may be sufficient for diagnosis. Inflammation may be seen histologically, with pleomorphic cellular infiltrates and segmental transmural necrosis leading to aneurysm formation.

Neuritis from nerve infarction occurs in 60% of patients, and GI complications in up to 50%.[215] Additionally, renal involvement is found in 40%, and manifests as microaneurysms within the kidney or segmental infarctions. Cardiac disease is a rare finding except at autopsy, where thickened, diseased coronary arteries may be seen, as well as patchy myocardial necrosis. Patients may succumb to renal failure, intestinal hemorrhage, or perforation. End-organ ischemia from vascular occlusion or aneurysm rupture can be disastrous complications with high mortality rates. The mainstay of treatment is steroid and cytotoxic agent therapy. Up to 50% of patients with active PAN will experience remission with high dosing.[215]

Radiation-Induced Arteritis

Radiation-induced arteritis results from progressive stenosis due to endothelial damage that leads to cellular proliferation and fibrosis. These are well-described complications of combined irradiation and chemotherapy for the treatment of head and neck malignancy. Arterial lesions are known complications of radiation and are similar to those found in atherosclerotic occlusive disease. A history of therapeutic irradiation to the neck can complicate the management of carotid artery occlusive disease. Radiation-induced damage to blood vessels has been well studied. The small capillaries and sinusoids are most susceptible to radiation effects, as endothelial cells are the most radiosensitive cells. The radiation effects on the medium and large-sized arteries include myointimal proliferation, with or without lipid deposits, and thrombosis. Characteristically, irregular, spindle-shaped cells are seen replacing the normal endothelial cells in the healing phase. Occlusive lesions develop in the irradiated carotid arteries, and are either the result of vessel wall fibrosis, or, more commonly, due to accelerated atherosclerosis. Neurologic complications related to radiation-induced carotid artery disease are similar to those due to nonirradiated atherosclerotic occlusive disease.

Rupture of the carotid artery has been reported following neck irradiation, and is likely related to local wound complication and superimposed infection. The diagnosis of radiation arteritis is based on the clinical history and confirmation of the occlusive lesion by duplex ultrasound, MRA, CTA, or subtraction angiography. Irradiated lesions can be confined to the irradiated segment of the ICA with the remaining part of the vessel spared of disease. Characteristically, the radiation-induced atherosclerotic lesion does not involve the carotid bulb, unlike the nonradiated atherosclerotic lesions. The indications for intervention in radiation-induced carotid lesions are the same for atherosclerotic carotid occlusive lesions as previously discussed in the "Treatment of Carotid Occlusive Disease" section. However, asymptomatic irradiated carotid artery lesions should be considered for intervention because they can be more prone to progression and development of neurologic complications. Endovascular treatment with carotid angioplasty/stenting has become the treatment of choice for radiation-induced lesions, although surgical endarterectomy and bypass have been shown to be safe. The rate of recurrent stenosis is higher in radiation-induced carotid lesions, whether stented or surgically treated.

Raynaud's Syndrome

First described in 1862 by Maurice Raynaud, the term *Raynaud's syndrome* applies to a heterogeneous symptom array associated with peripheral vasospasm, more commonly occurring in the upper extremities. The characteristically intermittent vasospasm classically follows exposure to various stimuli, including cold tempera-

tures, tobacco, or emotional stress. Formerly, a distinction was made between Raynaud's "disease" and Raynaud's "phenomenon" for describing a benign disease occurring in isolation or a more severe disease secondary to another underlying disorder, respectively. However, many patients develop collagen vascular disorders at some point after the onset of vasospastic symptoms; progression to a connective tissue disorder ranges from 11 to 65% in reported series.[211,216] Therefore, the term *Raynaud's syndrome* is now used to encompass both the primary and secondary conditions.

Characteristic color changes occur in response to the arteriolar vasospasm, ranging from intense pallor to cyanosis to redness as the vasospasm occurs. The digital vessels then relax, eventually leading to reactive hyperemia. The majority of patients are young women <40 years of age. Up to 70 to 90% of reported patients are women, although many patients with only mild symptoms may never present for treatment. Geographic regions located in cooler, damp climates such as the Pacific Northwest and Scandinavian countries have a higher reported prevalence of the syndrome. Certain occupational groups, such as those that use vibrating tools, may be more predisposed to Raynaud's syndrome or digital ischemia. The exact pathophysiologic mechanism behind the development of such severe vasospasm remains elusive, and much attention has focused on increased levels of alpha$_2$-adrenergic receptors and their hypersensitivity in patients with Raynaud's syndrome, as well as abnormalities in the thermoregulatory response, which is governed by the sympathetic nervous system.[211]

The diagnosis of severe vasospasm may be made using noninvasive measurements in the vascular laboratory. Angiography is usually reserved for those who have digital ulceration and an embolic or obstructive cause is believed to be present and potentially surgically correctable. Different changes in digital BP will occur in patients with Raynaud's syndrome. Normal individuals will show only a slight decrease in digital BP in response to external cold stimuli, whereas those with Raynaud's syndrome will show a similar curve until a critical temperature is reached.[211] It is at this point that arterial closure acutely occurs.

There is no cure for Raynaud's syndrome, thus all treatments mainly palliate symptoms and decrease the severity and, perhaps, frequency of attacks. Conservative measures predominate, including the wearing of gloves, use of electric or chemically activated hand warmers, avoiding occupational exposure to vibratory tools, abstinence from tobacco, or relocating to a warmer, dryer climate. The majority (90%) of patients will respond to avoidance of cold and other stimuli. The remaining 10% of patients with more persistent or severe syndromes can be treated with a variety of vasodilatory drugs, albeit with only a 30 to 60% response rate. Calcium-channel blocking agents such as diltiazem and nifedipine are the drugs of choice. The selective serotonin reuptake inhibitor fluoxetine has been shown to reduce the frequency and duration of vasospastic episodes.[211] IV infusions of prostaglandins have been reserved for nonresponders with severe symptoms.

Surgical therapy is limited to débridement of digital ulcerations and amputation of gangrenous digits, which are rare complications. Upper extremity sympathectomy may provide relief in 60 to 70% of patients; however, the results are short lived with a gradual recurrence of symptoms in 60% within 10 years.[211,216]

Fibromuscular Dysplasia

Fibromuscular dysplasia (FMD) is a vasculopathy of uncertain etiology that is characterized by segmental arterial involvement. Histologically, fibrous tissue proliferation, smooth muscle cell hyperplasia, and elastic fiber destruction alternate with mural thinning.[213] The characteristic beaded appearance of FMD is due to areas of medial thinning alternating with areas of stenosis. Most commonly affected are medium-sized arteries, including the internal carotid, renal, vertebral, subclavian, mesenteric, and iliac arteries. The ICA is the second most common site of involvement after the renal arteries. FMD occurs most frequently in women (90%) and is recognized at approximately 55 years of age. Only 10% of patients with FMD will have complications attributable to the disease.[213] Pathologically, FMD is a heterogeneous group of four distinct types of lesions that are subgrouped, based on the predominant site of involvement within the vessel wall. Of the four types (medial fibroplasia, intimal fibroplasia, medial hyperplasia, and perimedial dysplasia), medial fibroplasia is the most common pathologic type, affecting the ICA and the renal artery, and occurring in 85% of reported cases.[213]

The two main clinical syndromes associated with FMD are transient ischemic attacks from disease in the ICA, and hypertension from renal artery involvement. Symptoms produced by FMD are generally secondary to associated arterial stenosis, and are clinically indistinguishable from those caused by atherosclerotic disease. Often, asymptomatic disease is found incidentally on conventional angiographic studies being performed for other reasons. Within the ICA, FMD lesions tend to be located higher in the extracranial segment than with atherosclerotic lesions, and may not be readily demonstrated by duplex scan.

Clinically, symptoms are due to encroachment on the vessel lumen and a reduction in flow. Additionally, thrombi may form in areas of mural dilatation from a stagnation of flow, leading to distal embolization. Surgical treatment has been favored for symptomatic patients with angiographically proven disease. Owing to the distal location of FMD lesions in the extracranial carotid artery, resection and repair is not usually feasible. Instead, graduated luminal dilatation under direct vision has been used successfully in patients, with antiplatelet therapy continued postoperatively. Percutaneous transluminal angioplasty (PTA) has been used effectively in patients with FMD-induced hypertension. Several series have documented a high technical success rate, with recurrence rates of 8 to 23% at more than 1 year.[217] However, the therapeutic effect of BP control may continue to be observed despite restenosis. Surgical reconstruction of the renal arteries for FMD has good long-term results and is recommended for recurrent lesions after angioplasty.[217] Open balloon angioplasty of the ICA has been described, which allows for precise fluoroscopic guidance, rather than blind dilatation with calibrated metal probes, and back-bleeding after dilatation to eliminate cerebral embolization.[218] Distal neuroprotective devices may allow this procedure to be performed completely percutaneously, by lessening the threat of cerebral emboli.

Non-Atherosclerotic Disease Affecting the Popliteal Artery Disease

There are three distinct non-atherosclerotic disease entities that may result in LE claudication that predominantly occur in 40- to 50-year-old men. Adventitial cystic disease, popliteal artery entrapment syndrome, and Buerger's disease should be considered in any young patients presenting with intermittent claudication.

Adventitial Cystic Disease of the Popliteal Artery

The first successful operative repair of popliteal artery occlusion caused by a cyst arising from the adventitia was reported in 1954 by Ejrup and Hierton.[218] Adventitial cystic disease is a rare arterial condition occurring at an incidence of 0.1%, usually in the popliteal artery. This disease affects men in a ratio of approximately 5:1 and appears predominantly in the fourth and fifth decades. The incidence is approximately one in 1200 cases of claudication or one in 1000 peripheral arteriograms.[218] The predominance of reported cases is found in Japan and Europe. However, this disease may affect other vascular sites such as the femoral, external iliac, radial, ulnar, and brachial arteries. Besides claudication as a symptom, this diagnosis should be considered in young patients who have a mass in a nonaxial vessel in proximity to a related joint. These synovial-like, mucin-filled cysts reside in the subadventitial layer of the vessel wall and have a similar macroscopic appearance to ganglion cysts. Despite this similarity and suggestion of a joint origin for these lesions, histochemical markers have failed to link the cystic lining to synovium.

Patients presenting at a young age with bilateral LE claudication and minimal risk factors for atheroma formation should be evaluated for adventitial cystic disease, as well as the other two non-atherosclerotic vascular lesions described herein. Because of luminal encroachment and compression, peripheral pulses may be present in the limb when extended, but then can disappear during knee joint flexion. Noninvasive studies may suggest arterial stenosis with elevated velocities. Color flow duplex scanning followed by T2-weighted MRI now appears to be the best diagnostic choice. Angiography will demonstrate a smooth, well-defined, crescent-shaped filling defect, the classic "scimitar" sign.[218] There may be associated calcification in the cyst wall and no other evidence of atherosclerotic occlusive disease.

Various therapeutic methods have been described for the treatment of adventitial cystic disease. The recommended treatments are excision of the cyst with the cystic wall, enucleation, or simple aspiration when the artery is stenotic. Retention of the cystic lining leads to continued secretion of the cystic fluid and recurrent lesions. In 30% of patients who have an occluded artery, resection of the affected artery, followed by an interposition graft using autogenous saphenous vein, is recommended.

Popliteal Artery Entrapment Syndrome

Love and colleagues first coined the term *popliteal artery entrapment* in 1965 to describe a syndrome combining muscular involvement with arterial ischemia occurring behind the knee, with the successful surgical repair having taken place 6 years earlier.[214] This is a rare disorder with an estimated prevalence of 0.16% that occurs with a male-to-female ratio of 15:1. Five types of anatomic entrapment have been defined, according to the position of the medial head of the gastrocnemius muscle, abnormal muscle slips or tendinous bands, or the course of the popliteal artery itself (Table 23-29). Concomitant popliteal vein impingement occurs in up to 30%. Twenty-five percent of cases are bilateral.

The typical patient presents with swelling and claudication of isolated calf muscle groups following vigorous physical activity. Various differential diagnoses must be considered when encountering patients with symptoms and signs suggestive of popliteal artery entrapment syndrome (Table 23-30). In a large series of 240 patients reported by Turnipseed, the median age for surgical treatment was 28.5 years.[214] Noninvasive studies with ankle-brachial indices should be performed with the knee extended and the foot in a neutral, forced plantar, and dorsiflexed position. A drop in pressure of 50% or greater or dampening of the plethysmographic waveforms in plantar or dorsiflexion is a classic finding. Contraction of the gastrocnemius should compress the entrapped popliteal artery. The sudden onset of signs and symptoms of acute ischemia with absent distal pulses is consistent with popliteal artery occlusion secondary to entrapment. Other conditions resulting from entrapment are thrombus formation with distal emboli or popliteal aneurysmal degeneration. Although CT and MRI have been used, angiography remains the most widely used test. Angiography performed with the foot in a neutral position may demonstrate classical medial deviation

TABLE 23-29	Classification of popliteal entrapment syndrome

Type	Description
I	Popliteal artery is displaced medially around a normal medial head of the gastrocnemius
II	Medial head of gastrocnemius, which arises lateral to popliteal artery
III	Popliteal artery is compressed by an accessory slip of muscle form medial head of gastrocnemius
IV	Entrapment by a deeper popliteus muscle
V	Any of the above plus popliteal vein
VI	Functional entrapment

TABLE 23-30	Differential diagnosis for popliteal entrapment syndrome

Vascular etiologies
Atherosclerosis
Buerger's disease
Trauma
Popliteal aneurysm
Adventitial cystic disease
Extrinsic compression
Cardiac embolism
Deep vein thrombosis
Venous entrapment
Musculoskeletal etiologies
Gastrocnemius or soleus strain
Periostitis
Compartment syndrome
Stress fractures
Tibialis posterior tendonitis
Muscular anomalies
General neurologic etiologies
Spinal stenosis

of the popliteal artery or normal anatomic positioning. Coexisting abnormalities may include stenosis, luminal irregularity, delayed flow, aneurysm, or complete occlusion. Diagnostic accuracy is increased with the use of ankle stress view–active plantar flexion and passive dorsiflexion.

The treatment of popliteal artery entrapment consists of surgical decompression of the impinged artery with possible arterial reconstruction. Division of the anomalous musculotendinous insertion site with or without saphenous vein interposition grafting to bypass the damaged arterial segment has been described to be the procedure of choice. The natural history of entrapment is progressive arterial degeneration, leading to complete arterial thrombosis. In such instances, thrombolytic therapy is needed with subsequent release of the functional arterial impairment. Lysis will improve distal runoff and may improve limb-salvage and bypass patency rates.

Buerger's Disease (Thromboangiitis Obliterans)

Buerger's disease, also known as *thromboangiitis obliterans*, is a progressive non-atherosclerotic segmental inflammatory disease that most often affects small and medium-sized arteries, veins, and nerves of the upper and lower extremities.[219] The clinical and pathologic findings of this disease entity were published in 1908 by Leo Buerger in a description of 11 amputated limbs.[219] The typical age range for occurrence is 20 to 50 years old, and the disorder is more frequently found in males who smoke. The upper extremities may be involved, and a migratory superficial phlebitis may be present in up to 16% of patients, thus indicating a systemic inflammatory response. In young adults presenting to the Mayo Clinic (1953–1981) with lower limb ischemia, Buerger's disease was diagnosed in 24%.[219] Conversely, the diagnosis was made in 9% of patients with ischemic finger ulcerations. The cause of thromboangiitis obliterans is unknown; however, use of or exposure to tobacco is essential to both the diagnosis and progression of the disease.

Pathologically, thrombosis occurs in small to medium-sized arteries and veins with associated dense polymorphonuclear leukocyte aggregation, microabscesses, and multinucleated giant cells. The chronic phase of the disease shows a decrease in the hypercellularity and frequent recanalization of the vessel lumen. End-stage lesions demonstrate organized thrombus and blood vessel fibrosis. Although the disease is common in Asia, North American males do not appear to have any particular predisposition, as the diagnosis is made in less than 1% of patients with severe limb ischemia.

Buerger's disease typically presents in young male smokers, with symptoms beginning before age 40 years old. Patients initially present with foot, leg, arm, or hand claudication, which may be mistaken for joint or neuromuscular problems. Progression of the disease leads to calf claudication and eventually ischemic rest pain and ulcerations on the toes, feet, or fingers. A complete history should exclude diabetes, hyperlipidemia, or autoimmune disease as possible etiologies for the occlusive lesions. Because it is likely that multiple limbs are involved, angiography should be performed of all four limbs. Even if symptoms are not yet present in a limb, angiographic findings may be demonstrated. Characteristic angiographic findings show disease confinement to the distal circulation, usually infrapopliteal and distal to the brachial artery. The occlusions are segmental and show "skip" lesions with extensive collateralization, the so-called "corkscrew collaterals."

The treatment of thromboangiitis obliterans revolves around strict smoking cessation. In patients who are able to abstain, disease remission is impressive and amputation avoidance is increased. In the experience reported from the Oregon Health Sciences Center, no disease progression with associated tissue loss occurred after discontinuation of tobacco. The role of surgical intervention is minimal in Buerger's disease, as there is often no acceptable target vessel for bypass. Furthermore, autogenous vein conduits are limited secondary to coexisting migratory thrombophlebitis. Mills and associates reported their results of 31% limb loss in 26 patients over 15 years, thus authenticating the virulence of Buerger's disease involving the lower extremities.[219] In addition, others have described a significant discrepancy in limb loss in patients that continued to smoke vs. those who discontinued tobacco use (35 vs. 67%).

REFERENCES

Entries highlighted in bright blue are key references.

1. Hooi JD, Stoffers HE, Kester AD, et al: Peripheral arterial occlusive disease: Prognostic value of signs, symptoms, and the ankle-brachial pressure index. *Med Decis Making* 22:99, 2002.
2. Norgren L, Hiatt WR, Dormandy JA, et al: Inter-Society Consensus for the Management of Peripheral Arterial Disease (TASC II). *Eur J Vasc Endovasc Surg* 33:S1, 2007.
3. Jones DN, Rutherford RB: Peripheral vascular assessment and its role in predicting wound healing potential. *Clin Podiatr Med Surg* 8:909, 1991.
4. Favaretto E, Pili C, Amato A, et al: Analysis of agreement between Duplex ultrasound scanning and arteriography in patients with lower limb artery disease. *J Cardiovasc Med (Hagerstown)* 8:337, 2007.
5. Jakobs TF, Wintersperger BJ, Becker CR: MDCT-imaging of peripheral arterial disease. *Semin Ultrasound CT MR* 25:145, 2004.
6. Maintz D, Kugel H, Schellhammer F: In vitro evaluation of intravascular stent artifacts in three-dimensional MR angiography. *Invest Radiol* 36:218, 2001.
7. Eagle KA, Coley CM, Newell JB, et al: Combining clinical and thallium data optimizes preoperative assessment of cardiac risk before major vascular surgery. *Ann Intern Med* 110:859, 1989.
8. Hertzer NR, Beven EG, Young JR, et al: Coronary artery disease in peripheral vascular patients. A classification of 1000 coronary angiograms and results of surgical management. *Ann Surg* 199:223, 1984.
9. McFalls EO, Ward HB, Moritz TE, et al: Predictors and outcomes of a perioperative myocardial infarction following elective vascular surgery in patients with documented coronary artery disease: Results of the CARP trial. *Eur Heart J* 29:394, 2008.
10. Brady AR, Gibbs JS, Greenhalgh RM, et al: Perioperative beta-blockade (POBBLE) for patients undergoing infrarenal vascular surgery: Results of a randomized double-blind controlled trial. *J Vasc Surg* 41:602, 2005.
11. Daumerie G, Fleisher LA: Perioperative beta-blocker and statin therapy. *Curr Opin Anaesthesiol* 21:60, 2008.
12. Austin D, Pell JP, Oldroyd KG: Drug-eluting stents: A review of current evidence on clinical effectiveness and late complications. *Scott Med J* 53:16, 2008.
13. Parodi JC, Marin ML, Veith FJ: Transfemoral, endovascular stented graft repair of an abdominal aortic aneurysm. *Arch Surg* 130:549, 1995.

14. Criado FJ, Fairman RM, Becker GJ: Talent LPS AAA stent graft: Results of a pivotal clinical trial. *J Vasc Surg* 37:709, 2003.

15. Tanquilut EM, Ouriel K: Current outcomes in endovascular repair of abdominal aortic aneurysms. *J Cardiovasc Surg (Torino)* 44:503, 2003.

16. Zarins CK, White RA, Moll FL, et al: The AneuRx stent graft: Four-year results and worldwide experience 2000. *J Vasc Surg* 33:S135, 2001.

17. Donnan GA, Fisher M, Macleod M, et al: Stroke. *Lancet* 371:1612, 2008.

18. Chaer RA, DeRubertis B, Patel S, et al: Current management of extracranial carotid artery disease. *Rev Recent Clin Trials* 1:293, 2006.

19. Grant EG, Benson CB, Moneta GL, et al: Carotid artery stenosis: Grayscale and Doppler ultrasound diagnosis—Society of Radiologists in Ultrasound consensus conference. *Ultrasound Q* 19:190, 2003.

20. Wardlaw JM, Chappell FM, Stevenson M, et al: Accurate, practical and cost-effective assessment of carotid stenosis in the UK. *Health Technol Assess* 10:iii, 2006.

21. Saba L, Mallarini G: MDCTA of carotid plaque degree of stenosis: Evaluation of interobserver agreement. *AJR Am J Roentgenol* 190:W41, 2008.

22. Price TR, Psaty B, O'Leary D, et al: Assessment of cerebrovascular disease in the Cardiovascular Health Study. *Ann Epidemiol* 3:504, 1993.

23. Chen ZM, Sandercock P, Pan HC, et al: Indications for early aspirin use in acute ischemic stroke: A combined analysis of 40,000 randomized patients from the Chinese acute stroke trial and the international stroke trial. On behalf of the CAST and IST collaborative groups. *Stroke* 31:1240, 2000.

24. Kita MW: Carotid endarterectomy in symptomatic carotid stenosis: NASCET comparative results at 30 months of follow-up. *J Insur Med* 24:42, 1992.

25. Warlow CP: Symptomatic patients: The European Carotid Surgery Trial (ECST). *J Mal Vasc* 18:198, 1993.

26. Strandness DE, Eikelboom BC: Carotid artery stenosis—where do we go from here? *Eur J Ultrasound* 7:S17, 1998.

27. Rothwell PM, Eliasziw M, Gutnikov SA, et al: Analysis of pooled data from the randomised controlled trials of endarterectomy for symptomatic carotid stenosis. *Lancet* 361:107, 2003.

28. Topakian R, Strasak AM, Sonnberger M, et al: Timing of stenting of symptomatic carotid stenosis is predictive of 30-day outcome. *Eur J Neurol* 14:672, 2007.

29. Roederer GO, Langlois YE, Jager KA, et al: The natural history of carotid arterial disease in asymptomatic patients with cervical bruits. *Stroke* 15:605, 1984.

30. Fisher M, Martin A, Cosgrove M, et al: The NASCET-ACAS plaque project. North American Symptomatic Carotid Endarterectomy Trial. Asymptomatic Carotid Atherosclerosis Study. *Stroke* 24:I24; discussion I31, 1993.

31. Halliday A, Mansfield A, Marro J, et al: Prevention of disabling and fatal strokes by successful carotid endarterectomy in patients without recent neurological symptoms: Randomised controlled trial. *Lancet* 363:1491, 2004.

32. Coward LJ, Featherstone RL, Brown MM: Safety and efficacy of endovascular treatment of carotid artery stenosis compared with carotid endarterectomy: A Cochrane systematic review of the randomized evidence. *Stroke* 36:905, 2005.

33. Lin PH, Barshes NR, Annambhotla S, et al: Prospective randomized trials of carotid artery stenting versus carotid endarterectomy: An appraisal of the current literature. *Vasc Endovascular Surg* 42:5, 2008.

34. Crawford RS, Chung TK, Hodgman T, et al: Restenosis after eversion vs patch closure carotid endarterectomy. *J Vasc Surg* 46:41, 2007.

35. Organ N, Walker PJ, Jenkins J, et al: 15 year experience of carotid endarterectomy at the Royal Brisbane and Women's Hospital: Outcomes and changing trends in management. *Eur J Vasc Endovasc Surg* 35:273, 2008.

36. Zhou W, Felkai DD, Evans M, et al: Ultrasound criteria for severe in-stent restenosis following carotid artery stenting. *J Vasc Surg* 47:74, 2008.

37. Lin PH, Zhou W, Kougias P, et al: Factors associated with hypotension and bradycardia after carotid angioplasty and stenting. *J Vasc Surg* 46:846; discussion 853, 2007.

38. Plouin PF, Perdu J, La Batide-Alanore A, et al: Fibromuscular dysplasia. *Orphanet J Rare Dis* 2:28, 2007.

39. Zhou W, Lin PH, Bush RL, et al: Carotid artery aneurysm: Evolution of management over two decades. *J Vasc Surg* 43:493; discussion 497, 2006.

40. Athanasiou A, Liappis CD, Rapidis AD, et al: Carotid body tumor: Review of the literature and report of a case with a rare sensorineural symptomatology. *J Oral Maxillofac Surg* 65:1388, 2007.

41. Hoornweg LL, Storm-Versloot MN, Ubbink DT, et al: Meta analysis on mortality of ruptured abdominal aortic aneurysms. *Eur J Vasc Endovasc Surg* 35:558, 2008.

42. Dotter CT, Judkins MP, Rosch J: Transluminal angioplasty in arteriosclerotic obstruction of the lower extremities. *Med Times* 97:95, 1969.

43. Fleming C, Whitlock EP, Beil TL, et al: Screening for abdominal aortic aneurysm: A best-evidence systematic review for the U.S. Preventive Services Task Force. *Ann Intern Med* 142:203, 2005.

44. Lederle FA, Johnson GR, Wilson SE, et al: Yield of repeated screening for abdominal aortic aneurysm after a 4-year interval. Aneurysm Detection and Management Veterans Affairs Cooperative Study Investigators. *Arch Intern Med* 160:1117, 2000.

45. Ouriel K. Endovascular therapies: an update on aortic aneurysm repair and carotid endarterectomy. *J Am Coll Surg* 195:549, 2002.

46. Humphreys WV, Byrne J, James W: Elective abdominal aortic aneurysm operations—the results of a single surgeon series of 243 consecutive operations from a district general hospital. *Ann R Coll Surg Engl* 82:64, 2000.

47. Hausegger KA, Schedlbauer P, Deutschmann HA, et al: Complications in endoluminal repair of abdominal aortic aneurysms. *Eur J Radiol* 39:22, 2001.

48. Magennis R, Joekes E, Martin J, et al: Complications following endovascular abdominal aortic aneurysm repair. *Br J Radiol* 75:700, 2002.

49. Zarins CK, White RA, Fogarty TJ: Aneurysm rupture after endovascular repair using the AneuRx stent graft. *J Vasc Surg* 31:960, 2000.

50. Lin PH, Bush RL, Chaikof EL, et al: A prospective evaluation of hypogastric artery embolization in endovascular aortoiliac aneurysm repair. *J Vasc Surg* 36:500, 2002.

51. Bush RL, Lin PH, Reddy PP, et al: Epidural analgesia in patients with chronic obstructive pulmonary disease undergoing transperitoneal abdominal aortic aneurysmorraphy—a multi-institutional analysis. *Cardiovasc Surg* 11:179, 2003.

52. Greenhalgh RM, Brown LC, Kwong GP, et al: Comparison of endovascular aneurysm repair with open repair in patients with abdominal aortic aneurysm (EVAR trial 1), 30-day operative mortality results: Randomised controlled trial. *Lancet* 364:843, 2004.

53. Prinssen M, Verhoeven EL, Buth J, et al: A randomized trial comparing conventional and endovascular repair of abdominal aortic aneurysms. *N Engl J Med* 351:1607, 2004.

54. Matsumura JS, Brewster DC, Makaroun MS, et al: A multicenter controlled clinical trial of open versus endovascular treatment of abdominal aortic aneurysm. *J Vasc Surg* 37:262, 2003.

55. Greenberg RK, Chuter TA, Sternbergh WC 3rd, et al: Zenith AAA endovascular graft: Intermediate-term results of the US multicenter trial. *J Vasc Surg* 39:1209, 2004.

56. Zarins CK: The US AneuRx Clinical Trial: 6-year clinical update 2002. *J Vasc Surg* 37:904, 2003.

57. Criado FJ, Clark NS, McKendrick C, et al: Update on the Talent LPS AAA stent graft: Results with "enhanced talent." *Semin Vasc Surg* 16:158, 2003.

58. Bertges DJ, Zwolak RM, Deaton DH, et al: Current hospital costs and medicare reimbursement for endovascular abdominal aortic aneurysm repair. *J Vasc Surg* 37:272, 2003.

59. Seiwert AJ, Wolfe J, Whalen RC, et al: Cost comparison of aortic aneurysm endograft exclusion versus open surgical repair. *Am J Surg* 178:117, 1999.

60. Angle N, Dorafshar AH, Moore WS, et al: Open versus endovascular repair of abdominal aortic aneurysms: what does each really cost? *Ann Vasc Surg* 18:612, 2004.

61. Baum RA, Stavropoulos SW, Fairman RM, et al: Endoleaks after endovascular repair of abdominal aortic aneurysms. *J Vasc Interv Radiol* 14:1111, 2003.

62. Buth J, Harris PL, Van Marrewijk C, et al: Endoleaks during follow-up after endovascular repair of abdominal aortic aneurysm. Are they all dangerous? *J Cardiovasc Surg (Torino)* 44:559, 2003.

63. Dubenec SR, White GH, Pasenau J, et al: Endotension. A review of current views on pathophysiology and treatment. *J Cardiovasc Surg (Torino)* 44:553, 2003.

64. Lin PH, Bush RL, Katzman JB, et al: Delayed aortic aneurysm enlargement due to endotension after endovascular abdominal aortic aneurysm repair. *J Vasc Surg* 38:840, 2003.

65. Criado FJ, Wilson EP, Fairman RM, et al: Update on the Talent aortic stent-graft: A preliminary report from United States phase I and II trials. *J Vasc Surg* 33:S146, 2001.

66. Harris PL, Vallabhaneni SR, Desgranges P, et al: Incidence and risk factors of late rupture, conversion, and death after endovascular repair of infrarenal aortic aneurysms: The EUROSTAR experience. European Collaborators on Stent/graft techniques for aortic aneurysm repair. *J Vasc Surg* 32:739, 2000.

67. Krohg-Sorensen K, Brekke M, Drolsum A, et al: Periprosthetic leak and rupture after endovascular repair of abdominal aortic aneurysm: The significance of device design for long-term results. *J Vasc Surg* 29:1152, 1999.

68. May J, White GH, Yu W, et al: Endoluminal repair of abdominal aortic aneurysms: Strengths and weaknesses of various prostheses observed in a 4.5-year experience. *J Endovasc Surg* 4:147, 1997.

69. Kougias P, Lin PH, Dardik A, et al: Successful treatment of endotension and aneurysm sac enlargement with endovascular stent graft reinforcement. *J Vasc Surg* 46:124, 2007.

70. Teufelsbauer H, Prusa AM, Prager M, et al: Endovascular treatment of a multimorbid patient with late AAA rupture after stent-graft placement: 1-year follow-up. *J Endovasc Ther* 9:896, 2002.

71. Yasuhara H: Acute mesenteric ischemia: The challenge of gastroenterology. *Surg Today* 35:185, 2005.

72. Zelenock GB, Graham LM, Whitehouse WM Jr., et al: Splanchnic arteriosclerotic disease and intestinal angina. *Arch Surg* 115:497, 1980.

73. Karwowski J, Arko F: Surgical management of mesenteric ischemia. *Tech Vasc Interv Radiol* 7:151, 2004.

74. Moneta GL, Lee RW, Yeager RA, et al: Mesenteric duplex scanning: A blinded prospective study. *J Vasc Surg* 17:79; discussion 85, 1993.

75. Mitchell EL, Moneta GL: Mesenteric duplex scanning. *Perspect Vasc Surg Endovasc Ther* 18:175, 2006.

76. Kougias P, El Sayed HF, Zhou W, et al: Management of chronic mesenteric ischemia. The role of endovascular therapy. *J Endovasc Ther* 14:395, 2007.

77. Gloviczki P, Duncan AA: Treatment of celiac artery compression syndrome: Does it really exist? *Perspect Vasc Surg Endovasc Ther* 19:259, 2007.

78. Kougias P, Lau D, El Sayed HF, et al: Determinants of mortality and treatment outcome following surgical interventions for acute mesenteric ischemia. *J Vasc Surg* 46:467, 2007.

79. Park WM, Cherry KJ Jr., Chua HK, et al: Current results of open revascularization for chronic mesenteric ischemia: A standard for comparison. *J Vasc Surg* 35:853, 2002.

80. Silva JA, White CJ, Collins TJ, et al: Endovascular therapy for chronic mesenteric ischemia. *J Am Coll Cardiol* 47:944, 2006.

81. AbuRahma AF, Stone PA, Bates MC, et al: Angioplasty/stenting of the superior mesenteric artery and celiac trunk: Early and late outcomes. *J Endovasc Ther* 10:1046, 2003.

82. Furrer J, Gruntzig A, Kugelmeier J, et al: Treatment of abdominal angina with percutaneous dilatation of an arteria mesenterica superior stenosis. Preliminary communication. *Cardiovasc Intervent Radiol* 3:43, 1980.

83. Atkins MD, Kwolek CJ, LaMuraglia GM, et al: Surgical revascularization versus endovascular therapy for chronic mesenteric ischemia: A comparative experience. *J Vasc Surg* 45:1162, 2007.

84. Kasirajan K, O'Hara PJ, Gray BH, et al: Chronic mesenteric ischemia: Open surgery versus percutaneous angioplasty and stenting. *J Vasc Surg* 33:63, 2001.

85. Textor SC: Atherosclerotic renal artery stenosis: Overtreated but underrated? *J Am Soc Nephrol* 19:656, 2008.

86. Klassen PS, Svetkey LP: Diagnosis and management of renovascular hypertension. *Cardiol Rev* 8:17, 2000.

87. Chade AR, Rodriguez-Porcel M, Grande JP, et al: Distinct renal injury in early atherosclerosis and renovascular disease. *Circulation* 106:1165, 2002.

88. Vuong PN, Desoutter P, Mickley V, et al: Fibromuscular dysplasia of the renal artery responsible for renovascular hypertension: A histological presentation based on a series of 102 patients. *Vasa* 33:13, 2004.

89. Cherr GS, Hansen KJ, Craven TE, et al: Surgical management of atherosclerotic renovascular disease. *J Vasc Surg* 35:236, 2002.

90. Hansen KJ, Cherr GS, Craven TE, et al: Management of ischemic nephropathy: Dialysis-free survival after surgical repair. *J Vasc Surg* 32:472; discussion 481, 2000.

91. Guzman RP, Zierler RE, Isaacson JA, et al: Renal atrophy and arterial stenosis. A prospective study with duplex ultrasound. *Hypertension* 23:346, 1994.

92. van de Ven PJ, Kaatee R, Beutler JJ, et al: Arterial stenting and balloon angioplasty in ostial atherosclerotic renovascular disease: A randomised trial. *Lancet* 353:282, 1999.

93. Surowiec SM, Sivamurthy N, Rhodes JM, et al: Percutaneous therapy for renal artery fibromuscular dysplasia. *Ann Vasc Surg* 17:650, 2003.

94. van Jaarsveld BC, Krijnen P: Prospective studies of diagnosis and intervention: The Dutch experience. *Semin Nephrol* 20:463, 2000.

95. White CJ, Ramee SR, Collins TJ, et al: Renal artery stent placement: Utility in lesions difficult to treat with balloon angioplasty. *J Am Coll Cardiol* 30:1445, 1997.

96. Blum U, Krumme B, Flugel P, et al: Treatment of ostial renal-artery stenoses with vascular endoprostheses after unsuccessful balloon angioplasty. *N Engl J Med* 336:459, 1997.

97. Watson PS, Hadjipetrou P, Cox SV, et al: Effect of renal artery stenting on renal function and size in patients with atherosclerotic renovascular disease. *Circulation* 102:1671, 2000.

98. Harden PN, MacLeod MJ, Rodger RS, et al: Effect of renal-artery stenting on progression of renovascular renal failure. *Lancet* 349:1133, 1997.

99. Bush RL, Najibi S, MacDonald MJ, et al: Endovascular revascularization of renal artery stenosis: Technical and clinical results. *J Vasc Surg* 33:1041, 2001.

100. Dorros G, Jaff M, Mathiak L, et al: Four-year follow-up of Palmaz-Schatz stent revascularization as treatment for atherosclerotic renal artery stenosis. *Circulation* 98:642, 1998.

101. Henry M, Amor M, Henry I, et al: Stents in the treatment of renal artery stenosis: Long-term follow-up. *J Endovasc Surg* 6:42, 1999.

102. Iannone LA, Underwood PL, Nath A, et al: Effect of primary balloon expandable renal artery stents on long-term patency, renal function, and blood pressure in hypertensive and renal insufficient patients with renal artery stenosis. *Cathet Cardiovasc Diagn* 37:243, 1996.

103. Rundback JH, Gray RJ, Rozenblit G, et al: Renal artery stent placement for the management of ischemic nephropathy. *J Vasc Interv Radiol* 9:413, 1998.

104. Shannon HM, Gillespie IN, Moss JG: Salvage of the solitary kidney by insertion of a renal artery stent. *AJR Am J Roentgenol* 171:217, 1998.

105. Leertouwer TC, Gussenhoven EJ, Bosch JL, et al: Stent placement for renal arterial stenosis: Where do we stand? A meta-analysis. *Radiology* 216:78, 2000.

106. Dormandy JA, Rutherford RB: Management of peripheral arterial disease (PAD). TASC Working Group. TransAtlantic Inter-Society Consensus (TASC). *J Vasc Surg* 31:S1, 2000.

107. Ameli FM: Aortobifemoral bypass—an enduring operation. *Can J Surg* 35:237, 1992.

108. Martin D, Katz SG: Axillofemoral bypass for aortoiliac occlusive disease. *Am J Surg* 180:100, 2000.

109. Criado E, Burnham SJ, Tinsley EA Jr., et al: Femorofemoral bypass graft: Analysis of patency and factors influencing long-term outcome. *J Vasc Surg* 18:495; discussion 504, 1993.

110. Patel A, Taylor SM, Langan EM 3rd, et al: Obturator bypass: A classic approach for the treatment of contemporary groin infection. *Am Surg* 68:653; discussion 658, 2002.

111. Sautner T, Niederle B, Herbst F, et al: The value of obturator canal bypass. A review. *Arch Surg* 129:718, 1994.

112. Brewster DC, Cambria RP, Darling RC, et al: Long-term results of combined iliac balloon angioplasty and distal surgical revascularization. *Ann Surg* 210:324; discussion 331, 1989.

113. van den Akker PJ, van Schilfgaarde R, Brand R, et al: Long term success of aortoiliac operation for arteriosclerotic obstructive disease. *Surg Gynecol Obstet* 174:485, 1992.

114. Szilagyi DE, Elliott JP Jr., Smith RF, et al: A thirty-year survey of the reconstructive surgical treatment of aortoiliac occlusive disease. *J Vasc Surg* 3:421, 1986.

115. Sagic D, Grujicic S, Peric M, et al: "Kissing-balloon" technique for abdominal aorta angioplasty. Initial results and long term outcome. *Int Angiol* 14:364, 1995.

116. Insall RL, Loose HW, Chamberlain J: Long-term results of double-balloon percutaneous transluminal angioplasty of the aorta and iliac arteries. *Eur J Vasc Surg* 7:31, 1993.

117. Mendelsohn FO, Santos RM, Crowley JJ, et al: Kissing stents in the aortic bifurcation. *Am Heart J* 136:600, 1998.

118. Haulon S, Mounier-Vehier C, Gaxotte V, et al: Percutaneous reconstruction of the aortoiliac bifurcation with the "kissing stents" technique: Long-term follow-up in 106 patients. *J Endovasc Ther* 9:363, 2002.

119. Palmaz JC, Laborde JC, Rivera FJ, et al: Stenting of the iliac arteries with the Palmaz stent: Experience from a multicenter trial. *Cardiovasc Intervent Radiol* 15:291, 1992.

120. Sapoval MR, Long AL, Pagny JY, et al: Outcome of percutaneous intervention in iliac artery stents. *Radiology* 198:481, 1996.

121. Uberoi R, Tsetis D: Standards for the endovascular management of aortic occlusive disease. *Cardiovasc Intervent Radiol* 30:814, 2007.

122. Mousa AY, Beauford RB, Flores L, et al: Endovascular treatment of iliac occlusive disease: Review and update. *Vascular* 15:5, 2007.

123. Tetteroo E, van der Graaf Y, Bosch JL, et al: Randomised comparison of primary stent placement versus primary angioplasty followed by selective stent placement in patients with iliac-artery occlusive disease. Dutch Iliac Stent Trial Study Group. *Lancet* 351:1153, 1998.

124. Piffaretti G, Tozzi M, Lomazzi C, et al: Mid-term results of endovascular reconstruction for aorto-iliac obstructive disease. *Int Angiol* 26:18, 2007.

125. Bosiers M, Iyer V, Deloose K, et al: Flemish experience using the Advanta V12 stent-graft for the treatment of iliac artery occlusive disease. *J Cardiovasc Surg (Torino)* 48:7, 2007.

126. Harris RA, Hardman DT, Fisher C, et al: Aortic reconstructive surgery for limb ischaemia: Immediate and long-term follow-up to provide a standard for endovascular procedures. *Cardiovasc Surg* 6:256, 1998.

127. Becker GJ, Cikrit DF, Lalka SG, et al: Early experience with the Palmaz stent in human iliac angioplasty. *Indiana Med* 82:286, 1989.

128. Tsetis D, Uberoi R: Quality improvement guidelines for endovascular treatment of iliac artery occlusive disease. *Cardiovasc Intervent Radiol* 31:238, 2008.

129. Powell RJ, Fillinger M, Bettmann M, et al: The durability of endovascular treatment of multisegment iliac occlusive disease. *J Vasc Surg* 31:1178, 2000.

130. Timaran CH, Stevens SL, Grandas OH, et al: Influence of hormone replacement therapy on the outcome of iliac angioplasty and stenting. *J Vasc Surg* 33:S85, 2001.

131. Bosch JL, Hunink MG: Meta-analysis of the results of percutaneous transluminal angioplasty and stent placement for aortoiliac occlusive disease. *Radiology* 204:87, 1997.

132. Park KB, Do YS, Kim JH, et al: Stent placement for chronic iliac arterial occlusive disease: The results of 10 years experience in a single institution. *Korean J Radiol* 6:256, 2005.

133. Leville CD, Kashyap VS, Clair DG, et al: Endovascular management of iliac artery occlusions: Extending treatment to TransAtlantic Inter-Society Consensus class C and D patients. *J Vasc Surg* 43:32, 2006.

134. McDaniel MD, Cronenwett JL: Basic data related to the natural history of intermittent claudication. *Ann Vasc Surg* 3:273, 1989.

135. Leng GC, Papacosta O, Whincup P, et al: Femoral atherosclerosis in an older British population: Prevalence and risk factors. *Atherosclerosis* 152:167, 2000.

136. Schroll M, Munck O: Estimation of peripheral arteriosclerotic disease by ankle blood pressure measurements in a population study of 60-year-old men and women. *J Chronic Dis* 34:261, 1981.

137. Stoffers HE, Rinkens PE, Kester AD, et al: The prevalence of asymptomatic and unrecognized peripheral arterial occlusive disease. *Int J Epidemiol* 25:282, 1996.

138. Ouriel K: Peripheral arterial disease. *Lancet* 358:1257, 2001.

139. Koelemay MJ, den Hartog D, Prins MH, et al: Diagnosis of arterial disease of the lower extremities with duplex ultrasonography. *Br J Surg* 83:404, 1996.

140. Eiberg JP, Hansen MA, Jensen F, et al: Ultrasound contrast-agent improves imaging of lower limb occlusive disease. *Eur J Vasc Endovasc Surg* 25:23, 2003.

141. Nehler MR, McDermott MM, Treat-Jacobson D, et al: Functional outcomes and quality of life in peripheral arterial disease: Current status. *Vasc Med* 8:115, 2003.

142. Ouriel K: The use of glycoprotein IIb/IIIa antagonists in peripheral arterial occlusion. *Tech Vasc Interv Radiol* 4:107, 2001.

143. Ouriel K: Current status of thrombolysis for peripheral arterial occlusive disease. *Ann Vasc Surg* 16:797, 2002.

144. Lin PH, Barshes NR, Annambhotla S, et al: Advances in endovascular interventions for deep vein thrombosis. *Expert Rev Med Devices* 5:153, 2008.

145. Lin PH, Zhou W, Dardik A, et al: Catheter-direct thrombolysis versus pharmacomechanical thrombectomy for treatment of symptomatic lower extremity deep venous thrombosis. *Am J Surg* 192:782, 2006.

146. Ouriel K: Comparison of surgical and thrombolytic treatment of peripheral arterial disease. *Rev Cardiovasc Med* 3:S7, 2002.

147. Conte MS, Belkin M, Upchurch GR, et al: Impact of increasing comorbidity on infrainguinal reconstruction: A 20-year perspective. *Ann Surg* 233:445, 2001.

148. Hunink MG, Donaldson MC, Meyerovitz MF, et al: Risks and benefits of femoropopliteal percutaneous balloon angioplasty. *J Vasc Surg* 17:183; discussion 192, 1993.

149. Johnston KW: Femoral and popliteal arteries: Reanalysis of results of balloon angioplasty. *Radiology* 183:767, 1992.

150. Hunink MG, Wong JB, Donaldson MC, et al: Patency results of percutaneous and surgical revascularization for femoropopliteal arterial disease. *Med Decis Making* 14:71, 1994.

151. Lofberg AM, Karacagil S, Ljungman C, et al: Percutaneous transluminal angioplasty of the femoropopliteal arteries in limbs with chronic critical lower limb ischemia. *J Vasc Surg* 34:114, 2001.

152. Varty K, Bolia A, Naylor AR, et al: Infrapopliteal percutaneous transluminal angioplasty: A safe and successful procedure. *Eur J Vasc Endovasc Surg* 9:341, 1995.

153. Bolia A, Sayers RD, Thompson MM, et al: Subintimal and intraluminal recanalisation of occluded crural arteries by percutaneous balloon angioplasty. *Eur J Vasc Surg* 8:214, 1994.

154. London NJ, Srinivasan R, Naylor AR, et al: Subintimal angioplasty of femoropopliteal artery occlusions: The long-term results. *Eur J Vasc Surg* 8:148, 1994.

155. Lipsitz EC, Ohki T, Veith FJ, et al: Does subintimal angioplasty have a role in the treatment of severe lower extremity ischemia? *J Vasc Surg* 37:386, 2003.

156. Treiman GS, Whiting JH, Treiman RL, et al: Treatment of limb-threatening ischemia with percutaneous intentional extraluminal recanalization: A preliminary evaluation. *J Vasc Surg* 38:29, 2003.

157. Ingle H, Nasim A, Bolia A, et al: Subintimal angioplasty of isolated infragenicular vessels in lower limb ischemia: Long-term results. *J Endovasc Ther* 9:411, 2002.

158. Becquemin JP, Favre JP, Marzelle J, et al: Systematic versus selective stent placement after superficial femoral artery balloon angioplasty: A multicenter prospective randomized study. *J Vasc Surg* 37:487, 2003.

159. Gray BH, Sullivan TM, Childs MB, et al: High incidence of restenosis/reocclusion of stents in the percutaneous treatment of long-segment superficial femoral artery disease after suboptimal angioplasty. *J Vasc Surg* 25:74, 1997.

160. Mewissen MW: Self-expanding nitinol stents in the femoropopliteal segment: Technique and mid-term results. *Tech Vasc Interv Radiol* 7:2, 2004.

161. Laird JR: Interventional options in SFA. *Endovascular Today* 9, 2004.

162. Ansel GM, Silver MJ, Botti CF Jr., et al: Functional and clinical outcomes of nitinol stenting with and without abciximab for complex superficial femoral artery disease: A randomized trial. *Catheter Cardiovasc Interv* 67:288, 2006.

163. Duda SH, Poerner TC, Wiesinger B, et al: Drug-eluting stents: Potential applications for peripheral arterial occlusive disease. *J Vasc Interv Radiol* 14:291, 2003.

164. Bauermeister G: Endovascular stent-grafting in the treatment of superficial femoral artery occlusive disease. *J Endovasc Ther* 8:315, 2001.

165. Kedora J, Hohmann S, Garrett W, et al: Randomized comparison of percutaneous Viabahn stent grafts vs prosthetic femoral-popliteal bypass in the treatment of superficial femoral arterial occlusive disease. *J Vasc Surg* 45:10; discussion 16, 2007.

166. Ramaiah V, Gammon R, Kiesz S, et al: Midterm outcomes from the TALON Registry: Treating peripherals with SilverHawk: Outcomes collection. *J Endovasc Ther* 13:592, 2006.

167. Laird JR Jr., Reiser C, Biamino G, et al: Excimer laser assisted angioplasty for the treatment of critical limb ischemia. *J Cardiovasc Surg (Torino)* 45:239, 2004.

168. Scheinert D, Laird JR Jr., Schroder M, et al: Excimer laser-assisted recanalization of long, chronic superficial femoral artery occlusions. *J Endovasc Ther* 8:156, 2001.

169. Steinkamp HJ, Rademaker J, Wissgott C, et al: Percutaneous transluminal laser angioplasty versus balloon dilation for treatment of popliteal artery occlusions. *J Endovasc Ther* 9:882, 2002.

170. Clark TW, Groffsky JL, Soulen MC: Predictors of long-term patency after femoropopliteal angioplasty: Results from the STAR registry. *J Vasc Interv Radiol* 12:923, 2001.

171. Axisa B, Fishwick G, Bolia A, et al: Complications following peripheral angioplasty. *Ann R Coll Surg Engl* 84:39, 2002.

172. Yilmaz S, Sindel T, Yegin A, et al: Subintimal angioplasty of long superficial femoral artery occlusions. *J Vasc Interv Radiol* 14:997, 2003.

173. Desgranges P, Boufi M, Lapeyre M, et al: Subintimal angioplasty: Feasible and durable. *Eur J Vasc Endovasc Surg* 28:138, 2004.

174. Fava M, Loyola S, Polydorou A, et al: Cryoplasty for femoropopliteal arterial disease: Late angiographic results of initial human experience. *J Vasc Interv Radiol* 15:1239, 2004.

175. Jahnke T, Andresen R, Muller-Hulsbeck S, et al: Hemobahn stent-grafts for treatment of femoropopliteal arterial obstructions: Midterm results of a prospective trial. *J Vasc Interv Radiol* 14:41, 2003.

176. Grubnic S, Heenan SD, Buckenham TM, et al: Evaluation of the pullback atherectomy catheter in the treatment of lower limb vascular disease. *Cardiovasc Intervent Radiol* 19:152, 1996.

177. Savader SJ, Venbrux AC, Mitchell SE, et al: Percutaneous transluminal atherectomy of the superficial femoral and popliteal arteries: Long-term results in 48 patients. *Cardiovasc Intervent Radiol* 17:312, 1994.

178. Albers M, Battistella VM, Romiti M, et al: Meta-analysis of polytetrafluoroethylene bypass grafts to infrapopliteal arteries. *J Vasc Surg* 37:1263, 2003.

179. Hamsho A, Nott D, Harris PL: Prospective randomised trial of distal arteriovenous fistula as an adjunct to femoro-infrapopliteal PTFE bypass. *Eur J Vasc Endovasc Surg* 17:197, 1999.

180. Davies AH, Hawdon AJ, Sydes MR, et al: Is duplex surveillance of value after leg vein bypass grafting? Principal results of the Vein Graft Surveillance Randomised Trial (VGST). *Circulation* 112:1985, 2005.

181. Baldwin ZK, Pearce BJ, Curi MA, et al: Limb salvage after infrainguinal bypass graft failure. *J Vasc Surg* 39:951, 2004.

182. Stone PA, Flaherty SK, Aburahma AF, et al: Factors affecting perioperative mortality and wound-related complications following major lower extremity amputations. *Ann Vasc Surg* 20:209, 2006.

183. Holzenbein TJ, Pomposelli FB Jr., Miller A, et al: The upper arm basilic-cephalic loop for distal bypass grafting: Technical considerations and follow-up. *J Vasc Surg* 21:586; discussion 592, 1995.

184. Dosluoglu HH, Kittredge J, Cherr GS: Use of cryopreserved femoral vein for in situ replacement of infected femorofemoral prosthetic artery bypass. *Vasc Endovascular Surg* 42:74, 2008.

185. Dardik H, Wengerter K, Qin F, et al: Comparative decades of experience with glutaraldehyde-tanned human umbilical cord vein graft for lower limb revascularization: An analysis of 1275 cases. *J Vasc Surg* 35:64, 2002.

186. Johnson WC, Lee KK: A comparative evaluation of polytetrafluoroethylene, umbilical vein, and saphenous vein bypass grafts for femoral-popliteal above-knee revascularization: A prospective randomized Department of Veterans Affairs cooperative study. *J Vasc Surg* 32:268, 2000.

187. Fahner PJ, Idu MM, van Gulik TM, et al: Systematic review of preservation methods and clinical outcome of infrainguinal vascular allografts. *J Vasc Surg* 44:518, 2006.

188. Gupta SK, Veith FJ, Kram HB, et al: Prospective, randomized comparison of ringed and nonringed polytetrafluoroethylene femoropopliteal bypass grafts: A preliminary report. *J Vasc Surg* 13:163, 1991.

189. Stonebridge PA, Prescott RJ, Ruckley CV: Randomized trial comparing infrainguinal polytetrafluoroethylene bypass grafting with and without vein interposition cuff at the distal anastomosis. The Joint Vascular Research Group. *J Vasc Surg* 26:543, 1997.

190. Klinkert P, van Dijk PJ, Breslau PJ: Polytetrafluoroethylene femorotibial bypass grafting: 5-year patency and limb salvage. *Ann Vasc Surg* 17:486, 2003.

191. Panneton JM, Hollier LH, Hofer JM: Multicenter randomized prospective trial comparing a pre-cuffed polytetrafluoroethylene graft to a vein cuffed polytetrafluoroethylene graft for infragenicular arterial bypass. *Ann Vasc Surg* 18:199, 2004.

192. Bellosta R, Luzzani L, Carugati C, et al: Which distal anastomosis should be used in PTFE femoro-tibial bypass? *J Cardiovasc Surg (Torino)* 46:499, 2005.

193. Begovac PC, Thomson RC, Fisher JL, et al: Improvements in GORE-TEX vascular graft performance by Carmeda BioActive surface heparin immobilization. *Eur J Vasc Endovasc Surg* 25:432, 2003.

194. Devine C, Hons B, McCollum C: Heparin-bonded Dacron or polytetrafluoroethylene for femoropopliteal bypass grafting: A multicenter trial. *J Vasc Surg* 33:533, 2001.

195. Walluscheck KP, Bierkandt S, Brandt M, et al: Infrainguinal ePTFE vascular graft with bioactive surface heparin bonding. First clinical results. *J Cardiovasc Surg (Torino)* 46:425, 2005.

196. Duda SH, Bosiers M, Lammer J, et al: Drug-eluting and bare nitinol stents for the treatment of atherosclerotic lesions in the superficial femoral artery: Long-term results from the SIROCCO trial. *J Endovasc Ther* 13:701, 2006.

197. Ferreira M, Lanziotti L, Monteiro M, et al: Superficial femoral artery recanalization with self-expanding nitinol stents: Long-term follow-up results. *Eur J Vasc Endovasc Surg* 34:702, 2007.

198. Schillinger M, Sabeti S, Dick P, et al: Sustained benefit at 2 years of primary femoropopliteal stenting compared with balloon angioplasty with optional stenting. *Circulation* 115:2745, 2007.

199. Bosiers M, Deloose K, Verbist J, et al: Nitinol stenting for treatment of "below-the-knee" critical limb ischemia: 1-year angiographic outcome after Xpert stent implantation. *J Cardiovasc Surg (Torino)* 48:455, 2007.

200. Kickuth R, Keo HH, Triller J, et al: Initial clinical experience with the 4-F self-expanding XPERT stent system for infrapopliteal treatment of patients with severe claudication and critical limb ischemia. *J Vasc Interv Radiol* 18:703, 2007.

201. Wolf GL, Wilson SE, Cross AP, et al: Surgery or balloon angioplasty for peripheral vascular disease: A randomized clinical trial. Principal investigators and their Associates of Veterans Administration Cooperative Study Number 199. *J Vasc Interv Radiol* 4:639, 1993.

202. Adam DJ, Beard JD, Cleveland T, et al: Bypass versus angioplasty in severe ischaemia of the leg (BASIL): Multicentre, randomised controlled trial. *Lancet* 366:1925, 2005.

203. Nolan B, Finlayson S, Tosteson A, et al: The treatment of disabling intermittent claudication in patients with superficial femoral artery occlusive disease—decision analysis. *J Vasc Surg* 45:1179, 2007.

204. Maffei S, Di Renzo M, Bova G, et al: Takayasu's arteritis: A review of the literature. *Intern Emerg Med* 1:105, 2006.

205. Davies JE, Sundt TM: Surgery insight: The dilated ascending aorta—indications for surgical intervention. *Nat Clin Pract Cardiovasc Med* 4:330, 2007.

206. Chassaing N, Martin L, Calvas P, et al: Pseudoxanthoma elasticum: A clinical, pathophysiological and genetic update including 11 novel ABCC6 mutations. *J Med Genet* 42:881, 2005.

207. Yeung RS: Pathogenesis and treatment of Kawasaki's disease. *Curr Opin Rheumatol* 17:617, 2005.

208. Baxter BT: Heritable diseases of the blood vessels. *Cardiovasc Pathol* 14:185, 2005.

209. Cikrit DF, Glover JR, Dalsing MC, et al: The Ehlers-Danlos specter revisited. *Vasc Endovascular Surg* 36:213, 2002.

210. Ho NC, Tran JR, Bektas A: Marfan's syndrome. *Lancet* 366:1978, 2005.

211. Herrick AL: Pathogenesis of Raynaud's phenomenon. *Rheumatology (Oxford)* 44:587, 2005.

212. Krause I, Weinberger A: Behcet's disease. *Curr Opin Rheumatol* 20:82, 2008.

213. Das CJ, Neyaz Z, Thapa P, et al: Fibromuscular dysplasia of the renal arteries: A radiological review. *Int Urol Nephrol* 39:233, 2007.

214. di Marzo L, Cavallaro A: Popliteal vascular entrapment. *World J Surg* 29:S43, 2005.

215. Pettigrew HD, Teuber SS, Gershwin ME: Polyarteritis nodosa. *Compr Ther* 33:144, 2007.

216. Stoyneva Z, Lyapina M, Tzvetkov D, et al: Current pathophysiological views on vibration-induced Raynaud's phenomenon. *Cardiovasc Res* 57:615, 2003.

217. Gray BH: Intervention for renal artery stenosis: endovascular and surgical roles. *J Hypertens Suppl* 23:S23, 2005.

218. Pannone A, Di Cesare F, Bartolucci R, et al: Cystic adventitial disease of the popliteal artery. A case report and review of the literature. *Chir Ital* 60:153, 2008.

219. Paraskevas KI, Liapis CD, Briana DD, et al: Thromboangiitis obliterans (Buerger's disease): Searching for a therapeutic strategy. *Angiology* 58:75, 2007.

Venous and Lymphatic Disease

Timothy K. Liem and Gregory L. Moneta

VENOUS ANATOMY

Veins are part of a dynamic and complex system that returns venous blood to the heart against the force of gravity in an upright individual. Venous blood flow is dependent on multiple factors such as gravity, venous valves, the cardiac and respiratory cycles, blood volume, and the calf muscle pump. Alterations in the intricate balance of these factors can result in venous pathology.

Structure of Veins

Veins are thin-walled, highly distensible, and collapsible structures. Their structure specifically supports their two primary functions of transporting blood toward the heart and serving as a reservoir to prevent intravascular volume overload. The venous intima is composed of a nonthrombogenic endothelium with an underlying basement membrane and an elastic lamina. The endothelium produces endothelium-derived relaxing factor and prostacyclin, which help maintain a nonthrombogenic surface through inhibition of platelet aggregation and promotion of platelet disaggregation.[1] Circumferential rings of elastic tissue and smooth muscle located in the media of the vein allow for changes in vein caliber with minimal changes in venous pressure. When an individual is upright and standing still, the veins are maximally distended and their diameter may be several times greater than that in the supine position.

Unidirectional blood flow is achieved with multiple venous valves. The number of valves is greatest below the knee and fewest in the more proximal veins. Each valve is made of two thin cusps consisting of a fine connective tissue skeleton covered by endothelium. Venous valves close in response to cephalad-to-caudal blood flow at a velocity of at least 30 cm/s.[2] The inferior vena cava (IVC), common iliac veins, portal venous system, and cranial sinuses are valveless.

Lower Extremity Veins

The nomenclature relating to venous anatomy recently has been revised. Lower extremity veins are divided into superficial, deep, and perforating veins. The superficial venous system lies above the uppermost fascial layer of the leg and thigh, and consists of the great saphenous vein (GSV) and small saphenous vein (SSV) and their tributaries. The GSV originates from the dorsal pedal venous arch and courses cephalad, anterior to the medial malleolus, entering the common femoral vein approximately 4 cm inferior and lateral to the pubic tubercle. The saphenous nerve accompanies the GSV medially and supplies cutaneous sensation to the medial leg and ankle. The SSV originates laterally from the dorsal pedal venous arch and courses cephalad in the posterior calf. Most often, it penetrates the popliteal fossa, between the medial and lateral heads of the gastrocnemius muscle, to join the popliteal vein. The termination of the SSV may be quite variable, however, with a proximal extension of the SSV (the vein of Giacomini) frequently connecting

with the deep femoral vein or GSV. The sural nerve accompanies the SSV laterally along its course and supplies cutaneous sensation to the lateral malleolar region.

The deep veins follow the course of major arteries in the extremities. In the lower leg, paired veins parallel the course of the anterior tibial, posterior tibial, and peroneal arteries, and join behind the knee to form the popliteal vein. Venous bridges connect the paired veins in the lower leg. The popliteal vein continues through the adductor hiatus to become the femoral vein. In the proximal thigh, the femoral vein joins with the deep femoral vein to form the common femoral vein, becoming the external iliac vein at the inguinal ligament.

Multiple perforator veins traverse the deep fascia to connect the superficial and deep venous systems. Clinically important perforator veins are the Cockett and Boyd perforators. The Cockett perforator veins drain the medial lower leg and are relatively constant. They connect the posterior arch vein (a tributary to the GSV) and the posterior tibial vein. They may become varicose or incompetent in venous insufficiency states. The Boyd perforator veins connect the GSV to the deep veins approximately 10 cm below the knee and 1 to 2 cm medial to the tibia.

Venous sinuses are thin-walled, large veins located within the substance of the soleus and gastrocnemius muscles. These sinuses are valveless and are linked by valved, small venous channels that prevent reflux. A large amount of blood can be stored in the venous sinuses. With each contraction of the calf muscle bed, blood is pumped out through the venous channels into the main conduit veins to return to the heart.

Upper Extremity Veins

As in the lower extremity, there are deep and superficial veins in the upper extremity. Deep veins of the upper extremity are paired and follow the named arteries in the arm. Superficial veins of the upper extremity are the cephalic and basilic veins and their tributaries. The cephalic vein originates at the lateral wrist and courses over the ventral surface of the forearm. In the upper arm, the cephalic vein terminates in the infraclavicular fossa, piercing the clavipectoral fascia to empty into the axillary vein. The basilic vein runs medially

KEY POINTS

1. Deep vein thrombosis (DVT) and pulmonary embolism are frequent complications after major abdominal and orthopedic procedures. The risk is further increased in patients with malignancy and a history of venous thromboembolism. Options for DVT prophylaxis include intermittent pneumatic compression, use of graduated compression stockings, and administration of low-dose unfractionated heparin, low molecular weight heparin, fondaparinux, and vitamin K antagonists. However, prophylaxis should be stratified based on the patient's level of risk.

2. In patients with established DVT, unfractionated heparin, low molecular weight heparin, and fondaparinux are options for *initial* antithrombotic therapy. The duration and type of *long-term* anticoagulation should be stratified based on the provoked or unprovoked nature of the DVT, the location of the DVT, previous occurrence of DVT, and presence of concomitant malignancy.

3. Thrombolytic therapy, surgical thrombectomy, and placement of inferior vena cava filters are adjunc-

tive treatments that may be indicated in patients with extensive and complicated venous thromboembolism.

4. Saphenous vein stripping, endovenous laser treatment, and radiofrequency ablation are effective therapies for patients with saphenous vein valvular insufficiency. Concomitant varicose veins may be managed with compression therapy, sclerotherapy (for smaller varices), and phlebectomy.

5. The mainstay of treatment for chronic venous insufficiency is compression therapy. Sclerotherapy, perforator vein ligation, and venous reconstruction may be indicated in patients in whom conservative management fails.

6. Lymphedema is categorized as primary (with early or delayed onset) or secondary. The goals of treatment are to minimize edema and prevent infection. Lymphatic massage, sequential pneumatic compression, use of compression garments, and limb elevation are effective forms of therapy.

along the forearm and penetrates the deep fascia as it courses past the elbow in the upper arm. It then joins with the deep brachial veins to become the axillary vein. The median cubital vein joins the cephalic and the basilic veins on the ventral surface of the elbow.

The axillary vein becomes the subclavian vein at the lateral border of the first rib. At the medial border of the scalenus anterior muscle, the subclavian vein joins with the internal jugular vein to become the brachiocephalic vein, with the subclavian vein coursing anterior to the scalenus anterior muscle. The left and right brachiocephalic veins join to become the superior vena cava, which empties into the right atrium.

EVALUATION OF THE VENOUS SYSTEM

Clinical Evaluation

The evaluation of the venous system begins with a detailed history and physical examination. Risk factors for acute and chronic venous disease are identified. They include increased age, history of venous thromboembolism (VTE), malignancy, trauma and spinal cord injury, hospitalization and immobilization, obesity, nephrotic syndrome, pregnancy and the recently postpartum state, oral contraceptive use or hormone replacement therapy, varicose veins, and hypercoagulable states, as well as the postoperative state. Venous pathology is often, but not always, associated with visible or palpable signs that can be identified during the physical examination. There is variation among individuals in the prominence of superficial veins when the person is standing. The superficial veins of a lean athletic person, even when normal, will appear large and easily visualized, but these veins will be far less obvious in the obese individual. Possible signs of superficial venous abnormalities are listed in Table 24-1. The deep veins cannot be directly assessed clinically, and abnormalities within them can only be inferred indirectly from changes found on clinical examination.

Chronic venous insufficiency (CVI) may lead to characteristic changes in the skin and subcutaneous tissues in the affected limb. CVI results from incompetence of venous valves, venous obstruction, or both. Most CVI involves venous reflux, and severe CVI often reflects a combination of reflux and venous obstruction. It is important to remember that although CVI originates with abnormalities of the veins, the target organ of CVI is the skin. A typical leg affected by CVI will be edematous, with edema increasing over the course of the day (Fig. 24-1). The leg may also be indurated and pigmented with eczema and dermatitis. These changes are due to excessive proteinaceous capillary exudate and deposition of a pericapillary fibrin cuff that may limit nutritional exchange. In addition, an increase in white blood cell trapping within the skin microcirculation in CVI patients may lead to microvascular congestion and thrombosis. Subsequently, white blood cells may migrate into the interstitium and release necrotizing lysosomal enzymes, which results in tissue destruction and eventual ulceration.

Fibrosis occurs from impaired nutrition, chronic inflammation, and fat necrosis (lipodermatosclerosis). Hemosiderin deposition due to the exudation of red cells and subsequent lysis in the skin causes the characteristic pigmentation of chronic venous disease (Fig. 24-2). Ulceration can develop with longstanding venous hypertension and is associated with alterations in microcirculatory

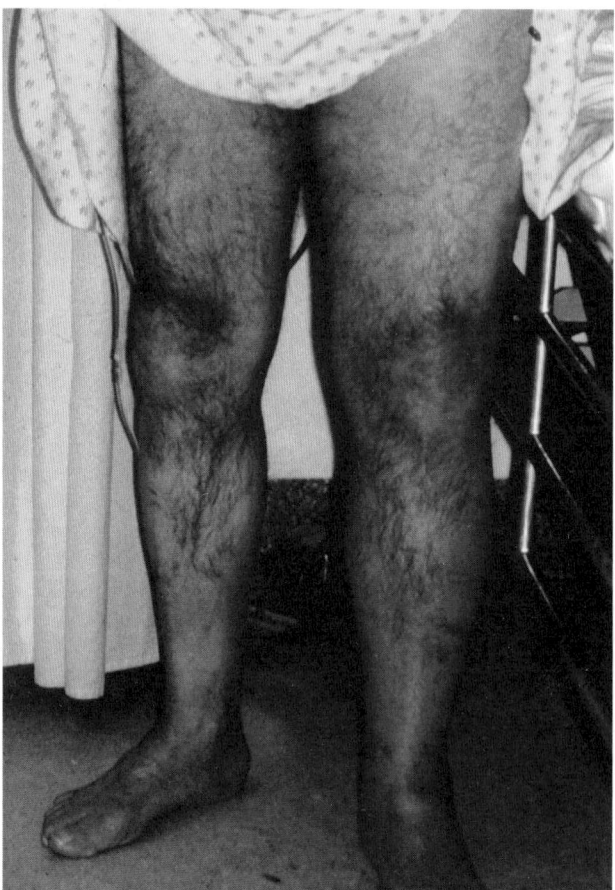

FIG. 24-1. Edematous left leg of a patient with chronic venous insufficiency.

and cutaneous lymphatic anatomy and function. The most common location of venous ulceration is approximately 3 cm proximal to the medial malleolus (Fig. 24-3).

Trendelenburg's test is a clinical test that can help determine whether incompetent valves are present and in which of the three venous systems (superficial, deep, or perforator) the valves are abnormal. There are two components to this test. First, with the patient supine, the leg is elevated 45 degrees to empty the veins, and the GSV is occluded with the examiner's hand or with a rubber tourniquet. With the GSV still occluded, the patient stands and the superficial veins are observed for blood filling. Then compression on the GSV is released and the superficial veins are observed for increased filling with blood. A negative result, indicating no clinically evident venous reflux, is the gradual filling of the veins from arterial inflow. A positive result is the sudden filling of veins with standing in the first part of the test or with release of GSV compression in the second part of the test. The perforator veins are thought to be normal with competent valves if the result of the first component of the test is negative. If the result of this part of the test is positive, there are theoretically incompetent valves in both the deep and perforator veins. The GSV valves are competent if the second component of the test gives a negative result, and the GSV valves are incompetent if the second component of the test yields a positive result. Interpretation of the findings of Trendelenburg's test is obviously subjective. The test has therefore been largely supplanted by the more objective noninvasive vascular laboratory tests to localize sites of venous reflux.

Noninvasive Evaluation

Before the development of vascular ultrasound, noninvasive techniques to evaluate the venous system were based on plethysmographic techniques. Although a variety of plethysmographic techniques are

TABLE 24-1	Possible signs of superficial venous abnormalities

Tortuosity
Varicosity
Venous saccule
Distended subdermal venules (corona phlebectatica)
Distended intradermal venules (spider angiomata)
Warmth, erythema, tenderness (superficial thrombophlebitis)

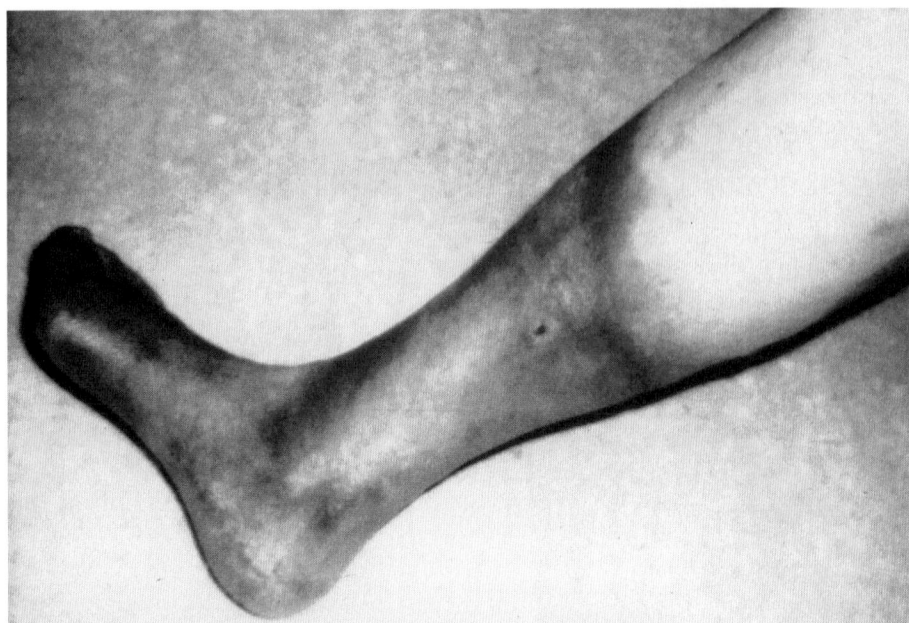

FIG. 24-2. Characteristic hyperpigmentation of chronic venous insufficiency.

used in the evaluation of both acute and chronic venous disease, they are all based on the detection of volume changes in the limb in response to blood flow.

Duplex ultrasonography (DUS) augmented by color flow imaging is now the most important noninvasive diagnostic method in the evaluation of the venous system. DUS has become standard for the detection of infrainguinal deep vein thrombosis (DVT), with near 100% sensitivity and specificity in symptomatic patients.[3] It is also the preferred method of evaluation for upper extremity venous thrombosis and is useful in the evaluation of CVI by documenting the presence of valvular reflux and venous obstruction.

Invasive Evaluation

With the improved accuracy of noninvasive techniques for diagnostic purposes, the use of invasive procedures has become more selective. Venography is now primarily used as an adjunct to percutaneous or operative treatment of venous disorders. Because the pelvic veins often cannot be visualized with DUS because of overlying bowel gas or body habitus, venography is often used to evaluate iliofemoral vein thrombosis in preparation for endovascular treatment or open surgical treatment.

Venography is performed by direct venipuncture with injection of contrast material. As with any invasive procedure, there are inherent risks associated with venography. Local effects include pain and local thrombosis at the puncture site and possible formation of a hematoma if larger veins are used for access. Pain is significantly lower with nonionic low-osmolality contrast media than with conventional contrast agents (with 18% vs. 44% of patients experiencing discomfort, respectively).[4] Systemic effects of iodinated contrast media include allergic reaction and risk of renal failure. Postvenography venous

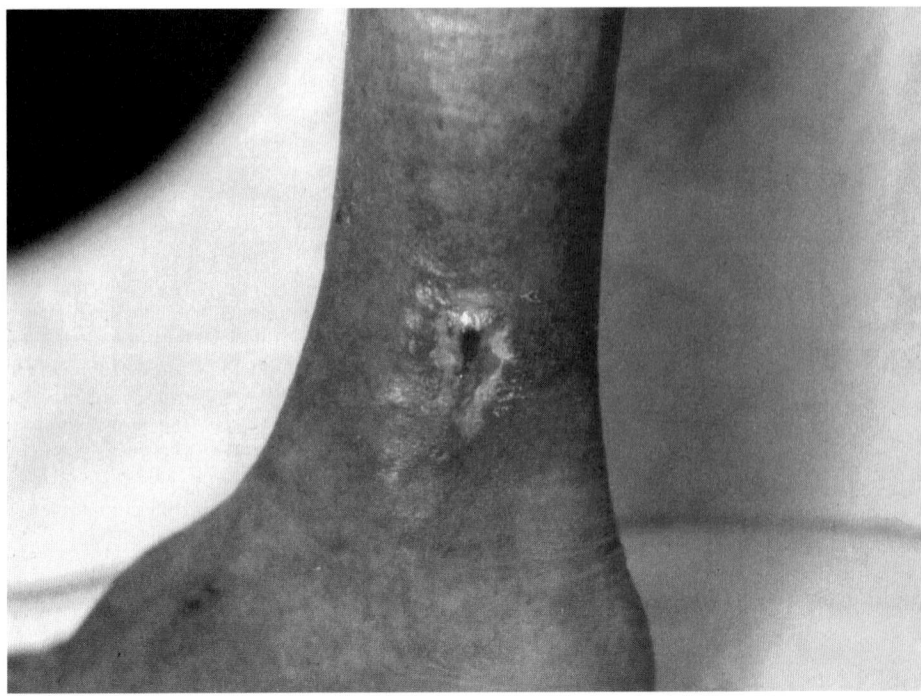

FIG. 24-3. Venous ulceration located proximal to the medial malleolus.

thrombosis occurs distal to the puncture site in 1 to 9% of patients undergoing venography and results from vein intimal damage from the IV contrast agent.[4]

VENOUS THROMBOEMBOLISM

Epidemiology

Despite increased awareness and use of prophylactic modalities, DVT and pulmonary embolism (PE) remain important preventable sources of morbidity and mortality. The incidence of DVT ranges between 5 and 9 per 10,000 person-years in the general population, and the incidence of VTE (DVT and PE combined) is approximately 14 per 10,000 person-years.[5,6] The resultant number of new cases of VTE may be over 275,000 per year in the United States.[7] Not only does VTE pose an immediate threat to life, it also can cause long-term impairment due to resultant venous insufficiency. The 20-year cumulative incidence rates are 26.8 and 3.7% for the development of venous stasis changes and venous ulcers, respectively, after an episode of DVT.[8]

Risk Factors

Three conditions, first described by Rudolf Virchow in 1862, contribute to VTE formation: stasis of blood flow, endothelial damage, and hypercoagulability. Of these risk factors, relative hypercoagulability appears most important in most cases of *spontaneous* DVT, whereas stasis and endothelial damage likely play a greater role in *secondary* DVT after immobilization, surgical procedures, and trauma. Identifiable risk factors for VTE relate to one of the conditions described by Virchow, and often more than one factor is present. Specific risk factors for VTE are listed in Table 24-2.

The more common acquired risk factors include advanced age, hospitalization and immobilization, hormone replacement and oral contraceptive therapy, pregnancy and the recently postpartum state, prior VTE, malignancy, major surgery, obesity, nephrotic syndrome, trauma and spinal cord injury, long-haul travel (>6 hours), varicose veins, antiphospholipid syndrome, myeloproliferative disorders, and polycythemia. Heritable risk factors include factor V Leiden; prothrombin 20210A gene variant; antithrombin, protein C, and protein S deficiencies; and dysfibrinogenemias. In some patients, the cause of the thrombophilia may have both a heritable and an acquired component. These mixed causes include homocysteinemia; factor VII, VIII, IX, and XI elevation; hyperfibrinogenemia; and activated protein C resistance in the absence of factor V Leiden.[9]

When multiple inherited and acquired risk factors are present in the same patient, a synergistic effect may occur, depending on the thrombophilia in question. For example, patients who are heterozygous for factor V Leiden are at only moderately increased risk for VTE (fourfold to eightfold). However, when this genetic risk is combined with the additional risk of oral contraceptive use, the risk for VTE increases approximately 35-fold, the same order of magnitude as for someone who is homozygous for factor V Leiden. The interaction between other common risk factors also was demonstrated in the Women's Health Initiative investigation.[10] The concomitant presence of obesity, advancing age, or factor V Leiden increased the thrombosis risk associated with hormone replacement therapy. However, not all risk factors have the same synergistic effect. Hyperhomocysteinemia and the most common genotype associated with elevated homocysteine levels (MTHFR 677TT) do not appear to interact with the presence of factor V Leiden to further increase the risk for venous thrombosis.[11]

Other factors associated with venous thrombosis include traditional cardiovascular risk factors (obesity, hypertension, diabetes), and there is a racial predilection for whites and African Americans, compared with Asians and Native Americans.[12,13] Certain gene variants (single nucleotide polymorphisms) are associated with a mildly increased risk for DVT, and their presence may interact with other risk factors to increase the overall risk for venous thrombosis.[14] However, testing for these polymorphisms is not common in clinical practice.

Diagnosis
Clinical Evaluation

Early in the course of DVT development, venous thrombosis is thought to begin in an area of relative stasis, such as a soleal sinus vein or immediately downstream of the cusps of a venous valve in the axial calf veins. Isolated proximal DVT without tibial vein thrombosis is unusual. Early in the course of a DVT, there may be no or few clinical findings such as pain or swelling. Even extensive DVT may sometimes be present without signs or symptoms. History and physical examination are therefore unreliable in the diagnosis of DVT. In addition, symptoms and signs generally associated with DVT, such as extremity pain and/or swelling, are nonspecific. In large studies, DVT has been found by venography or DUS in ≤50% of patients in whom it was clinically suspected.[15,16] Objective studies are therefore required to confirm a diagnosis of DVT or to exclude the presence of DVT.

Clinical symptoms may worsen as DVT propagates and involves the major proximal deep veins. Massive DVT that obliterates the major deep venous channel of the extremity with relative sparing of collateral veins causes a condition called *phlegmasia alba dolens* (Fig. 24-4). This condition is characterized by pain, pitting edema, and blanching. There is no associated cyanosis. When the thrombosis extends to the collateral veins, massive fluid sequestration and more significant edema ensues, resulting in a condition known as *phlegmasia cerulea dolens.*[17] Phlegmasia cerulea dolens is preceded by phlegmasia alba dolens in 50 to 60% of patients. The affected extremity in phlegmasia cerulea dolens is extremely painful, edematous, and cyanotic, and arterial insufficiency or compartment syndrome may be present. If the condition is left untreated, venous gangrene can ensue, leading to amputation.

Vascular Lab and Radiologic Evaluation

Duplex Ultrasound DUS is now the most commonly performed test for the detection of infrainguinal DVT, both above and below the knee, and has a sensitivity and specificity of >95% in symptomatic patients.[3] DUS combines real-time B-mode ultrasound with pulsed Doppler capability. Color flow imaging is useful in more technically difficult examinations, such as in the evaluation of possible calf vein DVT. This combination offers the ability to noninvasively visualize the venous anatomy, detect occluded and partially occluded venous segments, and demonstrate physiologic flow characteristics using a mobile self-contained device.

In the supine patient, normal lower extremity venous flow is phasic (Fig. 24-5), decreasing with inspiration in response to in-

| TABLE 24-2 | Risk factors for venous thromboembolism |

Acquired	Inherited
Advanced age	Factor V Leiden
Hospitalization/immobilization	Prothrombin 20210A
Hormone replacement therapy and oral contraceptive use	Antithrombin deficiency
	Protein C deficiency
Pregnancy and puerperium	Protein S deficiency
Prior venous thromboembolism	Factor XI elevation
Malignancy	Dysfibrinogenemia
Major surgery	**Mixed Etiology**
Obesity	Homocysteinemia
Nephrotic syndrome	Factor VII, VIII, IX, XI elevation
Trauma or spinal cord injury	Hyperfibrinogenemia
Long-haul travel (>6 h)	Activated protein C resistance without factor V Leiden
Varicose veins	
Antiphospholipid antibody syndrome	
Myeloproliferative disease	
Polycythemia	

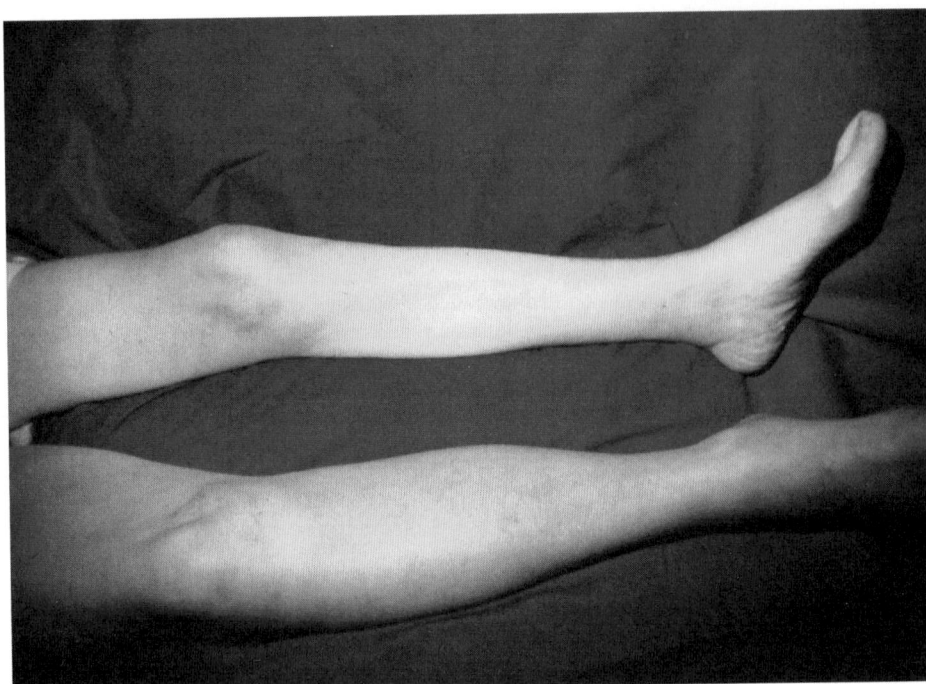

FIG. 24-4. Phlegmasia alba dolens of the right leg. Note the blanching and edema.

creased intra-abdominal pressure with the descent of the diaphragm and then increasing with expiration. When the patient is upright, the decrease in intra-abdominal pressure with expiration cannot overcome the hydrostatic column of pressure existing between the right atrium and the calf. Muscular contractions of the calf, along with the one-way venous valves, are then required to promote venous return to the heart. Flow also can be increased by leg elevation or compression and decreased by sudden elevation of intra-abdominal pressure (Valsalva's maneuver). In a venous DUS examination performed with the patient supine, spontaneous flow, variation of flow with respiration, and response of flow to Valsalva's maneuver are all assessed. However, the primary method of detecting DVT with ultrasound is

demonstration of the lack of compressibility of the vein with probe pressure on B-mode imaging. Normally, in transverse section, the vein walls should coapt with pressure. Lack of coaptation indicates thrombus.

The examination begins at the ankle and continues proximally to the groin. Each vein is visualized, and the flow signal is assessed with distal and proximal compression. Lower extremity DVT can be diagnosed by any of the following DUS findings: lack of spontaneous flow (Fig. 24-6), inability to compress the vein (Fig. 24-7), absence of color filling of the lumen by color flow DUS, loss of respiratory flow variation, and venous distention. Again, lack of venous compression on B-mode imaging is the primary diagnostic variable. Several studies

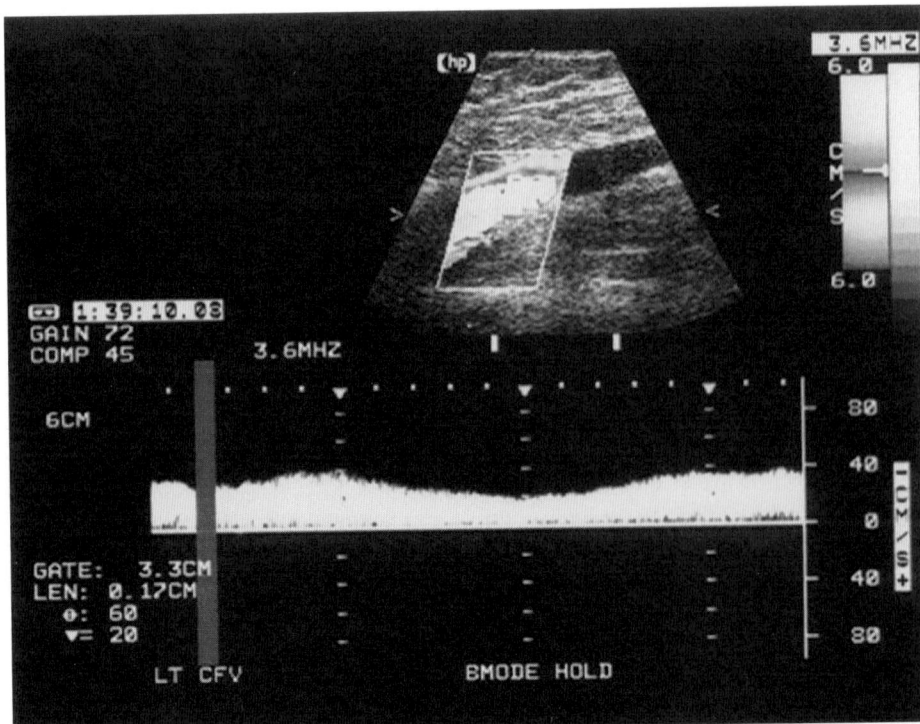

FIG. 24-5. Duplex ultrasound scan of a normal femoral vein with phasic flow signals.

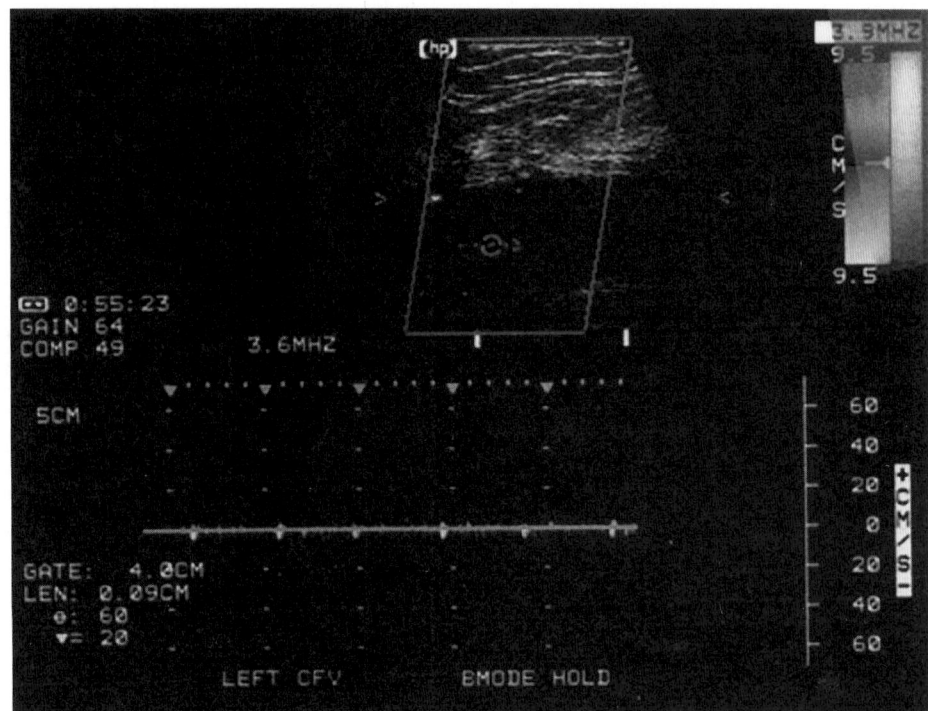

FIG. 24-6. Duplex ultrasound of a femoral vein containing thrombus demonstrating no flow within the femoral vein.

comparing B-mode ultrasound to venography for the detection of femoropopliteal DVT in patients clinically suspected to have DVT report sensitivities of >91% and specificities of >97%.[18,19] The ability of DUS to assess isolated calf vein DVT varies greatly, with sensitivities ranging from 50 to 93% and specificities approaching 100%.[20,21]

Impedance Plethysmography Impedance plethysmography (IPG) was the primary noninvasive method of diagnosing DVT before the widespread use of DUS but is infrequently used today. IPG is based on

the principle that resistance to the flow of electricity between two electrodes, or electrical impedance, occurs as the volume of the extremity changes in response to blood flow. Two pairs of electrodes containing aluminum strips are placed circumferentially around the leg approximately 10 cm apart and a low-level current is delivered to the two outer electrodes. A pneumatic cuff is inflated over the thigh for venous outflow obstruction and then rapidly deflated. Changes in electrical resistance resulting from lower extremity blood volume changes are quantified. IPG is less accurate than DUS for the detection

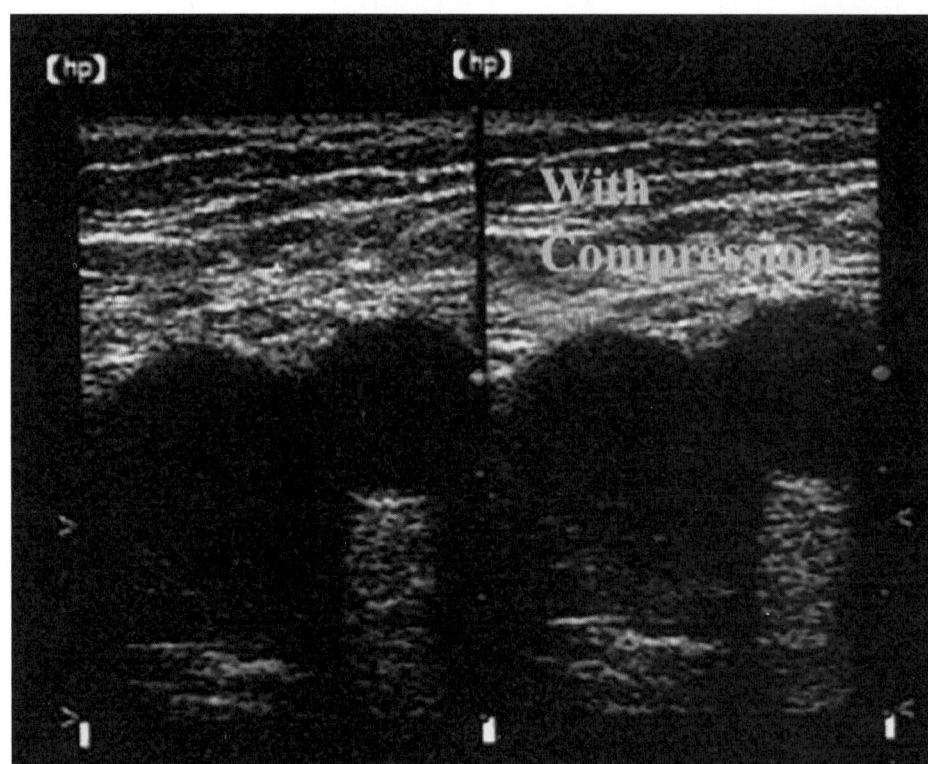

FIG. 24-7. B-mode ultrasound of the femoral vein in cross-section. The femoral vein does not collapse with external compression.

of proximal DVT, with an 83% sensitivity in symptomatic patients. It is a poor detector of calf vein DVT.[22]

Iodine 125 Fibrinogen Uptake Iodine 125 fibrinogen uptake (FUT) is a seldom used technique that involves IV administration of radioactive fibrinogen and monitoring for increased uptake in fibrin clots. An increase of 20% or more in one area of a limb indicates an area of thrombus.[23] FUT can detect DVT in the calf, but high background radiation from the pelvis and the urinary tract limits its ability to detect proximal DVT. It also cannot be used in an extremity that has recently undergone surgery or has active inflammation. In a prospective study, FUT had a sensitivity of 73% and specificity of 71% for identification of DVT in a group of symptomatic and asymptomatic patients.[22] Currently, FUT is primarily a research tool of historic interest.

Venography Venography is the most definitive test for the diagnosis of DVT in both symptomatic and asymptomatic patients. It is the gold standard to which other modalities are compared. This procedure involves placement of a small catheter in the dorsum of the foot and injection of a radiopaque contrast agent. Radiographs are obtained in at least two projections. A positive study result is failure to fill the deep system with passage of the contrast medium into the superficial system or demonstration of discrete filling defects (Fig. 24-8). A normal study result virtually excludes the presence of DVT. In a study of 160 patients with a normal venogram followed for 3 months, only two patients (1.3%) subsequently developed DVT and no patients experienced symptoms of PE.[24]

Venography is not routinely used for the evaluation of lower extremity DVT because of the associated complications discussed

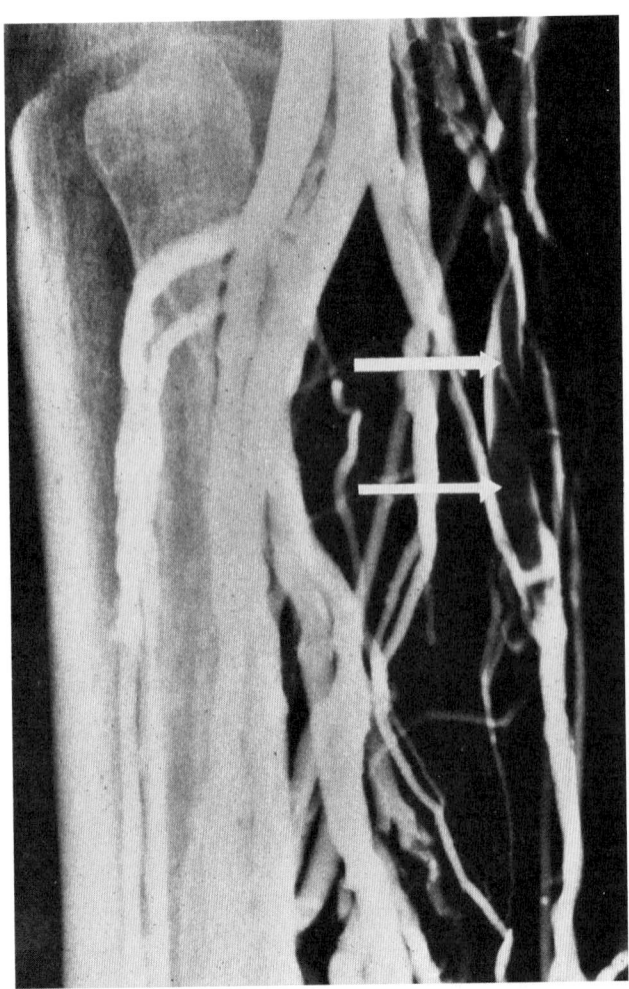

FIG. 24-8. Venogram showing a filling defect in the popliteal vein (*arrows*).

previously. Currently, venography is reserved for imaging before operative venous reconstruction and catheter-based therapy. It does, however, remain the procedure of choice in research studies evaluating methods of prophylaxis for DVT.

Treatment

Once the diagnosis of VTE has been made, antithrombotic therapy should be initiated promptly. If clinical suspicion for VTE is high, it may be prudent to start treatment while the diagnosis is being objectively confirmed. The theoretic goals of VTE treatment are the prevention of mortality and morbidity associated with PE and the prevention of the postphlebitic syndrome. However, the only proven benefit of anticoagulant treatment for DVT is the prevention of death from PE. Treatment regimens may include antithrombotic therapy, vena caval interruption, catheter-directed or systemic thrombolytic therapy, and operative thrombectomy.

Antithrombotic Therapy

Antithrombotic therapy may be initiated with IV or SC unfractionated heparin, SC low molecular weight heparin, or SC fondaparinux (a synthetic pentasaccharide). This initial therapy usually is continued for at least 5 days, while oral vitamin K antagonists are being simultaneously administered. The initial therapy typically is discontinued when the international normalized ratio (INR) is ≥2.0 for 24 hours.[25]

Unfractionated heparin (UFH) binds to antithrombin via a specific 18-saccharide sequence, which increases its activity over 1000-fold. This antithrombin-heparin complex primarily inhibits factor IIa (thrombin) and factor Xa and, to a lesser degree, factors IXa, XIa, and XIIa. In addition, UFH also binds to tissue factor pathway inhibitor, which inhibits the conversion of factor X to Xa, and factor IX to IXa. Finally, UFH catalyzes the inhibition of thrombin by heparin cofactor II via a mechanism that is independent of antithrombin.

UFH therapy is most commonly administered with an initial IV bolus of 80 units/kg or 5000 units. Weight-based UFH dosages have been shown to be more effective than standard fixed boluses in rapidly achieving therapeutic levels.[26] The initial bolus is followed by a continuous IV drip, initially at 18 units/kg per hour or 1300 units per hour. The half-life of IV UFH ranges from 45 to 90 minutes and is dose dependent. The level of antithrombotic therapy should be monitored every 6 hours using the activated partial thromboplastin time (aPTT), with the goal range of 1.5 to 2.5 times control values. This should correspond with plasma heparin anti-Xa activity levels of 0.3 to 0.7 IU/mL.

Initial anticoagulation with UFH may be administered SC, although this route is less commonly used. Adjusted-dose therapeutic SC UFH is initiated with 17,500 units, followed by 250 units/kg twice daily, and dosing is adjusted to an aPTT goal range similar to that for IV UFH. Fixed-dose unmonitored SC UFH is started with a bolus of 333 units/kg, followed by 250 units/kg twice daily.[25]

Hemorrhage is the primary complication of UFH therapy. The rate of major hemorrhage (fatal, intracranial, retroperitoneal, or requiring transfusion of >2 units of packed red blood cells) is approximately 5% in hospitalized patients undergoing UFH therapy (1% in medical patients and 8% in surgical patients).[27] For patients with UFH-related bleeding complications, cessation of UFH is required, and anticoagulation may be reversed with protamine sulfate. Protamine sulfate binds to UFH and forms an inactive salt compound. Each milligram of protamine neutralizes 90 to 115 units of heparin, and the dosage should not exceed 50 mg IV over any 10-minute period. Side effects of protamine sulfate include hypotension, pulmonary edema, and anaphylaxis. Patients with prior exposure to protamine-containing insulin (NPH) and patients with allergy to fish may have an increased risk of hypersensitivity, although no direct relationship has been established. The protamine infusion should be terminated if any side effects occur.

In addition to hemorrhage, heparin also has unique complications. Heparin-induced thrombocytopenia (HIT) results from heparin-associated antiplatelet antibodies (HAAbs) directed against platelet factor 4 complexed with heparin.[28] HIT occurs in 1 to 5% of patients being treated with heparin.[29,30] In patients with repeat heparin exposure (such as vascular surgery patients), the incidence of HAAb may be as high as 21%.[31] HIT occurs most frequently in the second week of therapy and may lead to disastrous venous or arterial thrombotic complications. Therefore, platelet counts should be monitored periodically in patients receiving continuous heparin therapy. All forms of heparin should be stopped if there is a high clinical suspicion or confirmation of HIT [usually accompanied by an unexplained thrombocytopenia (<100,000/μL) or platelet count decrease of 30 to 50%]. Fortunately, direct thrombin inhibitors (recombinant hirudin, argatroban, bivalirudin) now are available as alternative antithrombotic agents (see later). Another complication of prolonged high-dose heparin therapy is osteopenia, which results from impairment of bone formation and enhancement of bone resorption by heparin.

Low molecular weight heparins (LMWHs) are derived from the depolymerization of porcine UFH. Like UFH, LMWHs bind to antithrombin via a specific pentasaccharide sequence to expose an active site for the neutralization of factor Xa. However, LMWHs lack the sufficient number of additional saccharide units (18 or more), which results in less inactivation of thrombin (factor IIa). In comparison to UFH, LMWHs have increased bioavailability (>90% after SC injection), longer half-lives (approximately 4 to 6 hours), and more predictable elimination rates. Weight-based once- or twice-daily SC LMWH injections, for which no monitoring is needed, provide a distinct advantage over continuous IV infusions of UFH for treatment of VTE.

Most patients who receive therapeutic LMWH do not require monitoring. Patients who do require monitoring include those with significant renal insufficiency or failure, pediatric patients, obese patients of >120 kg, and patients who are pregnant. Monitoring may be performed using anti-Xa activity assays. However, the therapeutic anti-Xa goal range will depend on the type of LMWH and the frequency of dosing. Numerous LMWHs are commercially available. The various preparations differ in their anti-Xa and anti-IIa activities, and the treatment dosing for one LMWH cannot be extrapolated for use with another. The action of LMWHs may be partially reversed (approximately 60%) with protamine sulfate.

Numerous well-designed trials comparing SC LMWH with IV and SC UFH for the treatment of DVT have been critically evaluated in several meta-analyses.[32–34] The more recent studies demonstrate a decrease in thrombotic complications, bleeding, and mortality with LMWHs. LMWHs also are associated with a decreased rate of HAAb formation and HIT (<2%) compared with UFH (at least in prophylactic doses).[29] However, patients with established HIT should not subsequently receive LMWHs due to significant rates of cross reactivity.[35] A major benefit of LMWHs is the ability to treat patients with VTE as outpatients.[36,37] In a randomized study comparing IV UFH and the LMWH nadroparin calcium,[36] there was no significant difference in recurrent thromboembolism (8.6% for UFH vs. 6.9% for LMWH) or major bleeding complications (2.0% for UFH vs. 0.5% for LMWH). There was a 67% reduction in mean days in the hospital for the LMWH group.

A patient with VTE should meet several criteria before receiving outpatient LMWH therapy. First, the patient should not require hospitalization for any associated conditions. The patient should not require monitoring of the LMWH therapy (which is necessary in patients with severe renal insufficiency, pediatric patients, obese patients, and pregnant patients). The patient should be hemodynamically stable with a low suspicion of PE and have a low bleeding risk. An established outpatient system to administer LMWH and warfarin, as well as to monitor for recurrent VTE and bleeding complications, should be present. In addition, the patient's symptoms of pain and edema should be controllable at home.

Fondaparinux currently is the only synthetic pentasaccharide that has been approved by the U.S. Food and Drug Administration (FDA) for the initial treatment of DVT and PE. Its five-polysaccharide ride sequence binds and activates antithrombin, causing specific inhibition of factor Xa. In two large noninferiority trials, fondaparinux was compared with the LMWH enoxaparin for the initial treatment of DVT and with IV UFH for the initial treatment of PE.[38,39] The rates of recurrent VTE ranged from 3.8 to 5%, with rates of major bleeding of 2 to 2.6%, for all treatment arms. The drug is administered SC once daily with a weight-based dosing protocol: 5 mg, 7.5 mg, or 10 mg for patients weighing <50 kg, 50 to 100 kg, or >100 kg, respectively. The half-life of fondaparinux is approximately 17 hours in patients with normal renal function. There are rare case reports of fondaparinux-induced thrombocytopenia.[40]

Direct-thrombin inhibitors (DTIs) include recombinant hirudin, argatroban, and bivalirudin. These antithrombotic agents bind to thrombin, inhibiting the conversion of fibrinogen to fibrin as well as thrombin-induced platelet activation. These actions are independent of antithrombin. The direct thrombin inhibitors should be reserved for (a) patients in whom there is a high clinical suspicion or confirmation of HIT, and (b) patients who have a history of HIT or test positive for heparin-associated antibodies. In patients with established HIT, DTIs should be administered for at least 7 days, or until the platelet count normalizes. Warfarin may then be introduced slowly, overlapping therapy with a DTI for at least 5 days.[41] Because bivalirudin is approved primarily for patients with or without HIT who undergo percutaneous coronary intervention, it is not discussed here in further detail.

Commercially available hirudin is manufactured using recombinant DNA technology. It is indicated for the prophylaxis and treatment of patients with HIT. In patients with normal renal function, recombinant hirudin is administered in an IV bolus dose of 0.4 mg/kg, followed by a continuous IV infusion of 0.15 mg/kg per hour. The half-life ranges from 30 to 60 minutes. The aPTT is monitored, starting approximately 4 hours after initiation of therapy, and dosage is adjusted to maintain an aPTT of 1.5 to 2.5 times the laboratory normal value. The less commonly used ecarin clotting time is an alternative method of monitoring. Because recombinant hirudin is eliminated via renal excretion, significant dosage adjustments are required in patients with renal insufficiency.

Argatroban is indicated for the prophylaxis and treatment of thrombosis in HIT. It also is approved for patients with, or at risk for, HIT who undergo percutaneous coronary intervention. Antithrombotic prophylaxis and therapy are initiated with a continuous IV infusion of 2 μg/kg per minute, without the need for a bolus. The half-life ranges from 39 to 51 minutes, and the dosage is adjusted to maintain an aPTT of 1.5 to 3 times normal. Large initial boluses and higher rates of continuous infusion are reserved for patients with coronary artery thrombosis and myocardial infarction. In these patients, therapy is monitored using the activated clotting time. Argatroban is metabolized by the liver, and the majority is excreted via the biliary tract. Significant dosage adjustments are needed in patients with hepatic impairment. There is no reversal agent for argatroban.

Vitamin K antagonists, which include warfarin and other coumarin derivatives, are the mainstay of long-term antithrombotic therapy in patients with VTE. Warfarin inhibits the γ-carboxylation of vitamin K–dependent procoagulants (factors II, VII, IX, X) and anticoagulants (proteins C and S), which results in the formation of less functional proteins. Warfarin usually requires several days to achieve its full effect, because normal circulating coagulation proteins must first undergo their normal degradation. Factors X and II have the longest half-lives, in the range of 36 and 72 hours, respectively. In addition, the steady-state concentration of warfarin is usually not reached for 4 to 5 days.

Warfarin therapy usually is monitored by measuring the INR, calculated using the following equation:

$$INR = (\text{patient prothrombin time/laboratory normal prothrombin time})^{ISI}$$

where *ISI* is the international sensitivity index. The ISI describes the strength of the thromboplastin that is added to activate the extrinsic

TABLE 24-3	Summary of American College of Chest Physicians recommendations regarding duration of long-term antithrombotic therapy for deep vein thrombosis (DVT)

Clinical Subgroup	Antithrombotic Treatment Duration
First episode DVT/transient risk	VKA for 3 mo
First episode DVT/unprovoked	VKA for at least 3 mo
	Consider for long-term therapy if:
	• Proximal DVT
	• Minimal bleeding risk
	• Stable coagulation monitoring
Distal DVT/unprovoked	VKA for 3 mo
Second episode DVT/unprovoked	VKA long-term therapy
DVT and cancer	LMWH 3–6 mo
	Then VKA or LMWH indefinitely until cancer resolves

LMWH = low molecular weight heparin; VKA = vitamin K antagonist.
Source: Adapted with permission from Kearon C, Kahn SR, Agnelli G, et al: Antithrombotic therapy for venous thromboembolic disease: American College of Chest Physicians Evidence-Based Clinical Practice Guidelines (8th edition). *Chest* 133:454S, 2008.

coagulation pathway. The therapeutic target INR range is usually 2.0 to 3.0, but the response to warfarin is variable and depends on liver function, diet, age, and concomitant medications. In patients receiving anticoagulation therapy without concomitant thrombolysis or venous thrombectomy, the vitamin K antagonist may be started on the same day as the initial parenteral anticoagulant, usually at doses ranging from 5 to 10 mg. Smaller initial doses may be needed in older and malnourished patients, in those with liver disease or congestive heart failure, and in those who have recently undergone major surgery.[42]

The recommended duration of warfarin antithrombotic therapy is increasingly being stratified based on whether the DVT was provoked or unprovoked, whether it was the first or a recurrent episode, where the DVT is located, and whether malignancy is present. Current American College of Chest Physicians (ACCP) recommendations for duration of warfarin therapy are summarized in Table 24-3. In patients with proximal DVT, several randomized clinical trials have demonstrated that shorter-term antithrombotic therapy (4 to 6 weeks) is associated with a higher rate of recurrence than 3 to 6 months of anticoagulation.[43–45] In these trials, most of the patients with transient risk factors had a low rate of recurrent VTE; most of the recurrences were in patients with continuing risk factors. These studies support the ACCP recommendation that 3 months of anticoagulation is sufficient to prevent recurrent VTE in patients whose DVT occurred around the time of a transient risk factor (e.g., hospitalization, orthopedic or major general surgery).

In contrast to patients with thrombosis related to transient risk factors, patients with idiopathic VTE are much more likely to develop recurrence (rates as high as 40% at 10 years). In this latter group of patients, numerous clinical trials have compared 3 to 6 months of anticoagulation therapy with extended-duration warfarin therapy, both at low intensity (INR of 1.5 to 2.0) and at conventional intensity (INR of 2.0 to 3.0).[46–49] In patients with idiopathic DVT, extended-duration antithrombotic therapy is associated with a relative reduction in the rate of recurrent VTE by 75% to >90%. In addition, conventional-intensity warfarin reduces the risk even further compared with low-intensity warfarin (0.7 events per 100 person-years vs. 1.9 events per 100 person-years), but the rate of bleeding complications is no different.[49]

In patients with VTE in association with a hypercoagulable condition, the optimal duration of anticoagulation therapy is influenced more by the clinical circumstances at the time of the VTE (idiopathic vs. secondary) than by the actual presence or absence of the more common thrombophilic conditions. In patients with VTE related to malignancy, increasing evidence suggests that longer-term therapy with LMWH (up to 6 months) is associated with a lower VTE recurrence rate than treatment using conventional vitamin K antagonists.[50,51]

The primary complication of warfarin therapy is hemorrhage, and the risk is related to the magnitude of INR prolongation. Depending on the INR and the presence of bleeding, warfarin anticoagulation may be reversed by (a) omitting or decreasing subsequent dosages, (b) administering oral or parenteral vitamin K, or (c) administering fresh-frozen plasma, prothrombin complex concentrate, or recombinant factor VIIa.[42] Warfarin therapy rarely may be associated with the development of skin necrosis and limb gangrene. These conditions occur more commonly in women (4:1), and the most commonly affected areas are the breast, buttocks, and thighs. This complication, which usually occurs in the first days of therapy, is occasionally, but not exclusively, associated with protein C or S deficiency and malignancy. Patients who require continued anticoagulation may restart low-dose warfarin (2 mg) while receiving concomitant therapeutic heparin. The warfarin dosage is then gradually increased over a 1- to 2-week period.[42]

Systemic and Catheter-Directed Thrombolysis

Patients with extensive proximal DVT may benefit from systemic thrombolysis or catheter-directed thrombolysis, which can potentially reduce acute symptoms more rapidly than anticoagulation alone. These techniques also may decrease the development of postthrombotic syndrome. Several thrombolysis preparations are available, including streptokinase, urokinase, alteplase (recombinant tissue plasminogen activator), reteplase, and tenecteplase. All these agents share the ability to convert plasminogen to plasmin, which leads to the degradation of fibrin. They differ with regard to their half-lives, their potential for inducing fibrinogenolysis (generalized lytic state), their potential for antigenicity, and their FDA-approved indications for use.

Streptokinase is purified from beta-hemolytic *Streptococcus* and is approved for the treatment of acute myocardial infarction, PE, DVT, arterial thromboembolism, and occluded central lines and arteriovenous shunts. It is not specific for fibrin-bound plasminogen, however, and its use is limited by its significant rates of antigenicity. Fevers and shivering occur in 1 to 4% of patients. Urokinase is derived from human neonatal kidney cells, grown in tissue culture. Currently, it is only approved for lysis of massive PE or PE associated with unstable hemodynamics. Alteplase, reteplase, and tenecteplase all are recombinant variants of tissue plasminogen activator. Alteplase is indicated for the treatment of acute myocardial infarction, acute ischemic stroke, and acute massive PE. However, it often is used for catheter-directed thrombolysis of DVT. Reteplase and tenecteplase are indicated only for the treatment of acute myocardial infarction.

Systemic thrombolysis was evaluated in numerous older prospective and randomized clinical trials, and its efficacy was summarized in a recent Cochrane Review.[52] In 12 studies involving over 700 patients, systemic thrombolysis was associated with significantly more clot lysis [relative risk (RR) 0.24 to 0.37] and significantly less postthrombotic syndrome (RR 0.66). However, venous function was not significantly improved. In addition, more bleeding complications did occur (RR 1.73), but the incidence appears to have decreased in later studies, probably due to improved patient selection.

In an effort to minimize bleeding complications and increase efficacy, catheter-directed thrombolytic techniques have been developed for the treatment of symptomatic DVT. With catheter-directed therapy, venous access may be achieved through percutaneous catheterization of the ipsilateral popliteal vein, retrograde catheterization through the contralateral femoral vein, or retrograde cannulation from the internal jugular vein. Multi–side-hole infusion catheters, with or without infusion wires, are used to deliver the lytic agent directly into the thrombus.

The efficacy of catheter-directed urokinase for the treatment of symptomatic lower extremity DVT has been reported in a large multicenter registry.[53] Two hundred twenty-one patients with iliofemoral DVT and 79 patients with femoropopliteal DVT were treated with catheter-directed urokinase for a mean of 53 hours. Complete lysis was seen in 31% of the limbs, 50 to 99% lysis in 52% of the limbs, and <50% lysis in 17%. Overall, 1-year primary patency was 60%. Patency was higher in patients with iliofemoral DVT than in patients with femoropopliteal DVT (64% vs. 47%, P <.01). In addition, patients with acute symptoms (≤10 days) had a greater likelihood of complete lysis (34%) than patients with chronic symptoms (>10 days; 19%). Major bleeding occurred in 11%, but neurologic involvement and mortality were rare (both 0.4%). Adjunctive stent placement to treat residual stenosis and/or short segment occlusion was required in 103 limbs.

One small randomized trial and numerous other retrospective studies have demonstrated similar rates of thrombolysis, with some also showing improved valve preservation and quality of life.[25,54,55] Combining thrombolysis with percutaneous thrombus fragmentation and extraction has the added benefit of decreasing the infusion time, the hospital stay, and the overall cost of treatment.[56] These studies, as well as the current ACCP guidelines, suggest that catheter-directed thrombolysis (with adjunctive angioplasty, venous stenting, and pharmacomechanical fragmentation and extraction) may be useful in selected patients with extensive iliofemoral DVT. Patients should have a recent onset of symptoms (<14 days), good functional status, decent life expectancy, and low bleeding risk.

Inferior Vena Caval Filters

Since the introduction of the Kimray-Greenfield filter in the United States in 1973, numerous vena caval filters have been developed. Although the designs are variable, they all prevent pulmonary emboli, while allowing continuation of venous blood flow through the IVC. Early filters were placed surgically through the femoral vein. Currently, less invasive techniques allow percutaneous filter placement through a femoral vein, internal jugular vein, or small peripheral vein under fluoroscopic or ultrasound guidance. Complications associated with IVC filter placement include insertion site thrombosis, filter migration, erosion of the filter into the IVC wall, and IVC thrombosis. The rate of fatal complications is <0.12%.[57]

Placement of an IVC filter is indicated for patients who develop recurrent DVT (significant propagation of the original thrombus or proximal DVT at a new site) or PE despite adequate anticoagulation therapy and for patients with pulmonary hypertension who experience recurrent PE. In patients who receive IVC filters for these indications, therapeutic anticoagulation should be continued. The duration of anticoagulation is determined by the underlying VTE and not by the presence of the IVC filter itself. Practically speaking, however, many patients who require an IVC filter for recurrent VTE are the same ones who would benefit most from indefinite anticoagulation. The other major indication for placement of an IVC filter is a contraindication to, or complication of, anticoagulation therapy in the presence of an acute proximal DVT. In patients who are not able to receive anticoagulants due to recent surgery or trauma, the clinician should continually reassess if antithrombotic agents may be started safely at a later date. Even some patients who develop anticoagulation-associated bleeding complications may be able to restart therapy at a lower intensity of anticoagulation later in the hospital course. As before, the clinical circumstances surrounding the VTE should determine the duration of anticoagulation.

Placement of permanent IVC filters has been evaluated as an adjunct to routine anticoagulation in patients with proximal DVT.[58] In this study, routine IVC filter placement did not prolong early or late survival in patients with proximal DVT but did decrease the rate of PE (hazard ratio, 0.22; 95% confidence interval, 0.05 to 0.90). An increased rate of recurrent DVT was seen in patients with IVC filters (hazard ratio, 1.87; 95% confidence interval, 1.10 to 3.20). More controversial indications for IVC filter placement include prophy-

laxis against PE in patients receiving catheter-directed thrombolysis and in high-risk patients without established DVT or PE.

Operative Venous Thrombectomy

In patients with acute iliofemoral DVT, surgical therapy is generally reserved for patients who worsen with anticoagulation therapy and those with phlegmasia cerulea dolens and impending venous gangrene. If the patient has phlegmasia cerulea dolens, a fasciotomy of the calf compartments is first performed. In iliofemoral DVT, a longitudinal venotomy is made in the common femoral vein and a venous balloon embolectomy catheter is passed through the thrombus into the IVC and pulled back several times until no further thrombus can be extracted. The distal thrombus in the leg is removed by manual pressure beginning in the foot. This is accomplished by application of a tight rubber elastic wrap beginning at the foot and extending to the thigh. If the thrombus in the femoral vein is old and cannot be extracted, the vein is ligated. For a thrombus that extends into the IVC, the IVC is exposed transperitoneally and the IVC is controlled below the renal veins. The IVC is opened and the thrombus is removed by gentle massage. An intraoperative completion venogram is obtained to determine if any residual thrombus or stenosis is present. If a residual iliac vein stenosis is present, intraoperative angioplasty and stenting can be performed. In most cases, an arteriovenous fistula is then created by anastomosing the great saphenous vein (GSV) end to side with the superficial femoral artery in an effort to maintain patency of the thrombectomized iliofemoral venous segment. Heparin is administered postoperatively for several days. Warfarin anticoagulation is maintained for at least 6 months after thrombectomy. Complications of iliofemoral thrombectomy include PE in up to 20% of patients[59] and death in <1% of patients.[60]

One study[61] followed 77 limbs for a mean of 8.5 years after thrombectomy for acute iliofemoral DVT. In limbs with successful thrombectomies, valvular competence in the thrombectomized venous segment was 80% at 5 years and 56% at 10 years. More than 90% of patients had minimal or no symptoms of postthrombotic syndrome. There were 12 (16%) early thrombectomy failures. Patients were required to wear compression stockings for at least 1 year after thrombectomy.

Survival rates for surgical pulmonary embolectomy have improved over the past 20 years with the addition of cardiopulmonary bypass. Emergency pulmonary embolectomy for acute PE is rarely indicated. Patients with preterminal massive PE (Fig. 24-9) for whom thrombolysis has failed or who have contraindications to thrombolytics may be candidates for this procedure. Open pulmonary artery embolectomy is performed through a posterolateral thoracotomy with direct visualization of the pulmonary arteries. Mortality rates range between 20 and 40%.[62-64]

Percutaneous catheter-based techniques for removal of a PE involve mechanical thrombus fragmentation or embolectomy using suction devices. Mechanical clot fragmentation is followed by catheter-directed thrombolysis. Results of catheter-based fragmentation are based on small case series. In a study in which a fragmentation device was used in 10 patients with acute massive PE, fragmentation was successful in 7 patients with a mortality rate of 20%.[65] Transvenous catheter pulmonary suction embolectomy has also been performed for acute massive PE with a reported 76% successful extraction rate and a 30-day survival of 70%.[66]

Prophylaxis

Patients who undergo major general surgical, gynecologic, urologic, and neurosurgical procedures without thromboprophylaxis have a significant incidence of perioperative DVT (15 to 40%). The incidence is even higher with major trauma (40 to 80%), hip and knee replacement surgery (40 to 60%), and spinal cord injury (60 to 80%).[67] The goal of prophylaxis is to reduce the mortality and morbidity associated with VTE. The first manifestation of VTE may

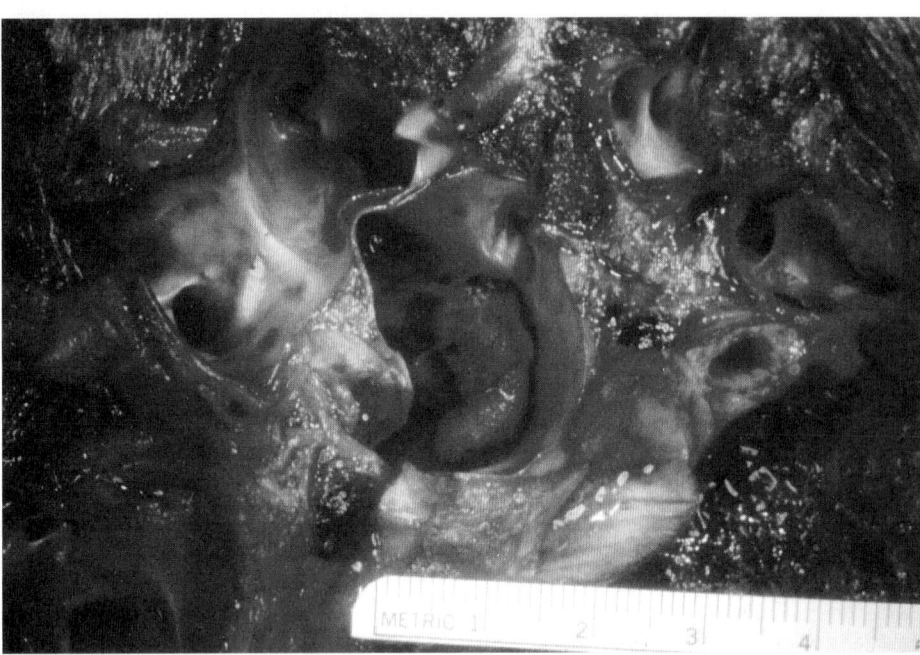

FIG. 24-9. Autopsy specimen showing a massive pulmonary embolism.

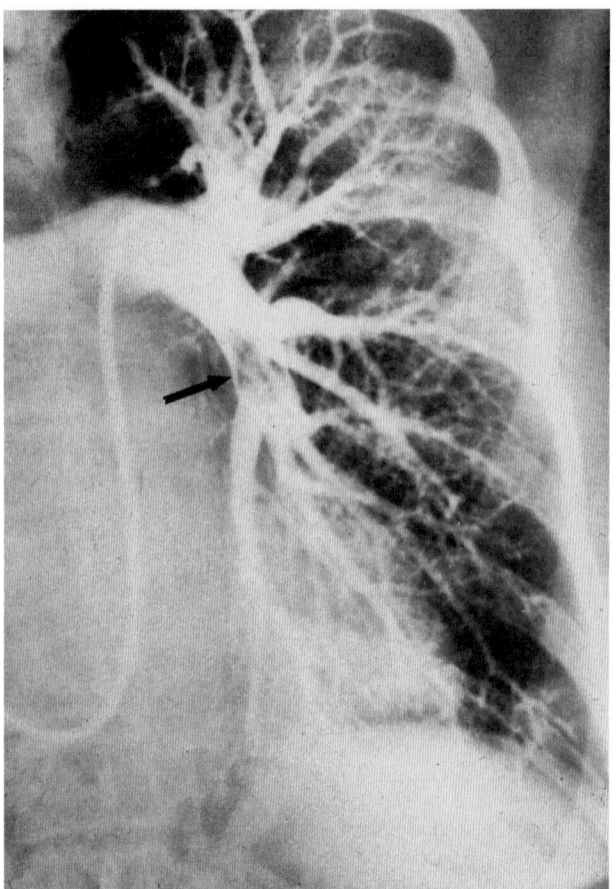

FIG. 24-10. Pulmonary angiogram showing a pulmonary embolism (*arrow*).

be a life-threatening PE (Fig. 24-10), and as indicated earlier, clinical evaluation to detect DVT before PE is unreliable.

Effective methods of VTE prophylaxis involve the use of one or more pharmacologic or mechanical modalities. Currently available pharmacologic agents include low-dose UFH, LMWH, synthetic pentasaccharides, and vitamin K antagonists. Mechanical methods include intermittent pneumatic compression (IPC) and graduated compression stockings. Aspirin therapy alone is not adequate for DVT prophylaxis. These prophylaxis methods vary with regard to their efficacy, and the 2008 ACCP Clinical Practice Guidelines stratify their uses according to the patient's level of risk (Table 24-4).

Venous Thromboembolism Prophylaxis in General Surgery

The risk for VTE in general surgery depends on the type of operation, the type of anesthesia, the duration of surgery, and other risk factors, including patient age, presence of cancer, prior VTE, obesity, and presence of infection. Patients at low risk who undergo minor procedures do not require pharmacologic or mechanical prophylaxis. Patients at moderate risk who undergo major procedures should receive low-dose UFH, LMWH, or fondaparinux. These prophylactic options also are effective for patients at high risk, but the UFH requires more frequent dosing (5000 units SC, tid) to achieve a similar level of prevention. The patients at highest risk with multiple VTE risk factors benefit from a combination of pharmacologic and mechanical prophylaxis (IPC and/or graduated compression stockings). Thromboprophylaxis should continue until discharge, except in select high-risk patients with malignancy in whom extended-duration prophylaxis (up to 28 days) may be beneficial. Patients with significant risk for bleeding should receive mechanical prophylaxis until this risk subsides.[67]

Overall, low-dose UFH and LMWH reduce the risk for symptomatic and nonsymptomatic VTE by 60 to 70%. The risks for bleeding differ, depending on the dosage. Lower dosages of LMWH appear to be associated with less bleeding risk than low-dose UFH, but the latter produces less bleeding risk than higher prophylactic dosages of LMWH.[68] Other advantages of LMWH include once-daily dosing protocols and a lower rate of heparin-associated antibody formation.

Fondaparinux has been compared with the LMWH dalteparin in patients who undergo high-risk major abdominal surgery. It also has been compared with IPC alone in patients undergoing non–high-risk abdominal surgery.[69,70] The pentasaccharide had rates of VTE prevention, bleeding complications, and mortality similar to those of LMWH. It was more beneficial than IPC alone

TABLE 24-4	Thromboembolism risk and recommended thromboprophylaxis in surgical patients

Level of Risk	Approximate DVT Risk without Thromboprophylaxis (%)	Suggested Thromboprophylaxis Options
Low risk	<10	No specific thromboprophylaxis
Minor surgery in mobile patients		Early and "aggressive" ambulation
Moderate risk	10–40	LMWH (at recommended doses), LDUH bid or tid, fondaparinux
Most general, open gynecologic, or urologic surgery		Mechanical thromboprophylaxis
Moderate VTE risk plus high bleeding risk		
High risk	40–80	LMWH (at recommended doses), fondaparinux, oral vitamin K antagonist (INR 2–3)
Hip or knee arthroplasty, hip fracture surgery		
Major trauma, spinal cord injury		Mechanical thromboprophylaxis
High VTE risk plus high bleeding risk		

DVT = deep vein thrombosis; INR = International Normalized Ratio; LDUH = low-dose unfractionated heparin; LMWH = low molecular weight heparin; VTE = venous thromboembolism.

Source: Adapted with permission from Geerts WH, Bergqvist D, Pineo GF, et al: Prevention of venous thromboembolism: American College of Chest Physicians Evidence-Based Clinical Practice Guidelines (8th edition). *Chest* 133:381, 2008.

in reducing VTE but at the cost of a higher rate of bleeding (1.6% vs. 0.2%).

Prophylactic insertion of IVC filters has been suggested for VTE prophylaxis in high-risk trauma patients and in some patients with malignancy who have contraindications for LMWH therapy.[71] Trauma patients at a higher risk than the general trauma population include those with severe head injuries, spinal cord injuries, and severe fractures of the pelvis or long bones. A 5-year study of prophylactic IVC filter placement in 132 trauma patients at high risk of PE reported a 0% incidence of symptomatic PE in patients with a correctly positioned IVC filter.[72] In 47 patients with a malpositioned IVC filter (strut malposition or filter tilt) there was a 6.3% incidence of symptomatic PE with three deaths. DVT occurred at the insertion site in 3.1% of the patients. IVC patency was 97.1% at 3 years by life table analysis.

Fatal and nonfatal PE can still occur in a patient with prophylactic vena cava interruption. Long-term complications associated with permanent IVC filters include IVC thrombosis and DVT. Currently, the ACCP recommends that IVC filters be placed only if a proximal DVT is present and anticoagulation therapy is contraindicated. IVC filter insertion is not recommended for primary prophylaxis, although this is widely done.

In an attempt to avoid long-term complications associated with permanent IVC filters, retrievable IVC filters have been developed for use in patients with a temporarily increased risk of PE (Fig. 24-11).[73] Depending on the device, the filter may be removed at anywhere from 4 weeks to 6 months after insertion, assuming the period of increased PE risk has passed and no significant emboli are trapped by the filter. The best patient groups for retrievable filter placement may include young trauma patients with transient immobility, patients undergoing surgical procedures associated with a high risk of PE, and patients with hypercoagulable states who cannot receive anticoagulation therapy for a short period of time. If the device traps a significant embolus, it may be left in place as a permanent filter.

Venous Thromboembolism Prophylaxis in Laparoscopic Surgery

There are significant discrepancies in the recommendations regarding the optimal use of thromboprophylaxis around the time of laparoscopic procedures. The ACCP guidelines recommend against routine thromboprophylaxis, other than early and frequent ambulation, in patients at low risk who undergo entirely laparoscopic procedures.[67] In patients with additional VTE risk factors, the guidelines recommend prophylaxis with one or more of the following: LMWH, low-dose UFH, fondaparinux, IPC, or graduated compression stockings. The Society of American Gastrointestinal Endoscopic Surgeons recently revised its guidelines based on the magnitude of the laparoscopic procedure and the presence of additional venous thrombosis risk factors.[74]

OTHER VENOUS THROMBOTIC DISORDERS

Superficial Vein Thrombophlebitis

Superficial vein thrombophlebitis (SVT) most commonly occurs in varicose veins but can occur in normal veins. When SVT recurs at variable sites in normal superficial veins, it may signify a hidden visceral malignancy or a systemic disease such as a blood dyscrasia and/or a collagen vascular disease. This condition is known as *thrombophlebitis migrans*. SVT also frequently occurs as a complication of indwelling catheters, with or without associated extravasation of injected material. Upper extremity vein thrombosis has been reported to occur in 38% of patients with peripherally inserted central catheters; 57% of these developed in the cephalic vein (Fig. 24-12).[75] Finally, suppurative SVT may occur in veins with indwelling catheters and may be associated with generalized sepsis.

Clinical signs of SVT include redness, warmth, and tenderness along the distribution of the affected veins, often associated with a palpable cord. Patients with suppurative SVT may have fever and leukocytosis. DUS should be performed in patients with signs and symptoms of acute SVT to confirm the diagnosis and to determine if any associated DVT is present. Concomitant DVT may be present in 5 to 40% of patients with SVT; most occur in patients with SVT within 1 cm of the saphenofemoral junction. A follow-up DUS should be performed in 5 to 7 days in patients with SVT in the proximal GSV but without deep vein involvement. Approximately 10 to 20% of patients with SVT involving the proximal GSV experience progression to deep venous involvement within 1 week.[76,77]

Treatment of SVT is quite variable. A recent Cochrane review reported that LMWHs and NSAIDs both reduce the rate of SVT extension or recurrence. Topical medications appear to improve local symptoms. Surgical treatment, combined with the use of graduated compression stockings, is associated with a lower rate of VTE and SVT progression.[78] The treatment is individualized and depends on the location of the thrombus and the severity of symptoms. In patients with SVT not within 1 cm of the saphenofemoral junction, treatment consists of compression and administration of an anti-inflammatory medication such as indomethacin. In patients with suppurative SVT, removal of any existing indwelling catheters is mandatory, and excision of the vein may be necessary. If the SVT extends proximally to within 1 cm of the saphenofemoral junction, extension into the common femoral vein is more likely to occur. In these patients, anticoagulation therapy for 6 weeks and GSV ligation appear equally effective in preventing thrombus extension into the deep venous system.[79,80]

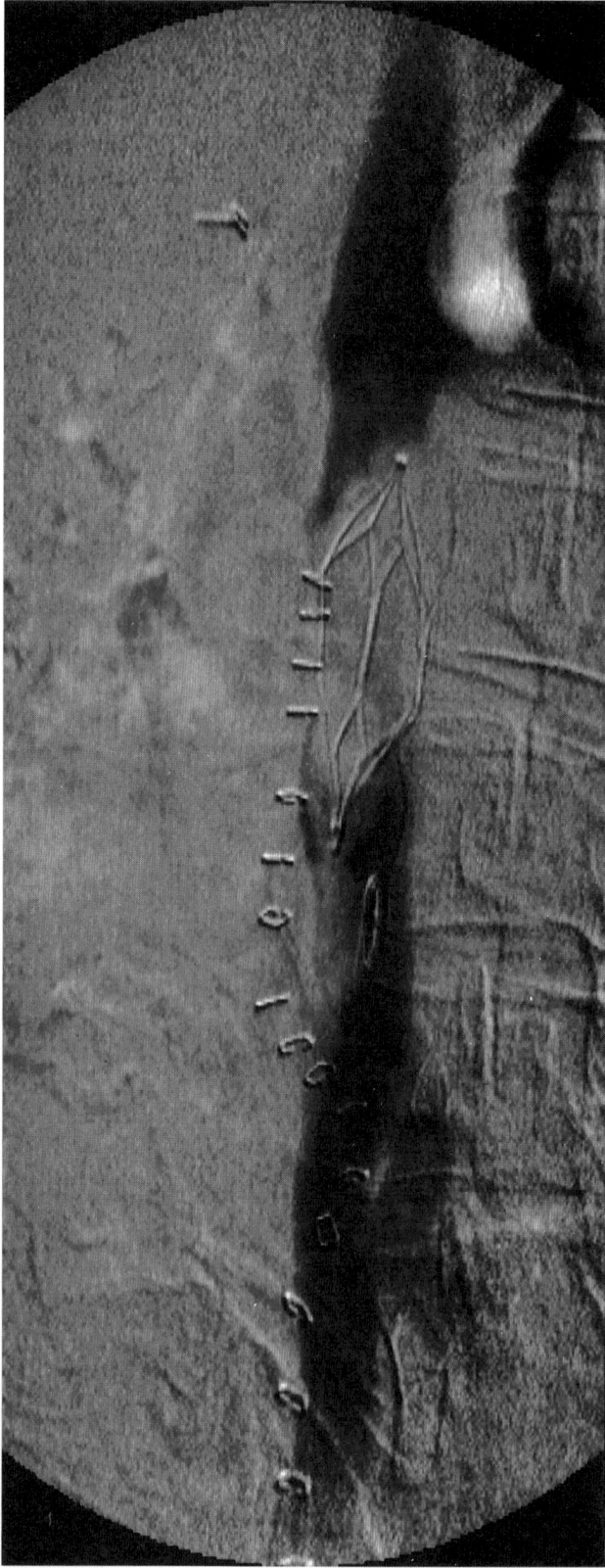

FIG. 24-11. Carbon dioxide venogram of emboli trapped within a retrievable inferior vena caval filter. The filter was not retrieved.

Upper Extremity Vein Thrombosis

Axillary-subclavian vein thromboses (ASVT) are classified into two forms. Primary ASVT occurs in only a small minority of all patients with ASVT. In the primary form, no clear cause for the thrombosis is readily identifiable at initial evaluation. Patients with primary ASVT often give a history of performing prolonged, repetitive motion activ-

ities, which results in damage to the subclavian vein, usually where it passes between the head of the clavicle and the first rib. This condition is also known as *venous thoracic outlet syndrome, effort thrombosis,* and *Paget-Schroetter syndrome.* Secondary ASVT is more common and is associated with an easily identified cause such as an indwelling catheter or a hypercoagulable state. Over 30% of patients with tunneled subclavian vein access devices develop ASVT.[81]

A patient with ASVT may be asymptomatic or may present with varying degrees of upper extremity edema and tenderness. DUS can be performed initially to confirm the diagnosis. Anticoagulation therapy should be initiated once ASVT is diagnosed to prevent PE and decrease symptoms. Patients presenting with acute symptomatic primary ASVT may be candidates for catheter-directed thrombolytic therapy. Venography is performed through a catheter placed using an ultrasound-guided percutaneous basilic vein approach to document the extent of the thrombus (Fig. 24-13). A guidewire is traversed through the thrombus and a catheter is placed within the thrombus. Typically, tissue plasminogen activator is administered through a multi–side-hole infusion catheter. Heparin is administered concurrently with the urokinase infusion. After completion of thrombolytic therapy, a follow-up venogram is obtained to identify any correctable anatomic abnormalities. Adjuvant procedures after thrombolytic therapy may include cervical or first rib resection for thoracic outlet abnormalities, surgical venous reconstruction, and balloon angioplasty for residual venous stenosis.[82]

Mesenteric Vein Thrombosis

Five to 15% of cases of acute mesenteric ischemia occur as a result of mesenteric vein thrombosis (MVT). Mortality rates in patients with MVT are as high as 50%.[83] The major presenting symptom is nonspecific abdominal pain, followed by diarrhea, nausea, and vomiting.[84] Peritoneal signs are present in fewer than half of MVT patients. MVT is more common in patients with a hypercoagulable state and malignancy.[84]

Plain abdominal radiographs are usually obtained in patients with abdominal pain. Free air suggestive of a perforated viscus should be ruled out. In most patients with MVT, plain abdominal radiographs show a nonspecific bowel gas pattern and are generally nondiagnostic. Currently, contrast-enhanced abdominal computed tomographic (CT) scanning is the diagnostic study of choice in patients suspected of having MVT. In addition to revealing MVT, CT scanning can accurately detect portal and ovarian vein thrombosis. In one series, contrast-enhanced abdominal CT scanning was diagnostic for MVT in 90% of patients.[84]

Patients with MVT should undergo adequate fluid resuscitation and receive anticoagulation therapy with heparin. Urgent laparotomy is undertaken in patients presenting with peritoneal findings. Broad-spectrum antibiotics are administered perioperatively. Findings at laparotomy consist of edema and cyanotic discoloration of the mesentery and bowel wall with thrombus involving the distal mesenteric veins. Complete thrombosis of the superior mesenteric vein is rare, occurring in only 12% of patients undergoing laparotomy for suspected MVT.[85] The arterial supply to the involved bowel is usually intact. Nonviable bowel is resected, and primary anastomoses can be performed. If the viability of the remaining bowel is in question, a second-look operation is performed within 24 to 48 hours.

In patients without peritoneal findings, anticoagulation with IV UFH is promptly initiated. Patients are maintained on bowel rest and undergo fluid resuscitation. Close clinical observation is warranted with serial abdominal examinations. Once the patient's clinical status improves, oral intake can be carefully started. The patient is transitioned to oral anticoagulation over 3 to 4 days and is usually maintained on lifelong oral anticoagulation therapy.

VARICOSE VEINS

Varicose veins are a common medical condition present in at least 10% of the general population.[86] The findings of varicose veins may

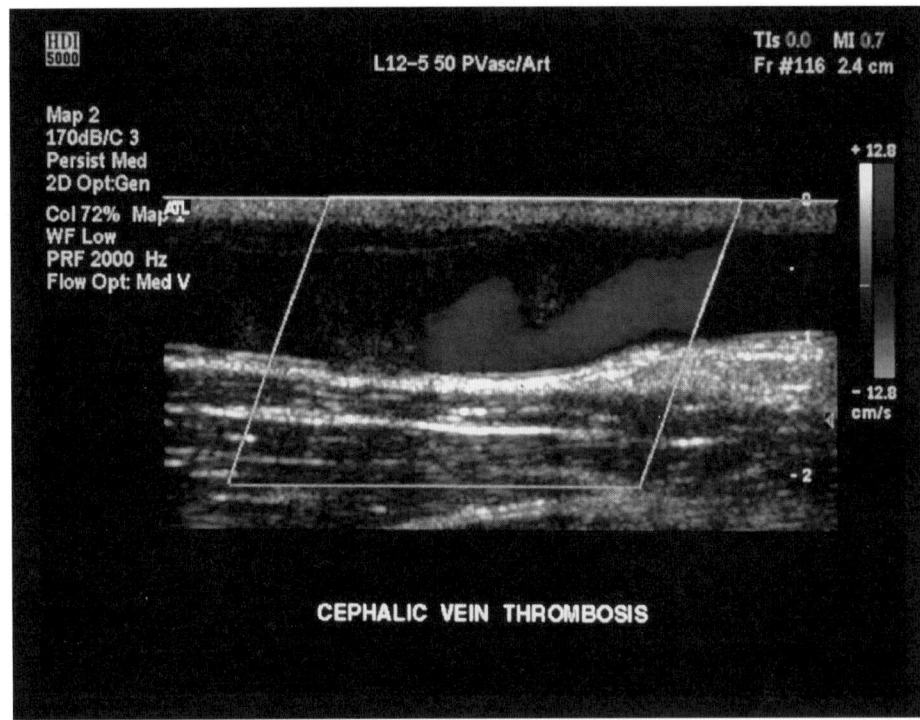

FIG. 24-12. Duplex ultrasound of a cephalic vein containing thrombus.

include dilated and tortuous veins, telangiectasias, and fine reticular varicosities. Risk factors for varicose veins include obesity, female sex, inactivity, and family history.[87] Varicose veins can be classified as primary or secondary. Primary varicose veins result from intrinsic abnormalities of the venous wall, whereas secondary varicose veins are associated with deep and/or superficial venous insufficiency.

In addition to noting the unsightly appearance, patients with varicose veins may complain of aching, heaviness, pruritus, and early fatigue of the affected leg. These symptoms worsen with prolonged standing and sitting and are relieved by elevation of the leg above the level of the heart. A mild amount of edema is often present. More severe signs include thrombophlebitis, hyperpigmentation, lipodermatosclerosis, ulceration, and bleeding from attenuated vein clusters.

An important component of treatment for patients with varicose veins is the use of elastic compression stockings. Patients may be prescribed elastic stockings with compression ranging from 20 to 30, 30 to 40, or even 40 to 50 mmHg. Stockings range in length from knee high to waist high, and they should be able to cover the symptomatic varices. The majority of patients may be managed without additional therapy.

Additional interventions are warranted in patients whose symptoms worsen or are unrelieved despite compression therapy or who have signs of lipodermatosclerosis. Cosmetic concerns also often lead to intervention. Varicose veins may be managed by injection sclerotherapy or surgical therapy or a combination of both techniques. Injection sclerotherapy can be successful in varicose veins <3 mm in diameter and in telangiectatic vessels. Sclerotherapy acts by destroying the venous endothelium. Sclerosing agents include hypertonic saline, sodium tetradecyl sulfate, and polidocanol. Concentrations of 11.7 to 23.4% hypertonic saline, 0.125 to 0.250% sodium tetradecyl sulfate, and 0.5% polidocanol are used for telangiectasias. Larger varicose veins require higher concentrations: 23.4% hypertonic saline, 0.50 to 1% sodium tetradecyl sulfate, and 0.75 to 1.0% polidocanol.[83] Elastic bandages are wrapped around the leg after injection and worn continuously for 3 to 5 days to produce apposition of the inflamed vein walls and prevent thrombus formation. After the bandages are removed, elastic compression stockings should be worn for a minimum of 2 weeks. Complications from sclerotherapy include allergic reaction, pigmentation, thrombophlebitis, DVT, and possible skin necrosis.

Patients with symptomatic great or small saphenous vein reflux may be treated with endovenous ablation techniques or surgical removal. Endovenous laser treatment and radiofrequency ablation (RFA) have gained in popularity in the past several years. With either technique, the distal thigh or proximal calf GSV is punctured with a 21-gauge needle under ultrasound guidance. A sheath is placed over a guidewire, and the laser fiber or RFA catheter is advanced until it is near to, but not at, the saphenofemoral junction. Tumescent anesthetic is administered around the GSV, and the vein is treated as the catheter is withdrawn. Endovenous laser treatment and RFA result in durable ablation of the GSV, with rates of varicose vein recurrence

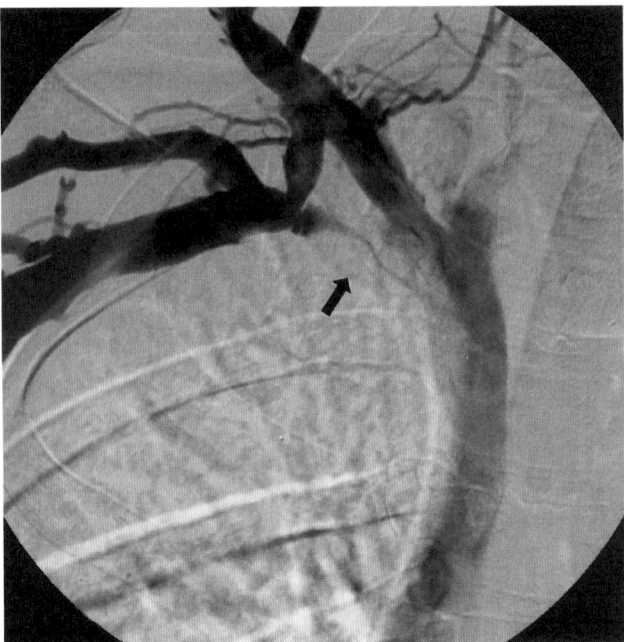

FIG. 24-13. Upper extremity venogram showing stenosis of the right subclavian vein (*arrow*).

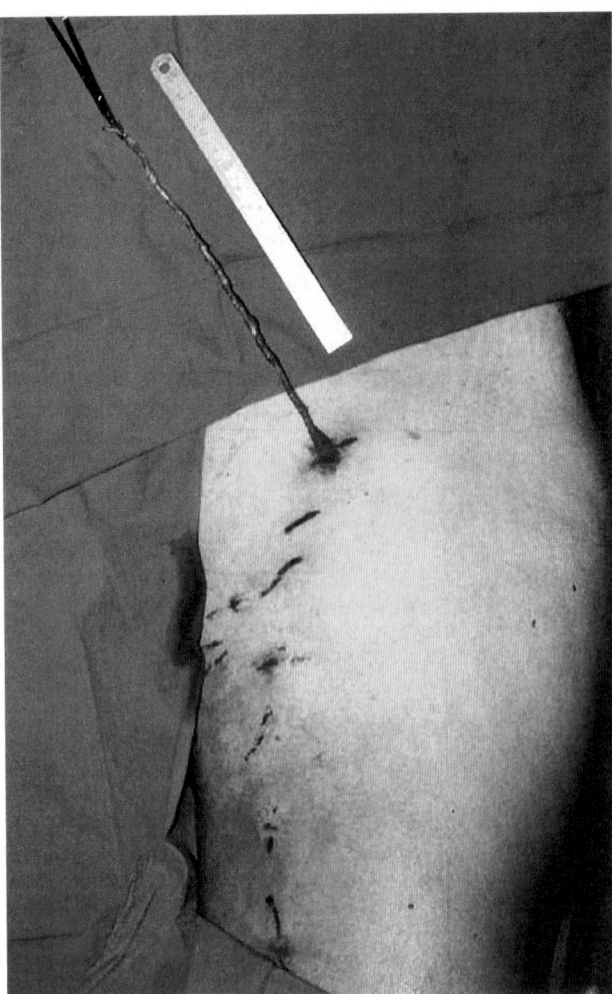

FIG. 24-14. Removal of varicose veins via stab avulsions.

and clinical severity scores comparable to those seen with open surgery.[88,89] Risks of endovenous ablation include DVT, ecchymosis, and saphenous nerve injury.

Saphenous vein ligation and stripping is still the more commonly performed procedure worldwide, and it may be the preferred therapy for patients with GSVs of very large diameter (>2 cm). Surgical removal of the GSV usually is performed via small incisions placed medially in the groin and just below the knee. The GSV is removed using a blunt tip catheter or an invagination pin stripper. Complications associated with GSV stripping include ecchymosis, lymphocele formation, DVT, infection, and saphenous nerve injury. GSV stripping is associated with a lower rate of recurrence of varicose veins and a better quality of life than saphenofemoral junction ligation alone.

Larger varicose veins are best treated by surgical excision using the "stab avulsion" technique. Stab avulsions are performed by making 2-mm incisions directly over branch varicosities, and the varicosity is dissected from the surrounding subcutaneous tissue as far proximally and distally as possible through the small incisions (Fig. 24-14). In most cases the vein is simply avulsed with no attempt at ligation. Bleeding is easily controlled with leg elevation, manual compression, and preprocedure tumescent anesthesia.

CHRONIC VENOUS INSUFFICIENCY

Chronic venous insufficiency (CVI) is a major and costly medical problem, affecting an estimated 600,000 people in the United States.[90] Patients complain of leg fatigue, discomfort, and heaviness. Signs of CVI may include varicose veins, pigmentation, lipodermatosclerosis,

and venous ulceration. Importantly, severe CVI can be present without varicose veins. Chronic venous ulcers carry significant negative physical, financial, and psychologic implications. A quality-of-life study reported that 65% of patients with chronic leg ulcers had severe pain, 81% had decreased mobility, and 100% experienced a negative impact of their disease on their work capacity.[91] The socioeconomic impact of chronic venous leg ulcers is staggering, with an estimated 2 million workdays lost per year.[92] The annual health care cost in the United States to treat CVI is estimated at $1 billion.[93]

The signs and symptoms of CVI can be attributed to venous reflux, venous obstruction, calf muscle pump dysfunction, or a combination of these factors, as well as loss of venous wall elasticity.[94] In the majority of patients with CVI, the most important factor appears to be venous reflux. Venous reflux results from abnormalities of the venous valve and can be classified as primary or secondary. Primary valvular reflux or incompetence is diagnosed when there is no known underlying cause of valvular dysfunction. Secondary valvular reflux is diagnosed when an identifiable cause is present. The most frequent secondary cause is DVT, which can lead to the dysfunction of venous valves. Signs of CVI include edema, hyperpigmentation, and ulceration.

Evaluation of Venous Insufficiency

Early diagnostic studies to evaluate CVI required invasive measurements of ambulatory venous pressure (AVP) and venous recovery time (VRT). To measure AVP and VRT, a needle is inserted into a dorsal foot vein and connected to a pressure transducer. Pressures measured in the dorsal veins of the foot are thought to reflect those in the deep veins of the calf. Once the needle is placed, the patient is asked to perform 10 tiptoe exercises. Initially there is often a slight upward deflection of pressure with the onset of exercise. With each subsequent tiptoe maneuver, the measured pressure should decrease. After approximately 10 tiptoes, the measured pressure stabilizes and reflects a balance of venous inflow and outflow. The pressure at this point is the AVP, which is measured in millimeters of mercury. The patient is then asked to stop exercising to allow the vein to fill with return of the venous pressure to baseline. The time required for the venous pressure to return from the AVP level to 90% of baseline pressure is referred to as the *VRT*. Elevations of AVP indicate the presence of venous hypertension. The magnitude of AVP reflects the severity of CVI. There is an 80% incidence of venous ulceration in patients with an AVP of >80 mmHg.[95]

Plethysmography in Venous Insufficiency

Noninvasive plethysmographic methods based on the measurement of volume changes in the leg have been used to evaluate CVI. Venous photoplethysmography indirectly evaluates venous function through the use of infrared light. A light-emitting diode is placed just above the medial malleolus and the patient then performs a series of tiptoe maneuvers. Photoplethysmography does not give accurate AVP measurements but does provide adequate VRT determinations. In limbs with CVI, VRT is shortened compared with that in a normal limb. AVP and VRT are measures of overall function in the lower extremity venous system. They cannot localize the site of reflux or evaluate the function of the calf pump in patients with CVI.

Air plethysmography can be used to assess calf pump function as well as venous reflux and overall lower extremity venous function.[96] An air-filled plastic pressure bladder is placed on the calf to detect volume changes in the leg during a standard set of maneuvers. The patient is first supine and then the leg is elevated and the minimum volume of venous blood recorded. The patient is then asked to assume an upright position with the examined leg nonweightbearing. The venous volume in the examined leg is determined when the volume curve flattens out. The venous filling index (VFI) is calculated by dividing the maximum venous volume by the time required to achieve maximum venous volume. The VFI is a measure of reflux. Next, the patient performs a single tiptoe maneuver and the ejection fraction (EF) is determined. The EF is the volume change between the recorded volume before and after the tiptoe maneuver and is a

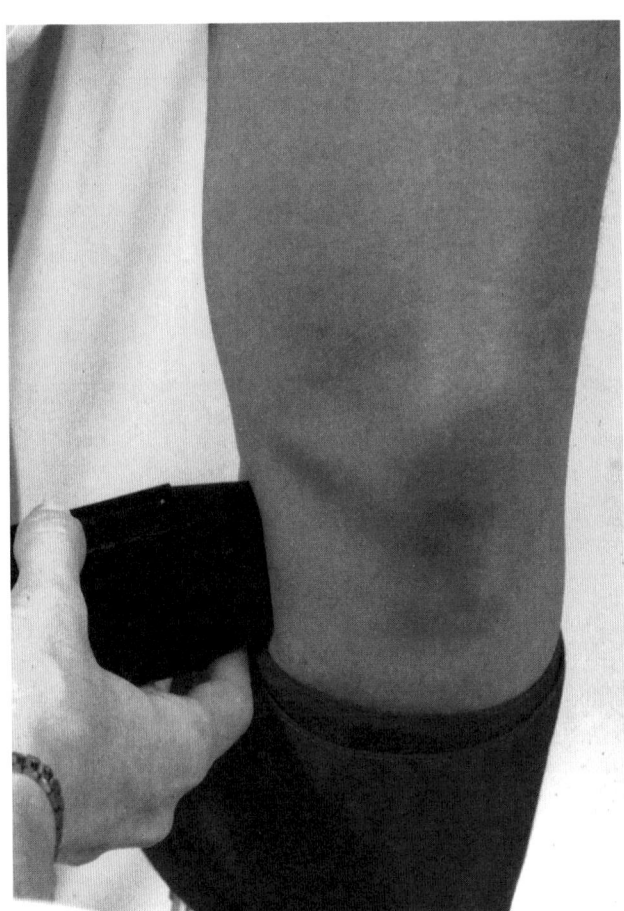

FIG. 24-15. Evaluation of a patient with chronic venous insufficiency with duplex ultrasonography.

measure of calf pump function. At this point, the veins of the leg are allowed to refill. The patient then performs 10 tiptoe maneuvers, and the residual volume fraction is calculated by dividing the venous volume in the leg after 10 tiptoe exercises by the venous volume present before the exercises. The residual volume fraction is a reflection of overall venous function. Theoretically, patients with increased VFIs and normal EFs (indicating the presence of reflux with normal calf pump function) would benefit from antireflux surgery, whereas patients with normal VFIs and diminished EFs would not.

Venous Duplex Ultrasound

In addition to identifying patients with DVT, DUS can be used to evaluate reflux in individual venous segments of the leg. The examination is performed with the patient in the standing position and the examined leg in a nonweightbearing position. Pneumatic pressure cuffs of appropriate size are placed around the thigh, calf, and forefoot. The ultrasound transducer is positioned over the venous segment to be examined, just proximal to the pneumatic cuff (Fig. 24-15). The cuff is then inflated to a standard pressure for 3 seconds and then rapidly deflated. Ninety-five percent of normal venous valves close within 0.5 second.[97] The presence of reflux for >0.5 second is considered abnormal. Typically, the common femoral, femoral, popliteal, and posterior tibial veins, as well as the great and small saphenous veins, are evaluated in a complete examination.

Nonoperative Treatment of Chronic Venous Insufficiency
Compression Therapy

Compression therapy is the mainstay of CVI management. Compression can be achieved using a variety of techniques, including elastic compression stockings, paste gauze boots (Unna's boots), multilayer elastic wraps or dressings (Fig. 24-16), and pneumatic compression devices. The exact mechanism by which compression therapy can improve CVI remains uncertain. An improvement in skin and subcutaneous tissue microcirculatory hemodynamics as well as a direct effect on subcutaneous pressure have been hypothesized as the mechanism of compression therapy.[98] Clinically, routine use of elastic and nonelastic bandages reduces lower extremity edema in patients with CVI. In addition, supine perimalleolar subcutaneous pressure has been demonstrated to increase with elastic compression.[99] With edema reduction, cutaneous metabolism may improve due to enhanced diffusion of oxygen and other nutrients to the cellular elements of skin and subcutaneous tissues. Increases in subcutaneous tissue pressure with elastic compression bandages may counteract transcapillary Starling forces, which favor leakage of fluid out of the capillary.

Before the initiation of therapy for CVI, patients must be educated about their chronic disease and the need to comply with their treatment plan to heal ulcers and prevent recurrence. A definitive diagnosis of venous ulceration must be made before treatment is initiated. A detailed history should be obtained from a patient presenting with lower extremity ulcerations, including medications used and associated medical conditions that may promote lower extremity ulceration. Arterial insufficiency is assessed by physical examination or noninvasive studies. In addition, systemic conditions that affect wound healing and leg edema, such as diabetes mellitus, immunosuppression, malnutrition, and congestive heart failure, should be improved as much as possible.

Compression therapy is most commonly achieved with graduated elastic compression stockings. Graduated elastic compression stockings, initially developed by Conrad Jobst in the 1950s, were made to simulate the gradient of hydrostatic forces exerted by water in a swimming pool. Elastic compression stockings are available in various compositions, strengths, and lengths, and can be customized for a particular patient.

The benefits of elastic compression stocking therapy for the treatment of CVI and healing of ulcerations have been well documented.[100–103] In a retrospective study involving 113 venous ulcer patients,[101] the use of below-knee, 30- to 40-mmHg elastic compression stockings, after edema and cellulitis were first resolved if present, resulted in 93% healing. Complete ulcer healing occurred in

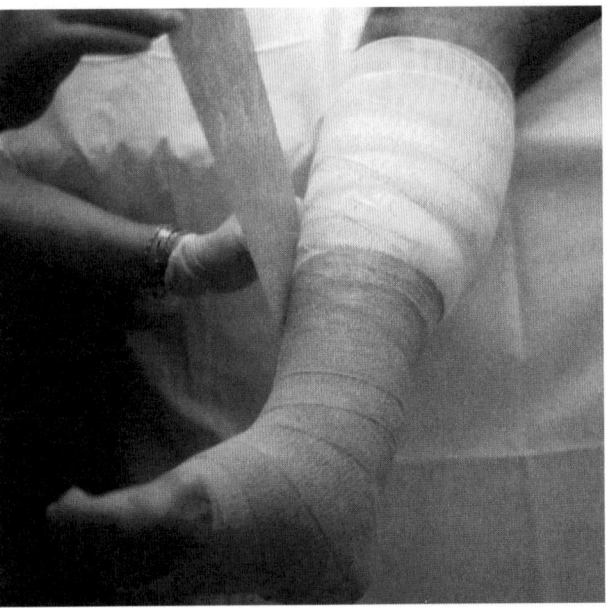

FIG. 24-16. Multilayered dressing for treatment of chronic venous insufficiency.

99 of 102 patients (97%) who were compliant with stocking use vs. 6 of 11 patients (55%) who were noncompliant (*P* <.0001). The mean time to ulcer healing was 5 months. The rate of ulcer recurrence was lower in patients who were compliant with their compression therapy. By life table analysis, ulcer recurrence was 29% at 5 years for compliant patients and 100% at 3 years for noncompliant patients. In more recent studies, the reported rate of venous ulcer healing with compression therapy is approximately 40 to 50% at 6 months.[104,105]

In addition to promoting ulcer healing, elastic compression therapy can also improve quality of life in patients with CVI. In one prospective study,[106] 112 patients with CVI documented by DUS were administered a questionnaire to quantify the symptoms of swelling, pain, skin discoloration, cosmesis, activity tolerance, depression, and sleep alterations. Patients were treated with 30- to 40-mmHg elastic compression stockings. There were overall improvements in symptom severity scores at 1 month after initiation of treatment. Further improvements were noted at 16 months after treatment.

Patient compliance with compression therapy is crucial in treating venous leg ulcers. Many patients are initially intolerant of compression in areas of hypersensitivity adjacent to an active ulcer or at sites of previously healed ulcers. They may also have difficulty applying elastic stockings. To improve compliance, patients should be instructed to wear their stockings initially only as long as it is easily tolerated and then gradually to increase the amount of time the stockings are worn. Alternatively, patients can be fitted with lower-strength stockings initially followed by introduction of higher-strength stockings over a period of several weeks. Many commercially available devices, such as silk inner toe liners, stockings with zippered sides (Fig. 24-17), and metal fitting aids (Fig. 24-18), are available to assist patients in applying elastic stockings.

Another method of compression was developed by the German dermatologist Paul Gerson Unna in 1896. Unna's boot has been used for many years to treat venous ulcers and is available in many versions. A typical Unna's boot consists of a three-layer dressing and requires application by trained personnel. A rolled gauze bandage impregnated with calamine, zinc oxide, glycerin, sorbitol, gelatin, and magnesium aluminum silicate is first applied with graded compression from the forefoot to just below the knee. The next layer consists of a 4-in-wide continuous gauze dressing followed by an outer layer of elastic wrap, also applied with graded compression. The bandage becomes stiff after drying and the rigidity may aid in preventing

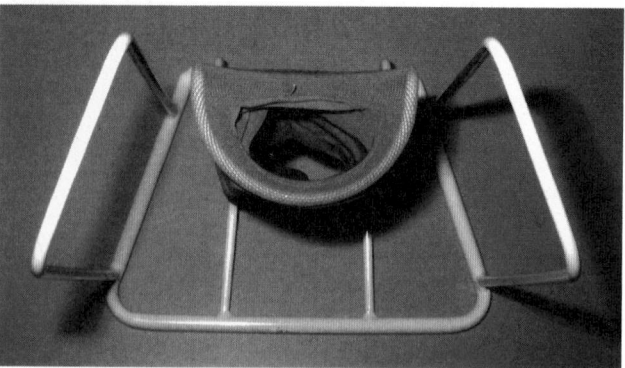

FIG. 24-18. Metal fitting aid to assist in placement of elastic compression stockings.

edema formation. Unna's boot is changed weekly, or sooner if the patient experiences significant drainage from the ulcer bed.

Once applied, Unna's boot requires minimal patient involvement and provides continuous compression and topical therapy. However, Unna's boot has several disadvantages. It is uncomfortable to wear because of its bulkiness, which may affect patient compliance. In addition, the ulcer cannot be monitored after the boot is applied, the technique is labor intensive, and the degree of compression provided is operator dependent. Occasionally, patients may develop contact dermatitis to the components of Unna's boot, which may require discontinuation of therapy.

The efficacy of Unna's dressing has been studied. A retrospective 15-year survey encompassing 998 patients with one or more venous ulcers treated weekly with Unna's dressing[107] reported that 73% of ulcers healed in patients who returned for more than one treatment. The median time to healing for individual ulcers was 9 weeks. Unna's dressing has been compared to other forms of treatment. A randomized, prospective study[108] comparing Unna's boot to polyurethane foam dressing in 36 patients with venous ulcers demonstrated superior healing over 12 months in patients treated with Unna's boot (94.7% vs. 41.2%).

Other forms of compression dressing available to treat CVI include multilayered dressings and legging orthoses. The purported advantages of multilayered dressings include maintenance of compression for a longer period of time, more even distribution of compression, and better absorption of wound exudates. However, the efficacy of multilayered dressings depends on the wrapping technique of health care personnel. A commercially available legging orthosis consisting of multiple adjustable loop-and-hook closure compression bands provides compression similar to that of Unna's boot and can be applied daily by the patient.[109]

Skin Substitutes

Several types of skin substitutes are commercially available or under clinical study in the United States.[92] Bioengineered skin ranges in composition from acellular skin substitutes to partial living skin substitutes. Their mechanism of action in healing venous ulcers is uncertain; however, they may serve as delivery vehicles for various growth factors and cytokines important in wound healing.

Apligraf is a commercially available bilayered living skin construct that closely approximates human skin for use in the treatment of venous ulcers. It contains a protective stratum corneum and a keratinocyte-containing epidermis overlying a dermis consisting of dermal fibroblasts in a collagen matrix.[110] Apligraf is between 0.5 mm and 1.0 mm thick and is supplied as a disk of living tissue on an agarose gel nutrient medium. It must be used within 5 days of release from the manufacturer[110] (Fig. 24-19). The disk is easily handled and applied, and easily conforms to irregularly contoured ulcer beds.

A prospective randomized study comparing multilayer compression therapy alone to treatment with Apligraf in addition to multi-

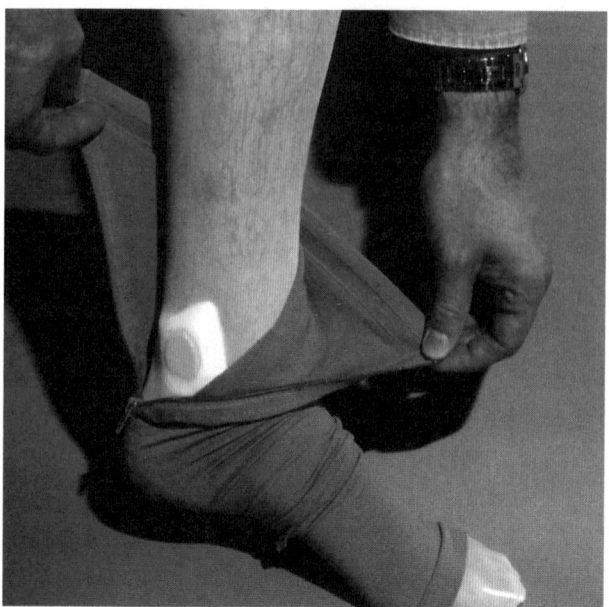

FIG. 24-17. Elastic compression stocking with zippered side to facilitate treatment of chronic venous insufficiency.

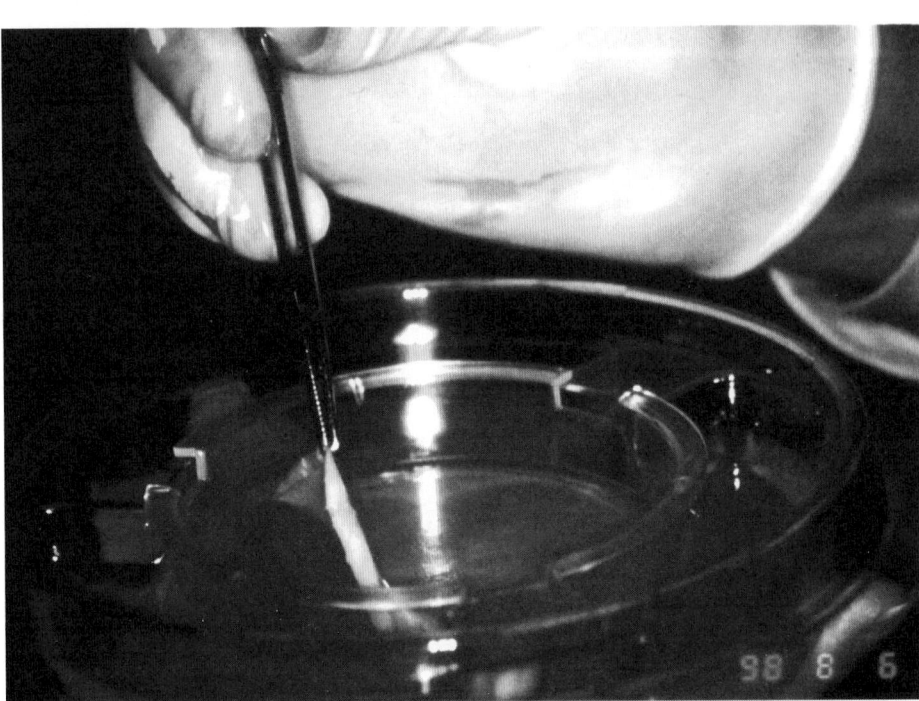

FIG. 24-19. Apligraf skin graft material supplied as a disk on an agarose gel nutrient medium.

layered compression therapy has been performed to assess the efficacy of Apligraf in the treatment of venous ulcers.[104] More patients treated with Apligraf had ulcer healing at 6 months (63% vs. 49%, $P = .02$). The median time to complete ulcer closure was significantly shorter in patients treated with Apligraf (61 days vs. 181 days, $P = .003$). The ulcers that showed the greatest benefit with the living skin construct were ones that were large and deep (>1000 mm^2) or were longstanding (>6 months). No evidence of rejection or sensitization has been reported in response to Apligraf application.

Surgical Treatment of Chronic Venous Insufficiency

Perforator Vein Ligation

Incompetence of the perforating veins connecting the superficial and deep venous systems of the lower extremities has been implicated in the development of venous ulcers. The classic open technique described by Linton in 1938 for perforator vein ligation has a high incidence of wound complications and has largely been abandoned.[111] A minimally invasive technique termed *subfascial endoscopic perforator vein surgery* (SEPS) has evolved with the improvement in endoscopic equipment.

DUS is performed preoperatively in patients undergoing SEPS to document deep venous competence and to identify perforating veins in the posterior compartment. The patient is positioned on the operating table with the affected leg elevated at 45 to 60 degrees. An Esmarch bandage and a thigh tourniquet are used to exsanguinate the limb. The knee is then flexed, and two small incisions are made in the proximal medial leg away from areas of maximal induration at the ankle. Laparoscopic trocars are then positioned, and the subfascial dissection is performed with a combination of blunt and sharp dissection. Carbon dioxide is then used to insufflate the subfascial space. The thigh tourniquet is inflated to prevent air embolism. The perforators are then identified and doubly clipped and divided. After completion of the procedure, the leg is wrapped in a compression bandage for 5 days postoperatively.

In a report from a large North American registry of 146 patients undergoing SEPS[112] (Fig. 24-20), healing was achieved in 88% of ulcers (75 of 85) at 1 year. Adjunctive procedures, primarily superficial vein stripping, were performed in 72% of patients. Ulcer recurrence was predicted to be 16% at 1 year and 28% at 2 years by life table analysis. The efficacy of the technique has not been confirmed in a randomized trial.

Venous Reconstruction

In the absence of significant deep vein valvular incompetence, saphenous vein stripping and perforator vein ligation can be effective in the treatment of CVI. However, in patients with a combination of superficial and deep vein valvular incompetence, the addition of deep vein valvular reconstruction theoretically may improve ulcer healing.[113] Numerous techniques of deep vein valve correction have been reported. These techniques consist of repair of existing valves, transplant of venous segments from the arm, and transposition of an incompetent vein onto an adjacent competent vein. A method in which cryopreserved venous valve allografts are placed below incompetent vein segments surgically or percutaneously is currently in the early phases of development but does not seem effective.[114]

Successful long-term outcomes of 60 to 80% have been reported for venous valve reconstructions by internal suture repair.[113,115,116] However, among patients who initially had ulceration, 40 to 50% still had persistence or recurrence of ulcers in the long term.[115,116] Valve transplantation involves replacement of a segment of incompetent femoral vein or popliteal vein with a segment of axillary or brachial vein with competent valves. Early results are similar to those for venous valve reconstruction.[113,115,116] However, in the long term, the transplanted venous segments tend to develop incompetence, and long-term outcomes are poorer than those for venous valve reconstructions. The outcomes for venous transposition are similar to those for valve transplantation.

LYMPHEDEMA

Pathophysiology

Lymphedema is extremity swelling that results from a reduction in lymphatic transport, with resultant pooling of lymph within the interstitial space. It is caused by anatomic problems such as lymphatic hypoplasia, functional insufficiency, or absence of lymphatic valves.

The original classification system, described by Allen, is based on the cause of the lymphedema. Primary lymphedema is further subdi-

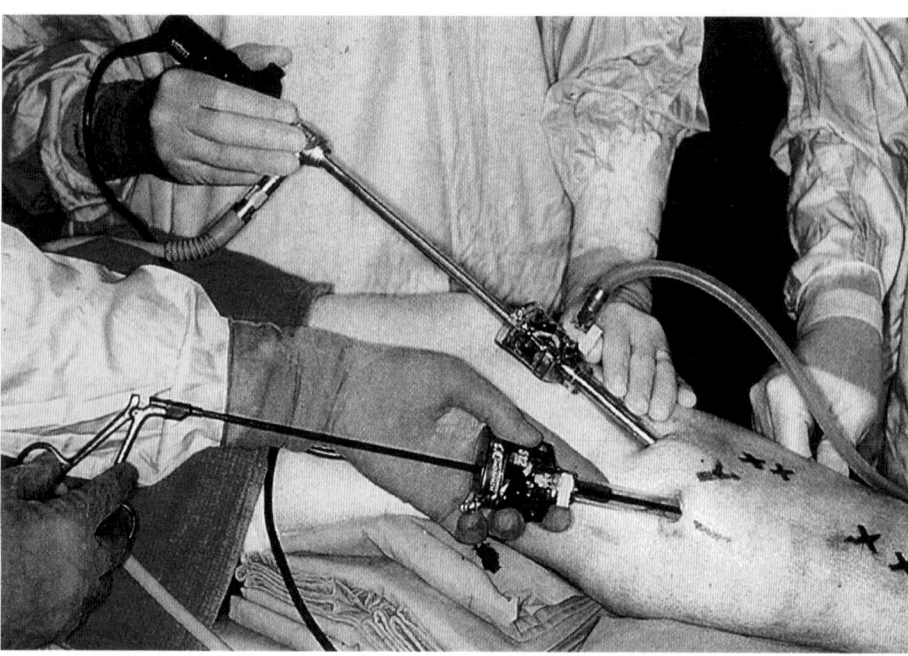

FIG. 24-20. Trocar placement for subfascial endoscopic perforator vein surgery.

vided into congenital lymphedema, lymphedema praecox, and lymphedema tarda. *Congenital lymphedema* may involve a single lower extremity, multiple limbs, the genitalia, or the face. The edema typically develops before 2 years of age and may be associated with specific hereditary syndromes (Turner syndrome, Milroy syndrome, Klippel-Trénaunay-Weber syndrome). *Lymphedema praecox* is the most common form of primary lymphedema, accounting for 94% of cases. Lymphedema praecox is far more common in women, with the gender ratio favoring women 10:1. The onset is during childhood or the teenage years, and the swelling involves the foot and calf. *Lymphedema tarda* is uncommon, accounting for <10% of cases of primary lymphedema. The onset of edema is after 35 years of age.

Secondary lymphedema is far more common than primary lymphedema. Secondary lymphedema develops as a result of lymphatic obstruction or disruption. Axillary node dissection leading to lymphedema of the arm is the most common cause of secondary lymphedema in the United States. Other causes of secondary lymphedema include radiation therapy, trauma, infection, and malignancy. Globally, filariasis (caused by *Wuchereria bancrofti*, *Brugia malayi*, and *Brugia timori*) is the most common cause of secondary lymphedema.

Clinical Diagnosis

In most patients the diagnosis of lymphedema can be made based on the history and physical examination alone. Patients commonly complain of heaviness and fatigue in the affected extremity. The limb size increases throughout the day and decreases over the course of the night when the patient is in bed. The limb, however, never completely normalizes. In the lower extremity the swelling involves the dorsum of the foot, and the toes have a squared-off appearance. In advanced cases, hyperkeratosis of the skin develops, and fluid weeps from lymph-filled vesicles (Fig. 24-21).

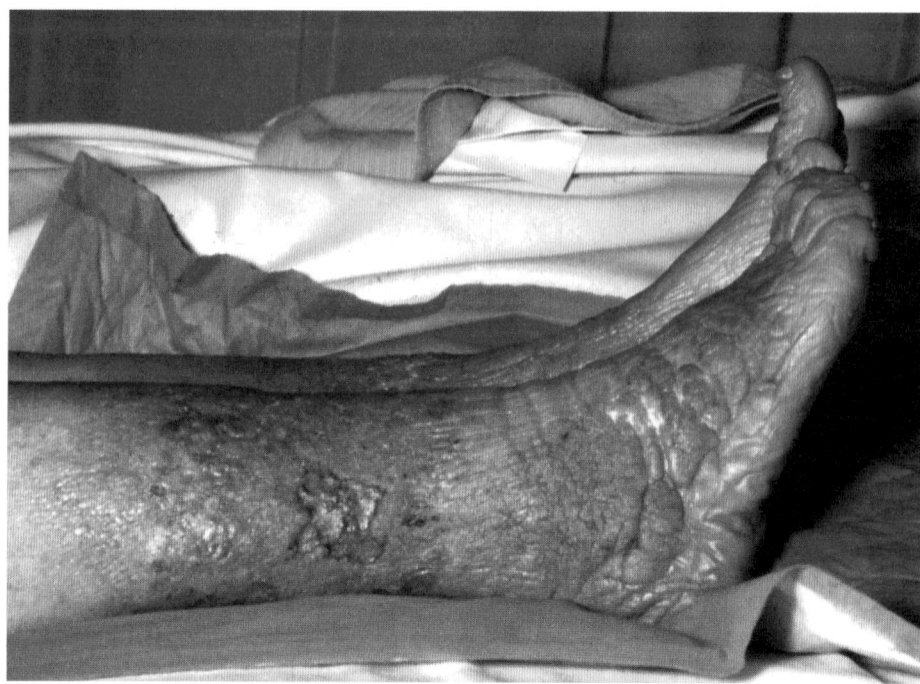

FIG. 24-21. Hyperkeratosis of the skin in a patient with longstanding lymphedema.

Recurrent cellulitis is a common complication of lymphedema. Repeated infection results in further lymphatic damage, worsening existing disease. The clinical presentation of cellulitis ranges from subtle erythema and worsening of edema to a rapidly progressive soft tissue infection with systemic toxicity.

Many medical conditions can cause edema. If the symptoms are mild, distinguishing lymphedema from other causes of leg swelling can be difficult. Venous insufficiency is often confused with lymphedema. However, patients with advanced venous insufficiency typically have lipodermatosclerosis in the gaiter region, skin ulceration, and/or varicose veins. Bilateral pitting edema is typically associated with congestive heart failure, renal failure, or a hypoproteinemic state.

Radiologic Diagnosis
Duplex Ultrasound

When a patient is evaluated for edema, it is often difficult to distinguish the early stages of lymphedema from venous insufficiency. Duplex ultrasound of the venous system can determine if there is concomitant venous thrombosis or venous reflux, perhaps contributing to extremity edema. The diagnostic modalities discussed in the following sections have limited use in clinical practice. They are invasive and tedious, and rarely change the management of a patient with lymphedema. Most physicians rely on the patient's history and physical examination alone to make the diagnosis of lymphedema.

Lymphoscintigraphy

Lymphoscintigraphy has become the most commonly used diagnostic test to identify lymphatic abnormalities. It has largely replaced lymphangiography. A radiolabeled sulfur colloid (technetium 99m sulfur colloid) is injected into the subdermal, interdigital region of the affected limb. The lymphatic transport is monitored with a whole body gamma camera, and major lymphatics and nodes can be visualized (Fig. 24-22). In normal individuals, tracer activity may be detected in the inguinal region within 15 to 60 minutes. Within 3 hours, uptake should be present in the pelvic and abdominal lymph nodes. In patients with lymphedema, various patterns may be seen on lymphoscintigraphy. There may be delayed or absent transport to the inguinal nodes. Increased cutaneous collaterals may be seen with obstruction of the primary axial channels. There may be localized regions of reduced uptake in patients with prior node dissection or radiation therapy.

Lymphangiography

Radiologic lymphology is performed by first visualizing the lymphatics by injecting colored dye into the hand or foot. The visualized lymphatic segment is exposed through a small incision and cannulated with a 27- to 30-gauge needle. An oil-based dye is then injected slowly into the lymphatics over several hours. The lymphatic channels and nodes are then visualized with traditional radiographs (Figs. 24-23 and 24-24). Lymphangiography is reserved for patients with lymphangiectasia or lymphatic fistulas, and patients who are being considered for microvascular reconstruction.

Management

An important aspect of the management of lymphedema is patient understanding that there is no cure for lymphedema. The primary goals of treatment are to minimize swelling and to prevent recurrent infections. Controlling the chronic limb swelling can improve discomfort, heaviness, and tightness, and potentially reduce the progression of disease.[117]

Compression Garments

Graded compression stockings are widely used in the treatment of lymphedema. The stockings reduce the amount of swelling in the

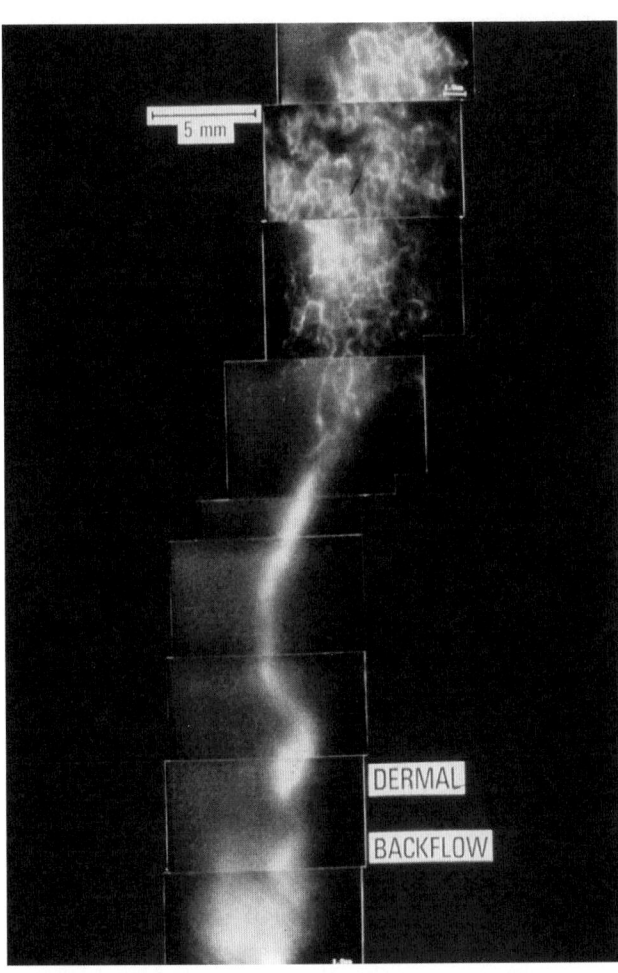

FIG. 24-22. Lymphoscintigraphy of the lower extremity.

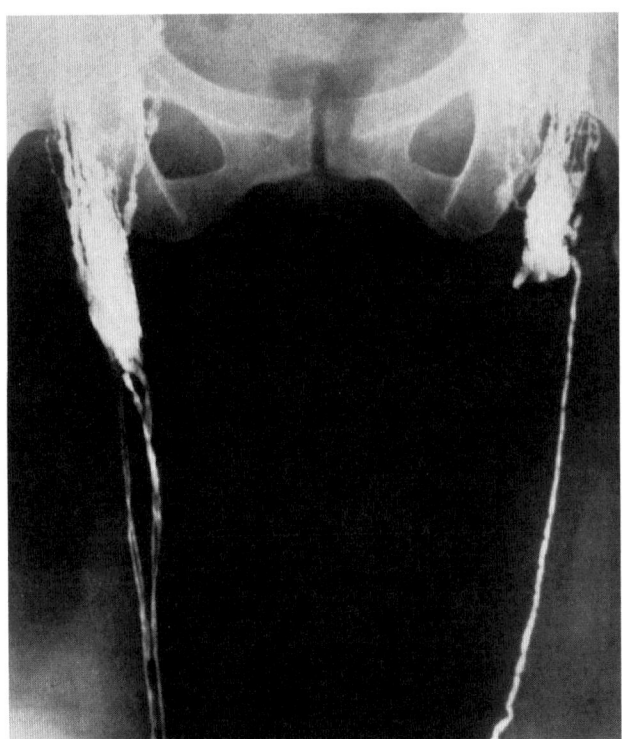

FIG. 24-23. Normal lymphangiogram of the pelvis.

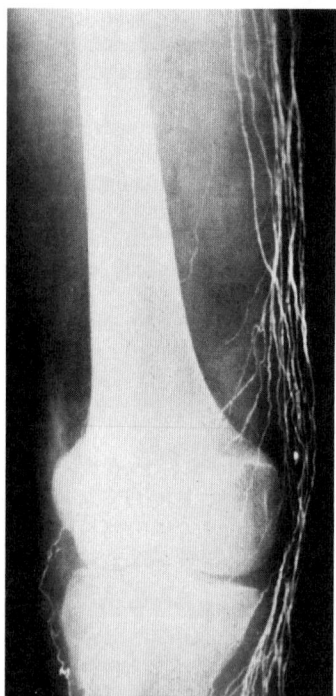
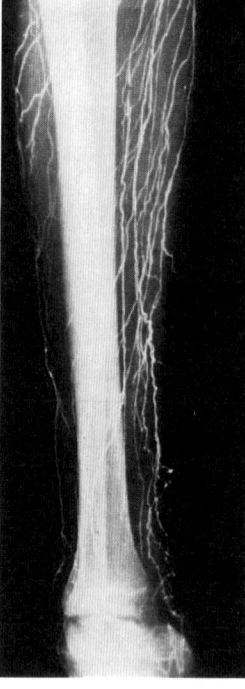

FIG. 24-24. Normal lymphangiogram of the thigh and lower leg.

involved extremity by preventing the accumulation of edema while the extremity is dependent. When worn daily, compression stockings have been associated with long-term maintenance of reduced limb circumference.[118] They may also protect the tissues against chronically elevated intrinsic pressures, which lead to thickening of the skin and subcutaneous tissue.[119] Compression stockings also offer a degree of protection against external trauma.

The amount of compression required for controlling lymphedema ranges from 20 to 60 mmHg and varies among patients. The stockings can be custom made or prefabricated and are available in above- and below-knee lengths. The stockings should be worn during waking hours. The garments should be replaced approximately every 6 months when they lose elasticity.

Bedrest and Leg Elevation

Elevation is an important aspect of controlling lower extremity swelling and is often the first recommended intervention. However, continuous elevation throughout the day can interfere with quality of life more than lymphedema itself. Elevation is an adjunct to lymphedema therapy but is not the mainstay of treatment.

Sequential External Pneumatic Compression

The use of intermittent pneumatic compression with a single-chamber or multichamber pump temporarily reduces edema and provides another adjunct to the use of compression stockings. These devices have been shown to be effective in reducing limb volume[120,121]; however, use of compression stockings is necessary to maintain the volume reduction when the patient is no longer supine. Typically, intermittent pneumatic compression is used for 4 to 6 hours per day at home when the patient is supine.

Lymphatic Massage

Manual lymphatic drainage is a form of massage developed by Vodder[122] that is directed at reducing edema. In combination with the use of compression stockings, manual lymphatic drainage is associated with a long-term reduction in edema and fewer infections per patient per year.[123]

Antibiotic Therapy

Patients with lymphedema are at increased risk of developing cellulitis in the affected extremity. Recurrent infection can damage the lymphatics, aggravating the edema. *Staphylococcus* and beta-hemolytic *Streptococcus* are the most common organisms causing soft tissue infection. Aggressive antibiotic therapy is recommended at the earliest signs or symptoms of cellulitis. The drug of choice is penicillin, usually 500 mg orally three to four times per day. Patients with a history of lymphedema and recurrent cellulitis should be prescribed antibiotics that they can keep at home and begin taking at the first sign of infection.

Surgery

A variety of surgical procedures have been devised for the treatment of lymphedema. Surgical treatment involves either excision of extra tissue[124] or anastomosis of a lymphatic vessel to another lymphatic or vein.[125] In excisional procedures, part or all of the edematous tissue is removed. This does not improve lymphatic drainage but debulks redundant tissue. The microsurgical procedures involve the creation of a lymphaticolymphatic or lymphaticovenous anastomosis, which theoretically improves lymphatic drainage. No long-term follow-up data are available for these interventions, and therefore operative therapy for lymphedema is not well accepted worldwide. Furthermore, operative intervention can further obliterate lymphatic channels, worsening the edema.[126]

Summary

Lymphedema is a chronic condition caused by ineffective lymphatic transport, which results in edema and skin damage. Lymphedema is not curable, but the symptoms can be controlled with a combination of elastic compression stockings, limb elevation, pneumatic compression, and massage. Controlling the edema protects the skin and potentially prevents cellulitis.

REFERENCES

Entries highlighted in bright blue are key references.

1. Moncada S, Radomski MW, Palmer RM: Endothelium-derived relaxing factor. Identification as nitric oxide and role in the control of vascular tone and platelet function. *Biochem Pharmacol* 37:2495, 1988.
2. van Bemmelen PS, Beach K, Bedford G, et al: The mechanism of venous valve closure. Its relationship to the velocity of reverse flow. *Arch Surg* 125:617, 1990.
3. Moneta GL, Strandness DE Jr.: Basic data concerning noninvasive vascular testing. *Ann Vasc Surg* 3:190, 1989.
4. Bettman MA, Robbins A, Braun SD, et al: Contrast venography of the leg: Diagnostic efficacy, tolerance, and complication rates with ionic and nonionic contrast medial. *Radiology* 165:113, 1987.
5. Fowkes FJ, Price JF, Fowkes FG: Incidence of diagnosed deep vein thrombosis in the general population: Systematic review. *Eur J Vasc Endovasc Surg* 25:1, 2003.
6. Naess IA, Christiansen SC, Romundstad P, et al: Incidence and mortality of venous thrombosis: A population based study. *J Thromb Haemost* 5:692, 2007.
7. Heit JA: The epidemiology of venous thromboembolism in the community: Implications for prevention and management. *J Thromb Thrombolysis* 21:23, 2006.
8. Mohr DN, Silverstein MD, Heit JA, et al: The venous stasis syndrome after deep venous thrombosis or pulmonary embolism: A population-based study. *Mayo Clin Proc* 75:1249, 2000.
9. Rosendaal FR: Risk factors for venous thrombotic disease. *Thromb Haemost* 82:610, 1999.
10. Cushman M, Kuller L, Prentice R, et al: Estrogen plus progestin and risk of venous thrombosis. *JAMA* 292:1573, 2004.
11. Keijzer MB, Borm GF, Blom HJ, et al: No interaction between factor V Leiden and hyperhomocysteinemia or MTHFR 677TT genotype in venous thrombosis. Results of a meta-analysis of published studies and a large case-only study. *Thromb Haemost* 97:32, 2007.

12. Ageno W, Becattini C, Brighton T, et al: Cardiovascular risk factors and venous thromboembolism: A meta-analysis. *Circulation* 117:93, 2008.

13. White R, Zhou H, Romano P: Incidence of idiopathic deep venous thrombosis and secondary thromboembolism among ethnic groups in California. *Ann Intern Med* 128:737, 1998.

14. Bezemer ID, Bare LA, Doggen CJM, et al: Gene variants associated with deep vein thrombosis. *JAMA* 299:106, 2008.

15. Markel A, Manzo RA, Bergelin RO, et al: Pattern and distribution of thrombi in acute venous thrombosis. *Arch Surg* 127:305, 1992.

16. Nicolaides AN, Kakkar VV, Field ES, et al: The origin of deep vein thrombosis: A venographic study. *Br J Radiol* 44:653, 1971.

17. Brockman SK, Vasko JS: The pathologic physiology of phlegmasia cerulea dolens. *Surgery* 59:997, 1966.

18. Lensing AW, Prandoni P, Brandjes D, et al: Detection of deep-vein thrombosis by real-time B-mode ultrasonography. *N Engl J Med* 320:342, 1989.

19. O'Leary DH, Kane RA, Chase BM: A prospective study of the efficacy of B-scan sonography in the detection of deep venous thrombosis in the lower extremities. *J Clin Ultrasound* 16:1, 1988.

20. Mussurakis S, Papaioannou S, Voros D, et al: Compression ultrasonography as a reliable imaging monitor in deep venous thrombosis. *Surg Gynecol Obstet* 171:233, 1990.

21. Habscheid W, Hohmann M, Wilhelm T, et al: Real-time ultrasound in the diagnosis of acute deep venous thrombosis of the lower extremity. *Angiology* 41:599, 1990.

22. Comerota AJ, Katz ML, Grossi RJ, et al: The comparative value of noninvasive testing for diagnosis and surveillance of deep vein thrombosis. *J Vasc Surg* 7:40, 1988.

23. Gomes AS, Webber MM, Buffkin D: Contrast venography vs. radionuclide venography: A study of discrepancies and their possible significance. *Radiology* 142:719, 1982.

24. Hull R, Hirsh J, Sackett DL, et al: Clinical validity of a negative venogram in patients with clinically suspected venous thrombosis. *Circulation* 64:622, 1981.

25. Kearon C, Kahn SR, Agnelli G, et al: Antithrombotic therapy for venous thromboembolic disease: American College of Chest Physicians Evidence-Based Clinical Practice Guidelines (8th edition). *Chest* 133:454S, 2008.

26. Raschke RA, Reilly BM, Guidry JR, et al: The weight-based heparin dosing nomogram compared with a standard care nomogram. A randomized controlled trial. *Ann Intern Med* 119:874, 1993.

27. Hylek EM, Regan S, Henault LE, et al: Challenges to the effective use of unfractionated heparin in the hospitalized management of acute thrombosis. *Arch Intern Med* 163:621, 2003.

28. Amiral J, Bridey F, Dreyfus M, et al: Platelet factor 4 complexed to heparin is the target for antibodies generated in heparin-induced thrombocytopenia. *Thromb Haemost* 68:95, 1992.

29. Warkentin TE, Levine MN, Hirsh J, et al: Heparin-induced thrombocytopenia in patients treated with low-molecular-weight heparin or unfractionated heparin. *N Engl J Med* 332:1330, 1995.

30. Warkentin TE, Kelton JG: Heparin and platelets. *Hematol Oncol Clin North Am* 4:243, 1990.

31. Calaitges JG, Liem TK, Spadone D, et al: The role of heparin-associated antiplatelet antibodies in the outcome of arterial reconstruction. *J Vasc Surg* 29:779, 1999.

32. Gould MK, Dembitzer AD, Doyle RL, et al: Low-molecular-weight heparins compared with unfractionated heparin for treatment of acute deep venous thrombosis: A meta-analysis of randomized, controlled trials. *Ann Intern Med* 130:800, 1999.

33. Dolovich LR, Ginsberg JS, Douketis JD, et al: A meta-analysis comparing low-molecular-weight heparins with unfractionated heparin in the treatment of venous thromboembolism: Examining some unanswered questions regarding location of treatment, product type, and dosing frequency. *Arch Intern Med* 160:181, 2000.

34. Van Dongen CJJ, van der Belt AGM, Prins MH, et al: Fixed dose subcutaneous low molecular weight heparins versus adjusted dose unfractionated heparin for venous thromboembolism. *Cochrane Database Syst Rev* Issue 4:CD001100, 2004. doi:10.1002/14651858.CD001100.pub2.

35. Kikta MJ, Keller MP, Humphrey PW, et al: Can low molecular weight heparins and heparinoids be safely given to patients with heparin-induced thrombocytopenia syndrome? *Surgery* 114:705, 1993.

36. Koopman MM, Prandoni P, Piovella F, et al: Treatment of venous thrombosis with intravenous unfractionated heparin administered in the hospital as compared with subcutaneous low-molecular-weight heparin administered at home. The Tasman Study Group. *N Engl J Med* 334:682, 1996.

37. Levine M, Gent M, Hirsh J, et al: A comparison of low-molecular-weight heparin administered primarily at home with unfractionated heparin administered in the hospital for proximal deep-vein thrombosis. *N Engl J Med* 334:677, 1996.

38. Büller HR, Davidson BL, Decousus H, et al: Fondaparinux or enoxaparin for the initial treatment of symptomatic deep venous thrombosis: A randomized trial. *Ann Intern Med* 140:867, 2004.

39. The Matisse Investigators: Subcutaneous fondaparinux versus intravenous unfractionated heparin in the initial treatment of pulmonary embolism. *N Engl J Med* 349:1695, 2003.

40. Warkentin TE, Maurer BT, Aster RH: Heparin-induced thrombocytopenia associated with fondaparinux. *N Engl J Med* 356:2653, 2007.

41. Kelton JG: The pathophysiology of heparin-induced thrombocytopenia: Biological basis for treatment. *Chest* 127:9, 2005.

42. Ansell J, Hirsh J, Hylek E, et al: Pharmacology and management of the vitamin K antagonists: American College Of Chest Physicians Evidence-Based Clinical Practice Guidelines (8th edition). *Chest* 133:160S, 2008.

43. Schulman S, Rhedin A-S, Lindmarker P, et al: A comparison of six weeks with six months of oral anticoagulant therapy after a first episode of venous thromboembolism. *N Engl J Med* 332:1661, 1995.

44. Research Committee of the British Thoracic Society: Optimal duration of anticoagulation for deep vein thrombosis and pulmonary embolism. *Lancet* 340:873, 1992.

45. Levine MN, Hirsh J, Gent M, et al: Optimal duration of oral anticoagulant therapy: A randomized trial comparing four weeks with three months of warfarin in patients with proximal deep vein thrombosis. *Thromb Haemost* 74:606, 1995.

46. Kearon C, Gent M, Hirsh J, et al: A comparison of three months of anticoagulation with extended anticoagulation for a first episode of idiopathic venous thromboembolism. *N Engl J Med* 340:901, 1999.

47. Agnelli G, Prandoni P, Santamaria MG, et al: Three months versus one year of oral anticoagulant therapy for idiopathic deep venous thrombosis. *N Engl J Med* 345:165, 2001.

48. Ridker PM, Goldhaber SZ, Danielson E, et al: Long-term, low-intensity warfarin therapy for the prevention of recurrent venous thromboembolism. *N Engl J Med* 348:1425, 2003.

49. Kearon C, Ginsber JS, Kovacs MJ, et al: Comparison of low-intensity warfarin therapy with conventional-intensity warfarin therapy for long-term prevention of recurrent venous thromboembolism. *N Engl J Med* 349:631, 2003.

50. Lee AYY, Levine MN, Baker RI, et al: Low-molecular-weight heparin versus a coumarin for the prevention of recurrent venous thromboembolism in patients with cancer. *N Engl J Med* 349:146, 2003.

51. Akl EA, Barba M, Rohilla S, et al: Anticoagulation for the long term treatment of venous thromboembolism in patients with cancer. *Cochrane Database Syst Rev* Issue 2:CD006650, 2008. doi:10.1002/14651858.

52. Watson LI, Armon MP: Thrombolysis for treatment of acute deep vein thrombosis. *Cochrane Database Syst Rev* Issue 4:CD002783, 2004. doi:10.1002/14651858.CD002783.pub2.

53. Mewissen MW, Seabrook GR, Meissner MH, et al: Catheter-directed thrombolysis for lower extremity deep venous thrombosis: Report of a national multicenter registry. *Radiology* 211:39, 1999.

54. Elsharawy M, Elzayat E: Early results of thrombolysis vs anticoagulation in iliofemoral venous thrombosis: A randomised clinical trial. *Eur J Vasc Endovasc Surg* 24:209, 2002.

55. Comerota AJ, Throm RC, Mathias SD, et al: Catheter-directed thrombolysis for iliofemoral deep venous thrombosis improves health-related quality of life. *J Vasc Surg* 32:130, 2000.

56. Lin PH, Zhou W, Dardik A, et al : Catheter-directed thrombolysis versus pharmacomechanical thrombectomy for treatment of symptomatic lower extremity deep venous thrombosis. *Am J Surg* 192:782, 2006.

57. Becker DM, Philbrick JT, Selby JB: Inferior vena cava filters. Indications, safety, effectiveness. *Arch Intern Med* 152:1985, 1992.

58. Decousus H, Leizorovicz A, Parent F, et al: A clinical trial of vena caval filters in the prevention of pulmonary embolism in patients with proximal deep-vein thrombosis. Prévention du Risque d'Embolie Pulmonaire par Interruption Cave Study Group. *N Engl J Med* 338:409, 1998.

59. Plate G, Ohlin P, Eklof B: Pulmonary embolism in acute iliofemoral venous thrombosis. *Br J Surg* 72:912, 1985.

60. Eklof B, Kistner RL, Masuda EM: Surgical treatment of acute iliofemoral deep venous thrombosis, in Gloviczki P, Yao JST (eds): *Handbook of Venous Disorders*. New York: Arnold, 2001, p 202.

61. Juhan CM, Alimi YS, Barthelemy PJ, et al: Late results of iliofemoral venous thrombectomy. *J Vasc Surg* 25:417, 1997.

62. Schmid C, Zietlow S, Wagner TO, et al: Fulminant pulmonary embolism: Symptoms, diagnostics, operative technique, and results. *Ann Thorac Surg* 52:1102, 1991.

63. Kieny R, Charpentier A, Kieny MT: What is the place of pulmonary embolectomy today? *J Cardiovasc Surg* 32:549, 1991.

64. Gulba DC, Schmid C, Borst HG, et al: Medical compared with surgical treatment for massive pulmonary embolism. *Lancet* 343:576, 1994.

65. Schmitz-Rode T, Janssens U, Schild HH, et al: Fragmentation of massive pulmonary embolism using a pigtail rotation catheter. *Chest* 114:1427, 1998.

66. Greenfield LJ, Proctor MC, Williams DM, et al: Long-term experience with transvenous catheter pulmonary embolectomy. *J Vasc Surg* 18:450, 1993.

67. Geerts WH, Bergqvist D, Pineo GF, et al: Prevention of venous thromboembolism: American College of Chest Physicians Evidence-Based Clinical Practice Guidelines (8th edition). *Chest* 133:381S, 2008.

68. Mismetti P, Laporte S, Darmon JY, et al: Meta-analysis of low molecular weight heparin in the prevention of venous thromboembolism in general surgery. *Br J Surg* 88:913, 2001.

69. Agnelli G, Bergqvist D, Cohen AT, et al: Randomized clinical trial of postoperative fondaparinux versus perioperative dalteparin for prevention of venous thromboembolism in high-risk abdominal surgery. *Br J Surg* 92:1212, 2005.

70. Turpie AG, Bauer KA, Caprini JA, et al: Fondaparinux combined with intermittent pneumatic compression versus intermittent pneumatic compression alone for prevention of venous thromboembolism after abdominal surgery: A randomized, double-blind comparison. *J Thromb Haemost* 5:1854, 2007.

71. Rogers FB, Shackford SR, Ricci MA, et al: Routine prophylactic vena cava filter insertion in severely injured trauma patients decreases the incidence of pulmonary embolism. *J Am Coll Surg* 180:641, 1995.

72. Rogers FB, Strindberg G, Shackford SR, et al: Five-year follow-up of prophylactic vena cava filters in high-risk trauma patients. *Arch Surg* 133:406, 1998.

73. Millward SF, Oliva VL, Bell SD, et al: Gunther Tulip retrievable vena cava filter: Results from the Registry of the Canadian Interventional Radiology Association. *J Vasc Intervent Radiol* 12:1053, 2001.

74. Society of American Gastrointestinal and Endoscopic Surgeons: *Guidelines for deep venous thrombosis prophylaxis during laparoscopic surgery*. SAGES publication No. 0016. Los Angeles: SAGES, revised October 2006.

75. Allen AW, Megargell JL, Brown DB, et al: Venous thrombosis associated with the placement of peripherally inserted central catheters. *J Vasc Intervent Radiol* 11:1309, 2000.

76. Chengelis DL, Bendick PJ, Glover JL, et al: Progression of superficial venous thrombosis to deep vein thrombosis. *J Vasc Surg* 24:745, 1996.

77. Lutter KS, Kerr TM, Roedersheimer LR, et al: Superficial thrombophlebitis diagnosed by duplex scanning. *Surgery* 110:42, 1991.

78. Di Nisio M, Wichers IM, Middeldorp S: Treatment of superficial thrombophlebitis of the leg. *Cochrane Database Syst Rev* Issue 2:CD004982, 2007. doi:10.1002/14651858.

79. Lohr JM, McDevitt DT, Lutter KS, et al: Operative management of greater saphenous thrombophlebitis involving the saphenofemoral junction. *Am J Surg* 164:269, 1992.

80. Ascer E, Lorensen E, Pollina RM, et al: Preliminary results of a nonoperative approach to saphenofemoral junction thrombophlebitis. *J Vasc Surg* 22:616, 1995.

81. Horne MK 3rd, May DJ, Alexander HR, et al: Venographic surveillance of tunneled venous access devices in adult oncology patients. *Ann Surg Oncol* 2:174, 1995.

82. Landry GL, Liem TK: Endovascular management of Paget-Schroetter syndrome. *Vascular* 15:290, 2007.

83. Rhee RY, Gloviczki P, Jost C, et al: Acute mesenteric venous thrombosis, in Gloviczki P, Yao JST (eds): *Handbook of Venous Disorders*. New York: Arnold, 2001, p 244.

84. Morasch MD, Ebaugh JL, Chiou AC, et al: Mesenteric venous thrombosis: A changing clinical entity. *J Vasc Surg* 34:680, 2001.

85. Rhee RY, Gloviczki P, Mendonca CT, et al: Mesenteric venous thrombosis: Still a lethal disease in the 1990s. *J Vasc Surg* 20:688, 1994.

86. Burkitt DP: Varicose veins, deep vein thrombosis, and haemorrhoids: Epidemiology and suggested aetiology. *Br Med J* 2:556, 1972.

87. Brand FN, Dannenberg AL, Abbott RD, et al: The epidemiology of varicose veins: The Framingham Study. *Am J Prev Med* 4:96, 1988.

88. Lurie F, Creton D, Eklof B, et al: Prospective randomized study of endovenous radiofrequency obliteration (closure) versus ligation and vein stripping (EVOLVeS): Two-year follow-up. *Eur J Vasc Endovasc Surg* 29:67, 2005.

89. Darwood RJ, Theivacumar N, Dellagrammaticas D, et al: Randomized clinical trial comparing endovenous laser ablation with surgery for the treatment of primary great saphenous varicose veins. *Br J Surg* 95:294, 2008.

90. Falanga V: Venous ulceration. *J Dermatol Surg Oncol* 19:764, 1993.

91. Phillips T, Stanton B, Provan A, et al: A study of the impact of leg ulcers on quality of life: Financial, social, and psychologic implications. *J Am Acad Dermatol* 31:49, 1994.

92. Skin Substitute Consensus Development Panel: Nonoperative management of venous ulcers: Evolving role of skin substitutes. *Vasc Surg* 33:197, 1999.

93. Abenhaim L, Kurz X: The VEINES study (VEnous Insufficiency Epidemiologic and Economic Study): An international cohort study on chronic venous disorders of the leg. VEINES Group. *Angiology* 48:59, 1997.

94. Clarke H, Smith SR, Vasdekis SN, et al: Role of venous elasticity in the development of varicose veins. *Br J Surg* 76:577, 1989.

95. Nicolaides AN, Hussein MK, Szendro G, et al: The relation of venous ulceration with ambulatory venous pressure measurements. *J Vasc Surg* 17:414, 1993.

96. Christopoulos DG, Nicolaides AN, Szendro G, et al: Air-plethysmography and the effect of elastic compression on venous hemodynamics of the leg. *J Vasc Surg* 5:148, 1987.

97. van Bemmelen PS, Bedford G, Beach K, et al: Quantitative segmental evaluation of venous valvular reflux with duplex ultrasound scanning. *J Vasc Surg* 10:425, 1989.

98. Nehler MR, Porter JM: The lower extremity venous system. Part II: The pathophysiology of chronic venous insufficiency. *Perspect Vasc Surg* 5:81, 1992.

99. Nehler MR, Moneta GL, Woodard DM, et al: Perimalleolar subcutaneous tissue pressure effects of elastic compression stockings. *J Vasc Surg* 18:783, 1993.

100. Dinn E: Treatment of venous ulceration by injection sclerotherapy and compression hosiery: A 5-year study. *Phlebology* 7:23, 1992.

101. Mayberry JC, Moneta GL, Taylor LM Jr., et al: Fifteen-year results of ambulatory compression therapy for chronic venous ulcers. *Surgery* 109:575, 1991.

102. Kitahama A, Elliott LF, Kerstein MD, et al: Leg ulcer. Conservative management or surgical treatment? *JAMA* 247:197, 1982.

103. Anning S: Leg ulcers: The results of treatment. *Angiology* 7:505, 1956.

104. Falanga V, Margolis D, Alvarez O, et al: Rapid healing of venous ulcers and lack of clinical rejection with an allogeneic cultured human skin equivalent. Human Skin Equivalent Investigators Group. *Arch Dermatol* 134:293, 1998.

105. Phillips TJ: New skin for old: Developments in biological skin substitutes [editorial; comment]. *Arch Dermatol* 134:344, 1998.

106. Motykie GD, Caprini JA, Arcelus JI, et al: Evaluation of therapeutic compression stockings in the treatment of chronic venous insufficiency. *Dermatol Surg* 25:116, 1999.

107. Lippmann HI, Fishman LM, Farrar RH, et al: Edema control in the management of disabling chronic venous insufficiency. *Arch Phys Med Rehabil* 75:436, 1994.

108. Rubin JR, Alexander J, Plecha EJ, et al: Unna's boot vs. polyurethane foam dressings for the treatment of venous ulceration. A randomized prospective study. *Arch Surg* 125:489, 1990.

109. Vernick SH, Shapiro D, Shaw FD: Legging orthosis for venous and lymphatic insufficiency. *Arch Phys Med Rehabil* 68:459, 1987.

110. Sibbald RG: Apligraf living skin equivalent for healing venous and chronic wounds. *J Cutan Med Surg* 3(Suppl 1):S124, 1998.

111. Linton R: The communicating veins of the lower leg and the operative technique for their ligation. *Ann Surg* 107:582, 1938.

112. Gloviczki P, Bergan JJ, Rhodes JM, et al: Mid-term results of endoscopic perforator vein interruption for chronic venous insufficiency: Lessons learned from the North American Subfascial Endoscopic Perforator Surgery registry. The North American Study Group. *J Vasc Surg* 29:489, 1999.

113. Sottiurai VS: Surgical correction of recurrent venous ulcer. *J Cardiovasc Surg* 32:104, 1991.

114. Dalsing MC, Raju S, Wakefield TW, et al: A multicenter, phase I evaluation of cryopreserved venous valve allografts for the treatment of chronic deep venous insufficiency. *J Vasc Surg* 30:854, 1999.

115. Raju S, Fredericks R: Valve reconstruction procedures for nonobstructive venous insufficiency: Rationale, techniques, and results in 107 procedures with two- to eight-year follow-up. *J Vasc Surg* 7:301, 1988.

116. Masuda EM, Kistner RL: Long-term results of venous valve reconstruction: A four- to twenty-one-year follow-up. *J Vasc Surg* 19:391, 1994.

117. Rockson SG, Miller LT, Senie R, et al: American Cancer Society Lymphedema Workshop. Workgroup III: Diagnosis and management of lymphedema. *Cancer* 83:2882, 1998.

118. Yasuhara H, Shigematsu H, Muto T: A study of the advantages of elastic stockings for leg lymphedema. *Int Angiol* 15:272, 1996.

119. Grabois M: Breast cancer. Postmastectomy lymphedema. State of the art review. *Phys Med Rehabil Rev* 8:267, 1994.

120. Miranda F Jr., Perez MC, Castiglioni ML, et al: Effect of sequential intermittent pneumatic compression on both leg lymphedema volume and on lymph transport as semi-quantitatively evaluated by lymphoscintigraphy. *Lymphology* 34:135, 2001.

121. Richmand DM, O'Donnell TF Jr., Zelikovski A: Sequential pneumatic compression for lymphedema. A controlled trial. *Arch Surg* 120:1116, 1985.

122. Vodder E: *Le drainage lymphatique, une novelle méthode thérapeutique.* Paris: Santé pour tous, 1936.

123. Ko DS, Lerner R, Klose G, et al: Effective treatment of lymphedema of the extremities. *Arch Surg* 133:452, 1998.

124. Miller TA, Wyatt LE, Rudkin GH: Staged skin and subcutaneous excision for lymphedema: A favorable report of long-term results. *Plast Reconstr Surg* 102:1486, 1998.

125. Baumeister RG, Siuda S: Treatment of lymphedemas by microsurgical lymphatic grafting: What is proved? *Plast Reconstr Surg* 85:64, 1990.

126. Bernas MJ, Witte CL, Witte MH: The diagnosis and treatment of peripheral lymphedema: Draft revision of the 1995 Consensus Document of the International Society of Lymphology Executive Committee for discussion at the September 3–7, 2001, XVIII International Congress of Lymphology in Genoa, Italy. *Lymphology* 34:84, 2001.

CHAPTER 24 Venous and Lymphatic Disease

CHAPTER 25

Esophagus and Diaphragmatic Hernia

Blair A. Jobe, John G. Hunter,
and Jeffrey H. Peters

SURGICAL ANATOMY

The esophagus is a muscular tube that starts as the continuation of the pharynx and ends as the cardia of the stomach. When the head is in a normal anatomic position, the transition from pharynx to esophagus occurs at the lower border of the sixth cervical vertebra. Topographically this corresponds to the cricoid cartilage anteriorly and the palpable transverse process of the sixth cervical vertebra laterally (Fig. 25-1). The esophagus is firmly attached at its upper end to the cricoid cartilage and at its lower end to the diaphragm; during swallowing, the proximal points of fixation move craniad the distance of one cervical vertebral body.

The esophagus lies in the midline, with a deviation to the left in the lower portion of the neck and upper portion of the thorax, and returns to the midline in the midportion of the thorax near the bifurcation of the trachea (Fig. 25-2). In the lower portion of the

thorax, the esophagus again deviates to the left and anteriorly to pass through the diaphragmatic hiatus.

Three normal areas of esophageal narrowing are evident on the barium esophagogram or during esophagoscopy. The uppermost narrowing is located at the entrance into the esophagus and is caused by the cricopharyngeal muscle. Its luminal diameter is 1.5 cm, and it is the narrowest point of the esophagus. The middle narrowing is due to an indentation of the anterior and left lateral esophageal wall caused by the crossing of the left main stem bronchus and aortic arch. The luminal diameter at this point is 1.6 cm. The lowermost narrowing is at the hiatus of the diaphragm and is caused by the gastroesophageal sphincter mechanism. The luminal diameter at this point varies somewhat, depending on the distention of the esophagus by the passage of food, but has been measured at 1.6 to 1.9 cm. These normal constrictions tend to hold up swallowed foreign objects, and the overlying mucosa is subject to

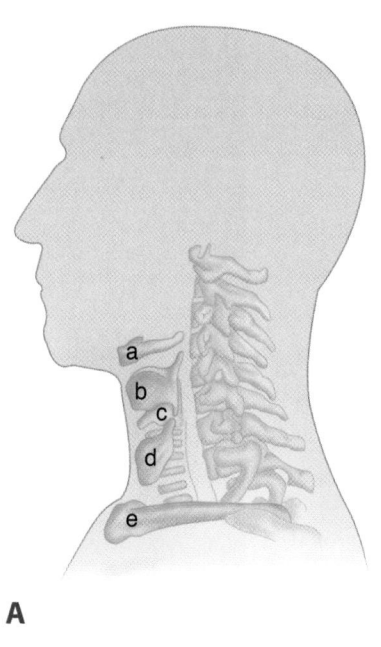

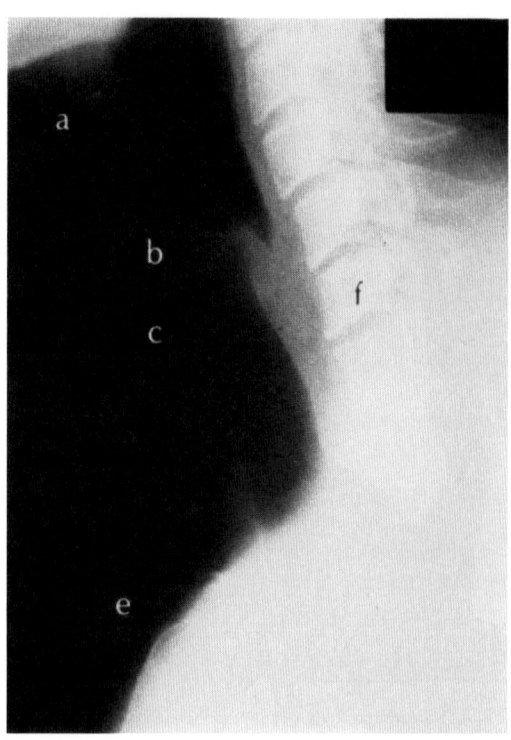

FIG. 25-1. A. Topographic relationships of the cervical esophagus: (*a*) hyoid bone, (*b*) thyroid cartilage, (*c*) cricoid cartilage, (*d*) thyroid gland, (*e*) sternoclavicular. **B.** Lateral radiographic appearance with landmarks identified as labeled in **A**. The location of C6 is also included (*f*). [*Reproduced with permission from Rothberg M, DeMeester TR: Surgical anatomy of the esophagus, in Shields TW (ed): General Thoracic Surgery, 3rd ed. Philadelphia: Lea & Febiger, 1989, p 77.*]

A

B

injury by swallowed corrosive liquids due to their slow passage through these areas.

Figure 25-3 shows the average distance in centimeters measured during endoscopic examination between the incisor teeth and the cricopharyngeus, aortic arch, and cardia of the stomach. Manometrically, the length of the esophagus between the lower border of the cricopharyngeus and upper border of the lower sphincter varies according to the height of the individual.

The pharyngeal musculature consists of three broad, flat, overlapping fan-shaped constrictors (Fig. 25-4). The opening of the esophagus is collared by the cricopharyngeal muscle, which arises from both sides of the cricoid cartilage of the larynx and forms a continuous transverse muscle band without interruption by a median raphe. The fibers of this muscle blend inseparably with those of the inferior pharyngeal constrictor above and the inner circular muscle fibers of the esophagus below. Some investigators believe that the cricopharyngeus is part of the inferior constrictor; that is, that the inferior constrictor has two parts, an upper or retrothyroid portion having diagonal fibers, and a lower or retrocricoid portion having transverse fibers. Keith in 1910 showed that these two parts of the same muscle serve totally different functions. The retrocricoid portion serves as the upper sphincter of the esophagus and relaxes when the retrothyroid portion contracts, to force the swallowed bolus from the pharynx into the esophagus.

The cervical portion of the esophagus is approximately 5 cm long and descends between the trachea and the vertebral column, from the level of the sixth cervical vertebra to the level of the interspace between the first and second thoracic vertebrae posteriorly, or the level of the suprasternal notch anteriorly. The recurrent laryngeal nerves lie in the right and left grooves between the trachea

KEY POINTS

1. Objective esophageal physiology testing is cornerstone to making the diagnosis of benign esophageal disorders and in developing an individualized treatment plan for patients.

2. While most esophageal procedures can be performed using either a videoscopic or flexible endoscopic approach, the surgeon must be familiar with the surgical anatomy and open approaches to the esophagus along its entire length.

3. Laparoscopic cardiomyotomy is now considered the most effective treatment for achalasia and should include division of the gastric collar sling musculature.

4. While esophageal replacement is most commonly performed with the tubularized stomach, the surgeon should be familiar with the anatomy and techniques which enable the use of colon and jejunum.

5. Giant paraesophageal hernia should be repaired surgically in patients with symptoms, anemia, or signs of strangulation.

6. The cornerstone to esophageal cancer clinical staging includes the use of endoscopy, CT, PET, and endoscopic ultrasound.

7. In surgical candidates with esophageal cancer confined to the posterior mediastinum, esophagectomy represents the best possible chance for cure.

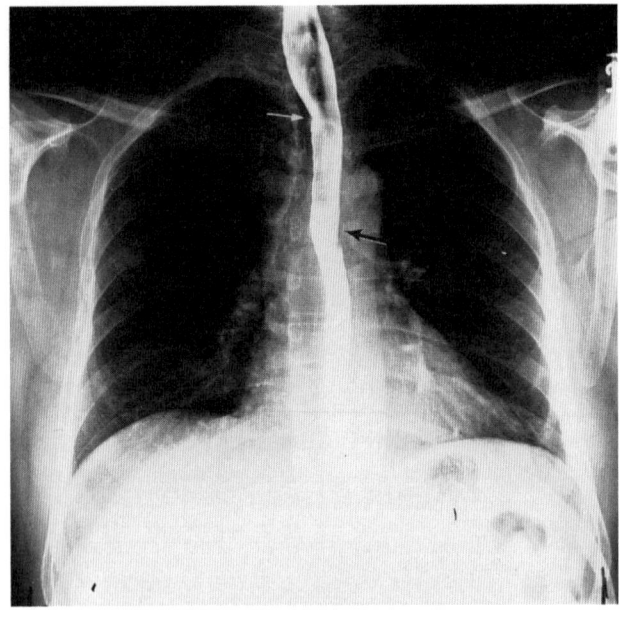

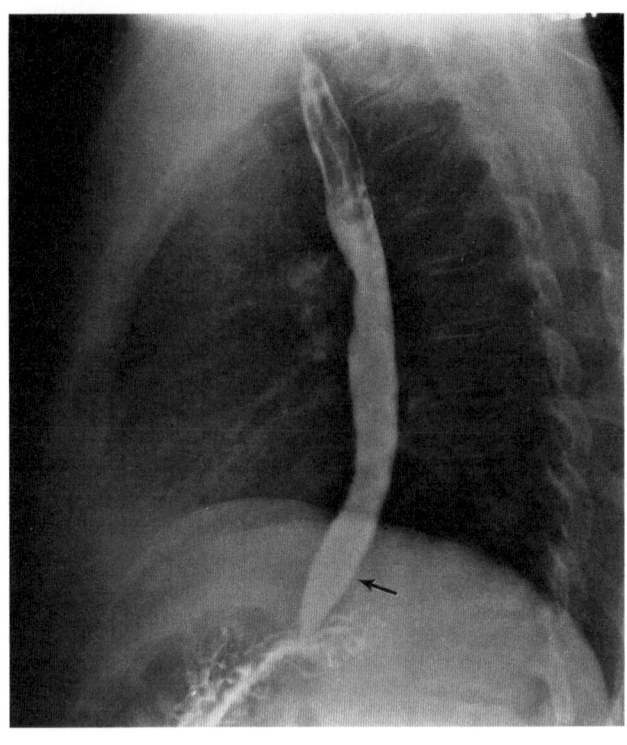

FIG. 25-2. Barium esophagogram. **A.** Posterior-anterior view. *White arrow* shows deviation to left. *Black arrow* shows return to midline. **B.** Lateral view. *Black arrow* shows anterior deviation. *[Reproduced with permission from Rothberg M, DeMeester TR: Surgical anatomy of the esophagus, in Shields TW (ed):* General Thoracic Surgery, *3rd ed. Philadelphia: Lea & Febiger, 1989, p 77.]*

and the esophagus. The left recurrent nerve lies somewhat closer to the esophagus than the right, owing to the slight deviation of the esophagus to the left, and the more lateral course of the right recurrent nerve around the right subclavian artery. Laterally, on the left and right sides of the cervical esophagus are the carotid sheaths and the lobes of the thyroid gland.

The thoracic portion of the esophagus is approximately 20 cm long. It starts at the thoracic inlet. In the upper portion of the thorax,

FIG. 25-3. Important clinical endoscopic measurements of the esophagus in adults. *[Reproduced with permission from Rothberg M, DeMeester TR: Surgical anatomy of the esophagus, in Shields TW (ed):* General Thoracic Surgery. *Philadelphia: Lea & Febiger, 1989, p 78.]*

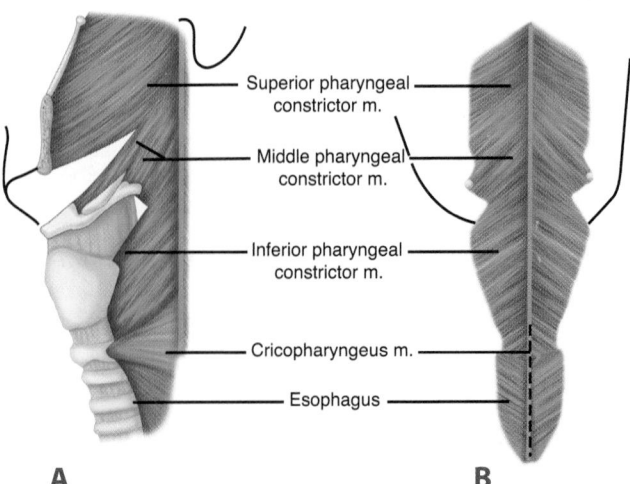

FIG. 25-4. External muscles of the pharynx. **A.** Posterolateral view. **B.** Posterior view. *Dotted line* represents usual site of myotomy. *[Reproduced with permission from Rothberg M, DeMeester TR: Surgical anatomy of the esophagus, in Shields TW (ed):* General Thoracic Surgery, *3rd ed. Philadelphia: Lea & Febiger, 1989, p 78.]*

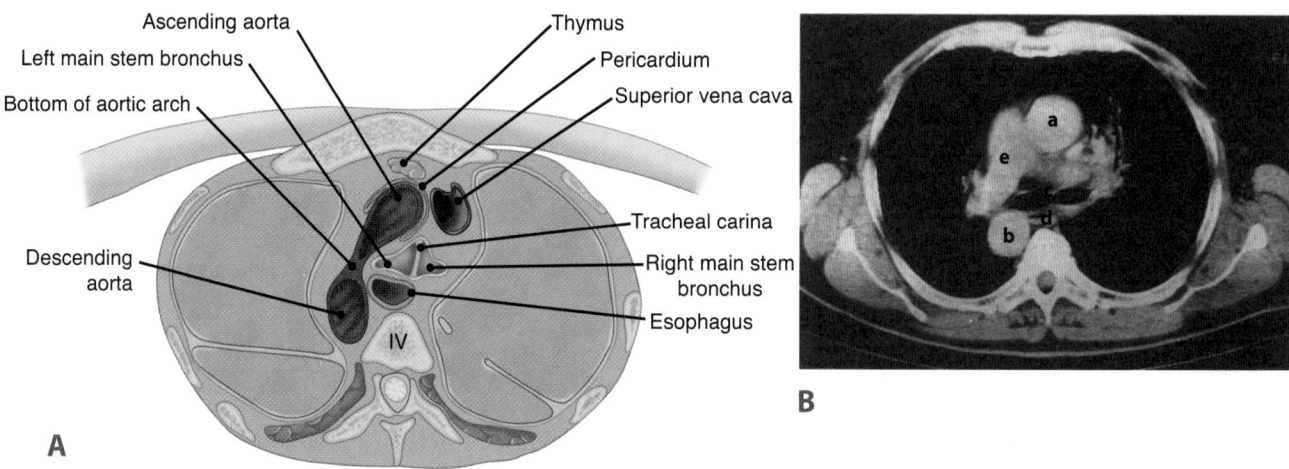

FIG. 25-5. A. Cross-section of the thorax at the level of the tracheal bifurcation. **B.** Computed tomographic scan at same level viewed from above: (*a*) ascending aorta, (*b*) descending aorta, (*c*) tracheal carina, (*d*) esophagus, (*e*) pulmonary artery. [*Reproduced with permission from Rothberg M, DeMeester TR: Surgical anatomy of the esophagus, in Shields TW (ed):* General Thoracic Surgery, *3rd ed. Philadelphia: Lea & Febiger, 1989, p 81.*]

it is in intimate relationship with the posterior wall of the trachea and the prevertebral fascia. Just above the tracheal bifurcation, the esophagus passes to the right of the aorta. This anatomic positioning can cause a notch indentation in its left lateral wall on a barium swallow radiogram. Immediately below this notch, the esophagus crosses both the bifurcation of the trachea and the left main stem bronchus, owing to the slight deviation of the terminal portion of the trachea to the right by the aorta (Fig. 25-5). From there down, the esophagus passes over the posterior surface of the subcarinal lymph nodes (LNs), and then descends over the pericardium of the left atrium to reach the diaphragmatic hiatus (Fig. 25-6). From the bifurcation of the trachea downward, both the vagal nerves and the esophageal nerve plexus lie on the muscular wall of the esophagus.

Dorsally, the thoracic esophagus follows the curvature of the spine and remains in close contact with the vertebral bodies. From the eighth thoracic vertebra downward, the esophagus moves vertically away from the spine to pass through the hiatus of the diaphragm. The thoracic duct passes through the hiatus of the diaphragm on the anterior surface of the vertebral column behind the aorta and under the right crus. In the thorax, the thoracic duct lies dorsal to the esophagus between the azygos vein on the right and the descending thoracic aorta on the left.

The abdominal portion of the esophagus is approximately 2 cm long and includes a portion of the lower esophageal sphincter (LES) (Fig. 25-7). It starts as the esophagus passes through the diaphragmatic hiatus and is surrounded by the phrenoesophageal membrane, a fibroelastic ligament arising from the subdiaphragmatic fascia as a continuation of the transversalis fascia lining the abdomen (Fig. 25-8). The upper leaf of the membrane attaches itself in a circumferential fashion around the esophagus, about 1 to 2 cm above the level of the hiatus. These fibers blend in with the elastic-containing adventitia of the abdominal esophagus and the cardia of the stomach. This portion of the esophagus is subjected to the positive-pressure environment of the abdomen.

The musculature of the esophagus can be divided into an outer longitudinal and an inner circular layer. The upper 2 to 6 cm of the

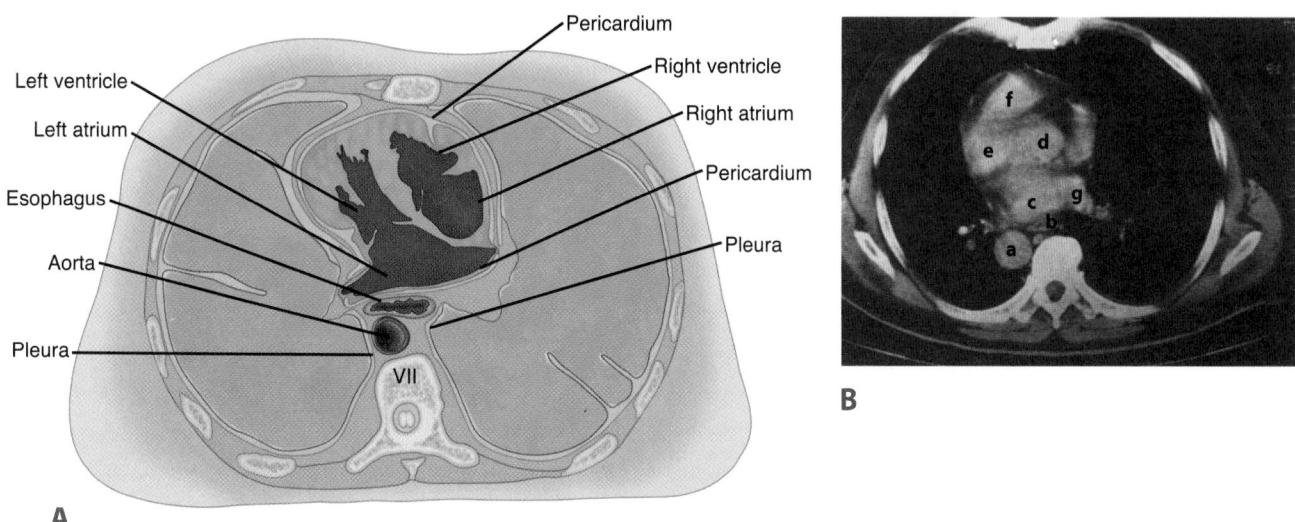

FIG. 25-6. A. Cross-section of the thorax at the midleft atrial level. **B.** Computed tomographic scan at same level viewed from above: (*a*) aorta, (*b*) esophagus, (*c*) left atrium, (*d*) right atrium, (*e*) left ventricle, (*f*) right ventricle, (*g*) pulmonary vein. [*Reproduced with permission from Rothberg M, DeMeester TR: Surgical anatomy of the esophagus, in Shields TW (ed):* General Thoracic Surgery, *3rd ed. Philadelphia: Lea & Febiger, 1989, p 82.*]

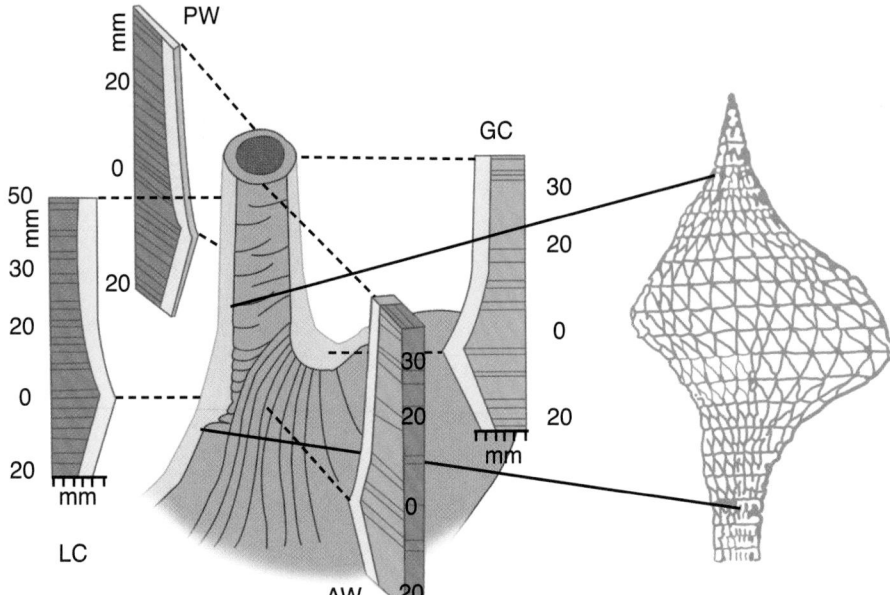

FIG. 25-7. Schematic drawing shows correlation between radial muscle thickness (*left*) and three-dimensional manometric pressure image (*right*) at human gastroesophageal junction. Muscle thickness across the gastroesophageal junction at the posterior gastric wall (PW), greater curvature (GC), anterior gastric wall (AW), and lesser curvature (LC) is shown in millimeters. Radial pressures at gastroesophageal junction (in millimeters of mercury) are plotted around an axis representing atmospheric pressure. *(Reproduced with permission from Stein HJ, Liebermann-Meffert D, DeMeester TR, et al: Three-dimensional pressure image and muscular structure of the human lower esophageal sphincter. Surgery 117:692, 1995. Copyright Elsevier.)*

esophagus contains only striated muscle fibers. From there on, smooth muscle fibers gradually become more abundant. Most clinically significant esophageal motility disorders involve only the smooth muscle in the lower two thirds of the esophagus. When a surgical esophageal myotomy is indicated, the incision needs to extend only this distance.

The longitudinal muscle fibers originate from a cricoesophageal tendon arising from the dorsal upper edge of the anteriorly located cricoid cartilage. The two bundles of muscle diverge and meet in the midline on the posterior wall of the esophagus about 3 cm below the cricoid (see Fig. 25-4). From this point on, the entire circumference of the esophagus is covered by a layer of longitudinal muscle fibers. This configuration of the longitudinal muscle fibers around the most proximal part of the esophagus leaves a V-shaped area in the posterior wall covered only with circular muscle fibers. Contraction of the longitudinal muscle fibers shortens the esophagus. The circular muscle layer of the esophagus is thicker than the outer longitudinal layer. In situ, the geometry of the circular muscle is helical and makes the peristalsis of the esophagus assume a worm-like drive, as opposed to segmental and sequential squeezing. As a consequence, severe motor abnormalities of the esophagus assume a corkscrew-like pattern on the barium swallow radiogram.

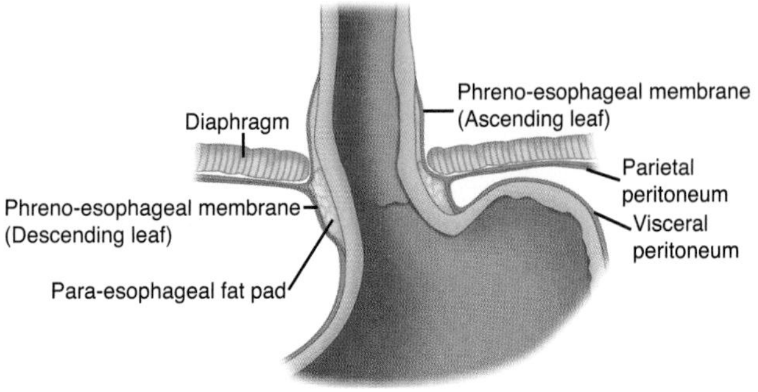

The cervical portion of the esophagus receives its main blood supply from the inferior thyroid artery. The thoracic portion receives its blood supply from the bronchial arteries, with 75% of individuals having one right-sided and two left-sided branches. Two esophageal branches arise directly from the aorta. The abdominal portion of the esophagus receives its blood supply from the ascending branch of the left gastric artery and from inferior phrenic arteries (Fig. 25-9). On entering the wall of the esophagus, the arteries assume a T-shaped division to form a longitudinal plexus,

FIG. 25-8. Attachments and structure of the phrenoesophageal membrane. Transversalis fascia lies just above the parietal peritoneum. *[Reproduced with permission from Rothberg M, DeMeester TR: Surgical anatomy of the esophagus, in Shields TW (ed): General Thoracic Surgery, 3rd ed. Philadelphia: Lea & Febiger, 1989, p 83.]*

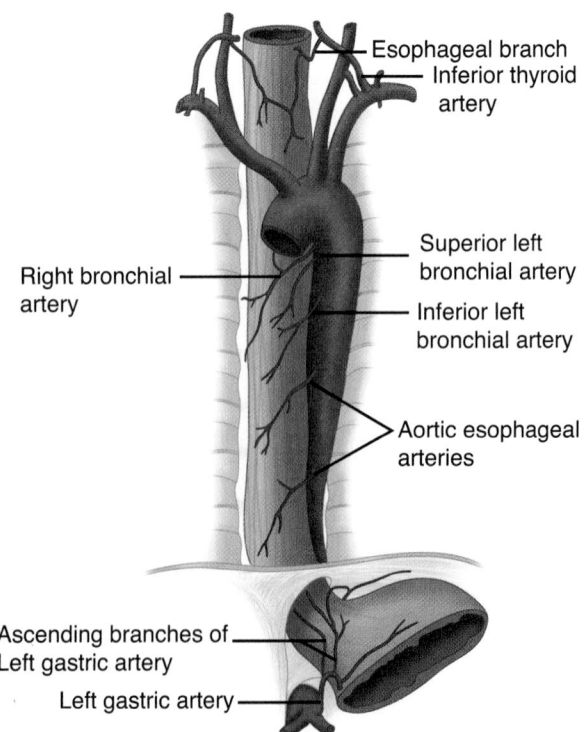

FIG. 25-9. Arterial blood supply of the esophagus. *[Reproduced with permission from Rothberg M, DeMeester TR: Surgical anatomy of the esophagus, in Shields TW (ed): General Thoracic Surgery, 3rd ed. Philadelphia: Lea & Febiger, 1989, p 84.]*

giving rise to an intramural vascular network in the muscular and submucosal layers. As a consequence, the esophagus can be mobilized from the stomach to the level of the aortic arch without fear of devascularization and ischemic necrosis. Caution should be exercised as to the extent of esophageal mobilization in patients who have had a previous thyroidectomy with ligation of the inferior thyroid arteries proximal to the origin of the esophageal branches.

Blood from the capillaries of the esophagus flows into a submucosal venous plexus, and then into a periesophageal venous plexus from which the esophageal veins originate. In the cervical region, the esophageal veins empty into the inferior thyroid vein; in the thoracic region, they empty into the bronchial, azygos, or hemiazygos veins; and in the abdominal region, they empty into the coronary vein (Fig. 25-10). The submucosal venous networks of the esophagus and stomach are in continuity with each other, and, in patients with portal venous obstruction, this communication functions as a collateral pathway for portal blood to enter the superior vena cava via the azygos vein.

The parasympathetic innervation of the pharynx and esophagus is provided mainly by the vagus nerves. The constrictor muscles of the pharynx receive branches from the pharyngeal plexus, which is on the posterior lateral surface of the middle constrictor muscle, and is formed by pharyngeal branches of the vagus nerves with a small contribution from cranial nerves IX and XI (Fig. 25-11). The cricopharyngeal sphincter and the cervical portion of the esophagus receive branches from both recurrent laryngeal nerves, which originate from the vagus nerves—the right recurrent nerve at the lower margin of the subclavian artery and the left at the lower margin of the aortic arch. They are slung dorsally around these vessels and ascend in the groove between the esophagus and trachea, giving branches to each. Damage to these nerves interferes not only with the function of the vocal cords, but also with the function of the cricopharyngeal sphincter and the motility of the cervical esophagus, predisposing the individual to pulmonary aspiration on swallowing.

Afferent visceral sensory pain fibers from the esophagus end without synapse in the first four segments of the thoracic spinal

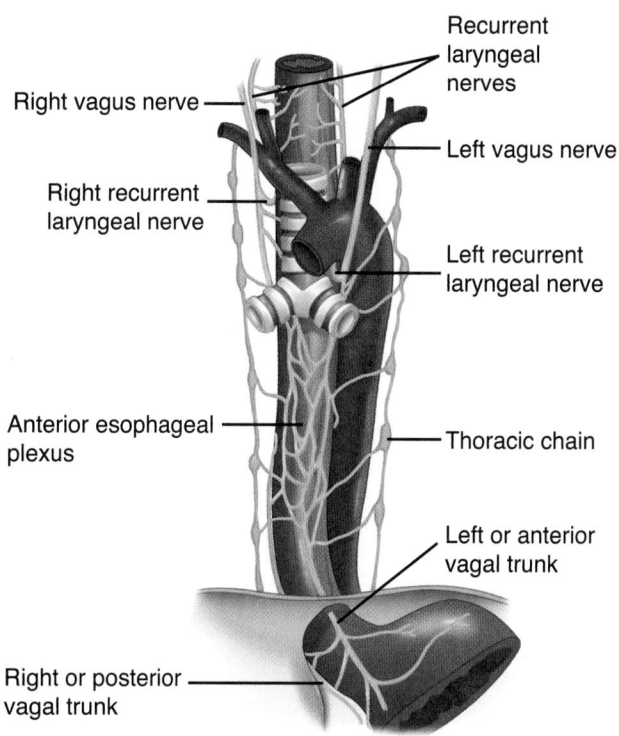

FIG. 25-11. Innervation of the esophagus. *[Reproduced with permission from Rothberg M, DeMeester TR: Surgical anatomy of the esophagus, in Shields TW (ed):* General Thoracic Surgery, *3rd ed. Philadelphia: Lea & Febiger, 1989, p 85.]*

cord, using a combination of sympathetic and vagal pathways. These pathways are also occupied by afferent visceral sensory fibers from the heart; hence, both organs have similar symptomatology.

The lymphatics located in the submucosa of the esophagus are so dense and interconnected that they constitute a single plexus (Fig. 25-12). There are more lymph vessels than blood capillaries in the submucosa. Lymph flow in the submucosal plexus runs in a

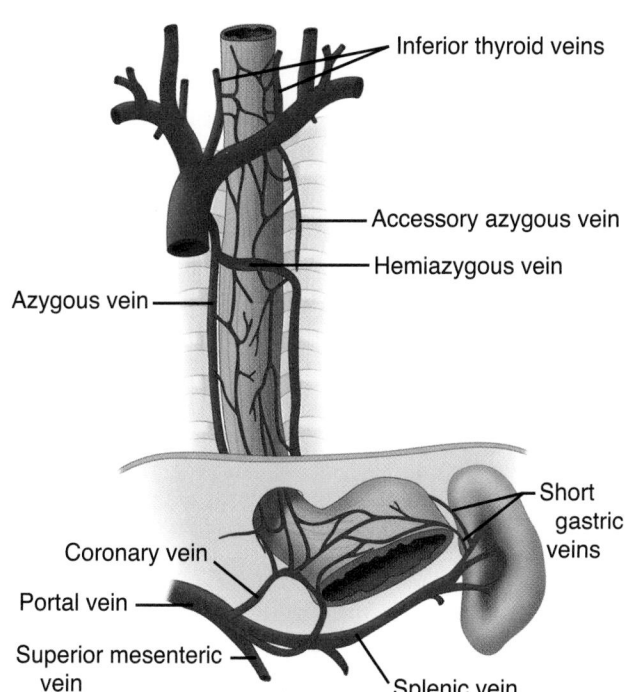

FIG. 25-10. Venous drainage of the esophagus. *[Reproduced with permission from Rothberg M, DeMeester TR: Surgical anatomy of the esophagus, in Shields TW (ed):* General Thoracic Surgery, *3rd ed. Philadelphia: Lea & Febiger, 1989, p 85.]*

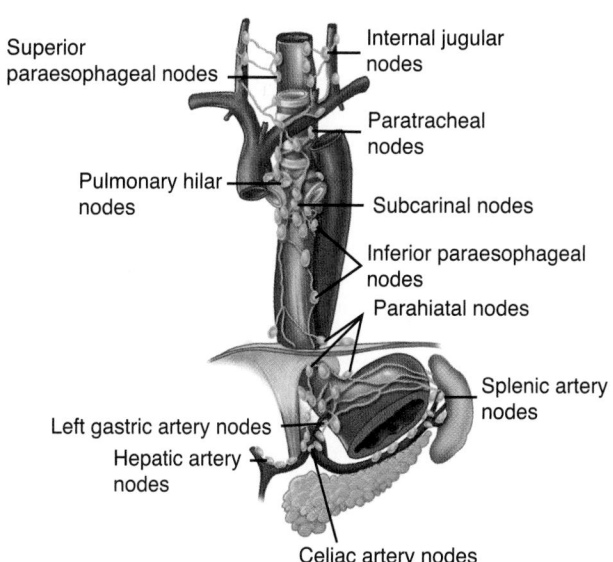

FIG. 25-12. Lymphatic drainage of the esophagus. *(Reproduced with permission from DeMeester TR, Barlow AP: Surgery and current management for cancer of the esophagus and cardia: Part I.* Curr Probl Surg *25:498, 1988. Copyright Elsevier.)*

longitudinal direction, and, on injection of a contrast medium, the longitudinal spread is seen to be about six times that of the transverse spread. In the upper two-thirds of the esophagus, the lymphatic flow is mostly cephalad, and, in the lower third, caudad. In the thoracic portion of the esophagus, the submucosal lymph plexus extends over a long distance in a longitudinal direction before penetrating the muscle layer to enter lymph vessels in the adventitia. As a consequence of this nonsegmental lymph drainage, a primary tumor can extend for a considerable length superiorly or inferiorly in the submucosal plexus. Consequently, free tumor cells can follow the submucosal lymphatic plexus in either direction for a long distance before they pass through the muscularis and on into the regional LNs. The cervical esophagus has a more direct segmental lymph drainage into the regional nodes, and, as a result, lesions in this portion of the esophagus have less submucosal extension and a more regionalized lymphatic spread.

The efferent lymphatics from the cervical esophagus drain into the paratracheal and deep cervical LNs, and those from the upper thoracic esophagus empty mainly into the paratracheal LNs. Efferent lymphatics from the lower thoracic esophagus drain into the subcarinal nodes and nodes in the inferior pulmonary ligaments. The superior gastric nodes receive lymph not only from the abdominal portion of the esophagus, but also from the adjacent lower thoracic segment.

PHYSIOLOGY

Swallowing Mechanism

The act of alimentation requires the passage of food and drink from the mouth into the stomach. One third of this distance consists of the mouth and hypopharynx, and two thirds is made up by the esophagus. To comprehend the mechanics of alimentation, it is useful to visualize the gullet as a mechanical model in which the tongue and pharynx function as a piston pump with three valves, and the body of the esophagus and cardia function as a worm-drive pump with a single valve. The three valves in the pharyngeal cylinder are the soft palate, epiglottis, and cricopharyngeus. The valve of the esophageal pump is the LES. Failure of the valves or the pumps leads to abnormalities in swallowing—that is, difficulty in food propulsion from mouth to stomach—or regurgitation of gastric contents into the esophagus or pharynx.

Food is taken into the mouth in a variety of bite sizes, where it is broken up, mixed with saliva, and lubricated. Once initiated, swallowing is entirely a reflex act. When food is ready for swallowing, the tongue, acting like a piston, moves the bolus into the posterior oropharynx and forces it into the hypopharynx (Fig. 25-13). Concomitantly with the posterior movement of the tongue, the soft palate is elevated, thereby closing the passage between the oropharynx and nasopharynx. This partitioning prevents pressure generated in the oropharynx from being dissipated through the nose. When the soft palate is paralyzed, for example, after a cerebrovascular accident, food is commonly regurgitated into the nasopharynx. During swallowing, the hyoid bone moves upward and anteriorly, elevating the larynx and opening the retrolaryngeal space, bringing the epiglottis under the tongue (see Fig. 25-13). The backward tilt of the epiglottis covers the opening of the larynx to prevent aspiration. The entire pharyngeal part of swallowing occurs within 1.5 seconds.

During swallowing, the pressure in the hypopharynx rises abruptly, to at least 60 mmHg, due to the backward movement of the tongue and contraction of the posterior pharyngeal constrictors. A sizable pressure difference develops between the hypopharyngeal pressure and the less-than-atmospheric midesophageal or intrathoracic pressure (Fig. 25-14). This pressure gradient speeds the movement of food from the hypopharynx into the esophagus when the cricopharyngeus or upper esophageal sphincter relaxes. The bolus is both propelled by peristaltic contraction of the posterior pharyngeal constrictors and sucked into the thoracic esophagus. Critical to

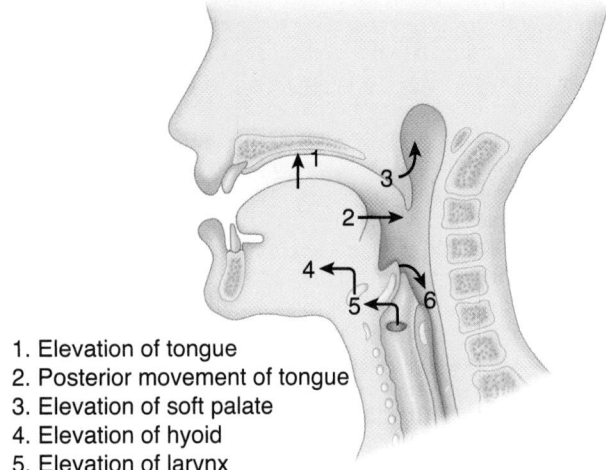

1. Elevation of tongue
2. Posterior movement of tongue
3. Elevation of soft palate
4. Elevation of hyoid
5. Elevation of larynx
6. Tilting of epiglottis

FIG. 25-13. Sequence of events during the oropharyngeal phase of swallowing. *[Reproduced with permission from DeMeester TR, Stein HJ, Fuchs KH: Physiologic diagnostic studies, in Zuidema GD, Orringer MB (eds): Shackelford's Surgery of the Alimentary Tract, 3rd ed., Vol. I. Philadelphia: W.B. Saunders, 1991, p 95. Copyright Elsevier.]*

receiving the bolus is the compliance of the cervical esophagus; when compliance is lost due to muscle pathology, dysphagia can result. The upper esophageal sphincter closes within 0.5 second of the initiation of the swallow, with the immediate closing pressure reaching approximately twice the resting level of 30 mmHg. The postrelaxation contraction continues down the esophagus as a peristaltic wave (Fig. 25-15). The high closing pressure and the initiation of the peristaltic wave prevents reflux of the bolus from

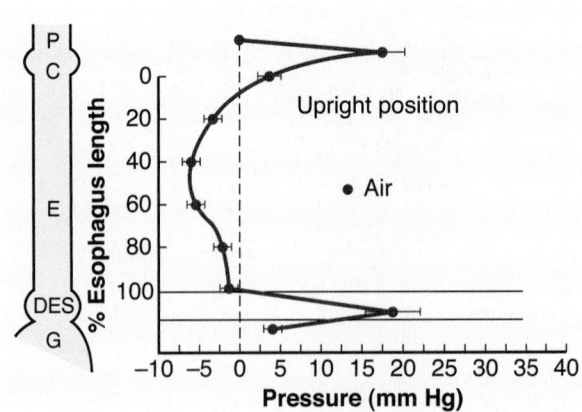

FIG. 25-14. Resting pressure profile of the foregut showing the pressure differential between the atmospheric pharyngeal pressure (*P*) and the less-than-atmospheric midesophageal pressure (*E*) and greater-than-atmospheric intragastric pressure (*G*), with the interposed high pressure zones of the cricopharyngeus (*C*) and distal esophageal sphincter (*DES*). The necessity for relaxation of the cricopharyngeus and DES pressure to move a bolus into the stomach is apparent. Esophageal work occurs when a bolus is pushed from the midesophageal area (*E*), with a pressure less than atmospheric, into the stomach, which has a pressure greater than atmospheric (*G*). *(Reproduced with permission from Waters PF, DeMeester TR: Foregut motor disorders and their surgical management.* Med Clin North Am *65:1237, 1981. Copyright Elsevier.)*

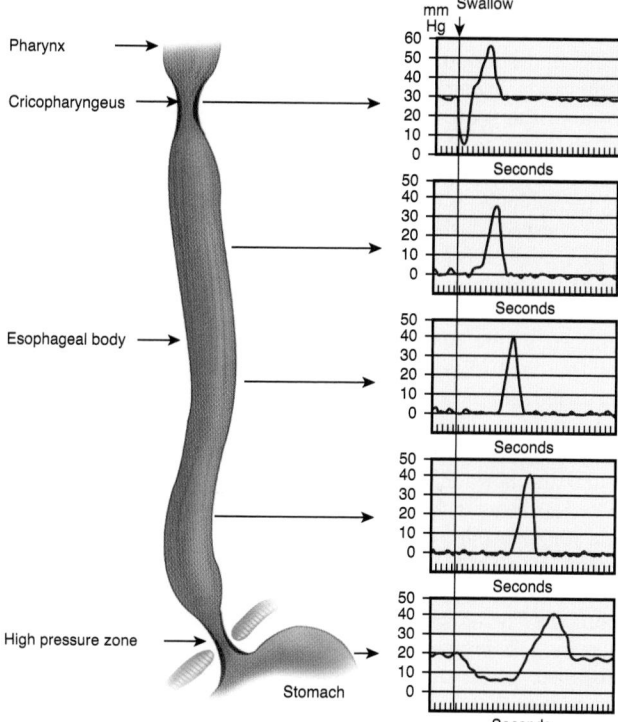

FIG. 25-15. Intraluminal esophageal pressures in response to swallowing. *(Reproduced with permission from Waters PF, DeMeester TR: Foregut motor disorders and their surgical management.* Med Clin North Am *65:1238, 1981. Copyright Elsevier.)*

the esophagus back into the pharynx. After the peristaltic wave has passed farther down the esophagus, the pressure in the upper esophageal sphincter returns to its resting level.

Swallowing can be started at will, or it can be reflexively elicited by the stimulation of areas in the mouth and pharynx, among them the anterior and posterior tonsillar pillars or the posterior lateral walls of the hypopharynx. The afferent sensory nerves of the pharynx are the glossopharyngeal nerves and the superior laryngeal branches of the vagus nerves. Once aroused by stimuli entering via these nerves, the swallowing center in the medulla coordinates the complete act of swallowing by discharging impulses through cranial nerves V, VII, X, XI, and XII, as well as the motor neurons of C1 to C3. Discharges through these nerves occur in a rather specific pattern and last for approximately 0.5 second. Little is known about the organization of the swallowing center, except that it can trigger swallowing after a variety of different inputs, but the response is always a rigidly ordered pattern of outflow. Following a cerebrovascular accident, this coordinated outflow may be altered, causing mild to severe abnormalities of swallowing. In more severe injury, swallowing can be grossly disrupted, leading to repetitive aspiration.

The striated muscles of the cricopharyngeus and the upper one third of the esophagus are activated by efferent motor fibers distributed through the vagus nerve and its recurrent laryngeal branches. The integrity of innervation is required for the cricopharyngeus to relax in coordination with the pharyngeal contraction, and resume its resting tone once a bolus has entered the upper esophagus. Operative damage to the innervation can interfere with laryngeal, cricopharyngeal, and upper esophageal function, and predispose the patient to aspiration.

The pharyngeal activity in swallowing initiates the esophageal phase. The body of the esophagus functions as a worm-drive propulsive pump due to the helical arrangement of its circular muscles, and is responsible for transferring a bolus of food into the stomach. The esophageal phase of swallowing represents esoph-

ageal work done during alimentation, in that food is moved into the stomach from a negative-pressure environment of –6 mmHg intrathoracic pressure, to a positive-pressure environment of 6 mmHg intra-abdominal pressure, or over a gradient of 12 mmHg (see Fig. 25-14). Effective and coordinated smooth muscle function in the lower one third of the esophagus is therefore important in pumping the food across this gradient.

The peristaltic wave generates an occlusive pressure varying from 30 to 120 mmHg (see Fig. 25-15). The wave rises to a peak in 1 second, lasts at the peak for about 0.5 second, and then subsides in about 1.5 seconds. The whole course of the rise and fall of occlusive pressure may occupy one point in the esophagus for 3 to 5 seconds. The peak of a primary peristaltic contraction initiated by a swallow (primary peristalsis) moves down the esophagus at 2 to 4 cm/s and reaches the distal esophagus about 9 seconds after swallowing starts (see Fig. 24-15). Consecutive swallows produce similar primary peristaltic waves, but when the act of swallowing is rapidly repeated, the esophagus remains relaxed and the peristaltic wave occurs only after the last movement of the pharynx. Progress of the wave in the esophagus is caused by sequential activation of its muscles, initiated by efferent vagal nerve fibers arising in the swallowing center.

Continuity of the esophageal muscle is not necessary for sequential activation if the nerves are intact. If the muscles, but not the nerves, are cut across, the pressure wave begins distally below the cut as it dies out at the proximal end above the cut. This allows a sleeve resection of the esophagus to be done without destroying its normal function. Afferent impulses from receptors within the esophageal wall are not essential for progress of the coordinated wave. Afferent nerves, however, do go to the swallowing center from the esophagus, because, if the esophagus is distended at any point, a contractual wave begins with a forceful closure of the upper esophageal sphincter and sweeps down the esophagus. This secondary contraction occurs without any movements of the mouth or pharynx. Secondary peristalsis can occur as an independent local reflex to clear the esophagus of ingested material left behind after the passage of the primary wave. Current studies suggest that secondary peristalsis is not as common as once thought.

Despite the powerful occlusive pressure, the propulsive force of the esophagus is relatively feeble. If a subject attempts to swallow a bolus attached by a string to a counterweight, the maximum weight that can be overcome is 5 to 10 g. Orderly contractions of the muscular wall and anchoring of the esophagus at its inferior end are necessary for efficient aboral propulsion to occur. Loss of the inferior anchor, as occurs with a large hiatal hernia, can lead to inefficient propulsion.

The LES provides a pressure barrier between the esophagus and stomach and acts as the valve on the worm-drive pump of the esophageal body. Although an anatomically distinct LES has been difficult to identify, microdissection studies show that, in humans, the sphincter-like function is related to the architecture of the muscle fibers at the junction of the esophageal tube with the gastric pouch (Fig. 25-16). The sphincter actively remains closed to prevent reflux of gastric contents into the esophagus and opens by a relaxation that coincides with a pharyngeal swallow (see Fig. 25-15). The LES pressure returns to its resting level after the peristaltic wave has passed through the esophagus. Consequently, reflux of gastric juice that may occur through the open valve during a swallow is cleared back into the stomach.

If the pharyngeal swallow does not initiate a peristaltic contraction, then the coincident relaxation of the LES is unguarded and reflux of gastric juice can occur. This may be an explanation for the observation of spontaneous lower esophageal relaxation, thought by some to be a causative factor in gastroesophageal reflux disease (GERD). The power of the worm-drive pump of the esophageal body is insufficient to force open a valve that does not relax. In dogs, a bilateral cervical parasympathetic blockade abolishes the relaxation of the LES that occurs with pharyngeal swallowing or distention of the esophagus. Consequently, vagal function appears to be important in coordinating the relaxation of the LES with esophageal contraction.

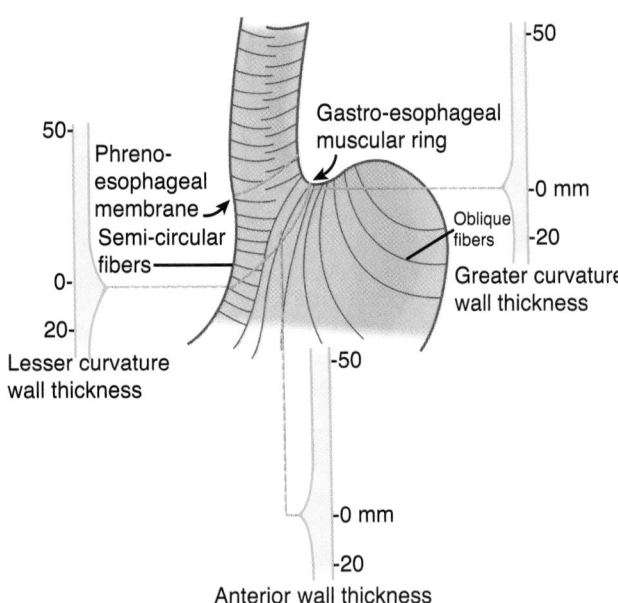

FIG. 25-16. Wall thickness and orientation of fibers on microdissection of the cardia. At the junction of the esophageal tube and gastric pouch, there is an oblique muscular ring composed of an increased muscle mass inside the inner muscular layer. On the lesser curve side of the cardia, the muscle fibers of the inner layer are oriented transversely and form semicircular muscle clasps. On the greater curve side of the cardia, these muscle fibers form oblique loops that encircle the distal end of the cardia and gastric fundus. Both the semicircular muscle clasps and the oblique fibers of the fundus contract in a circular manner to close the cardia. [Reproduced with permission from DeMeester TR, Skinner DB: Evaluation of esophageal function and disease, in Glenn WWL (ed): Thoracic and Cardiovascular Surgery, 4th ed. Norwalk, CT: Appleton-Century-Crofts, 1983, p 461.]

The antireflux mechanism in human beings is composed of three components: a mechanically effective LES, efficient esophageal clearance, and an adequately functioning gastric reservoir. A defect of any one of these three components can lead to increased esophageal exposure to gastric juice and the development of mucosal injury.

Physiologic Reflux

On 24-hour esophageal pH monitoring, healthy individuals have occasional episodes of gastroesophageal reflux. This physiologic reflux is more common when awake and in the upright position than during sleep in the supine position. When reflux of gastric juice occurs, normal subjects rapidly clear the acid gastric juice from the esophagus regardless of their position.

There are several explanations for the observation that physiologic reflux in normal subjects is more common when they are awake and in the upright position than during sleep in the supine position. First, reflux episodes occur in healthy volunteers primarily during transient losses of the gastroesophageal barrier, which may be due to a relaxation of the LES or intragastric pressure overcoming sphincter pressure. Gastric juice can also reflux when a swallow-induced relaxation of the LES is not protected by an oncoming peristaltic wave. The average frequency of these "unguarded moments" or of transient losses of the gastroesophageal barrier is far less while asleep and in the supine position than while awake and in the upright position. Consequently, there are fewer opportunities for reflux to occur in the supine position. Second, in the upright position, there is a 12-mmHg pressure gradient between the resting, positive intra-abdominal pressure measured in the stomach and the most negative intrathoracic pressure measured in the esophagus at

midthoracic level. This gradient favors the flow of gastric juice up into the thoracic esophagus when upright. The gradient diminishes in the supine position. Third, the LES pressure in normal subjects is significantly higher in the supine position than in the upright position. This is due to the apposition of the hydrostatic pressure of the abdomen to the abdominal portion of the sphincter when supine. In the upright position, the abdominal pressure surrounding the sphincter is negative compared with atmospheric pressure, and, as expected, the abdominal pressure gradually increases the more caudally it is measured. This pressure gradient tends to move the gastric contents toward the cardia and encourages the occurrence of reflux into the esophagus when the individual is upright. By contrast, in the supine position, the gastroesophageal pressure gradient diminishes, and the abdominal hydrostatic pressure under the diaphragm increases, causing an increase in sphincter pressure and a more competent cardia.

The LES has intrinsic myogenic tone, which is modulated by neural and hormonal mechanisms. Alpha-adrenergic neurotransmitters or beta blockers stimulate the LES, and alpha blockers and beta stimulants decrease its pressure. It is not clear to what extent cholinergic nerve activity controls LES pressure. The vagus nerve carries both excitatory and inhibitory fibers to the esophagus and sphincter. The hormones gastrin and motilin have been shown to increase LES pressure; and cholecystokinin, estrogen, glucagon, progesterone, somatostatin, and secretin decrease LES pressure. The peptides bombesin, l-enkephalin, and substance P increase LES pressure; and calcitonin gene-related peptide, gastric inhibitory peptide, neuropeptide Y, and vasoactive intestinal polypeptide decrease LES pressure. Some pharmacologic agents such as antacids, cholinergics, agonists, domperidone, metoclopramide, and prostaglandin F_2 are known to increase LES pressure; and anticholinergics, barbiturates, calcium channel blockers, caffeine, diazepam, dopamine, meperidine, prostaglandin E_1 and E_2, and theophylline decrease LES pressure. Peppermint, chocolate, coffee, ethanol, and fat are all associated with decreased LES pressure and may be responsible for esophageal symptoms after a sumptuous meal.

ASSESSMENT OF ESOPHAGEAL FUNCTION

A thorough understanding of the patient's underlying anatomic and functional deficits before making therapeutic decisions is fundamental to the successful treatment of esophageal disease. The diagnostic tests, as presently used, may be divided into four broad groups: (a) tests to detect structural abnormalities of the esophagus; (b) tests to detect functional abnormalities of the esophagus; (c) tests to detect increased esophageal exposure to gastric juice; and (d) tests of duodenogastric function as they relate to esophageal disease.

Tests to Detect Structural Abnormalities

Radiographic Evaluation

The first diagnostic test in patients with suspected esophageal disease should be a barium swallow including a full assessment of the stomach and duodenum. Esophageal motility can be assessed by observing several individual swallows of barium traversing the entire length of the organ, with the patient in the horizontal position. Hiatal hernias are best demonstrated with the patient prone because the increased intra-abdominal pressure produced in this position promotes displacement of the esophagogastric junction above the diaphragm. To detect lower esophageal narrowing, such as rings and strictures, fully distended views of the esophagogastric region are crucial. The density of the barium used to study the esophagus can potentially affect the accuracy of the examination. Esophageal disorders shown clearly by a full-column technique include circumferential carcinomas, peptic strictures, large esophageal ulcers, and hiatal hernias. A small hiatal hernia is usually not associated with significant symptoms or illness, and its presence is an irrelevant finding unless the hiatal hernia is large (Fig. 25-17), the hiatal opening is narrow and interrupts the flow of

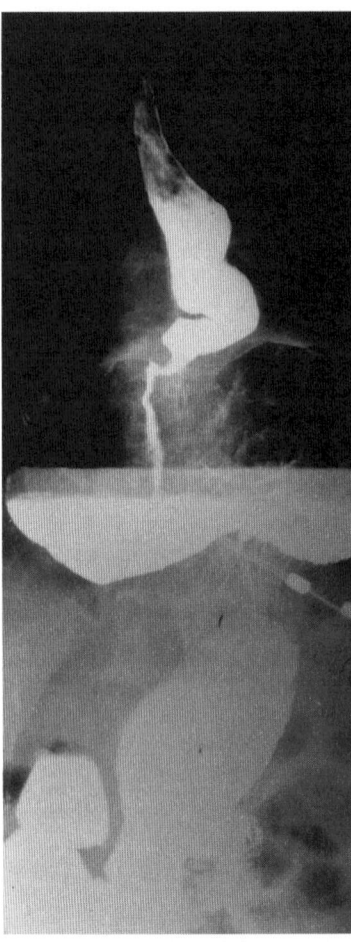

FIG. 25-17. Radiogram of an intrathoracic stomach. This is the end stage of a large hiatal hernia, regardless of its initial classification. *[Reproduced with permission from DeMeester TR, Stein HJ, Fuchs KH: Physiologic diagnostic studies, in Zuidema GD, Orringer MB (eds): Shackelford's Surgery of the Alimentary Tract, 3rd ed, Vol. I. Philadelphia: W. B. Saunders, 1991, p 111. Copyright Elsevier.]*

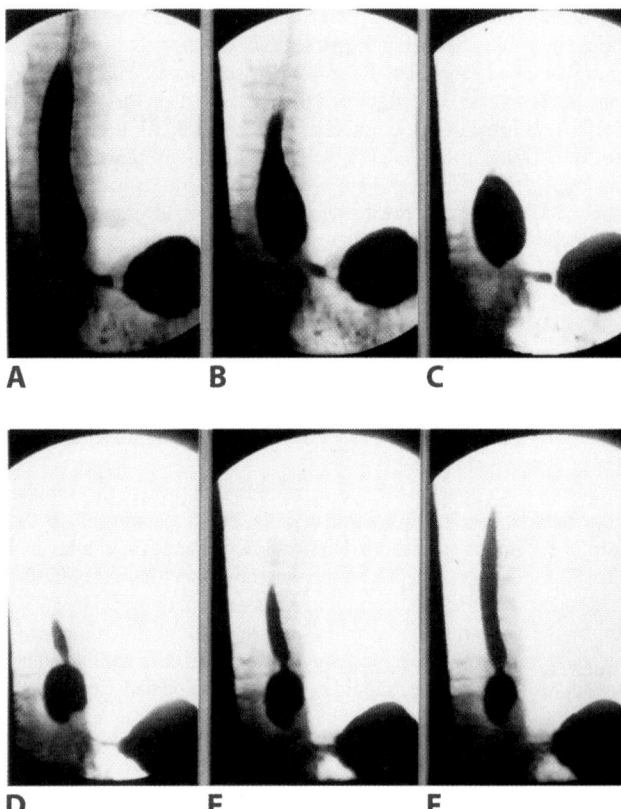

FIG. 25-18. Radiographic barium study showing a primary esophageal wave propelling liquid barium into the supradiaphragmatic portion of the stomach in a patient with a hiatal hernia (**A** and **B**). The diaphragmatic impingement on the stomach and the lack of contraction of the supradiaphragmatic stomach prevent passage of the bolus into the distal stomach (**C**). As a consequence, the contents in the supradiaphragmatic portion of the stomach are regurgitated into the thoracic esophagus (**D, E,** and **F**). The patient experiences dysphagia and regurgitation. On endoscopy, no anatomic abnormality other than a hiatal hernia was found, and on 24-hour pH monitoring, the patient had normal esophageal acid exposure. Symptoms of dysphagia and regurgitation were relieved by hiatal herniorrhaphy. *(Reproduced with permission from Kaul BJ, DeMeester TR, Oka M, et al: The cause of dysphagia in uncomplicated sliding hiatal hernia and its relief by hiatal herniography. A roentgenographic manometric and clinical study. Ann Surg 211:409, 1990.)*

barium into the stomach (Fig. 25-18), or the hernia is of the paraesophageal variety. Lesions extrinsic but adjacent to the esophagus can be reliably detected by the full-column technique if they contact the distended esophageal wall. Conversely, a number of important disorders may go undetected if this is the sole technique used to examine the esophagus. These include small esophageal neoplasms, mild esophagitis, and esophageal varices. Thus, the full-column technique should be supplemented with mucosal relief or double-contrast films to enhance detection of these smaller or more subtle lesions.

Motion-recording techniques greatly aid in evaluating functional disorders of the pharyngoesophageal and esophageal phases of swallowing. The technique and indications for cine- and videoradiography will be discussed in the section entitled Video- and Cineradiography, as they are more useful to evaluate function and seldom used to detect structural abnormalities.

The radiographic assessment of the esophagus is not complete unless the entire stomach and duodenum have been examined. A gastric or duodenal ulcer, partially obstructing gastric neoplasm, or scarred duodenum and pylorus may contribute significantly to symptoms otherwise attributable to an esophageal abnormality.

When a patient's complaints include dysphagia and no obstructing lesion is seen on the barium swallow, it is useful to have the patient swallow a barium-impregnated marshmallow, a barium-soaked piece of bread, or a hamburger mixed with barium. This test may bring out a functional disturbance in esophageal transport that can be missed when liquid barium is used.

Endoscopic Evaluation

In any patient complaining of dysphagia, esophagoscopy is indicated, even in the face of a normal radiographic study. A barium study obtained before esophagoscopy is helpful to the endoscopist by directing attention to locations of subtle change, and alerting the examiner to such potential danger spots as a cervical vertebral osteophyte, esophageal diverticulum, a deeply penetrating ulcer, or a carcinoma. Regardless of the radiologist's interpretation of an abnormal finding, each structural abnormality of the esophagus should be confirmed visually.

For the initial endoscopic assessment, the flexible fiber-optic esophagoscope is the instrument of choice because of its technical ease, patient acceptance, and the ability to simultaneously assess the stomach and duodenum. Rigid endoscopy may be required in specific instances and should be part of the armamentarium of the endoscopist. The rigid esophagoscope may be an essential instrument when deeper biopsies are required or the cricopharyngeus and cervical esophagus need closer assessment.

When GERD is the suspected diagnosis, particular attention should be paid to detecting the presence of esophagitis and Barrett's columnar-lined esophagus (CLE). When endoscopic esophagitis is seen, severity and the length of esophagus involved are recorded. Grade I esophagitis is defined as small, circular, nonconfluent erosions. Grade II esophagitis is defined by the presence of linear erosions lined with granulation tissue that bleeds easily when touched. Grade III esophagitis represents a more advanced stage, in which the linear erosions coalesce into circumferential loss of the epithelium and the mucosa may take a "cobblestone" appearance. Grade IV esophagitis is the presence of a stricture. Its severity can be assessed by the ease of passing a 36F endoscope. When a stricture is observed, the severity of the esophagitis above it should be recorded. The absence of esophagitis above a stricture suggests a chemical-induced injury or a neoplasm as a cause. The latter should always be considered and is ruled out only by evaluation of a tissue biopsy of adequate size.

Barrett's esophagus (BE) is a condition in which the tubular esophagus is lined with columnar epithelium, as opposed to the normal squamous epithelium. Histologically, it appears as intestinal metaplasia (IM). It is suspected at endoscopy when there is difficulty in visualizing the squamocolumnar junction at its normal location, and by the appearance of a redder, more luxuriant mucosa than is normally seen in the lower esophagus. Its presence is confirmed by biopsy. Multiple biopsies should be taken in a cephalad direction to determine the level at which the junction of Barrett's epithelium with normal squamous mucosa occurs. BE is susceptible to ulceration, bleeding, stricture formation, and, most important, malignant degeneration. The earliest sign of the latter is severe dysplasia or intramucosal adenocarcinoma (Fig. 25-19). These dysplastic changes have a patchy distribution, so a minimum of four biopsy samples spaced 2 cm apart should be taken from the Barrett's-lined portion of the esophagus. Changes seen in one biopsy are significant. Nishimaki has determined that the tumors occur in an area of specialized columnar epithelium near the squamocolumnar junction in 85% of patients, and within 2 cm of the squamocolumnar junction in virtually all patients. Particular attention should be focused on this area in patients suspected of harboring a carcinoma.

Abnormalities of the gastroesophageal flap valve can be visualized by retroflexion of the endoscope. Hill has graded the appearance of the gastroesophageal valve from I to IV according to the degree of unfolding or deterioration of the normal valve architecture (Fig. 25-20). The appearance of the valve correlates with the presence of increased esophageal acid exposure, occurring predominantly in patients with grade III and IV valves.

A hiatal hernia is endoscopically confirmed by finding a pouch lined with gastric rugal folds lying 2 cm or more above the margins of the diaphragmatic crura, identified by having the patient sniff. A prominent sliding hiatal hernia frequently is associated with increased esophageal exposure to gastric juice. When a paraesoph-

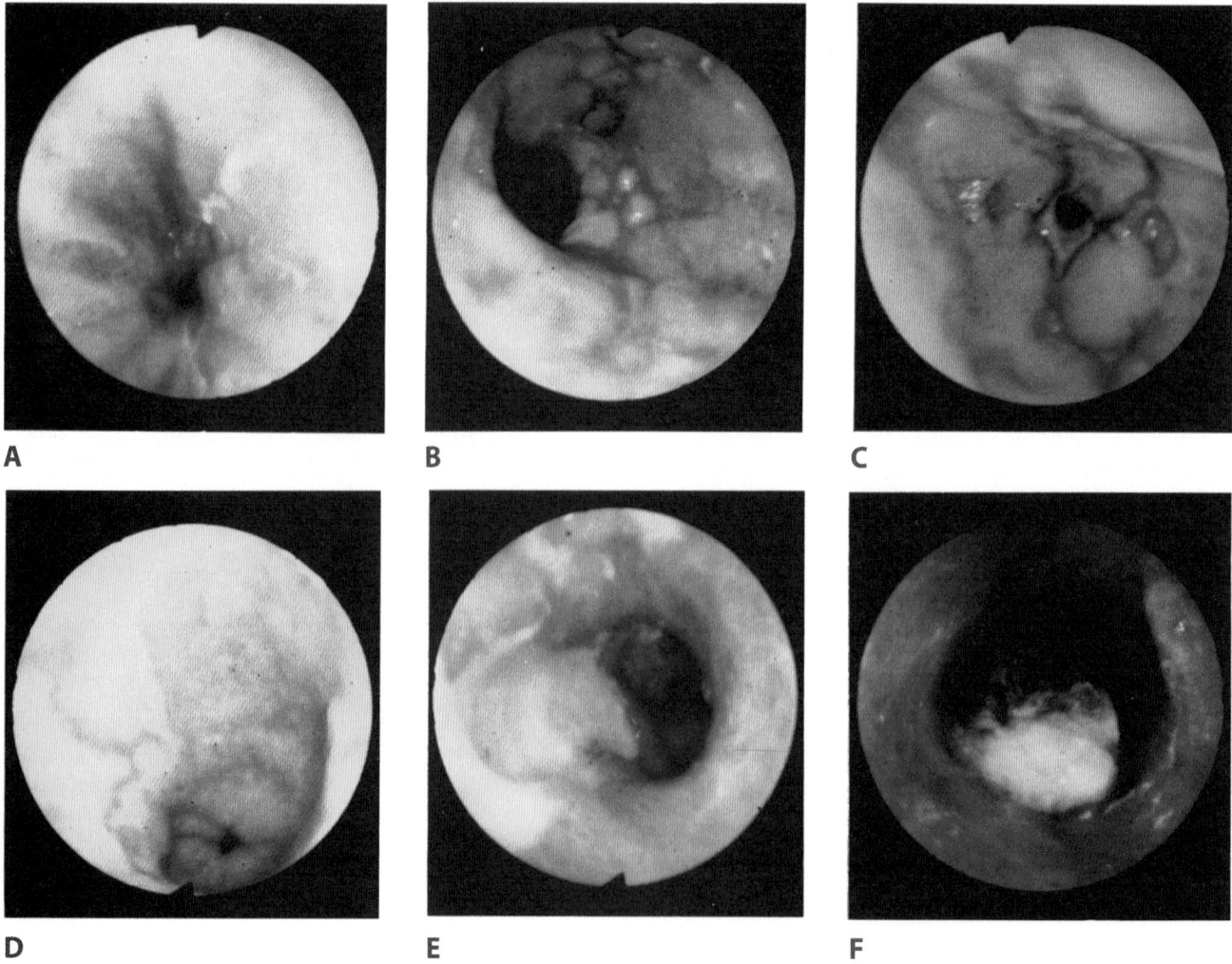

FIG. 25-19. Complications of reflux disease as seen on endoscopy. **A.** Linear erosion of grade II esophagitis. **B.** Cobblestone mucosa of grade III esophagitis. **C.** Stricture associated with grade III esophagitis. **D.** Uncomplicated Barrett's mucosa. **E.** Large ulcer in Barrett's mucosa. **F.** Adenocarcinoma arising in Barrett's mucosa.

ageal hernia (PEH) is observed, particular attention is taken to exclude a gastric ulcer or gastritis within the pouch. The intragastric retroflex or J maneuver is important in evaluating the full circumference of the mucosal lining of the herniated stomach.

When an esophageal diverticulum is seen, it should be carefully explored with the flexible endoscope to exclude ulceration or neopla-sia. When a submucosal mass is identified, biopsies are usually not performed. At the time of surgical resection, a submucosal leiomy-oma or reduplication cyst can generally be dissected away from the intact mucosa, but if a biopsy sample is taken, the mucosa may become fixed to the underlying abnormality. This complicates the surgical dissection by increasing the risk of mucosal perforation.

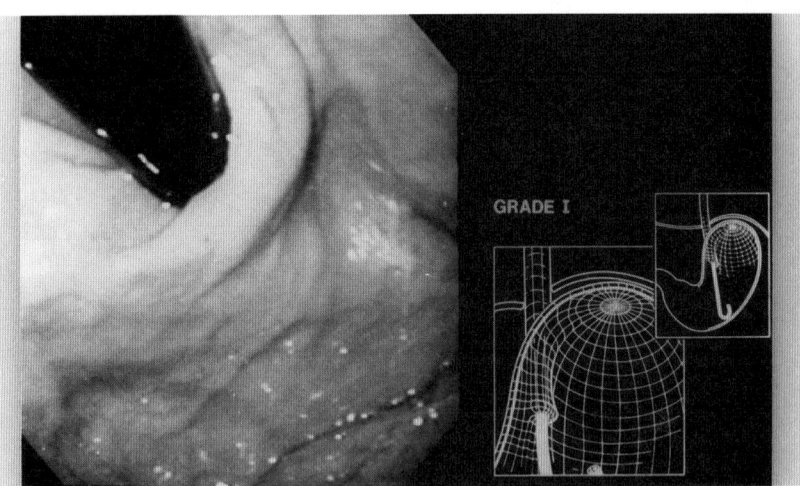

A

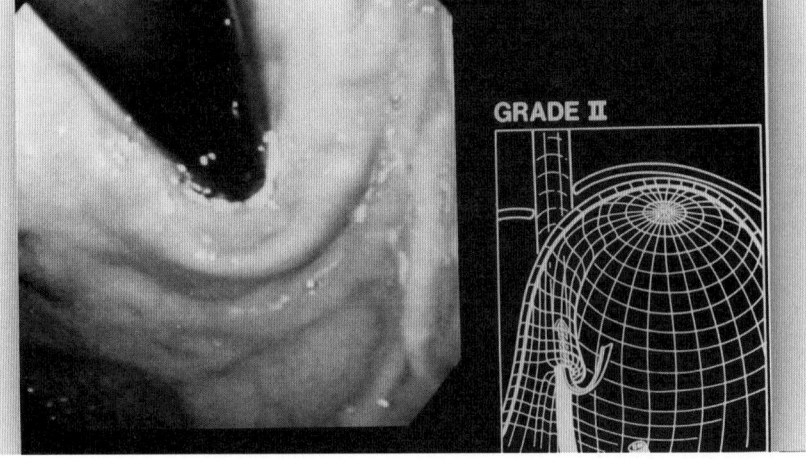

B

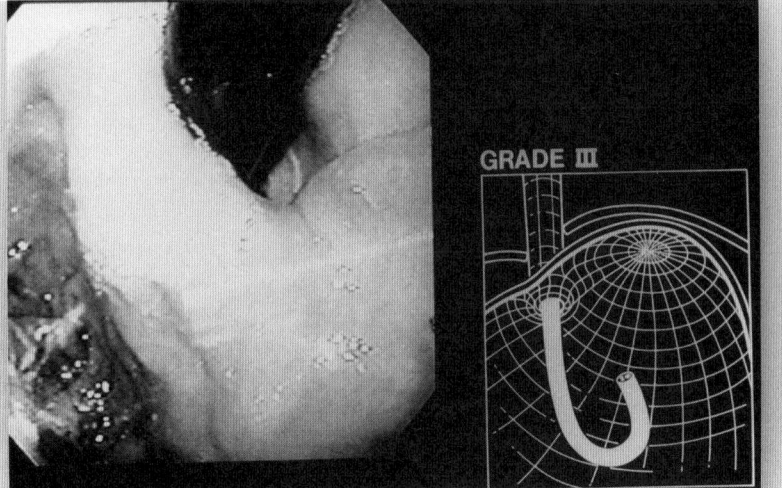

C

FIG. 25-20. **A.** Grade I flap valve appearance. Note the ridge of tissue that is closely approximated to the shaft of the retroflexed endoscope. It extends 3–4 cm along the lesser curve. **B.** Grade II flap valve appearance. The ridge is slightly less well defined than in grade I and it opens rarely with respiration and closes promptly. **C.** Grade III flap valve appearance. The ridge is barely present, and there is often failure to close around the endoscope. It is nearly always accompanied by a hiatal hernia. (*Continued*)

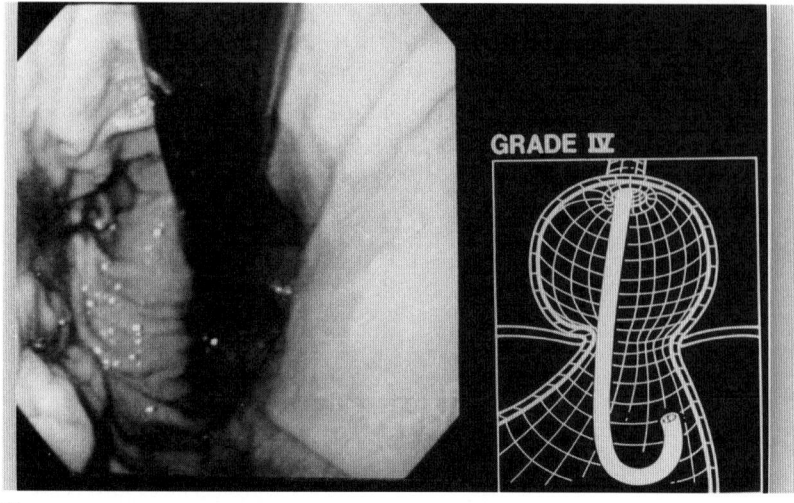

D

FIG. 25-20. (*Continued*) **D.** Grade IV flap valve appearance. There is no muscular ridge at all. The gastroesophageal valve stays open all the time, and squamous epithelium can often be seen from the retroflexed position. A hiatal hernia is always present. (*Reproduced with permission from Hill LD, Kozarek RA, et al: The gastroesophageal flap valve. In vitro and in vivo observations. Gastrointest Endosc 44:541, 1996. Copyright Elsevier.*)

Tests to Detect Functional Abnormalities

In many patients with symptoms of an esophageal disorder, standard radiographic and endoscopic evaluation fails to demonstrate a structural abnormality. In these situations, esophageal function tests are necessary to identify a functional disorder.

Stationary Manometry

Esophageal manometry is a widely used technique to examine the motor function of the esophagus and its sphincters. Manometry is indicated whenever a motor abnormality of the esophagus is suspected on the basis of complaints of dysphagia, odynophagia, or noncardiac chest pain, and the barium swallow or endoscopy does not show a clear structural abnormality. Esophageal manometry is particularly necessary to confirm the diagnosis of specific primary esophageal motility disorders [i.e., achalasia, diffuse esophageal spasm (DES), nutcracker esophagus, and hypertensive LES]. It also identifies nonspecific esophageal motility abnormalities and motility disorders secondary to systemic disease such as scleroderma, dermatomyositis, polymyositis, or mixed connective tissue disease. In patients with symptomatic GERD, manometry of the esophageal body can identify a mechanically defective LES, and evaluate the adequacy of esophageal peristalsis and contraction amplitude. Manometry has become an essential tool in the preoperative evaluation of patients before antireflux surgery, allowing selection of the appropriate procedure based upon the patient's underlying esophageal function.

Esophageal manometry is performed using electronic, pressure-sensitive transducers located within the catheter, or water-perfused catheters with lateral side holes attached to transducers outside the body. The traditional catheter consists of a train of five pressure transducers or five or more water-perfused tubes bound together. The transducers or lateral openings are placed at 5-cm intervals from the tip and oriented radially at 72° from each other around the circumference of the catheter. A special catheter assembly consisting of four lateral openings at the same level, oriented at 90° to each other, is of special use in measuring the three-dimensional vector volume of the LES. Other specially designed catheters can be used to assess the upper sphincter.

As the pressure-sensitive station is brought across the gastroesophageal junction (GEJ), a rise in pressure above the gastric baseline signals the beginning of the LES. The respiratory inversion point is identified when the positive excursions that occur in the abdominal cavity with breathing change to negative deflections in the thorax. The respiratory inversion point serves as a reference point at which the amplitude of LES pressure and the length of the sphincter exposed to abdominal pressure are measured. As the pressure-sensitive station

is withdrawn into the body of the esophagus, the upper border of the LES is identified by the drop in pressure to the esophageal baseline. From these measurements, the pressure, abdominal length, and overall length of the sphincter are determined (Fig. 25-21). To account for the asymmetry of the sphincter (Fig. 25-22), the pressure profile is repeated with each of the five radially oriented transducers, and the average values for sphincter pressure above gastric baseline, overall sphincter length, and abdominal length of the sphincter are calculated.

Table 25-1 shows the values for these parameters in 50 normal volunteers without subjective or objective evidence of a foregut disorder. The level at which a deficiency in the mechanics of the LES occurs was defined by comparing the frequency distribution of these values in the 50 healthy volunteers with a population of similarly studied patients with symptoms of GERD. The presence of increased esophageal exposure to gastric juice was documented by 24-hour esophageal pH monitoring. Based on these studies, a mechanically defective sphincter is identified by having one or more of the following characteristics: an average LES pressure of <6 mmHg, an average length exposed to the positive-pressure environment in the abdomen of 1 cm or less, and/or an average overall sphincter length of 2 cm or less. Compared with the normal volunteers, these values are below the 2.5 percentile for sphincter pressure and overall length and for abdominal length.

To assess the relaxation and postrelaxation contraction of the LES, a pressure transducer is positioned within the high-pressure

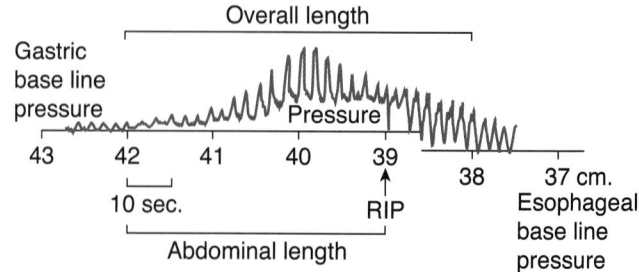

RIP = Respiratory inversion point

FIG. 25-21. Manometric pressure profile of the lower esophageal sphincter. The distances are measured from the nares. (*Reproduced with permission from: Zaninotto G, DeMeester TR, et al: The lower esophageal sphincter in health and disease. Am J Surg 155:105, 1988. Copyright Elsevier.*)

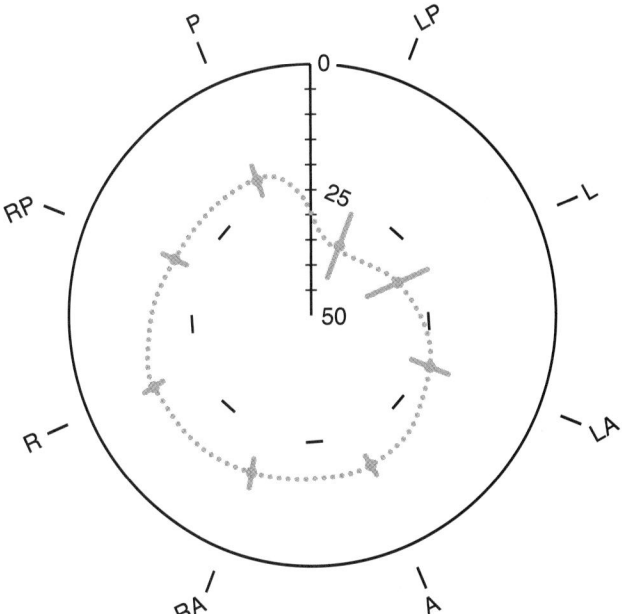

FIG. 25-22. Radial configuration of the lower esophageal sphincter. A = anterior; L = left; LA = left anterior; LP = left posterior; P = posterior; R = right; RA = right anterior; RP = right posterior. *(Reproduced with permission from Winans CS: Manometric asymmetry of the lower esophageal high pressure zone. Dig Dis 22:348, 1977. With kind permission from Springer Science+Business Media.)*

zone, with the distal transducer located in the stomach and the proximal transducer within the esophageal body. Ten wet swallows (5 mL water each) are performed. The normal pressure of the LES should drop to the level of gastric pressure during each wet swallow.

The function of the esophageal body is assessed with the five pressure transducers located in the esophagus. The standard procedure is to locate the most proximal pressure transducer 1 cm below the well-defined cricopharyngeal sphincter, allowing a pressure response throughout the whole esophagus to be obtained on one swallow. Ten wet swallows are recorded. Amplitude, duration, and morphology of contractions following each swallow are calculated at all recorded levels of the esophageal body. The delay between the onset or peak of esophageal contractions at the various levels of the esophagus is used to calculate the speed of wave propagation. The relationship of the esophageal contractions following a swallow is classified as peristaltic or simultaneous. The data are used to identify motor disorders of the esophagus.

TABLE 25-1	Normal manometric values of the distal esophageal sphincter, $n = 50$		
		Percentile	
	Median	**2.5**	**97.5**
Pressure (mmHg)	13	5.8	27.7
Overall length (cm)	3.6	2.1	5.6
Abdominal length (cm)	2	0.9	4.7
	Mean	**Mean – 2 SD**	**Mean +2 SD**
Pressure (mmHg)	13.8 ± 4.6	4.6	23.0
Overall length (cm)	3.7 ± 0.8	2.1	5.3
Abdominal length (cm)	2.2 ± 0.8	0.6	3.8

SD = standard deviation.
Source: Reproduced with permission from DeMeester TR, et al: Gastroesophageal reflux disease, in Moody FG, Carey LC, et al (eds): *Surgical Treatment of Digestive Disease.* Chicago: Year Book Medical, 1990, p 89. Copyright Elsevier.

The position, length, and pressure of the cricopharyngeal sphincter are assessed with a stationary pull-through technique similar to that used for the LES. The manometric catheter is withdrawn in 0.5-cm intervals from the upper esophagus through the upper esophageal sphincter region into the pharynx. The relaxation of the upper esophageal sphincter is studied by straddling the eight pressure transducers across the sphincter so that some are in the pharynx and some are in the upper esophagus. High-speed graphic recordings (50 mm/s) are necessary to obtain an assessment of the coordination of cricopharyngeal relaxation with hypopharyngeal contraction. It has been difficult to consistently demonstrate a motility abnormality in patients with pharyngoesophageal disorders.

High-Resolution Manometry

Esophageal manometry was introduced into clinical practice in the 1970s and, until recently, has changed little. In 1991, Ray Clouse introduced the concept of improving conventional manometry by increasing the number of recording sites and adding a three-dimensional assessment. This "high-resolution manometry" is a variant of the conventional manometry in which multiple, circumferential recording sites are used, in essence creating a "map" of the esophagus and its sphincters. High-resolution catheters contain 36 miniaturized pressure sensors positioned every centimeter along the length of the catheter. The vast amount of data generated by these sensors is then processed and presented in traditional linear plots or as a visually enhanced spatiotemporal video tracing that is readily interpreted (Fig. 25-23).

Simultaneous acquisition of data for the upper esophageal sphincter, esophageal body, LES, and gastric pressure minimizes the movement artifacts and study time associated with conventional esophageal manometry. Powerful, computer-based, and easy-to-use tools give unprecedented data analysis capability. This technology significantly enhances esophageal diagnostics, bringing it into the realm of "image" based studies. High-resolution manometry may allow the identification of focal motor abnormalities previously overlooked. It has enhanced the ability to predict bolus propagation and increased sensitivity in the measurement of pressure gradients.

Esophageal Impedance

New technology recently introduced into the clinical realm allows measurement of esophageal function and gastroesophageal reflux in a way that has heretofore not been possible. An intraluminal electrical impedance catheter has recently been developed for the measurement of GI function. *Impedance* is the ratio of voltage to current, and is a measure of the electrical conductivity of a hollow organ and its contents. Intraluminal electrical impedance is inversely proportional to the electrical conductivity of the luminal contents and the cross-sectional area of the lumen. Air has a very low electrical conductivity and, therefore, high impedance. Saliva and food cause an impedance decrease because of their increased conductivity. Luminal dilatation results in a decrease in impedance, whereas luminal contraction yields an impedance increase. Investigators have established the impedance waveform characteristics that define esophageal bolus transport. This allows for the characterization of both esophageal function, via quantification of bolus transport, and gastroesophageal reflux (Fig. 25-24). The probe measures impedance between adjacent electrodes, with measuring segments located at 2, 4, 6, 8, 14, and 16 cm from the distal tip. An extremely low electric current of 0.00025 μW is transmitted across the electrodes at a frequency of 1 to 2 kHz and is limited to 8 μA. This is below the stimulation threshold for nerves and muscles, and is three orders of magnitude below the threshold of cardiac stimulation. A standard pH electrode is located 5 cm from the distal tip, so that the acidic or nonacidic nature of refluxate can be correlated with the number of reflux events.

Esophageal impedance has been validated as an appropriate method for the evaluation of GI function and is becoming increasingly used for the diagnosis of gastroesophageal reflux. It has been

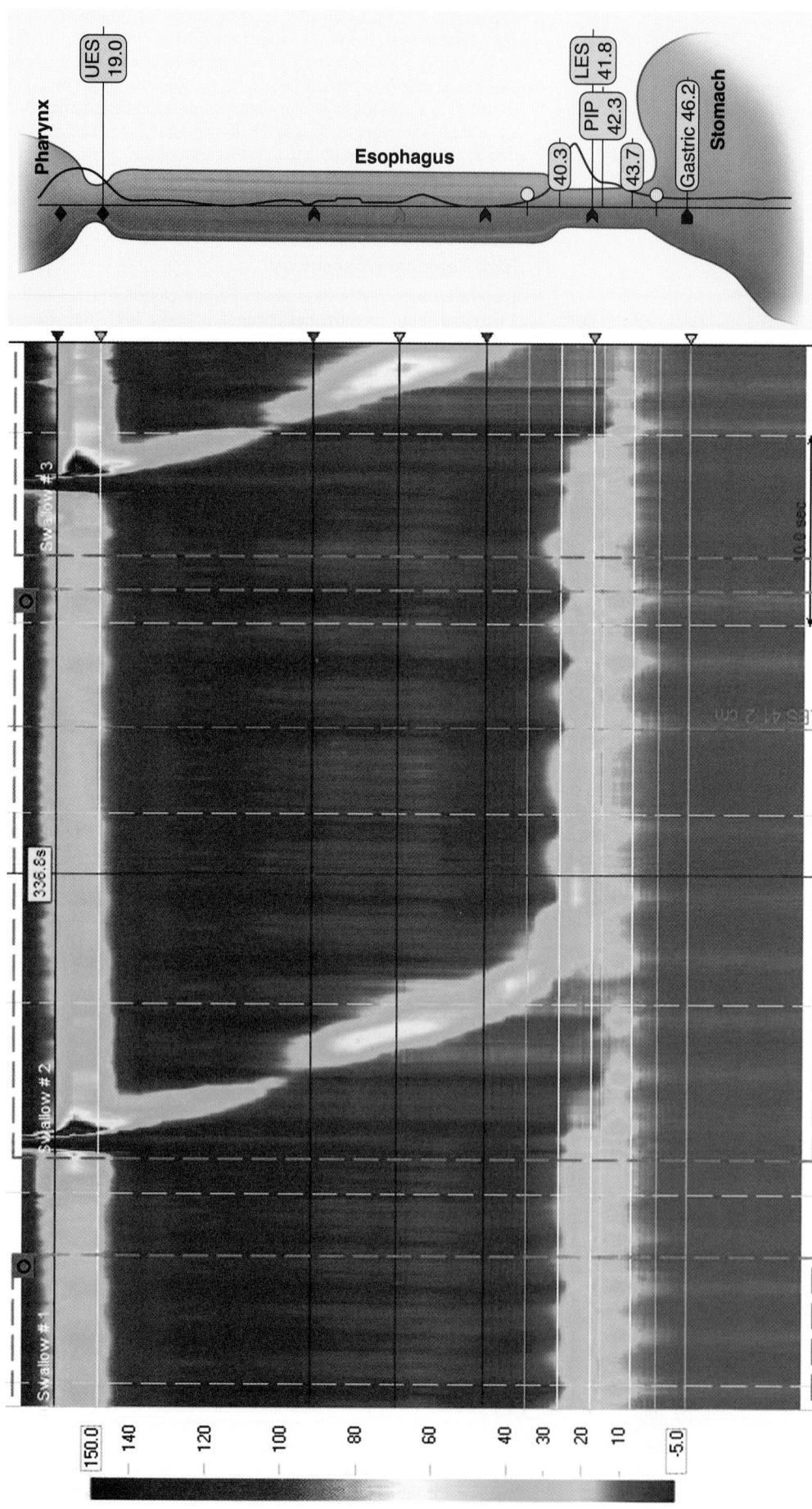

FIG. 25-23. High-resolution manometry motility study. Pressure measurements are recorded with color coding (red = high; blue = low). LES = lower esophageal sphincter; PIP = pressure inversion point; UES = upper esophageal sphincter. (*Continued*)

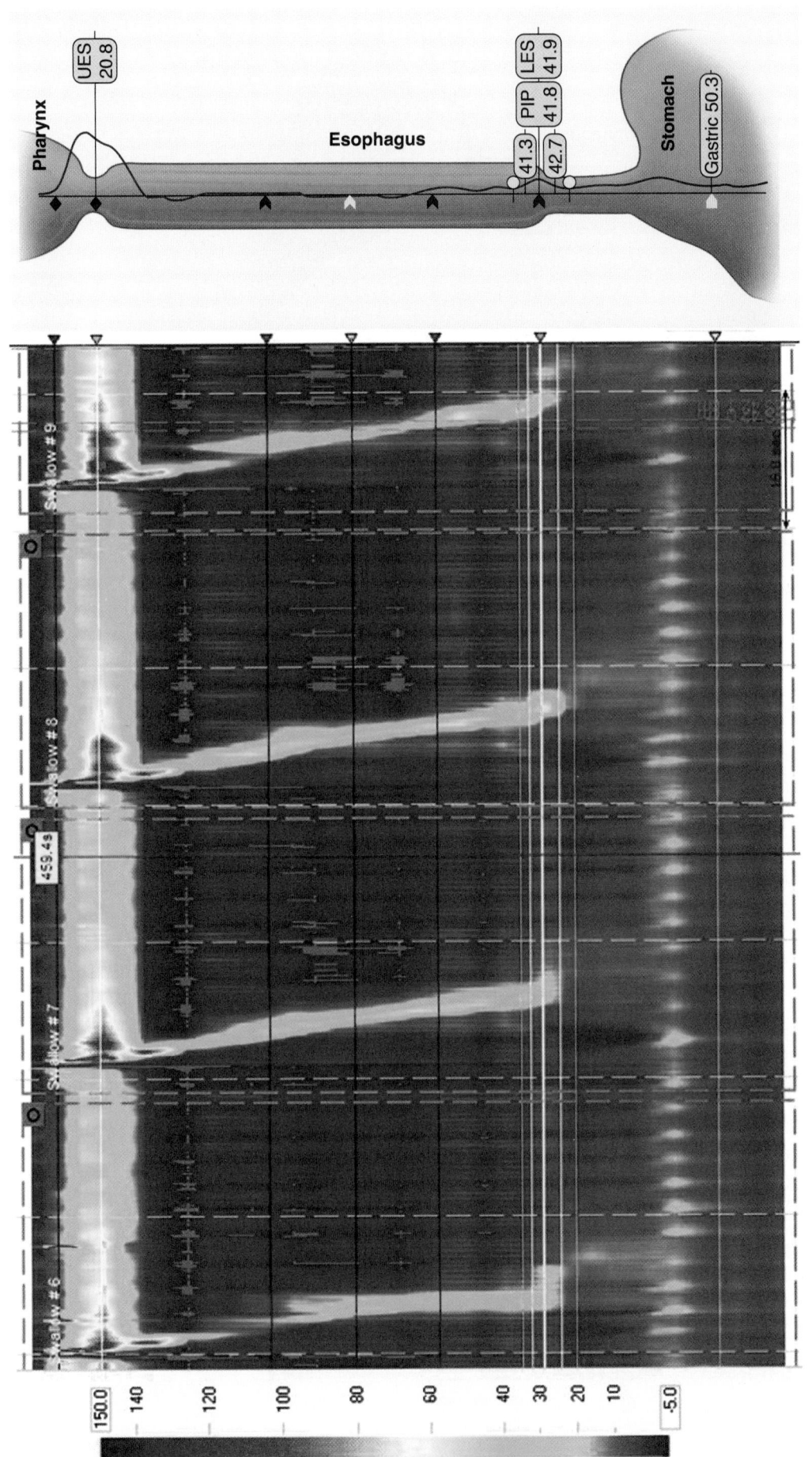

FIG. 25-23. (*Continued*)

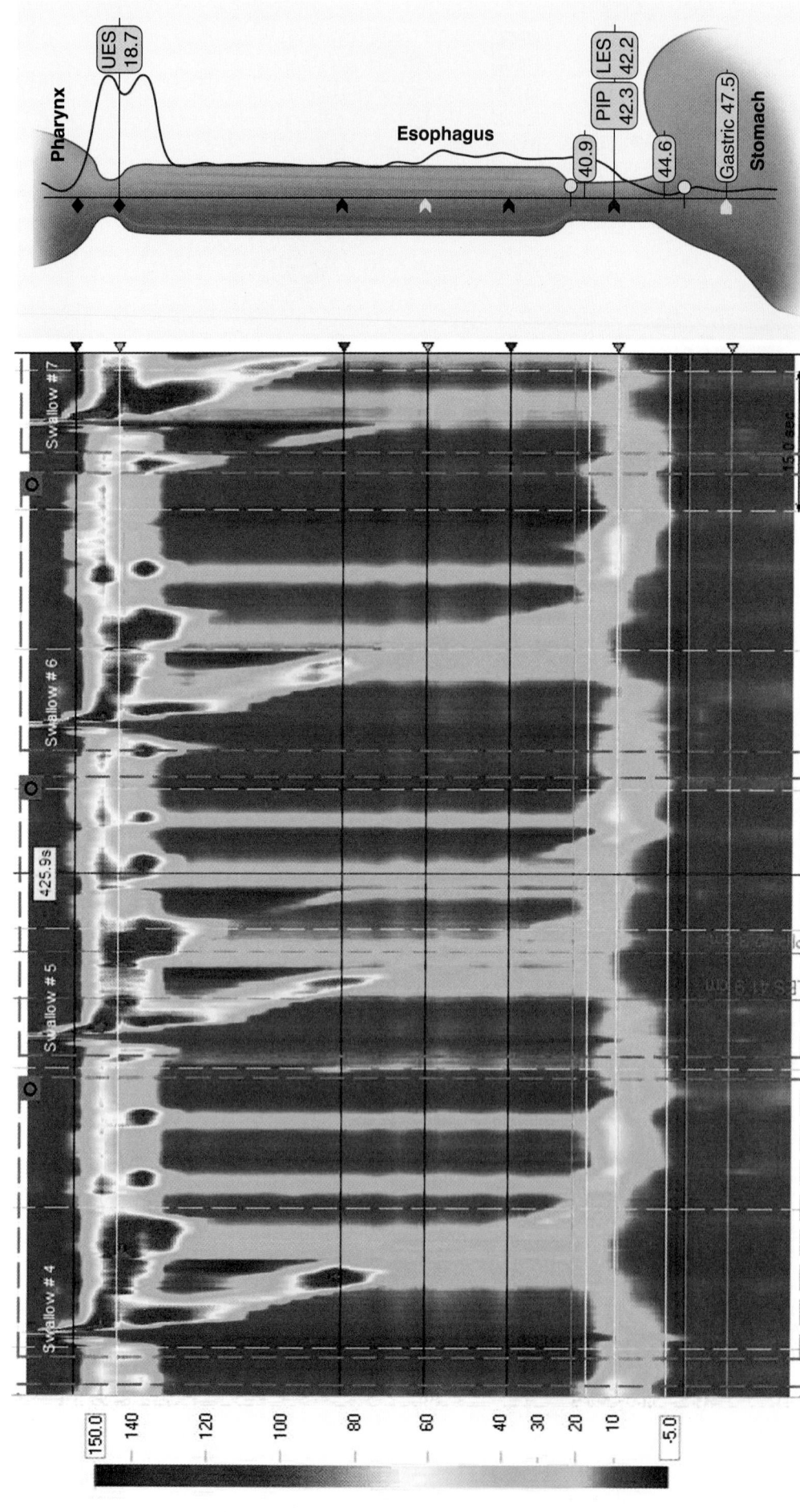

FIG. 25-23. (*Continued*)

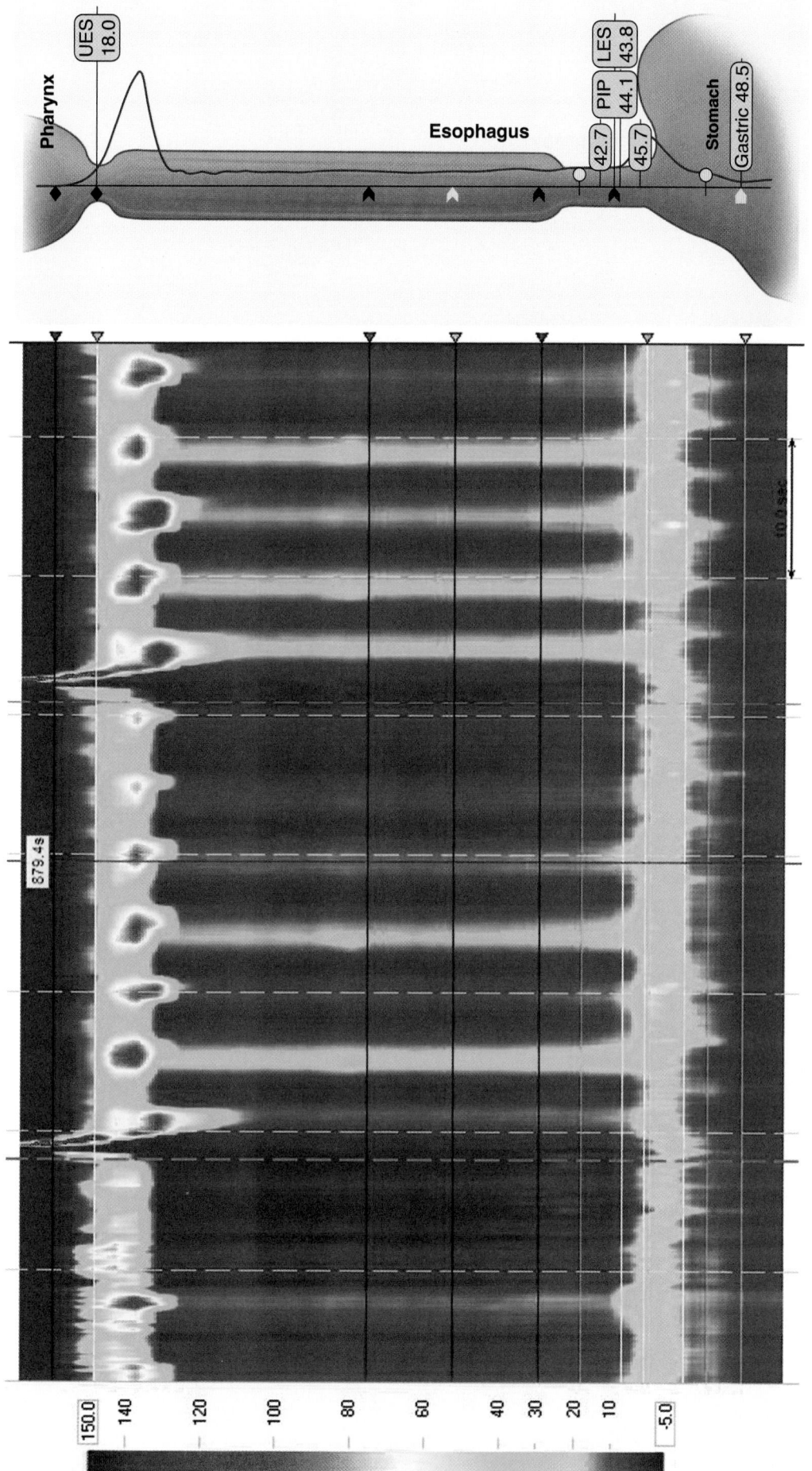

FIG. 25-23. *(Continued)*

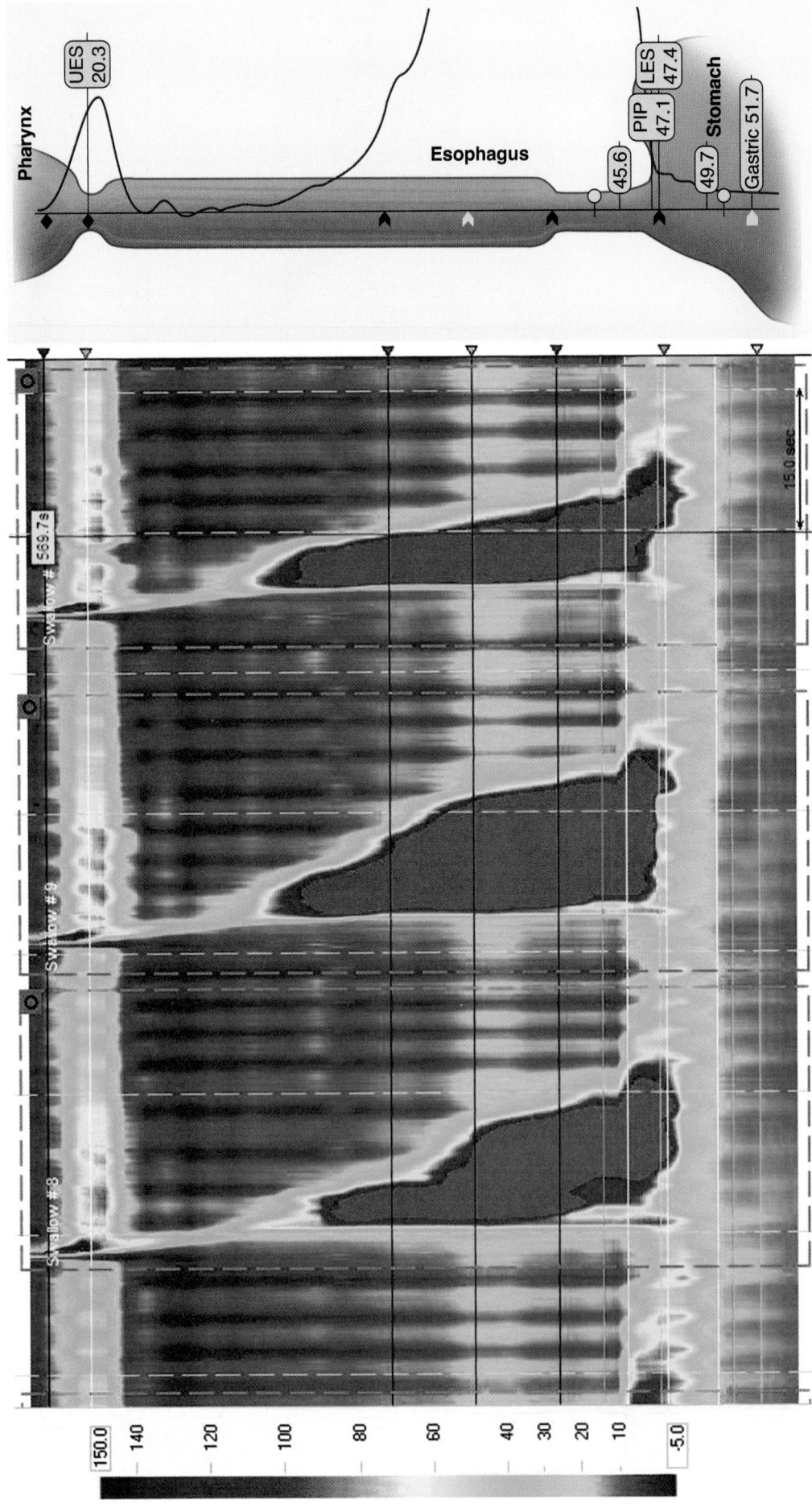

FIG. 25-23. (Continued)

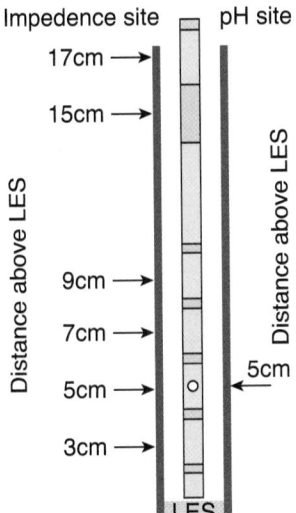

FIG. 25-24. Esophageal impedance probe measures electrical resistance between evenly spaced electrodes. LES = lower esophageal sphincter.

effectively "blinds" the test to reflux occurring at higher pH values. Furthermore, in patients with persistent symptoms on proton pump inhibitor (PPI) therapy, pH monitoring has limited use as it can only detect abnormal acid reflux (pH <4), the occurrence of which has been altered by the antisecretory medication. Given that PPI anti-secretory therapy is highly effective in neutralizing gastric acid, the question of whether persistent symptoms are a result of persistent acid reflux, nonacid reflux, or are not reflux related becomes a key issue in surgical decision making. Until recently, this differentiation could not be made. A reliable method for detecting both acid and nonacid reflux has potential to define these populations of patients and thus improve patient selection for antireflux surgery. The recent introduction of multichannel intraluminal impedance technology allows the measurement of both acid and nonacid reflux, with potential to significantly enhance diagnostic accuracy.

Using this technology, Balaji and colleagues showed that most gastroesophageal reflux remains despite acid suppression. Imped-ance pH may be particularly useful in evaluating patients with persistent symptoms despite PPI treatment, patients with respiratory symptoms, and postoperative patients who are having symptoms that are elusive to diagnosis.

Esophageal Transit Scintigraphy

The esophageal transit of a 10-mL water bolus containing techne-tium-99m (^{99m}Tc) sulfur colloid can be recorded with a gamma camera. Using this technique, delayed bolus transit has been shown in patients with a variety of esophageal motor disorders, including achalasia, scleroderma, DES, and nutcracker esophagus.

Video- and Cineradiography

High-speed cinematic or video recording of radiographic studies allows re-evaluation by reviewing the studies at various speeds. This technique is more useful than manometry in the evaluation of the pharyngeal phase of swallowing. Observations suggesting oropha-ryngeal or cricopharyngeal dysfunction include misdirection of barium into the trachea or nasopharynx, prominence of the cri-copharyngeal muscle, a Zenker's diverticulum, a narrow pharyn-goesophageal segment, and stasis of the contrast medium in the valleculae or hypopharyngeal recesses (Fig. 25-25). These findings are usually not specific, but rather common manifestations of

compared to cineradiography showing that impedance waves correspond well with actual bolus transport illustrated by radiography. Bolus entry, transit, and exit can be clearly identified by impedance changes in the corresponding measuring segments. Preliminary studies comparing standard esophageal manometry with imped-ance measurements in healthy volunteers have been performed, and have validated the ability of esophageal impedance to correlate with peristaltic wave progression and bolus length. Clinical investigators are beginning to examine and validate impedance measurement in the evaluation of esophageal and small intestinal pathophysiology.

It is increasingly recognized that 24-hour pH monitoring as the historical gold standard for diagnosing and quantifying gastroesoph-ageal reflux has significant limitations. With 24-hour ambulatory pH testing, reflux is defined as a drop in the pH below 4, which

FIG. 25-25. Esophagograms from a patient with cricopharyngeal achalasia. **A.** Anteroposterior film showing retention of the contrast medium at the level of the vallecula and piriform recesses, with no barium passing into the esophagus. **B.** Lateral film, taken opposite the C5–C6 vertebrae, showing posterior indentation of the cri-copharyngeus, retention in the hypopharynx, and tracheal aspiration. *[Reproduced with permission from Lafontaine E: Pharyngeal dysphagia, in DeMeester TR, Matthews H (eds):* International Trends in General Thoracic Surgery, Vol. 3. Benign Esophageal Disease. *St. Louis: Mosby, 1987, p 345. Copyright Elsevier.]*

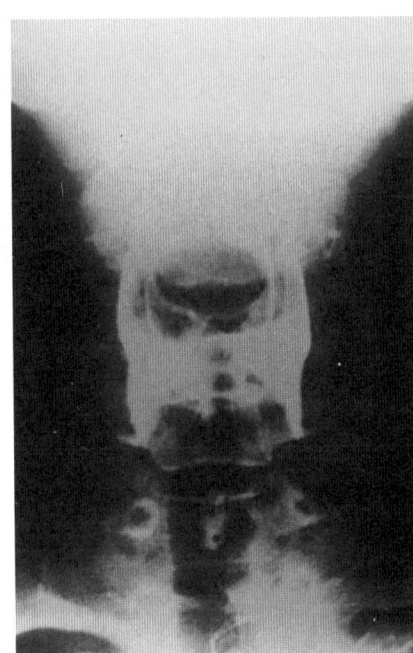

A

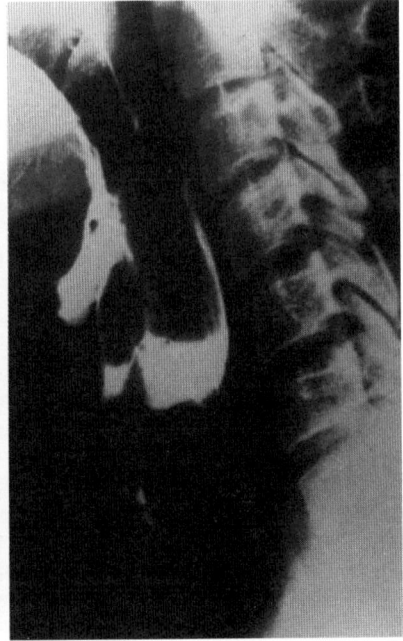

B

neuromuscular disorders affecting the pharyngoesophageal area. Studies using liquid barium, barium-impregnated solids, or radiopaque pills aid the evaluation of normal and abnormal motility in the esophageal body. Loss of the normal stripping wave or segmentation of the barium column with the patient in the recumbent position correlates with abnormal motility of the esophageal body. In addition, structural abnormalities such as small diverticula, webs, and minimal extrinsic impressions of the esophagus may be recognized only with motion-recording techniques. The simultaneous computerized capture of videofluoroscopic images and manometric tracings is now available, and is referred to as *manofluorography*. Manofluorographic studies allow precise correlation of the anatomic events, such as opening of the upper esophageal sphincter, with manometric observations, such as sphincter relaxation. Manofluorography, although not widely available, is presently the best means available to evaluate complex functional abnormalities.

Tests to Detect Increased Exposure to Gastric Juice
24-Hour Ambulatory pH Monitoring

The most direct method of measuring increased esophageal exposure to gastric juice is by an indwelling pH electrode, or, more recently, via a radiotelemetric pH monitoring capsule that can be clipped to the esophageal mucosa. The latter consists of an antimony pH electrode fitted inside a small, capsule-shaped device accompanied by a battery and electronics that allow 48-hour monitoring and transmission of the pH data via transcutaneous radio telemetry to a waist-mounted data logger. The device can be introduced either transorally or transnasally, and clipped to the esophageal mucosa using endoscopic fastening techniques. It passes spontaneously within 1 to 2 weeks. Prolonged monitoring of esophageal pH is performed by placing the pH probe or telemetry capsule 5 cm above the manometrically measured upper border of the distal sphincter for 24 hours. It measures the actual time the esophageal mucosa is exposed to gastric juice, measures the ability of the esophagus to clear refluxed acid, and correlates esophageal acid exposure with the patient's symptoms. A 24- to 48-hour period is necessary so that measurements can be made over one or two complete circadian cycles. This allows measuring the effect of physiologic activity, such as eating or sleeping, on the reflux of gastric juice into the esophagus (Fig. 25-26).

The 24-hour esophageal pH monitoring should not be considered a test for reflux, but rather a measurement of the esophageal exposure to gastric juice. The measurement is expressed by the time the esophageal pH was below a given threshold during the 24-hour period. This single assessment, although concise, does not reflect how the exposure has occurred; that is, did it occur in a few long episodes or several short episodes? Consequently, two other assessments are necessary: the frequency of the reflux episodes and their duration.

The units used to express esophageal exposure to gastric juice are (a) cumulative time the esophageal pH is below a chosen threshold, expressed as the percentage of the total, upright, and supine monitored time; (b) frequency of reflux episodes below a chosen threshold, expressed as number of episodes per 24 hours; and (c) duration of the episodes, expressed as the number of episodes >5 minutes per 24 hours, and the time in minutes of the longest episode recorded. Table 25-2 shows the normal values for these components of the 24-hour record at the whole-number pH threshold derived from 50 normal asymptomatic subjects. The upper limits of normal were established at the ninety-fifth percentile. Most centers use pH 4 as the threshold.

The components' 24-hour pH record are then combined into one expression of the overall esophageal acid exposure below a pH threshold; the pH score is calculated by using the standard deviation (SD) of the mean of each of the six components measured in the 50 normal subjects as a weighting factor. By accepting an abstract zero level two SDs below the mean, the data measured in normal subjects could be treated as though they had a normal distribution. Thus,

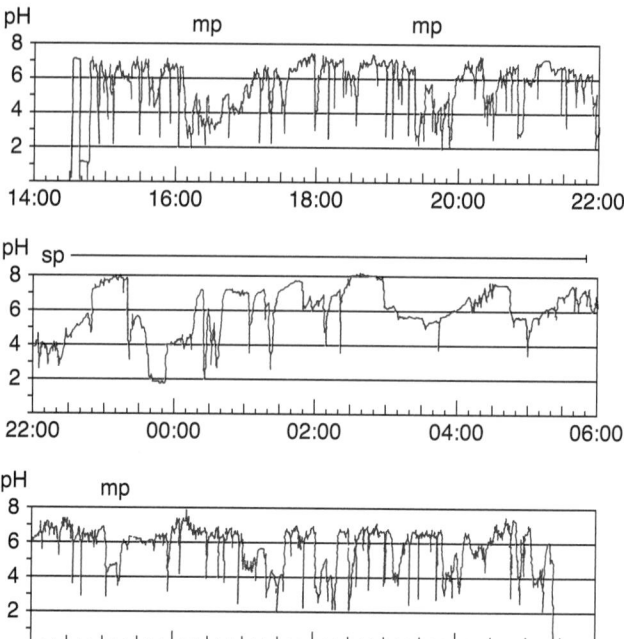

FIG. 25-26. Strip chart display of a 24-hour esophageal pH monitoring study in a patient with increased esophageal acid exposure. mp = meal period; sp = supine period. *[Reproduced with permission from DeMeester TR, Stein HJ, Fuchs KH: Physiologic diagnostic studies, in Zuidema GD, Orringer MB (eds):* Shackelford's Surgery of the Alimentary Tract, *3rd ed, Vol. I. Philadelphia: W.B. Saunders, 1991, p 119. Copyright Elsevier.]*

any measured patient value could be referenced to this zero point, and, in turn, be awarded points based on whether it was below or above the normal mean value for that component, according to this formula:

$$\text{Component score} = \frac{\text{Point value} - \text{mean}}{\text{SD} + 1}$$

The upper limits of normal for the composite score for each whole-number pH threshold are shown in Table 25-3.

The detection of increased esophageal exposure to acid gastric juice is more dependable than the detection of increased exposure to alkaline gastric juice. The latter is suggested by an increased alkaline exposure time above pH 7 or 8. Increased exposure in this pH range can be caused by abnormal calibration of the pH recorder; dental infection, which increases salivary pH; esophageal obstruction, which results in static pools of saliva with an increase in pH secondary to bacterial overgrowth; or regurgitation of alkaline gastric juice into the esophagus. Using a properly calibrated probe, in the absence of dental

TABLE 25-2	Normal values for esophageal exposure to pH <4 (n = 50)		
Component	**Mean**	**SD**	**95%**
Total time	1.51	1.36	4.45
Upright time	2.34	2.34	8.42
Supine time	0.63	1.0	3.45
No. of episodes	19.00	12.76	46.90
No. >5 min	0.84	1.18	3.45
Longest episode	6.74	7.85	19.80

SD = standard deviation.
Source: Reproduced with permission from DeMeester TR, et al: Gastroesophageal reflux disease, in Moody FG, Carey LC, et al (eds): *Surgical Treatment of Digestive Disease*. Chicago: Year Book Medical, 1990, p 68. Copyright Elsevier.

TABLE 25-3	Normal composite score for various pH thresholds: upper level of normal value
pH Threshold	**95th Percentile**
<1	14.2
<2	17.37
<3	14.10
<4	14.72
<5	15.76
<6	12.76
>7	14.90
>8	8.50

Source: Reproduced with permission from DeMeester TR, et al: Gastroesophageal reflux disease, in Moody FG, Carey LC, et al (eds): *Surgical Treatment of Digestive Disease*. Chicago: Year Book Medical, 1990, p 69. Copyright Elsevier.

infections or esophageal obstruction, the percentage of time the pH is measured above 7 correlates with the concentration of bile acids continuously aspirated over a 24-hour period.

When done in a test population with an equal distribution of normal healthy subjects and patients with the classic reflux symptoms and a defective sphincter, 24-hour esophageal pH monitoring had a sensitivity and specificity of 96%. (*Sensitivity* is the ability to detect a disease when known to be present; *specificity* is the ability to exclude the disease when known to be absent.) This gave a predictive value of a positive and negative test of 96%, and an overall accuracy of 96%. Based on these studies and extensive clinical experience, 24-hour esophageal pH monitoring has emerged as the gold standard for the diagnosis of GERD.

Catheter-based, 24-hour, ambulatory, esophageal pH monitoring does have a significant drawback of the physical presence of a transnasal catheter that must be worn for 24 hours. Although most doctors ask patients to go about their normal activities of daily living, many do not comply due to embarrassment about the catheter or from discomfort. The recent development of a wireless capsule, which can be implanted in the esophagus and record pH data for 48 hours, has significantly changed patient satisfaction with the procedure.

The Bravo pH Capsule (Medtronics, Minneapolis, Minn) measures pH levels in the esophagus and transmits continuous esophageal pH readings to a receiver worn on the patient's belt or waistband (Fig. 25-27). Symptoms that the patient experiences are recorded in a diary and/or by pressing buttons on the receiver unit. Generally, 48 hours of pH data are measured with this probe. A recent study has shown that the addition of a second day of pH monitoring increased the sensitivity of pH measurement by 22%. The capsule eventually detaches and passes through the digestive tract in 5 to 7 days.

Radiographic Detection of Gastroesophageal Reflux

The definition of radiographic gastroesophageal reflux varies depending on whether reflux is spontaneous or induced by various maneuvers. In only about 40% of patients with classic symptoms of GERD is spontaneous reflux (i.e., reflux of barium from the stomach into the esophagus with the patient in the upright position) observed by the radiologist. In most patients who show spontaneous reflux on radiography, the diagnosis of increased esophageal acid exposure is confirmed by 24-hour esophageal pH monitoring. Therefore, the radiographic demonstration of spontaneous regurgitation of barium into the esophagus in the upright position is a reliable indicator that reflux is present. Failure to see this does not indicate the absence of disease.

Tests of Duodenogastric Function

Esophageal disorders are frequently associated with abnormalities of duodenogastric function. Abnormalities of the gastric reservoir or increased gastric acid secretion can be responsible for increased esophageal exposure to gastric juice. Reflux of alkaline duodenal juice, including bile salts, pancreatic enzymes, and bicarbonate, is thought to have a role in the pathogenesis of esophagitis and complicated Barrett's esophagus. Furthermore, functional disorders of the esophagus are often not confined to the esophagus alone, but are associated with functional disorders of the rest of the foregut (i.e., stomach and duodenum). Tests of duodenogastric function that are helpful to investigate esophageal symptoms include gastric emptying studies, gastric acid analysis, and cholescintigraphy (for the diagnosis of pathologic duodenogastric reflux). The single test of 24-hour gastric pH monitoring can be used to identify gastric hypersecretion and imply the presence of duodenogastric reflux and delayed gastric emptying.

Gastric Emptying

Gastric emptying studies are performed with radionuclide-labeled meals. Emptying of solids and liquids can be assessed simultaneously when both phases are marked with different tracers. After ingestion of a labeled standard meal, gamma camera images of the stomach are obtained at 5- to 15-minute intervals for 1.5 to 2 hours. After correction for decay, the counts in the gastric area are plotted as the percentage of total counts at the start of the imaging. The resulting emptying curve can be compared with data obtained in normal volunteers. In general, normal subjects will empty 59% of a meal within 90 minutes.

Gastric Acid Analysis

The gastric secretory state is usually evaluated by determination of the titratable gastric acid in aspirated gastric juice. Interdigestive or basal gastric acid secretion is measured in the fasting state, and varies between 0 and 5 mmol/h in normal volunteers. The maximal acid secretory capacity of the stomach, which reflects the available parietal cell mass, is calculated following stimulation of gastric acid secretion with pentagastrin or histamine. Acid hypersecretors have a basal gastric acid secretory capacity of >5 mmol/h and a maximal acid secretory capacity of more than 30 mmol/h.

Cholescintigraphy

Scintigraphic hepatobiliary imaging is performed after IV injection of 5 μCi of ^{99m}Tc iminodiacetic acid derivatives such as disofenin (^{99m}Tc-DISIDA). Gamma camera images of the upper abdomen, including the gallbladder and stomach, are obtained at 5-minute intervals for 60 minutes. Imaging is continued for an additional 30 minutes after stimulation of gallbladder contraction with 20 mg/kg of synthetic C-terminal octapeptide of cholecystokinin. Duodenogastric reflux is demonstrated as an increase of radioactivity in the stomach in the sequential images. The clinical value of this test is limited due to its short duration and a relatively high false-positive rate in normal volunteers.

24-Hour Gastric pH Monitoring

Monitoring is performed over a complete circadian cycle with a pH electrode placed 5 cm below the manometrically located LES. The patient is fully ambulatory during the test and is encouraged to perform normal daily activity. The gastric pH profile is assessed separately for the meal, postprandial period, and fasting period. The latter is divided into the time spent upright and supine.

The interpretation of continuous gastric pH recordings is more difficult than that of esophageal pH recordings. This is because the gastric pH environment is determined by a complex interplay of acid secretion; mucus secretion; ingested food; swallowed saliva; regurgitated duodenal, pancreatic, and biliary secretions; and the effectiveness of the mixing and evacuation of the chyme. Using 24-hour gastric pH monitoring to evaluate the gastric secretory state is based on studies that have shown that a good correlation exists between increased basal acid output on standard gastric acid analysis, and a left shift on the frequency distribution graph of gastric pH recordings during the supine fasting period. The evaluation of gastric emptying by 24-hour gastric pH monitoring is based on studies

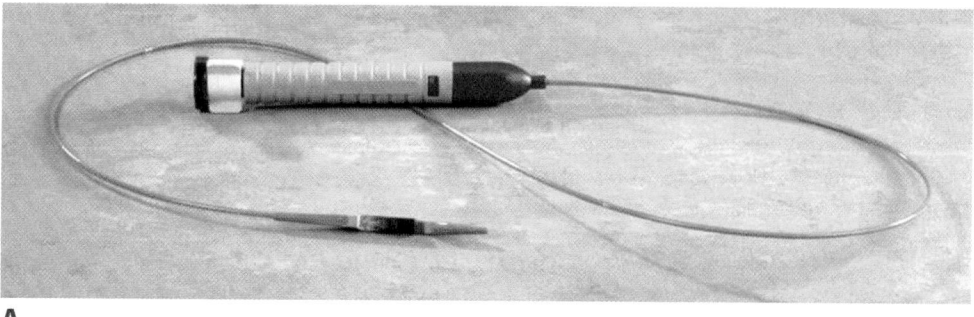

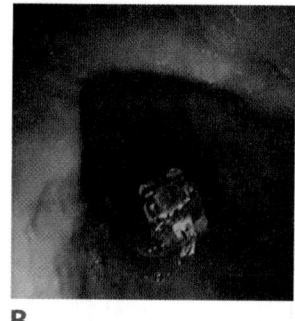

FIG. 25-27. Wireless pH monitoring. **A.** Delivery device. **B.** Capsule engaged in the wall of the esophagus.

demonstrating a good correlation between the emptying of a solid meal and the duration of the postprandial plateau and decline phase of the gastric pH record.

Using 24-hour gastric pH monitoring to evaluate duodenogastric reflux is based on the observation that reflux of alkaline duodenal juice into the stomach can alkalinize the gastric pH environment. The measurement is not straightforward because of the effect of meals, and reduction in acid secretion can result in changes in gastric pH that mimic alkaline reflux episodes. To overcome this problem, computerized measurements of the number and height of alkalinizing peaks, the baseline pH, the postprandial pH plateau, and the pattern of pH decline from the plateau can

be used to identify the probability of duodenogastric reflux. The results are presented as an overall score that indicates the likelihood of pathologic duodenogastric reflux. Initial data indicate that this approach has a higher sensitivity and specificity for the diagnosis of pathologic duodenogastric reflux than scintigraphic methods do.

Combined 24-hour esophageal and gastric pH monitoring can identify excessive alkaline duodenogastric and alkaline gastroesophageal reflux in symptomatic patients. The combined tracings can often identify simultaneous gastric and esophageal alkalinization, suggesting a duodenal origin for the esophageal alkaline exposure (Fig. 25-28).

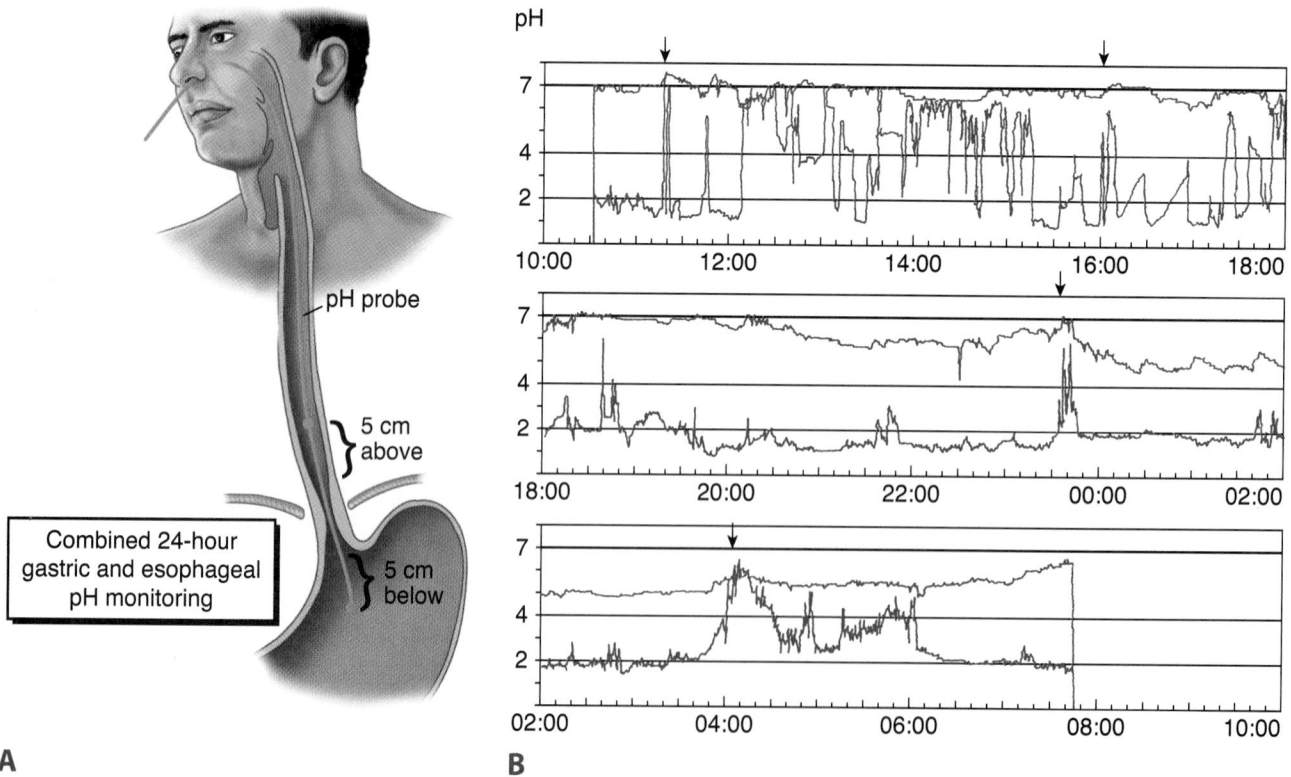

FIG. 25-28. A. Combined esophageal and gastric pH monitoring showing position of probes in relation to the lower esophageal sphincter. **B.** Combined ambulatory esophageal (*upper tracing*) and gastric (*lower tracing*) pH monitoring showing duodenogastric reflux (*arrows*) with propagation of the alkaline juice into the esophagus of a patient with complicated Barrett's esophagus. The gastric tracing (*lower*) is taken from a probe lying 5 cm below the upper esophageal sphincter. The esophageal tracing (*upper*) is taken from a probe lying 5 cm above the lower esophageal sphincter. Note that in only a small proportion of time does duodenogastric reflux move the pH of the esophagus above the threshold of 7, causing the iceberg effect. [*Reproduced with permission from DeMeester TR, Stein HJ, Fuchs KH: Physiologic diagnostic studies, in Zuidema GD, Orringer MB (eds): Shackelford's Surgery of the Alimentary Tract, 3rd ed., Vol. I. Philadelphia: W.B. Saunders, 1991, p 123. Copyright Elsevier.*]

GASTROESOPHAGEAL REFLUX DISEASE

GERD was not recognized as a significant clinical problem until the mid-1930s and was not identified as a precipitating cause for esophagitis until after World War II. In the early twenty-first century, it has grown to be a very common problem and now accounts for a majority of esophageal pathology. It is recognized as a chronic disease, and when medical therapy is required, it is often lifelong. Recent efforts at the development of various endoscopic antireflux interventions, although innovative, have not been successful in consistently controlling gastroesophageal reflux. Antireflux surgery is an effective and long-term therapy and is the only treatment that is able to restore the gastroesophageal barrier. Despite the common prevalence of GERD, it can be one of the most challenging diagnostic and therapeutic problems in clinical medicine. A contributing factor to this is the lack of a universally accepted definition of the disease.

The most simplistic approach is to define the disease by its symptoms. However, symptoms thought to be indicative of GERD, such as heartburn or acid regurgitation, are very common in the general population and many individuals consider them to be normal and do not seek medical attention. Even when excessive, these symptoms are not specific for gastroesophageal reflux. They can be caused by other diseases such as achalasia, DES, esophageal carcinoma, pyloric stenosis, cholelithiasis, gastritis, gastric or duodenal ulcer, and coronary artery disease.

A thorough, structured evaluation of the patient's symptoms is essential before any therapy, particularly any form of esophageal surgery. The presence and severity of both typical symptoms of heartburn, regurgitation, and dysphagia, and atypical symptoms of cough, hoarseness, chest pain, asthma, and aspiration should be discussed with the patient in detail. Many of these atypical symptoms may not be esophageal related and hence will not improve and may even worsen with antireflux surgery.

Heartburn is generally defined as a substernal burning-type discomfort, beginning in the epigastrium and radiating upward. It is often aggravated by meals, spicy or fatty foods, chocolate, alcohol, and coffee and can be worse in the supine position. It is commonly, although not universally, relieved by antacid or antisecretory medications. Epidemiologic studies have shown that heartburn occurs monthly in as many as 40 to 50% of the Western population. The occurrence of heartburn at night and its effect on quality of life have recently been highlighted by a Gallup poll conducted by the American Gastroenterologic Society (Table 25-4).

Regurgitation, the effortless return of acid or bitter gastric contents into the chest, pharynx, or mouth, is highly suggestive of foregut pathology. It is often particularly severe at night when supine or when bending over and can be secondary to either an incompetent or obstructed GEJ. With the later, as in achalasia, the regurgitant is often bland, as if food was put into a blender. When questioned, most patients can distinguish the two. It is the regurgitation of gastric contents that may result in associated pulmonary symptoms, including cough, hoarseness, asthma, and recurrent pneumonia. Bronchospasm can be precipitated by esophageal acid-ification and cough by either acid stimulation or distention of the esophagus.

Dysphagia, or *difficulty swallowing*, is a relatively nonspecific term but arguably the most specific symptom of foregut disease. It is often a sign of underlying malignancy and should be aggressively investigated until a diagnosis is established. Dysphagia refers to the sensation of difficulty in the passage of food from the mouth to the stomach and can be divided into oropharyngeal and esophageal etiologies. Oropharyngeal dysphagia is characterized by difficulty transferring food out of the mouth into the esophagus, nasal regurgitation, and/or aspiration. Esophageal dysphagia refers to the sensation of food sticking in the lower chest or epigastrium. This may or may not be accompanied by pain (odynophagia) that will be relieved by the passage of the bolus.

Chest pain, although commonly and appropriately attributed to cardiac disease, is frequently secondary to esophageal pathology as well. As early as 1982, DeMeester and associates showed that nearly 50% of patients with severe chest pain, normal cardiac function, and normal coronary arteriograms had positive 24-hour pH studies, implicating gastroesophageal reflux as the underlying etiology. Exercise-induced gastroesophageal reflux is well known to occur, and may result in exertional chest pain similar to angina. It can be quite difficult, if not impossible, to distinguish between the two etiologies, particularly on clinical grounds alone. Nevens and colleagues evaluated the ability of experienced cardiologists to differentiate pain of cardiac vs. esophageal origin. Of 248 patients initially seen by cardiologists, 185 were thought to have typical angina and 63 atypical chest pain. Forty eight (26%) of those thought to have classic angina had normal coronary angiograms and 16 of the 63 with atypical pain had abnormal angiogram. Thus, the cardiologists' clinical impression was wrong 25% of the time. Finally, Pope and associates investigated the ultimate diagnosis in 10,689 patients presenting to an emergency room with acute chest pain. Seventeen percent were found to have acute ischemia, 6% stable angina, 21% other cardiac causes and 55% had noncardiac causes. They concluded that the majority of people presenting to the emergency room with chest pain do not have an underlying cardiac etiology for their symptoms. Chest pain precipitated by meals, occurring at night while supine, nonradiating, responsive to antacid medication, or accompanied by other symptoms suggesting esophageal disease such as dysphagia or regurgitation should trigger the thought of possible esophageal origin. Further, the distinction between heartburn and chest pain is also difficult and largely dependent upon the individual patient. One person's heartburn is another's chest pain.

The precise mechanisms accounting for the generation of symptoms secondary to esophageal pathology remain unclear. Considerable insight has been acquired, however. Investigations into the effect of luminal content, esophageal distention and muscular function, neural pathways, and brain localization have provided a basic understanding of the stimuli responsible for symptom generation. It is also clear that the visceroneural pathways of the foregut are complexly intertwined with that of the tracheobronchial tree and heart. This fact accounts for the common overlap of clinical presentations with diverse disease processes in upper GI, cardiac, and pulmonary systems.

The Human Antireflux Mechanism and the Pathophysiology of Gastroesophageal Reflux Disease

There is a high-pressure zone located at the esophagogastric junction in humans. Although this is typically referred to as the lower esophageal "sphincter," there are no distinct anatomical landmarks which define its beginning and end. Architecturally speaking, there is a specialized thickening in this region that is made up of the collar sling musculature and the clasp fibers. The collar sling is located on the greater curvature side of the junction, and the clasp fibers are located on the lesser curvature side. These muscles remain in tonic opposition until the act of swallowing, whereupon receptive relax-

TABLE 25-4	American Gastroenterologic Association Gallup poll on nighttime gastroesophageal reflux disease symptoms

- 50 million Americans have nighttime heartburn at least 1/wk
- 80% of heartburn sufferers had nocturnal symptoms—65% both day & night
- 63% report that it affects their ability to sleep and impacts their work the next day
- 72% are on prescription medications
- Nearly half (45%) report that current remedies do not relieve all symptoms

ation occurs allowing passage of a food bolus into the stomach. In addition, the LES will also open when the gastric fundus is distended with gas and liquid, thus resulting in an unfolding of the valve and enabling venting of gas (a belch). Whether physiologic or pathologic, the common denominator for most episodes of gastroesophageal reflux is the loss of the high-pressure zone and thus a decrease in the resistance it imparts to the retrograde flow of gastric juice into the esophageal body. The primary cause of GERD is secondary to the permanent attenuation of the collar sling musculature, with a resultant opening of the gastric cardia and loss of the high-pressure zone as measured with esophageal manometry.

The Lower Esophageal Sphincter

As defined by esophageal manometry, there are three characteristics of the LES that work in unison to maintain its barrier function. These characteristics include the resting LES pressure, its overall length, and the intra-abdominal length that is exposed to the positive pressure environment of the abdomen (Table 25-5). The resistance to gastroesophageal reflux is a function of both the resting LES pressure and length over which this pressure is exerted. Thus, as the sphincter becomes shorter, a higher pressure will be required in order to prevent a given amount of reflux (Fig. 25-29). Much like the neck of a balloon as it is inflated, as the stomach fills and distends, sphincter length decreases. Therefore, if the overall length of the sphincter is permanently short from repeated distention of the fundus secondary to large volume meals, then with minimal episodes of gastric distention and pressure, there will be insufficient sphincter length for the barrier to remain competent, and reflux will occur.

A third characteristic of the LES that impacts its ability to prevent reflux is its position about the diaphragm. It is important that a portion of the total length of the LES be exposed to the effects of intra-abdominal pressure. That is, during periods of elevated intra-abdominal pressure, the resistance of the barrier would be overcome if pressure were not applied equally to both the LES and stomach simultaneously. Thus, in the presence of a hiatal hernia, the sphincter resides entirely within the chest cavity and cannot respond to an increase in intra-abdominal pressure because the pinch valve mechanism is lost and gastroesophageal reflux is more liable to occur.

Therefore, a permanently defective sphincter is defined by one or more of the following characteristics: An LES with a mean resting pressure of less than 6 mmHg, an overall sphincter length of <2 cm, and intra-abdominal sphincter length of <1 cm. When compared to normal subjects without GERD these values are below the 2.5 percentile for each parameter. The most common cause of a defective sphincter is an inadequate abdominal length.

Once the sphincter is permanently defective, this condition is irreversible, and although esophageal mucosal injury may be healed with antisecretory medication, reflux will continue to occur. Additionally, the presence of a defective LES may be associated with reduced esophageal body function and thus decreased clearance times of refluxed material. In addition, with the progressive loss of effective esophageal clearance the patient may be predisposed to severe mucosal injury, volume regurgitation, aspiration, and pulmonary failure. Reflux may occur in the face of a normal LES resting pressure. This condition is usually due to a functional

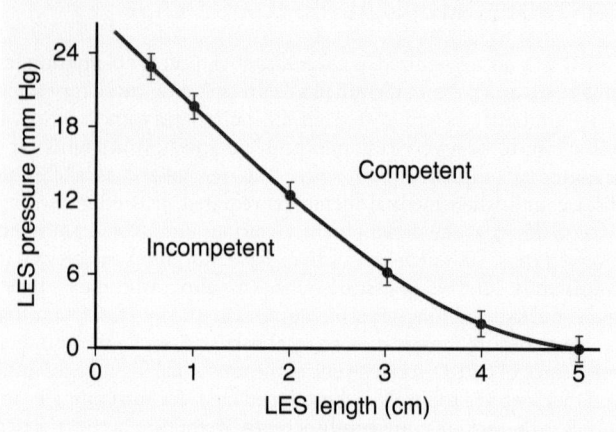

FIG. 25-29. As the esophageal sphincter becomes shorter, increased pressure is necessary to maintain competence. LES = lower esophageal sphincter.

problem of gastric emptying or excessive air swallowing. These conditions may lead to gastric distention, increased intra-gastric pressure, a resultant shortening or unfolding of the LES, and subsequent reflux. The mechanism by which gastric distention contributes to LES unfolding provides a mechanical explanation for "transient LES relaxation." It is thought that with repeated gastric distention secondary to large meal volume or chronic air swallowing, there is repeated unfolding of the LES and subsequent attenuation of the collar sling musculature. It is at this point that the physiologic and normal mechanism of gastric venting is replaced with pathologic and severe postprandial reflux disease. In addition, patients with GERD will increase the frequency of swallowing in an effort to neutralize the refluxed acid with their saliva (pH 7.0). This phenomenon leads to increased air swallowing and further gastric distention thus compounding the problem. Therefore GERD may have its origins in the stomach secondary to gastric distention due to over-eating, and this may be further compounded by the ingestion of fatty meals, which result in delayed gastric emptying.

Relationship between Hiatal Hernia and Gastroesophageal Reflux Disease

As the collar sling musculature and clasp fibers become attenuated with repeated gastric distention, the esophagogastric junction begins to assume an "upside down funnel" appearance, with progressive opening of the acute angle of His. This in turn may result in attenuation and stretching of the phrenoesophageal ligament, with subsequent enlargement of the hiatal opening and axial herniation. There is a high degree of correlation between reflux threshold and the degree of hiatal herniation (Fig. 25-30).

It is believed that the source of postprandial esophageal acid exposure results from a "pocket of acid" at the esophageal gastric junction that is unaffected by the buffering action of the meal. This same process is thought to occur in patients with endoscopy-negative dyspepsia and normal conventional esophageal pH monitoring at a location of 5 cm proximal to the upper boarder of the LES.

Summary

It is believed that GERD has its origins within the stomach. Distention of the fundus occurs because of over-eating and delayed gastric emptying secondary to a high-fat diet. The resultant distention causes "unrolling" of the sphincter by the expanding fundus, and this subsequently exposes the squamous epithelium in the region of the distal LES to gastric juice. Repeated exposure results in inflammation and the development of columnar epithelium at the cardia. This is the initial step of the development of carditis and

Parameter	Median Value	2.5th Percentile	97.5th Percentile
TABLE 25-5	Normal manometric values of the distal esophageal sphincter, n = 50		
Pressure (mmHg)	13	5.8	27.7
Overall length (cm)	3.6	2.1	5.6
Abdominal length (cm)	2	0.9	4.7

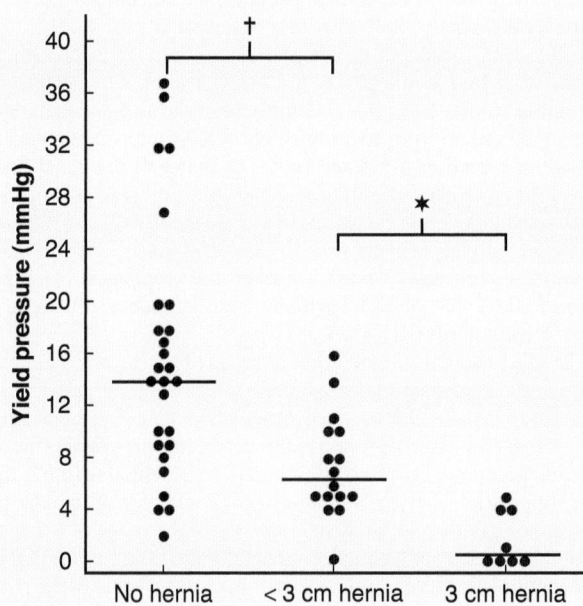

FIG. 25-30. Yield pressure of the lower esophageal sphincter decreases as hiatal hernia size increases.

TABLE 25-6	Complications of gastroesophageal reflux disease: 150 consecutive cases with proven gastroesophageal reflux disease (24-hour esophageal pH monitoring endoscopy, and motility)

Complication	No.	Structurally Normal Sphincter (%)	Structurally Defective Sphincter (%)
None	59	58	42
Erosive esophagitis	47	23	77[a]
Stricture	19	11	89
Barrett's esophagus	25	0	100
Total	150		

[a]Grade more severe with defective cardia.
Source: Reproduced with permission from DeMeester TR, et al: Gastroesophageal reflux disease, in Moody FG, Carey LC, et al (eds): *Surgical Treatment of Digestive Disease*. Chicago: Year Book Medical, 1990, p 81. Copyright Elsevier.

explains why in early disease esophagitis is mild and commonly limited to the very distal aspect of the esophagus. The patient attempts to compensate for this by increased swallowing, allowing the saliva to neutralize the refluxed gastric juice and thus alleviate the discomfort induced by the reflux event. The increased swallowing results in aerophagia, bloating, and belching. This in turn creates a viscous cycle of increased gastric distention and thus further exposure and repetitive injury to the distal esophagus. The development of carditis explains the complaint of epigastric pain often experienced by patients with early reflux disease. Additionally this process can lead to a fibrotic mucosal ring located at the squamocolumnar junction, which is termed a "Schatzki ring," and may result in dysphagia. This inflammatory process may extend into muscularis propria and thus result in a progressive loss in the length and pressure of the LES. This explanation for the pathophysiology of GERD is supported by the observation that severe esophagitis is almost always associated with a defective LES.

Complications Associated with Gastroesophageal Reflux Disease

The complications of gastroesophageal reflux disease may result from the direct injurious effects of gastric fluid on the mucosa, larynx, or respiratory epithelium. Complications due to repetitive reflux are esophagitis, stricture, and BE; repetitive aspiration may lead to progressive pulmonary fibrosis. The severity of the complications is directly related to the prevalence of a structurally defective sphincter (Table 25-6). The observation that a structurally defective sphincter

occurs in 42% of patients without complications (most of whom have one or two components failed) suggests that disease may be confined to the sphincter due to compensation by a vigorously contracting esophageal body. Eventually, all three components of the sphincter fail, allowing unrestricted reflux of gastric juice into the esophagus and overwhelming its normal clearance mechanisms. This leads to esophageal mucosal injury with progressive deterioration of esophageal contractility, as is commonly seen in patients with strictures and BE. The loss of esophageal clearance increases the potential for regurgitation into the pharynx with aspiration.

The potential injurious components that reflux into the esophagus include gastric secretions such as acid and pepsin, as well as biliary and pancreatic secretions that regurgitate from the duodenum into the stomach. There is a considerable body of experimental evidence to indicate that maximal epithelial injury occurs during exposure to bile salts combined with acid and pepsin. These studies have shown that acid alone does minimal damage to the esophageal mucosa, but the combination of acid and pepsin is highly deleterious. Similarly, the reflux of duodenal juice alone does little damage to the mucosa, although the combination of duodenal juice and gastric acid is particularly noxious (Table 25-7).

Experimental animal studies have shown that the reflux of duodenal contents into the esophagus enhances inflammation, increases the prevalence of Barrett's esophagus, and results in the development of esophageal adenocarcinoma. The component of duodenal juice thought to be most damaging is bile acids. For bile acids to injure mucosal cells, it is necessary that they be both soluble and un-ionized, so that the un-ionized, nonpolar form may enter mucosal cells. Before the entry of bile into the GI tract, 98% of bile acids are conjugated with either taurine or glycine in a ratio of about 3:1. Conjugation increases the solubility and ionization of bile acids by lowering their pK_a. At the normal duodenal pH of approximately 7, over 90% of bile salts are in solution and completely ionized. At pH ranges from 2 to 7, there is a mixture of the ionized salt and the lipophilic, nonionized acid. Acidification of bile to below pH 2

TABLE 25-7	Relation of the type of reflux to injury

	No Injury	Esophagitis	Uncomplicated Barrett's	Complicated Barrett's
Gastric reflux	15 (54%)	13 (38%)	8 (32%)	1 (8%)
Gastroduodenal reflux	13 (38%)	21 (62%)	17 (68%)	12 (92%)

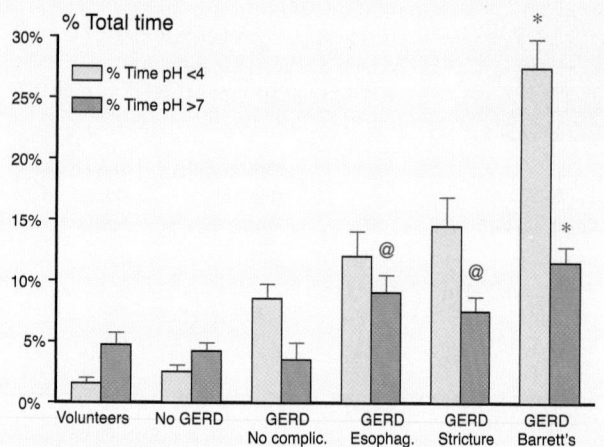

FIG. 25-31. Esophageal acid and alkaline exposure expressed as percentage of total time pH <4 and pH >7. * = *P* <.01 vs. gastroesophageal reflux disease (GERD) patients with no complication. @ = *P* <.05 vs. GERD patients with no complications. (*Reproduced with permission from Stein HJ, Barlow AP, et al: Complications of gastroesophageal reflux disease: Role of the lower esophageal sphincter, esophageal acid and acid/alkaline exposure, and duodenogastric reflux. Ann Surg 216:39, 1992.*)

predisposing factors: a mechanically defective LES and an increased esophageal exposure to fluid with a pH of <4 and >7 (Fig. 25-31). The duodenal origin of esophageal contents in patients with an increased exposure to a pH >7 has been confirmed by esophageal aspiration studies (Fig. 25-32). Studies have clarified and expanded these observations by measuring esophageal bilirubin exposure over a 24-hour period as a marker for the presence of duodenal juice. Direct measurement of esophageal bilirubin exposure as a marker for duodenal juice has shown that 58% of patients with GERD have increased esophageal exposure to duodenal juice, and that this exposure occurs most commonly when the esophageal pH is between 4 and 7 (Fig. 25-33). Furthermore, it is associated with more severe mucosal injury (Fig. 25-34).

The fact that the combination of refluxed gastric and duodenal juice is more noxious to the esophageal mucosa than gastric juice alone may explain the repeated observation that 25% of patients with reflux esophagitis develop recurrent and/or progressive mucosal damage, often despite medical therapy. A potential reason is that acid suppression therapy is unable to consistently maintain the pH of refluxed gastric and duodenal juice above the range of 6. Lapses into pH ranges from 2 to 6 encourage the formation of undissociated, nonpolarized, soluble bile acids, which are capable of penetrating the cell wall and injuring mucosal cells. To assure that bile acids

results in an irreversible bile acid precipitation. Consequently, under normal physiologic conditions, bile acids precipitate and are of minimal consequence when an acid gastric environment exists. On the other hand, in a more alkaline gastric environment, such as occurs with excessive duodenogastric reflux and after acid suppression therapy or vagotomy and partial or total gastrectomy, bile salts remain in solution, are partially dissociated, and when refluxed into the esophagus can cause severe mucosal injury by crossing the cell membrane and damaging the mitochondria.

Complications of gastroesophageal reflux such as esophagitis, stricture, and Barrett's metaplasia occur in the presence of two

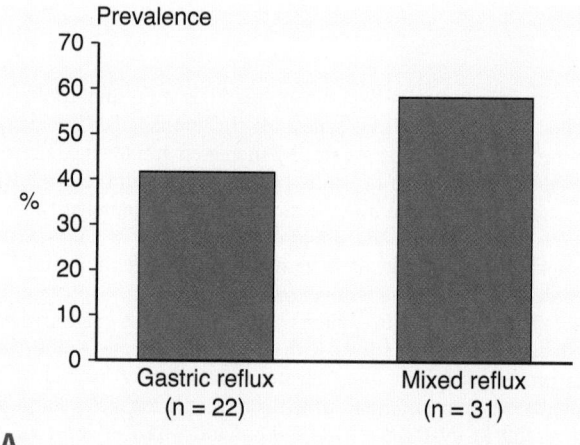

A

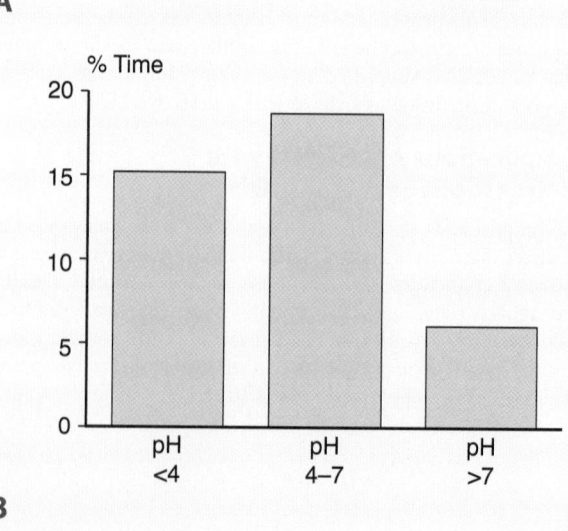

B

FIG. 25-33. A. Prevalence of reflux types in 53 patients with gastroesophageal reflux disease. **B.** Esophageal luminal pH during bilirubin exposure. (*Reproduced with permission from Kauer WK, Peters JH, DeMeester TR, et al: Mixed reflux of gastric juice is more harmful to the esophagus than gastric juice alone: The need for surgical therapy reemphasized. Ann Surg 222:525, 1995.*)

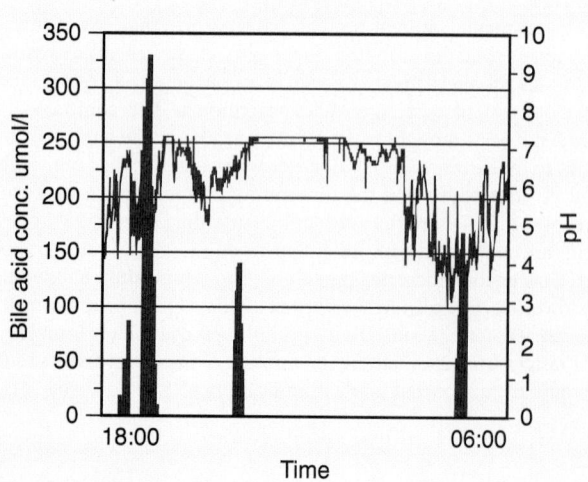

FIG. 25-32. Sample bile acid concentration and esophageal pH plotted against time to obtain detailed profiles; in this case showing both significant bile acid (*vertical bars*) and acid (*linear plot*) reflux. (*Reproduced with permission from Nehra D, Watt P, Pye JK, et al: Automated oesophageal reflux sampler: A new device used to monitor bile acid reflux in patients with gastroesophageal reflux disease. J Med Engr Tech 21:1, 1997.*)

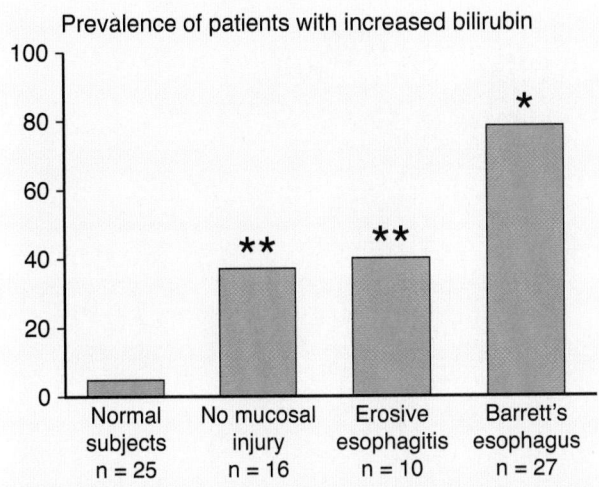

FIG. 25-34. Prevalence of abnormal esophageal bilirubin exposure in healthy subjects and in patients with gastroesophageal reflux disease with varied degrees of mucosal injury. (*P <.03 vs. all other groups; **P <.03 vs. healthy subjects.) *(Reproduced with permission from Kauer WK, Peters JH, DeMeester TR, et al: Mixed reflux of gastric juice is more harmful to the esophagus than gastric juice alone: The need for surgical therapy reemphasized. Ann Surg 222:525, 1995.)*

remain completely ionized in their polarized form, and thus unable to penetrate the cell, requires that the pH of the refluxed material be maintained above 7, 24 hours a day, 7 days a week, for the patient's lifetime. In practice, this would not only be impractical but likely impossible, unless very high doses of medications were used. The use of lesser doses would allow esophageal mucosal damage to occur while the patient was relatively asymptomatic. Antireflux operative procedures re-establish the barrier between stomach and esophagus, protecting the esophagus from damage in patients with mixed gastroesophageal reflux.

If reflux of gastric juice is allowed to persist and sustained or repetitive esophageal injury occurs, two sequelae can result. First, a luminal stricture can develop from submucosal and eventually intramural fibrosis. Second, the tubular esophagus may become replaced with columnar epithelium. The columnar epithelium is resistant to acid and is associated with the alleviation of the complaint of heartburn. This columnar epithelium often becomes intestinalized, identified histologically by the presence of goblet cells. This specialized IM is currently required for the diagnosis of BE. Endoscopically, BE can be quiescent or associated with complications of esophagitis, stricture, Barrett's ulceration, and dysplasia. The complications associated with BE may be due to the continuous irritation from refluxed duodenogastric juice. This continued injury is pH dependent and may be modified by medical therapy. The incidence of metaplastic Barrett's epithelium becoming dysplastic and progressing to adenocarcinoma is approximately 1% per year.

An esophageal stricture can be associated with severe esophagitis or BE. In the latter situation, it occurs at the site of maximal inflammatory injury (i.e., the columnar-squamous epithelial interface). As the columnar epithelium advances into the area of inflammation, the inflammation extends higher into the proximal esophagus, and the site of the stricture moves progressively up the esophagus. Patients who have a stricture in the absence of Barrett's esophagus should have the presence of gastroesophageal reflux documented before the presence of the stricture is ascribed to reflux esophagitis. In patients with normal acid exposure, the stricture may be due to cancer or a drug-induced chemical injury, the latter resulting from the lodgment of a capsule or tablet in the distal

esophagus. In such patients, dilation usually corrects the problem of dysphagia. Heartburn, which may have occurred only because of the chemical injury, need not be treated. It is also possible for drug-induced injuries to occur in patients who have underlying esophagitis and a distal esophageal stricture secondary to gastroesophageal reflux. In this situation, a long, string-like stricture progressively develops as a result of repetitive caustic injury from capsule or tablet lodgment on top of an initial reflux stricture. These strictures are often resistant to dilation.

Metaplastic (Barrett's Esophagus) and Neoplastic (Adenocarcinoma) Complications

The condition whereby the tubular esophagus is lined with columnar epithelium rather than squamous epithelium was first described by Norman Barrett in 1950. He incorrectly believed it to be congenital in origin. It is now realized that it is an acquired abnormality, occurs in 10 to 15% of patients with GERD, and represents the end stage of the natural history of this disease. It is also distinctly different from the congenital condition in which islands of gastric fundic epithelium are found in the upper half of the esophagus.

The definition of BE has evolved considerably over the past decade. Traditionally, BE was identified by the presence of columnar mucosa extending at least 3 cm into the esophagus. It is now recognized that the specialized, intestinal-type epithelium found in the Barrett's mucosa is the only tissue predisposed to malignant degeneration. Consequently, the diagnosis of BE is presently made given any length of endoscopically identifiable columnar mucosa that proves, on biopsy, to show IM. Although long segments of columnar mucosa without IM do occur, they are uncommon and are probably congenital in origin.

The hallmark of IM is the presence of intestinal goblet cells. There is a high prevalence of biopsy-demonstrated IM at the cardia, on the gastric side of the squamocolumnar junction, in the absence of endoscopic evidence of a CLE. Evidence is accumulating that these patches of what appears to be Barrett's in the cardia have a similar malignant potential as in the longer segments, and are precursors for carcinoma of the cardia.

The long-term relief of symptoms remains the primary reason for performing antireflux surgery in patients with BE. Healing of esophageal mucosal injury and the prevention of disease progression are important secondary goals. In this regard, patients with BE are no different than the broader population of patients with gastroesophageal reflux. They should be considered for antireflux surgery when patient data suggest severe disease or predict the need for long-term medical management. Most patients with BE are symptomatic. Although it has been argued that some patients with BE may not have symptoms, careful history taking will reveal the presence of symptoms in most, if not all, patients.

Patients with BE have a spectrum of disease ranging from visually identifiable but short segments, to long segments of classic BE. In general, however, they represent a relatively severe stage of gastroesophageal reflux, usually with markedly increased esophageal acid exposure, deficient LES characteristics, poor esophageal body function, and a high prevalence of duodenogastroesophageal reflux. Gastric hypersecretion occurs in 44% of patients. Most will require long-term PPI therapy for relief of symptoms and control of coexistent esophageal mucosal injury. Given such profound deficits in esophageal physiology, antireflux surgery is an excellent means of long-term control for most patients with BE. In years past, referral for antireflux surgery was reserved for patients with associated complications such as stricture, ulceration, or progression of the metaplastic segment. The advent of laparoscopic fundoplication and its successful control of gastroesophageal reflux in more than 90% of patients has lowered the threshold for referral. Patients with quiescent, uncomplicated BE, particularly young patients, are now considered by many to be excellent candidates for antireflux surgery.

The typical complications in BE include ulceration in the columnar-lined segment, stricture formation, and a dysplasia-cancer se-

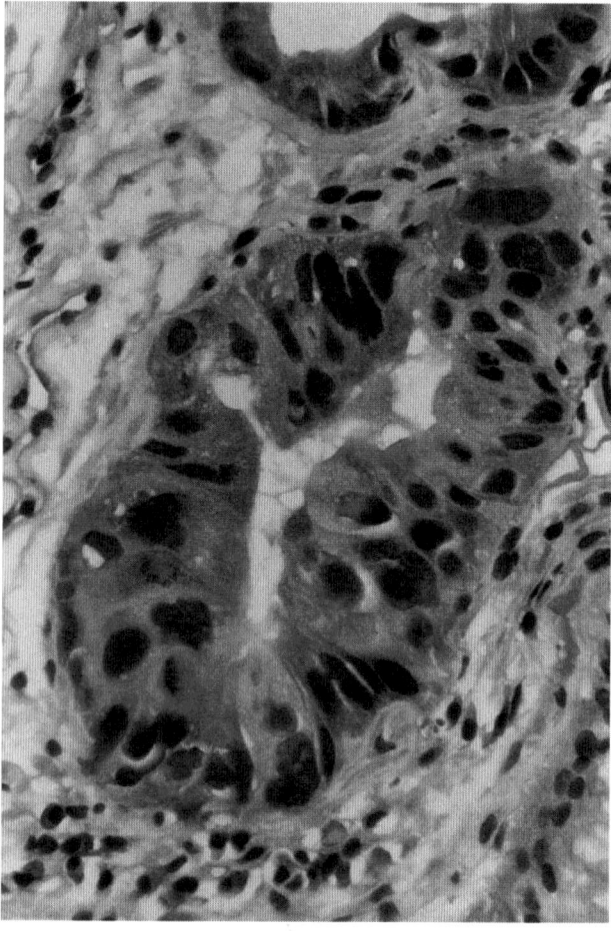

A

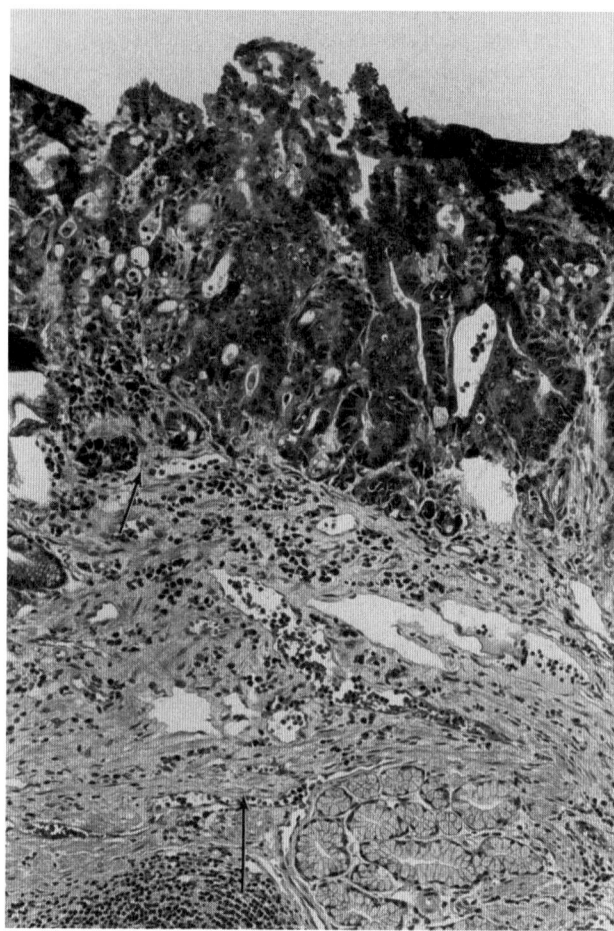

B

FIG. 25-35. Photomicrographs. **A.** Barrett's epithelium with severe dysplasia. (×200.) Note nuclear irregularity, stratification, and loss of polarity. **B.** Barrett's epithelium with intramucosal carcinoma. (×66.) Note malignant cells in the mucosa (*upper arrow*), but not invading the muscularis mucosae (*bottom arrow*). [*Reproduced with permission from DeMeester TR, Stein HJ, Fuchs KH: Physiologic diagnostic studies, in Zuidema GD, Orringer MB (eds):* Shackelford's Surgery of the Alimentary Tract, *3rd ed, Vol. I. Philadelphia: W.B. Saunders, 1991, p 113. Copyright Elsevier.*]

quence. Barrett's ulceration is unlike the erosive ulceration of reflux esophagitis in that it more closely resembles peptic ulceration in the stomach or duodenum, and has the same propensity to bleed, penetrate, or perforate. The strictures found in BE occur at the squamocolumnar junction, and are typically higher than peptic strictures in the absence of BE. Ulceration and stricture in association with BE were commonly reported before 1975, but, with the advent of potent acid suppression medication, they have become less common. In contrast, the complication of adenocarcinoma developing in Barrett's mucosa has become more common. Adenocarcinoma developing in Barrett's mucosa was considered a rare tumor before 1975. Today, it occurs in approximately one in every 100 patient-years of follow-up, which represents a risk 40 times that of the general population. Most, if not all, cases of adenocarcinoma of the esophagus arise in Barrett's epithelium (Fig. 25-35). About one third of all patients with BE present with malignancy.

The long-term risk of progression to dysplasia and adenocarcinoma, although not the driving force behind the decision to perform antireflux surgery, is a significant concern for both patient and physician. Although to date, there have been no prospective randomized studies documenting that antireflux surgery has an effect on the risk of progression to dysplasia and carcinoma, complete control of reflux of gastric juice into the esophagus is clearly a desirable goal. As data accumulate regarding the relative impact of medical and surgical therapy on the natural history of Barrett's metaplasia, the risk of progression may play a larger role in therapeutic decisions.

Respiratory Complications

A significant proportion of patients with GERD will have associated respiratory symptoms. These patients may have laryngopharyngeal reflux-type symptoms, adult-onset asthma, or even idiopathic pulmonary fibrosis. These symptoms and organ injury may occur in isolation or in conjunction with typical reflux symptoms such as heartburn and regurgitation. Several studies have demonstrated that up to 50% of patients with asthma have either endoscopically evident esophagitis or abnormal distal esophageal acid exposure. These findings support a causal relationship between GERD and aerodigestive symptoms and complications in a proportion of patients.

Etiology of Reflux-Induced Respiratory Symptoms

There are two mechanisms that have been proposed as the cause of reflux-induced respiratory symptoms. The *reflux theory* suggests that these symptoms are the direct result of laryngopharyngeal exposure and aspiration of gastric contents. The *reflex theory* suggests that the vagal-mediated afferent fibers result in bronchoconstriction during episodes of distal esophageal acidification. The evidence supporting a mechanism of direct exposure to the aerodigestive system is based in clinical studies that have documented a strong correlation between idiopathic pulmonary fibrosis and hiatal hernia. In addition, the presence of GERD was demonstrated to be highly associated with several pulmonary diseases in a recent

Department of Veteran Affairs multivariate analysis. Next, with ambulatory pH testing, acid exposure within the proximal esophagus is more frequently identified in patients with gastroesophageal reflux and respiratory symptoms than in patients who have gastroesophageal reflux symptoms alone. These findings are supported by scintigraphic studies, which have demonstrated aspiration of ingested radioisotope in patients with both gastroesophageal reflux and pulmonary symptoms. In animal studies, tracheal instillation of acid has been demonstrated to profoundly increase airway resistance. Finally, in patients who have undergone multichannel intraluminal impedance testing with a catheter configured to detect laryngopharyngeal reflux, a correlation between proximal fluid movement and laryngopharyngeal symptoms, such as cough, can be demonstrated.

The reflex mechanism is supported by the bronchoconstriction that occurs with the infusion of acid into the distal esophagus. There is a shared embryologic origin of the tracheoesophageal tract and vagus nerve, and this reflex is thought to be an afferent fiber–mediated reflex that protects the aerodigestive system from the aspiration of refluxate. In patients with respiratory symptoms and documented gastroesophageal reflux without proximal esophageal acid exposure, pulmonary symptoms will often times significantly improve or completely resolve after undergoing laparoscopic fundoplication. It is likely that both of the proposed mechanisms work simultaneously to cause these symptoms in the face of GERD.

The most difficult clinical challenge in formulating a treatment plan for reflux-associated respiratory symptoms resides in establishing the diagnosis. Although the diagnosis made be straightforward in patients with predominately typical reflux symptoms and secondary respiratory complaints, a substantial number of patients will have respiratory symptoms that dominate the clinical scenario. Typical gastroesophageal reflux symptoms, such as heartburn and regurgitation, may often be completely absent only to be uncovered with objective esophageal physiology testing. Traditionally, the diagnosis of reflux-induced respiratory injury is established using ambulatory dual probe pH monitoring, with one probe positioned within the distal esophagus and the other at a proximal location. Proximal probe positioning has included multiple locations such as the trachea, pharynx, and proximal esophagus. Although ambulatory esophageal pH monitoring allows a direct correlation between esophageal acidification and respiratory symptoms, sensitivity of this testing modality is poor, and the temporal relationship between laryngeal or pulmonary symptoms and reflux events is complex. In addition, as the refluxed gastric fluid travels proximally, it may be neutralized by saliva and therefore go undetected with pH monitoring. Impedance testing is a novel technology that may be used more to detect the movement of fluid throughout the entire esophageal column regardless of pH content.

Treatment

Once the diagnosis is established, treatment may be initiated with either PPI therapy or antireflux surgery. A trial of high-dose PPI therapy may help establish the fact that reflux is partly or completely responsible for the respiratory symptoms. It is important to note that the persistence of symptoms in the face of aggressive PPI treatment does not necessarily rule out reflux as a possible cofactor or sole etiology. The algorithm suggested in Fig. 25-36 represents a useful starting point for the diagnostic evaluation in this patient population.

Although there is most likely some elements of a placebo effect, relief of respiratory symptoms can be anticipated in up to 50% of patients with reflux-induced asthma treated with antisecretory medications. However, when examined objectively, <15% of patients can be expected to have improvement in their pulmonary function with medical therapy. In properly selected patients, antireflux surgery improves respiratory symptoms in nearly 90% of children and 70% of adults with asthma and reflux disease. Improvements in pulmonary function can be demonstrated in around 30% of patients. Uncontrolled studies of the two forms of therapy (PPI and surgery) and the evidence from the two randomized

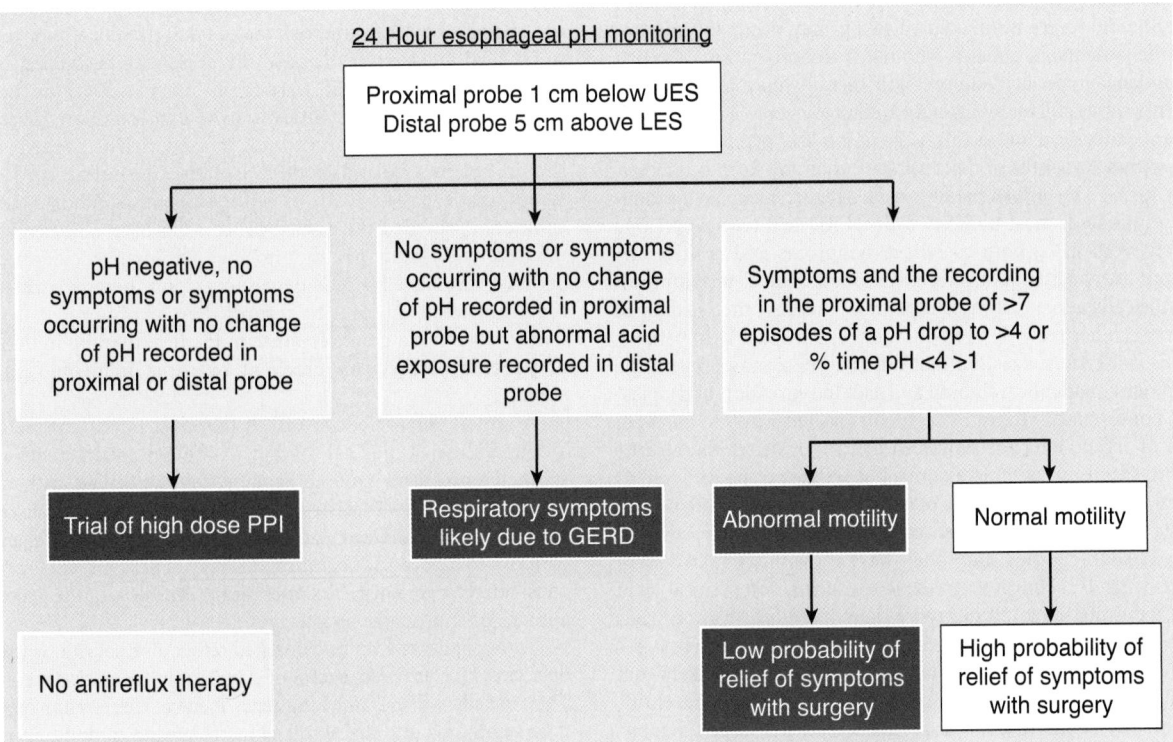

FIG. 25-36. Correlation of symptoms with pH measurements predict the likelihood that reflux symptoms are caused directly by acid reflux. GERD = gastroesophageal reflux disease; LES = lower esophageal sphincter; PPI = proton pump inhibitor; UES = upper esophageal sphincter.

controlled trials of medical vs. surgical therapy indicate that surgical valve reconstruction is the most effective therapy for reflux-induced asthma. The superiority of the surgery over PPI is most noticeable in the supine position, which corresponds with the nadir of PPI blood levels and resultant acid breakthrough and is the time in the circadian cycle when asthma symptoms are at their worst.

In asthmatic patients with an esophageal motility disorder, performing an antireflux operation will not prevent the regurgitation and possible aspiration of swallowed liquid or food "upstream" to the valve reconstruction. It is critical that esophageal body function be considered prior to surgical intervention in this patient population.

Medical Therapy for Gastroesophageal Reflux Disease

With the widespread availability of over-the-counter antisecretory medications, most patients with mild or moderate symptoms will carry self-medication. When initially identified with mild symptoms of uncomplicated GERD, patients can be placed on 12 weeks of simple antacids before diagnostic testing is initiated. This approach may successfully and completely resolve the symptoms. Patients should be counseled to elevate the head of the bed; avoid tight-fitting clothing; eat small, frequent meals; avoid eating the nighttime meal immediately prior to bedtime; and avoid alcohol, coffee, chocolate, and peppermint, which are known to reduce resting LES pressure and may aggravate symptoms.

Used in combination with simple antacids, alginic acid may augment the relief of symptoms by creating a physical barrier to reflux, as well as by acid reduction. Alginic acid reacts with sodium bicarbonate in the presence of saliva to form a highly viscous solution that floats like a raft on the surface of the gastric contents. When reflux occurs, this protective layer is refluxed into the esophagus, and acts as a protective barrier against the noxious gastric contents. Medications to promote gastric emptying, such as metoclopramide or domperidone, are beneficial in early disease, but of little value in more severe disease.

In patients with persistent symptoms, the mainstay of medical therapy is acid suppression. High-dosage regimens of hydrogen potassium PPIs, such as omeprazole (up to 40 mg/d), can reduce gastric acidity by as much as 80 to 90%. This usually heals mild esophagitis. In severe esophagitis, healing may occur in only one half of the patients. In patients who reflux a combination of gastric and duodenal juice, acid-suppression therapy may give relief of symptoms, while still allowing mixed reflux to occur. This can allow persistent mucosal damage in an asymptomatic patient. Unfortunately, within 6 months of discontinuation of any form of medical therapy for GERD, 80% of patients have a recurrence of symptoms.

Once initiated, most patients with GERD will require lifelong treatment with PPIs, both to relieve symptoms and control any coexistent esophagitis or stricture. Although control of symptoms has historically served as the endpoint of therapy, the wisdom of this approach has recently been questioned, particularly in patients with BE. Evidence suggesting that reflux control may prevent the development of adenocarcinoma and lead to regression of dysplastic and nondysplastic Barrett's segments has led many to consider control of reflux, and not symptom control, a better therapeutic endpoint. However, complete control of reflux can be difficult, as has been highlighted by studies of acid breakthrough while on PPI therapy, and of persistent reflux following antireflux surgery. Castell, Triadafilopoulos, and others have shown that 40 to 80% of patients with BE continue to have abnormal esophageal acid exposure despite up to 20 mg twice daily of PPIs. Ablation trials have shown that mean doses of 56 mg of omeprazole were necessary to normalize 24-hour esophageal pH studies. It is likely that antireflux surgery results in more reproducible and reliable elimination of reflux of both acid and duodenal contents, although long-term outcome studies suggest that as many as 25% of post-Nissen patients will have persistent pathologic esophageal acid exposure confirmed by positive 24-hour pH studies.

Suggested Therapeutic Approach

The traditional stepwise approach to the therapy of GERD should be re-examined in view of a more complete understanding of the pathophysiology of gastroesophageal reflux, the rising incidence of BE, and the increasing mortality rates associated with end-stage reflux disease. The approach should be to identify risk factors for persistent and progressive disease early in the course of the disease, and encourage surgical treatment when these factors are present. The following approach is suggested.

Medical therapy for most patients will be started with H_2 blockade. Failure of this medication, or the immediate return of symptoms after stopping treatment, suggests either that the patient may have relatively severe disease or a non-GERD cause for his or her symptoms. Endoscopic examination at this stage of the patient's evaluation is recommended and will provide the opportunity to assess the degree of mucosal injury and screening for BE and esophageal adenocarcinoma. In addition, the measurement of esophageal acid exposure via 24-hour pH or impedance monitoring should also be obtained at this point. The status of the LES and esophageal body function with esophageal manometry should also be performed. These studies will serve to establish the diagnosis and characterize the severity and patterns of gastroesophageal reflux such as the supine reflux, esophageal body dysfunction, erosive esophagitis, or BE, bile reflux, and a defective LES. Patients who present with these risk factors should be offered laparoscopic antireflux surgery as a primary therapy, with the expectation of long-term control of symptoms and prevention of GERD-related complications.

Surgical Therapy for Gastroesophageal Reflux Disease
Selection of Patients for Surgery

Studies of the natural history of GERD indicate that most patients have a relatively benign form of the disease that is responsive to lifestyle changes and dietary and medical therapy, and do not need surgical treatment. Approximately 25 to 50% of the patients with GERD have persistent or progressive disease, and it is this patient population that is best suited to surgical therapy. These patients are identified by the same risk factors that predict a poor response to medical therapy. In the past, the presence of esophagitis and a structurally defective LES were the primary indications for surgical treatment, and many internists and surgeons were reluctant to recommend operative procedures in their absence. However, one should not be deterred from considering antireflux surgery in a symptomatic patient with or without esophagitis or a defective sphincter, provided the disease process has been objectively documented by 24-hour pH monitoring. This is particularly true in patients who have become dependent upon therapy with PPIs, or require increasing doses to control their symptoms. It is important to note that a good response to medical therapy in this group of patients predicts an excellent outcome following antireflux surgery.

A structurally defective LES is the most important factor predicting failure of medical therapy. Although patients with normal sphincter pressures tend to remain well controlled with medical therapy, patients with a structurally defective LES do not respond well to medical therapy, usually developing recurrent symptoms within 1 to 2 years of beginning therapy. These patients should be considered for an antireflux operation, regardless of the presence or absence of endoscopic esophagitis.

Young patients with documented reflux disease with or without a defective LES are also excellent candidates for antireflux surgery. They usually will require long-term medical therapy for control of their symptoms, and many will go on to develop complications of the disease. An analysis of the cost of therapy based on data from the Veterans Administration Cooperative trial indicates that surgery has a cost advantage over medical therapy in patients <49 years of age.

Severe endoscopic esophagitis in a symptomatic patient with a structurally defective LES is also an indication for early surgical therapy. These patients are prone to breakthrough of their symptoms while receiving medical therapy. Symptoms and mucosal injury can be controlled in such patients, but careful monitoring is required, and increasing dosages of PPIs are necessary. In everyday clinical practice, however, such treatment can be both difficult and impractical, and, in such cases, antireflux surgery should be considered early as a therapeutic option.

The development of a stricture in a patient represents a failure of medical therapy, and is also an indication for a surgical antireflux procedure. In addition, strictures are often associated with a structurally defective sphincter and loss of esophageal contractility. Before proceeding with surgical treatment, malignancy and a drug-related etiology of the stricture should be excluded, and the stricture progressively dilated up to a 60F bougie. When the stricture is fully dilated, the relief of dysphagia is evaluated and esophageal manometry is performed to determine the adequacy of peristalsis in the distal esophagus. If dysphagia is relieved and the amplitude of esophageal contractions is adequate, an antireflux procedure should be performed; if there is a global loss of esophageal contractility, caution should be exercised in performing an antireflux procedure with a complete fundoplication, and a partial fundoplication should be considered.

Barrett's CLE is commonly associated with a severe structural defect of the LES and often poor contractility of the esophageal body. Patients with BE are at risk of progression of the mucosal abnormality up the esophagus, formation of a stricture, hemorrhage from a Barrett's ulcer, and the development of an adenocarcinoma. An antireflux procedure may arrest the progression of the disease, heal ulceration, and resolve strictures. Evidence is accumulating that surgical treatment also reduces the risk of progression to cancer. If severe dysplasia or intramucosal carcinoma is found on mucosal biopsy specimens, an esophageal resection should be done.

The majority of patients requiring treatment have a relatively mild form of disease and will respond to antisecretory medications. Patients with more severe forms of disease, particularly those with risk factors predictive of medical failure and those who develop persistent or progressive disease, should be considered for early definitive therapy. Laparoscopic Nissen fundoplication will provide a long-term cure in the majority of these patients, with minimal discomfort and an early return to normal activity. If the disease has resulted in global failure of esophageal contractility, Barrett's metaplasia with high-grade dysplasia, or esophageal adenocarcinoma, an esophagectomy may be the best surgical treatment option.

Preoperative Evaluation

Before proceeding with an antireflux operation, several factors should be evaluated. First, the propulsive force of the body of the esophagus should be evaluated by esophageal manometry to determine if it has sufficient power to propel a bolus of food through a newly reconstructed valve. Patients with normal peristaltic contractions do well with a 360° Nissen fundoplication. When peristalsis is absent a partial fundoplication may be the procedure of choice, but only if achalasia has been ruled out.

Second, anatomic shortening of the esophagus can compromise the ability to do an adequate repair without tension, and lead to an increased incidence of breakdown or thoracic displacement of the repair. Esophageal shortening is identified on a barium swallow roentgenogram by a sliding hiatal hernia that will not reduce in the upright position, or that measures larger than 5 cm between the diaphragmatic crura and GEJ on endoscopy. When esophageal shortening is present, the motility of the esophageal body must be carefully evaluated, and, if inadequate, a gastroplasty should be performed. In patients who have a global absence of contractility, more than 50% interrupted or dropped contractions, or a history

of several failed previous antireflux procedures, esophageal resection should be considered as an alternative.

Third, the surgeon should specifically query the patient for complaints of nausea, vomiting, and loss of appetite. In the past, these symptoms were accepted as part of the reflux syndrome, but we now realize that they can be due to excessive duodenogastric reflux or gastric pathology. This problem is most pronounced in patients who have had previous upper GI surgery, particularly cholecystectomy, although this is not always the case. In such patients, these symptoms may persist after an antireflux procedure, and patients should be given this information before the operation. In these patients, 24-hour bilirubin monitoring and gastric emptying studies can be performed to detect and quantify duodenogastric abnormalities. Antireflux surgery alone may influence these symptoms by improving the efficiency of gastric emptying.

Fourth, approximately 30% of patients with proven gastroesophageal reflux on 24-hour pH monitoring will have hypersecretion on gastric analysis, and 2 to 3% of patients who have an antireflux operation will develop a gastric or duodenal ulcer. The presence of *Helicobacter pylori* should be assessed in these patients and treated if present.

Principles of Surgical Therapy

The primary goal of antireflux surgery is to safely restore the structure of the sphincter or to prevent its shortening with gastric distention, while preserving the patient's ability to swallow normally, to belch to relieve gaseous distention, and to vomit when necessary. Regardless of the choice of the procedure, this goal can be achieved if attention is paid to five principles in reconstructing the cardia. First, the operation should restore the pressure of the distal esophageal sphincter to a level twice the resting gastric pressure (i.e., 12 mmHg for a gastric pressure of 6 mmHg), and its length to at least 3 cm. This not only augments sphincter characteristics in patients in whom they are reduced before surgery, but prevents unfolding of a normal sphincter in response to gastric distention (Fig. 25-37). Preoperative and postoperative esophageal manometry measurements have shown that the resting sphincter pressure and the overall sphincter length can be surgically augmented over preoperative values, and that the change in the former is a function of the degree of gastric wrap around the esophagus (Fig. 25-38).

Second, the operation should place an adequate length of the distal esophageal sphincter in the positive-pressure environment of the abdomen by a method that ensures its response to changes in intra-abdominal pressure. The permanent restoration of 1.5 to 2 cm of abdominal esophagus in a patient whose sphincter pressure has been augmented to twice resting gastric pressure will maintain the competency of the cardia over various challenges of intra-abdominal pressure. All three of the popular antireflux procedures

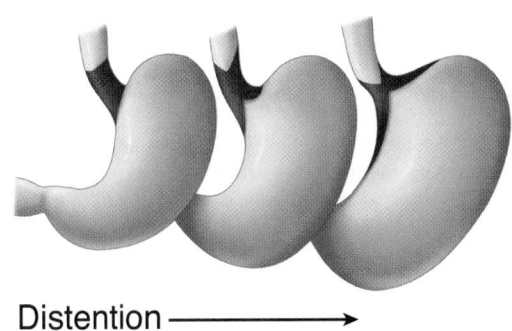

Distention ⟶

FIG. 25-37. A graphic illustration of the shortening of the lower esophageal sphincter that occurs as the sphincter is "taken up" by the cardia as the stomach distends.

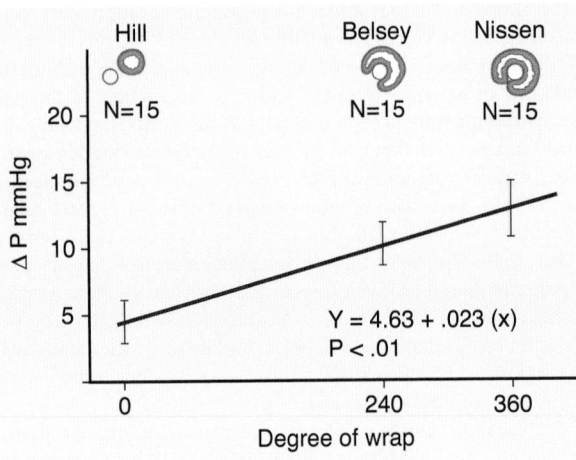

FIG. 25-38. The relationship between the augmentation of sphincter pressure over preoperative pressure (ΔP) and the degree of gastric fundic wrap in three popular antireflux procedures. *(Reproduced with permission from O'Sullivan GC, et al: Interaction of lower esophageal pressure and length of sphincter in the abdomen as detriments of gastroesophageal competence. Am J Surg 143:43, 1982. Copyright Elsevier.)*

increase the length of the sphincter exposed to abdominal pressure by an average of 1 cm. When poorly performed, however, an operation may result in a reduction of the length of abdominal sphincter. Increasing the length of sphincter exposed to abdominal pressure will improve competency only if it is acted on by challenges of intra-abdominal pressure. The creation of a conduit that will ensure the transmission of intra-abdominal pressure changes around the abdominal portion of the sphincter is a necessary aspect of surgical repair. The fundoplication in the Nissen and Belsey repairs serves this purpose.

Third, the operation should allow the reconstructed cardia to relax on deglutition. In normal swallowing, a vagally mediated relaxation of the distal esophageal sphincter and the gastric fundus occurs. The relaxation lasts for approximately 10 seconds and is followed by a rapid recovery to the former tonicity. To ensure relaxation of the sphincter, three factors are important: (a) Only the fundus of the stomach should be used to buttress the sphincter, because it is known to relax in concert with the sphincter; (b) the gastric wrap should be properly placed around the sphincter and not incorporate a portion of the stomach or be placed around the stomach itself, because the body of the stomach does not relax with swallowing; and (c) damage to the vagal nerves during dissection of the thoracic esophagus should be avoided because it may result in failure of the sphincter to relax.

Fourth, the fundoplication should not increase the resistance of the relaxed sphincter to a level that exceeds the peristaltic power of the body of the esophagus. The resistance of the relaxed sphincter depends on the degree, length, and diameter of the gastric fundic wrap, and on the variation in intra-abdominal pressure. A 360° gastric wrap should be no longer than 2 cm and constructed over a 60F bougie. This will ensure that the relaxed sphincter will have an adequate diameter with minimal resistance. This is not necessary when constructing a partial wrap.

Fifth, the operation should ensure that the fundoplication can be placed in the abdomen without undue tension, and maintained there by approximating the crura of the diaphragm above the repair. Leaving the fundoplication in the thorax converts a sliding hernia into a PEH, with all the complications associated with that condition. Maintaining the repair in the abdomen under tension predisposes to an increased incidence of recurrence. This can occur in patients who have a stricture or BE, and is due to shortening of the

esophagus from the inflammatory process. This problem can be resolved by lengthening the esophagus by gastroplasty and constructing a partial fundoplication.

Procedure Selection

A laparoscopic approach is used in patients with normal esophageal contractility and length. Patients with questionable esophageal length may be best approached transthoracically, where full esophageal mobilization serves as a lengthening procedure. Those with a failed esophagus characterized by absent esophageal contractions and/or absent peristalsis such as those with scleroderma are best treated either medically or with a partial fundoplication to avoid the increased outflow resistance associated with a complete fundoplication. If the esophagus is short after it is mobilized from diaphragm to aortic arch, a Collis gastroplasty is done to provide additional length and avoid placing the repair under tension. In the majority of patients who have good esophageal contractility and normal esophageal length, the laparoscopic Nissen fundoplication is the procedure of choice for a primary antireflux repair. Experience and randomized studies have shown that the Nissen fundoplication is an effective and durable antireflux repair with minimal side effects that provides long-lasting relief of reflux symptoms in over 90% of patients.

Primary Antireflux Repairs
Nissen Fundoplication

The most common antireflux procedure is the Nissen fundoplication. The procedure can be performed through an abdominal or a chest incision, as well as through a laparoscope. Rudolph Nissen described the procedure as a 360° fundoplication around the lower esophagus for a distance of 4 to 5 cm. Although this provided good control of reflux, it was associated with a number of side effects that have encouraged modifications of the procedure as originally described. These include using only the gastric fundus to envelop the esophagus in a fashion analogous to a Witzel jejunostomy, sizing the fundoplication with a 60F bougie, and limiting the length of the fundoplication to 1 to 2 cm. The essential elements necessary for the performance of a transabdominal fundoplication are common to both the laparoscopic and open procedures and include the following:

1. Crural dissection and preservation of both vagi along their entire length
2. Circumferential esophageal mobilization
3. Posterior crural closure
4. Division of short gastric vessels and posterior fundus
5. Creation of a short and floppy fundoplication over an esophageal dilator

The Laparoscopic Approach

Laparoscopic fundoplication has become commonplace and has replaced the open abdominal Nissen fundoplication as the procedure of choice. Five 10-mm ports are used (Fig. 25-39). Dissection is begun by an incision of the portion of the gastrohepatic omentum above the hepatic branch of the anterior vagus nerve. The circumference of the diaphragmatic crura is dissected and the esophagus is mobilized by careful dissection of the anterior and posterior soft tissues within the hiatus. The esophagus is held anterior and to the left and the crura approximated with three to four interrupted 0 silk sutures, starting just above the aortic decussation and working anterior. Complete fundic mobilization allows construction of a tension-free fundoplication. Short gastric vessels along the upper one third of the greater curvature are sequentially dissected and divided. Following complete mobilization, the posterior wall of the fundus is gently brought behind the esophagus to the right side. The anterior wall of the fundus is brought anterior to the esophagus, and the fundic lips are manipulated to allow the fundus to envelop the esophagus without twisting (Fig. 25-40). A 60F bougie is passed to properly size the fundopli-

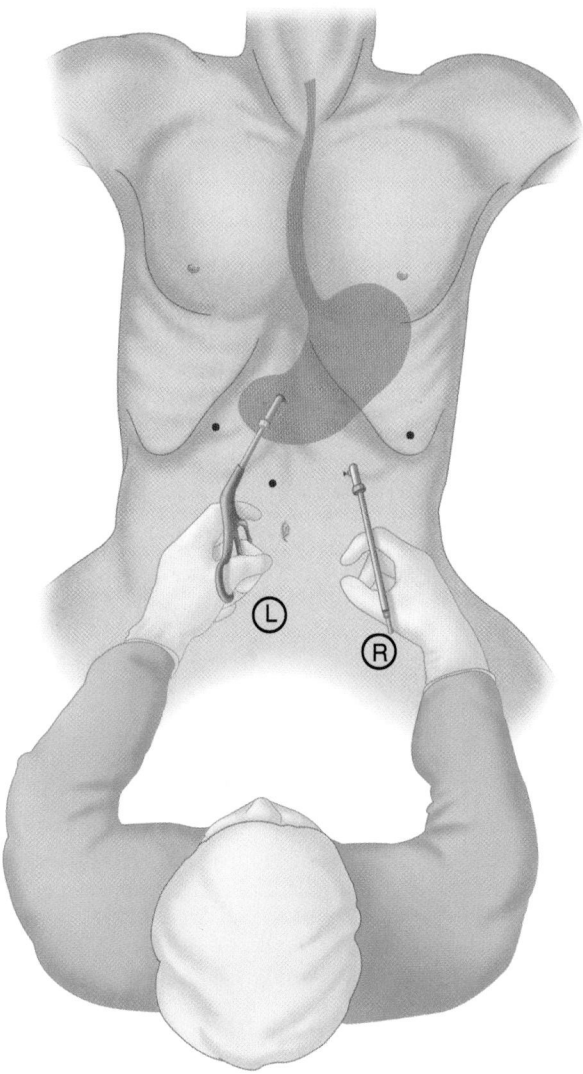

FIG. 25-39. Patient positioning and trocar placement for laparoscopic antireflux surgery. The patient is placed with the head elevated 45° in the modified lithotomy position. The surgeon stands between the patient's legs, and the procedure is completed using five abdominal access ports.

cation, and it is sutured by using a single U stitch of 2-0 polypropylene buttressed with felt pledgets (Fig. 25-41).

Transthoracic Nissen Fundoplication

The indications for performing an antireflux procedure by a transthoracic approach are as follows:

1. A patient has had a previous hiatal hernia repair. In this situation, a peripheral circumferential incision in the diaphragm is made to provide simultaneous exposure of the upper abdomen. This allows safe dissection of the previous repair from both the abdominal and thoracic sides of the diaphragm.
2. A patient who requires a concomitant esophageal myotomy for achalasia or diffuse spasm.
3. A patient who has a short esophagus. This is usually associated with a stricture or BE. In this situation, the thoracic approach is preferred to allow maximum mobilization of the esophagus, and to perform a Collis gastroplasty to place the repair without tension below the diaphragm.
4. A patient with a sliding hiatal hernia that does not reduce below the diaphragm during a roentgenographic barium study

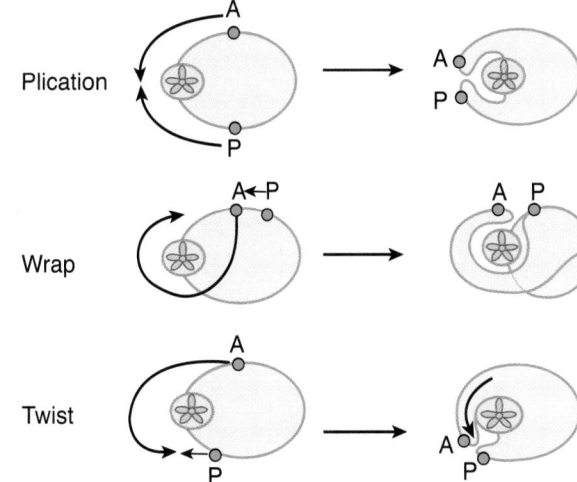

FIG. 25-40. Schematic representations of the various possibilities of orientation of a Nissen fundoplication. The top box represents the preferred approach; it can be seen that the approach shown in the bottom two boxes results in twisting of the fundoplication. A = anterior; P = posterior.

in the upright position. This can indicate esophageal shortening, and again, a thoracic approach is preferred for maximum mobilization of the esophagus, and, if necessary, the performance of a Collis gastroplasty.
5. A patient who has associated pulmonary pathology. In this situation, the nature of the pulmonary pathology can be evaluated and the proper pulmonary surgery, in addition to the antireflux repair, can be performed.
6. An obese patient. In this situation, the abdominal repair is difficult because of poor exposure, particularly in men, in whom the intra-abdominal fat is more abundant.

When employing the thoracic approach, the hiatus is exposed through a left posterior lateral thoracotomy incision in the sixth intercostal space. The diaphragm can be incised circumferentially and laterally for a distance of approximately 10 to 15 cm. The esophagus is circumferentially mobilized from the level of the diaphragm to the aortic arch. The proximal stomach is then freed from below the diaphragm and the fundus and part of the body of the stomach are drawn up through the hiatus into the chest cavity. The gastroesophageal fat pad is then excised. A crural closure is then performed, and the fundoplication is constructed by enveloping the fundus around the distal esophagus. When complete, the fundoplication is placed into the abdomen.

Laparoscopic Toupet and Belsey Mark IV Partial Fundoplications

In the presence of severely altered esophageal motility, where the propulsive force of the esophagus is not sufficient to overcome the outflow obstruction of a complete fundoplication, a partial fundoplication is indicated. A partial fundoplication may be performed laparoscopically, a Toupet fundoplication, or transthoracically, a Belsey Mark IV repair. Both consist of a 270° gastric fundoplication around the distal 4 cm of esophagus, performed either laparoscopically or through a left chest incision (Fig. 25-42).

In patients with a short esophagus secondary to a stricture, BE, or a large hiatal hernia, the esophagus is lengthened with a Collis gastroplasty (see Fig. 25-42). The esophagus is lengthened by constructing a gastric tube along the lesser curvature. This allows a tension-free constriction of a Belsey Mark IV or Nissen fundoplication around the newly formed gastric tube, with placement of the repair in the abdo-

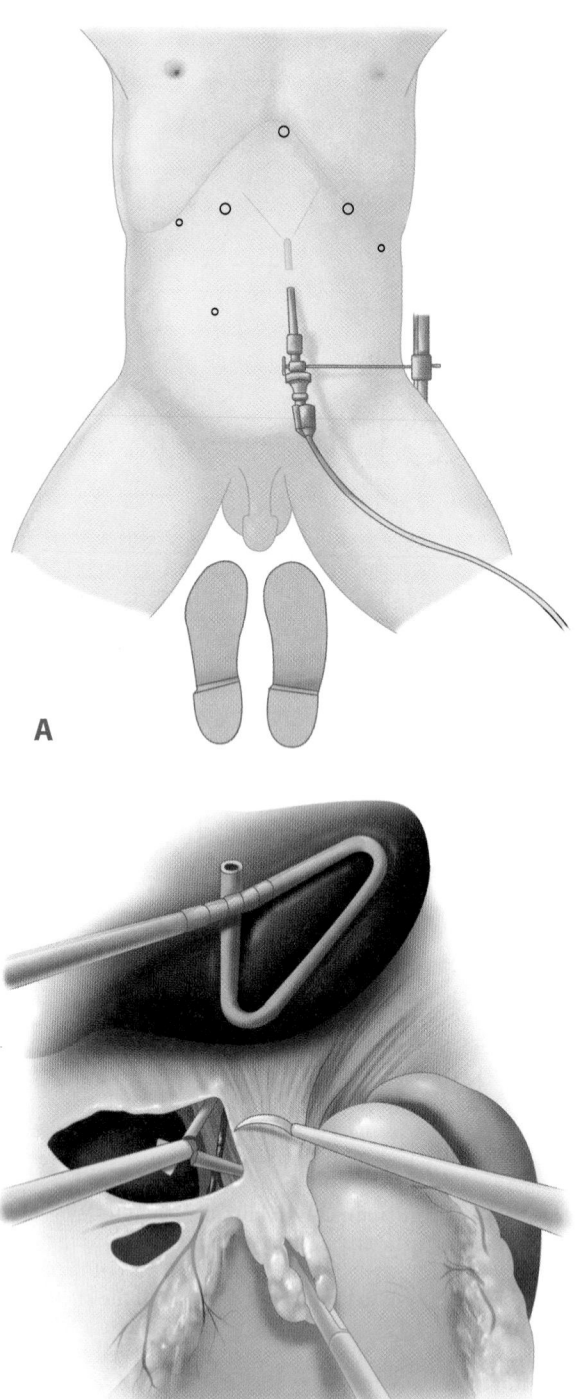

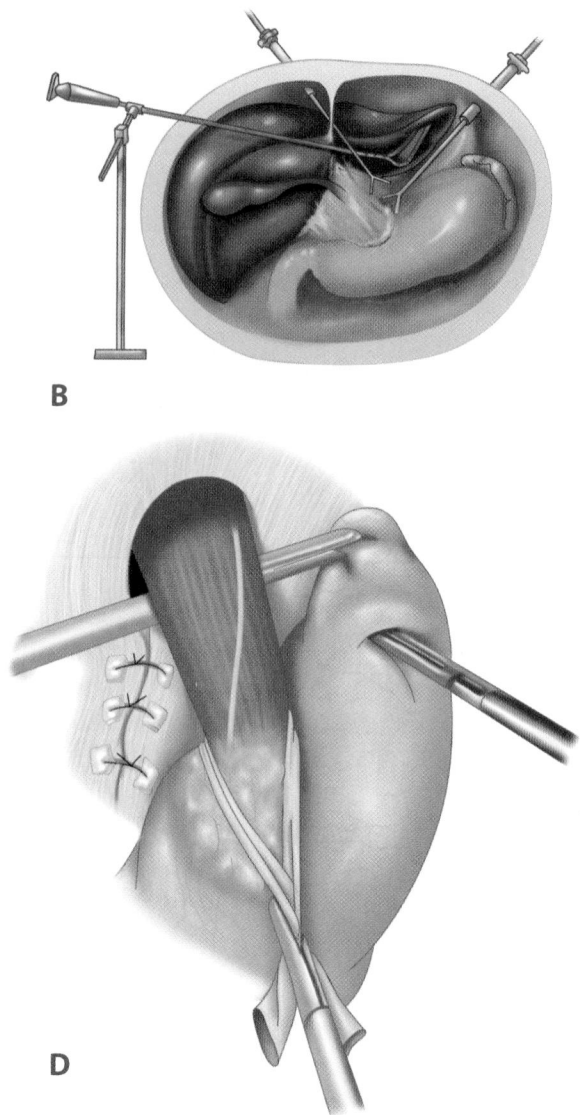

FIG. 25-41. A. Laparoscopic Nissen fundoplication is performed with a five-trocar technique. **B.** The liver retractor is affixed to a mechanical arm to hold it in place throughout the operation. **C.** After division of the gastrohepatic omentum above the hepatic branch of the vagus (pars flaccida), the surgeon places a blunt atraumatic grasper beneath the phrenoesophageal ligament. **D.** After completion of the crural closure, an atraumatic grasper is placed right to left behind the gastroesophageal junction. The grasper is withdrawn, pulling the posterior aspect of the gastric fundus behind the esophagus. (*Continued*)

men. Because a short esophagus is commonly associated with a reduction in esophageal contraction amplitude and the gastric tube is inert, most surgeons prefer to combine the gastroplasty procedure with a 280° Belsey Mark IV fundoplication rather than a 360° Nissen fundoplication.

Outcome after Fundoplication

Studies of long-term outcome following both open and laparoscopic fundoplication document the ability of laparoscopic fundoplication to relieve typical reflux symptoms (heartburn, regurgitation, and dysphagia) in more than 90% of patients at follow-up intervals averaging 2 to 3 years and 80 to 90% of patients 5 years or more following surgery. This includes evidence-based reviews of antireflux surgery, prospective randomized trials comparing antireflux surgery to PPI therapy and open to laparoscopic fundoplication and analysis of U.S. national trends in use and outcomes. Laparoscopic fundoplication results in a significant increase in LES pressure and length, generally restoring these values to normal. Postoperative pH studies indicate that more than 90% of patients will normalize their pH tracings. The results of laparoscopic fundoplication compare favorably with those of the "modern" era of open fundoplication. They also indicate the less predictable outcome of atypical reflux symptoms (cough, asthma, laryngitis) after surgery, being relieved in only two thirds of patients.

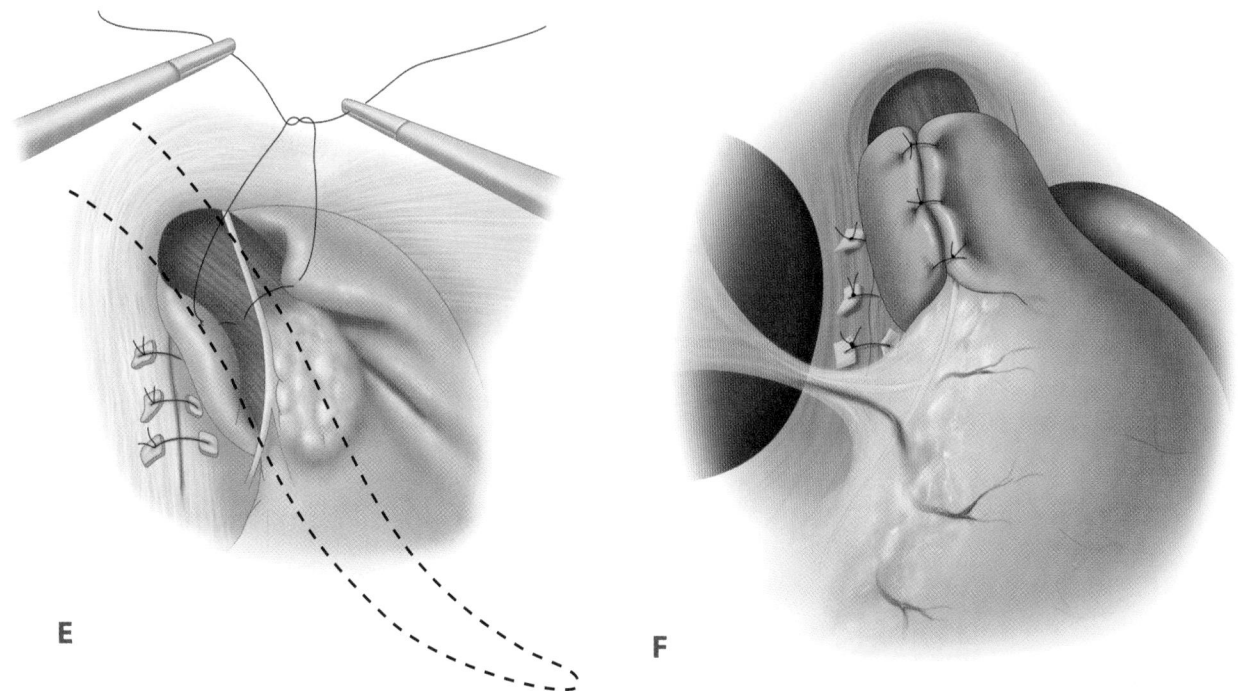

FIG. 25-41. (*Continued*) **E.** Once the suture positions are chosen, the first stitch (2-0 silk, 20 cm long) is introduced through the 10-mm trocar, and the needle is passed first through the left limb of the fundus, then the esophagus (2.5 cm above the gastroesophageal junction), then through the right limb of the fundus. **F.** Final position of the fundoplication.

The goal of surgical treatment for GERD is to relieve the symptoms of reflux by re-establishing the gastroesophageal barrier. The challenge is to accomplish this without inducing dysphagia or other untoward side effects. Dysphagia, existing before surgery, usually improves following laparoscopic fundoplication. Temporary dysphagia is common after surgery and generally resolves within 3 months. Dysphagia persisting beyond 3 months has been reported in up to 10% of patients. In the authors' experience, dysphagia, manifest by occasional difficulty swallowing solids, was present in 7% of patients at 3 months, 5% at 6 months, 2% at 12 months, and in a single patient at 24 months following surgery. Others have observed a similar improvement in postoperative dysphagia with time. Induced dysphagia is usually mild, does not require dilatation, and is temporary. It can be induced by technical misjudgments, but this explanation does not hold in all instances. In experienced hands, its prevalence should be <3% at 1 year. Other side effects common to antireflux surgery include the inability to vomit and increased flatulence. Most patients cannot vomit through an intact wrap, though this is rarely clinically relevant. Hyperflatulence is a common and noticeable problem, likely related to increased air swallowing that is present in most patients with reflux disease.

Quality-of-life analyses have become an important part of surgical outcome assessment, with both generic and disease-specific questionnaires in use, in an attempt to quantitate quality of life before and after surgical intervention. In general, these measures relate the effect of disease management to the overall well being of the patient. Most studies have used the Short Form 36 instrument, as it is rapidly administered and well validated. This questionnaire measures 12 different health-related quality-of-life parameters encompassing mental and physical well-being. Data generally indicate significant improvements in scores for most areas of the general health index.

Outcome of Antireflux Surgery in Patients with Barrett's Esophagus

Few studies have focused on the alleviation of symptoms after antireflux surgery in patients with BE (Table 25-8). Those that are available document excellent to good results in 72 to 95% of patients at 5 years following surgery. Several studies have compared medical and surgical therapy. Attwood and associates, in a prospective but nonrandomized study, reported on 45 patients undergoing either medical (26) or surgical (19) treatment of BE. The groups were similar in age, length of Barrett's segment, the percentage of time during which pH was <4, and length of follow-up. Improvement of symptoms was dramatic after antireflux surgery. Symptoms of heartburn or dysphagia recurred in 88% of patients treated with medical therapy alone, and 21% after antireflux surgery. Complications, most commonly the development of an esophageal stricture, occurred in 38% of medically treated patients and 16 percent of surgically treated patients (P <.05) over the 3-year follow-up period. One patient in each group developed esophageal adenocarcinoma. It was concluded that antireflux surgery was superior to acid suppression for both the control of symptoms and the prevention of complications in patients with BE. Other nonrandomized comparisons of medical and surgical therapy have reported similar results. Parrilla and colleagues recently reported an update of a study originally published in the *British Journal of Surgery* in 1996. The study enrolled 101 patients over 18 years (1982 to 2000). Median follow-up was 6 years. Medical therapy consisted of 20 mg of omeprazole (PPI) twice daily since 1992 in all medically treated patients. Surgical therapy consisted of an open 1.5 to 3.0 cm Nissen, over a 48 to 50F bougie, with division of the short gastric arteries in 39% of patients, and crural closure in all. Symptomatic outcome in the two groups was nearly identical, although esophagitis and/or stricture persisted in 20% of the medically treated patients, compared to only 3 to 7% of patients following antireflux surgery. Fifteen percent of patients had abnormal acid exposure after surgery. Although pH data were not routinely collected in patients on PPI therapy, in the subgroup of 12 patients that did have 24-hour monitoring on treatment, three of 12 (25%) had persistently high esophageal acid exposure, and most (75%) had persistently high bilirubin exposure.

The outcome of laparoscopic Nissen fundoplication in patients with BE has been assessed at 1 to 3 years after surgery. Hofstetter and

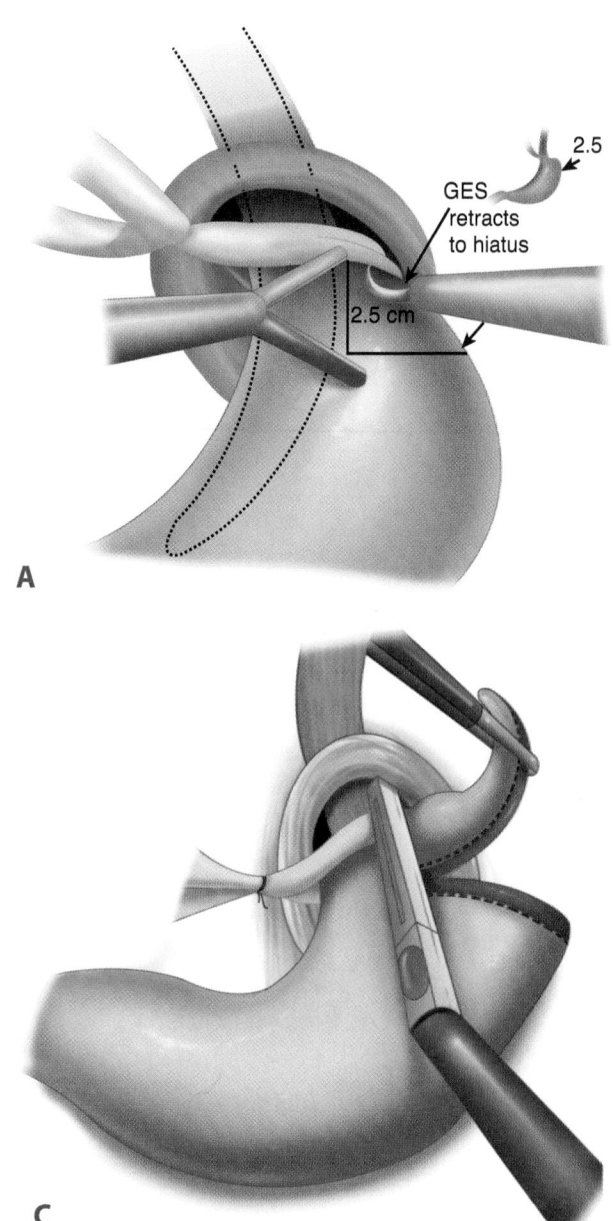

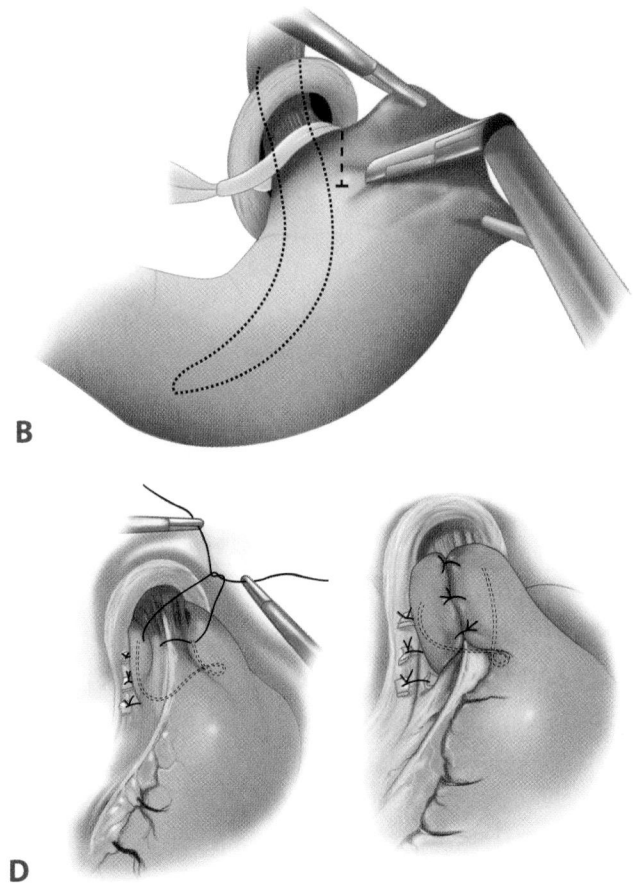

FIG. 25-42. A. After removal of the fat pad and release of tension on the Penrose drain, the gastroesophageal junction (GES) retracts to the level of the hiatus. The interior end of the staple line is marked $^2/_5$ cm below the angle of His. **B.** The first horizontal firing of the stapler occurs by maximally articulating the stapler to the left, aiming toward the previously marked spot adjacent to the dilator. **C.** The vertical staple line is created by a single firing of the GIA placed parallel and flush against the 48F dilator. **D.** The highest Nissen fundoplication suture is placed on the native esophagus, and the second suture tucks in the apex of the staple line.

colleagues reported the experience at the University of Southern California with 85 patients with BE at a median of 5 years after surgery. Fifty-nine patients had long- and 26 had short-segment Barrett's; 50 had a laparoscopic approach. Reflux symptoms were absent in 67 of 85 patients (79%). Eighteen (20%) developed recurrent symptoms, while four patients were back on daily acid-suppressive medication. Seven patients underwent a secondary repair and were asymptomatic, raising the eventual successful outcome to 87%. Postoperative 24-hour pH was normal in 17 of 21 patients (81%). Ninety-nine percent of the patients considered themselves cured (77%) or improved (22%), and 97% were satisfied with the surgery.

Farrell and associates also reported symptomatic outcome of laparoscopic Nissen fundoplication in 50 patients with both long- and short-segment BE. Mean scores for heartburn, regurgitation, and dysphagia all improved dramatically post-Nissen. Importantly, there was no significant decrement in symptom scores when 1-year results were compared to those at 2 to 5 years postoperatively. They did find a higher prevalence of "anatomic" failures requiring reoperation in patients with BE when compared to non-Barrett's patients with GERD. Others have reported similar results. Taken together these

studies document the ability of antireflux surgery to provide long-term symptomatic relief in patients with BE.

Three relevant questions arise concerning the fate, over time, of the metaplastic tissue found in BE: (a) Does antireflux surgery cause

| TABLE 25-8 | Symptomatic outcome of surgical therapy for Barrett's esophagus |

Author	Year	No. of Patients	% Excellent to Good Response	Mean Follow-Up, Years
Starnes	1984	8	75	2
Williamson	1990	37	92	3
DeMeester	1990	35	77	3
McDonald	1996	113	82.2	6.5
Ortiz	1996	32	90.6	5

regression of Barrett's epithelium? (b) Does it prevent progression? and (c) Can the development of Barrett's metaplasia be prevented by early antireflux surgery in patients with reflux disease?

The common belief that Barrett's epithelium cannot be reversed is likely false. DeMeester and associates reported that, after antireflux surgery, loss of IM in patients with visible BE was rare, but occurred in 73% of patients with inapparent IM of the cardia. This suggests that the metaplastic process may indeed be reversible if reflux is eliminated early in its process, that cardiac mucosa is dynamic, and that, as opposed to IM extending several centimeters into the esophagus, IM of the cardia is more likely to regress following antireflux surgery. Gurski and colleagues reviewed pre- and posttreatment endoscopic biopsies from 77 Barrett's patients treated surgically and 14 treated with PPIs. Posttreatment histology was classified as having regressed if two consecutive biopsies taken more than 6 months apart, plus all subsequent biopsies, showed loss of IM or loss of dysplasia. Histopathologic regression occurred in 28 of 77 patients (36.4%) following antireflux surgery, and in one of 14 (7.1%) patients treated with PPIs alone (P <.03). After surgery, regression from low-grade dysplastic to nondysplastic BE occurred in 17 of 25 (68%) patients and from IM to no IM in 11 of 52 (21.2%) patients. Both types of regression were significantly more common in short- (<3 cm) compared to long-segment (>3 cm) BE. Eight patients progressed; five from IM alone to low-grade dysplasia, and three from low- to high-grade dysplasia. All those who progressed had long-segment BE. On multivariate analysis, the presence of short-segment Barrett's and the type of treatment were significantly associated with regression; age, sex, and surgical procedure, and preoperative LES and pH characteristics were not. The median time of biopsy-proven regression was 18.5 months after surgery, with 95% occurring within 5 years. Similar findings have been reported by the University of Washington group and Hunter and colleagues. Although these studies do not conclusively prove the ability of antireflux surgery to reverse the changes of early BE, they do provide encouragement that, given early changes, the process may indeed be reversible.

Recent evidence suggests that the development of BE may even be preventable. Although a very difficult hypothesis to study, Oberg and coworkers followed a cohort of 69 patients with short-segment, nonintestinalized, CLE over a median of 5 years of surveillance endoscopy. Forty-nine of the patients were maintained on PPI therapy and 20 had antireflux surgery. Patients with antireflux surgery were 10 times less likely to develop IM in these CLE segments over a follow-up span of nearly 15 years than those on medical therapy. This rather remarkable observation supports the two-step hypothesis of the development of BE (cardiac metaplasia followed by IM), and suggests that the second step can be prevented if reflux disease is recognized and treated early and aggressively.

Current data indicate that patients with BE should remain in an endoscopic surveillance program following antireflux surgery. Biopsy specimens should be reviewed by a pathologist with expertise in the field. If low-grade dysplasia is confirmed, biopsies should be repeated after 12 weeks of high-dose acid suppression therapy. If high-grade dysplasia is evident on more than one biopsy specimen, esophageal resection is advisable because of the more than 50% probability that an invasive cancer is already present. Early detection and resection have been shown to decrease the mortality rate from esophageal cancer in these patients. Because BE results from chronic, uncontrolled gastroesophageal reflux, and esophageal adenocarcinoma is virtually always associated with IM, there are strong theoretical grounds for halting the progression toward malignancy by permanently and effectively stopping reflux of gastric contents. Thus, prevention of progression, not regression, becomes the central issue. Although some cancers have developed after antireflux surgery, the absence of pre-existent dysplasia before surgery or the efficacy of the operative procedure in reducing 24-hour esophageal acid exposure to normal has not been documented. If the dysplasia is reported as lower grade or indetermi-

nant, then inflammatory change that is often confused with dysplasia should be suppressed by a course of acid suppression therapy in high doses for 2 to 3 weeks, followed by rebiopsy of the Barrett's segment.

There is a growing body of evidence to attest to the ability of fundoplication to protect against dysplasia and invasive malignancy. Three studies suggest that an effective antireflux procedure can impact the natural history of BE in this regard. Two prospective randomized studies found less adenocarcinoma in the surgically treated groups. Parrilla and associates reported that, although the development of dysplasia and adenocarcinoma was no different overall, the subgroup of surgical patients with normal postoperative pH studies developed significantly less dysplasia and had no adenocarcinoma. Spechler identified one adenocarcinoma 11 to 13 years after antireflux surgery, compared to four following medical treatment. Most of these authors concluded that there is a critical need for future trials exploring the role of antireflux surgery in protecting against the development of dysplasia in patients with BE.

Data from the Mayo Clinic strongly suggest that antireflux surgery impacts the development of adenocarcinoma in patients with BE. The authors reviewed the outcome of 118 patients with BE undergoing antireflux surgery between 1960 and 1990. Three cancers occurred over an 18.5-year follow-up period, all within the first 3 years after surgery. The fact that the development of adenocarcinoma was clustered in the early years after antireflux surgery, and not randomly dispersed throughout the follow-up period, suggests that antireflux surgery altered the natural history of the disease. Hammeetman has shown that once dysplasia has developed, carcinoma ensues in an average of 3 years. The occurrence of all observed cancers in the first few years suggests that the point of no return in the dysplasia-cancer sequence had already occurred before the time of antireflux surgery.

Reoperation for Failed Antireflux Repairs

Failure of an antireflux procedure occurs when, after the repair, the patient is unable to swallow normally, experiences upper abdominal discomfort during and after meals, or has recurrence or persistence of reflux symptoms. The assessment of these symptoms and the selection of patients who need further surgery are challenging problems. Functional assessment of patients who have recurrent, persistent, or emergent new symptoms following a primary antireflux repair is critical to identifying the cause of the failure. Analysis of patients requiring reoperation after a previous antireflux procedure shows that placement of the wrap around the stomach is the most frequent cause for failure after open procedures, while herniation of the repair into the chest is the most frequent cause of failure after a laparoscopic procedure. Partial or complete breakdown of the fundoplication and construction of a too-tight or too-long wrap of a fundoplication occurs with both open and closed procedures. The fact that 10% of these patients had an undiagnosed underlying esophageal motor disorder underlines the critical role of preoperative esophageal function tests before the initial procedure.

Patients who have recurrence of heartburn and regurgitation without dysphagia and have good esophageal motility are most amenable to reoperation, and can be expected to have an excellent outcome. When dysphagia is the cause of failure, the situation is more difficult to manage. If the dysphagia occurred immediately following the repair, it is usually due to a technical failure, most commonly a misplaced fundoplication around the upper stomach, and reoperation is usually satisfactory. When dysphagia is associated with poor motility and multiple previous repairs, serious consideration should be given to esophageal resection and replacement. With each reoperation the esophagus is damaged further, and the chances of preserving function become less. Also, blood supply is reduced, and ischemic necrosis of the esophagus can occur after several previous mobilizations.

GIANT DIAPHRAGMATIC (HIATAL) HERNIAS

With the advent of clinical radiology, it became evident that a diaphragmatic hernia was a relatively common abnormality and was not always accompanied by symptoms. Three types of esophageal hiatal hernia were identified: (a) the sliding hernia, type I, characterized by an upward dislocation of the cardia in the posterior mediastinum (Fig. 25-43A); (b) the rolling or PEH, type II, characterized by an upward dislocation of the gastric fundus alongside a normally positioned cardia (Fig. 25-43B); and (c) the combined sliding-rolling or mixed hernia, type III, characterized by an upward dislocation of both the cardia and the gastric fundus (Fig. 25-43C). The end stage of type I and type II hernias occurs when the whole stomach migrates up into the chest by rotating 180° around its longitudinal axis, with the cardia and pylorus as fixed points. In this situation the abnormality is usually referred to as an intrathoracic stomach (Fig. 25-43D). In some taxonomies, a type IV hiatal hernia is declared when an additional organ, usually the colon, herniates as well.

Incidence and Etiology

The true incidence of a hiatal hernia is difficult to determine because of the absence of symptoms in a large number of patients who are subsequently shown to have a hernia. When radiographic examinations are done in response to GI symptoms, the incidence of a sliding hiatal hernia is seven times higher than that of a PEH. The PEH is also known as the *giant hiatal hernia*. Over time the pressure gradient between the abdomen and chest enlarges the hiatal hernia. In many cases the type 1 sliding hernia will evolve into a type III mixed hernia. Type II hernias are quite rare. The age distribution of patients with PEHs is significantly different from that observed in sliding hiatal hernias. The median age of the former is 61 years old; of the latter, 48 years old. PEHs are more likely to occur in women by a ratio of 4:1.

Structural deterioration of the phrenoesophageal membrane over time may explain the higher incidence of hiatal hernias in the older age group. These changes involve thinning of the upper fascial layer of the phrenoesophageal membrane (i.e., the supradiaphragmatic continuation of the endothoracic fascia) and loss of elasticity in the lower fascial layer (i.e., the infradiaphragmatic continuation of the transversalis fascia). Consequently, the phrenoesophageal membrane yields to stretching in the cranial direction due to the persistent intra-abdominal pressure and the tug of esophageal shortening on swallowing. Interestingly, the stretching and thinning occurs more anteriorly and posteriorly, with fixation of the left crus of the diaphragm to the stomach at the 3 o'clock position, as viewed from the foot. This creates an anterior and posterior hernia sac, the latter of which is often filled with epiphrenic and retroperitoneal fat. These observations point to the conclusion that the development of a hiatal hernia is an age-related phenomenon secondary to repetitive upward stretching of the phrenoesophageal membrane.

Clinical Manifestations

The clinical presentation of a giant hiatal (paraesophageal) hernia differs from that of a sliding hernia. There is usually a higher

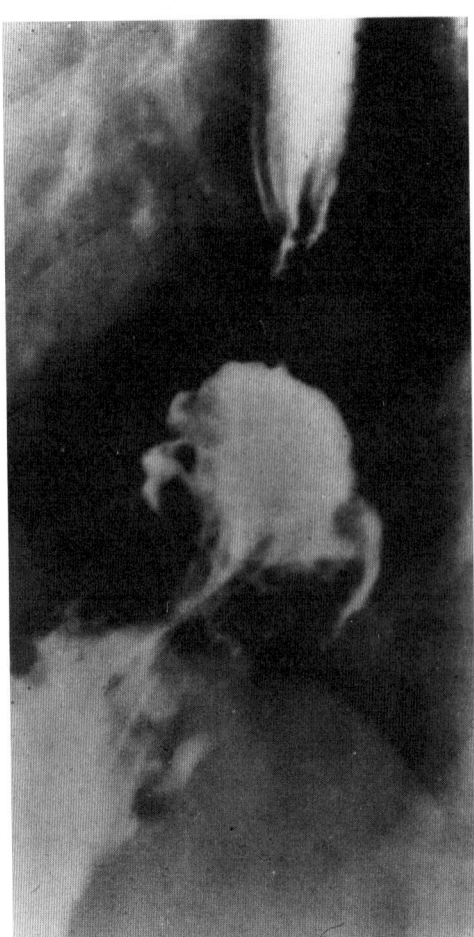

A

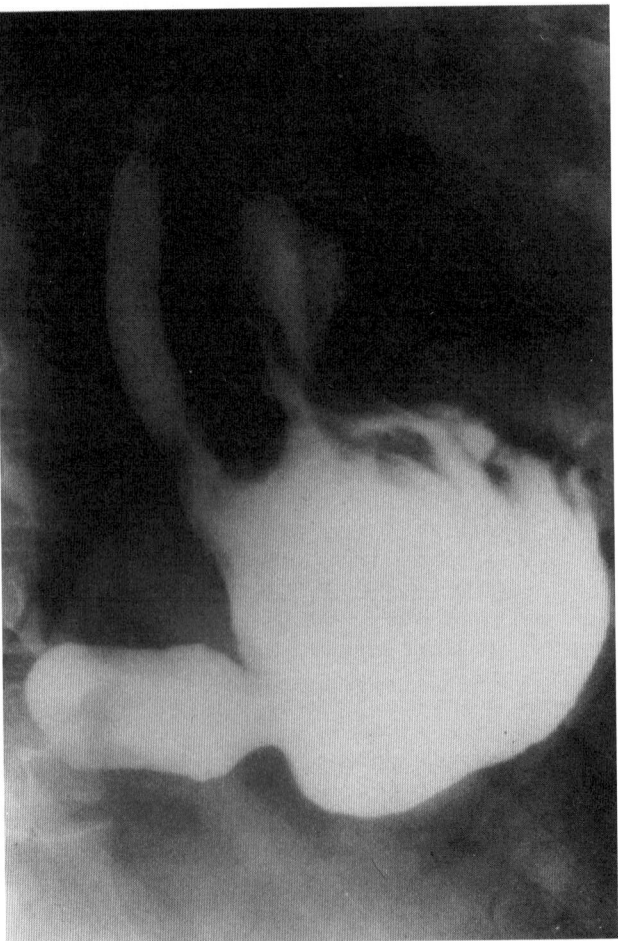

B

FIG. 25-43. **A.** Radiogram of a type I (sliding) hiatal hernia. **B.** Radiogram of a type II (rolling or paraesophageal) hernia. *(Continued)*

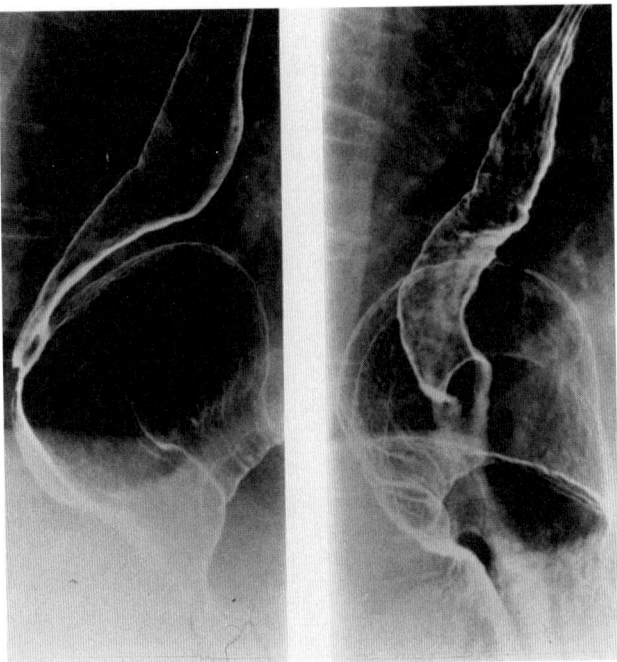

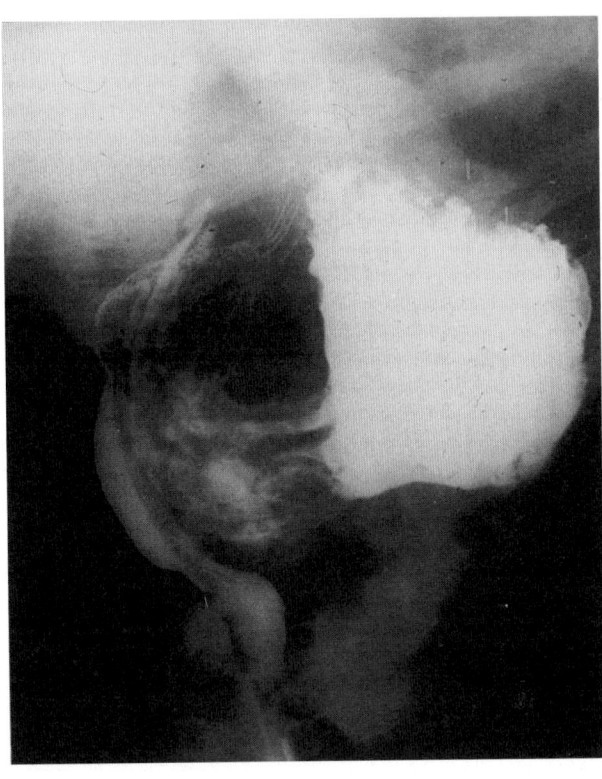

FIG. 25-43. (*Continued*) **C.** Radiogram of a type III (combined sliding-rolling or mixed) hernia. **D.** Radiogram of an intrathoracic stomach. This is the end stage of a large hiatal hernia regardless of its initial classification. Note that the stomach has rotated 180° around its longitudinal axis, with the cardia and pylorus as fixed points. [*Reproduced with permission from DeMeester TR, Bonavina L: Paraesophageal hiatal hernia, in Nyhus LM, Condon RE (eds): Hernia, 3rd ed. Philadelphia: Lippincott, 1989, p 684.*]

prevalence of symptoms of dysphagia and postprandial fullness with PEHs, but the typical symptoms of heartburn and regurgitation present in sliding hiatal hernias can also occur. Both are caused by gastroesophageal reflux secondary to an underlying mechanical deficiency of the cardia. The symptoms of dysphagia and postprandial fullness in patients with a PEH are explained by the compression of the adjacent esophagus by a distended cardia, or twisting of the GEJ by the torsion of the stomach that occurs as it becomes progressively displaced in the chest. Many patients with sliding hernias and reflux symptoms will lose the reflux symptoms when the hernia evolves into the paraesophageal variety. This can be explained by the re-creation of the cardiophrenic angle when the stomach herniates alongside the GEJ or becomes twisted in the sac. Repair of the hernia without addressing the reflux can create extremely bothersome heartburn. Respiratory complications are frequently associated with a PEH, and consist of dyspnea from mechanical compression and recurrent pneumonia from aspiration.

Approximately one third of patients with a PEH are found to be anemic, which is due to recurrent bleeding from ulceration of the gastric mucosa in the herniated portion of the stomach, even if ulcerations are not detected at the time of endoscopy. The association of anemia and PEH is best proven by fixing the hernia. Anemia is corrected in >90% of patients with this condition. With time, more and more stomach migrates into the chest and can cause intermittent foregut obstruction due to the rotation that has occurred. In contrast, many patients with paraesophageal hiatal hernia are asymptomatic or complain of minor symptoms. However, the presence of a PEH can be life threatening in that the hernia can lead to sudden catastrophic events, such as excessive bleeding or volvulus with acute gastric obstruction or infarction. With mild dilatation of the stomach, the gastric blood supply can be markedly reduced, causing gastric ischemia, ulceration, perforation, and sepsis. The

probability of incarceration is not well known, although recent analysis using mathematical modeling suggests the risk is small.

The symptoms of sliding hiatal hernias are usually due to functional abnormalities associated with gastroesophageal reflux and include heartburn, regurgitation, and dysphagia. These patients have a mechanically defective LES, giving rise to the reflux of gastric juice into the esophagus and the symptoms of heartburn and regurgitation. The symptom of dysphagia occurs from the presence of mucosal edema, Schatzki's ring, stricture, or the inability to organize peristaltic activity in the body of the esophagus as a consequence of the disease.

There is a group of patients with sliding hiatal hernias not associated with reflux disease who have dysphagia without any obvious endoscopic or manometric explanation. Video barium radiograms have shown that the cause of dysphagia in these patients is an obstruction of the swallowed bolus by diaphragmatic impingement on the herniated stomach. Manometrically, this is reflected by a double-humped high-pressure zone at the GEJ. The first pressure rise is due to diaphragmatic impingement on the herniated stomach, and the second to the true distal esophageal sphincter. These patients usually have a mechanically competent sphincter, but the impingement of the diaphragm on the stomach can result in propelling the contents of the supradiaphragmatic portion of the stomach up into the esophagus and pharynx, resulting in complaints of pharyngeal regurgitation and aspiration. Consequently, this abnormality is often confused with typical GERD. Surgical reduction of the hernia results in relief of the dysphagia in 91% of patients.

Diagnosis

A radiogram of the chest with the patient in the upright position can diagnose a hiatal hernia if it shows an air-fluid level behind the cardiac shadow. This is usually caused by a PEH or an intrathoracic stomach. The accuracy of the upper GI barium study in detecting a paraesophageal hiatal hernia is greater than for a sliding hernia because the latter can often spontaneously reduce. The paraesophageal hiatal hernia is a permanent herniation of the stomach into the thoracic cavity, so a barium swallow provides the diagnosis in virtually every case. Attention should be focused on the position of the GEJ, when seen, to differentiate it from a type II hernia (see Fig. 25-43B and C). Fiber-optic esophagoscopy is useful in the diagnosis and classification of a hiatal hernia because the scope can be retroflexed. In this position, a sliding hiatal hernia can be identified by noting a gastric pouch lined with rugal folds extending above the impression caused by the crura of the diaphragm, or measuring at least 2 cm between the crura, identified by having the patient sniff, and the squamocolumnar junction on withdrawal of the scope (Fig. 25-44). A PEH is identified on retroversion of the scope by noting a separate orifice adjacent to the GEJ into which gastric rugal folds ascend. A sliding-rolling or mixed hernia can be identified by noting a gastric pouch lined with rugal folds above the diaphragm, with the GEJ entering about midway up the side of the pouch.

Pathophysiology

Physiologic testing with 24-hour esophageal pH monitoring has shown increased esophageal exposure to acid gastric juice in 60% of the patients with a paraesophageal hiatal hernia, compared with the observed 71% incidence in patients with a sliding hiatal hernia. It is now recognized that paraesophageal hiatal hernia can be associated with pathologic gastroesophageal reflux.

Physiologic studies have also shown that the competency of the cardia depends on an interrelationship between distal esophageal sphincter pressure, the length of the sphincter that is exposed to the positive-pressure environment of the abdomen, and the overall

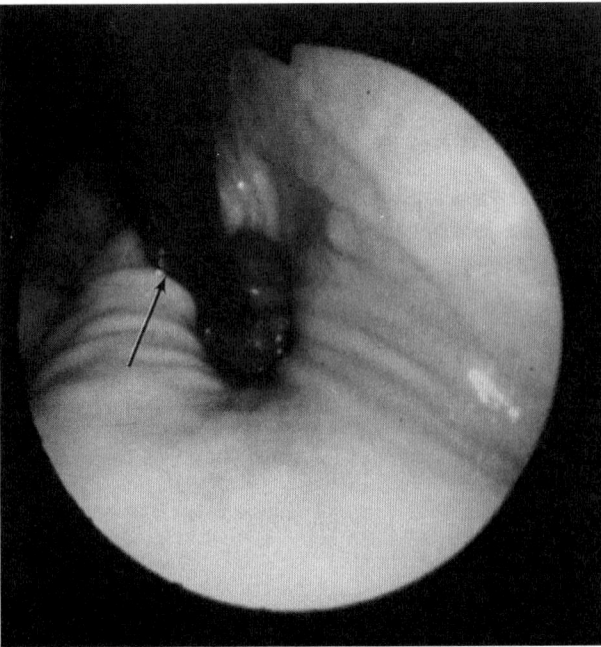

FIG. 25-44. Endoscopic view through a retroflexed fiber-optic gastroscope showing the shaft of the scope (*arrow*) coming down through a sliding hernia. Note the gastric rugal folds extending above the impression caused by the crura of the diaphragm. *[Reproduced with permission from DeMeester TR, Bonavina L: Paraesophageal hiatal hernia, in Nyhus LM, Condon RE (eds):* Hernia, *3rd ed. Philadelphia: Lippincott, 1989, p 689.]*

length of the sphincter. A deficiency in any one of these manometric characteristics of the sphincter is associated with incompetency of the cardia regardless of whether a hernia is present. Patients with a PEH who have an incompetent cardia have been shown to have a distal esophageal sphincter with normal pressure, but a shortened overall length and displacement outside the positive-pressure environment of the abdomen. One might expect esophageal body function to be diminished with the esophagus "accordianed" up into the chest. Surprisingly, esophageal peristalsis in patients with PEH is normal in 88%.

Treatment

The treatment of paraesophageal hiatal hernia is largely surgical. Controversial aspects include (a) indications for repair, (b) surgical approach, and (c) role of fundoplication.

Indications

The presence of a paraesophageal hiatal hernia has traditionally been considered an indication for surgical repair. This recommendation is largely based upon two clinical observations. First, retrospective studies have shown a significant incidence of catastrophic, life-threatening complications of bleeding, infarction, and perforation in patients being followed with known paraesophageal herniation. Second, emergency repair carries a high mortality. In the classic report of Skinner and Belsey, six of 21 patients with a PEH, treated medically because of minimal symptoms, died from the complications of strangulation, perforation, exsanguinating hemorrhage, or acute dilatation of the herniated intrathoracic stomach. These catastrophes occurred for the most part without warning. Others have reported similar findings.

Recent studies suggest that catastrophic complications may be somewhat less common. Allen and colleagues followed 23 patients for a median of 78 months with only four patients progressively worsening. There was a single mortality secondary to aspiration that occurred during a barium swallow examination to investigate progressive symptoms. Although emergency repairs had a median hospital stay of 48 days compared to a stay of 9 days in those having elective repair, there were only three cases of gastric strangulation in 735 patient-years of follow-up.

If surgery is delayed and repair is done on an emergency basis, operative mortality is high, compared to <1% for an elective repair. With this in mind, patients with a PEH are generally counseled to have elective repair of their hernia, particularly if they are symptomatic. Watchful waiting of asymptomatic PEHs may be an acceptable option.

Surgical Approach

The surgical approach to repair of a paraesophageal hiatal hernia may be either transabdominal (laparoscopic or open) or transthoracic. Each has its advantages and disadvantages. A transthoracic approach facilitates complete esophageal mobilization but is rarely used because the access trauma and postoperative pain are significantly greater than a laparoscopic approach.

The transabdominal approach facilitates reduction of the volvulus that is often associated with PEHs. Although some degree of esophageal mobilization can be accomplished transhiatally, complete mobilization to the aortic arch is difficult or impossible without risk of injury to the vagal nerves.

Laparoscopic repair of PEH would appear to have become the standard approach; however, a recent review of large national databases suggests that most giant hernias are still repaired through an open approach. Laparoscopic repair of a pure type II, or mixed type III PEH is an order of magnitude more difficult than a standard laparoscopic Nissen fundoplication. Most would recommend that these procedures are best avoided until the surgeon has accumulated considerable experience with laparoscopic antireflux surgery. There are several reasons for this. First, the vertical and horizontal volvulus of the stomach often associated with PEHs makes identification of the anatomy, in particular the location of the esophagus, difficult. Second, dissection of a large PEH sac may result in significant bleeding if the surgeon deviates from the correct plane of dissection between the peritoneal sac and the endothoracic fascia. Finally, redundant tissue present at the GEJ following dissection of the sac frustrates the creation of a fundoplication, which these authors believe should accompany the repair of all PEHs. Mindful of these difficulties, and given appropriate experience, patients with PEH may be approached laparoscopically, with expectation of success in the majority.

Giant PEH can be associated with a short esophagus in up to 5 to 20% of patients as a result of chronic cephalad displacement of the GEJ. The presence of a short esophagus increases the difficulty of laparoscopic PEH repair. Up to 10 to 20% of surgical failures with PEH repair is due to the lack of recognition of a short esophagus. Preoperative results of barium swallow and esophagogastroduodenoscopy may provide an indication of short esophagus, but no combination of preoperative clinical variables reliably predict the presence of short esophagus, defined as the failure to achieve 2.5 cm of intra-abdominal esophagus with standard mediastinal dissection techniques. Hence, the diagnosis of this entity continues to be made definitively only in the operating room. Collis gastroplasty achieves esophageal lengthening by creation of a neoesophagus using the gastric cardia. The totally laparoscopic approach to the short esophagus has evolved from a method using an end-to-end anastomosis circular stapler to the current approach that uses a linear stapler creating a stapled wedge gastroplasty. Elements of importance in fashioning the fundoplication after Collis gastroplasty include placement of the initial suture of the fundoplication on the esophagus, immediately above the GEJ to ensure that acid-secreting (gastric) mucosa does not reside above the fundoplication. A second element that ensures safety and avoids wrap deformation is to place the gastric portion of the staple line against the neoesophagus, such that the tip of the gastric staple line sits adjacent to the middle suture of the fundoplication on the right side of the esophagus.

It has been shown that PEH repair has a relatively high incidence of recurrence (10 to 40%) when the crura is closed primarily with permanent suture. Recently, there has been an interest in using a biomaterial as a reinforcement of the standard crural closure. Randomized control studies have demonstrated a reduction in PEH recurrence rate when a synthetic mesh was used. However, the use of a nonabsorbable mesh at the hiatus is not universally accepted because of a potential risk of esophagus or gastric erosion and mesh infection. There is also a higher incidence of postoperative dysphagia when a nonabsorbable mesh is used, as it stimulates a more intense inflammatory reaction and subsequent fibrosis. The associated postoperative dysphagia may not be amenable to endoscopic dilatation. A biomaterial like the porcine small intestinal submucosa is an acellular xenograft consisting primarily of type I collagen. This biomaterial generally degrades rapidly intracorporeally and yet allows the remodeling tissue to be incorporated into the native tissue, providing a better tensile strength. A recent multicenter, prospective randomized study demonstrated that adding this type of mesh to the primarily closed hiatus in patients with PEH repair can result in a 2.5-fold reduction of hiatal hernia recurrence in 6 months in the absence of any mesh-related complication. This form of repair appears to be safe, but the long-term durability of this mesh-based reinforcement of the hiatus in PEH repair is yet to be validated.

Role of Fundoplication in Giant Hiatal Hernia Repair

Controversy remains as to whether to perform an antireflux procedure at all, in selected cases only, or in all patients. The case against an antireflux procedure rests on the frequency of significant postoperative complications secondary to the fundoplication, as well as the slightly longer operative time and increased cost that additional surgery entails. Most advocate the routine addition of an antireflux procedure following repair of the hernia defect. There are several reasons for this. Physiologic testing with 24-hour esophageal pH monitoring has shown increased esophageal exposure to acid gastric juice in 60 to 70% of patients with a paraesophageal hiatal hernia, nearly identical to the observed 71% incidence in patients with a sliding hiatal hernia. Furthermore, there is no relation between the symptoms experienced by the patient with a PEH and the competency of the cardia. Finally, dissection of the gastroesophageal esophagus may lead to postoperative reflux despite a negative preoperative pH score.

Results

Most outcome studies report relief of symptoms following surgical repair of PEHs in more than 90% of patients. The current literature suggests that laparoscopic repair of a paraesophageal hiatal hernia can be successful. Most authors report symptomatic improvement in 80 to 90% of patients, and <10 to 15% prevalence of recurrent hernia. However, the problem of recurrent hernia following PEH repair, open or laparoscopic, is becoming increasingly appreciated. Recurrent hiatal hernia is now the most common cause of anatomic failure following laparoscopic Nissen fundoplication done for GERD (5 to 10%), but this risk is compounded for the giant hernia where radiologic recurrence is detected in 25 to 40% of patients, when mesh is not used. It appears that optimal results with open or laparoscopic giant hiatal hernia repair should include options for mesh buttressing of hiatal closure and selective esophageal lengthening with one of the many techniques developed for the creation of a Collis gastroplasty.

SCHATZKI'S RING

Schatzki's ring is a thin submucosal circumferential ring in the lower esophagus at the squamocolumnar junction, often associated with a hiatal hernia. Its significance and pathogenesis are unclear (Fig. 25-45). The ring was first noted by Templeton, but Schatzki and Gary defined it as a distinct entity in 1953. Its prevalence varies from

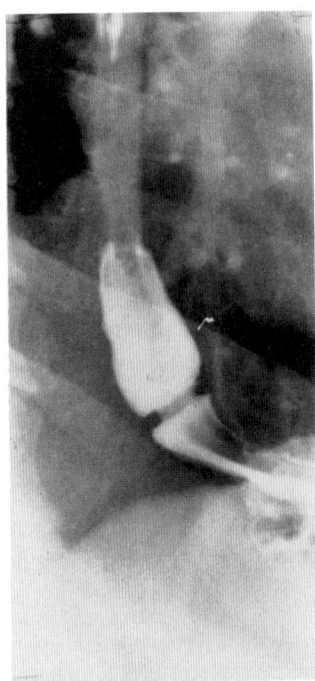

FIG. 25-45. Barium esophagogram showing Schatzki's ring (i.e., a thin circumferential ring in the distal esophagus at the squamocolumnar junction). Below the ring is a hiatal hernia.

0.2 to 14% in the general population, epending on the technique of diagnosis and the criteria used. Stiennon believed the ring to be a pleat of mucosa formed by infolding of redundant esophageal mucosa due to shortening of the esophagus. Others believe the ring to be congenital, and still others suggest it is an early stricture resulting from inflammation of the esophageal mucosa caused by chronic reflux.

Schatzki's ring is a distinct clinical entity having different symptoms, upper GI function studies, and response to treatment when compared with patients with a hiatal hernia, but without a ring. Twenty-four-hour esophageal pH monitoring has shown that patients with a Schatzki's ring have a lower incidence of reflux than hiatal hernia controls. They also have better LES function. This, together with the presence of a ring, could represent a protective mechanism to prevent gastroesophageal reflux.

Symptoms associated with Schatzki's ring are brief episodes of dysphagia during hurried ingestion of solid foods. Its treatment has varied from dilation alone to dilation with antireflux measures, antireflux procedure alone, incision, and even excision of the ring. Little is known about the natural progression of Schatzki's rings. Using radiologic techniques, Chen and colleagues showed progressive stenosis of rings in 59% of patients, whereas Schatzki found that the rings decreased in diameter in 29% of patients and remained unchanged in the rest.

Symptoms in patients with a ring are caused more by the presence of the ring than by gastroesophageal reflux. Most patients with a ring but without proven reflux respond to one dilation, while most patients with proven reflux require repeated dilations. In this regard, the majority of Schatzki's ring patients without proven reflux have a history of ingestion of drugs known to be damaging to the esophageal mucosa. Bonavina and associates have suggested drug-induced injury as the cause of stenosis in patients with a ring, but without a history of reflux. Because rings also occur in patients with proven reflux, it is likely that gastroesophageal reflux also plays a part. This is supported by the fact that there is less drug ingestion in the history of these patients. Schatzki's ring is probably an acquired lesion that can lead to stenosis from chemical-induced injury by pill lodgment in the distal esophagus, or from reflux-induced injury to the lower esophageal mucosa.

The best form of treatment of a symptomatic Schatzki's ring in patients who do not have reflux consists of esophageal dilation for relief of the obstructive symptoms. In patients with a ring who have proven reflux and a mechanically defective sphincter, an antireflux procedure is necessary to obtain relief and avoid repeated dilation.

SCLERODERMA

Scleroderma is a systemic disease accompanied by esophageal abnormalities in approximately 80% of patients. In most, the disease follows a prolonged course. Renal involvement occurs in a small percentage of patients and signals a poor prognosis. The onset of the disease is usually in the third or fourth decade of life, occurring twice as frequently in women as in men.

Small vessel inflammation appears to be an initiating event, with subsequent perivascular deposition of normal collagen, which may lead to vascular compromise. In the GI tract, the predominant feature is smooth muscle atrophy. Whether the atrophy in the esophageal musculature is a primary effect or occurs secondary to a neurogenic disorder is unknown. The results of pharmacologic and hormonal manipulation, with agents that act either indirectly via neural mechanisms or directly on the muscle, suggest that scleroderma is a primary neurogenic disorder. Methacholine, which acts directly on smooth muscle receptors, causes a similar increase in LES pressure in normal controls and in patients with scleroderma. Edrophonium, a cholinesterase inhibitor that enhances the effect of acetylcholine when given to

patients with scleroderma, causes an increase in LES pressure that is less marked in these patients than in normal controls, suggesting a neurogenic rather than a myogenic etiology. Muscle ischemia due to perivascular compression has been suggested as a possible mechanism for the motility abnormality in scleroderma. Others have observed that in the early stage of the disease, the manometric abnormalities may be reversed by reserpine, an agent that depletes catecholamines from the adrenergic system. This suggests that, in early scleroderma, an adrenergic overactivity may be present that causes a parasympathetic inhibition, supporting a neurogenic mechanism for the disease. In advanced disease manifested by smooth muscle atrophy and collagen deposition, reserpine no longer produces this reversal. Consequently, from a clinical perspective, the patient can be described as having a poor esophageal pump and a poor valve.

The diagnosis of scleroderma can be made manometrically by the observation of normal peristalsis in the proximal striated esophagus, with absent peristalsis in the distal smooth muscle portion (Fig. 25-46). The LES pressure is progressively weakened as the disease advances. Because many of the systemic sequelae of the disease may be nondiagnostic, the motility pattern is frequently used as a specific diagnostic indicator. Gastroesophageal reflux commonly occurs in patients with scleroderma, because they have both hypotensive sphincters and poor esophageal clearance. This combined defect can lead to severe esophagitis and stricture formation. The typical barium swallow shows a dilated, barium-filled esophagus, stomach, and duodenum, or a hiatal hernia with distal esophageal stricture and proximal dilatation (Fig. 25-47).

Traditionally, esophageal symptoms have been treated with PPIs, antacids, elevation of the head of the bed, and multiple dilations for strictures, with generally unsatisfactory results. The degree of esophagitis is usually severe and may lead to marked esophageal shortening as well as stricture. Scleroderma patients have frequently had numerous dilations before they are referred to the surgeon. The surgical management is somewhat controversial,

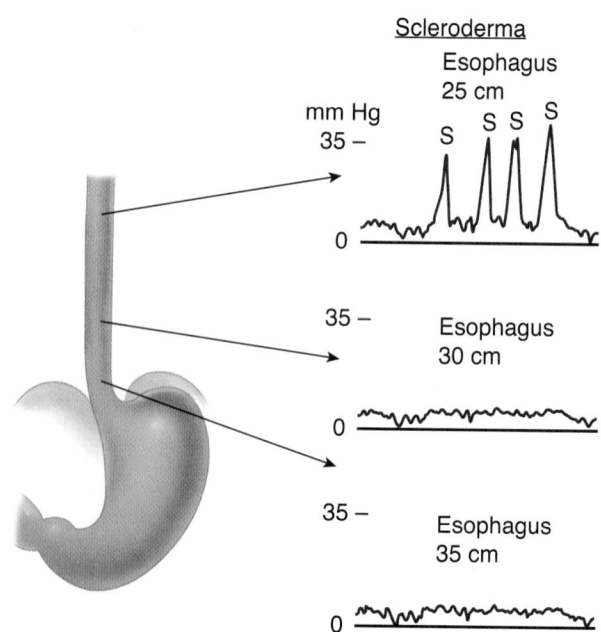

FIG. 25-46. Esophageal motility record in a patient with scleroderma showing aperistalsis in the distal two thirds of the esophageal body with peristalsis in the proximal portion. *(Reproduced with permission from Waters PF, DeMeester TR: Foregut motor disorders and their surgical management. Med Clin North Am 65:1252, 1981. Copyright Elsevier.)*

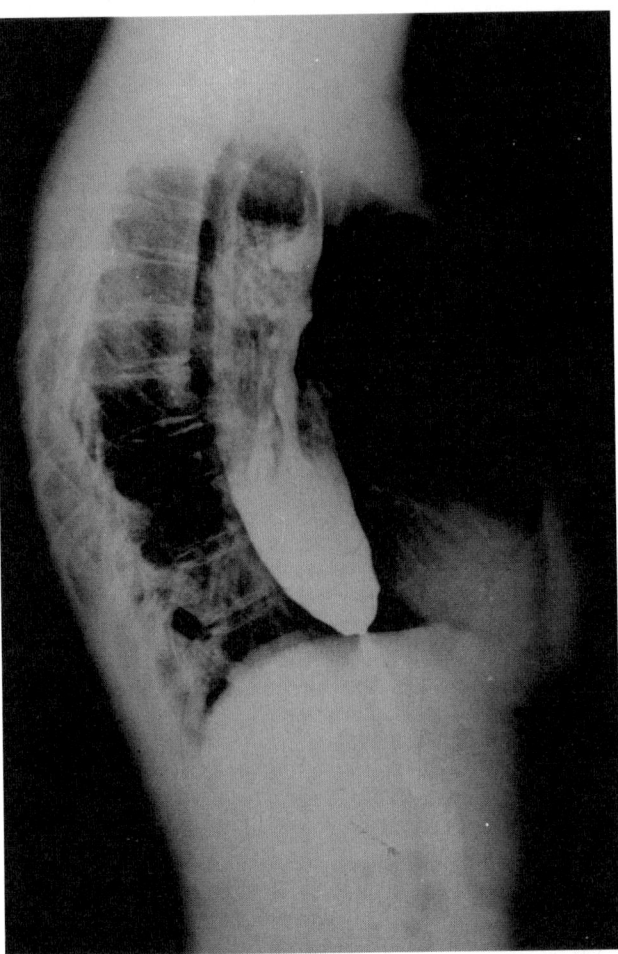

FIG. 25-47. Barium esophagogram of a patient with scleroderma and stricture. Note the markedly dilated esophagus and retained food material. *(Reproduced with permission from Waters PF, DeMeester TR: Foregut motor disorders and their surgical management.* Med Clin North Am *65:1253, 1981. Copyright Elsevier.)*

but the majority of opinion suggests that a partial fundoplication (anterior or posterior) performed laparoscopically is the procedure of choice. The need for a partial fundoplication is dictated by the likelihood of severe dysphagia if a total fundoplication is performed in the presence of aperistalsis. Esophageal shortening may require a Collis gastroplasty in combination with a partial fundoplication. Surgery reduces esophageal acid exposure, but does not return it to normal because of the poor clearance function of the body of the esophagus. Only 50% of the patients have a good-to-excellent result. If the esophagitis is severe, or there has been a previous failed antireflux procedure and the disease is associated with delayed gastric emptying, a gastric resection with Roux-en-Y gastrojejunostomy has proved the best option.

MOTILITY DISORDERS OF THE PHARYNX AND ESOPHAGUS

Clinical Manifestations

Dysphagia (i.e., difficulty in swallowing) is the primary symptom of esophageal motor disorders. Its perception by the patient is a balance between the severity of the underlying abnormality causing the dysphagia, and the adjustment made by the patient in altering eating habits. Consequently, any complaint of dysphagia must include an assessment of the patient's dietary history. It

must be known whether the patient experiences pain, chokes, or vomits with eating; whether the patient requires liquids with the meal, is the last to finish, or is forced to interrupt or avoid a social meal; and whether he or she has been admitted to the hospital for food impaction. These assessments, plus an evaluation of the patient's nutritional status, help to determine how severe the dysphagia is and judge the need for surgical intervention, rather than more conservative (and usually less effective) methods of treating dysphagia.

Motility Disorders of the Pharyngoesophageal Segment

Disorders of the pharyngoesophageal phase of swallowing result from a discoordination of the neuromuscular events involved in chewing, initiation of swallowing, and propulsion of the material from the oropharynx into the cervical esophagus. They can be categorized into one or a combination of the following abnormalities: (a) inadequate oropharyngeal bolus transport; (b) inability to pressurize the pharynx; (c) inability to elevate the larynx; (d) discoordination of pharyngeal contraction and cricopharyngeal relaxation; and (e) decreased compliance of the pharyngoesophageal segment secondary to neuromuscular disease. The latter may result in incomplete anatomic relaxation of the cricopharyngeus and cervical esophagus.

Pharyngoesophageal swallowing disorders are usually congenital or due to acquired disease involving the central and peripheral nervous system. This includes cerebrovascular accidents, brain stem tumors, poliomyelitis, multiple sclerosis, Parkinson's disease, pseudobulbar palsy, peripheral neuropathy, and operative damage to the cranial nerves involved in swallowing. Pure muscular diseases such as radiation-induced myopathy, dermatomyositis, myotonic dystrophy, and myasthenia gravis are less common causes. Rarely, extrinsic compression by thyromegaly, cervical lymphadenopathy, or hyperostosis of the cervical spine can cause pharyngoesophageal dysphagia.

Diagnostic Assessment of the Cricopharyngeal Segment

Abnormalities of pharyngoesophageal swallowing are difficult to assess with standard manometric techniques because of the rapidity of the oropharyngeal phase of swallowing, the elevation of the larynx, and the asymmetry of the cricopharyngeus. Video- or cineradiography is currently the most objective test to evaluate oropharyngeal bolus transport, pharyngeal compression, relaxation of the pharyngoesophageal segment, and the dynamics of airway protection during swallowing. It readily identifies a diverticulum (Fig. 25-48), stasis of the contrast medium in the valleculae, a cricopharyngeal bar, and/or narrowing of the pharyngoesophageal segment. These are anatomic manifestations of neuromuscular disease, and result from the loss of muscle compliance in portions of the pharynx and esophagus composed of skeletal muscle.

Careful analysis of video- or cineradiographic studies combined with manometry using specially designed catheters can identify the cause of a pharyngoesophageal dysfunction in most situations (Fig. 25-49). Motility studies may demonstrate inadequate pharyngeal pressurization, insufficient or lack of cricopharyngeal relaxation, marked discoordination of pharyngeal pressurization, cricopharyngeal relaxation and cervical esophageal contraction, or a hypopharyngeal bolus pressure suggesting decreased compliance of the skeletal portion of the cervical esophagus.

In many patients with cricopharyngeal dysfunction, including those with Zenker's diverticulum, it has been difficult to consistently demonstrate a motility abnormality or discoordination of pharyngoesophageal events. The abnormality most apt to be present is a loss of compliance in the pharyngoesophageal segment manifested by an increased bolus pressure. Cook and colleagues have demonstrated an increased resistance to the movement of a bolus through what appears on manometry to be a completely relaxed cricopharyngeal sphincter. Using simultaneous manome-

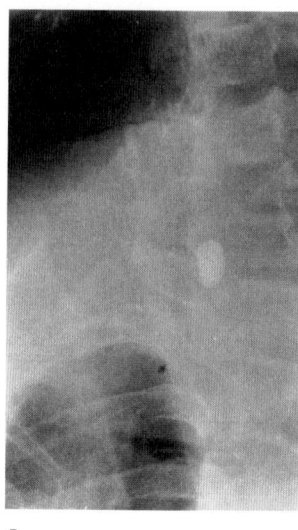 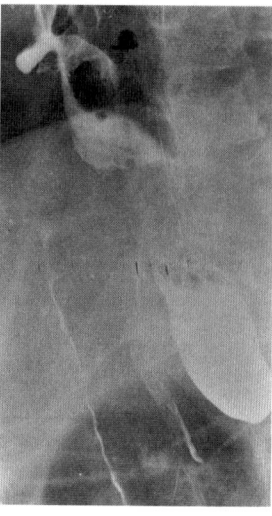

A   **B**

FIG. 25-48. A. Zenker's diverticulum, initially discovered 15 years ago and left untreated. **B.** Note its marked enlargement and evidence of laryngeal inlet aspiration on recent esophagogram. *(Reproduced with permission from Waters PF, DeMeester TR: Foregut motor disorders and their surgical management. Med Clin North Am 65:1257, 1981. Copyright Elsevier.)*

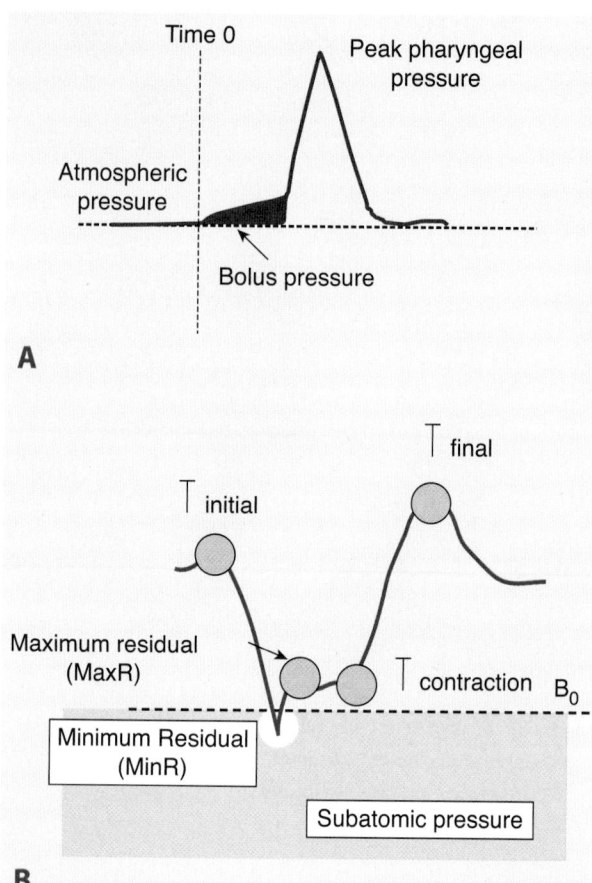

FIG. 25-49. A. Schematic drawing of a pharyngeal pressure wave indicating the presence of the bolus pressure. **B.** Schematic drawing of the manometric recording typically seen during cricopharyngeal sphincter relaxation.

try and videofluoroscopy, they showed that, in these patients, the cricopharyngeus is only partially relaxed; that is, the sphincter is relaxed enough to allow a drop of its pressure to esophageal baseline on manometry, but insufficiently relaxed to allow unimpaired passage of the bolus into the esophagus. This incomplete relaxation is due to a loss of compliance of the muscle in the pharyngoesophageal segment, and may be associated with a cricopharyngeal bar or Zenker's diverticulum. This decreased compliance of the cricopharyngeal sphincter can be recognized on esophageal manometry by a "shoulder" on the pharyngeal pressure wave, the amplitude of which correlates directly with the degree of outflow obstruction (Fig. 25-50). Increasing the diameter of this noncompliant segment reduces the resistance imposed on the passage of a bolus. Consequently, patients with low pharyngeal pressure (i.e., poor piston function of the pharynx), or patients with increased resistance of the pharyngocervical esophageal segment from loss of skeletal muscle compliance, are improved by a pharyngocricocervical esophageal myotomy. This enlarges the pharyngoesophageal segment and reduces outflow resistance. Esophageal muscle biopsy specimens from patients with Zenker's diverticulum have shown histologic evidence of the restrictive myopathy in the pharyngoesophageal segment. These findings correlate well with the observation of a decreased compliance of the upper esophagus demonstrated by videoradiography and the findings on detailed manometric studies of the pharynx and cervical esophagus. They suggest that the diverticulum develops as a consequence of the outflow resistance to bolus transport through the noncompliant muscle of the pharyngoesophageal segment.

The requirements for a successful pharyngoesophageal myotomy are (a) adequate oropharyngeal bolus transport; (b) the presence of an intact swallowing reflex; (c) reasonable coordination of pharyngeal pressurization with cricopharyngeal relaxation; and (d) a cricopharyngeal bar, Zenker's diverticulum, or a narrowed pharyngoesophageal segment on videoesophagogram and/or the presence of excessive pharyngoesophageal shoulder pressure on motility study.

Zenker's Diverticulum

In the past, the most common recognized sign of pharyngoesophageal dysfunction was the presence of a Zenker's diverticulum, originally described by Ludlow in 1769. The eponym resulted from Zenker's classic clinicopathologic descriptions of 34 cases published in 1878. Pharyngoesophageal diverticula have been reported to occur in 1 of 1000 routine barium examinations, and classically occur in elderly, white males. Zenker's diverticula tend to enlarge progressively with time due to the decreased compliance of the skeletal portion of the cervical esophagus that occurs with aging.

Presenting symptoms include dysphagia associated with the spontaneous regurgitation of undigested, bland material, often interrupting eating or drinking. On occasion, the dysphagia can be severe enough to cause debilitation and significant weight loss. Chronic aspiration and repetitive respiratory infection are common associated complaints. Once suspected, the diagnosis is established by a barium swallow. Endoscopy is usually difficult in the presence of a cricopharyngeal diverticulum, and potentially dangerous, owing to obstruction of the true esophageal lumen by the diverticulum and the attendant risk of diverticular perforation.

Cricopharyngeal Myotomy

The low morbidity and mortality associated with cricopharyngeal and upper esophageal myotomy have encouraged a liberal approach toward its use for almost any problem in the oropharyngeal phase of swallowing. This attitude has resulted in an overall success rate in the relief of symptoms of only 64%. When patients are selected for surgery using radiographic or motility markers of disease, a much higher proportion will benefit. Two methods of cricopharyngoesophageal myotomy are in common use, one using traditional

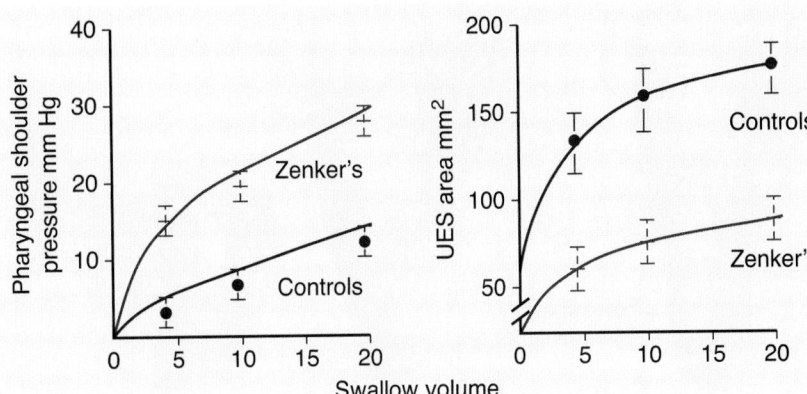

FIG. 25-50. Pharyngeal shoulder pressures and diameter of the pharyngoesophageal segment in controls and patients with Zenker's diverticulum. UES = upper esophageal sphincter. *(Data from Cook IJ, et al: Zenker's diverticulum: Evidence for a restrictive cricopharyngeal myopathy.* Gastroenterology 96:A98, 1989.)

surgical approaches, and one using rigid laryngoscopy and a linear cutting stapler.

Open Cricopharyngeal Myotomy, Diverticulopexy, and Diverticulectomy

The myotomy can be performed under local or general anesthesia through an incision along the anterior border of the left sternocleidomastoid muscle. The pharynx and cervical esophagus are exposed by retracting the sternocleidomastoid muscle and carotid sheath laterally, and the thyroid, trachea, and larynx medially (Fig. 25-51). When a pharyngoesophageal diverticulum is present, localization of the pharyngoesophageal segment is easy. The diverticulum is carefully freed from the overlying areolar tissue to expose its neck, just below the inferior pharyngeal constrictor and above the cricopharyngeus muscle. It can be difficult to identify the cricopharyngeus muscle in the absence of a diverticulum. A benefit of local anesthesia is that the patient can swallow and demonstrate an area of persistent narrowing at the pharyngoesophageal junction. Furthermore, before closing the incision, gelatin can be fed to the patient to ascertain whether the symptoms have been relieved, and to inspect the opening of the previously narrowed pharyngoesophageal segment. Under general anesthesia, and in the absence of a diverticulum, the placement of a nasogastric tube to the level of the manometrically determined cricopharyngeal sphincter helps in localization of the structures. The myotomy is extended cephalad by dividing 1 to 2 cm of inferior constrictor muscle of the pharynx, and caudad by dividing the cricopharyngeal muscle and the cervical esophagus for a length of 4 to 5 cm. The cervical wound is closed only when all oozing of blood has ceased, because a hematoma after this procedure is common, and is often associated with temporary dysphagia while the hematoma absorbs. Oral alimentation is started the day after surgery. The patient is usually discharged on the first or second postoperative day.

If a diverticulum is present and is large enough to persist after a myotomy, it may be sutured in the inverted position to the prevertebral fascia using a permanent suture (i.e., diverticulopexy) (Fig. 25-52). If the diverticulum is excessively large so that it would be redundant if suspended, or if its walls are thickened, a diverticulectomy should be performed. This is best performed under general anesthesia by placing a Maloney dilator (48F) in the esophagus, after controlling the neck of the diverticulum and after myotomy. A linear stapler is placed across the neck of the diverticulum and the diverticulum is excised distal to the staple line. The security of this staple line and effectiveness of the myotomy may be tested before hospital discharge with a water soluble contrast esophagogram. Postoperative complications include fistula formation, abscess, hematoma, recurrent nerve paralysis, difficulties in phonation, and Horner's syndrome. The incidence of the first two can be reduced by performing a diverticulopexy rather than diverticulectomy.

Endoscopic Cricopharyngotomy

Endoscopic stapled cricopharyngotomy and diverticulotomy recently has been described. This procedure is most effective for larger diverticula (>2 cm), and may be impossible to perform for

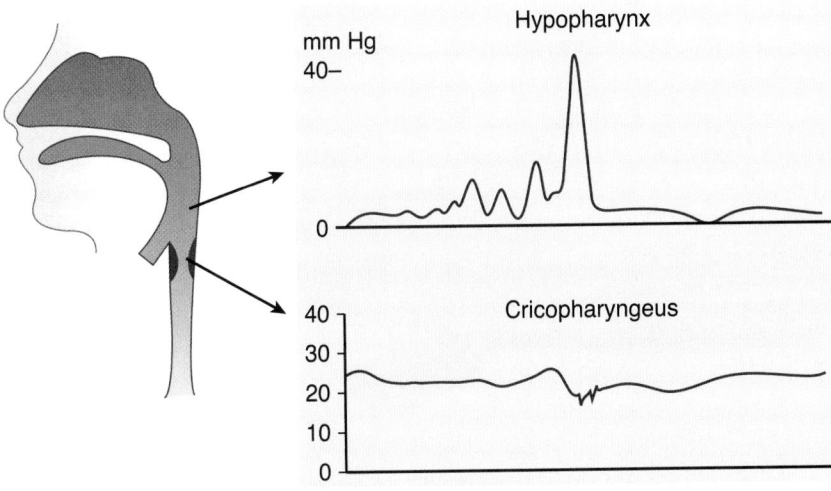

FIG. 25-51. Cross-section of the neck at the level of the thyroid isthmus that shows the surgical approach to the hypopharynx and cervical esophagus. *(Reproduced with permission from Waters PF, DeMeester TR: Foregut motor disorders and their surgical management.* Med Clin North Am 65:1257, 1981. Copyright Elsevier.)

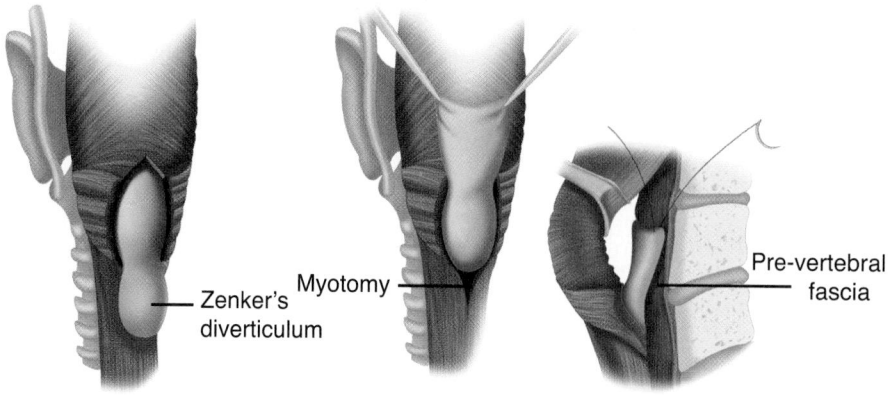

Zenker's diverticulum

Myotomy

Pre-vertebral fascia

FIG. 25-52. Posterior of the anatomy of the pharynx and cervical esophagus showing pharyngoesophageal myotomy and pexing of the diverticulum to the prevertebral fascia.

the small diverticulum. The procedure uses a specialized "diverticuloscope" with two retractable valves passed into the hypopharynx. The lips of the diverticuloscope are positioned so that one lip lies in the esophageal lumen and the other in the diverticular lumen. The valves of the diverticuloscope are retracted appropriately so as to visualize the septum interposed between the diverticulum and the esophagus. An endoscopic linear stapler is introduced into the diverticuloscope and positioned against the common septum with the anvil in the diverticulum and the cartridge in the esophageal lumen. Firing of the stapler divides the common septum between the posterior esophageal and the diverticular wall over a length of 30 mm, placing three rows of staples on each side. More than one stapler application may be needed, depending on the size of the diverticulum (Fig. 25-53). The patient is allowed to resume liquid feeds immediately, and is usually discharged the day after surgery. Complications are rare and may include perforation at the apex of the diverticulum, and failure to relieve dysphagia resulting from incomplete myotomy. The former complication can usually be treated with antibiotics, but may rarely require neck drainage.

Recurrence of a Zenker's diverticulum occurs late, and is more common after diverticulectomy without myotomy, presumably due to persistence of the underlying loss of compliance of the cervical esophagus when a myotomy is not performed. After endoscopic cricopharyngotomy lateral residual "pouches" may be seen on radiographs, but are rarely responsible for residual or recurrent symptoms if the myotomy has been complete.

Postoperative motility studies have shown that the peak pharyngeal pressure generated on swallowing is not affected, the resting cricopharyngeal pressure is reduced but not eliminated, and the cricopharyngeal sphincter length is shortened. Consequently, after myotomy, there is protection against esophagopharyngeal regurgitation.

Motility Disorders of the Esophageal Body and Lower Esophageal Sphincter

Disorders of the esophageal phase of swallowing result from abnormalities in the propulsive pump action of the esophageal body or the relaxation of the LES. These disorders result from either primary esophageal abnormalities, or from generalized neural, muscular, or collagen vascular disease (Table 25-9). The use of standard and high-resolution esophageal manometry techniques has allowed specific primary esophageal motility disorders to be identified out of a pool of nonspecific motility abnormalities. Primary esophageal motor disorders include achalasia, DES, nutcracker esophagus, and the hypertensive LES. The manometric characteristics of these disorders are shown in Table 25-10.

The boundaries between the primary esophageal motor disorders are vague, and intermediate types exist, some of which may combine more than one type of motility pattern. These findings indicate that esophageal motility disorders should be looked at as a spectrum of abnormalities that reflects various stages of destruction of esophageal motor function.

Achalasia

The best known and best understood primary motility disorder of the esophagus is achalasia, with an incidence of six per 100,000 population per year. Although complete absence of peristalsis in the esophageal body has been proposed as the major abnormality, present evidence indicates achalasia is a primary disorder of the LES. This is based on 24-hour outpatient esophageal motility monitoring, which shows that, even in advanced disease, up to 5%

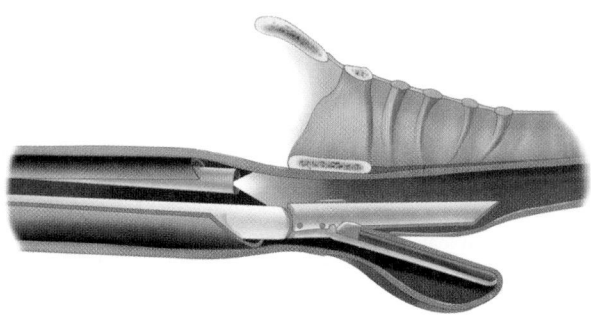

FIG. 25-53. The technique for transoral cricopharyngotomy and Zenker's diverticulotomy.

TABLE 25-9	Esophageal motility disorders

Primary esophageal motility disorders

Achalasia, "vigorous" achalasia
Diffuse and segmental esophageal spasm
Nutcracker esophagus
Hypertensive lower esophageal sphincter
Nonspecific esophageal motility disorders

Secondary esophageal motility disorders

Collagen vascular diseases: progressive systemic sclerosis, polymyositis and dermatomyositis, mixed connective tissue disease, systemic lupus erythematosus, et al
Chronic idiopathic intestinal pseudo-obstruction
Neuromuscular diseases
Endocrine and metastatic disorders

TABLE 25-10	Manometric characteristics of the primary esophageal motility disorders

Achalasia

Incomplete lower esophageal sphincter (LES) relaxation (<75% relaxation)

Aperistalsis in the esophageal body

Elevated LES pressure ≤26 mmHg

Increased intraesophageal baseline pressures relative to gastric baseline

Diffuse esophageal spasm (DES)

Simultaneous (nonperistaltic contractions) (>20% of wet swallows)

Repetitive and multipeaked contractions

Spontaneous contractions

Intermittent normal peristalsis

Contractions may be of increased amplitude and duration

Nutcracker esophagus

Mean peristaltic amplitude (10 wet swallows) in distal esophagus ≥180 mmHg

Increased mean duration of contractions (>7.0 s)

Normal peristaltic sequence

Hypertensive lower esophageal sphincter

Elevated LES pressure (≥26 mmHg)

Normal LES relaxation

Normal peristalsis in the esophageal body

Ineffective esophageal motility disorders

Decreased or absent amplitude of esophageal peristalsis (<30 mmHg)

Increased number of nontransmitted contractions

Source: Reproduced with permission from DeMeester TR, et al: Physiologic diagnostic studies, in Zuidema GD, Orringer MB (eds): *Shackelford's Surgery of the Alimentary Tract*, 3rd ed, Vol. I. Philadelphia: W.B. Saunders, 1991, p 115. Copyright Elsevier.

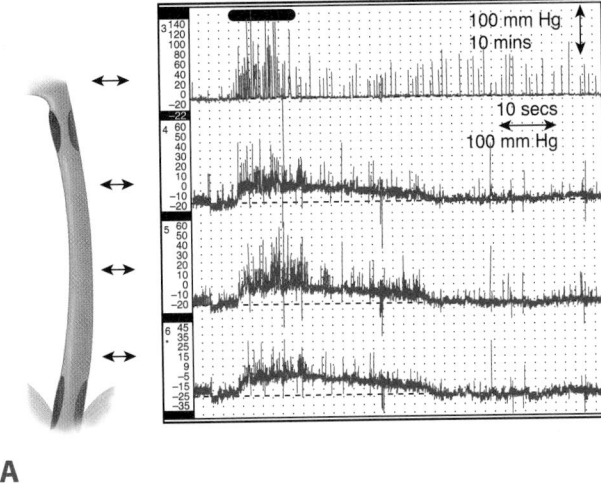

A

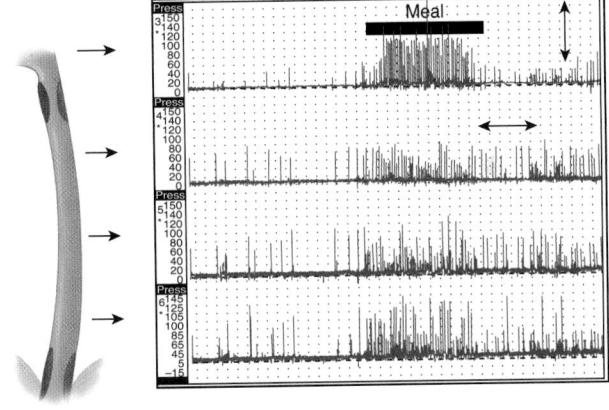

B

FIG. 25-54. Pressurization of esophagus: Ambulatory motility tracing of a patient with achalasia. **A.** Before esophageal myotomy. **B.** After esophageal myotomy. The tracings have been compressed to exaggerate the motility spikes and baseline elevations. Note the rise in esophageal baseline pressure during a meal represented by the rise off the baseline to the left of panel **A**. No such rise occurs postmyotomy (panel **B**).

of contractions can be peristaltic. Simultaneous esophageal waves develop as a result of the increased resistance to esophageal emptying caused by the nonrelaxing LES. This conclusion is supported by experimental studies in which a band placed loosely around the GEJ in experimental models did not change sphincter pressures, but resulted in impaired relaxation of the LES and outflow resistance. This led to a markedly increased frequency of simultaneous waveforms and a decrease in contraction amplitude. The changes were associated with radiographic dilation of the esophagus and were reversible after removal of the band. Observations in patients with pseudoachalasia due to tumor infiltration, a tight stricture in the distal esophagus, or an antireflux procedure that is too tight also provide evidence that dysfunction of the esophageal body can be caused by the increased outflow obstruction of a nonrelaxing LES. The observation that esophageal peristalsis can return in patients with classic achalasia following dilation or myotomy provides further support that achalasia is a primary disease of the LES.

The pathogenesis of achalasia is presumed to be a neurogenic degeneration, which is either idiopathic or due to infection. In experimental animals, the disease has been reproduced by destruction of the nucleus ambiguus and the dorsal motor nucleus of the vagus nerve. In patients with the disease, degenerative changes have been shown in the vagus nerve and in the ganglia in the myenteric plexus of the esophagus itself. This degeneration results in hypertension of the LES, a failure of the sphincter to relax on swallowing, elevation of intraluminal esophageal pressure, esophageal dilatation, and a subsequent loss of progressive peristalsis in the body of the esophagus. The esophageal dilatation results from the combination of a nonrelaxing sphincter, which causes a functional retention of ingested material in the esophagus, and elevation of intraluminal pressure from repetitive pharyngeal air swallowing (Fig. 25-54). With time, the functional disorder results in anatomic alterations seen on radiographic studies, such as a dilated esophagus with a tapering, "bird's beak"–like narrowing of the distal end (Fig. 25-55). There is usually an air-fluid level in the

esophagus from the retained food and saliva, the height of which reflects the degree of resistance imposed by the nonrelaxing sphincter. As the disease progresses, the esophagus becomes massively dilated and tortuous.

A subgroup of patients with otherwise typical features of classic achalasia has simultaneous contractions of their esophageal body that can be of high amplitude. This manometric pattern has been termed *vigorous achalasia*, and chest pain episodes are a common finding in these patients. Differentiation of vigorous achalasia from DES can be difficult. In both diseases, videoradiographic examination may show a corkscrew deformity of the esophagus and diverticulum formation.

Diffuse and Segmental Esophageal Spasm

DES is characterized by substernal chest pain and/or dysphagia. DES differs from classic achalasia in that it is primarily a disease of the esophageal body, produces a lesser degree of dysphagia, causes more chest pain, and has less effect on the patient's general condition. Nonetheless, it is impossible to differentiate achalasia from DES on the basis of symptoms alone. Esophagogram and esophageal manometry are required to distinguish these two entities. True symptomatic DES is a rare condition, occurring about five times less frequently than achalasia.

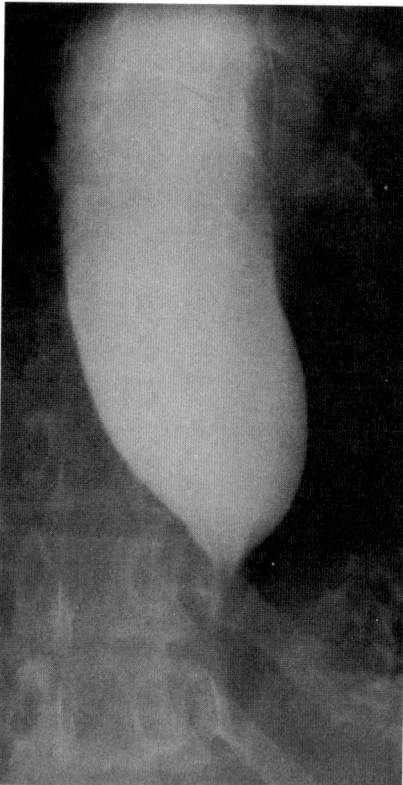

FIG. 25-55. Barium esophagogram showing a markedly dilated esophagus and characteristic "bird's beak" in achalasia. *(Reproduced with permission from Waters PF, DeMeester TR: Foregut motor disorders and their surgical management. Med Clin North Am 65:1244, 1981. Copyright Elsevier.)*

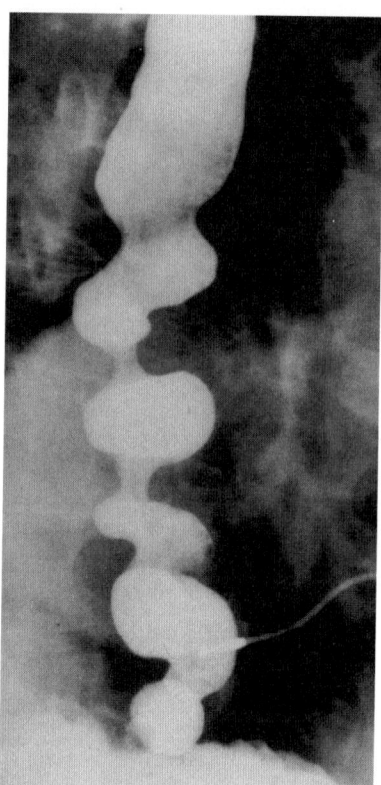

FIG. 25-56. Barium esophagogram of patient with diffuse spasm showing the corkscrew deformity.

The causation and neuromuscular pathophysiology of DES are unclear. The basic motor abnormality is rapid wave progression down the esophagus secondary to an abnormality in the latency gradient. Hypertrophy of the muscular layer of the esophageal wall and degeneration of the esophageal branches of the vagus nerve have been observed in this disease, although these are not constant findings. Manometric abnormalities in DES may be present over the total length of the esophageal body, but usually are confined to the distal two thirds. In *segmental esophageal spasm*, the manometric abnormalities are confined to a short segment of the esophagus.

The classic manometric findings in these patients are characterized by the frequent occurrence of simultaneous waveforms and multipeaked esophageal contractions, which may be of abnormally high amplitude or long duration. Key to the diagnosis of DES is that there remain some peristaltic waveforms in excess of those seen in achalasia. A criterion of 30% or more peristaltic waveforms out of 10 wet swallows has been used to differentiate DES from vigorous achalasia. However, this figure is arbitrary and often debated.

The LES in patients with DES usually shows a normal resting pressure and relaxation on swallowing. A hypertensive sphincter with poor relaxation may also be present. In patients with advanced disease, the radiographic appearance of tertiary contractions appears helical, and has been termed *corkscrew esophagus* or *pseudodiverticulosis* (Fig. 25-56). Patients with segmental or diffuse esophageal spasm can compartmentalize the esophagus and develop an epiphrenic or midesophageal diverticulum between two areas of high pressure occurring simultaneously (Fig. 25-57).

Nutcracker Esophagus

The disorder, termed *nutcracker* or *supersqueezer esophagus*, was recognized in the late 1970s. Other terms used to describe this entity are *hypertensive peristalsis* or *high-amplitude peristaltic contractions*. It is the most common of the primary esophageal motility disorders. By definition the so-called *nutcracker esophagus* is a manometric abnormality in patients who are characterized by peristaltic esophageal contractions with peak amplitudes greater than two SDs above the normal values in individual laboratories. Contraction amplitudes in these patients can easily be above 400 mmHg. At the lower end of peak pressure, it is unclear whether nutcracker esophagus causes any symptoms. In fact, chest pain symptoms in nutcracker esophagus patients may be related to GERD rather than intraluminal hypertension. Treatment in these patients should be aimed at the treatment of GERD. At the high end (peak pressures >300 mmHg) chest pain may be the result of the nutcracker physiology, as treatment directed at reducing intraluminal pressure is more effective than when used for those with lower peak pressures.

Hypertensive Lower Esophageal Sphincter

Hypertensive LES in patients with chest pain or dysphagia was first described as a separate entity by Code and associates. This disorder is characterized by an elevated basal pressure of the LES with normal relaxation and normal propulsion in the esophageal body. About one half of these patients, however, have associated motility disorders of the esophageal body, particularly hypertensive peristalsis and simultaneous waveforms. In the remainder, the disorder exists as an isolated abnormality. Dysphagia in these patients may be caused by a lack of compliance of the sphincter, even in its relaxed state. Myotomy of the LES may be indicated in patients not responding to medical therapy or dilation.

Secondary Esophageal Motility Disorders

Connective tissue disease, particularly scleroderma and the CREST syndrome, exhibits severe esophageal motility disorders. Additionally, patients treated as infants for esophageal atresia will often develop secondary motility disorders manifest later in life. Symp-

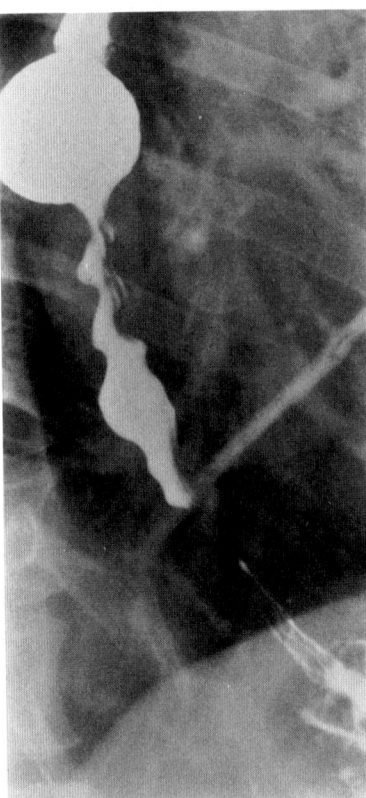

FIG. 25-57. Barium esophagogram showing a high epiphrenic diverticulum in a patient with diffuse esophageal spasm. *[Reproduced with permission from DeMeester TR, Stein HJ: Surgery for esophageal motor disorders, in Castell DO (ed): The Esophagus. Boston: Little, Brown, 1992, p 415.]*

toms of these disorders are heartburn and dysphagia. The latter may be a result of a peptic stricture rather than the esophageal dysmotility. An esophageal motility study will usually show severely reduced or absent peristalsis with severely reduced or absent LES pressure. The role of antireflux surgery in these conditions is controversial, but, if performed, should be limited to partial fundoplication, as full (Nissen) fundoplication may result in severe dysphagia.

Nonspecific Esophageal Motor Disorders and Ineffective Esophageal Motility

Many patients complaining of dysphagia or chest pain of noncardiac origin demonstrate a variety of wave patterns and contraction amplitudes on esophageal manometry that are clearly out of the normal range, but do not meet the criteria of a primary esophageal motility disorder. Esophageal motility in these patients frequently shows an increased number of multipeaked or repetitive contractions, contractions of prolonged duration, nontransmitted contractions, an interruption of a peristaltic wave at various levels of the esophagus, or contractions of low amplitude. These motility abnormalities have been termed *nonspecific esophageal motility disorders*. Their significance in the causation of chest pain or dysphagia is still unclear. Surgery plays no role in the treatment of these disorders unless there is an associated diverticulum.

A clear distinction between primary esophageal motility disorders and nonspecific esophageal motility disorders is often not possible. Patients diagnosed as having nonspecific esophageal motility abnormalities on repeated studies will occasionally show abnormalities consistent with nutcracker esophagus. Similarly, progression from a nonspecific esophageal motility disorder to classic DES has been demonstrated. Therefore, the finding of a nonspecific esophageal motility disorder may represent only a manometric marker of an intermittent, more severe esophageal motor abnormality. Combined ambulatory 24-hour esophageal pH and motility monitoring has shown that an increased esophageal exposure to gastric juice is common in patients diagnosed as having a nonspecific esophageal motility disorder. In some situations, the motor abnormalities may be induced by the irritation of refluxed gastric juice; in other situations, it may be a primary event unrelated to the presence of reflux. High-amplitude peristalsis (nutcracker esophagus) and low-amplitude peristalsis (ineffective esophageal motility) are frequently associated with GERD.

Diverticula of the Esophageal Body

Diverticula of the esophagus may be characterized by their location in the esophagus (proximal, mid-, or distal esophagus), or by the nature of concomitant pathology. Diverticula associated with motor disorders are termed *pulsion diverticula* and those associated with inflammatory conditions are termed *traction diverticula*. Pulsion diverticula occur most commonly with nonspecific motility disorders, but can occur with all of the primary motility disorders. In the latter situation, the motility disorder is usually diagnosed before the development of the diverticulum. When associated with achalasia, the development of a diverticulum may temporarily alleviate the symptom of dysphagia by becoming a receptacle for ingested food, and substitute the symptom of dysphagia for postprandial pain and regurgitation of undigested food. If a motility abnormality of the esophageal body or LES cannot be identified, a traction or congenital cause for the diverticulum should be considered.

Because development in radiology preceded development in motility monitoring, diverticula of the esophagus were considered historically to be a primary abnormality, the cause, rather than the consequence, of motility disorders. Consequently, earlier texts focused on them as specific entities based upon their location.

Epiphrenic diverticula arise from the terminal third of the thoracic esophagus and are usually found adjacent to the diaphragm. They have been associated with distal esophageal muscular hypertrophy, esophageal motility abnormalities, and increased luminal pressure. They are "pulsion" diverticula, and are associated with diffuse spasm, achalasia, or nonspecific motor abnormalities in the body of the esophagus.

Whether the diverticulum should be surgically resected or suspended depends on its size and proximity to the vertebral body. When diverticula are associated with esophageal motility disorders, esophageal myotomy from the distal extent of the diverticulum to the stomach should be combined with diverticulectomy. If diverticulectomy alone is performed, one can expect a high incidence of suture line rupture due to the same intraluminal pressure that initially gave rise to the diverticulum. If the diverticulum is suspended to the prevertebral fascia of the thoracic vertebra, a myotomy is begun at the neck of the diverticulum and extended across the LES. If the diverticulum is excised by dividing the neck, the muscle is closed over the excision site and a myotomy is performed on the opposite esophageal wall, starting at the level of diverticulum. If complete, the myotomy will cross the LES, reducing distal esophageal peak pressure, and will increase the likelihood that dysphagia will be replaced with GERD symptoms. Increasingly, partial fundoplication (anterior or posterior) is performed after LES myotomy to decrease the frequency of disabling GERD developing after myotomy and diverticulectomy. When a large diverticulum is associated with a hiatal hernia, then hiatal hernia repair is added. All these procedures may be performed with traditional or minimally invasive techniques.

Midesophageal or traction diverticula were first described in the nineteenth century (Fig. 25-58). At that time, they were frequently noted in patients who had mediastinal LN involvement with tuberculosis. It was theorized that adhesions formed between the inflamed mediastinal nodes and the esophagus. By contraction, the adhesions exerted traction on the esophageal wall and led to a

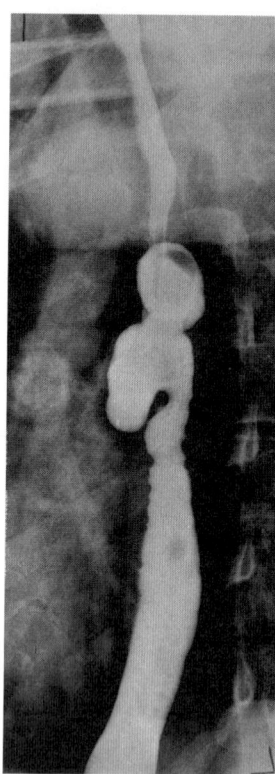

FIG. 25-58. Barium esophagogram showing a midesophageal diverticulum. Despite the anatomic distortion, the patient was asymptomatic. *(Reproduced with permission from Waters PF, DeMeester TR: Foregut motor disorders and their surgical management. Med Clin North Am 65:1255, 1981. Copyright Elsevier.)*

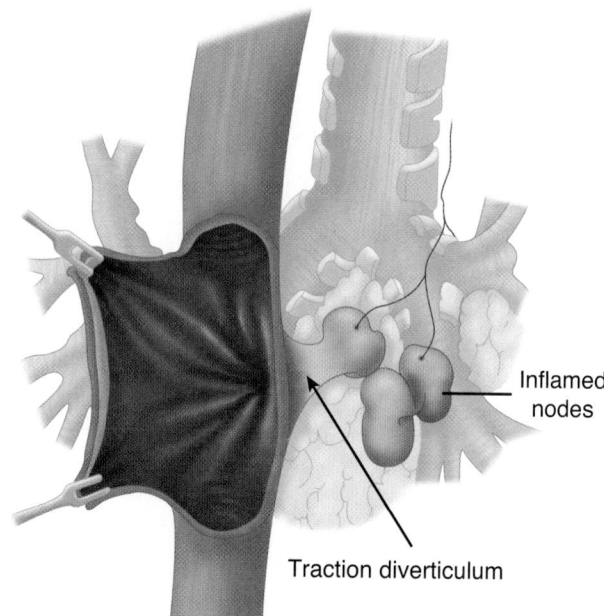

Inflamed nodes

Traction diverticulum

FIG. 25-59. Illustration of the pathophysiology of midesophageal diverticulum showing traction on the esophageal wall from adhesions to inflamed subcarinal lymph nodes.

localized diverticulum (Fig. 25-59). This theory was based on the findings of early dissections, where adhesions between diverticula and LNs were commonly found. Other conditions associated with mediastinal lymphadenopathy, such as pulmonary fungal infections (e.g., aspergillosis), lymphoma, or sarcoid, may create traction esophageal diverticula after successful treatment. Rarely, when no underlying inflammatory pathology is identified, a motility disorder may be identified.

Most midesophageal diverticula are asymptomatic and incidentally discovered during investigation for nonesophageal complaints. In such patients, the radiologic abnormality may be ignored. Patients with symptoms of dysphagia, regurgitation, chest pain, or aspiration, in whom a diverticulum is discovered, should be thoroughly investigated for an esophageal motor abnormality. Occasionally, a patient will present with a bronchoesophageal fistula manifested by a chronic cough on ingestion of meals. The diverticulum in such patients is most likely to have an inflammatory etiology.

The indication for surgical intervention is dictated by the degree of symptomatic disability. Usually, midesophageal diverticula can be suspended due to their proximity to the spine. If a motor abnormality is documented, a myotomy should be performed as described for an epiphrenic diverticulum.

OPERATIONS FOR ESOPHAGEAL MOTOR DISORDERS AND DIVERTICULA

Long Esophageal Myotomy for Motor Disorders of the Esophageal Body

A long esophageal myotomy is indicated for dysphagia caused by any motor disorder characterized by segmental or generalized simultaneous waveforms in a patient whose symptoms are not relieved by medical therapy. Such disorders include diffuse and segmental esophageal spasm, vigorous achalasia, and nonspecific motility disorders associated with a mid- or epiphrenic esophageal diverticulum. However, the decision to operate must be made by a balanced evaluation of the patient's symptoms, diet, lifestyle adjustments, and nutritional status, with the most important factor being the possibility of improving the patient's swallowing disability. The symptom of chest pain alone is not an indication for a surgical procedure.

The identification of patients with symptoms of dysphagia and chest pain who might benefit from a surgical myotomy is difficult. Ambulatory motility studies have shown that when the prevalence of "effective contractions" (i.e., peristaltic waveforms consisting of contractions with an amplitude above 30 mmHg) drops below 50% during meals, the patient is likely to experience dysphagia (Fig. 25-60). This would suggest that relief from the symptom can be expected with an improvement of esophageal contraction amplitude or amelioration of nonperistaltic waveforms. Prokinetic agents may increase esophageal contraction amplitude, but do not alter the prevalence of simultaneous waveforms. Patients in whom the efficacy of esophageal propulsion is severely compromised because of a high prevalence of simultaneous waveforms usually receive little benefit from medical therapy. In these patients, a surgical myotomy of the esophageal body can improve the patients' dysphagia, provided the loss of contraction amplitude in the remaining peristaltic waveforms, caused by the myotomy, has less effect on swallowing function than the presence of the excessive simultaneous contractions. This situation is reached when the prevalence of effective waveforms during meals drops below 30%, (i.e., 70% of esophageal waveforms are ineffective).

In patients selected for surgery, preoperative manometry is essential to determine the proximal extent of the esophageal myotomy. Most surgeons extend the myotomy distally across the LES to reduce outflow resistance. Consequently, some form of antireflux protection is needed to avoid gastroesophageal reflux if there has been extensive dissection of the cardia. In this situation, most authors prefer a partial, rather than a full, fundoplication, in order not to add back-resistance that will further interfere with the ability of the myotomized esophagus to empty (Fig. 25-61). If the symptoms of

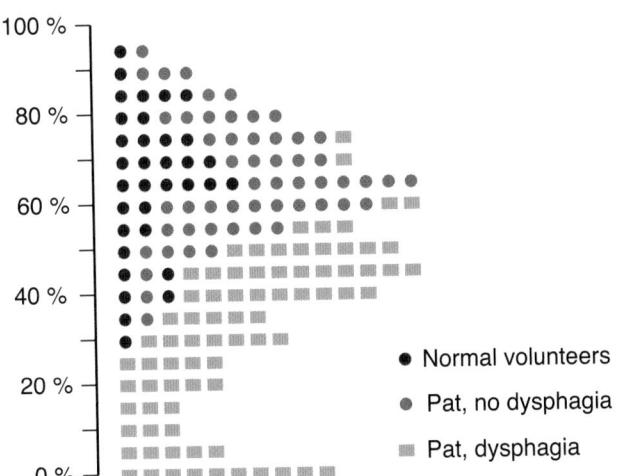

FIG. 25-60. Prevalence of effective contractions, (i.e., peristaltic contractions with an amplitude >30 mmHg) during meal periods in individual normal volunteers, patients (Pat) without dysphagia, and patients with nonobstructive dysphagia.

reflux are present preoperatively, 24-hour pH monitoring is required to confirm its presence.

The procedure may be performed either open or via thoracoscopy. The open technique is performed through a left thoracotomy in the sixth intercostal space (Fig. 25-62). An incision is made in the posterior mediastinal pleura over the esophagus, and the left lateral wall of the esophagus is exposed. The esophagus is not circumferentially dissected unless necessary. A 2-cm incision is made into the abdomen through the parietal peritoneum at the midportion of the left crus. A tongue of gastric fundus is pulled into the chest. This exposes the GEJ and its associated fat pad. The latter is excised to give a clear view of the junction. A myotomy is performed through all muscle layers, extending distally over the stomach 1 to 2 cm below the GEJ, and proximally on the esophagus over the distance of the manometric abnormality. The muscle layer is dissected from the mucosa laterally for a distance of 1 cm. Care is taken to divide all minute muscle ibands, particularly in the area

of the GEJ. The gastric fundic tongue s sutured to the margins of the myotomy over a distance of 3 to 4 cm and replaced into the abdomen. This maintains separation of the muscle and acts as a partial fundoplication to prevent reflux.

If an epiphrenic diverticulum is present, it is excised by dividing the neck with a stapler sized for the thickness of the diverticulum (2.0- to 4.8-mm staple leg length) followed by a closure of the muscle over the staple line, when possible. The myotomy is then performed on the opposite esophageal wall. If a midesophageal diverticulum is present, the myotomy is made so that it includes the muscle around the neck, and the diverticulum is suspended by attaching it to the paravertebral fascia of the thoracic vertebra above the level of the diverticular neck. Before performing any operation for an esophageal diverticulum, it is wise to endoscope the patient to wash all food and other debris from the diverticulum.

The results of myotomy for motor disorders of the esophageal body have improved in parallel with the improved preoperative diagnosis afforded by manometry. Previous published series report between 40 and 92% improvement of symptoms, but interpretation is difficult due to the small number of patients involved and the varying criteria for diagnosis of the primary motor abnormality. When myotomy is accurately done, 93% of the patients have effective palliation of dysphagia after a mean follow-up of 5 years, and 89% would have the procedure again, if it was necessary. Most patients gain or maintain rather than lose weight after the operation. Postoperative motility studies show that the myotomy reduces the amplitude of esophageal contractions to near zero and eliminates simultaneous peristaltic waves. If the benefit of obliterating the simultaneous waves exceeds the adverse effect on bolus propulsion caused by the loss of peristaltic waveforms, the patient's dysphagia is likely to be improved by the procedure. If not, the patient is likely to continue to complain of dysphagia and to have little improvement as a result of the operation.

The thoracoscopic technique is complicated by the fact that it requires complete retraction of the lung anteriorly to expose the esophagus. Proper positioning of the patient is critical to achieving this exposure. A prone position is ideal, allowing the left lung to fall forward away from the esophagus. Because of the possibility of open thoracotomy, however, it is best to place the patient in the right lateral decubitus position with the left thorax up, and then to roll the patient anteriorly 45° toward prone. A beanbag secured to the table is used to hold the patient. The table can be rotated a further 30 to 40° so that the patient ends up nearly prone. Should thoracotomy become necessary, the table can be rotated back to the horizontal position and a thoracotomy performed without difficulty. Prone positioning is the key element in providing exposure for long myotomy. Four thoracoscopic ports in the left chest are used. With suitable lung retraction, the myotomy is performed through all esophageal muscle layers, extending distally to the endoscopic GEJ, and proximally over the distance of the manometric abnormality.

Few reports exist concerning the minimally invasive technique for performing long esophageal myotomy. Cuschieri has reported a preliminary experience with a thoracoscopically performed long esophageal myotomy for the treatment of nutcracker esophagus. Three patients with symptoms of chest pain and high-amplitude esophageal contractions and peristaltic waveforms were operated on. No major morbidity was encountered. Nasogastric tubes were removed the first postoperative day and oral feeding was started on the second postoperative day. Two patients were discharged on postoperative day 4 and one patient on day 5. All had symptomatic relief on short-term follow-up.

Epiphrenic diverticula are more frequently addressed with laparoscopic access, in combination with a laparoscopic division of the LES (Heller myotomy) (Fig. 25-63). If the diverticulum can be completely mobilized through the hiatus, it may be safely excised from below. The neck of the diverticulum is transected with a GIA

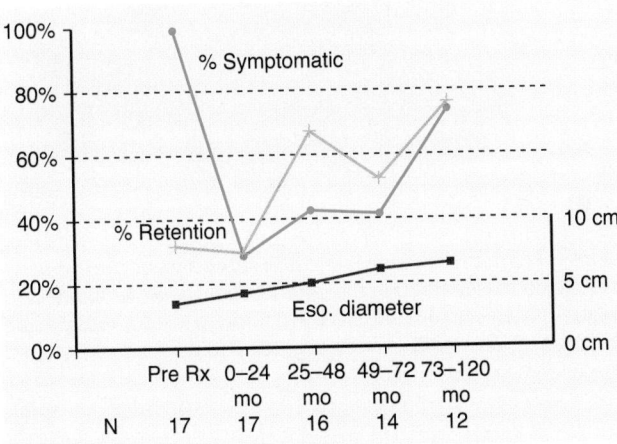

FIG. 25-61. Esophageal (Eso.) diameter, dysphagia, and esophageal retention in patients with achalasia treated with myotomy and Nissen fundoplication, 10 years after treatment (Rx). *(Based on Topart P, et al: Long-term effect of total fundoplication on the myotomized esophagus. Ann Thorac Surg 54:1046, 1992.)*

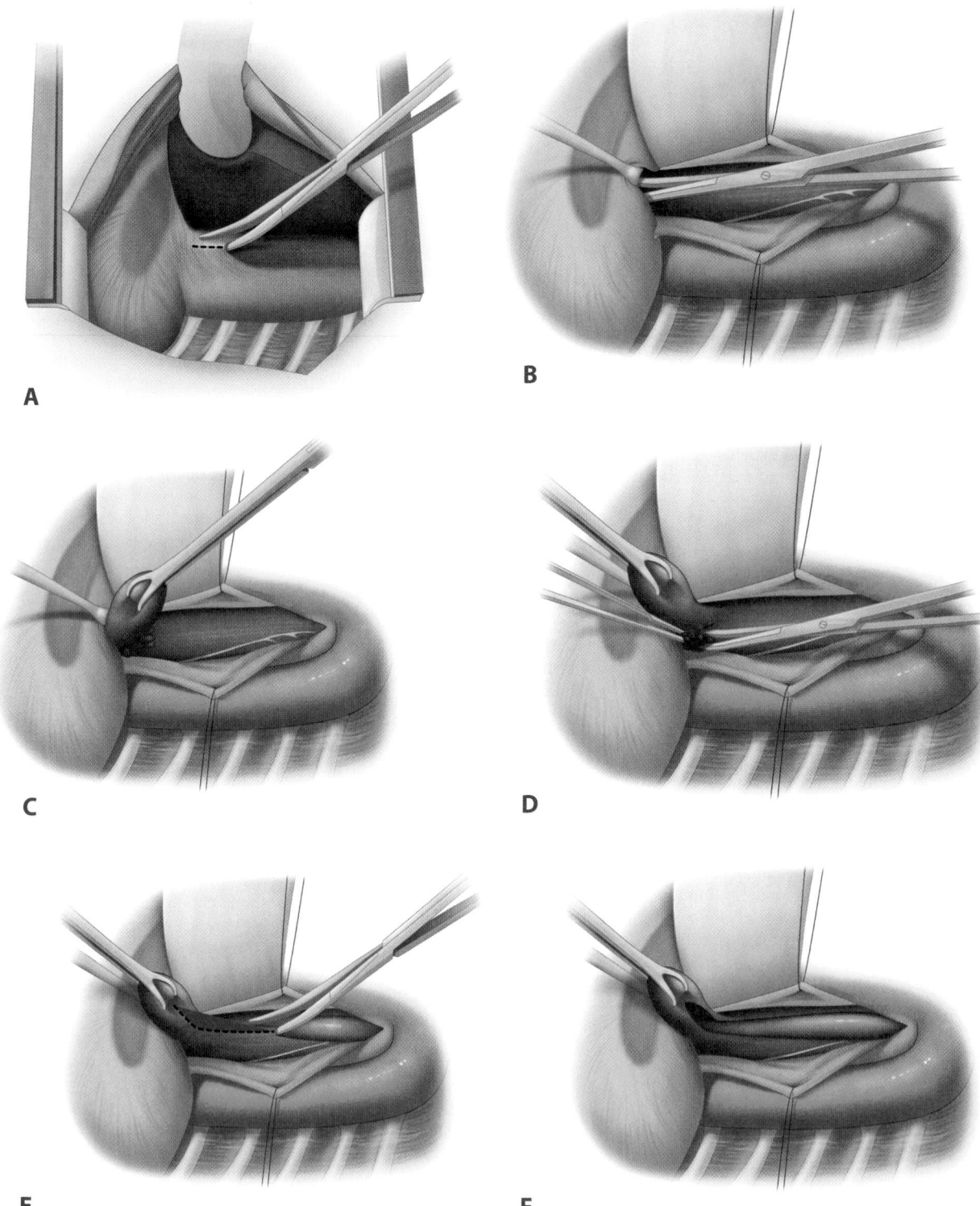

FIG. 25-62. Technique of long myotomy: **A.** Exposure of the lower esophagus through the left sixth intercostal space and incision of the mediastinal pleura in preparation for surgical myotomy. **B.** Location of a 2-cm incision made through the phrenoesophageal membrane into the abdomen along the midlateral border of the left crus. **C.** Retraction of tongue of gastric fundus into the chest through the previously made incision. **D.** Removal of the gastroesophageal fat pad to expose the gastroesophageal junction. **E.** A myotomy down to the mucosa is started on the esophageal body. **F.** Completed myotomy extending over the stomach for 1 cm. (*Continued*)

stapler after passage of a 48F dilator. Not infrequently, the diverticulum is sufficiently large that access to the neck of the diverticulum across the hiatus is quite difficult. Additionally, the inflammatory reaction to the diverticulum may further make the transhiatal dissection difficult. Under these circumstances, it is safer to perform the diverticulectomy through a right thoracoscopic approach either at the time of the initial procedure or at a later date, depending upon the frailty of the patient. Following diverticulectomy, it is

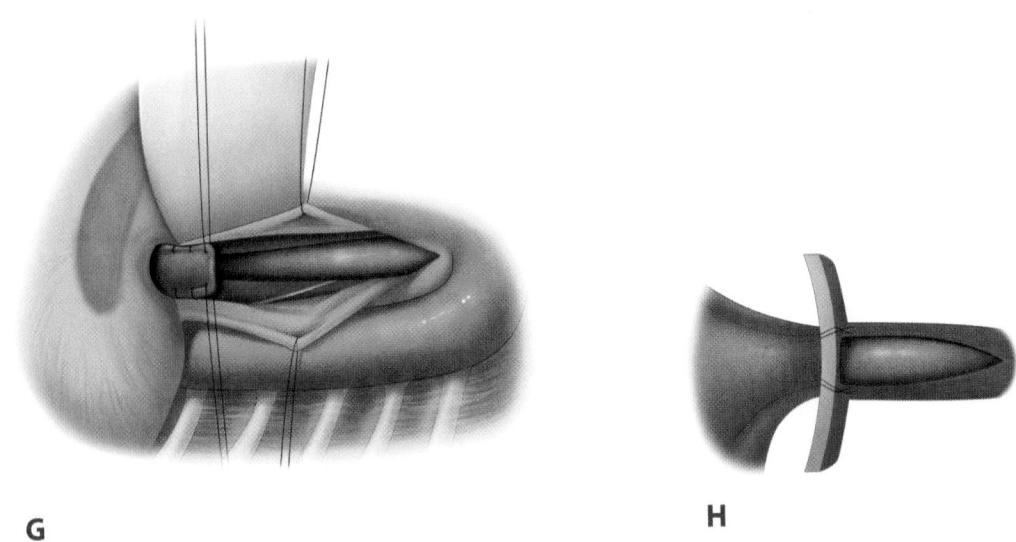

G   **H**

FIG. 25-62. (*Continued*) **G.** Reconstruction of the cardia after a myotomy, illustrating the position of the sutures used to stitch the gastric fundic flap to the margins of the myotomy. **H.** Reconstruction of the cardia after a myotomy, illustrating the intra-abdominal position of the gastric tongue covering the distal 4 cm of the myotomy.

critical that the esophageal staple line be treated with a great deal of care. Closure of the muscle over the staple line is preferable. Additionally, the patient kept NPO for 3 to 5 days and obtained a contrast study before initiating clear liquids. Solid foods are withheld for 2 weeks to decrease the likelihood of staple line leak. Buttressing or sealing the staple line with fibrin glue is also an attractive option.

Myotomy of the Lower Esophageal Sphincter (Heller Myotomy)

Second only to reflux disease, achalasia is the most common functional disorder of the esophagus to require surgical intervention. The goal of treatment is to relieve the functional outflow obstruction secondary to the loss of relaxation and compliance of the LES. This requires disrupting the LES muscle. When performed adequately (i.e., reducing sphincter pressure to <10 mmHg), and done early in the course of disease, LES myotomy results in symptomatic improvement with the occasional return of esophageal peristalsis. Reduction in LES resistance can be accomplished intraluminally by hydrostatic balloon dilation, which ruptures the sphincter muscle, by botulinum toxin injection, or by a surgical myotomy that cuts the sphincter. The difference between these three methods appears to be the greater likelihood of reducing sphincter pressure to <10 mmHg by surgical myotomy as compared with hydrostatic balloon dilation. However, patients whose sphincter pressure has been reduced by hydrostatic balloon dilation to <10 mmHg have an outcome similar to those after surgical myotomy (Fig. 25-64). Botulinum toxin injection may achieve similar results, but has a duration of action that may be measured in weeks or months, rather than years. Botulinum toxin injection may best be used as a diagnostic tool, when it is not clear whether a hypertensive LES is the primary cause of dysphagia. Responsiveness to botulinum toxin injection may predict a good response to Heller myotomy.

The therapeutic decisions regarding the treatment of patients with achalasia center around four issues. The first issue is the question of whether newly diagnosed patients should be treated with pneumatic dilation or a surgical myotomy. Long-term follow-up studies have shown that pneumatic dilation achieves adequate relief of dysphagia and pharyngeal regurgitation in 50 to 60% of patients (Fig. 25-65). Close follow-up is required, and if dilation fails, myotomy is indicated. For those patients who have a dilated

and tortuous esophagus or an associated hiatal hernia, balloon dilation is dangerous and surgery is the better option The outcome of the one controlled randomized study (38 patients) comparing the two modes of therapy suggests that surgical myotomy as a primary treatment gives better long-term results. Several randomized trials comparing laparoscopic cardiomyotomy with balloon dilation or botulinum toxin injection have favored the surgical approach as well. Although it has been reported that a myotomy after previous balloon dilation is more difficult, this has not been the experience of these authors unless the cardia has been ruptured in a sawtooth manner. In this situation, operative intervention, either immediately or after healing has occurred, can be difficult. Similarly, myotomy after botulinum toxin injection has reported to be more difficult, but this is largely a function of the submucosal inflammatory response, which may be a bit unpredictable, and is most intense in the first 6 to 12 weeks after injection. It is important to wait at least 3 months after botulinum toxin injection to perform cardiomyotomy to minimize the risk of encountering dense inflammation.

The second issue is the question of whether a surgical myotomy should be performed through the abdomen or the chest. Myotomy of the LES can be accomplished via either an abdominal or thoracic approach. In the absence of a previous upper abdominal surgery, most surgeons prefer the abdominal approach to LES myotomy as laparoscopy results in less pain and a shorter length of stay than thoracoscopy. In addition, it is a bit easier to assure a long gastric myotomy when the approach is transabdominal.

The third issue—and one that has been long debated—is the question of whether an antireflux procedure should be added to a surgical myotomy. Excellent results have been reported following meticulously performed myotomy without an antireflux component. Retrospective studies, with long-term follow-up of large cohorts of patients undergoing Heller myotomy demonstrated that, after 10 years, more than 50% of patients had reflux symptoms without a fundoplication. In a recent randomized clinical trial, 7% of patients undergoing Dor fundoplication following LES myotomy had abnormal 24-hour pH probes, and 42% of patients with a myotomy only had abnormal reflux profiles. If an antireflux procedure is used as an adjunct to esophageal myotomy, a complete 360° fundoplication should be avoided. Rather, a 270° Belsey fundoplication, a Toupet posterior 180° fundoplication, or a Dor anterior 180° fundoplication should be used to avoid the long-term esophageal

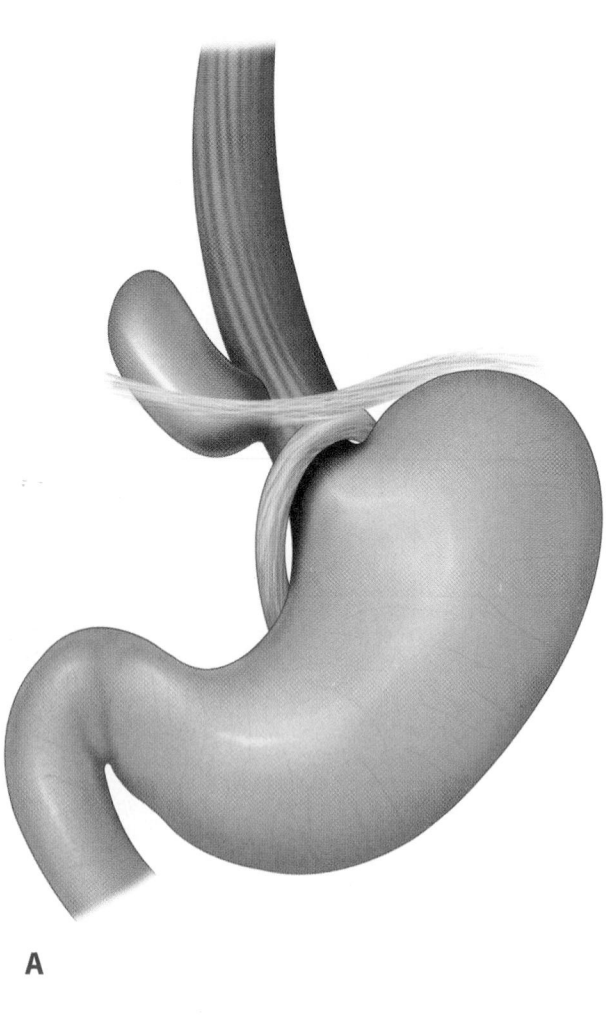

A

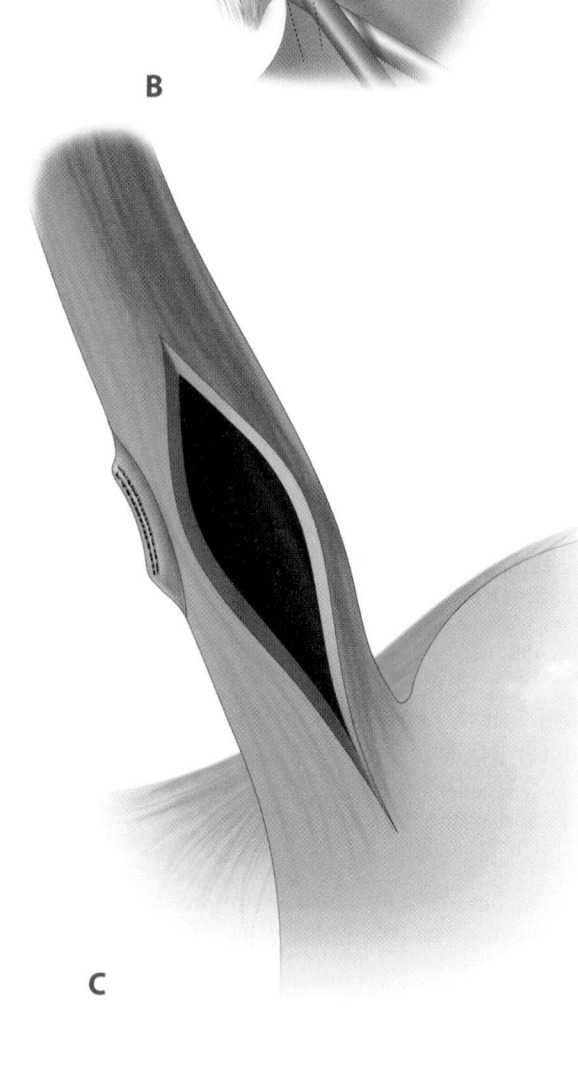

B

C

FIG. 25-63. A. Epiphrenic diverticula are situated above the lower esophageal sphincter on right side of esophagus. **B.** Stapler amputates neck of diverticulum. **C.** Muscle reapproximated over staple line, and Heller myotomy is performed.

dysfunction secondary to the outflow obstruction afforded by the fundoplication itself.

The fourth issue centers on whether or not a cure of this disease is achievable. Long-term follow-up studies after surgical myotomy have shown that late deterioration in results occurs after this procedure, regardless of whether an antireflux procedure is done, and also after balloon dilation, even when the sphincter pressure is reduced to below 10 mmHg. It may be that, even though a myotomy or balloon rupture of the LES muscle reduces the outflow obstruction at the cardia, the underlying motor disorder in the body of the esophagus persists and deteriorates further with the passage of time, leading to increased impairment of esophageal emptying. The earlier an effective reduction in outflow resistance can be accomplished, the better the outcome will be, and the more likely some esophageal body function can be restored.

In performing a surgical myotomy of the LES, there are four important principles: (a) complete division of all circular and collar-sling muscle fibers, (b) adequate distal myotomy to reduce outflow resistance, (c) "undermining" of the muscularis to allow wide

separation of the esophageal muscle, and (d) prevention of postoperative reflux. In the past, the drawback of a surgical myotomy was the need for an open procedure, which often deterred patients from choosing the best treatment option for achalasia. With the advent of minimally invasive surgical techniques two decades ago, laparoscopic cardiomyotomy (Heller myotomy) has become the treatment of choice for most patients with achalasia.

Open Esophageal Myotomy

Open techniques of distal esophageal myotomy are rarely used outside of reoperations. Primary procedures can almost always be successfully completed via laparoscopy. A modified Heller myotomy can be performed through a left thoracotomy incision in the sixth intercostal space along the upper border of the seventh rib. The esophagus and a tongue of gastric fundus are exposed as described for a long myotomy. A myotomy through all muscle layers is performed, extending distally over the stomach to 1 to 2 cm below the junction, and proximally on the esophagus for 4 to 5 cm.

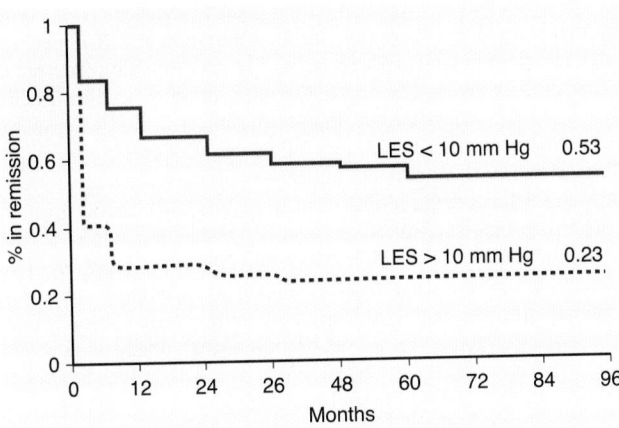

FIG. 25-64. Prevalence of clinical remission in 122 patients stratified according to postdilatation lower esophageal sphincter (LES) pressures greater than or <10 mmHg. (*Reproduced with permission from Ponce J, Garrigues V, Pertejo V, et al: Individual prediction of response to pneumatic dilation in patients with achalasia. Dig Dis Sci 41:2138, 1996. With kind permission from Springer Science+Business Media.*)

The cardia is reconstructed by suturing the tongue of gastric fundus to the margins of the myotomy, to prevent rehealing of the myotomy site, and to provide reflux protection in the area of the divided sphincter. If an extensive dissection of the cardia has been done, a more formal Belsey repair is performed. The tongue of gastric fundus is allowed to retract into the abdomen. Traditionally, nasogastric drainage is maintained for 6 days to prevent distention of the

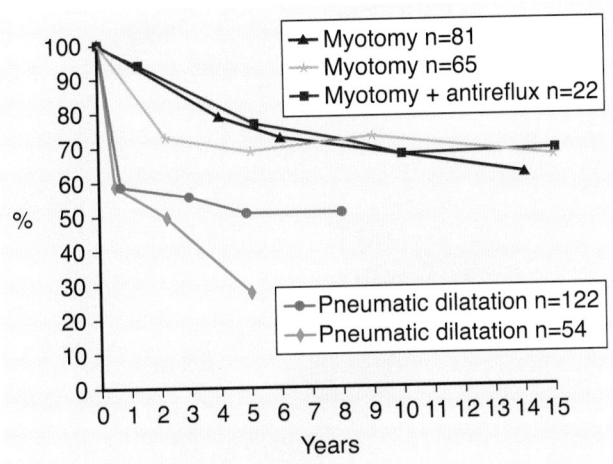

FIG. 25-65. Summary of long-term studies reporting the proportion of patients with complete relief or minimal dysphagia (stage 0–1) stratified according to type of treatment. (*Data reproduced from:*
← *Ellis FH Jr.: Oesophagomyotomy for achalasia: A 22-year experience. Br J Surg 80:882, 1993.*
← *Goulbourne IA, Walbaum PR: Long-term results of Heller's operation for achalasia. J Royal Coll Surg 30:101, 1985.*
← *Malthaner RA, Todd TR, Miller L, et al: Long-term results in surgically managed esophageal achalasia. Ann Thorac Surg 58:1343, 1994.*
← *Ponce J, Garrigues V, Pertejo V, et al: Individual prediction of response to pneumatic dilation. Dig Dis Sci 41:2135, 1996.*
← *Eckardt V, Aignherr C, Bernhard G: Predictors of outcome in patients with achalasia treated by pneumatic dilation. Gastroenterol 103:1732, 1992.*)

stomach during healing. An oral diet is resumed on the seventh day, after a barium swallow study shows unobstructed passage of the bolus into the stomach without extravasation.

In a randomized, long-term follow-up by Csendes and colleagues of 81 patients treated for achalasia, either by forceful dilation or by surgical myotomy, myotomy was associated with a significant increase in the diameter at the GEJ and a decrease in the diameter at the middle third of the esophagus on follow-up radiographic studies. There was a greater reduction in sphincter pressure and improvement in the amplitude of esophageal contractions after myotomy. Thirteen percent of patients regained some peristalsis after dilation, compared with 28% after surgery. These findings were shown to persist over a 5-year follow-up period, at which time 95% of those treated with surgical myotomy were doing well. Of those who were treated with dilation, only 54% were doing well, while 16% required redilation and 22% eventually required surgical myotomy to obtain relief.

If simultaneous esophageal contractions are associated with the sphincter abnormality, the so-called *vigorous achalasia*, then the myotomy should extend over the distance of the abnormal motility as mapped by the preoperative motility study. Failure to do this will result in continuing dysphagia and a dissatisfied patient. The best objective evaluation of improvement in the patient following either balloon dilation or myotomy is a scintigraphic measurement of esophageal emptying time. A good therapeutic response improves esophageal emptying toward normal. However, some degree of dysphagia may persist despite improved esophageal emptying, due to disturbances in esophageal body function. When an antireflux procedure is added to the myotomy, it should be a partial fundoplication. A 360° fundoplication is associated with progressive retention of swallowed food, regurgitation, and aspiration to a degree that exceeds the patient's preoperative symptoms.

Laparoscopic Cardiomyotomy

More commonly known as a *laparoscopic Heller myotomy*, after Ernst Heller, a German surgeon who described a "double myotomy" in 1913, the laparoscopic approach is similar to the Nissen fundoplication in terms of the trocar placement and exposure and dissection of the esophageal hiatus (Fig. 25-66). The procedure begins by division of the short gastric vessels in preparation for fundoplication. Exposure of the GEJ via removal of the gastroesophageal fat pad follows. The anterior vagus nerve is swept right laterally along with the fat pad. Once completed, the GEJ and distal 4 to 5 cm of esophagus should be bared of any overlying tissue, and generally follows dissection of the GEJ. A distal esophageal myotomy is performed. It is generally easiest to begin the myotomy 1 to 2 cm above the GEJ, in an area above that of previous botulinum toxin injections or balloon dilation. Either scissors or a hook-type electrocautery can be used to initiate the incision in the longitudinal and circular muscle. Distally, the myotomy is carried across the GEJ and onto the proximal stomach for approximately 2 to 3 cm. After completion, the muscle edges are separated bluntly from the esophageal mucosa for approximately 50% of the esophageal circumference. An antireflux procedure follows completion of the myotomy. Either an anterior hemifundoplication augmenting the angle of His (Dor) or posterior partial fundoplication (Toupet) can be performed. The Dor type fundoplication is slightly easier to perform, and does not require disruption of the normal posterior gastroesophageal attachments (a theoretical advantage in preventing postoperative reflux).

Outcome Assessment of the Therapy for Achalasia

Critical analysis of the results of therapy for motor disorders of the esophagus requires objective measurement. The use of symptoms alone as an endpoint to evaluate therapy for achalasia may be misleading. The propensity for patients to unconsciously modify their diet to avoid difficulty swallowing is underestimated, making an assessment of results based on symptoms unreliable. Insufficient reduction in outflow resistance may allow progressive esophageal dilation to develop slowly, giving the impression of improvement because the volume of food able to be ingested with comfort increases. A variety of objective measurements may be used to assess success, including LES pressure, esophageal baseline pressure, and scintigraphic assessment of esophageal emptying time. Esophageal baseline pressure is usually negative when compared to gastric pressure. Given that the goal of therapy is to eliminate the outflow resistance of a nonrelaxing sphincter, measurement of improvements in esophageal baseline pressure and scintigraphic transit time may be better indicators of success, but are rarely reported.

Eckardt and associates investigated whether the outcome of pneumatic dilation in patients with achalasia could be predicted on the basis of objective measurements. Postdilation LES pressure was the most valuable measurement for predicting long-term clinical response. A postdilatation sphincter pressure <10 mmHg predicted a good response. Fifty percent of the patients studied had postdilatation sphincter pressures between 10 and 20 mmHg, with a 2-year remission rate of 71%. Importantly, 16 of 46 patients were left with a postdilatation sphincter pressure of >20 mmHg, and had an unacceptable outcome. Overall, only 30% of patients dilated remained in symptomatic remission at 5 years.

Bonavina and colleagues reported good to excellent results with transabdominal myotomy and Dor fundoplication in 94% of patients after a mean follow-up of 5.4 years. No operative mortality occurred in either of these series, attesting to the safety of the procedure. Malthaner and Pearson reported the long-term clinical results in 35 patients with achalasia, having a minimum follow-up of 10 years (Table 25-11). Twenty-two of these patients underwent primary esophageal myotomy and Belsey hemifundoplication at the Toronto General Hospital. Excellent to good results were noted in 95% of patients at 1 year, declining to 68, 69, and 67% at 10, 15, and 20 years, respectively. Two patients underwent early reoperation for an incomplete myotomy, and three underwent an esophagectomy for progressive disease. They concluded that there was a deterioration of the initially good results after surgical myotomy and hiatal repair for achalasia, which is due to late complications of gastroesophageal reflux.

Ellis reported his lifetime experience with transthoracic short esophageal myotomy without an antireflux procedure. One hundred seventy-nine patients were analyzed at a mean follow-up of 9 years, ranging from 6 months to 20 years. Overall, 89% of patients were improved at the 9-year mark. He also observed that the level of improvement deteriorated with time, with excellent results (patients continuing to be symptom free) decreasing from 54% at 10 years to 32% at 20 years. He concluded that a short

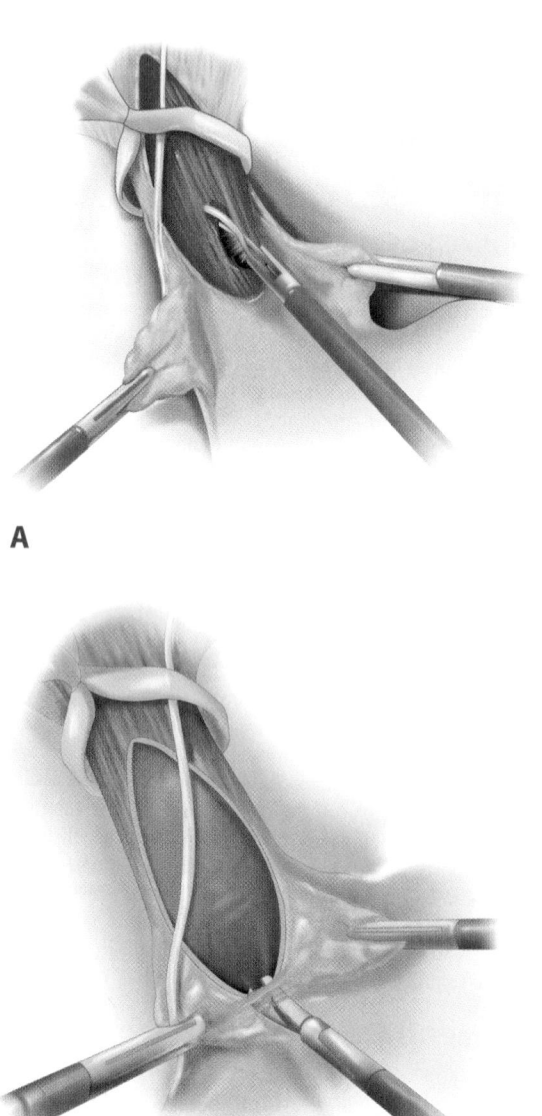

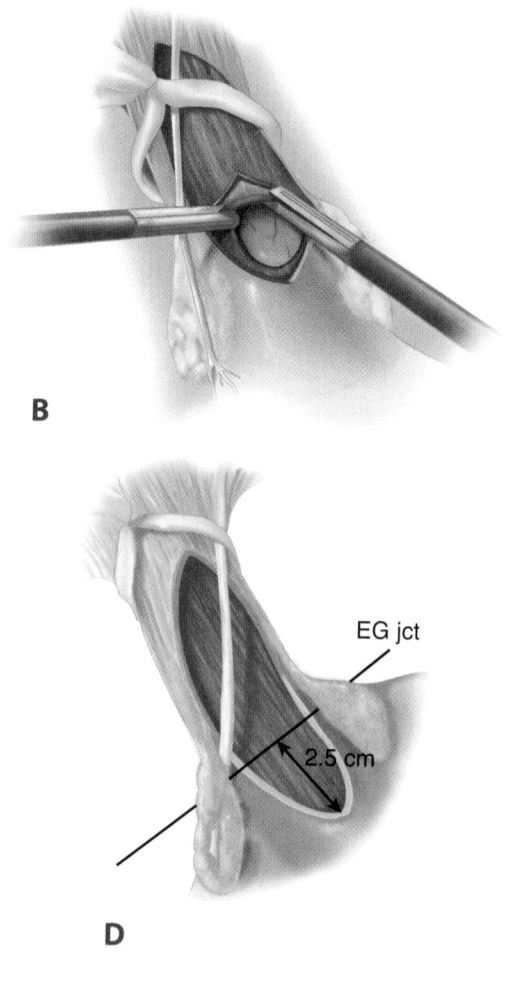

FIG. 25-66. A. Longitudinal muscle is divided. **B.** Mechanical disruption of lower esophageal sphincter muscle fibers. **C.** Myotomy must be carried across gastroesophageal junction. **D.** Gastric extension should equal 2 to 3 cm. (*Continued*)

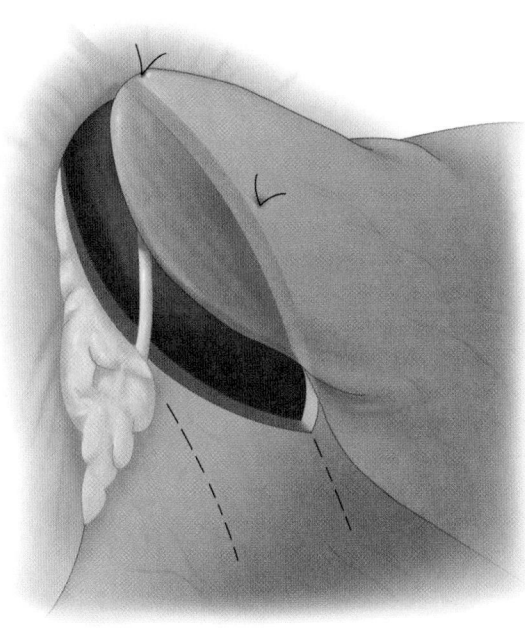

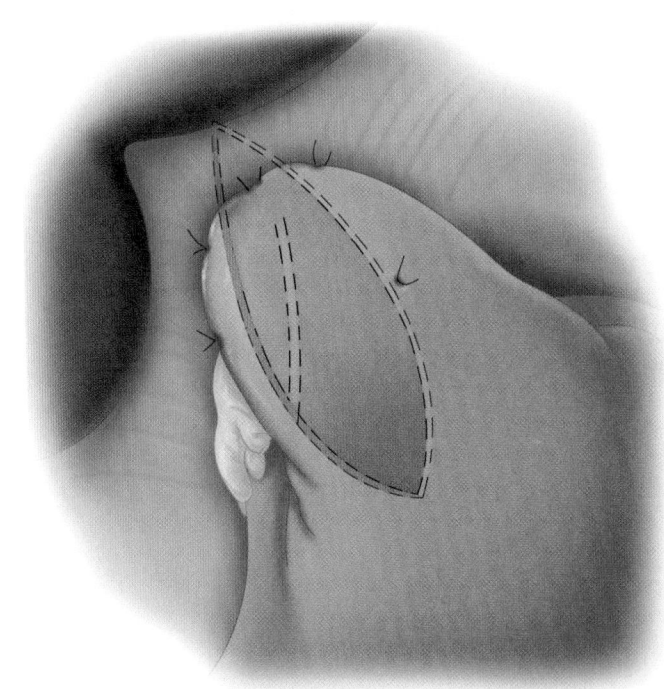

E

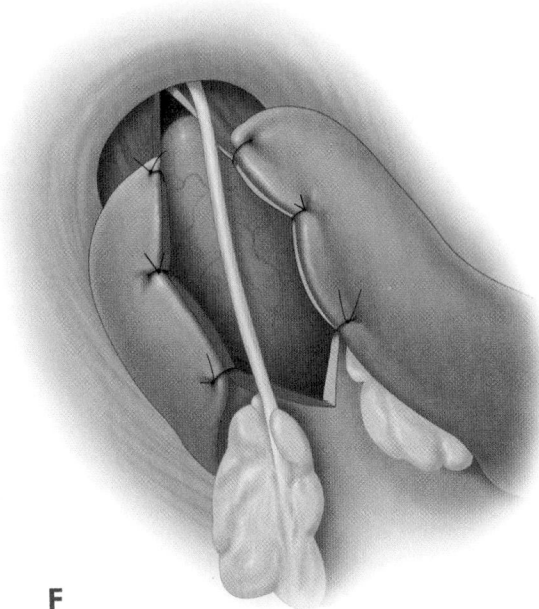

FIG. 25-66. (*Continued*) **E.** Anterior (Dor) fundoplication is sutured to the diaphragmatic arch. **F.** Posterior (Toupet) fundoplication is sutured to cut edges of myotomy. EG jct = esophagogastric junction.

F

transthoracic myotomy without an antireflux procedure provides excellent long-term relief of dysphagia, and, contrary to Malthaner and Pearson's experience, does not result in complications of gastroesophageal reflux. Both studies document nearly identical results 10 to 15 years following the procedure, and both report deterioration over time, probably due to progression of the underlying disease. The addition of an antireflux procedure if the operation is performed transthoracically has no significant effect on the outcome.

The outcome of laparoscopic myotomy and hemifundoplication has been well documented. Two reports of over 100 patients have documented relief of dysphagia in 93% of patients. Richter and coworkers reviewed published reports to date, including 254 patients with an average success rate of 93% at 2.5 years. Conversion to an open procedure occurs in 0 to 5% of patients. Complications are uncommon, occurring in <5% of patients. Intraoperative complications consist largely of mucosal perforation, and have been more likely to occur after botulinum toxin injection. The incidence of objective reflux disease as evidenced by abnormal acid exposure is <10%.

A number of randomized clinical trials in the past decade have compared the outcomes of laparoscopic Heller myotomy to pneumatic dilation and to botulinum toxin injection. In each of these trials, laparoscopic Heller myotomy and partial fundoplication was superior to the alternative treatment. Lastly, a randomized clinical trial examining the need for fundoplication following Heller myotomy demonstrated a great deal more reflux in patients without fundoplication, and no better swallowing in the Heller-only group. The best treatment for achalasia is a laparoscopic Heller myotomy and partial fundoplication.

TABLE 25-11 Reasons for failure of esophageal myotomy

| | Author, Procedure (n) | | |
Reason	Ellis, Myotomy Only (n = 81)	Goulbourne, Myotomy Only (n = 65)	Malthaner, Myotomy + Antireflux (n = 22)
Reflux	4%	5%	18%
Inadequate myotomy	2%	—	9%
Megaesophagus	2%	—	—
Poor emptying	4%	3%	—
Persistent chest pain	1%	—	—

Source: Data from Malthaner RA, et al: Long-term results in surgically managed esophageal achalasia. *Ann Thorac Surg* 58:1343, 1994; Ellis FH Jr.: Oesophagomyotomy for achalasia: A 22-year experience. *Br J Surg* 80:882, 1993; and Goulbourne IA, et al: Long-term results of Heller's operation for achalasia. *J Royal Coll Surg* 30, 1985.

Esophageal Resection for End-Stage Motor Disorders of the Esophagus

Patients with dysphagia and long-standing benign disease, whose esophageal function has been destroyed by the disease process or multiple previous surgical procedures, are best managed by esophagectomy. Fibrosis of the esophagus and cardia can result in weak contractions and failure of the distal esophageal sphincter to relax. The loss of esophageal contractions can result in the stasis of food, esophageal dilatation, regurgitation, and aspiration. The presence of these abnormalities signals end-stage motor disease. In these situations esophageal replacement is usually required to establish normal alimentation. Before proceeding with esophageal resection for patients with end-stage benign disease, the choice of the organ to substitute for the esophagus (i.e., stomach, jejunum, or colon) should be considered. The choice of replacement is affected by a number of factors, as described later in the section on Techniques of Esophageal Reconstruction.

CARCINOMA OF THE ESOPHAGUS

Squamous carcinoma accounts for the majority of esophageal carcinomas worldwide. Its incidence is highly variable, ranging from approximately 20 per 100,000 in the United States and Britain, to 160 per 100,000 in certain parts of South Africa and the Honan Province of China, and even 540 per 100,000 in the Guriev district of Kazakhstan. The environmental factors responsible for these localized high-incidence areas have not been conclusively identified, though additives to local foodstuffs (nitroso compounds in pickled vegetables and smoked meats) and mineral deficiencies (zinc and molybdenum) have been suggested. In Western societies, smoking and alcohol consumption are strongly linked with squamous carcinoma. Other definite associations link squamous carcinoma with long-standing achalasia, lye strictures, tylosis (an autosomal dominant disorder characterized by hyperkeratosis of the palms and soles), and human papillomavirus.

Adenocarcinoma of the esophagus, once an unusual malignancy, is diagnosed with increasing frequency (Fig. 25-67), and now accounts for more than 50% of esophageal cancer in most Western countries. The shift in the epidemiology of esophageal cancer from predominantly squamous carcinoma seen in association with smoking and alcohol, to adenocarcinoma in the setting of BE, is one of the most dramatic changes that have occurred in the history of human neoplasia. Although esophageal carcinoma is a relatively uncommon malignancy, its prevalence is exploding, largely secondary to the well-established association between gastroesophageal reflux, BE, and esophageal adenocarcinoma. Once a nearly uni-

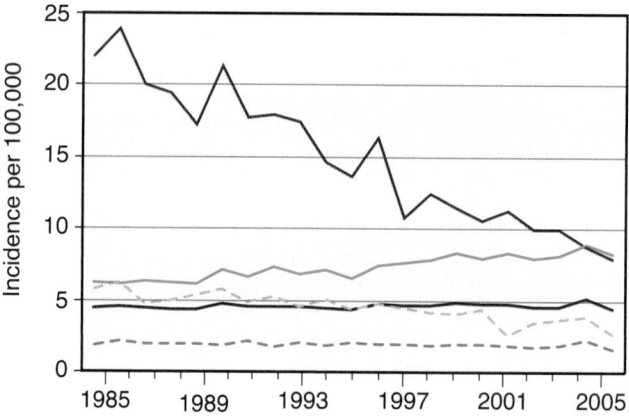

U.S. esophageal cancer incidence

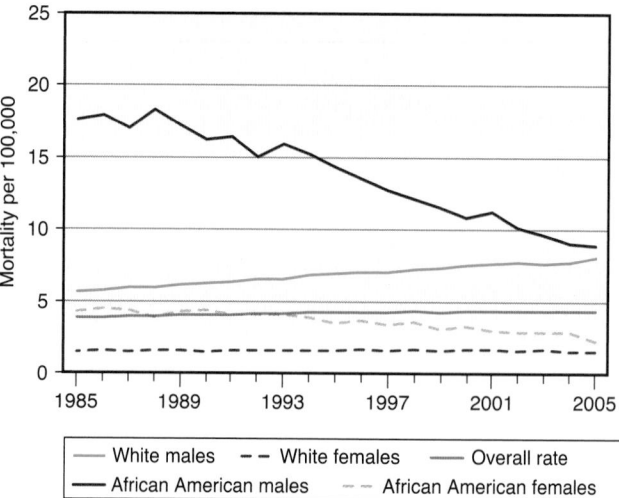

U.S. esophageal cancer mortality

—— White males   – – White females   —— Overall rate
—— African American males   – – African American females

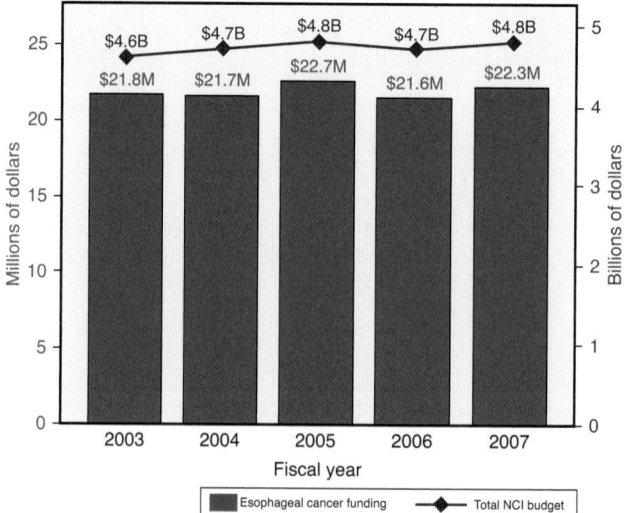

NCI esophageal cancer research investment

FIG. 25-67. Incidence and mortality rate trends for esophageal cancer. NCI = National Cancer Institute. *(Reproduced with permission from the National Cancer Institute. Last updated September, 2008.)*

formly lethal disease, survival is improving because of advances in the understanding of its molecular biology, screening and surveillance practices, improved staging, minimally invasive surgical techniques, and neoadjuvant therapy.

Furthermore, the clinical picture of esophageal adenocarcinoma is changing. It now occurs not only considerably more frequently, but in younger patients, and is often detected at an earlier stage. These facts support rethinking the traditional approach of assuming palliation is appropriate in all patients. The historical focus on palliation of dysphagia in an elderly patient with comorbidities should change when dealing with a young patient with dependent children and a productive life ahead. The potential for cure becomes of paramount importance.

The gross appearance resembles that of squamous cell carcinoma. Microscopically, adenocarcinoma almost always originates in metaplastic Barrett's mucosa, and resembles gastric cancer. Rarely, it arises in the submucosal glands, and forms intramural growths that resemble the mucoepidermal and adenoid cystic carcinomas of the salivary glands.

The most important etiologic factor in the development of primary adenocarcinoma of the esophagus is a metaplastic columnar-lined or Barrett's esophagus, which occurs as a complication in approximately 10 to 15% of patients with GERD. When studied prospectively, the incidence of adenocarcinoma in a patient with BE is one in 100 to 200 patient-years of follow-up (i.e., for every 100 patients with BE followed for 1 year, one will develop adenocarcinoma). Although this risk appears to be small, it is at least 40 to 50 times that expected for a similar population without BE. This risk is similar to the risk for developing lung cancer in a person with a 20-pack-per-year history of smoking. Endoscopic surveillance for patients with BE is recommended for two reasons: (a) At present there is no reliable evidence that medical therapy removes the risk of neoplastic transformation, and (b) malignancy in BE is curable if detected at an early stage.

Clinical Manifestations

Esophageal cancer generally presents with dysphagia, although increasing numbers of relatively asymptomatic patients are now identified on surveillance endoscopy, or present with nonspecific upper GI symptoms and undergo upper endoscopy. Extension of the primary tumor into the tracheobronchial tree can cause stridor, and, if a tracheoesophageal fistula develops, coughing, choking, and aspiration pneumonia result. Rarely, severe bleeding from the primary tumor or from erosion into the aorta or pulmonary vessels occurs. Either vocal cord may be invaded, causing paralysis, but most commonly, paralysis is caused by invasion of the left recurrent laryngeal nerve by the primary tumor or LN metastasis. Systemic organ metastases are usually manifested by jaundice or bone pain. The situation is different in high-incidence areas where screening is practiced. In these communities, the most prominent early symptom is pain on swallowing rough or dry food.

Dysphagia usually presents late in the natural history of the disease, because the lack of a serosal layer on the esophagus allows the smooth muscle to dilate with ease. As a result, the dysphagia becomes severe enough for the patient to seek medical advice only when more than 60% of the esophageal circumference is infiltrated with cancer. Consequently, the disease is usually advanced if symptoms herald its presence. Tracheoesophageal fistula may be present in some patients on their first visit to the hospital, and more than 40% will have evidence of distant metastases. With tumors of the cardia, anorexia and weight loss usually precede the onset of dysphagia. The physical signs of esophageal tumors are those associated with the presence of distant metastases.

General Approach to Esophageal Cancer

Therapy of esophageal cancer is dictated by the stage of the cancer at the time of diagnosis. Put simply, one needs to determine if the disease is confined to the esophagus, (T1–T2, N0), locally advanced (T1–3, N1), or disseminated (any T, any N, M1). If cancer is confined to the esophagus, removal of the tumor with adjacent LNs may be curative. Very early tumors confined to the mucosa (T in situ, T1a, intramucosal cancer) may be addressed with endoscopic treatment.

When the tumor is locally aggressive, modern therapy dictates a multimodality approach in a surgically fit patient. Multimodality therapy is either chemotherapy followed by surgery or radiation and chemotherapy followed by surgery. When given before surgery, these treatments are referred to as *neoadjuvant* or *induction therapy*. For disseminated cancer, treatment is aimed at palliation of symptoms. If the patient has dysphagia, as many do, the most rapid form of palliation is the placement of an expandable esophageal stent, endoscopically. For palliation of GEJ cancer, radiation may be the first choice, as stents placed across the GEJ create a great deal of gastroesophageal reflux.

Staging of Esophageal Cancer

Choosing the best therapy for an individual patient requires accurate staging. Staging starts with the history and physical. LN disease remote from the tumor, particularly in the cervical region, may be palpable on neck examination and generally indicates cancer dissemination. This is often referred to as *M1a disease*, indicating that these patients should not be treated with therapy directed toward locally advanced cancer. Other metastatic LNs are rarely palpable but are equally ominous, especially the umbilical LN in GEJ cancer.

Chest x-ray is the first step of staging, but is rarely informative. Computed tomographic (CT) scanning of the chest, abdomen, and pelvis provides information on local invasion of the primary cancer, LN involvement, or disseminated disease. The most common sites of esophageal cancer metastases are lung, liver, and peritoneal surfaces, including the omentum and small bowel mesentery. If masses are identified that are not characteristic for cancer or are in a location that precludes resection with the cancer specimen, positron emission tomography (PET) scanning may be able to tell whether the masses are metabolically active (likely to be cancer) or not. A PET active focus corresponding to a mass on CT scan outside of the field of esophageal resection should be biopsied before resection is performed.

The introduction of endoscopic ultrasound (EUS) has made it possible to identify patients who are potentially curable before surgical therapy. Using an endoscope, the depth of the wall penetration by the tumor and the presence of LN metastases can be determined with 80% accuracy. A curative resection should be encouraged if EUS indicates that the tumor has not invaded adjacent organs (T4), and/or fewer than five enlarged LNs are imaged. Thoracoscopic and laparoscopic staging of esophageal cancer may add benefit when the nature of enlarged LNs remote from the cancer cannot be determined, or when advanced imaging systems (PET and high-resolution spiral CT) are not available.

Occasionally, diagnostic laparoscopy and jejunostomy tube placement may proceed induction chemoradiation in the patient with severe dysphagia and weight loss from a locally advanced cancer. In summary, esophageal cancer is diagnosed with endoscopic biopsy and is staged with CT scanning of the chest and abdomen, EUS, and PET scan for all patients with CT or EUS evidence of advanced disease (T2 or greater, N1 or NX). Experience with esophageal resections in patients with early disease has identified characteristics of esophageal cancer that are associated with improved survival. A number of studies suggest that only metastasis to LNs and tumor penetration of the esophageal wall have a significant and independent influence on prognosis. Factors known to be important in the survival of patients with advanced disease, such as cell type, degree of cellular differentiation, or location of tumor in the esophagus, have no effect on survival of patients who have undergone resection for early disease. Studies also showed that patients having five or fewer LN metastases have a better outcome. Using these data, Skinner developed the wall penetration, LN, and distant organ metastases system for staging.

The wall penetration, LN, and distant organ metastases system differed somewhat from the previous efforts to develop a satisfactory staging criteria for carcinoma of the esophagus. Most surgeons agreed that the 1983 tumor, nodes, and metastasis system left much to be desired. In the third edition of the manual for Staging of Cancer

TABLE 25-12 Staging of cancer of the esophagus and cardia (AJCC 1988)

Stage	Classification			No. of Patients	% 5-Year Survival	P Value
0	Tis	N_0	M_0	16	100	NS
I	T_1	N_0	M_0	22	78.9	.0021
IIA	T_2	N_0	M_0	80	37.9	
	T_3	N_0	M_0			
IIB	T_1	N_1	M_0	39	27.3	NS
	T_2	N_1	M_0			
III	T_3	N_1	M_0	218	13.7	NS
	T_4	Any N	M_0			
IV	Any T	Any N	M_1	33/408	0	.0001

AJCC = American Joint Committee on Cancer; NS = not significant.
Source: Reproduced with permission from Ellis FH, et al: Esophagogastrectomy for carcinoma of the esophagus and cardia: A comparison of findings and results after standard resection in three consecutive 8 year time intervals, using improved staging criteria. *J Thorac Cardiovasc Surg* 113:836, 1997. Copyright Elsevier.

of the American Joint Committee on Cancer in 1988, an effort was made to provide a finer discrimination between stages than had been contained in the previous edition in 1983. Table 25-12 shows the definitions for the primary tumor, regional LNs, and distant metastasis, as listed in the 1988 manual. Further refinements of the staging system of esophageal cancer are underway and likely to be approved by the American Joint Committee on Cancer, recognizing the difference in survival afforded by resection of limited LN disease adjacent to the tumor, as compared to multilevel LN disease and positive LNs remote from the primary. In addition, the difference between intramucosal cancer and cancer extending to the submucosa (both currently T1 cancer) will be recognized.

Clinical Approach to Carcinoma of the Esophagus and Cardia

The selection of a curative vs. a palliative operation for cancer of the esophagus is based on the location of the tumor, the patient's age

and health, the extent of the disease, and preoperative staging. Figure 25-68 shows an algorithm of the clinical decisions important in the selection of curative or palliative therapy.

Tumor Location

The selection of surgical therapy for patients with carcinoma of the esophagus depends not only on the anatomic stage of the disease and an assessment of the swallowing capacity of the patient, but also on the location of the primary tumor.

It is estimated that 8% of the primary malignant tumors of the esophagus occur in the cervical portion (Fig. 25-69). They are almost always squamous cell lesions, with a rare adenocarcinoma arising from a congenital inlet patch of columnar lining. These tumors, particularly those in the postcricoid area, represent a separate pathologic entity for two reasons: (a) They are more common in females and appear to be a unique entity in this regard; and (b) The efferent lymphatics from the cervical esophagus drain completely differently from those of the thoracic esophagus. The latter drain directly into the paratracheal and deep cervical or internal jugular LNs with minimal flow in a longitudinal direction. Except in advanced disease, it is unusual for intrathoracic LNs to be involved.

Cervical esophageal cancer is frequently unresectable because of early invasion of the larynx, great vessels, or trachea. Radical surgery including esophagolaryngectomy may occasionally be performed for these lesions, but the ensuing morbidity makes this a less than desirable approach in the face of uncertain cure. Thus, for most patients with cervical esophageal cancer, stereotactic radiation with concomitant chemotherapy is the most desirable treatment.

Tumors that arise within the middle third of the esophagus are squamous carcinomas most commonly and are frequently associated with LN metastasis, which are usually in the thorax but may be in the neck or abdomen, and may skip areas in between. Although it is generally felt that individuals with midthoracic cancer and abdominal LN metastases are incurable with surgery, there are some emerging data that suggest that cervical LN metastases, if isolated, can be resected with benefit. Generally, T1 and T2 cancers without LN metastases are treated with resection only, but there is more and more data to suggest that LN involvement or transmural cancer (T3) warrants treatment with neoadjuvant chemoradiation therapy fol-

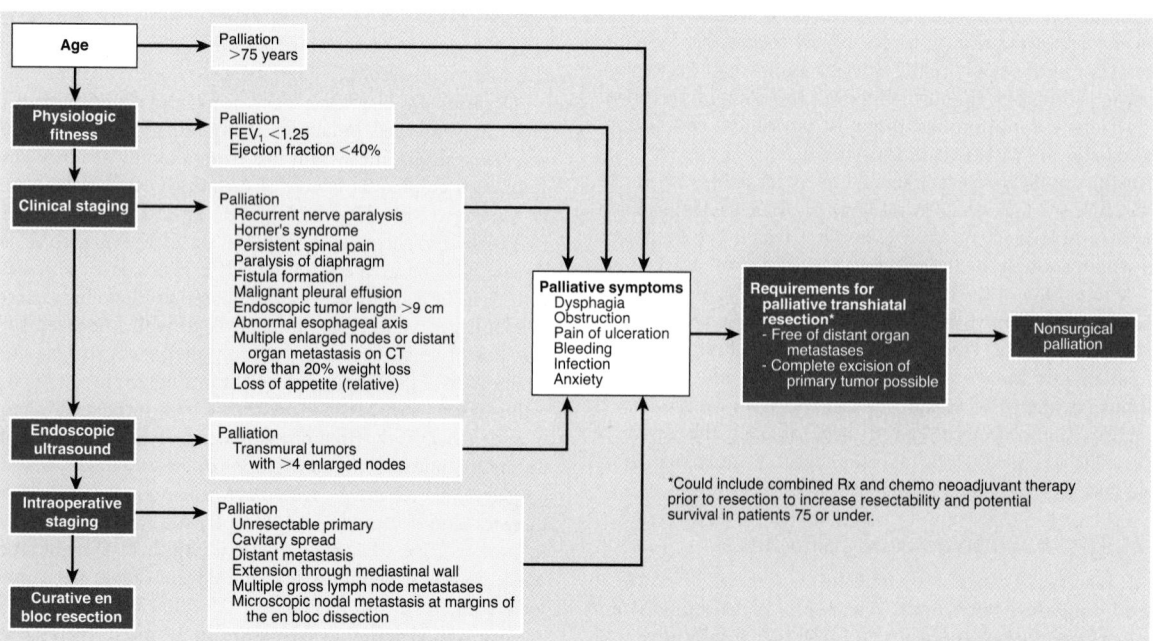

FIG. 25-68. Algorithm for the evaluation of esophageal cancer patients to select the proper therapy: curative en bloc resection, palliative transhiatal resection, or nonsurgical palliation. CT = computed tomography; FEV₁ = forced expiratory volume in 1 second. (*Reproduced with permission from DeMeester TR: Esophageal carcinoma: Current controversies. Sem Surg Oncol 13:217, 1997.*)

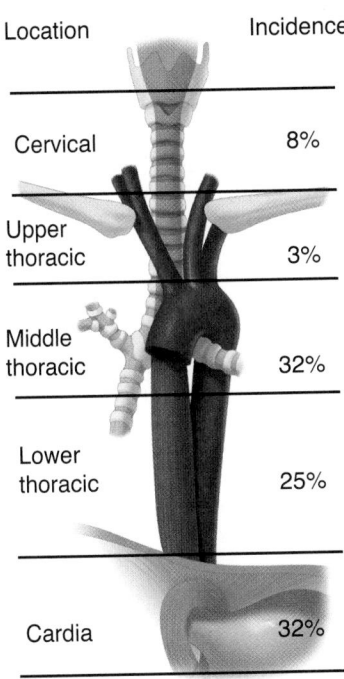

Location	Incidence
Cervical	8%
Upper thoracic	3%
Middle thoracic	32%
Lower thoracic	25%
Cardia	32%

FIG. 25-69. Incidence of carcinoma of the esophagus and cardia based on tumor location.

lowed by resection. Although some surgeons prefer a transhiatal esophagectomy for all tumor locations, most surgeons believe that resection of midesophageal cancer should be performed under direct vision with either thoracoscopy [video-assisted thoracic surgery (VATS)] or with thoracotomy.

Tumors of the lower esophagus and cardia are usually adenocarcinomas. Unless preoperative and intraoperative staging clearly demonstrate an incurable lesion, resection in continuity with a LN dissection should be performed. Because of the propensity of GI tumors to spread for long distances submucosally, long lengths of grossly normal GI tract should be resected The longitudinal lymph flow in the esophagus can result in skip areas, with small foci of tumor above the primary lesion, which underscores the importance of a wide resection of esophageal tumors. Wong has shown that local recurrence at the anastomosis can be prevented by obtaining a 10-cm margin of normal esophagus above the tumor. Anatomic studies have also shown that there is no submucosal lymphatic barrier between the esophagus and the stomach at the cardia, and Wong has shown that 50% of the local recurrences in patients with esophageal cancer who are resected for cure occur in the intrathoracic stomach along the line of the gastric resection. Considering that the length of the esophagus ranges from 17 to 25 cm, and the length of the lesser curvature of the stomach is approximately 12 cm, a curative resection requires a cervical division of the esophagus and a >50% proximal gastrectomy in most patients with carcinoma of the distal esophagus or cardia.

Age

Resection for cure of carcinoma of the esophagus in a patient older than 80 years is rarely indicated, because of the additional operative risk and the shorter life expectancy. Despite this general guideline, octogenarians with a high performance status and excellent cardiopulmonary reserve may be considered candidates for esophagectomy. It is in this group of patients that the lesser physiologic impact of minimally invasive surgery may reduce the morbidity and mortality associated with open two- or three-field esophagectomy.

Cardiopulmonary Reserve

Patients undergoing esophageal resection should have sufficient cardiopulmonary reserve to tolerate the proposed procedure. The respiratory function is best assessed with the forced expiratory volume in 1 second, which ideally should be 2 L or more. Any patient with a forced expiratory volume in 1 second of <1.25 L is a poor candidate for thoracotomy, because he or she has a 40% risk of dying from respiratory insufficiency within 4 years. In patients with poor pulmonary reserve, the transhiatal esophagectomy should be considered, as the pulmonary morbidity of this operation is less than is seen following thoracotomy. Clinical evaluation and electrocardiogram are not sufficient indicators of cardiac reserve. Echocardiography and dipyridamole thallium imaging provide accurate information on wall motion, ejection fraction, and myocardial blood flow. A defect on thallium imaging may require further evaluation with preoperative coronary angiography. A resting ejection fraction of <40%, particularly if there is no increase with exercise, is an ominous sign. In the absence of invasive testing, observed stair-climbing is an economical (albeit not quantitative) method of assessing cardiopulmonary reserve. Most individuals who can climb three flights of stairs without stopping will do well with two-field open esophagectomy, especially if an epidural catheter is used for postoperative pain relief.

Nutritional Status

The factor most predictive of postoperative complication is the nutritional status of the patient. Profound weight loss, more than 20 lb, associated with hypoalbuminemia (albumin <3.5 g/dL) is associated with a much higher rate of complications and mortality than patients who enter curative surgery in better nutritional condition. Because malnourished patients generally have locally advanced esophageal cancer, if not metastatic disease, one should consider the placement of a feeding tube before the beginning of induction chemoradiation therapy. Although mild amounts of dysphagia are improved by induction chemoradiation therapy, more pronounced dysphagia and associated malnutrition should be addressed before the initiation of chemoradiation. A laparoscopic jejunostomy tube can be placed prior to induction therapy or at the time of esophagectomy. There are emerging data that 5 days' pretreatment with immune-enhancing nutrition, rich in fish oils, decreases cardiac and other complications, following esophagectomy.

Clinical Staging

Clinical factors that indicate an advanced stage of carcinoma and exclude surgery with curative intent are recurrent nerve paralysis, Horner's syndrome, persistent spinal pain, paralysis of the diaphragm, fistula formation, and malignant pleural effusion. Factors that make surgical cure unlikely include a tumor >8 cm in length, abnormal axis of the esophagus on a barium radiogram, more than four enlarged LNs on CT, a weight loss more than 20%, and loss of appetite. Studies indicate that there are several favorable parameters associated with tumors <4 cm in length, there are fewer with tumors between 4 and 8 cm, and there are no favorable criteria for tumors >8 cm in length. Consequently, the finding of a tumor >8 cm in length should exclude curative resection; the finding of a smaller tumor should encourage an aggressive approach.

Preoperative Staging with Advanced Imaging

For years, clinical staging, contrast radiography, endoscopy, and CT scanning formed the backbone of esophageal cancer staging. More recently, preoperative decision making is guided by endoscopic ultrasonography and PET scanning.

EUS provides the most reliable method of determining depth of cancer invasion. In the absence of enlarged LNs, the degree of wall invasion dictates surgical therapy. If a small focus of esophageal cancer is seen to be confined to the mucosa, endoscopic mucosal resection (EMR) is a preferable option. If the tumor invades the submucosa, without visible lymph node involvement, most individuals would suggest esophagectomy with LN dissection, as positive nodes can be found in 20 to 25% of those with cancer limited to the mucosa and submucosa. If EUS demonstrates spread through the wall of the esophagus, especially if LNs are enlarged, then induction chemoradiation therapy (neoadjuvant therapy) should be strongly considered. Lastly, when the EUS demonstrates invasion of the trachea, bronchus, aorta, or pleura, especially with a pleural effusion, then surgical resection is rarely indicated. Thus, it can be seen that the therapy of esophageal cancer is largely driven by the finding of an endoscopic ultrasonography. It is difficult to provide modern treatment of esophageal cancer without access to this modality.

PET scanning, usually combined with an axial CT scan (CT-PET), usually is performed on patients with locally advanced cancer or questionable lesions on CT scan to determine whether metastases are present. The PET scan uses the injection of radiolabeled deoxyglucose, which is taken up in metabolically active tissues such as cancer. PET-positive areas must be correlated with the CT scan findings to assess the significance of "hot spots." CT-PET scanning has been especially useful before the initiation of chemoradiation therapy. An early response to chemoradiotherapy, by PET scan, improves the prognosis whether or not resection is ultimately performed. Conversely, if a PET-avid tumor shows no change in metabolic activity after 2 weeks of induction chemoradiation therapy, it is unlikely that further chemo or radiation therapy will be of any benefit. These patients have a worse prognosis, and may be referred for resection or palliation without incurring the morbidity or expense of a full course of chemo- and radiation therapy.

Palliation of Esophageal Cancer

Palliation of esophageal cancer is indicated for individuals with metastatic esophageal cancer or cancer invading adjacent organs (T4) who are unable to swallow, or individuals with fistulae into the tracheobronchial tree. Aortic esophageal fistulas are extremely rare and nearly 100% lethal. Dysphagia as a result of esophageal cancer can be graded from grade I, eating normally, to grade VI, unable to swallow saliva (Table 25-13). Grades I–III often can be managed with radiation therapy, usually in combination with chemotherapy. When surgical resection is not anticipated in the future, this is termed *definitive chemoradiation therapy* and usually is palliative. Radiation dose is increased from 45 Gy to 60 Gy administered over 8 weeks, rather than the 4 weeks given for chemoradiation induction therapy. In a small percentage of patients, a complete response to chemoradiation therapy will not only palliate the symptoms, but leave the patient with undetectable cancer of the esophagus. Although some of these patients are truly cured, cancer will recur in many either locally or systemically 1 to 5 years following definitive chemoradiation. In a few patients, definitive chemoradiation will be successful in all sites but the esophagus. After a 12-month wait from initial treatment and no other sites of tumor detectable except the esophagus, some of these patients may be candidates for salvage esophagectomy.

For individuals with dysphagia grades IV and higher, additional treatment generally is necessary. The mainstay of therapy is indwelling esophageal stents. Covered removable stents may be used to seal fistulae or when stent removal becomes desirable in the future. When large, locally invasive tumors or metastatic esophageal cancer precludes any future hope of resection, uncovered expandable metal stents are the treatment of choice. The major limitations to stenting exist in cancers at the GEJ. A stent placed across the GEJ will result in severe gastroesophageal reflux and heartburn that can be quite disabling. In cancers at this level, radiation therapy alone may be preferable. If feeding access is desirable, a laparoscopic jejunostomy is usually the procedure of choice.

Surgical Treatment

The surgical treatment of esophageal cancer is dependent upon the location of the cancer, the depth of invasion, LN metastases, the fitness of the patient for operation, and the culture and beliefs of the individuals and institutions in which the treatment is performed. In an ideal world, there would be a single, stage-specific method of treating esophageal cancer, because the evidence would be unassailable and noncontroversial. Randomized clinical trials and meta-analyses would prove beyond a shadow of a doubt the value of surgery vs. nonoperative therapy and would dictate the type and extent of surgery that would optimally balance immediate morbidity and mortality with duration and quality of life conferred by the procedure and the perioperative management of the esophagectomy patient. Despite many noble attempts to establish this high level of evidence, many questions relating to the appropriate therapy of esophageal cancer remain controversial. About the only area of complete agreement is that esophagectomy should not be performed if an R0 resection is not possible. In other words, if the surgeon does not believe he or she can remove all LNs invaded by cancer and provide a tumor-free radial margin and esophagus and stomach margins that are tumor free, then a resection should not be performed.

Mucosally Based Cancer

In patients with BE, and especially those with high-grade dysplasia, subcentimeter nodules are frequently discovered. Nodules should be resected in entirety, as they often harbor adenocarcinoma. Five years ago, such resection was performed with a transhiatal esophagectomy, but greater comfort by therapeutic endoscopists with EMR offers another method for removing intramucosal cancer. Ideally, EMR starts with a very high-resolution EUS that can differentiate between nodules invading the submucosa and those confined to the mucosa. Tumors invading the submucosa are generally not felt amenable to endoscopic mucosal resection because of the high-frequency (20 to 25%) concurrent finding of positive LNs, which cannot be removed without esophagectomy. On the other hand, intramucosal cancers have little risk of spreading to regional LNs, as the esophageal lymphatics reach only to the level of the submucosa.

For this reason, small intramucosal carcinomas may be removed with EMR in the following manner: The area beneath the nodule is infiltrated with saline through a sclerotherapy needle. A specialized suction cap is mounted on the end of the endoscope and the nodule is drawn up into the cap, following which a snare is applied to resect the tissue. Alternatively, a rubber band can be delivered and the snare can be used to resect above the level of the rubber band. This specimen is then removed and sent to pathology. As long as the tumor is found to be confined to the mucosa and all margins are negative, the resection is complete. A positive margin or involvement of the submucosa warrants esophagectomy. Most importantly, these patients are at high risk for developing small nodular carcinomas elsewhere in their Barrett's segment, and routine surveillance on a 3- to 6-month basis must be continued indefinitely. Alternatively, one can consider radiofrequency ablation of the remainder of the high-grade dysplasia after careful surveillance biopsies demonstrate

TABLE 25-13	Functional grades of dysphagia	
Grade	**Definition**	**Incidence at Diagnosis (%)**
I	Eating normally	11
II	Requires liquids with meals	21
III	Able to take semisolids but unable to take any solid food	30
IV	Able to take liquids only	40
V	Unable to take liquids, but able to swallow saliva	7
VI	Unable to swallow saliva	12

Source: Modified with permission from Takita H, et al: Squamous cell carcinoma of the esophagus: A study of 153 cases. *J Surg Oncol* 9:547, 1977.

no further sign of cancer. This approach to the early esophageal cancer should not be used when there is any suspicion of mediastinal or abdominal lymphadenopathy. Although it is currently rare that EMR provides definitive therapy of small nodular esophageal cancers, this may become more of the norm as greater surveillance reveals earlier cancers, and proficiency of the technique by surgeons and gastroenterologists increases. In addition, EMR allows a "large-particle biopsy," which may be helpful in directing surgical therapy, and targeted therapies "personalized" for the genotype and phenotype of each individual tumor.

Minimally Invasive Transhiatal Esophagectomy

Minimally invasive transhiatal esophagectomy is an increasingly popular procedure; however, the number of these operations performed around the world remains small. Mini-invasive surgery (MIS) transhiatal esophagectomy was first performed by Aureo DePaula in Brazil and has been modified and adopted by many individuals around the world. This operation combines the advantages of transhiatal esophagectomy at minimizing pulmonary complications with the advantages of laparoscopy (less pain, quicker rehabilitation). Several variations of MIS transhiatal esophagectomy have been developed. For the earliest lesions, such as high-grade dysplasia or intramucosal carcinoma, a vagal sparing procedure can be entertained. In such a procedure, the vagal trunks are separated from the esophagus at the level of the diaphragm and the lesser curvature dissection of the stomach allows the vagus and left gastric pedicle to remain intact. Clearly, this dissection, which hugs the stomach and esophagus, provides no LN staging and is thus inadequate for all high-grade dysplasia and intramucosal cancer.

MIS transhiatal esophagectomy is usually performed through five or six small incisions in the upper abdomen and a transverse cervical incision for removing the specimen and performing the cervical esophagogastrostomy. To remove the esophagus from the posterior mediastinum, especially the area behind the pulmonary vessels and the tracheal bifurcation, which cannot be visualized even with a long laparoscope placed in the posterior mediastinum, it is preferred to use a vein stripping "inversion" technique (Fig. 25-70A). The details of this operation are too lengthy to include in this text, but include the laparoscopic creation of a 4-cm neoesophagus (gastric conduit) along the greater curvature of the stomach using the right gastroepiploic artery as the primary vascular pedicle. The conduit can be created through a mini-laparotomy or laparoscopically. A Kocher maneuver releases the duodenum, and a pyloroplasty may be performed (optional). Retrograde esophageal stripping is performed by dividing the esophagus below the GEJ and sliding a vein stripper from the neck down into the abdomen followed by an inversion of the esophagus in the posterior mediastinum and removal through the neck (Fig. 25-70B). This technique is reserved for patients with high-grade dysplasia and only microscopically detectable cancer. For small cancers at the GEJ, the esophagus can be stripped in an antegrade fashion by sliding the vein stripper down from the cervical incision and out the tail of the lesser curvature (Fig. 25-70C). The tail of the lesser curvature is pulled out a port site high in the epigastrium and used as a wound protector while the esophagus is inverted on itself. For GEJ cancers, a wide celiac access LN dissection, splenic artery, hepatic artery, and posterior mediastinal LN dissection can be performed as well or better than through a laparotomy. The gastric conduit is pulled up to the neck with a chest tube and anastomosed to the cervical esophagus in an end-to-side fashion using a surgical stapler or with a handsewn anastomosis. This method of esophagogastrectomy may mitigate the need for intensive care unit care, and shorten the hospitalization to the time necessary for anatomic healing. Complications of this technique have been rare and primarily limited to leak from the esophagogastric anastomosis, which is self-limited and usually heals within 1 to 3 weeks, spontaneously.

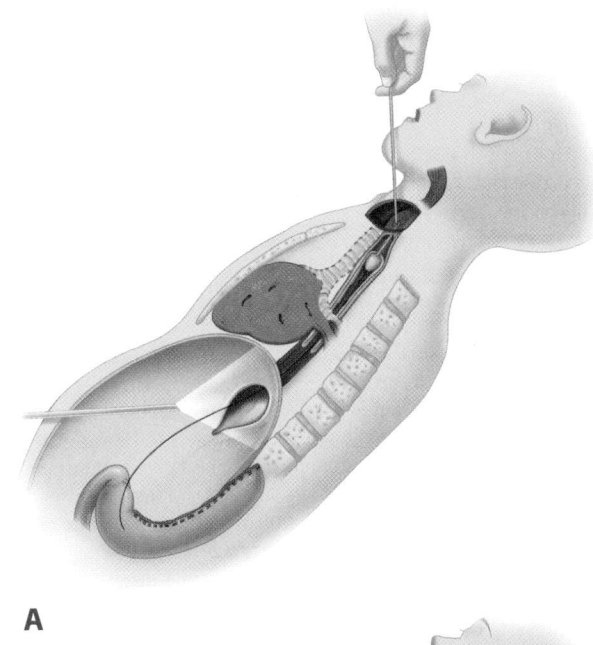

A

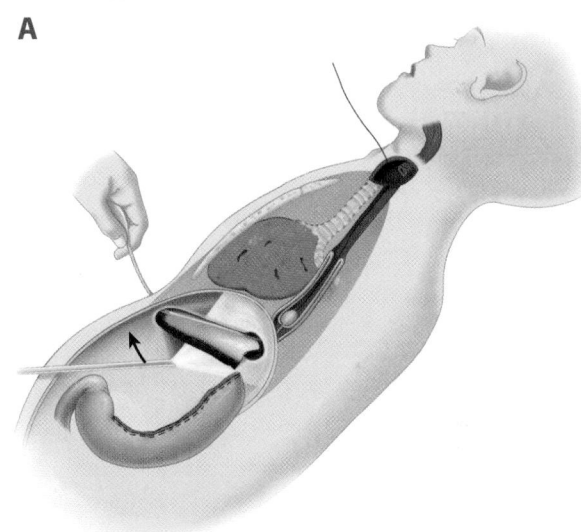

B

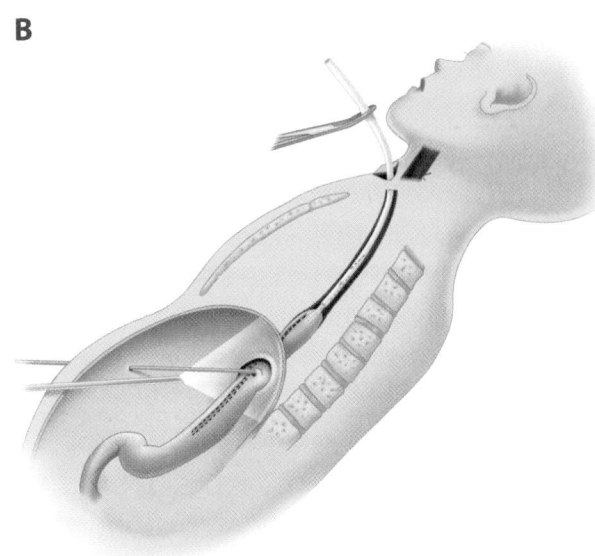

C

FIG. 25-70. A. Laparoscopic retrograde inversion. **B.** Laparoscopic antegrade inversion. A silk suture holds the tunnel after the esophagus is removed. **C.** The esophageal conduit is returned to the neck after passing a chest tube down the tunnel and suturing the conduit to the chest tube.

Open Transhiatal Esophagectomy

Transhiatal esophagectomy, also known as *blunt esophagectomy* or *esophagectomy without a thoracotomy*, was first performed in 1933 by a British surgeon, but was popularized in the last quarter of the twentieth century by Mark Orringer from the University of Michigan. Although this operation may violate many of the principles of cancer resection, including extended radical LN dissection, this operation has performed as well as any of the more radical procedures in randomized trials, and in large database analyses. With transhiatal esophagectomy, the elements of dissection are similar to that described in the section entitled Minimally Invasive Transhiatal Esophagectomy including the creation of the gastric tube and the posterior mediastinal dissection through the hiatus. Because this dissection is performed with the fingertips rather than under direct vision with surgical instruments, it requires an enlargement of the diaphragmatic hiatus. The lower mediastinal LN basins can be resected as can the upper abdominal LNs, making this an attractive option for GEJ cancers. The mediastinal LNs above the inferior pulmonary vein are not removed with this technique, but rarely result in a point of isolated cancer recurrence.

Of all procedures for esophageal cancer, this operation is the quickest to perform in experienced hands and lies in an intermediate position between minimally invasive esophagectomy and the Ivor Lewis procedure with respect to complications and recovery.

Minimally Invasive Two- and Three-Field Esophagectomy

After a rocky start, minimally invasive esophagectomy using a thoracic dissection through VATS has become reasonably popular. In general, this operation is performed with an anastomosis created in the neck (three-field), but may be performed with the anastomosis stapled in the high thorax (two-field). Both procedures will be described.

With a minimally invasive three-field esophagectomy, the patient is placed in the left lateral decubitus position. Double lumen intubation is required. Videoscopic access to the thorax is obtained in the midaxillary line in the ninth intercostal space and an angled telescope illuminates the chest superiorly. A mini-thoracotomy at about the sixth intercostal space anteriorly allows introduction of conventional surgical instruments, and a high trocar allows retraction of the lung away from the esophagus. In a three-field approach, the esophagus is dissected out along its length to include division of the azygos vein and harvesting of the LNs in the upper, middle, and lower posterior mediastinum. Hilar, aortopulmonary window, and posterior mediastinal nodes are all removed and sent with the specimen or individually. The thoracic duct is divided at the level of the diaphragm and removed with the specimen.

Following complete intrathoracic dissection, the patient is placed in the supine position and five laparoscopic ports are placed as with the MIS transhiatal esophagectomy. The abdominal portions of the operation are identical to those described previously in the section entitled Minimally Invasive Transhiatal Esophagectomy, and the gastric conduit is then sewn to the tip of the fully mobilized GEJ and lesser curvature sleeve. A feeding tube is placed and the pyloroplasty may be performed laparoscopically if the surgeon feels so inclined. A transverse cervical incision and dissection between the sternomastoid and the anterior strap muscles allows access to the cervical esophagus. Great care is made to avoid stretching the recurrent laryngeal nerve. The esophagus and proximal stomach is then pulled up into the neck with the gastric conduit following. Cervical anastomosis is then performed.

The MIS transthoracic two-field esophagectomy is slightly different. In this operation, the abdominal portions of the operation are done first, including placement of the feeding tube, the creation of the conduit, and the sewing of the tip of the conduit to the fully dissected GEJ. The patient is then rolled into the left lateral decubitus position and, through right thoracoscopy, the esophagus is dissected out and divided 10 cm above the tumor. Once freed, the specimen is pulled out through the mini-thoracotomy and an end-to-end anastomosis stapler is introduced through the high corner of the gastric conduit and out a stab wound along the greater curvature. The anvil of the stapler is placed in the proximal esophagus and held with a purse-string, the stapler is docked, the anastomosis is created, and a gastrotomy is then closed with another firing of the GIA stapler. The three-field esophagectomy has the advantage of placing the anastomosis in the neck where leakage is unlikely to create a severe systemic consequence. On the other hand, placement of the anastomosis in the high chest minimizes the risks of injury to structures in the neck, particularly the recurrent laryngeal nerve. Although the leak of the intrathoracic anastomosis may be more likely to bear septic consequences, the incidence of leak is diminished. Other complications of this approach relate to pulmonary and cardiac status. In many series, the most common complication is pneumonia, the second is atrial fibrillation, and the third is anastomotic leak.

Ivor Lewis (En Bloc) Esophagectomy

The theory behind radical transthoracic esophagectomy is that greater removal of LNs and periesophageal tissues diminishes the chance of a positive radial margin and LN recurrence. Although there are no randomized data demonstrating this to be superior to other forms of esophagectomy, there are many retrospective data demonstrating improved survival with greater numbers of LNs harvested. A recent study from Sloan-Kettering demonstrates a direct relationship between the number of negative nodes harvested and long-term survival. Although such a survival advantage may be related to the completeness of resection, extended radical resections may also be a surrogate for experienced surgeons working in great institutions. As a time-honored operation, there is no doubt that en bloc esophagectomy is the standard to which less radical techniques must be compared.

Generally, this operation is started in the abdomen with an upper midline laparotomy and extensive LN dissection in and about the celiac access and its branches, extending into the porta hepatis and along the splenic artery to the tail of the pancreas. All LNs are removed en bloc with the lesser curvature of the stomach. Unless the tumor extends into the stomach, reconstruction is performed with a greater curvature gastric tube. For GEJ cancers extending significantly into the gastric cardia or fundus, the proximal stomach is removed and reconstruction is performed with an isoperistaltic section of left colon between the upper esophagus and the remnant stomach, or the colon is connected to a Roux-en-Y limb of jejunum, if total gastrectomy is necessary. In the majority of cases, colon interposition is unnecessary, and a 4-cm gastric conduit is used.

Following closure of the abdominal incision, the patient is placed in the left lateral decubitus position and an anterolateral thoracotomy is performed through the sixth intercostal space. The azygos vein is divided and the posterior mediastinum is entirely cleaned out to include the thoracic duct, all periaortic tissues, and all tissue in the upper mediastinum along the course of the current laryngeal nerves and in the peribronchial, hilar, and tracheal LN stations. The proximal stomach is pulled up into the thorax where a conduit is created (if not performed previously) and a handsewn or stapled anastomosis is made between the upper thoracic esophagus and the gastric conduit or transverse colon. Chest tubes are placed, and the patient is taken to the intensive care unit.

Because this is the most radical of dissections, complications are most common, including pneumonia, respiratory failure, atrial fibrillation, chylothorax, anastomotic leak, conduit necrosis, gastrocutaneous fistula, and, if dissection is too near the recurrent laryngeal nerves, hoarseness or other vocal cord dysfunction. Tracheobronchial injury resulting in fistulas between the bronchus and conduit may also occur, however rarely. Although this procedure and three-field esophagectomy are fraught with the highest complication rate, the long-term outcome of this procedure provides the greatest survival in many single-center series and retrospective reviews.

Three-Field Open Esophagectomy

Three-field open esophagectomy is very similar to a minimally invasive three-field except that all access is through open incisions.

This procedure is preferred by certain Japanese surgeons and LN counts achieved through this kind of operation may run from 45 to 60 LNs. Most Western surgeons question the benefit of such radical surgery when it is hard to define a survival advantage. Nonetheless, high intrathoracic cancers probably deserve such an aggressive approach if cure is the goal.

Salvage Esophagectomy

"Salvage esophagectomy" is the nomenclature applied to esophagectomy performed after failure of definitive radiation and chemotherapy. The most frequent scenario is one in which distant disease (bone, lung, brain, or wide LN metastases) renders the patient nonoperable at initial presentation. Then, systemic chemotherapy, usually with radiation of the primary tumor, destroys all foci of metastasis, as demonstrated by CT and CT-PET, but the primary remains present and symptomatic. Following a period of observation, to make sure no new disease will "pop up," salvage esophagectomy is performed, usually with an open two-field approach. Surprisingly, the cure rate of salvage esophagectomy is not inconsequential. One in four patients undergoing this operation will be disease free 5 years later, despite the presence of residual cancer in the operative specimen. Because of the dense scarring created by radiation treatment, this procedure is the most technically challenging of all esophagectomy techniques.

Comparative Studies of Esophagectomy Technique
Transthoracic vs. Transhiatal Esophagectomy

There has been a great debate as to whether en bloc esophagectomy will provide a greater long-term benefit and cure rate in esophageal cancer than transhiatal esophagectomy. In a recent 7-year follow-up of a Dutch study addressing GEJ and lower esophageal cancers, there does not appear to be any benefit to the more extensive dissection despite higher morbidity and mortality. In a subgroup analysis of those with one to eight positive LNs, it did appear that the en bloc transthoracic resection may add to longevity. In another large database analysis of the Surveillance, Epidemiology, and End Results database, transthoracic and transhiatal esophagectomy were compared. In this study, the transhiatal esophagectomy had a greater long-term survival, but, when adjusted by cancer stage, this survival benefit disappeared. The mortality and morbidity after transhiatal esophagectomy appeared to be less. Suffice it to say that this debate over the best procedure for esophagectomy remains an open question.

The role of the minimally invasive surgical procedures for a cancer cure will require further study and longer follow-up. It would appear from preliminary analysis that the transhiatal esophagectomy, like its open cousin, may be performed with less morbidity and mortality than the VATS procedure. Long-term survival analyses will require careful follow-up for at least 5 to 10 years after cancer treatment.

Alternative Therapies
Radiation Therapy

Primary treatment with radiation therapy does not produce results comparable with those obtained with surgery. Currently, the use of radiotherapy is restricted to patients who are not candidates for surgery, and is usually combined with chemotherapy. Radiation alone is used for palliation of dysphagia but the benefit is short lived, lasting only 2 to 3 months. Furthermore, the length and course of treatment are difficult to justify in patients with a limited life expectancy.

Adjuvant Chemotherapy

The proposal to use adjuvant chemotherapy in the treatment of esophageal cancer began when it became evident that most patients develop postoperative systemic metastasis without local recurrence. This observation led to the hypothesis that undetected systemic micrometastasis had been present at the time of diagnosis, and, if

effective systemic therapy was added to local regional therapy, survival should improve.

Recently, this hypothesis has been supported by the observation of epithelial tumor cells in the bone marrow in 37% of patients with esophageal cancer who were resected for cure. These patients had a greater prevalence of relapse at 9 months after surgery compared to those patients without such cells. Such studies emphasize that hematogenous dissemination of viable malignant cells occurs early in the disease, and that systemic chemotherapy may be helpful if the cells are sensitive to the agent. On the other hand, systemic chemotherapy may be a hindrance, because of its immunosuppressive properties, if the cells are resistant. Unfortunately, current technology is not able to test tumor cell sensitivity to chemotherapeutic drugs. This requires that the choice of drugs be made solely on the basis of their clinical effectiveness against grossly similar tumors.

The decision to use preoperative rather than postoperative chemotherapy was based on the ineffectiveness of chemotherapeutic agents when used after surgery, and animal studies suggesting that agents given before surgery were more effective. The claim that patients who receive chemotherapy before resection are less likely to develop resistance to the drugs is unsupported by hard evidence. The claim that drug delivery is enhanced because blood flow is more robust before patients undergo surgical dissection is similarly flawed, due to the fact that if enough blood reaches the operative site to heal the wound or anastomosis, then the flow should be sufficient to deliver chemotherapeutic drugs. There are, however, data supporting the claim that preoperative chemotherapy in patients with esophageal carcinoma can, if effective, facilitate surgical resection by reducing the size of the tumor. This is particularly beneficial in the case of squamous cell tumors above the level of the carina. Reducing the size of the tumor may provide a safer margin between the tumor and the trachea, and allow an anastomosis to a tumor-free cervical esophagus just below the cricopharyngeus. Involved margin at this level usually requires a laryngectomy to prevent subsequent local recurrence.

Preoperative Chemotherapy

Eight randomized prospective studies of neoadjuvant chemotherapy vs. surgery alone have demonstrated mixed results. For adenocarcinomas of the distal esophagus and proximal stomach, preoperative neoadjuvant 5-fluorouracil (5-FU) and cisplatin chemotherapy has been shown to provide a survival advantage over surgery alone in a well-powered study from the United Kingdom (MRC trial). This trial is one of the few to include enough patients (800) to detect small differences. The trial had a 10% absolute survival benefit at 2 years for the neoadjuvant chemotherapy group. In a second trial from the United Kingdom (MAGIC trial) of distal esophageal and proximal gastric adenocarcinomas, the use of epirubicin in combination with cisplatin and 5-FU also demonstrated a survival advantage for the induction chemotherapy arm with 4 years median follow-up, As a result of these two trials, standard treatment of locally advanced adenocarcinoma in Europe calls for neoadjuvant chemotherapy with one of these two regimens. Most failures are due to distant metastatic disease, underscoring the need for improved systemic therapy. Postoperative septic and respiratory complications may be more common in patients receiving chemotherapy.

Preoperative Combination Chemo- and Radiotherapy

Preoperative chemoradiotherapy using cisplatin and 5-FU in combination with radiotherapy has been reported by several investigators to be beneficial in both adenocarcinoma and squamous cell carcinoma of the esophagus. There have been 10 randomized prospective studies (Table 25-14). A recent meta-analysis of these trials demonstrates a 13% survival advantage for neoadjuvant chemoradiation therapy, which is more pronounced for patients with adenocarcinoma than for those with squamous carcinoma (Table 25-15). It was also observed that the benefit for chemotherapy alone (7%) was not as dramatic as for chemoradiotherapy used in the neoadjuvant setting.

TABLE 25-14 Randomized trials of neoadjuvant chemoradiotherapy vs. surgery, or neoadjuvant chemotherapy vs. surgery

Year Activated	Treatment Schedule (Radiotherapy)	Treatment Schedule (Chemotherapy)	Concurrent or Sequential	Tumor Type	Sample Size	Median Follow-Up (Mo)
Chemoradiotherapy						
1983	35 Gy, 1.75 Gy/fraction over 4 wk	Two cycles: cisplatin 20 mg/m² d 1–5; bleomycin 5 mg/m² d 1–5	Sequential	SCC	78	18[a]
1986	40 Gy, 2 Gy/fraction over 4 wk	Two cycles: cisplatin 100 mg/m² d 1; 5-fluorouracil 1000 mg/m² days 1–4	Concurrent	SCC	69	12[a]
1988	20 Gy, 2 Gy/fraction over 12 d	Two cycles: cisplatin 100 mg/m² d 1; 5-fluorouracil 600 mg/m² d 2–5, 22–25	Sequential	SCC	86	12[a]
1989	45 Gy, 1.5 Gy/fraction over 3 wk	Two cycles: cisplatin 20 mg/m² d 1–5; 5-fluorouracil 300 mg/m² d 1–21; vinblastine 1 mg/m² d 1–4	Concurrent	SCC and adeno-carcinoma	100	98
1989	37 Gy, 3.7 Gy/fraction over 2 wk	Two cycles: cisplatin 80 mg/m² d 0–2	Sequential	SCC	293	55
1990	40 Gy, 2.7 Gy/fraction over 3 wk	Two cycles: cisplatin 75 mg/m² d 7; 5-fluorouracil 15 mg/kg d 1–5	Concurrent	Adenocarcinoma	113	24
1990	40 Gy, 2.7 Gy/fraction over 3 wk	Two cycles: cisplatin 75 mg/m² d 7; 5-fluorouracil 15 mg/kg d 1–5	Concurrent	SCC	61	10
1994	35 Gy, 2.3 Gy/fraction over 3 wk	One cycle: cisplatin 80 mg/m² d 1; 5-fluorouracil 800 mg/m² d 2–5	Concurrent	SCC and adeno-carcinoma	256	65
2006	50.4 Gy, 1.8 Gy/fraction over 5.6 wk	Two cycles: cisplatin 60 mg/m² d 1; 5-fluorouracil 1000 mg/m² d 3–5	Concurrent	SCC and adeno-carcinoma	56	60
1999	45.6 Gy, 1.2 Gy/fraction over 28 d	Two cycles: cisplatin 60 mg/m² d 1; 5-fluorouracil 1000 mg/m² d 3–5	Concurrent	SCC	101	25
Chemotherapy						
1982	—	Two cycles: cisplatin 120 mg/m² d 1; vindesine 3 mg/m² d 1, 8; bleomycin 10 U/m² d 3–6	—	SCC	39	20
1983	—	Two cycles: cisplatin 20 mg/m² d 1–5; bleomycin 5 mg/m² d 1–5	—	SCC	106	18[a]
1988[c]	—	Three cycles: cisplatin 20 mg/m² d 1–5; 5-fluorouracil 1000 mg/m² d 1–5	—	SCC	46	75
1988	—	Two cycles: cisplatin 100 mg/m² d 1; bleomycin 10 mg/m² d 3–8; vinblastine 3 mg/m² d 1, 8	—	SCC	46	17[a]
1989	—	Two cycles: cisplatin 100 mg/m² d 1; 5-fluorouracil 1000 mg/m² d 1–5	—	SCC	147	17
1990	—	Two cycles: cisplatin 80 mg/m² d 1; etoposide 200 mg/m² d 1–5	—	SCC	160	19[a]
1990	—	Three cycles: cisplatin 100 mg/m² 1; 5-fluorouracil 1000 mg/m² days 1–5	—	SCC and adeno-carcinoma	467	56
1992	—	Two cycles: cisplatin 100 mg/m² d 1; 5-fluorouracil 1000 mg/m² d 1–5	—	SCC	96	24
1992	—	Two cycles: cisplatin 80 mg/m² d 1; 5-fluorouracil 1000 mg/m² d 1–4	—	SCC and adeno-carcinoma	802	37

[a]Estimated as median survival.
[b]Unpublished thesis.
[c]Year of activation not reported, but imputed.
[d]Only available as an abstract.
SCC = squamous cell carcinoma.
Source: Reproduced with permission from Gebski V, et al for the Australasian Gastro-Intestinal Trials Group (eds): Survival benefits from neoadjuvant chemoradiotherapy or chemotherapy in oesophageal carcinoma: A meta-analysis. *Lancet Oncol* 8:226, 2007. Table 1, p 228. Copyright Elsevier.

Additionally, other work has demonstrated the importance of obtaining an R0 (tumor-free) resection as the most important variable determining long-term survival. Although there are not direct, randomized comparisons between chemotherapy and chemoradiation therapy, it appears that the addition of radiation may improve local response of the tumor, and may allow a greater opportunity for the surgeon to obtain an R0 resection.

The timing of surgery after chemoradiation induction is generally felt to be optimal between 6 and 8 weeks following the completion of induction therapy. Earlier than this time, active inflammation may make the resection hazardous, and the patients have not had time to recover fully from the chemoradiation. After 8 weeks, edema in the periesophageal tissue starts to turn to scar tissue, making dissection more difficult.

With chemoradiation, the complete response rates for adenocarcinoma range from 17 to 24% (Table 25-16). No tumor is detected in the specimen after esophagectomy. Patients demonstrating a complete response to chemoradiation have a better survival rate than those without complete response, but distant failure remains common.

At present, the strongest predictors of outcome of patients with esophageal cancer are the anatomic extent of the tumor at diagnosis and the completeness of tumor removal by surgical resection. After incomplete resection of an esophageal cancer, the 5-year survival

TABLE 25-15	Results of the meta-analysis applied to effects of preoperative chemoradiotherapy and chemotherapy on 2-y survival for patients with various levels of risk

| | | Expected 2-y Mortality | | | |
Risk Group	2-y Survival Rate (%)	Control (%)	Treated[a] (%)	ARR (%)	NNT
Chemoradiotherapy					
High	20	80	64.8	15.2	7
Medium	35	65	52.7	12.3	8
Low	50	50	40.5	9.5	10
Chemotherapy					
High	20	80	72.0	12.0	8
Medium	35	65	58.5	6.5	15
Low	50	50	45.0	5.0	20

[a]Based on a 19% relative mortality reduction for those receiving concurrent chemoradiotherapy and a 10% relative mortality reduction for those receiving chemotherapy.
ARR = absolute risk reduction; NNT = number needed to treat to prevent one death.
Source: Reproduced with permission from Gebski V, et al for the Australasian Gastro-Intestinal Trials Group (eds): Survival benefits from neoadjuvant chemoradiotherapy or chemotherapy in oesophageal carcinoma: A meta-analysis. *Lancet Oncol* 8:226, 2007. Table 2, p 231. Copyright Elsevier.

rates are 0 to 5%. In contrast, after complete resection, independent of stage of disease, 5-year survival ranges from 15 to 40%, according to selection criteria and stage distribution. The importance of early recognition and adequate surgical resection cannot be overemphasized. Figure 25-71 is a global algorithm for the management of esophageal carcinoma.

SARCOMA OF THE ESOPHAGUS

Sarcomas and carcinosarcomas are rare neoplasms, accounting for approximately 0.1 to 1.5% of all esophageal tumors. They present with the symptom of dysphagia, which does not differ from the dysphagia associated with the more common epithelial carcinoma. Tumors located within the cervical or high thoracic esophagus can cause symptoms of pulmonary aspiration secondary to esophageal obstruction. Large tumors originating at the level of the tracheal bifurcation can produce symptoms of airway obstruction and syncope by direct compression of the tracheobronchial tree and heart (Fig. 25-72). The duration of dysphagia and age of the patients affected with these tumors are similar to those with carcinoma of the esophagus.

A barium swallow usually shows a large polypoid intraluminal esophageal mass, causing partial obstruction and dilatation of the esophagus proximal to the tumor (Fig. 25-73). The smooth polypoid nature of the lesion, although not diagnostic, is distinctive enough to suggest the presence of a sarcoma rather than the more common ulcerating, stenosing carcinoma.

Esophagoscopy commonly shows an intraluminal necrotic mass. When biopsy is attempted, it is important to remove the necrotic tissue until bleeding is seen on the tumor's surface. When this is not done, the biopsy specimen will show only tissue necrosis. Even when viable tumor is obtained on biopsy, it has been these authors' experience that it cannot be definitively identified as carcinoma, sarcoma, or carcinosarcoma on the basis of the histology of the portion biopsied. Biopsy results cannot be totally relied on to identify the presence of sarcoma, and it is often the polypoid nature of the lesion that arouses suspicion that it may be something other than carcinoma.

Polypoid sarcomas of the esophagus, in contrast to infiltrating carcinomas, remain superficial to the muscularis propria and are less likely to metastasize to regional LNs. In one series of 14 patients, local extension or tumor metastasis would have prevented a potentially curative resection in only five. Thus, the presence of a large polypoid tumor should not deter the surgeon from resecting the lesion.

Sarcomatous lesions of the esophagus can be divided into epidermoid carcinomas with spindle cell features, such as carcinosarcoma, and true sarcomas that arise from mesenchymal tissue, such as leiomyosarcoma, fibrosarcoma, and rhabdomyosarcoma. Based on current histologic criteria for diagnosis, fibrosarcoma and rhabdomyosarcoma of the esophagus are extremely rare lesions and may not, in fact, exist.

TABLE 25-16	Results of neoadjuvant therapy in adenocarcinoma of the esophagus

Institution	Year	No. of Patients	Regimen	Complete Pathologic Response (%)	Survival
M. D. Anderson	1990	35	P, E, 5-FU	3	42% at 3 y
SLMC	1992	18	P, 5-FU, RT	17	40% at 3 y
Vanderbilt	1993	39	P, E, 5-FU, RT	19	47% at 4 y
Michigan	1993	21	P, VBL, 5-FU, RT	24	34% at 5 y
MGH	1994	16	P, 5-FU	0	42% at 4 y
MGH	1994	22	E, A, P	5	58% at 2 y

A = doxorubicin; E = etoposide; 5-FU = 5-fluorouracil; MGH = Massachusetts General Hospital; P = cisplatin; RT = radiation therapy; SLMC = St. Louis University Medical Center; VBL = vinblastine.
Source: Reproduced with permission from Wright CD, et al: Evolution of treatment strategies for adenocarcinoma of the esophagus and gastroesophageal junction. *Ann Thorac Surg* 58:1574, 1994. Copyright Elsevier.

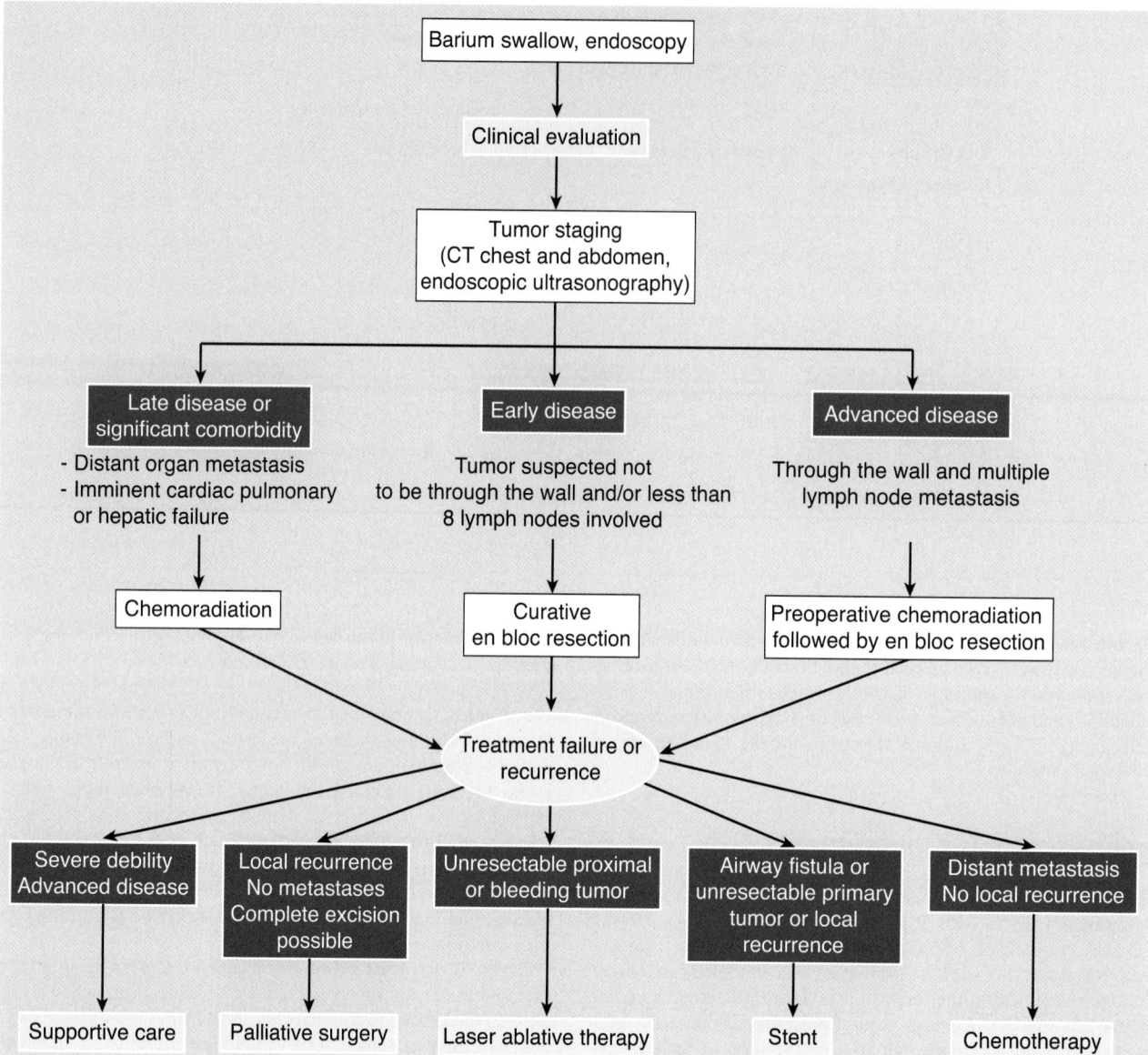

FIG. 25-71. Suggested global algorithm for the management of carcinoma of the esophagus. CT = computed tomography.

Surgical resection of polypoid sarcoma of the esophagus is the treatment of choice, because radiation therapy has little success and the tumors remain superficial, with local invasion or distant metastases occurring late in the course of the disease. As with carcinoma, the absence of both wall penetration and LN metastases is necessary for curative treatment, and surgical resection is consequently responsible for the majority of the reported 5-year survivals. Resection also provides an excellent means of palliating the patient's symptoms. The surgical technique for resection and the subsequent restoration of the GI continuity is similar to that described for carcinoma.

In these authors' experience, four of the eight patients with carcinosarcoma survived for 5 years or longer. Even though this number is small, it suggests that resection produces better results in epithelial carcinoma with spindle cell features than in squamous cell carcinoma of the esophagus. Similarly, with leiomyosarcoma of the esophagus, the same scattered reports exist with little information on survival. Of seven patients with leiomyosarcoma, two died from their disease—one in 3 months and the other 4 years and 7 months after resection. The other five patients were reported to have survived more than 5 years.

It is difficult to evaluate the benefits of resection for leiomyoblastoma of the esophagus, due to the small number of reported patients with tumors in this location. Most leiomyoblastomas occur in the stomach, and 38% of these patients succumb to the cancer in 3 years. Fifty-five percent of patients with extragastric leiomyoblastoma also die from the disease, within an average of 3 years. Consequently, leiomyoblastoma should be considered a malignant lesion and apt to behave like a leiomyosarcoma. The presence of nuclear hyperchromatism, increased mitotic figures (more than one per high-power field), tumor size larger than 10 cm, and clinical symptoms of longer than 6 months' duration are associated with a poor prognosis.

BENIGN TUMORS AND CYSTS

Benign tumors and cysts of the esophagus are relatively uncommon. From the perspectives of both the clinician and the pathologist, benign tumors may be divided into those that are within the muscular wall and those that are within the lumen of the esophagus.

Intramural lesions are either solid tumors or cysts, and the vast majority are leiomyomas. They are made up of varying portions of smooth muscle and fibrous tissue. Fibromas, myomas, fibromyomas, and lipomyomas are closely related and occur rarely. Other histologic types of solid intramural tumors have been described,

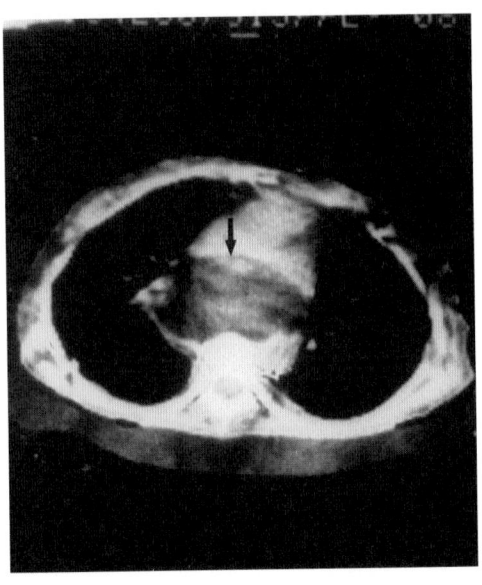

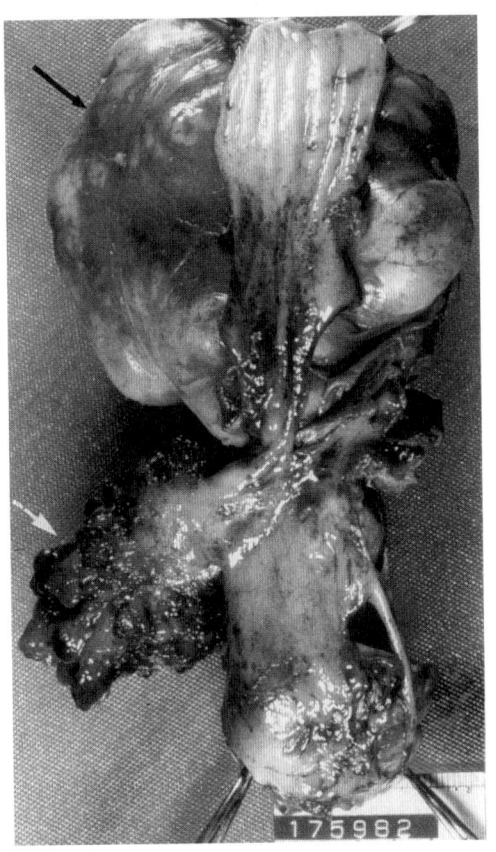

FIG. 25-72. **A.** Computed tomographic scan of a leiomyosarcoma (*black arrow*) that caused compression of the heart and symptoms of syncope. **B.** Surgical specimen of leiomyosarcoma shown in **A** with a pedunculated luminal lesion (*white arrow*) and a large extraesophageal component (*black arrow*). There was no evidence of lymph node metastasis at the time of operation.

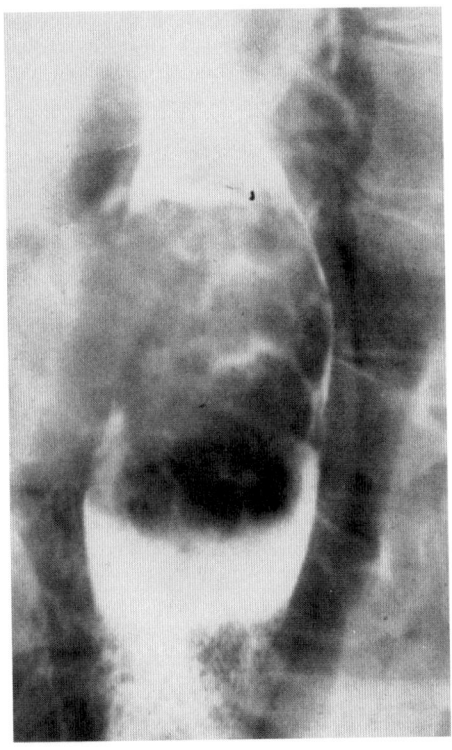

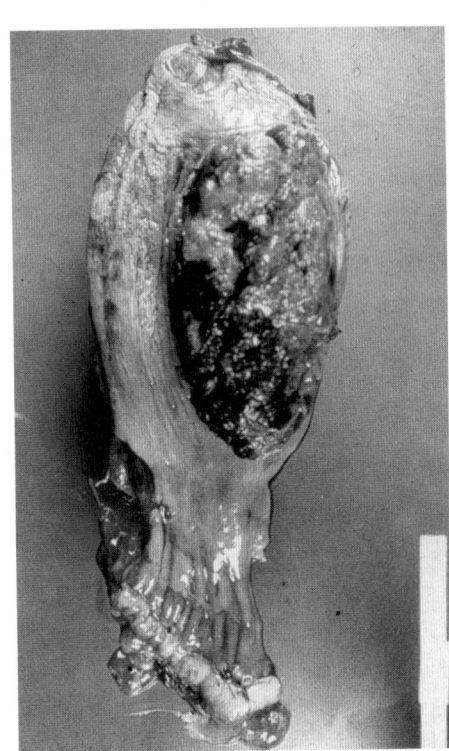

FIG. 25-73. **A.** Barium swallow showing a large polypoid intraluminal esophageal mass causing partial obstruction and dilation of the proximal esophagus. **B.** Operative specimen showing 9-cm polypoid leiomyoblastoma.

such as lipomas, neurofibromas, hemangiomas, osteochondromas, granular cell myoblastomas, and glomus tumors, but they are medical curiosities.

Intraluminal lesions are polypoid or pedunculated growths that usually originate in the submucosa, develop mainly into the lumen, and are covered with normal stratified squamous epithelium. The majority of these tumors are composed of fibrous tissue of varying degrees of compactness with a rich vascular supply. Some are loose and myxoid (e.g., myxoma and myxofibroma), some are more collagenous (e.g., fibroma), and some contain adipose tissue (e.g., fibrolipoma). These different types of tumor are frequently collectively designated as fibrovascular polyps, or simply as polyps. Pedunculated intraluminal tumors should be removed. If the lesion is not too large, endoscopic removal with a snare is feasible.

Leiomyoma

Leiomyomas constitute more than 50% of benign esophageal tumors. The average age at presentation is 38, which is in sharp contrast to that seen with esophageal carcinoma. Leiomyomas are twice as common in males. Because they originate in smooth muscle, 90% are located in the lower two thirds of the esophagus. They are usually solitary, but multiple tumors have been found on occasion. They vary greatly in size and shape. Tumors as small as 1 cm in diameter and as large as 10 lb have been removed.

Typically, leiomyomas are oval. During their growth, they remain intramural, having the bulk of their mass protruding toward the outer wall of the esophagus. The overlying mucosa is freely movable and normal in appearance. Neither their size nor location correlates with the degree of symptoms. Dysphagia and pain are the most common complaints, the two symptoms occurring more frequently together than separately. Bleeding directly related to the tumor is rare, and when hematemesis or melena occurs in a patient with an esophageal leiomyoma, other causes should be investigated.

A barium swallow is the most useful method to demonstrate a leiomyoma of the esophagus (Fig. 25-74). In profile, the tumor appears as a smooth, semilunar, or crescent-shaped filling defect that moves with swallowing, is sharply demarcated, and is covered and surrounded by normal mucosa. Esophagoscopy should be performed to exclude the reported observation of a coexistence with carcinoma. The freely movable mass, which bulges into the lumen,

should not be biopsied because of an increased chance of mucosal perforation at the time of surgical enucleation.

Despite their slow growth and limited potential for malignant degeneration, leiomyomas should be removed unless there are specific contraindications. The majority can be removed by simple enucleation. If, during removal, the mucosa is inadvertently entered, the defect can be repaired primarily. After tumor removal, the outer esophageal wall should be reconstructed by closure of the muscle layer. The location of the lesion and the extent of surgery required will dictate the approach. Lesions of the proximal and middle esophagus require a right thoracotomy, whereas distal esophageal lesions require a left thoracotomy. Videothoracoscopic approaches have been reported. The mortality rate associated with enucleation is <2%, and success in relieving the dysphagia is near 100%. Large lesions or those involving the GEJ may require esophageal resection.

Esophageal Cyst

Cysts may be congenital or acquired. Congenital cysts are lined wholly or partly by columnar ciliated epithelium of the respiratory type, by glandular epithelium of the gastric type, by squamous epithelium, or by transitional epithelium. In some, epithelial lining cells may be absent. Confusion over the embryologic origin of congenital cysts has led to a variety of names, such as enteric, bronchogenic, and mediastinal cysts. Acquired retention cysts also occur, probably as a result of obstruction of the excretory ducts of the esophageal glands.

Enteric and bronchogenic cysts are the most common, and arise as a result of developmental abnormalities during the formation and differentiation of the lower respiratory tract, esophagus, and stomach from the foregut. During its embryologic development, the esophagus is lined successively with simple columnar, pseudostratified ciliated columnar, and, finally, stratified squamous epithelium. This sequence probably accounts for the fact that the lining epithelium may be any or a combination of these; the presence of cilia does not necessarily indicate a respiratory origin.

Cysts vary in size from small to very large, and are usually located intramurally in the middle to lower third of the esophagus. Their symptoms are similar to those of a leiomyoma. The diagnosis similarly depends on radiographic and endoscopic findings. Surgical excision by enucleation is the preferred treatment. During removal, a fistulous tract connecting the cysts to the airways should be sought, particularly in patients who have had repetitive bronchopulmonary infections.

ESOPHAGEAL PERFORATION

Perforation of the esophagus constitutes a true emergency. It most commonly occurs following diagnostic or therapeutic procedures. Spontaneous perforation, referred to as *Boerhaave's syndrome*, accounts for only 15% of cases of esophageal perforation, foreign bodies for 14%, and trauma for 10%. Pain is a striking and consistent symptom and strongly suggests that an esophageal rupture has occurred, particularly if located in the cervical area following instrumentation of the esophagus, or substernally in a patient with a history of resisting vomiting. If subcutaneous emphysema is present, the diagnosis is almost certain.

Spontaneous rupture of the esophagus is associated with a high mortality rate because of the delay in recognition and treatment. Although there usually is a history of resisting vomiting, in a small number of patients, the injury occurs silently, without any antecedent history. When the chest radiogram of a patient with an esophageal perforation shows air or an effusion in the pleural space, the condition is often misdiagnosed as a pneumothorax or pancreatitis. An elevated serum amylase caused by the extrusion of saliva through the perforation may fix the diagnosis of pancreatitis in the mind of an unwary physician. If the chest radiogram is normal, a mistaken diagnosis of myocardial infarction or dissecting aneurysm is often made.

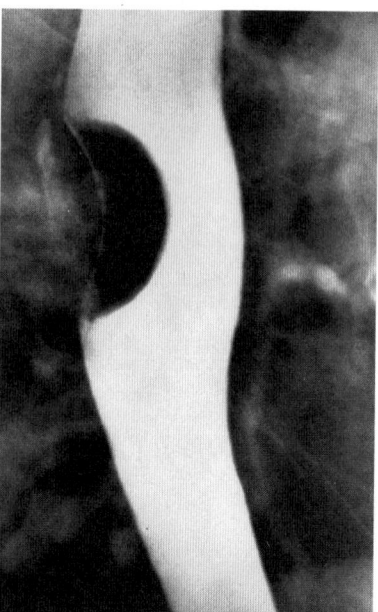

FIG. 25-74. Barium esophagogram showing a classical, smooth, contoured, punched-out defect of a leiomyoma.

Spontaneous rupture usually occurs into the left pleural cavity or just above the GEJ. Fifty percent of patients have concomitant GERD, suggesting that minimal resistance to the transmission of abdominal pressure into the thoracic esophagus is a factor in the pathophysiology of the lesion. During vomiting, high peaks of intragastric pressure can be recorded, frequently exceeding 200 mmHg, but because extragastric pressure remains almost equal to intragastric pressure, stretching of the gastric wall is minimal. The amount of pressure transmitted to the esophagus varies considerably, depending on the position of the GEJ. When it is in the abdomen and exposed to intra-abdominal pressure, the pressure transmitted to the esophagus is much less than when it is exposed to the negative thoracic pressure. In the latter situation, the pressure in the lower esophagus will frequently equal intragastric pressure if the glottis remains closed. Cadaver studies have shown that when this pressure exceeds 150 mmHg, rupture of the esophagus is apt to occur. When a hiatal hernia is present and the sphincter remains exposed to abdominal pressure, the lesion produced is usually a Mallory-Weiss mucosal tear, and bleeding rather than perforation is the problem. This is due to the stretching of the supradiaphragmatic portion of the gastric wall. In this situation, the hernia sac represents an extension of the abdominal cavity, and the GEJ remains exposed to abdominal pressure.

Diagnosis

Abnormalities on the chest radiogram can be variable and should not be depended upon to make the diagnosis. This is because the abnormalities are dependent on three factors: (a) the time interval between the perforation and the radiographic examination, (b) the site of perforation, and (c) the integrity of the mediastinal pleura. Mediastinal emphysema, a strong indicator of perforation, takes at least 1 hour to be demonstrated, and is present in only 40% of patients. Mediastinal widening secondary to edema may not occur for several hours. The site of perforation also can influence the radiographic findings. In cervical perforation, cervical emphysema is common and mediastinal emphysema rare; the converse is true for thoracic perforations. Frequently, air will be visible in the erector spinae muscles on a neck radiogram before it can be palpated or seen on a chest radiogram (Fig. 25-75). The integrity of the mediastinal pleura influences the radiographic abnormality in that rupture of the pleura results in a pneumothorax, a finding that is seen in 77% of patients. In two thirds of patients, the perforation is on the left side; in one fifth, it is on the right side; and in one tenth, it is bilateral. If pleural integrity is maintained, mediastinal emphysema (rather than a pneumothorax) appears rapidly. A pleural effusion secondary to inflammation of the mediastinum occurs late. In 9% of patients, the chest radiogram is normal.

The diagnosis is confirmed with a contrast esophagogram, which will demonstrate extravasation in 90% of patients. The use of a water-soluble medium such as Gastrografin is preferred. Of concern is that there is a 10% false-negative rate. This may be due to obtaining the radiographic study with the patient in the upright position. When the patient is upright, the passage of water-soluble contrast material can be too rapid to demonstrate a small perforation. The studies should be done with the patient in the right lateral decubitus position (Fig. 25-76). In this , the contrast material fills the entire length of the esophagus, allowing the actual site of perforation and its interconnecting cavities to be visualized in almost all patients.

Management

The key to optimum management is early diagnosis. The most favorable outcome is obtained following primary closure of the perforation within 24 hours, resulting in 80 to 90% survival. Figure 25-77 is an operative photograph taken through a left thoracotomy of an esophageal rupture following a pneumatic dilation for achalasia. The most common location for the injury is the left lateral wall of the esophagus, just above the GEJ. To get adequate exposure of the injury, a dissection similar to that described for esophageal

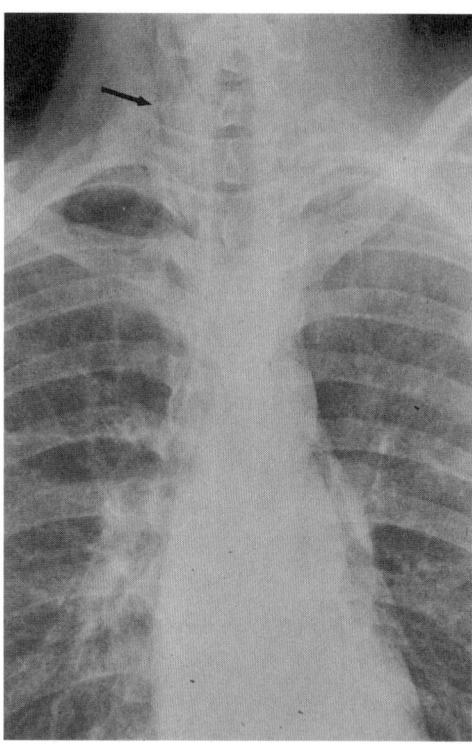

FIG. 25-75. Chest radiogram showing air in the deep muscles of the neck following perforation of the esophagus (*arrow*). This is often the earliest sign of perforation and can be present without evidence of air in the mediastinum.

myotomy is performed. A flap of stomach is pulled up and the soiled fat pad at the GEJ is removed. The edges of the injury are trimmed and closed using a modified Gambee stitch (Fig. 25-78). The closure is reinforced by the use of a pleural patch or construction of a Nissen fundoplication.

Mortality associated with immediate closure varies between 8 and 20%. After 24 hours, survival decreases to <50%, and is not influenced by the type of operative therapy (i.e., drainage alone or

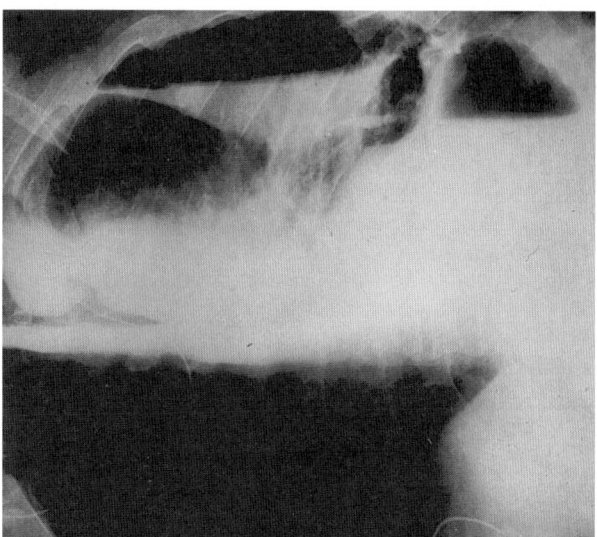

FIG. 25-76. Radiographic study of a patient with a perforation of the esophagus using water-soluble contrast material. The patient is placed in the lateral decubitus position with the left side up to allow complete filling of the esophagus and demonstration of the defect.

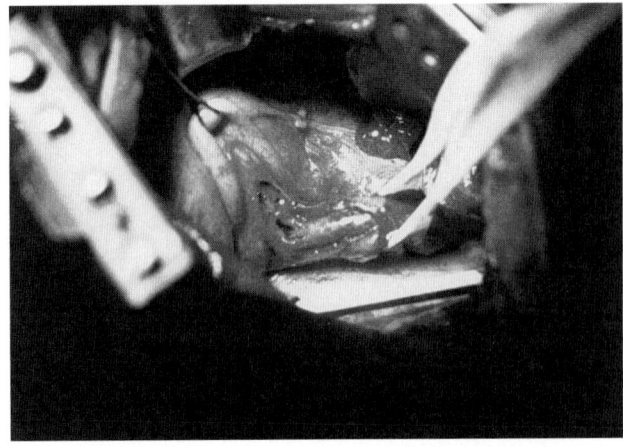

FIG. 25-77. Left thoracotomy in a patient with an esophageal rupture at the gastroesophageal junction following forceful dilation of the lower esophagus for achalasia (the surgical clamp is on the stomach, and the Penrose drain encircles the esophagus). The injury consists of a mucosal perforation and extensive splitting of the esophageal muscle from just below the Penrose drain to the stomach.

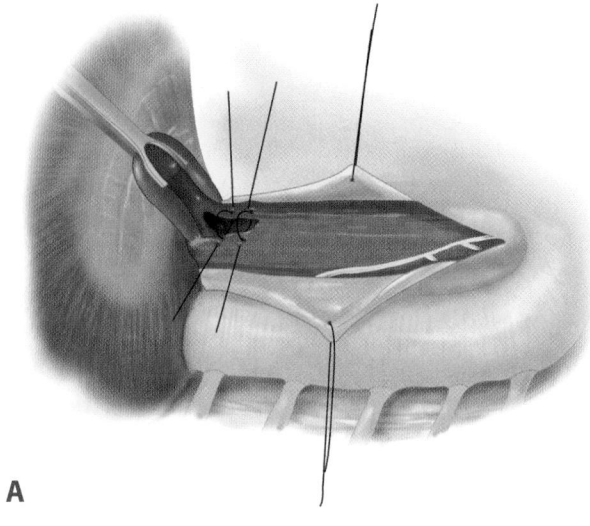

A

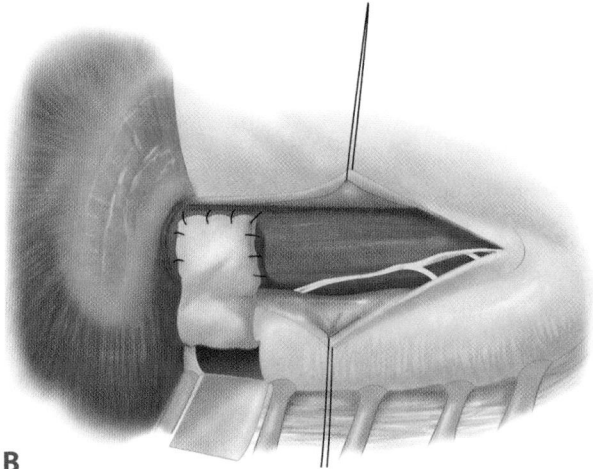

B

FIG. 25-78. The technique of closure of an esophageal perforation through a left thoracotomy. **A.** A tongue of stomach is pulled up through the esophageal hiatus, and the gastroesophageal fat pad is removed; the edges of the mucosal injury are trimmed and closed using interrupted modified Gambee stitches. **B.** Reinforcement of the closure with a parietal pleural patch.

drainage plus closure of the perforation). If the time delay before closing a perforation approaches 24 hours and the tissues are inflamed, division of the cardia and resection of the diseased portion of the esophagus are recommended. The remainder of the esophagus is mobilized, and as much normal esophagus as possible is saved and brought out as an end cervical esophagostomy. In some situations, the retained esophagus may be so long that it loops down into the chest. The contaminated mediastinum is drained and a feeding jejunostomy tube is inserted. The recovery from sepsis is often immediate, dramatic, and reflected by a marked improvement in the patient's condition over a 24-hour period. On recovery from the sepsis, the patient is discharged and returns on a subsequent date for reconstruction with a substernal colon interposition. Failure to apply this aggressive therapy can result in a mortality rate in excess of 50% in patients in whom the diagnosis has been delayed.

Nonoperative management of esophageal perforation has been advocated in select situations. The choice of conservative therapy requires skillful judgment and necessitates careful radiographic examination of the esophagus. This course of management usually follows an injury occurring during dilation of esophageal strictures or pneumatic dilations of achalasia. Conservative management should not be used in patients who have free perforations into the pleural space. Cameron proposed three criteria for the nonoperative management of esophageal perforation: (a) The barium swallow must show the perforation to be contained within the mediastinum and drain well back into the esophagus (Fig. 25-79), (b) symptoms should be mild, and (c) there should be minimal evidence of clinical sepsis. If these conditions are met, it is reasonable to treat the patient with hyperalimentation, antibiotics, and cimetidine to decrease acid secretion and diminish pepsin activity. Oral intake is resumed in 7 to 14 days, dependent on subsequent radiographic examinations.

MALLORY-WEISS SYNDROME

In 1929, Mallory and Weiss described four patients with acute upper GI bleeding who were found at autopsy to have mucosal tears at the GEJ. This syndrome, characterized by acute upper GI bleeding following repeated vomiting, is considered to be the cause of up to 15% of all severe upper GI bleeds. The mechanism is similar to spontaneous esophageal perforation: an acute increase in intra-abdominal pressure against a closed glottis in a patient with a hiatal hernia.

Mallory-Weiss tears are characterized by arterial bleeding, which may be massive. Vomiting is not an obligatory factor, as there may be other causes of an acute increase in intra-abdominal pressure, such as paroxysmal coughing, seizures, and retching. The diagnosis requires a high index of suspicion, particularly in the patient who develops upper GI bleeding following prolonged vomiting or retching. Upper endoscopy confirms the suspicion by identifying one or more longitudinal fissures in the mucosa of the herniated stomach as the source of bleeding.

In the majority of patients, the bleeding will stop spontaneously with nonoperative management. In addition to blood replacement, the stomach should be decompressed and antiemetics administered, as a distended stomach and continued vomiting aggravate further bleeding. A Sengstaken-Blakemore tube will not stop the bleeding, as the pressure in the balloon is not sufficient to overcome arterial pressure. Endoscopic injection of epinephrine may be therapeutic if bleeding does not stop spontaneously. Only occasionally will surgery be required to stop blood loss. The procedure consists of laparotomy and high gastrotomy with oversewing of the linear tear. Mortality is uncommon, and recurrence is rare.

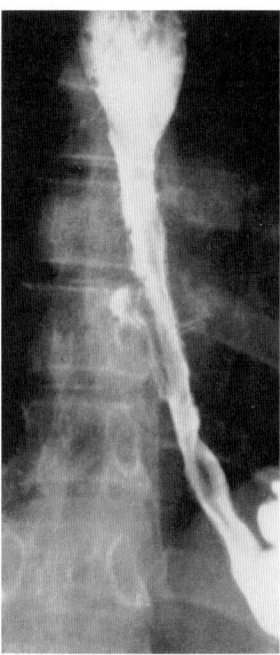

FIG. 25-79. Barium esophagogram showing a stricture and a contained perforation following dilation. The injury meets Cameron criteria: It is contained within the mediastinum and drawn back into the esophagus, the patient had mild symptoms, and there was no evidence of clinical sepsis. Nonoperative management was successful.

CAUSTIC INJURY

Accidental caustic lesions occur mainly in children, and, in general, rather small quantities of caustics are taken. In adults or teenagers, the swallowing of caustic liquids is usually deliberate, during suicide attempts, and greater quantities are swallowed. Alkalies are more frequently swallowed accidentally than acids, because strong acids cause an immediate burning pain in the mouth.

Pathology

The swallowing of caustic substances causes an acute and a chronic injury. During the acute phase, care focuses on controlling the immediate tissue injury and the potential for perforation. During the chronic phase, the focus is on treatment of strictures and disturbances in pharyngeal swallowing. In the acute phase, the degree and extent of the lesion are dependent on several factors: the nature of the caustic substance, its concentration, the quantity swallowed, and the time the substance is in contact with the tissues.

Acids and alkalies affect tissue in different ways. Alkalies dissolve tissue, and therefore penetrate more deeply, while acids cause a coagulative necrosis that limits their penetration. Animal experiments have shown that there is a correlation between the depth of the lesion and the concentration of sodium hydroxide solution. When a solution of 3.8% comes into contact with the esophagus for 10 seconds, it causes necrosis of the mucosa and the submucosa, but spares the muscular layer. A concentration of 22.5% penetrates the whole esophageal wall and into the periesophageal tissues. Cleansing products can contain up to 90% sodium hydroxide. The strength of esophageal contractions varies according to the level of the esophagus, being weakest at the striated muscle–smooth muscle interface. Consequently, clearance from this area may be somewhat slower, allowing caustic substances to remain in contact with the mucosa longer. This explains why the esophagus is preferentially and more severely affected at this level than in the lower portions.

The lesions caused by lye injury occur in three phases. First is the acute necrotic phase, lasting 1 to 4 days after injury. During this period, coagulation of intracellular proteins results in cell necrosis, and the living tissue surrounding the area of necrosis develops an intense inflammatory reaction. Second is the ulceration and granulation phase, starting 3 to 5 days after injury. During this period, the superficial necrotic tissue sloughs, leaving an ulcerated, acutely inflamed base, and granulation tissue fills the defect left by the sloughed mucosa. This phase lasts 10 to 12 days, and it is during this period that the esophagus is the weakest. Third is the phase of cicatrization and scarring, which begins the third week following injury. During this period, the previously formed connective tissue begins to contract, resulting in narrowing of the esophagus. Adhesions between granulating areas occur, resulting in pockets and bands. It is during this period that efforts must be made to reduce stricture formation.

Clinical Manifestations

The clinical picture of an esophageal burn is determined by the degree and extent of the lesion. In the initial phase, complaints consist of pain in the mouth and substernal region, hypersalivation, pain on swallowing, and dysphagia. The presence of fever is strongly correlated with the presence of an esophageal lesion. Bleeding can occur, and frequently, the patient vomits. These initial complaints disappear during the quiescent period of ulceration and granulation. During the cicatrization and scarring phase, the complaint of dysphagia reappears and is due to fibrosis and retraction, resulting in narrowing of the esophagus. Of the patients who develop strictures, 60% do so within 1 month, and 80% within 2 months. If dysphagia does not develop within 8 months, it is unlikely that a stricture will occur. Serious systemic reactions such as hypovolemia and acidosis resulting in renal damage can occur in cases in which the burns have been caused by strong acids. Respiratory complications such as laryngospasm, laryngoedema, and occasionally pulmonary edema can occur, especially when strong acids are aspirated.

Inspection of the oral cavity and pharynx can indicate that caustic substances were swallowed, but does not reveal that the esophagus has been burned. Conversely, esophageal burns can be present without apparent oral injuries. Because of this poor correlation, early esophagoscopy is advocated to establish the presence of an esophageal injury. To lessen the chance of perforation, the scope should not be introduced beyond the proximal esophageal lesion. The degree of injury can be graded according to the criteria listed in Table 25-17. Even if the esophagoscopy is normal, strictures may appear later. Radiographic examination is not a reliable means to identify the presence of early esophageal injury, but is important in later follow-up to identify strictures. The most common locations of caustic injuries are shown in Table 25-18.

Treatment

Treatment of a caustic lesion of the esophagus is directed toward management of both the immediate and late consequences of the injury. The immediate treatment consists of limiting the burn by administering neutralizing agents. To be effective, this must be done within the first hour. Lye or other alkali can be neutralized with half-strength vinegar, lemon juice, or orange juice. Acid can be neutralized with milk, egg white, or antacids. Sodium bicarbonate is not used because it generates carbon dioxide, which might increase the

TABLE 25-17	Endoscopic grading of corrosive esophageal and gastric burns

First degree: Mucosal hyperemia and edema

Second degree: Limited hemorrhage, exudate ulceration, and pseudomembrane formation

Third degree: Sloughing of mucosa, deep ulcers, massive hemorrhage, complete obstruction of lumen by edema, charring, and perforation

TABLE 25-18	Location of caustic injury (n = 62)
Pharynx	10%
Esophagus	70%
Upper	15%
Middle	65%
Lower	2%
Whole	18%
Stomach	20%
Antral	91%
Whole	9%
Both stomach and esophagus	14%

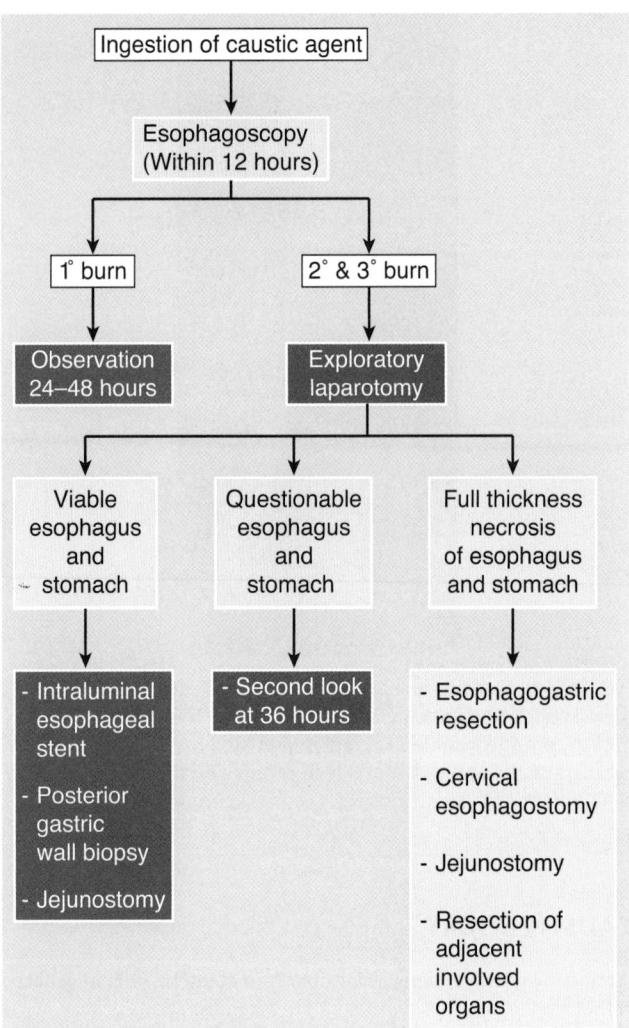

FIG. 25-80. Algorithm summarizing the management of acute caustic injury.

danger of perforation. Emetics are contraindicated, because vomiting renews the contact of the caustic substance with the esophagus and can contribute to perforation if too forceful. Hypovolemia is corrected and broad-spectrum antibiotics are administered to lessen the inflammatory reaction and prevent infectious complications. If necessary, a feeding jejunostomy tube is inserted to provide nutrition. Oral feeding can be started when the dysphagia of the initial phase has regressed.

In the past, surgeons waited until the appearance of a stricture before starting treatment. Currently, dilations are started the first day after the injury, with the aim of preserving the esophageal lumen by removing the adhesions that occurred in the injured segments. However, this approach is controversial in that dilations can traumatize the esophagus, causing bleeding and perforation, and there are data indicating that excessive dilations cause increased fibrosis secondary to the added trauma. The use of steroids to limit fibrosis has been shown to be effective in animals, but their effectiveness in human beings is debatable.

Extensive necrosis of the esophagus frequently leads to perforation, and is best managed by resection. When there is extensive gastric involvement, the esophagus is nearly always necrotic or severely burned, and total gastrectomy and near-total esophagectomy are necessary. The presence of air in the esophageal wall is a sign of muscle necrosis and impending perforation and is a strong indication for esophagectomy.

Management of acute injury is summarized in the algorithm in Fig. 25-80. Some authors have advocated the use of an intraluminal esophageal stent (Fig. 25-81) in patients who are operated on and found to have no evidence of extensive esophagogastric necrosis. In these patients, a biopsy of the posterior gastric wall should be performed to exclude occult injury. If, histologically, there is a question of viability, a second-look operation should be done within 36 hours. If a stent is inserted, it should be kept in position for 21 days, and removed after a satisfactory barium esophagogram. Esophagoscopy should be done, and, if strictures are present, dilations initiated.

Once the acute phase has passed, attention is turned to the prevention and management of strictures. Both antegrade dilation with a Hurst or Maloney bougie and retrograde dilation with a Tucker bougie have been satisfactory. Occasionally, particularly with severe strictures, the patient is instructed to swallow a string, over which metal Sippy dilators are passed until an adequate lumen can be obtained for passage of a mercury bougie. In a series of 1079 patients, early dilations started during the acute phase gave excellent results in 78%, good results in 13%, and poor results in 2%. Fifty-five patients died during the treatment. In contrast, of 333 patients whose strictures were dilated when they became symptomatic, only 21% had excellent results, 46% good, and 6% poor, with three dying during the process. The length of time the surgeon should persist with dilation before consideration of esophageal resection is problematic. An adequate lumen should be re-established within 6 months to 1 year, with progressively longer intervals between dilations. If, during the course of treatment, an adequate lumen cannot

be established or maintained (i.e., smaller bougies must be used), operative intervention should be considered. Surgical intervention is indicated when there is (a) complete stenosis in which all attempts from above and below have failed to establish a lumen, (b) marked irregularity and pocketing on barium swallow, (c) the development of a severe periesophageal reaction or mediastinitis with dilatation, (d) a fistula, (e) the inability to dilate or maintain the lumen above a 40F bougie, or (f) a patient who is unwilling or unable to undergo prolonged periods of dilation.

The variety of abnormalities seen requires that creativity be used when considering esophageal reconstruction. Skin tube esophagoplasties are now used much less frequently than they were in the past, and are mainly of historical interest. Currently, the stomach, jejunum, and colon are the organs used to replace the esophagus, through either the posterior mediastinum or the retrosternal route. A retrosternal route is chosen when there has been a previous esophagectomy or there is extensive fibrosis in the posterior mediastinum. When all factors are considered, the order of preference for an esophageal substitute is (a) colon, (b) stomach, and (c) jejunum. Free jejunal grafts based on the superior thyroid artery have provided excellent results. Whatever method is selected, it must be emphasized that these procedures cannot be taken lightly; minor errors of judgment or technique may lead to serious or even fatal complications.

Critical in the planning of the operation is the selection of cervical esophagus, pyriform sinus, or posterior pharynx as the site

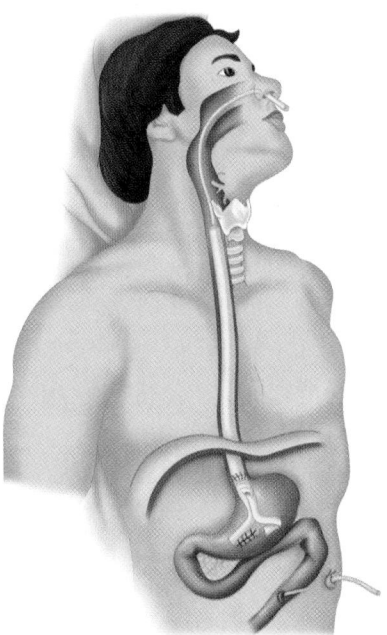

FIG. 25-81. The use of an esophageal stent to prevent stricture. The stent is constructed from a chest tube and placed in the esophagus at the time of an exploratory laparotomy. A Penrose drain is placed over the distal end as a flap valve to prevent reflux. The stent is supported at its upper end by attaching it to a suction catheter that is secured to the nares. Continuous suction removes saliva and mucus trapped in the pharynx and upper esophagus.

for proximal anastomosis. The site of the upper anastomosis depends on the extent of the pharyngeal and cervical esophageal damage encountered. When the cervical esophagus is destroyed and a pyriform sinus remains open the anastomosis can be made to the hypopharynx (Fig. 25-82). When the pyriform sinuses are com-

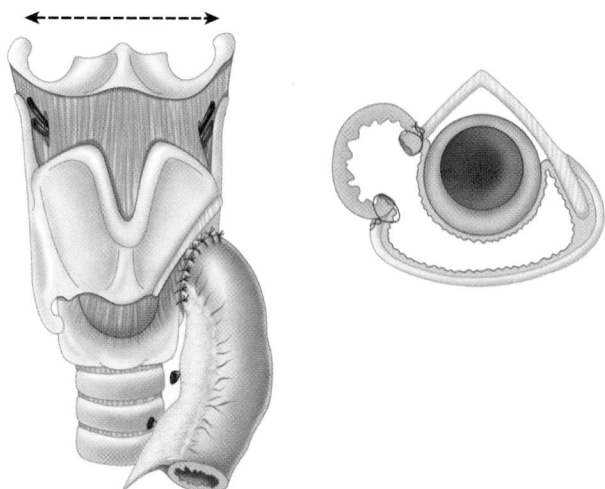

FIG. 25-82. Anastomosis of the bowel to a preserved pyriform sinus. To identify the site, a finger is inserted into the free pyriform sinus through a suprahyoid incision (*dotted line*). This requires removing the lateral inferior portion of the thyroid cartilage as shown in cross-section. (*Reproduced with permission from Tran Ba Huy P, Celerier M: Management of severe caustic stenosis of the hypopharynx and esophagus by ileocolic transposition via suprahyoid or transepiglottic approach. Analysis of 18 cases. Ann Surg 207:439, 1988.*)

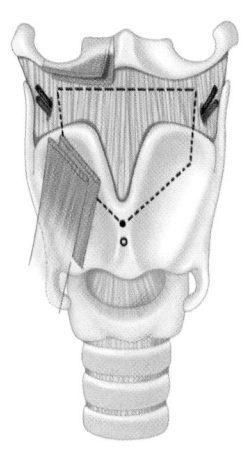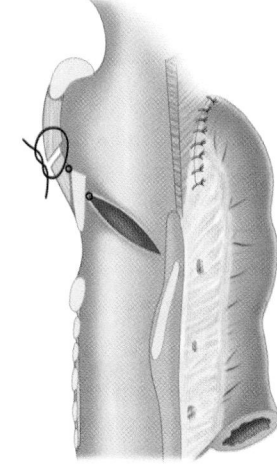

FIG. 25-83. Anastomosis of the bowel to the posterior oropharynx. The anastomosis is done through an inverted trapezoid incision above the thyroid cartilage (*dotted line*). A triangle-shaped piece of the upper half of the cartilage is resected. Closure of the oropharynx is done so that the larynx is pulled up (sagittal section). (*Reproduced with permission from Tran Ba Huy P, Celerier M: Management of severe caustic stenosis of the hypopharynx and esophagus by ileocolic transposition via suprahyoid or transepiglottic approach. Analysis of 18 cases. Ann Surg 207:439, 1988.*)

pletely stenosed, a transglottic approach is used to perform an anastomosis to the posterior oropharyngeal wall (Fig. 25-83). This allows excision of supraglottic strictures and elevation and anterior tilting of the larynx. In both of these situations, the patient must relearn to swallow. Recovery is long and difficult and may require several endoscopic dilations, and often reoperations. Sleeve resections of short strictures are not successful because the extent of damage to the wall of the esophagus can be greater than realized, and almost invariably the anastomosis is carried out in a diseased area.

The management of a bypassed damaged esophagus after injury is problematic. If the esophagus is left in place, ulceration from gastroesophageal reflux or the development of carcinoma must be considered. The extensive dissection necessary to remove the esophagus, particularly in the presence of marked periesophagitis, is associated with significant morbidity. Leaving the esophagus in place preserves the function of the vagus nerves, and, in turn, the function of the stomach. On the other hand, leaving a damaged esophagus in place can result in multiple blind sacs and subsequent development of mediastinal abscesses years later. Most experienced surgeons recommend that the esophagus be removed unless the operative risk is unduly high.

ACQUIRED FISTULA

The esophagus lies in close contact with the membranous portion of the trachea and left bronchus, predisposing to the formation of fistula to these structures. Most acquired esophageal fistulas are to the tracheobronchial tree, and secondary to either esophageal or pulmonary malignancy. Traumatic fistulas and those associated with esophageal diverticula account for the remainder. Fistulas associated with traction diverticula are usually due to mediastinal inflammatory disease, and traumatic fistulas usually occur secondary to penetrating wounds, lye ingestion, or iatrogenic injury.

These fistulas are characterized by paroxysmal coughing following the ingestion of liquids, and by recurrent or chronic pulmonary infections. The onset of cough immediately after swallowing suggests aspiration, whereas a brief delay (30 to 60 seconds) suggests a fistula.

Spontaneous closure is rare, owing to the presence of malignancy or a recurrent infectious process. Surgical treatment of benign fistulas consists of division of the fistulous tract, resection of irreversibly damaged lung tissue, and closure of the esophageal defect. To prevent recurrence, a pleural flap should be interposed. Treatment of malignant fistulas is difficult, particularly in the presence of prior irradiation. Generally, only palliative treatment is indicated. This can best be done by using a specially designed esophageal endoprosthesis that bridges and occludes the fistula, allowing the patient to eat. Rarely, esophageal diversion, coupled with placement of a feeding jejunostomy, can be used as a last resort.

TECHNIQUES OF ESOPHAGEAL RECONSTRUCTION

Options for esophageal substitution include gastric advancement, colonic interposition, and either jejunal free transfer or advancement into the chest. Rarely, combinations of these grafts will be the only possible option. The indications for esophageal resection and substitution include malignant and end-stage benign disease. The latter includes reflux- or drug-induced stricture formation that cannot be dilated without damage to the esophagus, a dilated and tortuous esophagus secondary to severe motility disorders, lye-induced strictures, and multiple previous antireflux procedures. The choice of esophageal substitution has significant impact upon the technical difficulty of the procedure, and influences the long-term outcome.

Partial Esophageal Resection

Low-lying benign lesions, with preserved proximal esophageal function, are best treated with the interposition of a segment of proximal jejunum into the chest and primary anastomosis. A jejunal interposition can reach to the inferior border of the pulmonary hilum with ease, but the architecture of its blood supply rarely allows the use of the jejunum above this point. Because the anastomosis is within the chest, a thoracotomy is necessary.

The jejunum is a dynamic graft and contributes to bolus transport, whereas the stomach and colon function more as a conduit. The stomach is a poor choice in this circumstance because of the propensity for the reflux of gastric contents into the upper esophagus following an intrathoracic esophagogastrostomy. It is now well recog-

nized that this occurs, and can lead to incapacitating symptoms and esophageal destruction in some patients. Short segments of colon, on the other hand, lack significant motility and have a propensity for the development of esophagitis above the anastomosis.

Replacement of the cervical portion of the esophagus, while preserving the distal portion, is occasionally indicated in cervical esophageal or head and neck malignancy, and following the ingestion of lye. Free transfer of a portion of jejunum to the neck has become a viable option and is successful in the majority of cases. Revascularization is achieved via use of the internal mammary artery and the internal mammary or innominate vein. Removal of the sternoclavicular joint aids in performing the vascular and distal esophageal anastomosis (Fig. 25-84).

Reconstruction after Total Esophagectomy

Neither the intrathoracic stomach nor the intrathoracic colon functions as well as the native esophagus after an esophagogastrectomy. The choice between these organs will be influenced by several factors, such as the adequacy of their blood supply and the length of resected esophagus that they are capable of bridging. If the stomach shows evidence of disease, or has been contracted or reduced by previous gastric surgery, the length available for esophageal replacement may not be adequate. The presence of diverticular disease, unrecognized carcinoma, or colitis prohibits the use of the colon. The blood supply of the colon is more affected by vascular disease than the blood supply of the stomach, which may prevent its use. Of the two, the colon provides the longest graft. The stomach can usually reach to the neck if the amount of lesser curvature resected does not interfere with the blood supply to the fundus. Gastric interposition has the advantage that only one anastomosis is required. On the other hand, there is greater potential for aspiration of gastric juice or stricturing of the cervical anastomosis from chronic reflux when stomach is used for replacement.

Following an esophagogastrectomy, patients may have discomfort during or shortly after eating. The most common symptom is a postprandial pressure sensation or a feeling of being stuffed, which probably results from the loss of the gastric reservoir. This symptom is less common when the colon is used as an esophageal substitute, probably because the distal third of the stomach is retained in the

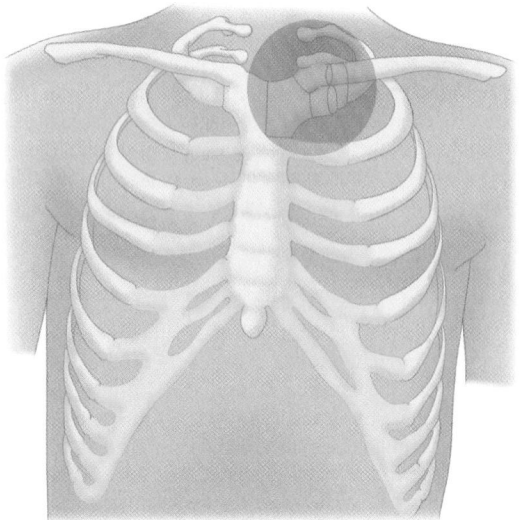

A

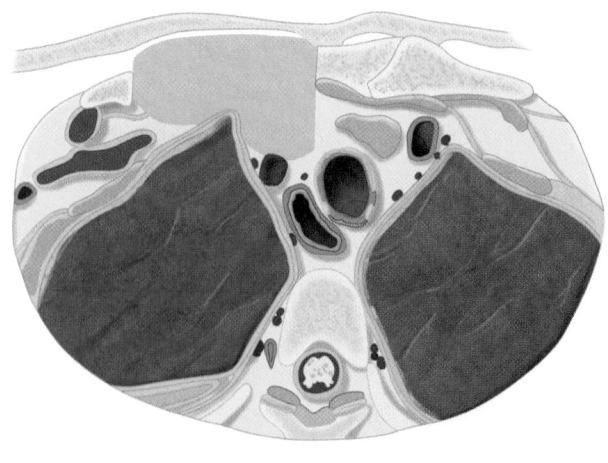

B

FIG. 25-84. A. The portion of the thoracic inlet to be resected to provide space for a free jejunal graft and access to the internal mammary artery (*shaded area*). **B.** Cross-section showing the space available after resection of the sternoclavicular joint and one half of the manubrium. *[Reproduced with permission from Rothberg M, DeMeester TR: Exposure of the cervical esophagus, in Shields TW (ed):* General Thoracic Surgery, *3rd ed. Philadelphia: Lea & Febiger, 1989, p 419.]*

abdomen and the interposed colon provides an additional reservoir function.

King and Hölscher have reported a 40 and 50% incidence of dysphagia after re-establishing GI continuity with the stomach following esophagogastrectomy. This incidence is similar to Orringer's results after using the stomach to replace the esophagus in patients with benign disease. More than one-half of the patients experienced dysphagia postoperatively; two-thirds of this group required postoperative dilation and one-fourth had persistent dysphagia and required home dilation. By contrast, dysphagia is uncommon and the need for dilation is rare following a colonic interposition. Isolauri reported on 248 patients with colonic interpositions and noted a 24% incidence of dysphagia 12 months after the operation. When it occurred, the most common cause was recurrent mediastinal tumor. The high incidence of dysphagia with the use of the stomach is probably related to the esophagogastric anastomosis in the neck and the resulting difficulty of passing a swallowed bolus.

Another consequence of the transposition of the stomach into the chest is the development of postoperative duodenogastric reflux, probably due to pyloric denervation, and adding a pyloroplasty may worsen this problem. Following gastric advancement, the pylorus lies at the level of the esophageal hiatus, and a distinct pressure differential develops between the intrathoracic gastric and intra-abdominal duodenal lumina. Unless the pyloric valve is extremely efficient, the pressure differential will encourage reflux of duodenal contents into the stomach. Duodenogastric reflux is less likely to occur following colonic interposition, because there is sufficient intra-abdominal colon to be compressed by the abdominal pressure, and the pylorus and duodenum remain in their normal intra-abdominal position.

Although there is general acceptance of the concept that an esophagogastric anastomosis in the neck results in less postoperative esophagitis and stricture than one at a lower level, reflux esophagitis following a cervical anastomosis does occur, albeit at a slower rate than when the anastomosis is at a lower level. Most patients undergo cervical esophagogastrostomy for malignancy; thus the long-term sequelae of an esophagogastric anastomosis in the neck are not of concern. However, patients who have had a cervical esophagogastrostomy for benign disease may develop problems associated with the anastomosis in the fourth or fifth postoperative year that are severe enough to require anastomotic revision. This is less likely in patients who have had a colonic interposition for esophageal replacement. Consequently, in patients who have a benign process or a potentially curable carcinoma of the esophagus or cardia, a colonic interposition is used to obviate the late problems associated with a cervical esophagogastrostomy. Colonic interposition for esophageal substitution is a more complex procedure than gastric advancement, with the potential for greater perioperative morbidity, particularly in inexperienced hands.

Composite Reconstruction

Occasionally, a combination of colon, jejunum, and stomach is the only reconstructive option available. This situation may arise when there has been previous gastric or colonic resection, when dysphagia has recurred after a previous esophageal resection, or following postoperative complications such as ischemia of an esophageal substitute. Although not ideal, combinations of colon, jejunum, and stomach used to restore GI continuity function surprisingly well, and allow alimentary reconstruction in an otherwise impossible situation.

Vagal Sparing Esophagectomy with Colon Interposition

Traditional esophagectomy typically results in bilateral vagotomy and its attendant consequences. It is likely that symptoms such as dumping, diarrhea, early satiety, and weight loss seen in 15 to 20% of patients postesophagectomy are at least in part, if not completely,

due to vagal interruption. The technique of vagal sparing esophagectomy with colon interposition has been described in an effort to avoid the morbidities associated with standard esophagectomy.

Through an upper midline abdominal incision, the right and left vagal nerves are identified, circled with a tape, and retracted to the right. A limited, highly selective proximal gastric vagotomy is performed along the cephalad 4 cm of the lesser curvature. The stomach is divided with an Endo-GIA stapler just below the GEJ. The colon is prepared to provide an interposed segment as previously described. A neck incision is made along the anterior border of the left sternocleidomastoid muscle, and the strap muscles are exposed. The omohyoid muscle is divided at its pulley, and the sternohyoid and sternothyroid muscles are divided at their manubrial insertion. The left carotid sheath is retracted laterally and the thyroid and trachea medially. The left inferior thyroid artery is ligated laterally as it passes under the left common carotid artery. The left recurrent laryngeal nerve is identified and protected. The esophagus is dissected out circumferentially in an inferior direction, from the left neck to the apex of the right chest, to avoid injury to the right recurrent laryngeal nerve. The esophagus is divided at the level of the thoracic inlet, leaving about 3 to 4 cm of cervical esophagus. The proximal esophagus is retracted anteriorly and to the right with the use of two sutures to keep saliva and oral contents from contaminating the neck wound.

Returning to the abdomen, the proximal staple line of the gastric division is opened and the esophagus is flushed with povidone-iodine solution. A vein stripper is passed up the esophagus into the neck wound. The distal portion of the esophagus in the neck is secured tightly around the stripping cable with "endoloops" and an umbilical tape for a trailer. The tip of the stripper is exchanged for a mushroom head, and the stripper is pulled back into the abdomen, inverting the esophagus as it transverses the posterior mediastinum. This maneuver strips the branches of the esophageal plexus off the longitudinal muscle of the esophagus, preserving the esophageal plexus along with the proximal vagal nerves and the distal vagal nerve trunks. In patients with end-stage achalasia, only the mucosa is secured around the stripping cable, so that it alone is stripped and the dilated muscular wall of the esophagus, with its enriched blood supply, remains. The resulting mediastinal tunnel, or in the case of achalasia the muscular tube, is dilated with a Foley catheter containing 90 mL of fluid in the balloon. The previously prepared interposed portion of the transverse colon is passed behind the stomach and up through the mediastinal tunnel into the neck. An end-to-end anastomosis is performed to the cervical esophagus using a single layer technique. The colon is pulled taut and secured to the left crus with four or five interrupted sutures. Five centimeters below the crura, an opening is made in the mesentery adjacent to the colon along its mesenteric border, through which an Endo-GIA stapler is passed and the colon is divided. The proximal end, which is the distal end of the interposed colon, is anastomosed high on the posterior fundic wall of the stomach, using a triangular stapling anastomotic technique. This is done by stapling longitudinally the stomach and colon together with a 75-mm Endo-GIA stapler, spreading the base of the incision apart, and closing it with a T-55 stapler. Colonic continuity is re-established by bringing the proximal right colon to the distal staple line in the left colon and performing an end-to-end anastomosis using a double layer technique.

Although conceptually appealing, preservation of vagal nerve integrity or the gastric reservoir function after vagal sparing esophagectomy only recently has been validated. Banki and associates compared patients undergoing vagal sparing esophagectomy to those with conventional esophagectomy and colon or gastric interposition. This study showed that vagal sparing esophagectomy preserved gastric secretion, gastric emptying, meal capacity, and body mass index, when compared to esophagogastrectomy with colon interposition or standard esophagectomy with gastric pull-up. Vagal sparing esophagectomy patients functioned, for the most part, similarly to normal subjects, allowing them to eat a normal meal, free of dumping or diarrhea. These results indicate that the vagal sparing esophagectomy procedure does indeed preserve the vagal nerves, and may be considered in the treatment of benign and early malignant lesions requiring esophagectomy.

BIBLIOGRAPHY

Entries highlighted in bright blue are key references.

General References

Balaji B, Peters JH: Minimally invasive surgery for esophageal motor disorders. *Surg Clin North Am* 82:763, 2002.

Bremner CG, DeMeester TR, Bremner RM: *Esophageal Motility Testing Made Easy.* St. Louis: Quality Medical Publishing, 2001.

Castel DW, Richter J (eds): *The Esophagus.* Boston: Little, Brown & Co., 1999.

DeMeester SR, Peters JH, DeMeester TR: Barrett's esophagus. *Curr Probl Surg* 38:549, 2001.

Demeester SR (ed): Barrett's esophagus. *Problems in General Surgery*, Vol. 18, no. 2. Hagerstown, MD: Lippincott Williams & Wilkins, 2001.

DeMeester TR, Peters JH, Bremner CG, et al: Biology of gastroesophageal reflux disease; pathophysiology relating to medical and surgical treatment. *Annu Rev Med* 50:469, 1999.

Hunter JG, Pellagrini CA: Surgery of the esophagus. *Surg Clin North Am* 77:959, 1997.

McFadyen BV, Arregui ME, Eubanks S, et al: *Laparoscopic Surgery of the Abdomen.* New York: Springer, 2003.

Surgical Anatomy

Daffner RH, Halber MD, Postlethwait RW, et al: CT of the esophagus. II. Carcinoma. *AJR Am J Roentgenol* 133:1051, 1979.

Gray SW, Rowe JS Jr., Skandalakis JE: Surgical anatomy of the gastroesophageal junction. *Am Surg* 45:575, 1979.

Liebermann-Meffert D: The pharyngoesophageal segment: Anatomy and innervation. *Dis Esophagus* 8:242, 1995.

Liebermann-Meffert D, Siewert JR: Arterial anatomy of the esophagus: A review of the literature with brief comments on clinical aspects. *Gullet* 2:3, 1992.

Liebermann-Meffert DM, Meier R, Siewert JR: Vascular anatomy of the gastric tube used for esophageal reconstruction. *Ann Thorac Surg* 54:1110, 1992.

Liebermann-Meffert DM, Walbrun B, Hiebert CA, et al: Recurrent and superior laryngeal nerves: A new look with implications for the esophageal surgeon. *Ann Thorac Surg* 67:217, 1999.

Physiology

Barlow AP, DeMeester TR, et al: The significance of the gastric secretory state in gastroesophageal reflux disease. *Arch Surg* 124:937, 1989.

DeMeester TR, Lafontaine E, et al: The relationship of a hiatal hernia to the function of the body of the esophagus and the gastroesophageal junction. *J Thorac Cardiovasc Surg* 82:547, 1981.

Helm JF, Dodds WJ, et al: Effect of esophageal emptying and saliva on clearance of acid from the esophagus. *N Engl J Med* 310:284, 1984.

Joelsson BE, DeMeester TR, et al: The role of the esophageal body in the antireflux mechanism. *Surgery* 92:417, 1982.

Johnson LF, DeMeester TR: Evaluation of elevation of the head of the bed, bethanechol, and antacid foam tablets on gastroesophageal reflux. *Dig Dis Sci* 26:673, 1981.

Kahrilas PJ, Dodds WJ, Hogan WJ: Effect of peristaltic dysfunction on esophageal volume clearance. *Gastroenterology* 94:73, 1988.

McCallum RW, Berkowitz DM, Lerner E: Gastric emptying in patients with gastroesophageal reflux. *Gastroenterology* 80:285, 1981.

Mittal RK, Lange RC, McCallum RW: Identification and mechanism of delayed esophageal acid clearance in subjects with hiatus hernia. *Gastroenterology* 92:130, 1987.

Rao SSC, Madipalli RS, Mujica VR, et al: Effects of age and gender on esophageal biomechanical properties and sensation. *Am J Gastroenterol* 98:1688, 2003.

Tseng D, Rizvi AZ, Fennerty MB, et al: Forty-eight-hour pH monitoring increases sensitivity in detecting abnormal esophageal acid exposure. *J Gastrointest Surg* 9:1043; discussion 1051, 2005.

Zaninotto G, DeMeester TR, Schwizer W, et al: The lower esophageal sphincter in health and disease. *Am J Surg* 155:104, 1988.

Assessment of Esophageal Function

Adamek RJ, Wegener M, et al: Long-term esophageal manometry in healthy subjects: Evaluation of normal values and influence of age. *Dig Dis Sci* 39:2069, 1994.

Barish CF, Castell DO, Richter JE: Graded esophageal balloon distention: A new provocative test for non-cardiac chest pain. *Dig Dis Sci* 31:1292, 1986.

Battle WS, Nyhus LM, Bombeck CT: Gastroesophageal reflux: Diagnosis and treatment. *Ann Surg* 177:560, 1973.

Bechi P: Fiberoptic measurement of "alkaline" gastro-esophageal reflux: Technical aspects and clinical indications. *Dis Esophagus* 131, 1994.

Bernstein IM, Baker CA: A clinical test for esophagitis. *Gastroenterology* 34:760, 1958.

DeMeester TR, Johnson LF, et al: Patterns of gastroesophageal reflux in health and disease. *Ann Surg* 184:459, 1976.

DeMeester TR, Wang CI, et al: Technique, indications and clinical use of 24-hour esophageal pH monitoring. *J Thorac Cardiovasc Surg* 79:656, 1980.

Dodds WJ: Current concepts of esophageal motor function: Clinical implications for radiology. *AJR Am J Roentgenol* 128:549, 1977.

Fein M, Fuchs KH, Bohrer T, et al: Fiberoptic technique for 24-hour bile reflux monitoring. Standards and normal values for gastric monitoring. *Dig Dis Sci* 41:216, 1996.

Fuchs KH, DeMeester TR, Albertucci M: Specificity and sensitivity of objective diagnosis of gastroesophageal reflux disease. *Surgery* 102:575, 1987.

Iascone C, DeMeester TR, et al: Barrett's esophagus: Functional assessment, proposed pathogenesis and surgical therapy. *Arch Surg* 118:543, 1983.

Johnson LF, DeMeester TR: Development of 24-hour intraesophageal pH monitoring composite scoring. *J Clin Gastroenterol* 8:52, 1986.

Johnson LF, DeMeester TR: Twenty-four-hour pH monitoring of the distal esophagus: A quantitative measure of gastroesophageal reflux. *Am J Gastroenterol* 62:325, 1974.

Kauer WK, Burdiles P, Ireland A, et al: Does duodenal juice reflux into the esophagus in patients with complicated GERD? Evaluation of a fiberoptic sensor for bilirubin. *Am J Surg* 169:98, 1995.

Kramer P, Hollander W: Comparison of experimental esophageal pain with clinical pain of angina pectoris and esophageal disease. *Gastroenterology* 29:719, 1955.

Pandolfino JE, Richter JE, Ours T, et al: Ambulatory esophageal pH monitoring using a wireless system. *Am J Gastroenterol* 98:740, 2003.

Reid BJ, Weinstein WM, et al: Endoscopic biopsy can detect high-grade dysplasia or early adenocarcinoma in Barrett's esophagus without grossly recognizable neoplastic lesions. *Gastroenterology* 94:81, 1988.

Schwizer W, Hinder RA, DeMeester TR: Does delayed gastric emptying contribute to gastroesophageal reflux disease? *Am J Surg* 157:74, 1989.

Stein HJ, DeMeester TR, et al: Three-dimensional imaging of the LES in gastroesophageal reflux disease. *Ann Surg* 214:374, 1991.

Tutuian R, Vela MF, Balaji NS, et al: Esophageal function testing with combined multichannel intraluminal impedance and manometry; multicenter study in healthy volunteers. *Clin Gastroenterol Hepatol* 1:174, 2003.

Wickremesinghe PC, Bayrit PQ, et al: Quantitative evaluation of bile diversion surgery utilizing 99mTc HIDA scintigraphy. *Gastroenterology* 84:354, 1983.

Gastroesophageal Reflux Disease

Allison PR: Hiatus hernia: A 20 year retrospective survey. *Ann Surg* 178:273, 1973.

Allison PR: Peptic ulcer of the esophagus. *J Thorac Surg* 15:308, 1946.

Allison PR: Reflux esophagitis, sliding hiatus hernia and the anatomy of repair. *Surg Gynecol Obstet* 92:419, 1951.

Barlow AP, DeMeester TR, et al: The significance of the gastric secretory state in gastroesophageal reflux disease. *Arch Surg* 124:937, 1989.

Bonavina L, DeMeester TR, et al: Drug-induced esophageal strictures. *Ann Surg* 206:173, 1987.

Bremner RM, DeMeester TR, Crookes PF, et al: The effect of symptoms and non-specific motility abnormalities on surgical therapy for gastroesophageal reflux disease. *J Thorac Cardiovasc Surg* 107:1244, 1994.

Castell DO: Nocturnal acid breakthrough in perspective: Let's not throw out the baby with the bathwater. *Am J Gastroenterol* 98:517, 2003.

Chandrasoma P, Barrett N: So close, yet 50 years from the truth. *J Gastrointest Surg* 3:7, 1999.

Clark GW, Ireland AP, Peters JH, et al: Short segments of Barrett's esophagus: A prevalent complication of gastroesophageal reflux disease with malignant potential. *J Gastrointest Surg* 1:113, 1997.

DeMeester SR, Campos GM, DeMeester TR, et al: The impact of an antireflux procedure on intestinal metaplasia of the cardia. *Ann Surg* 228:547; 1998.

DeMeester TR, Bonavina L, Albertucci M: Nissen fundoplication for gastroesophageal reflux disease: Evaluation of primary repair in 100 consecutive patients. *Ann Surg* 204:9, 1986.

DeMeester TR, Bonavina L, et al: Chronic respiratory symptoms and occult gastroesophageal reflux. *Ann Surg* 211:337, 1990.

DeMeester SR, DeMeester TR: Columnar mucosa and intestinal metaplasia of the esophagus: Fifty years of controversy. *Ann Surg* 231:303, 2000.

DeMeester TR, Johansson KE, et al: Indications, surgical technique, and long-term functional results of colon interposition or bypass. *Ann Surg* 208:460, 1988.

Desai KM, Klingensmith ME, Winslow ER, et al: Symptomatic outcomes of laparoscopic antireflux surgery in patients eligible for endoluminal therapies. *Surg Endosc* 16:1669, 2002.

Donahue PE, Samelson S, et al: The floppy Nissen fundoplication: Effective long-term control of pathologic reflux. *Arch Surg* 120:663, 1985.

Farrell TM, Richardson WS, Halkar R, et al: Nissen fundoplication improves gastric motility in patients with delayed gastric emptying. *Surg Endosc* 15:271, 2001.

Farrell TM, Richardson WS, Trus TL, et al: Response of atypical symptoms of gastroesophageal reflux antireflux surgery. *Br J Surg* 88:1649, 2001.

Farrell TM, Smith CD, Metreveli RE, et al: Fundoplication provides effective and durable symptom relief in patients with Barrett's esophagus. *Am J Surg* 178:18, 1999.

Fass R: Epidemiology and pathophysiology of symptomatic gastroesophageal reflux disease. *Am J Gastroenterol* 98:S2, 2003.

Fiorucci S, Santucci L, et al: Gastric acidity and gastroesophageal reflux patterns in patients with esophagitis. *Gastroenterology* 103:855, 1992.

Fletcher J, Wirz A, Young J, et al: Unbuffered highly acidic gastric juice exists at the gastroesophageal junction after a meal. *Gastroenterology* 121:775, 2001.

Fuchs KH, DeMeester TR, et al: Computerized identification of pathologic duodenogastric reflux using 24-hour gastric pH monitoring. *Ann Surg* 213:13, 1991.

Gerson LB, Shetler K, Triadafilopoulos G: Prevalence of Barrett's esophagus in asymptomatic individuals. *Gastroenterology* 123:461, 2002.

Gillen P, Keeling P, et al: Implication of duodenogastric reflux in the pathogenesis of Barrett's oesophagus. *Br J Surg* 75:540, 1988.

Graham DY: The changing epidemiology of GERD: Geography and *Helicobacter pylori*. *Am J Gastroenterol* 98:1462, 2003.

Gurski RR, Peters JH, Hagen JA, et al: Barrett's esophagus can and does regress following antireflux surgery: A study of prevalence and predictive features. *J Am Coll Surg* 196:706, 2003.

Henderson RD, Henderson RF, Marryatt GV: Surgical management of 100 consecutive esophageal strictures. *J Thorac Cardiovasc Surg* 99:1, 1990.

Hill LD, Kozarek RA, et al: The gastroesophageal flap valve. In vitro and in vivo observations. *Gastroeintest Endosc* 44:541, 1996.

Hinder RA, et al: Relationship of a satisfactory outcome to normalization of delayed gastric emptying after Nissen fundoplication. *Ann Surg* 210:458, 1989.

Hirota WK, Loughney TM, Lazas DJ, et al: Specialized intestinal metaplasia, dysplasia and cancer of the esophagus and esophagogastric junction: Prevalence and clinical data. *Gastroenterology* 116:277, 1999.

Hofstetter WA, Peters JH, DeMeester TR, et al: Long term outcome of antireflux surgery in patients with Barrett's esophagus. *Ann Surg* 234:532, 2001.

Ireland AP, Clark GWB, et al: Barrett's esophagus: The significance of p53 in clinical practice. *Ann Surg* 225:17, 1997.

Isolauri J, Luostarinen M, et al: Long-term comparison of antireflux surgery versus conservative therapy for reflux esophagitis. *Ann Surg* 225:295, 1997.

Jamieson JR, Hinder RA, et al: Analysis of 32 patients with Schatzki's ring. *Am J Surg* 158:563, 1989.

Johnson WE, Hagen JA, DeMeester TR, et al: Outcome of respiratory symptoms after antireflux surgery on patients with gastroesophageal reflux disease. *Arch Surg* 131:489, 1996.

Kahrilas PJ: Diagnosis of symptomatic gastroesophageal reflux disease. *Am J Gastroenterol* 98:S15, 2003.

Kahrilas PJ: Radiofrequency therapy of the lower esophageal sphincter for treatment of GERD. *Gastroint Endosc* 57:723; 2003.

Kaul BK, DeMeester TR, et al: The cause of dysphagia in uncomplicated sliding hiatal hernia and its relief by hiatal herniorrhaphy: A roentgenographic, manometric, and clinical study. *Ann Surg* 211:406, 1990.

Khaitan L, Ray WA, Holzman MD, et al: Health care utilization after medical and surgical therapy for gastroesophageal reflux disease. *Arch Surg* 138:1356, 2003.

Labenz J, Tillenburg B, et al. *Helicobacter pylori* augments the pH-increasing effect of omeprazole in patients with duodenal ulcer. *Gastroenterology* 110:725, 1996.

Lin KM, Ueda RK, et al: Etiology and importance of alkaline esophageal reflux. *Am J Surg* 162:553, 1991.

Little AG, Ferguson MK, Skinner DB: Reoperation for failed antireflux operations. *J Thorac Cardiovasc Surg* 91:511, 1986.

Liu JY, Finlayson SRG, Laycock WS, et al: Determining the appropriate threshold for referral to surgery for gastroesophageal reflux disease. *Surgery* 133:5, 2003.

Lundell L, Miettinen P, Myrvold HE, et al: Long-term management of gastro-oesophageal reflux disease with omeprazole or open antireflux surgery: Results of a prospective randomized trial. *Eur J Gastroenterol Hepatol* 12:879, 2000.

Marshall RE, Anggiansah A, Owen WJ: Bile in the esophagus: Clinical relevance and ambulatory detection. *Br J Surg* 84:21, 1997.

Morgenthal CB, Shane MD, Stival A, et al: The durability of laparoscopic Nissen fundoplication: 11-year outcomes. *J Gastrointest Surg* 11:693, 2007.

Narayani RI, Burton MP, Young GS: Utility of esophageal biopsy in the diagnosis of non-erosive reflux disease. *Dis Esophagus* 16:187, 2003.

Nissen R: Eine einfache operation zur beeinflussung der refluxoesophagitis. *Schweiz Med Wochenschr* 86:590, 1956.

Nissen R: Gastropexy and fundoplication in surgical treatment of hiatus hernia. *Am J Dig Dis* 6:954, 1961.

Oberg S, Johansson H, Wenner J, et al: Endoscopic surveillance of columnar lined esophagus: Frequency of intestinal metaplasia detection and impact of antireflux surgery. *Ann Surg* 234:619, 2001.

Orlando RC: The pathogenesis of gastroesophageal reflux disease: The relationship between epithelial defense, dysmotility, and acid exposure. *Am J Gastroenterol* 92:3S, 1997.

Orringer MB, Skinner DB, Belsey RHR: Long-term results of the Mark IV operation for hiatal hernia and analyses of recurrences and their treatment. *J Thorac Cardiovasc Surg* 63:25, 1972.

Parrilla P, Martinez de Haro LF, Ortiz A, et al: Long term results of a randomized prospective study comparing medical and surgical treatment in Barrett's esophagus. *Ann Surg* 237:291, 2003.

Patti MG, Debas HT, et al: Esophageal manometry and 24-hour pH monitoring in the diagnosis of pulmonary aspiration secondary to gastroesophageal reflux. *Am J Surg* 163:401, 1992.

Pearson FG, Cooper JD, et al: Gastroplasty and fundoplication for complex reflux problems. *Ann Surg* 206:473, 1987.

Pelligrini CA, DeMeester TR, et al: Gastroesophageal reflux and pulmonary aspiration: Incidence, functional abnormality, and results of surgical therapy. *Surgery* 86:110, 1979.

Peters JH, Heimbucher J, Incarbone R, et al: Clinical and physiologic comparison of laparoscopic and open Nissen fundoplication. *J Am Coll Surg* 180:385, 1995.

Provenzale D, Kemp JA, et al: A guide for surveillance of patients with Barrett's esophagus. *Am J Gastroenterol* 89:670, 1994.

Richter JE: Long-term management of gastroesophageal reflux disease and its complications. *Am J Gastroenterol* 92:30S, 1997.

Romagnuolo J, Meier MA, Sadowski DC: Medical or surgical therapy for erosive reflux esophagitis: Cost utility analysis using a Markov model. *Ann Surg* 236:191, 2002.

Schwizer W, Hinder RA, DeMeester TR: Does delayed gastric emptying contribute to gastroesophageal reflux disease? *Am J Surg* 157:74, 1989.

Shaker R, Castell DO, Schoenfeld PS, et al: Nighttime heartburn is an underappreciated clinical problem that impacts sleep and daytime function: The results of a Gallup survey conducted on behalf of the American Gastroenterologic Association. *Am J Gastroenterol* 98:1487, 2003.

Siewert JR, Isolauri J, Feussuer M: Reoperation following failed fundoplication. *World J Surg* 13:791, 1989.

Smith CD, McClusky DA, Rajhad MA, et al: When fundoplication fails: Redo? *Ann Surg* 241:861, 2005.

Sontag SJ, O'Connell S, Khandelwal S, et al: Asthmatics with gastroesophageal reflux: Long term results of a randomized trial of medical and surgical antireflux therapies. *Am J Gastroenterol* 98:987, 2003.

Spechler SJ, Department of Veterans Affairs Gastroesophageal Reflux Disease Study Group: Comparison of medical and surgical therapy for complicated gastroesophageal reflux disease in veterans. *N Engl J Med* 326:786, 1992.

Spechler SJ, Lee E, Ahmen D: Long term outcome of medical and surgical therapies for gastroesophageal reflux disease: Follow-up of a randomized controlled trial. *JAMA* 285:2331, 2001.

Spivak H, Farrell TM, Trus TL, et al: Laparoscopic fundoplication for dysphagia and peptic esophageal stricture. *J Gastrointest Surg* 2:555, 1998.

Stein HJ, Barlow AP, et al: Complications of gastroesophageal reflux disease: Role of the LES, esophageal acid and acid/alkaline exposure, and duodenogastric reflux. *Ann Surg* 216:35, 1992.

Stein HJ, Bremner RM, et al: Effect of Nissen fundoplication on esophageal motor function. *Arch Surg* 127:788, 1992.

Terry M, Smith CD, Branum GD, et al: Outcomes of laparoscopic fundoplication for gastroesophageal reflux disease and paraesophageal hernia: Experience with 1000 consecutive cases. *Surg Endosc* 15:691, 2001.

Terry ML, Vernon A, Hunter JG: Stapled-wedge Collis gastroplasty for the shortened esophagus. *Am J Surg* 188:195, 2004.

Trus TL, Laycock WS, Waring JP, et al: Improvement in quality of life measures after laparoscopic antireflux surgery. *Ann Surg* 229:331, 1999.

Tseng D, Rizvi AZ, Fennerty MB, et al: Forty-eight-hour pH monitoring increases sensitivity in detecting abnormal esophageal acid exposure. *J Gastrointest Surg* 9:1043, 2005.

Van Den Boom G, Go PM, et al: Cost effectiveness of medical versus surgical treatment in patients with severe or refractory gastroesophageal reflux disease in the Netherlands. *Scand J Gastroenterol* 31:1, 1996.

Watson DI, Baigrie RJ, Jamieson GG: A learning curve for laparoscopic fundoplication. Definable, avoidable, or a waste of time? *Ann Surg* 224:198, 1996.

Wattchow DA, Jamieson GG, et al: Distribution of peptide-containing nerve fibers in the gastric musculature of patients undergoing surgery for gastroesophageal reflux. *Ann Surg* 290:153, 1992.

Weston AP, Krmpotich P, et al: Short segment Barrett's esophagus: Clinical and histological features, associated endoscopic findings, and association with gastric intestinal metaplasia. *Am J Gastroenterol* 91:981, 1996.

Williamson WA, Ellis FH Jr., et al: Effect of antireflux operation on Barrett's mucosa. *Ann Thorac Surg* 49:537, 1990.

Wright TA: High-grade dysplasia in Barrett's oesophagus. *Br J Surg* 84:760, 1997.

Zaninotto G, DeMeester TR, et al: Esophageal function in patients with reflux-induced strictures and its relevance to surgical treatment. *Ann Thorac Surg* 47:362, 1989.

Diaphragmatic Hernias

Bombeck TC, Dillard DH, Nyhus LM: Muscular anatomy of the gastroesophageal junction and role of the phrenoesophageal ligament. *Ann Surg* 164:643, 1966.

Casbella F, Sinanan M, et al: Systematic use of gastric fundoplication in laparoscopic repair of paraesophageal hernias. *Am J Surg* 171:485, 1996.

Dalgaard JB: Volvulus of the stomach. *Acta Chir Scand* 103:131, 1952.

DeMeester TR, Lafontaine E, et al: The relationship of a hiatal hernia to the function of the body of the esophagus and the gastroesophageal junction. *J Thorac Cardiovasc Surg* 82:547, 1981.

Eliska O: Phreno-oesophageal membrane and its role in the development of hiatal hernia. *Acta Anat* 86:137, 1973.

Frantzides CT, Madan AK, Carlson MA, et al: A prospective, randomized trial of laparoscopic polytetrafluoroethylene (PTFE) patch repair vs simple cruroplasty for large hiatal hernia. *Arch Surg* 137:649, 2002.

Fuller CB, Hagen JA, et al: The role of fundoplication in the treatment of type II paraesophageal hernia. *J Thorac Cardiovasc Surg* 111:655, 1996.

Gangopadhyay N, Perrone JM, Soper NJ, et al: Outcomes of laparoscopic paraesophageal hernia repair in elderly and high-risk patients. *Surgery.* 140:491; discussion 498, 2006. Epub 2006 Sep 6.

Granderath FA, Schweiger UM, Kamolz T, et al: Laparoscopic Nissen fundoplication with prosthetic hiatal closure reduces postoperative intrathoracic wrap herniation: Preliminary results of a prospective randomized functional and clinical study. *Arch Surg* 140:40, 2005.

Hashemi M, Peters JH, DeMeester TR, et al: Laparoscopic repair of large type III hiatal hernia: Objective follow-up reveals high recurrence rate. *J Am Coll Surg* 190:539, 2000.

Kahrilas PJ, Wu S, et al: Attenuation of esophageal shortening during peristalsis with hiatus hernia. *Gastroenterology* 109:1818, 1995.

Kleitsch WP: Embryology of congenital diaphragmatic hernia. I. Esophageal hiatus hernia. *Arch Surg* 76:868, 1958.

Mattar SG, Bowers SP, Galloway KD, et al: Long-term outcome of laparoscopic repair of paraesophageal hernia. *Surg Endosc* 16:745, 2002.

Menguy R: Surgical management of large paraesophageal hernia with complete intrathoracic stomach. *World J Surg* 12:415, 1988.

Myers GA, Harms BA, et al: Management of paraesophageal hernia with a selective approach to antireflux surgery. *Am J Surg* 170:375, 1995.

Oddsdottir M, Franco AL, Laycock WS, et al: Laparoscopic repair of paraesophageal hernia: New access, old technique. *Surg Endosc* 9:164, 1995.

Oelschlager BK, Pellegrini CA, Hunter J, et al: Biologic prosthesis reduces recurrence after laparoscopic paraesophageal hernia repair: A multicenter, prospective, randomized trial. *Ann Surg* 244:481, 2006.

Patti MG, Goldberg HI, et al: Hiatal hernia size affects LES function, esophageal acid exposure, and the degree of mucosal injury. *Am J Surg* 171:182, 1996.

Pierre AF, Luketich JD, Fernando HC, et al: Results of laparoscopic repair of giant paraesophageal hernias: 200 consecutive patients. *Ann Thorac Surg* 74:1909, 2002.

Skinner DB, Belsey RH: Surgical management of esophageal reflux and hiatus hernia: Long-term results with 1030 patients. *J Thorac Cardiovasc Surg* 53:33, 1967.

Stylopoulos N, Gazelle GS, Ratner DW: Paraesophageal hernias: Operation or observation. *Ann Surg* 236:492, 2002.

Trus TL, Bax T, Richardson WS, et al: Complications of laparoscopic paraesophageal hernia repair. *J Gastrointest Surg* 1:221; discussion 228, 1997.

Wo JM, Branum GD, Hunter JG, et al: Clinical features of type III (mixed) paraesophageal hernia. *Am J Gastroenterol* 91:914, 1996.

Miscellaneous Esophageal Lesions

Burdick JS, Venu RP, Hogan WJ: Cutting the defiant lower esophageal ring. *Gastrointest Endosc* 39:616, 1993.

Burt M, Diehl W, et al: Malignant esophagorespiratory fistula: Management options and survival. *Ann Thorac Surg* 52:1222, 1991.

Chen MYM, Ott DJ, Donati DL: Correlation of lower esophageal mucosal ring and LES pressure. *Dig Dis Sci* 39:766, 1994.

D'Haens G, Rutgeerts P, et al: The natural history of esophageal Crohn's disease. Three patterns of evolution. *Gastrointest Endosc* 40:296, 1994.

Eckhardt VF, Kanzler G, Willems D: Single dilation of symptomatic Schatzki rings. A prospective evaluation of its effectiveness. *Dig Dis Sci* 37:577, 1992.

Klein HA, Wald A, et al: Comparative studies of esophageal function in systemic sclerosis. *Gastroenterology* 102:1551, 1992.

Mathisen DJ, Grillo HC, et al: Management of acquired nonmalignant tracheoesophageal fistula. *Ann Thorac Surg* 52:759, 1991.

Poirier NC, Taillefer R, et al: Antireflux operations in patients with scleroderma. *Ann Thorac Surg* 58:66, 1994.

Soudah HC, Hasler WL, Owyang C: Effect of octreotide on intestinal motility and bacterial overgrowth in scleroderma. *N Engl J Med* 325:1461, 1991.

Toskes PP: Hope for the treatment of intestinal scleroderma (Letter to the Editor). *N Engl J Med* 325:1508, 1991.

Wilcox CM, Straub RF: Prospective endoscopic characterization of cytomegalovirus esophagitis in AIDS. *Gastrointest Endosc* 40:481, 1994.

Motility Disorders of the Pharynx and Esophagus

Achem SR, Crittenden J, et al: Long-term clinical and manometric follow-up of patients with nonspecific esophageal motor disorders. *Am J Gastroenterol* 87:825, 1992.

Andreollo NA, Earlam RJ: Heller's myotomy for achalasia: Is an added antireflux procedure necessary? *Br J Surg* 74:765, 1987.

Anselmino M, Perdikis G, et al: Heller myotomy is superior to dilatation for the treatment of early achalasia. *Arch Surg* 132:233, 1997.

Bianco A, Cagossi M, et al: Appearance of esophageal peristalsis in treated idiopathic achalasia. *Dig Dis Sci* 90:978, 1986.

Bonavina L, Nosadinia A, et al: Primary treatment of esophageal achalasia: Long-term results of myotomy and Dor fundoplication. *Arch Surg* 127:222, 1992.

Chen LQ, Chughtau T, Sideris L, et al: Long term effects of myotomy and partial fundoplication for esophageal achalasia. *Dis Esophagus* 15:171, 2002.

Code CF, Schlegel JF, et al: Hypertensive gastroesophageal sphincter. *Mayo Clin Proc* 35:391, 1960.

Cook IJ, Blumbergs P, et al: Structural abnormalities of the cricopharyngeus muscle in patients with pharyngeal (Zenker's) diverticulum. *J Gastroenterol Hepatol* 7:556, 1992.

Cook IJ, Gabb M, et al: Pharyngeal (Zenker's) diverticulum is a disorder of upper esophageal sphincter opening. *Gastroenterology* 103:1229, 1992.

Csendes A, Braghetto I, et al: Late results of a prospective randomized study comparing forceful dilatation and oesophagomyotomy in patients with achalasia. *Gut* 30:299, 1989.

DeMeester TR, Johansson KE, et al: Indications, surgical technique and long-term functional results of colon interposition or bypass. *Ann Surg* 208:460, 1988.

DeMeester TR, Lafontaine E, et al: The relationship of a hiatal hernia to the function of the body of the esophagus and the gastroesophageal junction. *J Thorac Cardiovasc Surg* 82:547, 1981.

Eckardt V, Aignherr C, Bernhard G: Predictors of outcome in patients with achalasia treated by pneumatic dilation. *Gastroenterology* 103:1732, 1992.

Ekberg O, Wahlgren L: Dysfunction of pharyngeal swallowing: A cineradiographic investigation in 854 dysphagial patients. *Acta Radiol Diagn* 26:389, 1985.

Ellis FH: Long esophagomyotomy for diffuse esophageal spasm and related disorders: An historical overview. *Dis Esophagus* 11:210; 1998.

Ellis FH Jr.: Oesophagomyotomy for achalasia: A 22-year experience. *Br J Surg* 80:882, 1993.

Evander A, Little AG, et al: Diverticula of the mid and lower esophagus. *World J Surg* 10:820, 1986.

Ferguson TB, Woodbury JD, Roper CL: Giant muscular hypertrophy of the esophagus. *Ann Thorac Surg* 8:209, 1969.

Foker JE, Ring WE, Varco RL: Technique of jejunal interposition for esophageal replacement. *J Thorac Cardiovasc Surg* 83:928, 1982.

Gutschow CA, Hamoir M, Rombaux P, et al: Management of pharyngo-esophageal (Zenker's) diverticulum: Which technique? *Ann Thorac Surg* 74:1677, 2002.

Hirano I, Tatum RP, Shi G, et al: Manometric heterogeneity in patients with idiopathic achalasia. *Gastroenterology* 120:789, 2001.

Jeansonne LO, White BC, Pilger KE, et al: Ten-year follow-up of laparoscopic Heller myotomy for achalasia shows durability. *Surg Endosc* 21:1498, 2007. Epub 2007 Jul 11.

Jobe BA, Kim CY, Minjarez RC, et al: Simplifying minimally invasive transhiatal esophagectomy with the inversion approach: Lessons learned from the first 20 cases.: *Arch Surg* 141:857; discussion 865, 2006.

Kahrilas PJ, Logemann JA, et al: Pharyngeal clearance during swallowing: A combined manometric and videofluoroscopic study. *Gastroenterology* 103:128, 1992.

Kostic S, Kjellin A, Ruth M, et al: Pneumatic dilation or laparoscopic cardiomyotomy in the management of newly diagnosed idiopathic achalasia. Results of a randomized controlled trial. *World J Surg* 31:470, 2007.

Lam HG, Dekker W, et al: Acute noncardiac chest pain in a coronary care unit. *Gastroenterology* 102:453, 1992.

Mellow MH: Return of esophageal peristalsis in idiopathic achalasia. *Gastroenterology* 70:1148, 1976.

Meshkinpour H, Haghighat P, et al: Quality of life among patients treated for achalasia. *Dig Dis Sci* 41:352, 1996.

Migliore M, Payne H, et al: Pathophysiologic basis for operation on Zenker's diverticulum. *Ann Thorac Surg* 57:1616, 1994.

Moser G, Vacariu-Granser GV, et al: High incidence of esophageal motor disorders in consecutive patients with globus sensation. *Gastroenterology* 101:1512, 1991.

Moses PL, Ellis LM, Anees MR, et al: Antineural antibodies in idiopathic achalasia and gastro-oesophageal reflux disease. *Gut* 52:629, 2003.

Nehra D, Lord RV, DeMeester TR, et al: Physiologic basis for the treatment of epiphrenic diverticulum. *Ann Surg* 235:346, 2002.

Oelschlager BK, Chang L, Pellegrini CA: Improved outcome after extended gastric myotomy for achalasia. *Arch Surg* 138:490, 2003.

O'Rourke RW, Seltman AK, Chang EY, et al: A model for gastric banding in the treatment of morbid obesity: The effect of chronic partial gastric outlet obstruction on esophageal physiology. *Ann Surg* 244:723, 2006.

Patti MG, Fisichella PM, Peretta S, et al: Impact of minimally invasive surgery on the treatment of esophageal achalasia: A decade of change. *J Am Coll Surg* 196:698, 2003.

Pellegrini C, Wetter LA, et al: Thoracoscopic esophagomyotomy: Initial experience with a new approach for the treatment of achalasia. *Ann Surg* 216:291, 1992.

Peters JH: An antireflux procedure is critical to the long-term outcome of esophageal myotomy for achalasia. *J Gastrointest Surg* 5:17, 2001.

Peters JH, Kauer WK, Ireland AP, et al: Esophageal resection with colon interposition for end-stage achalasia. *Arch Surg* 130:632, 1995.

Ponce J, Garrigues V, Pertejo V, et al: Individual prediction of response to pneumatic dilation in patients with achalasia. *Dig Dis Sci* 41:2135, 1996.

Richards WO, Torquati A, Holzman MD, et al: Heller myotomy versus Heller myotomy with Dor fundoplication for achalasia: A prospective randomized double-blind clinical trial. *Ann Surg* 240:405; discussion 412, 2004.

Shoenut J, Duerksen D: A prospective assessment of gastroesophageal reflux before and after treatment of achalasia patients: Pneumatic dilation versus transthoracic limited myotomy. *Am J Gastroenterol* 92:1109, 1997.

Spechler S, Castell DO: Classification of oesophageal motility abnormalities. *Gut* 49:145, 2001.

Streitz JM Jr., Glick ME, Ellis FH Jr.: Selective use of myotomy for treatment of epiphrenic diverticula: Manometric and clinical analysis. *Arch Surg* 127:585, 1992.

Vaezi MF, Baker ME, Achkar E, et al: Timed barium oesophogram: Better predictor of long term success after pneumatic dilation in achalasia than symptom assessment. *Gut* 50:765, 2002.

Verne G, Sallustio JE, et al: Anti-myenteric neuronal antibodies in patients with achalasia: A prospective study. *Dig Dis Sci* 42:307, 1997.

Williams RB, Grehan MJ, Andre J, et al: Biomechanics, diagnosis, and treatment outcome in inflammatory myopathy presenting as oropharyngeal dysphagia. *Gut* 52:471, 2003.

Zaninotto G, Annese V, Costantini M, et al: Randomized controlled trial of botulinum toxin versus laparoscopic Heller myotomy for esophageal achalasia. *Ann Surg* 239:364, 2004.

Zhao X, Pasricha PJ: Botulinum toxin for spastic GI disorders: A systematic review. *Gastrointest Endosc* 57:219, 2003.

Carcinoma of the Esophagus

Akiyama H: Surgery for carcinoma of the esophagus. *Curr Probl Surg* 17:53, 1980.

Akiyama H, Tsurumaru M: Radical lymph node dissection for cancer of the thoracic esophagus. *Ann Surg* 220:364, 1994.

Altorki N, Skinner D: Should en-bloc esophagectomy be the standard of care for esophageal carcinoma? *Ann Surg* 234:581, 2001.

Badwe RA, Sharma V, Bhansali MS, et al: The quality of swallowing for patients with operable esophageal carcinoma: A randomized trial comparing surgery with radiotherapy. *Cancer* 85:763, 1999.

Baker JW Jr., Schechter GL: Management of paraesophageal cancer by blunt resection without thoracotomy and reconstruction with stomach. *Ann Surg* 203:491, 1986.

Blazeby JM, Williams MH, et al: Quality of life measurement in patients with oesophageal cancer. *Gut* 37:505, 1995.

Borrie J: Sarcoma of esophagus: Surgical treatment. *J Thorac Surg* 37:413, 1959.

Cameron AJ, Ott BJ, Payne WS: The incidence of adenocarcinoma in columnar-lined (Barrett's) esophagus. *N Engl J Med* 313:857, 1985.

Chang AC, Ji H, Birkmeyer NJ, et al: Outcomes after transhiatal and transthoracic esophagectomy for cancer. *Ann Thorac Surg* 85:424, 2008.

Chang EY, Morris CD, Seltman AK, et al: The effect of antireflux surgery on esophageal carcinogenesis in patients with Barrett's esophagus: A systematic review. *Ann Surg* 246:11, 2007.

Clark GWB, Peters JH, Hagen JA, et al: Nodal metastases and recurrence patterns after en-bloc esophagectomy for adenocarcinoma. *Ann Thorac Surg* 58:646, 1994.

Clark GW, Smyrk TC, et al: Is Barrett's metaplasia the source of adenocarcinomas of the cardia? *Arch Surg* 129:609, 1994.

Collin CF, Spiro RH: Carcinoma of the cervical esophagus: Changing therapeutic trends. *Am J Surg* 148:460, 1984.

Corley DA, Kerlikowske K, Verma R, et al: Protective association of aspirin/NSAIDs and esophageal cancer: A systematic review and meta-analysis. *Gastroenterology* 124:47, 2003.

Cunningham D, Allum WH, Stenning SP, et al: Perioperative chemotherapy versus surgery alone for resectable gastroesophageal cancer. *N Engl J Med* 6;355:11, 2006.

Dallal HJ, Smith GD, Grieve DC, et al: A randomized trial of thermal ablative therapy versus expandable metal stents in the palliative treatment of patients with esophageal carcinoma. *Gastrointest Endosc* 54:549, 2001.

DeMeester TR, Skinner DB: Polypoid sarcomas of the esophagus. *Ann Thorac Surg* 20:405, 1975.

Duhaylongsod FG, Wolfe WG: Barrett's esophagus and adenocarcinoma of the esophagus and gastroesophageal junction. *J Thorac Cardiovasc Surg* 102:36, 1991.

Ell C, May A, Gossner L, et al: Endoscopic mucosal resection of early cancer and high grade dysplasia in Barrett's esophagus. *Gastroenterology* 118:670, 2001.

Ellis FH, Heatley GJ, Krosna MJ, et al: Esophagogastrectomy for carcinoma of the esophagus and cardia: A comparison of findings and results after standard resection in three consecutive 8 year time intervals, using improved staging criteria. *J Thorac Cardiovasc Surg* 113:836, 1997.

Frenken M: Best palliation in esophageal cancer; surgery, stenting, radiation or what? *Dis Esophagus* 14:120, 2001.

Fujita H, Kakegawa T, et al: Mortality and morbidity rates, postoperative course, quality of life, and prognosis after extended radical lymphadenectomy for esophageal cancer. *Ann Surg* 222:654, 1995.

Gebski V, Burmeister B, Smithers BM, et al: Survival benefits from neoadjuvant chemoradiotherapy or chemotherapy in oesophageal carcinoma: A meta-analysis. *Lancet* 8:226, 2007.

Greenstein AJ, Litle VR, Swanson SJ, et al: Effect of the number of lymph nodes sampled on postoperative survival of lymph node-negative esophageal cancer. *Cancer* 112:1239, 2008.

Hagen JA, DeMeester TR, Peters JH, et al: Curative resection for esophageal adenocarcinoma analysis of 100 en bloc esophagectomies. *Ann Surg* 234:520, 2001.

Hofstetter W, Swisher SG, Correa AM: Treatment outcomes of resected esophageal cancer. *Ann Surg* 236:376, 2002.

Hulscher JB, Van Sandick JW, de Boer AG, et al: Extended transthoracic resection compared with limited transhiatal resection for adenocarcinoma of the esophagus. *N Engl J Med* 347:1662, 2002.

Iijima K, Henrey E, Moriya A, et al: Dietary nitrate generates potentially mutagenic concentrations of nitric oxide at the gastroesophageal junction. *Gastroenterology* 122:1248, 2002.

Ikeda M, Natsugoe S, Ueno S, et al: Significant host and tumor related factors for predicting prognosis in patients with esophageal carcinoma. *Ann Surg* 238:197, 2003.

Jankowski JA, Wight NA, Meltzer SJ, et al: Molecular evolution of the metaplasia-dysplasia-adenocarcinoma sequence in the esophagus. *Am J Pathol* 154:965, 1999.

Jobe BA, Kim CY, Minjarez RC, et al: Simplifying minimally invasive transhiatal esophagectomy with the inversion approach: Lessons learned from the first 20 cases. *Arch Surg* 141:857; discussion 865.

Johansson J, DeMeester TR, Hoger JA, et al: En bloc is superior to transhiatal esophagectomy for T3 N1 adenocarcinoma of the distal esophagus and GE junction. *Arch Surg* 139:627, 2004.

Kaklamanos IG, Walker GR, Ferry K, et al: Neoadjuvant treatment for resectable cancer of the esophagus and the gastroesophageal junction: A meta-analysis of randomized clinical trials. *Ann Surg Oncol* 10:754, 2003.

Kelsen DP, Winter KA, Gunderson LL, et al: Long-term results of RTOG trial 8911 (USA Intergroup 113): A random assignment trial comparison of chemotherapy followed by surgery compared with surgery alone for esophageal cancer. *J Clin Oncol* 25:3719, 2007.

Krasna MJ, Reed CE, Nedzwiecki D, et al: CALBG 9380: A prospective trial of the feasibility of thoracoscopy/laparoscopy in staging esophageal cancer. *Ann Thorac Surg* 71:1073, 2001.

Kirby JD: Quality of life after esophagectomy: The patients' perspective. *Dis Esophagus* 12:168, 1999.

Lagergren J, Bergstrom R, Lindgren A, et al: Symptomatic gastroesophageal reflux as a risk factor for esophageal adenocarcinoma. *N Engl J Med* 340:825, 1999.

Lavin P, Hajdu SI, Foote FW Jr.: Gastric and extragastric leiomyoblastomas. *Cancer* 29:305, 1972.

Law SYK, Fok M, Wong J: Pattern of recurrence after oesophageal resection for cancer: Clinical implications. *Br J Surg* 83:107, 1996.

Law SYK, Fok M, et al: A comparison of outcomes after resection for squamous cell carcinomas and adenocarcinomas of the esophagus and cardia. *Surg Gynecol Obstet* 175:107, 1992.

Law S, Kwong DL, Kwok KF, et al: Improvement in treatment results and long term survival of patients with esophageal cancer: Impact of chemoradiation and change in treatment strategy. *Ann Surg* 238:339, 2003.

Lerut T, Coosemans W, et al: Surgical treatment of Barrett's carcinoma. Correlations between morphologic findings and prognosis. *J Thorac Cardiovasc Surg* 107:1059, 1994.

Leuketich JD, Alvelo-Rivera M, Buenaventura PO, et al: Minimally invasive esophagectomy: Outcomes in 222 patients. *Ann Surg* 238:486, 2003.

Levine DS, Reid BJ: Endoscopic diagnosis of esophageal neoplasms. *Gastrointest Clin North Am* 2:395, 1992.

Lewis I: The surgical treatment of carcinoma of the esophagus with special reference to a new operation for the growths of the middle third. *Br J Surg* 34:18, 1946.

Logan A: The surgical treatment of carcinoma of the esophagus and cardia. *J Thorac Cardiovasc Surg* 46:150, 1963.

Manner H, May A, Pech O, et al: Early Barrett's carcinoma with "low-risk" submucosal invasion: Long-term results of endoscopic resection with a curative intent. *Am J Gastroenterol* 103:2589, 2008. Epub 2008 Sep 10.

McCort JJ: Esophageal carcinosarcoma and pseudosarcoma. *Radiology* 102:519, 1972.

Medical Research Council Oesophageal Working Party: Surgical resection with or without preoperative chemotherapy in oesophageal cancer: A randomized controlled trial. *Lancet* 359:1727, 2002.

Naunheim KS, Petruska PJ, et al: Preoperative chemotherapy and radiotherapy for esophageal carcinoma. *J Thorac Cardiovasc Surg* 103:887, 1992.

Nicks R: Colonic replacement of the esophagus. *Br J Surg* 54:124, 1967.

Nigro JJ, Hagen JA, DeMeester TR, et al: Occult esophageal adenocarcinoma: Extent of disease and implications for effective therapy. *Ann Surg* 230:433, 1999.

Omloo JM, Lagarde SM, Hulscher JB, et al: Extended transthoracic resection compared with limited transhiatal resection for adenocarcinoma of the mid/distal esophagus: Five year survival of a randomized clinical trial. *Ann Surg* 246:992, 2007.

Orringer MB, Marshall B, Iannettoni MD: Transhiatal esophagectomy: Clinical experience and refinements. *Ann Surg* 230:392, 1999.

Orringer MB, Marshall B, Chang AC, et al: Two thousand transhiatal esophagectomies: changing trends, lessons learned. *Ann Surg* 246:363; discussion 372, 2007.

Ott K, Herrmann K, Lordick F, et al: Early metabolic response evaluation by fluorine-18 fluorodeoxyglucose positron emission tomography allows in vivo testing of chemosensitivity in gastric cancer: long-term results of a prospective study. *Clin Cancer Res* 14:2012, 2008.

Pacifico RJ, Wang KK, Wongkeesong LM, et al: Combined endoscopic mucosal resection and photodynamic therapy versus esophagectomy for management of early adenocarcinoma of the esophagus. *Clin Gastroenterol Hepatol* 1:252, 2003.

Pera M, Cameron AJ, et al: Increasing incidence of adenocarcinoma of the esophagus and esophagogastric junction. *Gastroenterology* 104:510, 1993.

Pera M, Trastek VF, et al: Barrett's esophagus with high-grade dysplasia: An indication for esophagectomy? *Ann Thorac Surg* 54:199, 1992.

Pera M, Trastek VF, et al: Influence of pancreatic and biliary reflux on the development of esophageal carcinoma. *Ann Thorac Surg* 55:1386, 1993.

Peters JH, Clark GWB, et al: Outcome of adenocarcinoma arising in Barrett's esophagus in endoscopically surveyed and non-surveyed patients. *J Thorac Cardiovasc Surg* 108:813, 1994.

Peters JH, Hoeft SF, et al: Selection of patients for curative or palliative resection of esophageal cancer based on preoperative endoscopic ultrasound. *Arch Surg* 129:534, 1994.

Peters JH: Surgical treatment of esophageal adenocarcinoma: Concepts in evolution. *J Gastrointest Surg* 6:518, 2002.

Rasanen JV, Sihvo EIT, Knuuti J, et al: Prospective analysis of accuracy of proton emission tomography, computed tomography and endoscopic ultrasonography in staging of adenocarcinoma of the esophagus and esophagogastric junction. *Ann Surg Oncol* 10:954, 2003.

Ravitch M: *A Century of Surgery*. Philadelphia: Lippincott, 1981, p 56.

Reed CE: Comparison of different treatments for unresectable esophageal cancer. *World J Surg* 19:828, 1995.

Reid BJ, Weinstein WM, et al: Endoscopic biopsy can detect high-grade dysplasia or early adenocarcinoma in Barrett's esophagus without grossly recognizable neoplastic lesions. *Gastroenterology* 94:81, 1988.

Ribeiro U Jr., Posner MC, et al: Risk factors for squamous cell carcinoma of the oesophagus. *Br J Surg* 83:1174, 1996.

Rice TW, Boyce GA, et al: Esophageal ultrasound and the preoperative staging of carcinoma of the esophagus. *J Thorac Cardiovasc Surg* 101:536, 1991.

Robertson CS, Mayberry JF, Nicholson JA: Value of endoscopic surveillance in the detection of neoplastic changes in Barrett's esophagus. *Br J Surg* 75:760, 1988.

Rösch T, Lorenz R, et al: Endosonographic diagnosis of submucosal upper gastrointestinal tract tumors. *Scand J Gastroenterol* 27:1, 1992.

Rosenberg JC, Budev H, et al: Analysis of adenocarcinoma in Barrett's esophagus utilizing a staging system. *Cancer* 55:1353, 1985.

Ruol A, Portale G, Castoro C, et al: Effects of neoadjuvant therapy on perioperative morbidity in elderly patients undergoing esophagectomy for esophageal cancer. *Ann Surg Oncol* 14:3243, 2007.

Skinner DB, Dowlatshahi KD, DeMeester TR: Potentially curable carcinoma of the esophagus. *Cancer* 50:2571, 1982.

Skinner DB, Ferguson MK, Little AG: Selection of operation for esophageal cancer based on staging. *Ann Surg* 204:391, 1986.

Smithers BM, Cullinan M, Thomas JM, et al: *Dis Esophagus* 20:471, 2007.

Sonnenberg A, Fennerty MB: Medical decision analysis of chemoprevention against esophageal adenocarcinoma. *Gastroenterology* 124:1758, 2003.

Streitz JM Jr., Ellis FH Jr., et al: Adenocarcinoma in Barrett's esophagus. *Ann Surg* 213:122, 1991.

Turnbull AD, Rosen P, et al: Primary malignant tumors of the esophagus other than typical epidermoid carcinoma. *Ann Thorac Surg* 15:463, 1973.

Urschel JD, Ashiku S, Thurer R, et al: Salvage or planned esophagectomy after chemoradiation for locally advanced esophageal cancer: A review. *Dis Esophagus* 16:60, 2003.

Vigneswaran WT, Trastek VK, et al: Extended esophagectomy in the management of carcinoma of the upper thoracic esophagus. *J Thorac Cardiovasc Surg* 107:901, 1994.

Walsh TN, Noonan N, et al: A comparison of multimodal therapy and surgery for esophageal adenocarcinoma. *N Engl J Med* 335:462, 1996.

Watson WP, Pool L: Cancer of the cervical esophagus. *Surgery* 23:893, 1948.

Benign Tumors and Cysts

Bardini R, Segalin A, et al: Videothoracoscopic enucleation of esophageal leiomyoma. *Am Thorac Surg* 54:576, 1992.

Bonavina L, Segalin A, et al: Surgical therapy of esophageal leiomyoma. *J Am Coll Surg* 181:257, 1995.

Esophageal Perforation

Brewer LA III, Carter R, et al: Options in the management of perforations of the esophagus. *Am J Surg* 152:62, 1986.

Bufkin BL, Miller JI Jr., Mansour KA: Esophageal perforation. Emphasis on management. *Ann Thorac Surg* 61:1447, 1996.

Chang C-H, Lin PJ, et al: One-stage operation for treatment after delayed diagnosis of thoracic esophageal perforation. *Ann Thorac Surg* 53:617, 1992.

Engum SA, Grosfeld JL, et al: Improved survival in children with esophageal perforation. *Arch Surg* 131:604, 1996.

Gouge TH, Depan HJ, Spencer FC: Experience with the Grillo pleural wrap procedure in 18 patients with perforation of the thoracic esophagus. *Ann Surg* 209:612, 1989.

Jones WG II, Ginsberg RJ: Esophageal perforation: A continuing challenge. *Ann Thorac Surg* 53:534, 1992.

Pate JW, Walker WA, et al: Spontaneous rupture of the esophagus: A 30-year experience. *Ann Thorac Surg* 47:689, 1989.

Reeder LB, DeFilippi VJ, Ferguson MK: Current results of therapy for esophageal perforation. *Am J Surg* 169:615, 1995.

Salo JA, Isolauri JO, et al: Management of delayed esophageal perforation with mediastinal sepsis. Esophagectomy or primary repair? *J Thorac Cardiovasc Surg* 106:1088, 1993.

Sawyer R, Phillips C, Vakil N: Short- and long-term outcome of esophageal perforation. *Gastrointest Endosc* 41:130, 1995.

Segalin A, Bonavina L, et al: Endoscopic management of inveterate esophageal perforations and leaks. *Surg Endosc* 10:928, 1996.

Weiman DS, Walker WA, et al: Noniatrogenic esophageal trauma. *Ann Thorac Surg* 59:845, 1995.

Whyte RI, Iannettoni MD, Orringer MB: Intrathoracic esophageal perforation. The merit of primary repair. *J Thorac Cardiovasc Surg* 109:140, 1995.

Caustic Injury

Anderson KD, Rouse TM, Randolph JG: A controlled trial of corticosteroids in children with corrosive injury of the esophagus. *N Engl J Med* 323:637, 1990.

Ferguson MK, Migliore M, et al: Early evaluation and therapy for caustic esophageal injury. *Am J Surg* 157:116, 1989.

Lahoti D, Broor SL, et al: Corrosive esophageal strictures. Predictors of response to endoscopic dilation. *Gastrointest Endosc* 41:196, 1995.

Popovici Z: About reconstruction of the pharynx with colon in extensive corrosive strictures. *Kurume Med J* 36:41, 1989.

Sugawa C, Lucas CE: Caustic injury of the upper gastrointestinal tract in adults: A clinical and endoscopic study. *Surgery* 106:802, 1989.

Wu M-H, Lai W-W: Surgical management of extensive corrosive injuries of the alimentary tract. *Surg Gynecol Obstet* 177:12, 1993.

Zargar SA, Kochhar R, et al: The role of fiberoptic endoscopy in the management of corrosive ingestion and modified endoscopic classification of burns. *Gastrointest Endosc* 37:165, 1991.

Techniques of Esophageal Reconstruction

Akiyama H: Esophageal reconstruction. Entire stomach as esophageal substitute. *Dis Esophagus* 8:7, 1995.

Banki F, Mason RJ, DeMeester SR, et al: Vagal sparing esophagectomy: A more physiologic alternative. *Ann Surg* 236:324, 2002.

Burt M, Scott A, et al: Erythromycin stimulates gastric emptying after esophagectomy with gastric replacement. A randomized clinical trial. *J Thorac Cardiovasc Surg* 111:649, 1996.

Cheng W, Heitmiller RF, Jones BJ: Subacute ischemia of the colon esophageal interposition. *Ann Thorac Surg* 57:899, 1994.

DeMeester TR, Johansson KE, et al: Indications, surgical technique, and long-term functional results of colon interposition or bypass. *Ann Surg* 208:460, 1988.

DeMeester TR, Kauer WK: Esophageal reconstruction. The colon as an esophageal substitute. *Dis Esophagus* 8:20, 1995.

Dexter SPL, Martin IG, McMahon MJ: Radical thoracoscopic esophagectomy for cancer. *Surg Endosc* 10:147, 1996.

Ellis FH Jr., Gibb SP: Esophageal reconstruction for complex benign esophageal disease. *J Thorac Cardiovasc Surg* 99:192, 1990.

Finley RJ, Lamy A, et al: Gastrointestinal function following esophagectomy for malignancy. *Am J Surg* 169:471, 1995.

Fok M, Cheng SW, Wong J: Pyloroplasty versus no drainage in gastric replacement of the esophagus. *Am J Surg* 162:447, 1991.

Gossot D, Cattan P, Fritsch S: Can the morbidity of esophagectomy be reduced by the thoracoscopic approach? *Surg Endosc* 9:1113, 1995.

Honkoop P, Siersema PD, et al: Benign anastomotic strictures after transhiatal esophagectomy and cervical esophagogastrostomy. Risk factors and management. *J Thorac Cardiovasc Surg* 111:1141, 1996.

Liebermann-Meffert DMI, Meier R, Siewert JR: Vascular anatomy of the gastric tube used for esophageal reconstruction. *Ann Thorac Surg* 54:1110, 1992.

Maier G, Jehle EC, Becker HD: Functional outcome following oesophagectomy for oesophageal cancer. A prospective manometric study. *Dis Esophagus* 8:64, 1995.

Naunheim KS, Hanosh J, et al: Esophagectomy in the septuagenarian. *Ann Thorac Surg* 56:880, 1993.

Nishihira T, Oe H, et al: Esophageal reconstruction. Reconstruction of the thoracic esophagus with jejunal pedicled segments for cancer of the thoracic esophagus. *Dis Esophagus* 8:30, 1995.

Peters JH, Kronson J, Bremner CG, et al: Arterial anatomic considerations in colon interposition for esophageal replacement. *Arch Surg* 130:858, 1995.

Stark SP, Romberg MS, et al: Transhiatal versus transthoracic esophagectomy for adenocarcinoma of the distal esophagus and cardia. *Am J Surg* 172:478, 1996.

Valverde A, Hay JM, Fingerhut A, et al: Manual versus mechanical esophagogastric anastomosis after resection for carcinoma. A controlled trial. French Associations for Surgical Research. *Surgery* 120:476, 1996.

Watson T, DeMeester TR, Kauer WK, et al: Esophagectomy for end stage benign esophageal disease. *J Thorac Cardiovasc Surg* 115:1241, 1998.

Wu M-H, Lai W-W: Esophageal reconstruction for esophageal strictures or resection after corrosive injury. *Ann Thorac Surg* 53:798, 1992.

Stomach

Daniel T. Dempsey

HISTORY

The stomach is a remarkable organ with important digestive, nutritional, and endocrine functions. The stomach stores and facilitates the digestion and absorption of ingested food, and it helps regulate appetite. Treatable diseases of the stomach are common, and it is accessible and relatively forgiving. Thus, the stomach is a favorite therapeutic target. To provide intelligent diagnosis and treatment, the physician and surgeon must understand gastric anatomy, physiology, and pathophysiology. This includes a sound understanding of the mechanical, secretory, and endocrine processes through which the stomach accomplishes its important functions. It also includes a familiarity with the common benign and malignant gastric disorders of clinical significance. The purpose of this chapter is to enhance the reader's current understanding and familiarity with these concepts and topics. Some important milestones in the history of gastric surgery[1-6] are listed in Table 26-1.

ANATOMY

Anatomic Relationships and Gross Morphology

The stomach is readily recognizable as the asymmetrical, pear-shaped, most proximal abdominal organ of the digestive tract (Fig. 26-1).[7] The part of the stomach attached to the esophagus is called the cardia. Just proximal to the cardia at the gastroesophageal (GE) junction is the anatomically indistinct but physiologically demonstrable lower esophageal sphincter. At the distal end, the pyloric sphincter connects the stomach to the proximal duodenum. The stomach is relatively fixed at these points, but the large midportion is quite mobile.

The superior-most part of the stomach is the distensible floppy fundus, bounded superiorly by the diaphragm and laterally by the spleen. The angle of His is where the fundus meets the left side of the GE junction. Generally, the inferior extent of the fundus is considered to be the horizontal plane of the GE junction, where the body (corpus) of the stomach begins. The body of the stomach contains most of the parietal (oxyntic) cells, some of which are also present in the cardia and fundus. The body is bounded on the right by the relatively straight lesser curvature and on the left by the more curved greater curvature. At the angularis incisura, the lesser curvature turns rather abruptly to the right, marking the anatomic beginning of the antrum, which comprises the distal 25 to 30% of the stomach.

The organs that commonly abut the stomach are the liver, colon, spleen, pancreas, and occasionally the kidney (Fig. 26-2). The left lateral segment of the liver usually covers a large part of the anterior stomach. Inferiorly, the stomach is attached to the transverse colon by the gastrocolic omentum. The lesser curvature is tethered to the liver by the hepatogastric ligament, also referred to as the lesser omentum or pars flaccida. Posterior to the stomach is the lesser omental bursa and the pancreas.

Arterial and Venous Blood Supply

The stomach is the most richly vascularized portion of the alimentary tube. Both the quantity of blood delivered to the stomach and the richness of the intramural gastric vascular anastomotic network are impressive. The large majority of the gastric blood supply is from the celiac axis via four named arteries (Fig. 26-3). The left and right gastric arteries form an anastomotic arcade along the lesser curvature, and the right and left gastroepiploic arteries form an arcade along the greater gastric curvature. The consistently largest artery to the stomach is the left gastric artery, which usually arises directly from the celiac trunk and divides into an ascending and descending branch along the lesser gastric curvature. Approximately 15% of the time, the left gastric artery supplies an aberrant vessel that travels in the gastrohepatic ligament (lesser omentum) to the left side of the liver. Rarely, this is the only arterial blood supply to this part of the liver, and inadvertent ligation may lead to clinically significant hepatic ischemia in this unusual circumstance. The more common smaller aberrant left hepatic artery may usually be ligated without significant consequences.

The second largest artery to the stomach is the right gastroepiploic artery, which arises consistently from the gastroduodenal artery behind the first portion of the duodenum. The left gastroepiploic artery arises from the splenic artery, and, together with the right gastroepiploic artery, forms the rich gastroepiploic arcade along the greater curvature. The right gastric artery usually arises from the hepatic artery near the pylorus and hepatoduodenal ligament, and runs proximally along the distal stomach. In the fundus along the proximal greater curvature, the short gastric arteries and veins arise from the splenic circulation. There also may be additional vascular branches to the proximal stomach from the phrenic and splenic circulation.

The veins draining the stomach generally parallel the arteries. The left gastric (coronary vein) and right gastric veins usually drain into the portal vein, though occasionally the coronary vein drains into the splenic vein. The right gastroepiploic vein drains into the superior mesenteric vein near the inferior border of the pancreatic neck, and the left gastroepiploic vein drains into the splenic vein.

The richness of the gastric blood supply and the extensiveness of the anastomotic connections have some important clinical implications. Erosion of a peptic ulcer or gastric cancer into a large perigastric vessel may cause life-threatening hemorrhage. Because of the rich venous interconnections in the stomach, a distal splenorenal shunt, which connects the distal end of the divided splenic vein to the side of the left renal vein, can effectively decompress esophagogastric varices in patients with portal hypertension.[8] Finally, at least two of the four named gastric arteries may be occluded or ligated with impunity. This is done routinely when the stomach is mobilized and pedicled on the

TABLE 26-1 Historic milestones in gastric surgery

Date	Event	Date	Event
350 B.C. – 201 A.D.	Existence of gastric ulceration was acknowledged by Diocles of Carystos (350 B.C.), Celsus, and Galen (131–201 A.D.).	1886	Heineke performs pyloroplasty.
1363	Guy de Chauliac describes closure of gastric wound.	1888	Mikulicz performs similar operation.
1586	Marcellus Donatus of Mantua describes gastric ulcer at autopsy.	1892	Jaboulay describes bypassing the intact pylorus with gastroduodenostomy.
1600–1700	Reports of surgeons cutting stomach to remove foreign bodies.	1902	Finney from Baltimore describes pyloroplasty technique.
1688	Muralto describes duodenal ulcer at autopsy.	1891–1913	Different techniques of gastrostomy are described by Witzel (1891), Stamm (1894), and Janeway (1913).
1737	Morgagni describes both gastric and duodenal ulcer at autopsy.	1920–1950	Subtotal gastrectomy grows popular as an operation for peptic ulcer. Von Haberer and Finsterer proponents.
1833	William Beaumont reports data recorded during his care of Alexis St. Martin who developed a gastric fistula from a left upper quadrant musket wound.	1943	Dragstedt and Owen describe transthoracic truncal vagotomy to treat peptic ulcer disease. By the early 1950s, it is well recognized that some patients developed gastric stasis after this procedure, and transabdominal truncal vagotomy and drainage (pyloroplasty or gastrojejunostomy) become a standard ulcer operation.
1869	Maury reportedly performs feeding gastrostomy to palliate esophageal stricture following consultation with Samuel D. Gross.		
1875	Sidney Jones in London publishes the first successful gastrostomy for feeding.	1952	Farmer and Smithwick describe good results with truncal vagotomy and hemigastrectomy for peptic ulcer.
1879	Paen performed distal gastrectomy and gastroduodenostomy. The patient died 5 d later.	1953	Edwards and Herrington (Nashville) describe truncal vagotomy and antrectomy for peptic ulcer.
1880	Rydygier resected a distal gastric cancer, and the patient died 12 h later.	1955	Zollinger and Ellison describe the eponymous syndrome.
1880	Billroth resects distal gastric cancer and performs gastroduodenostomy (Billroth I). Patient Therese Heller recovers and survives 4 mo.	1957	Griffith and Harkins (Seattle) describe parietal cell vagotomy (highly selective vagotomy) for the elective treatment of peptic ulcer disease.
1881	Anton Wolfler performs loop gastrojejunostomy to palliate an obstructing distal gastric cancer.	1980–2000	Japanese surgeons and other surgical groups from East Asia demonstrate that more aggressive lymphadenectomy may improve survival in patients with gastric cancer.
1884	Rydygier reports an unsuccessful gastrojejunostomy for benign gastric outlet obstruction.	1990–current	Evolving role of laparoscopic techniques in the treatment of surgical gastric disease.
1885	Billroth performs a successful distal gastrectomy and gastrojejunostomy (Billroth II) for gastric cancer.	1995–current	Dramatic increase in bariatric operations.
		2000–current	Development of natural orifice translumenal endoscopic surgery.

right gastric and right gastroepiploic vessels to reach into the neck as an esophageal replacement (see Chap. 25).[9]

Lymphatic Drainage

Generally speaking, the gastric lymphatics parallel the blood vessels (Fig. 26-4).[10] The cardia and medial half of the corpus commonly drain to nodes along the left gastric and celiac axis. The lesser curvature side of the antrum usually drains to the right gastric and pyloric nodes, while the greater curvature half of the distal stomach drains to the nodes along the right gastroepiploic chain. The proximal greater curvature side of the stomach usually drains into nodes along the left gastroepiploic or splenic hilum. The nodes along both the greater and lesser curvature commonly drain into the celiac nodal basin. There is a rich anastomotic network of lymphatics that drain the stomach, often in a somewhat unpredictable fashion. Thus, a tumor arising in the distal stomach may give rise to positive lymph nodes in the splenic hilum. The rich intramural plexus of lymphatics

KEY POINTS

1. Any patient admitted to a hospital because of peptic ulcer disease should be placed on lifelong acid suppression.

2. Patients who regularly take NSAIDs or aspirin should take concomitant acid suppressive medication if they are more than age 60 years old, or on anticoagulants, or if they have multiple medical comorbidities.

3. Lifelong acid suppressive medication may be equivalent to surgical vagotomy in preventing recurrent peptic ulcer or ulcer complications.

4. Gastric resection for peptic ulcer should be avoided in the asthenic or high-risk patient.

5. Many patients with locally advanced gastric cancer (T2b, T3, T4) are cured by an oncologically sound operation that includes wide margins and adequate lymphadenectomy.

6. Most patients with primary gastric lymphoma can be treated without gastric resection.

7. Gastric carcinoids should usually be removed either endoscopically or surgically. The surgeon should treat gastric carcinoid without hypergastrinemia (type 3) as if it were malignant.

8. Roux-en-Y gastrojejunostomy should be avoided unless more than half of the stomach has been removed. Otherwise marginal ulceration and/or gastric stasis (Roux syndrome) may become problematic.

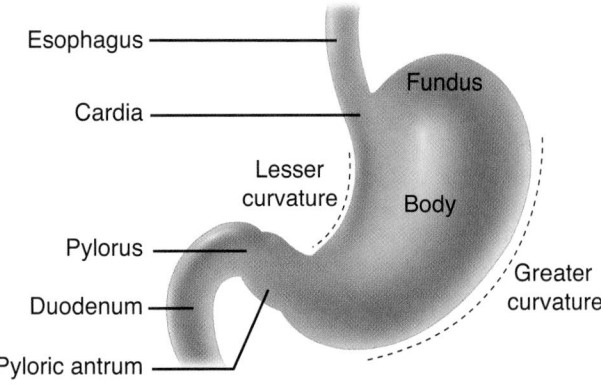

FIG. 26-1. Anatomic regions of the stomach. *[Reproduced with permission from Mercer DW, Liu TH, Castaneda A: Anatomy and physiology of the stomach, in Zuidema GD, Yeo CJ (eds): Shackelford's Surgery of the Alimentary Tract, 5th ed., Vol. II. Philadelphia: Saunders, 2002, p 3. Copyright Elsevier.]*

and veins accounts for the fact that there can be microscopic evidence of malignant cells in the gastric wall at a resection margin that is several centimeters away from palpable malignant tumor. It also helps explain the not infrequent finding of positive lymph nodes which may be many centimeters away from the primary tumor, with closer nodes that remain negative.

Extensive and meticulous lymphadenectomy is considered by many surgeons to be an important part of the operation for gastric cancer. Surgeons and pathologists have numbered the primary and secondary lymph node groups to which the stomach drains (see Fig. 26-4).[11,12]

Innervation

Both the extrinsic and intrinsic innervation of the stomach play an important role in gastric secretory and motor function.[13] The vagus nerves provide the extrinsic parasympathetic innervation to the stomach, and acetylcholine is the most important neurotransmitter.

From the vagal nucleus in the floor of the fourth cerebral ventricle, the vagus traverses the neck in the carotid sheath and enters the mediastinum, where it gives off the recurrent laryngeal nerve and divides into several branches around the esophagus. These branches come together again above the esophageal hiatus and form the *left* (*anterior*) and *right* (*posterior*) vagal trunks (mnemonic LARP). Near the GE junction the anterior vagus sends a branch (or branches) to the liver in the gastrohepatic ligament, and continues along the lesser curvature as the anterior nerve of Latarjet (Fig. 26-5). Similarly, the posterior vagus sends branches to the celiac plexus and continues along the posterior lesser curvature. The nerves of Latarjet send segmental branches to the body of the stomach before they terminate near the angularis incisura as the "crow's foot," sending branches to the antropyloric region. There may be additional branches to the distal stomach and pylorus that travel near the right gastric and/or gastroepiploic arteries. In 50% of patients, there are more than two vagal nerves at the esophageal hiatus. The branch that the posterior vagus sends to the posterior fundus is termed the *criminal nerve of Grassi*. This branch typically arises above the esophageal hiatus and is easily missed during truncal or highly selective vagotomy (HSV). Vagal fibers originating in the brain synapse with neurons in Auerbach's myenteric plexus and Meissner's submucosal plexus. Although clinicians are accustomed to thinking about the vagus nerves as important efferent nerves (i.e., carrying stimuli to the viscera), it is important to consider the fact that fully 75% of the axons contained in the vagal trunks are afferent (i.e., carrying stimuli from the viscera to the brain).

The extrinsic sympathetic nerve supply to the stomach originates at spinal levels T5 through T10 and travels in the splanchnic nerves to the celiac ganglion. Postganglionic sympathetic nerves then travel from the celiac ganglion to the stomach along the blood vessels.

Neurons in the myenteric and submucosal plexuses constitute the intrinsic nervous system of the stomach. There may be more intrinsic gastric neurons than extrinsic neurons, but their function is poorly understood.

It is obviously an oversimplification (and incorrect) to think exclusively of the vagus as the cholinergic system and the sympathetic system as the adrenergic system of innervation. Although

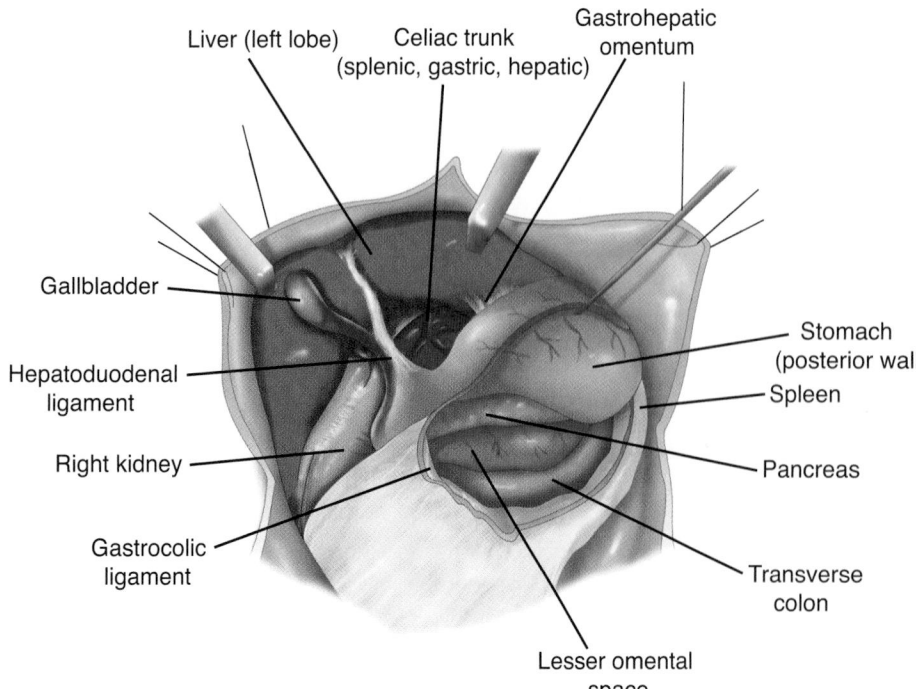

FIG. 26-2. Anatomic relationships of the stomach. *[Reproduced with permission from Mercer DW, Liu TH, Castaneda A: Anatomy and physiology of the stomach, in Zuidema GD, Yeo CJ (eds): Shackelford's Surgery of the Alimentary Tract, 5th ed., Vol. II. Philadelphia: Saunders, 2002, p 3. Copyright Elsevier.]*

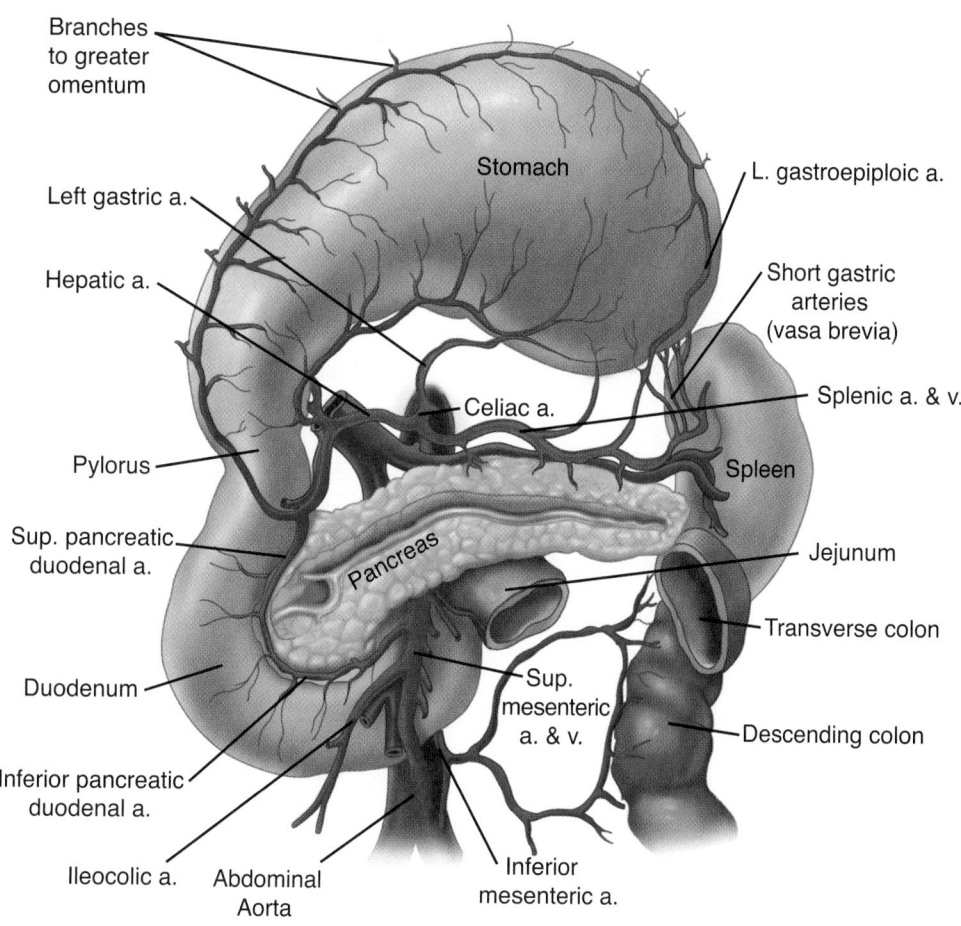

FIG. 26-3. Arterial blood supply to the stomach. a. = artery; v. = vein. *[Reproduced with permission from Mercer DW, Liu TH, Castaneda A: Anatomy and physiology of the stomach, in Zuidema GD, Yeo CJ (eds):* Shackelford's Surgery of the Alimentary Tract, *5th ed., Vol. II. Philadelphia: Saunders, 2002, p 3. Copyright Elsevier.]*

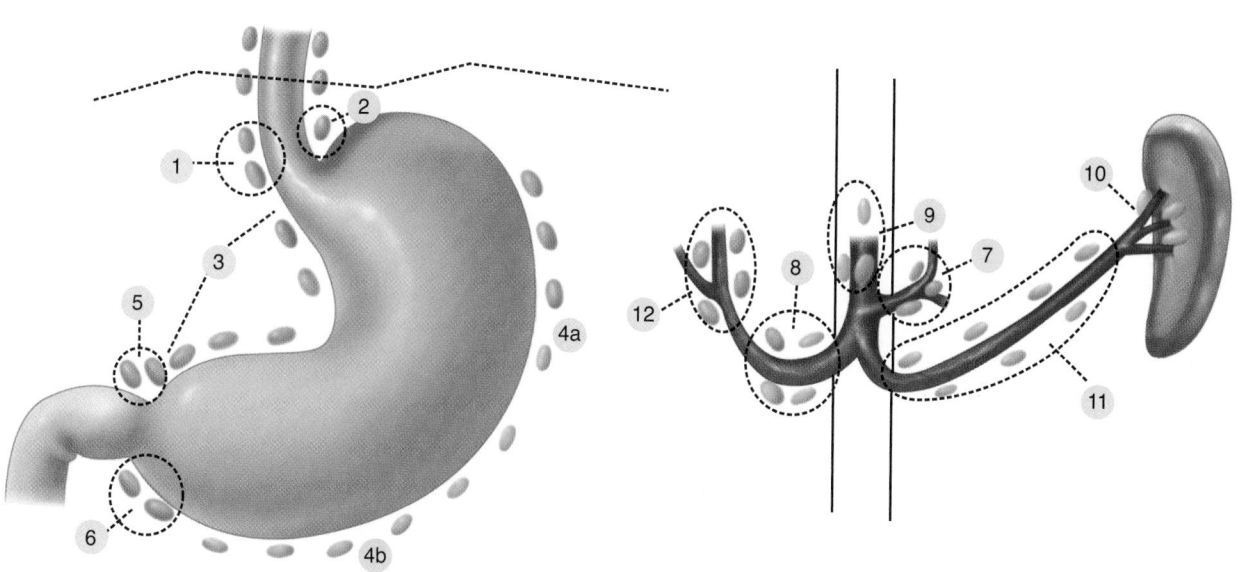

FIG. 26-4. Lymph node stations draining the stomach according to the Japanese Research Society for Gastric Cancer. Stations 3–6 are commonly removed with D1 gastrectomy. Stations 1, 2, and 7–12 are commonly removed with D2 gastrectomy. *[Reproduced with permission from Hermanek P, et al (eds):* TNM Atlas: Illustrated Guide to the TNM/pTNM Classification of Malignant Tumours, *4th ed. Berlin: Springer-Verlag, 1997, p 82–83. Copyright 1997, with kind permission of Springer Science + Business Media.]*

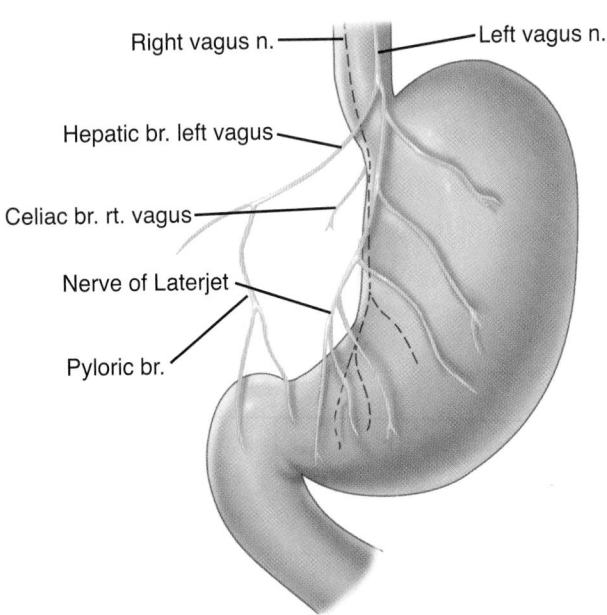

FIG. 26-5. Vagal innervation of the stomach. br. = branch; n. = nerve; rt. = right. *[Reproduced with permission from Anatomy and physiology of the stomach, in Menguy R: Surgery of Peptic Ulcer. Philadelphia: Saunders, 1976, p 8. Copyright Elsevier.]*

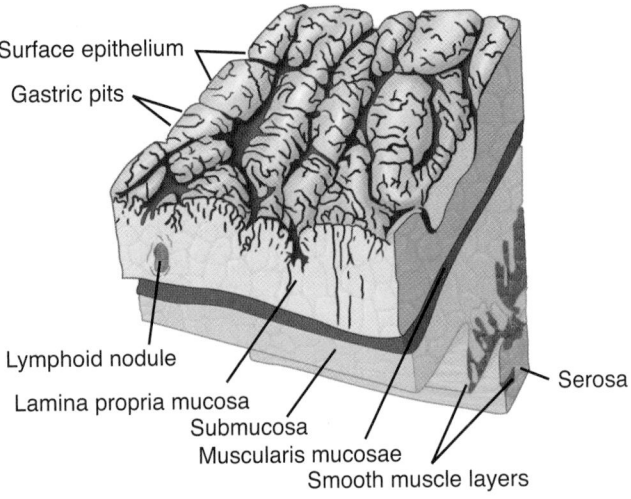

FIG. 26-6. Layers of the gastric wall. *[Reproduced with permission from The esophagus and stomach, in Fawcett DW: Bloom and Fawcett's Textbook of Histology, 11th ed. Philadelphia: Saunders, 1986, p 625. Copyright Elsevier.]*

acetylcholine is an important neurotransmitter mediating vagal function, and epinephrine is important in the sympathetic nerves, both systems (as well as the intrinsic neurons) have various and diverse neurotransmitters including cholinergic, adrenergic, and peptidergic (e.g., substance P and somatostatin).

Histology

There are four distinct layers of the gastric wall: mucosa, submucosa, muscularis propria, and serosa (Fig. 26-6).[7] The inner layer of the stomach is the mucosa, which is lined with columnar epithelial cells

of various types. Beneath the basement membrane of the epithelial cells is the lamina propria, which contains connective tissue, blood vessels, nerve fibers, and inflammatory cells. Beneath the lamina propria is a thin muscle layer called the *muscularis mucosa*, the deep boundary of the mucosal layer of the gut. The epithelium, lamina propria, and muscularis mucosa constitute the mucosa (Fig. 26-7).[14] The epithelium of the gastric mucosa is columnar glandular. A scanning electron micrograph shows a smooth mucosal carpet punctuated by the openings of the gastric glands. The gastric glands are lined with different types of epithelial cells, depending upon their location in the stomach (Fig. 26-8, Table 26-2).[15,16] There are also endocrine cells present in the gastric glands. Progenitor cells at the base of the glands differentiate and replenish sloughed cells on

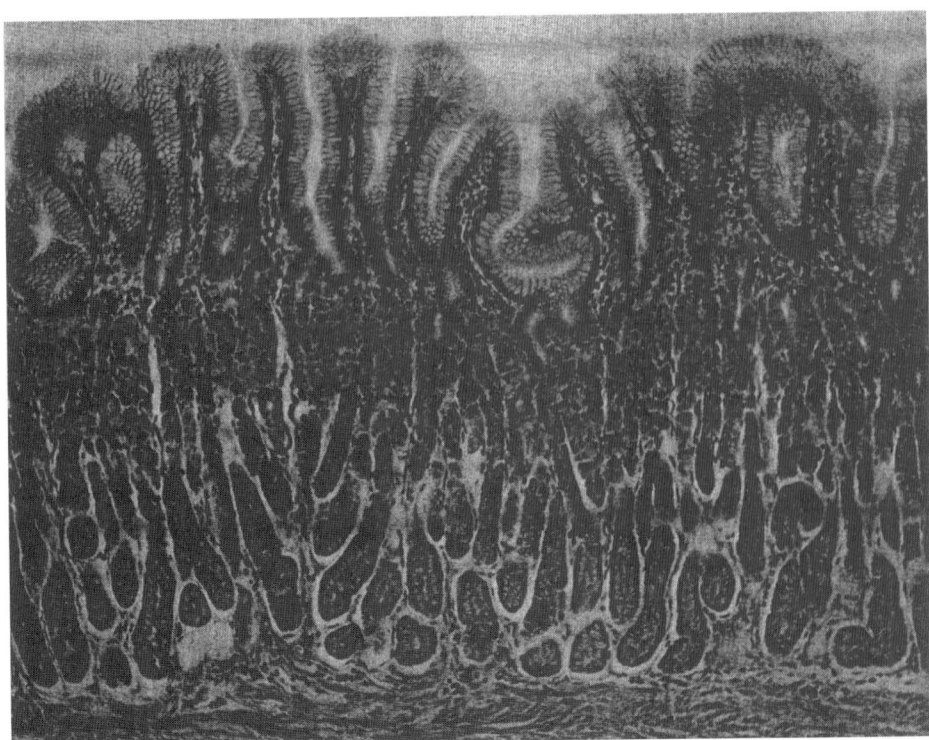

FIG. 26-7. Gastric mucosa. *(Reproduced with permission from Bloom W, Fawcett DW: A Textbook of Histology. Philadelphia: Saunders, 1975, p 639.)*

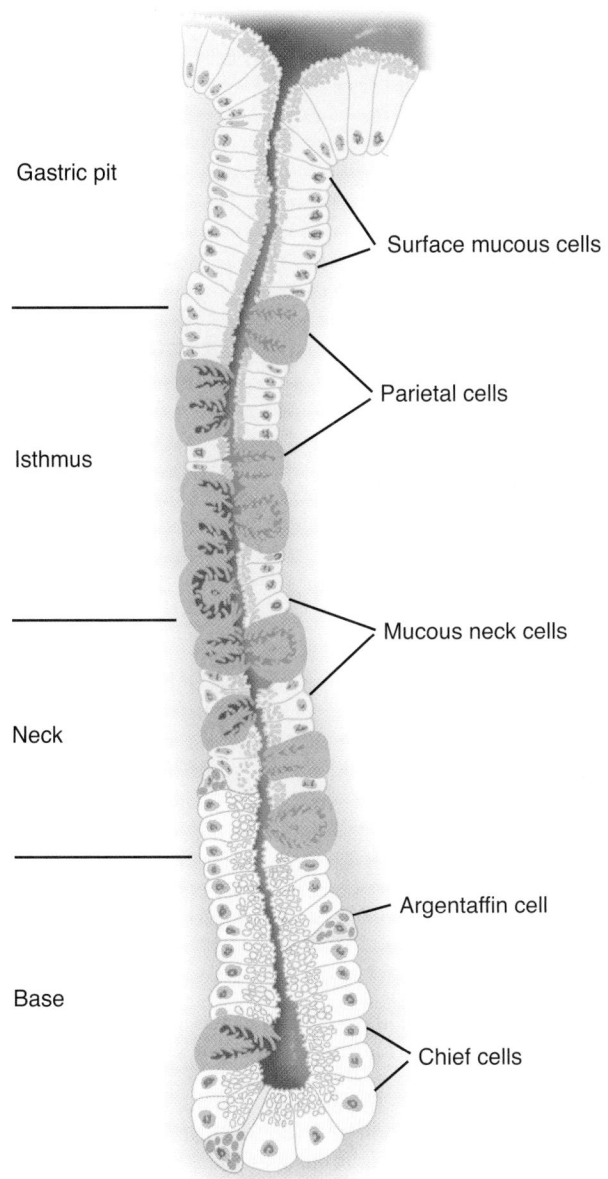

Gastric pit

Surface mucous cells

Parietal cells

Isthmus

Mucous neck cells

Neck

Argentaffin cell

Base

Chief cells

FIG. 26-8. Mammalian gastric gland from the body of the stomach. *[Reproduced with permission from Ito S, Winchester RJ: The fine structure of the gastric muscosa in the bat. J Cell Biol 16:541, 1963. By copyright permission of The Rockefeller University Press.]*

a regular basis. Throughout the stomach, the carpet consists primarily of mucus-secreting surface epithelial cells (SECs) that extend down into the gland pits for variable distances. These cells also secrete bicarbonate and play an important role in protecting the stomach from injury due to acid, pepsin, and/or ingested irritants. In fact, all epithelial cells of the stomach (except the endocrine cells) contain carbonic anhydrase and are capable of producing bicarbonate.

In the cardia, the gastric glands are branched and secrete primarily mucus and bicarbonate, but not much acid. In the fundus and body, the glands are more tubular and the pits are deep. Parietal and chief cells are common in these glands (Fig. 26-9). Histamine-secreting enterochromaffin-like (ECL) cells and somatostatin-secreting D cells are also found. Parietal cells secrete acid and intrinsic factor into the gastric lumen, and bicarbonate into the intercellular space. They have a characteristic ultrastructural appearance with secretory canaliculi (deep invaginations of the surface membrane), and cytoplasmic tubulovesicles containing the acid-producing apparatus H+/K+-ATPase (proton pump) (see Fig. 26-9). There are numerous mitochondria; in fact the parietal cell is the most mitochondria rich cell in the body. When the parietal cell is stimulated, the cytoplasmic tubulovesicles fuse with the membrane of the secretory canaliculus; when acid production ceases, the process is reversed. Arguably, parietal cells produce the only truly essential substance produced by the stomach (i.e., intrinsic factor). Parietal cells tend to occupy the midportion of the gastric glands found in the corpus of the stomach.

Chief cells (also called *zymogenic cells*) secrete pepsinogen I, which is maximally activated at a pH of 2.5. They tend to be clustered toward the base of the gastric glands and have a low columnar shape. Ultrastructurally, chief cells have the characteristics of protein-synthesizing cells: basal granular endoplasmic reticulum, supranuclear Golgi apparatus, and apical zymogen granules (Fig. 26-10). When stimulated, the chief cells produce two immunologically distinct proenzyme forms of pepsinogen: predominantly pepsinogen I and some pepsinogen II, most of which is produced by SECs. These proenzymes are activated in an acidic luminal environment.

In the antrum, the gastric glands are again more branched and shallow, parietal cells are rare, and gastrin-secreting G cells and somatostatin-secreting D cells are present. A variety of hormone-secreting cells are present in various proportions throughout the gastric mucosa (Fig. 26-11).[17] Histologic analysis suggests that in the normal stomach, 13% of the epithelial cells are oxyntic (parietal) cells, 44% are chief (zymogenic) cells, 40% are mucous cells, and 3% are endocrine cells. In general, the antrum produces gastrin but not acid, and the proximal stomach produces acid but not gastrin. The

TABLE 26-2	Epithelial cells of the stomach	
Cell Type	**Distinctive Ultrastructural Features**	**Major Functions**
Surface-foveolar mucous cells	Apical stippled granules up to 1 μm in diameter	Production of neutral glycoprotein and bicarbonate to form a gel on the gastric luminal surface; neutralization of hydrochloric acid[a]
Mucous neck cell	Heterogeneous granules 1–2 μm in diameter dispersed throughout the cytoplasm	Progenitor cell for all other gastric epithelial cells; glycoprotein production; production of pepsinogens I and II
Oxyntic (parietal) cell	Surface membrane invaginations (canaliculi); tubulovesicle structures; numerous mitochondria	Production of hydrochloric acid; production of intrinsic factor; production of bicarbonate
Chief cell	Moderately dense apical granules up to 2 μm in diameter; prominent supranuclear Golgi apparatus; extensive basolateral granular endoplasmic reticulum	Production of pepsinogens I and II, and of lipase
Cardiopyloric mucous cell	Mixture of granules like those in mucous neck and chief cells; extensive basolateral granular endoplasmic reticulum	Production of glycoprotein; production of pepsinogen II
Endocrine cells	See Figure 26-11	

[a]Bicarbonate is probably produced by other gastric epithelial cells in addition to surface-foveolar mucous cells.
Source: From Antonioli et al,[16] with permission.

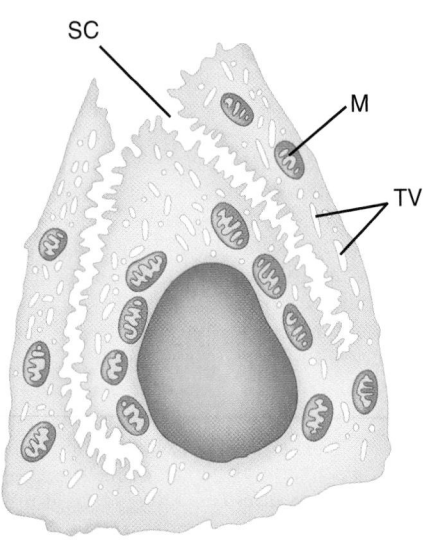

FIG. 26-9. Ultrastructural features of the parietal (oxyntic) cell. SC = secretory canaliculus; M = mitochondria; TV = tubulovesicle. *[Reproduced with permission from Antonioli DA, Madara JL: Functional anatomy of the gastrointestinal tract, in Ming S-C, Goldman H (eds):* Pathology of the Gastrointestinal Tract, *2nd ed. Baltimore: Williams & Wilkins, 1998, p 13.]*

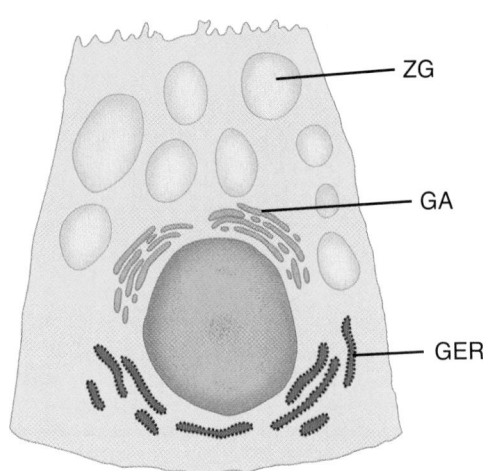

FIG. 26-10. Ultrastructural features of the chief (zymogenic) cell. GA = Golgi apparatus; GER = granular endoplasmic reticulum; ZG = zymogen granule. *[Reproduced with permission from Antonioli DA, Madara JL: Functional anatomy of the gastrointestinal tract, in Ming S-C, Goldman H (eds):* Pathology of the Gastrointestinal Tract, *2nd ed. Baltimore: Williams & Wilkins, 1998, p 13.]*

border between the corpus and antrum migrates proximally with age (especially on the lesser curvature side of the stomach).

Deep to the muscularis mucosa is the submucosa, which is rich in branching blood vessels, lymphatics, collagen, various inflammatory cells, autonomic nerve fibers, and ganglion cells of Meissner's autonomic submucosal plexus. The collagen-rich submucosa gives strength to GI anastomoses. The mucosa and submucosa are folded into the grossly visible gastric rugae, which tend to flatten out as the stomach becomes distended.

Below the submucosa is the thick muscularis propria (also referred to as the *muscularis externa*), which consists of an incomplete inner oblique layer, a complete middle circular layer (continuous with the esophageal circular muscle and the circular muscle of the pylorus), and a complete outer longitudinal layer (continuous with the longitudinal layer of the esophagus and duodenum). Within the muscularis propria is the rich network of autonomic ganglia and nerves that make up Auerbach's myenteric plexus. Specialized pacemaker cells, the interstitial cells of Cajal (ICC), also are present.

The outer layer of the stomach is the serosa, also known as the *visceral peritoneum*. This layer provides significant tensile strength to gastric anastomoses. When tumors originating in the mucosa pene-

trate and breach the serosa, microscopic or gross peritoneal metastases are common, presumably from shedding of tumor cells that would not have occurred if the serosa had not been penetrated. In this way, the serosa may be thought of as an outer envelope of the stomach.

PHYSIOLOGY

The stomach stores food and facilitates digestion through a variety of secretory and motor functions. Important secretory functions include the production of acid, pepsin, intrinsic factor, mucus, and a variety of GI hormones. Important motor functions include food storage (receptive relaxation and accommodation), grinding and mixing, controlled emptying of ingested food, and periodic interprandial "housekeeping."

Acid Secretion

Hydrochloric acid in the stomach hastens both the physical and (with pepsin) the biochemical breakdown of ingested food. In an acidic environment, pepsin and acid facilitate proteolysis. Gastric acid also inhibits the proliferation of ingested pathogens, which

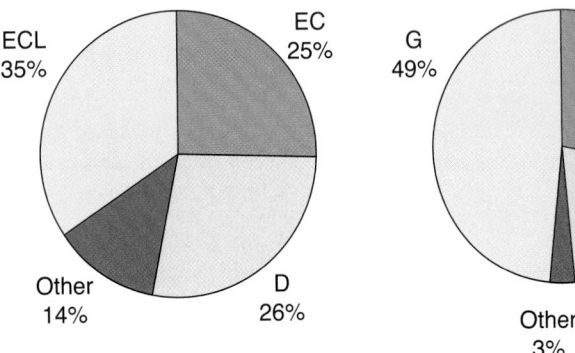

Oxyntic mucosa   **Pyloric mucosa**

FIG. 26-11. Endocrine cells of the stomach. D = d cell (somatostatin); EC = enterochrommafin cell; ECL = enterochrommafin-like cell (histamine); G = g cell (gastrin). *[Reproduced with permission from Feldman M: Gastric secretion, in Feldman M, et al (eds):* Sleisenger and Fordtran's Gastrointestinal and Liver Disease, *7th ed. Philadelphia: Saunders, 2002, p 715. Copyright Elsevier.]*

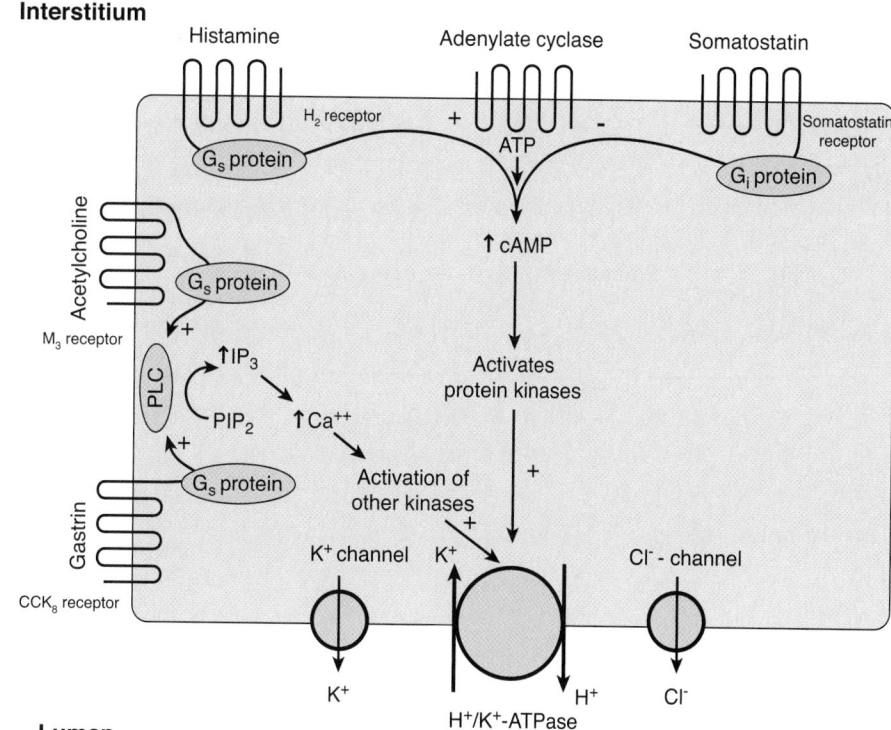

Interstitium

Lumen

FIG. 26-12. Control of acid secretion in the parietal cell. ATP = adenosine triphosphate; cAMP = cyclic adenosine monophosphate; CCK = cholecystokinin; H_2 = histamine 2; IP_3 = inositol trisphosphate; PIP_2 = phosphatidylinositol 4,5-bisphosphate; PLC = phospholipase C. [*Reproduced with permission from Mercer DW, Liu TH, Castaneda A: Anatomy and physiology of the stomach, in Zuidema GD, Yeo CJ (eds): Shackelford's Surgery of the Alimentary Tract, 5th ed., Vol. II. Philadelphia: Saunders, 2002, p 3. Copyright Elsevier.]*

protects against both infectious gastroenteritides and intestinal bacterial overgrowth. Long-term acid suppression with proton pump inhibitors (PPIs) has been associated with an increased risk of community acquired *Clostridium difficile* colitis and other gastroenteritides, presumably because of the absence of this protective germicidal barrier.[18,19]

Parietal Cell

The parietal cell is stimulated to secrete acid (Fig. 26-12) when one or more of three membrane receptor types is stimulated by acetylcholine (from vagal nerve fibers), gastrin (from D cells), or histamine (from ECL cells).[7,20,21] The enzyme H^+/K^+-ATPase is the proton pump. It is stored within the intracellular tubulovesicles and is the final common pathway for gastric acid secretion. When the parietal cell is stimulated, there is a cytoskeletal rearrangement and fusion of the tubulovesicles with the apical membrane of the secretory canaliculus. The heterodimer assembly of the enzyme subunits into the microvilli of the secretory canaliculus results in acid secretion, with extracellular potassium being exchanged for cytosolic hydrogen. Although electro-neutral, this is an energy requiring process because the hydrogen is secreted against a gradient of at least 1 million-fold, which explains why the parietal cell is packed with energy producing mitochondria. During acid production, potassium and chloride are also secreted into the secretory canaliculus through separate channels, providing potassium for the H^+/K^+-ATPase, and chloride for the secreted hydrogen.

The normal human stomach contains approximately 1 billion parietal cells, and total gastric acid production is proportional to parietal cell mass. The potent acid-suppressing PPI drugs irreversibly interfere with the function of the H^+/K^+-ATPase molecule. These agents must be incorporated into the activated enzyme to be effective, and thus work best when taken before or during a meal (when the parietal cell is stimulated). When PPI therapy is stopped, acid secretory capability gradually returns (within days) as new H^+/K^+-ATPase is synthesized.

Gastrin, acetylcholine, and histamine stimulate the parietal cell to secrete hydrochloric acid (see Fig. 26-12). Gastrin binds to type B cholecystokinin (CCK) receptors, and acetylcholine binds to M_3

muscarinic receptors. Both stimulate phospholipase C via a G-protein–linked mechanism leading to increased production of inositol trisphosphate from membrane bound phospholipids. Inositol trisphosphate stimulates the release of calcium from intracellular stores, which leads to activation of protein kinases and activation of H^+/K^+-ATPase. Histamine binds to the histamine 2 (H_2) receptor, which stimulates adenylate cyclase, also via a G-protein–linked mechanism. Activation of adenylate cyclase results in an increase in intracellular cyclic adenosine monophosphate which activates protein kinases, leading to increased levels of phosphoproteins and activation of the proton pump. Somatostatin from mucosal D cells binds to membrane receptors and inhibits the activation of adenylate cyclase through an inhibitory G protein.

Physiologic Acid Secretion

Food ingestion is the physiologic stimulus for acid secretion (Fig. 26-13). The acid secretory response that occurs after a meal is traditionally described in three phases: cephalic, gastric, and intestinal.[22,23] The cephalic or vagal phase begins with the thought, sight, smell, and/or taste of food. These stimuli activate several cortical and hypothalamic sites (e.g., tractus solitarius, dorsal motor nucleus, and dorsal vagal complex), and signals are transmitted to the stomach by the vagal nerves. Acetylcholine is released, leading to stimulation of ECL cells and parietal cells. Although the acid secreted per unit of time in the cephalic phase is greater than in the other two phases, the cephalic phase is shorter. Thus, the cephalic phase accounts for no more than 30% of total acid secretion in response to a meal. Sham feeding (chewing and spitting) stimulates gastric acid secretion only via the cephalic phase, and results in acid secretion that is about half of that seen in response to IV pentagastrin or histamine.

When food reaches the stomach, the gastric phase of acid secretion begins. This phase lasts until the stomach is empty, and accounts for about 60% of the total acid secretion in response to a meal. The gastric phase of acid secretion has several components. Amino acids and small peptides directly stimulate antral G cells to secrete gastrin, which is carried in the bloodstream to the parietal cells and stimulates acid secretion in an endocrine fashion. In addition, proximal gastric distention stimulates acid secretion via a

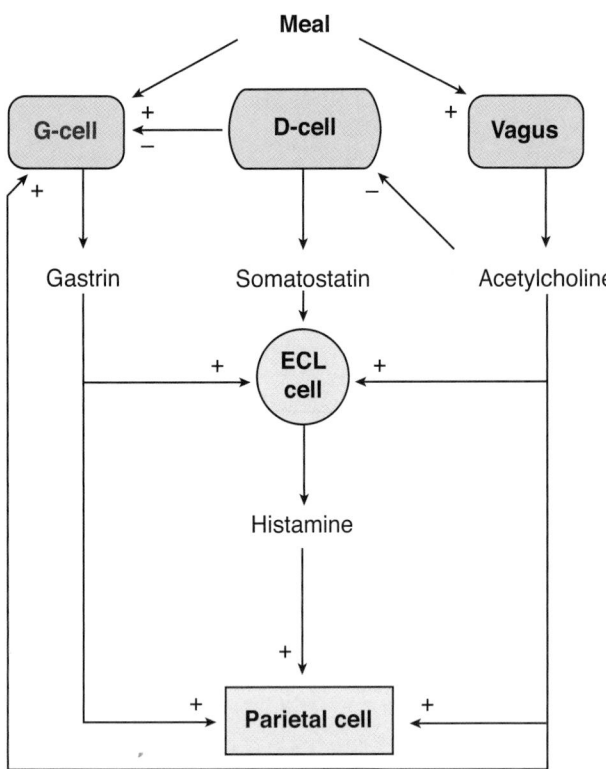

FIG. 26-13. Physiologic control of acid secretion. ECL = enterochromaffin-like. [*Reproduced with permission from Mercer DW, Liu TH, Castaneda A: Anatomy and physiology of the stomach, in Zuidema GD, Yeo CJ (eds):* Shackelford's Surgery of the Alimentary Tract, *5th ed., Vol. II. Philadelphia: Saunders, 2002, p 3. Copyright Elsevier.*]

vagovagal reflex arc, which is abolished by truncal or HSV. Antral distention also stimulates antral gastrin secretion. Acetylcholine stimulates gastrin release and gastrin stimulates histamine release from ECL cells.

The intestinal phase of gastric secretion is poorly understood. It is thought to be mediated by a hormone yet to be discovered that is released from the proximal small bowel mucosa in response to luminal chyme. This phase starts when gastric emptying of ingested food begins, and continues as long as nutrients remain in the proximal small intestine. It accounts for about 10% of meal-induced acid secretion.

Interprandial basal acid secretion is 2 to 5 mEq hydrochloric acid per hour, about 10% of maximal acid output (MAO), and it is greater at night. Basal acid secretion probably contributes to the relatively low bacterial counts found in the stomach. Basal acid secretion is reduced 75 to 90% by vagotomy or H_2 receptor blockade.

The pivotal role that ECL cells play in the regulation of gastric acid secretion is emphasized in Fig. 26-13. A large part of the acid stimulatory effects of both acetylcholine and gastrin are mediated by histamine released from mucosal ECL cells. This explains why the histamine 2 receptor antagonists (H_2RAs) are such effective inhibitors of acid secretion, even though histamine is only one of three parietal cell stimulants. The mucosal D cell, which releases somatostatin, is also an important regulator of acid secretion. Somatostatin inhibits histamine release from ECL cells and gastrin release from antral G cells. The function of D cells is inhibited by *Helicobacter pylori* infection, and this leads to an exaggerated acid secretory response (see below under *Helicobacter pylori* Infection).

Pepsinogen Secretion

The most potent physiologic stimulus for pepsinogen secretion from chief cells is food ingestion; acetylcholine is the most impor-

tant mediator. Somatostatin inhibits pepsinogen secretion. Pepsinogen I is produced by chief cells in acid producing glands, whereas pepsinogen II is produced by SECs in both acid producing and gastrin producing (i.e., antral) glands. Pepsinogen is cleaved to the active pepsin enzyme in an acidic environment and is maximally active at pH 2.5, and inactive at pH >5, although pepsinogen II may be activated over a wider pH range than pepsinogen I. Pepsin catalyzes the hydrolysis of proteins and is denatured at alkaline pH.

Intrinsic Factor

Activated parietal cells secrete intrinsic factor in addition to hydrochloric acid. Presumably the stimulants are similar, but acid secretion and intrinsic factor secretion may not be linked. Intrinsic factor binds to luminal vitamin B_{12}, and the complex is absorbed in the terminal ileum via mucosal receptors. Vitamin B_{12} deficiency can be life threatening, and patients with total gastrectomy or pernicious anemia (i.e., patients with no parietal cells) require B_{12} supplementation by a nonenteric route. Some patients develop vitamin B_{12} deficiency following gastric bypass, presumably because there is insufficient intrinsic factor present in the small proximal gastric pouch. Under normal conditions, a significant excess of intrinsic factor is secreted, and acid-suppressive medication does not appear to inhibit intrinsic factor production and release.

Gastric Mucosal Barrier

The stomach's durable resistance to autodigestion by caustic hydrochloric acid and active pepsin is intriguing. Some of the important elements of gastric barrier function and cytoprotection are listed in Table 26-3.[24,25] When these defenses break down, ulceration occurs. A variety of factors are important in maintaining an intact gastric mucosal layer. The mucus and bicarbonate secreted by SECs form an unstirred mucous gel with a favorable pH gradient. Cell membranes and tight junctions prevent hydrogen ions from gaining access to the interstitial space. Hydrogen ions that do break through are buffered by the alkaline tide created by basolateral bicarbonate secretion from stimulated parietal cells. Any sloughed or denuded SECs are rapidly replaced by migration of adjacent cells, a process known as *restitution*. Mucosal blood flow plays a crucial role in maintaining a healthy mucosa, providing nutrients and oxygen for the cellular functions involved in cytoprotection. "Back-diffused" hydrogen is buffered and rapidly removed by the rich blood supply. When "barrier breakers" such as bile or aspirin lead to increased back-diffusion of hydrogen ions from the lumen into the lamina propria and submucosa, there is a protective increase in mucosal

TABLE 26-3	Important components and mediators of mucosal defenses in the stomach

Components
Mucous barrier
Bicarbonate secretion
Epithelial barrier
    Hydrophobic phospholipids
    Tight junctions
    Restitution
Microcirculation (reactive hyperemia)
Afferent sensory neurons
Mediators
Prostaglandins
Nitric oxide
Epidermal growth factor
Calcitonin gene-related peptide
Hepatocyte growth factor
Histamine
Gastrin-releasing peptide

blood flow. If this protective response is blocked, gross ulceration can occur. Important mediators of these protective mechanisms include prostaglandins, nitric oxide, intrinsic nerves, and peptides (e.g., calcitonin gene-related peptide, gastrin-releasing peptide [GRP], and gastrin). Misoprostol is a commercially available prostaglandin E analogue that has been shown to prevent gastric mucosal damage in chronic users of NSAIDs. More commonly used is sucralfate, which acts locally to enhance mucosal defenses. Some protective reflexes involve afferent sensory neurons, and can be blocked by the application of topical anesthetics to the gastric mucosa, or the experimental destruction of the afferent sensory nerves. In addition to these local defenses, there are important protective factors in saliva, duodenal secretions, and pancreatic or biliary secretions.

Gastric Hormones
Gastrin

Gastrin is produced by antral G cells and is the major hormonal stimulant of acid secretion during the gastric phase. Gastrin is also trophic to GI epithelial and enterochromaffin cells. A variety of molecular forms exist: big gastrin (34 amino acids; G_{34}), little gastrin (17 amino acids; G_{17}), and minigastrin (14 amino acids; G_{14}). The large majority of gastrin released by the human antrum is G_{17}. The biologically active pentapeptide sequence at the C-terminal end of gastrin is identical to that of CCK. Luminal peptides and amino acids are the most potent stimulants of gastrin release, and luminal acid is the most potent inhibitor of gastrin secretion. The latter effect is predominantly mediated in a paracrine fashion by somatostatin released from antral D cells. Gastrin-stimulated acid secretion is significantly blocked by H_2 antagonists, suggesting that the principal mediator of gastrin-stimulated acid production is histamine from mucosal ECL cells (see Fig. 26-13). In fact, chronic hypergastrinemia such as that seen with pernicious anemia or long-term use of potent acid suppressants or gastrinoma is associated with hyperplasia of gastric ECL cells and, rarely, gastric carcinoid. Gastrin also is trophic to gastric parietal cells and to other GI mucosal cells. Important causes of hypergastrinemia include pernicious anemia, acid-suppressive medication, gastrinoma, retained antrum following distal gastrectomy and Billroth II surgery, and vagotomy.

Somatostatin

Somatostatin is produced by D cells located throughout the gastric mucosa. The predominant form in humans is somatostatin 14, though somatostatin 28 is present as well. The major stimulus for somatostatin release is antral acidification; acetylcholine from vagal nerve fibers inhibits its release. Somatostatin inhibits acid secretion from parietal cells and gastrin release from G cells. It also decreases histamine release from ECL cells. The proximity of the D cells to these target cells suggests that the primary effect of somatostatin is mediated in a paracrine fashion, but an endocrine (i.e., bloodstream) effect also is possible.

Gastrin-Releasing Peptide

GRP is the mammalian equivalent of bombesin, a hormone discovered more than two decades ago in an extract of skin from a frog. In the antrum, GRP stimulates both gastrin and somatostatin release by binding to receptors on the G and D cells. There are nerve terminals ending near the mucosa in the gastric body and antrum, which are rich in GRP immunoreactivity. When GRP is given peripherally, it stimulates acid secretion, but when it is given centrally into the cerebral ventricles of animals, it inhibits acid secretion, apparently via a pathway involving the sympathetic nervous system. GRP is a mediator of gastroprotective increased mucosal blood flow in response to luminal irritants.

Leptin

Leptin is a protein primarily synthesized in adipocytes. It is also made by chief cells in the stomach, the main source of leptin in the GI tract.[26] Leptin works at least in part via vagally mediated pathways to decrease food intake in animals. Not surprisingly, leptin, a satiety signal hormone, and ghrelin, a hunger signal hormone, are both primarily synthesized in the stomach, an organ increasingly recognized as central to the mechanisms of appetite control.[26,27]

Ghrelin

Ghrelin is a small peptide described in 1999 that is produced primarily in the stomach.[28] Ghrelin is a potent secretagogue of pituitary growth hormone (but not adrenocorticotropic hormone, follicle-stimulating hormone, luteinizing hormone, prolactin, or thyroid-stimulating hormone). Ghrelin appears to be an orexigenic regulator of appetite (i.e., when ghrelin is elevated, appetite is stimulated, and when it is suppressed, appetite is suppressed). Resection of the primary source of this hormone (i.e., the stomach) may partly account for the anorexia and weight loss seen in some patients following gastrectomy (Fig. 26-14).[29] The gastric bypass operation, a very effective treatment for morbid obesity, has been shown by some investigators to be associated with suppression of plasma ghrelin levels (and appetite) in humans (Fig. 26-15A).[30]

Other groups have failed to show a significant decrease in ghrelin levels following gastric bypass but have found such decreases following sleeve gastrectomy, another effective weight loss operation (Fig. 26-15B).[31] Obviously appetite control is complex with redundant and overlapping orexigenic and anorexigenic pathways and signals.[26,27]

Gastric Motility and Emptying

Gastric motor function has several purposes.[32–34] Interprandial motor activity clears the stomach of undigested debris, sloughed cells, and mucus. When feeding begins, the stomach relaxes to accommodate the meal. Regulated motor activity then breaks down the food into small particles and controls the output into the

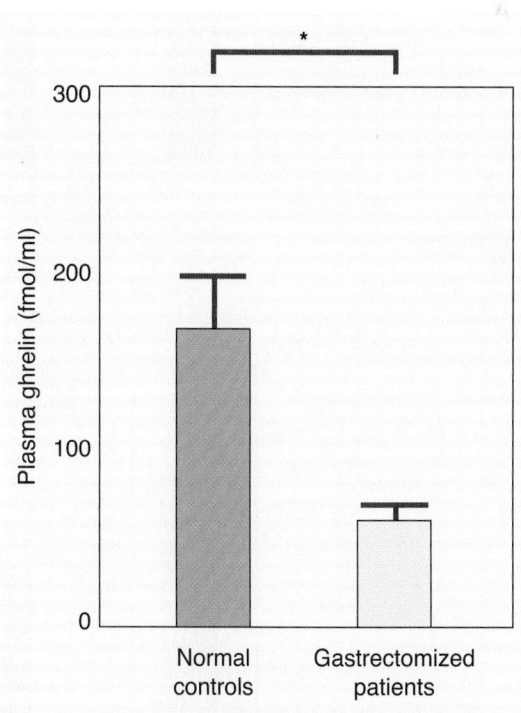

FIG. 26-14. Ghrelin levels are decreased after gastrectomy. *(Reproduced with permission from Ariyasu H, Takaya K, Tagami T, et al: Stomach is a major source of circulating ghrelin, and feeding state determines plasma ghrelin-like immunoreactivity levels in humans.* J Clin Endocrinol Metab *86:4753, 2001.)*

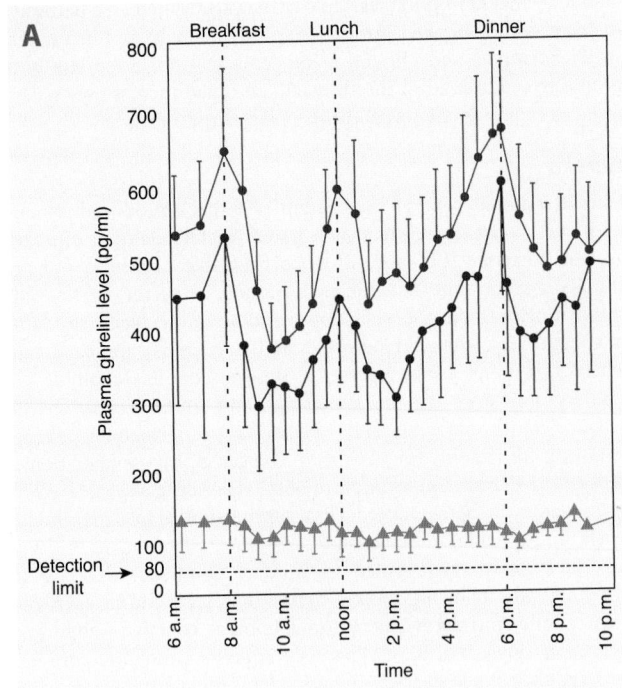

FIG. 26-15. **A** and **B.** Ghrelin secretion after bariatric surgery. Some investigators have suggested that ghrelin secretion is dramatically decreased after gastric bypass. Other groups have shown statistically insignificant changes in ghrelin levels after gastric bypass, but significant decreases after sleeve gastrectomy. **A:** green = gastric bypass; blue = obese controls; red = normal weight controls; **B:** blue = fasting; pink = postprandial. *(Fig. 26-15A reproduced with permission from Cummings DE, et al: Plasma ghrelin levels after diet-induced weight loss or gastric bypass surgery. N Engl J Med 346:1623, 2002. Copyright ©2002 Massachusetts Medical Society. All rights reserved. Fig. 26-15B reproduced with permission from Karamanakos SN, et al: Weight loss, appetite suppression, and changes in fasting and postprandial ghrelin and peptide-YY levels after Roux-en-Y gastric bypass and sleeve gastrectomy: A prospective, double blind study. Ann Surg 247:401, 2008.)*

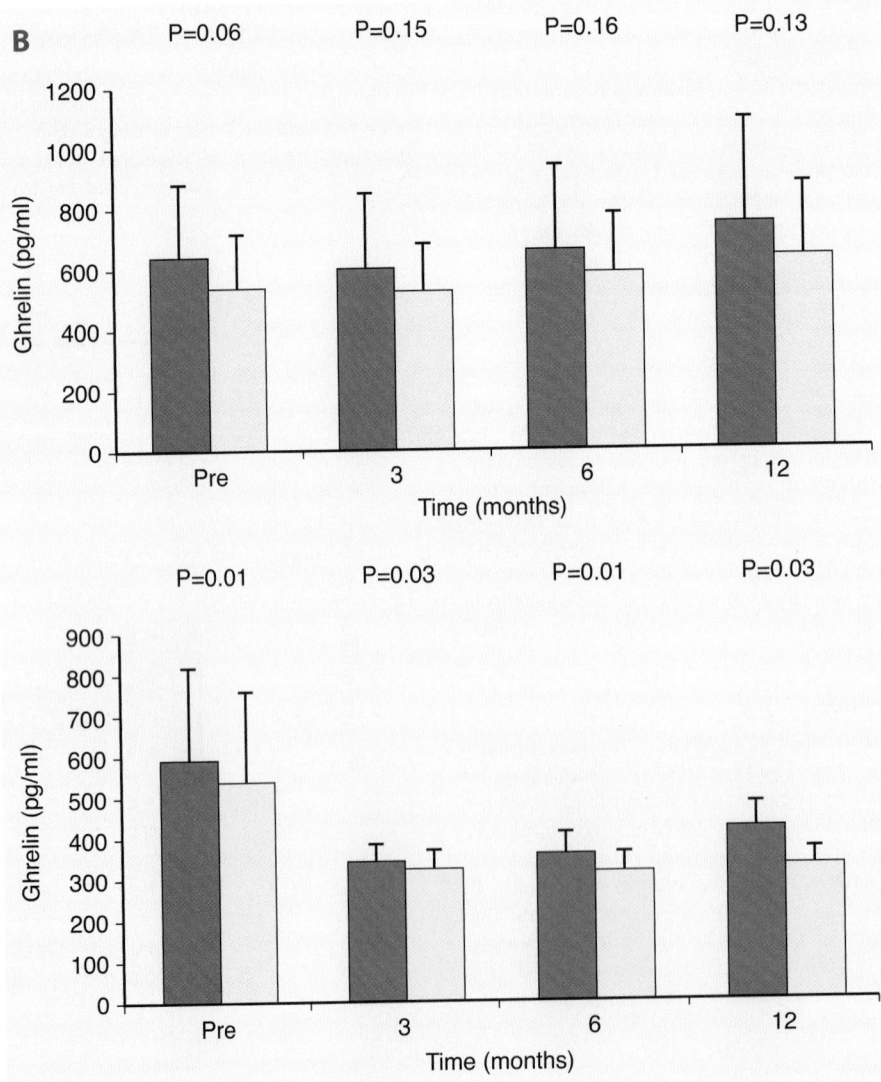

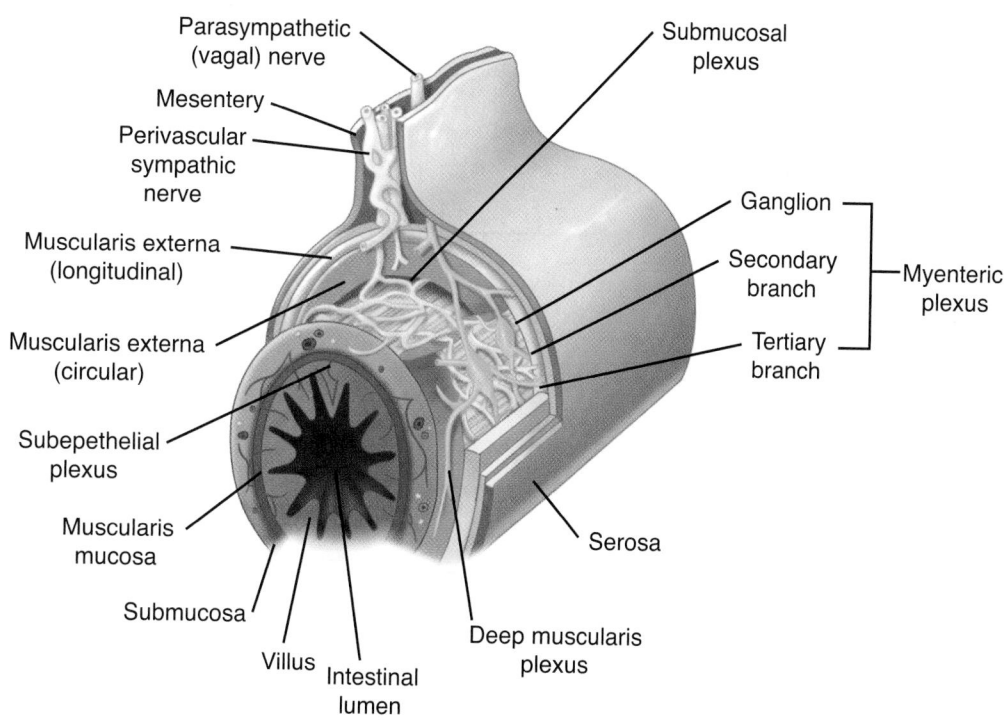

Parasympathetic
(vagal) nerve

Mesentery

Perivascular
sympathic
nerve

Muscularis externa
(longitudinal)

Muscularis externa
(circular)

Subepethelial
plexus

Muscularis
mucosa

Submucosa

Villus

Intestinal
lumen

Submucosal
plexus

Ganglion

Secondary
branch

Tertiary
branch

Myenteric
plexus

Serosa

Deep muscularis
plexus

FIG. 26-16. Enteric nervous system. *[Reproduced with permission from Chial HJ, Camilleri M: Motility disorders of the stomach and small intestine, in Friedman SL, McQuaid KR, Grendell JH (eds):* Current Diagnosis and Treatment in Gastroenterology, *2nd ed. New York: McGraw-Hill, 2003, p 355.]*

duodenum. The stomach accomplishes these functions by coordinated smooth muscle relaxation and contraction of the various gastric segments (proximal, distal, and pyloric). Smooth muscle myoelectric potentials are translated into muscular activity, which is modulated by extrinsic and intrinsic innervation and hormones. The mechanisms by which gastric distention is translated into a neurohormonal satiety signal have only been partially elucidated.[26,27]

Intrinsic Gastric Innervation

The extrinsic parasympathetic and sympathetic gastric innervation was discussed above under Innervation. The intrinsic innervation consists of ganglia and nerves that constitute the enteric nervous system (Fig. 26-16).[35] There are a variety of neurotransmitters, which are generally grouped as excitatory (augment muscular activity) and inhibitory (decrease muscular activity). Important excitatory neurotransmitters include acetylcholine, the tachykinins, substance P, and neurokinin A. Important inhibitory neurotransmitters include nitric oxide (NO) and vasoactive intestinal peptide (VIP). Serotonin has been shown to modulate both contraction and relaxation. A variety of other molecules affect motility, including GRP, histamine, neuropeptide Y, norepinephrine, and endogenous opioids.

Specialized cells in the muscularis propria also are important modulators of GI motility. These cells, called *interstitial cells of Cajal*, are distinguishable histologically from neurons and myocytes, and appear to amplify both cholinergic excitatory and nitrergic inhibitory input to the smooth muscle of the stomach and intestine.[36] They are thought either to share a common stem cell of origin with, or to be the cell of origin for, gastrointestinal stromal tumors (GISTs) which are the most common mesenchymal neoplasm in the GI tract.

Segmental Gastric Motility

In general, the proximal stomach serves as short-term food storage function and helps regulate basal intragastric tone, and the distal stomach mixes and grinds the food. The pylorus helps the latter process when closed, facilitating retropulsion of the solid food bolus

back into the body of the stomach for additional breakdown. The pylorus opens intermittently to allow metered emptying of liquids and small solid particles into the duodenum.

Most of the motor activity of the proximal stomach consists of slow tonic contractions and relaxations, lasting up to 5 minutes. This activity is the main determinant of basal intragastric pressure, an important determinant of liquid emptying. Rapid phasic contractions may be superimposed on the slower tonic motor activity. When food is ingested, intragastric pressure falls as the proximal stomach relaxes. This proximal relaxation is mediated by two important vagovagal reflexes: receptive relaxation and gastric accommodation. Receptive relaxation refers to the reduction in proximal gastric tone associated with the act of swallowing. This occurs before the food reaches the stomach, and can be reproduced by mechanical stimulation of the pharynx or esophagus. Gastric accommodation refers to the proximal gastric relaxation associated with distention of the stomach. Accommodation is mediated through stretch receptors in the gastric wall and does not require esophageal or pharyngeal stimulation. Because both of these reflexes are mediated by afferent and efferent vagal fibers, they are significantly altered by truncal and HSV. Both these operations result in decreased gastric compliance, shifting the volume/pressure curve to the left. That is, interference with normal receptive relaxation and/or accommodation results in decreased gastric compliance, such that for any given amount of food or liquid ingested, the intragastric pressure is greater. This may increase the rate of liquid emptying, perhaps contributing to dumping symptoms in some patients after vagotomy.

NO and VIP are the principal mediators of proximal gastric relaxation. But a variety of other agents increase proximal gastric relaxation and compliance, including dopamine, gastrin, CCK, secretin, GRP, and glucagon. Proximal gastric tone also is decreased by duodenal distention, colonic distention, and ileal perfusion with glucose (ileal brake).

The distal stomach breaks up solid food and is the main determinant of gastric emptying of solids. Slow waves of myoelectric depolarization sweep down the distal stomach at a rate of about three per minute. These waves originate from the proximal gastric

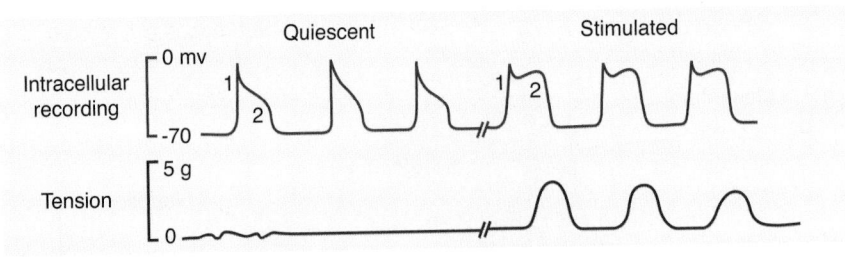

FIG. 26-17. The relationship between intracellular electrical activity and muscle cell contraction. Note that contractile activity is always associated with electrical activity, but the converse is not so. During mechanical quiescence, there are regular depolarizations that do not reach threshold. In the stimulated state, the threshold for contraction is reached, and motor activity is demonstrable. *[Reproduced with permission from Kim CH: Electrical activity of the stomach: clinical implications. Mayo Clin Proc 61:205, 1986.]*

pacemaker, high on the greater curvature. The pacing cells may be ICC, which have been shown to have a similar function in the small intestine and colon. Most of these myoelectric waves are below the threshold for smooth muscle contraction in the quiescent state, and thus are associated with negligible changes in pressure. Neural and/or hormonal input, which increases the plateau phase of the action potential, can trigger muscle contraction, resulting in a peristaltic wave associated with the electrical slow wave, and of the same frequency (three per minute) (Fig. 26-17). It is possible that implantable gastric pacemakers benefit some patients with gastroparesis by favorably impacting this myoelectric coupling.

During fasting, distal gastric motor activity is controlled by the migrating motor complex (MMC), the "gastrointestinal housekeeper" (Fig. 26-18). The purported function of the MMC is to sweep along any undigested food, debris, sloughed cells, and mucus after the fed phase of digestion is complete. The MMC lasts approximately 100 minutes (longer at night, shorter during daytime) and is divided into four phases. Phase I (about half the length of the entire cycle) is a period of relative motor inactivity. High-amplitude muscular contractions do not occur in phase I of the MMC. Phase II (about 25% of the entire MMC cycle) consists of some irregular, high-amplitude, generally nonpropulsive contractions. Phase III, a period of intense, regular, (about three per minute) propulsive contractions, only lasts

about 5 to 10 minutes. Most phase III complexes of the GI MMC begin in the stomach, and the frequency approximates that of the myoelectric gastric slow wave. Phase IV is a transition period.

Neurohormonal control of the MMC is poorly understood, but it appears that different phases are regulated by different mechanisms. For example, vagotomy abolishes phase II of the gastric MMC but has little influence on phase III. In fact, phase III persists in the autotransplanted stomach, totally devoid of extrinsic neural input. This suggests that phase III is regulated by intrinsic nerves and/or hormones. Indeed, the initiation of phase III of the MMC in the distal stomach corresponds temporally to elevation in serum levels of motilin, a hormone produced in the duodenal mucosa. Resection of the duodenum abolishes distal gastric phase III in dogs. Resection of the duodenum in humans (e.g., with pancreaticoduodenectomy, the Whipple procedure) commonly results in early postoperative delayed gastric emptying sometimes responsive to erythromycin, a motilin agonist.[37] There are clearly motilin receptors on antral smooth muscle and nerves. Other modulators of gastric MMC activity include NO, endogenous opioids, intrinsic cholinergic and adrenergic nerves, and duodenal pH (MMC phase III does not occur if the duodenal pH is below 7).

Feeding abolishes the MMC and leads to the fed motor pattern. The fed motor pattern of gastric activity starts within 10 minutes of food ingestion and persists until all the food has left the stomach. The

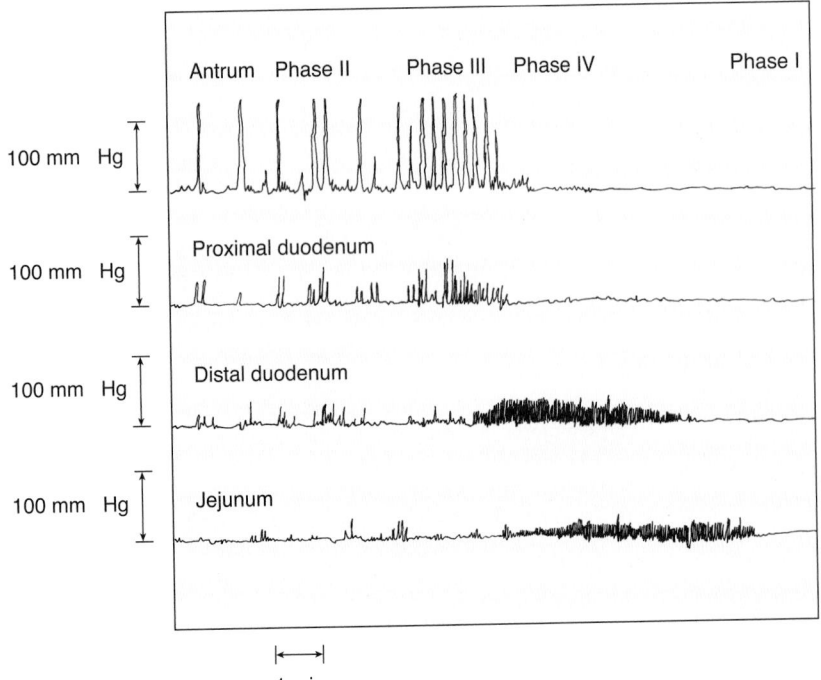

FIG. 26-18. Migrating motor complex, the fasting pattern of GI activity. During phase III of the migrating motor complex, effective peristaltic waves progress from the stomach to the distal small intestine. *[Reproduced with permission from Rees WDW, et al: Human interdigestive and postprandial gastrointestinal motor and gastrointestinal hormone patterns. Dig Dis Sci 27(4):321, 1982. Copyright 1982, with kind permission of Springer Science + Business Media.]*

neurohormonal initiator of this change is unknown, but CCK and the vagus appear to play some role: Sham feeding transiently induces antral motor activity resembling the fed motor pattern, and this is blocked by the CCK receptor antagonist loxiglumide. Gastric motility during the fed pattern resembles phase II of the MMC, with irregular but continuous phasic contractions of the distal stomach. During the fed state, about half of the myoelectric slow waves are associated with strong distal gastric contractions. Some are prograde and some are retrograde, serving to mix and grind the solid components of the meal. The magnitude of gastric contractions and the duration of the pattern is influenced by the consistency and composition of the meal.

The pylorus functions as an effective regulator of gastric emptying and an effective barrier to duodenogastric reflux. Bypass, transection, or resection of the pylorus may lead to uncontrolled gastric emptying of food and the dumping syndrome (see below under Postgastrectomy Problems). Pyloric dysfunction or disruption may also result in uncontrolled entry of duodenal contents into the stomach. Perfusion of the duodenum with lipids, glucose, amino acids, hypertonic saline, or hydrochloric acid results in closure of the pylorus and decreased transpyloric flow. Ileal perfusion with fat has the same effect. A variety of neurohumoral pathways are involved with these physiologic responses, and there is evidence that different pathways may be involved for different stimuli.

The pylorus is readily apparent grossly as a thick ring of muscle and connective tissue. The density of nerve tissue in the pyloric smooth muscle is severalfold higher than in the antrum, with increased numbers of neurons staining positive for substance P, neuropeptide Y, VIP, and galanin. ICC are more closely associated with pyloric myocytes, and the myoelectric slow wave of the pylorus has the same frequency as that seen in the distal stomach. The motor activity of the pylorus is both tonic and phasic. During phase III of the MMC, the pylorus is open as gastric contents are swept into the duodenum. During the fed phase, the pylorus is closed most of the time. It relaxes intermittently, usually in synchronization with lower-amplitude, minor antral contractions. The higher-amplitude, more major antral contractions are usually met with a closed pylorus, facilitating retropulsion and further grinding of food.

Modulation of pyloric motor activity is complex. There is evidence of both inhibitory and excitatory vagal pathways. Some contractile vagal effects are mediated by opioid pathways, because they are blocked by naloxone. Electrical stimulation of the duodenum causes the pylorus to contract, whereas electrical stimulation of the antrum causes pyloric relaxation. Generally, NO mediates pyloric relaxation; NO donors lead to pyloric relaxation and decreased resistance to flow in a variety of models, whereas NO synthetase inhibitors have the opposite effect. Other molecules that may play a physiologic role in controlling pyloric smooth muscle include serotonin, VIP, prostaglandin E$_1$, and galanin (pyloric relaxation); and histamine, CCK, and secretin (pyloric contraction).

Gastric Emptying

The control of gastric emptying is complex. In general, gastric emptying is slowed by increasing caloric content or osmolarity, increased fat content, and increased particle size; liquid emptying is faster than solid emptying. Osmolarity, acidity, caloric content, and nutrient composition are important modulators. Stimulation of duodenal osmoreceptors, glucoreceptors, and pH receptors clearly inhibits gastric emptying by a variety of neurohumoral mechanisms. CCK has been consistently shown to inhibit gastric emptying at physiologic doses (Fig. 26-19). Recently, it has been noted that the anorexigenic hormone leptin, secreted mostly by fat but also by gastric mucosa, inhibits gastric emptying, perhaps through the same pathway as CCK (which also has properties of a satiety hormone). The orexigenic hormone ghrelin has the opposite effect.

Liquid Emptying

The gastric emptying of water or isotonic saline follows first-order kinetics, with a half emptying time around 12 minutes. Thus, if one

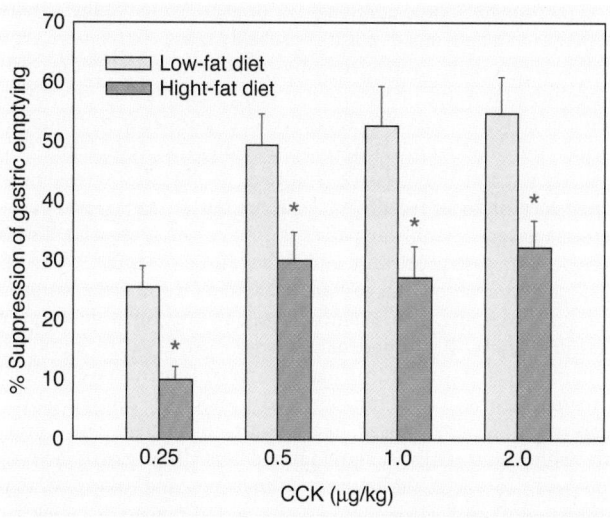

FIG. 26-19. Cholecystokinin (CCK) inhibits gastric emptying. *[Reproduced with permission from Covasa M, Ritter RC: Adaptation to high-fat diet reduces inhibition of gastric emptying by CCK and intestinal oleate. Am J Physiol Regulatory Integrative Comp Physiol 278:R166, 2000.]*

drinks 200 mL of water, about 100 mL enters the duodenum by 12 minutes, whereas if one drinks 400 mL of water, about 200 mL enters the duodenum by 12 minutes. This emptying pattern of liquids is modified considerably as the caloric density, osmolarity, and nutrient composition of the liquid changes (Fig. 26-20). Up to an osmolarity of about 1 M, liquid emptying occurs at a rate of about 200 kcal per hour. Duodenal osmoreceptors and hormones (e.g., secretin and VIP) are important modulators of liquid gastric emptying. Generally, liquid emptying is delayed in the supine position.

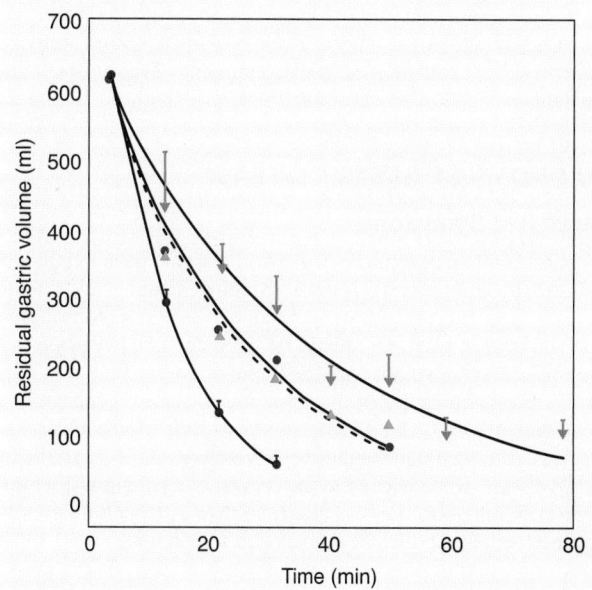

FIG. 26-20. Nutrient composition and caloric density affect liquid gastric emptying. Glucose solution (solid circles), the least calorically dense, emptied the fastest. Other more calorically dense solutions, such as milk protein (solid triangles) and peptide hydrolysates (open circles and solid triangles), emptied slower. *[Reproduced with permission from Calbet JA, MacLean DA: Role of caloric content on gastric emptying in humans. J Physiol 498:533, 1997.]*

Traditionally, liquid emptying has been attributed to the activity of the proximal stomach, but it is probably more complicated than previously thought. Clearly, receptive relaxation and gastric accommodation play a role in gastric emptying of liquids. Patients with a denervated (e.g., vagotomized), resected, or plicated (e.g., fundoplication) proximal stomach have decreased gastric compliance and may show accelerated gastric emptying of liquids. A swallowed liquid meal induces receptive relaxation, but the same meal delivered via nasogastric tube bypasses this reflex and is associated with a higher intragastric pressure and accelerated emptying.

Some observations suggest an active role for the distal stomach in liquid emptying. For instance even if the proximal intragastric pressure is lower than duodenal pressure, normal gastric emptying of liquids can occur. Also, diabetic patients may have normal proximal gastric motor function and profoundly delayed gastric emptying of liquids. Indeed, antral contractile activity does correlate with liquid gastric emptying, and this distal gastric activity appears to vary with the nutrient composition and caloric content of the liquid meal. Depending on the circumstances, distal gastric motor activity can promote or inhibit gastric emptying of liquids. Distal gastrectomy and pyloric stenting both obviously interfere with distal gastric motor activity, and both accelerate the initial rapid phase of liquid gastric emptying.

Solid Emptying

Normally, the half-time of solid gastric emptying is <2 hours. Unlike liquids, which display an initial rapid phase followed by a slower linear phase of emptying, solids have an initial lag phase during which little emptying of solids occurs. It is during this phase that much of the grinding and mixing occurs. A linear emptying phase follows, during which the smaller particles are metered out to the duodenum. Solid gastric emptying is a function of meal particle size, caloric content, and composition (especially fat). When liquids and solids are ingested together, the liquids empty first. Solids are stored in the fundus and delivered to the distal stomach at constant rates for grinding. Liquids also are sequestered in the fundus, but they appear to be readily delivered to the distal stomach for early emptying. The larger the solid component of the meal, the slower the liquid emptying. Patients bothered by dumping syndrome are advised to limit the amount of liquid consumed with the solid meal, taking advantage of this effect. Three prokinetic agents are commonly used to treat delayed gastric emptying. Typical doses and mechanism of action are shown in Table 26-4.

DIAGNOSIS OF GASTRIC DISEASE

Signs and Symptoms

The most common symptoms of gastric disease are pain, weight loss, early satiety, and anorexia. Nausea, vomiting, bloating, and anemia also are frequent complaints. Several of these symptoms (pain, bloating, nausea, and early satiety) are often described by physicians as dyspepsia, synonymous with the common nonmedical term *indigestion*. Common causes of dyspepsia include gastroesophageal reflux disease (GERD) and disorders of the stomach, gallbladder, and pancreas. Although none of the above symptoms alone is specific for gastric disease, when elicited in the context of a careful history and physical examination, they can clearly point to a probable differential diagnosis, which can then be refined with certain tests.

TABLE 26-4	Drugs that accelerate gastric emptying	
Agent	**Typical Adult Dose**	**Mechanism of Action**
Metoclopramide	10 mg PO qid	Dopamine antagonist
Erythromycin	250 mg PO qid	Motilin agonist
Domperidone	10 mg PO qid	Dopamine antagonist

TABLE 26-5	Alarm symptoms that indicate the need for upper endoscopy

Weight loss
Recurrent vomiting
Dysphagia
Bleeding
Anemia

Diagnostic Tests
Esophagogastroduodenoscopy

Patients with one or more of the alarm symptoms listed in Table 26-5 should undergo expeditious upper endoscopy. Esophagogastroduodenoscopy (EGD) is a safe and accurate outpatient procedure performed under conscious sedation.[38] Smaller flexible scopes with excellent optics and a working channel are easily passed transnasally in the unsedated patient. Following an 8-hour fast, the flexible scope is advanced under direct vision into the esophagus, stomach, and duodenum. The fundus and GE junction are inspected by retroflexing the scope. To rule out cancer with a high degree of accuracy, all patients with gastric ulcer diagnosed on upper GI series or found at EGD should have multiple biopsies of the base and rim of the lesion. Brush cytology also should be considered. Gastritis should be biopsied both for histologic examination and for a tissue urease test to rule out the presence of *H. pylori*. If *Helicobacter* infection is detected, it should probably be treated because of the etiologic association with peptic ulcers, mucosa-associated lymphoid tissue (MALT), and gastric cancer. The most serious complications of EGD are perforation (which is rare, but can occur anywhere from the cervical esophagus to the duodenum), aspiration, and respiratory depression from excessive sedation. Although EGD is a more sensitive test than double-contrast upper GI series, these modalities should be considered complementary rather than mutually exclusive.

Radiologic Tests

Plain abdominal x-rays may be helpful in the diagnosis of gastric perforation (pneumoperitoneum) or delayed gastric emptying (large air-fluid level).

Double-contrast upper GI series may be better than EGD at elucidating the following: diverticula, fistula, tortuosity or stricture location, and size of hiatal hernia. Although there are radiologic characteristics of ulcers that suggest the presence or absence of malignancy, it must be reiterated that gastric ulcers require adequate biopsy.

Computed Tomographic Scanning and Magnetic Resonance Imaging

Most cases of significant gastric disease can be diagnosed without these sophisticated imaging studies. However, one or the other should be part of the routine staging work-up for most patients with a malignant gastric tumor. Magnetic resonance imaging (MRI) may prove clinically useful as a quantitative test for gastric emptying, and may even hold some promise for the analysis of myoelectric derangements in patients with gastroparesis. Advanced processing of high-resolution helical computed tomography (CT) and MRI data has made virtual endoscopy a reality.[39-41] Currently a research tool, it may have potential as a screening tool for gastric disease because it is noninvasive and does not require a physician on site to perform. Digital transmission allows the images to be analyzed remotely.

In specialized centers, impressive virtual endoscopic images are obtained with CT scan or MRI (Fig. 26-21). Of course suspicious lesions discovered by such techniques require endoscopic evaluation. And, before screening at-risk populations with these noninvasive modalities for gastric disease, the false-negative rates would have to be shown to be acceptably low.

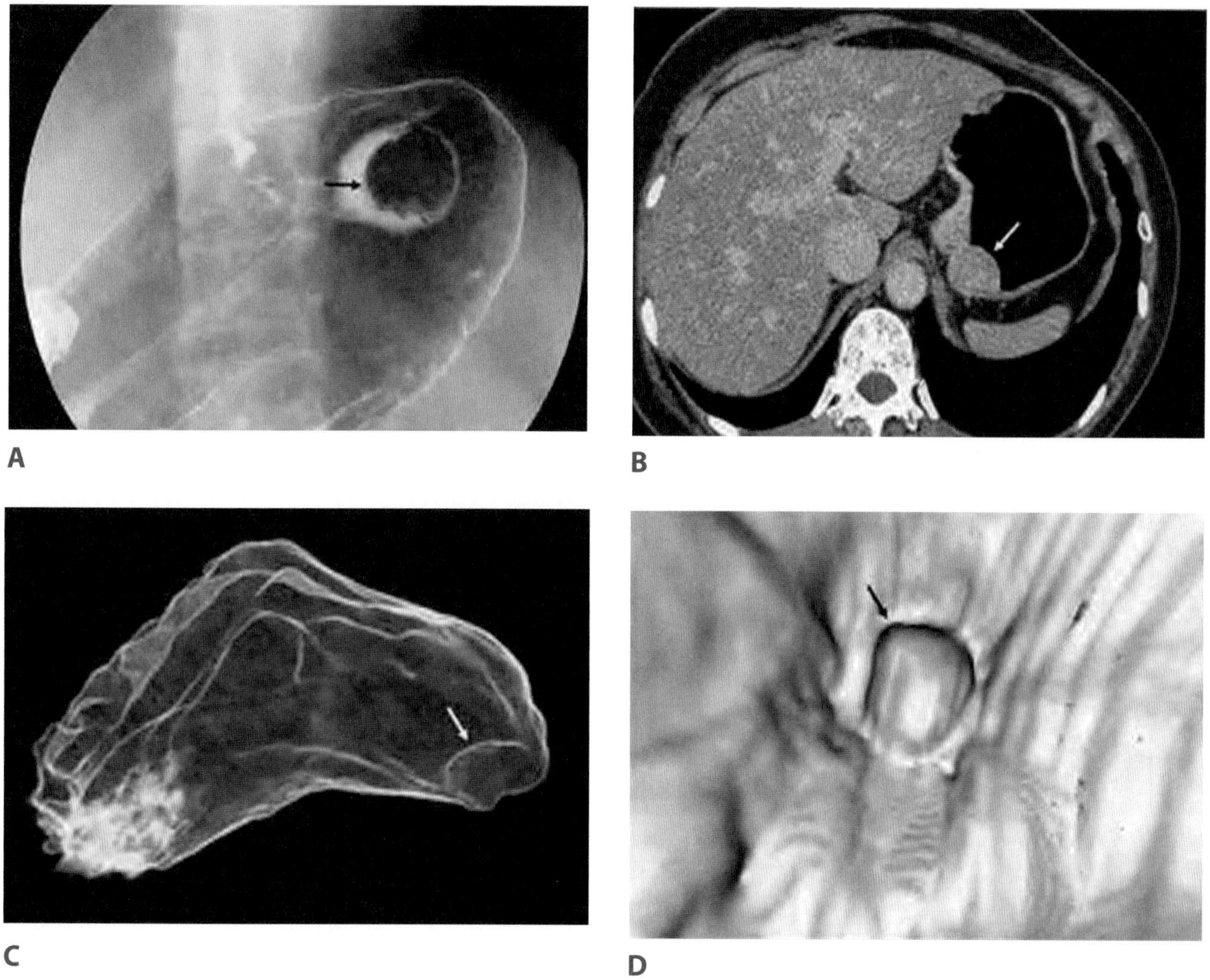

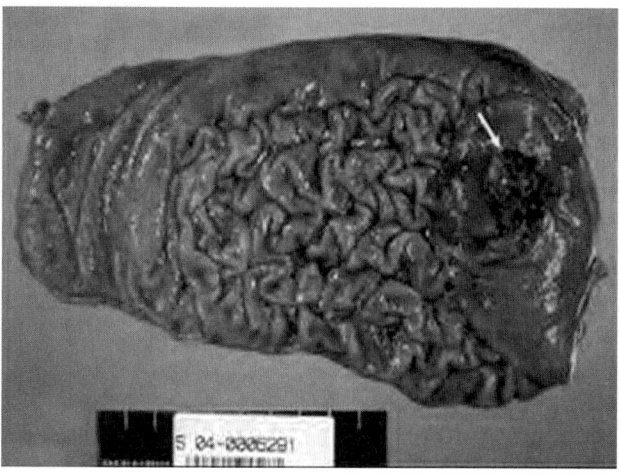

FIG. 26-21. Conventional double-contrast barium study (**A**) shows a focal protruding mass (*arrow*) on the gastric fundus. Axial computed tomographic scan (**B**) also shows a protruding polyp (*arrow*). The three dimensional computed tomographic gastrographic images in the transparent (**C**) and virtual endoscopic (**D**) modes show an elevated lesion on the gastric fundus (*arrows*). Photograph of the total gastrectomy specimen (**E**) shows a well-demarcated polypoid mass (*arrow*); this lesion was confirmed as early gastric carcinoma type I on microscopic examination (not shown). *(Reproduced with permission from Shin KS, et al: Three-dimensional MDCT gastrography compared with axial CT for the detection of early gastric cancer.* J Comput Assist Tomogr *31:741, 2007.)*

Arteriography rarely is necessary or useful in the diagnosis of gastric disease. It may be helpful in the occasional poor-risk patient with exsanguinating gastric hemorrhage, or in the patient with occult gastric bleeding that is difficult to diagnose. Extravasation of contrast indicates the location of the bleeding vessel, and embolization or selective infusion of vasopressin may be therapeutic. Occasionally, empiric embolization of the suspected but unproven

bleeding vessel helps. Arteriovenous malformations have a characteristic angiographic appearance.

Endoscopic Ultrasound

Endoscopic ultrasound (EUS) is useful in the evaluation and management of some gastric lesions.[42–44] Local staging of gastric adenocarcinoma with EUS is quite accurate, and this modality can be used to plan therapy. At some centers, patients with transmural and/or node positive adenocarcinoma of the stomach are considered for preoperative (neoadjuvant) chemoradiation therapy. EUS is the best way to clinically stage these patients locoregionally. Suspicious nodes can be sampled with EUS-guided endoscopic needle biopsy. Malignant tumors that are confined to the mucosa on EUS may be amenable to endoscopic mucosal resection (EMR). EUS also can be used to assess tumor response to chemotherapy. Submucosal masses are commonly discovered during routine EGD. Large submucosal masses should be resected because of the risk of malignancy, but observation may be appropriate for some small submucosal masses (e.g., lipoma or small GIST). There are endoscopic characteristics of benign and malignant mesenchymal tumors, and thus, EUS can provide reassurance, but no guarantee, that small lesions under observation are probably benign. Submucosal varices also can be assessed by EUS.

Gastric Secretory Analysis

Analysis of gastric acid output requires gastric intubation, and it is performed infrequently nowadays. This test may be useful in the evaluation of patients with hypergastrinemia, including the Zollinger-Ellison syndrome (ZES), patients with refractory ulcer or GERD, and patients with recurrent ulcer after operation. Historically, gastric analysis was performed most commonly to test for the adequacy of vagotomy in postoperative patients with recurrent or persistent ulcer. Now this can be done by assessing peripheral pancreatic polypeptide levels in response to sham feeding.[45] A 50% increase in pancreatic polypeptide within 30 minutes of sham feeding suggests vagal integrity.

Gastric analysis is performed in the fasted state with the semirecumbent patient in the left lateral position. After the position of the nasogastric tube is verified, the tube is hand aspirated every 5 minutes. Four successive 15-minute samples are created by pooling 5-minute aliquots. An IV stimulant of acid secretion may then be administered (typically pentagastrin) or, more commonly, the patient is sham fed ("chew and spit"), and the process repeated. Samples are analyzed by titration. Normal basal acid output (BAO) is <5 mEq/h. MAO is the average of the two final stimulated 15-minute periods and is usually 10 to 15 mEq/h. Peak acid output is defined as the highest of the four stimulated periods. Patients with a gastrinoma commonly have a high BAO, often above 30 mEq/h, but consistently above 15 mEq/h unless there has been previous vagotomy or gastric resection. In patients with gastrinoma, the ratio of BAO to MAO exceeds 0.6. Normal acid output in the patient prescribed acid-suppressive medication usually means that the patient is noncompliant. To assess acid-secretory capacity in the absence of medication effect, H_2 blockers and PPIs should be withheld for a week before gastric analysis.

Scintigraphy

Nuclear medicine tests can be helpful in the evaluation of gastric emptying and duodenogastric reflux. The standard scintigraphic evaluation of gastric emptying involves the ingestion of a test meal with one or two isotopes, and scanning the patient under a gamma camera. A curve for liquid and solid emptying is plotted, and the half-time calculated. Normal standards exist for each facility. Duodenogastric reflux can be quantitated by the IV administration of hepatobiliary iminodiacetic acid, which is concentrated and excreted by the liver into the duodenum. Software allows a semiquantitative assessment of how much of the isotope refluxes into the stomach. Positron emission tomography (PET) scan or CT/PET scan may be useful in certain patients with gastric malignancy.

Tests for Helicobacter pylori

Over the past two decades, *H. pylori* infection has emerged as a significant human pathogen. It is present in most patients with peptic ulcer disease (PUD), and has been associated with gastric lymphoma and adenocarcinoma. A variety of tests can help the clinician to determine whether the patient has active *H. pylori* infection.[46] The predictive value (positive and negative) of any of these tests when used as a screening tool depends on the prevalence of *H. pylori* infection in the screened population. *A positive test is quite accurate in predicting* H. pylori *infection, but a negative test is characteristically unreliable.* Thus, in the appropriate clinical setting, treatment for *H. pylori* should be initiated on the basis of a positive test, but not necessarily withheld if the test is negative. Because of the association between *H. pylori* infection and gastric lymphoma and carcinoma, many clinicians recommend treating *Helicobacter* infection when the diagnosis is made.

A positive serologic test is presumptive evidence of active infection if the patient has never been treated for *H. pylori*. Histologic examination of an antral mucosal biopsy using special stains is the gold standard test. Other sensitive tests include commercially available rapid urease tests, which assay for the presence of urease in mucosal biopsies (strong presumptive evidence of infection). Urease is an omnipresent enzyme in *H. pylori* strains that colonize the gastric mucosa. The labeled carbon-13 urea breath test has become the standard test to confirm eradication of *H. pylori* following appropriate treatment.[47] In this test, the patient ingests urea labeled with nonradioactive ^{13}C. The labeled urea is acted upon by the urease present in the *H. pylori* and converted into ammonia and carbon dioxide. The radiolabeled carbon dioxide is excreted from the lungs and can be detected in the expired air (Fig. 26-22). It also can be detected in a blood sample. The fecal antigen test also is quite sensitive and specific

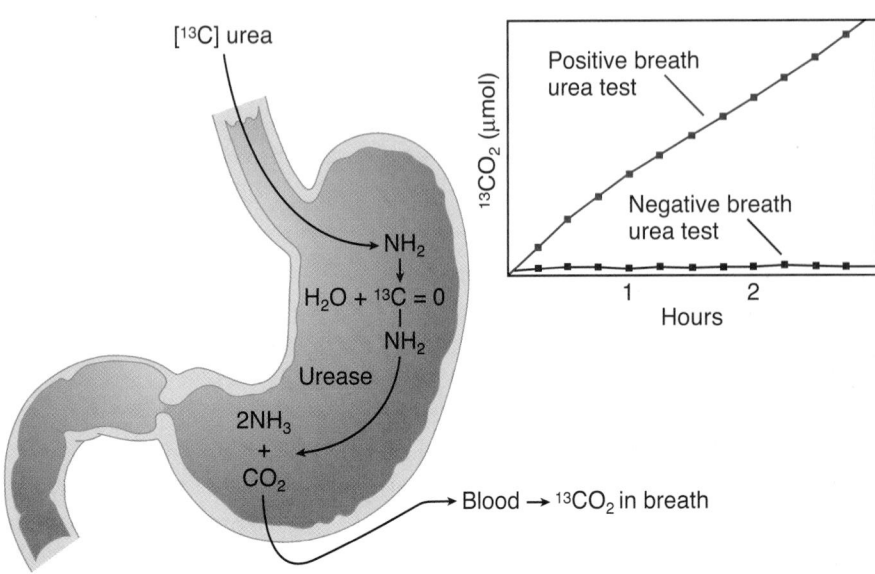

FIG. 26-22. Labeled urea breath test to detect *Helicobacter* infection. *(Reproduced with permission from Walsh JH, Peterson WL: The treatment of* Helicobacter pylori *infection in the management of peptic ulcer disease. N Engl J Med 333:984, 1995. Copyright ©1995 Massachusetts Medical Society. All rights reserved.)*

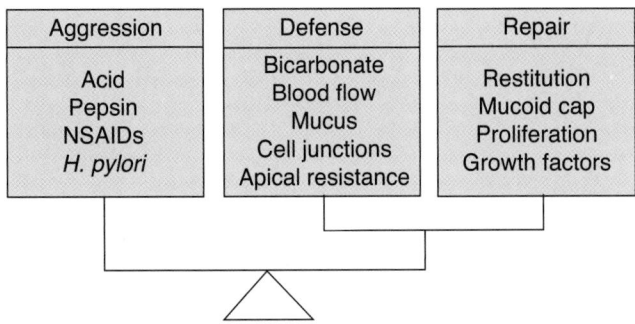

FIG. 26-23. Balance of aggressive and defensive factors in the gastric mucosa. *(Reproduced with permission from Mertz HR, Walsh JH: Peptic ulcer pathophysiology. Med Clin North Am 75:799, 1991. Copyright Elsevier.)*

for active *H. pylori* infection and may prove more practical in confirming a cure.

Antroduodenal Motility Testing and Electrogastrography

Antroduodenal motility testing and electrogastrography (EGG) are performed in specialized centers and may be useful in the evaluation of the patient with anomalous epigastric symptoms. EGG consists of the transcutaneous recording of gastric myoelectric activity. Antroduodenal motility testing is done with a tube placed transnasally or transorally into the distal duodenum. There are pressure-recording sensors extending from the stomach to the distal duodenum. The combination of these two tests together with scintigraphy provides a thorough assessment of gastric motility.

PEPTIC ULCER DISEASE

Peptic ulcers are focal defects in the gastric or duodenal mucosa that extend into the submucosa or deeper. They may be acute or chronic and, ultimately, are caused by an imbalance between mucosal defenses and acid/peptic injury (Fig. 26-23).[48,49] Peptic ulcer remains a common outpatient diagnosis, but the number of physician visits, hospital admissions, and elective operations for PUD has decreased steadily and dramatically over the past three decades. Interestingly, the start of these trends all predated the use of H_2 receptor blockers, fiber-optic endoscopy, and HSV. However, the incidence of emergency surgery and the death rate associated with peptic ulcers has not decreased nearly so dramatically. These epidemiologic changes probably represent the net effect of several factors, including (beneficially) decreased prevalence of *H. pylori* infection, better medical therapy, and increased outpatient management; and (detrimentally) the use of NSAIDs and aspirin (with and without ulcer prophylaxis) in an aging population with multiple risk factors.

PUD is one of the most common GI disorders in the United States with a prevalence of about 2%, and a lifetime cumulative prevalence of about 10%, peaking around age 70 years.[50] The costs of PUD, including lost work time and productivity, are estimated to be above $8 billion per year in the United States. In 1998, approximately 1.5% of all Medicare hospital costs were spent treating PUD, and the crude mortality rate for peptic ulcer was 1.7 per 100,000 individuals. Gastric ulcer has a higher mortality than duodenal ulcer because of its increased prevalence in the elderly. Recent studies have shown an increase in the rates of hospitalization and mortality in elderly patients for the peptic ulcer complications of bleeding and perforation. Presumably, this is due to the increasingly common use of NSAIDs and aspirin in this elderly cohort, many of whom also have *H. pylori* infection.

Pathophysiology and Etiology

A variety of factors may contribute to the development of PUD. Although it is now recognized that the large majority of duodenal and gastric ulcers are caused by *H. pylori* infection and/or NSAID use[17,51] (Fig. 26-24), the final common pathway to ulcer formation is acid-peptic injury of the gastroduodenal mucosal barrier. Thus, the adage "no acid, no ulcer" remains true even today. Acid suppression remains a mainstay in healing both duodenal and gastric ulcers and in preventing recurrence. It generally is thought that *H. pylori* predisposes to ulceration, both by acid hypersecretion, and by compromise of mucosal defense mechanisms including damage to SECs. NSAID use is thought to lead to PUD predominantly by compromise of mucosal defenses. Duodenal ulcer has typically been viewed as a disease of increased acid-peptic action on the duodenal mucosa, whereas gastric ulcer has been thought of as a disease of weakened mucosal defenses in the face of relatively normal or even decreased acid-peptic activity. However, an increased understanding of peptic ulcer pathophysiology has blurred this overly simplistic distinction. Clearly, weakened mucosal defenses play a role in many duodenal and most gastric ulcers (e.g., duodenal ulcer in an *H. pylori*–negative patient on NSAIDs or a patient with a typical type I gastric ulcer with acid hyposecretion), whereas increased aggressive activity of peptic acid may result in a duodenal or gastric ulcer in the setting of normal mucosal defenses (e.g., a duodenal ulcer in a patient with ZES, or a gastric ulcer in a patient with gastric outlet obstruction, antral stasis, and acid hypersecretion).

Elimination of *H. pylori* infection or NSAID use is important for optimal ulcer healing, and perhaps is even more important in pre-

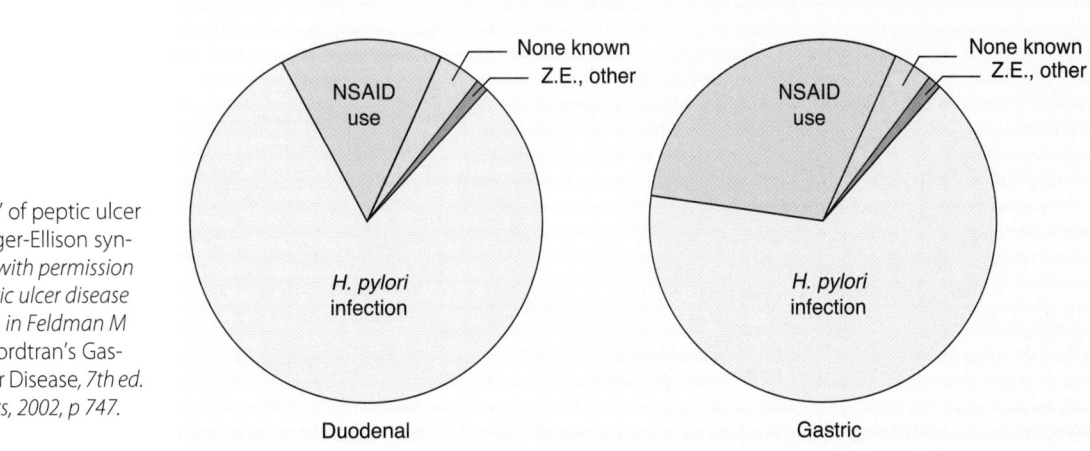

Conditions associated with peptic ulcer

FIG. 26-24. "Causes" of peptic ulcer disease. Z.E. = Zollinger-Ellison syndrome. *[Reproduced with permission from Spechler SJ: Peptic ulcer disease and its complications, in Feldman M (ed): Sleisinger and Fordtran's Gastrointestinal and Liver Disease, 7th ed. Philadelphia: Saunders, 2002, p 747. Copyright Elsevier.]*

venting ulcer recurrence and/or complications. A variety of other diseases are known to cause peptic ulcer, including ZES (gastrinoma), antral G-cell hyperfunction and/or hyperplasia, systemic mastocytosis, trauma, burns, and major physiologic stress. Other causative agents include drugs (all NSAIDs, aspirin, and cocaine), smoking, alcohol, and psychologic stress. In the United States, probably more than 90% of serious peptic ulcer complications can be attributed to *H. pylori* infection, NSAID use, and/or cigarette smoking.

Helicobacter pylori *Infection*

With specialized flagella and a rich supply of urease, *H. pylori* is uniquely equipped for survival in the hostile environment of the stomach.[52–55] Fifty percent of the world's population is infected with *H. pylori*, a major cause of chronic gastritis. The same sequence of inflammation to metaplasia to dysplasia to carcinoma, that is well known to occur in the esophagus from reflux-induced inflammation (and in the colon from inflammatory bowel disease), is now increasingly well recognized to occur in the stomach with *Helicobacter*-induced gastritis. The influence of prolonged acid suppression with PPIs or H₂RAs on these esophagogastric processes is largely unknown. *Helicobacter* also clearly has an etiologic role in the development of gastric lymphoma.

The organism possesses the enzyme urease, which converts urea into ammonia and bicarbonate, thus creating an environment around the bacteria that buffers the acid secreted by the stomach. The ammonia is damaging to the SECs. Mutant strains of *H. pylori* that do not produce urease are unable to colonize the stomach. The organism lives in the mucus layer atop the gastric SECs, and some attach to these cells (Fig. 26-25).[53,54] Apparently *Helicobacter* strains that lack flagella are unable to navigate through the unstirred mucus layer to get to the apical membrane of the SEC for attachment, and are nonpathogenic. One of the mechanisms by which *Helicobacter* causes gastric injury may be through a disturbance in gastric acid secretion. This is due, in part, to the inhibitory effect that *H. pylori* exerts on antral D cells that secrete somatostatin, a potent inhibitor of antral G-cell gastrin production. *H. pylori* infection is associated with decreased levels of somatostatin, decreased somatostatin messenger RNA production, and fewer somatostatin-producing D cells. These effects are probably mediated by *H. pylori*–induced local alkalinization of the antrum (antral acidification is the most potent antagonist to antral gastrin secretion), and *H. pylori*–mediated increases in other local mediators and cytokines. The end result is hypergastrinemia and acid hypersecretion (Fig. 26-26).[49] This hypergastrinemia presumably leads to the parietal cell hyperplasia seen in many patients with duodenal ulcer. The acid hypersecretion and the antral gastritis are thought to lead to antral epithelial metaplasia in the postpyloric duodenum. This duodenal metaplasia allows *H. pylori* to colonize the duodenal mucosa and, in these patients, the risk of developing a duodenal ulcer increases 50-fold. When *H. pylori* colonizes the duodenum, there is a significant decrease in acid-stimulated duodenal bicarbonate release. When *H. pylori* infection is successfully treated, acid secretory physiology tends to normalize. Other mechanisms whereby *H. pylori* can induce gastroduodenal mucosal injury include the production of toxins (vacA and cagA), local elaboration of cytokines (particularly interleukin-8) by infected mucosa, recruitment of inflammatory cells and release of inflammatory mediators, recruitment and activation of local immune factors, and increased apoptosis (Fig. 26-27).[54,55] The net effect is a weakening of mucosal defenses.

The evidence supporting the central role of *H. pylori* in the pathophysiology of PUD is strong. Patients with *H. pylori* infection and antral gastritis are three and one-half times more likely to develop PUD than patients without *H. pylori* infection. Up to 90% of patients with duodenal ulcers, and 70 to 90% of patients with gastric ulcers, have *H. pylori* infection. It is clear from multiple randomized prospective studies that curing *H. pylori* infection dramatically alters the natural history of PUD, decreasing the recurrent ulcer rate from more than 75% in patients treated with a course of acid-suppressive therapy

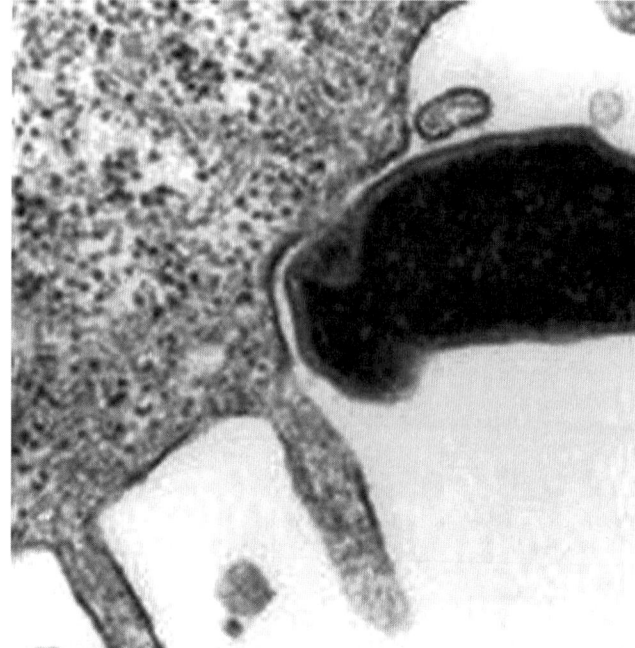

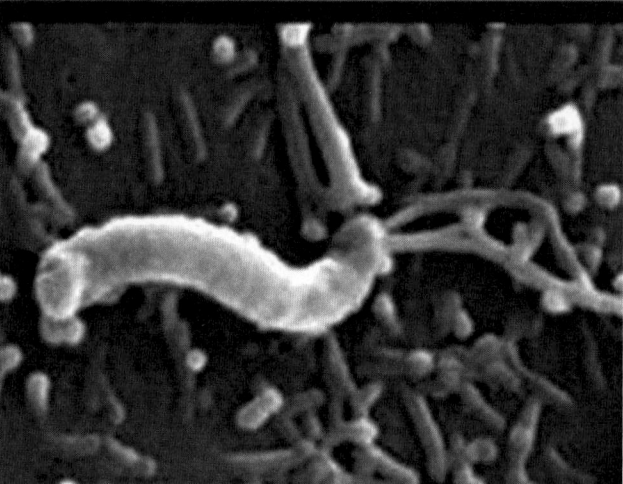

FIG. 26-25. *Helicobacter pylori* closely adherent to the cell membrane (*top*), and spiral-shaped *H. pylori* attached to epithelial surface and surrounding microvilli (*bottom*). In the image on the bottom, the bacterial flagella can be seen arising from the upper pole of the bacterium. *(From Parsonnet J: Clinician-discoverers—Marshall, Warren, and* H. pylori. *N Engl J Med 353:2421, 2005. Photomicrographs courtesy of Dr. Manuel Amieva, Stanford University.)*

alone (in whom *H. pylori* is not eradicated) to less than 20% in patients treated with a course of antibacterial therapy (Fig. 26-28).[56]

Obviously, other factors are involved in the etiology of PUD because everyone who has *H. pylori* (up to 50% of the adult population in some areas of the United States) does not get PUD. Only about 10 to 15% of patients colonized with *H. pylori* will develop PUD over their lifetime. Many patients on aspirin and NSAIDs develop PUD without *H. pylori* infection. These observations notwithstanding, it is clear from a variety of well-designed laboratory, clinical, and epidemiologic studies that *H. pylori* is indubitably an important factor in the development and recurrence of PUD. *H. pylori* also plays an etiologic role in gastric cancer and lymphoma.[54]

Acid Secretion and Peptic Ulcer

A variety of abnormalities related to mucosal acid exposure have been described in patients with duodenal ulcer (Fig. 26-29).[57] As a

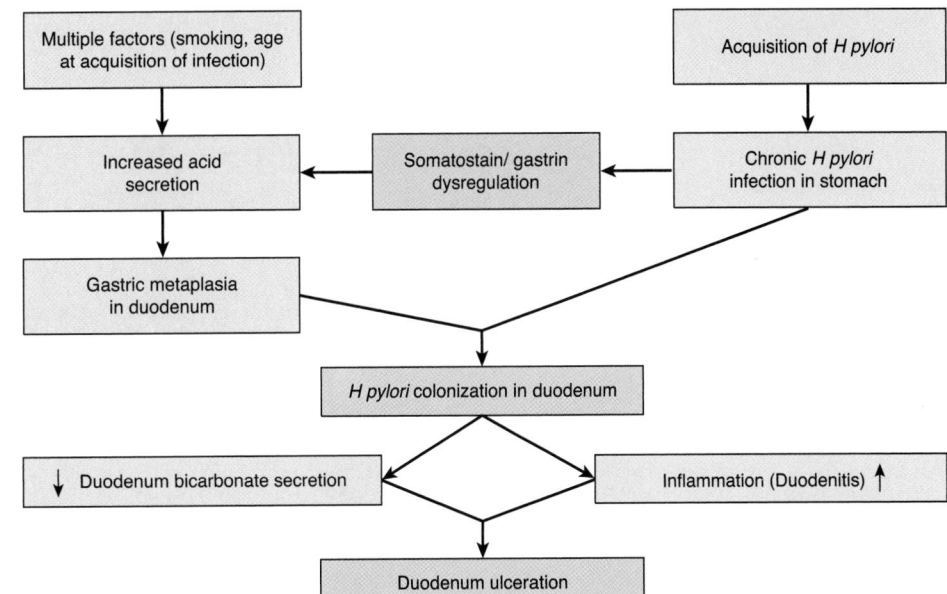

FIG. 26-26. Model of *Helicobacter* effects on duodenal ulcer pathogenesis. *(Reproduced with permission from Peek RM Jr., Blaser MJ: Pathophysiology of* Helicobacter pylori-*induced gastritis and peptic ulcer disease. Am J Med 102:200, 1997. Copyright Elsevier.)*

rule, duodenal ulcer patients secrete more acid than patients with gastric ulcer. It has long been recognized that duodenal ulcer patients as a group have a higher mean BAO and also a higher mean MAO compared to normal controls. Nocturnal acid secretion is more commonly elevated than daytime secretion. However, many duodenal ulcer patients have basal and peak acid outputs in the normal range, and there is no correlation between acid secretion and the severity of the ulcer disease. Duodenal ulcer patients produce more acid than normal controls in response to any known secretory stimulus for gastric acid output. Although duodenal ulcer patients usually have normal fasting gastrin concentrations, they often produce more gastric acid at any given dose of gastrin than controls. Considering that many duodenal ulcer patients do produce excessive gastric acid, it has been argued that a "normal" fasting gastrin level in these patients is inappropriately high, and that there is an impaired feedback mechanism, especially in light of the apparently increased sensitivity of the parietal cell mass to gastrin. Many of these long-standing observations now seem reasonable in light of recently gained understanding of the perturbations in acid and gastrin secretion associated with *H. pylori* infection. Some patients with duodenal ulcer also have increased rates of gastric emptying that deliver an increased acid load per unit of time to the duodenum. Finally, the buffering capacity of the duodenum in many patients with duodenal ulcer is compromised due to decreased duodenal bicarbonate secretion.

In patients with gastric ulcer, acid secretion is variable. Currently, five types of gastric ulcer are described, although the original Johnson classification contained three types (Fig. 26-30).[58] The most common, Johnson type I gastric ulcer, is typically located near the angularis incisura on the lesser curvature, close to the border between the antrum and the body of the stomach. Patients with type I gastric ulcer usually have normal or decreased acid secretion. Type II gastric ulcer is associated with active or quiescent duodenal ulcer disease, and type III gastric ulcer is prepyloric ulcer disease. Both type II and type III gastric ulcers are associated with normal or increased gastric acid secretion. Type IV gastric ulcers occur near the GE junction, and acid secretion is normal or below normal. Type V gastric ulcers are medication induced and may occur anywhere in the stomach. Patients with gastric ulcers may have weak mucosal defenses that permit an abnormal amount of injurious acid backdiffusion into the mucosa. Duodenogastric reflux may play a role in weakening the gastric mucosal defenses, and a variety of components in duodenal juice, including bile, lysolecithin, and pancreatic juice, have been shown to cause injury and inflammation in the gastric mucosa. NSAIDs and aspirin have similar effects. Although chronic gastric ulcer usually is associated with surrounding gastritis, it is unproven that the latter leads to the former.

Nonsteroidal Anti-Inflammatory Drugs in Peptic Ulcer Disease

NSAIDs (including aspirin) are inextricably linked to PUD.[59] Patients with rheumatoid arthritis and osteoarthritis who take NSAIDs have a 15 to 20% annual incidence of peptic ulcer, and the prevalence of peptic ulcer in chronic NSAID users is about 25% (15% gastric and 10% duodenal). Complications of PUD (specifically hemorrhage and perforation) are much more common in patients taking NSAIDs. More than half of patients who present with peptic ulcer hemorrhage or perforation report the recent use of NSAIDs, including aspirin. Many of these patients remain asymptomatic until they develop these life-threatening complications.

The overall risk of significant serious adverse GI events in patients taking NSAIDs is more than three times that of controls (Table 26-6). This risk increases to five times in patients more than age 60 years old. In elderly patients taking NSAIDs, the likelihood that they will require an operation related to a GI complication is 10 times that of the control group, and the risk that they will die from a GI cause is about four and one-half times higher. This problem is put into perspective when one realizes that approximately 20 million patients in the United States take NSAIDs on a regular basis; perhaps as many regularly take aspirin. Persons who take NSAIDs also have a higher hospitalization rate for serious GI events than those who do not.

Factors that clearly put patients at increased risk for NSAID-induced GI complications include age >60, prior GI event, high NSAID dose, concurrent steroid intake, and concurrent anticoagulant intake. *Any patient taking NSAIDs or aspirin who has one or more of these risk factors should receive concomitant acid suppressive medication* (Table 26-7).[60]

Smoking, Stress, and Other Factors

Epidemiologic studies suggest that smokers are about twice as likely to develop PUD as nonsmokers. Smoking increases gastric acid secretion and duodenogastric reflux. Smoking decreases both gastroduodenal prostaglandin production and pancreaticoduodenal bicarbonate production. These observations may be related, and any or all could explain the observed association between smoking and PUD.

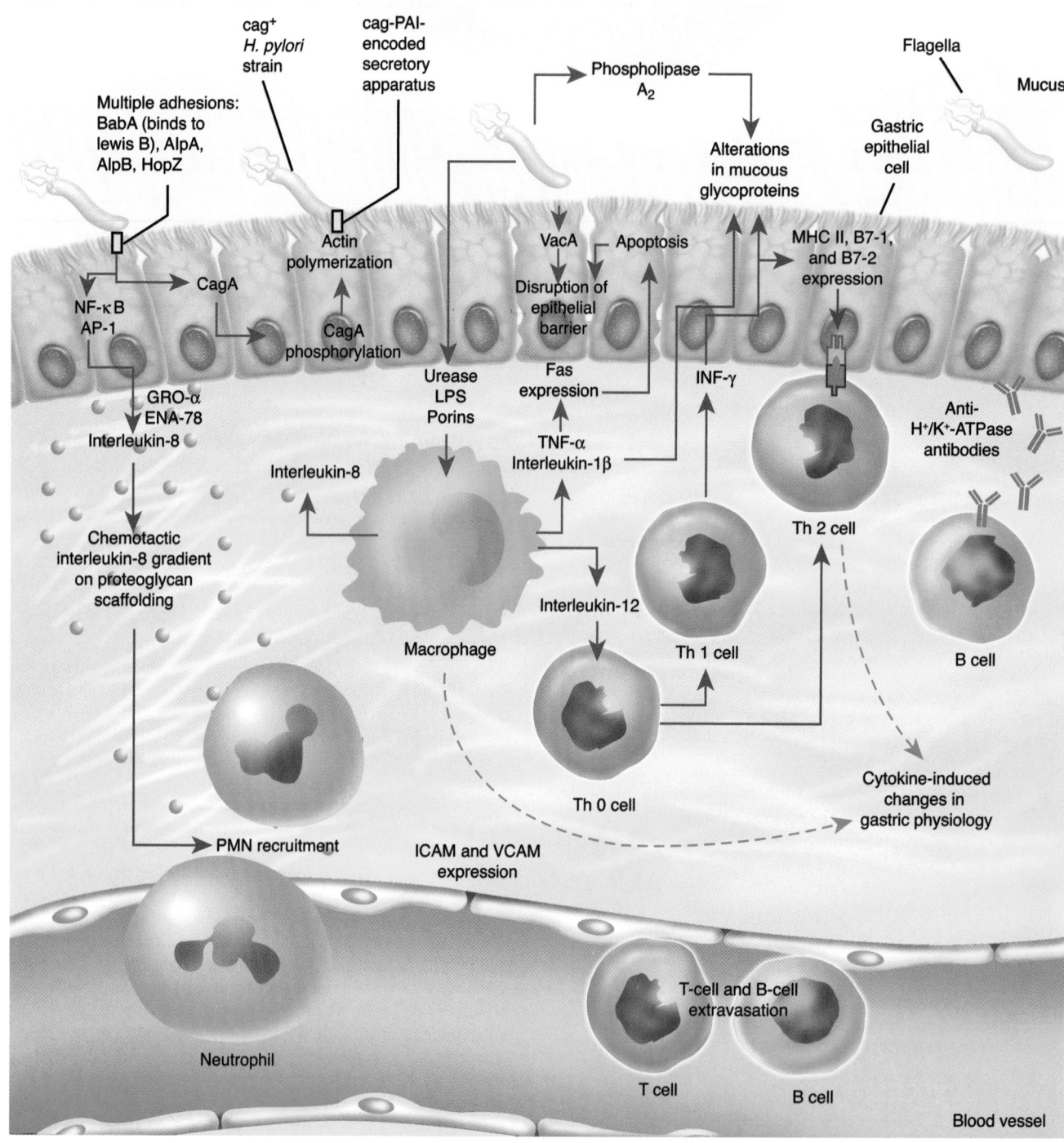

FIG. 26-27. Pathogen-host interactions in the pathogenesis of *Helicobacter pylori* infection. ICAM = intercellular adhesion molecule-1; INF-γ = interferon-γ; LPS = lipopolysaccharide; NF-κB = nuclear factor κB; PAI = pathogenicity island; PMN = polymorphonuclear neutrophil; TNF-α = tumor necrosis factor alpha; VCAM = vascular cell adhesion molecule. *(Reproduced with permission from Suerbaum S, Michetti P:* Helicobacter pylori *infection.* N Engl J Med *347:1175, 2002. Copyright ©2002 Massachusetts Medical Society. All rights reserved.)*

Although difficult to measure, both physiologic and psychologic stress undoubtedly play a role in the development of peptic ulcer in some patients. In 1842, Curling described duodenal ulcer and/or duodenitis in burn patients. Decades later, Cushing described the appearance of acute peptic ulceration in patients with head trauma (Cushing's ulcer). Even the ancients recognized the undeniable links between PUD and stress. Patients still present with ulcer complications (bleeding, perforation, and obstruction) that are seemingly exacerbated by stressful life events. The use of crack cocaine has been linked to juxtapyloric peptic ulcers with a propensity to perforate. Alcohol is commonly mentioned as a risk factor for PUD, but confirmatory data are lacking.

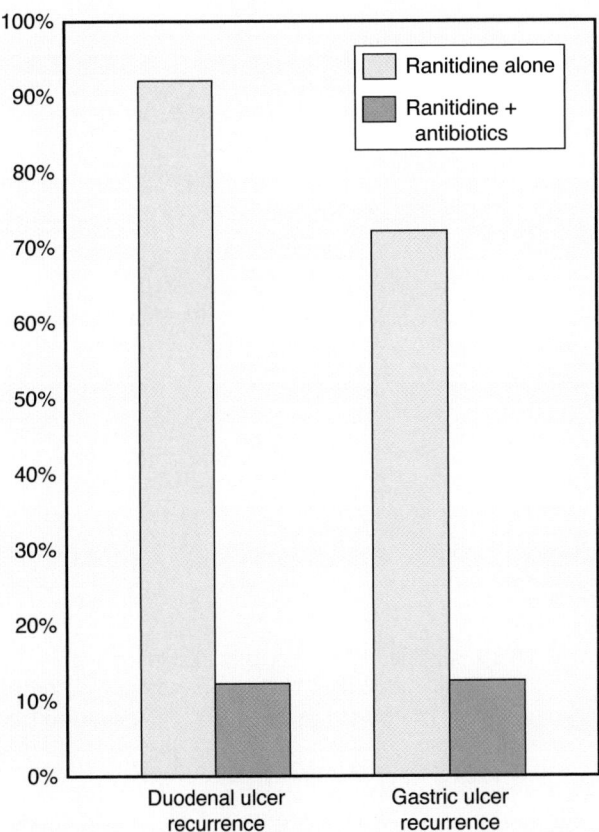

FIG. 26-28. *Helicobacter* treatment dramatically decreases the recurrence rate of duodenal and gastric ulcer. *(Data from Graham DY, Lew GM, Klein PD, et al: Effect of treatment of* Helicobacter pylori *infection on the long-term recurrence of gastric or duodenal ulcer. A randomized controlled study.* Ann Intern Med *116:705, 1992.)*

Clinical Manifestations

More than 90% of patients with PUD complain of abdominal pain. The pain is typically nonradiating, burning in quality, and located in the epigastrium. The mechanism of the pain is unclear. Patients with duodenal ulcer often experience pain 2 to 3 hours after a meal and at night. Two thirds of patients with duodenal ulcers will complain of pain that awakens them from sleep. The pain of gastric ulcer more commonly occurs with eating and is less likely to awaken the patient at night. A history of PUD, use of NSAIDs, over-the-counter antacids, or antisecretory drugs is suggestive of the diagnosis. Other signs and symptoms include nausea, bloating, weight loss, stool positive for occult blood, and anemia. Duodenal ulcer is about twice as common in men compared to women, but the incidence of gastric ulcer is similar in men and women. On average, gastric ulcer patients are 10 years older than duodenal ulcer patients, and the incidence is increasing in the elderly, probably because of increasing NSAID use in this cohort with a high incidence of *H. pylori* infection.

Diagnosis

In the young patient with dyspepsia and/or epigastric pain, it may be appropriate to initiate empiric PPI therapy for PUD without confirmatory testing. In such cases, it is prudent to discuss with the patient the small possibility of an alternative diagnosis, including malignancy, even if symptoms improve with the initiation of therapy. All patients more than 45 years old with the above symptoms should have an upper endoscopy, and all patients, regardless of age, should have this study if any alarm symptoms (see Table 26-5) are present. A double-contrast upper GI x-ray study may be useful. Once an ulcer has been confirmed endoscopically or radiologically, obvious possible causes (*Helicobacter*, NSAIDs, gastrinoma, cancer) should always be considered. All gastric ulcers should be adequately biopsied, and any sites of gastritis should be biopsied to rule out *H. pylori*, and for histologic evaluation. Additional testing for *H. pylori* may be indicated. It is not unreasonable to test all peptic ulcer patients for *H. pylori* (Table 26-8).[61] A baseline serum gastrin level is appropriate to rule out gastrinoma.

Complications

The three most common complications of PUD, in decreasing order of frequency, are bleeding, perforation, and obstruction.[62–64] Most peptic ulcer–related deaths in the United States are due to bleeding. Bleeding peptic ulcers are by far the most common cause of upper GI bleeding in patient admitted to hospital (Fig. 26-31).[65] Patients with a bleeding peptic ulcer typically present with melena and/or hematemesis. Nasogastric aspiration is usually confirmatory of the upper GI bleeding. Abdominal pain is quite uncommon. Shock may be present, necessitating aggressive resuscitation and blood transfusion. Early endoscopy is important to diagnose the cause of the bleeding and to assess the need for hemostatic therapy.

Three fourths of the patients who come to the hospital with bleeding peptic ulcer will stop bleeding if given acid suppression and nothing by mouth. However, one fourth will continue to bleed or will rebleed after an initial quiescent period, and virtually all the

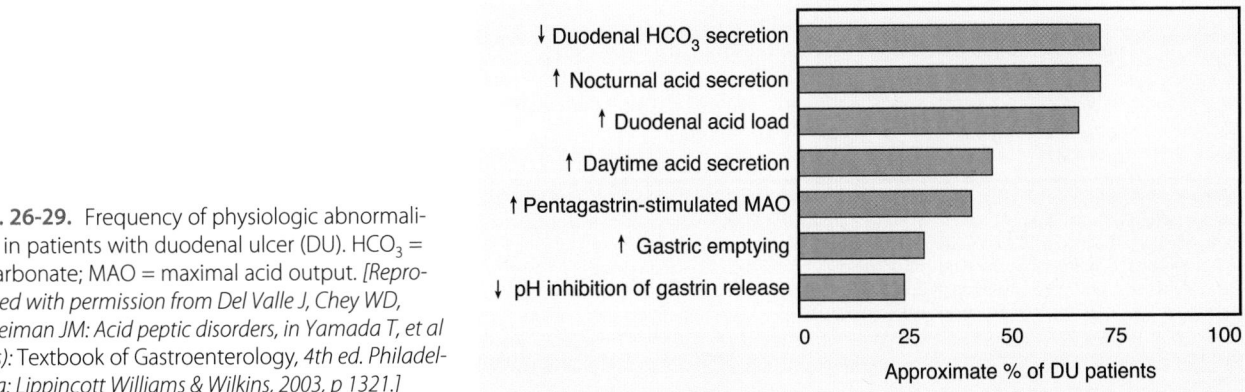

FIG. 26-29. Frequency of physiologic abnormalities in patients with duodenal ulcer (DU). HCO_3 = bicarbonate; MAO = maximal acid output. *[Reproduced with permission from Del Valle J, Chey WD, Scheiman JM: Acid peptic disorders, in Yamada T, et al (eds):* Textbook of Gastroenterology, *4th ed. Philadelphia: Lippincott Williams & Wilkins, 2003, p 1321.]*

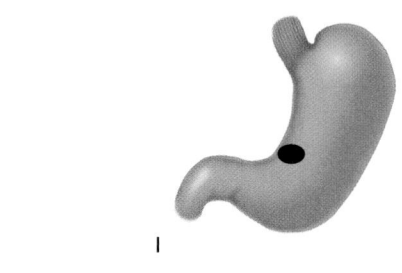

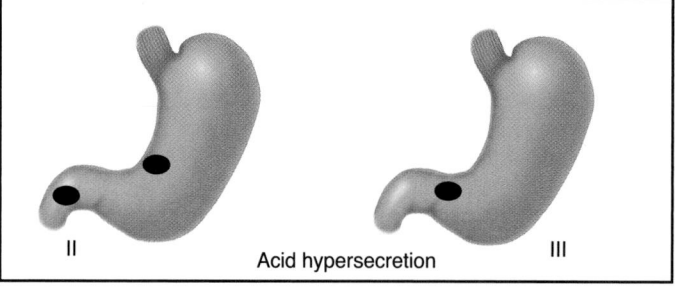

Acid hypersecretion

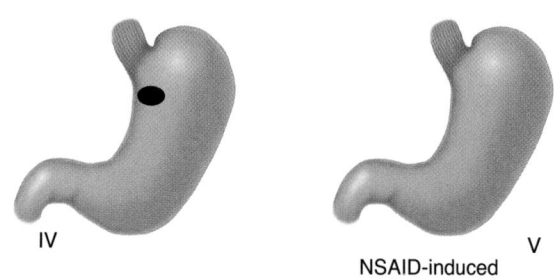

NSAID-induced

FIG. 26-30. Modified Johnson classification for gastric ulcer. I. Lesser curve, incisura. II. Body of stomach, incisura + duodenal ulcer (active or healed). III. Prepyloric. IV. High on lesser curve, near gastroesophageal junction. V. Medication-induced (NSAID/acetylsalicylic acid), anywhere in stomach. *[Reproduced with permission from Fisher WE, Brunicardi FC: Benign gastric ulcer, in Cameron JL (ed):* Current Surgical Therapy, *9th ed. Philadelphia: Mosby Elsevier, 2008, p 81. Copyright Elsevier.]*

mortalities (and all the operations for bleeding) occur in this group. This group can be fairly well delineated based on clinical factors related to the magnitude of the hemorrhage, comorbidities, age, and endoscopic findings. Shock, hematemesis, transfusion requirement exceeding four units in 24 hours, and certain endoscopic stigmata (active bleeding or visible vessel) define this high-risk group. Two widely used risk stratification tools have proven useful in predicting

rebleeding and death: the Blatchford and Rockall scores (Table 26-9).[66] High-risk patients benefit from endoscopic therapy to stop the bleeding. The most common endoscopic hemostatic modalities used are injection with epinephrine, and electrocautery. Persistent bleeding or rebleeding after endoscopic therapy is an indication for operation, although repeat endoscopic treatment has been successful in treating rebleeding. Elderly patients and patients with multiple

TABLE 26-6 Hospitalization rates for GI events with and without NSAID use in selected large populations

| | Therapies Used | | Annualized Incidence[b] | | | |
| | | | Clinical Upper GI Events[c] | | Complicated Upper GI Events[d] | |
Study[a]	NSAID Control	Study Drugs	Control	Study Drug	Control	Study Drug
MUCOSA	10 NSAIDs (n = 4439)	Misoprostol 200 μg qid + NSAID (n = 4404)	3.1%	1.6%	1.5%	0.7%
CLASS	Ibuprofen 800 mg tid, diclofenac 75 mg bid (n = 3987)	Celecoxib 400 mg bid (n = 3995)	3.5%	2.1%	1.5%	0.8%
			(No aspirin[e]: 2.9%)	1.4%	1.3%	0.4%
VIGOR	Naproxen 500 mg bid (n = 4047)	Rofecoxib 50 mg qd (n = 4029)	4.5%	2.1%	1.4%	0.6%

[a]MUCOSA and VIGOR trials included only rheumatoid arthritis patients; CLASS trial included osteoarthritis (73%) and rheumatoid arthritis (27%).
[b]Incidence for MUCOSA trial represents doubling of results provided at 6 months (although median follow-up was <6 months). Incidences for VIGOR and CLASS trials represent rates per 100 patient-years, although VIGOR median follow-up was 9 months and CLASS data include only the first 6 months of the study.
[c]Includes perforations, obstructions, bleeding, and uncomplicated ulcers discovered on clinically indicated work-up.
[d]Includes perforation, obstruction, bleeding (documented due to ulcer or erosions in MUCOSA and CLASS; major bleeding in VIGOR).
[e]21% of patients in CLASS study were taking low-dose aspirin.
Note: All differences between controls and study drugs were significant except clinical upper GI events in overall CLASS study (P = .09).
Source: Reproduced with permission from Laine L: Approaches to nonsteroidal anti-inflammatory drug use in the high-risk patient. *Gastroenterology* 120:594, 2001. Copyright Elsevier.

TABLE 26-7	Patients taking NSAIDs or aspirin need concomitant acid suppressing medication if any of the following risk factors is present

- Age over 60
- History of acid/peptic disease
- Concurrent steroid intake
- Concurrent anticoagulant intake
- High-dose NSAID or acetylsalicylic acid

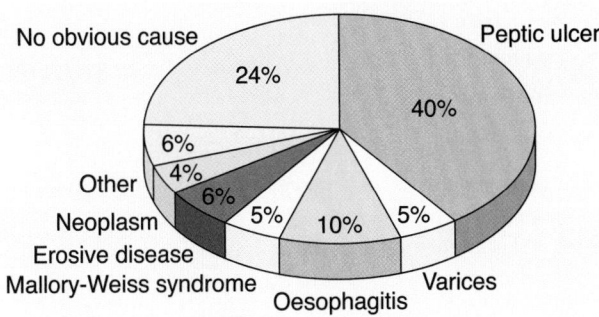

FIG. 26-31. Causes of upper GI bleeding. *(Reproduced with permission from Dallal HJ, Palmer KR: Clinical Review: Upper gastrointestinal hemorrhage. BMJ 323:1115, 2001. With permission from the BMJ Publishing Group.)*

comorbidities do not tolerate repeated episodes of hemodynamically significant hemorrhage, and may benefit from early elective operation after initially successful endoscopic treatment, especially if they have one or more of the risk factors mentioned above or a high-risk ulcer. Planned surgery under controlled circumstances often yields better outcomes than emergent surgery performed in the middle of the night. Deep bleeding ulcers on the posterior duodenal bulb or lesser gastric curvature are high-risk lesions, because they often erode large arteries not amenable to nonoperative treatment, and early operation should be considered.

Perforated peptic ulcer usually presents as an acute abdomen. The patient can often give the exact time of onset of the excruciating abdominal pain. Initially, a chemical peritonitis develops from the gastric and/or duodenal secretions, but within hours a bacterial peritonitis supervenes. Fluid sequestration into the third space of the inflamed peritoneum can be impressive, and fluid resuscitation is mandatory. The patient is in obvious distress, and the abdominal examination shows peritoneal signs. Usually, marked involuntary guarding and rebound tenderness is evoked by a gentle examination. Upright chest x-ray shows free air in about 80% of patients (Fig. 26-32). Once the diagnosis has been made, the patient is given analgesia and antibiotics, resuscitated with isotonic fluid, and taken to the operating room. Sometimes, the perforation has sealed spontaneously by the time of presentation, and surgery can be avoided if the patient is doing well. Nonoperative management is appropriate only if there is objective evidence that the leak has sealed (i.e., radiologic contrast study), and in the absence of clinical peritonitis.

Gastric outlet obstruction occurs in no more than 5% of patients with PUD. It is usually due to duodenal or prepyloric ulcer disease, and may be acute (from inflammatory swelling and peristaltic dysfunction) or chronic (from cicatrix). Patients typically present with nonbilious vomiting and may have a profound hypokalemic hypochloremic metabolic alkalosis. Pain or discomfort is common. Weight loss may be prominent, depending on the duration of symp-

toms. A succussion splash may be audible with stethoscope placed in the epigastrium. Initial treatment is nasogastric suction, IV hydration and electrolyte repletion, and antisecretory medication. The diagnosis is confirmed by endoscopy. Most patients admitted to the hospital nowadays with obstructing ulcer disease require intervention, either balloon dilation or operation. Cancer must be ruled out because most patients who present with the symptoms of gastric outlet obstruction will have a pancreatic, gastric, or duodenal malignancy.

Medical Treatment of Peptic Ulcer Disease

PPIs are the mainstay of medical therapy for PUD, but high dose H_2RAs are also quite effective. Patients hospitalized for ulcer complications should receive PPI by continuous IV infusion and, when discharged, should be considered for lifelong PPIs unless the definitive cause is eliminated or a definitive operation performed. Peptic ulcer patients should stop smoking and avoid alcohol and NSAIDs (including aspirin). Patients who require NSAIDs or aspirin to treat other medical conditions should always take concomitant PPIs or high dose H_2 receptor blockers. If *H. pylori* infection is documented, it should be treated with one of several acceptable regimens (Table 26-10).[61] Infectious disease consultation may be helpful in the compliant, symptomatic patient with persistent *H. pylori* infection following treatment, or another regimen could be tried (e.g., quadruple therapy). If initial *H. pylori* testing is negative and ulcer symptoms persist, an empiric trial of anti-*H. pylori* therapy is reasonable (false-negative *H. pylori* tests are common). Generally, antisecretory therapy can be stopped after 3 months if the ulcerogenic stimulus (usually *H. pylori*, NSAIDs, or aspirin) has been removed. However, long-term maintenance PPI therapy should be considered in all patients admitted to hospital with ulcer complications, all high-risk patients on NSAIDs or aspirin (the elderly or debilitated), and all patients with a history of recurrent ulcer or bleeding. Consideration should be given to maintenance therapy in refractory smokers with a history of peptic ulcer. Misoprostol, sucralfate, and acid suppression may be quite comparable in many patient groups; occasionally treatment with more than one agent is useful. Misoprostol may cause diarrhea and cramps, and cannot be used in women of childbearing age because of its abortifacient properties. For these reasons, it is not widely used to treat PUD. Sucralfate acts locally and is well tolerated.

Surgical Treatment of Peptic Ulcer Disease

The indications for surgery in PUD are bleeding, perforation, obstruction, and intractability or nonhealing.[67,68] Gastric cancer must always be considered in patients with gastric ulcer or gastric outlet obstruction.

Today, most patients undergoing operation for PUD have simple oversewing of a bleeding ulcer, or simple patch of a perforated ulcer, or distal gastrectomy. Simultaneous performance of vagot-

TABLE 26-8	Indications for diagnosis and treatment of *Helicobacter pylori*

Established
- Active peptic ulcer disease (gastric or duodenal ulcer)
- Confirmed history of peptic ulcer disease (not previously treated for *H. pylori*)

Gastric mucosa-associated lymphoid tissue lymphoma (low grade)
- After endoscopic resection of early gastric cancer
- Uninvestigated dyspepsia (depending on *H. pylori* prevalence)

Controversial
- Nonulcer dyspepsia
- Gastroesophageal reflux disease
- Persons using NSAIDS
- Unexplained iron deficiency anemia
- Populations at higher risk for gastric cancer

Source: From Chey et al,[61] with permission.

TABLE 26-9 Risk-stratification tools for upper gastrointestinal hemorrhage[a]

A. Blatchford Score

At Presentation	Points
Systolic blood pressure	
100–109 mmHg	1
90–99 mmHg	2
<90 mmHg	3
Blood urea nitrogen	
6.5–7.9 mmol/L	2
8.0–9.9 mmol/L	3
10.0–24.9 mmol/L	4
≥25 mmol/L	6
Hemoglobin for men	
12.0–12.9 g/dL	1
10.0–11.9 g/dL	3
<10.0 g/dL	6
Hemoglobin for women	
10.0–11.9 g/dL	1
<10.0 g/dL	6
Other variables at presentation	
Pulse ≥100 beats/min	1
Melena	1
Syncope	2
Hepatic disease	2
Cardiac failure	2

B. Rockall Score

	Variable	Points
Complete Rockall Score { **Clinical Rockall Score** {	Age	
	<60 y	0
	60–79 y	1
	≥80 y	2
	Shock	
	Heart rate >100 beats/min	1
	Systolic blood pressure <100 mmHg	2
	Coexisting illness	
	Ischemic heart disease, congestive heart failure, other major illness	2
	Renal failure, hepatic failure, metastatic cancer	3
	Endoscopic diagnosis	
	No lesions observed, Mallory-Weiss syndrome	0
	Peptic ulcer, erosive disease, esophagitis	1
	Cancer of the upper GI tract	2
	Endoscopic stigmata of recent hemorrhage	
	Clean base ulcer, flat pigmented spot	0
	Blood in upper GI tract, active bleeding, visible vessel, clot	2

[a]Panel A shows the values used in the Blatchford risk-stratification score, which ranges from 0 to 23, with higher scores indicating higher risk. Panel B shows the Rockall score, with point values assigned for each of three clinical variables (age and the presence of shock and coexisting illnesses) and two endoscopic variables (diagnosis and stigmata of recent hemorrhage). The complete Rockall score ranges from 0 to 11, with higher scores indicating higher risk. Patients with a clinical Rockall score of 0 or a complete Rockall score of 2 or less are considered to be at low risk for rebleeding or death.

Source: Reproduced with permission from Gralnek IM et al: Management of acute bleeding from peptic ulcer. *N Engl J Med* 359:928, 2008. Copyright ©2008 Massachusetts Medical Society. All rights reserved.

omy either truncal or highly selective is increasingly uncommon, probably due to surgeon unfamiliarity with the procedure and reliance on postoperative PPIs to decrease acid secretion.

Unfortunately, the data from many excellent randomized clinical trials evaluating elective operation for peptic ulcer over the last several decades may be irrelevant to most patients presenting for ulcer surgery today.[67] The large majority of these excellent studies were done in the pre-PPI, pre-*Helicobacter*, pre-NSAID era, and focused on elective operation for intractable disease, an unusual indication in the modern era. Thus, today's surgeon should take great care in applying this literature to inform surgical decision making.

Classically, in the previous era, the vast majority of peptic ulcers were adequately treated by a variant of one of the three basic operations: HSV, vagotomy and drainage (V+D), and vagotomy

and distal gastrectomy. Recurrence rates were lowest but morbidity highest with the latter procedure, while the opposite was true for HSV (Table 26-11).[67–69]

HSV, also called *parietal cell vagotomy* or *proximal gastric vagotomy*, is safe (mortality risk <0.5%) and causes minimal side effects. The operation severs the vagal nerve supply to the proximal two thirds of the stomach, where essentially all the parietal cells are located, and preserves the vagal innervation to the antrum and pylorus, and the remaining abdominal viscera (Fig. 26-33). Thus, the operation decreases total gastric acid secretion by about 75%, and GI side effects are rare. Elective HSV has largely been supplanted by long-term PPI treatment, but the operation, which has a learning curve, may still be useful in the patient (elective or emergent) who is noncompliant with, intolerant of, or cannot afford medical treat-

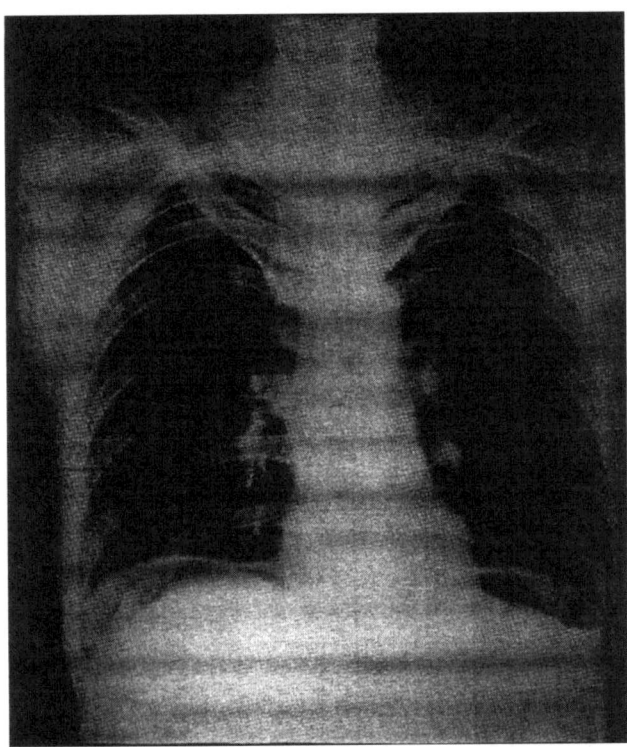

FIG. 26-32. Pneumoperitoneum on upright chest x-ray in patient with perforated ulcer.

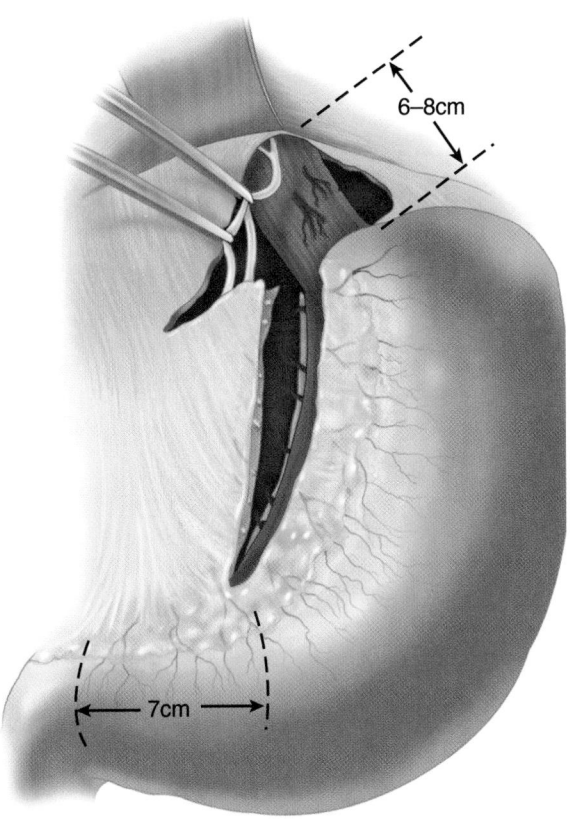

FIG. 26-33. Highly selective vagotomy. *[Reproduced with permission from Zinner MJ et al (eds):* Maingot's Abdominal Operations, *10th ed., Vol. I. Stamford, Connecticut: Appleton & Lange, 1997, p 987.]*

TABLE 26-10	Treatment regimens for *Helicobacter pylori*
Medications/Dose/Frequency	**Duration**
PPI + clarithromycin 500 mg bid + amoxicillin 1000 mg bid	10–14 d
PPI + clarithromycin 500 bid + metronidazole 500 bid	10–14 d
PPI + amoxicillin 1000 mg bid, then	5 d
PPI + clarithromycin 500 mg bid + tinidazole 500 mg bid	5 d
Salvage regimens for patients who fail one of the above initial regimens:	
Bismuth subsalicylate 525 mg qid + metronidazole 250 mg qid + tetracycline 500 mg qid + PPI	10–14 d
PPI + amoxicillin 1000 mg bid + levofloxacin 500 mg daily	10 d

PPI = proton pump inhibitor.
Source: Data from Chey et al.[61]

TABLE 26-11	Clinical results of surgery for duodenal ulcer		
	Parietal Cell Vagotomy	**Truncal Vagotomy and Pyloroplasty**	**Truncal Vagotomy and Antrectomy**
Operative mortality rate (%)	0	<1	1
Ulcer recurrence rate (%)	5–15	5–15	<2
Dumping (%)			
Mild	<5	10	10–15
Severe	0	1	1–2
Diarrhea (%)			
Mild	<5	25	20
Severe	0	2	1–2

Source: Modified from Mulholland et al,[68] with permission. Copyright Elsevier.

ment. Historically, HSV has not performed particularly well for type II (gastric and duodenal) and III (prepyloric) gastric ulcer, perhaps because of hypergastrinemia caused by gastric outlet obstruction and persistent antral stasis. The Taylor procedure consists of a posterior truncal vagotomy and anterior seromyotomy (but anterior HSV is probably equivalent), and is an attractive and simple alternative to HSV with similar results.

Truncal vagotomy and pyloroplasty, and truncal vagotomy and gastrojejunostomy are the paradigmatic *vagotomy and drainage procedures*. HSV may be substituted for truncal vagotomy. The advantage of V+D is that it can be performed safely and quickly by the experienced surgeon. The main disadvantages are the side effect profile (10% of patients have significant dumping and/or diarrhea). During truncal vagotomy (Fig. 26-34), care must be taken not to perforate the esophagus, a potentially lethal complication. Intraoperative frozen section confirmation of at least two vagal trunks is prudent; additional vagal trunks are common. Unlike HSV, V+D is widely accepted as a successful operation for complicated PUD. It has been described as a useful part of the operative treatment for bleeding duodenal and gastric ulcer, perforated duodenal and gastric ulcer, and obstructing duodenal and gastric (type II and III) ulcer. When applied to gastric ulcer, the ulcer should be excised or biopsied.

Truncal vagotomy denervates the antropyloric mechanism, and therefore, some sort of procedure is necessary to ablate or bypass the pylorus. Gastrojejunostomy is a good choice in patients with gastric outlet obstruction or a severely diseased proximal duodenum. The anastomosis is done between the proximal jejunum and the most dependent portion of the greater gastric curvature, in either an antecolic or retrocolic fashion (Fig. 26-35). Marginal ulceration is a potential complication. Pyloroplasty is useful in patients who require a pyloroduodenotomy to deal with the ulcer

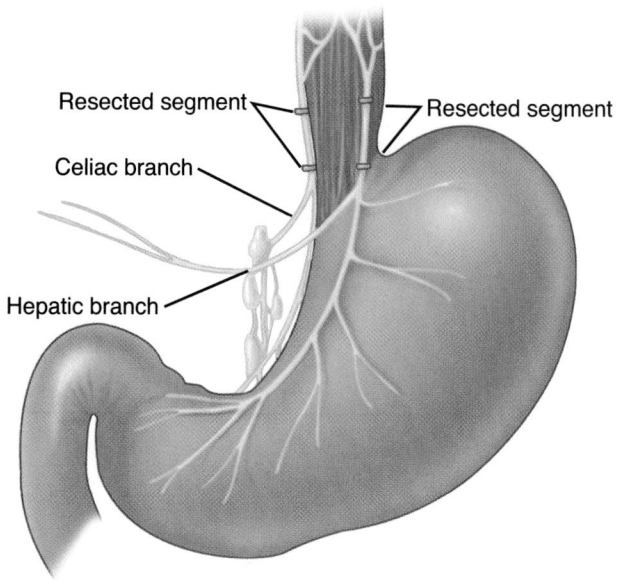

FIG. 26-34. Truncal vagotomy. *[Reproduced with permission from Zollinger RM Jr., Zollinger RM Sr. (eds):* Zollinger's Atlas of Surgical Operations, *8th ed. New York: McGraw-Hill, 2003, p 45.]*

complication (e.g., posterior bleeding duodenal ulcer), in those with limited or focal scarring in the pyloric region, or when gastrojejunostomy is technically difficult. The most commonly performed pyloroplasty is the Heineke-Mikulicz type (Fig 26-36). Other occasionally useful techniques include the Finney (Fig. 26-37) and the Jaboulay pyloroplasties (Fig. 26-38). These more extensive pyloroplasty techniques may make subsequent distal gastric resection more difficult and/or hazardous.

The advantages of *vagotomy and antrectomy* (V+A) are the extremely low ulcer recurrence rate and the applicability of the operation to many patients with complicated PUD (e.g., bleeding duodenal and gastric ulcer, obstructing peptic ulcer, nonhealing gastric ulcer, and recurrent ulcer). When applied to gastric ulcer disease, the resection is usually extended far enough proximally to include the ulcer. The disadvantage of V+A is the higher operative

mortality risk (when compared with HSV or V+D), and its irreversibility. Following antrectomy, GI continuity may be re-established with a Billroth I gastroduodenostomy (Fig. 26-39) or a Billroth II loop gastrojejunostomy (Fig. 26-40). Since antrectomy routinely leaves a 60 to 70% gastric remnant, reconstruction as a Roux-en-Y gastrojejunostomy should be avoided (Fig. 26-41). Although the Roux-en-Y operation is an excellent procedure for keeping duodenal contents out of the stomach and esophagus, in the presence of a large gastric remnant, this reconstruction will predispose to marginal ulceration and/or gastric stasis.

V+A should be avoided in hemodynamically unstable patients, and in patients with extensive inflammation and/or scarring of the proximal duodenum, because secure anastomosis (Billroth I) or duodenal closure (Billroth II) may be difficult.

Distal gastrectomy without vagotomy (usually about a 50% gastrectomy to include the ulcer) has traditionally been the procedure of choice for type I gastric ulcer. The addition of vagotomy should be considered for type II and III gastric ulcers (because the pathophysiology is more analogous to duodenal ulcer), or if the patient is believed to be at increased risk for recurrent ulcer, or perhaps even if Billroth II reconstruction is contemplated (to decrease the chance of marginal ulcer). Subtotal gastrectomy (75% distal gastrectomy) without vagotomy is rarely used to treat PUD today, although it was the most popular ulcer operation at the middle of the last century.

Choice of Operation for Peptic Ulcer

The choice of operation for the individual patient with PUD depends on a variety of factors, including the type of ulcer (duodenal, gastric, recurrent, or marginal), the indication for operation, and the condition of the patient, among others. Other important considerations are intra-abdominal factors (duodenal scarring/inflammation, adhesions, or difficult exposure), the ulcer diathesis status of the patient, the surgeon's experience and personal preference, whether *H. pylori* infection is present, the need for NSAID therapy, previous treatment, and the likelihood of future compliance with treatment. Table 26-12 shows the surgical options for managing various aspects of PUD. In general, resective procedures have a lower ulcer recurrence rate, but a higher operative morbidity and mortality rate (see Table 26-11) when compared to nonresective ulcer operations. Because ulcer recurrence often is related to *H. pylori* and/or NSAIDs, it is usually managed adequately without reoperation. Thus, gastric resection to minimize recurrence in duodenal ulcer disease is often not justified today; resection for gastric ulcer remains the standard because of the risk of

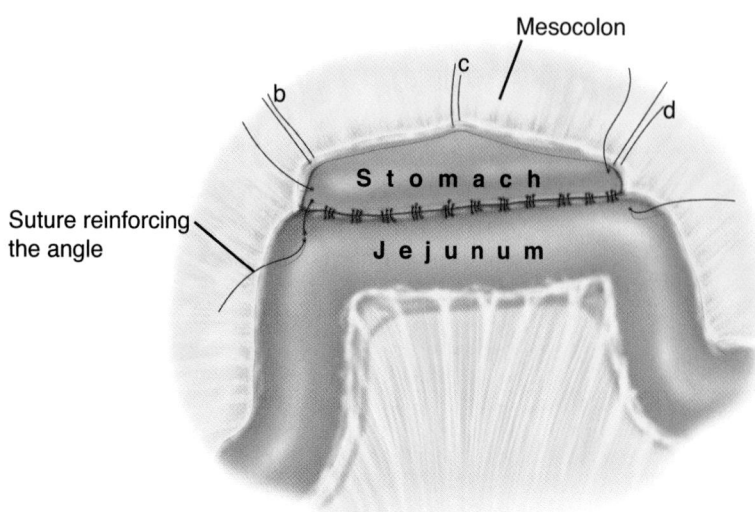

FIG. 26-35. Retrocolic gastrojejunostomy. Note mesocolon sutured to stomach (*b, c, d*). *[Reproduced with permission from Vagotomy and drainage, in Zuidema GD, Yeo CJ (eds):* Shackleford's Surgery of the Alimentary Tract, *5th ed. Vol. II. Philadelphia: Saunders, 2002, p 129. Copyright Elsevier.]*

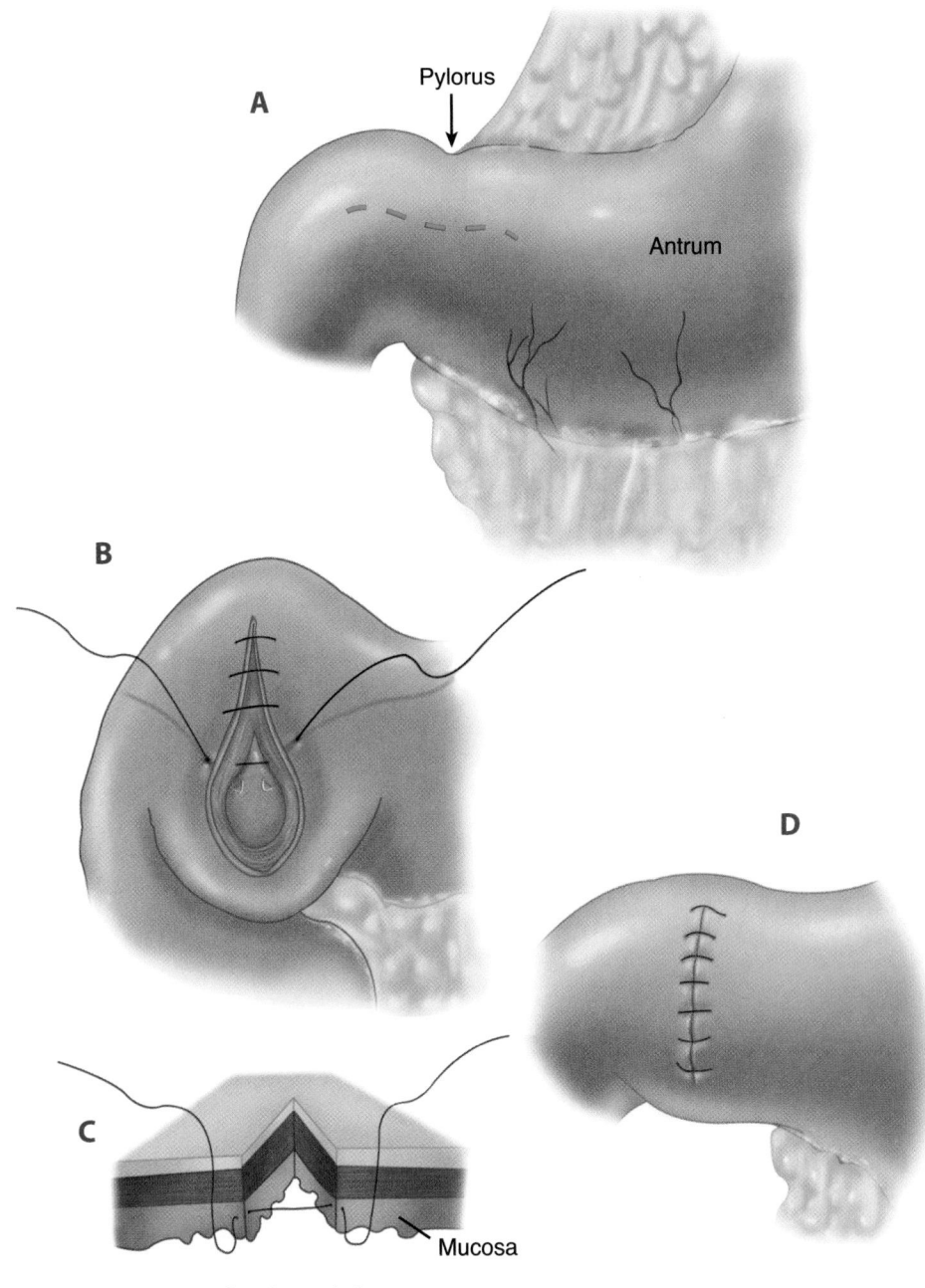

FIG. 26-36. A through **D.** Heineke-Mikulicz pyloroplasty. *[Reproduced with permission from Zinner MJ (ed): Atlas of Gastric Surgery. New York: Churchill Livingstone, 1992, p 17. Copyright Elsevier.]*

cancer. Clearly, the modern trend in peptic ulcer operation could be described as "less is more."[70,71] Vagotomy as a component of emergency ulcer surgery is increasingly uncommon.

Bleeding Peptic Ulcer

Bleeding is the most common cause of ulcer-related death, but most patients admitted to hospital with bleeding gastric or duodenal ulcer today will not require an operation. The success of endoscopic treatment and medical therapy in treating and preventing bleeding PUD has resulted in the selection of a subgroup of high-risk patients for today's surgeon. It is likely that patients currently coming to operation for bleeding PUD are at higher risk for a poor outcome than ever before. The surgical options for treating bleeding PUD include suture ligation of the bleeder; suture ligation and definitive nonresective ulcer operation (HSV or V+D); and gastric resection (usually including vagotomy and ulcer excision). Gastric ulcer requires biopsy if not resected.

The management of bleeding peptic ulcer is summarized in the algorithm provided in Fig. 26-42. All patients admitted to hospital with bleeding peptic ulcer should be adequately resuscitated and started on continuous IV PPI.[72] Seventy-five percent of patients will stop bleeding with these measures alone, but 25% will continue to bleed or will rebleed in hospital. It is important to identify this high-risk group early with clinical and endoscopic parameters because, essentially, all the deaths from bleeding ulcer occur in this group. Surgical consultation is mandatory, and endoscopic hemostatic therapy (cautery, epinephrine injection, clipping) is indicated and usually successful in these high-risk patients.[73,74] Indications for operation include massive hemorrhage unresponsive to endoscopic control, and transfusion requirement of more than four to six units of blood, despite attempts at endoscopic control. Lack of availability of a therapeutic endoscopist, recurrent hemorrhage after one or more attempts at endoscopic control, lack of availability of blood for transfusion, repeat hospitalization for bleeding ulcer, and concurrent

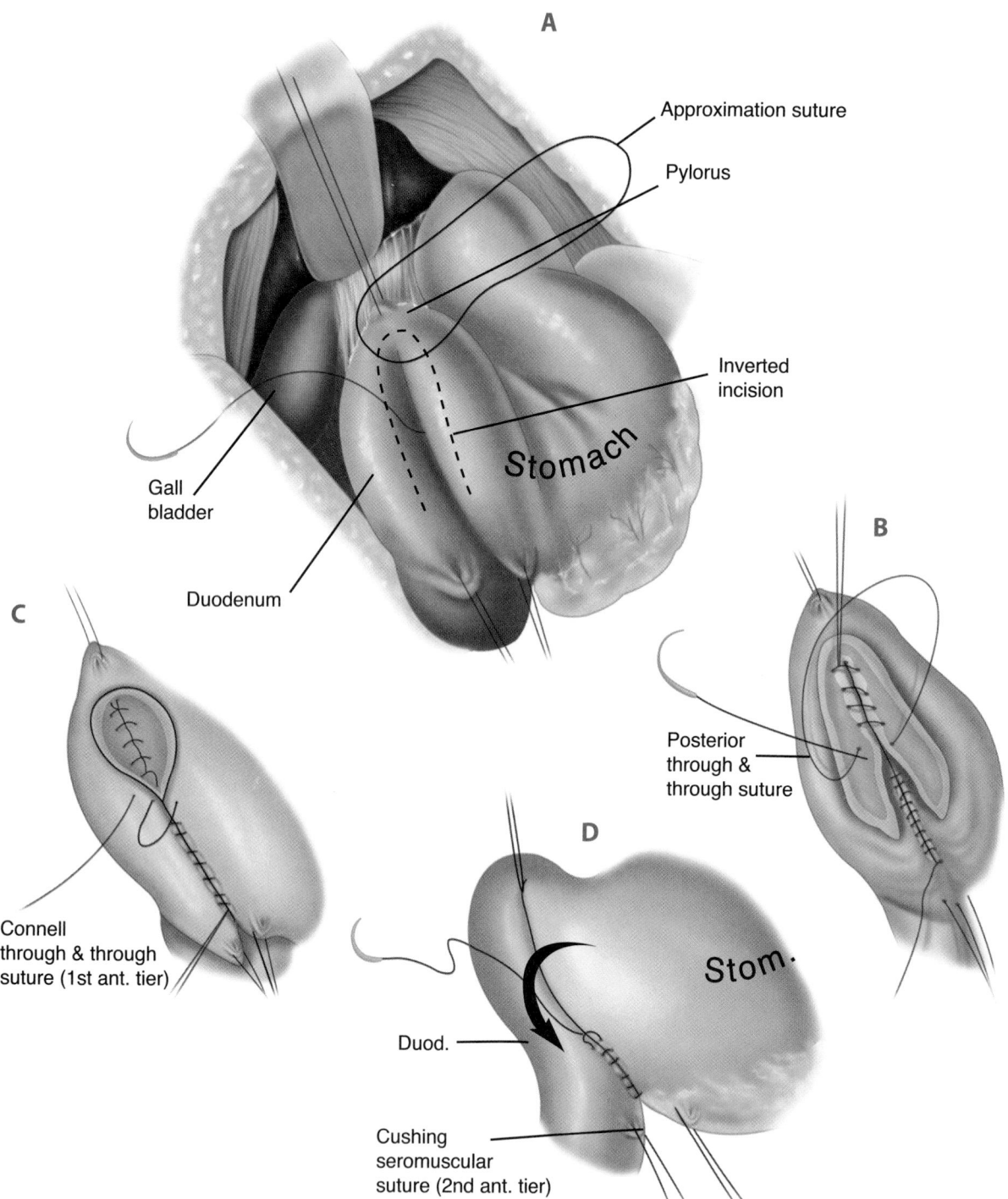

FIG. 26-37. A through **D.** Finney pyloroplasty. ant. = anterior; Duod. = duodenum; Stom. = stomach. *[Reproduced with permission from Sawyers JL: Vagotomy and pyloroplasty, in Zuidema GD (ed): Shackelford's Surgery of the Alimentary Tract, 4th ed. Philadelphia: Saunders, 1996, p 150. Copyright Elsevier.]*

indications for surgery such as perforation or obstruction, are also indications for surgery. Patients with massive bleeding from high-risk lesions (e.g., posterior duodenal ulcer with erosion of gastroduodenal artery, or lesser curvature gastric ulcer with erosion of left gastric artery or branch) should be considered for early operation. Early operation should also be considered in patients more than 60 years of age, those presenting in shock, those requiring more than four units of blood in 24 hours or eight units of blood in 48 hours, those with rebleeding, and those with

ulcers >2 cm in diameter. The mortality rate for surgery for bleeding peptic ulcer is 10 to 20%.

Operation for Bleeding Peptic Ulcer (Fig. 26-43)

The two operations most commonly used for bleeding duodenal ulcer are oversewing of the ulcer usually without vagotomy,[70] or V+A. Oversewing alone results in a higher rebleeding rate but a lower operative mortality rate. When the mortality for reoperation for rebleeding is considered, the overall mortality is probably

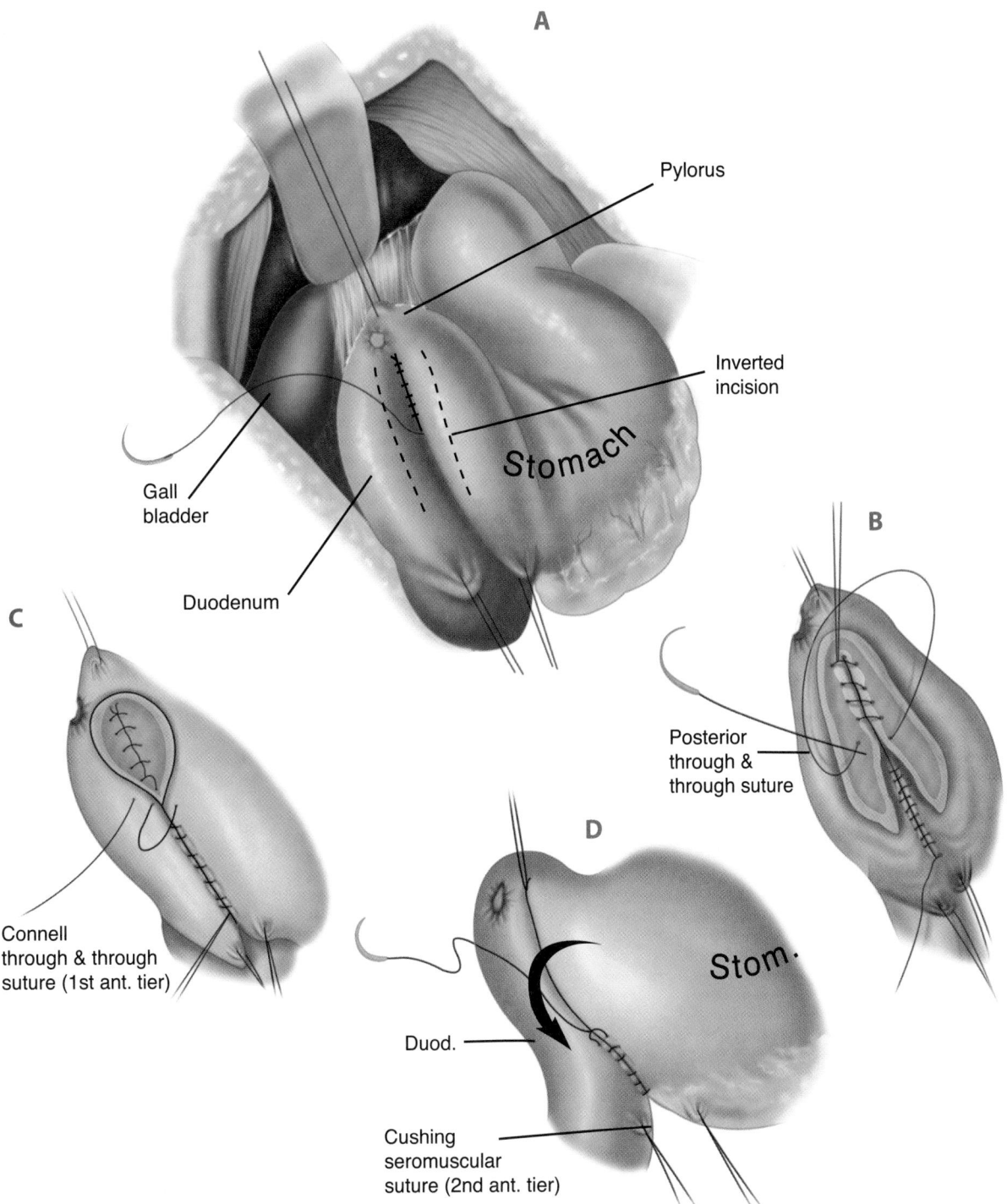

FIG. 26-38. A through **D.** Jaboulay pyloroplasty. ant. = anterior; Duod. = duodenum; Stom. = stomach. *[Reproduced with permission from Sawyers JL: Vagotomy and pyloroplasty, in Zuidema GD (ed): Shackelford's Surgery of the Alimentary Tract, 4th ed. Philadelphia: Saunders, 1996, p 150. Copyright Elsevier.]*

comparable for the two approaches. Patients who are in shock or medically unstable should not have gastric resection.

An initial pyloromyotomy incision allows access to the bleeding posterior duodenal ulcer, and an expeditious Kocher maneuver allows the surgeon to control the hemorrhage with the left hand if necessary. Heavy suture material on a stout needle is used to place figure-of-eight sutures or a U-stitch to secure the bleeding vessel at the base of the posterior duodenal ulcer. Multiple sutures are usually necessary. Once the surgeon is unequivocally convinced that hemostasis is secure, a pyloroplasty can be performed. If the patient is

stable, vagotomy may be added. If the patient is not a high operative risk and V+A is selected, smaller duodenal ulcers are resected with the specimen; larger bleeding duodenal ulcers must often be left behind in the duodenal stump. In this situation, suture hemostasis must be attained and a secure duodenal closure accomplished. The anterior wall of the open duodenum can be sutured to either the proximal or distal lip of the posterior ulcer once the bleeding vessel has been sutured. The duodenal closure can be buttressed with omentum and the duodenum should be decompressed, either with a lateral duodenostomy or retrograde duodenostomy tube via the

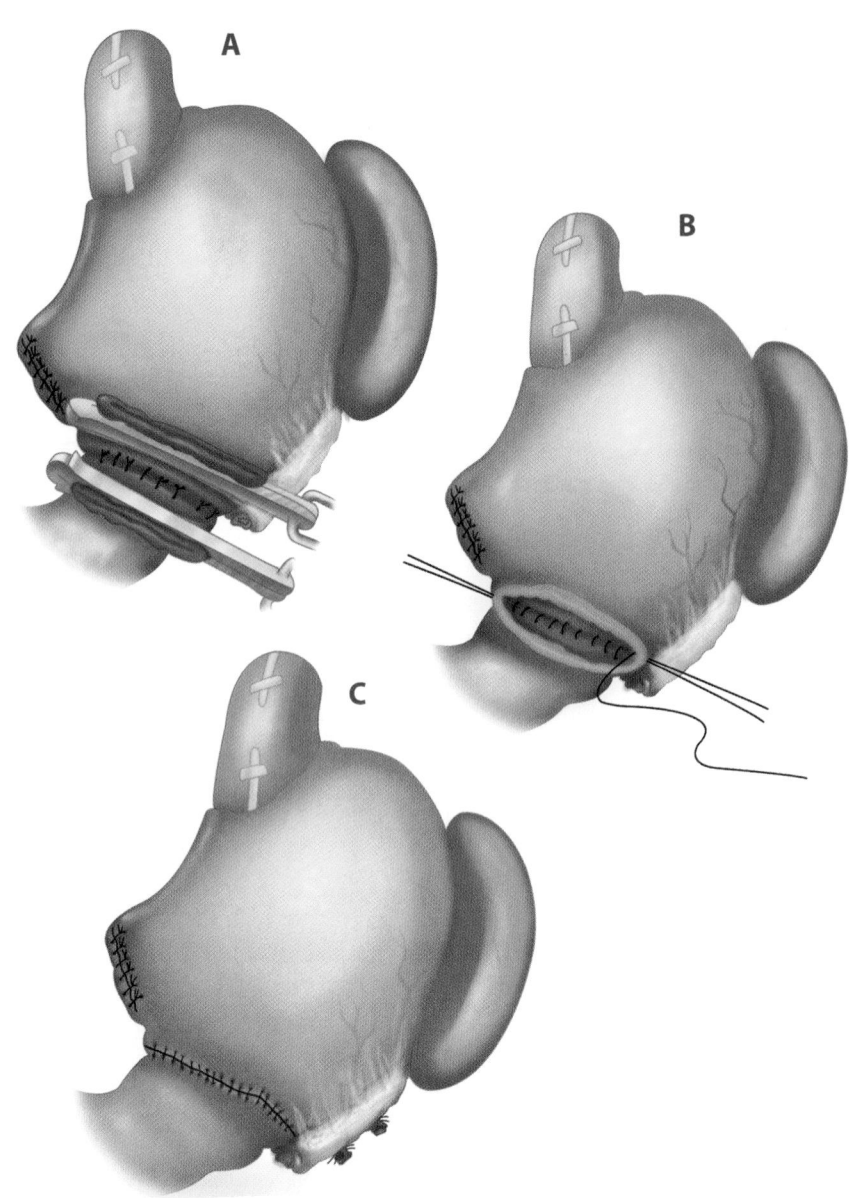

FIG. 26-39. A though C. Billroth I gastroduodenostomy. *[Reproduced with permission from Zinner MJ (ed):* Atlas of Gastric
Surgery. *New York: Churchill Livingstone,
1992, p 35. Copyright Elsevier.]*

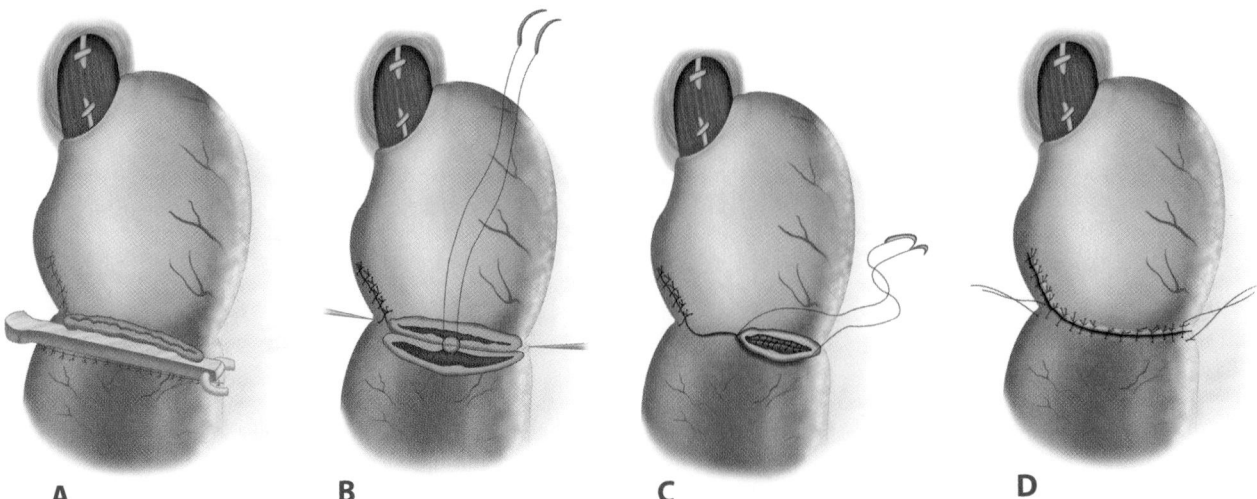

FIG. 26-40. A through D. Billroth II antecolic gastrojejunostomy. *[Reproduced with permission from Soybel DI, Zinner MJ: Stomach and duodenum: Operative procedures, in Zinner MJ et al (eds):* Maingot's Abdominal Operations, *10th ed., Vol. I. Stamford, Connecticut: Appleton & Lange, 1997,
p 1112.]*

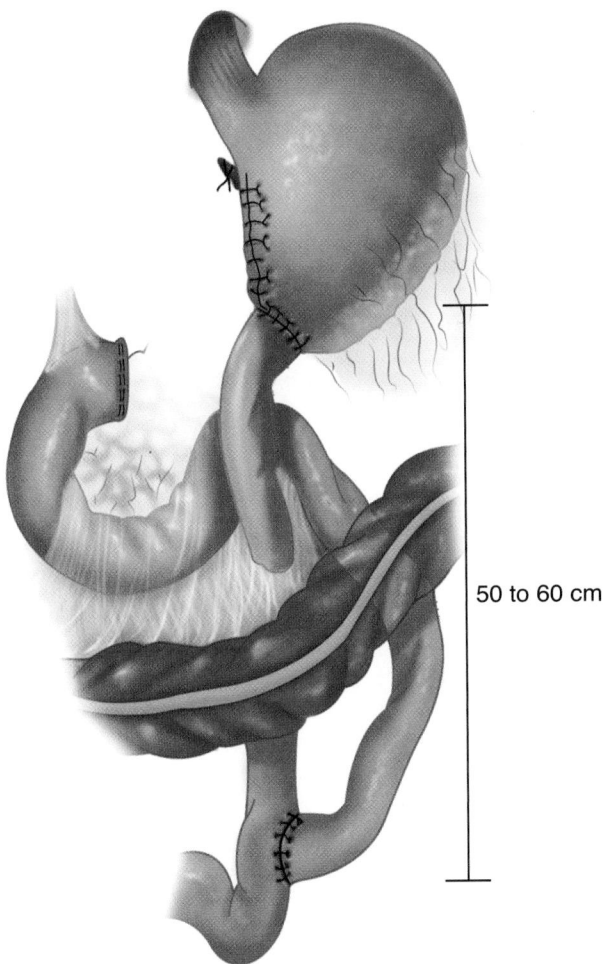

FIG. 26-41. Roux-en-Y gastrojejunostomy. [*Reproduced with permission from Ritchie WP Jr.: Benign diseases of the stomach and duodenum, in Ritchie WP, Steele G, Dean RH (eds):* General Surgery. *Philadelphia: Lippincott, 1995, p 117.*]

50 to 60 cm

Indication	Duodenal	Gastric
Bleeding	1. Oversew[a]	1. Oversew and biopsy[a]
	2. Oversew, V+D	2. Oversew, biopsy, V+D
	3. V+A	3. Distal gastrectomy[b]
Perforation	1. Patch[a]	1. Biopsy and patch[a]
	2. Patch, HSV[b]	2. Wedge excision, V+D
	3. Patch, V+D	3. Distal gastrectomy[b]
Obstruction	1. HSV + GJ	1. Biopsy; HSV + GJ
	2. V+A	2. Distal gastrectomy[b]
Intractability/ nonhealing	1. HSV[b]	1. HSV and wedge excision
	2. V+D	2. Distal gastrectomy
	3. V+A	

TABLE 26-12 Surgical options in the treatment of duodenal and gastric ulcer

[a]Unless the patient is in shock or moribund, a definitive procedure should be considered.
[b]Operation of choice in low-risk patient.
GJ = gastrojejunostomy; HSV = highly selective vagotomy; V+A = vagotomy and antrectomy; V+D = vagotomy and drainage.

proximal jejunum or nasogastric route. Right upper quadrant closed suction peritoneal drainage is important. Use of a feeding jejunostomy is also considered. A Billroth II anastomosis is preferred.

The initial management of bleeding gastric ulcers and the indications for operation are similar to those for bleeding duodenal ulcer. These lesions tend to occur in older and/or medically complicated patients, and this fact may increase the operative risk. Although this has been used by some as an excuse not to operate early on these patients, experience shows that planned surgery in a resuscitated patient results in a better operative survival rate than emergent operation in a patient who has rebled and is in shock. Distal gastric resection to include the bleeding ulcer is the procedure of choice for bleeding gastric ulcer. Second best is V+D with oversewing and biopsy of the ulcer to rule out cancer. Oversewing of the bleeder followed by long-term acid suppression is a reasonable alternative in high-risk or unstable patients.

Perforated Peptic Ulcer (Fig. 26-44)

Perforation is the second most common complication of peptic ulcer. As with bleeding ulcer, NSAID and/or aspirin use have been inextricably linked with perforated PUD, especially in the elderly population.[75] Well over 20% of patients over the age of 60 years old presenting with a perforated ulcer are taking NSAIDs at the time of perforation. Surgery is almost always indicated, although occasionally nonsurgical treatment can be used in the stable patient without peritonitis in whom radiologic studies document a sealed perforation. Patients with acute perforation and GI blood loss (either chronic or acute) should be suspected of having a second ulcer.

The options for surgical treatment of perforated duodenal ulcer are simple patch closure, patch closure and HSV, or patch closure and V+D. Simple patch closure alone should be done in patients with hemodynamic instability and/or exudative peritonitis signifying a perforation >24 hours old. In all other patients, the addition of HSV may be considered because numerous studies have reported a negligible mortality with this approach.[63,67] However, in the United States and Western Europe, there is clearly a trend away from definitive operation for perforated duodenal ulcer, probably because of the ready availability of PPI, and surgeon unfamiliarity with definitive operation in this setting.[70]

Perforated gastric ulcer results in a higher mortality rate than perforated duodenal ulcer (10 to 40%) due to the following: patients' more advanced age, increased medical comorbidities, delay in seeking medical attention, and the larger size of gastric ulcers. In the stable patient without multiple operative risk factors, perforated gastric ulcers are best treated by distal gastric resection. Vagotomy is usually added for type II and III gastric ulcers. Patch closure with biopsy; or local excision and closure; or biopsy, closure, truncal vagotomy, and drainage are alternative operations in the unstable or high-risk patient, or in the patient with a perforation in an inopportune location (e.g., juxtapyloric). All perforated gastric ulcers, even those in the prepyloric position, should be biopsied if they are not removed at surgery.

Obstructing Peptic Ulcer

Currently, gastric outlet obstruction is the least common indication for operation in PUD. Acute ulcers associated with obstruction due to edema and/or motor dysfunction may respond to intensive antisecretory therapy and nasogastric suction. But most patients with significant obstruction from chronic ulceration will require some sort of more substantial intervention. Endoscopic balloon dilation can often transiently improve obstructive symptoms, but many of these patients ultimately fail and come to operation.[76]

The most common operations for obstructing PUD are V+A and V+D. HSV and gastrojejunostomy is comparable to V+A in this setting[77] and is an appealing operation for obstruction, both because it can readily be done using laparoscopic techniques, and because it does not complicate future resection, should this be needed. However, potentially curable gastric or duodenal cancers can be missed with this approach.

Intractable or Nonhealing Peptic Ulcer

This should indeed be a rare indication for surgery performed today. Arguably, the patient referred for surgical evaluation because

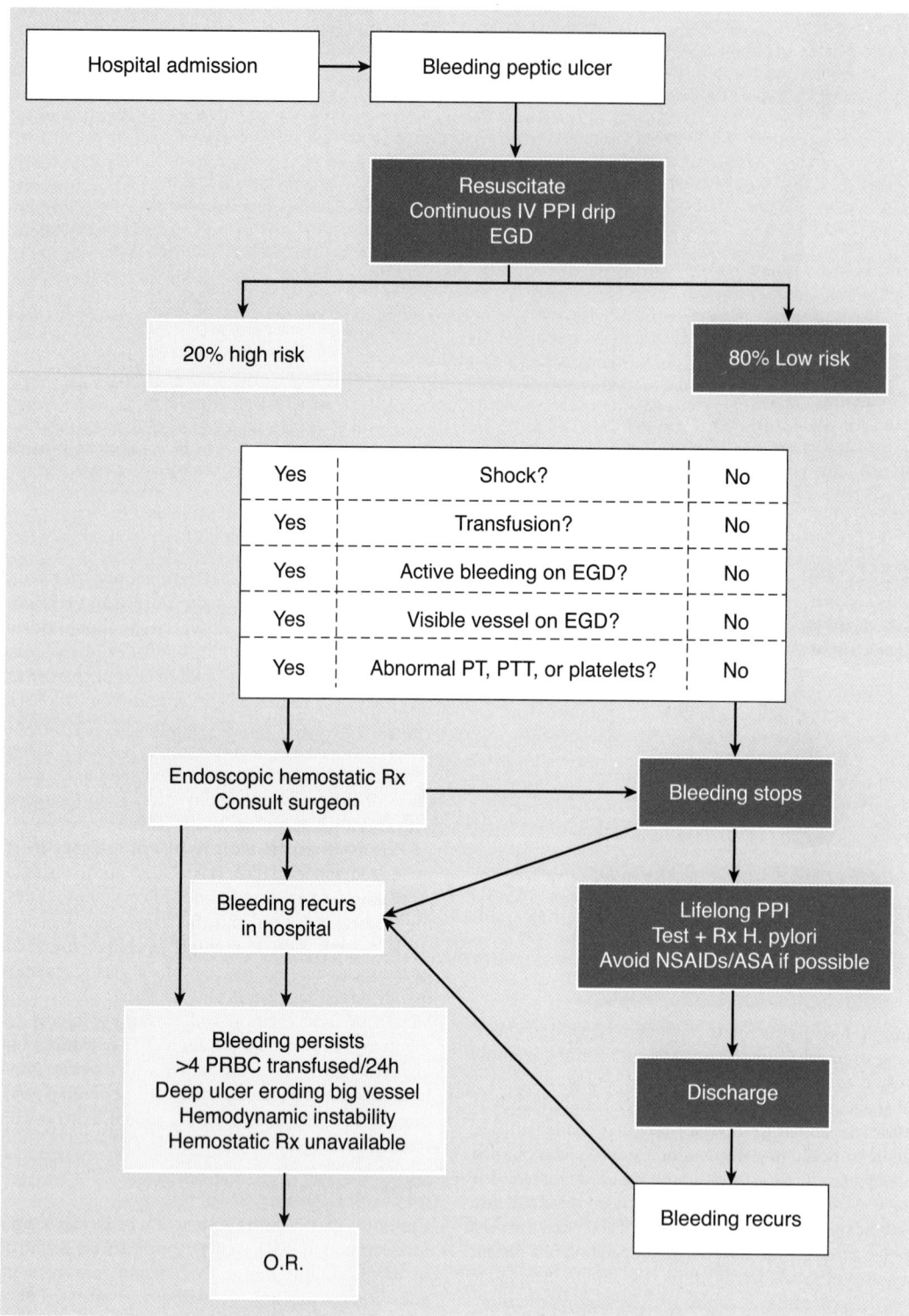

FIG. 26-42. Algorithm for the treatment of bleeding peptic ulcer. ASA = acetylsalicylic acid; EGD = esophagogastroduodenoscopy; O.R. = operating room; PPI = proton pump inhibitor; PRBC = unit of packed red blood cells; PT = prothrombin time; PTT = partial thromboplastin time; Rx = treatment.

of intractable PUD should raise red flags for the surgeon: Maybe the patient has a missed cancer; maybe the patient is noncompliant (not taking prescribed PPI, still taking NSAIDs, still smoking); maybe the patient has *Helicobacter* despite the presence of a negative test or previous treatment. Because acid secretion can be totally blocked and *H. pylori* eradicated with modern medication, the question remains: "Why does the patient have a persistent ulcer diathesis?" The surgeon should review the differential diagnosis of nonhealing ulcer before any consideration of operative treatment (Table 26-13).

Surgical treatment should be considered in patients with non-healing or intractable PUD who have multiple recurrences, large ulcers (>2 cm), complications (obstruction, perforation, or hemorrhage), or suspected malignancy. Definitive operation, particularly gastric resection, should be considered most cautiously in the thin or marginally nourished individual.

It is important that the surgeon not fall into the trap of performing a large, irreversible operation on these patients, based on the unproven theory that if all other methods have failed to heal the ulcer, a

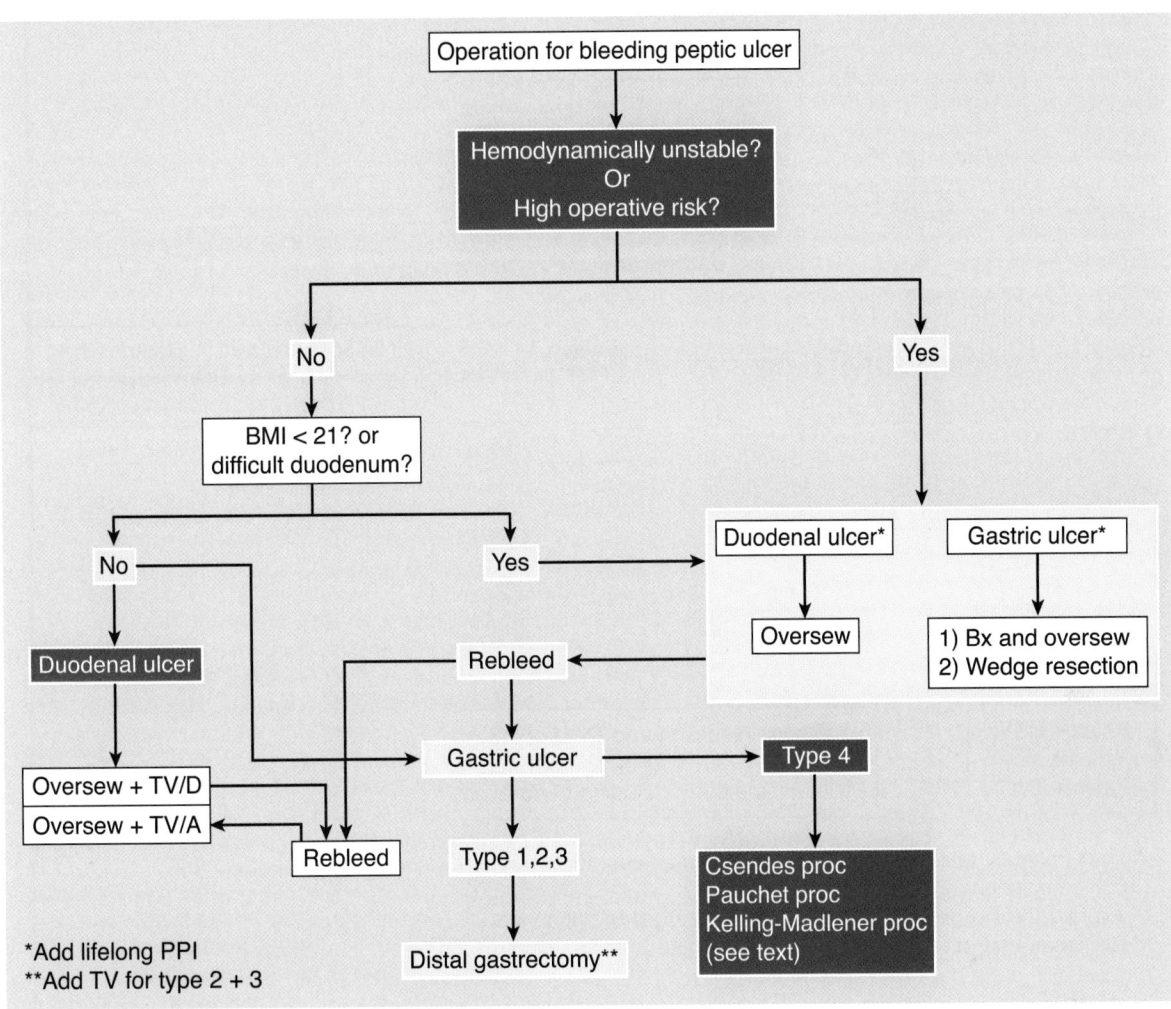

FIG. 26-43. Algorithm for operation for bleeding peptic ulcer. BMI = body mass index; Bx = biopsy; PPI = proton pump inhibitor; proc = procedure; TV = truncal vagotomy; TV/A = truncal vagotomy and antrectomy; TV/D = truncal vagotomy and drainage.

large operation is required. Although there is a large quantity of very good data in the surgical literature suggesting that the large majority of patients do well after the larger elective ulcer operations, these data may not be particularly relevant to the modern patient.[67] Candidates for ulcer operation today are different than those of three or four decades ago. One might argue that current medical care has healed the minor ulcers, and that patients presenting with true intractability or nonhealing will be more difficult to treat and are likely to have chronic problems after a major ulcer operation.

If surgery is necessary, a lesser operation may be preferable. It is the practice of this author never to perform a gastrectomy as the initial elective operation for intractable duodenal ulcer in the thin or asthenic patient. Instead, the preferred operation for this group of patients is HSV. In patients with nonhealing gastric ulcer, wedge resection with HSV should be considered in thin or frail patients. Otherwise, distal gastrectomy (to include the ulcer) is recommended. It is unnecessary to add a vagotomy in patients with type I or type IV (juxtaesophageal) gastric ulcers because they are usually associated with acid hyposecretion. Type IV gastric ulcers may be difficult to resect as part of a distal gastrectomy, and a variety of surgical techniques have been described to treat these more proximal lesions (Fig. 26-45).

Zollinger-Ellison Syndrome[78–81]

ZES is caused by the uncontrolled secretion of abnormal amounts of gastrin by a duodenal or pancreatic neuroendocrine tumor (i.e.,

gastrinoma). Most cases (80%) are sporadic, but 20% are inherited. The inherited or familial form of gastrinoma is associated with multiple endocrine neoplasia type 1 (MEN1), which consists of parathyroid, pituitary, and pancreatic (or duodenal) tumors. Gastrinoma is the most common pancreatic tumor in patients with MEN I. Patients with MEN I usually have multiple gastrinoma tumors, and surgical cure is unusual. Sporadic gastrinomas are more often solitary and amenable to surgical cure. Currently, about 50 to 60% of gastrinomas are malignant, with lymph node, liver, or other distant metastases at operation. Five-year survival in patients presenting with metastatic disease is approximately 40%. The larger the primary gastrinoma, the higher the likelihood of metastatic disease. More than 90% of patients with sporadically, completely resected gastrinoma will be cured.

The most common symptoms of ZES are epigastric pain, GERD, and diarrhea. More than 90% of patients with gastrinoma have peptic ulcer. Most ulcers are in the typical location (proximal duodenum), but atypical ulcer location (distal duodenum, jejunum, or multiple ulcers) should prompt an evaluation for gastrinoma. Gastrinoma also should be considered in the differential diagnosis of recurrent or refractory peptic ulcer, secretory diarrhea, gastric rugal hypertrophy, esophagitis with stricture, bleeding or perforated ulcer, familial ulcer, peptic ulcer with hypercalcemia, and gastric carcinoid. The majority of patients with ZES have been symptomatic for several years before definitive diagnosis and, in general, patients with ZES and MEN1 are diagnosed in their 20s and 30s, while those with sporadic ZES more typically are diagnosed in their 40s and 50s.

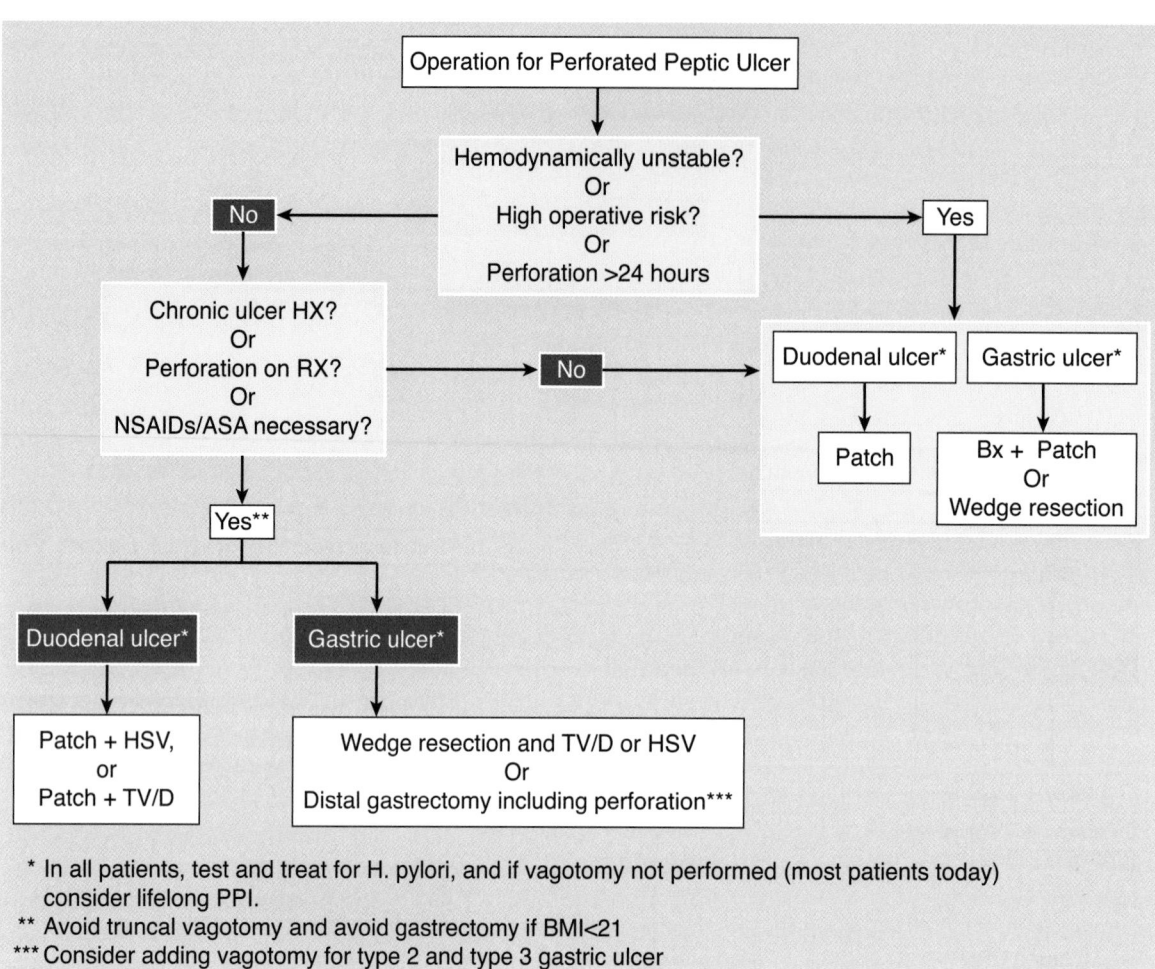

FIG. 26-44. Algorithm for operation for perforated peptic ulcer. ASA = acetylsalicylic acid; BMI = body mass index; Bx = biopsy; HSV = highly selective vagotomy; Hx = history; PPI = proton pump inhibitor; Rx = treatment; TV/D = truncal vagotomy and drainage.

ZES is an important part of the differential diagnosis of hypergastrinemia (Fig. 26-46). All patients with gastrinoma have an elevated gastrin level, and hypergastrinemia in the presence of elevated BAO strongly suggests gastrinoma. Patients with gastrinoma usually have a BAO >15 mEq/h or >5 mEq/h if they have had a previous procedure for peptic ulcer. Acid secretory medications should be held for several days before gastrin measurement, because acid suppression may falsely elevate gastrin levels. Causes of hypergastrinemia can be divided into those associated with hyperacidity and those associated

with hypoacidity (see Fig. 26-46). The diagnosis of ZES is confirmed by the secretin stimulation test. An IV bolus of secretin (2 U/kg) is given and gastrin levels are checked before and after injection. An increase in serum gastrin of 200 pg/mL or greater suggests the presence of gastrinoma. Patients with gastrinoma should have serum calcium and parathyroid hormone levels determined to rule out MEN1 and, if present, parathyroidectomy should be considered before resection of gastrinoma.

Eighty percent of primary tumors are found in the gastrinoma triangle (Fig. 26-47), and many tumors are small (<1 cm), making preoperative localization difficult. Transabdominal ultrasound is quite specific, but not very sensitive. CT will detect most lesions >2 cm in size and MRI is comparable. EUS is more sensitive than these other noninvasive imaging tests, but it still misses many of the smaller lesions, and may confuse normal lymph nodes for gastrinomas. Currently, the preoperative imaging study of choice for gastrinoma is somatostatin receptor scintigraphy (the octreotide scan). When the pretest probability of gastrinoma is high, the sensitivity and specificity of this modality approach 100%. Gastrinoma cells contain type 2 somatostatin receptors that bind the indium-labeled somatostatin analogue (octreotide) with high affinity, making imaging with a gamma camera possible (Fig. 26-48). Currently, angiographic localization studies are infrequently performed for gastrinoma. Both diagnostic angiography and transhepatic selective venous sampling of the portal system have been supplanted by selective secretin infusion, which helps to localize the tumor as inside or outside the gastrinoma triangle.

In this test, an arterial catheter is selectively placed in a named vessel supplying the pancreas (e.g., gastroduodenal or splenic), and a

TABLE 26-13	Differential diagnosis of intractability or nonhealing peptic ulcer disease

Cancer
    Gastric
    Pancreatic
    Duodenal
Persistent *Helicobacter pylori* infection
    Tests may be false-negative
    Consider empiric treatment
Noncompliant patient
    Failure to take prescribed medication
    Surreptitious use of NSAIDs
Motility disorder
Zollinger-Ellison syndrome

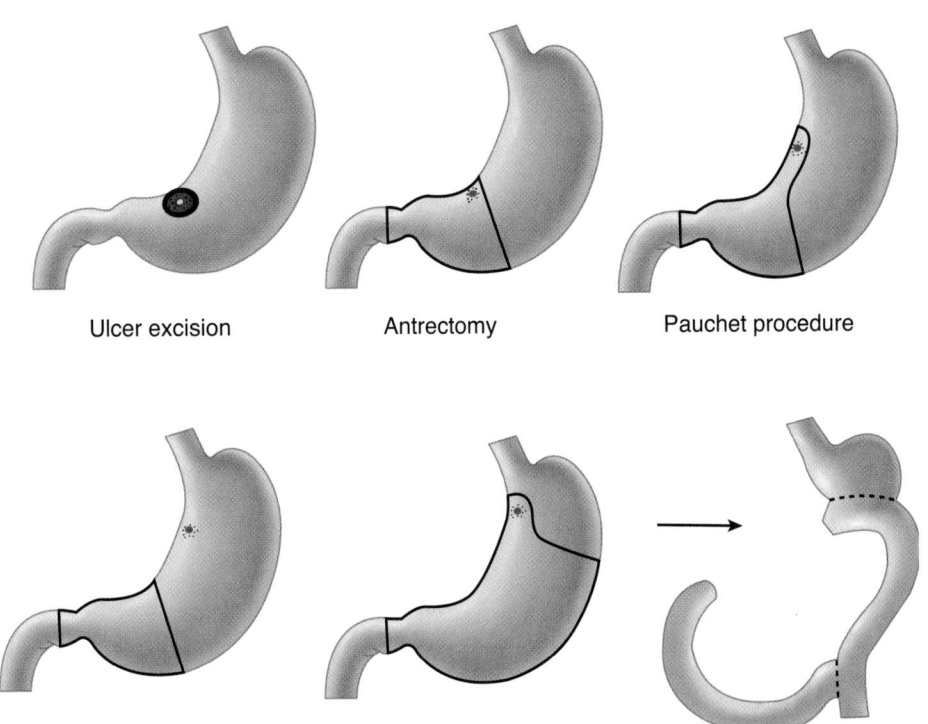

Ulcer excision   Antrectomy   Pauchet procedure

Kelling-Madlener procedure   Subtotal gastrectomy Roux-en-Y esophagogastrojejunostomy   Sendes procedure

FIG. 26-45. Operations for gastric ulcer. *[Reproduced with permission from Seymour NE: Operations for peptic ulcer and their complications, in Feldman M, Sharschmidt BF, Sleisenger MH (eds): Gastrointestinal and Liver Disease, 6th ed. Philadelphia: Saunders, 1998, p 702. Copyright Elsevier.]*

venous catheter is placed in a hepatic vein. Secretin is injected into the visceral artery and gastrin is sampled in the hepatic vein. A significant elevation in hepatic venous gastrin indicates that the tumor is supplied by the injected artery. This test should be performed if pancreaticoduodenectomy is contemplated. Probably the most important means of locating gastrinomas is intraoperative exploration.

All patients with sporadic (nonfamilial) gastrinoma should be considered for surgical resection and possible cure. The lesions should be located in 90% of patients, and the large majority is cured by extirpation of the gastrinoma(s). A thorough intraoperative exploration of the gastrinoma triangle and pancreas is essential, but other sites (i.e., liver, stomach, small bowel, mesentery, and pelvis) should be evaluated as part of a thorough intra-abdominal evaluation to find the primary tumor, which is usually solitary. The duodenum and pancreas should be extensively mobilized and intraoperative ultrasound should be used. Intraoperative EGD with transillumination should be considered. If the tumor cannot be located, generous longitudinal duodenotomy with inspection and palpation of the duodenal wall should be considered. Lymph nodes from the portal, peripancreatic, and celiac drainage basins should be sampled. Ablation or resection of hepatic metastases should be considered.

The management of gastrinoma in patients with MEN1 is controversial because the patients are rarely cured by operation, and the tumors tend to be small and multiple. If the tumor can be imaged preoperatively, operation by an experienced gastrinoma surgeon is reasonable.

Acid hypersecretion in patients with gastrinoma can always be managed with high-dose PPIs. Highly selective vagotomy may make management easier in some patients and should be considered in those with surgically untreatable or unresectable gastrinoma. Gastrectomy for ZES is no longer indicated.

GASTRITIS AND STRESS ULCER

Pathogenesis and Prevention

Gastritis is mucosal inflammation. The gross endoscopic diagnosis of gastritis correlates poorly with histologic findings, and is thus rela-

tively useless as a diagnosis without confirmatory biopsy. Additionally, there is poor correlation between symptoms and histologic gastritis. The most common cause of gastritis is *H. pylori*. Other causes of gastritis include alcohol, NSAIDs, Crohn's disease, tuberculosis, and bile reflux (primary or secondary). These agents cause injury by a variety of different mechanisms. In general, the infectious and inflammatory causes result in immune cell infiltration and cytokine production which damage mucosal cells. The chemical agents (alcohol, aspirin, and bile) generally work to disrupt the mucosal barrier, allowing mucosal damage by back diffusion of luminal hydrogen ions.

Stress gastritis is a peculiar entity that has all but disappeared from the clinical (if not endoscopic) lexicon, largely due to better critical care and acid suppression or cytoprotective agents (e.g., sucralfate) in the intensive care unit (ICU). Stress gastritis and stress ulcer are probably due to inadequate gastric mucosal blood flow during periods of intense physiologic stress. Adequate mucosal blood flow is important to maintain the mucosal barrier, and to buffer any back-diffused hydrogen ions. When blood flow is inadequate, these processes fail and mucosal breakdown occurs. Modern intensive care, with emphasis on adequate tissue perfusion and oxygenation, has undoubtedly decreased the severity of gastric mucosal injury seen in the ICU today. Although it is still common to see small mucosal erosions when performing upper endoscopy in the ICU, it is rare for these lesions to coalesce into the larger bleeding erosions that plagued the ICU patient 30 to 40 years ago. The rationale for routine acid suppression in the ICU, supported by excellent data from clinical trials[82] and the laboratory,[83] is that less mucosal injury will be caused in the potentially weakened gastric mucosa if there is less luminal acid. There are some studies suggesting that routine acid suppression leads to overgrowth of gastric bacteria, which increases the incidence and/or severity of aspiration pneumonia in the ICU. Nevertheless, acid suppression, particularly in the severely ill patient, remains an important part of clinical pathways in most ICUs.[84] In the extraordinarily rare patient requiring operation today for hemorrhagic stress gastritis, the surgical options include V+D with oversewing of the major bleeding lesions, or near total gastrectomy. Angiographic embolization and endoscopic hemostatic treatment should be considered as well.

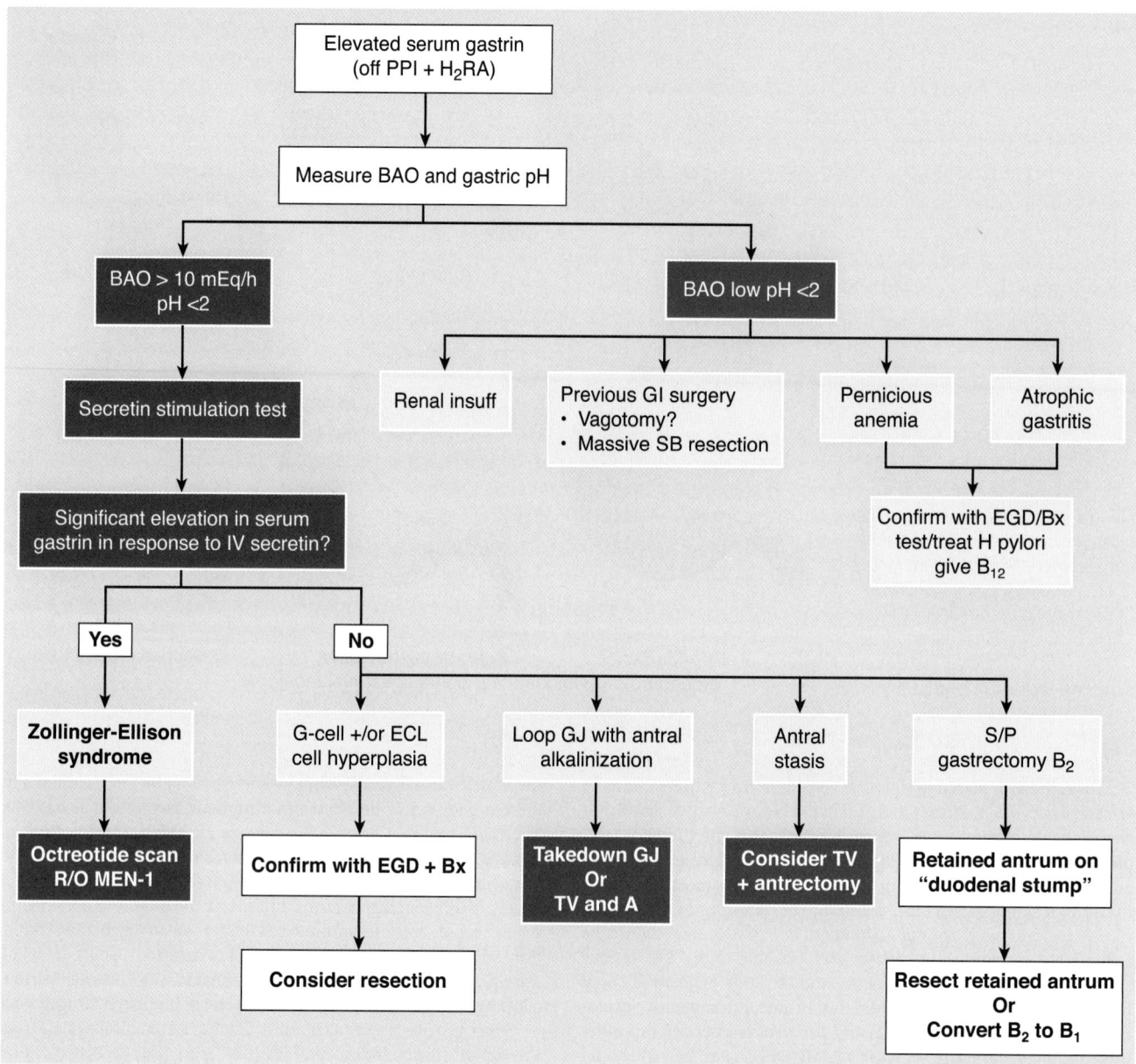

FIG. 26-46. Algorithm for diagnosis and management of hypergastrinemia. BAO = basal acid output; B₁ = Billroth 1; B₂ = Billroth 2; Bx = biopsy; ECL = enterochromaffin-like; EGD = esophagogastroduodenoscopy; GJ = gastrojejunostomy; H₂RA = histamine 2 receptor antagonist; insuff = insufficiency; MEN1 = multiple endocrine neoplasia type 1; PPI = proton pump inhibitor; R/O = rule out; SB = small bowel; S/P = status post; TV = truncal vagotomy; TV and A = truncal vagotomy and antrectomy.

MALIGNANT NEOPLASMS OF THE STOMACH

The three most common primary malignant gastric neoplasms are adenocarcinoma (95%), lymphoma (4%), and malignant GIST (1%) (Table 26-14). Other rare primary malignancies include carcinoid, angiosarcoma, carcinosarcoma, and squamous cell carcinoma. Occasionally the stomach is the site of hematogenous metastasis from other sites (e.g., melanoma or breast). More commonly, malignant tumors from adjacent organs invade the stomach by direct extension (e.g., colon or pancreas) or by peritoneal seeding (e.g., ovary).

Adenocarcinoma
Epidemiology

In 1930 in the United States, gastric cancer was the leading cause of cancer death among men and the third leading cause of cancer death among women. Today, it is not even included among the top 10 causes. Over the past several decades, there has been a dramatic decrease in the gastric cancer incidence and death rate in the United States as well as in most Western industrialized countries (Fig. 26-49). This decrease has been mostly in the so-called *intestinal form* rather than in the *diffuse form* of gastric cancer. Worldwide, especially in Asia and Eastern Europe, gastric cancer remains a leading cause of cancer death. In 2007 in the United States, there were approximately 21,500 new cases of stomach cancer (13,190 in men and 8310 in women), and 10,848 deaths from this disease (6418 men and 4430 women).[85] The estimated 5-year survival rate is 22%, up from about 15% in 1975.

In general, gastric cancer is a disease of the elderly, and it is twice as common in blacks as in whites. In younger patients, tumors are more often of the diffuse variety and tend to be large, aggressive, and more poorly differentiated, sometimes infiltrating the entire stomach (linitis plastic). Gastric cancer has a higher incidence in groups of lower socioeconomic status.

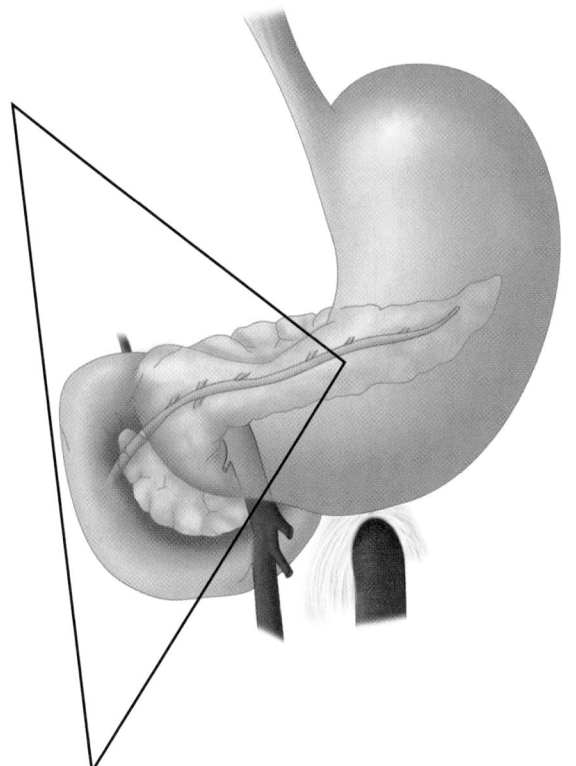

FIG. 26-47. Gastrinoma triangle. *[Reproduced with permission from Ritchie WP Jr.: Benign diseases of the stomach and duodenum, in Ritchie WP, Steele G, Dean RH (eds):* General Surgery. *Philadelphia: Lippincott, 1995, p 117.]*

Tumor Type	No. of Cases	Percent
Malignant tumors	4199	93.0
Carcinoma	3970	87.9
Lymphoma	136	3.0
Leiomyosarcoma	77	1.7
Carcinoid	11	0.3
Others	5	0.1
Benign tumors	315	7.0
Polyp	140	3.1
Leiomyoma	92	2.0
Inflammatory lesions	30	0.7
Heterotopic pancreas	20	0.4
Others	33	0.8

TABLE 26-14 Frequency of gastric tumors

Source: Modified with permission from Ming S-C (ed): Tumors of the Esophagus and Stomach, *AFIP Atlas of Tumor Pathology,* Second Series, Fascicle 7. Washington DC: American Registry of Pathology, 1973, p 82, Table VI.

Etiology

Gastric cancer is more common in patients with pernicious anemia, blood group A, or a family history of gastric cancer. When patients migrate from a high-incidence region to a low-incidence region, the risk of gastric cancer decreases in the subsequent generations born in the new region. This strongly suggests an environmental influence on the development of gastric cancer. Environmental factors appear to be more related etiologically to the intestinal form of gastric cancer than the more aggressive diffuse form. The commonly accepted risk factors for gastric cancer are listed in Table 26-15.

Diet and Drugs Typically, a starchy diet high in pickled, salted, or smoked food is found in many regions of high gastric cancer risk. Dietary nitrates have been impugned as a possible cause of gastric cancer. Gastric bacteria (more common in the achlorhydric stomach of patients with atrophic gastritis, a risk factor for gastric cancer) convert nitrate into nitrite, a proven carcinogen. A diet high in fresh fruits and vegetables and rich in vitamin C and E has been shown to decrease the population's risk of gastric cancer. The reduced consumption of nitrate-rich preserved foods seen with the growth of refrigeration has been suggested as a cause of the dramatic decrease in gastric cancer seen in North America and Western Europe. Tobacco use probably increases the risk of stomach cancer, and alcohol use probably has no effect. Regular aspirin use may be protective.

Helicobacter pylori[54,86] The risk of gastric cancer in patients with chronic *H. pylori* infection is increased about threefold. When compared to uninfected patients, patients with a history of gastric ulcer are more likely to develop gastric cancer (incidence ratio 1.8, 95% confidence interval 1.6 to 2.0), and patients with a history of duodenal ulcer are at decreased risk for gastric cancer (incidence ratio 0.6, 95% confidence interval 0.4 to 0.7). As diagrammed in Fig. 26-50, this may be due to the fact that some patients develop antral-predominant disease (predisposing to duodenal ulcer and somehow protecting against gastric cancer), while other patients develop corpus-predominant gastritis, resulting in hypochlorhydria and somehow predisposing to gastric ulcer and gastric cancer.[87] The theoretical sequence for development of gastric adenocarcinoma is diagrammed in Fig. 26-51.[54,87] Recently, it has been demonstrated that bone marrow–derived stem cells play a key role in the pathogenesis of gastric adenocarcinoma in patients with chronic *H. pylori* infection.[54] However, it must be recognized that gastric adenocarcinoma is a multifactorial disease. Not all patients with gastric cancer have *H. pylori*, and there are some geographic areas with a high prevalence of chronic *H. pylori* infection and a low prevalence of gastric cancer (the "African enigma"). Finally, *H. pylori*–infected patients seem to be at decreased risk for the development of adenocarcinoma of the distal esophagus

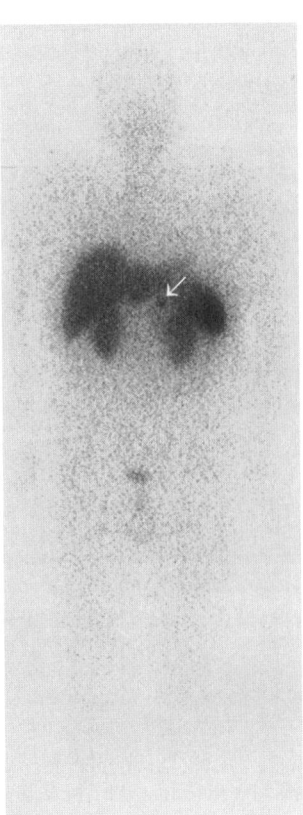

FIG. 26-48. Positive octreotide scan in patient with gastrinoma. *(Courtesy of Dr. Alan Maurer.)*

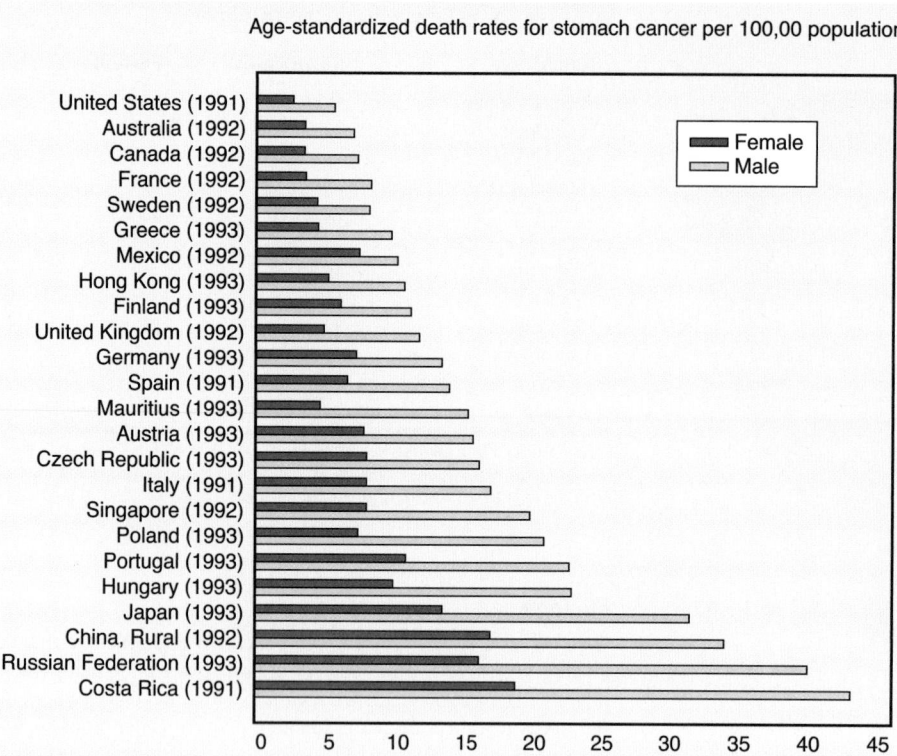

Age-standardized death rates for stomach cancer per 100,00 population

FIG. 26-49. Death rates for gastric cancer in different countries. *[Reproduced with permission from Ming S-C, Hirota T: Malignant epithelial tumors of the stomach, in Ming S-C, Goldman H (eds): Pathology of the Gastrointestinal Tract, 2nd ed. Baltimore: Williams & Wilkins, 1998, p 607.]*

and cardia region.[88] Perhaps the corporeal gastritis decreases acid secretion, creating a less damaging refluxate and thus reducing the risk for Barrett's esophagus, the precursor lesion for these tumors.

Epstein-Barr Virus About 10% of gastric adenocarcinomas carry the EBV virus. This amounts to about 50 to 75,000 cases worldwide. Recently it has been suggested that EBV infection is a rather late step in gastric carcinogenesis, since EBV transcripts are present in cancer cells but not in the metaplastic cells of precursor epithelium.[89]

Genetic Factors A variety of genetic abnormalities have been described in gastric cancer (Table 26-16). Most gastric cancers are aneuploid. The most common genetic abnormalities in sporadic gastric cancer affect the *p53* and *COX-2* genes. Over two thirds of gastric cancers have deletion or suppression of the important tumor-suppressor gene *p53*. Additionally, approximately the same proportion have overexpression of *COX-2*. In the colon, tumors with

upregulation of this gene have suppressed apoptosis, more angiogenesis, and higher metastatic potential. Gastric tumors that overexpress *COX-2* are more aggressive tumors. Recently, a germline mutation in the CDH1 gene encoding for E-cadherin was shown to be associated with hereditary diffuse gastric cancer. Prophylactic total gastrectomy should be considered in patients with these mutations.[90]

Premalignant Conditions of the Stomach Figure 26-52 shows the prevalence of some premalignant conditions associated with the development of early gastric cancer in a series of 1900 cases from Tokyo. By far the most common precancerous lesion is atrophic gastritis.

Polyps There are five types of gastric epithelial polyps: inflammatory, hamartomatous, heterotopic, hyperplastic, and adenoma. The first three types have negligible malignant potential. Adenomas can lead to carcinoma, just like in the colon, and should be removed when diagnosed. Occasionally, hyperplastic polyps can be associated with carcinoma. Patients with familial adenomatous polyposis have a high prevalence of gastric adenomatous polyps (about 50%), and are 10 times more likely to develop adenocarcinoma of the stomach than the general population.[91] Screening EGD is indicated in these families. Patients with hereditary nonpolyposis colorectal cancer may also be at risk for gastric cancer.[92]

Atrophic Gastritis Chronic atrophic gastritis (Fig. 26-53) is by far the most common precursor for gastric cancer, particularly the intestinal subtype (see Fig. 26-52). The prevalence of atrophic gastritis is higher in older age groups, but it is also common in younger people in areas with a high incidence of gastric cancer. In many patients, it is likely that *H. pylori* is involved in the pathogenesis of atrophic gastritis. Correa described three distinct patterns of chronic atrophic gastritis: autoimmune (involves the acid-secreting proximal stomach), hypersecretory (involving the distal stomach), and environmental (involving multiple random areas at the junction of the oxyntic and antral mucosa).[86]

Intestinal Metaplasia Gastric carcinoma often occurs in an area of intestinal metaplasia. Furthermore, an individual's risk of gastric cancer is proportional to the extent of intestinal metaplasia of the gastric mucosa. These observations strongly suggest that intestinal metaplasia is a precursor lesion to gastric cancer. There are different

TABLE 26-15	Factors increasing or decreasing the risk of gastric cancer

Increase risk
  Family history
  Diet (high in nitrates, salt, fat)
  Familial polyposis
  Gastric adenomas
  Hereditary nonpolyposis colorectal cancer
  Helicobacter pylori infection
    Atrophic gastritis, intestinal metaplasia, dysplasia
  Previous gastrectomy or gastrojejunostomy (>10 y ago)
  Tobacco use
  Ménétrier's disease
Decrease risk
  Aspirin
  Diet (high fresh fruit and vegetable intake)
  Vitamin C

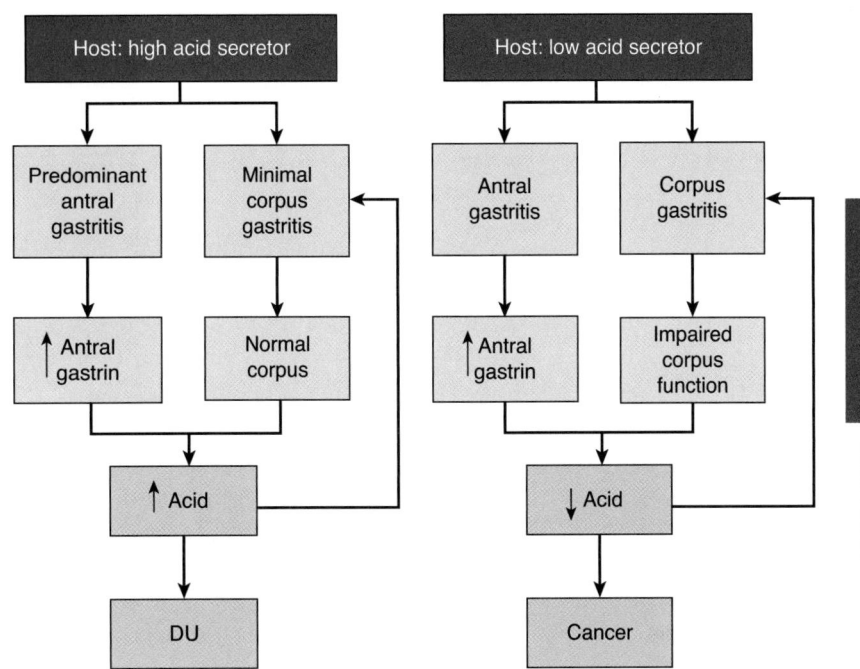

FIG. 26-50. *Helicobacter* and gastritis, and the pathogenesis of duodenal ulcer (DU) or gastric cancer. *[Reproduced with permission from Leung WK, Ng EKW, Sung JJY: Tumors of the stomach, in Yamada T et al (eds):Textbook of Gastroenterology, 4th ed. Philadelphia: Lippincott, Williams & Wilkins, 2003, p 1416.]*

pathologic subtypes of intestinal metaplasia in the stomach, based upon the histologic and biochemical characteristics of the changed mucosal glands. In the complete type of intestinal metaplasia, the glands are completely lined with goblet cells and intestinal absorptive cells (Fig. 26-54). These cells are indistinguishable histologically and biochemically from their small bowel counterparts, and are not seen in the normal stomach. There is evidence that eradication of *H. pylori* infection leads to significant regression of intestinal metaplasia and improvement in atrophic gastritis. Therefore, treatment of *H. pylori* infection is a reasonable recommendation for patients with these pathologic diagnoses and *H. pylori* infection.

Benign Gastric Ulcer Although once considered a premalignant condition, it is likely that the older literature was confounded by mistakenly labeling inadequately biopsied ulcers and healing ulcers as "benign," when, in fact, they were malignant to begin with. It is now generally recognized that all gastric ulcers are cancer until proven otherwise with adequate biopsy and follow-up. Even today, carcinomas are occasionally found when adequately biopsied "benign" ulcers are resected for nonhealing. It is more than likely that the factors just discussed above are more significant etiologically in the development of gastric cancer than the history of a benign gastric ulcer.

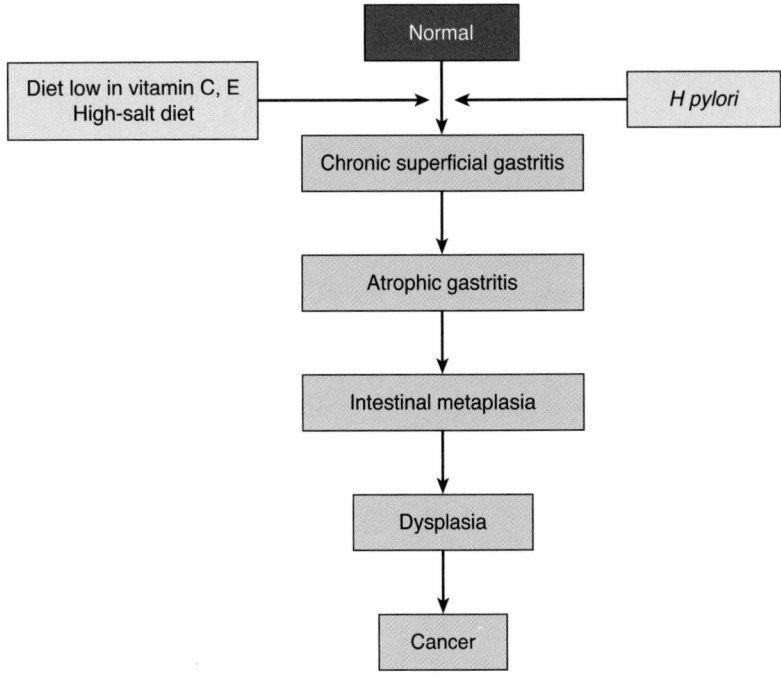

FIG. 26-51. Gastric carcinogenesis. *[Reproduced with permission from Leung WK, Ng EKW, Sung JJY: Tumors of the stomach, in Yamada T, et al (eds): Textbook of Gastroenterology, 4th ed. Philadelphia: Lippincott, Williams & Wilkins, 2003, p 1416.]*

TABLE 26-16 Genetic abnormalities in gastric cancer

Abnormalities	Gene	Approximate Frequency %
Deletion/suppression	p53	60–70
	FHIT	60
	APC	50
	DCC	50
	E-cadherin	<5
Amplification/overexpression	COX-2	70
	HGF/SF	60
	VEGF	50
	c-met	45
	AIB-1	40
	β-catenin	25
	k-sam	20
	ras	10–15
	c-erb B-2	5–7
Microsatellite instability		25–40
DNA aneuploidy		60–75

Source: Reproduced with permission from Koh TJ, Wang TC: Tumors of the stomach, in Feldman M et al (eds): *Sleisenger & Fordtran's Gastrointestinal and Liver Diseases*, 7th ed. Philadelphia: Saunders, 2002. Copyright Elsevier.

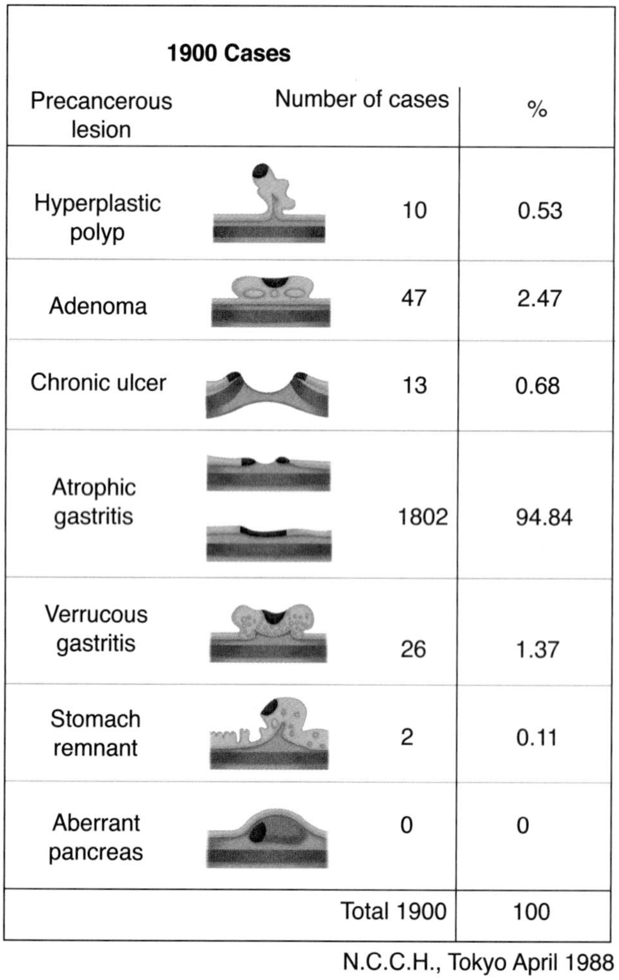

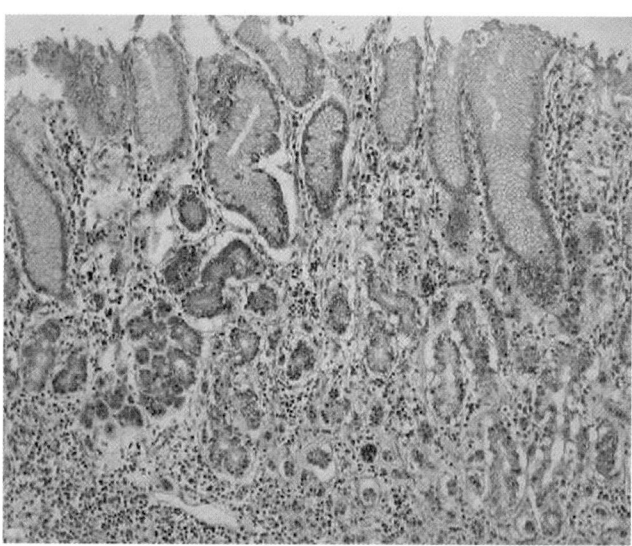

FIG. 26-53. Chronic atrophic gastritis. *(Reproduced with permission from* http://www.epathologies.com.*)*

Gastric Remnant Cancer It has long been recognized that stomach cancer can develop in the gastric remnant, usually years following distal gastrectomy for PUD. The risk is controversial, but the phenomenon is real. Most tumors develop >10 years following the initial operation, and they usually arise in an area of chronic gastritis, metaplasia, and dysplasia. This is often near the stoma, but many of these tumors are quite large at presentation, and are equally divided between intestinal and diffuse subtypes. Most cases have been reported following Billroth II gastroenterostomy, but there also have been cases following Billroth I gastroduodenostomy. Whether simple loop gastrojejunostomy increases a patient's risk of gastric cancer, and whether a Roux-en-Y anastomosis following gastric resection lowers their risk of gastric cancer is unknown. Stage for stage, the prognosis for gastric stump cancer is similar to proximal gastric cancer.[93]

Other Premalignant States A mutated E-cadherin gene is associated with hereditary diffuse gastric cancer. Prophylactic total gastrectomy should be considered.[90] Obviously, a myriad of genetic and

1900 Cases		
Precancerous lesion	Number of cases	%
Hyperplastic polyp	10	0.53
Adenoma	47	2.47
Chronic ulcer	13	0.68
Atrophic gastritis	1802	94.84
Verrucous gastritis	26	1.37
Stomach remnant	2	0.11
Aberrant pancreas	0	0
Total	1900	100

N.C.C.H., Tokyo April 1988

FIG. 26-52. Precancerous lesions of the stomach. *[Reproduced with permission from Ming S-C, Hirota T: Malignant epithelial tumors of the stomach, in Ming S-C, Goldman H (eds):* Pathology of the Gastrointestinal Tract, *2nd ed. Baltimore: Williams & Wilkins, 1998, p 607.]*

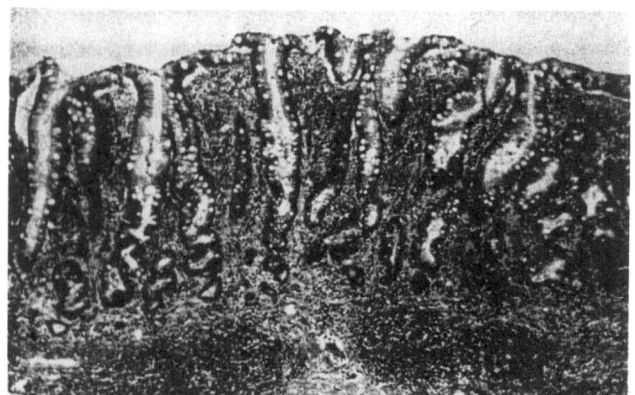

FIG. 26-54. Complete intestinal metaplasia of the stomach. Note intestinal type crypts lined with goblet cells and intestinal absorptive cells. *[Reproduced with permission from Ming S-C, Hirota T: Malignant epithelial tumors of the stomach, in Ming S-C, Goldman H (eds):* Pathology of the Gastrointestinal Tract, *2nd ed. Baltimore: Williams & Wilkins, 1998, p 607.]*

environmental factors will affect members of the same family, and up to 10% of gastric cancer cases appear to be familial without a clear-cut genetic diagnosis. First-degree relatives of patients with gastric cancer have a two- to threefold increased risk of developing the disease. Patients with hereditary nonpolyposis colorectal cancer have a 10% risk of developing gastric cancer, predominantly the intestinal subtype. The mucous cell hyperplasia of Ménétrier's disease is generally considered to carry a 5 to 10% risk of adenocarcinoma. Periodic surveillance EGD is prudent in all the above conditions. The glandular hyperplasia associated with gastrinoma is not premalignant, but ECL hyperplasia and/or carcinoid tumors can occur.

Pathology

Dysplasia It is generally accepted that gastric dysplasia is the universal precursor to gastric adenocarcinoma. Patients with severe dysplasia should be considered for gastric resection if the abnormality is widespread or multifocal, or EMR if the severe dysplasia is localized. Patients with mild dysplasia should be followed with endoscopic biopsy surveillance, and *Helicobacter* eradication.

Early Gastric Cancer Early gastric cancer is defined as adenocarcinoma limited to the mucosa and submucosa of the stomach, regardless of lymph node status. The entity is common in the Orient, where gastric cancer is a common cause of cancer death, and where aggressive surveillance programs have therefore been established. Approximately 10% of patients with early gastric cancer will have lymph node metastases. There are several types and subtypes of early gastric cancer (Table 26-17 and Fig. 26-55). Approximately 70% of early gastric cancers are well differentiated, and 30% are poorly differentiated. The overall cure rate with adequate gastric resection and lymphadenectomy is 95%. In some Japanese centers, 50% of the gastric cancers treated are early gastric cancer. In the United States, less than 20% of resected gastric adenocarcinomas are early gastric cancer. Small intramucosal lesions can be treated with EMR.[94]

Gross Morphology and Histologic Subtypes There are four gross forms of gastric cancer: polypoid, fungating, ulcerative, and scirrhous. In the first two, the bulk of the tumor mass is intraluminal. Polypoid tumors are not ulcerated; fungating tumors are elevated intraluminally, but also ulcerated. In the latter two gross subtypes, the bulk of the tumor mass is in the wall of the stomach. Ulcerative tumors are self-descriptive; scirrhous tumors infiltrate the entire thickness of the stomach and cover a very large surface area. Scirrhous tumors (linitis plastica) have a particularly poor prognosis, and commonly involve the entire stomach. Although these latter lesions may be technically resectable with total gastrectomy, it is common for both the esophageal and duodenal margins of resection to show microscopic evidence of tumor infiltration. Death from recurrent disease within 6 months is common.

The location of the primary tumor in the stomach is important in planning the operation. Several decades ago, the large majority of gastric cancers were in the distal stomach. Recently, there has been a proximal migration of tumors, so that currently, the distribution is closer to 40% distal, 30% middle, and 30% proximal.

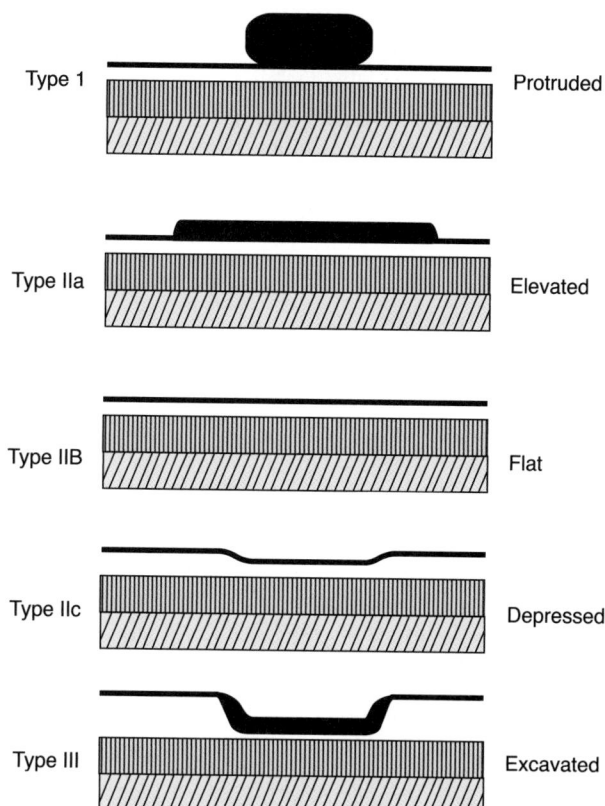

FIG. 26-55. Pathologic types of early gastric cancer. *[Reproduced with permission from Fenoglio-Preiser CM et al: Pathologic and phenotypic features of gastric cancer.* Semin Oncol *23(3):292, 1996. Copyright Elsevier.]*

Histology The most important prognostic indicators in gastric cancer are both histologic: lymph node involvement and depth of tumor invasion. Tumor grade (degree of differentiation: well, moderately, or poorly) is also important prognostically.

There are several histologic classifications of gastric cancer. The World Health Organization recognizes several histologic types (Table 26-18). The Japanese classification is similar but more detailed. The commonly used Lauren classification separates gastric cancers into intestinal type (53%), diffuse type (33%), and unclassified (14%). The intestinal type is associated with chronic atrophic gastritis, severe intestinal metaplasia, and dysplasia, and tends to be less aggressive than the diffuse type. The diffuse type of gastric cancer is more likely to be poorly differentiated and is associated

---

TABLE 26-17 Early gastric cancer

Type I	Exophytic lesion extending into the gastric lumen
Type II	Superficial variant
II A	Elevated lesions with a height no more than the thickness of the adjacent mucosa
IIB	Flat lesions
IIC	Depressed lesions with an eroded but not deeply ulcerated appearance
Type III	Excavated lesions that may extend into the muscularis propria without invasion of this layer by actual cancer cells

---

TABLE 26-18 World Health Organization histologic typing of gastric cancer

Adenocarcinoma
  Papillary adenocarcinoma
  Tubular adenocarcinoma
  Mucinous adenocarcinoma
  Signet-ring cell carcinoma
Adenosquamous carcinoma
Squamous cell carcinoma
Small cell carcinoma
Undifferentiated carcinoma
Others

Source: Reproduced with permission from Ming S-C, Hirota T: Malignant epithelial tumors of the stomach, in Ming S-C, Goldman H (eds): *Pathology of the Gastrointestinal Tract,* 2nd ed. Baltimore: Williams & Wilkins, 1998.

with younger patients and proximal tumors. The Ming classification also is useful and easy to remember, with only two types—expanding (67%) and infiltrative (33%).

Pathologic Staging Ultimately, prognosis is related to pathologic stage. The most widespread system for staging of gastric cancer is the tumor-node-metastasis (TNM) staging system based on depth of tumor invasion, extent of lymph node metastases, and presence of distant metastases. This system was developed by the American Joint Committee on Cancer and the International Union Against Cancer, and has undergone several modifications since it was originally conceived (Table 26-19).

Clinical Manifestations

Most patients who are diagnosed with gastric cancer in the United States have advanced stage III or IV disease at the time of diagnosis. The most common symptoms are weight loss and decreased food intake due to anorexia and early satiety. Abdominal pain (usually not severe and often ignored) also is common. Other symptoms include nausea, vomiting, and bloating. Acute GI bleeding is somewhat unusual (5%), but chronic occult blood loss is common and manifests as iron deficiency anemia and heme-positive stool. Dysphagia is common if the tumor involves the cardia of the stomach. Paraneoplastic syndromes such as Trousseau's syndrome (thrombophlebitis), acanthosis nigricans (hyperpigmentation of the axilla and groin), or peripheral neuropathy are rarely present.

TABLE 26-19	TNM staging of gastric cancer by the International Union Against Cancer and American Joint Committee on Cancer

T: Primary tumor

Tis	Carcinoma in situ; intraepithelial tumor without invasion of lamina propria
T1	Tumor invades lamina propria or submucosa
T2	Tumor invades muscularis propria or subserosa
T3	Tumor penetrates serosa (visceral peritoneum) without invasion of adjacent structures
T4	Tumor invades adjacent structures

N: Regional lymph node

N0	No regional lymph node metastasis
N1	Metastasis in 1 to 6 regional lymph nodes
N2	Metastasis in 7 to 15 lymph nodes
N3	Metastasis in more than 15 regional lymph nodes

M: Distant metastasis

M0	No distant metastasis
M1	Distant metastasis

Stage grouping

Stage	T	N	M
0	Tis	N0	M0
IA	T1	N0	M0
IB	T1	N1	M0
	T2	N0	M0
II	T1	N2	M0
	T2	N1	M0
	T3	N0	M0
IIIA	T2	N2	M0
	T3	N1	M0
	T4	N0	M0
IIIB	T3	N2	M0
IV	T4	N1–3	M0
	T1–3	N3	M0
	Any T	Any N	M1

Source: Used with the permission of the American Joint Committee on Cancer (AJCC), Chicago, Illinois. The original source for this material is the *AJCC Cancer Staging Manual*, Sixth Edition (2002) published by Springer Science and Business Media LLC, *www.springerlink.com*.

Physical examination usually is normal. Other than signs of weight loss, specific physical findings usually indicate incurability. A focused examination in a patient in whom gastric cancer is a likely part of the differential diagnosis should include an examination of the neck, chest, abdomen, rectum, and pelvis. Cervical, supraclavicular (on the left referred to as Virchow's node), and axillary lymph nodes may be enlarged, and today can be sampled in the office with fine-needle aspiration cytology. There may be a metastatic pleural effusion, or aspiration pneumonitis in a patient with vomiting and/or obstruction. An abdominal mass could indicate a large (usually T4 incurable) primary tumor, liver metastases, or carcinomatosis (including Krukenberg's tumor of the ovary). A palpable umbilical nodule (Sister Joseph's nodule) is pathognomonic of advanced disease, or there may be evidence on exam of malignant ascites. Rectal exam may reveal heme-positive stool and hard nodularity extraluminally and anteriorly, indicating so-called *drop metastases*, or rectal shelf of Blumer in the pouch of Douglas.

Diagnostic Evaluation

Distinguishing between peptic ulcer and gastric cancer on clinical grounds alone is usually impossible. Patients over the age of 45 years old who have new-onset dyspepsia, as well as all patients with dyspepsia and alarm symptoms (weight loss, recurrent vomiting, dysphagia, evidence of bleeding, or anemia) or with a family history of gastric cancer should have *prompt upper endoscopy and biopsy* if a mucosal lesion is noted. Essentially, all patients in whom gastric cancer is part of the differential diagnosis should have endoscopy and biopsy. If suspicion for cancer is high and the biopsy is negative, the patient should be re-endoscoped and more aggressively biopsied. In some patients with gastric tumors, upper GI series can be helpful in planning treatment. Although a good *double-contrast barium upper GI examination* is sensitive for gastric tumors (up to 75% sensitive), in most centers, endoscopy has become the gold standard for the diagnosis of gastric malignancy.

Preoperative staging of gastric cancer is best accomplished with abdominal/pelvic CT scanning with IV and oral contrast. MRI is probably comparable. The best way to stage the tumor locally is via EUS, which gives fairly accurate (80%) information about the depth of tumor penetration into the gastric wall, and can usually show enlarged (>5 mm) perigastric and celiac lymph nodes. In some centers, if the tumor is transmural (T3) or involves lymph nodes (enlarged nodes can usually be needled under ultrasound guidance), preoperative (neoadjuvant) chemotherapy is given. However, there are limitations to tumor staging with EUS. It largely is operator dependent and may underestimate lymph node involvement because normal-sized nodes (<5 mm) can harbor metastases. EUS is most accurate in distinguishing early gastric cancer (T1) from more advanced tumors.

Positron Emission Tomography Scanning Whole-body PET scanning uses the principle that tumor cells preferentially accumulate positron-emitting ^{18}F-fluorodeoxyglucose. This modality is most useful in the evaluation of distant metastasis in gastric cancer but can also be useful in locoregional staging. PET scan is most useful when combined with spiral CT (PET-CT)[95] and should be considered before major surgery in patients with particularly high-risk tumors or multiple medical comorbidities.

Staging Laparoscopy and Peritoneal Cytology To some extent, the usefulness of these modalities depends on the individual patient's situation as well as the treatment philosophy of the cancer team. The fundamental question is "will it make a difference to this patient's management?" Patients with gastric cancer who undergo R0 resection (i.e., no gross residual disease) and are found to have positive peritoneal cytology (no gross carcinomatosis) have a much worse prognosis than the cytology negative group (median survival 14.8 months vs. 98.5 months).[96] It is controversial how much this information adds prognostically to that of pathologic staging (TNM). Whether this poor prognosis can be improved postresection with aggressive adjuvant treatment (systemic, or local intraperitoneal hyperthermic chemotherapy) is unknown. Unfortunately, it is also unclear how much these patients benefit from gastric resection. Currently peritoneal cytology information is unlikely to change the treatment of patients with gastric cancer, and most patients without detectable distant metastases will have (and should have) gastric resection regardless of the peritoneal cytology results. A quick laparoscopic examination can occasionally reveal small peritoneal implants or liver metastases that were not detected on preoperative imaging studies and, in some patients (e.g., high risk for surgery or impressive carcinomatosis), this will change the operative plan and avoid a major but futile surgical procedure. Laparoscopy may be most useful in patients with proximal tumors or with adenopathy on spiral CT scan.[97] An extensive laparoscopic staging procedure, although quite accurate, has not been widely adopted.

Treatment

Surgical resection is the only curative treatment for gastric cancer[98,99] and most patients with clinically resectable locoregional disease should have gastric resection. Obvious exceptions include patients who cannot tolerate an abdominal operation, and patients with overwhelming metastatic disease.

The goal of curative surgical treatment is resection of all tumor (i.e., R0 resection). Thus, all margins (proximal, distal, and radial) should be negative and an adequate lymphadenectomy performed. Generally, the surgeon strives for a grossly negative margin of at least 5 cm. Some gastric tumors, particularly the diffuse variety, are quite infiltrative and tumor cells can extend well beyond the tumor mass; thus, gross margins beyond 5 cm may be desirable. Frozen section confirmation of negative margins is important when performing operation for cure, but it is less important in patients with nodal metastases beyond the N1 nodal basin. It should be strongly emphasized that many patients with positive lymph nodes are cured by adequate surgery. It should also be stressed that often lymph nodes that appear to be grossly involved with tumor turn out to be benign or reactive on pathologic examination. More than 15 resected lymph nodes are required for adequate staging.[100] Therapeutic nihilism should be avoided and, in the low-risk patient, an aggressive attempt to resect all tumor should be made. The primary tumor may be resected en bloc with adjacent involved organs (e.g., distal pancreas, transverse colon, or spleen) during the course of curative gastrectomy. Palliative gastrectomy may be indicated in some patients with obviously incurable disease, but most patients presenting with stage IV gastric cancer can be managed without major operation.[99,101]

Extent of Gastrectomy The standard operation for gastric cancer is radical subtotal gastrectomy. Unless required for R0 resection, total gastrectomy confers no additional survival benefit and may have adverse nutritional or quality-of-life consequences, and higher perioperative morbidity and mortality.[98,99] Subtotal gastric resection typically entails ligation of the left and right gastric and gastroepiploic arteries at the origin, as well as the en bloc removal of the distal 75% of the stomach, including the pylorus and 2 cm of duodenum, the greater and lesser omentum, and all associated lymphatic tissue (Fig. 26-56). Reconstruction is usually by Billroth II gastrojejunostomy, but if a small gastric remnant is left (<20%), a Roux-en-Y reconstruction is considered. The operative mortality is around 2 to 5%. Radical subtotal gastrectomy is generally deemed to be an adequate cancer operation in most Western countries, provided that the contingencies stated result in tumor-free margins, >15 lymph nodes, and the resection of all gross tumor. In the absence of involvement by direct extension, the spleen and pancreatic tail are not removed.

Total gastrectomy with Roux-en-Y esophagojejunostomy may be required for R0 resection (Fig. 26-57), and may be the best operation for patients with proximal gastric adenocarcinoma. The construction of a jejunal pouch may be beneficial nutritionally, particularly for those patients with a good prognosis.[102] Proximal subtotal gastric resection, a technically feasible alternative to total gastrectomy for some proximal gastric tumors, requires an esophagogastrostomy to

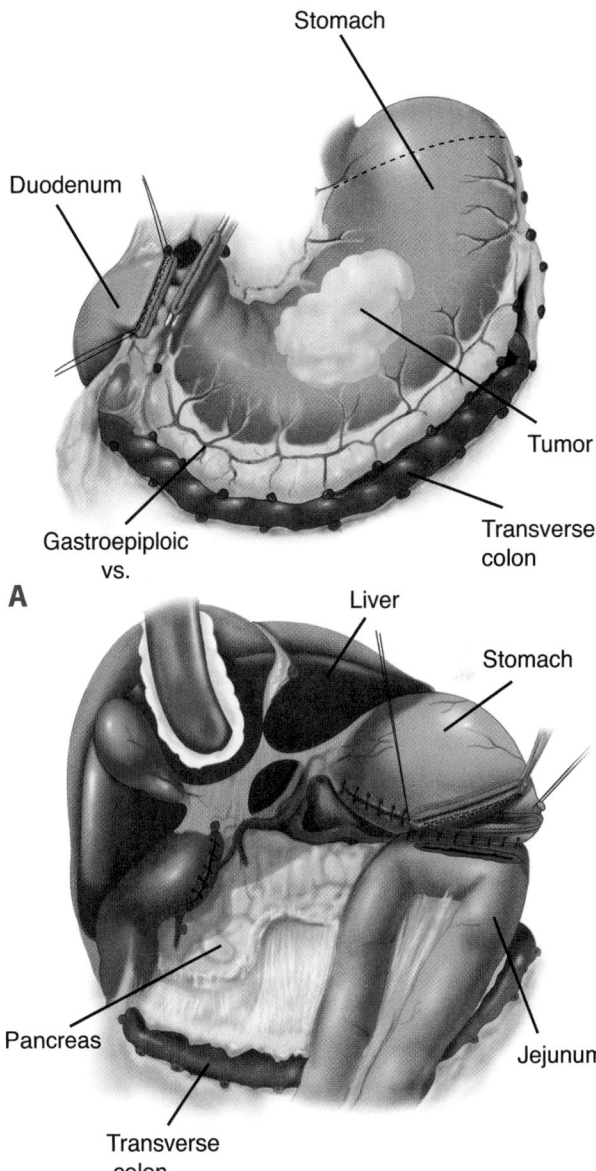

FIG. 26-56. A and **B.** Radical subtotal gastrectomy. vs. = vessels. *[Reproduced with permission from Daly JM, Cady B, Low DW (eds):* Atlas of Surgical Oncology. *St. Louis: Mosby-Year Book, 1993, p 231. Copyright Elsevier.]*

a vagotomized distal gastric remnant. Pyloroplasty in this setting virtually guarantees bile esophagitis, and if the pylorus is left intact, gastric emptying may be problematic. An isoperistaltic jejunal interposition (Henley loop) between the esophagus and antrum could be considered as an alternative reconstruction, but, all things considered, total gastrectomy usually results in superior functional, if not oncologic, results for most patients with proximal gastric cancer.

Extent of Lymphadenectomy The Japanese Research Society for Gastric Cancer has numbered the lymph node stations that potentially drain the stomach (see Fig. 26-4). Generally these are grouped into level D1 (i.e., stations 3 to 6), level D2 (i.e., stations 1, 2, 7, 8, and 11), and level D3 (i.e., stations 9, 10, and 12) nodes. Generally, D1 nodes are perigastric, D2 nodes are along the hepatic and splenic arteries, and D3 nodes are the most distant. The operation described above (radical subtotal gastrectomy in the Extent of Gastrectomy section), which is by far the most commonly performed procedure in the United States for gastric cancer, is called a D1 resection because it

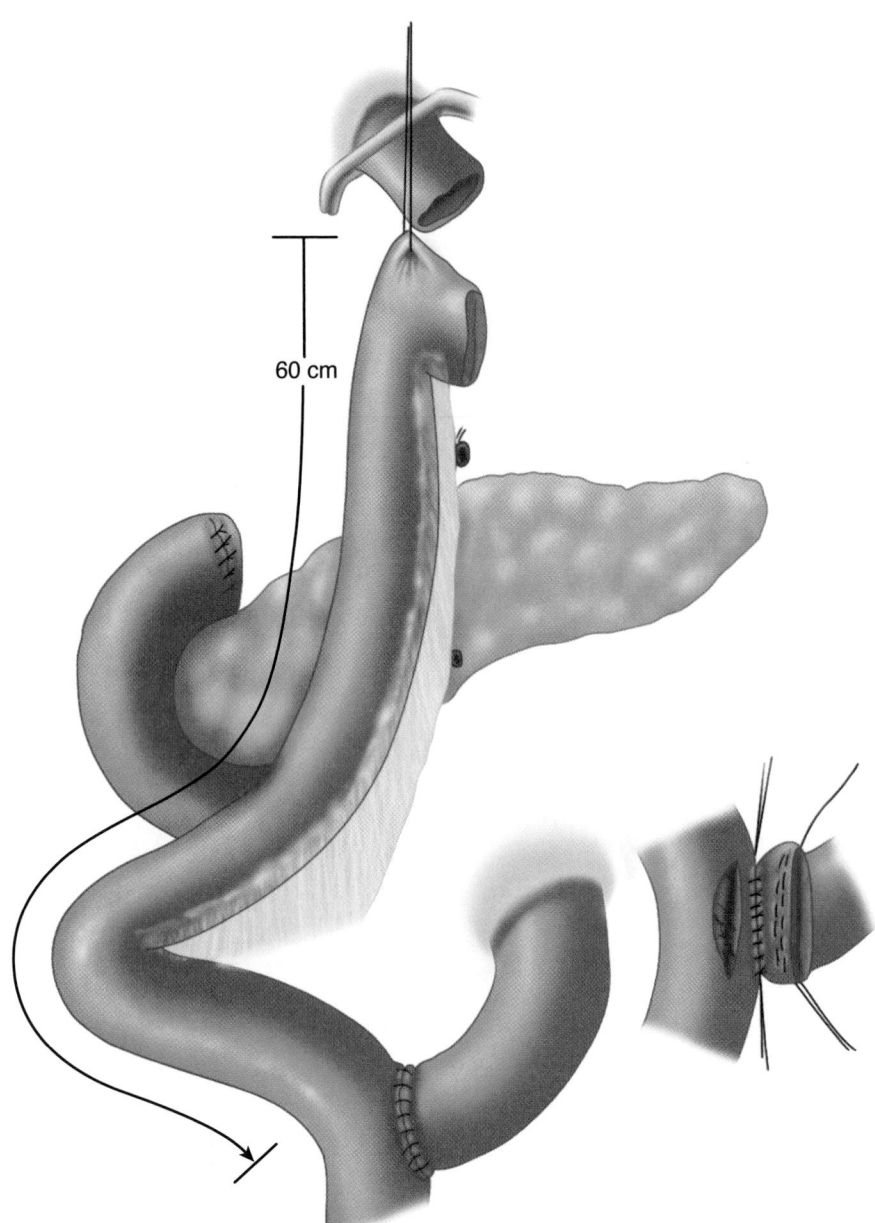

60 cm

FIG. 26-57. Reconstruction after total gastrectomy. Jejunal pouch (not shown here) should be considered. *[Reproduced with permission from Zinner MJ (ed):* Atlas of Gastric Surgery. *New York: Churchill Livingstone, 1992, p 167. Copyright Elsevier.]*

removes the tumor and the perigastric D1 nodes. The standard operation for gastric cancer in Asia and specialized U.S. centers is the D2 gastrectomy, which involves a more extensive lymphadenectomy (removal of the D1 and D2 nodes). In addition to the tissue removed in a D1 resection, the standard D2 gastrectomy removes the peritoneal layer over the anterior mesocolon and selectively over the pancreas, along with nodes along the hepatic and splenic arteries, and the crural nodes. Splenectomy and distal pancreatectomy are not routinely performed, because this clearly has been shown to increase the morbidity of the operation. The purported survival advantage of D2 gastrectomy in gastric cancer is shown in Table 26-20, which shows the 5-year survival rates for gastric cancer stratified by pathologic stage for the United States and Japan. Unfortunately, the randomized prospective trials that have been performed have not confirmed this survival advantage, but the morbidity and mortality in the D2 group was higher (Table 26-21).[103,104] This was mostly attributable to the splenectomy and distal pancreatectomy, which are no longer routinely done as part of the D2 gastrectomy.

Some experts have argued that the D2 operation is simply a better staging procedure, and that the apparent improved survival with this more extensive dissection is simply an epiphenomenon of improved pathologic staging. This stage shift suggests that many patients in the U.S. series treated with D1 gastrectomy really had metastatic nodes at the D2 level that went unresected and undetected. Therefore, in the U.S. series, there were patients classified as stage I, who, if they had

TABLE 26-20 Gastric cancer 5-year survival and operative mortality in the USA and Japan

	Maruyama (Japan), 1971–1985	American College of Surgeons, 1982–1987	Memorial Sloan Kettering, 1985–1994
No. patients	3176	18,365	675
Stage I	91%	50%	84%
Stage II	72%	29%	61%
Stage III	44%	13%	29%
Stage IV	9%	3%	25%
Operative mortality	1%	7%	3%

TABLE 26-21 Randomized trials comparing D1 and D2 gastrectomy for gastric cancer

Authors	Number of Patients	Type of Surgery	Postoperative Complications (%)	Postoperative Mortality (%)	5-Year Survival (%)
Bonenkamp et al.	711	D1	25	4	45
		D2	43	10	47
Cuschieri et al.	400	D1	28	6.5	35
		D2	46	13	33

Source: Data from Bonenkamp JJ, Hermans J, Sasako M, et al: Extended lymph node dissection for gastric cancer. *N Engl J Med* 340:908, 1999; and Cuschieri A, Fayers P, Fielding J, et al: Postoperative morbidity and mortality after D1 and D2 resections for gastric cancer: Preliminary results of the MRC randomized controlled surgical trial. The Surgical Cooperative Group. *Lancet* 347:995, 1996.

undergone a D2 gastrectomy, would be classified as stage II; and there were patients classified as stage II, who, if they had undergone a D2 gastrectomy, would be classified as stage III. The stage I survival in the United States would then actually be closer to the (more accurately staged) stage II survival in Japan, because this group includes some patients who really *are* stage II, but the nodes were not found in the D1 resection. All experts would agree that to avoid understaging of gastric cancer, a minimum of 15 nodes should be resected with the gastrectomy specimen.

Chemotherapy and Radiation for Gastric Cancer In general, the actuarial 5-year survival for resected gastric adenocarcinoma stages 1, 2, and 3 is about 75%, 50%, and 25%, respectively. Because most surgical patients have stage 2 disease or greater, it is common to refer gastric cancer patients postoperatively to a medical and/or radiation oncologist. Unfortunately, the existing data suggest that the incremental survival benefit attendant to adjuvant treatment is marginal, particularly in those patients who have had an adequate resection.[98,99] In one prospective randomized study, adjuvant treatment with chemotherapy (5-fluorouracil and leucovorin) and radiation (4500 cGy) has demonstrated a survival benefit in resected patients with stage II and III adenocarcinoma of the stomach.[105] Unfortunately, only 10% of patients entered in the study actually had D2 gastrectomy, and most (54%) had less than an adequate D1 gastrectomy. Because adequacy of lymphadenectomy has clearly been shown to impact survival, particularly in patients with stage III gastric cancer,[99,100] it has been suggested that the benefits of adjuvant chemoradiation shown in this study would be vitiated by an adequate operation. Clearly further studies are needed.

A recently published study from the Japan Clinical Oncology Group showed a 69% overall 5-year survival rate in patients with clinically curable T2b, T3, and T4 gastric cancer, treated with D2 gastrectomy alone (no chemotherapy).[106] There was no incremental benefit from para-aortic lymph node dissection. There is no indication for the routine use of radiation alone in the adjuvant setting, but in certain patients, it can be effective palliation for bleeding or pain. In patients with gross unresectable, metastatic, or recurrent disease, palliative chemotherapy has not been demonstrated to conclusively prolong survival, but occasionally, a patient has a dramatic response. These patients should be considered for clinical trials. Agents that have shown activity against gastric cancer include 5-fluorouracil, cisplatin, doxorubicin, and methotrexate. Neoadjuvant treatment of gastric adenocarcinoma is being evaluated, particularly in patients with clinical T3 or N1 disease.

Endoscopic Resection It has been demonstrated initially at numerous East Asian centers that some patients with early gastric cancer can be adequately treated by an EMR. Small tumors (<3 cm) confined to the mucosa have an extremely low chance of lymph node metastasis (3%), which approaches the operative mortality rate for gastrectomy. If the resected specimen demonstrates no ulceration, no penetration of the muscularis mucosae, no lymphatic invasion, and size <3 cm, then the risk of lymph node metastases is less than 1%. Thus, some patients with early gastric cancer might be better treated with the endoscopic technique. Currently, this should

be limited to patients with tumors <2 cm in size that are node negative and confined to the mucosa on EUS, in the absence of other gastric lesions. The addition of laparoscopic lymph node sampling may be considered in selected patients.

Prognosis

The 5-year survival for gastric adenocarcinoma has increased from 15 to 22% in the United States over the past 25 years. Survival is dependent on pathologic stage (TNM stage) and degree of tumor differentiation. Other important prognostic factors are sex, age, primary gastric site, tumor size, and tumor depth.

Palliative gastrectomy may be indicated in some patients with obviously incurable disease, but most patients presenting with stage IV gastric cancer can be managed without major operation.[99,101]

Screening for Gastric Cancer

In Japan, it clearly has been shown that patients participating in gastric cancer screening programs have a significantly decreased risk of dying from gastric cancer. Thus screening is effective in a high-risk population. Screening the general population in the United States (a low-risk country) does not make sense, but patients clearly at risk for gastric cancer probably should have periodic endoscopy and biopsy. This includes patients with familial adenomatous polyposis, hereditary nonpolyposis colorectal cancer, gastric adenomas, Ménétrier's disease, intestinal metaplasia or dysplasia, and remote gastrectomy or gastrojejunostomy.

Gastric Lymphoma

Gastric lymphomas generally account for about 4% of gastric malignancies. Over half of patients with non-Hodgkin's lymphoma have involvement of the GI tract. The stomach is the most common site of primary GI lymphoma, and over 95% are non-Hodgkin's type. Most are B-cell type, thought to arise in MALT, although most high-grade gastric lymphomas are without any characteristics of the low-grade MALT neoplasm.[107] About half of gastric lymphomas are histologically low grade, and about half are high grade. Interestingly, the normal stomach is relatively devoid of lymphoid tissue. However, in the setting of chronic gastritis, the stomach acquires MALT, which can undergo malignant degeneration. Again, *H. pylori* is thought to be the culprit. In populations with a high incidence of gastric lymphoma, there is a high incidence of *H. pylori* infection; patients with gastric lymphoma also usually have *H. pylori* infection.

Low-grade MALT lymphoma, essentially a monoclonal proliferation of B cells, presumably arises from a background of chronic gastritis associated with *H. pylori*. These relatively innocuous tumors then undergo degeneration to high-grade lymphoma, which is the usual variety seen by the surgeon. Remarkably, when the *H. pylori* is eradicated and the gastritis improves, the low-grade MALT lymphoma often disappears. Thus low-grade MALT lymphoma is not a surgical lesion. Careful follow-up is necessary particularly in those lesions with a t(11:18) translocation, thought to be a risk factor for a more aggressive MALT lesion. If low-grade lymphoma persists after *H. pylori* eradication, radiation should be considered for disease

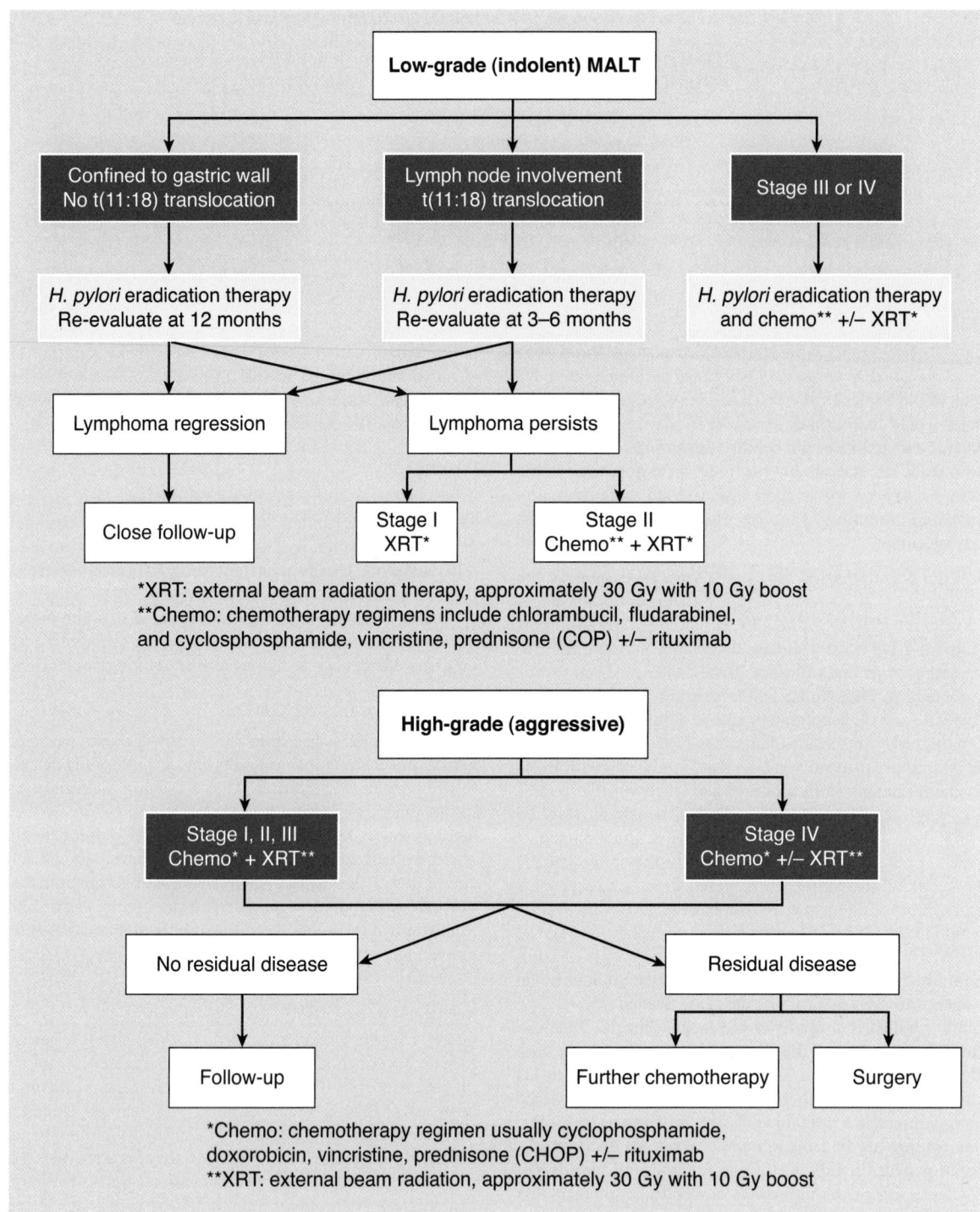

FIG. 26-58. Algorithm for the treatment of gastric lymphoma. MALT = mucosa-associated lymphoid tissue. *(Reproduced with permission from Yoon SS, Coit DG, Portlock CS, et al: The diminishing role of surgery in the treatment of gastric lymphoma. Ann Surg 240:28, 2004.)*

clinically confined to the stomach (stage I), while chemotherapy with or without radiation is used for more advanced lesions (Fig. 26-58).

Patients with high-grade gastric lymphoma require aggressive oncologic treatment for cure and present with many of the same symptoms as gastric cancer patients. However, systemic symptoms such as fever, weight loss, and night sweats occur in about 50% of patients with gastric lymphoma. The tumors may bleed and/or obstruct. Lymphadenopathy and/or organomegaly suggest systemic disease. Diagnosis is by endoscopy and biopsy. Much of the tumor may be submucosal, and an assiduous attempt at biopsy is neces-

sary. Primary lymphoma is usually nodular with enlarged gastric folds. A diffusely infiltrative process akin to linitis plastica is more suggestive of secondary gastric involvement by lymphoma. A diligent search for extragastric disease is necessary before the diagnosis of localized primary gastric lymphoma is made. This includes EUS; CT scanning of the chest, abdomen, and pelvis; and bone marrow biopsy. Most patients with high-grade gastric lymphoma are currently treated with chemotherapy and radiation, without surgical resection. Treatment-related perforation or bleeding is unusual but recognized. For disease limited to the stomach and regional nodes, radical subtotal D2 gastrectomy may be performed, especially for bulky tumors with bleeding and/or obstruction. Palliative gastrectomy for tumor complications also has a role. Certainly, a multidisciplinary team should be involved with the treatment plan for patients with primary gastric lymphoma.

Gastrointestinal Stromal Tumor

GISTs arise from interstitial cells of Cajal (ICC) and are distinct from leiomyoma and leiomyosarcoma, which arise from smooth muscle.[108,109] Prognosis in patients with GIST tumors depends mostly on tumor size and mitotic count, and metastasis, when it occurs, is typically by the hematogenous route. Any lesion >1 cm can behave in a malignant fashion and may recur. Thus, all GISTs are best resected along with a margin of normal tissue. Almost all GISTs (and almost no smooth muscle tumors) express c-KIT (CD117) or the related PDGFRA, as well as CD34; almost all smooth muscle tumors (and almost no GISTs) express actin and desmin. These markers can often be detected on specimens obtained by fine-needle aspiration[110]and are useful in differentiating between GIST and smooth muscle tumor histopathologically. Lesions that are definitively leiomyoma by current histopathologic criteria are adequately treated by enucleation. Lesions that are definitively GIST or leiomyosarcoma are best treated by resection with negative margins. Most equivocal lesions should be resected provided that the patient is a reasonable operative risk.

Two thirds of all GISTs occur in the stomach. Epithelial cell stromal GIST is the most common cell type arising in the stomach, and cellular spindle type is the next most common. The glomus tumor type is seen only in the stomach.

GISTs are submucosal tumors that are slow growing. Smaller lesions are usually found incidentally, although they occasionally may ulcerate and cause impressive bleeding. Larger lesions generally produce symptoms of weight loss, abdominal pain, fullness, early satiety, and bleeding. An abdominal mass may be palpable. Metastasis is by the hematogenous route, often to liver and/or lung, although positive lymph nodes are occasionally seen in resected specimens.

Diagnosis is by endoscopy and biopsy, although the interpretation of the latter may be problematic. EUS may be helpful, but symptomatic tumors and tumors >1 cm in size should be removed. Metastatic work-up entails CT of the chest, abdomen, and pelvis (chest x-ray may suffice in lieu of CT of the chest). Most gastric GISTs occur in the body of the stomach, but they also can occur in the fundus or antrum. They are almost always solitary. Wedge resection with clear margins is adequate surgical treatment. True invasion of adjacent structures by the primary tumor is evidence of malignancy. If safe, en bloc resection of involved surrounding organs is appropriate to remove all tumor when the primary is large and invasive. Five-year survival following resection for GIST is about 50%. Most patients with low-grade lesions are cured (80% 5-year survival), but most patients with high-grade lesions are not (30% 5-year survival).

GISTs are usually positive for the protooncogene, c-kit, a characteristic shared with the ICC. Imatinib (Gleevec), a chemotherapeutic agent that blocks the activity of the tyrosine kinase product of c-kit, yields excellent results in many patients with metastatic or unresectable GIST. Up to 50% of treated patients develop resistance to imatinib by 2 years, and several newer agents show promise for patients with refractory disease. An algorithm for the treatment of patients with GIST is shown in Fig. 26-59.

Gastric Carcinoid Tumors[111–113]

Compared to midgut and hindgut locations, carcinoid tumors of the stomach are rather unusual. Gastric carcinoids comprise about

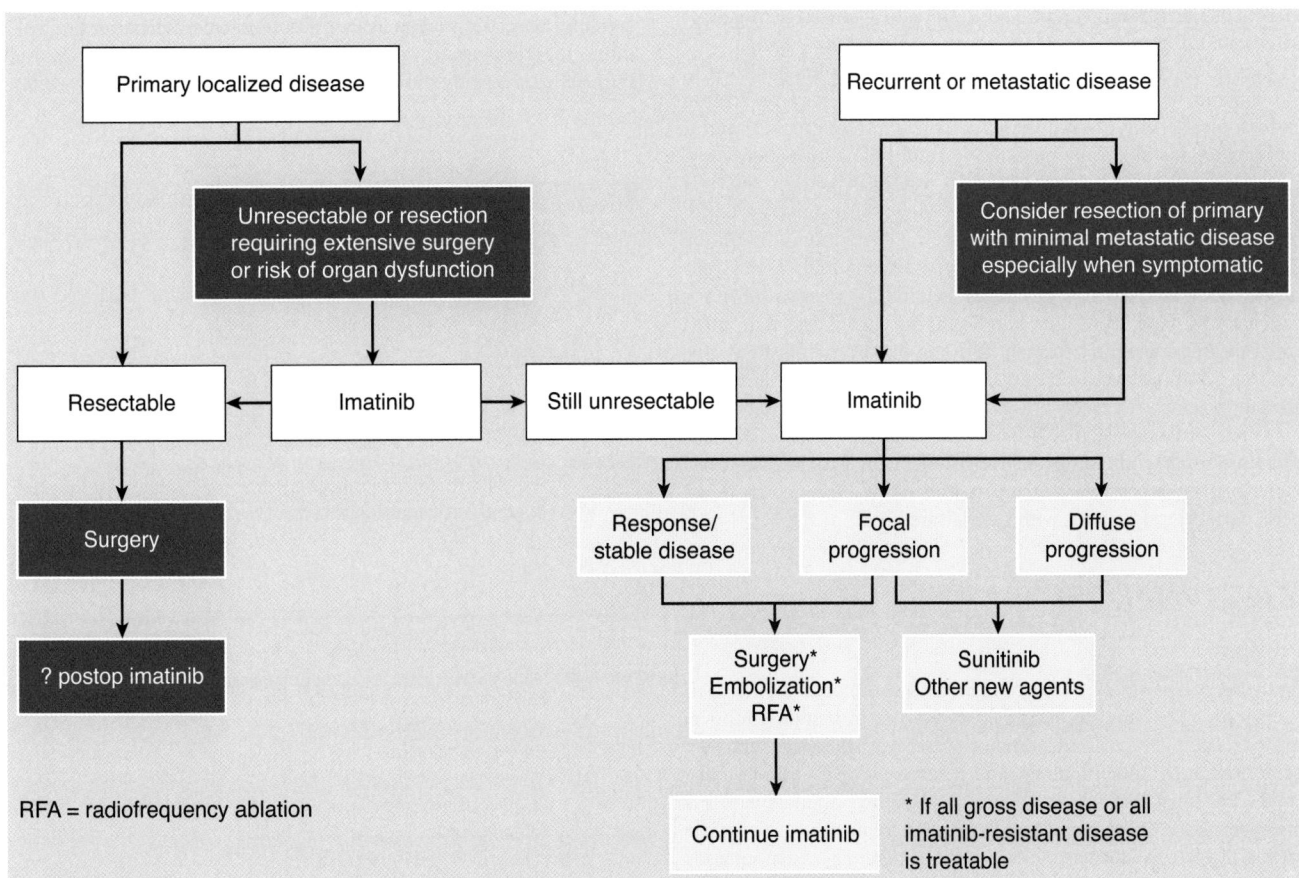

FIG. 26-59. Algorithm for the treatment of gastrointestinal stromal tumor. *(Reproduced with permission from Gold JS, DeMatteo RP: Combined surgical and molecular therapy: The gastrointestinal stromal tumor model. Ann Surg 244:176, 2006.)*

1% of all carcinoid tumors and less than 2% of gastric neoplasms. They arise from gastric enterochromaffin-like (ECL) cells and clearly have malignant potential. The apparent incidence of gastric carcinoids is increasing, perhaps related to the more common use of upper endoscopy and/or the increasing use of acid suppressive medication. The latter may cause hypergastrinemia, and gastrin has a recognized trophic effect on gastric ECL cells.

Gastric carcinoids are classified into one of three different types. Type I is the most common type of gastric carcinoid, accounting for about 75% of patients. Type I carcinoids occur in patients with chronic hypergastrinemia secondary to pernicious anemia or chronic atrophic gastritis. These lesions occur more frequently in women, are often multiple and small, and have low malignant potential (<5% metastasize). The role of long-term acid suppression with resultant hypergastrinemia in the pathogenesis of type I gastric carcinoids is unclear.

Type II gastric carcinoids are associated with MEN1 and ZES. These lesions also tend to be small and multiple, but have a somewhat higher malignant potential than type I lesions (10% metastasize). Type II gastric carcinoids are more strongly associated with MEN1; they are quite uncommon in patients with sporadic ZES without MEN1. Gastric acid hypersecretion, hypergastrinemia, and gastric carcinoid imply gastrinoma until proven otherwise.

Type III gastric carcinoids are sporadic tumors. They are usually solitary (usually >2 cm) and occur more commonly in men. They are not associated with hypergastrinemia and biopsy shows a heterogeneous cell population. Most patients have nodal or distant metastases at the time of diagnosis, and some present with symptoms of carcinoid syndrome.

Gastric carcinoids are usually diagnosed with endoscopy and biopsy. Some tumors are submucosal and may be quite small. They are often confused with heterotopic pancreas or small leiomyomas. Biopsy may be difficult because of the submucosal location, and EUS can be helpful in defining the size and depth of the lesion. Plasma chromogranin A levels are elevated in patients with gastric carcinoid. CT scan and octreotide scan are useful for staging.

Gastric carcinoids should be resected. Small lesions confined to the mucosa (typically type I or type II lesions) may be treated endoscopically with EMR if there are only a few lesions (<5) and if margins are histologically negative. Careful follow-up is necessary. Larger lesions should be removed by D1 or D2 gastrectomy. Survival is excellent for node-negative patients (>90% 5-year survival); node-positive patients have a 50% 5-year survival. Gastrinoma should be resected if located in patients with type II carcinoid. The 5-year survival for patients with type I gastric carcinoid is close to 100%; for patients with type III lesions, the 5-year survival is less than 50%. Somatostatin analogue treatment is useful in controlling the symptoms of carcinoid syndrome but apparently does not prolong survival in patients with metastatic gastric carcinoid. Surgical debulking may have a role in selected patients with metastatic disease. Because somatostatin has an antiproliferative effect on gastric ECL cells, there may be a possible primary treatment role for octreotide in poor-risk surgical patients with gastric carcinoid.

BENIGN GASTRIC NEOPLASMS

Polyps

Epithelial polyps are the most common benign tumor of the stomach (Table 26-22). There are essentially five types of benign epithelial polyps (Table 26-23): adenomatous, hyperplastic (regenerative), hamartomatous, inflammatory, and heterotopic (e.g., ectopic pancreas). The most common gastric polyp (about 75% in most series) is the hyperplastic or regenerative polyp, which frequently occurs in the setting of gastritis and has a low malignant potential. Adenomatous polyps may undergo malignant transformation, similarly to adenomas in the colon. They constitute about 10 to 15% of gastric polyps. Hamartomatous, inflammatory, and heterotopic polyps have negligi-

ble malignant potential (including fundic gland polyps). Polyps that are symptomatic, >2 cm, or adenomatous should be removed, usually by endoscopic snare polypectomy. Consideration should also be given to removing hyperplastic polyps, especially if large. Repeat EGD for surveillance should be done following removal of adenomatous polyps, and, perhaps, after removal of hyperplastic polyps as well.

Leiomyoma

The typical leiomyoma is submucosal and firm. If ulcerated, it has an umbilicated appearance and may bleed. Histologically, these lesions appear to be of smooth muscle origin. Lesions <2 cm are usually asymptomatic and benign. Larger lesions have greater malignant potential and a greater likelihood to cause symptoms such as bleeding, obstruction, or pain. Asymptomatic lesions <2 cm may be carefully observed or enucleated if fine-needle aspiration and immune markers confirm smooth muscle tumor; larger lesions and symptomatic lesions should be removed by wedge resection (often

TABLE 26-22 Benign polypoid lesions of the stomach

Type of Lesion	Total Number	Percent
Epithelial polyp	252	40.9
Leiomyoma	230	37.3
Inflammatory polyp	29	4.7
Heterotopic tissue	25	4.1
Lipoma	21	3.4
Neurogenic tumor	19	3.1
Vascular tumor	13	2.1
Eosinophilic granuloma	12	1.9
Fibroma	9	1.5
Miscellaneous lesions	6	1.0
Total	616	100.0

Source: Modified with permission from Ming S-C (ed): Tumors of the Esophagus and Stomach, *AFIP Atlas of Tumor Pathology,* Second Series, Fascicle 7. Washington DC: American Registry of Pathology, 1973, p 82, Table VIII.

TABLE 26-23 Histology of gastric epithelial polyps

I. Neoplastic polyp
  A. Benign: adenoma
    1. Flat (tubular) adenoma
    2. Papillary (villous) adenoma
  B. Malignant
    1. Primary polypoid carcinoma and carcinoid
    2. Secondary epithelial tumors
II. Non-neoplastic polyp
  A. Hyperplastic polyp
    1. Focal (polypoid) foveolar hyperplasia
    2. Hyperplastic (regenerative) polyp
    3. Hyperplastic polyp with dysplastic (adenomatous) lesion
  B. Hamartomatous polyp
    1. Peutz-Jeghers polyp
    2. Juvenile polyp
    3. Fundic gland polyp
  C. Inflammatory polyp
    1. Inflammatory pseudopolyp
    2. Inflammatory (retention) polyp
    3. Heterotopic polyp
  D. Ectopic pancreatic tissue
    1. Brunner gland hyperplasia
    2. Adenomyoma
  E. Nodular mucosal remnants

Source: Reproduced with permission from Ming S-C, Hirota T: Malignant epithelial tumors of the stomach, in Ming S-C, Goldman H (eds): *Pathology of the Gastrointestinal Tract,* 2nd ed. Baltimore: Williams & Wilkins, 1998.

possible laparoscopically). When lesions thought to be leiomyoma are observed rather than resected, the patient should be made aware of their presence and the small possibility for malignancy.

Lipoma

Lipomas are benign submucosal fatty tumors that are usually asymptomatic, found incidentally on upper GI series or EGD. Endoscopically, they have a characteristic appearance; there also is a characteristic appearance on EUS. Excision is unnecessary unless the patient is symptomatic.

Gastric Motility Disorders

Gastric motility disorders include delayed gastric emptying (gastroparesis), rapid gastric emptying, and motor and sensory abnormalities (e.g., functional dyspepsia). Surgically relevant secondary disorders of gastric motility (e.g., dumping, gastric stasis, and Roux syndrome) are discussed below under Postgastrectomy Problems. Gastroparesis is the most surgically relevant primary disorder of gastric motility.[114,115]

Most patients with primary gastroparesis present with nausea and vomiting. Bloating, early satiety, and abdominal pain are common. Eighty percent of these patients are women; some are diabetic. Postprandial vomiting significantly complicates the management in the latter group: Frequently, the patient takes parenteral insulin, eats and then vomits, becoming dangerously hypoglycemic. In patients with gastroparesis, it is important to rule out mechanical gastric outlet obstruction, and small-bowel obstruction. An upper GI series may suggest slow gastric emptying and relative atony, or it may be normal. EGD may show bezoars, but is frequently normal. Gastric emptying scintigraphy shows delayed solid emptying, and often delayed liquid emptying. Gastroparesis can be a manifestation of a variety of problems (Table 26-24). Medical treatment includes promotility agents, antiemetics, and, perhaps, botulinum injection into the pylorus.

Surgeons need to understand the role of surgery in primary gastroparesis. If appropriate, the patient with severe diabetic gastroparesis should be evaluated for pancreas transplant before any invasive abdominal procedure, because some patients improve substantially after pancreas transplant. If the diabetic gastroparetic patient is not a candidate for pancreas transplant, both gastrostomy (for decompression) and jejunostomy tubes (for feeding and prevention of hypoglycemia) can be effective. Infection and wound problems are more common in diabetics with transabdominal tubes than in nondiabetics. Other surgical options include implantation of a gastric pacemaker, and gastric resection. Generally, gastric resection should be done infrequently, if at all, for primary gastroparesis.

Massive Upper Gastrointestinal Bleeding

Although there have been arbitrary definitions of "massive" upper GI bleeding put forth, perhaps the most practical definition in the current era would be acute bleeding proximal to the ligament of Treitz, which requires blood transfusion. In multiple series, the stomach and proximal duodenum is by far the most common source of pathology associated with this diagnosis.[65,116] The most common causes of acute GI bleeding in emergency room or hospitalized patients are peptic ulcer, gastritis, Mallory-Weiss syndrome, and esophagogastric varices. Less common causes include benign or malignant neoplasm, angiodysplasia, Dieulafoy's lesion, portal gastropathy, Ménétrier's disease, and watermelon stomach. Arterioenteric fistula should always be considered in the patient who has an aortic graft or who has undergone repair of a visceral artery aneurysm.

The most important issues in the early hospital management of patients with acute upper GI bleeding are resuscitation and risk stratification. Large-bore IV access and Foley catheterization is accomplished, and nasogastric intubation is considered. Risk stratification is essentially accomplished by answering the following questions:

1. What is the magnitude and acuity of the hemorrhage? Hypotension, tachycardia, oliguria, low hematocrit, pallor, altered menta-

TABLE 26-24 Etiology of gastroparesis

Idiopathic
Endocrine or metabolic
  Diabetes mellitus
  Thyroid disease
  Renal insufficiency
After gastric surgery
  After resection
  After vagotomy
Central nervous system disorders
  Brain stem lesions
  Parkinson's disease
Peripheral neuromuscular disorders
  Myotonia dystrophica
  Duchenne muscular dystrophy
Connective tissue disorders
  Scleroderma
  Polymyositis/dermatomyositis
Infiltrative disorders
  Lymphoma
  Amyloidosis
Diffuse gastrointestinal motility disorder
  Chronic intestinal pseudo-obstruction
Medication-induced
Electrolyte imbalance
  Potassium, calcium, magnesium
Miscellaneous conditions
  Infections (especially viral)
  Paraneoplastic syndrome
  Ischemic conditions
  Gastric ulcer

Source: Reproduced with permission from Parkman HP, Fisher RS: Disorders of gastric emptying, in Yamada T et al (eds): *Textbook of Gastroenterology*, 4th ed. Philadelphia: Lippincott Williams & Wilkins, 2003, p 1297.

tion, and/or hematemesis suggest a large blood loss that has occurred over a short period of time. This is a high-risk situation.
2. Does the patient have significant chronic disease, particularly lung, liver, kidney, and/or heart disease, which compromises physiologic reserve? If yes, this is a high-risk situation.
3. Is the patient anticoagulated, or immunosuppressed? If yes, this is a high-risk situation.
4. On endoscopy, is the patient bleeding from varices, or is there active bleeding, or is there a visible vessel, or is there a deep ulcer overlying a large vessel (e.g., posterior duodenal ulcer overlying the gastroduodenal artery)? Could the patient be bleeding from an arterioenteric fistula? If yes, this is a high-risk situation.

If judged to be low risk, most patients will stop bleeding with supportive treatment and IV PPI. Selected patients may be discharged from the emergency room and managed on an outpatient basis.

If the patient is judged to be high risk based on one or more of the questions above, then the following should be done immediately:

1. Type and crossmatch for transfusion of blood products.
2. Admit to ICU or monitored bed in specialized unit.
3. Consult surgeon.
4. Consult gastroenterologist.
5. Start continuous infusion of PPI.
6. Perform upper endoscopy within 12 hours, after resuscitation and correction of coagulopathy. Endoscopic hemostasis should be considered in most high-risk patients with acute upper GI bleeding.

Although the surgeon should be involved early in the hospital course of all high-risk patients with acute upper GI bleeding, most of these patients will be adequately managed without operation. Mucosal lesions can usually be controlled with endoscopic hemotherapy and medical management. Occasionally, arteriography can be helpful.[117] Operation for bleeding ulcer is discussed above (see Operation for Bleeding Peptic Ulcer and Fig. 26-43).

Isolated Gastric Varices

Isolated gastric varices are those that occur in the absence of esophageal varices and are classified as type 1 (fundic) or type 2 (distal to fundus including proximal duodenum).[118] The presence of isolated gastric varices is usually associated with portal hypertension or splenic vein thrombosis. Although there is a significant bleeding risk from isolated gastric varices on long-term follow-up, there is no indication for the routine application of prophylactic measures.

Patients with acute upper GI bleeding from isolated gastric varices should be considered high risk. Although data are limited, octreotide and/or vasopressin infusion may decease bleeding, if tolerated. Balloon tamponade with a Sengstaken-Blakemore tube may provide temporary control of exsanguinating hemorrhage from type 1 isolated gastric varices, but if this is used, endotracheal intubation for airway protection is prudent. Endoscopic treatment with sclerotherapy or varix ligation is less successful than in esophageal varices, but should be considered. Interventional radiology should be consulted and balloon occluded retrograde transvenous obliteration considered. A transjugular intrahepatic portosystemic shunt may be useful if there is nonsegmental portal hypertension. If the patient has splenic vein thrombosis and left-sided (sinistral) or segmental portal hypertension, splenectomy is quite effective in controlling bleeding from isolated gastric varices. The operative mortality is 5%. Liver transplantation should always be considered in the cirrhotic patient before any abdominal operation.

Hypertrophic Gastropathy (Ménétrier's Disease)

There are two clinical syndromes characterized by epithelial hyperplasia and giant gastric folds: ZES and Ménétrier's disease. The latter is characteristically associated with protein-losing gastropathy and hypochlorhydria. There are large rugal folds in the proximal stomach, and the antrum is usually spared. Mucosal biopsy shows diffuse hyperplasia of the surface mucus-secreting cells and usually decreased parietal cells (Fig. 26-60). It has recently been suggested that Ménétrier's disease is caused by local overexpression of transforming growth factor alpha in the gastric mucosa, which stimulates the epidermal growth factor receptor, a receptor tyrosine kinase, on gastric SECs. This results in the selective expansion of surface mucous cells in the gastric body and fundus. A few patients with this unusual disease have been successfully treated with the epidermal growth factor receptor blocking monoclonal antibody cetuximab.[119]

Most patients with Ménétrier's disease are middle-aged men who present with epigastric pain, weight loss, diarrhea, and hypoproteinemia. There may be an increased risk of gastric cancer. Sometimes, the disease regresses spontaneously. Gastric resection may be indicated for bleeding, severe hypoproteinemia, or cancer.

Watermelon Stomach (Gastric Antral Vascular Ectasia)

The parallel red stripes atop the mucosal folds of the distal stomach give this rare entity its sobriquet. Histologically, gastric antral vascular ectasia is characterized by dilated mucosal blood vessels that often contain thrombi, in the lamina propria. Mucosal fibromuscular hyperplasia and hyalinization often are present (Fig. 26-61). The histologic appearance can resemble portal hypertensive gastropathy, but the latter usually affects the proximal stomach, whereas watermelon stomach predominantly affects the distal stomach. Beta blockers and nitrates, useful in the treatment of portal hypertensive gastropathy, are ineffective in patients with gastric antral vascular ectasia. Patients with the latter diagnosis are usually elderly women with chronic GI blood loss requiring transfusion. Most have an associated autoimmune connective tissue disorder, and at least 25% have chronic liver disease. Nonsurgical treatment options include estrogen and progesterone, and endoscopic treatment with the neodymium yttrium-aluminum garnet (Nd:YAG) laser or argon plasma coagulator.[120] Antrectomy may be required to control blood loss, and this operation is quite effective but carries increased morbidity in this elderly patient group. Patients with portal hypertension and antral vascular ectasia should be considered for transjugular intrahepatic portosystemic shunt.

Dieulafoy's Lesion

Dieulafoy's lesion is a congenital arteriovenous malformation characterized by an unusually large tortuous submucosal artery. If this artery is eroded, impressive pulsatile bleeding may occur. To the operating surgeon, this appears as a stream of arterial blood emanating from what appears grossly to be a normal gastric mucosa. The lesion typically occurs in middle-aged or elderly men and may be more common in patients with liver disease.[121] Patients typically present with upper GI bleeding, which may be intermittent, and endoscopy can miss the lesion if it is not actively bleeding. Treatment options include endoscopic hemostatic therapy, angiographic embolization, or operation. At surgery, the lesion may be oversewn or resected.

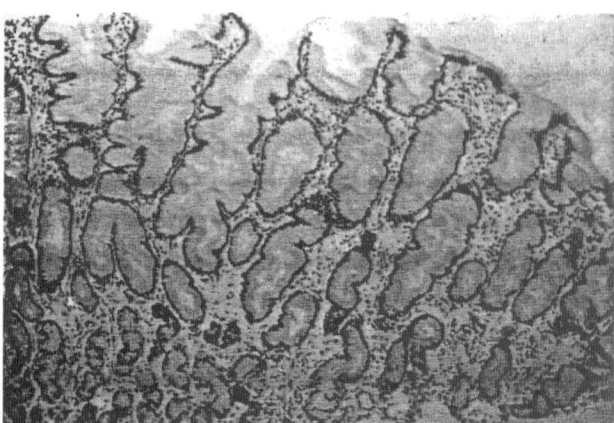

FIG. 26-60. Mucosal biopsy in Ménétrier's disease. *[Reproduced with permission from Goldman H: Mucosal hypertrophy and hyperplasia of the stomach, in Ming S-C, Goldman H (eds): Pathology of the Gastrointestinal Tract, 2nd ed. Baltimore: Williams & Wilkins, 1998, p 577.]*

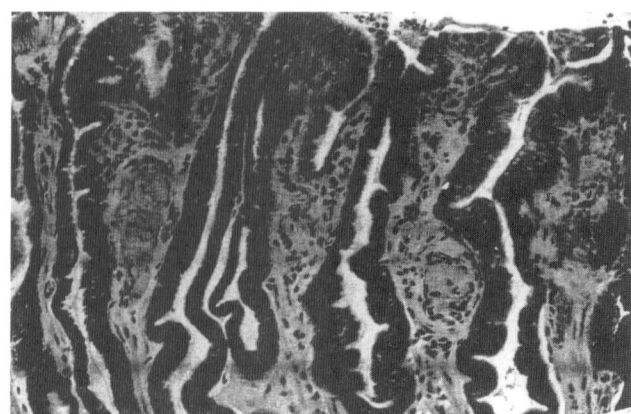

FIG. 26-61. Gastric antral vascular ectasia (watermelon stomach). *[Reproduced with permission from Goldman H: Mucosal hypertrophy and hyperplasia of the stomach, in Ming S-C, Goldman H (eds): Pathology of the Gastrointestinal Tract, 2nd ed. Baltimore: Williams & Wilkins, 1998, p 577.]*

Bezoars/Diverticula

Bezoars are concretions of undigestible matter that accumulate in the stomach. Trichobezoars, composed of hair, occur most commonly in young women who swallow their hair (Fig. 26-62). Phytobezoars are composed of vegetable matter and, in the United States, are usually seen in association with gastroparesis or gastric outlet obstruction. They also are associated with persimmon ingestion. Most commonly, bezoars produce obstructive symptoms, but they may cause ulceration and bleeding. Diagnosis is suggested by upper GI series and confirmed by endoscopy. Treatment options include enzyme therapy (papain, cellulase, or acetylcysteine), endoscopic disruption and removal, or surgical removal.

Gastric diverticula are usually solitary and may be congenital or acquired. Congenital diverticula are true diverticula and contain a full coat of muscularis propria, whereas acquired diverticula (perhaps caused by pulsion) usually have a negligible outer muscle layer. Most gastric diverticula occur in the posterior cardia or fundus (Fig. 26-63). Most of the time gastric diverticula are asymptomatic. However, they can become inflamed and may produce pain or bleeding. Perforation is rare. Asymptomatic diverticula do not require treatment, but symptomatic lesions should be removed. This can often be done laparoscopically.

Foreign Bodies

Ingested foreign bodies are usually asymptomatic. Removal of sharp or large objects should be considered. This can usually be done endoscopically, with an overtube technique. Recognized dangers include aspiration of the foreign body during removal, and rupture of drug-containing bags in "body packers." Both complications can be fatal. Surgical removal is recommended in body packers, and in patients with large jagged objects. Corrosive objects (e.g., watch batteries) should be removed promptly.

Mallory-Weiss Syndrome

The Mallory-Weiss lesion is a longitudinal tear in the mucosa of the GE junction.[122] It is presumably caused by forceful vomiting and/or

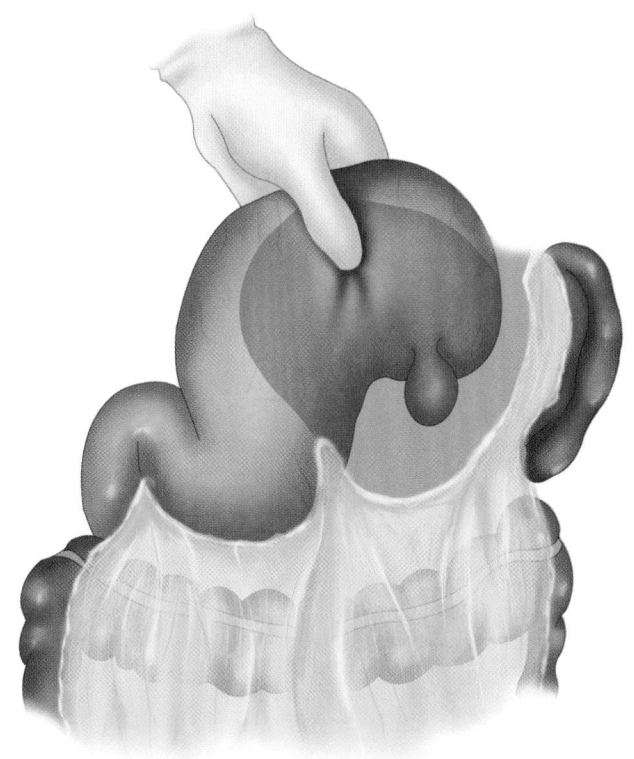

FIG. 26-63. Gastric diverticulum. *[Reproduced with permission from Ellis H: Diverticula, volvulus, superior mesenteric artery syndrome, and foreign bodies, in Schwartz SL, Ellis H, Husser WC (eds):* Maingot's Abdominal Operations, *9th ed. East Norwalk, Connecticut: Appleton & Lange, 1989, p 577.]*

retching, and is commonly seen in alcoholics. It commonly presents with impressive upper GI bleeding, often with hematemesis. Endoscopy confirms the diagnosis and may be useful in controlling the bleeding, but 90% of patients stop bleeding spontaneously. Other options to control the bleeding include balloon tamponade, angiographic embolization, or selective infusion of vasopressin, systemic vasopressin, and operation. Surgical treatment consists of oversewing the bleeding lesion through a long gastrotomy.

Volvulus

Gastric volvulus is a twist of the stomach that usually occurs in association with a large hiatal hernia. It also can occur in patients with an unusually mobile stomach without hiatal hernia. Typically, the stomach twists along its long axis (organoaxial volvulus), and the greater curvature flips up (Fig. 26-64C). If the stomach twists around the transverse axis, it is called *mesenteroaxial rotation* (Fig. 26-64A and Fig. 26-64B). Usually, volvulus is a chronic condition that can be surprisingly asymptomatic. In these instances, expectant nonoperative management is usually advised, especially in the elderly. The risk of strangulation and infarction has been overestimated in asymptomatic patients. Symptomatic patients should be considered for operation, especially if the symptoms are severe and/or progressive. Patients usually present with symptoms of pain and pressure related to the intermittently distending and poorly emptying twisted stomach. Pressure on the lung may produce dyspnea, pressure on the pericardium may produce palpitations, and pressure on the esophagus may produce dysphagia. Symptoms are often relieved with vomiting or passage of a nasogastric tube. Gastric infarction is a surgical emergency, and the patient often presents moribund. Elective operation for gastric volvulus usually involves reduction of the stomach and repair of hiatal hernia, with or without gastropexy. Gastropexy alone may be considered for high-risk patients. A laparoscopic approach should be considered and, if possible, the herniated portion of the stomach should be reduced and secured in the abdomen.

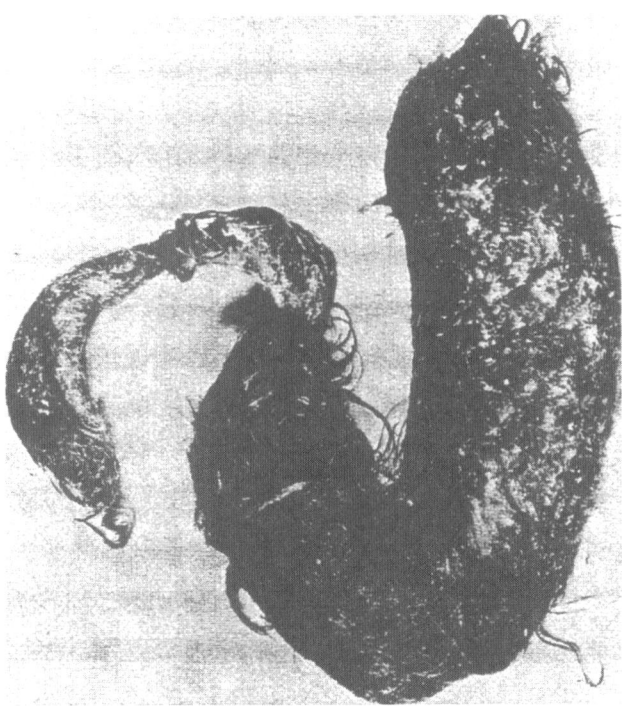

FIG. 26-62. Trichobezoar forming cast of stomach and duodenum; removed from 15-year-old girl. *[Reproduced with permission from DeBakey M, Ochsner A: Bezoars and concretions.* Surgery 4:934, 1938. Copyright Elsevier.]*

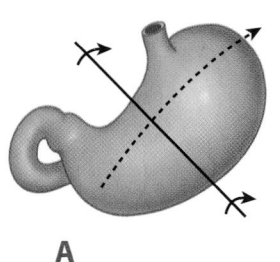 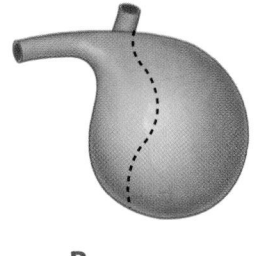 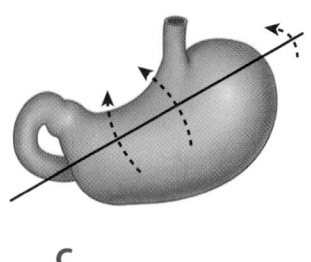

A   **B**   **C**

FIG. 26-64. A through C. Gastric volvulus. *[Reproduced with permission from Buchanan J: Volvulus of the stomach.* Br J Surg *18:99, 1930.]*

GASTROSTOMY

A gastrostomy is performed either for alimentation or for gastric drainage/decompression. Gastrostomy may be done percutaneously, laparoscopically, or via open technique.[123,124] Currently, percutaneous endoscopic gastrostomy is the most common method used. The open techniques include the Stamm method (Fig. 26-65), the Witzel method (Fig. 26-66), and the Janeway method (Fig. 26-67). The latter is meant to create a permanent stoma that can be intubated as needed, but does not drain spontaneously. The Janeway gastrostomy is more complicated than the other open techniques, and is rarely necessary. By far the most common technique is the Stamm gastrostomy, which can be performed open or laparoscopically.

Complications of gastrostomy include infection, dislodgment, and aspiration pneumonia. Although gastrostomy tubes usually do prevent tense gastric dilatation, they may not adequately drain the stomach, especially when the patient is bedridden.

Postgastrectomy Problems[125,126]

A variety of abnormalities affect some patients after a gastric operation that has usually been performed because of ulcer or tumor or severe obesity. Some of the more common disorders result from disturbance of the normal anatomic and physiologic mechanisms that control gastric motor function, and a discussion of these follows.

Dumping Syndrome

Dumping is a phenomenon caused by the destruction or bypass of the pyloric sphincter.[127] However, other factors undoubtedly play a role because dumping can occur after operations that preserve the pylorus,

such as parietal cell vagotomy. The appropriate stimulus can provoke dumping symptoms, even in some patients who have not undergone surgery. Clinically significant dumping occurs in 5 to 10% of patients after pyloroplasty, pyloromyotomy, or distal gastrectomy, and consists of a constellation of postprandial symptoms ranging in severity from annoying to disabling. The symptoms are thought to be the result of the abrupt delivery of a hyperosmolar load into the small bowel. This usually is due to ablation of the pylorus, but decreased gastric compliance with accelerated emptying of liquids (e.g., after highly selective vagotomy) is another accepted mechanism. About 15 to 30 minutes after a meal, the patient becomes diaphoretic, weak, light-headed, and tachycardic. These symptoms may be ameliorated by recumbence or saline infusion. Crampy abdominal pain is not uncommon and diarrhea often follows. This is referred to as *early dumping*, and should be distinguished from postprandial (reactive) hypoglycemia, also called *late dumping*, which usually occurs later (2 to 3 hours following a meal), and is relieved by the administration of sugar. A variety of hormonal aberrations have been observed in early dumping, including increased VIP, CCK, neurotensin, peripheral hormone peptide YY, renin-angiotensin-aldosterone, and decreased atrial natriuretic peptide. Late dumping is associated with hypoglycemia and hyperinsulinemia.

The medical therapy for the dumping syndrome consists of dietary management and somatostatin analogue (octreotide). Often, symptoms improve if the patient avoids liquids during meals. Hyperosmolar liquids (e.g., milk shakes) may be particularly troublesome. There is some evidence that adding dietary fiber compounds at mealtime may improve the syndrome. If dietary manipulation fails, the patient is started on octreotide, 100 μg subcutaneously twice daily. This can be increased up to 500 μg twice daily if necessary. The long-acting depot octreotide preparation is useful. Octreotide not only

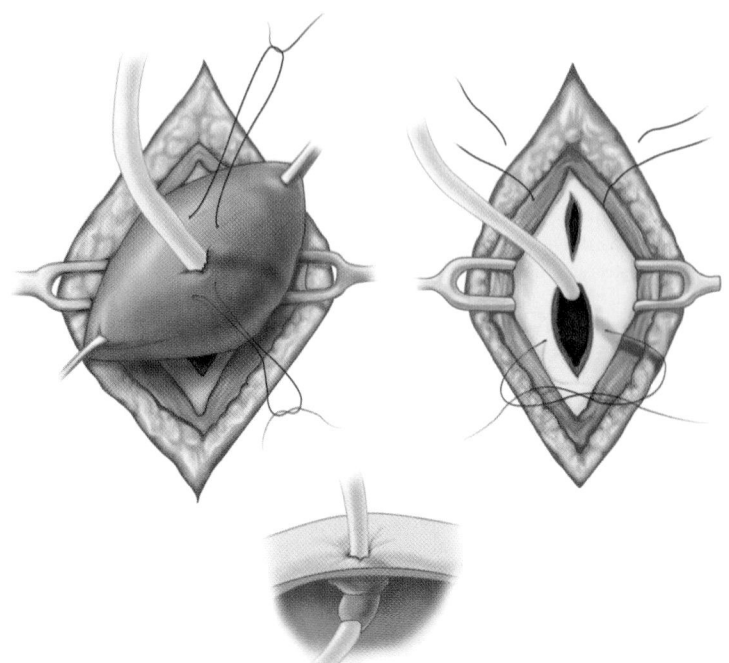

FIG. 26-65. Stamm gastrostomy. *[Reproduced with permission from Tatum RP, Joehl RJ: Intubation of the stomach and small intestine, in Zuidema GD, Yeo CJ (eds):* Shackelford's Surgery of the Alimentary Tract, *5th ed., Vol. II. Philadelphia: Saunders, 2002, p 46.]*

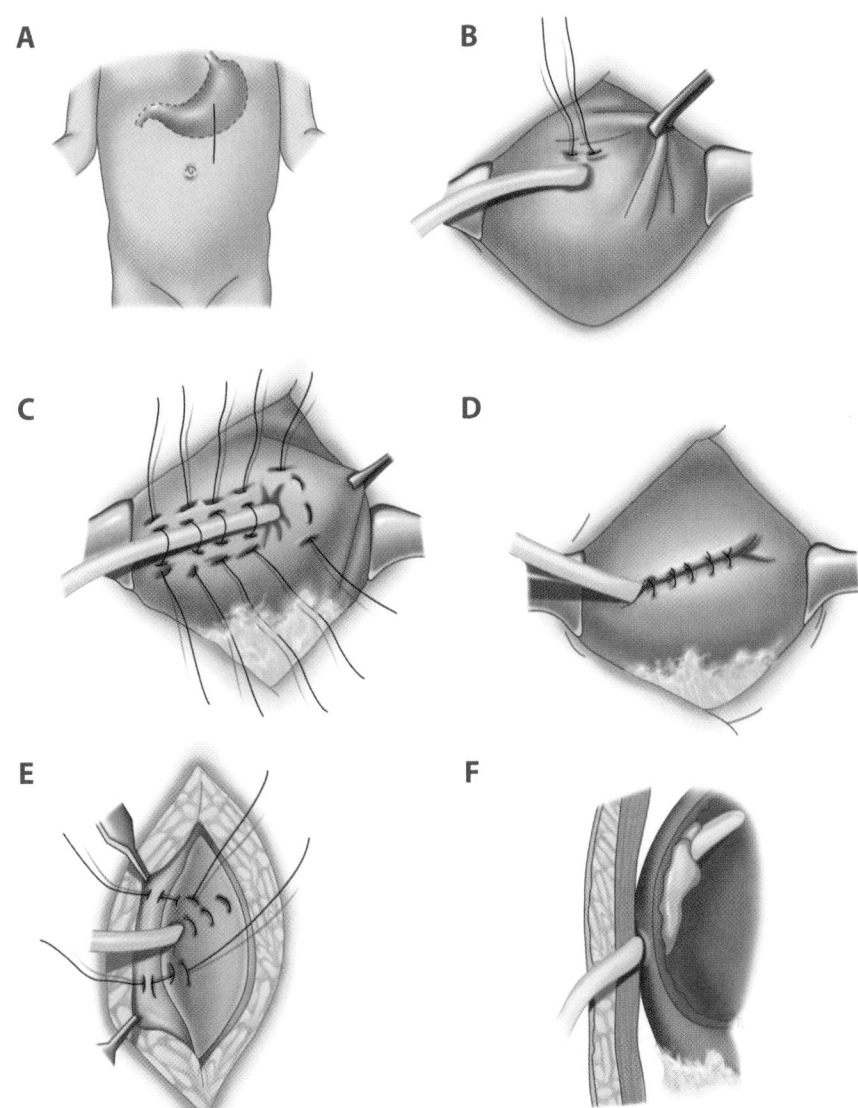

FIG. 26-66. A through **F.** Witzel gastrostomy. *[Reproduced with permission from Tatum RP, Joehl RJ: Intubation of the stomach and small intestine, in Zuidema GD, Yeo CJ (eds):* Shackelford's Surgery of the Alimentary Tract, *5th ed., Vol. II. Philadelphia: Saunders, 2002, p 46.]*

ameliorates the abnormal hormonal pattern seen in patients with dumping symptoms, but also promotes restoration of a fasting motility pattern in the small intestine (i.e., restoration of the MMC). The α-glucosidase inhibitor acarbose may be particularly helpful in ameliorating the symptoms of late dumping.

Only a small percentage of patients with dumping symptoms ultimately require surgery. Most patients improve with time (months and even years), dietary management, and medication. Therefore, the surgeon should not rush to reoperate on the patient with dumping symptoms. Multidisciplinary nonsurgical management must be optimized first. Before reoperation, a period of inhospital observation is useful to define the severity of the patient's symptoms. Patient compliance with dietary and medical therapy also can be assessed.

The results of remedial operation for dumping are variable and unpredictable. There are a variety of surgical approaches, none of which work consistently well. Additionally, there is not a great deal of experience reported in the literature with any of these methods. Long-term follow-up is rare. Operations performed to treat disabling dumping syndrome include pyloric reconstruction, takedown of gastrojejunostomy, interposition of a 10-cm reversed intestinal segment between the stomach and duodenum, conversion of Billroth II to Billroth I anastomosis, and conversion to Roux-en-Y anastomosis.

Patients with disabling dumping after gastrojejunostomy can be considered for simple takedown of this anastomosis provided that there is some vagal innervation to the antrum, and the pyloric channel is open endoscopically. The reversed intestinal segment is rarely used today—and rightly so. This operation interposes a 10-cm

reversed segment of intestine between the stomach and the proximal small bowel. This slows gastric emptying, but often leads to obstruction, requiring reoperation. Isoperistaltic interposition (Henley loop) has not been successful in ameliorating severe dumping over the long term. The Roux-en-Y gastrojejunostomy is associated with delayed gastric emptying, probably on the basis of disordered motility in the Roux limb. Taking advantage of this disordered physiology, surgeons have used this operation successfully in the management of the dumping syndrome. Although this is probably the procedure of choice in the small group of patients requiring operation for severe dumping following gastric resection, gastric stasis may result, particularly if a large gastric remnant is left. In the presence of significant gastric acid secretion, marginal ulceration is common after both jejunal interposition and Roux-en-Y procedures; thus concomitant vagotomy and hemigastrectomy should be considered. The theoretical possibility of treating postpyloroplasty dumping with a Roux-en-Y to the proximal duodenum (the duodenal switch, a potentially reversible operation) has not been reported (Fig. 26-68). Because pyloric ablation seems to be the dominant factor in the etiology of dumping, it is not surprising that conversion of Billroth II to Billroth I anastomosis has not been successful in the treatment of dumping.

Diarrhea

Diarrhea following gastric surgery may be the result of truncal vagotomy, dumping, or malabsorption. Truncal vagotomy is associated with clinically significant diarrhea in 5 to 10% of patients. It occurs

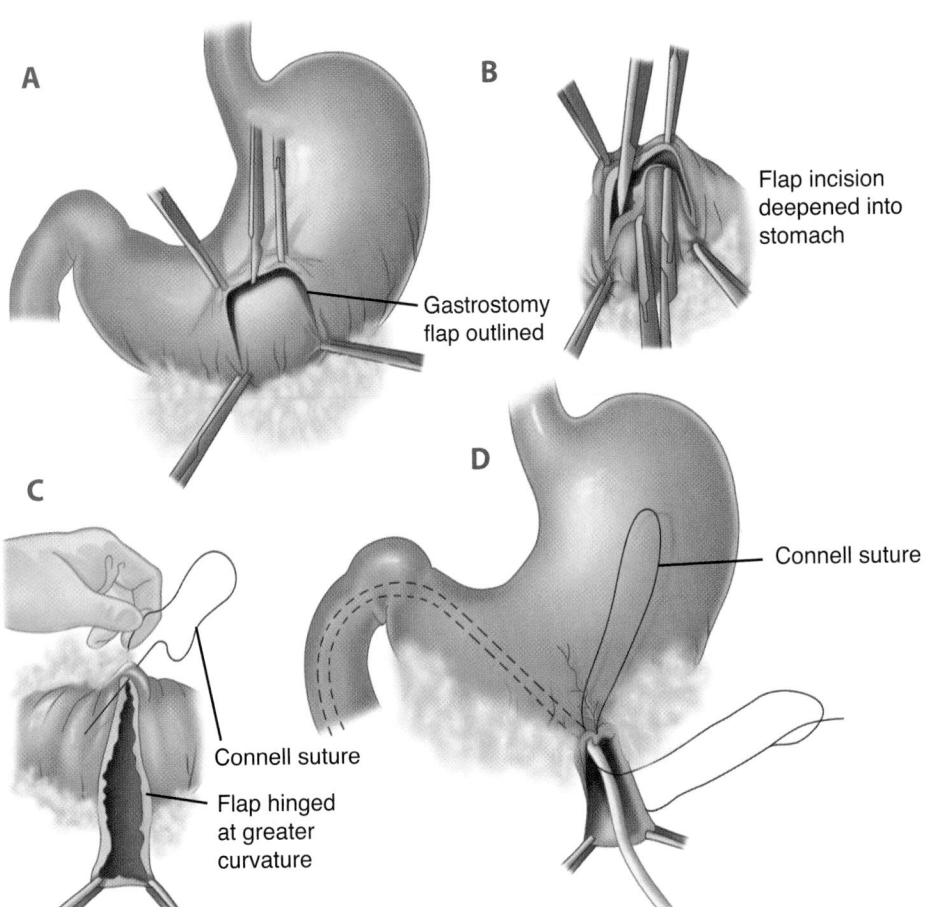

A

B

Flap incision
deepened into
stomach

Gastrostomy
flap outlined

C

D

Connell suture

Connell suture

Flap hinged
at greater
curvature

FIG. 26-67. **A** through **D.** Janeway gastrostomy. [*Reproduced with permission from Tatum RP, Joehl RJ: Intubation of the stomach and small intestine, in Zuidema GD, Yeo CJ (eds): Shackelford's Surgery of the Alimentary Tract, 5th ed., Vol. II. Philadelphia: Saunders, 2002, p 46.*]

soon after surgery and usually is not associated with other symptoms, a fact that helps to distinguish it from dumping. The diarrhea may be a daily occurrence, or there may be significant periods of relatively normal bowel function. The symptoms tend to improve over the months and years after the index operation. The cause of postvagotomy diarrhea is unclear. Possible mechanisms include intestinal dysmotility and accelerated transit, bile acid malabsorption, rapid gastric emptying, and bacterial overgrowth. The latter problem is facilitated by decreased gastric acid secretion and (even small) blind loops. Although bacterial overgrowth can be confirmed with the hydrogen breath test, a simpler test is an empirical trial of oral antibiotics. Some patients with postvagotomy diarrhea respond to cholestyramine, while in others codeine or loperamide may be useful. Another theoretical cause of diarrhea following gastric surgery is fat malabsorption due to acid inactivation of pancreatic enzymes or poorly coordinated mixing of food and digestive juices. This can be confirmed with a qualitative test for fecal fat and treated with acid suppression. Postvagotomy diarrhea usually does not respond to treatment with pancreatic enzymes. In the rare patient who is debilitated by postvagotomy diarrhea that is unresponsive to medical management, the operation of choice is a 10-cm reversed jejunal interposition placed in continuity 100 cm distal to the ligament of Treitz. Another option is the onlay antiperistaltic distal ileal graft. Both operations can cause obstructive symptoms and/or bacterial overgrowth.

Gastric Stasis[128,129]

Gastric stasis following surgery on the stomach may be due to a problem with gastric motor function or be caused by an obstruction. The gastric motility abnormality may have been pre-existing and unrecognized by the operating surgeon. Alternatively, it may be secondary to deliberate or unintentional vagotomy, or resection of the dominant gastric pacemaker. An obstruction may be mechanical

(e.g., anastomotic stricture, efferent limb kink from adhesions or constricting mesocolon, or a proximal small-bowel obstruction) or functional (e.g., retrograde peristalsis in a Roux limb). Gastric stasis presents with vomiting (often of undigested food), bloating, epigastric pain, and weight loss.

The evaluation of a patient with suspected postoperative gastric stasis includes EGD, upper GI series, gastric emptying scan, and

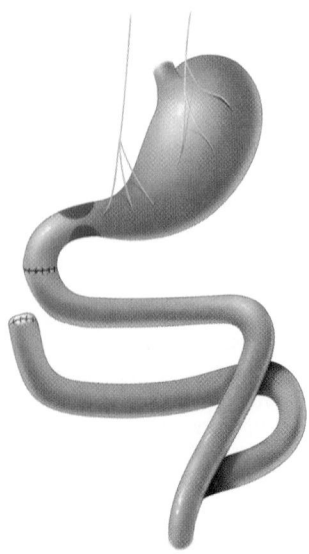

FIG. 26-68. Duodenal switch operation. [*Reproduced with permission from Hinder RA: Duodenal switch: A new form of pancreaticobiliary diversion. Surg Clin North Am 72:487, 1992. Copyright Elsevier.*]

gastric motor testing. Endoscopy shows gastritis and retained food or bezoar. The anastomosis and efferent limb should be evaluated for stricture or narrowing. Endoscopy may be facilitated by reviewing a recent upper GI series to help define the anatomy and to look for an area of obstruction. A dilated efferent limb suggests chronic stasis, either from a motor abnormality (e.g., Roux syndrome) or mechanical obstruction (e.g., chronic adhesion). Gastric emptying is best quantified clinically with scintigraphic techniques, which give a half-time for liquid and solid emptying. The former may be fairly normal, while the latter is profoundly delayed. If the problem is thought to be primarily a disorder of intrinsic motor function, newer techniques such as EGG and GI manometry should be considered. It should, however, be remembered that chronic mechanical obstruction may result in disordered motility in the proximal organ.

Once mechanical obstruction has been ruled out, medical treatment is successful in most cases of motor dysfunction following previous gastric surgery. This consists of dietary modification and promotility agents. Intermittent oral antibiotic therapy may be helpful in treating bacterial overgrowth, with its attendant symptoms of bloating, flatulence, and diarrhea.

Gastroparesis following V+D may be treated with subtotal (75%) gastrectomy. Billroth II anastomosis with Braun enteroenterostomy may be preferable to Roux-en-Y reconstruction. This latter option may be associated with persistent emptying problems that will subsequently require near-total or total gastrectomy, a nutritionally unattractive option. Delayed gastric emptying following ulcer surgery (V+D or V+A) may represent an anastomotic stricture (often due to recurrent ulcer), or proximal small bowel obstruction. The latter should be dealt with at reoperation. Recurrent ulcer usually responds to medical therapy. Endoscopic dilation is occasionally helpful. Gastroparesis following subtotal gastric resection is best treated with near-total (95%) or total gastric resection and Roux-en-Y reconstruction. If total gastrectomy is performed, a jejunal reservoir should be fashioned. Gastric pacing is promising, but it has not achieved widespread clinical usefulness in the treatment of postoperative gastric atony.

Bile Reflux Gastritis

Most patients who have undergone ablation or resection of the pylorus have bile in the stomach on endoscopic examination, along with some degree of gross or microscopic gastric inflammation. Therefore, attributing postoperative symptoms to bile reflux is problematic because most asymptomatic patients have bile reflux as well. However, it is generally accepted that a small subset of patients have bile reflux gastritis, and present with nausea, bilious vomiting, and epigastric pain, and *quantitative evidence* of excess enterogastric reflux. Curiously, symptoms often develop months or years after the index operation. The differential diagnosis includes afferent or efferent loop obstruction, gastric stasis, and small-bowel obstruction. Plain abdominal x-rays, upper endoscopy, upper GI series, abdominal CT scan, and gastric emptying scans are helpful in evaluating these possibilities.

Bile reflux may be quantified with gastric analysis or, more commonly, with scintigraphy (bile reflux scan). Typically, enterogastric reflux is greatest after Billroth II gastrectomy or gastrojejunostomy, and least after vagotomy and pyloroplasty, with Billroth I gastrectomy giving intermediate values. Patients who are well into the abnormal range may be considered for remedial surgery if symptoms are severe. Remedial surgery will eliminate the bile from the vomitus and may improve the epigastric pain, but it is quite unusual to render these patients completely asymptomatic, especially if they are narcotic dependent.

Bile reflux gastritis after distal gastric resection may be treated by one of the following options: Roux-en-Y gastrojejunostomy; interposition of a 40-cm isoperistaltic jejunal loop between the gastric remnant and the duodenum (Henley loop); or Billroth II gastrojejunostomy with Braun enteroenterostomy. To avoid bile reflux into the stomach, the Roux limb should be at least 45 cm long. The Braun enteroenterostomy should be placed a similar distance from the stomach. Excessively long limbs may be associated with obstruction

or malabsorption. All operations can result in marginal ulceration on the jejunal side of the gastrojejunostomy, and thus are combined with a generous distal gastrectomy. If this has already been done at a previous operation, the Roux or Braun operations may be attractively simple. Whether truncal vagotomy is necessary is controversial in the current era of excellent acid-suppressing medications. The benefits of decreased acid secretion following vagotomy may be outweighed by problems with vagotomy-associated dysmotility in the gastric remnant. The Roux operation may be associated with an increased risk of emptying problems compared to the other two options, but controlled data are lacking. Patients with debilitating bile reflux after gastrojejunostomy can be considered for simple takedown of this anastomosis provided that (a) there is some vagal innervation to the antrum and (b) the pyloric channel is open.

Primary bile reflux gastritis (i.e., no previous operation) is rare, and may be treated with the duodenal switch operation, essentially an end-to-end Roux-en-Y to the proximal duodenum (see Fig. 26-68). The Achilles' heel of this operation is, not surprisingly, marginal ulceration. Thus, it should be combined with highly selective vagotomy, and/or acid suppressive medication.

Roux Syndrome

A subset of patients who have had distal gastrectomy and Roux-en-Y gastrojejunostomy will have great difficulty with gastric emptying in the absence of mechanical obstruction. These patients present with vomiting, epigastric pain, and weight loss. This clinical scenario has been labeled the *Roux syndrome*. Endoscopy may show bezoar formation, dilation of the gastric remnant, and/or dilation of the Roux limb. An upper GI series confirms these findings and may show delayed gastric emptying. This is better quantified by a gastric emptying scan, which always shows delayed solid emptying, and may show delayed liquid emptying as well.

GI motility testing shows abnormal motility in the Roux limb, with propulsive activity toward, rather than away from, the stomach.[130] Gastric motility also may be abnormal. Presumably, the disordered motility in the Roux limb occurs in all patients with this operation. Why only a subset develops the Roux syndrome is unclear. Perhaps those patients with disordered gastric motility are at most risk. The disorder seems to be more common in patients with a generous gastric remnant. Truncal vagotomy also has been implicated.

Medical treatment consists of promotility agents. Surgical treatment consists of paring down the gastric remnant. If gastric motility is severely disordered, 95% gastrectomy should be done. The Roux limb should be resected if it is dilated and flaccid, unless doing so puts the patient at risk for short bowel problems. GI continuity may be reestablished with another Roux, a Billroth II with Braun enteroenterostomy, or an isoperistaltic jejunal interposition between the stomach and the duodenum (Henley loop). Truncal vagotomy should probably not be done. Long-term acid suppression may be necessary.

Gallstones

Gallstone formation following gastric surgery generally is thought to be secondary to vagal denervation of the gallbladder with attendant gallbladder dysmotility. Presumably, vagotomy causes stasis of gallbladder bile with subsequent sludge and stone formation. Other possible but incompletely investigated possibilities include postoperative ampullary dysfunction and changes in bile composition. It is unclear whether simply dividing the hepatic branches of the anterior vagal trunk (as is frequently done during antireflux and bariatric operations, as well as subtotal gastric resection) increases gallstone formation. Although prophylactic cholecystectomy is not justified with most gastric surgery, it should be considered if the gallbladder appears abnormal, especially if subsequent cholecystectomy is likely to be difficult. If preoperative evaluation reveals sludge or gallstones, or if intraoperative evaluation reveals stones, cholecystectomy should be done if it appears straightforward and the gastric operation has gone well.

Weight Loss

Patients who have an operation on the stomach commonly lose weight. In the case of bariatric surgery, this is intentional and meant to be a permanent effect of the operation. In antireflux surgery, this is usually transient, and attributed to the temporary dietary modification required in the first few postoperative weeks as the patient compensates for mild dysphagia and early satiety. Severe (>10% ideal body weight) or permanent weight loss after antireflux surgery indicates a significant problem and should prompt a diagnostic work-up. Possible causes include a tight or slipped wrap, gastric stasis (due to vagal injury or a missed motor disorder), bacterial overgrowth and malabsorption, or an unrecognized preoperative problem (commonly a motor disorder).

Weight loss is common in patients who have had a vagotomy and/or gastric resection. The degree of weight loss tends to parallel the magnitude of the operation. It may be insignificant in the large person, or devastating in the asthenic female. The surgeon should always consider the possible consequences before performing a gastric resection for benign disease in a thin female. The causes of weight loss after gastric surgery generally fall into one of two categories: altered dietary intake or malabsorption. If a stool stain for fecal fat is negative, it is likely that decreased caloric intake is the cause. This is the most common cause of weight loss after gastric surgery, and may be due to small stomach syndrome, postoperative gastroparesis, or self-imposed dietary modification because of dumping and/or diarrhea. Consultation with an experienced dietitian may prove invaluable.

Anemia

Iron absorption takes place primarily in the proximal GI tract, and is facilitated by an acidic environment. Intrinsic factor, essential for the enteric absorption of vitamin B_{12}, is made by the parietal cells of the stomach. Vitamin B_{12} bioavailability also is facilitated by an acidic environment.

With this as background, it is easy to understand why patients who have had a gastric operation are at risk for anemia. Anemia is the most common metabolic side effect in patients who have had a gastric bypass for morbid obesity. It also occurs in up to one third of patients who have had a vagotomy and/or gastric resection. Iron deficiency is the most common cause, but vitamin B_{12} or folate deficiency also occurs, even in patients who have not had total gastrectomy. Of course, patients who have had a total gastrectomy will all develop B_{12} deficiency without parenteral vitamin B_{12}. Gastric bypass patients should be given oral iron supplements, and monitored for iron, B_{12}, and folate deficiency. Patients who have had a vagotomy and/or gastrectomy should be similarly monitored with periodic determination of hematocrit, red blood cell indices, iron and transferrin levels, B_{12}, and folate levels. Marginal nutrient status should be corrected with oral and/or parenteral supplementation.

Bone Disease

Gastric surgery sometimes disturbs calcium and vitamin D metabolism. Calcium absorption occurs primarily in the duodenum, which is bypassed with gastrojejunostomy. Fat malabsorption may occur because of blind loop syndrome and bacterial overgrowth, or because of inefficient mixing of food and digestive enzymes. This can significantly affect the absorption of vitamin D, a fat-soluble vitamin. Both abnormalities of calcium and vitamin D metabolism can contribute to metabolic bone disease in patients following gastric surgery. The problems usually manifest as pain and/or fractures years after the index operation. Musculoskeletal symptoms should prompt a study of bone density. Dietary supplementation of calcium and vitamin D may be useful in preventing these complications. Routine skeletal monitoring of patients at high-risk (e.g., elderly males and females and postmenopausal females) may prove useful in identifying skeletal deterioration that may be stopped with appropriate treatment.

LAPAROSCOPIC GASTRIC OPERATIONS

Perhaps the most common laparoscopic gastric operations performed today are for GERD and obesity (see Chap. 27, The Surgical Management of Obesity). However, all of the gastric operations described here can be performed with minimally invasive techniques.[131] Some are technically difficult (e.g., partial or total gastric resection) or are of debatable merit. The operations described in this chapter that lend themselves most readily to minimally invasive techniques are highly selective vagotomy, vagotomy and gastrojejunostomy, and gastrostomy. Laparoscopic wedge resection often is possible for GI stromal tumors, lipomas, or gastric diverticula. Combined endoscopic and laparoscopic techniques occasionally are useful. Diagnostic laparoscopy may prevent a futile laparotomy in some patients with gastric cancer. Robotic gastric operations have been described, but have not yet been widely adopted.[132] The transgastric route figures prominently in animal models of natural orifice translumenal endoscopic surgery,[6] but the clinical future of this new frontier is unclear.

REFERENCES

Entries highlighted in bright blue are key references.

1. Beaumont W: *Experiments and Observations on the Gastric Juice and the Physiology of Digestion.* Plattsburgh, NY: PP Allen, 1833.
2. Wangensteen OH, Wangensteen SD: Gastric surgery, in *The Rise of Surgery.* Minneapolis: University of Minnesota Press, 1978.
3. Herrington JL: Historical aspects of gastric surgery, in Scott HW Jr., Sawyers JL (eds): *Surgery of the Stomach, Duodenum, and Small Intestine,* 2nd ed. Boston: Blackwell, 1992.
4. Dragstedt LR: Vagotomy for the gastroduodenal ulcer. *Ann Surg* 122:973, 1945.
5. Zollinger RM, Ellison EH: Primary peptic ulcerations of the jejunum associated with islet cell tumors of the pancreas. *Ann Surg* 142:709, 1955.
6. Flora ED, Wilson TG, Martin IJ, et al: A review of natural orifice translumenal endoscopic surgery (NOTES) for intra-abdominal surgery: Experimental models, techniques, and applicability to the clinical setting. *Ann Surg* 247:583, 2008.
7. Mercer DW, Liu TH, Castaneda A: Anatomy and physiology of the stomach, in Zuidema GD, Yeo CJ (eds): *Shackelford's Surgery of the Alimentary Tract,* 5th ed, Vol. II. Philadelphia: Saunders, 2002, p 3.
8. Warren WD, Zeppa R, Fomon JJ: Selective trans-splenic decompression of gastroesophageal varices by distal splenorenal shunt. *Ann Surg* 166:437, 1967.
9. Orringer MB, Marshall B, Chang AC, et al: Two thousand transhiatal esophagectomies: Changing trends, lessons learned. *Ann Surg* 246:363, 2007.
10. Leung WK, et al: Tumors of the stomach, in Yamada T, et al (eds): *Textbook of Gastroenterology,* 4th ed. Philadelphia: Lippincott, Williams & Wilkins, 2003, p 1416.
11. Kajitani T: Japanese Research Society for the Study of Gastric Cancer: The general rules for gastric cancer study in surgery and pathology. *Japn J Surg* 11:127, 1981.
12. Jansen EPM, Boot H, Verheij M, et al: Optimal locoregional treatment in gastric cancer. *J Clin Oncol* 23:4509, 2005.
13. Johnson L, et al: *Physiology of the Gastrointestinal Tract,* 4th ed. Academic Press, 2006.
14. Bloom W, Fawcett DW: *A Textbook of Histology.* Philadelphia: Saunders, 1975, p 639.
15. Ashley SW, Evoy D, Daly JM: Stomach, in Schwartz SI (ed): *Principles of Surgery,* 7th ed. New York: McGraw-Hill, 1999, p 1181.
16. Antonioli DA, Madara JL: Functional anatomy of the gastrointestinal tract, in Ming S-C, Goldman H (eds): *Pathology of the Gastrointestinal Tract,* 2nd ed. Baltimore: Williams & Wilkins, 1998, p 13.
17. Feldman M: Gastric secretion, in Feldman M (ed): *Sleisenger and Fordtran's Gastrointestinal and Liver Disease,* 7th ed. Philadelphia: Saunders, 2002, p 715.
18. Cadle RM, Mansouri MD, Logan N, et al: Association of proton-pump inhibitors with outcomes in *Clostridium difficile* colitis. *Am J Health Syst Pharm* 64:2359, 2007.
19. Williams C, McColl KEL: Proton pump inhibitors and bacterial overgrowth. *Aliment Pharmacol Ther* 23:3, 2006.

20. Mössner J, Caca K: Developments in the inhibition of gastric acid secretion. *Eur J Clin Invest* 35:469, 2005.

21. Wolfe MM, Soll AH: The physiology of gastric acid secretion. *N Engl J Med* 319:707, 1988.

22. Lloyd KCK, Debas HT: Hormonal and neural regulation of gastric acid secretion, in Johnson LR (ed): *Physiology of the Gastrointestinal Tract*, 3rd ed. New York: Raven, 1993.

23. Del Valle J, Todisco A: Gastric secretion, in Yamada T, et al (eds): *Textbook of Gastroenterology*, 4th ed. Philadelphia: Lippincott, Williams & Wilkins, 2003, p 266.

24. Wallace JL: Gastric resistance to acid: Is the "mucus-bicarbonate barrier" functionally redundant? *Am J Physiol* 256:31, 1989.

25. Allen A, Flemstrom G, et al: Gastroduodenal mucosal protection. *Physiol Rev* 73:823, 1993.

26. Cummings DE, Overduin J: Gastrointestinal regulation of food intake. *J Clin Invest* 117:13, 2007.

27. Badman MK, Flier JS: The gut and energy balance: Visceral allies in the obesity wars. *Science* 307:1909, 2005.

28. Murray CD, Kamm MA, Bloom SR, et al: Ghrelin for the gastroenterologist: History and potential. *Gastroenterology* 125:1492, 2003.

29. Ariyasu H, Takaya K, Tagami T, et al: Stomach is a major source of circulating ghrelin, and feeding state determines plasma ghrelin-like immunoreactivity levels in humans. *J Clin Endocrinol Metab* 86:4753, 2001.

30. Cummings DE, Weigle DS, Frayo RS, et al: Plasma ghrelin levels after diet-induced weight loss or gastric bypass surgery. *N Engl J Med* 346:1623, 2002.

31. Karamanakos SN, Vagenas K, Kalfarentzos F, et al: Weight loss, appetite suppression, and changes in fasting and postprandial ghrelin and peptide-YY levels after Roux-en-Y gastric bypass and sleeve gastrectomy: a prospective, double blind study. *Ann Surg* 247:401, 2008.

32. Sanjeevi A: Gastric motility. *Curr Opin Gastroenterol* 23:625, 2007.

33. Cullen JJ, Kelly KA: Gastric motor physiology and pathophysiology. *Surg Clin North Am* 73:1145, 1993.

34. Hasler WL: Physiology of gastric motility and gastric emptying, in Yamada T, et al (eds): *Textbook of Gastroenterology*, 4th ed. Philadelphia: Lippincott, Williams & Wilkins, 2003, p 195.

35. Chial HJ, Camilleri M: Motility disorders of the stomach and small intestine, in Friedman SL, McQuaid KR, Grendell JH (eds): *Current Diagnosis and Treatment in Gastroenterology*, 2nd ed. New York: McGraw-Hill, 2003, p 355.

36. Farrugia G: Interstitial cells of Cajal in health and disease. *Neurogastroenterol Motil* 20 Suppl 1:54, 2008.

37. Yeo CJ, Barry MK, Sauter PK, et al: Erythromycin accelerates gastric emptying after pancreaticoduodenectomy. A prospective, randomized, placebo-controlled trial. *Ann Surg* 218:229, 1993.

38. Marks JM, Ponsky JL: Diagnostic and therapeutic endoscopy of the stomach and small bowel, in Yeo CJ, et al (eds): *Shackelford's Surgery of the Alimentary Tract*, 6th ed. Philadelphia: Saunders, 2007.

39. Ezzeddine D, Ezzeddine B, McKenzie R, et al: Virtual gastroscopy: Initial attempt in North American patients. *J Gastroenterol Hepatol* 21:219, 2006.

40. Scheibl K, Schreyer AG, Kullmann F, et al: Magnetic resonance imaging gastrography: Evaluation of the dark lumen technique compared with conventional gastroscopy in patients with malignant gastric disease. *Invest Radiol* 40:164, 2005.

41. Shin KS, Kim SH, Han JK, et al: Three-dimensional MDCT gastrography compared with axial CT for the detection of early gastric cancer. *J Comput Assist Tomogr* 31:741, 2007.

42. Caddy GR, Chen RY: Current clinical applications of endoscopic ultrasound. *ANZ J Surg* 77:101, 2007.

43. Raj M, Chen RY: Interventional applications of endoscopic ultrasound. *J Gastroenterol Hepatol* 21:348, 2006.

44. Jones DB: Role of endoscopic ultrasound in staging upper gastrointestinal cancers. *ANZ J Surg* 77:166, 2007.

45. Balaji NS, Crookes PF, Banki F, et al: A safe and noninvasive test for vagal integrity revisited. *Arch Surg* 137:954, 2002.

46. Vaira D, Gatta L, Ricci C, et al: Review article: Diagnosis of *Helicobacter pylori* infection. *Aliment Pharmacol Ther* 16:16, 2002.

47. Walsh JH, Peterson WL: The treatment of *Helicobacter pylori* infection in the management of peptic ulcer disease. *N Engl J Med* 333:984, 1995.

48. Mertz HR, Walsh JH: Peptic ulcer pathophysiology. *Med Clin North Am* 75:799, 1991.

49. Peek RM Jr., Blaser MJ: Pathophysiology of *Helicobacter pylori*-induced gastritis and peptic ulcer disease. *Am J Med* 102:200, 1997.

50. Brock J, Sauaia A, Ahnen D, et al: Process of care and outcomes for elderly patients hospitalized with peptic ulcer disease: Results from a quality improvement project. *JAMA* 286:1985, 2001.

51. Spechler SJ: Peptic ulcer disease and its complications, in Feldman M (ed): *Sleisinger and Fordtran's Gastrointestinal and Liver Disease*, 7th ed. Philadelphia: Saunders, 2002, p 747.

52. Parsonnet J: Clinician-discoverers—Marshall, Warren, and *H. pylori*. *N Engl J Med* 353:2421, 2005.

53. Blaser MJ, Atherton JC: *Helicobacter pylori* persistence: Biology and disease. *J Clin Invest* 113:321, 2004.

54. Fox JG, Wang TC: Inflammation, atrophy, and gastric cancer. *J Clin Invest* 117:60, 2007.

55. Suerbaum S, Michetti P: *Helicobacter pylori* infection. *N Engl J Med* 347:1175, 2002.

56. Graham DY, Lew GM, Klein PD, et al: Effect of treatment of *Helicobacter pylori* infection on the long-term recurrence of gastric or duodenal ulcer: A randomized controlled study. *Ann Intern Med* 116:705, 1992.

57. Del Valle J, Chey WD, Scheiman JM: Acid peptic disorders, in Yamada T, et al (eds): *Textbook of Gastroenterology*, 4th ed. Philadelphia: Lippincott, Williams & Wilkins, 2003, p 1321.

58. Fisher WE, Brunicardi FC: Benign gastric ulcer, in Cameron JL (ed): *Current Surgical Therapy*, 9th ed. Philadelphia: Mosby Elsevier, 2008, p 81.

59. Laine L: Approaches to nonsteroidal anti-inflammatory drug use in the high-risk patient. *Gastroenterology* 120:594, 2001.

60. Bjorkman DJ: Current status of nonsteroidal anti-inflammatory drug (NSAID) use in the United States: Risk factors and frequency of complications. *Am J Med* 107:3S, 1999.

61. Chey WD, Wong BCY, Practice Parameters Committee of the American College of Gastroenterology: American College of Gastroenterology Guideline on the Management of *Helicobacter pylori* Infection. *Am J Gastroenterol* 102:1808, 2007.

62. Blatchford O, Murray WR: A risk score to predict need for treatment for upper gastrointestinal hemorrhage. *Lancet* 356:1318, 2000.

63. Boey J, Wong J: Perforated duodenal ulcers. *World J Surg* 11:319, 1987.

64. Dempsey DT: Peptic ulcer disease—obstruction, in Bland KI (ed): *The Practice of General Surgery*. Philadelphia: Saunders, 2001.

65. Dallal HJ, Palmer KR: Clinical review: Upper gastrointestinal hemorrhage. *BMJ* 323:1115, 2001.

66. Gralnek IM, Barkun AN, Bardou M: Management of acute bleeding from peptic ulcer. *N Engl J Med* 359:928, 2008.

67. Harbison SP, Dempsey DT: Peptic ulcer disease. *Curr Probl Surg* 42:346, 2005.

68. Mulholland MW, Debas HT: Chronic duodenal and gastric ulcer. *Surg Clin North Am* 67:489, 1987.

69. Tavakkolizadeh A, Ashley SW: Operations for peptic ulcer, in Yeo CJ, et al (eds): *Shackelford's Surgery of the Alimentary Tract*, 6th ed. Philadelphia: Saunders, 2007, p 791.

70. Gilliam AD, Speake WJ, Lobo DN, et al: Current practice of emergency vagotomy and *Helicobacter pylori* eradication for complicated peptic ulcer in the United Kingdom. *Brit J Surg* 90:88, 2003.

71. Reuben BC, Neumayer LA: Variations reported in surgical practice for bleeding duodenal ulcers. *Am J Surg* 192:e42, 2006

72. Lau JYW, Sung JJY, Lee KKC, et al: Effect of intravenous omeprazole on recurrent bleeding after endoscopic treatment of bleeding peptic ulcers. *N Engl J Med* 343:310, 2000.

73. Lau JYW, Sung JJY, Lam Y-H, et al: Endoscopic retreatment compared with surgery in patients with recurrent bleeding after initial endoscopic control of bleeding ulcers. *N Engl J Med* 340:751, 1999.

74. Kahi CJ, Jensen DM, Sung JJ, et al: Endoscopic therapy versus medical therapy for bleeding peptic ulcer with adherent clot: A meta-analysis. *Gastroenterology.* 129:855, 2005.

75. Gabriel SE, Jaakkimainen L, Bombardier C: Risk for serious gastrointestinal complications related to use of nonsteroidal anti-inflammatory drugs—a meta-analysis. *Ann Intern Med* 115:787, 1991.

76. Yusuf TE, Brugge WR: Endoscopic therapy of benign pyloric stenosis and gastric outlet obstruction. *Curr Opin Gastroenterol* 22:570, 2006.

77. Csendes A, Maluenda F, Braghetto I, et al: Prospective randomized study comparing three surgical techniques for the treatment of gastric outlet obstruction secondary to duodenal ulcer. *Am J Surg* 166:45, 1993.

78. Norton JA, Fraker DL, Alexander HR, et al: Surgery to cure the Zollinger-Ellison syndrome. *N Engl J Med* 341:635, 1999.

79. Gibril F, Schumann M, Pace A, et al: Multiple endocrine neoplasia type 1 and Zollinger-Ellison syndrome: A prospective study of 107 cases and comparison with 1009 cases from the literature. *Medicine* 83:43, 2004.

80. Dolan JP, Norton JA: Zollinger-Ellison Syndrome, in Yeo CJ, et al (eds): *Shackelford's Surgery of the Alimentary Tract*, 6th ed. Philadelphia: Saunders/Elsevier, 2007, p 862.

81. Orlando LA, Lenard L, Orlando RC: Chronic hypergastrinemia: Causes and consequences. *Dig Dis Sci* 52:2482, 2007.

82. Ying L, Harris A, Ying M, et al: Prophylaxis for stress-related gastrointestinal bleeding. Cochrane Upper Gastrointestinal and Pancreatic Diseases Group Cochrane Database of Systematic Reviews. 3, 2008.

83. Helmer KS, West SD, Shipley GL, et al: Gastric nitric oxide synthase expression during endotoxemia: implications in mucosal defense in rats. *Gastroenterology* 123:173, 2002.

84. Tablan OC, Anderson LJ, Besser R, et al: Healthcare Infection Control Practices Advisory Committee. Guidelines for preventing health-care–associated pneumonia, 2003: recommendations of CDC and the Healthcare Infection Control Practices Advisory Committee. *MMWR Recomm Rep* 53:1, 2004.

85. Jemal A, Siegel R, Ward E, et al: Cancer Statistics 2008. *Cancer J Clin* 58:71, 2008.

86. Correa P, Houghton J: Carcinogenesis of *Helicobacter pylori*. *Gastroenterology* 133:659, 2007.

87. Leung WK, Ng EKW, Sung JJY: Tumors of the stomach, in Yamada T, et al (eds): *Textbook of Gastroenterology*, 4th ed. Philadelphia: Lippincott, Williams & Wilkins, 2003.

88. McColl KE, Watabe H, Derakhshan MH: Role of gastric atrophy in mediating negative association between *Helicobacter pylori* infection and reflux oesophagitis, Barrett's oesophagus and oesophageal adenocarcinoma. *Gut* 57:721, 2008.

89. Zur Hausen A, van Rees BP, van Beek J, et al: Epstein-Barr virus in gastric carcinomas and gastric stump carcinomas: A late event in gastric carcinogenesis. *J Clin Pathol* 57:487, 2004.

90. Norton JA, Ham CM, Dam JV, et al: CDH1 truncating mutations in the E-cadherin gene: An indication for total gastrectomy to treat hereditary diffuse gastric cancer. *Ann Surg* 245:873, 2007.

91. Shimoyama S, Aoki F, Kawahara M, et al: Early gastric cancer development in a familial adenomatous polyposis patient. *Dig Dis Sci* 49:260, 2004.

92. Gylling A, Abdel-Rahman WM, Juhola M, et al: Is gastric cancer part of the tumour spectrum of hereditary non-polyposis colorectal cancer? A molecular genetic study. *Gut* 56:926, 2007.

93. Schaefer N, Sinning C, Standop J, et al: Treatment and prognosis of gastric stump carcinoma in comparison with primary proximal gastric cancer. *Am J Surg* 194:63, 2007.

94. Ono H, Kondo H, Gotoda T, et al: Endoscopic mucosal resection for treatment of early gastric cancer. *Gut* 48:225, 2001.

95. Chen J, Cheong JH, Yun MJ, et al: Improvement in preoperative staging of gastric adenocarcinoma with positron emission tomography. *Cancer* 103:2383, 2005.

96. Bentrem D, Wilton A, Mazumdar M, et al: The value of peritoneal cytology as a preoperative predictor in patients with gastric carcinoma undergoing a curative resection. *Ann Surg Oncol* 12:347, 2005.

97. Sarela AI, Lefkowitz R, Brennan MF, et al: Selection of patients with gastric adenocarcinoma for laparoscopic staging. *Am J Surg* 191:134, 2006.

98. Dicken BJ, Bigam DL, Cass C, et al: Gastric adenocarcinoma: Review and considerations for future directions. *Ann Surg* 241:27, 2005.

99. Cho CS, Brennan MF: Gastric adenocarcinoma, in Cameron JL (ed): *Current Surgical Therapy*, 9th ed. Philadelphia: Mosby, 2008.

100. Karpeh MS, Leon L, Klimstra D, et al: Lymph node staging in gastric cancer: Is location more important than number? An analysis of 1,038 patients. *Ann Surg* 232:362, 2000.

101. Saidi RF, ReMine SG, Dudrick PS, et al: Is there a role for palliative gastrectomy in patients with stage IV gastric cancer? *World J Surg* 30:21, 2006.

102. Fein M, Fuchs KH, Thalheimer A, et al: Long-term benefits of Roux-en-Y pouch reconstruction after total gastrectomy: A randomized trial. *Ann Surg* 247:759, 2008.

103. Bonenkamp JJ, Hermans J, Sasako M, et al: Extended lymph node dissection for gastric cancer. *N Engl J Med* 340:908, 1999.

104. Cuschieri A, Fayers P, Fielding J, et al: Postoperative morbidity and mortality after D1 and D2 resections for gastric cancer: Preliminary results of the MRC randomised controlled surgical trial. The Surgical Cooperative Group. *Lancet* 347:995, 1996.

105. Macdonald JS, Smalley SR, Benedetti J, et al: Chemoradiotherapy after surgery compared with surgery alone for adenocarcinoma of the stomach or gastroesophageal junction. *N Engl J Med* 345:725, 2001.

106. Sasako M, Sano T, Yamamoto S, et al: D2 lymphadenectomy alone or with para-aortic nodal dissection for gastric cancer. *N Engl J Med* 359:453, 2008.

107. Yoon SS, Coit DG, Portlock CS, et al: The diminishing role of surgery in the treatment of gastric lymphoma. *Ann Surg* 240:28, 2004.

108. Gold JS, DeMatteo RP: Combined surgical and molecular therapy: The gastrointestinal stromal tumor model. *Ann Surg* 244:176, 2006.

109. Rubin BP, Heinrich MC, Corless CL: Gastrointestinal stromal tumour. *Lancet* 369:1731, 2007.

110. Stelow EB, Murad FM, Debol SM, et al: A limited immunocytochemical panel for the distinction of subepithelial gastrointestinal mesenchymal neoplasms sampled by endoscopic ultrasound-guided fine-needle aspiration. *Am J Clin Pathol* 129:219, 2008

111. Raut CP, Kulke MH, Glickman JN, et al: Carcinoid tumors. *Curr Probl Surg* 43:383, 2006.

112. Modlin IM, Kidd M, Latich I, et al: Current status of gastrointestinal carcinoids. *Gastroenterology* 128:1717, 2005.

113. Mulkeen A, Cha C: Gastric carcinoid. *Curr Opin Oncol* 17:1, 2005.

114. Parkman HP, Hasler WL, Fisher RS: American Gastroenterological Association technical review on the diagnosis and treatment of gastroparesis. *Gastroenterology* 127:1592, 2004.

115. Yin J, Chen JD: Implantable gastric electrical stimulation: Ready for prime time? *Gastroenterology* 134:665, 2008.

116. Cappell MS, Friedel: Initial management of acute upper gastrointestinal bleeding-from initial evaluation to gastrointestinal endoscopy. *Med Clin North Am* 92:491, 2008.

117. Dempsey DT, Burke DR, Reilly RS, et al: Angiography in poor-risk patients with massive nonvariceal upper gastrointestinal bleeding. *Am J Surg* 159:282, 1990.

118. Zaman A: Portal hypertension related bleeding-management of difficult cases. *Clin Liver Dis* 10:353, 2006.

119. Coffey RJ, Washington MK, Corless CL, et al: Ménétrier disease and gastrointestinal stromal tumors: Hyperproliferative disorders of the stomach. *J Clin Invest* 117:70, 2007.

120. Sebastian S, O'Morain CA, Buckley MJ: Current therapeutic options for gastric antral vascular ectasia. *Aliment Pharmacol Ther* 18:157, 2003.

121. Akhras J, Patel P, Tobi M: Dieulafoy's lesion-like bleeding: An under-recognized cause of upper gastrointestinal hemorrhage in patients with advanced liver disease. *Dig Dis Sci* 52:722, 2007.

122. Harbison SP, Dempsey DT: Mallory-Weiss syndrome, in Cameron JL (ed): *Current Surgical Therapy*, 9th ed. Philadelphia: Mosby, 2008.

123. Schrag SP, Sharma R, Jaik NP, et al: Complications related to percutaneous endoscopic gastrostomy (PEG) tubes. A comprehensive clinical review. *J Gastrointestin Liver Dis* 16:407, 2007.

124. McClave SA: Critical care nutrition: Getting involved as a gastrointestinal endoscopist. *J Clin Gastroenterol* 40:870, 2006.

125. Dempsey DT: Reoperative gastric surgery and postgastrectomy syndromes, in Zuidema GD, Yeo CJ (eds): *Shackelford's Surgery of the Alimentary Tract*, 5th ed., Vol. II. Philadelphia: Saunders, 2002, p 161.

126. Meilahn JE, Dempsey DT: Postgastrectomy problems: Remedial operations and therapy, in Cameron JL (ed): *Current Surgical Therapy*, 8th ed. Philadelphia: Elsevier Mosby, 2004.

127. Ukleja A: Dumping syndrome: Pathophysiology and treatment. *Nutr Clin Pract* 20:517, 2005.

128. Forster-Barthell AW, Murr MM, Nitecki S, et al: Near-total completion gastrectomy for severe postvagotomy gastric stasis: Analysis of early and long-term results in 62 patients. *J Gastrointest Surg* 3:15, 1999.

129. Jones MP, Maganti K: A systematic review of surgical therapy for gastroparesis. *Am J Gastroenterol* 98:2122, 2003.

130. Van der Milje HC, Kleibeuker JH, Limburg AJ, et al: Manometric and scintigraphic studies of the relation between motility disturbances in the Roux limb and the Roux-en-Y syndrome. *Am J Surg* 166:11, 1993.

131. Farrell TM, Hunter JG: Laparoscopic surgery of the stomach and duodenum, in Zuidema GD, Yeo CJ (eds): *Shackelford's Surgery of the Alimentary Tract*, 5th ed., Vol. II. Philadelphia: Saunders, 2002, p 202.

132. Anderson C, Ellenhorn J, Hellan M, et al: Pilot series of robot-assisted laparoscopic assisted subtotal gastrectomy with extended lymphadenectomy for gastric cancer. *Surg Endosc* 21:1662, 2007.

THE DYNAMIC FIELD OF BARIATRIC SURGERY

The focus of this chapter is the surgical treatment of obesity. Bariatric surgery has been a dynamic surgical field, and changes have continued in recent years. The most substantial change is now the focus within the field on the recognized ability of surgical therapy to treat the metabolic consequences of obesity and not just obesity itself. Although the goal of bariatric surgery has always been to improve the medical condition of all patients for whom it is performed, a major emphasis is now being placed on the fact that resolution of the metabolic conditions that in severe obesity cause a variety of medical problems is as important as the actual amount of weight lost. This emphasis has been publicly recognized by the renaming of the professional society in the United States focusing on the surgical treatment of obesity from the American Society for Bariatric Surgery to the American Society for Metabolic and Bariatric Surgery.

Other major changes in the field of bariatric surgery in the United States since the last edition of this text include the increased popularity of the laparoscopic adjustable gastric banding procedure, the introduction of the sleeve gastrectomy as a primary weight loss operation, and the solidification of the laparoscopic approach to bariatric surgery as the optimal approach. The bariatric surgery community also has focused on improvement of outcomes and treatment for patients as well as documentation of the efficacy of bariatric surgery. A number of very important studies in front-line journals that have generated considerable public and medical attention have further confirmed the efficacy of bariatric surgery for producing durable long-term weight loss, improved survival, and improved resolution of comorbid medical problems compared with medical therapy. In an effort to encourage optimal outcomes at centers performing bariatric surgery, establishment of a "center of excellence" designation for institutions evolved from concept to reality. The process of institutional application for such center of excellence status has served to emphasize that many centers are now achieving outstanding outcomes for their bariatric operations, outcomes that are characterized by considerably lower rates of morbidity and mortality than were found in many studies whose results were previously published in the literature.

THE DISEASE OF OBESITY

Obesity is the second leading cause of preventable death in the United States, currently outranked only by smoking. However, this statement itself demonstrates the still incomplete appreciation of obesity as a disease entity, a concept that is still poorly understood. Obesity *is* a disease, and as such is in many respects not preventable. The components of this disease likely include a combination of environmental and genetic factors. The recent rapid rise in the incidence of obesity in less than a generation's time suggests that genetic causes alone cannot be responsible for the disease. Nevertheless, the multifactorial contributions to the disease increase the difficulty in understanding its causes.

The degrees of obesity are defined by body mass index, or BMI (calculated as weight in kilograms divided by height in meters squared), which correlates body weight with height. Patients are classified as overweight, obese, or severely obese (sometimes referred to as *morbidly obese*) (Table 27-1). Severely obese individuals generally exceed ideal body weight by 100 lb or more or are 100% over ideal body weight. A more metric, internationally accepted definition of severe or morbid obesity is a BMI of ≥ 35 kg/m^2. *Superobese* is a term sometimes used to describe individuals who have a BMI of >50 kg/m^2.

Prevalence and Contributing Factors

Severe obesity is reaching epidemic proportions in the United States. Since 1960, surveys of the prevalence of obesity have been

TABLE 27-1	Classification of obesity by body mass index (BMI)
Classification	**BMI Range (kg/m^2)**
Normal weight	20–25
Overweight	26–29
Obese	30–34
Severely obese	35–49
Superobese	≥ 50

KEY POINTS

1. Surgical therapy is the only effective and proven therapy for patients with severe obesity (body mass index of ≥ 35 kg/m^2). Bariatric operations prolong survival and resolve comorbid medical conditions associated with severe obesity.

2. Bariatric surgery is also metabolic surgery, treating the varied metabolic consequences of the comorbid diseases arising from severe obesity. Some operations are particularly effective treatments for such metabolic consequences, such as gastric bypass for type 2 diabetes.

3. Bariatric operations involve either restriction of caloric intake or malabsorption of nutrients, or both. Long-term follow-up is essential before the merits of an operation can be confirmed.

4. During the years 1999 to 2003, here called the *bariatric revolution*, the availability of a laparoscopic approach for bariatric operations caused major changes in the field, including a major increase in the number of procedures performed as well as an increased public and professional awareness and understanding of the field.

5. Laparoscopic gastric bypass is the most common procedure in the United States. The laparoscopic adjustable gastric band procedure is the most popular procedure performed outside the United States and is increasing in popularity in the United States.

6. Patients who develop a bowel obstruction after laparoscopic gastric bypass require surgical and not conservative therapy due to the high incidence of internal hernias and the potential for bowel infarction.

7. Malabsorptive operations are highly effective in producing durable weight loss but have considerable nutritional side effects. Patients undergoing such procedures require close follow-up and must take appropriate nutritional supplements.

8. All bariatric operations are tools that serve to allow the patient to lose weight, become healthier, and improve quality of life. These changes are maintained long term especially if the patient permanently adopts the new eating patterns and exercise habits that are taught and expected in the early year(s) after surgery.

conducted every decade by the National Center for Health Statistics. Obesity statistics have been updated annually since 1985. Twenty-five percent of adult Americans were overweight in 1980; by 1990 that number had risen to 34%. By 2004, 32.2% of adults were *obese*.[1] In 1990, conservative estimates put the number of Americans with a BMI between 35 and 40 kg/m² at 4 million, with an additional 4 million having a BMI exceeding 40 kg/m². Current estimates suggest that the population of patients with severe obesity (BMI >35 kg/m²) is greater than 15 million. Despite the expenditure of more than $30 billion annually on weight loss products, the prevalence of obesity is dramatically increasing. Obesity is most common in minorities, low-income groups, rural populations, and women, but is increasing in all socioeconomic groups.

The increase in obesity is multifactorial. Genetics plays an important role in the development of obesity. Although the children of parents of normal weight have a 10% chance of becoming obese, the children of two obese parents have an 80 to 90% chance of developing obesity by adulthood. The weight of adopted children correlates strongly with the weight of their birth parents. Furthermore, concordance rates for obesity in monozygotic twins are double those in dizygotic twins.[2]

Diet and culture are important factors as well. These environmental factors contribute significantly to the epidemic of obesity in the United States, because the rapid increase in obesity during the past two decades cannot be explained by any genetic cause.

Other factors appear to contribute significantly to severe obesity. Intermittent or consistent excessive caloric intake occurs. The lack of satiety, on a consistent or intermittent basis, appears to be strongly correlated with such episodes of excessive caloric ingestion. As yet the physiologic basis for such a lack of satiety is not understood. Other factors commonly suggested to play a role in the disease of obesity include decreased energy expenditure from reduced metabolic activity, reduction in the thermogenic response to meals, an abnormally high set point for body weight, and a decrease in the loss of heat energy. Another factor that may influence absorption of ingested food is the composition of the intraluminal bacteria of the intestinal tract. Recent studies have documented a difference in the composition of the intestinal flora of obese individuals compared with those of normal weight.[3]

Obese individuals have excessive adipose cells, in both size and number. The number of such cells often is determined early in life; adult-onset obesity is largely a product of an increase in adipose cell size. In children, however, weight gain results from increase in adipose cell size and cell number. Adipose tissue may be deposited in large quantities in the subcutaneous layer of the abdominal wall or the viscera. Males tend to have central visceral fat distribution, whereas females more often have a peripheral or gluteal fat distribution. Central or visceral fat distribution is associated with metabolic diseases such as diabetes, hypertension, and the metabolic syndrome.[4]

Concurrent Medical and Social Problems

The severely obese patient often has chronic weight-related problems, detailed later. However, the single most difficult aspect of the disease of severe obesity for those who have it is the discrimination they face from the rest of the population in terms of social stigmatization. This prejudice against obesity remains the last type of discrimination without legislative remedy. Obese individuals are routinely discriminated against in terms of employment. The design of public facilities often does not allow them to participate in activities. Examples include the inadequate size of airline seats and bathrooms, the lack of availability of appropriate clothing options, and the insufficient size of automobile cabins. Severely obese individuals are thought of by much of the public as being lazy or gluttonous and lacking self-discipline. They often endure not only discrimination and prejudice but also outright ridicule and disrespect. Consequently, the stigma of severe obesity has a major impact on social function and emotional well-being. Psychologic diseases such as depression therefore have an extraordinarily high incidence

in this population compared with the general public. Poor self-image is almost universal among these individuals as well.

Significant comorbidities, defined as medical problems associated with or caused by obesity, are numerous. The most prevalent and acknowledged of these include degenerative joint disease, low back pain, hypertension, obstructive sleep apnea, gastroesophageal reflux disease (GERD), cholelithiasis, type 2 diabetes, hyperlipidemia, hypercholesterolemia, asthma, hypoventilation syndrome of obesity, fatal cardiac arrhythmias, right-sided heart failure, migraine headaches, pseudotumor cerebri, venous stasis ulcers, deep vein thrombosis, fungal skin rashes, skin abscesses, stress urinary incontinence, infertility, dysmenorrhea, depression, abdominal wall hernias, and an increased incidence of various cancers such as those of the uterus, breast, colon, and prostate.[5]

Rarely conditions other than exogenous obesity cause excess body weight. Among these is Cushing's syndrome, which is associated with hirsutism, skin lesions, and wound-healing problems, and in rare cases has remained undiagnosed and is identified as the cause of obesity when the patient is evaluated for surgical therapy. After finding no elevated cortisol levels in obese patients in 15 years, we abandoned this screening blood test as being cost inefficient. In children, intractable eating can be associated with Prader-Willi syndrome. This syndrome has been refractory to all known bariatric operations.

Prognosis

Obesity has a profound effect on overall health and life expectancy, largely secondary to weight-related comorbidities. It is estimated that a man who is severely obese at age 21 will live 12 years less than a nonobese individual, and a severely obese woman will live 9 years less. The incidence of severe obesity in the population is comparable for females younger and older than 50 years of age, whereas for men the incidence of severe obesity declines above age 50. This is largely due to the fact that severely obese men often are dead of comorbid medical conditions, especially cardiac arrhythmias and coronary artery disease, by age 50. A study carried out by the Veterans Administration showed a 12-fold increase in mortality among 200 morbidly obese men aged 25 to 34 years and a 6-fold increase among those aged 35 to 44 years over a 7-year follow-up period.[6] Decreased quality of life also results from severe obesity. Most patients seeking surgical treatment of severe obesity do so because of the medical issues they face from comorbid conditions or the decreased quality of life they are experiencing as a result of severe obesity. As will be shown later, bariatric surgery can significantly prolong the life span of a severely obese individual as well as improve the quality of his or her life.

MEDICAL MANAGEMENT

Medical treatment for severe obesity is aimed at reducing body weight through a combination of decreased caloric intake and accompanying increases in energy expenditure from moderate exercise. This method of weight loss is the safest possible and may work well for obese individuals who have modest amounts of weight to lose to regain normal body weight or to return to being simply overweight instead of obese. For the severely obese individual, however, who usually must lose at least 75 lb or more to achieve elimination of obesity, this is a daunting and extremely difficult task. The success rate among severely obese patients who try dieting and exercise as a means of losing enough weight to no longer be obese and maintaining that weight loss is only approximately 3%.

Although success rates are limited with diet and exercise alone, all severely obese individuals are asked to attempt this route of weight loss before undertaking any surgical therapy. There are two main reasons for this. The first is to allow those who can achieve such weight loss through the safest possible means to do so. The second, and by far the more practical, is to have the severely obese individual begin to appreciate and practice the lifestyle changes that must ultimately become routine once weight loss is achieved, by whatever means. The adjustment of the patient's lifestyle to include these measures is valuable to long-term success with any bariatric operation.

The treatment of severe obesity should begin with simple lifestyle changes, including moderate reduction of caloric intake and initiation of an exercise plan. Walking is the most common choice of exercise in this population of patients, who may be unable to perform extremely vigorous exercise initially. Medical comorbidities must be identified and treated. Usually the patient's primary care physician will have already accomplished this, but we do at times identify obesity-related comorbidities on initial history taking and physical examination in our clinic.

The severely obese patient will usually have been given dietary counseling by his or her primary care physician and often will have been placed on a medically supervised diet. Most patients also have attempted commercially sponsored diets and diet plans. Success after starting such a program is not unusual, but sustained weight loss for more than a year after stopping the program is rare. Although primary care physicians usually do an outstanding job of identifying and treating comorbid medical problems, their offices usually do not have the related support staff of nutritionists and psychologists who often are very helpful in providing services to severely obese patients undergoing significant lifestyle changes.

Lifestyle changes involving diet, exercise, and behavior modification constitute the first tier of therapy for obesity. Dietary restriction and exercise can each independently create a caloric deficit. A daily energy deficit so created of 500 kcal/d, resulting in a weekly deficit of 3500 kcal, results in the loss of 1 lb of fat weekly. It has been shown that low-calorie diets (800 to 1500 kcal/d) are as effective as very-low-calorie diets at 1 year but result in a lower rate of nutritional deficiencies.[7] Such diets may produce an average of 8% body weight loss over a 6-month period. Longer follow-up shows recidivism. Moderate daily physical activity can produce a 2 to 3% body weight loss.[8]

A behavioral modification program that provided desirable rewards for meeting short-term dietary or exercise requirements, used in combination with diet and exercise, produced as much as a 10% weight loss at 6 months in one study. This weight loss was only sustained in 60% of patients at 40 weeks,[9] and at 1 year the average sustained weight loss was decreased to 8.6%.[10]

Dietary, exercise, or behavior modification therapy is appropriate treatment for patients who are overweight (BMI <30 kg/m^2) and is highly recommended for patients with a BMI between 30 and 35 kg/m^2. Most of the studies looking at dietary therapy do not include a patient population that is largely obese (BMI >30 kg/m^2). Dietary therapy can be effective in producing improvements in comorbid conditions such as diabetes mellitus, with weight loss of 2.3 to 3.7% influencing the disease.[11] Thus lifestyle changes can be effective in improving the health of the nonobese. Efficacy for the obese population is not as well documented, and there are no studies published to date that demonstrate significant, long-term efficacy of medical therapy for the severely obese.

Pharmacologic therapy is also an option for patients attempting to lose weight. Unfortunately, the number of effective pharmacologic agents is small compared with the number of products sold with assertions that they will promote or support weight loss. Pharmacotherapy is normally used only after lifestyle changes and dietary therapies have failed. It is used either alone as the primary therapy or in conjunction with simultaneous diet and exercise therapy. Currently there are only two drugs approved by the U.S. Food and Drug Administration for the treatment of obesity that promote weight loss. Sibutramine is a noradrenaline and 5-hydroxytryptamine reuptake inhibitor that works as an appetite suppressant. Orlistat inhibits gastric and pancreatic lipase enzymes that promote lipid absorption in the intestine.[12] Either of these drugs may produce a weight loss of between 6 and 10% of body weight after 1 year, but cessation of the drug usually results in prompt regaining of lost weight.[13] Pharmacotherapy is recommended as an adjunctive or supplementary therapy to lifestyle changes, including diet and exercise or behavioral therapy, by the National Institutes of Health (NIH) consensus guidelines for treatment of obesity.[14]

Because medical therapies are almost uniformly ineffective for patients with severe obesity, the severely obese patient tends to continue to gain weight. The number and strength of prescribed medications slowly increases as the medical comorbidities become increasingly worse. Unfortunately, for the majority of severely obese patients, this process continues unabated until death results eventually from the comorbidities. Until recently, <1% of severely obese patients underwent surgical treatment for obesity annually. That number has now increased but still is not over 2% of individuals. Even when one counts patients referred for surgery and felt to be poor candidates, it is likely that <5% of patients with severe obesity are referred on an annual basis. Part of the issue may be patient aversion to surgical therapy. Because of societal messages, the patient may feel self-blame for being obese and hence feel that surgery is either too drastic or an admission of weakness.

The recent national advertising campaign for laparoscopic adjustable gastric banding has produced an increased interest in surgery on the part of the severely obese patient population. Most of this interest is based on the belief that this procedure is less invasive than other bariatric surgeries. Not surprisingly, minimally invasive therapy has proven to be a more attractive surgical option to individuals with severe obesity. Over the past two decades, lack of information about bariatric surgery as an option for the severely obese patient has decreased dramatically as a reason why patients would not seek surgical therapy. It is difficult to say whether the persistent lack of attraction of surgical therapy or the currently limited access to surgical care is the more important factor preventing individuals with severe obesity from obtaining surgical therapy. Limited access to care is a result of either a patient's lack of health insurance or the insurance carrier's elimination of coverage for bariatric surgery from the policy. In states where such an elimination is unlawful, such as Virginia, insurance companies have successfully circumvented the intention of the law by attaching riders imposing severe financial penalties to the policies of employers who wish their employees to receive the benefits of coverage for bariatric surgery. Despite endorsement of bariatric surgery as standard of care treatment for severe obesity by many scientific and government organizations (Table 27-2), a majority of private insurance carriers in the U.S. do not provide coverage for bariatric surgery as a standard benefit.

OVERVIEW OF BARIATRIC SURGERY

Bariatric operations produce weight loss through two mechanisms. The most common is restriction of intake. Malabsorption of ingested food

TABLE 27-2	Government agencies and scientific societies that endorse bariatric surgery as standard of care treatment for severe obesity

Centers for Medicare and Medicaid Services
National Institute of Health
US Department of Veteran Affairs
US Department of Defense
The Obesity Society
American College of Physicians
American Diabetes Association
American Dietetic Association
American Association of Clinical Endocrinology
Association for Metabolic and Bariatric Surgery
American College of Surgeons
Society for Surgery of the Alimentary Tract
Society of American Gastrointestinal and Endoscopic Surgeons

TABLE 27-3	Types of commonly performed bariatric operations by mechanism of action

Restrictive
    Laparoscopic adjustable gastric banding (LAGB)
    Sleeve gastrectomy (SG)
    Vertical banded gastroplasty (VBG)[a]
Malabsorptive
    Biliopancreatic diversion (BPD)
    Jejunoileal bypass (JIB)[a]
Combined restrictive and malabsorptive
    Roux-en-Y gastric bypass (RYGB)
    BPD with duodenal switch (DS)

[a]Now rarely performed and of historic interest only.

is the second mechanism. Restrictive operations may include no or only a modest malabsorptive component. Malabsorptive operations may have some restrictive component, but it is secondary to the malabsorptive aspect of the operation. Table 27-3 describes the common currently performed operations listed by mechanism of action.

This chapter focuses on the operations listed in Table 27-3 regardless of whether they are done using a laparoscopic or an open incision approach. Although other procedures are known and available, they are performed very infrequently or are not yet approved for coverage by insurance providers, so they are not discussed in detail. Sleeve gastrectomy is now included because the operation has been shown to have medium-range efficacy, and its safety and effectiveness are now supported by a number of studies published in the literature.[15] In 2008 the American Society for Metabolic and Bariatric Surgery declared sleeve gastrectomy to be an appropriate first-line surgical therapy for weight loss. Vertical banded gastroplasty, although still one of the approved operations for the surgical treatment of severe obesity based on the NIH Consensus Conference of 1991,[14] is now so infrequently performed, and has such poor results on long-term follow-up,[16] that it is of historic interest only and has therefore been eliminated from this basic text as a standard of surgical care.

Evolution of Bariatric Surgery

During the 1950s, operations were first performed to treat severe hyperlipidemia with associated obesity.[17] These were ileocolic bypass operations to limit absorption and were associated with severe nutritional complications and liver failure postoperatively. The jejunoileal bypass was then devised and popularized in the mid-1970s.[18] It was also a malabsorptive operation but bypassed only a portion of the small intestine. Complications after this procedure were slower to manifest themselves but included severe diarrhea, electrolyte disturbances, protein/calorie malnutrition, renal stones, and liver failure.

In 1969, Mason and Ito performed the first gastric bypass, in which a loop of jejunum was connected to a transverse proximal gastric pouch.[19] Bile reflux esophagitis was severe postoperatively, which caused Griffin to develop the Roux-en-Y modification of the gastric bypass in 1977.[20] The gastric pouch was altered from transverse to vertical using the upper lesser curvature as well.

During the 1970s, the dismal failure of the jejunoileal bypass resulted in a very bad reputation in general for bariatric surgery among general surgeons who had performed the procedure or cared for patients experiencing its complications. Its reputation was not enhanced by the many variations of gastric stapling which then became commonplace during that time and in the early 1980s. Such operations often consisted of placing a few rows of staples partially across the upper stomach for restrictive purposes. Because the procedure was easily done, some surgeons performed it in prolific numbers. Staple breakdown predictably occurred months to years later, with subsequent regaining of weight. These procedures added to the string of failures of bariatric operations.[18]

In 1980, Mason[21] described vertical banded gastroplasty (VBG), a restrictive procedure in which stapling was used to create a proximal

gastric pouch of the upper lesser curvature of the stomach, with placement of a restrictive band to form its outlet to the rest of the stomach. This operation produced excellent initial weight loss (50% of excess weight or more) with low morbidity and mortality. It rapidly became the most commonly performed bariatric operation in the United States during the 1980s. By the early 1990s, however, it had become clear that patients who underwent VBG tended to adopt a diet of high-calorie liquids and regained weight.[22] A significant incidence of stenosis at the band was also a problem. Long-term weight loss was poor,[16] and by the 1990s in the United States Roux-en-Y gastric bypass (RYGB) became the procedure of choice for bariatric surgery.

In Italy, in the meantime, Scopinaro had developed and popularized the biliopancreatic diversion (BPD) procedure in the late 1970s.[23] This procedure, described in more detail later, along with its modification to include a duodenal switch (DS), has been the only major malabsorptive operation to enjoy long-term success. BPD and DS are both still used by a fairly select few surgeons throughout the world and both in the past and today represent <5% of operations performed in the United States.

Fixed banding of the stomach, aside from the VBG procedure, was also reported by other surgeons in the 1980s and 1990s. Kuzmak is credited with describing the fixed gastric band procedure that later led to the development of the adjustable gastric banding operation.[24]

The laparoscopic approach to bariatric surgery became available in the 1990s. Belachew and colleagues performed the first laparoscopic adjustable gastric banding (LAGB) operation in 1994.[25] Wittgrove and Clark performed the first laparoscopic Roux-en-Y gastric bypass (LRYGB) the same year.[26] Because the former operation is technically much easier than the latter, it was not surprising that it became very popular and was frequently performed in Europe and Australia during the late 1990s. In 2001 LAGB was approved for use in the United States by the U.S. Food and Drug Administration. Since then it has represented an increasingly larger percentage of bariatric operations performed in this country, with 2007 estimated figures suggesting that it accounts for at least 25% if not a higher percentage of bariatric operations performed. Its popularity seems to have been rapidly increasing due to significant national advertising campaigns. In the period since 1994, LRYGB, a much more technically difficult operation, saw a very slow adoption into common practice. Four years after the initial report, only a handful of medical centers had any significant experience with the procedure.

The Bariatric Revolution

The *bariatric revolution* is the term applied to the 5-year period from 1998 to 2003 in which the number of gastric bypass operations performed in the United States, membership in American Society for Metabolic and Bariatric Surgery, and public recognition and interest in and professional respect for the field dramatically increased. Few medical centers in the United States offered a laparoscopic approach to bariatric surgery before 1998, but many bariatric surgeons at that point were interested in learning to perform bariatric operations laparoscopically. Several centers, then began numerous programs to teach many bariatric surgeons the procedure.

General surgeons had demonstrated throughout the 1990s the improvements in outcomes that could result from performing operations laparoscopically rather than using an open incision. Bariatric surgeons were eager to extend laparoscopy to bariatric surgery. Once limitations in the availability of laparoscopic instruments for bariatric procedures had been overcome, and once the procedure was taught to leading bariatric surgeons at bariatric surgery centers (more than a few newly formed), the field literally exploded in terms of growth. Figure 27-1 illustrates the volume of RYGB procedures performed during the years before and during the bariatric revolution. The number of bariatric procedures recorded increased by nearly eightfold, and membership in the American Society for Bariatric Surgery tripled during these years. The number of fellowships in minimally invasive surgery offered to graduating residents, most of which included bariatric surgical procedures as a major component of the

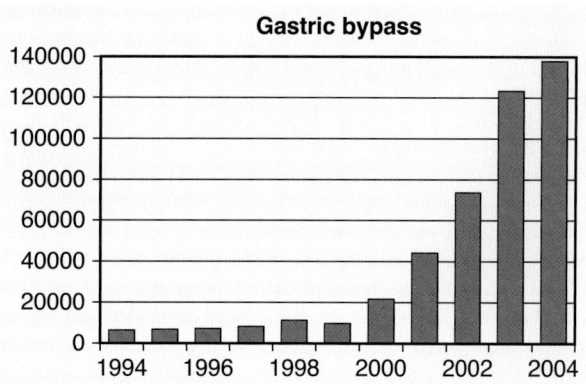

Gastric bypass

FIG. 27-1. Number of Roux-en-Y gastric bypass operations performed in the United States by year. *(Data from the Nationwide Inpatient Sample database.)*

case load, increased from a few to 125 during these years. Public recognition of the procedure markedly increased because some public figures in the media underwent bariatric surgery. The wide availability of the Internet to prospective patients allowed much more information to be relayed. Patients who had or were contemplating surgery were able to communicate via the Internet. Videos of bariatric operations became available through several media outlets, including television and the Internet. Many U.S. surgical departments that had previously shunned the field of bariatric surgery recruited bariatric surgeons and set up programs. Hospitals without programs recruited surgeons so they could offer the service. Bariatric surgery presentations at national surgical meetings became commonplace instead of rare or limited to bariatric meetings. In just 5 years, the field experienced greater growth than the field of general surgery had experienced during the introduction of laparoscopy a decade earlier—and underwent just as absolute a change.

Indications

The indications for performing bariatric surgery remain as described by the NIH Consensus Conference of 1991.[14] The only major difference is in which procedures are now recognized as standard procedures. The standard procedures were defined by the Centers for Medicare and Medicaid Services in 2005 as those listed in Table 27-3, with the exception of sleeve gastrectomy. The latter, although still often not covered by insurance policies in many areas, seems destined to take its place, among the available options for bariatric surgery. Vertical banded gastroplasty, although still listed as a standard procedure and still covered by many insurance policies, has fallen from favor. For this reason, as noted earlier, a detailed description of it has been eliminated from this text. The indications for performing bariatric surgery are summarized in Table 27-4.

Contraindications

Of all the reasons preventing a patient who desires bariatric surgery from having an operation, inadequate insurance coverage, or lack

thereof, is the most common. Assuming that the patient does have insurance coverage or the financial means to qualify for surgery, then application of the NIH criteria is the next step. Once a patient qualifies according to those criteria, then medical, social, and psychologic issues are considered to identify any possible reasons to avoid surgical therapy.

The NIH criteria do not set limits for age, and surgeon opinion on this issue varies widely. One of us (BS) observes a general upper limit of about 60 years of age for LRYGB and at most 65 years for LAGB. Rare exceptions are made for patients who appear younger than their chronologic age. However, most patients who are severely obese have been that way for decades, with concurrent deterioration of major vital organ systems as a result. Thus few of them are physiologically "younger" than their chronologic age, and the reverse is more often true. The rationale for age restriction is twofold: a large number of younger patients are interested in and eligible for bariatric surgery, and there is a greater likelihood of a longer period of postoperative benefit in terms of improved quality of life and longevity with younger patients. Although this represents something of a triage approach, until the vast majority of patients who qualify for surgery can obtain it, this approach can be justified. More details on bariatric surgery for both the old and the young are provided later in this chapter.

Medical issues that preclude patients from being good surgical candidates include the presence of American Society of Anesthesiologists class IV disease of a type that makes surgical therapy associated with an extraordinarily high risk. Psychologic instability or the inability to understand the implications of the proposed operation and what changes will result from it in terms of the patient's lifestyle is also a contraindication. Known and documented drug or alcohol addiction is a contraindication to surgery. Smoking is a relative contraindication, and the requirement for cessation of smoking varies by surgical practice. An ongoing eating disorder, especially bulimia, is also a contraindication to surgery. Nonambulatory status is a relative contraindication to surgery, especially if it results from such severe obesity that the patient cannot normally perform self-care or would not likely be able to do so after surgery. In our experience, not only do such patients have excessive morbidity, but placement in care facilities postoperatively after recovery from surgery is often difficult due to their size and limitations of physical ability. Some patients view the bariatric operation as a "magic bullet" for which they must only show up and after which they will not be required to make any substantive changes in eating or lifestyle. Although it may be hard to detect this attitude in a single visit, an accumulation of evidence suggests that such a view on the part of the patient is a very valid reason to deny surgery. Similarly, inappropriate, uncooperative, or intimidating behavior during the preoperative interval often is a harbinger of postoperative problems and may constitute a reason to deny surgical care. Finally, the lack of sufficient social support, an extremely poor or unsupportive home environment, or hostile spouse or relatives can be contraindications to surgical care, because a supportive environment is important to optimize outcomes once the patient is discharged from the hospital. Table 27-5 summarizes relative contraindications for surgery.

PREOPERATIVE ISSUES

Patient Selection

Patient selection for surgery should be based on a multidisciplinary team evaluation. The patient has usually been screened by his or her primary care physician before referral, with major medical issues addressed before referral. Determining whether the patient meets the NIH criteria and whether insurance coverage is available can be handled by office administrators and confirmed and documented before the first appointment.

The preoperative assessment of the patient for bariatric surgery must include input from the nutritionist as an important independent evaluation. Careful assessment of the patient's eating habits, knowledge, self-awareness, and insight are important. An estimation

TABLE 27-4	Indications for bariatric surgery

Patient must:
1. Have body mass index (weight in kilograms/height in square meters) of ≥40 with or without comorbid medical conditions associated with obesity
2. Have body mass index of 35–40 with comorbid medical conditions

In addition it is expected that patients:
3. Have failed attempt at other weight loss treatments
4. Be psychologically stable

Source: Adapted from 1991 NIH Concensus Conference.[14]

TABLE 27-5	Relative contraindications for bariatric surgery[a]

1. Severe medical disease that makes anesthesia or surgery prohibitively risky (American Society of Anesthesiologists class IV)
2. Mental incompetence that prevents the patient from understanding the procedure
3. Inability or unwillingness of the patient to change lifestyle postoperatively
4. Drug, alcohol, or other substance addiction
5. Uncontrolled bulimia or other eating disorder
6. Psychologic instability
7. Nonambulatory status
8. Patient view of surgery as a "magic bullet"
9. Antagonistic family, unsupportive home environment
10. Noncompliant behavior

[a]These relative contraindications should be weighed against the potential benefits of surgery which may be the only treatment likely to yield significant weight loss and clinical improvement in the high-risk patient.

of the patient's motivation to change eating habits is important. An experienced bariatric nutritionist can be helpful in predicting which patients will be compliant or noncompliant with recommended lifestyle changes postoperatively. Specific nutritional counseling and education is required based on the operation to be performed.

Psychologic assessment is required by some insurance carriers. In our opinion, the major benefit of the psychologic assessment is to determine how the patient views the operation and whether the patient has a realistic understanding of the changes in lifestyle that are needed for optimal outcomes. The psychologist or psychiatrist often diagnoses previously unappreciated depression, which is detected in nearly 40% of our preoperative patients when they are carefully screened. Treatment of the depression is felt to improve postoperative outcomes.

Most of the patients referred to us for surgery who have been screened for qualification according to the NIH standards are appropriate candidates for bariatric surgery. Some will decide against the procedure after completing thorough educational and counseling sessions. We advocate detailed written information and a multihour verbal presentation by our multidisciplinary team to educate patients preoperatively regarding bariatric surgical procedures and expected outcomes and potential complications. Informed and prepared patients will be much more compliant with requested perioperative and postoperative behavioral and eating changes. Some patients who decide against the procedure will return for re-evaluation in the future after their obesity comorbidities worsen.

Preoperative Preparation

Preoperatively, current comorbidities and other medical problems are reviewed and optimized. Potentially undiagnosed medical problems are recognized and treated. Screening for hidden diseases such as coronary artery disease in patients >50 years of age is important. For such patients, or those with known cardiovascular disease, we advocate a preoperative cardiology consultation. Such consultation usually involves electrocardiography, echocardiography, stress test, and perhaps even cardiac catheterization. Another condition often underdiagnosed preoperatively in the severely obese patient population is obstructive sleep apnea. Patients who give a history of loud snoring, morning tiredness on waking, and falling asleep easily while driving or sitting likely have obstructive sleep apnea. A diagnostic sleep study is indicated. One report suggests that the incidence of sleep apnea in severely obese patients, when all routinely undergo sleep studies, may approach 80%.[27] Once diagnosed with sleep apnea, patients should use a positive airway pressure device as treatment. Use of this system in the immediately postoperative period is especially important to prevent episodes of hypoxia and the cardiac arrhythmias that can potentially result. Asthma and hypoventilation syndrome of obesity are other significant pulmonary diseases often requiring preoperative management. Hypoventilation syndrome of obesity is defined as a resting

partial pressure of arterial oxygen of <55 mmHg and a resting partial pressure of arterial carbon dioxide of >47 mmHg, with accompanying pulmonary hypertension and polycythemia. Pulmonary consultation is indicated for patients with hypoventilation syndrome. Postoperative intensive care unit hospitalization, rarely used after bariatric surgery, is usually indicated for these patients in our opinion.

For patients with active GERD taking medication, a preoperative screening upper endoscopy to rule out Barrett's esophagus and intrinsic lesions of the stomach or duodenum is recommended. This is especially true for patients planning LRYGB, in which the distal stomach and duodenum will be precluded from easy inspection postoperatively. Several studies have documented the considerable incidence of preoperative pathology identified on flexible upper endoscopy in this patient population, as well as a small but not insignificant incidence of pathology resulting in alteration of the originally planned surgical procedure.[28,29] At the University of Virginia Medical Center, our experience was that such pathology was found on 4.6% of examinations.[30]

In patients who are taking anticoagulants for prosthetic cardiac valves or recent venous thromboembolism, anticoagulation therapy must be managed perioperatively. Options include total cessation of oral warfarin therapy 5 days before surgery, then administration of subcutaneous low molecular weight heparin until resumption of warfarin postoperatively. Alternatively, one can proceed with preoperative hospital admission for IV heparin anticoagulation therapy, which is then stopped 6 hours before surgery.

Patients who have a strong history of venous thromboembolism or who are felt to have multiple risk factors for postoperative venous thromboembolism are potential candidates for preoperative placement of a temporary inferior vena cava filter. Such filters are placed the day before surgery by our interventional radiology colleagues and removed 3 to 6 weeks postoperatively. Our results with such therapy have been excellent, with little morbidity and effective prevention of any significant pulmonary embolism in such patients.

We routinely perform screening ultrasound of the abdomen in patients planning to undergo LRYGB who have an intact gallbladder to rule out the presence of gallstones. Should gallstones be discovered, we currently recommend simultaneous laparoscopic cholecystectomy. Another approach is to defer cholecystectomy until after LRYGB if the patient is symptomatic. Recent analysis of our experience with this approach at the University of Virginia has shown an average increase in operative time of approximately 30 minutes for both LRYGB and RYGB with no increase in hospitalization time or morbidity.[31] An earlier study at Pittsburgh did demonstrate an increased length of hospitalization for patients undergoing simultaneous cholecystectomy.[32] When a patient does not have gallstones as determined by preoperative ultrasound, we have followed the recommendations of a previous study which showed that prophylactic administration of ursodiol at a dosage of 300 mg bid will decrease the incidence of gallstone formation after RYGB to approximately 4%.[33] Controversy currently exists as to the proper role of simultaneous laparoscopic cholecystectomy at the time of LAGB. The conservative approach is not to perform such an operation, given the small potential for gallbladder bile spillage, which can result in infection of the prosthesis. Insufficient data have been published on the subject for a more evidence-based recommendation to be made. Another value of preoperative ultrasound of the abdomen is the assessment of liver size and composition. An ultrasound finding of a large fatty liver in a patient planning to undergo either LAGB or LRYGB should alert the surgeon to the high potential for technical difficulty in liver retraction and exposure. We have converted to an open procedure and even deferred persisting with the operation altogether when confronted with an excessively large liver. Knowledge of this before surgery allows the patient to follow a low-calorie diet to shrink the liver preoperatively.

Some surgeons require patients to follow a low-calorie diet in the immediately preoperative period, insisting on weight loss before proceeding with surgery. Some data indicate that preoperative weight loss by patients may improve outcomes. Such studies suffer from the fact that the patients who are most compliant and lose weight preoperatively may also be the most compliant postoperatively, which may account for the improved outcomes. Preoperative weight loss is not necessary to achieve good outcomes from surgery, because many practices do not require such preoperative weight loss and still achieve good outcomes. Requiring preoperative weight loss raises the dilemma of whether patients who do not achieve weight loss should then be denied the benefit of surgical therapy.

Other routine preparation for surgery in our practice includes measurement of baseline arterial blood gas values. This is especially important in any patient with significant pulmonary disease or hypoventilation syndrome of obesity, because a baseline value of "normal" *for that patient* must be known if ventilator management is necessary postoperatively.

Baseline evaluation of thyroid function is recommended preoperatively, because hypothyroidism is not uncommon in this patient population. Serum chemical analysis, liver function tests, and the usual screening blood tests are performed. Blood tests to determine baseline nutritional parameters commonly reveal abnormally low iron and vitamin D levels. The former finding is common in the menstruating female population, obese or not, whereas the latter has also been noted.[34] Whether to treat low vitamin D levels preoperatively is unclear, because its influence on clinical outcomes remains undefined.

Preoperative patient education is important to re-emphasize important events of the perioperative period, expected postoperative course, and instructions for postoperative activity and diet. Expectations we have for patients include ambulating on the day of surgery, adhering to postoperative dietary instructions, taking recommended vitamin and mineral supplements, and following a regular exercise plan.

Anesthesiology Issues

A preoperative anesthesiology assessment is indicated for all patients undergoing bariatric surgery. This assessment confirms that ongoing comorbid medical problems are being optimally evaluated and managed. It also includes the aforementioned cardiopulmonary evaluation to identify any underlying pathology that requires preoperative treatment to decrease perioperative morbidity from cardiopulmonary complications.

It is important that the anesthesiologist for the bariatric surgical procedure be experienced in carrying out general anesthesia management for the bariatric patient. There is no question that the consistent participation of a few selected and experienced anesthesiologists who specialize in the care of the bariatric patient will minimize morbidity in surgical outcomes. Perioperative and intraoperative communication between the anesthesiology team and the surgical team is particularly important during bariatric operations to facilitate the smooth flow of the operation and avoid complications from the procedure.

Two major difficulties the anesthesiologist faces when administering a general anesthetic to a severely obese patient are vascular access and airway management. Both are significantly more difficult in the obese patient population than in the normal-weight population. Central venous access is at times the only available route for establishment of reliable IV access. Access to both arms during the procedure is standard in our operating rooms; this allows for additional larger-bore IV access should an episode of intra-abdominal hemorrhage occur. Jugular cannulation is often very difficult due to neck adipose tissue. Subclavian access is used when other central access routes are not feasible.

Management of the airway in the severely obese patient is often a major challenge for the anesthesiologist and must be done well to avoid potentially significant morbidity. Videotelescopic intubation systems are successfully used in some institutions to accomplish difficult airway intubation. Fiber-optic laryngoscopy is more commonly used for difficult intubations should standard laryngoscopy

provide an inadequate view. For the most difficult class IV or even class III airways, fiberoptically guided intubation is used. Experience again is key in accomplishing smooth intubation of this patient population. Significant preoxygenation for 3 minutes or longer before intubation is performed in the severely obese patient to provide a longer safe duration for intubation should difficulties be encountered. However, desaturation must be addressed immediately with re-establishment of oxygenated ventilation, because this patient group does not tolerate any prolonged desaturation without potential adverse cardiopulmonary consequences.

The anesthesiologist must be adept at understanding and managing alterations in cardiopulmonary function from the use of a pneumoperitoneum during laparoscopic bariatric procedures. These alterations include the effects of carbon dioxide absorption on required minute ventilation, the potential for bradyarrhythmias, and the potential for decreased systemic pH with longer procedures in patients with pre-existing cardiopulmonary disease. Arterial monitoring of the latter group of patients by the anesthesiology team is necessary, and placement of a radial arterial line is standard for such patients.[35]

Drug pharmacokinetics differ in severely obese patients as well. Factors affecting changes in volume of distribution include smaller-than-normal fraction of total body water, greater adipose tissue content, altered protein binding, and increased blood volume. Possible changes in renal function and hepatic function must be considered when administering drugs.

Alterations in the metabolism of specific anesthetic drugs in the severely obese include a larger volume of distribution of thiopentone, which results in a prolonged effect of the drug. The dosage should be calculated based on lean body weight. Benzodiazepines also exhibit a prolonged elimination phase, which causes persistence of their effects. Increased pseudocholinesterase activity is present in the severely obese patient, so that increased dosages of pancuronium are required. Enflurane metabolism is increased over that in the average-sized person, so that a lower dosage of this agent must be used.

BARIATRIC SURGICAL PROCEDURES

Laparoscopic vs. Open Procedures

The procedures described later use the laparoscopic approach as the default or typical approach. The Roux-en-Y gastric bypass (RYGB), the biliopancreatic diversion (BPD), and the duodenal switch (DS) are often still performed using an open approach, and such an approach has been well documented to be safe and effective. Decreased wound complications, as well as earlier hospital discharge and lower 30-day complication rates, have all been demonstrated for the laparoscopic approach, which clearly favors the use of this approach when feasible.[36–38] In addition, the logical assumption that avoiding the major tissue trauma associated with a long abdominal wall incision is beneficial to patient recovery has been confirmed. Most importantly, patient interest in bariatric surgery increased dramatically once a laparoscopic approach was available for these procedures, especially RYGB. In the United States, the annual number of RYGB procedures in the 1990s was just under 20,000 but by 2003 had reached 130,000 (see Fig. 27-1).[39] In the twenty-first century, most prospective bariatric surgery patients are informed enough about the options for surgery to seek out a surgeon who performs laparoscopic bariatric surgery if such a surgeon is available within a reasonable distance of their home.

When an open surgical approach is used for any of these procedures, an upper midline incision is the most commonly used approach. Some surgeons have had excellent success with a left subcostal incision for performing RYGB.[40] Mechanical retractors afford additional exposure for open surgery, and their use is indicated. Wound closure for midline incisions usually is performed using heavy monofilament suture for the midline fascia, but surgeon preferences vary. Thorough hemostasis and irrigation of the subcutaneous tissues is indicated before secure skin closure. The use of drains has been shown to increase wound infections. We have found that leaving skin staples in place for a longer interval is beneficial to prevent premature skin dehiscence, which in turn can lead to more severe wound infection. Any worrisome drainage from a postoperative open surgical incision line requires opening of the wound in that area to confirm that a more severe deep-seated fascial tissue infection does not exist.

Laparoscopy is the most commonly used approach for bariatric surgical procedures at this time. Table 27-3 lists the operations that are discussed in later sections by mechanism of action. As implied by the name *laparoscopic adjustable gastric banding (LAGB)*, virtually all gastric banding procedures are performed using this approach. The same is true for sleeve gastrectomy, although the nomenclature for that operation does not include the word *laparoscopic*. The majority of gastric bypass operations are now done laparoscopically (LRYGB). BPD and DS, both malabsorptive operations, are performed with relative infrequency in the United States. When performed, they often are still done using an open approach, but some centers do use a laparoscopic approach as well.

Laparoscopic surgery requires a core set of knowledge and skills that have now become a standard part of surgical training. Successful completion of the Fundamentals of Laparoscopic Surgery unit developed by the Society of Gastrointestinal and Endoscopic Surgeons[41] has now become a mandatory requirement for all surgical residents in the United States who wish to become certified by the American Board of Surgery.

Laparoscopy begins with the safe creation of a pneumoperitoneum, often a difficult step in the bariatric patient. We have found the use of a tracheostomy hook inserted through a trocar-sized incision to elevate the fascia in the left subcostal region to be of great assistance in facilitating the insertion of a Veress needle into an appropriate location for pneumoperitoneum creation. In general, the use of a Hasson approach for creating a pneumoperitoneum in the bariatric population is problematic because of the thick body wall. In the patient with an extremely thick body wall, extra long trocar ports can be used for laparoscopic surgery.

The pneumoperitoneum pressure that is used when performing bariatric surgical procedures is generally in the 15- to 18-mmHg range. A high-flow insufflator is mandatory to maintain the pneumoperitoneum for adequate and safe visualization. Use of an angled telescope is quite helpful. Instrumentation for performing laparoscopic bariatric surgery has dramatically improved in the past 15 years and continues to improve. We now favor using certain laparoscopic instruments, such as the staplers and Harmonic scalpel ultrasonic cutting and coagulating device, even if conversion to an open approach is necessary.

Conversion to an open incision is appropriate in circumstances in which patient safety would potentially be compromised by persisting with a laparoscopic approach. Table 27-6 lists appropriate reasons for conversion to an open incision as well as certain conditions that, if known beforehand, are grounds for beginning with open surgery, such as an existing large upper abdominal incisional hernia or known severe intra-abdominal adhesions. Conversion to an open incision should not be viewed as a failure by the surgeon, nor should such an attitude bias the surgeon in favor of persisting with a laparoscopic approach if the operation is not progressing or if a complication is worsening when it could be corrected more quickly using an open approach. Patient safety is the gold standard for determining the timing and appropriateness of conversion. Usually, if conversion is needed, it is best to do so as early in the course of the operation as possible.

Some bariatric surgeons have adopted a hand-assisted approach to performing bariatric surgery. In some cases this technique has been used as a bridge when a surgeon experienced at performing open surgery is transitioning to performing laparoscopic bariatric surgery.[42] Most bariatric surgeons have found the discomfort of the

TABLE 27-6	Indications for conversion from laparoscopic to open surgery

1. Failure to establish an adequate pneumoperitoneum
2. Hemodynamic adverse reaction to pneumoperitoneum
3. Intra-abdominal adhesions precluding safe access or presenting excessive difficulty in accessing abdomen
4. Hepatomegaly such that retraction is not feasible or organ visualization is obscured even with retraction
5. Intraoperative complications such as hemorrhage that are best managed with an open approach
6. Exceedingly thick body wall precluding adequate trocar access or manipulation
7. Existing large upper abdominal wall hernia that optimally can be repaired at the same time using the same incision

thick abdominal wall on the forearm of the operating surgeon, the potential for infections and incisional hernias at the hand port site, and the lack of superiority in results compared with those of a total laparoscopic approach to be reasons not to use this approach routinely.

Postoperative Follow-Up

Short-term follow-up is defined as follow-up of up to 2 years. Such follow-up is expected of most if not all of one's bariatric surgical patients. Unfortunately, even in the best of practices in the United States, because of the lack of a centralized health system or registry, 1-year follow-up of 90% or greater is a laudable achievement and is rarely reported in most case series. Recommendations for bariatric centers wishing to be centers of excellence are that 75% of patients be followed for 5 years after restrictive operations and 90% after malabsorptive operations. Those recommendations, however, assume the presence of a system that attempts maximum possible follow-up and therefore should be able to produce such results. Although a system may be in place that generates multiple attempts to have the patient return for postoperative checkups, without patient compliance all such systems are fallible.

The goals of short-term follow-up are to maximize care of the patient in the postoperative period; assist the patient in adjusting to new eating, exercise, and lifestyle patterns; provide early identification of postoperative complications; and recommend measures to limit such complications. Objective data that should be obtained after all bariatric operations include weight loss, change in BMI, resolution or improvement in medical comorbidities, and any adverse events or complications that occur. Optimally, a measure of quality of life, such as the Short Form-36 General Health Survey questionnaire, is also used to help gauge efficacy. Short-term follow-up data give a good reflection of the safety of the procedure, but they provide only an estimate of its efficacy with regard to weight loss and effect on the resolution of medical comorbidities.

Medium-term follow-up, defined as follow-up for 2 to 5 years, and long-term follow-up, defined as that for >5 years, are the only means by which the true long-term efficacy of bariatric surgical operations can be assessed. Operations that initially appeared quite promising, such as VBG or even jejunoileal bypass, were shown with long- and medium-length follow-up, respectively, to have significant deficiencies in efficacy (for the VBG[16]) and safety (for the jejunoileal bypass[20]). Other stapled gastroplasty procedures similarly did not demonstrate efficacy on medium-term follow-up.[18]

Unfortunately, to date there has been no standardized method of reporting outcomes after bariatric surgery. The ideal publication includes the number of patients; description of the operative technique; rate of conversion to an open procedure if applicable; number of patients included in follow-up data per year; percentage of patients lost to follow-up; weight loss (usually expressed as percentage of excess weight); initial and subsequent BMI; information on complications, mortality, and resolution of medical comorbidities; and any quality-of-life data. Not all publications have included all these elements. There are also only a few studies that have conducted a prospective randomized comparison either between bariatric surgery and medical management or between different bariatric surgical operations or approaches (e.g., laparoscopic vs. open). Improvement in study design and reporting of more complete data in future publications is needed.

Postoperative follow-up for the various operations to be described later has some common overall themes. These include an initial visit soon after surgery to determine wound healing, tolerance of oral intake, adjustment to the operation, and return to activity, and to confirm the postoperative nutrition and exercise plan. Periodic follow-up is indicated for all procedures, with the goal of documenting the previously listed items for optimal outcomes reporting. A multidisciplinary team approach is as essential postoperatively for follow-up as it was preoperatively, if not more so. Regular counseling sessions with the nutritionist are indicated for at least the first year after surgery. Psychologic support should be available as needed to assist the patient in adjusting to major life changes. Patient-oriented support groups can add significant value to preparation for surgery and adjustment afterward. Geographic proximity to the hospital improves patients' ability to attend such sessions.

Our combined experience of several decades in performing bariatric surgery has led us to conclude that *regardless of what operation is performed, patients can achieve long-term success if they embrace the eating and lifestyle changes that the operation allows them to adopt.* Continuation of exercise as part of the daily lifestyle is associated with a high rate of preservation of weight loss. Diligence to avoid snacking and returning to other poor eating habits is also important. The majority of patients do embrace the metamorphosis that their bariatric operation produces so that they maintain their new eating, lifestyle, and exercise habits to the benefit of their continued improved health, self-image, and well-being. Whether the patient achieves this behavior pattern is, in the opinion of one of us (BS), the main factor that determines the appropriateness of considering any revisional or additional surgery in response to weight gain.

Laparoscopic Adjustable Gastric Banding
Background

Laparoscopic adjustable gastric banding (LAGB) involves placement of an inflatable silicone band around the proximal stomach. The band is attached to a reservoir system that allows adjustment of the tightness of the band. This reservoir system is accessed through a subcutaneously placed port, similar in concept to the ports used for chemotherapy via central venous catheters. Figure 27-2 shows the LAGB apparatus in place.

Two major types of bands have been used for this procedure. The original Lap-Band Adjustable Gastric Banding System, most recently marketed by Allergan, has been used most frequently. The Swedish adjustible gastric band, now remarketed as the Realize Adjustable Gastric Band by Ethicon, is slightly wider than the Lap-Band.[43] The two both work with a port system, but the ports have differences in profile and method of attachment to the fascia.

Technique

Port placement for LAGB has varied among surgeons. Usually some combination of two ports for the surgeon's hands, one or two for the assistant, a port for the telescope, and a liver retractor site are needed.

With the patient placed in reverse Trendelenburg's position, the procedure begins with division of the peritoneum at the angle of His, then division of the gastrohepatic ligament in its avascular area (the pars flaccida) to expose the base of the right crus of the diaphragm. If a hiatal hernia is present, it must be repaired at this point, and a standard posterior esophageal dissection is used to expose the crura and perform suture repair. A grasper (Lap-Band)

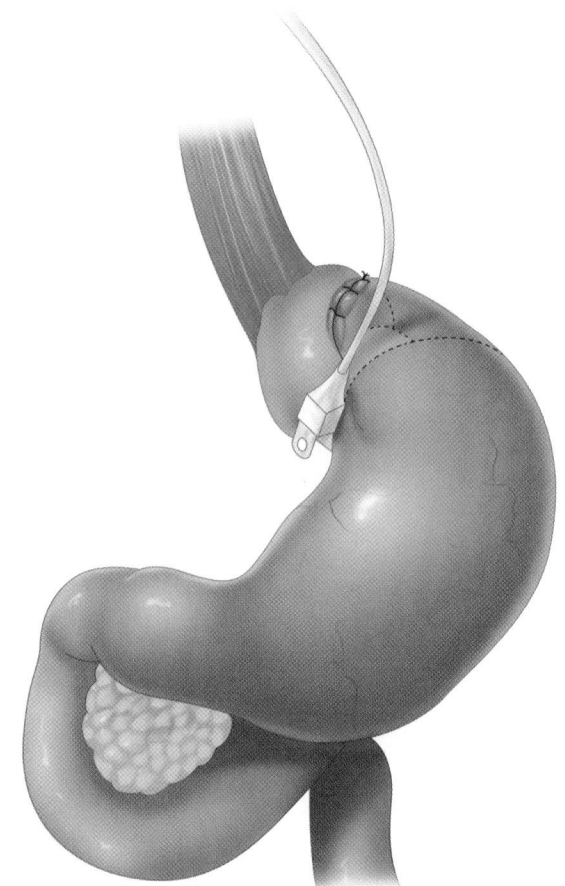

FIG. 27-2. Laparoscopic adjustable banding overall scheme. *[Reproduced with permission from Austrheim-Smith I, et al: Evolution of bariatric minimally invasive surgery, in Schauer PR, et al (eds): Minimally Invasive Bariatric Surgery, 1st ed. New York: Springer, 2007, p 21.]*

or specially devised instrument (Realize band) is inserted along the base of the anterior surface of the diaphragmatic crura, from right to left, emerging at the angle of His in the area of the divided peritoneum (Fig. 27-3). The device is then used to pull the band underneath the posterior surface of the gastroesophageal junction. Use of this technique, in which the band is passed through some fibrous tissue in this plane, serves to anchor the band more securely posteriorly. During the initial years of band placement, a retrogastric location of the posterior half of the band in the free space of the lesser sac caused an unacceptably high incidence of slippage and prolapse of the band. The adoption of the pars flaccida technique decreased the incidence of such slippage.[44]

Once the band is passed around the proximal stomach, it is locked into its ring configuration through its own self-locking mechanism. This involves passing the tubing end through the orifice of the buckle for the Lap-Band, and passing through the suture on the end of the flanged end of the band site for the Realize band. Once the band is securely locked in place, the buckle portion of the band is located on the lesser curvature of the stomach (Fig. 27-4A and 27-4B). Now the anterior surface of the fundus and proximal stomach is imbricated over the band using several sutures (Fig. 27-5).

The tubing of the band system is brought out through the desired site for placement of the port portion of the system. Usually this is a trocar site near the upper abdomen or xiphoid region to allow placement of the port most superficially so that it can be palpated postoperatively. The port is secured to the anterior abdominal wall

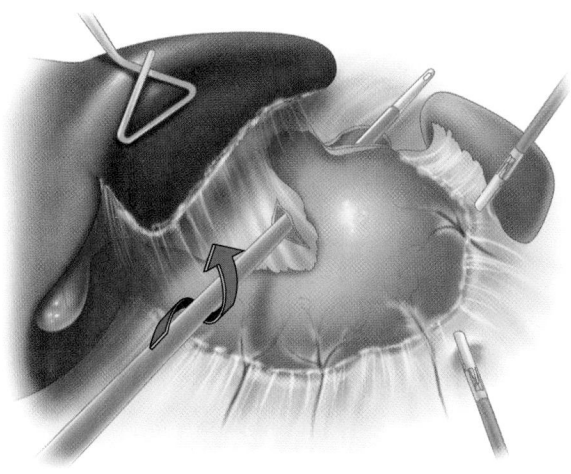

FIG. 27-3. Grasper being passed through under the stomach to grasp tubing during placement. *[Reproduced with permission from O'Brien PE, et al: Laparoscopic adjustable gastric banding: Technique, in Schauer PR, et al (eds): Minimally Invasive Bariatric Surgery, 1st ed. New York: Springer, 2007, p 184.]*

fascia. Access to the port for subsequent addition of fluid to the band system is gained percutaneously using a Huber or noncutting-type needle. The band is initially placed in the fully deflated state.

Patient Selection and Preparation

Most LAGB procedures are done on an outpatient basis. Technically the operation is not as difficult as the other operations described later. Because the GI tract is not violated, the relative risk of the procedure is lower than that of most other bariatric operations, which makes this procedure more suitable to offer to older, more medically ill, or higher-risk patient populations. However, efficacy of the operation in the superobese (BMI >50 kg/m^2) is less impressive, with average BMI remaining >40 kg/m^2 after 5- to 8-year follow-up.[45] It has been our impression that optimal results occur with this operation in patients who are motivated, need to lose <50 kg to achieve a BMI of <30 kg/m^2, are willing and able to exercise regularly, are amenable to changing eating patterns as recommended, and live within a geographic area close enough for easy follow-up. Patients who are impatient to lose weight, are immobile, are unable to exercise, are confirmed "grazers" or nibblers on high-calorie sweets, and expect to be able to continue their dietary habits without great alteration are not good candidates for this operation. Similarly, patients who have had previous upper gastric surgery, such as a Nissen fundoplication, are relatively poor

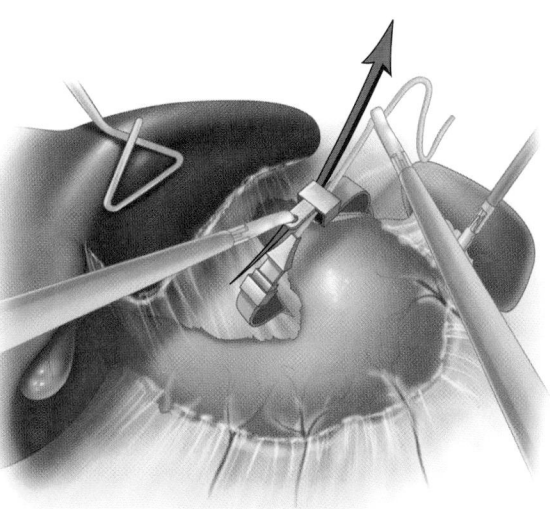

A

FIG. 27-4. A. Lap-Band adjustable gastric band in place around stomach. *[Reproduced with permission from O'Brien PE, et al: Laparoscopic adjustable gastric banding: Technique, in Schauer PR, et al (eds): Minimally Invasive Bariatric Surgery, 1st ed. New York: Springer, 2007, p 186.]* **B.** Realize Adjustable Gastric Band (Swedish adjustible gastric band) in place around stomach.

B

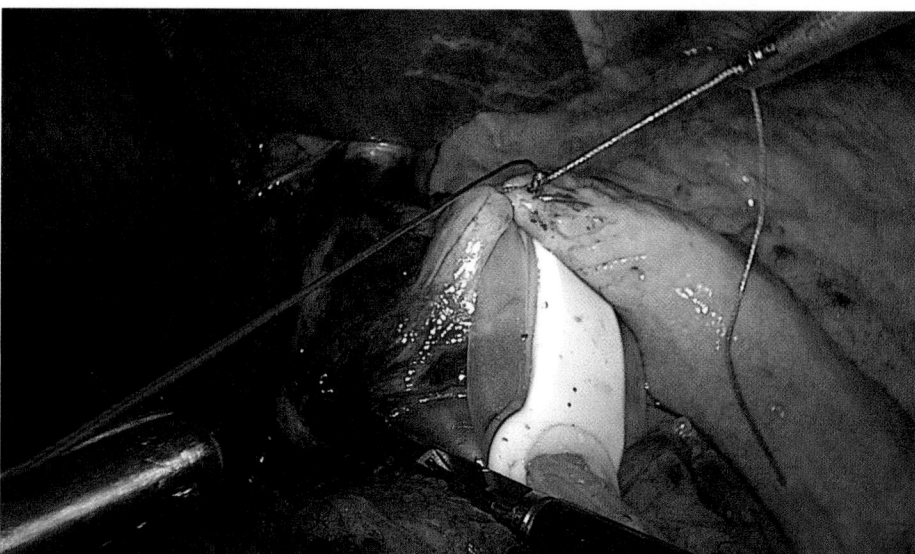

FIG. 27-5. Stomach imbricated over band.

candidates for LAGB due to the potential tissue compromise in taking down the wrap to place the band.

Important points of preoperative preparation specific to the procedure include placing the patient on nil per os status, providing appropriate venous thromboembolism prophylaxis preoperatively, administering appropriate broad-spectrum IV antibiotics, and ensuring appropriate IV access and monitoring. A Foley catheter is inserted into the bladder and an orogastric tube into the stomach. These preoperative measures are indicated for all the procedures described later as well.

Postoperative Care and Follow-Up

As noted earlier, the majority of LAGB procedures are performed on an outpatient basis. Insurance requirements and pre-existing medical issues are usually the only reason for overnight hospitalization. Instructions regarding diet, wound care, pain medications, and the time schedule for resuming preoperative medications should be explained to the patient as well as to a family member (who has not just undergone general anesthesia) before discharge. In addition, arrangements should be made for a postoperative follow-up visit, and phone numbers to call in emergencies should be provided, along with an explanation of the indications that should prompt such calls.

We usually see our LAGB patients 2 weeks after surgery. By this time they have begun to tire of the blenderized diet recommended, are often eager to return to work if they have not already done so, and are amenable to discussions of an exercise plan and diet progression plan. Wounds are assessed, as are medical problems, oral intake, and adherence to the prescribed diet. Because LAGB does not preclude absorption of any specific nutrients, we recommend only a multivitamin for patients whose preoperative laboratory results were normal. We have not routinely recommended ursodiol (300 mg bid) for gallstone prophylaxis, because weight loss often does not occur as rapidly after LAGB as after gastric bypass, and data regarding gallstone formation after LAGB are lacking. However, many surgeons do recommend gallstone prophylaxis after LAGB.

Band adjustments and postoperative support group sessions are extremely important for good outcomes after LAGB. Band adjustments are paramount as part of the operation. The actual performance of the LAGB procedure is really just one part of the care of the patient. Frequent postoperative visits, band adjustments as necessary, and participation in an appropriate exercise program are all important for postoperative success for these patients. Recommendations for the timing of band adjustments vary from practice to practice. In general, there is agreement that losing <2 lb/wk is an indication to increase the restriction of the band by adding fluid. Patients who can easily eat most solid foods and have little satiety and a fairly pronounced appetite need additional restriction from the band.

Band fills usually are accomplished in the outpatient clinic setting. Occasionally fluoroscopic radiology is needed to assist in accessing the port, based on the depth of the port from the skin and its ease of palpation. Experience by the person doing the band fill is an important factor in increasing the percentage of patients whose ports can be accessed in the clinic without radiologic assistance. A careful record should be maintained of the amount of fluid in each patient's band. Some surgeons withdraw all the fluid at each fill, reinserting the desired amount. Many just add additional fluid as indicated. The amount of fluid added is based on hunger, weight loss, and ability to eat meat or bread. Figure 27-6 shows an in office algorithm adjustment scheme used by Ren.[46] Ideally, adjustments are performed over an approximately 2-year period after surgery.

An optimal situation for LAGB success is a program in which patients all live within an easy drive of the center, will and do participate in frequently available support groups and use exercise facilities supplied by the program, have access to band adjustment visits as needed, and are carefully selected for appropriateness and motivation for the procedure preoperatively.

Outcomes

Medium- to long-term (8-year follow-up) outcomes have been reported for LAGB by Weiner and colleagues.[47] Published studies have shown that, on average, at 5 and 7 years after LAGB patients had lost 60% and 58% of excess weight, respectively.[48] The authors point out that the weight loss curve for LAGB approaches that for RYGB after 3 years, because LAGB patients often continue to lose weight for at least 2 and often 3 years after operation, whereas gastric bypass patients lose weight the first year then tend to regain weight with the passage of time. Resolution of comorbidities after LAGB has been reported as very good overall, with hypertension resolving in 55% of patients at 1 year,[48] observed sleep apnea decreasing from 33 to 2%,[49] GERD improving in >50% of cases,[50] and asthma,[51] depression,[52] and quality of life[53] improving for patients after LAGB. Dixon and associates[54] published a landmark article describing the vastly superior results of LAGB over optimal medical treatment in managing patients with diabetes. Resolution of diabetes was 13% in the medical group vs. 73% in the surgical group after a 2-year follow-up.

Results of large institutional series of LAGB have been published by centers in Europe and Australia reporting excellent results for the Lap-Band.[55,56] Similarly excellent results have been published for the Swedish adjustable band.[57] Buchwald and colleagues[58] performed a

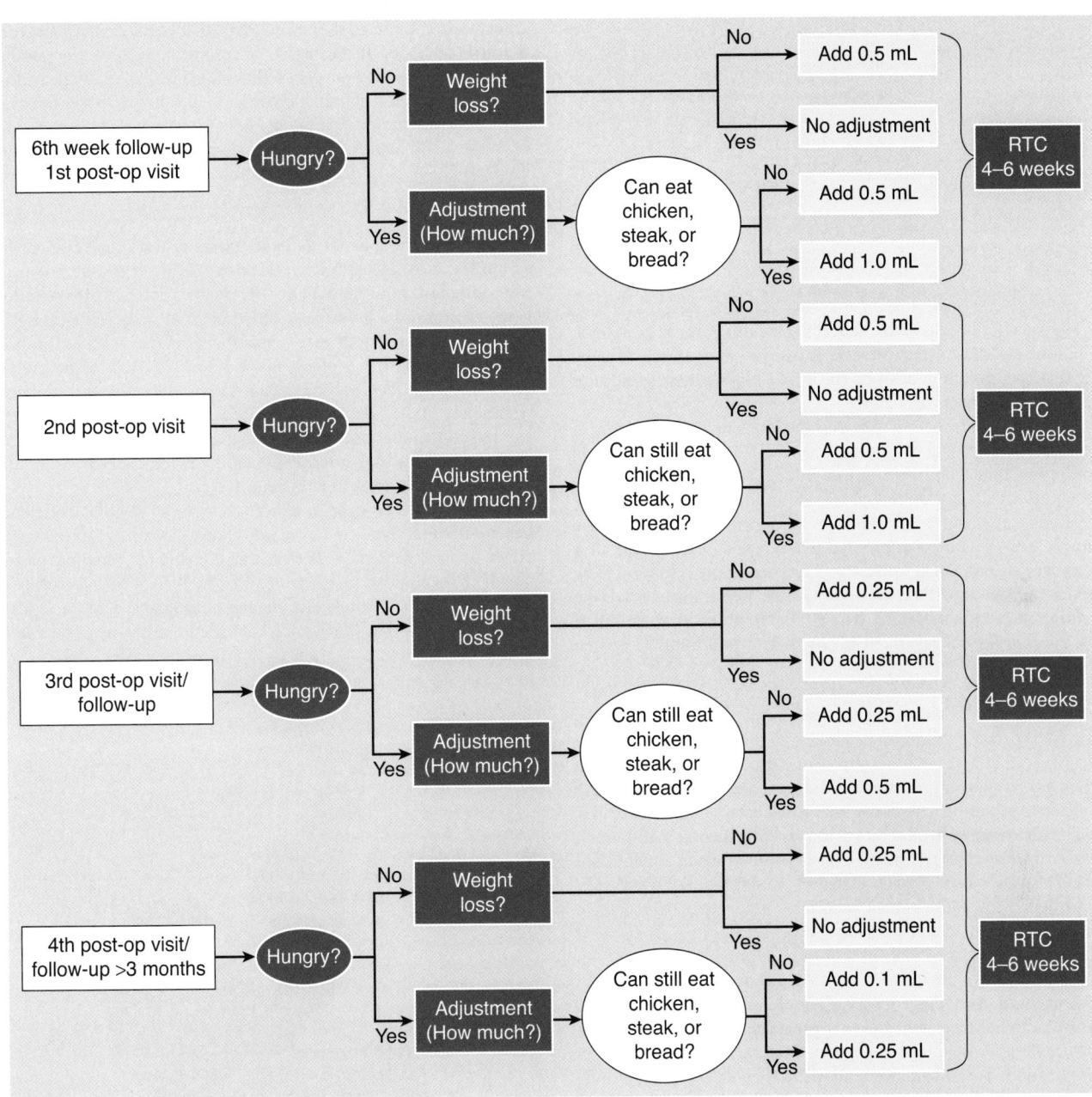

FIG. 27-6. Algorithm for postoperative band adjustment. RTC = return to clinic. The band capacity for this algorithm was 5.0 ml. New bands have larger capacities, and the recommended adjustment amounts should be altered proportionately according to the increased band capacity. *[Reproduced with permission from Ren CJ: Laparoscopic adjustable gastric banding: Postoperative management and nutritional evaluation, in Schauer PR, et al (eds): Minimally Invasive Bariatric Surgery, 1st ed. New York: Springer, 2007, p 200.]*

meta-analysis of all bariatric surgical papers published from 1990 to 2003. Overall mortality for LAGB was given as 0.1%. Table 27-7 shows the data from this paper for weight loss, morbidity, and mortality for LAGB compared with RYGB and the malabsorptive procedures. Table 27-8 also shows the findings of Buchwald and colleagues[58] on the percentage of resolution of four major comorbidities associated with obesity after the most common types of bariatric operations, including LAGB. Another contemporary meta-analysis shows similar outcomes for LAGB compared to other bariatric operations.[59]

Specific complications that may occur after LAGB include prolapse, slippage, erosion, and port and tubing complications. In addition, just plain failure to lose weight is more commonly seen with this procedure than with other common bariatric procedures.

Prolapse is perhaps the most common emergent complication that requires reoperation after LAGB. The incidence is generally in the 3% range. Postoperative vomiting predisposes to this problem, because the lower stomach can be pushed upward and trapped within the lumen of the band. Typical patient symptoms include immediate dysphagia, vomiting, and inability to take oral food or liquid. Either anterior or posterior prolapse may occur.[60] Reoperation laparoscopically to reduce the prolapse and resuture the band imbrication is indicated.

TABLE 27-7 Outcomes for bariatric operations

	LAGB	RYGB	BPD/DS
Excess weight loss (%)	47.5	61.6	70.1
Mortality (%)	0.1	0.5	1.1
Morbidity (%)	10–25	13–38	27–33
Nutritional morbidity (%)	0–10	15–25	40–77

BPD/DS = biliopancreatic diversion with duodenal switch; LAGB = laparoscopic adjustable gastric banding; RYGB = Roux-en-Y gastric bypass.
Source: Data from Buchwald et al.[58]

962

TABLE 27-8	Effect of bariatric surgery on comorbid medical conditions	
Condition	% Resolved	% Improved
Diabetes	76.8	85.4
Hypertension	61.7	78.5
Sleep apnea	83.6	85.7
Hyperlipidemia	70.0	96.9

Source: Data from Buchwald et al.[58]

Slippage has been greatly reduced by the use of the pars flaccida technique and now occurs in <3% of cases in most series. Laparoscopic reoperation to reposition the band in the optimal location is the treatment for this problem.

Band erosion is uncommon, reported in 1 to 2% of patients in most series. The patient usually becomes ill but not floridly ill, developing either a port site infection or systemic fever and signs or symptoms suggesting low-grade abdominal inflammatory sepsis. Endoscopy can be diagnostic. The presence of otherwise unexplained free air on computed tomographic scan should alert the surgeon to this diagnosis as well. Laparoscopic removal of the band is indicated, with repair of any gastric perforation. Often the perforation is already sealed by an inflammatory process, but if not, appropriate management of the gastric perforation must be undertaken.[60]

Port and tubing problems occur in approximately 5% of patients undergoing LAGB. These require revision of the port and tubing system to correct perforation or kinking of the tubing or turning of the port so that access to the surface of the port for adding fluid is precluded. Usually a procedure under local anesthesia is all that is required to repair or realign the tubing or port.

The incidence of band removal because of patient dissatisfaction or lack of weight loss is difficult to assess, due to a lack of published data. The figure also is likely related to patient follow-up and may be artificially low if the patient seeks a second surgeon to remove a band. The true incidence probably varies widely, from almost zero in some practices to possibly as high as >10% in others.

An overview of the outcomes of LAGB should note the safety of the procedure. Although complications are now rare, most of them involve non–life-threatening events. Most reoperations can and are performed laparoscopically or under local anesthesia. Nutritional complications are uncommon and easily treated. Based on worldwide data, the results appear to be optimal in those practices and centers in which continued optimal follow-up and encouragement of appropriate behavioral lifestyle changes preserve the excellent weight loss enabled by such conditions. In centers in which suboptimal conditions exist for support and follow-up, the rate of band failure in terms of poor overall weight loss can be significant. Reports in the literature tend to include only those patients who still have their bands in place and to exclude patients who have had their bands removed due to failure to lose weight. Although the number of patients in the latter group probably varies widely from center to center, the trend in many European centers now to perform more LRYGB and fewer LAGB procedures than 5 years ago suggests that the outcomes for LAGB may rest as much on the postoperative support setting as on the operation itself. Centers should reassess their ability to provide such optimal follow-up and should do so if possible for the best long-term results after this operation.

Laparoscopic Roux-en-Y Gastric Bypass
Background

The laparoscopic approach to gastric bypass (LRYGB) was first described in 1994,[26] but by 1998 only a few centers had accumulated any significant experience with the procedure. Many training programs were conducted in the late 1990s that enabled many surgeons to learn and adopt the laparoscopic approach. By 2001, the number of minimally invasive surgery fellowships had exploded, providing an opportunity for young surgeons to work in an apprentice-type setting for the bariatric surgeons doing laparoscopic bariatric and GI surgery. By 2003, >130,000 gastric bypasses were performed in the United States, with more than half of them being done laparoscopically.

RYGB had been done since the 1960s, and the evolution of that procedure to the current general configuration of LRYGB is described later in the discussion of open RYGB. Figure 27-7 depicts the configuration of the RYGB. The major feature of the operation is the creation of a proximal gastric pouch of small size (often <20 mL) that is totally separated from the stomach. A Roux limb of proximal jejunum is brought up and anastomosed to the pouch. The pathway of that limb can be anterior to the colon and stomach, posterior to both, or posterior to the colon and anterior to the stomach. The length of the biliopancreatic limb from the ligament of Treitz to the distal enteroenterostomy is from 20 to 50 cm, and the length of the Roux limb is 75 to 150 cm.

Although it is an oversimplification, one can say that experience has resolved several controversies about gastric bypass, whereas others are still debated. It is clear that creating the proximal gastric pouch by totally dividing it from the distal stomach is superior to open techniques of simply stapling the stomach, because the latter is associated with a high incidence of staple breakdown.[61] The size of

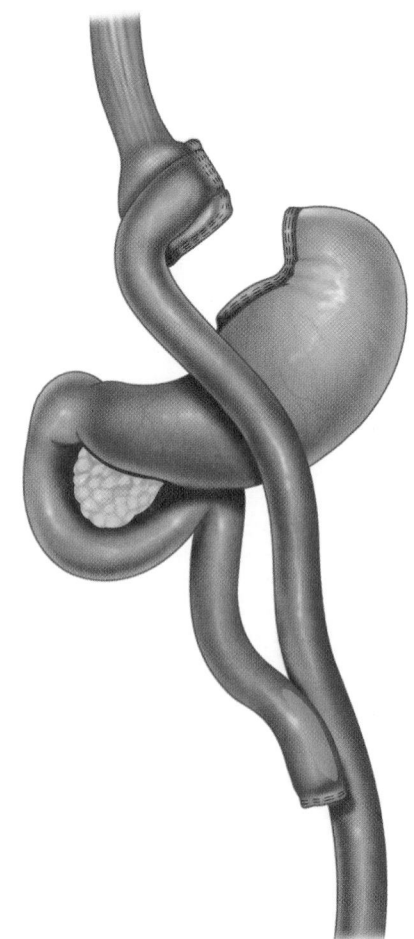

FIG. 27-7. Configuration of gastric bypass. [Reproduced with permission from Austrheim-Smith I, et al: Evolution of bariatric minimally invasive surgery, in Schauer PR, et al (eds): Minimally Invasive Bariatric Surgery, 1st ed. New York: Springer, 2007, p 22.]

the proximal gastric pouch must be small (<20 mL) to create adequate restriction, and it should exclude the fundus of the stomach to prevent dilation over time. Longer length of the Roux limb is associated with higher short-term weight loss,[62] but this difference becomes insignificant on long-term follow-up.[63] Some surgeons doing LRYGB create a longer (150-cm) Roux limb for patients with a BMI of >60 kg/m² or even >50 kg/m². Antecolic position of the Roux limb was associated with a lower incidence of internal hernias leading to obstruction in most early series.[64] However, follow-up reports suggest that the incidence of late internal hernia may increase with an antecolic approach.[65] Despite the overabundance of enthusiasm for reoperative endoscopic narrowing of the gastrojejunostomy opening,[66,67] there are not yet any good long-term data to confirm what size of gastrojejunostomy can be related to weight loss. The gastrojejunal anastomosis can be constructed in a variety of ways. Smaller-diameter circular stapling (21 mm vs. 25 mm) is associated with a higher incidence of postoperative stenosis, and linear stapling is associated with a lower incidence of stenosis than circular stapling.[68,69]

Technique

The operation generally is performed using five ports plus a site for a liver retractor. Both the surgeon, who stands on the patient's right, and the first assistant, who stands on the patient's left, have two ports for instruments. The telescope requires a port, usually in the supraumbilical region. The assistant's ports are in the left subcostal and flank areas, whereas both of the surgeon's ports may be in the right upper quadrant (Cleveland approach) or one may be on each side of the camera (Virginia approach, Fig. 27-8). Division of the proximal jejunum at 40 to 50 cm distal to the ligament of Treitz is performed with the linear stapler using the white (2.8-mm) stapler cartridge. Further division of the mesentery at that location is performed either with the stapler or the Harmonic scalpel, so that adequate mobilization of the Roux limb is achieved. A Penrose drain is sutured to the proximal Roux limb (Fig. 27-9).

The length of the Roux limb to be created (usually 100 to 150 cm) is now measured. A jejunojejunostomy is then created to the proximal end of the biliopancreatic limb at the above-determined location along the Roux limb. A side-to-side stapled anastomosis is performed (Fig. 27-10). Either single- or double-fired staple technique (the latter using a stapler fired in each direction) is used. The stapler defect is optimally closed with sutures but can be closed with a stapler if great care is taken not to narrow the lumen of the alimentary tract at this location. Once the stapler defect is closed, the mesenteric defect is then also closed with running permanent suture.

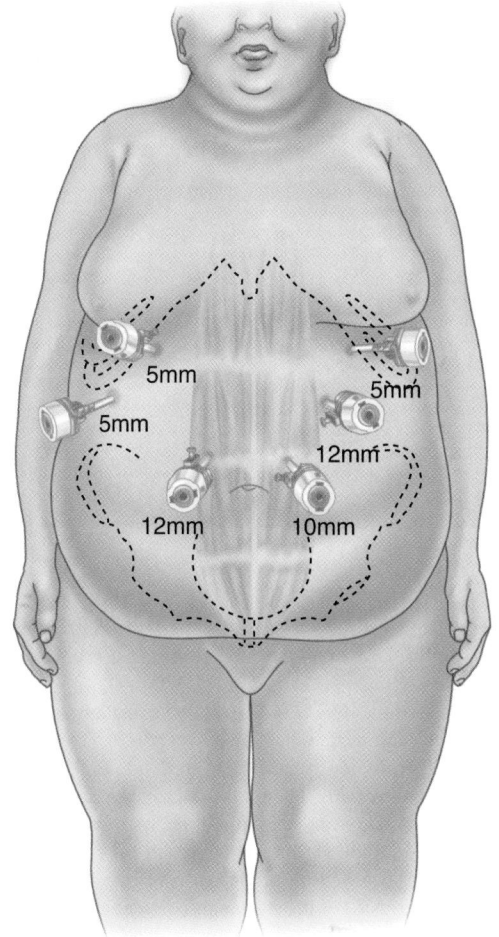

FIG. 27-8. Port scheme for laparoscopic gastric bypass. *[Reproduced with permission from Thodiyil PA, et al: Linear stapled technique for gastrojejunal anastomosis, in Schauer PR, et al (eds): Minimally Invasive Bariatric Surgery, 1st ed. New York: Springer, 2007, p 263.]*

Passage of the Roux limb toward the stomach is now performed. If an antecolic route is to be used, the end of the Roux limb is brought up so as to confirm its ability to reach the stomach. If a retrocolic route is to be used, a defect is made in the transverse colon mesentery

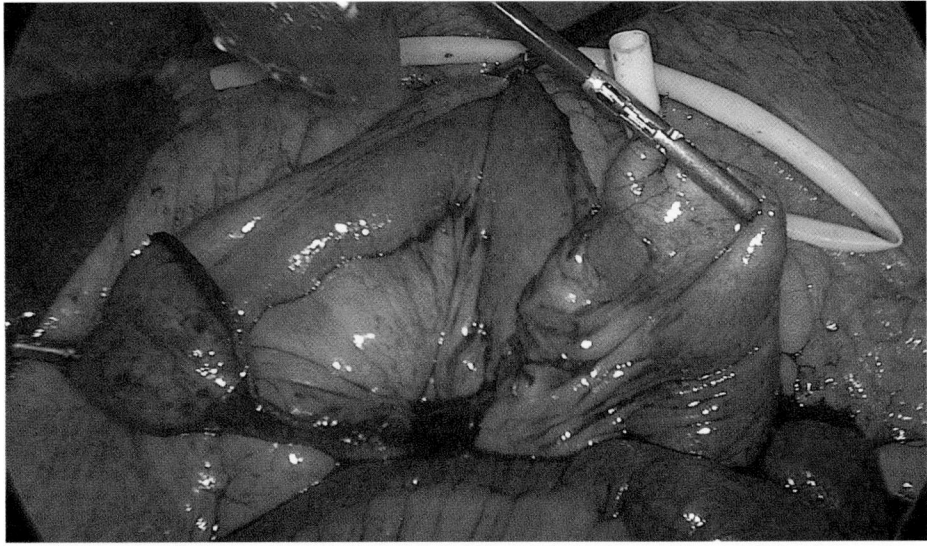

FIG. 27-9. Creation of the Roux limb during laparoscopic gastric bypass.

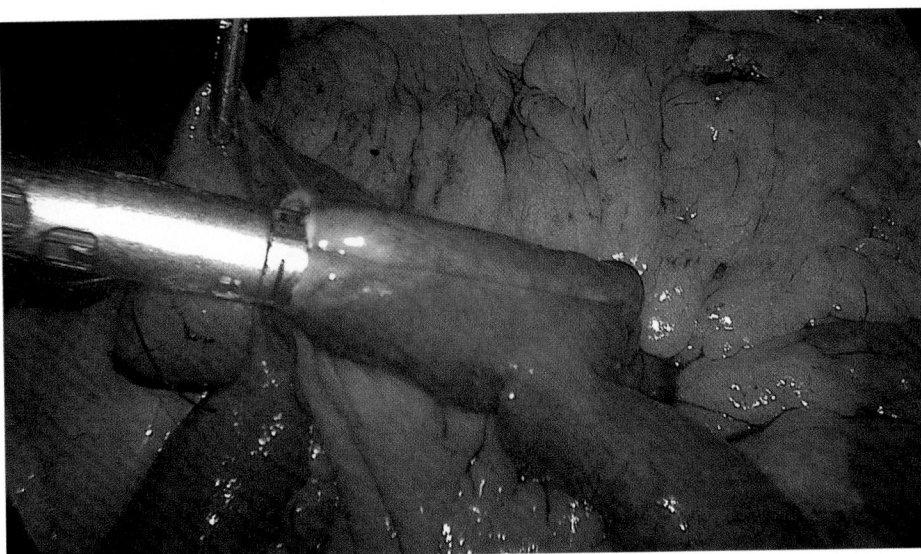

FIG. 27-10. Enteroenterostomy of laparoscopic Roux-en-Y gastric bypass.

just to the left and slightly above the ligament of Treitz. The Penrose drain and the proximal end of the Roux limb are placed into the retrogastric space (Fig. 27-11).

The left lobe of the liver is now retracted using any one of several retractor types. The patient is moved to reverse Trendelenburg's position. The Harmonic scalpel is used to divide the peritoneum in the area of the angle of His. Then it is used to open an area along the lesser curvature of the stomach approximately 3 cm down from the gastroesophageal junction. Another approach for creating access to the lesser curvature of the stomach is to use a white or gray (2.0-mm) cartridge (vascular load) of the stapler and divide the lesser curvature vessels up to the surface of the stomach. Then a blue (3.8-mm) cartridge of the stapler is fired one time transversely from the lesser curvature side partially across the stomach; this is followed by multiple subsequent firings of the stapler upward in the direction of the angle of His to completely separate the proximal gastric pouch from the remainder of the stomach (Fig. 27-12). Use of a Ewald tube passed

by the anesthesiologist and maneuvered to lie against the lesser curvature of the proximal stomach can help calibrate the pouch size.

Once the pouch is created, the Roux limb is brought up to the proximal gastric pouch. For the linear stapled anastomosis, the proximal end of the Roux limb is aligned with the distal gastric pouch end, and the sides of the organs are sutured together to maintain their side-by-side position. A blue stapler cartridge is introduced through a gastrotomy and an enterotomy for the two legs of the stapler, and the anastomosis is created (Fig. 27-13). The stapler defect is closed with sutures and often reinforced with a second layer of sutures. At this point the gastrojejunostomy is tested for security either by injecting methylene blue under pressure through the Ewald tube or by performing flexible upper endoscopy intraoperatively to test for air leakage from the anastomosis. The latter technique has been clearly shown to decrease the incidence and seriousness of anastomotic leaks postoperatively.[70] The final step of the operation involves suture closure of all mesenteric defects using permanent suture.

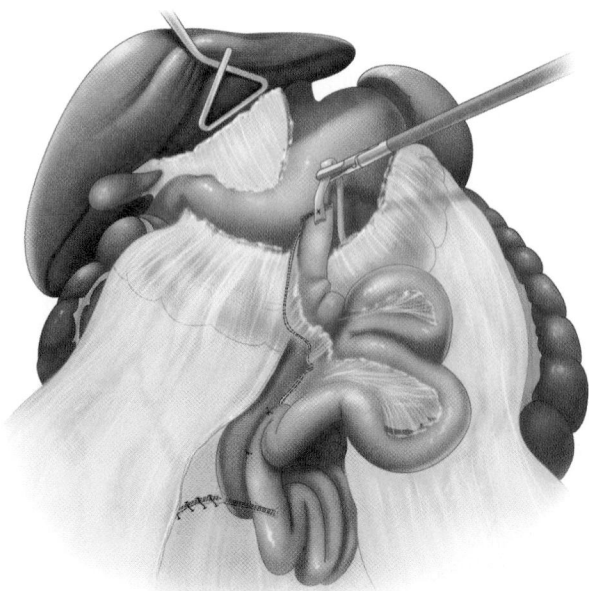

FIG. 27-11. Passage of Roux limb. *[Reproduced with permission from Thodiyil PA, et al: Linear stapled technique for gastrojejunal anastomosis, in Schauer PR, et al (eds): Minimally Invasive Bariatric Surgery, 1st ed. New York: Springer, 2007, p 266.]*

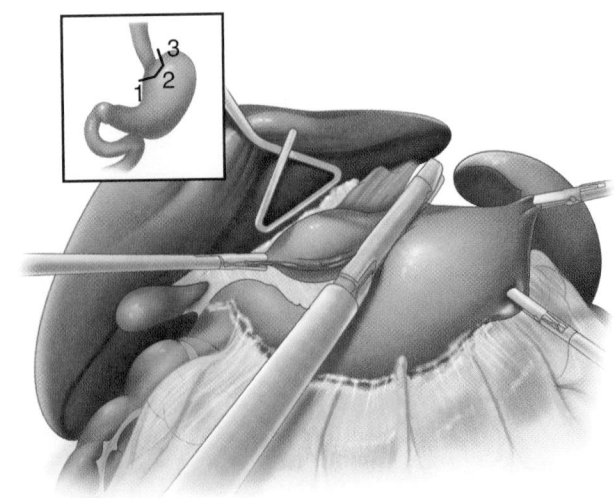

FIG. 27-12. Creation of gastric pouch for laparoscopic Roux-en-Y gastric bypass. *[Reproduced with permission from Thodiyil PA, et al: Linear stapled technique for gastrojejunal anastomosis, in Schauer PR, et al (eds): Minimally Invasive Bariatric Surgery, 1st ed. New York: Springer, 2007, p 266.]*

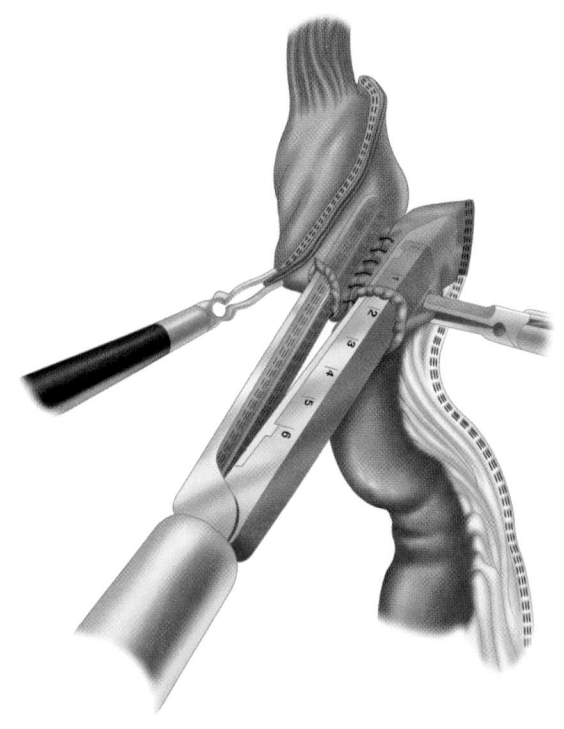

FIG. 27-13. Gastrojejunostomy in laparoscopic Roux-en-Y gastric bypass. *[Reproduced with permission from Thodiyil PA, et al: Linear stapled technique for gastrojejunal anastomosis, in Schauer PR, et al (eds): Minimally Invasive Bariatric Surgery, 1st ed. New York: Springer, 2007, p 267.]*

Circular anastomosis for the gastrojejunostomy is accomplished by placing the anvil of the stapler through the anterior wall of the proximal gastric pouch. This is done either by pulling the anvil transorally via an endoscopically placed guidewire (Fig. 27-14),

making a gastrotomy in the pouch that is later closed, or by creating a gastrotomy in the lower stomach before completing gastric division to form the pouch, which allows the anvil to be placed into the lumen of the stomach and then be brought through the anterior stomach in an area that is subsequently included in the proximal gastric pouch (Fig. 27-15).

A hand-sewn gastrojejunostomy is usually created using two layers of absorbable suture to anastomose an approximately 1-cm gastrotomy and enterotomy.

Patient Selection and Preparation

LRYGB is an appropriate operation to consider for most patients eligible for bariatric surgery. Relative contraindications to LRYGB include previous gastric surgery, previous antireflux surgery, severe iron deficiency anemia, distal gastric or duodenal lesions that require ongoing future surveillance, and Barrett's esophagus with severe dysplasia. Contraindications to a laparoscopic approach to RYGB should cause the surgeon to choose an open RYGB or other open procedure instead.

Preoperative flexible upper endoscopy for all patients contemplating RYGB is advocated by some to rule out lesions of the stomach or duodenum noted earlier. Preoperative consumption of a low-calorie diet by patients with hepatomegaly can decrease liver size and thereby improve the chances of completing the operation laparoscopically. We use a mechanical bowel preparation to decrease bowel weight and protect against complications due to an inadvertent tear caused by the laparoscopic graspers.

Postoperative Care and Follow-Up

Patients undergoing LRYGB usually are hospitalized for 2 to 3 days. Major concerns on the night of surgery include adequate analgesia, adequate fluid resuscitation to provide adequate urine output, and early ambulation. We routinely perform a postoperative oral contrast study on the first postoperative day to rule out a leak. Some studies have advocated abandoning this practice due to its lack of accuracy and cost effectiveness, while others have shown that it can lead to

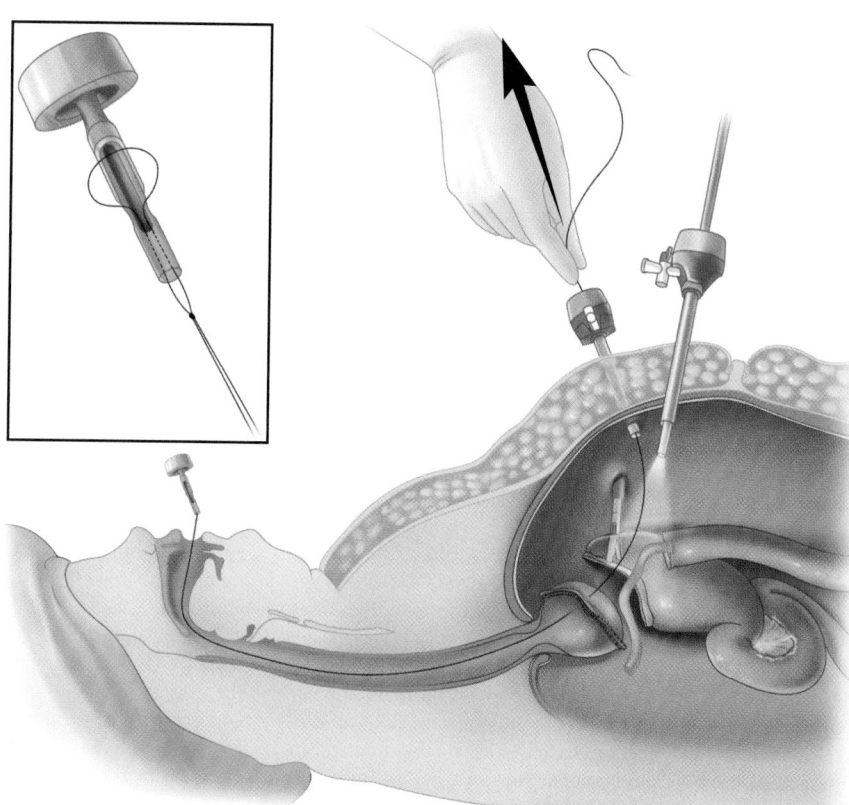

FIG. 27-14. Oral passage of circular stapler to create a gastrojejunostomy for laparoscopic Roux-en-Y gastric bypass. *[Reproduced with permission from Wittgrove A, et al: Circular stapler technique for gastroenterostomy, in Schauer PR, et al (eds): Minimally Invasive Bariatric Surgery, 1st ed. New York: Springer, 2007, p 240.]*

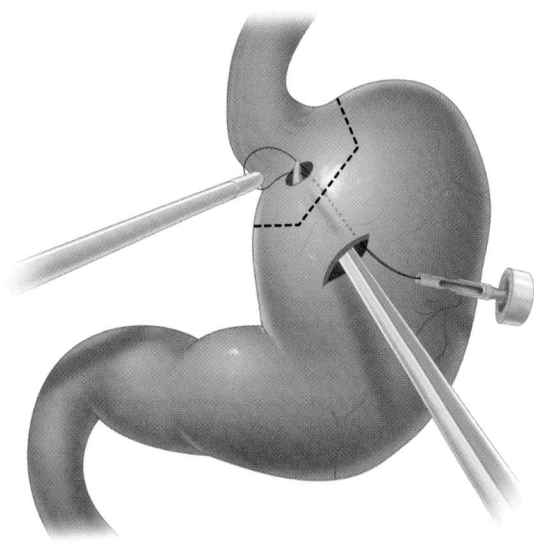

FIG. 27-15. Transgastric passage of circular stapler to create a gastrojejunostomy for laparoscopic Roux-en-Y gastric bypass. *[Reproduced with permission from Schneider BE, et al: Circular stapled transabdominal technique, in Schauer PR, et al (eds): Minimally Invasive Bariatric Surgery, 1st ed. New York: Springer, 2007, p 248.]*

TABLE 27-9	Complications for which patients undergoing laparoscopic Roux-en-Y gastric bypass require urgent surgical intervention

Small-bowel obstruction
Early postoperative vomiting with signs and symptoms suggesting obstruction
Early postoperative hematemesis with signs and symptoms suggesting obstruction

earlier identification of leaks.[71–73] The study's value to us has been to alert us to an early asymptomatic leak or to edema or stenosis of the enteroenterostomy or to any other obstructive pattern of the proximal bowel. Obstruction of the enteroenterostomy or beyond can result in distal gastric dilatation over a period as short as several hours, which if untreated can cause distal gastric staple line rupture with fatal consequences.

In addition to early ambulation, postoperative prophylaxis against venous thromboembolism includes use of compression devices and SC administration of low molecular weight heparin. Discharge on a blenderized diet is standard for our practice.

Diet advancement occurs after the first clinic visit, usually approximately 3 weeks after surgery. At that time an exercise plan is initiated if not already started.

Patients taking insulin for type 2 diabetes and those taking antihypertensive medications should be monitored to determine if reduction of their medication is indicated. Subsequent follow-up visits are usually scheduled for 3 months, 6 months, and 1 year after surgery, then annually after that. The focus of later postoperative visits is documentation of outcomes and testing for postoperative nutritional deficiencies.

Outcomes

Patients undergoing LRYGB usually lose between 60 and 80% of excess body weight during the first year after surgery. This has held true since the earliest large series of this operation was reported.[74] Resolution of comorbidities varies depending on the disease but is >90% for GERD and venous stasis ulcers, and >80% for type 2 diabetes of <5 years' duration. Hyperlipidemias are almost always improved and resolve totally in approximately 70% of cases. Hypertension is resolved in 50 to 65% of cases (Table 27-8). Even superobese patients who do not achieve an ultimate BMI of <35 kg/m² can experience significant improvements in comorbidities after LRYGB or open RYGB.[75]

Mortality after LRYGB is consistently <1% in most large reported series. Recent data from centers applying to be bariatric surgery centers of excellence show a mortality of approximately 0.3% overall.[76]

Overall morbidity after LRYGB has been acceptably low and in non–Veterans Administration National Surgical Quality Improvement Program centers generally is reported in the 15% range.[77]

plications that do occur include anastomotic leak (1 to 2% incidence), venous thromboembolism (1 to 3% incidence with a <1% incidence of pulmonary embolism), wound infections or problems (3 to 5% incidence), marginal ulcers (3 to 15% incidence), bowel obstruction (an approximately 7% incidence), need for postoperative transfusion (a 4% incidence), and anastomotic stenosis (1 to 19% incidence based on the type of anastomosis created).

Postoperative nutritional complications after LRYGB include iron deficiency in 20 to 40% of patients, iron deficiency anemia in 20%, vitamin B₁₂ deficiency in 15%, and vitamin D deficiency in at least 15%, which usually is present preoperatively.

Several complications that are specific to the LRYGB procedure must be emphasized. The most important is small-bowel obstruction. This complication must be treated differently from obstruction in the average general surgery patient, in whom it is usually caused by adhesions and often will resolve with conservative, nonoperative therapy. Patients who have undergone LRYGB who have symptoms of obstruction *require surgical therapy on an emergent basis* (see Table 27-9). This is because the cause of the bowel obstruction after LRYGB is often an internal hernia from inadequate closure or nonclosure of the mesenteric defects by the surgeon at the time of operation. Treatment for these patients therefore differs from that for most patients with small-bowel obstruction. The *single most important point* made in this chapter is to caution general surgeons to be aware of the need to operate emergently on patients who present with small-bowel obstruction after LRYGB. Currently centers that perform small-bowel transplantation are finding that the leading patient group referred for that procedure is patients who had small-bowel obstruction after LRYGB, developed infarction of most of the bowel from the internal hernia, and have short-gut syndrome. Patients for whom surgery is delayed and in whom the bowel infarcts often do not survive. When the surgeon does encounter bowel obstruction after LRYGB, he or she can expect to see proximally dilated bowel. Cutoff of passage of contrast medium on computed tomographic scan at the enteroenterostomy is particularly suggestive of this diagnosis (Fig. 27-16). If this particular problem is addressed early in the course of the obstruction, the surgical treatment can be performed laparoscopically. The surgeon must place a trocar for the telescope low enough in the abdomen to adequately survey most of the small intestine. The cecum and terminal ileum are identified, and the bowel is followed in a retrograde direction from the terminal ileum to determine the anatomy. Often much of the small bowel is herniated through a mesenteric defect, and only this technique allows the surgeon to reliably identify the bowel and decompress it appropriately. If the bowel is viable, suturing the mesenteric defect is all that is required for treatment. It should be emphasized that this complication can occur with either an antecolic or retrocolic placement of the Roux limb, because internal hernias can arise with either approach.

Marginal ulcers are another complication relatively specific to RYGB, either LRYGB or open RYGB. The patient presents with pain in the epigastric region that is not altered by eating. Diagnosis is by endoscopy. Treatment is medical with administration of proton pump inhibitors, which are effective in 90% of cases. Only those with a gastrogastric fistula to the distal stomach or severe stenosis of the lumen of the gastrojejunostomy or non-healing ulcers require surgical therapy.

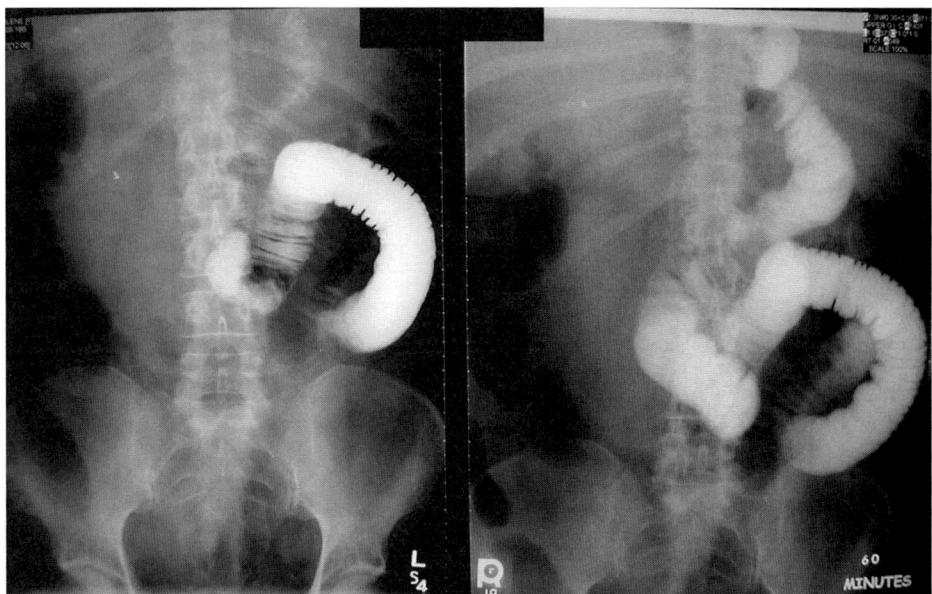

FIG. 27-16. Obstruction of passage of contrast medium at enteroenterostomy with small-bowel obstruction from internal hernia after laparoscopic Roux-en-Y gastric bypass.

In our experience stenosis of the gastrojejunostomy has been markedly reduced by the use of a linear stapling technique.[68] Symptoms of stenosis most commonly appear between 6 and 12 weeks postoperatively but can also occur later. Diagnosis is by upper endoscopy. Treatment is balloon dilatation. Resolution normally occurs with one or two treatments. Fewer than 10% of patients require reoperation, and these are almost always patients with concurrent marginal ulcers.[78]

In the immediately postoperative period, anastomotic leak is the single most feared complication after RYGB, either open or laparoscopic. Careful vigilance and a high index of suspicion for this problem is the only appropriate approach. The presentation of anastomotic leak may be insidious and the patient's demise sudden if the condition is untreated. Tachycardia, tachypnea, fever, and oliguria are the most common symptoms that arouse suspicion of this problem. The treatment is surgical except in circumstances in which a drain is already in place, no hemodynamic or clinical deterioration is present, and the leak is contained.[73] Surgical treatment involves oversewing and repair of the leak as feasible along with drainage. A gastrostomy tube in the diverted stomach can provide a reliable feeding access and decompression.

In the first few hours or day after surgery, hematemesis often indicates bleeding from the gastrojejunostomy unless proven otherwise. The dangers to the patient include aspiration, life-threatening hemorrhage, or, more commonly, intraluminal hematoma of the Roux limb and enteroenterostomy, which then causes an obstruction of the biliopancreatic limb leading to distal gastric staple line rupture. In fact, any obstructive symptoms in the first few weeks after surgery or any signs of obstruction of the biliopancreatic limb due to stenosis of the enteroenterostomy on postoperative swallow studies require immediate attention and possible surgical intervention to prevent rupture of the distal gastric staple line. Some reports show that percutaneous decompression of the distal stomach can ameliorate the danger. We have preferred operative therapy to decompress the stomach and treat the obstructive problem.

Overall, LRYGB has the significant advantages over open RYGB of avoiding incisional hernias and severe wound infections. Table 27-10 shows the data on these problems, comparing outcomes for laparoscopic vs. open procedures performed at the University of Virginia. Compared with other bariatric surgical procedures, the LRYGB offers a reliable and powerful operation to allow the severely obese patient to lose weight. The more reliable and greater weight loss after RYGB is accompanied by a higher rate of severe complications than with LAGB. However, recently reported data from scores

of medical centers around the United States suggest that the incidence of LRYGB-related morbidity is decreasing. RYGB is particularly effective in resolving the comorbidities of GERD and type 2 diabetes when compared with LAGB.

Open Roux-en-Y Gastric Bypass
Background

As mentioned earlier, Mason and Itoh[19] first described gastric bypass and Griffin and colleagues[20] described the Roux limb modification. The RYGB procedure has been the most time tested and proven of all bariatric operations. Open RYGB is now done in virtually the same manner as LRYGB, the only difference being the access route to perform it. Experienced bariatric surgeons who do not perform laparoscopic surgery still perform this operation with excellent overall outcomes.[40] Open RYGB was the most popular bariatric operation performed in the United States in the 1990s but is now far exceeded by LRYGB and LAGB in terms of volume, likely due largely to the preference of patients to undergo a laparoscopic rather than an open procedure. However, for the patient for whom a laparoscopic approach fails, open RYGB must be an operation that the bariatric surgeon can perform with skill.

Technique

Open RYGB is performed in essentially the same way as LRYGB. Some surgeons who use an open approach prefer to create the gastric pouch

| TABLE 27-10 | Outcomes for laparoscopic vs. open Roux-en-Y gastric bypass, University of Virginia, 1994–2004 |

Characteristics	LRYGB	ORYGB	P Value
Preoperative body mass index (kg/m²)	50.9 ± 0.3[a]	57.5 ± 0.5[a]	<.001
Number of comorbidities	2.7 ± 0.1[a]	3.6 ± 0.1[a]	<.001
30-day mortality	2 (0.3%)	6 (1.7%)	<.02
Overall complications	111 (14.5 %)	208 (57.3%)	<.001
Reoperations	67 (8.8%)	150 (41.3%)	<.001
Incisional hernias	13 (1.7%)	123 (33.9%)	<.001
Wound infections	14 (1.8%)	27 (7.4%)	<.001

[a]Values indicate mean ± standard deviation.
LRYGB = laparoscopic Roux-en-Y gastric bypass; ORYGB = open Roux-en-Y gastric bypass.

as the first part of the procedure, but in essence the basic procedure is the same. Access for open RYGB is usually through an upper midline incision, although a left subcostal incision has been reported to furnish adequate access as well. Closure of the midline wound is performed using a running monofilament suture. Subcutaneous tissues are thoroughly irrigated, and the skin is closed with a skin stapler.

Patient Selection and Preparation

Patient selection for open RYGB is essentially the same as for LRYGB, because the operation is the same. Extraordinarily large patients or those who have previously undergone multiple abdominal operations, particularly previous gastric surgery, left colectomy, and splenectomy, often require an open incision to perform RYGB. An especially thick abdominal wall and large liver size are other factors that may require an open incision approach. Patients who have an existing large midline incisional hernia are also candidates for an open approach.

Preparation for open RYGB is identical to that for LRYGB.

Postoperative Care and Follow-Up

The postoperative care of the patient undergoing open RYGB is very similar to that of the patient undergoing LRYGB. Larger volumes for fluid resuscitation and often more narcotic analgesics are required the day of surgery and frequently the next as well. Greater attention must be paid to the incision site to check for potential infection, because an inadequately treated wound infection in these patients can extend easily to the fascial level and cause significant tissue loss before it is fully diagnosed. The perioperative care of patients undergoing open RYGB is usually more intense, often because such patients are very large and have severe comorbidities, which puts them at higher risk overall for complications of all types. It is interesting, though, that since the era of LRYGB, patients who still undergo open RYGB (usually due to intraoperative conversion) in our practice often are discharged within 1 day of the laparoscopic patients. The overall length of stay has decreased for our RYGB patients based on the use of postoperative pathways geared toward LRYGB.

Postoperative follow-up visits are similar to those for LRYGB patients, with the first visit being timed appropriately for removal of skin staples. Other visits, follow-up schedule, and blood testing are identical to those for LRYGB.

Outcomes

The weight loss statistics and patterns for open RYGB are comparable to those for LRYGB, as would be expected. Postoperative deaths are slightly higher with open RYGB, but this isin part due to the patient population, who are often among the most severely medically compromised preoperatively. Flum and Dellinger[79] showed that in a patient population with Medicare insurance and hence largely disabled, RYGB had an across-the-board mortality rate of 2.0%. This is considerably higher than the 0.3 to 0.4% incidence that has been reported on average the past 2 years for programs applying for qualification as bariatric centers of excellence and is due in large part to the patient population. Interestingly, in Flum and Dellinger's report, surgeons with the most experience had a patient mortality rate of <1.0% for this patient population, which suggests that surgeon experience and perhaps also patient selection by experienced surgeons influences mortality for RYGB.

One of the most important population studies showing the benefit of bariatric surgery was done in patients undergoing RYGB. Christou and colleagues[80] showed that, in a 5-year follow-up, mortality was lower among >1000 patients undergoing RYGB than among >5000 severely obese individuals who did not have surgery (0.68 vs. 6.17%). This represents a reduction of 89% in the death rate.

The incidence of postoperative complications is higher for open RYGB than for LRYGB. The major types of increased morbidity are incisional hernias and other wound-related problems. Table 27-10 presents data recently submitted for publication drawn from the Virginia experience after 10 years of follow-up. Findings included a very high incidence of incisional hernias after open RYGB as well as a lower

rate of wound infections for LRYGB than for open RYGB. The marked difference in reoperation rates for the laparoscopic and open procedures was due almost exclusively to incisional hernia repairs. However, when considering these data one must keep in mind that the patients undergoing LRYGB also were smaller and had fewer comorbidities during these years. Except for the higher rate of incisional hernias, the long-term results for patients undergoing open RYGB are similar to those for patients undergoing LRYGB with regard to nutritional complications, weight loss, and overall resolution of comorbidities.

Two randomized controlled trials with 5-year follow-up have compared LRYGB with LAGB. Both demonstrate a higher rate of postoperative morbidity for RYGB compared to LAGB (21 vs. 7%) but superior weight loss for RYGB compared to LABG (67–68 vs. 41–46% EWL). Failure to achieve significant weight greater for LAGB compared to RYGB (17-35 vs. 0-4%).[81,82]

Biliopancreatic Diversion and Duodenal Switch
Background

Biliopancreatic diversion (BPD) was first described by, and remains championed by, Scopinaro and colleagues in Italy.[23] The operation, which is pictured in Fig. 27-17, involves resection of the distal half to two thirds of the stomach and creation of an alimentary tract of the most distal 200 cm of ileum, which is anastomosed to the stomach. The biliopancreatic limb is anastomosed to the alimentary tract either 75 or 100 cm proximal to the ileocecal valve, depending on the protein content of the patient's diet. This operation met with limited international popularity, probably due to the technical difficulty of performing it combined with the significant percentage of nutritional complications that arise postoperatively. However, the procedure did develop a devoted following among a few bariatric surgeons.

One complication that plagued BPD was the high incidence of marginal ulcers postoperatively. Hess and colleagues[83] and Marceau and associates[84] separately described the adaptation of the duodenal switch (DS) operation, originally proposed by DeMeester and colleagues[85] for the treatment of bile reflux gastritis, to replace the gastric portion of the BPD. This new procedure was originally called *biliopancreatic diversion with duodenal switch*. For ease of description, the term *duodenal switch* is used to indicate this procedure. It is illustrated in Fig. 27-18. Currently BPD and DS together represent <5% of bariatric operations performed in the United States and perhaps as little as 2 to 3%. The lack of a significant number of surgeons offering the operation, especially via a laparoscopic approach, probably has a great deal to do with that statistic. BPD and DS are recognized as standard bariatric operations, however, and are approved for coverage by most insurance companies at this time.

Technique

The technique for BPD is described for the open approach, but the laparoscopic approach essentially reproduces what is done with the open approach using different access. Laparoscopic BPD and DS are very technically challenging operations, which is perhaps another factor contributing to the relatively low numbers of surgeons offering these operations.

The BPD operation begins with performance of a distal subtotal gastrectomy. A residual 200-mL gastric pouch is created for super-obese patients and a slightly larger pouch for patients with a BMI of <50 kg/m². The terminal ileum is identified and divided 250 cm proximal to the ileocecal valve. The distal end of that divided ileum is then anastomosed to the stomach, creating a 2- to 3-cm stoma. The proximal end of the ileum is then anastomosed side to side to the terminal ileum approximately 100 cm proximal to the ileocecal valve. Some surgeons perform the anastomosis only 50 cm proximal to the valve, but in these patients the likelihood of good protein intake postoperatively should be high. Prophylactic cholecystectomy is performed due to the high incidence of gallstone formation with the malabsorption of bile salts.

The DS procedure differs from BPD only in the proximal gut portion of the operation. Instead of a distal gastrectomy, a resection

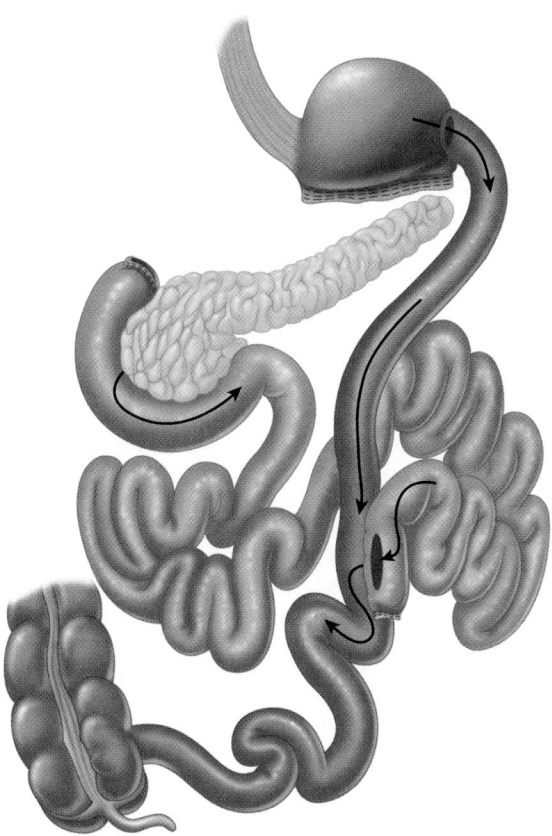

FIG. 27-17. Configuration of biliopancreatic diversion. *[Reproduced with permission from Austrheim-Smith I, et al: Evolution of bariatric minimally invasive surgery, in Schauer PR, et al (eds):* Minimally Invasive Bariatric Surgery, *1st ed. New York: Springer, 2007, p 21.]*

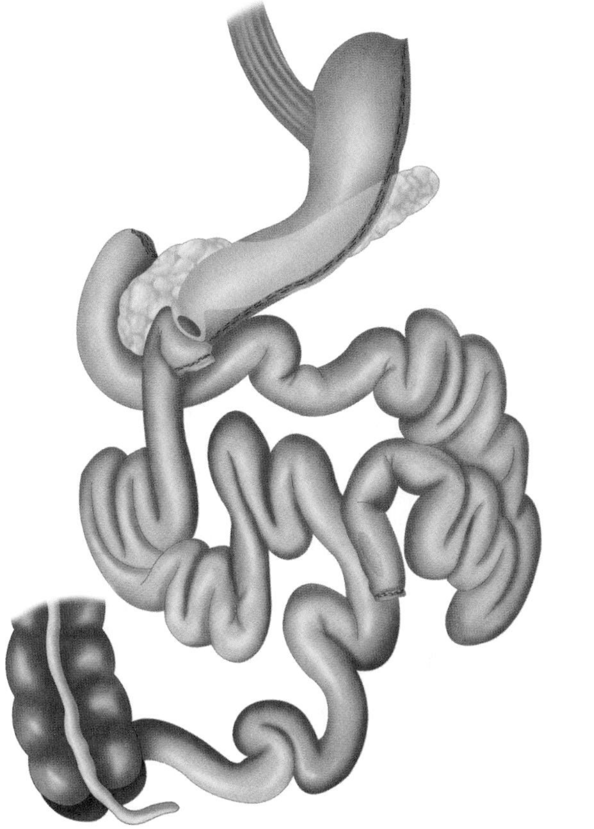

FIG. 27-18. Configuration of the duodenal switch. *[Reproduced with permission from Austrheim-Smith I, et al: Evolution of bariatric minimally invasive surgery, in Schauer PR, et al (eds):* Minimally Invasive Bariatric Surgery, *1st ed. New York: Springer, 2007, p 22.]*

of all the stomach except for a narrow lesser curvature tube is performed. The diameter of this tube is calibrated with a dilator and, if limited to an approximately 32F (11-mm) diameter, produces the optimal amount of weight loss while still allowing adequate oral intake. The duodenum is now divided in its first portion and an approximately 2-cm length of duodenum is left intact beyond the pylorus. This end of the duodenum is then anastomosed to the distal 250 cm of ileum. This anastomosis is often done in an end-to-end fashion with a circular stapler. It is the most difficult portion of the DS procedure, and leak rates are slightly higher than with other types of anastomosis. The distal bowel configuration and cholecystectomy are similar to those for BPD.

Patient Selection and Preparation

Patients who undergo either BPD or DS must be prepared for the consequences of a malabsorptive operation. The occurrence of diarrhea after any large amount of oral intake is a given. Patients who undergo this procedure must be willing to accept that and will also usually modify their eating pattern to restrict intake if access to a bathroom will prove difficult. Patients who undergo either operation must be followed closely *by the surgeon*. Internists and family physicians may not appreciate the problems related to protein-calorie malabsorption if they occur and treat the patients instead for congestive heart failure. Results may then be disastrous. Patients must also have the financial means to afford the large number of vitamin and mineral supplements that must be taken to avoid nutritional problems in this patient population. One unofficial estimate from a surgeon who performs these procedures is that the cost of such supplements may be approximately $1500 per year.

Given the higher incidence of postoperative nutritional and other complications compared with any of the restrictive opera-

tions, BPD and DS usually are recommended only for those patients who are superobese or for whom it is reasonable to believe that they will not succeed in meeting the diet and exercise requirements that form the basis for long-term success with restrictive operations. Patients for whom a restrictive operation has failed and who are considering reoperation are candidates for these procedures.

Contraindications to the procedure include significant geographic distance from the surgeon, lack of financial means to afford supplements, and pre-existing deficiencies of calcium, iron, or other vitamins or minerals.

Postoperative Care and Follow-Up

Patients undergoing BPD or DS must be followed closely and with absolute completeness for nutritional issues long term. Postoperatively, BPD and DS patients face the same potential complications as seen after RYGB. Anastomotic leaks, pulmonary compromise and complications, GI bleeding, anastomotic stenosis or obstruction, and infections are all potential concerns during the index hospitalization. The long gastric staple line and the duodenoileostomy of the DS and the duodenal stump and gastroileostomy of the BPD are all areas of anatomic concern postoperatively. Distal anastomotic problems can occur with either as well. Thorough preoperative and postoperative counseling by a nutritionist well versed in the operation and potential associated nutritional deficiencies is essential. Vitamin and mineral supplements, including oral supplements of iron, calcium, and B$_{12}$ and a multivitamin, must be taken regularly on follow-up. Fat-soluble vitamins must be supplemented in parenteral form. Careful monitoring of protein intake and serum albumin level is necessary. More frequent follow-up is needed than after RYGB. Checkups at 2-month intervals for the first year and semiannual or more frequent visits thereafter is an appropriate schedule.

Outcomes

Weight loss results after BPD or DS are both excellent and are comparable. The losses also are very durable. One 18-year follow-up of patients after BPD showed a mean excess weight loss of 70% persisting for that duration.[86]

Although most of the results reported for BPD or DS are for open operations, one report of laparoscopic DS showed that for 40 patients with an average BMI of 60 kg/m² the mean hospital stay was 4 days, the average operating room time was 3.5 hours, and mean excess weight loss at 9 months was 58%.[87]

Buchwald and colleagues[58] showed that the average excess weight loss after BPD and DS reported in the literature was >70%; the mortality rate was 1.1%, the complication rate was 27 to 33%, and the nutritional complication rate was 40 to 77% (see Table 27-7).

Complications that occur after BPD include those seen after RYGB, in which intestinal anastomoses and gastric division create potential problems. Scopinaro and associates[86] reported complication rates of 1.2% for obstruction, a similar rate for wound infections, and 2.8% for marginal ulcers. However, others found the incidence of marginal ulcers to be higher after BPD, which led to the adoption of the DS procedure. Preservation of the pylorus drastically reduces the incidence of significant dumping after BPD (poorly quantitated in most series). The duodenoileostomy of DS also is associated with a very low rate of stomal ulcer, unlike the gastroileostomy of BPD.

Nutritional complications are by far the most frequent and worrisome after both these operations, particularly on long-term follow-up. Scopinaro and colleagues[86] reported a protein malnutrition rate of 7%, an iron deficiency anemia rate of <5%, and a bone demineralization rate at 5 years of 53%. Other problems that may arise include alopecia from inadequate protein absorption, night blindness from a lack of vitamin A, and gallstones if the gallbladder is not removed. Of all these nutritional complications, however, protein-calorie malnutrition is the most severe and life-threatening. When it is diagnosed, the treatment is parenteral nutrition. The occurrence of two episodes in which parenteral nutrition is required is usually considered an adequate indication to lengthen the common channel of ileum—the section of ileum between the ileoileostomy connecting the biliopancreatic limb to the alimentary tract and the ileocecal valve. The amount by which the surgeon should lengthen the common channel is poorly documented, but most surgeons will lean toward making it long enough to be certain to avoid recurrence of the problem, such as doubling the length of the common channel, even if it decreases weight loss somewhat.

It cannot be emphasized enough that patients who undergo either BPD or DS must be compliant with the required regimen and understand that lifetime nutritional supplementation and lifetime follow-up are essential to the preservation of good health after one of these operations.

Sleeve Gastrectomy

Background

Sleeve gastrectomy (SG) was originally conceived by Gagner's group after they reviewed their results with laparoscopic DS procedures.[85] Because candidates for DS tended to be superobese and often had significant risk factors for surgery, it was not surprising that a somewhat high mortality rate was seen in this series. Demonstrating that mortality was confined to the patients at very high risk, Gagner recommended doing the procedure in two stages for these patients. The gastric resection, for which the term *sleeve gastrectomy* was coined, was performed as an initial stand-alone procedure for high-risk patients. These patients then underwent the remainder of the DS procedure after they had lost significant amounts of weight from the SG. Mortality was decreased with this two-step operation.[88]

Other surgeons subsequently began to use SG as a primary weight loss operation. Insurance approval was problematic, because until recently few insurance companies would reimburse for this operation unless it was part of a staged DS procedure. Reports in the literature of the success and excellent weight loss after SG have been accumu-lating for the past few years.[89,90] One recent report described 750 patients who underwent SG as a primary weight loss procedure.[91]

The American Society of Metabolic and Bariatric Surgery recently officially recommended that SG be used in selected patients for whom the results of other weight loss operations were not superior or as part of a staged DS procedure. It thus recognized SG as a standard weight loss operation.

Technique

SG is performed laparoscopically under most circumstances, although the word *laparoscopic* is omitted from its description in this chapter. It is assumed that this is the approach. Placement of surgical team members is similar to that for LRYGB. Port placement is comparable or altered slightly to improve the angle of placement of the stapler along the lesser curvature of the stomach. Once a liver retractor is placed, the operation begins with passage by the anesthesiologist of a 32F bougie. The bougie is aligned along the lesser curvature of the stomach and used to size the sleeve pouch. Alternatively, some surgeons use an endoscope (approximately 30F) instead of a bougie to size the sleeve. The surgeon begins the gastric resection by dividing the vessels along the greater curvature of the stomach using the Harmonic scalpel. Division is begun 2 to 3 cm proximal to the pylorus and continued to the angle of His. Clips may be used to additionally secure named vessels. Once the greater curvature of the stomach is completely devascularized, gastric division begins. The stomach is divided approximately 2 to 3 cm proximal to the pylorus starting on the greater curvature side. The stapler is initially equipped with a green (4.5-mm) staple cartridge due to the thickness of the stomach wall in this location. The stapler is fired repeatedly toward the angle of His; after the first or second firing it is placed directly adjacent to the dilator along the lesser curvature to limit sleeve diameter (Fig. 27-19). This spacing continues all the way up the stomach to the angle of His. The specimen is removed in a bag, and the staple line is checked for integrity and hemostasis. Figure 27-20 shows the completed operation.

Patient Selection and Preparation

Patients undergoing SG tend to fall into two groups. One group is high-risk superobese patients considering eventually undergoing the second procedure to complete the DS operation. The other group is

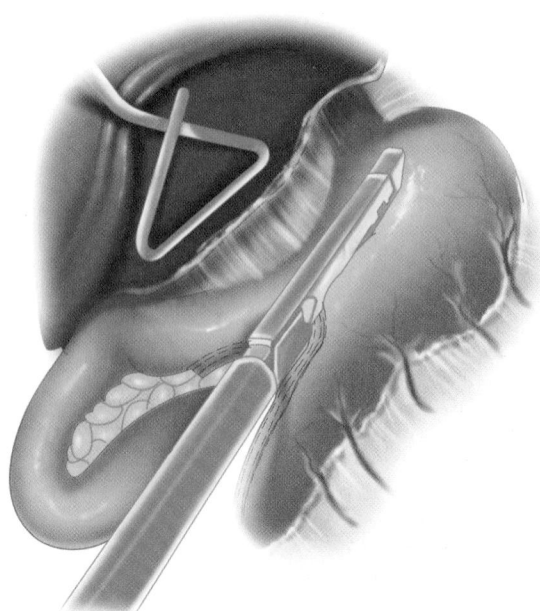

FIG. 27-19. Performance of sleeve gastrectomy. *[Reproduced with permission from Sherman V, et al: Laparoscopic sleeve gastrectomy, in Schauer PR, et al (eds): Minimally Invasive Bariatric Surgery, 1st ed. New York: Springer, 2007, p 174.]*

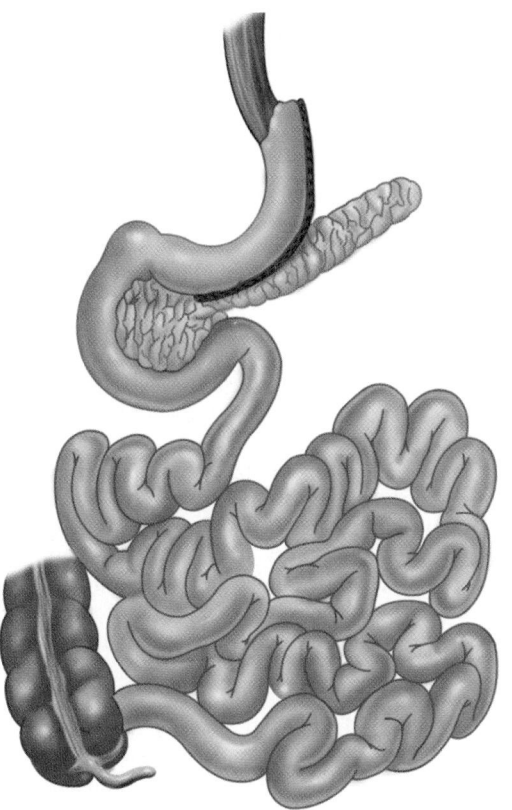

FIG. 27-20. Completed sleeve gastrectomy. *[Reproduced with permission from Sherman V, et al: Laparoscopic sleeve gastrectomy, in Schauer PR, et al (eds): Minimally Invasive Bariatric Surgery, 1st ed. New York: Springer, 2007, p 174.]*

patients who have a BMI of <50 kg/m² and have decided that they prefer the SG operation. Reasons usually include surgeon preference and recommendation, the presence of gastric lesions that require monitoring and have potential consequences (adenomatous polyps), or a desire to undergo a relatively simple restrictive operation not requiring the placement of a foreign body. Preoperative preparation is similar to that for LRYGB. Bowel preparation is not needed, however. Whether or not preoperative upper endoscopy should routinely be performed has yet to be determined.

Postoperative Care and Follow-Up

SG usually is performed with an overnight stay after surgery. Longer hospitalizations are indicated for patients with more severe medical problems. Absence of signs of bleeding and a documented intact staple line with good gastric emptying are required before discharge. Routine meglumine diatrizoate (Gastrografin) swallow on the first day after surgery is ordered by many surgeons, but its efficacy and cost effectiveness have yet to be documented. Follow-up is similar to that after LRYGB. Few nutritional complications occur unless the patient has difficulty taking in enough nutrients or protein or vitamins due to edema or tightness of the sleeve lumen. Multivitamins are usually prescribed to avert any other potential shortages from dietary vagaries.

Outcomes

SG results in excellent short-term weight loss. Depending on body size, weight loss is in the range of 45–50% of excess weight for patients with a BMI of >60 kg/m², but for patients with a BMI of 35 to 50 kg/m² with a 32F pouch size, excess weight loss at 3 years was recently reported as being 60%.[91] A report of >1000 operations by this same center described a hospital stay averaging 1.7 days, an operative time <80 minutes, and no conversions to open procedures or mortality. The rate of severe complications was <5%. A recent systematic review

by Brethauer and colleagues of sleeve gastrectomy outcomes involving over 2500 patients (mean BMI = 51.2 kg/m²) with up to 5-year follow-up demonstrated a mean excess weight loss of approximately 55%, a complication rate of approximately 8%, and mortality rate of 0.19%. In half of these studies, SG was used as a staging procedure for high BMI, high-risk patients while in the remainder it was used as a primary procedure.[15]

Sleeve gastrectomy is becoming a more commonly accepted bariatric operation either as a staging operation or a stand-alone procedure.

SPECIAL ISSUES RELATING TO THE BARIATRIC PATIENT

Bariatric Procedures in the Adolescent and the Elderly Patient

The incidence of obesity in the U.S. population has risen dramatically during the past 2 decades. This increase has been seen in children and adolescents as well. The incidence of obesity (BMI >30 kg/m²) is estimated to exceed 25% in the adolescent population. Factors felt to contribute to the rise of obesity among adolescents include decreased participation in physical sports and activities, increased time spent playing computer and screen games, and increased consumption of fast food and processed foods.

Obese adolescents have a high likelihood of being obese adults. In one study 75% of adolescents above the 85th percentile for weight were obese as adults.[92] The social stigmatization of the severely obese adolescent is often brutal. Comorbid medical problems, including hypertension and type 2 diabetes, may already be present in severely obese adolescents. The overwhelming likelihood that a severely obese adolescent will face a lifetime of severe obesity as an adult also implies that an average of 12 years of life for males and 9 years of life for females will be lost due to this medical problem.

The major controversies with regard to performing bariatric surgery in adolescents include the general aversion to subjecting an adolescent to surgery as well as concern about the secondary side effects of bariatric surgery on remaining growth and development. Clearly, the younger the patient, the more relevant the latter concern becomes.

The literature to date regarding the outcomes of bariatric surgery in adolescents is generally quite favorable. However, the data are still limited. Sugerman and colleagues[93] reported results for 33 adolescents, 30 of whom underwent RYGB. There were two late deaths at 2 and 6 years of follow-up unrelated to surgery. Complications both early and late numbered 20, including six incisional hernias and five wound infections. Significant weight loss was maintained in the majority of patients for up to 14 years after surgery. Most comorbidities resolved at 1 year after surgery. Self-image was greatly enhanced and social stigmatization greatly decreased. Capella and Capella[94] reported on 19 adolescent patients treated using a modified version of RYGB in which a vertical band was added to the pouch. After an average of 5.5 years of follow-up, average BMI for the group was 28 kg/m². No deaths occurred, but two patients required revisional surgery. No mortality or morbidity was reported, and all comorbidities resolved. Abu-Abeid and colleagues[95] treated 11 adolescents with LAGB. No late complications occurred, and after a 4-year follow-up average BMI went from 46.4 to 32.1 kg/m².

The elderly patient population certainly includes those with severe obesity. However, data on the effect of conservative therapies in treating this patient population are lacking. Similarly, it is likely that a patient who becomes obese late in life has a significantly different prognosis from that of an individual who has been severely obese for many years and manages to survive to an older age despite the resulting comorbidities.

There has been an increasing tendency to offer bariatric surgery to patients >60 years of age. Studies have documented that this patient population can enjoy the same good outcomes and resolution of comorbidities as younger patients.[96] Nehoda and associates[97] reported equally excellent results for LAGB in patients >50 years of age and those <50 years of age. Excess weight loss of 68%, a reoperation rate of 10%, and a 97% rate of improvement in comorbidities were reported for this age group (>50 years).

Although these data show that in selected older patients excellent results can be obtained, surgeons must be careful to determine which patients have been severely obese for decades and therefore have essentially end-stage organ function in many cases as a result of the comorbid medical conditions that have been present for those years. Flum and Dellinger[79] showed that the older patient population, especially those few patients >70 years undergoing bariatric surgery, did have an increased incidence of mortality and morbidity after RYGB.

The concept that bariatric surgery confers to patients receiving it an improved quality of life, a longer life, and a life without as many associated medical problems leads to the logical conclusion that the benefits of the operation will be more fully realized the younger the patient. In view of the large number of unserved patients, this philosophy does justify setting age limits for individual surgical practices. Although we do have such age limits, patients near or just over the age limit are often evaluated on an individual basis to determine their appropriateness for surgery. Accumulation of data may also change these limits in the future.

Bariatric Procedures in the Female Patient: Pregnancy and Gynecologic Issues

Hormonal levels in female patients are related to body weight. Obesity alters the levels of estrogen and progesterone available for normal ovulation, which results in abnormal ovulation patterns, amenorrhea, and difficulty conceiving. Should an obese woman become pregnant, the increased chances of gestational diabetes and hypertension make the pregnancy high risk. Macrosomia is increased. There is a twofold to threefold increase in the rate of cesarean sections, with more complications. Fetal mortality does not appear to be changed when maternal weight gain is limited.[98] With obesity, there is an increased risk for breast and endometrial cancer in the postpartum mother.

Infertility compounds the difficulties of the obese woman who wishes to have an uncomplicated pregnancy and delivery. The same hormonal alterations that cause an increased incidence of cancer, such as increased circulating estrogen levels, also cause infertility. If a severely obese woman becomes pregnant, pregnancy management is made more difficult by the body habitus and the need for more frequent ultrasound imaging as opposed to physical examination, which yields limited information.

Women who become pregnant soon after undergoing bariatric surgery can be at risk due to the ongoing weight loss produced by the operation. However, if the pregnancy is quickly recognized and appropriately managed, patients who have undergone bariatric surgery may actually have a better prognosis than if they had not had surgery. Wittgrove and colleagues[99] showed that patients who had undergone RYGB had a lower incidence of diabetes, macrosomia, and cesarean section than those who had not had surgery. Iron replacement, though, was cited as a critical need for these pregnant women. Despite these good results, there are issues for the female patient undergoing RYGB who becomes pregnant during the rapid weight loss phase after surgery. Special attention is needed to ensure adequate intake of vitamins and essential nutrients during what otherwise would be a period of rapid weight loss. In our practice, patients undergoing RYGB are cautioned to practice strict birth control during the first year after surgery to avoid becoming pregnant.

Patients who become pregnant after LAGB would seem to have even less likelihood of significant risk to their pregnancy, because the band can be adjusted to allow more food intake during the pregnancy but also limit weight gain to a healthy amount. Dixon and associates[100] wrote that morbidly obese women do have higher risks during pregnancy but that LAGB allows weight loss which reduces such risk. The adjustability of the band makes this an ideal operation for the woman planning to become pregnant.

Weight loss after bariatric surgery can correct the gynecologic problems that occur at high incidence in women with severe obesity.

Deitel and associates[101] found menstrual irregularities in >40% of patients preoperatively, but menstruation became normal in >95% of patients postoperatively. Infertility problems were present preoperatively in 29% of patients, and medical problems were frequent during previous pregnancies, including hypertension in 26.7%, preeclampsia in 12.8%, diabetes in 7%, and deep vein thrombosis in 7%. These problems were virtually eliminated after weight loss. The rate of stress urinary incontinence in the female patients in that study decreased from 61.2% before surgery to 11.6% after bariatric surgery.

Polycystic ovary syndrome is another common hormonal dysfunction associated with severe obesity. It is characterized by infertility, hyperandrogenism, dyslipidemia, anovulation, insulin resistance, and abnormal menses as well as obesity.[102]

Stress urinary incontinence is a frequent problem in the severely obese woman and must be specifically solicited in history taking. The increased intra-abdominal pressure from severe obesity contributes to the high incidence of this problem in the severely obese population. Obesity may also alter the neuromuscular function of the genitourinary tract, contributing to incontinence. Studies have confirmed the increased incidence of obesity in patients with both true stress incontinence and detrusor instability.[103] Weight loss alone relieves symptoms in many patients with obesity, but if symptoms persist, surgical therapy is still effective for this problem even in the obese patient.

Metabolic Surgery

Probably the single most prominent change in the field of bariatric surgery since the last version of this text is the increased emphasis on and attention to the metabolic aspects of surgery for weight loss. As noted earlier, the obvious indication of this emphasis is the changing of the name of the American Society for Bariatric Surgery to the American Society for Metabolic and Bariatric Surgery, effective as of June 2007. International meetings on the topic of bariatric surgery and its effects on diabetes have been convened during the last few years as well. The entire field of bariatric surgery is now much more focused on the metabolic effects and benefits of bariatric surgery.

Although many comorbidities are improved by bariatric surgery and the resultant weight loss, the metabolic diseases that are most particularly affected are type 2 diabetes, the hyperlipidemias, and the metabolic syndrome. Hypertension and cardiovascular disease are also improved indirectly through metabolic benefits as well as directly through weight loss effects.

Type 2 Diabetes

There has been a dramatic increase in the potential application of surgical therapy to treat type 2 diabetes. Much of this stems from the original observations of surgeons performing RYGB that patients who had undergone the operation showed improvement or near resolution of type 2 diabetes well before they had achieved maximum weight loss. Hickey and colleagues[104] highlighted these observations in a landmark paper which confirmed that RYGB was an effective treatment for type 2 diabetes, resolving the condition in 85% of patients who had developed it within the 5 years before surgery. MacDonald and associates,[105] also from the same institution, showed that the use of RYGB to treat patients with type 2 diabetes resulted in a longer life span. Schauer and colleagues[106] showed that the improvement in type 2 diabetes after LRYGB is comparable to that seen in Pories's original work, with fasting insulin levels and glycosylated hemoglobin levels returning to normal values in 83% and improving markedly in 17%.[106] RYGB has been shown to decrease overall long-term mortality related to diabetes in several large population studies.[107,108]

These results, as well as the observation that type 2 diabetes resolved quickly after RYGB, led to the general belief that the enteric hormonal component of glucose metabolism has an important influence on the disease. Rubino and Marescaux[109] reported the resolution of diabetes in an obese rat model with surgical diversion of the food stream from the duodenum and proximal jejunum. Reversal of the operation led to return of the disease state. The extension of Rubino and Marescaux's findings to humans has now occurred: A duodenojejunal exclusion operation has now been performed and has shown initial safety and efficacy in a small group of patients.[110] Although the majority of patients who have type 2 diabetes are obese, approximately 10% of patients with this disease are not obese, and these data from South America may confirm that the resolution of the disease through enteric diversion is not based on associated weight loss.[111]

Surgical therapy that produces weight loss without diversion of the enteric stream also can be quite effective in resolving type 2 diabetes. Dixon and associates[54] reported that 73% of patients who underwent LAGB and were followed for 2 years experienced resolution of their type 2 diabetes, compared with only 13% in a control group of medically treated patients. An editorial accompanying the article by Dixon and associates advocated that treatment for diabetes be reshaped to include consideration of surgical therapy as an option for patients, especially severely obese patients.[112]

Despite these data, there has been resistance from endocrinologists and internists specializing in the medical treatment of diabetes to accept the use of surgical therapy as an optimal treatment for the disease.[113] Only recently have these medical groups shown any recognition of the role of surgery in treating diabetes. However, in recent years there have been an increasing number of joint symposia and meetings between internists and basic scientists, including surgeons, on the topic of the treatment of diabetes. The first International Diabetes Surgery Summit was convened in Rome in 2007. That meeting documented the considerable benefits of surgical therapy for diabetes as well as the reluctance on the part of major groups such as the American Diabetes Association to include surgery as a common treatment option for diabetic patients. In 2009, the American Diabetes Association included bariatric surgery in their position statement on standards of medical care in diabetes. The guideline indicates that "bariatric surgery should be considered for adults with BMI ≥35 kg/m^2 and type 2 diabetes, especially if the diabetes is difficult to control with lifestyle and pharmacologic therapy."[114]

That surgical therapy is the single best treatment to resolve type 2 diabetes in 80% of severely obese patients who have it is a powerful fact that one would think would cause a rapid adoption of this treatment. Reasons for its slow penetration may include the stigma associated with obesity and obesity surgery. Obesity currently remains one of the last unaddressed areas of discrimination within society. It must be inferred that some of the bias against obesity is due to the slow acceptance of obesity surgery as a treatment for the diseases common to obesity. The bariatric surgery community is only now beginning to recognize that gastric bypass may best be described to the public and the insurance industry as an operation that corrects the metabolic diseases of severe obesity, such as diabetes.

Metabolic Syndrome

Metabolic syndrome is characterized by central obesity, glucose intolerance, dyslipidemia, and hypertension. Metabolic syndrome is a common finding in patients with severe obesity, occurring in 52% of individuals in one report.[115] All the associated metabolic problems of metabolic syndrome respond to surgical therapy to produce weight loss. Basic scientists attribute the occurrence of this associated array of diseases to an enhanced inflammatory state in the body resulting from the increased production of cytokines by the adipocyte. These cytokines in turn produce a mild inflammatory reaction that promotes the production of these diseases.

Diabetes and pre-diabetes (fasting plasma glucose of 100–124 mg/dL) are effectively treated by both RYGB and LAGB, as discussed earlier. These operations also are effective in treating the other components of metabolic syndrome. RYGB produced a resolution of metabolic syndrome in 98% of patients 1 year after surgery.[116]

Dyslipidemias improve in >70% of patients undergoing RYGB. The rate of resolution is >90% after any of the malabsorptive operations (see Table 27-8). Overall lipid profiles also are improved. The degree to which this occurs is in part related to the exercise levels of individuals as well as genetic components of the disease.

Cardiovascular Disease

Hypertension, a component of metabolic syndrome, is one of the cardiovascular diseases that are increased in the setting of obesity. Elevated arterial pressure in patients with obesity-related hypertension is associated with increased cardiac output and total peripheral resistance. The elevated output is related to expanded intravascular volume, which increases cardiopulmonary volume, venous return, and left ventricular preload; the elevated pressure and total peripheral resistance increase afterload. This dual ventricular overload promotes a dimorphic, concentric, and eccentric hypertrophy in response to the volume and pressure overload. Increased myocardial oxygen demand results from the elevated tension in the left ventricular wall, reflecting its increased diameter and pressure, and provides a physiologic rationale for the greater potential for coronary arterial insufficiency and cardiac failure. There is higher renal blood flow and lower renal vascular resistance in patients with obesity-related hypertension at any level of arterial pressure. This may be offset by an increased renal filtration fraction, which may favor protein deposition and glomerulosclerosis.[116]

Weight loss results in decreased intravascular volume, decreased cardiac output, and decreased arterial pressure. These manifestations occur after all the various bariatric operations that produce weight loss.

Heart failure also is increased in the setting of severe obesity. Much of the risk is secondary to the processes described earlier that produce hypertension and cardiac hypertrophy. Hypertension and obesity each have significant independent associations with left ventricular hypertrophy and cardiac wall thickness. Obesity is particularly strongly associated with left ventricular internal diameter.[117]

Resolution of Other Comorbid Medical Problems

Bariatric surgery can produce resolution of many if not all of the comorbid medical problems associated with obesity and present at the time of surgery. This is true to some extent for all bariatric procedures, although some are more efficient at reversing specific comorbid problems than others.

Gastroesophageal reflux disease (GERD) is symptomatically present in approximately half of patients with severe obesity and has been objectively proven to be present in 21%.[75] Unfortunately, obese patients with GERD have a higher chance of failing to obtain symptomatic relief from standard antireflux surgery. The recurrence of symptoms is higher, likely due to a higher incidence of wrap herniation into the mediastinum and other mechanical failure of the fundoplication, which in turn is likely affected by the increased intra-abdominal pressure occurring in the obese condition. A patient with a BMI of >35 kg/m^2 who has GERD has a better chance of eliminating symptoms by undergoing LRYGB, which is approximately 95 to 97% effective in the elimination of GERD.[118] LRYGB creates such a small gastric pouch that it has a very limited volume for acid production. LAGB also improves GERD but to a considerably lesser extent than RYGB.

Obstructive sleep apnea is a disturbance of sleep associated with obesity. It is a measurable problem, quantitated by polysomnography. In one recent study, of 349 patients considering bariatric surgery who were referred and tested, only 17% had no sleep apnea, whereas 32% had mild, 18% had moderate, and 33% had severe sleep apnea. At a mean time of 11 months after RYGB, the mean Respiratory Disturbance Index for all patients decreased from 51 to 15 (P <.01). Of 83 patients requiring continuous positive airway pressure or bilevel positive airway pressure preoperatively, only 31 still required it after surgery and machine settings could be decreased.[119] This study illustrates the results generally reported in the literature regarding resolution of this problem after bariatric operations.

Another pulmonary disorder that is commonly seen in severely obese patients is asthma. This comorbidity has been poorly quantitated and studied in this population to date. Observation from our practice shows that, with good weight loss, most nonallergic-type asthma symptoms, possibly related to dyspnea of exertion and secondary mild bronchospasm, do resolve.

Nonalcoholic fatty liver disease (NAFLD) is a metabolically related problem associated with obesity. The disease is a spectrum of liver abnormalities including steatosis, steatohepatitis, and fibrosis and cirrhosis of the liver. It is estimated that 20% of U.S. adults have NAFLD, largely because of the high incidence of obesity. NAFLD is present in an estimated 85% of patients with severe obesity.[120] Due to the high incidence of this disease, some authorities have advocated routine liver biopsy at the time of bariatric operations. Because the treatment of the disease is weight loss, however, patients with mild forms of the disease need no further treatment or follow-up. Patients whose biopsy report shows any degree of fibrosis should generally undergo further follow-up with a hepatologist. Histologic evaluation of liver biopsies before and after bariatric surgery have demonstrated significant improvements in degrees of steatosis, inflammation, and in some cases even fibrosis.[121] It has also been shown that RYGB does decrease the metabolic abnormalities involved in the pathogenesis of NAFLD and decreases the expression of factors involved in the progression of liver fibrosis.[122]

Musculoskeletal problems, especially degenerative joint disease and low back pain, are among the most common complaints and comorbid problems of the severely obese population. Quantitation of their severity is often difficult, however, which makes resolution or improvement equally difficult. Symptoms usually improve and often resolve in patients who experience significant weight loss. This is likely a combined effect of the directly decreased workload and some secondary resolution of the inflammatory process in the joints brought on directly and indirectly by obesity.

Plastic Surgery after Weight Loss

Patients who have undergone bariatric surgery are often left with large amounts of hanging skin or rolls of skin and subcutaneous tissue as a result of the weight loss. Related additional problems that arise include skin rashes; maceration under folds in the pannus,

thighs, and breasts; body odor; and poorly fitting clothes. Excess skin can be a limiting factor in exercise and sexual activity.

Most such patients wish to be rid of the extra skin and its associated problems. However, the major problem these patients face in accomplishing this is obtaining insurance approval for surgical removal of the excess skin. Most insurance companies consider this "cosmetic" surgery and will not authorize coverage. A few, with appropriate documentation of the conditions and problems caused by excess skin, do provide coverage for surgery. Plastic surgeons who are experienced in abdominoplasty and body contouring can offer these patients an excellent surgical treatment for the problems of excessive skin.

Reconstructive surgery requires careful preoperative planning and is based on the patient's deformities and priorities. Excess tissue of the lower torso is the most common deformity for which patients undergo surgical intervention. A standard abdominoplasty to remove this excessive tissue is performed. More radical body contouring can include a circumferential abdominoplasty and lower body lift.[123] This procedure involves excision of tissue from the buttocks and lateral thighs, with skin undermining down the thighs. Circumferential abdominoplasty removes redundant skin of the lower abdomen, flattens the abdomen, and incorporates the lower body lift. It requires central undermining to the xiphoid and minimal lateral undermining of the superior flap. The central abdominal fascia often requires imbrication. If simultaneous abdominal hernia repair is performed, this serves the function of fascial imbrication by creating a repair with some degree of fascial tension. The closure of the superior flap to the inferior skin edge incorporates lateral tension to narrow the waist and advance the anterolateral thighs. Medial thighplasty also may be needed for patients with significant excess medial thigh skin. This is done transversely.

Excess skin distal to the mid-thighs requires long vertical medial excision of skin. Mid-back and epigastric rolls, along with sagging breasts, are corrected with an upper body lift. The upper body lift is a reverse abdominoplasty, removal of mid-torso excessive skin, and reshaping of the breasts. For highly selected individuals, and with a well-organized team, a single-stage total body lift, which includes a circumferential abdominoplasty, lower body lift, medial thighplasty, upper body lift, and breast reshaping, can be performed safely in <8 hours (Figs. 27-21 and 27-22).[124] Although many bariatric surgery programs do not have the accompanying volume, experience, and

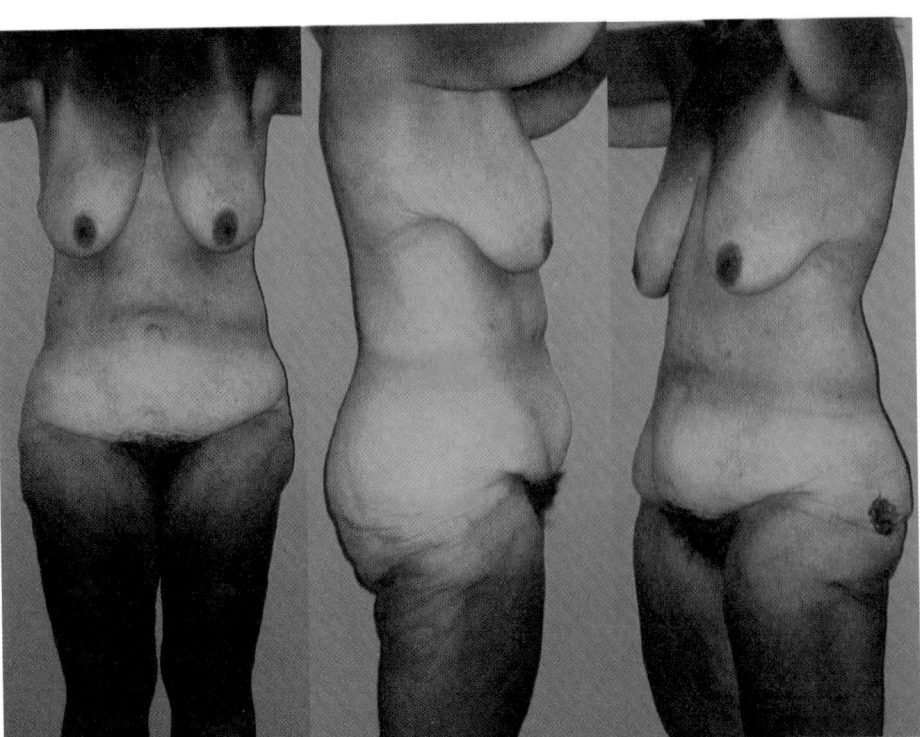

FIG. 27-21. Preoperative frontal, right lateral, and left anterior oblique views of a 36-year-old, 150-lb, 5'6" woman who lost 120 lb 2 years after a laparoscopic Roux-en-Y bypass procedure. She desired a one-stage total body lift and bilateral brachioplasties, which were performed in the manner described in the text. *(Courtesy of Dennis Hurwitz, MD, Clinical Professor of Plastic Surgery, University of Pittsburgh.)*

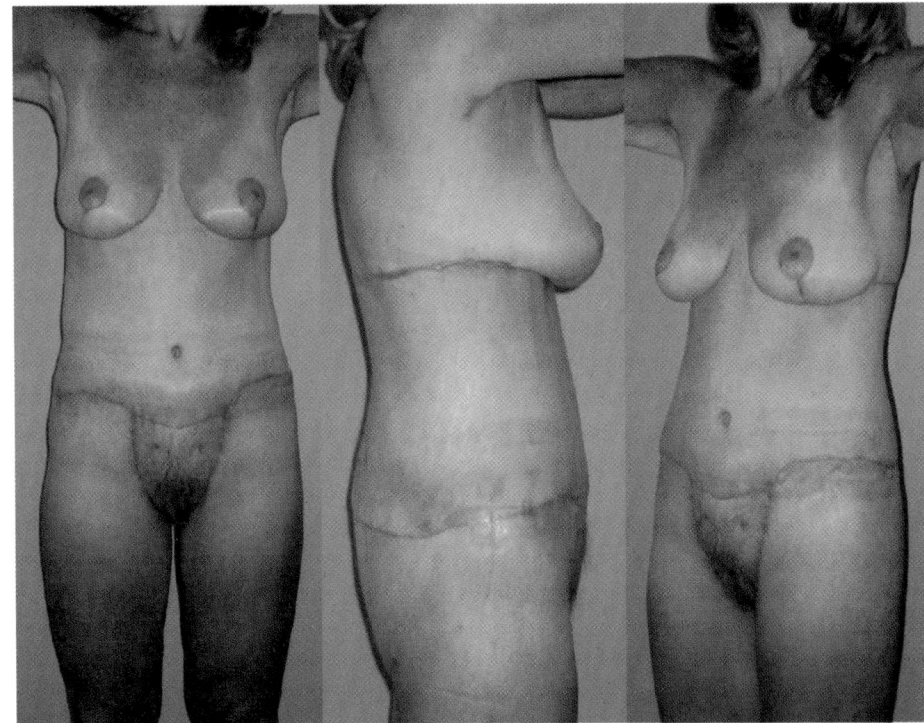

FIG. 27-22. Frontal, right lateral, and left anterior oblique views 6 weeks after surgery for the woman in Fig. 27-21. The scars indicate the circumferential abdominoplasty, lower body lift, upper body lift, breast reshaping, and autoaugmentation through a keyhole pattern and bilateral brachioplasties. All redundant skin has been removed, leaving well-positioned scars and feminine features. *(Courtesy of Dennis Hurwitz, MD, Clinical Professor of Plastic Surgery, University of Pittsburgh.)*

interest to offer such an extensive single-stage operation, most programs do have plastic surgery expertise available for abdominoplasty and removal of excess skin of the extremities as separate procedures. The rising numbers of patients undergoing bariatric surgery have provided an increased flow of patients requesting such services, which in turn should lead to improved outcomes with increasing experience for surgeons performing these procedures.

Endoscopic, Electric, and Other Experimental Procedures

Bariatric surgery has been a field in which a constant succession of procedures have been developed in an attempt to improve safety, minimize invasiveness, and offer better outcomes. Recent experimental procedures include electrical stimulation of the stomach and vagus nerves to produce weight loss.

The implantable gastric stimulation device, initially marketed by Transneuronix, Inc, in the early part of the twenty-first century, was a dual-lead implantable gastric electrical stimulator that theoretically interfered with the stomach's innate myoelectric pattern, causing decreased gastric emptying and nausea. A mean excess weight loss of 23% after implantation was reported at 16-month follow-up for the second U.S. trial study of the device.[125] Longer-term follow-up for the first European study has shown a 25% excess weight loss in 91 patients over a 2-year follow-up.[126] The disappointing aspect of this treatment is that a significant number of patients lose little weight, whereas a smaller group seem to respond well to the treatment. The ability to select those patients who will respond remains a challenge for this technology, which still is only a proposed potential operation for weight loss.

Vagal stimulation has recently been proposed as a means of stimulating the neural input to the stomach to achieve decrease in appetite, early satiety, at times nausea, and weight loss. Data to date have been sparse and very preliminary in showing any merits or potential efficacy for this approach.[127]

Endoscopic procedures to decrease gastric pouch size and to limit gastrojejunostomy anastomotic size are currently being performed at several medical centers.[67,128] These are currently reoperative procedures, not initial procedures for weight loss.

Intragastric balloon placement for weight loss has resurfaced on the bariatric scene in the past few years. The Garren-Edwards bubble of the late 1980s era[129] proved to be a disastrous failure. Now this concept has been reintroduced by one company, which has marketed a device of this type as a short-term bridge to weight loss to be followed by a more definitive procedure. Although there may be some limited application of this device for such purposes,[130] its ability to produce durable weight loss is unproven. It may have potential use only as a preliminary procedure before a more definitive one.

Prototype procedures undergoing trial include one that uses an endoscopically placed intraluminal sleeve to limit absorption.[110] The eventual ability to endoscopically create a gastric pouch and hence perform a restrictive operation completely endoscopically is being envisioned. Although these proposed procedures speak to the energy and innovation of today's bariatric surgery community, their actual creation has yet to occur.

REFERENCES

Entries highlighted in bright blue are key references.

1. Ogden CL, Carroll MD, Curtin LR, et al: Prevalence of overweight and obesity in the United States, 1999–2004. *JAMA* 295:1549, 2006.
2. Stunkard AJ, Foch TT, Hrubec Z: A twin study of human obesity. *JAMA* 256:51, 1986.
3. Woodard GA, Peraza J, Downey J, et al: Probiotics improve weight loss, GI-related quality of life and H-2 breath tests after gastric bypass surgery: A prospective randomized trial. Paper presented at: 49th Annual Meeting of the Society for Surgery of the Alimentary Tract; May 19, 2008; San Diego.
4. Timar O, Sestier F, Levy E: Metabolic syndrome X: A review. *Can J Cardiol* 16:779, 2000.
5. Garfinkel L: Overweight and cancer. *Ann Intern Med* 1103:1034, 1985.
6. Dreick EJ, Bale GS, Seltzer F, et al: Excessive mortality and causes of death in morbidly obese men. *JAMA* 243:443, 1980.
7. Wadden TA, Foster GD, Letizia KA: One-year behavioral treatment of obesity: Comparison of moderate and severe caloric restriction and the effects of weight maintenance therapy. *J Consult Clin Psychol* 62:165, 1994.
8. Wood PD, Stefanick ML, Dreon DM, et al: Changes in plasma lipids and lipoproteins in overweight men during weight loss through dieting as compared with exercise. *N Engl J Med* 319:1173, 1988.

9. Wing RR: Behavioral strategies to improve long-term weight loss and maintenance. *Med Health R I* 82:123, 1999.

10. Miller WC, Koxeja DM, Hamilton EJ: A meta-analysis of the past 25 years of weight loss research using diet, exercise or diet plus exercise intervention. *Int J Obes Relat Metab Disord* 21:941, 1987.

11. Eriksson KF, Lindgarde F: Prevention of type 2 (non–insulin-dependent) diabetes by diet and physical exercise. The 6-year Malmö feasibility study. *Diabetologia* 34:891, 1991.

12. Scheen AJ, Ernest P: New antiobesity agents in type 2 diabetes. Overview of clinical trials with sibutramine and orlistat. *Diabetes Metab* 28:437, 2002.

13. Bray GA: Drug treatment of obesity. *Rev Endocr Metab Disord* 2:403, 2001.

14. National Institutes of Health Consensus Conference. Gastrointestinal surgery for severe obesity. Consensus Development Conference Panel. *Ann Intern Med* 115:956, 1991.

15. Brethauer SA, Hammel JP, Schauer PR: A systematic review of sleeve gastrectomy as a staging and primary bariatric procedure. In Press. SOARD.

16. Balsinger BM, Poggio JL, Mai J, et al: Ten and more years after vertical banded gastroplasty as primary operation for morbid obesity. *J Gastrointest Surg* 4:598, 2000.

17. Kremen AJ, Linner JH, Nelson CH: An experimental evaluation of the nutritional importance of proximal and distal small intestine. *Ann Surg* 140:439, 1954.

18. Deitel M: Overview of operations for morbid obesity. *World J Surg* 22:913, 1998.

19. Mason EE, Ito C: Gastric bypass in obesity. *Surg Clin North Am* 47:1345, 1969.

20. Griffin WO, Young VL, Stevenson CC: A prospective comparison of gastric and jejunoileal bypass procedures for morbid obesity. *Ann Surg* 186:500, 1977.

21. Mason EE, Doherty C, Cullen JJ, et al: Vertical gastroplasty: Evolution of vertical banded gastroplasty. *World J Surg* 22:919, 1998.

22. Brolin RE, Robertson LB, Kenler HA, et al: Weight loss and dietary intake after vertical banded gastroplasty and Roux-en-Y gastric bypass. *Ann Surg* 220:782, 1994.

23. Scopinaro N, Gianetta E, Civalleri D, et al: Bilio-pancreatic bypass for obesity: II. Initial experience in man. *Br J Surg* 66:618, 1979.

24. Kuzmak LI: A review of seven years' experience with silicone gastric banding. *Obes Surg* 1:403, 1991.

25. Belachew M, Legrand MJ, Defechereux TH, et al: Laparoscopic adjustable silicone gastric banding in the treatment of morbid obesity. A preliminary report. *Surg Endosc* 8:1354, 1994.

26. Wittgrove AC, Clark WG, Tremblay LJ: Laparoscopic gastric bypass, Roux en-Y: Preliminary report of five cases. *Obes Surg* 4:353, 1994.

27. O'Keefe T, Patterson EJ: Evidence supporting routine polysomnography before bariatric surgery. *Obes Surg* 14:23, 2004.

28. Sharaf RN, Weinshel EH, Bini EJ, et al: Endoscopy plays an important preoperative role in bariatric surgery. *Obes Surg* 14:1367, 2004.

29. Verset D, Houben J-J, Gay F, et al: The place of upper gastrointestinal tract endoscopy before and after vertical banded gastroplasty for morbid obesity. *Dig Dis Sci* 42:2333, 1997.

30. Schirmer B, Erenoglu C, Miller A: Flexible endoscopy in the management of patients undergoing Roux-en-Y gastric bypass. *Obes Surg* 12:634, 2002.

31. Kim JJ, Schirmer B: Safety and efficacy of simultaneous cholecystectomy at the time of Roux-en-Y gastric bypass. *Surg Obes Relat Dis* 5:48, 2009.

32. Hamad GG, Ikramuddin S, Gourash WF, et al: Elective cholecystectomy during laparoscopic Roux-en-Y gastric bypass. Is it worth the wait? *Obes Surg* 13:76, 2003.

33. Sugerman HJ, Brewer WH, Shiffman ML, et al: A multicenter, placebo-controlled, randomized, double-blind prospective trial of prophylactic ursodiol for the prevention of gallstone formation following gastric-bypass-induced rapid weight loss. *Am J Surg* 169:91, 1995.

34. Buffington C, Walker B, Cowan GS Jr., et al: Vitamin D deficiency in the morbidly obese. *Obes Surg* 3:421, 1993.

35. Bogdonoff DL, Schirmer B: Laparoscopic surgery, in Stone DJ, Bogdonoff DL, Leisure GS, et al (eds): *Perioperative Care: Anesthesia, Medicine and Surgery,* 1st ed. St. Louis, Mo: Mosby, 1998, p 547.

36. Nguyen NT, Goldman C, Rosenquist CJ, et al: Laparoscopic versus open gastric bypass: A randomized study of outcomes, quality of life, and costs. *Ann Surg* 234:279, 2001.

37. Hutter M, Randall S, Khuri SF, et al: Laparoscopic versus open gastric bypass for morbid obesity. A multicenter, prospective, risk-adjusted analysis from the National Surgical Quality Improvement Program. *Ann Surg* 243:657, 2006.

38. Lujan JA, Frutos MD, Hernandez Q, et al: Laparoscopic versus open gastric bypass in the treatment of morbid obesity. *Ann Surg* 239:433, 2004.

39. Schirmer B: Laparoscopic bariatric surgery. *Surg Endosc* 20 Suppl:S450, 2006.

40. Jones KB Jr., Affram JD, Benotti PM, et al: Open versus laparoscopic Roux-en-Y gastric bypass: A comparative study of over 25,000 open cases and the major laparoscopic bariatric reported series. *Obes Surg* 16:721, 2006.

41. Swanstrom LL, Fried GM, Hoffman KI, et al: Beta test results of a new system assessing competence in laparoscopic surgery. *J Am Coll Surg* 202:62, 2006.

42. McGrath V, Needleman BJ, Melvin WS: Evolution of the laparoscopic gastric bypass. *J Laparoendosc Adv Surg Tech A* 13:221, 2003.

43. Wright TA, Kow L, Wilson T, et al: Early results of laparoscopic Swedish adjustable gastric banding for morbid obesity. *Br J Surg* 87:362, 2000.

44. Dargent J: Laparoscopic adjustable gastric banding: Lessons from the first 500 patients in a single institution. *Obes Surg* 9:446, 1999.

45. Favretti F, Segato G, DeLuca M, et al: Laparoscopic adjustable gastric banding: Revisional surgery, in Schauer PR, Schirmer BD, Brethauer SA (eds): *Minimally Invasive Bariatric Surgery.* New York: Springer, 2007, p 213.

46. Ren C: Laparoscopic adjustable gastric banding: Postoperative management and nutritional evaluation, in Schauer PR, Schirmer BD, Brethauer SA (eds): *Minimally Invasive Bariatric Surgery.* New York: Springer, 2007, p 200.

47. Weiner R, Blanco-Engert R, Weiner S, et al: Outcome after laparoscopic adjustable gastric banding—8 years' experience. *Obes Surg* 13:427, 2003.

48. Dixon JB, O'Brien PE: Laparoscopic adjustable gastric banding: Outcomes, in Schauer PR, Schirmer BD, Brethauer SA (eds): *Minimally Invasive Bariatric Surgery.* New York: Springer, 2007, p 189.

49. Dixon JB, Schachter LM, O'Brien PE: Predicting sleep apnea and excessive day sleepiness in the severely obese: Indicators for polysomnography. *Chest* 123:1134, 2003.

50. Angrisani L, Iovino P, Lorenzo M, et al: Treatment of morbid obesity and gastroesophageal reflux with hiatal hernia by Lap-Band. *Obes Surg* 9:396, 1999.

51. Dixon JB, Chapma L, O'Brie PE: Marked improvement in asthma after Lap-Band surgery for morbid obesity. *Obes Surg* 9:15, 1999.

52. Dixon JB, Dixon ME, O'Brien PE: Depression in association with severe obesity: Changes in weight loss. *Arch Intern Med* 163:2058, 2003.

53. Schok M, Geenen R, van Antwerpen T, et al: Quality of life after laparoscopic adjustable gastric banding for severe obesity: Postoperative and retrospective preoperative evaluations. *Obes Surg* 10:502, 2000.

54. Dixon JB, O'Brien PE, Playfair J, et al: Adjustable gastric banding and conventional therapy for type 2 diabetes. A randomized controlled trial. *JAMA* 299:316, 2008.

55. Favretti F, Cadiere GB, Segato G, et al: Laparoscopic banding: Selection and technique in 830 patients. *Obes Surg* 12:385, 2002.

56. Dixon JB, O'Brien PE: Changes in comorbidities and improvements in qualify of life after LAP-BAND placement. *Am J Surg* 184:S51, 2002.

57. Ceelen W, Walder J, Cardon A, et al: Surgical treatment of severe obesity with a low-pressure adjustable gastric band. Experimental data and clinical results in 625 patients. *Ann Surg* 237:10, 2003.

58. Buchwald H, Avidor Y, Braunwald E, et al: Bariatric surgery. A systematic review and meta-analysis. *JAMA* 292:1724, 2004.

59. Maggard MA, Shugarman LR, Suttorp M, et al: Meta-analysis: Surgical treatment of obesity. *Ann Intern Med* 142:547, 2005.

60. Allen JW, Lagardere AO: Laparoscopic adjustable gastric banding: Complications, in Schauer PR, Schirmer BD, Brethauer SA (eds): *Minimally Invasive Bariatric Surgery.* New York: Springer, 2007, p 205.

61. MacLean LD, Rhode BM, Nohr CW: Late outcome of isolated gastric bypass. *Ann Surg* 231:524, 2000.

62. Brolin RE: Long-limb gastric bypass in the super-obese. A prospective randomized trial. *Ann Surg* 215:387, 1992.

63. Choba PS, Flancbaum L: The effect of Roux limb lengths on outcome after Roux-en-Y gastric bypass: A prospective randomized clinical trial. *Obes Surg* 12:540, 2002.

64. Champion JK, Williams M: Small bowel obstruction and internal hernias after laparoscopic Roux-en-Y gastric bypass. *Obes Surg* 13:596, 2003.

65. Carmody B, DeMaria EJ, Jamal M, et al: Internal hernia after laparoscopic Roux-en-Y gastric bypass. *Surg Obes Rel Dis* 1:543, 2005.

66. Schweitzer M: Endoscopic intraluminal suture placation of the gastric pouch and stoma in postoperative Roux-en-Y gastric bypass patients. *J Laparoendosc Adv Surg Tech A* 14:223, 2004.

67. Thompson CC: Per-oral endoscopic reduction of dilated gastrojejunal anastomosis following Roux-en-Y gastric bypass: A possible new option for patients with weight regain. *Surg Obes Rel Disord* 1:223, 2005.

68. Schirmer BD, Lee SK, Northup CJ, et al: Gastrojejunal anastomosis stenosis is lower using linear rather than circular stapling during Roux-en-Y gastric bypass. Paper presented at: Society of American Gastrointestinal and Endoscopic Surgeons 2006 Scientific Session; Dallas, TX, April 2006.

69. Gonzalez R, Lin E, Venkatesh KR, et al: Gastrojejunostomy during laparoscopic gastric bypass: Analysis of three techniques. *Arch Surg* 138:181, 2003.

70. Sekhar N, Torquati A, Lufti R, et al: Endoscopic evaluation of the gastrojejunostomy in laparoscopic gastric bypass. A series of 340 patients without postoperative leak. *Surg Endosc* 20:199, 2006.

71. Singh R, Fisher BL: Sensitivity and specificity of postoperative upper GI series following gastric bypass. *Obes Surg* 13:73, 2003.

72. Ganci-Cerrud G, Herrera MF: Role of radiologic contrast studies in the early postoperative period after bariatric surgery. *Obes Surg* 9:532, 1999.

73. Thodiyil PA, Yenumula P, Rogula T, et al: Selective non operative management of leaks after gastric bypass: lessons learned from 2675 consecutive patients. *Ann Surg* 248:782, 2008.

74. Schauer PR, Ikramuddin S, Gourash W, et al: Outcomes after laparoscopic Roux-en-Y gastric bypass for morbid obesity. *Ann Surg* 232:515, 2000.

75. Bennett JC, Wang H, Schirmer BD, et al: Quality of life and resolution of comorbidities in super-obese patients remaining morbidly obese after Roux-en-Y gastric bypass. *Surg Obes Rel Dis* 3:387, 2007.

76. Pratt GM, Learn CA, Hughes GD, et al: Demographics and outcomes at American Society for Metabolic and Bariatric Surgery Centers of Excellence. *Surg Endosc* 23:795, 2009.

77. http://www.acsnsqip.org: National Surgical Quality Improvement Program database, 2008, American College of Surgeons. Comparison of University of Virginia to 15 other centers [accessed October 2006].

78. Vance PL, de Lange EE, Shaffer HA Jr., et al: Gastric outlet obstruction following surgery for morbid obesity: Effect of fluoroscopically guided balloon dilation. *Radiology* 222:70, 2002.

79. Flum DR, Dellinger EP: Impact of gastric bypass operation on survival: A population-based analysis. *J Am Coll Surg* 199:543, 2004.

80. Christou NV, Sampalis JS, Liberman M, et al: Surgery decreases long-term mortality, morbidity, and health care use in morbidly obese patients. *Ann Surg* 240:416, 2004.

81. Angrisani L, Lorenzo M, Borrelli V: Laparosocpic adjustable gastric banding versus Roux-en-Y gastric bypass: 5-year results of a prospective randomized trial. *Surgery for Obesity and Related Diseases* 3:127, 2007.

82. Nguyen NT, Slone J, Nguyen XT, et al: A prospective randomized trial of laparoscopic gastric bypass versus laparoscopic gastric banding for the treatment of morbid obesity: outcomes, cost, and quality of life. *Annals of Surgery* (in press).

83. Hess DS, Hess DW: Biliopancreatic diversion with a duodenal switch. *Obes Surg* 8:267, 1998.

84. Marceau P, Hould FS, Simard S, et al: Biliopancreatic diversion with a duodenal switch. *World J Surg* 22:947, 1998.

85. DeMeester TR, Fuchs KH, Ball CS, et al: Experimental and clinical results with proximal end-to-end duodenojejunostomy for pathologic duodenogastric reflux. *Ann Surg* 206:414, 1987.

86. Scopinaro N, Scopinaro N, Gianetta E, et al: Biliopancreatic diversion for obesity at eighteen years. *Surgery* 119:261, 1996.

87. Ren CJ, Patterson E, Gagner M: Early results of laparoscopic biliopancreatic diversion with duodenal switch: A case series of 40 consecutive patients. *Obes Surg* 10:514, 2000.

88. Almogy G, Crookes PF, Anthone GJ: Longitudinal gastrectomy as a treatment for the high-risk super-obese patient. *Obes Surg* 14:492, 2004.

89. Cottam D, Qureshi FG, Mattar SG, et al: Laparoscopic sleeve gastrectomy as an initial weight-loss procedure for high-risk patients with morbid obesity. *Surg Endosc* 20:859, 2006.

90. Baltasar A, Serra C, Perez N, et al: Laparoscopic sleeve gastrectomy: A multi-purpose bariatric operation. *Obes Surg* 15:1124, 2005.

91. Lee CM, Cirangle PT, Jossart GH: Laparoscopic vertical sleeve gastrectomy for morbid obesity: A report of a five-year experience with 750 patients. Paper presented at: 49th Annual Meeting of the Society for Surgery of the Alimentary Tract; May 19, 2008; San Diego. *J Gastrointest Surg*. In press.

92. Whitaker RC, Wright JA, Pepe MS, et al: Predicting obesity in young adulthood from childhood and parental obesity. *N Engl J Med* 337:869, 1997.

93. Sugerman HJ, Sugerman EL, DeMaria EJ, et al: Bariatric surgery for severely obese adolescents. *J Gastrointest Surg* 7:102, 2003.

94. Capella JF, Capella RF: Bariatric surgery in adolescence. Is this the best age to operate? *Obes Surg* 13:826, 2003.

95. Abu-Abeid S, Gavert N, Klausner JM, et al: Bariatric surgery in adolescence. *J Pediatr Surg* 38:1379, 2003.

96. Rossner S: Obesity in the elderly—a future matter of concern? *Obes Rev* 2:183, 2001.

97. Nehoda H, Hourmont K, Sauper T, et al: Laparoscopic gastric banding in older patients. *Arch Surg* 136:1171, 2001.

98. Bongain A, Isnard V, Gillet JY: Obesity in obstetrics and gynaecology. *Eur J Obstet Gynecol Reprod Biol* 77:217, 1998.

99. Wittgrove AC, Jester L, Wittgrove P, et al: Pregnancy following gastric bypass for morbid obesity. *Obes Surg* 8:461, 1998.

100. Dixon JB, Dixon ME, O'Brien PE: Pregnancy after Lap-Band surgery: Management of the band to achieve healthy weight outcomes. *Obes Surg* 11:59, 2001.

101. Deitel M, Stone E, Kassam HA, et al: Gynaecologic-obstetric changes after loss of massive excess weight following bariatric surgery. *J Am Coll Nutr* 7:147, 1988.

102. Gonzalez CA, Hernandez MI, Mendoza R, et al: Polycystic ovarian disease: Clinical and biochemical expression. *J Ginecol Obstet Mex* 71:253, 2003.

103. Subak LL, Johnson C, Whitcomb E, et al: Does weight loss improve incontinence in moderately obese women? *Int Urogynecol J Pelvic Floor Dysfunct* 13:40, 2002.

104. Hickey MS, Pories WJ, MacDonald KG Jr., et al: A new paradigm for type 2 diabetes mellitus. Could it be a disease of the foregut? *Ann Surg* 227:637, 1998.

105. MacDonald KG Jr., Long SD, Swanson MS, et al: The gastric bypass operation reduces the progression and mortality of non–insulin-dependent diabetes mellitus. *J Gastrointest Surg* 1:213, 1997.

106. Schauer PR, Burguera B, Ikramuddin S, et al: Effect of laparoscopic Roux-en-Y gastric bypass on type 2 diabetes mellitus. *Ann Surg* 238:467, 2003.

107. Sjöström L, Narbro K, Sjöström CD, et al: Effects of bariatric surgery on mortality in Swedish obese subjects. *N Engl J Med* 357:741, 2007.

108. Adams TD, Gress RE, Smith SC, et al: Long-term mortality after gastric bypass surgery. *N Engl J Med* 357:753, 2007.

109. Rubino F, Marescaux J: Effect of duodenal-jejunal exclusion in a nonobese animal model of type 2 diabetes: A new perspective for an old disease. *Ann Surg* 239:1, 2004.

110. Tarnoff M, Escalona A, Ibanez L, et al: Twenty-four-week followup of an open label, prospective, randomized controlled trial of endoscopic duodenal jejunal bypass sleeve (DJBS) versus low calorie diet for weight loss. Paper presented at: 25th Annual Meeting of the American Society for Metabolic and Bariatric Surgery; June 18, 2008; Washington, DC.

111. Cohen RV, Schiavon CA, Pinheiro JS, et al: Duodenal-jejunal bypass for treatment of type 2 diabetes in patients with body mass index of 22–34 kg/m2: A report of two cases. *Surg Obes Rel Dis* 3:195, 2007.

112. Cummings DE, Flum DR: Gastrointestinal surgery as a treatment for diabetes. *JAMA* 299:341, 2008.

113. Dixon JB, Pories WJ, O'Brien PE, et al: Surgery as an effective early intervention for diabesity: Why the reluctance? *Diabetes Care* 28:472, 2005.

114. American Diabetes Association: Standards of Medical Care in Diabetes—2009. *Diabetes Care* 32;513, 2009.

115. Lee W-J, Huang M-T, Wang W, et al: Effects of obesity surgery on the metabolic syndrome. *Arch Surg* 139:1088, 2004.

116. Frohlich ED: Obesity and hypertension. Hemodynamic aspects. *Ann Epidemiol* 1:287, 1991.

117. Lauer MS, Anderson KM, Levy D: Separate and joint influences of obesity and mild hypertension on left ventricular mass and geometry: The Framingham Heart Study. *J Am Coll Cardiol* 19:130, 1992.

118. Frezza EE, Ikramuddin S, Gourash W, et al: Symptomatic improvement in gastroesophageal reflux disease (GERD) following laparoscopic Roux-en-Y gastric bypass. *Surg Endosc* 16:1027, 2002.

119. Haines KL, Nelson LG, Gonzalez R, et al: Objective evidence that bariatric surgery improves obesity-related obstructive sleep apnea. *Surgery* 141:354, 2007.

120. Beymer C, Kowdley KV, Larson A, et al: Prevalence and predictors of asymptomatic liver disease in patients undergoing gastric bypass surgery. *Arch Surg* 138:1240, 2003.

121. Mattar SG, Velcu LM, Rebinovitz M, et al: Surgically-induced weight loss significantly improves nonalcoholic fatty liver disease and the metabolic syndrome. *Ann Surg* 242:610, 2005.

122. Klein S, Mittendorfer B, Eagon JC, et al: Gastric bypass surgery improves metabolic and hepatic abnormalities associated with nonalcoholic fatty liver disease. *Gastroenterology* 130:1564, 2006.

123. Hurwitz DJ, Zewert T: Body contouring surgery in the bariatric surgical patient. *Oper Tech Plast Surg Reconstr Surg* 8:87, 2002.

124. Hurwitz DJ: Single-staged total body lift after massive weight loss. *Ann Plast Surg* 52:435, 2004.

125. Shikora SA: Implantable gastric stimulation for weight loss. *J Gastrointest Surg* 8:408, 2004.

126. Miller K, Hoeller E, Aigner F: The implantable gastric stimulator for obesity: An update of the European Experience in the LOSS (Laparoscopic Obesity Stimulation Survey) Study. *Treat Endocrinol* 5:53, 2006.

127. Toouli J, Kow L, Kulseng B, et al: Vagal blocking for obesity control (VBLOCTM): Ongoing comparison of weight loss with two generations of an active, implantable medical device. Paper presented at: 25th Annual Meeting of the American Society for Metabolic and Bariatric Surgery; June 19, 2008; Washington, DC.

128. Thompson CC, Slattery J, Bundga ME, et al: Peroral endoscopic reduction of dilated gastrojejunal anastomosis after Roux-en-Y gastric bypass: A possible new option for patients with weight regain. *Surg Endosc* 20:1744, 2006.

129. Garren L: Garren gastric bubble. *Bariatr Surg* 3:14, 1985.

130. Genco A, Brui T, Doldi SB, et al: BioEnterics Intragastric Balloon: The Italian experience with 2,515 patients. *Obes Surg* 15:1161, 2005.

AN UNDERRATED ORGAN

The small intestine is the raison d'être of the GI tract as it is the principle site of nutrient digestion and absorption.[1] The small intestine is also the body's largest reservoir of immunologically active and hormone-producing cells, and hence can be conceptualized as the largest organ of the immune and endocrine systems, respectively. It achieves this diversity of action through unique anatomical features that provide it with a massive surface area, a diversity of cell types, and a complex neural network to coordinate these functions.

Despite its size and importance, diseases of the small intestine are relatively infrequent, and present diagnostic and therapeutic challenges. Treatments for common conditions such as postoperative ileus are hardly more effective than those used at the dawn of the last century. Mortality rates associated with acute mesenteric ischemia have not improved during the past 50 years.

Despite the introduction of novel imaging techniques such as capsule endoscopy and double balloon endoscopy, diagnostic tests lack sufficient predictive power to definitively guide clinical decision making for individual patients. Furthermore, few high-quality, controlled data on the efficacy of surgical therapies for small bowel diseases are available.

Therefore, sound clinical judgment and a thorough understanding of anatomy, physiology, and pathophysiology remain essential to the care of patients with intestinal disorders.

GROSS ANATOMY

The small intestine is a tubular structure that extends from the pylorus to the cecum. The estimated length of this structure varies depending on whether radiologic, surgical, or autopsy measurements are made. In the living, it is thought to measure 4 to 6 m.[2] The small intestine consists of three segments lying in series: the duodenum, jejunum, and ileum. The duodenum, the most proximal segment, lies in the retroperitoneum immediately adjacent to the head and inferior border of the body of the pancreas. The duodenum is demarcated from the stomach by the pylorus and from the jejunum by the ligament of Treitz. The jejunum and ileum lie within the peritoneal cavity and are tethered to the retroperitoneum by a broad-based mesentery. No distinct anatomic landmark demarcates the jejunum from the ileum; the proximal 40% of the jejunoileal segment is arbitrarily defined as the jejunum and the distal 60% as the ileum. The ileum is demarcated from the cecum by the ileocecal valve.

The small intestine contains mucosal folds known as *plicae circulares* or *valvulae conniventes* that are visible upon gross inspection. These folds are also visible radiographically and help in the distinction between small intestine and colon, which does not contain them, on abdominal radiographs. These folds are more prominent in the proximal intestine than in the distal small intestine. Other features evident on gross inspection that are more characteristic of the proximal than distal small intestine include a larger circumference, thicker wall, less fatty mesentery, and longer vasa recta (Fig. 28-1). Gross examination of the small intestinal mucosa also reveals aggregates of lymphoid follicles. Those follicles, located in the ileum, are the most prominent and are designated *Peyer's patches*.

Most of the duodenum derives its arterial blood from branches of both the celiac and the superior mesenteric arteries. The distal duodenum, the jejunum, and the ileum derive their arterial blood from the superior mesenteric artery. Their venous drainage occurs via the superior mesenteric vein. Lymph drainage occurs through lymphatic vessels coursing parallel to corresponding arteries. This lymph drains through mesenteric lymph nodes to the cisterna chyli, then through the thoracic duct, and ultimately into the left subclavian vein. The parasympathetic and sympathetic innervation of the small intestine is derived from the vagus and splanchnic nerves, respectively.

HISTOLOGY

The wall of the small intestine consists of four distinct layers: mucosa, submucosa, muscularis externa, and serosa (Fig. 28-2).

The mucosa is the innermost layer and it consists of three layers: epithelium, lamina propria, and muscularis mucosae. The epithelium is exposed to the intestinal lumen and is the surface through which absorption from and secretion into the lumen occurs. The lamina propria is located immediately external to the epithelium and consists of connective tissue and a heterogeneous population of cells. It is demarcated from the more external submucosa by the muscularis mucosae, a thin sheet of smooth muscle cells.

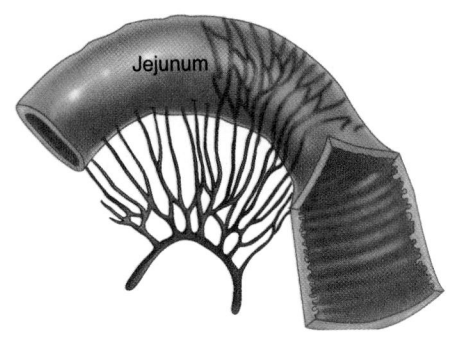
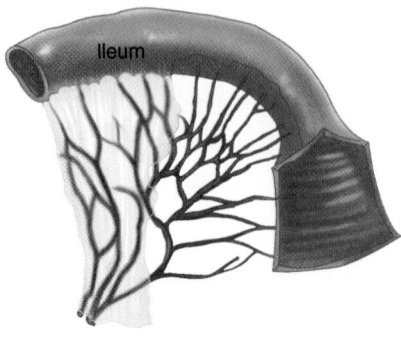

FIG. 28-1. Gross features of jejunum contrasted with those of ileum. Relative to the ileum, the jejunum has a larger diameter, thicker wall, more prominent plicae circulares, a less fatty mesentery, and longer vasa recta.

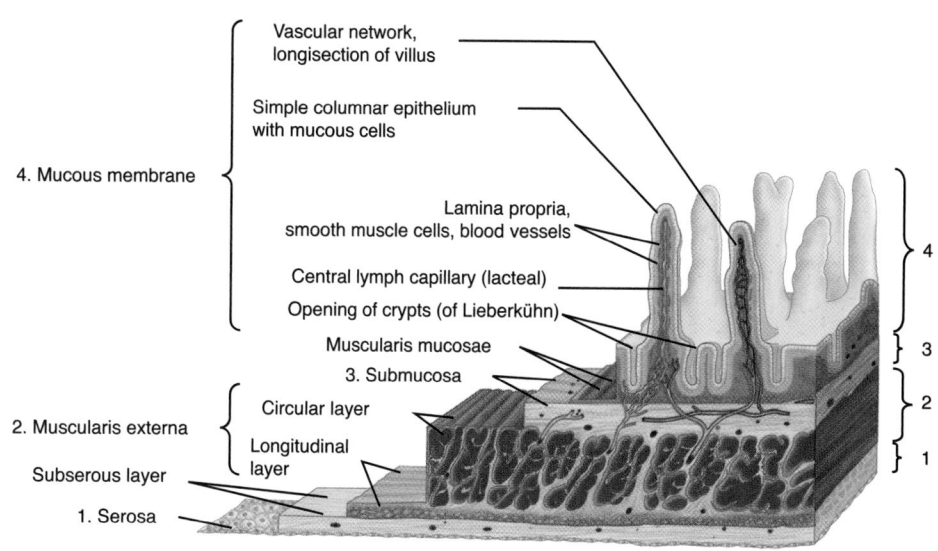

Vascular network,
longisection of villus

Simple columnar epithelium
with mucous cells

4. Mucous membrane

Lamina propria,
smooth muscle cells, blood vessels

Central lymph capillary (lacteal)

Opening of crypts (of Lieberkühn)

Muscularis mucosae

3. Submucosa

Circular layer

2. Muscularis externa

Longitudinal layer

Subserous layer

1. Serosa

FIG. 28-2. Layers of wall of the small intestine. The individual layers and their prominent features are represented schematically.

The mucosa is organized into villi and crypts (crypts of Lieberkühn). *Villi* are finger-like projections of epithelium and underlying lamina propria that contain blood and lymphatic (lacteals) vessels that extend into the intestinal lumen. Intestinal, epithelial cellular proliferation is confined to the *crypts*, each of which carries an average census of 250 to 300 cells. All epithelial cells in each crypt are derived from an unknown number of the yet uncharacterized multipotent stem cells located at or near the crypt's base. Their immediate descendants are amplified by undergoing several cycles of rapid division. These descendants then make a commitment to differentiate along one of four pathways that ultimately yield *enterocytes* and *goblet, enteroendocrine,* and *Paneth* cells. With the exception of Paneth cells, these lineages complete their terminal differentiation during an upward migration from each crypt to adjacent villi. The journey from the crypt to the villus tip is completed in 2 to 5 days and terminates with cells being removed by apoptosis and/or exfoliation. Thus, the small intestinal epithelium undergoes continuous renewal, making it one of the body's most dynamic tissues. The high cellular turnover rate contributes to mucosal resiliency but also makes the intestine uniquely susceptible to certain forms of injury such as that induced by radiation and chemotherapy.

Enterocytes are the predominant absorptive cell of the intestinal epithelium. Their apical (lumen-facing) cell membrane contains specialized digestive enzymes, transporter mechanisms, and microvilli that are estimated to increase the absorptive surface area of the small intestine by up to 40-fold. *Goblet cells* produce mucin believed to play a role in mucosal defense against pathogens. *Enteroendocrine cells* are characterized by secretory granules containing regulatory agents and are discussed in greater detail below in the Endocrine Function section. *Paneth cells* are located at the base of the crypt and contain secretory granules containing growth factors, digestive enzymes, and antimicrobial peptides. In addition, the intestinal epithelium contains microfold (M) cells and intraepithelial lymphocytes. These two components of the immune system are discussed below.

The submucosa consists of dense connective tissue and a heterogeneous population of cells, including leukocytes and fibroblasts. The submucosa also contains an extensive network of vascular and lymphatic vessels, nerve fibers, and ganglion cells of the submucosal (Meissner's) plexus.

The muscularis propria consists of an outer, longitudinally oriented layer and an inner, circularly oriented layer of smooth muscle fibers. Located at the interface between these two layers are ganglion cells of the myenteric (Auerbach's) plexus.

The serosa consists of a single layer of mesothelial cells and is a component of the visceral peritoneum.

DEVELOPMENT

The first recognizable precursor of the small intestine is the embryonic gut tube, formed from the endoderm during the fourth week of gestation. The gut tube is divided into foregut, midgut, and hindgut. Other than duodenum, which is a foregut structure, the rest of the small intestine is derived from the midgut. The gut tube initially communicates with the yolk sac; however, the communication between these two structures narrows by the sixth week to form the vitelline duct. The yolk sac and vitelline duct usually undergo obliteration by the end of gestation. Incomplete obliteration of the vitelline duct results in the spectrum of defects associated with Meckel's diverticula.

Also, during the fourth week of gestation, the mesoderm of the embryo splits. The portion of mesoderm that adheres to the endoderm forms the visceral peritoneum, while the portion that adheres to the ectoderm forms the parietal peritoneum. This mesodermal division results in the formation of a coelomic cavity that is the precursor of the peritoneal cavity.

KEY POINTS

1. The small intestine performs a diverse set of functions.
2. Small bowel obstruction is one of the most common surgical diagnoses.
3. Most cases of small bowel obstruction are due to adhesions from previous surgery.
4. If, following surgical resection, less than 200 cm of small bowel remains, patients are at risk of developing short bowel syndrome.
5. Tumors and malignancies of the small bowel are rare and difficult to diagnose.

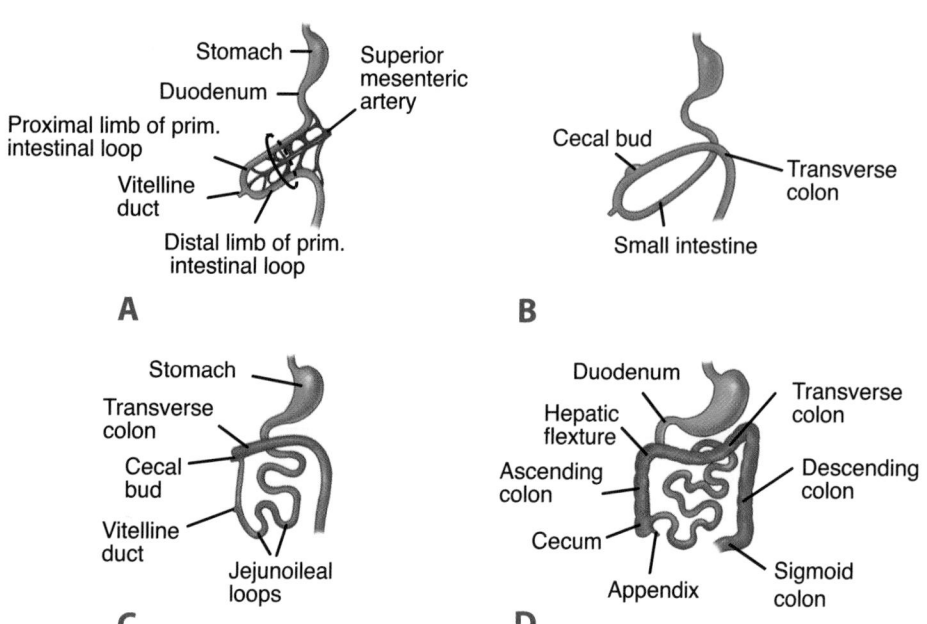

FIG. 28-3. Developmental rotation of the intestine. **A.** During the fifth week of gestation, the developing intestine herniates out of the coelomic cavity and begins to undergo a counterclockwise rotation about the axis of the superior mesenteric artery. **B** and **C.** Intestinal rotation continues, as the developing transverse colon passes anterior to the developing duodenum. **D.** Final positions of the small intestine and colon resulting from a 270° counterclockwise rotation of the developing intestine and its return into the abdominal cavity.

At approximately the fifth week of gestation, the bowel begins to lengthen to an extent greater than that which can be accommodated by the developing abdominal cavity, resulting in the extracoelomic herniation of the developing bowel. The bowel continues to lengthen during the subsequent weeks and is retracted back into the abdominal cavity during the tenth week of gestation. Subsequently, the duodenum becomes a retroperitoneal structure. Coincident with extrusion and retraction, the bowel undergoes a 270° counterclockwise rotation relative to the posterior abdominal wall. This rotation accounts for the usual locations of the cecum in the right lower quadrant and the duodenojejunal junction to the left of midline (Fig. 28-3).

The celiac and superior mesenteric arteries and veins are derived from the vitelline vascular system, which, in turn, is derived from blood vessels formed within the splanchnopleuric mesoderm during the third week of gestation. Neurons found in the small intestine are derived from neural crest cells that begin to migrate away from the neural tube during the third week of gestation. These neural crest cells enter the mesenchyme of the primitive foregut and subsequently migrate to the remainder of the bowel.

During the sixth week of gestation, the lumen of the developing bowel becomes obliterated as bowel epithelial proliferation accelerates. Vacuoles form within the bowel substance during the subsequent weeks and coalesce to form the intestinal lumen by the ninth week of gestation. Errors in this recanalization may account for defects such as intestinal webs and stenoses. Most intestinal atresias, however, are believed to be related to ischemic episodes occurring after organogenesis has been completed rather than to errors in recanalization.

During the ninth week of gestation, the intestinal epithelium develops intestine-specific features such as crypt-villus architecture. Organogenesis is complete by approximately the twelfth week of gestation.

Elucidation of the fundamental mechanisms regulating patterned intestinal development is an area of active investigation.

PHYSIOLOGY

Digestion and Absorption

The intestinal epithelium is the interface through which absorption and secretion occur. It has features characteristic of absorptive epithelia in general, including epithelial cells with cellular membranes possessing distinct apical (luminal) and basolateral (serosal) domains demarcated by intercellular tight junctions, and an asymmetric distribution of transmembrane transporter mechanisms that promotes vectorial transport of solutes across the epithelium.

Solutes can traverse the epithelium by active or passive transport. Passive transport of solutes occurs through diffusion or convection and is driven by existing electrochemical gradients. *Active transport* is the energy-dependent net transfer of solutes in the absence of or against an electrochemical gradient.

Active transport occurs through transcellular pathways (through the cell), whereas passive transport can occur through either transcellular or paracellular pathways (between cells through the tight junctions). Transcellular transport requires solutes to traverse the cell membranes through specialized membrane proteins, such as channels, carriers, and pumps. The molecular characterization of transporter proteins is evolving rapidly, with different transporter families, each containing many individual genes encoding specific transporters, now identified. Similarly, understanding of the paracellular pathway is evolving. In contrast to what was once believed, it is becoming apparent that paracellular permeability is substrate specific, dynamic, and subject to regulation by specific tight junction proteins.[3]

Water and Electrolyte Absorption and Secretion

Eight to 9 L of fluid enter the small intestine daily. Most of this volume consists of salivary, gastric, biliary, pancreatic, and intestinal secretions. Under normal conditions, the small intestine absorbs over 80% of this fluid, leaving approximately 1.5 L that enters the colon (Fig. 28-4). Small intestinal absorption and secretion are tightly regulated; derangements in water and electrolyte homeostasis characteristic of many of the disorders discussed in this chapter play an important role in contributing to their associated clinical features.

Water absorption is believed to be driven by osmotic gradients created primarily by active transepithelial Na^+ absorption. Intestinal water secretion, in contrast, is believed to be driven by osmotic gradients created primarily by transepithelial Cl^- secretion. Most intestinal water transport is believed to occur through the transcellular pathway.[4] The specific transport mechanisms mediating water absorption are incompletely characterized. Aquaporins (water channels) are expressed in the intestinal epithelium; however, their

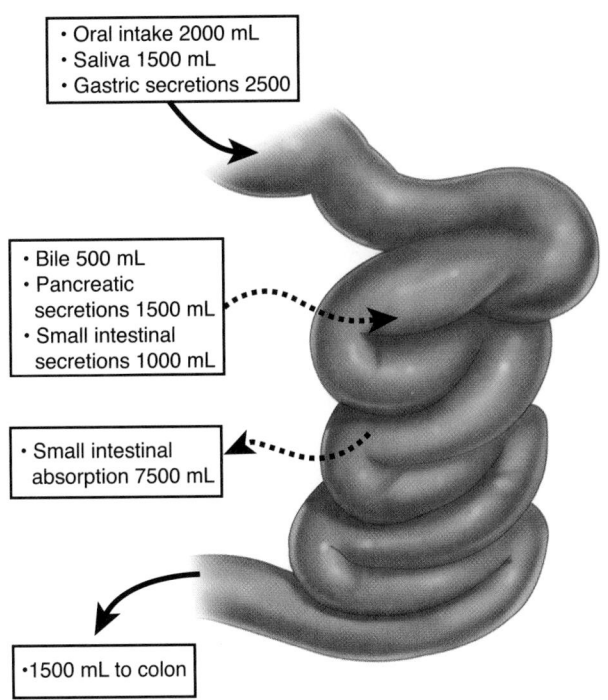

- Oral intake 2000 mL
- Saliva 1500 mL
- Gastric secretions 2500

- Bile 500 mL
- Pancreatic secretions 1500 mL
- Small intestinal secretions 1000 mL

- Small intestinal absorption 7500 mL

- 1500 mL to colon

FIG. 28-4. Small intestinal fluid fluxes. Typical quantities (in volume per day) of fluid entering and leaving the small intestinal lumen in a healthy adult are shown.

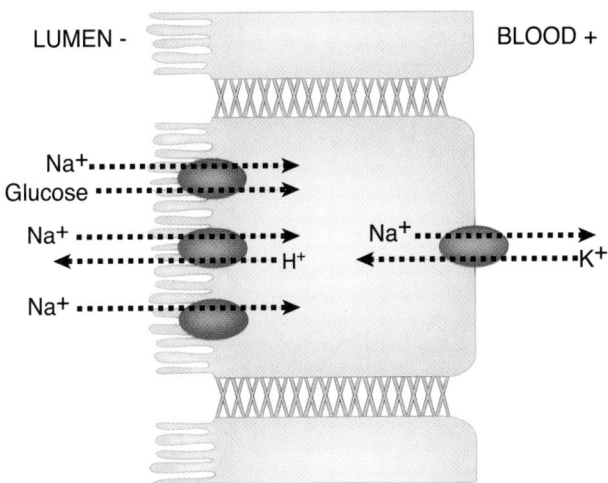

FIG. 28-5. Model of transepithelial sodium (Na^+) absorption. Na^+ traverses the apical membrane of enterocytes through a variety of mechanisms, including nutrient-coupled Na^+ transport, Na^+/H^+ exchange, and Na^+ channels. Activity of the Na^+/K^+ ATPase located on the basolateral membrane generates the electrochemical gradient that provides the driving force for Na^+ absorption.

contribution to overall intestinal water absorption appears to be relatively minor.[5]

The prevailing model for intestinal epithelial Na^+ absorption is shown in Fig. 28-5. Activity of the Na^+/K^+ ATPase enzyme, which is located in the basolateral membrane and exchanges three intracellular Na^+ for every two extracellular K^+ in an energy-dependent process, generates the electrochemical gradient that drives the transport of Na^+ from the intestinal lumen into the cytoplasm of enterocytes. Na^+ ions traverse the apical membrane through several distinct transporter mechanisms including nutrient-coupled sodium transport (e.g., sodium-glucose cotransporter-1, SGLT1), sodium channels, and sodium-hydrogen exchangers. Absorbed Na^+ ions are then extruded from enterocytes through the Na^+/K^+ ATPase located in the basolateral membrane. Similar mechanistic models that account for the transport of other common ions such as K^+ and HCO_3^- also exist.

Substantial heterogeneity, with respect to both crypt-villus and craniocaudal axes, exist for intestinal epithelial transport mechanisms. For example, nutrient-coupled Na^+ transporters are expressed in mature villus cells, but are absent in crypt cells. In contrast, the cystic fibrosis transmembrane regulator (a chloride channel) is expressed to a greater extent in crypt cells. This spatial distribution pattern is consistent with a model in which absorptive function resides primarily in the villus and secretory function in the crypt.

Intestinal absorption and secretion are subject to modulation under physiologic and pathophysiologic conditions by a wide array of hormonal, neural, and immune regulatory mediators (Table 28-1).

Carbohydrate Digestion and Absorption

Approximately 45% of energy consumption in the average Western diet consists of carbohydrates, approximately one half of which is in the form of starch (linear or branched polymers of glucose) derived from cereals and plants. Other major sources of dietary carbohydrates include sugars derived from milk (lactose), fruits and vegetables (fructose, glucose, and sucrose), or purified from sugar cane or beets (sucrose). Processed foods contain a variety of sugars including fructose, oligosaccharides, and polysaccharides.

Glycogen derived from meat contributes only a small fraction of dietary carbohydrate.

Pancreatic amylase is the major enzyme of starch digestion, although salivary amylase initiates the process. The terminal products of amylase-mediated starch digestion are oligosaccharides, maltotriose, maltose, and alpha-limit dextrins (Fig. 28-6). These products, as well as the major disaccharides in the diet (sucrose and lactose), are unable to undergo absorption in this form. They must first undergo hydrolytic cleavage into their constituent monosaccharides; these hydrolytic reactions are catalyzed by specific brush border membrane hydrolases that are expressed most abundantly in

TABLE 28-1	Regulation of intestinal absorption and secretion

Agents that stimulate absorption or inhibit secretion of water
- Aldosterone
- Glucocorticoids
- Angiotensin
- Norepinephrine
- Epinephrine
- Dopamine
- Somatostatin
- Neuropeptide Y
- Peptide YY
- Enkephalin

Agents that stimulate secretion or inhibit absorption of water
- Secretin
- Bradykinin
- Prostaglandins
- Acetylcholine
- Atrial natriuretic factor
- Vasopressin
- Vasoactive intestinal peptide
- Bombesin
- Substance P
- Serotonin
- Neurotensin
- Histamine

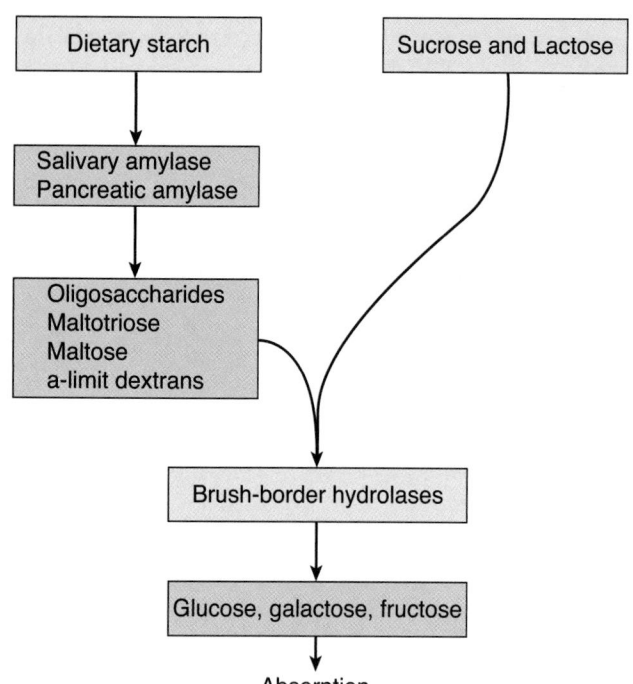

FIG. 28-6. Carbohydrate digestion. Dietary carbohydrates, including starch and the disaccharides sucrose and lactose, must undergo hydrolysis into constituent monosaccharides glucose, galactose, and fructose before being absorbed by the intestinal epithelium. These hydrolytic reactions are catalyzed by salivary and pancreatic amylase and by enterocyte brush border hydrolases.

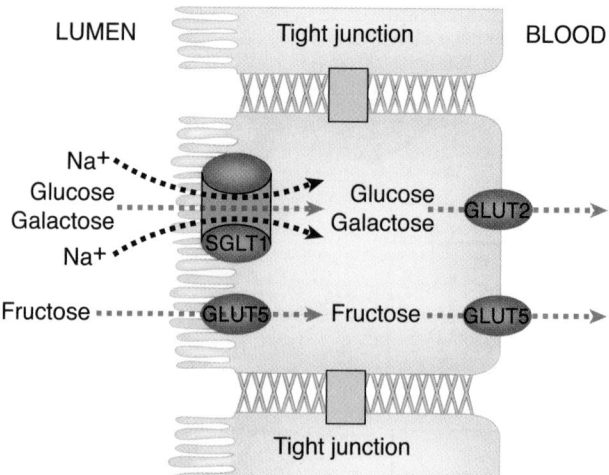

FIG. 28-7. Hexose transporters. Glucose and galactose enter the enterocyte through secondary active transport via the sodium-glucose cotransporter-1 (SGLT1) located on the apical (brush border) membrane. Fructose enters through facilitated diffusion via glucose transporter-5 (GLUT5). Glucose and galactose are extruded basolaterally through facilitated diffusion via glucose transporter-2 (GLUT2). Fructose is extruded basolaterally via GLUT5.

the villi of the duodenum and jejunum. The three major monosaccharides that represent the terminal products of carbohydrate digestion are glucose, galactose, and fructose.

Under physiologic conditions, most of these sugars are absorbed through the epithelium via the transcellular route. Glucose and galactose are transported through the enterocyte brush border membrane via intestinal SGLT1 (Fig. 28-7). Fructose is transported through the brush border membrane by facilitated diffusion via glucose transporter-5 (GLUT5, a member of the facilitative glucose transporter family). All three monosaccharides are extruded through the basolateral membrane by facilitated diffusion. Extruded monosaccharides diffuse into venules and ultimately enter the portal venous system.

There is evidence of overexpression of hexose transporters, specifically SGLT1, in disease states such as diabetes.[6] Several approaches aimed at down-regulation of these transporters are being investigated as a novel therapy for disease states such as diabetes and obesity.[7]

Protein Digestion and Absorption

Ten to 15% of energy consumption in the average Western diet consists of proteins. In addition to dietary proteins, approximately one half of the protein load that enters the small intestine is derived from endogenous sources including salivary and GI secretions and desquamated intestinal epithelial cells. Protein digestion begins in the stomach with action of pepsins. This is not, however, an essential step, because surgical patients who are achlorhydric, or have lost part or all their stomach, are still able to successfully digest proteins. Digestion continues in the duodenum with the actions of a variety of pancreatic peptidases. These enzymes are secreted as inactive proenzymes. This is in contrast to pancreatic amylase and lipase, which are secreted in their active forms. In response to the presence of bile acids, enterokinase is liberated from the intestinal brush border membrane to catalyze the conversion of trypsinogen to active trypsin;

trypsin, in turn, activates itself and other proteases. The final products of intraluminal protein digestion consist of neutral and basic amino acids and peptides two to six amino acids in length (Fig. 28-8). Additional digestion occurs through the actions of peptidases that exist in the enterocyte brush border and cytoplasm. Epithelial absorp-

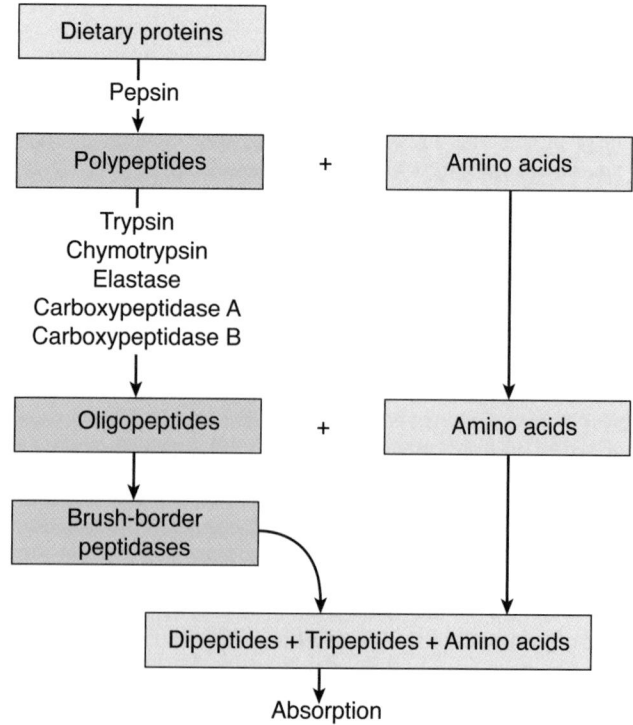

FIG. 28-8. Protein digestion. Dietary proteins must undergo hydrolysis into constituent single amino acids and di- and tripeptides before being absorbed by the intestinal epithelium. These hydrolytic reactions are catalyzed by pancreatic peptidases (e.g., trypsin) and by enterocyte brush border peptidases.

tion occurs for both single amino acids and di- or tripeptides via specific membrane-bound transporters. Absorbed amino acids and peptides then enter the portal venous circulation.

Of all amino acids, glutamine appears to be a unique, major source of energy for enterocytes. Active glutamine uptake into enterocytes occurs through both apical and basolateral transport mechanisms.

Fat Digestion and Absorption

Approximately 40% of the average Western diet consists of fat. Over 95% of dietary fat is in the form of long-chain triglycerides; the remainder includes phospholipids such as lecithin, fatty acids, cholesterol, and fat-soluble vitamins. Over 94% of the ingested fats are absorbed in the proximal jejunum.

Because fats are normally water insoluble, key to successful digestion of ingested fats is solubilization of them into an emulsion by the mechanical actions of mastication and antral peristalsis. Although lipolysis of triglycerides to form fatty acids and monoglycerides is initiated in the stomach by gastric lipase, its principal site is the proximal intestine, where pancreatic lipase is the catalyst (Fig. 28-9).

Bile acids act as detergents that help in solubilization of the lipolysis by forming mixed micelles. These micelles are polymolecular aggregates with a hydrophobic core of fat, and a hydrophilic surface that act as shuttles, delivering the products of lipolysis to the enterocyte brush border membrane, where they are absorbed. The bile salts, however, remain in the bowel lumen and travel to the terminal ileum, where they are actively resorbed. They enter the portal circulation and are resecreted into bile, thus completing the enterohepatic circulation.

Dissociation of lipids from the micelles occurs in a thin layer of water (50 to 500 μm thick) with an acidic microenvironment immediately adjacent to the brush border called the *unstirred water layer*. Most lipids are absorbed in the proximal jejunum, whereas bile salts are absorbed in the distal ileum through an active process. Fatty acid binding proteins are a family of proteins located on the brush border membrane, facilitating diffusion of long-chain fatty acids across the brush border membrane. Cholesterol crosses the brush border membrane through an active process that is yet to be completely characterized. Within the enterocytes, triglycerides are resynthesized and incorporated into chylomicrons that are secreted into the intestinal lymphatics and ultimately enter the thoracic duct. In these chylomicrons, lipoproteins serve a detergent-like role similar to that served by bile salts in the mixed micelles.

The steps described above are required for the digestion and absorption of triglycerides containing long-chain fatty acids. However, triglycerides containing short- and medium-chain fatty acids are more hydrophilic and are absorbed without undergoing intraluminal hydrolysis, micellular solubilization, mucosal re-esterification, and chylomicron formation. Instead, they are directly absorbed and enter the portal venous circulation rather than the lymphatics. This information provides the rationale for administering nutritional supplements containing medium-chain triglycerides to patients with GI diseases associated with impaired digestion and/or malabsorption of long-chain triglycerides.

Vitamin and Mineral Absorption

Vitamin B$_{12}$ (cobalamin) malabsorption can result from a variety of surgical manipulations. The vitamin is initially bound by saliva-derived R protein. In the duodenum, R protein is hydrolyzed by pancreatic enzymes, allowing free cobalamin to bind to gastric parietal cell-derived intrinsic factor. The cobalamin-intrinsic factor complex is able to escape hydrolysis by pancreatic enzymes, allowing it to reach the terminal ileum, which expresses specific receptors for intrinsic factor. Subsequent events in cobalamin absorption are poorly characterized, but the intact complex probably enters enterocytes through translocation. Because each of these steps is necessary for cobalamin assimilation, gastric resection, gastric bypass, and ileal resection can each result in vitamin B$_{12}$ insufficiency.

Other water-soluble vitamins for which specific carrier-mediated transport processes have been characterized include ascorbic acid, folate, thiamine, riboflavin, pantothenic acid, and biotin. Fat-soluble vitamins A, D, and E appear to be absorbed through passive diffusion. Vitamin K appears to be absorbed through both passive diffusion and carrier-mediated uptake.

Calcium is absorbed through both transcellular transport and paracellular diffusion. The duodenum is the major site for transcellular transport; paracellular transport occurs throughout the small intestine. A key step in transcellular calcium transport is mediated by calbindin, a calcium-binding protein located in the cytoplasm of enterocytes. Regulation of calbindin synthesis is the principal mechanism by which vitamin D regulates intestinal calcium absorption. Abnormal calcium levels are increasingly seen in surgical patients who have undergone a gastric bypass. Although usual calcium supplementation is in the form of calcium carbonate, which is cheap, in such patients with low acid exposure, calcium citrate is a better formulation for replacement therapy.

Iron and magnesium are each absorbed through both transcellular and paracellular routes. A divalent metal transporter capable of transporting Fe^{2+}, Zn^{2+}, Mn^{2+}, Co^{2+}, Cd^{2+}, Cu^{2+}, Ni^{2+}, and Pb^{2+} that has recently been localized to the intestinal brush border, may account for at least a portion of the transcellular absorption of these ions.[8]

Barrier and Immune Function

Although the intestinal epithelium allows for the efficient absorption of dietary nutrients, it must discriminate between pathogens and harmless antigens such as food proteins and commensal bacteria and it must resist invasion by pathogens. Factors contributing to epithelial defense include immunoglobulin A (IgA), mucins, and the relative impermeability of the brush border membrane and tight junctions to macromolecules and bacteria. Recently described factors likely to play important roles in intestinal mucosal defense include antimicrobial peptides such as the defensins.[9] The intestinal component of the immune system, known as the *gut-associated lymphoid tissue* (GALT), contains over 70% of the body's immune cells.

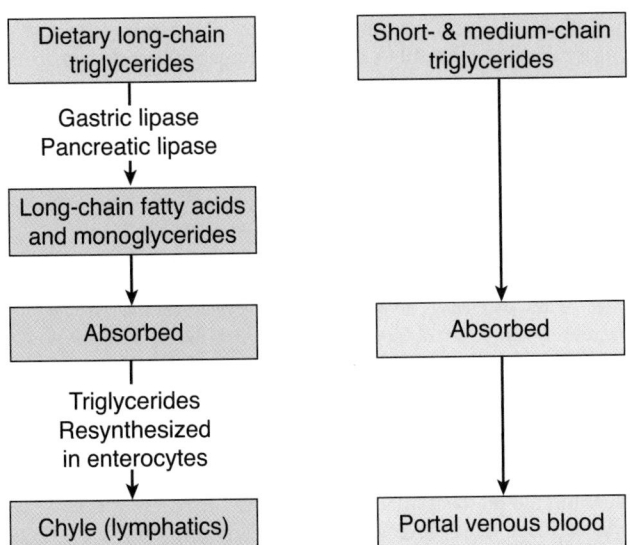

FIG. 28-9. Fat digestion. Long-chain triglycerides, which constitute the majority of dietary fats, must undergo lipolysis into constituent long-chain fatty acids and monoglycerides before being absorbed by the intestinal epithelium. These reactions are catalyzed by gastric and pancreatic lipases. The products of lipolysis are transported in the form of mixed micelles to enterocytes, where they are resynthesized into triglycerides, which are then packaged in the form of chylomicrons that are secreted into the intestinal lymph (chyle). Triglycerides composed of short- and medium-chain fatty acids are absorbed by the intestinal epithelium directly, without undergoing lipolysis, and are secreted into the portal venous circulation.

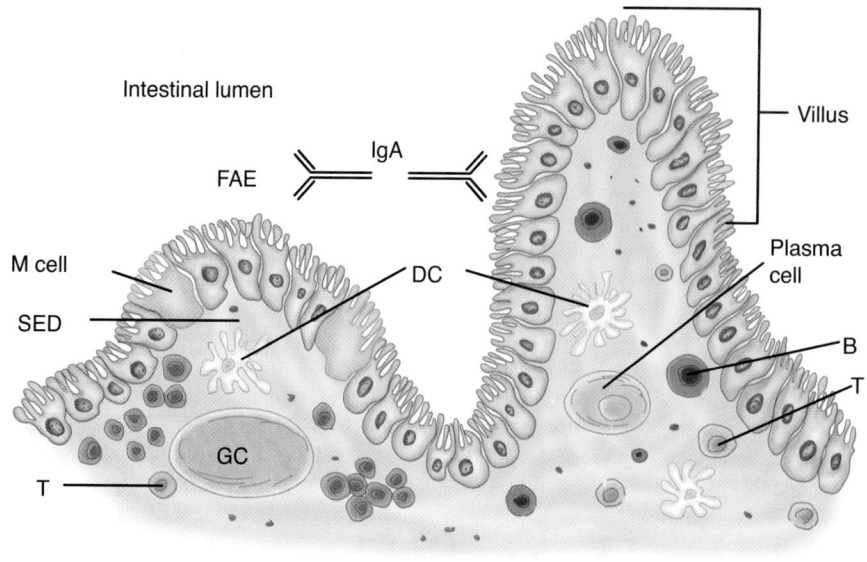

Intestinal lumen

IgA

FAE

M cell

SED

DC

Villus

Plasma cell

B

T

GC

T

Peyer's patch

Lamina propria

FIG. 28-10. Gut-associated lymphoid tissue. Select components of the gut-associated lymphoid tissue are schematically represented. Peyer's patches consist of a specialized follicle-associated epithelium (FAE) containing M cells, a subepithelial dome (SED) rich in dendritic cells (DC), and B-cell follicle containing germinal centers (GC). Plasma cells in the lamina propria produce immunoglobulin A (IgA), which is transported to the intestinal lumen where it serves as the first line of defense against pathogens. Other components of the gut-associated lymphoid tissue include isolated lymphoid follicles, mesenteric lymph nodes, and regulatory and effector lymphocytes. B = B cell; T = T cell.

The GALT is conceptually divided into inductive and effector sites.[10] Inductive sites include Peyer's patches, mesenteric lymph nodes, and smaller isolated lymphoid follicles scattered throughout the small intestine (Fig. 28-10). Peyer's patches are macroscopic aggregates of B-cell follicles and intervening T-cell areas found in the lamina propria of the small intestine, primarily the distal ileum. Overlying Peyer's patches is a specialized epithelium containing M cells. These cells possess an apical membrane with microfolds rather than microvilli, which is characteristic of most intestinal epithelial cells. Using transepithelial vesicular transport, M cells transfer microbes to underlying professional antigen-presenting cells, such as dendritic cells. Dendritic cells, in addition, may sample luminal antigens directly through their dendrite-like processes that extend through epithelial tight junctions. Antigen-presenting cells interact with and prime naïve lymphocytes, which then exit through the draining lymphatics to enter the mesenteric lymph nodes, where they undergo differentiation. These lymphocytes then migrate into the systemic circulation via the thoracic duct and ultimately accumulate in the intestinal mucosa at effector sites. Alternative induction mechanisms, such as antigen presentation within mesenteric lymph nodes, are also likely to exist.

Effector lymphocytes are distributed into distinct compartments. IgA-producing plasma cells are derived from B cells and are located in the lamina propria. CD4+ T cells are also located in the lamina propria. CD8+ T cells migrate preferentially to the epithelium, but are also found in the lamina propria. These T cells are central to immune regulation; in addition the CD8+ T cells have potent cytotoxic T lymphocyte activity. IgA is transported through the intestinal epithelial cells into the lumen, where it exists in the form of a dimer complexed with a secretory component. This configuration renders IgA resistant to proteolysis by digestive enzymes. IgA is believed to both help prevent the entry of microbes through the epithelium and to promote excretion of antigens or microbes that have already penetrated into the lamina propria.

Ineffective resistance to invasion by pathogens is hypothesized to play an etiologic role in sepsis by allowing translocation of bacteria and/or toxins into the systemic circulation. In contrast, overexuberant immune sensitivity or lack of tolerance to dietary antigens or commensal bacteria is believed to contribute to the pathogenesis of chronic inflammatory disorders such as celiac disease and Crohn's disease.[10]

Motility

Myocytes of the intestinal muscle layers are electrically and mechanically coordinated in the form of syncytia. Contractions of the muscularis propria are responsible for small intestinal peristalsis. Contraction of the outer longitudinal muscle layer results in bowel shortening; contraction of the inner circular layer results in luminal narrowing. Contractions of the muscularis mucosa contribute to mucosal or villus motility, but not to peristalsis.

Several distinctive patterns of muscularis propria activity have been observed to occur in the small intestine. These patterns include *ascending excitation* and *descending inhibition* in which muscular contraction occurs proximal to a stimulus, such as the presence of a bolus of ingested food, and muscular relaxation occurs distal to the stimulus (Fig. 28-11). These two reflexes are present even in the absence of any extrinsic innervation to the small intestine and contribute to peristalsis when they are propagated in a coordinated fashion along the length of the intestine. The *fed* or *postprandial pattern* begins within 10 to 20 minutes of meal ingestion and abates 4 to 6 hours afterward. *Rhythmic segmentations* or pressure waves traveling only short distances also are observed. This segmenting pattern is hypothesized to assist in mixing intraluminal contents and in facilitating their contact with the absorptive mucosal surface. The *fasting pattern* or *interdigestive motor cycle* (IDMC) consists of three phases. Phase I is characterized by motor quiescence, phase II by seemingly disorganized pressure waves occurring at submaximal rates, and phase III by sustained pressure waves occurring at maximal rates. This pattern is hypothesized to expel residual debris and bacteria from the small intestine. The median duration of the IDMC ranges from 90 to 120 minutes. At any given time, different portions of the small intestine can be in different phases of the IDMC.

The regulatory mechanisms driving small intestinal motility consist of both pacemakers intrinsic to the small intestine and external neurohumoral modulatory signals. The interstitial cells of Cajal are pleomorphic mesenchymal cells located within the muscularis propria of the intestine that generate the electrical slow wave (basic electrical rhythm or pacesetter potential) that plays a pacemaker role in setting the fundamental rhythmicity of small intestinal contractions. The frequency of the slow wave varies along the longitudinal axis of the intestine: It ranges from 12 waves per minute in the duodenum to 7 waves per minute in the distal ileum. Smooth muscle contraction occurs only when an electrical action potential (spike burst) is superimposed on the slow wave. Thus, the slow wave determines the maximum frequency of contractions; however, not every slow wave is associated with a contraction.

This intrinsic contractile mechanism is subject to neural and hormonal regulation. The enteric motor system (ENS) provides both inhibitory and excitatory stimuli. The predominant excitatory

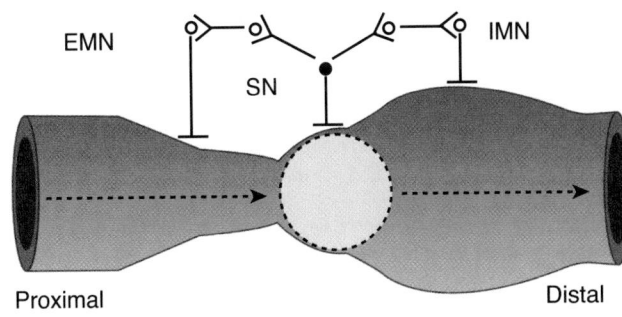

EMN   IMN

SN

Proximal   Distal

FIG. 28-11. Ascending excitation and descending inhibition. The presence of a food bolus within the intestinal lumen is sensed by a sensory neuron (SN) that relays signals to (a) excitatory motor neurons (EMN) that have projections to intestinal muscle cells located proximal to the food bolus and (b) inhibitory motor neurons (IMN) that have projections to intestinal muscle cells located distal to the food bolus. This stereotypical motor reflex is controlled by the enteric nervous system and occurs in the absence of extraintestinal innervations. It contributes to peristalsis.

transmitters are acetylcholine and substance P, and the inhibitory transmitters include nitric oxide, vasoactive intestinal peptide, and adenosine triphosphate. In general, the sympathetic motor supply is inhibitory to the ENS; therefore, increased sympathetic input into the intestine leads to decreased intestinal smooth muscle activity. The parasympathetic motor supply is more complex, with projections to both inhibitory and excitatory ENS motor neurons. Correspondingly, the effects of parasympathetic inputs into intestinal motility are more difficult to predict.

Endocrine Function

Endocrinology as a discipline was born with the discovery of secretin, an intestinal regulatory peptide that was the first hormone to be identified. The small intestine is now recognized to be the largest hormone-producing organ in the body, both with respect to the number of hormone-producing cells and the number of individual hormones produced.[11] Over 30 peptide hormone genes have been identified as being expressed in the GI tract. Because of differential posttranscriptional and posttranslational processing, over 100 distinct regulatory peptides are produced. In addition, monoamines, such as histamine and dopamine, and eicosanoids with hormone-like activities are produced in the intestine.

"Gut hormones" were previously conceptualized as peptides produced by the enteroendocrine cells of the intestinal mucosa that are released into the systemic circulation to reach receptors in target sites in the GI tract. Now it is clear that "gut hormone" genes are widely expressed throughout the body, not only in endocrine cells, but also in central and peripheral neurons.[12] The products of these genes are general intercellular messengers that can act as endocrine, paracrine, autocrine, or neurocrine mediators. Thus, they may act as true blood-borne hormones as well as through local effects.

There are notable homology patterns among individual regulatory peptides found in the GI tract. Based on these homologies, approximately one half of the known regulatory peptides can be classified into families.[12] For example, the secretin family includes secretin, glucagon, and glucagon-like peptides, glucose-dependent insulinotropic peptide, vasoactive intestinal polypeptide, peptide histidine isoleucine, growth hormone releasing hormone, and pituitary adenylyl cyclase-activating peptide. Other peptide families include those named for insulin, epidermal growth factor, gastrin, pancreatic polypeptide, tachykinin, and somatostatin.

Receptor subtype multiplicity and cell-specific expression patterns for these receptor subtypes that are characteristic of these

regulatory mediators make definition of their actions complex. Detailed description of these actions is beyond the scope of this chapter; however, examples of regulatory peptides produced by enteroendocrine cells of the small intestinal epithelium and their most commonly ascribed functions are summarized in Table 28-2. Some of these peptides or their analogues are used in routine clinical practice. For example, therapeutic applications of octreotide, a long-acting analogue of somatostatin, include the amelioration of symptoms associated with neuroendocrine tumors (e.g., carcinoid syndrome), postgastrectomy dumping syndrome, enterocutaneous fistulas, and the initial treatment of acute hemorrhage due to esophageal varices. The gastrin secretory response to secretin administration forms the basis for the standard test used to establish the diagnosis of Zollinger-Ellison syndrome. Cholecystokinin is used in evaluations of gallbladder ejection fraction, a parameter that may have use in patients who have symptoms of biliary colic but are not found to have gallstones. Of the peptides listed in Table 28-2, glucagon-like peptide 2 (GLP-2) has been identified as a specific and potent intestinotrophic hormone. GLP-2 both stimulates cellular proliferation and inhibits apoptosis in the intestinal epithelium. It has been demonstrated to induce intestinal regeneration and promote healing in numerous experimental models of intestinal disease. It is currently under clinical evaluation as an intestinotrophic agent in patients suffering from the short bowel syndrome, as discussed in the Short Bowel Syndrome section below.

Intestinal Adaptation

The small intestine has the capacity to adapt in response to varying demands imposed by physiologic and pathologic conditions. Of particular relevance to many of the diseases discussed in this chapter is the adaptation that occurs in the remnant intestine following surgical resection of a large portion of the small intestine (massive small bowel resection). Postresection intestinal adaptation has been studied extensively using animal models. Within a few hours after bowel resection, the remnant small intestine displays evidence of epithelial cellular hyperplasia. With additional time, villi lengthen, intestinal absorptive surface area increases, and digestive and absorptive functions improve. Postresection intestinal adaptation in human patients is less well studied, but seems to follow similar steps as that seen in experimental models, and takes 1 to 2 years to complete.[13]

The mechanisms responsible for inducing postresection intestinal adaptation are under active investigation. Several classes of effectors that stimulate intestinal growth include specific nutrients, peptide hormones and growth factors, pancreatic secretions, and

TABLE 28-2	Representative regulatory peptides produced in the small intestine	
Hormone	**Source**[a]	**Actions**
Somatostatin	D cell	Inhibits GI secretion, motility, and splanchnic perfusion
Secretin	S cell	Stimulates exocrine pancreatic secretion Stimulates intestinal secretion
Cholecystokinin	I cell	Stimulates pancreatic exocrine secretion Stimulates gallbladder emptying Inhibits sphincter of Oddi contraction
Motilin	M cell	Simulates intestinal motility
Peptide YY	L cell	Inhibits intestinal motility and secretion
Glucagon-like peptide 2	L cell	Stimulates intestinal epithelial proliferation
Neurotensin	N cell	Stimulates pancreatic and biliary secretion Inhibits small bowel motility Stimulates intestinal mucosal growth

[a]This table indicates which enteroendocrine cell types located in the intestinal epithelium produce these peptides. These peptides are also widely expressed in nonintestinal tissues.

some cytokines.[14] Nutritional components with intestinal growth-stimulating effects include fiber, fatty acids, triglycerides, glutamine, polyamines, and lectins. Peptide growth factors reported to induce growth include epidermal growth factor, transforming growth factor alpha, insulin-like growth factors I and II, keratinocyte growth factor, hepatocyte growth factor, gastrin, peptide YY, neurotensin, and bombesin. Cytokines that stimulate growth include interleukin (IL)-11, IL-3, and IL-15. The most recently characterized stimulator of enterocyte proliferation is GLP-2, which has potent trophic activity that is specific for the intestinal epithelium.[15] As serum concentrations of GLP-2 rise following massive small bowel resection and GLP-2 immunoneutralization inhibits postresection intestinal adaptation, GLP-2 is a promising candidate mediator of this response.

Postresection adaptation serves to compensate for the function of intestine that has been resected. Jejunal resection generally is better tolerated, as ileum shows better capacity to compensate. However, the magnitude of this response is limited. If enough small intestine is resected, a devastating condition known as the *short bowel syndrome* results. This condition is discussed in the Short Bowel Syndrome section at the end of this chapter.

SMALL BOWEL OBSTRUCTION

Epidemiology

Mechanical small bowel obstruction is the most frequently encountered surgical disorder of the small intestine. Although a wide range of etiologies for this condition exist, the obstructing lesion can be conceptualized according to its anatomic relationship to the intestinal wall as:

1. Intraluminal (e.g., foreign bodies, gallstones, or meconium)
2. Intramural (e.g., tumors, Crohn's disease–associated inflammatory strictures)
3. Extrinsic (e.g., adhesions, hernias, or carcinomatosis)

Intra-abdominal adhesions related to prior abdominal surgery account for up to 75% of the cases of small bowel obstruction. Over 300,000 patients are estimated to undergo surgery annually to treat adhesion-induced small bowel obstruction in the United States.[16]

Less prevalent etiologies for small bowel obstruction include hernias, malignant bowel obstruction, and Crohn's disease. The frequency with which obstruction related to these conditions is encountered varies according to the patient population and practice setting. Cancer-related small bowel obstructions are commonly due to extrinsic compression or invasion by advanced malignancies arising in organs other than the small bowel; few are due to primary small bowel tumors. The most commonly encountered etiologies of small bowel obstruction are summarized in Table 28-3. Although congenital abnormalities capable of causing small bowel obstruction usually become evident during childhood, they sometimes elude detection and are diagnosed for the first time in adult patients presenting with abdominal symptoms. For example, intestinal malrotation and midgut volvulus should not be forgotten when considering the differential diagnosis of adult patients with acute or chronic symptoms of small bowel obstruction, especially those without a history of prior abdominal surgery. A rare etiology of obstruction is the superior mesenteric artery syndrome, characterized by compression of the third portion of the duodenum by the superior mesenteric artery as it crosses over this portion of the duodenum. This condition should be considered in young asthenic individuals who have chronic symptoms suggestive of proximal small bowel obstruction.

Pathophysiology

With onset of obstruction, gas and fluid accumulate within the intestinal lumen proximal to the site of obstruction. The intestinal activity increases in an effort to overcome the obstruction, accounting for the colicky pain and the diarrhea that some experience even in the presence of complete bowel obstruction. Most of the gas that accumu-

TABLE 28-3	Small bowel obstruction: Common etiologies

Adhesions
Neoplasms
    Primary small bowel neoplasms
    Secondary small bowel cancer (e.g., melanoma-derived metastasis)
    Local invasion by intra-abdominal malignancy (e.g., desmoid tumors)
    Carcinomatosis
Hernias
    External (e.g., inguinal and femoral)
    Internal (e.g., following Roux-en-Y gastric bypass surgery)
Crohn's disease
Volvulus
Intussusception
Radiation-induced stricture
Postischemic stricture
Foreign body
Gallstone ileus
Diverticulitis
Meckel's diverticulum
Hematoma
Congenital abnormalities (e.g., webs, duplications, and malrotation)

lates originates from swallowed air, although some is produced within the intestine. The fluid consists of swallowed liquids and GI secretions (obstruction stimulates intestinal epithelial water secretion). With ongoing gas and fluid accumulation, the bowel distends and intraluminal and intramural pressures rise. The intestinal motility is eventually reduced with fewer contractions. With obstruction, the luminal flora of the small bowel, which is usually sterile, changes and a variety of organisms have been cultured from the contents. Translocation of these bacteria to regional lymph nodes has been demonstrated, although the significance of this process is not well understood. If the intramural pressure becomes high enough, intestinal microvascular perfusion is impaired, leading to intestinal ischemia, and, ultimately, necrosis. This condition is termed *strangulated bowel obstruction*.

With *partial small bowel obstruction*, only a portion of the intestinal lumen is occluded, allowing passage of some gas and fluid. The progression of pathophysiologic events described above tends to occur more slowly than with *complete small bowel obstruction*, and development of strangulation is less likely.

A particularly dangerous form of bowel obstruction is *closed loop obstruction*, in which a segment of intestine is obstructed both proximally and distally (e.g., with volvulus). In such cases, the accumulating gas and fluid cannot escape either proximally or distally from the obstructed segment, leading to a rapid rise in luminal pressure, and a rapid progression to strangulation.

Clinical Presentation

The symptoms of small bowel obstruction are colicky abdominal pain, nausea, vomiting, and obstipation. Vomiting is a more prominent symptom with proximal obstructions than distal. Character of vomitus is important as with bacterial overgrowth, the vomitus is more feculent, suggesting a more established obstruction (Fig. 28-12). Continued passage of flatus and/or stool beyond 6 to 12 hours after onset of symptoms is characteristic of partial rather than complete obstruction. The signs of small bowel obstruction include abdominal distention that is most pronounced if the site of obstruction is in the distal ileum, and may be absent if the site of obstruction is in the proximal small intestine. Bowel sounds may be hyperactive initially, but in late stages of bowel obstruction, minimal bowel sounds may be heard. Laboratory findings reflect intravascular volume depletion and consist of hemoconcentration and electrolyte abnormalities. Mild leukocytosis is common.

Features of strangulated obstruction include abdominal pain often disproportionate to the degree of abdominal findings, sugges-

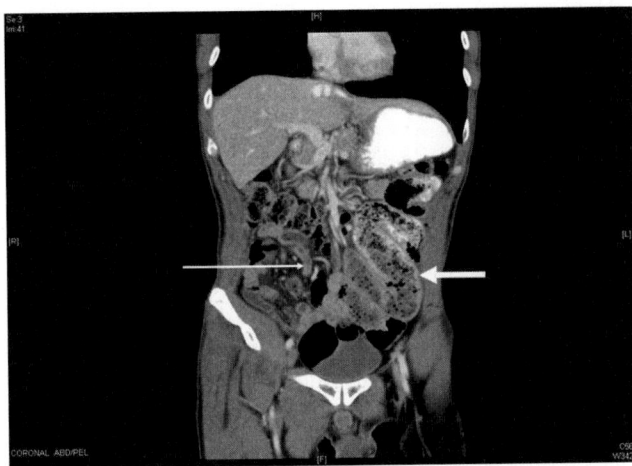

FIG. 28-12. Chronic partial small bowel obstruction. This patient presented with a several months' history of chronic abdominal pain, and intermittent vomiting. The coronal computed tomographic image shows grossly dilated loops of proximal small bowel on the left side (*wide arrow*), with decompressed loops of small bowel on the right side (*narrow arrow*). The dilated segment shows evidence of feculization of bowel contents, consistent with the chronic nature of the obstruction. Patient's vomitus had characteristic feculent smell and quality. At exploratory laparotomy, adhesive bands were identified and divided.

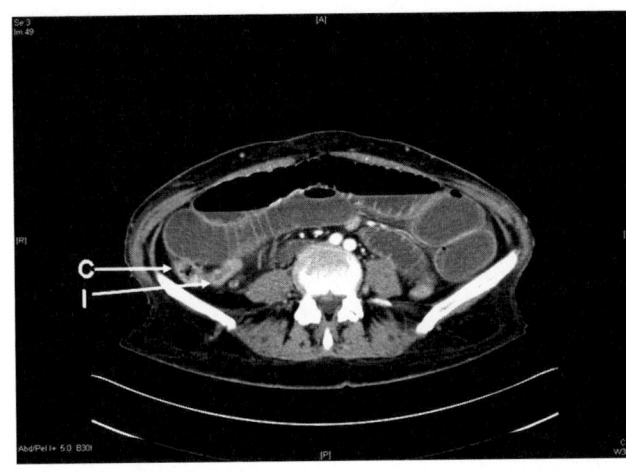

FIG. 28-13. Small bowel obstruction. A computed tomographic scan of a patient presenting with signs and symptoms of bowel obstruction. Image shows grossly dilated loops of small bowel, with decompressed terminal ileum (I) and ascending colon (C), suggesting a complete distal small bowel obstruction. At laparotomy, adhesive bands from a previous surgery were identified and divided.

tive of intestinal ischemia. Patients often have tachycardia, localized abdominal tenderness, fever, marked leukocytosis, and acidosis. Any of these findings should alert the clinician to the possibility of strangulation, and the need for early surgical intervention.

Diagnosis

The diagnostic evaluation should focus on the following goals: (a) distinguish mechanical obstruction from ileus, (b) determine the etiology of the obstruction, (c) discriminate partial from complete obstruction, and (d) discriminate simple from strangulating obstruction.

Important elements to obtain on history include prior abdominal operations (suggesting the presence of adhesions) and the presence of abdominal disorders (e.g., intra-abdominal cancer or inflammatory bowel disease) that may provide insights into the etiology of obstruction. Upon examination, a meticulous search for hernias (particularly in the inguinal and femoral regions) should be conducted. The stool should be checked for gross or occult blood, the presence of which is suggestive of intestinal strangulation.

The diagnosis of small bowel obstruction is usually confirmed with radiographic examination. The *abdominal series* consists of (a) a radiograph of the abdomen with the patient in a supine position, (b) a radiograph of the abdomen with the patient in an upright position, and (c) a radiograph of the chest with the patient in an upright position. The finding most specific for small bowel obstruction is the triad of dilated small bowel loops (>3 cm in diameter), air-fluid levels seen on upright films, and a paucity of air in the colon. The sensitivity of abdominal radiographs in the detection of small bowel obstruction ranges from 70 to 80%.[17] Specificity is low because ileus and colonic obstruction can be associated with findings that mimic those observed with small bowel obstruction. False-negative findings on radiographs can result when the site of obstruction is located in the proximal small bowel and when the bowel lumen is filled with fluid but no gas, thereby preventing visualization of air-fluid levels or bowel distention. The latter situation is associated with closed-loop obstruction. Despite these limitations, abdominal radiographs remain an important study in patients with suspected small bowel obstruction because of their widespread availability and low cost.

Computed tomographic (CT) scanning is 80 to 90% sensitive and 70 to 90% specific in the detection of small bowel obstruction.[17] The findings of small bowel obstruction include a discrete transition zone with dilation of bowel proximally, decompression of bowel distally, intraluminal contrast that does not pass beyond the transition zone, and a colon containing little gas or fluid (Fig. 28-13). CT scanning may also provide evidence for the presence of closed-loop obstruction and strangulation. Closed-loop obstruction is suggested by the presence of a U-shaped or C-shaped dilated bowel loop associated with a radial distribution of mesenteric vessels converging toward a torsion point. Strangulation is suggested by thickening of the bowel wall, pneumatosis intestinalis (air in the bowel wall), portal venous gas, mesenteric haziness, and poor uptake of IV contrast into the wall of the affected bowel (Fig. 28-14). CT scanning also offers a global evaluation of the abdomen and may therefore reveal the etiology of obstruction. This

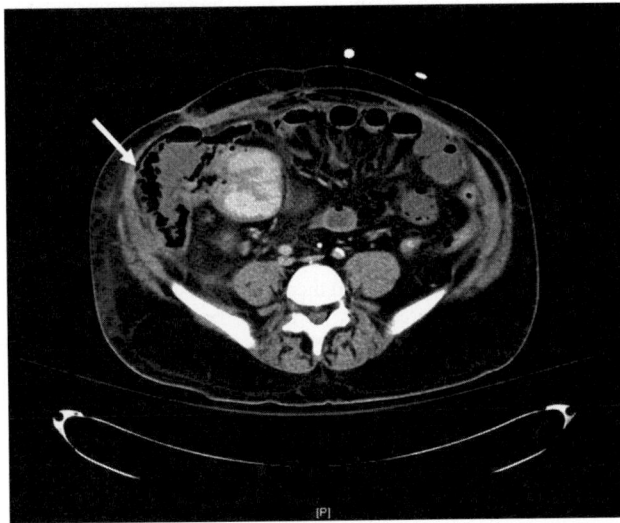

FIG. 28-14. Intestinal pneumatosis. This computed tomographic scan shows intestinal pneumatosis (*arrow*). The cause of this radiologic finding was intestinal ischemia. Patient was taken emergently to the operating room and underwent resection of an infarcted segment of small bowel.

feature is important in the acute setting when intestinal obstruction represents only one of many diagnoses in patients presenting with acute abdominal conditions.

The CT scan usually is performed after administration of oral water soluble contrast, or diluted barium. The water soluble contrast has been shown to have prognostic and therapeutic values too. Several studies and a subsequent meta-analysis have shown that appearance of the contrast in the colon within 24 hours is predictive of nonsurgical resolution of bowel obstruction.[18] Although use of oral contrast did not alter the rate of surgical intervention, it did reduce the overall length of hospital stay in those presenting with small bowel obstruction.

A limitation of CT scanning is its low sensitivity (<50%) in the detection of low-grade or partial small bowel obstruction. A subtle transition zone may be difficult to identify in the axial images obtained during CT scanning. In such cases, contrast examinations of the small bowel, either *small bowel series* (small bowel follow-through) or *enteroclysis*, can be helpful. For standard small bowel series, contrast is swallowed or instilled into the stomach through a nasogastric (NG) tube. Abdominal radiographs are then taken serially as the contrast travels distally in the intestine. Although barium can be used, water-soluble contrast agents, such as Gastrografin, should be used if the possibility of intestinal perforation exists. These examinations are more labor-intensive and less rapidly performed than CT scanning but may offer greater sensitivity in the detection of luminal and mural etiologies of obstruction, such as primary intestinal tumors. For enteroclysis, 200 to 250 mL of barium followed by 1 to 2 L of a solution of methylcellulose in water is instilled into the proximal jejunum via a long nasoenteric catheter. The double-contrast technique used in enteroclysis permits a better assessment of mucosal surface and detection of relatively small lesions, even through overlapping small bowel loops. Enteroclysis is rarely performed in the acute setting but offers greater sensitivity than small bowel series in the detection of lesions that may be causing partial small bowel obstruction. Recently, CT enteroclysis has been used, and reported to be superior to plain x-ray small bowel contrast studies.

Therapy

Small bowel obstruction is usually associated with a marked depletion of intravascular volume due to decreased oral intake, vomiting, and sequestration of fluid in bowel lumen and wall. Therefore, fluid resuscitation is integral to treatment. Isotonic fluid should be given intravenously and an indwelling bladder catheter placed to monitor urine output. Central-venous or pulmonary-artery catheter monitoring may be necessary to assist with fluid management, particularly in patients with underlying cardiac disease. Broad-spectrum antibiotics are given by some because of concerns that bacterial translocation may occur in the setting of small bowel obstruction; however, there are no controlled data to support this approach.

The stomach should be continuously evacuated of air and fluid using a NG tube. Effective gastric decompression decreases nausea, distention, and the risk of vomiting and aspiration. Longer nasoenteric tubes, with tips placed into the jejunum or ileum, were favored in the past but are rarely used today, as they are associated with higher complication rates than NG tubes, with no proven greater efficacy in several studies.

The standard therapy for *complete small bowel obstruction* generally has been expeditious surgery, although recently, some have advocated nonoperative approaches in management of these patients, providing closed loop obstruction is ruled out, and there is no evidence of intestinal ischemia. Such patients need to be observed closely and undergo serial exams. The rationale for those favoring early surgical intervention is to minimize the risk for bowel strangulation, which is associated with an increased risk for morbidity and mortality. Clinical signs and currently available laboratory tests and imaging studies do not reliably permit the distinction between pa-

tients with simple obstruction and those with strangulated obstruction before the onset of irreversible ischemia. Therefore, the goal is to operate before the onset of irreversible ischemia. Others note, however, that a period of observation and NG decompression, providing no tachycardia, tenderness, or an increase in white cell count is noted, is appropriate (see Fig. 28-15 for a proposed management algorithm).

Conservative therapy, in the form of NG decompression and fluid resuscitation is the initial recommendation for:

1. Partial small bowel obstruction
2. Obstruction occurring in the early postoperative period
3. Intestinal obstruction due to Crohn's disease
4. Carcinomatosis

In *partial obstruction*, progression to strangulation is unlikely to occur and an attempt at nonoperative resolution is warranted. Nonoperative management has been documented to be successful in 65 to 81% of patients with partial small bowel obstruction. Of those successfully treated nonoperatively, only 5 to 15% have been reported to have symptoms that were not substantially improved within 48 hours after initiation of therapy.[19] Therefore, most patients with partial small obstruction whose symptoms do not improve within 48 hours after initiation of nonoperative therapy should undergo surgery. Patients undergoing nonoperative therapy should be closely monitored for signs suggestive of peritonitis, the development of which would mandate urgent surgery. As stated before in the Diagnosis section above, the administration of hypertonic water-soluble contrast agents, such as Gastrografin used in upper GI and small bowel follow-through examinations, causes a shift of fluid into the intestinal lumen, thereby increasing the pressure gradient across the site of obstruction. This effect may accelerate resolution of partial small bowel obstruction; however, there is less evidence that administration of water-soluble contrast agents increases the probability of an episode of bowel obstruction being successfully managed nonoperatively.[18]

Obstruction presenting in *the early postoperative period* has been reported to occur in 0.7% patients undergoing laparotomy.[20] Patients undergoing pelvic surgery, especially colorectal procedures, have the greatest risk for developing early postoperative small bowel obstruction. The presence of obstruction should be considered if symptoms of intestinal obstruction occur after the initial return of bowel function or if bowel function fails to return within the expected 3 to 5 days after abdominal surgery. Plain radiographs may demonstrate dilated loops of small intestine with air-fluid levels but are interpreted as normal or nonspecific in up to one third of patients with early postoperative obstruction. CT scanning or small bowel series is often required to make the diagnosis. Obstruction that occurs in the early postoperative period is usually partial and only rarely is associated with strangulation. Therefore, a period of extended nonoperative therapy (2 to 3 weeks) consisting of bowel rest, hydration, and total parenteral nutrition (TPN) administration is usually warranted. However, if complete obstruction is demonstrated or if signs suggestive of peritonitis are detected, expeditious reoperation should be undertaken without delay.

Crohn's disease as a cause of small bowel obstruction is discussed in more detail below in the Crohn's Disease section.

Twenty-five to 33 percent of patients with a history of cancer who present with small bowel obstruction have adhesions as the etiology of their obstruction and therefore should not be denied appropriate therapy.[21] Even in cases in which the obstruction is related to recurrent malignancy, palliative resection or bypass can be performed. Patients with obvious carcinomatosis pose a difficult challenge, given their limited prognosis. Management must be tailored to an individual patient's prognosis and desires, and relief of the obstruction may be best achieved by a bypass procedure, avoiding a potentially difficult bowel resection.

The operative procedure performed for small bowel obstruction varies according to the etiology of the obstruction. For example, adhesions are lysed, tumors are resected, and hernias are reduced

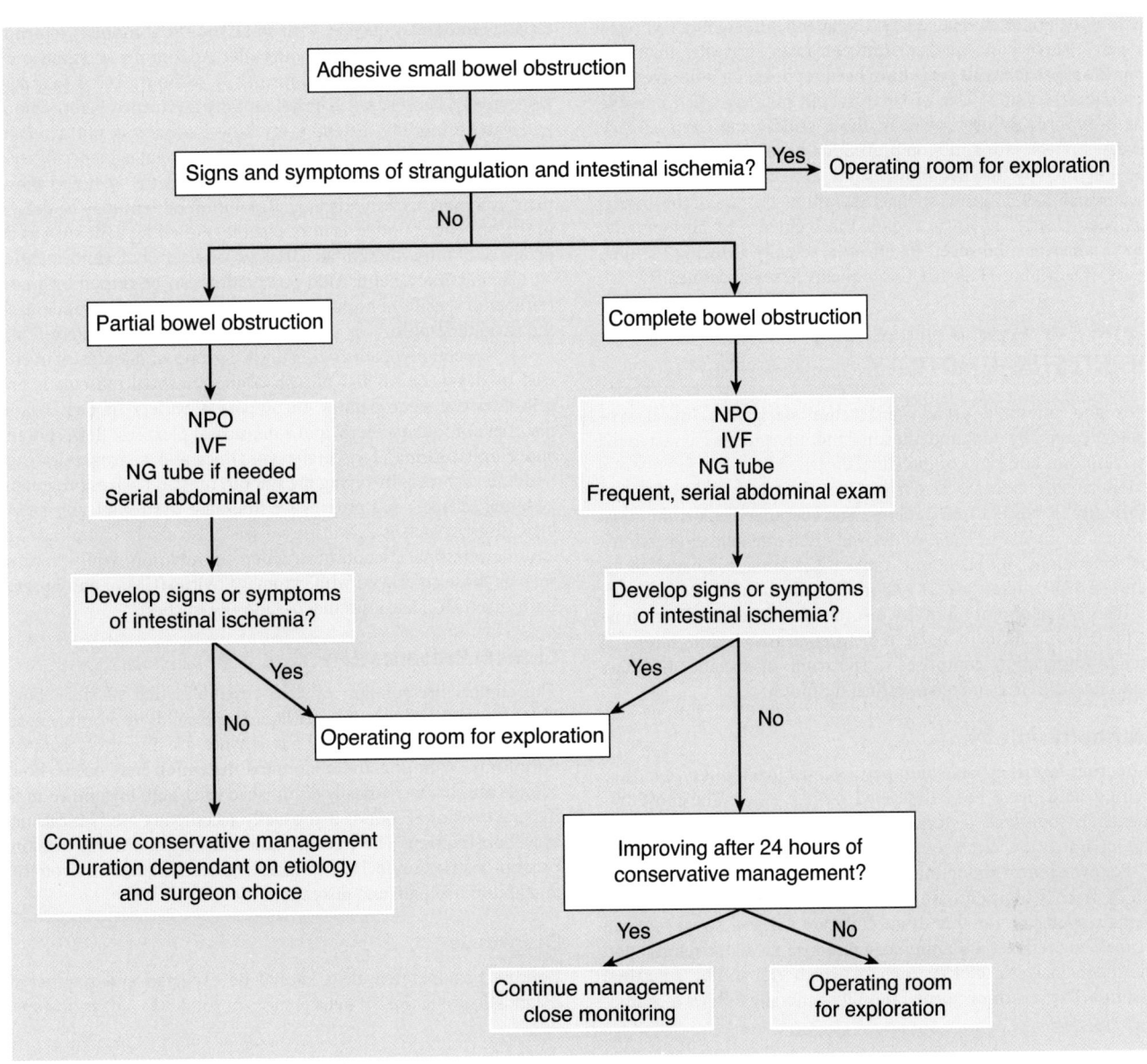

FIG. 28-15. Management algorithm of small bowel obstruction. IVF = intravenous fluid; NG = nasogastric; NPO = nothing by mouth.

and repaired. Regardless of the etiology, the affected intestine should be examined, and nonviable bowel resected. Criteria suggesting viability are normal color, peristalsis, and marginal arterial pulsations. Usually, visual inspection alone is adequate in judging viability. In borderline cases, a Doppler probe may be used to check for pulsatile flow to the bowel, and arterial perfusion can be verified by visualizing intravenously administered fluorescein dye in the bowel wall under ultraviolet illumination. Neither technique, however, has been found to be superior to clinical judgment. In general, if the patient is hemodynamically stable, short lengths of bowel of questionable viability should be resected and primary anastomosis of the remaining intestine performed. However, if the viability of a large proportion of the intestine is in question, a concerted effort to preserve intestinal tissue should be made. In such situations, the bowel of uncertain viability should be left intact and the patient re-explored in 24 to 48 hours in a "second-look" operation. At that time, definitive resection of nonviable bowel is completed.

Successful laparoscopic surgery for bowel obstruction is being reported with greater frequency.[22] Those that undergo successful laparoscopic procedure have a quicker recovery and less postoperative discomfort. Because distended loops of bowel can interfere with adequate visualization, early cases of proximal small bowel obstruction that are likely due to a single adhesive band are best suited for this approach. Presence of bowel distention and multiple adhesions can cause these procedures to be difficult and potentially hazardous. Conversion rate to open surgery can be as high as 33%.[22]

Outcomes

Prognosis is related to the etiology of obstruction. The majority of patients who are treated conservatively for adhesive small bowel obstruction do not require future readmissions; less than 20% of such patients will have a readmission over the subsequent 5 years with another episode of bowel obstruction.[23]

The perioperative mortality rate associated with surgery for nonstrangulating small bowel obstruction is less than 5%, with most deaths occurring in elderly patients with significant comorbidities. Mortality rates associated with surgery for strangulating obstruction range from 8 to 25%.

Prevention

With adhesive small bowel obstruction representing a large therapeutic burden, prevention of postoperative adhesions has become an area of great interest. Good surgical technique, careful handling of tissue, and minimal use and exposure of peritoneum to foreign bodies, form the cornerstone of adhesion prevention. These measures alone are often inadequate. In patients undergoing colorectal or pelvic surgery, hospital readmission rates of greater than 30% over the subsequent 10 years have been reported for adhesive small bowel obstruction.[24] Use of laparoscopic surgery, when possible, has been strongly promoted. In those undergoing open surgery, several strategies for adhesion prevention have been tried; however, the only therapy that has shown some success has been the use of hyaluronan-based agents, such as Seprafilm. The use of this barrier has been clearly shown to reduce the incidence of postoperative bowel adhesions; however, its effect in actually reducing the incidence of small bowel obstruction remains less well defined.[25]

ILEUS AND OTHER DISORDERS OF INTESTINAL MOTILITY

Ileus and intestinal pseudo-obstruction designate clinical syndromes caused by impaired intestinal motility and are characterized by symptoms and signs of intestinal obstruction in the absence of a lesion-causing mechanical obstruction. Ileus is a major cause of morbidity in hospitalized patients. Postoperative ileus is the most frequently implicated cause of delayed discharge following abdominal operations; its economic impact has been estimated to be between $750 million and $1 billion annually in the United States.[26]

Ileus is a temporary motility disorder that is reversed with time as the inciting factor is corrected. In contrast, chronic intestinal pseudo-obstruction comprises a spectrum of specific disorders associated with irreversible intestinal dysmotility.

Pathophysiology

Numerous factors capable of impairing intestinal motility, and thus inciting ileus, have been described (Table 28-4). The most frequently encountered factors are abdominal operations, infection and inflammation, electrolyte abnormalities, and drugs.

Following most abdominal operations or injuries, the motility of the GI tract is transiently impaired. Among the proposed mechanisms responsible for this dysmotility are surgical stress-induced sympathetic reflexes, inflammatory response mediator release, and anesthetic/analgesic effects; each of which can inhibit intestinal motility. The return of normal motility generally follows a characteristic temporal sequence, with small intestinal motility returning to normal within the first 24 hours after laparotomy and gastric and colonic motility returning to normal by 48 hours and 3 to 5 days, respectively. Because small bowel motility is returned before colonic and gastric motility, listening for bowel sounds is not a reliable indicator that ileus has fully resolved. Functional evidence of coordinated GI motility in the form of passing flatus or bowel movement is a more useful indicator. Resolution of ileus may be delayed in the presence of other factors capable of inciting ileus such as the presence of intra-abdominal abscesses or electrolyte abnormalities.

Chronic intestinal pseudo-obstruction can be caused by a large number of specific abnormalities affecting intestinal smooth muscle, the myenteric plexus, or the extraintestinal nervous system (Table 28-5). Visceral myopathies constitute a group of diseases characterized by degeneration and fibrosis of the intestinal muscularis propria. Visceral neuropathies encompass a variety of degenerative disorders of the myenteric and submucosal plexuses. Both sporadic and familial forms of visceral myopathies and neuropathies exist. Systemic disorders involving the smooth muscle, such as progressive systemic sclerosis and progressive muscular dystrophy, and neurologic diseases such as Parkinson's disease also can be complicated by chronic intestinal pseudo-obstruction. In addition, viral infections such as those associated with cytomegalovirus (CMV) and Epstein-Barr virus can cause intestinal pseudo-obstruction.

Clinical Presentation

The clinical presentation of ileus resembles that of small bowel obstruction. Inability to tolerate liquids and solids by mouth, nausea, and lack of flatus or bowel movements are the most common symptoms. Vomiting and abdominal distention may occur. Bowel sounds are characteristically diminished or absent, in contrast to the hyperactive bowel sounds that usually accompany mechanical small bowel obstruction. The clinical manifestations of chronic intestinal pseudo-obstruction include variable degrees of nausea and vomiting and abdominal pain and distention.

Diagnosis

Routine postoperative ileus should be expected and requires no diagnostic evaluation. If ileus persists beyond 3 to 5 days postoper-

---

TABLE 28-4	Ileus: Common etiologies

Abdominal surgery
Infection
  Sepsis
  Intra-abdominal abscess
  Peritonitis
  Pneumonia
Electrolyte abnormalities
  Hypokalemia
  Hypomagnesemia
  Hypermagnesemia
  Hyponatremia
Medications
  Anticholinergics
  Opiates
  Phenothiazines
  Calcium channel blockers
  Tricyclic antidepressants
Hypothyroidism
Ureteral colic
Retroperitoneal hemorrhage
Spinal cord injury
Myocardial infarction
Mesenteric ischemia

TABLE 28-5	Chronic intestinal pseudo-obstruction: Etiologies

Primary causes
  Familial types
    Familial visceral myopathies (types I, II, and III)
    Familial visceral neuropathies (types I and II)
    Childhood visceral myopathies (types I and II)
  Sporadic types
    Visceral myopathies
    Visceral neuropathies
Secondary causes
  Smooth muscle disorders
    Collagen vascular diseases (e.g., scleroderma)
    Muscular dystrophies (e.g., myotonic dystrophy)
    Amyloidosis
  Neurologic disorders
    Chagas' disease, Parkinson's disease, spinal cord injury
  Endocrine disorders
    Diabetes, hypothyroidism, hypoparathyroidism
  Miscellaneous disorders
    Radiation enteritis
  Pharmacologic causes
    (e.g., phenothiazines and tricyclic antidepressants)
  Viral infections

atively or occurs in the absence of abdominal surgery, diagnostic evaluation to detect specific underlying factors capable of inciting ileus and to rule out the presence of mechanical obstruction is warranted.

Patient medication lists should be reviewed for the presence of drugs, especially opiates, known to be associated with impaired intestinal motility. Measurement of serum electrolytes may demonstrate hypokalemia, hypocalcemia, hypomagnesemia, hypermagnesemia, or other electrolyte abnormalities commonly associated with ileus. Abdominal radiographs often are obtained, but the distinction between ileus and mechanical obstruction may be difficult based on this test alone. In the postoperative setting, CT scanning is the test of choice as it can demonstrate the presence of an intraabdominal abscess or other evidence of peritoneal sepsis that may be causing ileus and can exclude the presence of complete mechanical obstruction.

The diagnosis of chronic pseudo-obstruction is suggested by clinical features and confirmed by radiographic and manometric studies. Diagnostic laparotomy or laparoscopy with full-thickness biopsy of the small intestine may be required to establish the specific underlying cause.

Therapy

The management of ileus consists of limiting oral intake and correcting the underlying inciting factor. If vomiting or abdominal distention are prominent, the stomach should be decompressed using a NG tube. Fluid and electrolytes should be administered intravenously until ileus resolves. If the duration of ileus is prolonged, TPN may be required.

Given the frequency of postoperative ileus and its financial impact, a large number of investigations have been conducted to define strategies to reduce its duration. Although often recommended, the use of early ambulation and routine NG intubation has not been demonstrated to be associated with earlier resolution of postoperative ileus. There is some evidence that early postoperative feeding protocols are generally well tolerated, reduce postoperative ileus, and can result in a shorter hospital stay.[27] The administration of NSAIDs such as ketorolac and concomitant reductions in opioid dosing have been shown to reduce the duration of ileus in most studies. Similarly, the use of perioperative thoracic epidural anesthesia/analgesia with regimens containing local anesthetics combined with limitation or elimination of systemically administered opioids have been shown to reduce duration of postoperative ileus, although they have not reduced the overall length of hospital stay.[28] Interestingly, recent data have suggested that limiting intra and postoperative fluid administration can also result in reduction of postoperative ileus, and shortened hospital stay.[29] Table 28-6 summarizes some of the measures used to minimize postoperative ileus.

Most other pharmacologic agents, including prokinetic agents, are associated with efficacy-toxicity profiles that are too unfavorable to warrant routine use. Recently, administration of alvimopan, a novel peripherally active μ-opioid receptor antagonist with limited oral absorption, has been shown to reduce duration of postoperative ileus, hospital stay, and rate of readmissions in several prospective, randomized, placebo-controlled trials, and the subsequent meta-analysis.[30]

The therapy for patients with chronic intestinal pseudo-obstruction focuses on palliation of symptoms as well as fluid, electrolyte, and nutritional management. Surgery should be avoided, if at all possible. No standard therapies are curative or delay the natural history of any of the specific disorders causing intestinal pseudo-obstruction. Prokinetic agents, such as metoclopramide and erythromycin, are associated with poor efficacy. Cisapride has been associated with palliation of symptoms; however, because of cardiac toxicity and reported deaths, this agent is restricted to compassionate use.

Patients with refractory disease may require strict limitation of oral intake and long-term TPN administration. Despite these measures, some patients will continue to have severe abdominal pain or

TABLE 28-6	Measures to reduce postoperative ileus
Intraoperative measures
Minimize handling of the bowel
Laparoscopic approach, if possible
Avoid excessive intraoperative fluid administration
Postoperative measures
Early enteral feeding
Epidural anesthesia, if indicated
Avoid excessive IV fluid administration
Correct electrolyte abnormalities
Consider μ-opioid antagonists

such copious intestinal secretions that vomiting and fluid and electrolyte losses remain substantial. These patients may require a decompressive gastrostomy or an extended small bowel resection to remove abnormal intestine. Small intestinal transplantation has been applied in these patients with increasing frequency; the ultimate role of this modality remains to be defined.

CROHN'S DISEASE

Crohn's disease is a chronic, idiopathic transmural inflammatory disease with a propensity to affect the distal ileum, although any part of the alimentary tract can be involved. Estimates of the incidence of Crohn's disease in the United States have ranged from 3.6 to 8.8 per 100,000, with recent studies suggesting a prevalence of about 200 cases per 100,000.[31] A dramatic increase in incidence in the United States was observed to occur from the mid-1950s though the early 1970s. Incidence rates have been stable since the 1980s. Substantial regional variations in incidence have been observed, with the highest incidences reported to exist in northern latitudes. The incidence of Crohn's disease varies among ethnic groups within the same geographic region. For example, members of the Eastern European Ashkenazi Jewish population are at two- to fourfold higher risk of developing Crohn's disease than members of other populations living in the same location.

Most studies suggest that Crohn's disease is slightly more prevalent in females than in males. The mean age at which patients are diagnosed with Crohn's disease falls in the third decade of life years, with a second smaller peak in the sixth decade of life, giving it a bimodal distribution. The age at diagnosis can, however, range from early childhood through the entire life span.

Both genetic and environmental factors appear to influence the risk for developing Crohn's disease. The relative risk among first-degree relatives of patients with Crohn's disease is 14 to 15 times higher than that of the general population. Approximately one in five patients with Crohn's disease will report having at least one affected relative. The concordance rate among monozygotic twins is as high as 67%; however, Crohn's disease is not associated with simple mendelian inheritance patterns. Although there is a tendency within families for either ulcerative colitis or Crohn's disease to be present exclusively, mixed kindreds also occur, suggesting the presence of some shared genetic traits as a basis for both diseases.

Higher socioeconomic status is associated with an increased risk of Crohn's disease. Most studies have found breastfeeding to be protective against the development of Crohn's disease. Crohn's disease is more prevalent among smokers. Furthermore, smoking is associated with the increased risk for both the need for surgery and the risk of relapse after surgery for Crohn's disease.

Pathophysiology

Crohn's disease is characterized by sustained inflammation. Whether this inflammation represents an appropriate response to a yet unrecognized pathogen or an inappropriate response to a normally innocuous stimulus is unknown. Various hypotheses on the roles of environmental and genetic factors in the pathogenesis of Crohn's disease have been proposed. Many infectious agents have been suggested to be the causative organism of Crohn's disease. Candidate organisms have included chlamydia, *Listeria monocytogenes, Pseudomonas* species, reovirus, *Mycobacterium paratuberculosis*, and many others. There is no conclusive evidence that any of these organisms is the causative agent. Studies using animal models suggest that in a genetically susceptible host, nonpathogenic, commensal enteric flora are sufficient to induce a chronic inflammatory response resembling that associated with Crohn's disease. In these models, the sustained intestinal inflammation is the result of either abnormal epithelial barrier function or immune dysregulation. Poor barrier function is hypothesized to permit inappropriate exposure of lamina propria lymphocytes to antigenic stimuli derived from the intestinal lumen. In addition, a variety of defects in immune regulatory mechanisms, (e.g., over-responsiveness of mucosal T cells to enteric flora-derived antigens) can lead to defective immune tolerance and sustained inflammation.

Specific genetic defects associated with Crohn's disease in human patients are beginning to be defined. For example, the presence of a locus on chromosome 16 (the so-called *IBD1 locus*) has been linked to Crohn's disease. The IBD1 locus has been identified as the *NOD2* gene.[32,33] Persons with allelic variants on both chromosomes have a 40-fold relative risk of Crohn's disease compared to those without variant *NOD2* genes. The relevance of this gene to the pathogenesis of Crohn's disease is biologically plausible, as the protein product of the *NOD2* gene mediates the innate immune response to microbial pathogens. Other putative IBD loci have been identified on other chromosomes (IBD2 on chromosome 12q, and IBD3 on chromosome 6), and are under investigation.

Pathology

Although the pathologic hallmark of Crohn's disease is focal, transmural inflammation of the intestine, a spectrum of pathologic lesions can be present. The earliest lesion characteristic of Crohn's disease is the aphthous ulcer. These superficial ulcers are up to 3 mm in diameter and are surrounded by a halo of erythema. In the small intestine, aphthous ulcers typically arise over lymphoid aggregates. Granulomas are highly characteristic of Crohn's disease and are reported to be present in up to 70% of intestinal specimens obtained during surgical resection. These granulomas are noncaseating and can be found in both areas of active disease and apparently normal intestine, in any layer of the bowel wall, and in mesenteric lymph nodes.

As disease progresses, aphthae coalesce into larger, stellate-shaped ulcers. Linear or serpiginous ulcers may form when multiple ulcers fuse in a direction parallel to the longitudinal axis of the intestine. With transverse coalescence of ulcers, a cobblestoned appearance of the mucosa may arise.

With advanced disease, inflammation can be transmural. Serosal involvement results in adhesion of the inflamed bowel to other loops of bowel or other adjacent organs. Transmural inflammation also can result in fibrosis with stricture formation, intra-abdominal abscesses, fistulas, and, rarely, free perforation. Inflammation in Crohn's disease can affect discontinuous portions of intestine: so-called *skip lesions* that are separated by intervening normal appearing intestine.

A feature of Crohn's disease that is grossly evident and helpful in identifying affected segments of intestine during surgery is the presence of *fat wrapping*, which represents encroachment of mesenteric fat onto the serosal surface of the bowel (Fig. 28-16). This finding is virtually pathognomonic of Crohn's disease. The presence of fat wrapping correlates well with the presence of underlying acute and chronic inflammation.

Features that allow for differentiation between Crohn's disease of the colon and ulcerative colitis include the layers of the bowel wall affected (inflammation in ulcerative colitis is limited to the mucosa and submucosa but may involve the full thickness of the bowel wall in Crohn's disease) and the longitudinal extent of inflammation (inflammation is continuous and characteristically affects the rectum in ulcerative colitis but may be discontinuous and spare the rectum in Crohn's disease). In the absence of full expression of features of advanced disease, Crohn's colitis can sometimes be difficult to distinguish from ulcerative colitis. It is also important to remember that, although ulcerative colitis is a disease of the colon, it can be associated with inflammatory changes in the distal ileum (backwash ileitis).

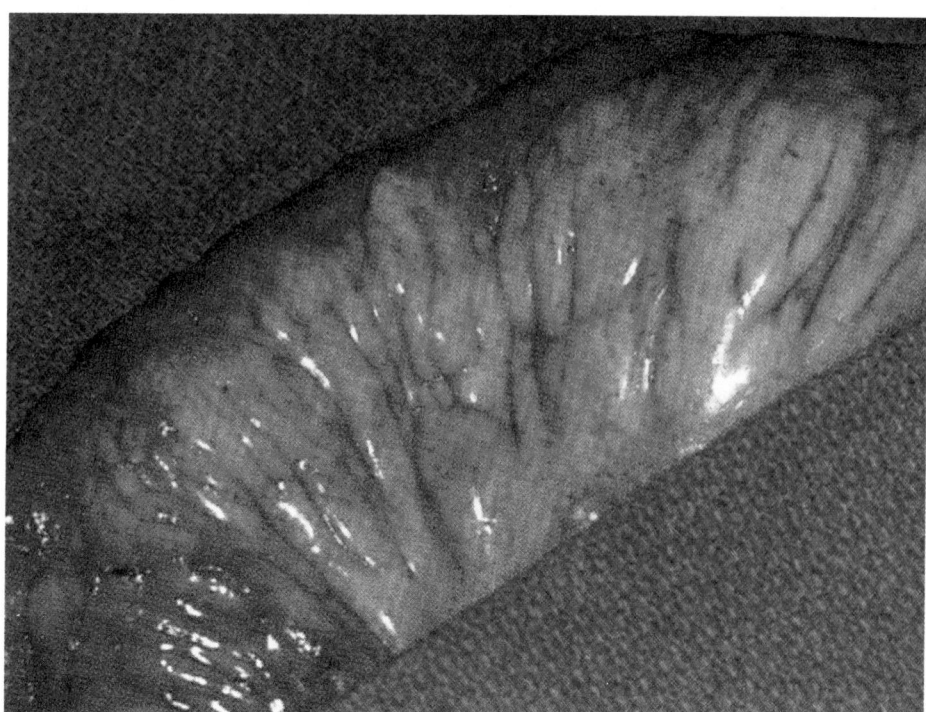

FIG. 28-16. Crohn's disease. This intraoperative photograph demonstrates encroachment of mesenteric fat onto the serosal surface of the intestine ("fat wrapping") that is characteristic of intestinal segments affected by active Crohn's disease.

Clinical Presentation

The most common symptoms of Crohn's disease are abdominal pain, diarrhea, and weight loss. However, the clinical features are highly variable among individual patients and depend on which segment(s) of the GI tract is (are) predominantly affected, the intensity of inflammation, and the presence or absence of specific complications. Patients with Crohn's disease can be classified by their predominant clinical manifestation as having primarily (a) fibrostenotic disease, (b) fistulizing disease, and (c) aggressive inflammatory disease. There is substantial overlap among these disease patterns in individual patients, however. The onset of symptoms is insidious, and, once present, their severity follows a waxing and waning course. Constitutional symptoms, particularly weight loss and fever, or growth retardation in children, may also be prominent and are occasionally the sole presenting features of Crohn's disease.

The disease affects the small bowel in 80% of cases, and colon alone in 20%. In those with small bowel disease, the majority have ileocecal disease. The small bowel alone is affected in 15 to 30% of patients. Isolated perineal and anorectal disease occurs in 5 to 10% of affected patients. Uncommon sites of involvement include the esophagus, stomach, and duodenum.

An estimated one fourth of all patients with Crohn's disease will have an extraintestinal manifestation of their disease. One fourth of those affected will have more than one manifestation. Many of these complications are common to both Crohn's disease and ulcerative colitis, although as a whole, they are more prevalent among patients with Crohn's disease than those with ulcerative colitis. The most common extraintestinal manifestations are listed in Table 28-7. The clinical severity of some of these manifestations, such as erythema nodosum and peripheral arthritis, is correlated with the severity of intestinal inflammation. The severity of other manifestations, such as pyoderma gangrenosum and ankylosing spondylitis, bears no apparent relationship to the severity of intestinal inflammation.

Diagnosis

The diagnosis usually is established with endoscopic findings in a patient with a compatible clinical history. The diagnosis should be considered in those presenting with acute or chronic abdominal pain, especially when localized to the right lower quadrant, chronic diarrhea, evidence of intestinal inflammation on radiography or endoscopy, the discovery of a bowel stricture or fistula arising from the bowel, and evidence of inflammation or granulomas on intestinal histology. Disorders associated with clinical presentations that resemble those of Crohn's disease include ulcerative colitis, functional bowel disorders such as irritable bowel syndrome, mesenteric ischemia, collagen vascular diseases, carcinoma and lymphoma, diverticular disease, and infectious enteritidis. These infectious enteritides are most frequently diagnosed in immunocompromised patients but can also occur in patients with normal immune function. Acute ileitis caused by *Campylobacter* and *Yersinia* species can be difficult to distinguish from that caused by an acute presentation of Crohn's disease. Typhoid enteritis caused by *Salmonella typhosa* can lead to overt intestinal bleeding and perforation, most often affecting the terminal ileum. The distal ileum and cecum are the most common sites of intestinal involvement by infection due to *Mycobacterium tuberculosis*. This condition can result in intestinal inflammation, strictures, and fistula formation, similar to those seen in Crohn's disease. CMV can cause intestinal ulcers, bleeding, and perforation.

No single symptom, sign, or diagnostic test establishes the diagnosis of Crohn's disease. Instead, the diagnosis is based on a complete assessment of the clinical presentation with confirmatory findings derived from radiographic, endoscopic, and, in most cases, pathologic tests. Colonoscopy with intubation of terminal ileum is the main diagnostic tool and can reveal focal ulcerations adjacent to areas of normal appearing mucosa along with polypoid mucosal changes that give a "cobblestone appearance." Skip areas of involvement are typical with segments of normal appearing bowel interrupted by large areas of obvious disease; this pattern is different from the continuous involve-

TABLE 28-7	Extraintestinal manifestations of Crohn's disease

Dermatologic
    Erythema nodosum
    Pyoderma gangrenosum
Rheumatologic
    Peripheral arthritis
    Ankylosing spondylitis
    Sacroiliitis
Ocular
    Conjunctivitis
    Uveitis/iritis
    Episcleritis
Hepatobiliary
    Hepatic steatosis
    Cholelithiasis
    Primary sclerosing cholangitis
    Pericholangitis
Urologic
    Nephrolithiasis
    Ureteral obstruction
Miscellaneous
    Thromboembolic disease
    Vasculitis
    Osteoporosis
    Endocarditis, myocarditis, pleuropericarditis
    Interstitial lung disease
    Amyloidosis
    Pancreatitis

ment in ulcerative colitis. Pseudopolyps, as seen in ulcerative colitis, are also often present. Contrast examinations of the small bowel and colon may reveal strictures or networks of ulcers and fissures. CT scanning may reveal intra-abdominal abscesses and is useful in acute presentations to rule out the presence of other intra-abdominal disorders. Esophagogastroduodenoscopy (EGD) is done for disease of the proximal alimentary tract. Because Crohn's disease often affects the small bowel, which is difficult to image, capsule endoscopy has been increasingly used to make this diagnosis (Fig. 28-17).[34]

Several antibodies also have been identified in patients with inflammatory bowel disease, which may have diagnostic value. The most commonly tested antibodies are perinuclear antineutrophil cytoplasmic antibody (pANCA) and anti–*Saccharomyces cerevisiae* antibody (ASCA). ASCA+/pANCA, is associated with a diagnosis of Crohn's disease, while ASCA–/pANCA+ is correlated with ulcerative colitis. Although these antibody tests are commercially available, their widespread use has been hampered by low test sensitivities.

Because of the insidious, and often, nonspecific presentation, the diagnosis of Crohn's disease typically is made only after symptoms have been present for several years. However, in acute presentations, the diagnosis is sometimes made intraoperatively or during surgical evaluation. The initial manifestation of Crohn's disease can consist of right lower quadrant abdominal mimicking the presentation of acute appendicitis. In patients with this presentation, Crohn's disease can be discovered for the first time during laparotomy or laparoscopy performed for presumed appendicitis. In some patients, the initial manifestation of Crohn's disease is an acute abdomen related to small bowel obstruction, intra-abdominal abscess, or free intestinal perforation. In other patients, perianal abscesses and fistulas requiring surgical therapy may be the first manifestation of Crohn's disease.

Therapy

Because no curative therapies are available for Crohn's disease, the goal of treatment is to palliate symptoms rather than to achieve cure. Medical therapy is used to induce and maintain disease

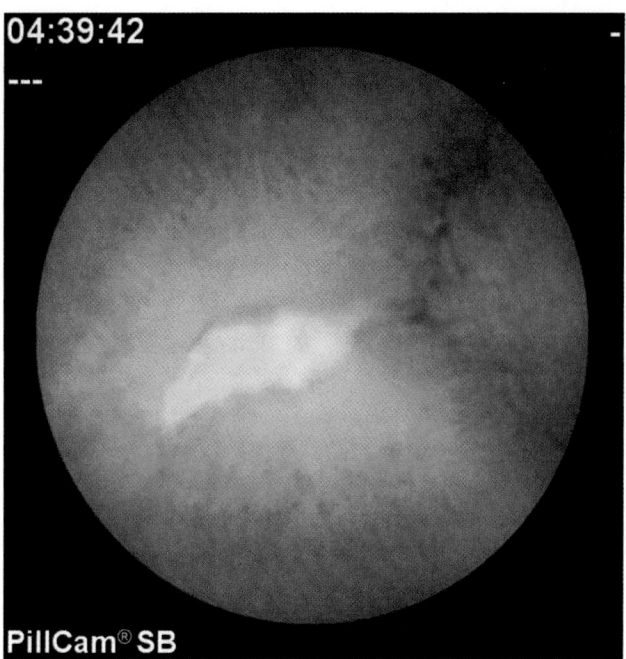

04:39:42

PillCam® SB

FIG. 28-17. Crohn's disease. This image was captured by a wireless capsule endoscope as it was traveling through the small intestine. It demonstrates a superficial ulceration in the small bowel consistent with Crohn's disease. (*Courtesy of Dr. Anne C. Travis, Division of Gastroenterology, Brigham and Women's Hospital.*)

remission. Surgery is reserved for specific indications described below in the Surgical Therapy section. In addition, nutritional support in the form of aggressive enteral regimens or, if necessary, parenteral nutrition, is used to manage the malnutrition that is common in patient's with Crohn's disease.

Medical Therapy

Pharmacologic agents used to treat Crohn's disease include antibiotics, aminosalicylates, corticosteroids, and immunomodulators. Antibiotics have an adjunctive role in the treatment of infectious complications associated with Crohn's disease. They also are used to treat patients with perianal disease, enterocutaneous fistulas, and active colonic disease.

Most studies have shown oral 5-aminosalicylic acid (5-ASA) drugs (e.g., mesalamine) to be superior to placebo in inducing disease remission. Its efficacy in the maintenance of remission is less clear. Aminosalicylates are associated with minimal toxicity and are available in a variety of formulations that allow for their delivery to specific regions of the alimentary tract. In Crohn's disease, sulfasalazine, the parent compound of 5-ASA and widely used in ulcerative colitis, has been shown to be less effective than 5-ASA.

Orally administered glucocorticoids are used to treat patients with mildly to moderately severe disease that does not respond to aminosalicylates. Patients with severe active disease usually require IV administration of glucocorticoids. Although glucocorticoids are effective in inducing remission, they are ineffective in preventing relapse and their adverse side-effect profile makes long-term use hazardous. Therefore, they should be tapered once remission is achieved. Some patients are unable to undergo glucocorticoid tapering without suffering recurrence of symptoms. Such patients are said to have *steroid dependence*. For these patients, along with those who do not respond to steroids at all (steroid resistant), use of immune modulators should be considered.

The thiopurine antimetabolites azathioprine and its active metabolite, 6-mercaptopurine, have demonstrated efficacy in inducing remission, in maintaining remission, and in allowing for glucocor-

ticoid tapering in glucocorticoid-dependent patients. A response to the medications is usually observed in 3 to 6 months. There is also some evidence that they decrease the risk of relapse after intestinal resection for Crohn's disease. These agents are relatively safe but can induce bone marrow suppression and promote infectious complications. For patients who do not respond to the thiopurines, methotrexate is an alternative that usually is given intramuscularly before switching to oral form after achieving symptomatic control. There is little role for cyclosporine in Crohn's disease; its efficacy/toxicity profile in this disease is poor.

Infliximab is a chimeric monoclonal anti–tumor necrosis factor alpha antibody that has been shown to have efficacy in inducing remission and in promoting closure of enterocutaneous fistulas.[35] It generally is used for patients resistant to standard therapy to help taper steroid dosage. Infliximab generally is well tolerated but should not be used in patients with ongoing septic processes, such as undrained intra-abdominal abscesses.

For patients with perianal disease, antibiotic therapy with metronidazole or ciprofloxacin is the primary step. Two to 4 weeks of therapy is needed before improvements are seen, and often long-term therapy is required to prevent relapse. In cases of relapse, azathioprine can be considered. In patients with fistulas, infliximab and azathioprine are drugs of choice.

Surgical Therapy

Fifty to 70% of patients with Crohn's disease will ultimately require at least one surgical intervention for their disease.[36,37] Surgery generally is reserved for patients whose disease is unresponsive to aggressive medical therapy or who develop complications of their disease (Table 28-8). Failure of medical management may be the indication for surgery if symptoms persist despite aggressive therapy for several months or if symptoms recur whenever aggressive therapy is tapered. Surgery should be considered if medication-induced complications arise, specifically corticosteroid-related complications, such as cushingoid features, cataracts, glaucoma, systemic hypertension, compression fractures, or aseptic necrosis of the femoral head. Growth retardation constitutes an indication for surgery in 30% of children with Crohn's disease.

One of the most common indications for surgical intervention is intestinal obstruction. Abscesses and fistulas frequently are encountered during operations performed for intestinal obstruction in these patients, but are rarely the only indication for surgery. Most abscesses are amenable to percutaneous drainage and fistulas unless associated with symptoms or metabolic derangements do not require surgical intervention. Less common complications that require surgical intervention are acute GI hemorrhage, perforations, and development of cancer.

Although most commonly, surgery for Crohn's disease is planned, an uncommon, but not rare, scenario is the intraoperative discovery

TABLE 28-8	Indications for surgical intervention in Crohn's disease

Acute onset of severe disease
    Crohn's colitis ± toxic megacolon (rare)
Failure of medical therapy
    Persistent symptoms despite long-term steroid use
    Recurrence of symptoms when high-dose steroids are tapered
    Drug induced complications (Cushing's disease, hypertension)
Development of disease complications
    Obstruction
    Perforation
    Complicated fistulas
    Hemorrhage
    Malignancy risk

of inflammation limited to the terminal ileum during operations performed for presumed appendicitis. This scenario can result from an acute presentation of Crohn's disease or from acute ileitis caused by bacteria such as *Yersinia* or *Campylobacter*. Both conditions should be treated medically; ileal resection is generally not indicated. However, the appendix, even if normal appearing, should be removed (unless the cecum is inflamed, increasing the potential morbidity of this procedure) to eliminate appendicitis from the differential diagnosis of abdominal pain in these patients, particularly those with Crohn's disease who may be destined to have recurring symptoms.

When the diagnosis of Crohn's disease is known and surgery planned, thorough examination of the entire intestine should be performed. The presence of active disease is suggested by thickening of the bowel wall, narrowing of the lumen, serosal inflammation and coverage by creeping fat, and thickening of the mesentery. Skip lesions are present in approximately 20% of cases and should be sought. The length of uninvolved small intestine should be noted.

Segmental intestinal resection of grossly evident disease followed by primary anastomosis is the usual procedure of choice. Microscopic evidence of Crohn's disease at the resection margins does not compromise a safe anastomosis, and frozen-section analysis of resection margins is unnecessary. In a randomized prospective trial, the effects of achieving 2-cm resection margins beyond grossly evident disease were compared with achieving 12-cm resection margins.[38] There were no evident differences with respect to clinical recurrence rates or anastomotic recurrences. Recurrence rates were similar whether margins were histologically free of or involved with Crohn's disease.

An alternative to segmental resection for obstructing lesions is stricturoplasty (Fig. 28-18). This technique allows for preservation of intestinal surface area and is especially well suited to patients with extensive disease and fibrotic strictures who may have undergone previous resection and are at risk for developing short bowel syndrome. In this technique, the bowel is opened longitudinally to expose the lumen. Any intraluminal ulcerations should be biopsied to rule out the presence of neoplasia. Depending on the length of the stricture, the reconstruction can be fashioned in a manner similar to the Heinecke-Mikulicz pyloroplasty (for strictures less than 12 cm in length) or the Finney pyloroplasty (for longer strictures as much as 25 cm in length). For longer strictures, variations on the standard stricturoplasty, namely the side-to-side isoperistaltic enteroenterostomy, have been advocated, and used for strictures with mean lengths of 50 cm.[39] Stricturoplasty sites should be marked with metallic clips to facilitate their identification on radiographs and during subsequent operations. Stricturoplasty is associated with recurrence rates that are no different from those associated with segmental resection. Because the affected bowel is left in situ rather than resected, there is the potential for cancer developing at the stricturoplasty site. However, as data on this complication are limited to anecdotes, this risk remains a theoretical one. Stricturoplasty is contraindicated in patients with intra-abdominal abscesses or intestinal fistulas. The presence of a solitary stricture relatively close to a segment for which resection is planned is a relative contraindication. In general, stricturoplasty is performed in cases where single or multiple strictures are identified in diffusely involved segments of bowel, or where previous resections have been performed, and maintenance of intestinal length is of great importance.

Intestinal bypass procedures are sometimes required in the presence of intramesenteric abscesses or if the diseased bowel is coalesced in the form of a dense inflammatory mass, making its mobilization unsafe. Bypass procedures (gastrojejunostomy) also are used in the presence of duodenal strictures, for which stricturoplasty and segmental resection can be technically difficult.

Since the 1990s, laparoscopic surgical techniques have been applied to patients with Crohn's disease. The inflammatory changes associated with Crohn's disease, such as thickened and foreshortened mesentery, obliterated tissue planes, and friable tissues with engorged vasculature, can make a laparoscopic approach challeng-

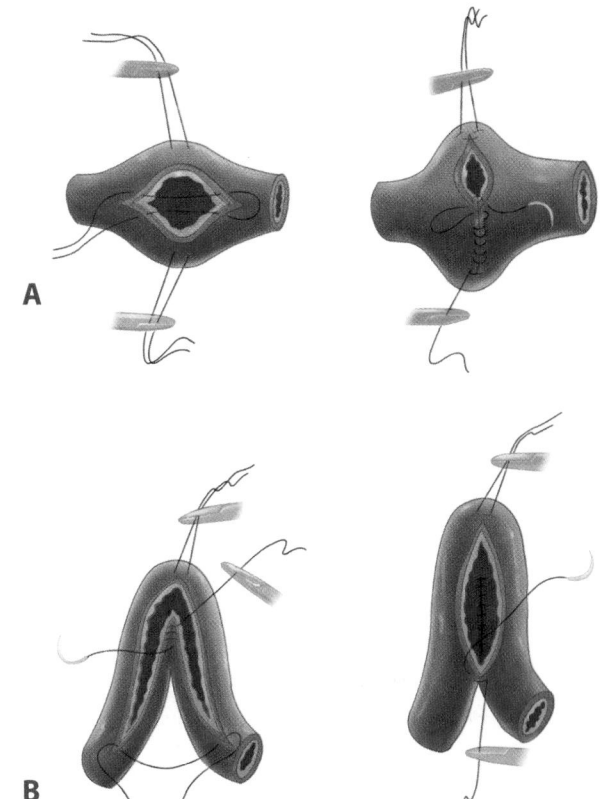

FIG. 28-18. Stricturoplasty. The wall of the strictured bowel is incised longitudinally. Reconstruction is performed by closing the defect transversely in a manner similar to the Heinecke-Mikulicz pyloroplasty for short strictures (**A**), or the Finney pyloroplasty for longer strictures (**B**).

ing. Theoretical advantages of laparoscopic surgery include less postoperative pain, earlier return of normal intestinal function that allows for shorter hospital stay, and superior cosmesis. In a prospective randomized trial comparing laparoscopic and open surgery for Crohn's disease conducted at a single institution, laparoscopic surgery was associated with faster recovery of pulmonary function, fewer complications, and shorter length of hospital stay.[40] A meta-analysis of subsequent studies has confirmed that laparoscopic surgery for Crohn's disease is associated with less postoperative pain, shorter duration of ileus, and a shorter hospital stay. The rates of disease recurrence were similar between the two groups.[41]

Outcomes

Overall complication rates following surgery for Crohn's disease range from 15 to 30%. Wound infections, postoperative intra-abdominal abscesses, and anastomotic leaks account for most of these complications.

Most patients whose disease is resected eventually develop recurrence. If recurrence is defined endoscopically, 70% recur within 1 year of a bowel resection and 85% by 3 years.[42] Clinical recurrence, defined as the return of symptoms confirmed as being due to Crohn's disease, affects 60% of patients by 5 years and 94% by 15 years after intestinal resection. Reoperation becomes necessary in approximately one third of patients by 5 years after the initial operation, with a median time to reoperation of 7 to 10 years.[43]

INTESTINAL FISTULAS

A *fistula* is defined as an abnormal communication between two epithelialized surfaces. The communication occurs between two parts of the GI tract or adjacent organs in an *internal fistula* (e.g., enterocolonic fistula or colovesicular fistula). An *external fistula* (e.g., enterocutaneous fistula or rectovaginal fistula) involves the skin or another external surface epithelium. Enterocutaneous fistulas that drain less than 200 mL of fluid per day are known as *low-output fistulas*, whereas those that drain more than 500 mL of fluid per day are known as *high-output fistulas*.

More than 80% of enterocutaneous fistulas represent iatrogenic complications that occur as the result of enterotomies or intestinal anastomotic dehiscences. Fistulas that arise spontaneously without antecedent iatrogenic injury are usually manifestations of progression of underlying Crohn's disease or cancer.

Pathophysiology

The manifestations of fistulas depend on which structures are involved. Low-resistance enteroenteric fistulas, which allow luminal contents to bypass a significant proportion of the small intestine, may result in clinically significant malabsorption. Enterovesicular fistulas often cause recurrent urinary tract infections. The drainage emanating from enterocutaneous fistulas are irritating to the skin and cause excoriation. The loss of enteric luminal contents, particularly from high-output fistulas originating from the proximal small intestine, results in dehydration, electrolyte abnormalities, and malnutrition.

Fistulas have the potential to close spontaneously. Factors inhibiting spontaneous closure, however, include malnutrition, sepsis, inflammatory bowel disease, cancer, radiation, obstruction of the intestine distal to the origin of the fistula, foreign bodies, high output, short fistulous tract (<2 cm), and epithelialization of the fistula tract (Table 28-9).

Clinical Presentation

Iatrogenic enterocutaneous fistulas usually become clinically evident between the fifth and tenth postoperative days. Fever, leukocytosis, prolonged ileus, abdominal tenderness, and wound infection are the initial signs. The diagnosis becomes obvious when drainage of enteric material through the abdominal wound or through existing drains occurs. These fistulas are often associated with intra-abdominal abscesses.

Diagnosis

CT scanning following the administration of enteral contrast is the most useful initial test. Leakage of contrast material from the intestinal lumen can be observed. Intra-abdominal abscesses should be sought and drained percutaneously. If the anatomy of the fistula is not clear on CT scanning, a small bowel series or enteroclysis examination can be obtained to demonstrate the fistula's site of origin in the bowel. This study also is useful to rule out the presence of intestinal obstruction distal to the site of origin. Occasionally, contrast administered into the intestine does not demonstrate the fistula tract. A *fistulogram*, in which contrast is injected under pressure through a catheter placed percutaneously into the fistula tract, may offer greater sensitivity in localizing the fistula origin.

Therapy

The treatment of enterocutaneous fistulas should proceed through an orderly sequence of steps.[44]

1. Stabilization. Fluid and electrolyte resuscitation is begun. Nutrition is provided, usually through the parenteral route initially. Sepsis is controlled with antibiotics and drainage of abscesses. The skin is protected from the fistula effluent with ostomy appliances or fistula drains.
2. Investigation. The anatomy of the fistula is defined using the studies described above in the Diagnosis section.
3. Decision. The available treatment options are considered, and a timeline for conservative measures determined.
4. Definitive management. This entails the surgical procedure, and requires appropriate preoperative planning and surgical experience.
5. Rehabilitation.

The overall objectives are to increase the probability of spontaneous closure. Nutrition and time are the key components of this approach. Most patients will require TPN; however, a trial of oral or enteral nutrition should be attempted in patients with low-output fistulas originating from the distal intestine. The somatostatin analogue octreotide is a useful adjunct, particularly in patients with high-output fistulas; its administration reduces the volume of fistula output, thereby facilitating fluid and electrolyte management. Further, octreotide may accelerate the rate at which fistulas close; however, its administration has not clearly been demonstrated to increase the probability of spontaneous closure.

Timing of Surgical Intervention

Most surgeons would pursue 2 to 3 months of conservative therapy before considering surgical intervention. This approach is based on evidence that 90% of fistulas that are going to close, close within a 5-week interval, and also that surgical interventions after this time period are associated with better outcomes and lower morbidity.[45]

If the fistula fails to resolve during this period, surgery may be required during which the fistula tract, together with the segment of intestine from which it originates, should be resected. Simple closure of the opening in the intestine from which the fistula originates is associated with high recurrence rates. Patients with intestinal fistulas typically have extensive and dense intra-abdominal adhesions. As a result, operations performed for nonhealing fistulas can present formidable challenges. Successful applications of alternative therapies to close intestinal fistulas, such as the use of biologic sealants, have been reported. The indications for their use remain to be defined.

Outcomes

Enterocutaneous fistulas are associated with a 10 to 15% mortality rate, mostly related to sepsis or underlying disease. Overall, 50% of intestinal fistulas close spontaneously. A useful mnemonic designates factors that inhibit spontaneous closure of intestinal fistulas: "FRIEND" (*F*oreign body within the fistula tract, *R*adiation enteritis, *I*nfection/Inflammation at the fistula origin, *E*pithelialization of the fistula tract, *N*eoplasm at the fistula origin, *D*istal obstruction of the intestine) (Table 28-10). Surgery for fistulas is associated with a greater than 50% morbidity rate, including a 10% recurrence rate.

TABLE 28-9	Factors negatively impacting enteric fistula closure

Patient factors
  Poor nutrition
  Medications such as steroids
Etiologic factors
  Malignant fistula
  Fistula related to Crohn's disease
  Fistula in radiated fields
Fistula site
  Gastric
  Duodenal
Local factors
  Persistence of local inflammation and sepsis
  Presence of a foreign body (e.g., meshes or sutures)
  Epithelialization of fistula tract
  Fistula tract <2 cm
  Distal obstruction to the fistula site

TABLE 28-10 Features of small intestinal malignancies

Tumor Type	Cell of Origin	Frequency[a]	Predominant Site
Adenocarcinoma	Epithelial cell	35–50%	Duodenum
Carcinoid	Enterochromaffin cell	20–40%	Ileum
Lymphoma	Lymphocyte	10–15%	Ileum
GIST	?Interstitial cell of Cajal	10–15%	—

[a]Frequencies given as percentages of small intestinal malignancies comprised by each of the tumor types. GI stromal tumors (GISTs) display no regional variation in prevalence within the small intestine.

SMALL BOWEL NEOPLASMS

Adenomas are the most common benign neoplasm of the small intestine. Other benign tumors include fibromas, lipomas, hemangiomas, lymphangiomas, and neurofibromas. The prevalence of small bowel tumors identified at autopsy is 0.2 to 0.3%, which is significantly higher than the rate of operation for small bowel tumors. This suggests that the majority of small bowel tumors are asymptomatic. These lesions are most frequently encountered in the duodenum as incidental findings during EGD examinations (Fig. 28-19). Their reported prevalence of duodenal polyps, as detected during EGD performed for other reasons, ranges from 0.3 to 4.6%.[46]

Benign neoplasms account for 30 to 50% of small bowel tumors and include adenomas, lipomas, hemartomas, and hemangiomas. Primary small bowel cancers are rare, with an estimated incidence of 5300 cases per year in the United States.[47] Among small bowel cancers, adenocarcinomas comprise 35 to 50% of all cases, carcinoid tumors comprise 20 to 40%, and lymphomas comprise approximately 10 to 15 percent. Gastrointestinal stromal tumors (GISTs) are the most common mesenchymal tumors arising in the small intestine and comprise up to 15% of small bowel malignancies. GISTs comprise the vast majority of tumors that were formerly

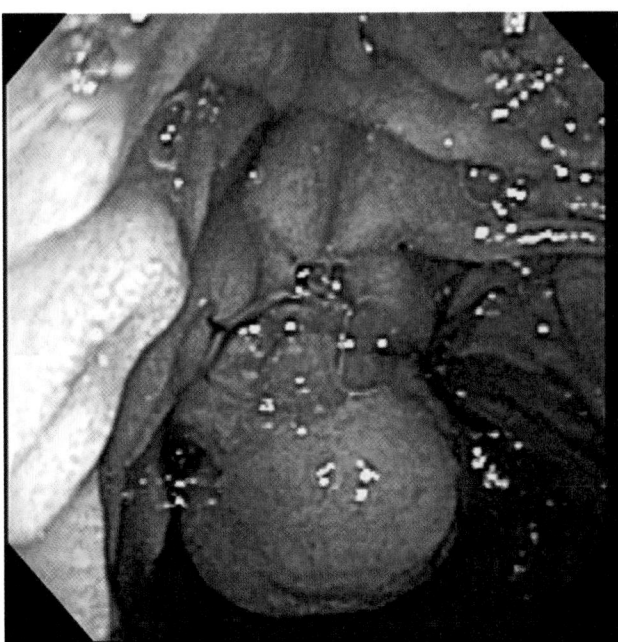

FIG. 28-19. Duodenal polyp. This polyp was incidentally encountered during esophagogastroduodenoscopy. It was biopsied and found to be an adenoma.

classified as leiomyomas, leiomyosarcomas, and smooth muscle tumors of the intestine. The small intestine is frequently affected by metastases from or local invasion by cancers originating at other sites. Melanoma, in particular, is associated with a propensity for metastasis to the small intestine.

Most patients with small intestinal cancers are in their fifth or sixth decade of life. Reported risk factors for developing small intestinal cancers include consumption of red meat, ingestion of smoked or cured foods, Crohn's disease, celiac sprue, hereditary nonpolyposis colorectal cancer, familial adenomatous polyposis (FAP), and Peutz-Jeghers syndrome.

Pathophysiology

The small intestine contains more than 90% of the mucosal surface area of the GI tract, but only 1.1 to 2.4% of all GI malignancies. Proposed explanations for the low frequency of small intestinal neoplasms include (a) dilution of environmental carcinogens in the liquid chyme present in the small intestinal lumen, (b) rapid transit of chyme, limiting the contact time between carcinogens and the intestinal mucosa, (c) a relatively low concentration of bacteria in small intestinal chyme and, therefore, a relatively low concentration of carcinogenic products of bacterial metabolism, (d) mucosal protection by secretory IgA and hydrolases such as benzpyrene hydroxylase that may render carcinogens less active, and (e) efficient epithelial cellular apoptotic mechanisms that serve to eliminate clones harboring genetic mutations.

Recent advances have begun to clarify the molecular pathogenesis of small intestinal adenocarcinomas and GISTs; there has been less progress with respect to the pathogenesis of the other small intestinal malignancies (see Table 28-10). Small intestinal adenocarcinomas are believed to arise from pre-existing adenomas through a sequential accumulation of genetic abnormalities in a model similar to that described for the pathogenesis of colorectal cancer. Adenomas are histologically classified as tubular, villous, and tubulovillous. Tubular adenomas have the least aggressive features. Villous adenomas have the most aggressive features and tend to be large, sessile, and located in the second portion of the duodenum. Malignant degeneration has been reported to be present in up to 45% of villous adenomas by the time of diagnosis. Patients with FAP have a nearly 100% cumulative lifetime risk of developing duodenal adenomas that have the potential to undergo malignant transformation. The risk of duodenal cancer in these patients is over 100-fold that in the general population. Indeed, duodenal cancer is the leading cause of cancer-related death among patients with FAP who have undergone colectomy. Patients with Peutz-Jeghers syndrome develop hamartomatous polyps; however, these polyps can contain adenomatous foci that can undergo malignant transformation (Fig. 28-20).

A defining feature of GISTs is their gain of function mutation of protooncogene KIT, a receptor tyrosine kinase. Pathologic KIT signal transduction is believed to be a central event in GIST pathogenesis.[48] The majority of GISTs have activating mutations in the *c-kit* protooncogene, which cause KIT to become constitutively activated, presumably leading to persistence of cellular growth or survival signals. Because the interstitial cells of Cajal normally express KIT, these cells have been implicated as the cell of origin for GISTs. KIT expression is assessed by staining the tissues for CD117 antigen, which is part of the KIT receptor, and present in 95% of GISTs.

Clinical Presentation

Most small intestinal neoplasms are asymptomatic until they become large. Partial small bowel obstruction, with associated symptoms of crampy abdominal pain and distention, nausea, and vomiting, is the most common mode of presentation. Obstruction can be the result of either luminal narrowing by the tumor itself or intussusception, with the tumor serving as the lead point. Hemorrhage, usually indolent, is the second most common mode of presentation.

Physical examination may be unrevealing. Up to 25% of patients with small intestinal malignancies are reported to have a palpable

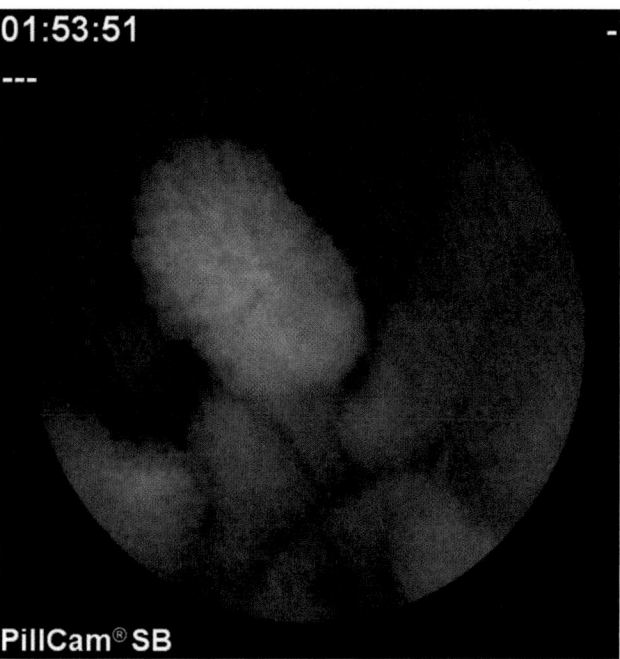

FIG. 28-20. Small bowel polyp in Peutz-Jeghers syndrome. This image was captured by a wireless capsule endoscope as it was traveling through the small intestine. It demonstrates a polyp in the small bowel. *(Courtesy of Dr. Anne C. Travis, Division of Gastroenterology, Brigham and Women's Hospital.)*

abdominal mass. Findings of intestinal obstruction are reported to be present in 25% of patients. Fecal occult blood test may be positive. Jaundice secondary to biliary obstruction or hepatic metastasis may be present. Cachexia, hepatomegaly, and ascites may be present with advanced disease.

Although the clinical presentation usually is not specific for tumor type, some general comments are appropriate. Adenocarcinomas, as well as adenomas (from which most are believed to arise), are most commonly found in the duodenum, except in patients with Crohn's disease, in whom most are found in the ileum. Lesions in the periampullary location can cause obstructive jaundice or pancreatitis. Adenocarcinomas located in the duodenum tend to be diagnosed earlier in their progression than those located in the jejunum or ileum, which are rarely diagnosed before the onset of locally advanced or metastatic disease.

Carcinoid tumors of the small intestine also are usually diagnosed after the development of metastatic disease. These tumors are associated with a more aggressive behavior than the more common appendiceal carcinoid tumors. Approximately 25 to 50% of patients

with carcinoid tumor-derived liver metastases will develop manifestations of the carcinoid syndrome. These manifestations include diarrhea, flushing, hypotension, tachycardia, and fibrosis of the endocardium and valves of the right heart. Candidate tumor-derived mediators of the carcinoid syndrome such as serotonin, bradykinin, and substance P undergo nearly complete metabolism during first passage through the liver. As a result, symptoms of carcinoid syndrome are rare in the absence of liver metastases.

Lymphoma may involve the small intestine primarily or as a manifestation of disseminated systemic disease. Primary small intestinal lymphomas are most commonly located in the ileum, which contains the highest concentration of lymphoid tissue in the intestine. Although partial small bowel obstruction is the most common mode of presentation, 10% of patients with small intestinal lymphoma present with bowel perforation.

Sixty to 70% of GISTs are located in the stomach. The small intestine is the second most common site, containing 25 to 35% of GISTs. There appears to be no regional variation in the prevalence of GISTs within the small intestine. GISTs have a greater propensity to be associated with overt hemorrhage than the other small intestinal malignancies (Fig. 28-21).

Metastatic tumors involving the small intestine can induce intestinal obstruction and bleeding.

Diagnosis

Because of the absent or nonspecific symptoms associated with most small intestinal neoplasms, these lesions rarely are diagnosed preoperatively. Laboratory tests are nonspecific, with the exception of elevated serum 5-hydroxyindole acetic acid levels in patients with the carcinoid syndrome. Elevated carcinoembryonic antigen levels are associated with small intestinal adenocarcinomas, but only in the presence of liver metastases.

Contrast radiography of the small intestine may demonstrate benign and malignant lesions. Enteroclysis is reported to have a sensitivity of over 90% in the detection of small bowel tumors and is the test of choice, particularly for tumors located in the distal small bowel. Upper GI with small bowel follow-through examinations have reported sensitivities ranging from only 30 to 44%.[49] CT scanning has low sensitivity for detecting mucosal or intramural lesions, but can demonstrate large tumors and is useful in the staging of intestinal malignancies. Tumors associated with significant bleeding can be localized with angiography or radioisotope-tagged red blood cell scans.

Tumors located in the duodenum can be visualized and biopsied on EGD. In addition, endoscopic ultrasonography can offer additional information such as the layers of the intestinal wall involved by the lesion. Occasionally, the distal ileum can successfully be visualized during colonoscopy. Intraoperative enteroscopy can be used to directly visualize small intestinal tumors beyond the reach of standard endoscopic techniques. Recently, capsule endoscopy and double-balloon endoscopy have been used to evaluate small bowel.

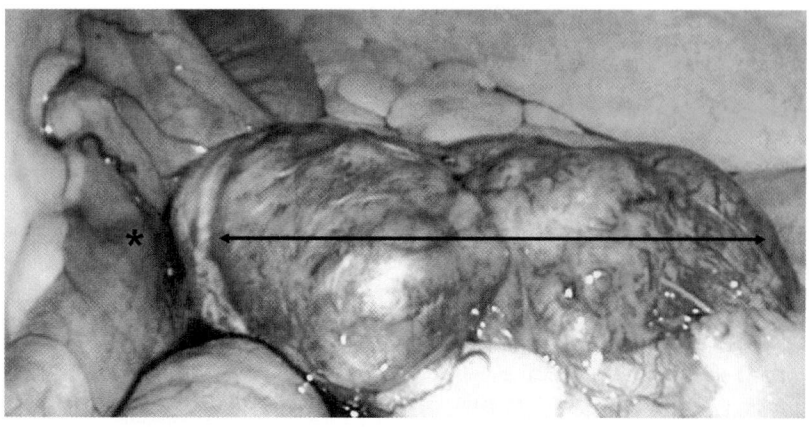

FIG. 28-21. Jejunal GI stromal tumor. This patient presented with overt obscure GI bleeding and was found to have a 7-cm jejunal GI stromal tumor. The picture represents the laparoscopic view of the mass *(black arrow)*, arising from the antimesenteric side of the small bowel *(*)*. He underwent a successful laparoscopic resection.

Therapy

Benign neoplasms of the small intestine that are symptomatic should be surgically resected or removed endoscopically, if feasible. Tumors located in the duodenum, including asymptomatic lesions incidentally found during EGD, can pose the greatest therapeutic challenges. These lesions should be biopsied; symptomatic tumors and adenomas, because of their malignant potential, should be removed. In general, duodenal tumors less than 1 cm in diameter are amenable to endoscopic polypectomy. Lesions greater than 2 cm in diameter are technically difficult to remove endoscopically and should therefore be removed surgically. Surgical options include transduodenal polypectomy and segmental duodenal resection. Tumors located in the second portion of the duodenum near the ampulla of Vater may require pancreaticoduodenectomy. Endoscopic ultrasonography may offer utility for duodenal tumors ranging in size between 1 and 2 cm in diameter, with those limited to the mucosa being amenable to endoscopic polypectomy.[50] Adenomas can recur; therefore, surveillance endoscopy is required after these procedures.

Duodenal adenomas occurring in the setting of FAP require an especially aggressive approach to management. Patients with FAP should undergo screening EGD starting sometime during their second or third decade of life. Adenomas detected should be removed endoscopically, if possible, followed by surveillance endoscopy in 6 months and yearly thereafter, in the absence of recurrence. If surgery is required, pancreaticoduodenectomy generally is necessary because adenomas in patients with FAP tend to be multiple and sessile, with a predilection for the periampullary region. Further, localized resections are complicated by high recurrence rates. Given the potential for recurrences in the duodenal remnant following pylorus preserving pancreaticoduodenectomy, there is a rationale for recommending the application of standard pancreaticoduodenectomy in these patients. However, recurrences have been reported even following this procedure; therefore, continuing surveillance is necessary. For most adenocarcinomas of the duodenum, except those in the distal duodenum, pancreaticoduodenectomy is required.

The surgical therapy of jejunal and ileal malignancies usually consists of wide local resection of the intestine harboring the lesion. For adenocarcinomas, a wide excision of corresponding mesentery is done to achieve regional lymphadenectomy, as is done for adenocarcinomas of the colon. In the presence of locally advanced or metastatic disease, palliative intestinal resection or bypass is performed. Chemotherapy has no proven efficacy in the adjuvant or palliative treatment of small intestinal adenocarcinomas.

The goal of surgical therapy for carcinoids is resection of all visible disease. Localized small intestinal carcinoid tumors should be treated with segmental intestinal resection and regional lymphadenectomy. Nodal metastases are unusual with tumors less than 1 cm in diameter but are present with 75 to 90% of tumors larger than 3 cm in diameter. In approximately 30% of cases, multiple small intestinal carcinoid tumors are present. Therefore, the entire small intestine should be examined before planning extent of resection. In the presence of metastatic disease, tumor debulking should be conducted as it can be associated with long-term survival and amelioration of symptoms of the carcinoid syndrome. Response rates of 30 to 50% have been reported to chemotherapy regimens based on agents such as doxorubicin, 5-fluorouracil, and streptozocin. However, none of these regimens is associated with a clearly demonstrable impact on the natural history of disease. Octreotide is the most effective pharmacologic agent for management of symptoms of carcinoid syndrome.

Localized small intestinal lymphoma should be treated with segmental resection of the involved intestine and adjacent mesentery. If the small intestine is diffusely affected by lymphoma, chemotherapy rather than surgical resection should be the primary therapy. The value to adjuvant chemotherapy after resection of localized lymphoma is controversial.

Small intestinal GISTs should be treated with segmental intestinal resection. If the diagnosis is known before resection, wide lymphadenectomy can be avoided as GISTs are rarely associated with lymph node metastases. GISTs are resistant to conventional chemotherapy agents. Imatinib (Gleevec) is a tyrosine kinase inhibitor with potent activity against tyrosine kinase KIT, and is used in those with metastatic disease. Recent clinical trials have shown that 80% of patients with unresectable or metastatic GISTs derive clinical benefit from the administration of imatinib, with 50 to 60% having objective evidence of reduction in tumor volume.[49] Imatinib has shown great promise as a neoadjuvant and adjuvant therapy of GISTs. Recent reports have emphasized the potential for development of tumor resistance to this agent. In this setting, an alternative tyrosine kinase inhibitor, sunitinib, has been used with good results.[51]

Metastatic cancers affecting the small intestine that are symptomatic should be treated with palliative resection or bypass except in the most advanced cases. Systemic therapy may be offered if effective chemotherapy exists for the primary cancer.

Outcomes

Complete resection of duodenal adenocarcinomas is associated with postoperative 5-year survival rates ranging from 50 to 60%. Complete resection of adenocarcinomas located in the jejunum or ileum is associated with 5-year survival rates of only 5 to 30%.[52] Five-year survival rates of 75 to 95% following resection of localized small intestinal carcinoid tumors have been reported. In the presence of carcinoid tumor-derived liver metastases, 5-year survival rates of 19 to 54% have been reported. The overall 5-year survival rate for patients diagnosed with intestinal lymphoma ranges from 20 to 40%. For patients with localized lymphoma amenable to surgical resection, the 5-year survival rate is 60%.

The recurrence rate following resection of GISTs averages 35%. The 5-year survival rate following surgical resection has been reported to range from 35 to 60%. Both tumor size and mitotic index are independently correlated with prognosis. Low-grade tumors (mitotic index <10 per high-power field) measuring less than 5 cm in diameter are associated with excellent prognosis.

RADIATION ENTERITIS

Radiation therapy is a component of multimodality therapy for many intra-abdominal and pelvic cancers such as those of the cervix, endometrium, ovary, bladder, prostate, and rectum. An undesired side effect of radiation therapy is radiation-induced injury to the small intestine, which can present clinically as two distinct syndromes: acute and chronic radiation enteritis. Acute radiation enteritis is a transient condition that occurs in approximately 75% of patients undergoing radiation therapy for abdominal and pelvic cancers. Chronic radiation enteritis is inexorable and develops in approximately 5 to 15% of these patients.

Pathophysiology

Radiation induces cellular injury directly and through the generation of free radicals. The principal mechanism of radiation-induced cell death is believed to be apoptosis resulting from free-radical–induced breaks in double-stranded DNA. Because radiation has its greatest impact on rapidly proliferating cells, the small intestinal epithelium is acutely susceptible to radiation-induced injury. Pathologic correlates of this acute injury include villus blunting and a dense infiltrate of leukocytes and plasma cells within the crypts. With severe cases, mucosal sloughing, ulceration, and hemorrhage are observed. The intensity of injury is related to the dose of radiation administered, with most cases occurring in patients who have received at least 4500 cGy. Risk factors for acute radiation enteritis include conditions that may limit splanchnic perfusion, such as hypertension, diabetes mellitus, coronary artery disease, and restricted mobility of the small intestine due to adhesions. Injury is potentiated by concomitant administration of chemotherapeutic agents such as doxorubicin, 5-fluorouracil, actinomycin D, and methotrexate that act as radiation-sensitizers. Because of the intestinal epithelium's capacity for regeneration, the mucosal injury that is characteristic of acute radiation enteritis resolves after the cessation of radiation therapy.

In contrast, chronic radiation enteritis is characterized by a progressive occlusive vasculitis that leads to chronic ischemia and fibrosis that affects all layers of the intestinal wall, rather than the mucosa alone. These changes can lead to strictures, abscesses, and fistulas, which are responsible for the clinical manifestations of chronic radiation enteritis.

Clinical Presentation

The most common manifestations of acute radiation enteritis are nausea, vomiting, diarrhea, and crampy abdominal pain. Symptoms generally are transient and subside after the discontinuation of radiation therapy. Because the diagnosis usually is obvious, given the clinical context, no specific diagnostic tests are required. However, if patients develop signs suggestive of peritonitis, CT scanning should be performed to rule out the presence of other conditions capable of causing acute abdominal syndromes.

The clinical manifestations of chronic radiation enteritis usually become evident within 2 years of radiation administration, although they can begin as early as several months or as late as decades afterward. The most common clinical presentation is one of partial small bowel obstruction with nausea, vomiting, intermittent abdominal distention, crampy abdominal pain, and weight loss being the most common symptoms. The terminal ileum is the most frequently affected segment. Other manifestations of chronic radiation enteritis include complete bowel obstruction, acute or chronic intestinal hemorrhage, and abscess or fistula formation.

Diagnosis

Evaluation of patients suspected of having chronic radiation enteritis should include review of the records of their radiation treatments for information on total radiation dose administered, fractionation, and volume of treatment. Areas that received high doses should be noted, as lesions subsequently found in imaging studies usually localize to areas that had received high radiation doses. Enteroclysis is the most accurate imaging test for diagnosing chronic radiation enteritis, with reported sensitivities and specificities of over 90% (Fig. 28-22). CT scan findings are neither very sensitive nor specific for chronic radiation enteritis. However, CT scanning should be obtained to rule out the presence of recurrent cancer because its clinical manifestations may overlap with those of chronic radiation enteritis.

Therapy

Most cases of acute radiation enteritis are self limited. Supportive therapy, including the administration of antiemetics, usually is sufficient. Patients with diarrhea-induced dehydration may require hospital admission and parenteral fluid administration. Rarely are symptoms severe enough to necessitate reduction in or cessation of radiation therapy.

In contrast, the treatment of radiation enteritis represents a formidable challenge. Surgery for this condition is difficult, is associated with high morbidity rates, and should be avoided in the absence of specific indications such as high-grade obstruction, perforation, hemorrhage, intra-abdominal abscesses, and fistulas. The goal of surgery is limited resection of diseased intestine with primary anastomosis between healthy bowel segments. However, the characteristically diffuse nature of fibrosis and dense adhesions among bowel segments can make limited resection difficult to achieve. Further, it is difficult to distinguish between normal and irradiated intestine intraoperatively by either gross inspection or even frozen section analysis. This distinction is important as anastomoses between irradiated segments of intestine have been associated with leak rates as high as 50%.[53] If limited resection is not achievable, an intestinal bypass procedure may be an option, except in cases for which hemorrhage is the surgical indication. There remain cases in which resections extensive enough to cause short

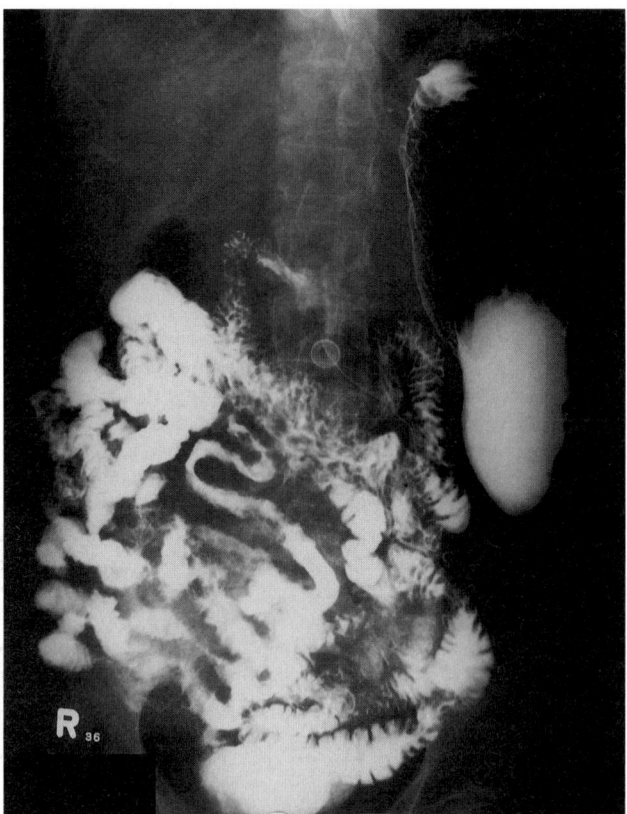

FIG. 28-22. Radiation enteritis. This contrast radiograph reveals widely separated loops of small bowel with luminal narrowing, loss of mucosal folds, and ulceration. This patient had received radiation therapy for a pelvic malignancy 8 years before this examination.

bowel syndrome are unavoidable. This condition is discussed in detail below in the Short Bowel Syndrome section.

Outcomes

Acute radiation injury to the intestine is self limited; its severity is not correlated with the probability of chronic radiation enteritis developing. Surgery for chronic radiation enteritis is associated with high morbidity rates and reported mortality rates averaging 10%.

Prevention

In view of significant morbidity associated with radiation enteritis, groups have studied possible measures to reduce or prevent such side effects. Keeping radiation exposure to below 5000 cGy is associated with minimal long-term side effects and recommended, where clinically possible.

Uses of multibeam radiation techniques to minimize the area of maximal radiation exposure, as well as tilt tables to move the bowel out of the pelvis during radiation are increasingly used. A few small studies have suggested that oral sulfasalazine may help reduce the incidence of acute radiation-induced enteritis.[54]

In patients undergoing pelvic surgery who are likely to require postoperative radiation therapy, surgical techniques that keep the small bowel out of the pelvis have been recommended. These measures include use of an absorbable mesh sling to separate the pelvis from the true abdominal cavity and prevent the small bowel from being exposed to pelvic radiation.[55]

MECKEL'S DIVERTICULUM

Meckel's diverticulum is the most prevalent congenital anomaly of the GI tract, affecting approximately 2% of the general population.[56]

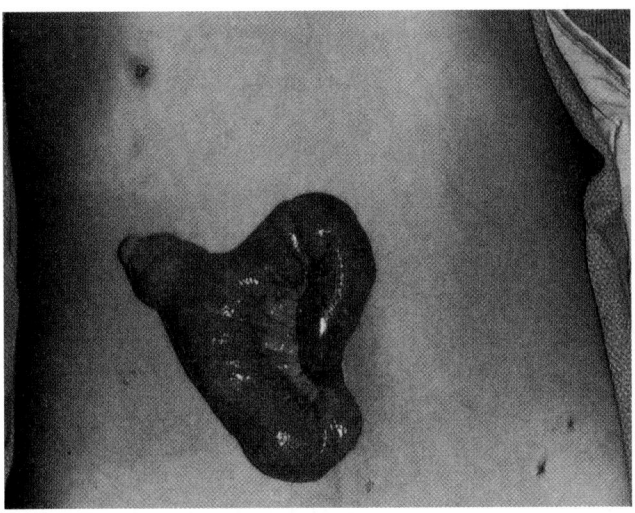

FIG. 28-23. Meckel's diverticulum. This intraoperative photograph shows Meckel's diverticulum in ileum that has been eviscerated.

A 3:2 male-to-female prevalence ratio has been reported. Meckel's diverticula are designated *true diverticula* because their walls contain all of the layers found in normal small intestine. Their location varies among individual patients, but they are usually found in the ileum within 100 cm of the ileocecal valve (Fig. 28-23). Approximately 60% of Meckel's diverticula contain heterotopic mucosa, of which over 60% consist of gastric mucosa. Pancreatic acini are the next most common; others include Brunner's glands, pancreatic islets, colonic mucosa, endometriosis, and hepatobiliary tissues. A useful, although crude, mnemonic describing Meckel's diverticula is the "rule of twos": 2% prevalence, 2:1 female predominance, location 2 ft proximal to the ileocecal valve in adults, and one half of those who are symptomatic are under 2 years of age.

Pathophysiology

During the eighth week of gestation, the omphalomesenteric (vitelline) duct normally undergoes obliteration. Failure or incomplete vitelline duct obliteration results in a spectrum of abnormalities, the most common of which is Meckel's diverticulum. Other abnormalities include omphalomesenteric fistula, enterocyst, and a fibrous band connecting the intestine to the umbilicus. A remnant of the left vitelline artery can persist to form a mesodiverticular band tethering a Meckel's diverticulum to the ileal mesentery.

Bleeding associated with Meckel's diverticulum is usually the result of ileal mucosal ulceration that occurs adjacent to acid-producing, heterotopic gastric mucosa located within the diverticulum. Intestinal obstruction associated with Meckel's diverticulum can result from several mechanisms:

1. Volvulus of the intestine around the fibrous band attaching the diverticulum to the umbilicus
2. Entrapment of intestine by a mesodiverticular band (Fig. 28-24)
3. Intussusception with the diverticulum acting as a lead point
4. Stricture secondary to chronic diverticulitis

Meckel's diverticula can be found in inguinal or femoral hernia sacs (known as *Littre's hernia*). These hernias, when incarcerated, can cause intestinal obstruction.

Clinical Presentation

Meckel's diverticula are asymptomatic unless associated complications arise. The lifetime incidence rate of complications arising in patients with Meckel's diverticula has been estimated to be approximately 4 to 6%.[56,57] Although initial data had suggested that the risk of developing a complication related to Meckel's diverticulum decreases with age, this has been now been questioned. In population-based reviews at Olmsted County, Minnesota, Cullen and colleagues showed that the risk of developing Meckel's-related complications does not change with age.[57]

The most common presentations associated with symptomatic Meckel's diverticula are bleeding, intestinal obstruction, and diverticulitis. Bleeding is the most common presentation in children with Meckel's diverticula, representing over 50% of Meckel's diverticulum-related complications among patients younger than 18 years of age. Bleeding associated with Meckel's diverticula is rare among patients older than 30 years of age.

Intestinal obstruction is the most common presentation in adults with Meckel's diverticula. Diverticulitis, present in 20% of patients with symptomatic Meckel's diverticula, is associated with a clinical syndrome that is indistinguishable from acute appendicitis. Neoplasms, most commonly carcinoid tumors, are present in 0.5 to 3.2% of symptomatic Meckel's diverticula that are resected.[56]

Diagnosis

Most Meckel's diverticula are discovered incidentally on radiographic imaging, during endoscopy, or at the time of surgery. In the absence of bleeding, Meckel's diverticula rarely are diagnosed before the time of surgical intervention. For those presenting with symptoms suggestive of a Meckel's diverticulum, confirmatory imaging can be challenging. The sensitivity of CT scanning for the detection of Meckel's

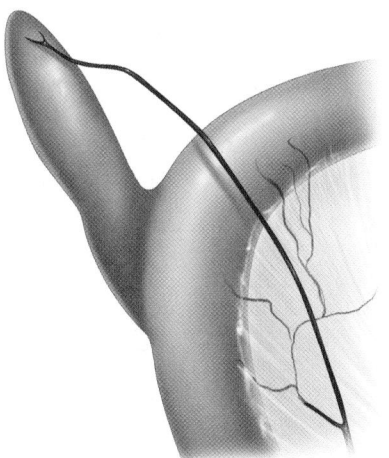
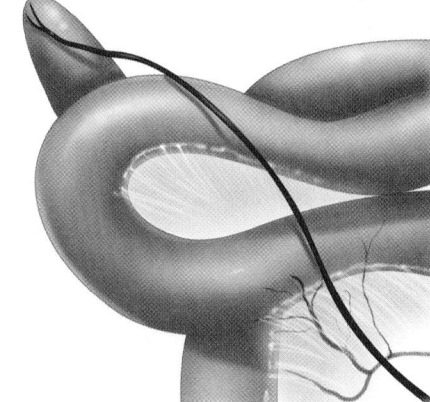

FIG. 28-24. A. Meckel's diverticulum with mesodiverticular band. **B.** One mechanism by which Meckel's diverticula can cause small bowel obstruction is entrapment of the intestine by a mesodiverticular band.

A   **B**

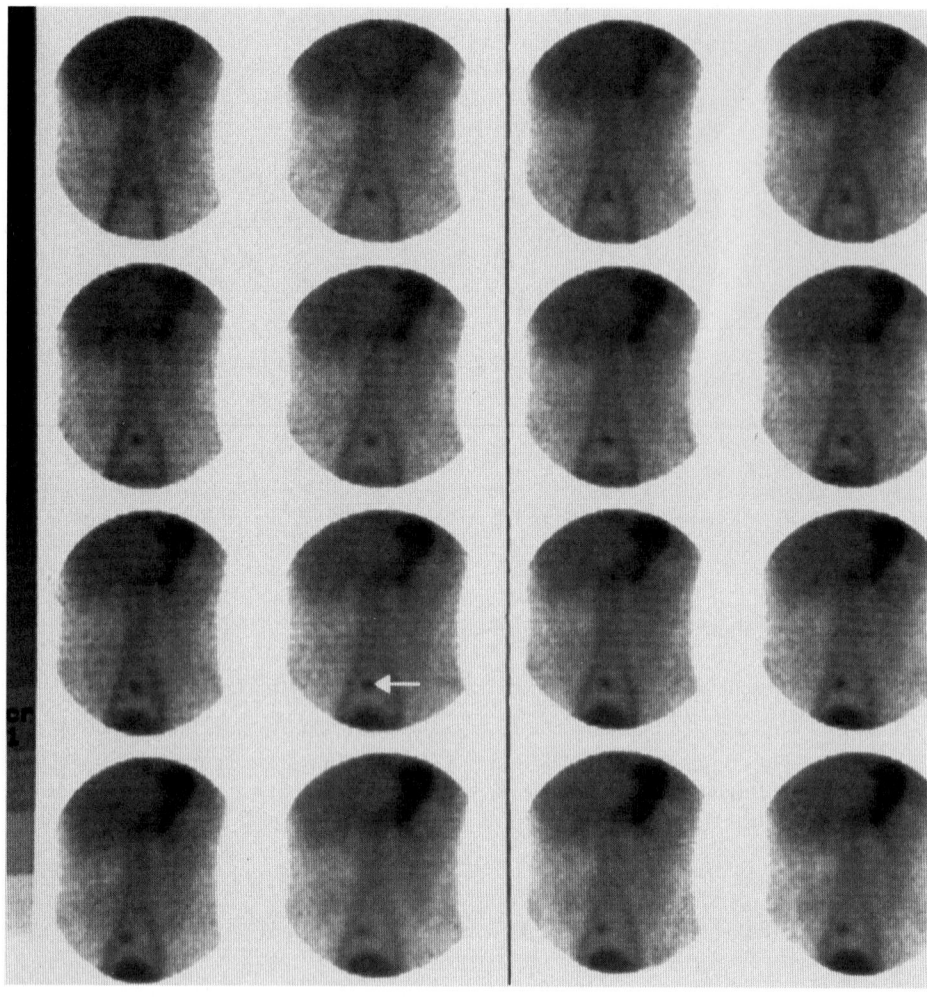

FIG. 28-25. Meckel's diverticulum with ectopic gastric tissue. The diagnosis was made in this patient using ^{99m}Tc-pertechnetate scintigraphy. The study revealed an abnormal focus of radiotracer accumulation in the right lower quadrant (*arrow*).

diverticula is too low to be clinically useful. Enteroclysis is associated with an accuracy of 75%, but usually is not applicable during acute presentations of complications related to Meckel's diverticula. Radionuclide scans (^{99m}Tc-pertechnetate) can be helpful in the diagnosis of Meckel's diverticulum; this test is, however, positive only when the diverticulum contains associated ectopic gastric mucosa that is capable of uptake of the tracer (Fig. 28-25). The accuracy of radionuclide scanning is reported to be 90% in pediatric patients but less than 50% in adults. Angiography can localize the site of bleeding during acute hemorrhage related to Meckel's diverticula.

Therapy

The surgical treatment of symptomatic Meckel's diverticula should consist of diverticulectomy with removal of associated bands connecting the diverticulum to the abdominal wall or intestinal mesentery. If the indication for diverticulectomy is bleeding, segmental resection of ileum that includes both the diverticulum and the adjacent ileal peptic ulcer should be performed. Segmental ileal resection may also be necessary if the diverticulum contains a tumor or if the base of the diverticulum is inflamed or perforated.

The management of incidentally found (asymptomatic) Meckel's diverticula is controversial. Until recently, most authors recommended against prophylactic removal of asymptomatic Meckel's diverticula, given the low lifetime incidence of complications. More recently, greater enthusiasm for prophylactic diverticulectomy has appeared in the literature.[57] Proponents of this approach cite the minimal morbidity associated with removing Meckel's diverticula and the possibility that previous estimates of the lifetime incidence of complications related to Meckel's diverticula may be erroneously low. Other authors have advocated a selective approach, with a recommendation to remove diverticula attached by bands and those with narrow bases, on the assumption that these diverticula are more likely to develop complications. No controlled data supporting or refuting these recommendations exist.

ACQUIRED DIVERTICULA

Acquired diverticula are designated *false diverticula* because their walls consist of mucosa and submucosa but lack a complete muscularis. Acquired diverticula are more common in the duodenum, and tend to be located near the ampulla; such diverticula are known as *periampullary*, *juxtapapillary*, or *peri-Vaterian diverticula*. Approximately 75% of juxtapapillary diverticula arise on the medial wall of the duodenum. Acquired diverticula in the jejunum or ileum are known as *jejunoileal diverticula*. Eighty percent of jejunoileal diverticula are localized to the jejunum, 15% to the ileum, and 5% to both jejunum and ileum. Diverticula in the jejunum tend to be large and accompanied by multiple other diverticula, whereas those in the ileum tend to be small and solitary.

The prevalence of duodenal diverticula, as detected on upper GI examinations (Fig. 28-26), has been reported to range from 0.16 to 6%.[58] Their prevalence, as detected during endoscopic retrograde cholangiography (ERCP) examinations, has been reported to range from 5 to 27%. A 23% prevalence rate has been reported in an autopsy series. The prevalence of duodenal diverticula increases with age; they are rare in patients under the age of 40 years. The mean age of diagnosis ranges from 56 to 76 years.

The prevalence of jejunoileal diverticula (Fig. 28-27) has been estimated to range from 1 to 5%.[59] Their prevalence increases with age; most patients diagnosed with these diverticula are in the sixth and seventh decades of life.

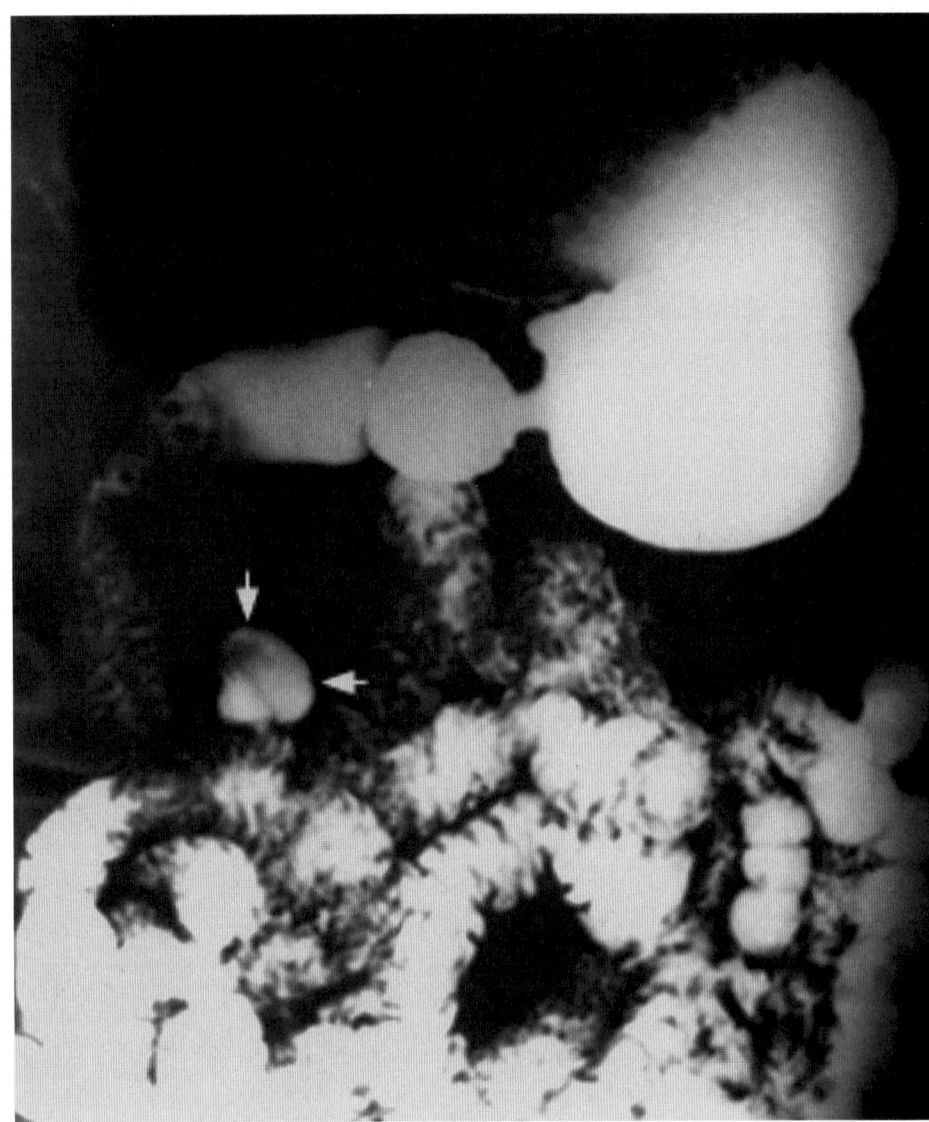

FIG. 28-26. Duodenal diverticulum. This contrast radiograph demonstrates a duodenal diverticulum (*arrows*) that extends medially into the substance of the head of the pancreas.

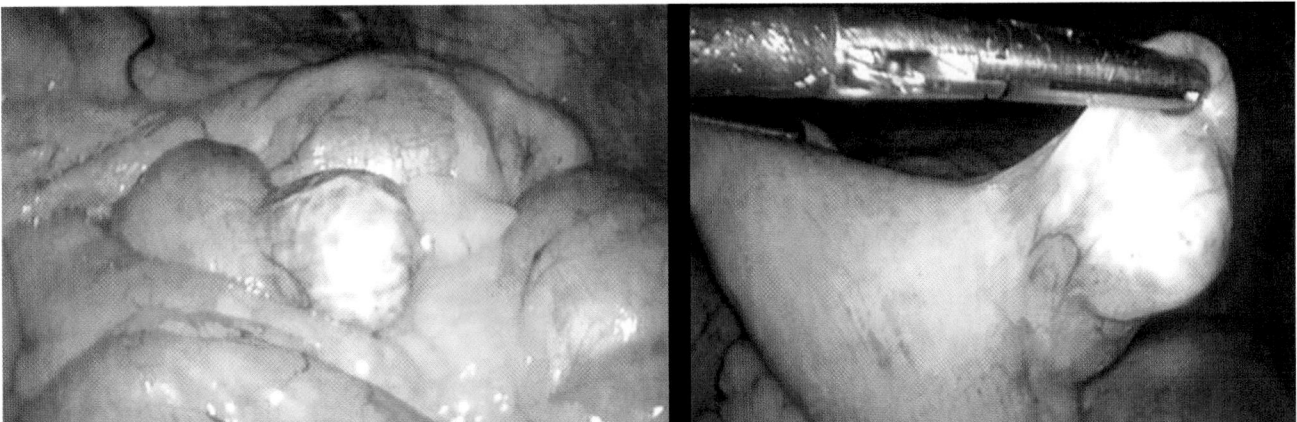

FIG. 28-27. Jejunoileal diverticula. This picture demonstrates incidental jejunal diverticula identified during a laparoscopic cholecystectomy. The diverticula are typically located on the mesenteric aspect of the jejunum. Resection was not indicated as the diverticula were asymptomatic.

Pathophysiology

The pathogenesis of acquired diverticula is hypothesized to be related to acquired abnormalities of intestinal smooth muscle or dysregulated motility, leading to herniation of mucosa and submucosa through weakened areas of muscularis.

Acquired diverticula can be associated with bacterial overgrowth, leading to vitamin B_{12} deficiency, megaloblastic anemia, malabsorption, and steatorrhea. Periampullary duodenal diverticula have been described to become distended with intraluminal debris and to compress the common bile duct or pancreatic duct, thus causing obstructive jaundice or pancreatitis, respectively. Jejunoileal diverticula also can cause intestinal obstruction through intussusception or compression of adjacent bowel.

Clinical Presentation

Acquired diverticula are asymptomatic unless associated complications arise. Such complications are estimated to occur in 6 to 10% of patients with acquired diverticula and include intestinal obstruction, diverticulitis, hemorrhage, perforation, and malabsorption. Periampullary duodenal diverticula may be associated with choledocholithiasis, cholangitis, recurrent pancreatitis, and sphincter of Oddi dysfunction. However, a clear link between the presence of the diverticula and the development of these conditions has not been demonstrated. Symptoms such as intermittent abdominal pain, flatulence, diarrhea, and constipation are reported to be present in 10 to 30% of patients with jejunoileal diverticula. The relationship between these symptoms and the presence of the diverticula is similarly unclear.

Diagnosis

Most acquired diverticula are discovered incidentally on radiographic imaging, during endoscopy, or at the time of surgery. On ultrasound and CT scanning, duodenal diverticula may be mistaken for pancreatic pseudocysts and fluid collections, biliary cysts, and periampullary neoplasms. These lesions can be missed on endoscopy, particularly with forward-viewing endoscopes, and are best diagnosed on upper GI radiographs. Enteroclysis is the most sensitive test for detecting jejunoileal diverticula.

Therapy

Asymptomatic acquired diverticula should be left alone. Bacterial overgrowth associated with acquired diverticula is treated with antibiotics. Other complications, such as bleeding and diverticulitis, are treated with segmental intestinal resection for diverticula located in the jejunum or ileum.

Bleeding and obstruction related to lateral duodenal diverticula generally are treated with diverticulectomy alone. These procedures can be technically difficult for medial duodenal diverticula that penetrate into the substance of the pancreas. Complications related to these medial duodenal diverticula should be managed nonoperatively if possible, using endoscopy. In emergent situations, bleeding related to medial duodenal diverticula can be controlled using a lateral duodenotomy and oversewing of the bleeding vessel. Similarly, perforation can be managed with wide drainage rather than complex surgery. Whether diverticulectomy should be done in patients with biliary or pancreatic symptoms is controversial and is not routinely recommended.[58]

MESENTERIC ISCHEMIA

Mesenteric ischemia can present as one of two distinct clinical syndromes: acute mesenteric ischemia and chronic mesenteric ischemia.

Four distinct pathophysiologic mechanisms can lead to acute mesenteric ischemia:

1. Arterial embolus
2. Arterial thrombosis
3. Vasospasm (also known as nonocclusive mesenteric ischemia)
4. Venous thrombosis

Embolus is the most common cause of acute mesenteric ischemia, and is responsible for more than 50% of cases. The embolic source is usually in the heart; most often the left atrial or ventricular thrombi or valvular lesions. Indeed, up to 95% of patients with acute mesenteric ischemia due to emboli will have a documented history of cardiac disease. Embolism to the superior mesenteric artery accounts for 50% of cases; most of these emboli become wedged and cause occlusion at branch points in the mid- to distal superior mesenteric artery, usually distal to the origin of the middle colic artery. In contrast, acute occlusions due to thrombosis tend to occur in the proximal mesenteric arteries, near their origins. Acute thrombosis is usually superimposed on pre-existing atherosclerotic lesions at these sites. Nonocclusive mesenteric ischemia is the result of vasospasm and usually is diagnosed in critically ill patients receiving vasopressor agents.

Mesenteric venous thrombosis accounts for 5 to 15% of cases of acute mesenteric ischemia and involves the superior mesenteric vein in 95% of cases.[60] The inferior mesenteric vein is only rarely involved. Mesenteric venous thrombosis is classified as primary if no etiologic factor is identifiable, or as secondary if an etiologic factor, such as heritable or acquired coagulation disorders, is identified.

Regardless of the pathophysiologic mechanism, acute mesenteric ischemia can lead to intestinal mucosal sloughing within 3 hours of onset and full-thickness intestinal infarction by 6 hours.

In contrast, *chronic mesenteric ischemia* develops insidiously, allowing for development of collateral circulation, and, therefore, rarely leads to intestinal infarction. Chronic mesenteric arterial ischemia results from atherosclerotic lesions in the main splanchnic arteries (celiac, superior mesenteric, and inferior mesenteric arteries). In most patients with symptoms attributable to chronic mesenteric ischemia, at least two of these arteries are either occluded or severely stenosed. A chronic form of mesenteric venous thrombosis can involve the portal or splenic veins and may lead to portal hypertension, with resulting esophagogastric varices, splenomegaly, and hypersplenism.

Severe abdominal pain, out of proportion to the degree of tenderness on examination, is the hallmark of acute mesenteric ischemia, regardless of the pathophysiologic mechanism. The pain typically is perceived to be colicky and most severe in the midabdomen. Associated symptoms can include nausea, vomiting, and diarrhea. Physical findings are characteristically absent early in the course of ischemia. With the onset of bowel infarction, abdominal distention, peritonitis, and passage of bloody stools occur.

Chronic mesenteric ischemia presents insidiously. Postprandial abdominal pain is the most prevalent symptom, producing a characteristic aversion to food ("food-fear") and weight loss. These patients are often thought to have a malignancy and suffer a prolonged period of symptoms before the correct diagnosis is made.

Most patients with chronic mesenteric venous thrombosis are asymptomatic because of the presence of extensive collateral venous drainage routes; this condition is usually discovered as an incidental finding on imaging studies. However, some patients with chronic mesenteric venous thrombosis present with bleeding from esophagogastric varices.

The diagnosis and management of these disorders that are of primary vascular origin are discussed in the section on Mesenteric Artery Disease in Chap. 23.

MISCELLANEOUS CONDITIONS

Obscure Gastrointestinal Bleeding

Up to 90% of lesions responsible for GI bleeding are within the reach of EGD and colonoscopy. *Obscure GI bleeding* refers to GI bleeding for which no source has been identified by routine endoscopic studies (EGD and colonoscopy). *Overt GI bleeding* refers to the presence of hematemesis, melena, or hematochezia. In contrast, *occult GI bleeding* occurs in the absence of overt bleeding and is identified on laboratory tests (e.g., iron-deficiency anemia) or examination of the stool (e.g., positive guaiac test). Obscure GI bleeding is occult in 20% of cases.[61]

Obscure bleeding can be frustrating for both the patient and the clinician, and particularly true for obscure-overt bleeding that cannot be localized despite aggressive diagnostic measures. One study from a tertiary referral center reported that the typical patient with obscure-overt bleeding had suffered intermittent episodes of hemorrhage for 26 months, had undergone up to 20 diagnostic tests, and had received an average of 20 units of blood before reaching a diagnosis.[62] Most of the small bowel is beyond the reach of these examinations and, hence, contains most lesions responsible for obscure GI bleeding. Small intestinal angiodysplasias account for approximately 75% of cases in adults, and neoplasms for approximately 10%. Meckel's diverticulum is the most common etiology of obscure GI bleeding in children. Other etiologies of obscure GI bleeding include Crohn's disease, infectious enteritides, NSAID-induced ulcers and erosions, vasculitis, ischemia, varices, diverticula, and intussusception.

The diagnostic evaluation of patients with obscure GI bleeding should be tailored to the severity to bleeding and to the availability of technology and expertise. Enteroscopy is playing an increasingly important role. Several endoscopic techniques for visualizing the small intestine are available: push enteroscopy, Sonde enteroscopy, intraoperative enteroscopy, double-balloon endoscopy, and wireless capsule enteroscopy.

Push enteroscopy entails advancing a long endoscope (such as a pediatric or adult colonoscope or a specialized instrument) beyond the ligament of Treitz into the proximal jejunum. This procedure can allow for visualization of approximately 60 cm of the proximal jejunum. Reported diagnostic yield rates in patients with obscure GI bleeding range from 3 to 65%. In addition to diagnosis, push enteroscopy allows for cauterization of bleeding sites.

In Sonde enteroscopy, a long, thin fiber-optic instrument is propelled through the intestine by peristalsis following inflation of a balloon at the instrument's tip. Visualization is done during instrument withdrawal; approximately 50 to 75% of the small intestinal mucosa can be examined. However, this instrument lacks biopsy or therapeutic capability. Further, it lacks tip deflection capability, limiting complete mucosal visualization, and therefore has been abandoned in favor of capsule endoscopy.

Wireless capsule enteroscopy relies on a radiotelemetry capsule enteroscope that is small enough to swallow and has no external wires, fiber-optic bundles, or cables. While the capsule is being propelled through the intestine by peristalsis, video images are transmitted using radiotelemetry to an array of detectors attached to the patient's body. These detectors capture the images and permit continuous triangulation of the capsule location in the abdomen, facilitating the localization of lesions detected. The entire system is portable, allowing the patient to be ambulatory during the entire examination. Capsule endoscopy is an excellent tool in the patient who is hemodynamically stable but continues to bleed. This technique has reported success rates as high as 90% in identifying a small bowel pathology.[61]

For patients in whom bleeding from an obscure GI source has apparently stopped, push enteroscopy or capsule enteroscopy is a reasonable initial study. If these examinations do not reveal a potential source of bleeding, then enteroclysis should be performed. Standard small bowel follow-through examinations are associated with a low diagnostic yield in this setting and should be avoided. If still no diagnosis has been made, a "watch-and-wait" approach is reasonable, although angiography should be considered if the prior episode of bleeding was overt. Angiography can reveal angiodysplasia and vascular tumors in the small intestine even in the absence of ongoing bleeding.

For persistent mild bleeding from an obscure GI source, push and capsule enteroscopy can be used. If these examinations are nondiagnostic, then ^{99m}Tc-labeled red blood cell scanning should be performed and, if positive, followed by angiography to localize the source of bleeding. ^{99m}Tc-pertechnetate scintigraphy to diagnose Meckel's diverticulum should be considered, although its yield in patients older than 40 years of age is extremely low. Patients who remain undiagnosed but continue to bleed and those with recurrent episodic bleeding significant enough to require blood transfusions should then undergo exploration with intraoperative enteroscopy.

Patients with persistent severe bleeding from an obscure source should undergo angiography to help localize the bleeding source. Therapy can be tailored based on the source. Push enteroscopy also can be attempted, but capsule enteroscopy is too slow to be applicable in this setting. If these examinations fail to localize the source of bleeding, exploratory laparoscopy or laparotomy with intraoperative enteroscopy is indicated. Intraoperative enteroscopy can be done during either laparotomy or laparoscopy. An endoscope (usually a colonoscope) is inserted into the small bowel through peroral intubation or through an enterotomy made in the small bowel or cecum. The endoscope is advanced by successively telescoping short segments of intestine onto the end of the instrument. In addition to the endoscopic image, the transilluminated bowel should be examined externally with the operating room lights dimmed, as this maneuver may facilitate the identification of angiodysplasias. Identified lesions should be marked with a suture placed on the serosal surface of the bowel; these lesions can be resected after completion of endoscopy. Examination should be performed during instrument insertion rather than withdrawal because instrument-induced mucosal trauma can be confused with angiodysplasias. Reported diagnostic rates, when applied to patients with obscure GI bleeding, range from 83 to 100%.

Figure 28-28 provides a diagnostic and management algorithm for patients with obscure GI bleeding.

Small Bowel Perforation

Before the 1980s, duodenal perforation due to peptic ulcer disease was the most common form of small bowel perforation. Today, iatrogenic injury incurred during GI endoscopy is the most common cause of small bowel perforation. Other etiologies of small bowel perforation include infections (especially tuberculosis, typhoid, and CMV), Crohn's disease, ischemia, drugs (e.g., potassium- and NSAID-induced ulcers), radiation-induced injury, Meckel's and acquired diverticula, neoplasms (especially lymphoma, adenocarcinoma, and melanoma), and foreign bodies.

Among iatrogenic injuries, duodenal perforation during ERCP with endoscopic sphincterotomy is the most common. This complication occurs in 0.3 to 2% of cases. Patients who have undergone Billroth II gastrectomy are at increased risk of duodenal perforations as well as free jejunal perforations during ERCP. Although ERCP-related duodenal perforations can result in a free perforation, most are retroperitoneal. Manifestations of such a contained duodenal perforation following ERCP can resemble those of ERCP-induced pancreatitis, including hyperamylasemia.

CT scanning is the most sensitive test for diagnosing duodenal perforations; positive findings include pneumoperitoneum for free perforations, but more commonly retroperitoneal air, contrast extravasation, and paraduodenal fluid collections. If all patients undergoing a therapeutic ERCP are imaged with a CT scan following the procedure, up to 30% will have evidence of air in the retroperitoneum, but the majority are asymptomatic. These patients do not require any specific therapy.[63]

True cases of retroperitoneal perforations of the duodenum can be managed nonoperatively, in the absence of progression and sepsis. However, intraperitoneal duodenal perforations require surgical repair with pyloric exclusion and gastrojejunostomy or tube duodenostomy. Iatrogenic small bowel perforation incurred during endoscopy, if immediately recognized, can sometimes be repaired using endoscopic techniques.

Perforation of the jejunum and ileum occurs into the peritoneal cavity and usually causes overt symptoms and signs, such as abdom-

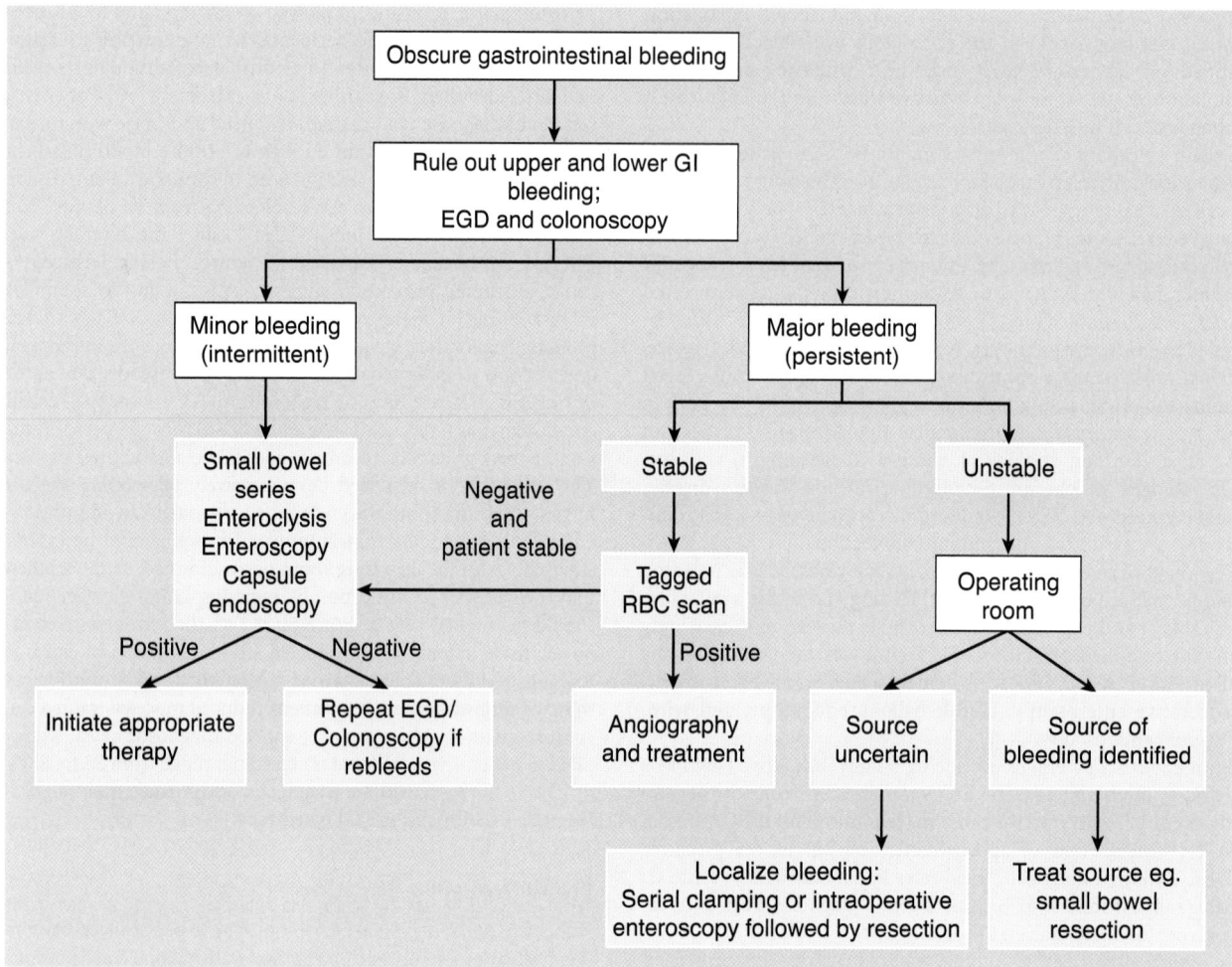

FIG. 28-28. Diagnostic and management algorithm for obscure GI bleeding. EGD = esophagogastroduodenoscopy; RBC = red blood cell.

inal pain, tenderness, and distention accompanied by fever and tachycardia. Plain abdominal radiographs may reveal free intraperitoneal air if intraperitoneal perforation has occurred. If perforation is suspected, but not clinically obvious, CT scanning should be performed. Jejunal and ileal perforations require surgical repair or segmental resection.

Chylous Ascites

Chylous ascites refers to the accumulation of triglyceride-rich peritoneal fluid with a milky or creamy appearance, caused by the presence of intestinal lymph in the peritoneal cavity. Chylomicrons, produced by the intestine and secreted into lymph during the absorption of long-chain fatty acids, account for the characteristic appearance and triglyceride content of chyle.

The most common etiologies of chylous ascites in Western countries are abdominal malignancies and cirrhosis. In Eastern and developing countries, infectious etiologies such as tuberculosis and filariasis account for most cases. Chylous ascites also can develop as a complication of abdominal and thoracic operations and trauma. Operations particularly associated with this complication include abdominal aortic aneurysm repair, retroperitoneal lymph node dissection, inferior vena cava resection, and liver transplantation. Other etiologies of chylous ascites include congenital lymphatic abnormalities (e.g., primary lymphatic hypoplasia), radiation, pancreatitis, and right-sided heart failure.

Three mechanisms have been postulated to cause chylous ascites: (a) exudation of chyle from dilated lymphatics on the wall of the bowel and in the mesentery caused by obstruction of lymphatic vessels at the base of the mesentery or the cisterna chili (e.g., by malignancies), (b) direct leakage of chyle through a lymphoperitoneal fistula (e.g., those that develop as a result of trauma or surgery), and (c) exudation of chyle through the wall of dilated retroperitoneal lymphatic vessels (e.g., in congenital lymphangiectasia or thoracic duct obstruction).

Patients with chylous ascites develop abdominal distention over a period of weeks to months. Postoperative chylous ascites can present acutely during the first postoperative week. Delayed presentations following surgery can occur if the mechanism of ascites formation is adhesion-induced lymphatic obstruction rather than lymphatic vessel disruption. Dyspnea may result if abdominal distention is severe enough.

Paracentesis is the most important diagnostic test. Chyle typically has a cloudy and turbid appearance; however, it may be clear in fasting patients (such as those in the immediate postoperative period). Fluid triglyceride concentrations above 110 mg/dL are diagnostic. CT scanning may be useful in identifying pathologic intra-abdominal lymph nodes and masses and in identifying the extent and localization of fluid. Lymphangiography and lymphoscintigraphy may help localize lymph leaks and obstruction; this information is particularly useful for surgical planning.

There are little data on optimal management of patients with chylous ascites. The general approach is to focus on evaluating and treating the underlying causes, especially for patients with infectious, inflammatory, or hemodynamic etiologies for this condition.

Most patients respond to administration of a high-protein and low-fat diet supplemented with medium-chain triglycerides. This regimen is designed to minimize chyle production and flow. Me-

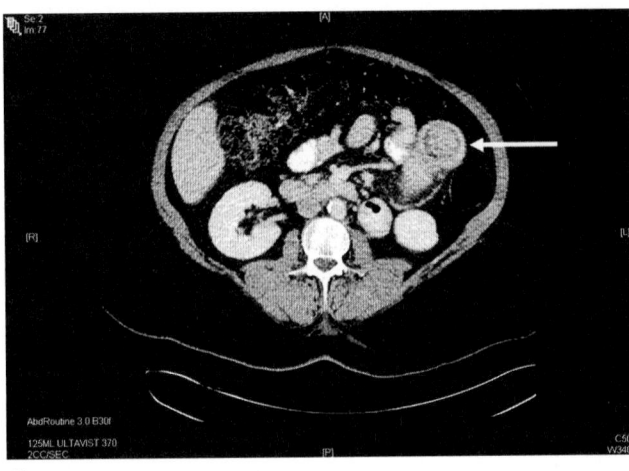
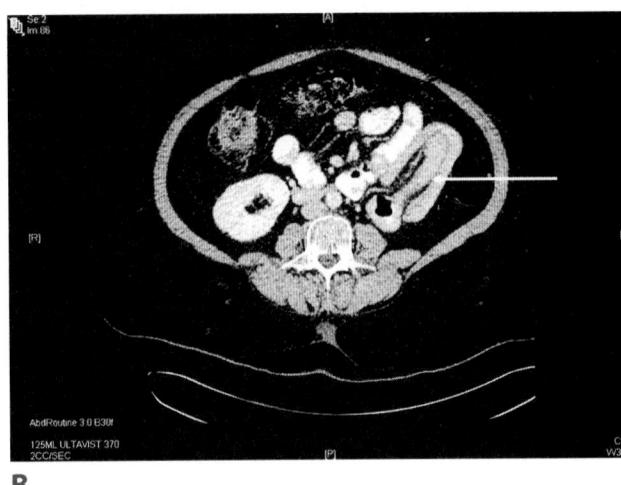

A

B

FIG. 28-29. Small bowel intussusception. Panel **A** demonstrates the target sign seen on computed tomographic scans in patients with small bowel intussusception (*arrow*). Panel **B** demonstrates the distal bowel clearly within the lumen of the proximal bowel (*arrow*).

dium-chain triglycerides are absorbed by the intestinal epithelium and are transported to liver through the portal vein; they do not contribute to chylomicron formation.

Patients who do not respond to this approach should fast and be placed on TPN. Octreotide can further decrease lymph flow. Paracentesis is indicated for respiratory difficulties related to abdominal distention. Overall, 60% of patients will respond to conservative therapy. However, 30% of patients will require surgical therapy for chylous ascites. In general, postoperative and trauma-related cases that fail to respond to initial nonoperative therapy are best managed by surgical repair. Lymphatic leaks are localized and repaired with fine nonabsorbable sutures. If extravasation of chyle is localized to the periphery of the small bowel mesentery, then a limited small bowel resection can be performed instead. For patients who are poor surgical candidates and do not respond to prolonged conservative therapy, peritoneovenous shunting may be an option. However, these shunts are associated with high rates of complications, including sepsis and disseminated intravascular coagulation. Because of the viscosity of chyle, these shunts are associated with a high occlusion rate.

Intussusception

Intussusception refers to a condition where one segment of the intestine becomes drawn in to the lumen of the proximal segment of the bowel. It usually is seen in the pediatric population, where the cecum intussuscepts in to the ileum (ileocolic intussusception). In children, it is often an idiopathic condition and treated nonsurgically by radiologic reduction.

Adult intussusceptions are far less common, and usually have a distinct pathologic lead point, which can be malignant in up to one half of cases.[64] They commonly present with a history of intermittent abdominal pain and signs and symptoms of bowel obstruction. CT scan is the investigation of choice, where a "target sign" may be seen (Fig. 28-29). Treatment is surgical resection of the involved segment and the lead point, which needs to undergo pathologic evaluation to rule out an underlying malignancy.

With increasing use of CT imaging, target signs are sometimes seen on CT scans of patients who do not have a clinical presentation indicative of bowel obstruction. In such cases, the finding is of little clinical significance and is probably related to normal peristalsis.

In patients who have undergone a Roux-en-Y gastric bypass surgery, an atypical form of intussusception has been increasingly described. In these cases, the proximal bowel is drawn in to the lumen of the distal bowel (retrograde intussusception). These intussusceptions usually are not associated with a lead point, and may

represent a motility disorder of the bowel following the Roux-en-Y reconstruction.[65] Surgical reductions without resection have been successfully reported in these patients.

Pneumatosis Intestinalis

Pneumatosis intestinalis indicates the presence of gas within the bowel wall. It may affect any region of the GI tract but is most commonly seen in the jejunum. Pneumatosis intestinalis is not a disease but merely a sign that can be idiopathic, or associated with many intestinal or nonintestinal disorders such as obstructive pulmonary disease and asthma. Most cases of pneumatosis intestinalis are secondary to an identifiable cause, and 15% are idiopathic. The pathogenesis of pneumatosis intestinalis is not fully understood.

The surgical interest in this finding is the association of it with bowel ischemia and infarction, both of which necessitate emergent surgical intervention (see Fig. 28-15). Thus, patients with this radiologic finding need to be fully evaluated and monitored closely to rule out such intra-abdominal catastrophes.

SHORT BOWEL SYNDROME

Intestinal resection is performed for many of the diseases discussed in this chapter and generally is associated with minimal morbidity. However, when the extent of resection is great enough, a devastating condition known as the *short bowel syndrome* may result. Short bowel syndrome has been arbitrarily defined as the presence of less than 200 cm of residual small bowel in adult patients.[66] A functional definition, in which insufficient intestinal absorptive capacity results in the clinical manifestations of diarrhea, dehydration, and malnutrition, is more broadly applicable.

In adults, the most common etiologies of short bowel syndrome are acute mesenteric ischemia, malignancy, and Crohn's disease. Seventy-five percent of cases result from resection of a large amount of small bowel at a single operation. Twenty-five percent of cases result from the cumulative effects of multiple operations during which small intestine is resected. This latter pattern is typical of patients with Crohn's disease who develop short bowel syndrome; the former is typical of patients with acute mesenteric ischemia who develop intestinal infarction. In pediatric patients, intestinal atresias, volvulus, and necrotizing enterocolitis are the most common etiologies of short bowel syndrome.

The prevalence of short bowel syndrome has been estimated to be as high as 2 million patients in the United States.[66] The most recent available data on chronic home TPN administration were obtained in 1992. At that time, approximately 40,000 patients were receiving TPN chronically at home. The most prevalent indication for TPN among these patients was short bowel syndrome; however, this estimate does not include patients with short bowel syndrome not receiving TPN at home. It also fails to include those who have been weaned off of TPN.

Pathophysiology

Resection of less than 50% of the small intestine is generally well tolerated. However, clinically significant malabsorption occurs when greater than 50 to 80% of the small intestine has been resected. Among adult patients who lack a functional colon, lifelong TPN dependence is likely to persist if there is less than 100 cm of residual small intestine. Among adult patients who have an intact and functional colon, lifelong TPN dependence is likely to persist if there is less than 60 cm of residual small intestine. Among infants with short bowel syndrome, weaning from TPN-dependence has been achieved with as little as 10 cm of residual small intestine.

Residual bowel length is not the only factor predictive of achieving independence from TPN (enteral autonomy), however. Other determinants of the severity of malabsorption include the presence or absence of an intact colon, as indicated in the paragraph above. The colon has the capacity to absorb large fluid and electrolyte loads. In addition, the colon can play an important, albeit small, role in nutrient assimilation by absorbing short-chain fatty acids. Second, an intact ileocecal valve is believed to be associated with decreased malabsorption. The ileocecal valve delays transit of chyme from the small intestine into the colon, thereby prolonging the contact time between nutrients and the small intestinal absorptive mucosa. Third, healthy, rather than diseased, residual small intestine is associated with decreased severity of malabsorption. Fourth, resection of jejunum is better tolerated than resection of ileum, as the capacity for bile salt and vitamin B_{12} absorption is specific to the ileum (Table 28-11).

During the first 1 to 2 years following massive small bowel resection, the remaining intestine undergoes compensatory adaptation, as discussed in the section on Intestinal Adaptation. Clinically, the period of adaptation is associated with reductions in volume and frequency of bowel movements, increases in the capacity for enteral nutrient assimilation, and reductions in TPN requirements. As this process completes, some patients are successfully weaned off TPN. Understanding the mechanisms mediating intestinal adaptation may suggest strategies for enhancing adaptation in patients with short bowel syndrome who are unable to achieve independence from TPN. To date, the phenomenon of intestinal adaptation in human patients remains poorly understood.[13]

Malabsorption in patients who have undergone massive small bowel resection is exacerbated by a characteristic hypergastrinemia-associated gastric acid hypersecretion that persists for 1 to 2 years postoperatively. The increased acid load delivered to the duodenum inhibits absorption by a variety of mechanisms, including the inhibition of digestive enzymes, most of which function optimally under alkaline conditions.

Therapy
Medical Therapy

For patients having undergone massive small bowel resection, the initial treatment priorities include management of the primary con-

---

TABLE 28-11	Risk factors for development of short bowel syndrome after massive small bowel resection

Small bowel length <200 cm
Absence of ileocecal valve
Absence of colon
Diseased remaining bowel (e.g., Crohn's disease)
Ileal resection

---

dition precipitating the intestinal resection and the repletion of fluid and electrolytes lost in the severe diarrhea that characteristically occurs. Most patients will require TPN, at least initially. Enteral nutrition should be gradually introduced, once ileus has resolved. High-dose histamine-2 receptor antagonists or proton pump inhibitors should be administered to reduce gastric acid secretion. Antimotility agents such as loperamide hydrochloride or diphenoxylate may be administered to delay small intestinal transit. Octreotide can be administered to reduce the volume of GI secretions, although, in animal models, its use is associated with an inhibition of intestinal adaptation.

During the period of adaptation, generally lasting 1 to 2 years postoperatively, TPN and enteral nutrition are titrated in an attempt to allow for independence from TPN. Patients who remain dependent on TPN face substantial TPN-associated morbidities including catheter sepsis, venous thrombosis, liver and kidney failure, and osteoporosis. Liver failure is a significant source of morbidity, and often leads to liver transplantation (always in combination with small bowel transplantation). Due to these complications, patients with short bowel syndrome on TPN have a reduced life expectancy with 5-year survival rates of 50 to 75%. Costs associated with chronic TPN administration are estimated to be as high as $150,000 per patient annually. Because of these problems, alternative therapies for short bowel syndrome are under investigation.

Nontransplant Surgical Therapy

Among patients with stomas, restoration of intestinal continuity should be performed whenever possible, to capitalize on the absorptive capacity of all residual intestine. Other forms of nontransplant surgery designed to improve intestinal absorption are associated with unclear efficacy and/or substantial morbidities and therefore should not be applied routinely.

The goal of these operations is to increase nutrient and fluid absorption by either slowing intestinal transit or increasing intestinal length. Operations designed to slow intestinal transit include segmental reversal of the small bowel, interposition of a segment of colon between segments of small bowel, construction of small intestinal valves, and electrical pacing of the small intestine.[67] Reported experience with these procedures is limited to case reports or series of a few cases. Objective evidence of increased absorption is lacking; further, these procedures are frequently associated with intestinal obstruction.

The intestinal lengthening operation for which there is the greatest experience is the longitudinal intestinal lengthening and tailoring procedure, first described by Bianchi in 1980.[68] Approximately 100 of these procedures have been reported in the literature. The procedure entails separation of the dual vasculature of the small intestine, followed by longitudinal division of the bowel with subsequent isoperistaltic end-to-end anastomosis. This procedure has the potential to double the length of small intestine to which it is applied. This procedure has generally been used for pediatric patients with *dilated* residual small bowel.

In 2003, the serial transverse enteroplasty procedure was described.[69] This procedure is designed to accomplish lengthening of dilated small intestine without the need for separating its dual vasculature (Fig. 28-30). Initial experimental studies and recent data from an international registry based in Boston have been promising.[70]

Intestinal Transplantation

This complex procedure is being increasingly performed to treat patients with short bowel syndrome. Approximately 1000 patients worldwide had undergone this procedure by 2003.[71] The currently accepted indication for intestinal transplantation is the presence of life-threatening complications attributable to intestinal failure and/or long-term TPN therapy. Specific complications for which intestinal transplantation is indicated include (a) impending or overt liver failure, (b) thrombosis of major central veins, (c) frequent episodes of catheter-related sepsis, and (d) frequent episodes of severe dehydration.

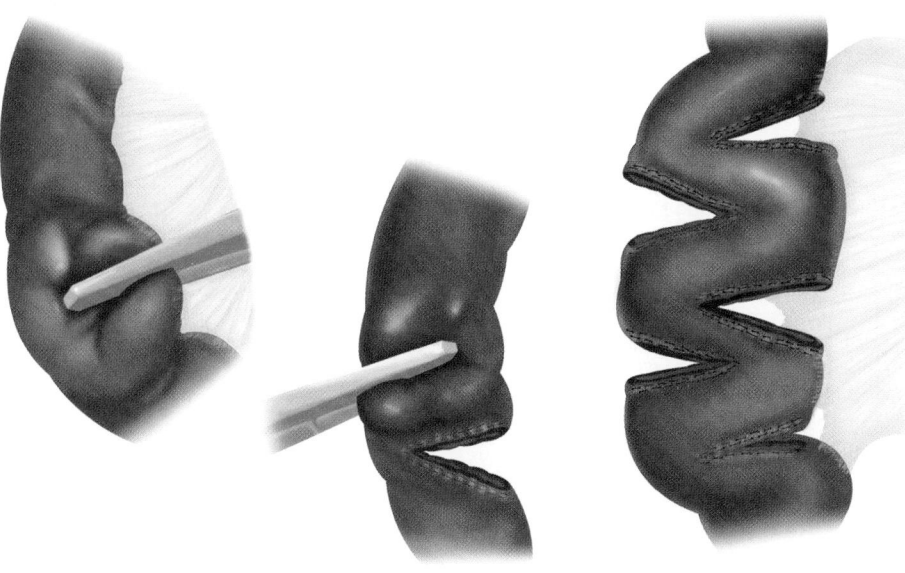

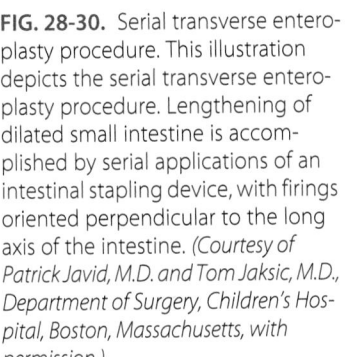

FIG. 28-30. Serial transverse entero-plasty procedure. This illustration depicts the serial transverse entero-plasty procedure. Lengthening of dilated small intestine is accomplished by serial applications of an intestinal stapling device, with firings oriented perpendicular to the long axis of the intestine. *(Courtesy of Patrick Javid, M.D. and Tom Jaksic, M.D., Department of Surgery, Children's Hospital, Boston, Massachusetts, with permission.)*

Currently, approximately 45% of transplants involving the small intestine are performed as isolated intestinal transplants, 40% as combined intestine/liver transplants, and 15% as multivisceral transplants.

Isolated intestinal transplantation is used for patients with intestinal failure who have no significant liver disease or failure of other organs. Combined intestine/liver transplantation is used for patients with both intestinal and liver failure. Multivisceral transplantation has been used for patients with giant desmoid tumors involving the vascular supply of the liver and pancreas as well as that of the intestine, for diffuse GI motility disturbances, and for diffuse splanchnic thrombosis.

Nearly 80% of survivors have full intestinal graft function with no need for TPN. However, morbidities associated with intestinal transplantation are substantial and include acute and chronic rejection, CMV infection, and posttransplant lymphoproliferative disease.

Alternative Therapies

Pharmacologic and biologic therapies designed to expand intestinal mucosal surface area or to enhance the efficiency of intestinal absorption are beginning to undergo clinical evaluation. Promising regimens include GLP-2 and the combination of glutamine and growth hormone with a modified, high-carbohydrate diet.[13]

Outcomes

Approximately 50 to 70% of patients with short bowel syndrome who initially require TPN are ultimately able to achieve independence from TPN.[66] Prognosis for achieving enteral autonomy is better among pediatric patients than among adults.

Information on survival among patients with short bowel syndrome is limited. In a study of 124 adults with short bowel syndrome due to nonmalignant etiologies, the survival rates at 2 and 5 years of follow-up were 86 and 45%, respectively.[72] Patients with end-enterostomies and those having less than 50 cm of residual small intestine had significantly worse survivals than those without these features.

No randomized trials comparing intestinal transplantation to chronic TPN administration among patients with short bowel syndrome have been reported. In the most recent United Network for Organ Sharing cohort evaluated, the 1-year patient and graft survival rates for isolated intestine recipients were 77 and 65%, respectively, and 50 and 49 percent, respectively, for intestine/liver recipients.[66] Five-year patient and graft survival rates for isolated intestine recipients were 50 and 38%, respectively, and for intestine/liver recipients, 37 and 36%, respectively.

REFERENCES

Entries highlighted in bright blue are key references.

1. Evers BM, Townsend CM, Thompson JC: Small intestine, in Schwartz S, Spencer F, Galloway A, et al (eds): *Principles of Surgery*, 7th ed. New York: McGraw-Hill, 1998, p 1217.
2. McMinn RMH: *Last's Anatomy—Regional and Applied*, 9th ed. Singapore: Churchill Livingstone, 1994, p 337.
3. Thomson ABR, Keelan M, Thiesen A, et al: Small bowel review: Normal physiology part 2. *Dig Dis Sci* 46:2588, 2001.
4. Lane JS, Whang EE, Rigberg DA, et al: Paracellular glucose transport plays a minor role in the unanesthetized dog. *Am J Physiol* 276:G276, 1999.
5. Ma T, Verkman AS: Aquaporin water channels in gastrointestinal physiology. *J Physiol* 517 (Pt 2):317, 1999.
6. Dyer J, Wood IS, Palejwala A, et al: Expression of monosaccharide transporters in intestine of diabetic humans. *Am J Physiol* 282:G241, 2002.
7. Vernaleken A, Veyhl M, Gorboulev V, et al: Tripeptides of RS1 (RSC1A1) inhibit a monosaccharide-dependent exocytotic pathway of Na+-D-glucose cotransporter SGLT1 with high affinity. *J Biol Chem* 282:28501, 2007.
8. Rolfs A, Hediger MA: Intestinal metal ion absorption: An update. *Curr Opin Gastroenterol* 17:177, 2001.
9. Nagler-Anderson C: Man the barrier! Strategic defenses in the intestinal mucosa. *Nat Rev Immunol* 1:59, 2001.
10. Mowat AM: Anatomical basis of tolerance and immunity to intestinal antigens. *Nat Rev Immunol* 3:331, 2003.
11. Ahlman H, Nilsson O: The gut as the largest endocrine organ in the body. *Ann Oncol* 12:S63, 2001.
12. Rehfeld JF: The new biology of gastrointestinal hormones. *Physiol Rev* 78:1087, 1998.
13. Tavakkolizadeh A, Whang EE: Understanding and augmenting human intestinal adaptation: A call for more clinical research. *J Parenter Enteral Nutr* 26:251, 2002.
14. Drucker DJ: Epithelial cell growth and differentiation. I. Intestinal growth factors. *Am J Physiol* 273:G3, 1997.
15. Drucker DJ: Gut adaptation and the glucagon-like peptides. *Gut* 50:428, 2002.
16. Ray NF, Denton WG, Thamer M, et al: Abdominal adhesiolysis: Inpatient care and expenditures in the United States in 1994. *J Am Coll Surg* 186:1, 1998.
17. Maglinte DD, Heitkamp DE, Howard TJ: Current concepts in imaging of small bowel obstruction. *Radiol Clin N Am* 41:263, 2003.
18. Abbas S, Bissett IP, Parry BR: Oral water soluble contrast for the management of adhesive small bowel obstruction. *Cochrane Database Syst Rev* 3:CD004651, 2007.

19. Brolin RE, Krasna MJ, Mast BA: Use of tubes and radiographs in the management of small bowel obstruction. *Ann Surg* 206:126, 1987.

20. Stewart RM, Page CP, Brender J, et al: The incidence and risk of early postoperative small bowel obstruction: A cohort study. *Am J Surg* 154:643, 1987.

21. Krouse RS, McCahill LE, Easson A, et al: When the sun can set on an unoperated bowel obstruction: Management of malignant bowel obstruction. *J Am Coll Surg* 195:117, 2002.

22. Ghosheh B, Salameh JR: Laparoscopic approach to acute small bowel obstruction: Review of 1061 cases. *Surg Endosc* 21:1945, 2007.

23. Foster NM, McGory ML, Zingmond DS, et al: Small bowel obstruction: A population-based appraisal. *J Am Coll Surg* 203:170, 2006.

24. Ellis H, Moran BJ, Thompson JN, et al: Adhesion-related hospital readmissions after abdominal and pelvic surgery: A retrospective cohort study. *Lancet* 353:1476, 1999.

25. Fazio VW, Cohen Z, Fleshman JW, et al: Reduction in adhesive small-bowel obstruction by Seprafilm adhesion barrier after intestinal resection. *Dis Colon Rectum* 49:1, 2006.

26. Lucky A, Livingstone E, Tache Y: Mechanisms and treatment of postoperative ileus. *Arch Surg* 138:206, 2003.

27. Charoenkwan K, Phillipson G, Vutyavanich T: Early versus delayed oral fluids and food for reducing complication after major abdominal gynecological surgery. *Cochrane Database Syst Rev* 4:CD004508, 2007.

28. Gendall KA, Kennedy RR, Watson AJ, et al: The effect of epidural analgesia on postoperative outcome after colorectal surgery. *Colorectal Dis* 9:584, 2007.

29. Noblett SE, Snowden CP, Shenton BK, et al: Randomized clinical trial assessing the effect of Doppler-optimized fluid management on outcome after elective colorectal resection. *Br J Surg* 93:1069, 2006.

30. Tan EK, Cornish J, Darzi AW, et al: Meta-analysis: Alvimopan vs. placebo in the treatment of post-operative ileus. *Aliment Pharmacol Ther* 25:47, 2007.

31. Loftus EV Jr., Schoenfeld P, Sandborn WJ: The epidemiology and natural history of Crohn's disease in population-based patient cohorts from North America: A systematic review. *Aliment Pharmacol Ther* 16:51, 2002.

32. Hugot JP, Chamaillard M, Zouali H, et al: Association of NOD leucin-rich repeat variants with susceptibility to Crohn's disease. *Nature* 411:599, 2001.

33. Ogura Y, Bonen DK, Inohara N, et al: A frameshift mutation in NOD2 associated with susceptibility to Crohn's disease. *Nature* 411:603, 2001.

34. Present DH, Rutgeerts P, Targan S, et al: Infliximab for the treatment of fistulas in patients with Crohn's disease. *N Engl J Med* 340:1398, 1999.

35. Nikolaus S, Schreiber S: Diagnosis of inflammatory bowel disease. *Gastroenterology* 133:1670, 2007.

36. Gardiner KR, Dasari BV: Operative management of small bowel Crohn's disease. *Surg Clin North Am* 87:587, 2007.

37. Solberg IC, Vatn MH, Hoie O, et al: Clinical course of Crohn's disease: Result of a Norwegian population-based ten-year follow up study. *Clin Gastroenterol Hepatol* 5:1430, 2007.

38. Fazio VW, Marchetti F, Church JM, et al: Effect of resection margins on the recurrence of Crohn's disease of the small bowel. *Ann Surg* 224:563, 1996.

39. Michelassi F, Upadhyay GA: Side-to-side isoperistaltic strictureplasty in the treatment of extensive Crohn's disease. *J Surg Res* 117:71, 2004.

40. Milsom JW, Hammerhofer KA, Bohm B, et al: Prospective, randomized trial comparing laparoscopic vs. conventional surgery for refractory ileocolic Crohn's disease. *Dis Colon Rectum* 44:1, 2001.

41. Tan JJ, Tjandra JJ: Laparoscopic surgery for Crohn's disease: A meta-analysis. *Dis Colon Rectum* 50:576, 2007.

42. Delaney CP, Fazio VW: Crohn's disease of the small bowel. *Surg Clin N Am* 81:137, 2001.

43. Penner RM, Madsen KL, Fedorak RN: Postoperative Crohn's disease. *Inflamm Bowel Dis* 11:765, 2005.

44. Evenson AR, Shrikhande G, Fischer JE: Abdominal abscess and enteric fistula, in Zinner MJ, Ashley SW (eds): *Maingot's Abdominal Operations*, 11th ed. New York: McGraw Hill, 2007, p 184.

45. Fazio VW, Coutsoftides T, Steiger E: Factors influencing the outcome of treatment of small bowel cutaneous fistula. *World J Surg* 7:481, 1983.

46. Jepsen JM, Persson M, Jakobsen NO, et al: Prospective study of prevalence and endoscopic and histopathologic characteristics of duodenal polyps in patients submitted to upper endoscopy. *Scand J Gastroenterol* 29:483, 1994.

47. Jemal A, Murray T, Sammuels A, et al: Cancer statistics, 2003. *CA Cancer J Clin* 53:5, 2003.

48. Hirota S, Isozaki K, Moriyama Y, et al: Gain-of-function mutations of *c-kit* in human gastrointestinal stromal tumors. *Science* 279:577, 1998.

49. Demetri GD, Mehren M, Blanke C, et al: Efficacy and safety of imatinib mesylate in advanced gastrointestinal stromal tumors. *N Engl J Med* 347:472, 2002.

50. Perez A, Saltzman JR, Carr-Locke DL, et al: Benign nonampullary duodenal neoplasms. *J Gastrointest Surg* 7:536, 2003.

51. Judson I, Demetri G: Advances in the treatment of gastrointestinal stromal tumors. *Ann Oncol* 18: S20, 2007.

52. Agrawal S, McCarron EC, Gibbs JF, et al: Surgical management and outcome in primary adenocarcinoma of the small bowel. *Ann Surg Onc* 14:2263, 2007.

53. Girvent M, Carlson GL, Anderson I, et al: Intestinal failure after surgery for complicated radiation enteritis. *Ann R Coll Surg Engl* 82:198, 2000.

54. Kiliç D, Egehan I, Ozenirler S, et al: Double-blinded, randomized, placebo-controlled study to evaluate the effectiveness of sulphasalazine in preventing acute gastrointestinal complications due to radiotherapy. *Radiother Oncol* 57:125, 2000.

55. Waddell BE, Lee RJ, Rodriguez-Bigas MA, et al: Absorbable mesh sling prevents radiation-induced bowel injury during "sandwich" chemoradiation for rectal cancer. *Arch Surg* 135:1212, 2000.

56. Yahchouchy EK, Marano AF, Etienne JC, et al: Meckel's diverticulum. *J Am Coll Surg* 192:654, 2001.

57. Cullen JJ, Kelly KA, Moir CR, et al: Surgical management of Meckel's diverticulum. An epidemiologic, population-based study. *Ann Surg* 220:564, 1994.

58. Lobo DN, Balfour TW, Iftikhar SY, et al: Periampullary diverticula and pancreaticobiliary disease. *Br J Surg* 86:588, 1999.

59. Chow DC, Babaian M, Taubin HL: Jejunoileal diverticula. *Gastroenterologist* 5:78, 1997.

60. Kumar S, Sarr MG, Kamath PS: Mesenteric venous thrombosis. *N Engl J Med* 345:1683, 2001.

61. Gralnek IM: Obscure-overt gastrointestinal bleeding. *Gastroenterology* 128:1424, 2005.

62. Szold A, Katz LB, Lewis BS: Surgical approach to occult gastrointestinal bleeding. *Am J Surg* 163:90, 1992.

63. Genzlinger JL, McPhee MS, Fisher JK, et al: Significance of retroperitoneal air after endoscopic retrograde cholangiopancreatography with sphincterotomy. *Am J Gastroenterol* 94:1267, 1999.

64. Nagorney DM, Sarr MG, McIlrath DC: Surgical management of intussusception in the adult. *Ann Surg* 193:230, 1981.

65. Duane TM, Wohlgemuth S, Ruffin K: Intussusception after Roux-en-Y gastric bypass. *Am J Surg* 66:82, 2000.

66. Buchman AL, Solapio J, Fryer J: AGA technical review on short bowel syndrome and intestinal transplantation. *Gastroenterology* 124:1111, 2003.

67. Thompson JS, Langnas AN: Surgical approaches to improving intestinal function in the short-bowel syndrome. *Arch Surg* 134:706, 1999.

68. Bianchi A: Intestinal loop lengthening—a technique for increasing small intestinal length: *J Pediatr Surg* 15:145, 1980.

69. Kim HB, Lee PW, Garza J, et al: Serial transverse enteroplasty for short bowel syndrome: A case report. *J Pedatr Surg* 38:881, 2003.

70. Modi BP, Javid PJ, Jaksic T, et al: First report of the international serial transverse enteroplasty data registry: Indications, efficacy, and complications. *J Am Coll Surg* 204:365, 2007.

71. Grant D, Abu-Elmagd K, Reyes J, et al: Intestine Transplant Registry 2003 report of the intestine transplant registry: A new era has dawned. *Ann Surg* 241:607, 2005.

72. Messing B, Crenn P, Beau P, et al: Long-term survival and parenteral nutrition dependence in adult patients with short bowel syndrome. *Gastroenterology* 117:1043, 1999.

CHAPTER 29

Colon, Rectum, and Anus

Kelli M. Bullard Dunn and David A. Rothenberger

EMBRYOLOGY AND ANATOMY

Embryology

The embryonic GI tract begins developing during the fourth week of gestation. The primitive gut is derived from the endoderm and divided into three segments: *foregut, midgut,* and *hindgut.* Both *midgut* and *hindgut* contribute to the colon, rectum, and anus.

The midgut develops into the small intestine, ascending colon, and proximal transverse colon, and receives blood supply from the superior mesenteric artery. During the sixth week of gestation, the midgut herniates out of the abdominal cavity, and then rotates 270° counterclockwise around the superior mesenteric artery to return to its final position inside the abdominal cavity during the tenth week of gestation.

The *hindgut* develops into the distal transverse colon, descending colon, rectum, and proximal anus, all of which receive their blood supply from the inferior mesenteric artery. During the sixth week of gestation, the distal-most end of the hindgut, the *cloaca,* is divided by the urorectal septum into the urogenital sinus and the rectum.

The distal anal canal is derived from ectoderm and receives its blood supply from the internal pudendal artery. The dentate line divides the endodermal hindgut from the ectodermal distal anal canal.

Anatomy

The large intestine extends from the ileocecal valve to the anus. It is divided anatomically and functionally into the *colon, rectum,* and *anal canal.* The wall of the colon and rectum comprise five distinct layers: mucosa, submucosa, inner circular muscle, outer longitudinal muscle, and serosa. In the colon, the outer longitudinal muscle is separated into three *teniae coli,* which converge proximally at the appendix and distally at the rectum, where the outer longitudinal muscle layer is circumferential. In the distal rectum, the inner smooth muscle layer coalesces to form the internal anal sphincter. The intraperitoneal colon and proximal one third of the rectum are covered by serosa; the mid and lower rectum lack serosa.

Colon Landmarks

The colon begins at the junction of the terminal ileum and cecum and extends 3 to 5 ft to the rectum. The rectosigmoid junction is found at approximately the level of the sacral promontory and is arbitrarily described as the point at which the three *teniae coli* coalesce to form the outer longitudinal smooth muscle layer of the rectum. The *cecum* is the widest diameter portion of the colon (normally 7.5 to 8.5 cm) and has the thinnest muscular wall. As a result, the cecum is most vulnerable to perforation and least vulnerable to obstruction. The ascending

colon usually is fixed to the retroperitoneum. The hepatic flexure marks the transition to the transverse colon. The intraperitoneal transverse colon is relatively mobile, but is tethered by the gastrocolic ligament and colonic mesentery. The greater omentum is attached to the anterior/superior edge of the transverse colon. These attachments explain the characteristic triangular appearance of the transverse colon observed during colonoscopy. The splenic flexure marks the transition from the transverse colon to the descending colon. The attachments between the splenic flexure and the spleen (the lienocolic ligament) can be short and dense, making mobilization of this flexure during colectomy challenging. The descending colon is relatively fixed to the retroperitoneum. The sigmoid colon is the narrowest part of the large intestine and is extremely mobile. Although the sigmoid colon usually is located in the left lower quadrant, redundancy and mobility can result in a portion of the sigmoid colon residing in the right lower quadrant. This mobility explains why volvulus is most common in the sigmoid colon and why diseases affecting the sigmoid colon, such as diverticulitis, may occasionally present as right-sided abdominal pain. The narrow caliber of the sigmoid colon makes this segment of the large intestine the most vulnerable to obstruction.

Colon Vascular Supply

The arterial supply to the colon is highly variable (Fig. 29-1). In general, the *superior mesenteric artery* branches into the *ileocolic artery* (absent in up to 20% of people), which supplies blood flow to the terminal ileum and proximal ascending colon, the *right colic artery,* which supplies the ascending colon, and the *middle colic artery,* which supplies the transverse colon. The *inferior mesenteric artery* branches into the *left colic artery,* which supplies the descending colon, several *sigmoidal branches,* which supply the sigmoid colon, and the *superior rectal artery,* which supplies the proximal rectum. The terminal branches of each artery form anastomoses with the terminal branches of the adjacent artery and communicate via the *marginal artery of Drummond.* This arcade is complete in only 15 to 20% of people.

Except for the *inferior mesenteric vein,* the veins of the colon parallel their corresponding arteries and bear the same terminology (Fig. 29-2). The inferior mesenteric vein ascends in the retroperitoneal plane over the psoas muscle and continues posterior to the pancreas to join the splenic vein. During a colectomy, this vein often is mobilized independently and ligated at the inferior edge of the pancreas.

Colon Lymphatic Drainage

The lymphatic drainage of the colon originates in a network of lymphatics in the muscularis mucosa. Lymphatic vessels and lymph nodes follow the regional arteries. Lymph nodes are found on the bowel wall

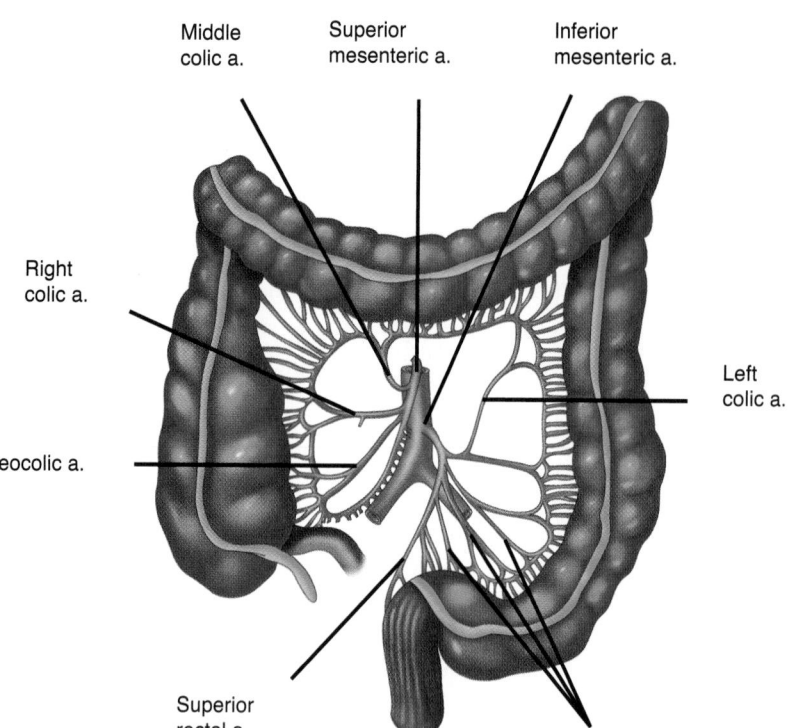

Middle
colic a.   Superior
mesenteric a.   Inferior
mesenteric a.

Right
colic a.

Left
colic a.

Ileocolic a.

Superior
rectal a.

Sigmoidal a.

FIG. 29-1. Arterial blood supply to the colon. a. = artery.

KEY POINTS

1. Resection principles: The mesenteric clearance technique dictates the extent of resection and is determined by the nature of the primary pathology, the intent of resection, the location of the lesion, and the condition of the mesentery.

2. Minimally invasive resection: Laparoscopic and/or hand-assisted laparoscopy has been shown to be both safe and efficacious for colorectal resection.

3. Function after resection: Bowel function is often compromised after colorectal resection, especially after low anterior resection. For this reason, it is important to obtain a history of prior anorectal trauma and/or incontinence before considering a low anastomosis.

4. Ostomies: Preoperative marking for a planned stoma is critical for a patient's quality of life. Ideally, a stoma should be located within the rectus muscle, in a location where the patient can easily see and manipulate the appliance, and away from previous scars, bony prominences, or abdominal creases.

5. Inflammatory bowel disease: Both Crohn's disease and ulcerative colitis are associated with an increased risk of colorectal carcinoma. Risk depends upon the amount of colon involved and the duration of disease.

6. Pathogenesis of colorectal cancer: A variety of mutations have been identified in colorectal cancer. Mutations may cause activation of oncogenes (K-ras) and/or inactivation of tumor-suppressor genes

[adenomatous polyposis coli (APC) < DCC (deleted in colorectal carcinoma), p53].

7. Early rectal cancer: Optimal treatment of very early rectal cancer (T1NXMX) is controversial. Transanal excision alone has been associated with a very high rate of local recurrence. In patients who will tolerate and accept radical surgery, this approach is probably appropriate. Chemoradiation either before or after transanal excision can also be considered, but has not been prospectively studied.

8. Anal epidermoid carcinoma: Unlike rectal adenocarcinoma, anal epidermoid carcinoma is treated primarily with chemoradiation. Surgery is reserved for patients with persistent or recurrent disease.

9. Rectal prolapse: Rectal prolapse occurs most commonly in elderly women. Transabdominal repair (rectopexy with or without resection) offers more durability than perineal proctosigmoidectomy, but carries greater operative risk.

10. Hemorrhoids: Hemorrhoids are cushions of submucosal tissue containing venules, arterioles, and smooth muscle fiber. They are thought o play a role in maintaining continence. Resection is only indicated for refractory symptoms.

11. Fistula in ano: Treatment of fistula in ano depends upon the location of the fistula, amount of anal sphincter involved in the fistula, and the underlying disease process.

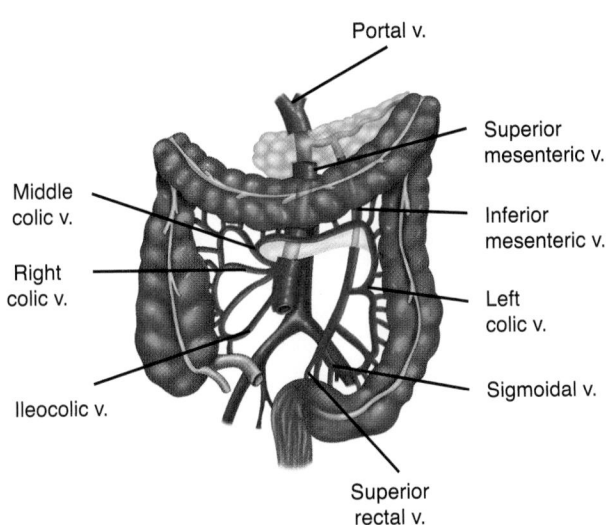

FIG. 29-2. Venous drainage of the colon. v. = vein. *[Reproduced with permission from Bell RH, Rikkers LF, Mulholland M (eds):* Digestive Tract Surgery: A Text and Atlas. *Philadelphia: Lippincott Williams & Wilkins, 1996, p 1459.]*

(epicolic), along the inner margin of the bowel adjacent to the arterial arcades (paracolic), around the named mesenteric vessels (intermediate), and at the origin of the superior and inferior mesenteric arteries (main). The *sentinel lymph nodes* are the first one to four lymph nodes to drain a specific segment of the colon, and are thought to be the first site of metastasis in colon cancer. The use of sentinel lymph node dissection and analysis in colon cancer remains controversial.

Colon Nerve Supply

The colon is innervated by both *sympathetic* (inhibitory) and *parasympathetic* (stimulatory) nerves, which parallel the course of

the arteries. Sympathetic nerves arise from T6–T12 and L1–L3. The parasympathetic innervation to the right and transverse colon is from the vagus nerve; the parasympathetic nerves to the left colon arise from sacral nerves S2–S4 to form the nervi erigentes.

Anorectal Landmarks

The rectum is approximately 12 to 15 cm in length. Three distinct submucosal folds, the *valves of Houston*, extend into the rectal lumen. Posteriorly, the *presacral fascia* separates the rectum from the presacral venous plexus and the pelvic nerves. At S4, the rectosacral fascia (*Waldeyer's fascia*) extends forward and downward and attaches to the fascia propria at the anorectal junction. Anteriorly, *Denonvilliers' fascia* separates the rectum from the prostate and seminal vesicles in men and from the vagina in women. The *lateral ligaments* support the lower rectum. The surgical anal canal measures 2 to 4 cm in length and generally is longer in men than in women. It begins at the anorectal junction and terminates at the anal verge. The *dentate* or *pectinate line* marks the transition point between columnar rectal mucosa and squamous anoderm. The 1 to 2 cm of mucosa just proximal to the dentate line shares histologic characteristics of columnar, cuboidal, and squamous epithelium and is referred to as the *anal transition zone*. The dentate line is surrounded by longitudinal mucosal folds, known as the *columns of Morgagni*, into which the anal crypts empty. These crypts are the source of cryptoglandular abscesses (Fig. 29-3).

In the distal rectum, the inner smooth muscle is thickened and comprises the *internal anal sphincter* that is surrounded by the *subcutaneous, superficial,* and *deep external sphincter*. The *deep external anal sphincter* is an extension of the *puborectalis muscle*. The *puborectalis, iliococcygeus,* and *pubococcygeus muscles* form the *levator ani muscle* of the pelvic floor (Fig. 29-4).

Anorectal Vascular Supply

The *superior rectal artery* arises from the terminal branch of the inferior mesenteric artery and supplies the upper rectum. The *middle rectal artery* arises from the internal iliac; the presence and size of these arteries are highly variable. The *inferior rectal artery* arises from

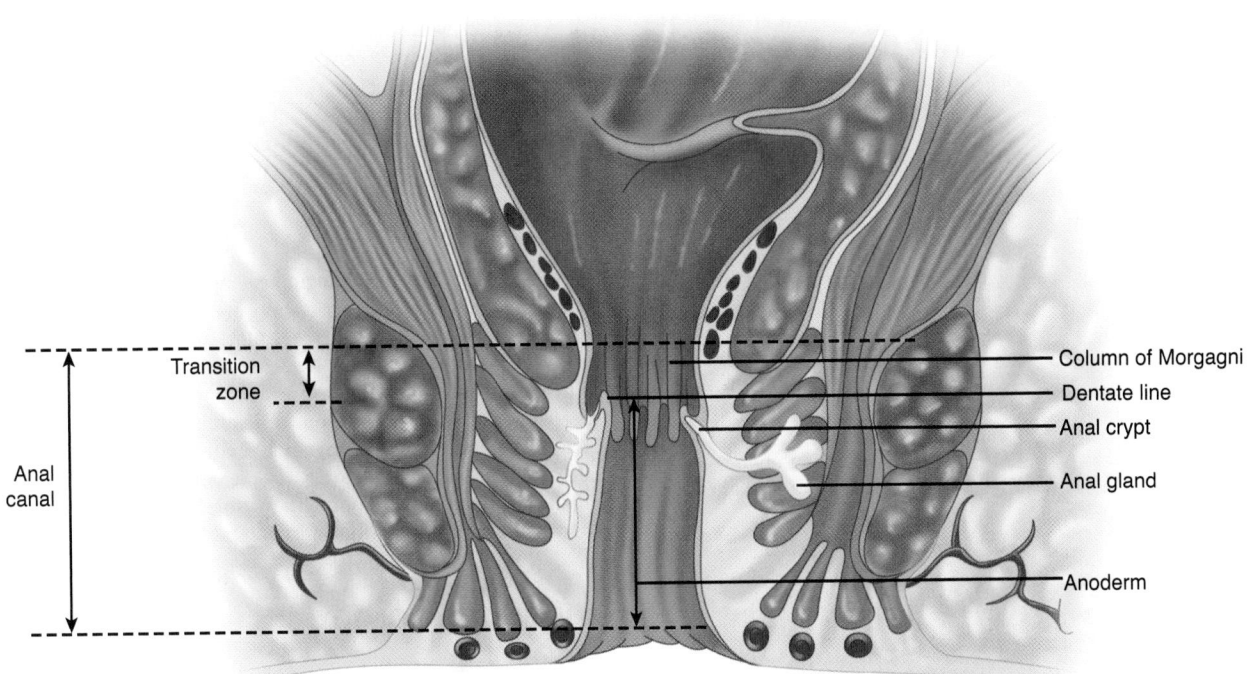

FIG. 29-3. The lining of the anal canal. *[From Goldberg SM, Gordon PH, Nivatvongs S (eds):* Essentials of Anorectal Surgery. *Philadelphia: J.B. Lippincott Company, 1980, p 4. Reproduced with permission from Stanley M. Goldberg, MD.]*

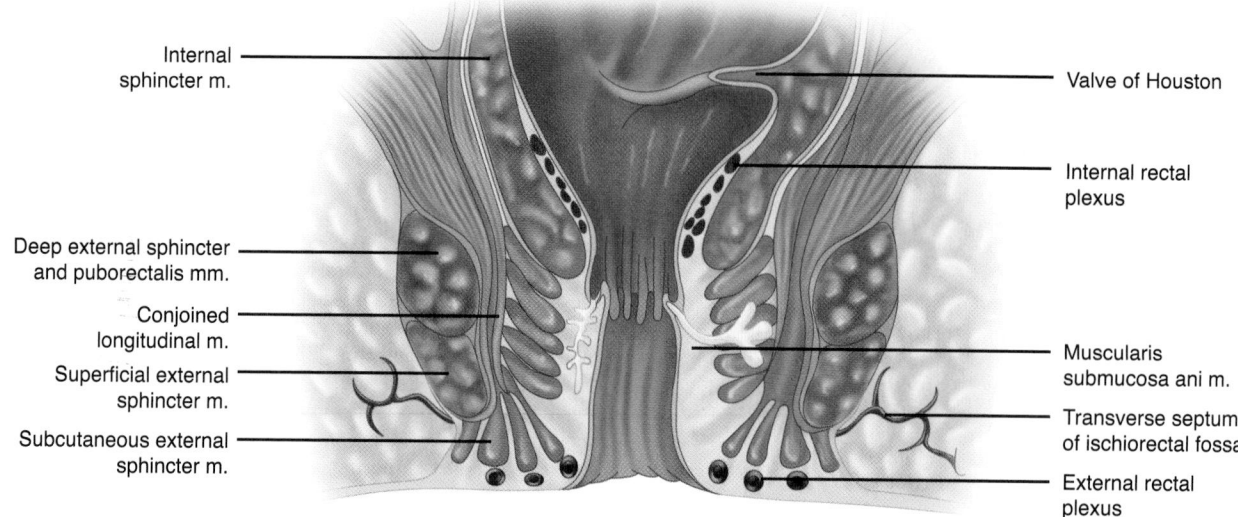

Internal
sphincter m.

Deep external sphincter
and puborectalis mm.

Conjoined
longitudinal m.

Superficial external
sphincter m.

Subcutaneous external
sphincter m.

Valve of Houston

Internal rectal
plexus

Muscularis
submucosa ani m.

Transverse septum
of ischiorectal fossa

External rectal
plexus

FIG. 29-4. The distal rectum and anal canal. m. = muscle.

the internal pudendal artery, which is a branch of the internal iliac artery. A rich network of collaterals connects the terminal arterioles of each of these arteries, thus making the rectum relatively resistant to ischemia (Fig. 29-5).

The venous drainage of the rectum parallels the arterial supply. The *superior rectal vein* drains into the portal system via the inferior mesenteric vein. The *middle rectal vein* drains into the internal iliac vein. The *inferior rectal vein* drains into the internal pudendal vein, and subsequently into the internal iliac vein. A submucosal plexus deep to the columns of Morgagni forms the *hemorrhoidal plexus* and drains into all three veins.

Anorectal Lymphatic Drainage

Lymphatic drainage of the rectum parallels the vascular supply. Lymphatic channels in the upper and middle rectum drain superiorly into the inferior mesenteric lymph nodes. Lymphatic channels in the lower rectum drain both superiorly into the inferior mesenteric lymph nodes and laterally into the internal iliac lymph nodes. The anal canal has a more complex pattern of lymphatic drainage. Proximal to the dentate line, lymph drains into both the inferior mesenteric lymph nodes and the internal iliac lymph nodes. Distal to the dentate

line, lymph primarily drains into the inguinal lymph nodes, but also can drain into the inferior mesenteric lymph nodes and internal iliac lymph nodes.

Anorectal Nerve Supply

Both sympathetic and parasympathetic nerves innervate the anorectum. Sympathetic nerve fibers are derived from L1–L3 and join the preaortic plexus. The preaortic nerve fibers then extend below the aorta to form the *hypogastric plexus*, which subsequently joins the parasympathetic fibers to form the pelvic plexus. Parasympathetic nerve fibers are known as the *nervi erigentes* and originate from S2–S4. These fibers join the sympathetic fibers to form the pelvic plexus. Sympathetic and parasympathetic fibers then supply the anorectum and adjacent urogenital organs.

The internal anal sphincter is innervated by sympathetic and parasympathetic nerve fibers; both types of fibers inhibit sphincter contraction. The external anal sphincter and puborectalis muscles are innervated by the *inferior rectal branch* of the *internal pudendal nerve*. The levator ani receives innervation from both the *internal pudendal nerve* and direct branches of S3 to S5. Sensory innervation to the anal canal is provided by the *inferior rectal branch* of the *pudendal nerve*. Although the rectum is relatively insensate, the anal canal below the dentate line is sensate.

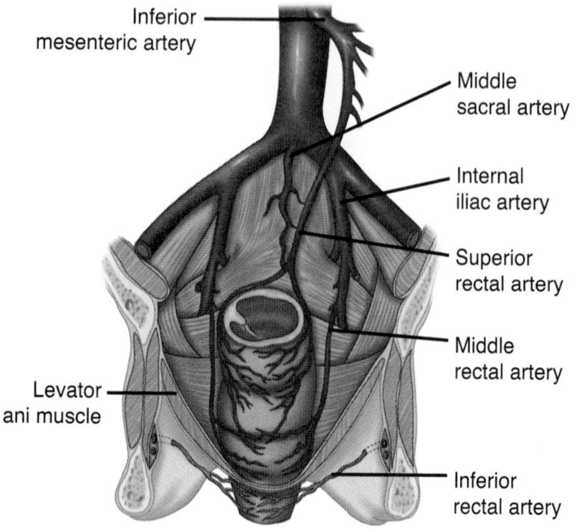

Congenital Anomalies

Perturbation of the embryologic development of the midgut and hindgut may result in anatomic abnormalities of the colon, rectum, and anus. Failure of the midgut to rotate and return to the abdominal cavity during the tenth week of gestation results in varying degrees of intestinal malrotation and colonic nonfixation. Failure of canalization of the primitive gut can result in colonic duplication. Incomplete descent of the urogenital septum may result in imperforate anus and associated fistulas to the genitourinary tract. Many infants with congenital anomalies of the hindgut have associated abnormalities in the genitourinary tract.

NORMAL PHYSIOLOGY

Fluid and Electrolyte Exchanges

The colon is a major site for water absorption and electrolyte exchange. Approximately 90% of the water contained in ileal fluid is absorbed in the colon (1000 to 2000 mL/d), and up to 5000 mL of

Inferior
mesenteric artery

Middle
sacral artery

Internal
iliac artery

Superior
rectal artery

Middle
rectal artery

Levator
ani muscle

Inferior
rectal artery

FIG. 29-5. Arterial supply to the rectum and anal canal.

fluid can be absorbed daily. Sodium is absorbed actively via a Na-K ATPase. The colon can absorb up to 400 mEq of sodium per day. Water accompanies the transported sodium and is absorbed passively along an osmotic gradient. Potassium is actively secreted into the colonic lumen and absorbed by passive diffusion. Chloride is absorbed actively via a chloride–bicarbonate exchange.

Bacterial degradation of protein and urea produces ammonia. Ammonia is subsequently absorbed and transported to the liver. Absorption of ammonia depends, in part, upon intraluminal pH. A decrease in colonic bacteria (e.g., broad-spectrum antibiotic usage) and/or a decrease in intraluminal pH (e.g., lactulose administration) will decrease ammonia absorption.

Short-Chain Fatty Acids

Short-chain fatty acids (acetate, butyrate, and propionate) are produced by bacterial fermentation of dietary carbohydrates. Short-chain fatty acids are an important source of energy for the colonic mucosa, and metabolism by colonocytes provides energy for processes such as active transport of sodium. Lack of a dietary source for production of short-chain fatty acids, or diversion of the fecal stream by an ileostomy or colostomy, may result in mucosal atrophy and "diversion colitis."

Colonic Microflora and Intestinal Gas

Approximately 30% of fecal dry weight is composed of bacteria (10^{11} to 10^{12} bacteria/g of feces). Anaerobes are the predominant class of microorganism, and *Bacteroides* species are the most common (10^{11} to 10^{12} organisms/mL). *Escherichia coli* are the most numerous aerobes (10^8 to 10^{10} organisms/mL). Endogenous microflora are crucial for the breakdown of carbohydrates and proteins in the colon and participate in the metabolism of bilirubin, bile acids, estrogen, and cholesterol. Colonic bacteria also are necessary for production of vitamin K. Endogenous bacteria also are thought to suppress the emergence of pathogenic microorganisms, such as *Clostridium difficile*. However, the high bacterial load of the large intestine may contribute to sepsis in critically ill patients and may contribute to intra-abdominal sepsis, abscess, and wound infection following colectomy.

Intestinal gas arises from swallowed air, diffusion from the blood, and intraluminal production. Nitrogen, oxygen, carbon dioxide, hydrogen, and methane are the major components of intestinal gas. Nitrogen and oxygen are largely derived from swallowed air. Carbon dioxide is produced by the reaction of bicarbonate and hydrogen ions, and by the digestion of triglycerides to fatty acids. Hydrogen and methane are produced by colonic bacteria. The production of methane is highly variable. The GI tract usually contains between 100 and 200 mL of gas and 400 to 1200 mL per day are released as flatus, depending upon the type of food ingested.

Motility, Defecation, and Continence
Motility

Unlike the small intestine, the large intestine does not demonstrate cyclic motor activity characteristic of the migratory motor complex. Instead, the colon displays intermittent contractions of either low or high amplitude. Low-amplitude, short-duration contractions occur in bursts and appear to move the colonic contents both antegrade and retrograde. It is thought that these bursts of motor activity delay colonic transit and thus increase the time available for absorption of water and exchange of electrolytes. High-amplitude contractions occur in a more coordinated fashion and create "mass movements." Bursts of "rectal motor complexes" also have been described. In general, cholinergic activation increases colonic motility.

Defecation

Defecation is a complex, coordinated mechanism involving colonic mass movement, increased intra-abdominal and rectal pressure, and relaxation of the pelvic floor. Distention of the rectum causes a reflex relaxation of the internal anal sphincter (the rectoanal inhibitory reflex) that allows the contents to make contact with the anal canal. This "sampling reflex" allows the sensory epithelium to distinguish solid stool from liquid stool and gas. If defecation does not occur, the rectum relaxes and the urge to defecate passes (the *accommodation response*). Defecation proceeds by coordination of increasing intra-abdominal pressure via the Valsalva maneuver, increased rectal contraction, relaxation of the puborectalis muscle, and opening of the anal canal.

Continence

The maintenance of fecal continence is at least as complex as the mechanism of defecation. Continence requires adequate rectal wall compliance to accommodate the fecal bolus, appropriate neurogenic control of the pelvic floor and sphincter mechanism, and functional internal and external sphincter muscles. At rest, the puborectalis muscle creates a "sling" around the distal rectum, forming a relatively acute angle that distributes intra-abdominal forces onto the pelvic floor. With defecation, this angle straightens, allowing downward force to be applied along the axis of the rectum and anal canal. The internal and external sphincters are tonically active at rest. The internal sphincter is responsible for most of the resting, involuntary sphincter tone (resting pressure). The external sphincter is responsible for most of the voluntary sphincter tone (squeeze pressure). Branches of the pudendal nerve innervate both the internal and external sphincter. Finally, the hemorrhoidal cushions may contribute to continence by mechanically blocking the anal canal. Thus, impaired continence may result from poor rectal compliance, injury to the internal and/or external sphincter or puborectalis, or nerve damage or neuropathy.

CLINICAL EVALUATION

Clinical Assessment

A complete history and physical examination is the starting point for evaluating any patient with suspected disease of the colon and rectum. Special attention should be paid to the patient's past medical and surgical history to detect underlying conditions that might contribute to a GI problem. If patients have had prior intestinal surgery, it is essential that one understand the resultant GI anatomy. A history of anorectal surgery may be critical for patients with either abdominal or anorectal complaints. Obstetric history in women is essential to suspect occult pelvic floor and/or anal sphincter damage. A family history of colorectal disease, especially inflammatory bowel disease, polyps, and colorectal cancer, is crucial. In addition to family history of colorectal disease, history of other malignancies may suggest the presence of a genetic syndrome. Medication use must be detailed as many drugs cause GI symptoms. Before recommending operative intervention, the adequacy of medical treatment must be ascertained. In addition to examining the abdomen, visual inspection of the anus and perineum and careful digital rectal exam are essential.

Endoscopy
Anoscopy

The anoscope is a useful instrument for examination of the anal canal. Anoscopes are made in a variety of sizes and measure approximately 8 cm in length. A larger anoscope provides better exposure for anal procedures such as rubber band ligation or sclerotherapy of hemorrhoids. The anoscope, with obturator in place, should be adequately lubricated and gently inserted into the anal canal. The obturator is withdrawn, inspection of the visualized anal canal is done, and the anoscope should then be withdrawn. It is rotated 90° and reinserted to allow visualization of all four quadrants of the canal. If the patient complains of severe perianal pain and cannot tolerate a digital rectal examination, anoscopy should not be attempted without anesthesia.

Proctoscopy

The rigid proctoscope is useful for examination of the rectum and distal sigmoid colon and occasionally is used therapeutically. The standard proctoscope is 25 cm in length and available in various diameters. Most often, a 15- or 19-mm diameter proctoscope is used for diagnostic examinations. The large (25-mm diameter) proctoscope is useful for procedures such as polypectomy, electrocoagulation, or detorsion of a sigmoid volvulus. A smaller "pediatric" proctoscope (11-mm diameter) is better tolerated by patients with anal stricture. Suction is necessary for an adequate proctoscopic examination.

Flexible Sigmoidoscopy and Colonoscopy

Video or fiber-optic flexible sigmoidoscopy and colonoscopy provide excellent visualization of the colon and rectum. Sigmoidoscopes measure 60 cm in length. Full depth of insertion may allow visualization as high as the splenic flexure, although the mobility and redundancy of the sigmoid colon often limit the extent of the examination. Partial preparation with enemas usually is adequate for sigmoidoscopy and most patients can tolerate this procedure without sedation. Colonoscopes measure 100 to 160 cm in length and are capable of examining the entire colon and terminal ileum. A complete oral bowel preparation usually is necessary for colonoscopy and the duration and discomfort of the procedure usually require conscious sedation. Both sigmoidoscopy and colonoscopy can be used diagnostically and therapeutically. Electrocautery generally should not be used in the absence of a complete bowel preparation because of the risk of explosion of intestinal methane or hydrogen gases. Diagnostic colonoscopes possess a single channel through which instruments such as snares, biopsy forceps, or electrocautery can be passed; this channel also provides suction and irrigation capability. Therapeutic colonoscopes possess two channels to allow simultaneous suction/irrigation and the use of snares, biopsy forceps, or electrocautery.

Capsule Endoscopy

Capsule endoscopy is an emerging technology that uses a small ingestible camera. After swallowing the camera, images of the mucosa of the GI tract are captured, transmitted by radiofrequency to a belt-held receiver, then downloaded to a computer for viewing and analysis. At present, capsule endoscopy largely has been used to detect small bowel lesions. However, it has been suggested that this technique might also be useful for diagnosing colorectal disease.[1–3] At present, the use of capsule endoscopy in the evaluation of colorectal disease remains unproven.

Imaging
Plain X-Rays and Contrast Studies

Despite advanced radiologic techniques, plain x-rays and contrast studies continue to play an important role in the evaluation of patients with suspected colon and rectal diseases. Plain x-rays of the abdomen (supine, upright, and diaphragmatic views) are useful for detecting free intra-abdominal air, bowel gas patterns suggestive of small or large bowel obstruction, and volvulus. Contrast studies are useful for evaluating obstructive symptoms, delineating fistulous tracts, and diagnosing small perforations or anastomotic leaks. While Gastrografin cannot provide the mucosal detail provided by barium, this water-soluble contrast agent is recommended if perforation or leak is suspected. Double-contrast barium enema has been reported to be 70 to 90% sensitive for the detection of mass lesions greater than 1 cm in diameter.[4] Detection of small lesions can be extremely difficult, especially in a patient with extensive diverticulosis. For this reason, a colonoscopy is preferred for evaluating nonobstructing mass lesions in the colon. Double-contrast barium enema has been used as a back-up examination if colonoscopy is incomplete.

Computed Tomography

Computed tomography (CT) is commonly used in the evaluation of patients with abdominal complaints. Its utility is primarily in the detection of extraluminal disease, such as intra-abdominal abscesses and pericolic inflammation, and in staging colorectal carcinoma, because of its sensitivity in detection of hepatic metastases. Extravasation of oral or rectal contrast also may confirm the diagnosis of perforation or anastomotic leak. Nonspecific findings such as bowel wall thickening or mesenteric stranding may suggest inflammatory bowel disease, enteritis/colitis, or ischemia. A standard CT scan is relatively insensitive for the detection of intraluminal lesions.

Virtual Colonoscopy/Computed Tomography Colography

Virtual colonoscopy (CT colography) is a new radiologic technique that is designed to overcome some of the limitations of traditional CT scanning. This technology uses helical CT and three-dimensional reconstruction to detect intraluminal colonic lesions. Oral bowel preparation, oral and rectal contrast, and colon insufflation are used to maximize sensitivity. Early evaluation of virtual colonoscopy suggests that accuracy may approach that of colonoscopy for detection of lesions 1 cm in diameter or greater.

Magnetic Resonance Imaging

The main use of magnetic resonance imaging (MRI) in colorectal disorders is in evaluation of pelvic lesions. MRI is more sensitive than CT for detecting bony involvement or pelvic sidewall extension of rectal tumors. MRI accurately determines the extent of spread of rectal cancer into the adjacent mesorectum and can reliably predict difficulty achieving radial margin clearance of a rectal cancer by surgery alone. When the radial margin is threatened, neoadjuvant chemoradiation generally is indicated. MRI also can be helpful in the detection and delineation of complex fistulas in ano. The use of an endorectal coil may increase sensitivity.

Positron Emission Tomography

Positron emission tomography (PET) is used for imaging tissues with high levels of anaerobic glycolysis, such as malignant tumors.[18] F-fluorodeoxyglucose is injected as a tracer; metabolism of this molecule then results in positron emission. PET has been used as an adjunct to CT in the staging of colorectal cancer and may prove useful in discriminating recurrent cancer from fibrosis. The combination of PET and CT technology recently has been introduced. By combining these modalities, anatomic correlation between regions of high isotope accumulation ("hot spots") on PET and abnormalities on CT can be determined. PET/CT increasingly is used to diagnose recurrent and/or metastatic colorectal cancer. However, the efficacy and use of this technology remains unproven.

Angiography

Angiography occasionally is used for the detection of bleeding within the colon or small bowel. To visualize hemorrhage angiographically, bleeding must be relatively brisk (approximately 0.5 to 1.0 mL per minute). If extravasation of contrast is identified, infusion of vasopressin or angiographic embolization can be therapeutic.

CT and MR angiography also are useful for assessing patency of visceral vessels. This technique uses three dimensional reconstruction to detect vascular lesions. If an abnormality is found, more traditional techniques (angiography, surgery) may then be used to further define and/or correct the problem.

Endorectal and Endoanal Ultrasound

Endorectal ultrasound is primarily used to evaluate the depth of invasion of neoplastic lesions in the rectum. The normal rectal wall appears as a five-layer structure (Fig. 29-6). Ultrasound can reliably differentiate most benign polyps from invasive tumors based upon the integrity of the submucosal layer. Ultrasound also can differentiate superficial T1–T2 from deeper T3–T4 tumors. Overall, the accuracy of ultrasound in detecting depth of mural invasion ranges between 81 and 94%.[5] This modality also can detect enlarged perirectal lymph nodes, which may suggest nodal metastases; accu-

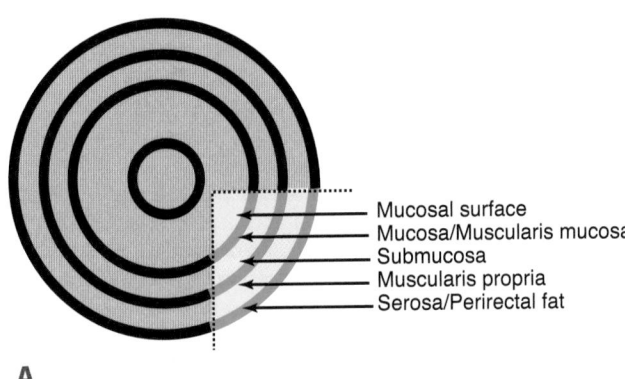

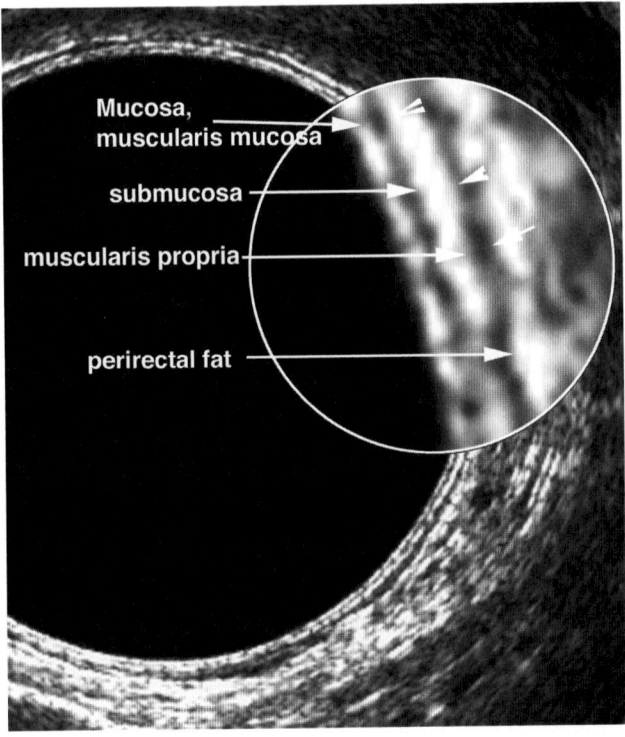

A

B

Mucosal surface
Mucosa/Muscularis mucosa
Submucosa
Muscularis propria
Serosa/Perirectal fat

Mucosa,
muscularis mucosa

submucosa

muscularis propria

perirectal fat

FIG. 29-6. **A.** Schematic of the layers of the rectal wall observed on endorectal ultrasonography. **B.** Normal endorectal ultrasonography. (*A. Courtesy of Charles O. Finne III, MD, Minneapolis, MN.*)

through the anal canal and pressures recorded. A balloon attached to the tip of the catheter also can be used to test anorectal sensation. The *resting pressure* in the anal canal reflects the function of the internal anal sphincter (normal: 40 to 80 mmHg), while the *squeeze pressure*, defined as the maximum voluntary contraction pressure minus the resting pressure, reflects function of the external anal sphincter (normal: 40 to 80 mmHg above resting pressure). The *high-pressure zone* estimates the length of the anal canal (normal: 2.0 to 4.0 cm). The *rectoanal inhibitory reflex* can be detected by inflating a balloon in the distal rectum; absence of this reflex is characteristic of Hirschsprung's disease.

Neurophysiology

Neurophysiologic testing assesses function of the pudendal nerves and recruitment of puborectalis muscle fibers. Pudendal nerve terminal motor latency measures the speed of transmission of a nerve impulse through the distal pudendal nerve fibers (normal: 1.8 to 2.2 milliseconds); prolonged latency suggests the presence of neuropathy. Electromyography (EMG) recruitment assesses the contraction and relaxation of the puborectalis muscle during attempted defecation. Normally, recruitment increases when a patient is instructed to "squeeze," and decreases when a patient is instructed to "push." Inappropriate recruitment is an indication of paradoxical contraction (nonrelaxation of the puborectalis). Needle EMG has been used to map both the pudendal nerves and the anatomy of the internal and external sphincters. However, this examination is painful and poorly tolerated by most patients. Needle EMG has largely been replaced by pudendal nerve motor-latency testing to assess pudendal nerve function and endoanal ultrasound to map the sphincters.

Rectal Evacuation Studies

Rectal evacuation studies include the balloon expulsion test and video defecography. Balloon expulsion assesses a patient's ability to expel an intrarectal balloon. Video defecography provides a more detailed assessment of defecation. In this test, barium paste is placed in the rectum and defecation is then recorded fluoroscopically. Defecography is used to differentiate nonrelaxation of the puborectalis, obstructed defecation, increased perineal descent, rectal prolapse and intussusception, rectocele, and enterocele. The addition of vaginal contrast and intraperitoneal contrast is useful in delineating complex disorders of the pelvic floor.

Laboratory Studies
Fecal Occult Blood Testing

Fecal occult blood testing (FOBT) is used as a screening test for colonic neoplasms in asymptomatic, average-risk individuals. The efficacy of this test is based upon serial testing because the majority of colorectal malignancies will bleed intermittently. FOBT has been a nonspecific test for peroxidase contained in hemoglobin; consequently, occult bleeding from any GI source will produce a positive result. Similarly, many foods (red meat, some fruits and vegetables, and vitamin C) will produce a false-positive result. Patients were counseled to eat a restricted diet for 2 to 3 days before the test. Increased specificity is now possible by using immunochemical FOBT. These tests rely on monoclonal or polyclonal antibodies to react with the intact globin portion of human hemoglobin. Because globin does not survive in the upper GI tract, the immunochemical tests are more specific for identifying occult bleeding from the colon or rectum. Dietary restrictions are not necessary. Any positive FOBT mandates further investigation, usually by colonoscopy.

Stool Studies

Stool studies often are helpful in evaluating the etiology of diarrhea. Wet-mount examination reveals the presence of fecal leukocytes, which may suggest colonic inflammation or the presence of an invasive organism such as invasive *E. coli* or *Shigella*. Stool cultures can detect pathogenic bacteria, ova, and parasites. *C. difficile* colitis

racy of detection of pathologically positive lymph nodes is 58 to 83%. Ultrasound may also prove useful for early detection of local recurrence after surgery.

Endoanal ultrasound is used to evaluate the layers of the anal canal. Internal anal sphincter, external anal sphincter, and puborectalis muscle can be differentiated. Endoanal ultrasound is particularly useful for detecting sphincter defects and for outlining complex anal fistulas.

Physiologic and Pelvic Floor Investigations

Anorectal physiologic testing uses a variety of techniques to investigate the function of the pelvic floor. These techniques are useful in the evaluation of patients with incontinence, constipation, rectal prolapse, obstructed defecation, and other disorders of the pelvic floor.

Manometry

Anorectal manometry is performed by placing a pressure-sensitive catheter in the lower rectum. The catheter is then withdrawn is diagnosed by detecting bacterial toxin in the stool.[6] Steatorrhea may be diagnosed by adding Sudan red stain to a stool sample.

Serum Tests

Specific laboratory tests that should be performed will be dictated by the clinical scenario. Preoperative studies generally include a complete blood count and electrolyte panel. The addition of coagulation studies, liver function tests, and blood typing/cross-matching depends upon the patient's medical condition and the proposed surgical procedure.

Tumor Markers

Carcinoembryonic antigen (CEA) may be elevated in 60 to 90% of patients with colorectal cancer. Despite this, CEA is not an effective screening tool for this malignancy. Many practitioners follow serial CEA levels after curative-intent surgery to detect early recurrence of colorectal cancer. However, this tumor marker is nonspecific, and no survival benefit has yet been proven. Other biochemical markers (ornithine decarboxylase, urokinase) have been proposed, but none has yet proven sensitive or specific for detection, staging, or predicting prognosis of colorectal carcinoma.[7]

Genetic Testing

Although familial colorectal cancer syndromes, such as familial adenomatous polyposis (FAP) and hereditary nonpolyposis colon cancer (HNPCC) are rare, information about the specific genetic abnormalities underlying these disorders has led to significant interest in the role of genetic testing for colorectal cancer.[8] Tests for mutations in the adenomatous polyposis coli (APC) gene responsible for FAP, and in mismatch repair genes responsible for HNPCC, are commercially available and extremely accurate in families with known mutations. However, in the absence of an identified mutation, a negative result is uninformative. For individuals from high-risk families without an identified mutation, increased surveillance is recommended.[9] Although many of these mutations also are present in sporadic colorectal cancer, the accuracy of genetic testing in average-risk individuals is considerably lower and these tests are not recommended for screening. Because of the potential psychosocial implications of genetic testing, it is strongly recommended that professional genetic counselors be involved in the care of any patient considering these tests.

Evaluation of Common Symptoms

Pain

Abdominal pain is a nonspecific symptom with a myriad of causes. Abdominal pain related to the colon and rectum can result from obstruction (either inflammatory or neoplastic), inflammation, perforation, or ischemia. Plain x-rays and judicious use of contrast studies and/or a CT scan often can confirm the diagnosis. Gentle retrograde contrast studies (barium or Gastrografin enema) may be useful in delineating the degree of colonic obstruction. Sigmoidoscopy and/or colonoscopy performed by an experienced endoscopist can assist in the diagnosis of ischemic colitis, infectious colitis, and inflammatory bowel disease. However, if perforation is suspected, colonoscopy and/or sigmoidoscopy generally are contraindicated. Evaluation and treatment of abdominal pain from a colorectal source should follow the usual surgical principles of a thorough history and physical examination, appropriate diagnostic tests, resuscitation, and appropriately timed surgical intervention.

Pelvic pain can originate from the distal colon and rectum or from adjacent urogenital structures. Tenesmus may result from proctitis or from a rectal or retrorectal mass. Cyclical pain associated with menses, especially when accompanied by rectal bleeding, suggests a diagnosis of endometriosis. Pelvic inflammatory disease also can produce significant abdominal and pelvic pain. The extension of a peridiverticular abscess or periappendiceal abscess into the pelvis may also cause pain. CT scan and/or MRI may be useful in differentiating these diseases. Proctoscopy (if tolerated) also can be helpful. Occasionally, laparoscopy will yield a diagnosis.

Anorectal pain is most often secondary to an anal fissure, perirectal abscess and/or fistula, or a thrombosed hemorrhoid. Physical examination usually can differentiate these conditions. Other, less common causes of anorectal pain include anal canal neoplasms, perianal skin infection, and dermatologic conditions. Proctalgia fugax results from levator spasm and may present without any other anorectal findings. Physical examination is critical in evaluating patients with anorectal pain. If a patient is too tender to examine in the office, an examination under anesthesia is necessary. MRI or other imaging studies may be helpful in select cases where the etiology of pain is elusive.

Lower Gastrointestinal Bleeding

The first goal in evaluating and treating a patient with GI hemorrhage is adequate resuscitation. The principles of ensuring a patent airway, supporting ventilation, and optimizing hemodynamic parameters apply and coagulopathy and/or thrombocytopenia should be corrected. The second goal is to identify the source of hemorrhage. Because the most common source of GI hemorrhage is esophageal, gastric, or duodenal, nasogastric aspiration should always be performed; return of bile suggests that the source of bleeding is distal to the ligament of Treitz. If aspiration reveals blood or nonbile secretions, or if symptoms suggest an upper intestinal source, esophagogastroduodenoscopy is performed. Anoscopy and/or limited proctoscopy can identify hemorrhoidal bleeding. A technetium-99–tagged red blood cell scan is extremely sensitive and is able to detect as little as 0.1 mL/h of bleeding; however, localization is imprecise. If the technetium-99–tagged red blood cell scan is positive, angiography can then be used to localize bleeding. Infusion of vasopressin or angioembolization may be therapeutic. Alternatively, a catheter can be left in the bleeding vessel to allow localization at the time of laparotomy. If the patient is hemodynamically stable, a rapid bowel preparation (over 4 to 6 hours) can be performed to allow colonoscopy. Colonoscopy may identify the cause of the bleeding, and cautery or injection of epinephrine into the bleeding site may be used to control hemorrhage. Colectomy may be required if bleeding persists despite these interventions. Intraoperative colonoscopy and/or enteroscopy may assist in localizing bleeding. If colectomy is required, a segmental resection is preferred if the bleeding source can be localized. "Blind" subtotal colectomy may very rarely be required in a patient who is hemodynamically unstable with ongoing colonic hemorrhage of an unknown source. In this setting, it is crucial to irrigate the rectum and examine the mucosa by proctoscopy to ensure that the source of bleeding is not distal to the resection margin (Fig. 29-7).

Occult blood loss from the GI tract may manifest as iron-deficiency anemia or may be detected with FOBT. Because colon neoplasms bleed intermittently and rarely present with rapid hemorrhage, the presence of occult fecal blood should always prompt a colonoscopy. Unexplained iron-deficiency anemia is also an indication for colonoscopy.

Hematochezia commonly is caused by hemorrhoids or fissure. Sharp, knife-like pain and bright-red rectal bleeding with bowel movements suggest the diagnosis of fissure. Painless, bright-red rectal bleeding with bowel movements often is secondary to a friable internal hemorrhoid that is easily detected by anoscopy. In the absence of a painful, obvious fissure, any patient with rectal bleeding should undergo a careful digital rectal examination, anoscopy, and proctosigmoidoscopy. Failure to diagnose a source in the distal anorectum should prompt colonoscopy.

Constipation and Obstructed Defecation

Constipation is an extremely common complaint, affecting more than 4 million people in the United States. Despite the prevalence of this problem, there is lack of agreement about an appropriate

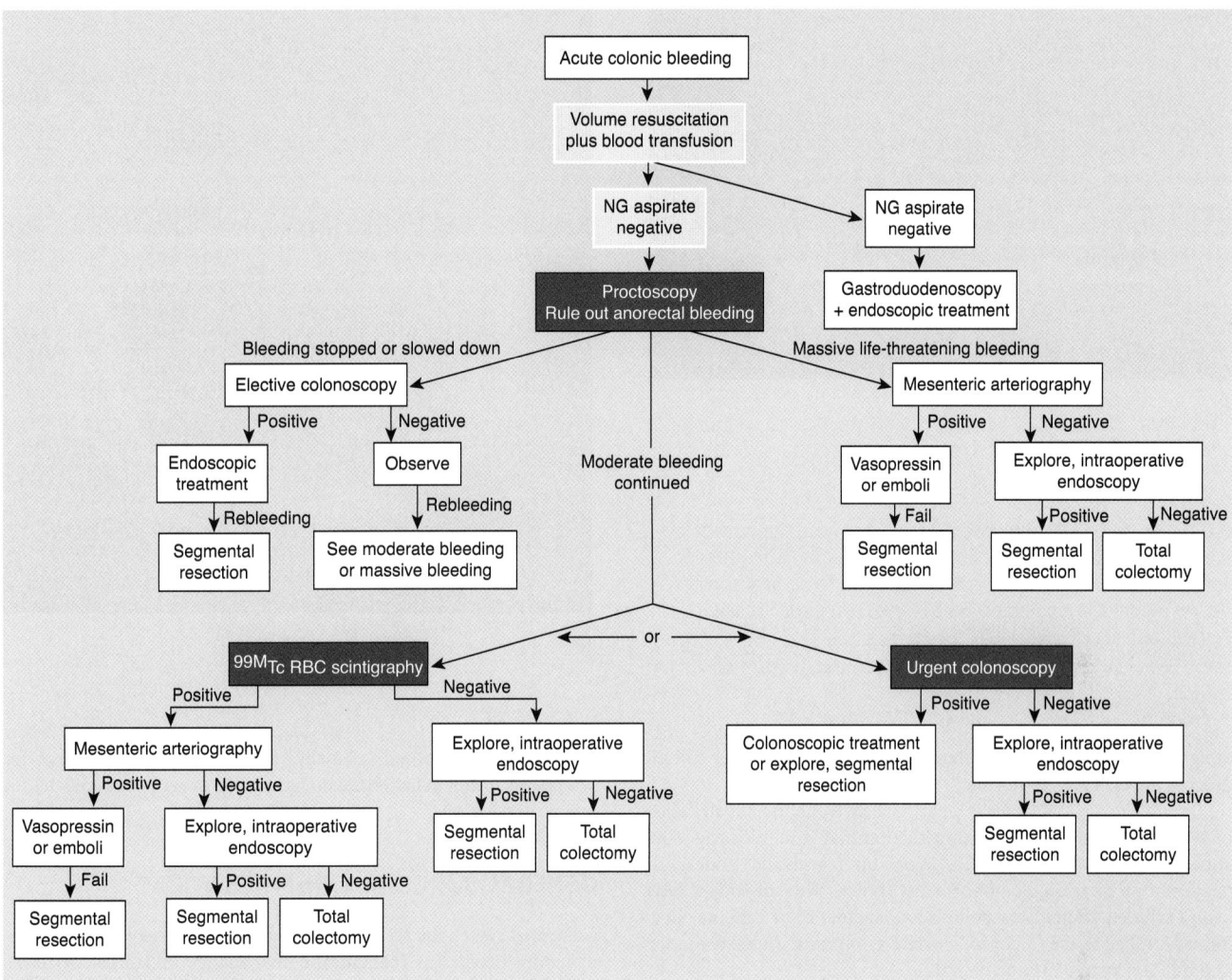

FIG. 29-7. Algorithm for treatment of colorectal hemorrhage. NG = nasogastric; ^{99m}Tc = technetium-99; RBC = red blood cell. *[Reproduced with permission from Gordon PH, Nivatvongs S (eds): Principles and Practice of Surgery for the Colon, Rectum, and Anus, 2nd ed. New York: Marcel Dekker, Inc., 1999, p 1279.]*

definition of constipation. Patients may describe infrequent bowel movements, hard stools, or excessive straining. A careful history of these symptoms often clarifies the nature of the problem.

Constipation has a myriad of causes. Underlying metabolic, pharmacologic, endocrine, psychological, and neurologic causes often contribute to the problem. A stricture or mass lesion should be excluded by colonoscopy or barium enema. After these causes have been excluded, evaluation focuses on differentiating *slow-transit constipation* from *outlet obstruction*. Transit studies, in which radiopaque markers are swallowed and then followed radiographically, are useful for diagnosing slow-transit constipation. Anorectal manometry and EMG can detect nonrelaxation of the puborectalis, which contributes to outlet obstruction. The absence of an anorectal inhibitory reflex suggests Hirschsprung's disease and may prompt a rectal mucosal biopsy. Defecography can identify rectal prolapse, intussusception, rectocele, or enterocele.

Medical management is the mainstay of therapy for constipation and includes fiber, increased fluid intake, and laxatives. Outlet obstruction from nonrelaxation of the puborectalis often responds to biofeedback.[10] Surgery to correct rectocele and rectal prolapse has a variable effect on symptoms of constipation, but can be successful in selected patients. Subtotal colectomy is considered only for patients with severe slow-transit constipation (colonic inertia) refractory to maximal medical interventions. Although this operation almost always increases bowel movement frequency, complaints of diarrhea,

incontinence, and abdominal pain are not infrequent, and patients should be carefully selected.[11]

Diarrhea and Irritable Bowel Syndrome

Diarrhea is also a common complaint and is usually a self-limited symptom of infectious gastroenteritis. If diarrhea is chronic or is accompanied by bleeding or abdominal pain, further investigation is warranted. Bloody diarrhea and pain are characteristic of colitis; etiology can be an infection (invasive *E. coli, Shigella, Salmonella, Campylobacter, Entamoeba histolytica,* or *C. difficile*), inflammatory bowel disease (ulcerative colitis or Crohn's colitis), or ischemia. Stool wetmount and culture often can diagnose infection. Sigmoidoscopy or colonoscopy can be helpful in diagnosing inflammatory bowel disease or ischemia. However, if the patient has abdominal tenderness, particularly with peritoneal signs, or any other evidence of perforation, endoscopy is contraindicated.

Chronic diarrhea may present a more difficult diagnostic dilemma. Chronic ulcerative colitis, Crohn's colitis, infection, malabsorption, and short-gut syndrome can cause chronic diarrhea. Rarely, carcinoid syndrome and islet cell tumors (vasoactive intestinal peptide-secreting tumor, somatostatinoma, gastrinoma) present with this symptom. Large villous lesions may cause secretory diarrhea. Collagenous colitis can cause diarrhea without any obvious mucosal abnormality. Along with stool cultures, tests for malabsorption, and metabolic investigations, colonoscopy can be invaluable in differenti-

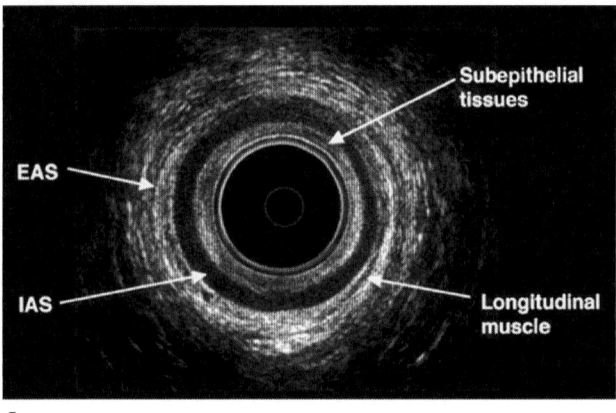

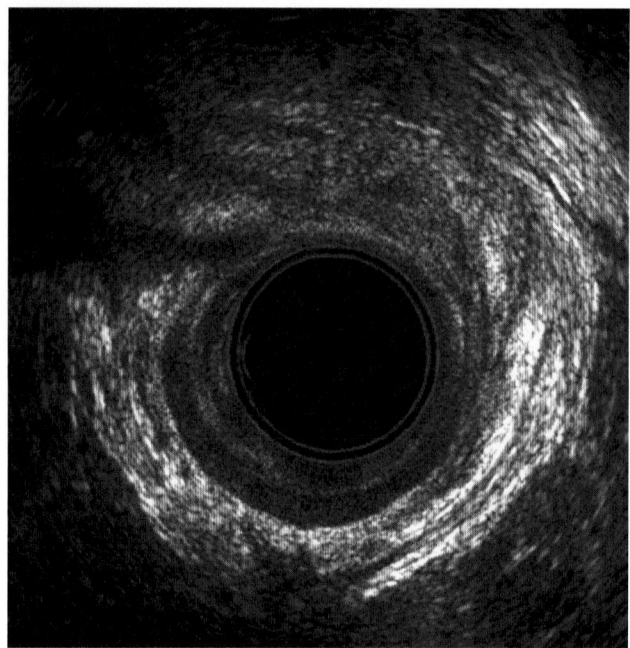

FIG. 29-8. A. Endoanal ultrasonography showing the normal layers of the anal canal. **B.** Endoanal ultrasonography with anterior sphincter defect from birthing injury. EAS = external anal sphincter; IAS = internal anal sphincter. *(Both images courtesy of Charles O. Finne III, MD, Minneapolis, MN.)*

ating these causes. Biopsies should be taken even if the colonic mucosa appears grossly normal.

Irritable bowel syndrome is a particularly troubling constellation of symptoms consisting of crampy abdominal pain, bloating, constipation, and urgent diarrhea. Work-up reveals no underlying anatomic or physiologic abnormality. Once other disorders have been excluded, dietary restrictions and avoidance of caffeine, alcohol, and tobacco may help to alleviate symptoms. Antispasmodics and bulking agents may be helpful.

Incontinence

The incidence of fecal incontinence has been estimated to occur in 10 to 13 individuals per 1000 people older than age 65 years. Incontinence ranges in severity from occasional leakage of gas and liquid stool to daily loss of solid stool. The underlying cause of incontinence is often multifactorial and diarrhea often is contributory. In general, causes of incontinence can be classified as *neurogenic* or *anatomic*. Neurogenic causes include diseases of the central nervous system and spinal cord along with pudendal nerve injury. Anatomic causes include congenital abnormalities, procidentia, overflow incontinence secondary to impaction or neoplasm, and trauma. The most common traumatic cause of incontinence is injury to the anal sphincter during vaginal delivery. Other causes include anorectal surgery, impalement, and pelvic fracture.

After a thorough medical evaluation to detect underlying conditions that might contribute to incontinence, evaluation focuses on assessment of the anal sphincter and pudendal nerves. Pudendal nerve terminal motor latency testing may detect neuropathy. Anal manometry can detect low resting and squeeze pressures. Defecography can detect rectal prolapse. Endoanal ultrasound is invaluable in diagnosing sphincter defects (Fig. 29-8).

Therapy depends upon the underlying abnormality. Diarrhea should be treated medically (fiber, antidiarrheal agents). Even in the absence of frank diarrhea, the addition of dietary fiber may improve continence. Some patients may respond to biofeedback. Many patients with a sphincter defect are candidates for an overlapping sphincteroplasty. Innovative technologies that focus on stimulating the sacral nerve roots via an implantable nerve stimulator or replacing a damaged or poorly functioning sphincter with an artificial sphincter are proving useful in patients who fail other interventions.[12,13] The delivery of radiofrequency energy to the anal canal (the Secca procedure)

also has been proposed.[14] Finally, a stoma can provide relief for severely incontinent patients who have failed or are not candidates for other interventions.[15]

GENERAL SURGICAL CONSIDERATIONS

Colorectal resections are performed for a wide variety of conditions, including neoplasms (benign and malignant), inflammatory bowel diseases, and other benign conditions. Although the indication and urgency for surgery will alter some of the technical details, the operative principles of colorectal resections, anastomoses, and use of ostomies are well established. These principles and general considerations for anesthesia and other operative preliminaries are outlined here.

Resections

The mesenteric clearance technique dictates the extent of colonic resection and is determined by the nature of the primary pathology (malignant or benign), the intent of the resection (curative or palliative), the precise location(s) of the primary pathology, and the condition of the mesentery (thin and soft or thickened and indurated). In general, a proximal mesenteric ligation will eliminate the blood supply to a greater length of colon and require a more extensive "colectomy." Curative resection of a colorectal cancer usually is accomplished best by performing a proximal mesenteric vessel ligation and radical mesenteric clearance of the lymphatic drainage basin of the tumor site with concomitant resection of the overlying omentum (Fig. 29-9). Resection of a benign process does not require wide mesenteric resection and the omentum can be preserved, if desired.

Emergency Resection

Emergency resection may be required because of obstruction, perforation, or hemorrhage. In this setting, the bowel is almost always unprepared and the patient may be unstable. The surgical principles described above in Resections apply and an attempt should be made to resect the involved segment along with its lymphovascular supply. If the resection involves the right colon or proximal transverse colon (right or extended right colectomy), a primary ileocolonic anastomosis usually can be performed safely as long as the remaining bowel appears healthy and the patient is stable. For left-sided tumors, the

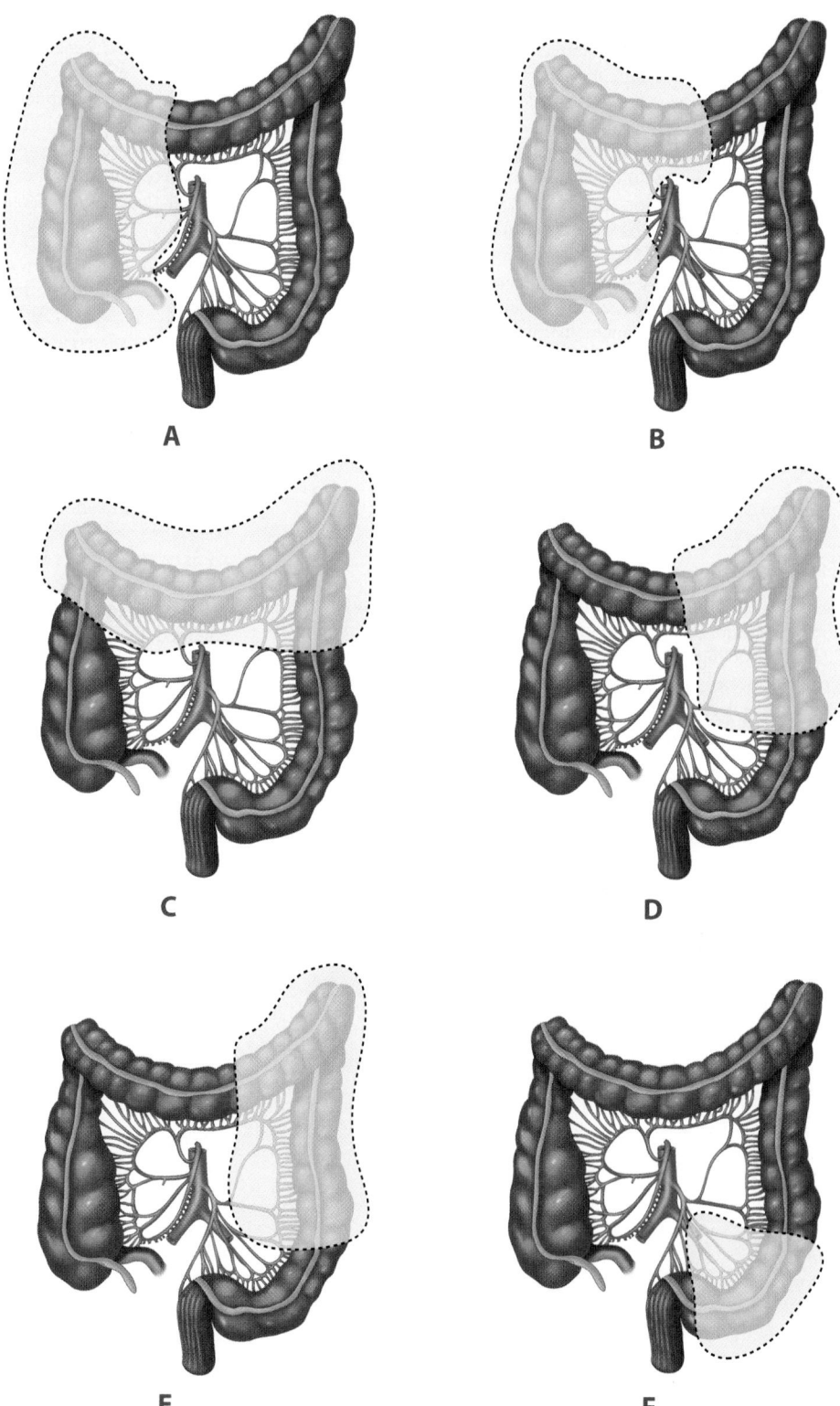

FIG. 29-9. Extent of resection for carcinoma of the colon. **A.** Cecal cancer. **B.** Hepatic flexure cancer. **C.** Transverse colon cancer. **D.** Splenic flexure cancer. **E.** Descending colon cancer. **F.** Sigmoid colon cancer.

traditional approach has involved resection of the involved bowel and end colostomy, with or without a mucus fistula. However, there is an increasing body of data to suggest that a primary anastomosis without a bowel preparation or with an on-table lavage, with or without a diverting ileostomy, may be equally safe in this setting. If the proximal colon looks unhealthy (vascular compromise, serosal tears, perforation), a subtotal colectomy can be performed with a small bowel to rectosigmoid anastomosis. Resection and diversion (ileostomy or colostomy) remains safe and appropriate if the bowel

looks compromised or if the patient is unstable, malnourished, or immunosuppressed.

Minimally Invasive Techniques of Resection

With advances in minimally invasive technology, many procedures that previously have required laparotomy can now be performed *laparoscopically* or *with hand-assisted laparoscopy*. Potential advantages of laparoscopy include improved cosmetic result, decreased postoperative pain, and earlier return of bowel function. Moreover, some experimental data suggest that minimally invasive operations have less immunosuppressive impact on the patient and thus might improve postoperative outcome and even long-term survival. To date, most studies have demonstrated equivalence between laparoscopic and open resection in terms of extent of resection. However, laparoscopic colon resections are technically demanding and consistently require longer operative time than do open procedures. Return of bowel function and length of hospital stay are highly variable. Long-term outcome has yet to be determined; however, short-term quality of life appears to be improved by laparoscopy.[16] As training in minimally invasive techniques improves, laparoscopic colon resection increasingly is gaining popularity.

The most recent advances in minimally invasive surgery involves use of robotics and telemanipulation in which the surgeon operates from a console remote from the patient. Robotic colectomy has been performed and appears to be technically feasible.[17] However, to date there has been no demonstrated advantage for robotic resection over laparoscopic resection.

Colectomy

A variety of terms are used to describe different types of colectomy (Fig. 29-10).

Ileocolic Resection An ileocolic resection describes a limited resection of the terminal ileum, cecum, and appendix. It is used to remove disease involving these segments of the intestine (e.g., ileocecal Crohn's disease) and benign lesions or incurable cancers arising in the terminal ileum, cecum, and, occasionally, the appendix. If curable malignancy is suspected, more radical resections, such as a right hemicolectomy, generally are indicated. The ileocolic vessels are ligated and divided. A variable length of small intestine may be resected, depending upon the disease process. A primary anastomosis is created between the distal small bowel and the ascending colon. It is technically difficult to perform an anastomosis at or just proximal to the ileocecal valve; therefore, if the most distal ileum needs to be resected, the cecum generally also is removed.

Right Colectomy A right colectomy is used to remove lesions or disease in the right colon and is oncologically the most appropriate operation for curative intent resection of proximal colon carcinoma. The ileocolic vessels, right colic vessels, and right branches of the middle colic vessels are ligated and divided. Approximately 10 cm of terminal ileum usually are included in the resection. A primary ileal-transverse colon anastomosis is almost always possible.

Extended Right Colectomy An extended right colectomy may be used for curative intent resection of lesions located at the hepatic flexure or proximal transverse colon. A standard right colectomy is extended to include ligation of the middle colic vessels at their base. The right colon and proximal transverse colon are resected, and a primary anastomosis is created between the distal ileum and distal transverse colon. Such an anastomosis relies on the marginal artery of Drummond. If the blood supply is questionable, the resection is extended to include the splenic flexure and the anastomosis of ileum is to the descending colon.

Transverse Colectomy Lesions in the mid and distal transverse colon may be resected by ligating the middle colic vessels and resecting the transverse colon, followed by a colocolonic anastomosis. However, an extended right colectomy with an anastomosis between the terminal ileum and descending colon may be a safer anastomosis with an equivalent functional result.

Left Colectomy For lesions or disease states confined to the distal transverse colon, splenic flexure, or descending colon, a left colectomy is performed. The left branches of the middle colic vessels, the left colic vessels, and the first branches of the sigmoid vessels are ligated. A colocolonic anastomosis usually can be performed.

Extended Left Colectomy An extended left colectomy is an option for removing lesions in the distal transverse colon. In this operation, the left colectomy is extended proximally to include the right branches of the middle colic vessels.

Sigmoid Colectomy Lesions in the sigmoid colon require ligation and division of the sigmoid branches of the inferior mesenteric artery. In general, the entire sigmoid colon should be resected to the level of the peritoneal reflection and an anastomosis created between the descending colon and upper rectum. Full mobilization of the splenic flexure often is required to create a tension-free anastomosis.

Total and Subtotal Colectomy Total or subtotal colectomy occasionally is required for patients with fulminant colitis, attenuated FAP (AFAP), or synchronous colon carcinomas. In this procedure, the ileocolic vessels, right colic vessels, middle colic vessels, and left colic vessels are ligated and divided. The superior rectal vessels are preserved. If it is desired to preserve the sigmoid, the distal sigmoid vessels are left intact and an anastomosis is created between the ileum and distal sigmoid colon (subtotal colectomy with ileosigmoid anastomosis). If the sigmoid is to be resected, the sigmoidal vessels are ligated and divided, and the ileum is anastomosed to the upper rectum (total abdominal colectomy with ileorectal anastomosis). If an anastomosis is contraindicated, an end-ileostomy is created and the remaining sigmoid or rectum is managed either as a mucus fistula or a Hartmann pouch.

Proctocolectomy

Total Proctocolectomy In this procedure, the entire colon, rectum, and anus are removed and the ileum is brought to the skin as a Brooke ileostomy.

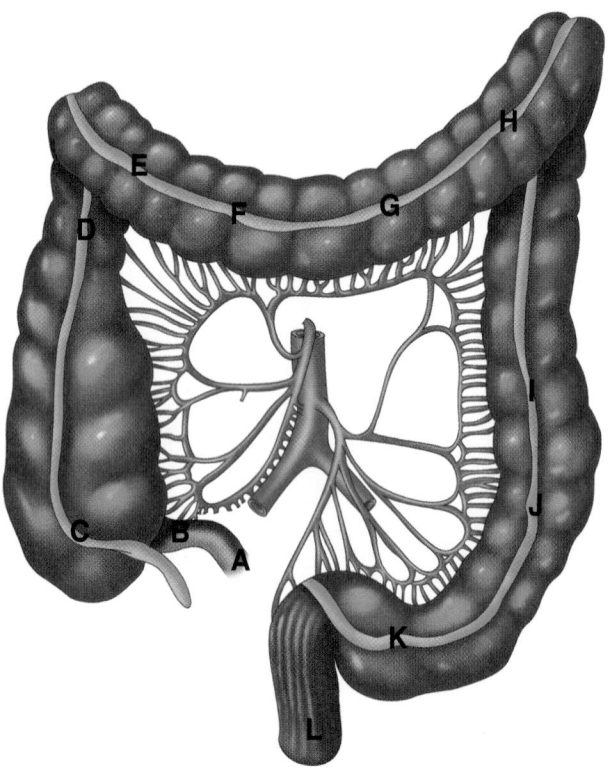

FIG. 29-10. Terminology of types of colorectal resections: A→C Ileocecectomy; + A + B→D Ascending colectomy; + A + B→F Right hemicolectomy; + A + B→G Extended right hemicolectomy; + E + F→G + H Transverse colectomy; G→I Left hemicolectomy; F→I Extended left hemicolectomy; J + K Sigmoid colectomy; + A + B→J Subtotal colectomy; + A + B→K Total colectomy; + A + B→L Total proctocolectomy. *[Reproduced with permission from Fielding LP, Goldberg SM (eds): Rob & Smith's Operative: Surgery of the Colon, Rectum, and Anus. UK: Elsevier Science Ltd., 1993, p 349.]*

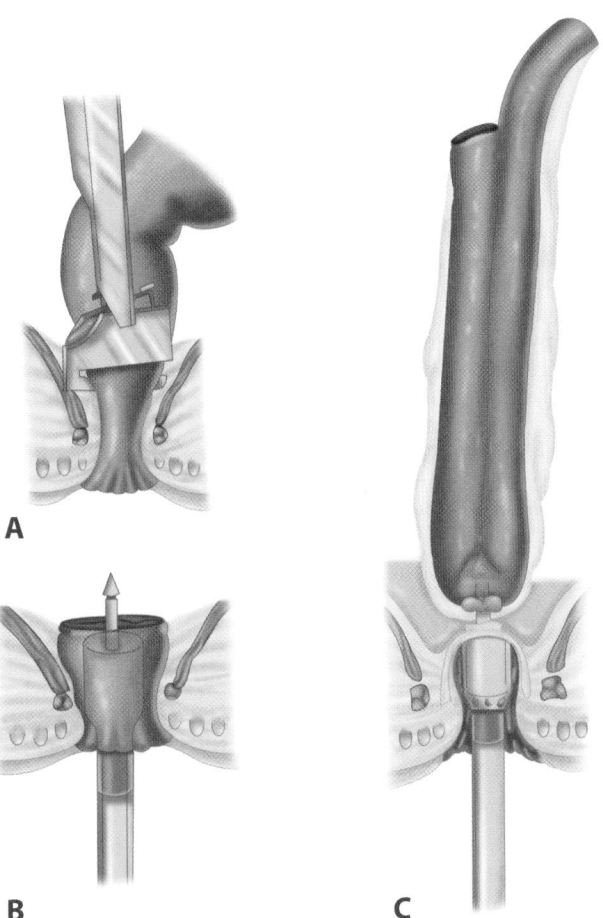

FIG. 29-11. After a total colectomy and resection of the rectum (**A**), the anal canal with a short cuff of transitional mucosa and sphincter muscles is preserved (**B**). An ileal J-pouch has been constructed and is anastomosed to the anal canal using a double-staple technique (**C**). *[Reproduced with permission from Bell RH, Rikkers LF, Mulholland M (eds): Digestive Tract Surgery: A Text and Atlas.* Philadelphia: Lippincott Williams & Wilkins, 1996, p 1527.]

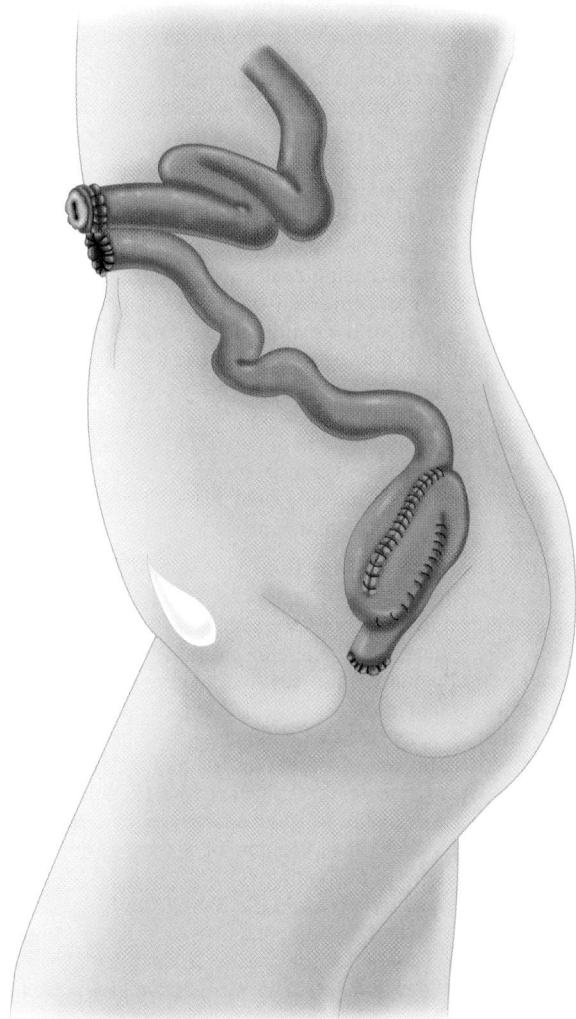

FIG. 29-12. Ileal S-pouch anal anastomosis with temporary loop ileostomy. *[Reproduced with permission from Bell RH, Rikkers LF, Mulholland M (eds):* Digestive Tract Surgery: A Text and Atlas. *Philadelphia: Lippincott Williams & Wilkins, 1996, p 1533.]*

Restorative Proctocolectomy (Ileal Pouch Anal Anastomosis)
The entire colon and rectum are resected, but the anal sphincter muscles and a variable portion of the distal anal canal are preserved. Bowel continuity is restored by anastomosis of an ileal reservoir to the anal canal. The original technique included a transanal mucosectomy and handsewn ileoanal anastomosis. Proponents of this technique argue that mucosectomy guarantees removal of all of the diseased mucosa, including the anal transition zone, and therefore decreases the risk of ongoing disease, dysplasia, and carcinoma.[18] Opponents cite the increased risk of incontinence after mucosectomy and argue that even meticulous technique invariably leaves behind mucosal "islands" that are subsequently hidden under the anastomosis. Moreover, the "double-staple" technique using the circular stapling devices is considerably simpler than mucosectomy and a handsewn anastomosis (Fig. 29-11).[19] Regardless of the anastomotic technique, many surgeons recommend that patients undergo annual surveillance of the anastomosis and/or anal transition zone by digital rectal exam and anoscopy or proctoscopy.

The neorectum is made by anastomosis of the terminal ileum aligned in a "J," "S," or "W" configuration. Because functional outcomes are similar and because the J-pouch is the simplest to construct, it has become the most used configuration. With increasing experience in laparoscopic colectomy, some centers have begun performing total proctocolectomy with ileal pouch anal reconstruction using minimally invasive surgical techniques. Most surgeons perform a proximal ileostomy to divert succus from the newly created pouch in an attempt to minimize the consequences of leak and sepsis, especially in patients who are malnourished or immunosuppressed (Fig. 29-12). The ileostomy is then closed 6 to 12 weeks later, after a contrast study confirms the integrity of the pouch. In low-risk patients, however, there are reports of successful creation of an ileoanal pouch without diverting stoma.[20]

Anterior Resection

Anterior resection is the general term used to describe resection of the rectum from an abdominal approach to the pelvis with no need for a perineal, sacral, or other incision. Three types of anterior resection have been described.

High Anterior Resection A high anterior resection is the term used to describe resection of the distal sigmoid colon and upper rectum and is the appropriate operation for benign lesions and disease at the rectosigmoid junction such as diverticulitis. The upper rectum is mobilized but the pelvic peritoneum is not divided and the rectum is not mobilized fully from the concavity of the sacrum. The inferior mesenteric artery is ligated at its base and the inferior mesenteric vein, which follows a different course than the artery, is ligated separately. A primary anastomosis (usually end-to-end) between the colon and rectal stump with a short cuff of peritoneum surrounding its anterior two thirds generally can be performed.

Low Anterior Resection A *low anterior resection* is used to remove lesions in the upper and midrectum. The rectosigmoid is mobilized, the pelvic peritoneum is opened, and the inferior mesenteric artery is ligated and divided either at its origin from the aorta or just distal to the takeoff of the left colic artery. The rectum is mobilized from the sacrum by sharp dissection under direct view within the endopelvic fascial plane. The dissection may be performed distally to the anorectal ring, extending posteriorly through the rectosacral fascia to the coccyx and anteriorly through Denonvilliers' fascia to the vagina in women or the seminal vesicles and prostate in men. The rectum and accompanying mesorectum are divided at the appropriate level, depending upon the nature of the lesion. A low rectal anastomosis usually requires mobilization of the splenic flexure and ligation and division of the inferior mesenteric vein just inferior to the pancreas. Circular stapling devices have greatly facilitated the conduct and improved the safety of the colon to extraperitoneal rectal anastomosis.

Extended Low Anterior Resection An *extended low anterior resection* is necessary to remove lesions located in the distal rectum, but several centimeters above the sphincter. The rectum is fully mobilized to the level of the levator ani muscle just as for a low anterior resection, but the anterior dissection is extended along the rectovaginal septum in women and distal to the seminal vesicles and prostate in men. After resection at this level, a *coloanal anastomosis* can be created using one of a variety of techniques described below in Anastomoses. Because the risk of an anastomotic leak and subsequent sepsis is higher when an anastomosis is created in the distal rectum or anal canal, creation of a temporary ileostomy should be considered in this setting.

Although an anastomosis may be technically feasible very low in the rectum or anal canal, it is important to note that postoperative function may be poor. Because the descending colon lacks the distensibility of the rectum, the reservoir function may be compromised. Pelvic radiation, prior anorectal surgery, and obstetric trauma may cause unsuspected sphincter damage. Finally, a very low anastomosis may involve and compromise the upper sphincter. Creation of a *colon J-pouch* improves function during the first postoperative year.[21] A history of sphincter damage or any degree of incontinence is a relative contraindication for a coloanal anastomosis. In such patients, an end colostomy may be a more satisfactory option.

Hartmann's Procedure and Mucus Fistula

Hartmann's procedure refers to a colon or rectal resection without an anastomosis in which a colostomy or ileostomy is created and the distal colon or rectum is left as a blind pouch. The term typically is used when the left or sigmoid colon is resected and the closed off rectum is left in the pelvis. If the distal colon is long enough to reach the abdominal wall, a *mucus fistula* can be created by opening the defunctioned bowel and suturing it to the skin.

Abdominoperineal Resection

An abdominoperineal resection (APR) involves removal of the entire rectum, anal canal, and anus with construction of a permanent colostomy from the descending or sigmoid colon. The abdominal-pelvic portion of this operation proceeds in the same fashion as described for an extended low anterior resection. The perineal dissection can be performed with the patient in lithotomy position (often by a second surgeon) or in the prone position after closure of the abdomen and creation of the colostomy. For cancer, the perineal dissection is designed to excise the anal canal with a wide circumferential margin. Primary wound closure usually is successful but the large perineal defect, especially if radiation has been used, may require a vascularized flap closure in some patients. For benign disease, proctectomy may be performed using an *intersphincteric dissection* between the internal and external sphincters. This ap-

proach minimizes the perineal wound making it easier to close because the levator muscle remains intact.

Anastomoses

Anastomoses may be created between two segments of bowel in a multitude of ways. The geometry of the anastomosis may be *end-to-end, end-to-side, side-to-end,* or *side-to-side.* The anastomotic technique may be *handsewn* (*single* or *double layer*) or *stapled* (Fig. 29-13). The submucosal layer of the intestine provides the strength of the bowel wall and must be incorporated in the anastomosis to assure healing. The choice of anastomosis depends upon the operative anatomy and surgeon preference. Although many surgeons advocate one method over another, none has been proven to be superior. Accurate approximation of two well-vascularized, healthy limbs of bowel without tension in a normotensive, well-nourished patient almost always results in a good outcome. Anastomoses at highest risk of leak or stricture are those that are in the distal rectal or anal canal, involve irradiated or diseased intestine, or are performed in malnourished, ill patients.

Anastomotic Configuration

End-to-End An end-to-end anastomosis can be performed when two segments of bowel are roughly the same caliber. This technique most often is used in rectal resections, but may be used for colocolostomy or small bowel anastomoses.

End-to-Side An end-to-side configuration is useful when one limb of bowel is larger than the other. This most commonly occurs in the setting of chronic obstruction.

Side-to-End A side-to-end anastomosis is used when the proximal bowel is of smaller caliber than the distal bowel. Ileorectal anastomoses commonly make use of this configuration. A side-to-end anastomosis may have a less tenuous blood supply than an end-to-end anastomosis.

Side-to-Side A side-to-side anastomosis allows a large, well-vascularized connection to be created on the antimesenteric side of two segments of intestine. This technique is commonly used in ileocolic and small bowel anastomoses.

Anastomotic Technique

Hand-Sutured Technique Any of the configurations described above under Anastomotic Configuration may be created using a hand-sutured or stapled technique. Hand-sutured anastomoses may be *single layer*, using either running or interrupted stitches, or *double layer*. A double-layer anastomosis usually consists of a continuous inner layer and an interrupted outer layer. Suture material may be either permanent or absorbable. After distal rectal or anal canal resection, a transanal, handsewn coloanal anastomosis may be necessary to restore bowel continuity. This can be done in conjunction with an anal canal mucosectomy to allow the anastomosis to be at the dentate line.

Stapled Techniques Linear cutter stapling devices are used to divide the bowel and to create side-to-side anastomoses. The anastomosis may be reinforced with interrupted sutures if desired. Circular stapling devices can create end-to-end, end-to-side, or side-to-end anastomoses. These instruments are particularly useful for creating low rectal or anal canal anastomoses where the anatomy of the pelvis makes a handsewn anastomosis technically difficult or impossible.

Following resection of the colorectum, a stapled end-to-end colorectal, coloanal canal, or ileal pouch anal canal anastomosis may be created by one of two techniques. With the open pursestring technique, the distal rectal stump pursestring is placed by hand and the assembled circular stapler is inserted into the anus and guided up to the rectal pursestring. The stapler is opened and the distal pursestring is tied. A pursestring is placed in the distal end of the proximal colon; the proximal colon is placed over the anvil

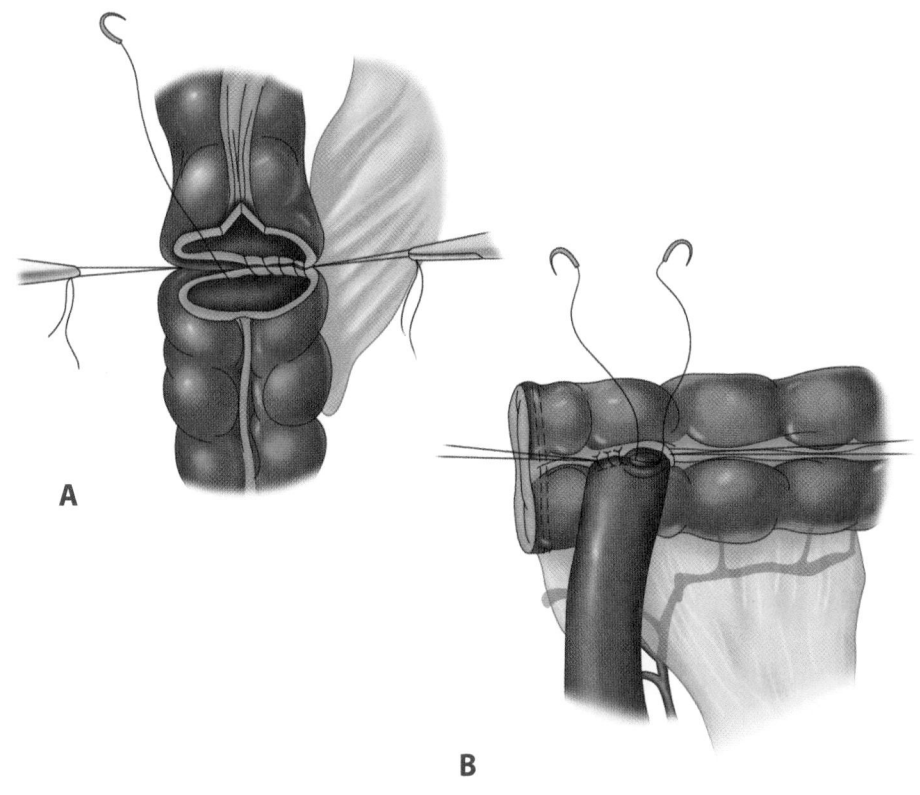

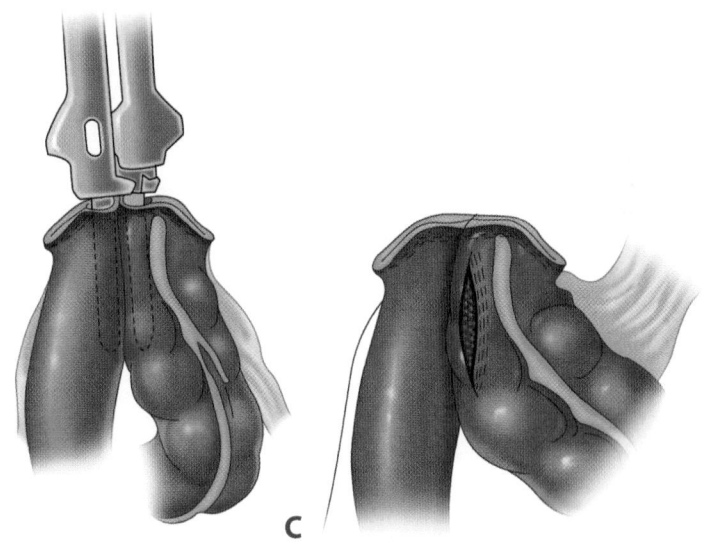

FIG. 29-13. A. Sutured end-to-end colocolic anastomosis. **B.** Sutured end-to-side ileocolic anastomosis. **C.** Stapled side-to-side, functional end-to-end ileocolic anastomosis. *[Reproduced with permission from Bell RH, Rikkers LF, Mulholland M (eds): Digestive Tract Surgery: A Text and Atlas. Philadelphia: Lippincott Williams & Wilkins, 1996, pp 1473, 1475, and 1479.]*

and the pursestring tightened. The stapler is closed and fired (Fig. 29-14). With the *alternative double-staple technique*, the distal rectum or anal canal is closed with a transverse staple line. The circular stapler is inserted through the anus without its anvil until the cartridge effaces the transverse staple line. The stapler is opened, causing the trocar to perforate through the rectal stump adjacent to the transverse staple line. A pursestring is placed in the distal end of the proximal colon or the end of the ileal pouch. The stapler anvil is inserted into the proximal colon or ileal pouch and the pursestring is tightened around the anvil. The anvil is mated to the trocar and the stapler closed and fired (see Fig. 29-11). After firing and removing the stapler, the resulting anastomotic rings should be inspected to ensure that they are intact. A gap in an anastomotic ring suggests that the circular staple line is incomplete and the anastomosis should be reinforced with suture circumferentially, if

technically feasible. A temporary proximal ileostomy may be indicated as well.

Ostomies

Depending upon the clinical situation, a stoma may be temporary or permanent. It may be end-on or a loop. However, regardless of the indication for a stoma, placement and construction are crucial for function. A stoma should be located within the rectus muscle to minimize the risk of a postoperative parastomal hernia. It also should be placed where the patient can see it and easily manipulate the appliance. The surrounding abdominal soft tissue should be as flat as possible to ensure a tight seal and prevent leakage. Preoperative evaluation by an enterostomal therapy (ET) nurse to identify the ideal stoma site and to counsel and educate the patient is invaluable (Fig. 29-15).

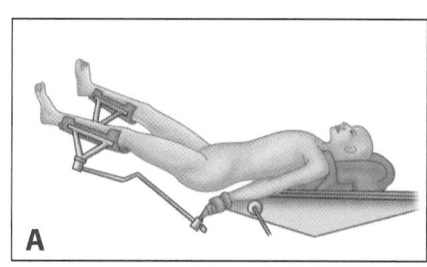

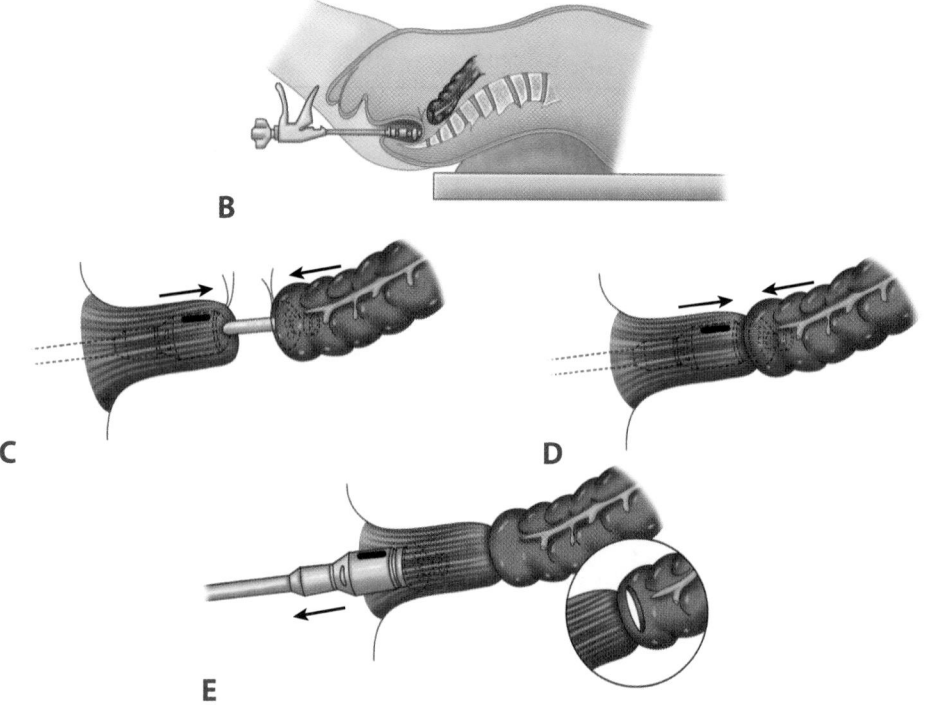

FIG. 29-14. Technique of end-to-end colorectal anastomosis using a circular stapler. **A.** The patient is in modified lithotomy position. **B.** After resection of the rectosigmoid and placement of purse-string sutures proximally and distally, the stapler is inserted into the anal canal and opened. **C.** Rectal purse-string suture is tied to secure the rectal stump to the rod of the stapler, and the colonic pursestring is tied to secure the colon to the anvil of the stapler. **D.** The stapler is closed and fired. **E.** The stapler is removed, leaving a circular stapled end-to-end anastomosis.

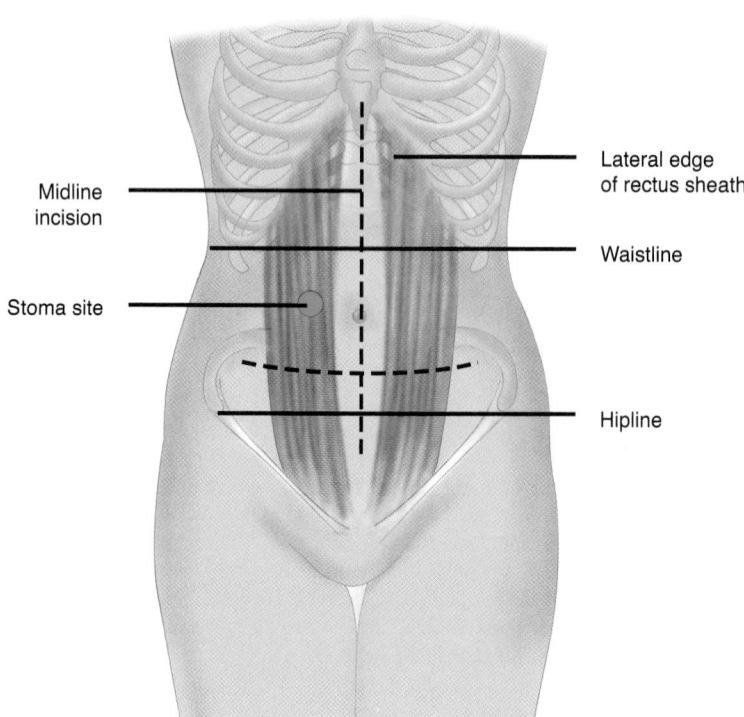

Midline incision

Lateral edge of rectus sheath

Waistline

Stoma site

Hipline

FIG. 29-15. Marking of an ideal site for ileostomy. *[Reproduced with permission from Bell RH, Rikkers LF, Mulholland M (eds):* Digestive Tract Surgery: A Text and Atlas. *Philadelphia: Lippincott Williams & Wilkins, 1996, p 1273.]*

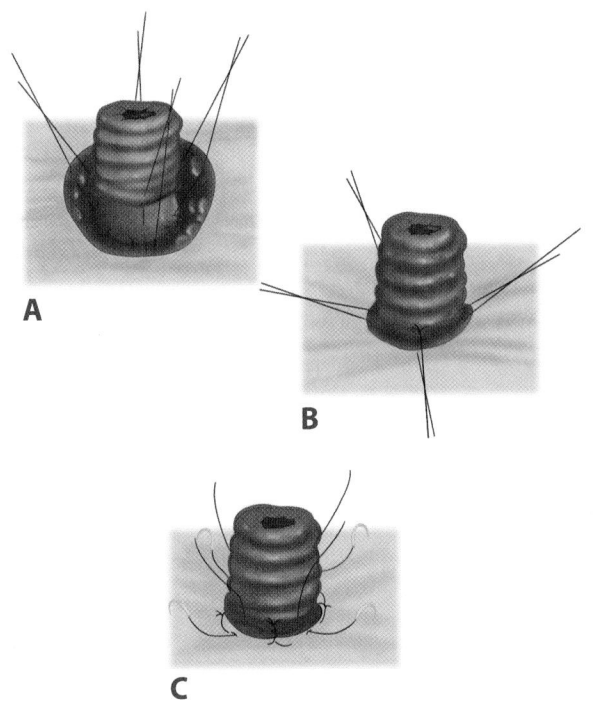

FIG. 29-16. Brooke ileostomy. **A.** Four sutures incorporating the cut end of the ileum, the seromuscular layer at the level of the anterior rectus fascia, and the subcuticular edge of the skin are placed at 90° to each other. **B.** The sutures are tied to produce stomal eversion, and (**C**) simple sutures from the cut edge of the bowel to the subcuticular tissue complete the maturation of the ileostomy. *[Reproduced with permission from Bell RH, Rikkers LF, Mulholland M (eds):* Digestive Tract Surgery: A Text and Atlas. *Philadelphia: Lippincott Williams & Wilkins, 1996, p 1278.]*

For all stomas, a circular skin incision is created and the subcutaneous tissue dissected to the level of the anterior rectus sheath. The anterior rectus sheath is incised in a cruciate fashion, the muscle fibers separated bluntly, and the posterior sheath identified and incised. The size of the defect depends upon the size of the bowel used to create the stoma, but should be as small as possible without compromising the intestinal blood supply (usually the width of two to three fingers). The bowel is then brought through the defect and secured. The abdominal incision is usually closed and dressed before maturing the stoma to avoid contaminating the wound. To make appliance use easier, a protruding nipple is fashioned by everting the bowel. Three or four interrupted absorbable sutures are placed through the edge of the bowel, then through the serosa, approximately 2 cm proximal to the edge, and then through the dermis (Brooke technique). After the stoma is everted, the mucocutaneous junction is sutured circumferentially with interrupted absorbable suture (Fig. 29-16).

Ileostomy

Temporary Ileostomy A temporary ileostomy often is used to "protect" an anastomosis that is at risk for leakage (low in the rectum, in an irradiated field, in an immunocompromised or malnourished patient, and in some emergency operations). In this setting, the stoma often is constructed as a *loop ileostomy* (see Fig. 29-12). A segment of distal ileum is brought through the defect in the abdominal wall as a loop. An enterotomy is created and the stoma matured as described above in Ostomies. The loop may be secured with or without an underlying rod. A *divided loop* may also be created by firing a linear cutter stapler across the distal limb of the loop flush with the skin followed by maturation of the proximal limb of the loop. This technique prevents incomplete diversion that occasionally occurs with a loop ileostomy.

The advantage of a loop or divided loop ileostomy is that subsequent closure often can be accomplished without a formal laparotomy. An elliptical incision is created around the stoma and the bowel gently dissected free of the subcutaneous tissues and fascia. A hand-sewn or stapled anastomosis can then be created and the intestine returned to the peritoneal cavity. This avoids a long laparotomy incision and generally is well tolerated. Timing of ileostomy closure should take into account anastomotic healing as well as the patient's overall condition. A flexible endoscopy exam and a contrast enema (Gastrografin) are recommended before closure to ensure that the anastomosis has not leaked and is patent. A patient's nutritional status should be optimized. In cancer patients receiving adjuvant chemotherapy, ileostomy closure should be delayed until chemotherapy is completed.

Permanent Ileostomy A permanent ileostomy sometimes is required after total proctocolectomy or in patients with obstruction. An *end ileostomy* is the preferred configuration for a permanent ileostomy because a symmetric protruding nipple can be fashioned more easily than with a loop ileostomy (see Fig. 29-16). The end of the small intestine is brought through the abdominal wall defect and matured. Stitches often are used to secure the bowel to the posterior fascia.

Complications of Ileostomy Stoma necrosis may occur in the early postoperative period and usually is caused by skeletonizing the distal small bowel and/or creating an overly tight fascial defect. Limited mucosal necrosis above the fascia may be treated expectantly, but necrosis below the level of the fascia requires surgical revision. Stoma retraction may occur early or late, and may be exacerbated by obesity. Local revision may be necessary. The creation of an ileostomy bypasses the fluid absorbing capability of the colon, and dehydration with fluid and electrolyte abnormalities is not uncommon. Ideally, ileostomy output should be maintained at less than 1500 mL/d to avoid this problem. Bulk agents and opioids (Lomotil, Imodium, tincture of opium) are useful. The somatostatin analogue, Octreotide, has been used with variable success in this setting. Skin irritation also can occur, especially if the stoma appliance fits poorly. Skin protecting agents and custom pouches can help to solve this problem. Obstruction may occur intra-abdominally or at the site where the stoma exits the fascia. Parastomal hernia is less common after an ileostomy than after a colostomy, but can cause poor appliance fitting, pain, obstruction, or strangulation. In general, symptomatic parastomal hernias should be repaired. Repair usually requires re-siting the stoma to the contralateral side of the abdomen. Prolapse is a rare, late complication and often is associated with a parastomal hernia. Valve slippage resulting in either leakage or obstruction is a common complication of a continent Kock pouch ileostomy.

Colostomy

Most colostomies are created as *end colostomies* rather than *loop colostomies* (Fig. 29-17). The bulkiness of the colon makes a loop colostomy awkward for an appliance, and prolapse is more likely with this configuration. Most colostomies are created on the left side of the colon. An abdominal wall defect is created and the end of the colon mobilized through it. Because a protruding stoma is considerably easier to pouch, colostomies also should be matured in a Brooke fashion. The distal bowel may be brought through the abdominal wall as a *mucus fistula* or left intra-abdominally as a *Hartmann's pouch.* Tacking the distal end of the colon to the abdominal wall or tagging it with permanent suture can make identification of the stump easier if the colostomy is closed at a later date. Closure of a colostomy usually requires laparotomy. The stoma is dissected free of the abdominal wall and the distal bowel identified. An end-to-end anastomosis is then created.

Complications of Colostomy *Colostomy necrosis* may occur in the early postoperative period and results from an impaired vascular supply (skeletonization of the distal colon or a tight fascial defect). Like ileostomy necrosis, limited suprafascial necrosis may be followed

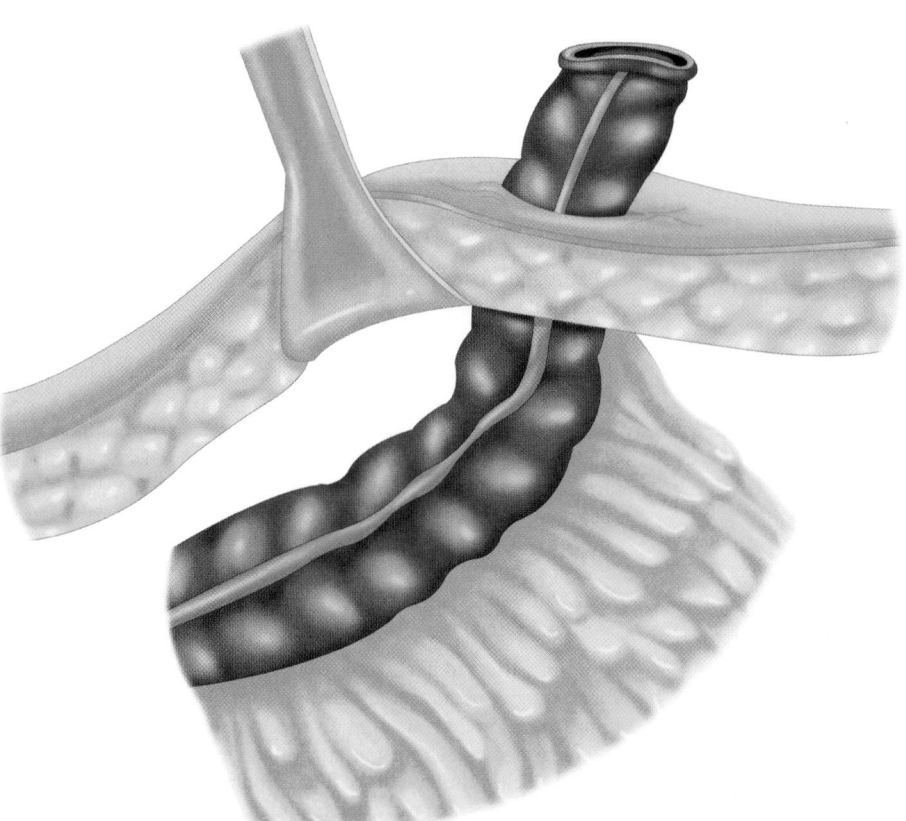

FIG. 29-17. Intraperitoneal end colostomy.

expectantly, but necrosis below the fascia requires surgery. *Retraction* may also occur, but is less problematic with a colostomy than with an ileostomy because the stool is less irritating to the skin than *succus entericus*. *Obstruction* is unusual, but may also occur. *Parastomal hernia* is the most common late complication of a colostomy and requires repair if it is symptomatic. *Prolapse* occurs rarely. Dehydration is rare after colostomy and skin irritation is less common than with ileostomy.

Functional Results

Function following segmental colonic resection and primary anastomosis generally is excellent. A small percentage of patients following subtotal or total colectomy and ileosigmoid or ileorectal anastomosis may experience diarrhea and bowel frequency. This is especially true if the patient is elderly, if significant length of small bowel has been resected, and if residual proctocolitis is poorly controlled. In general, the more distal the anastomosis, the more the risk of troublesome diarrhea and frequency.

Function following anterior resection is highly dependent on the level of anastomosis, the use of pre- or postoperative pelvic radiation, and underlying sphincter function. Following low anterior or extended low anterior resection, some surgeons prefer to construct a short (8 to 10 cm) colon-J-pouch to anastomose to the distal rectum or anal canal. The reservoir lessens urgency, frequency, and incontinence, but some patients have difficulty initiating defecation after construction of a colon-J-pouch.[21]

The physical and psychological problems associated with a permanent Brooke ileostomy led to development of the continent Kock pouch ileostomy. Unfortunately, complications, especially complications related to valve slippage, are common. Despite variations of technique designed to improve the function of the continent ileostomy, most surgeons have abandoned this operation and instead perform restorative proctocolectomy with ileal pouch anal anastomosis.

Although ileal pouch anal reconstruction is anatomically appealing, functional outcome is far from perfect.[22,23] Patients should be

counseled to expect eight to 10 bowel movements per day. Up to 50% have some degree of nocturnal incontinence. Pouchitis occurs in nearly 50% of patients, and small bowel obstruction is not uncommon. Other less common complications include difficulties with pouch evacuation, pouch–anal and/or pouch–vaginal fistula, and anal stricture. Pouch failure rate averages 5 to 10%. Patients who are subsequently diagnosed with Crohn's disease have a considerably higher pouch failure rate (approximately 50%), while patients with indeterminate colitis have an intermediate pouch failure rate (15 to 20%). Despite these drawbacks, the vast majority of patients are satisfied and prefer ileal pouch–anal reconstruction to permanent ileostomy.

Pouchitis is an inflammatory condition that affects both ileoanal pouches and continent ileostomy reservoirs. Incidence of pouchitis ranges from 30 to 55%. Symptoms include increased diarrhea, hematochezia, abdominal pain, fever, and malaise. Diagnosis is made endoscopically with biopsies. Differential diagnosis includes infection and undiagnosed Crohn's disease. The etiology of pouchitis is unknown. Some believe pouchitis results from fecal stasis within the pouch but emptying studies are not confirmatory. Antibiotics (metronidazole ± ciprofloxacin) are the mainstays of therapy and most patients will respond rapidly to either oral preparations or enemas.[24,25] Some patients develop chronic pouchitis that necessitates ongoing suppressive antibiotic therapy. Salicylate and corticosteroid enemas also have been used with some success. Reintroduction of normal flora by ingestion of *probiotics* has been suggested as a possible treatment in refractory cases. Occasionally, pouch excision is necessary to control the symptoms of chronic pouchitis.

Anesthesia Considerations
Local Anesthesia

Many anorectal procedures can be performed with local anesthetic alone. IV sedation often is provided to calm the patient. Injection of 0.5% lidocaine (short acting) and 0.25% bupivacaine (long acting) into the perianal skin, sphincter, and area around the pudendal nerves usually provides an adequate block. The addition of dilute epinephrine decreases bleeding and prolongs the anesthetic effect.

Regional Anesthesia

Epidural, spinal, and caudal anesthetics can be used for anorectal procedures and transanal resections. In patients with severe medical comorbidity, regional anesthesia occasionally may be used for laparotomy and colectomy. Postoperative epidural anesthesia provides excellent pain relief and improves pulmonary function.

General Anesthesia

General anesthesia is required for the vast majority of intra-abdominal procedures. Patients should undergo a thorough preoperative cardiovascular evaluation. In patients with significant co-morbid disease, preadmission and an anesthesia consultation may be appropriate.

Positioning

Most abdominal colectomies can be performed in the supine position. Anterior and APRs require lithotomy positioning. Adequate padding should be provided for the patient's sacrum and care should be taken to avoid stirrup pressure on the peroneal nerves.

Anorectal procedures may be performed in lithotomy but the prone jackknife position is preferred for most procedures, especially if the anterior quadrant needs to be seen well. Distal posterior lesions usually can be accessed from either position, but more proximal posterior lesions are better accessed in prone position.

Operative Preliminaries
Bowel Preparation

The rationale for bowel preparation is that decreasing the bacterial load in the colon and rectum will decrease the incidence of postoperative infection. *Mechanical bowel preparation* uses cathartics to rid the colon of solid stool the night before surgery.[26] The most commonly used regimens include polyethylene glycol (PEG) solutions or sodium phosphate. PEG solutions require patients to drink a large volume and may cause bloating and nausea. Sodium phosphate solutions generally are better tolerated, but are more likely to cause fluid and electrolyte abnormalities. PEG and sodium phosphate are equally efficacious in bowel cleansing. The preparatory formulations recently have been introduced in tablet form in an attempt to improve tolerance. However, these methods of bowel cleansing require ingestion of 40 or more tablets with water over several hours. To date, this has not proven superior to the more traditional products.[27] *Antibiotic prophylaxis* also is recommended. The addition of oral antibiotics to the preoperative mechanical bowel preparation is thought to decrease postoperative infection by further decreasing the bacterial load of the colon. A combination of three doses of neomycin (1 g) and erythromycin base (1 g) is most commonly used. Some surgeons substitute metronidazole (500 mg) for erythromycin to avoid GI upset. Ciprofloxacin also has been used in this setting. It is important to note, however, that although the majority of surgeons use oral antibiotic prophylaxis, this practice has never been proven to decrease postoperative infectious complications.[28,29] A broad-spectrum parenteral antibiotic(s) should be administered just before the skin incision. There is no proven benefit to using antibiotics postoperatively after an uncomplicated colectomy.

Despite widespread use of mechanical bowel preparation, the necessity of bowel cleansing before colectomy has been questioned. European surgeons in particular have advocated abandoning this practice. Several small studies suggest that a mechanical bowel preparation does not decrease the risk of postoperative wound infection or anastomotic dehiscence.[30–32] Larger prospective trials are needed to determine whether mechanical bowel preparation before colectomy is a necessity or a source of added morbidity that can be avoided.

Stoma Planning

The preoperative preparation of a patient who is expected to require a stoma should include a consultation with an *enterostomal therapy nurse*. ET nurses are specially trained and credentialed by the Wound, Ostomy and Continence Nurses Society. Preoperative planning includes counseling, education, and stoma siting. Postoperatively, the ET nurse assists with local skin care and pouching. Other considerations in stoma planning include evaluation of other medical conditions that may impact a patient's ability to manage a stoma (e.g., eyesight, manual dexterity).

Preoperative stoma siting is crucial for a patient's postoperative function and quality of life. A poorly placed stoma can result in leakage and skin breakdown. Ideally, a stoma should be placed in a location that the patient can easily see and manipulate, within the rectus muscle, and below the belt line (see Fig. 29-15). Because the abdominal landmarks in a supine, anesthetized patient may be dramatically different from those in an awake, standing, or sitting patient, the stoma site should always be marked with a tattoo, skin scratch, or permanent marker preoperatively, if possible. In an emergency operation where the stoma site has not been marked, an attempt should be made to place a stoma within the rectus muscle and away from both the costal margin and iliac crest. In emergencies, placement high on the abdominal wall is preferred to a low-lying site.

Ureteral Stents

Ureteral stents may be useful for identifying the ureters intraoperatively and are placed via cystoscopy after the induction of general anesthesia and removed at the end of the operation. Stents can be invaluable in reoperative pelvic surgery or when there is significant retroperitoneal inflammation (such as complicated diverticulitis). Lighted stents may be helpful in laparoscopic resections. Patients often have transient hematuria postoperatively but major complications are rare.

Multidisciplinary Teams

Patients with complex colorectal disease often benefit from a multidisciplinary approach. Patients with pelvic floor disorders (especially incontinence) often require evaluation by both a colorectal surgeon and a urologist or urogynecologist. Preoperative evaluation of cancer patients by a medical oncologist and/or radiation oncologist is crucial for planning either neoadjuvant or adjuvant therapy. Intraoperatively, complex pelvic resections often require the involvement of not only a colorectal surgeon but also a urologist, gynecologic oncologist, neurosurgeon, and/or plastic surgeon. Radiation oncologists should be involved in the operation if brachytherapy catheters are to be placed for intracavitary radiation or if intraoperative radiation therapy is planned. Rarely, psychiatric disorders may manifest as colorectal problems (especially functional disorders and chronic pain) and involvement of a psychiatrist or psychologist may be beneficial.

INFLAMMATORY BOWEL DISEASE

General Considerations
Epidemiology

Inflammatory bowel disease includes *ulcerative colitis*, *Crohn's disease*, and *indeterminate colitis*. Ulcerative colitis occurs in eight to 15 people per 100,000 in the United States and Northern Europe. The incidence is considerably lower in Asia, Africa, and South America, and among the nonwhite population in the United States. Ulcerative colitis incidence peaks during the third decade of life and again in the seventh decade of life. The incidence of Crohn's disease is slightly lower, one to five people per 100,000 population. Crohn's disease also affects Northern European and white populations disproportionately. Crohn's disease has a similar bimodal incidence, with most cases occurring between ages 15 to 30 years and ages 55 to 60 years. In 15% of patients with inflammatory bowel disease, differentiation between ulcerative colitis and Crohn's colitis is impossible; these patients are classified as having *indeterminate colitis.*

Etiology

Multiple etiologies for inflammatory bowel disease have been proposed, but none are proven. The consistent geographic differences in incidence suggest an environmental factor such as diet or infection. Smoking, alcohol, and oral contraceptive use also have been implicated. Family history may play a role because 10 to 30% of patients with inflammatory bowel disease report a family member with the same disease.[33] Other theories focus on an autoimmune mechanism and/or a defect in the intestinal immune system. Although there is general agreement that interaction among the immune system, the mucosal barrier of the gut, and a variety of infectious agents is involved in the pathogenesis of inflammatory bowel disease, the mechanism(s) by which these interactions produce disease is poorly understood.[34] Bacteria such as *Mycobacterium paratuberculosis* and *Listeria monocytogenes*, and viruses such as paramyxovirus and measles virus, have been suggested as etiologic agents in Crohn's disease. A defect in the gut mucosal barrier, which increases exposure to intraluminal bacteria, toxins, or proinflammatory substances, also has been suggested. Finally, an autoimmune mechanism has been postulated. Although there is no clear evidence linking an immunologic disorder to inflammatory bowel disease, the similarity of many of the extraintestinal manifestations to rheumatologic disorders has made this theory attractive. Regardless of the underlying cause of either ulcerative colitis or Crohn's disease, both disorders are characterized by intestinal inflammation and medical therapy is largely based upon reducing inflammation.

Pathology and Differential Diagnosis

Although ulcerative colitis and Crohn's colitis share many pathologic and clinical similarities, these conditions may be differentiated in 85% of patients. Ulcerative colitis is a mucosal process in which the colonic mucosa and submucosa are infiltrated with inflammatory cells. The mucosa may be atrophic and crypt abscesses are common. Endoscopically, the mucosa is frequently friable and may possess multiple inflammatory pseudopolyps. In long-standing ulcerative colitis, the colon may be foreshortened and the mucosa replaced by scar. In quiescent ulcerative colitis, the colonic mucosa may appear normal endoscopically and microscopically. Ulcerative colitis may affect the rectum (proctitis), rectum and sigmoid colon (proctosigmoiditis), rectum and left colon (left-sided colitis), or the rectum and entire colon (pancolitis). Ulcerative colitis does not involve the small intestine, but the terminal ileum may demonstrate inflammatory changes ("backwash ileitis"). A key feature of ulcerative colitis is the continuous involvement of the rectum and colon; rectal sparing or skip lesions suggest a diagnosis of Crohn's disease. Symptoms are related to the degree of mucosal inflammation and the extent of colitis. Patients typically complain of bloody diarrhea and crampy abdominal pain. Proctitis may produce tenesmus. Severe abdominal pain and fever raises the concern of *fulminant colitis* or *toxic megacolon*. Physical findings are nonspecific and range from minimal abdominal tenderness and distention to frank peritonitis. In the nonemergent setting, the diagnosis typically is made by colonoscopy and mucosal biopsy.

In contrast to ulcerative colitis, Crohn's disease is a transmural inflammatory process that can affect any part of the GI tract from mouth to anus. Mucosal ulcerations, an inflammatory cell infiltrate, and noncaseating granulomas are characteristic pathologic findings. Chronic inflammation may ultimately result in fibrosis, strictures, and fistulas in either the colon or small intestine. The endoscopic appearance of Crohn's colitis is characterized by deep serpiginous ulcers and a "cobblestone" appearance. Skip lesions and rectal sparing are common. Symptoms of Crohn's disease depend upon the severity of inflammation and/or fibrosis and the location of inflammation in the GI tract. Acute inflammation may produce diarrhea, crampy abdominal pain, and fever. Strictures may produce symp-

toms of obstruction. Weight loss is common, both because of obstruction and from protein loss. Perianal Crohn's disease may present with pain, swelling, and drainage from fistulas or abscesses. Physical findings are also related to the site and severity of disease.

In 15% of patients with colitis from inflammatory bowel disease, differentiation of ulcerative colitis from Crohn's colitis proves impossible either grossly or microscopically (indeterminate colitis). These patients typically present with symptoms similar to ulcerative colitis. Endoscopic and pathologic findings usually include features common to both diseases.

Further differential diagnoses include infectious colitides, especially *Campylobacter jejuni, Entamoeba histolytica, C. difficile, Neisseria gonococcus, Salmonella,* and *Shigella* species.

Extraintestinal Manifestations

The liver is a common site of extracolonic disease in inflammatory bowel disease. Fatty infiltration of the liver is present in 40 to 50% of patients and cirrhosis is found in 2 to 5%. Fatty infiltration may be reversed by medical or surgical treatment of colonic disease, but cirrhosis is irreversible. Primary sclerosing cholangitis is a progressive disease characterized by intra- and extrahepatic bile duct strictures. Forty to 60% of patients with primary sclerosing cholangitis have ulcerative colitis. Colectomy will not reverse this disease, and the only effective therapy is liver transplantation. Pericholangitis also is associated with inflammatory bowel disease and may be diagnosed with a liver biopsy. Bile duct carcinoma is a rare complication of long-standing inflammatory bowel disease. Patients who develop bile duct carcinoma in the presence of inflammatory bowel disease are, on average, 20 years younger than other patients with bile duct carcinoma.

Arthritis is also a common extracolonic manifestation of inflammatory bowel disease, and the incidence is 20 times greater than in the general population. Arthritis usually improves with treatment of the colonic disease. Sacroiliitis and ankylosing spondylitis are associated with inflammatory bowel disease, although the relationship is poorly understood. Medical and surgical treatment of the colonic disease does not impact symptoms.

Erythema nodosum is seen in 5 to 15% of patients with inflammatory bowel disease and usually coincides with clinical disease activity. Women are affected three to four times more frequently than men. The characteristic lesions are raised, red, and predominantly on the lower legs. Pyoderma gangrenosum is an uncommon but serious condition that occurs almost exclusively in patients with inflammatory bowel disease. The lesion begins as an erythematous plaque, papule, or bleb, usually located on the pretibial region of the leg and occasionally near a stoma. The lesions progress and ulcerate, leading to a painful, necrotic wound. Pyoderma gangrenosum may respond to resection of the affected bowel in some patients. In others, this disorder is unaffected by treatment of the underlying bowel disease.

Up to 10% of patients with inflammatory bowel disease will develop ocular lesions. These include uveitis, iritis, episcleritis, and conjunctivitis. They usually develop during an acute exacerbation of the inflammatory bowel disease. The etiology is unknown.

Principles of Nonoperative Management

Medical therapy for inflammatory bowel disease focuses on decreasing inflammation and alleviating symptoms, and many of the agents used are the same for both ulcerative colitis and Crohn's disease. In general, mild to moderate flares may be treated in the outpatient setting. More severe signs and symptoms mandate hospitalization. Pancolitis generally requires more aggressive therapy than limited disease. Because ulcerative proctitis and proctosigmoiditis are limited to the distal large intestine, topical therapy with salicylate and/or corticosteroid suppositories and enemas can be extremely effective. Systemic therapy rarely is required in these patients.

Salicylates Sulfasalazine (Azulfidine), 5-ASA, and related compounds are first-line agents in the medical treatment of mild to moderate inflammatory bowel disease. These compounds decrease inflammation by inhibition of cyclooxygenase and 5-lipoxygenase in the gut mucosa. They require direct contact with affected mucosa for efficacy. Multiple preparations are available for administration to different sites in the small intestine and colon [sulfasalazine, mesalamine (Pentasa), Asacol, Rowasa, Canasa].

Antibiotics Antibiotics often are used to decrease the intraluminal bacterial load in Crohn's disease. Metronidazole has been reported to improve Crohn's colitis and perianal disease, but the evidence is weak. Fluoroquinolones also may be effective in some cases. In the absence of fulminant colitis or toxic megacolon, antibiotics are not used to treat ulcerative colitis.

Corticosteroids Corticosteroids (either oral or parenteral) are a key component of treatment for an acute exacerbation of either ulcerative colitis or Crohn's disease. Corticosteroids are nonspecific inhibitors of the immune system and 75 to 90% of patients will improve with the administration of these drugs. However, corticosteroids have a number of serious side effects and use of these agents should be limited to the shortest course possible. In addition, corticosteroids should be used judiciously in children because of the potential adverse effect on growth. Failure to wean corticosteroids is a relative indication for surgery.

Because of the systemic effects of corticosteroids, an effort has been made to develop drugs that act locally and have limited systemic absorption. Newer agents such as budesonide, beclomethasone dipropionate, and tixocortol pivalate undergo rapid hepatic degradation that significantly decreases systemic toxicity. Budesonide is available as an oral preparation. Corticosteroid enemas provide effective local therapy for proctitis and proctosigmoiditis and have fewer side effects than systemic corticosteroids.

Immunosuppressive Agents Azathioprine and 6-mercaptopurine are antimetabolite drugs that interfere with nucleic acid synthesis and thus decrease proliferation of inflammatory cells. These agents are useful for treating ulcerative colitis and Crohn's disease in patients who have failed salicylate therapy or who are dependent upon or refractory to corticosteroids. It is important to note, however, that the onset of action of these drugs takes 6 to 12 weeks, and concomitant use of corticosteroids almost always is required.[34]

Cyclosporine is an immunosuppressive agent that interferes with T-cell function. Although cyclosporine is not routinely used to treat inflammatory bowel disease, up to 80% of patients with an acute flare of ulcerative colitis will improve with its use. However, the majority of these patients will ultimately require colectomy. Cyclosporine also occasionally is used to treat exacerbations of Crohn's disease and approximately two thirds of patients will note some improvement. Improvement generally is apparent within 2 weeks of beginning cyclosporine therapy. Long-term use of cyclosporine is limited by its significant toxicity.

Methotrexate is a folate antagonist that also has been used to treat inflammatory bowel disease. Although the efficacy of this agent is unproven, there are reports that more than 50% of patients will improve with administration of this drug.[35]

Infliximab (Remicade) is a monoclonal antibody against tumor necrosis factor alpha. IV infusion of this agent decreases inflammation systemically. More than 50% of patients with moderate to severe Crohn's disease will improve with infliximab therapy.[36] This agent also has been useful in treating patients with perianal Crohn's disease. Recurrence is common, however, and many patients require infusions on a bimonthly basis. Infliximab has not been used as extensively for treatment of ulcerative colitis; however, there are reports of efficacy in this setting.[37,38] Other monoclonal antibody agents have been developed and are now being used in clinical trials in patients with inflammatory bowel disease.

Nutrition Patients with inflammatory bowel disease often are malnourished. Abdominal pain and obstructive symptoms may decrease oral intake. Diarrhea can cause significant protein loss. Ongoing inflammation produces a catabolic physiologic state. Parenteral nutrition should be strongly considered early in the course of therapy for either Crohn's disease or ulcerative colitis. The nutritional status of the patient also should be considered when planning operative intervention and nutritional parameters such as serum albumin, prealbumin, and transferrin should be assessed. In extremely malnourished patients, especially those who also are being treated with corticosteroids, creation of a stoma often is safer than a primary anastomosis.

Ulcerative Colitis

Ulcerative colitis is a dynamic disease characterized by remissions and exacerbations. The clinical spectrum ranges from an inactive or quiescent phase to low-grade active disease to fulminant disease. The onset of ulcerative colitis may be insidious, with minimal bloody stools, or the onset can be abrupt, with severe diarrhea and bleeding, tenesmus, abdominal pain, and fever. The severity of symptoms depends upon the degree and extent of inflammation. Although anemia is common, massive hemorrhage is rare. Physical findings often are nonspecific.

Diagnosis of ulcerative colitis almost always is made endoscopically. Because the rectum is invariably involved, proctoscopy may be adequate to establish the diagnosis. The earliest manifestation is mucosal edema, which results in a loss of the normal vascular pattern. In more advanced disease, characteristic findings include mucosal friability and ulceration. Pus and mucus also may be present. Although mucosal biopsy often is diagnostic in the chronic phase of ulcerative colitis, biopsy in the acute phase often will reveal only nonspecific inflammation. A complete evaluation with colonoscopy or barium enema during an acute flare is contraindicated because of the risk of perforation.

Barium enema has been used to diagnose ulcerative colitis and to determine the extent of disease. However, this modality is less sensitive than colonoscopy and may not detect early disease. In long-standing ulcerative colitis, the colon is foreshortened and lacks haustral markings ("lead pipe" colon). Because the inflammation in ulcerative colitis is purely mucosal, strictures are highly uncommon. Any stricture diagnosed in a patient with ulcerative colitis must be presumed to be malignant until proven otherwise.

Indications for Surgery

Indications for surgery in ulcerative colitis may be emergent or elective. Emergency surgery is required for patients with massive life-threatening *hemorrhage, toxic megacolon,* or *fulminant colitis* who fail to respond rapidly to medical therapy. Patients with signs and symptoms of fulminant colitis should be treated aggressively with bowel rest, hydration, broad-spectrum antibiotics, and parenteral corticosteroids. Colonoscopy and barium enema are contraindicated, and antidiarrheal agents should be avoided. Deterioration in clinical condition or failure to improve within 24 to 48 hours mandates surgery.

Indications for elective surgery include intractability despite maximal medical therapy and high-risk development of major complications of medical therapy, such as aseptic necrosis of joints secondary to chronic steroid use. Elective surgery also is indicated in patients at significant risk of developing colorectal carcinoma. Risk of malignancy increases with pancolonic disease and the duration of symptoms is approximately 2% after 10 years, 8% after 20 years, and 18% after 30 years. Unlike sporadic colorectal cancers, carcinoma developing in the context of ulcerative colitis is more likely to arise from areas of *flat dysplasia* and may be difficult to diagnose at an early stage. For this reason, it is recommended that patients with long-standing ulcerative colitis undergo colonoscopic surveillance with multiple (40 to 50), random biopsies to identify dysplasia before invasive malignancy develops. However, the adequacy of this type of screening is controversial. Recently, magnifying chromoendoscopy has been used to improve sensitivity.[39,40] This technique uses topical dyes that are applied to the colonic mucosa at the time of endoscopy (Lugol's solution, methylene blue, indigo carmine, and others). These dyes highlight contrast between normal and dysplastic epithelium, allowing more precise biopsy of suspicious areas.[41] Surveillance is recommended annually after 8 years in patients with pancolitis, and annually after 15 years in patients with left-sided colitis. Although low-grade dysplasia was long thought to represent minimal risk, more recent studies show that invasive cancer may be present in up to 20% of patients with low-grade dysplasia. For this reason, any patient with dysplasia should be advised to undergo proctocolectomy. Controversy exists over whether prophylactic proctocolectomy should be recommended for patients who have had chronic ulcerative colitis for >10 years in the absence of dysplasia. Proponents of this approach note that surveillance colonoscopy with multiple biopsies samples only a small fraction of the colonic mucosa and dysplasia and carcinoma are often missed. Opponents cite the relatively low risk of progression to carcinoma if all biopsies have lacked dysplasia (approximately 2.4%). Neither approach has been definitively shown to decrease mortality from colorectal cancer.

Operative Management

Emergent Operation In a patient with fulminant colitis or toxic megacolon, total abdominal colectomy with end ileostomy, rather than total proctocolectomy, is recommended. Although the rectum is invariably diseased, most patients improve dramatically after an abdominal colectomy, and this operation avoids a difficult and time-consuming pelvic dissection in a critically ill patient. Rarely, a loop ileostomy and decompressing colostomy may be necessary if the patient is too unstable to withstand colectomy. Definitive surgery may then be undertaken at a later date once the patient has recovered. Complex techniques such as an ileal pouch anal reconstruction generally are contraindicated in the emergent setting. However, massive hemorrhage that includes bleeding from the rectum may necessitate proctectomy and either a permanent ileostomy or ileal pouch anal anastomosis.

Elective Operation In the past, *abdominal colectomy with ileorectal anastomosis* often was recommended for patients with relatively quiescent rectal disease. The risk of ongoing inflammation, the risk of malignancy, and the availability of restorative proctocolectomy have led most surgeons to now recommend elective operations that include resection of the rectum. Abdominal colectomy with ileorectal anastomosis is still an appropriate operation for a patient with indeterminate colitis and rectal sparing. *Total proctocolectomy with end ileostomy* has been the "gold standard" for patients with chronic ulcerative colitis. This operation removes the entire affected intestine and avoids the functional disturbances associated with ileal pouch–anal reconstruction. Most patients function well physically and psychologically after this operation. *Total proctocolectomy with continent ileostomy (Kock's pouch)* was developed to improve function and quality of life after total proctocolectomy, but morbidity is significant and restorative proctocolectomy generally is preferred today. Since its reintroduction in 1980, *restorative proctocolectomy with ileal pouch–anal anastomosis* has become the procedure of choice for most patients who require total proctocolectomy but wish to avoid a permanent ileostomy (see Figs. 29-11 and 29-12).[18]

Crohn's Disease

Like ulcerative colitis, Crohn's disease is characterized by exacerbations and remissions. Crohn's disease, however, may affect any portion of the intestinal tract, from mouth to anus. Diagnosis may be made by colonoscopy or esophagogastroduodenoscopy, or by barium small bowel study or enema, depending upon which part of the intestine is most affected. Skip lesions are key in differentiating Crohn's colitis from ulcerative colitis, and rectal sparing occurs in approximately 40% of patients. The most common site of involvement in Crohn's disease is the terminal ileum and cecum (*ileocolic Crohn's disease*), followed by the small bowel, and then by the colon

and rectum. Perianal and anal canal Crohn's disease manifest by complex anal fistulas and/or abscesses, anal ulcers, and large skin tags may be the initial site of presentation in up to 4% of cases.

Indications for Surgery

Because Crohn's disease can affect any part of the GI tract, the therapeutic rationale is fundamentally different from that of ulcerative colitis. Ulcerative colitis may be cured by removal of the affected intestinal segment (the colon and rectum). In Crohn's disease, it is impossible to remove all of the at-risk intestine; therefore, surgical therapy is reserved for complications of the disease.

Crohn's disease may present as an *acute inflammatory* process or as a *chronic fibrotic* process. During the acute inflammatory phase, patients may present with intestinal inflammation complicated by fistulas and/or intra-abdominal abscesses. Maximal medical therapy should be instituted, including anti-inflammatory medications, bowel rest, and antibiotics. Parenteral nutrition should be considered if the patient is malnourished. Most intra-abdominal abscesses can be drained percutaneously with the use of CT scan guidance. Although the majority of these patients will ultimately require surgery to remove the diseased segment of bowel, these interventions allow the patient's condition to stabilize, nutrition to be optimized, and inflammation to decrease before embarking upon a surgical resection.

Chronic fibrosis may result in strictures in any part of the GI tract. Because the fibrotic process is gradual, free perforation proximal to the obstructing stricture is rare, and, instead, adjacent structures "wall off" the site of perforation. The result often is development of enteric and colonic internal fistulas to other segments of intestine and other viscera (bladder, uterus, vagina) and retroperitoneal sites. Chronic strictures almost never improve with medical therapy. Optimal timing for surgery should take into account the patient's underlying medical and nutritional status. Strictures may be treated with *resection* or *strictureplasty*. Associated fistulas generally require resection of the segment of bowel with active Crohn's disease; the secondary sites of the fistula often are otherwise normal and generally do not require resection after division of the fistula. Simple closure of the secondary fistula site usually suffices.

Once an operation is undertaken for Crohn's disease, several principles should guide intraoperative decision making. In general, a laparotomy for Crohn's disease should be done through a *midline incision* because of the possible need for a stoma. *Laparoscopy* also is increasingly used in this setting. Because many patients with Crohn's disease will require multiple operations, *the length of bowel removed should be minimized*. Bowel should be resected to an area with *grossly normal margins*; frozen sections are not necessary. Finally, a primary anastomosis may be safely created if the patient is medically stable, nutritionally replete, and taking few immunosuppressive medications. *Creation of a stoma should be strongly considered* in any patient who is hemodynamically unstable, septic, malnourished, or receiving high-dose immunosuppressive therapy and in patients with extensive intra-abdominal contamination.

Ileocolic and Small Bowel Crohn's Disease

The terminal ileum and cecum are involved in Crohn's disease in up to 41% of patients; the small intestine is involved in up to 35% of patients. The most common indications for surgery are *internal fistula or abscess* (30 to 38% of patients) and *obstruction* (35 to 37% of patients). *Psoas abscess* may result from ileocolic Crohn's disease. Sepsis should be controlled with percutaneous drainage of abscess(es) and antibiotics, if possible. Parenteral nutrition may be necessary in patients with chronic obstruction. The extent of resection depends on the amount of involved intestine. Short segments of inflamed small intestine and right colon should be resected and a primary anastomosis created if the patient is stable, nutrition is adequate, and immunosuppression is minimal. Isolated chronic strictures also should be resected. In patients with multiple fibrotic strictures that would require extensive small bowel resection, *strictureplasty* is a safe and

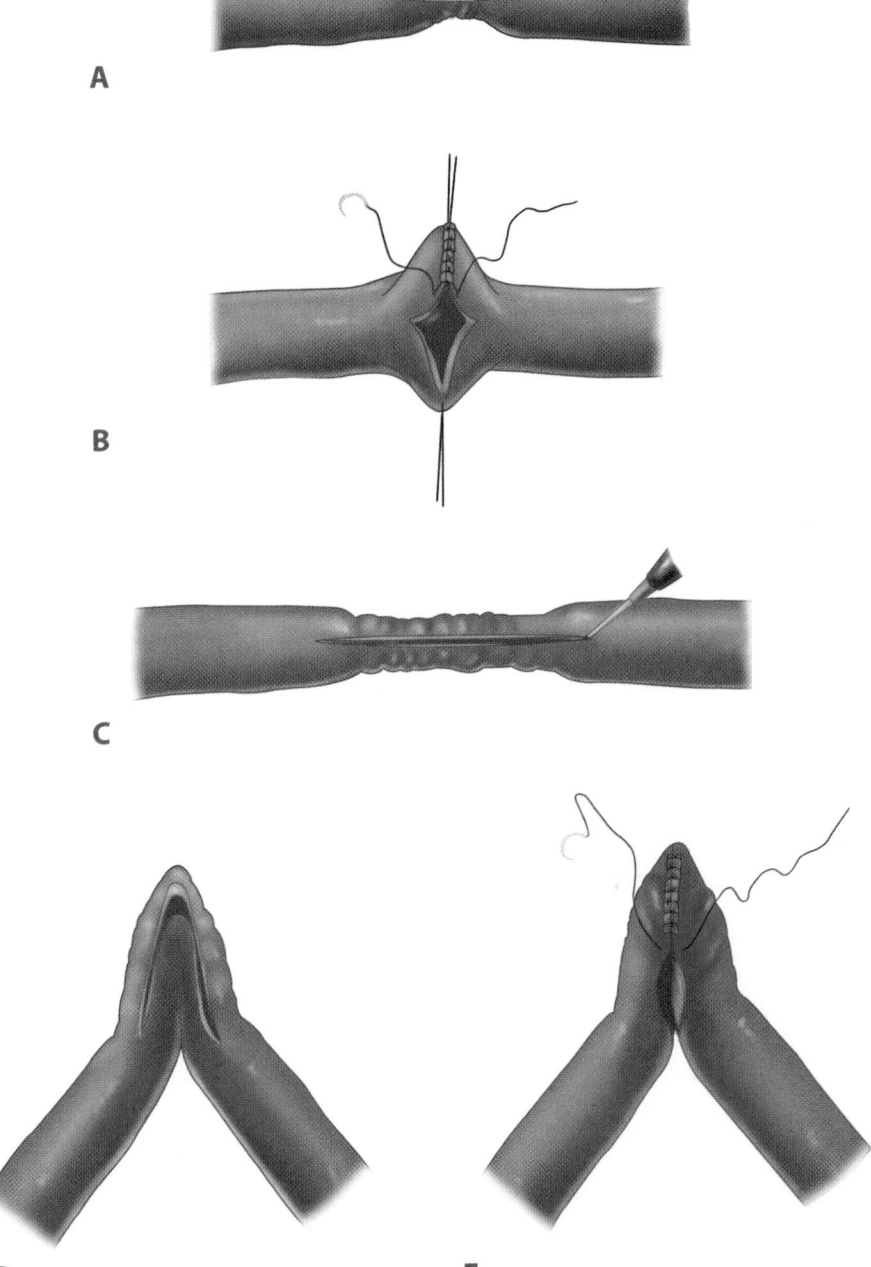

FIG. 29-18. Alternative stricturoplasty techniques. **A.** A short stricture is opened along the antimesenteric surface of the bowel wall. **B.** The enterotomy is closed transversely. **C.** A long stricture is opened along the antimesenteric surface of the bowel wall. **D.** The bowel is folded into an inverted "U." **E.** A side-to-side anastomosis is made. *(Reproduced with permission from Corman ML:* Colon & Rectal Surgery, *2nd ed. Philadelphia: Lippincott Williams & Wilkins, 1989, p 832.)*

effective alternative to resection. Short strictures are amenable to a transverse stricturoplasty, while longer strictures may be treated with a side-to-side small bowel anastomosis (Fig. 29-18).

Risk of recurrence after resection for ileocolic and small bowel Crohn's disease is high. More than 50% of patients will experience a recurrence within 10 years, and the majority of these will require a second operation.

Crohn's Colitis

Crohn's disease of the large intestine may present as *fulminant colitis* or *toxic megacolon*. In this setting, treatment is identical to treatment of fulminant colitis and toxic megacolon secondary to ulcerative colitis. Resuscitation and medical therapy with bowel rest, broad-spectrum antibiotics, and parenteral corticosteroids should be instituted. If the patient's condition worsens or fails to rapidly improve, total abdominal colectomy with end ileostomy is recommended. An elective proctectomy may be required if the patient has refractory

Crohn's proctitis. Alternatively, if the rectum is spared, an ileorectal anastomosis may be appropriate once the patient has recovered.

Other indications for surgery in chronic Crohn's colitis are *intractability, complications of medical therapy*, and *risk of or development of malignancy*. Unlike ulcerative colitis, Crohn's colitis may be segmental and rectal sparing often is observed. A segmental colectomy may be appropriate if the remaining colon and/or rectum appear normal. An isolated colonic stricture also may be treated by segmental colectomy. Although it was long thought that Crohn's disease did not increase the risk of colorectal carcinoma, it is now recognized that Crohn's colitis (especially pancolitis) carries nearly the same risk for cancer as ulcerative colitis. Annual surveillance colonoscopy with multiple biopsies is recommended for patients with long-standing Crohn's colitis (>7 years duration). As in ulcerative colitis, dysplasia is an indication for total proctocolectomy. Ileal pouch–anal reconstruction is not recommended in these patients because of the risk for development of Crohn's disease within the pouch and the high risk of complications—fistula, abscess, stricture, pouch dysfunction, and pouch failure.

Anal and Perianal Crohn's Disease

Anal and perianal manifestations of Crohn's disease are very common. Anal or perianal disease occurs in 35% of all patients with Crohn's disease. Isolated anal Crohn's disease is uncommon, affecting only 3 to 4% of patients. Detection of anal Crohn's disease, therefore, should prompt evaluation of the remainder of the GI tract.

The most common perianal lesions in Crohn's disease are *skin tags* that are minimally symptomatic. *Fissures* also are common. Typically, a fissure from Crohn's disease is particularly deep or broad and perhaps better described as an anal ulcer. They often are multiple and located in a lateral position rather than anterior or posterior midline as seen in an idiopathic fissure in ano. A classic appearing fissure in ano located laterally should raise the suspicion of Crohn's disease. *Perianal abscess* and *fistulas* are common and can be particularly challenging. Fistulas tend to be complex and often have multiple tracts (Fig. 29-19). *Hemorrhoids* are not more common in patients with Crohn's disease than in the general population, although many patients tend to attribute any anal or perianal symptom to "hemorrhoids."

Treatment of anal and perianal Crohn's disease focuses on alleviation of symptoms. Perianal skin irritation from diarrhea often responds to medical therapy directed at small bowel or colonic disease. In general, skin tags and hemorrhoids should *not* be excised unless they are extremely symptomatic because of the risk of creating chronic, nonhealing wounds. Fissures may respond to local or systemic therapy; sphincterotomy is relatively contraindicated because of the risk of creating a chronic, nonhealing wound, and because of

the increased risk of incontinence in a patient with diarrhea from underlying colitis or small bowel disease. Anal ulcers associated with Crohn's disease usually are not very painful unless there is an underlying abscess. Thus, in patients with significant anal pain, an examination under anesthesia is indicated to exclude an underlying abscess or fistula and to assess the rectal mucosa. In the absence of active Crohn's proctitis, one can proceed cautiously with a partial internal sphincterotomy if the examination under anesthesia reveals a classic-appearing posterior or anterior fissure and anal stenosis.

Recurrent abscess(es) or complex anal fistulas should raise the possibility of Crohn's disease. Treatment focuses on *control of sepsis, delineation of complex anatomy, treatment of underlying mucosal disease,* and *sphincter preservation.* Abscesses often can be drained locally, and mushroom catheters are useful for maintaining drainage. Endoanal ultrasound and pelvic MRI are useful for mapping complex fistulous tracts. Liberal use of setons can control many fistulas and avoid division of the sphincter. Many patients with anal Crohn's disease function well with multiple setons left in place for years. Endoanal advancement flaps may be considered for definitive therapy if the rectal mucosa is uninvolved. In 10 to 15% of cases, intractable perianal sepsis requires proctectomy.

Rectovaginal fistula can be a particularly difficult problem in these patients. A rectal or vaginal mucosal advancement flap may be used if the rectal mucosa appears healthy and scarring of the rectovaginal septum is minimal. Occasionally, proctectomy is the best option for women with highly symptomatic rectovaginal fistula. Although proximal diversion often is used to protect complex perianal reconstruction, there is no evidence that diversion alone increases healing of anal and perianal Crohn's disease.

Medical treatment of underlying proctitis with salicylate and/or corticosteroid enemas may be helpful; however, control of sepsis is the primary goal of therapy. Metronidazole also has been used with some success in this setting. Infliximab and other similar monoclonal antibody agents have shown some efficacy in healing chronic fistulas secondary to Crohn's disease. The success of infliximab has led to a concerted effort to identify other immunomodulators that might prove useful. Proinflammatory cytokines such as interleukin-12 and interferon-γ are potential targets. Inhibition of immune cell migration also has been suggested as an approach.[42] However, it is of paramount importance to drain any and all abscesses before initiating immunosuppressive therapy such as corticosteroids or infliximab.

Indeterminate Colitis

Approximately 15% of patients with inflammatory bowel disease manifest clinical and pathologic characteristics of both ulcerative colitis and Crohn's disease. Endoscopy, barium enema, and biopsy may be unable to differentiate ulcerative colitis from Crohn's colitis in this setting. The indications for surgery are the same as those for ulcerative colitis: *intractability, complications of medical therapy,* and *risk of or development of malignancy.* In the setting of indeterminate colitis in a patient who prefers a sphincter-sparing operation, a *total abdominal colectomy with end ileostomy* may be the best initial procedure. Pathologic examination of the entire colon may then allow a more accurate diagnosis. If the diagnosis suggests ulcerative colitis, an ileal pouch–anal anastomosis procedure can be performed. If the diagnosis remains in question, the safest surgical option is completion proctectomy with end ileostomy (similar to Crohn's colitis). Ileal pouch–anal reconstruction also may be considered with the understanding that the pouch failure rate is between 15 and 20%.

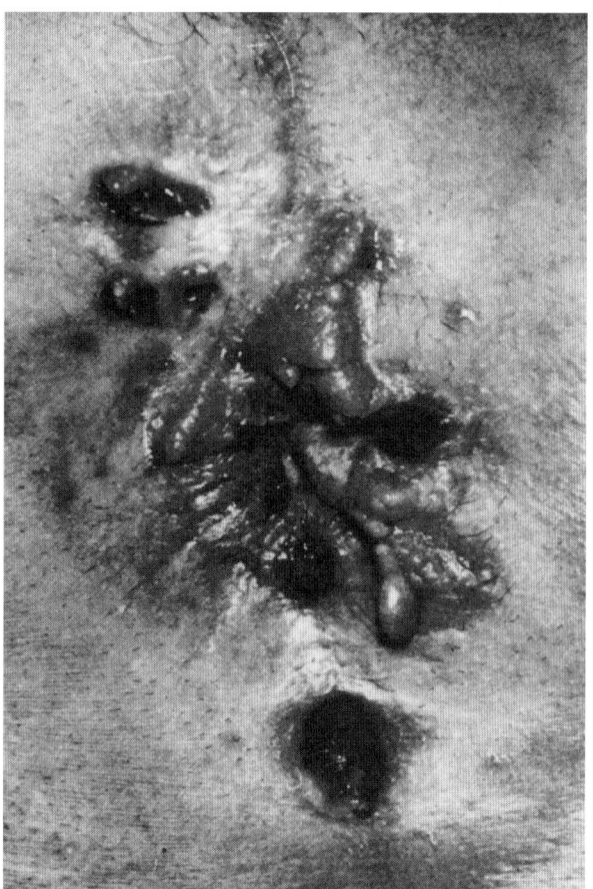

FIG. 29-19. Photograph of a patient with multiple perianal fistulas secondary to Crohn's disease. *[Reproduced with permission from Hamilton SR, Borson BC: Crohn's disease: Pathology, in Berk JE (ed): Bockus Gastroenterology, 4th ed. Philadelphia: Saunders, 1985, Fig. 127-5, p 2229. Copyright Elsevier.]*

DIVERTICULAR DISEASE

Diverticular disease is a clinical term used to describe the presence of symptomatic diverticula. *Diverticulosis* refers to the presence of diverticula without inflammation. *Diverticulitis* refers to inflammation and infection associated with diverticula. The majority of colonic diverticula are *false diverticula* in which the mucosa and

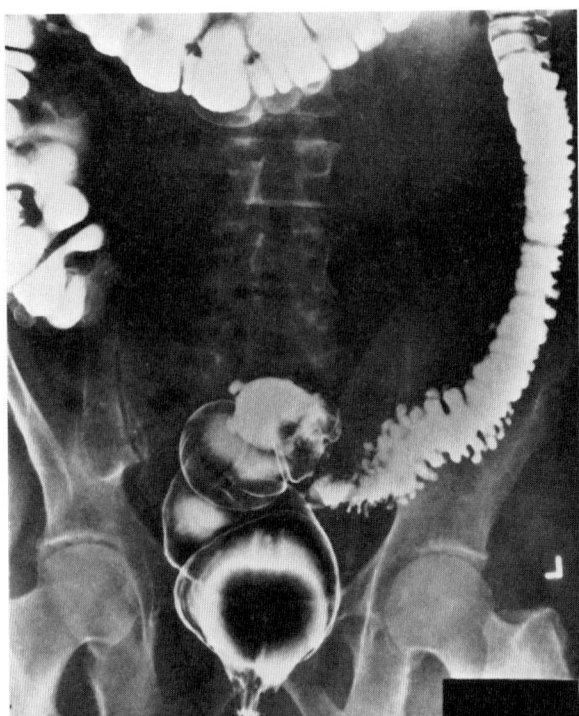

FIG. 29-20. Diverticulosis of sigmoid colon on barium enema. *[Reproduced with permission from Nivatvongs S, Becker ER: Colon, rectum and anal canal, in James EC, Corry RJ, Perry JCF Jr. (eds):* Basic Surgical Practice. *Philadelphia: Hanley & Belfus, 1987. Copyright Elsevier.]*

muscularis mucosa have herniated through the colonic wall. These diverticula occur between the taeniae coli, at points where the main blood vessels penetrate the colonic wall (presumably creating an area of relative weakness in the colonic muscle). They are thought to be *pulsion* diverticula resulting from high intraluminal pressure. *Diverticular bleeding* can be massive, but usually is self limited. *True diverticula*, which comprise all layers of the bowel wall, are rare and are usually congenital in origin.

Diverticulosis is extremely common in the United States and Europe. It is estimated that half of the population older than age 50 years has colonic diverticula. The sigmoid colon is the most common site of diverticulosis (Fig. 29-20). Diverticulosis is thought to be an acquired disorder, but the etiology is poorly understood. The most accepted theory is that a lack of dietary fiber results in smaller stool volume, requiring high intraluminal pressure and high colonic wall tension for propulsion. Chronic contraction then results in muscular hypertrophy and development of the process of segmentation in which the colon acts like separate segments instead of functioning as a continuous tube. As segmentation progresses, the high pressures are directed radially toward the colon wall rather than to development of propulsive waves that move stool distally. The high radial pressures directed against the bowel wall create pulsion diverticula. A loss of tensile strength and a decrease in elasticity of the bowel wall with age also have been proposed etiologies. While none of these theories has been proven, a high-fiber diet does appear to decrease the incidence of diverticulosis. Although diverticulosis is common, most cases are asymptomatic and complications occur in the minority of people with this condition.

Inflammatory Complications (Diverticulitis)

Diverticulitis refers to inflammation and infection associated with a diverticulum and is estimated to occur in 10 to 25% of people with diverticulosis. Peridiverticular and pericolic infection results from a perforation (either macroscopic or microscopic) of a diverticulum, which leads to contamination, inflammation, and infection. The spectrum of disease ranges from mild, uncomplicated diverticulitis that can be treated in the outpatient setting, to free perforation and

diffuse peritonitis that requires emergency laparotomy. Most patients present with left-sided abdominal pain, with or without fever, and leukocytosis. A mass may be present. Plain radiographs are useful for detecting free intra-abdominal air. CT scan is extremely useful for defining pericolic inflammation, phlegmon, or abscess. Contrast enemas and/or endoscopy are relatively contraindicated because of the risk of perforation. The differential diagnosis includes malignancy, ischemic colitis, infectious colitis, and inflammatory bowel disease.

Uncomplicated Diverticulitis

Uncomplicated diverticulitis is characterized by left lower quadrant pain and tenderness. CT findings include pericolic soft tissue stranding, colonic wall thickening, and/or phlegmon. Most patients with uncomplicated diverticulitis will respond to outpatient therapy with broad-spectrum oral antibiotics and a low-residue diet. Antibiotics should be continued for 7 to 10 days. About 10 to 20% of patients with more severe pain, tenderness, fever, and leukocytosis are treated in the hospital with parenteral antibiotics and bowel rest. Most patients improve within 48 to 72 hours. Failure to improve may suggest abscess formation. CT can be extremely useful in this setting and many pericolic abscesses can be drained percutaneously (see below in Complicated Diverticulititis). Deterioration in a patient's clinical condition and/or the development of peritonitis are indications for laparotomy.

Most patients with uncomplicated diverticulitis will recover without surgery, and 50 to 70% will have no further episodes. However, the risk of complications increases with recurrent disease. For this reason, elective sigmoid colectomy often is recommended after the second episode of diverticulitis, especially if the patient has required hospitalization. Resection often has been recommended after the first episode in very young patients and often is recommended after the first episode of *complicated diverticulitis*. These general guidelines have been questioned in recent years. Many surgeons now will not advise colectomy even after two documented episodes of diverticulitis assuming the patient is completely asymptomatic and that carcinoma has been excluded by colonoscopy. Immunosuppressed patients generally are still advised to undergo colectomy after a single episode of documented diverticulitis. Medical comorbidity should be considered when evaluating a patient for elective resection, and the risks of recurrent disease weighed against the risks of the operation. Because colon carcinoma may have an identical clinical presentation to diverticulitis (either complicated or uncomplicated), all patients must be evaluated for malignancy after resolution of the acute episode. Sigmoidoscopy or colonoscopy is recommended 4 to 6 weeks after recovery. Inability to exclude malignancy is another indication for resection.

In the elective setting, a *sigmoid colectomy with a primary anastomosis* is the procedure of choice. The resection should always be extended to the rectum distally because the risk of recurrence is high if a segment of sigmoid colon is retained. The proximal extent of the resection should include all thickened or inflamed bowel; however, resection of all diverticula is unnecessary. Increasingly, laparoscopy is being used for elective sigmoid colectomy for diverticular disease.

Complicated Diverticulitis

Complicated diverticulitis includes diverticulitis with abscess, obstruction, diffuse peritonitis (free perforation), or fistulas between the colon and adjacent structures. Colovesical, colovaginal, and coloenteric fistulas are long-term sequelae of complicated diverticulitis. *The Hinchey staging system* often is used to describe the severity of complicated diverticulitis: Stage I includes colonic inflammation with an associated pericolic abscess; stage II includes colonic inflammation with a retroperitoneal or pelvic abscess; stage III is associated with purulent peritonitis; and stage IV is associated with fecal peritonitis. Treatment depends on the patient's overall clinical condition and the degree of peritoneal contamination and infection. Small abscesses (<2 cm diameter) may be treated with parenteral antibiotics. Larger

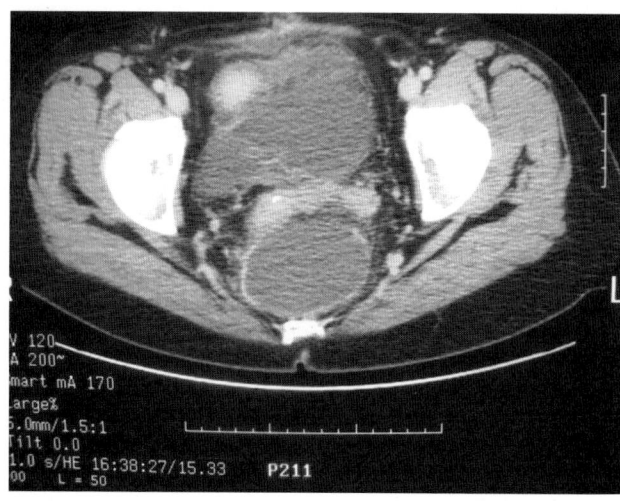

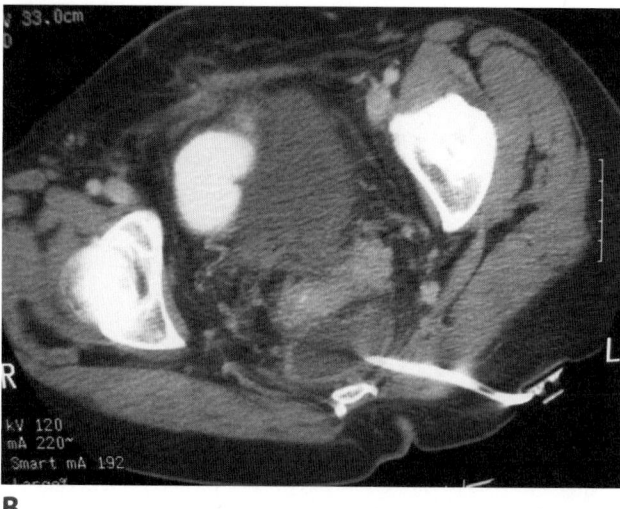

A   **B**

FIG. 29-21. A. Computed tomographic scan demonstrating pelvic abscess from perforated diverticular disease. **B.** Posterolateral computed tomographic–guided drainage of abdominal abscess from perforated diverticular disease. *(Both images courtesy of Charles O. Finne III, MD, Minneapolis, MN.)*

abscesses are best treated with CT-guided percutaneous drainage (Fig. 29-21).[43] The majority of these patients will ultimately require resection, but percutaneous drainage may allow a one-stage, elective procedure and may obviate the need for colectomy if full recovery follows the drainage.

Urgent or emergent laparotomy may be required if an abscess is inaccessible to percutaneous drainage, if the patient's condition deteriorates or fails to improve, or if the patient presents with free intra-abdominal air or peritonitis. In almost all cases, an attempt should be made to resect the affected segment of bowel. Patients with small, localized pericolic or pelvic abscesses (Hinchey stages I and II) may be candidates for a sigmoid colectomy with a primary anastomosis (a one-stage operation). In patients with larger abscesses, peritoneal soiling, or peritonitis, sigmoid colectomy with end colostomy and Hartmann pouch is the most commonly used procedure.[44,45] Success also has been reported after sigmoid colectomy, primary anastomosis, ± on-table lavage, and proximal diversion (loop ileostomy). This option may be appropriate in stable patients and offers the great advantage that the subsequent operation to restore bowel continuity is simpler than is takedown of a Hartmann pouch. The presence of inflammation and phlegmon may increase the risk of ureteral damage during mobilization of the sigmoid colon, and preoperative placement of ureteral catheters can be invaluable. In extremely unstable patients, or in the presence of such severe inflammation that resection would harm adjacent organs, proximal diversion and local drainage have been used. However, this approach generally is avoided because of high morbidity and mortality rates, along with the requirement for multiple operations.

Obstructive symptoms occur in approximately 67% of patients with acute diverticulitis, and complete obstruction occurs in 10%. Patients with incomplete obstruction often respond to fluid resuscitation, nasogastric suction, and gentle, low-volume water or Gastrografin enemas. Relief of obstruction allows full bowel preparation and elective resection. A high-volume oral bowel preparation is contraindicated in the presence of obstructive symptoms. Obstruction that does not rapidly respond to medical management mandates laparotomy. Sigmoid colectomy with end colostomy is the safest procedure to perform in this setting. However, colectomy and primary anastomosis, with or without on-table lavage (depending on extent of fecal load in the proximal colon), and proximal diversion may be appropriate if the patient is stable and the proximal and distal bowel appear healthy.

Approximately 5% of patients with complicated diverticulitis develop fistulas between the colon and an adjacent organ. *Colovesical*

fistulas are most common, followed by *colovaginal* and *coloenteric* fistulas. *Colocutaneous* fistulas are a rare complication of diverticulitis. Two key points in the evaluation of fistulas are to *define the anatomy of the fistula* and *exclude other diagnoses*. Contrast enema and/or small bowel studies are extremely useful in defining the course of the fistula. CT scan can identify associated abscesses or masses. The differential diagnosis includes *malignancy, Crohn's disease,* and *radiation-induced fistulas.* Although Crohn's disease and radiation injury may be suspected based upon the patient's medical history, colonoscopy or sigmoidoscopy usually is required to rule out malignancy. In addition, in a patient who has received radiation therapy, a fistula must be considered to be recurrent cancer until proven otherwise. Once the anatomy of the fistula has been defined and other diagnoses excluded, operative management should include resection of the affected segment of the colon involved with diverticulitis (usually with a primary anastomosis) and simple repair of the secondarily involved organ. Suspicion of carcinoma may mandate a wider, en bloc resection.

Hemorrhage

Bleeding from a diverticulum results from erosion of the peridiverticular arteriole and may result in massive hemorrhage. Most significant lower GI hemorrhage occurs in elderly patients in whom both diverticulosis and angiodysplasia are common. Consequently, the exact bleeding source may be difficult to identify. Fortunately, in 80% of patients, bleeding stops spontaneously. Clinical management should focus on resuscitation and localization of the bleeding site as described for lower GI hemorrhage. Colonoscopy may occasionally identify a bleeding diverticulum that may then be treated with epinephrine injection or cautery. Angiography may be diagnostic and therapeutic in this setting. In the rare instance in which diverticular hemorrhage persists or recurs, laparotomy and segmental colectomy may be required.

Giant Colonic Diverticulum

Giant colonic diverticula are extremely rare. Most occur on the antimesenteric side of the sigmoid colon. Patients may be asymptomatic or may present with vague abdominal complaints such as pain, nausea, or constipation. Plain radiographs may suggest the diagnosis. Barium enema usually is diagnostic. Complications of a giant diverticulum include perforation, obstruction, and volvulus. Resection of the involved colon and diverticulum is recommended.

Right-Sided Diverticula

The cecum and ascending colon infrequently are involved in diverticulosis coli. Even more uncommon is a true solitary diverticulum, which contains all layers of the bowel wall and is thought to be congenital in origin. Right-sided diverticula occur more often in younger patients than do left-sided diverticula, and are more common in people of Asian descent than in other populations. Most patients with right-sided diverticula are asymptomatic. However, diverticulitis does occur occasionally. Because patients are young and present with right lower quadrant pain, they often are thought to suffer from acute appendicitis, and the diagnosis of right-sided diverticulitis is subsequently made in the operating room. If there is a single large diverticulum and minimal inflammation, a diverticulectomy may be performed, but an ileocecal resection usually is the preferred operation in this setting. Hemorrhage rarely occurs and should be treated in the same fashion as hemorrhage from a left-sided diverticulum.

ADENOCARCINOMA AND POLYPS

Incidence

Colorectal carcinoma is the most common malignancy of the GI tract. Over 150,000 new cases are diagnosed annually in the United States and more than 52,000 patients die of this disease each year, making colorectal cancer the second most lethal cancer in the United States.[46] The incidence is similar in men and women and has remained fairly constant over the past 20 years. The widespread adoption of current national screening programs should dramatically decrease the incidence of this common and lethal disease. Early detection along with improvements in medical and surgical care are thought to be responsible for the decreasing mortality of colorectal cancer observed in recent years.

Epidemiology (Risk Factors)

Identification of risk factors for development of colorectal cancer is essential to establish screening and surveillance programs in appropriately targeted populations.

Aging

Aging is the dominant risk factor for colorectal cancer, with incidence rising steadily after age 50 years. More than 90% of cases diagnosed are in people older than age 50 years. This is the rationale for initiating screening tests of asymptomatic Americans at average risk of developing colorectal cancer at age 50 years. However, individuals of any age can develop colorectal cancer, so symptoms such as a significant change in bowel habits, rectal bleeding, melena, unexplained anemia, or weight loss require a thorough evaluation.

Hereditary Risk Factors

Approximately 80% of colorectal cancers occur sporadically, while 20% arise in patients with a known family history of colorectal cancer. Advances in the understanding of these familial disorders have led to interest in early diagnosis using genetic testing. Because of the medical, legal, and ethical considerations that are involved in this type of testing, all patients should be offered genetic counseling if a familial syndrome is suspected.

Environmental and Dietary Factors

The observation that colorectal carcinoma occurs more commonly in populations that consume diets high in animal fat and low in fiber has lead to the hypothesis that dietary factors contribute to carcinogenesis. A diet high in saturated or polyunsaturated fats increases risk of colorectal cancer, while a diet high in oleic acid (olive oil, coconut oil, fish oil) does not increase risk. Animal studies suggest that fats may be directly toxic to the colonic mucosa and thus may induce early malignant changes. In contrast, a diet high in *vegetable fiber* appears to be protective. A correlation between alcohol intake and incidence

of colorectal carcinoma also has been suggested. Ingestion of calcium, selenium, vitamins A, C, and E, carotenoids, and plant phenols may decrease the risk of developing colorectal cancer. Obesity and sedentary lifestyle dramatically increase cancer-related mortality in a number of malignancies, including colorectal carcinoma. This knowledge is the basis for primary prevention strategies to eliminate colorectal cancer by altering diet and lifestyle.[47,48]

Inflammatory Bowel Disease

Patients with long-standing colitis from inflammatory bowel disease are at increased risk for the development of colorectal cancer.[49] It is hypothesized that chronic inflammation predisposes the mucosa to malignant changes and there is some evidence that degree of inflammation influences risk. In general, the duration and extent of colitis correlate with risk. Other factors thought to increase risk include the presence of primary sclerosing cholangitis and family history of colorectal cancer. In ulcerative pancolitis, the risk of carcinoma is approximately 2% after 10 years, 8% after 20 years, and 18% after 30 years. Patients with Crohn's pancolitis have similar risk. Left-sided colitis carries somewhat less risk. For this reason, screening colonoscopy with multiple random mucosal biopsies has been recommended annually after 8 years of disease for patients with pancolitis and after 12 to 15 years of disease for patients with left-sided colitis. It is important to note, however, that intensive surveillance has not definitively been shown to improve survival, and some authors are questioning the efficacy of this approach.

Other Risk Factors

Cigarette smoking is associated with an increased risk of colonic adenomas, especially after more than 35 years of use. Patients with ureterosigmoidostomy are also at increased risk for both adenoma and carcinoma formation.[50] Acromegaly, which is associated with increased levels of circulating human growth hormone and insulin-like growth factor I, increases risk as well. Pelvic irradiation may increase the risk of developing rectal carcinoma, although it is unclear if this represents a direct effect of radiation damage or is instead a correlation between the development of rectal cancer and a history of another pelvic malignancy.

Pathogenesis of Colorectal Cancer
Genetic Defects

Over the past two decades, an intense research effort has focused on elucidating the genetic defects and molecular abnormalities associated with the development and progression of colorectal adenomas and carcinoma. Mutations may cause *activation of oncogenes* (K-ras) and/or *inactivation of tumor-suppressor genes* [APC, DCC (deleted in colorectal carcinoma), p53]. Colorectal carcinoma is thought to develop from adenomatous polyps by accumulation of these mutations (Fig. 29-22).

Defects in the APC gene were first described in patients with *FAP*. By investigating these families, characteristic mutations in the APC gene were identified. They are now known to be present in 80% of sporadic colorectal cancers as well.

The APC gene is a *tumor-suppressor gene*. Mutations in both alleles are necessary to initiate polyp formation. The majority of mutations are premature stop codons, which result in a truncated APC protein. In FAP, the site of mutation correlates with the clinical severity of the disease. For example, mutations in either the 3' or 5' end of the gene result in attenuated forms of FAP, while mutations in the center of the gene result in more virulent disease. Thus, knowledge of the specific mutation in a family may help guide clinical decision making.

APC inactivation alone does not result in a carcinoma. Instead, this mutation sets the stage for the accumulation of genetic damage that results in malignancy via mutations accumulated in the loss of heterozygosity (LOH) pathway. Additional mutations involved in this pathway include activation of the *K-ras* oncogene, and loss of the tumor-suppressor genes *DCC* and p53.

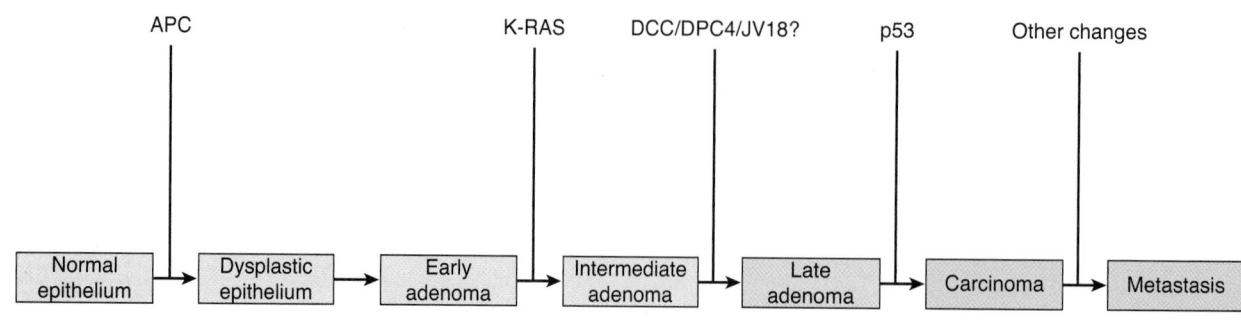

FIG. 29-22. Schematic showing progression from normal colonic epithelium to carcinoma of the colon.

K-ras is classified as a *proto-oncogene* because mutation of only one allele will perturb the cell cycle. The K-ras gene product is a G protein involved in intracellular signal transduction. When active, K-ras binds guanosine triphosphate (GTP); hydrolysis of GTP to guanosine diphosphate then inactivates the G protein. Mutation of K-ras results in an inability to hydrolyze GTP, thus leaving the G protein permanently in the active form. It is thought that this then leads to uncontrolled cell division.

In 2002, a new mutation in the MYH gene on chromosome 1p was found to be associated with an increased risk of colorectal cancer.[51] MYH is a base excision repair gene, and biallelic deletion results in changes in other downstream molecules. Since its discovery, MYH mutations have been associated with an AFAP phenotype in addition to sporadic cancers.[52] Unlike APC gene mutations that are expressed in an autosomal dominant pattern, the requirement for biallelic mutation in MYH results in an autosomal recessive pattern of inheritance.

DCC is a tumor-suppressor gene and loss of both alleles is required for malignant degeneration. The role of the DCC gene product is poorly understood. The main role of this molecule appears to be in the central nervous system, where it is involved in differentiation and axonal migration. This observation has led to the hypothesis that DCC may be involved in differentiation and cellular adhesion in colorectal cancer, but this theory remains unproven.[53] DCC mutations are present in more than 70% of colorectal carcinomas and may negatively impact prognosis.

The tumor-suppressor gene p53 has been well characterized in a number of malignancies. The p53 protein appears to be crucial for initiating apoptosis in cells with irreparable genetic damage. Mutations in p53 are present in 75% of colorectal cancers.

Genetic Pathways

Two major pathways for tumor initiation and progression have been described: the *LOH pathway* and the *replication error (RER) pathway*. The LOH pathway is characterized by chromosomal deletions and tumor aneuploidy. Eighty percent of colorectal carcinomas appear to arise from mutations in the LOH pathway. The remaining 20% of colorectal carcinomas are thought to arise from mutations in the RER pathway, which is characterized by errors in mismatch repair during DNA replication. A number of genes have been identified that appear to be crucial for recognizing and repairing DNA RERs. These *mismatch repair genes* include *hMSH2, hMLH1, hPMS1, hPMS2,* and *hMSH6/GTBP*. A mutation in one of these genes predisposes a cell to mutations, which may occur in proto-oncogenes or tumor-suppressor genes. Accumulation of these errors then leads to genomic instability and ultimately to carcinogenesis.

The RER pathway is associated with *microsatellite instability* (MSI). Microsatellites are regions of the genome in which short base-pair segments are repeated several times. These areas are particularly prone to RER. Consequently, a mutation in a mismatch repair gene produces variable lengths of these repetitive sequences, a finding that has been described as *microsatellite instability*. Approximately 15% of colorectal cancers are associated with MSI, but most do not have an MMR gene mutation per se. Instead, methylation of the gene promoter causes "silencing" of the gene, resulting in loss of the gene product and a phenotype similar to that present with a true gene mutation.[9]

Tumors associated with MSI appear to have different biologic characteristics than do tumors that result from the LOH pathway. Tumors with MSI are more likely to be right sided, possess diploid DNA, and are associated with a better prognosis than tumors that arise from the LOH pathway that are microsatellite stable. Tumors arising from the LOH pathway tend to occur in the more distal colon, often have chromosomal aneuploidy, and are associated with a poorer prognosis.

Deletion of the tumor suppressor phosphatase and tensin homolog (PTEN) appears to be involved in a number of hamartomatous polyposis syndromes. Deletions in PTEN have been identified in juvenile polyposis, Peutz-Jeghers syndrome, Cowden syndrome, and PTEN-hamartoma syndrome, in addition to multiple endocrine neoplasia IIB.[9]

Polyps

It is now well accepted that the majority of colorectal carcinomas evolve from adenomatous polyps; this sequence of events is the *adenoma–carcinoma sequence*. *Polyp* is a nonspecific clinical term that describes any projection from the surface of the intestinal mucosa regardless of its histologic nature. Colorectal polyps may be classified as *neoplastic (tubular adenoma, villous adenoma, tubulovillous adenomas), hamartomatous (juvenile, Peutz-Jeghers, Cronkite-Canada), inflammatory (pseudopolyp, benign lymphoid polyp),* or *hyperplastic*.

Neoplastic Polyps

Adenomatous polyps are common, occurring in up to 25% of the population older than 50 years of age in the United States. By definition, these lesions are dysplastic. The risk of malignant degeneration is related to both the size and type of polyp. Tubular adenomas are associated with malignancy in only 5% of cases, whereas villous adenomas may harbor cancer in up to 40%. Tubulovillous adenomas are at intermediate risk (22%). Invasive carcinomas are rare in polyps smaller than 1 cm; the incidence increases with size. The risk of carcinoma in a polyp larger than 2 cm is 35 to 50%. Although most neoplastic polyps do not evolve to cancer, most colorectal cancers originate as a polyp. It is this fact that forms the basis for secondary prevention strategies to eliminate colorectal cancer by targeting the neoplastic polyp for removal before malignancy develops.

Polyps may be *pedunculated* or *sessile*. Most pedunculated polyps are amenable to colonoscopic snare excision. Removal of sessile polyps often is more challenging. Special colonoscopic techniques, including saline lift and piecemeal snare excision, facilitate successful removal of many sessile polyps. For rectal sessile polyps, transanal operative excision is preferred because it produces an intact, single pathology specimen that can be used to determine the need for further therapy. Interpretation of the precise depth of invasion of a cancer arising in a sessile polyp after piecemeal excision often is impossible. The site of sessile polypectomies should be marked by injection of methylene blue or India ink to guide follow-up colonoscopy sessions to ensure that the polyp has been completely removed, and to facilitate identification of the involved bowel segment should operative resection be necessary. Colectomy is reserved for cases in which colonoscopic removal is impossible, such as large, flat lesions or if a focus of invasive cancer is confirmed in the specimen. These patients may be ideal candidates for laparoscopic colectomy.

Complications of polypectomy include *perforation* and *bleeding*. A small perforation (*microperforation*) in a fully prepared, stable patient may be managed with bowel rest, broad-spectrum antibiotics, and close observation. Signs of sepsis, peritonitis, or deterioration in clinical condition are indications for laparotomy. Bleeding may occur immediately after polypectomy or may be delayed. The bleeding usually will stop spontaneously, but colonoscopy may be required to re-snare a bleeding stalk or cauterize the lesion. Occasionally, angiography and infusion of vasopressin may be necessary. Rarely, colectomy is required.

Hamartomatous Polyps (Juvenile Polyps)

In contrast to adenomatous polyps, hamartomatous polyps (juvenile polyps) usually are not premalignant. These lesions are the characteristic polyps of childhood but may occur at any age. Bleeding is a common symptom and intussusception and/or obstruction may occur. Because the gross appearance of these polyps is identical to adenomatous polyps, these lesions should also be treated by polypectomy. In contrast to adenomatous polyposis syndromes, these conditions are often associated with mutation in PTEN.

Familial juvenile polyposis is an autosomal dominant disorder in which patients develop hundreds of polyps in the colon and rectum. Unlike solitary juvenile polyps, these lesions may degenerate into adenomas and, eventually, carcinoma. Annual screening should begin between the ages of 10 and 12 years. Treatment is surgical and depends, in part, upon the degree of rectal involvement. If the rectum is relatively spared, a total abdominal colectomy with ileorectal anastomosis may be performed with subsequent close surveillance of the retained rectum. If the rectum is carpeted with polyps, total proctocolectomy is the more appropriate operation. These patients are candidates for ileal pouch–anal reconstruction to avoid a permanent stoma.

Peutz-Jeghers syndrome is characterized by polyposis of the small intestine and, to a lesser extent, polyposis of the colon and rectum. Characteristic melanin spots often are noted on the buccal mucosa and lips of these patients. The polyps of Peutz-Jeghers syndrome generally are considered to be hamartomas and are not thought to be at significant risk for malignant degeneration. However, carcinoma may occasionally develop. Because the entire length of the GI tract may be affected, surgery is reserved for symptoms such as obstruction or bleeding or for patients in whom polyps develop adenomatous features. Screening consists of a baseline colonoscopy and upper endoscopy at age 20 years, followed by annual flexible sigmoidoscopy thereafter.

Cronkite-Canada syndrome is a disorder in which patients develop GI polyposis in association with alopecia, cutaneous pigmentation, and atrophy of the fingernails and toenails. Diarrhea is a prominent symptom, and vomiting, malabsorption, and protein-losing enteropathy may occur. Most patients die of this disease despite maximal medical therapy, and surgery is reserved for complications of polyposis, such as obstruction.

Cowden syndrome is an autosomal dominant disorder with hamartomas of all three embryonal cell layers. Facial trichilemmomas, breast cancer, thyroid disease, and GI polyps are typical of the syndrome. Patients should be screened for cancers. Treatment is otherwise based upon symptoms.

Inflammatory Polyps (Pseudopolyps)

Inflammatory polyps occur most commonly in the context of inflammatory bowel disease, but may also occur after amebic colitis, ischemic colitis, and schistosomal colitis. These lesions are not premalignant, but they cannot be distinguished from adenomatous polyps based upon gross appearance and therefore should be removed. Microscopic examination shows islands of normal, regenerating mucosa (the polyp) surrounded by areas of mucosal loss. Polyposis may be extensive, especially in patients with severe colitis, and may mimic FAP.

Hyperplastic Polyps

Hyperplastic polyps are extremely common in the colon. These polyps usually are small (<5 mm) and show histologic characteristics of hyperplasia without any dysplasia. They are not considered premalignant, but cannot be distinguished from adenomatous polyps colonoscopically and therefore often are removed. In contrast, large hyperplastic polyps (>2 cm) may have a slight risk of malignant degeneration. Moreover, large polyps may harbor foci of adenomatous tissue and dysplasia. *Hyperplastic polyposis* is a rare disorder in which multiple large hyperplastic polyps occur in young adults. These patients are at slightly increased risk for the development of colorectal cancer.

Inherited Colorectal Carcinoma

Many of the genetic defects originally described in hereditary cancers have subsequently been found in sporadic tumors. Although the majority of colorectal cancer is sporadic, several hereditary syndromes provide paradigms for the study of this disease. Insight gained from studying inherited colorectal cancer syndromes has led to better understanding of the genetics of colorectal carcinoma.

Familial Adenomatous Polyposis

This rare autosomal dominant condition accounts for only about 1% of all colorectal adenocarcinomas. Nevertheless, this syndrome has provided tremendous insight into the molecular mechanisms underlying colorectal carcinogenesis. The genetic abnormality in FAP is a mutation in the APC gene, located on chromosome 5q. Of patients with FAP, APC mutation testing is positive in 75% of cases. Although most patients with FAP will have a known family history of the disease, up to 25% present without other affected family members. Clinically, patients develop hundreds to thousands of adenomatous polyps shortly after puberty. The lifetime risk of colorectal cancer in FAP patients approaches 100% by age 50 years.

Flexible sigmoidoscopy of first-degree relatives of FAP patients beginning at age 10 to 15 years has been the traditional mainstay of screening. Today, following genetic counseling, APC gene testing may be used to screen family members, providing an APC mutation has been identified in a family member. If APC testing is positive in a relative of a patient with a known APC mutation, annual flexible sigmoidoscopy beginning at age 10 to 15 years is done until polyps are identified. If APC testing is negative, the relative can be screened starting at age 50 years per average-risk guidelines. If APC testing is refused, annual flexible sigmoidoscopy beginning at age 10 to 15 years is performed until age 24 years. Screening flexible sigmoidoscopy is then done every 2 years until age 34 years, every 3 years until age 44 years, and then every 3 to 5 years. If an APC mutation is not found in the family, either APC testing can be done for at-risk family members or traditional screening by flexible sigmoidoscopy can be initiated.

FAP patients also are at risk for the development of adenomas anywhere in the GI tract, particularly in the duodenum. Periampullary carcinoma is a particular concern. Upper endoscopy therefore is recommended for surveillance every 1 to 3 years beginning at age 25 to 30 years.

Once the diagnosis of FAP has been made and polyps are developing, treatment is surgical. Four factors affect the choice of operation: age of the patient; presence and severity of symptoms; extent of rectal polyposis; and presence and location of cancer or desmoid tumors. Three operative procedures can be considered: total proctocolectomy with either an end (Brooke) ileostomy or continent (Kock) ileostomy; total abdominal colectomy with ileorectal anastomosis;

and restorative proctocolectomy with ileal pouch–anal anastomosis with or without a temporary ileostomy. Most patients elect to have an ileal pouch–anal anastomosis in the absence of a distal rectal cancer, a mesenteric desmoid tumor that prevents the ileum from reaching the anus or poor sphincter function. Mucosectomy has been advocated in patients with FAP undergoing ileal pouch–anal anastomosis because of the risk of neoplasia in the anal transition zone, but the requirement for this procedure remains controversial. Although patient satisfaction with this procedure remains high, function may not be ideal, and up to 50% of patients experience some degree of incontinence. Total proctocolectomy with continent ileostomy (Kock pouch) has largely been abandoned because of the success of ileal pouch–anal reconstruction. Total abdominal colectomy with an ileorectal anastomosis is also an option in these patients, but requires vigilant surveillance of the retained rectum for development of rectal cancer.[54] There is increasing data suggesting that the administration of COX-2 inhibitors (celecoxib, sulindac) may slow or prevent the development of polyps.[55]

FAP may be associated with extraintestinal manifestations such as congenital hypertrophy of the retinal pigmented epithelium, desmoid tumors, epidermoid cysts, mandibular osteomas (Gardner's syndrome), and central nervous system tumors (Turcot's syndrome). Desmoid tumors in particular can make surgical management difficult and are a source of major morbidity and mortality in these patients. Desmoid tumors are often hormone responsive and growth may be inhibited in some patients with tamoxifen. COX-2 inhibitors and NSAIDs also may be beneficial in this setting.

Attenuated FAP

AFAP is a recently recognized variant of FAP associated with mutations at the 3' or 5' end of the APC gene. Patients present later in life with fewer polyps (usually 10 to 100) dominantly located in the right colon, when compared to classic FAP. Colorectal carcinoma develops in more than 50% of these patients, but occurs later (average age 55 years). Patients are also at risk for duodenal polyposis. However, in contrast to FAP, APC gene mutations are present in only about 30% of patients with AFAP. When present, these mutations are expressed in an autosomal dominant pattern.

Mutations in MYH also result in the AFAP phenotype, but are expressed in an autosomal recessive pattern. It has been suggested that MYH mutations may be responsible for AFAP in patients who do not have a detectable APC gene mutation.[53]

Genetic testing often is offered to patients with suspected AFAP. When positive, genetic counseling and testing may be used to screen at-risk family members. If the family mutation is unknown, screening colonoscopy is recommended beginning at age 13 to 15 years, then every 4 years to age 28 years, and then every 3 years. These patients are often candidates for a total abdominal colectomy with ileorectal anastomosis because the limited polyposis in the rectum can usually be treated by colonoscopic snare excision. Prophylaxis with COX-2 inhibitors also may be appropriate. Because of the more subtle phenotype in these patients, it is important to rule out other familial syndromes such as hereditary nonpolyposis colon cancer (HNPCC; Lynch syndrome) and more common familial colorectal cancer.[9]

Hereditary Nonpolyposis Colon Cancer (Lynch Syndrome)

HNPCC (or Lynch syndrome) is more common than FAP, but is still extremely rare (1 to 3%). The genetic defects associated with HNPCC arise from errors in *mismatch repair*, and study of this syndrome has elucidated many of the details of the RER pathway. HNPCC is inherited in an autosomal dominant pattern and is characterized by the development of colorectal carcinoma at an early age (average age: 40 to 45 years). Approximately 70% of affected individuals will develop colorectal cancer. Cancers appear in the proximal colon more often than in sporadic colorectal cancer and have a better prognosis regardless of stage. The risk of synchronous or metachronous colorectal carcinoma is 40%. HNPCC also

may be associated with extracolonic malignancies, including endometrial, which is most common, ovarian, pancreas, stomach, small bowel, biliary, and urinary tract carcinomas. The diagnosis of HNPCC is made based upon family history. The *Amsterdam criteria* for clinical diagnosis of HNPCC are three affected relatives with histologically verified adenocarcinoma of the large bowel (one must be a first-degree relative of one of the others) in two successive generations of a family with one patient diagnosed before age 50 years. The presence of other HNPCC-related carcinomas should raise the suspicion of this syndrome.[9] In a patient with an established diagnosis of colorectal cancer, tumor testing for presence of MMR gene products (immunohistochemistry) and/or MSI can sometimes serve as screening for this syndrome.

HNPCC results from mutations in mismatch repair genes, and, like FAP, specific mutations are associated with different phenotypes. For example, mutations in PMS2 or MSH6 result in a more attenuated form of HNPCC when compared to mutations in other genes. MSH6 inactivation also appears to be associated with a higher risk for endometrial cancer.[56] Further significance of these specific mutations remains to be determined.

Screening colonoscopy is recommended annually for at-risk patients beginning at either age 20 to 25 years or 10 years younger than the youngest age at diagnosis in the family, whichever comes first.[57] Because of the high risk of endometrial carcinoma, transvaginal ultrasound or endometrial aspiration biopsy also is recommended annually after age 25 to 35 years. Because there is a 40% risk of developing a second colon cancer, total colectomy with ileorectal anastomosis is recommended once adenomas or a colon carcinoma is diagnosed, or if prophylactic colectomy is decided upon. Annual proctoscopy is necessary because the risk of developing rectal cancer remains high. Similarly, prophylactic hysterectomy and bilateral salpingo-oophorectomy should be considered in women who have completed childbearing.

Familial Colorectal Cancer

Nonsyndromic familial colorectal cancer accounts for 10 to 15% of patients with colorectal cancer. The lifetime risk of developing colorectal cancer increases with a family history of the disease. The lifetime risk of colorectal cancer in a patient with no family history of this disease (average-risk population) is approximately 6%, but rises to 12% if one first-degree relative is affected and to 35% if two first-degree relatives are affected. Age of onset also impacts risk and a diagnosis before the age of 50 years is associated with a higher incidence in family members. Screening colonoscopy is recommended every 5 years beginning at age 40 years or beginning 10 years before the age of the earliest diagnosed patient in the pedigree. Although there are no specific genetic abnormalities that are associated with familial colorectal cancer, any of the defects found in either the LOH pathway or RER pathway may be present in these patients.

Prevention: Screening and Surveillance

Because the majority of colorectal cancers are thought to arise from adenomatous polyps, preventive measures focus upon identification and removal of these premalignant lesions. In addition, many cancers are asymptomatic and screening may detect these tumors at an early and curable stage (Table 29-1). Although screening for colorectal cancer decreases the incidence of cancer and cancer-related mortality, the optimal method of screening remains controversial. Screening guidelines are meant for *asymptomatic* patients.[58–60] Any patient with a GI complaint (bleeding, change in bowel habits, pain, etc.) requires a complete evaluation, usually by colonoscopy.

Fecal Occult Blood Testing

The University of Minnesota Colon Cancer Control Study, a large, prospective, randomized trial, was the first of several large studies to conclude that FOBT screening reduces colorectal cancer mortality by 33% and metastatic cases by 50%. However, FOBT is relatively

TABLE 29-1	Advantages and disadvantages of screening modalities for asymptomatic individuals

	Advantages	Disadvantages
Fecal occult blood testing	Ease of use and noninvasive Low cost Good sensitivity with repeat testing	May not detect most polyps Low specificity Colonoscopy required for positive result Poor compliance with serial testing
Sigmoidoscopy	Examines colon most at risk Very sensitive for polyp detection in left colon Does not require full bowel preparation (enemas only)	Invasive Uncomfortable Slight risk of perforation or bleeding May miss proximal lesions Colonoscopy required if polyp identified
Colonoscopy	Examines entire colon Highly sensitive and specific Therapeutic	Most invasive Uncomfortable and requires sedation Requires bowel preparation Risk of perforation or bleeding Costly
Double-contrast barium enema	Examines entire colon Good sensitivity for polyps >1 cm	Requires bowel preparation Less sensitivity for polyps <1 cm May miss lesions in the sigmoid colon Colonoscopy required for positive result
Computed tomographic colonography (virtual colonoscopy)	Examines entire colon Noninvasive Sensitivity may be as good as colonoscopy	Requires bowel preparation Insensitive for small polyps Minimal experience and data Colonoscopy required for positive result Costly

insensitive, missing up to 50% of cancers and the majority of adenomas. Its specificity is low because 90% of patients with positive tests do not have colorectal cancer. Compliance with annual testing is low and costs are significant if one includes the colonoscopy examinations done to evaluate patients with positive FOBT. Nonetheless, the direct evidence that FOBT screening is efficacious and decreases both the incidence and mortality of colorectal cancer is so strong that national guidelines recommend annual FOBT screening for asymptomatic, average-risk Americans older than 50 years of age as one of several accepted strategies. As noted earlier under Clinical Evaluation, newer immunohistochemical methods for detecting human globin may prove to be more sensitive and specific.[61] A positive FOBT test should be followed by colonoscopy.

Flexible Sigmoidoscopy

Screening by flexible sigmoidoscopy every 5 years may lead to a 60 to 70% reduction in mortality from colorectal cancer, chiefly by identifying high-risk individuals with adenomas. Presumed high cost has prohibited its use in mass screening in the past, but a randomized, multicenter, controlled trial of screening sigmoidoscopy was initiated by the National Cancer Institute in 1992, and data are currently undergoing analysis. Studies show that trained nurse endoscopists may achieve similar results in polyp detection as their physician colleagues, which may reduce costs considerably. Patients found to have a polyp, cancer, or other lesion on flexible sigmoidoscopy will require colonoscopy.

Fecal Occult Blood Testing and Flexible Sigmoidoscopy

The FOBT trials from Mandel and associates (University of Minnesota), Hardcastle and associates (England), and Kronberg and associates (Denmark) all showed that FOBT screening was least effective at detecting rectosigmoid cancers.[62,63] Two thirds of interval cancers arose in the rectosigmoid in the English series. This is precisely the area screened by flexible sigmoidoscopy; thus, the combination of the two tests has been suggested as a reasonable screening strategy. Winawer, in a study of 12,479 subjects, showed that the combination of FOBT annually with flexible sigmoidoscopy

every 5 years resulted in lower mortality from colorectal cancer and better survival in those patients with colorectal cancer.[64] Such data led to the American Cancer Society recommendations that one of the acceptable screening regimens for average-risk Americans is the combination of FOBT annually and flexible sigmoidoscopy every 5 years; this combination was preferred over either test alone.

Colonoscopy

Colonoscopy is currently the most accurate and most complete method for examining the large bowel.[60] This procedure is highly sensitive for detecting even small polyps (<1 cm) and allows biopsy, polypectomy, control of hemorrhage, and dilation of strictures. However, colonoscopy does require mechanical bowel preparation and the discomfort associated with the procedure requires conscious sedation in most patients. Colonoscopy also is considerably more expensive than other screening modalities and requires a well-trained endoscopist. The risk of a major complication after colonoscopy (perforation and hemorrhage) is extremely low (0.2 to 0.3%). Nevertheless, deaths have been reported.

Air-Contrast Barium Enema

Air-contrast barium enema also is highly sensitive for detecting polyps greater than 1 cm in diameter (90% sensitivity). Unfortunately, there are no studies proving its efficacy for screening large populations. Accuracy is greatest in the proximal colon but may be compromised in the sigmoid colon if there is significant diverticulosis. For this reason, barium enema often is combined with flexible sigmoidoscopy for screening purposes. The major disadvantages of barium enema are the need for mechanical bowel preparation and the requirement for colonoscopy if a lesion is discovered.

Computed Tomographic Colonography (Virtual Colonoscopy)

Advances in imaging technology have created a number of less invasive but highly accurate tools for screening. CT colonography makes use of helical CT technology and three-dimensional recon-

TABLE 29-2	Screening guidelines for colorectal cancer	
Population	**Initial Age**	**Recommended Screening Test**
Average risk	50 y	Annual FOBT or
		Flexible sigmoidoscopy every 5 y or
		Annual FOBT and flexible sigmoidoscopy every 5 y or
		Air-contrast barium enema every 5 y or
		Colonoscopy every 10 y
Adenomatous polyps	50 y	Colonoscopy at first detection; then colonoscopy in 3 y
		If no further polyps, colonoscopy every 5 y
		If polyps, colonoscopy every 3 y
		Annual colonoscopy for >5 adenomas
Colorectal cancer	At diagnosis	Pretreatment colonoscopy; then at 12 mo after curative resection; then colonoscopy after 3 y; then colonoscopy every 5 y, if no new lesions
Ulcerative colitis, Crohn's colitis	At diagnosis; then after 8 y for pancolitis, after 15 y for left-sided colitis	Colonoscopy with multiple biopsies every 1–2 y
FAP	10–12 y	Annual flexible sigmoidoscopy
		Upper endoscopy every 1–3 y after polyps appear
Attenuated FAP	20 y	Annual flexible sigmoidoscopy
		Upper endoscopy every 1–3 y after polyps appear
HNPCC	20–25 y	Colonoscopy every 1–2 y
		Endometrial aspiration biopsy every 1–2 y
Familial colorectal cancer first-degree relative	40 y or 10 y before the age of the youngest affected relative	Colonoscopy every 5 y
		Increase frequency if multiple family members are affected, especially before 50 y

FAP = familial adenomatous polyposis; FOBT = fecal occult blood testing; HNPCC = hereditary nonpolyposis colon cancer.
Sources: Data adapted from Smith et al,[4] Pignone et al,[58] and Levin et al.[61]

struction to image the intraluminal colon. Patients require a mechanical bowel preparation. The colon is then insufflated with air, a spiral CT is performed, and both two-dimensional and three-dimensional images are generated. In the hands of a qualified radiologist, sensitivity appears to be as good as colonoscopy for colorectal cancers and polyps greater than 1 cm in size.[65] Colonoscopy is required if a lesion is identified. CT colonography may also prove useful for imaging the proximal colon in cases of obstruction. Limitations of this technique include false-positive results from retained stool, diverticular disease, haustral folds, motion artifacts, and an inability to detect flat adenomas.

Guidelines for Screening

Current American Cancer Society guidelines advocate screening for the average-risk population (asymptomatic, no family history of colorectal carcinoma, no personal history of polyps or colorectal carcinoma, no familial syndrome) beginning at age 50 years.[4] Recommended procedures include yearly FOBT, flexible sigmoidoscopy every 5 years, FOBT and flexible sigmoidoscopy in combination, air-contrast barium enema every 5 years, or colonoscopy every 10 years. Patients with other risk factors should be screened earlier and more frequently (Table 29-2).

Routes of Spread and Natural History

Carcinoma of the colon and rectum arises in the mucosa. The tumor subsequently invades the bowel wall and eventually adjacent tissues and other viscera. Tumors may become bulky and circumferential, leading to colon obstruction. Local extension (especially in the rectum) may occasionally cause obstruction of other organs such as the ureter.

Regional lymph node involvement is the most common form of spread of colorectal carcinoma and usually precedes distant metastasis or the development of carcinomatosis. The likelihood of nodal metastasis increases with tumor size, poorly differentiated histology, lymphovascular invasion, and depth of invasion. The T stage (depth of invasion) is the single most significant predictor of lymph node spread. Carcinoma in situ (Tis) in which there is no penetration of the muscularis mucosa (basement membrane) also has been called *high-grade dysplasia* and should carry no risk of lymph node metastasis. Small lesions confined to the bowel wall (T1 and T2) are associated with lymph node metastasis in 5 to 20% of cases, while larger tumors that invade through the bowel wall or into adjacent organs (T3 and T4) are likely to have lymph node metastasis in more than 50% of cases. The number of lymph nodes with metastases correlates with the presence of distant disease and inversely with survival. Four or more involved lymph nodes predict a poor prognosis. In colon cancer, lymphatic spread usually follows the major venous outflow from the involved segment of the colon. Lymphatic spread from the rectum follows two routes. In the upper rectum, drainage ascends along the superior rectal vessels to the inferior mesenteric nodes. In the lower rectum, lymphatic drainage may course along the middle rectal vessels. Nodal spread along the inferior rectal vessels to the internal iliac nodes or groin is rare unless the tumor involves the anal canal or the proximal lymphatics are blocked with tumor (Fig. 29-23).

The most common site of distant metastasis from colorectal cancer is the liver. These metastases arise from hematogenous spread via the portal venous system. Like lymph node metastasis, the risk of hepatic metastasis increases with tumor size and tumor grade. However, even small tumors may produce distant metastasis. The lung is also a site of hematogenous spread for colorectal carcinoma. Pulmonary metastases rarely occur in isolation. Carcinomatosis (diffuse peritoneal metastases) occurs by peritoneal seeding and has a dismal prognosis.

Staging and Preoperative Evaluation
Clinical Presentation

Symptoms of colon and rectal cancers are nonspecific and generally develop when the cancer is locally advanced. The classic first symptoms are a change in bowel habits and rectal bleeding. Abdominal pain, bloating, and other signs of obstruction typically occur with larger tumors and suggest more advanced disease. Because of the caliber of the bowel and the consistency of the stool, left-sided tumors are more likely to cause obstruction than are right-sided tumors. Rectal tumors may cause bleeding, tenesmus, and pain. Alternatively, patients may be asymptomatic and/or present with unexplained anemia, weight loss, or poor appetite.

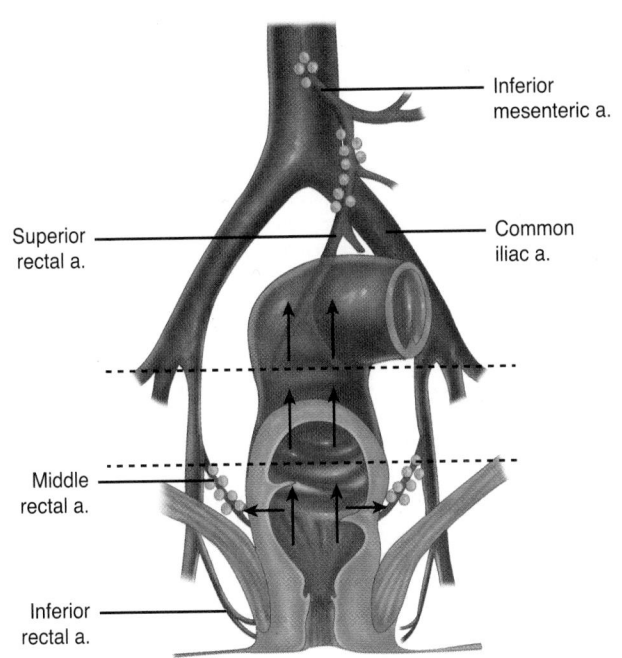

FIG. 29-23. Lymphatic drainage of the rectum. a. = artery.

Staging

Colorectal cancer staging is based upon tumor depth and the presence or absence of nodal or distant metastases. Older staging systems, such as the Dukes' Classification and its Astler-Coller modification, have been largely replaced by the tumor, nodes, and metastasis (TNM) staging system (Table 29-3).[66] Stage I disease includes adenocarcinomas that are invasive through the muscularis mucosa but are confined to the submucosa (T1) or the muscularis propria (T2) in the

TABLE 29-3   TNM staging of colorectal carcinoma

Tumor stage (T)	Definition
TX	Cannot be assessed
T0	No evidence of cancer
Tis	Carcinoma in situ
T1	Tumor invades submucosa
T2	Tumor invades muscularis propria
T3	Tumor invades through muscularis propria into serosa or into nonperitonealized pericolic or perirectal tissues
T4	Tumor directly invades other organs or tissues or perforates the visceral peritoneum of specimen

Nodal stage (N)	
NX	Regional lymph nodes cannot be assessed
N0	No lymph node metastasis
N1	Metastasis to one to three pericolic or perirectal lymph nodes
N2	Metastasis to four or more pericolic or perirectal lymph nodes
N3	Metastasis to any lymph node along a major named vascular trunk

Distant metastasis (M)	
MX	Presence of distant metastasis cannot be assessed
M0	No distant metastasis
M1	Distant metastasis present

Source: Adapted from Greene et al.[66] Used with the permission of the American Joint Committee on Cancer (AJCC), Chicago, Illinois. The original source for this material is the AJCC Cancer Staging Manual, Sixth Edition (2002) published by Springer Science and Business Media LLC, *www.springerlink.com.*

TABLE 29-4   TNM staging of colorectal carcinoma and 5-year survival

Stage	TNM	5-Y Survival (%)
I	T1–2, N0, M0	70–95
II	T3–4, N0, M0	54–65
III	*T*any, N1–3, M0	39–60
IV	*T*any, *N*any, M1	0–16

Source: Data from Greene et al.[66]

absence of nodal metastases. Stage II disease consists of tumors that invade through the bowel wall into the subserosa or nonperitonealized pericolic or perirectal tissues (T3) or into other organs or tissues or through the visceral peritoneum (T4) without nodal metastases. Stage III disease includes any T stage with nodal metastases, and stage IV disease denotes distant metastases.

The preoperative evaluation usually identifies stage IV disease. In colon cancer, differentiating stages I, II, and III depends upon examination of the resected specimen. In rectal cancer, endorectal ultrasound may predict the stage (ultrasound stage, u*TXNX*) preoperatively, but the final determination depends upon pathology examination of the resected tumor and adjacent lymph nodes (pathologic stage, p*TXNX*). Disease stage correlates with 5-year survival. Patients with stages I and II disease can expect excellent survival rates. The presence of nodal metastases (stage III) decreases survival to roughly 40% (Table 29-4). The 5-year survival rate with stage IV disease is less than 16%. In rectal cancer, staging has been further refined and outcomes suggest that subgroups of patients within each stage may have very different prognoses (Table 29-5).[67] If the mesorectum around a rectal cancer is involved or threatened (only 1 to 2 mm of clearance), there is a very high likelihood of local recurrence and a poor prognosis. This circumferential or radial margin is probably best assessed preoperatively by MRI. While nodal involvement is the single most important prognostic factor in colorectal carcinoma, tumor characteristics, such as degree of differentiation, mucinous or signet-ring cell histology, vascular invasion, and DNA aneuploidy, also affect prognosis.

Preoperative Evaluation

Once a colon or rectal carcinoma has been diagnosed, a staging evaluation should be undertaken. The colon must be evaluated for synchronous tumors, usually by colonoscopy. Synchronous disease will be present in up to 5% of patients. For rectal cancers, digital rectal examination and rigid proctoscopy with biopsy should be done to assess tumor size, location, morphology, histology, and fixation. Endorectal ultrasound can be invaluable in staging rectal cancer and is used to classify the ultrasound T and N stage of rectal cancers (Fig. 29-24). A chest/abdominal/pelvic CT scan should be obtained to evaluate for distant metastases. Pelvic CT scan, and sometimes MRI, can be invaluable in large rectal tumors and in

TABLE 29-5   American Joint Committee on Cancer staging

TNM	Stage	Local Recurrence (%)	Survival (%)
T1–2 N0	I	<5	90
T3 N0	IIA	8	74
T4 N0	IIB	15	65
T1–2 N1	IIIA	6	81
T1–2 N2	IIIB	8	69
T3 N1	IIIB	11	61
T3 N2	IIIC	15	48
T4 N1–2	IIIC	19–22	36

Source: From Gunderson et al.[67] Copyright Elsevier.

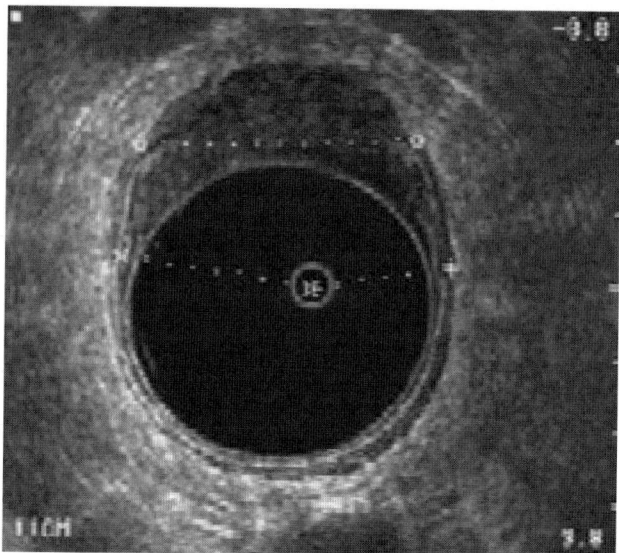

FIG. 29-24. Endorectal ultrasonography showing a T3 rectal carcinoma. The dotted line is being used to measure the diameter of the lesion. *(Courtesy of Charles O. Finne III, MD, Minneapolis, MN.)*

recurrent disease to determine the extent of local invasion. In patients with obstructive symptoms, a water-soluble contrast study (Gastrografin enema) may be useful for delineating the degree of obstruction. It is important to avoid mechanical bowel preparation (for either colonoscopy or surgery) in a patient who appears to be obstructed. PET scan may be useful in evaluating lesions seen on CT scan, and in patients in whom a risky or highly morbid operation is planned (pelvic exenteration, sacrectomy). Preoperative CEA often is obtained, and may be useful for postoperative follow-up.

Therapy for Colonic Carcinoma
Principles of Resection

The objective in treatment of carcinoma of the colon is to remove the primary tumor along with its lymphovascular supply. Because the lymphatics of the colon accompany the main arterial supply, the length of bowel resected depends upon which vessels are supplying the segment involved with the cancer. Any adjacent organ or tissue, such as the omentum, that has been invaded should be resected en bloc with the tumor. If all of the tumor cannot be removed, a palliative procedure should be considered.

The presence of synchronous cancers or adenomas or a strong family history of colorectal neoplasms suggests that the entire colon is at risk for carcinoma (often called a *field defect*) and a subtotal or total colectomy should be considered. Metachronous tumors (a *second primary colon cancer*) identified during follow-up studies should be treated similarly. However, the surgeon must be aware of which mesenteric vessels have been ligated at the initial colectomy because that may influence the choice of procedure.

The number of lymph nodes recovered in the surgical specimen has long served as a proxy for the oncologic adequacy of resection. A number of studies previously have suggested that a minimum of 12 lymph nodes in the resected specimen are necessary for adequate staging. In addition, patients in whom more nodes are harvested have better long-term outcome.[68] As such, a 12-node minimum has been suggested as an appropriate benchmark for assessing quality of care.[69] However, several investigators recently have called this into question, noting that the number of lymph nodes examined does not correlate with staging, use of adjuvant chemotherapy, or patient survival.[70] Others have suggested that the number of negative lymph nodes and/or the lymph node ratio (positive lymph nodes:total lymph nodes) may further improve staging.[71–73]

If unexpected metastatic disease is encountered at the time of a laparotomy, the primary tumor should be resected, if technically feasible and safe. Consideration can be given to a primary anastomosis if the bowel appears healthy, is not involved in carcinomatosis, and the patient is stable. In the rare instance in which the primary tumor is not resectable, a palliative procedure can be performed and usually involves a proximal stoma or bypass. Hemorrhage in an unresectable tumor can sometimes be controlled with angiographic embolization. External beam radiation also has been used for palliation.

Stage-Specific Therapy
Stage 0 (Tis, N0, M0) Polyps containing carcinoma in situ (high-grade dysplasia) carry no risk of lymph node metastasis. However, the presence of high-grade dysplasia increases the risk of finding an invasive carcinoma within the polyp. For this reason, these polyps should be excised completely and pathologic margins should be free of dysplasia. Most pedunculated polyps and many sessile polyps may be completely removed endoscopically. These patients should be followed with frequent colonoscopy to ensure that the polyp has not recurred and that an invasive carcinoma has not developed. In cases where the polyp cannot be removed entirely, a segmental resection is recommended.

Stage I: The Malignant Polyp (T1, N0, M0) Occasionally, a polyp that was thought to be benign will be found to harbor invasive carcinoma after polypectomy. Treatment of a *malignant polyp* is based upon the risk of local recurrence and the risk of lymph node metastasis.[58] The risk of lymph node metastases depends primarily upon the depth of invasion. Invasive carcinoma in the head of a pedunculated polyp with no stalk involvement carries a low risk of metastasis (<1%) and may be completely resected endoscopically. However, lymphovascular invasion, poorly differentiated histology, or tumor within 1 mm of the resection margin greatly increases the risk of local recurrence and metastatic spread. Segmental colectomy is then indicated. Invasive carcinoma arising in a sessile polyp extends into the submucosa and is usually best treated with segmental colectomy (Fig. 29-25).

Stages I and II: Localized Colon Carcinoma (T1–3, N0, M0) The majority of patients with stages I and II colon cancer will be cured with surgical resection. Few patients with completely resected stage I disease will develop either local or distant recurrence, and adjuvant chemotherapy does not improve survival in these patients. However, up to 46% of patients with completely resected stage II disease will ultimately die from colon cancer. For this reason, adjuvant chemotherapy has been suggested for selected patients with stage II disease

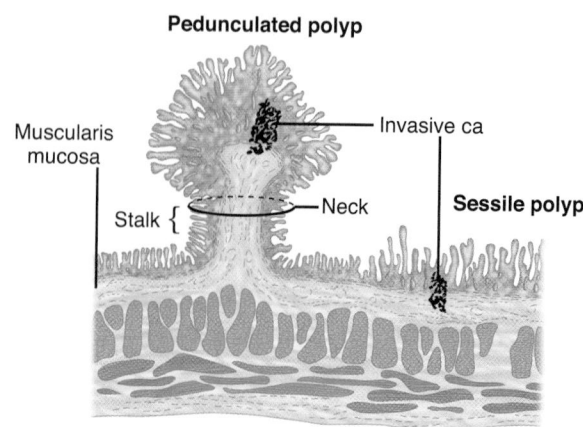

FIG. 29-25. Levels of invasive carcinoma in pedunculated and sessile polyps. ca = carcinoma.

(young patients, tumors with "high-risk" histologic findings). Data are controversial as to whether chemotherapy improves survival rates in these patients. Improved staging to detect micrometastases and/or more sensitive prognostic tumor markers may improve patient selection for adjuvant therapy.

Stage III: Lymph Node Metastasis (Tany, N1, M0) Patients with lymph node involvement are at significant risk for both local and distant recurrence, and adjuvant chemotherapy has been recommended routinely in these patients. 5-fluorouracil (5-FU)–based regimens (with levamisole or leucovorin) reduce recurrences and improve survival in this patient population. Newer chemotherapeutic agents such as capecitabine, irinotecan, oxaliplatin, angiogenesis inhibitors, and immunotherapy also show promise.

Stage IV: Distant Metastasis (Tany, Nany, M1) Survival is extremely limited in stage IV colon carcinoma. However, unlike many other malignancies, highly selected patients with isolated, resectable metastases may benefit from resection (metastasectomy). The most common site of metastasis is the liver. Of patients with systemic disease, approximately 15% will have metastases limited to the liver. Of these, 20% are potentially resectable for cure. Survival is improved in these patients (20 to 40% 5-year survival) when compared to patients who do not undergo resection. Hepatic resection of synchronous metastases from colorectal carcinoma may be performed as a combined procedure or in two stages. All patients require adjuvant chemotherapy. The second most common site of metastasis is the lung, occurring in approximately 20% of patients with colorectal carcinoma. Although very few of these patients will be potentially resectable, among those who are (about 1 to 2% of all colorectal cancer patients), long-term survival benefit can be expected in 30 to 40%.[74] There are limited reports of successful resection of metastases in other sites (ovary and retroperitoneum are most common).

The remainder of patients with stage IV disease cannot be cured surgically; and therefore, the focus of treatment should be palliation. Management of the primary tumor in the setting of systemic disease has been controversial. Traditionally, resection of the primary tumor has been recommended to prevent complications such as obstruction and bleeding. However, major abdominal surgery may delay definitive chemotherapy. Moreover, newer chemotherapeutic regimens have significantly improved response and tumor shrinkage. For this reason, some oncologists now advocate for chemotherapy without resection of the primary tumor in stage IV disease. Long-term outcome in this setting will require prospective study. Methods such as colonic stenting for obstructing lesions of the left colon also provide good palliation. More limited surgical intervention such as a diverting stoma may be appropriate in patients with stage IV disease who develop obstruction.

Therapy for Rectal Carcinoma
Principles of Resection

The biology of rectal adenocarcinoma is identical to the biology of colonic adenocarcinoma, and the operative principles of complete resection of the primary tumor, its lymphatic bed, and any other involved organ apply to surgical resection of rectal carcinoma. However, the anatomy of the pelvis and proximity of other structures (ureters, bladder, prostate, vagina, iliac vessels, and sacrum) make resection more challenging and often require a different approach than for colonic adenocarcinoma. Moreover, it is more difficult to achieve negative radial margins in rectal cancers that extend through the bowel wall because of the anatomic limitations of the pelvis. Therefore, local recurrence is higher than with similar stage colon cancers. However, unlike the intraperitoneal colon, the relative paucity of small bowel and other radiation-sensitive structures in the pelvis makes it easier to treat rectal tumors with radiation. Therapeutic decisions, therefore, are based upon the location and depth of the tumor and its relationship to other structures in the pelvis.

Local Therapy

The distal 10 cm of the rectum are accessible transanally. For this reason, several local approaches have been proposed for treating rectal neoplasms. *Transanal excision* (full thickness or mucosal) is an excellent approach for noncircumferential, benign, villous adenomas of the rectum. Although this technique can be used for selected T1 and, possibly, some T2 carcinomas, local excision does not allow pathologic examination of the lymph nodes, and might, therefore, understage patients. Local recurrence rates are high without the addition of adjuvant chemoradiation therapy. *Transanal endoscopic microsurgery* makes use of a specially designed proctoscope, magnifying system, and instruments similar to those used in laparoscopy to allow local excision of lesions higher in the rectum (up to 15 cm). Local excision of any rectal neoplasm should be considered an *excisional biopsy* because final pathologic examination of the specimen may reveal an invasive carcinoma that then mandates more radical therapy.

Ablative techniques such as electrocautery or endocavitary radiation also have been used. The disadvantage of these techniques is that no pathologic specimen is retrieved to confirm the tumor stage. Fulguration generally is reserved for extremely high-risk patients with a limited life span who cannot tolerate more radical surgery.

Radical Resection

Radical resection is preferred to local therapy for most rectal carcinomas. Radical resection involves removal of the involved segment of the rectum along with its lymphovascular supply. Although any microscopically negative margin has been suggested to be adequate, most surgeons still attempt to obtain a 2-cm distal mural margin for curative resections.

Total mesorectal excision (TME) is a technique that uses sharp dissection along anatomic planes to ensure complete resection of the rectal mesentery during low and extended low anterior resections. For upper rectal or rectosigmoid resections, a partial mesorectal excision of at least 5 cm distal to the tumor appears adequate. TME both decreases local recurrence rates and improves long-term survival rates. Moreover, this technique is associated with less blood loss and less risk to the pelvic nerves and presacral plexus than is blunt dissection. The principles of TME should be applied to all radical resections for rectal cancer.

Recurrence of rectal cancer generally has a poor prognosis. Extensive involvement of other pelvic organs (usually occurring in the setting of tumor recurrence) may require a *pelvic exenteration*. The rectal and perineal portions of this operation are similar to an abdominoperineal resection (APR) but en bloc resection of the ureters, bladder, and prostate or uterus and vagina also are performed. A permanent colostomy and an ileal conduit to drain the urinary tract may be necessary. The sacrum may also be resected if necessary (*sacrectomy*) up to the level of the S2–S3 junction. These operations are best performed in tertiary centers with multidisciplinary teams consisting of a colon and rectal surgeon, urologist, neurosurgeon, and plastic surgeon.

Stage-Specific Therapy (Fig. 29-26)

Pretreatment staging of rectal carcinoma often relies on endorectal ultrasound to determine the T and N status of a rectal cancer. Ultrasound is highly accurate at assessing tumor depth, but less accurate in diagnosing nodal involvement.[5] Ultrasound evaluation can guide choice of therapy in most patients. MRI is useful to assess mesorectal involvement. When the radial margin is threatened or involved, neoadjuvant chemoradiation is recommended.

Stage 0 (Tis, N0, M0) Villous adenomas harboring carcinoma in situ (high-grade dysplasia) are ideally treated with local excision. A 1-cm margin should be obtained. Rarely, radical resection will be necessary if transanal excision is not technically possible (large circumferential lesions).

Stage I: Localized Rectal Carcinoma (T1–2, N0, M0) Invasive carcinoma confined to the head of a pedunculated polyp carries a very

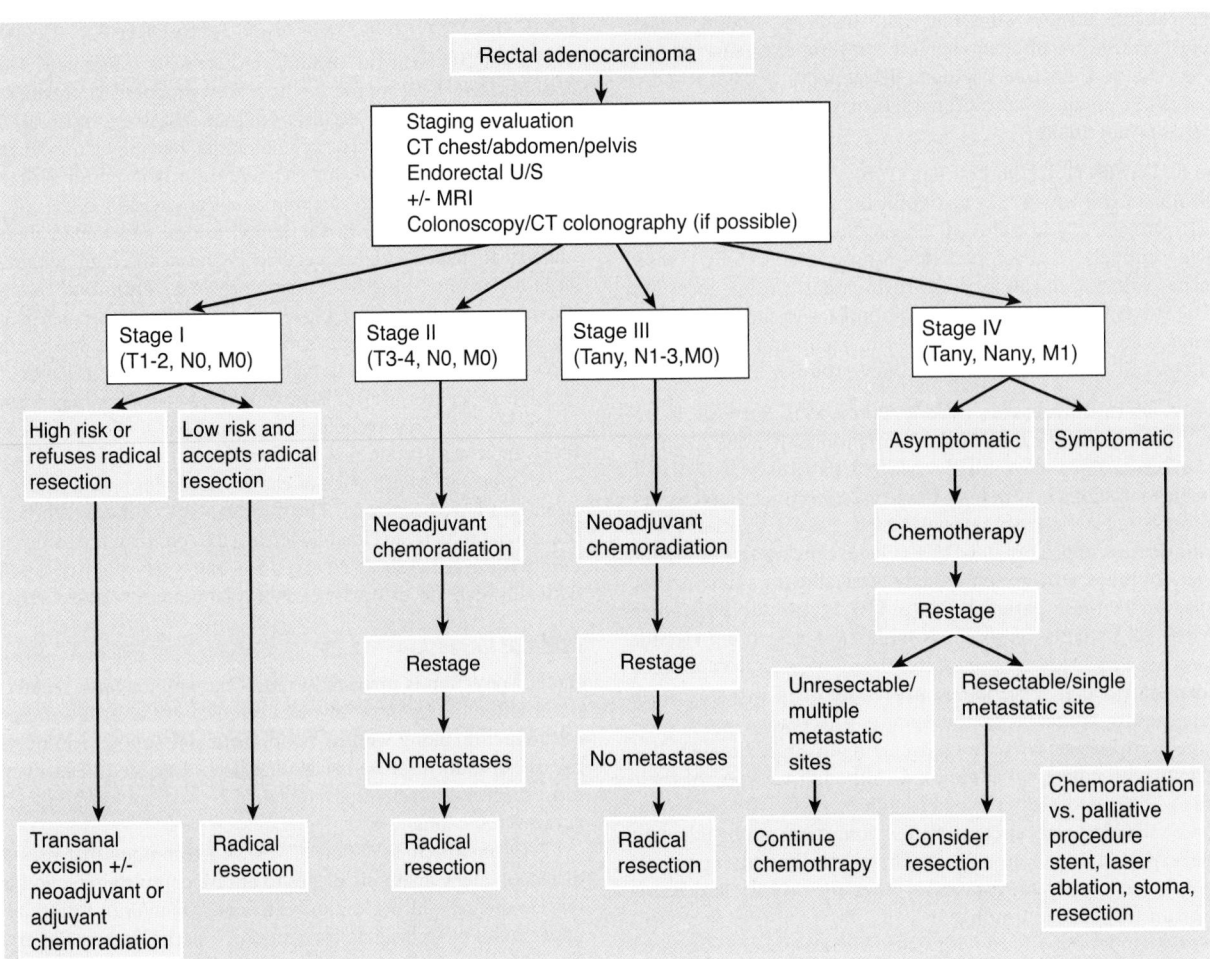

FIG. 29-26. Diagnostic algorithm for rectal cancer. CT = computed tomography; MRI = magnetic resonance imaging; U/S = ultrasound.

low risk of metastasis (<1%). Polypectomy with clear margins is appropriate therapy. Although local excision has been used for small, favorable sessile uT1N0 and uT2N0 rectal cancers, local recurrence rates may be as high as 20 and 40%, respectively.[61] For this reason, radical resection is strongly recommended in all good-risk patients. Lesions with unfavorable histologic characteristics and those located in the distal third of the rectum, in particular, are prone to recurrence. In high-risk patients and in those patients who refuse radical surgery because of the risk of need for a permanent colostomy, local excision may be adequate, but strong consideration should be given to adjuvant or neoadjuvant chemoradiation to improve local control. Uncontrolled studies suggest that the addition of such therapy improves outcome.[13–19]

Locally Advanced Rectal Cancer (Stages II and III) *Stage II: Localized Rectal Carcinoma (T3–4, N0, M0)* Larger rectal tumors, especially if located in the distal rectum, are more likely to recur locally. There are two schools of thought, each differing in their approach to control local recurrences. Advocates of total mesorectal resection suggest that optimization of operative technique will obviate the need for any adjuvant chemoradiation to control local recurrence after resection of stages I, II, and III rectal cancers. The opposing school suggests that stages II and III rectal cancers will benefit from chemoradiation. They argue that such therapy reduces local recurrences and prolongs survival whether given preoperatively or postoperatively. The advantages of preoperative chemoradiation include tumor shrinkage, increased likelihood of resection and of a sphincter-sparing procedure, tumor downstaging by treating locally involved lymph nodes, and decreased risk to the small intestine. Disadvantages include possible overtreatment of early stage tumors,

impaired wound healing, and pelvic fibrosis increasing the risk of operative complications. Postoperative radiation allows accurate pathologic staging of the resected tumor and lymph nodes, and avoids the wound healing problems associated with preoperative radiation. However, bulky tumors, tumors involving adjacent organs, and very low rectal tumors may be much more difficult to resect without preoperative radiation and may require a more extensive operation.

Stage III: Lymph Node Metastasis (Tany, N1, M0) Many surgeons now recommend chemotherapy and radiation either pre- or postoperatively for node-positive rectal cancers. The advantages and disadvantages are similar to those listed for stage II disease, except that the likelihood of overtreating an early stage lesion is considerably less.

Over the past two decades, a wide variety of studies have addressed the issue of adjuvant and neoadjuvant therapy for locally advanced rectal cancer. Many of these studies demonstrated both improved local control and prolonged survival, and resulted in the 1990 National Institutes of Health consensus conference recommendation for postoperative chemoradiation therapy in these patients. There is little controversy regarding chemoradiation therapy for stage III (node positive) disease. However, advances in surgical technique, such as TME, for locally advanced node negative cancers (T3–4, N0; stage II) have improved local control with surgery alone, prompting some authors to abandon adjuvant chemoradiation in these patients especially for those with proximally based rectal cancers. Although the data from these studies are intriguing, other reports have shown that chemoradiation improves local control and survival even in patients who undergo TME. Thus, most colorectal surgeons in the United States continue to recommend adjuvant or neoadjuvant therapy for patients with locally advanced disease. Many European surgeons now rely heavily on MRI staging to determine the need for neoadjuvant chemoradiation. They use neoadjuvant chemoradiation if the radial margin is threatened or involved by the cancer or if anal sphincter or other local organ invasion is present. In the United States, chemoradiation therapy still is recommended for all patients with stage III disease and the majority of patients with stage II disease. In well-selected patients with T3 tumors, favorable histology, and negative radial margins, chemoradiation may not be necessary, but larger prospective studies are required before this approach can be recommended.

Appropriate timing of chemoradiation for locally advanced rectal cancer has been debated. Historically, preoperative chemoradiation has been advocated based on tumor shrinkage/downstaging, improved resectability, and the possibility of performing a sphincter-sparing operation in some patients. In addition, the absence of small bowel adhesions in the pelvis may decrease toxicity. However, preoperative radiation therapy may increase operative complications and impairs wound healing. Although preoperative endorectal ultrasound and MRI have improved our ability to stage rectal cancer, clinical "overstaging" can be problematic, and neoadjuvant therapy may, therefore, overtreat patients with pT1–2, N0 tumors. Advocates of postoperative radiation therapy cite more accurate pathologic staging and fewer operative/postoperative complications. However, large, bulky tumors may be unresectable or require a more extensive operation (APR, pelvic exenteration) without preoperative therapy. In addition, postoperative pelvic radiation may compromise function of the neorectum.

Comparison of perioperative toxicity and oncologic outcome recently have been addressed by the German CAO/ARO/AIO-94 trial. In this study, pre- and postoperative chemoradiation were associated with equivalent acute toxicity and equivalent postoperative complication rate. Postoperative chemoradiation, however, doubled the risk of postoperative stricture formation. In addition, preoperative chemoradiation halved the risk of local recurrence (6% vs. 12%). Based upon these data, most surgeons consider preoperative chemoradiation to be the most appropriate therapy for locally advanced rectal cancer.[75]

Stage IV: Distant Metastasis (Tany, Nany, M1) As with stage IV colon carcinoma, survival is limited in patients with distant metastasis from rectal carcinoma. Isolated hepatic and/or pulmonary metastases are rare, but, when present, may be resected for cure in selected patients. Most patients will require palliative procedures. Radical resection may be required to control pain, bleeding, or tenesmus, but highly morbid procedures such as pelvic exenteration and sacrectomy should generally be avoided in this setting. Local therapy using cautery, endocavitary radiation, or laser ablation may be adequate to control bleeding or prevent obstruction. Intraluminal stents may be useful in the uppermost rectum, but often cause pain and tenesmus lower in the rectum. Occasionally, a proximal diverting colostomy will be required to alleviate obstruction. A mucus fistula should be created, if possible, to vent the distal colon.

Follow-Up and Surveillance

Patients who have been treated for one colorectal cancer are at risk for the development of recurrent disease (either locally or systemically) or metachronous disease (a second primary tumor). In theory, metachronous cancers should be preventable by using surveillance colonoscopy to detect and remove polyps before they progress to invasive cancer. For most patients, a colonoscopy should be performed within 12 months after the diagnosis of the original cancer (or sooner if the colon was not examined in its entirety before the original resection). If that study is normal, colonoscopy should be repeated every 3 to 5 years thereafter.

The optimal method of following patients for recurrent cancer remains controversial. The goal of close follow-up observation is to *detect resectable recurrence* and to *improve survival*. Re-resection of local recurrence and resection of distant metastasis to liver, lung, or other sites often is technically challenging and highly morbid, with only a limited chance of achieving long-term survival. Thus, only selected patients who would tolerate such an approach should be followed intensively. Because most recurrences occur within 2 years of the original diagnosis, surveillance focuses on this time period. Patients who have undergone local resection of rectal tumors also probably should be followed with frequent endorectal ultrasound examinations (every 4 months for 3 years, then every 6 months for 2 years). The role of endorectal ultrasound after radical resection is less clear. CEA often is followed every 2 to 3 months for 2 years. CT scans are not routinely used but may be useful if CEA is elevated. More intensive surveillance is appropriate in high-risk patients such as those with possible HNPCC syndrome or T3 N + cancers. Although intensive surveillance improves detection of resectable recurrences, it is important to note that a survival benefit has never been proven. Therefore, the risks and benefits of intensive surveillance must be weighed and treatment individualized.

Treatment of Recurrent Colorectal Carcinoma

Between 20 and 40% of patients who have undergone curative intent surgery for colorectal carcinoma will eventually develop recurrent disease. Most recurrences occur within the first 2 years after the initial diagnosis, but preoperative chemoradiation therapy may delay recurrence. Although most of these patients will present with distant metastases, a small proportion will have isolated local recurrence and may be considered for *salvage surgery*. Recurrence after colon cancer resection usually occurs at the local site within the abdomen or in the liver or lungs. Resection of other involved organs may be necessary. Recurrence of rectal cancer can be considerably more difficult to manage because of the proximity of other pelvic structures. If the patient has not received chemotherapy and radiation, then adjuvant therapy should be administered before salvage surgery. Radical resection may require extensive resection of pelvic organs (pelvic exenteration with or without sacrectomy). Ideally, the aim of a salvage operation should be to resect all of the tumor with negative margins. However, if the ability to achieve a negative margin is in question, the addition of intraoperative radiation therapy (usually brachytherapy) can help improve local control. Pelvic MRI is useful for identifying tumor extension that would prevent successful resection (extension of tumor into the pelvic sidewall, involvement of the iliac vessels or bilateral sacral nerves, sacral invasion above the S2–S3 junction). Patients should also undergo a thorough preoperative evaluation to identify distant metastases (CT of chest, abdomen, and pelvis, and PET scan) before undergoing such an extensive procedure. Nevertheless, radical salvage surgery can prolong survival in selected patients.

Sentinel Lymph Node Biopsy for Colorectal Carcinoma

The technique of sentinel lymph node biopsy has been applied to a number of malignancies and is commonly used in both breast cancer and melanoma. The goal of sentinel lymph node biopsy is to identify the first node(s) in the lymphatic basin because this site should be most likely to harbor metastases. Unlike sentinel lymph node biopsy in breast cancer and melanoma, the goal of this technique in colorectal carcinoma is not to avoid radical lymphadenectomy, but instead to improve staging.[68] Intensive pathologic examination of the sentinel node(s) with multiple histologic sections, immunohistochemistry, and reverse-transcriptase polymerase chain reaction can detect micrometastases in a significant number of patients who were thought to be node negative by conventional techniques. These patients may then be candidates for further adjuvant treatment. However, whether this increased sensitivity will translate into improved survival remains to be seen.

Minimally Invasive Techniques for Resection

Laparoscopic colectomy for cancer has been controversial. Early reports of high port site recurrence dampened enthusiasm for this technique.[76] The ability to perform an adequate oncologic resection for cancer also has been questioned. Several recent trials have laid to rest many of these fears. The Clinical Outcomes of Surgical Therapy Study Group (COST), the Colon Carcinoma Laparoscopic or Open Resection (COLOR) trial, and the United Kingdom Medical Research Council Conventional vs. Laparoscopic-Assisted Surgery in Colorectal Cancer (CLASSICC) trial have all shown oncologic equivalence between open and laparoscopic techniques. In these multi-institutional studies, the rates of cancer recurrence, survival, and quality of life were similar, suggesting that, in the hands of an appropriately trained surgeon, laparoscopic colectomy is appropriate for cancer.[77–79]

OTHER NEOPLASMS

Rare Colorectal Tumors

Carcinoid Tumors

Carcinoid tumors occur most commonly in the GI tract, and up to 25% of these tumors are found in the rectum. Most small rectal carcinoids are benign, and overall survival is greater than 80%. However, the risk of malignancy increases with size, and more than 60% of tumors greater than 2 cm in diameter are associated with distant metastases. Interestingly, rectal carcinoids appear to be less likely to secrete vasoactive substances than carcinoids in other locations, and carcinoid syndrome is uncommon in the absence of hepatic metastases. Small carcinoids can be locally resected, either transanally or using transanal endoscopic microsurgery. Larger tumors or tumors with obvious invasion into the muscularis require more radical surgery. Carcinoid tumors in the proximal colon are less common and are more likely to be malignant. Size also correlates with risk of malignancy, and tumors less than 2 cm in diameter rarely metastasize. However, the majority of carcinoid tumors in the proximal colon present as bulky lesions and up to two thirds will have metastatic spread at the time of diagnosis. These tumors usually should be treated with radical resection. Because carcinoid tumors are typically slow growing, patients with distant metastases may expect reasonably long survival. Symptoms of carcinoid syndrome often can be alleviated with somatostatin analogues (octreotide) and/or interferon-α. Tumor debulking can offer effective palliation in selected patients.

Carcinoid Carcinomas

Composite carcinoid carcinomas (adenocarcinoids) have histologic features of both carcinoid tumors and adenocarcinomas. The natural history of these tumors more closely parallels that of adenocarcinomas than carcinoid tumors, and regional and systemic metastases are common. Carcinoid carcinoma of the colon and rectum should be treated according to the same oncologic principles as followed for management of adenocarcinoma.

Lipomas

Lipomas occur most commonly in the submucosa of the colon and rectum. They are benign lesions, but rarely may cause bleeding, obstruction, or intussusception, especially when greater than 2 cm in diameter. Small asymptomatic lesions do not require resection. Larger lipomas should be resected by colonoscopic techniques or by a colotomy and enucleation or limited colectomy.

Lymphoma

Lymphoma involving the colon and rectum is rare, but accounts for about 10% of all GI lymphomas. The cecum is most often involved, probably as a result of spread from the terminal ileum. Symptoms include bleeding and obstruction, and these tumors may be clinically indistinguishable from adenocarcinomas. Bowel resection is the treatment of choice for isolated colorectal lymphoma. Adjuvant therapy may be given based upon the stage of disease.

Leiomyoma and Leiomyosarcoma

Leiomyomas are benign tumors of the smooth muscle of the bowel wall and occur most commonly in the upper GI tract. Most patients are asymptomatic, but large lesions can cause bleeding or obstruction. Because it is difficult to differentiate a benign leiomyoma from a malignant leiomyosarcoma, these lesions should be resected. Recurrence is common after local resection, but most small leiomyomas can be adequately treated with limited resection. Lesions larger than 5 cm should be treated with radical resection because the risk of malignancy is high.

Leiomyosarcoma is rare in the GI tract. When this malignancy occurs in the large intestine, the rectum is the most common site. Symptoms include bleeding and obstruction. A radical resection is indicated for these tumors.

Retrorectal/Presacral Tumors

Tumors occurring in the retrorectal space are rare. This region lies between the upper two thirds of the rectum and the sacrum above the rectosacral fascia. It is bound by the rectum anteriorly, the presacral fascia posteriorly, and the endopelvic fascia laterally (lateral ligaments). The retrorectal space contains multiple embryologic remnants derived from a variety of tissues (neuroectoderm, notochord, and hindgut). Tumors that develop in this space are often heterogeneous.

Congenital lesions are most common, comprising almost two thirds of retrorectal lesions. The remainder are classified as neurogenic, osseous, inflammatory, or miscellaneous lesions. Malignancy is more common in the pediatric population than in adults, and solid lesions are more likely to be malignant than are cystic lesions. Inflammatory lesions may be solid or cystic (abscess) and usually represent extensions of infection either in the perirectal space or in the abdomen.

Developmental cysts constitute the majority of congenital lesions and may arise from all three germ cell layers. Dermoid and epidermoid cysts are benign lesions that arise from the ectoderm. Enterogenous cysts arise from the primitive gut. Anterior meningocele and myelomeningocele arise from herniation of the dural sac through a defect in the anterior sacrum. A "scimitar sign" (sacrum with a rounded, concave border without any bony destruction) is the pathognomonic radiographic appearance of this condition.

Solid lesions include teratomas, chordomas, neurologic tumors, or osseus lesions. Teratomas are true neoplasms and contain tissue from each germ cell layer. They often contain both cystic and solid components. Teratomas are more common in children than in adults, but, when found in adults, 30% are malignant. Chordomas arise from the notochord and are the most common malignant tumor in this region. These are slow-growing, invasive cancers that show characteristic bony destruction. Neurogenic tumors include neurofibromas and sarcomas, neurilemomas, ependymomas, and ganglioneuromas. Osseous lesions include osteomas and bone cysts, as well as neoplasms such as osteogenic sarcoma, Ewing's tumor, chondromyxosarcoma, and giant cell tumor.

Patients may present with pain (lower back, pelvic, or lower extremity), GI symptoms, or urinary tract symptoms. Most lesions are palpable on digital rectal examination. While plain x-rays and CT scans often are used to evaluate these lesions, pelvic MRI is the most sensitive and specific imaging study. Myelogram occasionally is necessary if there is central nervous system involvement. Biopsy is not indicated, especially if the lesion appears to be resectable, because of the risk of infection and/or tumor seeding. Treatment is almost always surgical resection. The approach depends, in part, upon the nature of the lesion and its location. High lesions may be approached via a transabdominal route, whereas low lesions may be resected transsacrally. Intermediate lesions may require a combined abdominal and sacral operation. Although survival is excellent after resection of benign lesions, local recurrence is not uncommon. Prognosis after resection of malignant lesions is highly variable and reflects the biology of the underlying tumor. If a retrorectal tumor does not appear to be resectable, biopsy may be appropriate to direct further therapy (chemotherapy and/or radiation).[80]

Anal Canal and Perianal Tumors

Cancers of the anal canal are uncommon and account for approximately 2% of all colorectal malignancies. Neoplasms of the anal canal can be divided into those affecting the *anal margin* (distal to the dentate line) and those affecting the *anal canal* (proximal to the dentate line). Lymphatics from the anal canal proximal to the dentate line drain cephalad via the superior rectal lymphatics to the inferior mesenteric nodes and laterally along both the middle rectal vessels and inferior rectal vessels through the ischiorectal fossa to the internal iliac nodes. Lymph from the anal canal distal to the dentate line usually drains to the inguinal nodes. It can also drain to the superior rectal lymph nodes or along the inferior rectal lymphatics to the ischiorectal fossa if primary drainage routes are blocked with tumor (Fig. 29-27). In many cases, therapy depends upon whether the tumor is located in the anal canal or at the anal margin.

Anal Intraepithelial Neoplasia (Bowen's Disease)

Bowen's disease refers to squamous cell carcinoma in situ of the anus. Pathologically, carcinomas in situ and high-grade squamous intraepithelial dysplasia appear identical. The terms *high-grade squamous intraepithelial lesions* (HSILs) and *anal intraepithelial neoplasia* (AIN) recently have been used to describe these lesions. Like cervical intraepithelial neoplasia, AIN is a precursor to an invasive squamous cell carcinoma (epidermoid carcinoma), and generally is classified as AIN1 (least dysplastic), AIN2, or AIN3 (most dysplastic). AIN may appear as a plaque-like lesion, or may only be apparent with high-resolution anoscopy and application of acetic acid or Lugol's iodine solution. AIN is associated with infection with the human papillomavirus (HPV), especially HPV types 16 and 18. The incidence of both AIN and epidermoid carcinoma of the anus has increased dramatically among HIV-positive, homosexual men. This increase is thought to result from increased rates of HPV infection along with immunosuppression. Treatment of AIN is *ablation*. Because of a high recurrence and/or reinfection rate, these patients require extremely close surveillance. High-risk patients should be followed with frequent anal Papanicolaou smears every 3 to 6 months. An abnormal Papanicolaou smear should be followed by an examination under anesthesia and anal mapping using high-resolution anoscopy. High-resolution anoscopy shows areas with abnormal telangiectasias that are consistent with high-grade dysplasia (AIN3/HSIL). Many centers now consider this technique for ablation of AIN3 to be the optimal method for following these patients.[81] Rarely, extensive disease may require resection with flap closure. Medical therapy for HPV also has been proposed. Topical immunomodulators such as imiquimod (Aldara) have been shown to induce regression in some series.[82] Topical 5-FU also has been used in this setting. Finally, the recent introduction of a vaccine against HPV may help decrease the incidence of this disease in the future.

Epidermoid Carcinoma

Epidermoid carcinoma of the anus includes squamous cell carcinoma, cloacogenic carcinoma, transitional carcinoma, and basaloid carcinoma. The clinical behavior and natural history of these tumors is similar. Epidermoid carcinoma is a slow-growing tumor, and usually presents as an anal or perianal mass. Pain and bleeding may be present. Epidermoid carcinoma of the anal margin may be treated in a similar fashion as squamous cell carcinoma of the skin in other locations because adequate surgical margins usually can be achieved without resecting the anal sphincter. Wide local excision usually is adequate treatment for these lesions. Epidermoid carcinoma occurring in the anal canal or invading the sphincter cannot be excised locally, and first-line therapy relies upon chemotherapy and radiation (the *Nigro protocol*: 5-FU, mitomycin C, and 3000 cGy external beam radiation). More than 80% of these tumors can be cured by using this regimen. Recurrence usually requires radical resection (APR). Metastasis to inguinal lymph nodes is a poor prognostic sign.

Verrucous Carcinoma (Buschke-Lowenstein Tumor, Giant Condyloma Acuminata)

Verrucous carcinoma is a locally aggressive form of condyloma acuminata. Although these lesions do not metastasize, they can cause extensive local tissue destruction and may be grossly indistinguishable from epidermoid carcinoma. Wide local excision is the treatment of choice when possible, but radical resection may sometimes be required.

Basal Cell Carcinoma

Basal cell carcinoma of the anus is rare and resembles basal cell carcinoma elsewhere on the skin (raised, pearly edges with central ulceration). This is a slow-growing tumor that rarely metastasizes. Wide local excision is the treatment of choice, but recurrence occurs in up to 30% of patients. Radical resection and/or radiation therapy may be required for large lesions.

Adenocarcinoma

Adenocarcinoma of the anus is extremely rare, and usually represents downward spread of a low rectal adenocarcinoma. Adenocarcinoma may occasionally arise from the anal glands or may develop in a chronic fistula. Radical resection with or without adjuvant chemoradiation usually is required.

Extramammary perianal *Paget's disease* is *adenocarcinoma in situ* arising from the apocrine glands of the perianal area. The lesion is typically plaque-like and may be indistinguishable from Bowen's disease. Characteristic *Paget's cells* are seen histologically. These tumors often are associated with a synchronous GI adenocarcinoma, so a complete evaluation of the intestinal tract should be performed. Wide local excision is usually adequate treatment for perianal Paget's disease.

Melanoma

Anorectal melanoma is rare, comprising less than 1% of all anorectal malignancies and 1 to 2% of melanomas. Despite many advances

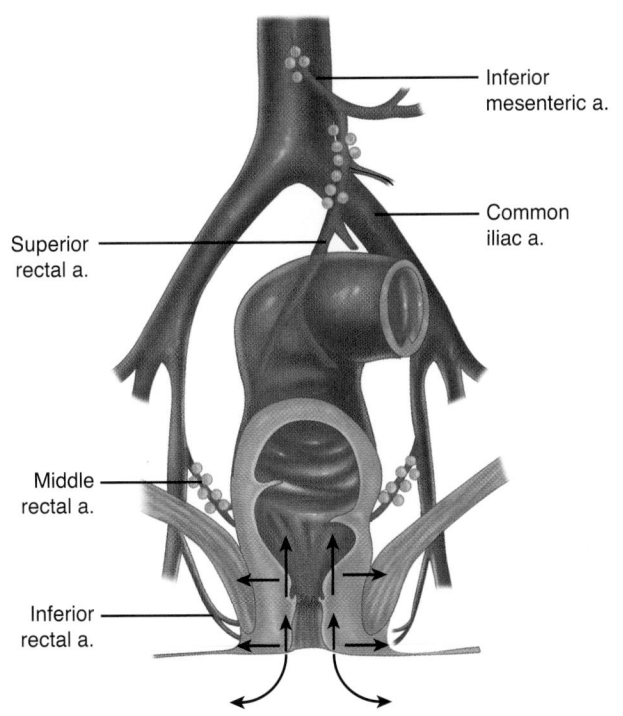

FIG. 29-27. Lymphatic drainage of the anal canal. a. = artery.

Inferior mesenteric a.

Common iliac a.

Superior rectal a.

Middle rectal a.

Inferior rectal a.

in the treatment of melanoma, prognosis for patients with anorectal disease remains poor. Overall 5-year survival is less than 10%, and many patients present with systemic metastasis and/or deeply invasive tumors at the time of diagnosis. A few patients with anorectal melanoma, however, present with isolated local or locoregional disease that is potentially resectable for cure, and both radical resection (APR) and wide local excision have been advocated. Recurrence is common and usually occurs systemically regardless of the initial surgical procedure. Local resection with free margins does not increase the risk of local or regional recurrence, and APR offers no survival advantage over local excision. Because of the morbidity associated with APR, wide local excision is recommended for initial treatment of localized anal melanoma.[83,84] In some patients, wide local excision may not be technically feasible and APR may be required if the tumor involves a significant portion of the anal sphincter or is circumferential. The addition of adjuvant chemotherapy, biochemotherapy, vaccines, or radiotherapy may be of benefit in some patients, but efficacy remains unproven.

OTHER BENIGN COLORECTAL CONDITIONS

Rectal Prolapse and Solitary Rectal Ulcer Syndrome

Rectal prolapse refers to a circumferential, full-thickness protrusion of the rectum through the anus and also has been called *first-degree prolapse*, *complete prolapse*, or *procidentia*.[85] Internal prolapse occurs when the rectal wall intussuscepts but does not protrude, and is probably more accurately described as internal intussusception. Mucosal prolapse is a partial-thickness protrusion often associated with hemorrhoidal disease and usually is treated with banding or hemorrhoidectomy.

In adults, this condition is far more common among women, with a female:male ratio of 6:1. Prolapse becomes more prevalent with age in women and peaks in the seventh decade of life. In men, prevalence is unrelated to age. Symptoms include tenesmus, a sensation of tissue protruding from the anus that may or may not spontaneously reduce, and a sensation of incomplete evacuation. Mucus discharge and leakage may accompany the protrusion. Patients also present with a myriad of functional complaints, from incontinence and diarrhea to constipation and outlet obstruction.

A thorough preoperative evaluation, including colonic transit studies, anorectal manometry, tests of pudendal nerve terminal motor latency, electromyography (EMG), and cinedefecography, may be useful. The colon should be evaluated by colonoscopy or air-contrast barium enema to exclude neoplasms or diverticular disease. Cardiopulmonary condition should be thoroughly evaluated because comorbidities may influence the choice of surgical procedure.

The primary therapy for rectal prolapse is surgery, and more than 100 different procedures have been described to treat this condition. Operations can be categorized as either *abdominal* or *perineal*. Abdominal operations have taken three major approaches: (a) reduction of the perineal hernia and closure of the cul-de-sac (*Moschcowitz's operation*); (b) fixation of the rectum, either with a prosthetic sling (*Ripstein* and *Wells rectopexy*) or by *suture rectopexy*; or (c) resection of redundant sigmoid colon (Fig. 29-28). In some cases, resection is combined with rectal fixation (*resection rectopexy*). Abdominal rectopexy with or without resection also is increasingly performed laparoscopically. Perineal approaches have focused on tightening the anus with a variety of prosthetic materials, reefing the rectal mucosa (*Delorme procedure*), or resecting the prolapsed bowel from the perineum (*perineal rectosigmoidectomy* or *Altemeier procedure*) (Fig. 29-29).

Because rectal prolapse occurs most commonly in elderly women, the choice of operation depends in part upon the patient's overall medical condition. Abdominal rectopexy (with or without sigmoid resection) offers the most durable repair, with recurrence occurring in fewer than 10% of patients. Perineal rectosigmoidectomy avoids an abdominal operation and may be preferable in high-risk patients, but is associated with a higher recurrence rate. Reefing the rectal mucosa is effective for patients with limited prolapse. Anal encirclement procedures generally have been abandoned.

Solitary rectal ulcer syndrome and colitis cystica profunda are commonly associated with internal intussusception. Patients may complain of pain, bleeding, mucus discharge, or outlet obstruction. In solitary rectal ulcer syndrome, one or more ulcers are present in the distal rectum, usually on the anterior wall. In colitis cystica profunda, nodules or a mass may be found in a similar location. Evaluation should include anorectal manometry, defecography, and either colonoscopy or barium enema to exclude other diagnoses. Biopsy of an ulcer or mass is mandatory to exclude malignancy. Nonoperative therapy (high-fiber diet, defecation training to avoid straining, and laxatives or enemas) is effective in the majority of patients. Biofeedback also has been reported to be effective in some patients. Surgery (either abdominal or perineal repair of prolapse as described above) is reserved for highly symptomatic patients for whom all other medical interventions have failed.[86]

Volvulus

Volvulus occurs when an air-filled segment of the colon twists about its mesentery. The sigmoid colon is involved in up to 90% of cases, but volvulus can involve the cecum (<20%) or transverse colon. A volvulus may reduce spontaneously, but more commonly produces bowel obstruction, which can progress to strangulation, gangrene, and perforation. Chronic constipation may produce a large, redundant colon (*chronic megacolon*) that predisposes to volvulus, especially if the mesenteric base is narrow.

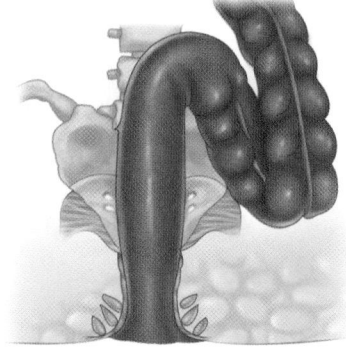

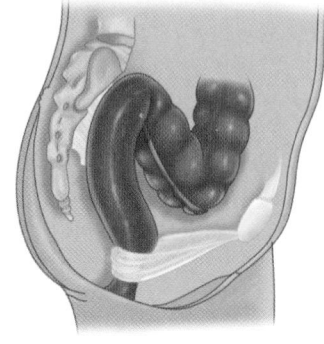

A   **B**

FIG. 29-28. Transabdominal proctopexy for rectal prolapse. The fully mobilized rectum is sutured to the presacral fascia. **A.** Anterior view. **B.** Lateral view. If desired, a sigmoid colectomy can be performed concomitantly to resect the redundant colon.

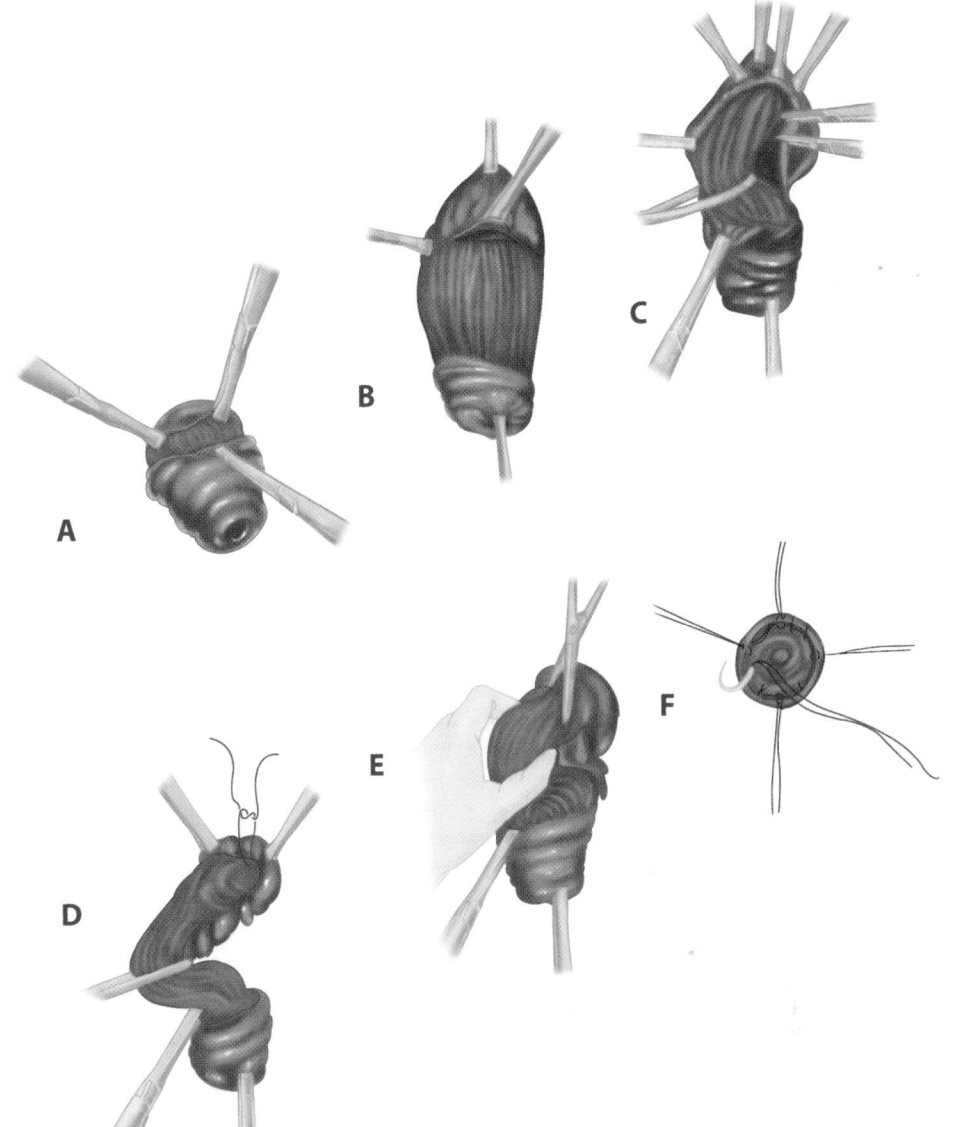

FIG. 29-29. Perineal rectosigmoidectomy shown in lithotomy position. **A.** A circular incision is made 2 cm proximal to the dentate line. **B.** The anterior peritoneal reflection is opened. **C.** The mesentery is divided and ligated. **D.** The peritoneum may be sutured to the bowel wall. **E.** The bowel is resected. **F.** A handsewn anastomosis is performed.

The symptoms of volvulus are those of acute bowel obstruction. Patients present with abdominal distention, nausea, and vomiting. Symptoms rapidly progress to generalized abdominal pain and tenderness. Fever and leukocytosis are heralds of gangrene and/or perforation. Occasionally, patients will report a long history of intermittent obstructive symptoms and distention, suggesting intermittent chronic volvulus.

Sigmoid Volvulus

Sigmoid volvulus often can be differentiated from cecal or transverse colon volvulus by the appearance of plain x-rays of the abdomen. Sigmoid volvulus produces a characteristic *bent inner tube* or *coffee bean* appearance, with the convexity of the loop lying in the right upper quadrant (opposite the site of obstruction). Gastrografin enema shows a narrowing at the site of the volvulus and a pathognomonic *bird's beak* (Fig. 29-30).

Unless there are obvious signs of gangrene or peritonitis, the initial management of sigmoid volvulus is resuscitation followed by endoscopic detorsion. Detorsion is usually most easily accomplished by using a rigid proctoscope, but a flexible sigmoidoscope or colonoscope might also be effective. A rectal tube may be inserted to maintain decompression. Although these techniques are successful in reducing sigmoid volvulus in the majority of patients, the risk

of recurrence is high (40%). For this reason, an elective sigmoid colectomy should be performed after the patient has been stabilized and undergone an adequate bowel preparation.

Clinical evidence of gangrene or perforation mandates immediate surgical exploration without an attempt at endoscopic decompression. Similarly, the presence of necrotic mucosa, ulceration, or dark blood noted on endoscopy examination suggests strangulation and is an indication for operation. If dead bowel is present at laparotomy, a sigmoid colectomy with end colostomy (Hartmann's procedure) may be the safest operation to perform.

Cecal Volvulus

Cecal volvulus results from nonfixation of the right colon. Rotation occurs around the ileocolic blood vessels and vascular impairment occurs early. Plain x-rays of the abdomen show a characteristic kidney-shaped, air-filled structure in the left upper quadrant (opposite the site of obstruction), and a Gastrografin enema confirms obstruction at the level of the volvulus.

Unlike sigmoid volvulus, cecal volvulus can almost never be detorsed endoscopically. Moreover, because vascular compromise occurs early in the course of cecal volvulus, surgical exploration is necessary when the diagnosis is made. Right hemicolectomy with a primary ileocolic anastomosis usually can be performed safely and

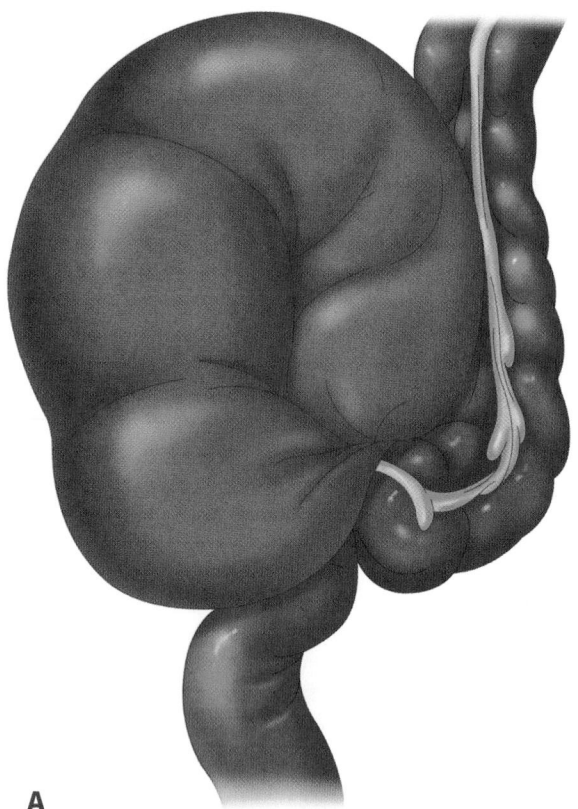

A

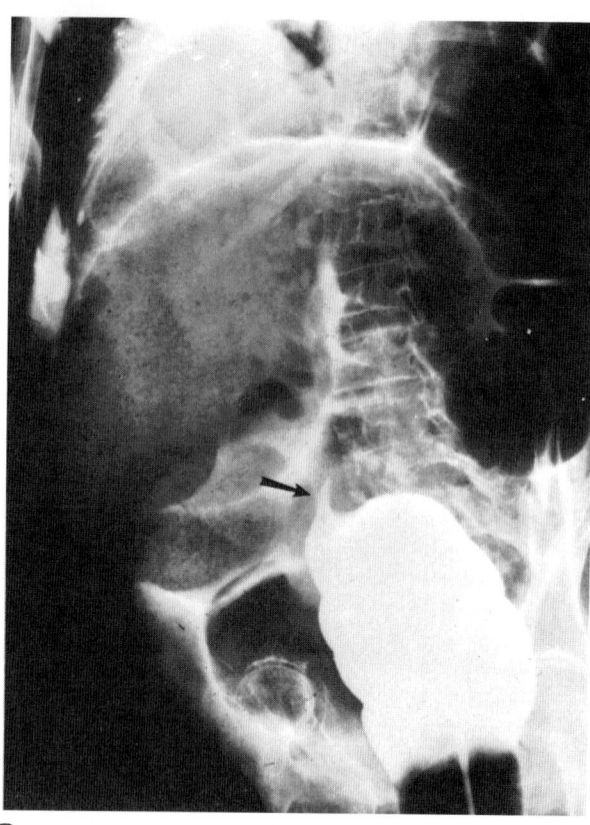

B

FIG. 29-30. Sigmoid volvulus: (**A**) Illustration and (**B**) Gastrografin enema showing "bird-beak" sign (*arrow*). [*B: Reproduced with permission from Nivatvongs S, Becker ER: Colon, rectum and anal canal, in James EC, Corry RJ, Perry JCF Jr. (eds): Basic Surgical Practice. Philadelphia: Hanley & Belfus, 1987. Copyright Elsevier.*]

prevents recurrence. Simple detorsion or detorsion and cecopexy are associated with a high rate of recurrence.

Transverse Colon Volvulus

Transverse colon volvulus is extremely rare. Nonfixation of the colon and chronic constipation with megacolon may predispose to transverse colon volvulus. The radiographic appearance of transverse colon volvulus resembles sigmoid volvulus, but Gastrografin enema will reveal a more proximal obstruction. Although colonoscopic detorsion is occasionally successful in this setting, most patients require emergent exploration and resection.

Megacolon

Megacolon describes a chronically dilated, elongated, hypertrophied large bowel. Megacolon may be congenital or acquired and usually is related to chronic mechanical or functional obstruction. In general, the degree of megacolon is related to the duration of obstruction. Evaluation must always include examination of the colon and rectum (either endoscopically or radiographically) to exclude a surgically correctable mechanical obstruction.

Congenital *megacolon* caused by Hirschsprung's disease results from the failure of migration of neural crest cells to the distal large intestine. The resulting absence of ganglion cells in the distal colon results in a failure of relaxation and causes a functional obstruction. The proximal, healthy bowel becomes progressively dilated. Surgical resection of the aganglionic segment is curative. Although Hirschsprung's disease is primarily a disease of infants and children, it occasionally presents later in adulthood, especially if an extremely short segment of the bowel is affected (*ultrashort-segment Hirschsprung's disease*).

Acquired megacolon may result from infection or chronic constipation. Infection with the protozoan *Trypanosoma cruzi* (*Chagas' disease*) destroys ganglion cells and produces both megacolon and

megaesophagus. Chronic constipation from slow transit or secondary to medications (especially anticholinergic medications) or neurologic disorders (paraplegia, poliomyelitis, amyotrophic lateral sclerosis, multiple sclerosis) may produce progressive colonic dilatation. Diverting ileostomy or subtotal colectomy with an ileorectal anastomosis is occasionally necessary in these patients.

Colonic Pseudo-Obstruction (Ogilvie's Syndrome)

Colonic pseudo-obstruction (Ogilvie's syndrome) is a functional disorder in which the colon becomes massively dilated in the absence of mechanical obstruction. Pseudo-obstruction most commonly occurs in hospitalized patients and is associated with the use of narcotics, bedrest, and comorbid disease. Pseudo-obstruction is thought to result from autonomic dysfunction and severe adynamic ileus. The diagnosis is made based upon the presence of massive dilatation of the colon (usually predominantly the *right* and *transverse* colon) in the absence of a mechanical obstruction. Initial treatment consists of cessation of narcotics, anticholinergics, or other medications that may contribute to ileus. Strict bowel rest and IV hydration are crucial. Most patients will respond to these measures. In patients who fail to improve, colonoscopic decompression often is effective. However, this procedure is technically challenging and great care must be taken to avoid causing perforation. Recurrence occurs in up to 40% of patients. IV neostigmine (an acetylcholinesterase inhibitor) also is extremely effective in decompressing the dilated colon and is associated with a low rate of recurrence (20%). However, neostigmine may produce transient but profound bradycardia and may be inappropriate in patients with cardiopulmonary disease. Because the colonic dilatation typically is greatest in the proximal colon, placement of a rectal tube is rarely effective. It is crucial to exclude mechanical obstruction (usually with a Gastrografin or barium enema) before medical or endoscopic treatment.

Ischemic Colitis

Intestinal ischemia occurs most commonly in the colon. Unlike small bowel ischemia, colonic ischemia is rarely associated with major arterial or venous occlusion. Instead, most colonic ischemia appears to result from low flow and/or small vessel occlusion. Risk factors include vascular disease, diabetes mellitus, vasculitis, and hypotension. In addition, ligation of the inferior mesenteric artery during aortic surgery predisposes to colonic ischemia. Occasionally, thrombosis or embolism may cause ischemia. Although the splenic flexure is the most common site of ischemic colitis, any segment of the colon may be affected. The rectum is relatively spared because of its rich collateral circulation.

Signs and symptoms of ischemic colitis reflect the extent of bowel ischemia. In mild cases, patients may have diarrhea (usually bloody) without abdominal pain. With more severe ischemia, intense abdominal pain (often out of proportion to the clinical examination), tenderness, fever, and leukocytosis are present. Peritonitis and/or systemic toxicity are signs of full-thickness necrosis and perforation.

The diagnosis of ischemic colitis is often based upon the clinical history and physical examination. Plain films may reveal *thumb printing*, which results from mucosal edema and submucosal hemorrhage. CT often shows nonspecific colonic wall thickening and pericolic fat stranding. Angiography is usually not helpful because major arterial occlusion is rare. Although sigmoidoscopy may reveal characteristic dark, hemorrhagic mucosa, the risk of precipitating perforation is high. For this reason, *sigmoidoscopy is relatively contraindicated* in any patient with significant abdominal tenderness. Contrast studies (Gastrografin or barium enema) are similarly contraindicated during the acute phase of ischemic colitis.

Treatment of ischemic colitis depends upon clinical severity. Unlike ischemia of the small bowel, the majority of patients with ischemic colitis can be treated medically. Bowel rest and broad-spectrum antibiotics are the mainstay of therapy, and 80% of patients will recover with this regimen. Hemodynamic parameters should be optimized, especially if hypotension and low flow appear to be the inciting cause. Long-term sequelae include stricture (10 to 15%) and chronic segmental ischemia (15 to 20%). Colonoscopy should be performed after recovery to evaluate strictures and to rule out other diagnoses such as inflammatory bowel disease or malignancy. Failure to improve after 2 to 3 days of medical management, progression of symptoms, or deterioration in clinical condition are indications for surgical exploration. In this setting, all necrotic bowel should be resected. Primary anastomosis should be avoided. Occasionally, repeated exploration (a *second-look operation*) may be necessary.

Infectious Colitis

Pseudomembranous Colitis (Clostridium difficile *Colitis*)

Pseudomembranous colitis is caused by *C. difficile*, a gram-positive bacillus. *C. difficile* colitis is extremely common and is the leading cause of nosocomially acquired diarrhea.[4,79] The spectrum of disease ranges from watery diarrhea to fulminant, life-threatening colitis. *C. difficile* is carried in the large intestine of many healthy adults. Colitis is thought to result from overgrowth of this organism after depletion of the normal commensal flora of the gut with the use of antibiotics. Although clindamycin was the first antimicrobial agent associated with *C. difficile* colitis, almost any antibiotic may cause this disease. Moreover, although risk of *C. difficile* colitis increases with prolonged antibiotic usage, even a single dose of an antibiotic may cause the disease. Immunosuppression, medical comorbidities, prolonged hospitalization or nursing home residence, and bowel surgery increase the risk.

The pathogenic changes associated with *C. difficile* colitis result from production of two toxins: *toxin A* (an enterotoxin) and *toxin B* (a cytotoxin). Diagnosis of this disease was traditionally made by culturing the organism from the stool. Recently, detection of one or both toxins (either by cytotoxic assays or by immunoassays) has

proven to be more rapid, sensitive, and specific. The diagnosis may also be made endoscopically by detection of characteristic ulcers, plaques, and pseudomembranes.

Management should include immediate cessation of the offending antimicrobial agent. Patients with mild disease (diarrhea but no fever or abdominal pain) may be treated as outpatients with a 10-day course of oral metronidazole. Oral vancomycin is a second-line agent used in patients allergic to metronidazole or in patients with recurrent disease. More severe diarrhea associated with dehydration and/or fever and abdominal pain is best treated with bowel rest, IV hydration, and oral metronidazole or vancomycin. Proctosigmoiditis may respond to vancomycin enemas. Recurrent colitis occurs in up to 20% of patients and may be treated by a longer course of oral metronidazole or vancomycin (up to 1 month). Reintroduction of normal flora by ingestion of *probiotics* has been suggested as a possible treatment for recurrent or refractory disease.[80] Fulminant colitis, characterized by septicemia and/or evidence of perforation, requires emergent laparotomy. A total abdominal colectomy with end ileostomy may be lifesaving.

Other Infectious Colitides

A variety of other infections with bacteria, parasites, fungi, or viruses may cause colonic inflammation. Common bacterial infections include enterotoxic *E. coli*, *Campylobacter jejuni*, *Yersinia enterocolitica*, *Salmonella typhi*, *Shigella*, and *Neisseria gonorrhoeae*. Less commonly, *Mycobacterium tuberculosis*, *Mycobacterium bovis*, *Actinomycosis israelii*, or *Treponema pallidum* (syphilis) may cause colitis or proctitis. Parasitic infections such as amebiasis, cryptosporidiosis, and giardiasis also are relatively common. Fungal infections (*Candida* species, histoplasmosis) are extremely rare in otherwise healthy individuals. The most common viral infections that produce colitic symptoms are the herpes simplex viruses, HIV, and cytomegalovirus (CMV).

Most symptoms are nonspecific and consist of diarrhea (with or without bleeding), crampy abdominal pain, and malaise. A thorough history may offer clues to the etiology (other medical conditions, especially immunosuppression; recent travel or exposures; and ingestions). Diagnosis usually is made by identification of a pathogen in the stool, either by microscopy or culture. Serum immunoassays may also be useful (amebiasis, HIV, CMV). Occasionally, endoscopy with biopsy may be required. Treatment is tailored to the infection.

ANORECTAL DISEASES

Any patient with anal/perianal symptoms requires a careful history and physical, including a digital rectal examination. Other studies such as defecography, manometry, CT scan, MRI, contrast enema, endoscopy, endoanal ultrasound, or examination under anesthesia may be required to arrive at an accurate diagnosis.

Hemorrhoids

Hemorrhoids are cushions of submucosal tissue containing venules, arterioles, and smooth-muscle fibers that are located in the anal canal (see Fig. 29-4). Three hemorrhoidal cushions are found in the left lateral, right anterior, and right posterior positions. Hemorrhoids are thought to function as part of the continence mechanism and aid in complete closure of the anal canal at rest. Because hemorrhoids are a normal part of anorectal anatomy, treatment is only indicated if they become symptomatic. Excessive straining, increased abdominal pressure, and hard stools increase venous engorgement of the hemorrhoidal plexus and cause prolapse of hemorrhoidal tissue. Bleeding, thrombosis, and symptomatic hemorrhoidal prolapse may result.

External hemorrhoids are located distal to the dentate line and are covered with anoderm. Because the anoderm is richly innervated, thrombosis of an external hemorrhoid may cause significant pain. It is for this reason that external hemorrhoids should not be ligated or excised without adequate local anesthetic. A *skin tag* is redundant fibrotic skin at the anal verge, often persisting as the residua of a thrombosed external hemorrhoid. Skin tags are often confused with symptomatic hemorrhoids. External hemorrhoids and skin tags may cause itching and difficulty with hygiene if they are large. Treatment of external hemorrhoids and skin tags are only indicated for symptomatic relief.

Internal hemorrhoids are located proximal to the dentate line and covered by insensate anorectal mucosa. Internal hemorrhoids may prolapse or bleed, but rarely become painful unless they develop thrombosis and necrosis (usually related to severe prolapse, incarceration, and/or strangulation). Internal hemorrhoids are graded according to the extent of prolapse. *First-degree hemorrhoids* bulge into the anal canal and may prolapse beyond the dentate line on straining. *Second-degree hemorrhoids* prolapse through the anus but reduce spontaneously. *Third-degree hemorrhoids* prolapse through the anal canal and require manual reduction. *Fourth-degree hemorrhoids* prolapse but cannot be reduced and are at risk for strangulation.

Combined internal and external hemorrhoids straddle the dentate line and have characteristics of both internal and external hemorrhoids. Hemorrhoidectomy often is required for large, symptomatic, combined hemorrhoids. *Postpartum hemorrhoids* result from straining during labor, which results in edema, thrombosis, and/or strangulation. Hemorrhoidectomy is often the treatment of choice, especially if the patient has had chronic hemorrhoidal symptoms. *Portal hypertension* was long thought to increase the risk of hemorrhoidal bleeding because of the anastomoses between the portal venous system (middle and upper hemorrhoidal plexuses) and the systemic venous system (inferior rectal plexuses). It is now understood that hemorrhoidal disease is no more common in patients with portal hypertension than in the normal population. *Rectal varices*, however, may occur and may cause hemorrhage in these patients. In general, rectal varices are best treated by lowering portal venous pressure. Rarely, suture ligation may be necessary if massive bleeding persists. Surgical hemorrhoidectomy should be avoided in these patients because of the risk of massive, difficult-to-control variceal bleeding.

Treatment

Medical Therapy Bleeding from first- and second-degree hemorrhoids often improves with the addition of dietary fiber, stool softeners, increased fluid intake, and avoidance of straining. Associated pruritus may often improve with improved hygiene. Many over-the-counter topical medications are desiccants and are relatively ineffective for treating hemorrhoidal symptoms.

Rubber Band Ligation Persistent bleeding from first-, second-, and selected third-degree hemorrhoids may be treated by rubber band ligation.

Mucosa located 1 to 2 cm proximal to the dentate line is grasped and pulled into a rubber band applier. After firing the ligator, the rubber band strangulates the underlying tissue, causing scarring and preventing further bleeding or prolapse (Fig. 29-31). In general, only one or two quadrants are banded per visit. Severe pain will occur if the rubber band is placed at or distal to the dentate line where sensory nerves are located. Other complications of rubber band ligation include *urinary retention*, *infection*, and *bleeding*. Urinary retention occurs in approximately 1% of patients and is more likely if the ligation has inadvertently included a portion of the internal sphincter. *Necrotizing infection* is an uncommon but life-threatening complication. Severe pain, fever, and urinary retention are early signs of infection and should prompt immediate evaluation of the patient usually with an examination under anesthesia. Treatment includes débridement of necrotic tissue, drainage of associated abscesses, and broad-spectrum antibiotics. *Bleeding* may occur approximately 7 to 10 days after rubber band ligation, at the time when the ligated pedicle necroses and sloughs. Bleeding is usually self limited, but persistent hemorrhage may require examination under anesthesia and suture ligation of the pedicle.

Infrared Photocoagulation Infrared photocoagulation is an effective office treatment for small first- and second-degree hemorrhoids. The instrument is applied to the apex of each hemorrhoid to coagulate the underlying plexus. All three quadrants may be treated during the same visit. Larger hemorrhoids and hemorrhoids with a significant amount of prolapse are not effectively treated with this technique.

Sclerotherapy The injection of bleeding internal hemorrhoids with sclerosing agents is another effective office technique for treatment of first-, second-, and some third-degree hemorrhoids. One to 3 mL of a sclerosing solution (phenol in olive oil, sodium morrhuate, or quinine urea) are injected into the submucosa of each hemorrhoid. Few complications are associated with sclerotherapy, but infection and fibrosis have been reported.

Excision of Thrombosed External Hemorrhoids Acutely thrombosed external hemorrhoids generally cause intense pain and a palpable perianal mass during the first 24 to 72 hours after thrombosis. The thrombosis can be effectively treated with an elliptical excision performed in the office under local anesthesia. Because the clot is usually loculated, simple incision and drainage is rarely effective. After 72 hours, the clot begins to resorb, and the pain resolves spontaneously. Excision is unnecessary, but sitz baths and analgesics often are helpful.

Operative Hemorrhoidectomy A number of surgical procedures have been described for elective resection of symptomatic hemorrhoids. All are based on decreasing blood flow to the hemorrhoidal plexuses and excising redundant anoderm and mucosa.

Closed Submucosal Hemorrhoidectomy The Parks or Ferguson hemorrhoidectomy involves resection of hemorrhoidal tissue and closure of the wounds with absorbable suture. The procedure may be performed in the prone or lithotomy position under local, regional, or general anesthesia. The anal canal is examined and an anal speculum inserted. The hemorrhoid cushions and associated redundant mucosa are identified and excised using an elliptical incision starting just distal to the anal verge and extending proximally to the anorectal ring. It is crucial to identify the fibers of the internal sphincter and carefully brush these away from the dissection to avoid injury to the sphincter. The apex of the hemorrhoidal plexus is then ligated and the hemorrhoid excised. The wound is then closed with a running absorbable suture. All three hemorrhoidal cushions may be removed using this technique; however, care should be taken to avoid resecting a large area of perianal skin to avoid postoperative anal stenosis (Fig. 29-32).

Open Hemorrhoidectomy This technique, often called the *Milligan and Morgan hemorrhoidectomy*, follows the same principles of excision described above in Submucosal Hemorrhoidectomy, but the wounds are left open and allowed to heal by secondary intention.

Whitehead's Hemorrhoidectomy Whitehead's hemorrhoidectomy involves circumferential excision of the hemorrhoidal cushions just proximal to the dentate line. After excision, the rectal mucosa is then advanced and sutured to the dentate line. Although some surgeons still use the Whitehead hemorrhoidectomy technique, most have abandoned this approach because of the risk of ectropion (*Whitehead's deformity*).

Procedure for Prolapse and Hemorrhoids/Stapled Hemorrhoidectomy Procedure for prolapse and hemorrhoids (PPH) has been proposed as an alternative surgical approach. The term *PPH* has largely replaced stapled hemorrhoidectomy because the procedure does not involve excision of hemorrhoidal tissue, but instead fixes the redundant mucosa above the dentate line. PPH removes a short circumferential segment of rectal mucosa proximal to the dentate line using a circular stapler. This effectively ligates the venules feeding the hemorrhoidal plexus and fixes redundant mucosa higher in the anal canal. Critics suggest that this technique is only appropriate for patients with large, bleeding, internal hemorrhoids, and is ineffective

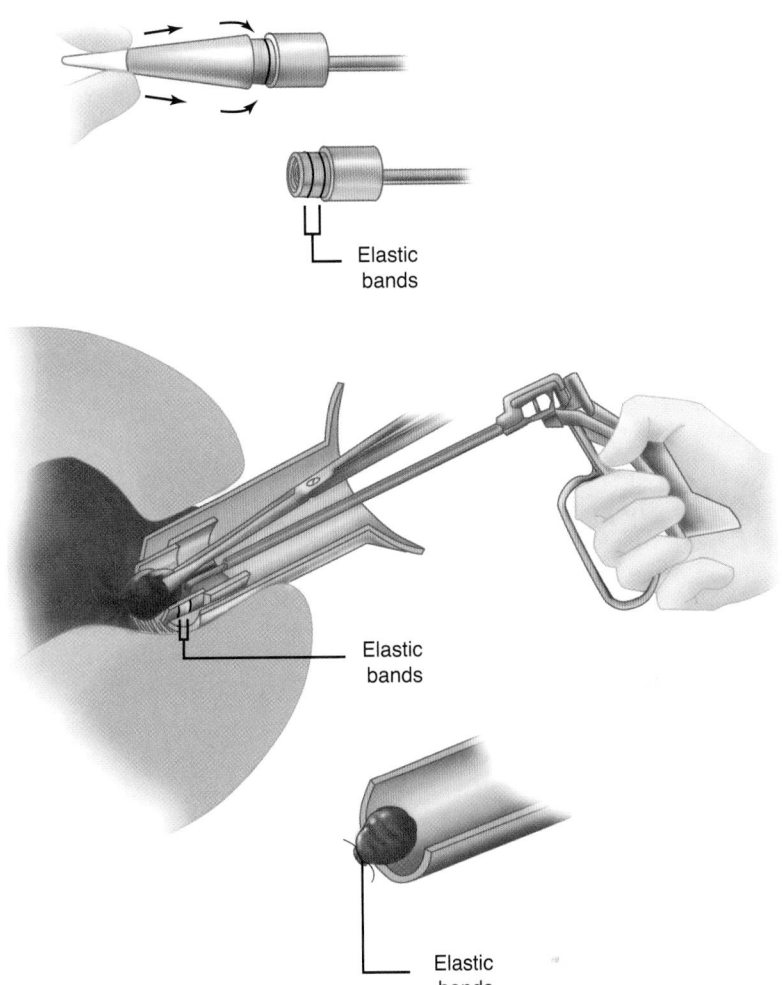

FIG. 29-31. Rubber band ligation of internal hemorrhoids. The mucosa just proximal to the internal hemorrhoids is banded.

in management of external or combined hemorrhoids. Nevertheless, several recent studies suggest that this procedure is safe and effective, is associated with less postoperative pain and disability, and has an equivalent risk of postoperative complications when compared to traditional hemorrhoidectomy.[87,88]

Complications of Hemorrhoidectomy Postoperative pain following excisional hemorrhoidectomy requires analgesia usually with oral narcotics. NSAIDs, muscle relaxants, topical analgesics, and comfort measures, including sitz baths, are often useful as well. Urinary retention is a common complication following hemorrhoidectomy and occurs in 10 to 50% of patients. The risk of urinary retention can be minimized by limiting intraoperative and perioperative IV fluids, and by providing adequate analgesia. Pain also can lead to *fecal impaction*. Risk of impaction may be decreased by preoperative enemas or a limited mechanical bowel preparation, liberal use of laxatives postoperatively, and adequate pain control. Although a small amount of *bleeding*, especially with bowel movements, is to be expected, massive hemorrhage can occur after hemorrhoidectomy. Bleeding may occur in the immediate postoperative period (often in the recovery room) as a result of inadequate ligation of the vascular pedicle. This type of hemorrhage mandates an urgent return to the operating room where suture ligation of the bleeding vessel will often solve the problem. Bleeding may also occur 7 to 10 days after hemorrhoidectomy when the necrotic mucosa overlying the vascular pedicle sloughs. Although some of these patients may be safely observed, others will require an examination under anesthesia to ligate the bleeding vessel or to oversew the wounds if no specific site of bleeding is identified. *Infection* is uncommon after hemorrhoidectomy; however, necrotizing soft tissue infection can occur

with devastating consequences. Severe pain, fever, and urinary retention may be early signs of infection. If infection is suspected, an emergent examination under anesthesia, drainage of abscess, and/or débridement of all necrotic tissue are required.

Long-term sequelae of hemorrhoidectomy include *incontinence, anal stenosis,* and *ectropion (Whitehead's deformity)*. Many patients experience transient incontinence to flatus, but these symptoms usually are short lived, and few patients have permanent fecal incontinence. Anal stenosis may result from scarring after extensive resection of perianal skin. Ectropion may occur after a Whitehead's hemorrhoidectomy. This complication is usually the result of suturing the rectal mucosa too far distally in the anal canal and can be avoided by ensuring that the mucosa is sutured at or just above the dentate line.

Anal Fissure

A fissure in ano is a tear in the anoderm distal to the dentate line. The pathophysiology of anal fissure is thought to be related to trauma from either the passage of hard stool or prolonged diarrhea. A tear in the anoderm causes spasm of the internal anal sphincter, which results in pain, increased tearing, and decreased blood supply to the anoderm. This cycle of pain, spasm, and ischemia contributes to development of a poorly healing wound that becomes a *chronic fissure*. The vast majority of anal fissures occur in the posterior midline. Ten to 15% occur in the anterior midline. Less than 1% of fissures occur off midline.

Symptoms and Findings

Anal fissure is extremely common.[88,89] Characteristic symptoms include tearing pain with defecation and hematochezia (usually

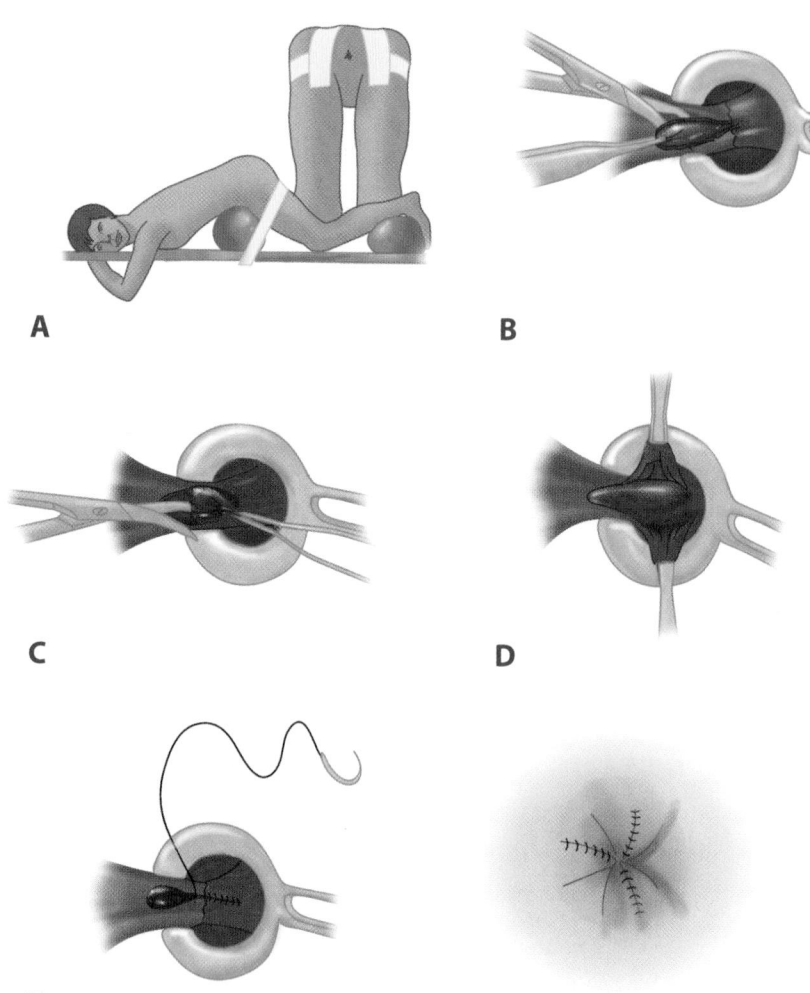

FIG. 29-32. Technique of closed submucosal hemorrhoidectomy. **A.** The patient is in prone jackknife position. **B.** A Fansler anoscope is used for exposure. **C.** A narrow ellipse of anoderm is excised. **D.** A submucosal dissection of the hemorrhoidal plexus from the underlying anal sphincter is performed. **E.** Redundant mucosa is anchored to the proximal anal canal, and the wound is closed with a running absorbable suture. **F.** Additional quadrants are excised to complete the procedure.

described as blood on the toilet paper). Patients also may complain of a sensation of intense and painful anal spasm lasting for several hours after a bowel movement. On physical examination, the fissure often can be seen in the anoderm by gently separating the buttocks. Patients are often too tender to tolerate digital rectal examination, anoscopy, or proctoscopy. An *acute fissure* is a superficial tear of the distal anoderm and almost always heals with medical management. *Chronic fissures* develop ulceration and heaped-up edges with the white fibers of the internal anal sphincter visible at the base of the ulcer. There often is an associated external skin tag and/or a hypertrophied anal papilla internally. These fissures are more challenging to treat and may require surgery. A lateral location of a chronic anal fissure may be evidence of an underlying disease such as Crohn's disease, HIV, syphilis, tuberculosis, or leukemia. If the diagnosis is in doubt or there is suspicion of another cause for the perianal pain, such as abscess or fistula, an examination under anesthesia may be necessary.

Treatment

Therapy focuses on breaking the cycle of pain, spasm, and ischemia thought responsible for development of fissure in ano. First-line therapy to minimize anal trauma includes bulk agents, stool softeners, and warm sitz baths. The addition of 2% lidocaine jelly or other analgesic creams can provide additional symptomatic relief. Nitroglycerin ointment (0.2%) has been used locally to improve blood flow but often causes severe headaches. Both oral and topical calcium channel blockers (diltiazem and nifedipine) also have been used to heal fissures and may have fewer side effects than topical nitrates. Newer agents, such as arginine (a nitric oxide donor) and

topical bethanechol (a muscarinic agonist), also have been used to treat fissures. Medical therapy is effective in most acute fissures, but will heal only approximately 50 to 60% of chronic fissures.

Botulinum toxin (Botox) causes temporary muscle paralysis by preventing acetylcholine release from presynaptic nerve terminals. Injection of botulinum toxin is used in some centers as an alternative to surgical sphincterotomy for chronic fissure. Although there are few long-term complications from the use of Botox, healing appears to be equivalent to other medical therapies.[90]

Surgical therapy traditionally has been recommended for chronic fissures that have failed medical therapy, and lateral internal sphincterotomy is the procedure of choice for most surgeons. The aim of this procedure is to decrease spasm of the internal sphincter by dividing a portion of the muscle. Approximately 30% of the internal sphincter fibers are divided laterally by using either an open (Fig. 29-33) or closed (Fig. 29-34) technique. Healing is achieved in more than 95% of patients by using this technique, and most patients experience immediate pain relief.[90] Recurrence occurs in less than 10% of patients and the risk of incontinence (usually to flatus) ranges from 5 to 15%.

Anorectal Sepsis and Cryptoglandular Abscess
Relevant Anatomy

The majority of anorectal suppurative disease results from infections of the anal glands (cryptoglandular infection) found in the intersphincteric plane. Their ducts traverse the internal sphincter and empty into the anal crypts at the level of the dentate line. Infection of an anal gland results in the formation of an abscess that

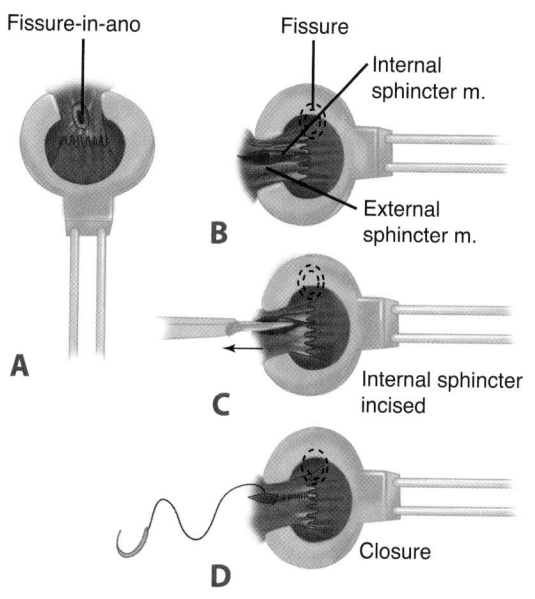

FIG. 29-33. A through **D.** Open lateral internal sphincterotomy for fissure in ano. m = muscle.

enlarges and spreads along one of several planes in the perianal and perirectal spaces. The *perianal space* surrounds the anus and laterally becomes continuous with the fat of the buttocks. The *intersphincteric space* separates the internal and external anal sphincters. It is continuous with the perianal space distally and extends cephalad into the rectal wall. The *ischiorectal space (ischiorectal fossa)* is located lateral and posterior to the anus and is bounded medially by the external sphincter, laterally by the ischium, superiorly by the levator ani, and inferiorly by the transverse septum. The ischiorectal space contains the inferior rectal vessels and lymphatics. The two ischiorectal spaces connect posteriorly above the anococcygeal ligament but below the levator ani muscle, forming the *deep postanal space*. The *supralevator spaces* lie above the levator ani on either side of the rectum and communicate posteriorly. The anatomy of these spaces influences the location and spread of cryptoglandular infection (Fig. 29-35).

As an abscess enlarges, it spreads in one of several directions. A *perianal abscess* is the most common manifestation and appears as a painful swelling at the anal verge. Spread through the external sphincter below the level of the puborectalis produces an *ischiorectal abscess*. These abscesses may become extremely large and may not be visible in the perianal region. Digital rectal exam will reveal a painful swelling laterally in the ischiorectal fossa. *Intersphincteric abscesses* occur in the intersphincteric space and are notoriously difficult to

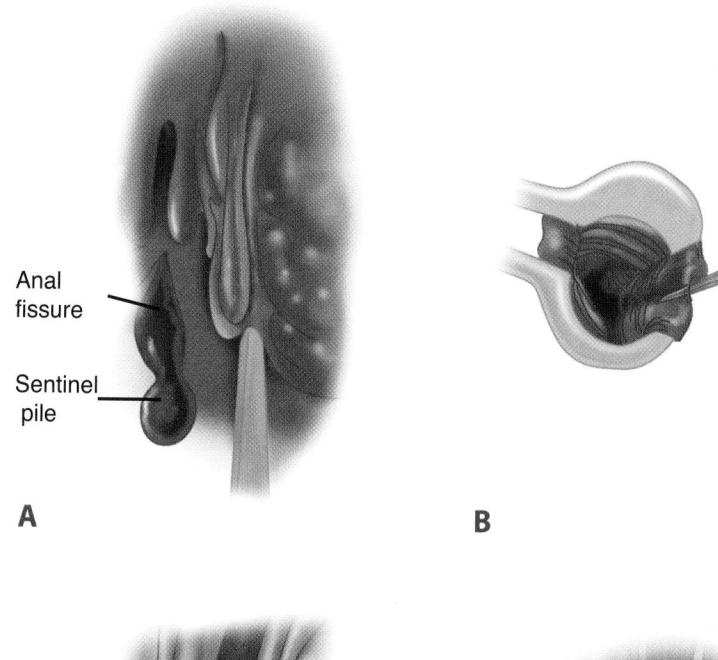

Anal fissure

Sentinel pile

A

B

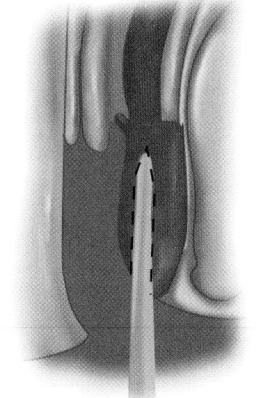

C

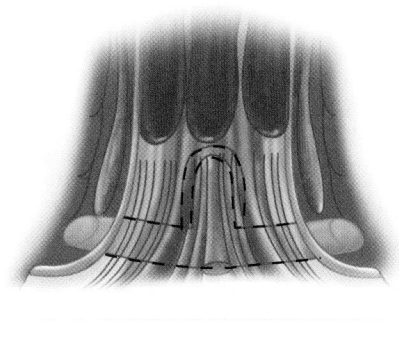

D

FIG. 29-34. A through **D.** Closed lateral internal sphincterotomy for fissure in ano.

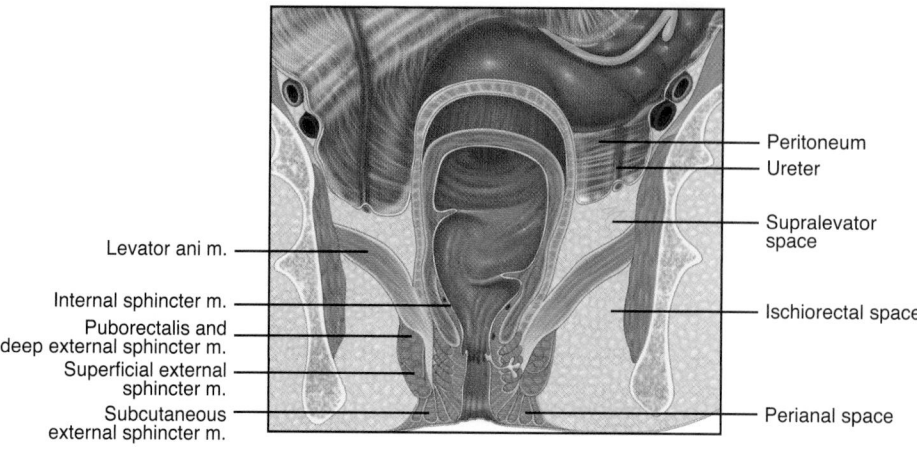

A

B

FIG. 29-35. Anatomy of perianorectal spaces. **A.** Anterior view and (**B**) lateral view. m = muscle.

diagnose, often requiring an examination under anesthesia. *Pelvic* and *supralevator abscesses* are uncommon and may result from extension of an intersphincteric or ischiorectal abscess upward, or extension of an intraperitoneal abscess downward (Fig. 29-36).

Diagnosis

Severe anal pain is the most common presenting complaint. Walking, coughing, or straining can aggravate the pain. A palpable mass often is detected by inspection of the perianal area or by digital rectal examination. Occasionally, patients will present with fever, urinary retention, or life-threatening sepsis. The diagnosis of a perianal or ischiorectal abscess usually can be made with physical examination alone (either in the office or in the operating room). However, complex or atypical presentations may require imaging studies such as CT or MRI to fully delineate the anatomy of the abscess.

Treatment

Anorectal abscesses should be treated by drainage as soon as the diagnosis is established. If the diagnosis is in question, an examination under anesthesia is often the most expeditious way both to confirm the diagnosis and to treat the problem. Delayed or inadequate treatment may occasionally cause extensive and life-threatening suppuration with massive tissue necrosis and septicemia. Antibiotics are only indicated if there is extensive overlying cellulitis or if the patient is immunocompromised, has diabetes mellitus, or

has valvular heart disease. Antibiotics alone are ineffective at treating perianal or perirectal infection.

Perianal Abscess

Most perianal abscesses can be drained under local anesthesia in the office, clinic, or emergency room. Larger, more complicated abscesses may require drainage in the operating room. A cruciate skin and subcutaneous incision is made over the most prominent part of the abscess and the "dog ears" are excised to prevent premature closure. No packing is necessary and sitz baths are started the next day (Fig. 29-37).

Ischiorectal Abscesses

An ischiorectal abscess causes diffuse swelling in the ischiorectal fossa that may involve one or both sides, forming a "horseshoe" abscess. Simple ischiorectal abscesses are drained through an incision in the overlying skin. Horseshoe abscesses require drainage of the deep postanal space and often require counterincisions over one or both ischiorectal spaces (Fig. 29-38).

Intersphincteric Abscess

Intersphincteric abscesses are notoriously difficult to diagnose because they produce little swelling and few perianal signs of infection. Pain is typically described as being deep and "up inside" the

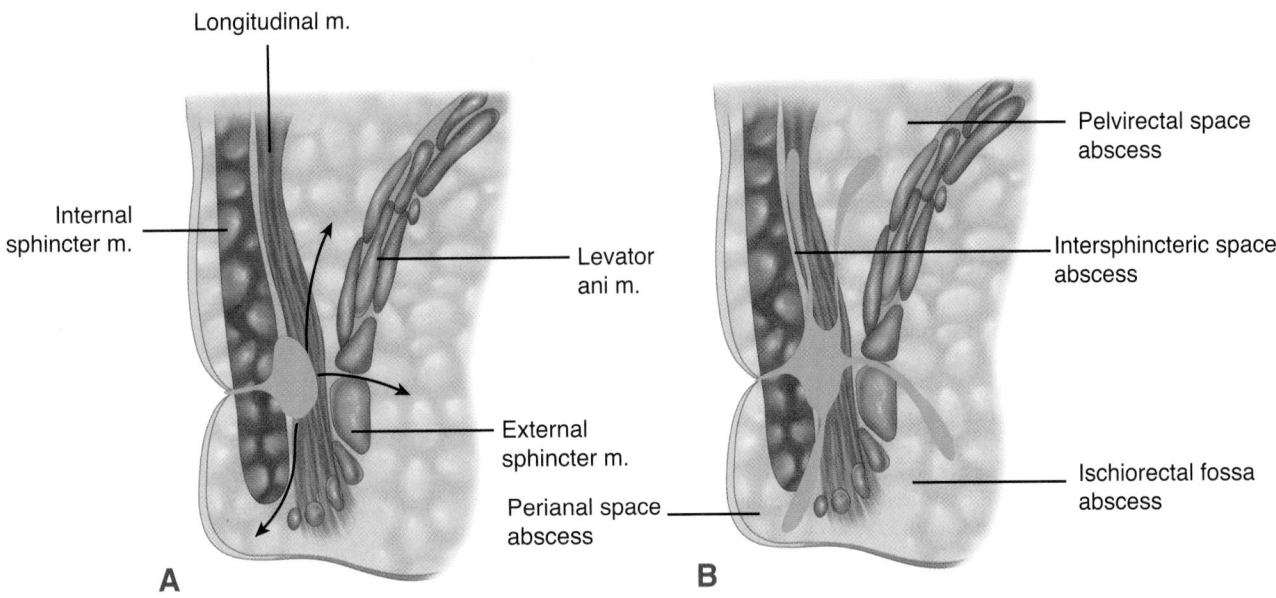

FIG. 29-36. A and **B.** Pathways of anorectal infection in perianal spaces. m = muscle.

anal area, and usually is exacerbated by coughing or sneezing. The pain is so intense that it usually precludes a digital rectal examination. The diagnosis is made based upon a high index of suspicion and usually requires an examination under anesthesia. Once identified, an intersphincteric abscess can be drained through a limited, usually posterior, internal sphincterotomy.

Supralevator Abscess

This type of abscess is uncommon and can be difficult to diagnose. Because of its proximity to the peritoneal cavity, supralevator abscesses can mimic intra-abdominal conditions. Digital rectal examination may reveal an indurated, bulging mass above the anorectal ring. It is essential to identify the origin of a supralevator abscess before treatment. If the abscess is secondary to an upward extension of an intersphincteric abscess, it should be drained through the rectum. If it is drained through the ischiorectal fossa, a complicated, suprasphincteric fistula may result. If a supralevator abscess arises

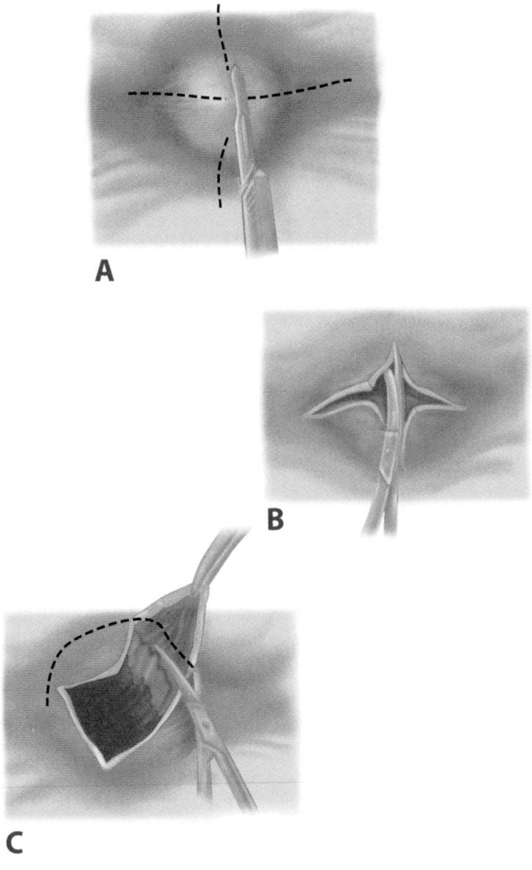

FIG. 29-37. A through **C.** Technique of drainage of perianal abscess.

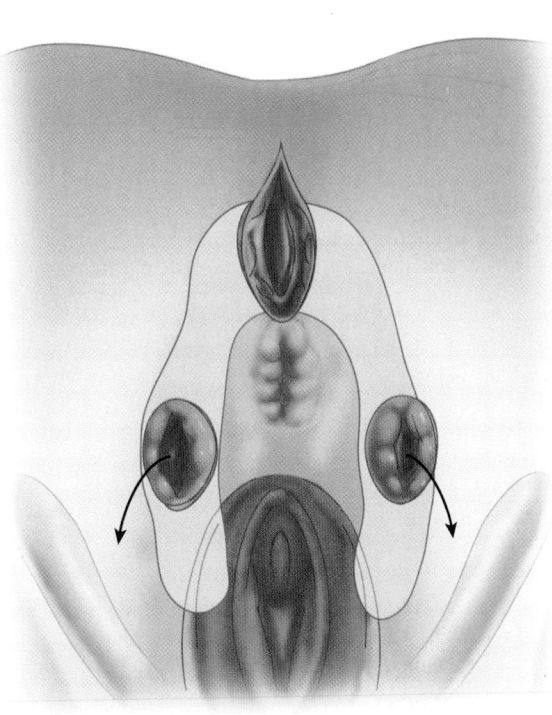

FIG. 29-38. Drainage of horseshoe abscess. The deep postanal space is entered, incising the anococcygeal ligament. Counter drainage incisions are made for each limb of the ischiorectal space.

from the upward extension of an ischiorectal abscess, it should be drained through the ischiorectal fossa. Drainage of this type of abscess through the rectum may result in an extrasphincteric fistula. If the abscess is secondary to intra-abdominal disease, the primary process requires treatment and the abscess is drained via the most direct route (transabdominally, rectally, or through the ischiorectal fossa).

Perianal Sepsis in the Immunocompromised Patient

The immunocompromised patient with perianal pain presents a diagnostic dilemma. Because of leukopenia, these patients may develop serious perianal infection without any of the cardinal signs of inflammation. Although broad-spectrum antibiotics may cure some of these patients, an examination under anesthesia should not be delayed because of neutropenia. An increase in pain or fever, and/or clinical deterioration mandates an examination under anesthesia. Any indurated area should be incised and drained, biopsied to exclude a leukemic infiltrate, and cultured to aid in the selection of antimicrobial agents.[91]

Necrotizing Soft Tissue Infection of the Perineum

Necrotizing soft tissue infection of the perineum is a rare, but lethal, condition. Most of these infections are polymicrobial and synergistic. The source of sepsis is commonly an undrained or inadequately drained cryptoglandular abscess or a urogenital infection. Occasionally, these infections may be encountered postoperatively (e.g., after inguinal hernia repair). Immunocompromised patients and diabetic patients are at increased risk.

Physical examination may reveal necrotic skin, bullae, or crepitus. Patients often have signs of systemic toxicity and may be hemodynamically unstable. A high index of suspicion is necessary because perineal signs of severe infection may be minimal and prompt surgical intervention can be lifesaving.

Surgical débridement of all nonviable tissue is required to treat all necrotizing soft tissue infections. Multiple operations may be necessary to ensure that all necrotic tissue has been resected. Broad-spectrum antibiotics are frequently used, but adequate surgical débridement remains the mainstay of therapy. Colostomy may be required if extensive resection of the sphincter is required or if stool contamination of the perineum makes wound management difficult. Despite early recognition and adequate surgical therapy, the mortality of necrotizing perineal soft tissue infections remains approximately 50%.

Fistula In Ano

Drainage of an anorectal abscess results in cure for about 50% of patients. The remaining 50% develop a persistent *fistula in ano*. The fistula usually originates in the infected crypt (*internal opening*) and tracks to the *external opening*, usually the site of prior drainage. The course of the fistula often can be predicted by the anatomy of the previous abscess.

Although the majority of fistulas are cryptoglandular in origin, trauma, Crohn's disease, malignancy, radiation, or unusual infections (tuberculosis, actinomycosis, and chlamydia) may also produce fistulas. A complex, recurrent, or nonhealing fistula should raise the suspicion of one of these diagnoses.

Diagnosis

Patients present with persistent drainage from the internal and/or external openings. An indurated tract often is palpable. Although the external opening is often easily identifiable, identification of the internal opening may be more challenging. Goodsall's rule can be used as a guide in determining the location of the internal opening (Fig. 29-39). In general, fistulas with an external opening *anteriorly* connect to the internal opening by a *short, radial tract*. Fistulas with an external opening *posteriorly* track in a *curvilinear fashion to the*

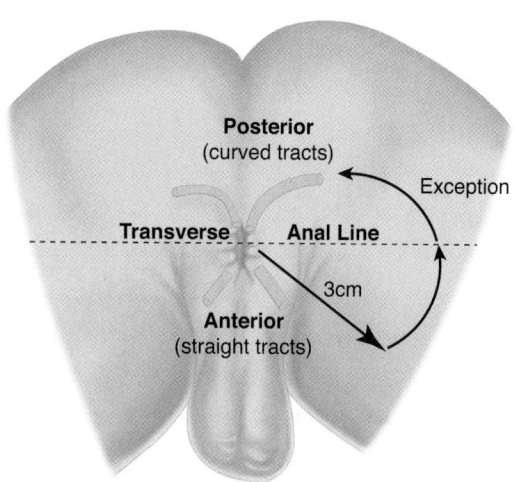

FIG. 29-39. Goodsall's rule to identify the internal opening of fistulas in ano.

posterior midline. However, exceptions to this rule often occur if an anterior external opening is greater than 3 cm from the anal margin. Such fistulas usually track to the posterior midline. Fistulas are categorized based upon their relationship to the anal sphincter complex, and treatment options are based upon these classifications. An *intersphincteric fistula* tracks through the distal internal sphincter and intersphincteric space to an external opening near the anal verge (Fig. 29-40A). A *transsphincteric fistula* often results from an ischiorectal abscess and extends through both the internal and external sphincters (Fig. 29-40B). A *suprasphincteric fistula* originates in the intersphincteric plane and tracks up and around the entire external sphincter (Fig. 29-40C). An *extrasphincteric fistula* originates in the rectal wall and tracks around both sphincters to exit laterally, usually in the ischiorectal fossa (Fig. 29-40D).

Treatment

The goal of treatment of fistula in ano is eradication of sepsis without sacrificing continence. Because fistulous tracks encircle variable amounts of the sphincter complex, surgical treatment is dictated by the location of the internal and external openings and the course of the fistula. The external opening usually is visible as a red elevation of granulation tissue with or without concurrent drainage. The internal opening may be more difficult to identify. Injection of hydrogen peroxide or dilute methylene blue may be helpful. Care must be taken to avoid creating an artificial internal opening (thus often converting a simple fistula into a complex fistula).

Simple intersphincteric fistulas often can be treated by *fistulotomy* (opening the fistulous tract), curettage, and healing by secondary intention (see Fig. 29-40A). *"Horseshoe" fistulas* usually have an internal opening in the posterior midline and extend anteriorly and laterally to one or both ischiorectal spaces by way of the deep postanal space. Treatment of a transsphincteric fistula depends upon its location in the sphincter complex. Fistulas that include less than 30% of the sphincter muscles often can be treated by sphincterotomy without significant risk of major incontinence (see Fig. 29-40B). High transsphincteric fistulas, which encircle a greater amount of muscle, are more safely treated by initial placement of a *seton* (see paragraph below). Similarly, suprasphincteric fistulas usually are treated with seton placement (see Fig. 29-40C). Extrasphincteric fistulas are rare, and treatment depends upon both the anatomy of the fistula and its etiology. In general, the portion of the fistula outside the sphincter should be opened and drained. A primary tract at the level of the dentate line may also be opened, if present. Complex fistulas with multiple tracts may require numerous procedures to control sepsis and facilitate healing. Liberal use of drains and setons is helpful.

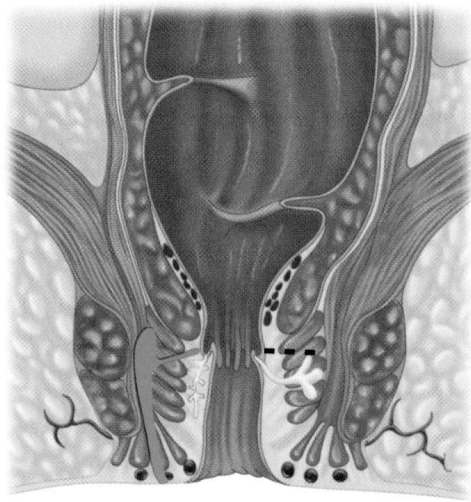

A

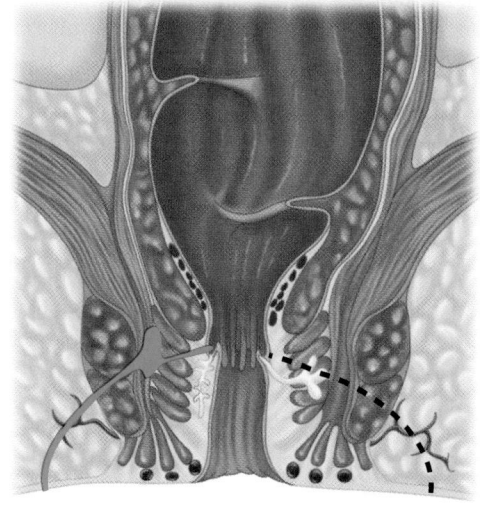

B

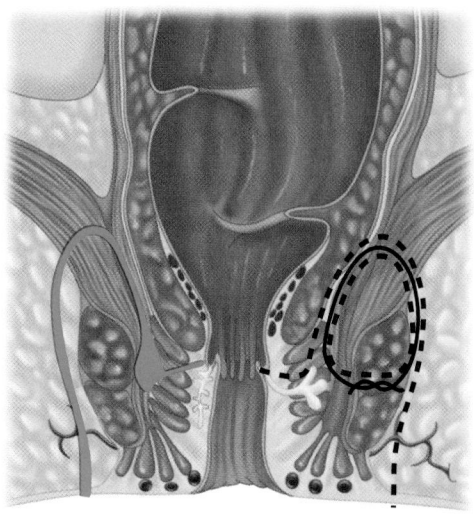

C

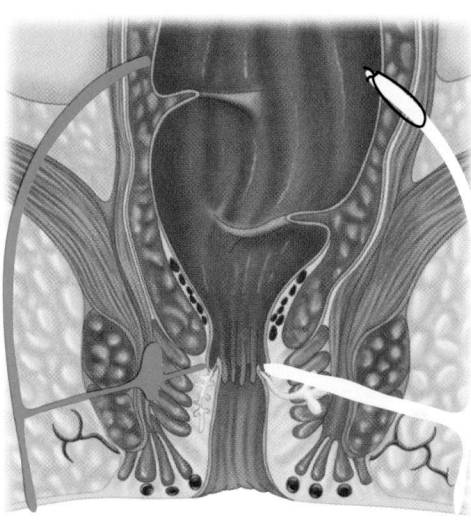

D

FIG. 29-40. The four major categories of fistula in ano (*left side of drawings*) and the usual operative procedure to correct the fistula (*right side of drawings*). **A.** Intersphincteric fistula with simple low tract. **B.** Uncomplicated transsphincteric fistula. **C.** Uncomplicated suprasphincteric fistula. **D.** Extrasphincteric fistula secondary to anal fistula. *[Reproduced with permission from Gordon PH, Nivatvongs S (eds): Principles and Practice of Surgery for the Colon, Rectum, and Anus, 2nd ed. New York: Marcel Dekker, Inc., 1999, pp 256–260.]*

Failure to heal may ultimately require fecal diversion (see Fig. 29-40D). Complex and/or nonhealing fistulas may result from Crohn's disease, malignancy, radiation proctitis, or unusual infection. Proctoscopy should be performed in all cases of complex and/or nonhealing fistulas to assess the health of the rectal mucosa. Biopsies of the fistula tract should be taken to rule out malignancy.

A *seton* is a drain placed through a fistula to maintain drainage and/or induce fibrosis. *Cutting setons* consist of a suture or a rubber band that is placed through the fistula and intermittently tightened in the office. Tightening the seton results in fibrosis and gradual division of the sphincter, thus eliminating the fistula while maintaining continuity of the sphincter. A *noncutting seton* is a soft plastic drain (often a vessel loop) placed in the fistula to maintain drainage. The fistula tract may subsequently be laid open with less risk of incontinence because scarring prevents retraction of the sphincter. Alternatively, the seton may be left in place for chronic drainage. Higher fistulas may be treated by an *endorectal advancement flap* (see below in Rectovaginal Fistula: Treatment). *Fibrin glue* and a variety of collagen-based plugs also have been used to treat persistent fistulas with variable results.

Rectovaginal Fistula

A rectovaginal fistula is a connection between the vagina and the rectum or anal canal proximal to the dentate line. Rectovaginal fistulas are classified as *low* (rectal opening close to the dentate line and vaginal opening in the fourchette), *middle* (vaginal opening between the fourchette and cervix), or *high* (vaginal opening near the cervix). Low rectovaginal fistulas are commonly caused by obstetric injuries or trauma from a foreign body. Midrectovaginal fistulas may result from more severe obstetric injury, but also occur after surgical resection of a midrectal neoplasm, radiation injury, or extension of an undrained abscess. High rectovaginal fistulas result from operative or radiation injury. Complicated diverticulitis may cause a colovaginal fistula. Crohn's disease can cause rectovaginal fistulas at all levels, as well as colovaginal and enterovaginal fistulas.

Diagnosis

Patients describe symptoms varying from the sensation of passing flatus from the vagina to the passage of solid stool from the vagina.

Most patients experience some degree of fecal incontinence. Contamination may result in *vaginitis*. Large fistulas may be obvious on anoscopic and/or vaginal speculum examination, but smaller fistulas may be difficult to locate. Occasionally, a barium enema or vaginogram may identify these fistulas. Endorectal ultrasound also may be useful. With the patient in the prone position, installation of methylene blue into the rectum while a tampon is in the vagina may confirm the presence of a small fistula.

Treatment

The treatment of rectovaginal fistula depends upon the size, location, etiology, and condition of surrounding tissues. Because up to

50% of fistulas caused by obstetric injury heal spontaneously, it is prudent to wait 3 to 6 months before embarking upon surgical repair in these patients. If the fistula was caused by a cryptoglandular abscess, drainage of the abscess may allow spontaneous closure. Low and midrectovaginal fistulas usually are best treated with an endorectal advancement flap. The principle of this procedure is based upon the advancement of healthy mucosa, submucosa, and circular muscle over the rectal opening (the high-pressure side of the fistula) to promote healing (Fig. 29-41). If a sphincter injury is present, an overlapping sphincteroplasty should be performed concurrently. Fecal diversion is rarely required. High rectovaginal, colovaginal, and enterovaginal fistulas are usually best treated via a transabdominal

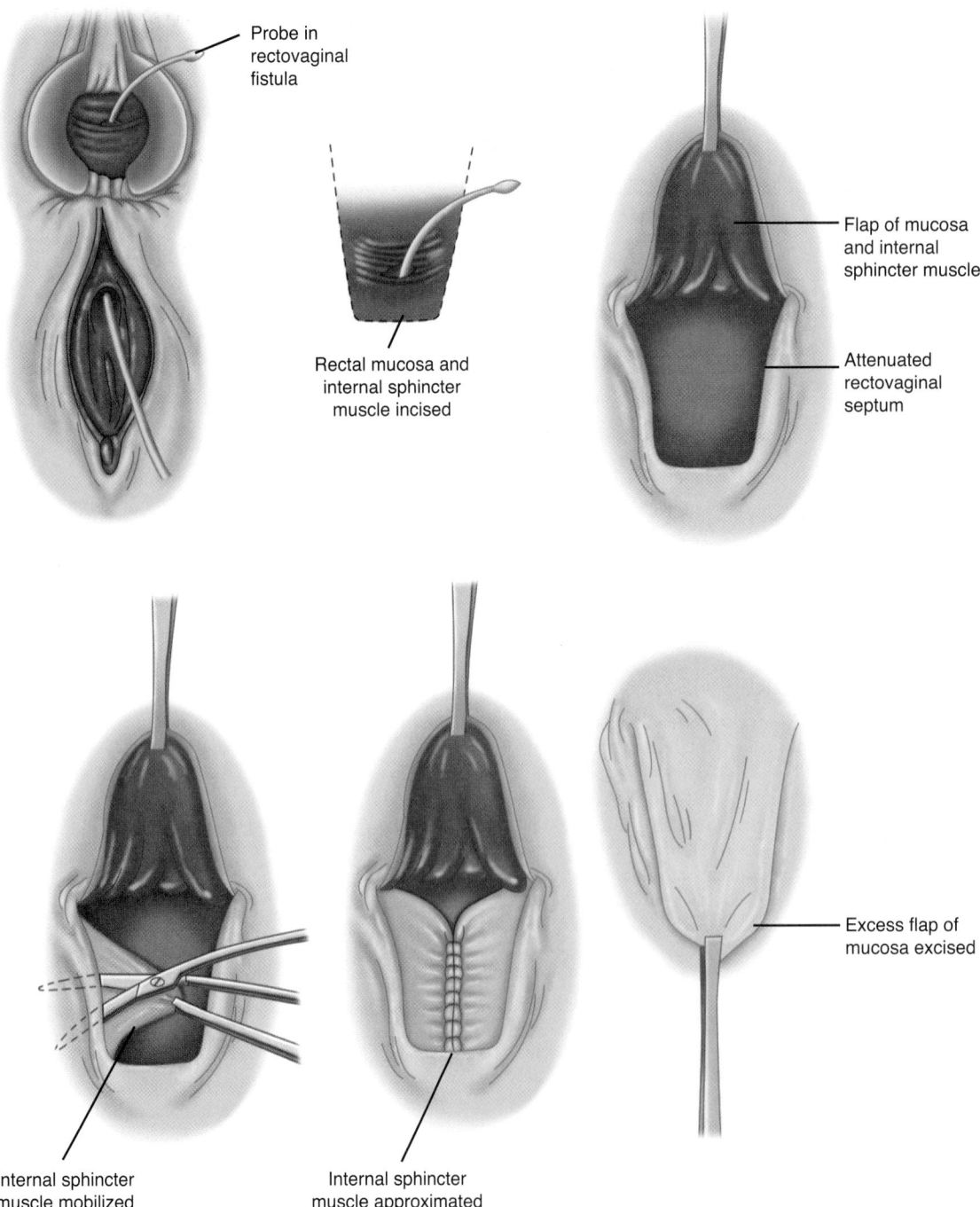

FIG. 29-41. Endorectal advancement flap for rectovaginal fistula. *[Reproduced with permission from Gordon PH, Nivatvongs S (eds): Principles and Practice of Surgery for the Colon, Rectum, and Anus, 2nd ed. New York: Marcel Dekker, Inc., 1999, p 412.]*

approach. The diseased tissue, which caused the fistula (upper rectum, sigmoid colon, or small bowel), is resected and the hole in the vagina closed. Healthy tissue such as omentum or muscle is frequently interposed between the bowel anastomosis and the vagina to prevent recurrence.

Rectovaginal fistulas caused by Crohn's disease, radiation injury, or malignancy almost never heal spontaneously. In Crohn's disease, treatment is based on adequate drainage of perianal sepsis and nutritional support. An endorectal advancement flap may be performed if the rectum is spared from active Crohn's disease. Fistulas resulting from radiation damage are not amenable to local repair with an advancement flap because of damage to the surrounding rectal and vaginal tissues. Mid- and high rectovaginal fistulas are occasionally repaired successfully with a transabdominal approach in which healthy tissue (omentum, muscle, or nonradiated bowel) is interposed between the damaged rectum and vagina. Fistulas caused by malignancy should be treated with resection of the tumor. Because differentiating radiation damage from malignancy can be extremely difficult, all fistulas resulting from radiation should be biopsied to rule out cancer.

Perianal Dermatitis

Pruritus Ani

Pruritus ani (severe perianal itching) is a common problem with a multitude of etiologies. Surgically correctable (anatomic) causes include prolapsing hemorrhoids, ectropion, fissure, fistula, and neoplasms. Perianal infection may also present with pruritus ani. Infections may be caused by fungus (*Candida* species, *Monilia*, and *Epidermophyton* organisms), parasites [*Enterobius vermicularis* (pinworms), *Pediculus pubis* (a louse), and *Sarcoptes scabiei* (scabies)], bacteria [*Corynebacterium minutissimum* (erythrasma) and *Treponema pallidum* (syphilis)], or viruses [HPV (condyloma acuminata)]. Antibiotic use may also cause itching, usually by precipitating fungal infection. Noninfectious dermatologic causes include seborrhea, psoriasis, and contact dermatitis. Contact dermatitis can be particularly troublesome because many over-the-counter topical agents used by patients to relieve itching may exacerbate the problem. Occasionally, systemic diseases such as jaundice and diabetes may present with pruritus ani.

Despite this myriad of causes, the majority of pruritus ani is idiopathic and probably related to local hygiene, neurogenic, or psychogenic causes. Treatment focuses on removal of irritants, improving perianal hygiene, dietary adjustments, and avoiding scratching. Biopsy and/or culture may be required to rule out an infectious or dermatologic cause. Hydrocortisone ointment 0.5 to 1.0% can provide symptomatic relief but should not be used for prolonged periods of time because of dermal atrophy. Skin barriers such as Calmoseptine also can provide relief. Systemic antihistamines or tricyclic antidepressants also have been used with some success.

Nonpruritic Lesions

Several perianal skin conditions may present with perianal skin changes. Leprosy, amebiasis, actinomycosis, and lymphogranuloma venereum produce characteristic perianal lesions. Neoplasms such as Bowen's disease, Paget's disease, and invasive carcinomas may also appear first in the perianal skin. Biopsy usually can distinguish these diagnoses.

Sexually Transmitted Diseases

Bacterial Infections

Proctitis is a common symptom of anorectal bacterial infection.[92,93] *N. gonorrhoeae* is the most common bacterial cause of proctitis and causes pain, tenesmus, rectal bleeding, and mucus discharge. *C. trachomatis* infection may be asymptomatic or may produce similar symptoms. *T. pallidum*, the microbe causing syphilis, causes a chancre at the site of inoculation, which may be asymptomatic or

may present as an atypical fissure (primary syphilis). Condyloma lata are characteristic of secondary syphilis. Chancroid, caused by *Haemophilus ducreyi*, is a disease manifested by multiple painful, bleeding lesions. Inguinal lymphadenopathy and fluctuant, draining lymph nodes are characteristic. *Donovania granulomatis* infection produces shiny, red masses on the perineum (granuloma inguinale). Diarrheal illnesses caused by organisms such as *Campylobacter* or *Shigella* also may be sexually transmitted. Treatment consists of antimicrobial agents directed against the infecting organism.

Parasitic Infections

Entamoeba histolytica is an increasingly common sexually transmitted disease. Amebas produce ulcerations in the GI mucosa and can infect any part of the gut. Symptoms include diarrhea, abdominal pain, and tenesmus. *Giardia lamblia* is also common and produces diarrhea, abdominal pain, and malaise.

Viral Infections

Herpes Simplex Virus Herpes proctitis is extremely common. Proctitis usually is caused by type II herpes simplex virus and less commonly by type I herpes simplex virus. Patients complain of severe, intractable perianal pain and tenesmus. Pain often precedes the development of characteristic vesicles, and these patients may require an examination under anesthesia to exclude another diagnosis such as an intersphincteric abscess. Diagnosis is confirmed by viral culture of tissue or vesicular fluid.

Human Papillomavirus HPV causes condyloma acuminata (anogenital warts) and is associated with AIN and squamous cell carcinoma (see Anal Canal and Perianal Tumors above). Condylomas occur in the perianal area or in the squamous epithelium of the anal canal. Occasionally, the mucosa of the lower rectum may be affected. There are approximately 30 serotypes of HPV. HPV types 16 and 18, in particular, appear to predispose to malignancy and often cause flat dysplasia in skin unaffected by warts. In contrast, HPV types 6 and 11 commonly cause warts, but do not appear to cause malignant degeneration.

Treatment of anal condyloma depends on the location and extent of disease. Small warts on the perianal skin and distal anal canal may be treated in the office with topical application of bichloracetic acid or podophyllin. Although 60 to 80% of patients will respond to these agents, recurrence and reinfection are common. Imiquimod (Aldara) is an immunomodulator that recently was introduced for topical treatment of several viral infections, including anogenital condyloma.[94] Initial reports suggest that this agent is highly effective in treating condyloma located on the perianal skin and distal anal canal.[95] Larger and/or more numerous warts require excision and/or fulguration in the operating room. Excised warts should be sent for pathologic examination to rule out dysplasia or malignancy. It is important to note that prior use of podophyllin may induce histologic changes that mimic dysplasia. The recent introduction of a vaccine against HPV holds promise for preventing anogenital condylomas.

Human Immunodeficiency Virus See The Immunocompromised Patient below.

Pilonidal Disease

Pilonidal disease (cyst, infection) consists of a hair-containing sinus or abscess occurring in the intergluteal cleft. Although the etiology is unknown, it is speculated that the cleft creates a suction that draws hair into the midline pits when a patients sits. These ingrown hairs may then become infected and present acutely as an abscess in the sacrococcygeal region. Once an acute episode has resolved, recurrence is common.

An acute abscess should be incised and drained as soon as the diagnosis is made. Because these abscesses are usually very superficial, this procedure often can be performed in the office, clinic, or emergency room under local anesthetic. Because midline wounds in the region heal poorly, some surgeons recommend using an incision *lateral* to the intergluteal cleft. A number of procedures have been proposed to treat a chronic pilonidal sinus. The simplest method involves unroofing the tract, curetting the base, and marsupializing the wound. The wound must then be kept clean and free of hair until healing is complete (often requiring weekly office visits for wound care). Alternatively, a small lateral incision can be created and the pit excised. This method is effective for most primary pilonidal sinuses. In general, extensive resection should be avoided. Complex and/or recurrent sinus tracts may require more extensive resection and closure with a Z-plasty, advancement flap, or rotational flap.

Hidradenitis Suppurativa

Hidradenitis suppurativa is an infection of the cutaneous apocrine sweat glands. Infected glands rupture and form subcutaneous sinus tracts. The infection may mimic complex anal fistula disease, but stops at the anal verge because there are no apocrine glands in the anal canal. Treatment involves incision and drainage of acute abscesses and unroofing of all chronically inflamed fistulas and débridement of granulation tissue. Radical excision and skin grafting is almost never necessary.

TRAUMA

Penetrating Colorectal Injury

Colorectal injury is common following penetrating trauma to the abdomen and has historically been associated with high mortality. In the first half of the twentieth century, the mortality rate from colorectal injury was as high as 90%. The introduction of exteriorization of colonic injuries and fecal diversion during World War II dramatically decreased mortality, and this principle has governed the management of large-bowel injury for over 50 years. Recently, however, this practice was challenged and trauma surgeons are increasingly performing primary repairs in selected patients.

Management of colonic injury depends upon the mechanism of injury, the delay between the injury and surgery, the overall condition and stability of the patient, the degree of peritoneal contamination, and the condition of the injured colon. A primary repair may be considered in hemodynamically stable patients with few additional injuries and minimal contamination if the colon appears otherwise healthy. Contraindications to primary repair include shock, injury to more than two other organs, mesenteric vascular damage, and extensive fecal contamination. A delay of greater than 6 hours between the injury and the operation also is associated with increased morbidity and mortality and is a relative contraindication to primary repair. Injuries caused by high-velocity gunshot wounds or blast injuries often are associated with multiple intra-abdominal injuries and tissue loss and therefore usually are treated by fecal diversion after débridement of all nonviable tissue. Patient factors, such as medical comorbidities, advanced age, and the presence of tumor or radiation injury, must also be considered (Table 29-6).

Like injuries to the intraperitoneal colon, penetrating trauma to the rectum traditionally has been associated with high morbidity and mortality. Primary repair of the rectum is more difficult than primary repair of the colon, however, and most rectal injuries are associated with significant contamination. For that reason, the majority of penetrating rectal injuries should be treated with proximal fecal diversion and copious irrigation of the rectum (distal rectal washout). If there is extensive fecal contamination, presacral drains may be useful. Small, clean rectal injuries may be closed primarily without fecal diversion in an otherwise stable patient. Intractable rectal bleeding may require angiographic embolization. Very rarely, hemorrhage or extensive tissue loss (especially if the anal sphincter is severely damaged) may require an emergent abdominoperineal resection. However, this operation should be

TABLE 29-6	Criteria for use of an ostomy

Injuring agent factors
  High-velocity bullet wounds
  Shotgun wounds
  Explosive blast wounds
  Crush injury
Patient factors
  Presence of tumor
  Radiated tissue
  Medical condition
  Advanced age
Injury factors
  Inflamed tissue
  Advanced infection
  Distal obstruction
  Local foreign body
  Impaired blood supply
  Mesenteric vascular damage
  Shock with blood pressure <80/60 mmHg
  Hemorrhage >1000 mL
  More than two organs (especially kidney) injured
  Interval to operation >6 h (pancreatic, splenic, hepatic)
  Extensive injury requiring resection
  Major abdominal wall loss
  Thoracoabdominal penetration

Source: Reproduced with permission from Gordon PH, Nivatvongs S (eds): *Principles and Practice of Surgery for the Colon, Rectum, and Anus*, 2nd ed. New York: Marcel Dekker, Inc., 1999, p 1249.

avoided, if at all possible, because of the morbidity associated with an extensive pelvic dissection in a severely injured patient.

Blunt Colorectal Injury

Blunt injury to the colon and rectum is considerably less common than penetrating injury. Nevertheless, blunt trauma can cause colon perforation, and shear injury to the mesentery can devascularize the intestine. Management of these injuries should follow the same principles outlined for management of penetrating injuries. Small perforations with little contamination in a stable patient may be closed primarily; more extensive injury requires fecal diversion. A serosal hematoma alone does not mandate resection, but the bowel should be carefully inspected to ensure that there is not an associated perforation or significant bowel ischemia.

Blunt injury to the rectum may result from significant trauma, such as a pelvic crush injury, or may result from local trauma caused by an enema or foreign body. Crush injuries, especially with an associated pelvic fracture, often are associated with significant rectal damage and contamination. These patients require débridement of all nonviable tissue, proximal fecal diversion, and a distal rectal washout, with or without drain placement. Blunt trauma from an enema or foreign body may produce a mucosal hematoma, which requires no surgical treatment if the mucosa is intact. Small mucosal tears may be closed primarily if the bowel is relatively clean and there is little contamination.

Iatrogenic Injury
Intraoperative Injury

The colon and rectum are at risk for inadvertent injury during other procedures, especially during pelvic operations. The key to managing these injuries is *early recognition*. The vast majority of iatrogenic colorectal injuries may be closed primarily if there is little contamination and if the patient is otherwise stable. Delayed recognition of colorectal injuries may result in significant peritonitis and life-threatening sepsis. In these cases, fecal diversion almost always is required and the patient may need repeated exploration for drainage of abscesses.

Injury from Barium Enema

Colorectal injury from a barium enema is an extremely rare complication associated with a high rate of morbidity and mortality. Perforation with spillage of barium, especially above the peritoneal reflection, may result in profound peritonitis, sepsis, and a systemic inflammatory response. If the perforation is recognized early, it may be closed primarily and the abdomen irrigated to remove stool and barium. However, if the patient has developed sepsis, fecal diversion (with or without bowel resection) is almost always required. Rarely, a small mucosal injury to the extraperitoneal rectum may be managed with bowel rest, broad-spectrum antibiotics, and close observation.

Colonoscopic Perforation

Perforation is the most common major complication after either diagnostic or therapeutic colonoscopy. Fortunately, this complication is rare and occurs in less than 1% of procedures. Perforation may result from trauma from the tip of the instrument, from shear forces related to the formation of a "loop" in the colonoscope, or from barotrauma from insufflation. Biopsy or fulguration also can cause perforation. Polypectomy using electrocautery may produce a full-thickness burn, resulting in *postpolypectomy syndrome*, in which a patient develops abdominal pain, fever, and leukocytosis without evidence of diffuse peritonitis.

Management of colonoscopic perforation depends on the *size of the perforation*, the *duration of time* since the injury, and the *overall condition of the patient*. A large perforation recognized during the procedure requires surgical exploration. Because the bowel almost always has been prepared before the colonoscopy, there is usually little contamination associated with these injuries and most can be repaired primarily. If there is significant contamination, if there has been a delay in diagnosis with resulting peritonitis, or if the patient is hemodynamically unstable, proximal diversion with or without resection is the safest approach. Occasionally, a patient will develop abdominal pain and localized signs of perforation after what was thought to be an uneventful colonoscopy. Many of these patients will have a "microperforation" that will resolve with bowel rest, broad-spectrum antibiotics, and close observation. Evidence of peritonitis or any deterioration in clinical condition mandates exploration. Similarly, free retroperitoneal or intraperitoneal air may be discovered incidentally after colonoscopy. In a completely asymptomatic patient, this finding is thought to result from barotrauma and dissection of air through tissue planes without a free perforation. Many of these patients can be successfully treated with bowel rest and broad-spectrum antibiotics. Surgical exploration is indicated for any clinical deterioration.

Anal Sphincter Injury and Incontinence

The most common cause of anal sphincter injury is obstetric trauma during vaginal delivery. The risk of sphincter injury is increased by a laceration that extends into the rectum (fourth-degree tear), infection of an episiotomy or laceration repair, prolonged labor, and possibly by use of a midline episiotomy. Sphincter damage also may result from hemorrhoidectomy, sphincterotomy, abscess drainage, or fistulotomy. Patients with incontinence and a suspected sphincter injury can be evaluated with anal manometry, EMG, and endoanal ultrasound. Mild incontinence, even in the presence of a sphincter defect, may respond to dietary changes and/or biofeedback. More severe incontinence may require surgical repair.

The anal sphincter also can be injured by penetrating or blunt mechanisms (impalement, blast injury, crush injuries of the pelvis). Because damage to the anal sphincter is not life threatening, definitive repair of the sphincter is often deferred until other injuries have been repaired and the patient's clinical condition is stable. Isolated sphincter injuries that do not involve the rectum may be repaired primarily. Rectal injury accompanied by sphincter injury should be treated with fecal diversion, distal rectal washout, and drain placement. Significant perineal tissue loss may require extensive débridement and a diverting colostomy.

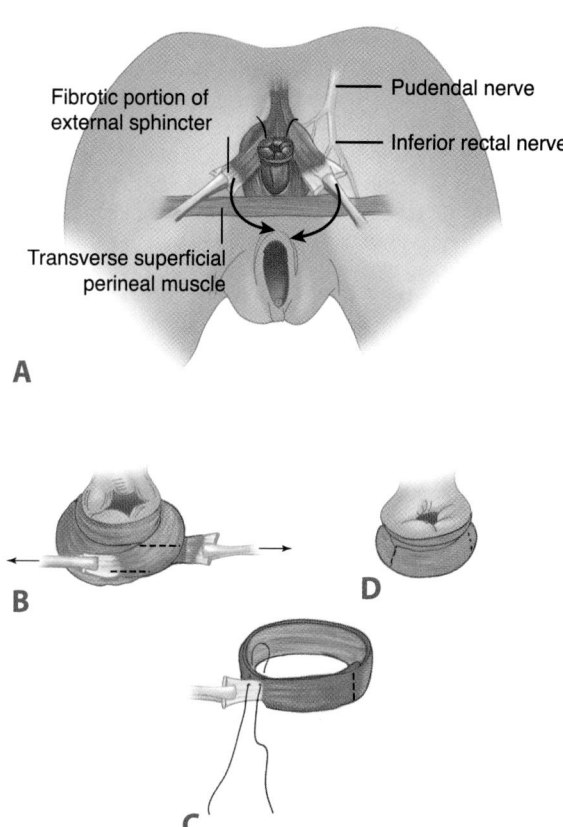

FIG. 29-42. Overlapping sphincteroplasty for incontinence from sphincter disruption. **A.** The external sphincter muscle with scar at site of injury is mobilized. **B.** The muscle edges are aligned in an overlapping fashion. **C.** Mattress sutures are used to approximate the muscle. **D.** The completed operation.

Surgical Repairs

The most common method of repair of the anal sphincter is a *wrap-around sphincteroplasty* (Fig. 29-42).[96] The procedure involves mobilization of the divided sphincter muscle and reapproximation without tension. The internal and external sphincters may be overlapped together or separately. *Postanal intersphincteric levatorplasty* is less commonly used to repair sphincter defects but may be useful for incontinence caused by prolapse and/or loss of the anorectal angle (see Continence above). The approach is via the intersphincteric plane posteriorly. It may be performed concomitantly with a perineal repair of rectal prolapse. The levator ani muscle is approximated to restore the anorectal angle and the puborectalis and external sphincter muscle are tightened with sutures. These elective procedures usually do not require a diverting colostomy.

In cases where there has been significant loss of sphincter muscle, or in which prior repairs have failed, more complex techniques, such as *gracilis muscle transposition* with or without chronic, low-frequency electrostimulation, have been used with some success.[97] In this procedure, the gracilis muscle is mobilized from the thigh, detached from its insertion on the tibial tuberosity, tunneled through the perineum, and wrapped around the anal canal. Another alternative in patients who have failed other repairs is the *artificial anal sphincter*. This device consists of an inflatable silastic cuff, a pressure-regulating balloon, and a control pump. Patients deflate the cuff manually to open the anal canal; the cuff then reinflates spontaneously to maintain closure of the anal canal. *Sacral nerve stimulation* via an implanted pulse generator is a new technique used for neurogenic incontinence when the sphincter is intact.[12,13] In some patients, an end stoma provides the best relief for intractable incontinence.[98]

Foreign Body

Foreign-body entrapment in the rectum is not uncommon. Depending upon the level of entrapment, a foreign body may cause damage to the rectum, rectosigmoid, or descending colon. Generalized abdominal pain suggests intraperitoneal perforation. Evaluation of the patient includes inspection of the perineum and a careful abdominal examination to detect any evidence of perforation. Plain films of the abdomen are mandatory to detect free intra-abdominal air.

Foreign bodies lodged low in the rectum may often be removed under conscious sedation with or without a local anesthetic block. Objects impacted higher in the rectum may require regional or general anesthesia for removal. Only rarely will a laparotomy be required to remove the object. After removal of the foreign body, it is crucial to evaluate the rectum and sigmoid colon for injury. Proctoscopy and/or flexible sigmoidoscopy should be performed. A hematoma without evidence of perforation requires no surgical treatment. Perforation of the rectum or sigmoid colon should be managed as described in the preceding section, Penetrating Colorectal Injury.

THE IMMUNOCOMPROMISED PATIENT

Human Immunodeficiency Virus

Patients infected with HIV may present with a myriad of GI symptoms. Diarrhea, in particular, is extremely common. The severity of GI disease depends, in part, upon the degree of immunosuppression; however, both ordinary and opportunistic pathogens may affect patients at any stage of the disease. Opportunistic infections with bacteria (*Salmonella, Shigella, Campylobacter, Chlamydia, and Mycobacterium species*), fungi (*Histoplasmosis, Coccidiosis, Cryptococcus*), protozoa (*Toxoplasmosis, Cryptosporidiosis, Isosporiasis*), and viruses (*CMV, herpes simplex virus*) can cause diarrhea, abdominal pain, and weight loss. CMV in particular may cause severe enterocolitis and is the most common infectious cause of emergency laparotomy in AIDS patients. *C. difficile* colitis is a major concern in these patients, especially because many patients are maintained on suppressive antibiotic therapy. The incidence of GI malignancy also is increased in patients with HIV infection.[99] Kaposi's sarcoma is the most common malignancy in AIDS patients and can affect any part of the GI tract. Patients may be asymptomatic or may develop bleeding or obstruction. GI lymphoma (usually non-Hodgkin's lymphoma) also is common. The incidence of colorectal carcinoma also may be increased in this population, although definitive data are lacking.

Perianal disease is extremely common in patients with HIV infection. Because HIV is sexually transmitted, it is common to find concomitant infection with other sexually transmitted diseases such as *Chlamydia, herpes simplex virus*, and *HPV (anal condyloma). Anal condyloma* in particular is very common and the incidence of dysplasia (AIN, HSIL) is high in the HIV-infected population.[100] Abscesses and fistulas may be more difficult to diagnose in these patients and may be complex. Many patients require an examination under anesthesia with biopsy and cultures to determine the etiology of many of these perianal problems. The introduction of highly active antiretroviral therapy has changed the natural history of HIV infection, but it remains to be seen how these medications will affect the incidence and outcome of colorectal disease in this patient population.

IMMUNOSUPPRESSION FOR TRANSPLANTATION

The GI tract is a common site for posttransplantation complications that are responsible for significant morbidity and mortality. In these patients, infection and medication are the most common causes of diarrhea. Immunosuppressant medications, in particular, may cause diarrhea. CMV infection is common and may be severe. *C. difficile* colitis also occurs commonly. Diverticulitis appears to be more common in some populations of transplant patients and may be more likely to present with abscess or free perforation. Elective resection after recovery from one episode of confirmed diverticulitis may be indicated in the transplant population. Graft-versus-host disease is unique to transplant patients and often requires endoscopy and biopsy to diagnose GI involvement. Patients are subject to the same opportunistic infections outlined above in Human Immunodeficiency Virus; however, sexually transmitted infections and Kaposi's sarcoma are somewhat less prevalent. Perianal disease is somewhat less common in the transplant population than in patients infected with HIV; however, similar infections may occur and immunosuppression often makes diagnosis challenging.

With increasing long-term survival among transplant recipients, the development of posttransplant malignancy has become a major concern. Posttransplant lymphoproliferative disease is increasingly common and may occur anywhere in the GI tract. The risk of colorectal carcinoma is increased in patients with predisposing conditions such as ulcerative colitis. However, immunosuppression alone does not appear to increase the incidence of colorectal cancer, and current screening recommendations are similar to those for the average risk population. In contrast, the incidence of anal squamous cell carcinoma is dramatically increased in transplant patients and patients with known HPV infection should undergo more vigorous screening.

THE NEUTROPENIC PATIENT

Neutropenic enterocolitis (typhlitis) is a life-threatening problem with a mortality rate of greater than 50%. This syndrome is characterized by abdominal pain and distention, fever, diarrhea (often bloody), nausea, and vomiting in a patient with fewer than 1000 neutrophils from any cause (bone marrow transplantation, solid organ transplantation, or chemotherapy). CT scan of the abdomen often shows a dilated cecum with pericolic stranding. However, a normal-appearing CT scan does not exclude the diagnosis. Some patients will respond to bowel rest, broad-spectrum antibiotics, parenteral nutrition, and granulocyte infusion or colony-stimulating factors. Evidence of perforation, generalized peritonitis, or deterioration in clinical condition is an indication for operation.

Neutropenic patients often develop perianal pain, and diagnosis may be difficult because of a lack of inflammatory response to infection. Although broad-spectrum antibiotics may cure some of these patients, an examination under anesthesia should not be delayed because of neutropenia. An increase in pain or fever, and/or clinical deterioration mandates an examination under anesthesia. Any indurated area should be incised and drained, biopsied to exclude a leukemic infiltrate, and cultured to aid in the selection of antimicrobial agents.

REFERENCES

Entries highlighted in bright blue are key references.

1. Tran K: Capsule colonoscopy: PillCam Colon. *Issues Emerg Health Technol* 106:1, 2007.
2. de Franchis R, Rondonotti E, Villa F: Capsule endoscopy—state of the art. *Dig Dis* 25:249, 2007.
3. Fireman Z, Kopelman Y: The colon—the latest terrain for capsule endoscopy. *Dig Liver Dis* 39:10, 2007.
4. Smith RA, von Eschenbach AC, Wender R, et al: American Cancer Society guidelines for the early detection of cancer: Update of early detection guidelines for prostate, colorectal, and endometrial cancers. Also: Update 2001—testing for early lung cancer detection. *CA Cancer J Clin* 51:38, 2001; quiz 77.
5. Garcia-Aguilar J, Pollack J, Lee SH, et al: Accuracy of endorectal ultrasonography in preoperative staging of rectal tumors. *Dis Colon Rectum* 45:10, 2002.
6. Turgeon DK, Novicki TJ, Quick J, et al: Six rapid tests for direct detection of *Clostridium difficile* and its toxins in fecal samples compared with the fibroblast cytotoxicity assay. *J Clin Microbiol* 41:667, 2003.
7. Qiu H, Sirivongs P, Rothenberger M, et al: Molecular prognostic factors in rectal cancer treated by radiation and surgery. *Dis Colon Rectum* 43:451, 2000.

8. Offit K: Genetic prognostic markers for colorectal cancer. *N Engl J Med* 342:124, 2000.

9. Lynch HT, Lynch JF, Lynch PM, et al: Hereditary colorectal cancer syndromes: Molecular genetics, genetic counseling, diagnosis and management. *Fam Cancer* 7:27, 2008.

10. Dailianas A, Skandalis N, Rimikis MN, et al: Pelvic floor study in patients with obstructive defecation: Influence of biofeedback. *J Clin Gastroenterol* 30:176, 2000.

11. FitzHarris GP, Garcia-Aguilar J, Parker SC, et al: Quality of life after subtotal colectomy for slow-transit constipation: Both quality and quantity count. *Dis Colon Rectum* 46:433, 2003.

12. Ganio E, Ratto C, Masin A, et al: Neuromodulation for fecal incontinence: Outcome in 16 patients with definitive implant. The initial Italian Sacral Neurostimulation Group (GINS) experience. *Dis Colon Rectum* 44:965, 2001.

13. Vaizey CJ, Kamm MA, Roy AJ, et al: Double-blind crossover study of sacral nerve stimulation for fecal incontinence. *Dis Colon Rectum* 43:298, 2000.

14. Takahashi T, Garcia-Osogobio S, Valdovinos MA, et al: Radio-frequency energy delivery to the anal canal for the treatment of fecal incontinence. *Dis Colon Rectum* 45:915, 2002.

15. Tjandra JJ, Dykes SL, Kumar RR, et al: Practice parameters for the treatment of fecal incontinence. *Dis Colon Rectum* 50:1497, 2007.

16. Weeks JC, Nelson H, Gelber S, et al: Short-term quality-of-life outcomes following laparoscopic-assisted colectomy vs open colectomy for colon cancer: A randomized trial. *JAMA* 287:321, 2002.

17. D'Annibale A, Morpurgo E, Fiscon V, et al: Robotic and laparoscopic surgery for treatment of colorectal diseases. *Dis Colon Rectum* 47:2162, 2004.

18. Regimbeau JM, Panis Y, Pocard M, et al: Handsewn ileal pouch-anal anastomosis on the dentate line after total proctectomy: Technique to avoid incomplete mucosectomy and the need for long-term follow-up of the anal transition zone. *Dis Colon Rectum* 44:43, 2001; discussion 50.

19. O'Riordain MG, Fazio VW, Lavery IC, et al: Incidence and natural history of dysplasia of the anal transitional zone after ileal pouch-anal anastomosis: Results of a five-year to ten-year follow-up. *Dis Colon Rectum* 43:1660, 2000.

20. Heuschen UA, Hinz U, Allemeyer EH, et al: One- or two-stage procedure for restorative proctocolectomy: Rationale for a surgical strategy in ulcerative colitis. *Ann Surg* 234:788, 2001.

21. Heah SM, Seow-Choen F, Eu KW, et al: Prospective, randomized trial comparing sigmoid vs. descending colonic J-pouch after total rectal excision. *Dis Colon Rectum* 45:322, 2002.

22. Farouk R, Pemberton JH, Wolff BG, et al: Functional outcomes after ileal pouch-anal anastomosis for chronic ulcerative colitis. *Ann Surg* 231:919, 2000.

23. Bullard KM, Madoff RD, Gemlo BT: Is ileoanal pouch function stable with time? Results of a prospective audit. *Dis Colon Rectum* 45:299, 2002.

24. Sandborn W, McLeod R, Jewell D: Pharmacotherapy for inducing and maintaining remission in pouchitis. *Cochrane Database Syst Rev* 2000:2, CD001176.

25. Stocchi L, Pemberton JH: Pouch and pouchitis. *Gastroenterol Clin North Am* 30:223, 2001.

26. Zmora O, Pikarsky AJ, Wexner SD: Bowel preparation for colorectal surgery. *Dis Colon Rectum* 2001:44, 1537.

27. Balaban DH, Leavell BS Jr, Oblinger MJ, et al: Low volume bowel preparation for colonoscopy: Randomized, endoscopist-blinded trial of liquid sodium phosphate versus tablet sodium phosphate. *Am J Gastroenterol* 98:827, 2003.

28. Solla JA, Rothenberger DA: Preoperative bowel preparation. A survey of colon and rectal surgeons. *Dis Colon Rectum* 33:154, 1990.

29. Nichols RL, Smith JW, Garcia RY, et al: Current practices of preoperative bowel preparation among North American colorectal surgeons. *Clin Infect Dis* 24:609, 1997.

30. Fa-Si-Oen P, Roumen R, Buitenweg J, et al: Mechanical bowel preparation or not? Outcome of a multicenter, randomized trial in elective open colon surgery. *Dis Colon Rectum* 48:1509, 2005.

31. Jansen JO, O'Kelly TJ, Krukowski ZH, et al: Right hemicolectomy: Mechanical bowel preparation is not required. *J R Coll Surg Edinb* 47:557, 2002.

32. Miettinen RP, Laitinen ST, Makela JT, et al: Bowel preparation with oral polyethylene glycol electrolyte solution vs. no preparation in elective open colorectal surgery: Prospective, randomized study. *Dis Colon Rectum* 43:669, 2000; discussion 675.

33. Bonen DK, Cho JH: The genetics of inflammatory bowel disease. *Gastroenterology* 124:521, 2003.

34. Yamamoto-Furusho JK: Genetic factors associated with the development of inflammatory bowel disease. *World J Gastroenterol* 13:5594, 2007.

35. Alfadhli AA, McDonald JW, Feagan BG: Methotrexate for induction of remission in refractory Crohn's disease. *Cochrane Database Syst Rev* 1:CD003459, 2003.

36. Hanauer SB, Feagan BG, Lichtenstein GR, et al: Maintenance infliximab for Crohn's disease: The ACCENT I randomised trial. *Lancet* 359:1541, 2002.

37. Actis GC, Bruno M, Pinna-Pintor M, et al: Infliximab for treatment of steroid-refractory ulcerative colitis. *Dig Liver Dis* 34:631, 2002.

38. Su C, Salzberg BA, Lewis JD, et al: Efficacy of anti-tumor necrosis factor therapy in patients with ulcerative colitis. *Am J Gastroenterol* 97:2577, 2002.

39. Matsumoto T, Iwao Y, Igarashi M, et al: Endoscopic and chromoendoscopic atlas featuring dysplastic lesions in surveillance colonoscopy for patients with long-standing ulcerative colitis. *Inflamm Bowel Dis* 2008:14, 259.

40. Kiesslich R, Neurath MF: Magnifying chromoendoscopy: Effective diagnostic tool for screening colonoscopy. *J Gastroenterol Hepatol* 22:1700, 2007.

41. Wong Kee Song LM, Adler DG, Chand B, et al: Chromoendoscopy. *Gastrointest Endosc* 66:639, 2007.

42. Bamias G, Cominelli F: Novel strategies to attenuate immune activation in Crohn's disease. *Curr Opin Pharmacol* 6:401, 2006.

43. Bernini A, Spencer MP, Wong WD, et al: Computed tomography-guided percutaneous abscess drainage in intestinal disease: Factors associated with outcome. *Dis Colon Rectum* 40:1009, 1997.

44. Wong WD, Wexner SD, Lowry A, et al: Practice parameters for the treatment of sigmoid diverticulitis—supporting documentation. The Standards Task Force. The American Society of Colon and Rectal Surgeons. *Dis Colon Rectum* 43:290, 2000.

45. Schilling MK, Maurer CA, Kollmar O, et al: Primary vs. secondary anastomosis after sigmoid colon resection for perforated diverticulitis (Hinchey Stage III and IV): A prospective outcome and cost analysis. *Dis Colon Rectum* 44:699, 2001; discussion 703.

46. http://www.cancer.org/downloads/STT/CAFF2007PWSecured.pdf: Cancer Facts & Figures 2007, American Cancer Society [accessed Jan. 5, 2009].

47. Janne PA, Mayer RJ: Chemoprevention of colorectal cancer. *N Engl J Med* 2000:342, 1960.

48. Calle EE, Rodriguez C, Walker-Thurmond K, et al: Overweight, obesity, and mortality from cancer in a prospectively studied cohort of U.S. adults. *N Engl J Med* 348:1625, 2003.

49. Eaden JA, Abrams KR, Mayberry JF: The risk of colorectal cancer in ulcerative colitis: A meta-analysis. *Gut* 48:526. 2001.

50. Woodhouse CR: Guidelines for monitoring of patients with ureterosigmoidostomy. *Gut* 51:V15, 2002.

51. Al-Tassan N, Chmiel NH, Maynard J, et al: Inherited variants of MYH associated with somatic G:C-->T:A mutations in colorectal tumors. *Nat Genet* 30:227, 2002.

52. Lefevre JH, Rodrigue CM, Mourra N, et al: Implication of MYH in colorectal polyposis. *Ann Surg* 244:874, 2006; discussion 879.

53. Martin M, Simon-Assmann P, Kedinger M, et al: DCC regulates cell adhesion in human colon cancer derived HT-29 cells and associates with ezrin. *Eur J Cell Biol* 85:769, 2006.

54. Bulow C, Vasen H, Jarvinen H, et al: Ileorectal anastomosis is appropriate for a subset of patients with familial adenomatous polyposis. *Gastroenterology* 119:1454, 2000.

55. Steinbach G, Lynch PM, Phillips RK, et al: The effect of celecoxib, a cyclooxygenase-2 inhibitor, in familial adenomatous polyposis. *N Engl J Med* 342:1946, 2000.

56. Hampel H, Frankel WL, Martin E, et al: Screening for the Lynch syndrome (hereditary nonpolyposis colorectal cancer). *N Engl J Med* 352:1851, 2005.

57. Jarvinen HJ, Aarnio M, Mustonen H, et al: Controlled 15-year trial on screening for colorectal cancer in families with hereditary nonpolyposis colorectal cancer. *Gastroenterology* 118:829, 2000.

58. Pignone M, Rich M, Teutsch SM, et al: Screening for colorectal cancer in adults at average risk: A summary of the evidence for the U.S. Preventive Services Task Force. *Ann Intern Med* 137:132, 2002.

59. Imperiale TF, Wagner DR, Lin CY, et al: Risk of advanced proximal neoplasms in asymptomatic adults according to the distal colorectal findings. *N Engl J Med* 343:169, 2000.

60. Lieberman DA, Weiss DG, Bond JH, et al: Use of colonoscopy to screen asymptomatic adults for colorectal cancer. Veterans Affairs Cooperative Study Group 380. *N Engl J Med* 343:162, 2000.

61. Levin B, Brooks D, Smith RA, et al: Emerging technologies in screening for colorectal cancer: CT colonography, immunochemical fecal occult blood tests, and stool screening using molecular markers. *CA Cancer J Clin* 53:44, 2003.

62. Mandel JS, Church TR, Bond JH, et al: The effect of fecal occult-blood screening on the incidence of colorectal cancer. *N Engl J Med* 343:1603, 2000.

63. Hardcastle JD, Armitage NC, Chamberlain J, et al: Fecal occult blood screening for colorectal cancer in the general population. Results of a controlled trial. *Cancer* 58:397, 1986.

64. Winawer SJ, Flehinger BJ, Schottenfeld D, et al: Screening for colorectal cancer with fecal occult blood testing and sigmoidoscopy. *J Natl Cancer Inst* 85:1311, 1993.

65. Yee J, Akerkar GA, Hung RK, et al: Colorectal neoplasia: Performance characteristics of CT colonography for detection in 300 patients. *Radiology* 219:685, 2001.

66. Greene FL PD, Fleming ID, Fritz A, et al: *AJCC Cancer Staging Manual*, 6th ed. New York: Springer, 2002.

67. Gunderson LL, Sargent DJ, Tepper JE, et al: Impact of T and N substage on survival and disease relapse in adjuvant rectal cancer: A pooled analysis. *Int J Radiat Oncol Biol Phys* 54:386, 2002.

68. Chang GJ, Rodriguez-Bigas MA, Skibber JM, et al: Lymph node evaluation and survival after curative resection of colon cancer: Systematic review. *J Natl Cancer Inst* 99:433, 2007.

69. http://www.qualityforum.org/pdf/cancer/txAppA-Specifications_web.pdf: Specifications of the National Voluntary Consensus Standards for Quality of Cancer Care, National Quality Forum [accessed Feb. 20, 2008].

70. Wong SL, Ji H, Hollenbeck BK, et al: Hospital lymph node examination rates and survival after resection for colon cancer. *JAMA* 298:2149, 2007.

71. Johnson PM, Porter GA, Ricciardi R, et al: Increasing negative lymph node count is independently associated with improved long-term survival in stage IIIB and IIIC colon cancer. *J Clin Oncol* 24:3570, 2006.

72. Ricciardi R, Madoff RD, Rothenberger DA, et al: Population-based analyses of lymph node metastases in colorectal cancer. *Clin Gastroenterol Hepatol* 4:1522, 2006.

73. Ricciardi R, Baxter NN: Association versus causation versus quality improvement: Setting benchmarks for lymph node evaluation in colon cancer. *J Natl Cancer Inst* 99:414, 2007.

74. Demmy TL, Dunn KB: Surgical and nonsurgical therapy for lung metastasis: Indications and outcomes. *Surg Oncol Clin N Am* 16:579, 2007.

75. Sauer R, Becker H, Hohenberger W, et al: Preoperative versus postoperative chemoradiation for rectal cancer. *N Engl J Med* 351:1731, 2004.

76. Berends FJ, Kazemier G, Bonjer HJ, et al: Subcutaneous metastases after laparoscopic colectomy. *Lancet* 344:58, 1994.

77. A comparison of laparoscopically assisted and open colectomy for colon cancer. *N Engl J Med* 350:2050, 2004.

78. Hazebroek EJ: COLOR: A randomized clinical trial comparing laparoscopic and open resection for colon cancer. *Surg Endosc* 16:949, 2002.

79. Jayne DG, Guillou PJ, Thorpe H, et al: Randomized trial of laparoscopic-assisted resection of colorectal carcinoma: 3-year results of the UK MRC CLASICC Trial Group. *J Clin Oncol* 25:3061, 2007.

80. Hobson KG, Ghaemmaghami V, Roe JP, et al: Tumors of the retrorectal space. *Dis Colon Rectum* 48:1964, 2005.

81. Berry JM, Palefsky JM, Welton M: Anal cancer and its precursors in HIV-positive patients: Perspectives and management. *Surg Oncol Clin N Amer* 13:355, 2004.

82. Wieland U, Brockmeyer NH, Weissenborn SJ, et al: Imiquimod treatment of anal intraepithelial neoplasia in HIV-positive men. *Arch Dermatol* 142:1438, 2006.

83. Bullard KM, Tuttle TM, Rothenberger DA, et al: Surgical therapy for anorectal melanoma. *J Am Coll Surg* 196:206, 2003.

84. Yeh JJ, Shia J, Hwu WJ, et al: The role of abdominoperineal resection as surgical therapy for anorectal melanoma. *Ann Surg* 244:1012, 2006.

85. Bullard K, Madoff R: *Rectal Prolapse and Intussusception*. New York: Marcel Dekker, 2003.

86. Torres C, Khaikin M, Bracho J, et al: Solitary rectal ulcer syndrome: Clinical findings, surgical treatment, and outcomes. *Int J Colorectal Dis* 22:11, 2007.

87. Tjandra JJ, Chan MK: Systematic review on the procedure for prolapse and hemorrhoids (stapled hemorrhoidopexy). *Dis Colon Rectum* 50:878, 2007.

88. Wong JC, Chung CC, Yau KK, et al: Stapled technique for acute thrombosed hemorrhoids: A randomized, controlled trial with long-term results. *Dis Colon Rectum* 51:397, 2008.

89. Madoff RD, Fleshman JW: AGA technical review on the diagnosis and care of patients with anal fissure. *Gastroenterology* 124:235, 2003.

90. Nelson R: Non surgical therapy for anal fissure. *Cochrane Database Syst Rev*, 4:CD003431, 2006.

91. North JH Jr, Weber TK, Rodriguez-Bigas MA, et al: The management of infectious and noninfectious anorectal complications in patients with leukemia. *J Am Coll Surg* 183:322, 1996.

92. Wexner SD: Sexually transmitted diseases of the colon, rectum, and anus. The challenge of the nineties. *Dis Colon Rectum* 33:1048, 1990.

93. Smith L: Sexually transmitted diseases, in Gordon P, Nivatvongs S, (eds): *Principles and Practice of Surgery for the Colon, Rectum, and Anus*. St. Louis: Quality Medical Publishing, 1999, p 341.

94. Stanley MA: Imiquimod and the imidazoquinolones: Mechanism of action and therapeutic potential. *Clin Exp Dermatol* 27:571, 2002.

95. Gunter J: Genital and perianal warts: New treatment opportunities for human papillomavirus infection. *Am J Obstet Gynecol* 189:S3, 2003.

96. Buie WD, Lowry AC, Rothenberger DA, et al: Clinical rather than laboratory assessment predicts continence after anterior sphincteroplasty. *Dis Colon Rectum* 44:1255, 2001.

97. Baeten CG, Bailey HR, Bakka A, et al: Safety and efficacy of dynamic graciloplasty for fecal incontinence: Report of a prospective, multicenter trial. Dynamic Graciloplasty Therapy Study Group. *Dis Colon Rectum* 43:743, 2000.

98. Tan EK, Vaizey C, Cornish J, et al: Surgical strategies for faecal incontinence—a decision analysis between dynamic graciloplasty, artificial bowel sphincter and end stoma. *Colorectal Dis* 10:577, 2008.

99. Cooksley CD, Hwang LY, Waller DK, et al: HIV-related malignancies: Community-based study using linkage of cancer registry and HIV registry data. *Int J STD AIDS* 10:795, 1999.

100. Palefsky JM: Anal squamous intraepithelial lesions: Relation to HIV and human papillomavirus infection. *J Acquir Immune Defic Syndr* 21:S42, 1999.

The Appendix

Bernard M. Jaffe and David H. Berger

ANATOMY AND FUNCTION

The appendix first becomes visible in the eighth week of embryologic development as a protuberance off the terminal portion of the cecum. During both antenatal and postnatal development, the growth rate of the cecum exceeds that of the appendix, so that the appendix is displaced medially toward the ileocecal valve. The relationship of the base of the appendix to the cecum remains constant, whereas the tip can be found in a retrocecal, pelvic, subcecal, preileal, or right pericolic position (Fig. 30-1). These anatomic considerations have significant clinical importance in the context of acute appendicitis. The three taeniae coli converge at the junction of the cecum with the appendix and can be a useful landmark to identify the appendix. The appendix can vary in length from <1 cm to >30 cm; most appendices are 6 to 9 cm long. Appendiceal absence, duplication, and diverticula have all been described.[1-4]

For many years, the appendix was erroneously viewed as a vestigial organ with no known function. It is now well recognized that the appendix is an immunologic organ that actively participates in the secretion of immunoglobulins, particularly immunoglobulin A. Although there is no clear role for the appendix in the development of human disease, recent studies demonstrate a potential correlation between appendectomy and the development of inflammatory bowel disease. There appears to be a negative age-related association between prior appendectomy and subsequent development of ulcerative colitis. In addition, comparative analysis clearly shows that prior appendectomy is associated with a more benign phenotype in ulcerative colitis and a delay in onset of disease. The association between Crohn's disease and appendectomy is less clear. Although earlier studies suggested that appendectomy increases the risk of developing Crohn's disease, more recent studies that carefully assessed the timing of appendectomy in relation to the onset of

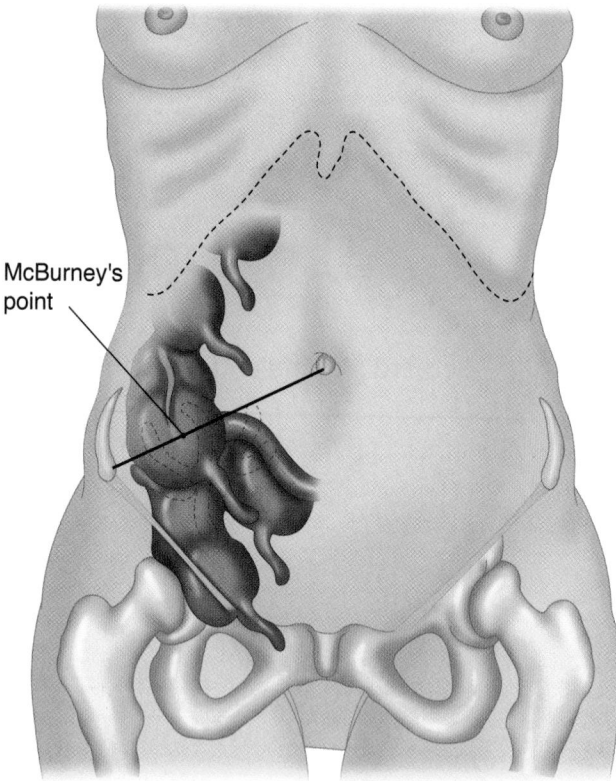

McBurney's point

FIG. 30-1. Various anatomic positions of the vermiform appendix.

Crohn's disease demonstrated a negative correlation. These data suggest that appendectomy may protect against the subsequent development of inflammatory bowel disease; however, the mechanism is unclear.[4]

Lymphoid tissue first appears in the appendix approximately 2 weeks after birth. The amount of lymphoid tissue increases throughout puberty, remains steady for the next decade, and then begins a steady decrease with age. After the age of 60 years, virtually no lymphoid tissue remains within the appendix, and complete obliteration of the appendiceal lumen is common.[1–4]

ACUTE APPENDICITIS

Historical Background

Although ancient texts have scattered descriptions of surgery being undertaken for ailments sounding like appendicitis, credit for performing the first appendectomy goes to Claudius Amyand, a surgeon at St. George's Hospital in London and Sergeant Surgeon to Queen Ann, King George I, and King George II. In 1736, he operated on an 11-year-old boy with a scrotal hernia and a fecal fistula. Within the hernial sac, Amyand found the appendix perforated by a pin. He successfully removed the appendix and repaired the hernia.[5]

The appendix was not identified as an organ capable of causing disease until the nineteenth century. In 1824, Louyer-Villermay presented a paper before the Royal Academy of Medicine in Paris. He reported on two autopsy cases of appendicitis and emphasized the importance of the condition. In 1827, François Melier, a French physician, expounded on Louyer-Villermay's work. He reported six autopsy cases and was the first to suggest the antemortem recognition of appendicitis.[5] This work was discounted by many physicians of the era, including Baron Guillaume Dupuytren. Dupuytren believed that inflammation of the cecum was the main cause of pathology of the right lower quadrant. The term *typhlitis* or *perityphlitis* was used to describe right lower quadrant inflammation. In 1839, a textbook authored by Bright and Addison entitled *Elements of Practical Medicine* described the symptoms of appendicitis and identified the primary cause of inflammatory processes of the right lower quadrant.[6] Reginald Fitz, a professor of pathologic anatomy at Harvard, is credited with coining the term *appendicitis*. His land-

KEY POINTS

1. Appendectomy for appendicitis is the most commonly performed emergency operation in the world.

2. Despite the increased use of ultrasonography, computed tomographic scanning, and laparoscopy, the rate of misdiagnosis of appendicitis has remained constant (15.3%), as has the rate of appendiceal rupture. The percentage of misdiagnosed cases of appendicitis is significantly higher among women than among men.

3. Appendicitis is a polymicrobial infection, with some series reporting up to 14 different organisms cultured in patients with perforation. The principal organisms seen in the normal appendix, in acute appendicitis, and in perforated appendicitis are *Escherichia coli* and *Bacteroides fragilis*.

4. Antibiotic prophylaxis is effective in the prevention of postoperative wound infection and intra-abdominal abscess. Antibiotic coverage is limited to 24 to 48 hours in cases of nonperforated appendicitis. For perforated appendicitis, 7 to 10 days of treatment is recommended.

5. Compared with younger patients, elderly patients with appendicitis often pose a more difficult diagnostic problem because of the atypical presentation, expanded differential diagnosis, and communication difficulty. These factors contribute to the disproportionately high perforation rate seen in the elderly.

6. The overall incidence of fetal loss after appendectomy is 4% and the risk of early delivery is 7%. Rates of fetal loss are considerably higher in women with complex appendicitis than in those with negative appendectomy and those with simple appendicitis. Removing a normal appendix is associated with a 4% risk of fetal loss and 10% risk of early delivery.

7. Recent data on appendiceal malignancies from the Surveillance, Epidemiology, and End Results program identified mucinous adenocarcinoma as the most frequent histologic diagnosis, followed by adenocarcinoma, carcinoid, goblet cell carcinoma, and signet-ring cell carcinoma.

mark paper definitively identified the appendix as the primary cause of right lower quadrant inflammation.[7]

Initial surgical therapy for appendicitis was primarily designed to drain right lower quadrant abscesses that occurred secondary to appendiceal perforation. It appears that the first surgical treatment for appendicitis or perityphlitis without abscess was carried out by Hancock in 1848. He incised the peritoneum and drained the right lower quadrant without removing the appendix. The first published account of appendectomy for appendicitis was by Krönlein in 1886. However, this patient died 2 days after operation. Fergus, in Canada, performed the first elective appendectomy in 1883.[5]

The greatest contributor to the advancement in the treatment of appendicitis was Charles McBurney. In 1889, he published his landmark paper in the *New York State Medical Journal* describing the indications for early laparotomy for the treatment of appendicitis. It is in this paper that he described the McBurney point as follows: "maximum tenderness, when one examines with the fingertips is, in adults, one half to two inches inside the right anterior spinous process of the ilium on a line drawn to the umbilicus."[8] McBurney subsequently published a paper in 1894 describing the incision that bears his name.[9] However, McBurney later credited McArthur with first describing this incision. Semm is widely credited with performing the first successful laparoscopic appendectomy in 1982.[10]

The surgical treatment of appendicitis is one of the great public health advances of the last 150 years. Appendectomy for appendicitis is the most commonly performed emergency operation in the world. Appendicitis is a disease of the young, with 40% of cases occurring in patients between the ages of 10 and 29 years.[11] In 1886, Fitz reported the associated mortality rate of appendicitis to be at least 67% without surgical therapy.[7] Currently, the mortality rate for acute appendicitis with treatment is reported to be <1%.[12]

Incidence

The lifetime rate of appendectomy is 12% for men and 25% for women, with approximately 7% of all people undergoing appendectomy for acute appendicitis during their lifetime. Over the 10-year period from 1987 to 1997, the overall appendectomy rate decreased in parallel with a decrease in incidental appendectomy.[11,13] However, the rate of appendectomy for appendicitis has remained constant at 10 per 10,000 patients per year.[14] Appendicitis is most frequently seen in patients in their second through fourth decades of life, with a mean age of 31.3 years and a median age of 22 years. There is a slight male:female predominance (1.2 to 1.3:1).[11,13]

Despite the increased use of ultrasonography, computed tomography (CT), and laparoscopy, the rate of misdiagnosis of appendicitis has remained constant (15.3%), as has the rate of appendiceal rupture. The percentage of misdiagnosed cases of appendicitis is significantly higher among women than among men (22.2 vs. 9.3%). The negative appendectomy rate for women of reproductive age is 23.2%, with the highest rates in women aged 40 to 49 years. The highest negative appendectomy rate is reported for women >80 years of age (Fig. 30-2).[13,14]

Etiology and Pathogenesis

Obstruction of the lumen is the dominant etiologic factor in acute appendicitis. Fecaliths are the most common cause of appendiceal obstruction. Less common causes are hypertrophy of lymphoid tissue, inspissated barium from previous x-ray studies, tumors, vegetable and fruit seeds, and intestinal parasites. The frequency of obstruction rises with the severity of the inflammatory process. Fecaliths are found in 40% of cases of simple acute appendicitis, in 65% of cases of gangrenous appendicitis without rupture, and in nearly 90% of cases of gangrenous appendicitis with rupture.

Traditionally the belief has been that there is a predictable sequence of events leading to eventual appendiceal rupture. The proximal obstruction of the appendiceal lumen produces a closed-loop obstruction, and continuing normal secretion by the appendiceal mucosa rapidly produces distention. The luminal capacity of the normal appendix is only 0.1 mL. Secretion of as little as 0.5 mL of fluid distal to an obstruction raises the intraluminal pressure to 60 cm H_2O. Distention of the appendix stimulates the nerve endings of visceral afferent stretch fibers, producing vague, dull, diffuse pain in the midabdomen or lower epigastrium. Peristalsis also is stimulated by the rather sudden distention, so that some cramping may be superimposed on the visceral pain early in the course of appendicitis. Distention increases from continued mucosal secretion and from rapid multiplication of the resident bacteria of the appendix. Distention of this magnitude usually causes reflex nausea and vomiting, and the diffuse visceral pain becomes more severe. As pressure in the organ increases, venous pressure is exceeded. Capillaries and venules are occluded, but arteriolar inflow continues, resulting in engorgement and vascular congestion. The inflammatory process soon involves the serosa of the appendix and in turn parietal peritoneum in the region, which produces the characteristic shift in pain to the right lower quadrant.

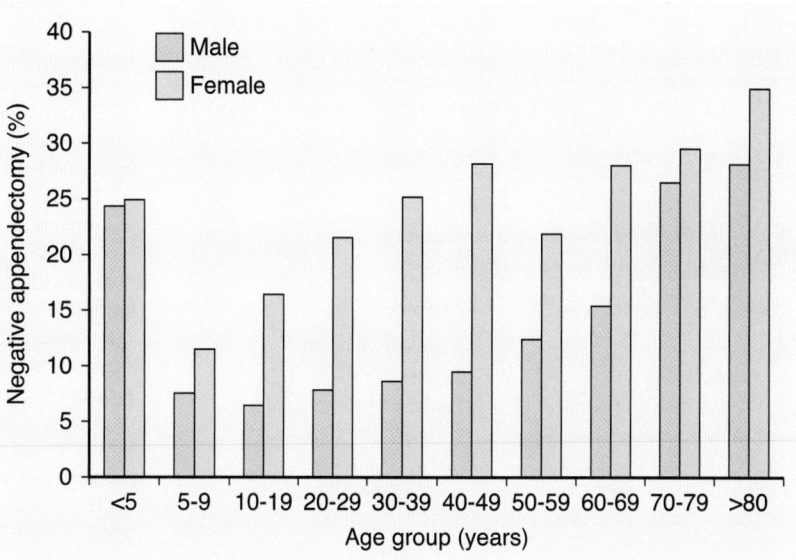

FIG. 30-2. Rate of negative appendectomy by age group. *(Adapted from Flum et al.[13,14])*

The mucosa of the GI tract, including the appendix, is susceptible to impairment of blood supply; thus its integrity is compromised early in the process, which allows bacterial invasion. As progressive distention encroaches on first the venous return and subsequently the arteriolar inflow, the area with the poorest blood supply suffers most: ellipsoidal infarcts develop in the antimesenteric border. As distention, bacterial invasion, compromise of vascular supply, and infarction progress, perforation occurs, usually through one of the infarcted areas on the antimesenteric border. Perforation generally occurs just beyond the point of obstruction rather than at the tip because of the effect of diameter on intraluminal tension.

This sequence is not inevitable, however, and some episodes of acute appendicitis apparently subside spontaneously. Many patients who are found at operation to have acute appendicitis give a history of previous similar, but less severe, attacks of right lower quadrant pain. Pathologic examination of the appendices removed from these patients often reveals thickening and scarring, suggesting old, healed acute inflammation.[15,16] The strong association between delay in presentation and appendiceal perforation supported the proposition that appendiceal perforation is the advanced stage of acute appendicitis; however, recent epidemiologic studies have suggested that nonperforated and perforated appendicitis may, in fact, be different diseases.[17]

Bacteriology

The bacterial population of the normal appendix is similar to that of the normal colon. The appendiceal flora remains constant throughout life with the exception of *Porphyromonas gingivalis*. This bacterium is seen only in adults.[18] The bacteria cultured in cases of appendicitis are therefore similar to those seen in other colonic infections such as diverticulitis. The principal organisms seen in the normal appendix, in acute appendicitis, and in perforated appendicitis are *Escherichia coli* and *Bacteroides fragilis*.[18–21] However, a wide variety of both facultative and anaerobic bacteria and mycobacteria may be present (Table 30-1). Appendicitis is a polymicrobial infection, with some series reporting the culture of up to 14 different organisms in patients with perforation.[18]

The routine culture of intraperitoneal samples in patients with either perforated or nonperforated appendicitis is questionable. As discussed earlier, the flora is known, and therefore broad-spectrum antibiotics are indicated. By the time culture results are available, the patient often has recovered from the illness. In addition, the number of organisms cultured and the ability of a specific laboratory to culture anaerobic organisms vary greatly. Peritoneal culture should be reserved for patients who are immunosuppressed, as a result of either illness or medication, and for patients who develop an abscess after the treatment of appendicitis.[20–22] Antibiotic prophylaxis is effective in the prevention of postoperative wound infection and intra-abdominal abscess.[23] Antibiotic coverage is limited to 24 to 48 hours in cases of nonperforated appendicitis. For perforated appendicitis, 7 to 10 days of therapy is recommended. IV antibiotics are usually given until the white blood cell count is

normal and the patient is afebrile for 24 hours. Antibiotic irrigation of the peritoneal cavity and the use of transperitoneal drainage through the wound are controversial.[24]

Clinical Manifestations

Symptoms

Abdominal pain is the prime symptom of acute appendicitis. Classically, pain is initially diffusely centered in the lower epigastrium or umbilical area, is moderately severe, and is steady, sometimes with intermittent cramping superimposed. After a period varying from 1 to 12 hours, but usually within 4 to 6 hours, the pain localizes to the right lower quadrant. This classic pain sequence, although usual, is not invariable. In some patients, the pain of appendicitis begins in the right lower quadrant and remains there. Variations in the anatomic location of the appendix account for many of the variations in the principal locus of the somatic phase of the pain. For example, a long appendix with the inflamed tip in the left lower quadrant causes pain in that area. A retrocecal appendix may cause principally flank or back pain; a pelvic appendix, principally suprapubic pain; and a retroileal appendix, testicular pain, presumably from irritation of the spermatic artery and ureter. Intestinal malrotation also is responsible for puzzling pain patterns. The visceral component is in the normal location, but the somatic component is felt in that part of the abdomen where the cecum has been arrested in rotation.

Anorexia nearly always accompanies appendicitis. It is so constant that the diagnosis should be questioned if the patient is not anorectic. Although vomiting occurs in nearly 75% of patients, it is neither prominent nor prolonged, and most patients vomit only once or twice. Vomiting is caused by both neural stimulation and the presence of ileus.

Most patients give a history of obstipation beginning before the onset of abdominal pain, and many feel that defecation would relieve their abdominal pain. Diarrhea occurs in some patients, however, particularly children, so that the pattern of bowel function is of little differential diagnostic value.

The sequence of symptom appearance has great significance for the differential diagnosis. In >95% of patients with acute appendicitis, anorexia is the first symptom, followed by abdominal pain, which is followed, in turn, by vomiting (if vomiting occurs). If vomiting precedes the onset of pain, the diagnosis of appendicitis should be questioned.

Signs

Physical findings are determined principally by what the anatomic position of the inflamed appendix is, as well as by whether the organ has already ruptured when the patient is first examined.

Vital signs are minimally changed by uncomplicated appendicitis. Temperature elevation is rarely >1°C (1.8°F) and the pulse rate is normal or slightly elevated. Changes of greater magnitude usually indicate that a complication has occurred or that another diagnosis should be considered.[25]

Patients with appendicitis usually prefer to lie supine, with the thighs, particularly the right thigh, drawn up, because any motion increases pain. If asked to move, they do so slowly and with caution.

The classic right lower quadrant physical signs are present when the inflamed appendix lies in the anterior position. Tenderness often is maximal at or near the McBurney point.[8] Direct rebound tenderness usually is present. In addition, referred or indirect rebound tenderness is present. This referred tenderness is felt maximally in the right lower quadrant, which indicates localized peritoneal irritation.[25] The Rovsing sign—pain in the right lower quadrant when palpatory pressure is exerted in the left lower quadrant—also indicates the site of peritoneal irritation. Cutaneous hyperesthesia in the area supplied by the spinal nerves on the right at T10, T11, and T12 frequently accompanies acute appendicitis. In patients with obvious appendicitis, this sign is superfluous, but in some early cases, it may be the first positive sign. Hyperesthesia is elicited either by needle prick or by gently picking up the skin between the forefinger and thumb.

TABLE 30-1	Common organisms seen in patients with acute appendicitis

Aerobic and Facultative	**Anaerobic**
Gram-negative bacilli	Gram-negative bacilli
Escherichia coli	*Bacteroides fragilis*
Pseudomonas aeruginosa	Other *Bacteroides* species
Klebsiella species	*Fusobacterium* species
Gram-positive cocci	Gram-positive cocci
Streptococcus anginosus	*Peptostreptococcus* species
Other *Streptococcus* species	Gram-positive bacilli
Enterococcus species	*Clostridium* species

Muscular resistance to palpation of the abdominal wall roughly parallels the severity of the inflammatory process. Early in the disease, resistance, if present, consists mainly of voluntary guarding. As peritoneal irritation progresses, muscle spasm increases and becomes largely involuntary, that is, true reflex rigidity due to contraction of muscles directly beneath the inflamed parietal peritoneum.

Anatomic variations in the position of the inflamed appendix lead to deviations in the usual physical findings. With a retrocecal appendix, the anterior abdominal findings are less striking, and tenderness may be most marked in the flank. When the inflamed appendix hangs into the pelvis, abdominal findings may be entirely absent, and the diagnosis may be missed unless the rectum is examined. As the examining finger exerts pressure on the peritoneum of Douglas' cul-de-sac, pain is felt in the suprapubic area as well as locally within the rectum. Signs of localized muscle irritation also may be present. The psoas sign indicates an irritative focus in proximity to that muscle. The test is performed by having the patient lie on the left side as the examiner slowly extends the patient's right thigh, thus stretching the iliopsoas muscle. The test result is positive if extension produces pain. Similarly, a positive obturator sign of hypogastric pain on stretching the obturator internus indicates irritation in the pelvis. The test is performed by passive internal rotation of the flexed right thigh with the patient supine.

Laboratory Findings

Mild leukocytosis, ranging from 10,000 to 18,000 cells/mm³, usually is present in patients with acute, uncomplicated appendicitis and often is accompanied by a moderate polymorphonuclear predominance. White blood cell counts are variable, however. It is unusual for the white blood cell count to be >18,000 cells/mm³ in uncomplicated appendicitis. White blood cell counts above this level raise the possibility of a perforated appendix with or without an abscess. Urinalysis can be useful to rule out the urinary tract as the source of infection. Although several white or red blood cells can be present from ureteral or bladder irritation as a result of an inflamed appendix, bacteriuria in a urine specimen obtained via catheter generally is not seen in acute appendicitis.[26]

Imaging Studies

Plain films of the abdomen, although frequently obtained as part of the general evaluation of a patient with an acute abdomen, rarely are helpful in diagnosing acute appendicitis. However, plain radiographs can be of significant benefit in ruling out other pathology. In patients with acute appendicitis, one often sees an abnormal bowel gas pattern, which is a nonspecific finding. The presence of a fecalith is rarely noted on plain films but, if present, is highly suggestive of the diagnosis. A chest radiograph is sometimes indicated to rule out referred pain from a right lower lobe pneumonic process.

Additional radiographic studies include barium enema examination and radioactively labeled leukocyte scans. If the appendix fills on barium enema, appendicitis is excluded. On the other hand, if the appendix does not fill, no determination can be made.[27] To date, there has not been enough experience with radionuclide scans to assess their utility.

Graded compression sonography has been suggested as an accurate way to establish the diagnosis of appendicitis. The technique is inexpensive, can be performed rapidly, does not require a contrast medium, and can be used even in pregnant patients. Sonographically, the appendix is identified as a blind-ending, nonperistaltic bowel loop originating from the cecum. With maximal compression, the diameter of the appendix is measured in the anteroposterior dimension. Scan results are considered positive if a noncompressible appendix ≥6 mm in the anteroposterior direction is demonstrated (Fig. 30-3). The presence of an appendicolith establishes the diagnosis. Thickening of the appendiceal wall and the presence of periappendiceal fluid is highly suggestive. Sonographic demonstration of a normal appendix, which is an easily compressible, blind-ending tubular structure measuring ≤5 mm in diameter, excludes the diagnosis of acute appendicitis. The study results are considered inconclusive if the appendix is not visualized and there is no pericecal fluid or mass. When the diagnosis of acute appendicitis is excluded by sonography, a brief survey of the remainder of the abdominal cavity should be performed to establish an alternative diagnosis. In females of childbearing age, the pelvic organs must be adequately visualized

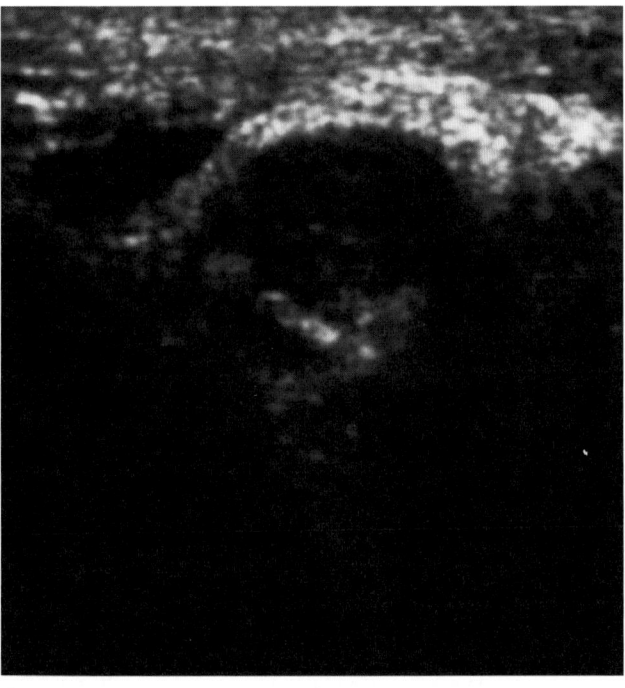

A

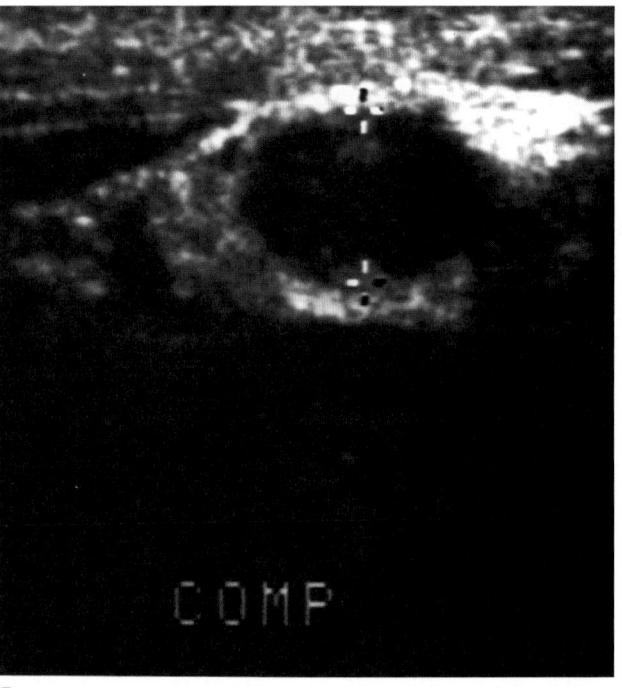

B

FIG. 30-3. Sonogram of a 10-year-old girl who presented with nausea, vomiting, and abdominal pain. The appendix measured 10.0 mm in maximal anteroposterior diameter in both the noncompression (**A**) and compression (**B**) views.

either by transabdominal or endovaginal ultrasonography to exclude gynecologic pathology as a cause of acute abdominal pain. The sonographic diagnosis of acute appendicitis has a reported sensitivity of 55 to 96% and a specificity of 85 to 98%.[28–30] Sonography is similarly effective in children and pregnant women, although its application is somewhat limited in late pregnancy.

Although sonography can easily identify abscesses in cases of perforation, the technique has limitations and results are user dependent. A false-positive scan result can occur in the presence of periappendicitis from surrounding inflammation, a dilated fallopian tube can be mistaken for an inflamed appendix, inspissated stool can mimic an appendicolith, and, in obese patients, the appendix may not be compressible because of overlying fat. False-negative sonogram results can occur if appendicitis is confined to the appendiceal tip, the appendix is retrocecal, the appendix is markedly enlarged and mistaken for small bowel, or the appendix is perforated and therefore compressible.[31]

Some studies have reported that graded compression sonography improved the diagnosis of appendicitis over clinical examination, specifically decreasing the percentage of negative explorations for appendectomies from 37 to 13%.[32] Sonography also decreases the time before operation. Sonography identified appendicitis in 10% of patients who were believed to have a low likelihood of the disease on physical examination.[33] The positive and negative predictive values of ultrasonography have impressively been reported as 91 and 92%, respectively. However, in a recent prospective multicenter study, routine ultrasonography did not improve diagnostic accuracy or rates of negative appendectomy or perforation compared with clinical assessment.

High-resolution helical CT also has been used to diagnose appendicitis. On CT scan, the inflamed appendix appears dilated (>5 cm) and the wall is thickened. There is usually evidence of inflammation, with "dirty fat," thickened mesoappendix, and even an obvious phlegmon (Fig. 30-4). Fecaliths can be easily visualized, but their presence is not necessarily pathognomonic of appendicitis. An important suggestive abnormality is the arrowhead sign. This is caused by thickening of the cecum, which funnels contrast agent toward the orifice of the inflamed appendix. CT scanning is also an excellent technique for identifying other inflammatory processes masquerading as appendicitis.

Several CT techniques have been used, including focused and nonfocused CT scans and enhanced and nonenhanced helical CT scanning. Nonenhanced helical CT scanning is important, because one of the disadvantages of using CT scanning in the evaluation of right lower quadrant pain is dye allergy. Surprisingly, all of these techniques have yielded essentially identical rates of diagnostic accuracy: 92 to 97% sensitivity, 85 to 94% specificity, 90 to 98% accuracy, and 75 to 95% positive and 95 to 99% negative predictive values.[34–36] The additional use of a rectally administered contrast agent did not improve the results of CT scanning.

A number of studies have documented improvement in diagnostic accuracy with the liberal use of CT scanning in the work-up of suspected appendicitis. CT lowered the rate of negative appendectomies from 19 to 12% in one study,[37] and the incidence of negative appendectomies in women from 24 to 5% in another.[38] The use of this imaging study altered the care of 24% of patients studied and provided alternative diagnoses in half of the patients with normal appendices on CT scan.[39]

Despite the potential usefulness of this technique, there are significant disadvantages. CT scanning is expensive, exposes the patient to significant radiation, and cannot be used during pregnancy. Allergy contraindicates the administration of IV contrast agents in some patients, and others cannot tolerate the oral ingestion of luminal dye, particularly in the presence of nausea and vomiting. Finally, not all studies have documented the utility of CT scanning in all patients with right lower quadrant pain.[40]

A number of studies have compared the effectiveness of graded compression sonography and helical CT in establishing the diagnosis of appendicitis. Although the differences are rather small, CT scanning has consistently proven superior. For example, in one study, 600 ultrasounds and 317 CT scans demonstrated sensitivity of 80 and 97%, specificity of 93 and 94%, diagnostic accuracy of 89 and 95%, positive predictive value of 91 and 92%, and negative predictive value of 88 and 98%, respectively.[30] In another study, ultrasound positively impacted the management of 19% of patients, compared with 73% of patients for CT. Finally, in a third study, the negative appendix rate was 17% for patients studied by ultrasonography compared with a negative appendix rate of 2% for patients who underwent helical CT scanning.[41] One concern about ultrasonography is the high intraobserver variability.[42]

One issue that has not been resolved is which patients are candidates for imaging studies.[43] This question may be moot, because CT scanning routinely is ordered by emergency physicians before surgeons are even consulted. The concept that all patients with right lower quadrant pain should undergo CT scanning has been strongly supported by two reports by Rao and his colleagues at the Massachusetts General Hospital. In one, this group documented that CT scanning led to a fall in the negative appendectomy rate from 20 to 7% and a decline in the perforation rate from 22 to 14%, as well as establishment of an alternative diagnosis in 50% of patients.[44] In the second study, published in the New England Journal of Medicine, Rao and associates documented that CT scanning prevented 13 unnecessary appendectomies, saved 50 inpatient hospital days, and lowered the per-patient cost by $447.[45] In contrast, several other studies failed to prove an advantage of routine CT scanning, documenting that surgeon accuracy approached that of the imaging study and expressing concern that the imaging studies could adversely delay appendectomy in affected patients.[46,47]

The rational approach is the selective use of CT scanning. This has been documented by several studies in which imaging was performed based on an algorithm or protocol.[48] The likelihood of appendicitis can be ascertained using the Alvarado scale (Table 30-2).[49] This scoring system was designed to improve the diagnosis of appendicitis and was devised by giving relative weight to specific clinical manifestation. Table 30-2 lists the eight specific indicators identified. Patients with scores of 9 or 10 are almost certain to have appendicitis; there is little advantage in further work-up, and they should go to the operating room. Patients with scores of 7 or 8 have a high likelihood of appendicitis, whereas scores of 5 or 6 are compatible with, but not diagnostic of, appendicitis. CT scanning is certainly appropriate for patients with Alvarado scores of 5 and 6, and a case can be built for imaging for those with scores of 7 and 8. On the other hand, it is difficult to justify the expense, radiation exposure, and possible complications of CT scanning in patients whose scores of 0 to 4 make it extremely unlikely (but not impossible) that they have appendicitis.

Selective CT scanning based on the likelihood of appendicitis takes advantage of the clinical skill of the experienced surgeon and, when indicated, adds the expertise of the radiologist and his or her imaging study. Figure 30-5 proposes a treatment algorithm addressing the rational use of diagnostic testing.[50]

Laparoscopy can serve as both a diagnostic and therapeutic maneuver for patients with acute abdominal pain and suspected acute appendicitis. Laparoscopy is probably most useful in the evaluation of females with lower abdominal complaints, because appendectomy is performed on a normal appendix in as many as 30 to 40% of these patients. Differentiating acute gynecologic pathology from acute appendicitis can be effectively accomplished using the laparoscope.

Appendiceal Rupture

Immediate appendectomy has long been the recommended treatment for acute appendicitis because of the presumed risk of progression to rupture. The overall rate of perforated appendicitis is 25.8%. Children <5 years of age and patients >65 years of age have the highest rates of perforation (45 and 51%, respectively) (Fig. 30-6).[14,15,51]

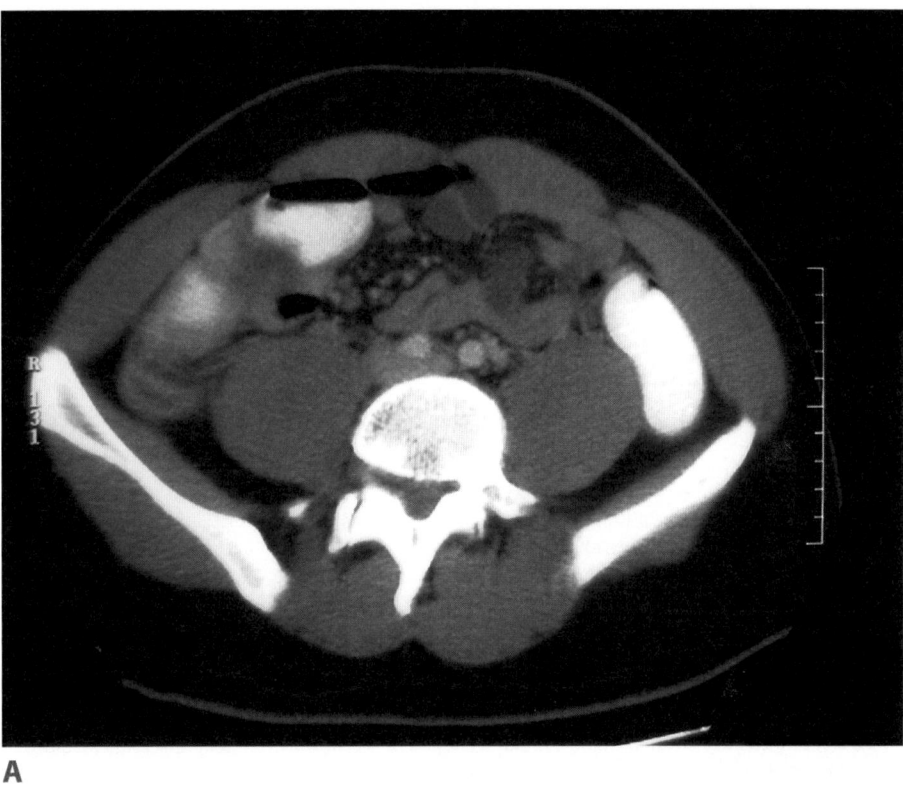

A

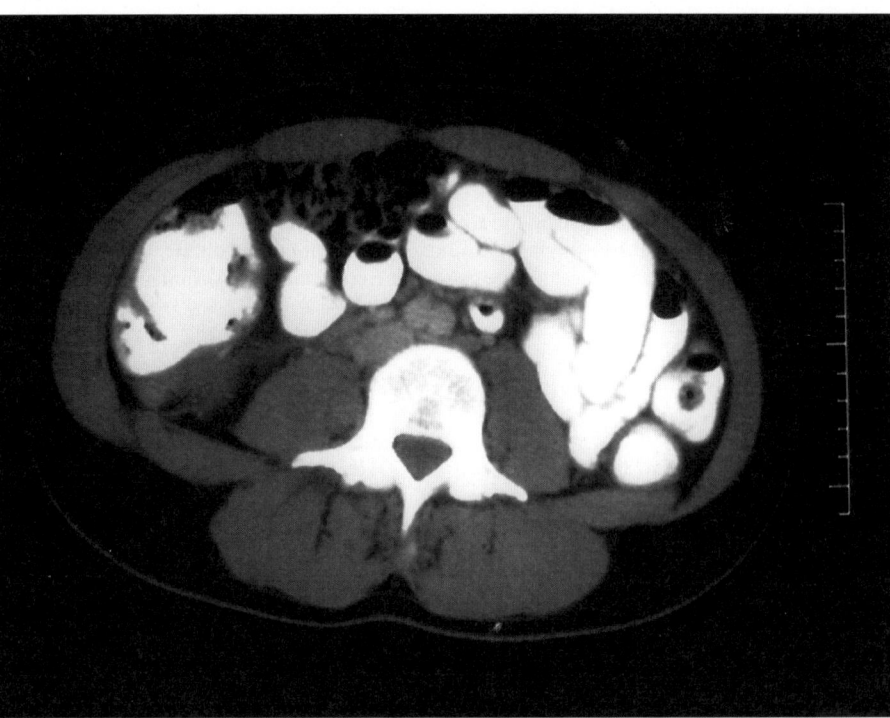

B

FIG. 30-4. Computed tomographic scans with findings positive for appendicitis. Note the thick-walled and dilated appendix (**A**) and mesenteric streaking and "dirty fat" (**B**).

It has been suggested that delays in presentation are responsible for the majority of perforated appendices. There is no accurate way of determining when and if an appendix will rupture before resolution of the inflammatory process. Recent studies suggest that, in selected patients, observation and antibiotic therapy alone may be an appropriate treatment for acute appendicitis.[17,52]

Appendiceal rupture occurs most frequently distal to the point of luminal obstruction along the antimesenteric border of the appendix. Rupture should be suspected in the presence of fever with

a temperature of >39°C (102°F) and a white blood cell count of >18,000 cells/mm³. In the majority of cases, rupture is contained and patients display localized rebound tenderness. Generalized peritonitis will be present if the walling-off process is ineffective in containing the rupture.

In 2 to 6% of cases, an ill-defined mass is detected on physical examination. This could represent a phlegmon, which consists of matted loops of bowel adherent to the adjacent inflamed appendix, or a periappendiceal abscess. Patients who present with a mass have

TABLE 30-2	Alvarado scale for the diagnosis of appendicitis	
	Manifestations	**Value**
Symptoms	Migration of pain	1
	Anorexia	1
	Nausea and/or vomiting	1
Signs	Right lower quadrant tenderness	2
	Rebound	1
	Elevated temperature	1
Laboratory values	Leukocytosis	2
	Left shift in leukocyte count	1
	Total points	10

Source: Reproduced with permission from Alvarado.[49]

experienced symptoms for a longer duration, usually at least 5 to 7 days. Distinguishing acute, uncomplicated appendicitis from acute appendicitis with perforation on the basis of clinical findings is often difficult, but it is important to make the distinction because their treatment differs. CT scan may be beneficial in guiding therapy. Phlegmons and small abscesses can be treated conservatively with IV antibiotics; well-localized abscesses can be managed with percutaneous drainage; complex abscesses should be considered for surgical drainage. If operative drainage is required, it should be performed using an extraperitoneal approach, with appendectomy reserved for cases in which the appendix is easily accessible. Interval appendectomy performed at least 6 weeks after the acute event has classically been recommended for all patients treated either nonoperatively or with simple drainage of an abscess.[53,54]

Differential Diagnosis

The differential diagnosis of acute appendicitis is essentially the diagnosis of the acute abdomen (see Chap. 35). This is because clinical manifestations are not specific for a given disease but are specific for disturbance of a given physiologic function or functions. Thus, an essentially identical clinical picture can result from a wide variety of acute processes within the peritoneal cavity that produce the same alterations of function as does acute appendicitis.

The accuracy of preoperative diagnosis should be approximately 85%. If it is consistently less, it is likely that some unnecessary operations are being performed, and a more rigorous preoperative differential diagnosis is in order. A diagnostic accuracy rate that is consistently >90% should also cause concern, because this may mean that some patients with atypical, but bona fide, cases of acute appendicitis are being "observed" when they should receive prompt surgical intervention. The Haller group, however, has shown that this is not invariably true.[55] Before that group's study, the perforation rate at the hospital at which the study took place was 26.7%, and acute appendicitis was found in 80% of the patients undergoing operation. By implementing a policy of intensive inhospital observation when the diagnosis of appendicitis was unclear, the group raised the rate of acute appendicitis found at operation to 94%, but the perforation rate remained unchanged at 27.5%.[55] The rate of false-negative appendectomies is highest in young adult females. A normal appendix is found in 32 to 45% of appendectomies performed in women 15 to 45 years of age.[14]

A common error is to make a preoperative diagnosis of acute appendicitis only to find some other condition (or nothing) at operation. Much less frequently, acute appendicitis is found after a preoperative diagnosis of another condition. The most common erroneous preoperative diagnoses—together accounting for >75% of cases—are, in descending order of frequency, acute mesenteric lymphadenitis, no organic pathologic condition, acute pelvic inflammatory disease, twisted ovarian cyst or ruptured graafian follicle, and acute gastroenteritis.

The differential diagnosis of acute appendicitis depends on four major factors: the anatomic location of the inflamed appendix; the stage of the process (i.e., simple or ruptured); the patient's age; and the patient's sex.[56–60]

Acute Mesenteric Adenitis

Acute mesenteric adenitis is the disease most often confused with acute appendicitis in children. Almost invariably, an upper respiratory tract infection is present or has recently subsided. The pain usually is diffuse, and tenderness is not as sharply localized as in appendicitis. Voluntary guarding is sometimes present, but true rigidity is rare.

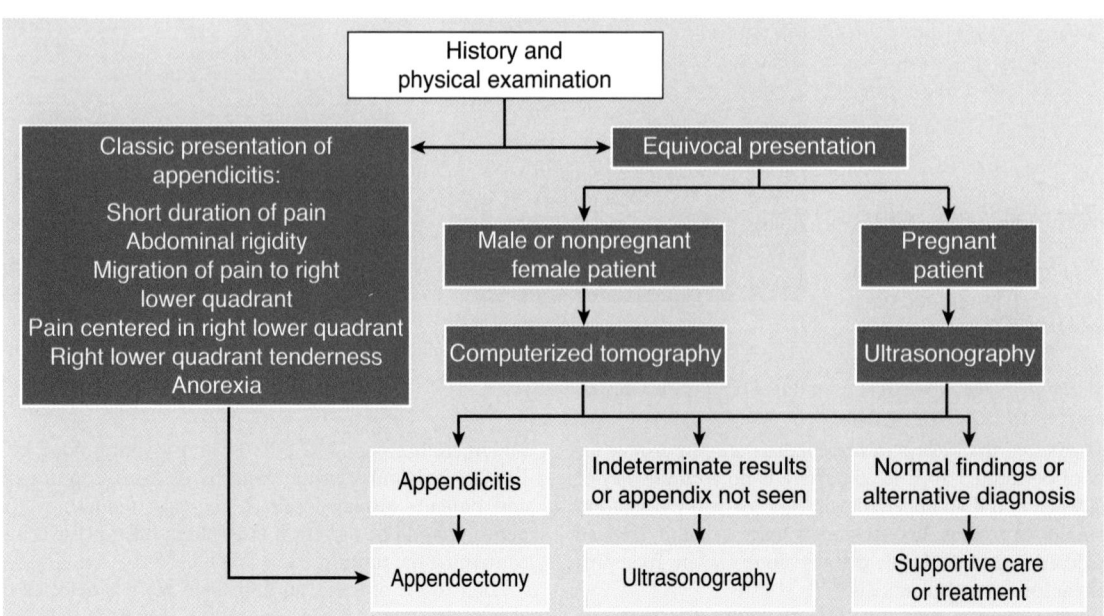

FIG. 30-5. Clinical algorithm for suspected cases of acute appendicitis. If gynecologic disease is suspected, a pelvic and endovaginal ultrasound examination is indicated. *(Reproduced with permission from Paulson et al.[50] Copyright © Massachusetts Medical Society. All rights reserved.)*

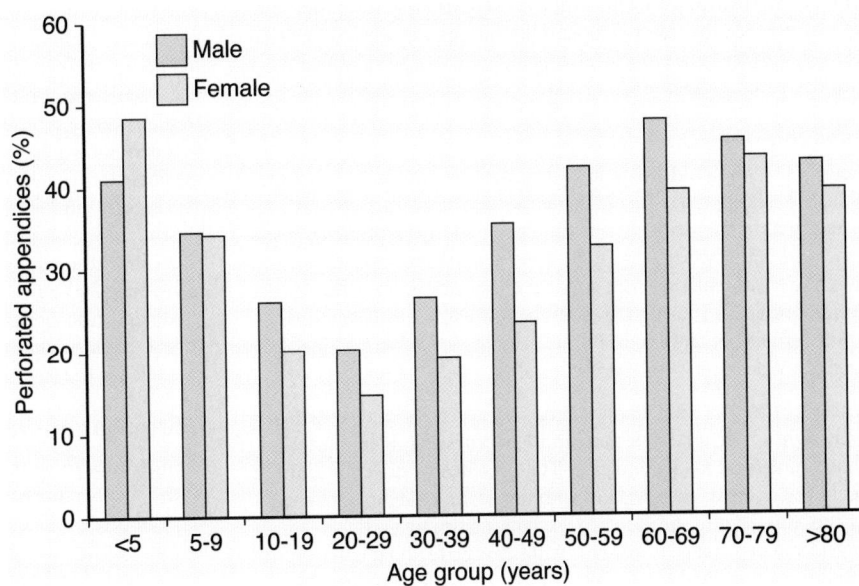

FIG. 30-6. Rate of appendiceal rupture by age group. (*Personal communication from David Flum, MD.*)

Generalized lymphadenopathy may be noted. Laboratory procedures are of little help in arriving at the correct diagnosis, although a relative lymphocytosis, when present, suggests mesenteric adenitis. Observation for several hours is in order if the diagnosis of mesenteric adenitis seems likely, because it is a self-limited disease. However, if the differentiation remains in doubt, immediate exploration is the safest course of action.

Human infection with *Yersinia enterocolitica* or *Yersinia pseudotuberculosis*, transmitted through food contaminated by feces or urine, causes mesenteric adenitis as well as ileitis, colitis, and acute appendicitis. Many of the infections are mild and self limited, but they may lead to systemic disease with a high fatality rate if untreated. The organisms are usually sensitive to tetracyclines, streptomycin, ampicillin, and kanamycin. A preoperative suspicion of the diagnosis should not delay operative intervention, because appendicitis caused by *Yersinia* cannot be clinically distinguished from appendicitis due to other causes. Approximately 6% of cases of mesenteric adenitis are caused by *Yersinia* infection.

Salmonella typhimurium infection causes mesenteric adenitis and paralytic ileus with symptoms similar to those of appendicitis. The diagnosis can be established by serologic testing. *Campylobacter jejuni* causes diarrhea and pain that mimics that of appendicitis. The organism can be cultured from stool.

Gynecologic Disorders

Diseases of the female internal reproductive organs that may erroneously be diagnosed as appendicitis are, in approximate descending order of frequency, pelvic inflammatory disease, ruptured graafian follicle, twisted ovarian cyst or tumor, endometriosis, and ruptured ectopic pregnancy.

Pelvic Inflammatory Disease In pelvic inflammatory disease the infection usually is bilateral but, if confined to the right tube, may mimic acute appendicitis. Nausea and vomiting are present in patients with appendicitis, but in only approximately 50% of those with pelvic inflammatory disease. Pain and tenderness are usually lower, and motion of the cervix is exquisitely painful. Intracellular diplococci may be demonstrable on smear of the purulent vaginal discharge. The ratio of cases of appendicitis to cases of pelvic inflammatory disease is low in females in the early phase of the menstrual cycle and high during the luteal phase. The careful clinical use of these features has reduced the incidence of negative findings on laparoscopy in young women to 15%.

Ruptured Graafian Follicle Ovulation commonly results in the spillage of sufficient amounts of blood and follicular fluid to produce brief, mild lower abdominal pain. If the amount of fluid is unusually copious and is from the right ovary, appendicitis may be simulated. Pain and tenderness are rather diffuse. Leukocytosis and fever are minimal or absent. Because this pain occurs at the midpoint of the menstrual cycle, it is often called *mittelschmerz*.

Twisted Ovarian Cyst Serous cysts of the ovary are common and generally remain asymptomatic. When right-sided cysts rupture or undergo torsion, the manifestations are similar to those of appendicitis. Patients develop right lower quadrant pain, tenderness, rebound, fever, and leukocytosis. If the mass is palpable on physical examination, the diagnosis can be made easily. Both transvaginal ultrasonography and CT scanning can be diagnostic if a mass is not palpable.

Torsion requires emergent operative treatment. If the torsion is complete or longstanding, the pedicle undergoes thrombosis, and the ovary and tube become gangrenous and require resection. Leakage of ovarian cysts resolves spontaneously, however, and is best treated nonoperatively.[24,56–61]

Ruptured Ectopic Pregnancy Blastocysts may implant in the fallopian tube (usually the ampullary portion) and in the ovary. Rupture of right tubal or ovarian pregnancies can mimic appendicitis. Patients may give a history of abnormal menses, either missing one or two periods or noting only slight vaginal bleeding. Unfortunately, patients do not always realize they are pregnant. The development of right lower quadrant or pelvic pain may be the first symptom. The diagnosis of ruptured ectopic pregnancy should be relatively easy. The presence of a pelvic mass and elevated levels of chorionic gonadotropin are characteristic. Although the leukocyte count rises slightly (to approximately 14,000 cells/mm³), the hematocrit level falls as a consequence of the intra-abdominal hemorrhage. Vaginal examination reveals cervical motion and adnexal tenderness, and a more definitive diagnosis can be established by culdocentesis. The presence of blood and particularly decidual tissue is pathognomonic. The treatment of ruptured ectopic pregnancy is emergency surgery.

Acute Gastroenteritis

Acute gastroenteritis is common but usually can be easily distinguished from acute appendicitis. Gastroenteritis is characterized by profuse diarrhea, nausea, and vomiting. Hyperperistaltic abdominal cramps precede the watery stools. The abdomen is relaxed between cramps, and there are no localizing signs. Laboratory values vary with the specific cause.

Other Intestinal Disorders

Meckel's Diverticulitis Meckel's diverticulitis gives rise to a clinical picture similar to that of acute appendicitis. Meckel's diverticulum is located within the distal 2 ft of the ileum. Meckel's diverticulitis is associated with the same complications as appendicitis and requires the same treatment—prompt surgical intervention. Resection of the segment of ileum bearing the diverticulum with end-to-end anastomosis can nearly always be done through a McBurney incision, extended if necessary, or laparoscopically.

Crohn's Enteritis The manifestations of acute regional enteritis—fever, right-lower quadrant pain and tenderness, and leukocytosis—often simulate acute appendicitis. The presence of diarrhea and the absence of anorexia, nausea, and vomiting favor a diagnosis of enteritis, but this is not sufficient to exclude acute appendicitis. In an appreciable percentage of patients with chronic regional enteritis, the diagnosis is first made at the time of operation for presumed acute appendicitis. In cases of an acutely inflamed distal ileum with no cecal involvement and a normal appendix, appendectomy is indicated. Progression to chronic Crohn's ileitis is uncommon.

Colonic Lesions Diverticulitis or perforating carcinoma of the cecum, or of that portion of the sigmoid that lies in the right side, may be impossible to distinguish from appendicitis. These entities should be considered in older patients. CT scanning is often helpful in making a diagnosis in older patients with right lower quadrant pain and atypical clinical presentations.

Epiploic appendagitis probably results from infarction of the colonic appendage(s) secondary to torsion. Symptoms may be minimal, or there may be continuous abdominal pain in an area corresponding to the contour of the colon, lasting several days. Pain shift is unusual, and there is no diagnostic sequence of symptoms. The patient does not look ill, nausea and vomiting are unusual, and appetite generally is unaffected. Localized tenderness over the site is usual and often is associated with rebound without rigidity. In 25% of reported cases, pain persists or recurs until the infarcted epiploic appendage is removed.

Other Diseases

Diseases or conditions not mentioned in the preceding sections that must be considered in the differential diagnosis include foreign body perforations of the bowel, closed-loop intestinal obstruction, mesenteric vascular infarction, pleuritis of the right lower chest, acute cholecystitis, acute pancreatitis, hematoma of the abdominal wall, epididymitis, testicular torsion, urinary tract infection, ureteral stone, primary peritonitis, and Henoch-Schönlein purpura.

Acute Appendicitis in the Young

The establishment of a diagnosis of acute appendicitis is more difficult in young children than in the adult. The inability of young children to give an accurate history, diagnostic delays by both parents and physicians, and the frequency of GI upset in children are all contributing factors.[62] In children the physical examination findings of maximal tenderness in the right lower quadrant, the inability to walk or walking with a limp, and pain with percussion, coughing, and hopping were found to have the highest sensitivity for appendicitis.[63]

The more rapid progression to rupture and the inability of the underdeveloped greater omentum to contain a rupture lead to significant morbidity rates in children. Children <5 years of age have a negative appendectomy rate of 25% and an appendiceal perforation rate of 45%. These rates may be compared with a negative appendectomy rate of <10% and a perforated appendix rate of 20% for children 5 to 12 years of age.[13,14] The incidence of major complications after appendectomy in children is correlated with appendiceal rupture.

The wound infection rate after the treatment of nonperforated appendicitis in children is 2.8% compared with a rate of 11% after the treatment of perforated appendicitis. The incidence of intra-abdominal abscess also is higher after the treatment of perforated appendicitis than after nonperforated appendicitis (6% vs. 3%).[23] The treatment regimen for perforated appendicitis generally includes immediate appendectomy and irrigation of the peritoneal cavity. Antibiotic coverage is limited to 24 to 48 hours in cases of nonperforated appendicitis. For perforated appendicitis IV antibiotics usually are given until the white blood cell count is normal and the patient is afebrile for 24 hours. The use of antibiotic irrigation of the peritoneal cavity and transperitoneal drainage through the wound are controversial. Laparoscopic appendectomy has been shown to be safe and effective for the treatment of appendicitis in children.[64]

Acute Appendicitis in the Elderly

Compared with younger patients, elderly patients with appendicitis often pose a more difficult diagnostic problem because of the atypical presentation, expanded differential diagnosis, and communication difficulty. These factors may be responsible for the disproportionately high perforation rate seen in the elderly. In the general population, perforation rates range from 20 to 30%, compared with 50 to 70% in the elderly.[65] In addition, the perforation rate appears to increase with age >80 years.[66]

Elderly patients usually present with lower abdominal pain, but on clinical examination, localized right lower quadrant tenderness is present in only 80 to 90% of patients. A history of periumbilical pain migrating to the right lower quadrant is reported infrequently. The usefulness of the Alvarado score appears to decline in the elderly. Fewer then 50% of the elderly with appendicitis have an Alvarado score of ≥7.[66] Although currently there are no criteria that definitively identify elderly patients with acute appendicitis who are at risk of rupture, prioritization should be given to patients with a temperature of >38°C (100.4°F) and a shift to the left in leukocyte count of >76%, especially if they are male, are anorectic, or have had pain of long duration before admission.[65]

As a result of increased comorbidities and an increased rate of perforation, postoperative morbidity, mortality, and hospital length of stay are increased in the elderly compared with younger populations with appendicitis. Although no randomized trials have been conducted, it appears that elderly patients benefit from a laparoscopic approach to treatment of appendicitis. The use of laparoscopy in the elderly has significantly increased in recent years. In general, laparoscopic appendectomy offers elderly patients with appendicitis a shorter length of hospital stay, a reduction in complication and mortality rates, and a greater chance of discharge to home (independent of further nursing care or rehabilitation).[67]

Acute Appendicitis during Pregnancy

Appendectomy for presumed appendicitis is the most common surgical emergency during pregnancy. The incidence is approximately 1 in 766 births. Acute appendicitis can occur at any time during pregnancy.[68] The overall negative appendectomy rate during pregnancy is approximately 25% and appears to be higher than the rate seen in nonpregnant women.[68,69] A higher rate of negative appendectomy is seen in the second trimester, and the lowest rate is in the third trimester. The diversity of clinical presentations and the difficulty in making the diagnosis of acute appendicitis in pregnant women is well established. This is particularly true in the late second trimester and the third trimester, when many abdominal symptoms may be considered pregnancy related. In addition, during pregnancy there are anatomic changes in the appendix (Fig. 30-7) and increased abdominal laxity that may further complicate clinical evaluation. *There is no association between appendectomy and subsequent fertility.*

Appendicitis in pregnancy should be suspected when a pregnant woman complains of abdominal pain of new onset. The most consistent sign encountered in acute appendicitis during pregnancy is pain in the right side of the abdomen. Seventy-four percent of patients

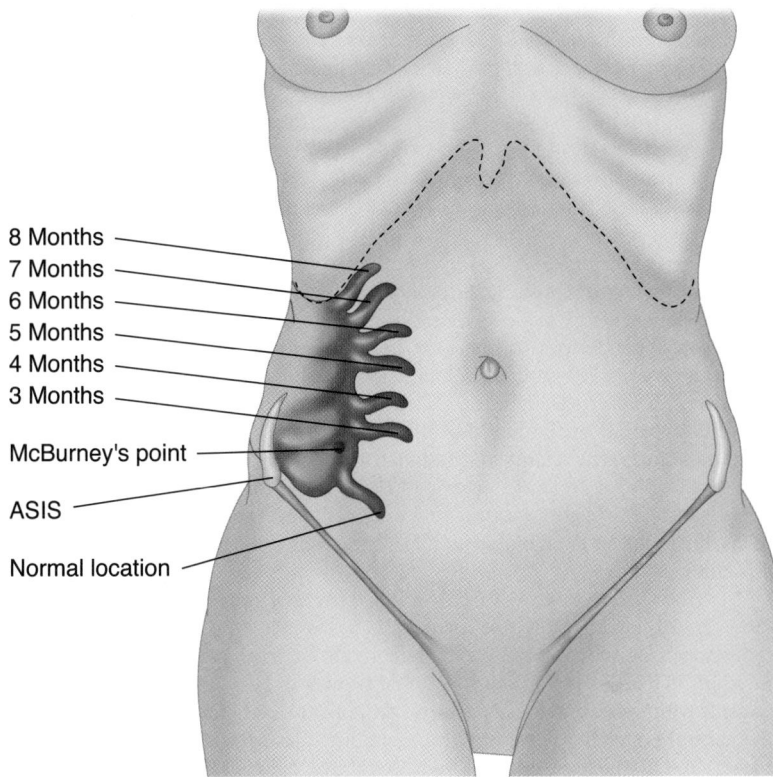

8 Months
7 Months
6 Months
5 Months
4 Months
3 Months

McBurney's point

ASIS

Normal location

FIG. 30-7. Location of the appendix during pregnancy. ASIS = anterior superior iliac spine. *[Reproduced with permission from Metcalf A: The appendix, in Corson JD, Williamson RCN (eds): Surgery. London: Mosby, 2001.]*

report pain located in the right lower abdominal quadrant, with no difference between early and late pregnancy. Only 57% of patients present with the classic history of diffuse periumbilical pain migrating to the right lower quadrant. Laboratory evaluation is not helpful in establishing the diagnosis of acute appendicitis during pregnancy. The physiologic leukocytosis of pregnancy has been defined as high as 16,000 cells/mm^3. In one series only 38% of patients with appendicitis had a white blood cell count of >16,000 cells/mm^3.[68] Recent data suggest that the incidence of perforated or complex appendicitis is not increased in pregnant patients.[69]

When the diagnosis is in doubt, abdominal ultrasound may be beneficial. Another option is magnetic resonance imaging, which has no known deleterious effects on the fetus. The American College of Radiology recommends the use of nonionizing radiation techniques for front-line imaging in pregnant women.[70] Laparoscopy has been advocated in equivocal cases, especially early in pregnancy; however laparoscopic appendectomy may be associated with an increase in pregnancy-related complications. In an analysis of outcomes in California using administrative databases, laparoscopy was found to be associated with a 2.31 increased odds of fetal loss over open surgery.[69]

The overall incidence of fetal loss after appendectomy is 4% and the risk of early delivery is 7%. Rates of fetal loss are considerably higher in women with complex appendicitis than in those with a negative appendectomy and with simple appendicitis. It is important to note that a negative appendectomy is not a benign procedure. Removing a normal appendix is associated with a 4% risk of fetal loss and 10% risk of early delivery. Maternal mortality after appendectomy is extremely rare (0.03%). Because the incidence of ruptured appendix is similar in pregnant and nonpregnant women and because maternal mortality is so low, it appears that the greatest opportunity to improve fetal outcomes is by improving diagnostic accuracy and reducing the rate of negative appendectomy.[68–71]

Appendicitis in Patients with AIDS or HIV Infection

The incidence of acute appendicitis in HIV-infected patients is reported to be 0.5%. This is higher than the 0.1 to 0.2% incidence

reported for the general population.[72] The presentation of acute appendicitis in HIV-infected patients is similar to that in noninfected patients. The majority of HIV-infected patients with appendicitis have fever, periumbilical pain radiating to the right lower quadrant (91%), right lower quadrant tenderness (91%), and rebound tenderness (74%). HIV-infected patients do not manifest an absolute leukocytosis; however, if a baseline leukocyte count is available, nearly all HIV-infected patients with appendicitis demonstrate a relative leukocytosis.[72,73]

The risk of appendiceal rupture appears to be increased in HIV-infected patients. In one large series of HIV-infected patients who underwent appendectomy for presumed appendicitis, 43% of patients were found to have perforated appendicitis at laparotomy.[74] The increased risk of appendiceal rupture may be related to the delay in presentation seen in this patient population.[72,74] The mean duration of symptoms before arrival in the emergency department has been reported to be increased in HIV-infected patients, with >60% of patients reporting the duration of symptoms to be longer than 24 hours.[72] In early series, significant hospital delay also may have contributed to high rates of rupture.[72] However, with increased understanding of abdominal pain in HIV-infected patients, hospital delay has become less prevalent.[72,75] A low CD4 count is also associated with an increased incidence of appendiceal rupture. In one large series, patients with nonruptured appendices had CD4 counts of 158.75 ± 47 cells/mm^3 compared with 94.5 ± 32 cells/mm^3 in patients with appendiceal rupture.[72]

The differential diagnosis of right lower quadrant pain is expanded in HIV-infected patients compared with the general population. In addition to the conditions discussed elsewhere in this chapter, opportunistic infections should be considered as a possible cause of right lower quadrant pain.[72–75] Such opportunistic infections include cytomegalovirus (CMV) infection, Kaposi's sarcoma, tuberculosis, lymphoma, and other causes of infectious colitis. CMV infection may be seen anywhere in the GI tract. CMV infection causes a vasculitis of blood vessels in the submucosa of the gut, which leads to thrombosis. Mucosal ischemia develops, leading to ulceration, gangrene of the bowel wall, and perforation. Spontaneous peritonitis may be caused by opportunistic pathogens, including CMV, *Mycobacterium avium-*

intracellulare complex, *Mycobacterium tuberculosis, Cryptococcus neoformans*, and *Strongyloides*. Kaposi's sarcoma and non-Hodgkin's lymphoma may present with pain and a right lower quadrant mass. Viral and bacterial colitis occur with a higher frequency in HIV-infected patients than in the general population. Colitis should always be considered in HIV-infected patients presenting with right lower quadrant pain. Neutropenic enterocolitis (typhlitis) should also be considered in the differential diagnosis of right lower quadrant pain in HIV-infected patients.[73,75]

A thorough history and physical examination is important when evaluating any patient with right lower quadrant pain. In the HIV-infected patient with classic signs and symptoms of appendicitis, immediate appendectomy is indicated. In those patients with diarrhea as a prominent symptom, colonoscopy may be warranted. In patients with equivocal findings, CT scan is usually helpful. The majority of pathologic findings identified in HIV-infected patients who undergo appendectomy for presumed appendicitis are typical. The negative appendectomy rate is 5 to 10%. However, in up to 25% of patients AIDS-related entities are found in the operative specimens, including CMV, Kaposi's sarcoma, and *M. avium-intracellulare* complex.[72,74]

In a retrospective study of 77 HIV-infected patients from 1988 to 1995, the 30-day mortality rate for patients undergoing appendectomy was reported to be 9.1%.[72] More recent series report 0% mortality in this group of patients.[75] Morbidity rates for HIV-infected patients with nonperforated appendicitis are similar to those seen in the general population. Postoperative morbidity rates appear to be higher in HIV-infected patients with perforated appendicitis. In addition, the length of hospital stay for HIV-infected patients undergoing appendectomy is twice that for the general population.[72,75] No series has been reported to date that addresses the role of laparoscopic appendectomy in the HIV-infected population.

Treatment

Despite the advent of more sophisticated diagnostic modalities, the importance of early operative intervention should not be minimized. Once the decision to operate for presumed acute appendicitis has been made, the patient should be prepared for the operating room. Adequate hydration should be ensured, electrolyte abnormalities should be corrected, and pre-existing cardiac, pulmonary, and renal conditions should be addressed. A large meta-analysis has demonstrated the efficacy of preoperative antibiotics in lowering the infectious complications in appendicitis.[23] Most surgeons routinely administer antibiotics to all patients with suspected appendicitis. If simple acute appendicitis is encountered, there is no benefit in extending antibiotic coverage beyond 24 hours. If perforated or gangrenous appendicitis is found, antibiotics are continued until the patient is afebrile and has a normal white blood cell count. For intra-abdominal infections of GI tract origin that are of mild to moderate severity, the Surgical Infection Society has recommended single-agent therapy with cefoxitin, cefotetan, or ticarcillin-clavulanic acid. For more severe infections, single-agent therapy with carbapenems or combination therapy with a third-generation cephalosporin, monobactam, or aminoglycoside plus anaerobic coverage with clindamycin or metronidazole is indicated.[24] The recommendations are similar for children.[76]

Open Appendectomy

For open appendectomy most surgeons use either a McBurney (oblique) or Rocky-Davis (transverse) right lower quadrant muscle-splitting incision in patients with suspected appendicitis. The incision should be centered over either the point of maximal tenderness or a palpable mass. If an abscess is suspected, a laterally placed incision is imperative to allow retroperitoneal drainage and to avoid generalized contamination of the peritoneal cavity. If the diagnosis is in doubt, a lower midline incision is recommended to allow a more extensive examination of the peritoneal cavity. This is especially relevant in older patients with possible malignancy or diverticulitis.

Several techniques can be used to locate the appendix. Because the cecum usually is visible within the incision, the convergence of the taeniae can be followed to the base of the appendix. A sweeping lateral to medial motion can aid in delivering the appendiceal tip into the operative field. Occasionally, limited mobilization of the cecum is needed to aid in adequate visualization. Once identified, the appendix is mobilized by dividing the mesoappendix, with care taken to ligate the appendiceal artery securely.

The appendiceal stump can be managed by simple ligation or by ligation and inversion with either a purse-string or Z stitch. As long as the stump is clearly viable and the base of the cecum is not involved with the inflammatory process, the stump can be safely ligated with a nonabsorbable suture. The mucosa is frequently obliterated to avoid the development of mucocele. The peritoneal cavity is irrigated and the wound closed in layers. If perforation or gangrene is found in adults, the skin and subcutaneous tissue should be left open and allowed to heal by secondary intent or closed in 4 to 5 days as a delayed primary closure. In children, who generally have little subcutaneous fat, primary wound closure has not led to an increased incidence of wound infection.

If appendicitis is not found, a methodical search must be made for an alternative diagnosis. The cecum and mesentery should first be inspected. Next, the small bowel should be examined in a retrograde fashion beginning at the ileocecal valve and extending at least 2 ft. In females, special attention should be paid to the pelvic organs. An attempt also should be made to examine the upper abdominal contents. Peritoneal fluid should be sent for Gram's staining and culture. If purulent fluid is encountered, it is imperative that the source be identified. A medial extension of the incision (Fowler-Weir), with division of the anterior and posterior rectus sheath, is acceptable if further evaluation of the lower abdomen is indicated. If upper abdominal pathology is encountered, the right lower quadrant incision is closed and an appropriate upper midline incision is made.[9]

Laparoscopic Appendectomy

Semm first reported successful laparoscopic appendectomy several years before the first laparoscopic cholecystectomy.[10] However, the laparoscopic approach to appendectomy did not come into widespread use until after the success of laparoscopic cholecystectomy. This may be due to the fact that appendectomy, by virtue of its small incision, is already a form of minimal-access surgery.[77]

Laparoscopic appendectomy is performed under general anesthesia. A nasogastric tube and a urinary catheter are placed before obtaining a pneumoperitoneum. Laparoscopic appendectomy usually requires the use of three ports. Four ports may occasionally be necessary to mobilize a retrocecal appendix. The surgeon usually stands to the patient's left. One assistant is required to operate the camera. One trocar is placed in the umbilicus (10 mm), and a second trocar is placed in the suprapubic position. Some surgeons place this second port in the left lower quadrant. The suprapubic trocar is either 10 or 12 mm, depending on whether or not a linear stapler will be used. The placement of the third trocar (5 mm) is variable and usually is either in the left lower quadrant, epigastrium, or right upper quadrant. Placement is based on location of the appendix and surgeon preference. Initially, the abdomen is thoroughly explored to exclude other pathology. The appendix is identified by following the anterior taeniae to its base. Dissection at the base of the appendix enables the surgeon to create a window between the mesentery and the base of the appendix (Fig. 30-8A). The mesentery and base of the appendix are then secured and divided separately. When the mesoappendix is involved with the inflammatory process, it is often best to divide the appendix first with a linear stapler and then to divide the mesoappendix immediately adjacent to the appendix with clips, electrocautery, Harmonic Scalpel, or staples (Fig. 30-8B and 30-8C). The base of the appendix is not inverted. The appendix is removed from the abdominal cavity through a trocar site or within a retrieval bag. The base of the appendix and the mesoappendix should be

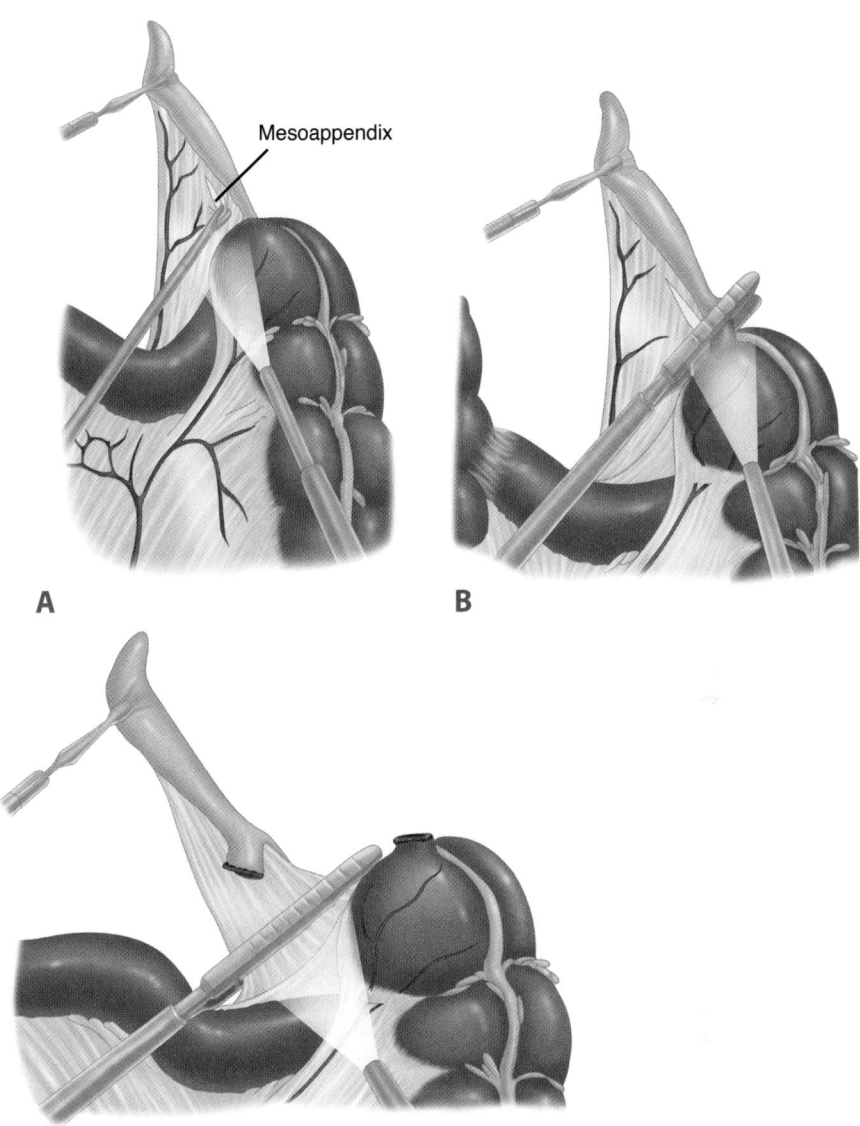

Mesoappendix

FIG. 30-8. Laparoscopic resection of the appendix. Occasionally, if the appendix and mesoappendix are extremely inflamed, it is easier to divide the appendix at its base before division of the mesoappendix. **A.** A window is created in the mesoappendix close to the base of the appendix. **B.** The linear stapler is then used to divide the appendix at its base. **C.** Finally the mesoappendix can be easily divided using the linear stapler. *[Reproduced with permission from Ortega JM, Ricardo AE: Surgery of the appendix and colon, in Moody FG (ed): Atlas of Ambulatory Surgery. Philadelphia: WB Saunders, 1999.]*

evaluated for hemostasis. The right lower quadrant should be irrigated. Trocars are removed under direct vision.[78,79]

The utility of laparoscopic appendectomy in the management of acute appendicitis remains controversial. Surgeons may be hesitant to implement a new technique because the conventional open approach already has proved to be simple and effective. A number of articles in peer-reviewed journals have compared laparoscopic and open appendectomy, including >20 randomized, controlled trials and 6 meta-analyses.[64,77,80–84] The overall quality of these randomized, controlled trials has been limited by the failure to blind patients and providers as to the treatment modality used. Furthermore, investigators have failed to perform prestudy sample size analysis for the outcomes studied.[64] The largest meta-analysis comparing open to laparoscopic appendectomy included 47 studies, 39 of which were studies of adult patients. This analysis demonstrated that the duration of surgery and costs of operation were higher for laparoscopic appendectomy than for open appendectomy. Wound infections were approximately half as likely after laparoscopic appendectomy as after open appendectomy. However, the rate of intra-abdominal abscess was three times higher after laparoscopic appendectomy than after open appendectomy.[64]

A principal proposed benefit of laparoscopic appendectomy has been decreased postoperative pain. Patient-reported pain on the first postoperative day is significantly less after laparoscopic appen-

dectomy. However, the difference has been calculated to be only 8 points on a 100-point visual analogue scale. This difference is below the level of pain that an average patient is able to perceive.[62] Hospital length of stay also is statistically significantly less after laparoscopic appendectomy. However, in most studies this difference is <1 day.[64,77] It appears that a more important determinant of length of stay after appendectomy is the pathology found at operation—specifically, whether a patient has perforated or nonperforated appendicitis. In nearly all studies, laparoscopic appendectomy is associated with a shorter period before return to normal activity, return to work, and return to sports.[64,77,80–84] However, treatment and subject bias may have a significant impact on the data. Although the majority of studies have been performed in adults, similar data have been obtained in children.[64]

There appears to be little benefit to laparoscopic appendectomy over open appendectomy in thin males between the ages of 15 and 45 years. In these patients, the diagnosis usually is straightforward. Open appendectomy has been associated with outstanding results for several decades. Laparoscopic appendectomy should be considered an option in these patients, based on surgeon and patient preference. Laparoscopic appendectomy may be beneficial in obese patients, in whom it may be difficult to gain adequate access through a small right lower quadrant incision. In a retrospective study of 116 patients with a mean body mass index of 35, postoperative length of stay was significantly shorter in the group undergoing laparoscopic appendectomy, and there were fewer open wounds. In all obese patients in whom the procedure was completed laparoscopically the incisions closed primarily, whereas the wounds closed primarily in only 58% of obese patients who underwent open appendectomy. There was no difference in rates of wound infection; intra-abdominal abscess rates were not reported.[85]

Diagnostic laparoscopy has been advocated as a potential tool to decrease the number of negative appendectomies performed. However, the morbidity associated with laparoscopy and general anesthesia is acceptable only if pathology requiring surgical treatment is present and is amenable to treatment using laparoscopic techniques. The question of leaving a normal appendix in situ is a controversial one. Seventeen to 26% of appendices that appear normal at exploration are found to have pathologic features on histologic analysis.[80] The availability of diagnostic laparoscopy may actually lower the threshold for exploration and thus adversely impact the negative appendectomy rate.[86] Fertile women with presumed appendicitis constitute the group of patients most likely to benefit from diagnostic laparoscopy. Up to one third of these patients do not have appendicitis at exploration. In most of the patients without appendicitis, gynecologic pathology is identified.[87] A large meta-analysis demonstrated that in fertile women in whom appendectomy was deemed necessary, diagnostic laparoscopy reduced the number of unnecessary appendectomies.[64] In addition, the number of women without a final diagnosis was smaller. It appears that leaving a normal-appearing appendix in fertile women with identifiable gynecologic pathology is safe.[87]

In summary, it has not been resolved whether laparoscopic appendectomy is more effective in treating acute appendicitis than the time-proven method of open appendectomy. It does appear that laparoscopic appendectomy is effective in the management of acute appendicitis. Laparoscopic appendectomy should be considered part of the surgical armamentarium available to treat acute appendicitis. The decision on how to treat a specific patient with appendicitis should be based on surgical skill, patient characteristics, clinical scenario, and patient preference. Additional well-controlled, prospective, blinded studies are needed to determine which subsets of patients may benefit from any given approach to the treatment of appendicitis.

Natural Orifice Transluminal Endoscopic Surgery

Natural orifice transluminal endoscopic surgery (NOTES) is a new surgical procedure using flexible endoscopes in the abdominal cavity. In this procedure, access is gained by way of organs that are reached through a natural, already-existing external orifice. The hoped-for advantages associated with this method include the reduction of postoperative wound pain, shorter convalescence, avoidance of wound infection and abdominal-wall hernias, and the absence of scars. The first case of transvaginal removal of a normal appendix has recently been reported.[88] Much work remains to determine if NOTES provides any additional advantages over the laparoscopic approach to appendectomy.

Antibiotics as Definitive Therapy

Traditional management of acute appendicitis has emphasized emergent surgical management. This approach has been based on the theory that, over time, simple appendicitis will progress to perforation, with resulting increases in morbidity and mortality. As a result, a relatively high negative appendectomy rate has been accepted to avoid the possibility of progression to perforation. Recent data suggest that acute appendicitis and acute appendicitis with perforation may be separate disease entities with distinct pathophysiology. A time series analysis performed on a 25-year data set did not find a significant negative relationship between the rates of negative appendectomy and perforation.[17] A study analyzing time to surgery and perforation demonstrated that risk of rupture is minimal within 36 hours of symptom onset. Beyond this point, there is about a 5% risk

of rupture in each ensuing 12-hour period. However, in many patients the disease will have an indolent course. In one study 10 of the 18 patients who did not undergo operation for ≥6 days after their symptoms began did not experience rupture.[89]

Many acute abdominal conditions such as acute diverticulitis and acute cholecystitis are managed with urgent but not emergent surgery. Moreover, evidence from submarine personnel who develop appendicitis suggests that nonoperative management of appendicitis may be a viable treatment option. Sailors who develop appendicitis while stationed on submarines do not have access to prompt surgical care. They are successfully treated with antibiotics and fluids days to weeks after the initial attack until the ship can surface and they can be transferred to a hospital for care.[90]

A randomized study comparing antibiotic treatment with immediate appendectomy has been completed. Two hundred and fifty-two men 18 to 50 years of age with the presumptive diagnosis of appendicitis were enrolled in the study between March 1996 and June 1999. For patients randomly assigned to antibiotic therapy, if symptoms did not improve within the first 24 hours, an appendectomy was performed. Participants were evaluated after 1 week, 6 weeks, and 1 year. Acute appendicitis was found in 97% of the 124 patients randomly assigned to surgery. Six patients (5%) had perforated appendices. The complication rate in the surgery group was 14% (17 of 124). Of the 128 patients enrolled in the antibiotic group, 15 patients (12%) underwent operation within the first 24 hours due to lack of improvement in symptoms and apparent local peritonitis. At operation seven patients (5%) had perforation. The rate of recurrence within 1 year was 15% (16 patients) in the group treated with antibiotics. In five of these patients a perforated appendix was found at operation.[52] Although it initially appears from these data that the use of antibiotics alone may be reasonable therapy for acute appendicitis, there are several issues to take into account. First, this study included only men between the ages of 18 and 50 and may not have broad applicability to all patients with appendicitis, especially those populations known to have higher perforation rates. Second, the incidence of perforation was 9% in the antibiotic group when patients requiring operation in both the acute and delayed settings are considered. This compares unfavorably with the perforation rate of 5% for those patients operated on immediately. In addition, the study follow-up was only 1 year, which suggests that patients receiving only antibiotic therapy may still be at risk for the development of appendicitis. Finally, when patients are treated with antibiotics alone it is possible that diagnoses of significant pathology such as carcinoid or carcinoma may be delayed.[16] Because no laboratory test or clinical investigation can reliably distinguish patients whose appendicitis is potentially amenable to conservative treatment, surgery still remains the gold standard of care for patients with acute appendicitis.

Interval Appendectomy

The accepted approach for the treatment of appendicitis associated with a palpable or radiographically documented mass (abscess or phlegmon) is conservative therapy with interval appendectomy 6 to 10 weeks later. This technique has been quite successful and produces much lower morbidity and mortality rates than immediate appendectomy. Unfortunately, this treatment is associated with greater expense and longer hospitalization time (8 to 13 days vs. 3 to 5 days).[91]

The initial treatment consists of IV antibiotics and bowel rest. Although this therapy is generally effective, there is a 9 to 15% failure rate, with operative intervention required at 3 to 5 days after presentation. Percutaneous or operative drainage of abscesses is not considered a failure of conservative therapy.

Although the second stage of this treatment plan, interval appendectomy, has usually been carried out, the need for subsequent operation has been questioned. The major argument against interval appendectomy is that approximately 50% of patients treated conservatively never develop manifestations of appendicitis, and those who do generally can be treated nonoperatively. In addition, pathologic examination of the resected appendix shows normal findings in 20 to 50% of cases.

On the other hand, the data clearly support the need for interval appendectomy. In a prospective series, 19 of 48 patients (40%) who were successfully treated conservatively needed appendectomy at an earlier time (mean of 4.3 weeks) than the 10 weeks planned because of bouts of appendicitis.[91] Overall, the rate of late failure as a consequence of acute disease averages 20%. An additional 14% of patients either continue to have, or redevelop, right lower quadrant pain. Although the appendix may occasionally be pathologically normal, persistent periappendiceal abscesses and adhesions are found in 80% of patients. In addition, almost 50% have histologic evidence of inflammation in the organ itself. Several neoplasms also have been detected in the resected appendices, even in those of children.[16]

The timing of interval appendectomy is somewhat controversial. Appendectomy may be required as early as 3 weeks after conservative therapy. Two thirds of the cases of recurrent appendicitis occur within 2 years, and this is the outside limit. Interval appendectomy is associated with a morbidity rate of ≤3% and a hospitalization time of 1 to 3 days. The laparoscopic approach has been used and has been successful in 68% of procedures.[92] In a more recent study in children, interval appendectomy was performed successfully using the laparoscopic approach in all 35 patients.[93]

Prognosis

The mortality from appendicitis in the United States has steadily decreased from a rate of 9.9 per 100,000 in 1939 to 0.2 per 100,000 today. Among the factors responsible are advances in anesthesia, antibiotics, IV fluids, and blood products. Principal factors influencing mortality are whether rupture occurs before surgical treatment and the age of the patient. The overall mortality rate in acute appendicitis with rupture is approximately 1%. The mortality rate of appendicitis with rupture in the elderly is approximately 5%—a fivefold increase from the overall rate. Death is usually attributable to uncontrolled sepsis—peritonitis, intra-abdominal abscesses, or gram-negative septicemia. Pulmonary embolism continues to account for some deaths.

Morbidity rates parallel mortality rates and are significantly increased by rupture of the appendix and, to a lesser extent, by old age. In one report, complications occurred in 3% of patients with nonperforated appendicitis and in 47% of patients with perforations. Most of the serious early complications are septic and include abscess and wound infection. Wound infection is common but is nearly always confined to the subcutaneous tissues and responds promptly to wound drainage, which is accomplished by reopening the skin incision. Wound infection predisposes the patient to wound dehiscence. The type of incision is relevant; complete dehiscence rarely occurs in a McBurney incision.

The incidence of intra-abdominal abscess secondary to peritoneal contamination from gangrenous or perforated appendicitis has decreased markedly since the introduction of potent antibiotics. The sites of predilection for abscesses are the appendiceal fossa, pouch of Douglas, the subhepatic space, and between loops of intestine. In the latter site abscesses are usually multiple. Transrectal drainage is preferred for an abscess that bulges into the rectum.

Fecal fistula is an annoying, but not particularly dangerous, complication of appendectomy that may be caused by sloughing of the portion of the cecum inside a constricting purse-string suture; by slipping of the ligature off a tied, but not inverted, appendiceal stump; or by necrosis from an abscess encroaching on the cecum.

Intestinal obstruction, initially paralytic but sometimes progressing to mechanical obstruction, may occur with slowly resolving peritonitis with loculated abscesses and exuberant adhesion formation. Late complications are quite uncommon. Adhesive band intestinal obstruction after appendectomy does occur, but much less frequently than after pelvic surgical therapy. The incidence of inguinal hernia is three times higher in patients who have had an appendectomy. Incisional hernia is like wound dehiscence in that infection predisposes to it, it rarely occurs in a McBurney incision, and it is not uncommon in a lower right paramedian incision.[94]

CHRONIC APPENDICITIS

Whether chronic appendicitis is a true clinical entity has been questioned for many years. However, clinical data document the existence of this uncommon disease.[95] Histologic criteria have been established. Characteristically, the pain lasts longer and is less intense than that of acute appendicitis but is in the same location. There is a much lower incidence of vomiting, but anorexia and occasionally nausea, pain with motion, and malaise are characteristic. Leukocyte counts are predictably normal and CT scans are generally nondiagnostic.

At operation, surgeons can establish the diagnosis with 94% specificity and 78% sensitivity. There is an excellent correlation between clinical symptomatology, intraoperative findings, and histologic abnormalities. Laparoscopy can be used effectively in the management of this clinical entity. Appendectomy is curative. Symptoms resolve postoperatively in 82 to 93% of patients. Many of those whose symptoms are not cured or recur are ultimately diagnosed with Crohn's disease.[95]

APPENDICEAL PARASITES

A number of intestinal parasites cause appendicitis. Although *Ascaris lumbricoides* is the most common, a wide spectrum of helminths have been implicated, including *Enterobius vermicularis*, *Strongyloides stercoralis*, and *Echinococcus granulosis*. The live parasites occlude the appendiceal lumen, causing obstruction. The presence of parasites in the appendix at operation makes ligation and stapling of the appendix technically difficult. Once appendectomy has been performed and the patient has recovered, therapy with helminthicide is necessary to clear the remainder of the GI tract.

Amebiasis also can cause appendicitis. Invasion of the mucosa by trophozoites of *Entamoeba histolytica* incites a marked inflammatory process. Appendiceal involvement is a component of more generalized intestinal amebiasis. Appendectomy must be followed by appropriate antiamebic therapy (metronidazole).

INCIDENTAL APPENDECTOMY

Decisions regarding the efficacy of incidental appendectomy should be based on the epidemiology of appendicitis. The best data were published by the Centers for Disease Control and Prevention based on the period from 1979 to 1984.[11] During this period, an average of 250,000 cases of appendicitis occurred annually in the United States. The highest annual incidence of appendicitis was in patients 9 to 19 years of age (23.3 per 10,000 population). Males were more likely to develop appendicitis than females. Accordingly, the incidence during teenage years was 27.6 in males and 20.5 in females per 10,000 population per year. Beyond age 19 years, the annual incidence fell. Among those >45 years of age, the annual incidence was 6 in 10,000 males and 4 in 10,000 females. When the life table technique was used, the data identified a lifetime risk of appendicitis of 8.6% in men and 6.7% in women. Although men were more likely to develop appendicitis, the preoperative diagnosis was correct in 91.2% of men and 78.6% of women. Similarly, perforation occurred more commonly in men than in women (19.2 vs. 17.8%). In contrast to the number of cases of appendicitis, 310,000 incidental appendectomies were performed between 1979 and 1984, 62% of the total appendectomies in men and 17.7% of those in women. Based on these data, 36 incidental appendectomies had to be performed to prevent one patient from developing appendicitis.[96]

The financial aspects of the decision to perform incidental appendectomy were assessed.[97] For open appendectomy, there was a financial disincentive to perform incidental appendectomy. On an annual basis, \$20,000,000 had to be spent to save the \$6,000,000 cost of appendicitis. With the laparoscopic approach, it was cost effective to perform incidental appendectomy only in patients <25 years of age and only if the reimbursement for surgeons was 10% of the usual and customary charges. At a higher rate of reimbursement, incidental appendectomy was not cost effective in any age group.

Although incidental appendectomy is generally neither clinically nor economically appropriate, there are some special patient groups in whom it should be performed during laparotomy or laparoscopy for other indications. These include children about to undergo chemotherapy, the disabled who cannot describe symptoms or react normally to abdominal pain, patients with Crohn's disease in whom the cecum is free of macroscopic disease, and individuals who are about to travel to remote places where there is no access to medical or surgical care.[98]

Appendectomy is routinely carried out during performance of Ladd's procedure for malrotation, because displacement of the cecum into the left upper quadrant would complicate the diagnosis of subsequent appendicitis.

TUMORS

Appendiceal malignancies are extremely rare. Primary appendiceal cancer is diagnosed in 0.9 to 1.4% of appendectomy specimens.[16] These tumors are only rarely suspected preoperatively. Fewer than 50% of cases are diagnosed at operation.[99] Most series report that carcinoid is the most common appendiceal malignancy, representing >50% of the primary lesions of the appendix.[16,98,99] A review from the National Cancer Institute's Surveillance, Epidemiology, and End Results (SEER) program found the age-adjusted incidence of appendiceal malignancies to be 0.12 cases per 1,000,000 people per year.[99] Data from the SEER program identified mucinous adenocarcinoma as the most frequent histologic diagnosis (38% of total reported cases), followed by adenocarcinoma (26%), carcinoid (17%), goblet cell carcinoma (15%), and signet-ring cell carcinoma (4%).[99] Five-year survival for appendiceal malignancies varies by tumor type. Patients with carcinoid tumors have the best 5-year survival (83%), whereas those with signet-ring cell cancers have the lowest (18%).[99,100]

Carcinoid

The finding of a firm, yellow, bulbar mass in the appendix should raise the suspicion of an appendiceal carcinoid. The appendix is the most common site of GI carcinoid, followed by the small bowel and then the rectum. Carcinoid syndrome is rarely associated with appendiceal carcinoid unless widespread metastases are present, which occur in 2.9% of cases. Symptoms attributable directly to the carcinoid are rare, although the tumor can occasionally obstruct the appendiceal lumen much like a fecalith and result in acute appendicitis.[16,100,101]

The majority of carcinoids are located in the tip of the appendix. Malignant potential is related to size, with tumors <1 cm rarely resulting in extension outside of the appendix or adjacent to the mass. The mean tumor size for carcinoids is 2.5 cm.[100] Carcinoid tumors usually present with localized disease (64%). Treatment for tumors ≤1 cm is appendectomy. For tumors larger than 1 to 2 cm located at the base or with lymph node metastases, right hemicolectomy is indicated (Fig. 30-9). Despite these recommendations, SEER data indicate that proper surgery for carcinoids is not performed at least 28% of the time.[100]

Adenocarcinoma

Primary adenocarcinoma of the appendix is a rare neoplasm with three major histologic subtypes: mucinous adenocarcinoma, colonic adenocarcinoma, and adenocarcinoid.[99] The most common mode of presentation for appendiceal carcinoma is that of acute appendicitis. Patients also may present with ascites or a palpable mass, or the neoplasm may be discovered during an operative procedure for an

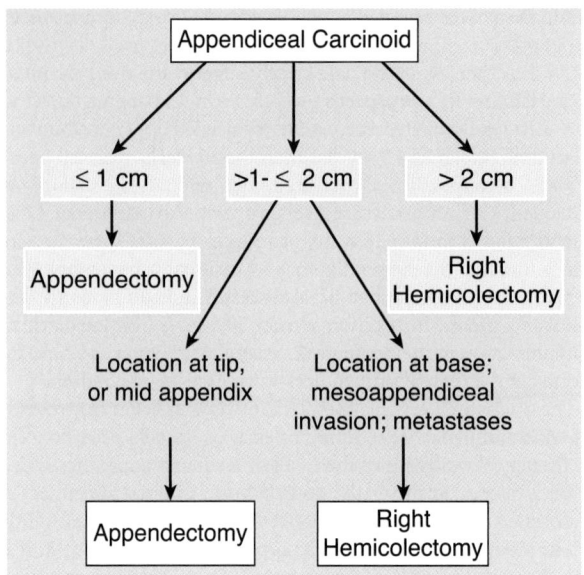

FIG. 30-9. Algorithm for the management of patients with appendiceal carcinoid.

unrelated cause. The recommended treatment for all patients with adenocarcinoma of the appendix is a formal right hemicolectomy. Appendiceal adenocarcinomas have a propensity for early perforation, although they are not clearly associated with a worsened prognosis.[101] Overall 5-year survival is 55% and varies with stage and grade. Patients with appendiceal adenocarcinoma are at significant risk for both synchronous and metachronous neoplasms, approximately half of which will originate from the GI tract.[99]

Mucocele

A mucocele of the appendix is an obstructive dilatation by intraluminal accumulation of mucoid material. Mucoceles may be caused by one of four processes: retention cysts, mucosal hyperplasia, cystadenomas, and cystadenocarcinomas. The clinical presentation of a mucocele is nonspecific, and often it is an incidental finding at operation for acute appendicitis. An intact mucocele presents no future risk for the patient; however, the opposite is true if the mucocele has ruptured and epithelial cells have escaped into the peritoneal cavity. As a result, when a mucocele is visualized at the time of laparoscopic examination, conversion to open laparotomy is recommended. Conversion from a laparoscopic approach to a laparotomy ensures that a benign process will not be converted to a malignant one through mucocele rupture. In addition, laparotomy allows for thorough abdominal exploration to rule out the presence of mucoid fluid accumulations.[99]

The presence of a mucocele of the appendix does not mandate performance of a right hemicolectomy. The principles of surgery include resection of the appendix, wide resection of the mesoappendix to include all the appendiceal lymph nodes, collection and cytologic examination of all intraperitoneal mucus, and careful inspection of the base of the appendix. Right hemicolectomy, or preferably cecectomy, is reserved for patients with a positive margin at the base of the appendix or positive periappendiceal lymph nodes. Recently, a more aggressive approach to ruptured appendiceal neoplasms has been advocated. This approach includes a thorough but minimally aggressive approach at initial laparotomy, as described earlier, with subsequent referral to a specialized center for consideration of re-exploration and hyperthermic intraperitoneal chemotherapy.[101]

Pseudomyxoma Peritonei

Pseudomyxoma peritonei is a rare condition in which diffuse collections of gelatinous fluid are associated with mucinous implants on peritoneal surfaces and omentum. Pseudomyxoma is two to three times more common in females than in males. Recent immunocytologic and molecular studies suggest that the appendix is the site of origin for the overwhelming majority of cases of pseudomyxoma. Pseudomyxoma is invariably caused by neoplastic mucus-secreting cells within the peritoneum. These cells may be difficult to classify as malignant because they may be sparse, widely scattered, and have a low-grade cytologic appearance. Patients with pseudomyxoma usually present with abdominal pain, distention, or a mass. Primary pseudomyxoma usually does not cause abdominal organ dysfunction. However, ureteral obstruction and obstruction of venous return can be seen.[102] Pseudomyxoma is a disease that progresses slowly and in which recurrences may take years to develop or become symptomatic.[102] In a series from the Mayo Clinic, 76% of patients developed recurrences within the abdomen.[103] Lymph node metastasis and distant metastasis are uncommon.

The use of imaging before surgery is advantageous to plan surgery. CT scanning is the preferred imaging modality. At surgery a variable volume of mucinous ascites is found together with tumor deposits involving the right hemidiaphragm, right retrohepatic space, left paracolic gutter, ligament of Treitz, and the ovaries in women. Peritoneal surfaces of the bowel are usually free of tumor. Thorough surgical debulking is the mainstay of treatment. All gross disease and the omentum should be removed. If not done previously, appendectomy is routinely performed. Hysterectomy with bilateral salpingo-oophorectomy is performed in women. Survival is better in patients who undergo R0 or R1 resection than in patients who undergo R2 resection (visible gross disease remaining).[104] *Because 5-year survival of mucinous appendiceal neoplasms is only 30%,* adjuvant intraperitoneal hyperthermic chemotherapy is advocated as a standard adjunct to radical cytoreductive surgery.[105] Cytoreductive surgery with intraperitoneal hyperthermic chemotherapy is a long, tedious procedure with operative times of 300 to 1020 minutes reported. In addition, morbidity (38%) and mortality (6%) are high. Cytoreductive surgery with intraperitoneal hyperthermic chemotherapy is associated with a 5-year survival of between 53 and 78%. Survival is associated with initial patient performance status.[104–106]

Any recurrence should be investigated completely. Recurrences are usually treated by additional surgery. It is important to note that surgery for recurrent disease is usually difficult and is associated with an increased incidence of unintentional enterotomies, anastomotic leaks, and fistulas.[102,103]

Lymphoma

Lymphoma of the appendix is extremely uncommon. The GI tract is the most frequently involved extranodal site for non-Hodgkin's lymphoma.[107] Other types of appendiceal lymphoma, such as Burkitt's, as well as leukemia, have also been reported.[108] Primary lymphoma of the appendix accounts for 1 to 3% of GI lymphomas. Appendiceal lymphoma usually presents as acute appendicitis and is rarely suspected preoperatively. Findings on CT scan of an appendiceal diameter ≥2.5 cm or surrounding soft tissue thickening should prompt suspicion of an appendiceal lymphoma. The management of appendiceal lymphoma confined to the appendix is appendectomy. Right hemicolectomy is indicated if tumor extends beyond the appendix onto the cecum or mesentery. A postoperative staging workup is indicated before initiating adjuvant therapy. Adjuvant therapy is not indicated for lymphoma confined to the appendix.[108,109]

REFERENCES

Entries highlighted in bright blue are key references.

1. Geboes K: Appendiceal function and dysfunction: What are the implications for inflammatory bowel disease? *Nat Clin Pract Gastroenterol Hepatol* 2:338, 2005.
2. Ajmani ML, Ajmani K: The position, length and arterial supply of vermiform appendix. *Anat Anz* 153:369, 1983.
3. Fitz RH: Persistent omphalo-mesenteric remains: Their importance in the causation of intestinal duplication, cyst formation, and obstruction. *Am J Med Sci* 88:30, 1884.
4. Radford-Smith GL, Edwards JE, Purdie DM, et al. Protective role of appendicectomy on onset and severity of ulcerative colitis and Crohn's disease. *Gut* 51:808, 2002.
5. Ellis H: Appendix, in Schwartz SI (ed): *Maingot's Abdominal Operations,* 8th ed, vol. 2. Norwalk, Conn: Appleton-Century-Crofts, 1985, p 1255.
6. Lewis F: Appendix, in Davis JH (ed): *Clinical Surgery,* 1st ed, vol. 1. St. Louis, Mo: Mosby, 1987, p 1581.
7. Fitz RH: Perforating inflammation of the vermiform appendix: With special reference to its early diagnosis and treatment. *Trans Assoc Am Physicians* 1:107, 1886.
8. McBurney C: Experience with early operative interference in cases of disease of the vermiform appendix. *N Y State Med J* 50:676, 1889.
9. McBurney C: The incision made in the abdominal wall in cases of appendicitis. *Ann Surg* 20:38, 1894.
10. Semm K: Endoscopic appendectomy. *Endoscopy* 15:59, 1983.
11. Addiss DG, Shaffer N, Fowler BS, et al: The epidemiology of appendicitis and appendectomy in the United States. *Am J Epidemiol* 132:910, 1990.
12. Hale DA, Molloy M, Pearl RH, et al: Appendectomy: A contemporary appraisal. *Ann Surg* 225:252, 1997.
13. Flum DR, Morris A, Koepsell T, et al: Has misdiagnosis of appendicitis decreased over time? A population-based analysis. *JAMA* 286:1748, 2001.
14. Flum DR, Koepsell T: The clinical and economic correlates of misdiagnosed appendicitis: Nationwide analysis. *Arch Surg* 137:799, 2002.
15. Burkitt DP: The aetiology of appendicitis. *Br J Surg* 58:695, 1971.
16. Marudanayagam R, Williams GT, Rees BI: Review of the pathological results of 2660 appendicectomy specimens. *J Gastroenterol* 41:745, 2006.
17. Livingston EH, Woodward WA, Sarosi GA, et al: Disconnect between incidence of nonperforated and perforated appendicitis: Implications for pathophysiology and management. *Ann Surg* 245:886, 2007.
18. Rautio M, Saxen H, Siitonen A, et al: Bacteriology of histopathologically defined appendicitis in children. *Pediatr Infect Dis J* 19:1078, 2000.
19. Allo MD, Bennion RS, Kathir K, et al: Ticarcillin/clavulanate versus imipenem/cilastatin for the treatment of infections associated with gangrenous and perforated appendicitis. *Am Surg* 65:99, 1999.
20. Soffer D, Zait S, Klausner J, et al: Peritoneal cultures and antibiotic treatment in patients with perforated appendicitis. *Eur J Surg* 167:214, 2001.
21. Kokoska ER, Silen ML, Tracy TF Jr., et al: The impact of intraoperative culture on treatment and outcome in children with perforated appendicitis. *J Pediatr Surg* 34:749, 1999.
22. Bilik R, Burnweit C, Shandling B: Is abdominal cavity culture of any value in appendicitis? *Am J Surg* 175:267, 1998.
23. Andersen BR, Kallehave FL, Andersen HK: Antibiotics versus placebo for prevention of postoperative infection after appendicectomy. *Cochrane Database Syst Rev* Issue 3:CD001439, 2005.
24. Mazuski JE, Sawyer RG, Nathens AB, et al: The Surgical Infection Society guidelines on antimicrobial therapy for intra-abdominal infections: An executive summary. *Surg Infect* 3:161, 2002.
25. Berry J, Malt RA: Appendicitis near its centenary. *Ann Surg* 200:567, 1984.
26. Bower RJ, Bell MJ, Ternberg JL: Diagnostic value of the white blood count and neutrophil percentage in the evaluation of abdominal pain in children. *Surg Gynecol Obstet* 152:424, 1981.
27. Smith DE, Kirchmer NA, Stewart DR: Use of the barium enema in the diagnosis of acute appendicitis and its complications. *Am J Surg* 138:829, 1979.
28. Douglas CD, Macpherson NE, Davidson PM, et al: Randomised controlled trial of ultrasonography in diagnosis of acute appendicitis, incorporating the Alvarado score. *Br Med J* 321:1, 2000.
29. Franke C, Bohner H, Yang Q, et al: Ultrasonography for diagnosis of acute appendicitis: Results of a prospective multicenter trial. *World J Surg* 23:141, 1999.
30. Kaiser S, Frenckner B, Jorulf HK: Suspected appendicitis in children: US and CT—A prospective randomized study. *Radiology* 223:633, 2002.
31. Jeffrey RB, Jain KA, Nghiem HV: Sonographic diagnosis of acute appendicitis: Interpretive pitfalls. *AJR Am J Roentgenol* 162:55, 1994.
32. Puig S, Hormann M, Rebhandl W, et al: US as a primary diagnostic tool in relation to negative appendectomy: Six years' experience. *Radiology* 226:101, 2003.

33. Rettenbacher T, Hollerweger A, Gritzmann N, et al: Appendicitis: Should diagnostic imaging be performed if the clinical presentation is highly suggestive of the disease? *Gastroenterology* 123:992, 2002.

34. Funaki B, Grosskreutz SR, Funaki CN: Using unenhanced helical CT with enteric contrast material for suspected appendicitis in patients treated at a community hospital. *AJR Am J Roentgenol* 171:997, 1998.

35. Raman SS, Lu DSK, Kadell BM, et al: Accuracy of nonfocused helical CT for the diagnosis of acute appendicitis: A 5-year review. *AJR Am J Roentgenol* 178:1319, 2002.

36. Stroman DL, Bayouth CV, Kuhn JA, et al: The role of computed tomography in the diagnosis of acute appendicitis. *Am J Surg* 178:485, 1999.

37. Weyant MJ, Eachempati SR, Maluccio MA, et al: Interpretation of computed tomography does not correlate with laboratory or pathologic findings in surgically confirmed acute appendicitis. *Surgery* 128:145, 2000.

38. Fuchs JR, Schlamberg JS, Shortsleeve MJ, et al: Impact of abdominal CT imaging on the management of appendicitis: An update. *J Surg Res* 106:131, 2002.

39. Walker S, Haun W, Clark J, et al: The value of limited computed tomography with rectal contrast in the diagnosis of acute appendicitis. *Am J Surg* 180:450, 2000.

40. Ujiki MB, Murayama KM, Cribbins AJ, et al: CT scan in the management of acute appendicitis. *J Surg Res* 105:119, 2002.

41. Applegate KE, Sivit CJ, Salvator AE, et al: Effect of cross-sectional imaging on negative appendectomy and perforation rates in children. *Radiology* 220:103, 2001.

42. Wise SW, Labuski MR, Kasales CJ, et al: Comparative assessment of CT and sonographic techniques for appendiceal imaging. *AJR Am J Roentgenol* 176:933, 2001.

43. Wilson EB, Cole JC, Nipper ML, et al: Computed tomography and ultrasonography in the diagnosis of appendicitis: When are they indicated? *Arch Surg* 136:670, 2001.

44. Rao PM, Rhea JT, Rattner DW, et al: Introduction of appendiceal CT: Impact on negative appendectomy and appendiceal perforation rates. *Ann Surg* 229:344, 1999.

45. Rao PM, Rhea JT, Novelline RA, et al: Effect of computed tomography of the appendix on treatment of patients and use of hospital resources. *N Engl J Med* 338:141, 1998.

46. Morris KT, Kavanagh M, Hansen P, et al: The rational use of computed tomography scans in the diagnosis of appendicitis. *Am J Surg* 183:547, 2002.

47. Lee SL, Walsh AJ, Ho HS: Computed tomography and ultrasonography do not improve and may delay the diagnosis and treatment of acute appendicitis. *Arch Surg* 136:556, 2001.

48. Garcia Pena BM, Taylor GA, Fishman SJ, et al: Effect of an imaging protocol on clinical outcomes among pediatric patients with appendicitis. *Pediatrics* 110:1088, 2002.

49. Alvarado A: A practical score for the early diagnosis of acute appendicitis. *Ann Emerg Med* 15:557, 1986.

50. Paulson EK, Kalady MF, Pappas TN: Clinical practice. Suspected appendicitis. *N Engl J Med* 348:236, 2003.

51. Owings MF, Kozak LJ: *Ambulatory and Inpatient Procedures in the United States, 1996.* National Center for Health Statistics Series 13, No. 139. Hyattsville, Md: Department of Health and Human Services, Centers for Disease Control and Prevention, National Center for Health Statistics, 2004.

52. Styrud J, Eriksson S, Nilsson I, et al: Appendectomy versus antibiotic treatment in acute appendicitis: A prospective multicenter randomized controlled trial. *World J Surg* 30:1033, 2006.

53. Tingstedt B, Bexe-Lindskog E, Ekelund M, et al: Management of appendiceal masses. *Eur J Surg* 168:579, 2002.

54. Willemsen PJ, Hoorntje LE, Eddes EH, et al: The need for interval appendectomy after resolution of an appendiceal mass questioned. *Dig Surg* 19:216, 2002.

55. Haller JA Jr., Shaker IJ, Donahoo JS, et al: Peritoneal drainage versus non-drainage for generalized peritonitis from ruptured appendicitis in children: A prospective study. *Ann Surg* 177:595, 1973.

56. Bongard F, Landers DV, Lewis F: Differential diagnosis of appendicitis and pelvic inflammatory disease. A prospective analysis. *Am J Surg* 150:90, 1985.

57. Jepsen OB, Korner B, Lauritsen KB, et al: *Yersinia enterocolitica* infection in patients with acute surgical abdominal disease. A prospective study. *Scand J Infect Dis* 8:189, 1976.

58. Knight PJ, Vassy LE: Specific diseases mimicking appendicitis in childhood. *Arch Surg* 116:744, 1981.

59. McDonald JC: Nonspecific mesenteric lymphadenitis: Collective review. *Surg Gynecol Obstet* 116:409, 1963.

60. Morrison JD: *Yersinia* and viruses in acute non-specific abdominal pain and appendicitis. *Br J Surg* 68:284, 1981.

61. Droegemueller W: Upper genital tract infections, in Herbst AL, Mishell DR, Stenchever MW, et al (eds): *Comprehensive Gynecology*, 2nd ed. St. Louis, Mo: Mosby–Year Book, 1992, p 691.

62. Bundy DG, Byerley JS, Liles EA, et al: Does this child have appendicitis? *JAMA* 298:438, 2007.

63. Colvin JM, Bachur R, Kharbanda A: The presentation of appendicitis in preadolescent children. *Pediatr Emerg Care* 23:849, 2007.

64. Sauerland S, Lefering R, Neugebauer EA: Laparoscopic versus open surgery for suspected appendicitis. *Cochrane Database Syst Rev* Issue 4:CD001546, 2004.

65. Sheu B-F, Chiu T-E, Chen J-C, et al: Risk factors associated with perforated appendicitis in elderly patients presenting with signs and symptoms of acute appendicitis. *ANZ J Surg* 77:662, 2007.

66. Young Y-R, Chiu T-F, Chen J-C, et al: Acute appendicitis in the octogenarians and beyond: A comparison with younger geriatric patients. *Am J Med Sci* 334:255, 2007.

67. Harrell AG, Lincourt AE, Novitsky YW, et al: Advantages of laparoscopic appendectomy in the elderly. *Am Surg* 72:474, 2006.

68. Andersen B, Nielsen TF: Appendicitis in pregnancy: Diagnosis, management and complications. *Acta Obstet Gynecol Scand* 78:758, 1999.

69. McGory ML, Zingmond DS, Tillou A, et al: Negative appendectomy in pregnant women is associated with a substantial risk of fetal loss. *J Am Coll Surg* 205:534, 2007.

70. Bree RL, Ralls PW, Bafle DM, et al: Evaluation of patients with acute right upper quadrant pain. American College of Radiology. ACR Appropriateness Criteria. *Radiology* 215 Suppl:153, 2000.

71. Bailey LE, Finley RK Jr., Miller SF, et al: Acute appendicitis during pregnancy. *Am Surg* 52:218, 1986.

72. Flum DR, Steinberg SD, Sarkis AY, et al: Appendicitis in patients with acquired immunodeficiency syndrome. *J Am Coll Surg* 184:481, 1997.

73. Mueller GP, Williams RA: Surgical infections in AIDS patients. *Am J Surg* 169(5A Suppl):34S, 1995.

74. Bova R, Meagher A: Appendicitis in HIV-positive patients. *Aust N Z J Surg* 68:337, 1998.

75. Lowy AM, Barie PS: Laparotomy in patients infected with human immunodeficiency virus: Indications and outcome. *Br J Surg* 81:942, 1994.

76. Nadler EP, Gaines BA: The Surgical Infection Society guidelines on antimicrobial therapy for children with appendicitis. *Surg Infect (Larchmt)* 9:75, 2008.

77. Golub R, Siddiqui F, Pohl D: Laparoscopic versus open appendectomy: A meta-analysis. *J Am Coll Surg* 186:545, 1998.

78. Hunter JG: Advanced laparoscopic surgery. *Am J Surg* 173:14, 1997.

79. Scott-Conner CE: Laparoscopic gastrointestinal surgery. *Med Clin North Am* 86:1401, 2002.

80. Fingerhut A, Millat B, Borrie F: Laparoscopic versus open appendectomy: Time to decide. *World J Surg* 23:835, 1999.

81. Hunter JG: Clinical trials and the development of laparoscopic surgery. *Surg Endosc* 15:1, 2001.

82. McCall JL, Sharples K, Jadallah F: Systematic review of randomized controlled trials comparing laparoscopic with open appendicectomy. *Br J Surg* 84:1045, 1997.

83. Ortega AE, Hunter JG, Peters JH, et al: A prospective, randomized comparison of laparoscopic appendectomy with open appendectomy. Laparoscopic Appendectomy Study Group. *Am J Surg* 169:208, 1995.

84. Pedersen AG, Petersen OB, Wara P, et al: Randomized clinical trial of laparoscopic versus open appendicectomy. *Br J Surg* 88:200, 2001.

85. Corneille MG, Steigelman MB, Myers, JG, et al: Laparoscopic appendectomy is superior to open appendectomy in obese patients. *Am J Surg* 194:877, 2007.

86. McGreevy JM, Finlayson SR, Alvarado R, et al: Laparoscopy may be lowering the threshold to operate on patients with suspected appendicitis. *Surg Endosc* 16:1046, 2002.

87. Borgstein PJ, Gordijn RV, Eijsbouts QA, et al: Acute appendicitis—a clear-cut case in men, a guessing game in young women. A prospective study on the role of laparoscopy. *Surg Endosc* 11:923, 1997.

88. Bernhardt J, Gerber B, Schober H-C, et al: NOTES—case report of a unidirectional flexible appendectomy. *Int J Colorectal Dis* 23:547, 2008.

89. Bickell NA, Aufses AA Jr., Rojas M, et al: How time affects the risk of rupture in appendicitis. *J Am Coll Surg* 202:401, 2006.

90. Campbell MR, Johnston, SL III, Marshburn T, et al: Nonoperative treatment of suspected appendicitis in remote medical care environments: Implications for future spaceflight medical care. *J Am Coll Surg* 198:822, 2004.

91. Samuel M, Hosie G, Holmes K: Prospective evaluation of nonsurgical versus surgical management of appendiceal mass. *J Pediatr Surg* 37:882, 2002.

92. Yamini D, Vargas H, Klein S, et al: Perforated appendicitis: Is it truly a surgical urgency? *Am Surg* 64:970, 1998.

93. Owen A, Moore O, Marven S, et al: Interval laparoscopic appendectomy in children. *J Laparoendosc Adv Surg Tech A* 16:308, 2006.

94. Cooperman M: Complications of appendectomy. *Surg Clin North Am* 63:1233, 1983.

95. Mussack T, Schmidbauer S, Nerlich A, et al: Chronic appendicitis as an independent clinical entity. *Chirurg* 73:710, 2002.

96. Wang HT, Sax HC: Incidental appendectomy in the era of managed care and laparoscopy. *J Am Coll Surg* 192:182, 2001.

97. Sugimoto T, Edwards D: Incidence and costs of incidental appendectomy as a preventive measure. *Am J Public Health* 77:471, 1987.

98. Fisher KS, Ross DS: Guidelines for therapeutic decision in incidental appendectomy. *Surg Gynecol Obstet* 171:95, 1990.

99. McCusker ME, Cote TR, Clegg LX, et al: Primary malignant neoplasms of the appendix: A population-based study from the Surveillance, Epidemiology and End Results program, 1973–1998. *Cancer* 94:3307, 2002.

100. McGory ML, Maggard MA, Kang H, et al: Malignancies of the appendix: Beyond case series reports. *Dis Colon Rectum* 48:2264, 2005.

101. Dhage-Ivatury S, Sugarbaker PH: Update on the surgical approach to mucocele of the appendix. *J Am Coll Surg* 202:680, 2006.

102. Hinson FL, Ambrose NS: Pseudomyxoma peritonei. *Br J Surg* 85:1332, 1998.

103. Gough DB, Donohue JH, Schutt AJ, et al: Pseudomyxoma peritonei. Long-term patient survival with an aggressive regional approach. *Ann Surg* 219:112, 1994.

104. Stewart JH IV, Shen P, Russell GB, et al: Appendiceal neoplasms with peritoneal dissemination: Outcomes after cytoreductive surgery and intraperitoneal hyperthermic chemotherapy. *Ann Surg Oncol* 13:624, 2006.

105. Sugarbaker PH: New standard of care for appendiceal epithelial neoplasms and pseudomyxoma peritonei syndrome? *Lancet Oncol* 7:69, 2006.

106. McQuellon RP, Russell GB, Shen P, et al: Survival and health outcomes after cytoreductive surgery with intraperitoneal hyperthermic chemotherapy for disseminated peritoneal cancer of appendiceal origin. *Ann Surg Oncol* 15:125, 2008.

107. Crump M, Gospodarowicz M, Shepherd FA: Lymphoma of the gastrointestinal tract. *Semin Oncol* 26:324, 1999.

108. Pickhardt PJ, Levy AD, Rohrmann CA Jr., et al: Non-Hodgkin's lymphoma of the appendix: Clinical and CT findings with pathologic correlation. *AJR Am J Roentgenol* 178:1123, 2002.

109. Muller G, Dargent JL, Duwel V, et al: Leukaemia and lymphoma of the appendix presenting as acute appendicitis or acute abdomen. Four case reports with a review of the literature. *J Cancer Res Clin Oncol* 123:560, 1997.

CHAPTER 30 The Appendix

CHAPTER 31

Liver

David A. Geller, John A. Goss, and Allan Tsung

HISTORY OF LIVER SURGERY

The ancient Greek myth of Prometheus reminds us that the liver is the only organ that regenerates. According to Greek mythology, Zeus was furious with the titan Prometheus because he gave fire to the mortals. In return, Zeus chained Prometheus to Mount Caucasus and sent his giant eagle to eat his liver during the day, only to have it regenerate at night. Although this is an exaggeration, the principles are correct that after hepatic resection, the remnant liver will hypertrophy over weeks to months to regain most of its original liver mass. It is interesting to note that the ancient Greeks seem to have been aware of this fact, because the Greek word for the liver, *hēpar*, derives from the verb *hēpaomai*, which means "mend" or "repair." Hence *hēpar* roughly translates as "repairable."[1] The importance of the liver dates back to even biblical times, for the Babylonians (c. 2000 B.C.) considered the liver to be the seat of the soul. There are scattered reports of liver surgery for battlefield injuries, but the first recorded elective hepatic resection was done in 1888 in Germany by Langenbuch. There followed reports of liver resections in the United States (Tiffany, 1890) and Europe (Lucke, 1891), as well as the first large series of hepatic resections by Keen in 1899.[2,3] In 1908, Pringle described in *Annals of Surgery* the "arrest of hepatic hemorrhage due to trauma" by compression of the porta hepatis, a maneuver that now bears his name.[4] Possibly due to the potential for massive hemorrhage during liver surgery, very little progress in surgical techniques was recorded for the next half-century. Work by Rex, Cantlie, and others laid the groundwork for experimental and clinical reports in the 1950s by Couinaud, Hjortsjo, Healey, Lortat-Jacob, and Starzl.[5,6] These seminal contributions paved the way for the modern era of hepatic resection surgery.

LIVER ANATOMY

The liver is the largest organ in the body, weighing approximately 1500 g. It sits in the right upper abdominal cavity beneath the diaphragm and is protected by the rib cage. It is reddish brown and is surrounded by a fibrous sheath known as *Glisson's capsule*. The liver is held in place by several ligaments (Fig. 31-1). The round ligament is the remnant of the obliterated umbilical vein and enters the left liver hilum at the front edge of the falciform ligament. The falciform ligament separates the left lateral and left medial segments along the umbilical fissure and anchors the liver to the anterior abdominal wall. Deep in the plane between the caudate lobe and the left lateral segment is the fibrous ligamentum venosum, which is the obliterated ductus venosus and is covered by the plate of Arantius. The left and right triangular ligaments secure the two sides of the liver to the diaphragm. Extending from the triangular ligaments anteriorly on the liver are the coronary ligaments. The right coronary ligament also extends from the right undersurface of the liver to the peritoneum overlying the right kidney, thereby anchoring the

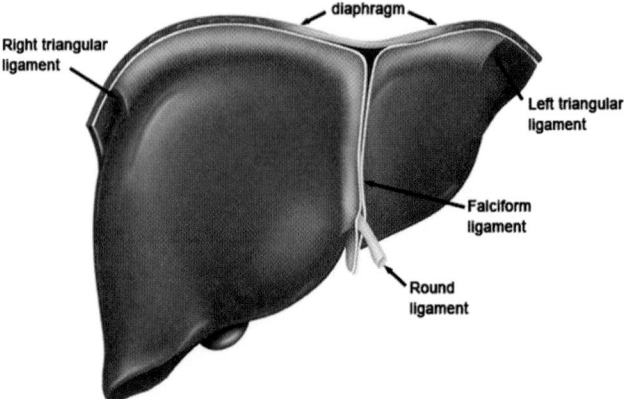

FIG. 31-1. Hepatic ligaments suspending the liver to the diaphragm and anterior abdominal wall.

liver to the right retroperitoneum. These ligaments (round, falciform, triangular, and coronary) can be divided in a bloodless plane to fully mobilize the liver to facilitate hepatic resection. Centrally and just to the left of the gallbladder fossa, the liver attaches via the hepatoduodenal and the gastrohepatic ligaments (Fig. 31-2). The hepatoduodenal ligament is known as the *porta hepatis* and contains the common bile duct, the hepatic artery, and the portal vein. From the right side and deep (dorsal) to the porta hepatis is the foramen of Winslow, also known as the *epiploic foramen* (see Fig. 31-2). This passage connects directly to the lesser sac and allows complete vascular inflow control to the liver when the hepatoduodenal ligament is clamped using the Pringle maneuver.

Segmental Anatomy

The liver is grossly separated into the right and left lobes by the plane from the gallbladder fossa to the inferior vena cava (IVC), known as *Cantlie's line.*[5] The right lobe typically accounts for 60 to 70% of the liver mass, with the left lobe (and caudate lobe) making up the remainder. The caudate lobe lies to the left and anterior of the IVC and contains three subsegments: the Spiegel lobe, the paracaval portion, and the caudate process.[7] The falciform ligament does not separate the right and left lobes, but rather it divides the left lateral segment from the left medial segment. The left lateral and left medial segments also are referred to as *sections* as defined in the Brisbane 2000 terminology, which is outlined later in the section "Hepatic Resection Techniques." A significant advance in our understanding of liver anatomy came from the cast work studies of the French surgeon and anatomist Couinaud in the early 1950s. Couinaud divided the liver into eight segments, numbering them in a clockwise direction beginning with the caudate lobe as segment I.[6] Segments II

and III comprise the left lateral segment, and segment IV is the left medial segment (Fig. 31-3). Thus, the left lobe is made up of the left lateral segment (Couinaud's segments II and III) and the left medial segment (segment IV). Segment IV can be subdivided into segment IVB and segment IVA. Segment IVA is cephalad and just below the diaphragm, spanning from segment VIII to the falciform ligament adjacent to segment II. Segment IVB is caudad and adjacent to the gallbladder fossa. Many anatomy textbooks also refer to segment IV as the *quadrate lobe*. *Quadrate lobe* is an outdated term, and the preferred term is *segment IV* or *left medial segment*. Most surgeons

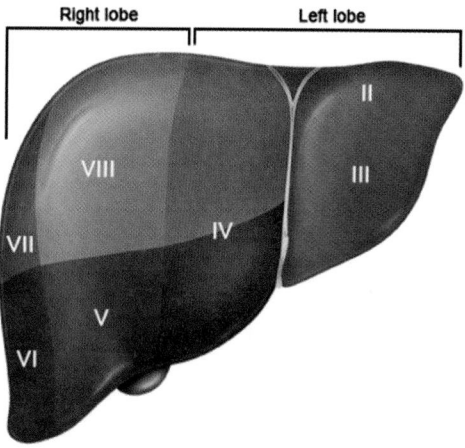

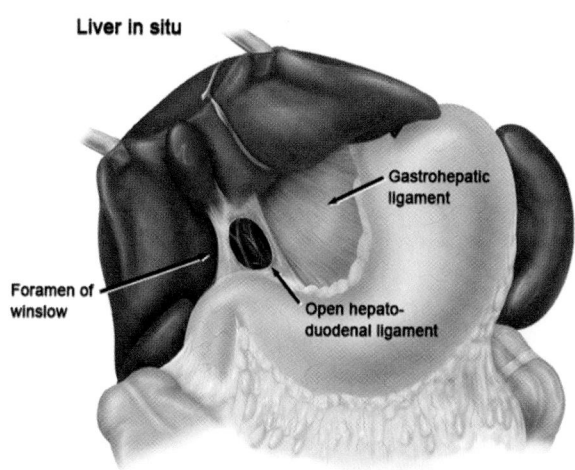

FIG. 31-2. In situ liver hilar anatomy with hepatoduodenal and gastrohepatic ligaments. Foramen of Winslow is depicted.

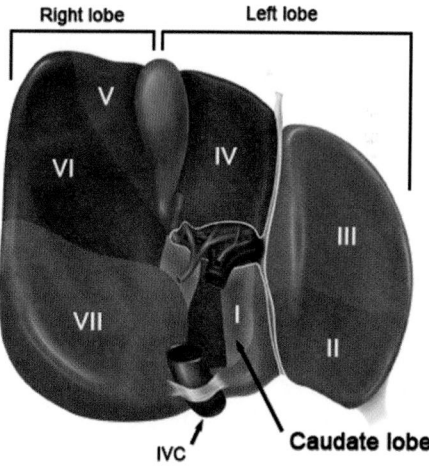

FIG. 31-3. Couinaud's liver segments (I through VIII) numbered in a clockwise manner. The left lobe includes segments II to IV, the right lobe includes segments V to VIII, and the caudate lobe is segment I. IVC = inferior vena cava.

KEY POINTS

1. Understand extrahepatic and intrahepatic liver anatomy and physiology.

2. Understand hepatic molecular signaling pathways.

3. Know the features of acute liver failure and cirrhosis, along with treatment options.

4. Formulate a plan for the work-up of an incidental liver lesion.

5. Understand the current treatment options for primary and metastatic liver cancer.

6. Describe the nomenclature and steps in performing an anatomic right or left hepatic resection.

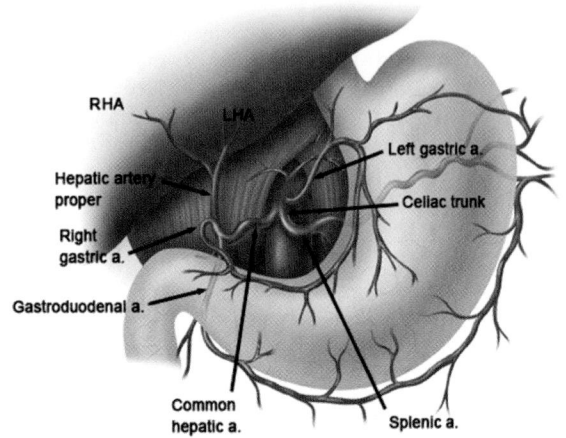

FIG. 31-4. Arterial anatomy of the upper abdomen and liver, including the celiac trunk and hepatic artery branches. a. = artery; LHA = left hepatic artery; RHA = right hepatic artery.

still refer to segment I as the *caudate lobe*, rather than segment I. The right lobe is comprised of segments V, VI, VII, and VIII, with segments V and VIII making up the right anterior lobe, and segments VI and VII the right posterior lobe.

Additional functional anatomy was highlighted by Bismuth based on the distribution of the hepatic veins. The three hepatic veins run in corresponding scissura (fissures) and divide the liver into four sectors.[8] The right hepatic vein runs along the right scissura and separates the right posterolateral sector from the right anterolateral sector. The main scissura contains the middle hepatic vein and separates the right

and left livers. The left scissura contains the course of the left hepatic vein and separates the left posterior and left anterior sectors. Although many other investigators contributed to the description of liver anatomy, it was clearly the work of Couinaud that provided the most detailed understanding of segmental liver anatomy. Couinaud devoted decades to understanding the anatomy of the liver—a PubMed search of "Couinaud C" and "liver" yields 72 publications.

Hepatic Artery

The liver has a dual blood supply consisting of the hepatic artery and the portal vein. The hepatic artery delivers approximately 25% of the blood supply, and the portal vein approximately 75%. The hepatic artery arises from the celiac axis (trunk), which gives off the left gastric, splenic, and common hepatic arteries (Fig. 31-4). The common hepatic artery then divides into the gastroduodenal artery and the hepatic artery proper. The right gastric artery typically originates off of the hepatic artery proper, but this is variable. The hepatic artery proper divides into the right and left hepatic arteries. This "classic" or standard arterial anatomy is present in only approximately 75% of cases, with the remaining 25% having variable anatomy. It is critical to understand the arterial (and biliary) anatomic variants to avoid surgical complications when operating on the liver, gallbladder, pancreas, or adjacent organs.

The most common hepatic arterial variants are shown (Fig. 31-5). The right hepatic artery is replaced coming off the superior mesenteric artery (SMA) 18 to 22% of the time. When there is a replacement or accessory right hepatic artery, it traverses posterior to the portal vein and then takes up a right lateral position before diving into the liver parenchyma. This can be recognized visually on a preoperative computed tomographic (CT) or magnetic resonance imaging (MRI) scan, and confirmed by palpation in the hilum where a separate right posterior pulsation is felt distinct from that of the hepatic artery proper that lies anteriorly in the hepatoduodenal ligament to the left

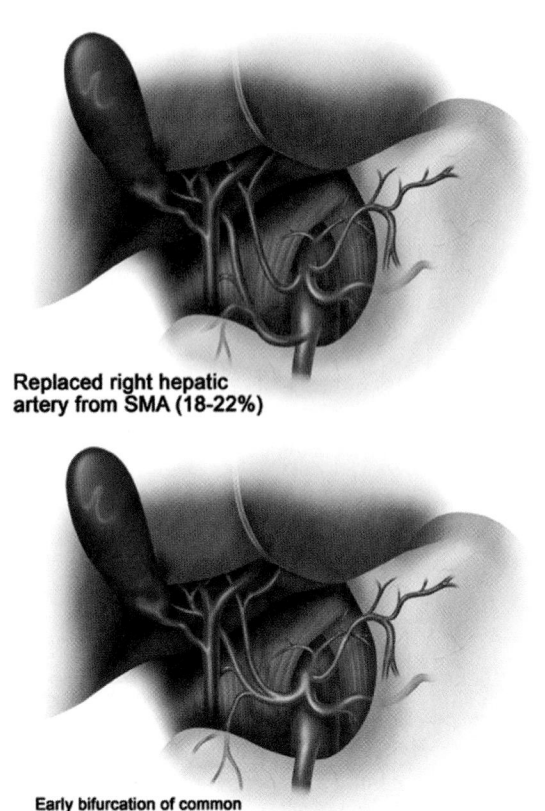

Replaced right hepatic artery from SMA (18-22%)

Early bifurcation of common hepatic artery (1-2%)

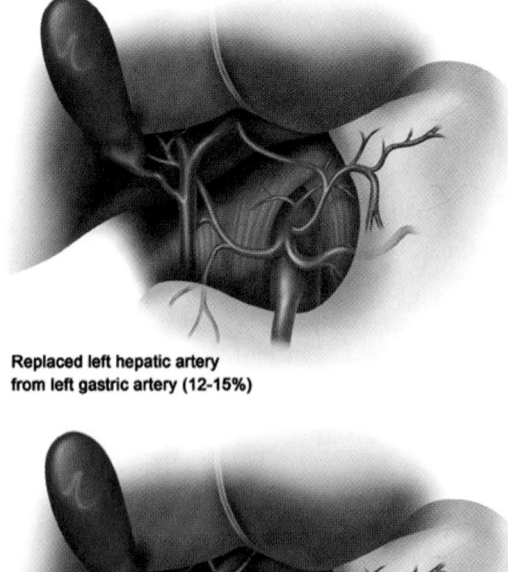

Replaced left hepatic artery from left gastric artery (12-15%)

Completely replaced common hepatic artery from SMA (1-2%)

FIG. 31-5. Common hepatic artery anatomic variants. SMA = superior mesenteric artery.

of the common bile duct. A replacement (or accessory) left hepatic artery comes off of the left gastric artery in 12 to 15% of cases and runs obliquely in the gastrohepatic ligament anterior to the caudate lobe before entering the hilar plate at the base of the umbilical fissure. Other less common variants (approximately 2% each) are an early bifurcation of the left and right hepatic arteries, as well as a completely replaced common hepatic artery coming off the SMA (see Fig. 31-5). Although not well demonstrated in the illustration, the clue for a completely replaced common hepatic artery coming off the SMA is the presence of a strong arterial pulsation to the right of the common bile duct, rather than the left side, in the porta hepatis. Another important point is that the right hepatic artery passes deep and posterior to the common bile duct approximately 88% of the time but crosses anterior to the common bile duct in approximately 12% of cases. The cystic artery feeding the gallbladder usually arises from the right hepatic artery in Calot's triangle.

Portal Vein

The portal vein is formed by the confluence of the splenic vein and the superior mesenteric vein. The inferior mesenteric vein usually drains into the splenic vein upstream from the confluence (Fig. 31-6). The main portal vein traverses the porta hepatis before dividing into the left and right portal vein branches. The left portal vein typically branches from the main portal vein outside of the liver with a sharp bend to the left and consists of the transverse portion followed by a 90-degree turn at the base of the umbilical fissure to become the umbilical portion before entering the liver parenchyma (Fig. 31-7). The left portal vein then divides to give off the segment III and II branches to the left lateral segment, as well as the segment IV feedback branches that supply the left medial segment. The left portal vein also provides the dominant inflow branch to the caudate lobe (although branches can arise from the main and right portal veins also), usually close to the bend between the transverse and umbilical portions. The division of the right portal vein is usually higher in the hilum and may be close to (or inside) the liver parenchyma at the hilar plate.

The portal vein drains the splanchnic blood from the stomach, pancreas, spleen, small intestine, and majority of the colon to the liver

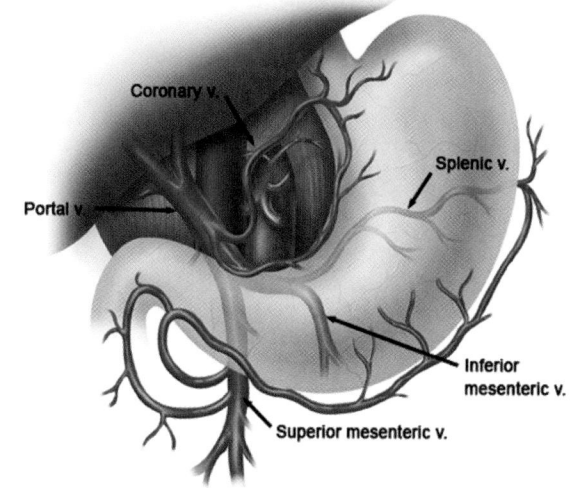

FIG. 31-6. Portal vein anatomy. The portal vein is formed by the confluence of the splenic and superior mesenteric veins. The inferior mesenteric vein drains into the splenic vein. The coronary (left gastric) vein drains into the portal vein in the vicinity of the confluence. v. = vein.

before returning to the systemic circulation. The portal vein pressure in an individual with normal physiology is low at 3 to 5 mmHg. The portal vein is valveless, however, and in the setting of portal hypertension, the pressure can be quite high (20 to 30 mmHg). This results in decompression of the systemic circulation through portocaval anastomoses, most commonly via the coronary (left gastric) vein, which produces esophageal and gastric varices with the propensity for major hemorrhage. Another branch of the main portal vein is the superior pancreaticoduodenal vein (which comes off low in an anterior lateral position and is divided during pancreaticoduodenectomy). Closer to the liver, the main portal vein typically gives off a short branch (posterior lateral) to the caudate process on the right side. It is

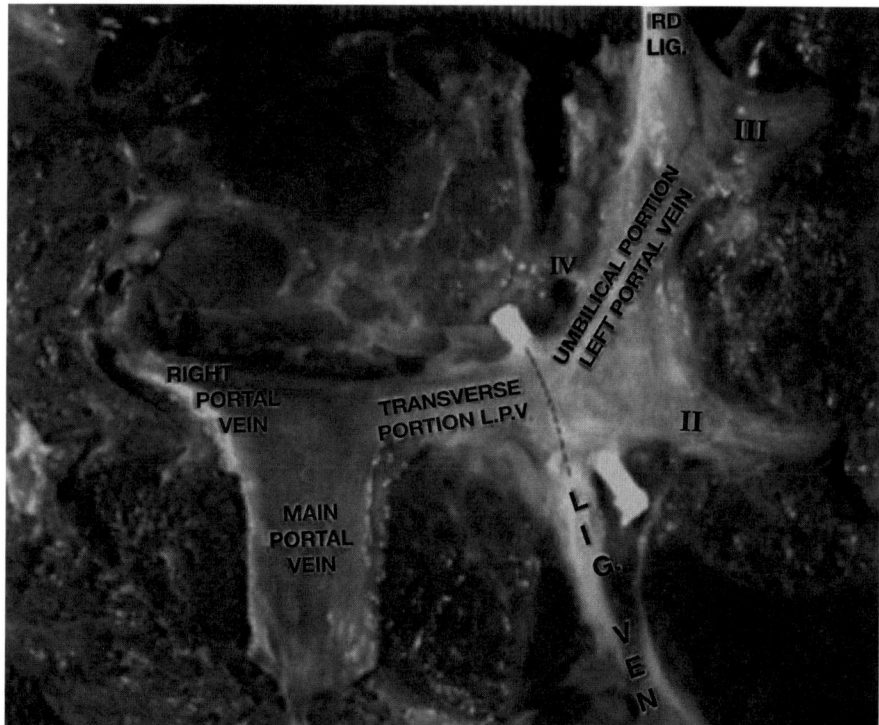

FIG. 31-7. Anatomy of the left portal vein (LPV). Cadaver cast shows the transverse and umbilical portions of the LPV. LIG. VEN = ligamentum venosum; RD LIG. = round ligament. *(Reproduced with permission from Botero AC, Strasberg SM: Division of the left hemiliver in man—segments, sectors, or sections.* Liver Transpl Surg *4:226, 1998.)*

important to identify this branch and ligate it during hilar dissection for anatomic right hemihepatectomy to avoid avulsion.

Hepatic Veins and Inferior Vena Cava

There are three hepatic veins (right, middle, and left) that pass obliquely through the liver to drain the blood to the suprahepatic IVC and eventually the right atrium (Fig. 31-8). The right hepatic vein drains segments V to VIII; the middle hepatic vein drains segment IV as well as segments V and VIII; and the left hepatic vein drains segments II and III. The caudate lobe is unique because its venous drainage feeds directly into the IVC. In addition, the liver usually has a few small, variable short hepatic veins that directly enter the IVC from the undersurface of the liver. The left and middle hepatic veins form a common trunk approximately 95% of the time before entering the IVC, whereas the right hepatic vein inserts separately (in an oblique orientation) into the IVC. There is a large inferior accessory right hepatic vein in 15 to 20% of cases that runs in the hepatocaval ligament. This can be a source of torrential bleeding if control is lost during right hepatectomy. The hepatic vein branches bisect the portal branches inside the liver parenchyma (i.e., the right hepatic vein runs between the right anterior and posterior portal veins; the middle hepatic vein passes between the right anterior and left portal vein; and the left hepatic vein crosses between the segment III and II branches of the left portal vein.

Bile Duct and Hepatic Ducts

Within the hepatoduodenal ligament, the common bile duct lies anteriorly and to the right. It gives off the cystic duct to the gallbladder and becomes the common hepatic duct before dividing into the right and left hepatic ducts. In general, the hepatic ducts follow the arterial branching pattern inside the liver. The bifurcation of the right anterior hepatic duct usually enters the liver above the hilar plate, whereas the right posterior duct dives behind the right portal vein and can be found on the surface of the caudate process before entering the liver. The left hepatic duct typically has a longer extrahepatic course before giving off segmental branches behind the left portal vein at the base of the umbilical fissure. Considerable variation exists, and in 30 to 40% of cases there is a nonstandard hepatic duct confluence with accessory or aberrant ducts (Fig. 31-9). The cystic duct itself also has a variable pattern of drainage into the common bile duct. This can lead to potential injury or postoperative bile leakage during cholecystectomy or hepatic resection, and the surgeon needs to expect these variants. The gallbladder sits adherent to hepatic segments IVB (left lobe) and V (right lobe) (see Chap. 32).

Neural Innervation and Lymphatic Drainage

The parasympathetic innervation of the liver comes from the left vagus, which gives off the anterior hepatic branch, and the right

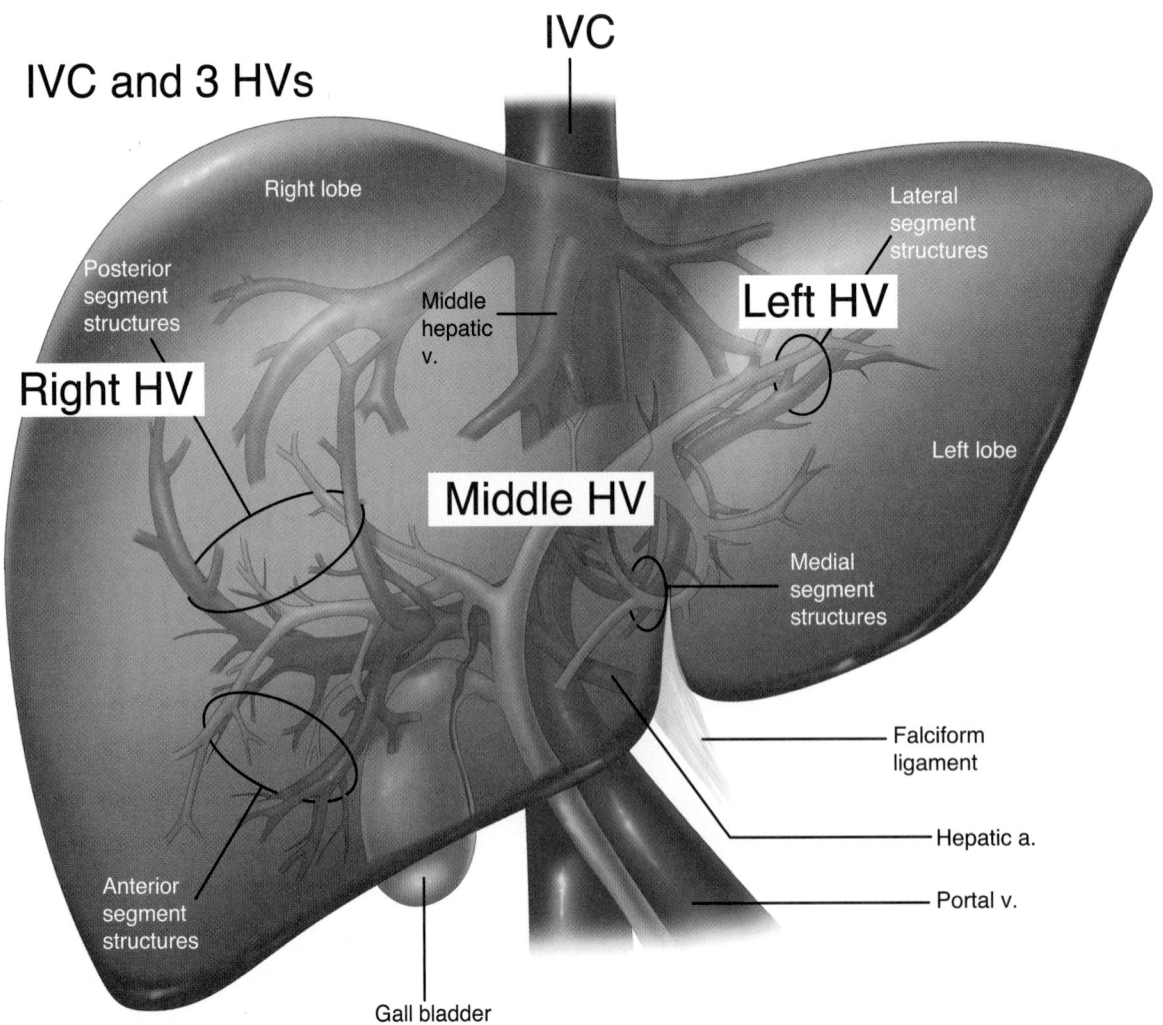

FIG. 31-8. Confluence of the three hepatic veins (HVs) and the inferior vena cava (IVC). Note that the middle and left hepatic veins (HVs) drain into a common trunk before entering the IVC. a. = artery; v. = vein. [*Adapted with permission from Cameron JL (ed):* Atlas of Surgery. Vol. I, Gallbladder and Biliary Tract, the Liver, Portasystemic Shunts, the Pancreas. *Toronto: BC Decker, 1990, p 153.*]

A: Normal bifurcation 57%
B: Trifurcation of 3 ducts 12%

C: R anterior (C1, 16%) or R posterior
(C2, 4%) duct draining into CHD

D: R posterior (D1, 5%) or R anterior
duct (D2, 1%) draining into the left
hepatic duct

E: Absence of hepatic duct
confluence 3%

F: Drainage of R posterior duct into
cystic duct 2%

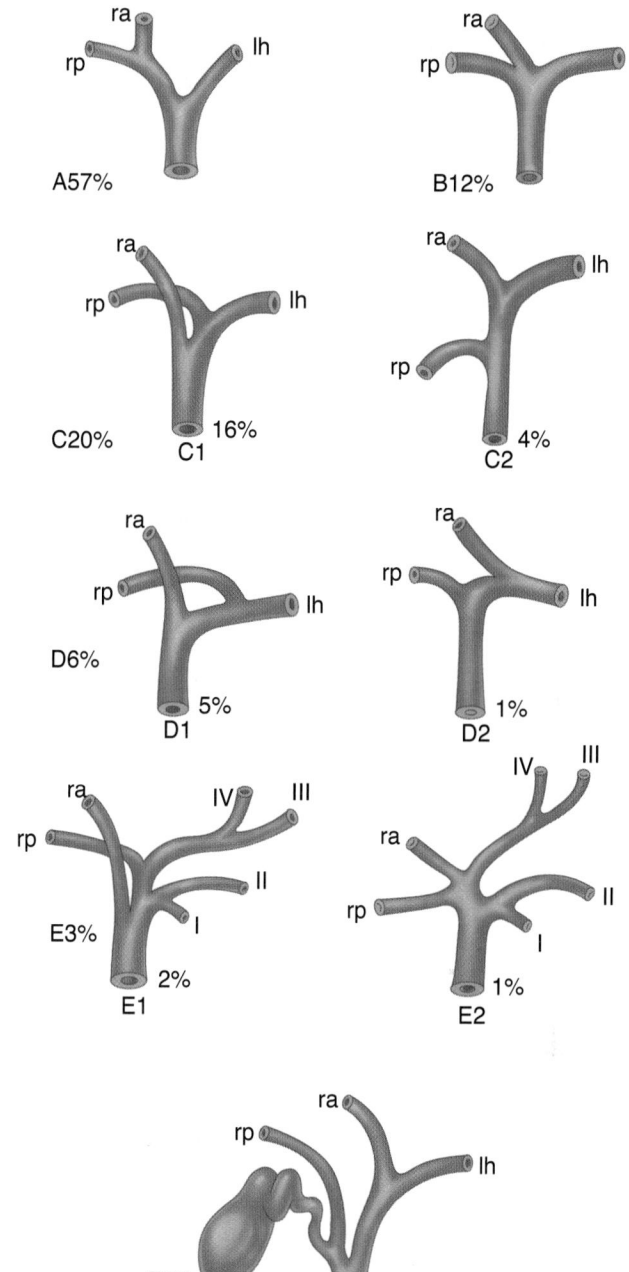

FIG. 31-9. Main variations of hepatic duct confluence. As described by Couinaud in 1957, the bifurcation of the hepatic ducts has a variable pattern in approximately 40% of cases. CHD = common hepatic duct; lh = left hepatic; R = right; ra = right anterior; rp = right posterior. *[Reproduced with permission from Blumgart LH, Fong Y (eds): Surgery of the Liver and Biliary Tract, 3rd ed, Vol. I. London: Elsevier Science, 2000. Copyright © Elsevier Science.]*

vagus, which gives off the posterior hepatic branch. The sympathetic innervation involves the greater thoracic splanchnic nerves and the celiac ganglia, although the function of these nerves is poorly understood. The denervated liver after hepatic transplantation seems to function with normal capacity. A common source of referred pain to the right shoulder and scapula as well as the right side or back is the right phrenic nerve, which is stimulated by tumors that stretch Glisson's capsule or by diaphragmatic irritation.

Lymph is produced within the liver and drains via the perisinusoidal space of Disse and periportal clefts of Mall to larger lymphatics that drain to the hilar cystic duct lymph node (Calot's triangle node), as well as the common bile duct, hepatic artery, and retropancreatic and celiac lymph nodes. This is particularly important for resection of hilar cholangiocarcinoma, which has a high incidence of lymph node metastases. The hepatic lymph also drains cephalad to the cardiophrenic lymph nodes and the latter can be pathologically identified on a staging CT or MRI scan.

LIVER PHYSIOLOGY

The liver is the largest gland in the body and has an extraordinary spectrum of functions. These many functions comprise processes such as storage, metabolism, production, and secretion. One crucial role is the processing of absorbed nutrients through the metabolism of glucose, lipids, and proteins. The liver maintains glucose concentrations in a normal range over both short and long periods by performing several important roles in carbohydrate metabolism. In the fasting state, the liver ensures a sufficient supply of glucose to the central nervous system. The liver can produce glucose by breaking down glycogen through glycogenolysis and by de novo synthesis of glucose through gluconeogenesis from noncarbohydrate precursors such as lactate, amino acids, and glycerol. In the postprandial state, excess circulating glucose is removed by glycogen synthesis or glycolysis and lipogenesis. The liver also plays a central role in lipid metabolism through the formation of bile and the production of cholesterol and fatty acids. Protein metabolism occurs in the liver through amino acid deamination resulting in the production of ammonia as well as the production of a variety of proteins. In addition to metabolism, the liver is also responsible for the synthesis of most circulating plasma proteins. Among these proteins are albumin, factors of the coagulation and fibrinolytic systems, and compounds of the complement cascade. Furthermore, the detoxification of many substances through drug metabolism occurs in the liver, as do immunologic responses through the many immune cells found in its reticuloendothelial system.[9]

Bilirubin Metabolism

Bilirubin is the breakdown product of normal heme catabolism. The bilirubin is bound to albumin in the circulation and sent to the liver. In the liver, it is conjugated to glucuronic acid in a reaction catalyzed by the enzyme glucuronyl transferase, which makes it soluble in water. Each bilirubin molecule reacts with two uridine diphosphoglucuronic acid molecules to form bilirubin diglucuronide. This glucuronide is then excreted into the bile canaliculi. A small amount of bilirubin glucuronide escapes into the blood and is then excreted in the urine. The majority of conjugated bilirubin is excreted in the intestine as waste, because the intestinal mucosa is relatively impermeable to conjugated bilirubin. However, it is permeable to unconjugated bilirubin and urobilinogens, a series of bilirubin derivatives formed by the action of bacteria. Thus, some of the bilirubin and urobilinogens are reabsorbed in the portal circulation; they are again excreted by the liver or enter the circulation and are excreted in the urine.[10]

Formation of Bile

Bile is a complex fluid containing organic and inorganic substances dissolved in an alkaline solution that flows from the liver through the biliary system and into the small intestine. The main components of bile are water, electrolytes, and a variety of organic molecules including bile pigments, bile salts, phospholipids (lecithin), and cholesterol. The two fundamental roles of bile are to aid in the digestion and absorption of lipids and lipid-soluble vitamins and to eliminate waste products (bilirubin and cholesterol) through secretion into bile and elimination in feces. Bile is produced by hepatocytes and secreted through the biliary system. In between meals, bile is stored in the gallbladder and concentrated through the absorption of water and electrolytes. Upon entry of food into the duodenum, bile is released from the gallbladder to aid in digestion. About 1 L of bile can be produced by the human liver daily. However, >95% of the bile salts secreted in bile are reabsorbed in the intestine and then excreted again by the liver (enterohepatic circulation).

Bile salts, in conjunction with phospholipids, are responsible for the digestion and absorption of lipids in the small intestine. Bile salts are sodium and potassium salts of bile acids conjugated to amino acids. The bile acids are derivatives of cholesterol synthesized in the hepatocyte. Cholesterol, ingested from the diet or derived from hepatic synthesis, is converted into the bile acids cholic acid and chenodeoxycholic acid. These bile acids are conjugated to either glycine or taurine before secretion into the biliary system. Bacteria in the intestine can remove glycine and taurine from bile salts. They can also convert some of the primary bile acids into secondary bile acids by removing a hydroxyl group, producing deoxycholic from cholic acid, and lithocholic from chenodeoxycholic acid.

Bile salts are amphipathic, containing both hydrophobic and hydrophilic domains. The amphipathic nature of bile salts allows for the emulsification of lipids, which results in the breakdown of fat globules into microscopic droplets. This greatly increases the surface area of lipids, which permits their digestion by lipases. Bile salts are also able to carry and solubilize lipids by forming micelles. Lipids collect in the micelles, with cholesterol in the hydrophobic center and amphipathic phospholipids with their hydrophilic heads on the outside and their hydrophobic tails in the center. The micelles play an important role in keeping lipids in solution and transporting them to the brush border of the intestinal epithelial cells, where they are absorbed.

Bile salts secreted into the intestine are efficiently reabsorbed and reused. Approximately 90 to 95% of the bile salts are absorbed from the small intestine at the terminal ileum. The remaining 5 to 10% enters the colon and is converted to the secondary salts of deoxycholic acid and lithocholic acid. The mixture of primary and secondary bile salts and bile acids is absorbed primarily by active transport in the terminal ileum. The absorbed bile salts are transported back to the liver in the portal vein and re-excreted in the bile. Those lost in the stool are replaced by synthesis in the liver. The continuous process of secretion of bile salts in the bile, their passage through the intestine, and their subsequent return to the liver is termed the *enterohepatic circulation*.[10]

Drug Metabolism

The liver plays an important role in providing mechanisms for ridding the body of foreign molecules (xenobiotics) that are absorbed from the environment. In most cases, a drug is relatively lipophilic to ensure good absorption. The liver participates in the elimination of these lipid-soluble drugs by transforming them into more readily excreted hydrophilic products. There are two main reactions that can occur in the liver important for drug metabolism. Phase I reactions include oxidation, reduction, and hydrolysis of molecules that result in metabolites that are more hydrophilic than the original chemicals. The cytochrome P-450 system is a family of hemoproteins important for oxidative reactions involving drug and toxic substances. Phase II reactions, also known as *conjugation reactions*, are synthetic reactions that involve addition of subgroups to the drug molecule. These subgroups include glucuronate, acetate, glutathione, glycine, sulfate, and methyl groups. These drug reactions occur mainly in the smooth endoplasmic reticulum of the hepatocyte.

Many factors can affect drug metabolism in the liver. When the rate of metabolism of a pharmacologically active metabolite is increased (i.e., enzyme induction), the duration of the drug action will decrease. However, when the metabolism of a drug is decreased (i.e., enzyme inhibition), then the drug will be metabolically active for a longer period of time. It is important to note that some drugs may be converted to active products by metabolism in the liver. An example is acetaminophen when taken in larger doses. Normally, acetaminophen is conjugated by the liver to harmless glucuronide and sulfate metabolites that are water soluble and eliminated in the urine. During an overdose, the normal metabolic pathways are overwhelmed, and some of the drug is converted to a reactive and toxic intermediate by the cytochrome P-450 system. Glutathione can normally bind to this intermediate and lead to the excretion of a harmless product. However, as glutathione stores are diminished, the reactive intermediate cannot be detoxified and it combines with lipid bilayers of hepatocytes, which results in cellular necrosis. Thus, treatment of acetaminophen overdoses consists of replacing glutathione with sulfhydryl compounds such as acetylcysteine.

Liver Function Tests

Liver function tests is a term frequently used to refer to measurement of the levels of a group of serum markers for evaluation of liver dysfunction. Most commonly, levels of aspartate transaminase (AST), alanine transaminase (ALT), alkaline phosphatase (AP), γ-glutamyltranspeptidase (GGTP), and bilirubin are included in this panel. This term is a misnomer, however, because most of these tests measure not liver function but rather cell damage. More accurate measurement of the liver's synthetic function is provided by serum albumin levels and prothrombin time. Although measuring liver enzyme levels is important in the assessment of a patient's liver disease, these test results can be nonspecific. Thus, evaluation of patients with suspected liver disease should always involve careful interpretation of abnormalities in these liver test results in the context of a thorough history and physical examination. The approach to evaluating abnormal laboratory values can also be simplified by categorizing the type of abnormality that predominates (hepatocellular damage, abnormal synthetic function, or cholestasis).

Hepatocellular Injury

Hepatocellular injury of the liver is usually indicated by abnormalities in levels of the liver aminotransferases AST and ALT. These enzymes participate in gluconeogenesis by catalyzing the transfer of amino groups from aspartic acid or alanine to ketoglutaric acid to produce oxaloacetic acid and pyruvic acid, respectively (these enzymes were formerly referred to as *glutamic-oxaloacetic transaminase* and *glutamic-pyruvic transaminase*). AST is found in the liver, cardiac muscle, skeletal muscle, kidney, brain, pancreas, lungs, and red blood cells and thus is less specific for disorders of the liver. ALT is predominately found in the liver and thus is more specific for liver disease. Hepatocellular injury is the trigger for release of these enzymes into the circulation. Common causes of elevated aminotransferase levels include viral hepatitis, alcohol abuse, medications, genetic disorders (Wilson's disease, hemochromatosis, alpha$_1$-antitrypsin deficiency), and autoimmune diseases.

The extent of serum aminotransferase elevations can suggest certain etiologies of the liver injury. However, the levels of the enzymes in these tests correlate poorly with the severity of hepatocellular necrosis, because they may not be significantly elevated in conditions of hepatic fibrosis or cirrhosis. In alcoholic liver disease, an AST:ALT ratio of >2:1 is common. Mild elevations of transaminase levels can be found in nonalcoholic fatty liver disease, chronic viral infection, or medication-induced injury. Moderate increases in the levels of these enzymes are common in acute viral hepatitis. In conditions of ischemic insults, toxin ingestions (i.e., acetaminophen), and fulminant hepatitis, AST and ALT levels can be elevated to the thousands.

Abnormal Synthetic Function

Albumin synthesis is an important function of the liver and thus can be measured to evaluate the liver's synthetic function. The liver produces approximately 10 g of albumin per day. However, albumin levels are dependent on a number of factors such as nutritional status, renal dysfunction, protein-losing enteropathies, and hormonal disturbances. In addition, level of albumin is not a marker of acute hepatic dysfunction due to albumin's long half-life of 15 to 20 days.

Most clotting factors (except factor VIII) are synthesized exclusively in the liver, and thus their levels can also be used as a measure of hepatic synthetic function. Measurements of the prothrombin time and international normalized ratio (INR) are one of the best tests of hepatic synthetic function. The prothrombin time measures the rate of conversion of prothrombin to thrombin. To standardize the reporting of prothrombin time and avoid interlaboratory variability, the INR was developed. The INR is the ratio of the patient's prothrombin time to the mean control prothrombin time. Because vitamin K is involved in the γ-carboxylation of factors used to measure prothrombin time (factors II, VII, IX, and X), values may be prolonged in other conditions such as vitamin K deficiency and warfarin therapy.

Cholestasis

Cholestasis is a condition in which bile flow from the liver to the duodenum is impaired. Disturbances in bile flow may be due to intrahepatic causes (hepatocellular dysfunction) or extrahepatic causes (biliary tree obstruction). Cholestasis often results in the release of certain enzymes and thus can be detected by measuring the serum levels of bilirubin, AP, and GGTP, which will be abnormal. Bilirubin is a breakdown product of hemoglobin metabolism. Unconjugated bilirubin is insoluble and thus is transported to the liver bound to albumin. In the liver, it is conjugated to allow excretion in bile. Measured total bilirubin levels can be low, normal, or high in patients with significant liver disease because of the liver's reserve ability to conjugate significant amounts of bilirubin. Thus, to help aid in the diagnosis of hyperbilirubinemia, fractionation of the total bilirubin is usually performed to distinguish between conjugated (direct) and unconjugated (indirect) bilirubin. *Indirect bilirubin* is a term frequently used to refer to unconjugated bilirubin in the circulation because the addition of another chemical is necessary to differentiate this fraction from the whole. Normally, >90% of serum bilirubin is unconjugated. The testing process for conjugated bilirubin, in contrast, is direct without the addition of other agents. The direct bilirubin test measures the levels of conjugated bilirubin and delta bilirubin (conjugated bilirubin bound to albumin).

The patterns of elevation of the different fractions of bilirubin provide important diagnostic clues as to the cause of cholestasis. In general, an elevated indirect bilirubin level suggests intrahepatic cholestasis and an elevated direct bilirubin level suggests extrahepatic obstruction. Mechanisms that can result in increases in unconjugated bilirubin levels include increased bilirubin production (hemolytic disorders and resorption of hematomas) or defects (inherited or acquired) in hepatic uptake or conjugation. The rate-limiting step in bilirubin metabolism is the excretion of bilirubin from hepatocytes, so conjugated hyperbilirubinemia can be seen in inherited or acquired disorders of intrahepatic excretion or extrahepatic obstruction. Conjugated bilirubin cannot be excreted and accumulates in the hepatocytes, which results in its secretion into the circulation. Because conjugated bilirubin is water soluble, it can be found in the urine of patients with jaundice.

AP is an enzyme with a wide tissue distribution but is found primarily in the liver and bones. In the liver, it is expressed by the bile duct epithelium. In conditions of biliary obstruction, levels rise as a result of increased synthesis and release into the serum. Because the half-life of serum AP is approximately 7 days, it may take several days for levels to normalize even after resolution of the biliary obstruction.

GGTP is another enzyme found in hepatocytes and released from the bile duct epithelium. Elevation of GGTP is an early marker and also a sensitive test for hepatobiliary disease. Like AP elevation, however, it is nonspecific and can be produced by a variety of disorders in the absence of liver disease. Increased levels of GGTP can be induced by certain medications, alcohol abuse, pancreatic disease, myocardial infarction, renal failure, and obstructive pulmonary disease. For this reason, elevated GGTP levels are often interpreted in conjunction with other enzyme abnormalities. For example, a raised GGTP level with increased AP level supports a liver source.

Jaundice

Jaundice refers to the yellowish staining of the skin, sclera, and mucous membranes with the pigment bilirubin. Hyperbilirubinemia is usually detectable as jaundice when blood levels rise above 2.5 to 3 mg/dL. Jaundice can be caused by a wide range of benign and malignant disorders. However, when present, it may indicate a serious condition, and thus knowledge of the differential diagnosis of jaundice and a systematic approach to the work-up of the patient is necessary. Work-up of a patient with jaundice is simplified by organizing the possible causes of the disorder into groups based on the location of bilirubin metabolism. As mentioned previously, bilirubin metabolism can take place in three phases: prehepatic, intrahepatic, and posthepatic. The prehepatic phase includes the production of bilirubin from the breakdown of heme products and its transport to the liver. The majority of the heme results from red blood cell metabolism and the rest from other heme-containing organic compounds such as myoglobin and cytochromes. In the liver, the insoluble unconjugated bilirubin is then conjugated to glucuronic acid to allow for solubility in bile and excretion. The posthepatic phase of bilirubin metabolism consists of excretion of soluble bilirubin through the biliary system into the duodenum. Dysfunction in any of these phases can lead to jaundice.[10]

Prehepatic

Jaundice as a result of elevated levels of unconjugated bilirubin occurs from faulty prehepatic metabolism and usually arises from conditions that interfere with proper conjugation of bilirubin in the hepatocyte. Insufficient conjugation is often seen in processes that result in excessive heme metabolism. Subsequently, the conjugation system is overwhelmed, which results in unconjugated hyperbilirubinemia. Causes of hemolysis include inherited and acquired hemolytic anemias. Inherited hemolytic anemias include genetic disorders of the red blood cell membrane (hereditary spherocytosis), enzyme defects (glucose-6-phosphate dehydrogenase deficiency), and defects in hemoglobin structure (sickle cell anemia and thalassemias). Hemolytic anemias can also be acquired, and these can be further divided into those with immune-mediated and those with non–immune-mediated causes. Immune-mediated hemolytic anemias result in a positive finding on a direct Coombs' test and have a variety of autoimmune and drug-induced causes. In contrast, direct Coombs' test results are negative in nonimmune hemolytic anemias. The causes in this latter category are varied and include drugs and toxins that directly damage red blood cells, mechanical trauma (heart valves), microangiopathy, and infections. Prehepatic dysfunction of bilirubin metabolism can also result from failure in the transport of unconjugated bilirubin to the liver by albumin in any condition that leads to plasma protein loss. A poor nutritional state or excess protein loss as seen in burn patients can lead to elevated levels of unconjugated bilirubin in the circulation and jaundice.

Intrahepatic

Intrahepatic causes of jaundice involve the intracellular mechanisms for conjugation and excretion of bile from the hepatocyte. The enzymatic processes in the hepatocytes can be affected by any condition that impairs hepatic blood flow and subsequent function of the liver (ischemic or hypoxic events). Furthermore, there are multiple inherited disorders of enzyme metabolism that can result in either unconjugated or conjugated hyperbilirubinemia. Gilbert syndrome is a genetic variant characterized by diminished activity of the enzyme glucuronyltransferase, which results in decreased conjugation of bilirubin to glucuronide. It is a benign condition that affects approximately 4 to 7% of the population. Typically, the disease results in transient mild increases in unconjugated bilirubin levels and jaundice during episodes of fasting, stress, or illness. These episodes are self limited and usually do not require further treatment. Another inherited disorder of bilirubin conjugation is Crigler-Najjar syndrome. It is a rare disease found in neonates and can result in neurotoxic sequelae from bilirubin encephalopathy.

In addition to defects in conjugation, disorders in bilirubin excretion in the hepatocyte can also lead to jaundice. Rotor's syndrome and Dubin-Johnson syndrome are two uncommon genetic disorders that disrupt transport of conjugated bilirubin from the hepatocyte and result in conjugated hyperbilirubinemia. There are also multiple acquired conditions that result in inflammation and intrahepatic cholestasis by affecting hepatocyte mechanisms for conjugation and excretion of bile. Viruses, alcohol abuse, sepsis, and autoimmune disorders can all result in inflammation in the liver with subsequent disruption of bilirubin transport in the liver. In addition, jaundice can also occur from the cytotoxic effects of many medications, including acetaminophen, oral contraceptives, and anabolic steroids.

Posthepatic

Posthepatic causes of jaundice are usually the result of intrinsic or extrinsic obstruction of the biliary duct system that prevents the flow of bile into the duodenum. There is a wide spectrum of pathologies that may present with obstructive jaundice. Intrinsic obstruction can occur from biliary diseases, including cholelithiasis, choledocholithiasis, benign and malignant biliary strictures, cholangiocarcinoma, cholangitis, and papillary disorders. Extrinsic compression of the biliary tree is commonly due to pancreatic disorders. Patients with pancreatitis, pseudocysts, and malignancies can present with jaundice due to external compression of the biliary system. Finally, with the growing armamentarium of endoscopic tools and minimally invasive surgical approaches, surgical complications are becoming more frequent causes of extrahepatic cholestasis. Misadventures with surgical clips, retained stones, and inadvertent ischemic insults to the biliary system can result in obstructive jaundice recognized immediately postoperatively or many years later.

MOLECULAR SIGNALING PATHWAYS IN THE LIVER

Acute Phase Reaction

The liver is the site of synthesis of acute phase proteins that consist of a group of plasma proteins that are rapidly released in response to inflammatory conditions elsewhere in the body. The synthesis of these proteins in the liver is influenced by a number of inflammatory mediators. Cytokines such as tumor necrosis factor alpha (TNF-α), interferon-γ, interleukin-1 (IL-1), interleukin-6 (IL-6), and interleukin-8 (IL-8) are released by inflammatory cells into the circulation at sites of injury and modulate the acute phase response. In response to these cytokines, the liver increases synthesis and release of a wide variety of proteins, including ceruloplasmin, complement factors, C-reactive protein, D-dimer protein, alpha$_1$-antitrysin, and serum amyloid A. There are proteins such as serum albumin and transferrin whose levels also decrease (negative acute phase proteins) in response to inflammation.

The acute phase response of the liver can be initiated in reaction to infection, trauma, or malignancy. The purpose of the release of these proteins from the liver is to contain infectious processes, prevent further tissue damage, and begin reparative and regeneration processes to restore body homeostasis. For example, products of the complement pathways can attach to microbes to allow for phagocytosis and act as chemoattractants to the areas of inflammation. C-reactive protein is an important acute phase protein that is also involved in the clearance of microorganisms by binding to their membranes and functioning as an opsonin to facilitate phagocytosis. Other proteins such as alpha$_1$-antitrypsin are protease inhibitors and restrict the protease activity of enzymes of inflammatory cells. Thus, the secretion of acute phase proteins from the liver during the acute phase response is an early defense measure against harmful stimuli before the full activation of the immune response.[11]

Lipopolysaccharide Signaling

The liver is a complex organ with an important function in immune surveillance and clearance of bacteria and their products. This function is facilitated by the fact that the liver receives all of the drainage of the GI tract via the portal blood flow, which makes it the last barrier preventing bacteria and their toxins from reaching the systemic circulation. The importance of preventing bacteria and their products from reaching the systemic bloodstream is evident in patients who are infected with gram-negative bacteria. Gram-negative bacterial infection produces an acute inflammatory reaction that can lead to septic shock and multiple organ failure. The complications of gram-negative sepsis are initiated by endotoxin (lipopolysaccharide, or LPS). LPS is a glycolipid constituent of the outer membranes of gram-negative bacteria composed of a hydrophilic polysaccharide portion and a hydrophobic domain called *lipid A*. The lipid A structure is the LPS component responsible for the biologic effects of LPS. Mere nanogram amounts of LPS injected into humans can result in the manifestations of septic shock. The profound effects of LPS are caused not only by the direct effect of LPS itself but also by activation of LPS-sensitive cells, which results in the excessive release of cytokines and other inflammatory mediators.

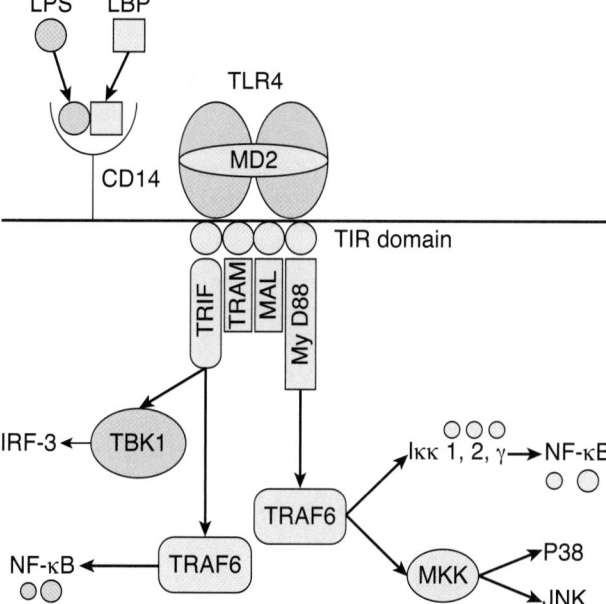

FIG. 31-10. Lipopolysaccharide (LPS) and toll-like receptor 4 (TLR4) signaling in the liver. Circulating LPS-binding protein (LBP) binds to LPS in the plasma and is recognized by CD14. LPS signaling requires the formation of a complex consisting of dimerized TLR4 receptors and the adaptor MD-2. Subsequent signals activated by TLR4 can be subdivided into those dependent on MyD88 and MAL and those independent of MyD88, which require the adaptors TRIF and TRAM. LPS signaling leads to the activation of multiple inflammatory pathways, including nuclear factor κB (NF-κB), interferon regulatory factor 3 (IRF-3), and mitogen-activated protein kinase kinase (MKK). Iκκ = inhibitor of κB kinase; JNK = c-Jun N-terminal kinase; MAL = MyD88-adaptor-like; MD-2 = myeloid differentiation-2; MyD88 = myeloid differentiation factor 88; TBK1 = TANK-binding kinase 1; TIR = toll/interleukin-1 receptor; TRAF6 = tumor necrosis factor receptor–associated factor 6; TRAM = TRIF-related adaptor molecule; TRIF = TIR domain–containing adaptor-inducing interferon-β.

Because sepsis from gram-negative bacterial infection continues to be a major cause of morbidity and mortality, significant efforts have been made to identify the molecules involved in LPS binding and signaling (Fig. 31-10). Lipopolysaccharide-binding protein (LBP), CD14, myeloid differentiation-2 (MD-2), and toll-like receptors all have been identified as important mediators in the pathway of LPS stimulation. LBP is an acute phase protein synthesized by hepatocytes that binds the lipid A moiety of LPS and forms a soluble LBP-LPS complex. This LBP-LPS complex then interacts with CD14, a receptor identified as important in LPS recognition, which results in the release of inflammatory cytokines and mediators.[12] Studies have shown that although LBP is important, it is not required for LPS to interact with CD14; however, its presence markedly decreases the concentration of LPS necessary for cellular activation. This may be important especially at the low concentrations of LPS found under physiologic conditions. CD14 exists in two forms: membrane form and soluble form. The interaction of LPS with membrane CD14 or soluble CD14 is important in host clearance of LPS. This interaction is also responsible for the toxic effects of LPS seen in the liver and systemic circulation after the release of inflammatory cytokines and mediators. Although membrane CD14 is a membrane protein found on the surface of cells of myeloid lineage and mediates the activation of these cells by LPS, soluble CD14 is found in the serum and enables responses to LPS by cells that do not express CD14. In addition to playing an important role in the release of LBP as an acute phase reactant during LPS-

mediated inflammatory insults, the liver is also one of the major sources of release of soluble CD14 into the circulation.

The binding of the LBP-LPS complex to CD14 is not enough to transduce an intracellular LPS signal.[12] Membrane CD14 is a glyco-sylphosphatidylinositol-anchored protein without a membrane-spanning domain. Thus, signaling further downstream of LPS requires additional elements. In studies using chemically modified, radiolabeled LPS capable of cross-linking to nearby proteins, LPS has been shown to cross-link specifically to two other molecules, TLR4 and MD-2. TLR4 is a member of the family of proteins called *toll-like receptors* and has been identified as the transmembrane coreceptor to CD14. TLR4 was originally identified as the molecular sensor for bacterial LPS when studies demonstrated that mutations in the tlr4 gene were responsible for defective LPS signaling in mutant mice. Thus, initiation of the LPS signaling cascade requires the interaction of LPS directly with the heteromeric receptor complex of CD14, TLR4, and MD-2. Activation of this complex senses the presence of bacterial LPS at the cell surface and then transmits a signal into the cytoplasm through two distinct pathways. One pathway is dependent on an adaptor known as *myeloid differentiation factor 88 (MyD88)*. The other pathway is MyD88 independent and relies on an adaptor known as *toll/IL-1 receptor domain–containing adaptor-inducing interferon-β (TRIF)*.

The liver is the main organ involved in the clearance of LPS from the bloodstream and so plays a critical role in the identification and processing of LPS.[13] Kupffer cells are the resident macrophages of the liver and have been shown to participate in LPS clearance. Studies have demonstrated that the majority of radiolabeled LPS injected IV is quickly cleared from the circulation and found in the liver, primarily localized to the Kupffer cells.[13] Kupffer cells also contribute to the inflammatory cascade by producing cytokines in response to LPS. Interestingly, hepatocytes, the parenchymal cells of the liver, also have all the components required for LPS recognition and signaling and can participate in the response to LPS and process LPS for clearance.

Although the liver is essential in the host response to gram-negative bacterial infection by contributing to LPS clearance and to the LPS-induced inflammatory reaction, evidence reveals that LPS may actually have a reciprocal role in the pathogenesis of liver disorders. A relationship between LPS and liver disease is not a novel concept. Early studies showed a correlation between the presence or absence of gut-derived LPS and the development of liver injury.[12] Attempts to eliminate gut-derived LPS have had protective effects in various animal models of liver injury, including models of alcohol-induced liver disease.[12] Other studies have shown the synergism between LPS and hepatotoxins in worsening liver injury. Strategies of endotoxin antagonism have been examined in animal models and clinical trials.[14]

In summary, the liver is essential in the clearance of LPS, but it can also contribute to the negative systemic effects seen in gram-negative bacterial sepsis by excessive activation of the LPS signaling pathway. In addition, there is evidence that this signaling pathway may participate in the pathogenesis of a variety of liver diseases. An understanding and characterization of the LPS pathway within the liver is an important step to understanding the molecular basis for the lethal effect of LPS during sepsis and liver disorders.

Nitric Oxide

Nitric oxide (NO) is a diffusible, free-radical gas that was first identified in 1980 as endothelium-derived relaxing factor. Its physiologic and pathophysiologic importance in the cardiovascular system was discovered with the identification of its vital role as a vasodilator. However, its mediation of a variety of other diverse biologic activities has since been recognized. In the liver, the influence of NO in normal physiology as well as in states of disease has been extensively studied. The activation of inflammatory cascades in the liver almost universally includes the upregulation of the inducible or inflammatory isoform of nitric oxide synthase (iNOS) and subsequent NO produc-

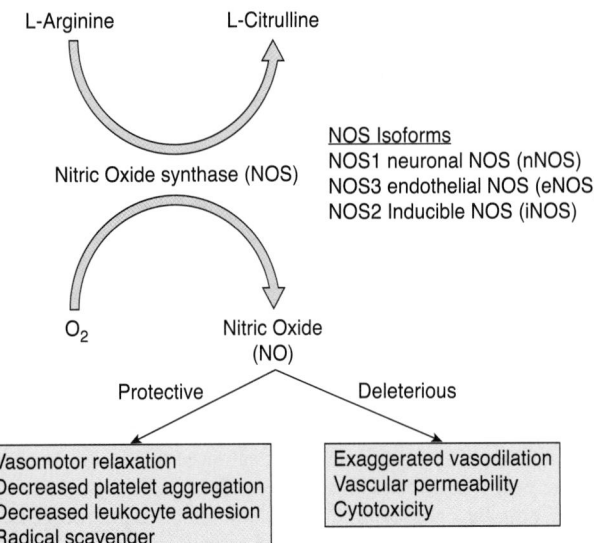

FIG. 31-11. The L-arginine/nitric oxide synthase (NOS)/nitric oxide (NO) pathway. NO is implicated in a wide range of regulatory mechanisms as well as inflammatory processes. L-Arginine is converted to NO by the enzyme NOS. NO has been found to have a dichotomous action in various inflammatory settings, mediating both protective and deleterious effects.

tion. The functions of iNOS and NO in the liver are complex, and a clear dichotomy in their roles in liver dysfunction, whether being protective or detrimental, has been demonstrated.

NO can be produced by one of three nitric oxide synthases (NOSs): neuronal NOS (nNOS), iNOS, and endothelial NOS (eNOS)[15] (Fig. 31-11). These enzymes catalyze the conversion of l-arginine to NO and l-citrulline. The enzymes nNOS and eNOS are constitutively expressed in a wide range of tissues. The activity of iNOS and eNOS is primarily controlled by calcium-mediated signaling that results in transient activation of these enzymes to produce small amounts of NO. As its name implies, iNOS is not normally expressed in resting states in most tissues but is upregulated by gene transcription under conditions of stress. In contrast to nNOS and eNOS, iNOS produces a large and sustained amount of NO. Although iNOS was first identified in macrophages, it has been shown to be expressed in most cell types if appropriately stimulated. Interestingly, studies of the liver with hepatocytes provided the first evidence that parenchymal cells could express iNOS. It is now known that iNOS can be expressed in all cell types of the liver, but hepatocyte expression appears to be the most prominent. Studies have shown that many inflammatory mediators, including cytokines, microbial products, and oxidative stress, are all capable of stimulating iNOS expression in the liver.[16]

The chemical action of NO in biologic systems has been difficult to study due to its short-lived nature. NO is highly reactive with other molecules due to its one unpaired electron. These interactions can result in either nitrosation or oxidation with subsequent varied effects on cellular processes. NO also can signal through cyclic nucleotides by activating the soluble isoform of guanylyl cyclase, which increases levels of cyclic guanosine monophosphate (cGMP). The functions of cGMP include acting as a second messenger that transmits signals by activating downstream kinases or cyclic nucleotide-gated channels. In addition to affecting cGMP signaling, NO also has been found to modulate the expression of many genes.

The role of NO in inflammatory states of the liver is complex and is at times conflicting.[16] Under physiologic conditions, NO is important in maintaining hepatic perfusion. However, under inflammatory conditions, such as ischemia/reperfusion (I/R), NO can play either a protective or harmful role depending on the enzymatic source (iNOS vs. eNOS) and the type of ischemia reperfusion (cold

vs. warm). It appears that the low level of constitutively expressed eNOS-derived NO is primarily beneficial in models of I/R injury, with vasodilation and subsequent improvement in hepatic microcirculation as the proposed mechanism of protection. Interestingly, activation of iNOS in similar models suggests a potentially harmful role for iNOS. NO, through its reaction with reactive nitrogen and oxygen intermediates generated in the course of reperfusion injury, can contribute to much of the hepatocellular damage, depending on the intracellular ratio of these intermediates to NO. The production of iNOS and NO are also closely tied to multiple other inflammatory mediators in the liver, and activation of these downstream signals may explain some of the detrimental effects of NO in I/R injury of the liver. Thus, given its diverse biologic effects as a signaling molecule, it is not surprising that NO plays both a protective and potentially harmful role in the setting of hepatic I/R injury. The final effect of NO varies in different liver diseases and depends on the overall hepatic environment. The potential use of NO pharmacologic manipulation to treat hepatic disease will require careful balance of the risks and benefits of this simple yet extremely complicated molecule.

Heme Oxygenase System

Heme oxygenase (HO) is the rate-limiting enzyme in the degradation of heme to yield biliverdin, carbon monoxide (CO), and free iron (Fig. 31-12). The HO system, which is activated in response to multiple cellular stresses, has been shown to be an endogenous cytoprotectant in a variety of inflammatory conditions. Currently three HO isozymes have been identified. HO-1 is the inducible form of HO, whereas HO-2 and HO-3 are constitutively expressed. The function of HO in heme degradation is essential due to the potentially toxic effects of heme. An excess of heme can cause cellular damage from oxidative stress due to its production of reactive oxygen species. Thus, the HO system is an important defense mechanism against free heme-mediated oxidative stress.

HO-1 has been shown to be induced in a variety of organs during diverse conditions such as hypoxia, endotoxemia, I/R, hyperthermia, and radiation exposure.[17] HO-1 is involved in maintaining redox homeostasis during cellular stress. In the liver, HO-1 is thought normally to modulate hepatic microvasculature tone through its generation of CO and, like NO, its activation of guanylyl cyclase. This important role is demonstrated in animal models of portal hypertension in which inhibition of HO-1 exacerbates hypertension. Because HO-1 is induced as a protective mechanism in response to various

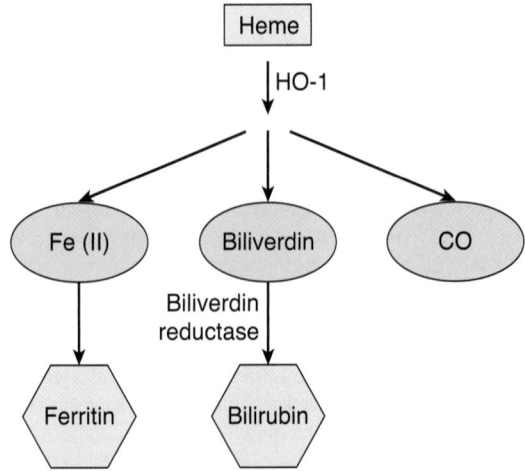

FIG. 31-12. Heme oxygenase 1 (HO-1) and carbon monoxide (CO) signaling. HO-1 is an enzyme involved in the degradation of heme. Its protective effects in settings of hepatic stress are mediated by the catalytic products of heme degradation: ferritin, bilirubin, and CO.

stimuli, targeted induction of HO-1 has been studied as a therapeutic strategy for protection against inflammatory processes. HO-1 overexpression exerts hepatoprotective effects in models of I/R injury, hemorrhagic shock and resuscitation, acetaminophen-induced hepatonecrosis, and sepsis-mediated liver injury.[17]

Although HO-1 has been shown to provide protective effects in a variety of inflammatory states, the specific mechanisms by which HO-1 mediates its protective effects remains to be fully elucidated.[17] Originally thought to be only potentially toxic waste, the by-products generated during heme catabolism now appear to play important roles in protecting against cellular stress. The well-known hazardous effects of high doses of CO are attributable to its ability to bind hemoglobin and myoglobin, which prevents the release of oxygen to tissues. However, only recently have the physiologic and beneficial roles of CO been identified. CO is produced in injured tissues via induction of HO-1 and contributes to the attenuation of proinflammatory processes. Similar to NO, CO plays an important role in maintaining the microcirculation through its activation of soluble guanylyl cyclase and subsequent elevation of intracellular cGMP. The signaling activities of cGMP lead to smooth muscle relaxation and inhibition and platelet aggregation. In addition, CO also has been shown to inhibit proinflammatory cytokines (TNF-α, IL-1) and chemokines while simultaneously inducing anti-inflammatory cytokines (IL-10). Exogenous low-dose CO has been shown to protect the liver from I/R injury and endotoxemia.

Biliverdin and bilirubin are other metabolites of heme that also are recognized as possible mediators of HO-1's protective function (see Fig. 31-12). The cytosolic enzyme biliverdin reductase catalyzes the reduction of biliverdin to bilirubin. Both biliverdin and bilirubin have important endogenous antioxidant properties. Free iron, the third by-product of heme oxidation, is known to be cytotoxic by catalyzing the production of hydroxyl radicals. However, HO-1 induction is associated with increased levels of ferritin, the free iron–sequestering protein. Thus, the increase in ferritin levels with the subsequent decrease in intracellular concentrations of free iron results in a net antioxidant effect. Importantly, both bilirubin and ferritin have been shown to protect against liver injury in a variety of I/R models.[17]

In summary, HO-1 is upregulated and protective in multiple conditions of hepatic stress. Until recently, the degradation products of the HO system were thought to be only potentially toxic waste. It now appears that CO, biliverdin and bilirubin, and ferritin are important in the maintenance of cellular redox homeostasis and may play a role in the mechanism of hepatoprotection in disease. Studies involving induction of HO-1 expression and use of its metabolic products hold therapeutic promise for novel agents to protect against disorders of hepatic inflammation.

Toll-Like Receptors

The liver is a central regulator of the systemic immune response after acute insults to the body. Not only does it play a crucial role in modulating the systemic inflammatory response to infection or injury, it is also subject to injury and dysfunction from these same processes. Recent advances in the study of mechanisms for the activation of the innate immune system have pointed to the TLRs as a common pathway for immune recognition of microbial invasion and tissue injury.[18] By recognizing either microbial products or endogenous molecules released from damaged sites, the TLR system is capable of alerting the host to danger by activating the innate immune system. Initially, this is manifested by the production of inflammatory mediators and the rapid uptake of invading microbes and their products. When excessive, this inflammatory response can contribute to organ damage and dysfunction.

To date, 13 TLRs have been described in mice and 10 in humans.[18] TLRs are a family of proteins that are mammalian homologues to the *Drosophila* Toll, a protein that functions in development and immunity. The cytoplasmic portion of TLRs is similar to that of the IL-1 receptor (IL-1R) family and is called the *toll/IL-1 receptor (TIR) domain*. Unlike the IL-1R extracellular portion that consists of an immunoglobulin-like domain, the TLRs have leucine-rich repeats in their extracellular portion. The TLRs have many structural similarities, both extracellularly and intracellularly, but they differ from each other in ligand specificities and expression patterns, and show some variability in the signaling pathways they activate.

The TLRs were initially identified as components of the innate immune system that acted as a front-line defense mechanism against infections. Their recognition of patterns on pathogens, such as microbial peptides, LPS, lipoteichoic acids, bacterial DNA, and single-stranded RNA, resulted in the activation of an inflammatory response meant for controlling the invading organisms. In situations of noninfectious inflammation such as seen in trauma, clinicians have long recognized similar activation of the same inflammatory pathways and systemic manifestations. This observation, among others, led to the hypothesis that the immune system is designed to recognize any threats, whether from pathogens or tissue damage, that may lead to disruption of homeostasis. Under conditions of sterile inflammation, the activation of immune cells is through the release of endogenous danger molecules, normal cell constituents released by damaged or dying cells, or components of the extracellular matrix, released by the action of proteases at the site of tissue damage. Recent observations show that both microbial products and endogenous danger molecules can be recognized through the TLR system.

Perhaps more than any of the other TLR family members, TLR4 sits at the interface of microbial and sterile inflammation. Whereas the role of TLR4 in the recognition of LPS is well established, only recently has it become apparent that TLR4 also participates in the recognition of endogenous danger molecules[18] (see Fig. 31-10). In vivo evidence for TLR4-mediated danger signaling comes from studies of acute tissue injury in hemorrhagic shock, trauma, and I/R models.[19] In each case, TLR4-mutant animals exhibited reduced injury or inflammation compared with wild-type controls. In efforts to identify the ligands responsible for TLR4-dependent signaling in noninfectious insults, multiple molecules have been suggested. These include heat shock proteins, fibrinogen, hyaluronic acid, heparin sulfate, and high mobility group box 1 (HMGB1). Although a central role for TLR4 in recognizing tissue injury is building, studies are beginning to suggest that other TLR family members may also participate in the recognition of endogenous molecules released by tissue injury.[19] The very recent realization that certain TLR family members also respond to endogenous molecules released from stressed or damaged tissues points to a molecular basis for a shared mechanism of innate immune activation by infection and injury.

RADIOLOGIC EVALUATION OF THE LIVER

Ultrasound

Abdominal ultrasound is a commonly applied imaging modality used to evaluate abdominal symptoms. Ultrasound technology is based on the pulse-echo principle. The ultrasound transducer converts electrical energy to high-frequency sound energy that is transmitted into tissue. Although some of the ultrasound waves are transmitted through the tissue, some are reflected back, and the ultrasound image is produced when the ultrasound receiver detects those reflected waves. This real-time gray scale (B-mode) imaging is augmented by Doppler flow imaging. Doppler ultrasound not only can detect the presence of blood vessels but also can determine the direction and velocity of blood flow. Ultrasonography is a useful initial imaging test of the liver because it is inexpensive, is widely available, involves no radiation exposure, and is well tolerated by patients. It is excellent for diagnosing biliary pathology and focal liver lesions. In addition, liver injury can be evaluated in trauma patients using the focused abdominal sonography for trauma examination. Limitations of ultrasound include incomplete imaging of the liver, most often at the dome or beneath ribs on the surface, and incomplete visualization of lesion boundaries. Moreover, obesity and overlying bowel gas also can interfere with image quality. Thus, ultrasonographically detected masses usually require further evaluation by other imaging modalities due to the lower sensitivity and specificity of ultrasound compared with CT and MRI.

The advent of contrast-enhanced ultrasound has improved the ability of this modality to differentiate among benign and malignant lesions. The injection of gas microbubble agents can increase the sensitivity and specificity of ultrasound in detecting and diagnosing liver lesions. Microbubbles are <10 μm and, when given IV, allow for more effective echo enhancement. Contrast-enhanced ultrasound imaging of the liver improves delineation of liver lesions through identification of dynamic enhancement patterns and the vascular morphology of the lesion. In addition, some agents exhibit a late liver-specific phase in which the bubbles are taken up by cells in the reticuloendothelial system and accumulate in normal liver parenchyma after the vascular enhancement has faded.

The use of intraoperative ultrasound of the liver has rapidly expanded over the years with the increasing number and complexity of hepatic resections being performed.[20] It has the ability to provide the surgeon with real-time accurate information useful for surgical planning. Intraoperative ultrasound is considered the gold standard for detecting liver lesions, and studies have shown that it can identify 20 to 30% more lesions than other preoperative imaging modalities. Importantly, it has been shown to influence surgical management in almost 50% of planned liver resections for malignancies. Applications for intraoperative ultrasound of the liver include tumor staging, visualization of intrahepatic vascular structures (Fig. 31-13), and guidance of resection plane by assessment of the relationship of a mass to the vessels. In addition, biopsy of lesions and ablation of tumors can be guided by intraoperative ultrasound.

Computed Tomography

Computed tomography (CT) produces a digitally processed cross-sectional image of the body from a large series of x-ray images. The introduction of helical (spiral) CT has tremendously improved the imaging capabilities of this technique compared to earlier conventional axial CT. This is especially true with regard to the liver. Helical CT scanners combine a continuous patient-table motion with continuous rotation of the CT gantry, which allows rapid acquisition of a volume of data within a single breath hold. This increased scan speed eliminates artifacts due to variations in inspiration and facilitates optimal contrast delivery.

Contrast medium is routinely used in CT evaluation of the liver because of the similar densities of most pathologic liver masses and normal hepatic parenchyma. A CT scan with a dual- or triple-phase bolus of IV contrast agent is performed to achieve the greatest enhancement of contrast between normal and pathologic tissues.[21] Ideally, contrast media should be selectively delivered to either the tumor or the liver, but not both. Radiologists use the dual blood supply of the liver and the hemodynamics of hepatic tumors to achieve this goal. The liver is unique in that it has a dual blood supply. The portal vein supplies approximately 75% of the blood flow and the hepatic artery the remaining 25%. However, many liver tumors receive the majority of their blood supply from the hepatic artery. After injection of the contrast agent, the rapid scan time of helical CT allows for CT sections through the liver in both the arterial dominant phase (20 to 30 seconds after the beginning of contrast delivery) and venous or portal dominant phase (60 to 70 seconds after contrast injection) (Fig. 31-14). Thus, many hepatic tumors that derive the majority of their blood supply from the hepatic artery as well as other hypervascular lesions are well delineated in the arterial phase. On the other hand, the portal phase provides optimal enhancement of the normal liver parenchyma because the majority of its blood supply is derived from the portal vein. This allows for detection of hypovascular lesions because they will appear hypoattenuated in relation to the brighter normal liver parenchyma.[21]

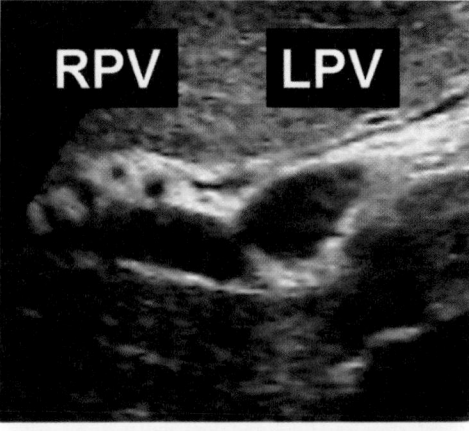

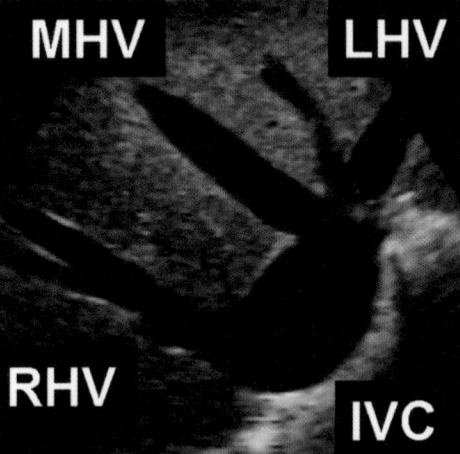

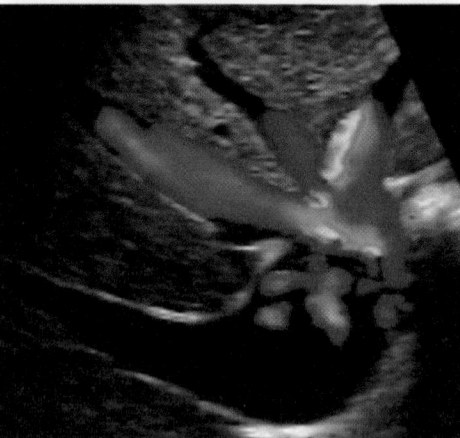

FIG. 31-13. Intraoperative liver ultrasound images of the portal veins, hepatic veins, and inferior vena cava (IVC). *Upper panel* shows the portal vein bifurcation with echogenic Glissonian sheath. The confluence of the three hepatic veins [right hepatic vein (RHV), middle hepatic vein (MHV), and left hepatic vein (LHV)] and the IVC is shown in the *middle panel.* An accessory LHV is present in this patient. *Lower panel* is a color Doppler image showing flow.

Magnetic Resonance Imaging

Magnetic resonance imaging (MRI) is a technique that produces images based on magnetic fields and radio waves. The MRI scanner creates a powerful magnetic field that aligns the hydrogen atoms in the body, and radio waves are used to alter the alignment of this magnetization. Different tissues absorb and release radio wave energy at different rates, and this information is used to construct an image of the body. Most tissues can be differentiated by differences in their characteristic T1 and T2 relaxation times. T1 is a measure of how

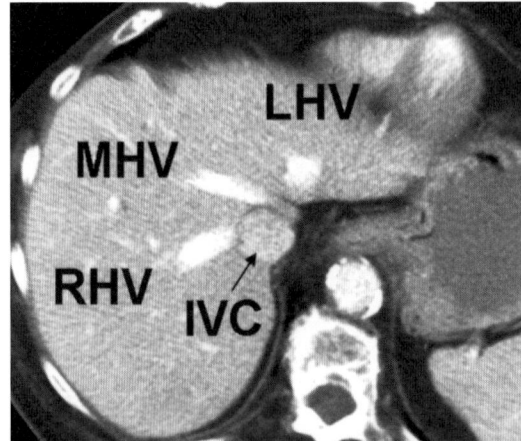

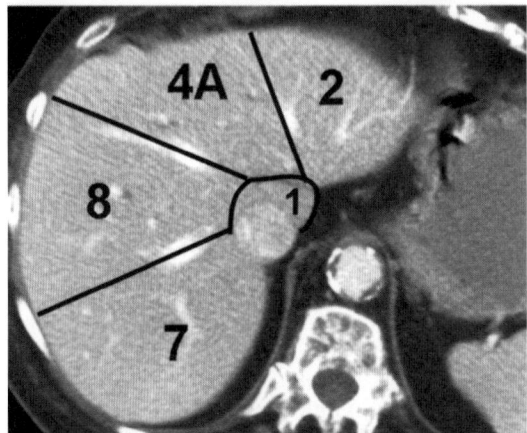

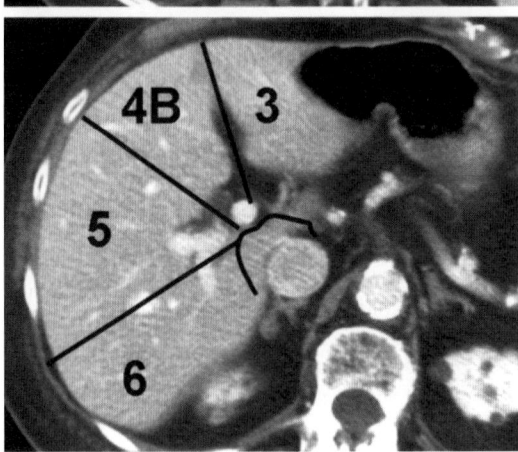

FIG. 31-14. Computed tomographic (CT) images of hepatic veins and Couinaud's liver segments. The images show the three hepatic veins and inferior vena cava (IVC) (*upper panel*), as well as Couinaud's liver segments (*lower panels*). LHV = left hepatic vein; MHV = middle hepatic vein; RHV = right hepatic vein.

contrast agent that behaves in a manner very similar to iodine in CT. Liver-specific MRI contrast agents also have been developed that rely on excretion by Kupffer cells (ferumoxides) or secretion in bile by hepatocytes (iminodiacetic acid–derivative radionuclides) to further improve the sensitivity and specificity of MRI.[22]

Positron Emission Tomography

Positron emission tomography (PET) is a nuclear medicine test that produces images of metabolic activity in tissues by detecting gamma rays emitted by a radioisotope incorporated into a metabolically active molecule. Fluorodeoxyglucose is the most common metabolic molecule used in PET imaging. Although traditional imaging such as CT, ultrasound, and MRI provide anatomic information, PET offers functional imaging of tissues with high metabolic activity, including most types of metastatic tumors. PET has emerged as another modality useful for detection of recurrent colorectal cancers. More than 20% of patients with colorectal cancer initially present with hepatic metastasis, and a large percentage of patients undergoing resection for their primary colorectal cancer eventually experience disease recurrence in the liver. Although hepatic resection of colorectal metastases provides survival rates nearing 50%, the presence of extrahepatic disease is a poor prognosticator and usually precludes aggressive surgical intervention. Thus, accurate information regarding the extent of the disease is necessary for management of patients with colorectal metastases. PET imaging is increasingly used as a tool in the diagnostic work-up of a patient with potentially resectable hepatic disease. In nonrandomized trials, PET demonstrated better sensitivity and specificity than CT scanning for both hepatic disease and extrahepatic disease.[23] Importantly, the information provided by PET resulted in changes to clinical management in up to 25% of cases. However, a disadvantage of images obtained from PET is the lack of exact localization of lesions due to poor resolution. For this reason, integrated PET and CT are increasingly available to potentially improve diagnostic accuracy over standard PET or CT alone. Although the benefit of a synergistic combination of PET and CT has yet to be fully established, this combined modality is rapidly becoming a valuable tool with its increasing availability and use for detection of recurrent colorectal cancer (Fig. 31-15).[23]

ACUTE LIVER FAILURE

Acute liver failure (ALF) occurs when the rate and extent of hepatocyte death exceeds the liver's regenerative capabilities. It was initially described as a specific disease entity in the 1950s. It also has been referred to as *fulminant hepatic failure*. ALF is a rare disorder affecting approximately 2000 patients annually in the United States. ALF has devastating consequences and is defined by the presence of hepatic encephalopathy occurring as the consequence of severe liver damage in a patient without a history of previous liver disease or portal hypertension.[24] The manifestations of ALF may include cerebral edema, hemodynamic instability, increased susceptibility to bacterial and fungal infections, renal failure, coagulopathy, and metabolic disturbances. Even with current medical care, ALF can progress rapidly to hepatic coma and death. The most common cause of death is intracranial hypertension due to cerebral edema, followed by sepsis and multisystem organ failure. The causes of ALF, which are the most important variables in determining outcome, are numerous and can include viral infection as well as drug overdose, reaction, and toxicity. It has been determined that the etiologic factor leading to ALF varies according to geographic location.[25] Before the introduction of orthotopic liver transplantation (OLT), the chance for survival was <20%. Currently, most series report survival rates of >65% for affected patients.[25,26]

Etiology

Differences in etiology, management, and patient outcomes have been described for various regions of the globe. In the East and

quickly a tissue can become magnetized, and T2 measures how quickly it loses its magnetization. As with CT technology, advances in MRI now provide the opportunity to perform single-breath T1-weighted imaging and respiration-triggered T2-weighted imaging. The development of breath-hold imaging techniques has eliminated many of the motion artifacts that previously limited the sensitivity and application of MRI for imaging of the liver. As with the iodinated contrast media use in CT scanning, multiple contrast agents have been developed for MRI to increase the difference in signal intensity between normal liver and pathologic lesion. Gadopentetate dimeglumine (salt of the gadolinium complex of diethylenetriamine pentaacetic acid) is an MRI

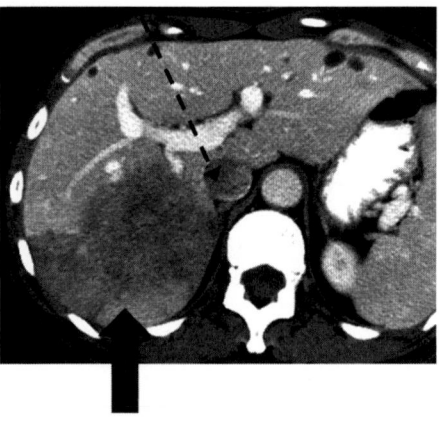 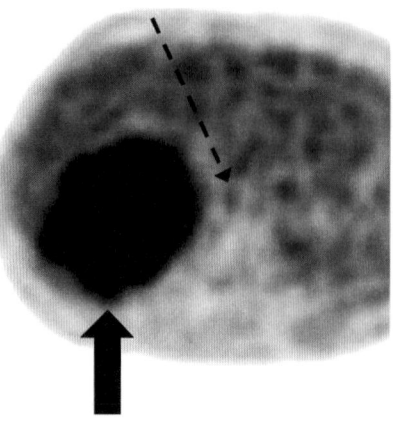 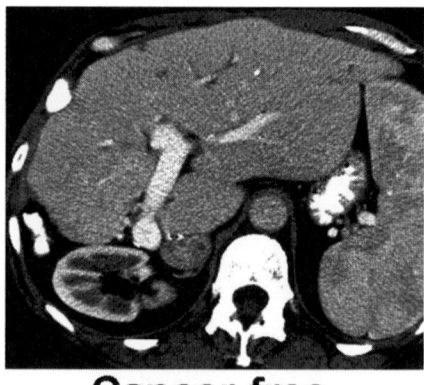

Cancer-free

FIG. 31-15. Computed tomography–positron emission tomography (CT-PET) scans before and after resection of liver metastasis from colorectal cancer in a 54-year-old patient. CT scan shows large 10-cm right lobe liver metastasis (*left panel*), and PET scan findings are strongly positive (*middle panel*). Two years after right hepatectomy, the patient has no evidence of recurrence and significant hypertrophy of the left lobe (*right panel*).

developing portions of the world, the most common causes of ALF are viral infections, primarily hepatitis B, A, and E.[24] In these areas there are a relatively small number of drug-induced cases. In contrast, 65% of cases of ALF in the West are thought to be due to drugs and toxins, with acetaminophen (paracetamol) being the most common etiologic agent in the United States, Australia, United Kingdom, and most of Europe. It is interesting that in France and Spain, where acetaminophen sales are restricted, the rate of acetaminophen-induced ALF is quite low.[27] Acetaminophen-induced ALF is also uncommon in South America. The U.S. Acute Liver Failure Study Group identified several other causes of ALF, including autoimmune hepatitis, hypoperfusion of the liver (in cardiomyopathy or cardiogenic shock), pregnancy-related conditions, and Wilson's disease.[28] Even with exhaustive efforts to identify a cause, approximately 20% of all cases of ALF remain indeterminate in origin.

Clinical Presentation

In a multicenter study involving 17 tertiary care centers and 308 patients in the United States, 73% of all patients with ALF were female, with a median age of 38 years.[26] The most common ethnic group affected was whites (74%), followed by Hispanics (9%) and African Americans (3%). Patients were ill for a median of 6 days before the onset of encephalopathy and had a median of 2 days between the onset of jaundice and the development of encephalopathy. Hepatic coma grade at presentation was approximately equally distributed across grades I to IV. Eighty-four percent of the patients in the study were referred from outside hospitals, 40% had a serum creatinine level exceeding 2.0 mg/dL, and 14% had an arterial pH of <7.30. In addition, 44% of the patients acquired a culture-proven infection.

Diagnosis and Clinical Management

When the medical history is obtained, it is important to address the possibility of exposure to viral infections, medications, and other possible toxins. The possibility of previous liver disease needs to be explored. The physical examination must assess and document the patient's mental status as well as attempt to identify findings of chronic liver disease. The initial laboratory examination must evaluate the severity of the ALF as well as attempt to identify the cause (Table 31-1). A liver biopsy should be performed if certain disease entities such as autoimmune hepatitis or lymphoma are a possibility. Because of the associated coagulopathy, if a liver biopsy is needed, it is usually safest to obtain the tissue via a transjugular approach. Patients with ALF should be admitted to the hospital and monitored frequently. Due to the rapidity with which this disease process may

progress, a liver transplant center should be contacted and the affected patient transferred to the center early in the evaluation period.

If acetaminophen overdose is suspected to have occurred within a few hours of presentation, administration of activated charcoal may be useful to reduce the volume of acetaminophen present in the GI tract. *N*-acetylcysteine (NAC), the clinically effective antidote for acetaminophen overdose, should be administered as early as possible to any patient with suspected acetaminophen-associated ALF.[29] NAC also should be administered to patients with ALF of unclear etiology, because glutathione stabilization may be beneficial in this patient population as well. NAC can be administered either orally (140 mg/kg initial dose, followed by 70 mg/kg every 4 hours × 17 doses) or via the intravenous route (loading dose of 150 mg/kg, followed by a maintenance dose of 50 mg/kg). For patients who are suspected of having drug-induced hepatotoxicity, it is important to obtain details regarding all prescription and nonprescription drugs, herbs, and dietary supplements that may have been taken in the previous year. Most instances of drug-induced hepatotoxicity occur in the first 6 months after drug initiation. Any suspected offending agent must be discontinued and an attempt should be made to administer only essential medications.

The majority of patients with ALF need to be monitored in the intensive care unit (ICU) setting, and specific attention needs to be

TABLE 31-1	Acute liver failure laboratory evaluation

Complete blood count
Complete metabolic panel
Amylase and lipase levels
Liver function tests
Prothrombin time/international normalized ratio
Factor V level
Factor VII level
Arterial blood gas concentrations
Arterial serum ammonia level
ABO typing
Acute hepatitis panel
Autoimmune marker levels
Ceruloplasmin level
Toxicology screening
Acetaminophen level
HIV screening
Pregnancy test (females)

given to fluid management, ulcer prophylaxis, hemodynamic monitoring, electrolyte management, and surveillance for and treatment of infection. Surveillance cultures should be performed to identify bacterial and fungal infections as early as possible. Serum phosphorus levels need to be monitored. Hypophosphatemia, which may indicate a higher likelihood of spontaneous recovery, needs to be corrected via IV administration of phosphorus. Sedation should be avoided, and the head of the bed should be elevated at least 30 degrees. Neurologic examinations should be performed frequently. Intracranial pressure monitoring is reserved for patients in whom a neurologic examination is no longer reliable. CT scans of the head should be performed only to rule out mass lesion or hemorrhage, because they provide limited information regarding increased intracranial pressure. The administration of blood products for thrombocytopenia and prolonged prothrombin time is recommended only in the setting of hemorrhage or before invasive procedures. Acute renal failure is a frequent complication in patients with ALF, and efforts should be made to protect renal function by maintaining sufficient perfusion and avoiding nephrotoxic medications. Should renal replacement therapy become necessary, continuous venovenous hemodialysis should be used rather than intermittent hemodialysis, because continuous venovenous hemodialysis provides better hemodynamic and intracranial stability. The most severely affected patients have a poor prognosis with medical management alone and require liver transplantation. To identify these patients early in the clinical course is important both to maximize the time available to obtain a donor liver allograft for those in need and to avoid transplant in those who will recover without it.

Prognosis

Accurate identification of those ALF patient who will recover spontaneously is important because of the severe shortage of donor liver allografts and the potential complications of lifelong nonspecific immunosuppression. The most widely applied prognostic scoring system is the King's College Hospital ALF criteria.[29] This scoring system has separate criteria predicting a poor medical management outcome for acetaminophen-related and non–acetaminophen-related forms of ALF (Table 31-2). Additional prognostic information may be gained from the Acute Physiology and Chronic Health Evaluation II (APACHE II) scores as well as the actin-free Gc-globulin serum concentration. Overall, prognostic scoring systems have proven to have acceptable specificity but low sensitivity in determining patient outcome and therefore should not replace the judgment of an experienced clinician.

Liver Transplantation

Despite advances in medical management, OLT remains the only definitive therapy for patients unable to regenerate sufficient hepatocyte mass in a timely manner. The advent of OLT has coincided with a rise in overall ALF survival rates from approximately 20% in the pretransplantation era to >65% at the present time. One-year posttransplantation survival for patients with ALF has been reported to be as high as 80 to 90%.[25] Although these improvements in survival rates are impressive, it most be noted that 10% of patients still die while awaiting OLT, which confirms that the potential for improved patient outcome still has not been realized because of the ongoing liver allograft shortage.

Extracorporeal Liver Support

As mentioned earlier, patient survival could be improved if additional time could be gained for the patient while awaiting liver replacement or hepatocyte regeneration. The development of a support device to replace the acutely failing liver has been a highly sought after (and elusive) goal. Several systems have been tested without definitive evidence of efficacy. Transient improvement in hepatic encephalopathy has been observed in several trials, but improvement in hepatocyte function and long-term benefit have not been realized with or

TABLE 31-2	King's College selection criteria for liver transplantation in acute liver failure
Cause	**Selection Criteria**
Acetaminophen	Arterial pH <7.30 irrespective of hepatic coma grade
	Or
	Prothrombin time >100 s + serum creatinine level >3.4 mg/dL + grade III or IV hepatic coma
Not acetaminophen	Prothrombin time >100 s irrespective of hepatic coma grade
	Or
	Any three of the following, irrespective of hepatic coma grade:
	Cryptogenic or drug-induced hepatitis
	Jaundice to coma interval >7 d
	Prothrombin time >50 s
	Serum bilirubin level >17.5 mg/dL
	Age <10 y or >40 y

without OLT. Liver support trials are difficult to perform due to access to liver replacement, the rarity of affected patients, and the heterogeneous causes and varying levels of disease severity. Therefore, additional data are necessary, and liver support systems should be used only as part of an approved clinical trial.

CIRRHOSIS AND PORTAL HYPERTENSION

Cirrhosis

Cirrhosis, the final sequela of chronic hepatic insult, is characterized by the presence of fibrous septa throughout the liver subdividing the parenchyma into hepatocellular nodules (Fig. 31-16).[30] Cirrhosis is the consequence of sustained wound healing in response to chronic liver injury. The etiology of liver injury includes viral, autoimmune, drug-induced, cholestatic, and metabolic diseases. The clinical manifestations of cirrhosis vary from no symptoms to liver failure. Approximately 40% of cirrhotic patients are asymptomatic, but progressive deterioration leading to the need for OLT or death is typical after the development of end-stage liver disease (ESLD). The complications of ESLD include progressive hyperbilirubinemia, malnutrition, decreased synthetic function of the liver, portal hypertension (i.e., ascites and varix-related GI bleeding), hepatic encephalopathy, and life-limiting fatigue. ESLD carries a 5-year mortality of 50%, with 70% of deaths due to liver failure.[31] In the United States, cirrhosis accounts for 30,000 deaths per year and is the most common non-neoplastic cause of death among patients with hepatobiliary and digestive diseases. An additional 10,000 to 12,000 deaths occur annually due to hepatocellular carcinoma (HCC), the most rapidly increasing neoplasm in the United States.[31]

An understanding of the fibrous septa that cause cirrhosis is essential, because fibrosis is felt to be the disease process leading to cirrhosis. Hepatic fibrosis is the accumulation of extracellular matrix or scar tissue in response to acute or chronic liver injury. It is postulated that the stellate cell is activated by hepatic necrosis; the production of cytokines, including IL-1, IL-6, and TNF-α; and the growth factors transforming growth factor beta1 and epidermal growth factor. Activation of the stellate cell is associated with pathologic matrix degeneration due to increased production of membrane-type matrix metalloproteinase-1, matrix metalloproteinase-2, and tissue inhibitors of metalloproteinases. The activated stellate cells undergo phenotypic changes, including proliferation, contraction, chemotaxis, retinoid loss, and proinflammatory responses that lead to the accumulation of extracellular matrix and cirrhosis. Activated stellate cells impede portal vein blood flow and increase portal resistance by constricting individual sinusoids and by contracting the cirrhotic liver. Endothelin-1, arginine vasopressin, adrenomedullin,

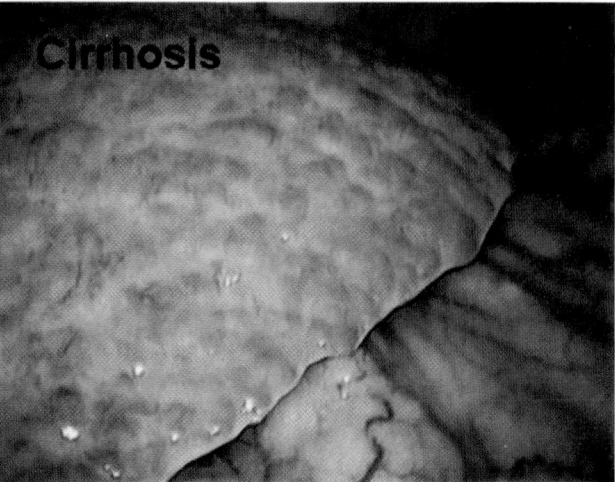

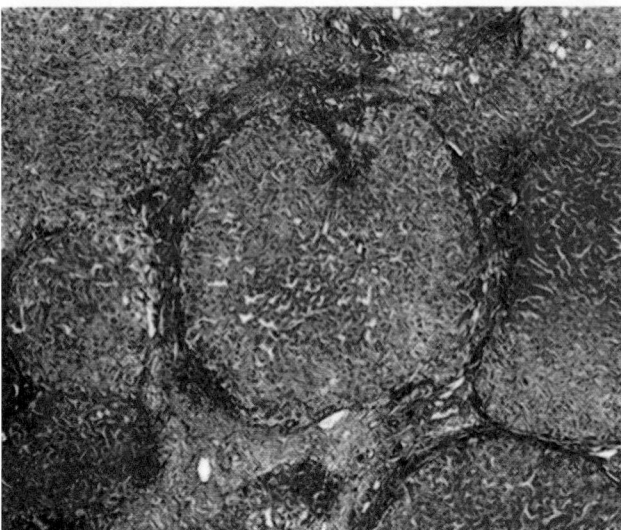

FIG. 31-16. Histology of cirrhotic liver with regenerating macro-nodules. *Upper panel:* Grossly cirrhotic liver. *Lower panel:* Regenerative nodules and bridging fibrosis representative of cirrhosis seen on standard light microscopy (hematoxylin and eosin stain).

and eicosanoids are all mediators of stellate cell contraction and appear to play a significant role in portal hypertension, as does a diminished production of NO by the endothelial cell.[32]

Classification of Cirrhosis

Morphologically, cirrhosis can be described as micronodular, macronodular, or mixed. Micronodular cirrhosis is characterized by thick regular septa, small uniform regenerative nodules, and involvement of virtually every hepatic lobule. Macronodular cirrhosis frequently has septa and regenerative nodules of varying sizes. The regenerative nodules consist of irregularly sized hepatocytes with large nuclei and cell plates of varying thickness. Mixed cirrhosis is present when regeneration is occurring in a micronodular liver and over time converts to a macronodular pattern. This morphologic categorization is limited, and cirrhosis is a dynamic process in which nodule size varies over time. The three patterns correlate poorly with etiology, and the same pattern can result from a variety of disease processes. Conversely, a single disease process can demonstrate several morphologic patterns. Irrespective of etiology and morphologic pattern, the cirrhotic liver frequently demonstrates right hepatic lobe atrophy, caudate lobe and left lateral segment hypertrophy, recanalization of the umbilical vein, a nodular surface contour, dilatation of the portal vein, gastroesophageal varices, and splenomegaly on radiographic evaluation.

Etiology and Clinical Manifestations of Cirrhosis

Cirrhosis can result from a wide range of disease processes (Table 31-3). Regardless of cause, cirrhosis leads to two consequences: hepatocellular failure and portal hypertension. Patients are then evaluated to determine if the cirrhosis is "compensated" (lacking manifestations of ESLD) or "decompensated" (with evidence of ESLD and certain clinicopathologic associations). Medical history and physical examination findings of cirrhosis are outlined (Table 31-4). Fat stores and muscle mass are reduced, and resting energy expenditure is increased. Muscle cramps occur frequently in the cirrhotic patient and are felt to correlate with ascites, low mean arterial pressure, and plasma renin activity. Cramps usually respond to administration of quinine sulfate and human albumin. Abdominal hernias are common with ascites and should be electively repaired only in patients with well-compensated cirrhosis; otherwise the hernia should be repaired at the time of or after the patient's OLT. HCC can occur in all forms of cirrhosis, and every cirrhotic patient should undergo screening for the development of HCC every 6 months via cross-sectional imaging and measurement of serum alpha-fetoprotein (AFP) level. It must be kept in mind that only 60 to 75% of HCCs produce AFP; therefore, a normal serum AFP level does not rule out HCC. Cirrhosis is associated with increased cardiac output and heart rate as well as decreased systemic vascular resistance and blood pressure. Cirrhotic patients are more prone to infections due to impaired phagocytic activity of the reticuloendothelial system. Bacterial infections, often of intestinal origin, are common and must be suspected in a patient with unexplained pyrexia or clinical deterioration. Spontaneous bacterial peritonitis also is seen in cases of cirrhosis with ascites. Intrinsic drug metabolism is reduced in the cirrhotic liver, and this fact needs to be recognized when prescribing medications.

Laboratory Findings Associated with Cirrhosis

Laboratory findings vary in the cirrhotic patient depending on the degree of compensation; however, in general a number of trends are seen. The cirrhotic patient usually has a mild normocytic normochromic anemia. The white blood cell and platelet counts are reduced, and the bone marrow is macronormoblastic. The prothrombin time is prolonged and does not respond to vitamin K therapy, and the serum albumin level is depressed. Urobilinogen is present and urinary sodium excretion is diminished in the presence of ascites. The serum levels of bilirubin, transaminases, and alkaline phosphatase may all be elevated. However, normal liver function test results do not eliminate the possibility of cirrhosis.

Liver Biopsy

Cirrhosis is identified by histopathologic examination of the liver; however, the diagnosis can be made in many cases from a constella-

TABLE 31-3	Etiology of cirrhosis

Viral hepatitis (hepatitis B, C, and D)
Cryptogenic
Alcohol abuse
Metabolic abnormalities
    Iron overload (hemochromatosis)
    Copper overload (Wilson's disease)
    Alpha$_1$-antitrypsin deficiency
    Glycogen storage disease (types IA, III, and IV)
    Tyrosinemia
    Galactosemia
Cholestatic liver disease
Hepatic vein outflow abnormalities
    Budd-Chiari syndrome
    Cardiac failure
Autoimmune hepatitis
Toxins and drugs

TABLE 31-4	Clinical history and physical examination findings associated with cirrhosis

History
  Life-limiting fatigue or weight loss
  Jaundice (icterus; skin, urine, and stool color)
  Anorexia and cachexia
  Abdominal pain
  Peripheral edema
  Ascites
  GI bleeding, hemorrhoids
  Loss of libido
  Loss of menstrual cycle
  Hepatic encephalopathy
Physical examination
  Malnutrition
  Fetor hepaticus
  Jaundiced skin, icteric sclera
  Spider angiomata
  Finger clubbing, white nail beds, palmar erythema, Dupuytren's contracture
  Gynecomastia, testicular atrophy
  Hyperdynamic cardiovascular status
  Parotid enlargement
  Ascites, pleural effusion
  Abdominal hernia
  Caput medusa
  Abnormal liver size
  Splenomegaly
  Temporal muscle wasting
  Asterixis

tion of clinical features, laboratory values, and radiographic findings. Liver biopsy, usually performed via a percutaneous approach, may be useful in determining the cause of the disease, disease activity, and disease progress. If there are contraindications to percutaneous liver biopsy, such as ascites or a coagulation defect, the transjugular approach should be used. If needed, ultrasound or CT guidance can be helpful in obtaining an adequate sample and avoiding other viscera.

Hepatic Reserve and Assessment of Surgical Risk in the Cirrhotic Patient

Assessing the hepatic reserve of the cirrhotic patient is important, because cirrhosis and portal hypertension can have a negative impact on the outcome of nontransplant surgical procedures. A number of laboratory tests have been used to assess hepatic reserve in patients with cirrhosis. Tests of indocyanine green, sorbitol, and galactose elimination capacity as well as the carbon 13 galactose breath test and carbon 13 aminopyrine breath test have all been disappointing clinically due to their dependence on flow to the liver as well as the unavailability and complexity of the tests. The monoethylglycinexylidide (MEGX) test, which measures MEGX formation after the administration of lidocaine, depends on the hepatic cytochrome P-450 3A4 isoenzyme and although approximately 80% sensitive and specific in determining cirrhosis, loses both sensitivity and specificity as the serum bilirubin level rises secondary to interference with the fluorescent readout system.

Child-Turcotte-Pugh Score The Child-Turcotte-Pugh (CTP) score was originally developed to evaluate the risk of portocaval shunt procedures secondary to portal hypertension and subsequently has been shown to be useful in predicting surgical risks of other intra-abdominal operations performed on cirrhotic patients (Table 31-5). Numerous studies have demonstrated overall surgical mortality rates of 10% for patients with class A cirrhosis, 30% for those with class B cirrhosis, and 75 to 80% for those with class C cirrhosis.[33] The CTP score is derived from five variables as shown in Table 31-5. The problems with the CTP score are the presence of subjective variables (encephalopathy and ascites), its narrow range (5 to 15 points), and the equal weighting given to each variable.

Model for End-Stage Liver Disease Scoring System The Model for End-Stage Liver Disease (MELD) is a linear regression model based on objective laboratory values (INR, bilirubin level, and creatinine level). It was originally developed as a tool to predict mortality after transjugular intrahepatic portosystemic shunt (TIPS) but has been validated and has been used as the sole method of liver transplant allocation in the United States since 2002. The MELD formula is as follows:

$$\text{MELD score} = 10\,[0.957\,\text{Ln}(SCr) + 0.378\,\text{Ln}(Tbil) + 1.12\,\text{Ln}(INR) + 0.643]$$

where SCr is serum creatinine level (in milligrams per deciliter) and Tbil is serum bilirubin level (in milligrams per deciliter).

A number of recent studies have examined the relative values of MELD and CTP scores in predicting postoperative mortality in cirrhotic patients undergoing nontransplant surgical procedures. Northup and colleagues demonstrated that MELD score was the only statistically significant predictor of 30-day mortality.[34] In this study, mortality increased by approximately 1% for each MELD point up to a score of 20 and by 2% for each MELD point above 20. It also has been demonstrated that cirrhotic patients who undergo emergent surgery or major surgical procedures have a greater risk of mortality.[35] In these studies, the relative risk of mortality increased by 14% for each 1-point increase in MELD score. The American Society of Anesthesiologists scoring system also has been shown to be useful in predicting 7-day mortality rates after surgery in cirrhotic patients.

Portal Hypertension

The portal venous system contributes approximately 75% of the blood and 72% of the oxygen supplied to the liver. The portal vein is formed by the confluence of the superior mesenteric vein and the splenic vein. In the average adult 1000 to 1500 mL/min of portal venous blood is supplied to the liver. However, this amount can be significantly increased in the cirrhotic patient. The portal venous system is without valves and drains blood from the spleen, pancreas, gallbladder, and abdominal portion of the alimentary tract into the liver. Tributaries of the portal vein communicate with veins draining directly into the systemic circulation. These communications occur at the gastroesophageal junction, anal canal, falciform ligament, splenic venous bed and left renal vein, and retroperitoneum (Fig. 31-17). The normal portal venous pressure is 5 to 10 mmHg, and at this pressure very little blood is shunted from the portal venous system into the systemic circulation. As portal venous pressure increases, however, the communications with the systemic

TABLE 31-5	Child-Turcotte-Pugh (CTP) score		
Variable	**1 Point**	**2 Points**	**3 Points**
Bilirubin level	<2 mg/dL	2–3 mg/dL	>3 mg/dL
Albumin level	>3.5 g/dL	2.8–3.5 g/dL	<2.8 g/dL
International normalized ratio	<1.7	1.7–2.2	>2.2
Encephalopathy	None	Controlled	Uncontrolled
Ascites	None	Controlled	Uncontrolled

Child-Turcotte-Pugh class

  Class A = 5–6 points
  Class B = 7–9 points
  Class C = 10–15 points

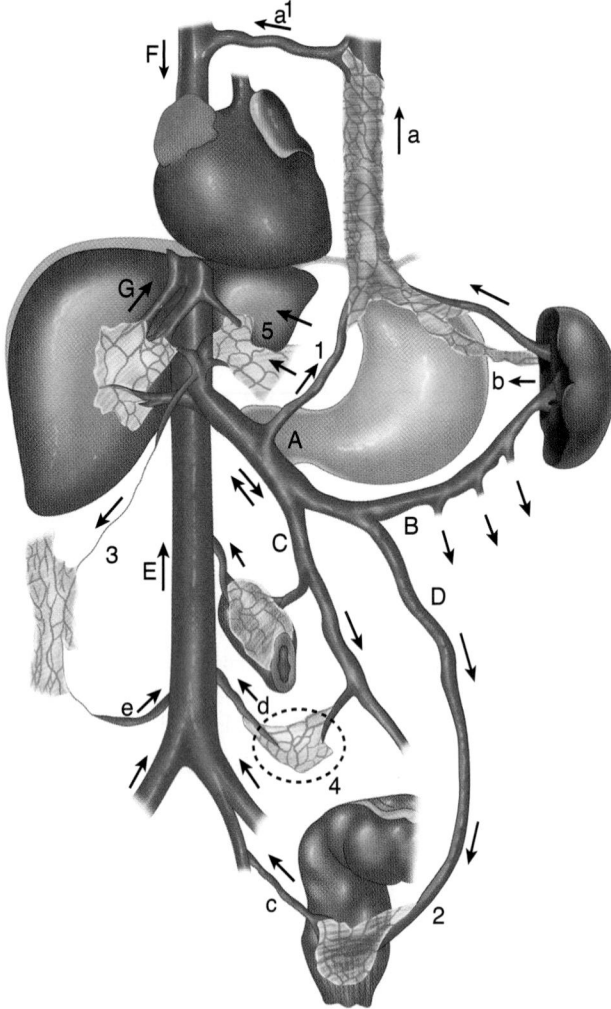

FIG. 31-17. Intra-abdominal venous flow pathways leading to engorged veins (varices) from portal hypertension. *1,* Coronary vein; *2,* superior hemorrhoidal veins; *3,* paraumbilical veins; *4,* Retzius' veins; *5,* veins of Sappey; *A,* portal vein; *B,* splenic vein; *C,* superior mesenteric vein; *D,* inferior mesenteric vein; *E,* inferior vena cava; *F,* superior vena cava; *G,* hepatic veins; *a,* esophageal veins; *a¹,* azygos system; *b,* vasa brevia; *c,* middle and inferior hemorrhoidal veins; *d,* intestinal; *e,* epigastric veins.

circulation dilate, and a large amount of blood may be shunted around the liver and into the systemic circulation. NO is believed to be an important mediator of this venous dilatation.

Imaging of the Portal Venous System and Measurement of Portal Venous Pressure

The patency of the portal vein and the nature of the collateral circulation should be established. An understanding of portal vein patency and anatomy is crucial before undertaking portosystemic shunts, hepatic resection, or hepatic transplantation. The simplest initial investigation is abdominal ultrasonography. A large portal vein suggests portal hypertension but is not diagnostic. Doppler ultrasound is capable of outlining the anatomy of the portal vein, ruling out thrombosis, and indicating portal venous flow direction. Doppler ultrasound also is useful in evaluating surgical shunt and TIPS flow. Abdominal CT arteriography and magnetic resonance angiography both are capable of revealing portal vein anatomy as well as patency. Visceral angiography and portal venography are reserved for cases that cannot be evaluated satisfactorily by noninvasive methods and require further clarification of portal patency or anatomy.

The most accurate method of determining portal hypertension is hepatic venography. The most commonly used procedure involves placing a balloon catheter directly into the hepatic vein and measuring the free hepatic venous pressure (FHVP) with the balloon deflated and the wedged hepatic venous pressure (WHVP) with the balloon inflated to occlude the hepatic vein. The hepatic venous pressure gradient (HVPG) is then calculated by subtracting the free from the wedged venous pressure (HVPG = WHVP − FHVP). The HVPG represents the pressure in the hepatic sinusoids and portal vein and is a measure of portal venous pressure.

Definition of Portal Hypertension

A WHVP or direct portal venous pressure that is >5 mmHg greater than the inferior vena cava (IVC) pressure, a splenic pressure of >15 mmHg, or a portal venous pressure measured at surgery of >20 mmHg is abnormal and indicates portal hypertension.[36] A portal pressure of >12 mmHg is necessary for varices to form and subsequently bleed.

Etiology and Clinical Features of Portal Hypertension

The causes of portal hypertension can be divided into three major groups: presinusoidal, sinusoidal, and postsinusoidal.[36] Although multiple disease processes can result in portal hypertension (Table 31-6), in the United States the most common cause of portal hypertension is usually an intrahepatic one, namely, cirrhosis. The most significant clinical finding associated with portal hypertension is the development of gastroesophageal varices. The major blood supply to gastroesophageal varices is the anterior branch of the left gastric or coronary vein. Portal hypertension also results in splenomegaly with enlarged, tortuous, and even aneurysmal splenic vessels. Splenomegaly frequently is associated with hypersplenism, causing leukopenia, thrombocytopenia, and anemia. The umbilical vein may recannulate and dilate, which leads to visible collaterals on the

---

TABLE 31-6   Etiology of portal hypertension

Presinusoidal
  Sinistral/extrahepatic
    Splenic vein thrombosis
    Splenomegaly
    Splenic arteriovenous fistula
  Intrahepatic
    Schistosomiasis
    Congenital hepatic fibrosis
    Nodular regenerative hyperplasia
    Idiopathic portal fibrosis
    Myeloproliferative disorder
    Sarcoid
    Graft-versus-host disease
Sinusoidal
  Intrahepatic
    Cirrhosis
      Viral infection
      Alcohol abuse
      Primary biliary cirrhosis
      Autoimmune hepatitis
      Primary sclerosing cholangitis
      Metabolic abnormality
Postsinusoidal
  Intrahepatic
    Vascular occlusive disease
  Posthepatic
    Budd-Chiari syndrome
    Congestive heart failure
    Inferior vena caval web
    Constrictive pericarditis

abdominal wall. If flow in the umbilical vein becomes great enough, a caput medusa will form and there may be an audible venous hum (Cruveilhier-Baumgarten murmur). Large spontaneous venous shunts may form between the portal venous system and the left renal vein. These shunts, however, are ineffective in reducing portal venous pressure and preventing upper GI bleeding from esophageal varices. Ascites occurs when portal hypertension is particularly high and when hepatic dysfunction is present. Anorectal varices are present in approximately 45% of cirrhotic patients, and incidence is increased in patients with bleeding from esophageal varices. Anorectal varices must be distinguished from hemorrhoids, which do not communicate with the portal system and are not present at increased incidence in patients with portal hypertension.

Portal hypertension is the consequence of both increased portal vascular resistance and increased portal flow. Increased portal resistance may be due to the abnormal architecture and nodularity of cirrhosis or an obstructed portal vein. Myofibroblasts, Ito cells, and sinusoidal endothelium all play a role in portal venous contraction. As portal venous collaterals develop, diverting blood into the systemic circulation, portal hypertension is maintained by increasing portal flow and splanchnic vasodilatation. This leads to a hyperdynamic portal venous circulation that seems to be related to the severity of the liver failure. Cardiac output increases, and there is a generalized vasodilation. Arterial blood pressure is normal to mildly depressed with a low systemic vascular resistance. The factors maintaining the hyperdynamic circulation are complex and only partially understood. There appears to be a complex interaction between vasodilators and vasoconstrictors that might be formed or fail to be inactivated by the hepatocyte or may be of gut origin. NO, endothelin-1, prostacyclin, and glucagon are all postulated to play a role in the hyperdynamic splanchnic circulation.

Management of Esophageal Varices

The most significant manifestation of portal hypertension and the leading cause of morbidity and mortality associated with portal hypertension is variceal bleeding. Approximately 30% of patients with compensated cirrhosis and 60% of patients with decompensated cirrhosis have esophageal varices. One third of all patients with varices experience variceal bleeding. Each episode of bleeding is associated with a 20 to 30% risk of mortality. Seventy percent of patients who survive the initial bleed will experience recurrent variceal hemorrhage within 1 year if left untreated.

Prevention of Variceal Bleeding Current measures aimed at preventing variceal bleeding include improvement of liver function (i.e., abstention from alcohol), avoidance of aspirin and NSAIDs, and administration of propranolol or nadolol, both of which are nonselective beta blockers. Meta-analyses have demonstrated that beta blockade reduces the index variceal bleed by approximately 45% and reduces bleeding mortality by 50%.[37] Approximately 20% of patients do not respond to beta blockade and another 20% cannot tolerate beta blockade due to medication side effects. It has recently been demonstrated that prophylactic endoscopic variceal ligation (EVL) is associated with a lower incidence of first variceal bleed.[38] EVL is recommended for patients with medium to large varices, performed every 1 to 2 weeks until obliteration, followed by esophagogastroduodenoscopy (EGD) 1 to 3 months later and surveillance EGD every 6 months to monitor for recurrence of varices.

Management of Acute Variceal Bleeding Patients with acute variceal hemorrhage should be admitted to an ICU for resuscitation and management. Blood resuscitation should be performed carefully to a hemoglobin level of approximately 8 g/dL. Overreplacment of packed red blood cells and the overzealous administration of saline can lead to both rebleeding and increased mortality. Administration of fresh-frozen plasma and platelets can be considered in patients with severe coagulopathy. Use of recombinant factor VIIa has not been shown to be more beneficial than standard therapy and therefore is not recommended at this time. Cirrhotic patients with variceal bleeding have a high risk of developing bacterial infections, which are associated with rebleeding and a higher mortality rate. The use of short-term prophylactic antibiotics has been shown both to decrease the rate of bacterial infections and to increase survival. Therefore, their use is recommended, and ceftriaxone 1 g/day IV is often given. Pharmacologic therapy for the variceal hemorrhage can be initiated as soon as the diagnosis of variceal bleeding is made. Vasopressin, administered IV at a dose of 0.2 to 0.8 units/min, is the most potent vasoconstrictor. However, its use is limited by its large number of side effects, and it should be administered for only a short period of time at high doses to prevent ischemic complications. Somatostatin and its analogue octreotide (initial bolus of 50 μg IV followed by continuous infusion of 50 μg/h) also cause splanchnic vasoconstriction. Octreotide has the advantage that it can be administered for 5 days or longer, and it is currently the preferred pharmacologic agent for initial management of acute variceal bleeding. In addition to pharmacologic therapy EGD should be carried out as soon as possible and EVL should be performed. This combination of pharmacologic and EVL therapy has been shown both to improve the initial control of bleeding and to increase the 5-day hemostasis rate.[38]

Even when aggressive pharmacologic and endoscopic therapies are initiated and these treatment options are maximized, 10 to 20% of patients with variceal bleeding will continue to bleed. Shunt therapy, with either surgical shunts or TIPS, has been shown to control refractory variceal bleeding in >90% of treated individuals. Shunt surgery usually is considered only in patients with preserved hepatic function (i.e., CTP class A); TIPS is used in patients with decompensated liver disease (i.e., CTP class B or C). However, the use of these treatment options is dependent on local expertise.

Balloon tamponade using a Sengstaken-Blakemore tube will control refractory variceal bleeding in >80% of patients. However, its application is limited due to the potential for complications, which include aspiration and esophageal perforation. Therefore, use of a Sengstaken-Blakemore tube should be limited to short-term therapy (<24 hours) in those patients awaiting definitive care.

Management of Gastric Varices

Gastric varices that occur along the lesser curvature of the stomach should be considered an extension of the patient's esophageal varices and treated in a manner similar to esophageal varices. Gastric varices along the greater curvature, however, require the evaluation of the splenic vein to assure patency. In the presence of cirrhosis and a patent splenic vein, greater curvature gastric varices can be managed with gastric variceal obturation using N-butyl-cyanoacrylate if available. If gastric variceal obturation is unavailable or if endoscopic therapy fails, the patient should be considered for TIPS, which will control variceal bleeding in >90% of cases.

Surgical Shunt

The need for surgical shunts has been reduced since the introduction of the TIPS procedure and hepatic transplantation. At this time the recommendation is that surgical shunts be considered only in patients who have MELD scores of <15, who are not candidates for hepatic transplantation, or who have limited access to TIPS therapy and the necessary follow-up. The aim of the surgical shunt is to reduce portal venous pressure, maintain total hepatic and portal blood flow, and avoid a high incidence of complicating hepatic encephalopathy. Patient survival is determined by hepatic reserve. The portacaval shunt, as first described by Eck in 1877, either joins the portal vein to the IVC in an end-to-side fashion and completely disrupts portal vein flow to the liver, or joins it in a side-to-side fashion and thereby maintains partial portal venous flow to the liver. Currently this shunt is rarely performed due to the high incidence of hepatic encephalopathy and decreased liver function resulting from the reduction of portal perfusion. The Eck fistula also makes subsequent hepatic transplantation much more technically difficult. The mesocaval shunt uses a Dacron graft of 8 to 10 mm in diameter and connects the superior mesenteric vein to the IVC. This procedure is technically easier and does not adversely affect subsequent hepatic transplantation. The shortcomings of this shunt include a higher incidence of shunt thrombosis and rebleeding. The surgical shunt currently used most often is the distal splenorenal or Warren shunt (Fig. 31-18). This shunt is technically the most difficult to perform. It requires division of the gastroesophageal collaterals and allows venous drainage of the stomach and lower esophagus through the short gastrosplenic veins into the spleen, and ultimately decompresses the left upper quadrant by allowing the splenic vein to drain directly into the left renal vein via an end-to-side splenic to left renal vein anastomosis. This shunt has the advantages of being associated with a lower rate of hepatic encephalopathy and decompensation, and not interfering with subsequent hepatic transplantation.

Transjugular Intrahepatic Portosystemic Shunt

The TIPS procedure involves implantation of a metallic stent between an intrahepatic branch of the portal vein and a hepatic vein radicle. The needle track is dilated until a portal pressure gradient of ≤12 mmHg is achieved. TIPS can be performed in 95% of patients by an experienced interventional radiologist, can control variceal bleeding in >90% of cases refractory to medical treatment, and should not affect subsequent hepatic transplantation. Possible complications include bleeding either intra-abdominally or via the biliary tree, infections, renal failure, decreased hepatic function, and hepatic encephalopathy, which occur in 25 to 30% of patients undergoing the TIPS procedure. After the TIPS procedure the hyperdynamic circulation of cirrhosis also can be worsened, and a patient with underlying cardiac problems can experience cardiac failure.

Nonshunt Surgical Management of Refractory Variceal Bleeding

In the patient with extrahepatic portal vein thrombosis and refractory variceal bleeding, the Sugiura procedure may be considered. The Sugiura procedure consists of extensive devascularization of the stomach and distal esophagus along with transection of the esophagus, splenectomy, truncal vagotomy, and pyloroplasty. As with performance of surgical shunts, patient survival is dependent on hepatic reserve at the time of the surgical procedure. Experience in Western countries is somewhat limited, and a number of modifications have been made to the original Sugiura procedure over time.

Hepatic Transplantation

Patients with cirrhosis, portal hypertension, and variceal bleeding usually die as a result of hepatic failure and not acute blood loss. Therefore, hepatic transplantation must be considered in the patient with ESLD, because it represents the patient's only chance for definitive therapy and long-term survival. Hepatic transplantation also can be considered for the patient with variceal bleeding refractory to all other forms of management. Survival after hepatic

transplantation is not affected adversely by the previous performance of EVL, TIPS, or splenorenal or mesocaval shunts. Previous creation of an Eck fistula, however, does make hepatic transplantation much more technically difficult, and therefore this procedure should be avoided in the transplantation candidate. In addition to saving the patient's life, hepatic transplantation reverses most of the hemodynamic and humoral changes associated with cirrhosis.

Budd-Chiari Syndrome

Budd-Chiari syndrome (BCS) is an uncommon congestive hepatopathy characterized by the obstruction of hepatic venous outflow. Patients may present with acute signs and symptoms of abdominal pain, ascites, and hepatomegaly or more chronic symptoms related to long-standing portal hypertension. The obstruction may be thrombotic or nonthrombotic anywhere along the venous outflow system from the hepatic venules to the right atrium. Variations in the level of obstruction is one of the factors explaining the heterogeneity of the disease. The incidence of BCS is 1 in 100,000 of the general population worldwide.[39]

BCS is defined as primary when the obstructive process involves an endoluminal venous thrombosis. BCS is considered as a secondary process when the veins are compressed or invaded by a neighboring lesion originating outside the vein. A thorough evaluation demonstrates one or more thrombotic risk factors in approximately 75 to 90% of patients with primary BCS. Twenty-five percent of primary BCS patients have two or more risk factors.[39] BCS remains poorly understood, however, and primary myeloproliferative disorders account for approximately 35 to 50% of the primary cases of BCS. In most cases the myeloproliferative disorder can be classified as essential thrombocythemia or polycythemia rubra, but forms that are more difficult to classify also occur. In >90% of affected patients the myeloproliferative disorder was not diagnosed before the development of BCS. Most patients (80%) are women of a relatively young age (mean age is 30 years). The diagnosis of myeloproliferative disorder is made by demonstrating clusters of dystrophic megakaryocytes in a bone marrow biopsy specimen or by demonstrating formation of spontaneous colonies in cultures of erythroid progenitors on erythropoietin-poor media.

All known inherited thrombophilias have been implicated in the development of BCS. Activated protein C resistance, generally related to heterozygous or homozygous factor V Leiden mutation, is seen in approximately 25% of patients with BCS. Factor V Leiden mutation is present in the majority of cases related to pregnancy or oral contraceptive use. Anticardiolipin antibodies and hyperhomocysteinemia are also risk factors for BCS. Protein S, protein C, and antithrombin III are all produced in the liver, and their levels are affected by liver dysfunction. Therefore, although levels of these proteins may be found to be low in patients with BCS, it is difficult to prove this as the causative factor. Oral contraceptive use has also been shown to be a risk factor for BCS.[39]

Clinically significant BCS is usually the result of obstruction of two or more of the major hepatic veins. The obstruction results in

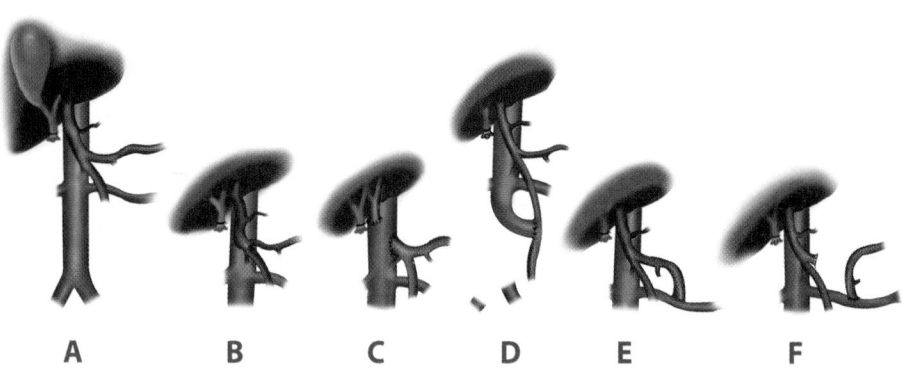

FIG. 31-18. Surgical shunts for portal hypertension. Types of portacaval anastomoses. **A.** Normal. **B.** Side to side. **C.** End to side. **D.** Mesocaval. **E.** Central splenorenal. **F.** Distal splenorenal (Warren). *[Reproduced with permission from Doherty GM, Way LW (eds): Current Surgical Diagnosis and Treatment, 12th ed. New York: McGraw-Hill, 2006.]*

increased sinusoidal pressure and decreased sinusoidal blood flow. Therefore, liver congestion, right upper quadrant pain, and ascites may occur. In addition, liver perfusion via the portal vein is decreased, and 70% of affected patients have noninflammatory centrilobular necrosis on biopsy. Acute liver failure is rare, and most patients go on to develop chronic portal hypertension and ascites. Within a few weeks of obstruction centrilobular fibrosis begins and is followed by progressive fibrosis, nodular regeneration, and cirrhosis. Caudate lobe hypertrophy occurs in approximately 50% of cases and is due to the fact that the caudate lobe has direct venous drainage into the IVC. This caudate lobe hypertrophy can result in obstruction of the IVC.

Abdominal ultrasonography is the initial investigation of choice and can demonstrate absence of hepatic vein flow, spiderweb hepatic veins, and collateral hepatic veins.[40] Abdominal ultrasonography has a sensitivity and specificity of approximately 85%. MRI of the abdomen also is capable of demonstrating hepatic vein thrombosis and evaluating the IVC but is limited in that it cannot show direction of blood flow. The definitive radiographic study to evaluate BCS is hepatic venography to determine the presence and extent of hepatic vein thrombus as well as IVC pressures. Hepatic venography with measurement of IVC pressures should be performed before undertaking TIPS or a surgical shunt. Liver biopsy specimens demonstrate congestion, hepatocyte loss, and centrilobular fibrosis. Liver biopsy is necessary to differentiate BCS from venoocclusive disease that is due to nonthrombotic obstruction of the hepatic venules by subendothelial swelling.

Initial treatment consists of diagnosing and medically managing the underlying disease process and preventing extension of the hepatic vein thrombosis through systemic anticoagulation. The BCS-associated portal hypertension and ascites are medically managed in a manner similar to that in most cirrhotic patients. Thrombolytic therapy alone for acute thrombosis may be attempted. However, the risk:benefit ratio is still unknown. Hepatic decompression aims to decrease sinusoidal pressure by restoring the outflow of blood from the liver via either medical therapy, recanalization of the obstructed hepatic veins, or side-to-side portacaval shunt. Radiographic and surgical intervention should be reserved for those patients whose condition is nonresponsive to medical therapy. Percutaneous angioplasty and TIPS, in combination with thrombolytic therapy, are currently preferred to surgical shunt because the procedural mortality is low and caudate lobe hypertrophy does not affect the outcome of these procedures. Side-to-side portacaval shunt attempts to turn the portal vein into a hepatic outflow tract. Usually a venous or prosthetic interposition graft is necessary. Patients with a hemodynamically significant IVC stricture due to caudate lobe hypertrophy require preshunt IVC stenting. Most patients with portacaval shunt show improvement in hepatic function and fibrosis at 1 year without significant hepatic encephalopathy.[40] However, the enthusiasm for this procedure has been curbed due to the relatively high rate of operative mortality and shunt dysfunction. Hepatic transplantation should be considered for patients with manifestations of ESLD and can be expected to produce a 10-year survival rate of 75%. Whether hepatic transplantation should be a primary treatment for BCS, should replace other hepatic decompressive treatment options, or should be used only as a rescue operation remains unclear and somewhat controversial. It must be noted that, irrespective of the nontransplantation treatment modality initially used, the manifestations of BCS may progress and ultimately require hepatic transplantation.

INFECTIONS OF THE LIVER

The liver contains the largest portion of the reticuloendothelial system in the human body and is therefore able to handle the continuous low-level exposure to enteric bacteria that it receives through the portal venous system. Due to the high level of reticuloendothelial cells in the liver, nonviral infections are unusual.

Pyogenic Liver Abscess

Pyogenic liver abscesses are the most common liver abscesses seen in the United States. Previously they were felt to be due to portal infection, often occurring in young patients secondary to acute appendicitis. However, with earlier diagnosis this cause of abscesses has decreased. Pyogenic liver abscesses also occur as a result of impaired biliary drainage, hematogenous infection arising from sources such as IV drug abuse and teeth cleaning, and local spread of infection (diverticulitis or Crohn's disease). Patients may also develop pyogenic abscess as a complication of subacute bacterial endocarditis and infected indwelling catheters. There appears to be an increasing incidence due to infection by opportunistic organisms among immunosuppressed patients, including transplant and chemotherapy recipients and the AIDS population. Pyogenic hepatic abscesses may be single or multiple and are more frequently found in the right lobe of the liver.[41] The abscess cavities are variable in size and, when multiple, may coalesce to give a honeycomb appearance. Approximately 40% of abscesses are monomicrobial, an additional 40% are polymicrobial, and 20% are culture negative. The most common infecting agents are gram-negative organisms. *Escherichia coli* is found in two thirds, and *Streptococcus faecalis*, *Klebsiella*, and *Proteus vulgaris* are also common. Anaerobic organisms such as *Bacteroides fragilis* are also seen frequently. *Staphylococcus* and *Streptococcus* are more common in patients with endocarditis and infected indwelling catheters.

Patients usually are symptomatic with right upper quadrant pain and fever. Jaundice occurs in up to one third of affected patients. A thorough history and physical examination are necessary to attempt to localize the primary causative site. Leucocytosis, an elevated sedimentation rate, and an elevated alkaline phosphatase (AP) level are the most common laboratory findings. Significant abnormalities in the results of the remaining liver function tests are unusual. Blood cultures reveal the causative organism in approximately 50% of cases. Ultrasound examination of the liver reveals pyogenic abscesses as round or oval hypoechoic lesions with well-defined borders and a variable number of internal echoes. CT scan is highly sensitive in the localization of pyogenic liver abscesses. The abscesses are hypodense and may contain air-fluid levels indicating a gas-producing infectious organism as well as peripheral enhancement (Fig. 31-19). MRI of the abdomen also can detect pyogenic abscesses with a high level of sensitivity but plays a limited role because of its inability to be used for image-guided diagnosis and therapy.

The current cornerstones of treatment include correction of the underlying cause, needle aspiration, and IV antibiotic therapy. On presentation, percutaneous aspiration and culture of the aspirate may be beneficial to guide subsequent antibiotic therapy. Initial antibiotic therapy needs to cover gram-negative as well as anaerobic organisms. Aspiration and placement of a drainage catheter is beneficial for only a minority of pyogenic abscesses, because most are quite viscous and drainage is ineffective. Antibiotic therapy must be continued for at least 8 weeks. Aspiration and IV antibiotic therapy can be expected to be effective in 80 to 90% of patients. If this initial mode of therapy fails, the patients should undergo surgical therapy, including laparoscopic or open drainage. Anatomic surgical resection can be performed in patients with recalcitrant abscesses. It must be kept in mind throughout the evaluation and treatment of the presumed pyogenic abscess that a necrotic hepatic malignancy must not be mistaken for a hepatic abscess. Therefore, early diagnosis and progression to surgical resection should be advocated for patients who do not respond to initial antibiotic therapy.

Amebic Abscess

Entamoeba histolytica is a parasite that is endemic worldwide, infecting approximately 10% of the world's population. Amebiasis is most common in subtropical climates, especially in areas with poor sanitation. *E. histolytica* exists in a vegetative form and as cysts capable of surviving outside the human body. The cystic form passes through the stomach and small bowel unharmed and then

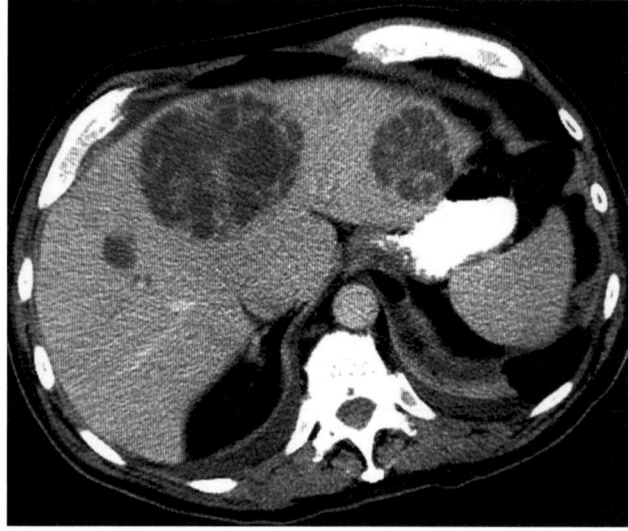

FIG. 31-19. Computed tomographic scan of pyogenic liver abscesses. Multiple hepatic abscesses are seen in a patient after an episode of diverticulitis. Note the loculated large central abscess as well as the left lateral segment abscess.

transforms into a trophozoite in the colon. Here it invades the colonic mucosa forming typical flask-shaped ulcers, enters the portal venous system, and is carried to the liver. Occasionally, the trophozoite will pass through the hepatic sinusoid and into the systemic circulation, which results in lung and brain abscesses.

Amebae multiply and block small intrahepatic portal radicles with consequent focal infarction of hepatocytes. They contain a proteolytic enzyme that also destroys liver parenchyma. The abscesses formed are variable in size and can be single or multiple. The amebic abscess is most commonly located in the superior-anterior aspect of the right lobe of the liver near the diaphragm and has a necrotic central portion that contains a thick, reddish brown, pus-like material. This material has been likened to anchovy paste or chocolate sauce. Amebic abscesses are the most common type of liver abscesses worldwide.

Amebiasis should be considered in patients who have traveled to an endemic area and present with right upper quadrant pain, fever, hepatomegaly, and hepatic abscess.[41] Leukocytosis is common, whereas elevated transaminase levels and jaundice are unusual. The most common biochemical abnormality is a mildly elevated AP level. Even though this disease process is secondary to a colonic infection, the presence of diarrhea is unusual. For most patients findings of the fluorescent antibody test for *E. histolytica* are positive, and results can remain positive for some time after a clinical cure. Amebiasis is unlikely to be present if the serologic test results are negative.

Ultrasound and CT scanning of the abdomen are both very sensitive but nonspecific for the detection of amebic abscesses.[41] CT scanning also is useful in detecting extrahepatic involvement. Amebic abscesses usually appear as well-defined low-density round lesions that have enhancement of the wall. They also usually appear somewhat ragged in appearance with a peripheral zone of edema. The central cavity may have septations as well as fluid levels.

Metronidazole 750 mg tid for 7 to 10 days is the treatment of choice and is successful in 95% of cases. Defervescence usually occurs in 3 to 5 days. The time necessary for the abscess to resolve depends on the initial size at presentation and varies from 30 to 300 days.[41] Both ultrasound and CT of the liver can be used as follow-up after the initiation of medical therapy. Aspiration of the abscess is rarely needed and should be reserved for patients with large abscesses, abscesses that do not respond to medical therapy, ab-

scesses that appear to be superinfected, and abscesses of the left lobe of the liver that may rupture into the pericardium.

Hydatid Disease

Hydatid disease is due to the larval or cyst stage of infection by the tapeworm *Echinococcus granulosus*, which lives in the dog.[42] Humans, sheep, and cattle are intermediate hosts. The dog is infected by eating the viscera of sheep that contain hydatid cysts. Scolices, contained in the cysts, adhere to the small intestine of the dog and become adult taenia, which attach to the intestinal wall. Each worm sheds approximately 500 ova into the bowel. The infected ova-containing feces of the dog contaminate grass and farmland, and the ova are ingested by sheep, pigs, and humans. The ova have chitinous envelopes that are dissolved by gastric juice. The liberated ovum burrows through the intestinal mucosa and is carried by the portal vein to the liver, where it develops into an adult cyst. Most cysts are caught in the hepatic sinusoids, and 70% of hydatid cysts form in the liver. A few ova pass through the liver and are held up in the pulmonary capillary bed or enter the systemic circulation, forming cysts in the lung, spleen, brain, or bones.

Hydatid disease is most common in sheep-raising areas, where dogs have access to infected offal. These include South Australia, New Zealand, Africa, Greece, Spain, and the Middle East. The disease is uncommon in Britain. Hydatid cysts commonly involve the right lobe of the liver, usually the anterior-inferior or poster-ior-inferior segments. The uncomplicated cyst may be silent and found only at autopsy or incidentally. Occasionally, the affected patient presents with dull right upper quadrant pain or abdominal distention. Cysts may become secondarily infected, involve other organs, or even rupture, which leads to an allergic or anaphylactic reaction.

The diagnosis of hydatid disease is based on the findings of an enzyme-linked immunosorbent assay (ELISA) for echinococcal antigens, and results are positive in approximately 85% of infected patients.[42] The ELISA results may be negative in an infected patient if the cyst has not leaked or does not contain scolices, or if the parasite is no longer viable. Eosinophilia of >7% is found is approximately 30% of infected patients. Ultrasonography and CT scanning of the abdomen are both quite sensitive for detecting hydatid cysts. The appearance of the cysts on images depends on the stage of cyst development. Typically, hydatid cysts are well-defined hypodense lesions with a distinct wall. Ring-like calcifications of the pericysts are present in 20 to 30% of cases. As healing occurs, the entire cyst calcifies densely, and a lesion with this appearance is usually dead or inactive. Daughter cysts generally occur in a peripheral location and are typically slightly hypodense compared with the mother cyst. MRI of the abdomen may be useful to evaluate the pericyst, cyst matrix, and daughter cyst characteristics.

Unless the cysts are small or the patient is not a suitable candidate for surgical resection, the treatment of hydatid disease is surgically based because of the high risk of secondary infection and rupture. Medical treatment with albendazole relies on drug diffusion through the cyst membrane. The concentration of drug achieved in the cyst is uncertain but is better than that of mebendazole, and albendazole can be used as initial treatment for small, asymptomatic cysts. For most cysts surgical resection involving laparoscopic or open complete cyst removal with instillation of a scolicidal agent is preferred and usually is curative. If complete cystectomy is not possible, then formal anatomic liver resection can be used. During surgical resection caution must be exercised to avoid rupture of the cyst with release of protoscolices into the peritoneal cavity. Peritoneal contamination can result in an acute anaphylactic reaction or peritoneal implantation of scolices with daughter cyst formation and inevitable recurrence.

Alveolar echinococcosis (caused by *Echinococcus multilocularis*) occurs in the Northern Hemisphere, produces a more generalized granulomatous reaction, and can present in a manner similar to that of a malignancy. Resection is the treatment of choice.

Ascariasis

Ascaris infection is particularly common in the Far East, India, and South Africa. Ova of the roundworm *Ascaris lumbricoides* arrive in the liver by retrograde flow in the bile ducts. The adult worm is 10 to 20 cm long and may lodge in the common bile duct, producing partial bile duct obstruction and secondary cholangitic abscesses. The ascaris may be a nucleus for the development of intrahepatic gallstones. The clinical presentation in an affected patient may include any of the following: biliary colic, acute cholecystitis, acute pancreatitis, or hepatic abscess.[43] Plain abdominal radiographs, abdominal ultrasound, and endoscopic retrograde cholangiography (ERCP) all can demonstrate the ascaris as linear filling defects in the bile ducts. Occasionally worms can be seen moving into and out of the biliary tree from the duodenum. Treatment consists of administration of piperazine citrate, mebendazole, or albendazole in combination with ERCP extraction of the worms. Failure of endoscopic extraction warrants surgical removal of the ascaris.

Schistosomiasis

Schistosomiasis affects >200 million people in 74 countries. Hepatic schistosomiasis is usually a complication of the intestinal disease, because emboli of schistosomiasis ova reach the liver via the mesenteric venous system. Eggs excreted in the feces hatch in water to release free-swimming embryos, which enter snails and develop into fork-tailed cercariae. They then re-enter human skin during contact within infected water. They burrow down to the capillary bed, and at that point there is widespread hematogenous dissemination. Those entering the intrahepatic portal system grow rapidly, and a granulomatous reaction occurs. The degree of resultant portal fibrosis is related to the adult worm load.

Schistosomiasis has three stages of clinical symptomatology: the first includes itching after the entry of cercariae through the skin; the second includes fever, urticaria, and eosinophilia; and the third involves hepatic fibrosis followed by presinusoidal portal hypertension. During this third phase the liver shrinks, the spleen enlarges, and the patient may develop complications of portal hypertension while hepatic function is maintained. Active infection is detected by stool examination. Serologic tests indicate past exposure without specifics regarding timing. A negative serologic test result rules out schistosomal infection. Serum levels of transaminases are usually normal, but the AP level may be mildly elevated. A decreased serum albumin level is usually the result of frequent GI bleeds and decreased nutrition.

Medical treatment of schistosomiasis includes education regarding hygiene and the avoidance of infected water. Treatment with praziquantel 40 to 75 mg/kg as a single dose is the treatment of choice for all forms of schistosomiasis and produces few side effects. GI bleeding usually is controlled by endoscopic variceal ligation. However, in a patient with refractory GI portal hypertensive bleeding, distal splenorenal shunt or gastric devascularization and splenectomy need to be considered.

Viral Hepatitis

The role of the surgeon in the management of viral hepatitis is somewhat limited. However, the disease entities of hepatitis A, B, and C need to be kept in mind during any evaluation for liver disease. The findings of hepatitis A in many cases will be acute, nonspecific, and similar to those associated with hepatic metastases, biliary obstruction, and cirrhosis. Hepatitis B and C can both lead to chronic liver disease, cirrhosis, and hepatocellular carcinoma (HCC). Current hepatitis B vaccination programs as well as treatment protocols involving nucleoside analogues and hepatitis B immunoglobulin have dramatically improved the treatment options for affected patients. The incidence of ESLD and HCC are both diminished by these protocols. Currently, the same therapeutic options are not available for hepatitis C, and although some patients

do maintain a sustained viral response after interferon-based therapy, many either do not respond or have recurrences of their disease. The unraveling of the crystal structures of all three major hepatitis C viral enzymes involved in replication has led to the development of several novel drugs, including protease inhibitors, polymerase inhibitors, and hepatitis C vaccines. Although early results are encouraging, longer-term data are required to determine the effectiveness of these new treatment options.

WORK-UP OF AN INCIDENTAL LIVER MASS

A liver mass often is identified incidentally during a radiologic imaging procedure performed for another indication. For example, a liver mass may be discovered during evaluation for gallbladder disease or kidney stones. In addition, with advances in imaging technology, previously undetected lesions are now identified. Although many of these lesions are benign and will require no further treatment, the concern for malignancy requires a thorough evaluation. Thus, an orderly approach should be taken to the work-up of an incidental liver lesion to minimize unnecessary testing.[44]

The evaluation of an incidental liver mass begins with a history and physical examination (Fig. 31-20). The patient should be asked about abdominal pain, weight loss, previous liver disease, cirrhosis, alcohol use, viral hepatitis, blood transfusions, tattoos, oral contraceptive use (in women), and personal or family history of cancer. On physical examination, jaundice, scleral icterus, hepatomegaly, splenomegaly, palpable mass, or stigmata of portal hypertension should be noted. After completion of the history and physical examination, blood work should be performed, including complete blood count; platelet count; measurement of levels of electrolytes, blood urea nitrogen, creatinine, glucose, and albumin; liver function tests; serum ammonia level; coagulation studies; hepatitis screen; and measurement of levels of the tumor markers carcinoembryonic antigen, alpha-fetoprotein, and cancer antigen 19-9.

The differential diagnosis for an incidental liver mass includes cysts, benign solid lesions, and primary or metastatic cancers (Table 31-7). Ultrasound or CT is commonly performed to evaluate respiratory or abdominal symptoms, and these scans are usually what leads to the discovery of an incidental liver lesion. Although hepatic ultrasound is inexpensive, technical limitations are often encountered due to interference by bowel gas, obesity, or overlying ribs; a mass seen on liver ultrasound should be further evaluated with a dedicated contrast helical CT or MRI scan.[21,22] Additional imaging studies should be performed as indicated. For example, if the working diagnosis is a liver hemangioma and the CT scan findings are not classical for this diagnosis, then a contrast liver MRI should be performed. If the MRI is inconclusive, then an old-fashioned nuclear medicine tagged red blood cell scan can be helpful. If the radiologic imaging results are classic for a benign hemangioma or focal nodular hyperplasia (FNH), then a liver biopsy is not indicated (and actually risks hemorrhage, because both lesions are hypervascular) and observation is warranted as long as the patient is asymptomatic.

If all imaging studies are inconclusive, then an image-guided percutaneous liver biopsy should be considered. If the lesion is too small to biopsy or cannot be well visualized or targeted for percutaneous biopsy, then options are either close follow-up imaging (e.g., 3 to 6 months) to document stability or laparoscopic liver biopsy. Laparoscopic liver biopsy also is indicated in cases of cirrhosis with ascites and coagulopathy, in which the bleeding risk is excessive by percutaneous route. If liver biopsy findings demonstrate adenocarcinoma, then the differential diagnosis narrows to metastatic adenocarcinoma from an unknown or occult primary; a primary liver adenocarcinoma, which also is known as *cholangiocarcinoma*; or bile duct cancer (see "Malignant Liver Tumors"). Although pathologic staining can provide clues to the origin, a primary liver cholangiocarcinoma is usually a diagnosis of exclusion after an occult extrahepatic primary malignancy is ruled out. In these cases the work-up for an occult

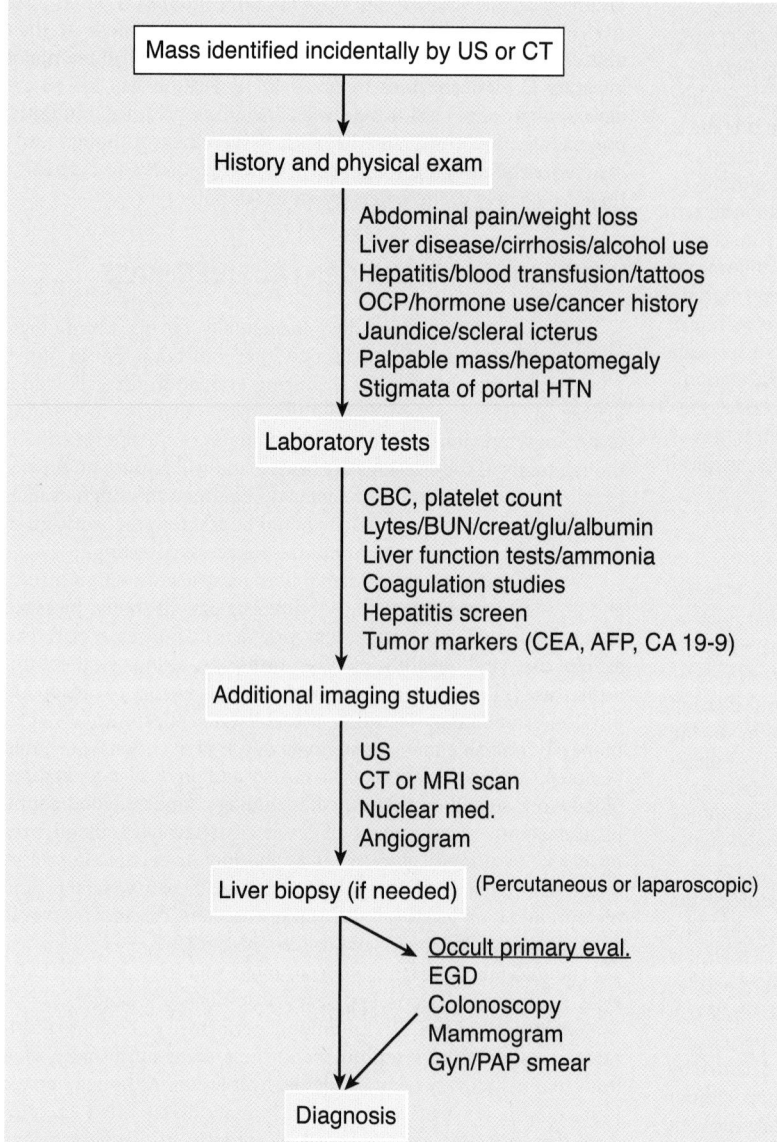

FIG. 31-20. Algorithm for diagnostic work-up of an incidental liver lesion. The evaluation includes history and physical examination, blood work, imaging studies, and liver biopsy (if needed). AFP = alphafetoprotein; BUN = blood urea nitrogen; CA 19-9 = cancer antigen 19-9; CEA = carcinoembryonic antigen; creat = creatinine; CBC = complete blood count; CT = computed tomography; EGD = esophagogastroduodenoscopy; glu = glucose; Gyn = gynecologic; HTN = hypertension; MRI = magnetic resonance imaging; OCP = oral contraceptive pill; PAP = Papanicolaou; US = ultrasound.

primary carcinoma should include colonoscopy; EGD (upper endoscopy); mammogram, gynecologic examination, and Papanicolaou smear (in women); and prostate-specific antigen testing and prostate evaluation (in men).

TABLE 31-7	Classification of liver lesions

Benign
  Cyst
  Hemangioma
  Focal nodular hyperplasia
  Adenoma
  Biliary hamartoma
  Abscess
Malignant
  Hepatocellular carcinoma
  Cholangiocarcinoma (bile duct cancer)
  Gallbladder cancer
  Metastatic colorectal cancer
  Metastatic neuroendocrine cancer (carcinoid)
  Other metastatic cancers

HEPATIC CYSTS

Congenital Cysts

The majority of hepatic cysts are asymptomatic. Hepatic cysts are usually identified incidentally and can occur at any time throughout life. The most common benign lesion found in the liver is the congenital or simple cyst. The exact prevalence of simple hepatic cysts in the U.S. population is not known, but the female:male ratio is approximately 4:1, and the prevalence is approximately 2.8 to 3.6%.[45] Simple cysts are the result of excluded hyperplastic bile duct rests. Simple cysts usually are identified in hepatic imaging studies as thin-walled, homogeneous, fluid-filled structures with few to no septations. The cyst epithelium is cuboidal and secretes a clear nonbilious serous fluid. With the exception of large cysts, simple cysts are usually asymptomatic. Large simple cysts may cause abdominal pain, epigastric fullness, and early satiety. Occasionally the affected patient presents with an abdominal mass. Asymptomatic simple cysts are best managed conservatively. The preferred treatment for symptomatic cysts is ultrasound- or CT-guided percutaneous cyst aspiration followed by sclerotherapy. This approach is approximately 90% effective in controlling symptoms and ablating the cyst cavity. If percutaneous treatment is unavailable or ineffective, treatment may include either laparoscopic or open surgical cysts fenestration. The laparoscopic approach is being used more frequently and is 90% effective. The excised cyst wall is sent for pathologic analysis to rule out carcinoma, and the remaining cyst wall must be carefully inspected for evidence of neoplastic change. If such change is present, complete resection is required, either by enucleation or formal hepatic resection.

Biliary Cystadenoma

Biliary cystadenomas are slow-growing, unusual, benign lesions that most commonly present as large lesions in the right lobe of the liver. Although these lesions are usually benign, they can undergo malignant transformation. Biliary cystadenomas usually present with abdominal pain. An abdominal mass occasionally can be identified on physical examination. In contrast to simple cysts, biliary cystadenomas have walls that appear thicker with soft tissue nodules and the cyst's septations usually enhance. The protein content of the fluid can be variable and can affect the radiographic images on CT and MRI. Surgical resection is the preferred mode of treatment.

Polycystic Liver Disease

Adult polycystic liver disease (ADPCLD) occurs as an autosomal dominant disease and usually presents in the third decade of life. Some 44 to 76% of affected families are found to have mutations of PKD1 and approximately 75% have mutations of PKD2.[46] The prevalence and number of hepatic cysts are higher in females and increase with advancing age and with increasing severity of renal cystic disease and renal dysfunction. At age 60 years, approximately 80% of ADPCLD patients will have hepatic cysts, with women having more and larger cysts. This gender difference may be due to the effects of estrogen. Patients with a small number of cysts or with small cysts (<2 cm) usually remain asymptomatic. In contrast, patients who develop many or large cysts, with a cyst:parenchymal volume ratio of >1, usually develop clinical symptoms, including abdominal pain, shortness of breath, and early satiety. Progressive ADPCLD will result in renal failure and the need for hemodialysis. In most patients, the liver parenchymal volume is preserved despite extensive cystic disease. Hepatic decompensation, variceal hemorrhage, ascites, and encephalopathy develop rarely in patients with ADPCLD and only in patients with massive cystic disease. The most common hepatologic complications associated with ADPCLD are intracystic hemorrhage, infection, and posttraumatic rupture. The most common abnormal biochemical test finding is a modestly elevated γ-glutamyltransferase level and the most useful imaging test is CT scanning of the abdomen, which will demonstrate the characteristic polycystic appearance. Other conditions that may be associated with ADPCLD include cerebral aneurysm, diverticulosis, mitral valve prolapse, and inguinal hernia. There is no effective medical therapy for ADPCLD. Cyst aspiration and sclerosis may be considered if the patient has one or a few dominant cysts; however, most patients have multiple cysts and do not improve when this technique is used. Cyst fenestration via an open or laparoscopic approach can be attempted in symptomatic patients; however, approximately 50% of treated patients will have recurrence of their symptoms.[47] The only definitive therapy for patients with symptomatic ADPCLD is orthotopic liver transplantation. If the patient has renal involvement (polycystic kidney disease) with renal failure, consideration should be given to combined liver-kidney transplantation. Because of the genetic basis of ADPCLD, living-donor transplantation should be considered only if the presence of ADPCLD in the donor can be ruled out.

Caroli's Disease

Caroli's disease is a syndrome of congenital ductal plate malformations of the intrahepatic bile ducts and is characterized by segmental cystic dilatation of the intrahepatic biliary radicals.[48] Caroli's disease also is associated with an increased incidence of biliary lithiasis, cholangitis, and biliary abscess formation. Caroli's disease usually occurs in the absence of cirrhosis and is associated with cystic renal disease.[48] The most common presenting symptoms include fever, chills, and abdominal pain. Most patients present by the age of 30 years, and males and females are affected equally. Rarely, patients can present later in life with complications secondary to portal hypertension. Approximately 33% of affected patients develop biliary lithiasis and 7% develop cholangiocarcinoma. The diagnosis of Caroli's disease is made based on imaging studies. Magnetic resonance cholangiopancreatography, ERCP, and percutaneous transhepatic cholangiography provide more detailed imaging of the biliary tree and confirm communication of the intrahepatic cysts with the biliary tree, which is necessary to solidify the diagnosis. Treatment consists of biliary drainage, with ERCP and percutaneous transhepatic cholangiography serving as first-line therapeutic modalities. If the disease is limited to a single lobe of the liver, hepatic resection can be beneficial. Liver resection can be considered in the patient with hepatic decompensation or unresponsive recurrent cholangitis and possibly in the patient with a small T1 or T2 cholangiocarcinoma.

BENIGN LIVER LESIONS

The liver is an organ that is commonly involved either primarily or secondarily with vascular, metabolic, infectious, and malignant processes. Many classification schemes are used to help narrow the differential diagnosis of liver lesions: solid or cystic, single or multiple, cell of origin (hepatocellular, cholangiocellular, or mesenchymal), and benign or malignant. The most common benign lesions are cysts, hemangiomas, FNH, and hepatocellular adenomas. Many of these lesions have typical features in imaging studies that help confirm the diagnosis.

Cyst

Hepatic cysts are the most frequently encountered liver lesion overall and are described in detail in the section "Hepatic Cysts." Cystic lesions of the liver can arise primarily (congenital) or secondarily from trauma (seroma or biloma), infection (pyogenic or parasitic), or neoplastic disease. Congenital cysts are usually simple cysts containing thin serous fluid and are reported to occur in 5 to 14% of the population, with higher prevalence in women. In most cases, congenital cysts are differentiated from secondary cysts (infectious or neoplastic origin) in that they have no visible wall or solid component and are filled with homogeneous, clear fluid. For benign solid liver lesions, the differential diagnosis includes hemangioma, adenoma, FNH, and bile duct hamartoma (see Table 31-7).

Hemangioma

Hemangiomas (also referred to as *hemangiomata*) are the most common solid benign masses that occur in the liver. They consist of large endothelial-lined vascular spaces and represent congenital vascular lesions that contain fibrous tissue and small blood vessels which eventually grow. They are more common in women and occur in 2 to 20% of the population. They can range from small (≤1 cm) to giant cavernous hemangiomas (10 to 25 cm). The most common symptom is pain, which often occurs with lesions larger than 5 to 6 cm. Spontaneous rupture (bleeding) is rare, and the main indication for resection is pain. Surgical resection can be accomplished by enucleation or formal hepatic resection, depending on the location and involvement of intrahepatic vascular structures and hepatic ducts.

The majority of hemangiomas can be diagnosed by liver imaging studies. On biphasic contrast CT scan, large hemangiomas show asymmetrical nodular peripheral enhancement that is isodense with large vessels and exhibit progressive centripetal enhancement fill-in over time (Fig. 31-21).[21] On MRI, hemangiomas are hypointense on T1-weighted images and hyperintense on T2-weighted images.[49] With gadolinium enhancement, hemangiomas show a pattern of peripheral nodular enhancement similar to that seen on contrast CT scans. Caution should be exercised in ordering a liver biopsy if the

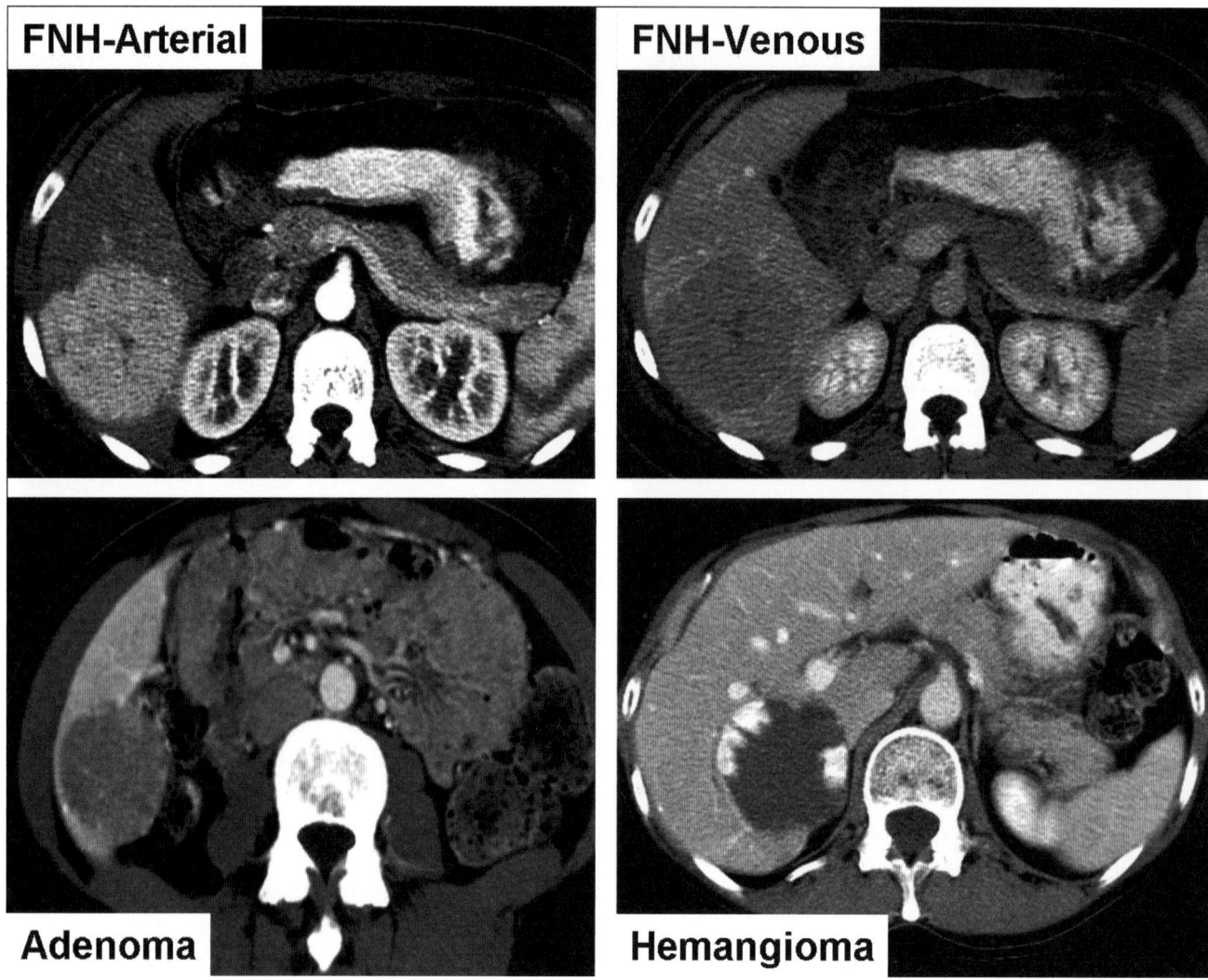

FIG. 31-21. Computed tomographic scans showing classic appearance of benign liver lesions. Focal nodular hyperplasia (FNH) is hypervascular on arterial phase, isodense to liver on venous phase, and has a central scar (*upper panels*). Adenoma is hypovascular (*lower left panel*). Hemangioma shows asymmetrical peripheral enhancement (*lower right panel*).

suspected diagnosis is hemangioma because of the risk of bleeding from the biopsy site, especially if the lesion is at the edge of the liver.

Adenoma

Hepatic adenomas are benign solid neoplasms of the liver. They are most commonly seen in young women (aged 20 years to the forties) and are typically solitary, although multiple adenomas also can occur. Prior or current use of estrogens (oral contraceptives) is a clear risk factor for development of liver adenomas, although they can occur even in the absence of oral contraceptive use. On gross examination, they appear soft and encapsulated and are tan to light brown. Histologically, adenomas lack bile duct glands and Kupffer cells, have no true lobules, and contain hepatocytes that appear congested or vacuolated due to glycogen deposition. On CT scan, adenomas usually have sharply defined borders and can be confused with metastatic tumors. With venous phase contrast, they can look hypodense or isodense in comparison with background liver, whereas on arterial phase contrast subtle hypervascular enhancement often is seen (see Fig. 31-21). On MRI scans, adenomas are hyperintense on T1-weighted images and enhance early after gadolinium injection. On nuclear medicine imaging, they typically appear as "cold," in contrast with FNH.

Hepatic adenomas carry a significant risk of spontaneous rupture with intraperitoneal bleeding. The clinical presentation may be abdominal pain, and in 10 to 25% of cases hepatic adenomas present with spontaneous intraperitoneal hemorrhage. Hepatic adenomas also have a risk of malignant transformation to a well-differentiated HCC. Therefore, it usually is recommended that a hepatic adenoma (once diagnosed) be surgically resected.[44]

Focal Nodular Hyperplasia

FNH is another solid, benign lesion of the liver. Similar to adenomas, they are more common in women of childbearing age, although the link to oral contraceptive use is not as clear as with adenomas. A good-quality biphasic CT scan usually is diagnostic of FNH, on which such lesions appear well circumscribed with a typical central scar (see Fig. 31-21). They show intense homogeneous enhancement on arterial phase contrast images and are often isodense or invisible compared with background liver on the venous phase. On MRI scans, FNH lesions are hypointense on T1-weighted images and isointense to hyperintense on T2-weighted images. After gadolinium administration, lesions are hyperintense but become isointense on delayed images. The fibrous septa extending from the central scar are also more readily seen with MRI. If CT or MRI scans do not show the classic appearance, radionuclide sulfur colloid imaging may be used to diagnose FNH based on select uptake by Kupffer cells. Unlike adenomas, FNH lesions usually do not rupture spontaneously and have no significant risk of malignant transformation. The main indication for surgical resection is abdominal pain. Oral contraceptive or estrogen use should be stopped when either FNH or adenoma is diagnosed.

Bile Duct Hamartoma

Bile duct hamartomas are typically small liver lesions, 2 to 4 mm in size, visualized on the surface of the liver at laparotomy. They are firm, smooth, and whitish yellow in appearance. They can be difficult to differentiate from small metastatic lesions, and excisional biopsy often is required to establish the diagnosis.

MALIGNANT LIVER TUMORS

Malignant tumors in the liver can be classified as primary (cancers that originate in the liver) or metastatic (cancers that spread to the liver from an extrahepatic primary site) (see Table 31-7). Primary cancers in the liver that originate from hepatocytes are known as *hepatocellular carcinomas* (HCCs or hepatomas), whereas cancers arising in the bile ducts are known as *cholangiocarcinomas.*

In the United States, approximately 150,000 new cases of colorectal cancer are diagnosed each year, and the majority of patients (approximately 60%) will develop hepatic metastases over their lifetime. Hence, the most common tumor seen in the liver is metastatic colorectal cancer. This compares with approximately 18,000 new cases of HCC diagnosed annually in the United States. Interestingly, in a Western series of 1000 consecutive new liver cancer patients seen at a university medical center, 47% were HCC, 17% were colorectal cancer metastases, 11% were cholangiocarcinomas, 7% were neuroendocrine metastases, and 18% were other tumors.[50] Although these figures do not reflect the incidence or prevalence of these liver cancers, they are indicative of referral patterns in a tertiary academic medical center with a large liver transplantation team and active hepatology clinic.

Hepatocellular Carcinoma

HCC is the fifth most common malignancy worldwide, with an estimated 1,000,000 new cases diagnosed annually. Major risk factors are viral hepatitis (B or C), alcoholic cirrhosis, hemochromatosis, and nonalcoholic steatohepatitis. In Asia, the risk is as high as 30 to 65 per 100,000 persons per year, whereas in the United States the risk is only 2 per 100,000 persons per year.[51] Although cirrhosis is not present in all cases, it has been estimated to be present 70 to 90% of the time. In a person with cirrhosis, the annual conversion rate to HCC is 3 to 6%. In patients with chronic hepatitis C virus infection, cirrhosis usually is present before the HCC develops; however, in cases of hepatitis C virus infection, HCC tumors can occur before the onset of cirrhosis. HCCs are typically hypervascular with blood supplied predominantly from the hepatic artery. Thus, the lesion often appears hypervascular during the arterial phase of CT studies (Fig. 31-22) and relatively hypodense during the delayed phases due to early washout of the contrast medium by the arterial blood. MRI imaging also is effective in characterizing HCC. HCC is variable on T1-weighted images and usually is hyperintense on T2-weighted images. As with contrast CT, HCC enhances in the arterial phase after gadolinium injection because of its hypervascularity and becomes hypointense in the delayed phases due to contrast washout. HCC has a tendency to invade the portal vein, and the presence of an enhancing portal vein thrombus is highly suggestive of HCC.

The treatment of HCC is complex and is best managed by a multidisciplinary liver transplant team. A complete algorithm for the evaluation and management of HCC is shown (Fig. 31-23).

For patients without cirrhosis who develop HCC, resection is the treatment of choice. For those patients with Child's class A cirrhosis with preserved liver function and no portal hypertension, resection also is considered. If resection is not possible because of poor liver function and the HCC meets the Milan criteria (one nodule <5 cm, or two or three nodules all <3 cm, no gross vascular invasion or extrahepatic spread), liver transplantation is the treatment of choice.[52]

The Barcelona-Clinic Liver Cancer Group has refined its HCC management strategy and has developed the American Association for the Study of Liver Diseases Practice Guidelines.[53,54] Manage-

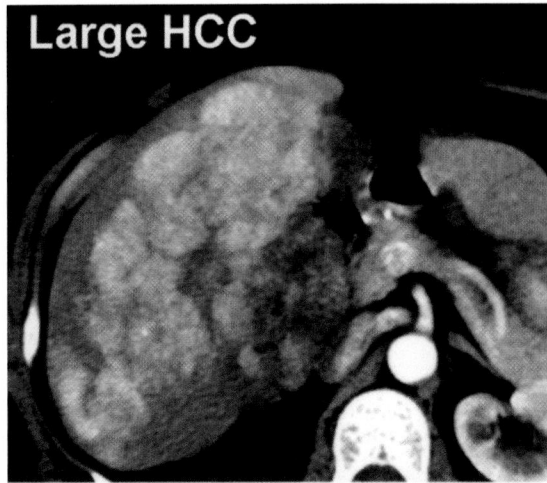
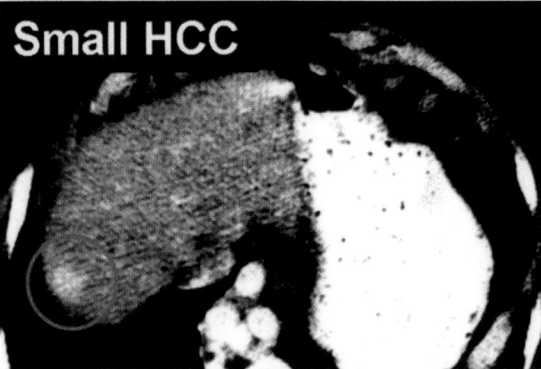
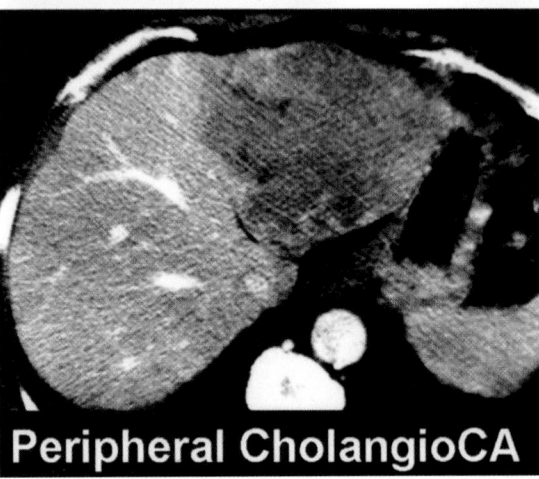

FIG. 31-22. Computed tomographic (CT) images of hepatocellular carcinoma (HCC) and peripheral cholangiocarcinoma. CT scans reveal a large (*upper panel*) and small (*middle panel*) hypervascular HCC. A hypovascular left lobe peripheral cholangiocarcinoma (Cholangio CA) is also shown (*lower panel*).

ment guidelines vary slightly in Asia, Europe, the United States, and other countries based in part on availability of organ donors for liver transplantation. Living-donor liver transplantation is also an alternative for patients with HCC awaiting transplantation to avoid dropout due to tumor progression.[52] Specific treatment options are described in the next section.

Cholangiocarcinoma (Bile Duct Cancer) (see also Chap. 32)

Cholangiocarcinoma, or bile duct cancer, is the second most common primary malignancy within the liver. Cholangiocarcinoma is

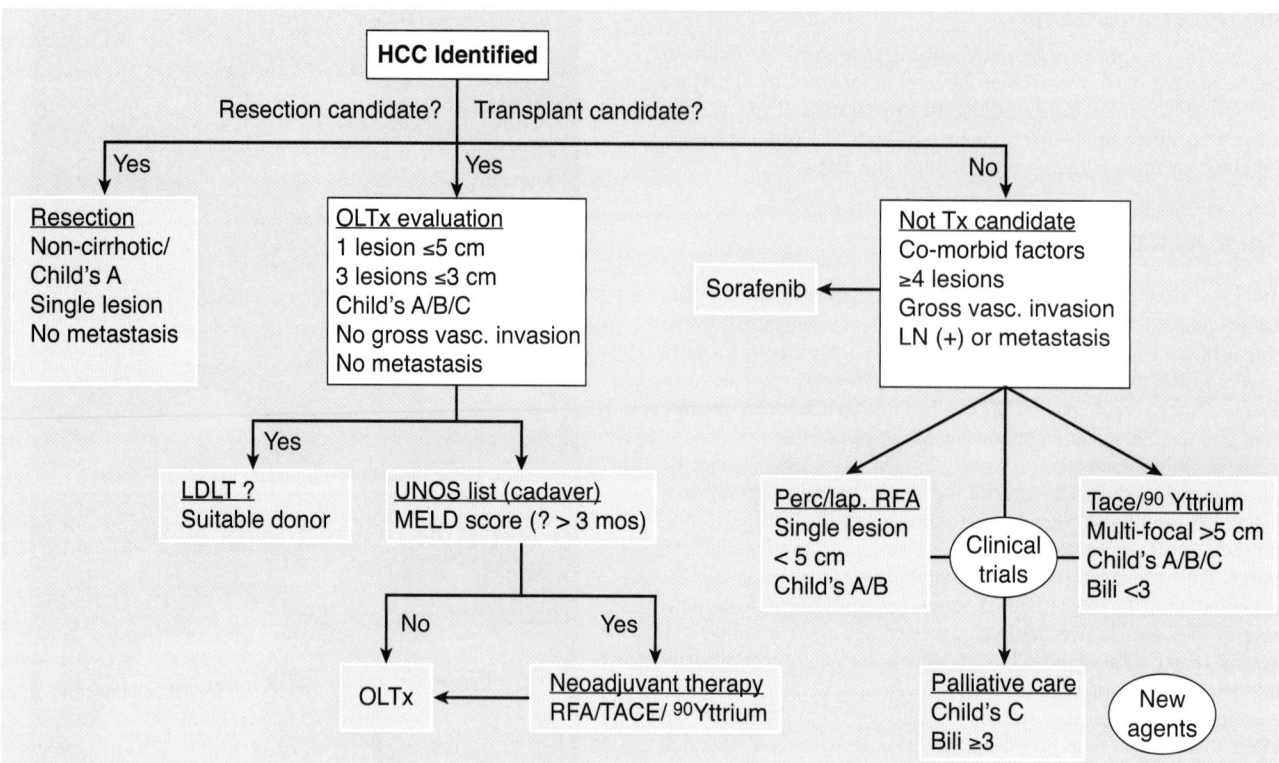

FIG. 31-23. Algorithm for the management of hepatocellular carcinoma (HCC). The treatment algorithm for HCC begins with determining whether the patient is a resection candidate or liver transplant candidate. Bili = bilirubin level (in milligrams per deciliter); Child's = Child-Turcotte-Pugh class; lap = laparoscopic; LDLT = living-donor liver transplantation; LN = lymph node; MELD = Model for End-Stage Liver Disease; OLTx = orthotopic liver transplantation; Perc = percutaneous; RFA = radiofrequency ablation; TACE = transarterial chemoembolization; Tx = transplantation; UNOS = United Network for Organ Sharing; vasc. = vascular.

an adenocarcinoma of the bile ducts that forms in the biliary epithelial cells and can be subclassified into peripheral (intrahepatic) bile duct cancer and central (extrahepatic) bile duct cancer. Extrahepatic bile duct cancer can be distally or proximally located. When proximal, it is referred to as a *hilar cholangiocarcinoma* (Klatskin's tumor). Hilar cholangiocarcinoma originates in the wall of the bile duct at the hepatic duct confluence and usually presents with obstructive jaundice rather than an actual liver mass. In contrast, a peripheral (or intrahepatic) cholangiocarcinoma represents a tumor mass within a hepatic lobe or at the periphery of the liver. A biopsy specimen from the cholangiocarcinoma will show adenocarcinoma, but the pathologist is often unable to differentiate metastatic adenocarcinoma to the liver from true primary bile duct adenocarcinoma. Therefore, a search for a primary site should be undertaken in cases in which an incidentally discovered liver lesion is proven to be an adenocarcinoma on biopsy.

Hilar cholangiocarcinoma is difficult to diagnose and typically presents as a stricture of the proximal hepatic duct causing painless jaundice. It preferentially grows along the length of the common bile duct, often involving the periductal lymphatics with frequent lymph node metastases. Surgical resection offers the only chance for cure of cholangiocarcinoma.[55,56] The location and extent of tumor dictates the operative approach. In one series of 225 patients with hilar cholangiocarcinoma, 29% were deemed to have unresectable tumors by initial imaging.[57] Of the remaining 160 patients who underwent exploratory surgery with curative intent, 50% were found to have inoperable tumors. Histologically negative margins, concomitant hepatic resection, and well-differentiated tumor histology were associated with improved outcome after resection. In another series of 61 patients undergoing surgical exploration for hilar cholangiocarcinoma, the 5-year actuarial survival rates for an

R0 or R1 resection were 45% and 26%, respectively.[58] In a large series reported by Nagino and colleagues, 132 patients with hilar cholangiocarcinoma underwent extended hepatectomy with resection of the caudate lobe and extrahepatic bile duct, and/or portal vein resection (*n* = 63) after portal vein embolization.[59] The 3- and 5-year survival rates were 41.7% and 26.8%, respectively.

In the absence of associated primary sclerosing cholangitis (PSC), surgical resection is the treatment of choice for hilar cholangiocarcinoma. However, approximately 10% of patients with cholangiocarcinoma have PSC.[60] Furthermore, cholangiocarcinoma in the setting of PSC is frequently multicentric and often is associated with underlying liver disease, with eventual cirrhosis and portal hypertension. As a result, experience has shown that resection of cholangiocarcinoma in patients with PSC yields dismal results. This led transplant centers to consider OLT for patients with hilar cholangiocarcinoma. The results of transplantation were disappointing, however, with high recurrence and overall 3-year survival rates of <30%.[61]

Because the growth of hilar cholangiocarcinoma indicates that this disease spreads in a locoregional manner, a rationale for the use of neoadjuvant chemoradiation was developed by the transplant team at the University of Nebraska in the late 1980s. This was adapted in 1993 by the transplant team at the Mayo Clinic, which led to the current Mayo Clinic protocol. The pretransplant Mayo protocol consists of external beam radiation therapy plus a protracted course of IV 5-fluorouracil followed by iridium 192 brachytherapy.[62] Patients then undergo an abdominal exploration and staging. If findings are negative, patients are given capecitabine for 2 of every 3 weeks until OLT. Even after restaging with CT/MRI and endoscopic ultrasonography, approximately 15 to 20% of patients will have positive findings on abdominal exploration for tumor.[60,62] The 5-year survival rate for those undergoing transplantation for cholangiocarcinoma at the Mayo Clinic is approximately 70% and compares favorably with the rate for resection.[60,62] Current eligibility criteria for this Mayo Clinic protocol include unresectable hilar cholangiocarcinoma or hilar cholangiocarcinoma with PSC. The tumor must have a radial dimension of ≤3 cm with no intrahepatic or extrahepatic metastases, and the patient must not have undergone prior radiation therapy or transperitoneal biopsy.[62] Whether these same outstanding results can be reproduced at other transplant centers remains unknown.

Peripheral, or intrahepatic, cholangiocarcinoma is less common than hilar cholangiocarcinoma. In a series of 53 patients at Memorial Sloan-Kettering Cancer Center who underwent surgical exploration for a diagnosis of intrahepatic cholangiocarcinoma, 33 (62%) were found to have resectable tumors.[63] Actuarial 3-year survival for patients undergoing resection was 55%. Factors predictive of poor survival included vascular invasion, histologically positive margins, and multiple tumors. In a large series in Taiwan, 373 patients with peripheral cholangiocarcinoma underwent surgical treatment from 1977 to 2001. Absence of mucobilia, nonpapillary tumor type, tumor of advanced stage, nonhepatectomy, and lack of postoperative chemotherapy were five independent prognostic factors that adversely affected overall survival.[64] Liver transplantation has been performed for peripheral cholangiocarcinoma[65]; however, most centers have abandoned this approach because of organ shortages and relatively high recurrence rates.

Gallbladder Cancer (see also Chap. 32)

Gallbladder cancer is a rare aggressive tumor with a very poor prognosis. Over 90% of patients have associated cholelithiasis. In one study examining the mode of presentation over a 10-year period from 1990 to 2000 in 44 patients diagnosed with gallbladder cancer, the diagnosis was found to be made preoperatively in 57%, intraoperatively in 11%, and incidentally after cholecystectomy in 32%.[66] Surgical approaches can be classified into (a) reoperation for an incidental finding of gallbladder cancer after cholecystectomy, and (b) radical resection in patients with advanced disease. The results are dismal for radical resection in patients with advanced disease and positive hilar lymph nodes.[67,68] For incidental gallbladder cancer beyond stage T1, reoperation with central liver resection, hilar lymphadenectomy, and evaluation of cystic duct stump is most commonly performed.[69,70] The role of formal lobectomy or extended lobectomy as well as common bile duct resection is more controversial. In a single-center study of 23 patients undergoing attempted curative treatment by surgical resection, survival was 85% at 1 year, 63% at 2 years, and 55% at 3 years.[70] In a multicenter study encompassing 115 patients with incidentally discovered gallbladder cancer who underwent reresection,[69] residual disease in the liver was identified in 46% of patients (0% of those with stage T1 disease, 10% of those with T2 tumors, and 36% of those with T3 disease). T stage also was associated with the risk of metastasis to locoregional lymph nodes (lymph node metastasis for T1 of 13%; for T2, 31%; and for T3, 46%). In another study, a German registry of incidental gallbladder cancer identified 439 patients. Patients with tumors staged as T2 or T3 after cholecystectomy had better survival if they underwent reoperation than if they were managed with observation.[71] Hence, reoperation should be considered for all patients who have T2 or T3 tumors or for whom the accuracy of staging is in question.

Metastatic Colorectal Cancer

Over 50% of patients diagnosed with colorectal cancer will develop hepatic metastases during their lifetime. Traditional teaching suggested that hepatic resection for metastatic colorectal cancer to the liver, if technically feasible, should be performed only for fewer than four metastases.[72] However, recent studies have challenged this paradigm. In a series of 235 patients who underwent hepatic resection for metastatic colorectal cancer, the 10-year survival rate of patients with four or more nodules was 29%, nearly comparable to the 32% survival rate of patients with only a solitary tumor metastasis.[73] In the

Memorial Sloan-Kettering Cancer Center series of 98 patients with four or more colorectal hepatic metastases who underwent resection between 1998 and 2002, the 5-year actuarial survival was 33%.[74] Furthermore, improved chemotherapeutic regimens and surgical techniques have produced aggressive strategies for the management of this disease. Many groups now consider volume of future liver remnant and the health of the background liver, and not actual tumor number, as the primary determinants in selection for an operative approach.[75,76] Hence, resectability is no longer defined by what is actually removed, but indications for hepatic resection now center on what will remain after resection.[77] Use of neoadjuvant chemotherapy, portal vein embolization, two-stage hepatectomy, simultaneous ablation, and resection of extrahepatic tumor in select patients have increased the number of patients eligible for a surgical approach.[78]

Neuroendocrine Cancer (Carcinoid Tumor)

Hepatic metastases from neuroendocrine tumors have a protracted natural history and commonly are associated with debilitating endocrinopathies. Several groups have advocated an aggressive surgical approach of cytoreductive surgery, both to control symptoms and to extend survival.[79,80] In a series of 170 patients undergoing resection of hepatic metastases from neuroendocrine tumors between 1977 and 1998 at the Mayo Clinic, overall survival was 61% and 35% at 5 and 10 years, respectively.[81] There was no difference in survival between patients with carcinoid tumors and those with islet cell tumors. Major hepatectomy was performed in 91 patients (54%), and recurrence rate was 84% at 5 years. Belghiti's group has described a two-stage strategy used in 41 patients with a primary neuroendocrine tumor and synchronous bilobar liver metastases.[82] In the first stage, the primary tumor is resected and limited resection of metastases in the left hemiliver, combined with right portal vein ligation, is performed. After 8 weeks of hypertrophy, a right or extended right hepatectomy is performed.[82] In patients treated using this strategy, the 2-, 5-, and 8-year Kaplan-Meier overall survival rates were 94%, 94%, and 79%, respectively, and disease-free survival rates were 85%, 50%, and 26%, respectively.

Other Metastatic Tumors

Nearly every cancer has the propensity to metastasize to the liver. Historically, enthusiasm was low for resecting metastases other than those from a colorectal cancer primary. This was due in part to the recognition that many other primary cancers (such as breast cancer) represent a systemic disease when liver metastases are present. However, more recent studies have shown acceptable 5-year survival rates in the 20 to 40% range for resection of hepatic metastases from breast, renal, and other GI tumors.[83–85] In a large study of hepatic resection for noncolorectal, nonendocrine liver metastases in 1452 patients, negative prognostic factors were nonbreast origin, age >60 years, disease-free interval of <12 months, need for major hepatectomy, performance of R2 resection, and presence of extrahepatic metastases.[86]

TREATMENT OPTIONS FOR LIVER CANCER

In general, the major treatment options for liver cancer can be categorized as shown in Table 31-8. The decision making for any given patient is complex and is best managed by a multidisciplinary liver and GI tumor board. The treatments listed in Table 31-8 are not mutually exclusive, and the important point is to select the most appropriate initial treatment after a complete evaluation. In general, surveillance imaging (CT or MRI) is performed every 3 to 4 months during the first year after diagnosis to observe for response, progression, or recurrence. The treatment plan is individualized and modified according to the response of the patient.

Hepatic Resection

For primary liver cancers or hepatic metastases, hepatic resection is the gold standard and treatment of choice. Although there are

| TABLE 31-8 | Treatment options for liver cancer |

Hepatic resection
Liver transplantation
Ablation techniques
- Radiofrequency ablation
- Ethanol ablation
- Cryoablation
- Microwave ablation
Regional liver therapies
- Chemoembolization/embolization
- Hepatic artery pump chemoperfusion
- Internal radiation therapy (yttrium 90 internal radiation)
External beam radiation therapy
- Stereotactic radiosurgery (CyberKnife, Trilogy, Synergy)
- Intensity-modulated radiation therapy
Systemic chemotherapy
Multimodality approach

anecdotal reports of long-term survival after ablation and other regional liver therapies, liver resection remains the only real option for cure. For HCC in the setting of cirrhosis, liver transplantation also offers the potential for long-term survival, albeit with the consequences of immunosuppression. Hepatic resection also has been advocated for HCC in select patients with cirrhosis before secondary liver transplantation,[87] although this approach remains controversial.[88] Many large series of patients undergoing major hepatectomy now report mortality rates of <5%.[89–92] Previously, a 1-cm tumor margin was considered desirable; however, recent studies have reported comparable survival rates with smaller margins.[93,94] The technical aspects of anatomic hepatic lobectomies are described later.

Liver Transplantation

The rationale supporting liver transplantation (OLT) for HCC includes the fact that most HCCs (>80%) arises in the setting of cirrhosis.[52,61] The cirrhotic liver often does not have enough reserve to tolerate a formal resection. Also, HCC tumors are commonly multifocal and are underestimated by current CT or MRI imaging. Further, recurrence rates are high at 5 years after resection (>50%). Hence, OLT is an appealing treatment, because it removes the cancer and the cirrhotic liver that leads to HCC. Approximately 6000 liver transplantations are performed each year in the United States, with 1-year survival rates approaching 90%. In April 2008, approximately 16,400 patients were on the waiting list for liver transplantation.[95]

Initial series of OLT for HCC reported in the 1990s included advanced cases of HCC, and the 5-year survival rates were only 20 to 50%.[61] This compared poorly with overall 5-year survival rates of 70 to 75% for OLT in the Organ Procurement and Transplantation Network/United Network for Organ Sharing (OPTN/UNOS) database. Mazzaferro and colleagues at Milan subsequently showed that survival rates were markedly improved when OLT was limited to patients with early-stage HCC (stage I or stage II) with one tumor ≤5 cm, or three tumors with the largest being ≤3 cm, along with an absence of gross vascular invasion or extrahepatic spread.[96,97] Multiple studies have validated these findings, although some groups have proposed an expansion of the Milan criteria.[52,61,98]

In 2002, OPTN/UNOS adopted the Model for End-Stage Liver Disease (MELD) score [a 6- to 40-point scale based on serum total bilirubin level, creatinine level, and international normalized ratio (INR)] for allocation of deceased donor liver organs in the United States. In an attempt to decrease the high mortality rate for patients with preserved liver function and progressive HCC, patients with stage II HCC were given priority points (currently 22 MELD points). This had a positive effect for HCC liver transplant candidates, leading to decreased waiting list dropout and increased transplant rates with excellent long-term outcomes.[99] The goal is to better equate death rates on the liver transplant waiting list for patients with stage II HCC with rates for patients with chronic liver disease without HCC.

Radiofrequency Ablation

In 1891, d'Arsonval discovered that radiofrequency (RF) waves delivered as an alternating electric current (>10 kHz) could pass through living tissue without causing pain or neuromuscular excitation. The resistance of the tissue to the rapidly alternating current produced heat. This discovery contributed to the development of the surgical application of electrocautery. In 1908, Beer used RF coagulation to destroy urinary bladder tumors. Cushing and Bovie later applied RF ablation to intracranial tumors. In 1961, Lounsberry studied the histologic changes of the liver after RFA in animal models. He found that RF caused local tissue destruction with uniform necrosis. In the early 1990s, two groups proposed that RFA can be an effective method for destroying unresectable malignant liver tumors.[100,101] Both groups found that RFA produced lesions with well-demarcated areas of necrosis without viable tumor cells present. Clinical reports after short-term follow-up suggested that RFA was safe and effective in the treatment of liver tumors.[102–104] However, Abdalla and colleagues examined data for 358 consecutive patients with colorectal liver metastases treated with curative intent over a 10-year period (1992 to 2002).[105] Liver-only recurrence after RFA was four times the rate after resection (44% vs. 11% of patients), and RFA alone or in combination with resection did not provide survival rates comparable to those with resection alone. Nonetheless, RFA remains a common procedure that can be performed by a percutaneous, minimally invasive laparoscopic, or open approach.[106,107] It also has been used successfully to ablate small HCCs as a bridge to liver transplantation.[108] Recently, results were reported for the first randomized clinical trial involving RFA treatment for HCC in 291 Chinese patients with three or fewer HCC tumors ranging in size from 3 to 7.5 cm.[109] Patients were randomly assigned to treatment arms of RFA alone (n = 100), transarterial chemoembolization (TACE) alone (n = 95), or combined TACE plus RFA (n = 96). At a median follow-up of 28.5 months, median survival was 22 months in the RFA group, 24 months in the TACE group, and 37 months in the TACE plus RFA group. Patients treated with TACE plus RFA had significantly better overall survival than those treated with TACE alone (P <.001) or RFA alone (P <.001).

Ethanol Ablation, Cryosurgery, and Microwave Ablation

Percutaneous ethanol injection has been shown to be a safe and effective treatment for small HCCs.[52] The ethanol usually is delivered by percutaneous injection under ultrasound or CT guidance. Percutaneous ethanol injection also is used to treat small HCC tumors as a bridge to liver transplantation in some centers to avoid patient dropout.[110] Although cryosurgery was used in the late 1980s and 1990s for ablation of liver tumors, many have abandoned this approach in favor of RFA because of the latter's fewer side effects and ease of use. Microwave ablation is the newest thermal ablative technique and is used in the management of unresectable liver tumors to produce a coagulation necrosis. A multicenter phase II U.S. trial was recently reported using a 915-MHz microwave generator.[111] Eighty-seven patients underwent 94 ablation procedures for 224 hepatic tumors. Forty-five percent of the procedures were performed using an open approach, 7% laparoscopically, and 48% percutaneously. The average tumor size was 3.6 cm (range, 0.5 to 9.0 cm). At a mean follow-up of 19 months, 47% of the patients were alive with no evidence of disease. Local recurrence at the ablation site occurred in 2.7% of tumors, and regional recurrence occurred in 43% of patients. There were no procedure-related deaths. Further studies are required to define the role of this technology in relation to the other ablation options available.

Chemoembolization and Hepatic Artery Pump Chemoperfusion

Chemoembolization is the process of injecting chemotherapeutic drugs combined with embolization particles into the hepatic artery that supplies the liver tumor using a percutaneous, transfemoral approach. It is most commonly used for treatment of unresectable HCC. Two randomized trials as well as a meta-analysis have shown a survival benefit with chemoembolization.[112-114] In a study by Lo and colleagues, 80 Asian patients were randomly assigned to receive either chemoembolization with cisplatin in lipiodol or symptomatic treatment only.[112] Chemoembolization resulted in a marked tumor response, and the actuarial survival was significantly better in the chemoembolization group (1- and 3-year survival of 57% and 26%, respectively) than in the control group (1- and 3-year survival of 32% and 3%, respectively). In another randomized trial, a Barcelona group compared chemoembolization with doxorubicin vs. supportive care and showed that chemoembolization significantly improved survival.[113] Finally, in a large prospective cohort study of 8510 patients with unresectable HCC in Japan who received transcatheter arterial lipiodol chemoembolization, the 5-year survival rate was 26% and median survival time was 34 months.[115] The TACE-related mortality rate after the initial therapy was 0.5%. Complications of TACE include liver dysfunction or liver failure, hepatic abscess, and hepatic artery thrombosis. Recent studies also have shown promising results for chemoembolization with drug-eluting beads (doxorubicin) in treatment of HCC.[116]

In the 1990s hepatic artery pump chemoperfusion with floxuridine for colorectal cancer metastases to the liver was used both for treatment of inoperable disease and in the adjuvant setting.[117] However, in the modern era of improved chemotherapeutic options, this treatment modality is seldom used outside of a clinical trial.

Yttrium 90 Microspheres

Selective internal radioembolization is a promising new treatment modality for patients with inoperable primary or metastatic liver tumors. The treatment is a minimally invasive transcatheter therapy in which radioactive microspheres are infused into the hepatic arteries via a transfemoral percutaneous approach. The yttrium 90 microspheres are directly injected into the hepatic artery branches that supply the tumor. Once infused, the microspheres deliver doses of high-energy, low-penetration radiation selectively to the tumor. The main indications are inoperable HCC[118] and colorectal cancer hepatic metastases for which systemic chemotherapy has failed.[119,120] In a recent study involving 137 patients with unresectable chemorefractory liver metastases treated with radioembolization, there was a response rate of 42.8% (2.1% complete response, 40.7% partial response) according to World Health Organization criteria.[120] One-year survival rate was 47.8% and 2-year survival rate was 30.9%. Median survival was 457 days for patients with colorectal tumor metastases, 776 days for those with neuroendocrine tumor metastases, and 207 days for those with noncolorectal, nonneuroendocrine tumor metastases. The two products available in the United States are SIR-Spheres and TheraSphere.

Stereotactic Radiosurgery

Although stereotactic radiosurgery (with CyberKnife and other systems) is in widespread use for brain and spinal tumors, body application to HCC or metastatic liver tumors has only recently occurred. In a phase I study, 31 patients with unresectable HCCs and 10 with unresectable cholangiocarcinomas completed a six-fraction course of stereotactic body radiotherapy.[121] The treatment was well tolerated, and median survival was 11.7 and 15.0 months for the two groups, respectively. A similar safety profile was observed in a study in the Netherlands.[122] Further clinical trials are required to define the future role of stereotactic radiosurgery in treatment of HCC and metastatic tumors.

Systemic Chemotherapy

A complete review of chemotherapy options for primary and metastatic liver cancers is beyond the scope of this chapter. For treatment of HCC, a phase II trial of the multikinase inhibitor sorafenib showed some efficacy,[123] and therefore a phase III randomized international multicenter trial (Sorafenib HCC Assessment Randomized Protocol, or SHARP) was initiated enrolling 602 patients with Child's class A cirrhosis and inoperable HCC. At interim analysis, the trial was discontinued because a survival benefit was found in the treatment group. Llovet and associates presented the findings at the 2007 American Society of Clinical Oncology annual meeting, which showed that sorafenib leads to a 44% improvement in overall survival compared with placebo.[124] The median overall survival for patients receiving sorafenib was 10.7 months vs. 7.9 months for patients in the control arm. Based on these findings, sorafenib received accelerated Food and Drug Administration approval for the treatment of advanced unresectable HCC. Future studies will likely examine the role of sorafenib in combination with other treatment modalities.

HEPATIC RESECTION SURGICAL TECHNIQUES

Nomenclature

Due to the confusion in language with regard to anatomic descriptions of hepatic resections, a common nomenclature was introduced at the International Hepato-Pancreato-Biliary Association meeting in Brisbane, Australia, in 2000 (Table 31-9).[125,126] The goal

TABLE 31-9   Brisbane 2000 liver terminology

Older hepatic resection terminology	Brisbane 2000 hepatic resection terminology
Right hepatic lobectomy	Right hepatectomy or right hemihepatectomy
Left hepatic lobectomy	Left hepatectomy or left hemihepatectomy
Right hepatic trisegmentectomy	Right trisectionectomy or extended right hepatectomy (or hemihepatectomy)
Left hepatic trisegmentectomy	
Left lateral segmentectomy	Left trisectionectomy or extended left hepatectomy (or hemihepatectomy)
Right posterior lobectomy	
Caudate lobectomy	Left lateral sectionectomy or bisegmentectomy 2, 3
	Right posterior sectionectomy
	Caudate lobectomy or segmentectomy 1
	Alternative "sector" terminology
	Right anterior sectorectomy
	Right posterior sectorectomy or right lateral sectorectomy
	Left medial sectorectomy or left paramedian sectorectomy (bisegmentectomy 3, 4)
	Left lateral sectorectomy (segmentectomy 2)

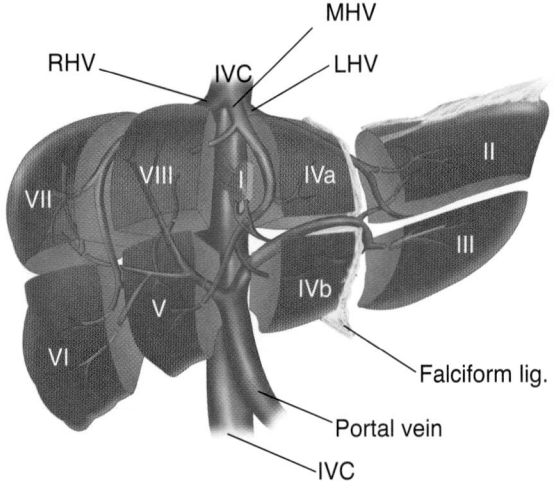

FIG. 31-24. Hepatic resection nomenclature and anatomy. Hepatic segments removed in the formal major hepatic resections are indicated. The International Hepato-Pancreato-Biliary Association (IHPBA) Brisbane 2000 terminology also is presented. IVC = inferior vena cava; LHV = left hepatic vein; MHV = middle hepatic vein; RHV = right hepatic vein.

was to provide universal terminology for liver anatomy and hepatic resections, because there was much overlap among the designations for hepatic lobes, sections, sectors, and segments used by surgeons worldwide (Fig. 31-24). The most common or prevailing anatomic pattern was used as the basis for naming liver anatomy, and the surgical procedure nomenclature adopted for hepatic resections was based on the assigned anatomic terminology.[127] Adoption of a common language should enable hepatic surgeons to better understand and interpret liver surgery publications from different continents and disseminate their knowledge to the next generation of hepatobiliary surgeons. Nonetheless, even today the literature is full of both old and new liver resection terminology, so the surgeon in training must be familiar with all the various classifications.

Techniques and Devices for Dividing the Hepatic Parenchyma

Hepatic resection surgery has evolved over the past 50 years. A better understanding of liver anatomy and physiology, coupled with improved anesthesia techniques and widespread use of intraoperative ultrasound, has led to virtually "bloodless" liver surgery in the modern era (the year 2000 to the present). Innovations in technology have expanded the list of liver parenchymal transection devices[128–130] and hemostatic agents (Table 31-10). Suffice it to say that each device or agent has a learning curve and that undoubtedly every experienced hepatic surgeon has his or her personal preferences.

One major advance was the application of vascular stapling devices for division of the hepatic and portal veins.[131–133] Based on early reports of successful stapling of extrahepatic vessels, stapling devices have now been used in the parenchymal transection phase, which remains a source of potential blood loss due to back bleeding from the middle hepatic vein.[134,135] One advantage of the stapling technique is the speed with which the transection can be performed, which minimizes surface bleeding and period of ischemia for the remnant liver. However, a major disadvantage of the stapling technique is the cost of multiple stapler cartridges. This is balanced by the decreased expenses reported with avoidance of ICU admission and blood transfusion, as well as shortened operating room time. Another consideration in the use of staplers for parenchymal transection is the potential for bile leaks. However, in a large series of 101 consecutive right hemihepatectomies performed using the

TABLE 31-10	Techniques and devices for dividing liver parenchyma and achieving hemostasis

Blunt fracture and clips
Monopolar cautery (Bovie)
Bipolar cautery
Argon beam coagulator
CUSA ultrasonic dissector
Hydro-Jet water-jet dissector
Harmonic Scalpel, AutoSonix ultrasonic transector-coagulator
LigaSure tissue fusion system
SurgRx EnSeal tissue sealing and transection system
Gyrus PK cutting forceps
Endovascular staplers
TissueLink sealing devices
Habib 4X Laparoscopic sealer
InLine bipolar linear coagulator
Topical agents (fibrin glues, Surgicel, Gelfoam, Avitene, Tisseel, Floseal, Crosseal)

stapling technique, there was only one reported bile leak (1%), which sealed after ERCP.[135]

Steps in Commonly Performed Hepatic Resections

A fundamental understanding of hepatic anatomy is vital for any surgeon with the desire to perform hepatobiliary surgery. Each hepatic resection surgery can be broken down into a series of orderly steps. The key to being a proficient hepatic surgeon is not to move one's hands swiftly but rather to accomplish the operation by completing the steps in an orchestrated fashion. The surgeon should not move to step 5 until steps 1 through 4 are complete. Mastery of the operative steps coupled with knowledge of liver anatomy and the common anatomic variants provides the foundation for safe hepatic surgery. (The same basic principle can be applied to any complex surgical procedure.) There are many different techniques and sequences for accomplishing each of the anatomic (and nonanatomic) hepatic operations. The authors present their preferred approach in a stepwise fashion for right hepatic lobectomy (right hemihepatectomy), left hepatic lobectomy (left hemihepatectomy), and left lateral segmentectomy (left lateral sectionectomy). Provision of a detailed approach for every type of liver resection is beyond the scope of this chapter, and readers are referred to several excellent descriptions.[136]

Steps Common to All Open Major Hepatic Resections

1. Make the skin incision—right subcostal with midline extension.
2. Open the abdomen and place a fixed table retractor (Thompson).
3. Take down the round and falciform ligaments, and expose the anterior surface of the hepatic veins.
4. For a left hepatectomy, divide the left triangular ligament; for a right hepatectomy, mobilize the right lobe from the right coronary and triangular ligaments.
5. Open the gastrohepatic ligament and assess for replaced hepatic arteries.
6. Perform an open cholecystectomy; leave the gallbladder with the cystic duct intact (until end of case).
7. Perform liver ultrasound and confirm the operation to be performed.

Right Hepatic Lobectomy (Right Hepatectomy or Hemihepatectomy)

8. Mobilize the liver from the inferior vena cava (IVC) in "piggyback" fashion; ligate the short hepatic veins up to the right hepatic vein (RHV).
9. Perform a right hilar dissection—gently lower the hilar plate, then doubly ligate and divide the right hepatic artery (RHA), staying high on the right side of the common bile duct.

10. Divide the inflow (right portal vein, or RPV) with a vascular stapler (white 2.5-mm cartridge), after taking the small lateral portal vein branch off the RPV to the caudate/right lobe.

11. Divide the outflow (right hepatic vein, or RHV) with the vascular stapler (white cartridge).

12. Notch or divide the caudate process crossing to the right hepatic lobe.

13. Make a counterincision at the right base of the gallbladder fossa; pass a large Kelly clamp deep to the hilar plate and emerge anterior to the IVC; place an umbilical tape in the tunnel behind the hilar plate.

14. Divide the right hilar plate with right hepatic ducts using the vascular stapler (white cartridge).

15. Repeat ultrasound and confirm the transection plane, staying just to the right of the middle hepatic vein (MHV).

16. Bovie down approximately 1 cm in the liver parenchyma, then switch to a LigaSure device.

17. Continue parenchymal division with a LigaSure device until segment V/VIII MHV branches are encountered.

18. Initiate the Pringle maneuver around the porta hepatis (Potts loop cinched up with right angle clamp).

19. Complete the parenchymal slice with sequential crushing vascular stapling (pretunnel with a large Kelly clamp), usually 4 to 6 minutes for the entire slice.

20. Check the cut edge for surgical bleeding; place a figure-of-eight suture if bleeding is encountered.

21. Release the Pringle maneuver and dry up the cut edge with a saline-cooled radiofrequency sealant device.

22. Inspect the IVC and right retroperitoneal space for hemostasis.

23. Perform completion ultrasound to confirm left portal vein (LPV) inflow and hepatic vein outflow.

24. Shoot a saline cholangiogram via the cystic duct stump to confirm that the cut edge is watertight.

25. Shoot a contrast fluoroscopic cholangiogram (optional) to confirm the patency of the proximal left hepatic duct and distal common bile duct; secure the cystic duct stump in the usual manner.

26. Tack the proximal falciform ligament back to the diaphragm side with a single figure-of-eight suture.

27. Place a Jackson-Pratt drain in the right subphrenic space and close the abdomen (Fig. 31-25).

Comments Although some liver surgeons advocate a one-step division of the entire intrahepatic Glissonian pedicle as described by Launois and Jamieson,[137] it is the authors' preference to divide the RHA and RPV in an extrahepatic fashion and restrict the intrahepatic maneuver for division of the right hilar plate with the right hepatic ducts. As for the transection plane, the key is to perform accurate ultrasound visualization and mapping of the MHV and to stay just to the right of it. Weaving in and out or bisecting the MHV can leading to torrential back bleeding. Also, for bulky right lobe tumors adherent to the diaphragm or retroperitoneum, an anterior approach with division of the parenchyma can be performed before right lobe mobilization.[138,139] The anterior approach also can be facilitated by use of the "hanging maneuver."[140]

Left Hepatic Lobectomy (Left Hepatectomy or Hemihepatectomy)

8. Widely open the gastrohepatic ligament flush with the undersurface of the left lateral section and the caudate lobe.

9. Doubly ligate and divide a replaced or accessory left hepatic artery (LHA) if present.

10. Clamp the round ligament (ligament teres) and pull it anteriorly as a handle to expose the left hilum.

11. Divide any existing parenchymal bridge between segments III and IVB.

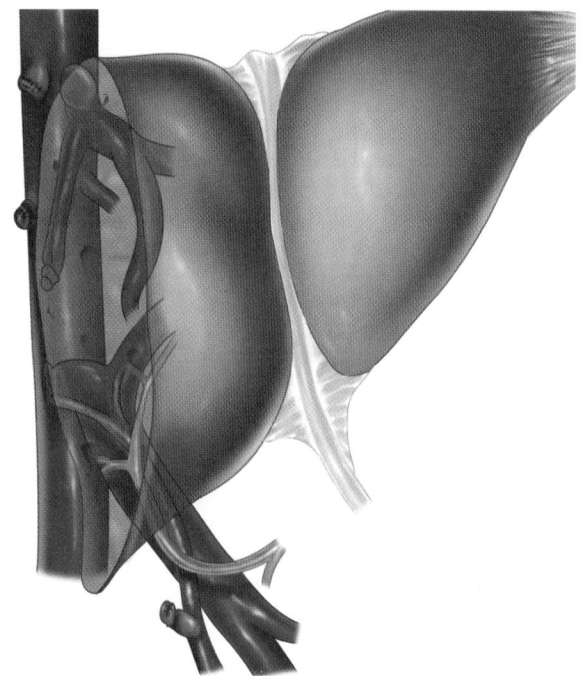

FIG. 31-25. Completed right hepatic lobectomy (right hepatectomy) with the right portal vein, right hepatic artery, and right bile duct ligated and divided. The right hepatic vein is ligated and divided with a vascular stapler. Middle hepatic vein branches inside the liver are divided with the vascular stapler.

12. Dissect the left hilum at the base of the umbilical fissure and lower the hilar plate anterior to the left portal pedicle.

13. Incise the peritoneum overlying the hilum from the left side and doubly ligate the LHA (after test clamping and confirming a palpable pulse in the RHA).

14. Dissect the portal vein at the base of the umbilical fissure (it will take a nearly 90-degree bend from the transverse to the umbilical portion).

15. Divide the LPV with a vascular stapler (white cartridge), staying just distal to (beyond) the take-off of the caudate inflow branch (if the caudate lobe is being preserved).

16. Divide the ligamentum venosum (Arantius' ligament) caudally.

17. Make a counterincision in segment IVB 1 cm above the base of the umbilical fissure and pass a blunt Kelly clamp behind the left hilar plate, aiming for the left lower quadrant and exiting just anterior (and superficial) to the caudate lobe.

18. Place an umbilical tape in the tunnel behind the left hilar plate.

19. Divide the left hilar plate and left hepatic duct with a vascular stapler (white cartridge).

20. Fold the left lateral segment up and back to the right, exposing the window at the base of the left hepatic vein (LHV) as it enters the IVC. This is facilitated by dividing any loose areolar tissue overlying the ligamentum venosum (Arantius' ligament), which is divided proximally.

21. Pass a large, blunt right-angle clamp in the window between the RHV and the MHV, and hug the back of the MHV, aiming for the deep edge of the LHV. *Do not force it or make a hole in the IVC or MHV.*

22. Pass an umbilical tape through this window and divide the LHV and MHV common trunk with a vascular stapler.

23. Repeat ultrasound and confirm the transection plane on the anterior surface, staying close to the demarcated line. Do not bisect the MHV as it passes tangentially from the left to the right lobe.

24. Bovie down approximately 1 cm in the liver parenchyma, then switch to a LigaSure device.

25. Continue parenchymal division with the LigaSure device until segment V/VIII MHV branches are encountered.

26. Initiate a Pringle maneuver around the porta hepatis (Potts loop cinched up with right angle clamp).

27. Complete the parenchymal slice with sequential crushing vascular stapling (pretunnel with a large Kelly clamp). As the slice is deepened, gradually carry the transection down to exit just anterior to the caudate at the level of Arantius' ligament.

28. Check the cut edge for surgical bleeding; place a figure-of-eight suture if bleeding is encountered.

29. Release the Pringle maneuver and dry up the cut edge with a saline-cooled radiofrequency sealant device.

30. Perform completion ultrasound to confirm RPV inflow and RHV outflow.

31. Shoot a saline cholangiogram via the cystic duct stump to confirm that the cut edge is watertight.

32. Shoot a contrast fluoroscopic cholangiogram (optional) to confirm the patency of the proximal right hepatic duct and the distal common bile duct; secure the cystic duct stump in the usual manner.

33. Place a Jackson-Pratt drain in the left subphrenic space and close the abdomen (Fig. 31-26).

Comments Because the right posterior duct comes off the left hepatic duct in approximately 20% of cases (see Fig. 31-9) and the right anterior duct comes off the left hepatic duct in approximately 5% of cases,[6] it is vital to divide the left hepatic duct at the base of the umbilical fissure and not more centrally in the hilum as it bifurcates. If the left hepatic duct were divided as it appears to bifurcate from the right hepatic duct, then approximately 20 to 25% of the time either the right posterior or right anterior duct would be transected. After the left hepatic duct is divided as described earlier (steps 17 through

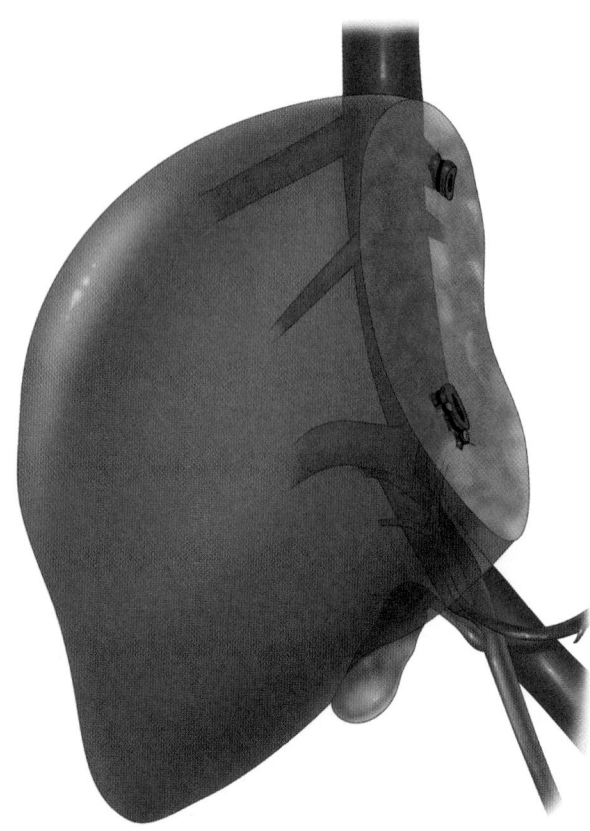

FIG. 31-26. Completed left hepatic lobectomy (left hepatectomy) resecting segments II, III, and IV.

19), the liver parenchyma is scored and divided horizontally approximately 1 cm above the left hilum; the surgeon thus assumes that an aberrant right anterior or posterior duct is coming off the left hepatic duct in the hilum and preserves it. Then as the parenchymal transection reaches the left side of the gallbladder fossa, the transection plane turns vertical to run parallel to Cantlie's line (or the left edge of the gallbladder bed). The left lobe of the liver will be well demarcated at this point (after the vascular inflow has been divided), which guides the transection plane on the anterior surface. In general, the transection plane should be close to the demarcation line to minimize the amount of devascularized liver remaining. When dividing the LHV and MHV, the surgeon should keep in mind that they have a common trunk approximately 90% of the time. If it is not easy to open the window deep to the MHV and LHV, then division of the MHV and LHV can be accomplished after the parenchymal transection.

Left Lateral Segmentectomy (Left Lateral Sectionectomy)

8. Widely open the gastrohepatic ligament flush with the undersurface of the left lateral section and the caudate lobe.

9. Doubly ligate and divide a replaced or accessory LHA if present.

10. Clamp the round ligament and pull it anteriorly as a handle to expose the left hilum.

11. Divide any existing parenchymal bridge between segments III and IVB.

12. Carry the dissection down from the end of the round ligament, and the segment III pedicle will be encountered.

13. Incise the peritoneal reflection on the left side of the round ligament as it inserts into the umbilical fissure. This will facilitate encircling the segment III and II pedicles, which can be divided separately with a vascular stapler. When encircling the segment II pedicle, take care to avoid injury to the caudate inflow vessels coming off the LPV.

14. Divide the liver parenchyma, staying flush on the left side of the falciform ligament using a Bovie cautery and/or LigaSure device.

15. Divide the LHV inside the liver parenchyma with a vascular stapler (white cartridge) as the parenchymal transection is complete.

16. A Pringle maneuver usually is not required for a left lateral sectionectomy because complete devascularization occurs before transection and little back bleeding is encountered.

Comments If the segment III and II LHA branches are large, they can be individually ligated in the left hilum before the pedicles (with portal vein and hepatic duct branches) are taken. If the tumor is more peripheral in the left lateral segment, then the segment III and II pedicles can be divided with a vascular stapler inside the liver during the parenchymal transection.

Pringle and Ischemic Preconditioning

Pringle described clamping of the portal triad a century ago in the landmark paper "Notes on the Arrest of Hepatic Hemorrhage Due to Trauma."[4] Although the Pringle maneuver was initially described for controlling bleeding due to traumatic liver injury, it is commonly used during elective hepatic resections.[141,142] The goal is to minimize blood loss and hypotension, which add significant morbidity to the operation. Further, intraoperative blood transfusion has been shown to be an independent risk factor for increased postoperative infection as well as worse patient survival in some studies. Therefore, all efforts should be made to minimize blood loss during hepatic resection.

Although the liver has been shown to tolerate up to 1 hour of warm ischemia, some technical variations of the Pringle maneuver include intermittent vascular occlusion with cycles of approximately 15 minutes on and 5 minutes off. Experimental and clinical studies have demonstrated the efficacy of intermittent vascular occlusion in decreasing ischemia/reperfusion injury compared with continuous vascular occlusion, with less elevation of postoperative liver enzyme levels.[143] Another variation is selective hemihepatic vascular occlusion, which can reduce the severity of visceral congestion and total liver ischemia. In one prospective trial of total vs. selective portal triad clamping, both techniques of inflow clamping were found to be equally effective for patients with normal livers, but greater liver damage was observed with total inflow occlusion in patients with cirrhotic livers.[144]

In an attempt to decrease the ischemic damage associated with inflow occlusion, some hepatic surgeons have advocated the use of ischemic preconditioning.[145] *Ischemic preconditioning* refers to the brief interruption of blood flow to an organ, followed by a short reperfusion period, and then a more prolonged period of ischemia. In a randomized clinical trial involving 100 patients undergoing major hepatic resection, Clavien and colleagues reported significantly less liver injury in the group who received ischemic preconditioning with a 10-minute clamp, a 10-minute reperfusion, and then a 30-minute clamp than in those who received a 30-minute clamp alone.[146] Patients with steatosis also were especially protected by ischemic preconditioning, and the mechanism was shown to be related in part to preservation of the adenosine triphosphate content of liver tissue.

Preoperative Portal Vein Embolization

The observation that tumor thrombosis of a major portal vein branch induced ipsilateral lobar atrophy and contralateral lobe hypertrophy led to the concept of intentional preoperative portal vein embolization (PVE) to induce compensatory hypertrophy of the remnant liver. This procedure was first described in the 1980s and is accomplished via a percutaneous, transhepatic route.[147,148] Numerous studies have subsequently confirmed that PVE is effective in inducing hypertrophy of nonembolized hepatic segments.[59,149] PVE usually is performed in the setting of a planned right or left trisectionectomy or extended hepatic lobectomy when it is thought that the patient's remnant liver will be too small to support liver function. The future liver remnant volume (e.g., the volume of segments II, III, and I) in a patient undergoing a planned right trisectionectomy can be directly measured by helical CT and then divided by the total estimated liver volume to calculate the percentage of the future liver remnant. If the future liver remnant is thought to be too small, then PVE should be considered to increase the size of the future liver remnant.[150] In general, surgery is planned approximately 4 weeks after PVE to allow adequate time for hypertrophy.

There is no universal agreement on what constitutes a future liver remnant adequate to avoid postoperative liver failure. It is thought that 25 to 30% of the total liver volume is adequate in patients with normal background liver.[151] Vauthey and associates reported that major postoperative complications were increased when the estimated future liver remnant was <25%.[152] Farges and colleagues conducted a prospective study to assess the benefits of PVE before right hepatectomy. They demonstrated that PVE had no beneficial effect on the postoperative course in patients with normal livers but significantly reduced postoperative complications in patients with chronic liver diseases.[153] A larger remnant may be necessary even in patients with normal livers when a complex hepatectomy is planned or when the background liver is steatotic.[154] This is especially relevant with the rise in fatty liver disease. A larger remnant may also be needed when patients have received preoperative chemotherapy. Some have suggested that 40% of the total hepatic volume should remain to minimize postoperative complications in patients who have underlying liver disease or who have received preoperative chemotherapy for colorectal cancer metastases.[155,156] In a recent study encompassing 112 patients who underwent PVE, major complications, hepatic insufficiency, length of hospital stay, and 90-day mortality rate were significantly greater in patients with a standardized future liver remnant of ≤20% or a degree of hypertrophy of <5% than in patients with higher values.[157] In another study, the authors performed PVE during neoadjuvant chemotherapy for colorectal cancer metastases. After a median wait of 30 days after PVE, patients receiving neoadjuvant chemotherapy showed median liver growth of 22% in the contralateral (nonembolized) lobe compared with 26% for those not receiving chemotherapy (not a statistically significant difference), which indicated that liver growth occurs after PVE even when cytotoxic chemotherapy is administered.[158] PVE-related complications occur at a relatively low rate and include bleeding, hemobilia, liver abscess, incomplete embolization, and small bowel obstruction.

Staged Hepatectomy and Repeat Hepatic Resection for Recurrent Liver Cancer

A two-stage hepatectomy is a sequential resection strategy to remove all metastatic liver tumors when it is impossible to resect all disease in a single operative procedure. The first-stage hepatectomy usually consists of clearance of the left hemiliver by nonanatomic resection, followed by right portal vein ligation or embolization to induce left lobe hypertrophy.[159,160] This is followed by a second-stage major right hepatectomy or extended right hepatectomy to resect the right liver metastases. This approach is most commonly used in cases of initially unresectable colorectal hepatic metastases and has yielded very good results.[160]

The majority of patients undergoing hepatic resection for colorectal cancer metastases experience a recurrence. For those with limited disease recurrence confined to the liver, repeat hepatectomy is a reasonable option and can be performed with low morbidity and mortality in experienced hands.[161] In one study, 126 patients who underwent a second liver resection for colorectal cancer metastases had 1-, 3-, and 5-year survival rates of 86%, 51%, and 34%, respectively. By multivariate analysis, the presence of more than one lesion and a tumor size of >5 cm were independent prognostic indicators of reduced survival.[162] In another study, 40 patients underwent a second hepatectomy for liver metastases from colorectal cancer and experienced a survival benefit similar to that from the first hepatectomy; however, the results suggested that this approach should be limited to those patients who do not have extrahepatic disease and for whom >1 year has elapsed since the first operation.[163] A meta-analysis of 21 studies examining clinical outcomes after first and second liver resections for colorectal cancer metastases showed that repeat hepatectomy was safe and provided a survival benefit equal to that from the first liver resection.[164]

Repeat hepatectomy also has been performed in patients with HCC. Nakajima and colleagues reported on follow-up of 94 patients who underwent curative liver resection for HCC from 1991 to 1996.[165] Of these, 57 patients had isolated recurrent disease in the liver. Twelve of these 57 patients underwent repeat hepatic resection, whereas the other 45 patients received ablation therapy. The overall survival rate in those undergoing a second hepatectomy was 90% at 2 years; however, the disease-free survival rate was only 31% at 2 years, significantly lower than the 62% rate after initial hepatectomy. Likewise, in another group of 84 patients who underwent second hepatectomy for recurrent HCC, the overall 5-year survival rate was 50%, but the recurrence-free survival rate was only 10%.[166] In a report of 67 patients undergoing a second resection for HCC, overall 1-, 3-, and 5-year survival rates were 93%, 70%, and 56%, respectively.[167] Multivariate analysis showed that absence of portal invasion at the second resection, single HCC at primary hepatectomy, and disease-free interval of ≥1 year after primary hepatectomy were independent prognostic factors after the second resection.

LAPAROSCOPIC LIVER RESECTION

Laparoscopic liver surgery has expanded from simple unroofing of hepatic cysts to resection of peripheral benign lesions to formal anatomic lobectomies for malignancy and more recently to laparoscopic hepatectomy for live donor liver transplantation. This evolution can been attributed largely to advances in technology as well as to a better understanding of hepatic anatomy and physiology. The result is

Pre-Op CT scan

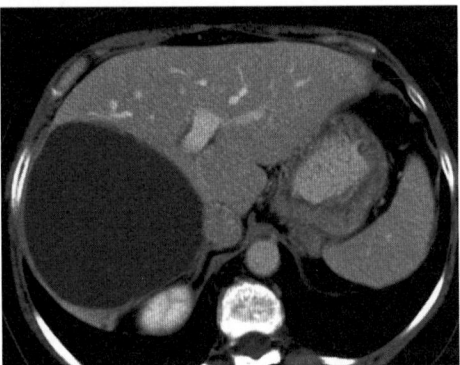

1 yr post-op scan

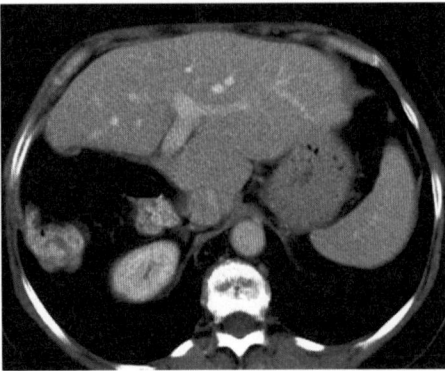

FIG. 31-27. Laparoscopic resection of a giant right lobe hepatic cyst. Preoperative and 1-year postoperative computed tomographic (CT) images show the liver before and after laparoscopic removal of the cyst.

a growing spectrum of hepatic lesions that can potentially be treated with a minimally invasive surgical approach. There is general agreement that surgeons getting started with the techniques should begin with cases involving giant hepatic cysts and peripheral (segment II and III or segment V and VI) benign lesions (Fig. 31-27).[168-171] Then, with experience, more difficult cases can be taken on, including cirrhotic livers, malignancies, and anatomic resections.[171-174] Large central lesions and bulky right lobe lesions with hepatic vein, IVC, or proximal hilar involvement are best addressed through an open approach. Also, there is consensus that laparoscopic liver resection should be performed by surgeons who are experienced in both open hepatic resection surgery and minimally invasive surgery.[171] Intraoperative laparoscopic liver ultrasonography is imperative to identify lesions and major vasculature to guide the operation. Technologies used to facilitate the parenchymal transection include the bipolar cautery, CUSA ultrasonic dissector, Harmonic Scalpel, LigaSure tissue fusion system, TissueLink wound-sealing devices, Habib 4X Laparoscopic sealer, SurgRx EnSeal sealer, and vascular stapling devices. These devices can be used for precoagulation, transection, and hemostasis, with each device having its strengths and weaknesses.

Results with laparoscopic liver resections have been excellent. Advantages of laparoscopic liver resection include decreased postoperative pain, faster return of GI function, shorter length of hospital stay, and quicker recovery time.[175] Although no randomized trials of laparoscopic liver resection for cancer have been performed, studies of laparoscopic surgery for HCC and colorectal cancer metastases yield overall and disease-free survival rates after short- and medium-term follow-up that are comparable to those for open surgical series.[176-178] A meta-analysis of eight nonrandomized studies (409 resections) compared laparoscopic hepatic resection (165 cases) with open resection (244 cases).[179] When matched for the presence of cancer and extent of resection, the laparoscopic cases showed no difference in oncologic clearance (margins), overall 5-year survival (61% for laparoscopic vs. 62% for open), or 5-year disease-free survival (31% for laparoscopic vs. 29% for open). The largest series reported to date consists of 335 hepatic resections, of which 105 were for malignancy.[171] Importantly, there was no perioperative mortality and no episodes of tumor seeding. In addition to the laparoscopic hepatic surgery for certain benign lesions and malignant tumors, Cherqui and colleagues described laparoscopic living-donor hepatectomy for liver transplantation in children,[180] and Koffron and colleagues recently reported laparoscopically assisted right lobe donor hepatectomy.[181]

REFERENCES

Entries highlighted in bright blue are key references.

1. *http://en.wikipedia.org/wiki/Prometheus*: Prometheus, Wikipedia: The free encyclopedia [accessed December 22, 2007].
2. Keen WW: Report of a case of resection of the liver for the removal of a neoplasm, with a table of seventy-six cases of resection of the liver for hepatic tumors. *Ann Surg* 30:267, 1899.
3. Fortner JG, Blumgart LH: A historic perspective of liver surgery for tumors at the end of the millennium. *J Am Coll Surg* 193:210, 2001.
4. Pringle JH: Notes on the arrest of hepatic hemorrhage due to trauma. *Ann Surg* 48:541, 1908.
5. Cantlie J: On a new arrangement of the right and left lobes of the liver. *Proc Anat Soc Great Britain Ireland* 32:4, 1897.
6. Couinaud C: Lobes de segments hépatiques: Notes sur l'architecture anatomique et chirurgical de foie. *Presse Méd* 62:709, 1954.
7. Abdalla EK, Vauthey JN, Couinaud C: The caudate lobe of the liver: Implications of embryology and anatomy for surgery [review]. *Surg Oncol Clin N Am* 11:835, 2002.
8. Bismuth H: Surgical anatomy and anatomical surgery of the liver. *World J Surg* 6:3, 1982.
9. Nordlie RC, Foster JD, Lange AJ: Regulation of glucose production by the liver. *Annu Rev Nutr* 19:379, 1999.
10. Merriman RB: Approach to the patient with jaundice, in Yamada T (ed): *Textbook of Gastroenterology*, 4th ed. Philadelphia: Lippincott Williams & Wilkins, 2003, p 911.
11. Ramadori G, Christ B: Cytokines and the hepatic acute-phase response. *Semin Liver Dis* 19:141, 1999.
12. Tsung A, Geller DA: CD14 and toll receptor, in Dufour JF, Clavien PA (eds): *Signaling Pathways in Liver Diseases*. Berlin: Springer, 2005, p 165.
13. Su GL: Lipopolysaccharides in liver injury: Molecular mechanisms of Kupffer cell activation. *Am J Physiol Gastrointest Liver Physiol* 283: G256, 2002.
14. Lazaron V, Dunn DL: Molecular biology of endotoxin antagonism [review]. *World J Surg* 26:790, 2002.
15. Geller DA, Billiar TR: Molecular biology of nitric oxide synthases. *Cancer Metastasis Rev* 17:7, 1998.
16. Prince JM, Billiar TR: Nitric oxide, in Dufour JF, Clavien PA (eds): *Signaling Pathways in Liver Diseases*. Berlin: Springer, 2005, p 299.
17. Tsuchihashi S, Busuttil RW, Kupiec-Weglinski JW: Heme oxygenase system, in Dufour JF, Clavien PA (eds): *Signaling Pathways in Liver Diseases*. Berlin: Springer, 2005, p 291.
18. Akira S, Takeda K: Toll-like receptor signalling. *Nat Rev Immunol* 4:499, 2004.
19. Mollen KP, Anand RJ, Tsung A, et al: Emerging paradigm: toll-like receptor 4-sentinel for the detection of tissue damage. *Shock* 26:430, 2006.
20. Kruskal JB, Kane RA: Intraoperative US of the liver: Techniques and clinical applications. *Radiographics* 26:1067, 2006.
21. Federle MP, Blachar A: CT evaluation of the liver. *Semin Liver Dis* 21:135, 2001.
22. Ros PR , Davis GL: The incidental focal liver lesion: Photon, proton, or needle? *Hepatology* 27:1183, 1998.
23. Wiering B, Krabbe PF, Jager GJ, et al: The impact of fluor-18-deoxyglucose-positron emission tomography in the management of colorectal liver metastases. *Cancer* 104:2658, 2005.
24. Polson J, Lee WM: Etiologies of acute liver failure: Location, location, location. *Liver Transpl* 13:1362, 2007.
25. Ascher NL, Lake JR, Emond JC, et al: Liver transplantation for fulminant hepatic failure. *Arch Surg* 128:677, 1993.

26. Ostapowicz GA, Fontana RJ, Schiodt FV, et al: Results of a prospective study of acute liver failure at 17 tertiary care centers in the United States. *Ann of Intern Med* 137:947, 2002.

27. Escorsell A, Mas A, de la Mata M; Spanish Group for the Study of Acute Liver Failure: Acute liver failure in Spain: Analysis of 267 cases. *Liver Transpl* 13:1389, 2007.

28. Larson AM, Fontana RJ, Davern TJ, et al; Acute Liver Failure Study Group: Acetaminophen-induced acute liver failure: Results of a United States multi-center, prospective study. *Hepatology* 42:1364, 2005.

29. O'Grady JG, Alexander GJM, Hayllar KM, et al: Early indicators of prognosis in fulminant hepatic failure. *Gastroenterology* 97:439, 1989.

30. Wanless IR, Nakashima E, Sherman M: Regression of human cirrhosis: Morphologic features and the genesis of incomplete septal cirrhosis. *Arch Pathol Lab Med* 124:1599, 2000.

31. Fattovich G, Giustina G, Degos F, et al: Morbidity and mortality in compensated cirrhosis type C: A retrospective follow-up of 384 patients. *Gastroenterology* 112:463, 1997.

32. Rockey DC: Vascular mediators in the injured liver. *Hepatology* 37:4, 2003.

33. Doberneck RC, Sterling WA Jr., Allison DC: Morbidity and mortality after operation in nonbleeding cirrhotic patients. *Am J Surg* 1146:306, 983.

34. Northup PG, Wanamaker RC, Lee VD, et al: Model for end-stage liver disease (MELD) predicts nontransplant surgical mortality in patient with cirrhosis. *Ann Surg* 242:244, 2005.

35. Farnsworth N, Fagan SP, Berger DH, et al: Child-Turcotte-Pugh versus MELD score as a predictor of outcome after elective and emergent surgery in cirrhotic patients. *Am J Surg* 188:580, 2004.

36. Shah V: Cellular and molecular basis of portal hypertension. *Clin Liver Disease* 5:629, 2001.

37. Poynard T, Cales P, Pasta L, et al: Beta-adrenergic-antagonistic drugs in the prevention of gastrointestinal bleeding in patients with cirrhosis and esophageal varices: An analysis of data and prognostic factors in 589 patients from four randomized clinical trials. Franco-Italian Multicenter Study Group. *N Engl J Med* 324:1532, 1991.

38. Garcia-Pagan JC, Bosch J: Endoscopic band ligation in the treatment of portal hypertension. *Nat Clin Pract Gastroenterol Hepatol* 2:526, 2005.

39. Valla DC: The diagnosis and management of Budd-Chiari syndrome: Consensus and controversies. *Hepatology* 38:793, 2003.

40. Henderson JM, Warren WD, Millikan WJ, et al: Surgical options, hematologic evaluation, and pathologic changes in Budd-Chiari syndrome. *Am J Surg* 159:41, 1990.

41. Barnes PF, Decock KM, Reynolds TN, et al: A comparison of amebic and pyogenic abscess of the liver. *Medicine* 66:472, 1987.

42. Pedrosa I, Saiz A, Arrazola J, et al: Hydatid disease: Radiologic and pathologic features and complications. *Radiographics* 20:795, 2000.

43. Khuroo MS, Zargar SA, Mahajan R: Hepatobiliary and pancreatic ascariasis in India. *Lancet* 335:1503, 1990.

44. Tsung A, Geller DA: Workup of the incidental liver lesion. *Adv Surg* 39:331, 2005.

45. Caremani M, Vincenti A, Benci A, et al: Ecographic epidemiology of non-parasitic hepatic cysts. *J Clin Ultrasound* 21:115, 1993.

46. Tahvanainen P, Tahvanainen E, Reijonen H, et al: Polycystic liver disease is genetically heterogenous: Clinical and linkage studies in eight Finnish families. *J Hepatology* 38:39, 2003.

47. Robinson TN, Stiegmann GV, Everson GT: Laparoscopic palliation of polycystic liver disease. *Surg Endosc* 19:130, 2005.

48. Caroli J: Disease of the intrahepatic biliary tree. *Clin Gastroenterol* 2:147, 1972.

49. Yoon SS, Charny CK, Fong Y, et al: Diagnosis, management, and outcomes of 115 patients with hepatic hemangioma. *J Am Coll Surg* 197:392, 2003.

50. Geller DA, Tsung A, Marsh JW, et al: Outcome of 1,000 liver cancer patients evaluated at the UPMC liver cancer center. *J Gastrointest Surg* 10:63, 2006.

51. El-Serag HB: Epidemiology of hepatocellular carcinoma in USA. *Hepatol Res* 37 Suppl 2:S88, 2007.

52. Schwartz M, Roayaie S, Konstadoulakis M: Strategies for the management of hepatocellular carcinoma [review]. *Nat Clin Pract Oncol* 4:424, 2007.

53. Bruix J, Sherman M; Practice Guidelines Committee, American Association for the Study of Liver Diseases. Management of hepatocellular carcinoma. *Hepatology* 42:1208, 2005.

54. Llovet JM, Fuster J, Bruix J; Barcelona-Clinic Liver Cancer Group. The Barcelona approach: Diagnosis, staging, and treatment of hepatocellular carcinoma. *Liver Transpl* 10:S115, 2004.

55. Madariaga JR, Iwatsuki S, Todo S, et al: Liver resection for hilar and peripheral cholangiocarcinomas: A study of 62 cases. *Ann Surg* 227:70, 1998.

56. Jonas S, Benckert C, Thelen A, et al: Radical surgery for hilar cholangiocarcinoma. *Eur J Surg Oncol* 34:263, 2008.

57. Jarnagin WR, Fong Y, DeMatteo RP, et al: Staging, resectability, and outcome in 225 patients with hilar cholangiocarcinoma. *Ann Surg* 234:507, 2001.

58. Hidalgo E, Asthana S, Nishio H, et al: Surgery for hilar cholangiocarcinoma: The Leeds experience. *Eur J Surg Oncol* 34:787, 2007. Epub November 22, 2007.

59. Nagino M, Kamiya J, Nishio H, et al: Two hundred forty consecutive portal vein embolizations before extended hepatectomy for biliary cancer: Surgical outcome and long-term follow-up. *Ann Surg* 243:364, 2006.

60. Gores GJ, Nagorney DM, Rosen CB: Cholangiocarcinoma: Is transplantation an option? For whom? *J Hepatol* 47:455, 2007.

61. Marsh JW, Geller DA, Finkelstein SD, et al: Role of liver transplantation for hepatobiliary malignant disorders. *Lancet Oncol* 5:480, 2004.

62. Hassoun Z, Gores GJ, Rosen CB: Preliminary experience with liver transplantation in selected patients with unresectable hilar cholangiocarcinoma. *Surg Oncol Clin N Am* 11:909, 2002.

63. Weber SM, Jarnagin WR, Klimstra D: Intrahepatic cholangiocarcinoma: Resectability, recurrence pattern, and outcomes. *J Am Coll Surg* 193:384, 2001.

64. Jan YY, Yeh CN, Yeh TS, et al: Prognostic analysis of surgical treatment of peripheral cholangiocarcinoma: Two decades of experience at Chang Gung Memorial Hospital. *World J Gastroenterol* 11:1779, 2005.

65. Casavilla FA, Marsh JW, Iwatsuki S, et al: Hepatic resection and transplantation for peripheral cholangiocarcinoma. *J Am Coll Surg* 185:429, 1997.

66. Smith G, Parks R, Madhavan K, et al: A 10-year experience in the management of gallbladder cancer. *HPB (Oxford)* 5:159, 2003.

67. Bartlett DL, Fong Y, Fortner JG, et al: Long-term results after resection for gallbladder cancer: Implications for staging and management [review]. *Ann Surg* 1224:639, 996.

68. Shoup M, Fong Y: Surgical indications and extent of resection in gallbladder cancer [review]. *Surg Oncol Clin N Am* 11:985, 2002.

69. Pawlik TM, Gleisner AL, Vigano L, et al: Incidence of finding residual disease for incidental gallbladder carcinoma: Implications for re-resection. *J Gastrointest Surg* 11:1478, 2007.

70. Chan SY, Poon RT, Lo CM, et al: Management of carcinoma of the gallbladder: A single-institution experience in 16 years. *J Surg Oncol* 97:156, 2008.

71. Goetze TO, Paolucci V: Benefits of reoperation of T2 and more advanced incidental gallbladder carcinoma: Analysis of the German registry. *Ann Surg* 247:104, 2008.

72. Poston G, Adam R, Vauthey JN: Downstaging or downsizing: Time for a new staging system in advanced colorectal cancer? *J Clin Oncol* 24:2702, 2006.

73. Minagawa M, Makuuchi M, Torzilli G, et al: Extension of the frontiers of surgical indications in the treatment of liver metastases from colorectal cancer: Long-term results. *Ann Surg* 231:487, 2000.

74. Kornprat P, Jarnagin WR, Gonen M, et al: Outcome after hepatectomy for multiple (four or more) colorectal metastases in the era of effective chemotherapy. *Ann Surg Oncol* 14:1151, 2007.

75. Charnsangavej C, Clary B, Fong Y, et al: Selection of patients for resection of hepatic colorectal metastases: Expert consensus statement. *Ann Surg Oncol* 13:1261, 2006.

76. Abdalla EK, Adam R, Bilchik AJ, et al: Improving resectability of hepatic colorectal metastases: Expert consensus statement. *Ann Surg Oncol* 13:1271, 2006.

77. Pawlik TM, Schulick RD, Choti MA: Expanding criteria for resectability of colorectal liver metastases [review]. *Oncologist* 13:51, 2008.

78. Adam R, Delvart V, Pascal G, et al: Rescue surgery for unresectable colorectal liver metastases downstaged by chemotherapy: A model to predict long-term survival. *Ann Surg* 240:644, 2004.

79. Que FG, Nagorney DM, Batts KP, et al: Hepatic resection for metastatic neuroendocrine carcinomas. *Am J Surg* 169:36, 1995.

80. Touzios JG, Kiely JM, Pitt SC, et al: Neuroendocrine hepatic metastases: Does aggressive management improve survival? *Ann Surg* 241:776, 2005.

81. Sarmiento JM, Heywood G, Rubin J, et al: Surgical treatment of neuroendocrine metastases to the liver: A plea for resection to increase survival. *J Am Coll Surg* 197:29, 2003.

82. Kianmanesh R, Sauvanet A, Hentic O, et al: Two-step surgery for synchronous bilobar liver metastases from digestive endocrine tumors: A safe approach for radical resection. *Ann Surg* 247:659, 2008.

83. Weitz J, Blumgart LH, Fong Y, et al: Partial hepatectomy for metastases from noncolorectal, nonneuroendocrine carcinoma. *Ann Surg* 241:269, 2005.

84. Adam R, Aloia T, Krissat J, et al: Is liver resection justified for patients with hepatic metastases from breast cancer? *Ann Surg* 244:897, 2006.

85. Reddy SK, Barbas AS, Marroquin CE, et al: Resection of noncolorectal nonneuroendocrine liver metastases: A comparative analysis. *J Am Coll Surg* 204:372, 2007.

86. Adam R, Chiche L, Aloia T, et al: Hepatic resection for noncolorectal nonendocrine liver metastases: Analysis of 1,452 patients and development of a prognostic model. *Ann Surg* 244:524, 2006.

87. Belghiti J, Cortes A, Abdalla EK, et al: Resection prior to liver transplantation for hepatocellular carcinoma. *Ann Surg* 238:885, 2003.

88. Adam R, Azoulay D, Castaing D, et al: Liver resection as a bridge to transplantation for hepatocellular carcinoma on cirrhosis: A reasonable strategy? *Ann Surg* 238:508, 2003.

89. Belghiti J, Hiramatsu K, Benoist S, et al: Seven hundred forty-seven hepatectomies in the 1990s: An update to evaluate the actual risk of liver resection. *J Am Coll Surg* 191:38, 2000.

90. Jarnagin WR, Gonen M, Fong Y, et al: Improvement in perioperative outcome after hepatic resection: Analysis of 1,803 consecutive cases over the past decade. *Ann Surg* 236:397, 2002.

91. Imamura H, Seyama Y, Kokudo N, et al: One thousand fifty-six hepatectomies without mortality in 8 years. *Arch Surg* 138:1198, 2003.

92. Mullen JT, Ribero D, Reddy SK, et al: Hepatic insufficiency and mortality in 1,059 noncirrhotic patients undergoing major hepatectomy. *J Am Coll Surg* 204:854, 2007.

93. Hamady ZZ, Cameron IC, Wyatt J, et al: Resection margin in patients undergoing hepatectomy for colorectal liver metastasis: A critical appraisal of the 1 cm rule. *Eur J Surg Oncol* 32:557, 2006.

94. Pawlik TM, Vauthey JN: Surgical margins during hepatic surgery for colorectal liver metastases: Complete resection not millimeters defines outcome. *Ann Surg Oncol* 15:677, 2008.

95. *http://www.optn.org*: Organ Procurement and Transplantation Network [accessed December 22, 2007].

96. Mazzaferro V, Chun YS, Poon RT, et al: Liver transplantation for hepatocellular carcinoma [review]. *Ann Surg Oncol* 15:1001, 2008.

97. Mazzaferro V, Regalia E, Doci R, et al: Liver transplantation for the treatment of small hepatocellular carcinomas in patients with cirrhosis. *N Engl J Med* 334:693, 1996.

98. Yao FY, Ferrell L, Bass NM, et al: Liver transplantation for hepatocellular carcinoma: Expansion of the tumor size limits does not adversely impact survival. *Hepatology* 33:1394, 2001.

99. Wiesner RH, Freeman RB, Mulligan DC: Liver transplantation for hepatocellular cancer: The impact of the MELD allocation policy. *Gastroenterology* 127:S261, 2004.

100. McGahan JP, Browning PD, Brock JM, et al: Hepatic ablation using radiofrequency electrocautery. *Invest Radiol* 25:267, 1990.

101. Rossi S, Fornari F, Pathies C, et al: Thermal lesions induced by 480 KHz localized current field in guinea pig and pig liver. *Tumori* 76:54, 1990.

102. Curley SA, Izzo F, Delrio P, et al: Radiofrequency ablation of unresectable primary and metastatic hepatic malignancies. *Ann Surg* 230:1, 1999.

103. Bilchik AJ, Wood TF, Allegra D, et al: Cryosurgical ablation and radiofrequency ablation for unresectable hepatic malignant neoplasms. *Arch Surg* 135:657, 2000.

104. Poon RT, Ng KK, Lam CM, et al: Learning curve for radiofrequency ablation of liver tumors: Prospective analysis of initial 100 patients in a tertiary institution. *Ann Surg* 239:441, 2004.

105. Abdalla EK, Vauthey JN, Ellis LM, et al: Recurrence and outcomes following hepatic resection, radiofrequency ablation, and combined resection/ablation for colorectal liver metastases. *Ann Surg* 239:818, 2004.

106. Sutherland LM, Williams JA, Padbury RT, et al: Radiofrequency ablation of liver tumors: A systematic review. *Arch Surg* 141:181, 2006.

107. Berber E, Siperstein AE: Perioperative outcome after laparoscopic radiofrequency ablation of liver tumors: An analysis of 521 cases. *Surg Endosc* 21:613, 2007.

108. Martin AP, Goldstein RM, Dempster J, et al: Radiofrequency thermal ablation of hepatocellular carcinoma before liver transplantation—a clinical and histological examination. *Clin Transpl* 20:695, 2006.

109. Cheng BQ, Jia CQ, Liu CT, et al: Chemoembolization combined with radiofrequency ablation for patients with hepatocellular carcinoma larger than 3 cm: A randomized controlled trial. *JAMA* 299:1669, 2008.

110. Schwartz M, Roayaie S, Uva P: Treatment of HCC in patients awaiting liver transplantation [review]. *Am J Transpl* 7:1875, 2007.

111. Iannitti DA, Martin RC, Simon CJ, et al: Hepatic tumor ablation with clustered microwave antennae: The US Phase II Trial. *HPB (Oxford)* 9:120, 2007.

112. Lo CM, Ngan H, Tso WK, et al: Randomized controlled trial of transarterial lipiodol chemoembolization for unresectable hepatocellular carcinoma. *Hepatology* 35:1164, 2002.

113. Llovet JM, Real MI, Montaña X, et al: Arterial embolisation or chemoembolisation versus symptomatic treatment in patients with unresectable hepatocellular carcinoma: A randomised controlled trial. *Lancet* 359:1734, 2002.

114. Llovet JM, Bruix J: Systematic review of randomized trials for unresectable hepatocellular carcinoma: Chemoembolization improves survival [review]. *Hepatology* 37:429, 2003.

115. Takayasu K, Arii S, Ikai I, et al: Prospective cohort study of transarterial chemoembolization for unresectable hepatocellular carcinoma in 8510 patients. *Gastroenterology* 131:461, 2006.

116. Poon RT, Tso WK, Pang RW, et al: A phase I/II trial of chemoembolization for hepatocellular carcinoma using a novel intra-arterial drug-eluting bead. *Clin Gastroenterol Hepatol* 5:1100, 2007.

117. Kemeny N, Huang Y, Cohen AM, et al: Hepatic arterial infusion of chemotherapy after resection of hepatic metastases from colorectal cancer. *N Engl J Med* 341:2039, 1999.

118. Ibrahim SM, Lewandowski RJ, Sato KT, et al: Radioembolization for the treatment of unresectable hepatocellular carcinoma: A clinical review. *World J Gastroenterol* 14:1664, 2008.

119. Gulec SA, Fong Y: Yttrium 90 microsphere selective internal radiation treatment of hepatic colorectal metastases [review]. *Arch Surg* 142:675, 2007.

120. Sato KT, Lewandowski RJ, Mulcahy MF, et al: Unresectable chemorefractory liver metastases: Radioembolization with ^{90}Y microspheres—safety, efficacy, and survival. *Radiology* 247:507, 2008. Epub March 18, 2008.

121. Tse RV, Hawkins M, Lockwood G, et al: Phase I study of individualized stereotactic body radiotherapy for hepatocellular carcinoma and intrahepatic cholangiocarcinoma. *J Clin Oncol* 26:657, 2008.

122. Méndez Romero A, Wunderink W, Hussain SM, et al: Stereotactic body radiation therapy for primary and metastatic liver tumors: A single institution phase I-II study. *Acta Oncol* 45:831, 2006.

123. Abou-Alfa GK, Schwartz L, Ricci S, et al: Phase II study of sorafenib in patients with advanced hepatocellular carcinoma. *J Clin Oncol* 24:4293, 2006.

124. Llovet J, Ricci S, Mazzaferro S, et al, for the SHARP Investigators Study Group: Sorafenib improves survival in advanced hepatocellular carcinoma (HCC): Results of a phase III randomized placebo-controlled trial (SHARP trial). American Society of Clinical Oncology annual meeting proceedings. *J Clin Oncol* 25 Suppl 18:LBA1, 2007.

125. *http://www.ahpba.org/resources/liver.asp*: IHPBA Brisbane liver terminology, American Hepato-Pancreato-Biliary Association [accessed December 22, 2007].

126. Terminology Committee of the International Hepato-Pancreato-Biliary Association: The Brisbane 2000 terminology of liver anatomy and resections. *HPB (Oxford)* 2:333, 2000.

127. Strasberg S: Nomenclature of hepatic anatomy and resections: A review of the Brisbane 2000 system. *J Hepatobiliary Pancreat Surg* 12:351, 2005.

128. Weber JC, Navarra G, Jiao LR, et al: New technique for liver resection using heat coagulative necrosis. *Ann Surg* 236:560, 2002.

129. Geller D, Tsung A, Maheshwari V, et al: Hepatic resection in 170 patients using saline-cooled radiofrequency coagulation. *HPB (Oxford)* 7:208, 2005.

130. Saiura A, Yamamoto J, Koga R, et al: Usefulness of LigaSure for liver resection: Analysis by randomized clinical trial. *Am J Surg* 192:41, 2006.

131. McEntee GP, Nagorney DM: Use of vascular staplers in major hepatic resections. *Br J Surg* 78:40, 1991.

132. Jurim O, Colonna JO 2nd, Colquhoun SD, et al: A stapling technique for hepatic resection. *J Am Coll Surg* 178:510, 1994.

133. Kaneko H, Otsuka Y, Takagi S, et al: Hepatic resection using stapling devices. *Am J Surg* 187:280, 2004.

134. Schemmer P, Friess H, Hinz U, et al: Stapler hepatecomy is a safe dissection technique: Analysis of 300 patients. *World J Surg* 30:419, 2006.

135. Balaa FK, Tsung A, Gamblin TC, et al: Right hepatic lobectomy using the staple technique in 101 patients. *J Gastrointest Surg* 12:338, 2008.

136. Blumgart LH: Liver resection for benign disease and for liver and biliary disease, in Blumgart LH, Fong Y (eds): *Surgery of the Liver and Biliary Tract*, 3rd ed. London: WB Saunders, 2000, p 1639.

137. Launois B, Jamieson GG: The importance of Glisson's capsule and its sheaths in the intrahepatic approach to resection of the liver. *Surg Gynecol Obstet* 174:7, 1992.

138. Azoulay D, Marin-Hargreaves G, Castaing D, et al: The anterior approach: The right way for right massive hepatectomy. *J Am Coll Surg* 192:412, 2001.

139. Liu CL, Fan ST, Cheung ST, et al: Anterior approach versus conventional approach right hepatic resection for large hepatocellular carcinoma: A prospective randomized controlled study. *Ann Surg* 244:194, 2006.

140. Ogata S, Belghiti J, Varma D, et al: Two hundred liver hanging maneuvers for major hepatectomy: A single-center experience. *Ann Surg* 245:31, 2007.

141. Makuuchi M, Mori T, Gunven P, et al: Safety of hemihepatic vascular occlusion during resection of the liver. *Surg Gynecol Obstet* 164:155, 1987.

142. Man K, Fan ST, Ng IOL, et al: Prospective evaluation of Pringle maneuver in hepatectomy for liver tumors by a randomized study. *Ann Surg* 226:704, 1997.

143. Belghiti J, Noun R, Malafosse R, et al: Continuous versus intermittent portal triad clamping for liver resection: A controlled study. *Ann Surg* 229:369, 1999.

144. Figueras J, Llado L, Ruiz D, et al: Complete versus selective portal triad clamping for minor liver resections: A prospective randomized trial. *Ann Surg* 241:582, 2005.

145. Clavien PA, Yadav S, Sindram D, et al: Protective effects of ischemic preconditioning for liver resection performed under inflow occlusion in humans. *Ann Surg* 232:155, 2000.

146. Clavien PA, Selzner M, Rudiger HA, et al: A prospective randomized study in 100 consecutive patients undergoing major liver resection with versus without ischemic preconditioning. *Ann Surg* 238:843, 2003.

147. Kinoshita H, Sakai K, Hirohashi K, et al: Preoperative portal vein embolization for hepatocellular carcinoma. *World J Surg* 10:803, 1986.

148. Makuuchi M, Thai BL, Takayasu K, et al: Preoperative portal embolization to increase safety of major hepatectomy for hilar bile duct carcinoma: A preliminary report. *Surgery* 107:521, 1990.

149. Abdalla EK, Hicks ME, Vauthey JN: Portal vein embolization: Rationale, technique and future prospects. *Br J Surg* 88:165, 2001.

150. Chun YS, Ribero D, Abdalla EK, et al: Comparison of two methods of future liver remnant volume measurement. *J Gastrointest Surg* 12:123, 2008.

151. Abdalla EK, Barnett CC, Doherty D, et al: Extended hepatectomy in patients with hepatobiliary malignancies with and without preoperative portal vein embolization. *Arch Surg* 137:675, 2002.

152. Vauthey JN, Chaoui A, Do KA, et al: Standardized measurement of the future liver remnant prior to extended liver resection: Methodology and clinical associations. *Surgery* 127:512, 2000.

153. Farges O, Belghiti J, Kianmanesh R, et al: Portal vein embolization before right hepatectomy: Prospective clinical trial. *Ann Surg* 237:208, 2003.

154. Hemming AW, Reed AI, Howard RJ, et al: Preoperative portal vein embolization for extended hepatectomy. *Ann Surg* 237:686, 2003.

155. Azoulay D, Castaing D, Smail A, et al: Resection of nonresectable liver metastases from colorectal cancer after percutaneous portal vein embolization. *Ann Surg* 231:480, 2000.

156. Kubota K, Makuuchi M, Kusaka K, et al: Measurement of liver volume and hepatic functional reserve as a guide to decision-making in resectional surgery for hepatic tumors. *Hepatology* 26:1176, 1997.

157. Ribero D, Abdalla EK, Madoff DC, et al: Portal vein embolization before major hepatectomy and its effects on regeneration, resectability and outcome. *Br J Surg* 94:1386, 2007.

158. Covey AM, Brown KT, Jarnagin WR, et al: Combined portal vein embolization and neoadjuvant chemotherapy as a treatment strategy for resectable hepatic colorectal metastases. *Ann Surg* 247:451, 2008.

159. Jaeck D, Oussoultzoglou E, Rosso E, et al: A two-stage hepatectomy procedure combined with portal vein embolization to achieve curative resection for initially unresectable multiple and bilobar colorectal liver metastases. *Ann Surg* 240:1037, 2004.

160. Adam R, Miller R, Pitombo M, et al: Two-stage hepatectomy approach for initially unresectable colorectal hepatic metastases. *Surg Oncol Clin N Am* 16:525, 2007.

161. Adam R, Bismuth H, Castaing D, et al: Repeat hepatectomy for colorectal liver metastases. *Ann Surg* 225:51, 1997.

162. Petrowsky H, Gonen M, Jarnagin W, et al: Second liver resections are safe and effective treatment for recurrent hepatic metastases from colorectal cancer: A bi-institutional analysis [review]. *Ann Surg* 235:863, 2002.

163. Sa Cunha A, Laurent C, Rault A, et al: A second liver resection due to recurrent colorectal liver metastases. *Arch Surg* 142:1144, 2007.

164. Antoniou A, Lovegrove RE, Tilney HS, et al: Meta-analysis of clinical outcome after first and second liver resection for colorectal metastases. *Surgery* 141:9, 2007.

165. Nakajima Y, Ko S, Kanamura T, et al: Repeat liver resection for hepatocellular carcinoma. *J Am Coll Surg* 192:339, 2001.

166. Itamoto T, Nakahara H, Amano H, et al: Repeat hepatectomy for recurrent hepatocellular carcinoma. *Surgery* 141:589, 2007.

167. Minagawa M, Makuuchi M, Takayama T, et al: Selection criteria for repeat hepatectomy in patients with recurrent hepatocellular carcinoma. *Ann Surg* 238:703, 2003.

168. Descottes B, Glineur D, Lachachi F, et al: Laparoscopic liver resection of benign liver tumors. *Surg Endosc* 17:23, 2003.

169. Are C, Fong Y, Geller DA: Laparoscopic liver resections. *Adv Surg* 39:57, 2005.

170. Buell J, Koffron A, Thomas M, et al: Laparoscopic liver resection. *J Am Coll Surg* 200:472, 2005.

171. Koffron A, Geller DA, Gamblin TC, et al: Laparoscopic liver surgery—shifting the management of liver tumors. *Hepatology* 44:1694, 2006.

172. Gigot JF, Glineur D, Santiago Azagra J, et al: Laparoscopic liver resection for malignant liver tumors: Preliminary results of a multicenter European study. *Ann Surg* 236:90, 2002.

173. Laurent A, Cherqui D, Lesurtel M, et al: Laparoscopic liver resection for subcapsular hepatocellular carcinoma complicating chronic liver disease. *Arch Surg* 138:763, 2003.

174. O'Rourke N, Fielding G: Laparoscopic right hepatectomy: Surgical technique. *J Gastrointest Surg* 8:213, 2004.

175. Koffron AJ, Auffenberg GB, Kung RD, et al: Evaluation of 300 minimally invasive liver resections at a single institution: Less is more. *Ann Surg* 246:385; discussion 392, 2007.

176. Vibert E, Perniceni T, Levard H, et al: Laparoscopic liver resection. *Br J Surg* 93:67, 2006.

177. Dagher I, Proske JM, Carloni A, et al: Laparoscopic liver resection: Results for 70 patients. *Surg Endosc* 21:619, 2007.

178. Cherqui D, Laurent A, Tayar C, et al: Laparoscopic liver resection for peripheral hepatocellular carcinoma in patients with chronic liver disease: Midterm results and perspectives. *Ann Surg* 243:499, 2006.

179. Simillis C, Constantinides VA, Tekkis PP, et al: Laparoscopic versus open hepatic resections for benign and malignant neoplasms—a meta-analysis. *Surgery* 141:203, 2007.

180. Cherqui D, Soubrane O, Husson E, et al: Laparoscopic living donor hepatectomy for liver transplantation in children. *Lancet* 359:392, 2002.

181. Koffron AJ, Kung R, Baker T, et al: Laparoscopic-assisted right lobe donor hepatectomy. *Am J Transplant* 6:2522, 2006.

CHAPTER 32

Gallbladder and the Extrahepatic Biliary System

Margrét Oddsdóttir, Thai H. Pham,
and John G. Hunter

ANATOMY

Gallbladder

The gallbladder is a pear-shaped sac, about 7 to 10 cm long, with an average capacity of 30 to 50 mL. When obstructed, the gallbladder can distend markedly and contain up to 300 mL.[1] The gallbladder is located in a fossa on the inferior surface of the liver. A line from this fossa to the inferior vena cava divides the liver into right and left liver lobes. The gallbladder is divided into four anatomic areas: the fundus, the corpus (body), the infundibulum, and the neck. The fundus is the rounded, blind end that normally extends 1 to 2 cm beyond the liver's margin. It contains most of the smooth muscles of the organ, in contrast to the body, which is the main storage area and contains most of the elastic tissue. The body extends from the fundus and tapers into the neck, a funnel-shaped area that connects with the cystic duct. The neck usually follows a gentle curve, the convexity of which may be enlarged to form the infundibulum or Hartmann's pouch. The neck lies in the deepest part of the gallbladder fossa and extends into the free portion of the hepatoduodenal ligament (Fig. 32-1).

The same peritoneal lining that covers the liver covers the fundus and the inferior surface of the gallbladder. Occasionally, the gallbladder has a complete peritoneal covering, and is suspended in a mesentery off the inferior surface of the liver and, rarely, it is embedded deep inside the liver parenchyma (an intrahepatic gallbladder).

The gallbladder is lined by a single, highly folded, tall columnar epithelium that contains cholesterol and fat globules. The mucus secreted into the gallbladder originates in the tubuloalveolar glands found in the mucosa lining the infundibulum and neck of the gallbladder, but are absent from the body and fundus. The epithelial lining of the gallbladder is supported by a lamina propria. The muscle layer has circular longitudinal and oblique fibers, but without well-developed layers. The perimuscular subserosa contains connective tissue, nerves, vessels, lymphatics, and adipocytes. It is covered by the serosa except where the gallbladder is embedded in the liver. The gallbladder differs histologically from the rest of the GI tract in that it lacks a muscularis mucosa and submucosa.

The cystic artery that supplies the gallbladder is usually a branch of the right hepatic artery (>90% of the time). The course of the cystic artery may vary, but it nearly always is found within the hepatocystic triangle, the area bound by the cystic duct, common hepatic duct, and the liver margin (triangle of Calot). When the cystic artery reaches the neck of the gallbladder, it divides into anterior and posterior divisions. Venous return is carried either through small veins that enter directly into the liver or, rarely, to a large cystic vein that carries blood back to the portal vein. Gallbladder lymphatics drain into nodes at the neck of the gallbladder. Frequently, a visible lymph node overlies the insertion of the cystic artery into the gallbladder wall. The nerves of the gallbladder arise from the vagus and from sympathetic branches that pass through the celiac plexus. The preganglionic sympathetic level is T8 and T9. Impulses from the liver, gallbladder, and the bile ducts pass by means of sympathetic afferent fibers through the splanchnic nerves and mediate the pain of biliary colic. The hepatic branch of the vagus nerve supplies cholinergic fibers to the gallbladder, bile ducts, and the liver. The vagal branches also have peptide-containing nerves containing agents such as substance P, somatostatin, enkephalins, and vasoactive intestinal polypeptide.[2]

Bile Ducts

The extrahepatic bile ducts consist of the right and left hepatic ducts, the common hepatic duct, the cystic duct, and the common bile duct or choledochus. The common bile duct enters the second portion of the duodenum through a muscular structure, the sphincter of Oddi.[3]

The left hepatic duct is longer than the right and has a greater propensity for dilatation as a consequence of distal obstruction. The two ducts join to form a common hepatic duct, close to their emergence from the liver. The common hepatic duct is 1 to 4 cm in length and has a diameter of approximately 4 mm. It lies in front of the portal vein and to the right of the hepatic artery. The common hepatic duct is joined at an acute angle by the cystic duct to form the common bile duct.

The length of the cystic duct is quite variable. It may be short or absent and have a high union with the hepatic duct, or long and run parallel, behind, or spiral to the main hepatic duct before joining it, sometimes as far as at the duodenum. Variations of the cystic duct and its point of union with the common hepatic duct are surgically important (Fig. 32-2). The segment of the cystic duct adjacent to the

---

KEY POINTS

1. The physiology of the gallbladder and sphincter of Oddi are regulated by a complex interplay of hormones and neuronal inputs designed to coordinate bile release with food consumption. Dysfunctions related to this activity are linked to the development of gallbladder pathologies described in this chapter.

2. In Western countries, the most common type of gallstones are cholesterol stones. The pathogenesis of these stones relates to supersaturation of bile with cholesterol and subsequent precipitation.

3. The main risk factor for gallbladder disease in Western countries is cholelithiasis. The main complications include cholecystitis, choledocholithiasis, cholangitis, and biliary pancreatitis. In addition, cholelithiasis plays the role as the major risk factor for the development of gallbladder cancer.

4. Laparoscopic cholecystectomy has been demonstrated to be a safe and effective alternative to open cholecystectomy and has become the treatment of choice for symptomatic gallstones. Knowledge of the various anatomic anomalies of the cystic duct and artery is helpful in guiding the dissection of these structures as well as avoiding injury to the common bile duct during cholecystectomy.

5. Common bile duct injuries, although uncommon, can be devastating to patients. Proper exposure of Calot's triangle and careful identification of the anatomic structures are keys to avoiding these injuries. Once a bile duct injury is diagnosed, the best outcomes are seen at large referral centers with experienced biliary surgeons.

6. Carcinoma of the gallbladder and bile duct generally have a poor prognosis because patients usually present late in the disease process and have poor response to chemo and radiation therapies. Surgery offers the best chance for survival and has good long-term survival in patients with early-stage disease.

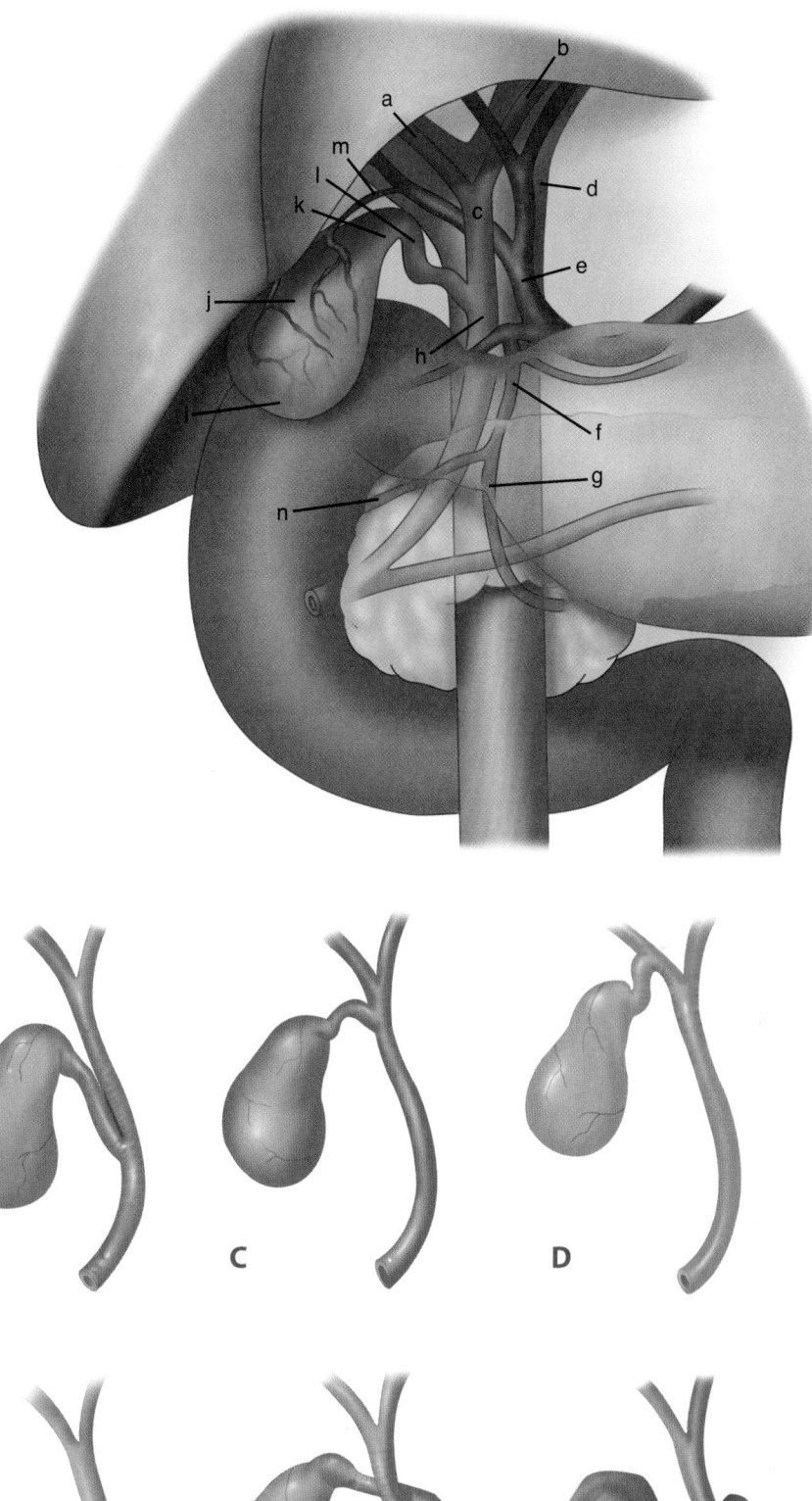

FIG. 32-1. Anterior aspect of the biliary anatomy. a = right hepatic duct; b = left hepatic duct; c = common hepatic duct; d = portal vein; e = hepatic artery; f = gastroduodenal artery; g = right gastroepiploic artery; h = common bile duct; i = fundus of the gallbladder; j = body of gallbladder; k = infundibulum; l = cystic duct; m = cystic artery; n = superior pancreaticoduodenal artery. Note: the situation of the hepatic bile duct confluence anterior to the right branch of the portal vein, the posterior course of the right hepatic artery behind the common hepatic duct.

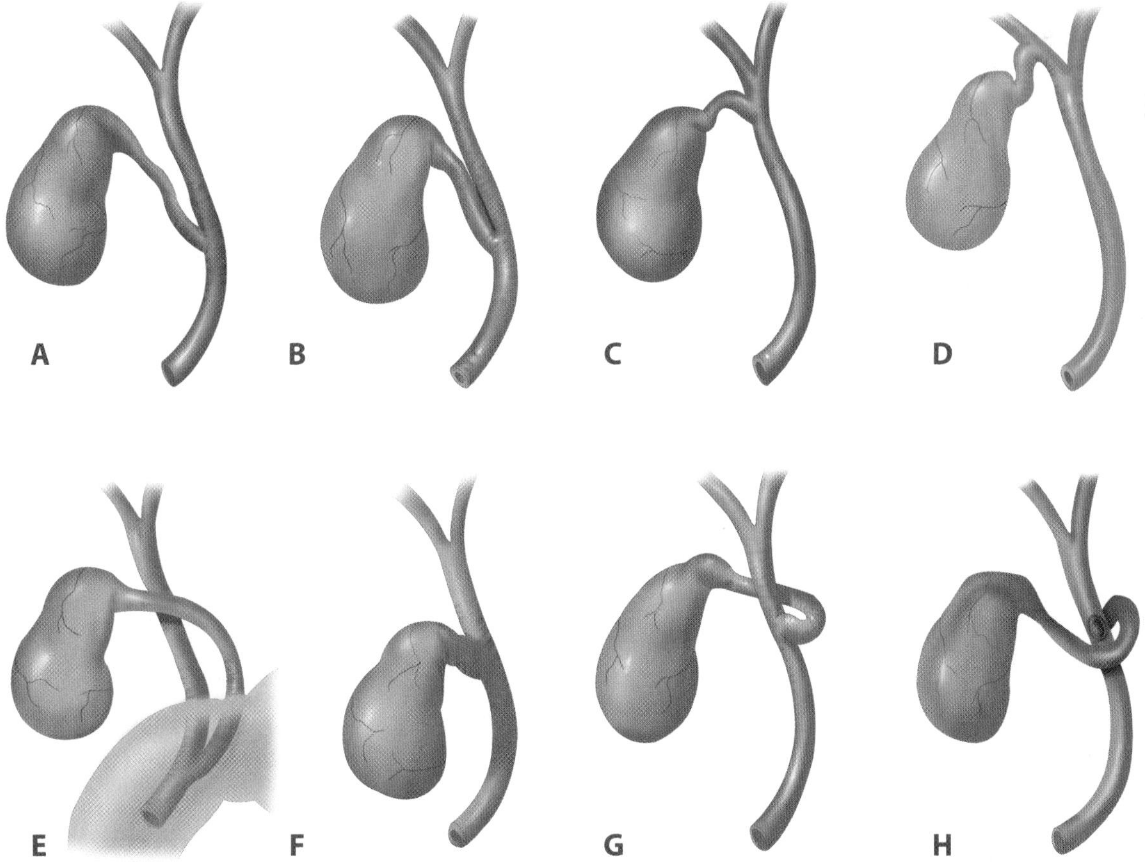

FIG. 32-2. Variations of the cystic duct anatomy. **A.** Low junction between the cystic duct and common hepatic duct. **B.** Cystic duct adherent to the common hepatic duct. **C.** High junction between the cystic and the common hepatic duct. **D.** Cystic duct drains into right hepatic duct. **E.** Long cystic duct that joins common hepatic duct behind the duodenum. **F.** Absence of cystic duct. **G.** Cystic duct crosses posterior to common hepatic duct and joins it anteriorly. **H.** Cystic duct courses anterior to common hepatic duct and joins it posteriorly.

gallbladder neck bears a variable number of mucosal folds called the *spiral valves of Heister.* They do not have any valvular function but may make cannulation of the cystic duct difficult.

The common bile duct is about 7 to 11 cm in length and 5 to 10 mm in diameter. The upper third (supraduodenal portion) passes downward in the free edge of the hepatoduodenal ligament, to the right of the hepatic artery and anterior to the portal vein. The middle third (retroduodenal portion) of the common bile duct curves behind the first portion of the duodenum and diverges laterally from the portal vein and the hepatic arteries. The lower third (pancreatic portion) curves behind the head of the pancreas in a groove, or traverses through it and enters the second part of the duodenum. There, the pancreatic duct frequently joins it. The common bile duct runs obliquely downward within the wall of the duodenum for 1 to 2 cm before opening on a papilla of mucous membrane (ampulla of Vater), about 10 cm distal to the pylorus. The union of the common bile duct and the main pancreatic duct follows one of three configurations. In about 70% of people, these ducts unite outside the duodenal wall and traverse the duodenal wall as a single duct. In about 20%, they join within the duodenal wall and have a short or no common duct, but open through the same opening into the duodenum. In about 10%, they exit via separate openings into the duodenum. The sphincter of Oddi, a thick coat of circular smooth muscle, surrounds the common bile duct at the ampulla of Vater (Fig. 32-3). It controls the flow of bile, and in some cases pancreatic juice, into the duodenum.

The extrahepatic bile ducts are lined by a columnar mucosa with numerous mucous glands in the common bile duct. A fibroareolar tissue containing scant smooth muscle cells surrounds the mucosa. A distinct muscle layer is not present in the human common bile duct. The arterial supply to the bile ducts is derived from the gastroduodenal and the right hepatic arteries, with major trunks running along the medial and lateral walls of the common duct (sometimes referred to as 3 o'clock and 9 o'clock). These arteries anastomose freely within the duct walls. The density of nerve fibers and ganglia increase near the sphincter of Oddi, but the nerve supply to the common bile duct and the sphincter of Oddi is the same as for the gallbladder.[1,2]

Anomalies

The classic description of the extrahepatic biliary tree and its arteries applies only in about one third of patients.[4] The gallbladder may have abnormal positions, be intrahepatic, be rudimentary, have anomalous forms, or be duplicated. Isolated congenital absence of the gallbladder is very rare, with a reported incidence of 0.03%. Before the diagnosis is made, the presence of an intrahepatic bladder or anomalous position must be ruled out. Duplication of the gallbladder with two separate cavities and two separate cystic ducts has an incidence of about one in every 4000 persons. This occurs in two major varieties: the more common form in which each gallbladder has its own cystic duct that empties independently into the same or different parts of the extrahepatic biliary tree, and as two cystic ducts that merge before they enter the common bile duct. Duplication is only clinically important when some pathologic processes affect one or both organs. A left-sided gallbladder with a cystic duct emptying into the left hepatic duct or the common bile duct and a retrodisplacement of the gallbladder are both extremely rare. A partial or totally intrahepatic gallbladder is associated with an increased incidence of cholelithiasis.

Small ducts (of Luschka) may drain directly from the liver into the body of the gallbladder. If present, but not recognized at the time of a cholecystectomy, a bile leak with the accumulation of bile (biloma) may occur in the abdomen. An accessory right hepatic duct occurs in about 5% of cases. Variations of how the common bile duct enters the duodenum are described in Bile Ducts above.

Anomalies of the hepatic artery and the cystic artery are quite common, occurring in as many as 50% of cases.[5] In about 5% of cases, there are two right hepatic arteries, one from the common hepatic artery and the other from the superior mesenteric artery. In about 20% of patients, the right hepatic artery comes off the superior mesenteric artery. The right hepatic artery may course anterior to the common duct. The right hepatic artery may be vulnerable during surgical procedures, in particular when it runs parallel to the cystic duct or in the mesentery of the gallbladder. The cystic artery arises from the right hepatic artery in about 90% of cases, but may arise from the left hepatic, common hepatic, gastroduodenal, or superior mesenteric arteries (Fig. 32-4).

PHYSIOLOGY

Bile Formation and Composition

The liver produces bile continuously and excretes it into the bile canaliculi. The normal adult consuming an average diet produces within the liver 500 to 1000 mL of bile a day. The secretion of bile is responsive to neurogenic, humoral, and chemical stimuli. Vagal stimulation increases secretion of bile, whereas splanchnic nerve stimulation results in decreased bile flow. Hydrochloric acid, partly digested proteins, and fatty acids in the duodenum stimulate the release of secretin from the duodenum that, in turn, increases bile production and bile flow. Bile flows from the liver through to the hepatic ducts, into the common hepatic duct, through the common bile duct, and finally into the duodenum. With an intact sphincter of Oddi, bile flow is directed into the gallbladder.

Bile is mainly composed of water, electrolytes, bile salts, proteins, lipids, and bile pigments. Sodium, potassium, calcium, and chlorine have the same concentration in bile as in plasma or extracellular fluid. The pH of hepatic bile is usually neutral or slightly alkaline, but varies with diet; an increase in protein shifts the bile to a more acidic pH. The primary bile salts, cholate and chenodeoxycholate, are synthesized in the liver from cholesterol. They are conjugated there with taurine and glycine, and act within the bile as anions (bile acids) that are balanced by sodium. Bile salts are excreted into the bile by the hepatocyte and aid in the digestion and absorption of fats in the intestines.[6] In the intestines, about 80% of the conjugated bile acids are absorbed in the terminal ileum. The remainder is dehydroxylated (deconjugated) by gut bacteria, form-

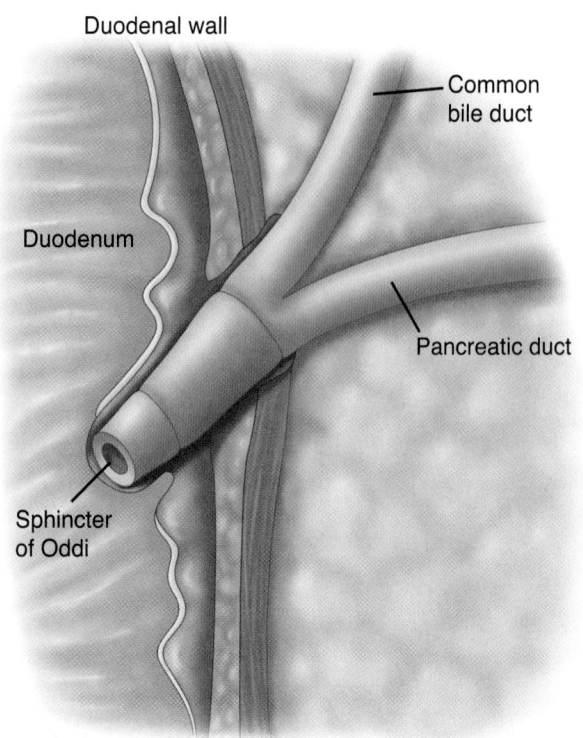

Duodenal wall

Common bile duct

Duodenum

Pancreatic duct

Sphincter of Oddi

FIG. 32-3. The sphincter of Oddi.

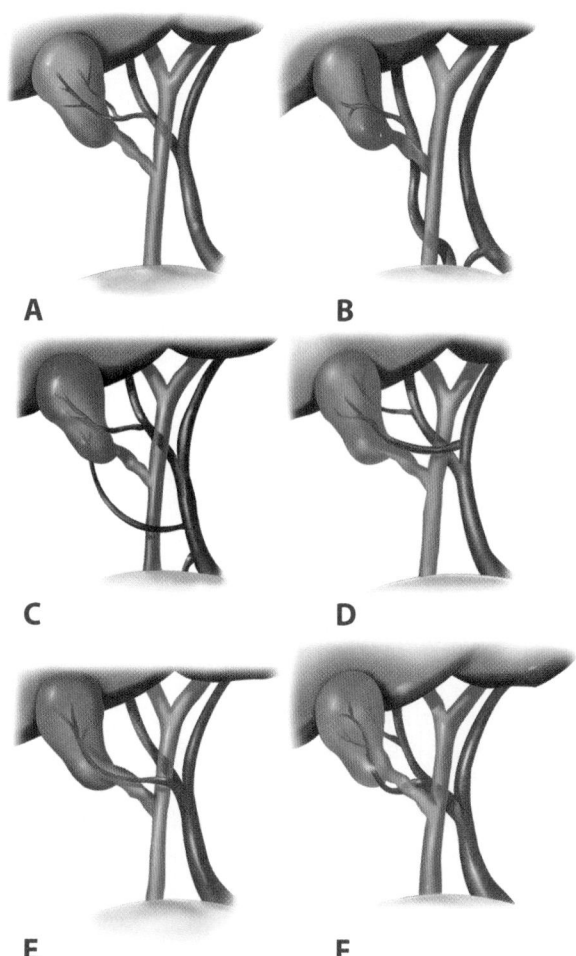

FIG. 32-4. Variations in the arterial supply to the gallbladder. **A.** Cystic artery from right hepatic artery, about 80–90%. **B.** Cystic artery from right hepatic artery (accessory or replaced) from superior mesenteric artery, about 10%. **C.** Two cystic arteries, one from the right hepatic, the other from the common hepatic artery, rare. **D.** Two cystic arteries, one from the right hepatic, the other from the left hepatic artery, rare. **E.** The cystic artery branching from the right hepatic artery and running anterior to the common hepatic duct, rare. **F.** Two cystic arteries arising from the right hepatic artery, rare.

ing secondary bile acids deoxycholate and lithocholate. These are absorbed in the colon, transported to the liver, conjugated, and secreted into the bile. Eventually, about 95% of the bile acid pool is reabsorbed and returned via the portal venous system to the liver, the so-called *enterohepatic circulation*. Five percent is excreted in the stool, leaving the relatively small amount of bile acids to have maximum effect.

Cholesterol and phospholipids synthesized in the liver are the principal lipids found in bile. The synthesis of phospholipids and cholesterol by the liver is, in part, regulated by bile acids. The color of the bile is due to the presence of the pigment bilirubin diglucuronide, which is the metabolic product from the breakdown of hemoglobin, and is present in bile in concentrations 100 times greater than in plasma. Once in the intestine, bacteria convert it into urobilinogen, a small fraction of which is absorbed and secreted into the bile.

Gallbladder Function

The gallbladder, the bile ducts, and the sphincter of Oddi act together to store and regulate the flow of bile. The main function of the gallbladder is to concentrate and store hepatic bile and to deliver bile into the duodenum in response to a meal.

Absorption and Secretion

In the fasting state, approximately 80% of the bile secreted by the liver is stored in the gallbladder. This storage is made possible because of the remarkable absorptive capacity of the gallbladder, as the gallbladder mucosa has the greatest absorptive power per unit area of any structure in the body. It rapidly absorbs sodium, chloride, and water against significant concentration gradients, concentrating the bile as much as 10-fold and leading to a marked change in bile composition. This rapid absorption is one of the mechanisms that prevent a rise in pressure within the biliary system under normal circumstances. Gradual relaxation as well as emptying of the gallbladder during the fasting period also plays a role in maintaining a relatively low intraluminal pressure in the biliary tree.

The epithelial cells of the gallbladder secrete at least two important products into the gallbladder lumen: glycoproteins and hydrogen ions. The mucosal glands in the infundibulum and the neck of the gallbladder secrete mucus glycoproteins that are believed to protect the mucosa from the lytic action of bile and to facilitate the passage of bile through the cystic duct. This mucus makes up the colorless "white bile" seen in hydrops of the gallbladder resulting from cystic duct obstruction. The transport of hydrogen ions by the gallbladder epithelium leads to a decrease in the gallbladder bile pH. The acidification promotes calcium solubility, thereby preventing its precipitation as calcium salts.[6]

Motor Activity

Gallbladder filling is facilitated by tonic contraction of the sphincter of Oddi, which creates a pressure gradient between the bile ducts and the gallbladder. During fasting, the gallbladder does not simply fill passively. In association with phase II of the interdigestive migrating myenteric motor complex in the gut, the gallbladder repeatedly empties small volumes of bile into the duodenum. This process is mediated at least in part by the hormone motilin. In response to a meal, the gallbladder empties by a coordinated motor response of gallbladder contraction and sphincter of Oddi relaxation. One of the main stimuli to gallbladder emptying is the hormone cholecystokinin (CCK). CCK is released endogenously from the duodenal mucosa in response to a meal.[7] When stimulated by eating, the gallbladder empties 50 to 70% of its contents within 30 to 40 minutes. Over the following 60 to 90 minutes, the gallbladder gradually refills. This is correlated with a reduced CCK level. Other hormonal and neural pathways also are involved in the coordinated action of the gallbladder and the sphincter of Oddi. Defects in the motor activity of the gallbladder are thought to play a role in cholesterol nucleation and gallstone formation.[8]

Neurohormonal Regulation

The vagus nerve stimulates contraction of the gallbladder, and splanchnic sympathetic stimulation is inhibitory to its motor activity. Parasympathomimetic drugs contract the gallbladder, whereas atropine leads to relaxation. Neurally mediated reflexes link the sphincter of Oddi with the gallbladder, stomach, and duodenum to coordinate the flow of bile into the duodenum. Antral distention of the stomach causes both gallbladder contraction and relaxation of the sphincter of Oddi.

Hormonal receptors are located on the smooth muscles, vessels, nerves, and epithelium of the gallbladder. CCK is a peptide that comes from epithelial cells of the upper GI tract and is found in the highest concentrations in the duodenum. CCK is released into the bloodstream by acid, fat, and amino acids in the duodenum.[9] CCK has a plasma half-life of 2 to 3 minutes and is metabolized by both the liver and the kidneys. CCK acts directly on smooth muscle receptors of the gallbladder and stimulates gallbladder contraction. It also relaxes the terminal bile duct, the sphincter of Oddi, and the duodenum. CCK stimulation of the gallbladder and the biliary tree also is mediated by cholinergic vagal neurons. In patients who have had a vagotomy, the response to CCK stimulation is diminished and the size and the volume of the gallbladder are increased.

Vasoactive intestinal polypeptide inhibits contraction and causes gallbladder relaxation. Somatostatin and its analogues are potent inhibitors of gallbladder contraction. Patients treated with somatostatin analogues and those with somatostatinoma have a high incidence of gallstones, presumably due to the inhibition of gallbladder contraction and emptying. Other hormones such as substance P and enkephalin affect gallbladder motility, but the physiologic role is unclear.[7]

Sphincter of Oddi

The sphincter of Oddi regulates flow of bile (and pancreatic juice) into the duodenum, prevents the regurgitation of duodenal contents into the biliary tree, and diverts bile into the gallbladder. It is a complex structure that is functionally independent from the duodenal musculature and creates a high-pressure zone between the bile duct and the duodenum. The sphincter of Oddi is about 4 to 6 mm in length and has a basal resting pressure of about 13 mmHg above the duodenal pressure. On manometry, the sphincter shows phasic contractions with a frequency of about four per minute and an amplitude of 12 to 140 mmHg.[8] The spontaneous motility of the sphincter of Oddi is regulated by the interstitial cells of Cajal through intrinsic and extrinsic inputs from hormones and neurons acting on the smooth muscle cells.[10] Relaxation occurs with a rise in CCK, leading to diminished amplitude of phasic contractions and reduced basal pressure, allowing increased flow of bile into the duodenum (Fig. 32-5). During fasting, the sphincter of Oddi activity is coordinated with the periodic partial gallbladder emptying and an increase in bile flow that occurs during phase II of the migrating myoelectric motor complexes.[11]

DIAGNOSTIC STUDIES

A variety of diagnostic modalities are available for the patient with suspected disease of the gallbladder and the bile ducts. In 1924 the diagnosis of gallstones was improved significantly by the introduction of oral cholecystography by Graham and Cole. For decades it was the mainstay of investigation for gallstones. In the 1950s biliary scintigraphy was developed, as well as intrahepatic and endoscopic retrograde cholangiography (ERC), allowing imaging of the biliary tract. Later ultrasonography, computed tomography (CT), and magnetic resonance imaging (MRI) vastly improved the ability to image the biliary tract.[12]

Blood Tests

When patients with suspected diseases of the gallbladder or the extrahepatic biliary tree are evaluated, a complete blood count and liver function tests are routinely requested. An elevated white blood cell (WBC) count may indicate or raise suspicion of cholecystitis. If associated with an elevation of bilirubin, alkaline phosphatase, and aminotransferase, cholangitis should be suspected. Cholestasis, an obstruction to bile flow, is characterized by an elevation of bilirubin (i.e., the conjugated form), and a rise in alkaline phosphatase. Serum aminotransferases may be normal or mildly elevated. In patients with biliary colic or chronic cholecystitis, blood tests will typically be normal.

Ultrasonography

An ultrasound is the initial investigation of any patient suspected of disease of the biliary tree.[13] It is noninvasive, painless, does not submit the patient to radiation, and can be performed on critically ill patients. It is dependent upon the skills and the experience of the operator, and it is dynamic (i.e., static images do not give the same information as those obtained during the ultrasound investigation itself). Adjacent organs can frequently be examined at the same time. Obese patients, patients with ascites, and patients with distended bowel may be difficult to examine satisfactorily with an ultrasound.

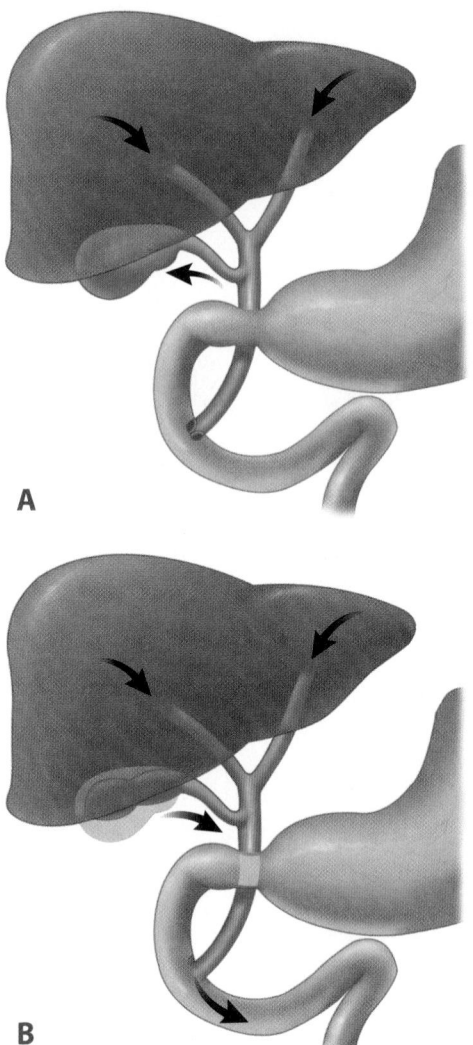

A

B

FIG. 32-5. The effect of cholecystokinin on the gallbladder and the sphincter of Oddi. **A.** During fasting, with the sphincter of Oddi contracted and the gallbladder filling. **B.** In response to a meal, the sphincter of Oddi relaxed and the gallbladder emptying.

Ultrasound will show stones in the gallbladder with sensitivity and specificity of >90%. Stones are acoustically dense and reflect the ultrasound waves back to the ultrasonic transducer. Because stones block the passage of sound waves to the region behind them, they also produce an acoustic shadow (Fig. 32-6). Stones move with changes in position. Polyps may be calcified and reflect shadows, but do not move with change in posture. Some stones form a layer in the gallbladder; others a sediment or sludge. A thickened gallbladder wall and local tenderness indicate cholecystitis. The patient has acute cholecystitis if a layer of edema is seen within the wall of the gallbladder or between the gallbladder and the liver in association with localized tenderness. When a stone obstructs the neck of the gallbladder, the gallbladder may become very large, but thin walled. A contracted, thick-walled gallbladder is indicative of chronic cholecystitis.

The extrahepatic bile ducts are also well visualized by ultrasound, except for the retroduodenal portion. Dilation of the ducts in a patient with jaundice establishes an extrahepatic obstruction as a cause for the jaundice. Frequently, the site and, sometimes, the cause of obstruction can be determined by ultrasound. Small stones in the common bile duct frequently get lodged at the distal end of it, behind the duodenum, and are, therefore, difficult to detect. A dilated common bile duct on ultrasound, small stones in the gallbladder,

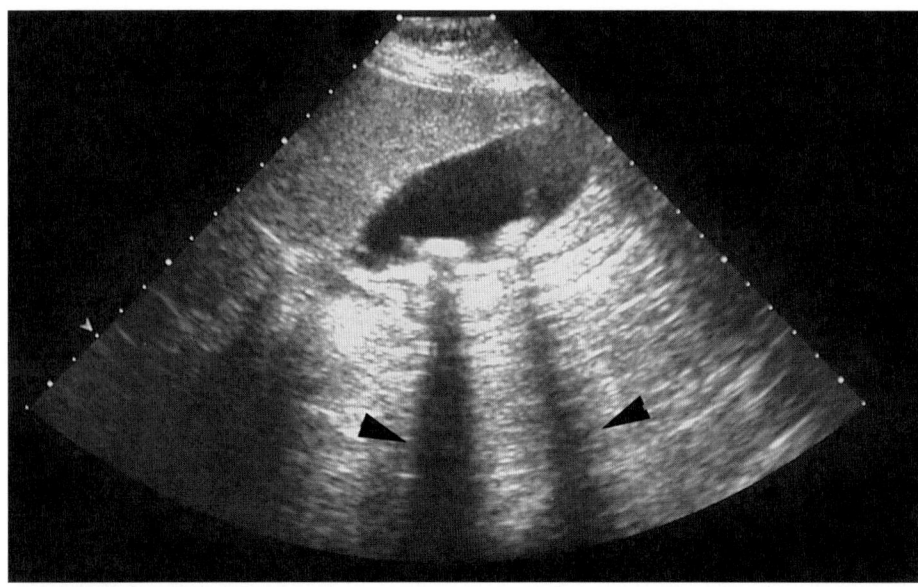

FIG. 32-6. An ultrasonography of the gallbladder. *Arrows* indicate the acoustic shadows from stones in the gallbladder.

and the clinical presentation allow one to assume that a stone or stones are causing the obstruction. Periampullary tumors can be difficult to diagnose on ultrasound, but beyond the retroduodenal portion, the level of obstruction and the cause may be visualized quite well. Ultrasound can be helpful in evaluating tumor invasion and flow in the portal vein, an important guideline for resectability of periampullary and pancreatic head tumors.[14]

Oral Cholecystography

Once considered the diagnostic procedure of choice for gallstones, oral cholecystography has largely been replaced by ultrasonography. It involves oral administration of a radiopaque compound that is absorbed, excreted by the liver, and passed into the gallbladder. Stones are noted on a film as filling defects in a visualized, opacified gallbladder. Oral cholecystography is of no value in patients with intestinal malabsorption, vomiting, obstructive jaundice, and hepatic failure.

Biliary Radionuclide Scanning (HIDA Scan)

Biliary scintigraphy provides a noninvasive evaluation of the liver, gallbladder, bile ducts, and duodenum with both anatomic and functional information. ^{99m}Technetium-labeled derivatives of dimethyl iminodiacetic acid (HIDA) are injected intravenously, cleared by the Kupffer cells in the liver, and excreted in the bile. Uptake by the liver is detected within 10 minutes, and the gallbladder, the bile ducts, and the duodenum are visualized within 60 minutes in fasting subjects. The primary use of biliary scintigraphy is in the diagnosis of acute cholecystitis, which appears as a nonvisualized gallbladder, with prompt filling of the common bile duct and duodenum. Evidence of cystic duct obstruction on biliary scintigraphy is highly diagnostic for acute cholecystitis. The sensitivity and specificity for the diagnosis are about 95% each. False-positive results are increased in patients with gallbladder stasis, as in critically ill patients and in patients receiving parenteral nutrition. Filling of the gallbladder and common bile duct with delayed or absent filling of the duodenum indicates an obstruction at the ampulla. Biliary leaks as a complication of surgery of the gallbladder or the biliary tree can be confirmed and frequently localized by biliary scintigraphy.[15]

Computed Tomography

Abdominal CT scans are inferior to ultrasonography in diagnosing gallstones. The major application of CT scans is to define the course and status of the extrahepatic biliary tree and adjacent structures. It is the test of choice in evaluating the patient with suspected malignancy

of the gallbladder, the extrahepatic biliary system, or nearby organs, in particular, the head of the pancreas. Use of CT scan is an integral part of the differential diagnosis of obstructive jaundice (Fig. 32-7). Spiral CT scanning provides additional staging information, including vascular involvement in patients with periampullary tumors.[16]

Percutaneous Transhepatic Cholangiography

Intrahepatic bile ducts are accessed percutaneously with a small needle under fluoroscopic guidance. Once the position in a bile duct has been confirmed, a guidewire is passed and, subsequently, a catheter is passed over the wire (Fig. 32-8). Through the catheter, a cholangiogram can be performed and therapeutic interventions done, such as biliary drain insertions and stent placements. Percutaneous transhepatic cholangiography (PTC) has little role in the management of patients with uncomplicated gallstone disease, but is particularly useful in patients with bile duct strictures and tumors, as it defines the anatomy of the biliary tree proximal to the affected segment. As with any invasive procedure, there are potential risks. For PTC, these are mainly bleeding, cholangitis, bile leak, and other catheter-related problems.[15]

Magnetic Resonance Imaging

Available since the mid-1990s, MRI provides anatomic details of the liver, gallbladder, and pancreas similar to those obtained from CT. Many MRI techniques (i.e., heavily T2-weighted sequences, pulse sequences with or without contrast materials) can generate high resolution anatomic images of the biliary tree and the pancreatic duct. It has a sensitivity and specificity of 95 and 89%, respectively, at detecting choledocholithiasis.[17] MRI with magnetic resonance cholangiopancreatography (MRCP) offers a single noninvasive test for the diagnosis of biliary tract and pancreatic disease[18] (Fig. 32-9).

Endoscopic Retrograde Cholangiography and Endoscopic Ultrasound

Using a side-viewing endoscope, the common bile duct can be cannulated and a cholangiogram performed using fluoroscopy (Fig. 32-10). The procedure requires IV sedation for the patient. The advantages of ERC include direct visualization of the ampullary region and direct access to the distal common bile duct, with the possibility of therapeutic intervention. The test is rarely needed for uncomplicated gallstone disease, but for stones in the common bile duct, in particular, when associated with obstructive jaundice, cholangitis, or gallstone pancreatitis, ERC is the diagnostic and often therapeutic procedure of choice. Once the endoscopic cholan-

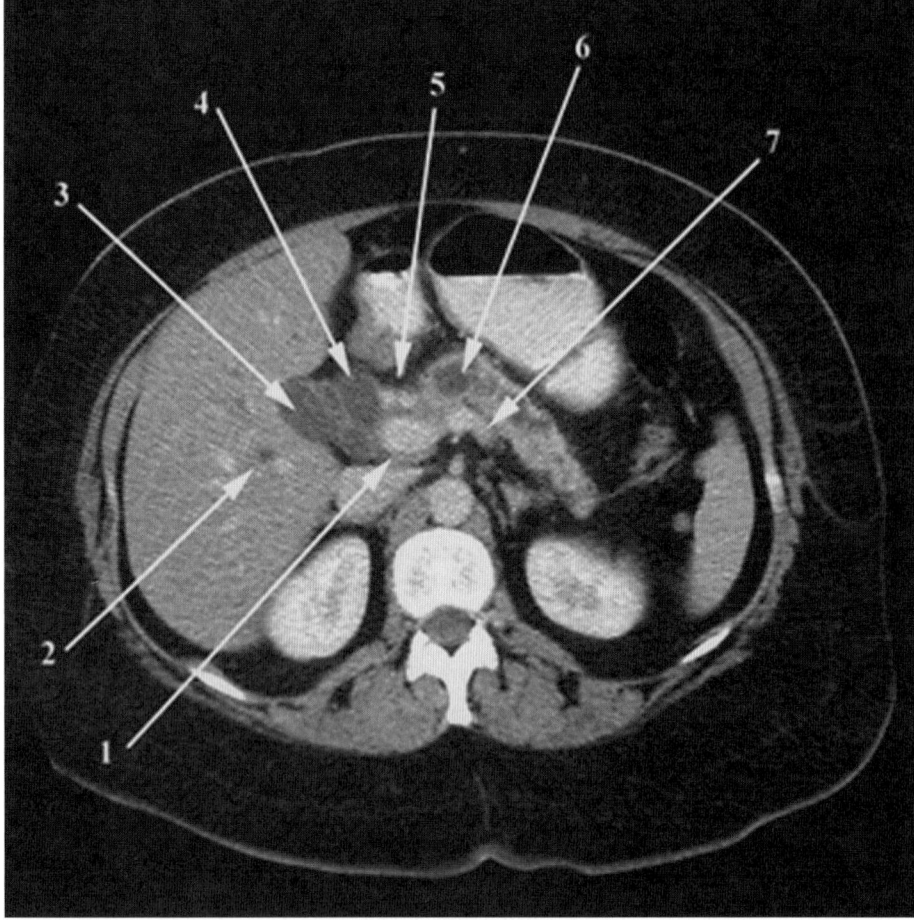

FIG. 32-7. Computed tomography scan of the upper abdomen from a patient with cancer of the distal common bile duct. The cancer obstructs the common bile duct as well as the pancreatic duct. 1 = the portal vein; 2 = a dilated intrahepatic bile duct; 3 = dilated cystic duct and the neck of the gallbladder; 4 = dilated common hepatic duct; 5 = the bifurcation of the common hepatic artery into the gastroduodenal artery and the proper hepatic artery; 6 = dilated pancreatic duct; 7 = the splenic vein.

giogram has shown ductal stones, sphincterotomy and stone extraction can be performed, and the common bile duct cleared of stones. In the hands of experts, the success rate of common bile duct cannulation and cholangiography is >90%. Complications of diagnostic ERC include pancreatitis and cholangitis, and occur in up to 5% of patients.[19] The development of small fiber-optic cameras that can be threaded through endoscopes used for endoscopic retrograde cholangiopancreatography (ERCP) has facilitated the development of intraductal endoscopy. By providing direct visualization of the biliary and pancreatic ducts, this technology has been shown to increase the effectiveness of ERCP in the diagnosis of certain biliary and pancreatic diseases.[20,21] Intraductal endoscopy has been shown to have therapeutic applications that include biliary stone lithotripsy and extraction in high-risk surgical patients.[22] As with most endoscopic procedures, intraductal endoscopy generally is considered safe, but there are no large trials that specifically address this issue. Typical complications such as bile duct perforation, minor bleeding from sphincterotomy or lithotripsy, and cholangitis have been described.[23] Further refinement of this technology will enhance ERCP as a diagnostic and therapeutic tool.

Endoscopic Ultrasound

An endoscopic ultrasound requires a special endoscope with an ultrasound transducer at its tip. The results are operator dependent, but offer noninvasive imaging of the bile ducts and adjacent structures. It is of particular value in the evaluation of tumors and their resectability. The ultrasound endoscope has a biopsy channel, allowing needle biopsies of a tumor under ultrasonic guidance. Endoscopic ultrasound also has been used to identify bile duct stones, and although it is less sensitive than ERC, the technique is less invasive.

GALLSTONE DISEASE

Prevalence and Incidence

Gallstone disease is one of the most common problems affecting the digestive tract. Autopsy reports have shown a prevalence of gallstones from 11 to 36%.[24] The prevalence of gallstones is related to many factors, including age, gender, and ethnic background. Certain conditions predispose to the development of gallstones. Obesity, pregnancy, dietary factors, Crohn's disease, terminal ileal resection, gastric surgery, hereditary spherocytosis, sickle cell disease, and thalassemia are all associated with an increased risk of developing gallstones.[8] Women are three times more likely to develop gallstones than men, and first-degree relatives of patients with gallstones have a twofold greater prevalence.[25]

Natural History

Most patients will remain asymptomatic from their gallstones throughout life. For unknown reasons, some patients progress to a symptomatic stage, with biliary colic caused by a stone obstructing the cystic duct. Symptomatic gallstone disease may progress to complications related to the gallstones.[26] These include acute cholecystitis, choledocholithiasis with or without cholangitis, gallstone pancreatitis, cholecystocholedochal fistula, cholecystoduodenal or cholecystoenteric fistula leading to gallstone ileus, and gallbladder carcinoma. Rarely, complication of gallstones is the presenting picture.

Gallstones in patients without biliary symptoms are commonly diagnosed incidentally on ultrasonography, CT scans, abdominal radiography, or at laparotomy. Several studies have examined the likelihood of developing biliary colic or developing significant complications of gallstone disease. Approximately 3% of asymptomatic individuals become symptomatic per year (i.e., develop bili-

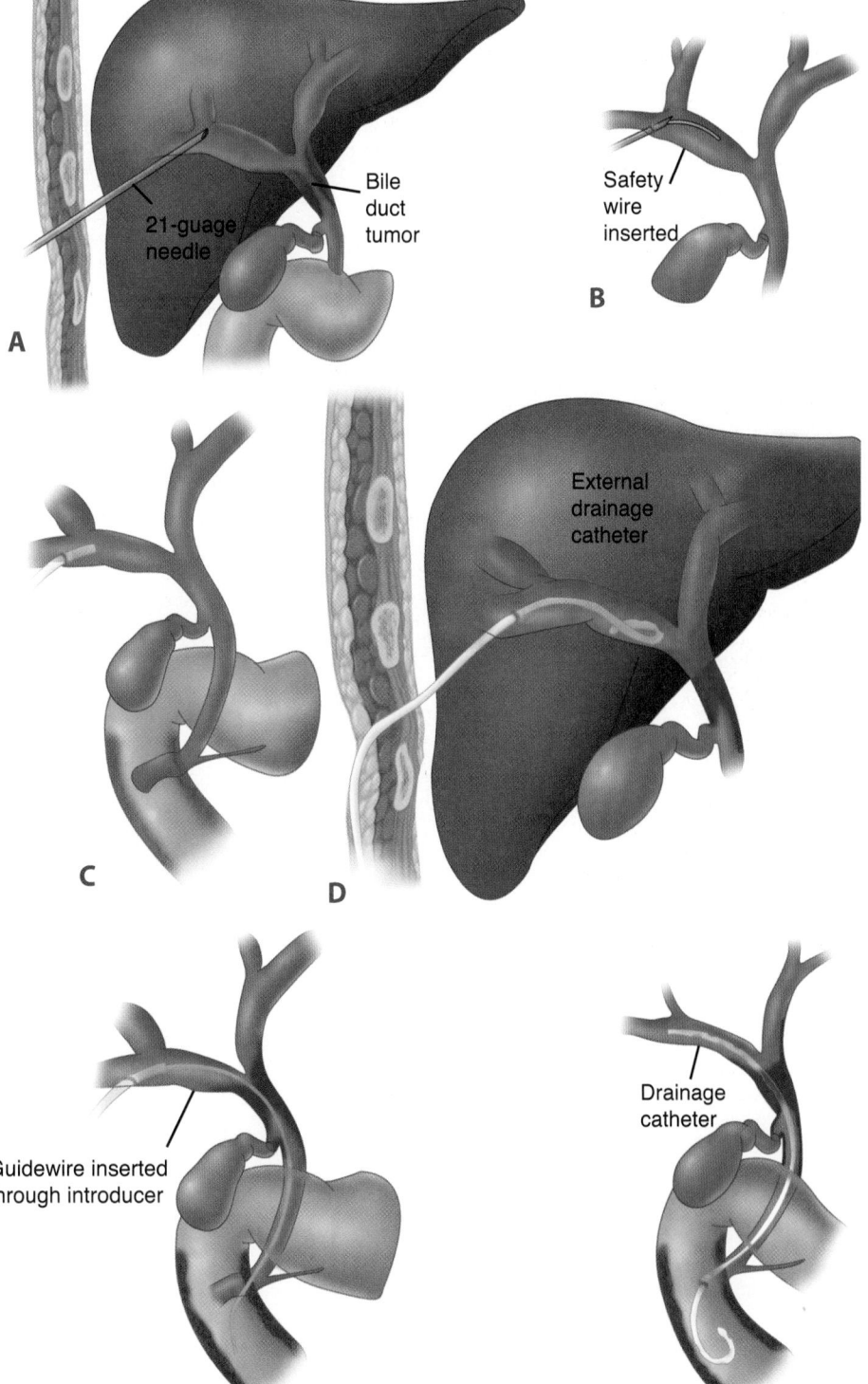

FIG. 32-8. Schematic diagram of percutaneous transhepatic cholangiogram and drainage for obstructing proximal cholangiocarcinoma. **A.** Dilated intrahepatic bile duct is entered percutaneously with a fine needle. **B.** Small guidewire is passed through the needle into the duct. **C.** A plastic catheter has been passed over the wire, and the wire is subsequently removed. A cholangiogram is performed through the catheter. **D.** An external drainage catheter in place. **E.** Long wire placed via the catheter and advanced past the tumor and into the duodenum. **F.** Internal stent has been placed through the tumor.

ary colic). Once symptomatic, patients tend to have recurring bouts of biliary colic. Complicated gallstone disease develops in 3 to 5% of symptomatic patients per year. Over a 20-year period, about two thirds of asymptomatic patients with gallstones remain symptom free.[27]

Because few patients develop complications without previous biliary symptoms, prophylactic cholecystectomy in asymptomatic persons with gallstones is rarely indicated. For elderly patients with diabetes, for individuals who will be isolated from medical care for extended periods of time, and in populations with increased risk of gallbladder cancer, a prophylactic cholecystectomy may be advis-

able. Porcelain gallbladder, a rare premalignant condition in which the wall of the gallbladder becomes calcified, is an absolute indication for cholecystectomy.

Gallstone Formation

Gallstones form as a result of solids settling out of solution. The major organic solutes in bile are bilirubin, bile salts, phospholipids, and cholesterol. Gallstones are classified by their cholesterol content as either cholesterol stones or pigment stones. Pigment stones can be further classified as either black or brown. In Western countries,

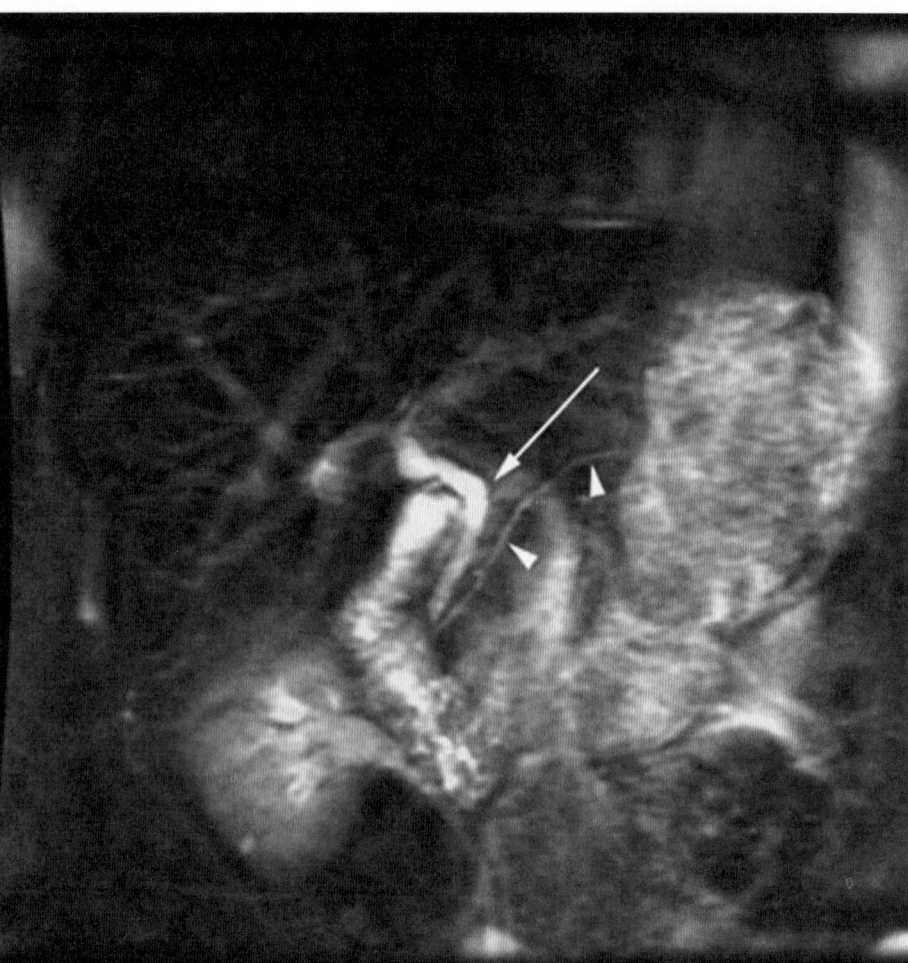

FIG. 32-9. Magnetic resonance cholangiopancreatography. This view shows the course of the extra-hepatic bile ducts (*arrow*) and the pancreatic duct (*arrowheads*).

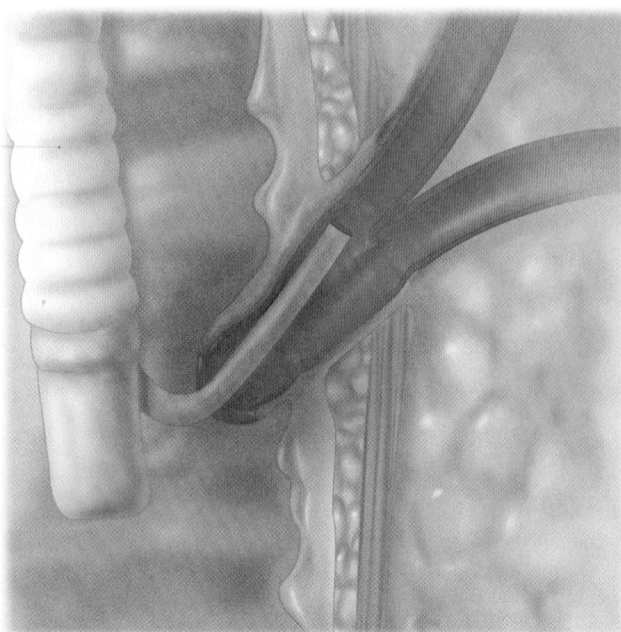

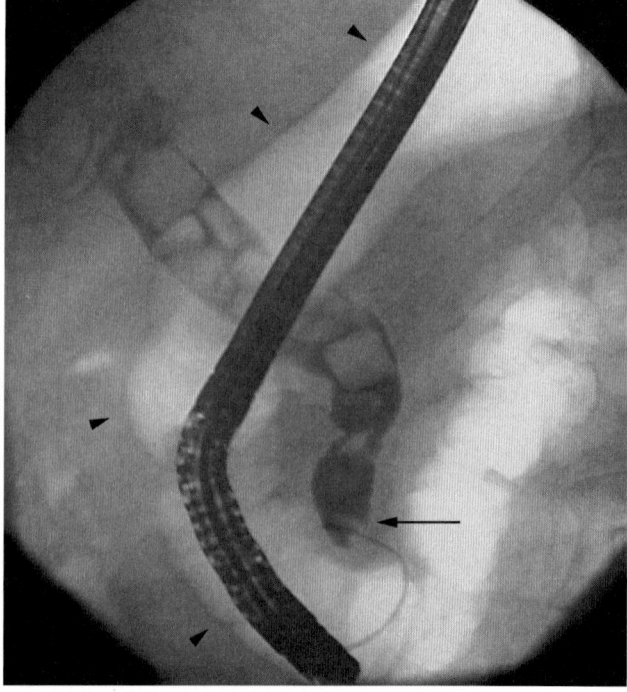

A   **B**

FIG. 32-10. Endoscopic retrograde cholangiography. **A.** A schematic picture showing the side-viewing endoscope in the duodenum and a catheter in the common bile duct. **B.** An endoscopic cholangiography showing stones in the common bile duct. The catheter has been placed in the ampulla of Vater (*arrow*). Note the duodenal shadow indicated with *arrowheads*.

about 80% of gallstones are cholesterol stones and about 15 to 20% are black pigment stones.[28] Brown pigment stones account for only a small percentage. Both types of pigment stones are more common in Asia.

Cholesterol Stones

Pure cholesterol stones are uncommon and account for <10% of all stones. They usually occur as single large stones with smooth surfaces. Most other cholesterol stones contain variable amounts of bile pigments and calcium, but are always >70% cholesterol by weight. These stones are usually multiple, of variable size, and may be hard and faceted or irregular, mulberry-shaped, and soft (Fig. 32-11). Colors range from whitish yellow and green to black. Most cholesterol stones are radiolucent; <10% are radiopaque. Whether pure or of mixed nature, the common primary event in the formation of cholesterol stones is supersaturation of bile with cholesterol. Therefore, high bile cholesterol levels and cholesterol gallstones are considered as one disease. Cholesterol is highly nonpolar and insoluble in water and bile. Cholesterol solubility depends on the relative concentration of cholesterol, bile salts, and lecithin (the main phospholipid in bile). Supersaturation almost always is caused by cholesterol hypersecretion rather than by a reduced secretion of phospholipid or bile salts.[2]

Cholesterol is secreted into bile as cholesterol-phospholipid vesicles. Cholesterol is held in solution by micelles, a conjugated bile salt-phospholipid-cholesterol complex, as well as by the cholesterol-phospholipid vesicles. The presence of vesicles and micelles in the same aqueous compartment allows the movement of lipids between the two. Vesicular maturation occurs when vesicular lipids are incorporated into micelles. Vesicular phospholipids are incorporated into micelles more readily than vesicular cholesterol. Therefore, vesicles may become enriched in cholesterol, become unstable, and then nucleate cholesterol crystals. In unsaturated bile, cholesterol enrichment of vesicles is inconsequential. In the supersaturated bile, cholesterol-dense zones develop on the surface of the cholesterol-enriched vesicles, leading to the appearance of cholesterol crystals. About one third of biliary cholesterol is transported in micelles, but the cholesterol-phospholipid vesicles carry the majority of biliary cholesterol[29] (Fig. 32-12).

Pigment Stones

Pigment stones contain <20% cholesterol and are dark because of the presence of calcium bilirubinate. Otherwise, black and brown pigment stones have little in common and should be considered as separate entities.

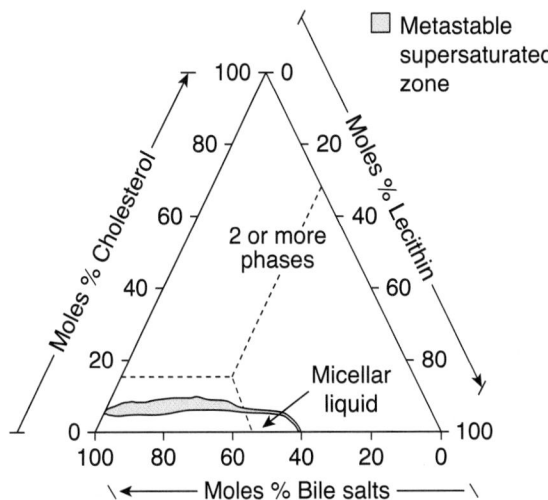

FIG. 32-12. The three major components of bile plotted on triangular coordinates. A given point represents the relative molar ratios of bile salts, lecithin, and cholesterol. The area labeled "micellar liquid" shows the range of concentrations found consistent with a clear micellar solution (single phase), where cholesterol is fully solubilized. The shaded area directly above this region corresponds to a metastable zone, supersaturated with cholesterol. Bile with a composition that falls above the shaded area has exceeded the solubilization capacity of cholesterol and precipitation of cholesterol crystals occurs. (*Reproduced with permission from Holzbach RT: Pathogenesis and medical treatment of gallstones, in Slesinger MH, Fordtran JS, eds: Gastrointestinal Diseases. Philadelphia: WB Saunders, 1989, p 1672.*)

Black pigment stones are usually small, brittle, black, and sometimes spiculated. They are formed by supersaturation of calcium bilirubinate, carbonate, and phosphate, most often secondary to hemolytic disorders such as hereditary spherocytosis and sickle cell disease, and in those with cirrhosis. Like cholesterol stones, they almost always form in the gallbladder. Unconjugated bilirubin is much less soluble than conjugated bilirubin in bile. Deconjugation of bilirubin occurs normally in bile at a slow rate. Excessive levels of conjugated bilirubin, as in hemolytic states, lead to an increased rate of production of unconjugated bilirubin. Cirrhosis may lead to increased secretion of unconjugated bilirubin. When altered conditions lead to increased levels of deconjugated bilirubin in bile, precipitation with calcium occurs. In Asian countries such as Japan, black stones account for a much higher percentage of gallstones than in the Western hemisphere.

Brown stones are usually <1 cm in diameter, brownish-yellow, soft, and often mushy. They may form either in the gallbladder or in the bile ducts, usually secondary to bacterial infection caused by bile stasis. Precipitated calcium bilirubinate and bacterial cell bodies compose the major part of the stone. Bacteria such as *Escherichia coli* secrete β-glucuronidase that enzymatically cleaves bilirubin glucuronide to produce the insoluble unconjugated bilirubin. It precipitates with calcium, and along with dead bacterial cell bodies, forms soft brown stones in the biliary tree.

Brown stones are typically found in the biliary tree of Asian populations and are associated with stasis secondary to parasite infection. In Western populations, brown stones occur as primary bile duct stones in patients with biliary strictures or other common bile duct stones that cause stasis and bacterial contamination.[2,30]

Symptomatic Gallstones
Chronic Cholecystitis (Biliary Colic)

About two thirds of patients with gallstone disease present with chronic cholecystitis characterized by recurrent attacks of pain,

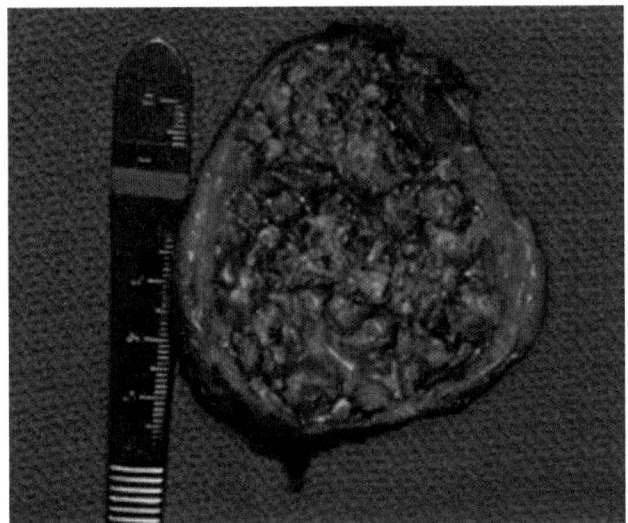

FIG. 32-11. Gallbladder with cholesterol stones. Note the different shapes and sizes.

often inaccurately labeled *biliary colic*. The pain develops when a stone obstructs the cystic duct, resulting in a progressive increase of tension in the gallbladder wall. The pathologic changes, which often do not correlate well with symptoms, vary from an apparently normal gallbladder with minor chronic inflammation in the mucosa, to a shrunken, nonfunctioning gallbladder with gross transmural fibrosis and adhesions to nearby structures. The mucosa is initially normal or hypertrophied, but later becomes atrophied, with the epithelium protruding into the muscle coat, leading to the formation of the so-called *Aschoff-Rokitansky sinuses*.

Clinical Presentation The chief symptom associated with symptomatic gallstones is pain. The pain is constant and increases in severity over the first half hour or so and typically lasts 1 to 5 hours. It is located in the epigastrium or right upper quadrant and frequently radiates to the right upper back or between the scapulae (Fig. 32-13). The pain is severe and comes on abruptly, typically during the night or after a fatty meal. It often is associated with nausea and sometimes vomiting. The pain is episodic. The patient suffers discrete attacks of pain, between which they feel well. Physical examination may reveal mild right upper quadrant tenderness during an episode of pain. If the patient is pain free, the physical examination is usually unremarkable. Laboratory values, such as WBC count and liver function tests, are usually normal in patients with uncomplicated gallstones.

Atypical presentation of gallstone disease is common. Association with meals is present in only about 50% of patients. Some patients report milder attacks of pain, but relate it to meals. The pain may be located primarily in the back or the left upper or lower right quadrant. Bloating and belching may be present and associated with the attacks of pain. In patients with atypical presentation, other conditions with upper abdominal pain should be sought out, even in the presence of gallstones. These include peptic ulcer disease, gastroesophageal reflux disease, abdominal wall hernias, irritable bowel disease, diverticular disease, liver diseases, renal calculi, pleuritic pain, and myocardial pain. Many patients with other conditions have gallstones.

When the pain lasts >24 hours, an impacted stone in the cystic duct or acute cholecystitis (see Acute Cholecystitis below) should be suspected. An impacted stone without cholecystis will result in what is called *hydrops of the gallbladder*. The bile gets absorbed, but the gallbladder epithelium continues to secrete mucus, and the gallbladder becomes distended with mucinous material. The gallbladder may be palpable but usually is not tender. Hydrops of the gallbladder may result in edema of the gallbladder wall, inflammation, infection, and perforation. Although hydrops may persist with few consequences, early cholecystectomy is generally indicated to avoid complications.

Diagnosis The diagnosis of symptomatic gallstones or chronic calculous cholecystitis depends on the presence of typical symptoms and the demonstration of stones on diagnostic imaging. An abdominal ultrasound is the standard diagnostic test for gallstones (see Ultrasonography above).[31] Gallstones are occasionally identified on abdominal radiographs or CT scans. In these cases, if the patient has typical symptoms, an ultrasound of the gallbladder and the biliary tree should be added before surgical intervention. Stones diagnosed incidentally in patients without symptoms should be left in place as discussed previously in Natural History. Occasionally, patients with typical attacks of biliary pain have no evidence of stones on ultrasonography. Sometimes only sludge in the gallbladder is demonstrated on ultrasonography. If the patient has recurrent attacks of typical biliary pain and sludge is detected on two or more occasions, cholecystectomy is warranted. In addition to sludge and stones, cholesterolosis and adenomyomatosis of the gallbladder may cause typical biliary symptoms and may be detected on ultrasonography. Cholesterolosis is caused by the accumulation of cholesterol in macrophages in the gallbladder mucosa, either locally or as polyps. It produces the classic macroscopic appearance of a "strawberry gallbladder." Adenomyomatosis or cholecystitis glandularis proliferans is characterized on microscopy by hypertrophic smooth muscle bundles and by the

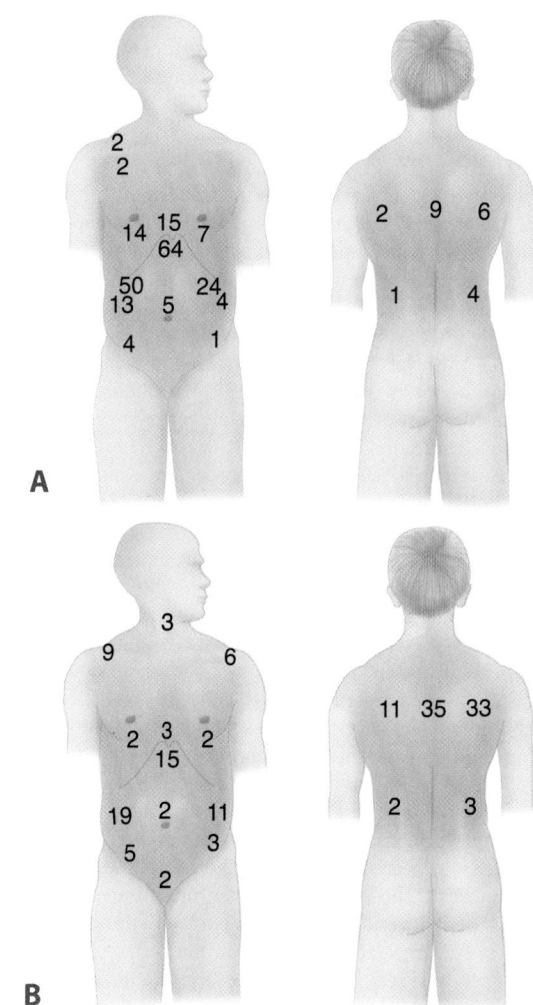

FIG. 32-13. **A.** Sites of the most severe pain during an episode of biliary pain in 107 patients with gallstones (% values add up to >100% because of multiple responses). The subxiphoid and right subcostal areas were the most common sites; note that the left subcostal area was not an unusual site of pain. **B.** Sites of pain radiation (%) during an episode of biliary pain in the same group of patients. *(Reprinted from Gunn A, Keddie N: Some clinical observations on patients with gallstones.* The Lancet *300(7771):239–241, Copyright 1972, with permission from Elsevier.)*

ingrowths of mucosal glands into the muscle layer (epithelial sinus formation). Granulomatous polyps develop in the lumen at the fundus, and the gallbladder wall is thickened and septae or strictures may be seen in the gallbladder. In symptomatic patients, cholecystectomy is the treatment of choice for patients with these conditions.[32]

Management Patients with symptomatic gallstones should be advised to have elective laparoscopic cholecystectomy. While waiting for surgery, or if surgery has to be postponed, the patient should be advised to avoid dietary fats and large meals. Diabetic patients with symptomatic gallstones should have a cholecystectomy promptly, as they are more prone to develop acute cholecystitis that is often severe. Pregnant women with symptomatic gallstones who cannot be managed expectantly with diet modifications can safely undergo laparoscopic cholecystectomy during the second trimester. Laparoscopic cholecystectomy is safe and effective in children as well as in the elderly.[33,34] Cholecystectomy, open or laparoscopic, for patients with symptomatic gallstones offers excellent long-term results. About 90% of patients with typical biliary symptoms and stones are rendered symptom free after cholecystectomy. For patients with atypical symptoms or dyspepsia (flatulence, belching, bloating, and dietary fat intolerance) the results are not as favorable.

Acute Cholecystitis

Pathogenesis Acute cholecystitis is secondary to gallstones in 90 to 95% of cases. Acute acalculous cholecystitis is a condition that typically occurs in patients with other acute systemic diseases (see Acalculous Cholecystitis section below). In <1% of acute cholecystitis, the cause is a tumor obstructing the cystic duct. Obstruction of the cystic duct by a gallstone is the initiating event that leads to gallbladder distention, inflammation, and edema of the gallbladder wall. Why inflammation develops only occasionally with cystic duct obstruction is unknown. It is probably related to the duration of obstruction of the cystic duct. Initially, acute cholecystitis is an inflammatory process, probably mediated by the mucosal toxin lysolecithin, a product of lecithin, as well as bile salts and platelet-activating factor. Increase in prostaglandin synthesis amplifies the inflammatory response. Secondary bacterial contamination is documented in 15 to 30% of patients undergoing cholecystectomy for acute uncomplicated cholecystitis. In acute cholecystitis, the gallbladder wall becomes grossly thickened and reddish with subserosal hemorrhages. Pericholecystic fluid often is present. The mucosa may show hyperemia and patchy necrosis. In severe cases, about 5 to 10%, the inflammatory process progresses and leads to ischemia and necrosis of the gallbladder wall. More frequently, the gallstone is dislodged and the inflammation resolves.[35]

When the gallbladder remains obstructed and secondary bacterial infection supervenes, an acute gangrenous cholecystitis develops, and an abscess or empyema forms within the gallbladder. Rarely, perforation of ischemic areas occurs. The perforation is usually contained in the subhepatic space by the omentum and adjacent organs. However, free perforation with peritonitis, intrahepatic perforation with intrahepatic abscesses, and perforation into adjacent organs (duodenum or colon) with cholecystoenteric fistula occur. When gas-forming organisms are part of the secondary bacterial infection, gas may be seen in the gallbladder lumen and in the wall of the gallbladder on abdominal radiographs and CT scans, an entity called an *emphysematous gallbladder*.

Clinical Manifestations About 80% of patients with acute cholecystitis give a history compatible with chronic cholecystitis. Acute cholecystitis begins as an attack of biliary colic, but in contrast to biliary colic, the pain does not subside; it is unremitting and may persist for several days. The pain is typically in the right upper quadrant or epigastrium, and may radiate to the right upper part of the back or the interscapular area. It is usually more severe than the pain associated with uncomplicated biliary colic. The patient is often febrile, complains of anorexia, nausea, and vomiting, and is reluctant to move, as the inflammatory process affects the parietal peritoneum. On physical examination, focal tenderness and guarding are usually present in the right upper quadrant. A mass, the gallbladder and adherent omentum, is occasionally palpable; however, guarding may prevent this. A Murphy's sign, an inspiratory arrest with deep palpation in the right subcostal area, is characteristic of acute cholecystitis.

A mild to moderate leukocytosis (12,000 to 15,000 cells/mm³) is usually present. However, some patients may have a normal WBC. A high WBC (above 20,000) is suggestive of a complicated form of cholecystitis such as gangrenous cholecystitis, perforation, or associated cholangitis. Serum liver chemistries are usually normal, but a mild elevation of serum bilirubin, <4 mg/mL, may be present along with mild elevation of alkaline phosphatase, transaminases, and amylase.[31] Severe jaundice is suggestive of common bile duct stones or obstruction of the bile ducts by severe pericholecystic inflammation secondary to impaction of a stone in the infundibulum of the gallbladder that mechanically obstructs the bile duct (Mirizzi's syndrome). In elderly patients and in those with diabetes mellitus, acute cholecystitis may have a subtle presentation resulting in a delay in diagnosis. The incidence of complications is higher in these patients, who also have approximately 10-fold the mortality rate compared to that of younger and healthier patients.

The differential diagnosis for acute cholecystitis includes a peptic ulcer with or without perforation, pancreatitis, appendicitis, hepatitis, perihepatitis (Fitz-Hugh–Curtis syndrome), myocardial ischemia, pneumonia, pleuritis, and herpes zoster involving the intercostal nerve.

Diagnosis Ultrasonography is the most useful radiologic test for diagnosing acute cholecystitis. It has a sensitivity and specificity of 95%. In addition to being a sensitive test for documenting the presence or absence of stones, it will show the thickening of the gallbladder wall and the pericholecystic fluid (Fig. 32-14). Focal tenderness over the gallbladder when compressed by the sonographic probe (sonographic Murphy's sign) also is suggestive of acute cholecystitis. Biliary radionuclide scanning (HIDA scan) may be of help in the atypical case. Lack of filling of the gallbladder after 4 hours indicates an obstructed cystic duct and, in the clinical setting of acute cholecystitis, is highly sensitive and specific for acute cholecystitis. A normal HIDA scan excludes acute cholecystitis. CT scan is frequently performed on patients with acute abdom-

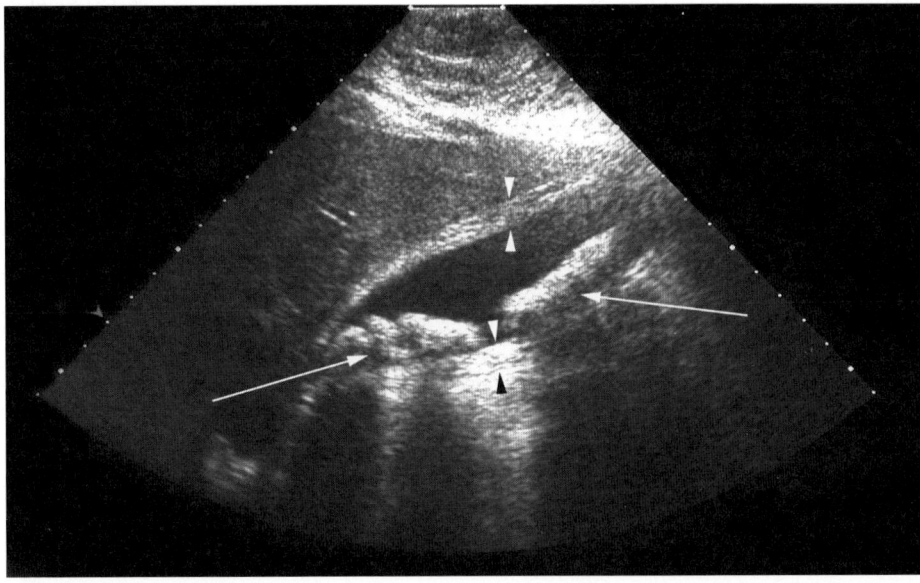

FIG. 32-14. Ultrasonography from a patient with acute cholecystitis. The *arrowheads* indicate the thickened gallbladder wall. There are several stones in the gallbladder (*arrows*) throwing acoustic shadows.

inal pain. It demonstrates thickening of the gallbladder wall, pericholecystic fluid, and the presence of gallstones as well as air in the gallbladder wall, but is less sensitive than ultrasonography.

Treatment Patients who present with acute cholecystitis will need IV fluids, antibiotics, and analgesia. The antibiotics should cover gram-negative aerobes as well as anaerobes. A third-generation cephalosporin with good anaerobic coverage or a second-generation cephalosporin combined with metronidazole is a typical regimen. For patients with allergies to cephalosporins, an aminoglycoside with metronidazole is appropriate. Although the inflammation in acute cholecystitis may be sterile in some patients, more than one half will have positive cultures from the gallbladder bile. It is difficult to know who is secondarily infected; therefore, antibiotics have become a part of the management in most medical centers.

Cholecystectomy is the definitive treatment for acute cholecystitis.[36] In the past, the timing of cholecystectomy has been a matter of debate. Early cholecystectomy performed within 2 to 3 days of the illness is preferred over interval or delayed cholecystectomy that is performed 6 to 10 weeks after initial medical treatment and recuperation. Several studies have shown that unless the patient is unfit for surgery, early cholecystectomy should be recommended, as it offers the patient a definitive solution in one hospital admission, quicker recovery times, and an earlier return to work.[37]

Laparoscopic cholecystectomy is the procedure of choice for acute cholecystitis. The conversion rate to an open cholecystectomy is higher (10 to 15%) in the setting of acute cholecystitis than with chronic cholecystitis. The procedure is more tedious and takes longer than in the elective setting. However, when compared to the delayed operation, early operation carries a similar complication rate.

When patients present late, after 3 to 4 days of illness, or if they are unfit for surgery, they can be treated with antibiotics with laparoscopic cholecystectomy scheduled for approximately 2 months later. Approximately 20% of patients will fail to respond to initial medical therapy and require an intervention. Laparoscopic cholecystectomy could be attempted, but the conversion rate is high and some prefer to go directly for an open cholecystectomy. For those unfit for surgery, a percutaneous cholecystostomy or an open cholecystostomy under local analgesia can be performed. Failure to improve after cholecystostomy usually is due to gangrene of the gallbladder or perforation. For these patients, surgery is unavoidable. For those who respond after cholecystostomy, the tube can be removed once cholangiography through it shows a patent ductus cysticus. Laparoscopic cholecystectomy may then be scheduled in the near future.[38] For the rare patients who can't tolerate surgery, the stones can be extracted via the cholecystostomy tube before its removal.[39]

Choledocholithiasis

Common bile duct stones may be small or large, single or multiple, and are found in 6 to 12% of patients with stones in the gallbladder. The incidence increases with age. About 20 to 25% of patients above the age of 60 with symptomatic gallstones have stones in the common bile duct as well as in the gallbladder.[40] The vast majority of ductal stones in Western countries are formed within the gallbladder and migrate down the cystic duct to the common bile duct. These are classified as secondary common bile duct stones, in contrast to the primary stones that form in the bile ducts. The secondary stones are usually cholesterol stones, whereas the primary stones are usually of the brown pigment type. The primary stones are associated with biliary stasis and infection and are more commonly seen in Asian populations. The causes of biliary stasis that lead to the development of primary stones include biliary stricture, papillary stenosis, tumors, or other (secondary) stones.

Clinical Manifestations Choledochal stones may be silent and often are discovered incidentally. They may cause obstruction, complete or incomplete, or they may manifest with cholangitis or gallstone pancreatitis. The pain caused by a stone in the bile duct is very similar to that of biliary colic caused by impaction of a stone in

the cystic duct. Nausea and vomiting are common. Physical examination may be normal, but mild epigastric or right upper quadrant tenderness as well as mild icterus are common. The symptoms may also be intermittent, such as pain and transient jaundice caused by a stone that temporarily impacts the ampulla but subsequently moves away, acting as a ball valve. A small stone may pass through the ampulla spontaneously with resolution of symptoms. Finally, the stones may become completely impacted, causing severe progressive jaundice. Elevation of serum bilirubin, alkaline phosphatase, and transaminases are commonly seen in patients with bile duct stones. However, in about one third of patients with common bile duct stones, the liver chemistries are normal.

Commonly, the first test, ultrasonography, is useful for documenting stones in the gallbladder (if still present), as well as determining the size of the common bile duct. As stones in the bile ducts tend to move down to the distal part of the common duct, bowel gas can preclude their demonstration on ultrasonography. A dilated common bile duct (>8 mm in diameter) on ultrasonography in a patient with gallstones, jaundice, and biliary pain is highly suggestive of common bile duct stones. Magnetic resonance cholangiography (MRC) provides excellent anatomic detail and has a sensitivity and specificity of 95 and 89%, respectively, at detecting choledocholithiasis >5mm in diameter.[18] Endoscopic cholangiography is the gold standard for diagnosing common bile duct stones. It has the distinct advantage of providing a therapeutic option at the time of diagnosis. In experienced hands, cannulation of the ampulla of Vater and diagnostic cholangiography are achieved in >90% of cases, with associated morbidity of <5% (mainly cholangitis and pancreatitis). Endoscopic ultrasound has been demonstrated to be as good as ERCP for detecting common bile duct stones (sensitivity of 91% and specificity of 100%), but it lacks therapeutic intervention and requires expertise, making it less available.[41] PTC is rarely needed in patients with secondary common bile duct stones but is frequently performed for both diagnostic and therapeutic reasons in patients with primary bile duct stones.

Treatment For patients with symptomatic gallstones and suspected common bile duct stones, either preoperative endoscopic cholangiography or an intraoperative cholangiogram will document the bile duct stones.[42] If an endoscopic cholangiogram reveals stones, sphincterotomy and ductal clearance of the stones is appropriate, followed by a laparoscopic cholecystectomy. An intraoperative cholangiogram at the time of cholecystectomy will also document the presence or absence of bile duct stones[43] (Fig. 32-15). Laparoscopic common bile duct exploration via the cystic duct or with formal choledochotomy allows the stones to be retrieved in the same setting (see Choledochal Exploration). If the expertise and/or the instrumentation for laparoscopic common bile duct exploration are not available, a drain should be left adjacent to the cystic duct and the patient scheduled for endoscopic sphincterotomy the following day. An open common bile duct exploration is an option if the endoscopic method has already been tried or is, for some reason, not feasible. If a choledochotomy is performed, a T tube is left in place. Stones impacted in the ampulla may be difficult for both endoscopic ductal clearance as well as common bile duct exploration (open or laparoscopic). In these cases the common bile duct is usually quite dilated (about 2 cm in diameter). A choledochoduodenostomy or a Roux-en-Y choledochojejunostomy may be the best option under this circumstance.[44]

Retained or recurrent stones following cholecystectomy are best treated endoscopically (Fig. 32-16). If the stones were deliberately left in place at the time of surgery or diagnosed shortly after the cholecystectomy, they are classified as *retained*; those diagnosed months or years later are termed *recurrent*. If a common bile duct exploration was performed and a T tube left in place, a T-tube cholangiogram is obtained before its removal. Retained stones can be retrieved either endoscopically or via the T-tube tract once it has matured (2 to 4 weeks). The T tube is then removed and a catheter passed through the tract into the common bile duct. Under fluoroscopic guidance, the

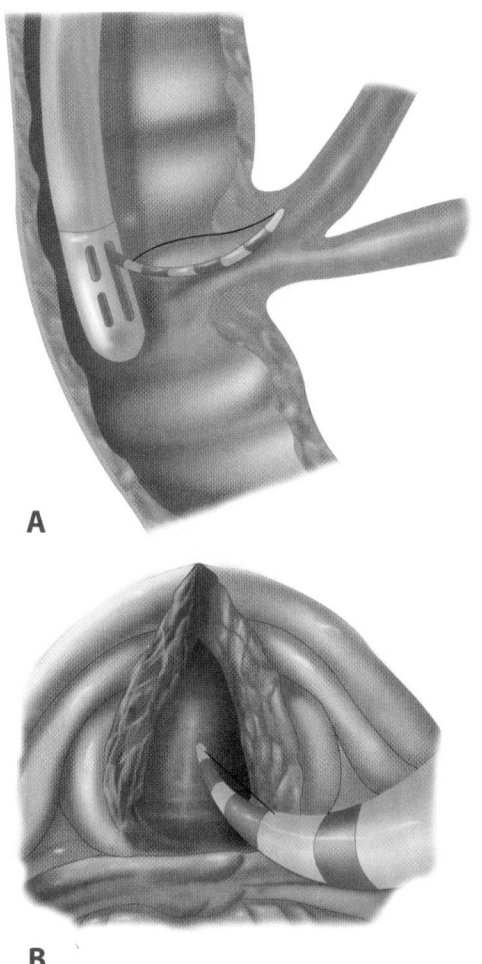

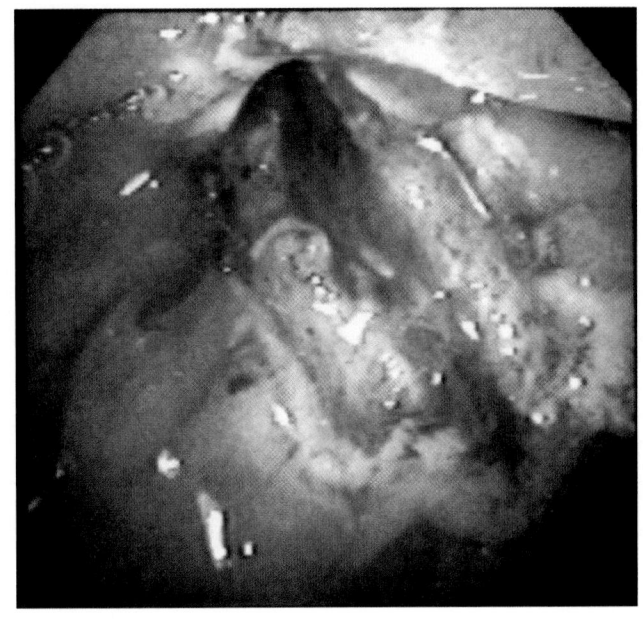

FIG. 32-15. An endoscopic sphincterotomy. **A.** The sphincterotome in place. **B.** Completed sphincterotomy. **C.** Endoscopic picture of completed sphincterotomy.

stones are retrieved with baskets or balloons. Recurrent stones may be multiple and large. A generous endoscopic sphincterotomy will allow stone retrieval as well as spontaneous passage of retained and recurrent stones. Patients >70 years old presenting with bile duct stones should have their ductal stones cleared endoscopically. Studies comparing surgery to endoscopic treatment have documented less morbidity and mortality for endoscopic treatment in this group of patients.[45] They do not need to be submitted for a cholecystectomy, as only about 15% will become symptomatic from their gallbladder stones, and such patients can be treated as the need arises by a cholecystectomy.[46]

Cholangitis

Cholangitis is one of the two main complications of choledochal stones, the other being gallstone pancreatitis. Acute cholangitis is an ascending bacterial infection in association with partial or complete obstruction of the bile ducts. Hepatic bile is sterile, and bile in the bile ducts is kept sterile by continuous bile flow and by the presence of antibacterial substances in bile, such as immunoglobulin. Mechanical hindrance to bile flow facilitates bacterial contamination. Positive bile cultures are common in the presence of bile duct stones as well as with other causes of obstruction. Biliary bacterial contamination alone does not lead to clinical cholangitis; the combination of both significant bacterial contamination and biliary obstruction is required for its development. Gallstones are the most common cause of obstruction in cholangitis; other causes are benign and malignant strictures, parasites, instrumentation of the ducts and indwelling stents, and partially obstructed biliary-enteric anastomosis. The most common organisms cultured from bile in patients with cholangitis include *E. coli*, *Klebsiella pneumoniae*, *Streptococcus faecalis*, Enterobacter, and *Bacteroides fragilis*.[47]

Clinical Presentation Cholangitis may present as anything from a mild, intermittent, and self-limited disease to a fulminant, potentially life-threatening septicemia. The patient with gallstone-induced cholangitis is typically older and female. The most common presentation is fever, epigastric or right upper quadrant pain, and jaundice. These classic symptoms, well known as *Charcot's triad*, are present in about two thirds of patients. The illness may progress rapidly with septicemia and disorientation, known as *Reynolds pentad* (e.g., fever, jaundice, right upper quadrant pain, septic shock, and mental status changes). However, the presentation may be atypical, with little if any fever, jaundice, or pain. This occurs most commonly in the elderly, who may have unremarkable symptoms until they collapse with septicemia. Patients with indwelling stents rarely become jaundiced. On abdominal examination, the findings are indistinguishable from those of acute cholecystitis.[48]

Diagnosis and Management Leukocytosis, hyperbilirubinemia, and elevation of alkaline phosphatase and transaminases are common and, when present, support the clinical diagnosis of cholangitis. Ultrasonography is helpful, as it will document the presence of gallbladder stones, demonstrate dilated ducts, and possibly pinpoint the site of obstruction; however, rarely will it elucidate the exact cause. The definitive diagnostic test is ERC. In cases in which ERC is not available, PTC is indicated. Both ERC and PTC will show the level and the reason for the obstruction, allow culture of the bile, possibly allow the removal of stones if present, and drainage of the bile ducts with drainage catheters or stents. CT scanning and MRI will show pancreatic and periampullary masses, if present, in addition to the ductal dilatation.

The initial treatment of patients with cholangitis includes IV antibiotics and fluid resuscitation. These patients may require inten-

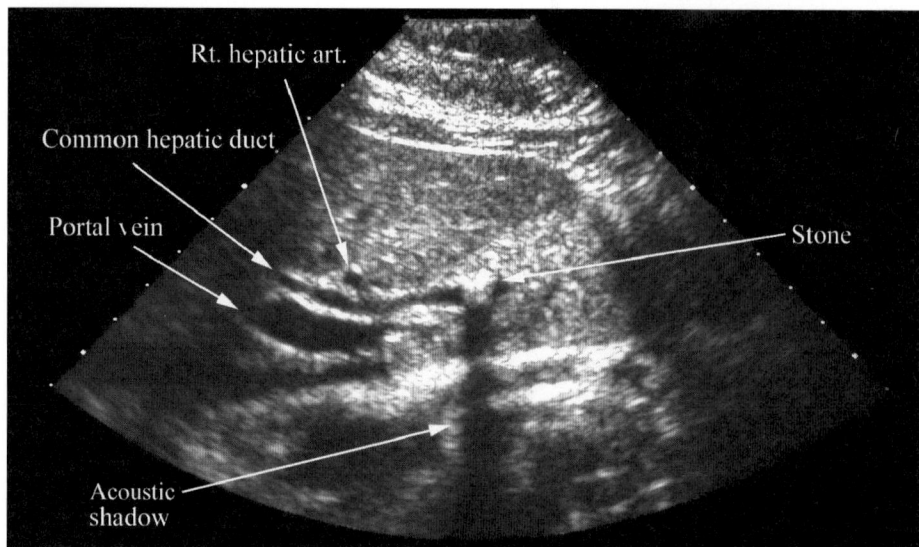

A

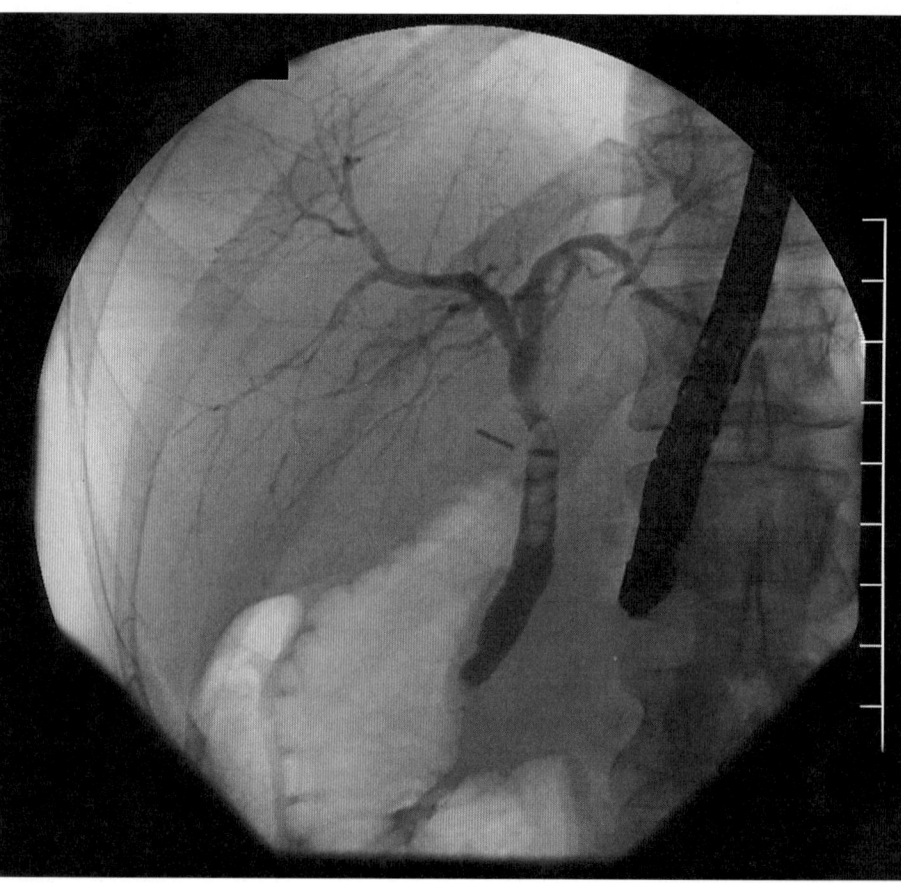

B

FIG. 32-16. Retained common bile duct stones. The patient presented 3 weeks after laparoscopic cholecystectomy. **A.** An ultrasound shows a normal or mildly dilated common bile duct with a stone. Note the location of the right hepatic artery anterior to the common hepatic duct (an anatomic variation). **B.** An endoscopic retrograde cholangiography from the same patient shows multiple stones in the common bile duct. Only the top one showed on ultrasound as the other stones lie in the distal common bile duct behind the duodenum.

sive care unit monitoring and vasopressor support. Most patients will respond to these measures. However, the obstructed bile duct must be drained as soon as the patient has been stabilized. About 15% of patients will not respond to antibiotics and fluid resuscitation, and an emergency biliary decompression may be required. Biliary decompression may be accomplished endoscopically, via the percutaneous transhepatic route, or surgically. The selection of procedure should be based on the level and the nature of the biliary obstruction. Patients with choledocholithiasis or periampullary malignancies are best approached endoscopically, with sphincterotomy and stone removal, or

by placement of an endoscopic biliary stent.[49] In patients in whom the obstruction is more proximal or perihilar, or when a stricture in a biliary-enteric anastomosis is the cause or the endoscopic route has failed, percutaneous transhepatic drainage is used. When neither ERC nor PTC is available, an emergent operation for decompression of the common bile duct with a T tube may be necessary and lifesaving. Definitive operative therapy should be deferred until the cholangitis has been treated and the proper diagnosis established. Patients with indwelling stents and cholangitis usually require repeated imaging and exchange of the stent over a guidewire.

Acute cholangitis is associated with an overall mortality rate of approximately 5%. When associated with renal failure, cardiac impairment, hepatic abscesses, and malignancies, the morbidity and mortality rates are much higher.

Biliary Pancreatitis

Gallstones in the common bile duct are associated with acute pancreatitis. Obstruction of the pancreatic duct by an impacted stone or temporary obstruction by a stone passing through the ampulla may lead to pancreatitis. The exact mechanism by which the obstruction of the pancreatic duct leads to pancreatitis is still not clear. An ultrasonogram of the biliary tree in patients with pancreatitis is essential. If gallstones are present and the pancreatitis is severe, an ERC with sphincterotomy and stone extraction may abort the episode of pancreatitis. Once the pancreatitis has subsided, the gallbladder should be removed during the same admission. When gallstones are present and the pancreatitis is mild and self-limited, the stone has probably passed. For these patients, a cholecystectomy and an intraoperative cholangiogram or a preoperative ERC is indicated.

Cholangiohepatitis

Cholangiohepatitis, also known as *recurrent pyogenic cholangitis*, is endemic to the Orient. It also has been encountered in the Chinese population in the United States, as well as in Europe and Australia. It affects both sexes equally and occurs most frequently in the third and fourth decades of life. Cholangiohepatitis is caused by bacterial contamination (commonly *E. coli*, *Klebsiella* species, *Bacteroides* species, or *Enterococcus* faecalis) of the biliary tree, and often is associated with biliary parasites such as *Clonorchis sinensis*, *Opisthorchis viverrini*, and *Ascaris lumbricoides*. Bacterial enzymes cause deconjugation of bilirubin, which precipitates as bile sludge. The sludge and dead bacterial cell bodies form brown pigment stones. The nucleus of the stone may contain an adult *Clonorchis* worm, an ovum, or an ascarid. These stones are formed throughout the biliary tree and cause partial obstruction that contributes to the repeated bouts of cholangitis. Biliary strictures form as a result of recurrent cholangitis and lead to further stone formation, infection, hepatic abscesses, and liver failure (secondary biliary cirrhosis).[50]

The patient usually presents with pain in the right upper quadrant and epigastrium, fever, and jaundice. Recurrence of symptoms is one of the most characteristic features of the disease. The episodes may vary in severity but, without intervention, will gradually lead to malnutrition and hepatic insufficiency. An ultrasound will detect stones in the biliary tree, pneumobilia from infection due to gas-forming organisms, liver abscesses, and, occasionally, strictures. The gallbladder may be thickened, but is inflamed in about 20% of patients, and rarely contains stones. MRCP and PTC are the mainstays of biliary imaging for cholangiohepatitis. They can detect obstructions, define strictures and stones, and allow emergent decompression of the biliary tree in the septic patient. Hepatic abscesses may be drained percutaneously. The long-term goal of therapy is to extract stones and debris and relieve strictures. It may take several procedures and require a Roux-en-Y hepaticojejunostomy to establish biliary-enteric continuity. Occasionally, resection of involved areas of the liver may offer the best form of treatment. Recurrences are common and the prognosis is poor once hepatic insufficiency has developed.[51]

OPERATIVE INTERVENTIONS FOR GALLSTONE DISEASE

Cholecystostomy

A cholecystostomy decompresses and drains the distended, inflamed, hydropic, or purulent gallbladder. It is applicable if the patient is not fit to tolerate an abdominal operation.[52] Ultrasound-guided percutaneous drainage with a pigtail catheter is the procedure of choice. The catheter is inserted over a guidewire that has

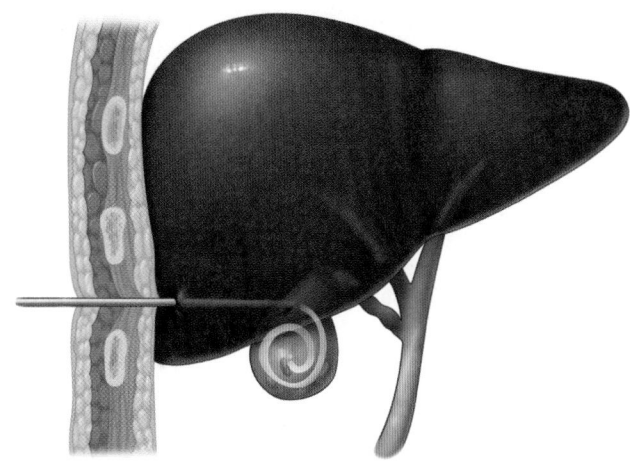

FIG. 32-17. Percutaneous cholecystostomy. A pigtail catheter has been placed through the abdominal wall, the right lobe of the liver, and into the gallbladder.

been passed through the abdominal wall, the liver, and into the gallbladder (Fig. 32-17). By passing the catheter through the liver, the risk of bile leak around the catheter is minimized.[53] The catheter can be removed when the inflammation has resolved and the patient's condition improved. The gallbladder can be removed later, if indicated, usually by laparoscopy. Surgical cholecystostomy with a large catheter placed under local anesthesia is rarely required today.

Cholecystectomy

Cholecystectomy is the most common major abdominal procedure performed in Western countries. Carl Langenbuch performed the first successful cholecystectomy in 1882, and for >100 years, it was the standard treatment for symptomatic gallbladder stones. Open cholecystectomy was a safe and effective treatment for both acute and chronic cholecystitis. In 1987, laparoscopic cholecystectomy was introduced by Philippe Mouret in France and quickly revolutionized the treatment of gallstones. It not only supplanted open cholecystectomy, but also more or less ended attempts for noninvasive management of gallstones, such as extracorporeal shock wave and bile salt therapy. Laparoscopic cholecystectomy offers a cure for gallstones with a minimally invasive procedure, minor pain and scarring, and early return to full activity. Today, laparoscopic cholecystectomy is the treatment of choice for symptomatic gallstones.

Absolute contraindications for the procedure are uncontrolled coagulopathy and end-stage liver disease. Rarely, patients with severe obstructive pulmonary disease or congestive heart failure (e.g., cardiac ejection fraction <20%) may not tolerate pneumoperitoneum with carbon dioxide and require open cholecystectomy. Conditions formerly believed to be relative contraindications such as acute cholecystitis, gangrene and empyema of the gallbladder, biliary-enteric fistulae, obesity, pregnancy, ventriculoperitoneal shunt, cirrhosis, and previous upper abdominal procedures are now considered risk factors for a potentially difficult laparoscopic cholecystectomy. When important anatomic structures cannot be clearly identified or when no progress is made over a set period of time, a conversion to an open procedure is usually indicated. In the elective setting, conversion to an open procedure is needed in about 5% of patients.[54] Emergent procedures may require more skill on the part of the surgeon and be needed in patients with complicated gallstone disease; the incidence of conversion is 10 to 30%. Conversion to an open procedure is not a failure, and the possibility should be discussed with the patient preoperatively.

Serious complications are rare. The mortality rate for laparoscopic cholecystectomy is about 0.1%. Wound infection and cardiopulmonary complication rates are considerably lower following laparoscopic cholecystectomy than are those for an open procedure. However, laparoscopic cholecystectomy is associated with a higher injury rate to the bile ducts (see section on Injury to the Biliary Tract below).[55]

Patients undergoing cholecystectomy should have a complete blood count and liver function tests preoperatively. Prophylaxis against deep venous thrombosis with either low molecular weight heparin or compression stockings is indicated. The patient should be instructed to empty their bladder before coming to the operating room. Urinary catheters are rarely needed. An orogastric tube is placed if the stomach is distended with gas and is removed at the end of the operation.

Laparoscopic Cholecystectomy

The patient is placed supine on the operating table with the surgeon standing at the patient's left side. Some surgeons prefer to stand between the patient's legs while doing laparoscopic procedures in the upper abdomen. The pneumoperitoneum is created with carbon dioxide gas, either with an open technique or by closed needle technique. Initially, a small incision is made in the upper edge of the umbilicus. With the closed technique, a special hollow insufflation needle (Veress needle) that is spring-loaded with a retractable cutting outer sheath is inserted into the peritoneal cavity and used for insufflation. Once an adequate pneumoperitoneum is established, a 10-mm trocar is inserted through the supraumbilical incision. With the open technique, the supraumbilical incision is carried through the fascia and into the peritoneal cavity. A special blunt cannula (Hasson cannula) is inserted into the peritoneal cavity and anchored to the fascia. The laparoscope with the attached video camera is passed through the umbilical port and the abdomen inspected. Three additional ports are placed under direct vision (Fig. 32-18). A 10-mm port is placed in the epigastrium, a 5-mm port in the middle of the clavicular line, and a 5-mm port in the right flank, in line with the gallbladder fundus. Occasionally, a fifth port is required for better visualization in patients recovering from pancreatitis or those with semi-acute cholecystitis, as well as in very obese patients.

Through the lateralmost port, a grasper is used to grasp the gallbladder fundus. It is retracted over the liver edge upward and toward the patient's right shoulder to expose the proximal gallbladder and the hilar area. Exposure of the hilar area may be facilitated by placing the patient in reverse Trendelenburg position with slight tilting of the table to bring the right side up. Through the midclavicular port a second grasper is used to grasp the gallbladder infundibulum and retract it laterally to expose the triangle of Calot. Before this, it may be necessary to take down any adhesions between the omentum, duodenum, or colon, and the gallbladder. Most of the dissection is carried out through the epigastric port using a dissector, hook cautery, or scissors.

The dissection starts at the junction of the gallbladder and the cystic duct. A helpful anatomic landmark is the cystic artery lymph node. The peritoneum, fat, and loose areolar tissue around the gallbladder and the cystic duct–gallbladder junction is dissected off toward the bile duct. This is continued until the gallbladder neck and the proximal cystic duct are clearly identified. The next step is the identification of the cystic artery, which usually runs parallel to and somewhat behind the cystic duct. A hemoclip is placed on the proximal cystic duct. If an intraoperative cholangiogram is to be performed, a small incision is made on the anterior surface of the cystic duct, just proximal to the clip, and a cholangiogram catheter is passed into the cystic duct. Once the cholangiogram is completed, the catheter is removed and two clips are placed proximal to the incision, and the cystic duct is divided. A wide cystic duct may be too big for clips, requiring the placement of a pre-tied loop ligature to close. The cystic artery is then clipped and divided.

Finally, the gallbladder is dissected out of the gallbladder fossa, using either a hook or scissors with electrocautery. Before the gallbladder is removed from the liver edge, the operative field is carefully searched for bleeding points and the placement of the clips

on the cystic duct and cystic artery is inspected. The gallbladder is removed through the umbilical incision. The fascial defect and skin incision may need to be enlarged if the stones are large. If the gallbladder is acutely inflamed or gangrenous, or if the gallbladder is perforated, it is placed in a retrieval bag before it is removed from the abdomen. Any bile or blood that has accumulated during the procedure is sucked away, and if stones were spilled, they are retrieved, placed inside a retrieval bag, and removed. If the gallbladder was severely inflamed, gangrenous, or if any bile or blood is expected to accumulate, a closed suction drain can be placed through one of the 5-mm ports and left underneath the right liver lobe close to the gallbladder fossa.

Open Cholecystectomy

The same surgical principles apply for laparoscopic and open cholecystectomies. Open cholecystectomy has become an uncommon procedure, usually performed either as a conversion from laparoscopic cholecystectomy or as a second procedure in patients who require laparotomy for another reason. After the cystic artery and cystic duct have been identified, the gallbladder is dissected free from the liver bed, starting at the fundus. The dissection is carried proximally toward the cystic artery and the cystic duct, which are then ligated and divided.

Intraoperative Cholangiogram or Ultrasound

The bile ducts are visualized under fluoroscopy by injecting contrast through a catheter placed in the cystic duct (Fig. 32-19A). Their size can then be evaluated, the presence or absence of common bile duct stones assessed, and filling defects confirmed, as the dye passes into the duodenum. Routine intraoperative cholangiography will detect stones in approximately 7% of patients, as well as outlining the anatomy and detecting injury[56,57] (Fig. 32-19B). A selective intraoperative cholangiogram can be performed when the patient has a history of abnormal liver function tests, pancreatitis, jaundice, a large duct and small stones, a dilated duct on preoperative ultrasonography, and if preoperative endoscopic cholangiography for the above reasons was unsuccessful. Laparoscopic ultrasonography is as accurate as intraoperative cholangiography in detecting common bile duct stones and it is less invasive; however, it requires more skill to perform and interpret.[58,59]

Choledochal Exploration

Common bile duct stones that are detected intraoperatively on intraoperative cholangiography or ultrasonography may be managed with laparoscopic choledochal exploration as a part of the laparoscopic cholecystectomy procedure. Patients with common bile duct stones detected preoperatively, but endoscopic clearance was either not available or unsuccessful, should also have their ductal stones managed during the cholecystectomy.

If the stones in the duct are small, they may sometimes be flushed into the duodenum with saline irrigation via the cholangiography catheter after the sphincter of Oddi has been relaxed with glucagon. If irrigation is unsuccessful, a balloon catheter may be passed via the cystic duct and down the common bile duct, where it is inflated and withdrawn to retrieve the stones. The next attempt is usually made with a wire basket passed under fluoroscopic guidance to catch the stones (Fig. 32-20). If needed, a flexible choledochoscope is the next step. The cystic duct may have to be dilated to allow its passage. Once in the common bile duct, the stones may be caught into a wire basket under direct vision or pushed into the duodenum. When the duct has been cleared, the cystic duct is ligated and cut and the cholecystectomy completed. Occasionally, a choledochotomy, an incision into the common bile duct itself, is necessary. The flexible choledochoscope is then passed into the duct for visualization and clearance of stones. The choledochotomy is sutured with a T tube left in the common bile duct with one end taken out through the abdominal wall for decompression of the bile ducts. By managing common bile

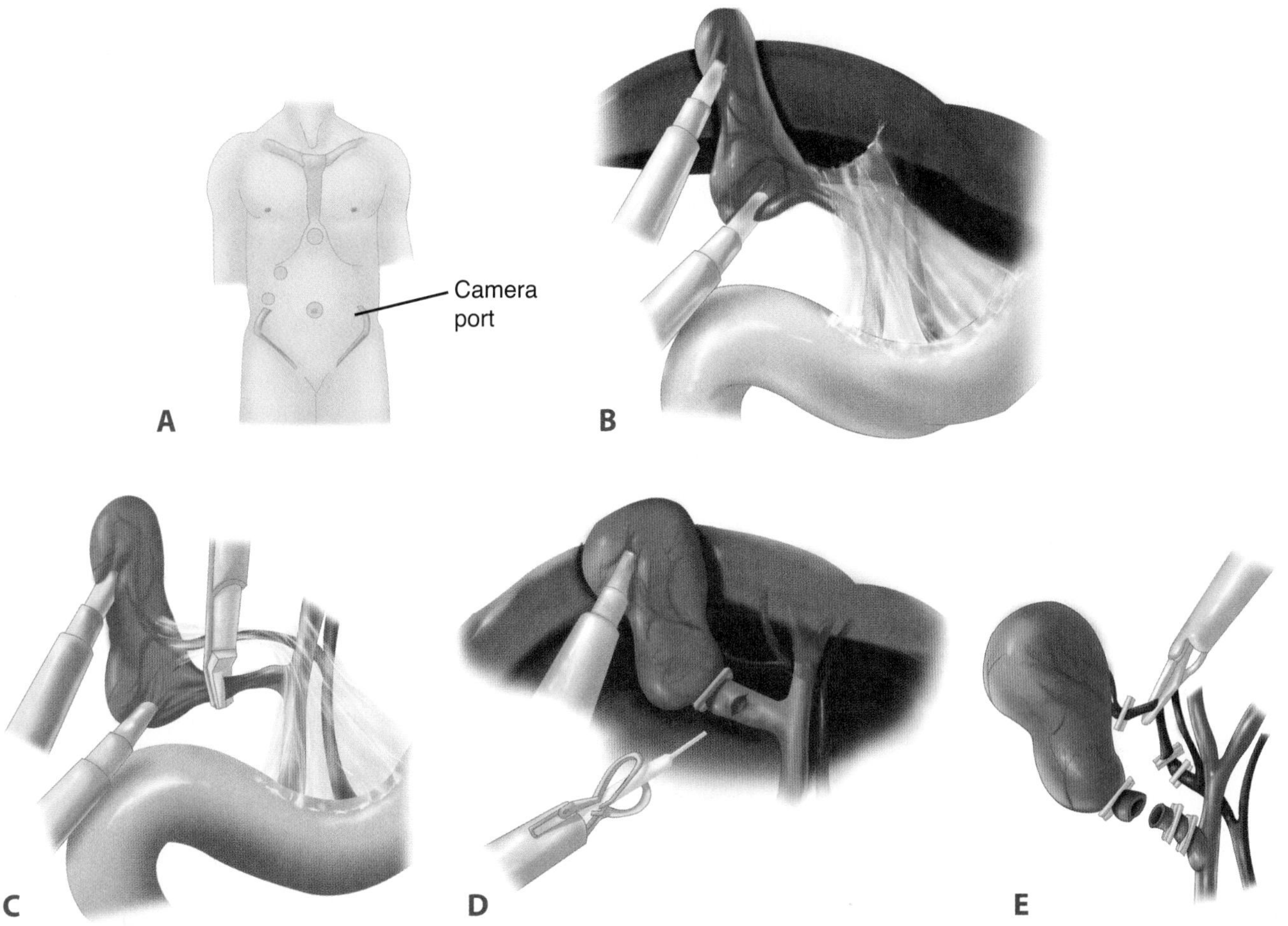

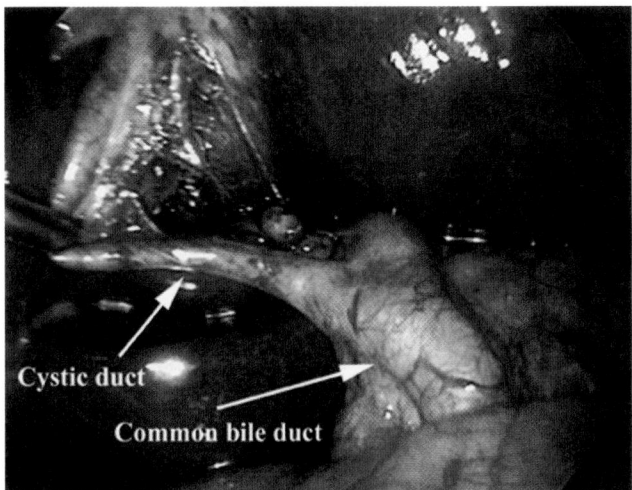

A

B

C

D

E

F

FIG. 32-18. Laparoscopic cholecystectomy. **A.** The trocar placement. **B.** The fundus has been grasped and retracted cephalad to expose the proximal gallbladder and the hepatoduodenal ligament. Another grasper retracts the gallbladder infundibulum posterolaterally to better expose the triangle of Calot (hepatocystic triangle bound by the common hepatic duct, cystic duct, and the liver margin). **C.** The triangle of Calot has been opened and the neck of the gallbladder and part of the cystic duct dissected free. A clip is being placed on the cystic duct–gallbladder junction. **D.** A small opening has been made into the cystic duct, and a cholangiogram catheter is to be inserted. **E.** The cystic duct has been divided, and the cystic artery is being divided. **F.** An intraoperative picture showing a grasper pulling the infundibulum of the gallbladder laterally, exposing the triangle of Calot that has been dissected. The cystic artery can be seen crossing the dissected area upward and to the left.

duct stones at the time of the cholecystectomy, the patients can have all of their gallstone disease treated with one invasive procedure. It does, however, depend on the available surgical expertise.[60]

Choledochal Drainage Procedures

Rarely, when the stones cannot be cleared and/or when the duct is very dilated (larger than 1.5 cm in diameter), a choledochal drainage procedure is performed (Fig. 32-21). Choledochoduodenostomy is performed by mobilizing the second part of the duodenum

(a Kocher maneuver) and anastomosing it side to side with the common bile duct.

A choledochojejunostomy is done by bringing up a 45-cm Roux-en-Y limb of jejunum and anastomosing it end to side to the choledochus.

Choledochojejunostomy or, more often, a hepaticojejunostomy, also can be used to repair common bile duct strictures or as a palliative procedure for malignant obstruction in the periampullary region. If the common bile duct has been transected or injured, it can be managed by an end-to-end choledochojejunostomy.

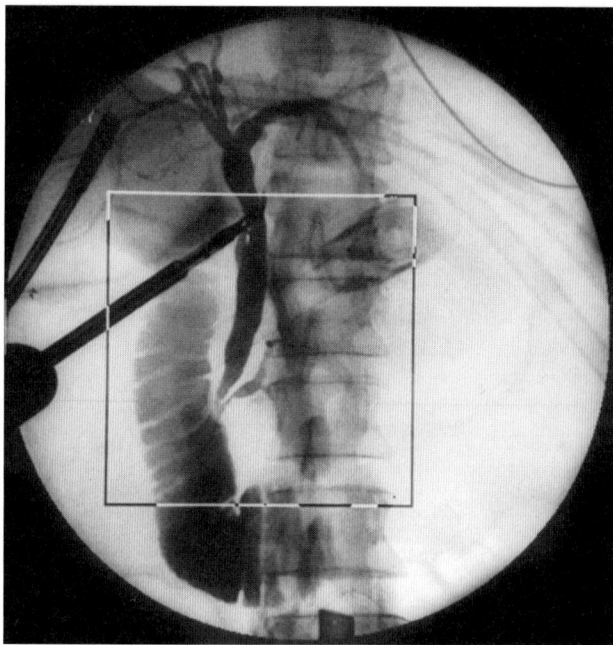

A

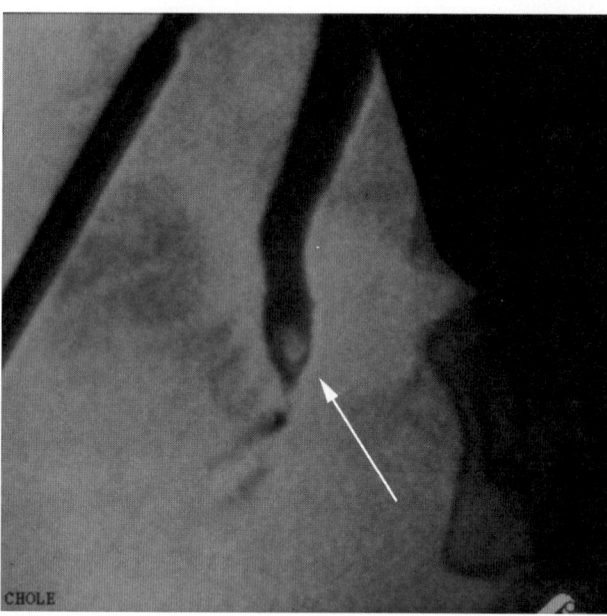

B

FIG. 32-19. A. An intraoperative cholangiogram. The bile ducts are of normal size, with no intraluminal filling defects. The left and the right hepatic ducts are visualized, the distal common bile duct tapers down, and the contrast empties into the duodenum. Cholangiography grasper that holds the catheter and the cystic duct stump partly projects over the common hepatic duct. **B.** An intraoperative cholangiogram showing common bile duct stone (*arrow*). A small amount of contrast has passed into the duodenum.

Transduodenal Sphincterotomy

In the majority of cases, endoscopic sphincterotomy has replaced open transduodenal sphincterotomy. If an open procedure for common bile duct stones is being done in which the stones are impacted, recurrent, or multiple, the transduodenal approach may be feasible. The duodenum is incised transversely. The sphincter then is incised at the 11 o'clock position to avoid injury to the pancreatic duct. The impacted stones are removed as are large stones from the duct. There is no need to fully clear the duct of stones, as they can pass spontaneously through the cut sphincter.

OTHER BENIGN DISEASES AND LESIONS

Acalculous Cholecystitis

Acute inflammation of the gallbladder can occur without gallstones. Acalculous cholecystitis typically develops in critically ill patients in the intensive care unit. Patients on parenteral nutrition with extensive burns, sepsis, major operations, multiple trauma, or prolonged illness with multiple organ system failure are at risk for developing acalculous cholecystitis. The cause is unknown, but gallbladder distention with bile stasis and ischemia has been implicated as causative factors. Pathologic examination of the gallbladder wall reveals edema of the serosa and muscular layers, with patchy thrombosis of arterioles and venules.[61,62]

The symptoms and signs depend on the condition of the patient, but in the alert patient, they are similar to acute calculous cholecystitis, with right upper quadrant pain and tenderness, fever, and leukocytosis. In the sedated or unconscious patient, the clinical features are often masked, but fever and elevated WBC count, as well as elevation of alkaline phosphatase and bilirubin are indications for further investigation.

Ultrasonography is usually the diagnostic test of choice, as it can be done bedside in the intensive care unit. It can demonstrate the distended gallbladder with thickened wall, biliary sludge, pericholecystic fluid, and the presence or absence of abscess formation. Abdominal CT scan can aid in the diagnosis of acalculous cholecystitis and additionally allows imaging of the abdominal cavity and chest to rule out other sources of infection. A HIDA scan can be useful and will show nonvisualization of the gallbladder, but it is a less sensitive test with high false-positive rates in patients who are fasting, on total parenteral nutrition, or have liver disease.[63] Acalculous cholecystitis requires urgent intervention. Percutaneous ultrasound- or CT-guided cholecystostomy is the treatment of choice for these patients, as they are usually unfit for surgery (see Fig. 32-17). If the diagnosis is uncertain, percutaneous cholecystostomy is both diagnostic and therapeutic. About 90% of patients will improve with the percutaneous cholecystostomy. However, if they do not improve, other steps, such as open cholecystostomy or cholecystectomy, may be required. If needed, cholecystectomy is performed after the patient has recovered from the underlying disease.

Biliary Cysts

Choledochal cysts are congenital cystic dilatations of the extrahepatic and/or intrahepatic biliary tree. They are rare—the incidence is between 1:100,000 and 1:150,000 in populations of Western countries—but are more commonly seen in populations of Eastern countries. Choledochal cysts affect females three to eight times more often than males. Although frequently diagnosed in infancy or childhood, as many as one half of the patients have reached adulthood when diagnosed. The cause is unknown. Weakness of the bile duct wall and increased pressure secondary to partial biliary obstruction are required for biliary cyst formation. More than 90% of patients have an anomalous pancreaticobiliary duct junction, with the pancreatic duct joining the common bile duct >1 cm proximal to the ampulla. This results in a long common channel that may allow free reflux of pancreatic secretions into the biliary tract, leading to inflammatory changes, increased biliary pressure, and cyst formation. Choledochal cysts are classified into five types (Fig. 32-22). The cysts are lined with cuboidal epithelium and can vary in size from 2 cm in diameter to giant cysts.

Adults commonly present with jaundice or cholangitis. Less than one half of patients present with the classic clinical triad of abdominal pain, jaundice, and a mass. Ultrasonography or CT scanning will confirm the diagnosis, but endoscopic, transhepatic,

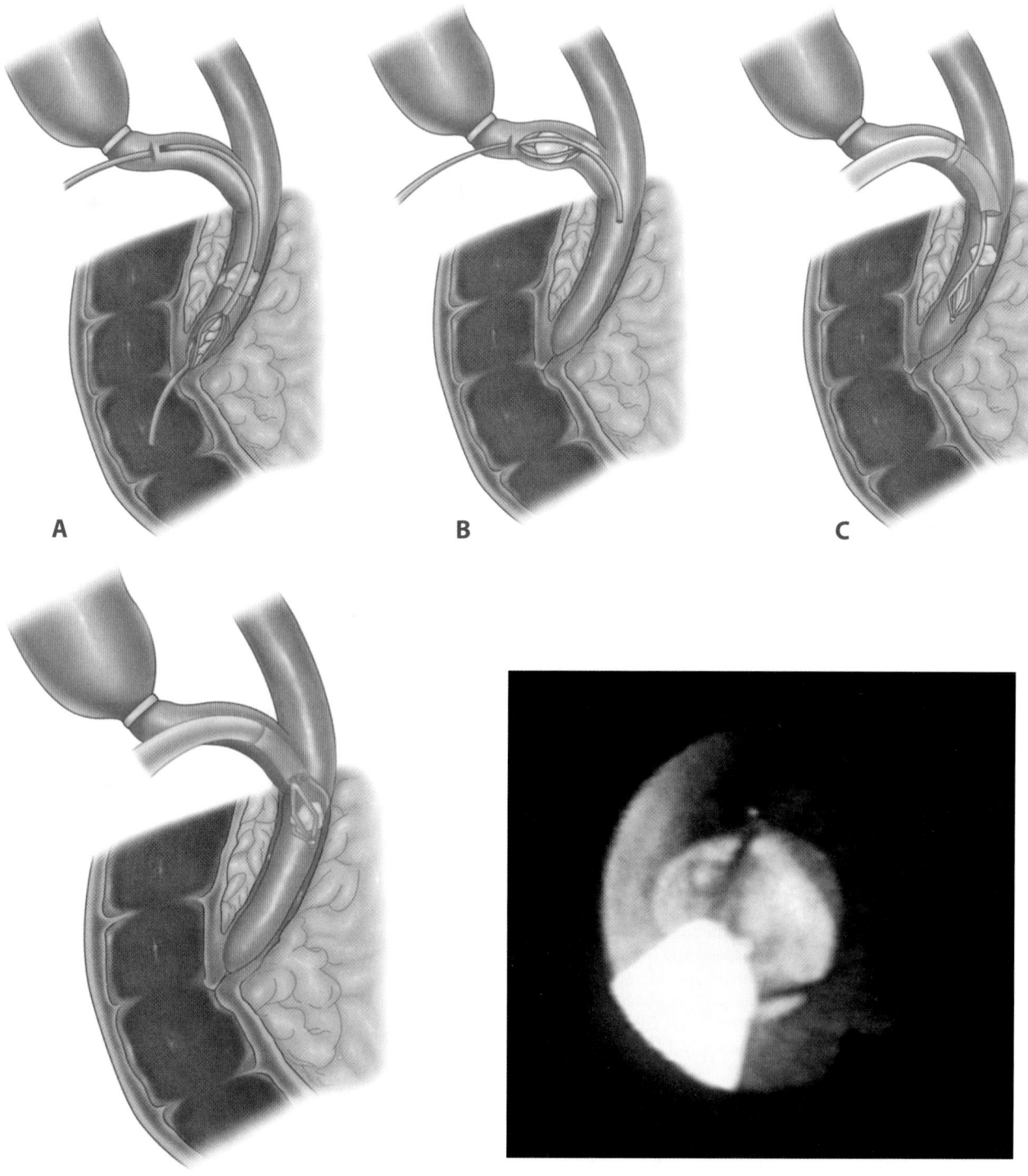

FIG. 32-20. Laparoscopic bile duct exploration. I. Transcystic basket retrieval using fluoroscopy. **A.** The basket has been advanced past the stone and opened. **B.** The stone has been entrapped in the basket, and together, they are removed from the cystic duct. II. Transcystic choledochoscopy and stone removal. **C.** The basket has been passed through the working channel of the scope, and the stone is entrapped under direct vision. **D.** Entrapped stone. **E.** A view from the choledochoscope. III. Choledochotomy and stone removal. (*Continued*)

or MRC is required to assess the biliary anatomy and to plan the appropriate surgical treatment. For types I, II, and IV, excision of the extrahepatic biliary tree, including cholecystectomy, with a Roux-en-Y hepaticojejunostomy are ideal. In type IV, additional segmental resection of the liver may be appropriate, particularly if intrahepatic stones, strictures, or abscesses are present, or if the dilatations are confined to one lobe. The risk of cholangiocarcinoma developing in choledochal cysts is as high as 15% in adults,

and supports complete excision when they are diagnosed. For type III, sphincterotomy is recommended.[64]

Sclerosing Cholangitis

Sclerosing cholangitis is an uncommon disease characterized by inflammatory strictures involving the intrahepatic and extrahepatic biliary tree. It is a progressive disease that eventually results in

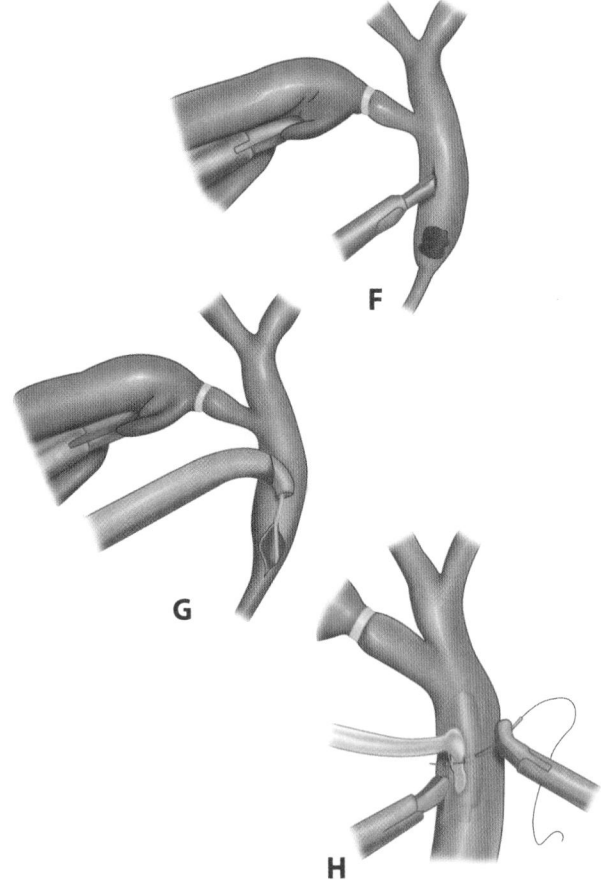

FIG. 32-20. (*Continued*) **F.** A small incision is made in the common bile duct. **G.** The common bile duct is cleared of stones. **H.** A T tube left in the common bile duct with one end taken out through the abdominal wall for decompression of the bile ducts.

secondary biliary cirrhosis. Sometimes, biliary strictures are clearly secondary to bile duct stones, acute cholangitis, previous biliary surgery, or toxic agents, and are termed *secondary sclerosing cholangitis*. However, primary sclerosing cholangitis is a disease entity of its own, with no known attributing cause. It is associated with ulcerative colitis in about two thirds of patients. Other diseases associated with sclerosing cholangitis include Riedel's thyroiditis and retroperitoneal fibrosis. Autoimmune reaction, chronic low-grade bacterial or viral infection, toxic reaction, and genetic factors have all been suggested to play a role in its pathogenesis. The human leukocyte antigen haplotypes HLA-B8, -DR3, -DQ2, and -DRw52A, commonly found in patients with autoimmune diseases, also are more frequently seen in patients with sclerosing cholangitis than in controls. Patients with sclerosing cholangitis are at risk for developing cholangiocarcinoma. Eventually, 10 to 20% of the patients will develop cancer. Cholangiocarcinoma can present at any time during the disease process and does not correlate with the extent of sclerosing cholangitis or the development of liver failure, but frequently follows an aggressive course.

The mean age of presentation is 30 to 45 years, and men are affected twice as commonly as women. The usual presentation is intermittent jaundice, fatigue, weight loss, pruritus, and abdominal pain. Symptoms of acute cholangitis are rare, without preceding biliary tract intervention or surgery. More than one half of patients are symptomatic when diagnosed. In several patients with ulcerative colitis, abnormal liver function tests found on routine testing lead to the diagnosis. The clinical course in sclerosing cholangitis is highly variable, but cyclic remissions and exacerbations are typical. However, some patients remain asymptomatic for years, while others

progress rapidly with the obliterative inflammatory changes leading to secondary biliary cirrhosis and liver failure. In patients with associated ulcerative colitis, the course of each disease seems independent of the other. Colectomy for the colitis makes no difference to the course of primary sclerosing cholangitis. The median survival for patients with primary sclerosing cholangitis from the time of diagnosis ranges from 10 to 12 years, and most die from hepatic failure.[65]

The clinical presentation and elevation of alkaline phosphatase and bilirubin may suggest the diagnosis, but ERC, revealing multiple dilatations and strictures (beading) of both the intra- and extrahepatic biliary tree, confirms it. The hepatic duct bifurcation is often the most severely affected segment. A liver biopsy may not be diagnostic, but is important to determine the degree of hepatic fibrosis and the presence of cirrhosis. Sclerosing cholangitis is followed by ERC and liver biopsies to provide appropriate management.

There is no known effective medical therapy for primary sclerosing cholangitis and no known curative treatment. Corticosteroids, immunosuppressants, ursodeoxycholic acid, and antibiotics have been disappointing. Biliary strictures can be dilated and stented either endoscopically or percutaneously. These measures have given short-term improvements in symptoms and serum bilirubin levels, and long-term improvements in only less than one half of the patients. Surgical management with resection of the extrahepatic biliary tree and hepaticojejunostomy has produced reasonable results in patients with extrahepatic and bifurcation strictures, but without cirrhosis or significant hepatic fibrosis.[66] In patients with sclerosing cholangitis and advanced liver disease, liver transplantation is the only option. It offers excellent results, with overall 5-year survival as high as 85%. Primary sclerosing cholangitis recurs in 10 to 20% of patients and may require retransplantation.[67,68]

Stenosis of the Sphincter of Oddi

A benign stenosis of the outlet of the common bile duct is usually associated with inflammation, fibrosis, or muscular hypertrophy. The pathogenesis is unclear, but trauma from the passage of stones, sphincter motility disorders, and congenital anomalies have been suggested. Episodic pain of the biliary type with abnormal liver function tests is a common presentation. However, recurrent jaundice or pancreatitis also may play a role. A dilated common bile duct that is difficult to cannulate with delayed emptying of the contrast are useful diagnostic features. Ampullary manometry and special provocation tests are available in specialized units. If the diagnosis is well established, endoscopic or operative sphincterotomy will yield good results.[69]

Bile Duct Strictures

Benign bile duct strictures can have numerous causes. However, the vast majority were caused by operative injury, most commonly by laparoscopic cholecystectomy (see the section on Injury to the Biliary Tract below). Other causes include fibrosis due to chronic pancreatitis, common bile duct stones, acute cholangitis, biliary obstruction due to cholecystolithiasis (Mirizzi's syndrome), sclerosing cholangitis, cholangiohepatitis, and strictures of a biliary-enteric anastomosis. Bile duct strictures that go unrecognized or are improperly managed may lead to recurrent cholangitis, secondary biliary cirrhosis, and portal hypertension.[70]

Patients with bile duct strictures most commonly present with episodes of cholangitis. Less commonly, they may present with jaundice without evidence of infection. Liver function tests usually show evidence of cholestasis. An ultrasound or a CT scan will show dilated bile ducts proximal to the stricture, as well as provide some information about the level of the stenosis. MRC will also provide good anatomic information about the location and the degree of dilatation. In patients with intrahepatic ductal dilatation, a percutaneous transhepatic cholangiogram will outline the proximal biliary tree, define the stricture and its location, and allow decompression of the biliary tree with transhepatic catheters or stents (Fig. 32-23). An endoscopic cholangiogram will outline the distal bile duct. Treatment

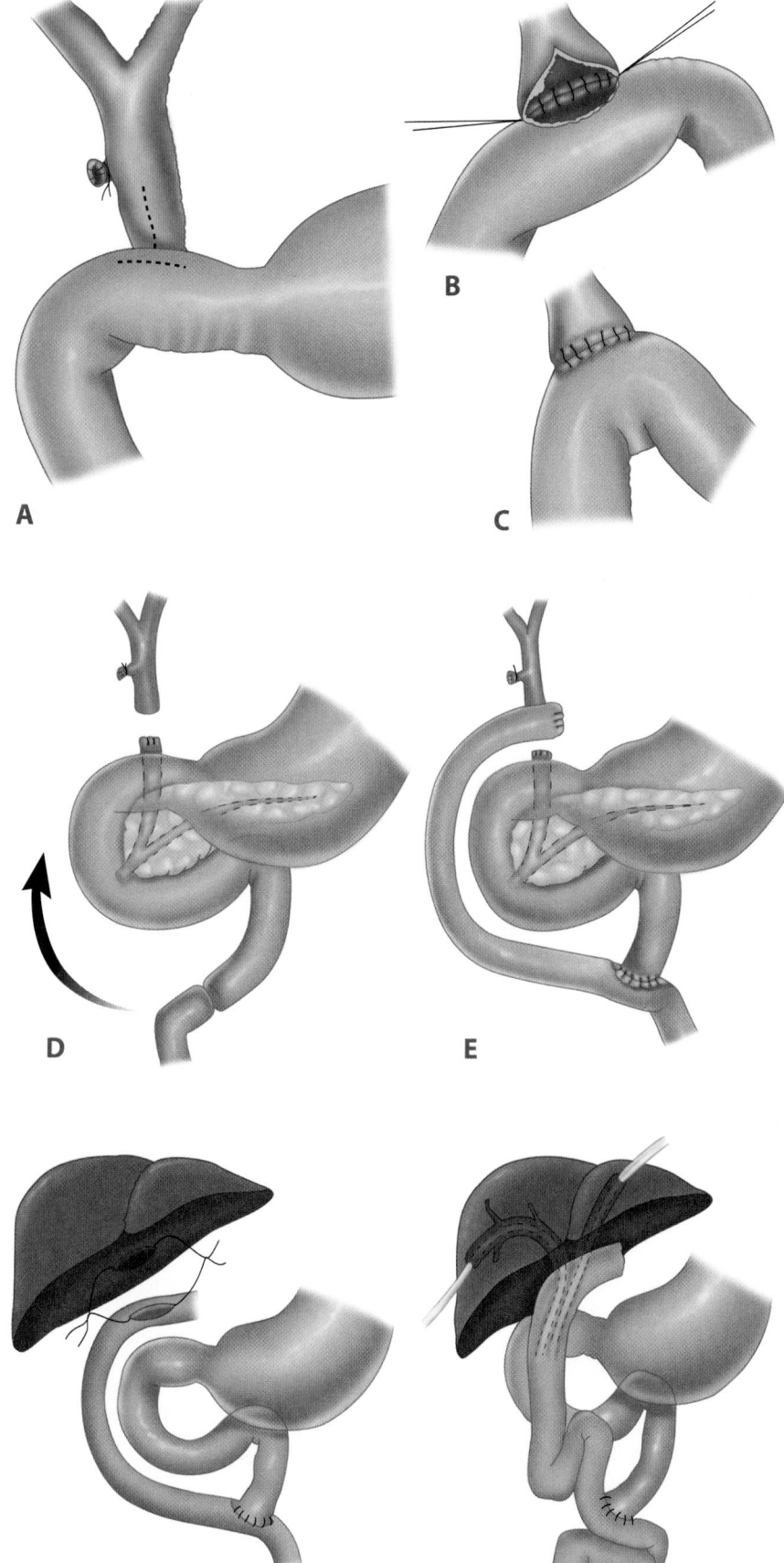

FIG. 32-21. Biliary enteric anastomoses. There are three types. I. Choledochoduodenostomy. **A.** The distal common bile duct is opened longitudinally, as is the duodenum. **B.** Interrupted sutures are placed between the common bile duct and the duodenum. **C.** Completed choledochoduodenostomy. II. Choledochojejunostomy. **D.** The common bile duct and small bowel are divided. **E.** A Roux-en-Y limb of jejunum is anastomosed to the choledochus. III. Hepaticojejunostomy. **F.** The entire extrahepatic biliary tree has been resected and the reconstruction done with a Roux-en-Y limb of jejunum. **G.** Percutaneous transhepatic stents are placed across hepaticojejunostomy.

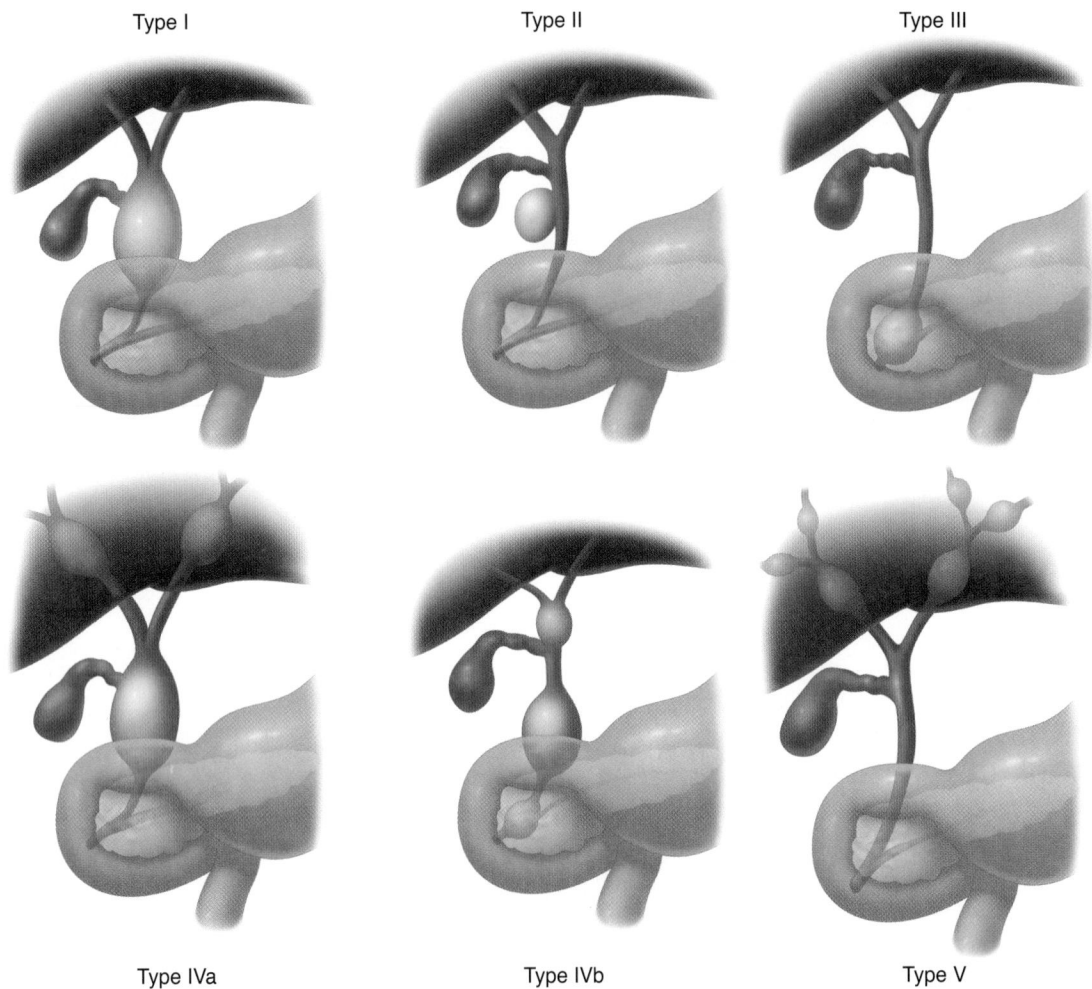

FIG. 32-22. Classification of choledochal cysts. Type I, fusiform or cystic dilations of the extrahepatic biliary tree, is the most common type, making up >50% of the choledochal cysts. Type II, saccular diverticulum of an extrahepatic bile duct. Rare, <5% of choledochal cysts. Type III, bile duct dilatation within the duodenal wall (choledochoceles), makes up about 5% of choledochal cysts. Type IVa and IVb, multiple cysts, make up 5–10% of choledochal cysts. Type IVa affects both extrahepatic and intrahepatic bile ducts while Type IVb cysts affect the extrahepatic bile ducts only. Type V, intrahepatic biliary cysts, is very rare and makes up 1% of choledochal cysts.

depends on the location and the cause of the stricture. Percutaneous or endoscopic dilatation and/or stent placement give good results in more than one half of patients. Surgery with Roux-en-Y choledochojejunostomy or hepaticojejunostomy is the standard of care with good or excellent results in 80 to 90% of patients.[71] Choledochoduodenostomy may be a choice for strictures in the distal-most part of the common bile duct.

INJURY TO THE BILIARY TRACT

Gallbladder

Injuries to the gallbladder are uncommon. Penetrating injuries are usually caused by gunshot wounds or stab wounds, and rarely by a needle biopsy procedure of the liver. Nonpenetrating trauma is extremely rare. These types of injury to the gallbladder include contusion, avulsion, laceration, rupture, and traumatic cholecystitis. The treatment of choice is cholecystectomy and the prognosis is directly related to the type and incidence of associated injury.

Extrahepatic Bile Ducts

Penetrating trauma to the extrahepatic bile ducts is rare and is usually associated with trauma to other viscera. The great majority

of injuries of the extrahepatic biliary duct system are iatrogenic, occurring in the course of laparoscopic or open cholecystectomies.[72] Less commonly, biliary injury is associated with common bile duct exploration, division or mobilization of the duodenum during gastrectomy, and dissection of the hepatic hilum during liver resections. The exact incidence of bile duct injury during cholecystectomy is unknown, but data suggest that during open cholecystectomy the incidence is relatively low (about 0.1 to 0.2%). However, the incidence during laparoscopic cholecystectomy, as derived from state and national databases, estimates the rate of major injury to range between 0.1% to 0.55%, and the incidence of minor injuries and bile leaks to be about 0.3%, a total of 0.85%. Limited view, difficult orientation and assessment of depth on a two-dimensional image, and the lack of tactile sensation and unusual manual skills that are needed have led to the rise in bile duct injury during laparoscopic cholecystectomy.[73]

A number of different factors are associated with bile duct injury during laparoscopic cholecystectomy. These include acute or chronic inflammation, obesity, anatomic variations, and bleeding. Surgical technique with inadequate exposure and failure to identify structures before ligating or dividing them are the most common cause of significant biliary injury. The bile ducts may be narrow and can be mistaken for the cystic duct. The cystic duct may run along side the common bile duct before joining it, leading the surgeon to the wrong

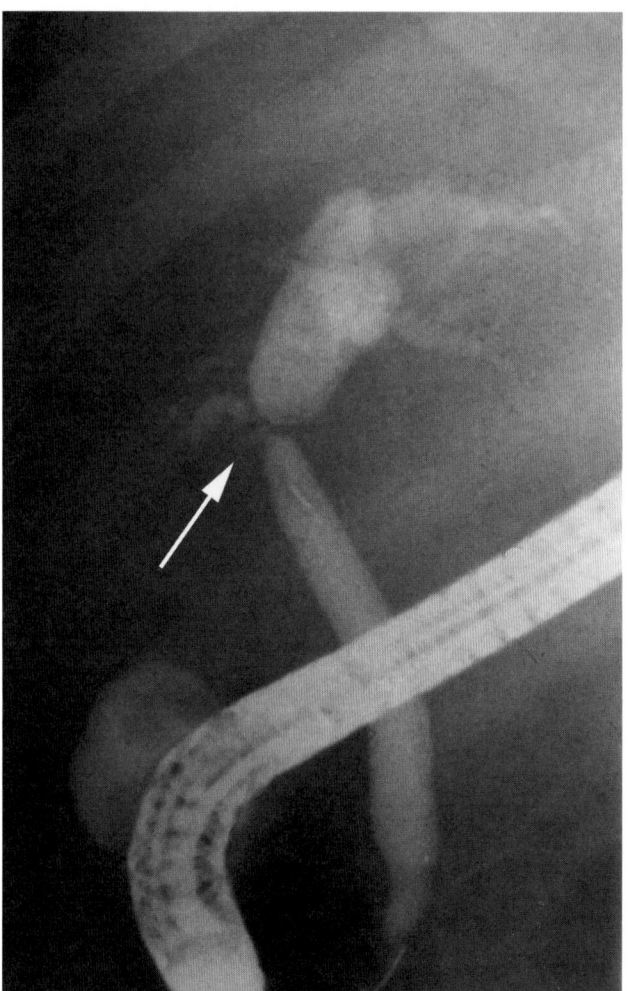

FIG. 32-23. An endoscopic retrograde cholangiography showing stricture of the common hepatic duct (*arrow*). The patient had recently had a laparoscopic cholecystectomy; clips from the operation can be seen projected over the common bile duct.

place. Additionally, the cystic duct may enter the right hepatic duct, and the right hepatic duct may run aberrantly, coursing through the triangle of Calot and entering the common hepatic duct. A number of intraoperative technical factors have been implicated in biliary injuries. Excessive cephalad retraction of the gallbladder may align the cystic duct with the common bile duct, and the latter is then mistaken for the cystic duct and clipped and divided. The use of an angled laparoscope instead of an end-viewing one will help visualize the anatomic structures, in particular those around the triangle of Calot. An angled scope also will aid in the proper placement of clips. Careless use of electrocautery may lead to thermal injury. Dissection deep into the liver parenchyma may cause injury to intrahepatic ducts, and poor clip placement close to the hilar area or to structures not well visualized can result in a clip across a bile duct.[74,75]

The routine use of intraoperative cholangiography to prevent bile duct injury is controversial.[76] It may limit the extent of injury but does not seem to prevent it. However, if a bile duct injury is suspected during cholecystectomy, a cholangiogram must be obtained to detect and identify the anatomic features. It is important to check that the whole biliary system fills with contrast and to be sure there are no leaks.

Diagnosis

Only about 25% of major bile duct injuries (common bile duct or hepatic duct) are recognized at the time of operation. Most com-

monly, intraoperative bile leakage, recognition of the correct anatomy, and an abnormal cholangiogram lead to the diagnosis of a bile duct injury. More than half of patients with biliary injury will present within the first postoperative month. The remainder will present months or years later, with recurrent cholangitis or cirrhosis from a remote bile duct injury. In the early postoperative period, patients present either with progressive elevation of liver function tests due to an occluded or a stenosed bile duct, or with a bile leak from an injured duct. Bile leak, most commonly from the cystic duct stump, a transected aberrant right hepatic duct, or a lateral injury to the main bile duct, usually presents with pain, fever, and a mild elevation of liver function tests. A CT scan or an ultrasound will show either a collection (biloma) in the gallbladder area or free fluid (bile) in the peritoneum (Fig. 32-24). Bilious drainage through operatively placed drains or through the wounds is abnormal. The site of the bile leak can be confirmed noninvasively with a HIDA scan. In patients with a surgical drain or a percutaneously placed catheter, injection of water-soluble contrast media through the drainage tract (sinogram) can often define the site of leakage and the anatomy of the biliary tree.[77]

CT scan and ultrasound also are important in the initial evaluation of the jaundiced patient, as they can demonstrate the dilated part of the biliary tree proximal to the stenosis or obstruction, and may identify the level of the extrahepatic bile duct obstruction. In the jaundiced patient with dilated intrahepatic ducts, a percutaneous cholangiogram will outline the anatomy and the proximal extent of the injury and allow decompression of the biliary tree with catheter or stent placements. An endoscopic cholangiogram demonstrates the anatomy distal to the injury and may allow the placement of stents across a stricture to relieve an obstruction (see Fig. 32-23). MRI cholangiography, if available, provides an excellent, noninvasive delineation of the biliary anatomy both proximal and distal to the injury.

Management

The management of bile duct injuries depends on the type, extent, and level of injury, and the time of its diagnosis. Initial proper treatment of bile duct injury diagnosed during the cholecystectomy can avoid the development of a bile duct stricture. If a major injury is discovered and an experienced biliary surgeon is not available, an external drain and, if necessary, transhepatic biliary catheters are placed, and the patient is transferred to a referral center.[73]

Transected bile ducts <3 mm or those draining a single hepatic segment can safely be ligated. If the injured duct is ≥4 mm, it is likely to drain multiple segments or an entire lobe, and thus needs to be reimplanted. Lateral injury to the common bile duct or the common hepatic duct, recognized at the time of surgery, is best managed with a T-tube placement. If the injury is a small incision in the duct, the T tube may be placed through it as if it were a formal choledochotomy. In more extensive lateral injuries, the T tube should be placed through a separate choledochotomy and the injury closed over the T-tube end to minimize the risk of subsequent stricture formation.

Major bile duct injuries such as transection of the common hepatic or common bile duct are best managed at the time of injury. In many of these major injuries, the bile duct has not only been transected, but a variable length of the duct removed. This injury usually requires a biliary enteric anastomosis with a jejunal loop. Either an end-to-side Roux-en-Y choledochojejunostomy, or more commonly a Roux-en-Y hepaticojejunostomy, should be performed. Transhepatic biliary catheters are placed through the anastomosis to stent it and to provide access to the biliary tract for drainage and imaging. Although rare, when the injury is to the distal common bile duct, a choledochoduodenostomy can be performed. If there is no or minimal loss of ductal length, a duct-to-duct repair may be done over a T tube that is placed through a separate incision. It is critical to perform a tension-free anastomosis to minimize the high risk of postoperative stricture formation.[66]

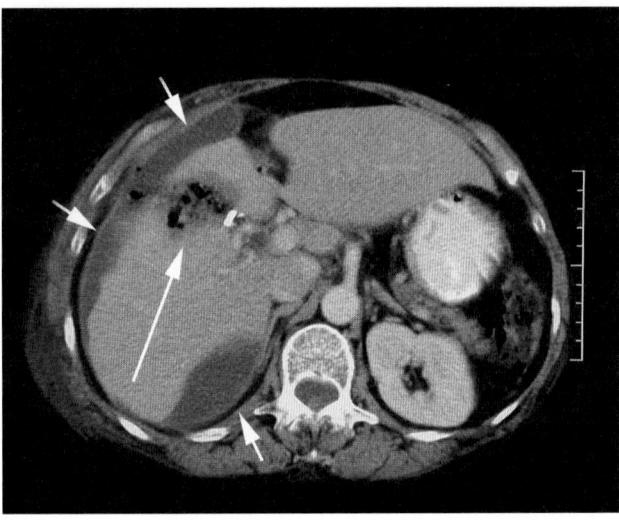

A

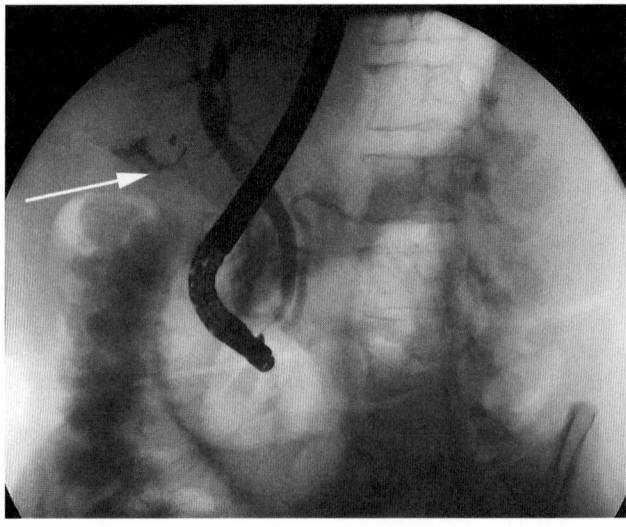

B

FIG. 32-24. A. Computed tomographic scan of a patient with bile leak after cholecystectomy. The *short arrows* indicate the intraperitoneal collections. Both air and bile are seen in the gallbladder bed (*long arrow*) as well as a surgical clip. **B.** An endoscopic retrograde cholangiography from the same patient showing a leak from the cystic duct stump (*arrow*). Note the filling of the pancreatic duct.

Cystic duct leaks can usually be managed with percutaneous drainage of intra-abdominal fluid collections followed by an endoscopic biliary stenting (see Fig. 32-24).

Major injuries diagnosed postoperatively require transhepatic biliary catheter placement for biliary decompression as well as percutaneous drainage of intra-abdominal bile collections, if any. When the acute inflammation has resolved 6 to 8 weeks later, operative repair is performed.

Patients with bile duct stricture from an injury or as a sequela of previous repair usually present with either progressive elevation of liver function tests or cholangitis. The initial management usually includes transhepatic biliary drainage catheter placement for decompression as well as for defining the anatomy and the location and the extent of the damage. These catheters will also serve as useful technical aids during subsequent biliary enteric anastomosis. An anastomosis is performed between the duct proximal to the injury and a Roux loop of jejunum. Balloon dilatation of a stricture usually requires multiple attempts and rarely provides adequate long-term relief. Self-expanding metal or plastic stents, placed either percutaneously or endoscopically across the stricture, can provide temporary drainage and, in the high-risk patient, permanent drainage of the biliary tree.

Outcome

Good results can be expected in 70 to 90% of patients with bile duct injuries.[78] The best results are obtained when the injury is recognized during the cholecystectomy and repaired by an experienced biliary tract surgeon. The operative mortality rate varies from 0 to almost 30% in various series, but commonly is about 5 to 8%. Common complications that are specific for bile duct repairs include cholangitis, external biliary fistula, bile leak, subhepatic and subphrenic abscesses, and hemobilia. Restenosis of a biliary enteric anastomosis occurs in about 10% of patients, and may manifest up to 20 years after the initial procedure. Approximately two thirds of recurrent strictures become symptomatic within 2 years after repair. The more proximal strictures are associated with a lower success rate than are distal ones. The worst results are in patients with many operative revisions and in those who have evidence of liver failure and portal hypertension. However, previous repair does not preclude successful outcome of repeated attempts, particularly in patients with good liver function. Patients with deteriorating liver function are candidates for liver transplants.

TUMORS

Carcinoma of the Gallbladder

Cancer of the gallbladder is a rare malignancy that occurs predominantly in the elderly. It is an aggressive tumor, with poor prognosis except when incidentally diagnosed at an early stage after cholecystectomy for cholelithiasis. The overall reported 5-year survival rate is about 5%.[79]

Incidence

Gallbladder cancer is the fifth most common GI malignancy in Western countries. However, it accounts for only 2 to 4% of all malignant GI tumors, with about 5000 new cases diagnosed annually in the United States. It is two to three times more common in females than males, and the peak incidence is in the seventh decade of life. Its occurrence in random autopsy series is about 0.4%, but approximately 1% of patients undergoing cholecystectomy for gallstone disease are found incidentally to have gallbladder cancer. The incidence of gallbladder cancer is particularly high in native populations of the United States, Mexico, and Chile. The annual incidence in Native American females with gallstones approaches 75 per 100,000, compared with the overall incidence of gallbladder cancer of 2.5 cases per 100,000 residents in the United States.[80]

Etiology

Cholithiasis is the most important risk factor for gallbladder carcinoma, and up to 95% of patients with carcinoma of the gallbladder have gallstones.[81] However, the 20-year risk of developing cancer for patients with gallstones is <0.5% for the overall population and 1.5% for high-risk groups. The pathogenesis has not been defined but is probably related to chronic inflammation. Larger stones (>3 cm) are associated with a 10-fold increased risk of cancer.[82] The risk of developing cancer of the gallbladder is higher in patients with symptomatic than asymptomatic gallstones.

Polypoid lesions of the gallbladder are associated with increased risk of cancer, particularly in polyps >10 mm.[83] The calcified "porcelain" gallbladder is associated with >20% incidence of gallbladder carcinoma. These gallbladders should be removed, even if the patients are asymptomatic. Patients with choledochal cysts have an increased risk of developing cancer anywhere in the biliary tree, but the incidence is highest in the gallbladder. Sclerosing cholangitis, anomalous pancreaticobiliary duct junction, and exposure to carcinogens (azotoluene, nitrosamines) also are associated with cancer of the gallbladder.

Pathology

Between 80 and 90% of the gallbladder tumors are adenocarcinomas. Squamous cell, adenosquamous, oat cell, and other anaplastic lesions occur rarely. The histologic subtypes of gallbladder adenocarcinomas include papillary, nodular, and tubular. Less than 10% are of the papillary type, but these are associated with an overall better outcome, as they are most commonly diagnosed while localized to the gallbladder. Cancer of the gallbladder spreads through the lymphatics, with venous drainage, and with direct invasion into the liver parenchyma. Lymphatic flow from the gallbladder drains first to the cystic duct node (Calot's), then the pericholedochal and hilar nodes, and finally the peripancreatic, duodenal, periportal, celiac, and superior mesenteric artery nodes. The gallbladder veins drain directly into the adjacent liver, usually segments IV and V, where tumor invasion is common (Fig. 32-25). The gallbladder wall differs histologically from the intestines in that it lacks a muscularis mucosa and submucosa. Lymphatics are present in the subserosal layer only. Therefore, cancers invading but not growing through the muscular layer have minimal risk of nodal disease. When diagnosed, about 25% of gallbladder cancers are localized to the gallbladder wall, 35% have regional nodal involvement and/or extension into adjacent liver, and approximately 40% have distant metastasis.[84]

Clinical Manifestations and Diagnosis

Signs and symptoms of carcinoma of the gallbladder are generally indistinguishable from those associated with cholecystitis and cholelithiasis. These include abdominal discomfort, right upper quadrant pain, nausea, and vomiting. Jaundice, weight loss, anorexia, ascites, and abdominal mass are less common presenting symptoms. More than one half of gallbladder cancers are not diagnosed before surgery. Common misdiagnoses include chronic cholecystitis, acute cholecystitis, choledocholithiasis, hydrops of the

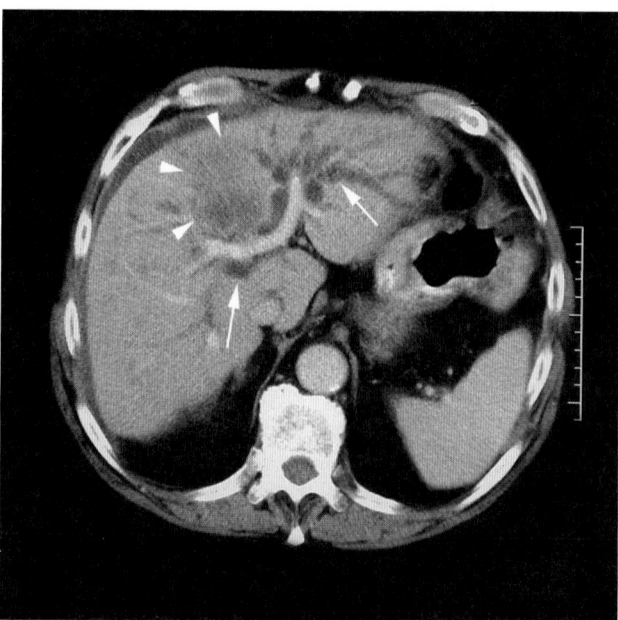

FIG. 32-25. Computed tomography scan of a patient with gallbladder cancer. The image shown is at the level of the liver hilum. The portal vein is bifurcating into the left and right portal branch. The tumor has invaded segment IV of the liver (*arrowheads*) and obstructed the common hepatic duct, resulting in intrahepatic ductal dilatation (*arrows*).

gallbladder, and pancreatic cancer. Laboratory findings are not diagnostic but, if abnormal, are most often consistent with biliary obstruction. Ultrasonography often reveals a thickened, irregular gallbladder wall or a mass replacing the gallbladder. Ultrasonography may visualize tumor invasion of the liver, lymphadenopathy, and a dilated biliary tree. The sensitivity of ultrasonography in detecting gallbladder cancer ranges from 70 to 100%. A CT scan is an important tool for staging and may identify a gallbladder mass or local invasion into adjacent organs. In addition, a spiral CT scan can demonstrate vascular invasion; however, CT scan is a poor method for identifying nodal spread. In jaundiced patients, a percutaneous transhepatic or endoscopic cholangiogram may be helpful to delineate the extent of biliary tree involvement, and typically shows a long stricture of the common bile duct. With newer MRI techniques, MRCP has evolved into a single noninvasive imaging method that allows complete assessment of biliary, vascular, nodal, hepatic, and adjacent organ involvement.[85] If diagnostic studies suggest that the tumor is unresectable, a CT scan or ultrasound-guided biopsy of the tumor can be obtained to provide a pathologic diagnosis.

Treatment

Surgery remains the only curative option for gallbladder cancer as well as for cholangiocarcinoma. However, palliative procedures for patients with unresectable cancer and jaundice or duodenal obstruction remain the most frequently performed surgery for gallbladder cancers. Today, patients with obstructive jaundice can frequently be managed with either endoscopic or percutaneously placed biliary stents. There are no proven effective options for adjuvant radiation or chemotherapy for patients with gallbladder cancer.

The pathologic stage of gallbladder cancer determines the operative treatment for patients with localized gallbladder cancer. Patients without evidence of distant metastasis warrant exploration for tissue diagnosis, pathologic staging, and possible curative resection.

Tumors limited to the muscular layer of the gallbladder (T1) are usually identified incidentally, after cholecystectomy for gallstone disease. There is near universal agreement that simple cholecystectomy is an adequate treatment for T1 lesions and results in a near 100% overall 5-year survival rate. When the tumor invades the perimuscular connective tissue without extension beyond the serosa or into the liver (T2 tumors), an extended cholecystectomy should be performed.[86] That includes resection of liver segments IVB and V, and lymphadenectomy of the cystic duct, and pericholedochal, portal, right celiac, and posterior pancreatoduodenal lymph nodes. One half of patients with T2 tumors are found to have nodal disease on pathologic examination. Therefore, regional lymphadenectomy is an important part of surgery for T2 cancers.[87] For tumors that grow beyond the serosa or invade the liver or other organs (T3 and T4 tumors), there is a high likelihood of intraperitoneal and distant spread. If no peritoneal or nodal involvement is found, complete tumor excision with an extended right hepatectomy (segments IV, V, VI, VII, and VIII) must be performed for adequate tumor clearance. An aggressive approach in patients who will tolerate surgery has resulted in an increased survival for T3 and T4 lesions.

Prognosis

Most patients with gallbladder cancer have unresectable disease at the time of diagnosis. The 5-year survival rate of all patients with gallbladder cancer is <5%, with a median survival of 6 months.[88] Patients with T1 disease treated with cholecystectomy have an excellent prognosis (85 to 100% 5-year survival rate). The 5-year survival rate for T2 lesions treated with an extended cholecystectomy and lymphadenectomy compared with simple cholecystectomy is >70% vs. 25 to 40%, respectively. Patients with advanced but resectable gallbladder cancer are reported to have 5-year survival rates of 20 to 50%. However, the median survival for patients with distant metastasis at the time of presentation is only 1 to 3 months.

Recurrence after resection of gallbladder cancer occurs most commonly in the liver or the celiac or retropancreatic nodes. The prognosis for recurrent disease is very poor. Death occurs most commonly secondary to biliary sepsis or liver failure. The main goal of follow-up is to provide palliative care. The most common problems are pruritus and cholangitis associated with obstructive jaundice, bowel obstruction secondary to carcinomatosis, and pain.

Bile Duct Carcinoma

Cholangiocarcinoma is a rare tumor arising from the biliary epithelium and may occur anywhere along the biliary tree. About two thirds are located at the hepatic duct bifurcation. Surgical resection offers the only chance for cure; however, many patients have advanced disease at the time of diagnosis. Therefore, palliative procedures aimed to provide biliary drainage to prevent liver failure and cholangitis are often the only therapeutic possibilities. Most patients with unresectable disease die within 1 year of diagnosis.[89]

Incidence

The autopsy incidence of bile duct carcinoma is about 0.3%. The overall incidence of cholangiocarcinoma in the United States is about 1.0 per 100,000 people per year, with about 3000 new cases diagnosed annually. The male to female ratio is 1.3:1, and the average age of presentation is between 50 and 70 years.

Etiology

Risk factors associated with cholangiocarcinoma include primary sclerosing cholangitis, choledochal cysts, ulcerative colitis, hepatolithiasis, biliary-enteric anastomosis, and biliary tract infections with *Clonorchis* or in chronic typhoid carriers. Features common to most risk factors include biliary stasis, bile duct stones, and infection. Other risk factors associated with cholangiocarcinoma are liver flukes, dietary nitrosamines, Thorotrast, and exposure to dioxin.[90,91]

Pathology

Over 95% of bile duct cancers are adenocarcinomas. Morphologically, they are divided into nodular (the most common type), scirrhous, diffusely infiltrating, or papillary. Anatomically, they are divided into distal, proximal, or perihilar tumors. Intrahepatic cholangiocarcinomas occur, but they are treated like hepatocellular

carcinoma, with hepatectomy when possible. About two thirds of cholangiocarcinomas are located in the perihilar location. Perihilar cholangiocarcinomas, also referred to as Klatskin tumors, are further classified based on anatomic location by the Bismuth-Corlette classification (Fig. 32-26). Type I tumors are confined to the common hepatic duct, but type II tumors involve the bifurcation without involvement of the secondary intrahepatic ducts. Type IIIa and IIIb tumors extend into the right and left secondary intrahepatic ducts, respectively. Type IV tumors involve both the right and left secondary intrahepatic ducts.

Clinical Manifestations and Diagnosis

Painless jaundice is the most common presentation. Pruritus, mild right upper quadrant pain, anorexia, fatigue, and weight loss also may be present. Cholangitis is the presenting symptom in about 10% of patients, but occurs more commonly after biliary manipulation in these patients. Except for jaundice, physical examination is usually normal in patients with cholangiocarcinoma. Occasionally, asymptomatic patients are found to have cholangiocarcinoma while being evaluated for elevated alkaline phosphatase and γ-glutamyltransferase levels. Tumor markers such CA 125 and carcinoembryonic antigen can be elevated in cholangiocarcinoma but tend to be nonspecific because they also increase in other GI and gynecologic malignancies or cholangiopathologies. The tumor marker most commonly used to aid the diagnosis of cholangiocarcinoma is CA 19-9, which has a sensitivity of 79% and specificity of 98% if the serum value is >129 U/mL.[92] However, mild elevations in CA 19-9 can be seen in cholangitis, other GI and gynecologic neoplasms, and in patients who lack the Lewis blood type antigen.[93]

The initial tests are usually ultrasound or CT scan. A perihilar tumor causes dilatation of the intrahepatic biliary tree, but normal or collapsed gallbladder and extrahepatic bile ducts distal to the tumor. Distal bile duct cancer leads to dilatation of the extra- and the intrahepatic bile ducts as well as the gallbladder. Ultrasound can establish the level of obstruction and rule out the presence of bile duct stones as the cause of the obstructive jaundice (Fig. 32-27). It is usually difficult to visualize the tumor itself on ultrasound or on a standard CT scan. Either ultrasound or spiral CT can be used to determine portal vein patency. The biliary anatomy is defined by

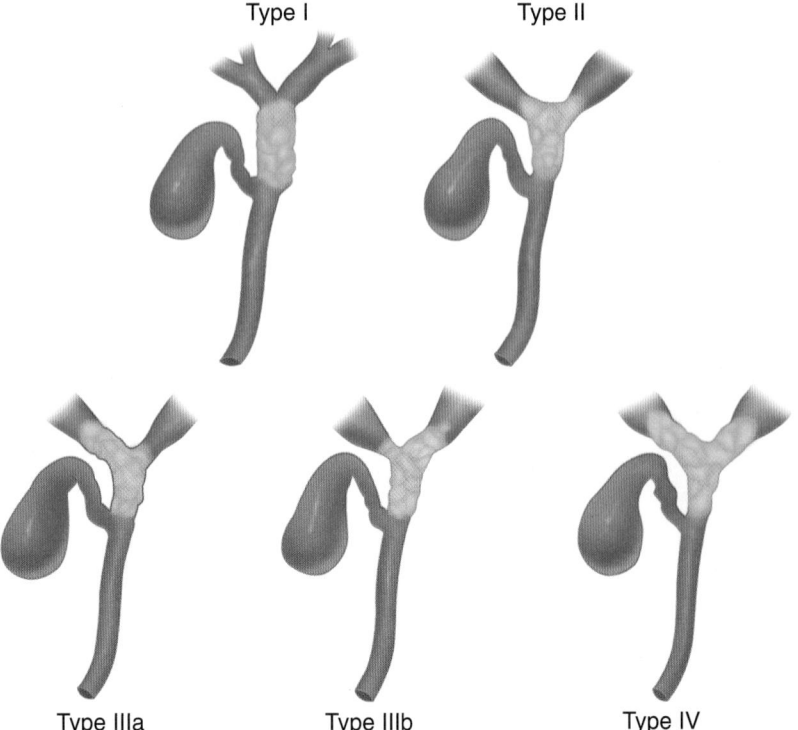

Type I

Type II

Type IIIa

Type IIIb

Type IV

FIG. 32-26. Bismuth-Corlette classification of bile duct tumors.

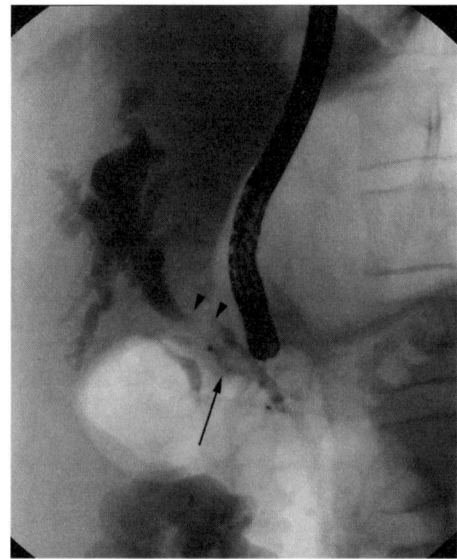 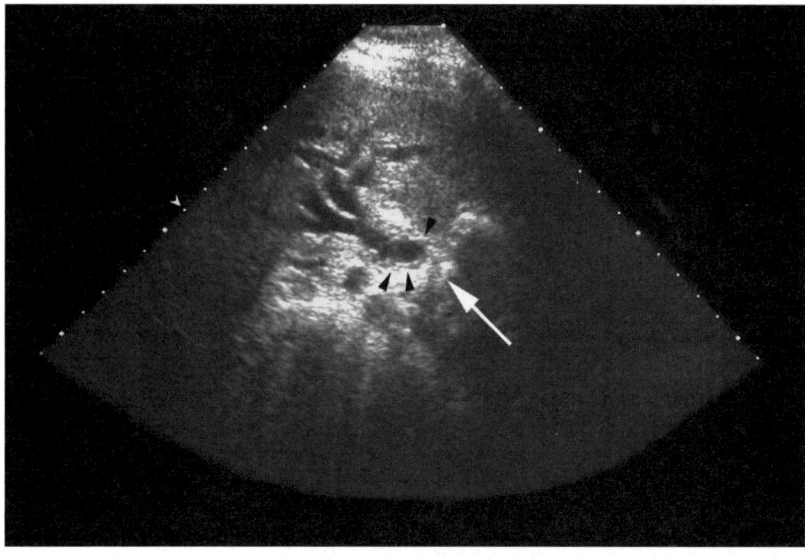

A **B**

FIG. 32-27. A. An endoscopic retrograde cholangiography from a patient with cancer of the common hepatic duct (*arrowheads*). The common bile duct is of normal size as is the cystic duct (*arrow*), but the proximal biliary tree is dilated. The gallbladder is not visualized because of tumor obstructing its neck. **B.** An ultrasound from the same patient showing dilated ducts and tumor obstructing the common hepatic duct (*arrow*). The walls of the bile ducts adjacent to the obstruction are thickened by tumor infiltration (*arrowheads*).

cholangiography. PTC defines the proximal extent of the tumor, which is the most important factor in determining resectability. ERC is used, particularly in the evaluation of distal bile duct tumors. For the evaluation of vascular involvement, celiac angiography may be necessary. With the newer types of MRI, a single noninvasive test has the potential of evaluating the biliary anatomy, lymph nodes, and vascular involvement, as well as the tumor growth itself.[94]

Tissue diagnosis may be difficult to obtain nonoperatively except in advanced cases. Percutaneous fine-needle aspiration biopsy, biliary brush or scrape biopsy, and cytologic examination have a low sensitivity in detecting malignancy. Patients with potentially resectable disease should, therefore, be offered surgical exploration based on radiographic findings and clinical suspicion.[95]

Treatment

Surgical excision is the only potentially curative treatment for cholangiocarcinoma. In the past one to two decades, improvements in surgical techniques have resulted in lower mortality and better outcome for patients undergoing aggressive surgical excision for cholangiocarcinoma.[96]

Patients should undergo surgical exploration if they have no signs of metastasis or locally unresectable disease. However, despite improvements in ultrasonography, CT scanning, and MRI, more than one half of patients who are explored are found to have peritoneal implants, nodal or hepatic metastasis, or locally advanced disease that precludes resection. For these patients, surgical bypass for biliary decompression and cholecystectomy to prevent the occurrence of acute cholecystitis should be performed.[97]

For unresectable perihilar cholangiocarcinoma, Roux-en-Y cholangiojejunostomy to either segment II or III bile ducts or to the right hepatic duct can be performed.

For curative resection, the location and local extension of the tumor dictates the extent of the resection. Perihilar tumors involving the bifurcation or proximal common hepatic duct (Bismuth-Corlette type I or II) with no signs of vascular involvement are candidates for local tumor excision with portal lymphadenectomy, cholecystectomy, common bile duct excision, and bilateral Roux-en-Y hepaticojejunostomies. If the tumor involves the right or left

hepatic duct (Bismuth-Corlette type IIIa or IIIb), right or left hepatic lobectomy, respectively, should also be performed. Frequently, resection of the adjacent caudate lobe is required because of direct extension into caudate biliary radicals or parenchyma.[95]

Distal bile duct tumors are more often resectable. They are treated with pylorus-preserving pancreatoduodenectomy (Whipple procedure). For patients with distal bile duct cancer found to be unresectable on surgical exploration, Roux-en-Y hepaticojejunostomy, cholecystectomy, and gastrojejunostomy to prevent gastric outlet obstruction should be performed.

Nonoperative biliary decompression is performed for patients with unresectable disease on diagnostic evaluation. Percutaneous placement of expandable metal stents or drainage catheters is usually the appropriate approach for proximal tumors. However, for distal bile duct tumors, endoscopic placement is often the preferred approach (Fig. 32-28). There is a significant risk of cholangitis with internal and external drainage, and stent occlusion is not uncommon. However, although surgical bypass offers improved patency and fewer episodes of cholangitis, an operative intervention is not warranted in patients with metastatic disease.[98]

There is no proven role for adjuvant chemotherapy in the treatment of cholangiocarcinoma. Adjuvant radiation therapy has also not been shown to increase either quality of life or survival in resected patients. Patients with unresectable disease often are offered treatment with 5-fluorouracil alone or in combination with mitomycin C and doxorubicin, but the response rates are low, <10% and <30%, respectively. The combination of radiation and chemotherapy may be more effective than either treatment alone for unresectable disease, but no data from randomized trials are available. Giving chemoradiation to these patients can be difficult because of the high incidence of cholangitis. External beam radiation has not been shown to be an effective treatment for unresected disease. The use of interstitial (intraoperative) radiation, brachytherapy with iridium 192 via percutaneous or endoscopic stents, and combined interstitial and external beam radiation for unresectable cholangiocarcinoma has been reported with some encouraging results. However, no randomized, prospective trials have been reported.[95] A palliative measure that has been shown effective in a

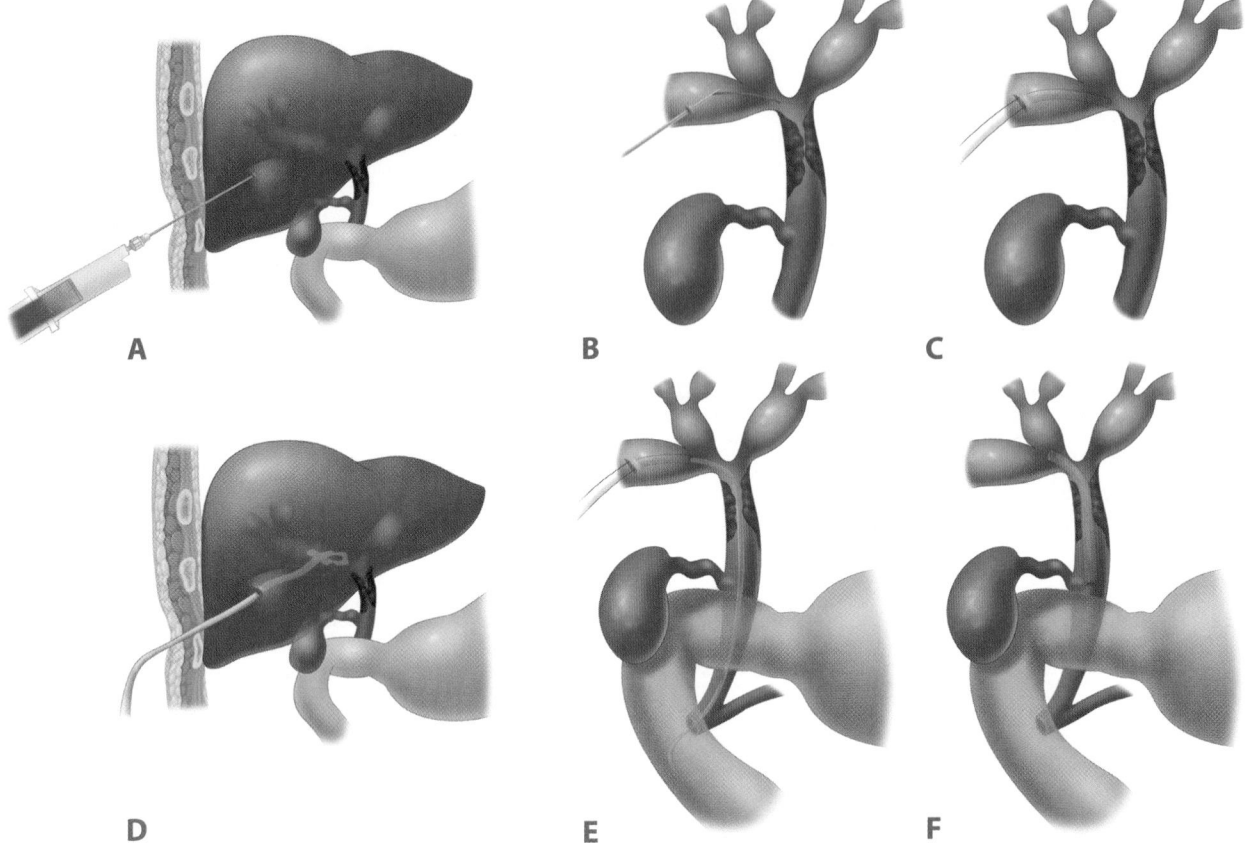

FIG. 32-28. A through **F**. Percutaneous transhepatic cholangiography and placement of a biliary drainage catheter. The catheter has been passed through the tumor area (distal cholangiocarcinoma) that is obstructing the distal common bile duct and into the duodenum.

multicenter randomized trial is photodynamic therapy. In this trial, patients with a diagnosis of unresectable cholangiocarcinoma were randomized to biliary stenting with photodynamic therapy or stenting alone. The authors found that photodynamic therapy prolonged survival by approximately 400 days and improved quality of life on standardized questionnaire.[99]

Prognosis

Most patients with perihilar cholangiocarcinoma present with advanced, unresectable disease. Patients with unresectable disease have a median survival between 5 and 8 months. The most common causes of death are hepatic failure and cholangitis. The overall 5-year survival rate for patients with resectable perihilar cholangiocarcinoma is between 10 and 30%, but for patients with negative margins, it may be as high as 40%. The operative mortality for perihilar cholangiocarcinoma is 6 to 8%. Patients with distal cholangiocarcinoma are more likely to have resectable disease and improved prognosis compared to perihilar cholangiocarcinoma. The overall 5-year survival rate for resectable disease is 30 to 50%, and the median survival is 32 to 38 months.

The greatest risk factors for recurrence after resection are the presence of positive margins and lymph node–positive tumors. Therapy for recurrent disease is palliation of symptoms. Surgery is not recommended for patients with recurrent disease.[94]

REFERENCES

Entries highlighted in bright blue are key references.

1. Clemente CD: *Gray's Anatomy*. Philadelphia: Lea & Febiger, 1985, p 132.
2. Klein AS, Lillemoe KD, Yeo CJ, et al: Liver, biliary tract, and pancreas, in O'Leary JP (ed): *Physiologic Basis of Surgery*. Baltimore: Williams & Wilkins, 1996, p 441.
3. Scott-Conner CEH, Dawson DL: *Operative Anatomy*. Philadelphia: JB Lippincott, 1993, p 388.
4. Molmenti EP, Pinto PA, Klein J, et al: Normal and variant arterial supply of the liver and gallbladder. *Pediatr Transplant* 7:80, 2003.
5. Chen TH, Shyu JF, Chen CH, et al: Variations of the cystic artery in Chinese adults. *Surg Laparosc Endosc Percutan Tech* 10:154, 2000.
6. Boyer J: Bile secretion—models, mechanisms, and malfunctions. A perspective on the development of modern cellular and molecular concepts of bile secretion and cholestasis. *J Gastroenterol* 31:475, 1996.
7. Geoghegan J, Pappas TN: Clinical uses of gut peptides. *Ann Surg* 225:145, 1997.
8. Al-Jiffry BO, Shaffer EA, Saccone GT, et al: Changes in gallbladder motility and gallstone formation following laparoscopic gastric banding for morbid obesity. *Can J Gastroenterol* 17:169, 2003.
9. McDonnell CO, Bailey I, Stumpf T, et al: The effect of cholecystectomy on plasma cholecystokinin. *Am J Gastroenterol* 97:2189, 2002.
10. Woods CM, Mawe GM, Saccone GTP: The sphincter of Oddi: Understanding its control and function. *Neurogastroenterol Motil* 17(Supp 1):31, 2005.
11. Yokohata K, Tanaka M: Cyclic motility of the sphincter of Oddi. *J Hepato-Biliary-Pancreatic Surg* 7:178, 2000.
12. Ahrendt SA: Biliary tract surgery. *Curr Gastroenterol Rep* 1:107, 1999.
13. Lee HJ, Choi BI, Han JK, et al: Three-dimensional ultrasonography using the minimum transparent mode in obstructive biliary diseases: Early experience. *J Ultrasound Med* 21:443, 2002.
14. Ralls PW, Jeffrey RB Jr., Kane RA, et al: Ultrasonography. *Gastroenterol Clin North Am* 31:801, 2002.
15. Wexler RS, Greene GS, Scott M: Left hepatic and common hepatic ductal bile leaks demonstrated by Tc-99m HIDA scan and percutaneous transhepatic cholangiogram. *Clin Nucl Med* 19:59, 1994.
16. Breen DJ, Nicholson AA: The clinical utility of spiral CT cholangiography. *Clin Radiol* 55:733, 2000.

17. Liu TH, Consorti ET, Kawashima A, et al: Patient evaluation and management with selective use of magnetic resonance cholangiography and endoscopic retrograde cholangiopancreatography before laparoscopic cholecystectomy. *Ann Surg* 234:33, 2001.

18. Magnuson TH, Bender JS, Duncan MD, et al: Utility of magnetic resonance cholangiography in the evaluation of biliary obstruction. *J Am Coll Surg* 189:63, 1999.

19. Washington M, Ghazi A: Complications of ERCP, in Scott-Conner CEH (ed): *The SAGES Manual*. New York: Springer-Verlag, 1999, p 516.

20. Tischendorf JJ, Kruger M, Trautwein C, et al: Cholangioscopic characterization of dominant bile duct stenoses in patients with primary sclerosing cholangitis. *Endoscopy* 38:665, 2006.

21. Tajiri H, Kobayashi M, Ohtsu A, et al: Peroral pancreatoscopy for the diagnosis of pancreatic diseases. *Pancreas* 16: 408, 1998.

22. Hui CK, Lai KC, Ng M, et al: Retained common bile duct stones: A comparison between biliary stenting and complete clearance of stones by electrohydraulic lithotripsy. *Aliment Pharmacol Ther* 17:289, 2003.

23. Tsuyuguchi T, Saisho H, Ishihara T, et al: Long-term follow-up after treatment of Mirizzi syndrome by peroral cholangioscopy. *Gastrointest Endosc* 52: 639, 2000.

24. Brett M, Barker DJ: The world distribution of gallstones. *Int J Epidemiol* 5:335, 1976.

25. Nakeeb A, Comuzzie AG, Martin L, et al: Gallstones: Genetics versus environment. *Ann Surg* 235:842, 2002.

26. Brasca A, Berli D, Pezzotto SM, et al: Morphological and demographic associations of biliary symptoms in subjects with gallstones: Findings from a population-based survey in Rosario, Argentina. *Dig Liver Dis* 34:577, 2002.

27. Attili AF, De Santis A, Capri R, et al: The natural history of gallstones: The GREPCO experience. The GREPCO Group. *Hepatology* 21:655, 1995.

28. Bellows CF, Berger DH, Crass RA: Management of gallstones. *Am Fam Physician* 72:637, 2005.

29. Strasberg SM: The pathogenesis of cholesterol gallstones a review. *J Gastrointest Surg* 2:109, 1998.

30. Stewart L, Oesterle AL, Erdan I, et al: Pathogenesis of pigment gallstones in Western societies: The central role of bacteria. *J Gastrointest Surg* 6:891, 2002.

31. Trowbridge RL, Rutkowski NK, Shojania KG: Does this patient have acute cholecystitis? *JAMA* 289:80, 2003.

32. Fletcher DR: Gallstones. Modern management. *Aust Fam Physician* 30:441, 2001.

33. Della Corte C, Falchetti D, Nebbia G, et al: Management of cholelithiasis in Italian children: A national multicenter study. *World J Gastroenterol* 14:1383, 2008.

34. Weber DM: Laparoscopic surgery: An excellent approach in elderly patients. *Arch Surg* 138:1083, 2003.

35. Strasberg SM: Cholelithiasis and acute cholecystitis. *Baillieres Clin Gastroenterol* 11:643, 1997.

36. Kiviluoto T, Siren J, Luukkonen P, et al: Randomised trial of laparoscopic versus open cholecystectomy for acute and gangrenous cholecystitis. *Lancet* 351:321, 1998.

37. Lo CM, Liu CL, Fan ST, et al: Prospective randomized study of early versus delayed laparoscopic cholecystectomy for acute cholecystitis. *Ann Surg* 227:461, 1998.

38. Chikamori F, Kuniyoshi N, Shibuya S, et al: Early scheduled laparoscopic cholecystectomy following percutaneous transhepatic gallbladder drainage for patients with acute cholecystitis. *Surg Endosc* 16:1704, 2002.

39. Patel M, Miedema BW, James MA, et al: Percutaneous cholecystostomy is an effective treatment for high-risk patients with acute cholecystitis. *Am Surg* 66:33, 2000.

40. Ko C, Lee S: Epidemiology and natural history of common bile duct stones and prediction of disease. *Gastrointest Endosc* 56:S165, 2002.

41. Amouyal P, Amouyal G, Levy P, et al: Diagnosis of choledocholithiasis by endoscopic ultrasonography. *Gastroenterology* 106:1062, 1994.

42. Tranter S, Thompson M: Comparison of endoscopic sphincterotomy and laparoscopic exploration of the common bile duct. *Br J Surg* 89:1495, 2002.

43. Hamy A, Hennekinne S, Pessaux P, et al: Endoscopic sphincterotomy prior to laparoscopic cholecystectomy for the treatment of cholelithiasis. *Surg Endosc* 17:872, 2003.

44. Lilly MC, Arregui ME: A balanced approach to choledocholithiasis. *Surg Endosc* 15:467, 2001.

45. Ross SO, Forsmark CE: Pancreatic and biliary disorders in the elderly. *Gastroenterol Clin North Am* 30:531, 2000.

46. Lai ECS, Mok FPT, Tan ESY, et al: Endoscopic biliary drainage for severe acute cholangitis. *N Engl J Med* 326:1582, 1992.

47. Lipsett PA, Pitt HA: Acute cholangitis. *Front Biosci* 8:S1229, 2003.

48. Lillemoe KD: Surgical treatment of biliary tract infections. *Am Surg* 66:138, 2000.

49. Rhodes M, Sussman L, Cohen L, et al: Randomised trial of laparoscopic exploration of common bile duct versus postoperative endoscopic retrograde cholangiography for common bile duct stones. *Lancet* 351:159, 1998.

50. Sperling RM, Koch J, Sandhu JS, et al: Recurrent pyogenic cholangitis in Asian immigrants to the United States: Natural history and role of therapeutic ERCP. *Dig Dis Sci* 42:865, 1997.

51. Thinh NC, Breda Y, Faucompret S, et al: Oriental biliary lithiasis. Retrospective study of 690 patients treated surgically over 8 years at Hospital 108 in Hanoi (Vietnam). *Med Trop (Mars)* 61:509, 2001.

52. Byrne MF, Suhocki P, Mitchell RM, et al: Percutaneous cholecystostomy in patients with acute cholecystitis: Experience of 45 patients at a US referral center. *J Am Coll Surg* 197:206, 2003.

53. Akhan O, Akinci D, Ozmen MN: Percutaneous cholecystostomy. *Eur J Radiol* 43:229, 2002.

54. Khaitan L, Apelgren K, Hunter J, et al: A report on the Society of American Gastrointestinal Endoscopic Surgeons (SAGES) Outcomes Initiative: What have we learned and what is its potential? *Surg Endosc* 17:365, 2003.

55. Richards C, Edwards J, Culver D, et al: Does using a laparoscopic approach to cholecystectomy decrease the risk of surgical site infection? *Ann Surg* 237:358, 2003.

56. Flum DR, Dellinger EP, Cheadle A, et al: Intraoperative cholangiography and risk of common bile duct injury during cholecystectomy. *JAMA* 289:1639, 2003.

57. Hunter JG: Acute cholecystitis revisited: Get it while it's hot. *Ann Surg* 227:468, 1998.

58. Biffl W, Moore E, Offner P, et al: Routine intraoperative ultrasonography with selective cholangiography reduces bile duct complications during laparoscopic cholecystectomy. *J Am Coll Surg* 193:272, 2001.

59. Halpin VJ, Dunnegan D, Soper NJ: Laparoscopic intracorporeal ultrasound versus fluoroscopic intraoperative cholangiography: After the learning curve. *Surg Endosc* 16:336, 2002.

60. Barwood NT, Valinsky LJ, Hobbs MS, et al: Changing methods of imaging the common bile duct in the laparoscopic cholecystectomy era in Western Australia: Implications for surgical practice. *Ann Surg* 235:41, 2002.

61. Pelinka LE, Schmidhammer R, Hamid L, et al: Acute acalculous cholecystitis after trauma: A prospective study. *J Trauma-Injury Infect Crit Care* 55:323, 2003.

62. Ryu JK, Ryu KH, Kim KH: Clinical features of acute acalculous cholecystitis. *J Clin Gastroenterol* 36:166, 2003.

63. Yasuda H, Takada T, Kawarada Y, et al: Unusual cases of acute cholecystitis and cholangitis: Tokyo Guidelines. *J Hepatobiliary Pancreat Surg* 14:98, 2007.

64. Lipsett PA, Pitt HA: Surgical treatment of choledochal cysts. *J Hepatobiliary Pancreat Surg* 10:352, 2003.

65. Ahrendt SA, Pitt HA, Nakeeb A, et al: Diagnosis and management of cholangiocarcinoma in primary sclerosing cholangitis. *J Gastrointest Surg* 3:357, 1999.

66. Ahrendt SA, Pitt HA, Kalloo AN, et al: Primary sclerosing cholangitis: Resect, dilate, or transplant? *Ann Surg* 227:412, 1998.

67. Goss JA, Shackleton CR, Farmer DG, et al: Orthotopic liver transplantation for primary sclerosing cholangitis. A 12-year single center experience. *Ann Surg* 225:472, 1997.

68. Ahrendt SA, Pitt HA: Surgical treatment for primary sclerosing cholangitis. *J Hepatobiliary Pancreat Surg* 6:366, 1999.

69. Linder JD, Klapow JC, Linder SD, et al: Incomplete response to endoscopic sphincterotomy in patients with sphincter of Oddi dysfunction: Evidence for a chronic pain disorder. *Am J Gastroenterol* 98:1738, 2003.

70. Lillemoe KD, Melton GB, Cameron JL, et al: Postoperative bile duct strictures: Management and outcome in the 1990s. *Ann Surg* 232:430, 2000.

71. Melton GB, Lillemoe KD: The current management of postoperative bile duct strictures. *Adv Surg* 36:193, 2002.

72. Archer SB, Brown DW, Smith CD, et al: Bile duct injury during laparoscopic cholecystectomy: Results of a national survey. *Ann Surg* 234:549, 2001.

73. Ahrendt SA, Pitt HA: Surgical therapy of iatrogenic lesions of biliary tract. *World J Surg* 25:1360, 2001.

74. Strasberg SM: Avoidance of biliary injury during laparoscopic cholecystectomy. *J Hepatobiliary Pancreat Surg* 9:543, 2002.

75. Way LW, Stewart L, Gantert W, et al: Causes and prevention of laparoscopic bile duct injuries: Analysis of 252 cases from a human factors and cognitive psychology perspective [Comment]. *Ann Surg* 237:460, 2003.

76. Flum DR, Flowers C, Veenstra DL: A cost-effectiveness analysis of intraoperative cholangiography in the prevention of bile duct injury during laparoscopic cholecystectomy. *J Am Coll Surg* 196:385, 2003.

77. Lee CM, Stewart L, Way LW: Postcholecystectomy abdominal bile collections. *Arch Surg* 135:538, 2000.

78. Melton GB, Lillemoe KD, Cameron JL, et al: Major bile duct injuries associated with laparoscopic cholecystectomy: Effect of surgical repair on quality of life. *Ann Surg* 235:888, 2002.

79. Grobmyer SR, Lieberman MD, Daly JM: Gallbladder cancer in the twentieth century: Single institution's experience. *World J Surg* 28:47, 2004.

80. Pandey M, Shukla VK: Diet and gallbladder cancer: A case-control study. *Eur J Cancer Prev* 11:365, 2002.

81. Serra I, Calvo A, Baez S, et al: Risk factors for gallbladder cancer. An international collaborative case control study. *Cancer* 78:1515, 1996.

82. Lowenfels AB, Walker AM, Althaus DP, et al: Gallstone growth, size, and risk of gallbladder cancer: An interracial study. *Int J Epidemiol* 18:50, 1998.

83. Csendes A, Burgos AM, Csendes P, et al: Late follow-up of polypoid lesions of the gallbladder smaller than 10 mm. *Ann Surg* 234:657, 2001.

84. Wagholikar G, Behari A, Krishnani N, et al: Early gallbladder cancer. *J Am Coll Surg* 194:137, 2002.

85. Kim JH, Kim TK, Eun HW: Preoperative evaluation of gallbladder carcinoma: Efficacy of combined use of MR imaging, MR cholangiography, and contrast-enhanced dual phase three dimensional MR angiography. *J Magn Reson Imaging* 16:676, 2002.

86. Bartlett DL, Fong Y, Fortner JG, et al: Long-term results after resection for gallbladder cancer. Implications for staging and management. *Ann Surg* 224:639, 1996.

87. Wakai T, Shirai Y, Hatakeyama K: Radical second resection provides survival benefit for patients with T2 gallbladder carcinoma first discovered after laparoscopic cholecystectomy. *World J Surg* 26:867, 2002.

88. Noshiro H, Chijiiwa K, Yamaguchi K, et al: Factors affecting surgical outcome for gallbladder carcinoma. *Hepatogastroenterology* 50:939, 2003.

89. Strasberg SM: Resection of hilar cholangiocarcinoma. *HPB Surg* 10:415, 1998.

90. Tocchi A, Mazzoni G, Liotta G, et al: Late development of bile duct cancer in patients who had biliary-enteric drainage for benign disease: A follow-up study of more than 1000 patients. *Ann Surg* 234:210, 2001.

91. Ahrendt SA, Rashid A, Chow JT, et al: p53 overexpression and K-ras gene mutations in primary sclerosing cholangitis-associated biliary tract cancer. *J Hepatobiliary Pancreat Surg* 7:426, 2000.

92. Nehls O, Gregor M, Klump B: Serum and bile markers for cholangiocarcinoma. *Semin Liver Dis* 24:139, 2004.

93. Siqueira E, Schoen RE, Silverman W, et al: Detecting cholangiocarcinoma in patients with primary sclerosing cholangitis. *Gastrointest Endosc* 56:40, 2005.

94. Ahrendt SA, Nakeeb A, Pitt HA: Cholangiocarcinoma. *Clin Liver Dis* 5:191, 2001.

95. Lillemoe KD, Cameron JL: Surgery for hilar cholangiocarcinoma: The Johns Hopkins approach. *J Hepatobiliary Pancreat Surg* 7:115, 2000.

96. Mulholland MW, Yahanda A, Yeo CJ: Multidisciplinary management of perihilar bile duct cancer. *J Am Coll Surg* 193:440, 2001.

97. Vollmer CM, Drebin JA, Middleton WD, et al: Utility of staging laparoscopy in subsets of peripancreatic and biliary malignancies [Comment]. *Ann Surg* 235:1, 2002.

98. Strasberg SM: ERCP and surgical intervention in pancreatic and biliary malignancies. *Gastrointest Endosc* 56:S213, 2002.

99. Ortner ME, Caca K, Berr F, et al: Successful photodynamic therapy for nonresectable cholangiocarcinoma: A randomized prospective study. *Gastroenterology.* 125:1355, 2003.

33

Pancreas

William E. Fisher, Dana K. Andersen,
Richard H. Bell Jr., Ashok K. Saluja,
and F. Charles Brunicardi

ANATOMY AND PHYSIOLOGY

The pancreas is perhaps the most unforgiving organ in the human body, leading most surgeons to avoid even palpating it unless necessary. Situated deep in the center of the abdomen, the pancreas is surrounded by numerous important structures and major blood vessels. Seemingly minor trauma to the pancreas can result in the release of pancreatic enzymes and cause life-threatening pancreatitis. Surgeons that choose to undertake surgery on the pancreas require a thorough knowledge of its anatomy. However, knowledge of the relationships of the pancreas and surrounding structures is also critically important for all surgeons to ensure that pancreatic injury is avoided during surgery on other structures.

Gross Anatomy

The pancreas is a retroperitoneal organ that lies in an oblique position, sloping upward from the C-loop of the duodenum to the splenic hilum (Fig. 33-1). In an adult, the pancreas weighs 75 to 100 g and is about 15 to 20 cm long. The fact that the pancreas is situated so deeply in the abdomen and is sealed in the retroperitoneum explains the poorly localized and sometimes ill-defined nature with which pancreatic pathology presents. Patients with pancreatic cancer without bile duct obstruction usually present after months of vague upper abdominal discomfort, or no antecedent symptoms at all. Due to its retroperitoneal location, pain associated with pancreatitis often is characterized as penetrating through to the back.

Regions of the Pancreas

Surgeons typically describe the location of pathology within the pancreas in relation to four regions: the head, neck, body, and tail. The head of the pancreas is nestled in the C-loop of the duodenum and is posterior to the transverse mesocolon. Just behind the head of the pancreas lie the vena cava, the right renal artery, and both renal veins. The neck of the pancreas lies directly over the portal vein. At the inferior border of the neck of the pancreas, the superior mesenteric vein joins the splenic vein and then continues toward the porta hepatis as the portal vein. The inferior mesenteric vein often joins the splenic vein near its junction with the portal vein. Sometimes, the inferior mesenteric vein joins the superior mesenteric vein or merges with the superior mesenteric portal venous junction to form a trifurcation (Fig. 33-2). The superior mesenteric artery lies parallel to and just to the left of the superior mesenteric vein. The uncinate process and the head of the pancreas wrap around the right side of the portal vein and end posteriorly near the space between the superior mesenteric vein and superior mesenteric artery. Venous branches draining the pancreatic head and uncinate process enter along the right lateral and posterior sides of the portal vein. There are usually no anterior venous tributaries, and a plane can usually be developed between the neck of the pancreas and the portal and superior mesenteric veins during pancreatic resection, unless the tumor is invading the vein anteriorly. The common bile duct runs in a deep groove on the posterior aspect of the pancreatic head until it passes through the pancreatic parenchyma to join the main pancreatic duct at the ampulla of Vater. The body and tail of the pancreas lie just anterior to the splenic artery and vein. The vein runs in a groove on the back of the pancreas and is fed by multiple fragile venous branches from the pancreatic parenchyma. These branches must be ligated to perform a spleen-sparing distal pancreatectomy. The splenic artery runs parallel and just superior to the vein along the posterior superior edge of the body and tail of the pancreas. The splenic artery often is tortuous. The anterior surface of the body of the pancreas is covered by peritoneum. Once the gastrocolic omentum is divided, the body and tail of the pancreas can be seen along the floor of the lesser sac, just posterior to the stomach.

Pancreatic pseudocysts commonly develop in this area, and the posterior aspect of the stomach can form the anterior wall of the pseudocyst, allowing drainage into the stomach. The base of the transverse mesocolon attaches to the inferior margin of the body and tail of the pancreas. The transverse mesocolon often forms the inferior wall of pancreatic pseudocysts or inflammatory processes, allowing surgical drainage through the transverse mesocolon. The body of the pancreas overlies the aorta at the origin of the superior mesenteric artery. The neck of the pancreas overlies the vertebral body of L1 and L2, and blunt anteroposterior trauma can compress the neck of the pancreas against the spine, causing parenchymal and, sometimes, ductal injury. The neck divides the pancreas into approximately two equal halves. The small portion of the pancreas anterior to the left kidney is referred to as the *tail* and is nestled in the hilum of the spleen near the splenic flexure of the left colon. Awareness of these anatomic relationships is important to avoid injury to the pancreatic tail during left colectomy or splenectomy.

Pancreatic Duct Anatomy

An understanding of embryology is required to appreciate the common variations in pancreatic duct anatomy. The pancreas is formed by the fusion of a ventral and dorsal bud. The duct from the smaller ventral bud, which arises from the hepatic diverticulum, connects directly to the common bile duct. The duct from the larger dorsal bud, which arises from the duodenum, drains directly into the duodenum. The duct of the ventral anlage becomes the duct of Wirsung, and the duct from the dorsal anlage becomes the duct of Santorini. With gut rotation, the ventral anlage rotates to the right and around the posterior side of the duodenum to fuse with the dorsal bud. The ventral anlage becomes the inferior portion of the pancreatic head and the uncinate process, while the dorsal anlage becomes the body and tail of the pancreas. The ducts from each anlage usually fuse together in the pancreatic head such that most of the pancreas drains through the duct of Wirsung, or main pancreatic duct, into the common channel formed from the bile duct and pancreatic duct. The length of the common channel is variable. In about one third of patients, the bile duct and pancreatic duct remain distinct to the end of the papilla, the two ducts merge at the end of the papilla in another one third, and in the remaining one third, a true common channel is present for a distance of several millimeters. Commonly, the duct from the dorsal anlage, the duct of Santorini, persists as the lesser pancreatic duct, and sometimes drains directly into the duodenum through the lesser papilla just proximal to the major papilla. In approximately 30% of patients, the duct of Santorini ends as a blind accessory duct and does not empty

KEY POINTS

1. Incomplete fusion of the dorsal and ventral pancreatic ducts results in pancreas divisum, but a variety of ductal anomalies can be seen. Magnetic resonance cholangiopancreatography as well as endoscopic retrograde cholangiopancreatography can identify these ductal anomalies, and clarification of the ductal pattern of the pancreas is important before attempts at interventions.

2. The "replaced right hepatic artery" occurs in 15% of patients and needs to be identified preoperatively to prevent inadvertent injury with resulting hepatic necrosis. Anomalous hepatic arterial anatomy can result in hepatic ischemia during dissection of the porta hepatis as well. "Thin cut" multidetector computed tomographic images are usually able to identify the relevant arterial and venous patterns around the pancreas.

3. Regardless of the etiology, the management of the early phase of acute pancreatitis is critical to achieve a successful outcome. "Resting the pancreas" means eliminating oral nutrients, and resumption of diet should be limited to liquids and low-fat/low-protein foods. Patients who do not improve spontaneously within 24 to 48 hours are at risk for developing severe disease with its risk of life-threatening sepsis.

4. Surgical intervention in acute pancreatitis is reserved for patients with infected collections or infected necrosis only, or to relieve an impacted gallstone in the ampulla if endoscopic or radiologic treatments are unavailable or unsuccessful. Infection is usually confirmed by a pattern of air in the retroperitoneum on computed tomographic scan, or by documentation of bacteria on Gram's stain or culture from fine-needle aspiration of a suspected infected fluid collection. Fine-needle aspiration of suspicious fluid collections should not be converted to percutaneous drainage unless infection is confirmed, and the consensus decision has been made that percutaneous drainage is appropriate for the individual patient.

5. The appearance of chronic pancreatitis on computed tomographic scan varies dramatically, and multiple diagnostic studies are usually needed to establish the extent of disease. Calcific pancreatitis is not a marker of alcoholic pancreatitis alone, and rarely indicates autoimmune pancreatitis. Endoscopic ultrasound provides a better assessment of the disease than computed tomography and is useful to disclose indolent or unsuspected cancer, which can occur in up to 10% of patients.

6. The nidus of inflammation in chronic pancreatitis due to any cause is the head of the gland. Therefore, treatment approaches that address the disease in the head have the best long-term results. The Whipple procedure, the Beger procedure, and the Frey procedure, with or without longitudinal duct drainage, are the best surgical options, as all three approaches remove all or most of the disease in the head of the gland.

7. The precursor lesion that probably leads to most cases of ductular adenocarcinoma is the ductal epithelial hyperplasia/dysplasia process described by the pancreatic intraepithelial neoplasia classification system. Pancreatic intraepithelial neoplasia 2 and pancreatic intraepithelial neoplasia 3 lesions may be associated with other, nonspecific changes in pancreatic morphology seen on imaging studies, or may only be seen histologically. Resection margins for pancreatic neoplasms should be examined for advanced pancreatic intraepithelial neoplasia stage patterns of ductal hyperplasia to ensure adequate resection status.

8. Intraductal papillary mucinous neoplasms are small macroscopic polypoid or plaque-like adenomas that develop in the main pancreatic duct or in side-branch ducts, and secrete mucin. They are often silent symptomatically, but cause characteristic appearances of small cyst-like collections of mucus, or diffuse dilatation of the main pancreatic duct with mucus. These premalignant lesions may be multifocal or single and can evolve into invasive adenocarcinoma in a similar pattern as with other adenomatous polypoid lesions of the gastrointestinal tract. They have been diagnosed with increasing frequency, and account for more than one third of pancreatic resections at some centers. Main-duct intraductal papillary mucinous neoplasms are an indication for resection; side-branch intraductal papillary mucinous neoplasms have a lower incidence of malignancy and are sometimes followed with serial imaging surveillance.

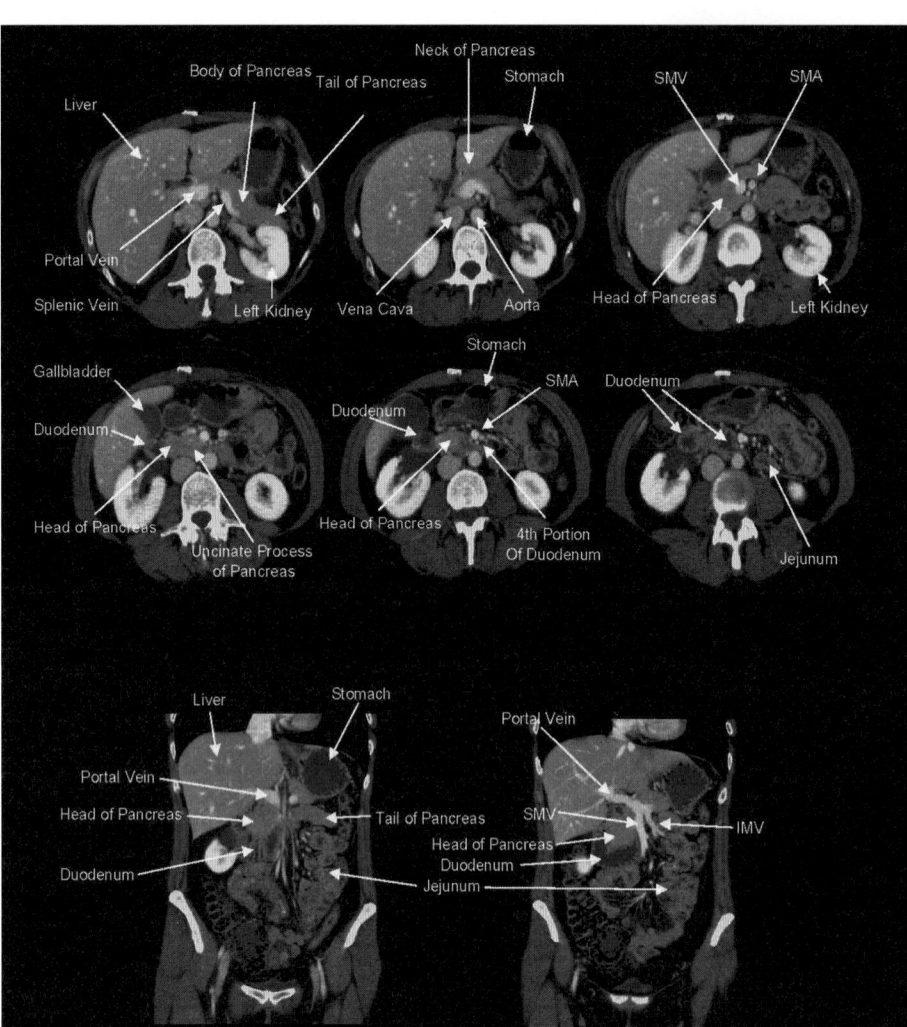

FIG. 33-1. Pancreatic anatomy as seen on computed tomography. Knowledge of the relationship of the pancreas with surrounding structures is important to ensure that injury is avoided during abdominal surgery. IMV = inferior mesenteric vein; SMA = superior mesenteric artery; SMV = superior mesenteric vein.

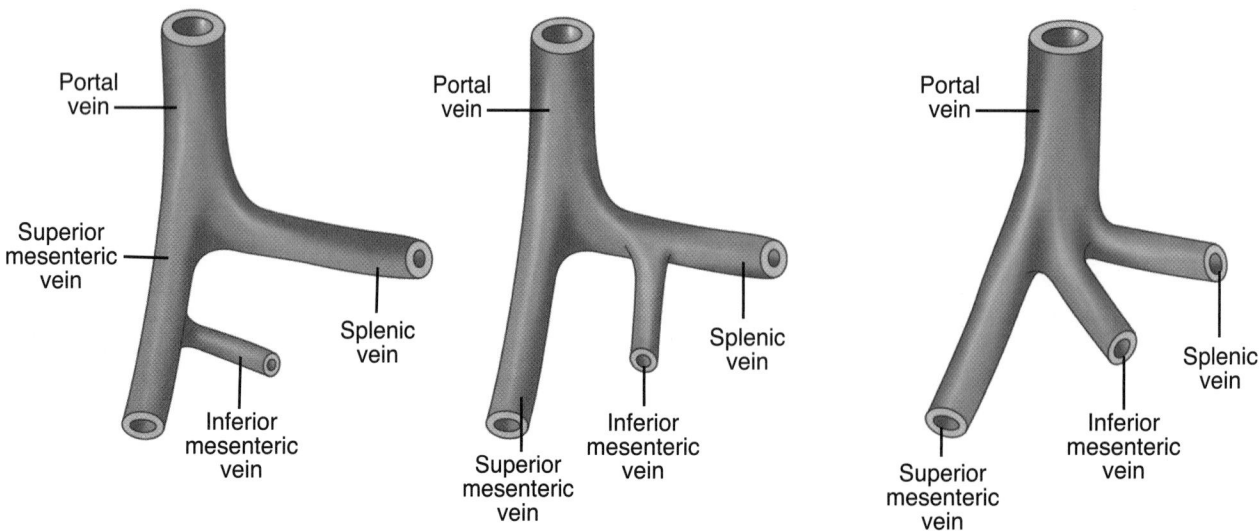

FIG. 33-2. Variations in portal venous anatomy. The superior mesenteric vein joins the splenic vein and then continues toward the porta hepatis as the portal vein. The inferior mesenteric vein often joins the splenic vein near its junction with the portal vein, but sometimes joins the superior mesenteric vein; or the three veins merge as a trifurcation to form the portal vein.

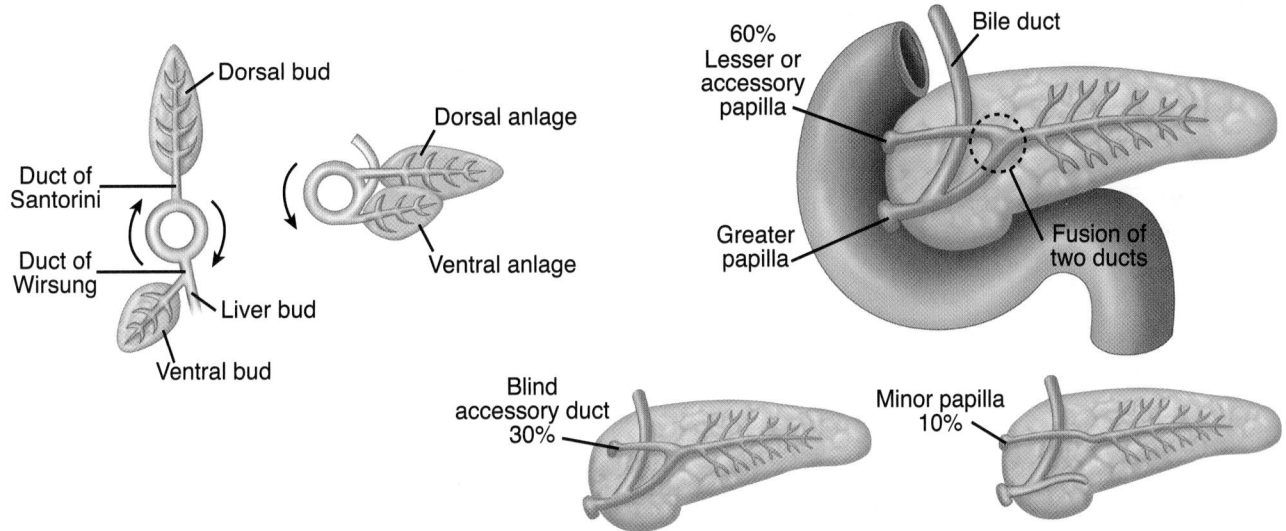

FIG. 33-3. Embryology of pancreas and duct variations. The duct of Wirsung from the ventral bud connects to the bile duct, while the duct of Santorini from the larger dorsal bud connects to the duodenum. With gut rotation, the two ducts fuse in most cases such that the majority of the pancreas drains through the duct of Wirsung to the major papilla. The duct of Santorini can persist as a blind accessory duct or drain through the lesser papilla. In a minority of patients, the ducts remain separate, and the majority of the pancreas drains through the duct of Santorini, a condition referred to as *pancreas divisum.*

into the duodenum. In 10% of patients, the ducts of Wirsung and Santorini fail to fuse.[1] This results in the majority of the pancreas draining through the duct of Santorini and the lesser papilla, while the inferior portion of the pancreatic head and uncinate process drains through the duct of Wirsung and major papilla. This normal anatomic variant, which occurs in one out of 10 patients, is referred to as *pancreas divisum* (Fig. 33-3). In a minority of these patients, the minor papilla can be inadequate to handle the flow of pancreatic juices from the majority of the gland. This relative outflow obstruction can result in pancreatitis and is sometimes treated by sphincteroplasty of the minor papilla.

The main pancreatic duct is usually only 2 to 3 mm in diameter and runs midway between the superior and inferior borders of the pancreas, usually closer to the posterior than to the anterior surface. Pressure inside the pancreatic duct is about twice that in the common bile duct, which is thought to prevent reflux of bile into the pancreatic duct. The main pancreatic duct joins with the common bile duct and empties at the ampulla of Vater or major papilla, which is located on the medial aspect of the second portion of the duodenum. The muscle fibers around the ampulla form the sphincter of Oddi, which controls the flow of pancreatic and biliary secretions into the duodenum. Contraction and relaxation of the sphincter is regulated by complex neural and hormonal factors. When the accessory pancreatic duct or lesser duct drains into the duodenum, a lesser papilla can be identified approximately 2 cm proximal to the ampulla of Vater.

Vascular and Lymphatic Anatomy

The blood supply to the pancreas comes from multiple branches from the celiac and superior mesenteric arteries (Fig. 33-4). The common hepatic artery gives rise to the gastroduodenal artery before continuing toward the porta hepatis as the proper hepatic artery. The gastroduodenal artery becomes the superior pancreaticoduodenal artery as it passes behind the first portion of the duodenum and branches into the anterior and posterior superior pancreaticoduodenal arteries. As the superior mesenteric artery passes behind the neck of the pancreas, it gives off the inferior pancreaticoduodenal artery at the inferior margin of the neck of the pancreas. This vessel quickly divides into the anterior and posterior inferior pancreaticoduodenal arteries. The superior and inferior pancreaticoduodenal arteries join together within the parenchyma of the anterior and posterior sides of the head of the pancreas along the medial aspect of the C-loop of the duodenum to form arcades that give off numerous branches to the duodenum and head of the pancreas. Therefore, it is impossible to resect the head of the pancreas without devascularizing the duodenum, unless a rim of pancreas containing the pancreaticoduodenal arcade is preserved. Variations in the arterial anatomy occur in one out of five patients. The right hepatic artery, common hepatic artery, or gastroduodenal arteries can arise from the superior mesenteric artery. In 15 to 20% of patients, the right hepatic artery will arise from the superior mesenteric artery and travel upwards toward the liver along the posterior aspect of the head of the pancreas (referred to as *replaced right hepatic artery*). It is important to look for this variation on preoperative computed tomographic (CT) scans and in the operating room so the replaced hepatic artery is recognized and injury is avoided. The body and tail of the pancreas are supplied by multiple branches of the splenic artery. The splenic artery arises from the celiac trunk and travels along the posterior-superior border of the body and tail of the pancreas toward the spleen. The inferior pancreatic artery usually arises from the superior mesenteric artery and runs to the left along the inferior border of the body and tail of the pancreas, parallel to the splenic artery. Three vessels run perpendicular to the long axis of the pancreatic body and tail and connect the splenic artery and inferior pancreatic artery. They are, from medial to lateral, the dorsal, great, and caudal pancreatic arteries. These arteries form arcades within the body and tail of the pancreas, and account for the rich blood supply of the organ.

The venous drainage of the pancreas follows a pattern similar to that of the arterial supply. The veins are usually superficial to the arteries within the parenchyma of the pancreas. There is an anterior and posterior venous arcade within the head of the pancreas. The superior veins drain directly into the portal vein just above the neck of the pancreas. The posterior inferior arcade drains directly into the inferior mesenteric vein at the inferior border of the neck of the pancreas. The anterior inferior pancreaticoduodenal vein joins the

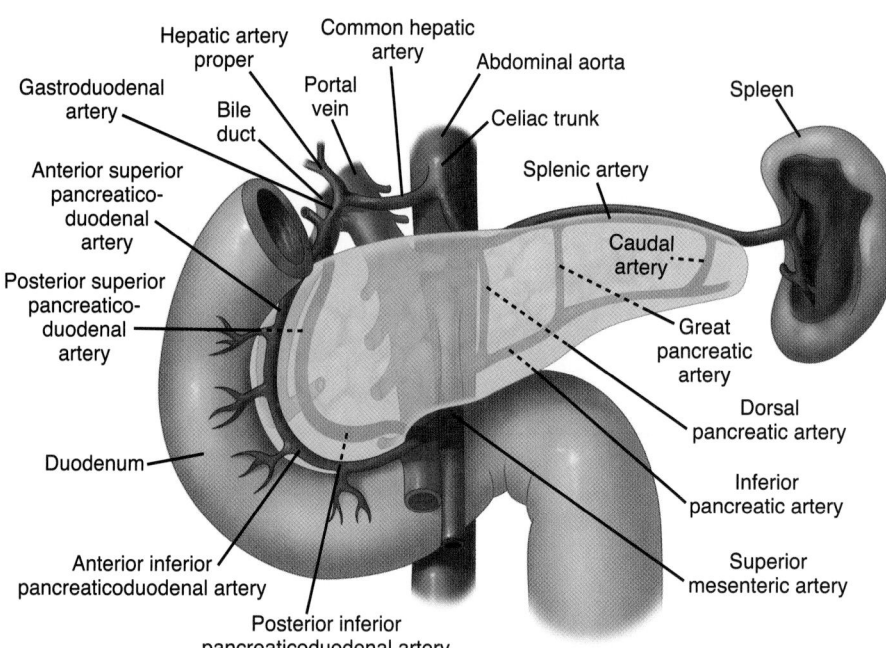

FIG. 33-4. Arterial supply to the pancreas. Multiple arcades in the head and body of the pancreas provide a rich blood supply. The head of the pancreas cannot be resected without devascularizing the duodenum unless a rim of pancreas containing the pancreaticoduodenal arcade is preserved.

right gastroepiploic vein and the middle colic vein to form a common venous trunk, which enters into the superior mesenteric vein. Traction on the transverse colon during colectomy can tear these fragile veins, which then retract into the parenchyma of the pancreas, making control tedious. There also are numerous small venous branches coming from the pancreatic parenchyma directly into the lateral and posterior aspect of the portal vein. Venous return from the body and tail of the pancreas drains into the splenic vein (Fig. 33-5).

The lymphatic drainage from the pancreas is diffuse and widespread. The profuse network of lymphatic vessels and lymph nodes

draining the pancreas provides egress to tumor cells arising from the pancreas. This diffuse lymphatic drainage contributes to the fact that pancreatic cancer often presents with positive lymph nodes and a high incidence of local recurrence after resection. Lymph nodes can be palpated along the posterior aspect of the head of the pancreas in the pancreaticoduodenal groove, where the mesenteric vein passes under the neck of the pancreas, along the inferior border of the body, along the hepatic artery ascending into the porta hepatis, and along the splenic artery and vein. The pancreatic lymphatics also communicate with lymph nodes in the transverse mesocolon and mesentery

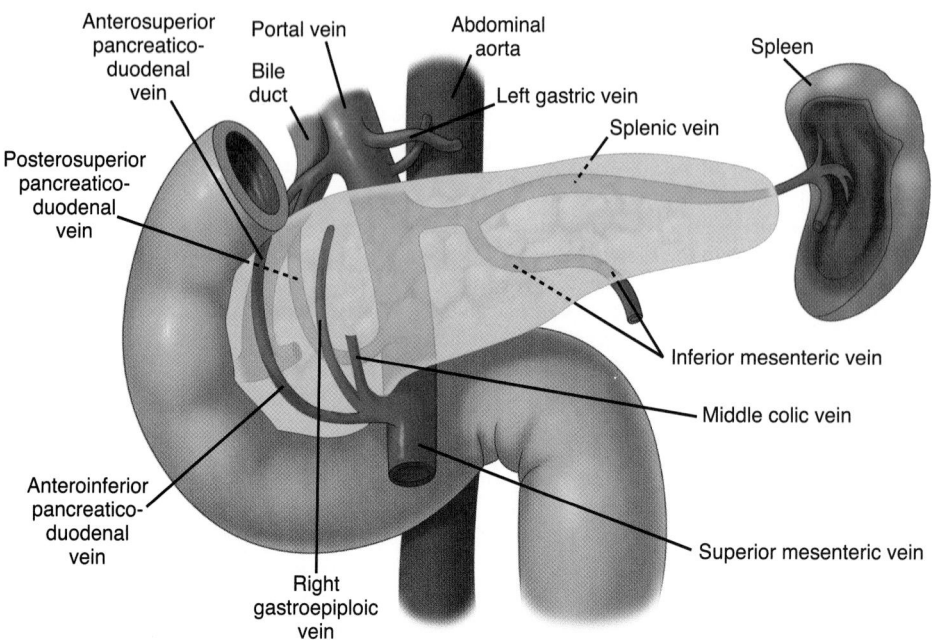

FIG. 33-5. Venous drainage from the pancreas. The venous drainage of the pancreas follows a pattern similar to the arterial supply, with the veins usually superficial to the arteries. Anterior traction on the transverse colon can tear fragile branches along the inferior border of the pancreas, which then retract into the parenchyma of the pancreas. Venous branches draining the pancreatic head and uncinate process enter along the right lateral and posterior sides of the portal vein. There are usually no anterior venous tributaries, and a plane can usually be developed between the neck of the pancreas and the portal and superior mesenteric veins.

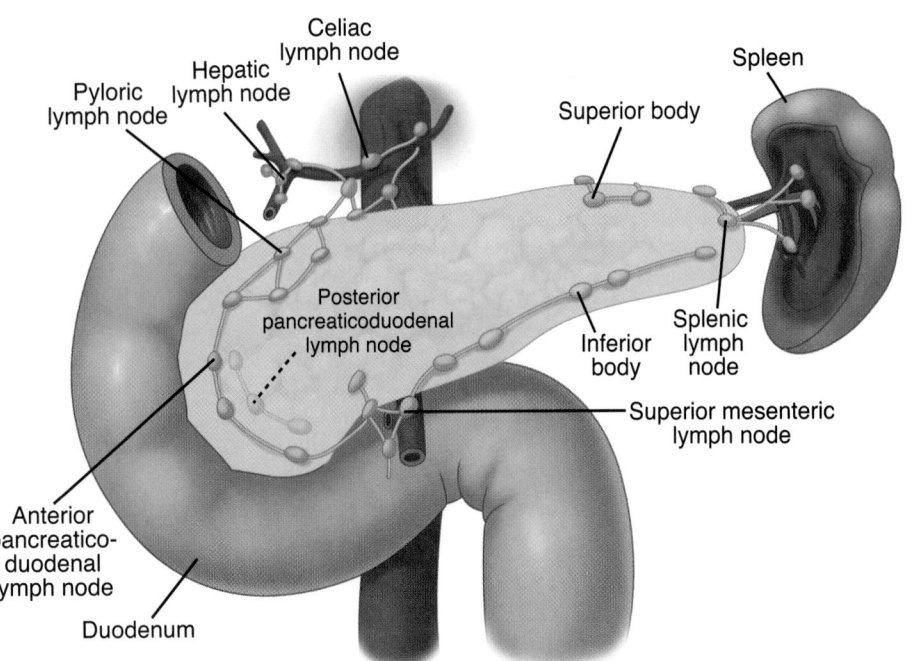

FIG. 33-6. Lymphatic supply to the pancreas. The lymphatic drainage from the pancreas is diffuse and widespread, which explains the high incidence of lymph node metastases and local recurrence of pancreatic cancer. The pancreatic lymphatics also communicate with lymph nodes in the transverse mesocolon and mesentery of the proximal jejunum. Tumors in the body and tail of the pancreas are often unresectable because they metastasize to these lymph nodes. *[Reproduced with permission from Bell RH Jr.: Atlas of pancreatic surgery, in Bell RH Jr., Rikkers LF, Mulholland MW (eds): Digestive Tract Surgery: A Text and Atlas. Philadelphia: Lippincott-Raven, 1996, p 969.]*

of the proximal jejunum. Tumors in the body and tail of the pancreas often metastasize to these nodes and lymph nodes along the splenic vein and in the hilum of the spleen (Fig. 33-6).

Neuroanatomy

The pancreas is innervated by the sympathetic and parasympathetic nervous systems. The acinar cells responsible for exocrine secretion, the islet cells responsible for endocrine secretion, and the islet vasculature are innervated by both systems. The parasympathetic system stimulates endocrine and exocrine secretion and the sympathetic

system inhibits secretion.[2] The pancreas is also innervated by neurons that secrete amines and peptides, such as somatostatin, vasoactive intestinal peptide (VIP), calcitonin gene-related peptide (CGRP), and galanin. The exact role of these neurons in pancreatic physiology is uncertain, but they do appear to affect both exocrine and endocrine function. The pancreas also has a rich supply of afferent sensory fibers, which are responsible for the intense pain associated with advanced pancreatic cancer, as well as acute and chronic pancreatitis. These somatic fibers travel superiorly to the celiac ganglia. Interruption of these somatic fibers can stop transmission of pain sensation (Fig. 33-7).

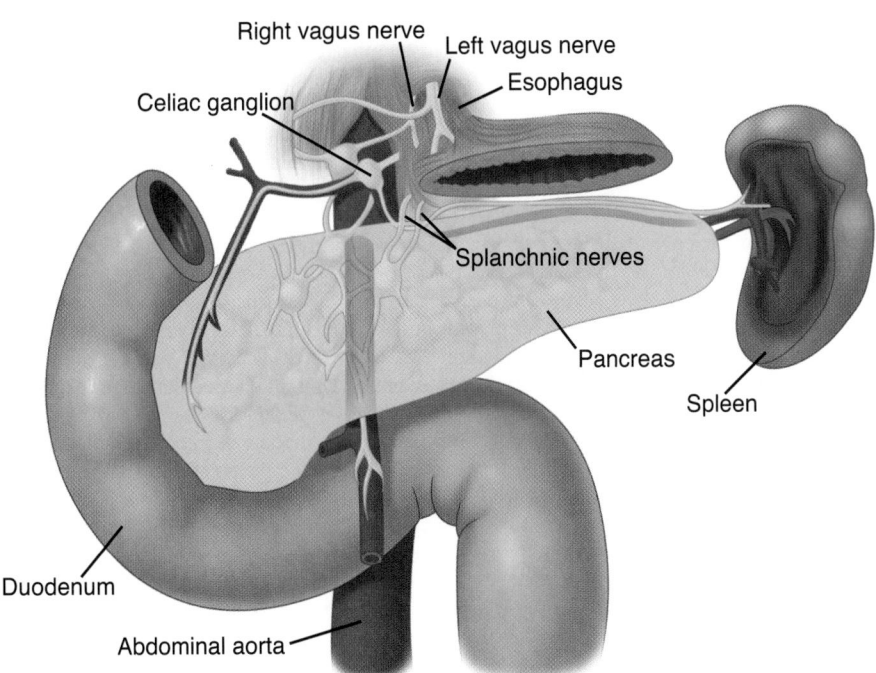

FIG. 33-7. Innervation of the pancreas. The pancreas has a rich supply of afferent sensory fibers that travel superiorly to the celiac ganglia. Interruption of these somatic fibers with a celiac plexus block can interfere with transmission of pancreatic pain. *[Reproduced with permission from Bell RH Jr.: Atlas of pancreatic surgery, in Bell RH Jr., Rikkers LF, Mulholland MW (eds): Digestive Tract Surgery: A Text and Atlas. Philadelphia: Lippincott-Raven, 1996, p 969.]*

HISTOLOGY AND PHYSIOLOGY

The exocrine pancreas accounts for about 85% of the pancreatic mass; 10% of the gland is accounted for by extracellular matrix, and 4% by blood vessels and the major ducts, whereas only 2% of the gland is comprised of endocrine tissue. The endocrine and exocrine pancreas are sometimes thought of as functionally separate, but these different components of the organ are coordinated to allow an elegant regulatory feedback system for digestive enzyme and hormone secretion. This complex system regulates the type of digestion, its rate, and the processing and distribution of absorbed nutrients. This coordination is facilitated by the physical approximation of the islets and the exocrine pancreas, the presence of specific islet hormone receptors on the plasma membranes of pancreatic acinar cells, and the existence of an islet-acinar portal blood system.

Although patients can live without a pancreas when insulin and digestive enzyme replacement are administered, the loss of this islet-acinar coordination leads to impairments in digestive function. Although only approximately 20% of the normal pancreas is required to prevent insufficiency, in many patients undergoing pancreatic resection, the remaining pancreas is not normal, and pancreatic endocrine and exocrine insufficiency can develop with removal of smaller portions of the gland.

Exocrine Pancreas

The pancreas secretes approximately 500 to 800 mL per day of colorless, odorless, alkaline, isosmotic pancreatic juice. Pancreatic juice is a combination of acinar cell and duct cell secretions. The acinar cells secrete amylase, proteases, and lipases, enzymes responsible for the digestion of all three food types: carbohydrate, protein, and fat. The acinar cells are pyramid-shaped, with their apices facing the lumen of the acinus. Near the apex of each cell are numerous enzyme-containing zymogen granules that fuse with the apical cell membrane (Fig. 33-8). Unlike the endocrine pancreas, where islet cells specialize in the secretion of one hormone type, individual acinar cells secrete all types of enzymes. However, the ratio of the different enzymes released is adjusted to the composition of digested food through nonparallel regulation of secretion.

Pancreatic amylase is secreted in its active form and completes the digestive process already begun by salivary amylase. Amylase is the only pancreatic enzyme secreted in its active form, and it hydrolyzes starch and glycogen to glucose, maltose, maltotriose, and dextrins. These simple sugars are transported across the brush border of the intestinal epithelial cells by active transport mechanisms. Gastric hydrolysis of protein yields peptides that enter the intestine and stimulate intestinal endocrine cells to release cholecystokinin (CCK)-releasing peptide, CCK, and secretin, which then stimulate the pancreas to secrete enzymes and bicarbonate into the intestine.

The proteolytic enzymes are secreted as proenzymes that require activation. Trypsinogen is converted to its active form, trypsin, by another enzyme, enterokinase, which is produced by the duodenal mucosal cells. Trypsin, in turn, activates the other proteolytic enzymes. Trypsinogen activation within the pancreas is prevented by the presence of inhibitors that are also secreted by the acinar cells. A failure to express a normal trypsinogen inhibitor, pancreatic secretory trypsin inhibitor (PSTI) or *SPINK1*, is a cause of familial pancreatitis. Inhibition of trypsinogen activation ensures that the enzymes within the pancreas remain in an inactive precursor state and are activated only within the duodenum. Trypsinogen is expressed in several isoforms, and a missense mutation on the cationic trypsinogen, or *PRSS1*, results in premature, intrapancreatic activation of trypsinogen. This accounts for about two-thirds of cases of hereditary pancreatitis. Chymotrypsinogen is activated to form chymotrypsin. Elastase, carboxypeptidase A and B, and phospholipase are also activated by trypsin. Trypsin, chymotrypsin, and elastase cleave bonds between amino acids within a target peptide chain, and carboxypeptidase A and B cleave amino acids at the end of peptide chains. Individual amino acids and small dipeptides are then actively

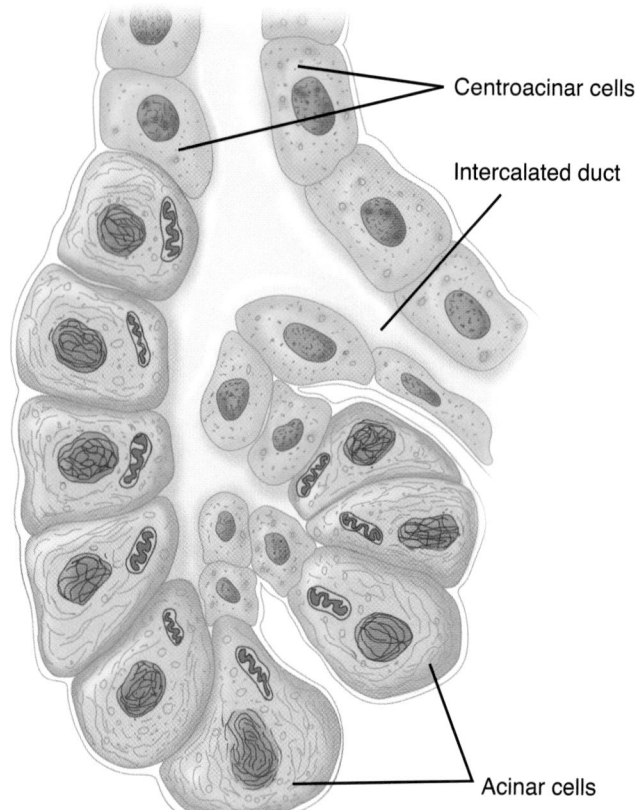

FIG. 33-8. Acinar cell. Zymogen granules fuse with the apical membrane and release multiple enzymes to digest carbohydrates, proteins, and fat. *[Reproduced with permission from Bloom W, Fawcett DW: A Textbook of Histology, 10th ed. Philadelphia: Saunders, 1975, p 738. Copyright Elsevier.]*

transported into the intestinal epithelial cells. Pancreatic lipase hydrolyzes triglycerides to 2-monoglyceride and fatty acid. Pancreatic lipase is secreted in an active form. Colipase is also secreted by the pancreas and binds to lipase, changing its molecular configuration and increasing its activity. Phospholipase A2 is secreted by the pancreas as a proenzyme that becomes activated by trypsin. Phospholipase A2 hydrolyzes phospholipids and, as with all lipases, requires bile salts for its action. Carboxylic ester hydrolase and cholesterol esterase hydrolyze neutral lipid substrates like esters of cholesterol, fat-soluble vitamins, and triglycerides. The hydrolyzed fat is then packaged into micelles for transport into the intestinal epithelial cells, where the fatty acids are reassembled and packaged inside chylomicrons for transport through the lymphatic system into the bloodstream (Table 33-1).

The centroacinar and intercalated duct cells secrete the water and electrolytes present in the pancreatic juice. About 40 acinar cells are arranged into a spherical unit called an *acinus*. Centroacinar cells are located near the center of the acinus and are responsible for fluid and electrolyte secretion. These cells contain the enzyme carbonic anhydrase, which is needed for bicarbonate secretion. The amount of bicarbonate secreted varies with the pancreatic secretory rate, with greater concentrations of bicarbonate being secreted as the pancreatic secretory rate increases. Chloride secretion varies inversely with bicarbonate secretion such that the sum of these two remains constant. In contrast, sodium and potassium concentrations are kept constant throughout the spectrum of secretory rates[3] (Fig. 33-9). The hormone secretin is released from cells in the duodenal mucosa in response to acidic chyme passing through the pylorus into the duodenum. Secretin is the major stimulant for bicarbonate secre-

TABLE 33-1	Pancreatic enzymes		
Enzyme		**Substrate**	**Product**
Carbohydrate			
Amylase (active)		Starch, glycogen	Glucose, maltose, maltotriose, dextrins
Protein			
Endopeptidases		Cleave bonds between amino acids	Amino acids, dipeptides
Trypsinogen (inactive) $\xrightarrow{\text{Enterokinase}}$ Trypsin (active)			
Chymotrypsinogen (inactive) $\xrightarrow[\text{Trypsin}]{\text{Enterokinase}}$ Chymotrypsin (active)			
Proelastase (inactive) $\xrightarrow[\text{Trypsin}]{\text{Enterokinase}}$ Elastase (active)			
Exopeptidases		Cleave amino acids from end of peptide chains	—
Procarboxy peptidase A&B (inactive) $\xrightarrow{\text{Enterokinase}}$ Carboxypeptidase A&B (active)			
Fat			
Pancreatic lipase (active)		Triglycerides	2-Monoglycerides fatty acids
Phospholipase A2 (inactive) $\xrightarrow{\text{Trypsin}}$ Phospholipase A2 (active)		Phospholipase	—
Cholesterol esterase		Neutral lipids	—

tion, which buffers the acidic fluid entering the duodenum from the stomach. CCK also stimulates bicarbonate secretion, but to a much lesser extent than secretin. CCK potentiates secretin-stimulated bicarbonate secretion. Gastrin and acetylcholine, both stimulants of gastric acid secretion, are also weak stimulants of pancreatic bicarbonate secretion.[4] Truncal vagotomy produces a myriad of complex effects on the downstream digestive tract, but the sum effect on the exocrine pancreas is a reduction in bicarbonate and fluid secretion.[5] The endocrine pancreas also influences the adjacent exocrine pancreatic secretions. Somatostatin, pancreatic polypeptide (PP), and glucagon are all thought to inhibit exocrine secretion.

The acinar cells release pancreatic enzymes from their zymogen granules into the lumen of the acinus, and these proteins combine with the water and bicarbonate secretions of the centroacinar cells. The pancreatic juice then travels into small inter-

calated ducts. Several small intercalated ducts join to form an interlobular duct. Cells in the interlobular ducts continue to contribute fluid and electrolytes to adjust the final concentrations of the pancreatic fluid. Interlobular ducts then join to form about 20 secondary ducts that empty into the main pancreatic duct. Destruction of the branching ductal tree from recurrent inflammation, scarring, and deposition of stones eventually contributes to destruction of the exocrine pancreas and exocrine pancreatic insufficiency.

Endocrine Pancreas

There are nearly 1 million islets of Langerhans in the normal adult pancreas. They vary greatly in size from 40 to 900 μm. Larger islets are located closer to the major arterioles and smaller islets are embedded more deeply in the parenchyma of the pancreas. Most islets contain 3000 to 4000 cells of five major types: alpha cells that secrete glucagon, β-cells that secrete insulin, delta cells that secrete somatostatin, epsilon cells that secrete ghrelin, and PP cells that secrete PP (Table 33-2).

Insulin is the best-studied pancreatic hormone. The discovery of insulin in 1920 by Frederick Banting, an orthopedic surgeon, and Charles Best, a medical student, was recognized with the awarding of the Nobel Prize in Physiology or Medicine. They produced diabetes in dogs by performing total pancreatectomy and then treated them with crude pancreatic extracts from dog and calf pancreata using techniques to prevent the breakdown of insulin by the proteolytic enzymes of the exocrine pancreas. Insulin was subsequently purified and found to be a 56-amino acid peptide with two chains, an α and a β chain, joined by two disulfide bridges and a connecting peptide, or C-peptide. Proinsulin is made in the endoplasmic reticulum and then is transported to the Golgi complex, where it is packaged into granules and the C-peptide is cleaved off. There are two phases of insulin secretion. In the first phase, stored insulin is released. This phase lasts about 5 minutes after a glucose challenge. The second phase of insulin secretion is a longer, sustained release due to ongoing production of new insulin. β-cell synthesis of insulin is regulated by plasma glucose levels, neural signals, and the paracrine influence of other islet cells. The diagnosis of diabetes is made by using glucose tolerance tests. Oral glucose tolerance tests and IV glucose tolerance tests are commonly used. Oral glucose not only enters the bloodstream but also stimulates the release of enteric hormones such as gastric inhibitory peptide (also known as *glucose-dependent insulinotropic polypeptide* or *GIP*), glucagon-like peptide-1 (GLP-1), and CCK, that augment the secretion of insulin, and are therefore referred to as *incretins*. Therefore

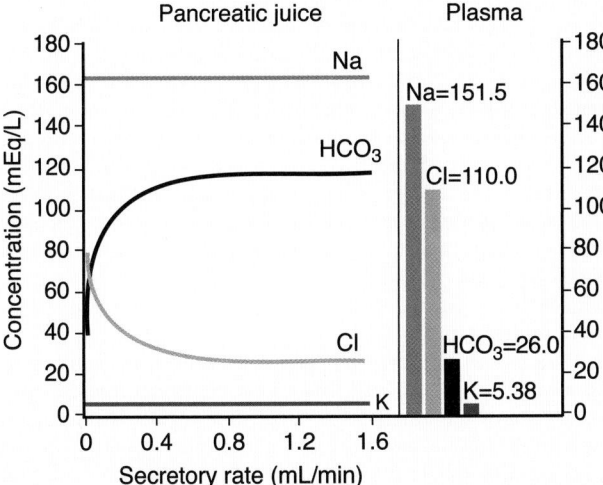

FIG. 33-9. Composition of pancreatic exocrine secretions. Greater concentrations of bicarbonate are secreted at higher secretory rates, and chloride secretion varies inversely with bicarbonate secretion. In contrast, sodium and potassium concentrations are independent of the secretory rate. (*Reproduced with permission from Bro-Rasmussen F et al: The composition of pancreatic juice as compared to sweat, parotid saliva, and tears. Acta Phys Scandinav 37:97–113, 1956.*)

TABLE 33-2	Pancreatic islet peptide products	
Hormones	**Islet Cell**	**Functions**
Insulin	β (beta cell)	Decreased gluconeogenesis, glycogenolysis, fatty acid breakdown, and ketogenesis
		Increased glycogenesis, protein synthesis
Glucagon	α (alpha cell)	Opposite effects of insulin; increased hepatic glycogenolysis and gluconeogenesis
Somatostatin	δ (delta cell)	Inhibits GI secretion
		Inhibits secretion and action of all GI endocrine peptides
		Inhibits cell growth
Pancreatic polypeptide	PP (PP cell)	Inhibits pancreatic exocrine secretion and section of insulin
		Facilitates hepatic effect of insulin
Amylin (IAPP)	β (beta cell)	Counterregulates insulin secretion and function
Pancreastatin	β (beta cell)	Decreases insulin and somatostatin release
		Increases glucagon release
		Decreases pancreatic exocrine secretion
Ghrelin	ε (epsilon cell)	Decreases insulin release and insulin action

IAPP = islet amyloid polypeptide.

oral glucose is a more vigorous stimulus to insulin secretion than IV glucose. In the oral glucose tolerance test, the patient is fasted overnight, and a basal glucose value is determined. Forty g/m² of glucose is given orally over 10 minutes. Blood samples are taken every 30 minutes for 2 hours. Normal values and criteria for diabetes vary by age, but essentially all values should be <200 mg/dL, and the 120-minute value should be <140 mg/dL.

Insulin secretion by the β-cell is also influenced by plasma levels of amino acids such as arginine, lysine, leucine, and free fatty acids. Glucagon, GIP, GLP-1, and CCK stimulate insulin release, while somatostatin, amylin, and pancreastatin inhibit insulin release.[6] Cholinergic fibers and beta sympathetic fibers stimulate insulin release, while alpha sympathetic fibers inhibit insulin secretion.

Insulin's function is to inhibit endogenous (hepatic) glucose production and to facilitate glucose transport into cells, thus lowering plasma glucose levels. Insulin also inhibits glycogenolysis, fatty acid breakdown, and ketone formation, and stimulates protein synthesis. There is a considerable amount of functional reserve in insulin secretory capacity. If the remaining portion of the pancreas is healthy, about 80% of the pancreas can be resected without the patient becoming diabetic.[7] In patients with chronic pancreatitis, or other conditions in which much of the gland is diseased, resection of a smaller fraction of the pancreas can result in diabetes. Insulin receptors are dimeric, tyrosine kinase–containing transmembrane proteins that are located on all cells. Insulin deficiency (type I diabetes) results in an overexpression or upregulation of insulin receptors, which causes an enhanced sensitivity to insulin. Type II diabetes is associated with a downregulation of insulin receptors and relative hyperinsulinemia, with resulting insulin resistance. Some forms of diabetes are associated with selected impairments of hepatic or peripheral insulin receptors, such as pancreatogenic diabetes or maturity-onset diabetes of the young.

Glucagon is a 29-amino-acid, single-chain peptide that promotes hepatic glycogenolysis and gluconeogenesis and counteracts the effects of insulin through its hyperglycemic action. Glucose is the primary regulator of glucagon secretion, as it is with insulin, but it has an inhibitory rather than stimulatory effect. Glucagon release is stimulated by the amino acids arginine and alanine. Gastric inhibitory peptide stimulates glucagon secretion at least in vitro, and GLP-1 inhibits glucagon secretion in vivo. Insulin and somatostatin inhibit glucagon secretion in a paracrine fashion within the islet. The same neural impulses that regulate insulin secretion also regulate glucagon secretion, so that the two hormones work together in a balance of actions to maintain glucose levels. Cholinergic and beta sympathetic fibers stimulate glucagon release, while alpha sympathetic fibers inhibit glucagon release.[8]

Although originally isolated from the hypothalamus, somatostatin is a peptide that is now known to have a wide anatomic distribution, not only in neurons but also in the pancreas, gut, and other tissues. It is a highly conserved peptide hormone, as it is found in lower vertebrates, and is now realized to be of fundamental importance in regulatory processes throughout the body. One gene encodes for a common precursor that is differentially processed to generate tissue-specific amounts of two bioactive products, somatostatin-14 and somatostatin-28. These peptides inhibit endocrine and exocrine secretion and affect neurotransmission, GI and biliary motility, intestinal absorption, vascular tone, and cell proliferation.

Five different somatostatin receptors (SSTRs) have been cloned and the biologic properties of each are being unraveled.[9] All five are G-protein-coupled receptors with seven highly conserved transmembrane domains and unique amino and carboxy termini. Phosphorylation sites located within the second and third intracellular loops and in the cytoplasmic C-terminal segment are thought to mediate receptor regulation. Although the naturally occurring peptides bind to all five receptors, somatostatin-28 is relatively selective for SSTR5. The hexapeptide and octapeptide analogues such as octreotide bind only to SSTR2, SSTR3, and SSTR5. These analogues have a longer serum half-life, and their potent inhibitory effect has been used clinically to treat both endocrine and exocrine disorders. For example, octreotide has been shown to decrease fistula output and speed the time it takes for enteric and pancreatic fistulas to close.[10]

Endocrine release of somatostatin occurs during a meal. The major stimulant is probably intraluminal fat. Acidification of the gastric and duodenal mucosa also releases somatostatin in isolated perfused organ preparations. Acetylcholine from the cholinergic neurons inhibits somatostatin release.

Pancreatic polypeptide (PP) is a 36-amino-acid, straight-chain peptide discovered by Kimmel in 1968 during the process of insulin purification. Protein is the most potent enteral stimulator of PP release, closely followed by fat, whereas glucose has a weaker effect.[11,12] Hypoglycemia, whether or not it is insulin induced, strongly stimulates PP secretion through cholinergic stimulation.[13] Phenylalanine, tryptophan, and fatty acids in the duodenum stimulate PP release, probably by inducing CCK and secretin release. In the isolated perfused pancreas, insulin and gastric inhibitory peptide stimulate PP release, while glucagon and somatostatin inhibit it. Vagal stimulation of the pancreas is the most important regulator of PP secretion. In fact, vagotomy eliminates the rise in PP levels usually seen after a meal. This can be used as a test for the completeness of a surgical vagotomy or for the presence of diabetic autonomic neuropathy.

PP is known to inhibit bile secretion, gallbladder contraction, and secretion by the exocrine pancreas. A number of studies suggest that PP's most important role is in glucose regulation through its regulation of hepatic insulin receptor gene expression. Deficiencies in PP secretion due to proximal pancreatectomy or severe chronic pancreatitis, are associated with diminished hepatic insulin sensitivity due to reduced hepatic insulin receptors.[14] These effects are reversed by PP administration.

Recent studies have shown that a fifth islet peptide, ghrelin, is secreted from a distinct population of islet cells, called *epsilon cells*.[15,16] Ghrelin also is present in the gastric fundus in large amounts and stimulates growth hormone secretion via growth hormone releasing hormone release from the pituitary. It is an orexigenic, or appetite-stimulating, peptide the plasma levels of which are increased in obesity. Ghrelin has also been shown to block insulin effects on the liver, and inhibits the β-cell response to incretin hormones and glucose.[17] Therefore, ghrelin secretion from and within the islet may modulate the responses of other islet cells to nutrient and hormonal stimuli.

In addition to the five main peptides secreted by the pancreas, there are a number of other peptide products of the islet cells, including amylin and pancreastatin, as well as neuropeptides such as VIP, galanin, and serotonin. Amylin or islet amyloid polypeptide (IAPP) is a 37-amino-acid polypeptide that was discovered in 1988. IAPP is predominantly expressed by the pancreatic β-cells, where it is stored along with insulin in secretory granules.[18] The function of IAPP seems to be the modulation or counterregulation of insulin secretion and function. Pancreastatin is a recently discovered pancreatic islet peptide product that inhibits insulin, and possibly somatostatin release, and augments glucagon release.[19,20] In addition to this effect on the endocrine pancreas, pancreastatin inhibits pancreatic exocrine secretion.[21]

INTRAISLET REGULATION

The β-cells are located in the central portion of each islet and make up about 70% of the total islet cell mass. The other cell types are located predominantly in the periphery. The delta cells are least plentiful, making up only 5%; the α-cells make up 10%, and the PP cells make up 15%.[22] In contrast to the acinar cells that secrete the full gamut of exocrine enzymes, the islet cells seem to specialize in the secretion of predominantly one hormone. However, individual islet cells can secrete multiple hormones. For example, the β-cells secrete both insulin and amylin, which counterregulates the actions of insulin. In reality, >20 different hormones are secreted by the islets, and the exact functions of this milieu are very complex. There is diversity among the islets depending on their location within the pancreas. In general, islets located closer to major arterioles are larger than islets located more deeply in the parenchyma of the pancreas. The β- and δ-cells are evenly distributed throughout the pancreas, but islets in the head and uncinate process (ventral anlage) have a higher percentage of PP cells and fewer α-cells, whereas islets in the body and tail (dorsal anlage) contain the majority of α-cells and few PP cells. This is clinically significant because pancreatoduodenectomy removes 95% of the PP cells in the pancreas. This may partially explain the higher incidence of glucose intolerance after the Whipple procedure than after distal pancreatectomy. In addition, chronic pancreatitis, which disproportionately affects the pancreatic head, is associated with PP deficiency and pancreatogenic diabetes.[23]

Control of islet secretion is complex and involves an interplay of neural signals, blood flow patterns, and autocrine, paracrine, and hormonal feedback loops. Although the pancreatic islets account for only 2% of the pancreatic mass, they receive about 20 to 30% of the pancreatic arteriolar flow. The manner in which the blood flows through an individual islet can affect islet function because the β-cells are located in the center and the other islet cells are located mostly in the periphery. Blood can flow into the center of the islet and then to the periphery, from the periphery to the center, or from one pole of the islet to the other. In rodents, in vivo microscopy has demonstrated blood flow from one pole to the other. In addition, sphincters at the feeding arteriole were observed regulating blood flow to the periphery or center of the islet as it passed from pole to pole. The sphincters are actually bulging endothelial cells of the afferent capillary. These sphincters seemed to be regulated by blood glucose concentrations, neural impulses, and nitric oxide. The predominant pattern of blood flow through the islets in the human pancreas is still conjectural. However, the peptide products of individual islet cells affect neighboring islet cells in a paracrine fashion. Experiments using isolated perfused pancreas and monoclonal antibodies to specific islet peptides have demonstrated that somatostatin from the δ-cells inhibits insulin secretion from the β-cells, glucagon secretion from the α-cells, and PP secretion from the PP cells. Somatostatin may have an important role in intraislet control of islet cell secretions[24] (Fig. 33-10). Islet hormone secretion also is regulated by endocrine feedback mechanisms. Insulin secretion, for example, is exquisitely sensitive to small increments in the arterial insulin concentration.

Although most of the blood supply to the exocrine pancreas comes directly from the pancreatic arterial flow, blood draining from the islet capillaries goes on to perfuse the exocrine pancreas. Perfusion of the acinar cells with venous blood from the islets allows the endocrine pancreas to influence the exocrine pancreas. For example, insulin release, stimulated by high levels of carbohydrates in the ingested meal, is thought to promote an amylase-rich exocrine secretion, which preferentially provides for digestion of starches and sugars.

ACUTE PANCREATITIS

Definition and Incidence

Acute pancreatitis is an inflammatory disease of the pancreas that is associated with little or no fibrosis of the gland. It can be initiated by several factors, including gallstones, alcohol, trauma, and infections, and, in some cases, it is hereditary. Very often, patients with acute pancreatitis develop additional complications such as sepsis,

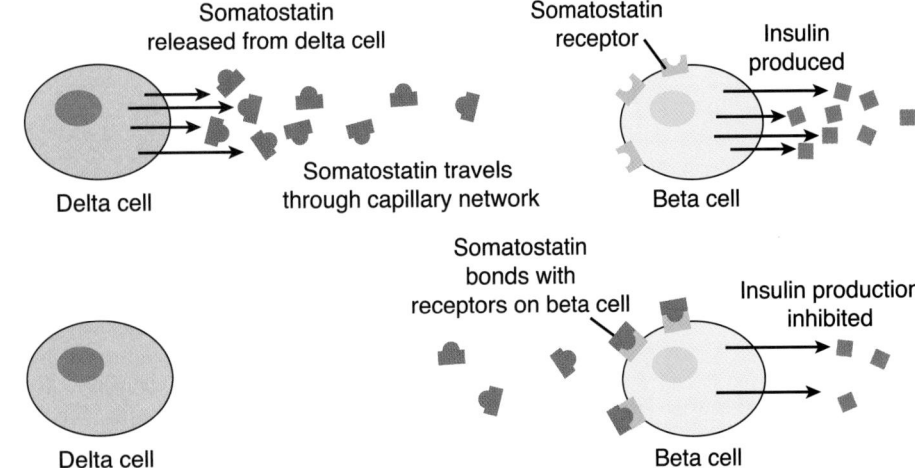

FIG. 33-10. δ- to β-cell axis. Somatostatin from the δ-cells may play an important role in intraislet paracrine control of insulin secretion from the β-cells.

shock, and respiratory and renal failure, resulting in considerable morbidity and mortality.[25] Approximately 300,000 cases occur in the United States each year, 10 to 20% of which are severe, leading to over 3000 deaths. Pancreatitis is a contributing factor in an additional 4000 deaths annually and inflicts a heavy economic burden, accounting for more than $2 billion in health costs annually in the United States.[26] Despite the considerable amount of research under way relating to this disease, its pathophysiologic mechanisms remain incompletely understood. This can be attributed, in part, to the relative inaccessibility of clinical material for experimental studies, which has led to the development of several models of experimental pancreatitis with which its etiology, pathophysiology, and treatment regimens are being explored.

Etiology

The etiology of acute pancreatitis is a complex subject because many different factors have been implicated in the causation of this disease, and sometimes there are no identifiable causes (Table 33-3). Two factors, biliary tract stone disease and alcoholism, account for 80 to 90% of the cases. The remaining 10 to 20 % is accounted for either by idiopathic disease or by a variety of miscellaneous causes including trauma, surgery, drugs, heredity, infection and toxins.

Biliary Tract Disease

Although acute pancreatitis is documented in association with acalculous biliary tract disease, bile duct stones (choledocholithiasis) represent the most common form of associated biliary abnormality. The mechanism by which a gallstone may cause pancreatitis is not entirely clear, although gallstones have been implicated ever since Opie made the seminal observation in 1901 of two patients who died of acute pancreatitis with stones impacted in their ampulla of Vater.[27] This led him to propose the "common-channel hypothesis," in which a blockage below the junction of the biliary and pancreatic ducts would cause bile to flow into the pancreas, which could then be damaged by the detergent action of bile salts.

Important objections to this theory include the anatomic reality that the majority of individuals have such a short common channel that a stone located there would block both the pancreatic and biliary ducts, effectively isolating the two systems. Furthermore,

hydrostatic pressure in the biliary tract is lower than in the pancreas, a condition that would favor abnormal flow of pancreatic juice into the bile duct rather than in the opposite direction. These reservations are bolstered by the observation that, in experimental animals, the flow of normal bile through an unobstructed pancreatic duct does not result in acute pancreatitis (although *forceful* retrograde injection of bile into the pancreas causes injury similar to that of acute pancreatitis).

Another proposed mechanism of causation postulates that passage of a gallstone through the sphincter of Oddi renders it momentarily incompetent, permitting the reflux of duodenal juice containing activated digestive enzymes into the pancreatic ductal system. However, it is questionable whether the transit time through the sphincter of Oddi is long enough to cause sufficient incompetence. Finally, the observation remains that procedures designed to render the sphincter incompetent, such as sphincterotomy, do not routinely cause pancreatitis.

Therefore, although it is reasonable to dismiss an incompetent sphincter of Oddi as an etiologic factor in acute pancreatitis, it is not as simple to dismiss the role of gallstones. A clinical study showed that 88% of patients with acute pancreatitis passed gallstones in their feces within 10 days of the attack. This is in contrast to only 11% of gallstone patients who did not have pancreatitis, suggesting that the process of passing a gallstone may be linked to the development of acute pancreatitis.

This information justifies searching for a more likely causative factor than abnormal bile or duodenal juice backflow into the pancreas. A common phenomenon shared by gallstone disease and other conditions causing acute pancreatitis, such as helminthic infestation of the pancreatic duct or its blockage by tumors, is ductal hypertension resulting from ongoing exocrine secretion into an obstructed pancreatic duct. A simple mechanical explanation has been proposed whereby elevated intraductal pressure causes rupture of the smaller ductules and leakage of pancreatic juice into the parenchyma. Although the pancreatic duct fluid pH is maintained in the range of 8 to 9 by the secretion of bicarbonate, the interstitial pH of 7 within the pancreatic tissue favors activation of proteases when transductal extravasation of fluid occurs. Although pancreatic ductal obstruction and hypertension are likely initiating factors in the etiology of acute pancreatitis, the mechanism by which ductal hypertension initiates pancreatic injury remains under investigation.[27] Although the mechanical factors that initiate the process are unclear, the *colocalization theory* of Steer and Saluja has gained acceptance as the cellular mechanism of acute pancreatitis.[28] In the normal pancreas, the inactive digestive zymogens and the lysosomal hydrolases are found separately in discrete organelles. However, in response to ductal obstruction, hypersecretion, or a cellular insult, these two classes of substances become improperly colocalized in a vacuolar structure within the pancreatic acinar cell. A cascade has been postulated in which trypsinogen colocalizes with cathepsin B to produce activated trypsin, which, in turn, activates the other digestive zymogens. These active digestive enzymes then begin autodigestion within the pancreatic acinar cells, leading to pancreatitis.

Alcohol

Although some patients show the symptoms of acute pancreatitis after little use or even a single exposure to alcohol, the disease commonly occurs in patients who have consumed alcohol for at least 2 years, and often much longer, up to 10 years. In a patient with an exposure history to ethanol and the total absence of other possible causative factors, a first attack of pancreatitis is considered alcohol-related acute pancreatitis. However, it is possible that a first attack of alcohol-related pancreatitis in the typical longstanding alcohol user is really the first manifestation of chronic pancreatitis. The disease can become recurrent with continued alcohol abuse. The nature of alcohol consumed (i.e., beer, wine, or hard liquor) is less significant than a daily intake of between 100 and 150 g of ethanol. Between 10 and 15% of individuals with this degree of alcohol intake go on to

---

TABLE 33-3	Etiologies of acute pancreatitis

Alcohol
Biliary tract disease
Hyperlipidemia
Hereditary
Hypercalcemia
Trauma
    External
    Surgical
    Endoscopic retrograde cholangiopancreatography
Ischemia
    Hypoperfusion
    Atheroembolic
    Vasculitis
Pancreatic duct obstruction
    Neoplasms
    Pancreas divisum
    Ampullary and duodenal lesions
Infections
Venom
Drugs
Idiopathic

Source: Reproduced with permission from Yeo CJ, Cameron JL: Exocrine pancreas, in Townsend CM et al (eds): *Sabiston's Textbook of Surgery*. Philadelphia: Saunders, 2000, p 1117. Copyright Elsevier.

develop pancreatitis, while a similar proportion develop cirrhosis of the liver.

Ethanol can induce pancreatitis by several methods. The "secretion with blockage" mechanism is possible because ethanol causes spasm of the sphincter of Oddi, and, more important, ethanol is a metabolic toxin to pancreatic acinar cells, where it can interfere with enzyme synthesis and secretion. The initial effect of ethanol is a brief secretory increase followed by inhibition. This can lead to elevation of enzyme proteins that can precipitate within the pancreatic duct. Calcium then can precipitate within this protein matrix, causing multiple ductal obstructions, while continued secretion can cause pressure buildup. Ethanol also increases ductal permeability, making it possible for improperly activated enzymes to leak out of the pancreatic duct into the surrounding tissue. The inappropriate activation of trypsin by ethanol has been demonstrated in vitro. Ethanol also transiently decreases pancreatic blood flow, possibly causing focal ischemic injury to the gland.[29,30]

There is evidence that alcoholics who develop pancreatitis have a diet richer in protein and fat than those who do not. Ethanol can alter lipid metabolism, and a transient hyperlipidemic state is sometimes seen during an attack of alcoholic pancreatitis, although the etiologic significance of this observation remains uncertain.

Tumors

A tumor should be considered in a nonalcoholic patient with acute pancreatitis who has no demonstrable biliary tract disease. Approximately 1 to 2% of patients with acute pancreatitis have pancreatic carcinoma, and an episode of acute pancreatitis can be the first clinical manifestation of a periampullary tumor. In both conditions, the pancreatitis possibly results from blockage of secreted juice and its upstream consequences.

Iatrogenic Pancreatitis

Acute pancreatitis can be associated with a number of surgical procedures, most commonly those performed on or close to the pancreas, such as pancreatic biopsy, biliary duct exploration, distal gastrectomy, and splenectomy. Acute pancreatitis is associated postoperatively with Billroth II gastrectomy and jejunostomy, in which increased intraduodenal pressure can cause backflow of activated enzymes into the pancreas. However, pancreatitis also can occur in association with surgery that uses low systemic perfusion, such as cardiopulmonary bypass and cardiac transplantation. Acute pancreatitis has been reported to be associated with severe hypothermia, and the hypothermia associated with cardiopulmonary bypass may be similarly causative. It also is possible that atheromatous emboli or ischemia may cause pancreatic injury. Most commonly, endoscopic retrograde cholangiopancreatography (ERCP) results in pancreatitis in 2 to 10% of patients, due to direct injury and/or intraductal hypertension.

Drugs

For practical reasons, it often is difficult to implicate a drug as the cause of pancreatitis. Many drugs can produce hyperamylasemia and/or abdominal pain, and a drug is considered suspect if the pancreatitis-like illness resolves with its discontinuation. Ethical considerations generally rule out rechallenge with the suspect drug, so the connection often remains vague. However, despite these limitations, certain drugs are known to be capable of causing acute pancreatitis. These include the thiazide diuretics, furosemide, estrogens, azathioprine, L-asparaginase, 6-mercaptopurine, methyldopa, the sulfonamides, tetracycline, pentamidine, procainamide, nitrofurantoin, dideoxyinosine, valproic acid, and acetylcholinesterase inhibitors.

Infections

Though mumps, coxsackievirus, and *Mycoplasma pneumoniae* are believed to be capable of inducing acute pancreatitis by infecting the acinar cells, none of these agents has been isolated from a diseased pancreas. The belief may have arisen from the observation that

antibody titers to mumps and coxsackievirus are elevated in approximately 30% of patients with acute pancreatitis with no other identified cause. However, this elevation may be an anamnestic or nonspecific response to pancreatitis.

Hyperlipidemia

It has been suggested that lipase can liberate large amounts of toxic fatty acids into the pancreatic microcirculation. This could lead to endothelial injury, sludging of blood cells, and consequent ischemic states. Patients with types I and V hyperlipoproteinemia often experience attacks of abdominal pain that are thought to indicate episodes of acute pancreatitis. These episodes are frequently associated with marked hypertriglyceridemia and lactescent serum and can be prevented by dietary modifications that restrict serum triglycerides.

Miscellaneous Causes

An episode of acute pancreatitis may be precipitated by several other factors. Hypercalcemic states arising from hyperparathyroidism can result in both acute and chronic pancreatitis; the mechanism most likely involves hypersecretion and the formation of calcified stones intraductally. Also implicated are infestations by *Ascaris lumbricoides* and the liver fluke *Clonorchis sinensis*, which is endemic to China, Japan, and Southeast Asia. These cause Oriental cholangitis, which is associated with cholangiocarcinoma obstructing the pancreatic duct. A dominant gene mutation following Mendelian inheritance is known to result in hereditary pancreatitis.[31] Whitcomb and associates described several families from various parts of the world who have mutations in their cationic trypsinogen gene *PRSS1*, which results in pancreatitis.[32] Additionally, 20 to 45% of patients with pancreas divisum (unfused ducts of Wirsung and Santorini) develop pancreatitis, but the failure of procedures to improve drainage of the lesser papilla in reducing attacks of pancreatitis, as well as the observed lack of ductal dilatation in such patients, argues against pancreas divisum as an etiologic factor, rendering the role of this condition as yet unclear. Other implicated factors include azotemia, vasculitis, and the sting of the Trinidadian scorpion *Tityus trinitatis*. This scorpion's venom has been shown to cause neurotransmitter discharge from cholinergic nerve terminals, leading to massive production of pancreatic juice. Poisoning with antiacetylcholinesterase insecticides has a similar effect. Finally, no apparent cause can be ascribed to some episodes of acute pancreatitis, and these constitute the group referred to as *idiopathic pancreatitis*. Some of these patients are eventually found to have gallstone-related pancreatitis, which calls for caution in labeling any episode "idiopathic."

Pathophysiology

Acute pancreatitis occurs in varying degrees of severity, the determinants of which are multifactorial. The generally prevalent belief today is that pancreatitis begins with the activation of digestive zymogens inside acinar cells, which cause acinar cell injury. Studies suggest that the ultimate severity of the resulting pancreatitis may be determined by the events that occur subsequent to acinar cell injury.[33] These include inflammatory cell recruitment and activation, as well as generation and release of cytokines and other chemical mediators of inflammation (Fig. 33-11).

Initial Events Leading to the Onset of Pancreatitis

Under physiologic conditions, the pancreas synthesizes a large amount of protein. A majority of these proteins consist of digestive enzymes. Because the exocrine pancreas produces several enzymes that are potentially injurious to itself, it prevents autodigestion by intracellularly assembling the inactive precursors of these enzymes, called *proenzymes* or *zymogens*, which are then transported and secreted outside of the gland. Their activation occurs safely in the duodenum, where the brush-border enzyme enteropeptidase (or enterokinase) activates the trypsinogen, and the resulting trypsin then activates the other zymogens in a cascade reaction.

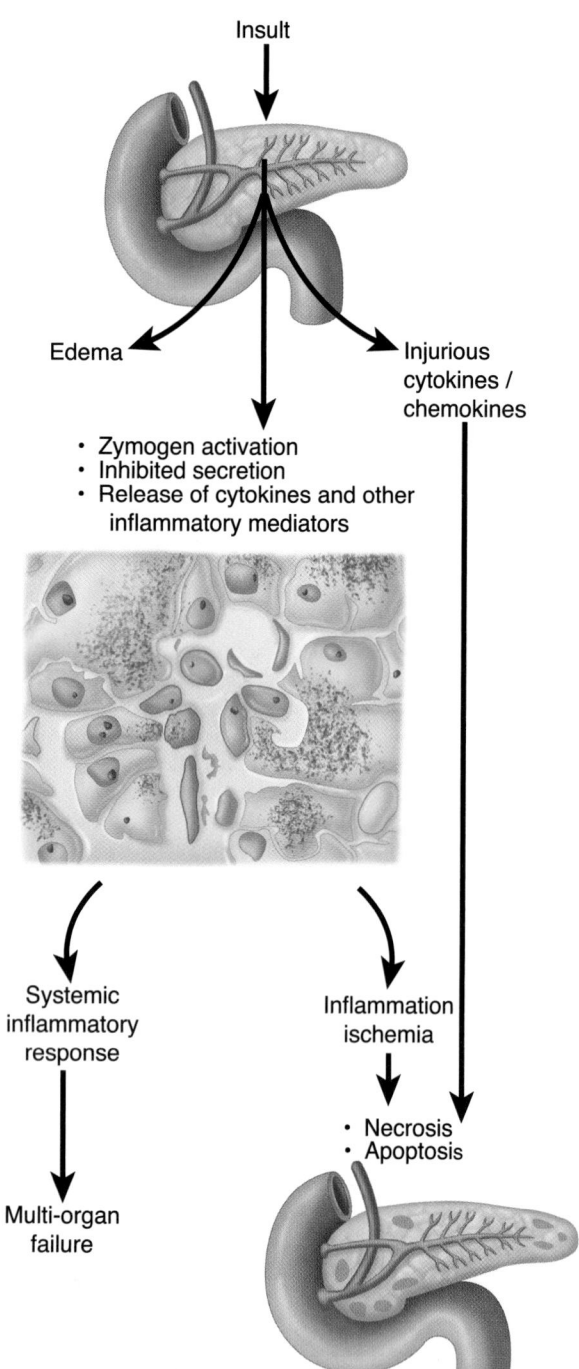

FIG. 33-11. Pathophysiology of acute pancreatitis.

coagulative necrosis. However, the mechanism(s) of erroneous activation are not fully understood.

Using several different models, recent research has focused intensively on the etiology of the activation mechanism. It was seen that the synthesis and intracellular transport of digestive enzymes are not affected during the development of pancreatitis, but that the secretory output of enzymes of the pancreas is markedly reduced.[34] Very early in the development of the disease (shortly after the onset, but before morphologic or biochemical changes are apparent), digestive enzymes are localized in cytoplasmic vacuoles that also contain the lysosomal hydrolase cathepsin B, which is known to activate trypsinogen. Furthermore, intracellular trypsinogen activation was found synchronously with the colocalization phenomenon. Further support for this hypothesis is provided by findings that inhibition of cathepsin B activity by the highly specific inhibitor, CA-074me, protects against intra-acinar cell trypsinogen activation and pancreatitis in two different models of experimental pancreatitis.[35] These studies strongly suggest that trypsinogen is activated because it erroneously colocalizes in cytoplasmic vacuoles with cathepsin B. The opportunity is therefore created for autodigestion, however, the mechanism by which the prematurely activated trypsin causes acinar cell injury and death is not well understood. Recent studies suggest that trypsin, once activated inside the colocalized vacuoles (which appear to be similar to those recently described as autophagic vacuoles,[36] mediates the permeability of these organelles, and causes them to release their contents into the cytosol. Cathepsin B is one of the enzymes released into the cytosol during pancreatitis. Once in the cytosol, it initiates apoptotic cell death by permeabilizing mitochondrial membranes, which allows cytochrome C to be released into the cytosol. This initiates the apoptotic cascade and results in the apoptotic death of the acinar cells (Fig. 33-12).[37]

Factors Determining the Severity of Pancreatitis

Clinically, the severity of acute pancreatitis varies significantly. Some patients experience a mild form of the disease that is self-limiting, while others suffer a more severe and sometimes lethal attack. The factors determining the severity of pancreatitis are multifactorial, but their identification is of considerable therapeutic importance, because their manipulation may decrease the morbidity and mortality associated with the disease. It generally is believed that pancreatitis begins with the intrapancreatic activation of digestive enzyme zymogens, acinar cell injury, and activation of transcription factors such as nuclear factor-κB (NF-κB) and activator protein 1.[38] This, in turn, leads to the production of proinflammatory factors, acinar cell necrosis, systemic inflammatory response syndrome, and distant organ dysfunction, including lung injury that frequently manifests as the acute respiratory distress syndrome (ARDS). The ultimate severity of acute pancreatitis depends on the extent of the systemic inflammatory response, as well as several cytokines and chemokines and their receptors that play a critical role in the activation and migration of inflammatory cells to the affected site.[39]

In addition to the cells of the immune system such as the neutrophils, the pancreatic acinar cells are also a source of inflammatory mediators during pancreatitis. Over the past few years, the list of factors associated with pancreatitis and associated lung injury has grown rapidly to include tumor necrosis factor alpha, monocyte chemotactic protein-1, Mob1, interleukin-1β (IL-1β), platelet activating factor (PAF), substance P, adhesion molecules [intercellular adhesion molecule-1 (ICAM-1) and selectins], IL-6, IL-8, IL-10, C5a, the CCR1 receptor and its ligands, granulocyte-macrophage colony-stimulating factor, macrophage migration inhibitory factor, COX-2, prostaglandin E$_1$, nitric oxide, and reactive oxygen species.[40] In addition, several studies have focused on the protective role played by heat shock proteins in pancreatitis.[41] The ultimate severity of pancreatitis and associated lung injury depends on the balance between the pro- and anti-inflammatory factors. Several therapeutic regimens aimed at reducing the inflammatory response have been tested and include anti–tumor necrosis factor alpha antibody, IL-1 receptor antagonist,

To further protect the pancreas from these potentially harmful digestive enzymes, they are segregated from the cytoplasmic space within acinar cells by being enclosed within membrane-bound organelles, referred to as *zymogen granules*. Another layer of protection is provided by the synthesis of trypsin inhibitors, which are transported and stored along with the digestive enzyme zymogens. These are available to inhibit small amounts of prematurely activated trypsinogen within pancreatic acinar cells. It is generally theorized that acute pancreatitis occurs when this process goes awry and the gland is injured by the erroneously activated enzymes that it produces. There are three reasons for this theory: (a) the pancreas is digestible by the activated enzymes of the duodenum; (b) activated digestive enzymes are found within the pancreas during pancreatitis, and (c) the histology of pancreatitis is suggestive of a

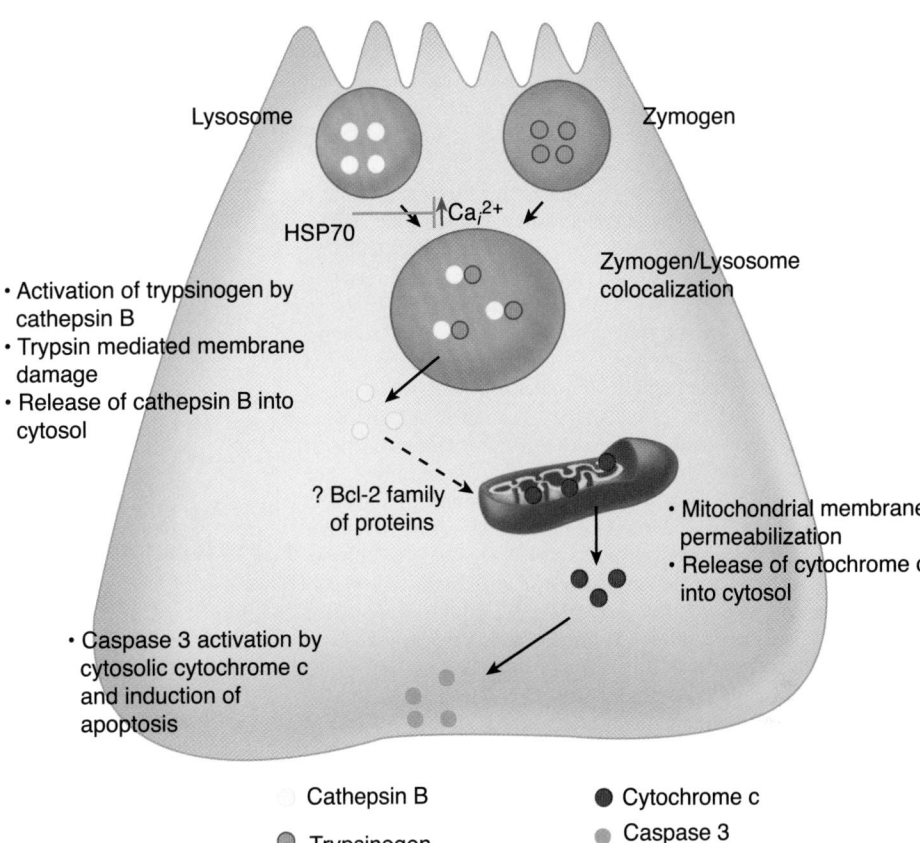

FIG. 33-12. Schematic representation of the overall pancreatitis hypothesis. When acinar cells are pathologically stimulated, their lysosomal and zymogen contents colocalize, whereupon trypsinogen is activated to trypsin by cathepsin B. Increased cytosolic calcium is required for colocalization. The active trypsin mediates the permeability of these colocalized organelles. Once trypsin has permeabilized the cells, cathepsin B and other contents of these colocalized organelles are released into the cytosol. Once in the cytosol, cathepsin B activates apoptosis by causing cytochrome c to be released from the mitochondria. Cathepsin B–induced activation of the Bcl-2 family of proteins may help release cytochrome c from the mitochondria. Heat shock protein 70 (HSP70) overexpression attenuates cytosolic calcium (Ca_i^{2+}), thus preventing colocalization and the subsequent events that lead to acinar cell injury and death.

anti–ICAM-1 and anti-CD3 antibodies, IL-10, recombinant PAF acetylhydrolase, and the calcineurin antagonist FK506. Recent studies also indicate that Toll-like receptor 4 (TLR4) is significant in determining the severity of acute pancreatitis. The TLR4 initiates a complex signaling pathway when it interacts with lipopolysaccharides that result in a proinflammatory response. Mice in which TLR4 is genetically deleted have significantly reduced pancreatitis; this suggests that TLR4 is a significant promoter of proinflammation. However, this effect appears independently of lipopolysaccharides and is probably mediated by a hitherto unknown TLR4 agonist. It is likely that TLR4 antagonists would be a good therapy against pancreatitis.[42]

An alternate approach to prevent or reduce the severity of pancreatitis is to inhibit the two early events in pancreatitis, intrapancreatic trypsinogen and NF-κB activation. Agents that specifically prevent an increase in trypsin activity, either by inhibiting trypsinogen activation and colocalization (e.g., low doses of wortmannin, water immersion, and thermal stress), or inhibiting the cathepsin B activity (E64d or CA074me), have been successful in reducing the severity of pancreatitis in experimental rodent models. Prior thermal (and arsenite) stress and water immersion stress, which upregulate heat shock proteins 70 and 60, respectively, not only prevent cerulein-induced trypsinogen activation, but also inhibit cerulein-induced NF-κB activation in the pancreas and protect against pancreatitis.[43] These studies await verification in a clinical setting.

Diagnosis

The clinical diagnosis of pancreatitis is one of exclusion. The other upper abdominal conditions that can be confused with acute pancreatitis include perforated peptic ulcer, a gangrenous small bowel obstruction, and acute cholecystitis. Because these conditions often have a fatal outcome without surgery, urgent intervention is indicated in the small number of cases in which doubt persists.

All episodes of acute pancreatitis begin with severe pain, generally following a substantial meal. The pain is usually epigastric, but can occur anywhere in the abdomen or lower chest. It has been described as "knifing" or "boring through" to the back, and may be relieved by the patient leaning forward. It precedes the onset of nausea and vomiting, with retching often continuing after the stomach has emptied. Vomiting does not relieve the pain, which is more intense in necrotizing than in edematous pancreatitis. An episode of acute pancreatic inflammation in a patient with known chronic pancreatitis has the same findings.

On examination, the patient may show tachycardia, tachypnea, hypotension, and hyperthermia. The temperature is usually only mildly elevated in uncomplicated pancreatitis. Voluntary and involuntary guarding can be seen over the epigastric region. The bowel sounds are decreased or absent. There are usually no palpable masses. The abdomen may be distended with intraperitoneal fluid. There may be pleural effusion, particularly on the left side.

With increasing severity of disease, the intravascular fluid loss may become life-threatening as a result of sequestration of edematous fluid in the retroperitoneum. Hemoconcentration then results in an elevated hematocrit. However, there also may be bleeding into the retroperitoneum or the peritoneal cavity. In some patients (about 1%), the blood from necrotizing pancreatitis may dissect through the soft tissues and manifest as a bluish discoloration around the umbilicus (Cullen's sign) or in the flanks (Grey Turner's sign). The severe fluid loss may lead to prerenal azotemia with elevated blood urea nitrogen and creatinine levels. There also may be hyperglycemia, hypoalbuminemia, and hypocalcemia sufficient in some cases to produce tetany.

Serum Markers

Because pancreatic acinar cells synthesize, store, and secrete a large number of digestive enzymes (e.g., amylase, lipase, trypsinogen, and elastase), the levels of these enzymes are elevated in the serum of most pancreatitis patients. Because of the ease of measurement, serum amylase levels are measured most often. Serum amylase concentration increases almost immediately with the onset of disease and peaks within several hours. It remains elevated for 3 to 5 days before returning to normal. There is no significant correlation between the magnitude of serum amylase elevation and severity of pancreatitis; in fact, a milder form of acute pancreatitis is often associated with higher levels of serum amylase as compared with that in a more severe form of the disease.

It is important to note that hyperamylasemia can also occur as a result of conditions not involving pancreatitis. For example, hyperamylasemia can occur in a patient with small bowel obstruction, perforated duodenal ulcer, or other intra-abdominal inflammatory conditions. In contrast, a patient with acute pancreatitis may have a normal serum amylase level, which could be due to several reasons. In patients with hyperlipidemia, values might appear to be normal because of interference by lipids with chemical determination of serum amylase. In many cases, urinary clearance of pancreatic enzymes from the circulation increases during pancreatitis; therefore, urinary levels may be more sensitive than serum levels. For these reasons, it is recommended that amylase concentrations also be measured in the urine. Urinary amylase levels usually remain elevated for several days after serum levels have returned to normal. In patients with severe pancreatitis associated with significant necrotic damage, the pancreas may not release large amounts of enzymes into the circulation. It is important to recognize that, in patients with severe pancreatitis, frequent measurement of serum enzymes is not needed. Patients with alcoholic pancreatitis, in general, have a smaller increase in serum amylase levels.

Because hyperamylasemia can be observed in many extrapancreatic diseases, measuring pancreatic-specific amylase (p-amylase) rather than total amylase, which also includes salivary amylase, makes the diagnosis more specific (88 to 93%).

Other pancreatic enzymes also have been evaluated to improve the diagnostic accuracy of serum measurements. Specificity of these markers ranges from 77 to 96%, the highest being for lipase. Measurements of many digestive enzymes also have methodologic limitations and cannot be easily adapted for quantitation in emergency labs. Because serum levels of lipase remain elevated for a

longer time than total or p-amylase, it is the serum indicator of highest probability of the disease.

Ultrasound

Abdominal ultrasound (US) examination is the best way to confirm the presence of gallstones in suspected biliary pancreatitis. It also can detect extrapancreatic ductal dilations and reveal pancreatic edema, swelling, and peripancreatic fluid collections (PFCs). However, in about 20% of patients, the US examination does not provide satisfactory results because of the presence of bowel gas, which may obscure sonographic imaging of the pancreas. A CT scan of the pancreas is more commonly used to diagnose pancreatitis (Fig. 33-13). CT scanning is used to distinguish milder (nonnecrotic) forms of the disease from more severe necrotizing or infected pancreatitis in patients whose clinical presentation raises the suspicion of advanced disease.[44]

Assessment of Severity

An early discrimination between mild edematous and severe necrotizing forms of the disease is of the utmost importance to provide optimal care to the patient. Several predictors of severity, including early prognostic signs, serum markers, and CT scans, are commonly used for this purpose.[45]

Early Prognostic Signs

In 1974, Ranson identified a series of prognostic signs for early identification of patients with severe pancreatitis.[46] Out of these 11 objective parameters, five are measured at the time of admission, whereas the remaining six are measured within 48 hours of admission (Table 33-4). Morbidity and mortality of the disease are directly related to the number of signs present. If the number of positive Ranson signs is less than two, the mortality is generally zero; with three to five positive signs, mortality is increased to 10 to 20%. The mortality rate increases to >50% when there are more than seven positive Ranson signs. Although prognostic signs are useful in

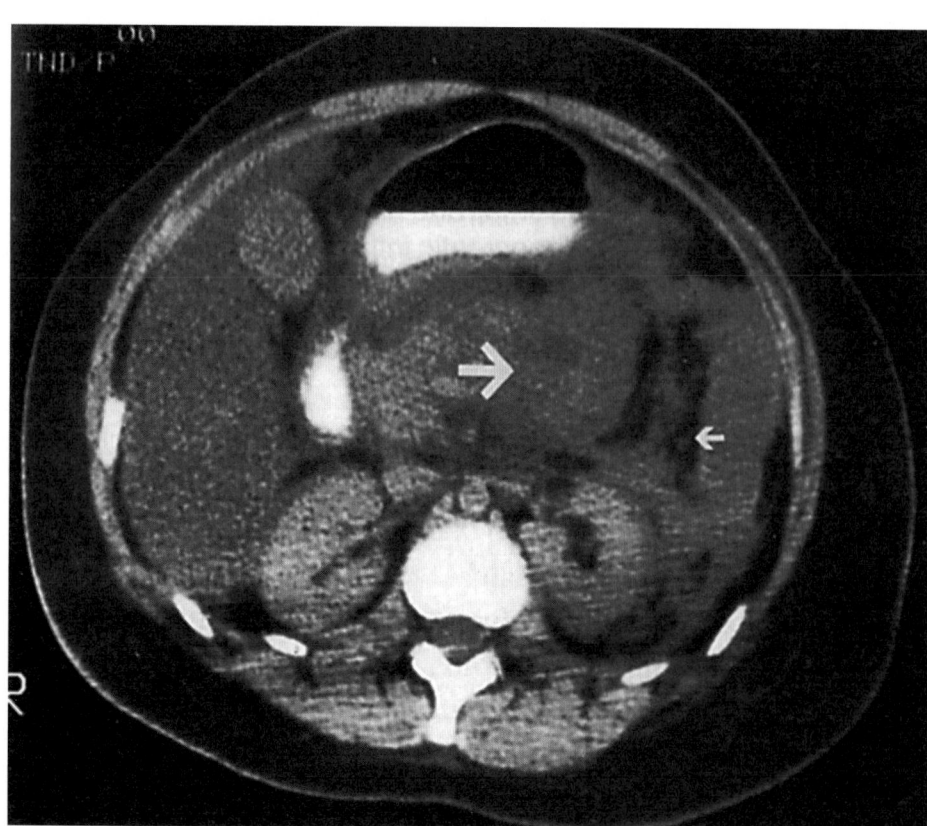

FIG. 33-13. Nonnecrotizing acute pancreatitis. The computed tomographic image reveals edema (*large arrow*) and fluid (*small arrow*) but intact vascularization of the pancreas overall.

TABLE 33-4 Ranson's prognostic signs of pancreatitis

Criteria for acute pancreatitis not due to gallstones

At admission	During the initial 48 h
Age >55 y	Hematocrit fall >10 points
WBC >16,000/mm^3	BUN elevation >5 mg/dL
Blood glucose >200 mg/dL	Serum calcium <8 mg/dL
Serum LDH >350 IU/L	Arterial Po_2 <60 mm Hg
Serum AST >250 U/dL	Base deficit >4 mEq/L
	Estimated fluid sequestration >6 L

Criteria for acute gallstone pancreatitis

At admission	During the initial 48 h
Age >70 y	Hematocrit fall >10 points
WBC >18,000/mm^3	BUN elevation >2 mg/dL
Blood glucose >220 mg/dL	Serum calcium <8 mg/dL
Serum LDH >400 IU/L	Base deficit >5 mEq/L
Serum AST >250 U/dL	Estimated fluid sequestration >4 L

AST = aspartate transaminase; BUN = blood urea nitrogen; LDH = lactate dehydrogenase; Po_2 = partial pressure of oxygen; WBC = white blood cell count.
Source: Data from Ranson JHC: Etiological and prognostic factors in human acute pancreatitis: A review. *Am J Gastroenterol* 77:633, 1982. From Macmillan Publishers Ltd. Ranson JH, Rifkind KM, Roses DF, et al: Prognostic signs and the role of operative management in acute pancreatitis. *Surg Gynecol Obstet* 139:69, 1974.

determining the severity of pancreatitis, there are several limitations to the value of these signs. One has to measure all 11 signs to achieve the best predictability of prognosis, and two full days are needed to complete the profile. A delay of 48 hours after admission merely for assessment may squander a valuable opportunity to prevent a complication during this time. It is important to realize that Ranson's prognostic signs are best used within the initial 48 hours of hospitalization and have not been validated for later time intervals. Although several investigators (Imrie, Banks, Agarwal-Pitchumoni, and others) have proposed modifications to simplify these prognostic criteria throughout the years since their inception, Ranson's original 11 signs are still the most commonly used.

Another set of criteria often used to assess the severity of pancreatitis is the *a*cute *p*hysiology *and* *c*hronic *h*ealth *e*valuation (APACHE-II) score. This grading system assesses severity on the basis of quantitative measures of abnormalities of multiple variables, including vital signs and specific laboratory parameters, coupled with the age and chronic health status of the patient. The main advantage of the APACHE-II scoring system is the immediate assessment of the severity of pancreatitis. A score of eight or more at admission is usually considered indicative of severe disease.[47]

Biochemical Markers

The ideal biochemical marker for prognosis of acute pancreatitis should not only have high specificity and sensitivity but also should be able to discriminate between mild (edematous) and severe (necrotic) disease on admission. Although serum enzymes such as amylase and lipase are helpful in the diagnosis of pancreatitis, these have no prognostic value. Several recent research studies have suggested additional markers that may have prognostic value, including acute phase proteins such as C-reactive protein (CRP), alpha$_2$-macroglobulin, polymorphonuclear neutrophil–elastase, alpha$_1$-antitrypsin, and phospholipase A2. Although CRP measurement is commonly available, many of the others are not. Therefore, at this time, CRP seems to be the marker of choice in clinical settings. The measurement of IL-6 has recently been shown to distinguish patients with mild or severe forms of the disease. However, these tests have to undergo large-scale evaluations before they can be recommended for routine use. Another prognostic marker under evaluation is urinary–trypsinogen activation peptide (TAP). TAP is a five- to seven-amino acid peptide that is released from the N-terminus of trypsinogen during its activation. In studies, Neoptolemos and colleagues have shown a good correlation between the severity of pancreatitis and concentrations of TAP in urine.[48] However, further testing and methodologic developments are needed before TAP can be used as a routine prognostic marker.

Computed Tomography Scan

CT scanning with bolus IV contrast has become the gold standard for detecting and assessing the severity of pancreatitis. Although clinically mild pancreatitis is usually associated with interstitial edema, severe pancreatitis is associated with necrosis. In interstitial pancreatitis, the microcirculation of the pancreas remains intact, and the gland shows uniform enhancement on IV contrast-enhanced CT scan (see Fig. 33-13). In necrotizing pancreatitis, however, the microcirculation is disrupted; therefore, the enhancement of the gland on contrast-enhanced CT scan is considerably decreased. The presence of air bubbles on a CT scan is an indication of infected necrosis or pancreatic abscess (Fig. 33-14). Currently, IV

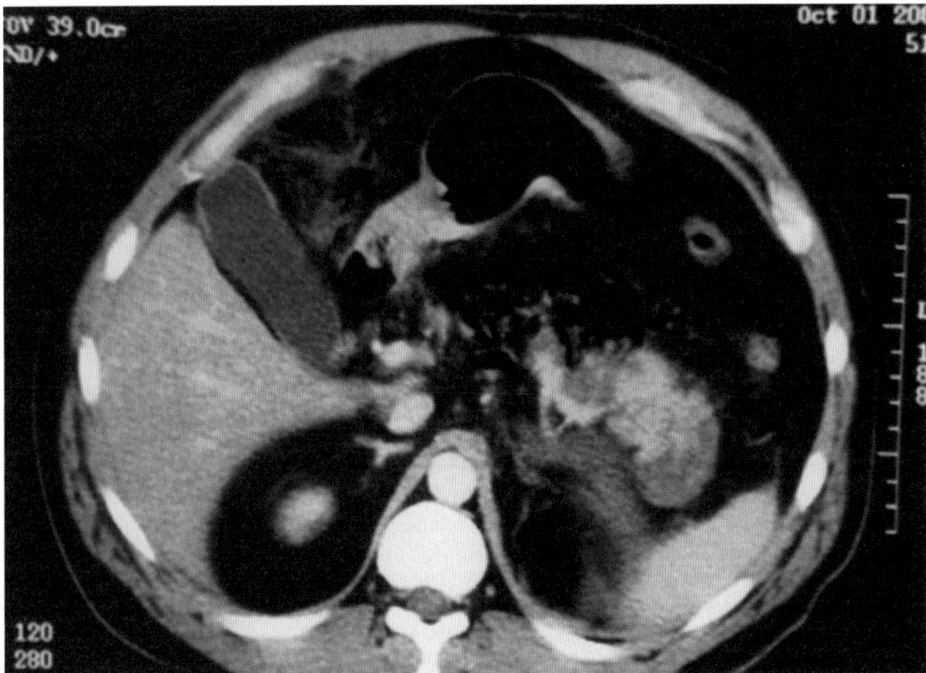

FIG. 33-14. Necrotizing (infected) acute pancreatitis. The computed tomographic image reveals areas of nonperfusion and the presence of gas in the region of severe necrosis, which indicates infection.

(bolus) contrast-enhanced CT scanning is routinely performed on patients who are suspected of harboring severe pancreatitis, regardless of their Ranson's or APACHE scores.[49]

Treatment

The severity of acute pancreatitis covers a broad spectrum of illness, ranging from the mild and self-limiting to the life-threatening necrotizing variety. Regardless of severity, hospitalization of the patient with suspected acute pancreatitis for observation and diagnostic study is usually mandatory. Upon confirmation of the diagnosis, patients with moderate to severe disease should be transferred to the intensive care unit for observation and maximal support. The most important initial treatment is conservative intensive care with the goals of oral food and fluid restriction, replacement of fluids and electrolytes parenterally as assessed by central venous pressure and urinary excretion, and control of pain. In severe acute pancreatitis, or when signs of infection are present, most experts recommend broad-spectrum antibiotics (e.g., imipenem) and careful surveillance for complications of the disease (Table 33-5).[49]

Mild Pancreatitis

Pancreatitis is classified as mild when the patient has no systemic complications, low APACHE-II scores and Ranson's signs, sustained clinical improvement, and when a CT scan rules out necrotizing pancreatitis. The treatment then is mostly supportive and has the important aim of *resting the pancreas* through restriction of oral food and fluids. Nasogastric suction and H$_2$-blockers have routinely been used in this connection, based on the reasoning that even the smallest amount of gastric acid reaching the duodenum could stimulate pancreatic secretion. However, these measures are of little value. The following secretion-inhibiting drugs have also been tried without notable success: atropine, calcitonin, somatostatin, glucagon, and fluorouracil.[50]

Pancreatitis is also an autodigestive process, and various protease-inhibiting drugs, including aprotinin, gabexate mesylate, camostate, and phospholipase A2 inhibitors, as well as fresh frozen plasma, have been tested to prevent proteolysis, but with little success. Because a significant component of the patient's distress arises from the inflammatory aspect of pancreatitis, various methods have been tried to alleviate inflammation, including indomethacin and the prostaglandin inhibitors; but again, these have not proved to be of much value. Some recent studies examined a different strategy, namely the use of PAF antagonists such as PAF acetylhydrolase and Lexipafant. These showed promising results in experimental animals and in initial clinical studies, but did not live up to their promise in larger-scale clinical trials.[51]

The current principles of treatment are physiologic monitoring, metabolic support, and maintenance of fluid balance, which can become dangerously disturbed even in mild acute pancreatitis because of fluid sequestration, vomiting, and sudoresis. Because hypovolemia can result in pancreatic and other visceral ischemia, fluid balance should be assessed at least every 8 hours initially.

The severe pain of acute pancreatitis prevents the patient from resting, and results in ongoing cholinergic discharge, which stimulates gastric and pancreatic secretion. Therefore, pain management is of great importance. Administration of buprenorphine, pentazocine, procaine hydrochloride, and meperidine are all of value in controlling abdominal pain. Morphine is to be avoided, due to its potential to cause sphincter of Oddi spasm. Antibiotic therapy has not proved to be of value in the absence of signs or documented sources of infection.

Cautious resumption of oral feeding consisting of small and slowly increasing meals is permissible after the abdominal pain and tenderness have subsided, serum amylase has returned to normal, and the patient experiences hunger. This usually occurs within a week of the onset of an attack of mild acute pancreatitis. A low-fat, low-protein diet is advocated as the initial form of nutrition following an attack of acute pancreatitis.

TABLE 33-5	Complications of acute pancreatitis

I. Local
  A. Pancreatic phlegmon
  B. Pancreatic abscess
  C. Pancreatic pseudocyst
  D. Pancreatic ascites
  E. Involvement of adjacent organs, with hemorrhage, thrombosis, bowel infarction, obstructive jaundice, fistula formation, or mechanical obstruction

II. Systemic
  A. Pulmonary
    1. Pneumonia, atelectasis
    2. Acute respiratory distress syndrome
    3. Pleural effusion
  B. Cardiovascular
    1. Hypotension
    2. Hypovolemia
    3. Sudden death
    4. Nonspecific ST-T wave changes
    5. Pericardial effusion
  C. Hematologic
    1. Hemoconcentration
    2. Disseminated intravascular coagulopathy
  D. GI hemorrhage
    1. Peptic ulcer
    2. Erosive gastritis
    3. Portal vein or splenic vein thrombosis with varices
  E. Renal
    1. Oliguria
    2. Azotemia
    3. Renal artery/vein thrombosis
  F. Metabolic
    1. Hyperglycemia
    2. Hypocalcemia
    3. Hypertriglyceridemia
    4. Encephalopathy
    5. Sudden blindness (Purtscher's retinopathy)
  G. Central nervous system
    1. Psychosis
    2. Fat emboli
    3. Alcohol withdrawal syndrome
  H. Fat necrosis
    1. Intra-abdominal saponification
    2. Subcutaneous tissue necrosis

Source: Reproduced with permission from Greenberger NJ, Toskes PP, Isselbacher KJ: Acute and chronic pancreatitis, in Isselbacher KJ et al (eds): *Harrison's Principles of Internal Medicine,* 13th ed. New York: McGraw-Hill, 1994, p 1524.

Severe Pancreatitis

Pancreatitis can be classified as severe based on predictors such as APACHE-II scores and Ranson's signs, and any evidence that the condition is severe mandates care of the patient in the intensive care unit. Such evidence may take various forms, such as the onset of encephalopathy, a hematocrit >50%, urine output <50 mL/h, hypotension, fever, or peritonitis. Elderly patients with three or more Ranson's criteria should also be monitored carefully despite the absence of severe pain.[52]

Patients may develop ARDS, and many patients who die during the early stages of severe acute pancreatitis have this complication. Until recently, the lung injury has been thought to be caused by the systemic release of phospholipase A2 and other enzymes that directly damage alveolar tissue and pulmonary capillaries. In addition, recent evidence implicates the cell adhesion molecule ICAM-1, neutrophils, PAF, substance P, and certain chemokines. The presence of ARDS usually requires assisted ventilation with positive

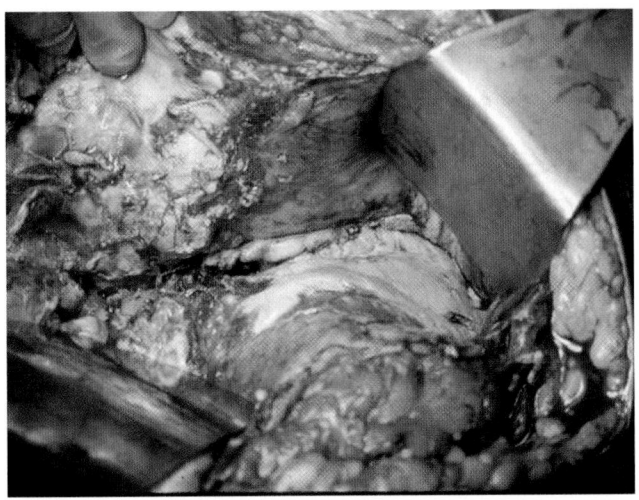

FIG. 33-15. Operative view of infected acute pancreatitis. Peripancreatic infection, characterized by mucopurulent exudate, extends far beyond the boundaries of the pancreas in the retroperitoneum.

suspected. A CT-guided, FNA then confirms or disproves infection, and in the latter instance, the patient can be managed medically. The last and most serious condition is that of the patient who appears to be very ill, has high APACHE-II and Ranson's scores, and shows evidence of systemic toxicity, including shock. Patients in this category have a poor chance of survival without aggressive débridement, and a decision may be made to proceed with exploration simply due to a relentless course of deterioration despite maximal medical therapy.[50] It must be emphasized that current opinion is against débridement in sterile necrosis unless it is accompanied by life-threatening systemic complications (Fig. 33-16).

Pancreatic Abscess

A pancreatic abscess occurs 2 to 6 weeks after the initial attack, in contrast to infected necrosis, which occurs in the first few hours or days. The mechanism of delayed infection is not clear, but the treatment consists of external drainage, whether established by surgical or by percutaneous catheter-based methods.

Nutritional Support

The guiding principle of resting the pancreas dictates that patients with acute pancreatitis not be fed orally until their clinical condition

end-expiratory pressure. The value of peritoneal lavage in removing enzyme-rich ascites remains unclear. It has been advocated in patients with deteriorating respiratory function and/or shock that is refractory to maximal management, but its effectiveness in reducing the mortality risk of severe acute pancreatitis remains unproven.

Acute pancreatitis may be accompanied by cardiovascular events such as cardiac arrhythmia, myocardial infarction, cardiogenic shock, and congestive heart failure. The conventional modalities of treatment apply in these cases in addition to the support described above.

Infections

Infection is a serious complication of acute pancreatitis and is the most common cause of death. It is caused most often by translocated enteric bacteria and is seen commonly in necrotizing rather than interstitial pancreatitis. If there is an indication of infection (e.g., retroperitoneal air on CT scan), then a CT- or US-guided fine-needle aspiration (FNA) should be performed for Gram's stain and culture of the fluid or tissue, and the indicated antibiotic therapy initiated. However, antibiotics alone may not be effective in infected necrosis, which has a mortality of nearly 50% unless débrided surgically (Fig. 33-15). The long-held opinion that antibiotic prophylaxis in necrotizing pancreatitis is of little use has been altered by studies showing a beneficial prophylactic effect with antibiotics such as metronidazole, imipenem, and third-generation cephalosporins.[53-55] Because *Candida* species are common inhabitants of the upper GI tract, *Candida* sepsis and secondary fungal infection of pancreatic necrosis is a risk in severe disease, and many surgeons advocate the use of empiric therapy with fluconazole in cases of severe acute pancreatitis.

Sterile Necrosis

Patients with sterile necrosis have a far better prognosis than those with infected necrosis, with a reported mortality of near zero in the absence of systemic complications. However, others report mortality rates as high as 38% in patients with a single systemic complication.

Treatment of sterile necrotic pancreatitis falls into three degrees of aggressiveness. At one end of the scale is the patient with no systemic complications and no concerns about secondary infections, who can be managed with the supportive care (see Mild Pancreatitis) and be cautiously brought back to refeeding. The area of sterile necrosis may evolve into a chronic pseudocyst or may resolve. An intermediate course is demonstrated by the patient who develops systemic complications, and in whom a secondary infection is

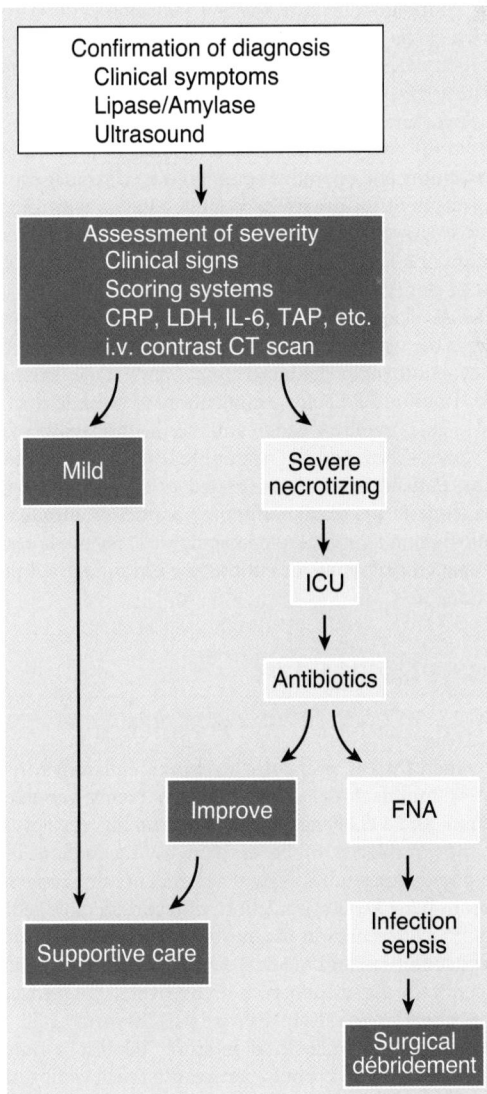

FIG. 33-16. Algorithm for managing acute pancreatitis. CRP = C-reactive protein; CT = computed tomography; FNA = fine-needle aspiration; ICU = intensive care unit; IL-6 = interleukin 6; LDH = lactate dehydrogenase; TAP = trypsinogen activation peptide.

improves. This generally occurs in 3 to 7 days in patients with mild pancreatitis, but the situation in patients with severe pancreatitis is more complicated, requiring nutritional support for several weeks. This can be provided by total parenteral nutrition (TPN) or by enteral nutrition through a jejunal tube.[56] There is some debate regarding the preferred route, because TPN is known to result in early atrophy of the gut mucosa, a condition that favors transmigration of luminal bacteria, and intrajejunal feeding still stimulates pancreatic exocrine secretion through the release of enteric hormones. Recent animal studies and preliminary clinical trials on humans suggest that, on balance, jejunal feeding may be superior to TPN, and a recent review of nasogastric feeding in acute pancreatitis indicated the safety of this technique even in patients with severe pancreatitis.[57]

Treatment of Biliary Pancreatitis

Gallstones are the most common cause of acute pancreatitis worldwide. Most patients pass the offending gallstone(s) during the early hours of acute pancreatitis, but have additional stones capable of inducing future episodes. This raises the question of the timing of surgical or endoscopic clearance of gallstones. The issue of when to intervene is controversial. Several studies have been aimed at resolving this controversy, but the issue is clouded by the fact that each position is open to some theoretical objection. Additional points of contention include varying inclusion criteria, years of observation of the studied groups, and a lack of uniformity regarding definitions. General consensus favors either urgent intervention (cholecystectomy) within the first 48 to 72 hours of admission, or briefly delayed intervention (after 72 hours, but during the initial hospitalization) to give an inflamed pancreas time to recover. Cholecystectomy and operative common duct clearance is probably the best treatment for otherwise healthy patients with obstructive pancreatitis. However, patients who are at high risk for surgical intervention are best treated by endoscopic sphincterotomy, with clearance of stones by ERCP.

In the case of acute biliary pancreatitis in which chemical studies suggest that the obstruction persists after 24 hours of observation, emergency endoscopic sphincterotomy and stone extraction is indicated. Routine ERCP for examination of the bile duct is discouraged in cases of biliary pancreatitis, as the probability of finding residual stones is low, and the risk of ERCP-induced pancreatitis is significant. Patients who are suspected of harboring a persistent impacted stone in the distal common bile duct or ampulla should have confirmation by radiologic imaging (CT, magnetic resonance cholangiopancreatography, or endoscopic ultrasonography) before intervention.

CHRONIC PANCREATITIS

Definition, Incidence, and Prevalence

Chronic pancreatitis is an incurable, chronic inflammatory condition that is multifactorial in its etiology, highly variable in its presentation, and a challenge to treat successfully. Autopsy studies indicate the prevalence to be as high as 5% in Scandinavia,[58] although population studies suggest a prevalence that ranges from 5 to 27 persons per 100,000 population, with considerable geographic variation.[59,60] Differences in diagnostic criteria, regional nutrition, alcohol consumption, and medical access account for variations in the frequency of the diagnosis, but the overall incidence of the disease has risen progressively over the past 50 years[61] (Fig. 33-17).

Autopsy data are difficult to interpret because a number of changes associated with chronic pancreatitis, such as fibrosis, duct ectasia, and acinar atrophy, are also present in asymptomatic elderly patients.[62] Although the prevalence of chronic pancreatitis in patients with alcoholic cirrhosis and fatty liver ranges from 9 to 34%, the prevalence of chronic pancreatitis among known alcoholics is only 5 to 15%.[61,63,64]

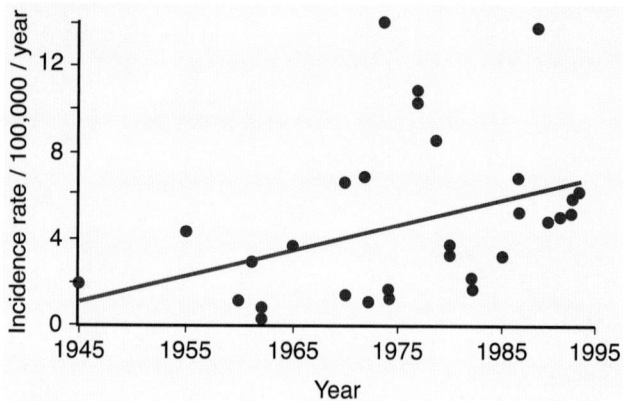

FIG. 33-17. Incidence of chronic pancreatitis. The reported incidence of chronic pancreatitis has increased steadily over the past 50 years. *(Reproduced with permission from Worning.[61])*

Etiology

Worldwide, alcohol consumption and abuse is associated with chronic pancreatitis in up to 70% of cases (Table 33-6). In 1878, Friedreich proposed that "a general chronic interstitial pancreatitis may result from excessive alcoholism (drunkard's pancreas).[65] Since that observation, numerous studies have shown that a causal relationship exists between alcohol and chronic pancreatitis, but the prevalence of this etiology of the disease in Western countries ranges widely, from 38 to 94%.[61] Other major causes worldwide include tropical (nutritional) and idiopathic disease, as well as hereditary causes.

Alcohol

There is a linear relationship between exposure to alcohol and the development of chronic pancreatitis.[66] The risk of disease is present in patients with even a low or occasional exposure to alcohol (1 to 20 g/d), so there is no threshold level of alcohol exposure below which there is no risk of developing chronic pancreatitis. Furthermore, although the risk of disease is dose related, and highest in heavy (150 g/d) drinkers, <15% of confirmed alcohol abusers suffer from chronic pancreatitis.[67,68] In a study of 247 patients with fatal acute alcoholic pancreatitis, 53% of patients had no autopsy evidence of chronic pancreatitis.[69] However, the duration of alcohol consumption is definitely associated with the development of pancreatic disease. The onset of disease typically occurs between ages 35 to 40, after 16 to 20 years of heavy alcohol consumption. Recurrent episodes of acute pancreatitis are typically followed by chronic symptoms after 4 or 5 years.[30,70]

Although the pattern of disease presentation is well known in those alcohol users who develop pancreatic disease, the pathophysiology of alcohol-induced pancreatic disease is still an area of active

TABLE 33-6	Etiology of chronic pancreatitis

Alcohol, 70%
Idiopathic (including tropical), 20%
Other, 10%
    Hereditary
    Hyperparathyroidism
    Hypertriglyceridemia
    Autoimmune pancreatitis
    Obstruction
    Trauma
    Pancreas divisum

Necrosis-fibrosis sequence

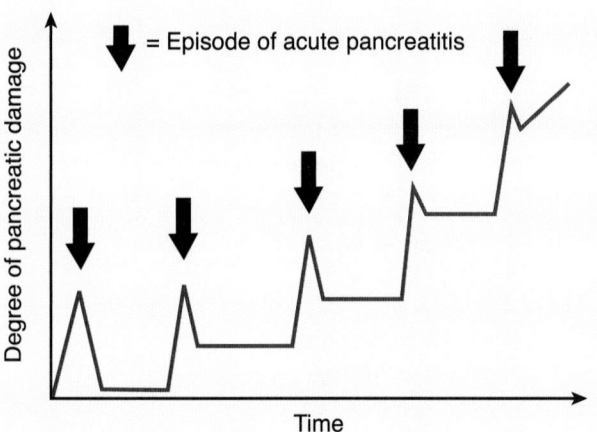

FIG. 33-18. "Multiple hit" theory of the etiology of acute pancreatitis. Multiple episodes of acute pancreatitis cause progressively more organized inflammatory changes that ultimately result in chronic inflammation and scarring. *(Reproduced with permission from Apte et al.[30] Copyright Elsevier.)*

investigation. In their 1946 classic study, Comfort, Gambrill, and Baggenstoss proposed that chronic pancreatitis was the result of multiple episodes of acute inflammation, with residual and progressively increasing chronic inflammation.[71] Subsequently, other investigators proposed that initial acute inflammation was not necessarily linked to chronic changes in the pancreas,[72] and Kondo and associates showed that other, additional factors were necessary for repeated exposure to alcohol to cause chronic pancreatitis.[73] Regardless of the requirement for other predisposing or facilitative factors, the concept that multiple episodes (or a prolonged course) of pancreatic injury ultimately leads to chronic disease is widely accepted as the pathophysiologic sequence[30] (Fig. 33-18). Laboratory studies in rodents reveal that repeated episodes of acute non–alcohol-induced pancreatitis results in findings of chronic pancreatitis,[74,75] and the induction of severe acute pancreatitis by a single intraductal infusion of oleic acid reproducibly results in chronic pancreatitis in rats.[76]

Alcohol-associated chronic pancreatitis is less common in Japan and India, where there is a lower per capita consumption of alcohol, and its incidence is otherwise quite variable with regard to geography, nutrition, and race.[72] Although alcohol exposure to the pancreatic ductal system, or elevated levels of alcohol in the bloodstream, has been shown to alter the integrity and function of pancreatic ducts and acini directly,[77,78] most investigators believe that alcohol metabolites such as acetaldehyde, combined with oxidant injury, result in local parenchymal injury that is preferentially targeted to the pancreas in predisposed individuals. Repeated or severe episodes of toxin-induced injury activate a cascade of cytokines, which, in turn, induces pancreatic stellate cells (PSCs) to produce collagen and cause fibrosis (Fig. 33-19). It remains to be determined whether alcohol sensitizes the pancreas of susceptible individuals to another cause of acute inflammation, or whether genetic or other factors predispose to direct alcohol-related injury.[30]

Since the discovery of specific genetic mutations and deletions associated with hereditary pancreatitis (see Hereditary Pancreatitis), many studies have been undertaken to determine whether specific genetic abnormalities are associated with alcoholic chronic pancreatitis.[79] No mutations of the major genetic abnormality associated with hereditary pancreatitis, the cationic trypsinogen gene or *PRSS1*,[31] have been identified in patients with alcoholic chronic pancreatitis. A

second genetic marker for hereditary pancreatitis, the PSTI, or *SPINK1* gene, has also been studied. Mutations in *SPINK1* are observed in the general population, and Witt and colleagues found a 5.8% rate of *SPINK1* mutations in patients with alcoholic pancreatitis, compared to a 0.8% rate in the control population.[80] Studies that have examined some of the known polymorphisms and mutations of the cystic fibrosis transmembrane receptor (*CFTR*) gene have thus far failed to demonstrate an association with alcoholic chronic pancreatitis. Therefore, a dominant hereditary cofactor for alcoholic pancreatitis remains to be elucidated.

Alcohol may interfere with the intracellular transport and discharge of digestive enzymes, and may contribute to the colocalization of digestive enzymes and lysosomal hydrolase within acinar cells, leading to autodigestion[81,82] (see section on Acute Pancreatitis). A high-protein, low-bicarbonate, low-volume secretory output is seen after chronic alcohol exposure[83] which may contribute to the precipitation of proteins in secondary ducts in the early stages of chronic pancreatitis.[84] Lithostathine, a protein found in pancreatic juice, inhibits the formation of calcium carbonate crystals,[85] and has been found to be decreased in the pancreatic duct fluid in alcoholic and nonalcoholic chronic pancreatitis patients[86] (see section on Stone Formation below). The zymogen membrane-associated protein GP2 is also found in protein precipitates within small ducts and may contribute to small duct obstruction in chronic pancreatitis.[87] Calcium is complexed to protein plugs in small ductules, secondary ducts, and, eventually, in the main ductal system, which causes ductal cell injury and obstruction of the secretory system, which further promotes an inflammatory response.

Cigarette smoking has been strongly associated with chronic pancreatitis and with the development of calcific pancreatitis.[88] Studies on the role of smoking in the development of alcoholic pancreatitis have been conflicting, although the risk of cancer in chronic pancreatitis is increased significantly by smoking. In hereditary pancreatitis, smoking has been found to lower the age of onset of carcinoma by about 20 years.[89] Smoking would therefore appear to be a definite risk factor for the late complications of alcoholic pancreatitis, if not an early cofactor.

Hyperparathyroidism

Hypercalcemia is a known cause of pancreatic hypersecretion,[90] and chronic hypercalcemia caused by untreated hyperparathyroidism is associated with chronic calcific pancreatitis.[91] Hypercalcemia is also a stimulant for pancreatic calcium secretion, which contributes to calculus formation and obstructive pancreatopathy. The treatment is correction of the hyperparathyroidism and assessment of any additional endocrinopathies.

Hyperlipidemia

In addition to the risk of acute pancreatitis, hyperlipidemia and hypertriglyceridemia predispose women to chronic pancreatitis when they receive estrogen replacement therapy.[92] Fasting triglyceride levels <300 mg/dL are below the threshold for this to occur, and the mechanism of estrogen potentiation of hyperlipidemia-induced chronic pancreatitis is unknown. It is assumed that chronic changes occur after repeated subclinical episodes of acute inflammation. Aggressive therapy of hyperlipidemia is therefore important in peri- or postmenopausal patients who are candidates for estrogen therapy.

Classification

A major impediment to an accurate accounting of the frequency and severity of chronic pancreatitis has been the difficulty with which investigators and clinicians have struggled to identify a useful classification system. Multiple classification systems have been proposed. In 1963, Henri Sarles organized a symposium in Marseille, France, and subsequent symposia were held in Cambridge (1983), Marseille (1984), and Rome (1998). A current classification system, as delineated by Singer and Chari, is shown in Table 33-7.[93]

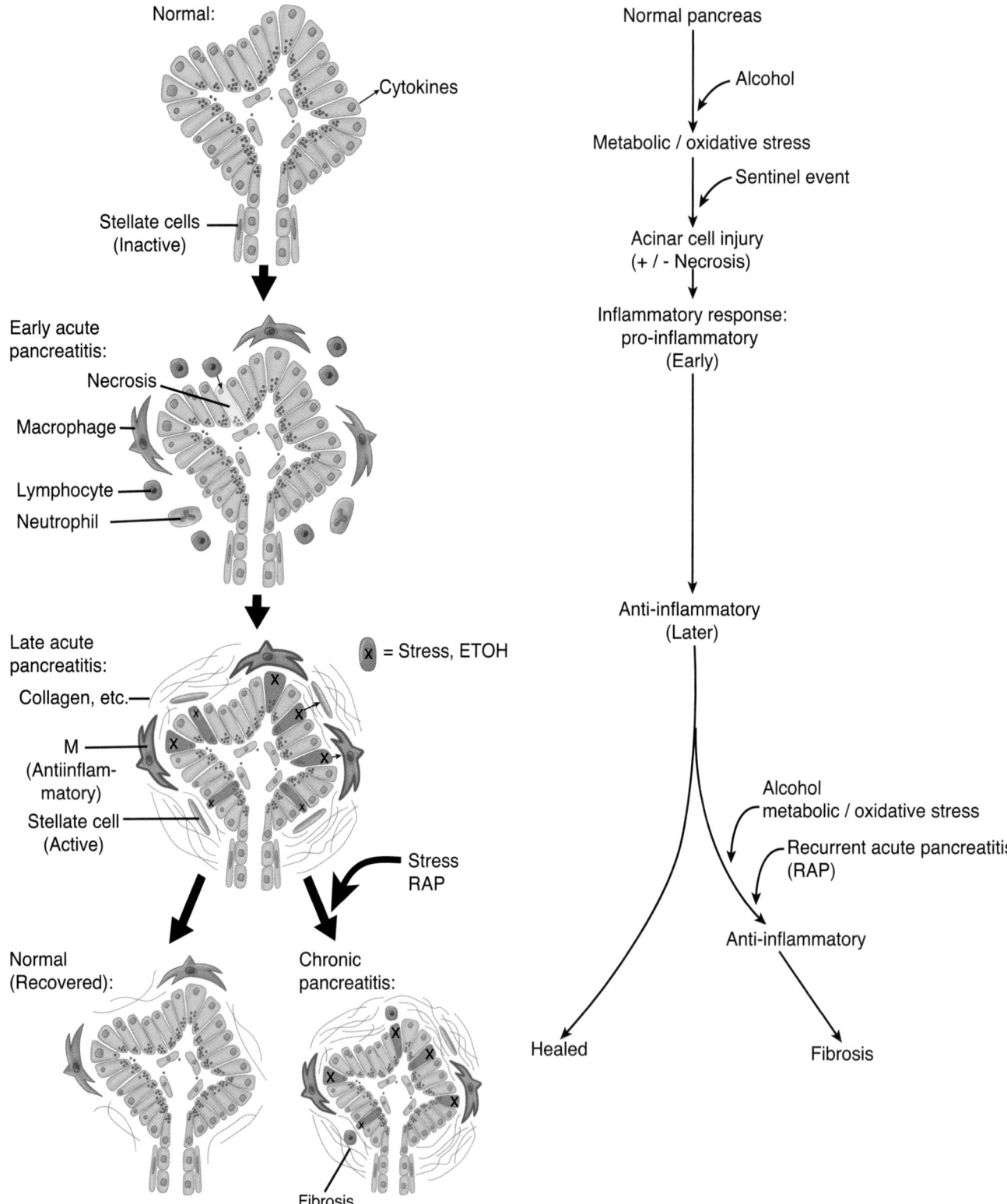

FIG. 33-19. The sentinel acute pancreatitis event (SAPE) hypothesis for the development of chronic pancreatitis. A critical episode of acute pancreatitis activates cytokine-induced transformation of pancreatic stellate cells, which results in collagen production and fibrosis. ETOH = ethyl alcohol. *(Reproduced with permission from Schneider et al.[127] Copyright Elsevier.)*

TABLE 33-7	Classification of chronic pancreatitis			
Chronic Calcific Pancreatitis	**Chronic Obstructive Pancreatitis**	**Chronic Inflammatory Pancreatitis**	**Chronic Autoimmune Pancreatitis**	**Asymptomatic Pancreatic Fibrosis**
Alcohol	Pancreatic tumors	Unknown	Associated with autoimmune disorders (e.g., primary sclerosing cholangitis)	Chronic alcoholic
Hereditary	Ductal stricture			Endemic in asymptomatic residents in tropical climates
Tropical	Gallstone- or trauma-induced pancreas divisum			
Hyperlipidemia			Sjögren's syndrome	
Hypercalcemia			Primary biliary cirrhosis	
Drug-induced				
Idiopathic				

Source: Reproduced with permission from Singer et al.[93]

Chronic Calcifying (Lithogenic) Pancreatitis

This type is the largest subgroup in the current classification scheme and includes patients with calcific pancreatitis of most etiologies. Although the majority of patients with calcific pancreatitis have a history of alcohol abuse, stone formation and parenchymal calcification can develop in a variety of etiologic subgroups; hereditary pancreatitis and tropical pancreatitis are particularly noteworthy for the formation of stone disease. The clinician should therefore avoid the assumption that calcific pancreatitis confirms the diagnosis of alcohol abuse.

Chronic Obstructive Pancreatitis

This refers to chronic inflammatory changes that are caused by the compression or occlusion of the proximal ductal system by tumor, gallstone, posttraumatic scar, or inadequate duct caliber (as in pancreas divisum). Obstruction of the main pancreatic duct by inflammatory (posttraumatic) or neoplastic processes can result in diffuse fibrosis, dilated main and secondary pancreatic ducts, and acinar atrophy. The patient may have little in the way of pain symptoms or may present with signs of exocrine insufficiency. Intraductal stone formation is rare, and both functional and structural abnormalities may improve when the obstructive process is relieved or removed. Trauma to the pancreas frequently results in duct injury and leakage, which may result in pseudocyst

formation as well as local scar formation. Inadequately treated pancreatic trauma may result in persistent inflammatory changes in the distal gland.[94]

Pancreas divisum represents a special case of obstructive pancreatitis. It is the most common congenital anomaly involving the pancreas and occurs in up to 10% of children. It is thought to predispose the pancreas to recurrent acute pancreatitis and chronic pancreatitis, due to functional obstruction of a diminutive duct of Santorini that fails to communicate with Wirsung's duct (Fig. 33-20). However, the classic picture of obstructive pancreatopathy with a dilated dorsal duct is unusual in pancreas divisum, so a decompressive operation or a lesser papilla sphincteroplasty is frequently not feasible or unsuccessful. Endoscopic stenting through the lesser papilla may result in temporary relief of symptoms, and this response would increase the possibility that a permanent surgical or endoscopic intervention will be successful. Although some authors emphasize the pathologic implications of pancreas divisum,[95,96] others express skepticism that it represents a true risk to pancreatic secretory capacity or contributes to the development of chronic pancreatitis.[97,98]

Chronic Inflammatory Pancreatitis

Chronic inflammatory pancreatitis is characterized by diffuse fibrosis and a loss of acinar elements with a predominant mononuclear cell infiltration throughout the gland.

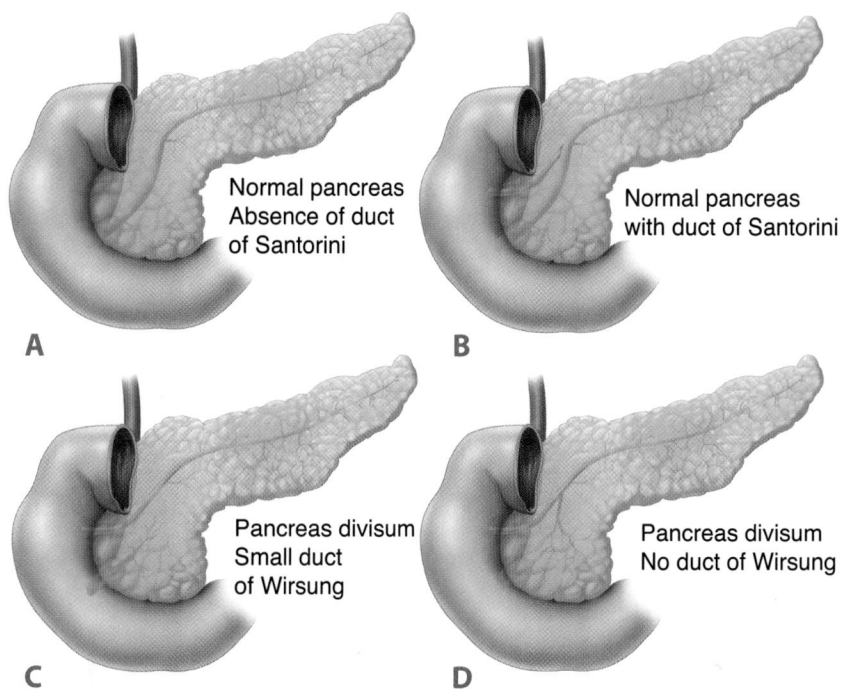

FIG. 33-20. Pancreas divisum. Normal pancreatic duct anatomy and the variations of partial or complete pancreas divisum are shown. *(Reproduced with permission from Warshaw.[96])*

Normal pancreas Absence of duct of Santorini

A

Normal pancreas with duct of Santorini

B

Pancreas divisum Small duct of Wirsung

C

Pancreas divisum No duct of Wirsung

D

Chronic Autoimmune Pancreatitis

A variant of chronic pancreatitis is a nonobstructive, diffusely infiltrative disease associated with fibrosis, a mononuclear cell (lymphocyte, plasma cell, or eosinophil) infiltrate, and an increased titer of one or more autoantibodies.[99] This type is associated with a variety of illnesses with suspected or proven autoimmune etiology, such as Sjögren's syndrome, rheumatoid arthritis, and type 1 diabetes mellitus.

Compressive stenosis of the intrapancreatic portion of the common bile duct is frequently seen, along with symptoms of obstructive jaundice. Increased levels of serum β-globulin or immunoglobulin G4 are also present. Steroid therapy is uniformly successful in ameliorating the disease, including any associated bile duct compression.[100] The differential diagnosis includes lymphoma, plasmacytoma ("pseudotumor" of the pancreas), and diffuse infiltrative carcinoma. Although the diagnosis is confirmed on pancreatic biopsy, presumptive treatment with steroids is usually undertaken, especially when clinical and laboratory findings support the diagnosis. Failure to obtain a cytologic specimen may lead to an unnecessary resectional procedure, and an untreated inflammatory component may cause sclerosis of the extrahepatic or intrahepatic bile ducts, with eventual liver failure.[101]

Tropical (Nutritional) Pancreatitis

Tropical chronic pancreatitis is highly prevalent among adolescents and young adults raised in Indonesia, southern India, and tropical Africa.[102] Abdominal pain develops in adolescence, followed by the development of a brittle form of pancreatogenic diabetes. Parenchymal and intraductal calcifications are seen, and the pancreatic duct stones may be quite large.[103] Many of the patients appear malnourished, some present with extreme emaciation, and a characteristic cyanotic coloration of the lips may be seen.[104] In addition to protein-caloric malnutrition, toxic products of some indigenous foodstuffs may also contribute to the disease. Cassava root is a starch (the origin of tapioca), which is a staple in the diet throughout the Afro-Asian region where tropical pancreatitis is prevalent. Cassava contains toxic glycosides, which form hydrocyanic acid when mixed with (gastric) hydrochloric acid.[105] Hydrocyanic acid is reduced to thiocyanate, which blocks a variety of enzymes, including superoxide dismutase. The simultaneous deficiency of dietary trace elements such as zinc, copper, and selenium could retard the detoxification of cyanogens and result in an increased susceptibility to free radical injury of the pancreas.

Clinically, tropical pancreatitis presents much like hereditary pancreatitis, and a familial pattern among cases is not unusual. An association with mutations of the PSTI or SPINK1 gene in patients with tropical pancreatitis has been reported.[106,107] The accelerated deterioration of endocrine and exocrine function, the chronic pain due to obstructive disease, and the recurrence of symptoms despite decompressive procedures characterize the course of disease.[104] As immigrants from the tropical regions increasingly find their way to all parts of the world, an awareness of this severe form of chronic pancreatitis is helpful for those who treat patients with pancreatic disease.

Hereditary Pancreatitis

In 1952, Comfort and Steinberg reported a kindred of "hereditary chronic relapsing pancreatitis" after treating the proband, a 24-year-old woman, at the Mayo Clinic.[108] Subsequently, familial patterns of chronic, nonalcoholic pancreatitis have been described worldwide, and a familiar pattern has emerged. Typically, patients first present in childhood or adolescence with abdominal pain and are found to have chronic calcific pancreatitis on imaging studies. Progressive pancreatic dysfunction is common, and many patients present with symptoms due to pancreatic duct obstruction. The risk of subsequent carcinoma formation is increased, reaching a prevalence, in some series, of 40%, but the age of onset for carcinoma is typically >50 years old.[109,110] The disorder is characterized by an autosomal dominant pattern of inheritance, with 80% penetrance and variable

expression. The incidence is equal in both sexes. Whitcomb and colleagues,[111] and separately LeBodic and associates,[112] performed gene linkage analysis and identified a linkage for hereditary pancreatitis to chromosome 7q35. Subsequently, the region was sequenced and revealed eight trypsinogen genes. Mutational analysis revealed a missense mutation resulting in an Arg to His substitution at position 117 of the cationic trypsinogen gene, or PRSS1, one of the primary sites for proteolysis of trypsin. This mutation prevents trypsin from being inactivated by itself or other proteases and results in persistent and uncontrolled proteolytic activity and autodestruction within the pancreas.[113] The position 117 mutation of PRSS1 and an additional mutation, now known collectively as the R122H and N291 mutations of PRSS1, account for about two-thirds of cases of hereditary pancreatitis. Recently, Masson and associates described a mutation in the anionic trypsinogen gene that may also be present in some cases.[114] Thus, hereditary pancreatitis results from one or more mutational defects that incapacitate an autoprotective process that normally prevents proteolysis within the pancreas.

Similarly, PSTI, also known as SPINK1, has been found to have a role in hereditary pancreatitis. SPINK1 specifically inhibits trypsin action by competitively blocking the active site of the enzyme. Witt and colleagues investigated 96 unrelated children with chronic pancreatitis in Germany and found a variety of SPINK1 mutations in 23% of the patients.[80] Several studies have now confirmed an association of SPINK1 mutations with familial and idiopathic forms of chronic pancreatitis, as well as tropical pancreatitis.[106,108,115,116] SPINK1 mutations are common in the general population as well, and the frequency of these mutations varies in different cohorts of idiopathic chronic pancreatitis, from 6.4% in France[101] to 25.8% in the United States.[115]

The CFTR gene contains over 4300 nucleotides, divided into 24 exons, which encode for a 1480-amino acid protein. Over 1000 polymorphisms have been reported, and many are common.[79] The severe CFTR mutation associated with the classic disease, F508, is rarely observed in chronic pancreatitis. But other minor CFTR mutations have been noted to be associated with chronic idiopathic pancreatitis in which the pulmonary, intestinal, and cutaneous manifestations of the disease are silent.[117,118] It is likely that many of the "idiopathic" forms of chronic pancreatitis, as well as some patients with the more common forms of the disease, will be found to have a genetic linkage or predisposition. The goal of this active area of research is to elucidate specific molecular abnormalities and provide strategies for treatment and prevention.

Asymptomatic Pancreatic Fibrosis

Asymptomatic pancreatic fibrosis is seen in some asymptomatic elderly patients, in tropical populations, or in asymptomatic alcohol users. There is diffuse perilobar fibrosis and a loss of acinar cell mass, but without a main ductular component.

A shortcoming of these clinical classification systems is the lack of histologic criteria of chronic inflammation due to the usual absence of a biopsy specimen. The differentiation of recurrent acute pancreatitis from chronic pancreatitis with exacerbations of pain can be difficult to establish and is not facilitated by the current system. Similarly, cystic fibrosis is known to cause fibrosis and acinar dysfunction but is not included in the classification despite increasing evidence for its possible role in idiopathic chronic pancreatitis.[119] Therefore, further refinements in the classification system for chronic pancreatitis are needed to allow a better prediction of its clinical course and a more accurate diagnosis of a likely etiologic agent.

Idiopathic Pancreatitis

When a definable cause for chronic pancreatitis is lacking, the term idiopathic is used to categorize the illness. Not surprisingly, as diagnostic methods and clinical awareness of disease improve, fewer patients fall into the idiopathic category. Classically, the idiopathic group includes young adults and adolescents who lack a family history of pancreatitis but who may represent individuals with spontaneous gene mutations encoding for regulatory proteins in the pancreas. In addition, the idiopathic group has included a large number of older patients for whom no obvious cause of recurrent or chronic pancreatitis can be found.[120] However, because the prevalence of biliary calculi increases steadily with age, it is not surprising that, as methods to detect biliary stone disease and microlithiasis have improved, a larger proportion of elderly "idiopathic" pancreatitis patients are found to have biliary tract disease.[121]

As noted in the section on Hereditary Pancreatitis above, an increasing number of mutations of the *CFTR* and *SPINK1* genes have been identified in association with idiopathic pancreatitis.[117,118,122] However, the role of genetic analysis in the management of these patients remains unclear, as guidelines have yet to be developed to allow physicians to use the data consistently. The clinical management of patients who harbor a minor *CFTR* mutation and chronic pancreatitis, for example, is still dictated by the manifestations of the pancreatitis. Any genetic counseling for the patient and his or her family has yet to be defined.[119]

Pathology
Histology

In early chronic pancreatitis, the histologic changes are unevenly distributed and are characterized by induration, nodular scarring, and lobular regions of fibrosis (Fig. 33-21). As the disease progresses, there is a loss of normal lobulation, with thicker sheets of fibrosis surrounding a reduced acinar cell mass, and dilatation of ductular structures (Fig. 33-22). The ductular epithelium is usually atypical and may display features of dysplasia, as evidenced by cuboidal cells with hyperplastic features, accompanied by areas of mononuclear cell infiltrates or patchy areas of necrosis. Cystic changes may be seen, but areas of relatively intact acinar elements and normal-appearing islets persist. In severe chronic pancreatitis, there is considerable replacement of acinar tissue by broad, coalescing areas of fibrosis, and the islet size and number are reduced (Fig. 33-23). Small arteries appear thickened and neural trunks become prominent.[123]

Tropical pancreatitis and hereditary pancreatitis are histologically indistinguishable from chronic alcoholic pancreatitis. In obstructive chronic pancreatitis, calculi are absent, although periacinar fibrosis and dilated ductular structures are prominent. In pancreatic lobular fibrosis seen in elderly subjects, small ducts are dilated, sometimes with small calculi trapped within. Hypertrophy of ductular epithelia is thought to cause this small-duct disease, which is accompanied by perilobular fibrosis.[124]

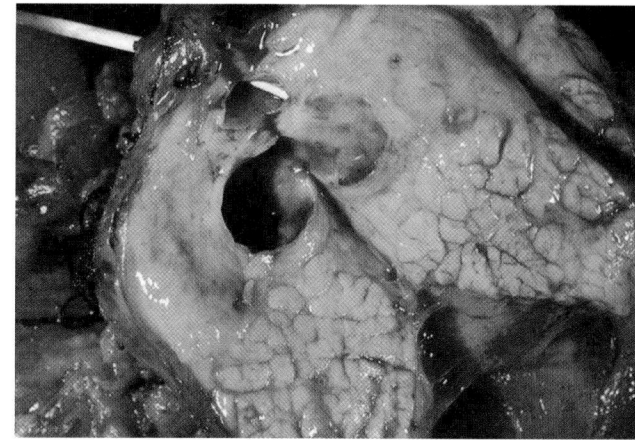

FIG. 33-22. Gross appearance of chronic pancreatitis. Areas of fibrosis and scarring are seen adjacent to other areas within the gland in which the lobar architecture is grossly preserved. A dilated pancreatic duct indicates the presence of downstream obstruction in this specimen removed from a patient with chronic pancreatitis. *(Courtesy of Dr. Rhonda Yantiss, Weill Cornell Medical College.)*

Fibrosis

A common feature of all forms of chronic pancreatitis is the perilobular fibrosis that forms surrounding individual acini, then propagates to surround small lobules, and eventually coalesces to replace larger areas of acinar tissue. The pathogenesis of this process involves the activation of PSCs that are found adjacent to acini and small arteries.[125] The extended cytoplasmic processes of PSCs encircle the acini but appear quiescent in the normal gland, where they contain lipid vacuoles and cytoskeletal proteins. In response to pancreatic injury, the PSCs become activated and proliferate (similarly to hepatic stellate cells), lose their lipid vesicles, and transform into myofibroblast-like cells. These cells respond to proliferative factors such as transforming growth factor beta, platelet-derived growth factor, and proinflammatory cytokines and synthesize and secrete type I and III collagen and fibronectin. Studies indicate that vitamin A metabolites, similar to those present in quiescent PSCs, can inhibit the collagen production of activated cultured PSCs.[126] This raises the

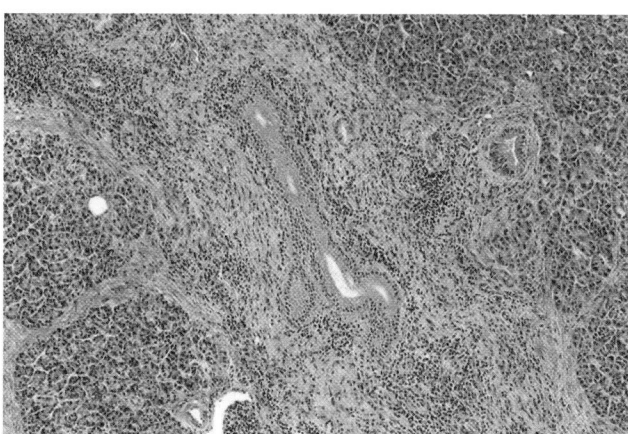

FIG. 33-21. Histology of early chronic pancreatitis. High-power microscopic (40×) histology of chronic pancreatitis shows an infiltration of mononuclear inflammatory cells throughout the interstitium of the pancreas, with little fibrosis. *(Courtesy of Dr. Rhonda Yantiss, Weill Cornell Medical College.)*

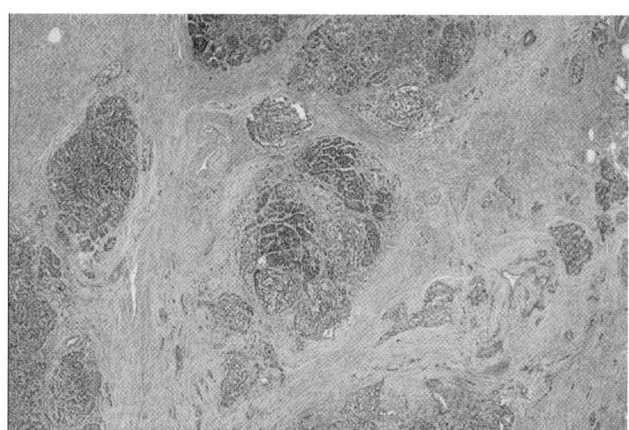

FIG. 33-23. Histology of severe chronic pancreatitis. High-power microscopic (40×) histologic appearance of advanced chronic pancreatitis shows extensive sheets of fibrosis and loss of acinar tissue, with preservation of islet tissue in scattered areas. *(Courtesy of Dr. Rhonda Yantiss, Weill Cornell Medical College.)*

possibility that early intervention may be possible to interrupt or prevent the fibrosis resulting from ongoing activation of PSCs.

The overall pathogenic sequence proposed by Schneider and Whitcomb[127] whereby alcohol induces acute pancreatitis and, with ongoing exposure, promotes the development of chronic fibrosis, is summarized in Fig. 33-19. Stellate cells surrounding the acinus are activated in acute pancreatitis but may be inactivated by anti-inflammatory cytokines and, in the absence of further injury, may revert to a quiescent state. The role of proinflammatory macrophages, cytokines, and stellate cells in models of acute and chronic pancreatitis represents an important area of current research.

Stone Formation

Pancreatic stones are composed largely of calcium carbonate crystals trapped in a matrix of fibrillar and other material.[128] The fibrillar center of most stones contains no calcium but rather a mixture of other metals. This suggests that stones form from an initial noncalcified protein precipitate, which serves as a focus for layered calcium carbonate precipitation. The same low-molecular-weight protein is present in stones and protein plugs and was initially named *pancreatic stone protein*, or PSP.[129] PSP comprises up to 14% of the protein content of mammalian pancreatic juice, and is secreted in four isoforms (PSP-S2, S3, S4, and S5), with molecular weights ranging from 16 to 20 kDa. PSP was found to be a potent inhibitor of calcium carbonate crystal growth and has subsequently been renamed *lithostathine*.[130] Independently, a 15-kDa fibrillar protein isolated from the pancreas was named *pancreatic thread protein*, and it has been shown to be homologous with lithostathine. Finally, a protein product of the *reg* gene, so named because it is expressed in association with regenerating islets in models of pancreatic injury, was isolated and called *reg* protein.[131] This also has been found to be homologous with lithostathine.[132] No overall homology has been found between lithostathine and other pancreatic proteins. The PSP/pancreatic thread protein/reg/lithostathine gene encodes for a 166-amino acid product that undergoes posttranslational modification to the S2 through S5 isoforms present in pancreatic juice. The protein is expressed in all rodents and mammals, both in the pancreas as well as in brain tissue, where it is found in particularly high concentrations in pyramidal neurons in Alzheimer's disease and Down syndrome. It is also found in the renal tubules, which is consistent with its biologic action of preventing calcium carbonate precipitation.[132]

Calcium and bicarbonate ions are normally present in pancreatic juice in high concentrations, and the solubility product of calcium carbonate is greatly exceeded under normal conditions. Microcrystals of calcium carbonate can be seen in normal pancreatic juice but are usually clinically silent. Lithostathine is a potent inhibitor of calcium carbonate crystal formation, at a concentration of only 0.1 μmol/L. However, lithostathine concentrations in normal pancreatic juice are in the range of 20 to 25 μmol/L, so a constant suppression of calcium carbonate crystal formation is present in the normal pancreas.

In alcoholics and in patients with alcoholic chronic pancreatitis, lithostathine expression and secretion are dramatically inhibited[132–134] (Fig. 33-24). In addition, elevated levels of precipitated lithostathine in the duct fluid in chronic pancreatitis patients suggests that the availability of the protein may be further reduced by the action of increased proteases and other proteins present in the duct fluid of alcoholic patients. Increased pancreatic juice protein levels in alcoholic men are reversible by abstinence from alcohol,[135] so the availability and effectiveness of lithostathine may be restored in patients with early-stage disease by timely intervention. Nevertheless, calcific stone formation represents an advanced stage of disease, which can further promote injury or symptoms due to mechanical damage to duct epithelium or obstruction of the ductular network.

Duct Distortion

Although calcific stone disease is normally a marker for an advanced stage of disease, parenchymal and ductular calcifications do

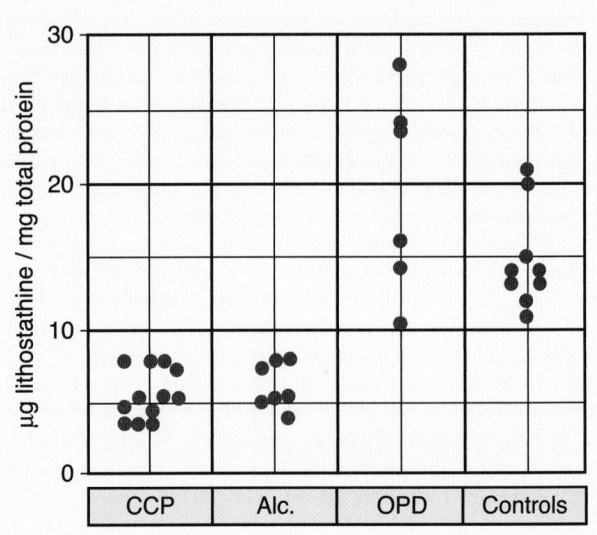

FIG. 33-24. Lithostathine levels in chronic calcific pancreatitis (CCP) patients, patients with alcohol abuse (Alc.), patients with other pancreatic disease (OPD), and controls. *(Reproduced with permission from Goggin et al.[132])*

not always correlate with symptoms. Obstructing main duct stones are commonly observed and are thought to be an indication for endoscopic or surgical removal. The ball-valve effect of a stone in a secreting system produces inevitable episodes of duct obstruction, usually accompanied by pain. But some patients with complete duct obstruction have prolonged periods of painlessness. Ductular hypertension has been documented in patients with proximal stenosis of the main pancreatic duct, and prolonged ductular distention after secretin administration is taken as a sign of ductular obstruction.[136] Although calculus disease and duct enlargement appear together as late stages of chronic pancreatitis, controversy persists over whether they are associated, are independent events, or are causally related.

Radiology

Radiologic imaging of chronic pancreatitis assists in four areas: (a) diagnosis, (b) the evaluation of severity of disease, (c) detection of complications, and (d) assistance in determining treatment options.[137] With the advent of cross-sectional imaging techniques such as CT and magnetic resonance imaging (MRI), the contour, content, ductal pattern, calcifications, calculi, and cystic disease of the pancreas are all readily discernible. Transabdominal ultrasonography is frequently used as a screening method for patients with abdominal symptoms or trauma, and the extension of ultrasonic imaging to include endoscopic ultrasound (EUS) and laparoscopic US have resulted in the highest-resolution images that are capable of detecting very small (<1 cm) abnormalities in the pancreas. EUS is now frequently used as a preliminary step in the evaluation of patients with pancreatic disease, and magnetic resonance cholangiopancreatography (MRCP) is increasingly being used to select patients who are candidates for the most invasive imaging method, ERCP. The staging of disease is important in the care of patients, and a combination of imaging methods is usually used (Table 33-8).

Ultrasonography is frequently used as an initial imaging method in patients with abdominal symptoms, and changes consistent with pancreatic duct dilatation, intraductal filling defects, cystic changes, and a heterogeneous texture are seen in chronic pancreatitis (Fig. 33-25). The sensitivity of transabdominal ultrasonography ranges from 48 to 96%, and is operator dependent.[138] However, the contour, texture, and ductal pattern are usually quite discernible, and it is a

TABLE 33-8 Cambridge classification of pancreatic morphology in chronic pancreatitis

Classification	ERCP Findings	CT and US Findings
Normal	No abnormal SBDs	Normal gland size, shape; homogeneous parenchyma
Equivocal	MPD normal	One of the following: less than three abnormal SBDs; MPD 2–4 mm; gland enlarged more than two times normal size; heterogeneous parenchyma
Mild	MPD normal	Two or more of the following: less than three abnormal SBDs; MPD 2–4 mm; slight gland enlargement; heterogeneous parenchyma
Moderate	MPD changes	Small cysts <10 mm; MPD irregularity
	SBD changes	Focal acute pancreatitis; increased echogenicity of MPD walls; gland-contour irregularity
Severe	Any of the above changes plus one or more of the following: Cysts <10 mm; intraductal filling defects; calculi; MPD obstruction or stricture; severe MPD irregularity; contiguous organ invasion	—

CT = computed tomography; ERCP = endoscopic retrograde cholangiopancreatography; MPD = main pancreatic duct; SBD = side-branch duct; US = ultrasound.
Source: Reproduced with permission from Freeney.[137]

reliable method for periodic re-examination to determine the efficacy of treatment.

EUS has heavily impacted the evaluation and management of patients with chronic pancreatitis. Although it is more operator dependent and less widely available than transabdominal ultrasonography, EUS provides not only imaging capability but adds the capacity to obtain cytologic and chemical samples of tissue and fluid aspirated with linear array monitoring (Fig. 33-26). EUS images obtained through a high-frequency (7.5- to 12.5-mHz) transducer are able to evaluate subtle changes in 2- to 3-mm structures within the pancreas and can detect indolent neoplasms in the setting of chronic inflammation. Small intraductal lesions, intraductal mucus, cystic lesions, and subtle ductular abnormalities are recognizable by EUS (Table 33-9). This allows ERCP to be reserved for these patients who require therapeutic maneuvers, or for the evaluation of more complex problems. EUS is comparable to ERCP in the detection of advanced changes in chronic pancreatitis[139] and may be more sensitive than ERCP in the detection of mild disease.[140]

CT scanning has affected the diagnosis of pancreatic disease more broadly than any other method. Before its widespread introduction in the early 1970s, pancreatic imaging was largely a matter of detecting the displacement of adjacent, contrast-filled viscera by mass lesions of the pancreas. Since the introduction of cross-sectional techniques, and with the advent of faster helical CT scanning and CT angiography, visualization of the nature, extent, location, and relative relationships of pancreatic structures and lesions is possible with great clarity. Duct dilatation, calculous disease, cystic changes, inflammatory events, and anomalies are all detectable with a resolution of 3 to 4 mm (Fig. 33-27). CT scanning has a false-negative rate of <10% for chronic pancreatitis, but early or mild chronic disease may go unde-

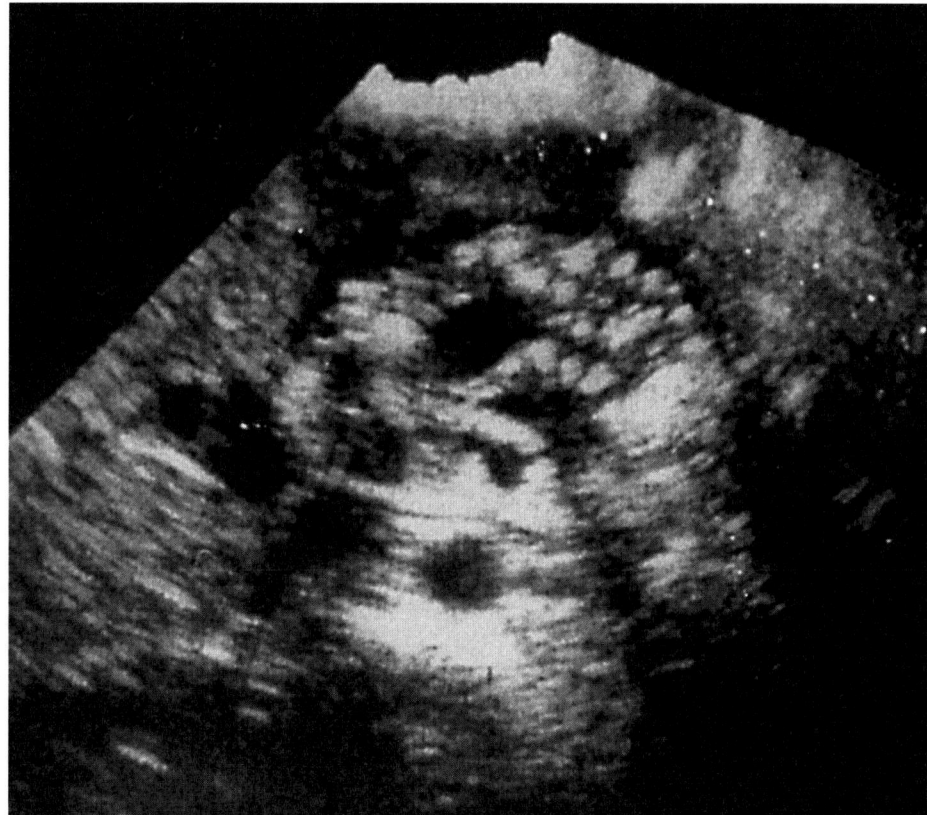

FIG. 33-25. Sonography in chronic pancreatitis. Transabdominal sonogram of patient with chronic pancreatitis demonstrates heterogeneity of the pancreatic parenchyma, dilated ductal systems, and cyst formation. *(Reproduced with permission from Bolondi et al.[138])*

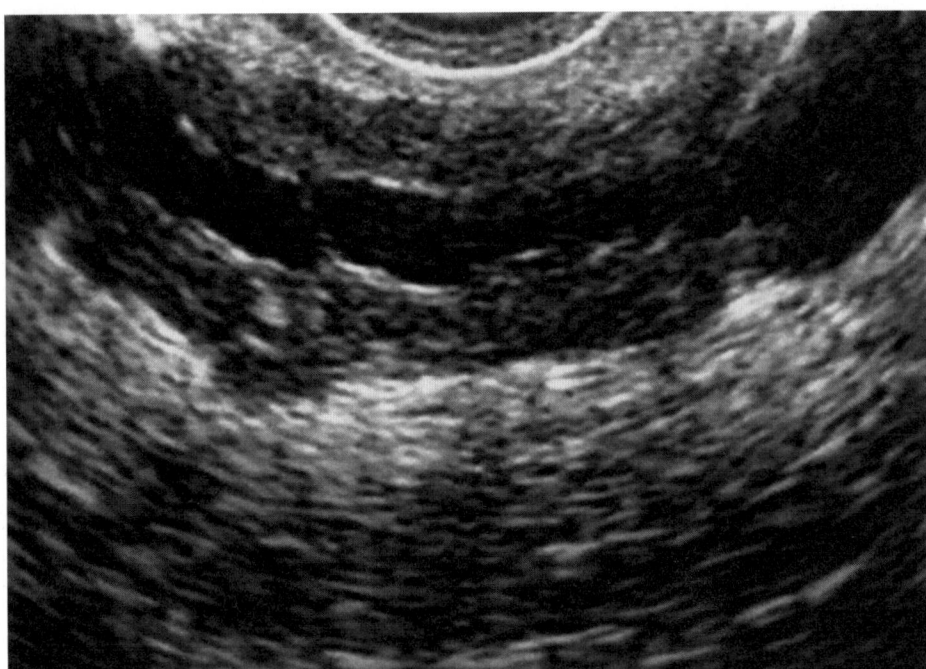

FIG. 33-26. Endoscopic ultrasound of chronic pancreatitis. The endoscopic ultrasound appearance of the parenchyma is heterogenous, and dilated ducts are seen, indicating early obstructive pancreatopathy. *(Courtesy of Dr. Mark Topazian, Division of Digestive Diseases, Department of Medicine, Mayo Clinic.)*

tected by CT imaging. The earliest changes are dilatation of secondary ducts and heterogeneous parenchymal changes, which are detectable by EUS and ERCP. Another drawback of CT scanning is its lower sensitivity for detecting small neoplasms, which are seen with increased frequency in chronic pancreatitis and may be invisible to all modalities except EUS.

MRI, in both the cross-sectional mode and the coronally oriented heavily weighted T2 or high spin ratio imaging (MRCP) that can disclose fluid-filled ducts and cystic lesions, has added greatly to the imaging options for chronic pancreatitis (Fig. 33-28). The resolution of cross-sectional MRI scanning is now approaching that of CT scanning, although the availability of MRI scanners and the complexity of the images produced have limited their large-scale use for routine imaging of the pancreas. MRCP has been shown to be an effective screening technique for disclosing ductal abnormalities that correlates closely with the contrast-filled ducts imaged by ERCP.[141] The advantages of MRCP include its noninvasive methodology and its ability to image obstructed ducts that are not opacified by ERCP injection. It is therefore a useful screening study to detect duct abnormalities and to confirm the need for interventional procedures. Oral, IV, and intraductal contrast are unnecessary for MRCP, and its lack of ionizing radiation makes this the safest method to image the ductal system in high-risk patients.

ERCP is considered to be the gold standard for the diagnosis and staging of chronic pancreatitis. It also serves as a vehicle that enables other diagnostic and therapeutic maneuvers, such as biopsy or brushing for cytology, or the use of stents to relieve obstruction or drain a pseudocyst (Fig. 33-29). Unfortunately, ERCP also carries a risk of procedure-induced pancreatitis that occurs in approximately 5% of patients.[142] Patients at increased risk include those with sphincter of Oddi dysfunction and those with a previous history of post-ERCP pancreatitis. Post-ERCP pancreatitis occurs after uncomplicated procedures, as well as after those that require prolonged manipulation. Severe pancreatitis and deaths have occurred after ERCP. This method should be reserved for patients in whom the diagnosis is unclear despite the use of other imaging methods, or in whom a diagnostic or therapeutic maneuver is specifically indicated.

Newer imaging methods are being evaluated that detect changes in metabolic activity, instead of radiologic behavior, as a means to analyze abnormal tissue. The positron emission tomographic scan measures focal changes in nutrient (e.g., glucose) metabolism to detect focal changes in tissue behavior. This method has shown usefulness in the detection of occult neoplasms of the brain and lung, and evaluations are currently ongoing to assess its role in pancreatic imaging.

Presentation, Natural History, and Complications
Presenting Signs and Symptoms

Pain is the most common symptom of chronic pancreatitis. It is usually midepigastric in location but may localize or involve either the left or right upper quadrant of the abdomen. Occasionally, it is perceived in the lower midabdomen but is frequently described as penetrating through to the back (Fig. 33-30). The pain is typically steady and boring, but not colicky. It persists for hours or days and may be chronic with exacerbations caused by eating or drinking alcohol. Chronic alcoholics also describe a steady, constant pain that is temporarily relieved by alcohol, followed by a more severe recurrence hours later.[143,144]

TABLE 33-9	Endoscopic ultrasound features of chronic pancreatitis

Endoscopic Ultrasound Feature	Implication
Ductal changes	
Duct size >3 mm	Ductal dilation
Tortuous pancreatic duct	Ductal irregularity
Intraductal echogenic foci	Stones or calcification
Echogenic duct wall	Ductal fibrosis
Side-branch ectasia	Periductal fibrosis
Parenchymal changes	
Inhomogeneous echo pattern	Edema
Reduced echogenic foci (1–3 mm)	Edema
Enhanced echogenic foci	Calcifications
Prominent interlobular septae	Fibrosis
Lobular outer gland margin	Fibrosis, glandular atrophy
Large, echo-poor cavities (>5 mm)	Pseudocyst

Source: Reproduced with permission from Catalano et al.[140] Copyright Elsevier.

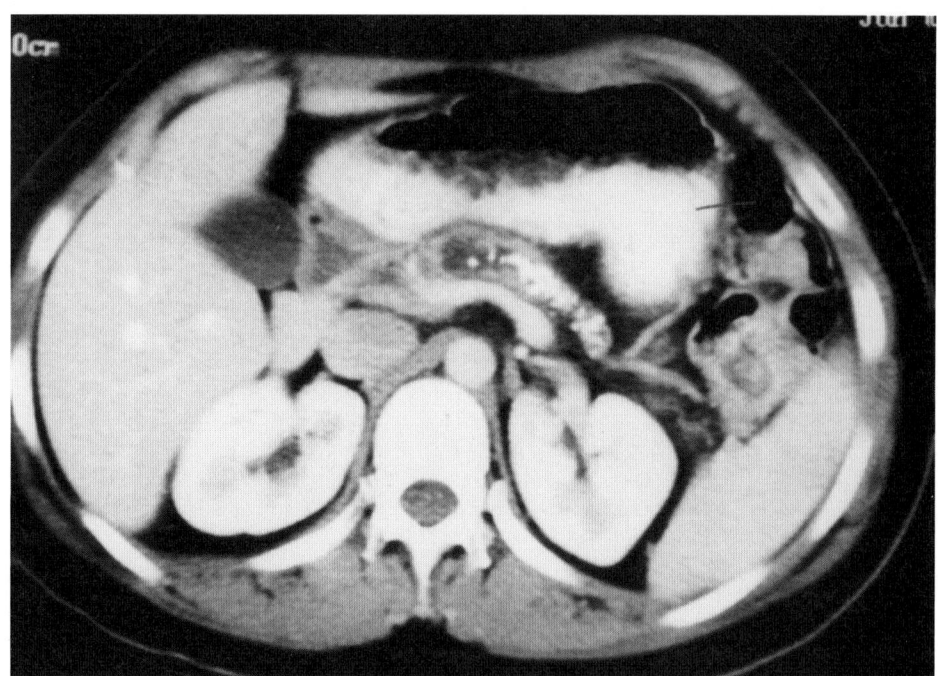

FIG. 33-27. Computed tomographic imaging of chronic pancreatitis. A dilated pancreatic duct is seen, with evidence of intraductal stones and parenchymal calcification.

Patients with chronic pancreatic pain typically flex their abdomen and either sit or lie with their hips flexed, or lie on their side in a fetal position. Unlike ureteral stone pain or biliary colic, the pain causes the patient to be still. Nausea or vomiting may accompany the pain, but anorexia is the most common associated symptom.

Pain from chronic pancreatitis has been ascribed to three possible etiologies. Ductal hypertension, due to strictures or stones, may predispose to pain that is initiated or exacerbated by eating. Chronic pain without exacerbation may be related to parenchymal disease or retroperitoneal inflammation with persistent neural involvement. Acute exacerbations of pain in the setting of chronic pain may be due to acute increases in duct pressure or recurrent episodes of acute inflammation in the setting of chronic parenchymal disease. Nealon and Matin have described these various pain syndromes as

being predictive of the response to various surgical procedures.[145] Pain that is found in association with ductal hypertension is most readily relieved by pancreatic duct decompression, through endoscopic stenting or surgical decompression.[143]

Ammann and colleagues also studied the pain patterns of patients with chronic pancreatitis and observed that the pain was commonly of relatively short (<10 days) duration, after which it was absent for long periods, or relentless or frequent, in which case it lasted for months.[146] Patients in the latter category frequently had other complications of pancreatitis, such as pseudocyst or duodenal compression.

The pain of chronic pancreatitis may decrease or disappear completely over a period of years, as symptoms of exocrine and endocrine deficiency become apparent.[147,148] This is referred to as

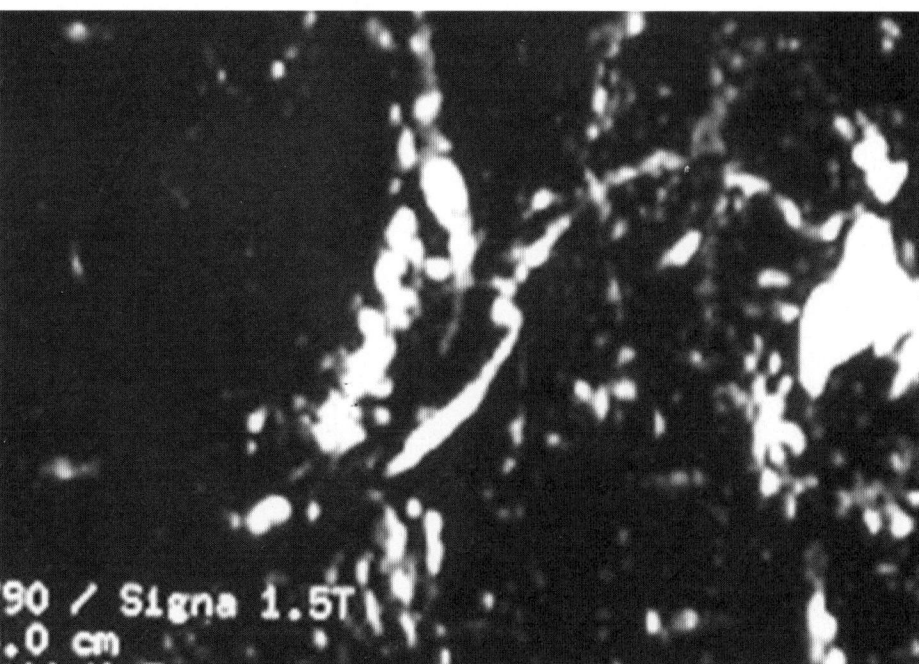

FIG. 33-28. Magnetic resonance cholangiopancreatography in chronic pancreatitis. A dilated pancreatic duct suggests obstructive pancreatopathy due to proximal scarring.

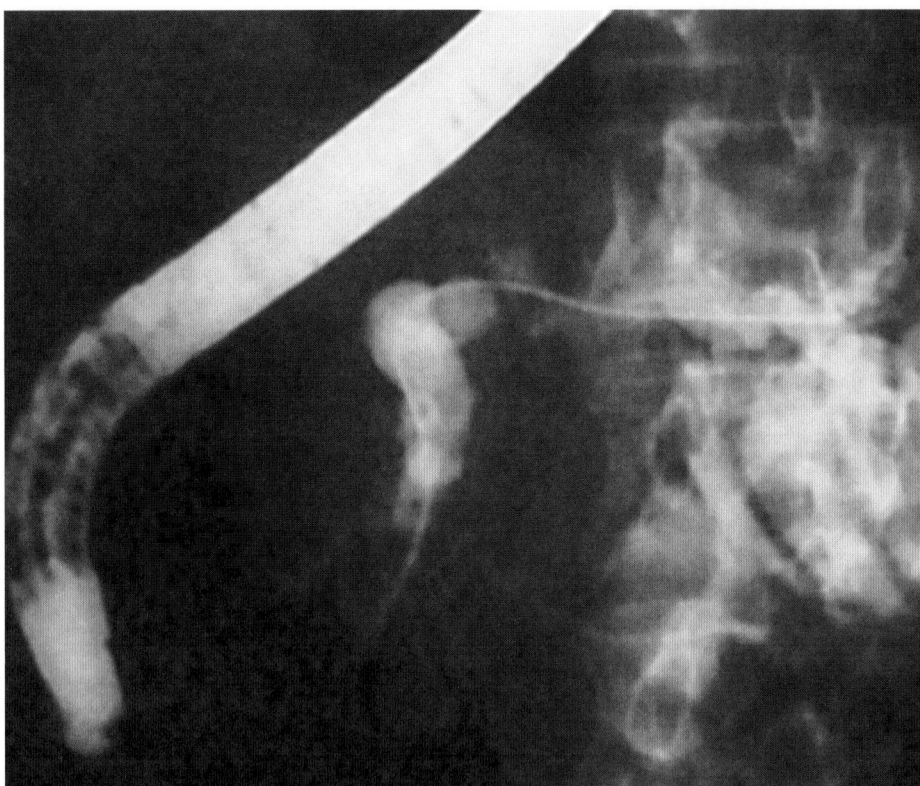

FIG. 33-29. Pancreatic duct stenting. At endoscopic retrograde cholangio-pancreatography, a stent is placed in the proximal pancreatic duct to relieve obstruction and reduce symptoms of pain. Pancreatic duct stents are left in place for only a limited time to avoid further inflammation.

burned out pancreatitis and correlates with the progression of disease from a mild or moderate stage to severe destruction of the pancreas.[149] Non-interventional approaches to the treatment of chronic pancreatitis are accompanied by the development of narcotic addiction, inability to work, and the sequelae of chronic illness.

Although increased ductal pressure, and therefore parenchymal pressure, is thought to be the cause of pain in chronic obstructive pancreatitis,[150] the role of chronic inflammation per se, and the development of actual nerve damage in the diseased gland, are also thought to contribute to pain.[151] Chronic inflammation results in the infiltration of tissue by macrophages, which secrete prostaglandins and other nociceptive agents that cause chronic stimulation of afferent neural fibers. Inflammatory damage to the perineurial layers surrounding the unmyelinated pancreatic nerves and a focal infiltration of inflammatory cells around nerves suggest that neural fibers are a target for the cellular response to inflammation in the pancreas.[152]

Strategies to relieve pain are therefore based on three approaches: (a) reducing secretion and/or decompress the secretory compartment, (b) resecting the focus of chronic inflammatory change, or (c) interrupting the transmission of afferent neural impulses through neural ablative procedures. A trial of antisecretory therapy or endoscopic duct drainage may select those patients who will benefit preferentially from a decompressive procedure.

Malabsorption and Weight Loss

When pancreatic exocrine capacity falls below 10% of normal, diarrhea and steatorrhea develop[153] (Fig. 33-31). Patients describe a bulky, foul-smelling, loose (but not watery) stool that may be pale

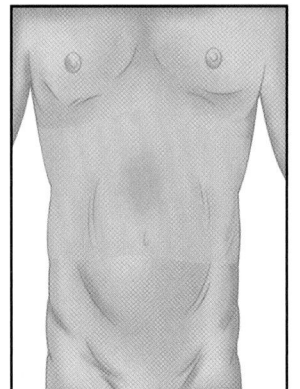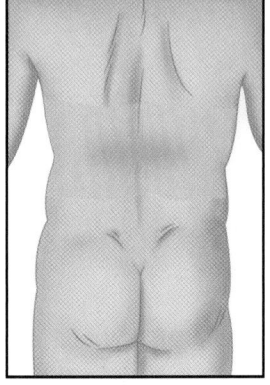

FIG. 33-30. Pain location in chronic pancreatitis. *(Reproduced with permission from Murayama et al.[144])*

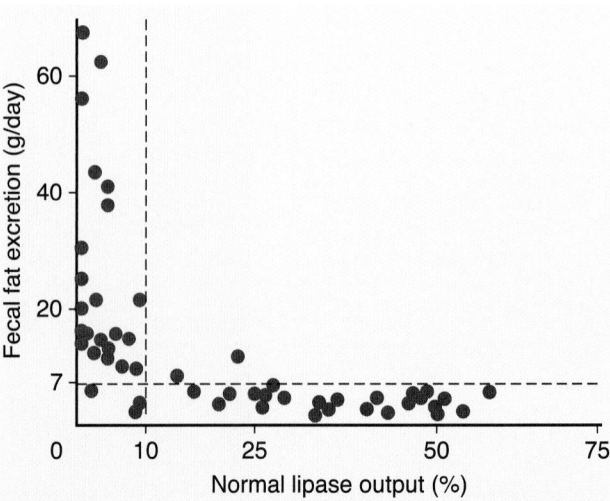

FIG. 33-31. Relationship of lipase output to fat malabsorption. Excess fecal fat appears when the pancreatic lipase output falls below 10% of normal secretory values. *(Reproduced with permission from DiMagno et al.[153])*

TABLE 33-10 Types of diabetes mellitus

Parameter	Type I IDDM Juvenile Onset	Type II NIDDM Adult Onset	Type III Apancreatic Postoperative Onset
Ketoacidosis	Common	Rare	Rare
Hyperglycemia	Severe	Usually mild	Mild
Hypoglycemia	Common	Rare	Common
Peripheral insulin sensitivity	Normal or increased	Decreased	Increased
Hepatic insulin sensitivity	Normal	Normal or decreased	Decreased
Insulin levels	Low	High	Low
Glucagon levels	Normal or high	Normal or high	Low
Pancreatic polypeptide levels	High	High	Low
Typical age of onset	Childhood or adolescence	Adulthood	Any

IDDM = insulin-dependent diabetes mellitus; NIDDM = non-insulin-dependent diabetes mellitus.
Source: Reproduced with permission from Slezak et al.[158] With kind permission from Springer Science + Business Media.

in color and float on the surface of toilet water. Frequently, patients will describe a greasy or oily appearance to the stool, or may describe an "oil slick" on the water's surface. In severe steatorrhea, an orange, oily stool is often reported.[58] As exocrine deficiency increases, symptoms of steatorrhea are often accompanied by weight loss. Patients may describe a good appetite despite weight loss, or diminished food intake due to abdominal pain.

In severe symptomatic chronic pancreatitis, anorexia or nausea may occur with or separate from abdominal pain. The combination of decreased food intake and malabsorption of nutrients usually results in chronic weight loss. As a result, many patients with severe chronic pancreatitis are below ideal body weight.

Lipase deficiency tends to manifest itself before trypsin deficiency,[154] so the presence of steatorrhea may be the first functional sign of pancreatic insufficiency. As pancreatic exocrine function deteriorates further, the secretion of bicarbonate into the duodenum is reduced, which causes duodenal acidification and further impairs nutrient absorption.[155]

Apancreatic Diabetes

The islets comprise only 2% of the mass of the pancreas, but they are preferentially conserved when pancreatic inflammation occurs. In chronic pancreatitis, acinar tissue loss and replacement by fibrosis is greater than the degree of loss of islet tissue, although islets are typically smaller than normal and may be isolated from their surrounding vascular network by the fibrosis. With progressive destruction of the gland, endocrine insufficiency commonly occurs. Frank diabetes is seen initially in about 20% of patients with chronic pancreatitis, and impaired glucose metabolism can be detected in up to 70% of patients. In a study of 500 patients with predominantly alcoholic chronic pancreatitis, diabetes developed in 83% within 25 years of the clinical onset of chronic pancreatitis, and more than half of the diabetic patients required insulin treatment.[156] Ketoacidosis and diabetic nephropathy are relatively uncommon in apancreatic (also termed *pancreatogenic*) diabetes (Table 33-10), but retinopathy and neuropathy are seen to occur with a similar frequency as in idiopathic diabetes.[157]

Apancreatic diabetes is more common after surgical resection for chronic pancreatitis.[156] Distal pancreatectomy and Whipple procedures have a higher incidence of diabetes than do drainage procedures, and the severity of diabetes is usually worse after subtotal or total pancreatectomy.[158]

The etiology and pathophysiology of apancreatic or type III diabetes is distinct from that of either insulin-dependent (type I) or non-insulin-independent (type II) diabetes. In apancreatic diabetes, due to the loss of functioning pancreatic tissue by disease or surgical removal, there is a global deficiency of all three glucoregulatory islet cell hormones: insulin, glucagon, and PP. In addition, there is a paradoxical combination of enhanced peripheral sensitivity to insulin and decreased hepatic sensitivity to insulin.[159] As a result, insulin therapy is frequently difficult; patients are hyperglycemic when insulin replacement is insufficient (due to unsuppressed hepatic glucose production) or hypoglycemic when insulin replacement is barely excessive (due to enhanced peripheral insulin sensitivity and a deficiency of pancreatic glucagon secretion to counteract the hypoglycemia). This form of diabetes is referred to as *brittle* diabetes and requires special attention.

Although the primary hormonal deficit is a loss of insulin secretory capacity, the additional deficiencies of glucagon and PP are pathognomonic for apancreatic diabetes. PP has recently been shown to be important in the regulation of insulin action.[160] The expression of the hepatic insulin receptor gene and the subsequent availability and action of insulin receptors on hepatocyte membranes are regulated by PP.[161] PP deficiency correlates with the severity of chronic pancreatitis, and impairments in the hepatic action of insulin are reversed in PP-deficient chronic pancreatitis patients by administration of PP[162] (Fig. 33-32).

Because PP cells are predominantly located in the posterior head and uncinate process of the pancreas,[163] proximal pancreatectomy

CHAPTER 33
Pancreas

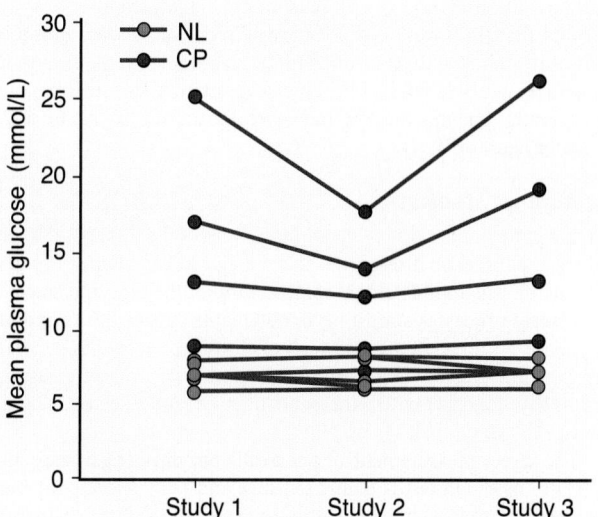

FIG. 33-32. Effect of pancreatic polypeptide replacement on plasma glucose levels. Main plasma glucose levels following ingestion of glucose (40 g/m² body surface area) before (study 1), immediately after (study 2), and 1 month after (study 3) an 8-hour infusion of bovine pancreatic polypeptide. NL represents normal control subjects (*n* = 6) and CP represents patients with chronic pancreatitis (*n* = 5), three of whom had an initial diabetic response. *(Reproduced with permission from Brunicardi et al.[162] Copyright 1996 The Endocrine Society.)*

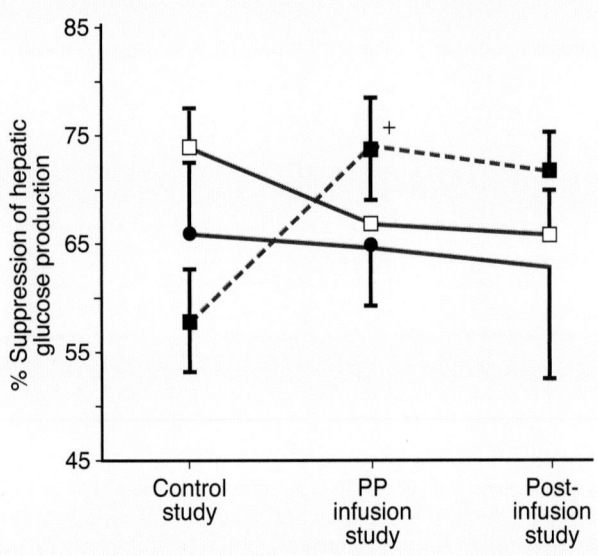

FIG. 33-33. Effect of pancreatic polypeptide (PP) infusion on insulin-induced suppression of hepatic glucose production. The percentage of suppression of hepatic glucose production (*Rah*) before (control study), during (PP infusion study), and 1 month after (postinfusion study) an 8-hour infusion of bovine PP, during a background infusion of insulin (0.25 mU/kg per minute). The results in normal subjects (*open boxes*), pancreatic resection patients with normal PP levels (*closed symbols, solid line*), and pancreatic resection patients with deficient PP levels (*closed symbols, dashed line*) are shown (+ = P <.02). (*Reproduced with permission from Seymour et al.[164] Copyright Elsevier.*)

is invariably associated with profound PP deficiency. Seymour and associates studied a group of nondiabetic young men who had previously undergone various pancreatic resections for trauma, and showed that those who were PP deficient had a measurable loss of hepatic insulin sensitivity, and that this was reversed by PP administration[164] (Fig. 33-33). In addition, Hanazaki and colleagues showed that the addition of PP to insulin delivered via a pump in pancreatectomized dogs resulted in decreased insulin requirements to achieve glucose control.[165] This suggests that the treatment of apancreatic diabetes may be improved by the use of PP or a PP receptor agonist.[166]

Laboratory Studies

Unlike chronic liver disease or abnormalities of the upper and lower GI tract, pancreatic disease presents a diagnostic challenge because a tissue biopsy and histologic confirmation of the type and stage of the disease process is almost never obtainable outside of the operating room. As a result, the diagnosis of chronic pancreatitis depends on the clinical presentation, a limited number of indirect measurements that correlate with pancreatic function, and selected imaging studies (Table 33-11).

The direct measurement of pancreatic enzymes (e.g., lipase and amylase) by blood test is highly sensitive and fairly specific in acute pancreatitis but is seldom helpful in the diagnosis of chronic pancreatitis. The pancreatic endocrine product that correlates most strongly with chronic pancreatitis is the PP response to a test meal (Fig. 33-34). Severe chronic pancreatitis is associated with a blunted or absent PP response to feeding but, as with many other tests, a normal PP response does not rule out the presence of early disease.[167]

The measurement of pancreatic exocrine secretion requires aspiration of pancreatic juice from the duodenum after nutrient (Lundh test meal) or hormonal (CCK or secretin) stimulation.[168,169] Direct aspiration of pancreatic juice by endoscopic cannulation of

TABLE 33-11	Tests for chronic pancreatitis

I. Measurement of pancreatic products in blood
  A. Enzymes
  B. Pancreatic polypeptide
II. Measurement of pancreatic exocrine secretion
  A. Direct measurements
    1. Enzymes
    2. Bicarbonate
  B. Indirect measurement
    1. Bentiromide test
    2. Schilling test
    3. Fecal fat, chymotrypsin, or elastase concentration
    4. [^{14}C]-olein absorption
III. Imaging techniques
  A. Plain film radiography of abdomen
  B. Ultrasonography
  C. Computed tomography
  D. Endoscopic retrograde cholangiopancreatography
  E. Magnetic resonance cholangiopancreatography
  F. Endoscopic ultrasonography

the duct has been proposed, but is not risk free, comfortable for the patient, or more sensitive than luminal intubation methods.[170]

Indirect tests of pancreatic exocrine function are based on the measurement of metabolites of compounds that are altered ("digested") by pancreatic exocrine products and can be quantified by serum or urine measurements. A commonly used indirect test is the bentiromide test, in which *N*-benzoyl-L-tyrosyl-p-aminobenzoic acid is ingested by the subject, and the urinary excretion of the proteolytic metabolite p-aminobenzoic acid (PABA) is measured. Free PABA is absorbed from the small intestine and excreted by the kidney in a linear correlation with the degree of chymotrypsin degradation of *N*-benzoyl-L-tyrosyl-p-aminobenzoic acid.[171] Although the sensitivity of the test is as high as 100% in patients with severe chronic pancreatitis, it identifies only 40 to 50% of patients with mild disease.[172] Furthermore, reduced PABA excretion is found in patients with a variety of other GI, hepatic, and renal diseases. Therefore, the test is of value not for the diagnosis of chronic pancreatitis but for determining the extent of exocrine pancreatic insufficiency in patients with known disease.

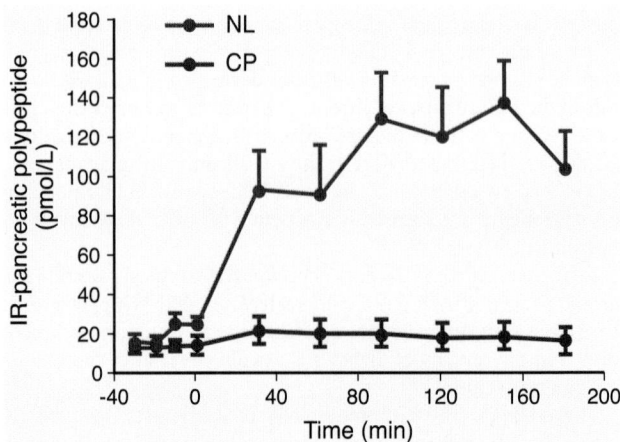

FIG. 33-34. Pancreatic polypeptide (PP) response to a test meal. Immunoreactive PP (IR-PP) responses in control subjects (NL, *n* = 6) and patients with severe chronic pancreatitis (CP) accompanied by PP deficiency (CP, *n* = 5) are shown. A test meal was administered at 0 minutes. Means ± standard error of the mean are shown. (*Reproduced with permission from Brunicardi et al.[162] Copyright 1996 The Endocrine Society.*)

Similarly, the absorption of vitamin B_{12} is adversely affected by pancreatic exocrine insufficiency, and the recovery of urinary cobalamin correlates with the functional impairment. This method is referred to as the *Schilling test* and has been modified by the addition of cobalamin binding agents such as intrinsic factor and R protein, which are differentially affected by exocrine secretion.[173] The test also is limited by poor sensitivity in patients with mild disease.

Fecal levels of chymotrypsin[174] and elastase[175] have been proposed as simpler, less expensive tests of exocrine function and correlate well with loss of pancreatic function. As with other test methods, however, these tests lose their sensitivity in patients with mild to moderate chronic pancreatitis and may be more sensitive for other causes of pancreatic dysfunction, including cystic fibrosis.

The quantification of stool fat has also been used as a measure of pancreatic lipase secretion, either through the direct measurement of total fecal fat levels while the subject consumes a diet of known fat content, or by the measurement of exhaled $^{14}CO_2$ after ingestion of [^{14}C]-triolein or [^{14}C]-olein. This so-called triolein breath test is less cumbersome than intubation methods, and avoids the necessity of stool collections and analysis, but also has a high false-negative rate.[176]

Radiologic imaging has become the principal method of diagnosis of chronic pancreatitis, with the codification of classification systems that correlate with proven disease. ERCP has been considered the most sensitive radiologic test for the diagnosis of chronic pancreatitis, with specific ERCP findings that are highly correlative with the degree or stage of chronic disease[177] (Table 33-12). CT scanning is sensitive for the diagnosis of chronic pancreatitis when calcification, duct dilatation, or cystic disease is present, but is not accurate in the absence of these findings. CT is helpful as a screening study to guide interventional therapy or other diagnostic modalites.[137] EUS has become a more widely used study for the diagnosis of pancreatic disease and offers the advantage of very-high-resolution images of the pancreatic parenchyma, the main and secondary ductal systems, cystic lesions, and calcific changes.[178] Although operator dependent and invasive, the technique is far safer than ERCP and, in experienced hands, is excellent for the diagnosis in moderate and severe stage disease[139] (Table 33-13). Most importantly, EUS is highly reliable in ruling out pancreatic carcinoma when EUS findings are normal.[179] Studies suggest that EUS may be more valuable than ERCP for the diagnosis of early chronic pancreatitis.[141]

Prognosis and Natural History

The prognosis for patients with chronic pancreatitis is dependent on the etiology of the disease, the development of complications, and on the age and socioeconomic status of the patient. The influence of treatment is less evident in long-term studies, although the general absence of randomized, prospective trials clouds the issue of whether specific forms of therapy alter the long-term outlook for patients with the disease.[180]

Several studies have demonstrated that, although symptoms of pain decrease over time in about half of the patients, this decline is also accompanied by a progression of exocrine and endocrine insufficiency.[147–149,181] In general, the likelihood of eventual pain relief is dependent upon the stage of disease at diagnosis, and the persistence of alcohol use in patients with alcoholic chronic pancreatitis. Miyake and colleagues found that pain relief was achieved in 60% of alcoholic patients who successfully discontinued drinking, but in only 26% who did not.[181]

The long-term survival of patients with chronic pancreatitis is less than for patients without pancreatitis. In an international multicenter study of >2000 patients, Lowenfels and colleagues found that the 10- and 20-year survival rates for patients with chronic pancreatitis were 70 and 45%, respectively, compared to 93 and 65% for patients without pancreatitis.[182] The mortality risk was found to be 1.6-fold higher in patients who continued to abuse alcohol, compared to those who did not (Fig. 33-35). Continued alcohol abuse has a similar effect on the response to surgical treatment (Fig. 33-36), and results in a twofold increase in mortality over a 10- to 14-year follow-up period.[183]

TABLE 33-13	Complications of chronic pancreatitis

Intrapancreatic complications
  Pseudocysts
    Duodenal or gastric obstruction
    Thrombosis of splenic vein
    Abscess
    Perforation
    Erosion into visceral artery
  Inflammatory mass in head of pancreas
    Bile duct stenosis
    Portal vein thrombosis
    Duodenal obstruction
  Duct strictures and/or stones
    Ductal hypertension and dilatation
  Pancreatic carcinoma
Extrapancreatic complications
  Pancreatic duct leak with ascites or fistula
  Pseudocyst extension beyond lesser sac into mediastinum, retroperitoneum, lateral pericolic spaces, pelvis, or adjacent viscera

TABLE 33-12	Cambridge classification of chronic pancreatitis by endoscopic retrograde cholangiopancreatography

Grade	Main Pancreatic Duct	Side Branches
Normal	Normal	Normal
Suggestive	Normal	<3 Abnormal
Mild	Normal	≥3 Abnormal
Moderate	Abnormal	>3 Abnormal
Severe	Abnormal plus at least one of the following:	
	Large cavity	
	Duct obstruction	
	Dilation or duct irregularity	
	Intraductal filing defects	

Source: Reproduced with permission from Axon ATR et al: Pancreatography in chronic pancreatitis: International definitions. *Gut* 25:1107, 1984. With permission from the BMJ Publishing Group.

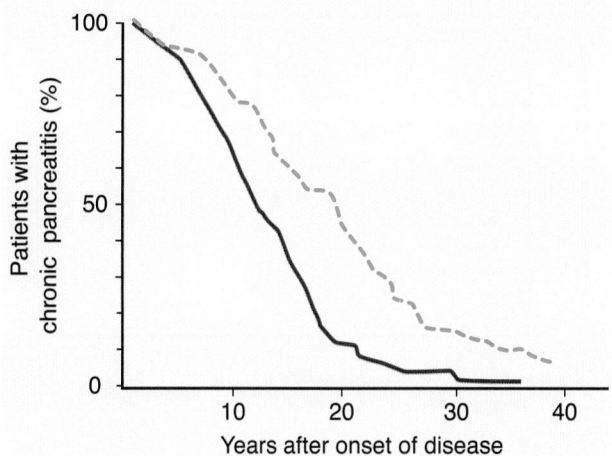

FIG. 33-35. Cumulative survival of patients with chronic pancreatitis. The overall survival rate for patients with chronic pancreatitis, with (*solid line*) or without (*dashed line*) continued alcohol abuse. (*Reproduced with permission from Lankisch.[180]*)

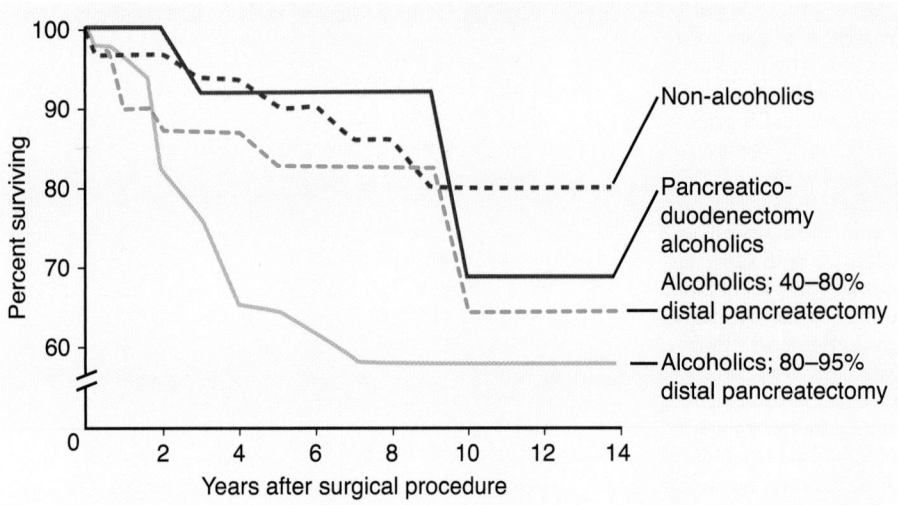

FIG. 33-36. Effect of alcohol use on survival after surgical procedures. The cumulative survival of patients with chronic pancreatitis following pancreaticoduodenectomy or distal pancreatectomy is shown for nonalcoholic and alcoholic patients. *(Reproduced with permission from Frey et al.[183])*

In addition to progressive endocrine and exocrine dysfunction, and the risk of the specific complications outlined below and in Table 33-13, the other significant long-term risk for the patient with chronic pancreatitis is the development of pancreatic carcinoma.[184] There is a progressive, cumulative increased risk of carcinoma development in patients with chronic pancreatitis, which continues throughout the subsequent lifetime of the patient (Fig. 33-37). The incidence of carcinoma in patients with chronic pancreatitis ranges from 1.5 to 2.7%,[148,149] which is at least 10-fold greater than that of patients of similar age seen in a hospital setting. In patients with advanced chronic pancreatitis referred for surgical therapy, the risk of indolent carcinoma can be as high as 10%.[185] The development of carcinoma in the setting of chronic pancreatitis is no doubt related to the dysregula-

tion of cellular proliferation and tissue repair processes in the setting of chronic inflammation, as is seen throughout the alimentary tract and elsewhere. In the setting of chronic pancreatitis, carcinoma development can be especially cryptic, and the diagnosis of early-stage tumors is particularly difficult. Awareness of this risk justifies close surveillance for cancer in patients with chronic pancreatitis. Periodic measurement of tumor markers such as CA19-9, and periodic imaging of the pancreas with CT scan and EUS are necessary to detect the development of carcinoma in the patient with chronic pancreatitis.

Complications
Pseudocyst

A chronic collection of pancreatic fluid surrounded by a nonepithelialized wall of granulation tissue and fibrosis is referred to as a *pseudocyst*. Pseudocysts occur in up to 10% of patients with acute pancreatitis, and in 20 to 38% of patients with chronic pancreatitis, and thus, they comprise the most common complication of chronic pancreatitis.[148,186,187] The identification and treatment of pseudocysts requires definition of the various forms of pancreatic fluid collections that occur (Table 33-14). In chronic pancreatitis, a pancreatic

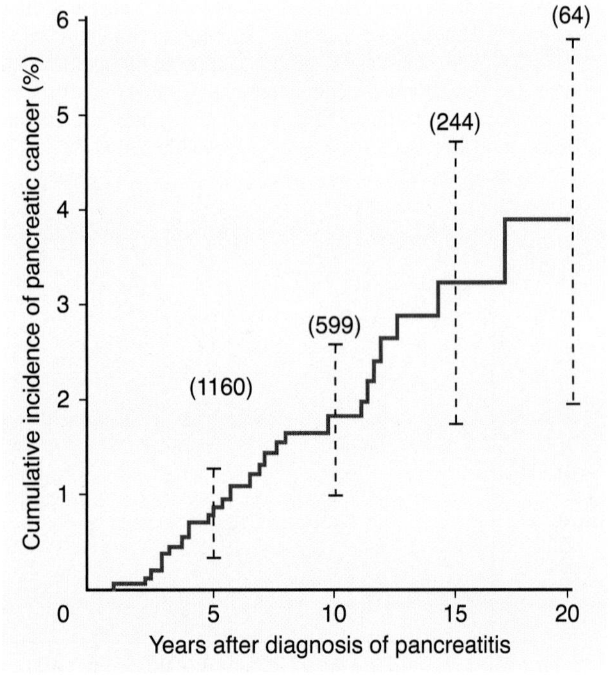

FIG. 33-37. Cumulative risk of pancreatic cancer in patients with chronic pancreatitis. The number of patients evaluated at different time intervals is shown in parentheses. *(Reproduced with permission from Lowenfels AB et al: Pancreatitis and the risk of pancreatic cancer. International Pancreatitis Study Group. N Engl J Med 328:1433, 1993. Copyright © 1993 Massachusetts Medical Society. All rights reserved.)*

TABLE 33-14	Definitions of pancreatic fluid collections
Term	**Definition**
Peripancreatic fluid collection	A collection of enzyme-rich pancreatic juice that occurs early in the course of acute pancreatitis, or that forms after a pancreatic duct leak; located in or near the pancreas; it lacks a well-organized wall of granulation or fibrous tissue
Early pancreatic (sterile) necrosis	A focal or diffuse area of nonviable pancreatic parenchyma, typically occupying >30% of the gland and containing liquefied debris and fluid
Late pancreatic (sterile) necrosis	An organized collection of sterile necrotic debris and fluid with a well-defined margin or wall within the normal domain of the pancreas
Acute pseudocyst	A collection of pancreatic juice enclosed within a perimeter of early granulation tissue, usually as a consequence of acute pancreatitis that has occurred within the preceding 3–4 wk
Chronic pseudocyst	A collection of pancreatic fluid surrounded by a wall of normal granulation and fibrous tissue, usually persisting for >6 wk
Pancreatic abscess	Any of the above in which gross purulence (pus) is present, with bacterial or fungal organisms documented to be present

Source: Modified with permission from Baron et al.[193] Copyright Elsevier.

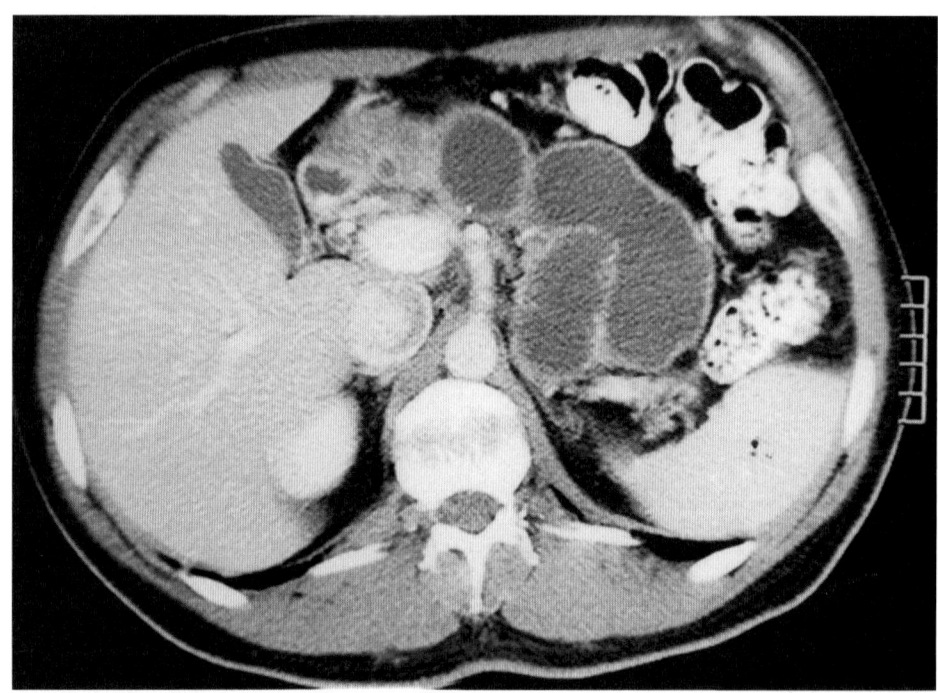

FIG. 33-38. Extensive pseudocyst disease. A computed tomographic scan in a patient with alcoholic chronic pancreatitis demonstrates multiloculated pseudocyst disease.

duct leak with extravasation of pancreatic juice results in a PFC. Over a period of 3 to 4 weeks, the PFC is sealed by an inflammatory reaction that leads to development of a wall of acute granulation tissue without much fibrosis. This is referred to as an *acute pseudocyst*. Acute pseudocysts may resolve spontaneously in up to 50% of cases, over a course of 6 weeks or longer.[186,187] Pseudocysts >6 cm resolve less frequently than smaller ones but may regress over a period of weeks to months. Pseudocysts are multiple in 17% of patients,[188] or may be multilobulated. They may occur intrapancreatically or extend beyond the region of the pancreas into other cavities or compartments (Fig. 33-38).

Pseudocysts may become secondarily infected, in which case they become abscesses. They can compress or obstruct adjacent organs or structures, leading to superior mesenteric-portal vein thrombosis or splenic vein thrombosis.[189] They can erode into visceral arteries and cause intracystic hemorrhage or pseudoaneurysms (Fig. 33-39). They also can perforate and cause peritonitis or intraperitoneal bleeding.[190]

Pseudocysts usually cause symptoms of pain, fullness, or early satiety. Asymptomatic pseudocysts can be managed expectantly and may resolve spontaneously or persist without complication.[187,191] Symptomatic or enlarging pseudocysts require treatment, and any presumed pseudocyst without a documented antecedent episode of acute pancreatitis requires investigation to determine the etiology of the lesion.[192] Although pseudocysts comprise roughly two thirds of all pancreatic cystic lesions, they resemble cystadenomas and

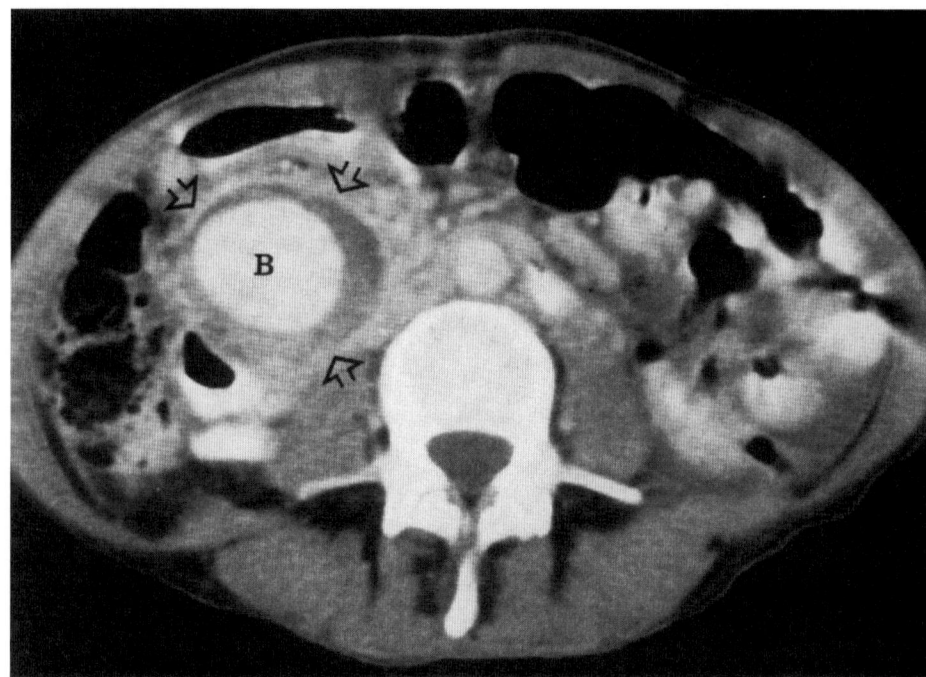

FIG. 33-39. Pseudoaneurysm of the gastroduodenal artery. A pseudocyst can erode into an adjacent artery, which results in contained hemorrhage otherwise known as a *pseudoaneurysm*. A contrast-injected computed tomographic scan reveals active bleeding (*B*) into a pseudocyst (*arrows*) as a result of this process. (*Reproduced with permission from Freeney.*[137])

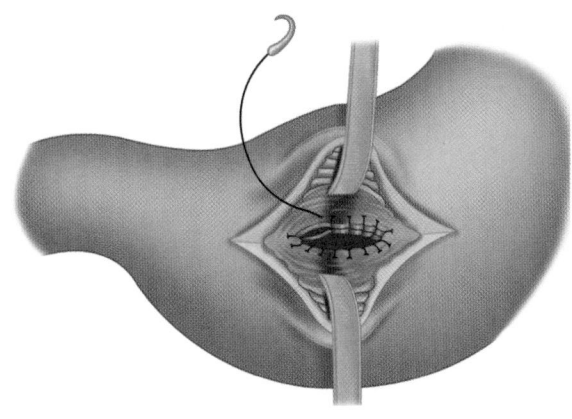

FIG. 33-40. Cystogastrostomy drainage of a retrogastric pancreatic pseudocyst. A larger opening is made through the common wall of a retrogastric pseudocyst, and a portion of the pseudocyst wall is submitted for histologic confirmation of the diagnosis. Suture reinforcement of the communication is performed to avoid the complication of bleeding. *(Reproduced with permission from Bell.[196])*

cystadenocarcinoma radiographically. An incidentally discovered cystic lesion should be examined by EUS and aspirated to determine whether it is a true neoplasm or a pseudocyst.

The timing and method of treatment requires careful consideration.[191,193] Pitfalls in the management of pseudocysts result from the incorrect (presumptive) diagnosis of a cystic neoplasm masquerading as a pseudocyst, a failure to appreciate the solid or debris-filled contents of a pseudocyst that appears to be fluid filled on CT scan, and a failure to document true adherence with an adjacent portion of the stomach before attempting transgastric internal drainage. Therefore, the management of a pseudocyst, as with other treatment decisions regarding chronic pancreatitis, should involve the multidisciplinary evaluation and selection of any given treatment strategy. Surgeons, therapeutic endoscopists, and interventional radiologists together offer all the expertise necessary to obtain the best possible outcome for a patient with pseudocystic disease. The challenge is to select the best approach for each individual patient, and this requires dedicated and experienced representatives from each specialty to participate in the decision making.

If infection is suspected, the pseudocyst should be aspirated (not drained) by CT- or US-guided FNA, and the contents examined for organisms by Gram's stain and culture.[194] If infection is present, and the contents resemble pus, external drainage is employed, using either surgical or percutaneous techniques.

If the pseudocyst has failed to resolve with conservative therapy, and symptoms persist, internal drainage is usually preferred to external drainage, to avoid the complication of a pancreaticocutaneous fistula. Pseudocysts communicate with the pancreatic ductal system in up to 80% of cases,[188,193] so external drainage creates a pathway for pancreatic duct leakage to and through the catheter exit site. Internal drainage may be performed with either percutaneous catheter-based methods (transgastric puncture and stent placement to create a cystogastrostomy), endoscopic methods (transgastric or transduodenal puncture and multiple stent placements, with or without a nasocystic irrigation catheter), or surgical methods (a true cystoenterostomy, biopsy of cyst wall, and evacuation of all debris and contents). Surgical options include a cystogastrostomy (Fig. 33-40), a Roux-en-Y cystojejunostomy, or a cystoduodenostomy. Cystojejunostomy is the most versatile method, and it can be applied to pseudocysts that penetrate into the transverse mesocolon, the paracolic gutters, or the lesser sac. Cystogastrostomy can be performed endoscopically[195] (Fig. 33-41), laparoscopically,[196] or by a combined laparoscopic-endoscopic method.[197]

Because pseudocysts often communicate with the pancreatic ductal system, two newer approaches to pseudocyst management are based on main duct drainage, rather than pseudocyst drainage per se. Transpapillary stents inserted at the time of ERCP may be directed into a pseudocyst through the ductal communication itself (Fig. 33-42), or can be left across the area of suspected duct leakage to facilitate decompression and cyst drainage, analogous to the use of common bile duct stents in the setting of a cystic duct leak.[195,197] In a surgical series of patients with chronic pancreatitis, ductal dilatation, and a coexisting pseudocyst, Nealon and Walser showed that duct drainage alone, without a separate cystoenteric anastomosis, was as successful as a combined drainage procedure.[198] Furthermore, the "duct drainage only" group enjoyed a shorter hospital stay and fewer complications than the group who underwent a separate cystoenterostomy. These observations suggest that transductal drainage may be a safe and effective approach to the management of pseudocystic disease. The endoscopic approach seems logical in the treatment of postoperative or posttraumatic pseudocysts when duct disruption is documented or in those patients with pseudocysts that communicate with the duct. Whether the technique will be as effective for chronic

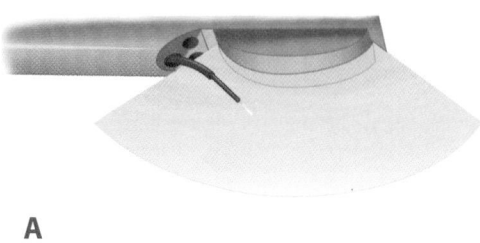

A

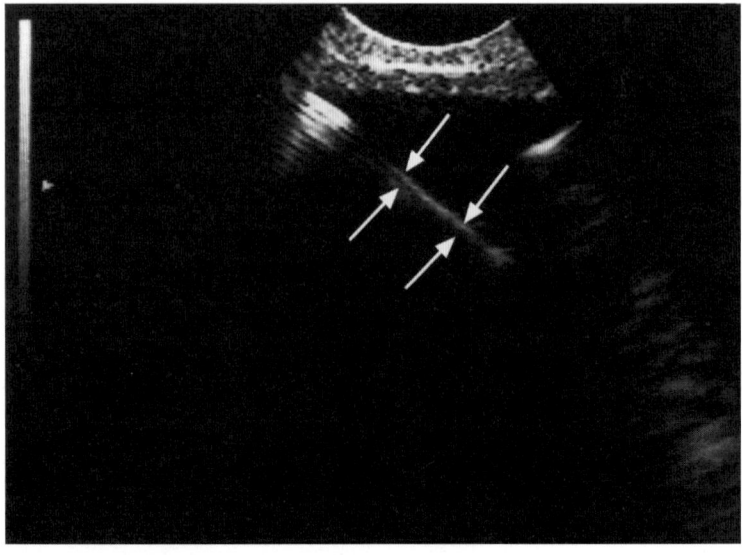

B

FIG. 33-41. Technique of endoluminal cystogastrostomy. **A.** A diagram of the linear-array endoscopic ultrasound probe that incorporates a needle-knife within the field of the ultrasound scan. **B.** Endoscopic ultrasound image showing extension of the needle-knife into the adjacent pseudocyst through the posterior gastric wall *(arrows)*. *(Reproduced with permission from Kozarek et al.[195])*

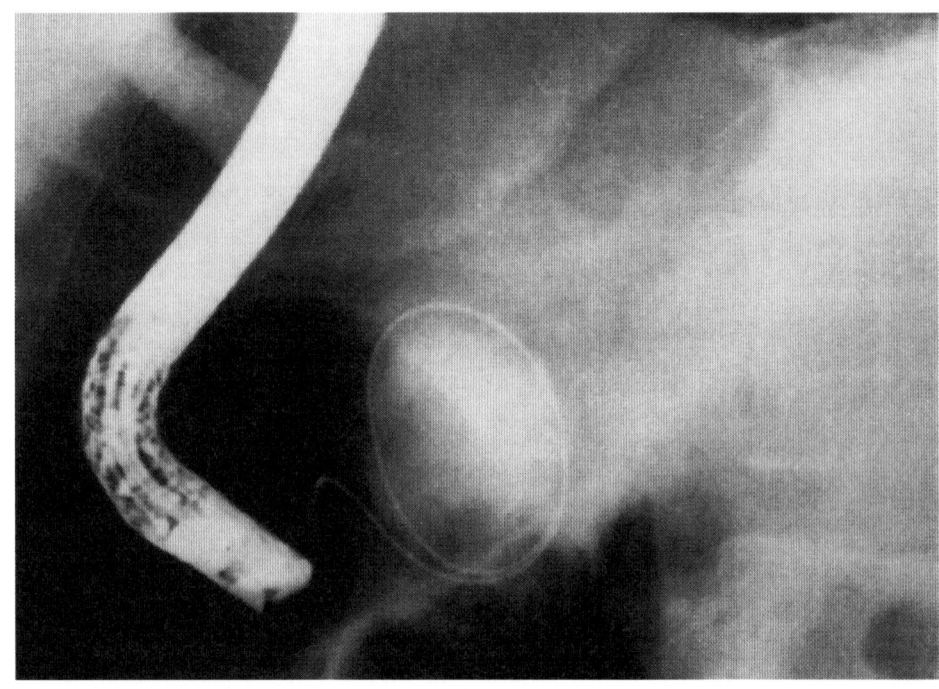

A

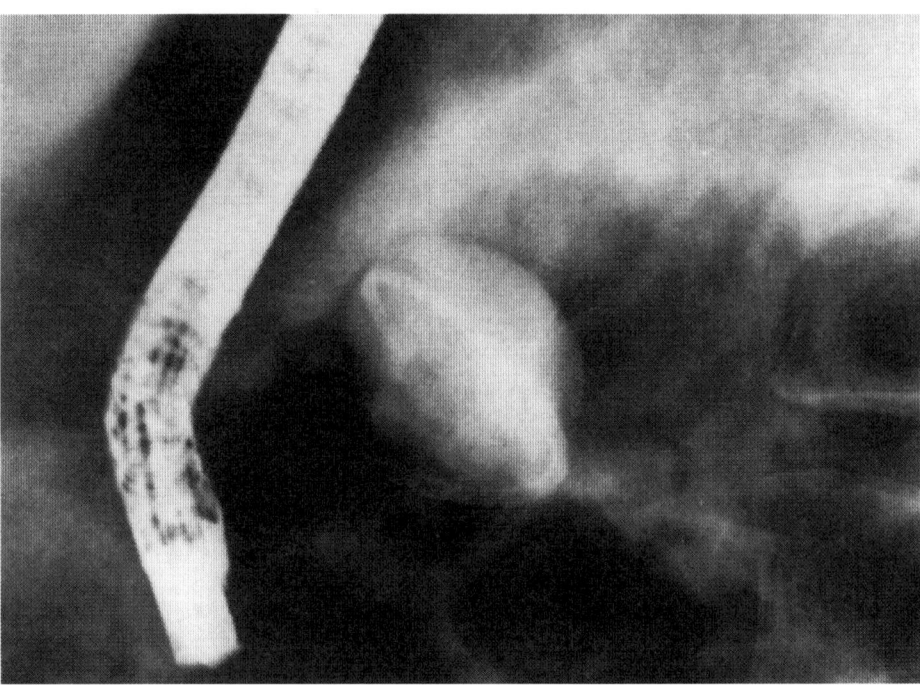

B

FIG. 33-42. Transpapillary drainage of a pancreatic pseudocyst. **A.** Endoscopic passage of a flexible wire through the major papilla, through the pancreatic duct, and into a communicating pseudocyst. **B.** Placement of a stent over the wire into the pseudocyst with transpapillary drainage. (*Reproduced with permission from Kozarek et al.*[195])

pseudocysts without demonstrable communication with the pancreatic duct remains open to investigation.

The complications of endoscopic or radiologic drainage of pseudocysts often require surgical intervention. Bleeding from the cystoenterostomy, and inoculation of a pseudocyst with failure of resolution and persistence of infection, may require surgical treatment. Bleeding risks may be lessened by the routine use of EUS in the selection of the site for transluminal stent placement.[199] Percutaneous and endoscopic treatment of pseudocysts requires large-bore catheters, multiple stents, and an aggressive approach to management for success to be achieved. Failure of nonsurgical therapy, with subsequent salvage procedures to remove infected debris and establish complete drainage,

is associated with increased risks for complications and death.[200,201] The most experienced therapeutic endoscopists report a complication rate of 17 to 19% for the treatment of sterile pseudocysts, and deaths as a result of endoscopic therapy have occurred.[193] The use of endoscopic methods to treat sterile or infected pancreatic necrosis has a higher complication rate and is limited to specialized centers.[199]

Resection of a pseudocyst is sometimes indicated for cysts located in the pancreatic tail, or when a midpancreatic duct disruption has resulted in a distally located pseudocyst. Distal pancreatectomy for removal of a pseudocyst, with or without splenectomy, can be a challenging procedure in the setting of prior pancreatitis. An internal drainage procedure of the communicating duct or of the

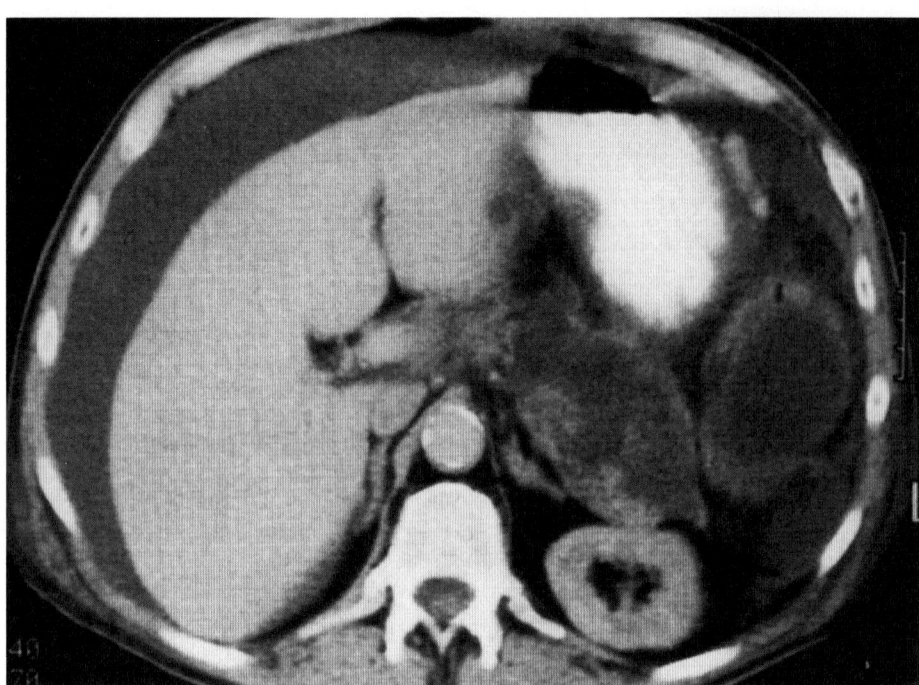

FIG. 33-43. Pancreatic ascites. Computed tomographic scan of a patient with a ruptured pancreatic pseudocyst resulting in intraperitoneal pancreatic fluid. (*Reproduced with permission from Lipsett et al.[203]*)

pseudocyst itself should be considered when distal resection is being contemplated.

Pancreatic Ascites

When a disrupted pancreatic duct leads to pancreatic fluid extravasation that does not become sequestered as a pseudocyst, but drains freely into the peritoneal cavity, pancreatic ascites occurs. Occasionally, the pancreatic fluid tracks superiorly into the thorax, and a pancreatic pleural effusion occurs. Referred to as *internal pancreatic fistulae*, both complications are seen more often in patients with chronic pancreatitis rather than after acute pancreatitis. Pancreatic ascites and pleural effusion occur together in 14% of patients, and 18% have a pancreatic pleural effusion alone.[202–204]

Patients demonstrate the general demographics of chronic pancreatitis and usually present with a subacute or recent history of progressive abdominal swelling despite weight loss. Pain and nausea are rarely present. The abdominal CT scan discloses ascites and the presence of chronic pancreatitis or a partially collapsed pseudocyst (Fig. 33-43). Paracentesis or thoracentesis reveals noninfected fluid with a protein level >25 g/L and a markedly elevated amylase level. Serum amylase may also be elevated, presumably from reabsorption across the parietal membrane. Serum albumin may be low, and patients may have coexisting liver disease. Paracentesis is therefore critical to differentiate pancreatic from hepatic ascites.

ERCP is most helpful to delineate the location of the pancreatic duct leak and to elucidate the underlying pancreatic ductal anatomy. Pancreatic duct stenting may be considered at the time of ERCP, but if nonsurgical therapy is undertaken and then abandoned, repeat imaging of the pancreatic duct is appropriate to guide surgical treatment.

Antisecretory therapy with the somatostatin analogue octreotide acetate, together with bowel rest and parenteral nutrition, is successful in more than half of patients.[205] Reapposition of serosal surfaces to facilitate closure of the leak is considered a part of therapy, and this is accomplished by complete paracentesis. For pleural effusions, a period of chest tube drainage may facilitate closure of the internal fistula.[202,205] Surgical therapy is reserved for those who fail to respond to medical treatment. If the leak originates from the central region of the pancreas, a Roux-en-Y pancreaticojejunostomy is performed to the site of duct leakage (Fig. 33-44). If the leak is in the tail, a distal pancreatectomy may be considered, or an internal

drainage procedure can be performed. The results of surgical treatment are usually favorable if the ductal anatomy has been carefully delineated preoperatively.

Pancreatic-Enteric Fistula

The erosion of a pancreatic pseudocyst into an adjacent hollow viscus can result in a pancreatic-enteric fistula. The most common site of

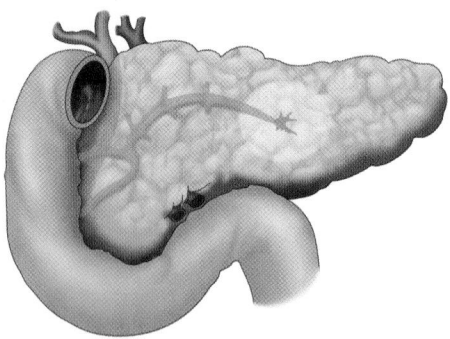

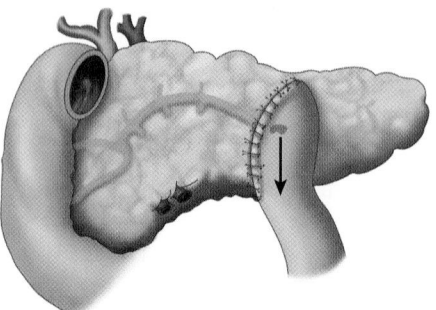

FIG. 33-44. Internal drainage for leaking pancreatic duct. A Roux-en-Y pancreaticojejunostomy is performed at the site of duct rupture to accomplish internal drainage of the pancreatic duct leak. (*Reproduced with permission from Cameron.[202]*)

| TABLE 33-15 | Signs and symptoms of chronic pancreatitis with and without a pancreatic head mass |

Signs and Symptoms	With Head Enlargement (n = 138) (%)	Without Head Enlargement (n = 141) (%)
Daily severe pain	67	40
Cholestasis	46	11
Slight to frequent pain	33	60
Duodenal obstruction	30	7
Diabetes mellitus	18	30
Vascular involvement	15	8

Source: Reproduced with permission from Beger et al.[207]

communication is the transverse colon or splenic flexure. The fistula usually presents with evidence of GI or colonic bleeding and sepsis. If the fistula communicates with the stomach or duodenum, it may close spontaneously or persist as a pancreatic-enteric fistula. When the fistula involves the colon, operative correction is usually required.[206]

Head-of-Pancreas Mass

In up to 30% of patients with advanced chronic pancreatitis, an inflammatory mass develops in the head of the pancreas.[207] The clinical presentation includes severe pain, and frequently includes stenosis of the distal common bile duct, duodenal stenosis, compression of the portal vein, and stenosis of the proximal main pancreatic duct (Table 33-15). In a series of 279 patients with chronic pancreatitis treated surgically at the University of Ulm in Germany, patients with pancreatic head enlargement represented half of the total group. The subgroup with pancreatic head enlargement appeared to have a lower incidence of endocrine and exocrine insufficiency, but a higher expression of epidermal growth factor and the c-erbB-2 protooncogene.[208] Mutations and polymorphisms of p53 were found in 3 and 8% of these patients, respectively, and a focus of ductular carcinoma was found in 3.7% of patients with pancreatic head enlargement. It was concluded that an accelerated transformation from hyperplasia to dysplasia exists in patients with pancreatic head enlargement, although the etiology for this process remains unclear. Treatment in the majority of cases consisted of the duodenum-preserving pancreatic head resection (DPPHR), with good results.

Splenic and Portal Vein Thrombosis

Vascular complications of chronic pancreatitis are fortunately infrequent, because they are difficult to treat successfully. Portal vein compression and occlusion can occur as a consequence of an inflammatory mass in the head of the pancreas, and splenic vein thrombosis occurs in association with chronic pancreatitis in 4 to 8% of cases.[209] Variceal formation can occur as a consequence of either portal or splenic venous occlusion, and splenic vein thrombosis with gastric variceal formation is referred to as *left-sided* or *sinistral portal hypertension*. Although bleeding complications are infrequent, the mortality risk of bleeding is >20%. When gastroesophageal varices are caused by splenic vein thrombosis, the addition of splenectomy to prevent variceal hemorrhage is prudent when surgery is otherwise indicated to correct other problems.

Treatment
Medical Therapy

The medical treatment of chronic or recurrent pain in chronic pancreatitis requires the use of analgesics, a cessation of alcohol use, oral enzyme therapy, and the selective use of antisecretory therapy. Interventional procedures to block visceral afferent nerve conduction or to treat obstructions of the main pancreatic duct are also an adjunct to medical treatment.

Analgesia

Oral analgesics are prescribed as needed, alone or with analgesia-enhancing agents such as gabapentin. Adequate pain control usually requires the use of narcotics, but these should be titrated to achieve pain relief with the lowest effective dose. Opioid addiction is common, and the use of long-acting analgesics by transdermal patch together with oral agents for pain exacerbations slightly reduces the sedative effects of high-dose oral narcotics.

It is essential for patients to abstain from alcohol. In addition to removing the causative agent, alcohol abstention results in pain reduction or relief in 60 to 75% of patients with chronic pancreatitis.[210] Despite this benefit, roughly half of alcoholic chronic pancreatitis patients continue to abuse alcohol.

Enzyme Therapy

Pancreatic enzyme administration serves to reverse the effects of pancreatic exocrine insufficiency and may reduce or alleviate the pain experienced by patients. The choice of enzyme supplement and the dose should be selected based on whether malabsorption or pain (or both) are the indications for therapy[211] (Table 33-16). Conventional (non–enteric-coated) enzyme preparations are partially degraded by gastric acid but are available within the duodenal and jejunal regions to bind to CCK-releasing peptide, and downregulate the release of CCK. This theoretically reduces the enteric signal for pancreatic exocrine secretion, which reduces the pressure within a partially or completely obstructed pancreatic duct.[212,213] Enteric-coated preparations result in little to no pain relief, presumably due to their reduced bioavailability in the proximal gut.[214] Due to the loss of pancreatic enzymes by acid hydrolysis and proteolysis, relatively large doses are required to achieve effective levels of enzyme within the proximal small bowel. Enteric-coated preparations are protected from acid degradation but are presumably not released in the critical proximal gut in sufficient quantity to inhibit the stimulus for endogenous pancreatic enzyme secretion. Nonalcoholic patients may experience more effective pain relief than alcoholic patients,[211] but it is recommended that all patients with chronic pancreatitis pain begin a trial of non–enteric-coated enzyme supplements for 1 month. If pain relief is achieved, therapy is continued. If enzyme therapy fails, further investigation of the pancreatic ductal system by ERCP guides the therapy based on the presence or absence of large duct (obstructive) disease (Fig. 33-45).

Antisecretory Therapy

Somatostatin administration has been shown to inhibit pancreatic exocrine secretion and CCK release.[215] The somatostatin analogue

| TABLE 33-16 | Pancreatic enzyme preparations |

Name	Dose[a]	Lipase/Protease (USP Units)
Conventional (non-enteric-coated) compounds[b]		
Viokase	8 tablets each time	8000/30,000
Ku-Zyme HP	8 tablets each time	8000/30,000
Enteric-coated compounds[c]		
Creon 10	2–3 capsules each time	10,000/37,500
Creon 20	2–3 capsules each time	20,000/75,000
Pancrease MT 10	2–3 capsules each time	10,000/30,000
Pancrease MT 16	2–3 capsules each time	16,000/48,000

[a]The dosing schedule is before meals; can also take a dose at night if patient experiences pain.
[b]Conventional enzymes are the treatment of choice for pain relief. If no improvement occurs with conventional enzymes alone, add H_2-blockers or proton pump inhibitors to decrease peptic acid inhibition of the enzymes.
[c]Enteric-coated preparations are treatment of choice for steatorrhea. Acid-suppressive therapy should not be given with enteric-coated preparations.
USP = United States Pharmacopeia.

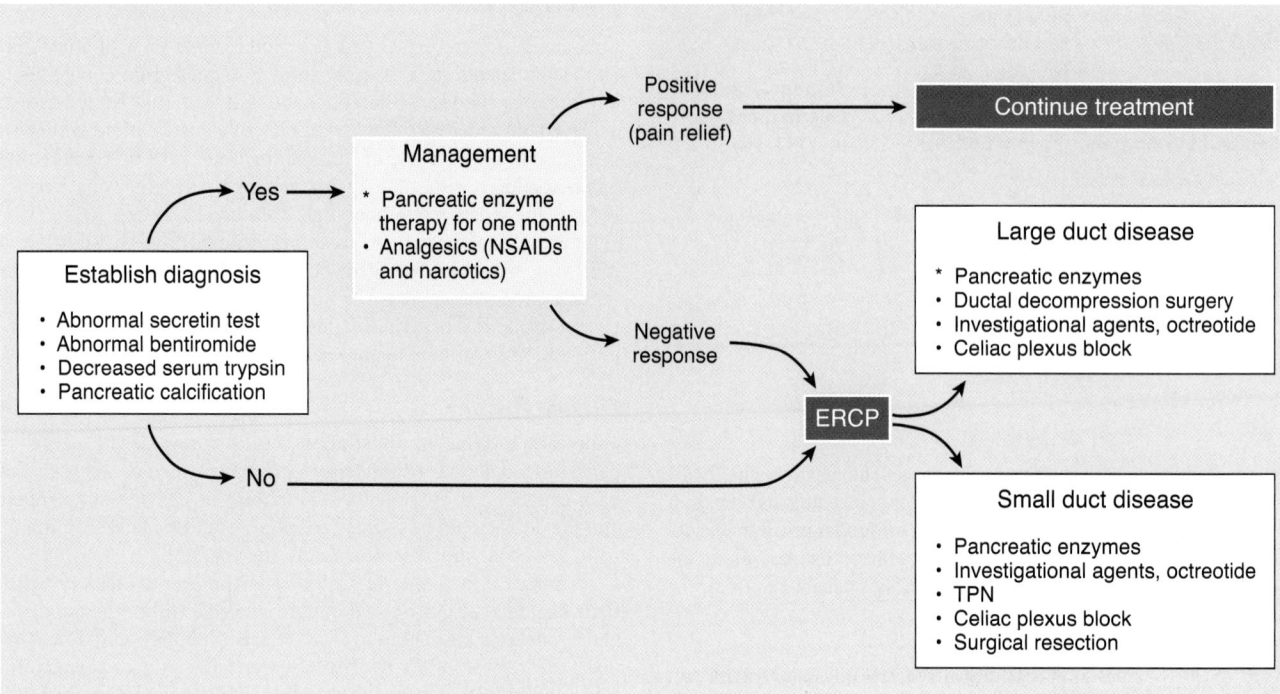

FIG. 33-45. Algorithm for the treatment of chronic pancreatitis pain. ERCP = endoscopic retrograde cholangiopancreatography; TPN = total parenteral nutrition. *(Reproduced with permission from Amann et al.[211])*

octreotide acetate has therefore been investigated for pain relief in patients with chronic pancreatitis.[216,217] In a double-blind, prospective, randomized 4-week trial, 65% of patients who received 200 μg of octreotide acetate subcutaneously three times daily reported pain relief, compared with 35% of placebo-treated subjects. Patients who had the best results were patients with chronic abdominal pain, suggestive of obstructive pancreatopathy. However, in another trial that used a 3-day duration of treatment, no significant pain relief was observed.[218] None of the studies published thus far have examined the sustained-release formulation of octreotide, and it remains unclear what subgroups of patients, or what dose of octreotide, might be beneficial in the treatment of pain. Anecdotal reports suggest that severe pain exacerbations in chronic pancreatitis can benefit from a combination of octreotide therapy and TPN, and trials are currently underway to assess the effectiveness of the sustained-release form of octreotide that requires only once-monthly administration.

Neurolytic Therapy

Celiac plexus neurolysis with alcohol injection has been an effective form of analgesic treatment in patients with pancreatic carcinoma. However, the use of radiologically- or endoscopically-guided celiac plexus blockade in chronic pancreatitis has been disappointing. Due to the risk of alcohol injury and the need for repeated injections, celiac plexus blockade in chronic pancreatitis has used short-acting analgesics or other drugs rather than 50% alcohol. A recent trial of EUS-guided celiac plexus blockade revealed successful pain relief in 55% of patients, but the benefit lasted beyond 6 months in only 10% of patients.[219] The procedure therefore appears safe, but the effect is short lived in those patients who obtain pain relief.

Endoscopic Management

The techniques of endoscopic treatment of pancreatic duct obstruction, stone disease, pseudocyst formation, pancreatic duct leak, and for the diagnosis and management of associated pancreatic tumors have expanded greatly over the past 10 years. Newer endoscopes with expanded therapeutic capabilities have been introduced, and the role of EUS and EUS-guided needle and catheter insertion has

expanded the ability of the therapeutic endoscopist in the diagnosis and treatment of chronic pancreatitis and its complications.[220]

Pancreatic duct stenting is used for treatment of proximal pancreatic duct stenosis, decompression of a pancreatic duct leak, and for drainage of pancreatic pseudocysts that can be catheterized through the main pancreatic duct (Fig. 33-46). Pancreatic duct stents can induce an inflammatory response within the duct, so prolonged stenting is usually avoided. Patients with sphincter of Oddi dyskinesia are at high risk for developing post-ERCP pancreatitis after biliary sphincterotomy, and a recent study demonstrated that the prophylactic placement of a pancreatic duct stent reduced the amylase level and development of pancreatitis after biliary sphincterotomy.[221] Pancreatic duct leaks were seen in 37% of patients with acute pancreatitis, and pancreatic duct stenting appeared to facilitate the resolution of the leak.[222] Similarly, pancreatic duct stenting has been used to treat postsurgical pancreatic duct leaks and posttraumatic leaks.[95,223,224]

Pancreas divisum (see Fig. 33-3) is thought to cause pain and chronic pancreatitis due to functional or mechanical obstruction of the dorsal duct draining exclusively, or predominantly, through the lesser papilla. A recent study from Marseille reported good long-term results in 24 patients after minor papilla sphincterotomy and dorsal duct stenting.[225] The number of patients with chronic pain decreased from 83% before stenting to 29% after stenting, but pancreatitis or recurrent papillary stenosis occurred in 38%. Patients that responded best were those with intermittent pain, and this subset may be preferentially treated with endoscopic therapy.

Idiopathic pancreatitis patients have been treated with endoscopic stenting, pancreatic duct sphincterotomy, and endoscopic stone removal with good results.[220,226] In a prospective randomized trial, 53% of idiopathic recurrent pancreatitis patients in the control group experienced continued episodes of pancreatitis, although only 11% of the treated patients had continued symptoms.[220]

Extracorporeal shock wave lithotripsy (ESWL) has been used for pancreatic duct stones, together with endoscopic stenting and stone removal.[227] A single ESWL session was used in 35 patients with pancreatic duct stones, together with 86 ERCP sessions to complete

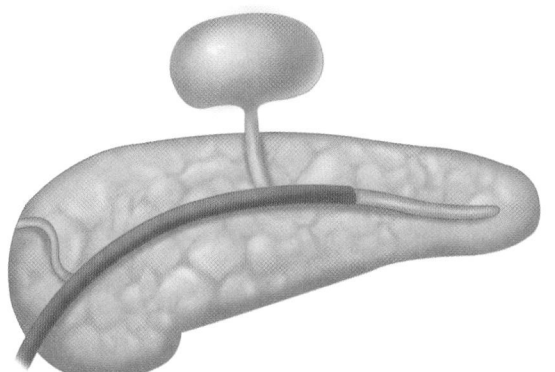

A

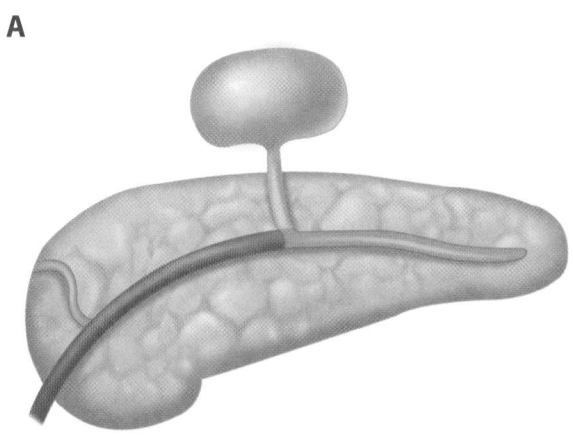

B

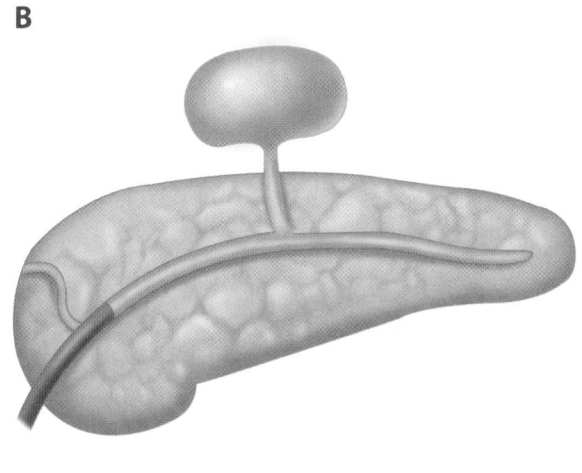

C

FIG. 33-46. Endoscopic decompression of a peripancreatic fluid collection through the pancreatic duct. Options for transpapillary placement include placement of the stent (**A**) beyond the point of duct disruption, (**B**) at the point of disruption, or (**C**) proximal to the point of duct disruption. Each of these locations may facilitate decompression of a peripancreatic fluid collection or pseudocyst caused by duct disruption, analogous to this successful treatment of a cystic duct leak by a common bile duct stent. *(Reproduced with permission from Hawes.[199])*

the stone removal process. After 2.4 years, 80% of patients had significant relief of symptoms (Fig. 33-47). However, due to the tendency for recurrent stone formation, the use of ESWL for long-term management of calcific pancreatitis remains uncertain.

Surgical Therapy

Indications and History The traditional approach to surgical treatment of chronic pancreatitis and its complications has maintained that surgery should be considered only when the medical therapy of symptoms has failed. Nealon and Thompson published a landmark study in 1993, however, that showed that the progression of chronic obstructive pancreatitis could be delayed or prevented by pancreatic duct decompression.[228] No other therapy has been shown to prevent the progression of chronic pancreatitis, and this study demonstrated the role of surgery in the early management of the disease (Table 33-17). Small-duct disease or the absence of a clear obstructive component are causes for uncertainty over the choice of operation. Major resections have a high complication rate, both early and late, in chronic alcoholic pancreatitis, and lesser procedures often result in symptomatic recurrence. So the choice of operation and the timing of surgery are based on each patient's pancreatic anatomy, the likelihood (or lack thereof) that further medical and endoscopic therapy will halt the symptoms of the disease, and the chance that a good result will be obtained with the lowest risk of morbidity and mortality. Finally, preparation for surgery should include restoration of protein-caloric homeostasis, abstinence from alcohol and tobacco, and a detailed review of the risks and likely outcomes to establish a bond of trust and commitment between the patient and the surgeon.

Historically, the surgery for chronic pancreatitis before the second half of the twentieth century was a true demonstration of trial and error, with little anatomic information available before operation. Excellent results before CT scans and ERCP were either the result of serendipity or due to the talent and creativity of the surgeon. In 1911, Link described an operation he devised on the spot, when a laparotomy in a young woman with abdominal pain revealed a fluctuant, obstructed pancreatic duct. After performing a dochotomy and evacuating multiple stones, he inserted a rubber tube, and exteriorized the pancreatostomy just above her navel.[229] He later described the operation as having been a success for the next 30 years of the patient's life, during which the patient managed the care of the drainage tube without apparent problems.[230]

With the demonstration in 1942 by Priestley that total pancreatectomy was technically feasible,[231] and the report in 1946 by Whipple that proximal pancreatic resection was beneficial in (three) patients with chronic pancreatitis,[232] the option of surgical resection as treatment for chronic pancreatitis was established. By the mid-1950s, however, growing disappointment with the high risk of resection and the lack of long-term benefit overshadowed the surgical treatment of chronic pancreatitis. The choice of resection vs. drainage was largely based on surgeon preference until the 1970s, when the widespread adoption of ERCP and CT scans provided the ability to preoperatively diagnose obstructive and sclerotic disease, and this resulted in the rational selection of operative procedures. During this period, the major drawbacks to surgical therapy remained the approximately 20% incidence of recurrent symptoms despite surgery, the corresponding development of an inflammatory (or malignant) mass in the undrained pancreatic head (Fig. 33-48), or the high morbidity and mortality of

TABLE 33-17	Effect of surgical drainage on progression of chronic pancreatitis
Treatment Group	**24-Month Evaluation**
Operated (*n* = 47)	Mild to moderate 48 (87%); severe 6 (13%)
Nonoperated (*n* = 36)	Mild to moderate 8 (22%); severe 28 (78%)

Eighty-three patients with chronic pancreatitis were evaluated by exocrine, endocrine, nutritional, and endoscopic retrograde cholangiopancreatography studies, and all had mild to moderate disease and dilated pancreatic ducts. A Puestow-type duct decompression procedure was performed in 47 patients, and all subjects were restaged by the same methods 24 months later.
Source: Reproduced with permission from Nealon et al.[228]

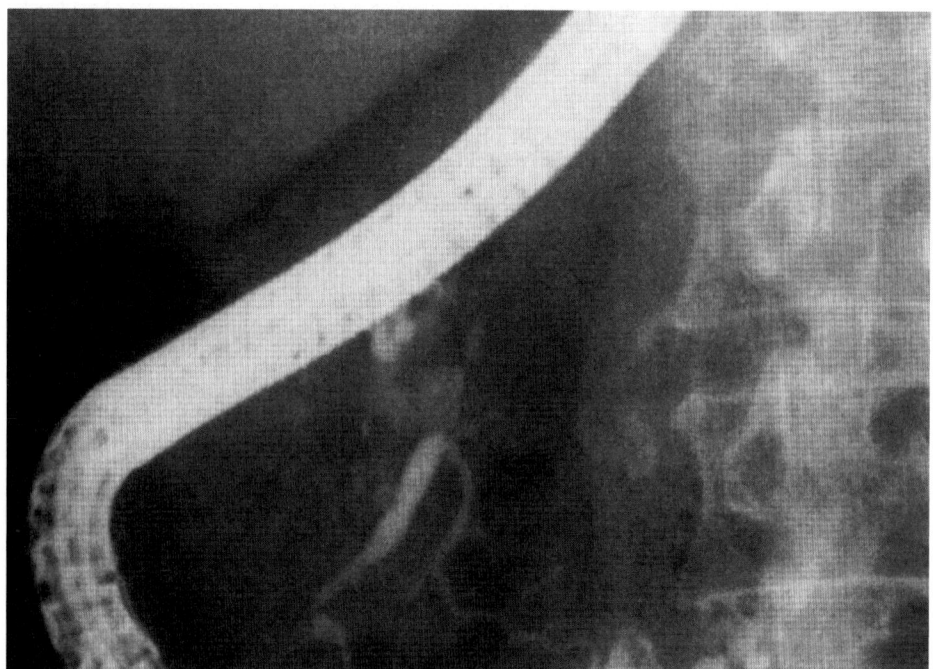

A

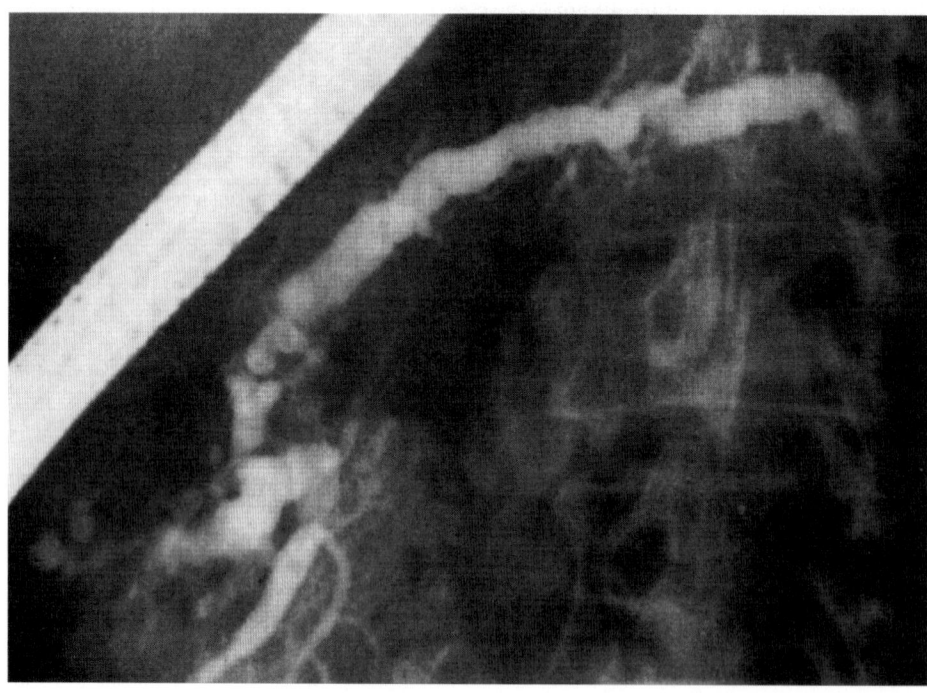

B

FIG. 33-47. Extracorporeal shock wave lithotripsy treatment of pancreatic duct stones. The endoscopic retrograde cholangiopancreatography images are shown (**A**) before and (**B**) after extracorporeal shock wave lithotripsy therapy of pancreatic duct obstruction due to calculus formation. *(Reproduced with permission from Kozarek et al.[227])*

major resectional procedures that seemed to predispose the patients to a cascade of metabolic problems.

Sphincteroplasty The sphincter of Oddi and the pancreatic duct sphincter serve as gatekeepers for the passage of pancreatic juice into the duodenum (Fig. 33-49). Stenosis of either sphincter (sclerosing papillitis), due to scarring from pancreatitis or from the passage of gallstones, may result in obstruction of the pancreatic duct and chronic pain.[233] As gallstone pancreatitis became a popular diagnosis in the 1940s and 1950s, attention was focused on the ampullary region as a possible cause of chronic symptoms, and surgical sphincteroplasty was advocated. Although endoscopic

techniques are now used routinely to perform sphincterotomy of either the common bile duct or pancreatic duct, a true (permanent) sphincteroplasty can only be performed surgically. Transduodenal sphincteroplasty with incision of the septum between the pancreatic duct and common bile duct appears to offer significant relief for patients with obstruction and inflammation isolated to this region[234] (Fig. 33-50).

Drainage Procedures After the early reports of success with pancreatostomy for the relief of symptoms of chronic pancreatitis,[229] Cattell described pancreaticojejunostomy for relief of pain in unresectable pancreatic carcinoma.[235] Shortly thereafter, Duval,[236] and

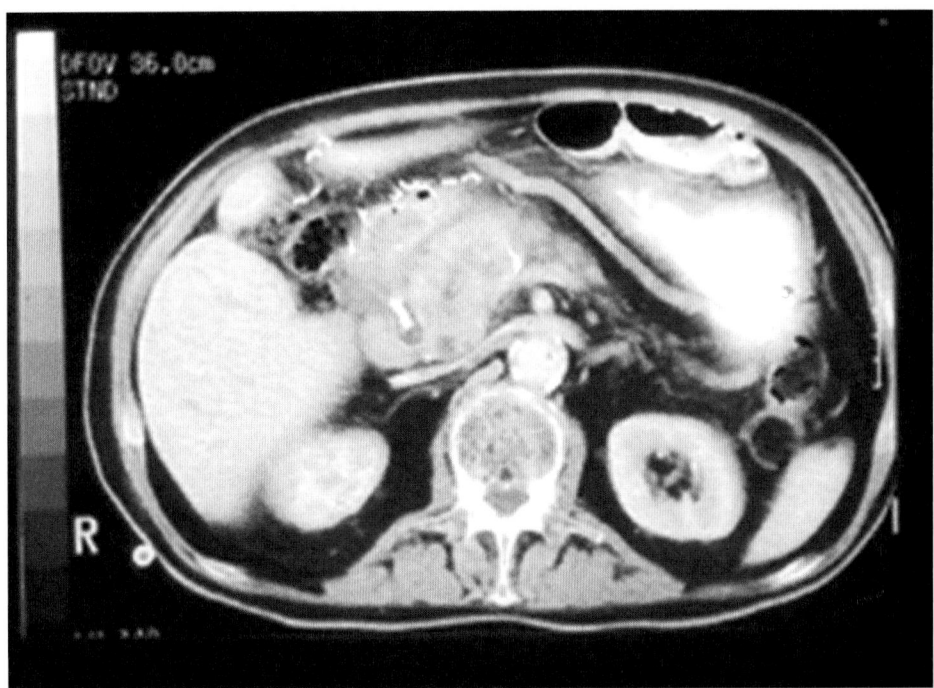

FIG. 33-48. Head-of-pancreas mass after Puestow procedure. The computed tomographic appearance of an inflammatory mass occupying the head of the pancreas, which developed 2 years after Puestow decompression of the body and tail of pancreas.

separately, Zollinger and associates,[237] described the caudal Roux-en-Y pancreaticojejunostomy for the treatment of chronic pancreatitis in 1954 (Fig. 33-51). The so-called Duval procedure was used for decades by some surgeons, but it almost invariably failed due to restenosis and segmental obstruction of the pancreas due to progressive scarring. In 1958, Puestow and Gillesby described these segmental narrowings and dilatations of the ductal system as a "chain of lakes," and proposed a longitudinal decompression of the body and tail of the pancreas into a Roux limb of jejunum[238]

(Fig 33-52). Four of Puestow and Gillesby's 21 initial cases were side-to-side anastomoses, and 2 years after their report, Partington and Rochelle described a much simpler version of the longitudinal, or side-to-side Roux-en-Y pancreaticojejunostomy that became universally known as the Puestow procedure[239] (Fig. 33-53).

The effectiveness of decompression of the pancreatic duct is dependent on the extent to which ductal hypertension is the etiologic agent for the disease. Thus, the diameter of the pancreatic duct is a surrogate for the degree of ductal hypertension, and the Puestow

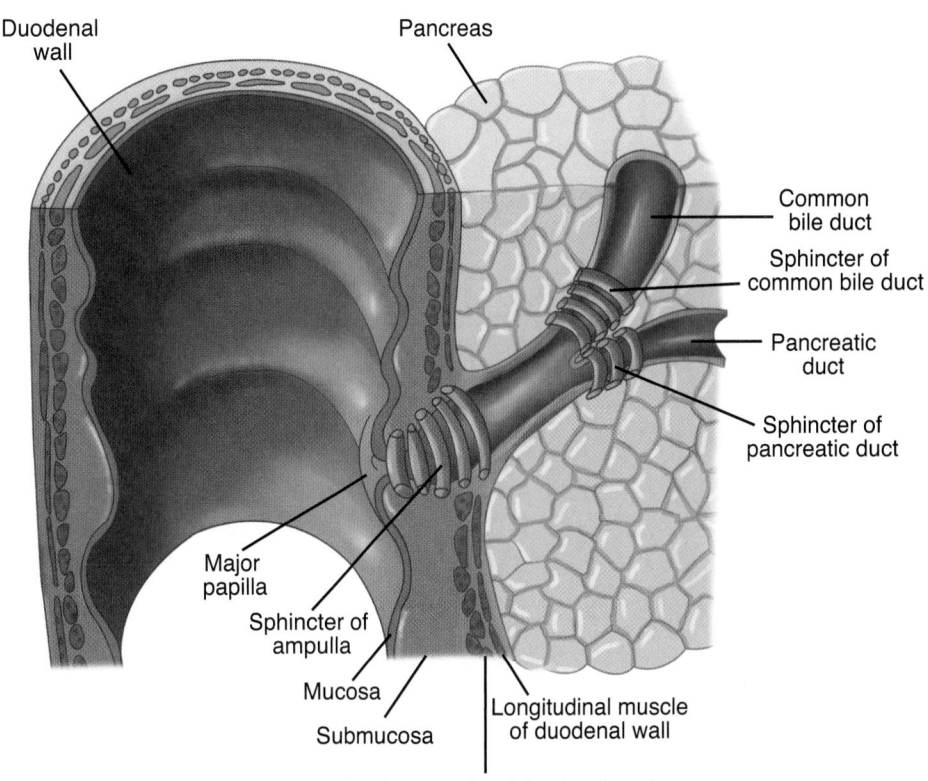

FIG. 33-49. Schematic diagram of the ampullary, biliary, and pancreatic duct sphincters. The point of merger of the bile duct and pancreatic duct is highly variable, and a true sphincter of the pancreatic duct may be poorly developed. [After Simeone DM: Gallbladder and biliary tract, in Yamada T et al (eds): Textbook of Gastroenterology, 4th ed. Philadelphia: Lippincott Williams & Wilkins, 2003, p 2173, with permission.]

Duodenal wall

Pancreas

Common bile duct

Sphincter of common bile duct

Pancreatic duct

Sphincter of pancreatic duct

Major papilla

Sphincter of ampulla

Mucosa

Submucosa

Longitudinal muscle of duodenal wall

Circular muscle of duodenal wall

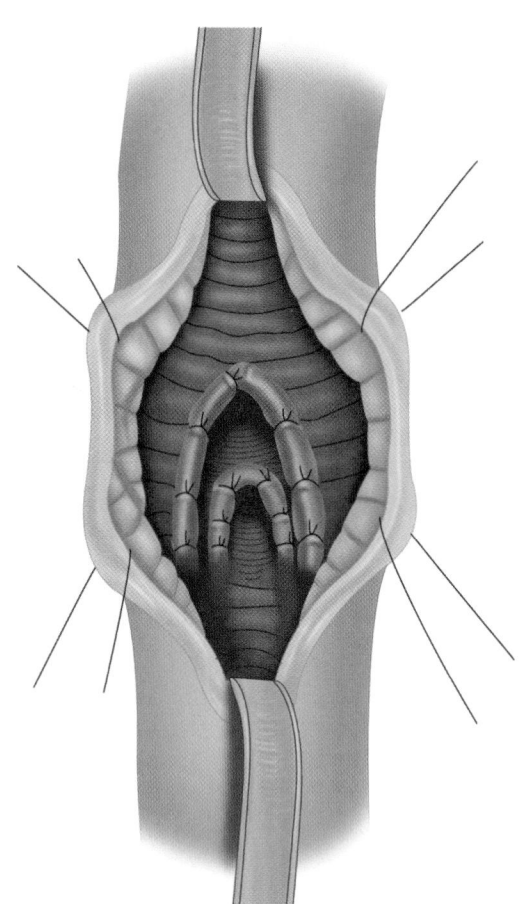

FIG. 33-50. Operative sphincteroplasty of the biliary and pancreatic duct. The ampullary and bile duct sphincters are divided, as is the pancreatic duct sphincter, with suture apposition of the mucosal edges of the incision. *(Adapted with permission from Moody et al.[234])*

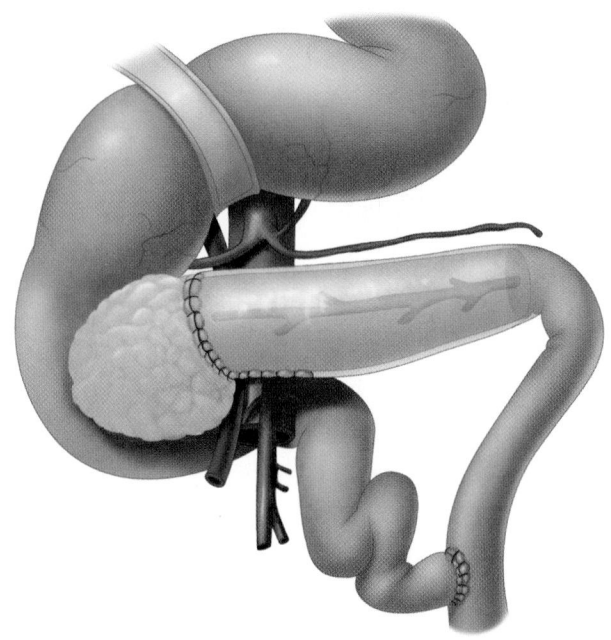

FIG. 33-52. Puestow and Gillesby's longitudinal pancreaticojejunostomy. Originally described as an invaginating anastomosis that drained the entire body and tail, the anastomosis was created after amputating the tail of the gland and opening the duct along the long axis of the gland. *[Reproduced with permission from Greenlee HB: The role of surgery for chronic pancreatitis and its complications, in Nyhus LM (ed): Surg Annu, Vol 15. Norwalk, Connecticut: Appleton-Century-Crofts, 1983, p 290.]*

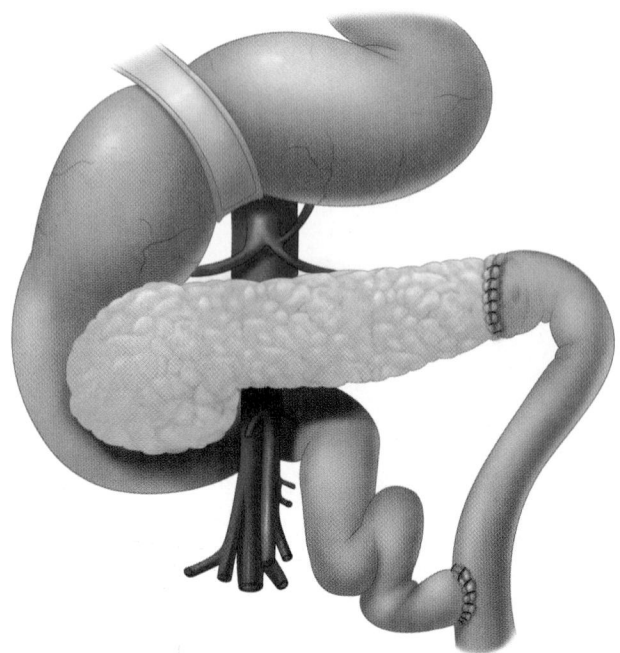

FIG. 33-51. Duval's caudal pancreaticojejunostomy. *[Reproduced with permission from Greenlee HB: The role of surgery for chronic pancreatitis and its complications, in Nyhus LM (ed): Surg Annu, Vol 15. Norwalk, Connecticut: Appleton-Century-Crofts, 1983, p 289.]*

procedure has been shown to be effective for pain relief when the maximum duct diameter is 6 mm. Results are less impressive in glands with smaller caliber ducts, although Izbicki and associates have described good results with a conization method that allows a longitudinal decompression of more normal caliber ducts.[240] Successful pain relief after the Puestow-type decompression procedure has been reported in 75 to 85% of patients for the first few years after surgery, but pain recurs in >20% of patients after 5 years,[149] even in patients who are abstinent from alcohol.

With the advent of therapeutic endoscopy and techniques for transluminal stone removal and lithotripsy, modern clinical series have reported the successful endoscopic treatment of pancreatic duct calculi, although the long-term outcomes of these efforts has been uneven.[241-244] Endoscopic removal of pancreatic duct stones is usually coupled to prolonged pancreatic duct stenting, which carries the risk of further inflammation.[245,246] Despite the risk of perioperative complications, the surgical management of pancreatic duct stones and stenosis has been shown to be superior to endoscopic treatment in randomized clinical trials in which the long, side-to-side technique of pancreaticojejunostomy is used.[247,248]

Resectional Procedures *Distal Pancreatectomy* For patients with focal inflammatory changes localized to the body and tail, or in whom no significant ductal dilatation exists, the technique of partial (40 to 80%) distal pancreatectomy has been advocated (Fig. 33-54). Although distal pancreatectomy is less morbid than more extensive resectional procedures, the operation leaves untreated a major portion of the gland, and is therefore associated with a significant risk of symptomatic recurrence.[140] It has been a more popular operation in British centers, where its success seems to be greater, perhaps due to the lower incidence of alcoholic chronic pancreatitis.[249] However, long-term outcomes reveal good pain relief in only 60% of patients, with completion pancreatectomy required for pain relief in 13% of patients.

Laparoscopic distal pancreatectomy has been shown to be feasible for the removal of focal lesions of the distal pancreas[250] but is more difficult in the setting of chronic pancreatitis.

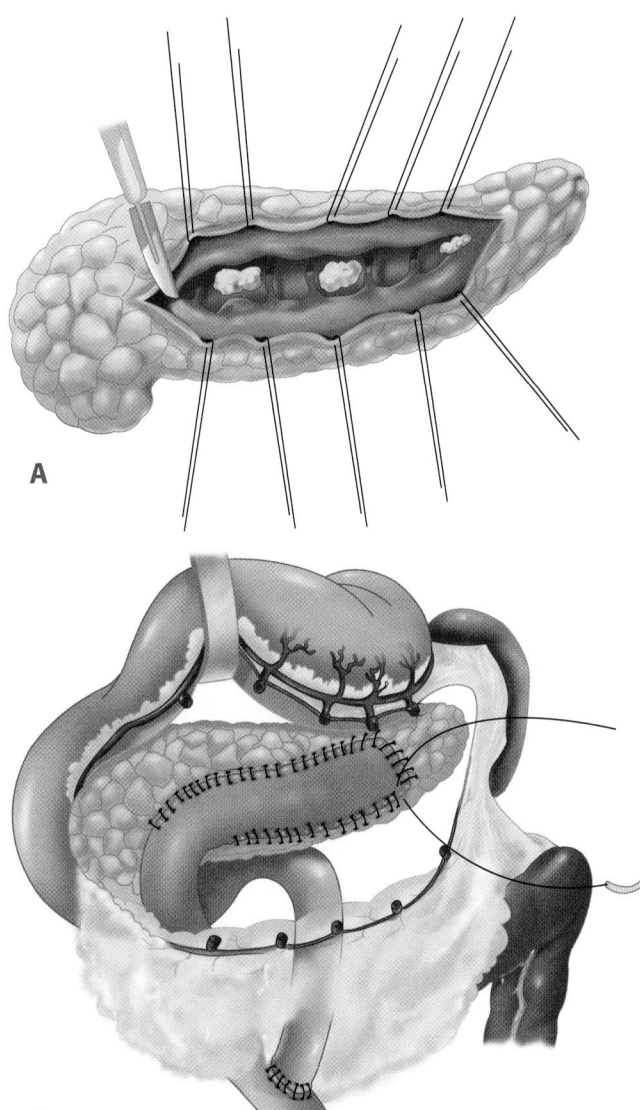

FIG. 33-53. Longitudinal dochotomy in obstructing calcific pancreatitis. A longitudinal pancreatotomy typically discloses segmental stenosis of the pancreatic duct and the presence of intraductal calculi in a patient with chronic calcific pancreatitis (**A**). Following mobilization of a Roux limb of jejunum, a longitudinal pancreaticojejunostomy is performed to permit extensive drainage of the pancreatic duct system (**B**). This technique, described by Partington and Rochelle, is the typical method used for the Puestow procedure. *(Reproduced with permission from Partington et al.[239])*

Ninety-Five Percent Distal Pancreatectomy In 1965, Fry and Child proposed the more radical 95% distal pancreatectomy, which was intended for patients with sclerotic (small duct) disease, and which attempted to avoid the morbidity of total pancreatectomy by preserving the rim of pancreas in the pancreaticoduodenal groove, along with its associated blood vessels and distal common bile duct.[233] The operation was found to be associated with pain relief in 60 to 77% of patients long term, but is accompanied by a high risk of brittle diabetes, hypoglycemic coma, and malnutrition.[251] Although the operation was the first attempt to resect the pancreatic head while preserving the duodenum and distal bile duct, the extensive degree of pancreatic removal led to its failure as viable treatment for the symptoms of pancreatic sclerosis.

Proximal Pancreatectomy In 1946, Whipple reported a series of five patients treated with either pancreaticoduodenectomy or total pancreatectomy for symptomatic chronic pancreatitis, with one operative death.[232] Subsequently, proximal pancreatectomy or pancreaticoduodenectomy, with or without pylorus preservation (Fig. 33-55), has been widely used for the treatment of chronic pancreatitis.[145,206,252] In the three largest modern (circa 2000) series of the treatment of chronic pancreatitis by the Whipple procedure, pain relief 4 to 6 years after operation was found in 71 to 89% of patients. However, mortality ranged from 1.5 to 3%, and major complications occurred in 25 to 38% of patients at the Johns Hopkins Hospital,[253] the Massachusetts General Hospital,[254] and the Mayo Clinic.[255] In follow-up, 25 to 48% of patients developed diabetes, and about the same percentage required exocrine therapy. Advocates of the Whipple procedure uniformly suggest that the high rate of symptomatic relief outweighs the metabolic consequences and the mortality risk of the procedure.

Total Pancreatectomy Priestley and associates first described successful total pancreatectomy in 1944 in a patient with hyperinsulinism,[231] and two of Whipple's original five cases of chronic pancreatitis reported in 1946 were treated with total pancreatectomy.[232] Subsequently, surgeons who used total pancreatectomy found that the operation produces no better pain relief for their patients than pancreaticoduodenectomy (about 80% to 85%). Moreover, the metabolic consequences of total pancreatectomy in the absence of islet cell transplantation are profound and life-threatening. The patients have a "brittle" form of diabetes in which avoidance of hyper- and hypoglycemia is problematic.[158,256-258] In addition, lethal episodes of hypoglycemia are common in severe apancreatic diabetes. These are due to hypoglycemic unresponsiveness, due to the absence of pancreatic glucagon, and to hypoglycemia unawareness, despite an ongoing need to treat with exogenous insulin.[259] In a series of >100 patients treated with total pancreatectomy, Gall and colleagues showed that half of all the late deaths after this operation were due to (iatrogenic) hypoglycemia.[260] Without adequate insulin treatment, patients with apancreatic diabetes become progressively more hyperglycemic and develop the same incidence of retinal and renal disease as type 1 diabetic patients.[157] Despite newer forms of insulin and insulin delivery systems, severe apancreatic diabetes is an adverse outcome, as complete prevention of the physiologic consequences of total pancreatectomy remains an unfulfilled goal.

Hybrid Procedures In 1980, Beger and associates described the DPPHR[261] (Fig. 33-56), and published long-term results with DPPHR for the treatment of chronic pancreatitis in 1985,[262] and more recently in 1999.[263] In 388 patients who were followed for an average of 6 years after DPPHR, pain relief was maintained in 91%, mortality was <1%, and diabetes developed in 21%, with 11% demonstrating a reversal of their preoperative diabetic status. These authors also compared the DPPHR procedure with the pylorus-sparing Whipple procedure in a randomized trial in 40 patients with chronic pancreatitis.[264] The mortality was zero in both groups, and the morbidity was also comparable. Pain relief (over 6 months) was seen in 94% of DPPHR patients, but in only 67% of Whipple patients. Furthermore, the insulin secretory capacity and glucose tolerance were noted to deteriorate in the Whipple group, but actually improved in the DPPHR patients.

The DPPHR requires the careful dissection of the gastroduodenal artery and the creation of two anastomoses (Fig. 33-57), and carries a similar complication risk as the Whipple procedure due to the risk of pancreatic leakage and intra-abdominal fluid collections.

In 1987, Frey and Smith described the local resection of the pancreatic head with longitudinal pancreaticojejunostomy (LR-LPJ), which included excavation of the pancreatic head including the ductal structures in continuity with a long dichotomy of the dorsal duct[265] (Fig. 33-58). The Frey procedure provides thorough decompression of the pancreatic head as well as the body and tail of the gland, and a long-term follow-up suggested that improved outcomes are associated with this more extensive decompressive procedure. Frey and Amikura reported their results in 50 patients

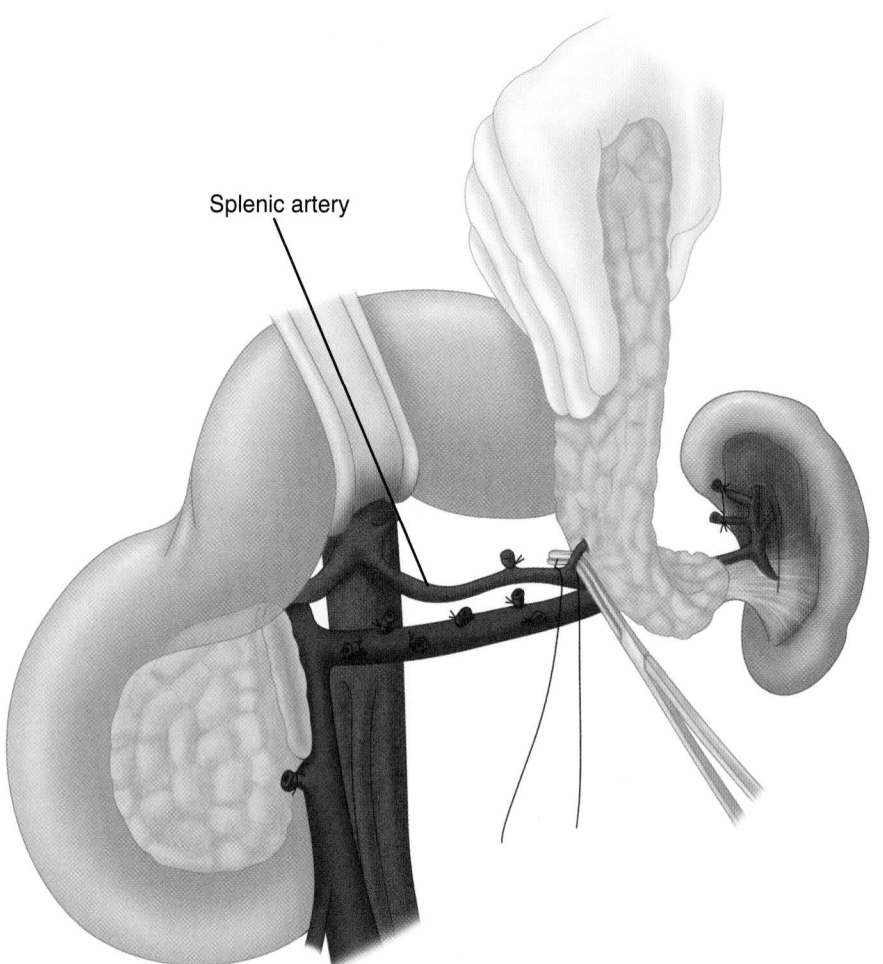

FIG. 33-54. Distal (spleen-sparing) pancreatectomy. A distal pancreatectomy for chronic pancreatitis is usually performed with en bloc splenectomy. In the presence of minimal inflammation, a spleen-sparing version can be performed, as shown here. *(Reproduced with permission from Bell.[196])*

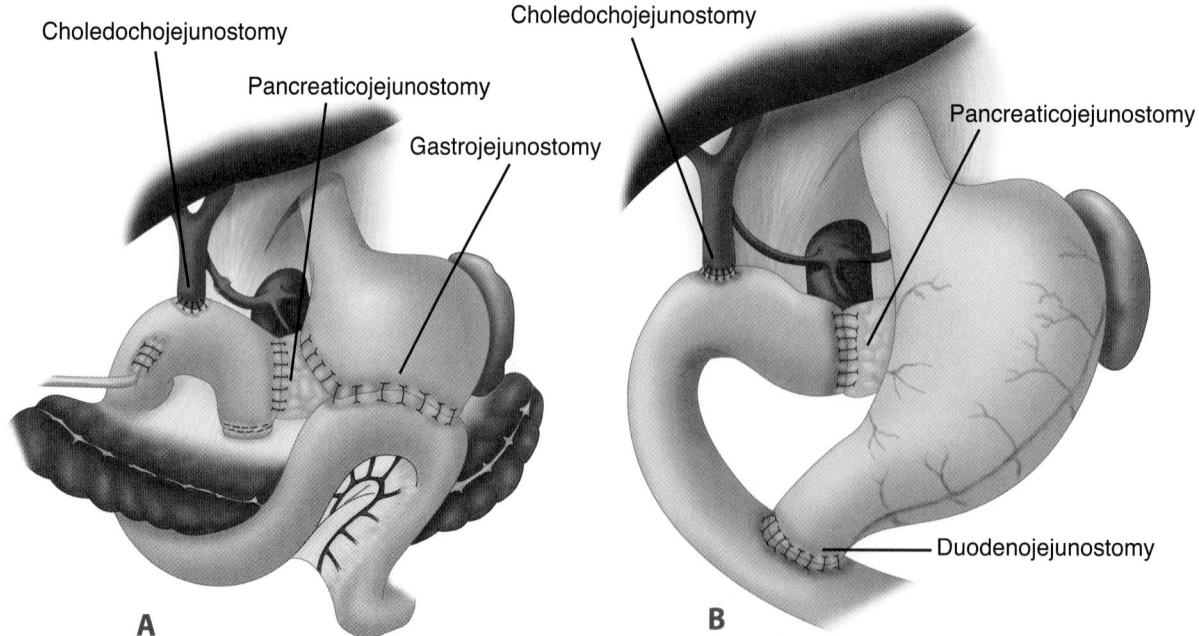

FIG. 33-55. The pancreaticoduodenectomy (Whipple procedure) can be performed either with the standard technique, which includes distal gastrectomy (**A**), or with preservation of the pylorus (**B**). The pylorus-sparing version of the procedure is used most commonly. *[Reproduced from Gaw JU, Andersen DK: Pancreatic surgery, in Wu GY, Aziz K, Whalen GF (eds): An Internist's Illustrated Guide to Gastrointestinal Surgery. Totowa, NJ: Humana Press, 2003, p 229, with permission.]*

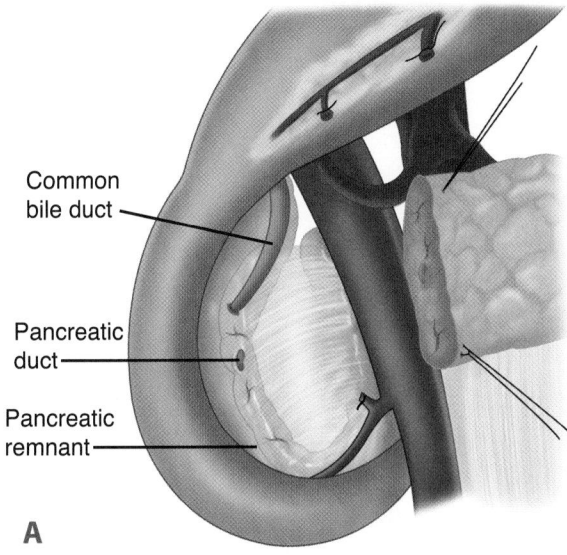

Common bile duct

Pancreatic duct

Pancreatic remnant

A

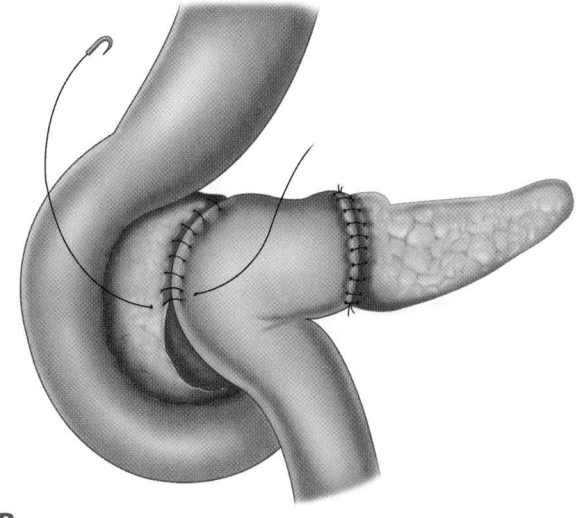

B

FIG. 33-56. The duodenum-preserving pancreatic head resection described by Beger and colleagues. **A.** The completed resection after transection of the pancreatic neck, and subtotal removal of the pancreatic head, with preservation of the distal common bile duct and duodenum. **B.** Completion of the reconstruction with anastomosis to the distal pancreas and to the proximal pancreatic rim by the same Roux limb of jejunum. *(Reproduced with permission from Bell.[196])*

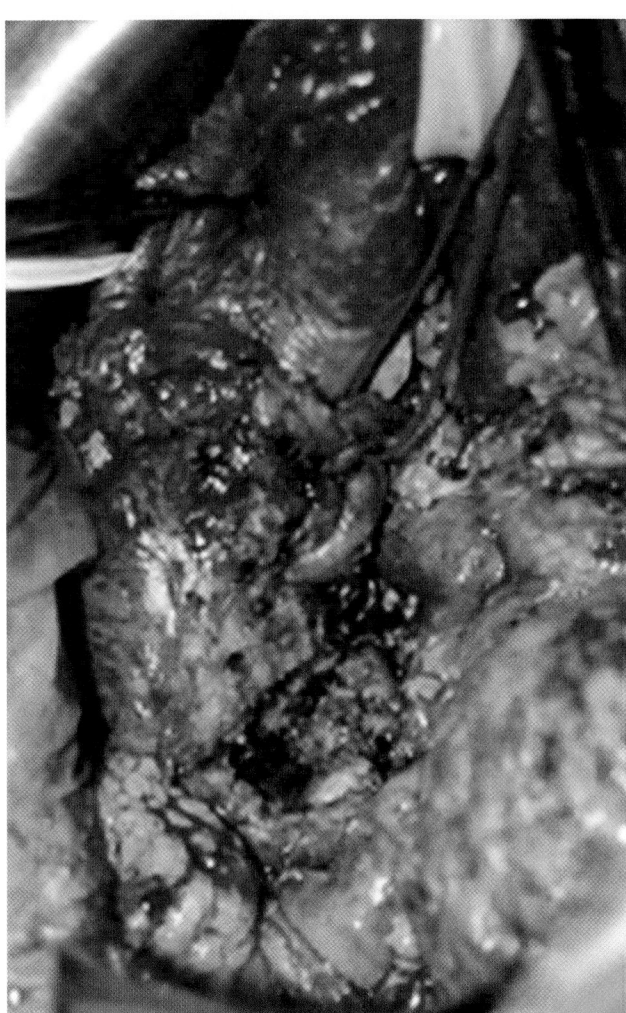

FIG. 33-57. Intraoperative view of the Beger procedure. The gastroduodenal artery is encircled by a vessel loop. Just below, the intrapancreatic portion of the common bile duct is exposed as it courses toward the ampulla. A rim of well-vascularized pancreatic tissue remains in the duodenal C-loop. Preservation of the posterior branch of the gastroduodenal artery is essential to preserve viability of these structures.

followed for >7 years, and found complete or substantial pain relief in 87% of patients. There was no operative mortality, but 22% of patients developed postoperative complications.[266]

Key steps in the performance of the LR-LPJ include preservation of the pancreatic neck as well as the capsule of the posterior pancreatic head. In the pancreaticoduodenectomy and the DPPHR, the pancreatic neck is freed up from the portal and superior mesenteric vein confluence and divided. In the LR-LPJ, the neck of the pancreas is preserved intact as are the body and tail of the pancreas. Not having to divide the pancreatic neck, as in the pancreaticoduodenectomy or DPPHR, reduces the risk of the operation, as it avoids intraoperative problems with the venous structures lying posterior to the gland. To reduce the risk of penetrating

the posterior capsule of the head, Frey recommended in his 1994 report that the posterior limit of resection be the back wall of the opened duct of Wirsung and duct to the uncinate (Fig. 33-59).

Subsequent to Frey's own modification of the technique, other surgeons have described modifications of the extent or technique of the LR-LPJ. Andersen and Topazian advocated performing the LR-LPJ as it was originally described, in which the entirety of the ducts are excised from the head (Fig. 33-60), and described the use of the ultrasonic aspirator and dissector for this purpose.[267] The use of this device permits precise removal of the ducts and adjacent tissue with good visualization and without complications. There is little pancreatic tissue behind these ducts and the pancreatic capsule is continuously palpated as the dissection proceeds to ensure a safe margin of resection. The intrapancreatic portion of the common bile duct is usually exposed, and avoiding injury to it is enhanced by the ultrasonic aspirator. The majority of the parenchyma of the uncinate process is spared, and the excavation of the pancreatic head is made contiguous with a generous dochotomy of the dorsal duct. Whether merely unroofing as opposed to removal of the proximal ducts contributes to better pain relief is not known and awaits a randomized trial to compare the two versions of the LR-LPJ. Izbicki and colleagues at the University of Hamburg also

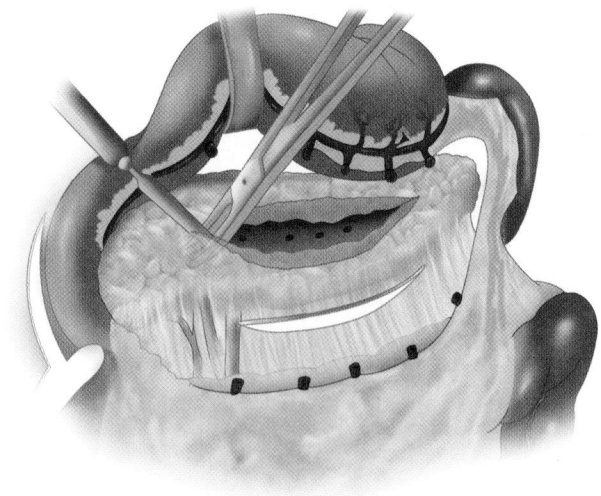

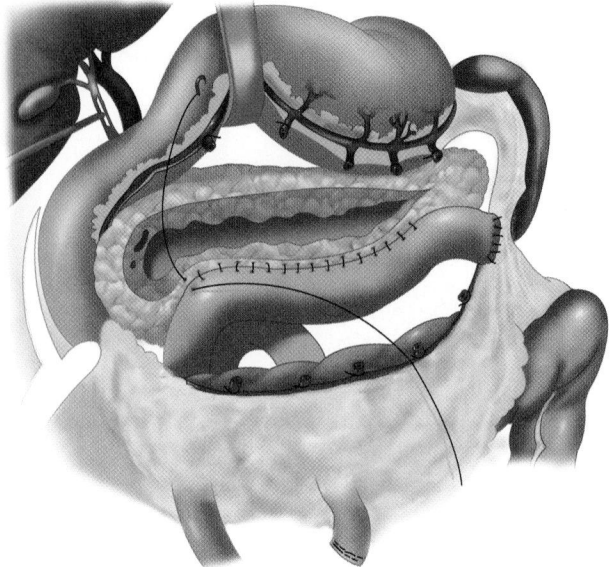

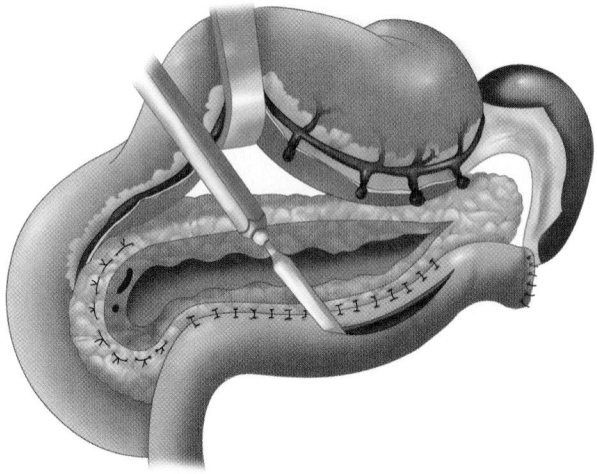

FIG. 33-58. Frey procedure. The local resection of the pancreatic head with longitudinal pancreaticojejunostomy (LR-LPJ) provides complete decompression of the entire pancreatic ductal system. Reconstruction is performed with a side-to-side Roux-en-Y pancreaticojejunostomy. *(Reproduced with permission from Bell.[196])*

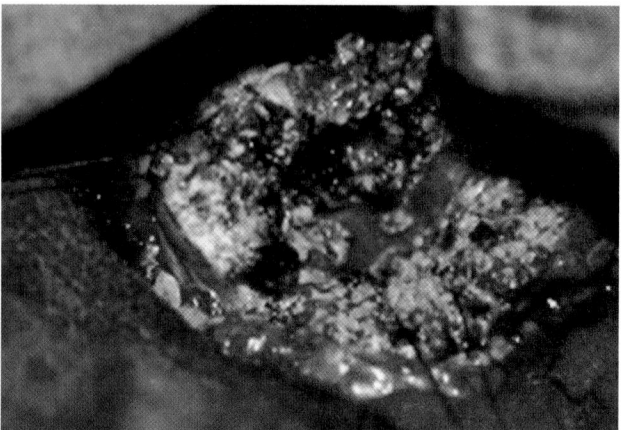

FIG. 33-59. Operative view of excavated head of the pancreas during the Frey procedure. The main pancreatic duct is opened widely down to the level of the ampulla, and the head of the pancreas is excavated in a conical fashion so as to allow complete decompression of the chronically obstructed and inflamed pancreatic ducts. *(Reproduced with permission from Aspelund G et al: Improved outcomes for benign disease with limited pancreatic head resection. J Gastrointest Surg 9:400, 2005. With kind permission from Springer Science + Business Media.)*

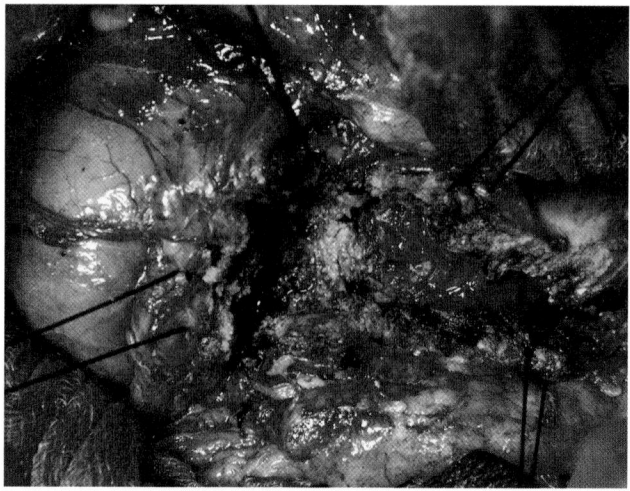

FIG. 33-60. Complete excavation of the pancreatic head and distal pancreatic dochotomy. A true excavation and removal of the proximal ductal system is combined with a distal pancreatic dochotomy. Reconstruction is performed with a single side-to-side Roux-en-Y pancreaticojejunostomy. *(Reproduced with permission from Andersen DK, Topazian MD: Pancreatic head excavation: A variation on the theme of duodenum-preserving pancreatic head resection. Arch Surg 139:375, 2004. Copyright © 2004 American Medical Association. All rights reserved.)*

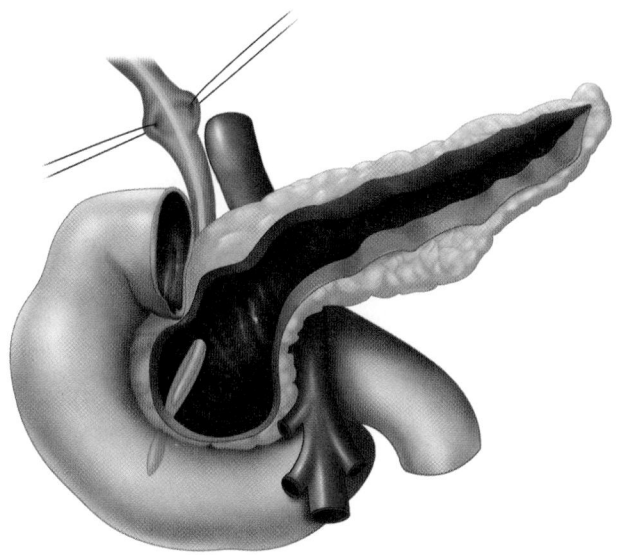

FIG. 33-61. The Hamburg modification of the local resection of the pancreatic head with longitudinal pancreaticojejunostomy. *(From Izbicki JR, Yekebas EE, Mann O: Shackelford's Surgery of the Alimentary Tract. New York: Saunders, 2007, p 1310.)*

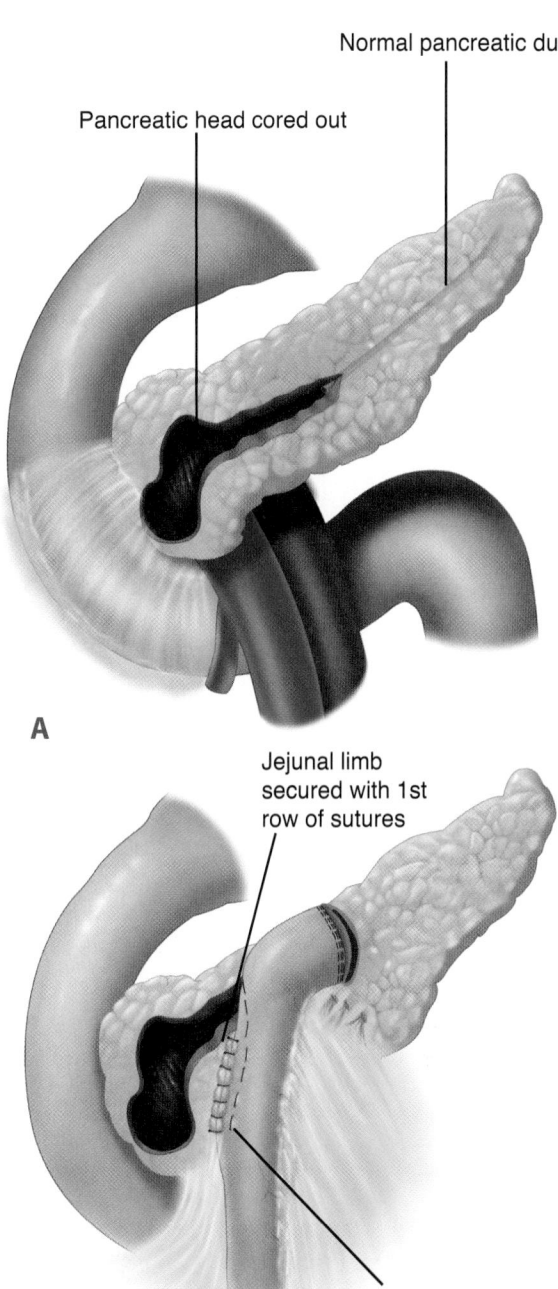

FIG 33-62. Excavation of pancreatic head without longitudinal pancreaticojejunostomy. *(From Ho HS, Frey CF: Arch Surg 136:1353, 2001.)*

recommend a more extensive excavation of the pancreatic head, and use a technique that they refer to as the *Hamburg modification* of the LR-LPJ[268] (Fig. 33-61). This wider excavation of the pancreatic head is created in continuity with the dorsal dochotomy, and is followed by a single, side-to-side pancreaticojejunostomy.

In 2001, Ho and Frey subsequently described merely excavating the core of the pancreatic head, and draining the excavation with a Roux-en-Y pancreaticojejunostomy, but without any effort to include the dorsal duct[269,270] (Fig. 33-62). In 2003, Farkas and colleagues described a similar excavation of the central portion of the pancreatic head without any effort to include the duct of the body in the lateral pancreaticojejunostomy,[271] and reported excellent results of what they termed an *organ-preserving pancreatic head resection* (OPPHR) in a randomized comparison to the pylorus-preserving pancreaticoduodenectomy (PPPD).[272]

This approach was advocated by Gloor and associates in Bern as an alternative to the DPPHR procedure in patients with portal hypertension,[273] and was described as the *Berne modification of the DPPHR* (Fig. 33-63). Most recently, Köninger and colleagues in Heidelberg published a randomized, controlled trial of the "Berne" version of the excavation method compared to the "classic" Beger procedure.[274] Operative times and length of stay were shorter in the group undergoing excavation of the pancreatic head, while long-term outcomes and quality-of-life scores were identical over 2 years postoperatively.

The common element of these variations on the theme of LR-LPJ remains the excavation or "coring out" of the central portion of the pancreatic head. It remains uncertain, however, whether and to what degree the dochotomy needs to be extended into the body and tail. The logical conclusion of all of these efforts is that the head of the pancreas is the nidus of the chronic inflammatory process in chronic pancreatitis, and that removal of the central portion of the head of the gland is the key to the successful resolution of pain long-term.

Complications Initial and long-term results of the LR-LPJ demonstrate pain relief that is equivalent to that of pancreaticoduodenectomy and the DPPHR.[275–277] The observed mortality rate has thus far been zero, and therefore, less than with the Whipple procedure. Major complications were less with the LR-LPJ (16%) than with

pancreaticoduodenectomy (40%) or DPPHR (25%) in one single-site series, and the incidence of new postoperative diabetes after LR-LPJ was 8% with an average follow-up of 3 years.[185]

Comparisons of the three operative procedures: Pancreaticoduodenectomy, DPPHR (Beger procedure), and LR-LPJ (Frey procedure) There has been considerable interest to apply evidence-based methods to the study of the three operations currently advocated for the treatment of chronic pancreatitis. The best studies, or level 1 data by the Strength of Recommendation Taxonomy, are prospective, randomized controlled trials comparing two or more operations from a single or multi-institutional study. Retrospective, cohort-based studies are regarded as level 2 data by the Strength of Recommendation Taxonomy criteria.

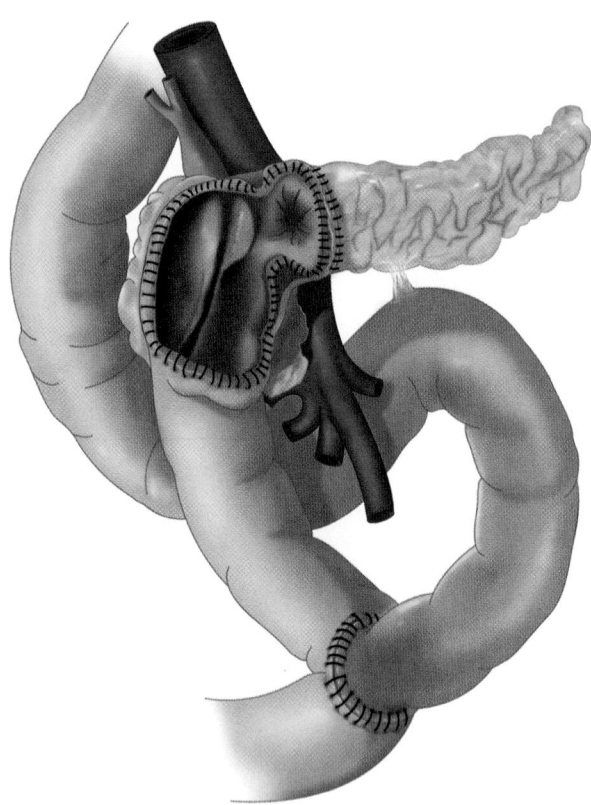

FIG. 33-63. The Berne modification of the local resection of the pancreatic head with longitudinal pancreaticojejunostomy. *(From Gloor B, Friess H, Uhl W, et al: A modified technique of the Beger and Frey procedure in patients with chronic pancreatitis. Dig Surg 18:21, 2001.)*

To date, six published level 1 studies have examined various comparisons between these three operations, and one level 2 study has examined all three procedures at a single institution. In the level 1 study of 43 patients by Klempa and colleagues,[278] DPPHR patients had a shorter hospital stay, greater weight gain, less postoperative diabetes, and exocrine dysfunction than standard Whipple patients over a 3- to 5-year follow-up. Pain control was similar between the two procedures. This was confirmed in a level 1 study of 40 patients by Buchler and associates,[279] in which DPPHR patients reported better pain relief, glucose tolerance, and weight gain compared to pylorus-preserving pancreaticoduodenectomy (PPPD) patients, however the follow-up averaged <1 year.

In a level 1 study of 61 patients randomized to PPPD or LR-LPJ, Izbicki and colleagues[276] found a lower postoperative complication rate associated with the Frey procedure (19%) compared to the PPPD group (53%), and better global quality-of-life scores (71 vs. 43%, respectively). Both operations were equally effective in controlling pain over a 2-year follow-up. More recently, the level 1 study by Farkas and associates[272] examined 40 patients randomized to PPPD or the method of excavation of the pancreatic head that their group described as an *organ-preserving pancreatic head resection* (OPPHR), and found that OPPHR was associated with a shorter operating time, less postoperative morbidity, shorter hospital stay, and better quality of life than PPPD. The degree of pain relief was equal over a 1- to 3-year follow-up. Operation times have been shown to be shorter with the LR-LPJ and DPPHR compared to the PPPD, and intraoperative blood loss and perioperative transfusion requirements are less with LR-LPJ and DPPHR procedures.[185,274,276,280]

Late Morbidity and Mortality In 1995, Izbicki and colleagues began a level 1 study of 42 patients randomized to the DPPHR or LR-LPJ. The study was continued and up dated in 1997[275] to include 74

patients. In 2005, the long-term results of these 74 patients with an average follow-up of 8.5 years were reported.[277] There were no significant differences between the groups with regard to global quality of life, pain scores, late mortality, and exocrine or endocrine insufficiency. The level 1 study by Köninger, which compared the classic DPPHR with excavation of the pancreatic head, showed identical outcomes at 2 years after an initial reduction in morbidity associated with the excavation procedure.[274] These results were echoed in the level 2 study by Aspelund and associates, which demonstrated fewer complications with both the DPPHR and LR-LPJ procedures compared to pancreaticoduodenectomy, a lower incidence of new diabetes (8%) for both DPPHR and LR-LPJ compared to the Whipple procedure (25%), but no significant differences in outcomes or pain relief between DPPHR and LR-LPJ.[185] Finally, level 2 data support the efficacy of both DPPHR and LR-LPJ in patients with dilated as well as nondilated ducts.[281,282]

Long-term exocrine and/or endocrine insufficiency in chronic pancreatitis patients treated surgically is a product of the surgical intervention as well as the progression of the underlying disease. Although the short-term (3-year) incidence of new diabetes after operation appears less with the LR-LPJ and DPPHR than with the PPPD, the late incidence of diabetes appears similar in all groups. After an average of 7 years of follow-up after LR-LPJ or PPPD, survival, pain relief, and pancreatic function were similar in both groups. The rate of diabetes was slightly lower after LR-LPJ (61%) than after PPPD (65%), but these had both more than doubled from their preoperative status.[277] Therefore, although the limited pancreatic procedures of DPPHR and LR-LPJ have a lower initial rate of endocrine dysfunction, the long-term risk of diabetes is more related to the progression of the underlying disease than to the effects of operation.

The decreased incidence of postoperative diabetes in the near-term after the duodenum-sparing operations may be the result of a preserved β-cell mass in the more conservative resections, and may also be due to the conservation of the PP-secreting cells localized to the posterior head and uncinate process.[158,164] Preservation of near-normal glucose metabolism and the avoidance of pancreatogenic diabetes is therefore a significant but time-limited benefit of the newer operative procedures.

Autotransplantation of Islets Islet cell transplantation for the treatment of diabetes is an attractive adjunct to pancreatic surgery in the treatment of benign pancreatic disease, but problems due to rejection of allotransplanted islets have plagued this method since its initial clinical application in the early 1970s. However, despite the difficulties in recovering islets from a chronically inflamed gland, Najarian and associates demonstrated the utility of autotransplantation of islets in patients with chronic pancreatitis in 1980.[283] Subsequently, through refinements in the methods of harvesting and gland preservation, and through standardization of the methods by which islets are infused into the portal venous circuit for intrahepatic engraftment, the success of autotransplantation has steadily increased to achieve insulin independence in the majority of patients treated in recent series.[284,285] Although 2 to 3 million islets are required for successful engraftment in an allogeneic recipient, the autotransplant recipient can usually achieve long-term, insulin-independent status after engraftment of only 300,000 to 400,000 islets.[286] However, the ability to recover a sufficient quantity of islets from a sclerotic gland is dependent on the degree of disease present, so the selection of patients as candidates for autologous islet transplantation is important. As success with autotransplantation increases, patients with nonobstructive, sclerotic pancreatitis may be considered for resection and islet autotransplantation earlier in their course, as end-stage fibrosis bodes poorly for transplant success.[287] As the necessary expertise with islet transplantation becomes more widespread, this therapy may become routine in the treatment of chronic pancreatitis.

Denervation Procedures In patients who have persistent and disabling pain, but who are poor candidates for resection or drainage

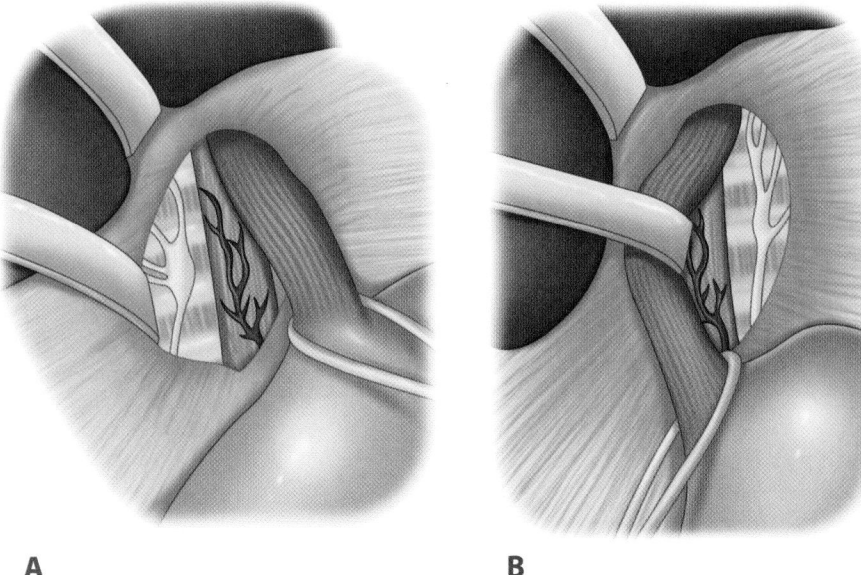

FIG. 33-64. Transhiatal splanchnicectomy. The transhiatal exposure of the right (**A**) and left (**B**) greater splanchnic nerves reveals the splanchnic ganglia, the esophagus, the aorta, and the vertebral column. *[Reproduced with permission from Klar E: Denervation procedures, in Beger HG et al (eds): The Pancreas. London: Blackwell Science, 1998, p 839.]*

A   **B**

procedures, a denervation procedure may provide symptomatic relief. As discussed above in "Presenting Signs and Symptoms" and Neurolytic Therapy," neural ablation is a valid treatment strategy to block afferent sympathetic nociceptive pathways. In addition to direct infiltration of the celiac ganglia with long-acting analgesics or neurolytic agents,[288] a variety of true denervation procedures have been described for symptomatic relief in chronic pancreatitis. These include operative celiac ganglionectomy or splanchnicectomy[289] transhiatal splanchnicectomy,[290] (Fig. 33-64), transthoracic splanchnicectomy with or without vagotomy,[291] and videoscopic transthoracic splanchnicectomy.[292] Mallet-Guy demonstrated long-term pain relief in 83% of 215 patients treated with operative celiac splanchnicectomy,[289] and Michotey and associates claimed pain relief in all 14 patients treated with (transabdominal) transhiatal splanchnicectomy of the lower mediastinal sympathetic tracts,[290] but both of these approaches represent major abdominal procedures. For the patient who is a poor candidate for an abdominal procedure, the transthoracic ablation of the sympathetic chain, either on the left side alone or bilaterally, has been shown to result in pain relief in 60 to 66% of patients. The application of videoscopic techniques to thoracic splanchnicectomy has further reduced the risks and discomfort of these procedures in chronically ill patients and provides a valuable alternative to a direct attack on the pancreas.

PANCREATIC NEOPLASMS

Neoplasms of the Endocrine Pancreas

Neoplasms of the endocrine pancreas are relatively uncommon but do occur with enough frequency (five cases per million population) that most surgeons will encounter them in an urban practice. The cells of the endocrine pancreas, or islet cells, originate from neural crest cells, also referred to as *amine precursor uptake and decarboxylation cells*. Multiple endocrine neoplasia (MEN) syndromes occur when these cells cause tumors in multiple sites. The MEN1 syndrome involves pituitary tumors, parathyroid hyperplasia, and pancreatic neoplasms. Some pancreatic endocrine neoplasms are functional, secreting peptide products that produce interesting clinical presentations. Neoplasms of the endocrine pancreas that are not associated with excess hormone levels and a recognizable clinical syndrome are considered nonfunctional. Special immunohistochemical stains allow pathologists to confirm the peptide products being produced within the cells of a pancreatic endocrine tumor. However, the histologic characteristics of these neoplasms do not predict their clinical behav-

ior, and malignancy is usually determined by the presence of local invasion and lymph node or hepatic metastases. Unfortunately, most pancreatic endocrine tumors are malignant, but the course of the disease is far more favorable than that seen with pancreatic exocrine cancer. The key to diagnosing these rare tumors is recognition of the classic clinical syndrome; confirmation is achieved by measuring serum levels of the elevated hormone. Localization of the tumor can be a challenging step, but once accomplished, the surgery is relatively straightforward. The goals of surgery range from complete resection, often accomplished with insulinomas, to controlling symptoms with debulking procedures. Unresectable disease in the liver is often addressed with chemoembolization.

As with pancreatic exocrine tumors, the initial diagnostic imaging test of choice for pancreatic endocrine tumors is a multidetector CT scan with four phases of contrast and fine cuts through the pancreas and liver. EUS also can be valuable in localizing these tumors, which can produce dramatic symptoms despite their small (<1 cm) size. In contrast to pancreatic exocrine tumors, many of the endocrine tumors have somatostatin receptors (SSTRs) that allow them to be detected by a radiolabeled octreotide scan. A radioactive somatostatin analogue is injected intravenously, followed by whole-body radionuclide scanning (Fig. 33-65). The success of this modality in localizing tumors and detecting metastases has decreased the use of older techniques such as angiography and selective venous sampling.

Insulinoma

Insulinomas are the most common pancreatic endocrine neoplasms and present with a typical clinical syndrome known as Whipple's triad. The triad consists of symptomatic fasting hypoglycemia, a documented serum glucose level <50 mg/dL, and relief of symptoms with the administration of glucose. Patients will often present with a profound syncopal episode and will admit to similar less severe episodes in the recent past. They also may admit to palpitations, trembling, diaphoresis, confusion or obtundation, and seizure, and family members may report that the patient has undergone a personality change.

Routine laboratory studies will uncover a low blood sugar, the cause of all of these symptoms. Serum insulin levels are elevated. C-peptide levels should also be elevated and rule out the unusual case of surreptitious administration of insulin or oral hypoglycemic agents, because excess endogenous insulin production leads to excess C-peptide. The diagnosis can be clinched with a monitored fast in which blood is sampled every 4 to 6 hours for glucose and insulin levels until the patient becomes symptomatic. However, this can be dangerous and must be done with close supervision.

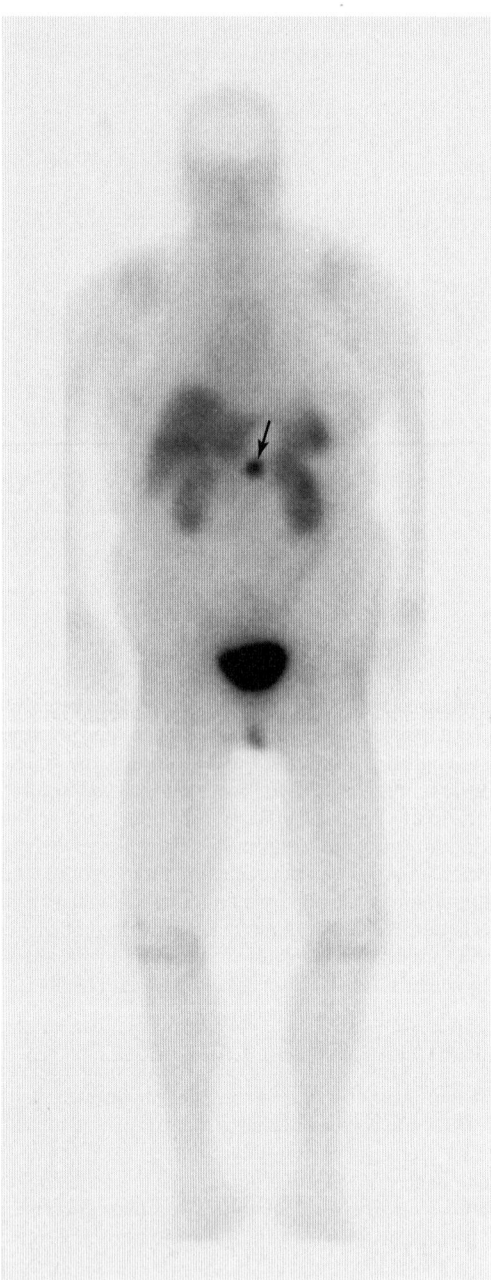

FIG. 33-65. Radioactive octreotide scan demonstrating pancreatic endocrine tumor in the body of the pancreas (*arrow*).

Insulinomas are usually localized with CT scanning and EUS. Technical advances in EUS have led to preoperative identification of >90% of insulinomas.[293] Visceral angiography with venous sampling is rarely required to accurately localize the tumor. Insulinomas are evenly distributed throughout the head, body, and tail of the pancreas.[294]

Unlike most endocrine pancreatic tumors, the majority (90%) of insulinomas are benign and solitary, and only 10% are malignant. They are typically cured by simple enucleation. However, tumors located close to the main pancreatic duct and large (>2 cm) tumors may require a distal pancreatectomy or pancreaticoduodenectomy. Intraoperative US is useful to determine the tumor's relation to the main pancreatic duct and guides intraoperative decision making. Enucleation of solitary insulinomas and distal pancreatectomy for insulinoma can sometimes be performed using a minimally invasive technique.

Ninety percent of insulinomas are sporadic, and 10% are associated with the MEN1 syndrome. Insulinomas associated with the

MEN1 syndrome are more likely to be multifocal and have a higher rate of recurrence.

Gastrinoma

Zollinger-Ellison syndrome (ZES) is caused by a *gastrinoma*, an endocrine tumor that secretes gastrin, leading to acid hypersecretion and peptic ulceration. Many patients with ZES present with abdominal pain, peptic ulcer disease, and severe esophagitis. However, in the era of effective antacid therapy, the presentation can be less dramatic. Although most of the ulcers are solitary, multiple ulcers in atypical locations that fail to respond to antacids should raise suspicion for ZES and prompt a work-up. Twenty percent of patients with gastrinoma have diarrhea at the time of diagnosis.

The diagnosis of ZES is made by measuring the serum gastrin level. It is important that patients stop taking proton pump inhibitors for this test. In most patients with gastrinomas, the level is >1000 pg/mL. Gastrin levels can be elevated in conditions other than ZES. Common causes of hypergastrinemia include pernicious anemia, treatment with proton pump inhibitors, renal failure, G-cell hyperplasia, atrophic gastritis, retained or excluded antrum, and gastric outlet obstruction. In equivocal cases, when the gastrin level is not markedly elevated, a secretin stimulation test is helpful.

In 70 to 90% of patients, the primary gastrinoma is found in Passaro's triangle, an area defined by a triangle with points located at the junction of the cystic duct and common bile duct, the second and third portion of the duodenum, and the neck and body of the pancreas (Fig. 33-66). However, because gastrinomas can be found almost anywhere, whole-body imaging is required. The test of choice is SSTR (octreotide) scintigraphy in combination with CT. The octreotide scan is more sensitive than CT, locating about 85% of gastrinomas and detecting tumors <1 cm. With the octreotide scan, the need for tedious and technically demanding selective angiography and measurement of gastrin gradients has declined. EUS is another new modality that assists in the preoperative localization of gastrinomas. It is particularly helpful in localizing tumors in the pancreatic head or duodenal wall, where gastrinomas are usually <1 cm in size. A combination of octreotide scan and EUS detects >90% of gastrinomas.

It is important to rule out MEN1 syndrome by checking serum calcium levels before surgery because resection of the gastrinoma(s) in these patients rarely results in normalization of serum gastrin concentrations or a prolongation of survival. Only one fourth of

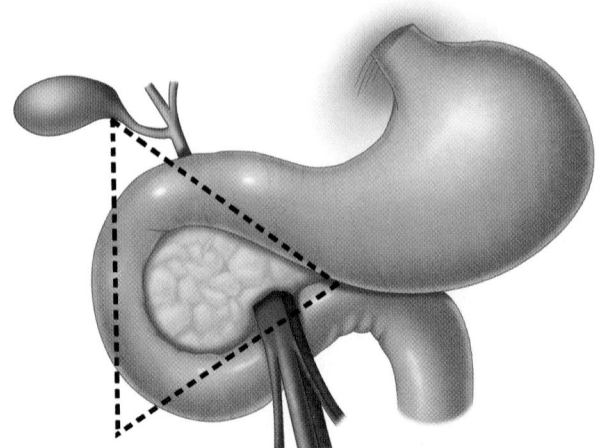

FIG. 33-66. Passaro's triangle. The typical location of a gastrinoma is described by this anatomic region, including the head of the pancreas, duodenum, and the lymphatic bed posterior and superior to the duodenum, as originally described by E. Passaro. (*Reproduced with permission from Bell.[196]*)

gastrinomas occur in association with the MEN1 syndrome. One half of patients with gastrinomas will have solitary tumors while the remainder will have multiple gastrinomas. Multiple tumors are more common in patients with MEN1 syndrome. Aggressive surgical treatment is justified in patients with sporadic gastrinomas. If patients have MEN1 syndrome, the parathyroid hyperplasia is addressed with total parathyroidectomy and implantation of parathyroid tissue in the forearm.

Fifty percent of gastrinomas metastasize to lymph nodes or the liver, and are therefore considered malignant. Patients who meet criteria for operability should undergo exploration for possible removal of the tumor. Although the tumors are submucosal, a full-thickness excision of the duodenal wall is performed if a duodenal gastrinoma is found. All lymph nodes in Passaro's triangle are excised for pathologic analysis. If the gastrinoma is found in the pancreas and does not involve the main pancreatic duct, it is enucleated. Pancreatic resection is justified for solitary gastrinomas with no metastases. A highly selective vagotomy can be performed if unresectable disease is identified or if the gastrinoma cannot be localized. This may reduce the amount of expensive proton pump inhibitors required. In cases in which hepatic metastases are identified, resection is justified if the primary gastrinoma is controlled and the metastases can be safely and completely removed. Debulking or incomplete removal of multiple hepatic metastases is probably not helpful, especially in the setting of MEN1. The application of new modalities such as radiofrequency ablation seems reasonable, but data to support this approach are limited.[295] Postoperatively, patients are followed with fasting serum gastrin levels, secretin stimulation tests, octreotide scans, and CT scans. In patients found to have inoperable disease, chemotherapy with streptozocin, doxorubicin, and 5-fluorouracil (5-FU) is used. Other approaches such as somatostatin analogues, interferon, and chemoembolization also have been used in gastrinoma with some success.

Unfortunately, a biochemical cure is achieved in only about one-third of the patients operated on for ZES. Despite the lack of success, long-term survival rates are good, even in patients with liver metastases. The 15-year survival rate for patients without liver metastases is about 80%, while the 5-year survival rate for patients with liver metastases is 20 to 50%. Pancreatic tumors are usually larger than tumors arising in the duodenum, and more often have lymph node metastases. In gastrinomas, liver metastases decrease survival rates, but lymph node metastases do not. The best results are seen after complete excision of small sporadic tumors originating in the duodenum. Large tumors associated with liver metastases, located outside of Passaro's triangle, have the worst prognosis.

Vasoactive Intestinal Peptide-Secreting Tumor

In 1958, Verner and Morrison first described the syndrome associated with a pancreatic neoplasm secreting VIP. The classic clinical syndrome associated with this pancreatic endocrine neoplasm consists of severe intermittent watery diarrhea leading to dehydration, and weakness from fluid and electrolyte losses. Large amounts of potassium are lost in the stool. The *vasoactive intestinal peptide-secreting tumor (VIPoma) syndrome* is also called the *WDHA syndrome* due to the presence of *w*atery *d*iarrhea, *h*ypokalemia, and *a*chlorhydria. The massive (5 L/d) and episodic nature of the diarrhea associated with the appropriate electrolyte abnormalities should raise suspicion of the diagnosis. Serum VIP levels must be measured on multiple occasions because the excess secretion of VIP is episodic, and single measurements might be normal and misleading. A CT scan localizes most VIPomas, although as with all islet cell tumors, EUS is the most sensitive imaging method. Electrolyte and fluid balance is sometimes difficult to correct preoperatively and must be pursued aggressively. Somatostatin analogues are helpful in controlling the diarrhea and allowing replacement of fluid and electrolytes. VIPomas are more commonly located in the distal pancreas and most have spread outside the pancreas. Palliative debulking operations can sometimes improve symptoms for a period, along with

somatostatin analogues. Hepatic artery embolization also has been reported as a potentially beneficial treatment.[296]

Glucagonoma

Diabetes in association with dermatitis should raise the suspicion of a glucagonoma. The diabetes usually is mild. The classic necrolytic migratory erythema manifests as cyclic migrations of lesions with spreading margins and healing centers typically on the lower abdomen, perineum, perioral area, and feet. The diagnosis is confirmed by measuring serum glucagon levels, which are usually >500 pg/mL. Glucagon is a catabolic hormone, and most patients present with malnutrition. The rash associated with glucagonoma is thought to be caused by low levels of amino acids. Preoperative treatment usually includes control of the diabetes, parenteral nutrition, and octreotide. Like VIPomas, glucagonomas are more often in the body and tail of the pancreas and tend to be large tumors with metastases. Again, debulking operations are recommended in good operative candidates to relieve symptoms.

Somatostatinoma

Because somatostatin inhibits pancreatic and biliary secretions, patients with a somatostatinoma present with gallstones due to bile stasis, diabetes due to inhibition of insulin secretion, and steatorrhea due to inhibition of pancreatic exocrine secretion and bile secretion. Most somatostatinomas originate in the proximal pancreas or the pancreatoduodenal groove, with the ampulla and periampullary area as the most common site (60%). The most common presentations are abdominal pain (25%), jaundice (25%), and cholelithiasis (19%).[297] This rare type of pancreatic endocrine tumor is diagnosed by confirming elevated serum somatostatin levels, which are usually >10 ng/mL. Although most reported cases of somatostatinoma involve metastatic disease, an attempt at complete excision of the tumor and cholecystectomy is warranted in fit patients.

Nonfunctioning Islet Cell Tumors

Although some pancreatic endocrine neoplasms secrete one or more hormones and are associated with interesting characteristic clinical syndromes, many are not associated with elevated serum hormone levels. After insulinoma, the most common islet cell tumor is the nonfunctioning islet cell neoplasm. Because it is clinically silent until its size and location produce symptoms, it is usually malignant when first diagnosed. Some presumably nonfunctional pancreatic endocrine neoplasms stain positive for pancreatic polypeptide (PP), and elevated PP levels are therefore a marker for the lesion. Because clinical manifestations are absent, the tumors are usually large and metastatic at the time of diagnosis, unless they are detected serendipitously on CT scan or sonogram. Nonfunctioning islet cell tumors are also seen in association with other multiple neoplasia syndromes, such as von Hippel-Lindau syndrome. The tumors grow slowly and 5-year survival is common, as opposed to pancreatic exocrine tumors, for which 5-year survival is extraordinarily rare.

Neoplasms of the Exocrine Pancreas

Epidemiology and Risk Factors

It is estimated that 37,680 patients were diagnosed with and 34,290 patients died of cancer of the pancreas in the United States in 2008.[298] Overall, pancreatic cancer has the worst prognosis of all malignancies with a 5% 5-year survival rate.[298] Despite its ubiquity, this disease is extremely difficult to treat, and its exact cause unknown. However, epidemiologic studies linking various environmental and host factors provide some clues. Recent discoveries using modern molecular biologic techniques have also improved our understanding of the causes of pancreatic cancer. The etiology of pancreatic cancer likely involves a complex interaction of genetic and environmental factors. Understanding these factors will become increasingly important as better diagnostic tools such as DNA sequencing become clinically available to screen populations at risk for developing pancreatic cancer.

Pancreatic cancer is more common in the elderly with most patients being >60 years old. Pancreatic cancer is more common in African Americans and slightly more common in men than women. The risk of developing pancreatic cancer is two to three times higher if a parent or sibling had the disease. Another risk factor that is consistently linked to pancreatic cancer is cigarette smoking. Smoking increases the risk of developing pancreatic cancer by at least twofold due to the carcinogens in cigarette smoke.[299] Coffee and alcohol consumption have been investigated as possible risk factors, but the data are inconsistent. As in other GI cancers, diets high in fat and low in fiber, fruits, and vegetables are thought to be associated with an increased risk of pancreatic cancer.

Diabetes has been known to be associated with pancreatic cancer for many years. In fact, glucose intolerance is present in 80% of patients with pancreatic cancer, and approximately 20% have overt diabetes, a much greater incidence than would be expected to occur by chance. Pre-existing type II diabetes may increase the risk for development of pancreatic cancer.[300] The new onset of diabetes also can be an early manifestation of otherwise occult pancreatic cancer. Thus, the new onset of diabetes or a sudden increase in insulin requirement in an elderly patient with pre-existing diabetes should provoke concern for the presence of pancreatic cancer.

Recent epidemiologic studies have confirmed the fact that patients with chronic pancreatitis, especially familial pancreatitis, have an increased risk of developing pancreatic cancer.[184] Large, retrospective cohort studies of patients with pancreatitis have revealed up to a 20-fold increase in risk for pancreatic cancer. This increased risk seems to be independent of the type of pancreatitis, a finding consistent with the fact that most studies have shown little effect of alcohol ingestion per se on the risk of pancreatic carcinoma. The mechanisms involved in carcinogenesis in patients with pre-existing pancreatitis are unknown. However, the mutated K-*ras* oncogene, which is present in most cases of pancreatic cancer, has been detected in the ductal epithelium of some patients with chronic pancreatitis.

Genetics of Pancreatic Cancer

Pancreatic carcinogenesis probably involves multiple mutations that are inherited and acquired throughout aging. The K-*ras* oncogene is currently thought to be the most commonly mutated gene in pancreatic cancer, with approximately 90% of tumors having a mutation.[301] This prevalent mutation is present in precursor lesions and is therefore thought to occur early and be essential to pancreatic cancer development. K-*ras* mutations can be detected in DNA from serum, stool, pancreatic juice, and tissue aspirates of patients with pancreatic cancer, suggesting that the presence of this mutation may provide the basis for diagnostic testing in select individuals. The HER-2/*neu* oncogene, homologous to the epidermal growth factor receptor (EGFr), is overexpressed in pancreatic cancers.[301] This receptor is involved in signal transduction pathways that lead to cellular proliferation. Multiple tumor-suppressor genes are deleted and/or mutated in pancreatic cancer, and include *p53*, *p16*, and *DPC4* (*Smad 4*), and in a minority of cases, *BRCA2*.[301] Most pancreatic cancers have three or more of the above mutations.

With the completion of the human genome project, comparison of the normal genome and the results of DNA sequencing of pancreatic and other cancers is an active area of research. Discovery of mutations in numerous other genes is likely in the near future and will hopefully lead to better diagnostic and therapeutic approaches.

It is estimated that up to 10% of pancreatic cancers occur as a result of an inherited genetic predisposition. A family history of pancreatic cancer in a first-degree relative increases the risk of pancreatic cancer by about twofold.[301] Rare familial cancer syndromes that are associated with an increased risk of pancreatic cancer include *BRCA2*, the familial atypical multiple mole–melanoma syndrome, hereditary pancreatitis, familial adenomatous polyposis (FAP), hereditary nonpolyposis colorectal cancer, Peutz-Jeghers syndrome, and ataxia-telangiectasia.[302]

In addition to mutations in oncogenes and tumor-suppressor genes, pancreatic cancers also are known to have aberrations in the expression of growth factors and their receptors. These growth factors include epidermal growth factor, fibroblast growth factor, transforming growth factor beta, insulin-like growth factor, hepatocyte growth factor, and vascular endothelial growth factor.[303]

The fact that many GI hormones and growth factors affect the growth of the normal exocrine pancreas suggests that these peptides also could affect the growth of pancreatic cancer, and some studies in cell culture and laboratory animals have supported this hypothesis.[303] Newer drugs such as erlotinib (Tarceva) and cetuximab (Erbitux), EGFr inhibitors, and bevacizumab (Avastin), a vascular endothelial growth factor inhibitor, and other drugs aimed at manipulation of growth factors, their receptors, and secondary messengers are the subject of ongoing clinical research. However, the combination of these drugs with standard chemotherapy in recent trials has not resulted in dramatic improvements in overall survival in pancreatic cancer.

Pathology

Pancreatic cancer probably arises through a stepwise progression of cellular changes, just as colon cancer progresses by stages from hyperplastic polyp to invasive cancer. Systematic histologic evaluation of areas surrounding pancreatic cancers has revealed the presence of precursor lesions that have been named *pancreatic intraepithelial neoplasia* (Fig. 33-67). Three stages of pancreatic intraepithelial neoplasia have been defined. These lesions demonstrate the same oncogene mutations and loss of tumor-suppressor genes found in invasive cancers, the frequency of these abnormalities increasing with progressive cellular atypia and architectural disarray.[304] The ability to detect these precursor lesions in humans at a stage where the cancer can still be prevented or cured is an important goal of current pancreatic cancer research.

About two thirds of pancreatic adenocarcinomas arise within the head or uncinate process of the pancreas; 15% are in the body, and 10% in the tail, with the remaining tumors demonstrating diffuse involvement of the gland. Tumors in the pancreatic body and tail are generally larger at the time of diagnosis, and therefore, less commonly resectable. Tumors in the head of the pancreas are typically diagnosed earlier because they cause obstructive jaundice. Ampullary carcinomas, carcinomas of the distal bile duct, and periampullary duodenal adenocarcinomas present in a similar fashion to pancreatic head cancer but have a slightly better prognosis, probably because early obstruction of the bile duct and jaundice leads to the diagnosis.

In addition to ductal adenocarcinoma, which makes up about 75% of nonendocrine cancers of the pancreas, there are a variety of less common types of pancreatic cancer. Adenosquamous carcinoma is a variant that has both glandular and squamous differentiation. The biologic behavior of this lesion is unfortunately no better than the typical ductal adenocarcinoma.[305] Acinar cell carcinoma is an uncommon type of pancreatic cancer that usually presents as a large tumor, often 10 cm in diameter or more, but the prognosis of patients with these tumors may be better than with ductal cancer.

Diagnosis and Staging

Exact pathologic staging of pancreatic cancer is important because it allows accurate quantitative assessment of results and comparisons between institutions. The *tumor-node-metastasis* (TNM) staging of pancreatic cancer is shown in Table 33-18.

T1 lesions are ≤2 cm in diameter and are limited to the pancreas. T2 lesions also are limited to the pancreas, but are >2 cm. T3 lesions extend beyond the pancreas but do not involve the celiac axis or superior mesenteric artery. T4 lesions involve the celiac axis or superior mesenteric artery and are not resectable. T1 and T2 tumors with no lymph node involvement are considered stage I disease (stage IA and IB). More extensive invasion, such as that associated with T3 tumors, indicates stage IIA disease. Any lymph node involvement

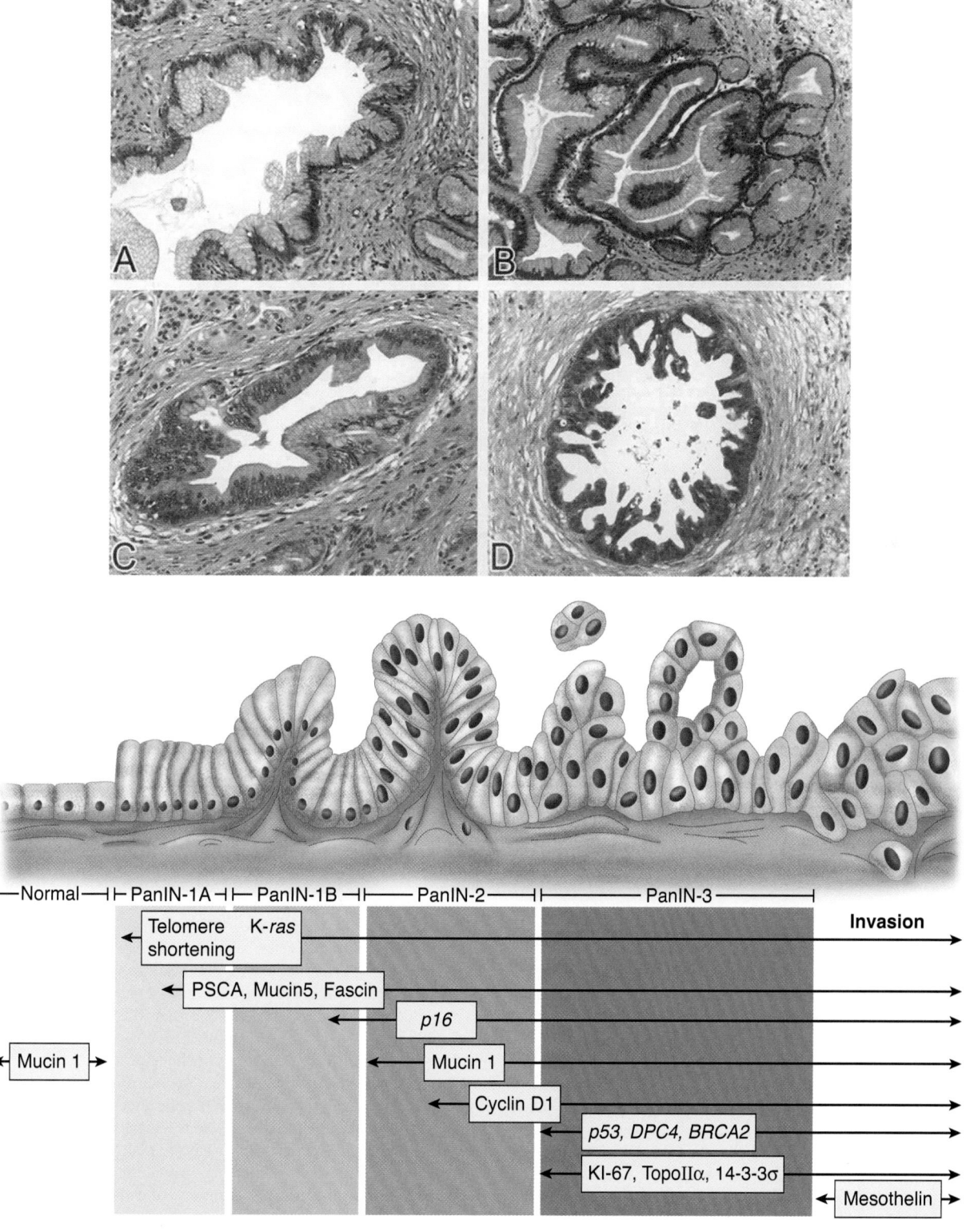

FIG. 33-67. Pancreatic intraepithelial neoplasia (PanIN). Histology (*top panel*) showing grades PanIN-1A (*A*), PanIN-1B (*B*), PanIN-2 (*C*), and PanIN-3 (*D*), and schema of correlation of histology with mutational events (*bottom panel*) showing cumulative abnormalities of tumor-promoter and tumor-suppressor factors such as kRAS, p53, etc, and their corresponding cellular phenotype. *(From Hruban RH, Takaori K, Klimstra DS, et al: An illustrated consensus on the classification of pancreatic intraepithelial neoplasia and intraductal papillary mucinous neoplasms. Am J Surg Pathol 28:977, 2004.)*

indicates stage IIB disease. Locally advanced unresectable tumors (T4) without metastatic disease are considered stage III while patients with metastases to distant sites such as the liver or lungs are stage IV.

Seven percent of pancreas cancer cases are diagnosed while the cancer is still confined to the primary site (localized stage); 26% are diagnosed after the cancer has spread to regional lymph nodes or directly beyond the primary site; 52% are diagnosed after the cancer has already metastasized (distant stage); and for the remaining 15%, the staging information was unknown. The corresponding 5-year relative survival rates were: 20.3% for localized, 8.0% for regional, 1.7% for distant, and 4.1% for unstaged. The overall 5-year relative survival rate for patients with pancreatic cancer for 1996 to 2003 from 17 Surveillance, Epidemiology and End Results geographic areas was 5%.[306]

TABLE 33-18 Staging of pancreatic cancer

Tumor (T)

TX: Primary tumor cannot be assessed

T0: No evidence of primary tumor

Tis: Carcinoma in situ

T1: Tumor is limited to the pancreas and is ≤2 cm in greatest dimension

T2: Tumor is limited to the pancreas and is >2 cm in greatest dimension

T3: Tumor extends beyond the pancreas but without involvement of the celiac axis or the superior mesenteric artery

T4: Tumor involves the celiac axis or the superior mesenteric artery (unresectable primary tumor)

Regional lymph nodes (N)

NX: Regional lymph nodes cannot be assessed

N0: No regional lymph node metastasis

N1: Regional lymph node metastasis

Distant metastasis (M)

MX: Distant metastasis cannot be assessed

M0: No distant metastasis

M1: Distant metastasis

Stage	T	N	M	Description
IA	1	0	0	Limited to pancreas ≤2 cm
IB	2	0	0	Limited to pancreas >2 cm
IIA	3	0	0	Extends beyond pancreas but does not involve arteries
IIB	1-3	1	0	Any tumor without artery involvement with lymph node involvement
III	4	Any	0	Tumor involves arteries (unresectable)
IV	Any	Any	1	Any tumor with distant metastases

Source: Exocrine pancreas, in: American Joint Committee on Cancer: *AJCC Cancer Staging Manual*, 6th ed. New York: Springer, 2002, p 157. Used with the permission of the American Joint Committee on Cancer (AJCC), Chicago, Illinois. The original source for this material is the AJCC Cancer Staging Manual, Sixth Edition (2002) published by Springer Science and Business Media LLC, *www.springerlink.com*.

The most critical deficit in the ability to treat pancreatic cancer effectively is the lack of tools for early diagnosis. The pancreas is situated deep within the abdomen, and the early symptoms of pancreatic cancer often are too vague to raise suspicion of the disease. Ultimately, the majority of patients present with pain and jaundice. On physical examination, weight loss is evident and the skin is icteric; a distended gallbladder is palpable in about one-fourth of patients. More fortunate patients have tumors situated such that biliary obstruction and jaundice occurs early and prompts diagnostic tests. Unfortunately, however, the vast majority of patients are not diagnosed until weight loss has occurred—a sign of advanced disease.

Although it is often taught that carcinoma of the pancreas presents with painless jaundice (to help distinguish it from choledocholithiasis), this aphorism is not accurate. Most patients do experience pain as part of the symptom complex of pancreatic cancer, and it is often the first symptom. Therefore, awareness of the way pancreatic pain is perceived may help clinicians suspect pancreatic cancer. The pain associated with pancreatic cancer is usually perceived in the epigastrium but can occur in any part of the abdomen, and often, but not always, penetrates to the back. When questioned in retrospect, patients often recall mild and vague pain for many months before diagnosis. A low threshold for ordering a CT scan with "pancreatic protocol" should be maintained for elderly patients with unexplained, persistent, although vague, abdominal pain. As mentioned above, new-onset diabetes in an elderly patient, especially if combined with vague abdominal pain, should prompt a search for pancreatic cancer.

Unfortunately, at this time there is no sensitive and specific serum marker to assist in the timely diagnosis of pancreatic cancer. With jaundice, direct hyperbilirubinemia and elevated alkaline phosphatase are expected but do not serve much of a diagnostic role other than to confirm the obvious. With long-standing biliary obstruction, the prothrombin time will be prolonged due to a depletion of vitamin K, a fat-soluble vitamin dependent on bile flow for absorption. CA19-9 is a mucin-associated carbohydrate antigen that can be detected in the serum of patients with pancreatic cancer. Serum levels are elevated in about 75% of patients with pancreatic cancer. However, CA19-9 is also elevated in about 10% of patients with benign diseases of the pancreas, liver, and bile ducts.[307] CA19-9 is thus neither sufficiently sensitive nor specific to allow an earlier diagnosis of pancreatic cancer. Despite the fact that many tumor markers such as CA19-9 have been studied in an attempt to facilitate early diagnosis, there are still no effective screening tests for pancreatic cancer. Research taking advantage of recent advances in genomics, gene expression analysis, and proteomics has demonstrated thousands of genes and corresponding proteins that are differentially expressed in pancreatic tumors that have potential for early detection of pancreatic cancer.[308] Some of these proteins would be expected to be expressed at the cell surface or in pancreatic juice and may become useful as biomarkers for pancreatic cancer in the future.

In patients presenting with jaundice, a reasonable first diagnostic imaging study is abdominal US. If bile duct dilation is not seen, hepatocellular disease is likely. Demonstration of cholelithiasis and bile duct dilation suggests a diagnosis of choledocholithiasis, and the next logical step would be ERCP to clear the bile duct. In the absence of gallstones, malignant obstruction of the bile duct is likely, and a CT scan rather than ERCP would be the next logical step. For patients suspected of having pancreatic cancer who present without jaundice, US is not appropriate, and a CT scan should be the first test.

The current diagnostic and staging test of choice for pancreatic cancer is a multidetector, dynamic, contrast-enhanced CT scan, and techniques are constantly improving (Fig. 33-68). The accuracy of CT scanning for predicting unresectable disease is about 90 to 95%.[309] CT findings that indicate a tumor is unresectable include invasion of the hepatic or superior mesenteric artery, enlarged lymph nodes outside the boundaries of resection, ascites, and distant metastases (e.g., liver). Invasion of the superior mesenteric vein or portal vein is not in itself a contraindication to resection as long as the veins are patent. In contrast, CT scanning is less accurate in predicting resectable disease. CT scanning will miss small liver metastases, and predicting arterial involvement is sometimes difficult.

Currently, CT is probably the single most versatile and cost-effective tool for the diagnosis of pancreatic cancer. Abdominal MRI is rapidly evolving but currently provides essentially the same

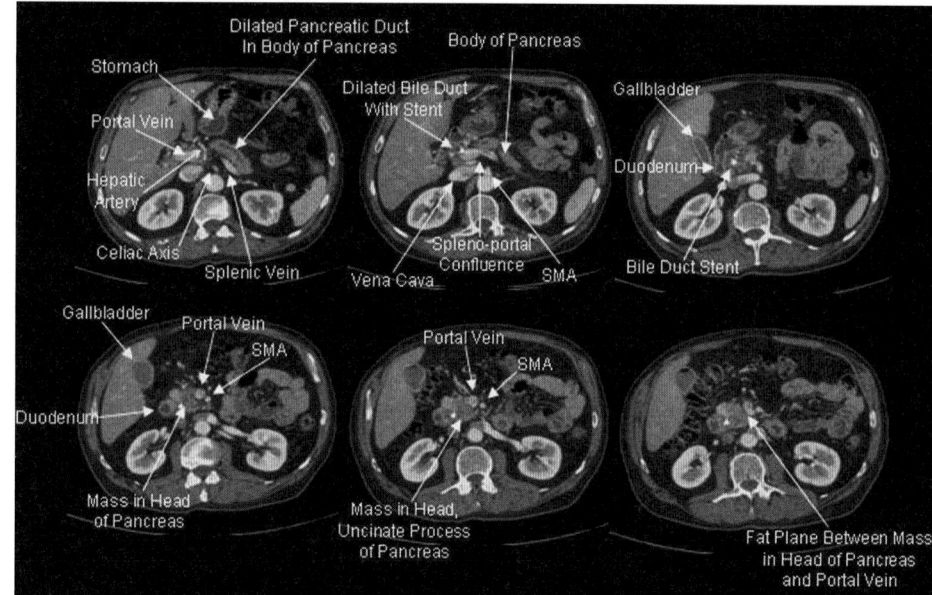

FIG. 33-68. Computed tomography scan demonstrating resectable pancreatic cancer. SMA = superior mesenteric artery.

information as CT scanning. Positron emission tomography scanning is becoming more widely available and may help distinguish chronic pancreatitis from pancreatic cancer. EUS can be used to detect small pancreatic masses that could be missed by CT scanning and is commonly used when there is a high suspicion for pancreatic cancer but no mass is identified by the CT scan. EUS has the added advantage of providing the opportunity for transluminal biopsy of pancreatic masses, although a tissue diagnosis before pancreaticoduodenectomy is not required. However, in specific patients a histologic diagnosis may be necessary such as for those in a neoadjuvant clinical trial or before chemotherapy in advanced tumors. EUS is a sensitive test for portal/superior mesenteric vein invasion, although it is somewhat less effective at detecting superior mesenteric artery invasion. When all of the current staging modalities are used, their accuracy in predicting resectability is reported to be about 80%, meaning that one in five patients brought to the operating room with the intent of a curative resection will be found at the time of surgery to have unresectable disease.[310]

In an attempt to avoid such futile laparotomies, preliminary laparoscopy has been advocated for patients with disease felt to be resectable by CT imaging (Fig. 33-69). Diagnostic laparoscopy with the use of US is reported to improve the accuracy of predicting resectability to about 98%.[310] The technique involves more than simple visualization with the scope and requires the placement of multiple ports and manipulation of the tissues. A general exploration of the peritoneal surfaces is carried out. The ligament of Treitz and the base of the transverse mesocolon are examined for tumor. The gastrocolic ligament is incised, and the lesser sac is examined. The US probe is used to examine the liver, porta hepatis, and the portal vein and superior mesenteric artery.

The percentage of patients in whom a positive laparoscopy helps avoid a nontherapeutic laparotomy varies from 10 to 30% in carcinoma of the head of the pancreas but may be as high as 50% in patients with tumors in the body and tail of the gland. As the quality of CT scanning has improved, the value of routine diagnostic laparoscopy has decreased. However, the morbidity of diagnostic laparoscopy is less than that of laparotomy, and the procedure can be performed on an outpatient basis. Patients who are found to have unresectable disease recover more rapidly from a laparoscopy than a laparotomy and can receive palliative chemotherapy and radiation sooner. The potential immunosuppressive effects of a major surgical procedure also are avoided, as well as the negative psychologic impact of a major painful operation with little benefit.

Biliary obstruction can be relieved with an endoscopic approach in almost all cases. When large (10F) plastic stents are used, most patients do not require replacement for about 3 months. Metallic wall stents last about 5 months on average and usually fail only with tumor ingrowth.[311] Keeping in mind that patients with unresectable pancreatic cancer usually live <1 year, the requirement for numerous stent changes is unlikely.

Diagnostic laparoscopy is possibly best applied to patients with pancreatic cancer on a selective basis. Diagnostic laparoscopy will have a higher yield in patients with large tumors (>4 cm), tumors located in the body or tail, patients with equivocal findings of metastasis or ascites on CT scan, and patients with other indications of advanced disease such as marked weight loss or markedly elevated CA19-9 (>1000 U/mL). An algorithm for the diagnosis, staging, and treatment of pancreatic cancer is shown in Fig. 33-70.

Palliative Surgery and Endoscopy

For the 85 to 90% of patients with pancreatic cancer who have disease that precludes surgical resection, appropriate and effective palliative treatment is critical to the quality of their remaining life. Because of the poor prognosis of the disease, it is not appropriate to

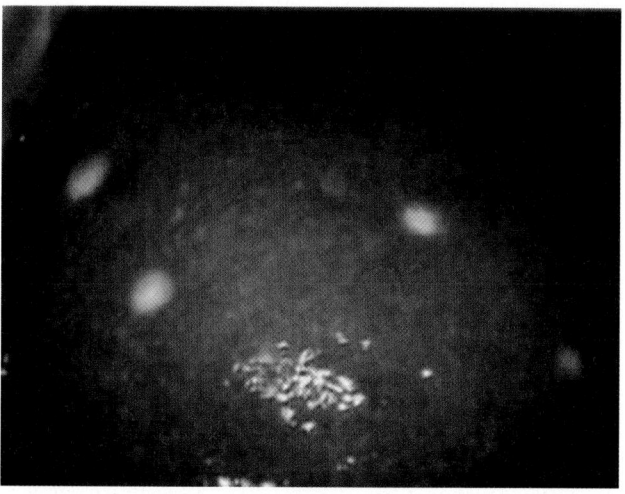

FIG. 33-69. Liver metastases identified at diagnostic laparoscopy.

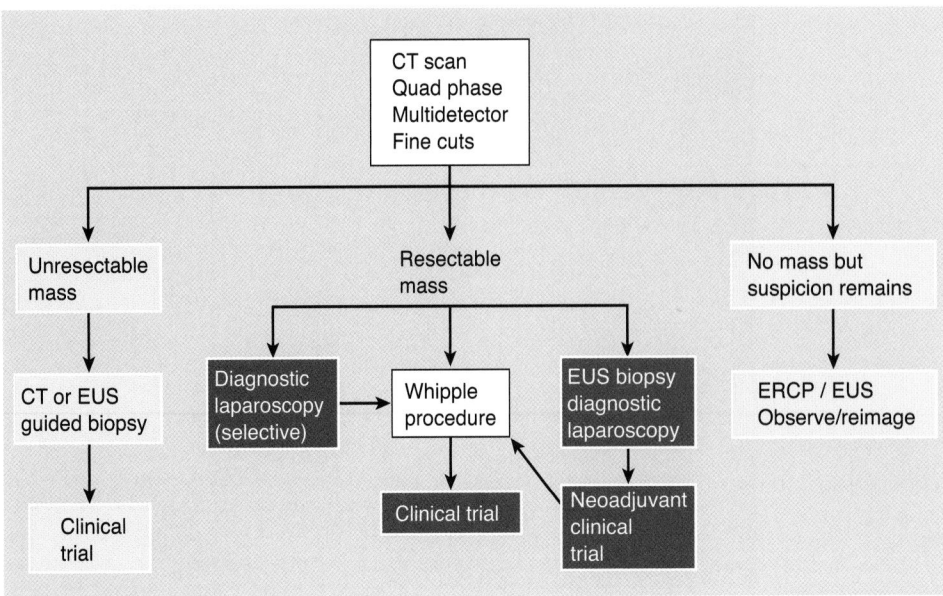

FIG. 33-70. Diagnostic and treatment algorithm for pancreatic cancer. If computed tomography (CT) scan demonstrates a potentially resectable tumor, patients are offered participation in a clinical trial after histologic confirmation by CT or endoscopic ultrasound (EUS)-guided biopsy. If CT scan demonstrates resectable disease, diagnostic laparoscopy is used selectively in patients with tumors in the body/tail, equivocal findings of metastasis or CT scan, ascites, high CA19-9, or marked weight loss. Patients also have diagnostic laparoscopy if they elect to participate in a neoadjuvant clinical trial. In cases where no mass is demonstrated on CT scan, but suspicion of cancer remains, EUS or endoscopic retrograde cholangiopancreatography (ERCP) with brushings are performed, and the CT may be repeated after an interval of observation.

use invasive and toxic regimens in patients with extremely advanced disease and poor performance status. When patients do desire antineoplastic therapy, it is important to encourage them to enroll in clinical trials so that therapeutic advances can be made.

In general, there are three clinical problems in advanced pancreatic cancer that require palliation: pain, jaundice, and duodenal obstruction. The mainstay of pain control is oral narcotics. Sustained-release preparations of morphine sulfate are frequently used. Invasion of retroperitoneal nerve trunks accounts for the severe pain experienced by patients with advanced pancreatic cancer. A celiac plexus nerve block can control pain effectively for a period of months, although the procedure sometimes needs to be repeated.

Jaundice is present in the majority of patients with pancreatic cancer, and the most troublesome aspect for the patient is the accompanying pruritus. Biliary obstruction may also lead to cholangitis, coagulopathy, digestive symptoms, and hepatocellular failure. In the past, surgeons traditionally performed a biliary bypass when unresectable disease was found at laparotomy. As many patients today already have a bile duct stent in place by the time of operation, it is not clear that operative biliary bypass is required. If an operative bypass is performed, choledochojejunostomy is the preferred approach. Although an easy procedure to perform, choledochoduodenostomy is felt to be unwise because of the proximity of the duodenum to tumor. Some have discouraged the use of the gallbladder for biliary bypass[311]; however, it is suitable as long as the cystic duct clearly enters the common duct well above the tumor.

Duodenal obstruction is usually a late event in pancreatic cancer and occurs in only about 20% of patients.[312] Therefore, in the absence of signs or symptoms of obstruction, such as a tumor that is already encroaching on the duodenum at the time of surgery, the routine use of prophylactic gastrojejunostomy when exploration reveals unresectable tumor is controversial. Although anastomotic leaks are uncommon, gastrojejunostomy is sometimes associated with delayed gastric emptying, the very symptom the procedure is designed to treat.

Whether performing both a biliary and enteric bypass or just a biliary bypass, the jejunum is brought anterior to the colon, if possible, rather than retrocolic, where the tumor potentially would invade the bowel sooner. Some surgeons use a loop of jejunum with a jejunojejunostomy to divert the enteric stream away from the biliary-enteric anastomosis. Others use a Roux-en-Y limb with the gastrojejunostomy located 50 cm downstream from the hepaticojejunostomy (Fig. 33-71). Potential advantages of the defunctionalized Roux-en-Y limb include the ease with which it will reach up to the hepatic hilum, probable decreased risk of cholangitis, and easier management of biliary anastomotic leaks. If a gastrojejunostomy is performed, it should be placed dependently and posterior along the greater curvature to improve gastric emptying, and a vagotomy should not be performed. If patients are explored laparoscopically and found to have unresectable disease, palliation of jaundice can be achieved in a minimally invasive fashion with ERCP and placement of a coated, expandable metallic endoscopic biliary stent (Fig. 33-72). Endoscopic stents are definitely not as durable as a surgical bypass. Recurrent obstruction and cholangitis is more common with stents and results in inferior palliation. However, this minimally invasive approach is associated with considerably less initial morbidity and mortality than surgical bypass. Newer, expandable metallic wall stents demonstrate improved patency and provide better palliation than plastic stents.

If an initial diagnostic laparoscopy reveals a contraindication to the Whipple procedure, such as liver metastases, it is not appropriate to perform a laparotomy simply to create a biliary bypass. In such a patient, it is better to place an endoscopic stent. In contrast, if a laparotomy has already been performed as part of the assessment of resectability and the Whipple procedure is not possible, a surgical bypass is usually performed. However, if the patient has a functioning endoscopic stent already in place, it may be reasonable to forego surgical bypass.

Palliative Chemotherapy and Radiation

In patients with unresectable pancreatic cancer, gemcitabine results in symptomatic improvement, improved pain control and performance status, and weight gain.[313] However, survival is improved by

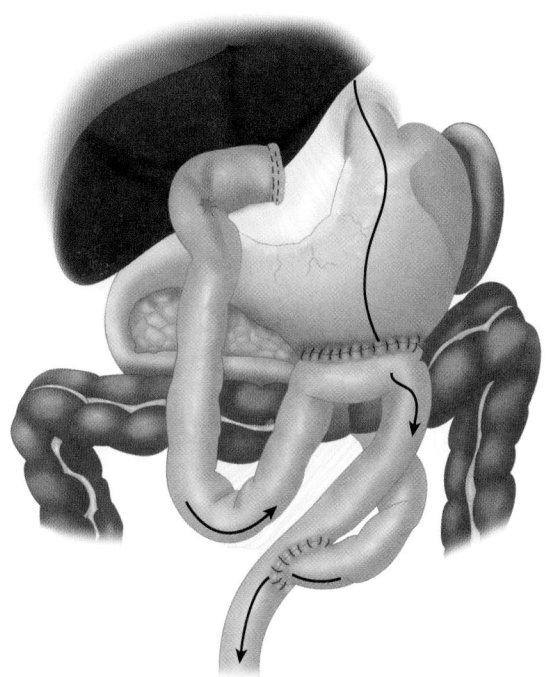

FIG. 33-71. Biliary-enteric bypass to palliate unresectable pancreatic cancer. *[Reproduced with permission from Bell RH Jr.: Atlas of pancreatic surgery, in Bell RH Jr., Rikkers LF, Mulholland MW (eds): Digestive Tract Surgery: A Text and Atlas. Philadelphia: Lippincott-Raven, 1996, p 1074.]*

only 1 to 2 months. Although these results may warrant treatment in patients who understand the benefits and risks, the lack of significant survival advantage should encourage physicians to refer motivated patients for experimental protocols, because it is only through continued clinical research that more meaningful treatments for pancreatic cancer will be developed.

Surgical Resection: Pancreaticoduodenectomy

In a patient with appropriate clinical and/or imaging indications of pancreatic cancer, a tissue diagnosis before performing a pancreaticoduodenectomy is not essential. Although percutaneous CT-guided biopsy is usually safe, complications such as hemorrhage, pancreatitis, fistula, abscess, and even death can occur. Tumor seeding along the subcutaneous tract of the needle is uncommon. Likewise, FNA under EUS guidance is safe and well tolerated. The problem with preoperative or even intraoperative biopsy is that

many pancreatic cancers are not very cellular and contain a significant amount of fibrous tissue, so a biopsy may be misinterpreted as showing chronic pancreatitis if it does not contain malignant glandular cells. In the face of clinical and radiologic preoperative indications of pancreatic cancer, a negative biopsy should not preclude resection. In patients who are not candidates for resection because of metastatic disease, biopsy for a tissue diagnosis becomes important because these patients may be candidates for palliative chemotherapy trials. It is especially important to make an aggressive attempt at tissue diagnosis before surgery in patients whose clinical presentation and imaging studies are more suggestive of alternative diagnoses such as pancreatic lymphoma or pancreatic islet cell tumors. These patients might avoid surgery altogether in the case of lymphoma or warrant an aggressive debulking approach in the case of islet cell carcinoma.

Pancreaticoduodenectomy can be performed through a midline incision from xiphoid to umbilicus or through a bilateral subcostal incision. The initial portion of the procedure is an assessment of resectability. The liver and visceral and parietal peritoneal surfaces are thoroughly assessed. The gastrohepatic omentum is opened, and the celiac axis area is examined for enlarged lymph nodes. The base of the transverse mesocolon to the right of the middle colic vessels is examined for tumor involvement.

The ascending and hepatic flexure of the colon are mobilized off the duodenum and head of the pancreas and reflected medially. A Kocher maneuver is performed by dissecting behind the head of the pancreas. The superior mesenteric vein is identified early in the case and dissected up toward the inferior border of the neck of the pancreas. The gastroepiploic vein and artery are ligated to prevent any traction injury. The relation of the tumor to the superior mesenteric vein and artery cannot be accurately assessed by palpation at this point and is not completely determined until later in the operation when the neck of the pancreas is divided and the surgeon is committed to resection. Mesenteric vascular involvement is best determined by a high quality preoperative CT scan.

It is important to assess for an aberrant right hepatic artery, which is present in 20% of patients. The aberrant artery arises from the superior mesenteric artery posterior to the pancreas and ascends parallel and adjacent to the superior mesenteric and portal veins. The presence of an aberrant right hepatic artery should be apparent on the preoperative CT scan and can be identified intraoperatively by palpation on the back side of the hepatoduodenal ligament, where a prominent pulse will be felt posterior and to the right of the portal vein.

The porta hepatis is examined. Enlarged or firm lymph nodes that can be swept down toward the head of the pancreas with the specimen do not preclude resection. If the assessment phase reveals no contraindications to the Whipple procedure (Table 33-19), the resection phase commences.

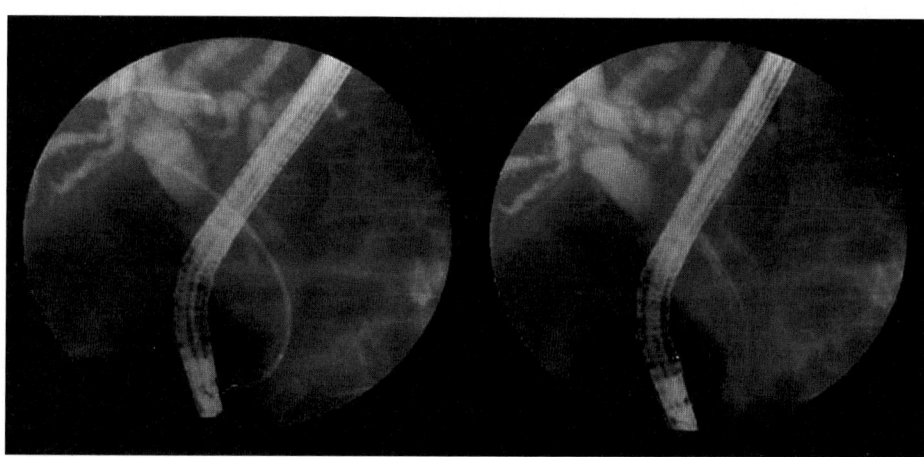

FIG. 33-72. Expandable metallic biliary stent.

TABLE 33-19 Findings at exploration

Findings contraindicating resection
   Liver metastases (any size)
   Celiac lymph node involvement
   Peritoneal implants
   Hepatic hilar lymph node involvement
Findings not contraindicating resection
   Invasion at duodenum or distal stomach
   Involved peripancreatic lymph nodes
   Involved lymph nodes along the porta hepatis that can be swept
     down with the specimen

If the pylorus is to be preserved, the stomach and proximal duodenum are mobilized off the pancreas, preserving the gastroepiploic vessels down to the pylorus. The proximal hepatic artery is identified usually by removing a lymph node that commonly lies just anterior to the artery. The hepatic artery is dissected and traced toward the porta hepatis. Small vessels in this area can be ligated with 3-0 or 4-0 silk ligatures to prevent bothersome hemorrhage later in the case that makes subsequent dissection more tedious. The gastroduodenal branch of the hepatic artery is identified. A test clamping is performed to assure that a strong pulse remains in the proper hepatic artery before division of the gastroduodenal artery. Once the gastroduodenal artery is divided, the hepatic artery is retracted medially and the common bile duct is retracted laterally to reveal the glistening anterior surface of the portal vein behind them. Dissection is performed only on the anterior surface of the vein. If there is no tumor involvement, the neck of the pancreas will separate from the vein easily. A large, blunt-tipped clamp is a safe instrument to use for this dissection. The tunnel under the neck of the pancreas can then be completed mostly under direct vision from inferior and superior.

The gallbladder is then mobilized from the liver, the cystic duct and artery are ligated, and the gallbladder is removed. The common hepatic duct is circumferentially dissected. Either the duodenum is divided 2 cm distal to the pylorus (PPPD) or the antrum is divided. The jejunum is divided beyond the ligament of Treitz, and the mesentery is ligated until the jejunum can be delivered posterior to the superior mesenteric vessels from left to right.

The common hepatic duct is then divided just above the entrance of the cystic duct, and the duct is dissected down to the superior margin of the duodenum. Inferior traction on the distal bile duct opens the plane to make visible the anterior portion of the portal vein. The pancreatic neck is divided anterior to the portal vein (Fig. 33-73). The pancreatic head and uncinate process then are dissected off of the right lateral aspect of the superior mesenteric vein, ligating the fragile branches draining the head and uncinate process into the portal vein (Fig. 33-74). The uncinate process is then dissected off of the posterior and lateral aspect of the superior mesenteric artery. This can be the most tedious portion of the operation, but thoroughly clearing all tissue from the mesenteric vessels helps avoid incomplete resection. The wound is irrigated and meticulous hemostasis is assured at this point because the view of the portal vein area and retroperitoneum is more difficult after the reconstruction phase is completed.

The reconstruction involves anastomoses of the pancreas first, then the bile duct, and, finally, the duodenum or stomach. There are various techniques for the pancreatic anastomoses, and all have equivalent outcomes. After the pancreatic anastomosis is completed, the choledochojejunostomy is performed about 10 cm down the jejunal limb from the pancreatic anastomosis. This is usually performed in an end-to-side fashion with one layer of interrupted sutures. The duodenojejunostomy or gastrojejunostomy is performed another 10 to 15 cm downstream from the biliary anastomosis, using a two-layer technique.

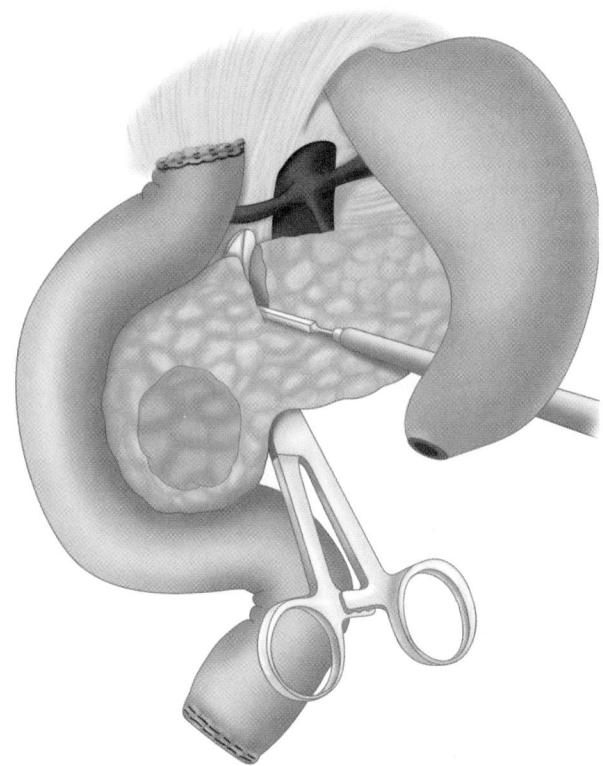

FIG. 33-73. Division of the pancreatic neck. The pancreatic neck is separated from the anterior surface of the portal vein and then divided. If there is no tumor involvement, the neck of the pancreas will separate from the vein easily. A large, blunt-tipped clamp is a safe instrument to use for this dissection. *[Reproduced with permission from Bell RH Jr.: Atlas of pancreatic surgery, in Bell RH Jr., Rikkers LF, Mulholland MW (eds): Digestive Tract Surgery: A Text and Atlas. Philadelphia: Lippincott-Raven, 1996, p 1054.]*

Variations and Controversies

The preservation of the pylorus has several theoretical advantages, including prevention of reflux of pancreaticobiliary secretions into the stomach, decreased incidence of marginal ulceration, normal gastric acid secretion and hormone release, and improved gastric function. Patients with pylorus-preserving resections have appeared to regain weight better than historic controls in some studies. Return of gastric emptying in the immediate postoperative period may take longer after the pylorus-preserving operation, and it is controversial whether there is any significant improvement in long-term quality of life with pyloric preservation.[314,315]

Techniques for the pancreaticojejunostomy include end-to-side or end-to-end and duct-to-mucosa sutures or invagination (Fig. 33-75). Pancreaticogastrostomy has also been investigated.

Some surgeons use stents, glue to seal the anastomosis, or octreotide to decrease pancreatic secretions. No matter what combination of these techniques is used, the pancreatic leakage rate is always about 10%. Therefore, the choice of techniques depends more on the surgeon's personal experience.

Traditionally, most surgeons place drains around the pancreatic and biliary anastomoses because disruption of the pancreaticojejunostomy cannot be avoided in one out of 10 patients. This complication can lead to the development of an upper abdominal abscess or can present as an external pancreatic fistula. Usually, a pure pancreatic leak is controlled by the drains and will eventually seal spontaneously. Combined pancreatic and biliary leaks are cause for concern because bile will activate the pancreatic enzymes. In its most virulent form, disruption leads to necrotizing retroperitoneal

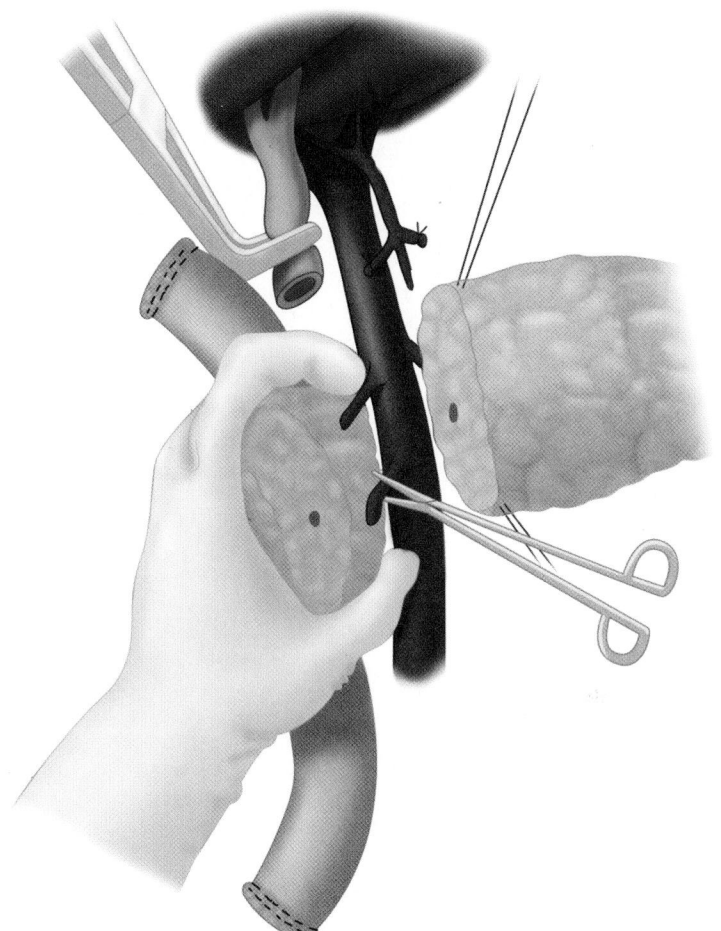

FIG. 33-74. Dissection of the pancreatic head and uncinate process. The pancreatic head and uncinate process are dissected off of the right lateral aspect of the superior mesenteric vein and portal vein by ligating the fragile venous branches. *[Reproduced with permission from Bell RH Jr.: Atlas of pancreatic surgery, in Bell RH Jr., Rikkers LF, Mulholland MW (eds): Digestive Tract Surgery: A Text and Atlas. Philadelphia: Lippincott-Raven, 1996, p 1056.]*

infection, which can erode major arteries and veins of the upper abdomen, including the exposed portal vein and its branches or the stump of the gastroduodenal artery. Impending catastrophe is often preceded by a small herald bleed from the drain site. Depending on the clinical situation, such an event is an indication to perform an angiogram or return the patient to the operating room to widely drain the pancreaticojejunostomy and to repair the involved blood vessel. Open packing may be necessary to control diffuse necrosis and infection. Some studies have questioned the practice of routine drain placement after pancreaticoduodenectomy. These studies indicated that most pancreatic leaks can be managed with percutaneous drainage.[316]

Many patients with pancreatic cancer are malnourished preoperatively and suffer from gastroparesis in the immediate postoperative period. Routine placement of a feeding jejunostomy tube and gastrostomy tube has become less common, and most surgeons use these tubes selectively. Gastrostomy tubes may decrease the length of stay in patients who might be predicted to have severe gastroparesis. Jejunostomy tubes are certainly not benign and can result in leaks and intestinal obstruction. However, parenteral nutrition is also associated with serious complications such as line sepsis, loss of gut mucosal integrity, and hepatic dysfunction.

Because of the high incidence of direct retroperitoneal invasion and regional lymph node metastasis at the time of surgery, it has been argued that the scope of resection for pancreatic cancer should be enlarged to include a radical regional lymphadenectomy and resection of areas of potential retroperitoneal invasion. The "radical pancreaticoduodenectomy" includes extension of the pancreatic resection to the middle body of the pancreas, segmental resection of the portal vein, if necessary, resection of retroperitoneal tissue along the right

perinephric area, and lymphadenectomy to the region of the celiac plexus. In the hands of experienced surgeons, these techniques are associated with greater blood loss but no increase in mortality; however, improved survival has not been demonstrated.[317] Total pancreatectomy has also been considered in the past. Although pancreatic leaks are eliminated, major morbidity from brittle diabetes and exocrine insufficiency outweigh any theoretical benefit.

Pancreatic cancer can recur locally after pancreaticoduodenectomy. Intraoperative radiotherapy (IORT) delivers a full therapeutic dose of radiation to the operative bed at the time of resection. Radiation to surrounding normal areas is minimized, but the radiation is delivered all in one setting, usually about 15 minutes, rather than in fractionated doses over time. IORT is best performed in a shielded, dedicated, operating room suite rather than by transporting the patient in the middle of an already long and complicated operation. IORT may improve local control and palliate symptoms after pancreaticoduodenectomy. However, IORT has not been shown to be superior to standard external beam radiation therapy, and further randomized trials are needed to determine how this modality should be utilized.[318]

Complications of Pancreaticoduodenectomy

The operative mortality rate for pancreaticoduodenectomy has decreased to <5% in "high volume" centers (where individual surgeons perform more than fifteen cases per year), suggesting that patients in rural areas would benefit from referral to large urban centers.[319,320] The most common causes of death are sepsis, hemorrhage, and cardiovascular events. Postoperative complications are unfortunately still very common, and include delayed gastric emptying, pancreatic fistula, and hemorrhage.

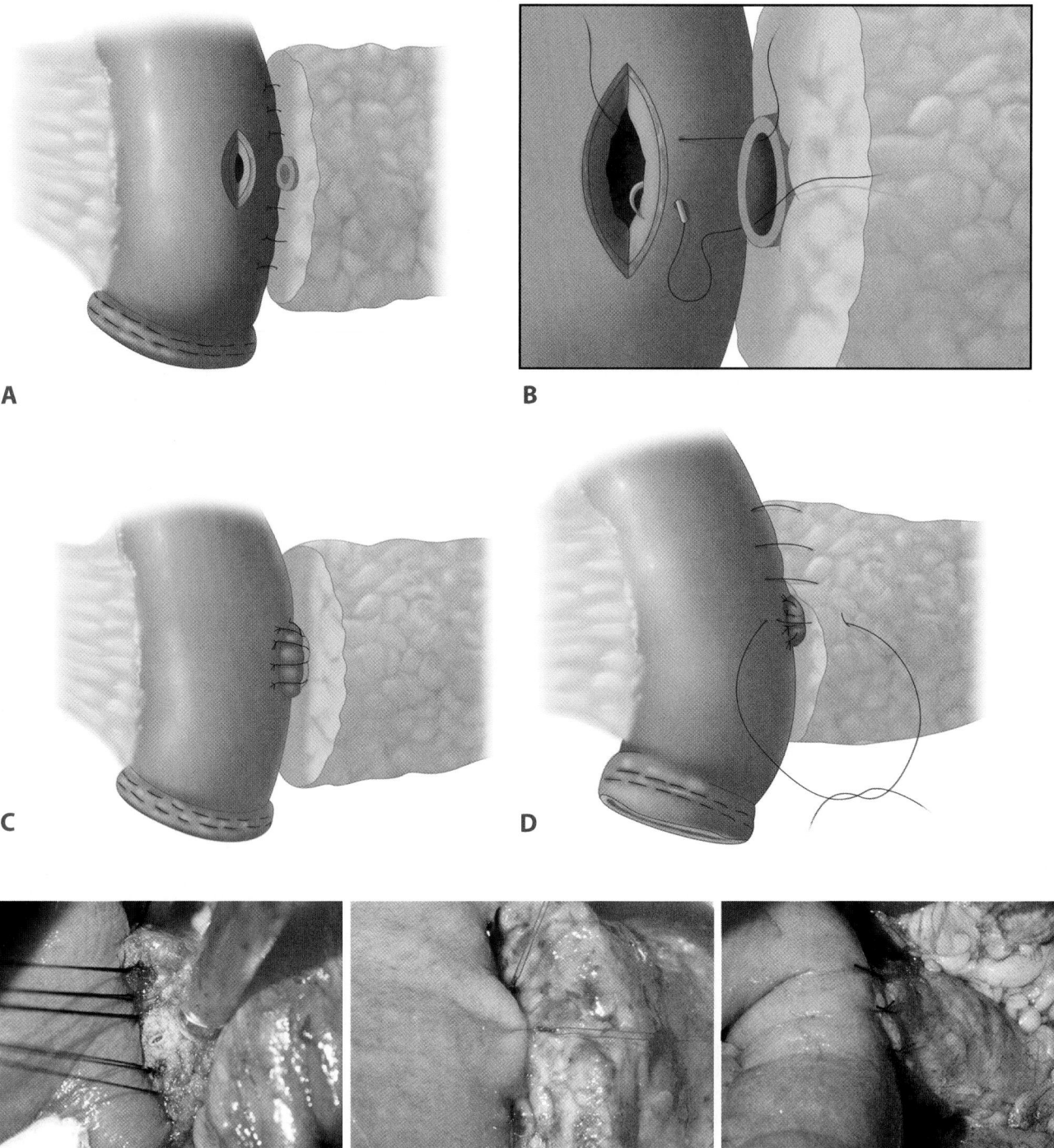

FIG. 33-75. Techniques for pancreaticojejunostomy. **A** to **D.** Duct-to-mucosa, end-to-side. **E.** Intraoperative photographs of end-to-side pancreaticojejunostomy. (*Continued*)

Delayed gastric emptying is common after pancreaticoduodenectomy and is treated conservatively as long as complete gastric outlet obstruction is ruled out by a contrast study. IV erythromycin may help in the acute phase, but the problem usually improves with time.

Considerable attention has been focused on the prevention of pancreatic leak after pancreas resection. Modifications of the anastomotic technique (end-to-side or end-to-end, duct-to-mucosa or invaginated), the use of jejunum or the stomach for drainage, the use of pancreatic duct stents, the use of octreotide, and various sealants have all been evaluated. Octreotide, a synthetic analogue of somatostatin with a longer half-life, has been evaluated as a pharmacologic therapy to reduce pancreatic secretion and the rate of

pancreatic fistula after pancreatic resection. European studies advocate the routine use of octreotide while North American trials conclude that octreotide is useless. European studies have demonstrated a significant reduction in the rate of postoperative pancreatic fistula with prophylactic preoperative octreotide injection.[321-323] However, recent randomized prospective studies in the United States showed that octreotide did not prevent postoperative pancreatic fistula when used following pancreatic resection.[206,324-330] However, a subgroup analysis done by Suc and colleagues[329] suggested that there may be a benefit to using octreotide in a high-risk group of patients undergoing pancreaticoduodenectomy who have a pancreatic duct measuring <3 mm. Some studies suggest a higher rate

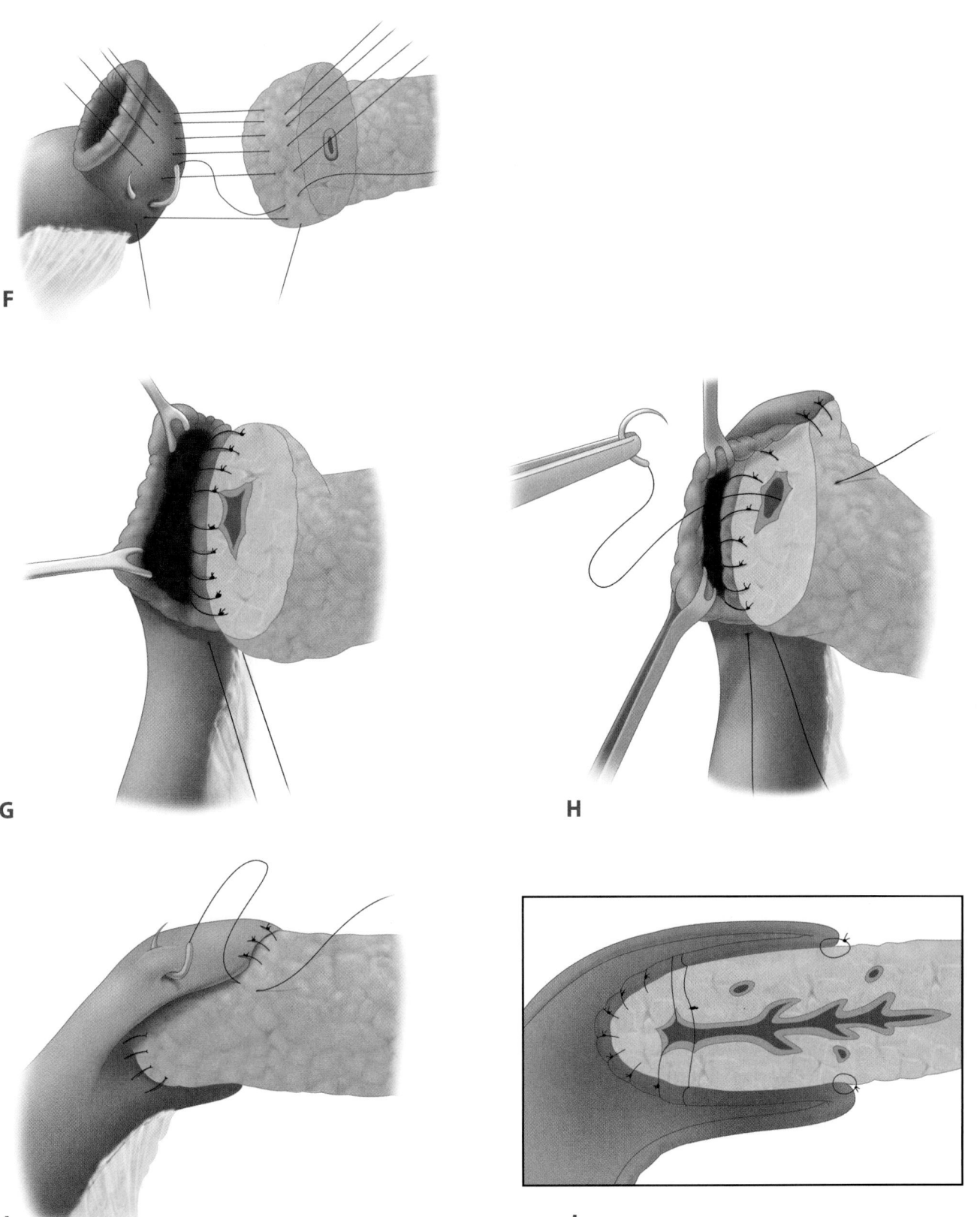

FIG. 33-75. (*Continued*) **F** to **J.** End-to-end invagination. (*Continued*)

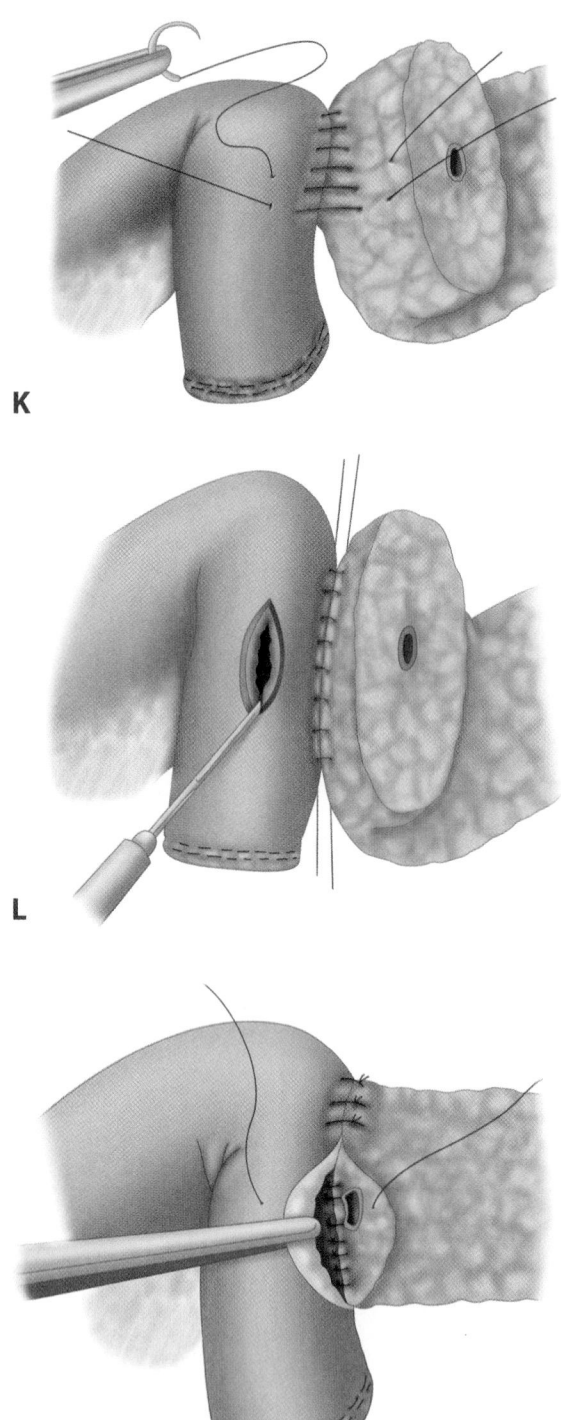

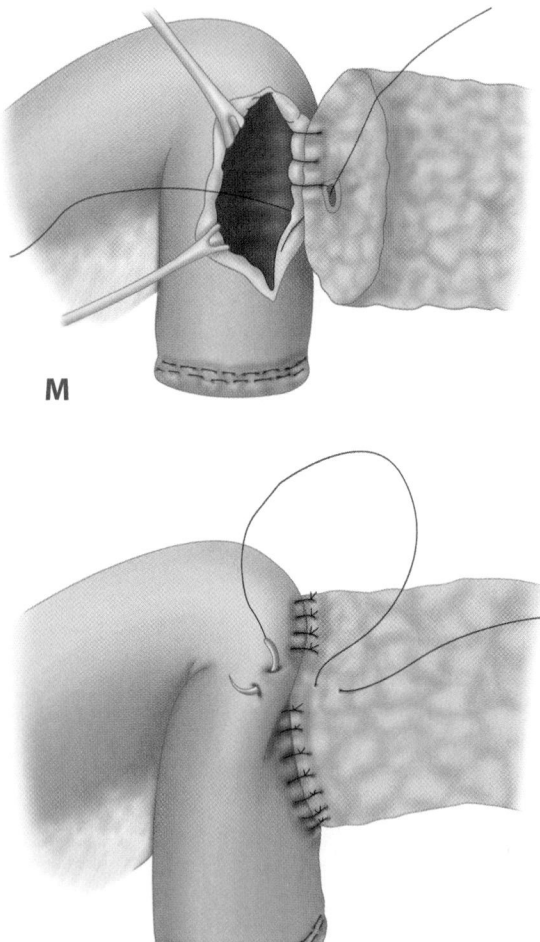

FIG. 33-75. (*Continued*) **K** to **O.** End-to-side invagination.

of complications[324,326] in patients who receive octreotide even though the difference was not statistically significant, while others report a significantly lower rate of complications with the use of octreotide.[322,323] Finally, the optimal dose, route (IV drip vs. subcutaneous injection), and timing (preoperative, intraoperative, or postoperative) of octreotide use is unclear.

Many technical modifications to the classic pancreaticoduodenectomy have been described. However, >70 technical variations to the pancreaticoenteric anastomosis have not clearly demonstrated an objective method to consistently decrease the rate of fistula, which varies from 0 to 40% depending on the definition of fistula.[324,325,330–338] Yeo compared the incidence of pancreatic fistula in patients who had a pancreaticoduodenectomy with reconstruction via a pancreatico-

gastrostomy or pancreaticojejunostomy.[338] There was no significant difference between the two techniques in the incidence of pancreatic fistula. A recent meta-analysis summarized the results of 16 trials comparing pancreaticogastrostomy to pancreaticojejunostomy. All of the observational clinical studies reported superiority of pancreaticogastrostomy over pancreaticojejunostomy, most likely influenced by publication bias. In contrast, all randomized prospective trials failed to show advantage of a particular technique, suggesting both techniques provide equally good results.[339]

Other options to consider when performing the pancreatic anastomosis are the duct-to-mucosa vs. the invagination techniques. Many surgeons choose the technique at the time of operation, depending on the size of the pancreatic duct and the texture of pancreas.[340] The duct-to-mucosa anastomosis results in a low pancreatic fistula rate[341] in patients with a large pancreatic duct and a fibrotic pancreas. However, the end-to-end invagination technique may be more secure in patients with a small duct and soft pancreas.

Even though there has been little convincing evidence for the use of a pancreatic duct stent, proponents suggest that a stent may discourage a pancreatic leak and aid in technical precision.[342,343] Both internal stenting as well as external stenting have been shown to reduce the incidence of pancreatic fistula in some clinical studies.[341]

Some studies[336,344] suggest that an isolated Roux-en-Y pancreaticoenteric anastomosis may be associated with a lower rate of postoperative pancreatic leak. The logic behind this technical modification is that the use of separate Roux-en-Y limbs for biliary and pancreatic secretions may protect the pancreatic anastomosis from activated pancreatic enzymes.

Avoiding the pancreatic anastomosis altogether by ductal ligation or occlusion has also been evaluated as a potential technique to reduce the rate of postoperative pancreatic fistula.[345] Ductal occlusion with neoprene or prolamine, which are nonresorbable glues, has been abandoned due to pancreatic atrophy and loss of exocrine function.[346] Another study by Tran and associates[347] comparing duct occlusion and pancreaticojejunostomy showed that duct occlusion significantly increases the risk of endocrine insufficiency without a decrease in the postoperative complication rate. To avoid long-term loss of function, absorbable glues, such as fibrin glue, have been evaluated to limit the action of pancreatic enzymes until the anastomosis is healed. Fibrin glue has been used for both duct occlusion and has also been applied to the surface of the pancreatic stump and anastomotic site without clear improvement in pancreatic fistula rate. The effect of BioGlue applied to the anastomotic surface after the Whipple procedure and pancreatic stump after distal pancreatectomy was recently evaluated in a retrospective cohort study. There were no statistically significant differences in the incidence or severity grades of postoperative pancreatic fistulas.[348]

If not combined with a biliary leak, pancreatic fistula, although serious, can usually be managed conservatively. In about 95% of cases, reoperation is not indicated and prolonged drainage, using drains placed in the original operation or percutaneously after resection, results in spontaneous closure of the fistula.[349]

Hemorrhage can occur either intraoperatively or postoperatively. Intraoperative hemorrhage typically occurs during the dissection of the portal vein. A major laceration of the portal vein can occur at a point in the operation at which the portal vein is not yet exposed. Temporary control of hemorrhage is generally possible in this situation by compressing the portal vein and superior mesenteric vein against the tumor with the surgeon's left hand behind the head of the pancreas. An experienced assistant is needed to divide the neck of the pancreas to the left of the portal vein and achieve proximal and distal control. Sometimes, the vein can be sutured closed with minimal narrowing. Other times, a segmental resection and interposition graft (internal jugular vein) may be needed.

Postoperative hemorrhage can occur from inadequate ligature of any one of numerous blood vessels during the procedure. Hemorrhage can also occur due to digestion of retroperitoneal blood vessels due to a combined biliary-pancreatic leak. Uncommonly, a stress ulcer, or later, a marginal ulcer, can result in GI hemorrhage. Typically, a vagotomy is not performed when pancreaticoduodenectomy is performed for pancreatic cancer, but patients are placed on proton pump inhibitors.

Outcome and Value of Pancreaticoduodenectomy for Cancer

Survival figures indicate that few, if any, patients are cured indefinitely of pancreatic cancer with pancreaticoduodenectomy. The tumor tends to recur locally with retroperitoneal and regional lymphatic disease. In addition, most patients also develop hematogenous metastases, usually in the liver. Malignant ascites, peritoneal implants, and malignant pleural effusions are all common. Median survival after pancreaticoduodenectomy is about 22 months. Even long-term (5-year) survivors often eventually die due to pancreatic cancer recurrence.

Although pancreaticoduodenectomy may be performed with the hope of the rare cure in mind, the operation more importantly provides better palliation than any other treatment, and is the only modality that offers any meaningful improvement in survival. If the procedure is performed without major complications, many months of palliation are usually achieved. It is the surgeon's duty to make sure patients and their families have a realistic understanding of the true goals of pancreaticoduodenectomy in the setting of pancreatic cancer.

Adjuvant Chemotherapy and Radiation

Small studies in the 1980s suggested that adjuvant chemotherapy with 5-FU combined with radiation improves survival by about 9 months after pancreatic resection for pancreatic adenocarcinoma.[350] Subsequent, noncontrolled studies have reinforced that concept; however, the data have been criticized due to the low number of patients and low dose of radiation therapy that was given. In addition, gemcitabine has recently replaced 5-FU as standard therapy in pancreatic cancer but is thought to be too toxic when given with radiotherapy at current doses. However, a recent large European multicenter trial concluded that there was no value to chemoradiotherapy, although the study suggested the possibility that chemotherapy alone might have survival benefit.[351] In contrast to that study, remarkable results in adjuvant therapy have been reported by the Virginia Mason Clinic with combination 5-FU, cisplatinum, interferon-α and external beam radiation. Although the toxicity is high (42% hospitalized for GI toxicity), the promising results prompted larger confirmatory studies. Unfortunately, one such study was stopped due to toxicity. Nevertheless, pending further study, it is typical in the United States for patients with acceptable functional status to receive adjuvant chemotherapy and radiotherapy after surgery.

Neoadjuvant Treatment

There are several potential advantages to the use of chemoradiation before an attempt at surgical resection. For example, it avoids the risk that adjuvant treatment is delayed by complications of surgery. Neoadjuvant treatment also may decrease the tumor burden at operation, increasing the rate of resectability and killing some tumor cells before they can be spread intraoperatively. Another potential advantage is that it allows patients with occult metastatic disease to avoid the morbidity of pancreatic resection. As many as 20% of patients treated with neoadjuvant chemoradiation develop metastatic disease detected by restaging CT and do not go on to surgery. Preoperative chemoradiation has been shown not to increase the perioperative morbidity or mortality of pancreaticoduodenectomy. It may even decrease the incidence of pancreatic fistula. However, level I data to support neoadjuvant over standard adjuvant chemoradiation in pancreatic cancer is lacking. Prospective randomized trials investigating this concept are ongoing but are difficult to complete due to the high number of patients who fail to complete or receive a full course of either therapy. Studies so far indicate that local or regional recurrence is decreased with this technique, but so far there is no generally accepted survival advantage compared to traditional postoperative therapy.[352]

Postoperative Surveillance

Recurrence after successful resection usually manifests as hepatic metastases. After adjuvant chemoradiation with 5-FU and external beam radiation, gemcitabine is usually administered on a weekly basis for 6 months. During this time period, patients are monitored with frequent physical examinations and laboratory tests, including CA19-9. CT scans are typically ordered after a course of chemotherapy is completed or when a rising CA19-9 or new symptoms suggest recurrence. Surgical therapy for recurrent disease is usually reserved for patients who remain reasonable operative candidates who develop symptomatic gastric outlet or bowel obstruction.

Future Therapy

With recent developments in molecular biology techniques and the mapping of the entire human genome, new therapies for pancreatic cancer are becoming available. Several strategies are possible, including immunotherapeutic gene therapy, replacement of tumor suppressor gene function, inactivation of oncogenes, and suicide gene therapy.[353] With immunotherapeutic gene therapy, the goal is to assist the immune system in recognizing the cancer cells. Cancer cells have been forced to express tumor-specific antigens and cytokines that activate the immune system and that may have antitumor effects. Because pancreatic cancer is a disease with multiple genetic aberrations, inactivated tumor suppressor genes have been replaced, and mutated oncogenes have been inactivated with gene therapy. In suicide gene therapy, a transgene is introduced that converts an inactive nontoxic drug into an active cytotoxic agent. The herpes simplex virus-thymidine kinase system has been the most extensively studied.[353] Various delivery systems, including viral vectors, liposomes, and protein-conjugated DNA, exist. With each of these strategies and delivery systems, tumor cell–specific delivery would be extremely desirable but awaits the discovery of effective tumor-specific promoters. Clinical trials for pancreatic cancer are ongoing and offer hope for more meaningful treatment.

Ampullary and Periampullary Cancer

Ampullary cancers need to be distinguished from periampullary cancers. The ampulla is the junction of the biliary and pancreatic ducts within the duodenum. Periampullary cancer includes tumors arising from the distal bile duct, duodenal mucosa, or pancreas just adjacent to the ampulla, and the ampulla can be overgrown by cancers that arise from these adjacent areas, making it impossible to determine the true site of origin. Clinically, the term *periampullary cancer* is, therefore, a nonspecific term used to refer to a variety of tumors arising at the intersection of these four sites. The term *ampullary cancer* is more specific and is reserved for tumors that arise at the ampulla. Based on their location, ampullary cancers are usually detected relatively early due to the appearance of jaundice and have a more favorable prognosis. The ampulla of Vater is lined by an epithelial layer that transitions from pancreatic and biliary ductal epithelium to duodenal mucosal epithelium. Ampullary adenocarcinomas can therefore have an intestinal and/or pancreaticobiliary histologic morphology, with the former having a better prognosis. Patients with ampullary cancer have a 10-year survival of about 35%, which is a much better prognosis than patients with pancreatic adenocarcinoma. The difference in survival is not entirely explained by an earlier presentation and lower incidence of lymph node metastases. There are probably biologic, particularly molecular, differences between ampullary and pancreatic adenocarcinoma of the pancreas. Intestinal type ampullary cancers have a lower incidence of EGFr and mutant p53 overexpression, and fewer activating K-*ras* mutations. These tumors are more likely to have genetic changes similar to colon cancer such as microsatellite instability and adenomatous polyposis coli mutations.

Management of Periampullary Adenomas

Benign tumors such as ampullary adenomas can also originate at the ampulla. The accuracy of endoscopic biopsy in distinguishing ampullary cancer from benign adenoma is poor with false negative rates from 25 to 56% even if sphincterotomy precedes the biopsy. However, benign villous adenomas of the ampullary region can be excised locally. This technique is applicable only for small tumors (approximately 2 cm or less) with no evidence of malignancy upon biopsy. EUS may help to accurately determine if there is invasion into the duodenal wall. In the absence of invasion, adenomas may be amenable to an endoscopic or transduodenal excision. A longitudinal duodenotomy is made and the tumor is excised with a 2- to 3-mm margin of normal duodenal mucosa. In some centers, small periampullary adenomas can also be removed endoscopically. A preoperative diagnosis of cancer is a contraindication to transduodenal excision, and pancreaticoduodenectomy should be performed. Likewise, if final pathologic examination of a locally excised tumor reveals invasive cancer, the patient should be returned to the operating room for a pancreaticoduodenectomy. An important subset of patients are those with FAP, who develop periam-

pullary or duodenal adenomas. These lesions have a high incidence of harboring carcinoma, and frequently recur unless the mucosa at risk is resected. A standard (not pylorus-sparing) Whipple is the procedure of choice in FAP patients with periampullary lesions.

Cystic Neoplasms of the Pancreas

A cystic neoplasm needs to be considered when a patient presents with a fluid-containing pancreatic lesion (Fig. 33-76). Cystic neoplasms of the pancreas may be more frequent than previously recognized and are being identified with increasing frequency as the use of abdominal CT scanning has increased. Most of these lesions are benign or slow growing, and the prognosis is significantly better than with pancreatic adenocarcinoma. However, some of these neoplasms slowly undergo malignant transformation and thus represent an opportunity for surgical cure, which is exceedingly uncommon in the setting of pancreatic adenocarcinoma. The dilemma for the surgeon is an accurate assessment of the risk-benefit ratio of resection vs. observation of these lesions in individual patients. Radiologic features including the size of the lesion and its growth rate, the density of the lesion, characteristics of the wall such as nodules, septations, or calcifications, and the relationship between the lesion and the pancreatic duct can help categorize these lesions. Although a thorough history and radiographic findings often suggest a particular diagnosis, EUS-guided FNA and analysis of cyst fluid or ERCP provide useful additional information to guide clinical decision making. Cysts that contain thick fluid with mucin, elevated carcinoembryonic antigen (CEA), or atypical cells must be treated as potentially malignant (Fig. 33-77).

Pseudocysts

The most common cystic lesion of the pancreas is the pseudocyst, which, of course, has no epithelial lining and is a nonneoplastic complication of pancreatitis or pancreatic duct injury. As discussed in "Complications of Chronic Pancreatitis," the diagnosis is usually straightforward from the clinical history. Although not usually necessary, analysis of pseudocyst fluid would reveal a high amylase content. The danger comes in mistaking a cystic pancreatic neoplasm for a pseudocyst and incorrectly draining a cystic neoplasm into the GI tract rather than resecting the neoplasm. For this reason, biopsy of the pseudocyst wall is a common step in the management of pancreatic pseudocysts.

Cystadenoma

Serous cystadenomas are essentially considered benign tumors without malignant potential. Serous cystadenocarcinoma has been reported very rarely (<1%). Therefore, malignant potential should not be

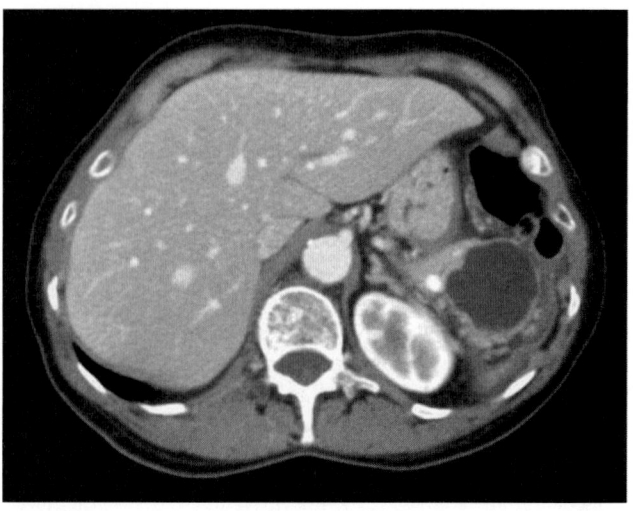

FIG. 33-76. Mucinous cystic neoplasm in tail of pancreas.

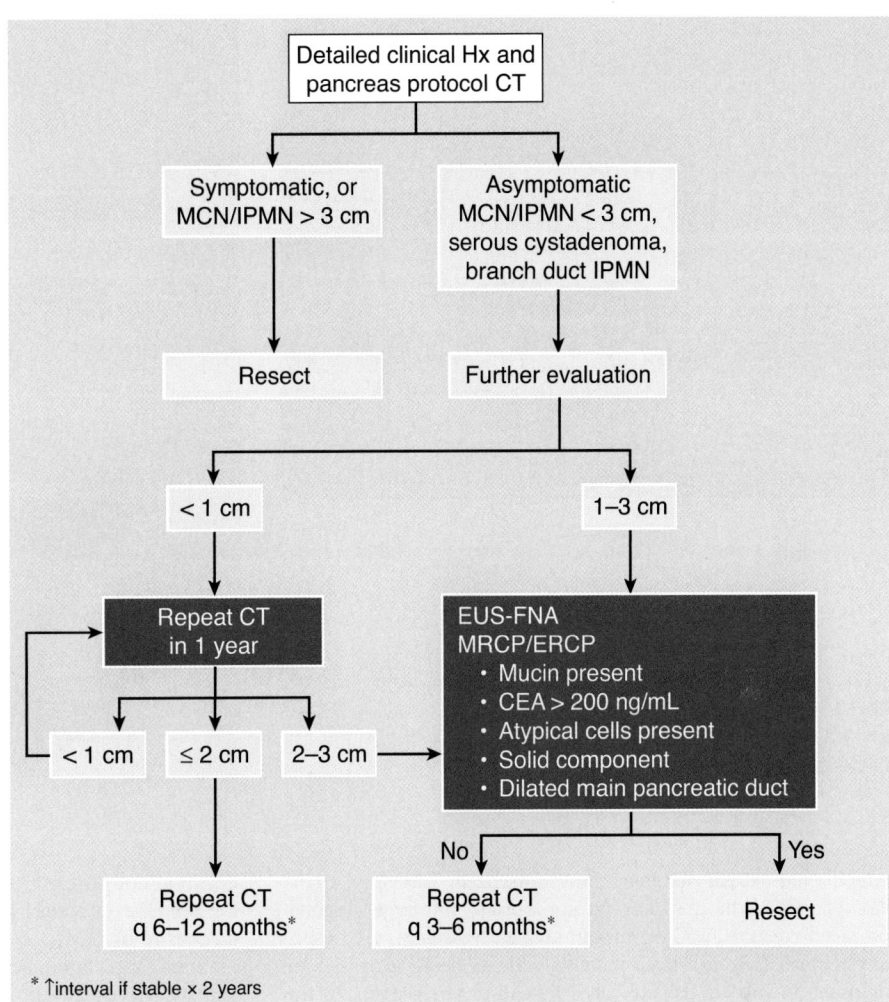

FIG. 33-77. Algorithm for management of pancreatic cystic neoplasms. CEA = carcinoembryonic antigen; CT = computed tomography; ERCP = endoscopic retrograde cholangiopancreatography; EUS = endoscopic ultrasound; FNA = fine-needle aspiration; Hx = history; IPMN = intraductal papillary mucinous neoplasm of the pancreas; MCN = mucinous cystic neoplasm; MRCP = magnetic resonance cholangiopancreatography.

used as an argument for surgical resection, and the majority of these lesions can be safely observed in the absence of symptoms due to mass effect or rapid growth. The average rate of growth is about 0.45 cm/y. About 50% of cystadenomas are asymptomatic and detected as an incidental finding. Most symptomatic patients have mild upper abdominal pain, epigastric fullness, or moderate weight loss. Occasionally, cystadenomas can grow to a size capable of producing jaundice or GI obstruction due to mass effect (Fig. 33-78). For symptomatic patients with serous cystadenoma, surgical resection is indicated. For lesions in the tail, splenectomy is not necessary, given the benign nature of the tumor. In appropriate candidates, a laparoscopic approach to distal pancreatectomy can be considered.[354,355] These cysts are frequently found in older women in which pancreatic resection for a benign neoplasm should be avoided in the absence of significant symptoms. All regions of the pancreas are affected, with half in the head/uncinate process, and half in the neck, body, or tail of the pancreas. They have a spongy appearance, and multiple small cysts (microcystic) are more common than larger cysts (macrocystic or oligocystic). These lesions contain thin serous fluid that does not stain positive for mucin and is low in CEA (<200 ng/mL). Typical imaging characteristics include a well-circumscribed cystic mass, small septations, fluid close to water density, and sometimes, a central scar with calcification. If a conservative management is adopted, it is important to be sure of the diagnosis. EUS-FNA should yield nonviscous fluid with low CEA and amylase levels, and if cells are obtained, which is rare, they are cuboidal and have a clear cytoplasm.

Mucinous Cystadenoma and Cystadenocarcinoma

Mucinous cystic neoplasms (MCNs) encompass a spectrum ranging from benign but potentially malignant to carcinoma with a very aggressive behavior (Table 33-20). There is often heterogeneity within the lesions with benign and malignant-appearing regions, making it impossible to exclude malignancy with biopsy. MCNs are commonly seen in perimenopausal women, and about two-thirds are located in the body or tail of the pancreas. Like cystadenomas, most MCNs are now incidental findings identified during imaging performed for other reasons. When symptoms are present, they are usually nonspecific and include upper abdominal discomfort or pain, early satiety, and weight loss. On imaging studies, the cysts have thick walls and do not communicate with the main pancreatic duct (see Fig. 33-76). There may be nodules or calcifications within the wall of the cyst. The cysts are lined by tall columnar epithelium that fills the cyst with viscous mucin. The submucosal layer consists of a highly cellular stroma of spindle cells with elongated nuclei similar to the "ovarian stroma," which is a key pathologic feature distinguishing these lesions. Elevated CEA levels in the fluid (>200 ng/mL) may suggest malignant transformation. Solid areas may contain atypical cells or invasive cancer, and extensive sampling of the specimen is necessary to accurately predict prognosis. Resection is the treatment of choice for most mucin-producing cystic tumors. Malignancy cannot be ruled out without removal and extensive sampling of the tumor. Current thinking is that all of these tumors will eventually evolve into cancer if left untreated. Malignant transformation is more common with larger tumors, and older patients, and there appears to be a stepwise accumulation of mutations (K-ras, p53). Because most MCNs are located in the body and tail of the pancreas, distal pancreatectomy is the most common treatment. For small lesions, it may be appropriate to preserve the spleen but splenectomy ensures removal of the lymph node basin that can potentially be involved. It is very important not to rupture the cyst during resection and the

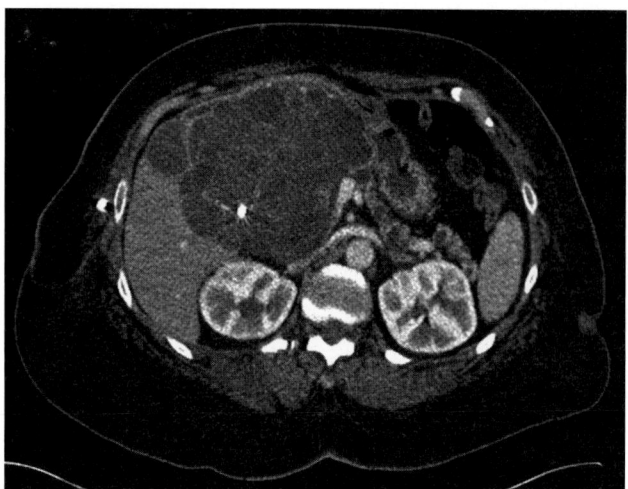

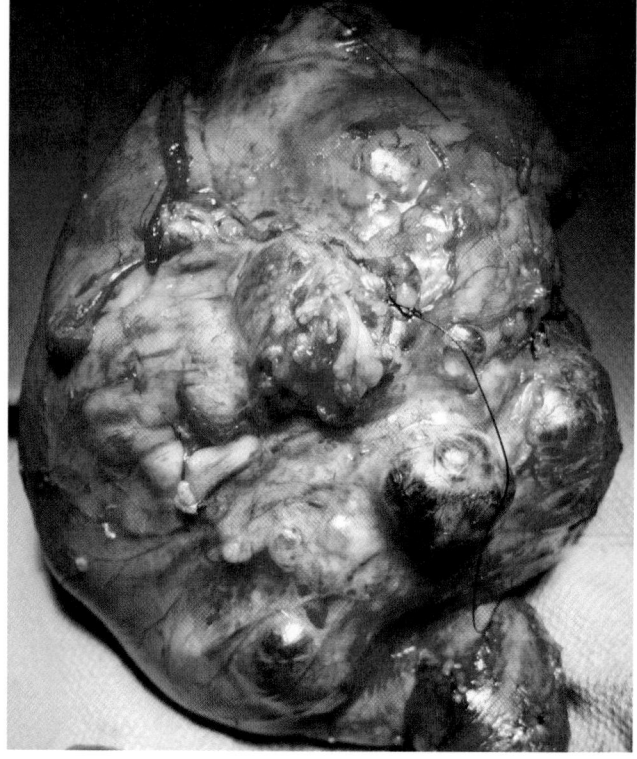

FIG. 33-78. Computed tomography appearance of massive multi-septated serous cystadenoma in head of pancreas with central stellate scar (*left*) and resected specimen (*right*).

tumor should be removed intact, not morselized. Therefore, a laparoscopic approach may not be appropriate for larger lesions. Completely resected MCNs without atypia are usually cured especially if small (<3 cm). Even patients with moderate dysplasia or carcinoma in situ are usually cured by complete resection. In the presence of invasive carcinoma, mucinous cystadenocarcinoma, the prognosis is dismal, similar to typical ductal adenocarcinoma of the pancreas.

Intraductal Papillary Mucinous Neoplasm

Intraductal papillary mucinous neoplasms (IPMNs) usually occur within the head of the pancreas and arise within the pancreatic ducts. The ductal epithelium forms a papillary projection into the duct, and mucin production causes intraluminal cystic dilation of the pancreatic ducts. Imaging studies demonstrate diffuse dilation of the pancreatic duct, and the pancreatic parenchyma is often atrophic due to chronic duct obstruction. However, classic features of chronic pancreatitis, such as calcification and a beaded appearance of the

TABLE 33-20	World Health Organization classification of primary tumors of the exocrine pancreas

A. Benign
  1. Serous cystadenoma (16%)
  2. Mucinous cystadenoma (45%)
  3. Intraductal papillary-mucinous adenoma (32%)
  4. Mature cystic teratoma
B. Borderline
  1. Mucinous cystic tumor with moderate dysplasia
  2. Intraductal papillary mucinous tumor with moderate dysplasia
  3. Solid pseudopapillary tumor
C. Malignant
  1. Ductal adenocarcinoma
  2. Serous/mucinous cystadenocarcinoma (29%)
  3. Intraductal mucinous papillary tumor

duct, are not present. At ERCP, mucin can be seen extruding from the ampulla of Vater, a so-called *fish-eye lesion*, that is virtually diagnostic of IPMN (Fig. 33-79). Initial reports suggested a male predominance, but more recent series indicate an equal distribution. Patients are usually in their seventh to eighth decade of life and present with abdominal pain or recurrent pancreatitis, thought to be caused by obstruction of the pancreatic duct by thick mucin. Some patients (5 to 10%) have steatorrhea, diabetes, and weight loss secondary to pancreatic insufficiency. Some IPMNs primarily involve the main pancreatic duct, while others involve the branch ducts (Figs. 33-80 and 33-81). Branch-duct type IPMNs are often found in the uncinate process, are sometimes asymptomatic, and are less frequently associated with malignant transformation. The surgical management of IPMNs is complicated by the fact that the lesion itself is small and preoperative imaging studies show a dilated pancreatic duct but not necessarily the mass. Mucus can dilate the duct proximal and distal to the lesion. Furthermore, these lesions can spread microscopically along the duct, and there can be skip areas of normal duct between the diseased portions.

Therefore, thorough preoperative imaging including EUS, MRCP, or ERCP, and sometimes pancreatic ductoscopy, which can also be repeated intraoperatively, is useful (see Fig. 33-79). The surgeon needs to be prepared to extend the resection, if necessary, based on intraoperative findings and frozen section of the margin. Extending the resection to the point of total pancreatectomy is controversial due to the morbidity of this operation. Like MCNs, the IPMNs require careful histologic examination of the entire specimen for an invasive component, which is present in about 35 to 40% of cases.

Survival of patients with IPMN, even when malignant and invasive, can be quite good. As with MCN, patients with borderline tumors or carcinoma in situ are usually cured. In IPMN associated with invasive carcinoma, the 5- and 10-year survival is 60% and 50%, which is much better than typical pancreatic adenocarcinoma.[356]

For this reason, if recurrence occurs in the remaining pancreas, further resection is warranted because several series have shown that some of these cases are salvageable. Patients with IPMN are also at risk for other malignancies and should undergo colonoscopy and close surveillance.

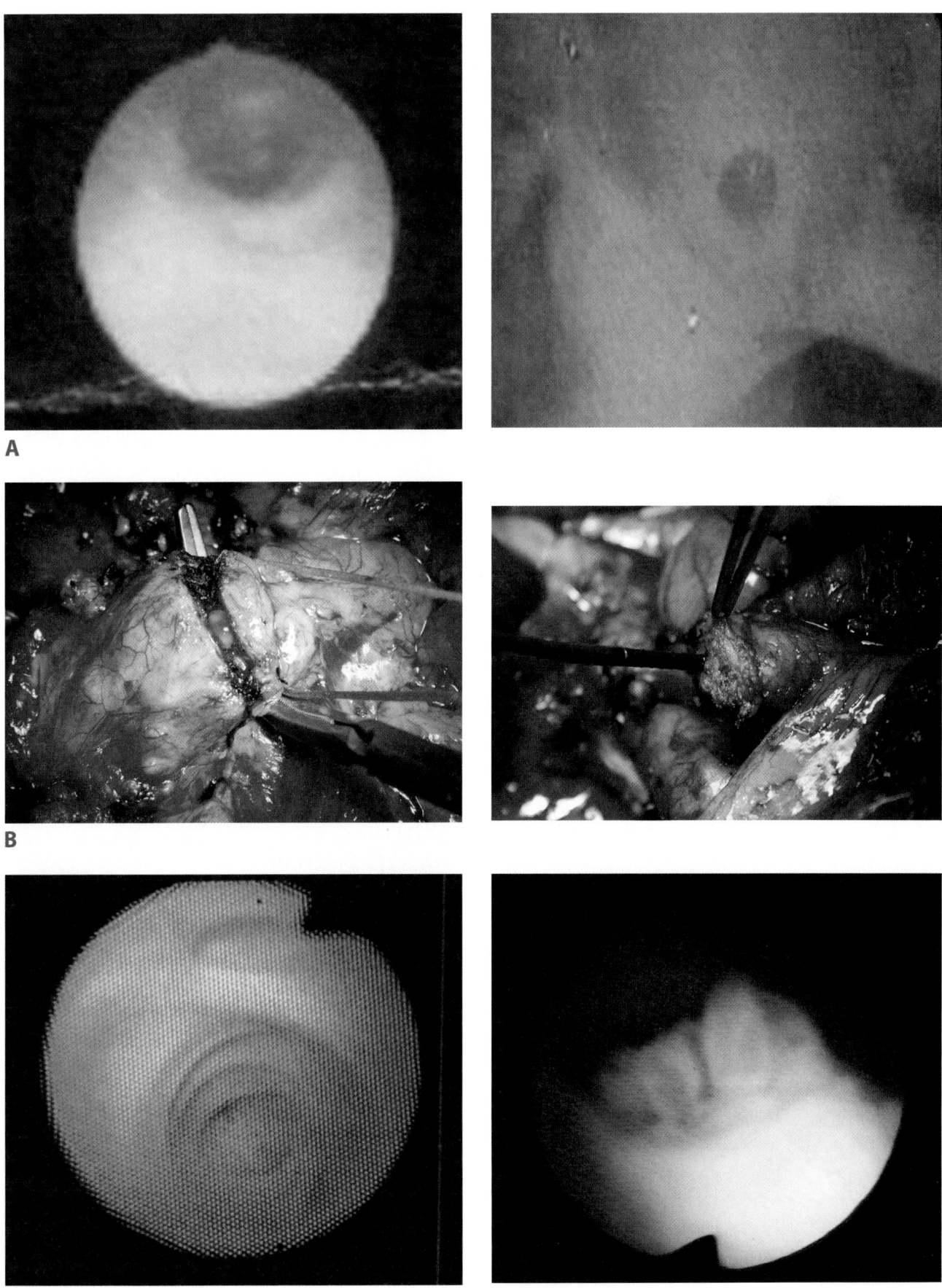

FIG. 33-79. Intraductal papillary mucinous neoplasm (IPMN). **A.** Examples of "fish-eye deformity" of IPMN. Mucin is seen extruding from the ampulla. **B.** Mucin coming from pancreatic duct when neck of pancreas is transected during Whipple procedure (*left*). Intraoperative pancreatic ductoscopy to assess the pancreatic tail (*right*). **C.** Views of pancreatic duct during ductoscopy; normal (*left*) and IPMN (*right*).

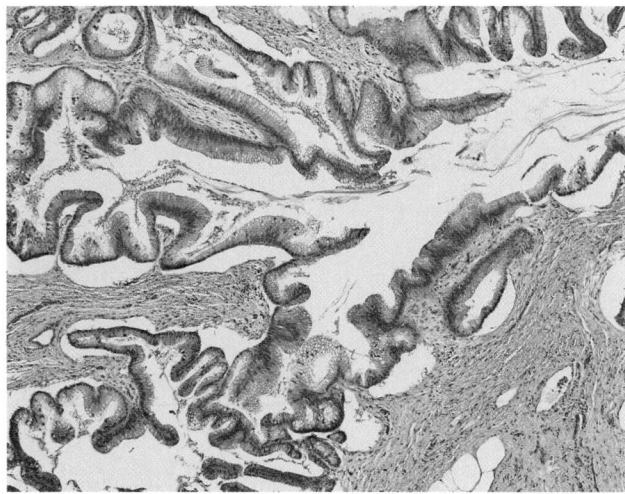

FIG. 33-80. Intraductal papillary mucinous neoplasm histology. Papillary projections of ductal epithelium resemble villous morphology and contain mucin-filled vesicles. *(From Asiyanbola B, Andersen DK: IPMN. Editorial Update. AccessSurgery, McGraw-Hill, 2008, with permission.)*

Solid-Pseudopapillary Tumor

Solid-pseudopapillary tumors are rare and typically occur in young women. Previous names for this entity include, *solid and cystic, solid and papillary, cystic and papillary,* and *papillary-cystic tumor.* They are typically well circumscribed on CT (Fig. 33-82). The cysts are not true epithelial-lined cysts but rather represent a necrotic/degenerative process. Histology may be similar to neuroendocrine tumors, but they do not stain positive for neuroendocrine markers such as chromogranin. Most are cured by resection but liver and peritoneal metastasis has been reported.

Other Cystic Neoplasms

Rarely, typical ductal adenocarcinoma of the pancreas may undergo cystic degeneration due to central necrosis. Occasionally, this will create difficulty in the proper preoperative diagnosis and should be kept in mind when deciding to conservatively follow a cystic pancreatic neoplasm. It is more common, 5 to 10%, for neuroendo-

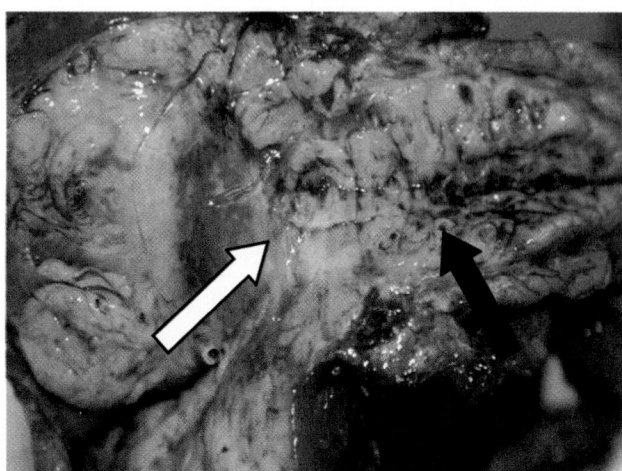

FIG. 33-81. Operative specimen of pancreas with multifocal intraductal papillary mucinous neoplasms *(black arrow)* and a focus of invasive adenocarcinoma *(white arrow). (From Asiyanbola B, Andersen DK: IPMN. Editorial Update. AccessSurgery, McGraw-Hill, 2008, with permission.)*

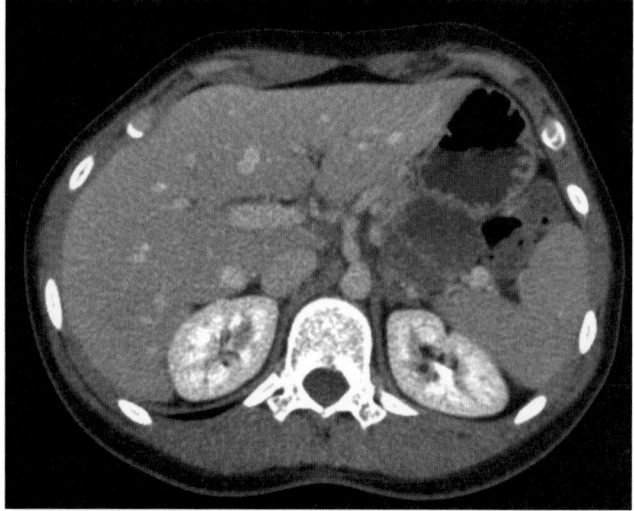

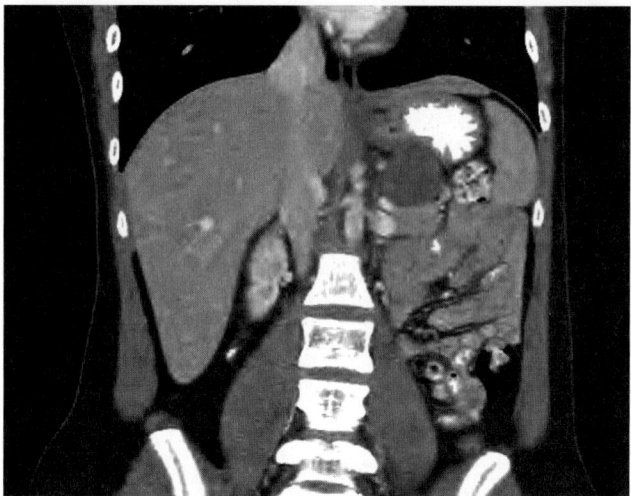

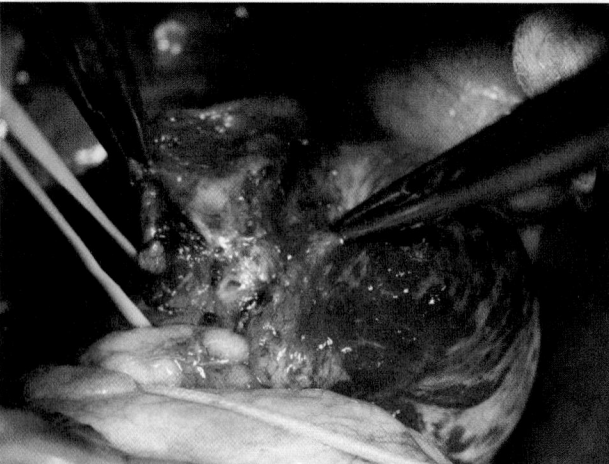

FIG. 33-82. Abdominal computed tomographic scan of a 25-year-old woman demonstrating a well-circumscribed cystic lesion with septation in body/tail of pancreas. At surgery, the tumor was adherent to the splenic artery. Pathologic diagnosis was solid-pseudopapillary carcinoma.

crine tumors of the pancreas to contain cysts. These cysts are filled with serosanguineous fluid rather than necrotic debris. Lymphoepithelial cysts of the pancreas usually occur in men in their fifth to sixth decade. These benign lesions may be unilocular or multilocular and vary widely in size. The contents of the cyst are also variable and may be thin serous fluid or cheesy/caseous material if there is increased keratin formation. A substantial number of patients with von Hippel-Lindau syndrome develop pancreatic cysts that resemble serous cystadenomas. There may be multiple lesions scattered throughout the pancreas. Patients with polycystic kidney and hepatic disease may also develop benign pancreatic cysts (cystadenomas). With all of these rare cystic neoplasms, careful clinical history, high-quality pancreatic imaging, and sampling of the cyst fluid for analysis will guide proper treatment.

Pancreatic Lymphoma

Lymphoma can affect the pancreas. Primary involvement of the pancreas with no disease outside the pancreas also occurs. The clinical presentation often is similar to pancreatic adenocarcinoma, with vague abdominal pain and weight loss. Identification of a large mass often involving the head and body of the pancreas should raise suspicion. Percutaneous or EUS-guided biopsy will confirm the diagnosis in most cases. If the diagnosis cannot be confirmed preoperatively, laparoscopic exploration and biopsy are indicated.[357] There is no role for resection in the management of pancreatic lymphoma. Endoscopic stenting to relieve jaundice followed by chemotherapy is the standard treatment, and long-term remission is often achieved.

REFERENCES

Entries highlighted in bright blue are key references.

1. Silen W: Surgical anatomy of the pancreas. *Surg Clin North Am* 44:1253, 1964.
2. Havel PJ, Taborsky GJ Jr.: The contribution of the autonomic nervous system to changes of glucagon and insulin secretion during hypoglycemic stress. *Endocr Rev* 10:332, 1989.
3. Davenport HW: Pancreatic secretion, in Davenport HN (ed): *Physiology of the Digestive Tract*, 5th ed. Chicago: Year Book Medical Publishers, 1982, p 143.
4. Valenzuela JE, Weiner K, Saad C: Cholinergic stimulation of human pancreatic secretion. *Dig Dis Sci* 31:615, 1986.
5. Konturek SJ, Becker HD, Thompson JC: Effect of vagotomy on hormones stimulating pancreatic secretion. *Arch Surg* 108:704, 1974.
6. Ebert R, Creutzfeldt W: Gastrointestinal peptides and insulin secretion. *Diabetes Metab Rev* 3:1, 1987.
7. Leahy JL, Bonner-Weir S, Weir GC: Abnormal glucose regulation of insulin secretion in models of reduced B-cell mass. *Diabetes* 33:667, 1984.
8. Brunicardi FC, Sun YS, Druck P, et al: Splanchnic neural regulation of insulin and glucagon secretion in the isolated perfused human pancreas. *Am J Surg* 153:34, 1987.
9. Yamada Y, Post SR, Wang K, et al: Cloning and functional characterization of a family of human and mouse somatostatin receptors expressed in brain, gastrointestinal tract, and kidney. *Proc Natl Acad Sci U S A* 89:251, 1992.
10. Voss M, Pappas T: Pancreatic fistula. *Curr Treat Options Gastroenterol* 5:345, 2002.
11. Feldman M, Richardson CT, Taylor IL, et al: Effect of atropine on vagal release of gastrin and pancreatic polypeptide. *J Clin Invest* 63:294, 1979.
12. Floyd JC Jr., Fajans SS, Pek S: Regulation in healthy subjects of the secretion of human pancreatic polypeptide, a newly recognized pancreatic islet polypeptide. *Trans Assoc Am Physicians* 89:146, 1976
13. Adrian TE, Bloom SR, Besterman HS, et al: Mechanism of pancreatic polypeptide release in man. *Lancet* 1:161, 1977.
14. Seymour NE, Andersen DK: Pancreatic polypeptide and glucose metabolism, in Greenly GH (ed): *Gastrointestinal Endocrinology*. Totowa, NJ: Humana Press, 1999, p 321.
15. Wierup N, Svensson H, Mulder H, et al: The ghrelin cell: A novel developmentally regulated islet cell in the human pancreas. *Regul Pept* 107:63, 2002.
16. Prado CL, Pugh-Bernard AE, Elghazi L, et al: Ghrelin cells replace insulin-producing beta cells in two mouse models of pancreas development. *Proc Natl Acad Sci U S A* 101:2924, 2004.
17. Sun Y, Asnicar M, Saha PK, et al: Ablation of ghrelin improves the diabetic but not obese phenotype of ob/ob mice. *Cell Metab* 3:379, 2006.
18. Westermark P, Wilander E, Westermark GT, et al: Islet amyloid polypeptide-like-immunoreactivity in the islet B-cells of type II (non-insulin-dependent) diabetic and non-diabetic individuals. *Diabetologia* 30:887, 1987.
19. Tatemoto K, Efendic S, Mutt V, et al: Pancreastatin, a novel pancreatic peptide that inhibits insulin secretion. *Nature* 324:476, 1986.
20. Efendic S, Tatemoto K, Mutt V, et al: Pancreastatin and islet hormone release. *Proc Natl Acad Sci U S A* 84:7257, 1987.
21. Funakoshi A, Miyasaka K, Nakamura R, et al: Inhibitory effect of pancreastatin on pancreatic exocrine secretion in the conscious rat. *Reg Peptides* 25:157, 1989.
22. Gorelick FS, Jamieson JD: Structure-function relationship of the pancreas, in Johnson LR (ed): *Physiology of the Gastrointestinal Tract*. New York: Raven Press, 1981, p 773.
23. Kennedy FP: Pathophysiology of pancreatic polypeptide secretion in human diabetes mellitus. *Diabetes Nutr Metab* 2:155, 1990.
24. Kleinman R, Ohning G, Wong H, et al: Regulatory role of intraislet somatostatin on insulin secretion in the isolated perfused human pancreas. *Pancreas* 9:172, 1994.
25. Pandol SJ, Saluja AK, Imrie CW, et al: Acute pancreatitis: Bench to the bedside. *Gastroenterology* 133:1056 e1, 2007.
26. Saluja AK, Bhagat L. Pancreatitis and associated lung injury: When MIF miffs. *Gastroenterology* 124:844, 2003.
27. Acosta JM, Ledesma CL: Gallstone migration as a cause of acute pancreatitis. *N Engl J Med* 290:484, 1974.
28. Steer ML, Saluja, AK: Pathogenesis and pathophysiology of acute pancreatitis, in Beger HG, Warshaw AL, Buchler MW, et al (ed): *The Pancreas*, Vol. 2. London: Blackwell Science Ltd, 1998, p 383.
29. Schneider A, Whitcomb DC, Singer MV: Animal models in alcoholic pancreatitis—what can we learn? *Pancreatology* 2:189, 2002.
30. Apte MV, Wilson JS. Alcohol-induced pancreatic injury. *Best Pract Res Clin Gastroenterol* 17:593, 2003.
31. Whitcomb DC, Gorry MC, Preston RA, et al: Hereditary pancreatitis is caused by a mutation in the cationic trypsinogen gene. *Nat Genet* 14:141, 1996.
32. Whitcomb DC, Ulrich CD, Lerch MM, et al: Third International Symposium on Inherited Diseases of the Pancreas. *Pancreatology* 1:423, 2001.
33. Saluja A, Steer M: Pathophysiology of pancreatitis. Role of cytokines and other mediators of inflammation. *Digestion* 60:27, 1999.
34. Saluja AK, Bhahat L: Experimental models of acute pancreatitis, in Johnson L (ed): *Encyclopedia of Gastroenterology*. San Diego: Elsevier, 2004, p 111.
35. Van Acker GJ, Saluja AK, Bhagat L, et al: Cathepsin B inhibition prevents trypsinogen activation and reduces pancreatitis severity. *Am J Physiol Gastrointest Liver Physiol* 283:G794, 2002.
36. Hashimoto D, Ohmuraya M, Hirota M, et al: Involvement of autophagy in trypsinogen activation within the pancreatic acinar cells. *J Cell Biol* 181:1065, 2008.
37. Dudeja V, Phillips P, Mujumdar N, et al: Heat shock protein 70 inhibits apoptosis in cancer cells by two simultaneous but independent mechanisms. *Gastroenterology* 2009 Feb 5 (Epub).
38. Rakonczay Z Jr., Hegyi P, Takacs T, et al: The role of NF-kappaB activation in the pathogenesis of acute pancreatitis. *Gut* 57:259, 2008.
39. Dawra R, Ku YS, Sharif R, et al: An improved method for extracting myeloperoxidase and determining its activity in the pancreas and lungs during pancreatitis. *Pancreas* 37:62, 2008.
40. Makhija R, Kingsnorth AN: Cytokine storm in acute pancreatitis. *J Hepatobiliary Pancreat Surg* 9:401, 2002.
41. Bhagat L, Singh VP, Hietaranta AJ, et al: Heat shock protein 70 prevents secretagogue-induced cell injury in the pancreas by preventing intracellular trypsinogen activation. *J Clin Invest* 106:81, 2000.
42. Sharif R, Dawra RK, Wasiluk K, et al: Impact on toll-like receptor 4 on the severity of acute pancreatitis and pancreatitis-associated lung injury in mice. *Gut* 2009 Feb 6 (Epub).
43. Hietaranta AJ, Singh VP, Bhagat L, et al: Water immersion stress prevents caerulein-induced pancreatic acinar cell nf-kappa b activation by attenuating caerulein-induced intracellular Ca2+ changes. *J Biol Chem* 276:18742, 2001.
44. Kraft M, Lerch MM: Gallstone pancreatitis: When is endoscopic retrograde cholangiopancreatography truly necessary? *Curr Gastroenterol Rep* 5:125, 2003.
45. Werner J, Hartwig W, Uhl W, et al: Useful markers for predicting severity and monitoring progression of acute pancreatitis. *Pancreatology* 3:115, 2003.

46. Ranson JHC: Acute pancreatitis: Surgical management, in Go VLW, DiMagno EP, Gardner JD et al (eds): *The Pancreas: Biology, Pathophysiology, and Disease*, 2nd ed. New York: Raven Press, 1993, p 637.

47. Banks PA: Epidemiology, natural history, and predictors of disease outcome in acute and chronic pancreatitis. *Gastrointest Endosc* 56:S226, 2002.

48. Neoptolemos JP, Kemppainen EA, Mayer JM, et al: Early prediction of severity in acute pancreatitis by urinary trypsinogen activation peptide: A multicentre study. *Lancet* 355:1955, 2000.

49. Balthazar EJ: Complications of acute pancreatitis: Clinical and CT evaluation. *Radiol Clin North Am* 40:1211, 2002.

50. Loser CH, Folsch UR: Acute pancreatitis: Medical and endoscopic treatment, in Lankisch PG, DiMagno EP (eds): *Pancreatic Disease*. Berlin: Springer-Verlag, 1999, p 66.

51. Johnson CD, Kingsnorth AN, Imrie CW, et al: Double blind, randomised, placebo controlled study of a platelet activating factor antagonist, lexipafant, in the treatment and prevention of organ failure in predicted severe acute pancreatitis. *Gut* 48:62, 2001.

52. Banks PA: Medical management of acute pancreatitis and complications, in Go VLW, DiMagno EP, Gardner JD et al (eds): *The Pancreas: Biology, Pathophysiology, and Disease*. 2nd ed. New York: Raven Press, 1993, p 593.

53. Runzi M, Layer P: Nonsurgical management of acute pancreatitis. Use of antibiotics. *Surg Clin North Am* 79:759, ix, 1999.

54. Buchler P, Reber HA: Surgical approach in patients with acute pancreatitis. Is infected or sterile necrosis an indication—in whom should this be done, when, and why? *Gastroenterol Clin North Am* 28:661, 1999.

55. Clancy TE, Ashley SW: Current management of necrotizing pancreatitis. *Adv Surg* 36:103, 2002.

56. Imrie CW, Carter CR, McKay CJ: Enteral and parenteral nutrition in acute pancreatitis. *Best Pract Res Clin Gastroenterol* 16:391, 2002.

57. Petrov MS, Correia MI, Windsor JA: Nasogastric tube feeding in predicted severe acute pancreatitis. A systematic review of the literature to determine safety and tolerance. *J Pancreas* 9:440, 2008.

58. Skyhoj J, Olsen T: The incidence and clinical relevance of chronic inflammation in the pancreas in autopsy material. *Acta Pathol Microbiol Scand* 86:361, 1978.

59. Copenhagen Pancreatitis Study: An interim report from a prospective epidemiological multicenter study. *Scand J Gastroenterol* 16:305, 1981.

60. Worning H: Incidence and prevalence of chronic pancreatitis, in Beger HG, Buchler M, Ditschuneit H (eds): *Chronic Pancreatitis*. Berlin: Springer-Verlag, 1990, p 8.

61. Worning H: Alcoholic chronic pancreatitis, in Beger HG et al (eds): *The Pancreas*, London: Blackwell-Sciences, 1998, p 672.

62. Zdankiewicz PD, Andersen DK: Pancreatitis in the elderly, in Rosenthal R, Katlic M, Zenilman ME (eds): *Principles and Practice of Geriatric Surgery*. New York: Springer-Verlag, 2001, p 740.

63. Pitchumoni CS: Pathogenesis of alcohol-induced chronic pancreatitis: Facts, perceptions, and misperceptions. *Surg Clin North Am* 81:379, 2001.

64. Strate T, Yekebas E, Knoefel WT, et al: Pathogenesis and the natural course of chronic pancreatitis. *Eur J Gastroenterol Hepatol* 14:929, 2002.

65. Friedreich N: Disease of the pancreas, in Ziemssen H (ed): *Cyclopedia of the Practice of Medicine*. New York: William Wood, 1878, p 549.

66. Durbec JP, Sarles H: Multicenter survey of the etiology of pancreatic diseases. Relationship between the relative risk of developing chronic pancreatitis and alcohol, protein and lipid consumption. *Digestion* 18:337, 1978.

67. Lankisch PG, Lowenfels AB, Maisonneuve P: What is the risk of alcoholic pancreatitis in heavy drinkers? *Pancreas* 25:411, 2002.

68. Dufour MC, Adamson MD: The epidemiology of alcohol-induced pancreatitis. *Pancreas* 27:286, 2003.

69. Renner IG, Savage WT 3rd, Pantoja JL, et al: Death due to acute pancreatitis. A retrospective analysis of 405 autopsy cases. *Dig Dis Sci* 30:1005, 1985.

70. Layer P, Yamamoto H, Kalthoff L, et al: The different courses of early- and late-onset idiopathic and alcoholic chronic pancreatitis. *Gastroenterology* 107:1481, 1994.

71. Comfort MW, Gambrill EE, Baggenstoss AH: Chronic relapsing pancreatitis: A study of twenty-nine cases without associated disease of the biliary or gastro-intestinal tract. *Gastroenterology* 6:376, 1946.

72. Ammann RW, Muellhaupt B, Meyenberger C, et al: Alcoholic nonprogressive chronic pancreatitis: Prospective long-term study of a large cohort with alcoholic acute pancreatitis (1976-1992). *Pancreas* 9:365, 1994.

73. Kondo T, Hayakawa T, Shibata T, et al: Aberrant pancreas is not susceptible to alcoholic pancreatitis. *Int J Pancreatol* 8:245, 1991.

74. Elsasser HP, Haake T, Grimmig M, et al: Repetitive cerulein-induced pancreatitis and pancreatic fibrosis in the rat. *Pancreas* 7:385, 1992.

75. Neuschwander-Tetri BA, Burton FR, Presti ME, et al: Repetitive self-limited acute pancreatitis induces pancreatic fibrogenesis in the mouse. *Dig Dis Sci* 45:665, 2000.

76. Seymour NE, Turk JB, Laster MK, et al: In vitro hepatic insulin resistance in chronic pancreatitis in the rat. *J Surg Res* 46:450, 1989.

77. Niebergall-Roth E, Harder H, Singer MV: A review: Acute and chronic effects of ethanol and alcoholic beverages on the pancreatic exocrine secretion in vivo and in vitro. *Alcohol Clin Exp Res* 22:1570, 1998.

78. Steer ML, Glazer G, Manabe T: Direct effects of ethanol on exocrine secretion from the in vitro rabbit pancreas. *Dig Dis Sci* 24:769, 1979.

79. Hanck C, Schneider A, Whitcomb DC: Genetic polymorphisms in alcoholic pancreatitis. *Best Pract Res Clin Gastroenterol* 17:613, 2003.

80. Witt H, Luck W, Hennies HC, et al: Mutations in the gene encoding the serine protease inhibitor, Kazal type 1 are associated with chronic pancreatitis. *Nat Genet* 25:213, 2000.

81. Lerch MM, Albrecht E, Ruthenburger M, et al: Pathophysiology of alcohol-induced pancreatitis. *Pancreas* 27:291, 2003.

82. Gorelick FS: Alcohol and zymogen activation in the pancreatic acinar cell. *Pancreas* 27:305, 2003.

83. Sahel J, Sarles H: Modifications of pure human pancreatic juice induced by chronic alcohol consumption. *Dig Dis Sci* 24:897, 1979.

84. Sarles H, Bernard JP, Johnson C: Pathogenesis and epidemiology of chronic pancreatitis. *Annu Rev Med* 40:453, 1989.

85. Yamadera K, Moriyama T, Makino I: Identification of immunoreactive pancreatic stone protein in pancreatic stone, pancreatic tissue, and pancreatic juice. *Pancreas* 5:255, 1990.

86. Multigner L, Sarles H, Lombardo D, et al: Pancreatic stone protein. II. Implication in stone formation during the course of chronic calcifying pancreatitis. *Gastroenterology* 89:387, 1985.

87. Freedman SD, Sakamoto K, Venu RP: GP2, the homologue to the renal cast protein uromodulin, is a major component of intraductal plugs in chronic pancreatitis. *J Clin Invest* 92:83, 1993.

88. Imoto M, DiMagno EP: Cigarette smoking increases the risk of pancreatic calcification in late-onset but not early-onset idiopathic chronic pancreatitis. *Pancreas* 21:115, 2000.

89. Lowenfels AB, Maisonneuve P, Whitcomb DC: Risk factors for cancer in hereditary pancreatitis. International Hereditary Pancreatitis Study Group. *Med Clin North Am* 84:565, 2000.

90. Goebell H, Steffen C, Baltzer G, et al: Stimulation of pancreatic secretion of enzymes by acute hypercalcaemia in man. *Eur J Clin Invest* 3:98, 1973.

91. Bess MA, Edis AJ, van Heerden JA: Hyperparathyroidism and pancreatitis. Chance or a causal association? *JAMA* 243:246, 1980.

92. Glueck CJ, Lang J, Hamer T, et al: Severe hypertriglyceridemia and pancreatitis when estrogen replacement therapy is given to hypertriglyceridemic women. *J Lab Clin Med* 123:59, 1994.

93. Singer MV, Chari ST: Classification of chronic pancreatitis, in Beger HG et al (eds): *The Pancreas*. London: Blackwell-Science, 1998, p 665.

94. Othersen HB Jr., Moore FT, Boles ET: Traumatic pancreatitis and pseudocyst in childhood. *J Trauma* 8:535, 1968.

95. Costamagna G, Mutignani M, Ingrosso M, et al: Endoscopic treatment of postsurgical external pancreatic fistulas. *Endoscopy* 33:317, 2001.

96. Warshaw AL: Pancreas divisum and pancreatitis, in Beger HG et al (eds): *The Pancreas*. London: Blackwell-Science, 1998, p 364.

97. Delhaye M, Engelholm L, Cremer M: Pancreas divisum: Congenital anatomic variant or anomaly? Contribution of endoscopic retrograde dorsal pancreatography. *Gastroenterology* 89:951, 1985.

98. Sugawa C, Walt AJ, Nunez DC, et al: Pancreas divisum: Is it a normal anatomic variant? *Am J Surg* 153:62, 1987.

99. Yoshida K, Toki F, Takeuchi T, et al: Chronic pancreatitis caused by an autoimmune abnormality. Proposal of the concept of autoimmune pancreatitis. *Dig Dis Sci* 40:1561, 1995.

100. Ito T, Nakano I, Koyanagi S, et al: Autoimmune pancreatitis as a new clinical entity. Three cases of autoimmune pancreatitis with effective steroid therapy. *Dig Dis Sci* 42:1458, 1997.

101. Stathopoulos G, Nourmand AD, Blackstone M, et al: Rapidly progressive sclerosing cholangitis following surgical treatment of pancreatic pseudotumor. *J Clin Gastroenterol* 21:143, 1995.

102. Shaper AG: Chronic pancreatic disease and protein malnutrition. *Lancet* 1:1223, 1960.

103. Mohan V, Pitchumoni CS: Tropical chronic pancreatitis, in Beger HG et al (eds): *The Pancreas*. London: Blackwell-Science, 1998, p 688.

104. GeeVarghese P: *Calcific Pancreatitis*. Bombay: Varghese Publishing House, 1985.

105. Pitchumoni CS, Jain NK, Lowenfels AB, et al: Chronic cyanide poisoning: Unifying concept for alcoholic and tropical pancreatitis. *Pancreas* 3:220, 1988.

106. Hassan Z, Mohan V, Ali L, et al: SPINK1 is a susceptibility gene for fibrocalculous pancreatic diabetes in subjects from the Indian subcontinent. *Am J Hum Genet* 71:964, 2002

107. Schneider A, Suman A, Rossi L, et al: SPINK1/PSTI mutations are associated with tropical pancreatitis and type II diabetes mellitus in Bangladesh. *Gastroenterology* 123:1026, 2002.

108. Comfort MW, Steinberg AG: Pedigree of a family with hereditary chronic relapsing pancreatitis. *Gastroenterology* 21:54, 1952.

109. Gross J: Hereditary pancreatitis, in Go VLW, Gardner JD, Brooks FP, et al (eds): *The Exocrine Pancreas: Biology, Pathophysiology and Diseases*. New York: Raven Press, 1986, p 829.

110. Tomsik H, Gress T, Adler G: Hereditary pancreatitis, in Beger HG et al (eds): *The Pancreas*. London: Blackwell-Science, 1998, p 355.

111. Whitcomb DC, Preston RA, Aston CE, et al: A gene for hereditary pancreatitis maps to chromosome 7q35. *Gastroenterology* 110:1975, 1996.

112. Le Bodic L, Bignon JD, Raguenes O, et al: The hereditary pancreatitis gene maps to long arm of chromosome 7. *Hum Mol Genet* 5:549, 1996.

113. Whitcomb DC: Hereditary diseases of the pancreas, in Yamada T, Alpers DH, Laine L, et al (eds): *Textbook of Gastroenterology*, 4th ed. Philadelphia: Lippincott Williams & Wilkins, 2002, p 2147.

114. Masson E, Le Marechal C, Delcenserie R, et al: Hereditary pancreatitis caused by a double gain-of-function trypsinogen mutation. *Hum Genet* 123:521, 2008.

115. Pfutzer RH, Barmada MM, Brunskill AP, et al: SPINK1/PSTI polymorphisms act as disease modifiers in familial and idiopathic chronic pancreatitis. *Gastroenterology* 119:615, 2000.

116. Chen JM, Mercier B, Audrezet MP, et al: Mutational analysis of the human pancreatic secretory trypsin inhibitor (PSTI) gene in hereditary and sporadic chronic pancreatitis. *J Med Genet* 37:67, 2000.

117. Cohn JA, Friedman KJ, Noone PG, et al: Relation between mutations of the cystic fibrosis gene and idiopathic pancreatitis. *N Engl J Med* 339:653, 1998.

118. Sharer N, Schwarz M, Malone G, et al: Mutations of the cystic fibrosis gene in patients with chronic pancreatitis. *N Engl J Med* 339:645, 1998.

119. Cohn JA, Bornstein JD, Jowell PS: Cystic fibrosis mutations and genetic predisposition to idiopathic chronic pancreatitis. *Med Clin North Am* 84:621, ix, 2000.

120. Layer P, Kalthoff L, Clain JE, et al: Nonalcoholic chronic pancreatitis: Two diseases? *Dig Dis Sci* 30:980, 1985.

121. Ammann RW: Chronic pancreatitis in the elderly. *Gastroenterol Clin North Am* 19:905, 1990.

122. Chen JM, Mercier B, Audrezet MP, et al: Mutations of the pancreatic secretory trypsin inhibitor (PSTI) gene in idiopathic chronic pancreatitis. *Gastroenterology* 120:1061, 2001.

123. Kloppel G, Maillet B: Pathology of chronic pancreatitis, in Beger HG et al (eds): *The Pancreas*. London: Blackwell-Science, 1998, p 720.

124. Nagai H, Ohtsubo K: Pancreatic lithiasis in the aged. Its clinicopathology and pathogenesis. *Gastroenterology* 86:331, 1984.

125. Apte MV, Wilson JS: Stellate cell activation in alcoholic pancreatitis. *Pancreas* 27:316, 2003.

126. McCarroll J, Phillips P, Santucci N, et al: Vitamin A induces quiescence in culture-activated pancreatic stellate cells—potential as an antifibrotic agent. *Pancreas* 27:396, 2003.

127. Schneider A, Whitcomb DC: Hereditary pancreatitis: A model for inflammatory diseases of the pancreas. *Best Pract Res Clin Gastroenterol* 16:347, 2002.

128. Bockman DE, Kennedy RH, Multigner L, et al: Fine structure of the organic matrix of human pancreatic stones. *Pancreas* 1:204, 1986.

129. Guy O, Robles-Diaz G, Adrich Z, et al: Protein content of precipitates present in pancreatic juice of alcoholic subjects and patients with chronic calcifying pancreatitis. *Gastroenterology* 84:102, 1983.

130. Sarles H, Dagorn JC, Giorgi D, et al: Renaming pancreatic stone protein as "lithostathine." *Gastroenterology* 99:900, 1990.

131. Watanabe T, Yonekura H, Terazono K, et al: Complete nucleotide sequence of human reg gene and its expression in normal and tumoral tissues. The reg protein, pancreatic stone protein, and pancreatic thread protein are one and the same product of the gene. *J Biol Chem* 265:7432, 1990.

132. Goggin P, Johnson C: Pancreatic stones, in Beger HG et al (eds): *The Pancreas*. London: Blackwell-Science, 1998, p 711.

133. Bernard JP, Barthet M, Gharib B, et al: Quantification of human lithostathine by high performance liquid chromatography. *Gut* 36:630, 1995.

134. Giorgi D, Bernard JP, Rouquier S, et al: Secretory pancreatic stone protein messenger RNA. Nucleotide sequence and expression in chronic calcifying pancreatitis. *J Clin Invest* 84:100, 1989.

135. Rinderknecht H, Renner IG, Koyama HH: Lysosomal enzymes in pure pancreatic juice from normal healthy volunteers and chronic alcoholics. *Dig Dis Sci* 24:180, 1979.

136. Warshaw AL, Simeone J, Schapiro RH, et al: Objective evaluation of ampullary stenosis with ultrasonography and pancreatic stimulation. *Am J Surg* 149:65, 1985.

137. Freeney P: Radiology, in Beger HG et al (eds): *The Pancreas*. London: Blackwell-Science, 1998, p 728.

138. Bolondi L, Li Bassi S, Gaiani S, et al: Sonography of chronic pancreatitis. *Radiol Clin North Am* 27:815, 1989.

139. Barish MA, Yucel EK, Soto JA, et al: MR cholangiopancreatography: efficacy of three-dimensional turbo spin-echo technique. *AJR Am J Roentgenol* 165:295, 1995.

140. Catalano MF, Lahoti S, Geenen JE, et al: Prospective evaluation of endoscopic ultrasonography, endoscopic retrograde pancreatography, and secretin test in the diagnosis of chronic pancreatitis. *Gastrointest Endosc* 48:11, 1998.

141. Kahl S, Glasbrenner B, Leodolter A, et al: EUS in the diagnosis of early chronic pancreatitis: a prospective follow-up study. *Gastrointest Endosc* 55:507, 2002.

142. Freeman ML, DiSario JA, Nelson DB, et al: Risk factors for post-ERCP pancreatitis: a prospective, multicenter study. *Gastrointest Endosc* 54:425, 2001.

143. Bradley EL 3rd: Pancreatic duct pressure in chronic pancreatitis. *Am J Surg* 144:313, 1982.

144. Murayama KM, Joehl RJ: Chronic pancreatitis, in Greenfield IJ, Mulholland M, Oldham KT et al (eds): *Surgery, Scientific Principles and Practice*, 3rd ed. Philadelphia: Lippincott Williams & Wilkins, 2001, p 873.

145. Nealon WH, Matin S: Analysis of surgical success in preventing recurrent acute exacerbations in chronic pancreatitis. *Ann Surg* 233:793, 2001.

146. Ammann RW, Muellhaupt B: The natural history of pain in alcoholic chronic pancreatitis. *Gastroenterology* 116:1132, 1999.

147. Ammann RW, Akovbiantz A, Largiader F, et al: Course and outcome of chronic pancreatitis. Longitudinal study of a mixed medical-surgical series of 245 patients. *Gastroenterology* 86:820, 1984.

148. Girdwood AH, Marks IN, Bornman PC, et al: Does progressive pancreatic insufficiency limit pain in calcific pancreatitis with duct stricture or continued alcohol insult? *J Clin Gastroenterol* 3:241, 1981.

149. Lankisch PG, Lohr-Happe A, Otto J, et al: Natural course in chronic pancreatitis. Pain, exocrine and endocrine pancreatic insufficiency and prognosis of the disease. *Digestion* 54:148, 1993.

150. Bockman DE, Buchler M: Pain mechanisms, in Beger HG et al (eds): *The Pancreas*. London: Blackwell-Science, 1998, p 698.

151. Bockman DE, Buchler M, Malfertheiner P, et al: Analysis of nerves in chronic pancreatitis. *Gastroenterology* 94:1459, 1988.

152. Ebbehoj N, Borly L, Bulow J, et al: Pancreatic tissue fluid pressure in chronic pancreatitis. Relation to pain, morphology, and function. *Scand J Gastroenterol* 25:1046, 1990.

153. DiMagno EP, Go VL, Summerskill WH: Relations between pancreatic enzyme outputs and malabsorption in severe pancreatic insufficiency. *N Engl J Med* 288:813, 1973.

154. DiMagno EP, Malagelada JR, Go VL: Relationship between alcoholism and pancreatic insufficiency. *Ann N Y Acad Sci* 252:200, 1975.

155. Dutta SK, Russell RM, Iber FL: Influence of exocrine pancreatic insufficiency on the intraluminal pH of the proximal small intestine. *Dig Dis Sci* 24:529, 1979.

156. Malka D, Hammel P, Sauvanet A, et al: Risk factors for diabetes mellitus in chronic pancreatitis. *Gastroenterology* 119:1324, 2000.

157. Couet C, Genton P, Pointel JP, et al: The prevalence of retinopathy is similar in diabetes mellitus secondary to chronic pancreatitis with or without pancreatectomy and in idiopathic diabetes mellitus. *Diabetes Care* 8:323, 1985.

158. Slezak LA, Andersen DK: Pancreatic resection: Effects on glucose metabolism. *World J Surg* 25:452, 2001.

159. Kono T, Wang XP, Fisher WE, et al: Pancreatic polypeptide (PP), in Martini L (ed): *Encyclopedia of Endocrine Diseases*, Vol. 3. San Diego: Elsevier, 2004, p 488.

160. Seymour NE, Volpert AR, Lee EL, et al: Alterations in hepatocyte insulin binding in chronic pancreatitis: Effects of pancreatic polypeptide. *Am J Surg* 169:105, discussion 110, 1995.

161. Spector SA, Frattini JC, Zdankiewicz PD, et al: Insulin receptor gene expression in chronic pancreatitis: The effects of pancreatic polypeptide. *Surg Forum* 48:168, 1997.

162. Brunicardi FC, Chaiken RL, Ryan AS, et al: Pancreatic polypeptide administration improves abnormal glucose metabolism in patients with chronic pancreatitis. *J Clin Endocrinol Metab* 81:3566, 1996.

163. Orci L: Macro- and micro-domains in the endocrine pancreas. *Diabetes* 31:538, 1982.

164. Seymour NE, Brunicardi FC, Chaiken RL, et al: Reversal of abnormal glucose production after pancreatic resection by pancreatic polypeptide administration in man. *Surgery* 104:119, 1988.

165. Hanazaki K, Nose Y, Brunicardi FC: Artificial endocrine pancreas. *J Am Coll Surg* 193:310, 2001.

166. Andersen DK: Mechanisms and emerging treatments of the metabolic complications of chronic pancreatitis. *Pancreas* 35:1, 2007.

167. Andersen D: The role of pancreatic polypeptide in glucose metabolism, in Thompson JC (ed): *Gastrointestinal Endocrinology Receptor and Post-Receptor Mechanisms*. San Diego: Academic Press, 1990, p 333.

168. Gyr K, Agrawal NM, Felsenfeld O, et al: Comparative study of secretin and Lundh tests. *Am J Dig Dis* 20:506, 1975.

169. Somogyi L, Cintron M, Toskes PP: Synthetic porcine secretin is highly accurate in pancreatic function testing in individuals with chronic pancreatitis. *Pancreas* 21:262, 2000.

170. Denyer ME, Cotton PB: Pure pancreatic juice studies in normal subjects and patients with chronic pancreatitis. *Gut* 20:89, 1979.

171. Tanner AR, Fisher D, Ward C, et al: An evaluation of the one-day NBT-PABA/14C-PABA in the assessment of pancreatic exocrine insufficiency. *Digestion* 29:42, 1984.

172. Ammann RW, Buhler H, Pei P: Comparative diagnostic accuracy of four tubeless pancreatic function tests in chronic pancreatitis. *Scand J Gastroenterol* 17:997, 1982.

173. Brugge W, Goff JS, Allen N: Development of a dual label Schilling test for pancreatic exocrine function based on the differential absorption of cobalamin malabsorption in pancreatic insufficiency. *J Clin Invest* 61:47, 1978.

174. Haverback B, Dyce B, Gutentag P: Measurement of trypsin and chymotrypsin in stool: A diagnostic test for pancreatic exocrine function. *Gastroenterology* 44:588, 1986.

175. Gullo L, Ventrucci M, Tomassetti P, et al: Fecal elastase 1 determination in chronic pancreatitis. *Dig Dis Sci* 44:210, 1999.

176. Goff JS: Two-stage triolein breath test differentiates pancreatic insufficiency from other causes of malabsorption. *Gastroenterology* 83:44, 1982.

177. Axon AT, Classen M, Cotton PB, et al: Pancreatography in chronic pancreatitis: International definitions. *Gut* 25:1107, 1984.

178. Brugge WR: The role of endoscopic ultrasound in pancreatic disorders. *Int J Pancreatol* 20:1, 1996.

179. Catanzaro A, Richardson S, Veloso H, et al: Long-term follow-up of patients with clinically indeterminate suspicion of pancreatic cancer and normal EUS. *Gastrointest Endosc* 58:836, 2003.

180. Lankisch PG: Prognosis, in Beger HG et al (eds): *The Pancreas*. London: Blackwell-Science, 1998, p 740.

181. Miyake H, Harada H, Kunichika K, et al: Clinical course and prognosis of chronic pancreatitis. *Pancreas* 2:378, 1987.

182. Lowenfels AB, Maisonneuve P, Cavallini G, et al: Prognosis of chronic pancreatitis: An international multicenter study. International Pancreatitis Study Group. *Am J Gastroenterol* 89:1467, 1994.

183. Frey CF, Child CG, Fry W: Pancreatectomy for chronic pancreatitis. *Ann Surg* 184:403, 1976.

184. Lowenfels AB, Maisonneuve P, Cavallini G, et al: Pancreatitis and the risk of pancreatic cancer. International Pancreatitis Study Group. *N Engl J Med* 328:1433, 1993.

185. Aspelund G, Topazian MD, Lee JH, et al: Improved outcomes for benign disease with limited pancreatic head resection. *J Gastrointest Surg* 9:400, 2005.

186. Sankaran S, Walt AJ: The natural and unnatural history of pancreatic pseudocysts. *Br J Surg* 62:37, 1975.

187. Yeo CJ, Bastidas JA, Lynch-Nyhan A, et al: The natural history of pancreatic pseudocysts documented by computed tomography. *Surg Gynecol Obstet* 170:411, 1990.

188. Goulet RJ, Goodman J, Schaffer R, et al: Multiple pancreatic pseudocyst disease. *Ann Surg* 199:6, 1984.

189. Vitas GJ, Sarr MG: Selected management of pancreatic pseudocysts: Operative versus expectant management. *Surgery* 111:123, 1992.

190. Warshaw AL, Jin GL, Ottinger LW: Recognition and clinical implications of mesenteric and portal vein obstruction in chronic pancreatitis. *Arch Surg* 122:410, 1987.

191. Warshaw AL, Rattner DW: Timing of surgical drainage for pancreatic pseudocyst. Clinical and chemical criteria. *Ann Surg* 202:720, 1985.

192. Pancreatitis: Pancreatic pseudocysts and their complications. *Gastroenterology* 73:593, 1977.

193. Baron TH, Harewood GC, Morgan DE, et al: Outcome differences after endoscopic drainage of pancreatic necrosis, acute pancreatic pseudocysts, and chronic pancreatic pseudocysts. *Gastrointest Endosc* 56:7, 2002.

194. Gerzof SG, Banks PA, Robbins AH, et al: Early diagnosis of pancreatic infection by computed tomography-guided aspiration. *Gastroenterology* 93:1315, 1987.

195. Kozarek RA, Brayko CM, Harlan J, et al: Endoscopic drainage of pancreatic pseudocysts. *Gastrointest Endosc* 31:322, 1985.

196. Bell RH Jr.: Atlas of pancreatic surgery, in Bell RH Jr., Rikkers LF, Mulholland MW (eds): *Digestive Tract Surgery. A Text and Atlas*. Philadelphia: Lippincott-Raven, 1996, p 963.

197. Park AE, Heniford BT: Therapeutic laparoscopy of the pancreas. *Ann Surg* 236:149, 2002.

198. Nealon WH, Walser: Duct drainage alone is sufficient in the operative management of pancreatic pseudocyst in patients with chronic pancreatitis. *Ann Surg* 237:614, discussion 620, 2003.

199. Hawes RH: Endoscopic management of pseudocysts. *Rev Gastroenterol Disord* 3:135, 2003.

200. Heider R, Meyer AA, Galanko JA, et al: Percutaneous drainage of pancreatic pseudocysts is associated with a higher failure rate than surgical treatment in unselected patients. *Ann Surg* 229:781, discussion 787, 1999.

201. Rao R, Fedorak I, Prinz RA: Effect of failed computed tomography-guided and endoscopic drainage on pancreatic pseudocyst management. *Surgery* 114:843, discussion 847, 1993.

202. Cameron J: Chronic pancreatic ascites and pancreatic pleural effusions. *Gastroenterology* 74:134, 1987.

203. Lipsett PA, Cameron JL: Internal pancreatic fistula. *Am J Surg* 163:216, 1992.

204. Uchiyama T, Suzuki T, Adachi A, et al: Pancreatic pleural effusion: Case report and review of 113 cases in Japan. *Am J Gastroenterol* 87:387, 1992.

205. Lipsett PA, Cameron JL: Treatment of ascites and fistulas, in Beger HG et al (eds): *The Pancreas*. London: Blackwell-Science, 1998, p 788.

206. Yeo C, Cameron J: Exocrine pancreas, in Townsend C, et al (eds): *Sabiston's Textbook of Surgery*. New York: Lippincott-Raven, 2000 p 1112.

207. Beger H, Schlosser W, Poch B, et al: Inflammatory mass in the head of the pancreas, in Beger HG et al (eds): *The Pancreas*. London: Blackwell-Science, 1998, p 757.

208. Friess H, Yamanaka Y, Buchler M, et al: A subgroup of patients with chronic pancreatitis overexpress the c-erb B-2 protooncogene. *Ann Surg* 220:183, 1994.

209. Sakorafas GH, Sarr MG, Farley DR, et al: The significance of sinistral portal hypertension complicating chronic pancreatitis. *Am J Surg* 179:129, 2000.

210. Trapnell JE: Chronic relapsing pancreatitis: A review of 64 cases. *Br J Surg* 66:471, 1979.

211. Amann ST, Toskes PP: Analgesic treatment, in Beger HG et al (eds): *The Pancreas*. London: Blackwell-Science, 1998, p 766.

212. Isaksson G, Ihse I: Pain reduction by an oral pancreatic enzyme preparation in chronic pancreatitis. *Dig Dis Sci* 28:97, 1983.

213. Ramo OJ, Puolakkainen PA, Seppala K, et al: Self-administration of enzyme substitution in the treatment of exocrine pancreatic insufficiency. *Scand J Gastroenterol* 24:688, 1989.

214. Halgreen H, Pedersen NT, Worning H: Symptomatic effect of pancreatic enzyme therapy in patients with chronic pancreatitis. *Scand J Gastroenterol* 21:104, 1986.

215. Hildebrand P, Ensinck JW, Gyr K, et al: Evidence for hormonal inhibition of exocrine pancreatic function by somatostatin 28 in humans. *Gastroenterology* 103:240, 1992.

216. Toskes PP, Forsmark CE, DeMeo MT, et al: A multicenter controlled trial of octreotide for pain of chronic pancreatitis. *Pancreas* 8:A774, 1993.

217. Toskes PP, Forsmark CE, DeMeo MT, et al: An open-label trial of octreotide for the pain of chronic pancreatitis. *Gastroenterology* 8:A326, 1994.

218. Malfertheiner P, Mayer D, Buchler M, et al: Treatment of pain in chronic pancreatitis by inhibition of pancreatic secretion with octreotide. *Gut* 36:450, 1995.

219. Gress F, Schmitt C, Sherman S, et al: Endoscopic ultrasound-guided celiac plexus block for managing abdominal pain associated with chronic pancreatitis: a prospective single center experience. *Am J Gastroenterol* 96:409, 2001.

220. Jacob L, Geenen JE, Catalano MF, et al: Prevention of pancreatitis in patients with idiopathic recurrent pancreatitis: A prospective non-blinded randomized study using endoscopic stents. *Endoscopy* 33:559, 2001.

221. Aizawa T, Ueno N: Stent placement in the pancreatic duct prevents pancreatitis after endoscopic sphincter dilation for removal of bile duct stones. *Gastrointest Endosc* 54:209, 2001.

222. Lau ST, Simchuk EJ, Kozarek RA, et al: A pancreatic ductal leak should be sought to direct treatment in patients with acute pancreatitis. *Am J Surg* 181:411, 2001.

223. Canty TG Sr., Weinman D: Management of major pancreatic duct injuries in children. *J Trauma* 50:1001, 2001.

224. Kim HS, Lee DK, Kim IW, et al: The role of endoscopic retrograde pancreatography in the treatment of traumatic pancreatic duct injury. *Gastrointest Endosc* 54:49, 2001.

225. Heyries L, Barthet M, Delvasto C, et al: Long-term results of endoscopic management of pancreas divisum with recurrent acute pancreatitis. *Gastrointest Endosc* 55:376, 2002.

226. Gabbrielli A, Mutignani M, Pandolfi M, et al: Endotherapy of early onset idiopathic chronic pancreatitis: Results with long-term follow-up. *Gastrointest Endosc* 55:488, 2002.

227. Kozarek RA, Brandabur JJ, Ball TJ, et al: Clinical outcomes in patients who undergo extracorporeal shock wave lithotripsy for chronic calcific pancreatitis. *Gastrointest Endosc* 56:496, 2002.

228. Nealon WH, Thompson JC: Progressive loss of pancreatic function in chronic pancreatitis is delayed by main pancreatic duct decompression. A longitudinal prospective analysis of the modified puestow procedure. *Ann Surg* 217:458, discussion 466, 1993.

229. Link G: The treatment of chronic pancreatitis by pancreatostomy: A new operation. *Ann Surg* 53:768, 1911.

230. Link G: Long term outcome of pancreatostomy for chronic pancreatitis. *Ann Surg* 101:287, 1935.

231. Priestley JT, Comfort MW, Radcliffe J: Total pancreatectomy for hyperinsulinism due to an islet-cell adenoma: Survival and cure at sixteen months after operation presentation of metabolic studies. *Ann Surg* 119:211, 1944.

232. Whipple AO: Radical surgery for certain cases of pancreatic fibrosis associated with calcareous deposits. *Ann Surg* 124:991, 1946.

233. Fry WJ, Child CG 3rd: Ninety-five per cent distal pancreatectomy for chronic pancreatitis. *Ann Surg* 162:543, 1965.

234. Moody FG, Calabuig R, Vecchio R, et al: Stenosis of the sphincter of Oddi. *Surg Clin North Am* 70:1341, 1990.

235. Cattell RB: Anastomosis of the duct of Wirsung in palliative operation for carcinoma of the head of the pancreas. *Surg Clin North Am* 27:636, 1947.

236. Duval MK Jr.: Caudal pancreatico-jejunostomy for chronic relapsing pancreatitis. *Ann Surg* 140:775, 1954.

237. Zollinger RM, Keith LM Jr., Ellison EH: Pancreatitis. *N Engl J Med* 251:497, 1954.

238. Puestow CB, Gillesby WJ: Retrograde surgical drainage of pancreas for chronic relapsing pancreatitis. *AMA Arch Surg* 76:898, 1958.

239. Partington PF, Rochelle RE: Modified Puestow procedure for retrograde drainage of the pancreatic duct. *Ann Surg* 152:1037, 1960.

240. Izbicki JR, Bloechle C, Broering DC, et al: Longitudinal V-shaped excision of the ventral pancreas for small duct disease in severe chronic pancreatitis: prospective evaluation of a new surgical procedure. *Ann Surg* 227:213, 1998.

241. Eleftheriadis N, Dinu F, Delhaye M: Long-term outcome after pancreatic stenting in severe chronic pancreatitis. *Endoscopy* 37:223, 2005.

242. Gabbrielli A, Pandolfi M, Mutignani M, et al: Efficacy of main pancreatic-duct endoscopic drainage in patients with chronic pancreatitis, continuous pain, and dilated duct. *Gastrointest Endosc* 61:576, 2005.

243. Morgan DE, Smith JK, Hawkins K, et al: Endoscopic stent therapy in advanced chronic pancreatitis: Relationships between ductal changes, clinical response, and stent patency. *Am J Gastroenterol* 98:821, 2003.

244. Rosch T, Daniel S, Scholz M, et al: Endoscopic treatment of chronic pancreatitis: a multicenter study of 1000 patients with long-term follow-up. *Endoscopy* 34:765, 2002.

245. Ponchon T, Bory RM, Hedelius F, et al: Endoscopic stenting for pain relief in chronic pancreatitis: Results of a standardized protocol. *Gastrointest Endosc* 42:452, 1995.

246. Vitale GC, Cothron K, Vitale EA, et al: Role of pancreatic duct stenting in the treatment of chronic pancreatitis. *Surg Endosc* 18:1431, 2004.

247. Bradley EL 3rd: Long-term results of pancreatojejunostomy in patients with chronic pancreatitis. *Am J Surg* 153:207, 1987.

248. Cahen DL, Gouma DJ, Nio Y, et al: Endoscopic versus surgical drainage of the pancreatic duct in chronic pancreatitis. *N Engl J Med* 356:676, 2007.

249. Aldridge MC, Williamson RC: Distal pancreatectomy with and without splenectomy. *Br J Surg* 78:976, 1991.

250. Khanna A, Koniaris LG, Nakeeb A, et al: Laparoscopic spleen-preserving distal pancreatectomy. *J Gastrointest Surg* 9:733, 2005.

251. Hess W: Surgical tactics in chronic pancreatitis, in Hess W, Berci G (eds): *Textbook of Bilio-Pancreatic Diseases*, Vol. 4. Paua: Piccin Nuova Libraria, 1997, p 2299.

252. Traverso LW, Longmire WP Jr.: Preservation of the pylorus in pancreaticoduodenectomy. *Surg Gynecol Obstet* 146:959, 1978.

253. Huang JJ, Yeo CJ, Sohn TA, et al: Quality of life and outcomes after pancreaticoduodenectomy. *Ann Surg* 231:890, 2000.

254. Sakorafas GH, Farnell MB, Nagorney DM, et al: Pancreatoduodenectomy for chronic pancreatitis: Long-term results in 105 patients. *Arch Surg* 135:517, discussion 523, 2000.

255. Jimenez RE, Fernandez-del Castillo C, Rattner DW, et al: Outcome of pancreaticoduodenectomy with pylorus preservation or with antrectomy in the treatment of chronic pancreatitis. *Ann Surg* 231:293, 2000.

256. Braasch JW, Vito L, Nugent FW: Total pancreatectomy of end-stage chronic pancreatitis. *Ann Surg* 188:317, 1978.

257. Cooper MJ, Williamson RC, Benjamin IS, et al: Total pancreatectomy for chronic pancreatitis. *Br J Surg* 74:912, 1987.

258. Mannell A, Adson MA, McIlrath DC, et al: Surgical management of chronic pancreatitis: Long-term results in 141 patients. *Br J Surg* 75:467, 1988.

259. Alberti M: Proceedings of the Post EASD International Symposium on Diabetes Secondary to Pancreatopathy, International Congress Series, Padova, 1987. Amsterdam: Excerpta Medica, 1988, p 211.

260. Gall FP, Muhe E, Gebhardt C: Results of partial and total pancreaticoduodenectomy in 117 patients with chronic pancreatitis. *World J Surg* 5:269, 1981.

261. Beger HG, Witte C, Krautzberger W, et al: [Experiences with duodenum-sparing pancreas head resection in chronic pancreatitis]. *Chirurg* 51:303, 1980.

262. Beger HG, Krautzberger W, Bittner R, et al: Duodenum-preserving resection of the head of the pancreas in patients with severe chronic pancreatitis. *Surgery* 97:467, 1985.

263. Beger HG, Schlosser W, Friess HM, et al: Duodenum-preserving head resection in chronic pancreatitis changes the natural course of the disease: A single-center 26-year experience. *Ann Surg* 230:512, discussion 519, 1999.

264. Buchler MW, Friess H, Muller MW, et al: Randomized trial of duodenum-preserving pancreatic head resection versus pylorus-preserving Whipple in chronic pancreatitis. *Am J Surg* 169:65, discussion 69, 1995.

265. Frey CF, Smith GJ: Description and rationale of a new operation for chronic pancreatitis. *Pancreas* 2:701, 1987.

266. Frey CF, Amikura K: Local resection of the head of the pancreas combined with longitudinal pancreaticojejunostomy in the management of patients with chronic pancreatitis. *Ann Surg* 220:492, discussion 504, 1994.

267. Andersen DK, Topazian MD: Pancreatic head excavation: A variation on the theme of duodenum-preserving pancreatic head resection. *Arch Surg* 139:375, 2004.

268. Izbicki JR, Strate T, Yekebas EE, et al: Chronic pancreatitis, in Yeo CJ, Dempsey DT, Klein AS, et al (eds): *Shackleford's Surgery of the Alimentary Tract.* 6th ed. New York: Saunders, 2007, p 1218.

269. Ho HS, Frey CF: The Frey procedure: Combined local resection of the head of the pancreas with longitudinal pancreaticojejunostomy. *Operat Tech Gen Surg* 4:153, 2001.

270. Ho HS, Frey CF: The Frey procedure: Local resection of pancreatic head combined with lateral pancreaticojejunostomy. *Arch Surg* 136:1353, 2001.

271. Farkas G, Leindler L, Daroczi M, et al: Organ-preserving pancreatic head resection in chronic pancreatitis. *Br J Surg* 90:29, 2003.

272. Farkas G, Leindler L, Daroczi M, et al: Prospective randomised comparison of organ-preserving pancreatic head resection with pylorus-preserving pancreaticoduodenectomy. *Langenbecks Arch Surg* 391:338, 2006.

273. Gloor B, Friess H, Uhl W, et al: A modified technique of the Beger and Frey procedure in patients with chronic pancreatitis. *Dig Surg* 18:21, 2001.

274. Koninger J, Seiler CM, Sauerland S, et al: Duodenum-preserving pancreatic head resection—a randomized controlled trial comparing the original Beger procedure with the Berne modification (ISRCTN No. 50638764). *Surgery* 143:490, 2008.

275. Izbicki JR, Bloechle C, Broering DC, et al: Extended drainage versus resection in surgery for chronic pancreatitis: A prospective randomized trial comparing the longitudinal pancreaticojejunostomy combined with local pancreatic head excision with the pylorus-preserving pancreatoduodenectomy. *Ann Surg* 228:771, 1998.

276. Izbicki JR, Bloechle C, Knoefel WT, et al: Duodenum-preserving resection of the head of the pancreas in chronic pancreatitis. A prospective, randomized trial. *Ann Surg* 221:350, 1995.

277. Strate T, Bachmann K, Busch P, et al: Resection vs drainage in treatment of chronic pancreatitis: Long-term results of a randomized trial. *Gastroenterology* 134:1406, 2008.

278. Klempa I, Spatny M, Menzel J, et al: [Pancreatic function and quality of life after resection of the head of the pancreas in chronic pancreatitis. A prospective, randomized comparative study after duodenum preserving resection of the head of the pancreas versus Whipple's operation]. *Chirurg* 66:350, 1995.

279. Buchler MW, Friess H, Bittner R, et al: Duodenum-preserving pancreatic head resection: Long-term results. *J Gastrointest Surg* 1:13, 1997.

280. Riediger H, Adam U, Fischer E, et al: Long-term outcome after resection for chronic pancreatitis in 224 patients. *J Gastrointest Surg* 11:949, discussion 959, 2007.

281. Ramesh H, Jacob G, Lekha V, et al: Ductal drainage with head coring in chronic pancreatitis with small-duct disease. *J Hepatobiliary Pancreat Surg* 10:366, 2003.

282. Shrikhande SV, Kleeff J, Friess H, et al: Management of pain in small duct chronic pancreatitis. *J Gastrointest Surg* 10:227, 2006.

283. Najarian JS, Sutherland DE, Baumgartner D, et al: Total or near total pancreatectomy and islet autotransplantation for treatment of chronic pancreatitis. *Ann Surg* 192:526, 1980.

284. Farney AC, Najarian JS, Nakhleh RE, et al: Autotransplantation of dispersed pancreatic islet tissue combined with total or near-total pancreatectomy for treatment of chronic pancreatitis. *Surgery* 110:427, discussion 437, 1991.

285. Robertson RP, Lanz KJ, Sutherland DE, et al: Prevention of diabetes for up to 13 years by autoislet transplantation after pancreatectomy for chronic pancreatitis. *Diabetes* 50:47, 2001.

286. Rastellini C: Donor and recipient selection in pancreatic islet transplantation. *Curr Opin Organ Transplant* 7:196, 2002.

287. Robertson GS, Dennison AR, Johnson PR, et al: A review of pancreatic islet autotransplantation. *Hepatogastroenterology* 45:226, 1998.

288. Lillemoe KD, Cameron JL, Kaufman HS, et al: Chemical splanchnicectomy in patients with unresectable pancreatic cancer. A prospective randomized trial. *Ann Surg* 217:447, discussion 456, 1993.

289. Mallet-Guy P: Bilan de 215 operations nerveuses, splanchnicectomies ou ganglietomies coeliaqus gauches, pour pancreatite chronique et recidivante. *Lyon Chir* 76:361, 1980.

290. Michotey G, Sastre B, Argeme M, et al: [Splanchnicectomy by Dubois' transhiatal approach. Technics, indications and results. Apropos of 25 nerve sections for visceral abdominal pain]. *J Chir* (Paris) 120:487, 1983.

291 Stone HH, Chauvin EJ: Pancreatic denervation for pain relief in chronic alcohol associated pancreatitis. *Br J Surg* 77:303, 1990.

292. Cuschieri A: Laparoscopic surgery of the pancreas. *J Roy Coll Surg Edinb* 39:178, 1994.

293. Richards ML, Gauger PG, Thompson NW, et al: Pitfalls in the surgical treatment of insulinoma. *Surgery* 132:1040, discussion 1049, 2002.

294. Howard TJ, Stabile BE, Zinner MJ, et al: Anatomic distribution of pancreatic endocrine tumors. *Am J Surg* 159:258, 1990.

295. Deol ZK, Frezza E, DeJong S, et al: Solitary hepatic gastrinoma treated with laparoscopic radiofrequency ablation. *JSLS* 7:285, 2003.

296. Case CC, Wirfel K, Vassilopoulou-Sellin R: Vasoactive intestinal polypeptide-secreting tumor (VIPoma) with liver metastases: Dramatic and durable symptomatic benefit from hepatic artery embolization, a case report. *Med Oncol* 19:181, 2002.

297. Tanaka S, Yamasaki S, Matsushita H, et al: Duodenal somatostatinoma: A case report and review of 31 cases with special reference to the relationship between tumor size and metastasis. *Pathol Int* 50:146, 2000.

298. *http://seer.cancer.gov/statfacts/html/pancreas.html*: SEER Stat Fact Sheets. [accessed March 20, 2009.]

299. Gold EB, Goldin SB: Epidemiology of and risk factors for pancreatic cancer. *Surg Oncol Clin N Am* 7:67, 1998.

300. Fisher WE: Diabetes: Risk factor for the development of pancreatic cancer or manifestation of the disease? *World J Surg* 25:503, 2001.

301. Jean M, Lowy A, Chiao P, et al: *The Molecular Biology of Pancreatic Cancer.* New York: Springer-Verlag, 2002.

302. Berger D, Fischer W: *Inherited Pancreatic Cancer Symdromes.* New York: Springer-Verlag, 2002.

303. Fisher WE, Muscarella P, Boros LG, et al: Gastrointestinal hormones as potential adjuvant treatment of exocrine pancreatic adenocarcinoma. *Int J Pancreatol* 24:169, 1998.

304. Biankin AV, Kench JG, Dijkman FP, et al: Molecular pathogenesis of precursor lesions of pancreatic ductal adenocarcinoma. *Pathology* 35:14, 2003.

305. Wilentz RE, Hruban RH: Pathology of cancer of the pancreas. *Surg Oncol Clin N Am* 7:43, 1998.

306. Ries L, Melbert D, Krapcho M, et al: SEER Cancer Statistics Review. National Cancer Institute 1975-2004.

307. Ritts R, Pitt H: CA29-9 in pancreatic cancer. *Surg Oncol Clin N Am* 7:93, 1998.

308. Iacobuzio-Donahue CA, Maitra A, Olsen M, et al: Exploration of global gene expression patterns in pancreatic adenocarcinoma using cDNA microarrays. *Am J Pathol* 162:1151, 2003.

309. Squillaci E, Fanucco E, Scuito F: Vascular involvement in pancreatic neoplasm: A comparison between spiral CT and DSA. *Dig Dis Sci* 48:449, 2003.

310. Kim HJ, Conlon KC: *Laparoscopic Staging.* New York: Springer-Verlag, 2002.

311. Shah RJ, Howell DA, Desilets DJ, et al: Multicenter randomized trial of the spiral Z-stent compared with the Wallstent for malignant biliary obstruction. *Gastrointest Endosc* 57:830, 2003.

312. Singh SM, Reber HA: Surgical palliation for pancreatic cancer. *Surg Clin North Am* 69:599, 1989.

313. Casper ES, Green MR, Kelsen DP, et al: Phase II trial of gemcitabine (2,2'-difluorodeoxycytidine) in patients with adenocarcinoma of the pancreas. *Invest New Drugs* 12:29, 1994.

314. Yamaguchi K, Kishinaka M, Nagai E, et al: Pancreatoduodenectomy for pancreatic head carcinoma with or without pylorus preservation. *Hepatogastroenterology* 48:1479, 2001.

315. Ohtsuka T, Yamaguchi K, Ohuchida J, et al: Comparison of quality of life after pylorus-preserving pancreatoduodenectomy and Whipple resection. *Hepatogastroenterology* 50:846, 2003.

316. Heslin MJ, Harrison LE, Brooks AD, et al: Is intra-abdominal drainage necessary after pancreaticoduodenectomy? *J Gastrointest Surg* 2:373, 1998.

317. Pedrazzoli S, DiCarlo V, Dionigi R, et al: Standard versus extended lymphadenectomy associated with pancreatoduodenectomy in the surgical treatment of adenocarcinoma of the head of the pancreas: A

multicenter, prospective, randomized study. Lymphadenectomy Study Group. *Ann Surg* 228:508, 1998.

318. Sindelar WF, Kinsella TJ: Studies of intraoperative radiotherapy in carcinoma of the pancreas. *Ann Oncol* 10:226, 1999.

319. Birkmeyer JD, Finlayson SR, Tosteson AN, et al: Effect of hospital volume on in-hospital mortality with pancreaticoduodenectomy. *Surgery* 125:250, 1999.

320. Gordon TA, Bowman HM, Tielsch JM, et al: Statewide regionalization of pancreaticoduodenectomy and its effect on in-hospital mortality. *Ann Surg* 228:71, 1998.

321. Buchler M, Friess H, Klempa I, et al: Role of octreotide in the prevention of postoperative complications following pancreatic resection. *Am J Surg* 163:125, discussion 130, 1992.

322. Montorsi M, Zago M, Mosca F, et al: Efficacy of octreotide in the prevention of pancreatic fistula after elective pancreatic resections: A prospective, controlled, randomized clinical trial. *Surgery* 117:26, 1995.

323. Pederzoli P, Bassi C, Falconi M, et al: Efficacy of octreotide in the prevention of complications of elective pancreatic surgery. Italian Study Group. *Br J Surg* 81:265, 1994.

324. Barnett SP, Hodul PJ, Creech S, et al: Octreotide does not prevent postoperative pancreatic fistula or mortality following pancreaticoduodenectomy. *Am Surg* 70:222, discussion 227, 2004.

325. Hesse UJ, DeDecker C, Houtmeyers P, et al: Prospectively randomized trial using perioperative low-dose octreotide to prevent organ-related and general complications after pancreatic surgery and pancreaticojejunostomy. *World J Surg* 29:1325, 2005.

326. Lowy AM, Lee JE, Pisters PW, et al: Prospective, randomized trial of octreotide to prevent pancreatic fistula after pancreaticoduodenectomy for malignant disease. *Ann Surg* 226:632, 1997.

327. Moon HJ, Heo JS, Choi SH, et al: The efficacy of the prophylactic use of octreotide after a pancreaticoduodenectomy. *Yonsei Med J* 46:788, 2005.

328. Srivastava S, Sikora SS, Pandey CM, et al: Determinants of pancreaticoenteric anastomotic leak following pancreaticoduodenectomy. *ANZ J Surg* 71:511, 2001.

329. Suc B, Msika S, Piccinini M, et al: Octreotide in the prevention of intra-abdominal complications following elective pancreatic resection: A prospective, multicenter randomized controlled trial. *Arch Surg* 139:288, discussion 295, 2004.

330. Aranha GV, Hodul PJ, Creech S, et al: Zero mortality after 152 consecutive pancreaticoduodenectomies with pancreaticogastrostomy. *J Am Coll Surg* 197:223, discussion 231, 2003.

331. Lillemoe KD, Cameron JL, Kim MP, et al: Does fibrin glue sealant decrease the rate of pancreatic fistula after pancreaticoduodenectomy? Results of a prospective randomized trial. *J Gastrointest Surg* 8:766, discussion 772, 2004.

332. Nakao A, Fujii T, Sugimoto H, et al: Is pancreaticogastrostomy safer than pancreaticojejunostomy? *J Hepatobiliary Pancreat Surg* 13:202, 2006.

333. Payne RF, Pain JA: Duct-to-mucosa pancreaticogastrostomy is a safe anastomosis following pancreaticoduodenectomy. *Br J Surg* 93:73, 2006.

334. Peng S, Mou Y, Cai X, et al: Binding pancreaticojejunostomy is a new technique to minimize leakage. *Am J Surg* 183:283, 2002.

335. Rosso E, Bachellier P, Oussoultzoglou E, et al: Toward zero pancreatic fistula after pancreaticoduodenectomy with pancreaticogastrostomy. *Am J Surg* 191:726, discussion 733, 2006.

336. Sutton CD, Garcea G, White SA, et al: Isolated Roux-loop pancreaticojejunostomy: A series of 61 patients with zero postoperative pancreaticoenteric leaks. *J Gastrointest Surg* 8:701, 2004.

337. Suzuki Y, Kuroda Y, Morita A, et al: Fibrin glue sealing for the prevention of pancreatic fistulas following distal pancreatectomy. *Arch Surg* 130:952, 1995.

338. Yeo CJ, Cameron JL, Maher MM, et al: A prospective randomized trial of pancreaticogastrostomy versus pancreaticojejunostomy after pancreaticoduodenectomy. *Ann Surg* 222:580, discussion 588, 1995.

339. Wente MN, Shrikhande SV, Muller MW, et al: Pancreaticojejunostomy versus pancreaticogastrostomy: Systematic review and meta-analysis. *Am J Surg* 193:171, 2007.

340. Suzuki Y, Fujino Y, Tanioka Y, et al: Selection of pancreaticojejunostomy techniques according to pancreatic texture and duct size. *Arch Surg* 137:1044, discussion 1048, 2002.

341. Reid-Lombardo KM, Farnell MB, Crippa S, et al: Pancreatic anastomotic leakage after pancreaticoduodenectomy in 1,507 patients: a report from the Pancreatic Anastomotic Leak Study Group. *J Gastrointest Surg* 11:1451, 2007.

342. Poon RT, Lo SH, Fong D, et al: Prevention of pancreatic anastomotic leakage after pancreaticoduodenectomy. *Am J Surg* 183:42, 2002.

343. Okamoto A, Tsuruta K: Fistulation method: simple and safe pancreaticojejunostomy after pancreatoduodenectomy. *Surgery* 127:433, 2000.

344. Yang YM, Tian XD, Zhuang Y, et al: Risk factors of pancreatic leakage after pancreaticoduodenectomy. *World J Gastroenterol* 11:2456, 2005.

345. Di Carlo V, Chiesa R, Pontiroli AE, et al: Pancreatoduodenectomy with occlusion of the residual stump by Neoprene injection. *World J Surg* 13:105, discussion 110, 1989.

346. Buchler MW, Friess H, Wagner M, et al: Pancreatic fistula after pancreatic head resection. *Br J Surg* 87:883, 2000.

347. Tran K, Van Eijck C, Di Carlo V, et al: Occlusion of the pancreatic duct versus pancreaticojejunostomy: A prospective randomized trial. *Ann Surg* 236:422, discussion 428, 2002.

348. Fisher WE, Chai C, Hodges SE, et al: Effect of BioGlue on the incidence of pancreatic fistula following pancreas resection. *J Gastrointest Surg* 12:882, 2008.

349. Kazanjian KK, Hines OJ, Eibl G, et al: Management of pancreatic fistulas after pancreaticoduodenectomy: Results in 437 consecutive patients. *Arch Surg* 140:849, discussion 854, 2005.

350. Group GTS: Further evidence of effective adjuvant combined radiation and chemotherapy following curative resection of pancreatic cancer. *Cancer* 59:2006, 1997.

351. Neoptolemos JP, Dunn JA, Stocken DD, et al: Adjuvant chemoradiotherapy and chemotherapy in resectable pancreatic cancer: A randomised controlled trial. *Lancet* 358:1576, 2001.

352. Pisters PW, Abbruzzese JL, Janjan NA, et al: Rapid-fractionation preoperative chemoradiation, pancreaticoduodenectomy, and intraoperative radiation therapy for resectable pancreatic adenocarcinoma. *J Clin Oncol* 16:3843, 1998.

353. Yazawa K, Fisher WE, Brunicardi FC: Current progress in suicide gene therapy for cancer. *World J Surg* 26:783, 2002.

354. Kiely JM, Nakeeb A, Komorowski RA, et al: Cystic pancreatic neoplasms: Enucleate or resect? *J Gastrointest Surg* 7:890, 2003.

355. Obermeyer R, Fisher W, Sweeney J, et al: Laparoscopic distal pancreatectomy for serous oligocystic adenoma. *Surg Rounds* 423, 2003.

356. Salvia R, Fernandez-del Castillo C, Bassi C, et al: Main-duct intraductal papillary mucinous neoplasms of the pancreas: Clinical predictors of malignancy and long-term survival following resection. *Ann Surg* 239:678, discussion 685, 2004.

357. Boni L, Benevento A, Dionigi G, et al: Primary pancreatic lymphoma. *Surg Endosc* 16:1107, 2002.

CHAPTER 34

Spleen

Adrian E. Park and Carlos D. Godinez Jr.

HISTORICAL BACKGROUND

The spleen has had a remarkable number of attributes and functions ascribed to it throughout history. In 350 B.C. Aristotle described how the "hot character" of the spleen aided in digestion. Writings dating back to the first century variously describe the spleen as the seat of laughter and also as the source of black bile giving rise to melancholy. Thus the term *spleen* came to be associated with the derivative meaning of "ill temper." Historically, credence was given to the idea of the spleen as a locus of conflicting emotions. In the midseventeenth century Blackmore characterized the spleen as the organ to which "Hypochondrial and Hysterical Affections" could be attributed. Throughout the centuries the spleen also has been considered an impediment to fleetness of foot for both man and beast. Until modern times, however, removal of the spleen usually resulted in the death of the patient.

Anecdotal reports of splenic surgery began to emerge in the sixteenth century. By the end of the eighteenth century, the vast majority of splenectomies performed were partial, with the majority of patients requiring surgical attention for left upper quadrant stab wounds resulting in partial or total splenic prolapse. By 1877 only 50 splenectomies had ever been performed, with a mortality rate of >70%. Yet by 1900, large series of splenectomies were reported with an operative mortality rate that had already dropped to <40%, and a 1920 report[1] of the Mayo Clinic experience with splenectomy noted an 11% mortality rate. Somewhat less dramatic progress has since occurred, with the largest series of laparoscopic splenectomies reporting ≤1% overall mortality.[2,3]

EMBRYOLOGY AND ANATOMY

Consisting of an encapsulated mass of vascular and lymphoid tissue, the spleen is the largest reticuloendothelial organ in the body. Arising from the primitive mesoderm as an outgrowth of the left side of the dorsal mesogastrium, by the fifth week of gestation the spleen is evident in an embryo 8 mm long. The organ continues its differentiation and migration to the left upper quadrant, where it comes to rest with its smooth, diaphragmatic surface facing posterosuperiorly.[3]

The most common anomaly of splenic embryology is the accessory spleen. Present in up to 20% of the population, one or more accessory spleens may also occur in up to 30% of patients with hematologic disease. Over 80% of accessory spleens are found in the region of the splenic hilum and vascular pedicle. Other locations for accessory spleens in descending order of frequency are the gastrocolic ligament, the pancreas tail, the greater omentum, the stomach's greater curve, the splenocolic ligament, the small and large bowel mesentery, the left broad ligament in women, and the left spermatic cord in men (Fig. 34-1).[4,5]

The abdominal surface of the diaphragm separates the spleen from the lower left lung and pleura and the ninth to eleventh ribs. The visceral surface faces the abdominal cavity and contains gastric, colic, renal, and pancreatic impressions. Spleen size and weight vary with age, with both diminishing in the elderly and in those with underlying pathologic conditions. The average adult spleen is 7 to 11 cm in length and weighs 150 g (range 70 to 250 g). Splenomegaly is described variably within the surgical literature as *moderate*, *massive*, and *hyper*, which reflects a lack of consensus. Most would agree, however, that *splenomegaly* applies to organs weighing ≥500 g and/or averaging ≥15 cm in length.

Massive splenomegaly similarly lacks a consensus definition but has been described variably as spleens >1 kg in mass or >22 cm in length (Fig. 34-2).[6] Spleens palpable below the left costal margin are thought to be at least double normal size, with an estimated weight of ≥750 g.[6]

The spleen's superior border separates the diaphragmatic surface from the gastric impression of the visceral surface and often contains one or two notches, which are particularly pronounced when the spleen is greatly enlarged.

Of particular clinical relevance, the spleen is suspended in position by several ligaments and peritoneal folds to the colon (splenocolic ligament), the stomach (gastrosplenic ligament), the diaphragm (phrenosplenic ligament), and the kidney, adrenal gland, and tail of the pancreas (splenorenal ligament) (Fig. 34-3). The gastrosplenic ligament contains the short gastric vessels; the remaining ligaments are avascular, with rare exceptions, such as in patients with portal hypertension. The relationship of the pancreas to the spleen also has important clinical implications. In cadaveric anatomic series, the tail of the pancreas has been demonstrated to lie within 1 cm of the splenic hilum 75% of the time and in 30% of patients actually to abut the spleen.[2]

The spleen derives most of its blood from the splenic artery, the longest and most tortuous of the three main branches of the celiac

KEY POINTS

1. The human spleen plays a key immunologic role in defense against a number of organisms, particularly encapsulated bacteria.

2. The spleen can cause significant morbidity and/or hematologic disturbance if it becomes hyperfunctioning (hypersplenism) or hypertrophied (splenomegaly).

3. There is a broad spectrum of nontraumatic diseases for which elective splenectomy can be curative or palliative. They can be broadly categorized as red blood cell disorders and hemoglobinopathies, white blood cell disorders, platelet disorders, bone marrow disorders, infections and abscesses, cysts and tumors, storage diseases and infiltrative disorders, and miscellaneous conditions.

4. Partial splenectomy may be a suitable alternative to total splenectomy for certain conditions of hypersplenism or splenomegaly, particularly in children in whom preservation of splenic immunologic function is especially important.

5. Preoperative splenic artery embolization for elective splenectomy has benefits and disadvantages.

It may be most suitable in cases of enlarged spleen. Conclusive evidence is lacking.

6. Overwhelming postsplenectomy infection (OPSI) is an uncommon but potentially grave disease. Children and those undergoing splenectomy for hematologic malignancy are at elevated risk.

7. Vaccination of the splenectomized patient remains the most effective prevention strategy against OPSI. Preoperative vaccination before elective splenectomy is most prudent.

8. Antibiotic prophylactic strategies against OPSI vary widely. Data regarding their use are lacking.

9. Laparoscopic splenectomy provides equal hematologic outcomes with decreased morbidity compared with the open operation. The laparoscopic approach has emerged as the standard for elective, nontraumatic splenectomy.

10. Inadvertent intraoperative splenic injury is a scenario for which every abdominal surgeon should be prepared. Availability of a predetermined algorithm, with emphasis on the patient's condition, facilitates intraoperative decision making.

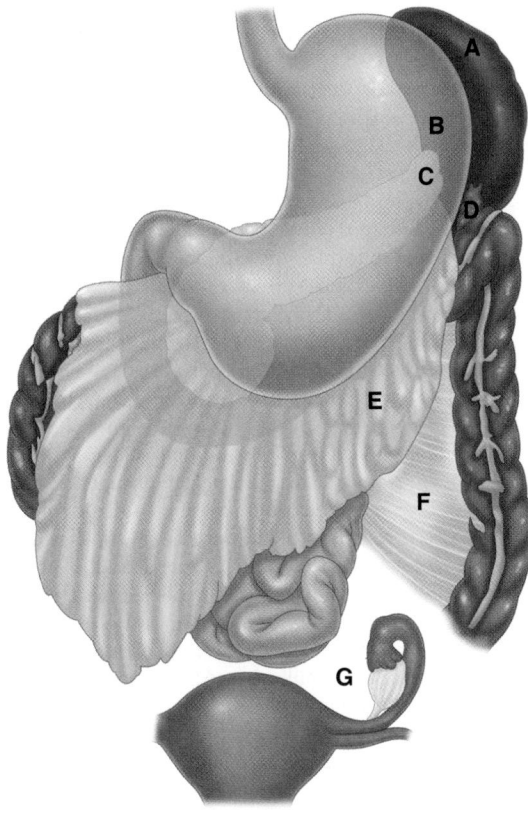

FIG. 34-1. Sites where accessory spleens are found in order of importance. *A*, Hilar region, 54%; *B*, pedicle, 25%; *C*, tail of pancreas, 6%; *D*, splenocolic ligament, 2%; *E*, greater omentum, 12%; *F*, mesentery, 0.5%; *G*, left ovary, 0.5%. *(Reproduced with permission from Poulin et al.[4])*

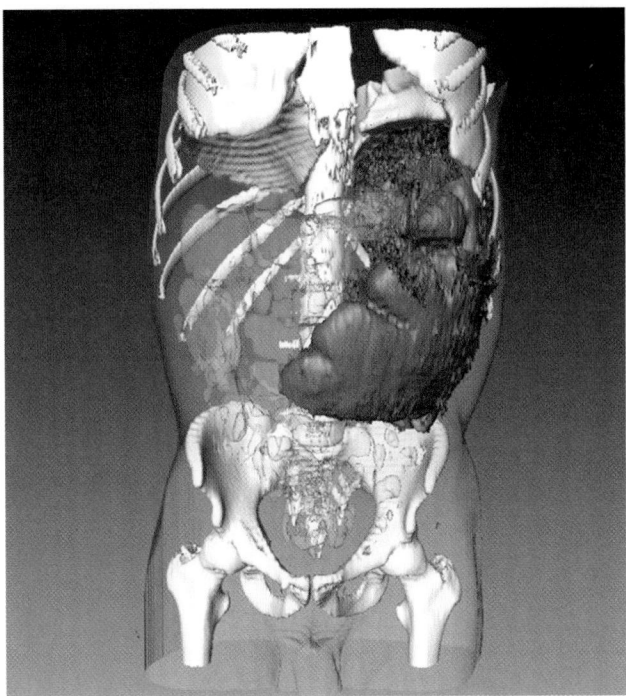

FIG. 34-2. Splenomegaly, shown in a three-dimensional reconstruction of computed tomographic scans. *(Courtesy of Ivan George, University of Maryland School of Medicine.)*

artery. The splenic artery can be characterized by the pattern of its terminal branches. The *distributed type* of splenic artery is the most common (70%) and is distinguished by a short trunk with many long branches entering over three fourths of the spleen's medial surface. The less common *magistral type* of splenic artery (30%) has a long main trunk dividing near the hilum into short terminal branches, and these enter over 25 to 30% of the spleen's medial surface. The spleen also receives some of its blood supply from the short gastric vessels that branch from the left gastroepiploic artery running within the gastrosplenic ligament. The splenic vein joins the superior mesenteric vein to form the portal vein and accommodates the major venous drainage of the spleen.

When a normal, freshly excised spleen is sectioned, the cut surface is finely granular and predominantly dark red with whitish nodules distributed liberally across its expanse. This gross observation reflects the spleen's microstructure. The splenic parenchyma is composed of two main elements: the red pulp, constituting approximately 75% of total splenic volume, and the white pulp (Fig. 34-4). At the interface between the red and white pulp is the narrow marginal zone.

The red pulp is comprised of large numbers of venous sinuses, which ultimately drain into tributaries of the splenic vein. The sinuses are surrounded and separated by the reticulum, a fibrocellular network of collagen fibers and fibroblasts. Within this network or mesh lie splenic macrophages. These intersinusoidal regions appear as *splenic cords.* The venous sinuses are lined by long, narrow endothelial cells that are variably in close apposition to one another or are separated by intercellular gaps in a configuration unique to the spleen. The red pulp serves as a dynamic filtration system, enabling macrophages to remove microorganisms, cellular debris, antigen-antibody complexes, and senescent erythrocytes from the circulation.

Around the terminal millimeters of splenic arterioles, a *periarticular lymphatic sheath* replaces the native adventitia of the vessel. The sheath is comprised of T lymphocytes and intermittent aggregations of B lymphocytes or lymphoid follicles. When antigenically stimulated, the follicles, serving as centers of lymphocyte proliferation, develop germinal centers, which regress as the stimulus or infection subsides. This white pulp consists of nodules that normally are ≤1 mm in size but can increase to several centimeters when nodules

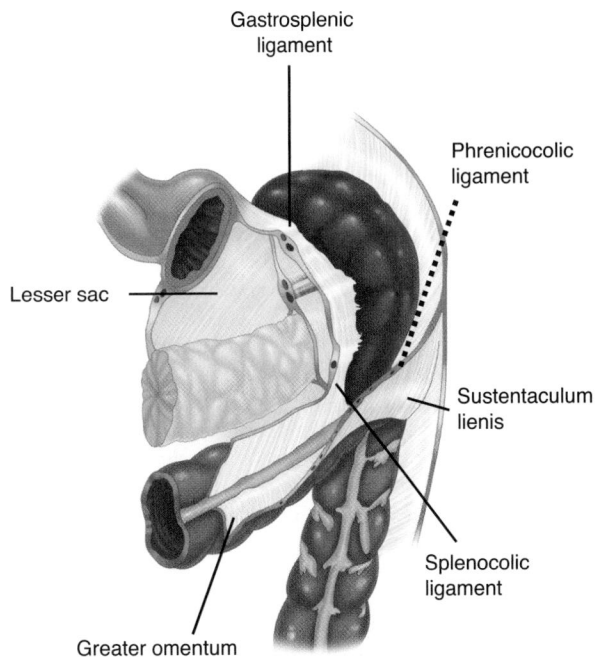

FIG. 34-3. Suspensory ligaments of the spleen. *(Reproduced with permission from Poulin et al.[4])*

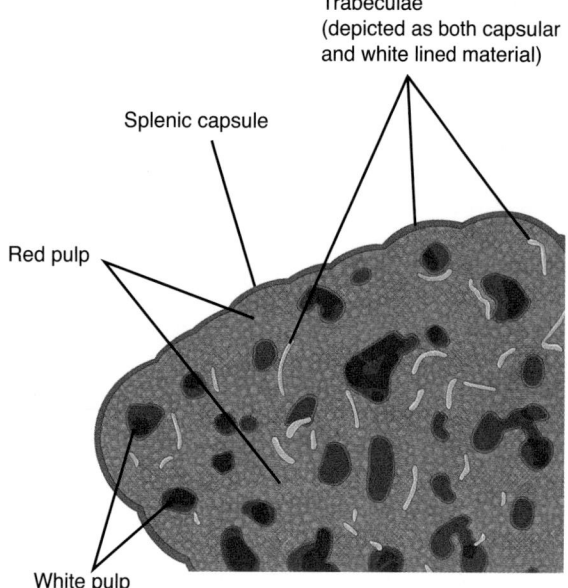

Trabeculae
(depicted as both capsular
and white lined material)

Splenic capsule

Red pulp

White pulp

FIG. 34-4. Splenic architecture. *(Courtesy of Ivan George, University of Maryland School of Medicine.)*

coalesce, as occurs in certain lymphoproliferative disorders. At the junction between the white and red pulp is the marginal zone, where lymphocytes are more loosely aggregated. Blood is delivered from this zone to the red pulp, where lymphocytes and locally produced immunoglobulins ultimately enter the systemic circulation.

PHYSIOLOGY AND PATHOPHYSIOLOGY

The spleen is contained by a 1- to 2-mm thick capsule. In humans, the capsule is rich in collagen and contains some elastin fibers. Many mammals have splenic capsules and trabeculae with abundant smooth muscle cells, which upon autonomic stimulation contract to expel large volumes of stored blood into the general circulation. Such spleens are descriptively characterized as *storage spleens*. The human splenic capsule and trabeculae, by contrast, contain few or no smooth muscle cells, and their function is largely related to immunologic protection. Thus the term *defense spleen* characterizes the human organ.[7] Historically the four splenic functions have been accurately noted as (a) filtration, (b) host defense, (c) storage, and (d) cytopoiesis. For the adult human, the most important, dominant functions are filtration and host defense.

Total splenic inflow of blood is approximately 250 to 300 mL/min. Blood flows through successively tapering arteries to arterioles, traverses the white pulp, crosses the marginal zone, and enters the red pulp. From that entry the flow rate through the spleen may vary greatly. Animal studies measuring the transit times of isotopically labeled blood through the spleen have revealed three distinct velocities of flow. Humans have long been recognized to have both a fast or closed circulation—with blood passing directly from arterioles into venous sinuses—and a slower or open circulation. Most of the spleen's filtration function occurs via the slower circulation. During open circulation, blood percolates through the reticular space and splenic cords, thus gaining access through gaps or slits in the endothelial cell lining to the sinuses. Flowing into and out of the venous sinuses through these gaps, the blood is exposed to extensive contact with splenic macrophages. In addition, because the passage of plasma through these spaces does not slow in a similar manner, a temporary and unique adhesive contact between blood cells and components of the splenic cord may occur. That there is a selective slowing of blood cell flow vs. plasma flow is

further evidenced by the fact that within the spleen the erythrocyte concentration (hematocrit) is twice that of the general circulation. During this contact with splenic macrophages, it is likely that the removal of both cellular debris and senescent blood cells occurs.

The process by which the spleen removes erythrocyte inclusions, such as Heinz bodies (intracellular altered hemoglobin) without cell lysis while red blood cells travel through the spleen is not well understood. The spleen acts as the major site for clearance from the blood of damaged or aged red blood cells and in addition has a part in the removal of abnormal white blood cells and platelets. A minimum of 2 days of the erythrocyte's 120-day life cycle is spent sequestered in the spleen. Daily, approximately 20 mL of aged red blood cells are removed. Evidence suggests that, as erythrocytes age, previously undetected antigens on their surfaces may attach to autoantibodies in the circulation; then macrophages may bind to the antibodies and initiate phagocytosis. It is probable that the erythrocyte is damaged over time by multiple passages through the spleen as well as delayed transit through the congested and relatively hypoxic and acidotic environment of the splenic cords.

The spleen plays a significant although not indispensable role in host defense, contributing to both humoral and cell-mediated immunity. Antigens, described earlier, are filtered in the white pulp and presented to immunocompetent centers within the lymphoid follicles. This gives rise to the elaboration of immunoglobulins (predominantly immunoglobulin M). After an antigen challenge, such an acute immunoglobulin M response results in the release of opsonic antibodies from the white pulp of the spleen. Antigen clearance is then facilitated by the splenic and hepatic reticuloendothelial systems.

The spleen also produces opsonins, tuftsin, and properdin. Circulating monocytes are converted within the red pulp into fixed macrophages that account for the spleen's remarkable phagocytic activity.

The spleen also appears to be a major source of the protein properdin, important in the initiation of the alternate pathway of complement activation. The splenic reticuloendothelial system is better able to clear bacteria that are poorly or inadequately opsonized from the circulation than is the hepatic reticuloendothelial system.[8] Encapsulated bacteria generally fit such a profile, hence the risk posed by pneumococcus and *Haemophilus influenzae* to an asplenic patient. There appears to be sufficient physiologic capacity within the complement cascade to withstand the loss of tuftsin and properdin production without an increase in patient vulnerability after splenectomy.[9]

In patients with chronic hemolytic disorders, splenic tissue may become permanently hypertrophied. The reticular spaces of the red pulp become distended with macrophages engorged with the products of erythrocyte breakdown, and splenomegaly can result. It is important to distinguish between *splenomegaly* and *hypersplenism*, two similar but distinct terms that it is critical to understand when discussing splenic pathology. *Splenomegaly* refers simply to abnormal enlargement of the spleen. There is not a single universally accepted standard, but most would agree that an ex vivo mass of >1 kg or a pole-to-pole length of >15 cm generally qualifies as splenomegaly. Hypersplenism often is found in association with splenomegaly but is not synonymous with it. Hypersplenism is defined as the presence of one or more cytopenias in the context of a normally functioning bone marrow.

Disorders causing hypersplenism can be categorized as either (a) those in which increased destruction of abnormal blood cells occurs in an intrinsically normal spleen (e.g., hemolytic anemias) or (b) primary disorders of the spleen resulting in increased sequestration and destruction of normal blood cells (e.g., infiltrative disorders).

The life cycles of cellular elements vary widely in human blood. A neutrophil in circulation has a normal half-life of approximately 6 hours. The spleen's role in the normal clearance of neutrophils is not well established. It is clear that hypersplenism may result in neutropenia through sequestration of normal white blood cells or the removal of abnormal ones. Platelets, on the other hand, generally survive in the circulation for 10 days. Under normal circumstances a third of the total platelet pool is sequestered in the spleen. Thrombocytopenia may result from excessive sequestration of platelets as well as accelerated platelet destruction in the spleen. Splenomegaly may result in sequestration of up to 80% of the platelet pool. The spleen may also contribute to the immunologic alteration of platelets, which leads to thrombocytopenia in the absence of splenomegaly (e.g., idiopathic thrombocytopenic purpura, or ITP).

The immunologic functions of the spleen are consistent with those of other lymphoid organs. It is a site of blood-borne antigen presentation and the initiation of T- and B-lymphocyte activities involved in humoral and cellular immune responses. Alteration of splenic immune function often gives rise to antibody production, which results in blood cell destruction.

Although the spleen contributes to the process of erythrocyte maturation, in adult humans there is little evidence of normal hematopoietic function. The spleen does have a minor role in hematopoiesis in the fourth month in the human fetus, and reactivation can occur in childhood if the bone marrow fails to meet the hematologic needs. Splenic hematopoiesis giving rise to abnormal red blood cells is seen in adults with myeloproliferative disorders. In addition, in response to some anemias, elements of the red pulp may revert to hematopoiesis.

IMAGING FOR EVALUATION OF SIZE AND PATHOLOGY

Imaging of the spleen is performed most frequently to assess its size before elective splenectomy. Other indications for splenic imaging include trauma, investigations of left upper quadrant pain, characterization of splenic lesions such as tumors, cysts, and abscesses, and guidance for percutaneous procedures.[10,11]

Ultrasound

Ultrasound is the least invasive mode of splenic imaging. It is rapid, easy to perform, and does not expose the patient to ionizing radiation. It is often the first imaging modality applied to the spleen during evaluation and resuscitation of the trauma patient, although questions of sensitivity and specificity remain.[12] In the elective setting, such as for routine diagnostic purposes or for preoperative planning, the sensitivity of ultrasound for detecting textural lesions of the spleen can be quite good in experienced hands. Percutaneous ultrasound-guided procedures for splenic disease (e.g., cyst aspiration, biopsy), historically avoided due to the risk of hemorrhage and other complications, are becoming more common as the safety of these procedures is being increasingly demonstrated.[10,11]

Computed Tomography

Computed tomography (CT) affords a high degree of resolution and detail of the splenic parenchyma. Modern-day CT is more automated and thus less operator dependent than ultrasound, which makes it the preferred imaging modality for many practitioners. CT has become an invaluable tool in the evaluation and management of the blunt trauma patient, and standardized scoring systems for splenic trauma based on CT images now aid in management decisions.[13] In the nontrauma setting, CT is extremely useful for assessment of splenomegaly, identification of solid and cystic lesions, and guidance of percutaneous procedures. The use of iodinated contrast material adds diagnostic clarity to CT imaging of the spleen, although at the cost of the small but real risks of renal impairment or allergic reaction.

Plain Radiography

Rarely is plain radiography used for primary splenic imaging. Plain films can indirectly provide an outline of the spleen in the left upper quadrant or suggest splenomegaly by revealing displacement of adjacent air-filled structures (e.g., the stomach or splenic flexure of the colon). Plain films may also demonstrate splenic calcifications.

Splenic calcifications often are found in association with splenomegaly but are otherwise a nonspecific finding. Splenic calcifications can indicate a number of benign, neoplastic, or infectious processes, including phlebolith, splenic artery aneurysm, sickle cell changes, tumors (e.g., hemangioma, hemangiosarcoma, lymphoma), echinococcosis, or tuberculosis.[14]

Magnetic Resonance Imaging

Although magnetic resonance imaging offers excellent detail and versatility in abdominal imaging, it is more expensive than CT scanning or ultrasound and offers no obvious advantage for primary imaging of the spleen. Magnetic resonance imaging can be a valuable adjunct to the more commonly used imaging techniques when splenic disease is suspected but not definitively diagnosed.[14,15]

Angiography

Angiography of the spleen most commonly refers to invasive arterial imaging, and when it is combined with therapeutic splenic arterial embolization (SAE), there are multiple applications for this procedure: localization and treatment of hemorrhage in select trauma patients[16]; delivery of a variety of therapies in patients with cirrhosis or portal and sinistral hypertension, and in transplant patients[17]; and adjunct (or, more controversially, as an alternative) to splenectomy for treatment of hematologic disorders such as ITP or hypersplenism.[18,19] Preoperative or intraoperative SAE for elective splenectomy is also a common, although not universal, practice. Few prospective data have been published in the last 5 years on preoperative SAE. Preoperative SAE is purported not only to facilitate operation but also possibly to allow a laparoscopic approach in patients whose spleens had previously been considered too large for, or otherwise not amenable to, laparoscopic resection. Limited success in using partial SAE as an alternative to therapeutic splenectomy in chronic ITP has been previously reported.[18,19] Its detractors argue that the need for increased analgesics and occasional extended hospital stay preoperatively, the possibility of pancreatitis, and the well-described risks of invasive arteriography negate any presumed benefits of preoperative SAE.

Nuclear Imaging

Radioscintigraphy with technetium Tc 99m sulfur colloid demonstrates splenic location and size. It may be especially helpful in locating accessory spleens after unsuccessful splenectomy for ITP and has recently proven useful in diagnosing splenosis.[20,21] Unfortunately, no conclusive outcome benefit has been shown for preoperative technetium scanning before splenectomy.[22]

Splenic Index

The splenic index (SI) is a useful concept, initially proposed by Cools and colleagues,[23] expressing the volume of the spleen in milliliters. The SI is obtained by multiplying the spleen's length, width, and height as determined by a reliable imaging modality and using these values in a specific standard ellipsoid volume and linear regression formula.[24] Normal values for SI range from 120 mL to 480 mL, and the normal ex vivo weight of the spleen is approximately 150 g.[23]

INDICATIONS FOR SPLENECTOMY

Splenectomy is therapeutic for a large host of conditions, which can be divided into the following broad categories: splenic rupture (trauma), red blood cell disorders and hemoglobinopathies, white blood cell disorders, platelet disorders, bone marrow disorders (myeloproliferative disorders), cysts and tumors, infections and abscesses, storage diseases and infiltrative disorders, and a number of miscellaneous disorders and lesions (Table 34-1).

Overall, the most common indication for splenectomy is trauma to the spleen, whether external trauma (blunt or penetrating) or iatro-

TABLE 34-1	Indications for and expected response to splenectomy in various diseases and conditions	
Disease/Condition	**Indications for Splenectomy**	**Response to Splenectomy**
Hereditary spherocytosis	Hemolytic anemia, recurrent transfusions, intractable leg ulcers	Improves or eliminates anemia
Hereditary elliptocytosis	Limited role for splenectomy	—
Pyruvate kinase deficiency	Only in severe cases, recurrent transfusions	Decreased transfusion requirement, palliative only
Glucose-6-phosphate dehydrogenase deficiency	None	
Warm-antibody autoimmune hemolytic anemia	Failure of medical (steroid) therapy	60–80% response rate, recurrences common
Sickle cell disease	History of acute sequestration crisis, splenic symptoms or infarction (consider concomitant cholecystectomy)	Palliative, variable response
Thalassemia	Excessive transfusion requirements, symptomatic splenomegaly or infarction	Diminished transfusion requirements, relief of symptoms
Acute myeloid leukemia (AML)	Intolerable symptomatic splenomegaly	Relief of abdominal pain and early satiety
Chronic myeloid leukemia	Symptomatic splenomegaly	Relief of abdominal pain and early satiety
Chronic myelomonocytic leukemia	Symptomatic splenomegaly	Relief of abdominal pain and early satiety
Essential thrombocythemia	Only for advanced disease (i.e., transformation to myeloid metaplasia or AML) with severe symptomatic splenomegaly	Relief of abdominal pain and early satiety
Polycythemia vera	Only for advanced disease (i.e., transformation to myeloid metaplasia or AML) with severe symptomatic splenomegaly	Relief of abdominal pain and early satiety
Myelofibrosis (agnogenic myeloid metaplasia)	Severe symptomatic splenomegaly	76% clinical response at 1 y, high risk of hemorrhagic, thrombotic, and infectious complications (26%)
Chronic lymphocytic leukemia	Cytopenias and anemia	75% response rate
Hairy cell leukemia	Cytopenias and symptomatic splenomegaly	40–70% response rate
Hodgkin's disease	Surgical staging in select cases	—
Non-Hodgkin's lymphoma	Cytopenias, symptomatic splenomegaly	Improved complete blood count values, relief of symptoms
Idiopathic thrombocytopenic purpura	Failure of medical therapy, recurrent disease	75–85% rate of long-term response
Thrombotic thrombocytopenic purpura	Excessive plasma exchange requirement	Typically curative
Abscesses of the spleen	Therapy of choice	Curative
Symptomatic parasitic cysts	Therapy of choice	Curative; exercise caution not to spill cyst contents
Symptomatic nonparasitic cysts	Partial splenectomy for small cysts; unroofing for large cysts	Curative
Gaucher's disease	Hypersplenism	Improves cytopenias; does not correct underlying disease
Niemann-Pick disease	Symptomatic splenomegaly	Improves symptoms; does not correct underlying disease
Amyloidosis	Symptomatic splenomegaly	Improves symptoms; does not correct underlying disease
Sarcoidosis	Hypersplenism or symptomatic splenomegaly	Improves symptoms and cytopenias; does not correct underlying disease
Felty's syndrome	Neutropenia	80% durable response rate
Splenic artery aneurysm	Splenectomy best for distal lesions near splenic hilum	Curative
Portal hypertension	Portal or sinistral hypertension due to splenic vein thrombosis	Palliative

genic injury (e.g., during operative procedures for other reasons). Inadvertent intraoperative injury to the spleen in the nontrauma patient is discussed in a later section. Management of splenic injury in the trauma patient is beyond the scope of this chapter. Regarding elective splenectomy, the most common indication in the past had been staging for Hodgkin's disease. More recent data suggest that ITP is now the most frequent indication for elective splenectomy.[2,25]

Red Blood Cell Disorders

Congenital

Hereditary Spherocytosis Hereditary spherocytosis (HS) results from an inherited dysfunction or deficiency in one of the erythrocyte membrane proteins (*spectrin, ankyrin, band 3 protein,* or *protein 4.2*). The resulting destabilization of the membrane lipid bilayer allows a pathologic release of membrane lipids. The red blood cell assumes a more spherical, less deformable shape, and the spherocytic erythrocytes are sequestered and destroyed in the spleen. Hemolytic anemia ensues; in fact, HS is the most common hemolytic anemia for which splenectomy is indicated.[26] HS is inherited primarily in an autosomal dominant fashion; the estimated prevalence in Western populations is 1 in 5000.

Patients with typical HS forms may have mild jaundice. Splenomegaly usually is present on physical examination. Laboratory examination reveals varying degrees of anemia: patients with mild forms of the disease may have no anemia; patients with severe forms may have hemoglobin levels as low as 4 to 6 g/dL. The mean corpuscular volume is typically low to normal or slightly decreased. For screening, a combined elevated mean corpuscular hemoglobin concentration and an elevated erythrocyte distribution width are an excellent predictor. Other laboratory indicators of HS include those providing evidence of rapid red blood cell destruction, including elevated reticulocyte count, elevated lactate dehydrogenase level, and increased level of unconjugated bilirubin. Spherocytes are readily apparent on peripheral blood film.

Dramatic clinical improvement—even despite persistent hemolysis—often occurs after splenectomy in patients with severe disease. Because children can be affected with HS, the timing of splenectomy is important and is aimed at reducing the quite small possibility of overwhelming postsplenectomy sepsis. Delaying such an operation until the patient is between the ages of 4 and 6—unless the anemia and hemolysis accelerate—is recommended by most.[26]

Gallstones are more likely to develop in patients with HS, and over half of patients between the ages of 10 and 30 with HS have cholelithiasis.[27] For children with cholelithiasis prophylactic cholecystectomy is recommended at the time of splenectomy.[28]

Hereditary elliptocytosis (HE) merits brief discussion to distinguish it from HS. Both HS and HE are conditions of the red blood cell membrane that result from genetic defects in skeletal membrane proteins. With the HE defect, the red blood cell elongates as it circulates, so that far fewer red blood cells are sequestered or destroyed when transiting the splenic parenchyma. Unless >50% of red blood cells are affected (a scenario that could permit development of a clinical syndrome like HS) HE may be considered harmless.

Red Blood Cell Enzyme Deficiencies Red blood cell enzyme deficiencies associated with hemolytic anemia may be classified into two groups: deficiencies of enzymes involved in glycolytic pathways, such as pyruvate kinase (PK) deficiency, and deficiencies of enzymes needed to maintain a high ratio of reduced to oxidized glutathione in the red blood cell, protecting it from oxidative damage, such as glucose-6-phosphate dehydrogenase (G6PD) deficiency.

Pyruvate Kinase Deficiency The most common red blood cell enzyme deficiency to cause congenital chronic hemolytic anemia is PK deficiency.[29] Its pathophysiology is unclear. PK deficiency affects people worldwide, with a slight preponderance among those of northern European or Chinese descent. Clinical manifestations of the disease vary widely, from transfusion-dependent severe anemia in early childhood to well-compensated mild anemia in adolescents or adults. Diagnosis is made either by a screening test or by detection of specific mutations at the complementary DNA or genomic level. Splenomegaly is common, and in severe cases splenectomy can alleviate transfusion requirements.[5] As with other disorders that cause hemolytic anemia in children, splenectomy should be delayed if possible to at least 4 years of age to reduce the risk of postsplenectomy infection.

Glucose-6-Phosphate Dehydrogenase Deficiency The most common red blood cell enzyme deficiency overall is G6PD deficiency. It is far more prevalent than PK deficiency with >400 million people affected worldwide, although most experience only moderate health risks and no longevity reduction.[30] Clinical manifestations—chronic hemolytic anemia, acute intermittent hemolytic episodes, or no hemolysis—depend on the variant of G6PD deficiency. The mainstay of therapy is avoidance of drugs known to precipitate hemolysis in patients with G6PD deficiency. Transfusions are given in cases of symptomatic anemia. Conventional wisdom is that splenectomy is not indicated in this disease,[5] and certainly the overwhelming majority of patients with G6PD deficiency will neither require nor benefit from splenectomy. However, one report described a small collection of cases of six symptomatic G6PD deficiency patients who had severe hemolytic anemia and required transfusion, all of whom were identified to share a common mutation at exon 10.[30] All underwent splenectomy. A complete response occurred in four patients (transfusion requirement eliminated) and a partial response in one (transfusion requirement reduced); no follow-up data were provided for the remaining patient. This study indicates that for a carefully select group of patients with severe hemolytic anemia attributable to G6PD deficiency, splenectomy may be of benefit, although more data must be collected before such a recommendation can be made.

Acquired

Warm-Antibody Autoimmune Hemolytic Anemia Autoimmune hemolytic anemias (AIHAs) are characterized by the destruction of red blood cells, whose erythrocyte life span is diminished by autoantibodies leveled against antigens. AIHA is classified as either primary or secondary, depending on whether an underlying cause, such as a disease or toxin, is identified. AIHA is also divided into "warm" and "cold" categories, based on the temperature at which the autoantibodies exert their effect. In cold-agglutinin disease severe symptoms are uncommon and splenectomy is almost never indicated; therefore, this entity is not discussed further in this section. However, warm-antibody AIHA has clinical consequences with which the surgeon should be familiar.

Warm-antibody AIHA, although occurring primarily in midlife, can affect individuals at all ages. The disorder is more common among women, and fully half of warm-antibody AIHA cases are idiopathic. Clinical presentation may be acute or gradual. Findings include mild jaundice and symptoms and signs of anemia. One third to one half of patients present with splenomegaly. Sometimes in such cases the spleen is palpable on physical examination. The diagnosis relies on demonstrating hemolysis as indicated by anemia, reticulocytosis, and/or products of red blood cell destruction, including bilirubin, in the blood, urine, and stool. A positive result on direct Coombs' test confirms the AIHA diagnosis by distinguishing autoimmune from other forms of hemolytic anemia.

Treatment of AIHA depends on the severity of the disease and whether it is primary or secondary. Severe symptomatic anemia demands prompt attention, often requiring red blood cell transfusion. The mainstay treatment for both primary and secondary forms of symptomatic, unstable AIHA is corticosteroids. Therapy should continue until a response is noted by a rise in hematocrit and fall in reticulocyte count, which generally occurs within 3 weeks.

Clinical response to splenectomy for AIHA varies, and the evidence from a number of small case series is conflicting. For example, one 2004 series reported a favorable response to splenectomy in patients with AIHA secondary to chronic lymphocytic leukemia,[31] whereas more recent series found no benefit from splenectomy in patients with AIHA secondary to systemic lupus erythematosus or inflammatory bowel disease.[32]

Favorable responses to splenectomy have been reported in patients with warm-antibody AIHA. Transient responses are more common, however, and many patients eventually experience hemolysis again despite splenectomy.[31,32] The decision regarding splenectomy in the case of AIHA should be individualized based on careful consideration of the clinical history and frank discussion with the patient.

Hemoglobinopathies Sickle cell disease is an inherited chronic hemolytic anemia that results from the mutant sickle cell hemoglobin (HbS) within the red blood cell and is inherited in an autosomal codominant fashion. Persons who inherit an HbS gene from one parent (heterozygous) are carriers; those who inherit an HbS gene from both parents (homozygous) have sickle cell anemia.

In sickle cell disease the underlying abnormality is the mutation of adenine to thymine in the sixth codon of the β-globin gene, which results in the substitution of valine for glutamic acid as the sixth amino acid of the β-globin chain. Mutant β chains included in the hemoglobin tetramer create HbS. Deoxygenated HbS is insoluble and becomes polymerized and sickled. The subsequent lack of deformability of the red blood cell, in addition to other processes, results in microvascular congestion, which may lead to thrombosis, ischemia, and tissue necrosis. The disorder is characterized by painful intermittent episodes.

Sequestration occurs in the spleen, with splenomegaly resulting early in the disease course. In most patients subsequent infarction of the spleen and autosplenectomy occur at some later time.[33] The most frequent indications for splenectomy in sickle cell disease are recurrent acute sequestration crises, hypersplenism, and splenic abscess.[34] The occurrence of one major acute sequestration crisis, characterized by rapid painful enlargement of the spleen and circulatory collapse, generally is considered sufficient grounds for splenectomy. Preoperative preparation should include special attention to adequate hydration and avoidance of hypothermia.

Splenectomy does not affect the sickling process, and therapy for sickle cell anemia remains largely palliative. Transfusions are indicated for anemia, for moderately severe episodes of acute chest syndrome (i.e., a new infiltrate on chest radiograph associated with new symptoms, such as fever, cough, sputum production, or hypoxia),[35] and preoperatively before splenectomy. Patients experiencing stroke or a severe crisis may require hydration and an exchange transfusion, which may be performed manually or with automated apheresis equipment. Hydroxyurea is an oral chemotherapeutic agent that upregulates fetal hemoglobin, which interferes with polymerization of HbS and thus reduces the sickling process.

Thalassemia *Thalassemia* is the term for a group of inherited disorders of hemoglobin synthesis prevalent among people of Mediterranean extraction and classified according to the hemoglobin chain (α, β, or γ) affected. As a group the thalassemias are the most common genetic diseases known to arise from a single gene defect.[36] Most forms of this disorder are inherited in Mendelian recessive fashion from asymptomatic carrier parents. In the so-called thalassemia belt that extends the shores of the Mediterranean as well as through the Arabian Peninsula, Turkey, Iran, India, and southeastern Asia the incidence of thalassemia is between 2.5 and 15%.[37] However, thalassemias have been found in people of all ethnic origins.[38]

In all forms of thalassemia the primary defect is absent or reduced production of hemoglobin chains. From this abnormality two significant consequences arise: (1) reduced functioning of hemoglobin tetramers, yielding hypochromia and microcytosis; and (2) unbalanced biosynthesis of individual α and β subunits, which results in insoluble red blood cells that cannot release oxygen normally and may precipitate with cell aging. Both underproduction of hemoglobin and excess production of unpaired hemoglobin subunits contribute to thalassemia-associated morbidity and mortality.

A diagnosis of thalassemia major (homozygous form) is made by demonstrating hypochromic microcytic anemia associated with randomly distorted red blood cells and nucleated erythrocytes (target cells) on peripheral blood smear.[5] Elevated reticulocyte count and white blood cell count are among the associated findings. Because α chains are needed to form both fetal hemoglobin and adult hemoglobin, α-thalassemia becomes symptomatic in utero or at birth. By contrast, β-thalassemia becomes symptomatic at 4 to 6 months, because β chains are involved only in adult hemoglobin synthesis.

The clinical spectrum of the thalassemias is wide. Heterozygous carriers of the disease are usually asymptomatic. Homozygous individuals, on the other hand, typically present before 2 years of age with pallor, growth retardation, jaundice, and abdominal swelling due to liver and spleen enlargement. Among other characteristics of thalassemia major are intractable leg ulcers, head enlargement, frequent infections, and the need for periodic blood transfusions. Untreated individuals usually die in late infancy or early childhood from severe anemia.[5]

Treatment for thalassemia involves red blood cell transfusions to maintain a hemoglobin level of >9 mg/dL, along with intensive parenteral chelation therapy with deferoxamine. Splenectomy is indicated for patients with excessive transfusion requirements (>200 mL/kg per year), discomfort due to splenomegaly, or painful splenic infarction.[5,39] Careful assessment of the risk:benefit ratio is essential. Thalassemia patients are at high risk for pulmonary hypertension after splenectomy; the precise etiology of this sequela is under investigation.[40] The increase in infectious complications is likely to be due to a coexisting immune deficiency, in large part brought about by iron overload, which may be associated both with the thalassemia itself and with transfusions. The disproportionately high rate of overwhelming postsplenectomy infection in thalassemia patients has led some investigators to consider partial splenectomy in children; some success in reducing mortality has been

reported.[41] However, splenectomy should be delayed until after the age of 4 years unless it is absolutely necessary.

White Blood Cell Disorders

The role of splenectomy in patients with white blood cell disorders varies. As for the myelogenous diseases mentioned previously, splenectomy for white blood cell disorders can be effective therapy for symptomatic splenomegaly and hypersplenism, improving some clinical parameters but generally not altering the course of the underlying disease. Historically, splenectomy has played a role during surgical staging for Hodgkin's disease, although this practice has become less common with the advent of advanced imaging technologies and less extensive biopsy strategies.[42] Careful consideration of the intended benefits of splenectomy must be weighed against the significant perioperative and postsplenectomy risks in this often complex patient population.[43]

Chronic Lymphocytic Leukemia

The main characteristic of chronic lymphocytic leukemia (CLL) is a progressive accumulation of long-lived but nonfunctional lymphocytes. Symptoms of CLL are nonspecific and include weakness, fatigue, fever without illness, night sweats, and frequent bacterial and viral infections. The most frequent finding is lymphadenopathy. When the spleen is enlarged, it may be massive or barely palpable below the costal margin. Splenectomy is indicated to improve cytopenias and was shown to be 75% effective in a combined group of patients who had either CLL or nonmalignant Hodgkin's disease.[44] Splenectomy may facilitate chemotherapy in patients whose cell counts were prohibitively low before spleen removal. Palliative splenectomy also is indicated for symptomatic splenomegaly.

Hairy Cell Leukemia

Hairy cell leukemia (HCL) is an uncommon blood disorder, representing only 2% of all adult leukemias. HCL is characterized by splenomegaly, pancytopenia, and large numbers of abnormal lymphocytes in the bone marrow. These lymphocytes contain irregular hair-like cytoplasmic projections identifiable on the peripheral smear. Many HCL patients have few symptoms and require no specific therapy. Splenectomy does not correct the underlying disorder but does return cell counts to normal in 40 to 70% of patients and alleviates symptoms of splenomegaly.[45,46]

Hodgkin's Disease

Hodgkin's disease (HD) is a disorder of the lymphoid system characterized by the presence of Reed-Sternberg cells (which actually form the minority of the Hodgkin's tumor). More than 90% of patients with HD present with lymphadenopathy above the diaphragm. Lymph nodes can become particularly bulky in the mediastinum, which may result in shortness of breath, cough, or obstructive pneumonia. Lymphadenopathy below the diaphragm is rare on presentation but can arise with disease progression. The spleen is often an occult site of spread, but massive splenomegaly is not common. In addition, large spleens do not necessarily signify involvement.

Four major histologic types exist: lymphocyte predominance type, nodular sclerosis type, mixed cellularity type, and lymphocyte depletion type. The histologic type, along with location of disease and symptomatology, influence survival for patients with HD. Stage I disease is limited to one anatomic region; stage II disease is defined by the presence of two or more contiguous or noncontiguous regions on the same side of the diaphragm; stage III disease involves disease on both sides of the diaphragm, but limited to lymph nodes, spleen, and Waldeyer's ring (the ring of lymphoid tissue formed by the lingual, palatine, and nasopharyngeal tonsils); stage IV disease includes involvement of the bone marrow, lung, liver, skin, GI tract, or any organ or tissue other than the lymph nodes or Waldeyer's ring.[47]

Staging laparotomy for HD is less commonly performed in the current era of minimally invasive surgery and advanced imaging techniques. More liberal use of chemotherapy for patients with HD has significantly reduced the indications for surgical staging. Current indications for surgical staging include clinical stage I or II disease of the nodular sclerosing type and no symptoms referable to HD.[5] The surgical staging procedure for HD includes a biopsy of the liver, splenectomy, and the removal of representative nodes in the retroperitoneum, mesentery, and hepatoduodenal ligament. An iliac marrow biopsy generally is included. Unlike in non-Hodgkin's lymphoma, studies have concluded that surgical staging has altered clinical staging in as many as 42% of cases (26 to 37% upgraded, 7 to 15% downgraded).[5] Staging information affects treatment, because patients with early-stage disease who have no splenic involvement may be candidates for radiotherapy alone. Those with splenic involvement generally require chemotherapy or multimodality therapy.

Non-Hodgkin's Lymphoma

Non-Hodgkin's lymphoma (NHL) encompasses all malignancies derived from the lymphoid system except classic HD. A proliferation of any one of the three predominant lymph cell types—natural killer cells, T cells, or B cells—may be included in the category of NHL. Because of the wide net cast by NHL, the clinical presentations of the disorders under its umbrella vary. The subentities of NHL may be clinically classified into nodal or extranodal, as well as indolent, aggressive, and very aggressive groups. Patients with indolent lymphomas may present with mild or no symptoms and seek medical attention for a swollen lymph node, whereas the aggressive and very aggressive lymphomas create easily noticeable symptoms, such as pain, swelling due to obstruction of vessels, fever, and night sweats. Surgical staging is no longer indicated for NHL, because the combination of history and physical examination, chest radiograph and abdominal/pelvic CT scan, biopsy of involved lymph nodes (including laparoscopically directed nodal and liver biopsies), and bone marrow biopsy is sufficient.[5] Splenomegaly exists in some, but not all, forms of NHL, and splenectomy is indicated for management of symptoms related to an enlarged spleen as well as for improvement of cytopenias.

Platelet Disorders

Idiopathic Thrombocytopenic Purpura

Idiopathic thrombocytopenic purpura (ITP), also called *immune thrombocytopenic purpura*, is an autoimmune disorder characterized by a low platelet count and mucocutaneous and petechial bleeding. The low platelet count stems from premature removal of platelets opsonized by antiplatelet immunoglobulin G autoantibodies produced in the spleen. This clearance occurs through the interaction of platelet autoantibodies with Fc receptors expressed on tissue macrophages, predominantly in the spleen and liver. The estimated incidence of ITP is 100 persons per million annually, about one half of whom are children.[48] Adult-onset and childhood-onset ITP are strikingly different in their clinical course and management.

Patients with ITP typically present with petechiae or ecchymoses, although some experience major bleeding from the outset. Bleeding may occur from mucosal surfaces in the form of gingival bleeding, epistaxis, menorrhagia, hematuria, or even melena. The severity of bleeding frequently corresponds to the deficiency in platelets: Patients with counts >50,000/mm^3 usually present with incidental findings; those with counts between 30,000 and 50,000/mm^3 often have easy bruising; those with platelet counts between 10,000 and 30,000/mm^3 may develop spontaneous petechiae or ecchymoses; and those with counts <10,000/mm^3 are at risk for internal bleeding.[48] The incidence of major intracranial hemorrhage is approximately 1%, and it usually occurs early in the disease course. The duration of the bleeding helps to distinguish acute from chronic forms of ITP. Children often present at a young age (peak age of approximately 5 years) with sudden onset of petechiae or purpura several days to weeks after an infectious illness. In contrast, adults experience a more chronic form of disease with an insidious onset. Splenomegaly is uncommon with ITP in both adults and children, and its occurrence

should prompt a search for a separate cause of thrombocytopenia. Up to 10% of children, however, have a palpable spleen tip.[48]

Diagnosis of ITP is based on exclusion of other possibilities in the presence of a low platelet count and mucocutaneous bleeding. Other diseases resulting in secondary forms of immune thrombocytopenic purpura, such as systemic lupus erythematosus, antiphospholipid syndrome, lymphoproliferative disorders, HIV infection, and hepatitis C should be identified and treated when present. In addition, any history of use of a drug known to cause thrombocytopenia, such as certain antimicrobials, anti-inflammatories, antihypertensives, and antidepressants, should be sought. In addition to low platelet count, another laboratory finding characteristic of ITP is the presence of large, immature platelets (megathrombocytes) on peripheral blood smear.

The usual first line of therapy is oral prednisone at a dosage of 1.0 to 1.5 mg/kg per day.[48] No consensus exists as to the optimal duration of steroid therapy, but most responses occur within the first 3 weeks. Response rates range from 50 to 75%, but relapses are common. IV immunoglobulin, given at 1.0 g/kg per day for 2 to 3 days, is indicated for internal bleeding when platelet counts remain <5000/mm^3 or when extensive purpura exists.[48] IV immunoglobulin is thought to impair clearance of immunoglobulin G–coated platelets by competing for binding to tissue macrophage receptors.[49] An immediate response is common but a sustained remission is not.[50] Splenectomy is indicated for failure of medical therapy, for prolonged use of steroids with undesirable effects, or for most cases of first relapse.[5] Prolonged use of steroids can be defined in various ways, but a persistent need for more than 10 to 20 mg/d for 3 to 6 months to maintain a platelet count of >30,000/mm^3 generally prompts referral for splenectomy.[48] Splenectomy provides a permanent response without subsequent need for steroids in 75 to 85% of patients (see "Splenectomy Outcomes" later). Responses usually occur within the first postoperative week. For patients with extremely low platelet counts (<10,000/mm^3) platelets should be available for surgery but should not be given preoperatively. Once the splenic pedicle is ligated, platelets are given to those who continue to bleed.

In children with ITP, the course is self limited, with durable and complete remission in >70% of patients regardless of therapy. Because of the good prognosis without treatment, the decision to intervene is controversial and is based largely on the fear of intracranial hemorrhage discussed earlier. Therefore children with typical ITP—and certainly those without hemorrhage—are managed principally by observation, with short-term therapy in select cases. Urgent splenectomy, in conjunction with aggressive medical therapy, may play a role in the rare circumstance of severe, life-threatening bleeding in both children and adults.

Thrombotic Thrombocytopenic Purpura

Thrombotic thrombocytopenic purpura (TTP) is a serious disorder characterized by thrombocytopenia, microangiopathic hemolytic anemia, and neurologic complications. Abnormal platelet clumping occurs in arterioles and capillaries, reducing the lumen of these vessels and predisposing the patient to microvascular thrombotic episodes. The reduced lumen size also causes shearing stresses on erythrocytes, which leads to deformed red blood cells subject to hemolysis. Hemolysis may be due in part to sequestration and destruction of erythrocytes in the spleen. Research has demonstrated that the underlying abnormality is likely related to the persistence of unusually large multimers of von Willebrand factor associated with platelet clumping in the patient's blood.[51]

TTP occurs in approximately 3.7 individuals per million,[52] but this rare disorder's dramatic clinical sequelae and favorable response to early therapy demand an understanding of its clinical presentation to ensure an early diagnosis. Clinical features of the disorder include petechiae, fever, neurologic symptoms, renal failure, and, infrequently, cardiac symptoms such as heart failure or arrhythmias. Petechial hemorrhages in the lower extremities are the most common presenting sign. Along with fever, patients may experience flu-like symptoms, malaise, or fatigue. Neurologic changes range from generalized headaches to altered mental status, seizures, and even coma. Generally, however, the mere presence of petechiae and thrombocytopenia are sufficient to lead to the diagnosis of TTP and consideration of treatment.

The diagnosis is confirmed by the peripheral blood smear, which shows schistocytes, nucleated red blood cells, and basophilic stippling. Although other conditions such as tight aortic stenosis or prosthetic valves may lead to the presence of schistocytes, these conditions generally are not accompanied by thrombocytopenia. TTP may be distinguished from autoimmune causes of thrombocytopenia, such as Evans syndrome (ITP and autoimmune hemolytic anemia) or systemic lupus erythematosus, by a negative result on Coombs' test.[51]

Plasma exchange is the first-line therapy for TTP. This treatment consists of the daily removal of a single volume of the patient's plasma and its replacement with fresh-frozen plasma until the thrombocytopenia, anemia, and associated symptoms are corrected. Therapy is then tapered over 1 to 2 weeks.[51] Splenectomy plays a key role for patients who experience relapse or who require multiple plasma exchanges to control symptoms, and generally is well tolerated without significant morbidity.[53]

Bone Marrow Disorders (Myeloproliferative Disorders)

The myeloproliferative disorders are characterized by an abnormal growth of cell lines in the bone marrow. They include chronic myeloid leukemia, acute myeloid leukemia, chronic myelomonocytic leukemia, essential thrombocythemia, polycythemia vera, and myelofibrosis, also known as *agnogenic myeloid metaplasia* [see "Myelofibrosis (Agnogenic Myeloid Metaplasia)" later in this chapter]. The common underlying problem leading to splenectomy in these disorders is symptomatic splenomegaly. Symptoms due to splenomegaly consist of early satiety, poor gastric emptying, heaviness or pain in the left upper quadrant, and even diarrhea. Hypersplenism, when it occurs in these conditions, usually is associated with splenomegaly. Splenectomy performed in the setting of the myeloproliferative disorders is generally for treatment of the pain, early satiety, and other symptoms of splenomegaly.

Splenomegaly can sometimes be treated nonsurgically by chemotherapeutic agents (busulfan, hydroxyurea, interferon-α) to achieve mild to moderate size reductions and some relief of symptoms, but discontinuation of treatment may result in rapid splenic regrowth. Radiation has been used since 1903 to treat symptomatic splenomegaly, but today it is principally used in situations in which splenectomy is not an option.

Chronic Myeloid Leukemia

Chronic myeloid leukemia (CML) is a disorder of the primitive pluripotent stem cell in the bone marrow that results in a significant increase in erythroid, megakaryotic, and pluripotent progenitors in the peripheral blood smear. The genetic hallmark is a transposition between the *bcr* gene on chromosome 9 and the *abl* gene on chromosome 22. CML accounts for 7 to 15% of all leukemias, with an incidence of 1.5 in 100,000 in the United States.[54] It is often asymptomatic, but CML can cause fatigue, anorexia, sweating, and left upper quadrant pain and early satiety secondary to splenomegaly. Enlargement of the spleen is found in roughly one half of patients with CML. Splenectomy is indicated to ease pain and early satiety.[55]

Acute Myeloid Leukemia

Like CML, acute myeloid leukemia (AML) involves the abnormal growth of stem cells in the bone marrow. Unlike CML, AML has a presentation that is more rapid and dramatic. The proliferation and accumulation of hematopoietic stem cells in the bone marrow and blood inhibit the growth and maturation of normal red blood cells, white blood cells, and platelets. Death usually results within weeks to months if AML goes untreated. The incidence of AML is

approximately 9200 new cases each year in the United States, and it accounts for 1.2% of all cancer deaths.[56] Patients with other myeloproliferative disorders, such as polycythemia vera, primary thrombocytosis, or myeloid metaplasia, are at increased risk for leukemic transformation to AML. Presenting signs and symptoms of AML include a viral-like illness with fever, malaise, and frequently bone pain due to the expansion of the medullary space. Splenectomy is indicated in AML only in the uncommon circumstance that left upper quadrant pain and early satiety become unbearable. The benefit must be weighed against the heightened risk of postsplenectomy infection in AML patients immunocompromised due to neutropenia and chemotherapy.

Chronic Myelomonocytic Leukemia

Like CML and AML, chronic myelomonocytic leukemia (CMML) is characterized by a proliferation of hematopoietic elements in the bone marrow and blood. CMML differs from CML in that it is associated with monocytosis in the peripheral smear ($>1 \times 10^3$ monocytes/mm^3) and in the bone marrow. Splenomegaly occurs in one half of these patients, and splenectomy can result in symptomatic relief.

Essential Thrombocythemia

Essential thrombocythemia (ET) represents abnormal growth of the megakaryocyte cell line, resulting in increased levels of platelets in the bloodstream. The diagnosis is made after the exclusion of other chronic myeloid disorders such as CML, polycythemia vera, and myelofibrosis that may also present with thrombocytosis.[57] Clinical manifestations of ET include vasomotor symptoms, thrombohemorrhagic events, recurrent fetal loss, and the transformation to myelofibrosis with myeloid metaplasia or AML. Hydroxyurea is used to reduce thrombotic events in ET but does not alter transformation to myelofibrosis or leukemia. Splenomegaly occurs in one third to one half of patients with ET. Splenectomy is not felt to be helpful in the early stages of ET and is best reserved for the later stages of disease, when myeloid metaplasia has developed.[57] Even in these circumstances, candidates should be chosen selectively, because significant bleeding has been reported to complicate splenectomy in these patients.

Polycythemia Vera

Polycythemia vera (PV) is a clonal, chronic, progressive myeloproliferative disorder characterized by an increase in red blood cell mass, frequently accompanied by leukocytosis, thrombocytosis, and splenomegaly. Patients with PV typically enjoy longer survival than those affected by hematologic malignancies but remain at risk for transformation to myelofibrosis or AML. The disease is rare, with an annual incidence of 5 to 17 cases per million population.[58] Physical findings include ruddy cyanosis, conjunctival plethora, hepatomegaly, splenomegaly, and hypertension. Treatment should be tailored to the risk status of the patient and ranges from phlebotomy and aspirin administration to the use of chemotherapeutic agents. As in ET, splenectomy is not helpful in the early stages of disease and is best reserved for patients with late-stage disease in whom myeloid metaplasia has developed and splenomegaly-related symptoms are severe.[55]

Myelofibrosis (Agnogenic Myeloid Metaplasia)

The term *myelofibrosis* may be used to describe either the generic condition of fibrosis of the bone marrow (which may be associated with a number of benign and malignant disorders) or a specific, chronic, malignant hematologic disease associated with splenomegaly, the presence of red blood cell and white blood cell progenitors in the bloodstream, marrow fibrosis, and extramedullary hematopoiesis, otherwise known as *agnogenic myeloid metaplasia (AMM)*. AMM also can be referred to as *myelosclerosis, idiopathic myeloid metaplasia,* and *osteosclerosis.* In this chapter the term *myelofibrosis* is synonymous with AMM.

In AMM fibrosis of the bone marrow is believed to be a response to a clonal proliferation of hematopoietic stem cells. Marrow failure is common. The true incidence of AMM is unknown due to the scarcity of epidemiologic data, but one study estimated its U.S. incidence at 1.46 per 100,000 population.[59] Excessive radiation exposure may play a role in the development of AMM, because persons within close proximity of the atomic bomb blasts in Japan, as well as those with a history of exposure to the contrast agent thorium dioxide (Thorotrast), have been shown to exhibit a higher incidence of AMM.

The diagnosis is made by a careful examination of the peripheral blood smear and bone marrow. Nucleated red blood cells and immature myeloid elements in the blood are present in 96% of cases and strongly suggest the diagnosis. Teardrop poikilocytosis is another frequent finding. Care must be taken, however, to exclude a history of a primary neoplasm (such as lymphoma or adenocarcinoma of the stomach, lung, prostate, or breast) or tuberculosis, because patients with these conditions may develop secondary myelofibrosis.

Treatment depends on symptoms: Asymptomatic patients are closely followed, whereas symptomatic patients undergo therapeutic intervention targeted to their symptoms.[60] Splenomegaly-related symptoms are best treated with splenectomy. Although some chemotherapeutic agents (busulfan, hydroxyurea, interferon-α) and low-dose radiation can reduce splenic size, their discontinuation usually results in rapid splenic regrowth.

A thorough preoperative work-up must precede splenectomy in patients with AMM. The candidate must possess acceptable cardiac, pulmonary, hepatic, and renal reserve for the operation. The coagulation system should be examined; testing should include measurement of coagulation factors V and VIII and fibrin split products, platelet count, and bleeding time. Low platelet counts may require administration of adrenal steroids and/or platelet transfusion at the time of surgery. Splenectomy provides durable, effective palliation for nearly all patients with AMM, although postoperative complications are more common in patients with AMM than in those with other hematologic indications.[5] The Mayo Clinic recently published its 30-year experience with 314 myelofibrosis patients who underwent splenectomy: nearly half of the operations (49%) were performed to alleviate the mechanical symptoms of splenomegaly; the remainder were undertaken to manage anemia, thrombocytopenia, or portal hypertension. Response to splenectomy was 76% overall at 1 year; overall complication rate was 28%, including 21 perioperative deaths.[61] Thrombosis, hemorrhage, and infection complications were common, with preoperative thrombocytopenia an independent predictor of mortality risk. These data underscore the severity of this malignancy and emphasize need for careful patient selection when considering splenectomy in AMM.

Infections and Abscesses

Primary infections of the spleen are infrequently reported. However, the potential effects of certain systemic infections on the spleen merit close attention, mostly because of the potential risk of spontaneous splenic rupture. Infectious mononucleosis due to either Epstein-Barr virus or cytomegalovirus infection imparts a small but often-discussed risk of spontaneous splenic rupture in both adults and children. The true incidence may be underreported, however. Recent case reports abound in the literature regarding spontaneous splenic rupture due to a variety of infectious causes (malaria, *Listeria* infection, fungal infections, dengue, and Q fever, to name a few) as well as a variety of neoplastic and other noninfectious causes (lymphoma, angiosarcoma, amyloidosis, pregnancy). The presumed pathophysiologic mechanism is infiltration of the splenic parenchyma with inflammatory cells, which distorts the architecture and fibrous support system of the spleen and thins the splenic capsule.[62] In this setting, splenic rupture can occur spontaneously or after a seemingly minor external trauma or even a Valsalva maneuver.[63]

Abscesses of the spleen are uncommon, with an incidence of 0.14 to 0.7% based on autopsy findings.[64] They occur more frequently in tropical locations, where they are associated with thrombosed splenic vessels and infarction in patients with sickle cell anemia. Five distinct mechanisms of splenic abscess formation have been described: (a) hematogenous infection; (b) contiguous infection; (c) hemoglobinopathy; (d) immunosuppression, including HIV infection and chemotherapy; and (e) trauma. Presentation frequently is delayed, with most patients enduring symptoms for 16 to 22 days before diagnosis. Clinical manifestations include fever, left upper quadrant pain, leukocytosis, and splenomegaly in about one third of patients. The diagnosis is confirmed by ultrasound or CT scan, which has a 95% sensitivity and specificity. Upon discovery of a splenic abscess, broad-spectrum antibiotics should be started, with adjustment to more specific therapy based on culture results and continuation of treatment for 14 days. Splenectomy is the operation of choice, but percutaneous and open drainage are options for patients who cannot tolerate splenectomy.[5] Percutaneous drainage is successful for patients with unilocular disease.

Cysts and Tumors

Splenic cysts can be categorized according to a number of criteria; one clinically relevant scheme is to characterize splenic cysts as either parasitic or nonparasitic.

Parasitic infection is the most common cause of splenic cysts worldwide, and the majority are due to *Echinococcus* species. Such cysts are more commonly found in areas where the pathogen is endemic. Symptoms, when present, generally are related to the presence of a mass lesion in the left upper quadrant or a lesion that impinges on the stomach. Ultrasound can establish the presence of a cystic lesion and occasionally incidentally detect asymptomatic lesions as well. Serologic testing for echinococcal antibodies can confirm or exclude the cystic lesion as parasitic, an important piece of information when planning operative therapy. Symptomatic parasitic cysts are best treated with splenectomy. Avoidance of spillage of parasitic cyst contents into the peritoneal cavity to avoid the possibility of anaphylactic shock is an important principle in surgical management.

Cysts resulting from trauma are termed *pseudocysts* due to their lack of cellular lining. Less common examples of nonparasitic cysts are dermoid, epidermoid, and epithelial cysts.[65] The treatment of nonparasitic cysts depends on whether or not they produce symptoms. Asymptomatic nonparasitic cysts may be observed with close follow-up by ultrasound to exclude significant expansion. Patients should be advised of the risk of cyst rupture with even minor abdominal trauma if they elect nonoperative management for large cysts. Small symptomatic nonparasitic cysts may be excised with splenic preservation, and large symptomatic nonparasitic cysts may be unroofed. Both of these operations may be performed laparoscopically.[66]

The most common primary tumor of the spleen is sarcoma. Autopsy studies reveal an approximately 0.6% rate of tumor metastasis to the spleen; most of these metastases are carcinomas.[67] Lung cancer is the tumor that most commonly spreads to the spleen.

Storage Diseases and Infiltrative Disorders

Gaucher's Disease

Gaucher's disease is an inherited lipid storage disorder characterized by the deposition of glucocerebroside in cells of the macrophage-monocyte system. The underlying abnormality is a deficiency in the activity of a lysosomal hydrolase. Abnormal glycolipid storage results in organomegaly, particularly hepatomegaly and splenomegaly.[68] Patients with Gaucher's disease frequently experience symptoms related to splenomegaly, including early satiety and abdominal discomfort, and to hypersplenism, including thrombocytopenia, normocytic anemia, and mild leukopenia. These latter findings occur as a result of excessive sequestration of formed blood elements in the spleen. Other symptoms in patients with Gaucher's disease include bone pain, pathologic fractures, and jaundice. Splenectomy alleviates hematologic abnormalities in patients with hypersplenism but it does not correct the underlying disease process. Partial splenectomy has been shown to be effective in children to correct both hematologic problems and symptoms due to splenomegaly without incurring the risk of overwhelming postsplenectomy sepsis.

Niemann-Pick Disease

Niemann-Pick disease is an inherited disorder of abnormal lysosomal storage of sphingomyelin and cholesterol in cells of the macrophage-monocyte system. Four types of the disease (A, B, C, and D) exist, with unique clinical presentations. Types A and B result from a deficiency in lysosomal hydrolase and are the forms most likely to demonstrate splenomegaly with its concomitant symptoms.

Amyloidosis

Amyloidosis is a disorder of abnormal extracellular protein deposition. There are multiple forms of amyloidosis, each with its own individual clinical presentation, and the severity of disease may range from asymptomatic to multiorgan failure. Patients with primary amyloidosis, associated with plasma cell dyscrasia, have splenic involvement in approximately 5% of cases. Secondary amyloidosis, associated with chronic inflammatory conditions, also may present with an enlarged spleen. Symptoms of splenomegaly are relieved by splenectomy.

Sarcoidosis

Sarcoidosis is an inflammatory disease of young adults characterized by noncaseating granulomas in affected tissues. Signs and symptoms of the disease range in severity and typically are nonspecific, such as fatigue and malaise. Any organ system may be involved. The most commonly involved organ is the lung, followed by the spleen. Splenomegaly occurs in approximately 25% of patients. Massive splenomegaly (>1 kg) is rare.[69] Other affected tissues include the lymph nodes, eyes, joints, liver, spleen, and heart. When splenomegaly occurs and causes symptoms related to size or hypersplenism, splenectomy effectively relieves symptoms and corrects hematologic abnormalities such as anemia and thrombocytopenia. Spontaneous splenic rupture has been reported in sarcoidosis.[70]

Miscellaneous Disorders and Lesions

Splenic Artery Aneurysm

Although splenic artery aneurysm is rare, it is the most common visceral artery aneurysm. Women are four times more likely to be affected than men. The aneurysm usually arises in the middle to distal portion of the splenic artery. In one series, mortality was significantly higher in patients with underlying portal hypertension (>50%) than in those without it (17%).[71] Indications for treatment include presence of symptoms, pregnancy, intention to become pregnant, and presence of pseudoaneurysms associated with inflammatory processes. Aneurysm resection or ligation alone is acceptable for amenable lesions in the midsplenic artery, but distal lesions in close proximity to the splenic hilum should be treated with concomitant splenectomy. An excellent prognosis follows elective treatment. Splenic artery embolization has been used to treat splenic artery aneurysm, but painful splenic infarction and abscess may follow.

Portal Hypertension

Portal hypertension can result from numerous causes but is usually due to cirrhosis. Splenomegaly and splenic congestion often accompany portal hypertension, which leads to sequestration and destruction of circulating cells in the spleen. Splenectomy is not indicated for hypersplenism per se in patients with portal hypertension, however, because no correlation exists between the degree of pancytopenia and long-term survival in these patients.[5] In rare circumstances in which splenectomy is required to reduce bleeding from esophageal varices exacerbated by thrombocytopenia, a concomitant splenorenal shunt procedure should be performed to decompress the portal system.[5]

Portal hypertension secondary to splenic vein thrombosis is potentially curable with splenectomy. Patients with bleeding from isolated gastric varices who have normal liver function test results, especially those with a history of pancreatic disease, should be examined for splenic vein thrombosis and treated with splenectomy if findings are positive.

Felty's Syndrome

The triad of rheumatoid arthritis, splenomegaly, and neutropenia is called *Felty's syndrome*. It exists in approximately 3% of all patients with rheumatoid arthritis, two thirds of whom are women. Immune complexes coat the surface of white blood cells, which leads to their sequestration and clearance in the spleen with subsequent neutropenia. This neutropenia (<2000 neutrophils/mm^3) increases the risk for recurrent infections and often drives the decision for splenectomy. The size of the spleen is variable, from nonpalpable in 5 to 10% of patients to massively enlarged in others. In Felty's syndrome the spleen is four times heavier than normal. Corticosteroids, hematopoietic growth factors, methotrexate, and splenectomy have all been used to treat the neutropenia of Felty's syndrome. Responses to splenectomy have been excellent, with >80% of patients showing a durable increase in white blood cell count. More than one half of patients who had infections before surgery did not have any infections after splenectomy.[72] Besides symptomatic neutropenia, other indications for splenectomy include transfusion-dependent anemia and profound thrombocytopenia.

PREOPERATIVE CONSIDERATIONS

Vaccination

Splenectomy imparts a small (<1 to 5%) but definite lifetime risk of fulminant, potentially life-threatening infection (see "Overwhelming Postsplenectomy Infection" for further discussion on the risk of infection). Therefore, when elective splenectomy is planned, vaccinations against encapsulated bacteria should be given at least 2 weeks before surgery to protect against such infection. The most common bacteria to cause serious infections in asplenic hosts are *Streptococcus pneumoniae*, *H. influenzae* type B, and meningococcus. Vaccinations against these bacteria are available and should be given.

If the spleen is removed emergently (e.g., for trauma), vaccinations should be given as soon as possible after surgery, with at least 1 to 2 days allowed for recovery. After splenectomy, annual influenza immunization is advisable. Splenectomized patients should be well educated regarding the potential consequences of overwhelming postsplenectomy infection and should be encouraged to maintain documentation of their own immunization status.[73]

Splenic Artery Embolization

The presumed advantages and disadvantages of SAE as a preoperative adjunct to elective splenectomy were discussed previously in the section "Imaging for Evaluation of Size and Pathology: Angiography." To reiterate, the purported advantages of preoperative SAE include reduced operative blood loss from a devascularized spleen[19] and reduced spleen size, which allows easier dissection and removal. Its detractors argue that equivalent splenectomy-related blood loss,[74] the need for more analgesics and occasionally an extended hospital stay preoperatively, the possibility of pancreatitis, and the well-described risks of invasive arteriography cancel out any presumed benefits of preoperative embolization.[75] No consensus exists at this time concerning the role of preoperative SAE with regard to elective splenectomy. It is the authors' practice to preoperatively embolize spleens measuring ≥20 cm in length; this has allowed even spleens >30 cm to be resected laparoscopically with an excellent conversion rate.

Deep Vein Thrombosis Prophylaxis

Deep vein thrombosis (DVT) after splenectomy is not infrequent, especially in cases involving splenomegaly and myeloproliferative disorders.[76] The risk of portal vein thrombosis (PVT) may reach 40% for patients presenting with both splenomegaly and myeloproliferative disorders. Postsplenectomy PVT typically presents with anorexia, abdominal pain, leukocytosis, and thrombocytosis. Effective PVT treatment is possible by maintaining a high index of suspicion, achieving early diagnosis with contrast-enhanced CT, and starting anticoagulation immediately. DVT prophylaxis, including use of sequential compression devices and SC administration of heparin (5000 U), should be initiated for patients undergoing splenectomy.[77] In the prevention of venous thromboembolism after splenectomy, no clear advantage has been confirmed for the use of low molecular weight heparin (LMWH) rather than low-dose unfractionated heparin.[78] Each patient's risk factors for DVT should be evaluated, and when elevated risk exists (obesity, history of prior venous thromboembolism, known hypercoagulable state, older age), a more aggressive antithrombotic regimen, including LMWH, may be pursued.

SPLENECTOMY TECHNIQUES

Patient Preparation

All patients undergoing elective splenectomy should be vaccinated at least 1 week preoperatively with polyvalent pneumococcal, meningococcal, and *Haemophilus* vaccines. Assessment of the potential need for transfusion of blood products and optimization of preoperative coagulation status are necessary. It is the authors' practice to order blood typing and antibody screening tests for normosplenic patients undergoing elective splenectomy. Anemic patients should be transfused before surgery to a hemoglobin level of 10 g/dL. In more complex cases, including patients with splenomegaly, at least 2 to 4 units of cross-matched blood should be available at the time of surgery. Thrombocytopenia may be transiently corrected with platelet transfusions. Thrombocytopenic patients preferably should not undergo transfusion before the day of surgery and ideally not before the intraoperative ligation of the splenic artery.

Patients who have been maintained on corticosteroid therapy preoperatively should receive parenteral corticosteroid therapy perioperatively. Bowel preparation is not routinely performed for patients undergoing elective splenectomy. All splenectomy patients do receive DVT prophylaxis, as discussed previously. After endotracheal intubation, a nasogastric (NG) tube is inserted for stomach decompression.

Open Splenectomy

Although laparoscopic surgery increasingly has achieved acceptance as the standard approach for normosplenic patients requiring splenectomy, open splenectomy (OS) is still widely practiced. Traumatic rupture of the spleen continues as the most common indication for OS. Several other clinical scenarios favor an OS approach, including massive splenomegaly, ascites, portal hypertension, multiple prior operations, extensive splenic irradiation, and possible splenic abscess.

During OS, the patient is placed in the supine position with the surgeon situated at the patient's right. A left subcostal incision paralleling the left costal margin and lying two fingerbreadths below it is preferred for most elective splenectomies. A midline incision is optimal for exposure when the spleen is ruptured or massively enlarged or when abdominal access is needed for a staging laparotomy for Hodgkin's disease. A thoracoabdominal incision, although rarely used, may be necessary for access to a challenging or significantly enlarged spleen.

The spleen is mobilized by dividing ligamentous attachments, usually beginning with the splenocolic ligament (Fig. 34-5). In patients with significant splenomegaly, once lesser sac access has been achieved through either the gastrosplenic or gastrohepatic attachments, ligating the splenic artery in continuity along the superior border of the pancreas may be preferable. This maneuver may serve several purposes: allowing safer manipulation of the spleen and dissection of the splenic hilum, facilitating some shrinkage of the spleen, and providing an autotransfusion of erythrocytes and platelets. Further medial mobilization of the spleen is achieved by incising its lateral peritoneal attachments, most notably the splenophrenic ligament. Then follows individual ligation and sequential division of the short gastric vessels, steps that if carefully executed reduce the risk of these vessels' retracting and bleeding. Splenic hilar dissection then takes place. Whenever possible, care should be taken to dissect and individually ligate the splenic artery and vein (in that order) before dividing them. As noted in the discussion of splenic anatomy, the tail of the pancreas lies within 1 cm of the splenic hilum in 75% of patients; therefore, during hilar dissection great care must be taken to avoid injuring the pancreas.

Once the spleen is excised, hemostasis is secured by irrigating, suctioning, and scrupulously inspecting the bed of dissection. The splenic bed is not routinely drained. A thorough search for accessory spleens must be undertaken when a hematologic disorder has occasioned splenectomy. At the completion of surgery, the nasogastric tube is removed.

Laparoscopic Splenectomy

Laparoscopic splenectomy (LS) has steadily supplanted OS as the approach of choice for most elective splenectomies. The benefits of LS for patients with normal-sized spleens were described first in case reports and then in large series. An ever-increasing amount of research confirms the value of LS, in appropriately experienced hands, for a growing number of patient groups: patients with splenomegaly, those with multiple prior abdominal operations, morbidly obese patients, those who need concomitant procedures, and even pregnant patients.[6]

Since the introduction of the lateral approach,[77] most LS procedures are now performed with the patient in the right lateral decubitus

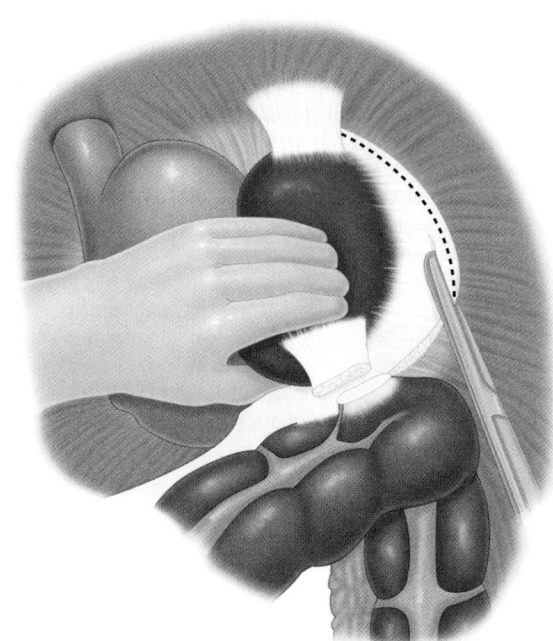

FIG. 34-5. Splenocolic ligament is divided at the beginning of open splenectomy.

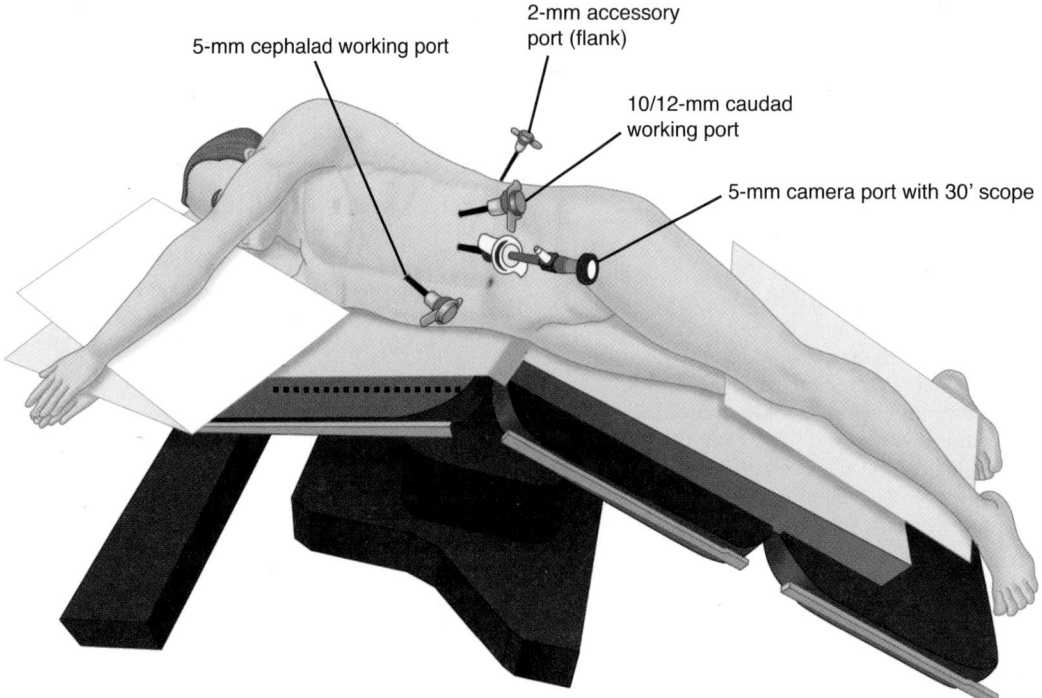

5-mm cephalad working port

2-mm accessory port (flank)

10/12-mm caudad working port

5-mm camera port with 30' scope

FIG. 34-6. Patient positioning and trocar placement for laparoscopic splenectomy.

position (Fig. 34-6). A midway "double-access" technique in which the patient is in a 45-degree right lateral decubitus position has also been advocated. This positioning permits concomitant surgery, such as laparoscopic cholecystectomy, more easily than does the lateral approach. The double-access technique requires the placement of five or six trocars. The lateral approach routinely involves the use of three or four trocars positioned as shown in Fig. 34-6. Use of an angled (30- or 45-degree) laparoscope (2 mm, 5 mm, or 10 mm) greatly facilitates the procedure. Exposure of the vital anatomy in a manner that allows for a more intuitive sequence of dissection, paralleling that of OS, may be considered an additional advantage of the lateral approach.

Placement of trocars in the left upper quadrant should be performed under laparoscopic visualization, particularly if any degree of splenomegaly exists, because the latter can significantly reduce the available operating space. As with OS, the splenocolic ligament and the lateral peritoneal attachments are divided with resultant medial mobilization of the spleen. The short gastric vessels may be divided by any number of methods, including individual application of clips, endovascular stapling, or, most commonly, use of hemostatic energy sources as in ultrasonic dissection, diathermy, or radiofrequency ablation. With the lower pole of the spleen gently retracted, the splenic hilum is accessible to further applications of clips or an endovascular stapling device. The splenic artery and vein are divided separately when possible (Fig. 34-7). Good long-term outcomes, however, are increasingly being achieved with mass hilar stapling (Fig. 34-8). Using the lateral approach with the spleen thus elevated, the surgeon can easily visualize the tail of the pancreas and avoid injury when placing the endovascular stapler.

Once excised, the spleen is placed in a durable ripstop nylon sack (Fig. 34-9), the neck of which is drawn through one of the 10-mm trocar sites. Morcellation of the spleen takes place within the sack and allows piecemeal extraction; a blunt instrument should be used to disrupt and remove the spleen to avoid the risk of sack rupture, spillage of contents, and subsequent splenosis (Fig. 34-10).

Hand-assisted LS has been suggested as a safer, more expeditiously performed procedure, especially in patients with splenomegaly. In this technique, which under direct laparoscopic visualization allows identification, retraction, and dissection of appropriate tissues

by palpation, the surgeon's left hand is completely introduced into the peritoneal cavity (left-handed surgeons would insert their right hands). Hemostasis is achieved by the use of clips, staples, and energy sources similar to those described earlier. The excised specimen is delivered via the hand access port. In cases in which normal-sized spleens are removed, the advantages of the hand-assisted approach may be lessened due to the size of the incision necessary to admit the surgeon's hand.

Partial Splenectomy

The past few decades have witnessed ever-widening endorsement for and practice of partial splenectomy. This technique, initially

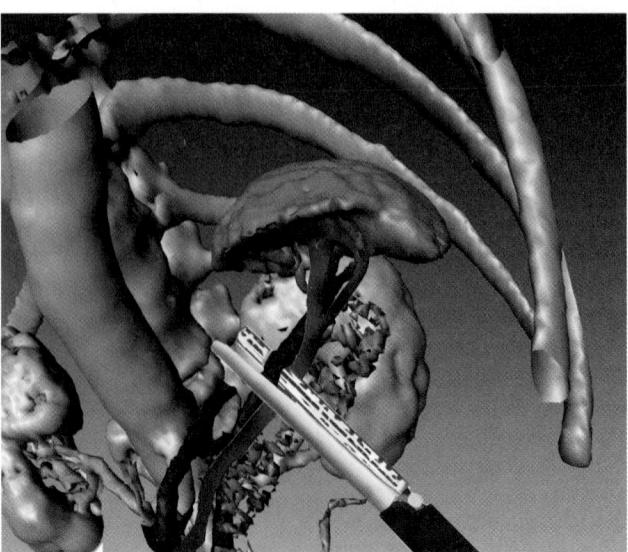

FIG. 34-7. Splenic artery and vein are ligated individually when the anatomy is favorable. (*Courtesy of Ivan George, University of Maryland School of Medicine.*)

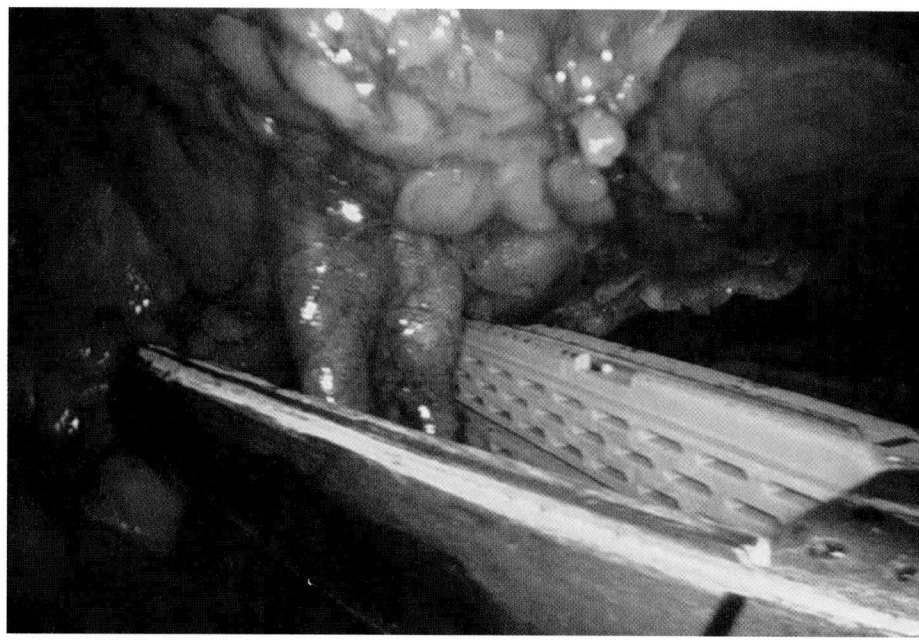

FIG. 34-8. Splenic hilum can be divided laparoscopically en masse.

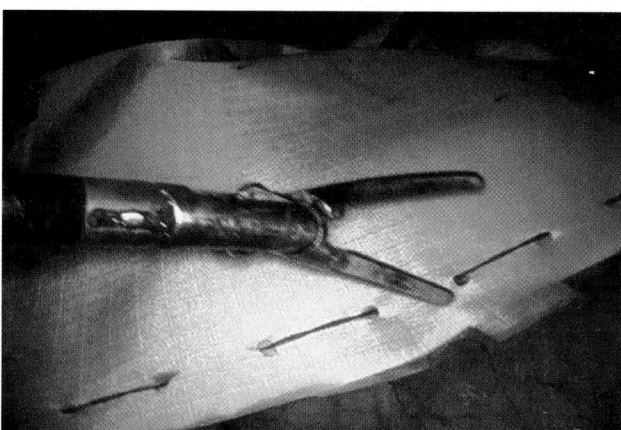

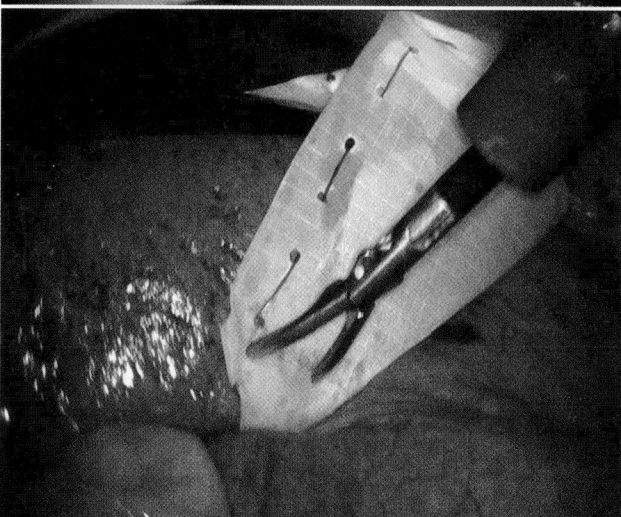

FIG. 34-9. Spleen is placed into a ripstop nylon bag before morcellation.

reported in the early eighteenth century, is particularly indicated to minimize the risk of postsplenectomy sepsis in children. Certain lipid storage disorders leading to splenomegaly (e.g., Gaucher's disease) and some forms of traumatic splenic injury (blunt and penetrating) are amenable to treatment with partial splenectomy. Both the laparoscopic and open approaches for partial splenectomy have been well described. The spleen must be adequately mobilized, and the splenic hilar vessels attached to the targeted segment ligated and divided. The devascularized segment of spleen is transected along an obvious line of demarcation. Bleeding from the cut surface of the spleen usually is limited and can be controlled by various methods, including cauterization, argon coagulation, or application of direct hemostatic agents such as cellulose gauze and fibrin glue.

Inadvertent Intraoperative Splenic Injury (Fig. 34-11)

Inadvertent intraoperative injury to the spleen is a noted occurrence in the surgical literature, familiar to and dreaded by the abdominal surgeon. The true incidence is unknown. It is likely underreported, although far from uncommon. The gravity of such injury is not to be underestimated. In addition to the risk of death, significant short-term morbidity is associated with injury to the spleen, including increased blood loss, need for transfusion, and prolonged hospital stay.[80]

Intraoperative injury to the spleen has been linked with numerous operations commonly performed by abdominal surgeons, such as gastric fundoplication, colectomy, paraesophageal hernia repair, nephrectomy, and abdominal and pelvic vascular surgery.[81-83] There are also reports of splenic injuries after endoscopic procedures, such as colonoscopy.[84-87]

Improper traction on the spleen against its peritoneal attachments is the most common mechanism of intraoperative injury. Capsular tears are the most common type of injury, but parenchymal lacerations and subcapsular hematomas also occur. The lower pole is more commonly injured, owing to its orientation as well as the greater concentration of peritoneal attachments found here.[88]

The time-honored surgical tenets of liberal exposure and visualization are particularly germane to the avoidance of splenic injury. Incisions and approaches must be tailored to both patient circumstances and surgeon experience. There is some evidence to support the assertion that use of the laparoscopic approach may reduce the incidence of splenic injury for certain operations.[89] An unexpected flow or pooling of blood from the left upper quadrant should raise suspicion of possible splenic injury. As with all hemorrhage, prompt temporary control of bleeding is required. Direct compression of the spleen itself, packing of the left upper quadrant, compression of

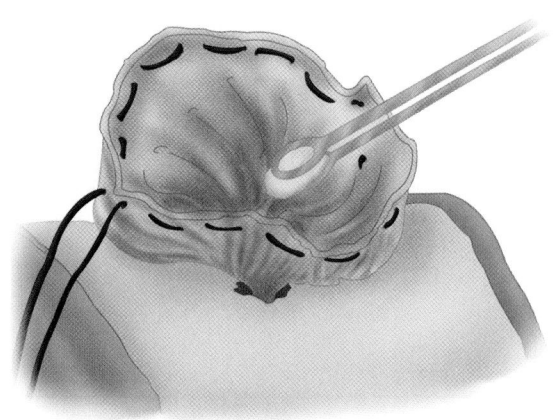 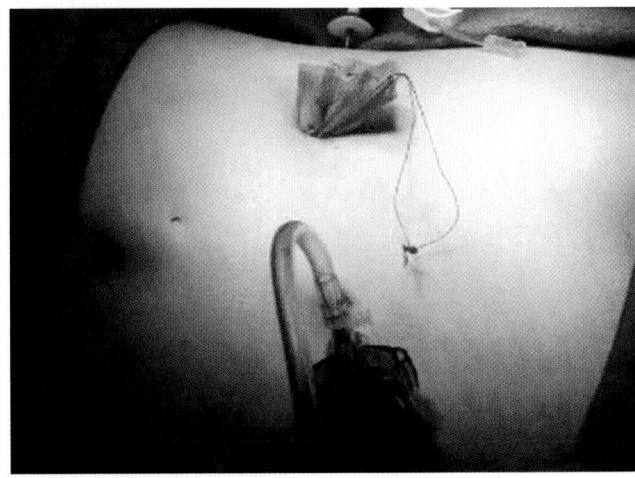

FIG. 34-10. Morcellation and extraction of the spleen with the nylon sack extending through the 10-mm trocar site. *(Illustration is reproduced with permission from Park A et al: Laparoscopic vs open splenectomy.* Arch Surg *134(11):1263, 1999. Copyright © 1999 American Medical Association. All rights reserved.)*

the vessels at the splenic hilum or pressure on the splenic artery at the superior pancreatic margin, or supraceliac compression of the aorta can slow or stop hemorrhage and allow more deliberate consideration of management options.

As the patient's condition is stabilized, the spleen is mobilized from its peritoneal attachments and the nature of the injury assessed. Overall, the patient's condition is the primary determinant of whether splenic salvage can be attempted. Hemodynamic instability, hemorrhage requiring transfusion, hypothermia, and coagulopathy are all situations more suited to prompt splenectomy and hemostasis. The type of injury plays a role as well; it has been suggested that hilar injury is best managed by splenectomy.[80] Barring these unfavorable circumstances, however, and recalling that the majority of intraoperative splenic injuries are capsular tears, it is reasonable to expect that splenic preservation can be achieved in many appropriately selected situations. Presented with one of these situations, the surgeon has at his or her disposal a number of useful and well-described splenorrhaphy techniques: application of topical hemostatics,[80] suture plication of disrupted parenchyma with or without omental buttress,[80,90] and the use of bioabsorbable mesh sheets sutured as buttressing "jackets," which compress the organ while simultaneously promoting clot formation at the level of the splenic capsule.[80,91]

SPLENECTOMY OUTCOMES

Changes in blood composition resulting from splenectomy include the appearance of Howell-Jolly bodies and siderocytes. After splenectomy leukocytosis and increased platelet counts are common as well. Although platelet counts most often rise within 2 days, they may not peak for several weeks in patients with preoperative thrombocytopenia (see "Hematologic Outcomes" later). Similarly, within 1 day after splenectomy the white blood cell count typically rises, and such elevation may continue for several months.

Complications

Complications of splenectomy may be classified as pulmonary, hemorrhagic, infectious, pancreatic, and thromboembolic. Left lower lobe atelectasis is the most common complication after OS; pleural effusion and pneumonia also can occur. Hemorrhage can occur intraoperatively or postoperatively, presenting as subphrenic hematoma. Transfusions have become less common since the advent of LS, although the indication for operation influences the likelihood of transfusion as well. Subphrenic abscess and wound infection are among the perioperative infectious complications. The

placement of a drain in the left upper quadrant may be associated with postoperative subphrenic abscess and is not routinely recommended. Pancreatitis, pseudocyst, and pancreatic fistula are among the pancreatic complications that may result from intraoperative trauma to the pancreas during dissection of the splenic hilum. Thromboembolic phenomena are well described in patients undergoing splenectomy; therefore DVT prophylaxis is routinely recommended. In patients with hemolytic anemia or myeloproliferative disorders and splenomegaly, thrombotic risk is heightened, particularly the risk of portal vein thrombosis.[76] Patients undergoing splenectomy for malignancy or myeloproliferative disorders should be strongly considered for perioperative pharmacoprophylaxis, either LMWH or unfractionated heparin.

Hematologic Outcomes

The results of splenectomy may be appraised according to the level of hematologic response (e.g., rise in platelet and hemoglobin levels) in those disorders in which the spleen contributes to the hematologic problem. Hematologic responses may be divided into initial and long-term responses. For thrombocytopenia, an initial response typically is defined as a rise in platelet count within several days of splenectomy. Reported series demonstrate the effectiveness of LS in providing a long-term platelet response in approximately 80% of individuals with ITP (Table 34-2). These results are consistent with the long-term success rate associated with OS.[105,108]

For chronic hemolytic anemias, a rise in hemoglobin levels to >10 g/dL without the need for transfusion signifies a successful response to splenectomy. By this criterion, splenectomy has been reported to be successful for the vast majority of patients with chronic hemolytic anemia. For hemolytic anemia due to spherocytosis, the success rate is usually higher, ranging from 90 to 100%.[109]

Splenectomy results also may be examined in terms of surgical and postsurgical characteristics, including operative time, recovery time, and morbidity and mortality rates, all of which tend to vary according to hematologic indication (Tables 34-3 and 34-4).

Results of few prospective, randomized trials comparing LS and OS have been published. In one prospective study investigators randomly assigned 28 thalassemia patients to undergo OS or LS.[100] There were no mortalities and no differences in complication rates in the two groups. Some differences were noted in operative times, transfusion requirements, and length of stay, but no hematologic outcome data have yet been published. Previously reported retrospective comparisons between LS and OS indicate that the laparoscopic approach typically results in longer operative times, shorter hospital stays, lower morbidity rates, similar blood loss, and similar mortality

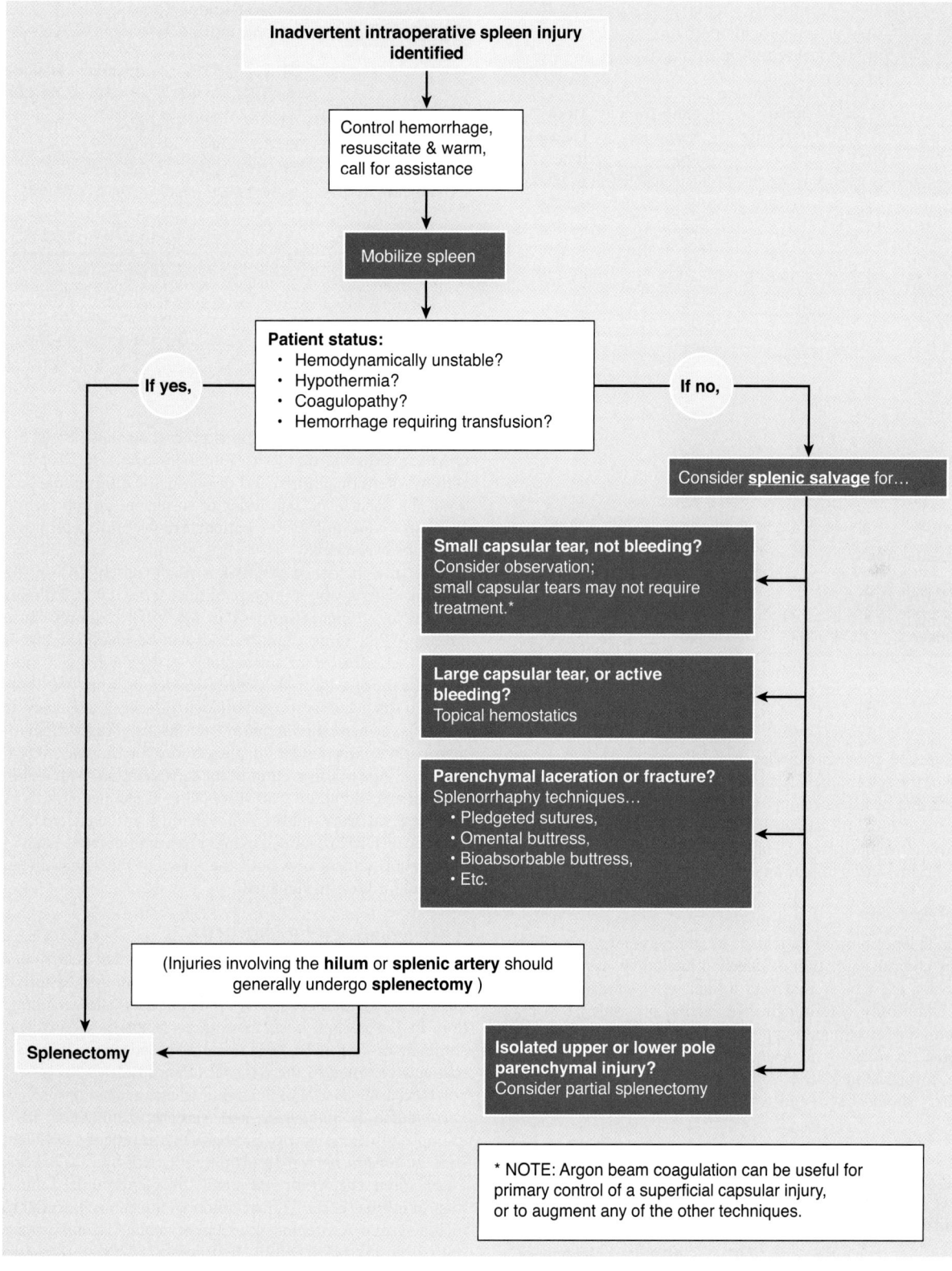

FIG. 34-11. Treatment algorithm for inadvertent intraoperative spleen injury.

rates compared with OS.[79,105] A meta-analysis of 51 series encompassing >2900 patients generally supports these observations, although there was a suggestion that hemorrhagic complications may be higher with the laparoscopic approach.[111] Questions of the cost effectiveness of LS persist, although analysis of this issue is hindered by a lack of universally accepted metrics as well as a paucity of recent objective data. Proponents of LS argue that the generally higher operating room charges are offset by the reduced hospital stay and presumably shorter time of lost productivity.[100] For those institutions with experienced personnel and technical capability, the laparoscopic approach has emerged as the standard for elective, nontraumatic splenectomy.

Overwhelming Postsplenectomy Infection

Asplenic patients bear an increased susceptibility to infection for the remainder of their lives. Although the overwhelming majority of

TABLE 34-2	Platelet response after laparoscopic splenectomy for idiopathic thrombocytopenic purpura			
Study	n	No. Showing Initial Response (%)	No. Showing Long-Term Response (%)	Mean Follow-Up (mo)
Vianelli et al[92]	402	86	66	57
Szold et al[93]	104	NA	84	36
Balague et al[94]	103	89	75	33
Katkhouda et al[2]	67	84	78	38
Wu et al[95]	67	83	74	23
Duperier et al[96]	67	NA	64	22
Berends et al[97]	50	86	64	35
Trias et al[98]	48	NA	88	30
Tanoue et al[99]	35	83	79	36
Friedman et al[100]	31	NA	93	2
Stanton[101]	30	89	89	30
Fass et al[102]	29	90	80	43
Bresler et al[103]	27	93	88	28
Harold et al[104]	27	92	85	20
Lozano-Salazar et al[105]	22	89	88	15
Meyer et al[106]	16	NA	86	14
Watson et al[107]	13	100	83	60
Total/mean	**1138**	**89**	**80**	**31**

NA = not available.

splenectomized patients experience no ill consequence from the absence of the spleen, the potentially catastrophic consequences of overwhelming postsplenectomy infection (OPSI) demand lifelong vigilance and intimate knowledge of the appropriate precautions and preventative measures. All involved—patient, family members, and physicians—need to play an active role.

Clinical Features

Sepsis in splenectomized patients is a medical emergency. Therefore, any clinical suggestion of infection, including seemingly isolated fevers, must be viewed with a high index of suspicion and treated empirically as thorough investigation proceeds. OPSI may begin with a relatively mild-appearing prodrome with nonspecific symptoms. In addition to fever, nonspecific symptoms such as malaise, myalgias, headache, vomiting, diarrhea, abdominal pain, and others should be viewed with alarm in the asplenic patient.

TABLE 34-3	Laparoscopic splenectomy results by hematologic indication (data from Rosen et al)			
	ITP (n = 65)	TTP (n = 9)	Anemia (n = 11)	Malignancy (n = 43)
OR time (min)	134	127	171	170
EBL (mL)	126	161	271	380
LOS (days)	2.8	8.3	2.6	4.3
Conversions from LS to OS	0	0	0	5
Complications	7	0	0	8
Response rate	85%	89%	91%	74%

EBL = estimated blood loss; ITP = idiopathic thrombocytopenic purpura; LOS = length of hospital stay; LS = laparoscopic splenectomy; OR = operating room; OS = open splenectomy; TTP = thrombotic thrombocytopenic purpura.
Source: Data from Rosen et al.[110]

TABLE 34-4	Laparoscopic splenectomy results by hematologic indication (data from Park et al)			
	ITP (n = 151)	TTP (n = 7)	Anemia (n = 40)	Malignancy (n = 28)
OR time (min)	128	146	149	165
EBL (mL)	137	96	116	238
LOS (days)	2.2	3.0	2.2	2.6
Conversions from LS to OS	3 (2%)	1 (14%)	1 (3%)	1 (4%)
Complications	14 (9%)	0	1 (3%)	3 (11%)

EBL = estimated blood loss; ITP = idiopathic thrombocytopenic purpura; LOS = length of hospital stay; LS = laparoscopic splenectomy; OR = operating room; OS = open splenectomy; TTP = thrombotic thrombocytopenic purpura.
Source: Data from Park A, McKinlay R: Spleen, in Brunicardi FC, Andersen DK, Billiar TR, et al (eds): *Schwartz's Principles of Surgery*, 8th ed. New York: McGraw-Hill, 2005, p 1312.

Absent the spleen, the infectious process signaled by such symptoms can progress rapidly to fulminant bacteremic septic shock, with hypotension, anuria, and disseminated intravascular coagulation. The need for a high index of suspicion, prompt action, and aggressive education of the patient, family, and medical provider cannot be overstated.

The true incidence of OPSI is not precisely known, because defining criteria vary among published series. Overall lifetime risk remains low, ranging from <1 to 5%.[73,112–114] Among those who develop OPSI, some characteristics can be identified that impart greater risk. Reason for splenectomy is the single most influential determinant of OPSI risk. Case series demonstrate that those who undergo splenectomy for hematologic disease (malignancy, myelodysplasia, or hemoglobinopathy) are far more susceptible to OPSI than patients who undergo splenectomy for trauma or iatrogenic reasons.[73] Age is also an important consideration, with children <5 years of age and adults >50 years being at elevated risk.[114] Finally, time interval from spleen removal must be considered. A large number of OPSI cases occur many years to decades later.[112] This observation underscores both the threat of this lethal disease and the need for lifelong vigilance.

Microbiology and Pathogenesis

Life-threatening infection in the asplenic patient is attributable to three factors: loss of splenic macrophages, diminished tuftsin production, and loss of the spleen's reticuloendothelial screening function. In the normal host, these three factors work in concert to eliminate opsonized bacteria from the bloodstream. This system is particularly suited to the removal of encapsulated bacteria, whose polysaccharide coating is a natural defense against opsonization (*S. pneumoniae*, *H. influenzae*, and *Neisseria meningitidis* are classic examples). Infections with protozoa that invade the red blood cell, such as *Babesia microti* (transmitted by tick bites), *Ehrlichia*, and *Plasmodium*, occur more frequently in splenectomized individuals than in normal hosts.[73] Other potential infectious bacterial sources include group A streptococci, *Capnocytophaga canimorsus* (transmitted by dog bites), group B streptococci, *Enterococcus* species, *Bacteroides* species, *Salmonella* species, and *Bartonella* species.[115] In the absence of the spleen, elimination of these pathogens from the bloodstream falls solely to the liver, a process that has been demonstrated to be less effective.[8]

Role of Vaccination

Mortality rates for OPSI in the prevaccination era are testimony to the importance of the vaccines available today. The use of currently available vaccines against pneumococcus and other encapsulated organisms has led to a drop in the overall incidence of OPSI to <1%.[112] The mechanism by which vaccination protects asplenic patients is not entirely understood. Serum antibody titers do not necessarily correspond to clinical immunity.[116] Moreover, antibody levels after pneumococcus vaccination decline steadily within 5 to 10 years. Revaccination is reasonably recommended for these patients, although the efficacy of this measure is not proven.[112] Timing of vaccination generally is accepted as a minimum of 2 weeks before planned elective splenectomy and within 7 to 10 days after unplanned or emergent splenectomy, although data supporting this practice are lacking.

Despite the current marked reduction in OPSI-related mortality, an alarming number of "vaccine failures" have been noted. OPSI developed in 41% of patients in one trauma series, despite the fact that these patients received the appropriate vaccines after splenectomy.[112] Nonetheless, vaccination of asplenic patients against encapsulated organisms has value when applied to the population as a whole. The most common causal organism, accounting for as many as 50 to 90% of all OPSI cases, remains pneumococcus. Meningococcus, *H. influenzae* type B, and group A streptococci follow in order of frequency.[115]

Antibiotics and the Asplenic Patient

Antibiotic therapy for the asplenic patient can be considered in three contexts: deliberate therapy for established or presumed infections, prophylaxis in anticipation of invasive procedures (e.g., dental procedures), and general prophylaxis. For the latter two indications, unfortunately, evidence supporting efficacy is scant, and guidelines for antibiotic prophylaxis are not uniform. Optimal duration of chemoprophylaxis in children is unclear. Daily doses of antibiotics until 5 years of age or at least 5 years after splenectomy are commonly recommended,[117] although some advocate continuation into at least young adulthood.[115] Concerns regarding compliance and bacterial resistance have been raised, which have led some authors to suggest that lifelong daily antibiotic prophylaxis be recommended only for those patients whose antibody titers fail to respond appropriately to vaccination or, alternately, that asplenic patients be advised to carry at all times a reserve supply of antibiotic to be self-administered at the earliest sign of infection.[118] Confounding the issue further, OPSI has been noted to occur even in appropriately vaccinated patients taking daily antibiotic prophylaxis at the time of infection.[118] Considering OPSI's grave consequences as well as its relatively low incidence, controlled trials resulting in meaningful data on this issue seem unlikely to be performed.

Several risk management strategies are commonly recommended to asplenic patients: wearing a medical bracelet, carrying a laminated medical alert card, possessing a medical letter with specific empiric therapy instructions (including drug names and dosages), and keeping a 5-day supply of stand-by antibiotics, particularly when travel is anticipated.[73] A recent review of the literature provides no reason to depart from these precautions.

REFERENCES

Entries highlighted in bright blue are key references.

1. Moynihan B: The surgery of the spleen. *Br J Surg* 8:307, 1920.
2. Katkhouda N, Hurwitz MG, Rivera RT, et al: Laparoscopic splenectomy: Outcome and efficacy in 103 consecutive patients. *Ann Surg* 228:1, 1998.
3. Morgenstern L, Skandalakis JE: Anatomy and embryology of the spleen, in Hiatt JR, Phillips EH, Morgenstern L (eds): *Surgical Diseases of the Spleen.* Berlin/Heidelberg: Springer-Verlag, 1997, p 15.
4. Poulin EC, Thibault C: The anatomical basis for laparoscopic splenectomy. *Can J Surg* 36:484, 1993.
5. Schwartz SI: Spleen, in Schwartz SI (ed): *Principles of Surgery: Specific Considerations,* 7th ed. New York: McGraw-Hill, 1999, p 1501.
6. Weiss CA, Kavic SM, Adrales GL, et al: Laparoscopic splenectomy: What barriers remain? *Surg Innov* 12:23, 2005.
7. Weiss L: Mechanisms of splenic clearance of the blood: A structural overview of the mammalian spleen, in Bowdler AJ (ed): *The Spleen. Structure, Function and Significance.* London: Chapman and Hall Medical, 1990, p 23.
8. Frank EL, Neu HC: Postsplenectomy infection. *Surg Clin North Am* 61:135, 1981.
9. Hosea SW: Role of the spleen in pneumococcal infection. *Lymphology* 16:115, 1983.
10. Lucey BC, Boland GW, Maher MM, et al: Percutaneous nonvascular splenic intervention: A 10-year review. *Am J Roentgenol* 179:1591, 2002.
11. Lieberman S, Libson E, Sella T, et al: Percutaneous image-guided splenic procedures: Update on indications, technique, complications, and outcomes. *Semin Ultrasound CT MR* 28:57, 2007.
12. Myers J: Focused assessment with sonography for trauma (FAST): The truth about ultrasound in blunt trauma. *J Trauma* 62(6 Suppl):S28, 2007.
13. Thompson BE, Munera F, Cohn SM, et al: Novel computed tomography scan scoring system predicts the need for intervention after splenic injury. *J Trauma* 60:1083, 2006.
14. Kamaya A, Weinstein S, Desser TS: Multiple lesions of the spleen: Differential diagnosis of cystic and solid lesions. *Semin Ultrasound CT MR* 27:389, 2006.
15. Karakas HM, Tuncbilek N, Okten OO: Splenic abnormalities: An overview on sectional images. *Diagn Interv Radiol* 11:152, 2005.
16. Dent D, Alsabrook G, Erickson BA, et al: Blunt splenic injuries: High nonoperative management rate can be achieved with selective embolization. *J Trauma* 56:1063, 2004.
17. Koconis KG, Singh H, Soares G: Partial splenic embolization in the treatment of patients with portal hypertension: A review of the English language literature. *J Trauma* 18:463, 2007.
18. Miyazaki M, Itoh H, Kaiho T, et al: Partial splenic embolization for the treatment of chronic idiopathic thrombocytopenic purpura. *Am J Roentgenol* 163:123, 1994.
19. Naoum JJ, Silberfein EJ, Zhou W, et al: Concomitant intraoperative splenic artery embolization and laparoscopic splenectomy versus laparoscopic splenectomy: Comparison of treatment outcome. *Am J Surg* 193:713, 2007.
20. Williams G, Rosen MP, Parker JA, et al: Splenic implants detected by SPECT images of Tc-99m labeled damaged red blood cells. *Clin Nucl Med* 31:467, 2006.
21. Lui EH, Lau KK: Intra-abdominal splenosis: How clinical history and imaging features averted an invasive procedure for tissue diagnosis. *Australas Radiol* 49:342, 2005.
22. Radaelli F, Faccini P, Goldaniga M, et al: Factors predicting response to splenectomy in adult patients with idiopathic thrombocytopenic purpura. *Haematologica* 85:1040, 2000.
23. Cools L, Osteaux M, Divano L, et al: Prediction of splenic volume by a simple CT measurement: A statistical study. *J Comp Assist Tomogr* 7:426, 1983.
24. Yetter EM, Acosta KB, Olson MC, et al: Estimating splenic volume: Sonographic measurements correlated with helical CT determination. *AJR Am J Roentgenol* 181:1615, 2003.
25. Schwartz SI, Cooper RA Jr.: Surgery in the diagnosis and treatment of Hodgkin's disease. *Adv Surg* 6:175, 1972.
26. Gallagher PG, Jarolim P: Red cell membrane disorders, in Hoffman R (ed): *Hematology: Basic Principles and Practice,* 3rd ed. New York: Churchill Livingstone, 2001, p 576.
27. Bates G, Brown C: Incidence of gallbladder disease in chronic hemolytic anemia (spherocytosis). *Gastroenterology* 21:104, 1952.
28. Sandler A, Winkel G, Kimura K, et al: The role of prophylactic cholecystectomy during splenectomy in children with hereditary spherocytosis. *J Pediatr Surg* 34:1077, 1999.
29. Prchal JT, Gregg XT: Red cell enzymopathies, in Hoffman R (ed): *Hematology: Basic Principles and Practice,* 3rd ed. New York: Churchill Livingstone, 2001, p 561.
30. Hamilton JW, Jones FGC: Glucose-6-phosphate dehydrogenase Guadalajara—a case of chronic non-spherocytic haemolytic anaemia responding to splenectomy and the role of splenectomy in this disorder. *Hematology* 9:307, 2004.
31. Hill J, Walsh RM, McHam S, et al: Laparoscopic splenectomy for autoimmune hemolytic anemia in patients with chronic lymphocytic leukemia: A case series and review of the literature. *Am J Hematol* 75:134, 2004.
32. Plikat K, Rogler G, Scholmerich J: Coombs-positive autoimmune hemolytic anemia in Crohn's disease. *Eur J Gastroenterol Hepatol* 17:661, 2005.
33. Schwartz SI: Role of splenectomy in hematologic disorders. *World J Surg* 20:1156, 1996.

34. al-Salem AH: Indications and complications of splenectomy for children with sickle cell disease. *J Pediatr Surg* 41:1909, 2006.

35. Vichinsky EP, Neumayr LD, Earles AN, et al: Causes and outcomes of the acute chest syndrome in sickle cell disease. National Acute Chest Syndrome Study Group. *N Engl J Med* 342:1855, 2000.

36. Lo L, Singer ST: Thalassemia: Current approach to an old disease. *Pediatr Clin North Am* 49:1165, 2002.

37. Rajabiani A, Heshmati P, Ghafouri M: Mean density of hemoglobin, a better discriminator of iron deficiency anemia from thalassemia. *MJIRC* 8:47, 2005.

38. Barrai I, Rosity A, Cappellozza G, et al: Beta-thalassemia in the Po delta: Selection, geography and population structure. *Am J Hum Genet* 36:1121, 1984.

39. al Hawsawi ZM, Hummaida TI, Ismail GA: Splenectomy in thalassaemia major: Experience at Madina Maternity and Children's Hospital, Saudi Arabia. *Ann Trop Paediatr* 21:155, 2001.

40. Phrommintikul A, Sukonthasarn A, Kanjanavanit R, et al: Splenectomy: A strong risk factor for pulmonary hypertension in patients with thalassaemia. *Heart* 92:1467, 2006.

41. Sheikha AK, Salih ZT, Kasnazan KH, et al: Prevention of overwhelming postsplenectomy infection in thalassemia patients by partial rather than total splenectomy. *Can J Surg* 50:382, 2007.

42. Casaccia M, Torelli P, Cavaliere D, et al: Laparoscopic lymph node biopsy in intra-abdominal lymphoma: High diagnostic accuracy achieved with a minimally invasive procedure. *Surg Laparosc Endosc Percutan Tech* 17:175, 2007.

43. Schellong G, Riepenhausen M: Late effects after therapy of Hodgkin's disease: Update 2003/04 on overwhelming post-splenectomy infections and secondary malignancies. *Klin Padiatr* 216:364, 2004.

44. Delpero JR, Houvenaeghel G, Gastaut JA, et al: Splenectomy for hypersplenism in chronic lymphocytic leukaemia and malignant non-Hodgkin's lymphoma. *Br J Surg* 77:443, 1990.

45. Golomb HM, Vardiman JW: Response to splenectomy in 65 patients with hairy cell leukemia: An evaluation of spleen weight and bone marrow involvement. *Blood* 61:349, 1983.

46. Magee MJ, McKenzie S, Filippa DA, et al: Hairy cell leukemia durability of response to splenectomy in 26 patients and treatment of relapse with androgens in 6 patients. *Cancer* 56:2557, 1985.

47. Schwartz SI, Cooper RA Jr.: Surgery in the diagnosis and treatment of Hodgkin's disease. *Adv Surg* 6:175, 1972.

48. Cines DB, Blanchette VS: Immune thrombocytopenic purpura. *N Engl J Med* 346:995, 2002.

49. Provan D, Newland A: Fifty years of idiopathic thrombocytopenic purpura (ITP): Management of refractory ITP in adults. *Br J Hematol* 188:933, 2002.

50. Huber MR, Kumar S, Tefferi A: Treatment advances in adult immune thrombocytopenic purpura. *Ann Hematol* 82:723, 2003.

51. Nabhan C, Kwaan HC: Current concepts in the diagnosis and treatment of thrombotic thrombocytopenic purpura. *Hematol Clin North Am* 17:177, 2003.

52. Torok TJ, Holman RC, Chorba TL: Increasing mortality from thrombotic thrombocytopenic purpura in the United States—analysis of national mortality data, 1968–1991. *Am J Hematol* 50:84, 1995.

53. Winslow GA, Nelson EW: Thrombotic thrombocytopenic purpura: Indications for results of splenectomy. *Am J Surg* 170:558, 1995.

54. Morrison VA: Chronic leukemias. *CA Cancer J Clin* 44:353, 1994.

55. Mesa RA, Elliott MA, Tefferi A: Splenectomy in chronic myeloid leukemia and myelofibrosis with myeloid metaplasia. *Blood Rev* 14:121, 2000.

56. Parker SL, Tang T, Bolden S, et al: Cancer statistics. *CA Cancer J Clin* 47:5, 1997.

57. Tefferi A, Murphy S: Current opinion in essential thrombocythemia: Pathogenesis, diagnosis, and management. *Blood Rev* 15:121, 2002.

58. Modan B: An epidemiological study of polycythemia vera. *Blood* 26:657, 1965.

59. Mesa RA, Silverstein MN, Jacobsen SJ, et al: Population-based incidence and survival figures in essential thrombocythemia and agnogenic myeloid metaplasia. An Olmsted County Study, 1976–1995. *Am J Hematol* 61:10, 1999.

60. Mesa RA: Myelofibrosis with myeloid metaplasia: Therapeutic options in 2003. *Curr Hematol Rep* 2:264, 2003.

61. Mesa RA, Nagorney DS, Schwager S, et al: Palliative goals, patient selection, and perioperative platelet management: Outcomes and lessons from three decades of splenectomy for myelofibrosis with myeloid metaplasia at the Mayo Clinic. *Cancer* 107:361, 2006.

62. Stephenson JT, DuBois JJ: Nonoperative management of spontaneous splenic rupture in infectious mononucleosis: A case report and review of the literature. *Pediatrics* 120:432, 2007.

63. Toubia NT, Tawk MM, Potts RM: Cough and spontaneous rupture of a normal spleen. *Chest* 128:1884, 2005.

64. Phillips G, Radosevich M, Lipsett P: Splenic abscess: Another look at an old disease. *Arch Surg* 132:1331, 1997.

65. Nakao A, Saito S, Yamano T, et al: Dermoid cyst of the spleen: Report of a case. *Surg Today* 29:660, 1999.

66. Comitalo JB: Laparoscopic treatment of splenic cysts. *JSLS* 5:313, 2001.

67. Lam KY, Tang V: Metastatic tumors to the spleen: A 25-year clinicopathologic study. *Arch Pathol Lab Med* 124:526, 2000.

68. Stone DL, Ginns EI, Krasnewich D, et al: Life-threatening splenic hemorrhage in two patients with Gaucher disease. *Am J Hematol* 64:140, 2000.

69. Xiao GQ, Zinberg JM, Unger PD: Asymptomatic sarcoidosis presenting as massive splenomegaly. *Am J Med* 113:698, 2002.

70. Nusair S, Kramer MR, Berkman N: Pleural effusion with splenic rupture as manifestations of recurrence of sarcoidosis following prolonged remission. *Respiration* 70:114, 2003.

71. Lee PC, Rhee RY, Gordon RY, et al: Management of splenic artery aneurysms: The significance of portal and essential hypertension. *J Am Coll Surg* 189:483, 1999.

72. Rashba EJ, Rowe JM, Packman CH: Treatment of the neutropenia of Felty syndrome. *Blood Rev* 10:177, 1996.

73. Davidson RN, Wall RA: Prevention and management of infections in patients without a spleen. *Clin Microbiol Infect* 7:657, 2001.

74. Farid H, O'Connell TX: Surgical management of massive splenomegaly. *Am Surg* 62:803, 1996.

75. Kimura F, Ito H, Shimizu H, et al: Partial splenic embolization for the treatment of hereditary spherocytosis. *Am J Roentgenol* 181:1021, 2003.

76. Winslow ER, Brunt LM, Drebin JA, et al: Portal vein thrombosis after splenectomy. *Am J Surg* 184:631, 2002.

77. Park AE, Gagner M, Pomp A: The lateral approach to laparoscopic splenectomy. *Am J Surg* 173:126, 1997.

78. Breddin HK: Low molecular weight heparins in the prevention of deep-vein thrombosis in general surgery. *Semin Thromb Hemost* 25(Suppl 3):83, 1999.

79. Park A, Marcaccio M, Sternbach M, et al: Laparoscopic vs. open splenectomy. *Arch Surg* 134:1263, 1999.

80. Cassar K, Munro A: Iatrogenic splenic injury. *J R Coll Surg Edinb* 47:731, 2002.

81. Biggs G, Hafron J, Feliciano J, et al: Treatment of splenic injury during laparoscopic nephrectomy with BioGlue, a surgical adhesive. *Urology* 66:882, 2005.

82. Eaton MA, Valentine J, Jackson MR, et al: Incidental splenic injury during abdominal vascular surgery: A case controlled analysis. *J Am Coll Surg* 190:58, 2000.

83. Hodge WA, DeWald RL: Splenic injury complicating the anterior thoracoabdominal surgical approach for scoliosis. *J Bone Joint Surg Am* 65:396, 1983.

84. Petersen CR, Adamsen S, Gocht-Jensen P: Splenic injury after colonoscopy. *Endoscopy* 40:76, 2008.

85. Badaoui R: Injury to the liver and spleen after diagnostic ERCP. *Can J Anesth* 49:755, 2002.

86. Cho CL, Yuen KK, Yeun CH, et al: Splenic laceration after endoscopic retrograde cholangiopancreatography. *Hong Kong Med J* 14:75, 2008.

87. Olenchock SA Jr., Lukaszczyk JJ, Reed J 3rd, et al: Splenic injury after intraoperative transesophageal echocardiography. *Ann Thorac Surg* 72:2141, 2001.

88. Hugh TB, Coleman MJ, Cohen A: Splenic protection in left upper quadrant operations. *Aust N Z J Surg* 56:925, 1986.

89. Hinder RA, Perdikis G, Klinger PJ, et al: The surgical option for gastroesophageal reflux disease. *Am J Med* 103:144S, 1997.

90. Feliciano DV, Bittondo CG, Mattox KL: A four-year experience with splenectomy versus splenorrhaphy. *Ann Surg* 201:5, 1985.

91. Tribble CG, Joob AW, Barone GW, et al: A new technique for wrapping the injured spleen with polyglactin mesh. *Am Surg* 53:661, 1987.

92. Vianelli N, Galli M, de Vivo A, et al: Efficacy and safety of splenectomy in immune thrombocytopenic purpura: Long-term results of 402 cases. *Haematologica* 90:72, 2005.

93. Szold A, Kais H, Keidar A, et al: Chronic idiopathic thrombocytopenic purpura (ITP) is a surgical disease. *Surg Endosc* 16:155, 2002.

94. Balague C, Vela S, Targarona EM, et al: Predictive factors for successful laparoscopic splenectomy in immune thrombocytopenic purpura: Study of clinical and laboratory data. *Surg Endosc* 20:1208, 2006.

95. Wu J, Lai R, Yuan R, et al: Laparoscopic splenectomy for idiopathic thrombocytopenic purpura. *Am J Surg* 187:720, 2004.

96. Duperier T, Brody F, Felsher J, et al: Predictive factors for successful laparoscopic splenectomy in patients with immune thrombocytopenic purpura. *Arch Surg* 139:61, 2004.

97. Berends FJ, Schep N, Cuesta MA, et al: Hematological long-term results of laparoscopic splenectomy for patients with idiopathic thrombocytopenic purpura: A case control study. *Surg Endosc* 18:766, 2004.

98. Trias M, Targarona EM, Espert JJ, et al: Impact of hematological diagnosis on early and late outcome after laparoscopic splenectomy: An analysis of 111 cases. *Surg Endosc* 14:556, 2000.

99. Tanoue K, Hashizume M, Morita M, et al: Results of laparoscopic splenectomy for immune thrombocytopenic purpura. *Am J Surg* 177:222, 1999.

100. Friedman RL, Fallas MJ, Carrol BJ, et al: Laparoscopic splenectomy for ITP. *Surg Endosc* 10:991, 1996.

101. Stanton CJ: Laparoscopic splenectomy for idiopathic thrombocytopenic purpura (ITP). A five-year experience. *Surg Endosc* 13:1083, 1999.

102. Fass SM, Hui TT, Lefor A, et al: Safety of laparoscopic splenectomy in elderly patients with idiopathic thrombocytopenic purpura. *Am Surg* 66:844, 2000.

103. Bresler L, Guerci A, Brunaud L, et al: Laparoscopic splenectomy for idiopathic thrombocytopenic purpura: Outcome and long-term results. *World J Surg* 26:111, 2002.

104. Harold KL, Schlinkert RT, Mann DK, et al: Long-term results of laparoscopic splenectomy for immune thrombocytopenic purpura. *Mayo Clin Proc* 74:37, 1999.

105. Lozano-Salazar RR, Herrera MF, Vargas-Vorackova F, et al: Laparoscopic versus open splenectomy for immune thrombocytopenic purpura. *Laparoscopy* 176:366, 1998.

106. Meyer G, Wichmann MW, Rau HG, et al: Laparoscopic splenectomy for idiopathic thrombocytopenic purpura. *Surg Endosc* 12:1348, 1998.

107. Watson DI, Conventry BJ, Chin T, et al: Laparoscopic versus open splenectomy for immune thrombocytopenic purpura. *Surgery* 121:18, 1997.

108. Cordera F, Long KH, Nagtorney DM, et al: Open versus laparoscopic splenectomy for idiopathic thrombocytopenia purpura: Clinical and economic analysis. *Surgery* 134:45, 2003.

109. Katkhouda N, Manhas S, Umbach TW: Laparoscopic splenectomy. *J Laparoendosc Adv Surg Tech* 11:383, 2001.

110. Rosen M, Brody F, Walsh RM, et al: Outcome of laparoscopic splenectomy based on hematologic indications. *Surg Endosc* 16:272, 2002.

111. Winslow E, Brunt M: Perioperative outcomes of laparoscopic versus open splenectomy: A meta-analysis with an emphasis on complications. *Surgery* 134:647, 2003.

112. Taylor MD, Genuit T, Napolitano LM: Overwhelming postsplenectomy sepsis and trauma: Time to consider revaccination? *J Trauma* 59:1482, 2005.

113. Weng J, Brown CV, Rhee P, et al: White blood cell and platelet counts can be used to differentiate between infection and the normal response after splenectomy for trauma: Prospective validation. *J Trauma* 59:1076, 2005.

114. Price VE, Blanchette MB, Ford-Jones EL, et al: The prevention and management of infections in children with asplenia or hyposplenia. *Infect Dis Clin North Am* 21:3, 2007.

115. Brigden ML, Pattullo AL: Prevention and management of overwhelming postsplenectomy infection—an update. *Crit Care Med* 27:836, 1999.

116. Reinert RR, Kaufhold A, Kühnemund O, et al: Serum antibody responses to vaccination with 23-valent pneumococcal vaccine in splenectomized patients. *Zentralbl Bakteriol* 281:481, 1994.

117. de Montalembert M, Lenoir G: Antibiotic prevention of pneumococcal infections in asplenic hosts: Admission of insufficiency. *Ann Hematol* 83:18, 2004.

118. Waghorn D: Overwhelming infection in asplenic patients: Current best practice preventive measures are not being followed. *J Clin Pathol* 54:214, 2001.

Abdominal Wall, Omentum, Mesentery, and Retroperitoneum

Neal E. Seymour and Robert L. Bell

ABDOMINAL WALL

General Considerations

The abdominal wall is defined superiorly by the costal margins, inferiorly by the symphysis pubis and pelvic bones, and posteriorly by the vertebral column. It serves to support and protect abdominal and retroperitoneal structures, and its complex muscular functions enable twisting and flexing motions of the trunk. Surgical implications of abdominal wall structure become apparent during the course of managing primary abdominal wall diseases or gaining access to the peritoneal cavity. A surgeon must have a thorough understanding of the arrangement of abdominal wall muscles and aponeuroses.

Surgical Anatomy

The abdominal wall is an anatomically complex, layered structure with segmentally derived blood supply and innervation (Fig. 35-1). It is mesodermal in origin and develops as bilateral migrating sheets that originate in the paravertebral region and envelop the future abdominal area. The leading edges of these structures develop into the rectus abdominis muscles, which eventually meet in the midline of the anterior abdominal wall. The muscle fibers of the rectus abdominis are arranged vertically and are encased within an aponeu-

rotic sheath, the anterior and posterior layers of which are fused in the midline at the *linea alba*. The rectus abdominis has insertions on the symphysis pubis and pubic bones, on the anteroinferior aspects of the fifth and sixth ribs, as well as on the seventh costal cartilages and the xiphoid process. The lateral border of the rectus muscles assumes a convex shape that gives rise to the surface landmark of the *linea semilunaris*. There usually are three tendinous intersections or inscriptions that cross the rectus muscles: one at the level of the xiphoid process, one at the level of the umbilicus, and one halfway between the xiphoid process and the umbilicus (see Fig. 35-1).

Lateral to the rectus sheath are three muscular layers with oblique fiber orientations relative to one another (Fig. 35-2). These layers are derived from the laterally migrating mesodermal tissues during the sixth to seventh week of fetal development, before fusion of the developing rectus abdominis muscles in the midline. The external oblique muscle runs inferiorly and medially, arising from the margins of the lowest eight ribs and costal cartilages. The external oblique muscle originates laterally on the latissimus dorsi and serratus anterior muscles, as well as on the iliac crest. Medially it forms a tendinous aponeurosis, which is contiguous with the anterior rectus sheath. The *inguinal ligament* is the inferior-most edge of the external oblique aponeurosis, reflected posteriorly in the area between the anterior superior iliac spine and pubic tubercle. The

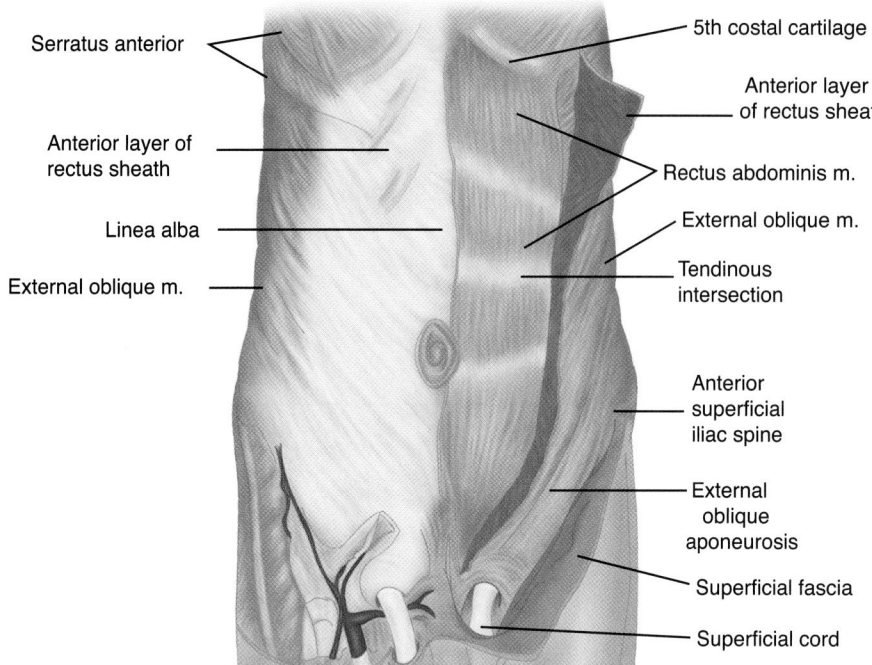

Serratus anterior

5th costal cartilage

Anterior layer
of rectus sheath

Anterior layer of
rectus sheath

Rectus abdominis m.

Linea alba

External oblique m.

External oblique m.

Tendinous
intersection

Anterior
superficial
iliac spine

External
oblique
aponeurosis

Superficial fascia

Superficial cord

FIG. 35-1. Anterior abdominal wall. The linea alba is the midline aponeurotic demarcation between the bellies of the rectus abdominis muscles. The rectus abdominis muscle and its tendinous intersections on the left are shown deep to the reflected anterior rectus sheath. Segmental cutaneous nerve branches also are shown. m. = muscle. [*Reproduced with permission from Moore KL, Dailey AF (eds):* Clinically Oriented Anatomy, *4th ed. Philadelphia: Lippincott Williams & Wilkins, 1999, p 181.*]

internal oblique muscle lies immediately deep to the external oblique muscle and arises from the lateral aspect of the inguinal ligament, the iliac crest, and the thoracolumbar fascia. Its fibers course superiorly and medially and form a tendinous aponeurosis that contributes components to both the anterior and posterior rectus sheath. The lower medial and inferior-most fibers of the internal oblique course may fuse with the lower fibers of the transversus abdominis muscle (the *conjoined area*). The inferior-most fibers of the internal oblique muscle are contiguous with the cremasteric muscle in the inguinal

canal. These relationships are of critical significance in the management of inguinal hernia. The transversus abdominis muscle is the deepest of the three lateral muscles and, as its name implies, runs transversely from the bilateral lowest six ribs, the lumbosacral fascia, and the iliac crest to the lateral border of the rectus abdominis musculoaponeurotic structures.

The complexities of the anterior and posterior aspects of the rectus sheath are best understood in their relationship to the *arcuate line* (semicircular line of Douglas), which lies roughly at the level of

KEY POINTS

1. Musculoaponeurotic anatomic features of the abdominal wall layers differ superior to and inferior to the arcuate line on the posterior aspect of the rectus sheath.

2. Defects of the complex process of abdominal wall development in the fetus can occur in several ways resulting in persistent midgut herniation (omphalocele and gastroschisis) or vitelline duct remnant abnormalities (Meckel's diverticulum, or vitelline duct fistula or cyst).

3. The management of rectus sheath hematomas consists of reversal of any anticoagulation or coagulopathy and observation, unless either hemodynamic instability or enlargement necessitates surgical evacuation.

4. Incisional hernias of the anterior abdominal wall may occur in up to 10–20% of prior abdominal operations of all types.

5. Primary suture repair of abdominal wall incisional hernias is associated with an unacceptably high incidence of hernia recurrence, and has prompted

the wide use of prosthetic mesh materials for hernia repair.

6. Laparoscopic incisional hernia repair offers important advantages over open repairs including reduced pain medication use, earlier return to normal function, and possibly superior protection from hernia recurrence.

7. Sclerosing mesenteritis is a poorly understood mesenteric process characterized by variable degrees of inflammation and fibrosis within mesenteric tissues of the small and large bowel, which frequently requires surgical biopsy to rule out neoplasm and to establish the correct diagnosis.

8. Retroperitoneal fibrosis is a primary or secondary fibroproliferative process in the retroperitoenum characterized by distortion of retroperitoneal structures, including the ureters and inferior vena cava.

9. Treatment of retroperitoneal fibrosis may include ureterolysis or ureteral stenting, and medical therapies such as corticosteroids or tamoxifen.

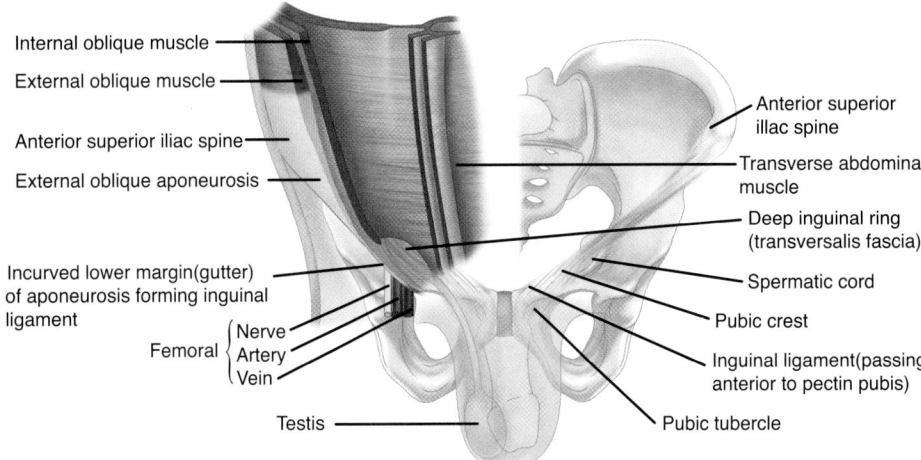

FIG. 35-2. The three muscular layers of the abdominal wall lateral to the rectus abdominis are the *external oblique, internal oblique,* and *transversus abdominis* muscles, shown here on the low abdomen, where the lower margin of the external oblique reflects posteriorly as the inguinal ligament. *[Reproduced with permission from Moore KL, Dailey AF (eds): Clinically Oriented Anatomy, 4th ed. Philadelphia: Lippincott Williams & Wilkins, 1999, p 181.]*

the anterior superior iliac spines (Fig. 35-3). Above the arcuate line, the anterior rectus sheath is formed by the external oblique aponeurosis and the external lamina of the internal oblique aponeurosis, whereas the posterior rectus sheath is formed by the internal lamina of the internal oblique aponeurosis, the transversus abdominis aponeurosis, and the transversalis fascia. Below the arcuate line, the anterior rectus sheath is formed by the external oblique aponeurosis, the laminae of the internal oblique aponeurosis, and the transversus abdominis aponeurosis. There is no aponeurotic posterior covering of this lower portion of the rectus muscles, although the transversalis fascia remains a contiguous structure on the posterior aspect of the abdominal wall in this area as well.

The majority of the blood supply to the muscles of the anterior abdominal wall is derived from the superior and inferior epigastric arteries (Fig. 35-4). The superior epigastric artery arises from the internal thoracic artery, whereas the inferior epigastric artery arises from the external iliac artery. A collateral network of branches of the subcostal and lumbar arteries also contributes to the abdominal wall blood supply. The lymphatic drainage of the abdominal wall is predominantly to the major nodal basins in the superficial inguinal and axillary areas.

Innervation of the anterior abdominal wall is segmentally related to specific spinal levels. The motor nerves to the rectus muscles, the internal oblique muscles, and the transversus abdominis muscles run from the anterior rami of spinal nerves at the T6 to T12 levels. The overlying skin is innervated by afferent branches of the T4 to L1 nerve roots, with the nerve roots of T10 subserving sensation of the skin around the umbilicus (Fig. 35-5).

Physiology

The rectus muscles, the external oblique muscles, and the internal oblique muscles work as a unit to flex the trunk anteriorly or laterally. Rotation of the trunk is achieved by the contraction of the external oblique muscle and the contralateral internal oblique muscle. For example, rotation of the trunk to the right is produced by contraction of the left external oblique muscle and the right internal oblique muscle. In addition, all four muscle groups (i.e., rectus muscles, external oblique muscles, internal oblique muscles, and transversus abdominis muscles) are involved in raising intra-abdominal pressure. If the diaphragm is relaxed when the abdominal musculature is contracted, the pressure exerted by the abdominal muscles results in expiration of air from the lungs or a cough if this contraction is forceful. Thus, these abdominal muscles are the primary muscles of expiration. If the diaphragm is contracted when the abdominal musculature is contracted (*Valsalva maneuver*) the increased abdominal pressure aids in processes such as micturition, defecation, and childbirth.

Abdominal Anatomy and Surgical Incisions

The abdominal wall can be viewed as a barrier to successful exposure of pathology in the deeper tissues. Surgeons must deal with this barrier every day to access sites of disease, and this engenders practical questions of where and how to make incisions. Structural characteristics of the abdominal wall are encountered with every abdominal incision used to gain entry to the peritoneal cavity or extraperitoneal tissues. Incisions for open surgery generally are

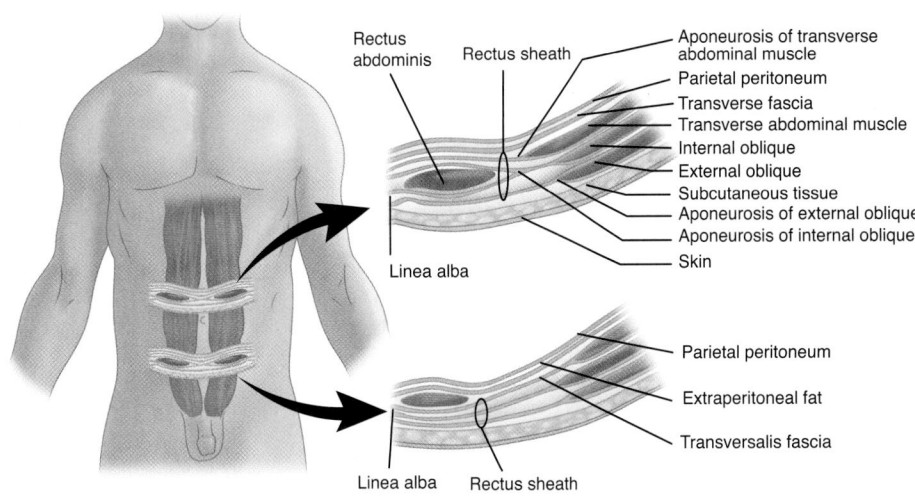

FIG. 35-3. Cross-sectional anatomy of the abdominal wall above and below the arcuate line of Douglas. The lower right abdominal wall segment shows clearly the absence of an aponeurotic covering of the posterior aspect of the rectus abdominis muscle inferior to the arcuate line. Superior to the arcuate line, there are both internal oblique and transversus abdominis aponeurotic contributions to the posterior rectus sheath. *[Reproduced with permission from Moore KL, Dailey AF (eds): Clinically Oriented Anatomy, 4th ed. Philadelphia: Lippincott Williams & Wilkins, 1999, p 185.]*

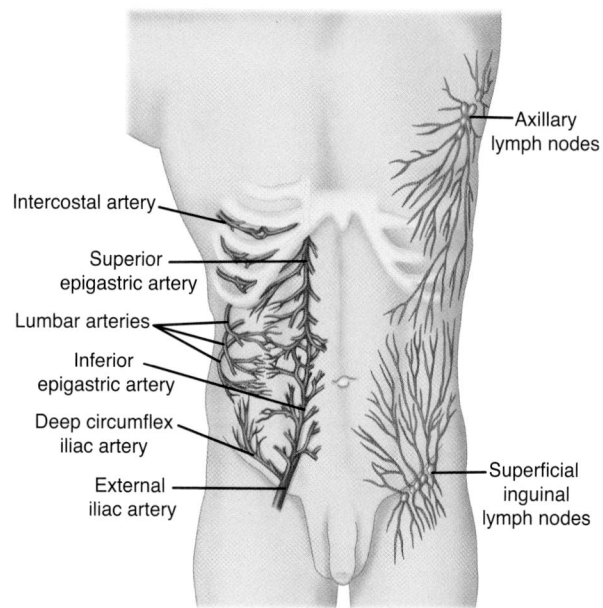

FIG. 35-4. The superior and inferior epigastric arteries form an anastomosing network of vessels in and around the rectus sheath, with collateralization to subcostal and lumbar vessels situated more laterally on the abdominal wall. Lymphatic drainage is via axially or inguinal nodal basins. *[Reproduced with permission from Moore KL, Dailey AF (eds):* Clinically Oriented Anatomy, *4th ed. Philadelphia: Lippincott Williams & Wilkins, 1999, p 86.]*

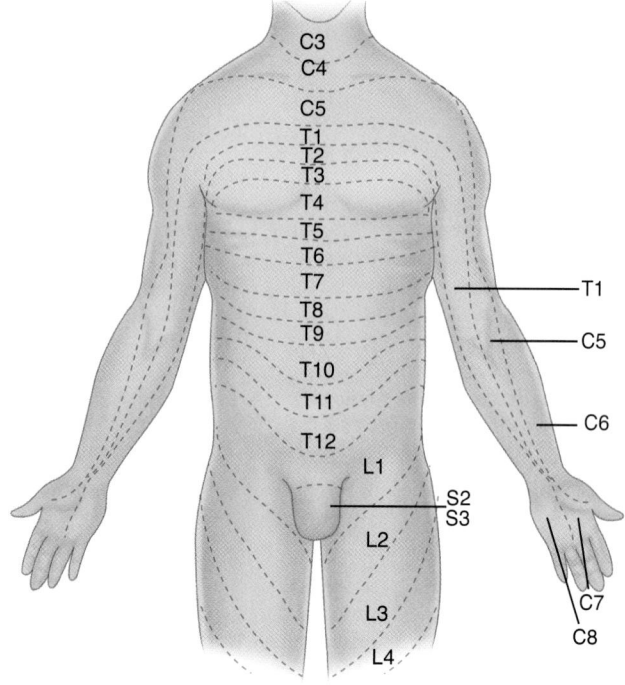

FIG. 35-5. Dermatomal sensory innervation of the abdominal wall. *[Reproduced with permission from Moore KL, Dailey AF (eds):* Clinically Oriented Anatomy, *4th ed. Philadelphia: Lippincott Williams & Wilkins, 1999, p 188.]*

located in proximity to the principal operative targets. Laparoscopic port site incisions might be remote from the site of interest and are carefully planned based on the anticipated instrument approach angles and necessary working distances both to the operative site and between ports. Orientation of the line of any incision may be determined based on expected quality of exposure; closure considerations, including cosmesis; avoidance of previous incision sites; and simple surgeon preference. In general, the incision for open peritoneal access can be longitudinal (in or off the midline), transverse (lateral to or crossing the midline), or oblique (directed either upward or downward toward the flank) (Fig. 35-6). Modifications of these general classes of incisions are numerous and can consist of various extensions that are intended to optimize exposure in specific clinical situations. In some infrequent situations, combinations of incision types may be used. For the majority of nonlaparoscopic procedures on the GI tract, midline incisions are used because of the flexibility offered by this approach in establishing adequate exposure. The incision in the fused midline aponeurotic tissue (linea alba) is simple and requires no division of skeletal muscle. Paramedian incisions are made longitudinally 3 cm off the midline, through the rectus abdominis sheath structures, and have largely been abandoned in favor of midline or nonlongitudinal access methods. Incisions lateral to the midline made with transverse or oblique orientations may divide the successive muscular layers or bluntly split them in the direction of their fibers. The latter muscle-splitting approach (exemplified by the classic McBurney incision for appendectomy) may be less destructive to tissue and thus allow healing with less scarring and tissue distortion but generally offers more limited exposure than other methods. Subcostal incisions on the right (Kocher incision for cholecystectomy) or left (for splenectomy) are archetypal muscle-dividing incisions that generally result in transection of some or all of the rectus abdominis muscle fibers and investing aponeuroses. These incisions generally are closed in two layers. The more superficial one incorporates the anterior aponeurotic sheath of the rectus muscle medially, transitioning to external oblique muscle and aponeurosis more laterally. The posterior,

deeper layer consists of internal oblique and transversus abdominis muscle. The anatomic considerations are the same for closure of transverse muscle-dividing incisions, either lateral to or crossing the midline. The Pfannenstiel incision, used commonly for pelvic proce-

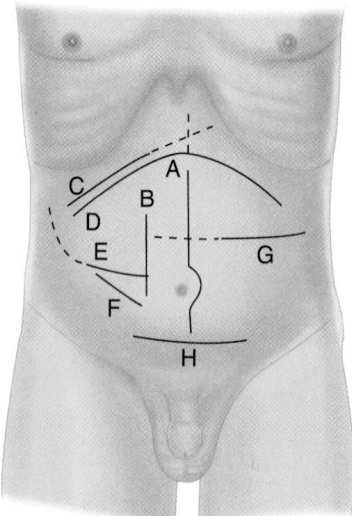

FIG. 35-6. Various anterior abdominal wall incisions for exposure of peritoneal structures. *A,* Midline incision; *B,* paramedian incision; *C,* right subcostal incision and "saber slash" extension to costal margin (*dashed line*); *D,* bilateral subcostal (also bucket handle, chevron, gable) incision, and "Mercedes Benz" extension (*dashed line*); *E,* Rocky-Davis incision and Weir extension (*dashed line*); *F,* McBurney incision; *G,* transverse incision and extension across midline (*dashed line*); and *H,* Pfannenstiel incision.

dures, is distinguished by transverse skin and anterior rectus sheath incisions, followed by rectus muscle retraction and longitudinal incision of the peritoneum. Irrespective of the incision type, suture apposition of abdominal wall tissues during closure ideally is accomplished without great tension and with great precision. The surgeon must appreciate all necessary anatomic distinctions to minimize the opportunity for defective healing.

Abdominal incisions are injuries inflicted under controlled circumstances that can lead to short- and long-term complications and patient disability. The question of how large an incision must be to allow safe operative maneuvers at the surgical site of interest has no simple answer. In general, it is prudent to make incisions no larger than is necessary to safely accomplish the operative goals. Efforts to deal with this issue have engendered surgical solutions intended both to reduce patient disability and to improve the overall ergonomics associated with smaller access sites. Laparoscopic surgery, and now natural orifice transluminal endoscopic surgery (NOTES), have owed their development largely to the belief that avoidance of surgical injury to the abdominal wall is of significant benefit to the patient. For open surgery, a variety of devices are available to retract the abdominal wall and facilitate peritoneal exposure without subjecting the patient to excessively large incisions or surgical personnel to exhausting retraction tasks (Fig. 35-7). Examples include the Bookwalter, Omni-Tract, and Thompson retractors.

Congenital Abnormalities

The abdominal wall layers begin to form in the first weeks after conception. Prominent in the early embryonic abdominal wall is a large central defect through which pass the vitelline (omphalomesenteric) duct and allantois. The vitelline duct connects the embryonic and fetal midgut to the yolk sac. During the sixth week of development, the abdominal contents grow too large for the abdominal wall to completely contain and the embryonic midgut herniates into the umbilical cord. Although outside the confines of the developing abdomen, it undergoes a 270-degree counterclockwise rotation and, at the end of the twelfth week, returns to the abdominal cavity. Defects in abdominal wall closure may lead to omphalocele or gastroschisis. In omphalocele, viscera protrude through an open umbilical ring and are covered by a sac derived from the amnion. In gastroschisis, the viscera protrude through a defect lateral to the umbilicus and no sac is present.

During the third trimester, the vitelline duct regresses. Persistence of a vitelline duct remnant on the ileal border results in *Meckel's diverticulum*. Complete failure of the vitelline duct to regress results in a *vitelline duct fistula*, which is associated with drainage of small intestine contents from the umbilicus. If both the intestinal and umbilical ends of the vitelline duct regress into fibrous cords, a central *vitelline duct (omphalomesenteric) cyst* may occur. Persistent vitelline duct remnants between the GI tract and the anterior abdominal wall may be associated with small intestine volvulus in neonates. When diagnosed, vitelline duct fistulas and cysts should be excised along with any accompanying fibrous cord.

The urachus is a fibromuscular, tubular extension of the allantois that develops with the descent of the bladder to its pelvic position. Persistence of urachal remnants can result in cysts as well as fistulas to the urinary bladder with drainage of urine from the umbilicus. These are treated by urachal excision and closure of any bladder defect that may be present.

Acquired Abnormalities
Rectus Abdominis Diastasis

Rectus abdominis diastasis (or diastasis recti) is a clinically evident separation of the rectus abdominis muscle pillars. This results in a characteristic bulging of the abdominal wall in the epigastrium that is sometimes mistaken for a ventral hernia despite the fact that the midline aponeurosis is intact and no hernia defect is present. Diastasis may be congenital, as a result of a more lateral insertion of the rectus muscles to the ribs and costochondral junctions, but is more typically an acquired condition, occurring with advancing age, in obesity, or after pregnancy. In the postpartum setting, rectus diastasis tends to occur in women who are of advanced maternal age, who have a multiple or twin pregnancy, or who deliver a high-birth-weight infant. Diastasis is usually easily identified on physical examination (Fig. 35-8). Computed tomographic (CT) scanning provides an accurate means of measuring the distance between the rectus pillars and can differentiate rectus diastasis from a true ventral hernia if clarification is required. Surgical correction of rectus diastasis by plication of the broad midline aponeurosis has been described for cosmetic indications and for alleviation of impaired abdominal wall muscular function. However, these approaches introduce the risk of an actual ventral hernia and are of questionable value in addressing pathology.

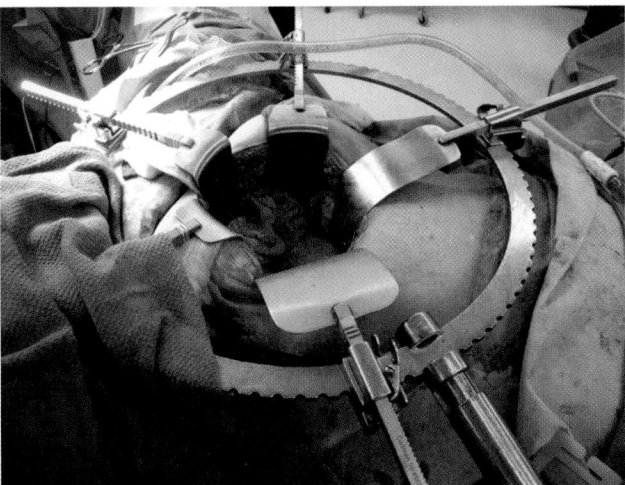

FIG. 35-7. Bookwalter retractor in use for exposure of peritoneal structures during abdominal surgery. Devices of this type are valuable exposure aids that reduce the physical demands on personnel in the operating room and allow more complete focus on the surgical site of interest.

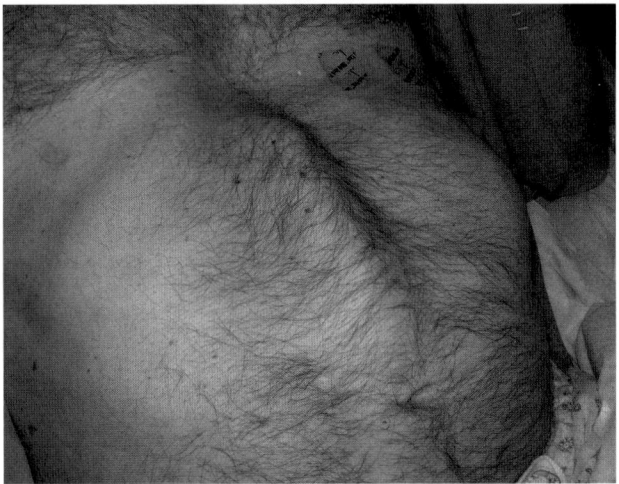

FIG. 35-8. Diastasis recti visible in the midepigastrium with Valsalva maneuver. The edges of the rectus abdominis muscle, rigid with voluntary contraction, are palpable along the entire length of the bulging area. This should not be mistaken for a ventral hernia.

Rectus Sheath Hematoma

The terminal branches of the superior and inferior epigastric arteries course deep to the posterior aspect of the left and right rectus abdominis muscles and enter the posterior rectus sheath. Hemorrhage from any of the network of collateralizing vessels within the rectus sheath and muscles can result in a rectus sheath hematoma. Although a history of major or minor blunt trauma may be elicited, less obvious events also have been reported to cause this condition, such as sudden contraction of the rectus muscles with coughing, sneezing, or any vigorous physical activity. Spontaneous rectus sheath hematomas have been described in the elderly and in those receiving anticoagulation therapy. Patients frequently describe the sudden onset of unilateral abdominal pain that may be confused with lateralized peritoneal disorders such as appendicitis. Below the arcuate line, a hematoma may cross the midline and cause bilateral lower quadrant pain.

History and physical examination alone may be diagnostic. Pain typically increases with contraction of the rectus muscles and a tender mass may be palpated. The ability to appreciate an intra-abdominal mass is ordinarily degraded with contraction of the rectus muscles. *Fothergill's sign* is a palpable abdominal mass that remains unchanged with contraction of the rectus muscles and is classically associated with rectus hematoma. Hemoglobin level and hematocrit should be measured and coagulation studies should be performed. Abdominal ultrasonography may show a solid or cystic mass within the abdominal wall depending on the chronicity of the bleeding. CT is the most definitive study to establish the correct diagnosis and to exclude other disorders (Fig. 35-9). Magnetic resonance imaging (MRI) also has been used for this purpose.

Specific treatment depends on the severity of the hemorrhage (Fig. 35-10). Small, unilateral, and stable hematomas may be observed without patient hospitalization. Bilateral or large hematomas will likely require hospitalization and possibly resuscitation. The need for transfusion or coagulation factor replacement is determined by the clinical circumstances. Reversal of warfarin (Coumadin) anticoagulation in the acute setting is frequently, but not always, necessary. Emergent operative intervention or angiographic embolization is required infrequently but may be necessary if hematoma enlargement, free bleeding, or clinical deterioration occur. Surgical therapy is used in the rare situations of failed angiographic treatment or hemodynamic instability that precludes any other options. The operative

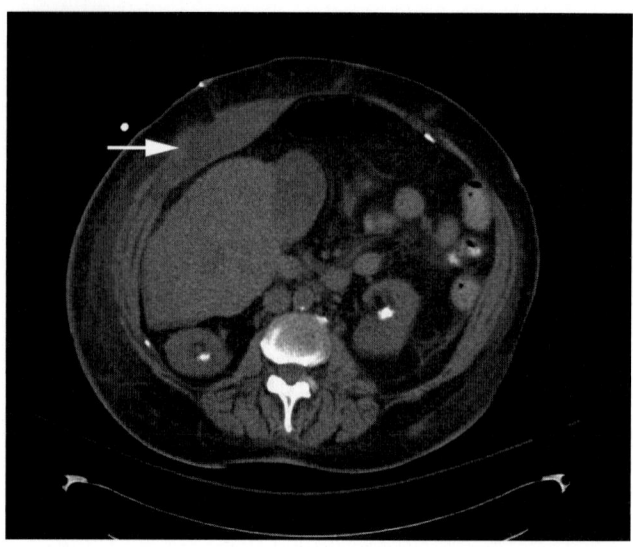

FIG. 35-9. Computed tomographic scan showing a medium-sized right rectus sheath hematoma. The hematoma occurred in an elderly patient without a clear history of trauma who was receiving anticoagulation therapy. Because of its size and the patient's slender body habitus, this hematoma was palpable and could be followed clinically.

goals are evacuation of the hematoma and ligation of any bleeding vessel identified. Mortality from this condition is rare but has been reported in elderly patients requiring surgical treatment.

Abdominal Wall Hernias

Hernias of the anterior abdominal wall, or *ventral* hernias, represent defects in the parietal abdominal wall fascia and muscle through which intra-abdominal or preperitoneal contents can protrude. Ventral hernias may be congenital or acquired. Acquired hernias may develop through slow architectural deterioration of the muscular aponeuroses or they may develop from failed healing of an anterior abdominal wall incision (*incisional hernia*). The most common finding is a mass or bulge on the anterior abdominal wall, which may increase in size with

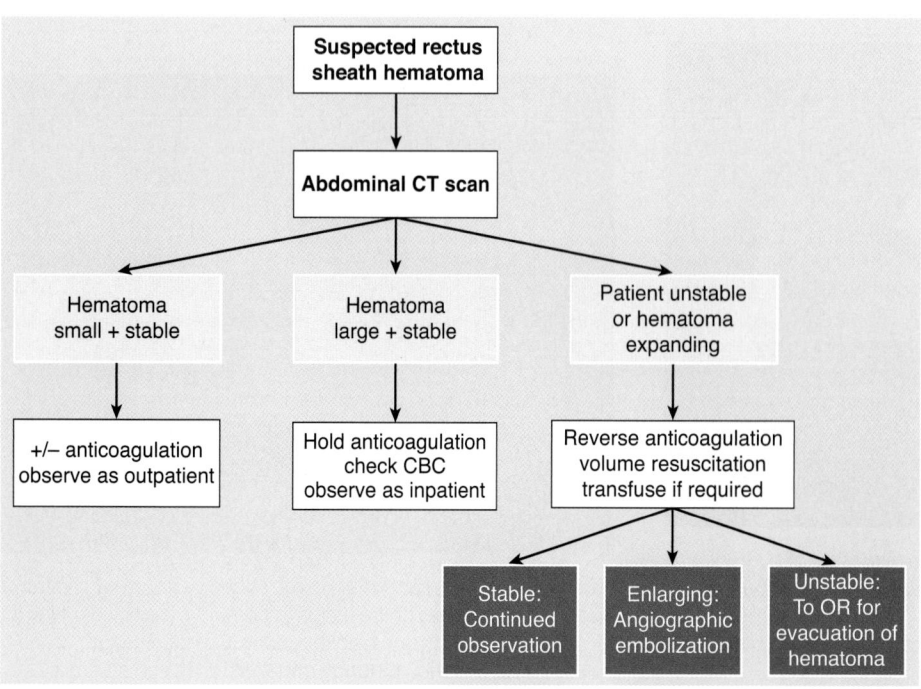

FIG. 35-10. Management algorithm for rectus sheath hematoma. Most patients present with a mass and/or pain and are managed without intervention. The potential for a rare catastrophic bleeding event must be recognized, however. Surgical evacuation is reserved for those circumstances in which clinical evidence of ongoing bleeding makes any other management option untenable. CBC = complete blood count; CT = computed tomography; OR = operating room.

a Valsalva maneuver. Ventral hernias may be asymptomatic or cause a considerable degree of discomfort, and generally enlarge over time. Physical examination reveals a bulge on the anterior abdominal wall that may reduce spontaneously, with recumbency, or with manual pressure. A hernia that cannot be reduced is described as *incarcerated* and requires emergent surgical correction. Incarceration of an intestinal segment may be accompanied by nausea, vomiting, and significant pain. Should the blood supply to the incarcerated bowel be compromised, the hernia is described as *strangulated*, and the localized ischemia may lead to infarction and perforation.

Primary ventral hernias (nonincisional) are also termed *true* ventral hernias. These are more properly named according to their anatomic location. *Epigastric* hernias are located in the midline between the xiphoid process and the umbilicus. They are generally small, may be multiple, and at elective repair are usually found to contain omentum or a portion of the falciform ligament. These may be congenital and due to defective midline fusion of developing lateral abdominal wall elements.

Umbilical hernias occur at the umbilical ring and may either be present at birth or develop gradually during the life of the individual. Umbilical hernias are present in approximately 10 percent of all newborns and are more common in premature infants. Most congenital umbilical hernias close spontaneously by age 5 years. If closure does not occur by this time, elective surgical repair usually is advised. Adults with small, asymptomatic umbilical hernias may be followed clinically. Surgical treatment is offered if a hernia is observed to enlarge, if it is associated with symptoms, or if incarceration occurs. Surgical treatment can consist of primary sutured repair or placement of prosthetic mesh for larger defects (>2 cm) using open or laparoscopic methods.

Spigelian hernias can occur anywhere along the length of the Spigelian line or zone—an aponeurotic band of variable width at the lateral border of the rectus abdominis. However, the most frequent location of these rare hernias is at or slightly above the level of the arcuate line. These are not always clinically evident as a bulge and may come to medical attention because of pain or incarceration.

Patients with advanced liver disease, ascites, and umbilical hernia require special consideration. Enlargement of the umbilical ring usually occurs in this clinical situation as a result of increased intra-abdominal pressure from uncontrolled ascites. The first line of therapy is aggressive medical correction of the ascites with diuretics, dietary management, and paracentesis for tense ascites with respiratory compromise. These hernias usually are filled with ascitic fluid, but omentum or bowel may enter the defect after large-volume paracentesis. Uncontrolled ascites may lead to skin breakdown on the protuberant hernia and eventual ascitic leak, which can predispose the patient to bacterial peritonitis. Patients with refractory ascites may be candidates for transjugular intrahepatic portocaval shunting or eventual liver transplantation. Umbilical hernia repair should be deferred until after the ascites is controlled.

Incisional Hernias

Approximately 4 million abdominal operations are performed every year and as many as 10 to 20% of these patients have been estimated to develop hernias at the abdominal incision sites. Any such occurrence is termed *incisional hernia* and can be regarded as a wound healing failure. The cause of incisional hernia in any given case can be difficult to determine, but obesity, primary wound healing defects, multiple prior procedures, prior incisional hernias, and technical errors during repair may all be contributory. Hernias can occur at sites of defective healing within the approximated incision or at the suture puncture sites created during the closure, or both. Repair of incisional hernias can be technically challenging, and a myriad of methods have been described. The most important distinctions in describing surgical management of incisional hernias are primary vs. mesh repair and open vs. laparoscopic repair.

Primary repair methods for incisional hernia include both simple suture closure and components separation, and are open procedures.

Simple suture approximation of fascial defect edges predictably results in a suture line under tension. Primary repair, even of small hernias (defects <3 cm), is associated with high reported hernia recurrence rates. In a randomized prospective study of open primary and open mesh incisional hernia repairs in 200 patients, investigators from the Netherlands found that after 3 years, recurrence rates were 43% and 24% for the two methods, respectively. Identified risk factors for recurrence were primary suture repair, postoperative wound infection, prostatism, and surgery for abdominal aortic aneurysm. These investigators concluded that mesh repair was superior to primary repair.

In an effort to decrease the suture line tension associated with primary repair, Ramirez first described the components separation technique. Components separation entails the creation of large subcutaneous flaps lateral to the fascial defect followed by incision of the external oblique muscles and, if necessary, incision of the posterior rectus sheath bilaterally. These fascial releases allow for primary apposition of the fascia under far less tension than in simple primary repair. Components separation hernia repair is associated with a high wound infection risk (20%) and a recurrence rate of 18.2% at 1 year. Components separation is most applicable for the repair of incisional hernias when there are converging needs to (a) avoid the use of prosthetic materials, and (b) achieve a definitive repair. Most commonly this occurs in the setting of a contaminated or potentially contaminated surgical field.

Mesh repair has become the gold standard in the elective management of most incisional hernias. Mesh repairs can be categorized according to the way in which the mesh is placed as well as its relationship to the abdominal wall fascia. Mesh can be placed as an underlay deep to the fascial defect (intraperitoneal or preperitoneal), as an interlay either bridging the gap between the defect edges or within the abdominal wall musculoaponeurotic layers (intraparietal), or as an onlay (superficial to the fascial defect). Laparoscopic repairs use an intraperitoneal underlay technique. Meshes can be characterized by type of material, each of which has a specified density, porosity, and strength. Broadly, these can be prosthetic or biologic. Permanent prosthetic mesh implants are made of materials that do not degrade over time, whereas absorbable meshes are degraded, primarily by hydrolytic enzyme activity. Biologic meshes are prepared from collagen-rich porcine, bovine, or human tissues from which all antigenic cellular materials are removed. These mesh materials can be chemically treated to cross-link collagen molecules, which increases strength and durability at the cost of some impairment in host cellular ingrowth. Over time, biologic mesh–derived collagen can be incorporated into the host tissue, remodeled, and eventually replaced by host collagen. Early in their use, biologic meshes were felt to represent a potentially definitive solution when used to bridge an abdominal wall defect. However, more recent reports show that hernia recurrence rates are excessive in this application. Jin and colleagues found that when human acellular dermis was used to bridge a complicated incisional hernia defect the recurrence rate was 73%, in sharp contrast to a 15% recurrence rate when the same material was used as an onlay or underlay in conjunction with primary closure. Blatnik and associates reported an 80% recurrence rate when human acellular dermis was used to bridge ventral hernia defects, at a cost of $5100 per patient for the mesh alone. Commonly used meshes for incisional hernia repair are listed in Table 35-1. The principal advantages of prosthetic meshes are ease of use, relatively low cost, and durability. Biologic meshes are useful in the setting of contaminated or potentially contaminated fields but are very expensive and, based on the most recent evidence, do not offer the durability of permanent prosthetic meshes unless combined with a primary repair. Absorbable meshes, composed of the same materials as polysaccharide-derived synthetic absorbable suture, provide relatively inexpensive solutions for temporary abdominal wall support in highly contaminated or infected fields. Use of these meshes leaves patients with recurrent ventral hernias that can be definitively repaired when permitted by improved local wound conditions.

TABLE 35-1	Meshes used in incisional hernia repair

Proprietary Name	Composition
Prosthetic meshes	
Parietex	Polyester/collagen film
Composix	Polypropylene/ePTFE
DualMesh, Dulex, MotifMESH	ePTFE
Prolene, Surgipro, ProLite	Polypropylene
Proceed	Polypropylene/polydioxanone
Sepramesh IP	Polypropylene/hyaluronate gel
C-Qur	Polypropylene/omega-3 fatty acid
TiMESH	Polypropylene/titanium
Proprietary Name	**Composition**
Biologic meshes	
Surgisis Gold	Porcine small intestine submucosa
AlloDerm	Human dermis
SurgiMend	Fetal bovine dermis
CollaMend	Porcine dermis
AlloMax	Human dermis
Proprietary Name	**Composition**
Absorbable meshes	
Gore Bio-A	Poly(glycolide:trimethylene carbonate)
Vicryl	Polyglactin
Dexon	Polyglycolate

ePTFE = expanded polytetrafluoroethylene.

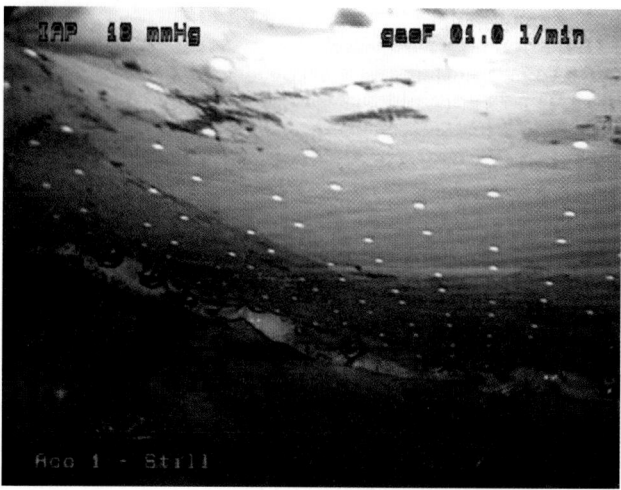

FIG. 35-11. Intraperitoneal view of polytetrafluoroethylene mesh used for laparoscopic ventral incisional hernia repair. The mesh is in place on the posterior aspect of the abdominal wall without apparent laxity due to the ongoing CO_2 insufflation. Once pneumoperitoneum is released, sufficient laxity is introduced to relieve any pull at the fixation points and to permit good apposition of mesh to the abdominal wall surface.

Open mesh repair of incisional hernias generally requires incision or excision of the previous laparotomy scar, with care taken to avoid injury to the underlying abdominal contents. The peritoneum and hernial sac are then dissected free from the abdominal wall fascia so that at least 3 to 4 cm of fascia is circumferentially exposed. The mesh can then be sutured into place using an underlay, onlay, interlay, or "sandwich-style" (both underlay and onlay) method. The most successful method is to extensively develop a preperitoneal space to accommodate a large sheet of polypropylene or woven polyester mesh. The mesh, which is isolated from the peritoneal contents, is then secured to the musculoaponeurotic tissues using interrupted nonabsorbable sutures. Tissue ingrowth within the interstices of these mesh types results in dense attachment to whatever tissues the mesh comes into contact with. This effect is desirable when the mesh is located in the preperitoneal position. However, exposure to the underlying bowel ought to be avoided whenever possible. Among the problems attributed to adherence of peritoneal contents to mesh are chronic pain, bowel obstruction, and fistulization to bowel. Polytetrafluoroethylene (PTFE) does not become incorporated into the surrounding tissues and is not associated with dense adhesions to the intraperitoneal structures. It is therefore commonly used for intraperitoneal applications. Irrespective of technique, the recurrence rate after open incisional hernia repair can be high. In two randomized trials of open mesh repair, one using an underlay technique and one using an onlay technique, the recurrence rates were 20% and 8%, respectively.

Laparoscopic incisional hernia repair was first described by LeBlanc and Booth in 1993. Since that time, many would argue, these procedures have become a new gold standard for abdominal wall reconstruction for ventral hernia. In 2000, data from 407 patients undergoing laparoscopic incisional hernia as part of a multicenter trial revealed a recurrence rate of only 3.4%, after a mean follow-up of >2 years. Of the recurrences noted, the overwhelming majority were felt to be secondary to technical errors committed early in the surgeons' experience that were avoided during the later cases. Recently, investigators at Washington University examined pooled data from 45 different series of laparoscopic and open ventral hernia repair. Use of the laparoscopic technique was associated with statistically fewer wound complications, fewer overall complications, and a lower recurrence rate than use of the open technique. These benefits

of the minimally invasive technique are achieved by eliminating the requisite large abdominal incision at a location where the abdominal wall blood supply has previously been compromised. In addition, with the laparoscopic technique, the entire undersurface of the abdominal wall can be examined, which often reveals multiple secondary defects that might not otherwise be appreciated.

The technique of laparoscopic incisional hernia repair generally involves laterally placed ports for midline defects and contralaterally placed ports for lateral defects. All adhesions to the anterior abdominal wall are divided, with great care taken not to injure the intestine either directly or with thermal or electrical energy. The contents of the hernial sac are completely reduced, but in contrast to open repairs, the sac itself is left in situ. Once the area encompassing all fascial defects is defined, a mesh is fashioned to allow for sufficient overlap (minimum of 3 to 4 cm) under the healthy abdominal wall. After insertion into the abdomen, the mesh is fixed into position with transfascial sutures placed circumferentially around the mesh and spiral tacks placed according to surgeon preference (Fig. 35-11). It has been proposed that transfascial sutures contribute to excessive postoperative pain, and some surgeons have eliminated them from the aforementioned technique, relying solely on spiral tacks for the strength of the repair. LeBlanc reviewed the usefulness of transfascial sutures and cautiously recommended a minimum 5-cm overlap of mesh from defect edge if transfascial sutures are not used.

OMENTUM

Surgical Anatomy

The greater omentum and lesser omentum are fibro-fatty aprons that provide support, coverage, and protection for peritoneal contents. These structures begin to develop during the fourth week of gestation. The greater omentum develops from the dorsal mesogastrium, which begins as a double-layered structure. The spleen develops in between the two layers, and later in development the two layers fuse, giving rise to the intraperitoneal spleen and the gastrosplenic ligament. The fused layers then hang from the greater curvature of the stomach and drape over the transverse colon, to which their posterior surface becomes fixed. The gastrocolic ligament and the gastrosplenic ligament are those segments of the greater omental apron that connect the named structures. In the adult, the greater omentum lies in between the anterior abdominal wall and the hollow viscera, and usually extends into the pelvis to the level of the symphysis pubis.

The lesser omentum, otherwise known as the *hepatoduodenal* and *hepatogastric ligaments*, develops from the mesoderm of the septum transversum, which connects the embryonic liver to the foregut. The common bile duct, portal vein, and hepatic artery are located in the inferolateral margin of the lesser omentum, which also forms the anterior margin of the foramen of Winslow.

The blood supply to the greater omentum is derived from the right and left gastroepiploic arteries. The venous drainage parallels the arterial supply to a great extent, with the left and right gastroepiploic veins ultimately draining into the portal system.

Physiology

In the early twentieth century, the British surgeon Rutherford Morison noted that the omentum tended to wall off areas of infection and limit the spread of intraperitoneal contamination. He termed the omentum the *abdominal policeman*. Shortly after his description was published, several reports suggested intrinsic hemostatic characteristics of the omentum. In 1996, researchers in the Netherlands demonstrated that the concentration of tissue factor in omentum is over twice the amount per gram of that found in muscle. This facilitates activation of coagulation at sites of inflammation, ischemia, infection, or trauma within the peritoneal cavity. The consequent local production of fibrin contributes to the ability of the omentum to adhere to areas of injury or inflammation.

Omental Infarction

Interruption of the blood supply to the omentum is a rare cause of an acute abdomen that may be secondary to torsion of the omentum around its vascular pedicle, thrombosis or vasculitis of the omental vessels, or omental venous outflow obstruction. Fewer than 100 cases have been reported, and the diagnosis is most likely to be made in male adults. Depending on the location of the infarcted omental tissue, this disease process may mimic appendicitis, cholecystitis, diverticulitis, perforated peptic ulcer, or ruptured ovarian cyst.

Patients typically present with localized right lower quadrant, right upper quadrant, or left lower quadrant pain. Although a mild degree of nausea may be present, patients do not usually have concomitant intestinal symptoms. Physical examination typically reveals a mild tachycardia and a low-grade fever. Abdominal examination may demonstrate a tender, palpable mass associated with guarding and rebound tenderness. The diagnosis is rarely made before abdominal imaging studies are performed. Either abdominal CT or ultrasonography will show a localized, inflammatory mass of fat density. Treatment of omental infarction depends on the certainty with which the diagnosis is made. In patients who are not toxic and whose abdominal imaging results are convincing, supportive care is sufficient. However, many cases are indistinguishable from surgical conditions with immediate surgical implications, such as appendicitis. In these instances, laparoscopic exploration offers the opportunity to establish an accurate diagnosis and determine the most appropriate treatment. Resection of the infarcted tissue results in rapid resolution of symptoms.

Omental Cysts

Cystic lesions of the omentum and mesentery are related disorders, likely resulting from either peritoneal inclusions or degeneration of lymphatic structures. Omental cysts are far less common than mesenteric cysts. Omental cysts may present as an asymptomatic abdominal mass or may cause abdominal pain with or without appreciable mass or distention. Physical examination may reveal a freely mobile intra-abdominal mass. Both CT and abdominal ultrasound reveal a well-circumscribed, cystic mass lesion arising from the greater omentum. Treatment involves resection of all symptomatic omental cysts. Resection of these benign lesions is readily accomplished using laparoscopic techniques.

Omental Neoplasms

Primary tumors of the omentum are uncommon. Benign tumors of the omentum include lipomas, myxomas, and desmoid tumors. Primary malignant tumors of the omentum are considered mesodermally derived stromal tumors, in which some of the associated immunohistochemical characteristics of GI stromal tumors have been described, including c-kit immunopositivity. Metastatic tumors of the omentum are common, with metastatic ovarian cancer showing the highest preponderance of omental involvement. Malignant tumors of the stomach, small intestine, colon, pancreas, biliary tract, uterus, and kidney may also metastasize to the omentum.

MESENTERY

Surgical Anatomy

The mesentery develops from mesenchyme that attaches the foregut, midgut, and hindgut to the posterior abdominal wall. During embryonic maturation, this mesenchyme forms the dorsal mesentery. In the region of the stomach, the dorsal mesentery becomes the greater omentum, whereas in the region of the jejunum and ileum the dorsal mesentery becomes the mesentery proper. In the region of the colon, the dorsal mesentery is known as the *mesocolon*. During embryonic development, after the 270-degree counterclockwise rotation of the herniated midgut, the reduced mesentery achieves its final fixation state. The segments at the duodenum, ascending colon, and descending colon become fixed to the retroperitoneum, whereas the small intestine mesentery, transverse colon mesentery, and, to a variable extent, the sigmoid colon mesentery remain mobile (Fig. 35-12). Defects in the normal developmental steps of intestinal rotation result in malrotation disorders.

The root of the small intestine mesentery wall normally courses in an oblique direction, from the left upper quadrant at the ligament of Treitz to the right lower quadrant at the ileocecal valve and the fixed cecum. The small and large intestine mesenteries serve as the major pathway for arterial, venous, lymphatic, and neural structures coursing to and from the bowel. Anatomic anomalies of the mesentery related to rotational disorders can lead to paraduodenal or mesocolic hernias (Fig. 35-13), which can present as chronic or acute intestinal obstruction in children or adults.

Sclerosing Mesenteritis

Sclerosing mesenteritis, also referred to as *mesenteric panniculitis* or *mesenteric lipodystrophy*, is a chronic inflammatory and fibrotic process that involves a portion of the intestinal mesentery. There is no gender or race predominance, but the condition is most commonly diagnosed in individuals >50 years of age.

The etiology of this process is unknown, but its cardinal feature is increased tissue density within the mesentery. This can be localized and associated with a discrete non-neoplastic mesenteric mass or more diffuse, sometimes involving large swaths of mesentery without well-defined borders. There may be varying relative degrees of fat tissue degeneration, inflammation, and fibrosis on histologic examination, which gives rise to the various terms used to describe this condition. *Mesenteric lipodystrophy* is used when the inflammatory and fibrotic components are small. *Mesenteric panniculitis* signifies an increased inflammatory component with replacement of degenerative fatty elements. *Sclerosing mesenteritis* signifies a major fibrotic component and is sometimes referred to as *retractile mesenteritis* to describe mesenteric retraction and shortening associated with scarring. It is not clear if these represent stages in a sequential process or variations in disease severity. A discrete mass may be up to 40 cm in diameter, and patients typically present with symptoms of a mass lesion. Abdominal pain is the most frequent presenting symptom, followed by the presence of a nonpainful mass or, more rarely, intestinal obstruction. However, many cases are discovered incidentally when imaging studies (most frequently abdominal CT

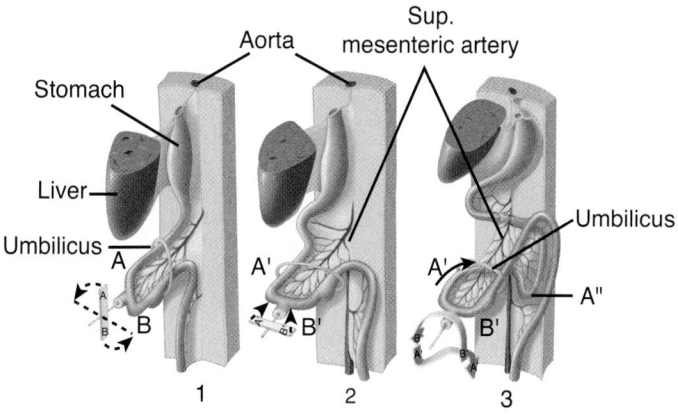

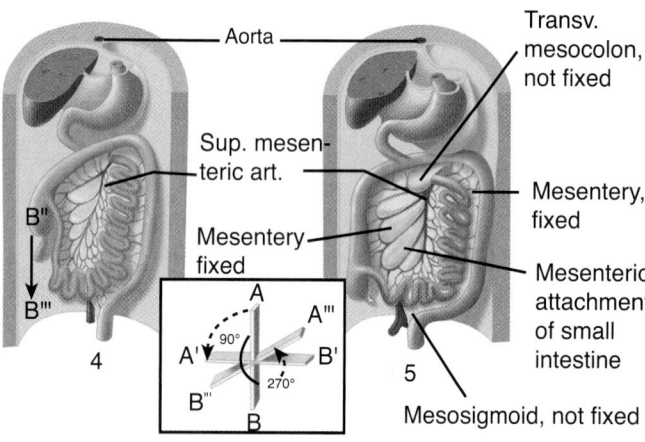

FIG. 35-12. Anatomic relationships of intestinal mesentery to the retroperitoneum after completion of intestinal rotation during fetal development. art. = artery; sup. = superior; transv. = transverse. *[Reproduced with permission from Healey JE, Hodge J (eds):* Surgical Anatomy, *2nd ed. Toronto: BC Decker, 1990, p 153.]*

scanning) are performed for unrelated reasons. This then raises diagnostic questions whose resolution is often pursued using invasive procedures.

CT of the abdomen can verify the presence of a mass lesion or area of the mesentery with a higher density than found in normal

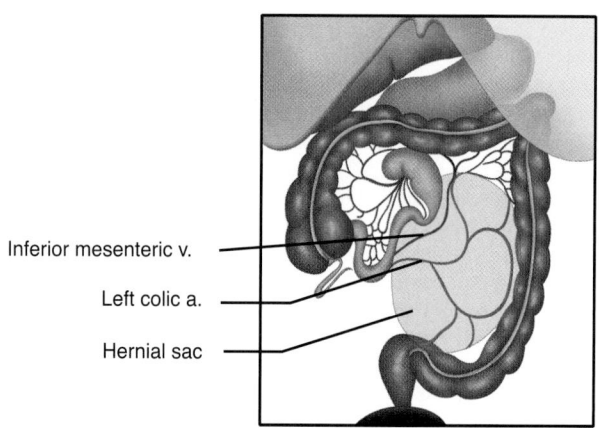

FIG. 35-13. Mesocolic hernia of small bowel into a retrocolic hernial sac posterior to the descending colon mesentery. Hernias of this type, as well as hernias into paraduodenal recesses, result from abnormal fixation of mesenteric structures during the course of intestinal rotation. a. = artery; v. = vein. *[Reproduced with permission from Healey JE, Hodge J (eds):* Surgical Anatomy, *2nd ed. Toronto: BC Decker, 1990, p 153.]*

mesenteric tissue. This may frequently involve the vascular structures in the mesenteric root (Fig. 35-14). Although CT cannot definitively distinguish sclerosing mesenteritis from a primary or secondary mesenteric tumor, identification of a "fat ring sign" or hypodense zone around the mass area has been suggested as a means of distinguishing sclerosing mesenteritis from lymphoma. The presence of a hyperattenuating stripe also has been suggested as a radiologic finding that would favor a diagnosis of mesenteritis (Fig. 35-15).

Surgery has been used most frequently to establish a diagnosis and to rule out a neoplastic process. The extent and location of mesenteric involvement defines, and in some cases limits, the options for surgical intervention. In addition to simple biopsy, bowel and mesenteric resection can be considered, particularly in cases in which it is technically feasible based on mass size and the ability to avoid injury to the small intestine blood supply (Fig. 35-16). Often, however, the involvement of the vascular structures at the mesenteric root makes resection unfeasible. In rare cases, an ostomy of some type for fecal diversion in the face of obstruction can be considered. The recent use of positron emission tomography with CT scanning has proven effective in ruling out neoplasia for focal mesenteric masses, which leaves the sclerosing mesenteritis diagnosis as one of exclusion. However, it is not clear that use of this newer modality will eliminate the need to obtain tissue for diagnostic purposes.

In most cases of sclerosing mesenteritis the process appears to be self-limited and may even demonstrate regression if followed with interval imaging studies. Clinical symptoms are very likely to improve without intervention, and therefore aggressive surgical treatments are generally not indicated. In clinically problematic cases that are not

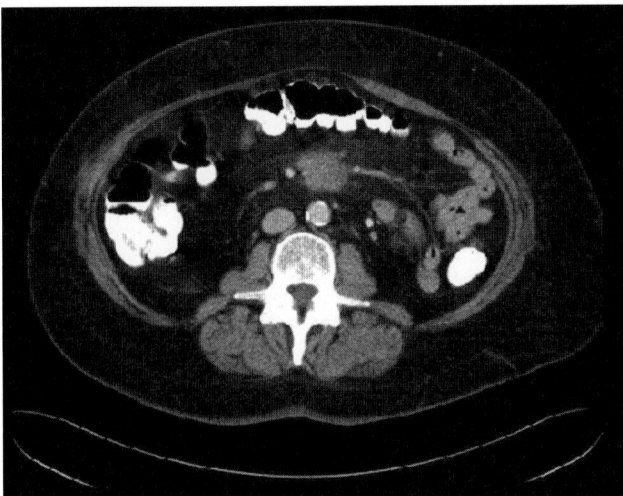

FIG. 35-14. Computed tomographic coronal section of a focus of sclerosing mesenteritis at the mesenteric root, straddling major proximal branches of the superior mesenteric artery. The location of the mass restricted surgical options to biopsy and confirmation of diagnosis.

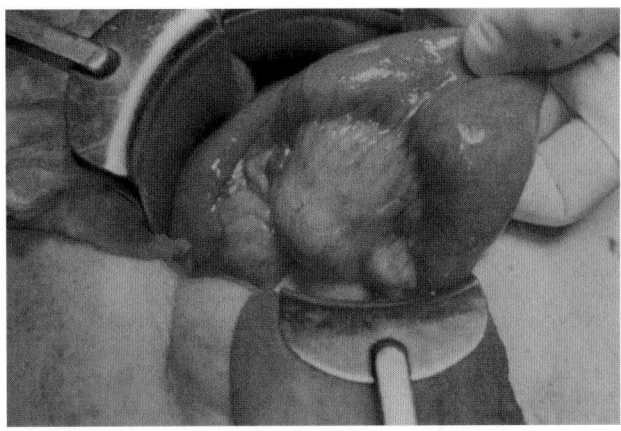

FIG. 35-16. Operative findings at the time of resection of what was believed to be a mesenteric tumor but which proved to be a focus of mesenteric lipodystrophy. In this case, the relatively small site of involvement and the peripheral location in the small intestine mesentery permitted management by resection en bloc with a segment of adjacent small bowel.

amenable to resection because of widespread mesenteric involvement or unfavorable location, medical treatment has been given to alleviate severe symptoms. Among the agents that have been used are corticosteroids, colchicine, tamoxifen, and cyclophosphamide.

Mesenteric Cysts

Cysts of the mesentery are benign lesions with an incidence of <1 in 100,000. Since the first description of such a cyst in 1507, approximately 1000 cases have been described in the literature. The etiology of such cysts remains unknown, but several theories regarding their

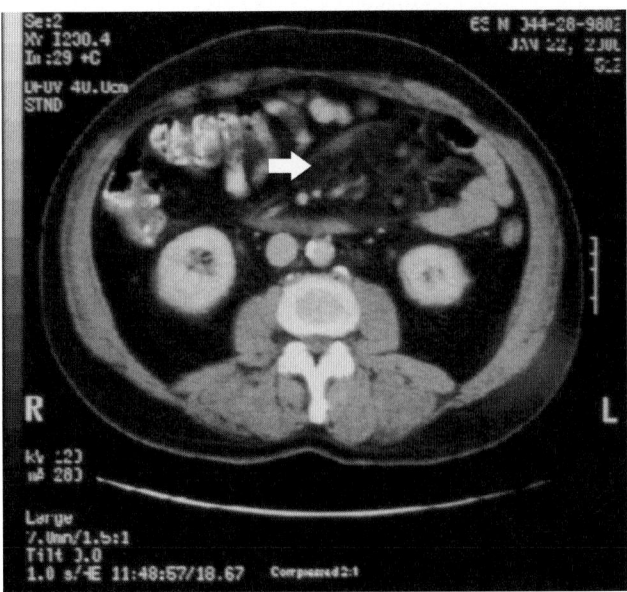

FIG. 35-15. Computed tomographic scan of sclerosing mesenteritis (mesenteric lipodystrophy). This condition cannot easily be distinguished from a neoplasm of the mesentery on radiologic study. In this case, the study showed "fatty mesenteric tumor with involvement of mesenteric vessels," and "mesenteric lipodystrophy" was demonstrated by biopsy findings at exploration. The finding of a hyperattenuating stripe around the lesion, as seen in this image, has been associated with the diagnosis of mesenteritis.

development have been put forward, including that they are caused by degeneration of the mesenteric lymphatics and that they simply arise as a congenital anomaly.

Mesenteric cysts may be asymptomatic or may cause symptoms of a mass lesion. Symptoms may be acute or chronic. Acute abdominal pain secondary to a mesenteric cyst is generally caused by rupture or torsion of the cyst or by acute hemorrhage into the cyst. Mesenteric cysts may also cause chronic intermittent abdominal pain secondary to compression of adjacent structures or spontaneous torsion followed by detorsion of the cyst. Mesenteric cysts can be the cause of nonspecific symptoms such as anorexia, nausea, vomiting, fatigue, and weight loss.

Physical examination may reveal a mass lesion that is mobile only from the patient's right to left or left to right (Tillaux's sign), in contrast to the findings with omental cysts, which should be freely mobile in all directions. Tillaux was the first to record this physical finding and, in 1850, the first to successfully remove a mesenteric cyst.

CT (Fig. 35-17), abdominal ultrasound, and MRI all have been used to evaluate patients with mesenteric cysts. Each of the aforementioned imaging modalities reveals a cystic structure without a solid component in the central abdomen. These structures are generally unilocular but may on occasion be multiple or multilocular. Irrespective of the imaging method used, it may be difficult to distinguish these cystic masses from rare solid mesenteric tumors with cystic components, such as a cystic stromal tumor or mesothelioma. Mesenteric cystic lymphangioma may present as numerous, often large cysts in the setting of abdominal pain. These can be difficult to treat and almost invariably recur after excision.

When symptomatic, simple mesenteric cysts are surgically excised either openly or laparoscopically when feasible. Cyst unroofing or marsupialization is not recommended, because mesenteric cysts have a high propensity to recur after drainage alone. On rare occasion, adjacent mesentery may be densely adherent to the cyst or mesenteric vessels must be sacrificed to achieve complete excision, in which case segmental bowel resection is performed.

Mesenteric Tumors

Primary tumors of the mesentery are rare. Benign tumors of the mesentery include lipoma, cystic lymphangioma, and desmoid tumors. Primary malignant tumors of the mesentery are similar to those described for the omentum. Liposarcomas, leiomyosarcomas, malignant fibrous histiocytomas, lipoblastomas, and lymphangiosar-

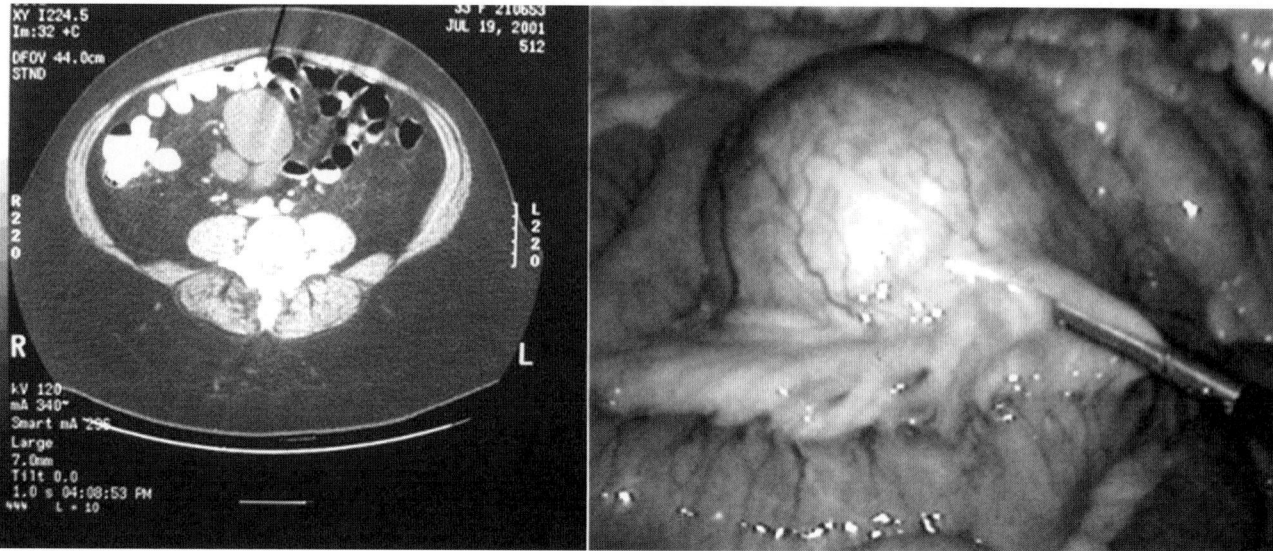

FIG. 35-17. Computed tomographic scan of a mesenteric cyst. The unilocular appearance without an associated solid component strongly suggests the diagnosis of benign cyst.

comas all have been described. Metastatic small intestine carcinoid in mesenteric lymph nodes may exceed the bulk of primary disease and compromise blood supply to the bowel. Treatment of mesenteric malignancies involves wide resection of the mass. Because of the proximity to the blood supply to the intestine, such resections may be technically unfeasible or involve loss of substantial lengths of bowel.

RETROPERITONEUM

Surgical Anatomy

Although there are ectodermal, mesodermal, and endodermal contributions to the contents of the retroperitoneum, embryonic mesoderm predominates in the developing retroperitoneal space. From the *intermediate* mesoderm arise the organs of the urinary and genital systems. The *lateral plate* mesoderm eventually divides into two layers, the parietal layer and the visceral layer. These layers eventually become the pleura, pericardium, peritoneum, and retroperitoneum.

The retroperitoneum is defined as the space between the posterior envelopment of the peritoneum and the posterior body wall (Fig. 35-18). The retroperitoneal space is bounded superiorly by the diaphragm, posteriorly by the spinal column and iliopsoas muscles, and inferiorly by the levator ani muscles. Although the retroperitoneum is technically bounded anteriorly by the posterior reflection of the peritoneum, the anterior border of the retroperitoneum is quite convoluted, extending into the spaces in between the mesenteries of the small and large intestine. Because of the rigidity of the superior, posterior, and inferior boundaries, and the compliance of the anterior margin, retroperitoneal tumors tend to expand anteriorly toward the peritoneal cavity. Table 35-2 lists the organs and structures that reside within the retroperitoneum.

Retroperitoneal Infections

The posterior reflection of the peritoneum limits the spread of most intra-abdominal infections to the peritoneum. Accordingly, the source of retroperitoneal infections is usually an organ contained within or abutting the retroperitoneum. Retrocecal appendicitis, perforated duodenal ulcers, pancreatitis, and diverticulitis may all lead to retroperitoneal infection with or without abscess formation. The substantial space and rather nondiscrete boundaries of the retroperitoneum allow some retroperitoneal abscesses to become quite large before diagnosis.

A patient with a retroperitoneal abscess usually presents with pain, fever, and malaise. The site of the patient's pain may be variable and can include the back, pelvis, or thighs. Clinical findings can include tachypnea and tachycardia. Erythema may be observed around the umbilicus or flank. This is analogous to the ecchymosis seen in these locations after massive retroperitoneal hemorrhage (Cullen's sign and Grey Turner's sign, respectively). A palpable flank or abdominal mass may be present. Laboratory evaluation usually reveals an elevated white blood cell count. The diagnostic imaging modality of choice is CT, which may demonstrate stranding of the retroperitoneal soft tissues and/or a unilocular or multilocular collection (Fig. 35-19).

Management of retroperitoneal infections includes identification and treatment of the underlying condition, IV administration of antibiotics, and drainage of all well-defined collections. Although unilocular abscesses may be drained percutaneously under CT guidance, multilocular collections usually require operative intervention for adequate drainage. Because of the large size of the retroperitoneal space, patients with retroperitoneal abscesses usually do not seek treatment until the abscess is advanced. Consequently, the mortality rate for retroperitoneal abscess, even when the abscess is drained, has been reported to be as high as 25%, or even higher in rare cases of necrotizing fasciitis of the retroperitoneum.

Retroperitoneal Fibrosis

Retroperitoneal fibrosis is a class of disorders characterized by hyperproliferation of fibrous tissue in the retroperitoneum. It may be a primary disorder as in idiopathic retroperitoneal fibrosis, also known as *Ormond disease*, or a secondary reaction to an inciting inflammatory process, malignancy, or medication. Idiopathic retroperitoneal fibrosis is a rare disorder, usually affecting 0.5 in 100,000 patients annually. Men are twice as likely to be affected as women, and no predilection for any particular ethnic group is seen. The disease primarily affects individuals in the fourth to the sixth decades of life.

An allergic or autoimmune mechanism has been postulated for this condition. Circulating antibodies to ceroid, a lipoproteinaceous by-product of vascular atheromatous plaque oxidation, are present in >90% of patients with retroperitoneal fibrosis. The relationship of this finding to the occurrence of fibrosis remains uncertain. The early inflammatory reaction involves predominantly helper T cells, plasma cells, and macrophages, but these are subsequently replaced by collagen-synthesizing fibroblasts. Microscopically, the infiltrate

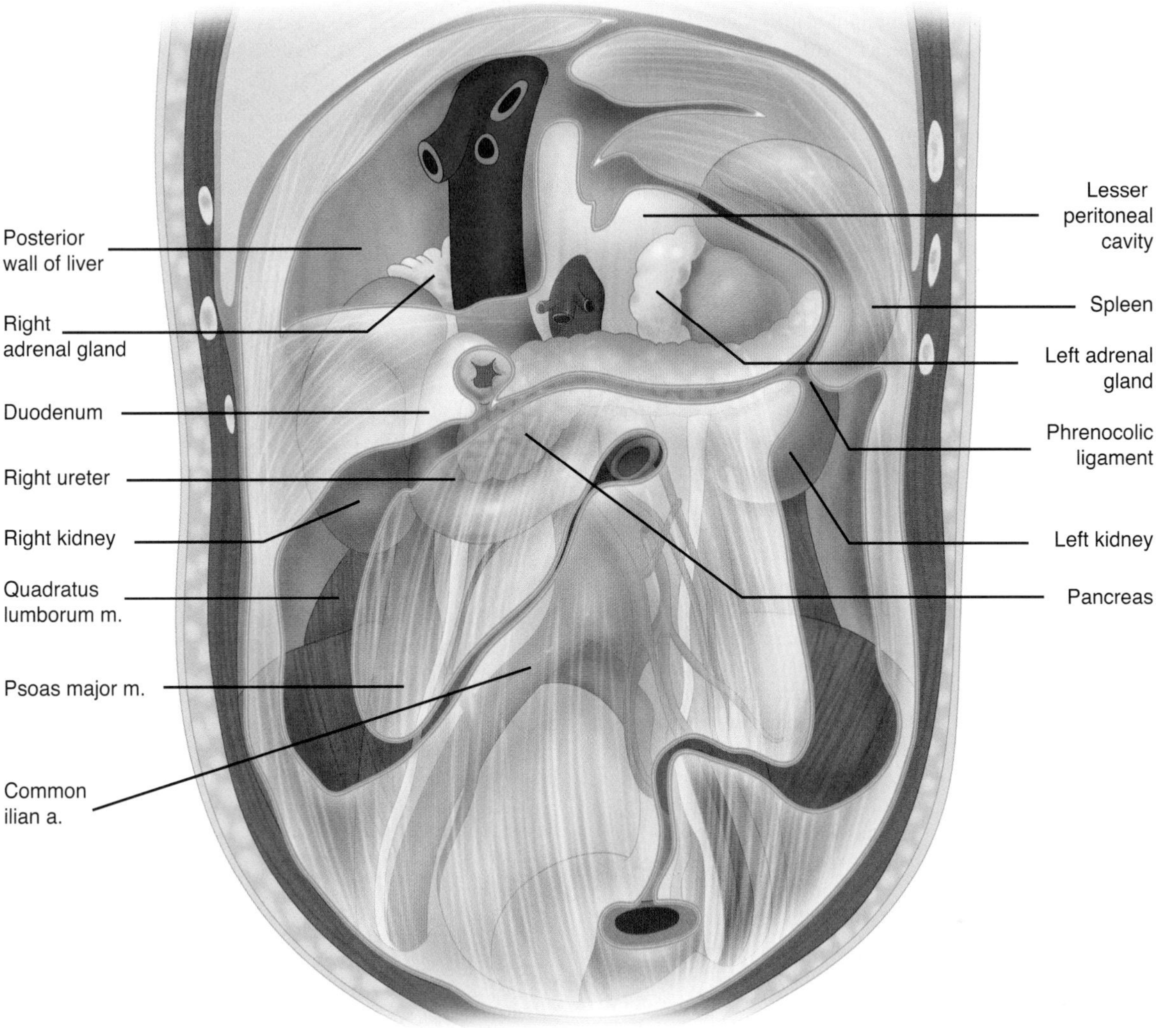

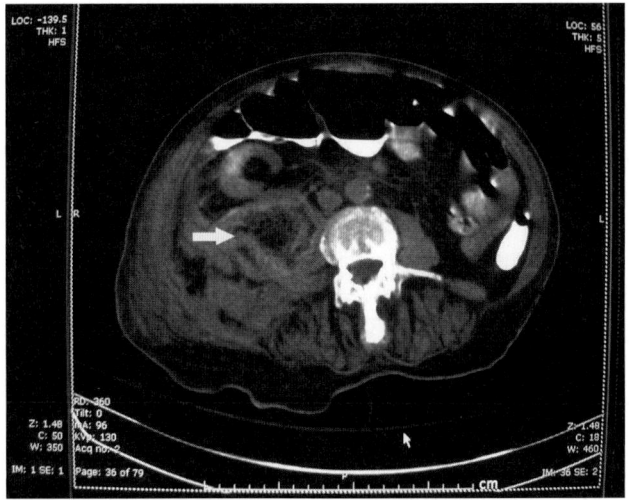

FIG. 35-18. Anatomy of the retroperitoneum. a. = artery; m. = muscle. *[Reproduced with permission from Healey JE, Hodge J (eds): Surgical Anatomy, 2nd ed. Toronto: BC Decker, 1990, p 201.]*

is indistinguishable from that seen with periadventitial involvement in aortic aneurysmal disease, Riedel's thyroiditis, sclerosing cholangitis, and Peyronie's disease. The fibrotic process begins in the retroperitoneum just below the level of the renal arteries. Fibrosis gradually expands, encasing the ureters, inferior vena cava, aorta, mesenteric vessels, or sympathetic nerves. Bilateral involvement is noted in 67% of cases.

Retroperitoneal fibrosis may also occur secondary to a variety of inflammatory conditions or as an allergic reaction to a medication. These conditions include abdominal aortic aneurysm, pancreatitis, histoplasmosis, tuberculosis, and actinomycosis. It is also associated with a variety of malignancies, including prostate, pancreatic, and gastric cancers as well as non-Hodgkin's lymphoma, stromal tu-

TABLE 35-2	Retroperitoneal structures	
Kidneys	Ureters	Bladder
Pancreas	Duodenum (D2 and D3)	Adrenal glands
Ascending colon	Descending colon	Rectum (upper two thirds)
Aorta	Inferior vena cava	Iliac vessels
Seminal vesicles	Vas deferens	Lymphatics (cisterna chyli)
Vagina (uppermost)	Ovaries	Nerves (lumbar sympathetics)

FIG. 35-19. Computed tomographic scan of a retroperitoneal abscess complicating complex, surgically treated retroperitoneal infection that had resulted from ampullary perforation at the time of endoscopic retrograde cholangiopancreatography. This pattern of infection may be difficult to treat and may result in multiple interventions, such as percutaneous drainage, before resolution.

mors, and carcinoid tumors. Retroperitoneal fibrosis has been described in association with autoimmune disorders, including ankylosing spondylitis, systemic lupus erythematosus, Wegener's granulomatosis, and polyarteritis nodosa. The strongest case for a causal relationship between medication and retroperitoneal fibrosis is made for methysergide, a semisynthetic ergot alkaloid used in the treatment of migraine headaches. Other medications that have been linked to retroperitoneal fibrosis include beta blockers, hydralazine, α-methyldopa, and entacapone, which inhibits catechol-O-methyltransferase and is used as an adjunct with levodopa in the treatment of Parkinson's disease. The retroperitoneal fibrosis regresses on discontinuation of these medications.

Presenting symptoms depend on the structure or structures affected by the fibrotic process. Initially, patients complain of the insidious onset of dull, poorly localized abdominal pain. Sudden-onset or severe abdominal pain may signify acute mesenteric ischemia. Other symptoms of retroperitoneal fibrosis include unilateral leg swelling, intermittent claudication, oliguria, hematuria, and dysuria.

As with the patient's symptomatology, findings on physical examination vary with the retroperitoneal structure involved. Consequently, findings may include hypertension, the palpation of an abdominal or flank mass, lower extremity edema (unilateral or bilateral), or diminished lower extremity pulses (unilateral or bilateral). Laboratory evaluation may reveal an elevated blood urea nitrogen and/or creatinine level. As with many autoimmune inflammatory processes, the erythrocyte sedimentation rate almost always is elevated in patients with retroperitoneal fibrosis.

Many imaging modalities have been used with varying sensitivity to diagnose retroperitoneal fibrosis. Abdominal and lower extremity ultrasonography is the least invasive imaging procedure, but results are technician dependent. It may be useful if iliocaval compressive or renal symptoms predominate. Lower extremity ultrasonography may show deep vein thrombosis, whereas abdominal ultrasonography may identify a mass lesion or hydronephrosis. IV pyelography, once the diagnostic procedure of choice, is less commonly used today. If the ureters are involved, the findings of IV pyelography will include ureteral compression, ureteral deviation toward the midline, and hydronephrosis.

Abdominopelvic CT with oral and IV contrast agents is the imaging procedure of choice and generally will allow the extent of the fibrotic process to be determined. If renal function is diminished so that the use of IV contrast agents must be avoided, the ability to characterize retroperitoneal tissue planes will be reduced. In this case, MRI may be used, because the signal intensity of the fibrotic process is discrete from that of muscle or fat. In addition, magnetic resonance angiography generally provides a good assessment of the degree of iliocaval involvement. Once a mass lesion is identified, biopsy of the mass should be performed to rule out a retroperitoneal malignancy. The specimen may be obtained using image-guided techniques or a surgical retroperitoneal biopsy procedure, which may be performed laparoscopically or during open laparotomy.

Once malignancy, drug effects, and infectious causes are ruled out, treatment of the retroperitoneal fibrotic process is instituted. Corticosteroids, with or without surgery, are the mainstay of medical therapy. Surgical treatment consists primarily of ureterolysis or ureteral stenting and is required in patients who present with moderate or massive hydronephrosis. Laparoscopic ureterolysis has been shown to be as efficacious as open surgery in addressing this problem. Patients with iliocaval thrombosis require anticoagulation, although the required duration of this therapy is unclear. Prednisone is initially administered at a relatively high dose (60 mg every other day for 2 months) and then gradually tapered over the next 2 months. Therapeutic efficacy is assessed on the basis of patient symptoms and interval imaging studies. Cyclosporin, tamoxifen, and azathioprine also have been used to treat patients who respond poorly to corticosteroids.

The overall prognosis in idiopathic retroperitoneal fibrosis is good, with 5-year survival rates of 90 to 100%. Because long-term recurrences have been described, lifelong follow-up is warranted.

BIBLIOGRAPHY

Entries highlighted in bright blue are key references.

General References

Burt BM, Tavakkolizaden A, Ferzoco SJ: Incisions, closures, and management of the abdominal wound, in Zinner MJ, Ashley SW (eds): *Maingot's Abdominal Operations*, 11th ed. New York: McGraw Hill, 2007, p 71.

Flament JB, Avisse C, Delattre JF: Anatomy of the abdominal wall, in Bendavid R, Abrahamson J, Arregui ME, et al (eds): *Abdominal Wall Hernias: Principles and Management*, 1st ed. New York: Springer-Verlag, 2001, p 39.

Voeller GR, Mangiante E: Laparoscopic repair of ventral/incisional hernias, in Fitzgibbons RJ Jr., Greenberg AG (eds): *Nyhus and Condon's Hernia*, 5th ed. Philadelphia: Lippincott William & Wilkins, 2001, p 373.

Abdominal Wall

Anthony T, Bergen PC, Kim LT, et al: Factors affecting recurrence following incisional herniorrhaphy. *World J Surg* 24:95, 2000.

Bendavid R: Composite mesh (polypropylene-e-PTFE) in the intraperitoneal position: A report of 30 cases. *Hernia* 1:5, 1997.

Blatnik J, Jin J, Rosen M: Abdominal hernia repair with bridging acellular dermal matrix—an expensive hernia sac. *Am J Surg* 196:47, 2008.

de Vries Reilingh TS, Bodegom ME, van Goor H, et al: Autologous tissue repair of large abdominal wall defects. *Br J Surg* 94:791, 2007.

Edlow JA, Juang P, Marglies S, et al: Rectus sheath hematoma. *Ann Emerg Med* 34:671, 1999.

Graves, EJ: Detailed diagnoses and procedures, National Hospital Discharge Survey, 1993. National Center for Health Statistics. *Vital Health Stat* 13(122):1, 1995.

Halm JA, de Wall LL, Steyerberg EW, et al: Intraperitoneal polypropylene mesh hernia repair complicates subsequent abdominal surgery. *World J Surg* 31:423, 2007.

Heniford BT, Park A, Ramshaw BJ, et al: Laparoscopic ventral and incisional hernia repair in 407 patients. *J Am Coll Surg* 190:645, 2000.

Hesselink VJ, Luijendijk R, de Wilt JH, et al: An evaluation of risk factors in incisional hernia recurrence. *Surg Gynecol Obstet* 176:228, 1993.

Jin J, Rosen MJ, Blatnik J, et al: Use of acellular dermal matrix for complicated hernia repair: Does technique affect outcome? *J Am Coll Surg* 205:654, 2007.

Klingler PJ, Wetcher G, Glaser K, et al: The use of ultrasound to differentiate rectus sheath hematoma from other acute abdominal disorders. *Surg Endosc* 13:1129, 1999.

Korenkov M, Sauerland S, Arndt M, et al: Randomized clinical trial of suture repair, polypropylene mesh or autodermal hernioplasty for incisional hernia. *Br J Surg* 89:50, 2002.

LeBlanc KA: Laparoscopic incisional hernia repair: Are transfascial sutures necessary? A review of the literature. *Surg Endosc* 21:508, 2007.

LeBlanc KA, Booth WV: Laparoscopic repair of incisional abdominal hernias using expanded polytetrafluoroethylene: Preliminary findings. *Surg Laparosc Endosc* 3:39, 1993.

Luijendijk RW, Hop WC, van den Tol MP, et al: A comparison of suture repair with mesh repair for incisional hernia. *N Engl J Med* 343:392, 2000.

Park A, Birch DW, Lovrics P: Laparoscopic and open incisional hernia repair: A comparison study. *Surgery* 124:816, 1998.

Perry CW, Phillips BJ: Rectus sheath hematoma: Review of an uncommon surgical complication. *Hosp Physician* 37:35, 2001.

Pierce RA, Spitler JA, Frisella MM, et al: Pooled data analysis of laparoscopic vs. open ventral hernia repair: 14 years of patient data accrual. *Surg Endosc* 21:378, 2007.

Ramirez OM, Ruas E, Dellon AL: "Components separation" method for closure of abdominal-wall defects: An anatomic and clinical study. *Plast Reconstr Surg* 86:519, 1990.

Stoppa R, Ralaimiaramanana F, Henry X, et al: Evolution of large ventral incisional hernia repair: The French contribution to a difficult problem. *Hernia* 3:1, 1999.

Zainea GG, Jordan F: Rectus sheath hematomas: Their pathogenesis, diagnosis, and management. *Am Surg* 54:630, 1988.

Omentum

Beelen RHJ: The greater omentum: Physiology and immunological concepts. *Neth J Surg* 43:145, 1991.

Fukatsu K, Saito H, Han I, et al: The greater omentum is the primary site of neutrophil exudation in peritonitis. *J Am Coll Surg* 183:450, 1996.

Goldsmith HS (ed): *The Omentum: Research and Clinical Applications*. New York: Springer-Verlag, 2000.

Liebermann-Meffert D: The greater omentum. Anatomy, embryology, and surgical applications. *Surg Clin North Am* 80:275, 2000.

Liebermann-Meffert D, White H (eds): *The Greater Omentum. Anatomy, Physiology, Pathology, Surgery with an Historical Survey*. New York: Springer-Verlag, 1983.

Logmans A, Schoenmakers CH, Haensel SM, et al: High tissue factor concentration in the omentum, a possible cause of its hemostatic properties. *Eur J Clin Invest* 26:82, 1996.

Morison R: Remarks on some functions of the omentum. *Br Med J* 1:76, 1906.

Nakagawa M, Akasaka Y, Kanai T, et al: Extragastrointestinal stromal tumor of the greater omentum: Case report and review of the literature. *Hepatogastroenterology* 50:691, 2003.

O'Leary DP: Use of the greater omentum in colorectal surgery. *Dis Colon Rectum* 42:533, 1999.

Powers JC, Fitzgerald JF, McAlvanah MJ: The anatomical basis for the surgical detachment of the greater omentum from the transverse colon. *Surg Gynecol Obstet* 143:105, 1976.

Saborido BP, Romero CJ, Medina ME, et al: Idiopathic segmental infarction of the greater omentum as a cause of acute abdomen. Report of two cases and review of the literature. *Hepatogastroenterology* 48:737, 2001.

Schwartz RW, Reames M, McGrath PC, et al: Primary solid neoplasms of the greater omentum. *Surgery* 109:543, 1990.

Sompayrac SW, Mindelzun RE, Silverman PM, et al: The greater omentum. *AJR Am J Roentgenol* 168:683, 1997.

Mesentery

Daskalogiannaki M, Voloudaki A, Prassopoulos P, et al: CT evaluation of mesenteric panniculitis: Prevalence and associated diseases. *AJR Am J Roentgenol* 174:427, 2000.

Durst AL, Freund H, Rosenmann E, et al: Mesenteric panniculitis: Review of the literature and presentation of cases. *Surgery* 81:203, 1977.

Egozi EI, Ricketts RR: Mesenteric and omental cysts in children. *Am Surg* 63:287, 1997.

Emory T, Monihan J, Carr NJ, et al: Sclerosing mesenteritis, mesenteric panniculitis, and mesenteric lipodystrophy. *Am J Surg Pathol* 21:392, 1997.

Genereau T, Bellin MF, Wechsler B, et al: Demonstration of efficacy of combining corticosteroids and colchicine in two patients with idiopathic sclerosing mesenteritis. *Dig Dis Sci* 41:684, 1996.

Hebra A, Brown MF, McGeehin KM, et al: Mesenteric, omental and retroperitoneal cysts in children: A clinical study of 22 cases. *South Med J* 86:173, 1993.

Kelly JK, Hwang WS: Idiopathic retractile (sclerosing) mesenteritis and its differential diagnosis. *Am J Surg Pathol* 13:513, 1989.

Kurtz RJ, Heimann TM, Holt J, et al: Mesenteric and retroperitoneal cysts. *Am J Surg* 40:462, 1974.

O'Brien MF, Winter DC, Lee G, et al: Mesenteric cysts—a series of six cases with a review of the literature. *Ir J Med Sci* 168:233, 1999.

Ogden WW, Bradburn DM, Rives JD: Panniculitis of the mesentery. *Ann Surg* 151:659, 1960.

Ros PR, Olmsted WW, et al: Mesenteric and omental cysts: Histologic classification with imaging correlation. *Radiology* 164:327, 1987.

Shamiyeh A, Rieger R, Schrenk P, et al: Role of laparoscopic surgery in treatment of mesenteric cysts. *Surg Endosc* 13:937, 1999.

Takiff H, Calabria R, Yin L, et al: Mesenteric cysts and intra-abdominal cystic lymphangiomas. *Arch Surg* 120:1266, 1985.

Zissen R, Metser U, Hain D, et al: Mesenteric panniculitis in oncologic patients: PET-CT findings. *Br J Radiol* 79:37, 2006.

Retroperitoneum

Cerfolio RJ, Morgan AS, Hirvela ER, et al: Idiopathic retroperitoneal fibrosis: Is there a role for postoperative steroids? *Curr Surg* 47:423, 1990.

Duchene DA, Winfield HN, Cadeddu JA, et al: Multi-institutional survey of laparoscopic ureterolysis for retroperitoneal fibrosis. *Urology* 69:1017, 2007.

Gilkeson GS, Allen NB: Retroperitoneal fibrosis. A true connective tissue disease. *Rheum Dis Clin North Am* 22:23, 1996.

Higgins PM, Bennett-Jones DN, Naish PF, et al: Non-operative management of retroperitoneal fibrosis. *Br J Surg* 75:573, 1988.

Kardar AH, Kattan S, Lindstedt E, et al: Steroid therapy for idiopathic retroperitoneal fibrosis: Dose and duration. *J Urol* 168:550, 2002.

Koep L, Zuidema GD: The clinical significance of retroperitoneal fibrosis. *Surgery* 81:250, 1977.

Kottra JJ, Reed DN: Retroperitoneal fibrosis. *Radiol Clin North Am* 34:1259, 1996.

Marzano A, Trapani A, Leone N, et al: Treatment of idiopathic retroperitoneal fibrosis using cyclosporine. *Ann Rheum Dis* 60:427, 2001.

Ormond JK: Bilateral ureteral obstruction due to envelopment and compression by an inflammatory process. *J Urol* 59:1072, 1948.

Pryor JP, Piotrowski E, Seltzer CW, et al: Early diagnosis of retroperitoneal necrotizing fasciitis. *Crit Care Med* 29:1071, 2001.

Rhee RY, Gloviczki P, Luthra HS, et al: Iliocaval complications of retroperitoneal fibrosis. *Am J Surg* 168:179, 1994.

Srinivasan AK, Richstone L, Permpongkosol S, et al: Comparison of laparoscopic with open approach for uterolysis in patients with retroperitoneal fibrosis. *J Urol* 179:1875, 2008.

Uchida K, Okazaki K, Asada M, et al: Case of chronic pancreatitis involving an autoimmune mechanism that extended to retroperitoneal fibrosis. *Pancreas* 26:92, 2003.

Woodburn KR, Ramsay G, Gillespie G, et al: Retroperitoneal necrotizing fasciitis. *Br J Surg* 79:342, 1992.

CHAPTER 35 Abdominal Wall, Omentum, Mesentery, and Retroperitoneum

Soft Tissue Sarcomas

Janice N. Cormier and Raphael E. Pollock

OVERVIEW

Incidence

Sarcomas are a heterogeneous group of tumors that arise predominantly from the embryonic mesoderm, but also can originate, as does the peripheral nervous system, from the ectoderm. In 2007, approximately 9220 new cases of soft tissue sarcoma were diagnosed in the United States with 3560 deaths attributable to disease.[1] These rare tumors account for less than 1% of cancers in adults and represent 7% of cancers in children. Several distinct groups of sarcomas are recognized; soft tissue sarcomas, the largest of these groups, are the focus of this chapter. Other groups include bone sarcomas (osteosarcomas and chondrosarcomas), Ewing's sarcomas, and peripheral primitive neuroectodermal tumors.

Soft tissue sarcomas can occur throughout the body and encompass more than 50 histiotypes (Table 36-1) with distinct histologic lines of differentiation. The most common histologic types of soft tissue sarcoma in adults (excluding Kaposi's sarcoma) are malignant fibrous histiocytoma (MFH, 28%), leiomyosarcoma (12%), liposarcoma (15%), synovial sarcoma (10%), and malignant peripheral nerve sheath tumors (6%).[2] Rhabdomyosarcoma is the most common soft tissue sarcoma of childhood. Most primary soft tissue sarcomas originate in an extremity (50 to 60%); the next most common sites are the trunk, retroperitoneum, and head and neck.

During the past 25 years, a multimodality treatment approach has been applied to patients with extremity sarcomas, which had led to modest improvements in both survival and quality of life. However, patients with abdominal sarcomas continue to have high rates of recurrence and poor overall survival. Overall 5-year survival rate for patients with all stages of soft tissue sarcoma is 50 to 60%. Of the patients who die of sarcoma, most will succumb to metastatic disease, which 80% of the time occurs within 2 to 3 years of the initial diagnosis.

Epidemiology

Except for malignant peripheral nerve sheath tumors in patients with neurofibromatosis, sarcomas do not seem to result from the progression or dedifferentiation of benign soft tissue tumors. Despite the variety of histologic subtypes, sarcomas have many common clinical and pathologic features. Overall, the clinical behavior of most soft tissue sarcomas is similar and is determined by anatomic location (depth), grade, and size. The dominant pattern of metastasis is hematogenous, primarily to the lungs. Lymph node metastases are rare (<5%) except for a few histologic subtypes such as epithelioid sarcoma, rhabdomyosarcoma, clear-cell sarcoma, synovial sarcoma, MFH, and angiosarcoma.[3]

TABLE 36-1	Relative frequency of histologic subtypes of soft tissue sarcoma[2]	
Histologic Subtypes	**n**	**%**
Malignant fibrous histiocytoma	349	28
Liposarcoma	188	15
Leiomyosarcoma	148	12
Unclassified sarcoma	140	11
Synovial sarcoma	125	10
Malignant peripheral nerve sheath tumor	72	6
Rhabdomyosarcoma	60	5
Fibrosarcoma	38	3
Ewing's sarcoma	25	2
Angiosarcoma	25	2
Osteosarcoma	14	1
Epithelioid sarcoma	14	1
Chondrosarcoma	13	1
Clear-cell sarcoma	12	1
Alveolar soft part sarcoma	7	1
Malignant hemangiopericytoma	5	0.4

Source: Data from Coindre et al.[2]

Radiation Exposure

External radiation therapy is a rare but well-established risk factor for soft tissue sarcoma. An eightfold to 50-fold increase in the incidence of sarcomas has been reported among patients treated for cancer of the breast, cervix, ovary, testes, and lymphatic system.[4,5] In a review of 160 patients with postirradiation sarcomas, the most common histologic types were osteogenic sarcoma, MFH, angiosarcoma, and lymphangiosarcoma.[4] In that study, the risk of developing a sarcoma increased with higher radiation doses, and the median latency period was 10 years. Postirradiation sarcomas usually are diagnosed at advanced stages and generally have a poor prognosis.

Occupational Chemicals

Exposure to some herbicides such as phenoxyacetic acids and wood preservatives containing chlorophenols has been linked to an increased risk of soft tissue sarcoma.[6] Several chemical carcinogens, including thorium oxide (Thorotrast), vinyl chloride, and arsenic have been associated with hepatic angiosarcomas.

Trauma

Although patients with sarcomas often report a history of trauma, no causal relationship has been established. More often, a minor

---

KEY POINTS

1. Sarcomas are a heterogeneous group of tumors that can occur throughout the body and encompass more than 50 subtypes with distinct histologic lines of differentiation.

2. These rare tumors account for less than 1% of cancers in adults (estimated 10,000 cases per year in the United States) and represent 7% of cancers in children.

3. Approximately two thirds of soft tissue sarcomas arise in the extremities; the remaining one third are distributed between the retroperitoneum, trunk, abdomen, and head and neck.

4. The treatment algorithm for soft tissue sarcomas depends on tumor stage, site, and histology.

5. Multimodality treatment including surgical resection, radiation therapy and, in selected cases, systemic chemotherapy, has been applied to patients with locally advanced, high-grade, extremity sarcomas.

6. Overall 5-year survival rate for patients with all stages of soft tissue sarcoma is 50 to 60%.

7. Of the patients who die of sarcoma, most will succumb to metastatic disease in the lungs, which 80% of the time occurs within 2 to 3 years of the initial diagnosis.

8. Progress in the understanding of soft tissue sarcoma biology is crucial for the development of new therapeutic targets.

injury calls attention to a pre-existing tumor that may be accentuated by edema or hematoma.

Chronic Lymphedema

In 1948, Stewart and Treves first described the association between chronic lymphedema after axillary dissection and subsequent lymphangiosarcoma.[7] Lymphangiosarcoma also has been reported as occurring after filarial infections and in the lower extremities of patients with congenital or heritable lymphedema.

Genetics

Molecular genetics, cytogenetics, and expression profiling have been used to investigate sarcomas, resulting in their classification into two main groups: those with defined diagnostic molecular events and those with variable histologic and genetic changes.[8] In general, the group of sarcoma patients with defined molecular events have been found to be younger with a defined histology, suggesting a clear line of differentiation. The defined molecular events include point mutations, a translocation causing overexpression of an autocrine growth factor or oncogenic fusion transcription factor. In contrast, sarcomas without currently identifiable genetic changes or expression profile signatures tend to occur in older patients exhibiting pleomorphic cytology and p53 dysfunction.[8]

Sarcomas occur more commonly within several hereditary cancer syndromes, including retinoblastoma, Li-Fraumeni syndrome, neurofibromatosis type I, and familial adenomatous polyposis.[9] Germline mutations have been identified as causal in only a limited number of these disorders. Developments in the field of molecular biology have led to a better understanding of some of the basic cellular processes governed by oncogenes and tumor suppressor genes.

Oncogene Activation

Oncogenes are genes that can induce malignant transformation and tend to drive cells toward proliferation. Several oncogenes have been identified in association with soft tissue sarcomas, including *MDM2*, *N-myc*, *c-erb*B-2, and members of the *ras* family. These oncogenes produce specific oncoproteins that either play a role in nuclear function and cellular signal transduction or function as growth factors or growth factor receptors. Amplification of these genes has been shown to correlate with adverse outcome in several soft tissue sarcomas.[10]

Cytogenetic analysis of soft tissue tumors has identified distinct chromosomal translocations that seem to encode for oncogenes associated with certain sarcoma histologic subtypes. These specific genetic changes result in the in-frame fusion of genes and fused product codes for the expression of oncoproteins functioning as transcriptional activators or repressors.[10,11] The best characterized gene rearrangements are found in Ewing's sarcoma (*EWS–FLI-1* fusion), clear-cell sarcoma (*EWS–ATF1* fusion), myxoid liposarcoma (*TLS–CHOP* fusion), alveolar rhabdomyosarcoma (*PAX3–FHKR* fusion), desmoplastic small round-cell tumor (*EWS–WT1* fusion), and synovial sarcoma (*SSX–SYT* fusion). It has been estimated that, in aggregate, fusion gene-related sarcomas may account for up to 30% of all sarcomas.[12] The oncogenic potential of many of these genes has been demonstrated in vitro and in vivo. These fusion genes provide not only specific diagnostic markers but encode chimeric proteins, both of which may be potential therapeutic targets.

Tumor Suppressor Genes

Tumor suppressor genes play a critical role in growth inhibition and can suppress growth in cancer cells. Inactivation of tumor suppressor genes (also known as *anti-oncogenes*) can occur through hereditary or sporadic mechanisms. The two genes that are most relevant to soft tissue tumors are the retinoblastoma (*Rb*) tumor suppressor gene and the p53 tumor suppressor gene. Mutations or deletions in *Rb* can lead to development of retinoblastoma or sarcomas of soft tissue and bone. Mutations in the p53 tumor suppressor gene are the most common mutations in human solid tumors and have been reported in 30 to 60% of soft tissue sarcomas.[13] Patients with germline mutations in the tumor suppressor gene p53 (the Li-Fraumeni syndrome) have a high incidence of sarcomas. Mutant p53 expression is thought to correlate with overall survival.[10] The p53 mutation also has been used as a therapeutic molecule in gene therapy strategies.

Neurofibromatosis is a neurocutaneous condition that exists in two forms. Neurofibromatosis type I, also known as *von Recklinghausen's disease*, occurs in approximately one of every 3000 people and is due to various mutations in the *NF-1* tumor suppressor gene located on chromosome 17. Patients with neurofibromatosis type I have an estimated 3 to 15% additional lifetime risk of malignant disease, including neurofibrosarcoma. Fifty percent of patients with neurofibrosarcomas have a mutation in *NF-1*.[14]

INITIAL ASSESSMENT

Clinical Presentation

Soft tissue sarcomas most commonly present as an asymptomatic mass. Another less common presentation of an extremity sarcoma may be a deep venous thrombosis, particularly in patients without significant risk factors for thrombosis.[15] Tumor size at presentation usually is associated with the location of the tumor. Smaller tumors generally are located in the distal extremities, whereas tumors in the proximal extremities and retroperitoneum can grow quite large before becoming apparent. Often, an extremity mass is discovered after a traumatic event that draws attention to a pre-existing lesion.

Soft tissue sarcomas often grow in a centrifugal fashion and compress surrounding normal structures. Infrequently, their impingement on bone or neurovascular bundles produces pain, edema, and swelling. Retroperitoneal soft tissue sarcomas almost always present as large asymptomatic masses. Less frequently, patients present with obstructive GI symptoms or neurologic symptoms related to compression of lumbar or pelvic nerves.

The differential diagnosis of a soft tissue mass includes benign lesions such as lipomas (100 times more common than sarcoma), lymphangiomas, leiomyomas, and neuromas. In addition to sarcomas, other malignant lesions such as primary or metastatic carcinomas, melanomas, or lymphomas must be considered. Small lesions that have not changed for several years by clinical history may be closely observed. All other tumors should be considered for biopsy to establish a definitive diagnosis.

Diagnostic Imaging

Pretreatment radiologic imaging serves several purposes: (a) defines the local extent of a tumor, (b) stages malignant disease, (c) assists in percutaneous biopsy procedures, and (d) aids in the diagnosis of soft tissue tumors (benign vs. malignant or low grade vs. high grade). Imaging studies are also crucial in monitoring tumor changes after treatment, especially preoperative chemotherapy or radiation therapy, and in detecting recurrences after surgical resection.

Radiographs provide useful information on primary bone tumors, but they are not useful in the evaluation of soft tissue sarcomas of the extremities unless underlying bone involvement from an adjacent soft tissue tumor is suspected. Chest radiography should be performed for patients with primary sarcomas to assess for lung metastases. For patients with high-grade lesions or tumors >5 cm (T2), computed tomography (CT) of the chest should be considered.

CT is the preferred technique for evaluating retroperitoneal sarcomas, whereas magnetic resonance imaging (MRI) often is favored for soft tissue sarcomas of the extremities.[16] Both ultrasonography and CT can assist in guiding fine-needle aspiration, core biopsy for initial diagnosis, and at recurrence.

Ultrasonography

Ultrasonography may have a diagnostic role for patients who cannot undergo MRI. Ultrasonography also can be a useful adjunct

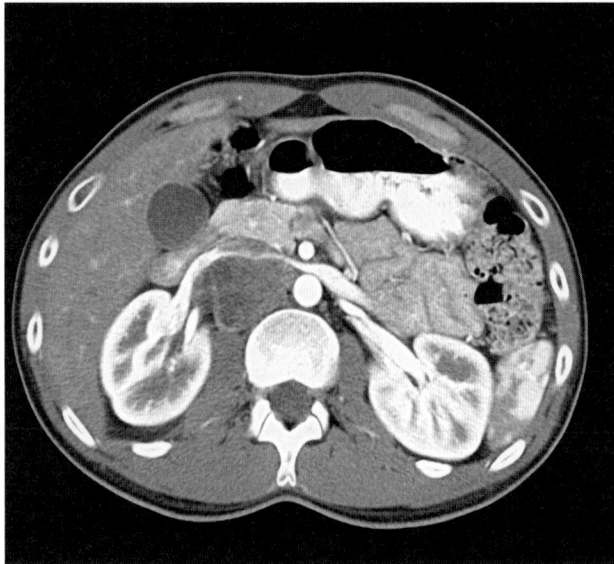

FIG. 36-1. A 27-year-old man presented with symptoms of back pain. Computed tomography of the abdomen demonstrating a 4.1 × 3.3 cm hypodense mass in the retrocaval region involving the inferior vena cava. Subsequent biopsy of the tumor confirmed leiomyosarcoma.

to MRI when findings are indeterminate and for delineating adjacent vascular structures.

Computed Tomography

Contrast-enhanced CT can assess the extent of soft tissue tumor burden and the proximity of the tumor to vital structures (Fig. 36-1). CT is the preferred imaging technique for evaluating retroperitoneal sarcomas.[16] Current CT techniques can provide a detailed survey of the abdomen and pelvis and can delineate adjacent organs and vascular structures. For extremity sarcomas, CT may be useful if MRI is not available or cannot be used. CT of the abdomen and pelvis should be done when histologic assessment of an extremity sarcoma reveals a myxoid liposarcoma, because this subtype is known to metastasize to the abdomen.[17]

Magnetic Resonance Imaging

MRI accurately delineates muscle groups and distinguishes among bone, vascular structures, and tumor. Sagittal and coronal views allow evaluation of anatomic compartments in three dimensions (Fig. 36-2). Soft tissue sarcomas of the extremities usually present on MRI as heterogeneous masses. Their signal intensity tends to be equal to or slightly higher than that of adjacent skeletal muscle on T1-weighted images and heterogeneous and high on T2-weighted images. Hemorrhagic, cystic, or necrotic changes also may be observed in the tumor. Special MRI techniques, including magnetic resonance angiography, may be performed if adjacent vascular structures must be delineated.

MRI has supplanted CT as the imaging technique of choice for evaluation of soft tissue sarcomas of the extremities. MRI also is valuable for assessing tumor recurrence after surgery (Fig. 36-3). A baseline image usually is obtained 3 months after surgery. Some clinicians believe that routine postoperative imaging of a primary extremity tumor site is not necessary for asymptomatic patients, citing the difficulties in detecting early recurrence in scarred, irradiated tissue.[16] Others advocate routine imaging every 6 months for the first 2 years.

MRI may be an important adjunct to cytologic analysis in distinguishing benign lesions such as lipomas, hemangiomas, schwannomas, neurofibromas, and intramuscular myxomas from their

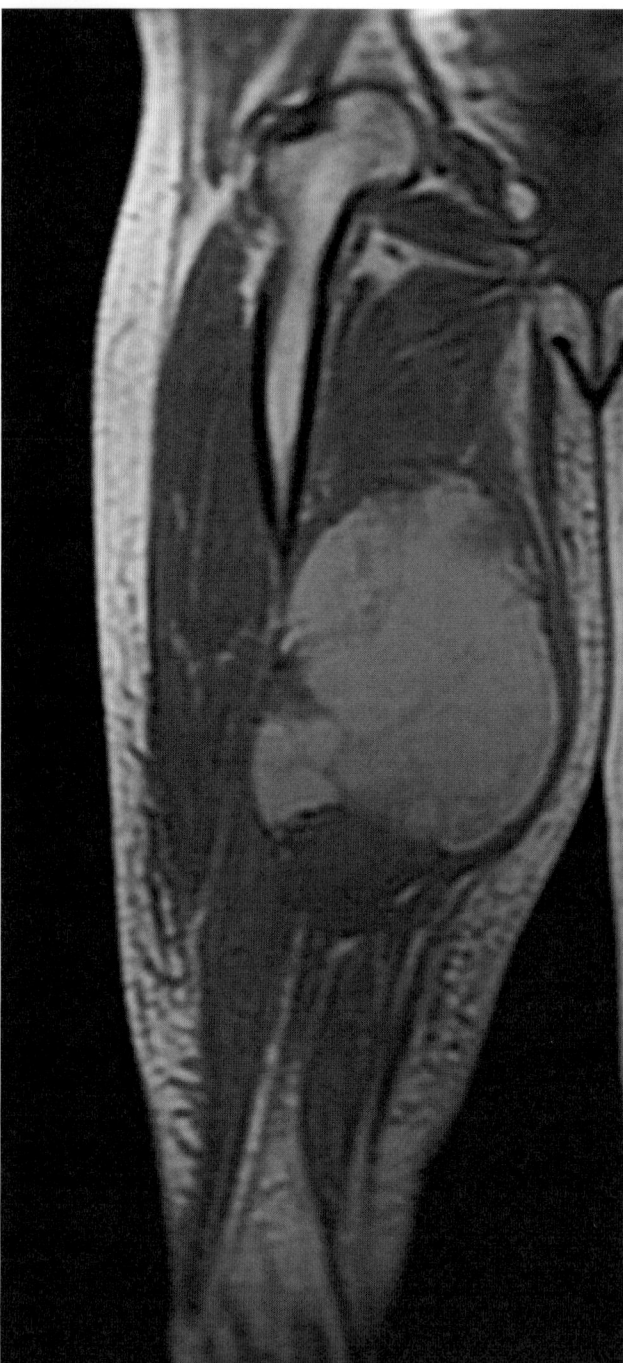

FIG. 36-2. A 55-year-old woman presented with right thigh pain and enlarging mass. Coronal image demonstrating an 18-cm mass within the adductor magnus musculature with evidence of necrosis and hemorrhage.

malignant counterparts. In the setting of preoperative chemotherapy, contrast-enhanced T1-weighted MRIs can be useful in evaluating intratumoral necrosis.

Biopsy Techniques
Fine-Needle Aspiration

Fine-needle aspiration is an acceptable method of diagnosing most soft tissue sarcomas, particularly when the results correlate closely with clinical and imaging findings.[18] However, fine-needle aspiration biopsy is indicated for primary diagnosis of soft tissue sarcomas only at centers where cytopathologists have experience with these types of tumors. Fine-needle aspiration biopsy is also the

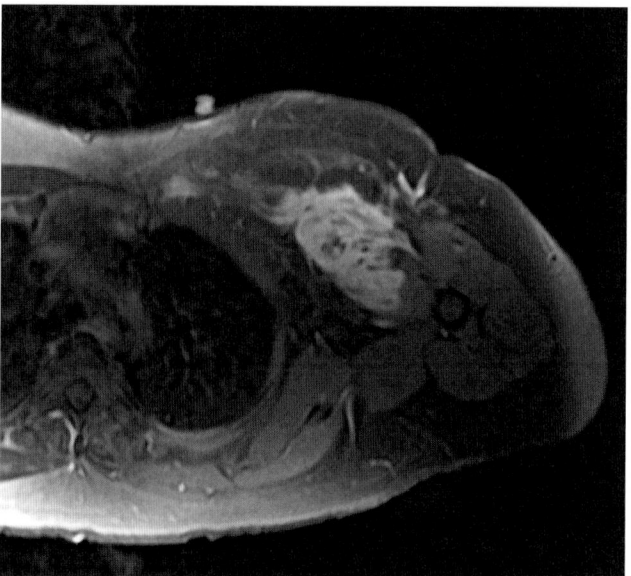

FIG. 36-3. A 51-year-old woman, 30 months status postexcision of desmoid tumor of the left breast and chest wall. Magnetic resonance imaging of the chest demonstrating a 5.2 × 7.7 cm mass with both T2 signal and postcontrast T1 signal indicating a recurrent desmoid tumor in the anterior aspect of the left upper arm and shoulder.

procedure of choice to confirm or rule out the presence of a metastatic focus or local recurrence. When tumor grading is essential for treatment planning, fine-needle aspiration biopsy is not the preferred technique.

Superficial lesions often are subjected to fine-needle aspiration biopsies in the clinic setting. Deeper tumors may require an interventional radiologist to perform the technique under sonographic or CT guidance. The technique generally involves the use of a 21- to 23-gauge needle that is introduced into the mass after appropriate cleansing of the skin and injection of local anesthetic. Negative pressure is applied, and the needle is pulled back and forth several times in various directions. After the negative pressure is released, the needle is withdrawn and the contents of the needle are used to prepare a smear.[19] A cytopathologist then examines the slides to determine whether sufficient diagnostic material is present. When insufficient diagnostic material is obtained, a core needle biopsy should be performed.

Diagnostic accuracy rates for fine-needle aspiration biopsy of primary tumors range from 60 to 96%. In general, the amount of material obtained from a fine-needle aspiration biopsy is small, and diagnostic accuracy clearly depends on the experience of the cytopathologist.

Core Needle Biopsy

Core needle biopsy is a safe, accurate, and economical procedure for diagnosing sarcomas. The tissue sample obtained from a core needle biopsy is usually sufficient for several diagnostic tests such as electron microscopy, cytogenetic analysis, and flow cytometry. The reported complication rate for core needle biopsy is less than 1%.[20]

CT guidance can enhance the positive yield rate of a core needle biopsy by more accurately pinpointing the location of the tumor. Precise localization in the tumor mass is particularly important to avoid sampling nondiagnostic necrotic or cystic areas of the tumor. CT guidance also permits access to tumors in otherwise inaccessible anatomic locations or when located near vital structures.

Dupuy and associates examined the accuracy of core needle biopsy in 221 patients with musculoskeletal neoplasms.[20] Core needle biopsy had an accuracy of 93% compared with the diagnosis

given at the time of definitive treatment. Only 8% of patients had nondiagnostic or insufficient specimens.

Incisional Biopsy

Open biopsy is a reliable diagnostic method that allows adequate tissue to be sampled for definitive and specific histologic identification of bone or soft tissue sarcomas. When adequate tissue for diagnosis cannot be obtained by fine-needle aspiration biopsy or core biopsy, an incisional biopsy is indicated for deep tumors and for superficial soft tissue tumors >3 cm. Incisional biopsies usually are performed as a last resort when fine-needle aspiration or core biopsy specimens are nondiagnostic. Open biopsies should be performed only by surgeons experienced in the management of soft tissue sarcomas. In a series of 107 patients with soft tissue sarcomas, planned surgical treatments had to be changed due to prior, poorly oriented biopsies in 25% of the cases.[21] Other series have reported complications in up to 16% of open biopsies.[19]

An open biopsy ideally should be performed in a designated treatment center and by the surgeon who will perform the definitive surgery. The biopsy incision should be oriented longitudinally along the extremity to allow a subsequent wide local excision that encompasses the biopsy site, scar, and tumor en bloc. A poorly oriented biopsy incision often mandates an excessively large surgical defect for a wide local excision. This, in turn, can result in a larger postoperative radiotherapy field to encompass all tissues at risk. Another mandate of surgical technique is that adequate hemostasis be achieved at the time of biopsy to prevent dissemination of tumor cells into adjacent tissue planes by hematoma.

An incisional or open biopsy is the most reliable of the diagnostic methods, providing accurate histologic diagnosis and grading in >95% of soft tissue sarcomas. In addition, the amount of tissue obtained often is sufficient for additional diagnostic studies if necessary.

Excisional Biopsy

Excisional biopsy can be performed for easily accessible (superficial) extremity or truncal lesions <3 cm. Excisional biopsy should not be done for lesions involving the hands and feet, because definitive re-excision may not be possible after the biopsy. Excisional biopsy results have a 30 to 40% rate of recurrence when margins are positive or uncertain. Excisional biopsies rarely provide any benefit over other biopsy techniques and may cause postoperative complications that could ultimately delay definitive therapy.

Pathologic Classification

Some experts have suggested that pathologic classification of soft tissue sarcomas has more prognostic significance than does tumor grade when other pretreatment variables are taken into account. Tumors with limited metastatic potential include desmoid, atypical lipomatous tumor (also called *well-differentiated liposarcoma*), dermatofibrosarcoma protuberans, and hemangiopericytoma. Tumors with an intermediate risk of metastatic spread usually have a large myxoid component and include myxoid liposarcoma and extraskeletal chondrosarcoma. Among the highly aggressive tumors that have substantial metastatic potential are angiosarcoma, clear-cell sarcoma, pleomorphic and dedifferentiated liposarcoma, leiomyosarcoma, rhabdomyosarcoma, and synovial sarcoma.

It recently has been noted that MFH is not associated with a distinct gene cluster, suggesting that MFH does not represent a separate tumor entity but rather a common morphologic appearance of various sarcoma subtypes.[22,23] For example, most tumors initially diagnosed as MFH in the retroperitoneum have been reclassified using genomic profiling as dedifferentiated liposarcomas.[24]

Expert sarcoma pathologists disagree about the specific histologic diagnoses and the criteria for defining tumor grade in 25 to 40% of individual cases.[25] The high rate of discordance emphasizes the need for more objective molecular and biochemical markers to improve conventional histologic assessment.

TABLE 36-2	Seventh Edition American Joint Committee on Cancer staging of soft tissue sarcoma[175]					
Primary tumor (T)						
T1	Tumor ≤5 cm					
		T1a		Superficial tumor		
		T1b		Deep tumor		
T2	Tumor >5 cm					
		T2a		Superficial tumor		
		T2b		Deep tumor		
Regional lymph nodes (N)						
N0	No regional lymph node metastasis					
N1	Regional lymph node metastasis					
Distance metastasis (M)						
M0	No distant metastasis					
M1	Distant metastasis					
Histologic grade (G)						
G1	Well differentiated					
G2	Moderately differentiated					
G3	Poorly differentiated					
Stage grouping						
Stage IA	T1a, T1b	N0	M0	G1	Low	
Stage IB	T2a	N0	M0	G1	Low	
Stage IIA	T1a, T1b	N0	M0	G2–G3	High	
Stage IIB	T2a	N0	M0	G2–G3	High	
Stage III	T2b	N0 or N1	M0	G2–G3	High	
Stage IV	Any T	Any N	M1	Any G	Any G	

Source: Used with the permission of the American Joint Committee on Cancer (AJCC), Chicago, Illinois. The original source for this material is the AJCC Cancer Staging Manual, Seventh Edition (in press) published by Springer Science and Business Media LLC, *www.springerlink.com*.[175]

Staging and Prognostic Factors

The newly revised Seventh Edition of the American Joint Committee on Cancer (AJCC) staging criteria for soft tissue sarcomas relies on histologic grade, tumor size, and depth, and the presence of nodal or distant metastases (Table 36-2).[26] This system does not apply to GI stromal tumor, fibromatosis (desmoid tumor), Kaposi's sarcoma, and infantile fibrosarcoma.

Histologic Grade

Histologic grade remains the most important prognostic factor for patients with sarcomas. For an accurate determination of tumor grade, an adequate tissue sample must be appropriately fixed, stained, and reviewed by an experienced sarcoma pathologist. The features that define grade are cellularity, differentiation, pleomorphism, necrosis, and the number of mitoses. Tumor grade has been shown to predict the development of metastases and overall survival.[27] The metastatic potentials have been estimated at 5 to 10% for low-grade lesions, 25 to 30% for intermediate-grade lesions, and 50 to 60% for high-grade tumors.

The number of grades varies according to the classification system used. The most common classification systems, those of the National Cancer Institute and the French Federation of Cancer Centers, use three tumor grades.[28] The National Cancer Institute system is based primarily on histologic tumor type, location, and amount of necrosis. The French Federation of Cancer Centers system generates a score based on tumor differentiation, mitotic rate, and the amount of tumor necrosis. A comparative analysis of the two grading systems suggested that the French Federation of Cancer Centers system may have better prognostic capability, predicting 5-year survival rates of 90%, 70%, and 40% for grade 1, 2, and 3 tumors, respectively.[28]

Following the recommendation of the College of American Pathologists, the 2008 AJCC staging system reformatted the newest staging system from a four grade to a three grade system.[29] The three tumor grades are designated: well differentiated (G1), moderately differentiated (G2), and poorly differentiated (G3). In this three-tiered system, grade 1 is considered "low grade," and grades 2 and 3 are considered "high grade."

Tumor Size

Tumor size has long been recognized to be an important prognostic variable in soft tissue sarcomas. Sarcomas have classically been stratified into two groups on the basis of size; T1 lesions are ≤5 cm, and T2 lesions are >5 cm. Some authors have suggested that further stratification of patients on the basis of tumor size can provide more accurate prognostic information. For example, when 316 patients with soft tissue sarcomas were examined and grouped into four tumor-size subgroups (<5 cm, 5 to 10 cm, 10 to 15 cm, and >15 cm), each subgroup was found to have a different prognosis, with 5-year survival of 84, 70, 50, and 33%, respectively.[30]

With respect to its association with the investing fascia of the extremity or trunk, anatomic tumor location was incorporated into the AJCC staging system in 1998. Soft tissue sarcomas above the superficial investing fascia of the extremity or trunk are designated "a" lesions in the T score, whereas tumors invading or deep to the fascia as well as all retroperitoneal, mediastinal, and visceral lesion tumors are designated "b" lesions.

Nodal Metastasis

Lymph node metastases arising from soft tissue sarcomas are rare.[3] A few histologic subtypes, including epithelioid sarcoma, rhabdomyosarcoma, clear-cell sarcoma, synovial sarcoma, MFH, and angiosarcoma, have a higher incidence of nodal involvement. In the newly revised AJCC staging system, nodal (N1) disease has been reclassified as stage III rather than stage IV disease.

A number of studies reporting better survival for patients with isolated regional lymph node metastases treated with radical lymphadenectomy compared to those with distant metastatic disease[3,31–33] prompted a change in the AJCC staging system. Results of these studies support the benefit of therapeutic lymphadenectomy, including axillary and ilioinguinal dissections, for extremity soft tissue sarcoma metastatic to regional lymph nodes.[31] Patients with clinically or radiologically suspicious regional nodes should have metastases confirmed by preoperative fine-needle aspiration before radical lymphadenectomy.

Distant Metastasis

Distant metastases occur most often in the lungs (Fig. 36-4). Selected patients with pulmonary metastases may survive for long periods after surgical resection and chemotherapy. Other potential sites of metastasis include bone, the brain, and the liver (Fig. 36-5). Visceral and retroperitoneal sarcomas have a higher incidence of liver and peritoneal metastases.

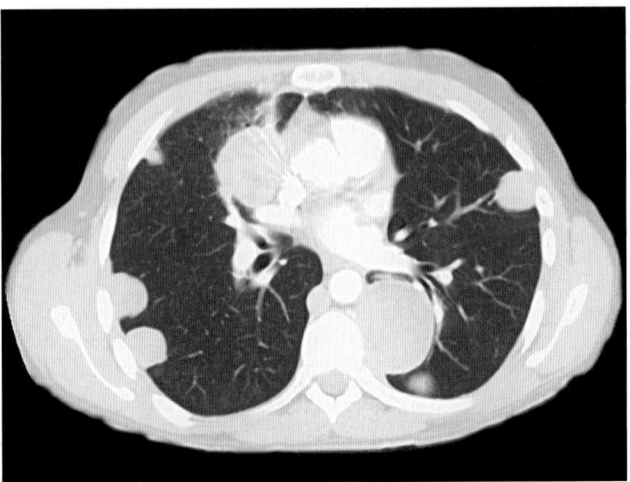

FIG. 36-4. A 29-year-old man with a history of a T1 leiomyosarcoma involving the inferior vena cava developed multiple lung metastases several months following surgical resection.

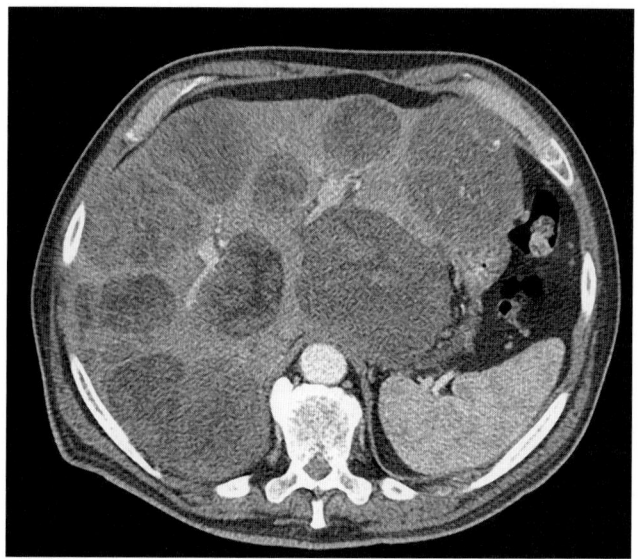

FIG. 36-5. A 69-year-old man with a history of a T2 pleomorphic liposarcoma of the thigh developed multiple liver metastases.

reported that Ki-67, a proliferation marker, is correlated with a poor clinical outcome in high-grade extremity sarcomas.[35,36] Others have investigated the correlation between expressions of various membrane proteins and clinical outcomes. E-cadherin and catenins, proteins essential for intercellular junctions, have been associated with poor outcome in patients with soft tissue sarcoma.[35] Similarly, higher CD100 expression in soft tissue sarcomas has been shown to correlate with higher proliferative potential and poorer outcome.[36]

Prognostic Nomograms

Nomograms have recently been introduced for a variety of malignancies[37–39] including soft tissue sarcoma[40] as a model in which identified prognostic factors can be combined and used to predict risk of disease-specific survival. One such nomogram was developed for 12-year disease-specific survival for general postoperative sarcoma and has been proposed as a useful tool for patient counseling, surveillance strategies, and consideration for clinical trials. This prognostic tool relies on patient age, tumor size, depth, site, grade, and histology. More recently, the same investigators developed a subtype-specific nomogram for patients with liposarcoma[41] and demonstrated that the nomogram was more accurate in predicting disease specific survival.

TREATMENT OF EXTREMITY SARCOMA (FIG. 36-6)

Accurate preoperative histologic diagnosis is critical when choosing a primary treatment strategy for soft tissue sarcomas. Presentation with gross disease after incisional biopsy, core-needle biopsy, or fine-needle aspiration biopsy allows the treatment planning team the best opportunity to evaluate the tumor's proximity to vital structures and the likelihood of being able to perform surgical resection with negative histologic margins. In addition, the tumor can serve as a biological marker of response if patients are to be enrolled in neoadjuvant treatment protocols.

In the past two decades, a multimodality treatment approach has improved survival and quality of life for patients with extremity sarcomas. For soft tissue sarcomas of the extremities, a multidisciplinary approach to management has resulted in local control rates

Prognostic Factors

Prognostic factors are important for identifying patients at high risk for recurrence and death from disease. Prognostic variables in soft tissue sarcoma include tumor characteristics such as size, grade, and depth, all of which have been incorporated into the staging system, as well as histology, tumor site, and locally recurrent presentation. Patient factors such as older age and gender also have been associated with recurrence and mortality in several studies.[34] A positive microscopic margin and early recurrence after resection of an extremity sarcoma have been shown to be associated with decreased survival.[34]

The expression of markers for cell kinetics and regulatory proteins of the cell cycle also have been investigated as potential prognostic factors for soft tissue sarcoma. Several groups have

CHAPTER 36

Soft Tissue Sarcomas

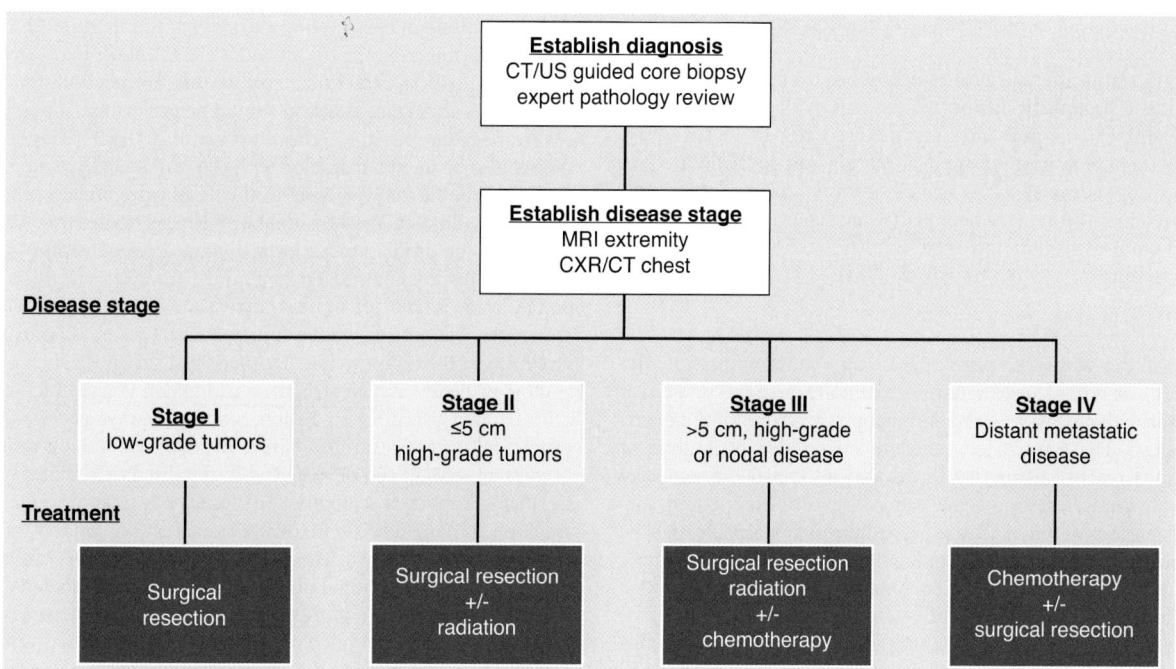

FIG. 36-6. Treatment algorithm of extremity soft tissue sarcoma. CT = computed tomography; CXR = chest x-ray; MRI = magnetic resonance imaging; US = ultrasound.

TABLE 36-3	Recommendations for the management of soft tissue masses

1. Soft tissue tumors that are enlarging or >3 cm should be evaluated with radiologic imaging [ultrasonography or computed tomography (CT)] and a tissue diagnosis made by core needle biopsy.

2. Once a sarcoma diagnosis is established, obtain imaging (magnetic resonance imaging for extremity lesions and CT for other anatomic locations) and evaluation for metastatic disease with chest CT for intermediate/high-grade or T2 tumors.

3. A wide local excision with 2-cm margins is adequate therapy for low-grade lesions and T1 tumors.

4. Radiation therapy plays a critical role in the management of large (T2) tumors.

5. Patients with recurrent high-grade sarcomas or distant metastatic disease should be evaluated for chemotherapy.

6. An aggressive surgical approach should be taken in the treatment of patients with an isolated local recurrence or resectable distant metastases.

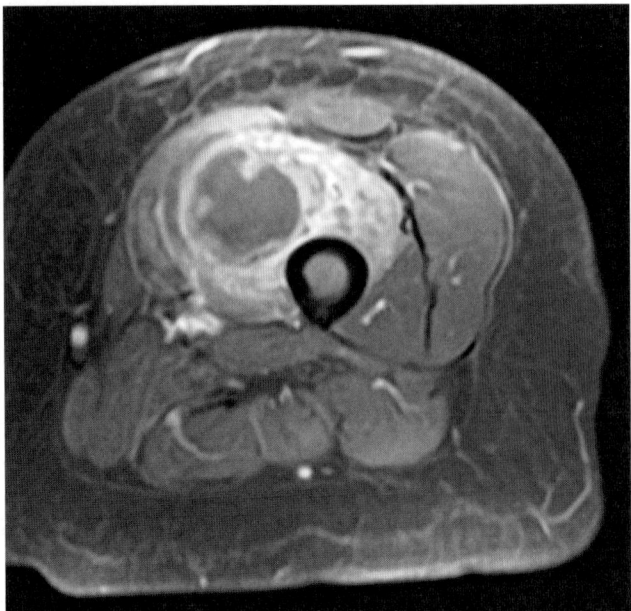

FIG. 36-7. Unclassified high-grade sarcoma of the left thigh measuring 21.7 × 7 × 5.2 cm abutting femoral cortex anteriorly and anteromedially with no evidence of medullary invasion.

up to and exceeding 90%. However, patients with abdominal sarcomas continue to have high rates of recurrence and poor overall survival. The overall 5-year survival for all stages of soft tissue sarcomas is 50 to 60%. Most patients die of metastatic disease, which becomes evident within 2 to 3 years of initial diagnosis in 80% of cases. A brief summary of the recommendations for the evaluation and management of patients presenting with soft tissue masses is presented in Table 36-3.

Surgery

Small (<5 cm) primary tumors with no evidence of distant metastatic disease are managed with local therapy consisting of surgery alone or in combination with radiation therapy, when wide pathologic margins are limited because of anatomic constraints. The type of surgical resection is determined by several factors, including tumor location, tumor size, depth of invasion, involvement of nearby structures, need for skin grafting or autogenous tissue reconstruction, and the patient's performance status. In 1985, the National Institutes of Health developed a consensus statement recommending limb-sparing surgery for most patients with high-grade extremity sarcomas.[42] However, for patients whose tumor cannot be grossly resected with a limb-sparing procedure and preservation of function (<5%), amputation remains the treatment of choice.

Margin status after surgical resection has been shown to be an independent prognostic factor.[43,44] Patients with microscopically positive surgical margins have an increased risk of local failure; however, neither a positive surgical margin nor local failure has been shown to adversely affect overall survival.[45] These data should be factored into the management plan when achieving clear surgical margins requires amputation or substantial functional compromise of an extremity.

Wide Local Excision

Wide local excision is the primary treatment strategy for extremity sarcomas. The goal of local therapy for extremity sarcomas is to resect the tumor with at least a 1- to 2-cm margin of surrounding normal soft tissue.[43] The tumors are generally surrounded by a zone of compressed reactive tissue that forms a pseudocapsule, which may mistakenly guide resection (enucleation) by an inexperienced surgeon. Extensions of tumor that go beyond the pseudocapsule must be considered in planning surgery and radiotherapy. In some anatomic areas, negative margins cannot be attained because of the tumor's proximity to vital structures. Soft tissue sarcomas abutting bone pose a particular dilemma in that obtaining a wide margin is not possible without excision of bone (Fig. 36-7). Although resection and reconstruction of skeletal defects is possible, the likelihood of postoperative complications may be increased and functional outcomes may not be

as favorable. A recent analysis by Lin and colleagues[46] of 55 patients with soft tissue sarcomas abutting bone reported that, in the absence of frank cortical bone penetration, periosteum is an adequate surgical margin for sarcomas treated with wide excision and radiation. Bone invasion from extremity soft tissue sarcoma, which generally can be identified using high-quality cross-sectional imaging such as MRI, has been estimated to occur in about 5% of patients.[47] In such cases, bone resection is required to obtain an adequate surgical margin and to achieve local control. Tumor invasion into bone is associated with a reduction in overall survival.[47]

Wide en bloc excision is seldom performed as a diagnostic procedure. When it is done for this purpose, the margin status often is not adequately evaluated in the pathologic assessment of the specimen. Unless detailed descriptions of the surgical procedure and the pathology specimen are provided, the margins should be classified as uncertain or unknown, a classification that carries the same prognosis as resection margins that are positive for tumor cells. In this setting, re-excision should be performed, if possible, to ensure negative margins. The biopsy site or tract (if applicable) should also be included en bloc with the re-resected specimen.

Soft tissue sarcomas arising in the distal extremities, particularly the hands and feet, present unique technical challenges. Although tumors of the distal extremities are often detected earlier (<5 cm) compared to proximal extremity tumors, resection and reconstruction techniques often are more complex, and preoperative planning is critical to obtaining favorable functional outcomes. Identifying the proximity of the tumor to underlying critical structures such as bone, tendon, or neurovascular structures using MRI is essential for surgical treatment planning. Radiation is almost always necessary as an adjunct to surgery, regardless of tumor size, given that it is rare that a 2- to 3-cm margin can be achieved in the distal extremities without sacrificing important structures. For locally advanced tumors, reconstruction of bone defects, vascular reconstruction, tendon transfers, and soft tissue reconstruction using regional or free flaps have resulted in good functional outcomes.[48] Amputation remains a reasonable treatment option for patients with soft tissue sarcomas of the distal extremities when oncologic or functional outcomes cannot be achieved using available limb salvage techniques.

A number of studies have reported improved survival for patients with isolated regional lymph node metastases treated with radical lymphadenectomy.[3,31-33] Patients with clinically or radiologically suspicious regional nodes should have metastases confirmed before radical lymphadenectomy. Current practice in our institution includes ultrasound evaluation with fine-needle aspiration biopsy of lymph nodes in selected patients with suspicious clinical or radiologic findings. The use of sentinel lymph node biopsy has been questioned for particular histologic subtypes of high-grade sarcoma with a propensity for lymph node metastases (e.g., epithelioid sarcoma, rhabdomyosarcoma, clear-cell sarcoma, synovial sarcoma, MFH, and angiosarcoma). However, there have been no prospective studies to adequately assess the sensitivity and specificity of sentinel lymph node biopsy techniques for these patients.

In the absence of appropriate surgery or combination treatment with surgery and radiation, the probability of local recurrence is >50%. With modern surgical and radiotherapy techniques, rates of limb preservation and local control have improved. A currently reported local failure rate of 10% after appropriate treatment is typical for soft tissue sarcomas of the extremity. Amputation is not required even for patients with locally advanced tumors involving major vascular structures, given that, in selected patients, vascular reconstruction has been shown to be feasible and often results in reasonable functional outcomes. In small series, en bloc tumor resection with vascular reconstruction resulted in increased postoperative complications. However, rates of local recurrence and 5-year survival were similar to those for patients who did not require vessel resection.[49,50]

Amputation

For the 5% of patients with primary or recurrent extremity tumors that cannot be grossly resected with a limb-sparing procedure and preservation of function, amputation is the treatment of choice. Historically, local excision of soft tissue sarcomas has resulted in local failure rates of 50 to 70%, even when a margin of normal tissue around the tumor was excised. As a consequence, radical resection or amputation has become the standard treatment. Because sarcomas usually spread along fascial planes or within muscle bundles, radical resection entails removal of all muscles in the involved compartment, along with nerves, vessels, and involved bone; it follows that this approach often requires amputation.

The addition of radiotherapy to less radical surgical resection has made limb salvage possible in many cases. A comparison of amputation vs. limb-sparing surgery followed by adjuvant radiation therapy was performed at the National Cancer Institute between 1975 and 1981.[51] Forty-three patients were randomized; 27 to the limb-sparing group and 16 to the amputation group. The median follow up was 4 years and 8 months. Four local recurrences were experienced in the limb-sparing group and none in patients in the amputation group. No statistically significant difference was noted in the local recurrence rates or in the overall survival rates of the two groups. Potter and colleagues[52] later reviewed the entire National Cancer Institute experience with 123 patients treated with conservative surgery plus radiotherapy and 83 treated with amputation. The difference in local control was statistically significant between groups with a local failure rate of 8% in the surgery and adjuvant radiotherapy group and no recurrences in the amputation group. However, survival rates did not differ significantly between the groups. Several large single-institution studies also have reported favorable local control rates with conservative resection combined with radiation therapy.[53-55]

Isolated Regional Perfusion

Isolated regional perfusion is an investigational approach for treating extremity sarcomas, and found its greatest support in Europe. It has been attempted mainly as a limb-sparing alternative for patients with locally advanced or locally recurrent soft tissue sarcomas, and for patients with multifocal sarcomas. Additionally, it has served as a palliative treatment to achieve local control for patients with distant metastatic disease.

Limb perfusion involves isolating the main artery and vein of the perfused limb from the systemic circulation. The choice of anatomic approach is determined by tumor site; external iliac vessels are used for thigh tumors, femoral or popliteal vessels for calf tumors, and axillary vessels for upper-extremity tumors. The vessels are dissected, and all collateral vessels are ligated. The vessels are then cannulated and connected to a pump oxygenator similar to that used in cardiopulmonary bypass. Either a tourniquet or Esmarch band is applied to the limb to achieve complete vascular isolation. For the lower limb, the Esmarch band is anchored at the anterior–superior iliac spine with the aid of a pin inserted into the pelvic bones. For the upper limb, the pin is anchored at the scapular and pectoral levels. Chemotherapeutic agents are then added to the perfusion circuit and circulated for 90 minutes. Systemic leakage from the perfused limb is monitored continuously with ^{99}Tc-radiolabeled human serum albumin injected into the perfusate, and radioactivity is recorded above the precordial area with a Geiger counter. The temperature of the perfused limb is maintained during the entire procedure by external heating and warming the perfusate to 40°C (104°F). At the end of the procedure, the limb is washed out, the cannulas are extracted, and the blood vessels are repaired.

Despite a 40-year history of the use of isolated limb perfusion to treat extremity sarcomas, many questions remain to be answered. The choice of chemotherapeutic agent in the perfusion circuit, the benefits of hyperthermia, and the effectiveness of hyperthermic perfusion in the neoadjuvant or adjuvant setting remain to be elucidated. Studies published to date have involved heterogeneous patient groups and diverse chemotherapeutic agents. Despite these limitations, favorable response rates ranging from 18 to 80% and overall 5-year survival rates of 50 to 70% have been reported.[56-60]

In 1974, McBride first reported results of 79 patients with extremity sarcomas who had been treated with isolated limb perfusion during the previous 14 years.[56] All patients had received melphalan and dactinomycin. The overall 5-year survival rate was 57%, and only 13 patients had subsequent amputation for recurrent disease. Over the next 20 years, isolated perfusion of the extremity to treat sarcoma fell out of favor for several reasons. Most notably, improved survival and decreased local recurrence rates could be obtained with less radical therapy. Conservative surgical excision was combined with radiation therapy or neoadjuvant chemotherapy to provide limb-sparing options to patients who were previously thought to require amputation. In view of the encouraging results of combination therapy, it is difficult to justify the technically challenging and expensive isolated perfusion procedure.

In 1992, a report by Lienard and associates[60] regenerated interest in isolated limb perfusion as a therapy for extremity tumors. Those investigators reported a 100% response rate among patients with extremity melanomas and sarcomas when high-dose recombinant tumor necrosis factor alpha plus interferon-γ and melphalan were given in an isolated perfusion circuit. This report led to larger studies geared specifically to patients with sarcoma. The largest of these studies, the European Multicenter Study, was reported by Eggermont and colleagues in 1996.[58] In that study of 186 patients, the overall tumor response rate was 82%. The clinical and pathologic complete response rate was 29%. Although all of the study participants were initially reported to be candidates for amputation, limb salvage following isolated limb perfusion was reported as 82%.[58]

A similar study evaluated the role of hyperthermic isolated limb perfusion with tumor necrosis factor and melphalan for patients with extremity sarcomas. A complete response was seen in 26% of the patients, and an additional 30% had a partial response. Fourteen patients (32%) underwent amputation for progressive tumors, while the other 68% were able to undergo limb salvage surgery after isolated limb perfusion.[59] The inferior results in the United States–based studies are thought to be due to patient selection biases and the degree of pretreatment before limb perfusion.

Although melphalan has been reported to have minimal activity against soft tissue sarcomas when used as a systemic agent, it can produce significant responses with minimal toxicity when used in the limb perfusion circuit. Doxorubicin has been the most effective systemic agent for soft tissue sarcomas, but concerns about potential locoregional toxicity have limited its use in isolated limb perfusion. Rossi and associates[61] performed a phase II trial of hyperthermic isolated limb perfusion with doxorubicin for 23 patients with extremity sarcomas. They reported a limb salvage rate of 91% and acceptable rates of grade 3 and 4 systemic (4%) and locoregional toxicity (22%).

Survival outcomes following isolated limb perfusion have not yet been directly compared with other more conventional treatment approaches, including wide local excision and radiation therapy or amputation.

Radiation Therapy

In the 1970s, 50% of patients presenting with extremity sarcomas underwent amputation for local control of their tumors. Despite a local recurrence rate of less than 10% after radical surgery, large numbers of patients died of metastatic disease. This realization prompted the development of local therapy involving conservative surgical excision combined with postoperative radiation therapy; these techniques offered local control rates of 80 to 90%. The evidence for adjunctive radiation therapy for patients eligible for conservative surgical resection comes from two randomized trials[62,63] and three large single-institution reports.[64–66] In a randomized trial by the National Cancer Institute, 91 patients with high-grade extremity tumors were treated with limb-sparing surgery followed by chemotherapy alone or radiation therapy plus adjuvant chemotherapy. A second group of 50 patients with low-grade tumors were treated with resection alone or with resection and radiation therapy. The 10-year rate of local control for all patients receiving radiation therapy was 98% compared with 70% for those not receiving radiation therapy ($P = .0001$).[62] Similarly, in a randomized trial from the Memorial Sloan-Kettering Cancer Center, 164 patients underwent observation or brachytherapy after conservative surgery. The 5-year local control rate for patients with high-grade tumors was 66% in the observation group and 89% in the brachytherapy group ($P = .003$).[63] No statistically significant difference was observed between treatment groups for patients with low-grade tumors.[67]

Until recently, the standard treatment guidelines required radiotherapy as an adjunct to surgery for all patients with intermediate or highly aggressive tumors of any size. However, small tumors (≤ 5 cm), in general, have not been associated with local recurrence, and radiation therapy may not be necessary. In a series of 174 patients reported by Geer and associates, postoperative radiation therapy did not improve 5-year local recurrence nor did it improve overall survival for patients with small soft tissue sarcomas.[68] Karakousis and colleagues reported a 5-year local recurrence rate of 6% for 80 patients with extremity sarcomas treated with wide local excision and observation, a rate similar to the 64 patients who underwent resection with more narrow surgical margins and adjuvant postoperative radiation.[69] These investigators argued that the high recurrence rates after less radical surgery were reported in the era before regular use of preoperative MRI and before the advent of improved surgical and pathologic techniques.

The optimal mode [external beam, brachytherapy, or intensity-modulated radiation therapy (IMRT)] and timing (preoperative, intraoperative, or postoperative) have yet to be defined. External-beam radiation therapy can be delivered by photons or particle beams (electrons, protons, pions, or neutrons). Conventional fractionation is usually 1.8 Gy to 2 Gy/d. CT is an integral part of radiation therapy. It is used to define the gross tumor volume and to estimate a margin of tissue at risk of microscopic tumor involvement. The optimal margin is not well defined; a radiation margin of 5 to 7 cm is standard, although some centers advocate wider margins for tumors >15 cm. At most institutions the typical *preoperative* dose is 50 Gy, given in 25 fractions. *Postoperative* radiation therapy

planning is based on tumor site, tumor grade, assessment of surgical margins, and on institutional preferences. The entire surgical scar and drain sites should be included in the field so that a near–full dose can be administered to the superficial skin. Metallic clips placed in the tumor bed during surgery can help define the limits of the resection and aid in radiation therapy planning. Doses of 60 to 70 Gy are usually necessary for postoperative treatment. Although postoperative radiation treatment of upper extremity sarcomas has been associated with a lower incidence of wound complications, the upper extremity site also is associated with a greater rate of local recurrence compared with the lower extremity.[70]

No consensus exists on the optimal sequence of radiation therapy and surgery. The available data come largely from single-institution, nonrandomized studies. Proponents of preoperative radiation therapy cite several advantages. Multidisciplinary planning with radiation oncologists, medical oncologists, and surgeons is facilitated early in the course of therapy if the tumor is in situ; moreover, lower doses of preoperative radiation can be delivered to an undisturbed tissue bed with improved tissue oxygenation. In addition, Nielsen and associates[71] demonstrated that the size of preoperative radiation fields is smaller and the number of joints included on those fields is fewer than in postoperative radiation fields, which may result in improved functional outcome. Critics of preoperative radiation therapy cite as deterrents the difficulty of pathologic assessment of margins and the increased rate of wound complications.[72] However, plastic surgery techniques with advanced tissue transfer procedures are being used more often in these high-risk wounds, and reportedly result in better outcomes.

The only randomized comparison of preoperative and postoperative radiation therapy conducted to date was performed by the National Cancer Institute of Canada Clinical Trial Canadian Sarcoma Group.[73] This trial was designed to compare complications and the functional outcome of patients treated with preoperative and postoperative external beam radiation therapy. The 190 patients enrolled from October 1994 to December 1997 were randomized to receive preoperative radiotherapy (50 Gy) or postoperative radiotherapy (66 Gy). With a median follow-up of 3.3 years, the recurrence and progression-free survival rates were similar between groups, with the only statistically significant difference being in the rates of wound complications. That is, the incidence of wound complications was 35% in the patients who received preoperative therapy but just 17% in the patients who received postoperative radiation therapy.[73] Late radiation toxicity was higher in the postoperative group compared to the preoperative radiation group (48.2 vs. 31.5%) with larger field sizes predicting greater rates of fibrosis, joint stiffness, and edema.[74]

Brachytherapy involves the placement of multiple catheters in the tumor resection bed. The primary benefit of brachytherapy is the shorter overall treatment time of 4 to 6 days compared with pre- or postoperative radiation therapy regimens, that can last 4 to 6 weeks. Brachytherapy produces less radiation scatter in critical anatomic regions (e.g., gonads or joints) and potentially improved function. A cost-analysis comparison of brachytherapy vs. external beam irradiation showed that costs were lower to undergo adjuvant irradiation with brachytherapy for soft tissue sarcomas.[75] Brachytherapy also can be used for recurrent disease previously treated with external beam radiation. Guidelines established at the Memorial Sloan-Kettering Cancer Center recommend spacing the afterloading catheters in 1-cm increments while leaving a 2-cm margin around the surgical bed.[63] After adequate wound healing is established, usually after the fifth postoperative day, the catheters are loaded with seeds containing iridium-192 that deliver 42 to 45 Gy of radiation to the tumor bed over 4 to 6 days. The primary disadvantage of brachytherapy is that it requires an extended inpatient stay and bed rest.

IMRT recently has been introduced as a radiation technique that delivers radiation more precisely to the tumor while sparing surrounding tissues. The proposed benefits of preoperative IMRT include treatment delivery to tumors while minimizing the dose to superficial tissues (i.e., skin), thereby reducing postoperative wound infections[76] and underlying bone complications (i.e., femur) by achieving concave dose distributions.[77] Theoretically, treatment with IMRT would result in a lower risk of long-term femur fractures. The long-term outcomes following IMRT have not yet been established.

Local toxicity from radiation therapy varies according to radiation dose, field size, and timing (pre- or postoperative). With preoperative radiotherapy, the most frequent wound complications are wound dehiscence, wound necrosis, persistent drainage, infection, seroma formation, ulceration, and cellulitis.[73] Postoperative radiation treatment of free flaps often is associated with wound complications, and patients should be advised that secondary surgical repair may be necessary. Wound complication rates of 13 to 37% have been reported for patients receiving preoperative radiation therapy as compared with 5 to 20% for patients receiving postoperative treatment.[78] If catheters are loaded after the fifth postoperative day, rates of wound complications following brachytherapy are similar to those reported after postoperative radiation therapy.

Long-term (chronic) effects of radiation therapy (those occurring more than 1 year after completion of therapy) generally are related to fibrosis/contracture, lymphedema, neurologic injury, osteitis, and fracture, all of which can cause substantial functional impairment.[78] Variables associated with poorer functional outcome following radiation therapy include treatment of larger tumors, use of higher doses of radiation (>63 Gy), longer radiation fields (>35 cm), poor radiation technique, neural sacrifice, postoperative fractures, and wound complications.[74,79] Additionally, complications of any kind are less likely following treatment for upper extremity sarcoma.[72,73]

Systemic Therapy

Despite improvements in local control rates, metastasis and death remain significant problems for patients with high-risk soft tissue sarcomas. Patients considered at high risk of death from sarcoma include those presenting with metastatic disease, presenting with localized sarcomas at nonextremity sites, or presenting with sarcomas of intermediate- or high-grade histology >5 cm (T2).[27,63] Treatment of patients with high-risk localized or metastatic disease often includes chemotherapy.

Results of conventional chemotherapy regimens have been poor for most patients with sarcoma. As a group, sarcomas include histologic subtypes that are responsive to cytotoxic chemotherapy and subtypes that are universally resistant to current agents. A spectrum of chemosensitivity has been demonstrated for various histologic subtypes. In particular, synovial sarcoma and fibrosarcoma have been noted to be highly sensitive to chemotherapy[80] and liposarcoma and myxofibrosarcoma as having intermediate sensitivity to chemotherapy; and GI stromal tumors and chondrosarcoma as being highly resistant to chemotherapy. Considering the variability of responses, it is not surprising that no overall survival benefit has been demonstrated.

Historically, only three drugs—doxorubicin, dacarbazine, and ifosfamide—have consistently demonstrated response rates of 20% or more for advanced soft tissue sarcomas. Doxorubicin and ifosfamide are the two most active agents, with consistently reported response rates of 20% or greater, and both agents have demonstrated positive dose-response curves.[81,82] Response rates to ifosfamide have been reported to range from 20 to 60% in single-institution series using higher-dose regimens or in combination with doxorubicin.[82] Over the last 5 years, several additional chemotherapeutic agents have been noted to be active. Single-agent response rates to gemcitabine in patients with advanced sarcoma have been reported to be 18%[83] except for the specific histologic subtype leiomyosarcoma, in which response rates as high as 53% have been reported both alone or in combination with docetaxel.[83,84] Gemcitabine combined with vinorelbine also has been associated with clinical benefit in patients with advanced sarcomas.[85] Other subtype-specific cytotoxic agents that have emerged include taxanes, docetaxel, and paclitaxel, which have been found to have specific activity in angiosarcomas.[86,87]

Integrating Multimodality Therapy

The primary objective of multimodality treatment is cure; when this endpoint is not possible, the goal is palliation of symptoms. Patients with a suspected diagnosis of soft tissue sarcoma should be referred to multidisciplinary centers that specialize in treating this disease.[88] Patients with a deep soft tissue mass should be referred, even before a biopsy is performed, to a tertiary treatment center that offers care by a team of specialists. Such multidisciplinary teams typically include oncologists from several disciplines (medicine, pediatrics [if applicable], surgery, and radiation therapy), as well as a pathologist, radiologist, and ancillary staff. An analysis by Gutierrez and colleagues[89] reported that soft tissue sarcoma patients treated at high-volume centers have significantly better survival and functional outcomes. They conclude that particularly those with large, high-grade, or truncal/retroperitoneal tumors should be treated exclusively at specialized centers.

Adjuvant Chemotherapy

The use of adjuvant chemotherapy for soft tissue sarcomas remains controversial. The average 5-year disease-free survival rate for patients initially presenting with localized disease is only about 50%. More than a dozen individual randomized trials of adjuvant chemotherapy have failed to demonstrate improvement in disease-free patients and overall survival in patients with soft tissue sarcomas. However, several limitations of these individual trials may explain the lack of observed improvement. First, the chemotherapy regimens used were suboptimal, relying on single-agent therapy (most commonly with doxorubicin) and insufficiently intensive dosing schedules. Second, the patient groups were not large enough to detect clinically significant differences in survival rates. Finally, most studies included patients at low risk of metastasis and death, namely those with small (<5 cm) and low-grade tumors.

The Sarcoma Meta-Analysis Collaboration analyzed 1568 patients from 14 trials of doxorubicin-based adjuvant chemotherapy to evaluate the effect of adjuvant chemotherapy on localized, resectable soft tissue sarcomas.[90] At a median follow-up of 9.4 years, doxorubicin-based chemotherapy significantly improved the time to local and distant recurrence and recurrence-free survival rates. However, the absolute benefit in overall survival for the sample was only 4%, which was not significant ($P = .12$). In a subset analysis, patients with extremity tumors had a 7% benefit in survival ($P = .029$).[90]

Subsequent to this meta-analysis, additional randomized controlled trials of more modern (drugs, dose, and schedule) anthracycline/ifosfamide combinations for relatively small numbers of patients have yielded conflicting results. In an Italian cooperative trial, apparent improvement was seen in median disease-free and overall survival times in patients with high-risk extremity soft tissue sarcomas.[91] In that study, 104 patients with high-grade tumors ≥5 cm were randomized to undergo definitive local therapy (surgery) vs. local therapy plus adjuvant chemotherapy consisting of epirubicin (60 mg/m[2] per day on day 1 and 2) and ifosfamide (1.8 g/m[2] per day on days 1 to 5) for five cycles. At a median follow-up of almost 5 years, disease-free survival times were 16 months in the surgery-alone group and 48 months in the combined-treatment group ($P = .04$), and median overall survival times were 46 months vs. 75 months ($P = .03$) for those treated with surgery vs. surgery plus chemotherapy, respectively.[91] However, several years later a convergence in both relapse rates (28 and 32% in chemotherapy and control groups respectively) and deaths (22 vs. 29%) was observed that resulted in statistically similar overall survival.[92] Other randomized studies have failed to confirm such benefit.

In an effort to further assess the role of chemotherapy in patients with stage III extremity sarcoma, a cohort analysis of the combined databases from both the University of Texas M. D. Anderson and Memorial Sloan-Kettering was recently performed. The data on 674 patients with stage III extremity sarcoma who received either preoperative or postoperative doxorubicin-based chemotherapy were reviewed to determine their outcomes (5-year disease-specific survival as well as 5-year local and distant recurrence rates) from systemic therapy. The 5-year disease-specific survival rate was 61%.[93] Cox regression analysis showed a time-varying effect of chemotherapy with an associated benefit during the first year. However, the clinical benefits of doxorubicin-based chemotherapy in patients with high-risk extremity sarcomas were not sustained beyond 1 year after therapy. Grobmyer and colleagues also compared the outcome of a cohort of patients treated at two institutions (1990 to 2001) with surgery only or neoadjuvant chemotherapy containing doxorubicin and ifosfamide. In this analysis, there was an improvement in 3-year disease-specific survival, which was most pronounced in patients with tumors >10 cm (62 vs. 83% for surgery alone vs. neoadjuvant chemotherapy and surgery, respectively).[94]

Because the evidence addressing treatment of stage III disease is inconclusive, considerable variation still exists in treatment standards. It may be that there are subsets of high-risk patients based on tumor size or histology with extremity soft tissue sarcoma who derive significant benefit from systemic chemotherapy. Specifically, retrospective cohort analyses have noted a benefit in disease-specific survival in patients with large (T2), high-grade liposarcomas and synovial sarcomas of the extremity treated with combination ifosfamide and doxorubicin compared with patients who received no chemotherapy.[95]

A major deterrent to the use of adjuvant chemotherapy has been the risk of adverse toxic effects in patients who do not respond to therapy. To optimize the use of doxorubicin and ifosfamide, investigators have tried to escalate the drug doses with combination regimens with the aim of maximizing tumor-cell kill. The ultimate goal is to achieve an incremental response rate and improve the quality of response sufficiently to influence survival. However, the limits to this approach are becoming apparent even when treatment includes support with hematopoietic growth factors. The advent of growth factors like granulocyte colony-stimulating factor and granulocyte-macrophage colony-stimulating factor has helped minimize the morbidity related to neutropenia; however, dose-limiting thrombocytopenia continues to pose a challenge for treatment. Use of high-dose doxorubicin has been limited by myelotoxicity, epithelial toxicity, painful hand-foot syndrome, and potentially severe cardiac toxicity. The toxicity profile for systemic regimens with gemcitabine has been mild, primarily related to hematologic toxicity. This regimen is of particular clinical interest for patients with limited options due to (a) prior exposure to full therapeutic doses of doxorubicin and ifosfamide, (b) advanced age, and (c) significant comorbidities.

Neoadjuvant/Preoperative Chemotherapy

The rationale for using neoadjuvant and preoperative chemotherapy for soft tissue sarcomas is the belief that only 30 to 50% of patients will respond to standard (postoperative) chemotherapy. Neoadjuvant chemotherapy enables oncologists to identify patients whose disease responds to chemotherapy by assessing that response while the primary tumor is in situ. Patients whose tumors do not respond to short courses of preoperative chemotherapy are, thus, spared the toxic effects of prolonged postoperative or adjuvant chemotherapy.

Treatment approaches that combine systemic chemotherapy with radiosensitizers and concurrent external beam radiation may improve disease-free survival by treating microscopic disease and enhancing the treatment of macroscopic disease. Concurrent chemoradiotherapy with doxorubicin-based regimens reportedly produces favorable local control rates for patients with sarcoma.[95] Since those findings were published, several groups have attempted to evaluate the optimal route of administration, alternative chemotherapeutic agents, and the toxicity of combined therapies.

Theoretical advantages of concurrent treatment notwithstanding, use of concurrent local and systemic therapy decreases the total treatment time for patients with high-risk sarcoma. This decrease represents a substantial advantage over current sequential combined-method treatment approaches, for which the total duration of treatment for radiation, chemotherapy, surgery, and rehabilitation frequently exceeds 6 to 9 months.

Surveillance

In general, it is believed that early recognition and treatment of recurrent local or distant disease can prolong survival in patients with soft tissue sarcoma. This is primarily based on a few reports involving small numbers of patients that have indicated salvage after recurrent local disease is possible by performing radical re-excision with or without radiation therapy.[96,97] Similarly, several groups have reported that survival can be prolonged after resection of pulmonary metastases. These limited data form the basis for use of aggressive surveillance strategies for all patients with soft tissue sarcoma.

History and physical examination are the most useful components of follow-up in evaluating for local recurrence after definitive treatment. CT and MRI are useful for evaluating less accessible regions, such as the retroperitoneum, and in assessing equivocal changes on examination. Most recurrences of soft tissue sarcomas occur in the first 2 years after completion of therapy. Patients should be evaluated with a complete history and physical examination and chest radiography every 3 to 6 months during the 2- to 3-year period of highest risk. Most experts recommend that the tumor site should be evaluated every 6 months by performing MRI for extremity tumors or CT for intra-abdominal or retroperitoneal tumors. Guidelines have been established for using MRI to distinguish recurrences from typical postsurgical changes. A discrete nodule with low signal intensity on T1-weighted images and higher signal intensity on T2-weighted images that enhances after administration of IV contrast is strongly suggestive of recurrence and should be sampled for biopsy. In some circumstances, ultrasonography can be used to assess recurrence of tumor in the extremities.

Recurrence after surgery for abdominal soft tissue sarcomas is common. CT is useful for detecting recurrences at primary and distant anatomic sites in the abdomen and pelvis. After surgery, cross-sectional imaging every 3 to 6 months during the first 2 years and every 6 months for 3 years thereafter has been recommended. However, many experienced surgeons are advocating less aggressive imaging for asymptomatic patients, particularly after a second recurrence of retroperitoneal sarcoma arguing that no evidence exists to suggest that survival is improved by earlier detection.

Because most metastases to distant sites occur within 2 to 3 years of initial diagnosis, general guidelines are that follow-up intervals can be lengthened to every 6 months, with annual imaging, for years 2 through 5. After 5 years, patients should be evaluated and undergo chest radiography annually.

Whooley and associates reviewed the efficacy of the surveillance strategy used at Roswell Park Cancer Institute for 174 patients with soft tissue sarcomas of the extremities.[98] Patients were evaluated every 3 months for the first 2 years, every 4 to 6 months during year 3, and every 6 months through year 5. Local recurrence occurred in 18% of patients at a median interval of 14 months, and all but one of the recurrences was detected by physical examination alone. Fifty-seven patients had distant recurrences (at a median of 18 months after treatment), of which 36 were asymptomatic and diagnosed by surveillance radiographic imaging. Those investigators determined that the positive predictive value of chest radiography in follow-up was 92%.[98] However, evaluation of the primary site by CT or MRI and routine laboratory assessment was ineffective in detecting recurrences. The authors of this report cautioned that their study did not conclusively demonstrate that CT and MRI should not be used. Rather, patient characteristics, location of the primary tumor, previous treatment, and physician familiarity with changes after surgery and radiation therapy should all be considered in determining the need for radiographic imaging.

Recurrent Sarcoma

The pattern of recurrence is related to the anatomic site of the primary tumor. Up to 20% of patients with extremity sarcoma develop locally recurrent disease. Patients with microscopically positive surgical margins are at increased risk of local recurrence. In a series of 179 patients with locally recurrent extremity soft tissue sarcoma at Memorial Sloan-Kettering Cancer Center, the median interval to local recurrence was noted to be 16 months; 65% developed a local recurrence by 2 years and 90% by 4 years.[96] The majority of patients (89%) were treated with additional limb-sparing surgery, and 73% received additional adjuvant therapy with a disease-specific survival of 55% at 4 years. Independent prognostic factors for disease-specific survival after local recurrence included histologic tumor grade, local recurrence size, and local recurrence-free interval. These data indicate that surveillance of patients for the first 4 years after resection of their primary extremity sarcoma is warranted.

An isolated local recurrence should be treated aggressively with margin-negative resection. For patients with extremity sarcomas, this frequently requires amputation. However, some patients with recurrent extremity sarcoma can undergo function-preserving resection combined with additional radiation therapy, with or without chemotherapy, with acceptable rates of local control.[99–101] Nori and colleagues reported a local control rate of 69% among 40 patients with recurrent tumors treated with re-excision and brachytherapy to a median dose of 45 Gy.[101] In a similar series, limb-sparing conservative surgery was possible in 24 of 36 patients (66%), and the 5-year local recurrence-free survival rate was 72%.[99]

The primary determinant of survival in patients with soft tissue sarcoma is development of distant metastases. Patients with extremity sarcomas generally have recurrence as distant pulmonary metastases, whereas patients with retroperitoneal or intra-abdominal sarcomas tend to have local recurrences.[98] Other less common sites of metastasis include bone (7%), liver (4%),[52] and lymph nodes.[3] Myxoid liposarcoma of the extremity is known to metastasize to the abdomen and pelvis and requires staging CT of these regions before definitive local therapy.[17]

Surgical Resection for Metastatic Sarcoma

The most common initial site of metastasis of soft tissue sarcomas is the lung. Selected patients with a limited number of pulmonary nodules (fewer than four), long disease-free intervals, and no endobronchial invasion may become long-term survivors after pulmonary resection (Fig. 36-8); 15 to 40% of patients with complete resection of metastatic disease confined to the lung are long-term survivors.[98,102] In a retrospective multi-institutional study of 255

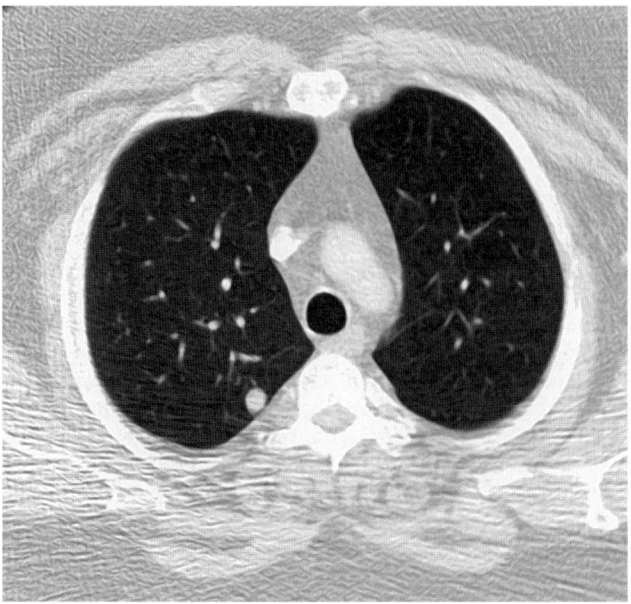

FIG. 36-8. A 58-year-old man with a history of a T2 unclassified sarcoma of the thigh developed a solitary lung metastasis 18 months following surgical resection.

patients, the 5-year overall survival rate after metastasectomy was reported to be 38%.[103] Favorable prognostic factors in that study included microscopically free margins, age younger than 40 years old, and grade I or II tumors.[103] For patients who are surgical candidates, pulmonary resection alone also has been shown to be the most cost-effective treatment strategy compared to no treatment, chemotherapy alone, and surgery combined with chemotherapy.[104]

Chemotherapy for Metastatic Sarcoma

The only available treatment for most patients with metastatic disease is chemotherapy. Historically, response rates for patients with stage IV soft tissue sarcoma have been low. Several prognostic factors have been defined for patients undergoing chemotherapy, including performance status, previous response to chemotherapy, younger age, absence of hepatic metastases, low-grade tumors, and long disease-free interval.[105] Isolated liver metastases, if stable over several months, may be amenable to resection, radiofrequency ablation, or chemoembolization.

Palliative Radiation Therapy

Definitive radiation therapy has been described as a treatment option to be considered in clinical situations where there is no acceptable surgical option available (e.g., patient with significant medical comorbidities). A window of therapeutic radiation dose benefit has been reported in this clinical setting in the range of 63 Gy to 67 Gy; higher radiation doses (greater than 63 Gy) yielded superior tumor control while doses over 68 Gy yielded increased rates of major complications.[106]

SPECIAL SITUATIONS

Myxoid Liposarcomas

Myxoid liposarcomas belong to the group of soft tissue sarcomas with lipomatous differentiation. However, these tumors have very distinct morphology with myxoid stroma and lipomatous differentiation and clinical behavior that differs from the other liposarcoma subtypes. Myxoid liposarcomas frequently present as slow-growing, deep tumors in the lower extremity. Distinct from other soft tissue sarcomas that metastasize to the lungs, metastases arising from myxoid liposarcoma often are detected in other soft tissue locations, including the retroperitoneum or extremities.[107,108] For this reason, CT of the chest, abdomen, and pelvis are recommended for the adequate staging and surveillance of patients with myxoid liposarcoma.

Specific chromosomal translocation has been identified in myxoid liposarcoma that consists of the fusion of the SUF and CHOP genes [(t12;16)(q13;p11)] in 90% of tumors and fusion of the EWS and CHOP [(t12;22)(q13;q12)] genes in greater than 5% of tumors.[109] These translocations can be detected using polymerase chain reaction techniques for diagnostic purposes.

Retroperitoneal Sarcomas

Most retroperitoneal tumors are malignant, and about one third are soft tissue sarcomas. Also included in the differential diagnosis are primary germ cell tumor, lymphoma, or metastatic testicular cancer. Ten to 15% of adult soft tissue sarcomas, or about 1000 new cases, of retroperitoneal sarcoma are diagnosed annually in the United States. The most common sarcomas occurring in the retroperitoneum are liposarcomas, MFHs, and leiomyosarcomas. In contrast to extremity sarcomas, many retroperitoneal sarcomas present as large tumor masses abutting or involving vital structures, making margin-free resection difficult. As a result, locoregional recurrence is common (72% at 5 years), and prognosis for patients with retroperitoneal sarcoma is poor with 5-year survival estimated at 36 to 58%.[110]

Retroperitoneal sarcomas generally present as large masses; nearly 50% are >20 cm at the time of diagnosis. They typically do not produce symptoms until they grow large enough to compress or invade contiguous structures. The evaluation for a patient with a retroperitoneal mass begins with an accurate history that should exclude signs and symptoms associated with lymphoma (e.g., fever and night sweats). Complete physical examination, with particular attention to all nodal basins and testicular examination in men, is critically important. Laboratory assessment can be helpful; an elevated lactate dehydrogenase level may suggest lymphoma, and elevated beta human chorionic gonadotropin levels or alpha-fetoprotein levels can indicate a germ cell tumor.

Radiologic assessment should include CT of the abdomen and pelvis to define the extent of the tumor and its relationship to surrounding structures, particularly vascular structures. Imaging should also encompass the liver for the presence of metastases, the abdomen for discontiguous disease, and the kidneys bilaterally for function. Angiography or magnetic resonance arteriography/venography also can be used to delineate vascular anatomy in selected patients when involvement of critical vascular structures is suspected. Thoracic CT is indicated to detect lung metastases. For patients presenting with an equivocal history, an unusual appearance of the mass, an unresectable tumor, or distant metastasis, CT guided core needle or laparoscopic biopsy is appropriate to obtain a sample for tissue diagnosis.

Complete surgical resection is the most effective treatment for primary or recurrent retroperitoneal sarcomas (Fig. 36-9). En bloc resections for these tumors often include sacrificing contiguous structures such as the small bowel, colon, kidney, inferior vena cava, and aorta. In a review of 141 patient who underwent resection of retroperitoneal sarcoma with major blood vessel involvement, postoperative morbidity and mortality were 36 and 4% respectively, and vessel patency rates were greater than 88% at a median follow-up of 19.3 months.[111] With favorable rates of local control and survival reported in their cohort of patients with tumor-free resection margins, the authors concluded that vascular resection is the treatment of choice in sarcomas that involve major blood vessels in the retroperitoneum.[111]

In several retrospective assessments of patients with retroperitoneal sarcoma, complete surgical excision was achieved in only 40 to 60% of patients.[112,113] In an analysis of 500 patients with retroperitoneal soft tissue sarcomas treated at Memorial Sloan-Kettering Cancer Center, the median survival time for those who underwent complete resection was 103 months vs. 18 months for those who underwent incomplete resection, or observation without resection.[114] In general, surgical resection should not be offered to patients unless radiographic evidence indicates the potential for complete resection, although palliative surgical procedures may be considered to reduce the symptoms of intestinal obstruction, pain, or bleeding.[115] In particular, patients with atypical lipomatous tumors, also termed *well-differentiated liposarcomas*, may benefit symptomatically from repeated tumor debulking.

Tumor stage at presentation, high histologic grade, unresectability, and grossly positive resection margins are strongly associated with rates of death from retroperitoneal sarcoma.[114,116,117] Survival rates at 5 years are typically reported to be 40 to 50%. The best chance for long-term survival for patients with retroperitoneal sarcoma is achieved with a margin-negative resection, however, this often is not possible. In one series, the 5-year disease-free survival rate was 50% for patients who had margin-negative resection as compared with 28% for patients undergoing incomplete resection.[112] In the series reported by Lewis and associates,[114] about 75% of patients died of locally recurrent disease without distant metastasis. As is true for extremity lesions, tumor grade is also a significant predictor of outcome for patients with retroperitoneal sarcoma. In the series reported by Jaques and colleagues,[113] patients with high-grade tumors ($n = 65$) had a median survival time of only 20 months compared with 80 months for patients with low-grade tumors ($n = 49$).

Adjuvant Therapy

Most studies have failed to show a survival advantage for adjuvant chemotherapy for retroperitoneal sarcomas.[118–120] However, adjuvant chemotherapy has been advocated for some of the more uncommon histologic variants of retroperitoneal sarcoma including dedifferentiated liposarcoma, MFHs, and primitive neuroectodermal tumors.[121,122]

Because of the high rates of local recurrence, adjuvant radiation therapy has been proposed as a potential means of treating microscopic residual disease following the surgical resection of retroperitoneal sarcomas. However, the optimal technique and timing of delivery continues to evolve as clinicians weigh the potential benefits with the increased risk of treatment-related toxicity. Treatment of retroperitoneal sarcomas is complex because tumors are usually large, requiring large fields, and due to the proximity of radiosensitive structures (i.e., bowel). Several techniques have been used, including preoperative and postoperative external beam radiation, intraoperative radiation therapy, and brachytherapy.[123] Preoperative radiotherapy is emerging as a technique that is feasible and well tolerated.

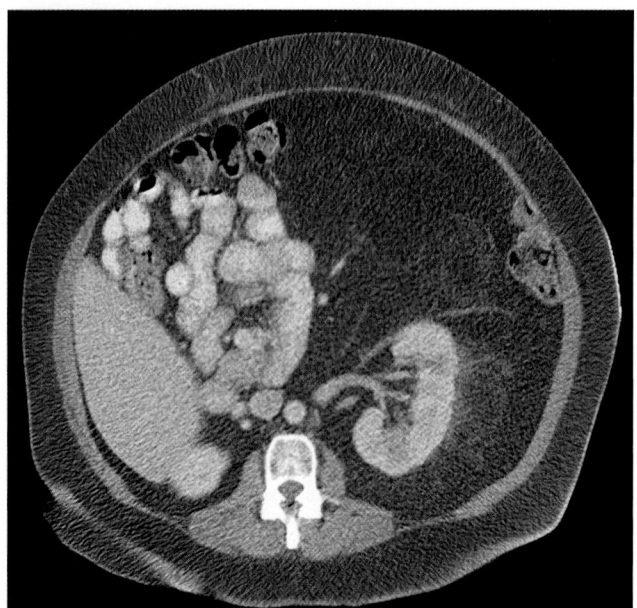

A

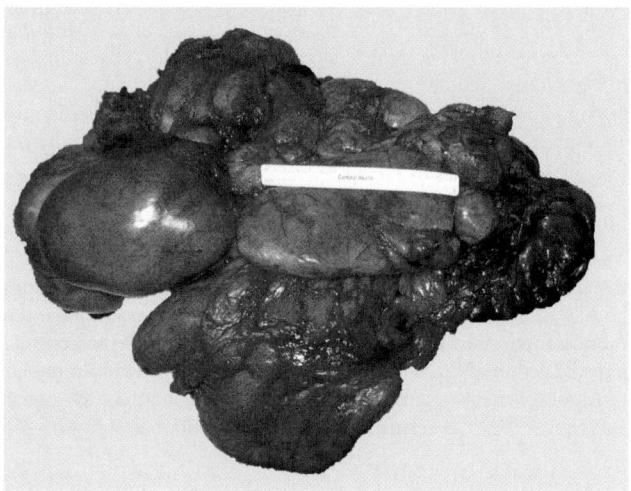

B

FIG. 36-9. **A.** Computed tomography image of the abdomen for a 50-year-old woman with a massive retroperitoneal tumor with anterior displacement of left kidney. **B.** Gross specimen, en bloc resection of retroperitoneal liposarcoma with spleen, left kidney, left adrenal gland, and transverse and sigmoid colon.

Toxicity may be lower with preoperative radiation given that (a) the tumor borders are definable, (b) the tumor acts as an expander, displacing radiosensitive viscera away from the treatment field, and (c) effective doses of radiation may be lower preoperatively.[124]

There are a number of studies that report favorable local control rates for intermediate and high-grade retroperitoneal sarcomas treated with preoperative radiotherapy plus complete resection compared to historical data.[123] However, most studies have failed to show a survival benefit for such patients.[125] This body of evidence prompted the initiation of a multicenter, randomized trial sponsored by the American College of Surgeon's Oncology Group to compare surgery alone with preoperative radiation therapy plus surgery (ACOSOG Z9031). Unfortunately, the study was closed prematurely in 2006 because of lack of patient accrual. There are no consensus guidelines for the use of radiation in patients with primary or recurrent retroperitoneal sarcomas. The optimal balance between acceptable radiation toxicity and effective local control is yet to be determined.

Current recommendations for radiation therapy for patients with retroperitoneal sarcoma at MDACC are based on presentation of disease.[117] For high-risk patients, defined as those with large, high-grade tumors or recurrent low-grade tumors, 50-Gy preoperative radiation therapy followed by surgical resection is recommended. In the preoperative setting, the tumor often displaces the bowel out of the field of radiation and treatment may be delivered with less toxicity. Postoperative radiation is discouraged unless the resected tumor bed is clearly away from dose-limiting structures.

Recurrences

Retroperitoneal sarcomas recur in two thirds of patients. In addition to recurring locally in the tumor bed and metastasizing to the lungs, retroperitoneal leiomyosarcomas frequently spread to the liver. Retroperitoneal sarcomas can also recur diffusely throughout the peritoneal cavity (sarcomatosis). The approach to resectable recurrent disease after the treatment of a retroperitoneal sarcoma is similar to the approach taken after the recurrence of an extremity sarcoma. However, the ability to resect a recurrent retroperitoneal sarcoma declines precipitously. In a large series of patients treated at Memorial Sloan-Kettering Cancer Center, the authors were able to resect recurrent tumors in 57% of patients with a first recurrence, but in only 20% after a second recurrence, and 10% after a third recurrence.[35] Of note is that in as many as 25% of patients, well-differentiated liposarcoma may recur in a poorly differentiated form or develop areas of dedifferentiation. Dedifferentiated retroperitoneal liposarcoma is more aggressive with a greater propensity for distant metastasis than its well-differentiated precursor.

Gastrointestinal Sarcomas

Patients with GI sarcomas most often present with nonspecific GI symptoms that are determined by the site of the primary tumor. In a series from Memorial Sloan-Kettering Cancer Center, early satiety and dyspepsia were noted in patients with upper GI tumors, whereas tenesmus and changes in bowel habits were common in those with tumors of the lower GI tract.[126] In a series of 80 patients with various smooth muscle tumors of the GI tract, Chou and associates[127] identified the most common presenting symptoms and signs as GI bleeding (44%), abdominal mass (38%), and abdominal pain (21%).

Establishing the diagnosis of a GI sarcoma preoperatively is often difficult. Radiologic assessment, including CT of the abdomen or pelvis, is sometimes useful to determine the anatomic location, size, and extent of disease. Patients with localized disease frequently present with a large intra-abdominal mass but no radiographic evidence of the regional lymph node metastases that would be typical of an adenocarcinoma of comparable size and anatomic location. In patients with advanced disease, CT may demonstrate disseminated intra-abdominal masses with or without concomitant ascites and possible invasion of tissue planes.

Endoscopy (esophagoduodenoscopy or colonoscopy) has become the mainstay for evaluating symptoms related to the GI tract. For tumors involving the stomach, upper endoscopy with endoscopic ultrasonography and biopsy are important diagnostic tests used to distinguish adenocarcinoma from GI sarcomas. This distinction is clinically significant because the extent of resection (local excision vs. gastrectomy) and the role of regional lymph node dissection differs for these two conditions. Lymphatic spread is not the primary route of metastasis for GI sarcomas. Consequently, lymphadenectomy is not routinely performed as part of resection. Based on published data and the primary pattern of distant (vs. local) failure, the general recommendation is to perform a margin-negative resection with a 2- to 4-cm margin of normal tissue. However, some cases may be technically challenging because of the tumor's anatomic location or size. For example, for gastric tumors located near the gastroesophageal junction, achieving adequate surgical margins may not be possible without a total or proximal subtotal gastrectomy. Similarly, large leiomyosarcomas arising from the stomach with invasion of adjacent organs should be resected together with the adjacent involved viscera en bloc.

Segmental bowel resection is the standard treatment for sarcomas of the small or large intestine. For the jejunum, ileum, and colon, the tumor is excised en bloc with the involved segment of intestine and its mesentery; radical mesenteric lymphadenectomy is not attempted. For sarcomas originating in the rectum, the technique used for tumor resection is based on the anatomic location and size of the tumor. For small, low rectal lesions, it may be possible to achieve clear margins with a transanal excision. Large or locally invasive lesions may require more extensive operations for complete tumor extirpation.[128,129] Meijer and colleagues[129] reviewed the experience with 50 patients with primary colorectal sarcoma at Memorial Sloan-Kettering Cancer Center. In 32 cases, the primary tumor was located in the rectum, and 18 tumors involved the colon. Of the rectal lesions, 15 were treated with abdominoperineal resection and 12 were treated with local excision. Distant metastasis was the first recurrence in 11 of the 32 patients who underwent curative resection.[129]

Gastrointestinal Stromal Tumor

Gastrointestinal stromal tumors (GISTs), which constitute the majority of GI sarcomas, have distinctive molecular features of GISTs that have been characterized over the last decade. These tumors share phenotypic similarities with the intestinal pacemaker cell known as the *interstitial cells of Cajal*.[130] The interstitial cells of Cajal and GIST cells express the hematopoietic progenitor cell marker CD34 and the growth factor receptor c-Kit (CD117).[131] c-Kit is a transmembrane glycoprotein receptor with an internal tyrosine kinase component that, when activated, triggers a cascade of intracellular signals regulating cell growth and survival.[132] The expression of the c-Kit gene protein product CD117 has emerged as an important defining feature of GISTs. Using these diagnostic criteria, the incidence of GIST has been estimated at 6–15 cases per 1 million population.[133–135]

Kit mutation site has emerged as a prognostic factor of progression-free and overall survival in patients with GIST. Patients with Kit exon 11 mutation have a superior progression-free and overall survival on imatinib therapy compared to those patients whose tumors have an exon 9 mutation or wild-type Kit. Current clinical practice in many centers is to perform mutation analysis of the Kit gene in all new patients for both prognostic and therapeutic consideration.

Radiologic Assessment

Positron emission tomography (PET) using ^{18}F-fluorodeoxyglucose has been reported as useful for preoperative staging of GISTs, as it may reveal early metastases and establish baseline metabolic activity. PET has been shown to be highly sensitive in detecting early response to imatinib treatment and predicting long-term response in patients with metastatic GIST. Because PET imaging is still not widely available and, in some lesions, insensitive, and because glucose uptake is not sufficient, predictive criteria for assessment of GISTs using CT imaging also have been proposed.[136]

Management of Localized Disease

Surgery remains the only potentially curative treatment for patients with localized GISTs. Complete resection with negative margins, even of locally advanced tumors, is associated with improved survival.[137] The extent of surgery required to produce a complete resection does not seem to influence survival. The 5-year survival rate for all patients with GISTs ranges from 20 to 44% and up to 75% for early-stage tumors that have been completely excised.[137] However, a more recent analysis of 200 patients by DeMatteo and colleagues noted a disease-specific survival rate of only 54% for patients in whom a grossly complete resection of primary GISTs had been achieved, and the median survival duration for patients with metastatic disease was only 20 months.[138]

As with other soft tissue sarcomas, tumor size has consistently been identified as an important prognostic factor for GISTs. Mitotic activity also has been identified as an important prognostic factor and is generally categorized as <5, 5 to 10, and 10 or more mitotic counts per high-power field. Based primarily on these prognostic variables, tumor size, and mitotic count, the National Institutes of Health[139] and the Armed Forces Institute of Pathology[140] have proposed prognostic criteria for the risk stratification (i.e., low risk, intermediate risk, high risk, and very high risk) for surgically treated localized primary GISTs. The Armed Forces Institute of Pathology also includes tumor site as a prognostic variable. Accurate risk stratification is essential to select patients most likely to benefit from adjuvant treatment.

Management of Locally Advanced or Metastatic Disease

Until recently, systemic treatment options for a patient with unresectable or metastatic GIST were of little therapeutic benefit. Treatment with imatinib (Gleevec, ST1571), a selective c-Kit inhibitor, has resulted in impressive clinical responses in a large percentage of patients with unresectable or metastatic GISTs. Based on the initial treatment results from a single patient with metastatic GIST, a phase I study was initiated by the European Organization for Research and Treatment of Cancer Soft Tissue and Bone Sarcoma Group to test the safety and efficacy of imatinib.[141] In that study, 53% of patients with GISTs had confirmed partial responses; investigators concluded that imatinib is safe and effective against GISTs.[141] A multicenter, international trial was begun in July of 2000 at four treatment centers: Dana-Farber Cancer Institute, Oregon Health Sciences University, Fox Chase Cancer Center, and University Hospital of Helsinki, Finland.[142] A total of 147 patients with unresectable or metastatic GISTs were randomized to receive one of two doses of imatinib (400 mg or 600 mg daily) for planned treatments of up to 24 months. Overall objective response was demonstrated in 79 patients (54%); all had partial responses and no significant difference was found between imatinib doses.[143] Fourteen percent of patients had disease progression. The toxicity profile was acceptable, with the predominant effects being GI toxicity and periorbital edema, cramps, and fatigue. However, 21% of patients experienced serious adverse events (grade 3 or 4 toxicity), including GI bleeding (5%) likely related to the rapid tumor response of mural lesions.

A phase III randomized Intergroup trial was simultaneously performed to assess the clinical activity of imatinib at two dose levels for patients with unresectable or metastatic GISTs expressing the c-Kit tyrosine kinase.[144] Between December 15, 2000, and September 1, 2001, 746 patients were accrued and randomized to receive low-dose (400 mg/d) or high-dose (800 mg/d) imatinib. The primary endpoint of the trial was survival. Preliminary toxicity data from 325 patients revealed a 23% incidence of grade 3 or 4 adverse events, including nausea and vomiting, GI bleeding, abdominal pain, edema, fatigue, and rash. The European Organization for Research and Treatment of Cancer Soft Tissue and Bone Sarcoma Group, in conjunction with the Italian Sarcoma Group and the

Australasian Gastro-Intestinal Trials Group, has accrued 753 patients with GISTs to another randomized phase III trial.[145] Response data from the trial are currently maturing.

In February 2002, the U.S. Food and Drug Administration approved imatinib for treatment of GISTs based on the results of these promising clinical trials. In addition, there continues to be little known about the optimal length of treatment, the duration of benefit, or the long-term toxicity of imatinib therapy. It has become evident that, when feasible, imatinib should be continued in the absence of disease progression. A randomized trial has reported worse progression-free survival in patients that stopped imatinib after 1 year of treatment compared to those who continued beyond 1 year (6 months vs. 18 months, respectively).[146] Less than 4% of patients with GISTs have experienced serious adverse events with imatinib. Mild GI toxicity is the most frequently reported adverse event, but GI tract hemorrhage, presumably from rapid tumor necrosis, also has been reported. Thus, all patients with GISTs treated on clinical protocols should be evaluated and followed by a team of medical professionals that includes a surgeon.

In 2006, sunitinib malate (Sutent, Pfizer), an inhibitor of a broad spectrum of tyrosine kinases, emerged as an alternative systemic treatment for patients unable to tolerate imatinib or with imatinib-refractory GIST. Sunitinib is a tyrosine kinase inhibitor that targets multiple kinases, including the vascular endothelial growth factor receptors, PDGFR-β, KIT, and FLt3. It has both antiangiogenic and antiproliferative activity. Oral administration as 50 mg daily for 4 weeks followed by no treatment for 2 weeks and then repeated as 6-week cycles for treatment of imatinib-resistant GISTs resulted in objective responses in 7% of patients while 58% had stable disease.[147] Many other tyrosine kinase inhibitors are in development, many of which target more than one family of protein kinases.[148] Among these include sorafenib, dasatinib, and AMG-706, which are actively being investigated for the treatment of imatinib-resistant GIST.[149] Several other new agents, everolimus (RAD001) and protein kinase C, are being investigated as synergistic agents that may maximize the extent and duration of response to imatinib by blocking potential pathways of resistance.

Multidisciplinary Approach

With the emergence of effective systemic treatment for GIST, so has the emergence of the multidisciplinary approach to managing locally advanced and metastatic disease. Although imatinib has improved survival of patients with advanced GISTs, most patients are not cured. There are groups of patients who develop secondary resistance to imatinib with one or more sites of disease progression after 6 months of clinical response. The mechanisms of imatinib resistance are areas of active investigation. Surgery has been shown to be of benefit for selected patients on imatinib with isolated progression of disease.[150–153] Surgical resection of residual metastatic disease responding to kinase inhibitor therapy also has been demonstrated to result in favorable progression-free survival in 70 to 96% of patients with imatinib- or sunitinib-sensitive GISTs.[152–154] The optimal timing of surgery for a patient with metastatic disease in relation to imatinib therapy remains to be determined. Comparison of nonrandomized outcomes for patients treated with kinase inhibitors alone to those treated with combination kinase inhibitors and surgical resection is not possible given the heterogeneity of patients and bias associated with those selected for surgical resection.

Given the promising results of imatinib therapy for metastatic or locally advanced GISTs, the logical next step is to study the efficacy of imatinib as adjuvant (postoperative) and neoadjuvant (preoperative) in patients with surgically resectable disease, particularly those who are at high risk for recurrence because of large tumor size or high mitotic count. The American College of Surgeons Oncology Group (ACOSOG Z9001) has conducted a phase III randomized double-blind study of adjuvant imatinib vs. placebo after complete resection of primary GISTs. Eligible patients included those with a primary c-Kit–expressing GIST 3 cm or larger, with tumor rupture before or during surgery, intraperitoneal hemorrhage, or one to four multifocal tumors. Patients were randomized to receive 400 mg/d imatinib or placebo for 1 year. The trial was suspended to accrual when an interim analysis demonstrated a relapse-free survival rate of 97% in the imatinib-treated group vs. 83% in the placebo group.[155] All placebo-treated patients were allowed to take imatinib. There are also two ongoing randomized trials in Europe in which imatinib is being given following surgical resection of GIST; the Scandinavian Sarcoma Group (SSG XVIII) is comparing 12 months vs. 36 months of imatinib and the European Organization for the Research and Treatment of Cancer (EORTC 62024) is comparing imatinib vs. no treatment for 24 months. A neoadjuvant trial also is being conducted by the Radiation Treatment Oncology Group (RTOG S0132), in which patients with potentially resection primary or recurrent tumors are being treated with imatinib for 8 to 10 weeks preoperatively and then 24 months postoperatively.[156]

Sarcomas of the Breast

Sarcomas of the breast are rare tumors, accounting for <1% of all breast malignancies and <5% of all soft tissue sarcomas. A variety of histologic subtypes have been reported to occur within the breast, including angiosarcoma, stromal sarcoma, fibrosarcoma, and MFH.

Angiosarcoma of the breast accounts for about 50% of all sarcomas of the breast and increasingly has been associated with radiation therapy for the treatment of primary breast cancer.[5] The latency period for radiation-associated sarcomas has been reported to range from 3 years to 20 years with an incidence of 0.3% at 10 years and 0.5% at 15 years.[157] In a retrospective study of 55 patients with angiosarcoma of the breast, patients with radiation therapy–associated angiosarcoma were on average 30 years older and less likely to present with distant metastatic disease than radiation-naïve patients. Clinically, angiosarcoma of the breast associated with radiation therapy may occur in the irradiated chest wall after mastectomy or in the remaining breast after breast conservation followed by radiation. The presentation of cutaneous angiosarcoma often includes an expanding erythematous patch, red papular eruptions, bluish-black lesions, or bruise-like discoloration overlying an area of induration. Mammography is often nonspecific. Diagnosis requires punch or incisional biopsy.

Cystosarcoma phyllodes generally are not considered to be sarcomas because these tumors are thought to originate from hormonally responsive stromal cells of the breast and the majority are benign. Tumors with infiltrating tumor margin, severe stromal overgrowth, atypia, and cellularity have been identified as high risk for metastases.[158]

As with sarcomas at other anatomic sites, the histopathologic grade and size of the tumor are important prognostic factors. Likewise, the likelihood of local recurrences increases as the tumor size increases; tumors <5 cm are associated with better overall survival. Local and distant recurrence are more common in patients with high-grade lesions. Complete excision with negative margins is the primary therapy. Simple mastectomy carries no additional benefit if complete excision can be accomplished by segmental mastectomy. Because of low rates of regional lymphatic spread, axillary dissection is not routinely indicated. Neoadjuvant chemotherapy or radiation therapy may be considered for patients with large, high-risk tumors.

Uterine Sarcomas

Sarcomas account for <5% of all uterine malignancies. They have been classified into three main histologic subgroups: endometrial stromal sarcoma, leiomyosarcoma, and mixed müllerian tumor. Five-year overall survival rates for patients with uterine sarcoma is poor at 30 to 50%.[159] Total abdominal hysterectomy is the treatment for local disease. Because of the rarity of the uterine sarcomas, the benefits of adjuvant therapy (e.g., radiation therapy to the pelvis, chemotherapy, and hormonal therapy) have not been adequately evaluated. Gemcitabine plus docetaxel has been noted to be well tolerated and highly active with a response rate of 53% in patients with unresectable leiomyosarcoma of the uterus.[84]

Endometrial stromal sarcomas comprise about 7 to 15% of uterine sarcomas. Mitotic count is used to classify tumors either as low-grade (<10 mitoses per 10 high-power field) or high-grade (>10 mitoses per 10 high-power field). In general, low-grade tumors demonstrate an indolent clinical course while high-grade tumors are more aggressive with a poorer prognosis. Distinct from other uterine sarcoma subtypes, endometrial stromal sarcomas express progesterone receptors and have been found to be responsive to hormonal manipulation as an adjuvant therapy or treatment of recurrent disease.[160,161]

Desmoids

Desmoid tumors are low-grade sarcomas that do not metastasize. Approximately half of these tumors arise in the extremities, with the remaining lesions located on the trunk or in the retroperitoneum. Abdominal wall desmoids are associated with pregnancy and are thought to arise as the result of hormonal influences. Patients with Gardner's syndrome may have retroperitoneal desmoids as an extracolonic manifestation of the disease. Surgical resection with wide local excision should be the primary therapy for desmoid tumors. Local recurrence may occur in up to one third of patients. Adjuvant radiation therapy has been associated with a reduced incidence of local recurrence.

Dermatofibrosarcoma Protuberans

Dermatofibrosarcoma protuberans (DFSP) is a rare, low-grade sarcoma arising in the dermis. The overall annual incidence has been estimated at 4.2 cases per million population[162] with a higher incidence among blacks than whites (6.5 vs. 3.9 per million). Approximately 40% arise on the trunk, with most of the remaining tumors distributed between the head and neck and extremities. The lesion presents as a nodular, cutaneous mass that shows slow and persistent growth. Satellite lesions may be found in patients with larger tumors. Standard treatment of DFSPs is wide local excision, with expected local recurrence rate of <10%. Although recurrence rates have been reported as high as 30 to 50% in population-based series, associated 5-year survival is >99%.[162]

The pathogenesis of DFSP arises from a specific chromosomal translocation involving chromosomes 17 and 22, in which the collagen1alpha1 gene is fused to the gene for platelet-derived growth factor (PDGF) β chain.[163] The resultant deregulated expression of PDGFβ leads to continuous activation of the PDGF receptor protein-tyrosine kinase that promotes DFSP tumor cell growth. The identification of this chromosomal translocation in >90% of DFSPs has led to the application of targeted therapy. Inhibiting PDGF receptors with imatinib has been shown to induce clinical and radiologic improvement in patients with unresectable DFSP.[8] These data have resulted in the approval by the U.S. Food and Drug Administration for imatinib treatment in patients with locally advanced DFSP.

Pediatric Sarcomas

Soft tissue sarcomas account for 7 to 8% of all pediatric cancers, totaling approximately 600 new cases per year.[164] Pediatric sarcomas traditionally have been divided into two groups: rhabdomyosarcoma and nonrhabdomyosarcoma soft tissue sarcomas. The most common nonrhabdomyosarcomas are synovial sarcoma, malignant peripheral nerve sheath tumor, and fibrosarcoma. Associated with skeletal muscle, rhabdomyosarcomas are the most common soft tissue tumors among children <15 years old and can occur at any site that has striated muscle. These tumors generally present as a painless enlarging mass; about 24% in the genitourinary system, 20% in the extremities, 20% in the head and neck, 16% in the parameningeal region, and 22% in miscellaneous other sites.[165] Regional lymphatic spread of tumor occurs frequently in extremity tumors and in paratesticular tumors. About 15 to 20% of cases have metastasis at presentation, most commonly (40 to 50%) involving the lungs, followed by bone marrow and bone. However, all patients are considered to have micrometastatic disease at presentation, which is the rationale for universal chemotherapy.

Rhabdomyosarcoma is classified as a small, round cell tumor that demonstrates muscle differentiation upon light microscopy and immunohistochemical analysis. Two primary histologic subtypes account for 90% of cases, an embryonal subtype (7%) and an alveolar (20%). Alveolar rhabdomyosarcoma is associated with cytogenetic translocation [t(2:13)(q35:q14)] in 85 to 90% of cases and [t(1:13)(p36:q14)] in 10% of cases.[166] These translocations affect biologic activity at the levels of protein function and gene expression affecting the control of cell growth, apoptosis, differentiation, and motility, ultimately contributing to tumorigenic behavior.[167] In contrast to the specific translocations found in alveolar rhabdomyosarcomas, most embryonal rhabdomyosarcomas have an allelic loss at chromosome 11p15.5 that is thought to inactivate a tumor suppressor gene.[167,168] Both of these distinct molecular subtypes of rhabdomyosarcomas are thought to affect similar downstream targets, such as the p53 and Rb pathways.[167] Further insight into these genetic alterations may lead to a better understanding of the pathogenesis of rhabdomyosarcoma and provide novel targets for therapeutic approaches.

Extent of disease is the strongest predictor of long-term outcome. Several staging systems for rhabdomyosarcoma are available; that of the Intergroup Rhabdomyosarcoma Study Group is based on surgical-pathologic groupings (Table 36-4). Multidisciplinary evaluation including pediatric oncologists, surgical subspecialists, and radiation oncologists is critical for treatment planning to achieve favorable long-term outcomes with the goal of maximizing local tumor control and minimizing long-term treatment effects.

Complete surgical resection is the treatment of choice for rhabdomyosarcoma, when function and cosmesis can be preserved. Patients who are able to undergo a complete tumor resection with negative (group I) or microscopic surgical margins (group II) are able to undergo less intensive systemic therapy with overall survival rates approaching 90%.[169] Given the morbidity associated with resections at some anatomic sites, in particular the head and neck and genitourinary systems, surgery often is not undertaken. Recent findings suggest that chemotherapy can adequately control several such tumors without additional local therapy. In the second International Society of Paediatric Oncology study of rhabdomyosarcoma (MMT84), the choice of local treatment was based on response to initial chemotherapy such that radical surgery and radiotherapy were avoided in 6% of patients. Among the patients who subsequently developed local relapse, the 5-year overall survival rate after salvage therapy was 46%.[169]

Unlike other soft tissue sarcomas, rhabdomyosarcomas have a high propensity for lymph node metastasis, with rates of up to 20 to 30% for sites such as the extremities, paratesticular nodes, and prostate. Lymph node sampling and, more recently, sentinel lymph node mapping have been used to evaluate regional node status in children with rhabdomyosarcoma.

Multiagent chemotherapy is recommended for all patients with rhabdomyosarcoma. Combination regimens including vincristine, actinomycin D, and cyclophosphamide continue to be the basis of effective curative therapy.[165] Although various combinations including doxorubicin, ifosfamide, cisplatin, and etoposide have been active against rhabdomyosarcoma, they have not improved outcomes.[169,170] Radiation therapy is given to most patients with microscopic residual disease (group II) after resection.

The prognosis for children with rhabdomyosarcomas is related to tumor site, surgical-pathologic grouping, and tumor histology. The 5-year, disease-free survival rate for all patients has been reported as 65%. Disease-free survival by group (see Table 36-4) has been reported as 84%, 74%, 62%, and 23% for groups I, II, III, and IV, respectively.[171]

RESEARCH PERSPECTIVES

Experimental Therapeutics

As the molecular alterations associated with various sarcoma subtypes are elucidated, many potential pathways for therapeutic development will become available. A wide variety of DNA alterations have been observed in sarcoma resulting in mutated genes encoding various proteins ranging from transcription factors, mutated tyrosine kinases, and mutated cytokines.[149] The challenge in identifying targets in sarcomas is to identify those that are specifically important to cellular function. The ideal therapeutic target has been described as one that is (a) a single molecule critical for pathogenesis, (b) expressed and active, (c) involved in a single pathway which is amenable to blockade (i.e., no alternative bypass pathways), and (d) critical for sarcoma cell survival.[12]

The translocations and mutations of tyrosine kinases have allowed the development of drugs targeting crucial proteins involved in the neoplastic transformation of sarcoma cells. Tyrosine kinases are enzymes that bind adenosine triphosphate and transfer phosphates from adenosine triphosphate to the tyrosine residues on substrate proteins. These enzymes have long been considered attractive targets for selective pharmacologic inhibition because many human cancers display deregulated kinase pathways.[172] In the early 1980s, it was recognized that constitutively activated tyrosine kinase is important in the pathogenesis of chronic myelogenous leukemia. The BCR-ABL gene, which is the result of a reciprocal exchange of genetic material between chromosomes 9 and 22, was identified as the causative molecular abnormality in chronic myelogenous leukemia. The genetic translocation was found to lead to the constitutive activation of a specific BCR-ABL tyrosine kinase protein, resulting in the malignant expansion of myeloid cells, disruption of regulatory control by stromal cells, and inhibition of apoptosis.[172] In the late 1980s, Ciba-Geigy identified a series of compounds with kinase inhibitory activity and subsequently developed a compound, [4=[(4-methyl-1-piperazinyl)methyl]-N-[4-methyl-3-[[4-(3-pyridinyl)-2-pyrimidinyl]amino]-phenyl]benzamide-methanesulfonate], that specifically blocked the tyrosine kinase activity of ABL.[173] Formerly referred to as STI571 (signal transduction inhibitor 571), imatinib mesylate, marketed as Gleevec, selectively inhibits several structurally similar tyrosine kinases, including all ABL tyrosine kinases, the PDGF receptor, and the c-Kit tyrosine kinase.

Mutations of c-Kit are common in GISTs, and most of the mutations result from an inframe deletion or a point mutation in exon 11 (the juxtamembrane domain). These mutations, which occur predominantly in malignant GISTs, lead to ligand-independent activation of the tyrosine kinase of c-Kit. The resulting constitutive c-Kit tyrosine kinase activity has been shown to promote tumor growth in vitro and may be the key molecular pathway in the

Clinical Group		Definition
TABLE 36-4		**Surgical-pathologic grouping of soft tissue sarcoma (Intergroup Rhabdomyosarcoma Study Group)**
I	a	Localized, completely resected, confined to site of origin
	b	Localized, completely resected, contiguous involvement beyond site of origin
II	a	Localized, grossly resected, microscopic residual tumor
	b	Regional disease, involved lymph nodes, completely resected
	c	Regional disease, involved lymph nodes, grossly resected but with evident of microscopic residual tumor
III	a	Local or regional grossly visible disease after biopsy only
	b	Grossly visible disease after >50% resection of primary tumor
IV		Distant metastases at diagnosis

pathogenesis of GISTs. Imatinib has been shown to selectively inhibit c-Kit tyrosine kinase activity, resulting in decreased GIST cellular proliferation and increased induction of apoptosis. These results have provided the rationale for clinical trials of imatinib for patients with solid tumors that are dependent on the activity of wild-type or mutant c-Kit for proliferation. GI stromal tumors are a rare subtype of sarcoma in which GIST cells harbor an activating mutation of the KIT resulting in tumor progression in 85% of cases.

Insight into the mechanisms of tumor resistance to imatinib, such as the acquisition of secondary mutation of the KIT and PDGF receptors, has provided insight for the development of many new agents.[174] There are a number of emerging second-generation receptor tyrosine kinase inhibitors, including sunitinib, sorafenib, nilotinib and AMG-706, that have shown therapeutic potential in imatinib-resistant patients.[174] Understanding of the molecular pathways and mediators with the introduction of new systemic treatments will hopefully improve survival for additional soft tissue sarcomas in the near future. It has become increasingly apparent that soft tissue sarcoma is a heterogeneous disease comprised of unique subtypes and the promise for future therapies is connecting specific sarcoma subtypes to novel therapeutics.

CONCLUSIONS

Soft tissue sarcomas are a family of rare tumors, constituting approximately 1% of adult malignancies. The etiology in the vast majority of patients is sporadic. The management of such diverse tumors is complex. Diagnosis by light microscopy is inexact. Molecular diagnosis, although still in its infancy, holds great promise for the future.

In spite of these confounding issues, the natural history of soft tissue sarcomas is well established. Approximately two thirds of cases arise in the extremities, whereas the remaining one third is distributed between the retroperitoneum, trunk, abdomen, and head and neck. The management algorithm for soft tissue sarcomas is complex and depends on tumor stage, site, and histology. The most common site of metastasis is the lungs and generally occurs within 3 years of diagnosis.

Progress in the understanding of soft tissue sarcoma biology is crucial for the development of new therapeutic targets. Drug engineering will enable molecular-based therapies to become increasingly incorporated into clinical trials and, with success, treatment strategies in the near future.

REFERENCES

Entries highlighted in bright blue are key references.

1. American Cancer Society: *Cancer Facts and Figures.* Philadelphia: Elsevier, 2007.
2. Coindre JM, Terrier P, Guillou L, et al: Predictive value of grade for metastasis development in the main histologic types of adult soft tissue sarcomas: A study of 1240 patients from the French Federation of Cancer Centers Sarcoma Group. *Cancer* 91:1914, 2001.
3. Fong Y, Coit DG, Woodruff JM, et al: Lymph node metastasis from soft tissue sarcoma in adults. Analysis of data from a prospective database of 1772 sarcoma patients. *Ann Surg* 217:72, 1993.
4. Brady MS, Gaynor JJ, Brennan MF: Radiation-associated sarcoma of bone and soft tissue. *Arch Surg* 127:1379, 1992.
5. Vorburger SA, Xing Y, Hunt KK, et al: Angiosarcoma of the breast. *Cancer* 104:2682, 2005.
6. Smith AH, Pearce NE, Fisher DO, et al: Soft tissue sarcoma and exposure to phenoxyherbicides and chlorophenols in New Zealand. *J Natl Cancer Inst* 73:1111, 1984.
7. Stewart FW, Treves N: Lymphangiosarcoma in post-mastectomy lymphedema. *Cancer* 1, 1948.
8. Wunder JS, Nielsen TO, Maki RG, et al: Opportunities for improving the therapeutic ratio for patients with sarcoma. *Lancet Oncol* 8:513, 2007.
9. Lynch HT, Deters CA, Hogg D, et al: Familial sarcoma: Challenging pedigrees. *Cancer* 98:1947, 2003.
10. Levine EA: Prognostic factors in soft tissue sarcoma. *Semin Surg Oncol* 17:23, 1999.
11. Sorensen PH, Triche TJ: Gene fusions encoding chimaeric transcription factors in solid tumours. *Semin Cancer Biol* 7:3, 1996.
12. Borden EC, Baker LH, Bell RS, et al: Soft tissue sarcomas of adults: State of the translational science. *Clin Cancer Res* 9:1941, 2003.
13. Hieken TJ, Das Gupta TK: Mutant p53 expression: A marker of diminished survival in well-differentiated soft tissue sarcoma. *Clin Cancer Res* 2:1391, 1996.
14. Karnes PS: Neurofibromatosis: a common neurocutaneous disorder. *Mayo Clin Proc* 73:1071, 1998.
15. Benns M, Dalsing M, Sawchuck A, et al: Soft tissue sarcomas may present with deep vein thrombosis. *J Vasc Surg* 43:788, 2006.
16. Heslin MJ, Smith JK: Imaging of soft tissue sarcomas. *Surg Oncol Clin N Am* 8:91, 1999.
17. Pearlstone DB, Pisters PW, Bold RJ, et al: Patterns of recurrence in extremity liposarcoma: implications for staging and follow-up. *Cancer* 85:85, 1999.
18. Kilpatrick SE, Geisinger KR: Soft tissue sarcomas: The usefulness and limitations of fine-needle aspiration biopsy. *Am J Clin Pathol* 110:50, 1998.
19. Ayala AG, Ro JY, Fanning CV, et al: Core needle biopsy and fine-needle aspiration in the diagnosis of bone and soft-tissue lesions. *Hematol Oncol Clin North Am* 9:633, 1995.
20. Dupuy DE, Rosenberg AE, Punyaratabandhu T, et al: Accuracy of CT-guided needle biopsy of musculoskeletal neoplasms. *AJR Am J Roentgenol* 171:759, 1998.
21. Huvos AG: The importance of the open surgical biopsy in the diagnosis and treatment of bone and soft-tissue tumors. *Hematol Oncol Clin North Am* 9:541, 1995.
22. Fletcher CD, Gustafson P, Rydholm A, et al: Clinicopathologic re-evaluation of 100 malignant fibrous histiocytomas: Prognostic relevance of subclassification. *J Clin Oncol* 19:3045, 2001.
23. Tschoep K, Kohlmann A, Schlemmer M, et al: Gene expression profiling in sarcomas. *Crit Rev Oncol Hematol* 63:111, 2007.
24. Coindre JM, Hostein I, Maire G, et al: Inflammatory malignant fibrous histiocytomas and dedifferentiated liposarcomas: Histological review, genomic profile, and MDM2 and CDK4 status favour a single entity. *J Pathol* 203:822, 2004.
25. Presant CA, Russell WO, Alexander RW, et al: Soft-tissue and bone sarcoma histopathology peer review: The frequency of disagreement in diagnosis and the need for second pathology opinions. The Southeastern Cancer Study Group experience. *J Clin Oncol* 4:1658, 1986.
26. AJCC Cancer Staging Manual. New York: Springer, 2002, p 221.
27. Coindre JM, Terrier P, Bui NB, et al: Prognostic factors in adult patients with locally controlled soft tissue sarcoma. A study of 546 patients from the French Federation of Cancer Centers Sarcoma Group. *J Clin Oncol* 14:869, 1996.
28. Guillou L, Coindre JM, Bonichon F, et al: Comparative study of the National Cancer Institute and French Federation of Cancer Centers Sarcoma Group grading systems in a population of 410 adult patients with soft tissue sarcoma. *J Clin Oncol* 15:350, 1997.
29. Rubin BP, Fletcher CD, Inwards C, et al: Protocol for the examination of specimens from patients with soft tissue tumors of intermediate malignant potential, malignant soft tissue tumors, and benign/locally aggressive and malignant bone tumors. *Arch Pathol Lab Med* 130:1616, 2006.
30. Ramanathan RC, A'Hern R, Fisher C, et al: Modified staging system for extremity soft tissue sarcomas. *Ann Surg Oncol* 6:57, 1999.
31. Atalay C, Altinok M, Seref B: The impact of lymph node metastases on survival in extremity soft tissue sarcomas. *World J Surg* 31:1433, 2007.
32. Riad S, Griffin AM, Liberman B, et al: Lymph node metastasis in soft tissue sarcoma in an extremity. *Clin Orthop Relat Res* 426:129, 2004.
33. Behranwala KA, A'Hern R, Omar AM, et al: Prognosis of lymph node metastasis in soft tissue sarcoma. *Ann Surg Oncol* 11:714, 2004.
34. Grobmyer SR, Brennan MF: Predictive variables detailing the recurrence rate of soft tissue sarcomas. *Curr Opin Oncol* 15:319, 2003.
35. Heslin MJ, Cordon-Cardo C, Lewis JJ, et al: Ki-67 detected by MIB-1 predicts distant metastasis and tumor mortality in primary, high grade extremity soft tissue sarcoma. *Cancer* 83:490, 1998.
36. Ch'ng E, Tomita Y, Zhang B, et al: Prognostic significance of CD100 expression in soft tissue sarcoma. *Cancer* 110:164, 2007.
37. Kattan MW, Heller G, Brennan MF: A competing-risks nomogram for sarcoma-specific death following local recurrence. *Stat Med* 22:3515, 2003.

38. Brennan MF, Kattan MW, Klimstra D, et al: Prognostic nomogram for patients undergoing resection for adenocarcinoma of the pancreas. *Ann Surg* 240:293, 2004.

39. Kattan MW, Karpeh MS, Mazumdar M, et al: Postoperative nomogram for disease-specific survival after an R0 resection for gastric carcinoma. *J Clin Oncol* 21:3647, 2003.

40. Kattan MW, Leung DH, Brennan MF: Postoperative nomogram for 12-year sarcoma-specific death. *J Clin Oncol* 20:791, 2002.

41. Dalal KM, Kattan MW, Antonescu CR, et al: Subtype specific prognostic nomogram for patients with primary liposarcoma of the retroperitoneum, extremity, or trunk. *Ann Surg* 244:381, 2006.

42. Limb-sparing treatment of adult soft-tissue sarcomas and osteosarcomas. *NIH Consens Statement* Dec 3–5. 5:1, 1984.

43. McKee MD, Liu DF, Brooks JJ, et al: The prognostic significance of margin width for extremity and trunk sarcoma. *J Surg Oncol* 85:68, 2004.

44. Herbert SH, Corn BW, Solin LJ, et al: Limb-preserving treatment for soft tissue sarcomas of the extremities. The significance of surgical margins. *Cancer* 72:1230, 1993.

45. Tanabe KK, Pollock RE, Ellis LM, et al: Influence of surgical margins on outcome in patients with preoperatively irradiated extremity soft tissue sarcomas. *Cancer* 73:1652, 1994.

46. Lin PP, Pino ED, Normand AN, et al: Periosteal margin in soft-tissue sarcoma. *Cancer* 109:598, 2007.

47. Ferguson PC, Griffin AM, O'Sullivan B, et al: Bone invasion in extremity soft-tissue sarcoma: Impact on disease outcomes. *Cancer* 106:2692, 2006.

48. Ferguson PC: Surgical considerations for management of distal extremity soft tissue sarcomas. *Curr Opin Oncol* 17:366, 2005.

49. Karakousis CP, Karmpaliotis C, Driscoll DL: Major vessel resection during limb-preserving surgery for soft tissue sarcomas. *World J Surg* 20:345; discussion 350, 1996.

50. Ghert MA, Davis AM, Griffin AM, et al: The surgical and functional outcome of limb-salvage surgery with vascular reconstruction for soft tissue sarcoma of the extremity. *Ann Surg Oncol* 12:1102, 2005.

51. Rosenberg SA, Tepper J, Glatstein E, et al: The treatment of soft-tissue sarcomas of the extremities: Prospective randomized evaluations of (1) limb-sparing surgery plus radiation therapy compared with amputation and (2) the role of adjuvant chemotherapy. *Ann Surg* 196:305, 1982.

52. Potter DA, Glenn J, Kinsella T, et al: Patterns of recurrence in patients with high-grade soft-tissue sarcomas. *J Clin Oncol* 3:353, 1985.

53. Lindberg RD, Martin RG, Romsdahl MM, et al: Conservative surgery and postoperative radiotherapy in 300 adults with soft-tissue sarcomas. *Cancer* 47:2391, 1981.

54. Suit HD, Proppe KH, Mankin HJ, et al: Preoperative radiation therapy for sarcoma of soft tissue. *Cancer* 47:2269, 1981.

55. Leibel SA, Tranbaugh RF, Wara WM, et al: Soft tissue sarcomas of the extremities: Survival and patterns of failure with conservative surgery and postoperative irradiation compared to surgery alone. *Cancer* 50:1076, 1982.

56. McBride CM: Sarcomas of the limbs. Results of adjuvant chemotherapy using isolation perfusion. *Arch Surg* 109:304, 1974.

57. Hoekstra HJ, Schraffordt Koops H, Molenaar WM, et al: Results of isolated regional perfusion in the treatment of malignant soft tissue tumors of the extremities. *Cancer* 60:1703, 1987.

58. Eggermont AM, Schraffordt Koops H, Klausner JM, et al: Isolated limb perfusion with tumor necrosis factor and melphalan for limb salvage in 186 patients with locally advanced soft tissue extremity sarcomas. The cumulative multicenter European experience. *Ann Surg* 224:756; discussion 764, 1996.

59. Fraker D, Alexander HR, Ross M: A phase II trial of isolated perfusion with high dose tumor necrosis factor and melphalan for unresectable extremity sarcomas, Society of Surgical Oncology Proceedings: Abstract #53, 1999.

60. Lienard D, Ewalenko P, Delmotte JJ, et al: High-dose recombinant tumor necrosis factor alpha in combination with interferon gamma and melphalan in isolation perfusion of the limbs for melanoma and sarcoma. *J Clin Oncol* 10:52, 1992.

61. Rossi CR, Vecchiato A, Foletto M, et al: Phase II study on neoadjuvant hyperthermic-antiblastic perfusion with doxorubicin in patients with intermediate or high grade limb sarcomas. *Cancer* 73:2140, 1994.

62. Yang JC, Chang AE, Baker AR, et al: Randomized prospective study of the benefit of adjuvant radiation therapy in the treatment of soft tissue sarcomas of the extremity. *J Clin Oncol* 16:197, 1998.

63. Pisters PW, Harrison LB, Leung DH, et al: Long-term results of a prospective randomized trial of adjuvant brachytherapy in soft tissue sarcoma. *J Clin Oncol* 14:859, 1996.

64. Suit HD, Spiro I: Role of radiation in the management of adult patients with sarcoma of soft tissue. *Semin Surg Oncol* 10:347, 1994.

65. Barkley HT Jr., Martin RG, Romsdahl MM, et al: Treatment of soft tissue sarcomas by preoperative irradiation and conservative surgical resection. *Int J Radiat Oncol Biol Phys* 14:693, 1988.

66. Wilson AN, Davis A, Bell RS, et al: Local control of soft tissue sarcoma of the extremity: The experience of a multidisciplinary sarcoma group with definitive surgery and radiotherapy. *Eur J Cancer* 30A:746, 1994.

67. Pisters PW, Harrison LB, Woodruff JM, et al: A prospective randomized trial of adjuvant brachytherapy in the management of low-grade soft tissue sarcomas of the extremity and superficial trunk. *J Clin Oncol* 12:1150, 1994.

68. Geer RJ, Woodruff J, Casper ES, et al: Management of small soft-tissue sarcoma of the extremity in adults. *Arch Surg* 127:1285, 1992.

69. Karakousis CP, Emrich LJ, Rao U, et al: Limb salvage in soft tissue sarcomas with selective combination of modalities. *Eur J Surg Oncol* 17:71, 1991.

70. Alektiar KM, Brennan MF, Singer S: Influence of site on the therapeutic ratio of adjuvant radiotherapy in soft-tissue sarcoma of the extremity. *Int J Radiat Oncol Biol Phys* 63:202, 2005.

71. Nielsen OS, Cummings B, O'Sullivan B, et al: Preoperative and postoperative irradiation of soft tissue sarcomas: effect of radiation field size. *Int J Radiat Oncol Biol Phys* 21:1595, 1991.

72. Tseng JF, Ballo MT, Langstein HN, et al: The effect of preoperative radiotherapy and reconstructive surgery on wound complications after resection of extremity soft-tissue sarcomas. *Ann Surg Oncol* 13:1209, 2006.

73. O'Sullivan B, Davis AM, Turcotte R, et al: Preoperative versus postoperative radiotherapy in soft-tissue sarcoma of the limbs: A randomised trial. *Lancet* 359:2235, 2002.

74. Davis AM, O'Sullivan B, Turcotte R, et al: Late radiation morbidity following randomization to preoperative versus postoperative radiotherapy in extremity soft tissue sarcoma. *Radiother Oncol* 75:48, 2005.

75. Janjan NA, Yasko AW, Reece GP, et al: Comparison of charges related to radiotherapy for soft-tissue sarcomas treated by preoperative external-beam irradiation versus interstitial implantation. *Ann Surg Oncol* 1:415, 1994.

76. Griffin AM, Euler CI, Sharpe MB, et al: Radiation planning comparison for superficial tissue avoidance in radiotherapy for soft tissue sarcoma of the lower extremity. *Int J Radiat Oncol Biol Phys* 67:847, 2007.

77. Hong L, Alektiar KM, Hunt M, et al: Intensity-modulated radiotherapy for soft tissue sarcoma of the thigh. *Int J Radiat Oncol Biol Phys* 59:752, 2004.

78. Cannon CP, Ballo MT, Zagars GK, et al: Complications of combined modality treatment of primary lower extremity soft-tissue sarcomas. *Cancer* 107:2455, 2006.

79. Stinson SF, DeLaney TF, Greenberg J, et al: Acute and long-term effects on limb function of combined modality limb sparing therapy for extremity soft tissue sarcoma. *Int J Radiat Oncol Biol Phys* 21:1493, 1991.

80. Ferrari A, Gronchi A, Casanova M, et al: Synovial sarcoma: A retrospective analysis of 271 patients of all ages treated at a single institution. *Cancer* 101:627, 2004.

81. O'Bryan RM, Baker LH, Gottlieb JE, et al: Dose response evaluation of adriamycin in human neoplasia. *Cancer* 39:1940, 1977.

82. Patel SR, Vadhan-Raj S, Papadopolous N, et al: High-dose ifosfamide in bone and soft tissue sarcomas: Results of phase II and pilot studies—dose-response and schedule dependence. *J Clin Oncol* 15:2378, 1997.

83. Patel SR, Gandhi V, Jenkins J, et al: Phase II clinical investigation of gemcitabine in advanced soft tissue sarcomas and window evaluation of dose rate on gemcitabine triphosphate accumulation. *J Clin Oncol* 19:3483, 2001.

84. Hensley ML, Maki R, Venkatraman E, et al: Gemcitabine and docetaxel in patients with unresectable leiomyosarcoma: Results of a phase II trial. *J Clin Oncol* 20:2824, 2002.

85. Dileo P, Morgan JA, Zahrieh D, et al: Gemcitabine and vinorelbine combination chemotherapy for patients with advanced soft tissue sarcomas: Results of a phase II trial. *Cancer* 109:1863, 2007.

86. Fata F, O'Reilly E, Ilson D, et al: Paclitaxel in the treatment of patients with angiosarcoma of the scalp or face. *Cancer* 86:2034, 1999.

87. Skubitz KM, Haddad PA: Paclitaxel and pegylated-liposomal doxorubicin are both active in angiosarcoma. *Cancer* 104:361, 2005.

88. Clark MA, Fisher C, Judson I, et al: Soft-tissue sarcomas in adults. *N Engl J Med* 353:701, 2005.

89. Gutierrez JC, Perez EA, Moffat FL, et al: Should soft tissue sarcomas be treated at high-volume centers? An analysis of 4205 patients. *Ann Surg* 245:952, 2007.

90. Adjuvant chemotherapy for localised resectable soft-tissue sarcoma of adults: Meta-analysis of individual data. Sarcoma Meta-analysis Collaboration. *Lancet* 350:1647, 1997.

91. Frustaci S, Gherlinzoni F, De Paoli A, et al: Adjuvant chemotherapy for adult soft tissue sarcomas of the extremities and girdles: Results of the Italian randomized cooperative trial. *J Clin Oncol* 19:1238, 2001.

92. Frustaci S, De Paoli A, Bidoli E, et al: Ifosfamide in the adjuvant therapy of soft tissue sarcomas. *Oncology* 65(Suppl 2):80, 2003.

93. Cormier JN, Huang X, Xing Y, et al: Cohort analysis of patients with localized, high-risk, extremity soft tissue sarcoma treated at two cancer centers: Chemotherapy-associated outcomes. *J Clin Oncol* 22:4567, 2004.

94. Grobmyer SR, Maki RG, Demetri GD, et al: Neo-adjuvant chemotherapy for primary high-grade extremity soft tissue sarcoma. *Ann Oncol* 15:1667, 2004.

95. Eilber FC, Tap WD, Nelson SD, et al: Advances in chemotherapy for patients with extremity soft tissue sarcoma. *Orthop Clin North Am* 37:15, 2006.

96. Eilber FC, Brennan MF, Riedel E, et al: Prognostic factors for survival in patients with locally recurrent extremity soft tissue sarcomas. *Ann Surg Oncol* 12:228, 2005.

97. Singer S, Antman K, Corson JM, et al: Long-term salvageability for patients with locally recurrent soft-tissue sarcomas. *Arch Surg* 127:548; discussion 553, 1992.

98. Whooley BP, Mooney MM, Gibbs JF, et al: Effective follow-up strategies in soft tissue sarcoma. *Semin Surg Oncol* 17:83, 1999.

99. Midis GP, Pollock RE, Chen NP, et al: Locally recurrent soft tissue sarcoma of the extremities. *Surgery* 123:666, 1998.

100. Karakousis CP, Proimakis C, Rao U, et al: Local recurrence and survival in soft-tissue sarcomas. *Ann Surg Oncol* 3:255, 1996.

101. Nori D, Schupak K, Shiu MH, et al: Role of brachytherapy in recurrent extremity sarcoma in patients treated with prior surgery and irradiation. *Int J Radiat Oncol Biol Phys* 20:1229, 1991.

102. Suri RM, Deschamps C, Cassivi SD, et al: Pulmonary resection for metastatic malignant fibrous histiocytoma: An analysis of prognostic factors. *Ann Thorac Surg* 80:1847, 2005.

103. van Geel AN, Pastorino U, Jauch KW, et al: Surgical treatment of lung metastases: The European Organization for Research and Treatment of Cancer-Soft Tissue and Bone Sarcoma Group study of 255 patients. *Cancer* 77:675, 1996.

104. Porter GA, Cantor SB, Walsh GL, et al: Cost-effectiveness of pulmonary resection and systemic chemotherapy in the management of metastatic soft tissue sarcoma: A combined analysis from the University of Texas M. D. Anderson and Memorial Sloan-Kettering Cancer Centers. *J Thorac Cardiovasc Surg* 127:1366, 2004.

105. Van Glabbeke M, van Oosterom AT, Oosterhuis JW, et al: Prognostic factors for the outcome of chemotherapy in advanced soft tissue sarcoma: An analysis of 2,185 patients treated with anthracycline-containing first-line regimens—a European Organization for Research and Treatment of Cancer Soft Tissue and Bone Sarcoma Group Study. *J Clin Oncol* 17:150, 1999.

106. Kepka L, Suit HD, Goldberg SI, et al: Results of radiation therapy performed after unplanned surgery (without re-excision) for soft tissue sarcomas. *J Surg Oncol* 92:39, 2005.

107. Spillane AJ, Fisher C, Thomas JM: Myxoid liposarcoma—the frequency and the natural history of nonpulmonary soft tissue metastases. *Ann Surg Oncol* 6:389, 1999.

108. Estourgie SH, Nielsen GP, Ott MJ: Metastatic patterns of extremity myxoid liposarcoma and their outcome. *J Surg Oncol* 80:89, 2002.

109. Panagopoulos I, Hoglund M, Mertens F, et al: Fusion of the EWS and CHOP genes in myxoid liposarcoma. *Oncogene* 12:489, 1996.

110. Porter GA, Baxter NN, Pisters PW: Retroperitoneal sarcoma: A population-based analysis of epidemiology, surgery, and radiotherapy. *Cancer* 106:1610, 2006.

111. Schwarzbach MH, Hormann Y, Hinz U, et al: Results of limb-sparing surgery with vascular replacement for soft tissue sarcoma in the lower extremity. *J Vasc Surg* 42:88, 2005.

112. Catton CN, O'Sullivan B, Kotwall C, et al: Outcome and prognosis in retroperitoneal soft tissue sarcoma. *Int J Radiat Oncol Biol Phys* 29:1005, 1994.

113. Jaques DP, Coit DG, Hajdu SI, et al: Management of primary and recurrent soft-tissue sarcoma of the retroperitoneum. *Ann Surg* 212:51, 1990.

114. Lewis JJ, Leung D, Woodruff JM, et al: Retroperitoneal soft-tissue sarcoma: Analysis of 500 patients treated and followed at a single institution. *Ann Surg* 228:355, 1998.

115. Yeh JJ, Singer S, Brennan MF, et al: Effectiveness of palliative procedures for intra-abdominal sarcomas. *Ann Surg Oncol* 12:1084, 2005.

116. Chiappa A, Zbar AP, Bertani E, et al: Primary and recurrent retroperitoneal soft tissue sarcoma: prognostic factors affecting survival. *J Surg Oncol* 93:456, 2006.

117. Ballo MT, Zagars GK, Pollock RE, et al: Retroperitoneal soft tissue sarcoma: An analysis of radiation and surgical treatment. *Int J Radiat Oncol Biol Phys* 67:158, 2007.

118. Tierney JF, Mosseri V, Stewart LA, et al: Adjuvant chemotherapy for soft-tissue sarcoma: Review and meta-analysis of the published results of randomised clinical trials. *Br J Cancer* 72:469, 1995.

119. Glenn J, Sindelar WF, Kinsella T, et al: Results of multimodality therapy of resectable soft-tissue sarcomas of the retroperitoneum. *Surgery* 97:316, 1985.

120. Singer S, Corson JM, Demetri GD, et al: Prognostic factors predictive of survival for truncal and retroperitoneal soft-tissue sarcoma. *Ann Surg* 221:185, 1995.

121. Eilber FC, Eilber KS, Eilber FR: Retroperitoneal sarcomas. *Curr Treat Options Oncol* 1:274, 2000.

122. Goss G, Demetri G: Medical management of unresectable, recurrent low-grade retroperitoneal liposarcoma: Integration of cytotoxic and non-cytotoxic therapies into multimodality care. *Surg Oncol* 9:53, 2000.

123. Pawlik TM, Ahuja N, Herman JM: The role of radiation in retroperitoneal sarcomas: a surgical perspective. *Curr Opin Oncol* 19:359, 2007.

124. Pawlik TM, Pisters PW, Mikula L, et al: Long-term results of two prospective trials of preoperative external beam radiotherapy for localized intermediate- or high-grade retroperitoneal soft tissue sarcoma. *Ann Surg Oncol* 13:508, 2006.

125. Tzeng CW, Fiveash JB, Heslin MJ: Radiation therapy for retroperitoneal sarcoma. *Expert Rev Anticancer Ther* 6:1251, 2006.

126. Conlon KC, Casper ES, Brennan MF: Primary GI sarcomas: Analysis of prognostic variables. *Ann Surg Oncol* 2:26, 1995.

127. Chou FF, Eng HL, Sheen-Chen SM: Smooth muscle tumors of the GI tract: Analysis of prognostic factors. *Surgery* 119:171, 1996.

128. Horowitz J, Spellman JE Jr., Driscoll DL, et al: An institutional review of sarcomas of the large and small intestine. *J Am Coll Surg* 180:465, 1995.

129. Meijer S, Peretz T, Gaynor JJ, et al: Primary colorectal sarcoma. A retrospective review and prognostic factor study of 50 consecutive patients. *Arch Surg* 125:1163, 1990.

130. Kindblom LG, Remotti HE, Aldenborg F, et al: GI pacemaker cell tumor (GIPACT): Gastrointestinal stromal tumors show phenotypic characteristics of the interstitial cells of Cajal. *Am J Pathol* 152:1259, 1998.

131. Hirota S, Isozaki K, Moriyama Y, et al: Gain-of-function mutations of c-kit in human GI stromal tumors. *Science* 279:577, 1998.

132. Williams DE, Eisenman J, Baird A, et al: Identification of a ligand for the c-kit proto-oncogene. *Cell* 63:167, 1990.

133. Nilsson B, Bumming P, Meis-Kindblom JM, et al: Gastrointestinal stromal tumors: The incidence, prevalence, clinical course, and prognostication in the preimatinib mesylate era—a population-based study in western Sweden. *Cancer* 103:821, 2005.

134. Rubio J, Marcos-Gragera R, Ortiz MR, et al: Population-based incidence and survival of gastrointestinal stromal tumours (GIST) in Girona, Spain. *Eur J Cancer* 43:144, 2007.

135. Tran T, Davila JA, El-Serag HB: The epidemiology of malignant GI stromal tumors: An analysis of 1,458 cases from 1992 to 2000. *Am J Gastroenterol* 100:162, 2005.

136. Choi H, Charnsangavej C, Faria SC, et al: Correlation of computed tomography and positron emission tomography in patients with metastatic gastrointestinal stromal tumor treated at a single institution with imatinib mesylate: Proposal of new computed tomography response criteria. *J Clin Oncol* 25:1753, 2007.

137. Ng EH, Pollock RE, Munsell MF, et al: Prognostic factors influencing survival in GI leiomyosarcomas. Implications for surgical management and staging. *Ann Surg* 215:68, 1992.

CHAPTER 36   Soft Tissue Sarcomas

138. DeMatteo RP, Lewis JJ, Leung D, et al: Two hundred GI stromal tumors: Recurrence patterns and prognostic factors for survival. *Ann Surg* 231:51, 2000.

139. Fletcher CD, Berman JJ, Corless C, et al: Diagnosis of gastrointestinal stromal tumors: A consensus approach. *Hum Pathol* 33:459, 2002.

140. Miettinen M, Lasota J: GI stromal tumors: Review on morphology, molecular pathology, prognosis, and differential diagnosis. *Arch Pathol Lab Med* 130:1466, 2006.

141. van Oosterom AT, Judson I, Verweij J, et al: Safety and efficacy of imatinib (STI571) in metastatic gastrointestinal stromal tumours: A phase I study. *Lancet* 358:1421, 2001.

142. Blanke CD, von Mehren M, Joensuu H, et al: Evaluation of the safety and efficacy of an oral molecularly-targeted therapy, ST1571, in patients with unresectable metastatic gastrointestinal stromal tumors (GISTs) expressing C-KIT (CD117). *Proc Am Soc Clin Oncol* 20:1, 2001.

143. von Mehren M, Blanke C, Joensuu H, et al: High incidence of durable responses induced by imatinib mesylate (Gleevec) in patients with unresectable and metastatic gastrointestinal stromal tumors. *Proc Am Soc Clin Oncol* 21:1608, 2002.

144. Demetri G, Rankin C, Fletcher C, et al: Phase III dose-randomized study of imatinib mesylate (Gleevec, ST1571) for GIST; intergroup S0033 early results. *Proc Am Soc Clin Oncol* 21:1651, 2002.

145. Casali PG, Verweij J, Zalcberg J, et al: Imatinib (Gleevec) 400 vs 800 mg daily patients with gastrointestinal stromal tumors (GIST) a randomized phase III trial from the EORTC Soft Tissue and Bone Sarcoma Group, the Italian Sarcoma Group (ISC), and the Australasian Gastro-Intestinal Trials Group (AGITG). A toxicity report. *Proc Am Soc Clin Oncol* 21:1650, 2002.

146. Blay JY, Le Cesne A, Ray-Coquard I, et al: Prospective multicentric randomized phase III study of imatinib in patients with advanced GI stromal tumors comparing interruption versus continuation of treatment beyond 1 year: The French Sarcoma Group. *J Clin Oncol* 25:1107, 2007.

147. Demetri GD, van Oosterom AT, Garrett CR, et al: Efficacy and safety of sunitinib in patients with advanced GI stromal tumour after failure of imatinib: A randomised controlled trial. *Lancet* 368:1329, 2006.

148. Boyar MS, Taub RN. New strategies for treating GIST when imatinib fails. *Cancer Invest* 25:328, 2007.

149. Cassier PA, Dufresne A, Fayette J, et al: Emerging drugs for the treatment of soft tissue sarcomas. *Expert Opin Emerg Drugs* 12:139, 2007.

150. Andtbacka RH, Ng CS, Scaife CL, et al: Surgical resection of gastrointestinal stromal tumors after treatment with imatinib. *Ann Surg Oncol* 14:14, 2007.

151. Desai J, Shankar S, Heinrich MC, et al: Clonal evolution of resistance to imatinib in patients with metastatic gastrointestinal stromal tumors. *Clin Cancer Res* 13:5398, 2007.

152. DeMatteo RP, Maki RG, Singer S, et al: Results of tyrosine kinase inhibitor therapy followed by surgical resection for metastatic gastrointestinal stromal tumor. *Ann Surg* 245:347, 2007.

153. Raut CP, Posner M, Desai J, et al: Surgical management of advanced gastrointestinal stromal tumors after treatment with targeted systemic therapy using kinase inhibitors. *J Clin Oncol* 24:2325, 2006.

154. Gronchi A, Fiore M, Miselli F, et al: Surgery of residual disease following molecular-targeted therapy with imatinib mesylate in advanced/metastatic GIST. *Ann Surg* 245:341, 2007.

155. DeMatteo RP, Owzar K, Maki RG, et al: Adjuvant imatinib mesylate increases recurrence free survival (RFS) in patients with completely resected localized primary gastrointestinal stromal tumor (GIST): North American Intergroup Phase III ACOSOG Z9001. Abstract 10079 Proceedings ASCO, 2007.

156. van der Zwan SM, DeMatteo RP: Gastrointestinal stromal tumor: 5 years later. *Cancer* 104:1781, 2005.

157. Kirova YM, Vilcoq JR, Asselain B, et al: Radiation-induced sarcomas after radiotherapy for breast carcinoma: A large-scale single-institution review. *Cancer* 104:856, 2005.

158. Chen WH, Cheng SP, Tzen CY, et al: Surgical treatment of phyllodes tumors of the breast: retrospective review of 172 cases. *J Surg Oncol* 91:185, 2005.

159. Denschlag D, Masoud I, Stanimir G, et al: Prognostic factors and outcome in women with uterine sarcoma. *Eur J Surg Oncol* 33:91, 2007.

160. Leunen M, Breugelmans M, De Sutter P, et al: Low-grade endometrial stromal sarcoma treated with the aromatase inhibitor letrozole. *Gynecol Oncol* 95:769, 2004.

161. Scribner DR Jr., Walker JL: Low-grade endometrial stromal sarcoma preoperative treatment with Depo-Lupron and Megace. *Gynecol Oncol* 71:458, 1998.

162. Criscione VD, Weinstock MA: Descriptive epidemiology of dermatofibrosarcoma protuberans in the United States, 1973 to 2002. *J Am Acad Dermatol* 56:968, 2007.

163. McArthur GA: Molecular targeting of dermatofibrosarcoma protuberans: A new approach to a surgical disease. *J Natl Compr Canc Netw* 5:557, 2007.

164. Grovas A, Fremgen A, Rauck A, et al: The National Cancer Data Base report on patterns of childhood cancers in the United States. *Cancer* 80:2321, 1997.

165. Meyer WH, Spunt SL: Soft tissue sarcomas of childhood. *Cancer Treat Rev* 30:269, 2004.

166. Barr FG, Chatten J, D'Cruz CM, et al: Molecular assays for chromosomal translocations in the diagnosis of pediatric soft tissue sarcomas. *JAMA* 273:553, 1995.

167. Xia SJ, Pressey JG, Barr FG: Molecular pathogenesis of rhabdomyosarcoma. *Cancer Biol Ther* 1:97, 2002.

168. Scrable H, Witte D, Shimada H, et al: Molecular differential pathology of rhabdomyosarcoma. *Genes Chromosomes Cancer* 1:23, 1989.

169. Flamant F, Rodary C, Rey A, et al: Treatment of non-metastatic rhabdomyosarcomas in childhood and adolescence. Results of the second study of the International Society of Paediatric Oncology: MMT84. *Eur J Cancer* 34:1050, 1998.

170. Crist WM, Anderson JR, Meza JL, et al: Intergroup rhabdomyosarcoma study-IV: Results for patients with nonmetastatic disease. *J Clin Oncol* 19:3091, 2001.

171. Crist WM, Garnsey L, Beltangady MS, et al: Prognosis in children with rhabdomyosarcoma: A report of the intergroup rhabdomyosarcoma studies I and II. Intergroup Rhabdomyosarcoma Committee. *J Clin Oncol* 8:443, 1990.

172. Savage DG, Antman KH: Imatinib mesylate—a new oral targeted therapy. *N Engl J Med* 346:683, 2002.

173. Mauro MJ, O'Dwyer M, Heinrich MC, et al: STI571: A paradigm of new agents for cancer therapeutics. *J Clin Oncol* 20:325, 2002.

174. Sankhala KK, Papadopoulos KP: Future options for imatinib mesilate-resistant tumors. *Expert Opin Investig Drugs* 16:1549, 2007.

175. AJCC *American Joint Committee on Cancer: Cancer Staging Manual*, in press (7th ed). New York: Springer.

CHAPTER 37

Inguinal Hernias

Vadim Sherman, James R. Macho,
and F. Charles Brunicardi

HISTORY

The treatment of inguinal hernias is integral to the history and current status of general surgery; evolution in the treatment of inguinal hernias has paralleled technologic developments in the field. The most significant advances to impact inguinal hernia repair have been the addition of prosthetic materials to conventional repairs and the introduction of laparoscopy to general surgical procedures.

Evidence of surgical repair of inguinal hernias can be traced back to civilizations of ancient Egypt and Greece.[1] Early management of inguinal hernias involved a conservative approach using trusses; however, the inefficacy of this approach prompted the initiation of a surgical approach to the problem. As a consequence of the primitiveness of the techniques, the treatment was often worse than the disease itself. Surgery often involved routine excision of the testicle, and wounds were closed with cauterization or left to granulate on their own. Considering these procedures were performed before the advent of the aseptic technique, it is safe to assume that mortality was quite high. For those that did survive the operation, recurrence of the hernia was commonplace.

Failure of these early techniques of hernia repair was based on inadequate knowledge of groin anatomy and poor understanding of the natural history of hernia formation. As the anatomy of the human body was described via dissection study, the anatomy of the groin became defined. From the late 1700s to the early 1800s, physicians such as Hasselbach, Cooper, Camper, Scarpa, Richter, and Gimbernat identified vital components of the inguinal region, and their contributions are reflected in the current nomenclature. The progress in anatomic understanding, coupled with the development of the aseptic technique, led surgeons such as Marcy, Kocher, and Lucas-Championnière to enter the inguinal canal and perform sac dissection, high ligation, and closure of the internal ring. Results had improved, but recurrence rates remained high with prolonged follow-up.

By demonstrating a comprehensive understanding of inguinal anatomy, Bassini (1844–1924) transformed inguinal hernia repair into a successful venture with minimal morbidity to the patient. His operation involved dissection of the layers of the inguinal canal to the transversalis fascia and then a reconstruction of the floor of the inguinal canal in several layers. The success of the Bassini repair over any of its predecessors ushered in an era of tissue-based repairs. Modifications of the Bassini repair were manifest in the McVay repair, as well as the Shouldice repair. All three of these techniques are currently practiced: the Shouldice repair, namely at the institution that bears its name (Shouldice Hernia Centre) and the McVay and Bassini in situations when prosthetic materials are contraindicated.

The era of tissue-based repairs was supplanted by tension-free repairs with the widespread acceptance of prosthetic materials for inguinal floor reconstruction. Initially described by Lichtenstein, the repair involved placement of a Marlex mesh over the entire floor of the inguinal canal. The repair capitalized on the concept of the myopectineal orifice of Fruchaud, which was based on the notion that whatever the type of inguinal hernia, the defect lay in the integrity of the transversalis fascia. This was superior to previous tissue-based repairs in that the weakness of the transversalis fascia could be restored by bridging the defect with mesh, rather than placing tension between tissues to close the defect. Superior results could be achieved by nonexpert hernia surgeons. The concept of prosthetic reconstruction of the inguinal floor was also furthered by Stoppa, Rives, and Wantz, who developed a preperitoneal mesh placement over the transversalis fascia.

With the advent of minimally invasive surgery, inguinal hernia repair underwent its most recent transformation. Laparoscopic inguinal hernia repair has added to the armamentarium of the general surgeon, providing a technique that lessens postoperative pain and improves recovery. Since the initial description by Ger, the laparoscopic method of hernia repair has become significantly more sophisticated. Refinements in approach and technique have led to the development of the intraperitoneal onlay mesh (Fitzgibbons and Toy 1990), the transabdominal preperitoneal (TAPP) repair (Arregui 1991), and the totally extraperitoneal (TEP) repair (Duluq 1991). Furthermore, an array of prosthetic materials has been introduced to further lower recurrence rates and provide the patient with the utmost quality of life.

Irrespective of the approach to hernia repair, be it open or laparoscopic, the current state of surgical treatment of inguinal hernia depends on a sound foundation of the inguinal anatomy. The application of current technologies to this anatomic knowledge has fostered successful treatment of inguinal hernias with minimal morbidity heretofore unknown to surgical practice.

EPIDEMIOLOGY

Inguinal hernia repair is one of the cornerstones of a general surgery practice and is one of the most commonly performed procedures in the United States, owing to a significant lifetime incidence and variety of successful treatment modalities. Although there are no exact figures totaling the number of inguinal hernia repairs performed annually, it has been estimated that approximately 800,000 cases were performed in 2003, not including recurrent or bilateral hernias.[2] A vast majority of these procedures were performed on an outpatient basis. Advancements in perioperative anesthesia and the increase in proportion of laparoscopic treatment of inguinal hernias have combined to increase the percentage of ambulatory inguinal hernias. In a survey of 17 states in 2003, 89% of the total number of inguinal hernia repairs were performed on an outpatient basis.[3] However, the preponderance of laparoscopic inguinal hernia repair is relatively low (14%) when compared to percentage of open inguinal hernia repair (86%).[4]

The majority of abdominal wall hernias occur in the groin, totaling approximately 75% of the total incidence. It is difficult to estimate the exact prevalence of inguinal hernias in the population, but an overwhelming majority of inguinal hernias occur in males vs. females. Of inguinal hernia repairs, 90% are performed in males and 10% in females. Approximately 70% of femoral hernia repairs are performed on female patients; however, females undergo nearly five times the number of inguinal hernia repairs as femoral hernia repairs. The most common type of groin hernia presenting in females remains the indirect inguinal hernia.[5]

Classical teaching has been that most unilateral hernias originate on the right side. However, it has been recognized that up to one third of patients that undergo unilateral inguinal hernia repair may develop a contralateral inguinal hernia. Physical examination, although dependable in confirming the presence of symptomatic hernias, is beset with limitations when a small hernia is present. Therefore, although patients were diagnosed with unilateral inguinal hernias, they may, in fact, have had bilateral hernias. With the advent of laparoscopic techniques, the contralateral side can be examined without additional incisions or trocars. In a study examining only patients with primary unilateral inguinal hernias, 22%

KEY POINTS

1. A proficient understanding of groin anatomy is essential to successful inguinal hernia treatment.

2. Conservative management of asymptomatic inguinal hernias is acceptable.

3. Elective repair of inguinal hernias can be undertaken using a laparoscopic or open approach.

4. Laparoscopic inguinal hernia repair results in less pain and faster recovery, yet requires specialized training and equipment.

5. The use of prosthetic mesh as a reinforcement significantly improves recurrence rates, whether the repair is open or laparoscopic.

6. Recurrence, pain, and quality of life are important outcome factors.

TABLE 37-1	Inguinal hernia prevalence by age					
Age (Y)	**25–34**	**35–44**	**45–54**	**55–64**	**65–74**	**75+**
Current prevalence (%)	12	15	20	26	29	34
Lifetime prevalence (%)	15	19	28	34	40	47

Current = repaired hernias excluded; Lifetime = repaired hernias included.

TABLE 37-2	Presumed causes of groin herniation

Coughing
Chronic obstructive pulmonary disease
Obesity
Straining
    Constipation
    Prostatism
Pregnancy
Birthweight <1500 g
Family history of a hernia
Valsalva's maneuvers
Ascites
Upright position
Congenital connective tissue disorders
Defective collagen synthesis
Previous right lower quadrant incision
Arterial aneurysms
Cigarette smoking
Heavy lifting
Physical exertion (?)

were found to have an occult contralateral hernia during laparoscopic inguinal hernia repair.[6] Although asymptomatic at time of diagnosis, these hernias have the potential to become clinically significant as the patient ages.

Incidence of inguinal hernias in males has a bimodal distribution with peaks before 1 year of age and then again after age 40. The age-dependence of inguinal hernias was demonstrated in an oft-cited study by Abramson. Males >25 years old (n = 1883) were studied and constituted 91% of the total males settled in western Jerusalem. Between the years 1969–71, the participants were first interviewed regarding the presence of an inguinal hernia and subsequently examined by a physician. A total of 459 men with 637 hernias between them were identified. The results were limited to those that had not previously undergone an inguinal hernia operation. The current prevalence rate was 18%, and the lifetime risk of developing an inguinal hernia was 24%. When subdivided into age groups, those aged 25 to 34 years had a lifetime prevalence rate of 15% whereas those aged 75 years and over had a rate of 47% (Table 37-1).[7] In a later study of California males aged 14 to 62, significantly decreased "current" prevalence rates were noted in most age groups; however, lifetime prevalence rates were largely similar between both studies. A notable drawback of this study was the reliance on self-reporting and the absence of physical examination to confirm findings.

ETIOLOGY

Inguinal hernias may be considered congenital or acquired diseases. Although there is debate, in all likelihood, inguinal hernias in the adult are acquired defects in the abdominal wall. A number of studies have attempted to delineate the precise causes of inguinal hernia formation; however, the risk factors are likely multifactorial, the common denominator being a weakness in the abdominal wall musculature (Table 37-2). Congenital hernias, which make up the majority of pediatric hernias, can be considered an impedance of normal development, rather than an acquired weakness. During the normal course of development, the testes descend from the intra-abdominal space into the scrotum in the third trimester. Their descent is preceded by the gubernaculum and a diverticulum of peritoneum, which protrudes through the inguinal canal and ultimately becomes the processus vaginalis. Between 36 and 40 weeks, the processus vaginalis closes and eliminates the peritoneal opening at the internal inguinal ring.[8] Failure of the peritoneum to close results in a patent processus vaginalis (PPV) and thus explains the high incidence of indirect inguinal hernias in preterm babies. It should be noted that the processus vaginalis continues to close as the child ages, with most closing within the first few months of life. Children with congenital indirect inguinal hernias will present with a PPV; however, its presence does not necessarily indicate an inguinal hernia (Fig. 37-1). In a study of nearly 600 adults undergoing laparoscopy for reasons not related to inguinal hernia repair, bilateral inspection of the internal inguinal rings revealed an incidence of 12% of PPV. None of these patients had clinically significant symptoms of a groin hernia.[9] However, in a group of 300

patients undergoing unilateral laparoscopic inguinal hernia repair, 12% were found to have a contralateral PPV. Over the next 5 years, they developed inguinal hernias at a rate four times more than counterparts that had a closed ring.[10]

The presence of a PPV likely predisposes the patient to the development of an inguinal hernia. This likelihood depends on the presence of other risk factors such as inherent tissue weakness, family

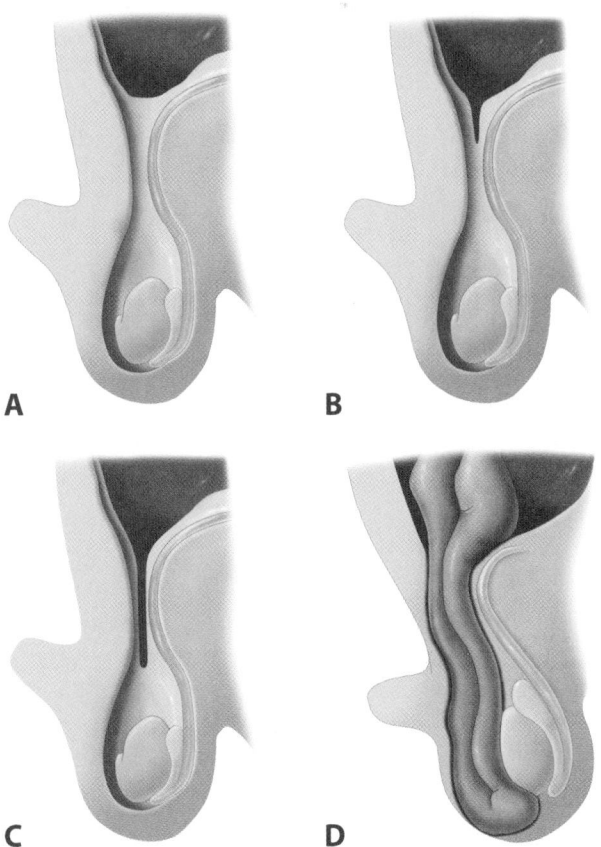

FIG. 37-1. Varying degrees of closure of the processus vaginalis (PV). **A.** Closed PV. **B.** Minimally patent PV. **C.** Moderately patent. **D.** Scrotal hernia.

history, and strenuous activity. Overall, there is limited data pertaining to the etiology of inguinal hernia development. Several studies have documented strenuous physical activity as a predisposing risk factor to acquiring an inguinal hernia.[11,12] Repeated physical exertion may increase intra-abdominal pressure; however, whether this process occurs in combination with a PPV or through age-related weakness of abdominal wall musculature is unknown. A case-controlled study of over 1400 male patients with inguinal hernia revealed that a positive family history was eight times as likely to lead to development of a primary inguinal hernia. Chronic obstructive pulmonary disease significantly increased the risk of direct inguinal hernias.[13] Interestingly, several studies have noted a protective effect of obesity. In a large, population-based prospective study of American individuals (First National Health and Nutrition Examination Survey), the risk of inguinal hernia development in obese men was only 50% that of normal weight males, while the risk in overweight males was 80% that of nonobese men. A possible explanation is the increased difficulty in detecting inguinal hernias in obese individuals.[14]

One of the most intriguing areas under study is the role of tissue biology in hernia formation. Epidemiologic studies have identified risk factors that may predispose to a hernia, but there are limited data specifically related to the molecular basis of these hernias. Early experiments involving iatrogenic laythirsm resulted in hernia formation. Furthermore, microscopic examination of skin of inguinal hernia patients demonstrated significantly decreased ratios of type I to type III collagen. Type III collagen does not contribute to wound tensile strength as significantly as type I collagen. Additional analyses of similar skin revealed disaggregated collagen tracts with decreased collagen fiber density.[15] Collagen disorders such as Ehlers-Danlos syndrome also are associated with an increased incidence of hernia formation (Table 37-3). Tissue analysis has revealed that there is a relationship between the aneurysmal component and hernias, owing to a pathologic extracellular matrix metabolism.[16] Although a significant amount of work remains to elicit the biologic nature of hernias, studies such as these provide compelling evidence for the presence of a genetic collagen defect.

TABLE 37-3	Connective tissue disorders associated with groin herniation

Osteogenesis imperfecta
Cutis laxa (congenital elastolysis)
Ehlers-Danlos syndrome
Hurler-Hunter syndrome
Marfan syndrome
Congenital hip dislocation in children
Polycystic kidney disease
Alpha$_1$-antitrypsin deficiency
Williams syndrome
Androgen insensitivity syndrome
Robinow's syndrome
Serpentine fibula syndrome
Alport's syndrome
Tel Hashomer camptodactyly syndrome
Leriche's syndrome
Testicular feminization syndrome
Rokitansky-Mayer-Küster syndrome
Goldenhar's syndrome
Morris syndrome
Gerhardt's syndrome
Menkes' syndrome
Kawasaki disease
Pfannenstiel syndrome
Beckwith-Wiedemann syndrome
Rubinstein-Taybi syndrome
Alopecia-photophobia syndrome

ANATOMY

It cannot be overstated that proficient knowledge of inguinal anatomy is necessary to produce a lasting surgical cure of the inguinal hernia. The groin region is a complex network of muscles, ligaments, and fascia that are interwoven in a multiplanar fashion. To understand the anatomy of the groin, it is best to first consider its components and then conceptualize them according to operative approach. Because the vast majority of inguinal hernias occur in men, general descriptions of groin anatomy contained herein will pertain to males. The inguinal canal is approximately 4 to 6 cm long and is situated in the anteroinferior portion of the pelvic basin (Fig. 37-2). Shaped like a cone, its base is at the superolateral margin of the basin, with its apex pointed inferomedially toward the symphysis pubis. The canal begins intra-abdominally on the deep aspect of the abdominal wall, where the spermatic cord passes through a hiatus in the transversalis fascia (in females, this is the round ligament). This hiatus is termed the *deep or internal inguinal ring*. The canal then concludes on the superficial aspect of the abdominal wall musculature at the superficial or external inguinal ring, the point at which the spermatic cord crosses the medial defect of the external oblique aponeurosis. In the normal situation, parietal peritoneum covers the intra-abdominal portion of the spermatic cord, as well as the internal ring. Anteriorly, the boundary of the canal is comprised of the external oblique aponeurosis and internal oblique muscle laterally. Posteriorly, the floor of the inguinal canal is formed by the fusion of the transversalis fascia and transversus abdominus muscle, although up to one fourth of subjects are found to have only the transversalis fascia forming the posterior floor. The superior boundary is an arch formed by the fibers of the internal oblique muscle. Lastly, the inferior margin consists of the inguinal ligament. The spermatic cord consists of three arteries, three veins, and two nerves. As well, it contains the pampiniform venous plexus anteriorly and the vas deferens posteriorly, with connective tissue and remnant of the processus vaginalis between. The cord is then enveloped in layers of spermatic fascia.

Additional structures that are important to the conceptualization of the inguinal canal include the inguinal ligament, Cooper's ligament, iliopubic tract, lacunar ligament, and conjoined area (Fig. 37-3). The inguinal ligament is also known as *Poupart's ligament* and is comprised of the inferior fibers of the external oblique aponeurosis. The ligament stretches from the anterior superior iliac spine to the pubic tubercle. The ligament serves an important purpose as a readily identifiable boundary of the inguinal canal, as well as a sturdy structure used in various hernia repairs. Cooper's ligament is otherwise known as the *pectineal ligament*, although controversy exists as to whether it is, in fact, a ligament at all. Its anatomic site predisposes the structure to varied explanations of its nature and relationships to contiguous structures. For all intents and purposes, it can be considered as the lateral portion of the lacunar ligament that is fused to the periosteum of the pubic tubercle. It also may include fibers from the transversus abdominus, iliopubic tract, internal oblique, and rectus abdominus. The iliopubic tract is an aponeurotic band that begins at the anterior superior iliac spine and inserts into Cooper's ligament from above. It often is confused with the inguinal ligament secondary to common origin and insertion points. However, the iliopubic tract forms on the deep side of the inferior margin of the transversus abdominus and transversalis fascia. The inguinal ligament is on the superficial side of the musculoaponeurotic layer of these structures. The shelving edge of the inguinal ligament is a structure that more or less connects the iliopubic tract to the inguinal ligament. The iliopubic tract helps form the inferior margin of the internal inguinal ring as it courses medially, where it continues as the anterior and medial border of the femoral canal. The lacunar ligament, or ligament of Gimbernat, is the triangular fanning out of the inguinal ligament as it joins the pubic tubercle. Controversy exists as to whether the lateral edge of the lacunar ligament forms the medial border of the femoral canal. Controversy also exists as to the nature

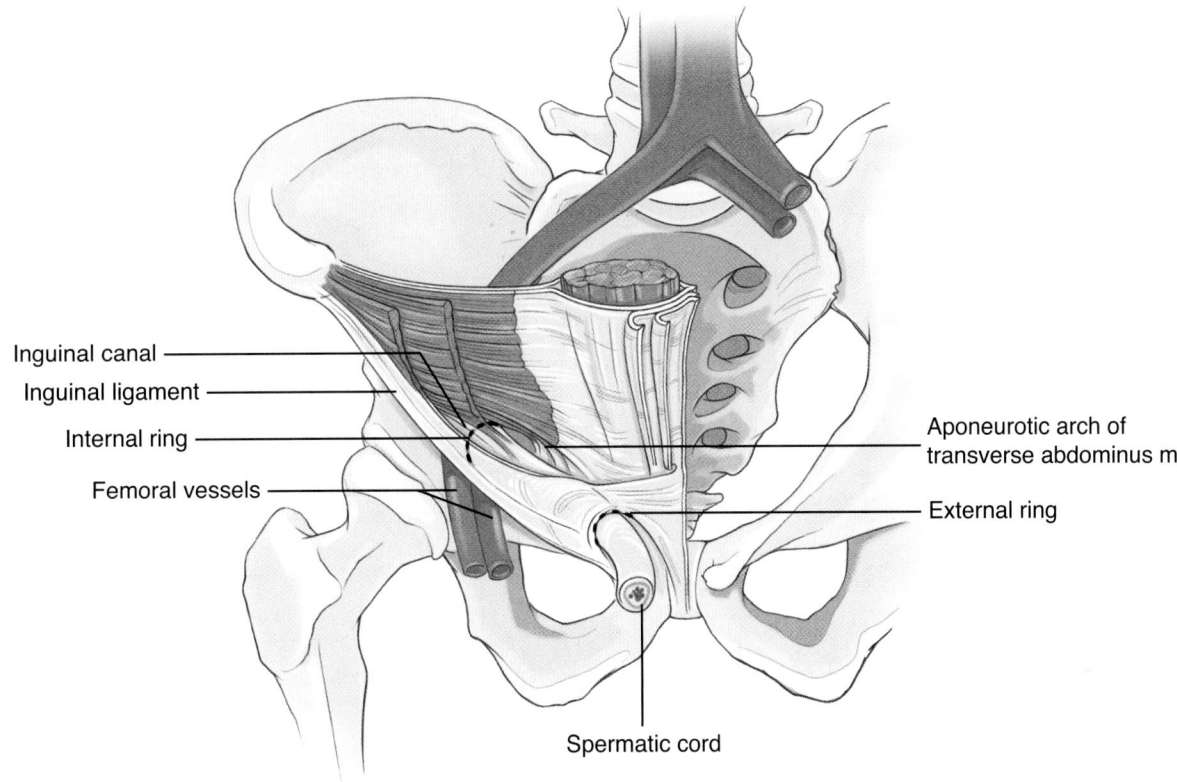

FIG. 37-2. Location and orientation of the inguinal canal within the pelvic basin. Boundaries of the canal include: posteriorly the transversus abdominus and transversalis fascia; superiorly the internal oblique muscle; anteriorly is the external oblique aponeurosis; inferiorly is the inguinal ligament. m. = muscle.

of the conjoined tendon. It is commonly described as the fusion of the inferior fibers of the internal oblique and transversus abdominus aponeurosis, at the point where they insert on the pubic tubercle. This exact anatomic entity is hard to describe consistently. More likely, the conjoined area is a combination of the transversus ab-

dominus aponeurosis, transversalis fascia, lateral edge of the rectus sheath, and internal oblique muscle or its fibers.

Nerves of interest in the inguinal region are the ilioinguinal, iliohypogastric, genitofemoral, and lateral femoral cutaneous nerve (Figs. 37-4 and 37-5). The ilioinguinal and iliohypogastric nerve arise

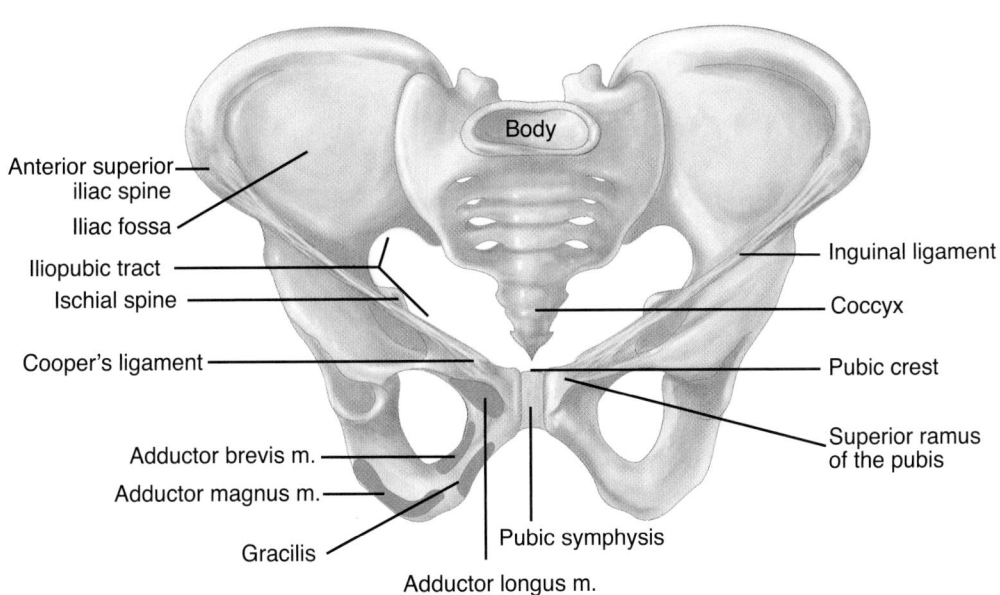

FIG. 37-3. Ligaments that contribute to the inguinal canal include the inguinal ligament, which spans the anterior superior iliac spine to the pubic bone. Cooper's ligament is seen as the lateral extension of the lacunar ligament, which is the fanning out of the inguinal ligament as it joins the pubic tubercle. The iliopubic tract originates and inserts in a similar fashion to the inguinal ligament, yet it is deep to it. m. = muscle.

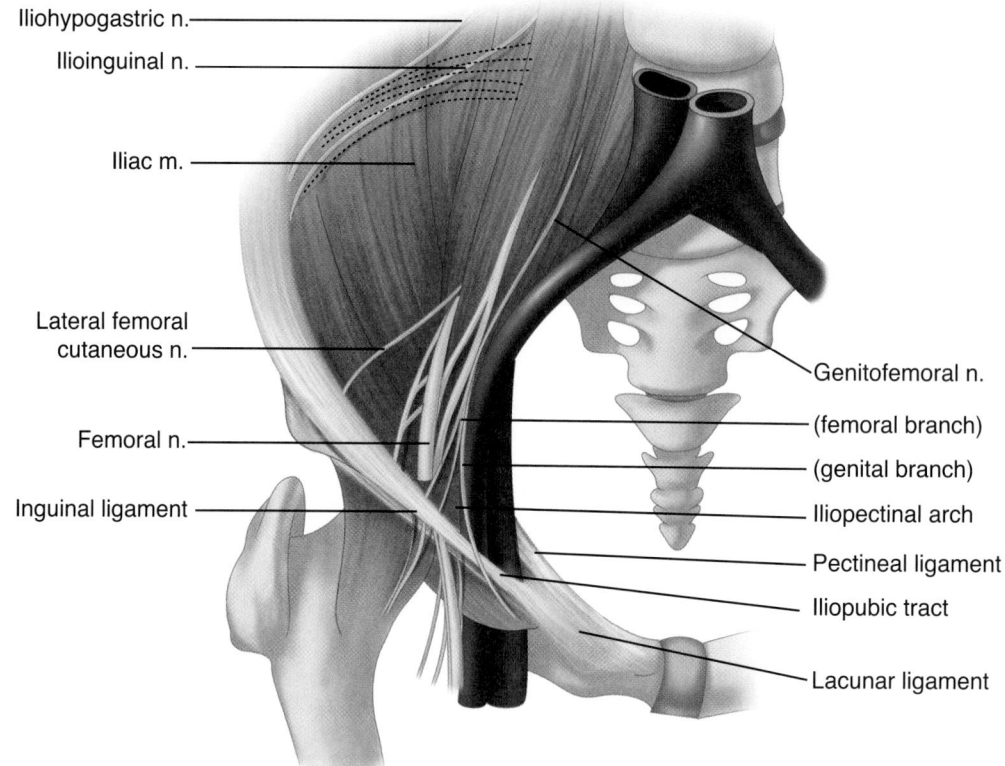

FIG. 37-4. Retroperitoneal view of major inguinal nerves and their courses: ilioinguinal, iliohypogastric, genitofemoral, lateral femoral cutaneous, and femoral. m. = muscle; n. = nerve.

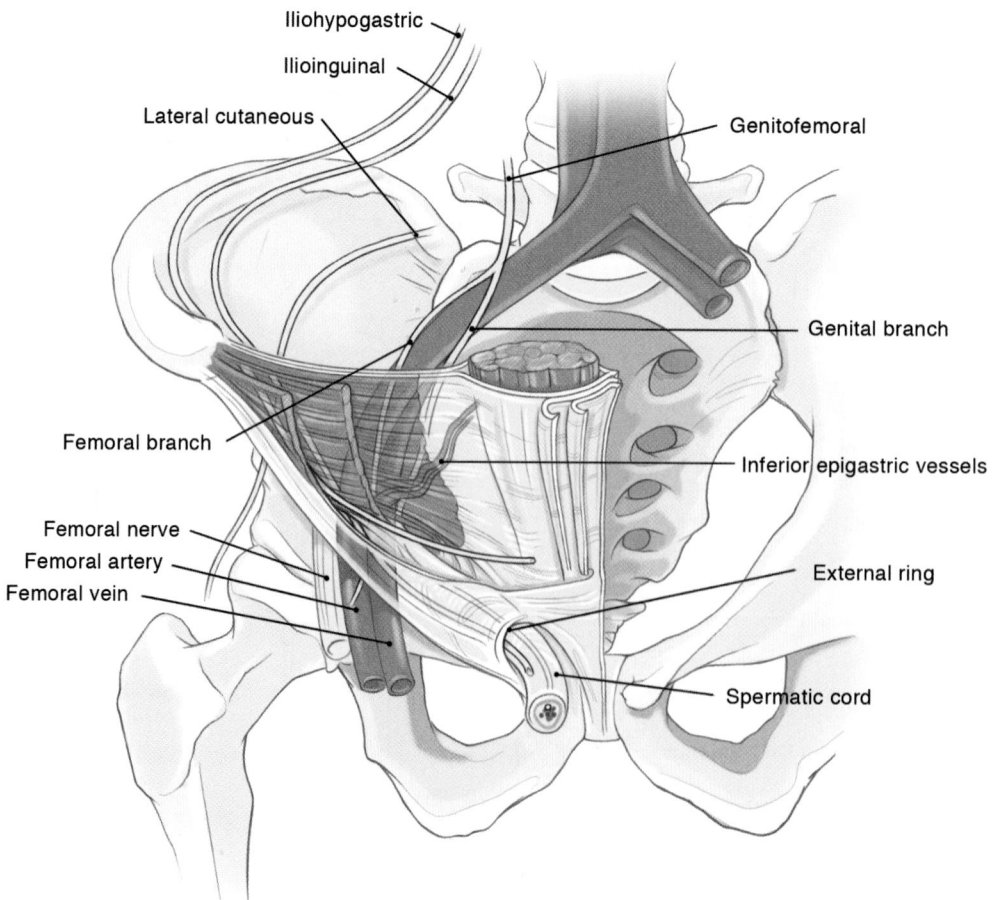

FIG. 37-5. Anterior view of the five major nerves of the inguinal region.

together from the first lumbar nerve (L1). The ilioinguinal nerve emerges from the lateral border of the psoas major and passes obliquely across the quadratus lumborum. At a point just medial to the anterior superior iliac spine, it crosses the internal oblique muscle to enter the inguinal canal between the internal and external oblique muscles and exits through the superficial inguinal ring. The nerve supplies the skin of the upper and medial thigh. In males, it also supplies the penis and upper scrotum, while supplying the mons pubis and labium majus in females. The iliohypogastric nerve arises from T12–L1 and follows the ilioinguinal nerve. After the iliohypogastric nerve pierces the deep abdominal wall in its downward course, it courses between the internal oblique and transversus abdominis, supplying both. It then branches into a lateral cutaneous branch and an anterior cutaneous branch, which pierces the internal oblique and then external oblique aponeurosis above the superficial inguinal ring. A common variant is for the iliohypogastric and ilioinguinal nerves to exit around the superficial inguinal ring as a single entity. The genitofemoral nerve arises from L1–L2, courses along the retroperitoneum, and emerges on the anterior aspect of the psoas. It then divides into the genital and femoral branches. The genital branch remains ventral to the iliac vessels and iliopubic tract as it enters the inguinal canal just lateral to the inferior epigastric vessels. In males, it travels through the superficial inguinal ring and supplies the scrotum and cremaster muscle. In females, it supplies the mons pubis and labia majora. The femoral branch courses along the femoral sheath, supplying the skin anterior to the upper part of the femoral triangle. The lateral femoral cutaneous nerve arises from L2–L3, but emerges from the lateral border of the psoas muscle at the level of L4. It crosses the iliacus muscle obliquely toward the anterior superior iliac spine. It then passes inferior to the inguinal ligament where it divides to supply the lateral aspect of the thigh (Fig. 37-6).

Anterior Perspective

The aforementioned borders of the inguinal canal can be readily appreciated when approaching an inguinal hernia in an open, anterior fashion. Once the subcutaneous tissue is passed, the oblique fibers of the external oblique aponeurosis are encountered. The external oblique muscle originates on the lower eight ribs (Fig. 37-7). The course of the fibers runs inferiorly from lateral to medial and is commonly referred to as *hands in the pockets* as they are parallel to one's fingers in this orientation. As the fibers approach the inguinal canal, they are no longer comprised of muscle, only tendinous aponeurosis. Once the aponeurosis is exposed, the superficial inguinal ring and inguinal ligament may be identified. The superficial ring consists of two crura. The medial crus is formed by the fibers of the external oblique aponeurosis and join with the lateral border of the rectus sheath. The inferior crus is formed by the inguinal ligament, which inserts into the pubic bone. The iliohypogastric nerve generally pierces the external oblique aponeurosis above the superficial inguinal ring. The spermatic cord, genitofemoral and ilioinguinal nerves are seen passing through the superficial inguinal ring. One layer deep to the external oblique aponeurosis, these same structures are visualized, as well as the deep inguinal ring. The inferior border of the internal inguinal ring is formed by the iliopubic tract, while the rest of the ring is formed by fibers of the transversalis fascia. Structures that are seen entering the internal inguinal ring include the spermatic cord and genital branch of the genitofemoral nerve.

The cord structures are enveloped by three fascial layers. The internal fascial layer is derived from the internal oblique muscle and contains the cremaster muscle. The external layer is adhered to the fascia of the external oblique muscle and must be dissected to mobilize the cord. The superficial fascia is also known as the *fascia of Gallaudet* or *innominate fascia*. Superior to the cord, the arch of the internal oblique muscle is seen fanning out to form the roof of the inguinal canal. The superior fibers are oriented perpendicular to the external oblique aponeurosis; however, the lower fibers run parallel with it, as they course toward the pubic bone (Fig. 37-8).

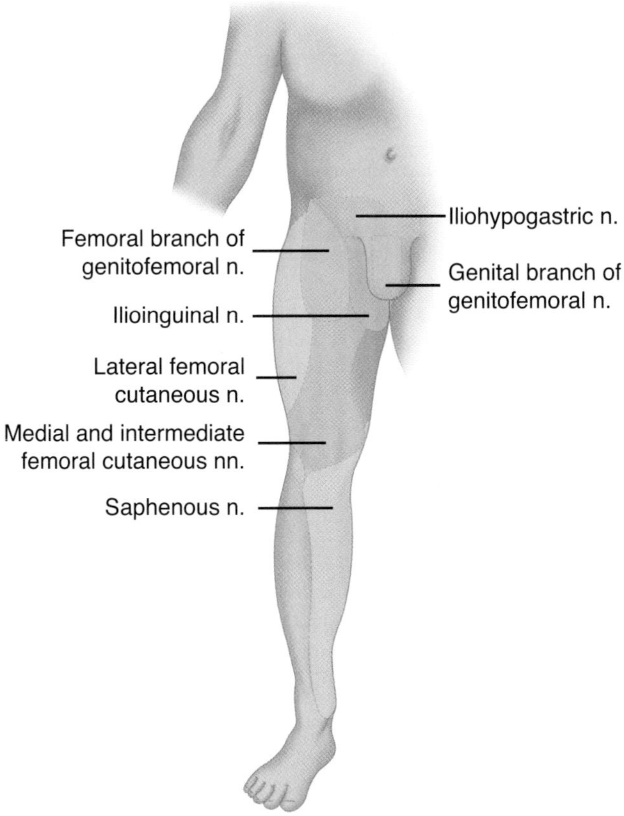

FIG. 37-6. Sensory distribution of the major nerves in the groin area. n. = nerve.

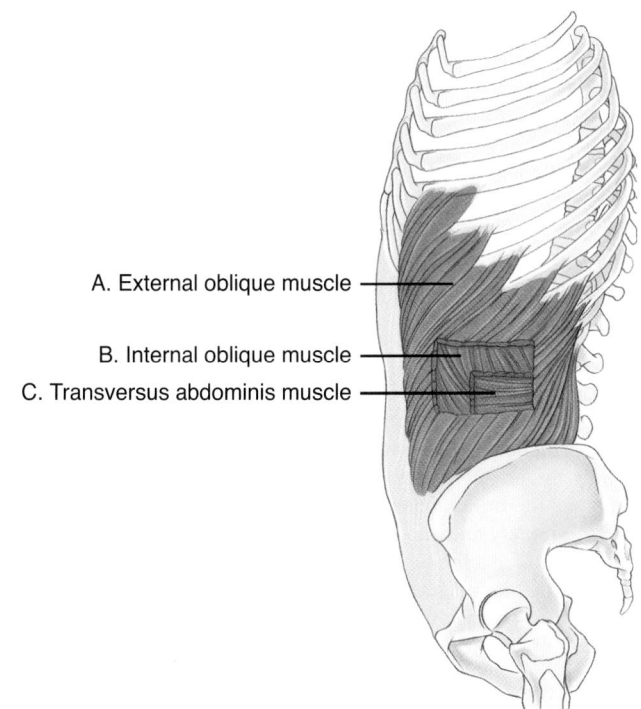

FIG. 37-7. The abdominal wall musculature. *A.* External oblique muscle. *B.* Internal oblique muscle. *C.* Transversus abdominis muscle.

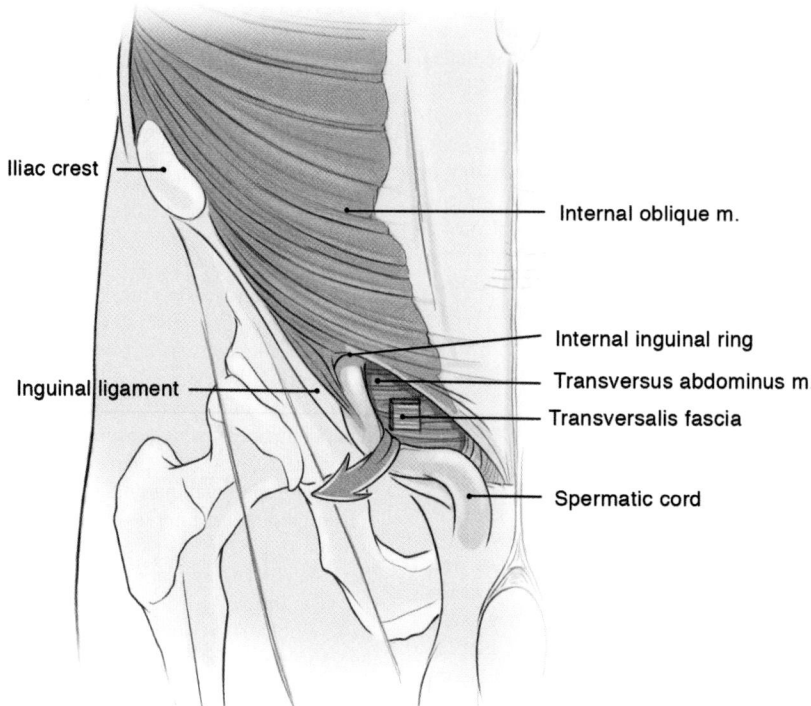

FIG. 37-8. Anterior perspective of posterior inguinal canal musculature. The external oblique aponeurosis has been removed to display the internal ring and inguinal canal floor. m. = muscle.

Continuing posteriorly through the inguinal canal, the transversus abdominis muscle is encountered deep to the inguinal ring. It arises from the iliac crest, iliopsoas fascia, thoracolumbar fascia, and lower six costal cartilages. Regardless of site of origin, the fibers run in a lateral to medial fashion and it becomes less muscular and more aponeurotic medial, where it contributes to the rectus sheath and falx inguinalis. It is a commonly held belief that the integrity of the transversus abdominis muscle is the most important determinant to hernia formation. As its fibers contract, the arch of the transversus abdominis closes off the internal inguinal ring, thereby serving as a shutter mechanism. One layer deep to the transversus abdominis is the anterior and posterior lamina of transversalis fascia. Inferior to the arcuate line, the posterior covering of the anterior abdominal wall consists only of transversalis fascia, as the fascia of the external and internal oblique muscles fans out anteriorly to constitute the anterior layer of the rectus sheath. Deep to the transversalis fascia, the next layer encountered is the preperitoneal areolar tissue and fat. Dissection of this tissue and progression through the next layer, the peritoneum, allows one to enter into the peritoneal space. Therefore, the preperitoneal space is in actuality a potential space, bordered by the peritoneum on the deep aspect and transversalis fascia superficially.

The inferior epigastric vessels are best visualized from a posterior approach. The inferior epigastric artery is responsible for the blood supply to the rectus abdominis and connects the vasculature of the upper extremity to the lower extremity. The internal thoracic artery offshoots to form the superior epigastric artery, which anastomoses with the inferior epigastric artery, and is derived from the external iliac artery. The epigastric veins run with the arteries within the rectus sheath, posterior to the rectus muscles. Inspection of the internal inguinal ring will reveal the deep location of the inferior epigastric vessels. Inguinal hernias that protrude lateral to the inferior epigastric vessels, through the deep inguinal ring, are referred to as *indirect inguinal hernias*. Direct hernias, on the contrary, are protrusions medial to the inferior epigastric vessels, in Hesselbach's triangle. The

borders of the triangle are as such: the inguinal ligament forms the inferior margin, the edge of rectus abdominis is the medial border, and the inferior epigastric vessels are the superior or lateral border.

From an anterior perspective, the femoral space can be visualized below the inguinal ligament. The iliopectineal arch is a fibrous band of fused iliac and psoas fascia that subdivides the space beneath the inguinal ligament into a lateral muscular space, housing the iliopsoas, femoral nerve, and lateral femoral cutaneous nerve, and a medial vascular space, containing the femoral vessels and femoral branch of the genitofemoral nerve. In addition to these components, the vascular space also houses a medial potential space known as the *femoral canal* and is the site of possible femoral hernia formation. The canal is shaped like a cone pointed inferiorly, extending to the fossa ovalis; the opening of the fascia latte for the great saphenous vein. The femoral ring is bordered by sturdy structures that lend to its inflexibility. The posterior boundary consists of the iliacus fascia and Cooper's ligament, and the anterior boundary is the iliopubic tract and inguinal ligament, internally and externally, respectively. Medially, the border is made up of the aponeurosis of transversus abdominis and the transversalis fascia and laterally, the canal is bordered by the femoral vein and its connective tissue. Normal contents of the femoral canal include areolar preperitoneal tissue and fat and lymph nodes, most notably the node of Cloquet at its upper end. The distal end of the canal is closed by fatty tissue called the *septum femorale*. Once the integrity of this septum is lost, femoral herniation occurs. Due to its small size and limited flexibility, the femoral ring is usually the site of incarceration. Reduction of incarcerated contents of a femoral hernia can thus be effected by splitting the inguinal ligament.

Posterior Perspective

Since laparoscopic procedures have been adapted as a treatment for inguinal hernias, surgeons have been required to reconceptualize the groin anatomy from the posterior perspective (Fig. 37-9). The large

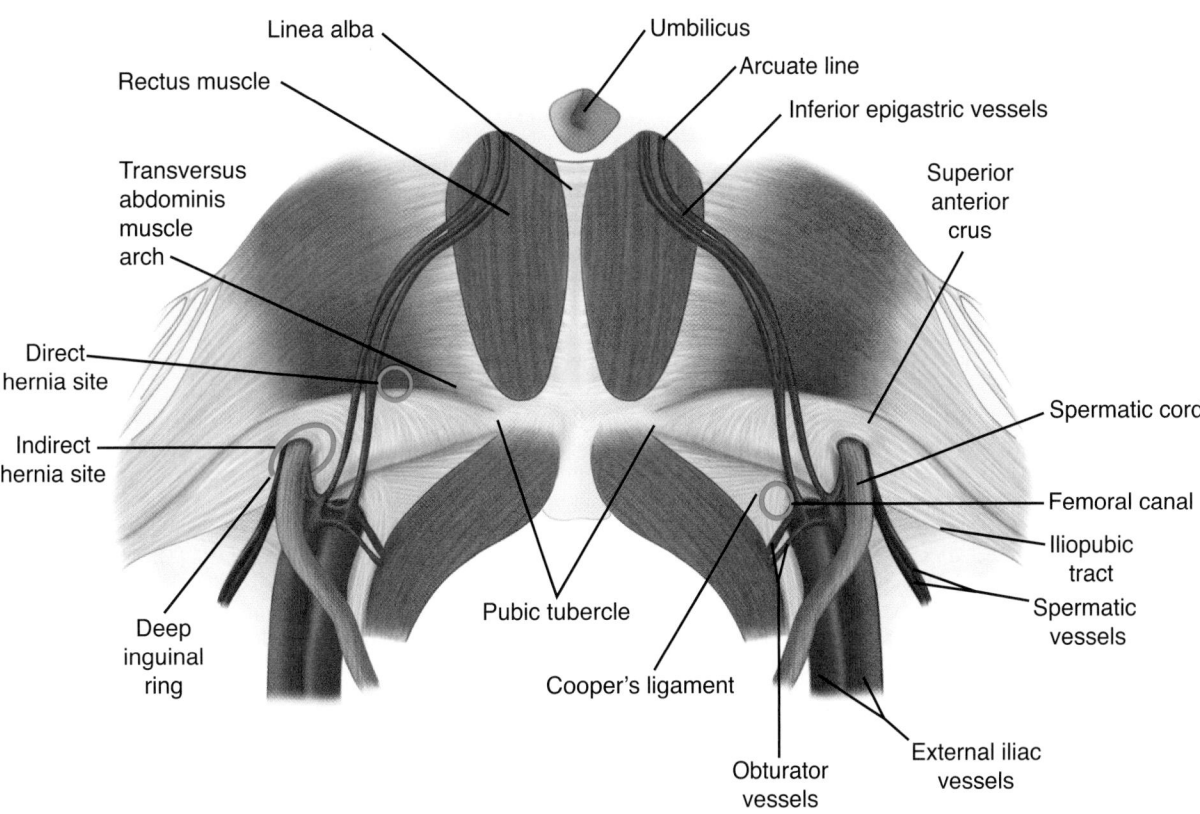

FIG. 37-9. Anatomy of the groin region from a posterior perspective.

visual field and familiarity with intra-abdominal anatomy result in easier identification of the posterior groin region when inguinal hernias are approached intraperitoneally compared to the preperitoneal approach. Initial points of reference intraperitoneally are the five peritoneal folds, bladder, inferior epigastric vessels, and psoas muscle (Fig. 37-10). Beginning at the midline, the median umbilical fold can be easily identified in the lower midline. The fold represents the fibrous remnant of the fetal allantois, but may persist in the adult as a patent urachus. As one follows the median peritoneal fold from the umbilicus inferiorly, one encounters the pubic symphysis and bladder. Radiating down bilaterally, just lateral to this fold, is the medial umbilical fold, which represents the obliterated portion of the fetal umbilical artery. Less likely, a superior vesicular artery will persist within this fold, supplying the superior and lateral edge of the bladder, which is often found immediately medial to the medial umbilical fold, adjacent to the lateral edge of the bladder. Lateral to the medial umbilical ligament, the paired lateral umbilical fold contains the inferior epigastric vessels. The inferior epigastric artery is the lateral border of Hesselbach's triangle and thus provides a useful landmark to differentiate between direct and indirect hernias. A defect medial to the inferior epigastric vessels is considered direct, whereas a lateral defect is an indirect hernia. The type of hernia also can be elucidated by referring to the series of depressions that exist between the peritoneal folds. Progressing from midline laterally, one can identify the supravesical, medial, and lateral fossae. The supravesical fossa is found between the median and medial umbilical ligaments and leads to hernias of the same name. The medial fossa is located between the medial and lateral umbilical folds and is the site of direct hernias. The lateral fossa is found lateral to the lateral umbilical ligament and is the site of the internal inguinal ring and thus the location for indirect inguinal hernias. The superficial inguinal ring is not visualized from the peritoneal perspective. Most laterally, the psoas muscle is seen coursing inferiorly along the retroperitoneum. The anterior superior iliac spine is not readily apparent, but may be elucidated by palpating outside the abdomen.

Identification of the internal inguinal ring then permits identification of the spermatic cord. Further inferior to the cord, the iliac vessels are identified deep to the peritoneum. Two potential spaces

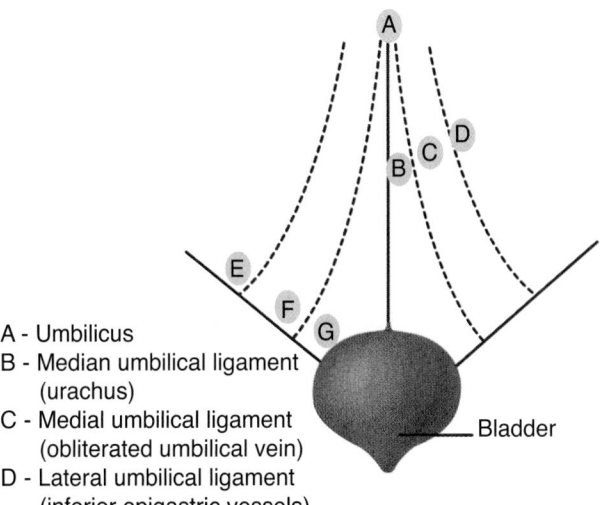

A - Umbilicus
B - Median umbilical ligament (urachus)
C - Medial umbilical ligament (obliterated umbilical vein)
D - Lateral umbilical ligament (inferior epigastric vessels)
E - Lateral fossa (indirect hernia)
F - Medial fossa (direct hernia)
G - Supravesical fossa

FIG. 37-10. Posterior view of intraperitoneal folds and associated fossa: *A.* Umbilicus. *B.* Median umbilical ligament. *C.* Medial umbilical ligament (obliterated umbilical vein). *D.* Lateral umbilical ligament (inferior epigastric vessels). *E.* Lateral fossa (indirect hernia). *F.* Medial fossa (direct hernia). *G.* Supravesical fossa. *(Modified with permission from Rowe JS Jr., Skandalakis JE, Gray SW: Multiple bilateral inguinal hernias. Am Surg 39:269, 1973.)*

exist deep to the peritoneum, and these are encountered once the peritoneal flap is created. Between the peritoneum and the posterior lamina of the transversalis fascia is Bogros's space. This area contains preperitoneal fat and areolar tissue. A less prominent space exists between the posterior and anterior laminae of the transversalis fascia termed the *vascular space*, as this is the location of the inferior epigastric vessels.

Once the peritoneum is reflected to expose Bogros's space, the pertinent structures of preperitoneal inguinal anatomy can be identified. The most medial aspect of the preperitoneal space, that which lies superior to the bladder, is alternately known as the *Retzius space*. The pubic symphysis is identified by its midline location, white periosteum, and rigidity to palpation. The vasculature of the groin is much more apparent from the posterior perspective than from the anterior perspective. The inferior epigastric vessels are found in the same longitudinal plane as the iliac vessels. A common finding is the corona mortis, which is found overlying Cooper's ligament and represents a connection between the inferior epigastric and obturator vessels. The deep circumflex iliac vessels arise from the external iliac vessels and must be protected, as they may be intimately associated with the medial portion of the iliopubic tract. Exposure of the iliac vessels allows identification of the genital branch of the genitofemoral nerve as it courses with the external iliac artery. At the internal inguinal ring, the nerve joins the spermatic cord as it enters the inguinal canal.

The femoral branch of the genitofemoral nerve is found lateral to the genital branch and is seen leaving the retroperitoneum underneath the iliopubic tract. Also found laterally, and sometimes in association with the femoral branch of the genitofemoral nerve, is the lateral cutaneous nerve of the thigh. After emerging from the lateral edge of the psoas muscle, it, too, leaves the retroperitoneum inferior to the iliopubic tract to innervate the anterolateral skin of the thigh. The femoral nerve is not routinely seen during laparoscopic inguinal hernia repair but can be demonstrated lateral to the external iliac vessels between the iliacus and psoas muscles. The nerve courses

beneath the iliopubic tract and inguinal ligament as it enters the thigh. The iliohypogastric and ilioinguinal nerves are more easily demonstrated via the anterior perspective because they do not cross into the operative space established by the preperitoneal approach.

The structures of the spermatic cord come together shortly before the cord enters through the internal inguinal ring. The vas deferens is of special note as it courses cephalad out from the pelvis and then crosses the inferior epigastric arteries to enter the spermatic cord inferomedially. Slightly inferior to the internal inguinal ring, the iliopubic tract is identified as it attaches to the iliac crest. On the medial side of the internal inguinal ring, Cooper's ligament can be demonstrated inserting inferolaterally into the pubic ramus. The pectineal ligament can also be identified on the medial aspect of the inferior epigastric vessels, along with the medial aspect of the femoral ring. The remainder of the boundaries of the femoral ring are also visualized. From the posterior perspective, this includes the iliopubic tract superiorly, Cooper's ligament inferiorly, and the femoral vein laterally.

The posterior perspective also allows excellent appreciation of the myopectineal orifice of Fruchaud (Fig. 37-11). The arch of the internal oblique muscle and transversus abdominis muscle constitute the superior margin, the iliopsoas muscle the lateral margin, the lateral edge of rectus abdominis medially, and the pubic pecten medially. The iliopubic tract divides the orifice into a superior portion housing the spermatic cord and an inferior portion containing the iliac vessels. The posterior perspective has also resulted in the characterization of important areas to avoid, known as the *triangle of doom*, *triangle of pain*, and the *circle of death* (Fig 37-12).[17] The triangle of doom is bordered medially by the vas deferens and laterally by the vessels of the spermatic cord, thereby pointing its apex superiorly. The contents of the space include the external iliac vessels, deep circumflex iliac vein, femoral nerve, and genital branch of the genitofemoral nerve. The triangle of pain can be conceptualized as the space bordered by the iliopubic tract and gonadal vessels. The structures within this space include nerves such as the lateral

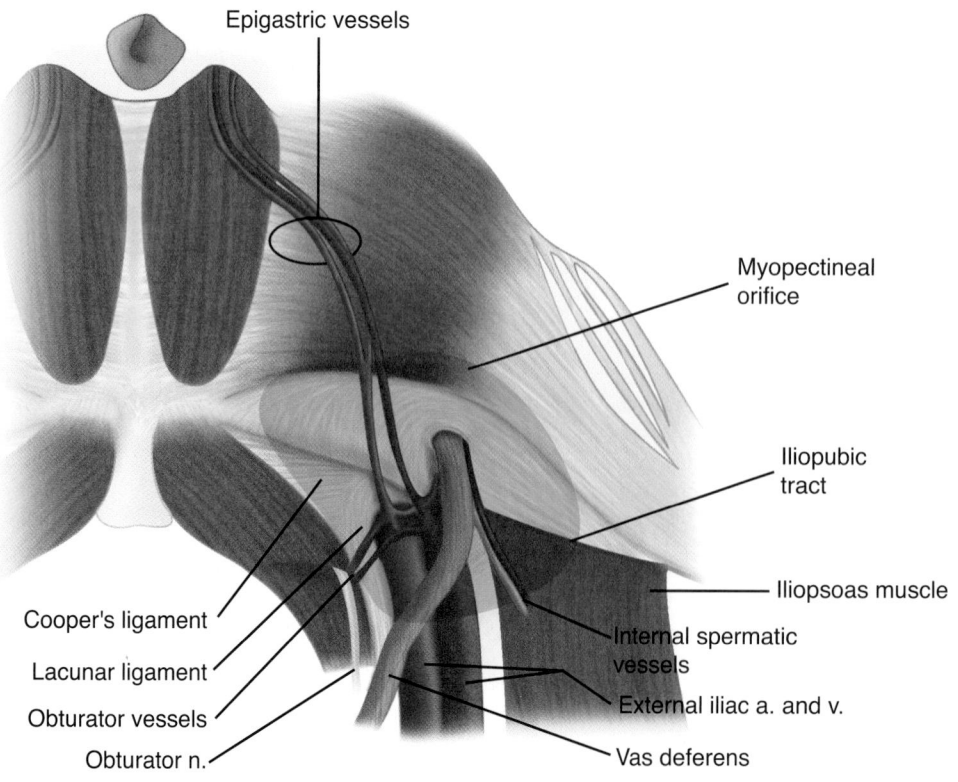

Epigastric vessels

Myopectineal orifice

Iliopubic tract

Iliopsoas muscle

Internal spermatic vessels

Cooper's ligament

Lacunar ligament

Obturator vessels

Obturator n.

External iliac a. and v.

Vas deferens

FIG. 37-11. Posterior view of the myopectineal orifice of Fruchaud. a. = artery; n. = nerve; v. = vein.

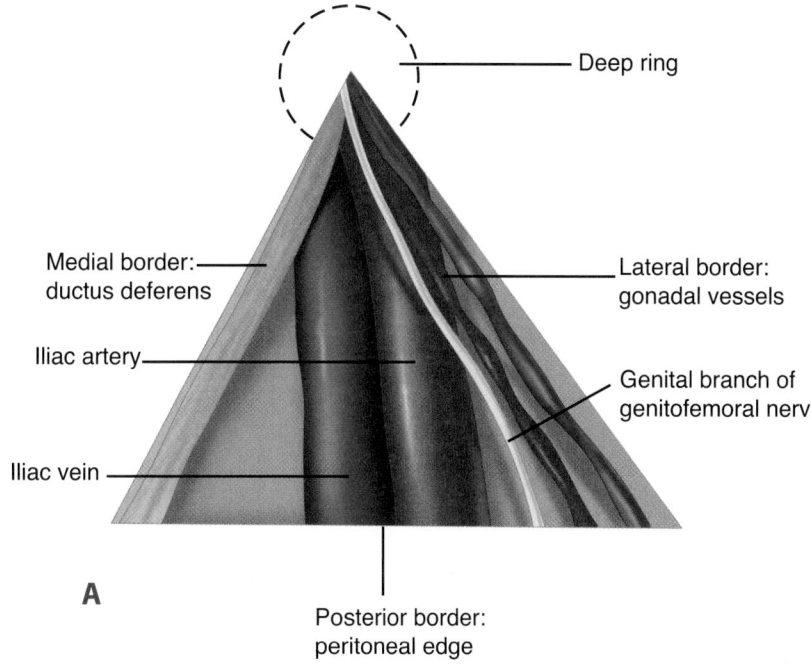

A

Deep ring

Medial border:
ductus deferens

Lateral border:
gonadal vessels

Iliac artery

Genital branch of
genitofemoral nerve

Iliac vein

Posterior border:
peritoneal edge

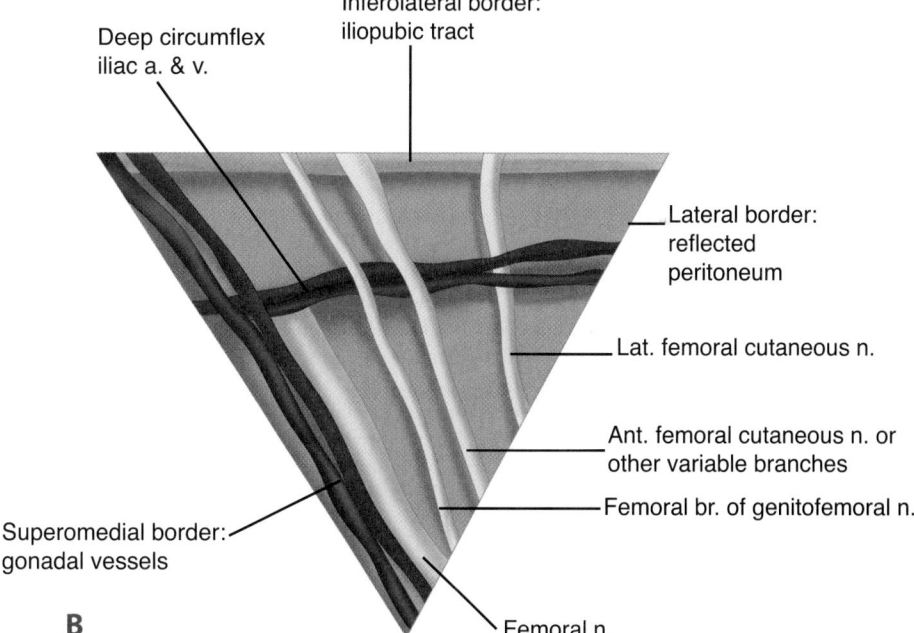

Deep circumflex
iliac a. & v.

Inferolateral border:
iliopubic tract

Lateral border:
reflected
peritoneum

Lat. femoral cutaneous n.

Ant. femoral cutaneous n. or
other variable branches

Femoral br. of genitofemoral n.

Superomedial border:
gonadal vessels

B

Femoral n.

FIG. 37-12. Borders and contents of the (**A**) triangle of doom and (**B**) triangle of pain. a. = artery; Ant. = anterior; br. = branch; Lat. = lateral; n. = nerve; v. = vein. *(Modified with permission from Colborn GL, Skandalakis JE: Laparoscopic cadaveric anatomy of the inguinal area. Probl Gen Surg 12:13, 1995.)*

femoral cutaneous, femoral branch of the genitofemoral, and femoral. The circle of death is a vascular continuation formed by the common iliac, internal iliac, obturator, aberrant obturator, inferior epigastric, and external iliac vessels. Basic knowledge of the boundaries of these triangles allows one to avert the dangers associated with injury to their contents.

CLASSIFICATION

A number of classification systems have been developed relating to inguinal hernias. The classification systems allow for standardization in comparing outcomes of various hernias, yet their clinical significance to date is limited. A common clinical classification system relates to location and subdivides hernias into indirect, direct, and

femoral, although this system does not take into account the complexity of the hernia. Even this system has undergone considerable transformation with the concept of the myopectineal orifice of Fruchaud. Instead of examining the various locations of herniation independently, Fruchaud determined that a common site of weakness, the transversalis fascia, predisposes to all three hernias. With hernia treatment directed at restoring the integrity of this area, recurrences of all three hernias can be reduced. An ideal classification system would also be able to preoperatively stratify hernias and allow for the most appropriate approach to repair, rather than making management decisions based on intraoperative findings. However, preoperative classification relies heavily upon physical examination and the inherent subjectivity of it. Intraoperative classification is also complicated by the fact that certain components of an inguinal hernia cannot be assessed via the laparoscopic method.

TABLE 37-4	Gilbert classification system
Type 1	Small, indirect
Type 2	Medium, indirect
Type 3	Large, indirect
Type 4	Entire floor, direct
Type 5	Diverticular, direct
Type 6	Combined (pantaloon)
Type 7	Femoral

A number of authors, including Rutkow, Robbins, Gilbert, Nyhus, and Schumpelick, have attempted to devise a standardized classification system. Gilbert's classification requires intraoperative assessment and divides hernias into five types, three indirect and two direct (Table 37-4). Type 1 hernias have a small internal ring, type 2 have a moderately dilated internal ring, and type 3 have a ring that is greater than two fingerbreadths. A type 4 direct hernia involved complete disruption of the inguinal floor, and type 5 represented direct hernias with a small diverticular opening of no more than one fingerbreadth.[18] Rutkow and Robbins further expanded the Gilbert classification to include a type 6 pantaloon hernia, which is a combination of a direct and indirect hernia sac, and type 7 femoral hernia.[19]

The Nyhus classification is more detailed and assesses not only the location and size of the defect, but also the integrity of the inguinal ring and inguinal floor (Table 37-5). Consequently, this is one of the most widely used classifications. The system divides hernias into four types, with three subgroups for type III. A type I hernia has a normal size and configuration of the internal ring and occurs primarily as a congenital hernia. Type II hernias have a distorted and enlarged internal ring, without encroachment into the inguinal floor, and small hernia sac. Type IIIA hernias include small- to moderate-sized direct hernias without any sac component through the internal ring. Type IIIB hernias consist of large indirect hernias with defects that encroach on the inguinal canal floor, usually secondarily affecting the structure of the floor. Femoral hernias are classified as type IIIC, and recurrent inguinal hernias are type IV, with A representing direct, B indirect, C femoral, and D any combination of the previous three.[20] Despite its general acceptance, the Nyhus classification scheme is limited by its subjectivity in assessment of distortion of the inguinal ring and posterior floor, especially laparoscopically.

A third major classification system was created by Schumpelick and enjoys greater application in Europe compared to North America. The major feature is the addition of orifice sizing to traditional systems. An L represents a lateral indirect site, M represents medial direct, and F for femoral. The defects are then graded according to size with type I being <1.5 cm in diameter, type II being 1.5 to 3 cm, and type III being >3 cm.[21] Although the system purports to be more objective, differences in the extent of abdominal distention during pneumoperitoneum may affect measurements. A significant amount of other classification systems exist, although no single system has been widely embraced by all surgeons. Future systems will have to take into account ease of use, objectivity, and account for varying anatomic perspectives between open and laparoscopic surgery.

DIAGNOSIS

History

Inguinal hernias present along a spectrum of scenarios. These range from incidental findings to symptomatic hernias to surgical emergencies such as incarceration and strangulation of hernia sac contents. Asymptomatic inguinal hernias are frequently diagnosed incidentally on physical examination or may be brought to the patient's attention as an abnormal bulge. In addition, these hernias can be identified intra-abdominally during laparoscopy. Inspection of the pelvis following mobilization of intestinal contents into the upper abdomen will reveal the myopectineal orifice and allow facile identification of the peritoneum herniating through the direct, indirect, or femoral space.

Patients who present with a symptomatic groin hernia will frequently present with groin pain. Less commonly, patients will present with extrainguinal symptoms such as change in bowel habits or urinary symptoms. Regardless of size, an inguinal hernia may impart pressure onto nerves in the proximity, leading to a range of symptoms. These include generalized pressure, local sharp pains, and referred pain. Pressure or heaviness in the groin is a common complaint, especially at the conclusion of the day, following prolonged activity. Sharp pains tend to indicate an impinged nerve and may not be related to the extent of physical activity performed by the patient. Lastly, neurogenic pains may be referred to the scrotum, testicle, or inner thigh. Questions also should be directed to elucidating the extrainguinal symptoms. A change in bowel habits or urinary symptoms may indicate a sliding hernia consisting of intestinal contents or involvement of the bladder within the hernia sac.

Important considerations of the patient's history include duration and progressiveness of the symptoms. Hernias will often increase in size and content over a protracted time. Much less commonly, a patient will present with a history of acute inguinal herniation following a strenuous activity. However, it is more likely that an asymptomatic, previously unknown, inguinal hernia became evident once the patient experienced symptoms associated with the circumstances of the acute event. Notwithstanding the type of presentation, specific questions should be focused as to whether the hernia is reducible. Oftentimes, patients will reduce the hernia by pushing the contents of the bulge back into the abdomen, thereby providing temporary relief. As the size of a hernia increases and a larger amount of intra-abdominal contents fill the hernia sac, the bulge may become harder to reduce.

Physical

Although the history may be tremendously indicative of an inguinal hernia, the physical examination is essential to forming the diagnosis. A significant drawback exists in morbidly obese patients, where delineation of external groin anatomy is difficult and may obscure the findings of a groin hernia. Ideally, the patient should be examined in a standing position, with the groin and scrotum fully exposed. The standing position has the advantage over the supine position in that intra-abdominal pressure is increased, and thereby, the hernia can be more easily elicited. Inspec-

TABLE 37-5	Nyhus classification system
Type I	Indirect hernia; internal abdominal ring normal; typically in infants, children, small adults
Type II	Indirect hernia; internal ring enlarged without impingement on the floor of the inguinal canal; does not extend to the scrotum
Type IIIA	Direct hernia; size is not taken into account
Type IIIB	Indirect hernia that has enlarged enough to encroach upon the posterior inguinal wall; indirect sliding or scrotal hernias are usually placed in this category because they are commonly associated with extension to the direct space; also includes pantaloon hernias
Type IIIC	Femoral hernia
Type IV	Recurrent hernia; modifiers A–D are sometimes added, which correspond to indirect, direct, femoral, and mixed, respectively

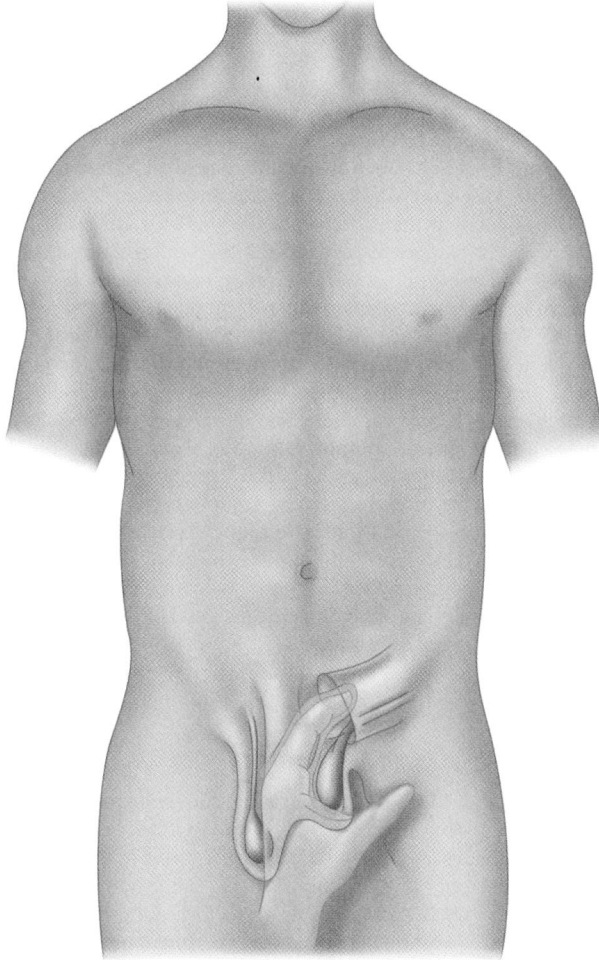

FIG. 37-13. Digital examination of the inguinal canal.

tion is performed first, with the goal of identifying an abnormal bulge along the groin or within the scrotum. If an obvious bulge is not detected, physical examination is performed to confirm the presence of the hernia.

Palpation is performed by placing the index finger into the scrotum, aiming it toward the external inguinal ring (Fig. 37-13). This allows the inguinal canal to be inspected. The patient is then asked to cough or bear down (i.e., Valsalva's maneuver) to protrude the hernia contents. Reproduction of patient symptoms, namely vague, generalized pressure sensations, will not usually be reproduced by these maneuvers, as they are a product of prolonged pressure on the cord contents. However, a Valsalva's maneuver will reveal an abnormal bulge and allow the clinician to determine whether the bulge is reducible or not. Examination of the contralateral side affords the clinician the opportunity to compare the extent of herniation between sides. This is especially useful in the case of a small hernia. The magnitude of the bulge on the affected side can be compared to the normal bulging of muscle on the nonaffected side, when the abdomen is placed under strain. However, the results may be misleading if there is a latent contralateral hernia that is discovered during this examination.

Certain techniques of the physical examination have classically been used to differentiate between direct and indirect hernias. The inguinal occlusion test involves placement of a finger over the internal inguinal ring and the patient is instructed to cough. If the cough impulse is controlled, then the hernia is indirect. If the cough impulse is still manifest, the hernia is direct. As well, with a finger in the inguinal canal, the cough impulse can be used to determine

the type of hernia. If the cough impulse is felt on the fingertip, the hernia is indirect; if felt on the dorsum of the finger, it is deemed direct. However, when results of clinical examination are compared against operative findings, there is a probability somewhat higher than chance (i.e., 50%) of correctly diagnosing the type of hernia.[22,23] Therefore, the utility of these tests should not be used to diagnose the type of inguinal hernia insomuch as they should be used to determine the presence or absence of one.

A further challenge to the physical examination is the identification of a femoral hernia. The anatomic position of a femoral hernia dictates that it should be palpable below the inguinal ligament, lateral to the pubic tubercle. As a consequence of increased subcutaneous tissue, a femoral hernia may be missed or misdiagnosed as a hernia of the inguinal canal. In contrast, a prominent fat pad in a thin patient may prompt an erroneous diagnosis of femoral hernia, otherwise known as a *femoral pseudohernia*.

In addition to inguinal hernia, a number of other diagnoses may be considered in the differential of a groin bulge (Table 37-6). The diagnosis is ambiguous; radiologic investigation may provide the answer.

Imaging

A number of situations can make the usually straightforward diagnosis of inguinal hernia ambiguous. These scenarios include obese patients, hernias that cannot be elicited on physical examination, and recurrent inguinal hernias. In these situations, radiologic investigations may be used as an adjunct to history and physical examination. The most common radiologic modalities include ultrasonography (US), computed tomography (CT), and magnetic resonance imaging (MRI). Each technique has certain advantages over physical examination alone; however, each also is associated with potential pitfalls.

Ultrasound is the least invasive technique and does not impart any radiation to the patient. Anatomic structures can be more easily identified by the presence of bony landmarks; however, because there are few in the inguinal canal, other structures such as the inferior epigastric vessels are used to define groin anatomy. Positive intra-abdominal pressure is used to elicit the herniation of abdominal contents. Movement of these contents is essential to making the diagnosis with US, and lack of this movement may lead to a false negative. In thin patients, normal movement of the spermatic cord

TABLE 37-6	Differential diagnosis of groin hernia

Malignancy
   Lymphoma
   Retroperitoneal sarcoma
   Metastasis
   Testicular tumor
Primary testicular
   Varicocele
   Epididymitis
   Testicular torsion
   Hydrocele
   Ectopic testicle
   Undescended testicle
Femoral artery aneurysm or pseudoaneurysm
Lymph node
Sebaceous cyst
Hidradenitis
Cyst of the canal of Nuck (female)
Saphenous varix
Psoas abscess
Hematoma
Ascites

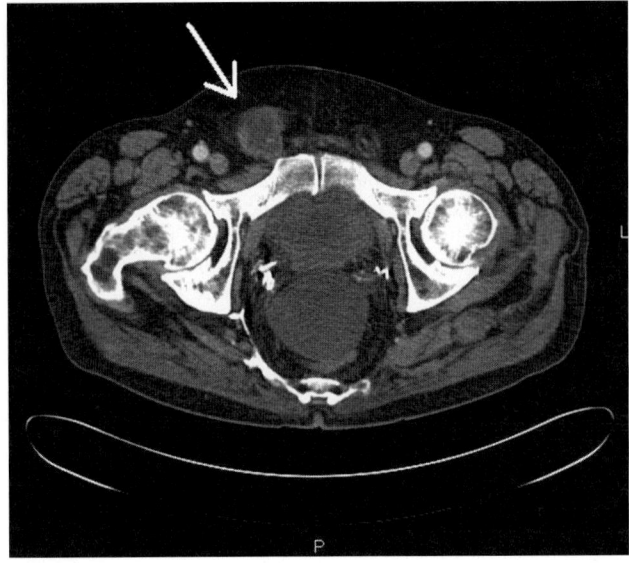

FIG. 37-14. Computed tomography scan depicting a large right inguinal hernia (*arrow*). A smaller left inguinal hernia is also visualized.

and posterior abdominal wall against the anterior abdominal wall may lead to false-positive diagnoses of hernia.[24]

CT and MRI provide static images that are able to delineate the groin anatomy and demonstrate not only the presence of groin hernias, but also rule out differential diagnoses that may cloud the clinical picture (Fig. 37-14). Although CT scan is useful in ambiguous clinical presentations, little data exist to support its routine use in diagnosis. The use of MRI in assessing groin hernias was examined in a group of 41 patients scheduled to undergo laparoscopic inguinal hernia repair. Preoperatively, all patients underwent US and MRI. Laparoscopic confirmation of the presence of inguinal hernia was deemed the gold standard. Physical examination was found to be the least sensitive, whereas MRI was found to be the most sensitive. False positives were low on physical examination and MRI (one finding), but higher with US (four findings). With further refinement of technology, radiologic techniques will continue to improve the sensitivity and specificity rates of diagnosis, thereby serving a supplementary role in cases of uncertain diagnosis.

ANESTHESIA

Local, regional, and general anesthesia are all viable options for open anterior hernia repairs. Laparoscopic repairs, on the other hand, usually are performed using general anesthesia for optimal abdominal expansion and patient comfort. This limitation of laparoscopic surgery becomes a consideration in high-risk patients that cannot tolerate general anesthesia and the effects of pneumoperitoneum. In contrast, there are relatively few side effects of local anesthesia, which can facilitate operative tolerance by the patient, especially when combined with an IV sedative or anxiolytic agent.

Local anesthesia is applied by the surgeon before the initial groin incision. Common anesthetic agents include lidocaine and the longer-acting bupivacaine, both with optional epinephrine. Patients with a history of coronary artery disease have a relative contraindication to epinephrine use. The maximum dose should be calculated according to the patient's weight during preparation of the injection. In advance of the initial incision, usually before the prep and drape, a variable amount of anesthetic is injected one fingerbreadth medial and inferior to the anterior superior iliac spine to block the

ilioinguinal nerve. In addition, anesthetic is injected along the cutaneous course of the skin incision and underlying subcutaneous tissue. The remaining amount is reserved for repeated applications to affected areas during the course of the operation. A combination of the two agents provides for a quick onset and prolonged control of pain, in the range of 18 hours.

Regional anesthesia, such as epidural, is another option reserved for patients that cannot tolerate general anesthesia. It also has a greater margin of patient comfort. Additional advantages of local and regional anesthesia include the ability of the patient to cough or Valsalva to test the repair. The versatility of anesthesia choices is a common argument for proponents of open inguinal hernia repairs. Nonetheless, the majority of procedures are performed using general anesthesia, which provides the greatest margin of patient comfort of all three choices. Advances in perioperative care have allowed for extensive general anesthesia use in an ambulatory surgery setting. Long- or short-acting local anesthetics can be applied to the incisions at the end of the procedure to prolong pain control. Common cardiorespiratory complications of anesthesia include myocardial depression, infarct, and aspiration pneumonia. The risk of these complications is reduced by using local anesthesia; however, anesthesiologists may prefer to completely sedate the patient and thereby control the airway. It should be noted that most procedures using only local anesthesia are performed at specialty hernia centers.

TREATMENT

The treatment of inguinal hernias can be subdivided according to approach (i.e., open vs. laparoscopic). Open inguinal hernias can be further subdivided according to whether the repair is performed anterior or posterior to the inguinal floor. A large number of open inguinal hernia repairs have been described over time; however, the most commonly performed and clinically pertinent procedures will be described herein.

Open Approach

Before the widespread use of prosthetic material, inguinal hernia repairs were based on restoring tissue strength through the use of sutures. Upon the introduction of prosthetics in the tension-free repair, these procedures came to be known as *tension repairs*; however, this would imply that these procedures do not adhere to basic surgical principles of avoiding tension between tissues. Therefore, these will be referred to as *tissue repairs*. Despite the advantages of the tension-free prosthetic repair, tissue repairs occupy an important place in the choice of inguinal hernia repair, especially in situations where prosthetic material is contraindicated. This includes a contaminated operative field or concern regarding possible azoospermia secondary to long-term effects of mesh on the vas deferens.[25]

Exposure of the inguinal region is common to open approaches to inguinal hernia repair. An oblique or horizontal incision is performed over the groin (Fig. 37-15). A point two fingerbreadths inferior and medial to the anterior superior iliac spine is chosen as the most lateral point of the incision. It is then progressed medially for approximately 6 to 8 cm. Electrocautery is then used to divide the subcutaneous tissue. Fascia of Camper is not routinely encountered; however, Scarpa's fascia generally is identified and then divided, thereby exposing the aponeurosis of the external oblique muscle. A vein coursing in a vertical fashion through the subcutaneous tissue frequently is encountered and is ligated and divided between hemostat clamps. The fibers of the external oblique muscle are then sharply divided parallel to the direction of fibers. Metzenbaum scissors are then advanced immediately beneath the fibers, laterally and then medially toward the external inguinal ring, and spread as they are retracted to create a space and avoid inadvertent dissection of the ilioinguinal nerve. The scissors are then used to

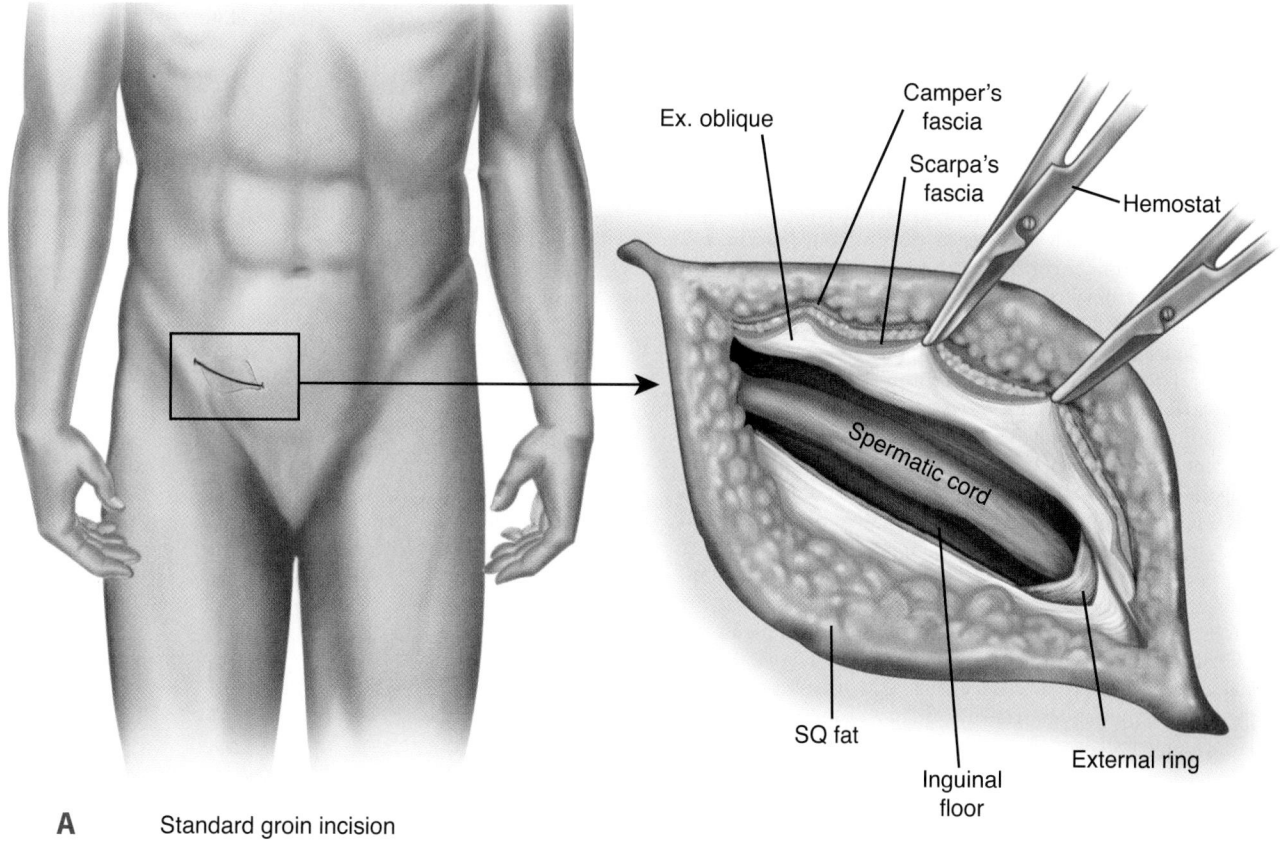

A Standard groin incision

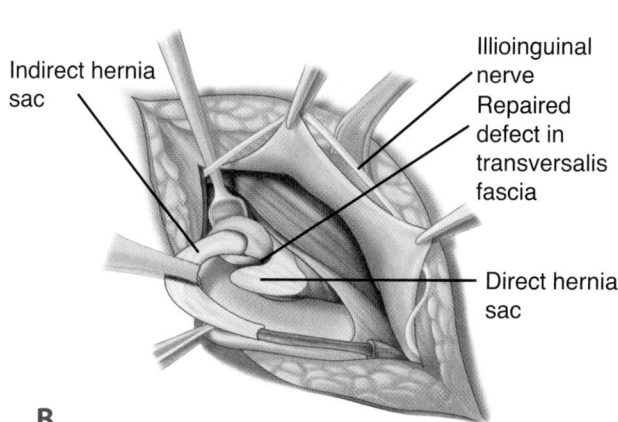

B

FIG. 37-15. A. Layers of the abdominal wall in an anterior open approach to hernia repair. **B.** Identification of indirect and direct hernia sacs once the spermatic cord has been isolated and the ilioinguinal nerve has been retracted away. Ex. = external; SQ = subcutaneous.

incise the aponeurosis, splitting the external inguinal ring, exposing the inguinal canal and its contents. The aponeurosis is divided superior to the inguinal ligament as consideration should be made for its reapproximation once the repair is complete.

Mobilization of the Cord Structures

Hemostat clamps are then applied to the superior and inferior edges of the aponeurosis and elevated from the inguinal canal. Blunt dissection is then performed to separate the superior flap of the external oblique aponeurosis from the internal oblique muscle. Likewise, the inferior flap of the external oblique aponeurosis is bluntly dissected to reveal the shelving edge of the inguinal ligament. The iliohypogastric and ilioinguinal nerves are identified and may be retracted from the operative field by placing a hemostat beneath their course and then grasping one of the edges of the aponeurosis. Some surgeons routinely divide these nerves to avoid possible entrapment; however, the sequelae involve permanent paresthesia to sites of their cutaneous distribution. The pubic

tubercle is then identified and the surgeon's index finger and thumb are placed around the cord as it passes the tubercle. A Penrose drain or metal cord ring may then be placed around the cord and its contents to permit its elevation from the floor of the inguinal canal. With the cord elevated at the external inguinal ring, cremasteric fibers are visualized connecting the floor of the inguinal canal to the posterior aspect of the cord. The cremasteric fibers can then be divided bluntly or through the use of electrocautery to initiate skeletonization of the cord. Once the cremasteric fibers are completely divided between the external and internal inguinal rings, the floor of the inguinal canal can be fully assessed for direct hernias. Care must be taken to avoid injury to cord structures during the division of the cremasteric muscle.

Identification and Reduction of the Sac

With the contents of the inguinal canal completely encircled, identification of cord contents and the hernia sac can be effected. Direct hernias will become evident as the floor of the inguinal canal is dissected. Even in tension-free repairs, the floor of the inguinal canal may be imbricated with stitches to reduce the direct hernia sac. An indirect hernia sac will generally be found on the anterolateral surface of the spermatic cord. In addition to sac identification, the vas deferens and vessels of the spermatic cord must be identified to allow dissection of the sac from the cord. At the leading edge of the sac, the two layers of peritoneum will fold upon themselves and reveal a white edge, which may help in the identification of the sac. This peritoneum can then be grasped with a tissue forceps and bluntly dissected from the cord. The dissection is carried proximally toward the deep inguinal ring.

The reduction of the hernia sac into the preperitoneal space is commonly known as *high ligation of the sac*. Some surgeons will routinely open the sac and inspect it to ensure there is no incarceration of intra-abdominal contents. As well, the decision must be made whether to excise the sac at the internal inguinal ring or simply invert it into the preperitoneum. Both methods are effective in reducing the sac; however, in a large prospective randomized study, patients undergoing high ligation and excision of the sac had significantly increased postoperative pain in the first week.[26] A densely adherent sac, which may result in injury to cord structures, does not necessarily deserve dissection; however, division at the internal inguinal ring is necessary. Likewise, an inguinal hernia sac that extends into the scrotum may require division within the inguinal canal. Attempts to reduce such sacs may be met with postoperative complications related to injury of the pampiniform plexus, including testicular atrophy and orchitis.

Wound Closure

Once the reconstruction of the inguinal canal is complete, the cord contents are returned to their anatomic position. The external oblique aponeurosis is then reapproximated. A useful starting position is at the external inguinal ring. Using an absorbable suture, the external inguinal ring is reconstructed and the external oblique fascia is then closed using a running stitch that progresses laterally. Avoidance of an overly constricting external ring will prevent compression of cord structures at that point. However, it should be small enough to contain the contents of the inguinal canal and prevent a future false-positive diagnosis of recurrent hernia. Scarpa's fascia may then be closed with a series of interrupted absorbable sutures. Lastly, skin is closed with a subcuticular stitch to preserve cosmesis of the incision.

Anterior Repairs, Nonprosthetic

Before the introduction of mesh prostheses, open anterior inguinal hernia repairs were performed by reapproximating tissue using only sutures. Despite their shortcomings, specific procedures such as the Bassini, Shouldice, and McVay repair continue to occupy a minor, yet important role in the overall treatment of inguinal hernias. The introduction of the Bassini repair was superior to previously performed procedures in that, not only was the hernia reduced and the defect oversewn, but now an attempt was made to reconstruct the site of weakness, although these tissue-based repairs tend to place tension on the reconstructed tissue. The Shouldice repair is an exception because the multilayer reconstruction distributes the tension, effectively resulting in a tension-free repair. Hernia exposure and reduction are common to all open anterior repairs; however, the mode of restoration of inguinal canal integrity differs according to procedure.

Bassini Repair The Bassini repair was a major advancement in the treatment of inguinal hernias owing to significantly reduced recurrence rates as compared to other operations of the day. Current use of the Bassini repair is limited because other tissue-based operations such as the Shouldice repair have demonstrated lower recurrence rates. The importance of the Bassini repair lies in the paradigm shift it promoted, which included dissection of the spermatic cord, dissection of the hernia sac with high ligation, and extensive reconstruc-

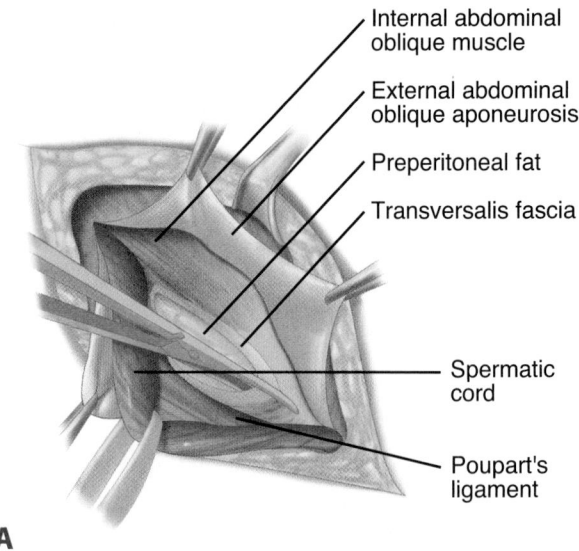

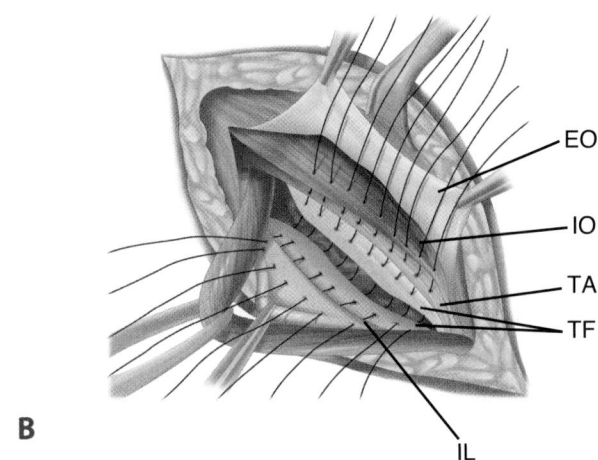

FIG. 37-16. Bassini repair. **A.** The transversalis fascia is opened from the internal inguinal ring to the pubic tubercle exposing the preperitoneal fat. **B.** Reconstruction of the posterior wall by suturing the transversalis fascia (TF), the transversus abdominis muscle (TA), and the internal oblique muscle (IO) (Bassini's famous "triple layer") medially to the inguinal ligament (IL) laterally. EO = external oblique aponeurosis.

tion of the floor of the inguinal canal (Fig. 37-16). Following division of the cremasteric muscle and ligation of the hernia sac deep to the internal inguinal ring, the transversalis fascia is incised from the pubic tubercle to the internal inguinal ring, thereby entering the preperitoneal space. Preperitoneal fat is bluntly dissected from the upper margin of the posterior side of the transversalis fascia to permit adequate tissue mobilization. A triple-layer repair is then performed to restore integrity to the floor. The medial tissues, including the internal oblique muscle, transversus abdominis muscle, and transversalis fascia, are fixed to the shelving edge of the inguinal ligament and pubic periosteum with interrupted sutures. The lateral border of the repair is the medial border of the internal inguinal ring, which subsequently is reinforced by the repair. Adoption of the Bassini technique in North America resulted in injury to neurovascular structures and high recurrence rates because the posterior floor was not routinely opened. Nevertheless, the significant advances promulgated by Bassini still resulted in a recurrence rate that could be further improved.

Numerous modifications of the technique by successive surgeons accomplished a lower recurrence rate, namely with the addition of the relaxing incision and the Shouldice technique. Current use of the Bassini technique is limited, although a modification may be useful in large direct hernias approached via an open approach. In these cases, imbrication of the posterior floor may be added to a tension-free repair with mesh.

Shouldice Repair The principles of the Bassini repair were revitalized within the Shouldice repair, resulting in superior recurrence rates. Although the Shouldice repair is generally grouped with open tissue-based repairs, its success rates are equivalent to that of tension-free repairs in many studies comparing the two approaches. As with the Bassini repair, the primary tenets of the procedure involve extensive dissection and reconstruction of inguinal canal anatomy. The use of a continuous suture in multiple layers resulted in the dual advantage of distributing tension over several layers and preventing subsequent herniation between interrupted sutures (Fig. 37-17). Original descriptions of the Shouldice technique involved the use of a stainless steel wire; however, modern modifications have resulted in the use of a synthetic nonabsorbable suture. With the posterior inguinal floor exposed, an incision in the transversalis fascia is performed between the pubic tubercle and internal ring. Care is taken to avoid injury to

any preperitoneal structures, and these are bluntly dissected to mobilize the upper and lower fascial flaps. The first layer of repair begins at the pubic tubercle where the iliopubic tract is sutured to the lateral edge of the rectus sheath, then progressing laterally. The inferior flap of the transversalis fascia, which includes the iliopubic tract, is sutured continuously to the posterior aspect of the superior flap of the transversalis fascia until the internal ring is encountered. At this point, the internal ring has been reconstituted. The suture is not tied here, but rather is continued back upon itself in the medial direction. At the internal ring, the second layer is the reapproximation of the superior edge of the transversalis fascia to the inferior fascial margin and the shelving edge of the inguinal ligament. The suture is then tied to the tail of the original stitch. A third suture is started at the tightened inguinal ring, joining the internal oblique and transversus abdominis aponeuroses to external oblique aponeurotic fibers just superficial to the inguinal ligament. This layer is continued to the pubic tubercle where it reverses upon itself to create a fourth suture line, which is similar and superficial to the third layer. Unique to this operation is the routine division of the genital branch of the genitofemoral nerve. The consequence of loss of skin sensation is countered by the observed decrease in recurrence rate at the pubic tubercle. The Shouldice technique is readily apparent in common practice, especially in specialized hospitals treating inguinal hernias.

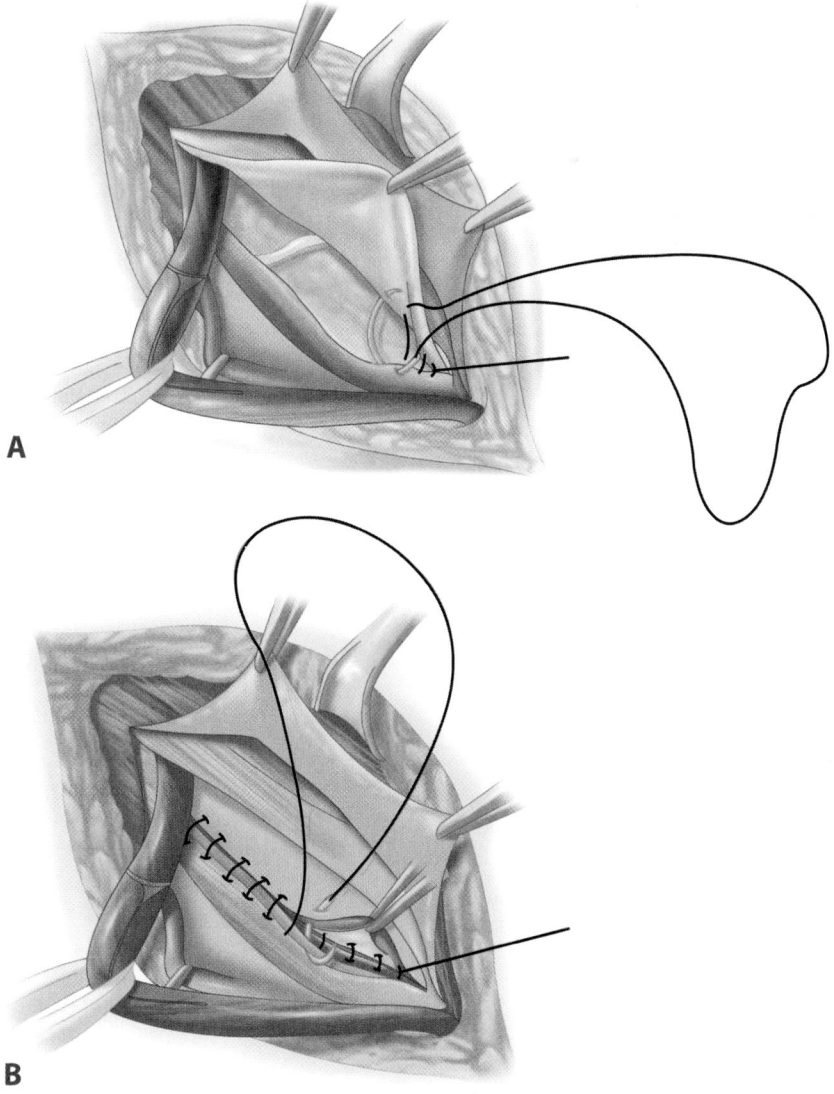

FIG. 37-17. The Shouldice repair. **A.** The iliopubic tract is sutured to the medial flap, which is made up of the transversalis fascia and the internal oblique and transverse abdominis muscles. **B.** This is the second of the four suture lines. After the stump of the cremaster muscle is picked up, the suture is reversed back toward the pubic tubercle approximating the internal oblique and transversus muscles to the inguinal ligament. Two more suture lines will eventually be created suturing the internal oblique and transversus muscles medially to an artificially created "pseudo" inguinal ligament developed from superficial fibers of the inferior flap of the external oblique aponeurosis parallel to the true ligament.

McVay Repair The advantage of the McVay (Cooper's ligament) repair is the ability to address both inguinal and femoral canal defects. Femoral hernias that are approached via a suprainguinal ligament approach, or situations where the use of prosthetic material is contraindicated, are amenable to this type of repair. The operation was popularized by McVay, who also added the concept of the relaxing incision as a tension reducing maneuver (Fig. 37-18). Once the cord has been isolated, a transverse incision is performed through the transversalis fascia, thereby entering the preperitoneal space. A small amount of dissection of the posterior aspect of the fascia is performed to allow mobilization of the upper margin of the transversalis fascia. The floor of the inguinal canal is then reconstructed to restore its strength. Cooper's ligament is identified medially, and it is bluntly dissected to expose its surface. The upper margin of the transversalis fascia is then sutured to Cooper's ligament. The repair is continued laterally along Cooper's ligament, occluding the femoral canal.

Once the femoral canal has been passed, a transition stitch is performed by now suturing the transversalis fascia to the inguinal ligament. The transition stitch helps obliterate the femoral canal, but more importantly, avoids injury to the femoral vessels. The transversalis fascia is subsequently sutured to the inguinal ligament, the lateral margin being the internal inguinal ring, which consequently undergoes transformation to a smaller, tighter ring. The repair can be performed using either interrupted sutures or a continuous stitch. An essential component of the procedure is the relaxing incision, which helps reduce the considerable amount of tension that normally results. Before suturing the transversalis fascia to Cooper's and the inguinal ligament, an incision in the anterior rectus sheath is made. The incision begins at the pubic tubercle and is extended superiorly for approximately 2 to 4 cm.

Potential consequences of the relaxing incision include increased postoperative pain and less likely herniation at the anterior abdominal wall. Disadvantages of routinely performing the McVay Cooper's ligament repair include elevated recurrence rates due to the tissue-based nature of the operation. Furthermore, the procedure requires extensive dissection and may result in injury to the underlying femoral vessels.

Anterior Repairs, Prosthetic

Outside of specialized centers dealing with inguinal hernias, recurrence rates of tissue-based repairs continued to be high, owing to the tension placed on reconstructed tissues. To circumvent this problem and adhere to no-tension principles of effective surgical repair, mesh herniorrhaphies were developed. The addition of a mesh prosthesis effected a reconstruction of the posterior inguinal canal, without placing tension on the floor itself, hence a tension-free repair, as championed by Lichtenstein. Further refinements have included the addition of a plug through the internal ring, resulting in the plug and patch repair. The consistently superior recurrence rates over the long-term, along with the ease of reproducibility of these techniques, resulted in the wide acceptance of tension-free repairs for inguinal hernias.

Lichtenstein Tension-Free Repair Initial exposure and mobilization of cord structures is identical to other open approaches. Particular attention must be paid to blunt dissection of the inguinal canal to expose the shelving edge of the inguinal ligament and pubic tubercle, as well as provide a large area for mesh placement. Unlike the tissue-based repairs, the Lichtenstein repair does not include routine division of the transversalis fascia, thereby preventing the identification of a latent femoral hernia. However, in the case where a clinically significant hernia is not visualized upon entrance into the inguinal canal, an argument can be made to enter the preperitoneal space and evaluate the femoral canal. The lack of inguinal floor division also indicates that the internal inguinal ring is not reconstructed using canal structures (Fig. 37-19). Instead, the floor and internal ring are reinforced through the application of the mesh.

The mesh is rectangular in shape, with a rounded edge at its apex, corresponding to the medial edge. At the other end, the mesh will be split to accommodate the spermatic cord. The mesh prosthesis must be large enough to adequately cover the posterior wall of the inguinal canal and can be sized accordingly when placed into the field. The rounded edge is attached to the anterior rectus sheath just medial to the pubic tubercle, ensuring that there is an adequate overlap medially to prevent recurrence. The suture is then continued in a running fashion to secure the mesh around the pubic tubercle. Care must be taken to avoid placing sutures directly into the periosteum of the pubic tubercle, which may result in persistent postoperative pain. The inferior margin of the mesh is then sutured to the shelving edge of the inguinal ligament, as the repair is continued laterally. The stitch is then tied at the internal ring. The mesh is then tailored to fit around the cord at the internal ring. The slit in the lateral end of the mesh may require expansion to accommodate the cord and prevent strangulation of cord contents. The superior and inferior flaps of the prosthesis are then placed around the base of the cord, lateral to the internal ring and near the anterior superior iliac spine, and sutured together with a single interrupted stitch. This allows the internal ring to be reinforced by a synthetic valve, helping to prevent recurrences of indirect inguinal hernias.

A flap closure that is too lose may lead to higher indirect hernia recurrences; however, one that is too tight may impart significant pressure on the spermatic cord, leading to the injury of its contents. The superior edge of the mesh is then fixed to the posterior aspect of the internal oblique aponeurosis and rectus sheath, using either interrupted or continuous sutures. Fixation of the upper and lower margin of the mesh too superficially to the internal and external oblique aponeuroses may shorten the superior and inferior flaps of the external oblique aponeurosis, making closure of the inguinal canal difficult. In the case of a femoral hernia, the inferior margin of the mesh is sutured to Cooper's ligament medially and inguinal ligament laterally, similar to McVay's repair. Nonabsorbable or long-term absorbable sutures generally are used with mesh repairs.

Plug and Patch Technique A modification of the Lichtenstein repair, known as the *plug and patch technique*, was developed by Gilbert and later popularized by Rutkow and Robbins.[27] In addition to placement of the prosthesis in a similar fashion to the Lichten-

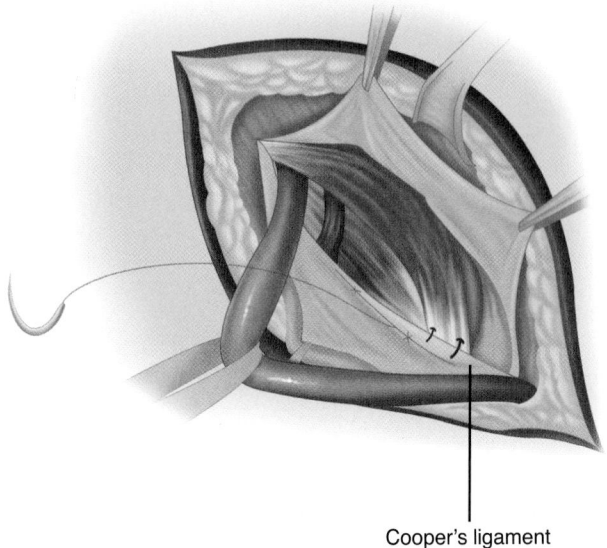

Cooper's ligament

FIG. 37-18. McVay Cooper ligament repair.

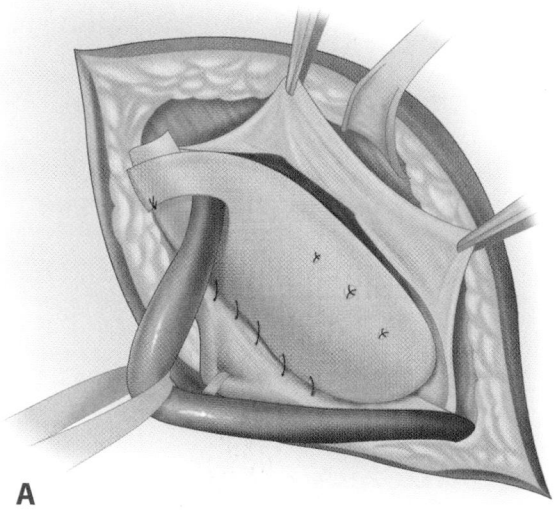

A

FIG. 37-19. Lichtenstein tension-free hernioplasty. **A.** Medially, the prosthesis (P) is sutured to the anterior rectus sheath 2 cm medial to the pubic tubercle. Laterally, a continuous suture is used to fix the prosthesis to the shelving edge of the inguinal ligament. The tails of the mesh are placed around the cord and secured with an interrupted suture. **B** and **C.** A lateral view demonstrates that the prosthesis is situated between the cord and the hernia defect (HD). The hernia defect has been imbricated to allow for facile prosthesis placement only (this does not affect the strength of the repair). EOA = external oblique aponeurosis.

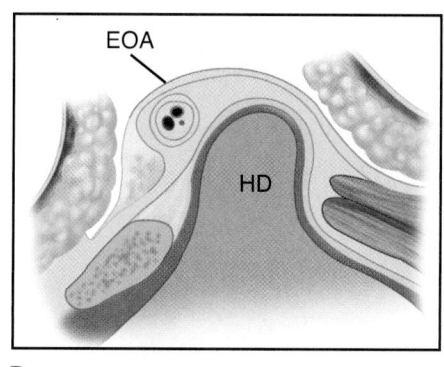

B

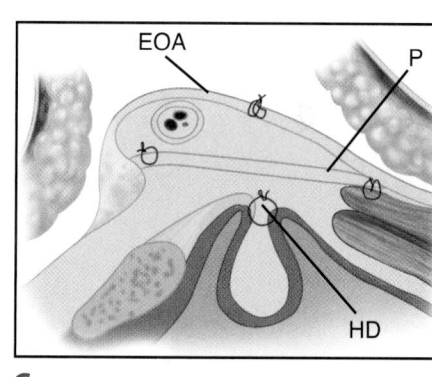

C

stein repair (i.e., the patch), the technique includes placement of a prosthesis (i.e., the plug) through the internal ring (Fig. 37-20). The internal ring is therefore reinforced by the leaflets of the patch as well as the plug. Initial technique described rolling a flat piece of polypropylene into a tight cylinder and placing it alongside the spermatic cord as it passes through the internal ring. Further modifications have involved shaping the plug into a flower or umbrella configuration, with the apex pointed intra-abdominally, in effect serving as a preperitoneal prosthesis. Increased abdominal pressure acts on the plug, opening its leaflets and creating a protective valve. Original descriptions of the plug and patch procedure emphasized a pure tension-free approach in that the plug and patch could be placed in their anatomic positions without sutures. Normal scarring would then fix the prostheses in place and provide reconstituted strength to the inguinal canal. Currently, preformed plugs in various sizes are available and are usually fixed to the margins of the internal ring with one or several interrupted sutures.[28] Direct defects may also be plugged; however, in the absence of inguinal floor division and dissection, suture fixation of the plug to the margins of the defect is necessary. In this case, the plug is fixed to Cooper's and the inguinal ligament inferiorly and the internal oblique aponeurosis superiorly. Numerous modifications of the plug and patch technique have occurred with various extents of prosthesis fixation. Considerations unique to the plug include intra-abdominal migration and erosion into contiguous structures.

Preperitoneal Repairs

As previously noted in the Bassini Repair section, the preperitoneal space can be entered using the anterior approach by dividing the transversalis fascia; however, wide exposure of the preperitoneal space is limited. Therefore, a number of surgeons have approached the preperitoneal space posterior to the transversalis fascia. Cheatle was the first to perform posterior preperitoneal repair of a groin hernias, usually through a lower midline and later using a Pfannenstiel incision. Nonprosthetic preperitoneal repairs were also described by Nyhus; however, the superior results achieved by mesh use lend them to historical significance only. The placement of a widely overlapping prosthesis in the preperitoneal space using the open approach eventually became the basis of laparoscopic surgery. The strength of the transversalis fascia is reinforced by the addition of the prosthesis deep to it. The perceived advantage of the preperitoneal approach is that the prosthesis can be placed between hernia contents and the hernia defect. Furthermore, increases in intra-abdominal pressure serve to push the mesh against the floor of the inguinal canal, unlike in anterior mesh placement where the mesh is pushed away. The posterior approach to preperitoneal repairs avoids entry into the inguinal canal and permits optional closure of the hernia defect. Therefore, nerves that course through the inguinal canal are avoided, and there is minimal manipulation of the spermatic cord. A Pfannenstiel or lower midline incision is generally used to gain access to the preperitoneal space, taking care not to disturb the peritoneum. The preperitoneal space can also be accessed intra-abdominally; however, this approach is optimal if a laparotomy is being performed for other purposes. A notable example is a laparotomy performed for bowel obstruction that results in the identification of an inguinal hernia as the cause of obstruction.

Read-Rives Repair The anterior approach to preperitoneal repairs, as described by Read and Rives, accesses the groin using a

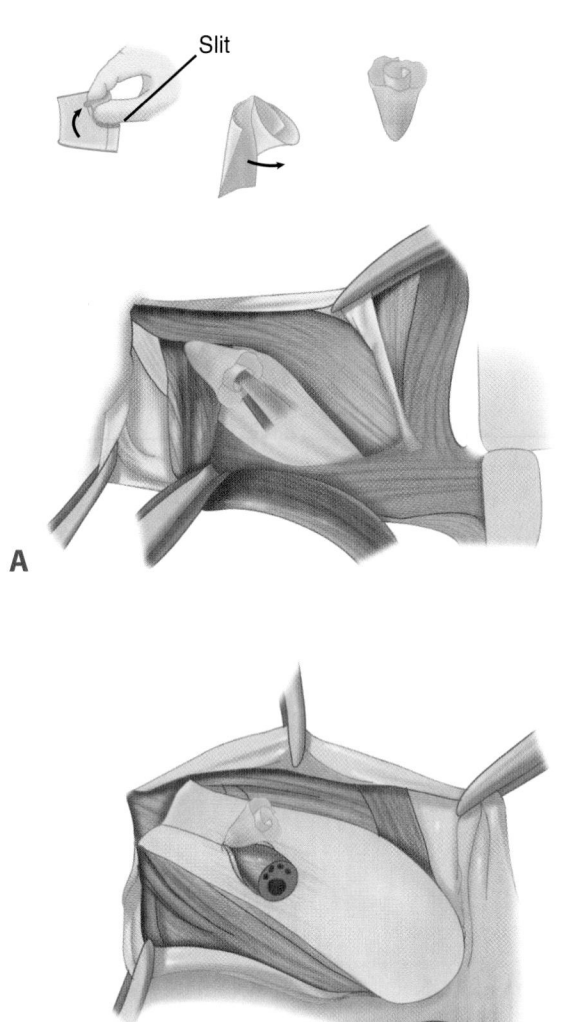

Slit

A

B

FIG. 37-20. **A.** A plug may be created from a flat piece of mesh, or a preformed, commercially available plug is placed in the internal ring. **B.** Final view of the repair following placement of the plug and patch. A common modification is to use the flat mesh to overlap the plug, after it is placed.

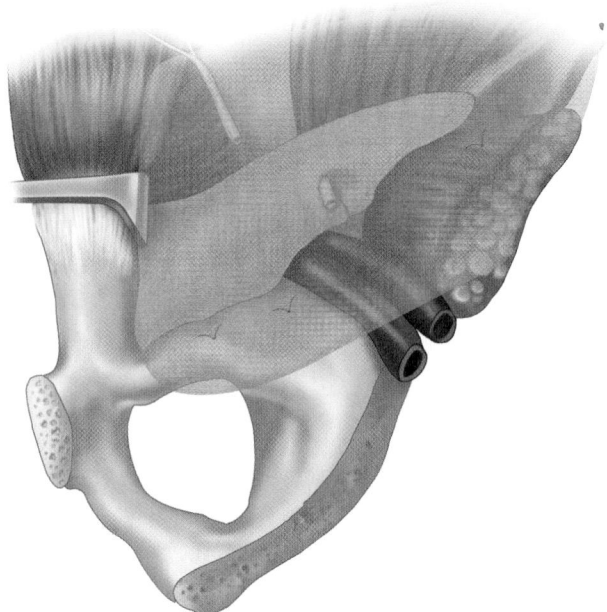

FIG. 37-21. View of mesh placement in posterior repairs. A large piece of mesh is used to overlap the myopectineal orifice. Sutures are placed at the pubic tubercle, Cooper's ligament, and psoas muscle.

standard groin incision (Fig. 37-21). The transversalis fascia is incised and a wide blunt dissection of the preperitoneal space is performed to accommodate a large prosthesis. The spermatic cord is identified at the internal ring and dissected from the peritoneum proximally to the pelvic portion of the vas deferens. The vas deferens is separated from the spermatic vessels during the course of cord parietalization. Cooper's ligament must also be identified medially and dissected free to expose its surface. Dissection to this extent frees the peritoneum from the iliac fossa and provides an adequate space for placement of a large prosthesis. An unsplit piece of mesh, approximately 16 × 12 cm is then placed in the preperitoneal space over the spermatic cord, ensuring overlap medial to Cooper's ligament, laterally to the anterior superior iliac spine and inferiorly to the margin of the preperitoneal dissection. The mesh is secured using three sutures, to Cooper's ligament, the pubic tubercle, and the psoas muscle. The transversalis fascia is then reclosed, and the inguinal canal is closed routinely as per the open approach.

Giant Prosthetic Reinforcement of the Visceral Sac The giant prosthetic reinforcement of the visceral sac is also known as the

Rives, Stoppa, or *Wantz* repair, although minor modifications exist between them. Ideal access is provided by a Pfannenstiel or lower transverse incision, which is more medial than a standard groin incision in anterior open approaches. The incision ranges 8 to 10 cm from the midline laterally, above the level of the internal ring. The intent is to expose the lateral aspect of the rectus sheath and divide it and the oblique muscles for a distance of 10 cm. Abdominal wall muscles are then retracted to expose the transversalis fascia, allowing it to be incised. The peritoneum is left intact to maintain the procedure within the preperitoneal space. Wide dissection is then performed posterior to the rectus sheath and inferior epigastric vessels (Fig. 37-22). The dissection begins on the contralateral side of the midline and continues laterally to beyond the anterior superior iliac spine. Inferiorly, the peritoneum is dissected to the division of the spermatic vessels and vas deferens. The posterior approach requires identification of Cooper's ligament medially and the iliopubic tract running laterally. A direct hernia will be identified and reduced during the course of initial dissection. Care must be taken to separate the hernia sac from the overlying transversalis fascia because an incorrect plane of dissection may be entered, resulting in dissection of the anterior abdominal wall. Direct defects can be ignored, or conversely, the defect can be imbricated or obliterated by suturing the transversalis fascia to Cooper's ligament. An indirect hernia will be identified at the internal ring and usually will require additional directed dissection. The advantage to the preperitoneal approach is minimal interaction with the spermatic cord. Therefore, in the case of large or densely adherent indirect hernia sacs that pose a problem during cord parietalization, ligation of the sac may be undertaken. The distal sac is left untouched, and the sac, at its insertion at the internal ring, is dissected from the spermatic cord. The resulting defect in the peritoneum is then closed to restore the peritoneal lining. Because the sac is bilayered, it can be opened on the side not adherent to the cord and dissected away until it can be circumferentially freed and divided.

A large mesh is then aseptically prepared for placement into the dissected space. The width of the mesh should span a distance between the umbilicus and anterior superior iliac spine, minus 1 cm,

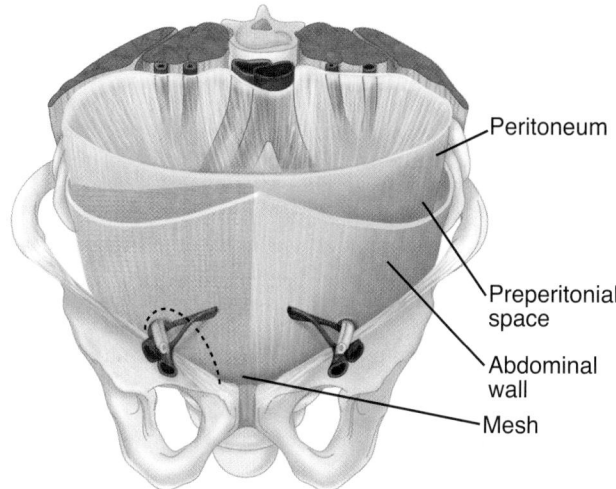

FIG. 37-22. Extensive dissection of the preperitoneal space on both sides will eventually accommodate the large prosthesis shown replacing the transversalis fascia.

preperitoneal structures such as the lateral femoral cutaneous nerve and inferior epigastric vessels. Wantz's technique advocates the placement of three absorbable sutures that attach the superior border of the mesh to the anterior abdominal wall above the level of the indirect or direct defect. The location of fixation sutures includes the linea alba, linea semilunaris, and anterior superior iliac spine. Long clamps placed along the inferior border of the prosthesis facilitate flat placement along the inferior margin of the preperitoneal space (Fig. 37-23). The clamps are placed along the lower corners of the mesh and one in between. The mesh should be placed in a flat, taut position, avoiding any scrolling of the inferior border. The medial clamp is directed into the space of Retzius, the middle clamp over the pubic ramus and iliac vessels, and the lateral clamp is placed into the iliac fossa to provide coverage of the spermatic cord. The clamps are removed as the peritoneal is brought into apposition with the prosthesis. In the case of bilateral hernias, Stoppa advocates the use of a single large mesh spanning the area between the two anterior superior iliac spines minus 2 cm. The height is the distance between the umbilicus and the pubis. The large mesh requires the application of eight clamps to the lower border to facilitate proper placement. Although the approach provides excellent coverage and reinforcement of the preperitoneal space, postoperative pain and recovery is a significant consideration (Fig. 37-24).

Iliopubic Tract Repair The iliopubic tract repair was popularized by Nyhus and Condon following extensive anatomic study detailing the importance of the iliopubic tract. The preperitoneal approach does not allow for visualization of the inguinal ligament; however, the iliopubic tract serves an analogous function in the preperitoneal space by providing a strong point of fixation. The repair combines a preperitoneal tissue-based repair with the implantation of mesh. Access to the preperitoneum is gained through a transverse abdomi-

and the height should be approximately 14 cm. Variations of mesh preparation include an intact mesh vs. a slit mesh. A slit in the lateral aspect accommodates the spermatic cord, similar to mesh placement in the Lichtenstein tension-free repair. Splitting of the mesh creates a small defect in its integrity, which may predispose it to a hernia recurrence. Proponents for a slit or keyhole argue that mesh positioning is optimal and obviates the need for fixation sutures. Fixation is an important consideration when avoiding

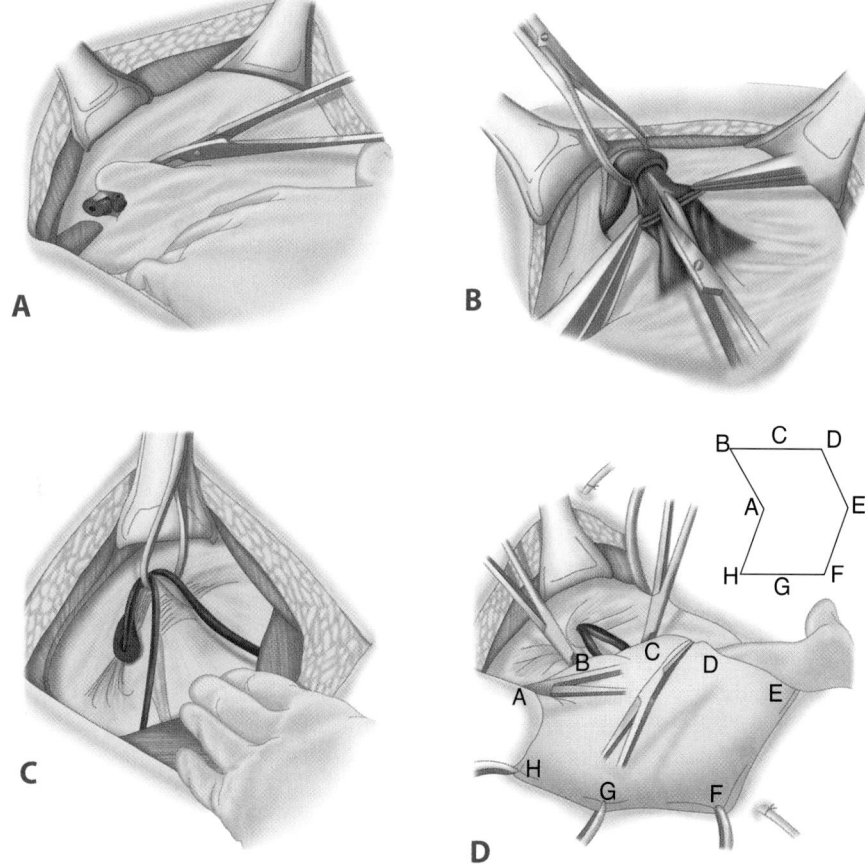

FIG. 37-23. A. A long indirect sac is isolated from the cord structures without disturbing the distal aspect. The sac is (**B**) divided, closed with sutures, and (**C**) dissected proximally from the cord structures. This allows the placement of the prosthesis deep in the preperitoneal space (**D**) without the possibility of roll-up.

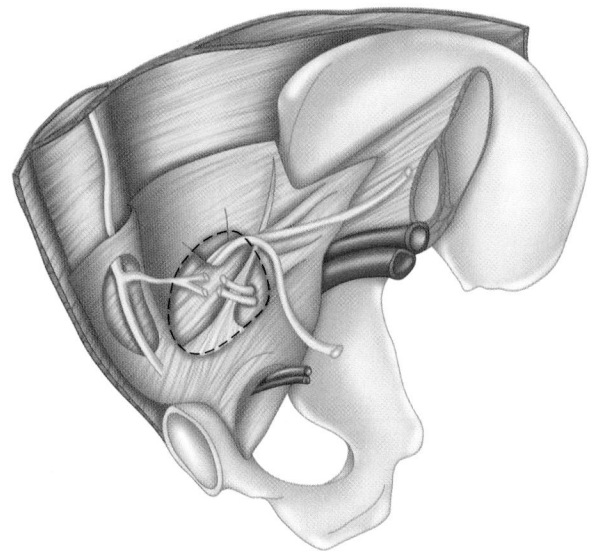

FIG. 37-24. Final appearance of Wantz's unilateral giant prosthetic reinforcement of the visceral sac.

nal incision two fingerbreadths above the pubic symphysis. The anterior rectus sheath is incised and the rectus abdominis is retracted medially to expose the posterior aspect of the sheath. The internal and external oblique muscles and the transversus abdominis muscle are also incised to reach the transversalis fascia (Fig. 37-25). The preperitoneal exposure and dissection is similar to other open preperitoneal techniques. Reconstruction of the inguinal floor is then enacted by suturing the transverse aponeurotic arch to Cooper's ligament and the iliopubic tract using interrupted sutures (Fig. 37-26). By suturing the transversalis fascia to Cooper's ligament, the femoral canal is obliterated. Around the internal ring, the leaflets of the transversalis fascia are sutured to the iliopubic tract to tighten the ring. The nature of the repair therefore specifically addresses femoral, direct, and indirect hernia defects. A mesh prosthesis is then implanted over the

posterior aspect of the transversalis fascia and fixed to Cooper's ligament and above the iliopubic tract.

Kugel Repair The Kugel repair aims to maximize on the preperitoneal approach while minimizing on the length of the skin and fascia incision.[29] An oblique skin incision is made approximately 2 to 3 cm above the internal ring, which is estimated to be halfway between the anterior superior iliac spine and the pubic tubercle. The 3- to 4-cm incision is made one third lateral and two thirds medial between these two structures. The abdominal wall is opened using a series of muscle splitting incisions similar to open appendectomy. The external oblique aponeurosis is incised, the internal oblique muscle is bluntly divided, and the transversalis fascia is opened vertically for 3 cm, avoiding the internal ring. Blunt dissection is then performed within the preperitoneal space, deep to the inferior epigastric vessels. Cooper's ligament, the pubic tubercle, the iliac vessels, and the hernia sac are palpated to aid in anatomic identification. Hernia sac dissection and division, if necessary, is similar to other open preperitoneal approaches. Similarly, dissection along the spermatic cord should be carried proximally enough to accommodate a mesh that will adequately cover the internal ring. In Kugel's view, placing the patch sufficiently posterior is the most critical part of preventing recurrences; however, the preperitoneal pocket should be dissected only up to the point that it barely accepts the mesh prosthesis. The pocket should extend 3 cm medial to the pubic tubercle and lateral to the lateral extent of the transversalis incision. The procedure is inextricably linked to a specially designed mesh. The 8×12 cm mesh is composed of two sheets of polypropylene, with a slit in the anterior layer that accommodates a single digit or instrument during mesh positioning. The mesh can be deformed to fit through the small incision, yet the self-retaining single monofilament fiber around the periphery of the mesh allows the mesh to spring open, assuming its normal shape. Additional features of the mesh promote anchoring and incorporation of tissue into the mesh. The mesh is oriented parallel to the inguinal ligament, with three fifths sitting above the level of the inguinal ligament. The transversalis fascia is closed with a single absorbable stitch, incorporating the anterior surface of the mesh to prevent migration. The remainder of the wound is closed in successive layers using absorbable sutures. Kugel's experience of nearly 1500 patients demonstrates excellent recurrence rates (0.4%); however, these have not been

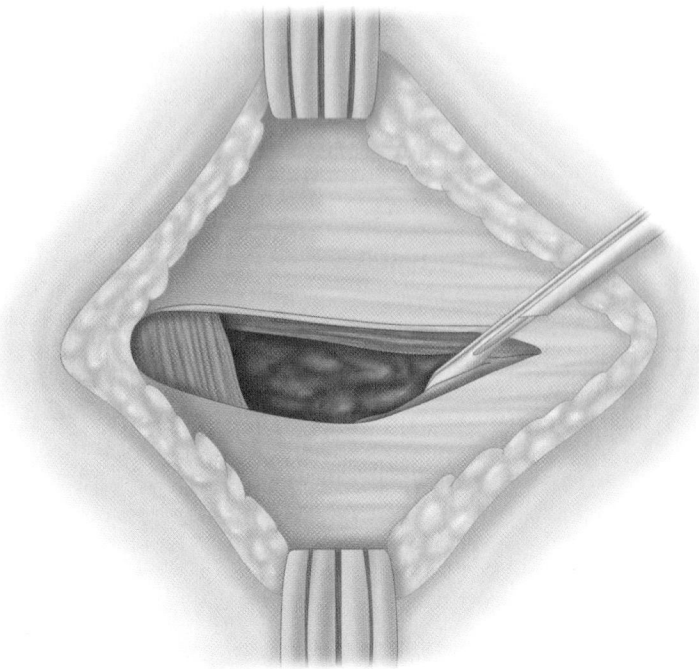

FIG. 37-25. Iliopubic tract repair. Initial incision. The lateral side of the anterior rectus sheath has been opened, and the rectus muscle is visible. The external oblique, internal oblique, and transversus abdominis muscles are incised to expose the transversalis fascia.

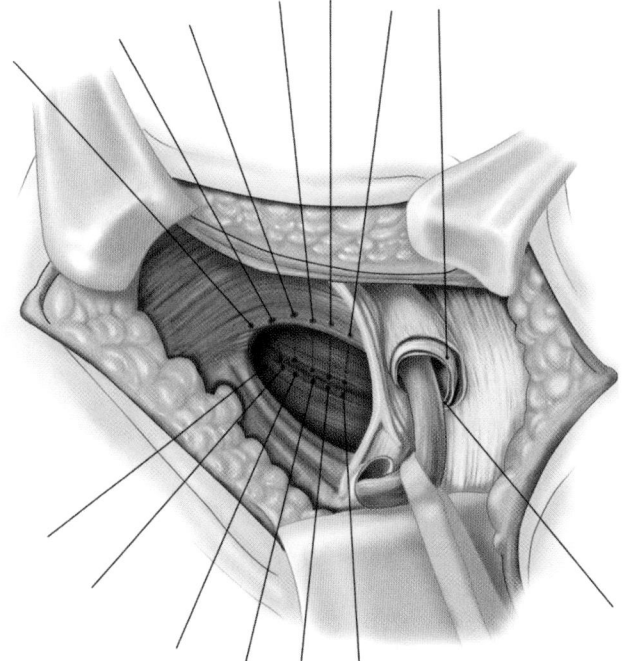

FIG. 37-26. Iliopubic tract repair. Direct hernia. The key to the repair is to suture the transverse aponeurotic arch to the iliopubic tract inferiorly. In this case, the internal ring is particularly large, so a suture is also placed lateral to the internal ring.

reproduced owing to a steep learning curve associated with blind placement of the patch.[30]

Prolene Hernia System The Prolene hernia system technology was constructed to take advantage of the benefits of the anterior and preperitoneal repair using an open approach. The mesh consists of two large flaps (an onlay and an underlay patch) with an intervening connector (Fig. 37-27). The underlay is positioned in the preperitoneal space while the overlay rests along the floor of the inguinal canal. Exposure of the inguinal canal is identical to standard open approaches. The preperitoneal space is entered according to the site of the defect. Indirect hernia sacs are dissected from the spermatic cord and sponge dissection of the preperitoneal space is subsequently performed through the internal ring. In the case of direct defects, the transversalis fascia is opened to provide for preperitoneal dissection. The underlay portion of the mesh is then placed through the hernia defect, thereby overlapping direct, indirect, and femoral site defects. The overlay flap reinforces the inguinal floor similar to a tension-free repair. Only the anterior layer of the mesh is secured, using three to four interrupted sutures to the pubic tubercle, inguinal

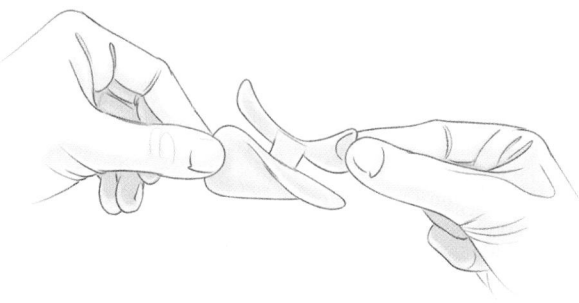

FIG. 37-27. The Prolene hernia system consists of two large flaps of mesh with an intervening connector.

ligament, and internal oblique muscle. As well, the overlay flap contains a slit to accommodate the spermatic cord. The bilayer connector prevents mesh migration and ensures correct positioning. The greatest advantage to this technique is that it adds a preperitoneal reinforcement to an otherwise open tension-free repair.

Laparoscopic

Laparoscopic inguinal hernia repairs capitalize on the preperitoneal approach using a series of small incisions. The predominant techniques include transabdominal preperitoneal (TAPP) and totally extraperitoneal (TEP) repair, with intraperitoneal only mesh (IPOM) performed the least. The operating room setup is identical for both TAPP and TEP procedures. Mobilization of intra-abdominal and preperitoneal contents is optimally achieved by placing the patient in a Trendelenburg position. To this end, the monitors are placed at the foot of the bed, allowing the surgeon and assistant to view the procedure in a direct line of sight with instrumentation. The surgeon generally is positioned on the contralateral side to the hernia in question, although bilateral hernias can be repaired from either side. An assistant will occupy a position opposite the surgeon. The patient's arms are tucked at their sides and efforts must be made to adequately secure the patient during mobilization to the Trendelenburg position. Before performing the surgical prep, the bed should be tested to ensure the patient is fully secured and can hemodynamically tolerate being in Trendelenburg during the procedure. The scrub nurse and instrumentation table can be positioned on either side of the bed or at the foot of the bed. Figure 37-28 demonstrates a typical operating room setup for laparoscopic inguinal hernia.

Transabdominal Preperitoneal Procedure

Unilateral or bilateral inguinal hernias can be assessed and repaired using a combination of three trocars. The authors' preference is for a 12-mm trocar in the umbilicus and one 5-mm trocar in each lower quadrant, slightly below the level of the umbilicus. Care must be taken to avoid injuring the inferior epigastric arteries when placing the 5-mm trocars (Fig. 37-29). Initially, a 12-mm trocar is placed through the umbilicus. The 12-mm trocar allows use of a 10-mm camera and allows for easy introduction of a prosthetic material into the abdominal cavity. A 12-mm vertical incision is performed through the umbilicus and sharp dissection is performed to clear the subcutaneous attachments around the umbilical ring. A Kelly hemostat is then inserted through the umbilical ring and gently widened to allow placement of a blunt 12-mm trocar. The surgeon's fifth finger is then swept circularly beneath the umbilical ring to ensure no adhesions or intestinal contents are present. Sutures are placed in the fascia around the umbilical ring to anchor the trocar. Once the trocar is fixed in place, pneumoperitoneum is instilled to a level of 15 mmHg. A 5-mm trocar is then placed in each lower quadrant. The patient is then placed in a Trendelenburg position and the pelvic anatomy is inspected.

Initial inspection relies on identification of the bladder, median and medial umbilical ligaments, external iliac, and inferior epigastric vessels. The inguinal hernia can then be identified in relation to this anatomy. The peritoneum at the medial umbilical ligament is then grasped and incised with endoscopic scissors. The incision should be at least 3 to 4 cm above the hernia defect to allow placement of a large mesh and allow for closure of the peritoneal defect at the conclusion of the procedure. The incision is then carried laterally along a horizontal plane until the anterior superior iliac spine is reached. The peritoneum is retracted inferiorly to reveal the areolar tissue of the preperitoneum. Sharp and blunt dissection is then performed to dissect free the preperitoneal space, the goal being to expose cord structures. Rarely is electrocautery necessary to aid in dissection. The symphysis pubis can then be used to identify Cooper's ligament lateral to it. Direct hernia sacs are reduced during the creation of the peritoneal flap. Indirect hernia sacs must be dissected free from the cord structures. Before handling the cord and hernia sac, the vessels of the spermatic cord and vas deferens must be identified. Care is

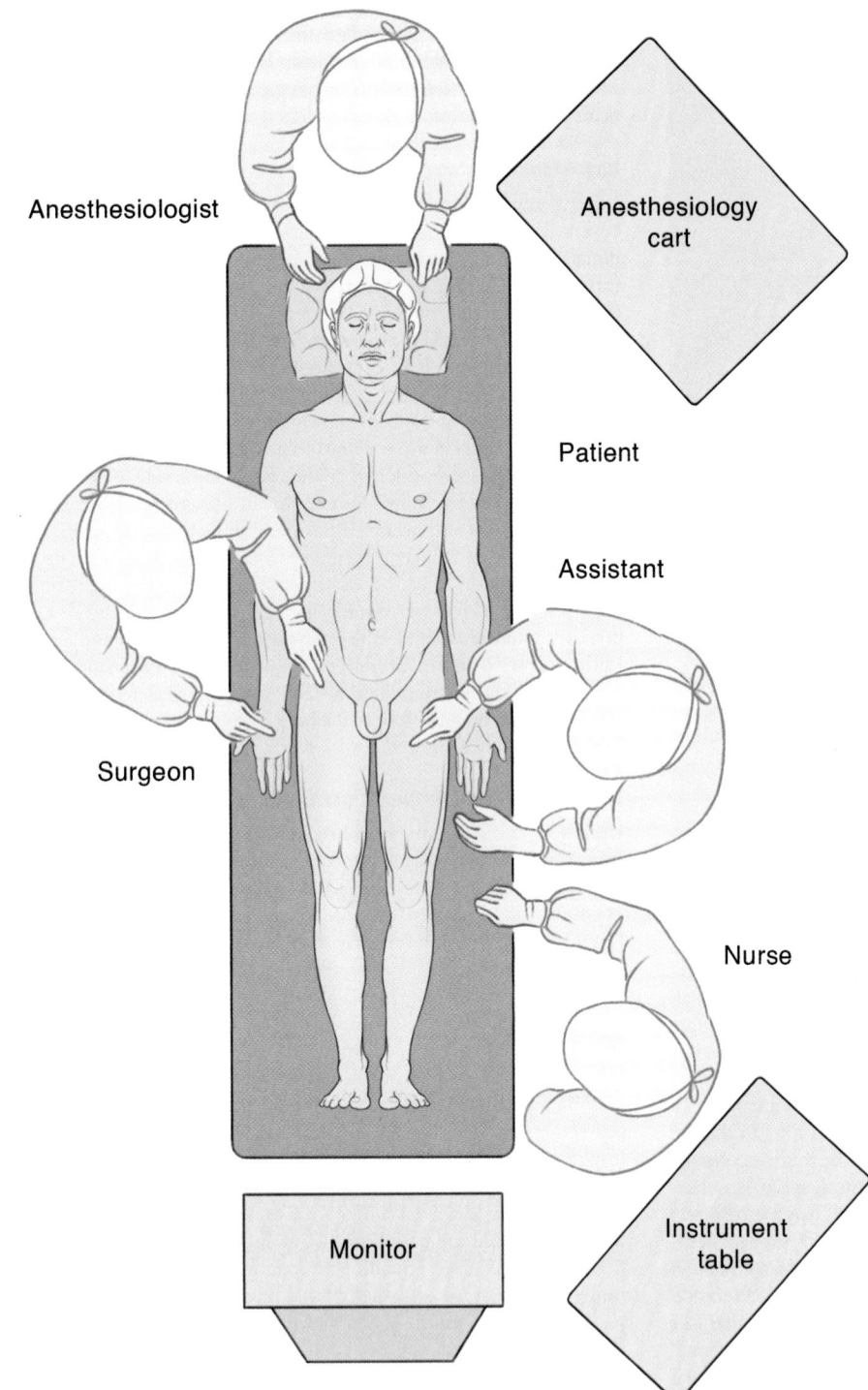

FIG. 37-28. Room setup and positioning of the patient and surgical team.

taken to avoid grasping these structures, as permanent injury may ensue. The hernia sac, which is usually located anterior to cord structures, is grasped and elevated superiorly from the cord. A space inferior to the cord is created through blunt dissection. The sac is then dissected from the cord and the cord is skeletonized, including removal of any lipomas of the cord. Densely adherent hernia sacs may need to be divided to avoid injury to cord structures. The peritoneum must be dissected inferiorly to the level of divergence of the vas deferens and spermatic vessels to allow a large, flat coverage of mesh.

Once the preperitoneum has been adequately dissected, the mesh prosthesis can be placed. The mesh usually measures 10 × 15 cm (4 × 6 in), to completely cover the myopectineal orifice, and can

be scrolled in a lengthwise fashion to facilitate easier handling. The mesh is then rolled lengthwise and placed through the 12-mm trocar with the aid of an instrument. The mesh is then unrolled in the preperitoneal space and secured to Cooper's ligament medially using a spiral tacker. The surgeon places the spiral tacker on the mesh and directs it into the abdominal wall. The other hand is able to palpate the end of the instrument and thus stabilizes the groin from the exterior. The mesh is then pulled relatively taut and fixed lateral to the anterior superior iliac spine, above the level of the iliopubic tract. The mesh can be further fixed along its superior edge, above the iliopubic tract, with great care taken to avoid fixation near the inferior epigastric vessels. Being able to palpate a spiral tacker with the surgeon's other hand avoids placement of

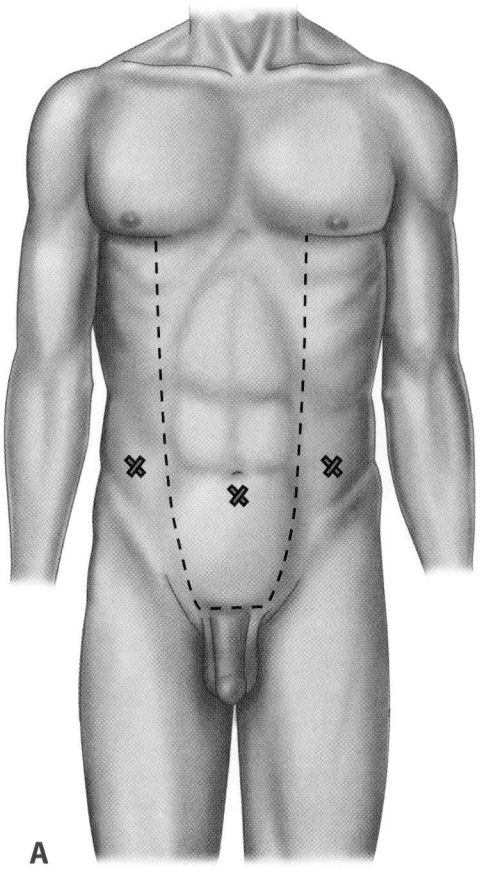 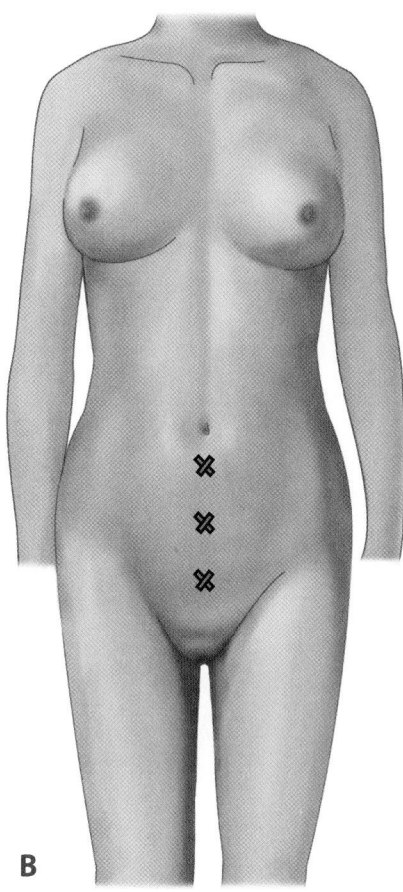

FIG. 37-29. Trocar placement for (**A**) transabdominal preperitoneal repair and (**B**) totally extraperitoneal repair.

spiral tacks below the iliopubic tract, thereby avoiding injury to the lateral cutaneous nerve of the thigh or the femoral branch of the genitofemoral nerve. Variations of this technique include the absence of fixation in situations where the mesh is preformed to the preperitoneal space or is very large. As well, some prostheses are fashioned with an extra amount of mesh to place around the cord structures, mimicking an open tension-free approach. The mesh can also be split by the surgeon if this is desired.

The mesh is then manipulated to lay flat within the preperitoneal space. The peritoneal edge is then grasped and returned to its normal anatomic position, while the mesh is stabilized. Closure of the peritoneal defect can be performed using intracorporeal suturing or through the use of spiral tacks. One of the greatest difficulties encountered in the TAPP procedure is the reapproximation of the peritoneum. Through the course of dissection, the peritoneum may become denuded and prevent complete reconstruction and complete coverage of the mesh implant. Any tears in the peritoneum, especially if the hernia sac was divided, should be repaired to avoid direct contact of mesh with intestinal contents or acute obstruction of intestinal contents within these defects. The abdomen is desufflated, the trocars are removed, and the umbilical ring is reconstructed to avoid future umbilical herniation.

Despite the shortcomings of the TAPP procedure, namely injury to intra-abdominal organs and difficulty in closing the peritoneal dissection, there are a number of clinical scenarios where the usefulness of the procedure is evident. These include the possibility of repairing an inguinal hernia during the course of a laparoscopic procedure for an unrelated ailment. Furthermore, large hernias, ambiguous diagnoses, and a history of lower abdominal procedure may make TAPP more attractive than TEP. Lastly, the inguinal anatomy associated with TAPP is more obvious than

that of its counterpart, TEP, and the presence of a large working space affords the surgeon a greater degree of motion.

Totally Extraperitoneal Procedure

The authors' preference is the TEP, as it is superior to TAPP on a number of levels. The TEP procedure allows the surgeon to work within the preperitoneal space, between the posterior aspect of the rectus abdominis and posterior rectus sheath, thereby circumventing penetration of the abdominal cavity. Inherent to this approach is a decrease in the possibility of injury to intra-abdominal organs and vascular structures. As well, the incidence of trocar site herniation is decreased owing to the preservation of the posterior rectus sheath. As importantly, TEP obviates the need for peritoneal closure and therefore may be performed faster than a TAPP. In situations involving large inguinal hernias or densely adherent tissue from previous abdominal operations, rents may result in the peritoneum, inadvertently exposing the intra-abdominal environment. These defects may be simply closed using tacks, sutures, or an endoloop. When the operation is wholly performed within the preperitoneal space, the incidence of bowel obstruction and mesh erosion into bowel in the proximity is insignificant compared to that of TAPP.

The preperitoneal dissection in TEP is identical to TAPP; however, access to the preperitoneal space is what makes the TEP unique and superior to TAPP. The initial incision is made horizontally, slightly inferior to the umbilicus. Subcutaneous tissue is dissected until the anterior rectus sheath is exposed. The anterior rectus sheath is opened away from the linea alba to expedite identification of the rectus abdominis. The muscle is then retracted laterally and superiorly to allow placement of a dissecting balloon. The balloon is advanced toward the symphysis pubis and then insufflated under direct vision, with the assistance of a 30° laparoscope. The dissecting

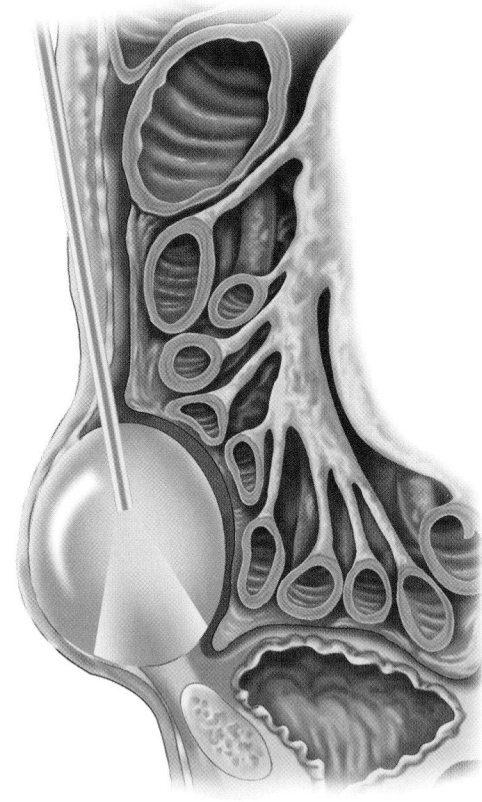

FIG. 37-30. Balloon dissection of the preperitoneal space in a totally extraperitoneal herniorrhaphy.

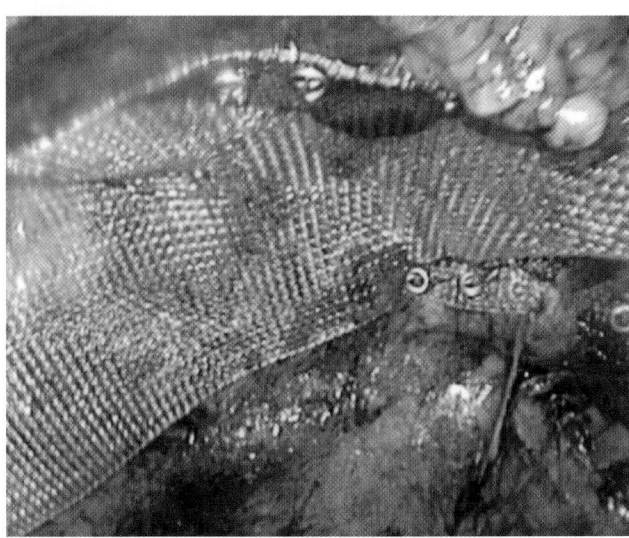

FIG. 37-32. Mesh placement using the totally extraperitoneal repair.

balloon is inflated slowly to provide the initial dissection of the preperitoneal space (Fig. 37-30). The dissecting balloon is then replaced with a 12-mm trocar containing a balloon that maintains pneumoperitoneum. Carbon dioxide is then insufflated to a level of 15 mmHg. Two additional 5-mm trocars are placed in the lower midline (see Fig. 37-29). One is placed suprapubically, while the other is placed immediately distal to the structural balloon. The patient is then placed in a Trendelenburg position and the operation proceeds in an identical fashion to a TAPP (Figs. 37-31 and 37-32). During the course of the operation, an inadvertent rent may result in the peritoneum leading to loss of working space. Usually, the intra-abdominal and preperitoneal pressure will equilibrate with no loss of

exposure. However, if the preperitoneal space becomes limited from billowing of the peritoneum, the defects may be closed using an endoloop. Alternatively, the operation can be converted to a TAPP; however, this is rarely necessary. The tears in the peritoneum should be repaired before conclusion of the operation to prevent mesh erosion or bowel obstruction. Following mesh placement, the preperitoneal space is desufflated slowly and in a deliberate manner under direct vision to ensure proper mesh positioning. Once trocars are removed, the anterior rectus sheath is reclosed with an interrupted suture.

Laparoscopic Bilateral Inguinal Hernia Repair

In the case of bilateral inguinal hernias approached via TAPP, two separate peritoneal incisions are advised, with a bridge of tissue remaining in the midline, in case of the presence of a patent urachus. In any case, adequate mobilization of tissue must still be performed in the midline, with placement and overlap of the mesh in the midline to prevent a recurrence. Bilateral inguinal hernias approached via TEP are exempt from this consideration, as the entire preperitoneum can more easily be exposed. The authors prefer to perform the TEP, with a bilateral dissection before placing mesh on either side.

Intraperitoneal Onlay Mesh Procedure

In contrast to TAPP and TEP, the IPOM allows for a laparoscopic approach without dissection of the preperitoneal space. Port placement and identification of the inguinal hernia is identical to TAPP. At this point, the hernia sac is not reduced, and the preperitoneal space is not cleared. Instead, a prosthesis is applied directly over the hernia defect and fixed in place with sutures or spiral tacks. The anchors are placed in much the same manner as in other laparoscopic approaches. Following its introduction in 1991, enthusiasm for the procedure was high, in that the procedure could be performed quickly and across a variety of laparoscopic skill levels. However, enthusiasm waned due to significant drawbacks of the operation. The lack of preperitoneal dissection, which significantly reduces operative time, resulted in increased neuralgias, secondary to nonidentification of the lateral cutaneous nerve of the thigh and genitofemoral nerve. As well, the early recurrence rate was unacceptably high at 11%.[31] In theory, intra-abdominal pressure would maintain the position of the mesh and prevent hernia recurrence; however, due to the nature of fixation, migration is a significant consideration.

The use of polypropylene mesh as the prosthetic device in IPOM added further postoperative risk such as bowel adherence and possible eventual erosion into contiguous structures. Recent ad-

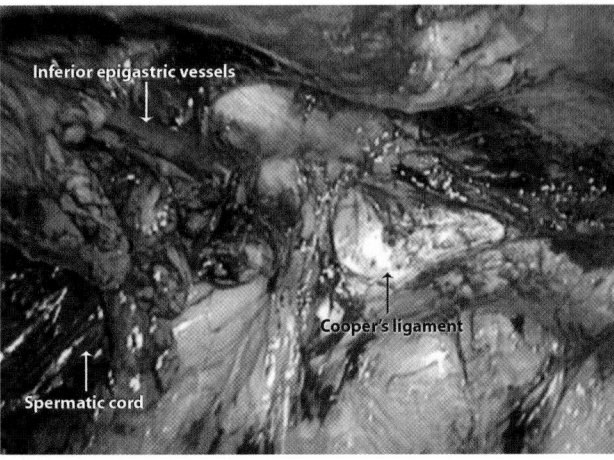

FIG. 37-31. Laparoscopic view of the preperitoneum following dissection.

vances in prosthetic material technology have attempted to circumvent this problem. The development of polyester mesh coated with porcine collagen on one surface allows for cellular integration on the polyester surface, while providing a barrier to intestinal contents on the other side until reperitonealization can take place. In a small study of IPOM using this mesh, no postoperative complications were reported in up to 2 years of follow-up. Recurrence rates also were found to be zero.[32] Although current evidence clearly favors TAPP and TEP as the preferred laparoscopic approaches to inguinal hernia, there is yet to be defined an important role for IPOM in situations where preperitoneal dissection cannot be safely accomplished. These situations include disruption of the preperitoneal space by previous procedures such as laparoscopic/robotic prostatectomy or laparoscopic inguinal hernia repair. The risks associated with preperitoneal dissection in a previously operated space may outweigh the risks inherent to IPOM, thereby making it an attractive procedure. As well, in the course of a laparoscopic prostatectomy and concurrent inguinal hernia repair, extensive peritoneal dissection may prohibit adequate closure of the peritoneal flap over the mesh prosthesis. In this case, mesh placement is akin to that of IPOM and considerations for mesh choice must take into account possible complications. To this end, an inert prosthesis such as expanded polytetrafluoroethylene may be useful, albeit considering the increased recurrence rates.[33]

Conservative Management

The definitive treatment of all hernias is surgical repair. A hernia defect will not decrease in size, but likely increase and possibly progress to incarceration or strangulation of the sac's contents. Surgery can be delayed or avoided in situations where the patient's medical status prohibits operative treatment. Conservative management is aimed at alleviating symptoms related to the inguinal hernia, such as pain, pressure, and protrusion of abdominal contents. Simple maneuvers include assuming a recumbent position, which aids in self-reduction of the hernia. A truss, an elastic belt or brief that aims to keep the hernia reduced, may also be worn; however, its use does not prevent hernia progression or incarceration. A truss may provide relief in up to 65% of patients; however, many will use it only intermittently as it does not provide continuous control of the hernia and may actually lead to an increased rate of hernia incarceration.[34]

More commonly, conservative management is applied to asymptomatic or minimally symptomatic inguinal hernias. Although surgery is the only definitive therapy for an inguinal hernia, there is debate concerning the need for surgical repair of all inguinal hernias. Of course, the main concern for asymptomatic hernias is their likelihood of incarceration or strangulation. The natural history of an inguinal hernia is not well known and has been minimally studied, thus making it difficult to quantify the number of inguinal hernias that will become emergencies. One study has calculated the cumulative probability of developing a strangulated hernia to be 2.8% at 3 months for an inguinal hernia, and rising to 4.5% after 2 years. The figures were much higher for development of a strangulated femoral hernia at 3 months and 2 years, 22 and 45%, respectively.[35] Although the cumulative probability continues to rise, it appears that the risk of incarceration per year decreases in the first year. This is likely due to the presence of a smaller hernia defect initially, which may hinder reduction of intestinal contents. As the size of the defect enlarges, reduction becomes easier, although incarceration can occur with large amounts of intra-abdominal contents and dense adherence to the hernia sac.

Historical data examining large populations of patients with inguinal hernias have provided limited data as to the risk of incarceration. One of the earliest studies from 1896 involved 8633 patients, of which 242 complications such as incarceration or strangulation were recorded. A number of medical conditions were also assessed within a large population of Colombians, including the risk of hernia complication. In both studies, the yearly risk of incarceration or

strangulation was calculated to be approximately 0.3%.[36] Perhaps the most compelling data to quantify the risk of hernia complication resulted from a randomized multicenter trial comparing 720 patients with asymptomatic or minimally symptomatic inguinal hernias. These patients were randomized to either receive surgical therapy (Lichtenstein tension-free repair) or undergo watchful waiting. At 2 years follow-up, pain and inability to perform usual activities, the primary outcomes, were found to be equal between both groups. More importantly, the safety of a watchful waiting strategy was confirmed by the incidence of incarceration (0.3%), concluding that conservative management of asymptomatic or mildly symptomatic hernias carried small risk.[37] However, the study was limited by relatively short-term follow-up, considering that lifetime risk of incarceration increases with age. Considering that nearly 40% of the study participants did not receive the therapy to which they were randomized, it is appropriate that results were based on an intention to treat analysis. In this manner, the study assesses the therapeutic strategy, rather than comparing two distinct forms of treatment. The study also determined that the risk of complications in the surgical group was similar to the conservatively managed group at 2-year follow-up. Therefore, not only is watchful waiting a safe and acceptable option, but the delay of surgical therapy does not place the patient at a higher risk for complications.

Emergent

The indications for emergent inguinal hernia repair are incarcerated and strangulated inguinal hernias, as well as sliding hernias. By definition, an incarcerated hernia is one that cannot be reduced. Reasons for incarceration include a large amount of intestinal contents within the hernia sac, dense and chronic adhesions of hernia contents to the sac, and a small neck of the hernia defect in relation to the sac contents. The common factor that predisposes these aforementioned hernia syndromes to emergent operation is compromise of intestinal contents.

An incarcerated inguinal hernia without the sequelae of a bowel obstruction is not necessarily a surgical emergency. However, once the patient demonstrates bowel obstruction secondary to incarceration or a sliding inguinal hernia, operative intervention becomes expedited. Patients will often present with vomiting, constipation, obstipation, a distended abdomen, or combination thereof. In a sliding hernia, only one wall of a hollow viscus is present within the hernia sac. Although the lumen of the intestine is initially patent, strangulation of the knuckle of bowel may progress to localized edema and subsequent obstruction of the entire lumen. Less commonly, a sliding hernia will result from a portion of the bladder present within the hernia.

The most common presentation of small-bowel obstruction is usually secondary to previous operation and presence of adhesions. However, in the case of a patient with small-bowel obstruction and virgin abdomen, the diagnosis of carcinoma and inguinal hernia incarceration should be considered first. Physical examination is generally directed to the affected abdomen; however, the inguinal regions must be examined to rule out the presence of an incarcerated hernia. In the case of an ambiguous physical examination, radiologic evaluation such as CT should be considered early to define the source of obstruction. Failing this, diagnostic laparoscopy should be undertaken with the dual aim of diagnosing and alleviating the source of obstruction.

For known incarcerated hernias, reduction should be attempted before definitive surgical intervention. Hernias that are not strangulated and do not reduce with gentle pressure should undergo taxis. The patient is sedated and placed in a Trendelenburg position. The hernia sac is grasped with both hands, elongated, and then milked back through the hernia defect. Pressure applied to the most distal portion of the sac will cause the contents to mushroom and prevent reduction. Before attempting taxis, the patient should be made aware of potential surgery in the case of failure of the maneuver. Laparoscopy can be considered initially in the algorithm of treatment; however, most surgeons would prefer to approach incarcerated hernias with a conventional open approach.

If the blood supply to incarcerated contents becomes compromised, an incarcerated hernia becomes a strangulated hernia. These pose a significant risk to life because the strangulated contents are ischemic and may quickly lose viability. Clinical signs that indicate strangulation include fever, leukocytosis, and hemodynamic instability. The hernia bulge usually is very tender, warm, and may exhibit red discoloration. Taxis should not be applied to strangulated hernias as a potentially gangrenous portion of bowel may be reduced into the abdomen without being addressed. Before proceeding with surgery, the patient should be hemodynamically resuscitated with electrolytes, undergo nasogastric tube placement, and consideration should be given to early prophylactic IV antibiotics. Strangulated inguinal hernias should be approached using a conventional open technique. Once the hernia sac is encountered, efforts must be made to control it and prevent its inadvertent reduction into the abdominal cavity. The sac is opened to assess the viability of its contents. If viable, the contents are reduced intra-abdominally. If viability is in question, the hernia defect is expanded to alleviate the pressure on the intestinal vasculature and allow the intestine to be mobilized into the operative field. The bowel is then wrapped in warm wet towels and reassessed. Bowel viability can be assessed by bowel color, temperature, presence of peristalsis, and the Woods fluorescein test. Entrapped bowel within a femoral hernia may necessitate division of the inguinal ligament to provide for reduction and mobilization of the bowel. If the bowel is clearly ischemic and nonrecoverable, a decision must be made to resect the affected intestinal portion using the groin incision or perform a lower midline incision to increase exposure. Ideally, the ischemic portion is resected and viable portions are anastomosed to restore intestinal continuity. If the procedure becomes clean-contaminated through the resection of bowel, or if the intestine has been significantly compromised, repair of the hernia should proceed without the use of prosthetics, for fear of contamination and infection of the mesh.

Not uncommonly, an incarcerated or strangulated inguinal hernia may reduce with the administration of general anesthesia. A suspected strangulated hernia sac that reduces inadvertently during anesthesia induction, or before visual inspection by the surgeon, usually necessitates the conversion of the procedure to a laparotomy or laparoscopy to fully assess the bowel for viability. The consequences of a retained portion of ischemic bowel may lead to dire consequences for the patient's life.

Rarely, a surgeon will discover that upon entering the inguinal canal during emergent hernia treatment that no inguinal hernia exists. In these situations, strong consideration should be given to the presence of a femoral hernia. The femoral canal, located inferior to the medial inguinal ligament, is assessed for presence of an incarcerated or strangulated hernia.

Elective

The most recent paradigm shift to affect general surgery has been the adoption of laparoscopic surgery. Nearly every abdominal procedure that was commonly performed using a long abdominal incision has been supplanted with a laparoscopic variation. As with the introduction of any new technology, debates have ensued challenging the benefits of laparoscopic surgery vs. open surgery. In regard to laparoscopic inguinal hernia repair, the controversy has endured. Despite numerous data attesting to the success of laparoscopic inguinal hernia repair, general surgeons continue to question the most appropriate approach to primary unilateral inguinal hernias, whether it should be by conventional open or laparoscopic approach. The benefits of laparoscopic inguinal hernia repair for bilateral and recurrent hernias are superior to open approaches. A detailed review of the literature suggests that laparoscopic repair of primary unilateral inguinal hernias can reproduce equivalent recurrence rates demonstrated by open, tension-free repairs, and further-

more, result in less postoperative pain, reduced recovery time, and faster return to normal activities (Table 37-7). The laparoscopic technique relies on advanced instrumentation and expertise, and has the potential for intra-abdominal complications not otherwise seen with the conventional open approach. The selection of the operative approach is therefore predicated on a number of factors.

Most surgeons would agree that the laparoscopic approach to bilateral or recurrent inguinal hernias is superior to that of the conventional open approach.[38] In regard to the treatment of recurrent hernias, the posterior approach afforded by laparoscopic surgery allows the surgeon to circumvent the previously scarred tissue resulting from the initial open approach. In effect, the surgeon is able to operate in virgin tissue planes, thereby greatly lessening the arduousness of the procedure. Likewise, bilateral inguinal hernias can be treated using the same number of incisions and trocars as a unilateral inguinal hernia, in contrast to the open anterior approach, which requires two separate groin incisions. Lastly, laparoscopic repair can be used concurrently during unrelated abdominal procedures such as laparoscopic prostatectomy.[39,40]

Nonetheless, there are several contraindications to the laparoscopic technique that must be taken into consideration. Because laparoscopy must be performed using general anesthesia, the patient must be able to hemodynamically tolerate both general anesthesia and the effects of pneumoperitoneum. As well, previous lower abdominal surgery, such as prostatectomy, or lower midline incisions for other abdominal procedures, are a relative contraindication to a laparoscopic approach secondary to the presence of scarred tissue in the preperitoneal space.

The successful outcomes of a hernia operation must be balanced against the potential adverse events of that procedure when choosing the most appropriate approach. Success can be measured by examining recurrence rates, level of postoperative pain, and return to normal activities. Outcomes of laparoscopic inguinal hernia repair can be compared against conventional open techniques using these outcome measures.

The greatest reduction in hernia recurrence rates has been accomplished through the use of the tension-free repair championed by Lichtenstein.[41] Similarly, when laparoscopic inguinal hernia repair is compared to open tissue repairs, there are significantly improved rates of recurrence, postoperative pain, and return to normal activities.[42] Detractors of the minimally invasive approach often cite studies that described the early experience of the laparoscopic technique and therefore demonstrated variable outcomes. In one such study, a significantly higher recurrence rate (12.5%) was seen in the TAPP group vs. 1.9% in the giant prosthetic reinforcement of the visceral sac group.[43] The authors described concerns about the learning curve associated with mastering the laparoscopic technique, but more importantly, the study was limited by its use of TAPP, which did not allow adequate coverage of mesh medially and therefore may have predisposed the patients to increased recurrence. Secondly, the mesh was not anchored, thereby allowing migration. As the laparoscopic techniques have undergone refinement and experience with them has increased, the multitude of randomized controlled trials comparing laparoscopic hernia repair with tension-free repairs have concluded similar recurrence rates exist between the two procedures. In a study of 168 patients randomized to either TEP or Lichtenstein repair, two recurrences were identified on physical examination at 1 year in the TEP group. Although no recurrences were identified in those treated with the open tension-free repair, the results were not statistically significant. In a later study, the 5-year recurrence rates of the same group of patients was examined. Overall, both the open and laparoscopic group demonstrated good long-term results with a low rate of recurrence (three recurrences in the TEP group and four in the open group).[44,45] Similarly, a study of 200 male patients randomized to either ambulatory TEP or Lichtenstein repair demonstrated no recurrences in either group at 1-year follow-up.[46]

The controversies associated with laparoscopic inguinal hernia repair were reignited in 2004 with the publication of a randomized

TABLE 37-7 Randomized controlled trials comparing open tension-free hernia repair to laparoscopic hernia repair

Study	Intervention	Y	No. of Pts.	No. of Hernias	Follow-Up	Complications	Analgesic Use	Pain Score	Recovery	Return to Work	Quality of Life	Comments
Lau et al[46]	TEP vs. TFR	2005	200	—	1 wk, 1 y	NS	NE	Yes	Yes	Yes	NE	Decreased chronic pain in the TEP group
Neumayer et al[47]	TEP/TAPP vs. TFR	2004	1983	—	2 wk, 3 mo, 2 y	Yes	NE	Yes	Yes	NE	NE	Higher complication and recurrence rates in laparoscopic group; decreased pain and shorter recovery in the laparoscopic group
Andersson et al[44]	TEP vs. TFR	2003	168	—	1 wk, 6 wk, 1 y	NS	Yes	NS	Yes	Yes	NE	
Douek et al[87]	TAPP vs. TFR	2003	403	—	5 y	—	—	—	—	—	—	Long-term study
Bringman et al[88]	TEP vs. TFR vs. P&P	2003	299	—	20 mo	NS	Yes	—	Yes	Yes	NE	Bilateral and recurrent only (Operating time less for laparoscopic hernia repair)
Colak et al[89]	TFR vs. TEP	2003	134	—	Short term	NS	NE	Yes	Yes	NE	NE	Bilateral inguinal hernias (Cost higher for laparoscopic hernia repair)
Sarli et al[31]	TAPP vs. TFR	2001	43	—	24 h, 48 h, 7 d, long term	NE	Yes	Yes	NE	Yes	NE	
Kumar et al[90]	TEP vs. TFR	1999	50	—	Short term	—	Yes	Yes	NE	NE	NE	Recurrent inguinal hernia only
Beets et al[43]	TAPP vs. GPRVS	1999	79	108	Mean = 34 mo	NS	Yes	NE	Yes	Yes	NE	All index hernias recurrent (Operating time greater and recurrence rate higher for the TAPP repair), recurrence rate for TAPP
MRC Trial Group[91]	TAPP, TEP vs. mainly TFR	1999	928	—	1 wk, 3 mo, 1 y	Yes	NE	Yes	Yes	NE	NE	Three serious with laparoscopy (Operating time longer for laparoscopic hernia repair)
Picchio et al[92]	TAPP vs. TFR	1999	105	—	Short term	NE	NS	No	No	No	NE	Half the time
Khoury[93]	TEP vs. P&P	1998	45	315	1 wk, q4mo × 3 y	Less	Yes	NE	Yes	Yes	NE	
Heikkinen et al[94]	TEP vs. TFR	1998	45	—	Short term	NE	NE	NE	NE	Yes	NE	All patients employed (Overall cost less for laparoscopic hernia repair, cost higher for laparoscopic hernia repair)
Wellwood et al[95]	TAPP (gen) vs. TFR (local)	1998	400	—	d 1–7, 2 wk, 1 & 3 mo	—	—	Yes	Yes	Yes	Yes	
Wright et al[96]	Laparoscopic vs. TFR, Stoppa	1996	120	—	Short term	Yes	Yes	Yes	NE	NE	NE	One half the hospital stay (Shorter hospital stay for laparoscopic hernia repair)
Payne et al[97]	TAPP vs. TFR	1994	100	100	1 wk, ?	—	Yes	—	Yes	Yes	NE	

GPRVS = giant prosthetic reinforcement of the visceral sac; MRC = Medical Research Council; NE = not evaluated; NS = no significant difference; P&P = plug and patch; TAPP = transabdominal extraperitoneal repair; TEP = totally extraperitoneal repair; TFR = tension-free repair.

controlled trial performed by the VA Cooperative Study. A total of 1983 patients underwent either a laparoscopic (TAPP or TEP) or open (Lichtenstein tension-free) operation. One of the most significant findings was a significantly increased recurrence rate of primary unilateral hernias at 2 years within the laparoscopic group vs. the open group (10.1% vs. 4.9%).[47] In addition, the overall complication rate was higher in the laparoscopic group vs. open (39% vs. 33.4%). The complications within the laparoscopic group were not subdivided according to whether a TAPP or TEP was performed. A larger proportion of intraoperative complications also were noted within the laparoscopic group, namely those related to general anesthesia and vascular injury. The laparoscopic group was found to have less pain on the operative day and 2 weeks later, as well as an earlier return to normal activities. A post-hoc evaluation of the surgeons' self-reported experience compared to recurrence rates demonstrated a statistically significant reduced recurrence rate for those that had performed >250 laparoscopic procedures. The complication rate was not included in this post-hoc evaluation. A review of the overall literature on the subject of laparoscopic vs. open hernia repair does conclude that both procedures are equivalent in their recurrence rates.[48] Much of the data, however, originates from highly specialized surgery centers and may not have widespread application to community hospital settings.

One of the greatest benefits of the tension-free repair has been the ease with which optimal outcomes can be reproduced by a wide array of surgeon experience and trainee level. The success of certain tissue repairs such as the Shouldice technique relies on the number of cases the surgeon has performed and the degree of specialization of the surgery center. With increasing experience, the recurrence rate for Shouldice repairs decreased from 9.4% to 2.5% after the performance of six procedures.[49] The VA cooperative study suggested that proficiency in laparoscopic inguinal hernia repair is achieved following completion of 250 procedures; however, much lower case volumes necessary to master the technique have been reported. One of the main edicts of a successful hernia repair is proficient knowledge of inguinal anatomy. Lal and colleagues proposed studying the posterior groin anatomy through the performance of open preperitoneal repair (Stoppa technique). After the performance of five cases, the remainder of the 61 patients were approached using a TEP technique. The first five laparoscopic inguinal hernia repairs resulted in a conversion to open Stoppa repair, with an additional conversion later in the study. Of the 50 laparoscopic inguinal hernia repairs that were completed successfully, no recurrences were identified in up to 2-year follow-up.[50] Retrospective reassessment of one group's 1700 TAPP procedures indicated that following the completion of 100 procedures, the recurrence rate decreased from 9 to 2.9%. Coinciding with this threshold of cases, the surgeons also adopted use of a much larger mesh.[51] Many would agree that routine use of laparoscopy is necessary to achieve and maintain optimal results. The training necessary to reach this level of expertise should be attained through a dedicated fellowship, specialized surgery center, or through repetition of the procedure.

In addition to recurrence rates, success of an inguinal hernia repair can be measured through degree of postoperative pain and return to normal activities. Although the VA Cooperative study described significantly less short-term postoperative pain in the laparoscopic group, the pain scores were equivalent between the open and laparoscopic group at 3 months. Nevertheless, a number of studies have demonstrated a significantly decreased incidence of chronic pain following laparoscopic repair. Overall, the incidence of chronic pain was approximately 11% in a pooled proportion meta-analysis. In randomized controlled trials comparing open to laparoscopic inguinal hernia repair, the presence of chronic pain was increased in the open cohorts.[52] Possible explanations for the difference may pertain to mode of mesh fixation. In open tension-free repairs, an extensive mesh fixation is necessary, including placement of sutures into the periosteum of the pubic symphysis. The problem of entrapment of the lateral cutaneous nerve of the thigh or the femoral branch of the genitofemoral nerve in laparoscopic procedures can be minimized by placement of sutures or tacks above the iliopubic tract.

Due to various socioeconomic and compensation factors, return to work has been an unreliable variable to assess success of inguinal hernia repair. Convalescence, which examines a patient's return to normal activities, has provided more sound evidence regarding recovery. In a systemic review of randomized controlled trials, the EU Hernia Trialists Collaboration reported a quicker return to various activities in the laparoscopic group in 24 trials and equal to the open group in one trial. Two trials showed a slower return to normal activity.[53] In the Cochrane Database of Systemic Reviews, all trials with said data demonstrated a faster return to normal activities in the laparoscopically treated group. This amounted to an absolute difference of 7 days shorter than in the open inguinal hernia repair group and was not limited to whether a TAPP or TEP was performed.[42] Due to the need for specialized instrumentation and longer operative times, the laparoscopic approach does entail more costs. However, considering the more rapid recovery and reduced postoperative pain, the potential financial benefit to society in the long-term may outweigh these deficiencies.

A number of effective operative therapies exist in the treatment of inguinal hernias. To attain and maintain consistent, successful outcomes, the general surgeon must have a proficient understanding of groin anatomy and be mindful of surgical principles. The application of prosthetics to effect a tension-free repair created an operation that was simple, effective, and reproducible across a range of operative experience, and reduced recurrence rates to a much lower level. Further advances in hernia treatment were part of the laparoscopic revolution, which has improved postoperative pain and shortened recovery time. Although laparoscopic repairs require more extensive training and equipment than open repairs, significant benefits can be imparted to the patient. Despite the controversies associated with laparoscopic inguinal hernia repair for primary unilateral inguinal hernias, the general surgeon must not only be cognizant, but also able to perform a variety of inguinal hernia repairs. By having more than one approach in one's armamentarium, the surgeon has the ability to choose the appropriate procedure for the problem at hand (Fig. 37-33).

RESULTS

Traditionally, the most important measure of success was the recurrence rate of the hernia, although newer measures focus on quality of life and return to normal activities. A repair that results in an asymptomatic recurrence may not be as clinically significant as a repair that imparts a significant amount of chronic pain, yet does not lead to recurrence. Recurrence rates of tissue-based repairs vary according to procedure; however, large-scale analyses continue to confirm the Shouldice repair as the most superior. Surgeons who perform a large volume of the Shouldice repair are able to demonstrate recurrence rates around 1%.[54] In less experienced hands, such low recurrence rates are not demonstrated, yet overall, recurrence rates for the Shouldice repair are consistently lower than those of the Bassini or McVay repair. Other comparative studies have demonstrated that the Shouldice repair, even with a recurrence rate near 6%, is superior to the Bassini repair (8.6% recurrence rate) and McVay repair (11.2%).[55] The introduction of the Lichtenstein tension-free repair radically reduced recurrence rates to a consistently low level. In a multi-institutional series, 3019 inguinal hernias were repaired using the Lichtenstein technique, with an overall recurrence rate of 0.2%.[56] Reports by other surgeons have confirmed the low recurrence rates, namely a 0.5% recurrence rate in 3175 patients with up to 5-year follow-up. Consistently low, easily reproducible recurrence rates eventually led to the widespread acceptance of the tension-free repair as the gold standard for open anterior approaches.[57] Discussion of recurrence rates for laparoscopic approaches is discussed in the Elective section of this chapter.

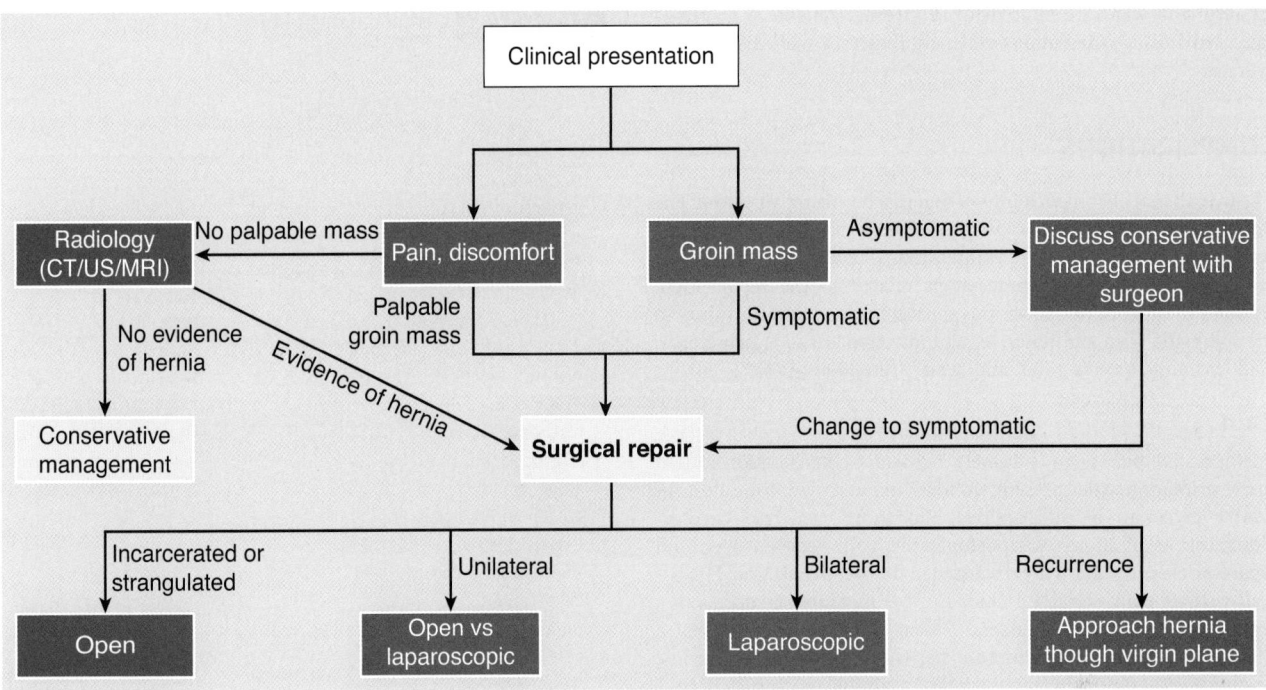

FIG. 37-33. Treatment algorithm for hernias. CT = computed tomography; MRI = magnetic resonance imaging; US = ultrasonography.

Common causes of hernia recurrence postrepair include patient, technical, and tissue factors. Patient factors that affect tissue healing include malnutrition, immunosuppression, diabetes, steroid use, and smoking. Technical factors include mesh size, prosthesis fixation, and technical proficiency of the surgeon. Tissue factors include wound infection, tissue ischemia, and increased tension within the surgical repair. Most recurrences are of the same type as the original hernia. A recurrence generally will present in a similar manner to the primary presentation of the inguinal hernia. The patient may notice the reappearance of a bulge or mass. Differential diagnosis of such a clinical presentation includes an exaggerated cough impulse, strength deficiency of the external oblique aponeurosis, persistent presence of a cord lipoma, or seroma. The lack of a bulge or mass does not exclude the possibility of a recurrence. In these cases, patients usually present with pain or pressure symptoms. It is important to delineate whether the pain is related to a recurrence or is related to a postherniorrhaphy pain syndrome because the treatment strategy is different. As with primary inguinal hernias, ambiguous physical findings can be further investigated through directed use of radiologic modalities such as ultrasound, CT, or MRI. The development of anterior and preperitoneal approaches to inguinal hernia repair has resulted in more effective treatment of recurrences. Before the introduction of laparoscopic or preperitoneal repairs, recurrence of open anterior approaches were dealt with in the same approach as the original operation. Recurrence rates of the second operation were high because dissection in scarred tissue does not allow for facile identification of the anatomic structures of the inguinal canal or the hernia recurrence.[58] Current teaching dictates that recurrent inguinal hernias should be approached via a virgin plane. That is, if the primary operation was performed using an anterior open approach, the second operation should be performed using a posterior peritoneal or laparoscopic procedure. Likewise, failed preperitoneal approaches are approached using an open anterior repair.

Difficulty arises when all approaches have been exhausted in successive repairs of the recurrent hernia. Re-entry into either space will be met with significant scarred tissue; therefore, surgeons will often approach these uncommon situations using techniques with which they are most comfortable. An advantage may be gained by using the laparoscopic approach because site of hernia recurrence can be easily visualized from the intra-abdominal perspective.[59] The hernia defect can be approached by opening peritoneum in a previously unscarred area and progressing the dissection into adhesed tissue. A decision must be made whether to attempt to remove the original prosthesis or leave it in place following hernia sac dissection. Extensive dissection of the original prosthesis may result in significant injury to the cord structures, bladder, vessels, and nerves in the vicinity. If the mesh is left in place, a second mesh may be placed as a new layer, ensuring adequate overlap of the pubic tubercle and myopectineal orifice. Oftentimes, creation of the peritoneal flap may cause it to shred and prevent it from adequately separating the new prosthesis from abdominal viscera. These situations may call for the creation of an omental flap. As well, the surgeon may choose to perform an IPOM with appropriate mesh, which effectively covers the defect and does not require peritoneal coverage, although one has to be cognizant of the increased recurrence rates associated with IPOM.

Quality of life is difficult to measure unless the study uses a validated scale. A patient's personal factors, socioeconomic status, occupation, and expectations are just some of the variables that make interpretation of quality of life measures more complicated. Quality of life, however, is invariably linked to the presence of chronic pain. Specific pain syndromes are discussed below under Pain; however, each can impact a patient's life well beyond the local effects of nerve damage. The use of pain scales such as the McGill Pain Questionnaire and University of California and San Francisco Pain Service patient questionnaire can be correlated against the short form 36 questionnaire to identify the impact of pain on functioning. In a study of 226 patients, chronic pain was found to impact social and recreational activities, as well as daily routine activities.[60] Return to work is more difficult to assess owing to varying patient motivations, occupations, secondary gain, and compensation issues. This is an extremely important issue because patients often will inquire when they can return to work. Advancements in perioperative management in anesthesia and surgical technique have dramatically reduced convalescence. The majority of hernia operations are performed on an outpatient basis, yet the average time to return to work still averages between 1 and 3 weeks.[61] Studies have attempted to compare hernia repair techniques; however, the factors responsible for return to work are multifactorial. Overall, patients with physically demanding occupations generally return to work beyond the average.

COMPLICATIONS

The overall risk of complications of inguinal hernia repair is low. The introduction of laparoscopic surgery to inguinal hernia repair has resulted in approach-specific complications, in addition to the general procedure-specific complications related to the repair itself. Complications common to various approaches include pain, injury to the spermatic cord and testes, wound infection, seroma, hematoma, bladder injury, osteitis pubis, and urinary retention (Table 37-8).

Pain

Postoperative pain is an extremely important consideration in that many primary hernias present without pain as a symptom. Postoperative pain can be subclassified into short term and chronic. Comparisons of short-term postoperative pain between open and laparoscopic procedures are discussed in the Elective section. Historically, either pain was not included in the measure of success of a repair or was difficult to assess. Recent evidence suggests that a majority of patients may indeed experience chronic pain. Chronic postherniorrhaphy pain lasts beyond 3 months and results secondary to nerve entrapment, scar tissue, or mesh adherence (Table 37-9). Identification of a specific nerve that sustained injury may be difficult to determine due to overlapping distributions. Regardless of the etiology or specific nerve, patients will usually present with common symptoms such as sharp localized pains, paresthesias, or numbness over the cutaneous distribution of the affected nerve. The ilioinguinal nerve is at considerable risk to injury during closure of the external oblique aponeurosis. The ilioinguinal, along with the iliohypogastric nerve, may also become entrapped within the mesh in tension-free repairs. Laparoscopically, the lateral femoral cutaneous nerve and the genital and femoral branches of the genitofemoral nerve are at risk when placing lateral fixation tacks below the iliopubic tract, yet the lateral femoral cutaneous nerve may too be affected by mesh entrapment. Such injury to the lateral femoral cutaneous nerve will lead to meralgia paresthetica, a "pins and needles" sensation over the lateral aspect of the thigh. It also may be associated with a specific paresthesia known as *formication*, a sensation of insects crawling on or under the skin. Routine nerve division has been advocated by some, namely within the Shouldice repair, while others continue to stress the need for nerve identification and protection. The sequelae of nerve division, such as numbness of the cutaneous distribution, may be better tolerated than the effects of nerve entrapment, such as sharp chronic pains.

A better understanding of postherniorrhaphy pain syndromes can be gained by classifying the pain into one of three syndromes: somatic, visceral, and neuropathic. *Somatic pain* is the most frequently encountered and usually is secondary to damage to ligaments and muscles. Pain that results from these injuries usually is reproduced with exertion or movement of the abdominal wall. *Visceral pain* refers to pain experienced during a visceral function such as ejaculation and may result from injury to a sympathetic nerve plexus. *Neuropathic pain* is usually a localized sharp pain that may impart a sensation of burning or tearing and indicates direct nerve damage or entrapment. Neuropathic pains may present as early as in the recovery room, where patients may complain of significant sharp pains. Somatic pains are usually treated with rest, NSAIDs, and reassurance. Neuropathic pains also are amenable to NSAIDs, but there is also a role for nerve-directed injections of steroids and anesthetics. Failing conservative management, neurectomy may be undertaken. In a series of 100 patients, of which the majority of patients experienced chronic pain following inguinal hernia repair, neurectomy at the internal ring was undertaken. The nerves were approached using an open anterior approach and then

TABLE 37-8	Complications of groin hernia repairs

Recurrence
Chronic groin pain
  Nociceptive
    Somatic
    Visceral
  Neuropathic
    Iliohypogastric
    Ilioinguinal
    Genitofemoral
    Lateral cutaneous
    Femoral
Cord and testicular
  Hematoma
  Ischemic orchitis
  Testicular atrophy
  Dysejaculation
  Division of vas deferens
  Hydrocele
  Testicular descent
Bladder injury
Wound infection
Seroma
Hematoma
  Wound
  Scrotal
  Retroperitoneal
Osteitis pubis
Prosthetic complications
  Contraction
  Erosion
  Infection
  Rejection
  Fracture
Laparoscopic
  Vascular injury
    Intra-abdominal
    Retroperitoneal
    Abdominal wall
    Gas embolism
  Visceral injury
    Bowel perforation
    Bladder perforation
  Trocar site complications
    Hematoma
    Hernia
    Wound infection
    Keloid
  Bowel obstruction
    Trocar or peritoneal closure site hernia
    Adhesions
  Miscellaneous
    Diaphragmatic dysfunction
    Hypercapnia
General
  Urinary
  Paralytic ileus
  Nausea and vomiting
  Aspiration pneumonia
  Cardiovascular and respiratory insufficiency

divided proximally as they pierced the internal oblique muscle. Symptoms such as pain radiating into the thigh and genital areas improved in 72%, with only 3% of patients reporting no improvement in symptoms.[62] More recently, neurectomies of nerves com-

TABLE 37-9	Conditions associated with chronic groin pain

Occult hernia (herniography only)
Muscle injury
Adductor strains
Tendon injury
Iliopsoas bursitis
Osteitis pubis
Pelvic stress fractures
Snapping hip syndrome
Lumbosacral disorders
Connective tissue disease
Nerve entrapment
Hip disorders
   Synovitis
   Avascular necrosis
   Osteoarthritis
   Legg-Calvé-Perthes disease
   Slipped femoral capital epiphysis
   Osteochondritis dissecans or avascular necrosis of the femoral head
   Acetabular labral tears
Prostatitis
Epididymitis
Nephrolithiasis
Urinary tract infection
Lymphadenitis
Intra-abdominal pathology
History of a previous herniorrhaphy

monly injured in inguinal hernia repairs have been attempted laparoscopically. With the patient in a lateral position, with the affected side up, the quadratus lumborum muscle is traced to the spine, where the junction of L1–L2 is identified with the assistance of fluoroscopy. Superficial dissection of the quadratus lumborum muscle leads to the identification of the proximal portion of the ilioinguinal and iliohypogastric nerves, which are then divided.[63]

Cord and Testes Injury

Injury to the spermatic cord and subsequently to the testicles is a very serious problem in the male patient. In the female, the round ligament, which occupies the inguinal canal, serves to maintain anteversion of the uterus. Injury to the artery of the round ligament or its division does not impart any clinically significant effects to the patient. The spermatic cord, on the other hand, is well vascularized and is prone to hematoma formation or ischemia with excessive handling. Male patients may experience a significant scrotal hematoma that results in a diffuse blue-black discoloration of the entire scrotum. These hematomas usually result from delayed bleeding from vascular cord structures and are self-limited. Patients should be reassured and counseled to aid resolution using intermittent warm and cold compresses.

More extensive injury to cord structures may result in ischemic orchitis or testicular atrophy. Ischemic orchitis usually presents within the first week following inguinal hernia repair. The patient may present with a low-grade fever, but more commonly with an enlarged, indurated, and painful testicle. This complication occurs in <1% of all herniorrhaphies, but increases in the reoperations for recurrent inguinal hernias.[64] Ischemic orchitis is likely caused by injury to the pampiniform plexus, not the testicular artery. Densely adherent or large hernia sacs that require extensive dissection may lead to injury of the pampiniform plexus. Reassurance, NSAIDs, and comfort measures are enacted to allow self-limited resolution of this complication. Long-term effects of ischemic orchitis are rare. Ultrasound will demonstrate the reduction of testicular blood flow to help determine whether it is testicular ischemia or necrosis. Emergent orchiectomy is rarely necessary except in the case of necrosis. Injury

to the testicular artery also may lead to testicular atrophy, which is manifest over a protracted period. Again, testicular atrophy is not a surgical emergency; however, the long-term implications to the patient are significant and irreversible. Similar to ischemic orchitis, surgery for hernia recurrence leads to increased rates of testicular atrophy. Injury to cord structures is minimized by using techniques of minimal handling of the spermatic cord and proximal ligation of large hernia sacs. Controversy exists as to whether the open distal hernia sac predisposes the patient to development of a hydrocele. Should a hydrocele result post–inguinal hernia repair, treatment is identical to primary hydroceles. Another less significant testicular complication is ptosis, secondary to the division of cremasteric muscle fibers. This complication is routinely averted in the Shouldice technique, which incorporates routine division of the cremaster muscle, by fixing the medial stump of the cremaster to the pubic tubercle.

In addition to vascular structures of the cord, complications include injury to the vas deferens, which may lead to infertility. Although transection of the vas deferens is rare, crushing or scarring of the vas deferens remains a possibility. In open inguinal hernia repairs, the vas deferens is isolated along with the cord structures using digital manipulation. The vas deferens is more likely grasped with instrumentation in the course of a laparoscopic approach and may result in a crushing injury. Transections of the vas deferens should be addressed with a urologic consult and possible early reanastomosis. Only in the case of a concurrent prostatectomy is injury to the vas deferens a minor consideration because it is otherwise divided in the course of that operation. Chronic scarring may lead to vas deferens obstruction, resulting in decreased fertility rates and a dysejaculation syndrome. The symptoms of pain and burning during ejaculation are usually self-limited and should be differentiated from other causes such as sexually transmitted diseases. Controversy exists as to whether placement of a prosthesis leads to decreased fertility rates because this complication is seen in both tension-free and tissue-based repairs.

Wound Infection

Primary inguinal hernias, which are considered clean cases, are subject to a low wound infection rate, usually 1 to 2%. Arguments have been made for the use of prophylactic antibiotics, especially in the era of the mesh repair. Owing to the large number of inguinal hernia repairs that are performed, some authors suggest that there is a significant lowering of the wound infection rate; however, it is not clinically significant. Large studies have compared wound infection rates with and without prophylactic antibiotics, with no apparent difference identified.[65,66] The goal of a recent Cochrane Database review of 6705 patients was to demonstrate the effectiveness of antibiotic prophylaxis in reducing postoperative wound infection rates in elective open inguinal hernia repair. The subgroup of patients treated with a mesh prosthesis experienced wound infection rates of 1.4 and 2.9% with and without prophylactic antibiotics, respectively. The authors cautioned that although the systematic review was not able to universally recommend the use of prophylactic antibiotics, they were also not against recommending them in situations where wound infection rates were increased.[67] Initial management of a wound infection is through use of antibiotics. Failure of medicinal treatment may necessitate incision and drainage of the wound. Polypropylene mesh is rarely removed and usually can be salvaged using conservative treatment.

Seroma

A seroma is a loculated fluid collection more commonly seen following prosthetic repairs, although seromas may result following repair of large hernias. It is perceived that the body attempts to encapsulate the foreign body through a normal reaction. In the case of large hernia sacs, the potential space that remains in the defect may fill with physiologic fluid postoperatively. Seromas will usually develop within the first week and may cause concern for the patient, who may perceive it as an early recurrence. Physical examination of the seroma will demonstrate a compressible bulge in the groin or scrotum. Seromas may be painful but are more likely uncomfortable. Aspiration of the seroma should be avoided unless it persists over a prolonged period because infection may be secondarily introduced. Warm compression may aid in resolution.

Hematoma

A hematoma may present as a localized collection or diffuse bruising over the operative site. In addition to scrotal hematomas, other sites of hematoma formation include the wound, retroperitoneum, and rectus sheath hematomas. Hematoma at the latter two sites is more commonly seen following laparoscopic repair; however, injury to the corona mortis or iliac vessels regardless of approach may present as a progressively expanding hematoma. Expansion of blood within the peritoneum or preperitoneal space is not tamponaded and may lead to a significant blood loss that is not readily apparent on physical examination. Large hematomas in the abdomin will present with pain and possibly ileus. The management of wound hematomas is expectant, yet they may rarely need to be opened for decompression.

Bladder Injury

Bladder injury may occur in open anterior inguinal hernia repairs but is a more important consideration in laparoscopic surgery. Instances where the bladder may be encountered in open surgery include sliding hernias including the bladder and previous lower abdominal surgeries such as prostate operations. Treatment involves primary closure in multiple layers with Foley catheter decompression of the bladder for 1 to 2 weeks. A confirmatory cystogram may be performed before catheter removal to confirm healing of the injury.

Osteitis Pubis

The placement of sutures or tacks within the periosteum of the pubic bone is generally avoided to prevent osteitis pubis, which is characterized by an inflammation of the pubic symphysis. Currently, the majority of cases of osteitis pubis are seen in athletes that perform repetitive kicking, jumping, or running. Outside the setting of postherniorrhaphy pubic pain, the condition can be categorized into either overload or biomechanical deficiency. Overload situations occur most commonly when an athlete exercises on hard concrete or uneven ground. Biomechanical deficiencies include muscular imbalances or gait deficiencies. The common pathogenesis involves excessive muscular physical strain on the bone that incites a lytic response. Patients usually will present with pain over the medial groin or symphysis, which is reproduced with adduction of the thigh. Diagnosis can be confirmed with a bone scan, but CT scan or MRI is usually used to rule out a possible hernia recurrence. Treatment is conservative and is aimed at symptom control. It consists of rest, ice, NSAIDs, physical therapy, and possibly, local corticosteroid injection. Rarely is surgery necessary to explore the pubic symphysis and remove a suture or tack as a possible cause of inflammation. In these cases, consultation with orthopedic surgery should be enacted for expertise with bone resection and curettage. Conservative management should be exhausted before the suggestion of an exploratory surgery. Regardless of treatment, the condition often takes a protracted course and may require 6 months to resolve.[68]

Urinary Retention

A common short-term complication of routine herniorrhaphy is urinary retention. A number of factors are responsible, the most common being choice of anesthesia. In a group of 880 patients undergoing inguinal hernia repair using only local anesthesia, the rate of urinary retention was 0.2%. In contrast, a similar group of 200 patients undergoing inguinal hernia repair using general or spinal anesthesia were found to have a 13% urinary retention rate.[69] Whereas open inguinal hernia repairs can be performed using either anesthesia, laparoscopic surgeries are dependent on general anesthesia. Other contributing factors include postoperative pain, narcotic analgesia, and bladder distention. The authors prefer to limit IV hydration, avoid prophylactic catheterization, and administer prophylactic tamsulosin. Initial treatment of urinary retention requires decompression of the bladder with short-term catheterization. Patients will generally require an overnight admission and trial of normal voiding before discharge. Failure to void normally requires reinsertion of the catheter for up to a week. Chronic requirement of a urinary catheter is rare, although prolonged catheterization is seen with advancing age.

Laparoscopic Complications

General complications of laparoscopic surgery include hypercapnia, gas embolism, pneumothorax, and paralytic ileus. In general, postoperative ileus is reduced in laparoscopic vs. open procedures. However, when considering inguinal hernia repair, the incidence of ileus is increased using the laparoscopic approach. The cause is unknown but may be secondary to the temperature of the insufflated gas or abdominal distention. Ileus also can present with complications such as a large rectus sheath hematoma or considerable pain. Treatment may require the use of a nasogastric tube. Unique laparoscopic complications of hernia repair include injuries to intra-abdominal viscera, vascular injuries, and bowel obstruction.

Visceral and Vascular Injury

The risk of visceral injury in inguinal hernia repairs was limited to hernia emergencies and sliding hernias when inguinal hernias were approached with an open anterior approach. The advent of laparoscopic inguinal hernia repair, coupled with a steep learning curve, initially increased the rate of visceral injury significantly. Increased experience and training have decreased the rates. Furthermore, by using the TEP approach, the intra-abdominal environment is avoided, and subsequently, visceral injury is reduced. Viscera at risk include small and large bowel as well as bladder. Previous lower abdominal surgeries may predispose to adhesions and thereby increase the risk of visceral injuries. A past surgical history including these types of procedures is a relative contraindication to laparoscopic inguinal hernia repair. Bowel injuries also result during the course of trocar placement. Strategies to reduce bowel injuries secondary to trocar placement include using an open Hasson technique when placing the umbilical trocar and visualization of trocars as they enter the intra-abdominal space. One of the main arguments against the use of laparoscopy for inguinal hernia repair is the need to cross into the intra-abdominal area, which otherwise would not occur in open repairs. Bowel injury also may occur secondary to arcing of electrocautery and instrument injury outside of the visual field. Because the laparoscopic view is limited, bowel injuries may present as missed injuries, which are associated with an increased mortality. If a bowel injury is suspected, the entire bowel should be inspected, possibly necessitating a conversion to open if repair is required.

Bladder injuries are less common than visceral injuries and are usually associated with a distended bladder or involvement in peritoneal adhesions. Suprapubic trocar placement in a TEP may also lead to bladder injury, but can be avoided using appropriate surgical principles. Rarely, a patent urachus will be divided during the course of peritoneal flap mobilization in a TAPP. Patient presentation is usually delayed with urine extravasation through a trocar site or peritonitis. As with bladder injuries encountered in open surgery, cystotomies must be repaired in several layers with prolonged catheterization. Preoperative prophylactic catheterization or patient-directed bladder emptying may be performed for laparoscopic cases, which decompresses the bladder and therefore places it away from contiguous structures such as Cooper's ligament and the spermatic cord. Controversy exists regarding prophylactic catheterization as the rare case of bladder injury may be outweighed by urinary retention and other urinary tract complications. Incomplete voiding secondary to benign prostatic hypertrophy may, however, necessitate catheterization.

An equally critical complication is vascular injury. Open surgery is not without vascular complications; however, the laparoscopic approach includes additional means for vascular injury such as trocar placement and dissection. Misplaced sutures in a tissue-based or tension-free repair may lead to iliac or femoral vessel injury. Laparoscopically, the most commonly injured vessels include the inferior epigastric and external iliac. Immediately inferior to the spermatic cord, the external iliac vessels can be easily identified with minimal dissection. During mesh fixation, the vessels may be difficult to visualize and become injured through placement of a tack or staple. Less likely, an inadvertent instrument injury during dissection can occur, leading to oozing or frank extravasation of blood. Inferior epigastric vessels may undergo injury during trocar placement in a TAPP. The lateral position of the two accessory trocars may coincide with the course of the inferior epigastrics. Identification of the vessels by direct visualization or transillumation should be performed to minimize the risk. Oftentimes, such an injury may go unnoticed as the trocar will tamponade bleeding. However, once the trocar is removed, a significant amount of blood can be lost. An indication of a significant vessel injury may include dripping of blood along the length of the trocar. Initial management of vascular injuries requires local compression. Definitive treatment may require conversion to open surgery, especially if a major vascular injury has occurred. Otherwise, the injury may be treated by laparoscopic clipping and division, depending on the skill of the surgeon. Inferior epigastric vessels may also be ligated with use of a percutaneous suture passer. Smaller vessels within the operative field usually respond to direct compression. The surgeon should be wary of the tamponading effects of pneumoperitoneum. If the pressure of the insufflated carbon dioxide is greater than the pressure within the vessel, bleeding will not be manifest until pneumoperitoneum is released. Such a situation is often seen with rectus sheath hematomas, where injury to the inferior epigastric vein results in a delayed presentation. Patients will present with significant diffuse pain and possible hypotension. Less severe vascular complications include trocar site and rectus sheath hematoma. Similar to open repairs, extensive dissection or injury to small vessels within the groin will lead to operative site hematomas that may extend into the scrotum.

Bowel Obstruction

Early in the course of development of the laparoscopic technique, an uncommon complication of bowel obstruction was seen, which is otherwise not evidenced in open inguinal hernia repairs. Bowel obstructions more commonly occur with TAPP, following an inadequate peritoneal closure, allowing bowel to herniate through a peritoneal defect. The theoretical advantage to TEP is the avoidance of the peritoneal space, although a missed peritoneal rent may rarely lead to a bowel obstruction. Similar to visceral injuries, bowel obstructions serve as another reason detractors of the laparoscopic approach cite to perform open inguinal hernia repairs. A second cause of bowel obstruction following laparoscopic inguinal hernia repair is umbilical trocar site herniation. The use of only a single 10- to 12-mm trocar has greatly reduced possible trocar site herniation, in addition to increased attention paid to closure of this fascial defect. The possibility of trocar site hernias using 5-mm trocars is greatly reduced. As well, the umbilical trocar in a TEP remains within the rectus sheath, which serves to protect against future herniation. The least common cause of bowel obstruction remains adherence to the implanted prosthesis. Again, incomplete peritoneal closure exposes the highly adherent mesh to intra-abdominal contents, predisposing to adhesions, obstructions, and possibly erosion.

PROSTHESIS CONSIDERATIONS

The purpose of a prosthetic in hernia repairs is to reconstitute strength to the weakened structures. Before the introduction of a mesh prosthesis for clinical use, tissue-based repairs were considered the gold standard. Refinements in mesh technology resulted in widespread application of mesh to tension-free anterior repairs, as well as preperitoneal repairs. Results of mesh-based hernia repairs have consistently been superior to that of tissue-based repairs, leading them to become the gold standard. Concerns related to mesh include rejection, carcinogenesis, and host reaction; however, the widespread implementation of mesh in hernia repairs has demonstrated that prosthesis use is safe, in addition to its effectiveness. Early hernia repairs, both open tension-free and preperitoneal procedures, suffered increased recurrence rates due to too small a prosthesis. Mesh prosthetics produced commercially now account for this by providing a larger size that may be trimmed if necessary. Controversy remains regarding the extent of mesh fixation necessary.

Mesh Choice

One of the most commonly used prosthetics in inguinal hernia repairs is polypropylene, first introduced by Usher in the 1950s. Since that time, numerous advances in mesh technology have led to a variety of prosthetics available for hernia repairs. These can be grouped according to their materials and subsequent bioreactivity, namely nonabsorbable, partially absorbable, and biologic. These factors alone do not account for the behavior of a mesh once it is implanted. Other considerations include its thickness, weight, architecture of fibers, and overall strength of the material. An ideal mesh should be easy to handle, provide adequate strength, be inert, resist contraction, avoid infection, place no restriction on patient function, and be simple and inexpensive to manufacture.[70] Current meshes have attempted to maximize on these ideals. Polypropylene is a synthetic nonabsorbable mesh that is hydrophobic, electrostatically neutral, and permanent. Common brand names include Marlex (Davol, Cranston, RI), Prolene (Ethicon, Somerville, NJ), and Pro-Lite (Covidien, Norwalk, Conn). Differences between them include the filament size, pore size, and weight. Recent advancements have included change from a heavyweight mesh to a lightweight mesh, with larger pores that promote a host scarring response. The end result is theorized to be better incorporation of the prosthetic into native tissue, without the deleterious effects such as chronic pain or discomfort that may result in the inflammatory response to the mesh. Polyester mesh is available commercially as Parietex (Covidien) and Mersilene (Ethicon). It promotes an inflammatory response similar to polypropylene and exhibits similar contracture rates. Polyester mesh is also woven and provides for transparency when fixing the mesh. Common to synthetic absorbable meshes is the concept of density, which combines fiber diameter, which relates to strength, and fiber number, which impacts pore size. This subdivides these materials into heavyweight and lightweight, depending on the extent of density. A healthy balance of density must be achieved for optimal results. Too heavy a density may lead to increased chronic pain whereas too lightweight of a mesh may lead to increased recurrences.

Polypropylene and polyester meshes are the most commonly used prosthetics in inguinal hernia repairs, although there is a limited role for expanded polytetrafluoroethylene, which is available as Gore-Tex (W.L. Gore and Associates, Flagstaff, Ariz). The mesh does not promote ingrowth into viscera and therefore makes it useful in IPOM or TAPP repairs where peritoneal closure is difficult. However, the lack of transparency makes fixation difficult. Compatibility of a synthetic nonabsorbable mesh with viscera may also be accomplished through the use of a coating agent. The coating is comprised of an absorbable or nonabsorbable layer that limits the inflammatory response on the side exposed to viscera, while maintaining the handling characteristics of the mesh. Absorbable coatings generally last beyond several months, allowing peritonealization to take place. A similar concept is the partially absorbable mesh, which combines a polypropylene mesh with an absorbable polymer. It is yet unclear whether an advantage is conferred to the patient by use of these materials. Biologic prosthetics do not have a role in routine herniorrhaphy at this time, their use being limited to contaminated fields. Choices include Surgisis (Cook Medical, Bloomington, Ind) and AlloDerm (LifeCell Corporation, Branchburg, NJ). Disadvantages to these materials include a decreased wound strength compared to native connective tissue and subsequently increased recurrence rates.[71]

In addition to mesh choice, there is the controversial issue of mesh fixation. Original descriptions of the plug and patch repair described no fixation of mesh in the anterior open approach. Mesh fixation in laparoscopic surgery is intended to prevent mesh migration and subsequent recurrence; however, the use of staples or tacks may also lead to chronic pain and injury to neurovascular structures. In a prospective randomized trial of fixation vs. no fixation in TEP repairs, a new pain was reported in 23% of patients where fixation was used. At the 6-month follow-up, no difference in recurrence was seen.[72] Studies using preformed mesh have yielded similar results, the theory being that mesh that is already conformed to the preperitoneal space has less tendency to migrate.[73] Fixation without tacks or staples has also been attempted with generally positive results. In these studies, mesh fixation has been attempted with fibrin glue. Long-term follow-up (1 to 2 years) has demonstrated that patients in whom fibrin glue is used experience less chronic pain than and equivalent recurrence rates to those in whom tack fixation is used.[74,75] Despite the encouraging, yet limited data concerning mesh fixation, general practice still involves the use of metal tack fixation of mesh in laparoscopic inguinal hernia repair. Technologic developments such as absorbable tacks may play a significant role in the future of mesh fixation.

SPORTS HERNIA

Groin pain may result from a number of conditions, including injuries to the spine, pelvis, abdomen, and genitourinary system. Despite a classical presentation, the absence of clinical findings makes the diagnosis of a hernia more dubious. Occult hernias such as these may, in fact, be a sports hernia, otherwise known as a *sportsman's hernia* or *athletic pubalgia*. They are commonly seen in athletes that perform repetitive kicking, twisting, or turning, as in hockey, soccer, and football, which results in a weakness or tearing of the posterior inguinal wall. A similar abrupt motion in a nonathlete also may lead to this condition. The hernia often is not identified until the time of surgical exploration, where a number of different anomalies may be visualized. These include tearing of the transversalis fascia or conjoined tendon, tearing of the internal oblique or avulsion of the internal oblique at the pubic tubercle, or tear of the external oblique aponeurosis or widened external ring. The lack of standardization in the literature makes analysis difficult because oftentimes groin pain of other origins is included in the discussion of sports hernias.

The presentation of a sports hernia may be acute, but more often, the deep groin pain presents in an insidious manner, gradually worsening with increasing activity. The pain is aggravated by movements and sudden increases in intra-abdominal pressure from coughing or sneezing. In the athlete, the pain is severe enough to limit optimal functioning during physical exertion. However, the physical examination will fail to identify a noticeable bulge or cough impulse. A dilated external ring may be palpable by a trained investigator, yet most patients will present with tenderness to palpation over the pubic bone and inguinal canal. Imaging generally fails to visualize a hernia or disruption of the inguinal canal but is useful to rule out differential diagnoses. A bone scan may be used to confirm osteitis pubis but will not be able to confirm the diagnosis of a sports hernia.

Initial treatment of a sports hernia is conservative, which also allows time to rule out other possible conditions such as muscle strain or osteitis pubis. Conservative therapy consists of rest, NSAIDs, deep tissue massage, and physiotherapy. Should the pain return upon gradual return to normal activities after 6 to 8 weeks of conservative management, surgical exploration often is necessary. Groin exploration is performed in the same approach as an open anterior inguinal herniorrhaphy. This allows the surgeon to fully assess the internal and external oblique musculature and aponeuro-

ses, inguinal rings, ligaments and tendons, and pubic tubercle. The most common finding is a deficiency of the floor of the inguinal canal, with a possible occult hernia. Reinforcement of the posterior wall can be performed in a tissue-based repair or using a laparoscopic preperitoneal mesh placement. Both techniques have yielded successful resolution of pain and return to physical activity. A deficiency of the laparoscopic method is the inability to assess the external oblique aponeurosis for any tears or distortions. Disruptions of the adductor tendon may also be considered with a concurrent tenotomy at time of the sports hernia repair.[76,77] The lack of a classification system makes treatment choices more difficult in this challenging group of patients. Repair of the posterior floor by open or laparoscopic approach is currently an effective strategy, yet improper treatment in professional athletes may impact not only quality of life, but also occupation.

PEDIATRIC HERNIAS

The incidence of inguinal hernias in children is between 0.8 and 44%, with a 10-fold increased incidence in boys vs. girls. The incidence also is significantly increased in low-birth-weight and premature infants, secondary to a patent processus vaginalis (PPV) in the latter. The difference in timing of testicular descent results in closure of the left processus vaginalis before the right. Consequently, right-sided hernias are more common than left-sided hernias, with approximately 10% of hernias presenting as bilateral. Repair of indirect inguinal hernias happens to be one of the most commonly performed procedures in children.[78,79] Diagnosis of a pediatric hernia is usually obvious to the clinician and supported by the parent's or caregiver's description. Physical examination by inspection alone will usually confirm the diagnosis. A Valsalva's maneuver is difficult to induce in infants, but the intra-abdominal pressure can be increased when crying. Differential diagnosis of a pediatric groin bulge commonly includes undescended testes, testicular mass, varicoceles, or hydroceles. Those hydroceles that present at birth do not necessarily increase the likelihood that a PPV is present and will usually resolve on their own. Conversely, hydroceles that present following birth may be more likely associated with a PPV that will not spontaneously close.[80]

Unlike in adults, pediatric hernias must be treated emergently, even if they are asymptomatic, to prevent the risk of incarceration. The risk of incarceration has been estimated to be up to 20%, with a significantly increased rate of complications when an incarcerated hernia must undergo surgical treatment.[81] Repairs are performed using an open approach using a groin incision over the internal ring. Once the inguinal canal is entered, the indirect hernia sac is identified, dissected, and ligated at the internal ring. A dilated internal ring can be repaired using the Marcy technique. With the cord structures retracted laterally, sutures are placed through the muscular and fascial layers constituting the inguinal ring. Mesh placement or floor reconstruction is unnecessary in uncomplicated indirect inguinal hernias as it may impart inflammatory changes in the vas deferens and testicles.[82] The classic repair including high ligation of the sac results in recurrence rates of approximately 1.2%, wound infection rates of 1.2%, and testicular atrophy at a rate of 0.3%.[83] Classical management of pediatric hernias involved routine exploration of the contralateral side. In up to one third of patients, a contralateral hernia was identified; however, these are usually the processus vaginalis that, if left untreated, is unlikely to lead to a hernia. Routine exploration continued until the last decade when the risks and benefits of contralateral exploration were questioned. Currently, most pediatric surgeons treat only the obvious hernia and avoid routine exploration of the contralateral side. However, the controversy with this treatment strategy continues because the possibility of metachronous hernia formation has been estimated to be 7.2% following a large-scale retrospective review of the literature.[84] The advent of laparoscopy has provided for a compromise in the debate because routine contralateral exploration can be accomplished with minimal morbidity. Laparoscopy can be performed through the hernia sac or using a separate umbilical incision. A normal internal ring obviates the need for added exploration, whereas an obvious contralateral inguinal hernia requires treatment. The difficulty in choosing management arises when a PPV is demonstrated. The majority of these are repaired, although only half of these are estimated to become clinically significant. Alternatively, the repair of a PPV reduces the incidence of metachronous hernia incarceration and the need for a second surgery in the future.[85] Another alternative includes ultrasound evaluation of the hernia and contralateral side, although the success of the imaging modality is heavily operator dependent.[86]

REFERENCES

Entries highlighted in bright blue are key references.

1. Johnson J, Roth JS, Hazey JW, et al: The history of open inguinal hernia repair. *Curr Surg* 61:49, 2004.
2. Rutkow IM: Demographic and socioeconomic aspects of hernia repair in the United States in 2003. *Surg Clin North Am* 83:1045, 2003.
3. www.ahrq.gov/data/hcup/factbk9: Russo CA, Owens P, Steiner C, et al: Ambulatory Surgery in U.S. Hospitals, 2003—HCUP Fact Book No. 9, 2003 [accessed January 28, 2009].
4. Awad SS, Fagan SP: Current approaches to inguinal hernia repair. *Am J Surg* 188:9S, 2004.
5. Rutkow IM: Epidemiologic, economic, and sociologic aspects of hernia surgery in the United States in the 1990s. *Surg Clin North Am* 78:941, 1998.
6. Bochkarev V, Ringley C, Vitamvas M, et al: Bilateral laparoscopic inguinal hernia repair in patients with occult contralateral inguinal defects. *Surg Endosc* 21:734, 2007.
7. Abramson JH, Gofin J, Hopp C, et al: The epidemiology of inguinal hernia. A survey in western Jerusalem. *J Epidemiol Community Health* 32:59, 1978.
8. Miltenburg DM, Nuchtern JG, Jaksic T, et al: Laparoscopic evaluation of the pediatric inguinal hernia—a meta-analysis. *J Pediatr Surg* 33:874, 1998.
9. van Wessem KJ, Simons MP, Plaisier PW et al: The etiology of indirect inguinal hernias: Congenital and/or acquired? *Hernia* 7:76, 2003.
10. van Veen RN, van Wessem KJ, Halm JA, et al: Patent processus vaginalis in the adult as a risk factor for the occurrence of indirect inguinal hernia. *Surg Endosc* 21:202, 2007.
11. Carbonell JF, Sanchez JL, Peris RT, et al: Risk factors associated with inguinal hernias: A case control study. *Eur J Surg* 159:481, 1993.
12. Flich J, Alfonso JL, Delgado F, et al: Inguinal hernia and certain risk factors. *Eur J Epidemiol* 8:277, 1992.
13. Lau H, Fang C, Yuen WK, et al: Risk factors for inguinal hernia in adult males: A case-control study. *Surgery* 141:262, 2007.
14. Ruhl CE, Everhart JE: Risk factors for inguinal hernia among adults in the US population. *Am J Epidemiol* 165:1154, 2007.
15. Klinge U, Binnebosel M, Mertens PR: Are collagens the culprits in the development of incisional and inguinal hernia disease? *Hernia* 10:472, 2006.
16. Franz MG: The biology of hernia formation. *Surg Clin North Am* 88:1, 2008.
17. Spaw AT, Ennis BW, Spaw LP: Laparoscopic hernia repair: The anatomic basis. *J Laparoendosc Surg* 1:269, 1991.
18. Gilbert AI: An anatomic and functional classification for the diagnosis and treatment of inguinal hernia. *Am J Surg* 157:331, 1989.
19. Rutkow IM, Robbins AW: "Tension-free" inguinal herniorrhaphy: A preliminary report on the "mesh plug" technique. *Surgery* 114:3, 1993.
20. Nyhus LM: Individualization of hernia repair: A new era. *Surgery* 114:1, 1993.
21. Zollinger RM Jr.: An updated traditional classification of inguinal hernias. *Hernia* 8:318, 2004.
22. Ralphs DN, Brain AJ, Grundy DJ, et al: How accurately can direct and indirect inguinal hernias be distinguished? *Br Med J* 280:1039, 1980.
23. Cameron AE: Accuracy of clinical diagnosis of direct and indirect inguinal hernia. *Br J Surg* 81:250, 1994.
24. Jamadar DA, Jacobson JA, Morag Y, et al: Sonography of inguinal region hernias. *AJR Am J Roentgenol* 187:185, 2006.
25. Shin D, Lipshultz LI, Goldstein M, et al: Herniorrhaphy with polypropylene mesh causing inguinal vasal obstruction: A preventable cause of obstructive azoospermia. *Ann Surg* 241:553, 2005.
26. Delikoukos S, Lavant L, Hlias G, et al: The role of hernia sac ligation in postoperative pain in patients with elective tension-free indirect inguinal hernia repair: A prospective randomized study. *Hernia* 11:425, 2007.
27. Gilbert AI: Sutureless repair of inguinal hernia. *Am J Surg* 163:331, 1992.
28. Millikan KW, Cummings B, Doolas A: The Millikan modified mesh-plug hernioplasty. *Arch Surg* 138:525; discussion 529, 2003.
29. Kugel RD: Minimally invasive, nonlaparoscopic, preperitoneal, and sutureless, inguinal herniorrhaphy. *Am J Surg* 178:298, 1999.
30. Kugel RD: The Kugel repair for groin hernias. *Surg Clin North Am* 83:1119, 2003.
31. Sarli L, Pietra N, Choua O, et al: Laparoscopic hernia repair: A prospective comparison of TAPP and IPOM techniques. *Surg Laparosc Endosc* 7:472, 1997.
32. Olmi S, Scaini A, Erba L, et al: Laparoscopic repair of inguinal hernias using an intraperitoneal onlay mesh technique and a Parietex composite mesh fixed with fibrin glue (Tissucol). Personal technique and preliminary results. *Surg Endosc* 21:1961, 2007.
33. Kingsley D, Vogt DM, Nelson MT, et al: Laparoscopic intraperitoneal onlay inguinal herniorrhaphy. *Am J Surg* 176:548, 1998.
34. Law NW, Trapnell JE: Does a truss benefit a patient with inguinal hernia? *BMJ* 304:1092, 1992.
35. Gallegos NC, Dawson J, Jarvis M, et al: Risk of strangulation in groin hernias. *Br J Surg* 78:1171, 1991.
36. Neutra R, Velez A, Ferrada R, et al: Risk of incarceration of inguinal hernia in Cell Colombia. *J Chronic Dis* 34:561, 1981.
37. Fitzgibbons RJ Jr., Giobbie-Harder A, Gibbs JO, et al: Watchful waiting vs repair of inguinal hernia in minimally symptomatic men: A randomized clinical trial. *JAMA* 295:285, 2006.
38. Voyles CR, Hamilton BJ, Johnson WD, et al: Meta-analysis of laparoscopic inguinal hernia trials favors open hernia repair with preperitoneal mesh prosthesis. *Am J Surg* 184:6, 2002.
39. Lee BC, Rodin DM, Shah KK, et al: Laparoscopic inguinal hernia repair during laparoscopic radical prostatectomy. *BJU Int* 99:637, 2007.
40. Antunes AA, Dall'oglio M, Crippa A, et al: Inguinal hernia repair with polypropylene mesh during radical retropubic prostatectomy: An easy and practical approach. *BJU Int* 96:330, 2005.
41. Lichtenstein IL, Shulman AG, Amid PK: Use of mesh to prevent recurrence of hernias. *Postgrad Med* 87:155, 1990.
42. McCormack K, Scott NW, Go PM, et al: Laparoscopic techniques versus open techniques for inguinal hernia repair. *Cochrane Database Syst Rev* 1:CD001785, 2003.
43. Beets GL, Dirksen CD, Go PM, et al: Open or laparoscopic preperitoneal mesh repair for recurrent inguinal hernia? A randomized controlled trial. *Surg Endosc* 13:323, 1999.
44. Andersson B, Hallen M, Leveau P, et al: Laparoscopic extraperitoneal inguinal hernia repair versus open mesh repair: A prospective randomized controlled trial. *Surgery* 133:464, 2003.
45. Hallen M, Bergenfelz A, Westerdahl J: Laparoscopic extraperitoneal inguinal hernia repair versus open mesh repair: Long-term follow-up of a randomized controlled trial. *Surgery* 143:313, 2008.
46. Lau H, Patil NG, Yuen WK: Day-case endoscopic totally extraperitoneal inguinal hernioplasty versus open Lichtenstein hernioplasty for unilateral primary inguinal hernia in males: a randomized trial. *Surg Endosc* 20:76, 2006.
47. Neumayer L, Giobbie-Harder A, Jonasson O, et al: Open mesh versus laparoscopic mesh repair of inguinal hernia. *N Engl J Med* 350:1819, 2004.
48. Fitzgibbons RJ Jr., Puri V: Laparoscopic inguinal hernia repair. *Am J Surg* 72:197, 2006.
49. Kingsnorth AN, Britton BJ, Morris PJ: Recurrent inguinal hernia after local anaesthetic repair. *Br J Surg* 68:273, 1981.
50. Lal P, Kajla RK, Chander J, et al: Laparoscopic total extraperitoneal (TEP) inguinal hernia repair: overcoming the learning curve. *Surg Endosc* 18:642, 2004.
51. Ridings P, Evans DS: The transabdominal pre-peritoneal (TAPP) inguinal hernia repair: A trip along the learning curve. *J R Coll Surg Edinb* 45:29, 2000.
52. Nienhuijs S, Staal E, Strobbe L, et al: Chronic pain after mesh repair of inguinal hernia: A systematic review. *Am J Surg* 194:394, 2007.

53. Collaboration EH: Laparoscopic compared with open methods of groin hernia repair: Systematic review of randomized controlled trials. *Br J Surg* 87:860, 2000.

54. Glassow F: The Shouldice Hospital technique. *Int Surg* 71:148, 1986.

55. Hay JM, Boudet MJ, Fingerhut A, et al: Shouldice inguinal hernia repair in the male adult: The gold standard? A multicenter controlled trial in 1578 patients. *Ann Surg*. 222:719, 1995.

56. Schulman A, Amid P, Lichtenstein I: The safety of mesh repair for primary inguinal hernias: Results of 3,019 operations from five diverse surgical sources. *Am Surg* 58:255, 1992.

57. Kark AE, Kurzer MN, Belsham PA: Three thousand one hundred seventy-five primary inguinal hernia repairs: Advantages of ambulatory open mesh repair using local anesthesia. *J Am Coll Surg* 186:447; discussion 456, 1998.

58. Bisgaard T, Bay-Nielsen M, Kehlet H: Re-recurrence after operation for recurrent inguinal hernia. A nationwide 8-year follow-up study on the role of type of repair. *Ann Surg* 247:707, 2008.

59. Felix EL: A unified approach to recurrent laparoscopic hernia repairs. *Surg Endosc* 15:969, 2001.

60. Poobalan AS, Bruce J, King PM, et al: Chronic pain and quality of life following open inguinal hernia repair. *Br J Surg* 88:1122, 2001.

61. Jones KR, Burney RE, Peterson M, et al: Return to work after inguinal hernia repair. *Surgery* 129:128, 2001.

62. Madura JA, Madura JA 2nd, Copper CM, et al: Inguinal neurectomy for inguinal nerve entrapment: An experience with 100 patients. *Am J Surg* 189:283, 2005.

63. Kim DH, Murovic JA, Tiel RL, et al: Surgical management of 33 ilioinguinal and iliohypogastric neuralgias at Louisiana State University Health Sciences Center. *Neurosurgery* 56:1013; discussion 1013, 2005.

64. Fong Y, Wantz GE: Prevention of ischemic orchitis during inguinal hernioplasty. *Surg Gynecol Obstet* 174:399, 1992.

65. Aufenacker TJ, van Geldere D, van Mesdag T, et al: The role of antibiotic prophylaxis in prevention of wound infection after Lichtenstein open mesh repair of primary inguinal hernia: A multicenter double-blind randomized controlled trial. *Ann Surg* 240:955; discussion 960, 2004.

66. Gilbert AI, Felton LL: Infection in inguinal hernia repair considering biomaterials and antibiotics. *Surg Gynecol Obstet* 177:126, 1993.

67. Sanchez-Manuel FJ, Lozano-Garcia J, Seco-Gil JL: Antibiotic prophylaxis for hernia repair. *Cochrane Database Syst Rev* 3:CD003769, 2007.

68. LeBlanc KE, LeBlanc KA: Groin pain in athletes. *Hernia* 7:68, 2003.

69. Finley RK Jr., Miller SF, Jones LM: Elimination of urinary retention following inguinal herniorrhaphy. *Am Surg* 57:486; discussion 488, 1991.

70. Earle DB, Romanelli J: Prosthetic materials for hernia: What's new. How to make sense of the multitude of mesh options for inguinal and ventral hernia repairs. *Contemporary Surgery* 63:63, 2007.

71. Earle DB, Mark LA: Prosthetic material in inguinal hernia repair: How do I choose? *Surg Clin North Am* 88:179, 2008.

72. Taylor C, Layani L, Liew V, et al: Laparoscopic inguinal hernia repair without mesh fixation, early results of a large randomised clinical trial. *Surg Endosc* 22:757, 2008.

73. Morrison JE Jr., Jacobs VR: Laparoscopic preperitoneal inguinal hernia repair using preformed polyester mesh without fixation: Prospective study with 1-year follow-up results in a rural setting. *Surg Laparosc Endosc Percutan Tech* 18:33, 2008.

74. Schwab R, Willms A, Kroger A, et al: Less chronic pain following mesh fixation using a fibrin sealant in TEP inguinal hernia repair. *Hernia* 10:272, 2006.

75. Canonico S, Santoriello A, Campitiello F, et al: Mesh fixation with human fibrin glue (Tissucol) in open tension-free inguinal hernia repair: A preliminary report. *Hernia* 9:330, 2005.

76. Ingoldby CJ: Laparoscopic and conventional repair of groin disruption in sportsmen. *Br J Surg* 84:213, 1997.

77. Van Der Donckt K, Steenbrugge F, Van Den Abbeele K, et al: Bassini's hernial repair and adductor longus tenotomy in the treatment of chronic groin pain in athletes. *Acta Orthop Belg* 69:35, 2003.

78. Manoharan S, Samarakkody U, Kulkarni M, et al: Evidence-based change of practice in the management of unilateral inguinal hernia. *J Pediatr Surg* 40:1163, 2005.

79. Brandt ML: Pediatric hernias. *Surg Clin North Am* 88:27, 2008.

80. Katz DA: Evaluation and management of inguinal and umbilical hernias. *Pediatr Ann* 30:729, 2001.

81. Stylianos S, Jacir NN, Harris BH: Incarceration of inguinal hernia in infants prior to elective repair. *J Pediatr Surg* 28:582, 1993.

82. Peiper C, Junge K, Klinge U, et al: Is there a risk of infertility after inguinal mesh repair? Experimental studies in the pig and the rabbit. *Hernia* 10:7, 2006.

83. Ein SH, Njere I, Ein A: Six thousand three hundred sixty-one pediatric inguinal hernias: A 35-year review. *J Pediatr Surg* 41:980, 2006.

84. Ron O, Eaton S, Pierro A: Systematic review of the risk of developing a metachronous contralateral inguinal hernia in children. *Br J Surg* 94:804, 2007.

85. Marulaiah M, Atkinson J, Kukkady A, et al: Is contralateral exploration necessary in preterm infants with unilateral inguinal hernia? *J Pediatr Surg* 41:2004, 2006.

86. Chen KC, Chu CC, Chou TY, et al: Ultrasonography for inguinal hernias in boys. *J Pediatr Surg* 33:1784, 1998.

87. Douek M, Smith G, Oshowo A, et al: Prospective randomised controlled trial of laparoscopic versus open inguinal hernia mesh repair: five year follow up. *BMJ* 326:1012, 2003.

88. Bringman S, Ramel S, Heikkinen TJ, et al: Tension-free inguinal hernia repair: TEP versus mesh-plug versus Lichtenstein: a prospective randomized controlled trial. *Ann Surg* 237:142, 2003.

89. Colak T, Akca T, Kanik A, et al: Randomized clinical trial comparing laparoscopic totally extraperitoneal approach with open mesh repair in inguinal hernia. *Surg Laparosc Endosc Percutan Tech* 13:191, 2003.

90. Kumar S, Nixon SJ, MacIntyre IM: Laparoscopic or Lichtenstein repair for recurrent inguinal hernia: one unit's experience. *J R Coll Surg Edinb* 44:301, 1999.

91. MRC Trial Group: Laparoscopic versus open repair of groin hernia: a randomised comparison. The MRC Laparoscopic Groin Hernia Trial Group. *Lancet* 354:185, 1999.

92. Picchio M, Lombardi A, Zolovkins A, et al: Tension-free laparoscopic and open hernia repair: randomized controlled trial of early results. *World J Surg* 23:1004; discussion 1008, 1999.

93. Khoury N: A randomized prospective controlled trial of laparoscopic extraperitoneal hernia repair and mesh-plug hernioplasty: a study of 315 cases. *J Laparoendosc Adv Surg Tech A* 8:367, 1998.

94. Heikkinen TJ, Haukipuro K, Koivukangas P, et al: A prospective randomized outcome and cost comparison of totally extraperitoneal endoscopic hernioplasty versus Lichtenstein hernia operation among employed patients. *Surg Laparosc Endosc* 8:338, 1998.

95. Wellwood J, Sculpher MJ, Stoker D, et al: Randomised controlled trial of laparoscopic versus open mesh repair for inguinal hernia: outcome and cost. *BMJ* 317:103, 1998.

96. Wright DM, Kennedy A, Baxter JN, et al: Early outcome after open versus extraperitoneal endoscopic tension-free hernioplasty: a randomized clinical trial. *Surgery* 119:552, 1996.

97. Payne JH Jr., Grininger LM, Izawa MT, et al: Laparoscopic or open inguinal herniorrhaphy? A randomized prospective trial. *Arch Surg* 129:973; discussion 979, 1994.

Thyroid, Parathyroid, and Adrenal

Geeta Lal and Orlo H. Clark

THYROID

Historical Background

Goiters (from the Latin *guttur*, throat), defined as an enlargement of the thyroid, have been recognized since 2700 B.C. even though the thyroid gland was not documented as such until the Renaissance period. In 1619, Hieronymus Fabricius ab Aquapendente recognized that goiters arose from the thyroid gland. The term *thyroid gland* (Greek *thyreoeides*, shield-shaped) is, however, attributed to Thomas Wharton in his *Adenographia* (1656). In 1776, the thyroid was classified as a ductless gland by Albrecht von Haller and was thought to have numerous functions ranging from lubrication of the larynx to acting as a reservoir for blood to provide continuous flow to the brain, to beautifying women's necks. Burnt seaweed was considered to be the most effective treatment for goiters.

The first accounts of thyroid surgery for the treatment of goiters were given by Roger Frugardi in 1170. In response to failure of medical treatment, two setons were inserted at right angles into the goiter and tightened twice daily until the goiter separated. The open wound was treated with caustic powder and left to heal. However, thyroid surgery continued to be hazardous with prohibitive mortality rates (>40%) until the latter half of the nineteenth century, when advances in general anesthesia, antisepsis, and hemostasis enabled surgeons to perform thyroid surgery with significantly reduced mortality and morbidity rates. The most notable thyroid surgeons were Emil Theodor Kocher (1841–1917) and C.A. Theodor Billroth (1829–1894), who performed thousands of operations with increasingly successful results. However, as more patients survived thyroid operations, new problems and issues became apparent. After total thyroidectomy, patients (particularly children) became myxedematous with cretinous features. Myxedema was first effectively treated in 1891 by George Murray using a subcutaneous injection of an extract of sheep's thyroid and later, Edward Fox demonstrated that oral therapy was equally effective. In 1909, Kocher was awarded the Nobel Prize for medicine in recognition "for his works on the physiology, pathology, and surgery of the thyroid gland."

Embryology

The thyroid gland arises as an outpouching of the primitive foregut around the third week of gestation. It originates at the base of the tongue at the foramen cecum. Endoderm cells in the floor of the pharyngeal anlage thicken to form the medial thyroid anlage (Fig. 38-1) that descends in the neck anterior to structures that form the hyoid bone and larynx. During its descent, the anlage remains connected to the foramen cecum via an epithelial-lined tube known as the *thyroglossal duct*. The epithelial cells making up the anlage give rise to the thyroid follicular cells. The paired lateral anlages originate from the fourth branchial pouch and fuse with the median anlage at approximately the fifth week of gestation. The lateral anlages are neuroectodermal in origin (ultimobranchial bodies) and provide the calcitonin producing parafollicular or C cells, which thus come to lie in the superoposterior region of the gland. Thyroid follicles are initially apparent by 8 weeks, and colloid formation begins by the eleventh week of gestation.

Developmental Abnormalities
Thyroglossal Duct Cyst and Sinus

Thyroglossal duct cysts are the most commonly encountered congenital cervical anomalies. During the fifth week of gestation, the thyro-

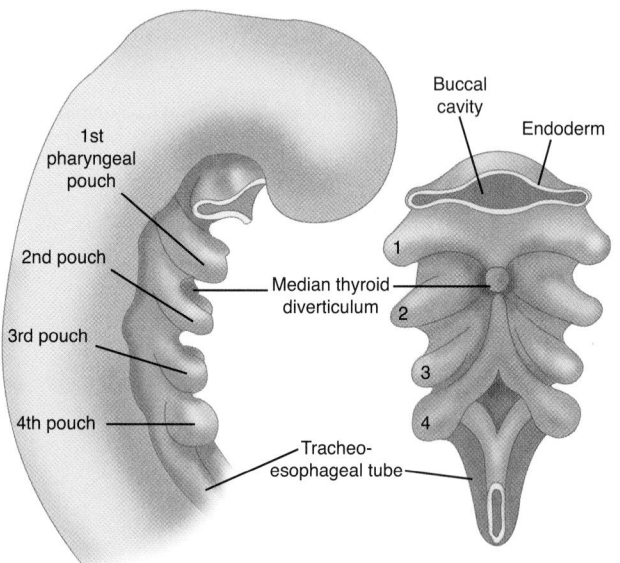

FIG. 38-1. Thyroid embryology—early development of the median thyroid anlage as a pharyngeal pouch. *[Reproduced with permission from Embryology and developmental abnormalities, in Cady B, Rossi R (eds):* Surgery of the Thyroid and Parathyroid Glands. *Philadelphia: WB Saunders, 1991, p 6.]*

glossal duct lumen starts to obliterate, and the duct disappears by the eighth week of gestation. Rarely, the thyroglossal duct may persist in whole, or in part. Thyroglossal duct cysts may occur anywhere along the migratory path of the thyroid although 80% are found in juxtaposition to the hyoid bone. They are usually asymptomatic but occasionally become infected by oral bacteria, prompting the patient to seek medical advice. Thyroglossal duct sinuses result from infection of the cyst secondary to spontaneous or surgical drainage of the cyst and are accompanied by minor inflammation of the surrounding skin. Histologically, thyroglossal duct cysts are lined by pseudostratified ciliated columnar epithelium and squamous epithelium, with heterotopic thyroid tissue present in 20% of cases.

The diagnosis usually is established by observing a 1- to 2-cm, smooth, well-defined midline neck mass that moves upward with protrusion of the tongue. Routine thyroid imaging is not necessary although thyroid scintigraphy and ultrasound have been performed to document the presence of normal thyroid tissue in the neck. Treatment involves the "Sistrunk operation," which consists of en bloc cystectomy and excision of the central hyoid bone to minimize recurrence. Approximately 1% of thyroglossal duct cysts are found to contain cancer, which is usually papillary (85%). The role of total thyroidectomy in this setting is controversial, but is advised in older patients with large tumors, particularly if there are additional thyroid nodules and evidence of cyst wall invasion or lymph node metastases.[1] Squamous, Hürthle cell, and anaplastic cancers also have been reported but are rare. Medullary thyroid cancers (MTCs) are, however, not found in thyroglossal duct cysts.

Lingual Thyroid

A lingual thyroid represents a failure of the median thyroid anlage to descend normally and may be the only thyroid tissue present. Intervention becomes necessary for obstructive symptoms such as choking, dysphagia, airway obstruction, or hemorrhage. Many of these patients develop hypothyroidism. Medical treatment options include administration of exogenous thyroid hormone to suppress thyroid-stimulating hormone (TSH) and radioactive iodine (RAI) ablation followed by hormone replacement. Surgical excision is rarely needed but, if required, should be preceded by an evaluation of normal thyroid tissue in the neck to avoid inadvertently rendering the patient hypothyroid.

Ectopic Thyroid

Normal thyroid tissue may be found anywhere in the central neck compartment, including the esophagus, trachea, and anterior mediastinum. Thyroid tissue has been observed adjacent to the aortic arch, in the aortopulmonary window, within the upper pericardium, or in the interventricular septum. Often, "tongues" of thyroid tissue are seen to extend off the inferior poles of the gland and are particularly apparent in large goiters. Thyroid tissue situated lateral to the carotid sheath and jugular vein, previously termed *lateral aberrant thyroid*, almost always represents metastatic thyroid cancer in lymph nodes, and not remnants of the lateral anlage that had failed to fuse with the main thyroid, as previously suggested by Crile. Even if not readily apparent on physical examination or ultrasound imaging, the ipsilateral thyroid lobe contains a focus of papillary thyroid cancer (PTC), which may be microscopic.

Pyramidal Lobe

Normally the thyroglossal duct atrophies, although it may remain as a fibrous band. In about 50% of individuals, the distal end that connects to the thyroid persists as a pyramidal lobe projecting up from the isthmus, lying just to the left or right of the midline. In the normal individual, the pyramidal lobe is not palpable, but in disorders resulting in thyroid hypertrophy (e.g., Graves' disease, diffuse nodular goiter, or lymphocytic thyroiditis), the pyramidal lobe usually is enlarged and palpable.

Thyroid Anatomy

The anatomic relations of the thyroid gland and surrounding structures are depicted in Fig. 38-2. The adult thyroid gland is brown in color and firm in consistency, and is located posterior to the strap muscles. The normal thyroid gland weighs approximately 20 g, but gland weight varies with body weight and iodine intake. The thyroid lobes are located adjacent to the thyroid cartilage and connected in the midline by an isthmus that is located just inferior to the cricoid cartilage. A pyramidal lobe is present in about 50% of patients. The thyroid lobes extend to the midthyroid cartilage superiorly and lie adjacent to the carotid sheaths and sternocleidomastoid muscles laterally. The strap muscles (sternohyoid, sternothyroid, and superior belly of the omohyoid) are located anteriorly and are innervated by the ansa cervicalis (ansa hypoglossi). The thyroid gland is enveloped by a loosely connecting fascia that is formed from the partition of the deep cervical fascia into anterior and posterior divisions. The true capsule of the thyroid is a thin, densely adherent fibrous layer that sends out septa that invaginate into the gland, forming pseudolobules. The thyroid capsule is condensed into the posterior suspensory or Berry's ligament near the cricoid cartilage and upper tracheal rings.

Blood Supply

The superior thyroid arteries arise from the ipsilateral external carotid arteries and divide into anterior and posterior branches at the apices of the thyroid lobes. The inferior thyroid arteries arise from the thyrocervical trunk shortly after their origin from the subclavian arteries. The inferior thyroid arteries travel upward in the neck posterior to the carotid sheath to enter the thyroid lobes at their midpoint. A thyroidea ima artery arises directly from the aorta or innominate in 1 to 4% of individuals to enter the isthmus or replace a missing inferior thyroid artery. The inferior thyroid artery

KEY POINTS

1. There has been a paradigm shift in the surgical management of Graves' disease with increased use of total or near-total thyroidectomy, rather than subtotal thyroidectomy.

2. Familial nonmedullary thyroid cancer is increasingly being recognized as a separate entity. Surgeons must be aware of the potential for false negative fine-needle aspiration biopsy in this setting.

3. Total thyroidectomy is the surgical treatment of choice for most thyroid cancers, provided complication rates are low.

4. The widespread use of positron emission tomography scanning for staging various malignancies and ultrasound for vascular screening is leading to an increased incidence of thyroid incidentalomas. Management should be based on assessment of the individual patient's risk following complete clinical and fine-needle aspiration biopsy evaluation.

5. Focused mini-incision parathyroidectomy, after appropriate localization, has become the procedure of choice for the treatment of sporadic primary hyperparathyroidism.

6. Parathyroidectomy has been shown to improve the classic and so-called *nonspecific symptoms* and metabolic complications of primary hyperparathyroidism.

7. Very high calcium and parathyroid hormone levels in a patient with primary hyperparathyroidism should alert the surgeon to the presence of a possible parathyroid carcinoma.

8. Subclinical Cushing's syndrome is characterized by subtle abnormalities in corticosteroid synthesis, and many of its manifestations appear to be treated by adrenalectomy.

9. Fine-needle aspiration biopsy has a very limited role in the evaluation of adrenal incidentalomas unless the patient has previously had a cancer and should only be performed after appropriate biochemical studies have been performed to rule out pheochromocytoma.

10. Adrenocortical cancer can be difficult to diagnose even on pathology examination so that continued follow-up of patients with resected seemingly benign tumors is advised.

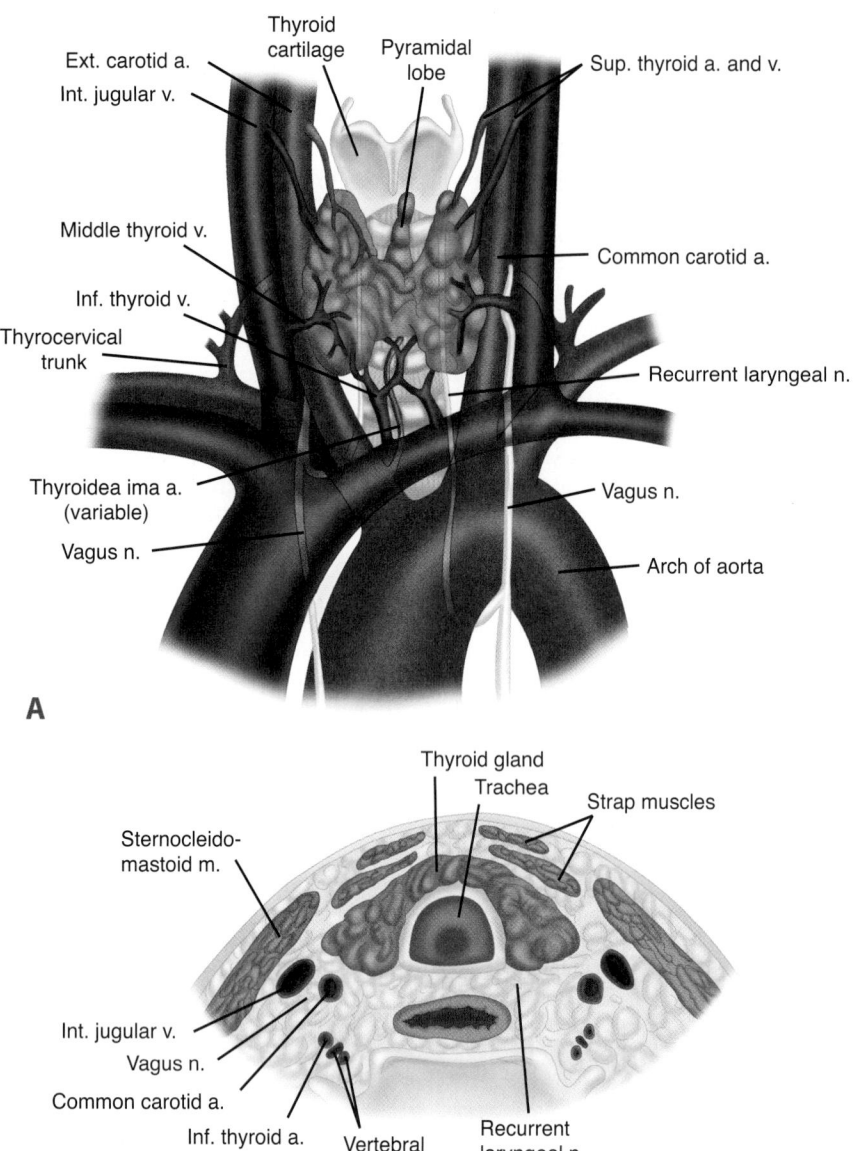

FIG. 38-2. Anatomy of the thyroid gland and surrounding structures, viewed anteriorly (**A**) and in cross-section (**B**). a. = artery; m. = muscle; n. = nerve; v. = vein.

crosses the recurrent laryngeal nerve (RLN), necessitating identification of the RLN before the arterial branches can be ligated. The venous drainage of the thyroid gland occurs via multiple small surface veins, which coalesce to form three sets of veins—the superior, middle, and inferior thyroid veins. The superior thyroid veins run with the superior thyroid arteries bilaterally. The middle vein or veins are the least consistent. The superior and middle veins drain directly into the internal jugular veins. The inferior veins often form a plexus, which drains into the brachiocephalic veins.

Nerves

The left RLN arises from the vagus nerve where it crosses the aortic arch, loops around the ligamentum arteriosum, and ascends medially in the neck within the tracheoesophageal groove. The right RLN arises from the vagus at its crossing with the right subclavian artery. The nerve usually passes posterior to the artery before ascending in the neck, its course being more oblique than the left RLN. Along their course in the neck, the RLNs may branch, and pass anterior, posterior, or interdigitate with branches of the inferior thyroid artery (Fig. 38-3). The right RLN may be nonrecurrent in 0.5 to 1% of individuals and often is associated with a vascular anomaly.[2] Nonrecurrent left RLNs are rare but have been reported in patients with situs inversus and a right-sided aortic arch. The RLN may branch in

its course in the neck and identification of a small nerve should alert the surgeon to this possibility. Identification of the nerves or their branches often necessitates mobilization of the most lateral and posterior extent of the thyroid gland, the tubercle of Zuckerkandl, at the level of the cricoid cartilage. The last segments of the nerves often course below the tubercle and are closely approximated to the ligament of Berry. Branches of the nerve may traverse the ligament in 25% of individuals, and are particularly vulnerable to injury at this junction. The RLNs terminate by entering the larynx posterior to the cricothyroid muscle.

The RLNs innervate all the intrinsic muscles of the larynx, except the cricothyroid muscles, which are innervated by the external laryngeal nerves. Injury to one RLN leads to paralysis of the ipsilateral vocal cord, which comes to lie in the paramedian or the abducted position. The paramedian position results in a normal, but weak voice, whereas the abducted position leads to a hoarse voice and an ineffective cough. Bilateral RLN injury may lead to airway obstruction, necessitating emergency tracheostomy, or loss of voice. If both cords come to lie in an abducted position, air movement can occur, but the patient has an ineffective cough and is at increased risk of repeated respiratory tract infections from aspiration.

The superior laryngeal nerves also arise from the vagus nerves. After their origin at the base of the skull, these nerves travel along the

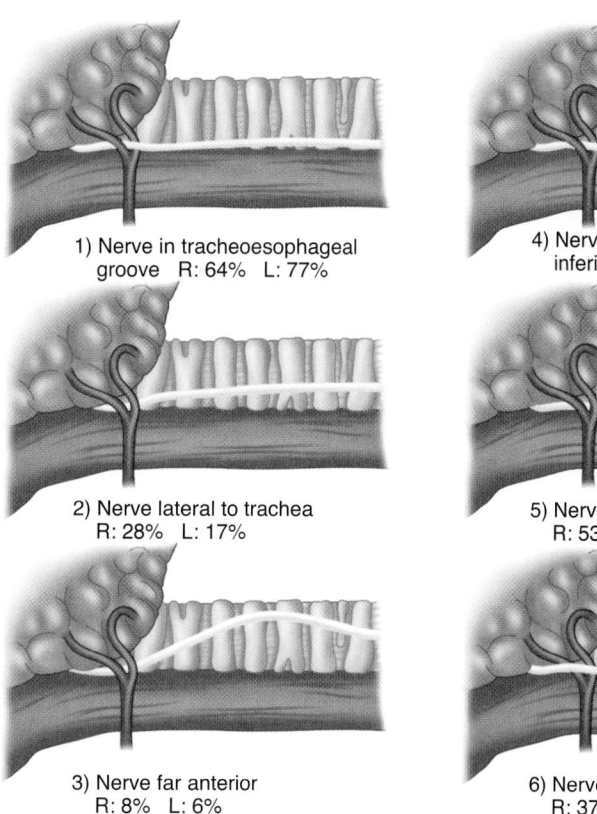

1) Nerve in tracheoesophageal groove   R: 64% L: 77%

2) Nerve lateral to trachea   R: 28%   L: 17%

3) Nerve far anterior   R: 8% L: 6%

4) Nerve between branches of inferior thyroid artery R: 7% L: 67%

5) Nerve posterior to artery   R: 53% L: 69%

6) Nerve anterior to artery   R: 37% L: 24%

7) Artery absent R: 3% L: 1%

FIG. 38-3. Relationship of recurrent laryngeal nerve to the inferior thyroid artery—the superior parathyroid is characteristically dorsal to the plane of the nerve, whereas the inferior gland is ventral to the nerve.

internal carotid artery and divide into two branches at the level of the hyoid bone. The internal branch of the superior laryngeal nerve is sensory to the supraglottic larynx. Injury to this nerve is rare in thyroid surgery, but its occurrence may result in aspiration. The external branch of the superior laryngeal nerve lies on the inferior pharyngeal constrictor muscle and descends alongside the superior thyroid vessels before innervating the cricothyroid muscle. Cernea and colleagues[3] proposed a classification system to describe the relationship of this nerve to the superior thyroid vessels (Fig. 38-4). The type 2a variant, in which the nerve crosses below the tip of the thyroid superior pole, occurs in up to 20% of individuals and places the nerve at a greater risk of injury. Therefore, the superior pole vessels should not be ligated en masse, but should be individually divided, low on the thyroid gland and dissected lateral to the cricothyroid muscle. Injury to this nerve leads to inability to tense the ipsilateral vocal cord and hence difficulty "hitting high notes," projecting the voice, and voice fatigue during prolonged speech.

Sympathetic innervation of the thyroid gland is provided by fibers from the superior and middle cervical sympathetic ganglia. The fibers enter the gland with the blood vessels and are vasomotor in action. Parasympathetic fibers are derived from the vagus nerve and reach the gland via branches of the laryngeal nerves.

Parathyroid Glands

The embryology and anatomy of the parathyroid glands is discussed in detail in the Parathyroid Gland section of this chapter. About 85% of individuals have four parathyroid glands that can be found within 1 cm of the junction of the inferior thyroid artery and the RLN. The superior glands are usually located dorsal to the RLN, whereas the inferior glands are usually found ventral to the RLN (Fig. 38-5).

Lymphatic System

The thyroid gland is endowed with an extensive network of lymphatics. Intraglandular lymphatic vessels connect both thyroid lobes through the isthmus and also drain to perithyroidal structures and lymph nodes. Regional lymph nodes include pretracheal, paratracheal, perithyroidal, RLN, superior mediastinal, retropharyngeal, esophageal, and upper, middle, and lower jugular chain nodes. These lymph nodes can be classified into seven levels as depicted in Fig. 38-6. The central compartment includes nodes located in the area between the two carotid sheaths, whereas nodes lateral to the vessels are present in the lateral compartment. Thyroid cancers may metastasize to any of these regions, although metastases to submaxillary nodes (level I) are rare (<1%). There also can be "skip" metastases to nodes in the ipsilateral neck.

Thyroid Histology

Microscopically, the thyroid is divided into lobules that contain 20 to 40 follicles (Fig. 38-7). There are about 3×10^6 follicles in the adult male thyroid gland. The follicles are spherical and average 30 μm in diameter. Each follicle is lined by cuboidal epithelial cells and contains a central store of colloid secreted from the epithelial cells under the influence of the pituitary hormone TSH. The second group of thyroid secretory cells is the C cells or parafollicular cells, which contain and secrete the hormone calcitonin. They are found as individual cells or clumped in small groups in the interfollicular stroma and located in the upper poles of the thyroid lobes.

Thyroid Physiology

Iodine Metabolism

The average daily iodine requirement is 0.1 mg, which can be derived from foods such as fish, milk, and eggs or as additives in bread or salt. In the stomach and jejunum, iodine is rapidly converted to iodide and absorbed into the bloodstream, and from there it is distributed uniformly throughout the extracellular space. Iodide is actively transported into the thyroid follicular cells by an adenosine triphosphate (ATP)–dependent process. The thyroid is

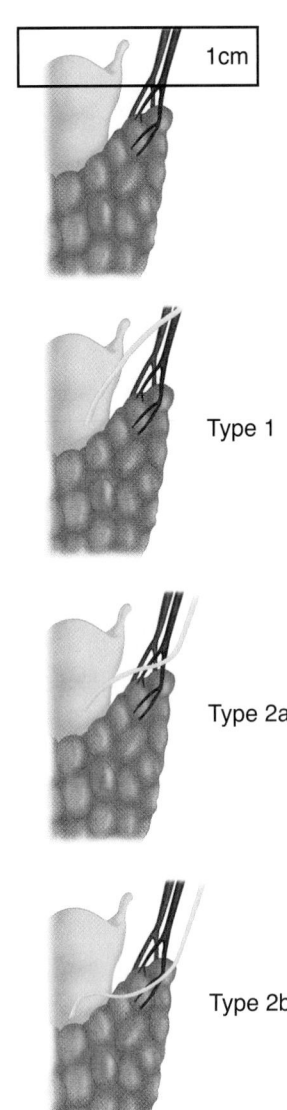

FIG. 38-4. Relationship of the external branch of the superior laryngeal nerve and superior thyroid artery originally described by Cernea and colleagues.[3] In type 1 anatomy, the nerve crosses the artery ≥1 cm above the superior aspect of the thyroid lobe. In type 2 anatomy, the nerve crosses the artery <1 cm above the thyroid pole (2a) or below (2b) it. *(Reproduced with permission from Bliss et al: Surgeon's approach to the thyroid gland: Surgical anatomy and the importance of technique.* World J Surg *24:893, 2000, Springer-Verlag.)*

the storage site of >90% of the body's iodine content and accounts for one third of the plasma iodine loss. The remaining plasma iodine is cleared via renal excretion.

Thyroid Hormone Synthesis, Secretion, and Transport

The synthesis of thyroid hormone consists of several steps (Fig. 38-8). The first, iodide trapping, involves active (ATP-dependent) transport of iodide across the basement membrane of the thyrocyte via an intrinsic membrane protein, the sodium/iodine (Na^+/I^-) symporter. Thyroglobulin (Tg) is a large (660 kDa) glycoprotein, which is present in thyroid follicles and has four tyrosyl residues. The second step in thyroid hormone synthesis involves oxidation of iodide to iodine and iodination of tyrosine residues on Tg, to form monoiodotyrosines (MIT) and diiodotyrosines (DIT). Both processes are catalyzed by thyroid peroxidase (TPO). A recently identified protein, pendrin, is thought to mediate iodine efflux at the apical membrane. The third

step leads to coupling of two DIT molecules to form tetra-iodothyronine or thyroxine (T_4), and one DIT molecule with one MIT molecule to form 3,5,3'-triiodothyronine (T_3) or 3,3',5'–triiodothyronine reverse (rT_3). When stimulated by TSH, thyrocytes form pseudopodia, which encircle portions of cell membrane containing Tg, which in turn, fuse with enzyme-containing lysosomes. In the fourth step, Tg is hydrolyzed to release free iodothyronines (T_3 and T_4) and mono- and diiodotyrosines. The latter are deiodinated in the fifth step to yield iodide, which is reused in the thyrocyte. In the euthyroid state, T_4 is produced and released entirely by the thyroid gland, whereas only 20% of the total T_3 is produced by the thyroid. Most of the T_3 is produced by peripheral deiodination (removal of 5'-iodine from the outer ring) of T_4 in the liver, muscles, kidney, and anterior pituitary, a reaction that is catalyzed by 5'-mono-deiodinase. Some T_4 is converted to rT_3, the metabolically inactive compound, by deiodination of the inner ring of T_4. In conditions such as Graves' disease, toxic multinodular goiter, or a stimulated thyroid gland the proportion of T_3 released from the thyroid may be dramatically elevated. Thyroid hormones are transported in serum bound to carrier proteins such as T_4-binding globulin, T_4-binding prealbumin, and albumin. Only a small fraction (0.02%) of thyroid hormone (T_3 and T_4) is free (unbound) and is the physiologically active component. T_3 is the more potent of the two thyroid hormones, although its circulating plasma level is much lower than that of T_4. T_3 is less tightly bound to protein in the plasma than T_4, and so it enters tissues more readily. T_3 is three to four times more active than T_4 per unit weight, with a half-life of about 1 day, compared to approximately 7 days for T_4.

The secretion of thyroid hormone is controlled by the hypothalamic-pituitary-thyroid axis (Fig. 38-9). The hypothalamus produces a peptide, the thyrotropin-releasing hormone (TRH), which stimulates the pituitary to release TSH or thyrotropin. TRH reaches the pituitary via the portovenous circulation. TSH, a 28-kDa glycopeptide, mediates iodide trapping, secretion, and release of thyroid hormones, in addition to increasing the cellularity and vascularity of the thyroid gland. The TSH receptor (TSH-R) belongs to a family of G-protein coupled receptors that have seven transmembrane-spanning domains and use cyclic adenosine monophosphate in the signal-transduction pathway. TSH secretion by the anterior pituitary is also regulated via a negative feedback loop by T_4 and T_3. Because the pituitary has the ability to convert T_4 to T_3, the latter is thought to be more important in this feedback control. T_3 also inhibits the release of TRH.

The thyroid gland also is capable of autoregulation, which allows it to modify its function independent of TSH. As an adaptation to low iodide intake, the gland preferentially synthesizes T_3 rather than T_4, thereby increasing the efficiency of secreted hormone. In situations of iodine excess, iodide transport, peroxide generation, and synthesis and secretion of thyroid hormones is inhibited. Excessively large doses of iodide may lead to initial increased organification, followed by suppression, a phenomenon called the *Wolff-Chaikoff effect*. Epinephrine and human chorionic gonadotrophin hormones stimulate thyroid hormone production. Thus, elevated thyroid hormone levels are found in pregnancy and gynecologic malignancies such as hydatidiform mole. In contrast, glucocorticoids inhibit thyroid hormone production. In severely ill patients, peripheral thyroid hormones may be reduced, without a compensatory increase in TSH levels, giving rise to the euthyroid sick syndrome.

Thyroid Hormone Function

Free thyroid hormone enters the cell membrane by diffusion or by specific carriers and is carried to the nuclear membrane by binding to specific proteins. T_4 is deiodinated to T_3 and enters the nucleus via active transport, where it binds to the thyroid hormone receptor. The T_3 receptor is similar to the nuclear receptors for glucocorticoids, mineralocorticoids, estrogens, vitamin D, and retinoic acid. In humans, two types of T_3 receptor genes (α and β) are located on chromosomes 3 and 17. Thyroid receptor expression depends upon peripheral concentrations of thyroid hormones and is tissue spe-

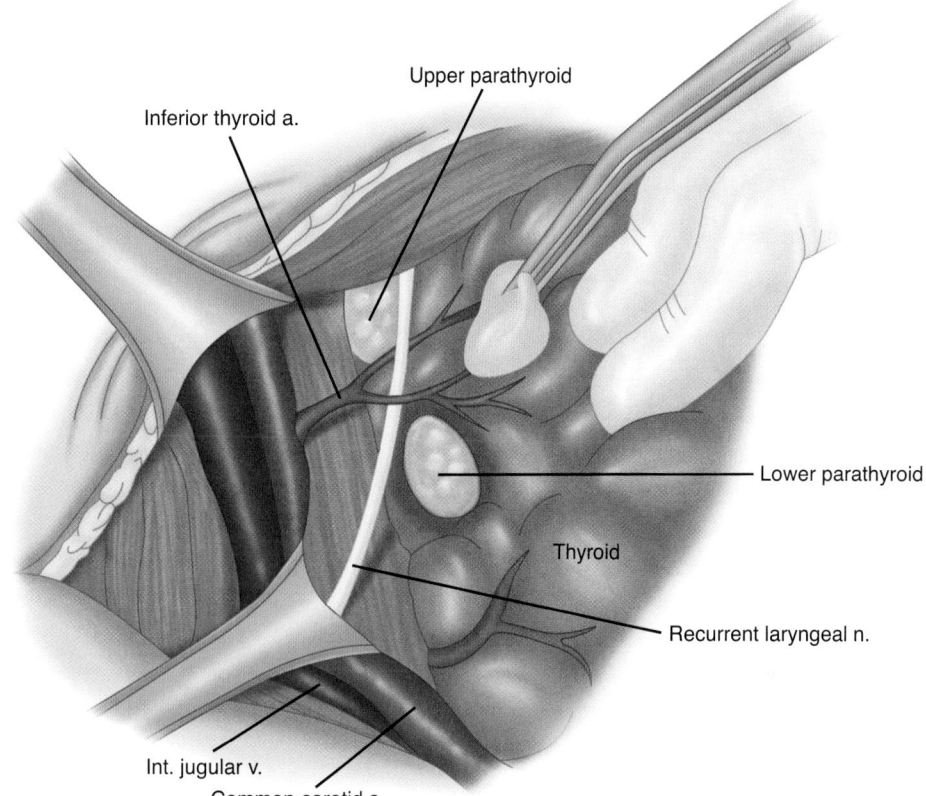

Upper parathyroid

Inferior thyroid a.

Lower parathyroid

Thyroid

Recurrent laryngeal n.

Int. jugular v.

Common carotid a.

FIG. 38-5. Relationship of the parathyroids to the recurrent laryngeal nerve. a. = artery; v. = vein.

cific—the α form is abundant in the central nervous system, whereas the β form predominates in the liver. Each gene product has a ligand-independent, amino-terminal domain; a ligand-binding, carboxy-terminal domain; and centrally located DNA-binding regions. Binding of thyroid hormone leads to the transcription and translation of specific hormone responsive genes.

Thyroid hormones affect almost every system in the body. They are important for fetal brain development and skeletal maturation. T_3 increases oxygen consumption, basal metabolic rate, and heat production by stimulation of Na^+/K^+ ATPase in various tissues. It also has positive inotropic and chronotropic effects on the heart by increasing transcription of the Ca^{2+} ATPase in the sarcoplasmic reticulum and increasing levels of beta-adrenergic receptors and concentration of G proteins. Myocardial alpha receptors are decreased and actions of catecholamines are amplified. Thyroid hormones are responsible for maintaining the normal hypoxic and hypercapnic drive in the respiratory center of the brain. They also increase GI motility, leading to diarrhea in hyperthyroidism and constipation in hypothyroidism. Thyroid hormones also increase bone and protein turnover and the speed of muscle contraction and relaxation. They also increase glycogenolysis, hepatic gluconeogenesis, intestinal glucose absorption, and cholesterol synthesis and degradation.

Evaluation of Patients with Thyroid Disease

Tests of Thyroid Function

A multitude of different tests are available to evaluate thyroid function. No single test is sufficient to assess thyroid function in all situations and the results must be interpreted in the context of the patient's clinical condition.[4] TSH is the only test necessary in most patients with thyroid nodules that clinically appear to be euthyroid.

Serum Thyroid-Stimulating Hormone (Normal 0.5–5 μU/mL) The tests for serum TSH are based on the following principle—monoclonal TSH antibodies are bound to a solid matrix and bind serum TSH. A second monoclonal antibody binds to a separate epitope on

TSH and is labeled with radioisotope, enzyme, or fluorescent tag. Therefore, the amount of serum TSH is proportional to the amount of bound secondary antibody (immunometric assay). Serum TSH levels reflect the ability of the anterior pituitary to detect free T_4 levels. There is an inverse relationship between the free T_4 level and the logarithm of the TSH concentration—small changes in free T_4 lead to a large shift in TSH levels. The ultrasensitive TSH assay has become the most sensitive and specific test for the diagnosis of hyper- and hypothyroidism and for optimizing T_4 therapy.

Total T_4 (Reference Range 55–150 nmol/L) and T_3 (Reference Range 1.5–3.5 nmol/L) Total T_4 and T_3 levels are measured by radioimmunoassay and measure both the free and bound components of the hormones. Total T_4 levels reflect the output from the thyroid gland, whereas T_3 levels in the nonstimulated thyroid gland are more indicative of peripheral thyroid hormone metabolism, and are, therefore, not generally suitable as a general screening test. Total T_4 levels are increased not only in hyperthyroid patients, but also in those with elevated Tg levels secondary to pregnancy, estrogen/progesterone use, or congenital diseases. Similarly, total T_4 levels decrease in hypothyroidism and in patients with decreased Tg levels due to anabolic steroid use and protein-losing disorders like nephrotic syndrome. Individuals with these latter disorders may be euthyroid if their free T_4 levels are normal. Measurement of total T_3 levels is important in clinically hyperthyroid patients with normal T_4 levels, who may have T_3 thyrotoxicosis. As discussed previously in Thyroid Hormone Synthesis, Secretion, and Transport, total T_3 levels often are increased in early hypothyroidism.

Free T_4 (Reference Range 12–28 pmol/L) and Free T_3 (3–9 pmol/L) These radioimmunoassay-based tests are a sensitive and accurate measurement of biologically active thyroid hormone. Free T_4 estimates are not performed as a routine screening tool in thyroid disease. Use of this test is confined to cases of early hyperthyroidism in which total T_4 levels may be normal but free T_4 levels are raised. In patients with end-organ resistance to T_4 (Refetoff syndrome), T_4

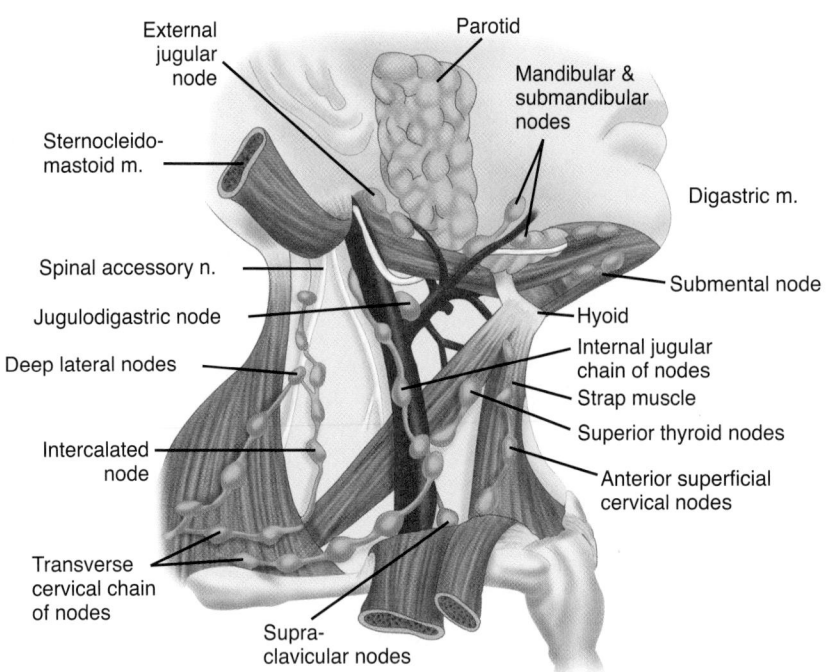

A

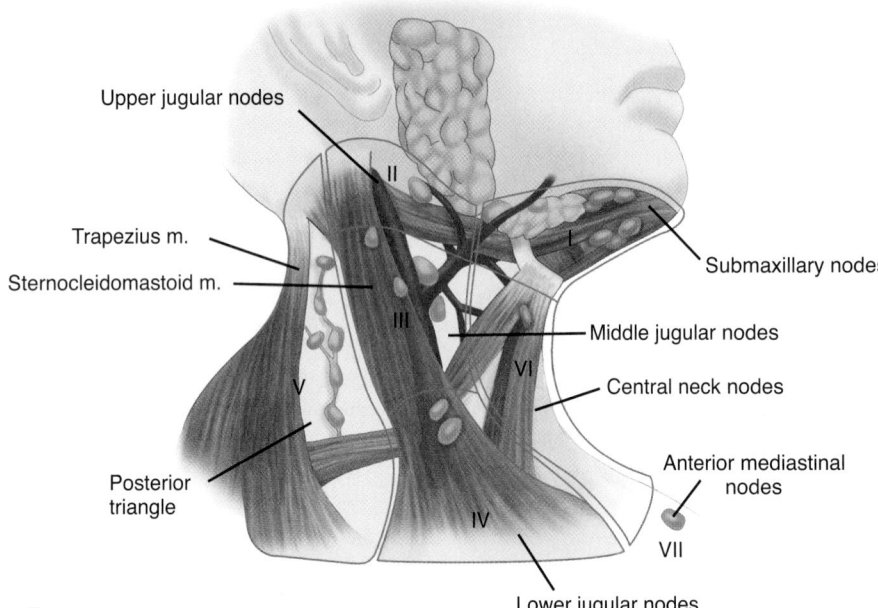

B

FIG. 38-6. A and **B.** Lymph nodes in the neck can be divided into six regions. Upper mediastinal nodes constitute level VII. m. = muscle; n. = nerve.

levels are increased, but TSH levels usually are normal. Free T_3 is most useful in confirming the diagnosis of early hyperthyroidism, in which levels of free T_4 and free T_3 rise before total T_4 and T_3. Free T_4 levels may also be measured indirectly using the T_3 resin-uptake test. If free T_4 levels are increased, fewer hormone binding sites are available for binding radiolabeled T_3 that has been added to the patient's serum. Therefore, more T_3 binds with an ion-exchange resin and the T_3-resin uptake is increased.

Thyrotropin-Releasing Hormone This test is useful to evaluate pituitary TSH secretory function and is performed by administering 500 μg of TRH intravenously and measuring TSH levels after 30 and 60 minutes. In a normal individual, TSH levels should increase at least 6 μIU/mL from the baseline. This test also was previously used to assess patients with borderline hyperthyroidism, but has largely been replaced by sensitive TSH assays for this purpose.

Thyroid Antibodies Thyroid antibodies include anti-Tg, antimicrosomal, or anti-TPO and thyroid-stimulating immunoglobulin (TSI). Anti-Tg and anti-TPO antibody levels do not determine thyroid function, but rather indicate the underlying disorder, usually an autoimmune thyroiditis. About 80% of patients with Hashimoto's thyroiditis have elevated thyroid antibody levels; however, levels may also be increased in patients with Graves' disease, multinodular goiter, and occasionally, with thyroid neoplasms.

Serum Thyroglobulin Tg is only made by normal or abnormal thyroid tissue. It normally is not released into the circulation in large amounts but increases dramatically in destructive processes of the thyroid gland, such as thyroiditis, or overactive states such as Graves' disease and toxic multinodular goiter. The most important use for serum Tg levels is in monitoring patients with differentiated thyroid cancer for recurrence, particularly after total thyroidectomy

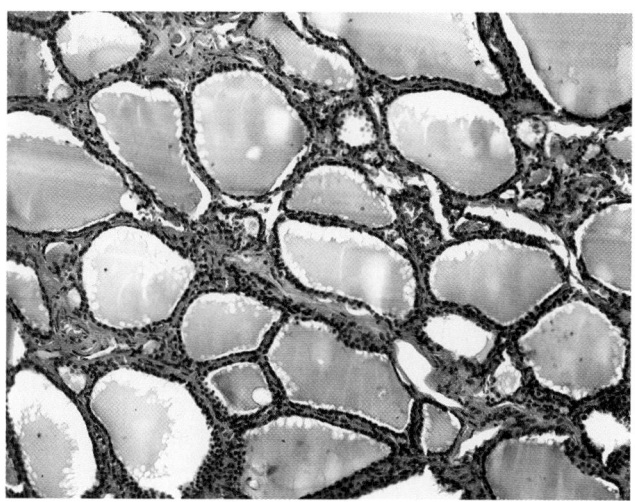

FIG. 38-7. Normal thyroid histology—follicular cells surround colloid.

and RAI ablation. Elevated anti-Tg antibodies can interfere with the accuracy of serum Tg levels and should always be measured when interpreting Tg levels.

Serum Calcitonin (0–4 pg/mL Basal) This 32-amino-acid polypeptide is secreted by the C cells and functions to lower serum calcium levels, although in humans, it has only minimal physiologic effects. It is also a sensitive marker of MTC.

Thyroid Imaging

Radionuclide Imaging Both iodine 123 (^{123}I) and iodine 131 (^{131}I) are used to image the thyroid gland. The former emits low-dose radiation, has a half-life of 12 to 14 hours, and is used to image lingual thyroids or goiters. In contrast, ^{131}I has a half-life of 8 to 10 days and leads to higher-dose radiation exposure. Therefore, this isotope is used to screen and treat patients with differentiated thyroid cancers for metastatic disease. The images obtained by these studies provide information not only about the size and shape of the gland, but also the distribution of functional activity. Areas that trap less radioactivity than the surrounding gland are termed *cold* (Fig. 38-10), whereas

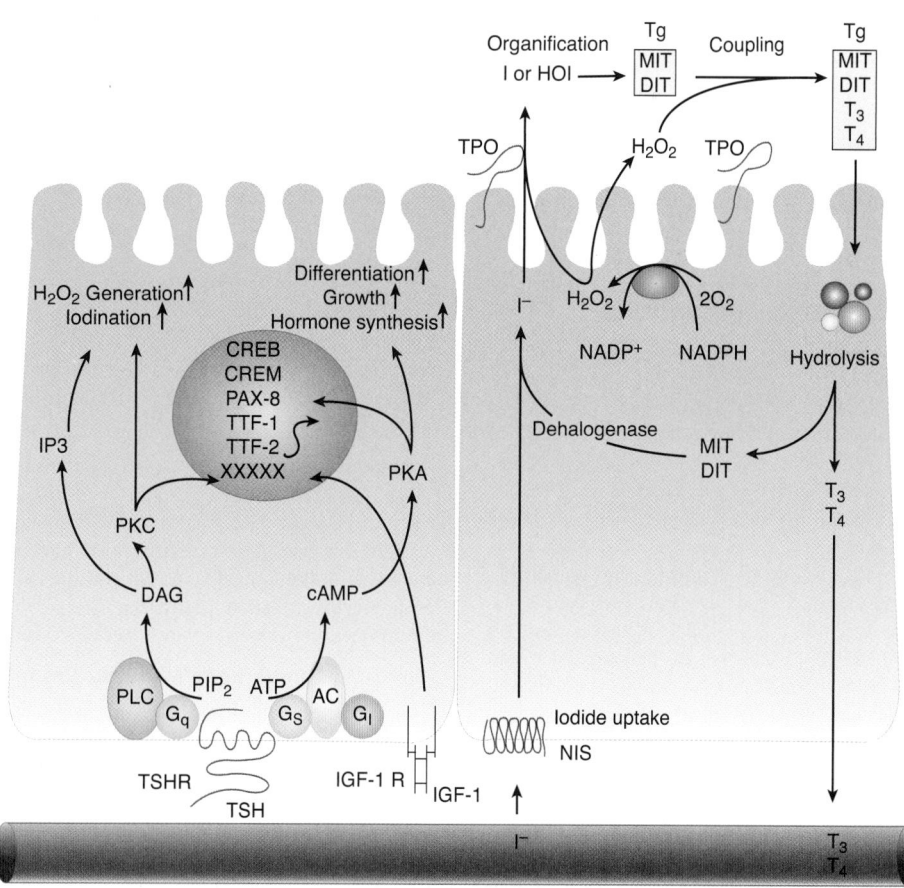

FIG. 38-8. Thyroid follicular cell showing the major signaling pathways involved in thyroid cell growth and function and key steps in thyroid hormone synthesis. The basal membrane of the cell in contact with the circulation and its apical surface contacts the thyroid follicle. Thyroid hormone synthesis is initiated by the binding of thyroid-stimulating hormone (TSH) to the TSH receptor (TSHR), a G-protein coupled transmembrane receptor, on the basal membrane. Activation leads to an increase in cyclic adenosine monophosphate (cAMP), phosphorylation of protein kinase A (PKA), and activation of target cytosolic and nuclear proteins. The protein kinase C (PKC) pathway is stimulated at higher doses of TSH. Iodide is actively transported into the cell via the Na/I symporter (NIS) and flows down an electrical gradient to the apical membrane. There, thyroid peroxidase (TPO) oxidizes iodide and iodinated tyrosyl residues on thyroglobulin (Tg) in the presence of peroxide (H_2O_2). Mono- and diiodotyrosyl (MIT, DIT) residues are also coupled to form T_4 and T_3 by TPO. Thyroglobulin carrying T_4 and T_3 is then internalized by pinocytosis and digested in lysosomes. Thyroid hormone is released into the circulation, while MIT and DIT are deiodinated and recycled. ATP = adenosine triphosphate; CREB = cAMP response element binding protein; CREM = cAMP response element modulator; DAG = diacylglycerol; IGF-1 = insulin-like growth factor; IP3 = inositol-3-phosphate; NADP+ = nicotinamide adenine dinucleotide phosphate, oxidized form; NADPH = nicotinamide adenine dinucleotide phosphate; PIP$_2$ = phosphatidylinostol; PLC = phospholipase C; T_3 = 3,5',3-triiodothyronine; T_4 = thyroxine. *(Reproduced with permission from Kopp P: Pendred's syndrome and genetic defects in thyroid hormone synthesis. Rev Endocr Metab Disord 1:114, 2000. Kluwer Academic Publishers.)*

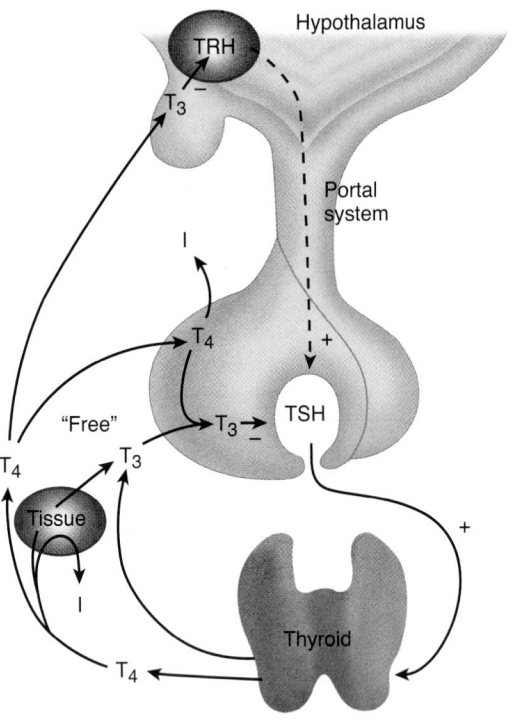

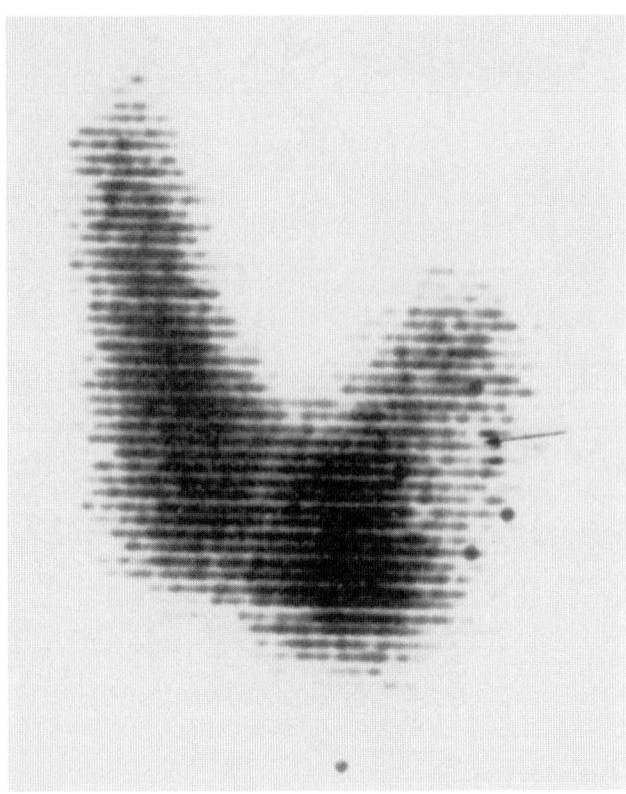

FIG. 38-9. Hypothalamic-pituitary-thyroid hormone axis. In both the hypothalamus and pituitary, 3,5',3-triiodothyronine (T_3) is primarily responsible for inhibition of thyrotropin-releasing hormone (TRH) and thyroid-stimulating hormone (TSH) secretion. T_4 = thyroxine. [*Reproduced with permission from Greenspan FS: The thyroid gland, in Greenspan FS, Gardner D (eds):* Basic and Clinical Endocrinology, *6th ed. New York: McGraw-Hill, 2001, p 217.*]

FIG. 38-10. Radioactive iodine scan of the thyroid, with the *arrow* showing an area of decreased uptake, a cold nodule.

areas that demonstrate increased activity are termed *hot*. The risk of malignancy is higher in "cold" lesions (20%) compared to "hot" or "warm" lesions (<5%). Technetium Tc 99m pertechnetate (^{99m}Tc) is taken up by the thyroid gland and is increasingly being used for thyroid evaluation. This isotope is taken up by the mitochondria, but is not organified. It also has the advantage of having a shorter half-life and minimizes radiation exposure. It is particularly sensitive for nodal metastases. More recently, ^{18}F-fluorodeoxyglucose positron emission tomography (FDG PET) is being increasingly used to screen for metastases in patients with thyroid cancer in whom other imaging studies are negative.[5] PET scans are not routinely used in the evaluation of thyroid nodules; however, they may show clinically occult

thyroid lesions. There are several recent reports of rates of malignancy in these lesions ranging from 14 to 63%. These incidentally discovered nodules should be worked up by ultrasound and fine-needle aspiration biopsy (FNAB).

Ultrasound Ultrasound is an excellent noninvasive and portable imaging study of the thyroid gland with the added advantage of no radiation exposure. It is helpful in the evaluation of thyroid nodules, distinguishing solid from cystic ones, and providing information about size and multicentricity. Ultrasound also can be used to assess for cervical lymphadenopathy (Fig. 38-11) and to guide FNAB. An experienced ultrasonographer is necessary for the best results.

Computed Tomography/Magnetic Resonance Imaging Scan

Computed tomography (CT) and magnetic resonance imaging (MRI) studies provide excellent imaging of the thyroid gland and

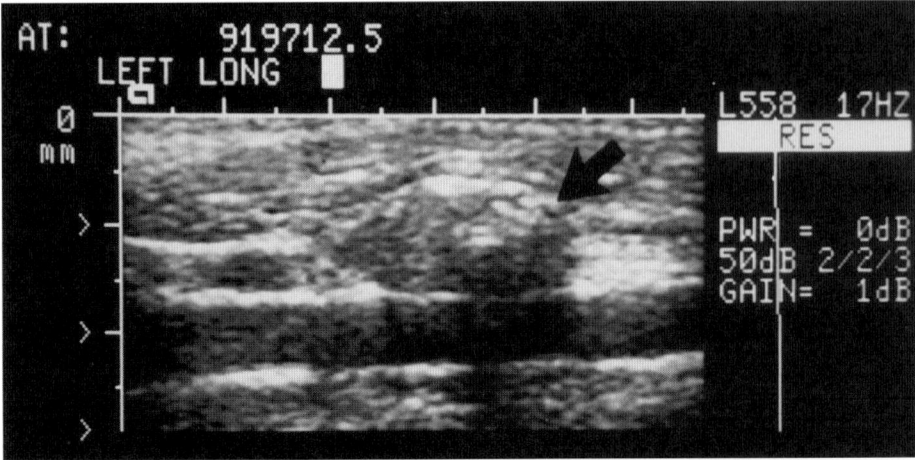

FIG. 38-11. Thyroid ultrasound showing a lymph node (*arrow*) along the carotid artery.

TABLE 38-1	Differential diagnosis of hyperthyroidism

Increased Hormone Synthesis (Increased RAIU)	**Release of Preformed Hormone (Decreased RAIU)**
Graves' disease (diffuse toxic goiter)	Thyroiditis—acute phase of Hashimoto's thyroiditis, subacute thyroiditis
Toxic multinodular goiter	
Plummer's disease (toxic adenoma)	Factitious (iatrogenic) thyrotoxicosis "Hamburger thyrotoxicosis"
Drug induced—amiodarone, iodine	
Thyroid cancer	
Struma ovarii	
Hydatidiform mole	
TSH-secreting pituitary adenoma	

RAIU = radioactive iodine uptake; TSH = thyroid-stimulating hormone.

adjacent nodes, and are particularly useful in evaluating the extent of large, fixed, or substernal goiters (which cannot be evaluated by ultrasound) and their relationship to the airway and vascular structures. Noncontrast CT scans should be obtained for patients who are likely to require subsequent RAI therapy. If contrast is necessary, therapy needs to be delayed by several months. Combined PET-CT scans are increasingly being used for Tg-positive, radioactive iodine–negative tumors.

Benign Thyroid Disorders
Hyperthyroidism

The clinical manifestations of hyperthyroidism result from an excess of circulating thyroid hormone. Hyperthyroidism may arise from a number of conditions that are listed in Table 38-1. It is important to distinguish disorders such as Graves' disease and toxic nodular goiters that result from increased production of thyroid hormone from those disorders that lead to a release of stored hormone from injury to the thyroid gland (thyroiditis) or from other nonthyroid gland–related conditions. The former disorders lead to an increase in radioactive iodine uptake (RAIU), whereas the latter group is characterized by low RAIU. Of these disorders, Graves' disease, toxic multinodular goiter, and solitary toxic nodule are most relevant to the surgeon.

Diffuse Toxic Goiter (Graves' Disease) Although originally described by the Welsh physician Caleb Parry in a posthumous article in 1825, this disorder is known as Graves' disease after Robert Graves, an Irish physician who described three patients in 1835. Graves' disease is by far the most common cause of hyperthyroidism in North America, accounting for 60 to 80% of cases. It is an autoimmune disease with a strong familial predisposition, female preponderance (5:1), and peak incidence between the ages of 40 to 60 years. Graves' disease is characterized by thyrotoxicosis, diffuse goiter, and extrathyroidal conditions including ophthalmopathy, dermopathy (pretibial myxedema), thyroid acropathy, gynecomastia, and other manifestations.

Etiology, Pathogenesis, and Pathology The exact etiology of the initiation of the autoimmune process in Graves' disease is not known. However, conditions such as the postpartum state, iodine excess, lithium therapy, and bacterial and viral infections have been suggested as possible triggers. Genetic factors also play a role, as haplotyping studies indicate that Graves' disease is associated with certain human leukocyte antigen (HLA) haplotypes—HLA-B8 and HLA-DR3 and HLADQA1*0501 in Caucasian patients whereas HLA-DRB1*0701 is protective against it. Polymorphisms of the cytotoxic T-lymphocyte antigen 4 (*CTLA-4*) gene also have been associated with Graves' disease development.[6] Once initiated, the process causes sensitized T-helper lymphocytes to stimulate B lymphocytes, which produce antibodies directed against the thyroid hormone receptor. TSIs or antibodies that stimulate the TSH-R, as well as TSH-binding inhibiting immunoglobulins or antibodies have

been described. The thyroid-stimulating antibodies stimulate the thyrocytes to grow and synthesize excess thyroid hormone, which is a hallmark of Graves' disease. Graves' disease also is associated with other autoimmune conditions such as type I diabetes mellitus, Addison's disease, pernicious anemia, and myasthenia gravis.

Macroscopically, the thyroid gland in patients with Graves' disease is diffusely and smoothly enlarged, with a concomitant increase in vascularity. Microscopically, the gland is hyperplastic, and the epithelium is columnar with minimal colloid present. The nuclei exhibit mitosis, and papillary projections of hyperplastic epithelium are common. There may be aggregates of lymphoid tissue, and vascularity is markedly increased.

Clinical Features The clinical manifestations of Graves' disease can be divided into those related to hyperthyroidism and those specific to Graves' disease. Hyperthyroid symptoms include heat intolerance, increased sweating and thirst, and weight loss despite adequate caloric intake. Symptoms of increased adrenergic stimulation include palpitations, nervousness, fatigue, emotional lability, hyperkinesis, and tremors. The most common GI symptoms include increased frequency of bowel movements and diarrhea. Female patients often develop amenorrhea, decreased fertility, and an increased incidence of miscarriages. Children experience rapid growth with early bone maturation, whereas older patients may present with cardiovascular complications such as atrial fibrillation and congestive heart failure.

On physical examination, weight loss and facial flushing may be evident. The skin is warm and moist and African American patients often note darkening of their skin. Tachycardia or atrial fibrillation is present with cutaneous vasodilation leading to a widening of the pulse pressure and a rapid falloff in the transmitted pulse wave (collapsing pulse). A fine tremor, muscle wasting, and proximal muscle group weakness with hyperactive tendon reflexes often are present.

Approximately 50% of patients with Graves' disease also develop clinically evident ophthalmopathy, and dermopathy occurs in 1 to 2% of patients. It is characterized by deposition of glycosaminoglycans leading to thickened skin in the pretibial region and dorsum of the foot (Fig. 38-12). Eye symptoms include lid lag (von Graefe's sign), spasm of the upper eyelid revealing the sclera above the corneoscleral limbus (Dalrymple's sign), and a prominent stare, due to catecholamine excess. True infiltrative eye disease results in periorbital edema, conjunctival swelling and congestion (chemosis), proptosis, limitation of upward and lateral gaze (from involvement of the inferior and medial rectus muscles, respectively), keratitis, and even blindness due to optic nerve involvement. The etiology of Graves' ophthalmopathy is not completely known; however, orbital fibroblasts and muscles are thought to share a common antigen, the TSH-R. Ophthalmopathy is thought to result from inflammation caused by cytokines released from sensitized killer T lymphocytes and cytotoxic antibodies. Gynecomastia is common in young men. Rare bony involvement leads to subperiosteal bone formation and swelling in the metacarpals (thyroid acropathy). Onycholysis, or separation of fingernails from their beds, is a more commonly observed finding. On physical examination, the thyroid usually is diffusely and symmetrically enlarged, as evidenced by an enlarged pyramidal lobe. There may be an overlying bruit or thrill and loud venous hum in the supraclavicular space.

Diagnostic Tests The diagnosis of hyperthyroidism is made by a suppressed TSH with or without an elevated free T_4 or T_3 level. If eye signs are present, other tests are generally not needed. However, in the absence of eye findings, an ^{123}I uptake and scan should be performed. An elevated uptake, with a diffusely enlarged gland, confirms the diagnosis of Graves' disease and helps to differentiate it from other causes of hyperthyroidism. If free T_4 levels are normal, free T_3 levels should be determined, as they often are elevated in early Graves' or Plummer's disease (T_3 toxicosis). Anti-Tg and anti-TPO antibodies are elevated in up to 75% of patients, but are not specific. Elevated TSH-R or thyroid-stimulating antibodies (TSAb)

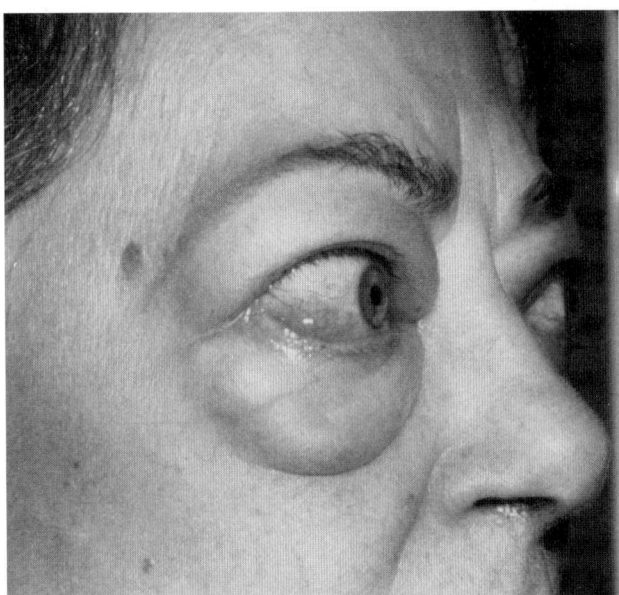

A

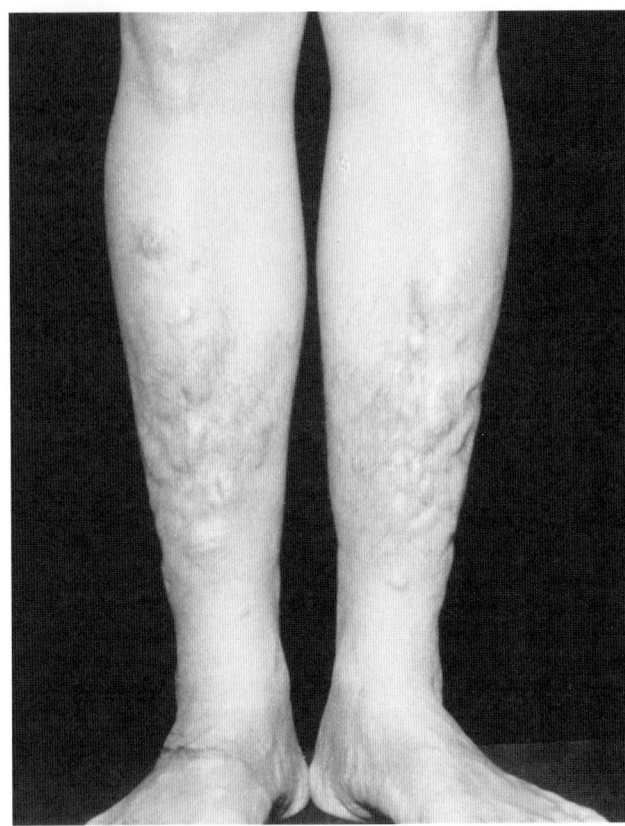

B

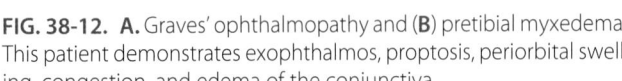

FIG. 38-12. A. Graves' ophthalmopathy and **(B)** pretibial myxedema. This patient demonstrates exophthalmos, proptosis, periorbital swelling, congestion, and edema of the conjunctiva.

are diagnostic of Graves' disease and are increased in about 90% of patients. MRI scans of the orbits are useful in evaluating Graves' ophthalmopathy.

Treatment Graves' disease may be treated by any of three treatment modalities—antithyroid drugs, thyroid ablation with radioactive ^{131}I, and thyroidectomy.[7] The choice of treatment depends upon several factors, as discussed in the following sections.

Antithyroid Drugs Antithyroid medications generally are administered in preparation for RAI ablation or surgery. The drugs commonly used are propylthiouracil (PTU, 100 to 300 mg three times daily) and methimazole (10 to 30 mg three times daily, then once daily). Methimazole has a longer half-life and can be dosed once daily. Both drugs reduce thyroid hormone production by inhibiting the organic binding of iodine and the coupling of iodotyrosines (mediated by TPO). In addition, PTU also inhibits the peripheral conversion of T_4 to T_3, making it useful for the treatment of thyroid storm. Both drugs can cross the placenta, inhibiting fetal thyroid function, and are excreted in breast milk, although PTU has a lower risk of transplacental transfer. Methimazole also has been associated with congenital aplasia; therefore, PTU is preferred in pregnant and breastfeeding women. Side effects of treatment include reversible granulocytopenia, skin rashes, fever, peripheral neuritis, polyarteritis, vasculitis, and, rarely, agranulocytosis and aplastic anemia. Patients should be monitored for these possible complications and should always be warned to stop PTU or methimazole immediately and seek medical advice should they develop a sore throat or fever. Treatment of agranulocytosis involves admission to the hospital, discontinuation of the drug, and broad-spectrum antibiotic therapy. Surgery should be postponed until the granulocyte count reaches 1000 cells/m³.

The dose of antithyroid medication is titrated as needed in accordance with TSH and T_4 levels. Most patients have improved symptoms in 2 weeks and become euthyroid in about 6 weeks. Some physicians use the block-replace regimen, by adding T_4 (0.05 to 0.10 mg) to prevent hypothyroidism and suppress TSH secretion, because some, but not all, studies suggest that this reduces recurrence rates. The length of therapy is debated. Treatment with antithyroid medications is associated with a high relapse rate when these drugs are discontinued, with 40 to 80% of patients developing recurrent disease after a 1- to 2-year course. Patients with small glands are less likely to recur so that treatment for curative intent is reserved for patients with (a) small, nontoxic goiters less than 40 g, (b) mildly elevated thyroid hormone levels, and (c) rapid decrease in gland size with antithyroid medications. The catecholamine response of thyrotoxicosis can be alleviated by administering beta-blocking agents. These drugs have the added effect of decreasing the peripheral conversion of T_4 to T_3. Propranolol is the most commonly prescribed medication in doses of about 20 to 40 mg four times daily. Higher doses are sometimes required due to increased clearance of the medication.

Radioactive Iodine Therapy (^{131}I) RAI forms the mainstay of Graves' disease treatment in North America. The major advantages of this treatment are the avoidance of a surgical procedure and its concomitant risks, reduced overall treatment costs, and ease of treatment. Antithyroid drugs are given until the patient is euthyroid and then discontinued to maximize drug uptake. The ^{131}I dose is calculated after a preliminary scan, and usually consists of 8 to 12 mCi administered orally. After standard treatment with RAI, most patients become euthyroid within 2 months. However, only about 50% of patients treated with RAI are euthyroid 6 months after treatment, and the remaining are still hyperthyroid or already hypothyroid.[8] After 1 year, about 2.5% of patients develop hypothyroidism each year. RAI also has been documented to lead to progression of Graves' ophthalmopathy (33% after RAI compared to 16% after surgery), and ophthalmopathy is more common in smokers. Although there is no evidence of long-term problems with infertility, and overall cancer incidence rates are unchanged, there is a small increased risk of nodular goiter, thyroid cancer[9] and hyperparathyroidism (HPT)[10] in patients who have been treated with RAI. Patients treated with RAI have an unexplained increase in their overall and cardiovascular mortality rates when compared to the general population.

RAI therapy is therefore most often used in older patients with small or moderate-sized goiters, those who have relapsed after medical or surgical therapy, and those in whom antithyroid drugs or surgery are contraindicated. Absolute contraindications to RAI include women who are pregnant or breastfeeding. Relative contraindications include young patients (i.e., especially children and adolescents), those with thyroid nodules, and those with ophthalmopathy. The higher the initial dose of ^{131}I, the earlier the onset and the higher the incidence of hypothyroidism.

Surgical Treatment In North America, surgery is recommended when RAI is contraindicated as in patients who (a) have confirmed cancer or suspicious thyroid nodules, (b) are young, (c) are pregnant or desire to conceive soon after treatment, (d) have had severe reactions to antithyroid medications, (e) have large goiters causing compressive symptoms, and (f) are reluctant to undergo RAI therapy. Relative indications for thyroidectomy include patients, particularly smokers, with moderate to severe Graves' ophthalmopathy, those desiring rapid control of hyperthyroidism with a chance of being euthyroid, and those demonstrating poor compliance to antithyroid medications. The goal of thyroidectomy for Graves' disease should be the complete and permanent control of the disease with minimal morbidity. Patients should be rendered euthyroid before operation with antithyroid drugs that should be continued up to the day of surgery. Lugol's iodide solution or saturated potassium iodide generally is administered beginning 7 to 10 days preoperatively (three drops twice daily) to reduce vascularity of the gland and decrease the risk of precipitating thyroid storm. The major action of iodine in this situation is to inhibit release of thyroid hormone.

The extent of thyroidectomy to be performed is controversial and is determined by the desired outcome (risk of recurrence vs. euthyroidism) and surgeon experience. Patients with coexistent thyroid cancer, and those who refuse RAI therapy or have severe ophthalmopathy or have life-threatening reactions to antithyroid medications (vasculitis, agranulocytosis, or liver failure) should undergo total or near-total thyroidectomy. Ophthalmopathy has been demonstrated to stabilize or improve in most patients after total thyroidectomy, presumably from removal of the antigenic stimulus. A subtotal thyroidectomy, leaving a 4- to 7-g remnant, is recommended for all remaining patients. Remnants <3 g are recommended for children. Remnants <4 g are associated with a 2 to 10% recurrence rate but a high (>40%) rate of hypothyroidism. During subtotal thyroidectomy, remnant tissue may be left on each side (bilateral subtotal thyroidectomy), or a total lobectomy can be performed on one side with a subtotal thyroidectomy on the other side (Hartley-Dunhill procedure). Results are similar with either procedure,[11] but the latter procedure is theoretically associated with fewer complications and requires re-entering only one side of the neck should recurrence require reoperation. Most studies, however, show no difference in the rates of complications with either approach. Recurrent thyrotoxicosis usually is managed by radioiodine treatment. Long-term follow-up should be maintained for all patients undergoing subtotal procedures, with clinical review and yearly TSH measurement to detect the possible late onset of hypothyroidism or recurrent hyperthyroidism.

Toxic Multinodular Goiter Toxic multinodular goiters usually occur in older individuals, who often have a prior history of a nontoxic multinodular goiter. Over several years, enough thyroid nodules become autonomous to cause hyperthyroidism. The presentation often is insidious in that hyperthyroidism may only become apparent when patients are placed on low doses of thyroid hormone suppression for the goiter. Some patients have T_3 toxicosis, whereas others may present only with atrial fibrillation or congestive heart failure. Hyperthyroidism also can be precipitated by iodide-containing drugs such as contrast media and the antiarrhythmic agent amiodarone (jodbasedow hyperthyroidism). Symptoms and signs of hyperthyroidism are similar to Graves' disease, but extrathyroidal manifestations are absent.

Diagnostic Studies Blood tests are similar to Graves' disease with a suppressed TSH level and elevated free T_4 or T_3 levels. RAI uptake also is increased, showing multiple nodules with increased uptake and suppression of the remaining gland.

Treatment Hyperthyroidism must be adequately controlled. Surgical resection is the preferred treatment of patients with toxic multinodular goiter with subtotal thyroidectomy being the standard procedure. Remnant size is not as crucial a concern because these patients require thyroid hormone suppression to prevent recurrence of the goiter. The Hartley-Dunhill procedure is preferred over a bilateral subtotal thyroidectomy for the reasons outlined earlier in Surgical Treatment. Care must be taken in identifying the RLN, which may be found laterally on the thyroid (rather than posterior) or stretched anteriorly over a nodule. Total thyroidectomy may sometimes be necessary if no normal thyroid tissue is present. RAI therapy is reserved for elderly patients who represent very poor operative risks, provided there is no airway compression from the goiter, and thyroid cancer is not a concern. However, because uptake is less than in Graves' disease, larger doses of RAI often are needed to treat the hyperthyroidism. Furthermore, RAI-induced thyroiditis has the potential to cause swelling and acute airway compromise, and leaves the goiter intact, with the possibility of recurrent hyperthyroidism.

Toxic Adenoma (Plummer's Disease) Hyperthyroidism from a single hyperfunctioning nodule typically occurs in younger patients who note recent growth of a long-standing nodule along with the symptoms of hyperthyroidism. Toxic adenomas are characterized by somatic mutations in the TSH-R gene, although G-protein stimulating gene (*gsp*) mutations may occur also.[12] Most hyperfunctioning or autonomous thyroid nodules have attained a size of at least 3 cm before hyperthyroidism occurs. Physical examination usually reveals a solitary thyroid nodule without palpable thyroid tissue on the contralateral side. RAI scanning shows a "hot" nodule with suppression the rest of the thyroid gland. These nodules are rarely malignant. Smaller nodules may be managed with antithyroid medications and RAI. Surgery (lobectomy and isthmusectomy) is preferred to treat young patients and those with larger nodules.

Thyroid Storm Thyroid storm is a condition of hyperthyroidism accompanied by fever, central nervous system agitation or depression, cardiovascular dysfunction that may be precipitated by infection, surgery, or trauma. Occasionally, thyroid storm may result from amiodarone administration. This condition was previously associated with high mortality rates but can be appropriately managed in an intensive care unit setting. Beta blockers are given to reduce peripheral T_4 to T_3 conversion and decrease the hyperthyroid symptoms. Oxygen supplementation and hemodynamic support should be instituted. Non-aspirin compounds can be used to treat pyrexia and Lugol's iodine or sodium ipodate (intravenously) should be administered to decrease iodine uptake and thyroid hormone secretion. PTU therapy blocks the formation of new thyroid hormone and reduces peripheral conversion of T_4 to T_3. Corticosteroids often are helpful to prevent adrenal exhaustion and block hepatic thyroid hormone conversion.

Hypothyroidism

Deficiency in circulating levels of thyroid hormone leads to hypothyroidism and, in neonates, to cretinism, which is characterized by neurologic impairment and mental retardation. Hypothyroidism also may occur in Pendred's syndrome (associated with deafness) and Turner's syndrome. Conditions that cause hypothyroidism are listed in Table 38-2.

TABLE 38-2	Causes of hypothyroidism		
Primary (Increased TSH Levels)	**Secondary (Decreased TSH Levels)**	**Tertiary**	
Hashimoto's thyroiditis	Pituitary tumor	Hypothalamic insufficiency	
RAI therapy for Graves' disease	Pituitary resection or ablation	Resistance to thyroid hormone	
Postthyroidectomy			
Excessive iodine intake			
Subacute thyroiditis			
Medications: antithyroid drugs, lithium			
Rare: iodine deficiency, dyshormogenesis			

RAI = radioactive iodine; TSH = thyroid-stimulating hormone.

Clinical Features Failure of thyroid gland development or function in utero leads to cretinism and characteristic facies similar to those of children with Down syndrome and dwarfism. Failure to thrive and severe mental retardation often are present. Immediate testing and treatment with thyroid hormone at birth can lessen the neurologic and intellectual deficits. Hypothyroidism developing in childhood or adolescence results in delayed development and may also lead to abdominal distention, umbilical hernia, and rectal prolapse. In adults, symptoms in general are nonspecific, including tiredness, weight gain, cold intolerance, constipation, and menorrhagia. Patients with severe hypothyroidism or myxedema develop characteristic facial features due to the deposition of glycosaminoglycans in the subcutaneous tissues, leading to facial and periorbital puffiness. The skin becomes rough and dry and often develops a yellowish hue from reduced conversion of carotene to vitamin A. Hair becomes dry and brittle, and severe hair loss may occur. There is also a characteristic loss of the outer two thirds of the eyebrows. An enlarged tongue may impair speech, which is already slowed, in keeping with the impairment of mental processes. Patients may also have nonspecific abdominal pain accompanied by distention and constipation. Libido and fertility are impaired in both sexes. Cardiovascular changes in hypothyroidism include bradycardia, cardiomegaly, pericardial effusion, reduced cardiac output, and pulmonary effusions. When hypothyroidism occurs as a result of pituitary failure, other features of hypopituitarism, such as pale, waxy skin; loss of body hair; and atrophic genitalia, may be present.

Laboratory Findings Hypothyroidism is characterized by low circulating levels of T_4 and T_3. Raised TSH levels are found in primary thyroid failure, whereas secondary hypothyroidism is characterized by low TSH levels that do not increase following TRH stimulation. Thyroid autoantibodies are highest in patients with autoimmune disease (Hashimoto's thyroiditis, Graves' disease) and may also be elevated in patients with nodular goiter and thyroid neoplasms. An electrocardiogram demonstrates decreased voltage with flattening or inversion of T waves.

Treatment T_4 is the treatment of choice and is administered in dosages varying from 50 to 200 μg per day, depending upon the patient's size and condition. Starting doses of 100 μg of T_4 daily are well tolerated; however, elderly patients and those with coexisting heart disease and profound hypothyroidism should be started on a considerably lower dose such as 25 to 50 μg daily because of associated hypercholesterolemia and atherosclerosis. The dose can be slowly increased over weeks to months to attain a euthyroid state. A baseline electrocardiogram should always be obtained in patients with severe hypothyroidism before treatment. T_4 dosage is titrated against clinical response and TSH levels, which should return to normal. The management of patients with subclinical hypothyroidism (normal T_4, slightly raised TSH) is controversial. Some evidence suggests that patients with subclinical hypothyroidism and increased antithyroid antibody levels should be treated, because they will subsequently develop hypothyroidism. Patients who present with myxedema coma may require initial emergency treatment with large doses of IV T_4 (300 to 400 μg), with careful monitoring in an intensive care unit setting.

Thyroiditis

Thyroiditis usually is classified into acute, subacute, and chronic forms, each associated with a distinct clinical presentation and histology.

Acute (Suppurative) Thyroiditis The thyroid gland is inherently resistant to infection due to its extensive blood and lymphatic supply, high iodide content, and fibrous capsule. However, infectious agents can seed it (a) via the hematogenous or lymphatic route, (b) via direct spread from persistent pyriform sinus fistulae or thyroglossal duct cysts, (c) as a result of penetrating trauma to the thyroid gland, or (d) due to immunosuppression. *Streptococcus* and anaerobes account for about 70% of cases; however, other species also have been cultured.[13] Acute suppurative thyroiditis is more common in children and often is preceded by an upper respiratory tract infection or otitis media. It is characterized by severe neck pain radiating to the jaws or ear, fever, chills, odynophagia, and dysphonia. Complications such as systemic sepsis, tracheal or esophageal rupture, jugular vein thrombosis, laryngeal chondritis, and perichondritis or sympathetic trunk paralysis may also occur.

The diagnosis is established by leukocytosis on blood tests and FNAB for Gram's stain, culture, and cytology. CT scans may help to delineate the extent of infection. A persistent pyriform sinus fistula should always be suspected in children with recurrent acute thyroiditis. A barium swallow demonstrates the anomalous tract with 80% sensitivity. Treatment consists of parenteral antibiotics and drainage of abscesses. Patients with pyriform sinus fistulae require complete resection of the sinus tract, including the area of the thyroid where the tract terminates, to prevent recurrence.

Subacute Thyroiditis Subacute thyroiditis can occur in the painful or painless forms. Although the exact etiology is not known, painful thyroiditis is thought to be viral in origin or result from a postviral inflammatory response. Genetic predisposition may also play a role, as manifested by its strong association with the HLA-B35 haplotype. One model of pathogenesis suggests that viral or thyroid antigens, when presented by macrophages in the context of HLA-B35, stimulate cytotoxic T lymphocytes and damage thyroid follicular cells.

Painful thyroiditis most commonly occurs in 30- to 40-year-old women and is characterized by the sudden or gradual onset of neck pain, which may radiate toward the mandible or ear. History of a preceding upper respiratory tract infection often can be elicited. The gland is enlarged, exquisitely tender, and firm. The disorder classically progresses through four stages. An initial hyperthyroid phase, due to release of thyroid hormone, is followed by a second, euthyroid phase. The third phase, hypothyroidism, occurs in about 20 to 30% of patients and is followed by resolution and return to the euthyroid state in >90% of patients. A few patients develop recurrent disease.

In the early stages of the disease, TSH is decreased, and Tg, T_4, and T_3 levels are elevated due to the release of preformed thyroid hormone from destroyed follicles. The erythrocyte sedimentation rate is typically >100 mm/h. RAIU also is decreased (<2% at 24 hours), even in euthyroid patients, due to the release of thyroid hormones from destruction of the thyroid parenchyma. Painful thyroiditis is self-limited, and therefore, treatment is primarily symptomatic. Aspirin and other NSAIDs are used for pain relief, but steroids may be indicated in more severe cases. Short-term thyroid replacement may be needed and may shorten the duration of symptoms. Thyroidectomy is reserved for the rare patient who has a prolonged course not responsive to medical measures or for recurrent disease.

Painless thyroiditis is considered to be autoimmune in origin and may occur sporadically or in the postpartum period; the latter typically occurs at about 6 weeks after delivery in women with high TPO antibody titers in early pregnancy. This timing is thought to coincide with a decrease in the normal immune tolerance of pregnancy and consequent rebound elevation of antibody titers.

Painless thyroiditis also is more common in women and usually occurs between 30 to 60 years of age. Physical examination demonstrates a normal sized or minimally enlarged, slightly firm, nontender gland. Laboratory tests and RAIU are similar to those in painful thyroiditis, except for a normal erythrocyte sedimentation rate. The clinical course also parallels painful thyroiditis. Patients with symptoms may require beta blockers and thyroid hormone replacement. Thyroidectomy or RAI ablation is only indicated for the rare patient with recurrent, disabling episodes of thyroiditis.

Chronic Thyroiditis *Lymphocytic (Hashimoto's) Thyroiditis* Lymphocytic thyroiditis was first described by Hashimoto in 1912 as *struma lymphomatosa*—a transformation of thyroid tissue to lymphoid tissue. It is the most common inflammatory disorder of the thyroid and the leading cause of hypothyroidism.

Etiology, Pathogenesis, and Pathology Hashimoto's thyroiditis is an autoimmune process that is thought to be initiated by the activation of CD4+ T (helper) lymphocytes with specificity for thyroid antigens. Once activated, T cells can recruit cytotoxic CD8+ T cells to the thyroid. Hypothyroidism results not only from the destruction of thyrocytes by cytotoxic T cells but by autoantibodies, which lead to complement fixation and killing by natural killer cells or block the TSH-R. Antibodies directed against three main antigens—Tg (60%), TPO (95%), the TSH-R (60%), and, less commonly, to the sodium/iodine symporter (25%). Apoptosis (programmed cell death) also has been implicated in the pathogenesis of Hashimoto's thyroiditis. Chronic thyroiditis also has been associated with increased intake of iodine and administration of medications such as interferon-α, lithium, and amiodarone. Support for an inherited predisposition includes an increased incidence of thyroid autoantibodies in first-degree relatives of patients with Hashimoto's thyroiditis compared to controls and the occurrence of the autoantibodies and hypothyroidism in patients with specific chromosomal abnormalities such as Turner's syndrome and Down syndrome. Associations with HLA-B8, DR3, and DR5 haplotypes of the major histocompatibility complex also have been described.

On gross examination, the thyroid gland is usually mildly enlarged throughout and has a pale, gray-tan cut surface that is granular, nodular, and firm. On microscopic examination, the gland is diffusely infiltrated by small lymphocytes and plasma cells and occasionally shows well-developed germinal centers. Thyroid follicles are smaller than normal with reduced amounts of colloid and increased interstitial connective tissue. The follicles are lined by Hürthle or Askanazy cells, which are characterized by abundant eosinophilic, granular cytoplasm.

Clinical Presentation Hashimoto's thyroiditis is also more common in women (male:female ratio 1:10 to 20) between the ages of 30 and 50 years old. The most common presentation is that of a minimally or moderately enlarged firm granular gland discovered on routine physical examination or the awareness of a painless anterior neck mass, although 20% of patients present with hypothyroidism, and 5% present with hyperthyroidism (Hashitoxicosis). In classic goitrous Hashimoto's thyroiditis, physical examination reveals a diffusely enlarged, firm gland, which also is lobulated. An enlarged pyramidal lobe often is palpable.

Diagnostic Studies When Hashimoto's thyroiditis is suspected clinically, an elevated TSH and the presence of thyroid autoantibodies usually confirm the diagnosis. FNAB is indicated in patients who present with a solitary suspicious nodule or a rapidly enlarging goiter. Thyroid lymphoma is a rare but well-recognized, ominous complication of chronic autoimmune thyroiditis and has a preva-

lence 80 times higher than expected frequency in this population than in a control population without thyroiditis. Recent studies of clonal similarity indicate that lymphoma may, in fact, evolve from Hashimoto's thyroiditis.[14]

Treatment Thyroid hormone replacement therapy is indicated in overtly hypothyroid patients, with a goal of maintaining normal TSH levels. The management of patients with subclinical hypothyroidism (normal T_4 and elevated TSH) is controversial. Treatment is advised especially for middle-aged patients with cardiovascular risk factors such as hyperlipidemia or hypertension and in pregnant patients.[15] Treatment also is indicated in euthyroid patients to shrink large goiters. Surgery may occasionally be indicated for suspicion of malignancy or for goiters causing compressive symptoms or cosmetic deformity.

Riedel's Thyroiditis Riedel's thyroiditis is a rare variant of thyroiditis also known as *Riedel's struma* or *invasive fibrous thyroiditis* that is characterized by the replacement of all or part of the thyroid parenchyma by fibrous tissue, which also invades into adjacent tissues. The etiology of this disorder is controversial, and it has been reported to occur in patients with other autoimmune diseases. This association, coupled with the presence of lymphoid infiltration and response to steroid therapy, suggests a primary autoimmune etiology. Riedel's thyroiditis also is associated with other focal sclerosing syndromes including mediastinal, retroperitoneal, periorbital, and retro-orbital fibrosis and sclerosing cholangitis, suggesting that it may, in fact, be a primary fibrotic disorder. The disease occurs predominantly in women between the ages of 30 to 60 years old. It typically presents as a painless, hard anterior neck mass, which progresses over weeks to years to produce symptoms of compression, including dysphagia, dyspnea, choking, and hoarseness. Patients may present with symptoms of hypothyroidism and hypoparathyroidism as the gland is replaced by fibrous tissue. Physical examination reveals a hard, "woody" thyroid gland with fixation to surrounding tissues. The diagnosis needs to be confirmed by open thyroid biopsy, because the firm and fibrous nature of the gland renders FNAB inadequate.

Surgery is the mainstay of the treatment. The chief goal of operation is to decompress the trachea by wedge excision of the thyroid isthmus and to make a tissue diagnosis. More extensive resections are not advised due to the infiltrative nature of the fibrotic process that obscures usual landmarks and structures. Hypothyroid patients are treated with thyroid hormone replacement. Some patients who remain symptomatic have been reported to experience dramatic improvement after treatment with corticosteroids and tamoxifen.[16]

Goiter

Any enlargement of the thyroid gland is referred to as a goiter. The causes of nontoxic goiters are listed in Table 38-3. Goiters may be diffuse, uninodular, or multinodular. Most nontoxic goiters are thought to result from TSH stimulation secondary to inadequate thyroid hormone synthesis and other paracrine growth factors.[17] Elevated TSH levels induce diffuse thyroid hyperplasia, followed by focal hyperplasia, resulting in nodules that may or may not concentrate iodine, colloid nodules, or microfollicular nodules. The TSH-dependent nodules progress to become autonomous. Familial goiters resulting from inherited deficiencies in enzymes necessary for thyroid hormone synthesis may be complete or partial. The term *endemic goiter* refers to the occurrence of a goiter in a significant proportion of individuals in a particular geographic region. In the past, dietary iodine deficiency was the most common cause of endemic goiter. This condition has largely disappeared in North America due to routine use of iodized salt and iodination of fertilizers, animal feeds, and preservatives. However, in areas of iodine deficiency, such as Central Asia, South America, and Indonesia, up to 90% of the population have goiters. Other dietary goitrogens that may participate in endemic goiter formation include kelp, cassava, and cabbage. In many sporadic goiters, no obvious cause can be identified.

TABLE 38-3	Etiology of nontoxic goiter
Classification	**Specific Etiology**
Endemic	Iodine deficiency, dietary goitrogens (cassava, cabbage)
Medications	Iodide, amiodarone, lithium
Thyroiditis	Subacute, chronic (Hashimoto's)
Familial	Impaired hormone synthesis from enzyme defects
Neoplasm	Adenoma, carcinoma
Resistance to thyroid hormone	—

Clinical Features Most patients with nontoxic goiters are asymptomatic, although patients often complain of a pressure sensation in the neck. As the goiters become very large, compressive symptoms such as dyspnea and dysphagia ensue. Patients also describe having to clear their throats frequently (catarrh). Dysphonia from RLN injury is rare, except when malignancy is present. Obstruction of venous return at the thoracic inlet from a substernal goiter results in a positive Pemberton's sign—facial flushing and dilatation of cervical veins upon raising the arms above the head (Fig. 38-13A). Sudden enlargement of nodules or cysts due to hemorrhage may cause acute pain. Physical examination may reveal a soft, diffusely enlarged gland (simple goiter) or nodules of various size and consistency in case of a multinodular goiter. Deviation or compression of the trachea may be apparent.

Diagnostic Tests Patients usually are euthyroid with normal TSH and low-normal or normal-free T_4 levels. If some nodules develop autonomy, patients have suppressed TSH levels or become hyperthyroid. RAI uptake often shows patchy uptake with areas of hot and cold nodules. FNAB is recommended in patients who have a dominant nodule or one that is painful or enlarging, as carcinomas have been reported in 5 to 10% of multinodular goiters. CT scans are helpful to evaluate the extent of retrosternal extension and airway compression (Fig. 38-13B).

Treatment Most euthyroid patients with small, diffuse goiters do not require treatment. Some physicians give patients with large goiters exogenous thyroid hormone to reduce the TSH stimulation of gland growth; this treatment may result in decrease and/or stabilization of goiter size and is most effective for small diffuse goiters. Endemic goiters are treated by iodine administration. Surgical resection is reserved for goiters that (a) continue to increase despite T_4 suppression, (b) cause obstructive symptoms, (c) have substernal extension, (d) have malignancy suspected or proven by FNAB, and (e) are cosmetically unacceptable. Subtotal thyroidectomy is the treatment of choice and patients require lifelong T_4 therapy to prevent recurrence.

Solitary Thyroid Nodule

Solitary thyroid nodules are present in approximately 4% of individuals in the United States, whereas thyroid cancer has a much lower incidence of 40 new cases per 1 million. Therefore, it is of utmost importance to determine which patients with solitary thyroid nodule would benefit from surgery.

History

Details regarding the nodule, such as time of onset, change in size, and associated symptoms such as pain, dysphagia, dyspnea, or choking, should be elicited. Pain is an unusual symptom and, when present, should raise suspicion for intrathyroidal hemorrhage in a benign nodule, thyroiditis, or malignancy. Patients with MTC may complain of a dull, aching sensation. A history of hoarseness is worrisome, as it may be secondary to malignant involvement of the

RLNs. Most importantly, patients should be questioned regarding risk factors for malignancy, such as exposure to ionizing radiation and family history of thyroid and other malignancies associated with thyroid cancer.

External Beam Radiation Low-dose therapeutic radiation has been used to treat conditions such as tinea capitis (6.5 cGy), thymic enlargement (100 to 400 cGy), enlarged tonsils and adenoids (750 cGy), acne vulgaris (200 to 1500 cGy), and other conditions such as hemangioma and scrofula. Radiation (approximately 4000 cGy) is also an integral part of the management of patients with Hodgkin's disease. It is now known that a history of exposure to low-dose ionizing radiation to the thyroid gland places the patient at increased risk for developing thyroid cancer. The risk increases linearly from 6.5 to 2000 cGy, beyond which the incidence declines as the radiation causes destruction of the thyroid tissue. The risk is maximum 20 to 30 years after exposure, but these patients require lifelong monitoring. During the nuclear fallout from Chernobyl in 1986, ^{131}I release was accompanied by a marked increase in the incidence of both benign and malignant thyroid lesions noted within 4 years of exposure, particularly in children.[18] Most thyroid carcinomas following radiation exposure are papillary, and some of these cancers with a solid type of histology and presence of *RET/PTC* translocations appear to be more aggressive. There is a 40% chance that patients presenting with a thyroid nodule and a history of radiation have thyroid cancer. Of those patients who have thyroid cancer, the cancer is located in the dominant nodule in 60% of patients, but in the remaining 40% of patients, the cancer is in another nodule in the thyroid gland.

Family History A family history of thyroid cancer is a risk factor for the development of both medullary and nonmedullary thyroid cancer. Familial MTCs occur in isolation or in association with other tumors as part of multiple endocrine neoplasia type 2 (MEN2) syndromes. Nonmedullary thyroid cancers can occur in association with other known familial cancer syndromes such as Cowden's syndrome, Werner's (adult progeroid syndrome), and familial adenomatous polyposis (Table 38-4). Nonmedullary thyroid cancers can also occur independently of these syndromes. Several candidate loci that predispose to these tumors have been identified, but they account for only a small proportion of families.[19]

Physical Examination

The thyroid gland is best palpated from behind the patient and with the neck in mild extension. The cricoid cartilage is an important landmark, as the isthmus is situated just below it. Nodules that are hard, gritty, or fixed to surrounding structures such as the trachea or strap muscles are more likely to be malignant. The cervical chain of lymph nodes should be assessed as well as the nodes in the posterior triangle.

Diagnostic Investigations

An algorithm for the work-up of a solitary thyroid nodule is shown in Fig. 38-14.

Fine-Needle Aspiration Biopsy FNAB has become the single most important test in the evaluation of thyroid masses and can be performed with or without ultrasound guidance.[20] Ultrasound guidance is recommended for nodules that are difficult to palpate and for cystic or solid-cystic nodules that recur after the initial aspiration. A 23-gauge needle is inserted into the thyroid mass, and several passes are made while aspirating the syringe. After releasing the suction on the syringe, the needle is withdrawn and the cells are immediately placed on prelabeled dry glass slides; some are immersed in a 70% alcohol solution while others are air dried. A sample of the aspirate is also placed in a 90% alcohol solution for cytospin or cell pellet. The slides are stained by Papanicolaou's or Wright's stains and examined under the microscope. If a bloody aspirate is obtained, the patient should be repositioned in a more

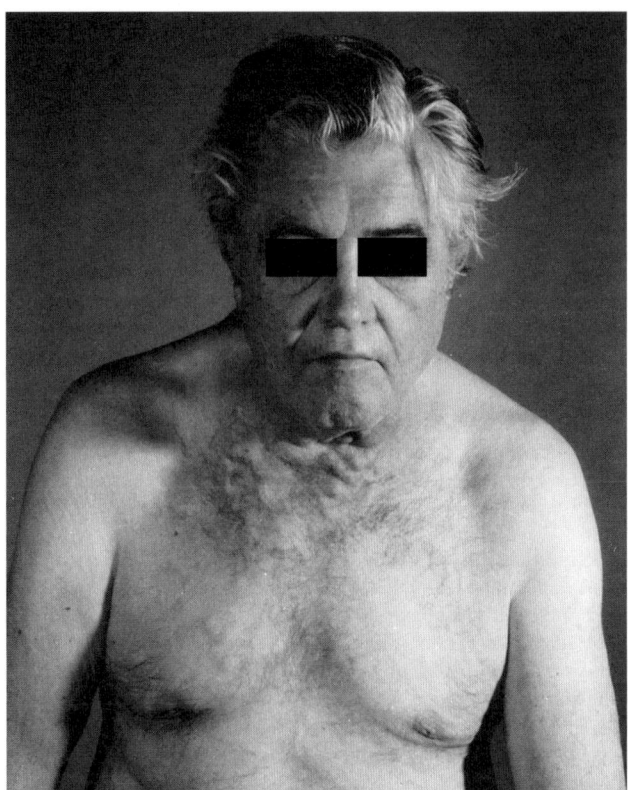

A

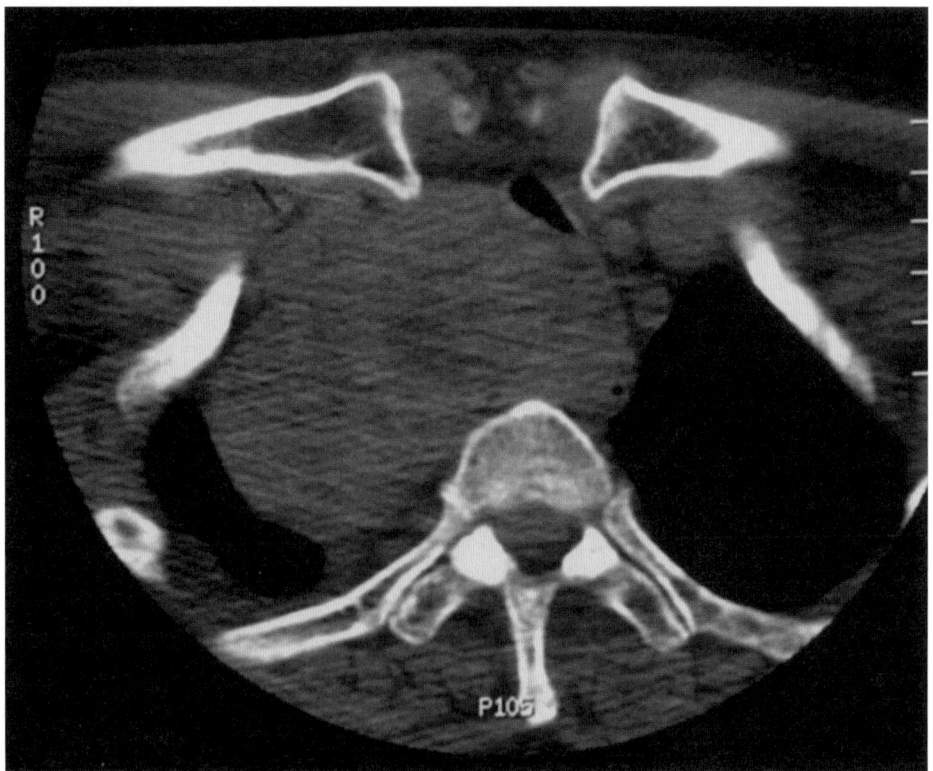

B

FIG. 38-13. A. Retrosternal extension of a large goiter may result in impeded flow in the superior vena cava, leading to dilated veins over the chest wall. This may become more prominent when patients raise their arms above the head—Pemberton's sign. **B.** Computed tomography scan demonstrating retrosternal extension and consequent tracheal deviation and compression from a large goiter.

upright position and the biopsy repeated with a finer (25- to 30-gauge) needle.

After FNAB, the majority of nodules can be categorized into the following groups: benign (65%), suspicious (20%), malignant (5%), and nondiagnostic (10%). The incidence of false-positive results is about 1% and false-negative results occur in approximately 3% of patients. If a biopsy is reported as nondiagnostic, it generally should be repeated. Benign lesions include cysts and colloid nodules. The risk of malignancy in this setting is <3%. The risk of malignancy in the setting of a suspicious cytology is about 20%. Most of these lesions

TABLE 38-4 Familial cancer syndromes involving nonmedullary thyroid cancer

Syndrome	Gene	Manifestation	Thyroid Tumor
Cowden's syndrome	PTEN	Intestinal hamartomas, benign and malignant breast tumors	FTC, rarely PTC and Hürthle cell tumors
FAP	APC	Colon polyps and cancer, duodenal neoplasms, desmoids	PTC cribriform growth pattern
Werner's syndrome	WRN	Adult progeroid syndrome	PTC, FTC, anaplastic cancer
Carney complex type 1	PRKAR1α	Cutaneous and cardiac myxomas, breast and adrenal tumors	PTC, FTC
McCune-Albright syndrome	GNAS1	Polyostotic fibrous dysplasia, endocrine abnormalities, café-au-lait spots	PTC clear cell

FAP = familial adenomatous polyposis; FTC = follicular thyroid cancer; PTC = papillary thyroid cancer.

are follicular or Hürthle cell neoplasms. In this situation, diagnosis of malignancy relies on demonstrating capsular or vascular invasion, features that cannot be determined via FNAB. FNAB also is less reliable in patients who have a history of head and neck irradiation or a family history of thyroid cancer, due to higher likelihood of multifocal lesions and occult cancer.

Laboratory Studies Most patients with thyroid nodules are euthyroid. Determining the blood TSH level is helpful. If a patient with a nodule is found to be hyperthyroid, the risk of malignancy is approximately 1%. Serum Tg levels cannot differentiate benign from malignant thyroid nodules unless the levels are extremely high, in which case metastatic thyroid cancer should be suspected. Tg levels are, however, useful in following patients who have undergone total thyroidectomy for thyroid cancer and also for serial evaluation of patients undergoing nonoperative management of thyroid nodules. Serum calcitonin levels should be obtained in patients with MTC or a family history of MTC or MEN2. All patients with MTC should be tested for *RET* oncogene mutations and have a 24-hour urine collection with measurement of levels of vanillylmandelic acid (VMA), metanephrine, and catechol-

amine to rule out a coexisting pheochromocytoma. About 10% of patients with familial MTC and MEN2A have de novo *RET* mutations, so that their children are at risk for thyroid cancer.

Imaging Ultrasound is helpful for detecting nonpalpable thyroid nodules, differentiating solid from cystic nodules, and identifying adjacent lymphadenopathy. Ultrasound evaluation can identify features of a nodule that increase the a priori risk of malignancy, such as fine stippled calcification and enlarged regional nodes; however, a tissue diagnosis is strongly recommended before thyroidectomy.[21] Ultrasound also provides a noninvasive and inexpensive method of following the size of suspected benign nodules diagnosed by FNAB and for identifying enlarged lymph nodes. CT and MRI are unnecessary in the routine evaluation of thyroid tumors except for large, fixed, or substernal lesions. Scanning the thyroid with ^{123}I or ^{99m}Tc is rarely necessary, and thyroid scanning currently is recommended in the assessment of thyroid nodules only in patients who have follicular thyroid nodules on FNAB and a suppressed TSH. As previously indicated in Thyroid Imaging, PET scanning does not play a major role in the primary evaluation of thyroid nodules.

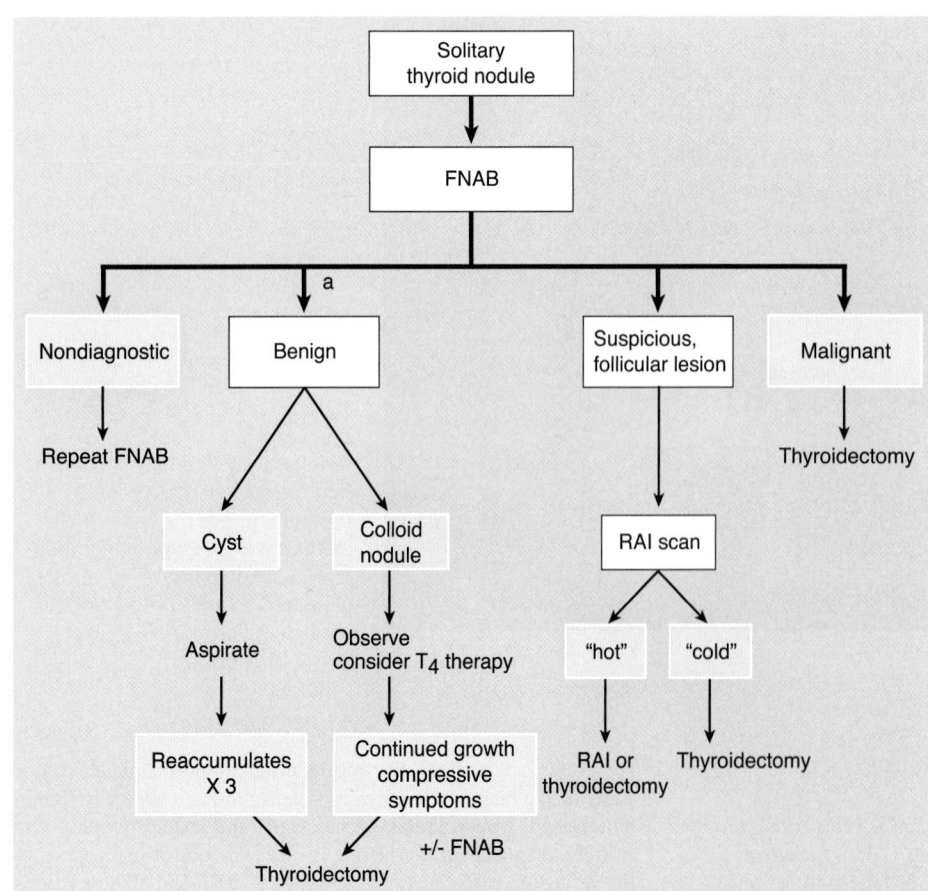

FIG. 38-14. Management of a solitary thyroid nodule. a = except in patients with a history of external radiation exposure or a family history of thyroid cancer; FNAB = fine-needle aspiration biopsy; RAI = radioactive iodine; T₄ = thyroxine.

Management

Malignant tumors are treated by thyroidectomy, as discussed later in this chapter in Surgical Treatment under Malignant Thyroid Disease. Simple thyroid cysts resolve with aspiration in about 75% of cases, although some require a second or third aspiration. If the cyst persists after three attempts at aspiration, unilateral thyroid lobectomy is recommended. Lobectomy also is recommended for cysts >4 cm in diameter or complex cysts with solid and cystic components, as the latter have a higher incidence of malignancy (15%). When FNAB is used in complex nodules, the solid portion should be sampled. If a colloid nodule is diagnosed by FNAB, patients should still be observed with serial ultrasound and Tg measurements. If the nodule enlarges, repeat FNAB often is indicated. Although controversial, L-thyroxine in doses sufficient to maintain a serum TSH level between 0.1 and 1.0 μU/mL may also be administered. Approximately 50% of these nodules decrease in size in response to the TSH suppression of this regimen, and others may not continue to grow, but it is most effective for nodules <3 cm. Thyroidectomy should be performed if a nodule enlarges on TSH suppression, causes compressive symptoms, or for cosmetic reasons. An exception to this general rule is the patient who has had previous irradiation of the thyroid gland or has a family history of thyroid cancer. In these patients, total or near-total thyroidectomy is recommended because of the high incidence of thyroid cancer and decreased reliability of FNAB in this setting.

Malignant Thyroid Disease

In the United States, thyroid cancer accounts for <1% of all malignancies (2% of women and 0.5% of men) and is the most rapidly increasing cancer in women. Thyroid cancer is responsible for six deaths per million persons annually. Most patients present with a palpable swelling in the neck, which initiates assessment through a combination of history, physical examination, and FNAB.

Molecular Genetics of Thyroid Tumorigenesis

Several oncogenes and tumor suppressor genes are involved in thyroid tumorigenesis,[22] as depicted in Table 38-5. The *RET* proto-oncogene (Fig. 38-15) plays a significant role in the pathogenesis of thyroid cancers. It is located on chromosome 10 and encodes a receptor tyrosine kinase, which binds several growth factors such as glial-derived neurotrophic factor and neurturin. The *RET* protein is expressed in tissues derived from the embryonic nervous and excretory systems. Therefore, *RET* disruption can lead to developmental abnormalities in organs derived from these systems, such as the enteric nervous system (Hirschsprung's disease) and kidney. Germ-line mutations in the *RET* proto-oncogene are known to predispose to MEN2A, MEN2B, and familial MTCs, and somatic mutations have been demonstrated in tumors derived from the neural crest, such as MTCs (30%) and pheochromocytomas. The tyrosine kinase domain of *RET* can fuse with other genes by rearrangement. These fusion products also function as oncogenes and have been implicated in the pathogenesis of PTCs. At least 15 *RET*/PTC rearrangements have been described and appear to be early events in tumorigenesis. Young age and radiation exposure seem to be independent risk factors for the development of *RET*/PTC rearrangements. Up to 70% of papillary cancers in children exposed to the radiation fallout from the 1986 Chernobyl disaster carry *RET*/PTC rearrangements, the most common being *RET*/PTC1 and *RET*/PTC3. These rearrangements confer constitutive activation of the receptor tyrosine kinases. *RET*/PTC3 is associated with a solid type of PTC that appears to present at a higher stage and to be more aggressive.[23] It has now been established that *RET*/PTC signaling involves the mitogen-activated protein kinase (MAPK) pathway via other signaling molecules such as *Ras*, Raf, and MEK. In normal cells, physiologic activation of Raf kinases occurs via direct interaction with guanosine triphosphate (GTP)-bound Ras, a membrane bound small G-protein. Activated Raf, a serine-threonine kinase, in turn phosphorylates MEK, another serine-threonine kinase. This leads to phosphorylation of ERK/MAPK, which phospho-

Gene	Function	Tumor
Oncogenes		
RET	Membrane receptor with tyrosine kinase activity	Sporadic and familial MTC, PTC (RET/PTC rearrangements)
MET	Same	Overexpressed in PTC
TRK1	Same	Activated in some PTC
TSH-R	Linked to heterotrimeric G protein	Hyperfunctioning adenoma
Gsα (gsp)	Signal transduction molecule (GTP binding)	Hyperfunctioning adenoma, follicular adenoma
Ras	Signal transduction protein	Follicular adenoma and carcinoma, PTC
PAX8/PPARγ1	Oncoprotein	Follicular adenoma, follicular carcinoma
B-Raf (BRAF)	Signal transduction	PTC, tall cell and poorly differentiated, anaplastic
Tumor suppressors		
p53	Cell cycle regulator, arrests cells in G₁, induces apoptosis	De-differentiated PTC, FTC, anaplastic cancers
p16	Cell cycle regulator, inhibits cyclin dependent kinase	Thyroid cancer cell lines
PTEN	Protein tyrosine phosphatase	Follicular adenoma and carcinoma

TABLE 38-5 Oncogenes and tumor-suppressor genes implicated in thyroid tumorigenesis

FTC = follicular thyroid cancer; GTP = guanosine triphosphate; MTC = medullary thyroid cancer; PTC = papillary thyroid cancer.

rylates regulatory molecules in the nucleus, thereby altering gene expression. Aberrant activation of the MAPK pathway leads to tumorigenesis. Aside from *RET*/PTC alterations, mutations in the *Ras* genes can also activate the MAPK pathway. Mutated *ras* oncogenes have been identified in up to 20 to 40% of thyroid follicular adenomas and carcinomas, multinodular goiters, and papillary and anaplastic carcinomas. There are three Raf kinases, A-Raf, B-Raf (*BRAF*), and C-Raf. Mutations in *BRAF* also have been implicated in aberrant MAPK pathway activation and tumorigenesis. Of the various identified *BRAF* mutations, T1799A (V600E amino acid substitution) is the most common and occurs frequently in thyroid cancers. Interestingly, *BRAF* mutations occur in papillary and anaplastic tumors (average prevalence of 44% and 22% respectively),[24] but not in follicular thyroid cancers, suggesting a role in the pathogenesis of these malignancies. Studies also show that *BRAF* mutations are associated with more aggressive clinicopathologic features, including larger tumor size, invasion, and lymphadenopathy, and may have a role as prognostic markers.

The *p53* gene is a tumor suppressor gene encoding a transcriptional regulator, which causes cell cycle arrest allowing repair of damaged DNA, thus helping to maintain genomic integrity. Mutations of *p53* are rare in PTCs, but are common in undifferentiated thyroid cancers and thyroid cancer cell lines. Other cell cycle regulators and tumor suppressors such as *p15* and *p16* are mutated more commonly in thyroid cancer cell lines than in primary tumors. An oncogene resulting from the fusion of the DNA binding domain of the thyroid-transcription factor *PAX8* gene to the peroxisome proliferator-activated receptor gamma 1 (PPARγ1) has been noted to play an important role in the development of follicular neoplasms, including follicular cancers.[25]

Specific Tumor Types

Papillary Carcinoma Papillary carcinoma accounts for 80% of all thyroid malignancies in iodine-sufficient areas and is the predomi-

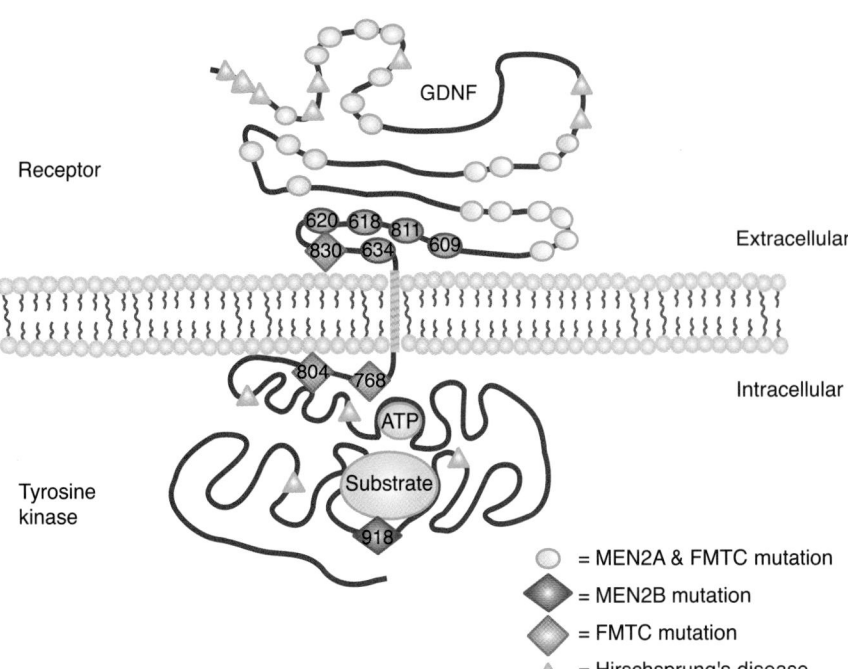

FIG. 38-15. Structure of the *RET* tyrosine kinase receptor. MEN2A, MEN2B, familial medullary thyroid cancer (FMTC), and Hirschsprung's disease result from germline mutations in the *RET* proto-oncogene. The extracellular domain binds the ligand glial-derived neurotrophic factor (GDNF) and contains 28 cysteine residues. Mutations in cysteine residues at codons 609, 611, 618, 620, and 634, which are in the juxtamembrane region of the receptor, are associated with MEN2A and FMTC. The ATP-binding site is located intracellularly near the site, which binds the substrate for the tyrosine kinase catalytic domain. Mutations at codon 918 (Met to Thr) alter the substrate binding pocket located in the intracellular region and cause MEN2B. FMTC is associated with mutations at codons 768 and 804. ATP = adenosine triphosphate. *(Reproduced with permission from Wells S and Franz C: Medullary carcinoma of the thyroid.* World J Surg *24:954, 2000, Springer-Verlag.)*

nant thyroid cancer in children and individuals exposed to external radiation. Papillary carcinoma occurs more often in women, with a 2:1 female-to-male ratio, and the mean age at presentation is 30 to 40 years. Most patients are euthyroid and present with a slow-growing painless mass in the neck. Dysphagia, dyspnea, and dysphonia usually are associated with locally advanced invasive disease. Lymph node metastases are common, especially in children and young adults, and may be the presenting complaint. "Lateral aberrant thyroid" almost always denotes a cervical lymph node that has been invaded by metastatic cancer. Suspicion of thyroid cancer often originates through physical examination of patients and a review of their history. Diagnosis is established by FNAB of the thyroid mass or lymph node. Once thyroid cancer is diagnosed on FNAB, a complete neck ultrasound is strongly recommended to evaluate the contralateral lobe and for lymph node metastases in the central and lateral neck compartments. Distant metastases are uncommon at initial presentation, but may ultimately develop in up to 20% of patients. The most common sites are lungs, followed by bone, liver, and brain.

Pathology On gross examination, PTCs generally are hard and whitish and remain flat on sectioning with a blade, in contrast to normal tissue or benign nodular lesions that tend to bulge. Macroscopic calcification, necrosis, or cystic change may be apparent. Histologically, papillary carcinomas may exhibit papillary projections (Fig. 38-16A), a mixed pattern of papillary and follicular structures, or a pure follicular pattern (follicular variant). The diagnosis is established by characteristic nuclear cellular features. Cells are cuboidal with pale, abundant cytoplasm, crowded nuclei that may demonstrate "grooving," and intranuclear cytoplasmic inclusions [leading to the designation of *Orphan Annie* nuclei (Fig. 38-16B)], which allow diagnosis by FNAB. Psammoma bodies, which are microscopic, calcified deposits representing clumps of sloughed cells, also may be present. Mixed papillary-follicular tumors and follicular variants of papillary carcinoma are classified as papillary carcinomas because they behave biologically as papillary carcinomas. Multifocality is common in papillary carcinoma and may be present in up to 85% of cases on microscopic examination. Multifocality is associated with an increased risk of cervical nodal metastases, and these tumors may rarely invade adjacent structures such as the trachea, esophagus, and RLNs. Other variants of papillary carcinoma include tall cell, insular, columnar, diffuse sclerosing, clear cell, trabecular, and poorly differentiated types.

These variants account for about 1% of all papillary carcinomas and are generally associated with a worse prognosis.

Minimal or occult/microcarcinoma refers to tumors of 1 cm or less in size with no evidence of local invasiveness through the thyroid capsule or angioinvasion, and that are not associated with lymph node metastases. They are nonpalpable and usually are incidental findings at operative, histologic, or autopsy examination. Studies have demonstrated occult PTC to be present in 2 to 36% of thyroid glands removed at autopsy. These tumors are also being identified more frequently due to the widespread use of ultrasound. These occult tumors are generally associated with a better prognosis than larger tumors, but they may be more aggressive than previously appreciated.[26]

Prognostic Indicators In general, patients with PTC have an excellent prognosis with a >95% 10-year survival rate. Several prognostic indicators have been incorporated into various staging systems, which enable patients to be stratified into low-risk and high-risk groups. Unfortunately, all of these classification systems rely on data that are not available preoperatively.

In 1987, Hay and colleagues[27] at the Mayo Clinic proposed the *AGES* scoring system, which incorporates *A*ge, histologic *G*rade, *E*xtrathyroidal invasion, and metastases and tumor *S*ize to predict the risk of dying from papillary cancer. Low-risk patients are young, with well-differentiated tumors, no metastases, and small primary lesions, whereas high-risk patients are older, with poorly differentiated tumors, local invasion, distant metastases, and large primary lesions. The *MACIS* scale is a postoperative system modified from the AGES scale. This scale incorporates distant *M*etastases, *A*ge at presentation (<40 or >40 years old), *C*ompleteness of original surgical resection, extrathyroidal *I*nvasion, and *S*ize of original lesion (in cm) and classifies patients into four risk groups based on their scores. Cady proposed the *AMES* system[28] to classify differentiated thyroid tumors into low- and high-risk groups using *A*ge (men <40 years old, women <50 years old), *M*etastases, *E*xtrathyroidal spread, and *S*ize of tumors (less than or >5 cm). Another classification systems is the *TNM* system, (*T*umor, *N*odal status, *M*etastases, Table 38-6), used by most medical centers in North America.[29] A simplified system by DeGroot and associates[30] uses four groups—class I (intrathyroidal), class II (cervical nodal metastases), class III (extrathyroidal invasion), and class IV (distant metastases) to determine prognosis.

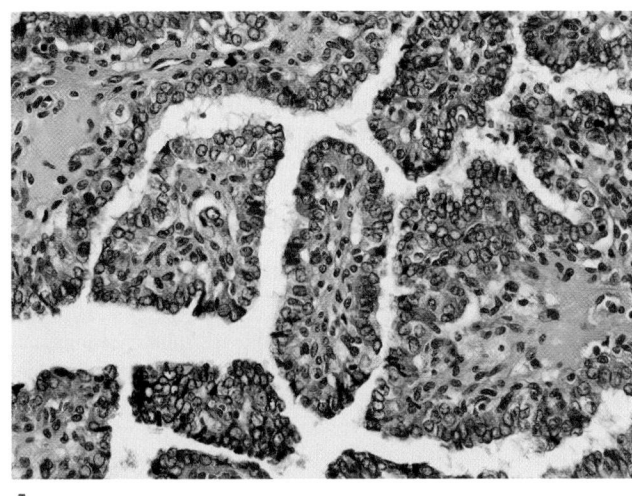
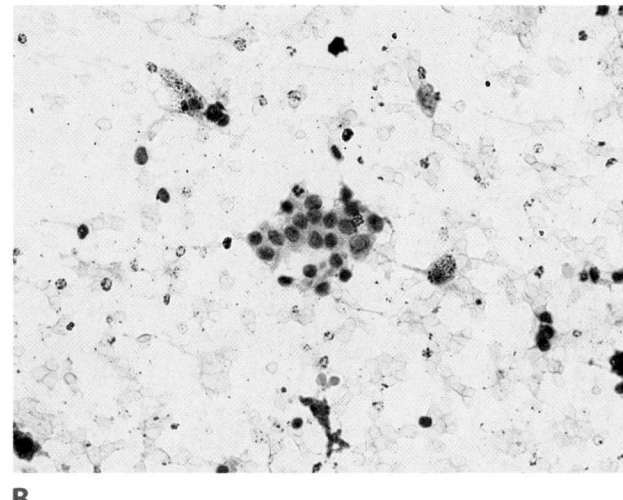

A   **B**

FIG. 38-16. **A.** Histomicrograph of a papillary thyroid cancer (hematoxylin-eosin stain). **B.** Fine-needle aspiration biopsy specimen from a papillary thyroid cancer showing typical intranuclear cytoplasmic inclusions in the center of the slide.

Several molecular and genetic markers such as tumor DNA aneuploidy, decreased cyclic adenosine monophosphate response to TSH, increased epidermal growth factor binding, presence of N-*ras* and *gsp* mutations, overexpression of c-*myc*, and presence of *p53* mutations also have been associated with a worse prognosis. The presence of *BRAF* mutations also has been demonstrated to be associated with lymph node metastasis and higher stage (III and IV) papillary tumors.[31]

Surgical Treatment Most authors agree that patients with high-risk tumors (judged by any of the classification systems discussed above in Prognostic Indicators) or bilateral tumors should undergo total or near-total thyroidectomy. When patients are found to have a minimal papillary thyroid carcinoma in a thyroid specimen removed for other reasons, unilateral thyroid lobectomy and isthmusectomy is usually considered to be adequate treatment, unless the tumor has evidence of angioinvasion, multifocality, or positive margins. The optimal surgical strategy in the majority of patients with low-risk (small, unilateral) cancers remains controversial. The focus of the debate centers around outcome data and risks associated with extent of thyroidectomy in this group of patients.

Proponents of total thyroidectomy argue that the procedure (a) enables the use of RAI to effectively detect and treat residual thyroid tissue or metastatic disease, (b) makes serum Tg level a more sensitive marker of recurrent or persistent disease, (c) eliminates contralateral occult cancers as sites of recurrence (because up to 85% of tumors are bilateral), (d) reduces the risk of recurrence and improves survival, (e) decreases the 1% risk of progression to undifferentiated or anaplastic thyroid cancer, and (f) reduces the need for reoperative surgery with its attendant risk of increased complication rates.

Investigators that favor lobectomy argue that (a) total thyroidectomy is associated with a higher complication rate than lobectomy, (b) recurrence in the remaining thyroid tissue is unusual (5%) and most are curable by surgery, (c) tumor multicentricity seems to have little prognostic significance, and (d) patients who have undergone lesser procedures such as lobectomy still have an excellent prognosis.

However, it is known that a significant proportion (33 to 50%) of patients who develop a recurrence die from their disease[32] and even though the data are retrospective, long-term, follow-up studies suggest that recurrence rates are lowered and that survival is improved in patients undergoing near-total or total thyroidectomy[30–36] (Fig. 38-17). In addition, diminished survival is noted in patients with low-risk disease (mortality rates of 5% at 10 to 20 years), and it is not possible to accurately risk stratify patients preoperatively. Given the above, it is recommended that even patients with low-risk

tumors undergo total or near-total thyroidectomy, provided complication rates are low (<2%).[37]

Thus, when PTC is diagnosed by FNAB, the definitive operation can be done without confirming the diagnosis by frozen section during the operation. Patients with a nodule that may be papillary cancer should be treated by thyroid lobectomy, isthmusectomy, and removal of any pyramidal lobe or adjacent lymph nodes. If intraoperative frozen-section examination of a lymph node or primary tumor confirms carcinoma, completion total or near-total thyroidectomy is performed. If a definitive diagnosis cannot be made or the surgeon is concerned about the viability of the parathyroid glands or the status of the RLN, the operation is terminated. When final histology confirms carcinoma, completion thyroidectomy usually is performed. For patients who have minimal PTCs (<1 cm) confined to the thyroid gland without angioinvasion, no further operative treatment is recommended.

During thyroidectomy, enlarged central neck nodes should be removed. Some investigators recommend routine bilateral central neck dissection due to the high incidence of microscopic metastases and data showing improved rates of recurrence and survival (compared to historic controls). However, these risks need to be balanced with the increased risk of hypoparathyroidism with routine central neck dissection. Biopsy-proven lymph node metastases detected clinically or by imaging in the lateral neck in patients with papillary carcinoma are managed with modified radical or functional neck dissection[37] as described later in this chapter in Thyroid Surgery. Dissection of the posterior triangle and suprahyoid dissection usually are not necessary unless there is extensive metastatic disease in levels 2, 3, and 4, but should be performed when appropriate.[38] Prophylactic lateral neck node dissection is not necessary in patients with PTC, because these cancers do not appear to metastasize systemically from lymph nodes, and micrometastases often can be ablated with RAI therapy.

Follicular Carcinoma Follicular carcinomas account for 10% of thyroid cancers and occur more commonly in iodine-deficient areas. The overall incidence of this tumor is declining in the United States, probably due to iodine supplementation and improved histologic classification. Women have a higher incidence of follicular cancer, with a female-to-male ratio of 3:1, and a mean age at presentation of 50 years old. Follicular cancers usually present as solitary thyroid nodules, occasionally with a history of rapid size increase, and long-standing goiter. Pain is uncommon, unless hemorrhage into the nodule has occurred. Unlike papillary cancers, cervical lymphadenopathy is uncommon at initial presentation (about 5%), although distant metastases may be present. In <1% of

TABLE 38-6 TNM classification of thyroid tumors[29]

Papillary or Follicular Tumors

Stage	TNM
<45 y	
I	Any T, any N, M0
II	Any T, any N, M1
≥45 y	
I	T1, N0, M0
II	T2, N0, M0
III	T3, N0, M0; T1–3, N1a, M0
IVA	T4a, N0–1a, M0; T1–4a, N1b, M0
IVB	T4b, any N, M0
IVC	Any T, any N, M1

Medullary Thyroid Cancer

Stage	TNM
I	T1, N0, M0
II	T2–3, N0, M0
III	T1–3, N1a, M0
IVA	T4a, N0–1a, M0; T1–4a, N1b, M0
IVB	T4b, any N, M0
IVC	Any T, any N, M1

Anaplastic Cancer

Stage	TNM
IVA	T4a, Any N, M0
IVB	T4b, Any N, M0
IVC	Any T, Any M, M1

Definitions:
Primary tumor (T)
TX = Primary tumor cannot be assessed
T0 = No evidence of primary tumor
T1 = Tumor ≤2 cm in diameter, limited to thyroid
T2 = Tumor >2 cm but <4 cm in diameter, limited to thyroid
T3 = Tumor >4 cm in diameter, limited to thyroid, or any tumor with minimal extrathyroidal invasion
T4a = Any size tumor extending beyond capsule to invade subcutaneous soft tissue, larynx, trachea, esophagus, or recurrent laryngeal nerve, or intrathyroidal anaplastic cancer
T4b = Tumor invading prevertebral fascia, or encasing carotid artery or mediastinal vessels; or extrathyroidal anaplastic cancer
Regional lymph nodes (N)—include central, lateral cervical, and upper mediastinal nodes
NX = Regional lymph nodes cannot be assessed
N0 = No regional lymph node metastasis
N1 = Regional lymph node metastasis
N1a = Metastases to level VI (pretracheal, paratracheal, and prelaryngeal/Delphian lymph nodes)
N1b = Metastases to unilateral, bilateral, or contralateral cervical or superior mediastinal lymph nodes
Distant metastasis (M)
MX = Distant metastases cannot be assessed
M1 = No distant metastasis
Source: Used with the permission of the American Joint Committee on Cancer (AJCC), Chicago, Illinois. The original source for this material is the AJCC Cancer Staging Manual, Sixth Edition (2002) published by Springer Science and Business Media LLC, *www.springerlink.com.*

cases, follicular cancers may be hyperfunctioning, leading patients to present with signs and symptoms of thyrotoxicosis. FNAB is unable to distinguish benign follicular lesions from follicular carcinomas. Therefore, preoperative clinical diagnosis of cancer is difficult unless distant metastases are present. Large follicular tumors (>4 cm) in older men are more likely to be malignant.

Due to the limitations inherent in the FNAB diagnosis, a number of studies have focused on identifying molecular markers to distinguish benign from malignant follicular lesions. Loss of heterozygosity (LOH) analysis compares normal and tumor tissue DNA at specific chromosomal loci for loss of one copy of a gene pair. LOH near the von Hippel-Lindau (VHL) locus of chromosome 3p25-26 has been reported to be a strong discriminant of benign from malignant follicular lesions.[39] Other studies have used complementary DNA microar-

rays to compare tumor tissue for differences in the expression of thousands of genes and have shown very promising results for the correct subsequent diagnosis of unknowns. These studies have identified combinations of three to six genes that appear to be useful in distinguishing benign from malignant follicular lesions.[40] Expression arrays also have been used to investigate the role of microRNAs, which are a new class of small, noncoding RNA that have been implicated in carcinogenesis. The specific microRNAs miR-197 and miR-364 are upregulated in follicular thyroid cancers.[41] Many of these genetic changes can be identified using tissue obtained during FNAB and have the potential to be used as diagnostic and possibly prognostic markers.

Pathology Follicular carcinomas usually are solitary lesions, and the majority are surrounded by a capsule. Histologically, follicles are present, but the lumen may be devoid of colloid. Architectural patterns depend on the degree of differentiation demonstrated by the tumor. Malignancy is defined by the presence of capsular and vascular invasion (Fig. 38-18). In general, minimally invasive tumors appear grossly encapsulated and have microscopic invasion through the tumor capsule without extension into the parenchyma and/or invasion into small- to medium-sized vessels (venous caliber) in or immediately outside the capsule, but not within the tumor.[42] On the other hand, widely invasive tumors demonstrate evidence of large vessel invasion and/or broad areas of tumor invasion through the capsule. They may, in fact, be unencapsulated. It is important to note that there is a wide variation of opinion among clinicians and pathologists with respect to the above definitions. Tumor infiltration and invasion, as well as tumor thrombus within the middle thyroid or jugular veins, may be apparent at operation.

Surgical Treatment and Prognosis Patients diagnosed by FNAB as having a follicular lesion should undergo thyroid lobectomy because at least 80% of these patients will have benign adenomas. Some surgeons recommend total thyroidectomy in older patients with follicular lesions >4 cm because of the higher risk of cancer in this setting (50%). Intraoperative frozen-section examination usually is not helpful, but should be performed when there is evidence of capsular or vascular invasion, or when adjacent lymphadenopathy is present. Total thyroidectomy should be performed when thyroid cancer is diagnosed. There is debate among experts about whether patients with minimally invasive follicular cancers should undergo completion thyroidectomy because the prognosis is so good in these patients. A diagnosis of frankly invasive carcinoma or follicular carcinoma with angioinvasion, with or without capsular invasion, necessitates completion of total thyroidectomy primarily so that ^{131}I can be used to detect and ablate metastatic disease. Prophylactic nodal dissection is unwarranted because nodal involvement is infrequent, but in the unusual patient with nodal metastases, therapeutic neck dissection is recommended. The cumulative mortality from follicular thyroid cancer is approximately 15% at 10 years and 30% at 20 years. Poor long-term prognosis is predicted by age over 50 years old at presentation, tumor size >4 cm, higher tumor grade, marked vascular invasion, extrathyroidal invasion, and distant metastases at the time of diagnosis.

Hürthle Cell Carcinoma Hürthle cell carcinomas account for approximately 3% of all thyroid malignancies and, under the World Health Organization classification, are considered to be a subtype of follicular thyroid cancer. Hürthle cell cancers also are characterized by vascular or capsular invasion and can, therefore, not be diagnosed by FNAB. Tumors contain sheets of eosinophilic cells packed with mitochondria, which are derived from the oxyphilic cells of the thyroid gland. Hürthle cell tumors differ from follicular carcinomas in that they are more often multifocal and bilateral (about 30%), usually do not take up RAI (about 5%), are more likely to metastasize to local nodes (25%) and distant sites, and are associated with a higher mortality rate (about 20% at 10 years). Hence, they are considered to be a separate class of tumors by some groups.

Management is similar to that of follicular neoplasms, with lobectomy and isthmusectomy being sufficient surgical treatment for unilateral Hürthle cell adenomas. When Hürthle cell neoplasms

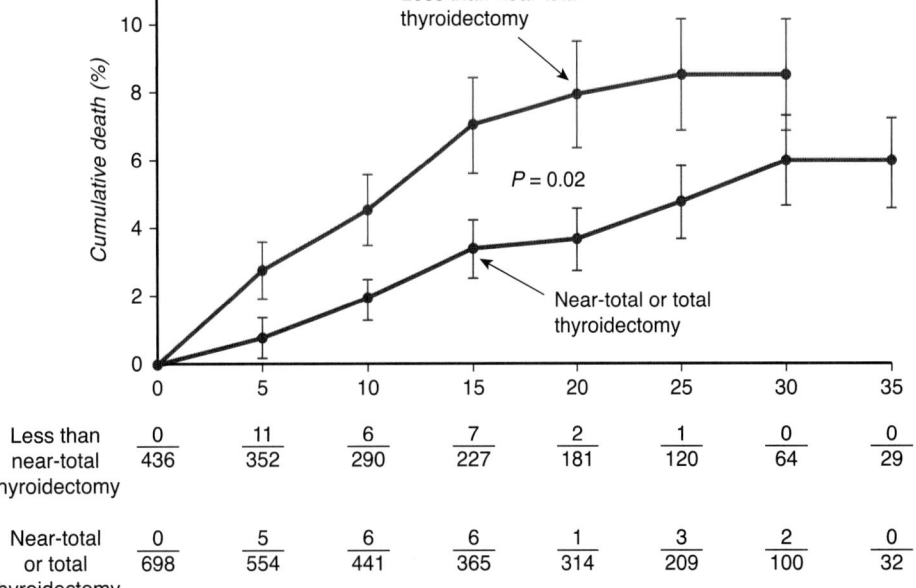

Less than near-total thyroidectomy	$\frac{0}{436}$	$\frac{11}{352}$	$\frac{6}{290}$	$\frac{7}{227}$	$\frac{2}{181}$	$\frac{1}{120}$	$\frac{0}{64}$	$\frac{0}{29}$
Near-total or total thyroidectomy	$\frac{0}{698}$	$\frac{5}{554}$	$\frac{6}{441}$	$\frac{6}{365}$	$\frac{1}{314}$	$\frac{3}{209}$	$\frac{2}{100}$	$\frac{0}{32}$

Years after initial therapy

FIG. 38-17. Improved survival in patients with papillary or follicular thyroid cancer following total or near-total thyroidectomy compared to those who underwent less than near-total thyroidectomy. *(Reproduced with permission from Mazzaferri E, Jhiang S: Long-term impact of initial surgical and medical therapy on papillary and follicular thyroid cancer. Am J Med 97:424, 1994. Copyright Elsevier.)*

are found to be invasive on definitive paraffin-section histology, then total thyroidectomy should be performed. These patients should also undergo routine central neck node removal, similar to patients with MTC, and modified radical neck dissection when lateral neck nodes are palpable. Although RAI scanning and ablation usually are ineffective, they probably should be considered to ablate any residual normal thyroid tissue and occasionally ablate tumors because there is no other good therapy. Redifferentiating therapies such as retinoic acid, PPARγ agonists have shown some utility in treating these tumors in vitro; however, the results of phase II clinical trials have been mixed.[43] Further research is needed to clarify the role of these treatments.

Postoperative Management of Differentiated Thyroid Cancer

Radioiodine Therapy The issue of whether RAI therapy offers any benefit to patients with differentiated thyroid cancer remains con-

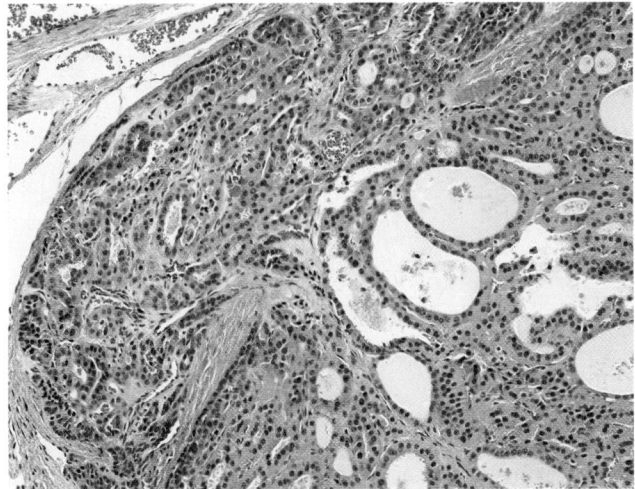

FIG. 38-18. Hematoxylin-eosin–stained section from follicular thyroid carcinoma showing capsular invasion.

troversial in the absence of prospective, randomized controlled trials. Long-term cohort studies by Mazzaferri and associates and DeGroot and colleagues demonstrate that postoperative RAI therapy reduces recurrence (Fig. 38-19) and provides a small improvement in survival, even in low-risk patients.[30,33] Screening with RAI is more sensitive than chest x-ray or CT scanning for detecting metastases; however, it is less sensitive than Tg measurements for detecting metastatic disease in most differentiated thyroid cancers except Hürthle cell tumors. Screening and treatment are facilitated by the removal of all normal thyroid tissue, which effectively competes for iodine uptake. Metastatic differentiated thyroid carcinoma can be detected and treated by ^{131}I in about 75% of patients. Multiple studies show that RAI effectively treats >70% of lung micrometastases that are detected by RAI scan in the presence of a normal chest x-ray, whereas the success rates drop to <10% with pulmonary macrometastases. Early detection therefore appears to be very important to improve prognosis. RAI ablation currently is recommended for all patients with stage III or IV disease, all patients with stage II disease younger than 45 years old, most patients 45 years or older with stage II disease, and patients with stage I disease who have aggressive histologies, nodal metastases, multifocal disease, and extrathyroid or vascular invasion.[37]

Generally, T4 therapy should be discontinued for approximately 6 weeks before scanning with [131]I. Patients should receive T3 during this time period to decrease the period if hypothyroidism. T3 has a shorter half-life than T4 (1 day vs. 1 week) and needs to be discontinued for 2 weeks to allow TSH levels to rise before treatment. Levels >30 mU/L are considered optimal, based on noncontrolled studies.[37] A low-iodine diet also is recommended during this 2-week period. The usual protocol involves administering a screening dose of 1 to 3 mCi of ^{123}I and measuring uptake 24 hours later. After a total thyroidectomy, this value should be <1%. A "hot" spot in the neck after initial screening usually represents residual normal tissue in the thyroid bed. Some investigators recommend omitting the scanning dose altogether to minimize thyrocyte "stunning" and subsequent requirement for higher treatment doses. Others recommend scanning only if the size of the remnant cannot be determined by the operative report or ultrasound, or if the results would alter the decision to treat or the dose to be administered. If there is significant uptake, then a therapeutic dose of ^{131}I, 30 to 100 mCi

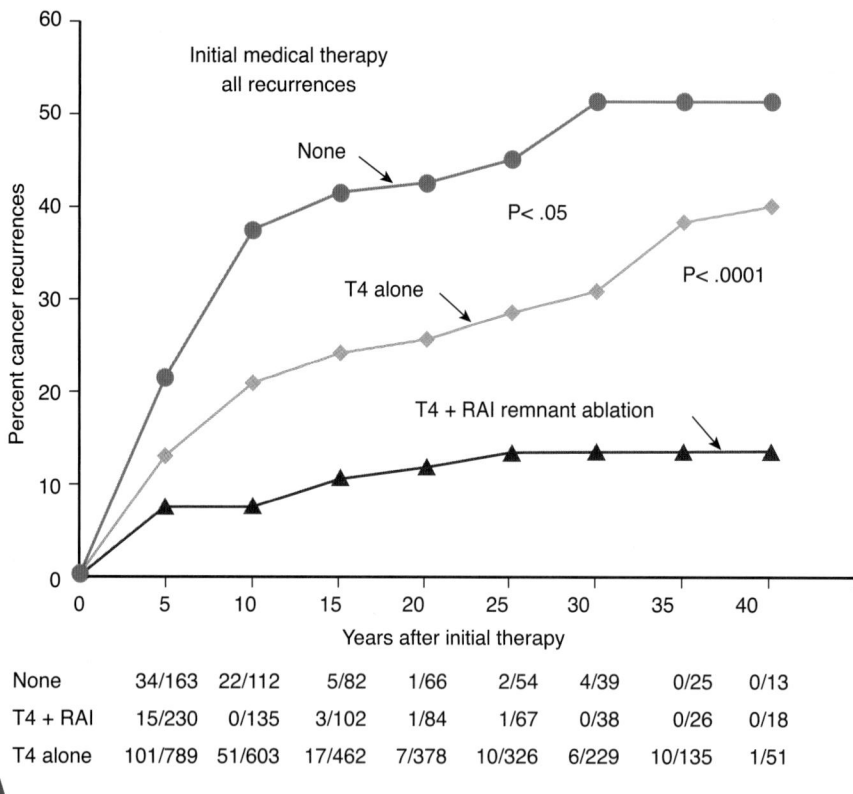

None	34/163	22/112	5/82	1/66	2/54	4/39	0/25	0/13
T4 + RAI	15/230	0/135	3/102	1/84	1/67	0/38	0/26	0/18
T4 alone	101/789	51/603	17/462	7/378	10/326	6/229	10/135	1/51

A

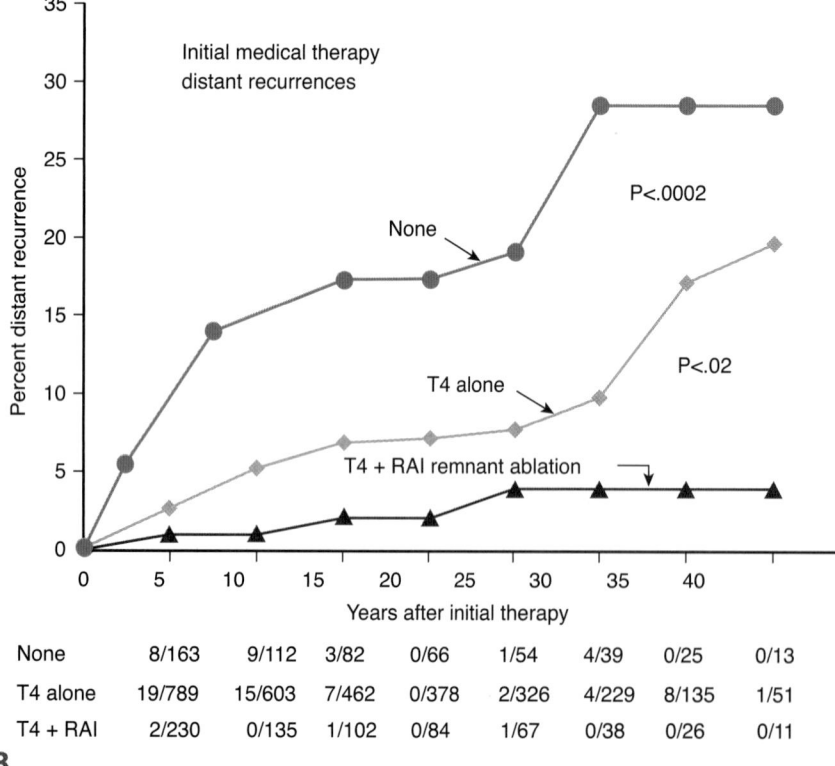

None	8/163	9/112	3/82	0/66	1/54	4/39	0/25	0/13
T4 alone	19/789	15/603	7/462	0/378	2/326	4/229	8/135	1/51
T4 + RAI	2/230	0/135	1/102	0/84	1/67	0/38	0/26	0/11

B

FIG. 38-19. Tumor recurrence at a median of 16.7 years after thyroid surgery. The numerator is the number of patients with recurrence, and the denominator is the number of patients in each time interval. The P values are derived from log-rank statistical analysis of 40-year life-table data. Figure shows that all recurrences (**A**) and distant metastases (**B**) were reduced in patients who received radioactive iodine (RAI) in addition to thyroxine (T4) therapy. *(Reproduced with permission from Mazzaferri E, Kloos R: Current approaches to primary therapy for papillary and follicular thyroid cancer. J Clin Endocrinol Metab 86:1453, 2001, Copyright by The Endocrine Society.)*

should be administered to low-risk patients and 100 to 200 mCi in high-risk patients. If patients have an elevated Tg level, but negative RAI scan, some physicians recommend treating once with 100 mCi of ^{131}I and repeating the imaging 1 to 2 weeks later. Approximately one third of these patients demonstrate uptake on posttreatment imaging, and Tg levels usually decrease in these patients, document-

ing therapeutic benefit. Patients with previously positive scans and patients with serum Tg levels >2 ng/mL usually need another ^{131}I treatment after 6 to 12 months until one or two negative scans are obtained. The follow-up scan can be done after hormone withdrawal or after recombinant TSH. The latter is more expensive but is preferred by patients. The maximum dose of radioiodine that can

TABLE 38-7	Complications of radioactive iodine therapy (^{131}I) and doses at which they are observed

Acute	Long-Term
Neck pain, swelling, and tenderness	Hematologic
Thyroiditis (if remnant present)	Bone marrow suppression
Sialadenitis (50–450 mCi), taste	(>500 mCi)
dysfunction	Leukemia (>1000 mCi)
Hemorrhage (brain metastases)	Fertility
Cerebral edema (brain metastases,	Ovarian/testicular damage,
200 mCi)	infertility
Vocal cord paralysis	Increased spontaneous abortion
Nausea and vomiting (50–450 mCi)	rate
Bone marrow suppression (200	Pulmonary fibrosis
mCi)	Chronic sialadenitis, nodules, taste
	dysfunction
	Increased risk of cancer
	Anaplastic thyroid cancer
	Gastric cancer
	Hepatocellular cancer
	Lung cancer
	Breast cancer (>1000 mCi)
	Bladder cancer
	Hypoparathyroidism

be administered at one time without performing dosimetry is approximately 200 mCi with a cumulative dose of 1000 to 1500 mCi. Up to 500 mCi can be given with proper pretreatment dosimetry. The early and delayed complications of RAI therapy are listed in Table 38-7.

External Beam Radiotherapy and Chemotherapy External beam radiotherapy is occasionally required to control unresectable, locally invasive or recurrent disease[44] and to treat metastases in support bones to decrease the risk of fractures. It also is of value for the treatment and control of pain from bony metastases when there is minimal or no RAIU. Single and multidrug chemotherapy has been used with little success in disseminated thyroid cancer, and there is no role for routine chemotherapy.[37] Doxorubicin (Adriamycin) and paclitaxel (Taxol) are the most frequently used agents. The former acts as a radiation sensitizer and should be considered in patients undergoing external beam radiation.

Thyroid Hormone T_4 is necessary not only as replacement therapy in patients after total or near-total thyroidectomy, but has the additional effect of suppressing TSH and reducing the growth stimulus for any possible residual thyroid cancer cells. TSH suppression reduces tumor recurrence rates. T_4 should be administered to ensure that the patient remains euthyroid, with circulating TSH levels at about 0.1 μU/L in low-risk patients, or <0.1 μU/mL in high-risk patients.[37] The risk of tumor recurrence must be balanced with the side effects

associated with prolonged TSH suppression, including osteopenia and cardiac problems, particularly in older patients.

Follow-Up of Patients with Differentiated Thyroid Cancer

Thyroglobulin Measurement Tg levels in patients who have undergone total thyroidectomy should be <2 ng/mL when the patient is taking T_4, and <5 ng/mL when the patient is hypothyroid. A Tg level >2 ng/mL is highly suggestive of metastatic disease or persistent normal thyroid tissue, especially if it increases when TSH levels increase when hypothyroid during preparation for RAI scanning or after recombinant TSH. Approximately 95% of patients with persistent or recurrent thyroid cancer of follicular cell origin will have Tg levels >2 ng/mL. Tg and anti-Tg antibody levels should be measured initially at 6-month intervals and then annually if the patient is clinically disease free.[37] More recently, Tg measurements in FNAB aspirates have been shown to be useful in the detection of nodal metastatic disease.[45]

Imaging After the first posttreatment scan, low-risk patients with negative TSH-stimulated Tg and cervical ultrasound do not require routine diagnostic whole body radioiodine scans. However, diagnostic whole body scans 6 to 12 months after remnant ablation may be of value in the follow-up of patients with high or intermediate risk of persistent disease. It also is recommended that cervical ultrasound to evaluate the thyroid bed and central and lateral cervical nodal compartments should be performed at 6 and 12 months postthyroidectomy and then annually for at least 3 to 5 years, depending on the patients' risk for recurrent disease and Tg status. If RAI and ultrasound scans are negative but Tg levels remain elevated, FDG PET scans can help to localize the disease.[37]

Medullary Carcinoma MTC accounts for about 5% of thyroid malignancies and arises from the parafollicular or C cells of the thyroid, which, in turn, are derived from the ultimobranchial bodies. These cells are concentrated superolaterally in the thyroid lobes, and this is where MTC usually develops. C cells secrete calcitonin, a 32-amino-acid polypeptide that functions to lower serum calcium levels, although its effects in humans are minimal. Most MTCs occur sporadically. However, approximately 25% occur within the spectrum of several inherited syndromes such as familial MTC, MEN2A, and MEN2B. All these variants are known to result secondary to germline mutations in the *RET* proto-oncogene. The syndromes also are characterized by genotype-phenotype correlations, with specific mutations leading to particular clinical manifestations. The salient clinical and genetic features of these syndromes are outlined in Table 38-8. Some clinical features of MEN2B patients are shown in Fig. 38-20.

Patients with MTC often present with a neck mass that may be associated with palpable cervical lymphadenopathy (15 to 20%). Pain or aching is more common in patients with these tumors, and local invasion may produce symptoms of dysphagia, dyspnea, or dysphonia. Distant blood-borne metastases to the liver, bone (frequently osteoblastic), and lung occur later in the disease. The female-to-male ratio is 1.5:1. Most patients present between 50 and 60 years

TABLE 38-8	Clinical and genetic features of medullary thyroid cancer syndromes	

Syndrome	Manifestations	*Ret* Mutations
MEN2A	MTC, pheochromocytoma, primary hyperparathyroidism, lichen planus amyloidosis	Exon 10—codons 609, 611, 618, 620 Exon 11—codon 634 (more commonly associated with pheochromocytoma and primary hyperparathyroidism)
MEN2B	MTC, pheochromocytoma, Marfanoid habitus, mucocutaneous ganglioneuromatosis	Exon 16—codon 918
Familial MTC	MTC	Codons 609, 611, 618, 620, and 634 Codons 768, 790, 791, or 804 (rare)
MEN2A and Hirschsprung's disease	MTC, pheochromocytoma, primary hyperparathyroidism, Hirschsprung's disease	Codons 609, 618, 620

MTC = medullary thyroid cancer.

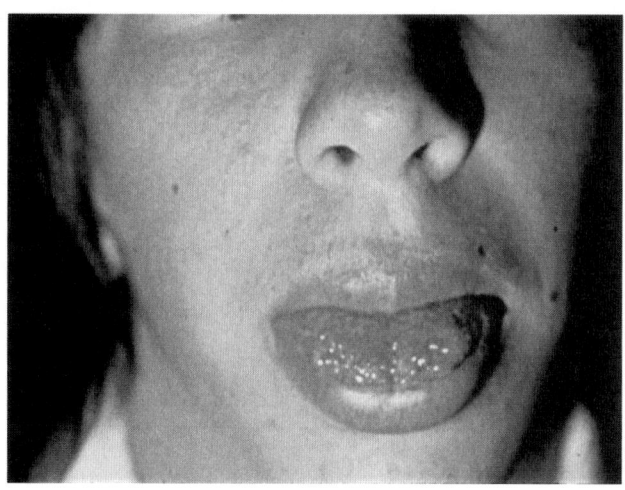

A

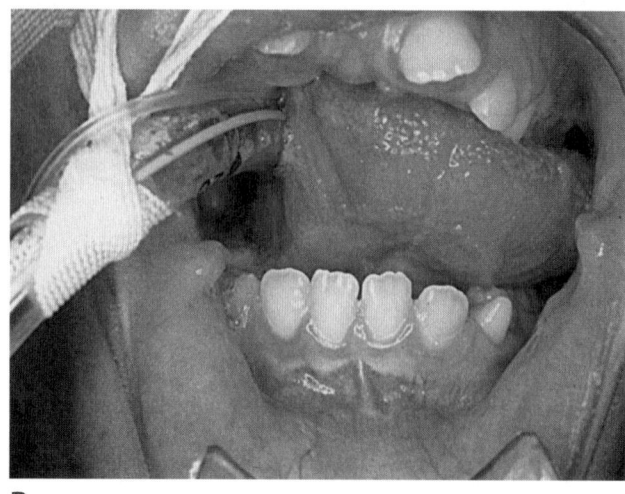

B

FIG. 38-20. Features of MEN2B: thickened lips (**A**) and mucosal neuromas (**A** and **B**).

old, although patients with familial disease present at a younger age. Medullary thyroid tumors secrete not only calcitonin and carcinoembryonic antigen (CEA), but also other peptides such as calcitonin gene–related peptide, histaminadases, prostaglandins E2 and $F_{2\alpha}$, and serotonin. Patients with extensive metastatic disease frequently develop diarrhea, which may result from increased intestinal motility and impaired intestinal water and electrolyte flux. About 2 to 4% of patients develop Cushing's syndrome as a result of ectopic production of adrenocorticotropic hormone (ACTH).

Pathology MTCs typically are unilateral (80%) in patients with sporadic disease and multicentric in familial cases, with bilateral tumors occurring in up to 90% of familial patients. Familial cases also are associated with C-cell hyperplasia, which is considered a premalignant lesion. Microscopically, tumors are composed of sheets of infiltrating neoplastic cells separated by collagen and amyloid. Marked heterogeneity is present; cells may be polygonal or spindle shaped. The presence of amyloid is a diagnostic finding, but immunohistochemistry for calcitonin is more commonly used as a diagnostic tumor marker. These tumors also stain positively for CEA and calcitonin gene–related peptide.

Diagnosis The diagnosis of MTC is established by history, physical examination, raised serum calcitonin, or CEA levels, and FNAB cytology of the thyroid mass. Attention to family history is important because about 25% of patients with MTC have familial disease. Because it is not possible to distinguish sporadic from familial disease at initial presentation, all new patients with MTC should be screened for *RET* point mutations, pheochromocytoma, and HPT. Screening of patients with familial MTC for *RET* point mutations has largely replaced using provocation testing with pentagastrin or calcium-stimulated calcitonin levels to make the diagnosis. Calcitonin and CEA are used to identify patients with persistent or recurrent MTC. Calcitonin is a more sensitive tumor marker, but CEA is a better predictor of prognosis.

Treatment If patients are found to have a pheochromocytoma, this must be operated on first. These tumors are generally (>50%) bilateral. Total thyroidectomy is the treatment of choice for patients with MTC because of the high incidence of multicentricity, the more aggressive course, and the fact that ^{131}I therapy usually is not effective. Central compartment nodes frequently are involved early in the disease process, so that a bilateral central neck node dissection should be routinely performed. In patients with palpable cervical nodes or involved central neck nodes, ipsilateral or bilateral, modified radical neck dissection is recommended. The role of prophylactic lateral neck dissection is controversial. However, in patients with

tumors >1 cm, ipsilateral prophylactic modified radical neck dissection is recommended because >60% of these patients have nodal metastases. If ipsilateral nodes are positive, a contralateral node dissection should be performed. In the case of locally recurrent or metastatic disease, tumor debulking is advised not only to ameliorate symptoms of flushing and diarrhea, but also to decrease risk of death from recurrent central neck or mediastinal disease. External beam radiotherapy is controversial, but is recommended for patients with unresectable residual or recurrent tumor. There is no effective chemotherapy regimen. Various targeted therapies are being investigated for the treatment of MTC. A tyrosine kinase inhibitor STI571 (imatinib) had shown promise in in vitro studies, but phase II clinical trials have been less encouraging.[46,47] Another tyrosine kinase inhibitor with activity against the vascular endothelial growth factor receptor 2, ZD6474 (Zactima) was more effective in that phase II studies have shown partial responses in 27% of patients, with reduction in both calcitonin and CEA levels. An anti-CEA monoclonal antibody (labetuzumab) also has shown antitumor response in a small group of patients.[48] Radiofrequency ablation done laparoscopically appears promising in the palliative treatment of liver metastases >1.5 cm.

In patients who have hypercalcemia at the time of thyroidectomy, only obviously enlarged parathyroid glands should be removed. The other parathyroid glands should be preserved and marked in patients with normocalcemia, as only about 20% of patients with MEN2A develop HPT. When a normal parathyroid cannot be maintained on a vascular pedicle, it should be removed, biopsied to confirm that it is a parathyroid, and then autotransplanted to the forearm of the nondominant arm. Total thyroidectomy is indicated in *RET* mutation carriers once the mutation is confirmed. The procedure should be performed before age 6 in MEN2A patients and before age 1 year old in MEN2B patients.[49,50] Central neck dissection can be avoided in children who are *RET*-positive and calcitonin-negative with a normal ultrasound examination. When the calcitonin is increased or the ultrasound suggests a thyroid cancer, a prophylactic central neck dissection is indicated.

Postoperative Follow-Up and Prognosis Patients are followed by annual measurements of calcitonin and CEA levels, in addition to history and physical examination. Other modalities used to localize recurrent disease include ultrasound, CT, MRI, and more recently, FDG PET scans. The latter have been reported to be superior to other radionuclide-based and routine morphologic imaging by some investigators.[51] Prognosis is related to disease stage. The 10-year survival rate is approximately 80% but decreases to 45% in patients with lymph node involvement. Survival also is significantly influenced by disease type. It is best in patients with non-MEN familial MTC, followed by those with MEN2A, and then those with sporadic disease. Prognosis is the worst (survival 35% at 10 years) in patients with MEN2B. Performing prophylactic surgery in *RET* oncogene mutation carriers not only improves survival rates but also renders most patients calcitonin free.

Anaplastic Carcinoma Anaplastic carcinoma accounts for approximately 1% of all thyroid malignancies in the United States and is declining in incidence. Women are more commonly affected, and the majority of tumors present in the seventh and eighth decade of life. The typical patient has a long-standing neck mass, which rapidly enlarges and may be painful. Associated symptoms such as dysphonia, dysphagia, and dyspnea are common. The tumor is large and may be fixed to surrounding structures or may be ulcerated with areas of necrosis (Fig. 38-21). Lymph nodes usually are palpable at presentation. Evidence of metastatic spread also may be present. Diagnosis is confirmed by FNAB revealing characteristic giant and multinucleated cells. Incisional biopsy occasionally is needed to confirm the diagnosis, and isthmusectomy with or without a tracheostomy may be needed to alleviate tracheal obstruction.

Pathology On gross inspection, anaplastic tumors are firm and whitish in appearance. Microscopically, sheets of cells with marked heterogeneity are seen. Cells may be spindle shaped, polygonal, or large, multinucleated cells. Foci of more differentiated thyroid tumors, either follicular or papillary, may be seen, suggesting that anaplastic tumors arise from more well-differentiated tumors. One should confirm that the tumor is not a MTC or a small cell lymphoma because the prognosis varies considerably.

Treatment and Prognosis This tumor is one of the most aggressive thyroid malignancies, with few patients surviving 6 months beyond diagnosis. All forms of treatment have been disappointing. If anaplastic carcinoma presents as a resectable mass, thyroidectomy may lead to a small improvement in survival, especially in younger individuals. Combined radiation and chemotherapy in an adjuvant setting in patients with resectable disease has been associated with prolonged survival,[52] although these agents are also being used in a neoadjuvant fashion. Tracheostomy may be needed to alleviate airway obstruction.

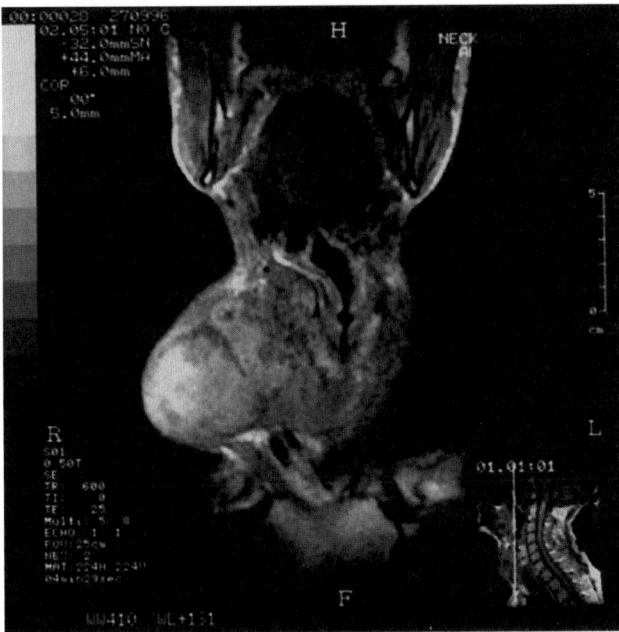

FIG. 38-21. Magnetic resonance imaging scan of a patient with anaplastic thyroid cancer. Note heterogeneity consistent with necrosis.

Lymphoma Lymphomas account for <1% of thyroid malignancies and most are of the non-Hodgkin's B-cell type. Although the disease can arise as part of a generalized lymphomatous condition, most thyroid lymphomas develop in patients with chronic lymphocytic thyroiditis. Chronic antigenic lymphocyte stimulation has been suggested to result in lymphocyte transformation. Patients usually present with symptoms similar to those of patients with anaplastic carcinoma, although the rapidly enlarging neck mass often is painless. Patients may present with acute respiratory distress. The diagnosis usually is suggested by FNAB, although needle-core or open biopsy may be necessary for definitive diagnosis. Staging studies should be obtained expeditiously to assess the extent of extrathyroidal spread.

Treatment and Prognosis Patients with thyroid lymphoma respond rapidly to chemotherapy (CHOP—cyclophosphamide, doxorubicin, vincristine, and prednisone), which also has been associated with improved survival. Combined treatment with radiotherapy and chemotherapy often is recommended. Thyroidectomy and nodal resection are used to alleviate symptoms of airway obstruction in patients who do not respond quickly to the above regimens or who have completed the regimen before diagnosis. Prognosis depends on the histologic grade of the tumor and whether the lymphoma is confined to the thyroid gland or is disseminated. The overall 5-year survival rate is about 50%; patients with extrathyroidal disease have markedly lower survival rates.

Metastatic Carcinoma The thyroid gland is a rare site of metastases from other cancers, including kidney, breast, lung, and melanoma. Clinical examination and a review of the patient's history often suggest the source of the metastatic disease, and FNAB usually provides definitive diagnosis. Resection of the thyroid, usually lobectomy, may be helpful in many patients, depending on the status of their primary tumor.

Thyroid Surgery

Conduct of Thyroidectomy Patients with any recent or remote history of altered phonation or prior neck surgery should undergo vocal cord assessment by direct or indirect laryngoscopy before thyroidectomy. The patient is positioned supine, with a sandbag between the scapulae. The head is placed on a donut cushion and the neck is extended to provide maximal exposure. A Kocher transverse collar incision, typically 4 to 5 cm in length, is placed in or parallel to a natural skin crease 1 cm below the cricoid cartilage (Fig. 38-22A), although longer incisions may be needed. The subcutaneous tissues and platysma are incised sharply and subplatysmal flaps are raised superiorly to the level of the thyroid cartilage and inferiorly to the suprasternal notch (Fig. 38-22B). The strap muscles are divided in the midline along the entire length of the mobilized flaps, and the thyroid gland is exposed. On the side to be approached first, the sternohyoid muscles are separated from the underlying sternothyroid muscle by blunt dissection until the internal jugular vein and ansa cervicalis nerve are identified. The strap muscles rarely need to be divided to gain exposure to the thyroid gland. If this maneuver is necessary, the muscles should be divided high to preserve their innervation by branches of the ansa cervicalis. If there is evidence of direct tumor invasion into the strap muscles, the portion of involved muscle should be resected en bloc with the thyroid gland. The sternothyroid muscle is then dissected off the underlying thyroid by a combination of sharp and blunt dissection, thus exposing the middle thyroid veins. The thyroid lobe is retracted medially and anteriorly and the lateral tissues are swept posterolaterally using a peanut sponge. The middle thyroid veins are ligated and divided (Fig. 38-22C). Attention is then turned to the midline where Delphian nodes and the pyramidal lobe are identified. The fascia just cephalad and caudad to the isthmus is divided. The superior thyroid pole is identified by retracting the thyroid first inferiorly and medially and then the upper pole of the thyroid is mobilized caudally and laterally. The dissection plane is

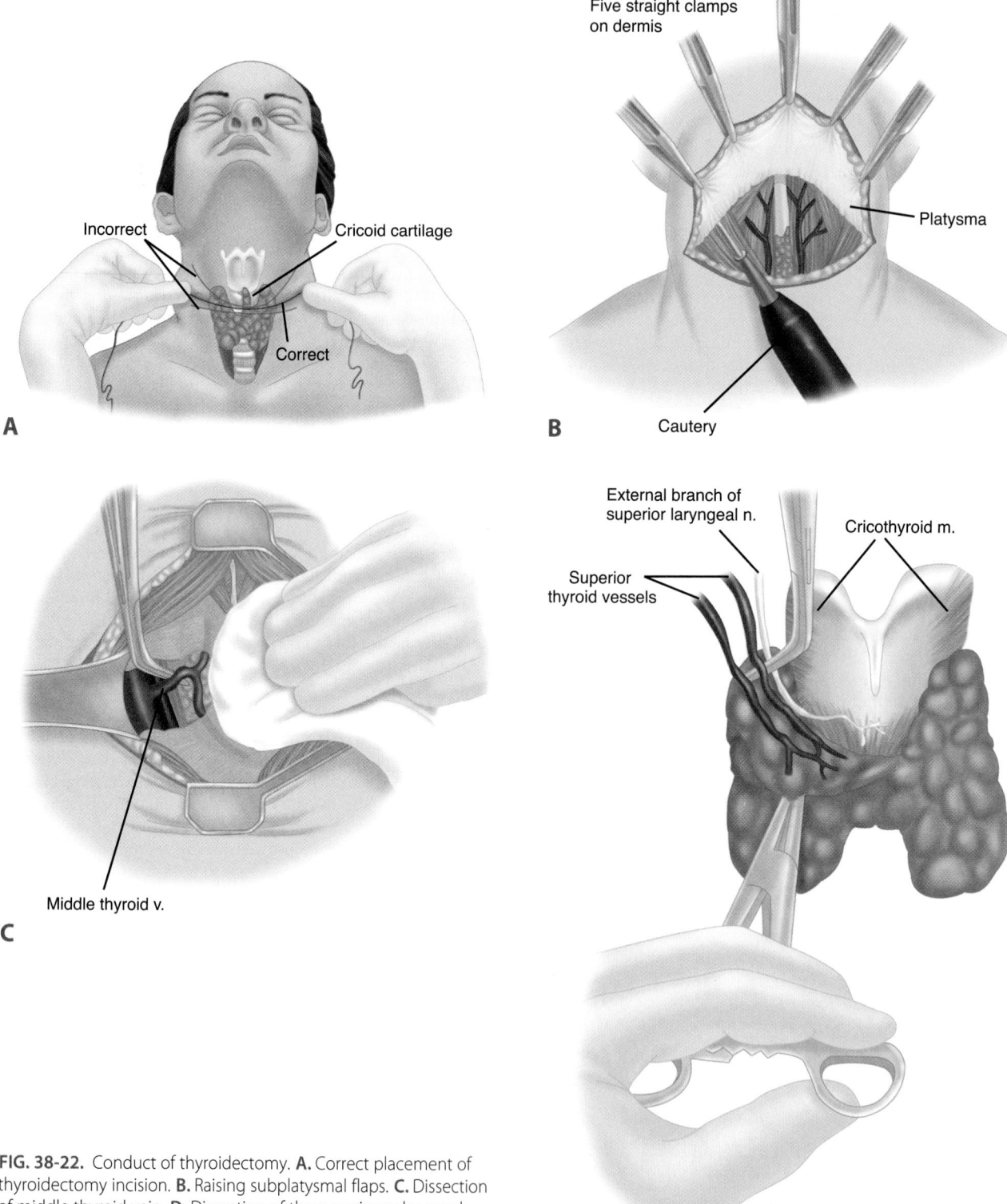

FIG. 38-22. Conduct of thyroidectomy. **A.** Correct placement of thyroidectomy incision. **B.** Raising subplatysmal flaps. **C.** Dissection of middle thyroid vein. **D.** Dissection of the superior pole vessels, which should be individually ligated. (*Continued*)

kept as close to the thyroid as possible and the superior pole vessels are individually identified, skeletonized, ligated, and divided low on the thyroid gland to avoid injury to the external branch of the superior laryngeal nerve (Fig. 38-22D). Once these vessels are divided, the tissues posterior and lateral to the superior pole can be swept from the gland in a posteromedial direction, to reduce the risk of damaging vessels supplying the upper parathyroid.

The RLNs should then be identified. The course of the right RLN is more oblique than the left RLN. The nerves can be most consistently identified at the level of the cricoid cartilage. The parathyroids usually can be identified within 1 cm of the crossing of the inferior thyroid artery and the RLN, although they also may be ectopic in location. The lower pole of the thyroid gland should be mobilized by gently sweeping all tissues dorsally. The inferior

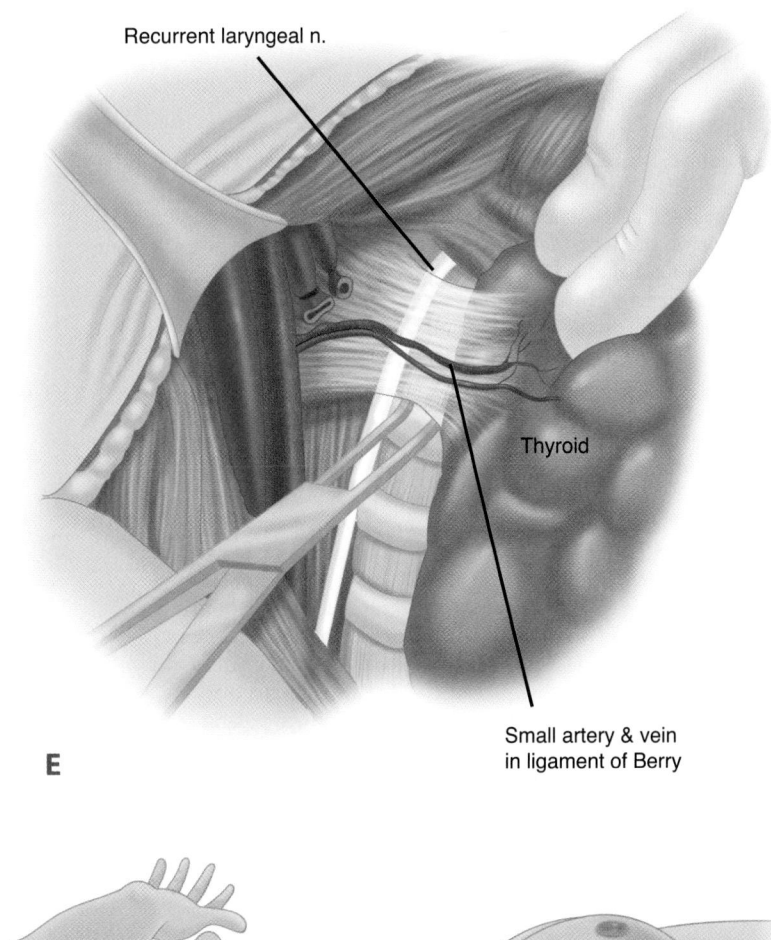

Recurrent laryngeal n.

Thyroid

Small artery & vein
in ligament of Berry

E

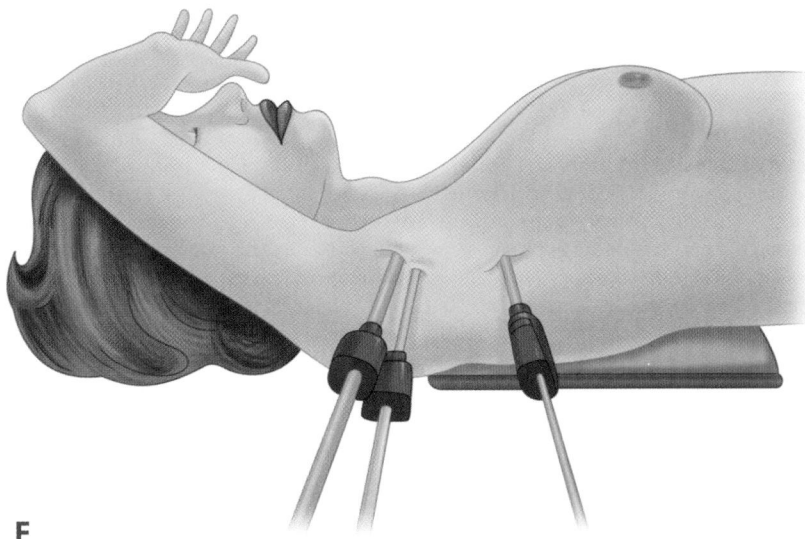

F

FIG. 38-22. (*Continued*) **E.** Dissection at the ligament of Berry. Note small artery and vein within the ligament and the recurrent laryngeal nerve coursing laterally. **F.** Endoscopic thyroidectomy via axillary incisions. m. = muscle; n. = nerve; v. = vein.

thyroid vessels are dissected, skeletonized, ligated, and divided as close to the surface of the thyroid gland as possible to minimize devascularization of the parathyroids (extracapsular dissection) or injury to the RLN. The RLN is most vulnerable to injury in the vicinity of the ligament of Berry. The nerve often passes through this structure along with small crossing arterial and venous branches (Fig. 38-22E). Any bleeding in this area should be controlled with gentle pressure before carefully identifying the vessel and ligating it. Use of the electrocautery should be avoided in proximity to the RLN. Once the ligament is divided, the thyroid can be separated from the underlying trachea by sharp dissection. The pyramidal lobe, if present, must be dissected in a cephalad direction to above the level of the notch in the thyroid cartilage or higher in continuity with the thyroid gland. If a lobectomy is to be performed, the isthmus is divided flush with the trachea on the contralateral

side and suture ligated. The procedure is repeated on the opposite side for a total thyroidectomy.

Parathyroid glands that are located anteriorly on the surface of the thyroid cannot be dissected from the thyroid with a good blood supply or that have been inadvertently removed during the thyroidectomy should be resected, confirmed as parathyroid tissue by frozen section, divided into 1-mm fragments, and reimplanted into individual pockets in the sternocleidomastoid muscle. The sites should be marked with silk sutures and a clip. If a subtotal thyroidectomy is to be performed, once the superior pole vessels are divided and the thyroid lobe mobilized anteriorly, the thyroid lobe is cross-clamped with a Mayo clamp, leaving approximately 4 g of the posterior portion of the thyroid. The thyroid remnant is suture ligated, taking care to avoid injury to the RLN. Routine drain placement rarely is necessary. After adequate hemostasis is obtained, the strap muscles are reapproximated in the midline. The platysma is approximated in a similar fashion. The skin can be closed with subcuticular sutures or clips.

Minimally Invasive Approaches Several approaches to minimally invasive thyroidectomy have been described. Mini-incision procedures use a small, 3-cm incision with no flap creation and minimal dissection to deliver the thyroid into the wound and then perform the pretracheal and paratracheal dissection. Video assistance can be used to improve the visualization via the small incision. Totally endoscopic approaches also have been described, via the supraclavicular, anterior chest, axillary, and breast approach. The axillary, anterior chest, and breast approaches eliminate the skin incision in the neck but are more invasive. All endoscopic thyroidectomies are performed under general anesthesia. For the axillary approach, a 30-mm skin incision is made in the axilla, and 12-mm and 5-mm trocars are inserted through this incision (Figure 38-22F). An additional 5-mm trocar is inserted adjacent to the incision. For the anterior chest approach, a 12-mm skin incision is made in the skin of the anterior chest approximately 3 to 5 cm below the border of the ipsilateral clavicle. Two additional 5-mm trocars are inserted by endoscopic guidance below the ipsilateral clavicle, and carbon dioxide (CO_2) is then insufflated up to a pressure of 4 mmHg to facilitate creation of a working space. The anterior border of the sternocleidomastoid muscle is then separated from the sternohyoid muscle to expose the sternothyroid muscle. The thyroid gland is exposed by splitting the sternothyroid muscle. The lower pole is retracted upward and dissected from the adipose tissue to identify the RLN. As the RLN is exposed, Berry's ligament is exposed and incised with a 5-mm clip or laparoscopic coagulating shears. The upper pole of the thyroid gland is separated from the cricothyroid muscle, and the external branch of the superior laryngeal nerve can be identified during this maneuver. The upper pole of the thyroid gland then is dissected free.

These methods are feasible, but clear benefits over the "traditional" open approach have not been established.

Surgical Removal of Intrathoracic Goiter A goiter is considered mediastinal if at least 50% of the thyroid tissue is located intrathoracically. Mediastinal goiters can be primary or secondary. Primary mediastinal goiters constitute approximately 1% of all mediastinal goiters and arise from accessory (ectopic) thyroid tissue located in the chest. These goiters are supplied by intrathoracic blood vessels and do not have any connection to thyroid tissue in the neck. The vast majority of mediastinal goiters are, however, secondary mediastinal goiters that arise from downward extension of cervical thyroid tissue along the fascial planes of the neck and derive their blood supply from the superior and inferior thyroid arteries. Virtually all intrathoracic goiters can be removed via a cervical incision. Patients who have (a) invasive thyroid cancers, (b) had previous thyroid operations and may have developed parasitic mediastinal vessels, or (c) primary mediastinal goiters with no thyroid tissue in the neck may require a median sternotomy for removal.[53] The chest, however, should be prepared in most cases in the event it is necessary to perform a median sternotomy to control mediastinal bleeding or completely remove an unsuspected invasive cancer. The goiter is approached via a neck incision. The superior pole vessels and the middle thyroid veins are identified and ligated first. Early division of the isthmus helps with subsequent mobilization of the substernal goiter from beneath the sternum. Placement of large 1-0 or 2-0 sutures deep into the goiter, when necessary, helps deliver it. For patients in whom thyroid cancer is suspected or demonstrated in an intrathoracic gland, attempts should be made to avoid rupture of the thyroid capsule. When sternotomy is indicated, the sternum usually should be divided to the level of the third intercostal space and then laterally on one side at the space between the third and fourth ribs (Fig. 36-23).

Central and Lateral Neck Dissection for Nodal Metastases Central compartment (medial to the carotid sheath) lymph nodes

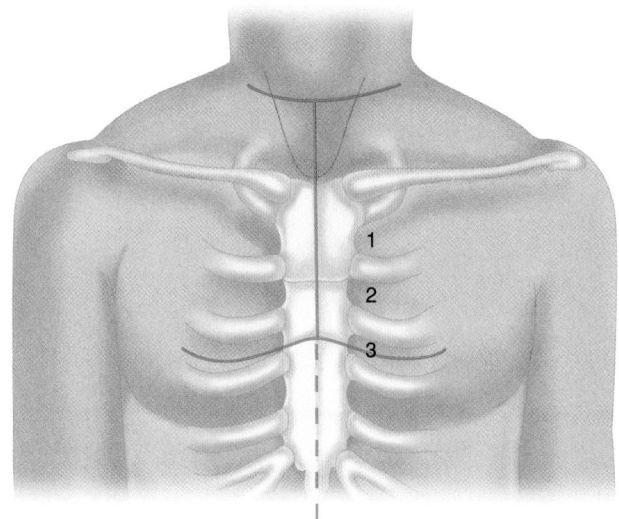

FIG. 38-23. Conduct of thyroidectomy. Incisions for a partial sternotomy.

frequently are involved in patients with papillary, medullary, and Hürthle cell carcinomas and should be removed at the time of thyroidectomy, preserving the RLNs and parathyroid glands. Central neck dissection is particularly important in patients with medullary and Hürthle cell carcinoma because of the high frequency of microscopic tumor spread and because these tumors cannot be ablated with ^{131}I. An ipsilateral modified radical neck dissection is indicated in the presence of palpable cervical lymph nodes or prophylactically in patients with medullary carcinoma when the thyroid lesion is >1 cm.

A modified radical (functional) neck dissection can be performed via the cervical incision used for thyroidectomy, which can be extended laterally (Fig. 38-24A) to the anterior margin of the trapezius muscle (MacFee extension). The procedure involves removal of all fibro-fatty tissue along the internal jugular vein (levels II, III, and IV) and the posterior triangle (level V). In contrast to a radical neck dissection, the internal jugular vein, the spinal accessory nerve, the cervical sensory nerves, and the sternocleidomastoid muscle are preserved unless they are adherent to or invaded by tumor. The procedure begins by opening the plane between the strap muscles medially and the sternocleidomastoid muscle laterally. The anterior belly of the omohyoid muscle is retracted laterally, and the dissection is carried posteriorly until the carotid sheath is reached. The internal jugular vein is retracted medially with a vein retractor and the fibro-fatty tissue and lymph nodes are dissected away from it by a combination of sharp and blunt dissection. The lateral dissection is carried along the posterior border of the sternocleidomastoid muscle, removing the tissue from the posterior triangle. The deep dissection plane is the anterior scalenus muscle, the phrenic nerve, the brachial plexus, and the medial scalenus muscle. The phrenic nerve is preserved on the scalenus anterior muscle, as are the cervical sensory nerves in most patients (Fig. 38-24B). Dissection along the spinal accessory nerve superiorly is most important because this is a frequent site of metastatic disease.

Complications of Thyroid Surgery Nerves, parathyroids, and surrounding structures are all at risk of injury during thyroidectomy. Injury to the RLN may occur by severance, ligation, or traction, but should occur in <1% of patients undergoing thyroidectomy by experienced surgeons. The RLN is most vulnerable to injury during the last 2 to 3 cm of its course, but also can be damaged if the surgeon is not alert to the possibility of nerve branches and the presence of a nonrecurrent nerve, particularly on the right side. If the injury is recognized intraoperatively, most surgeons advocate

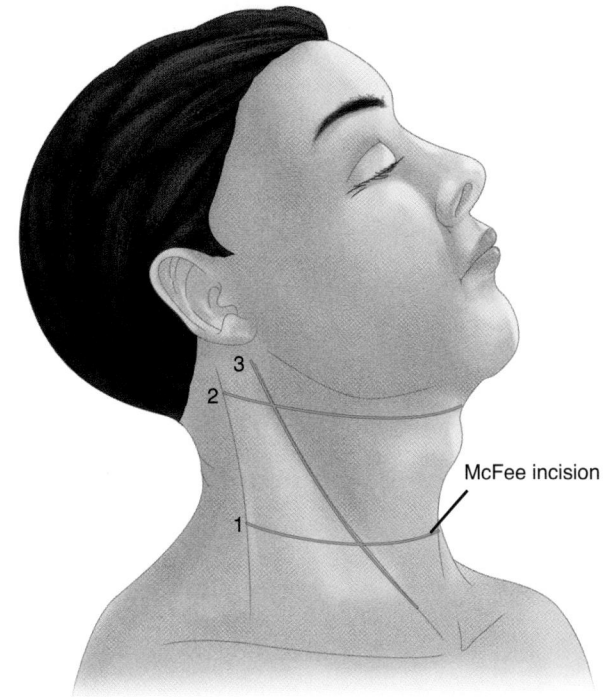

A

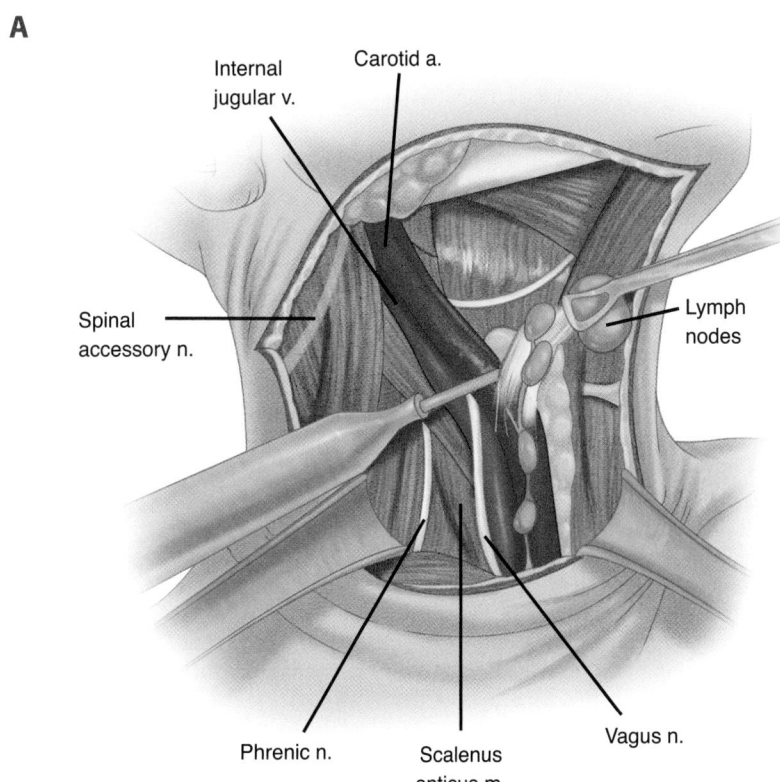

B

FIG. 38-24. Conduct of neck dissection. **A.** Incisions for modified radical neck dissection. **B.** Anatomic relations of structures identified during a modified radical neck dissection. a. = artery; m. = muscle; n. = nerve.

primary reapproximation of the perineurium using nonabsorbable sutures. Approximately 20% of patients are at risk of injury to the external branches of the superior laryngeal nerve, especially if superior pole vessels are ligated en masse. Intraoperative RLN and external laryngeal nerve monitoring techniques are being increasingly used during thyroid and parathyroid surgery. Both continuous monitoring using endotracheal tube electrodes and intermittent monitoring by periodic stimulation and laryngeal palpation are used. No large scale studies have shown that nerve monitoring

equivocally reduces nerve injury, particularly by experienced surgeons.[54] The cervical sympathetic trunk is at risk of injury in invasive thyroid cancers and retroesophageal goiters and may result in Horner's syndrome. Transient hypocalcemia (from surgical injury or inadvertent removal of parathyroid tissue) has been reported in up to 50% of cases, but permanent hypoparathyroidism occurs <2% of the time. Postoperative hypocalcemia is more likely in patients who undergo concomitant thyroidectomy, central and lateral neck dissection. Postoperative hematomas or bleeding may also complicate thyroidectomies and rarely necessitate emergency reoperation to evacuate the hematoma. Bilateral vocal cord dysfunction with airway compromises requires immediate reintubation and tracheostomy. Seromas may need aspiration to relieve patient discomfort. Wound cellulitis and infection, and injury to surrounding structures such as the carotid artery, jugular vein, and esophagus are infrequent.

PARATHYROID

Historical Background

In 1849, the curator of the London Zoological Gardens, Sir Richard Owen, provided the first accurate description of the normal parathyroid gland after autopsy examination of an Indian rhinoceros. However, human parathyroids were not grossly and microscopically described until 1879 by Ivar Sandström, a medical student in Uppsala, Sweden. He suggested that these glands be named the *glandulae parathyroideae*, although their function was not known.

The association of HPT and the bone disease osteitis fibrosa cystica (described by von Recklinghausen) was recognized in 1903. Calcium measurement became possible in 1909, and the association between serum calcium levels and the parathyroid glands was established. The first successful parathyroidectomy was performed in 1925 by Felix Mandl on a 38-year-old man who had severe bone pain secondary to advanced osteitis fibrosa cystica. The patient's condition dramatically improved after the operation, and he lived for another 7 years before dying of recurrent HPT or renal failure. In 1926, the first parathyroid operation was performed at Massachusetts General Hospital. Edward Churchill, assisted by an intern named Oliver Cope, operated on the famous sea captain Charles Martell for severe PHPT. It was not until his seventh operation, which included total thyroidectomy, that an ectopic adenoma was found substernally. Unfortunately, Captain Martell died 6 weeks later, likely due to laryngeal spasm and complications of renal stones and ureteral obstruction. The first successful parathyroidectomy for HPT in the United States was performed on a 56-year-old woman in 1928 by Isaac Y. Olch at the Barnes Hospital in St. Louis, Missouri. At operation, a parathyroid adenoma was found attached to the left lower lobe of the thyroid gland. Postoperatively, the patient developed tetany, requiring lifelong supplemental calcium.

Embryology

In humans, the superior parathyroid glands are derived from the fourth branchial pouch, which also gives rise to the thyroid gland. The third branchial pouches give rise to the inferior parathyroid glands and the thymus (Fig. 38-25). The parathyroids remain closely associated with their respective branchial pouch derivatives. The position of normal superior parathyroid glands is more consistent, with 80% of these glands being found near the posterior aspect of the upper and middle thyroid lobes, at the level of the cricoid cartilage.[55] Approximately 1% of normal upper glands may be found in the paraesophageal or retroesophageal space. Enlarged superior glands may descend in the tracheoesophageal groove and come to lie caudal to the inferior glands. Truly ectopic superior parathyroid glands are rare, but may be found in the middle or posterior mediastinum, or in the aortopulmonary window.[55] As the embryo matures, the thymus and inferior parathyroids migrate together caudally in the neck. The most common location for inferior glands is within a distance of 1 cm from a point centered where the inferior thyroid artery and RLN cross. Approximately 15% of inferior glands are found in the thymus. The position of the inferior glands, however, tends to be more variable due to their longer migratory path. Undescended inferior glands may be found near the skull base, angle of the mandible, or superior to the upper parathyroid glands along with an undescended thymus. The frequency of intrathyroidal glands is about 2%.

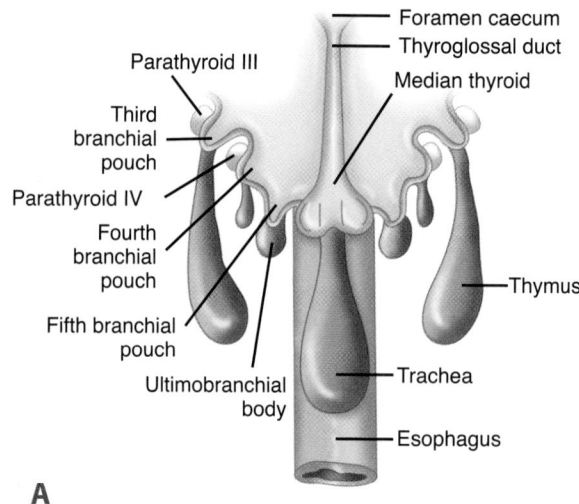

A

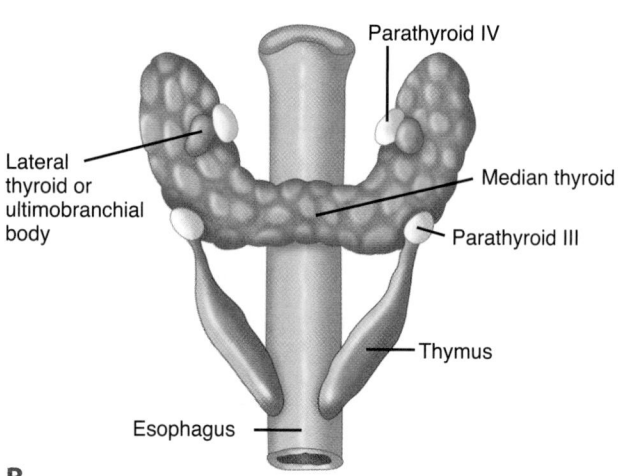

B

FIG. 38-25. Parathyroid embryology. Figure demonstrates a schematic view of the pharynx of an 8- to 10-mm embryo (**A**) and locations of the thyroid, parathyroid, and thymic tissues in a 13- to 14-mm embryo (**B**). The lower parathyroids are derived from the third branchial pouch and migrate with the thymus, whereas the upper parathyroids are derived from the fourth branchial pouch and lie in close proximity to the ultimobranchial bodies. *[Reproduced with permission from Henry J: Applied embryology of the thyroid and parathyroid glands, in Randolph G (ed): Surgery of the Thyroid and Parathyroid Glands. Philadelphia: WB Saunders Company, 2003. Copyright Elsevier.]*

Anatomy and Histology

Most patients have four parathyroid glands. The superior glands usually are dorsal to the RLN at the level of the cricoid cartilage, whereas the inferior parathyroid glands are located ventral to the nerve. Normal parathyroid glands are gray and semitransparent in newborns but appear golden yellow to light brown in adults. Parathyroid color depends on cellularity, fat content, and vascularity. Moreover, they often are embedded in and sometimes difficult to discern from surrounding fat. Normal parathyroid glands are located in loose tissue or fat and are ovoid. They measure up to 7 mm in size and weigh approximately 40 to 50 mg each. Parathyroid glands usually derive their blood supply from branches of the inferior thyroid artery, although branches from the superior thyroid artery supply at least 20% of upper glands. Branches from the

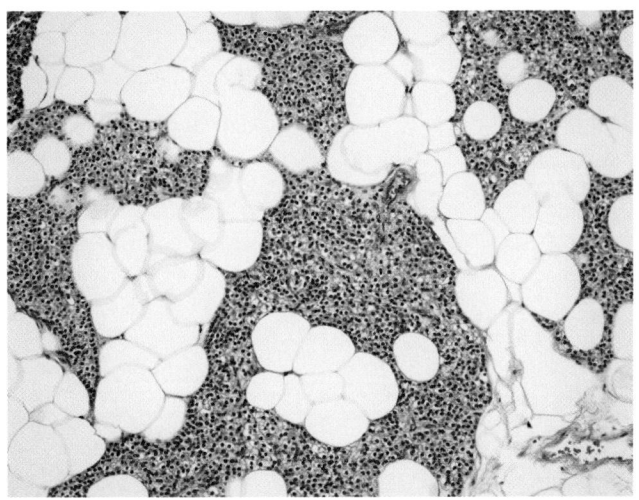

FIG. 38-26. Normal parathyroid histology showing chief cells interspersed with adipose cells.

thyroidea ima, and vessels to the trachea, esophagus, larynx, and mediastinum may also be found. The parathyroid glands drain ipsilaterally by the superior, middle, and inferior thyroid veins.

Akerström and colleagues,[55] in an autopsy series of 503 cadavers, found four parathyroid glands in 84% of cases. Supernumerary glands were present in 13% of patients, most commonly in the thymus. Only 3% of patients had less than four glands. Similar results were obtained in other dissection studies of 428 human subjects by Gilmour who reported a 6.7% incidence of supernumerary glands.[56]

Histologically, parathyroid glands are composed of chief cells and oxyphil cells arranged in trabeculae, within a stroma composed primarily of adipose cells (Fig. 38-26). The parathyroid glands of infants and children are composed mainly of chief cells, which produce parathyroid hormone (PTH). Acidophilic, mitochondria-rich oxyphil cells are derived from chief cells, can be seen around puberty, and increase in numbers in adulthood. A third group of

cells, known as *water-clear cells*, also are derived from chief cells, are present in small numbers, and are rich in glycogen. Although most oxyphil and water-clear cells retain the ability to secrete PTH, their functional significance is not known.

Parathyroid Physiology and Calcium Homeostasis

Calcium is the most abundant cation in human beings, and has several crucial functions. Extracellular calcium levels are 10,000-fold higher than intracellular levels, and both are tightly controlled. Extracellular calcium is important for excitation-contraction coupling in muscle tissues, synaptic transmission in the nervous system, coagulation, and secretion of other hormones. Intracellular calcium is an important second messenger regulating cell division, motility, membrane trafficking, and secretion. Calcium is absorbed from the small intestine in its inorganic form. Calcium fluxes in the steady state are depicted in Fig. 38-27.

Extracellular calcium (900 mg) accounts for only 1% of the body's calcium stores, the majority of which is sequestered in the skeletal system. Approximately 50% of the serum calcium is in the ionized form, which is the active component. The remainder is bound to albumin (40%) and organic anions such as phosphate and citrate (10%). The total serum calcium levels range from 8.5 to 10.5 mg/dL (2.1 to 2.6 mmol/L) and ionized calcium levels range from 4.4 to 5.2 mg/dL (1.1 to 1.3 mmol/L). Both concentrations are tightly regulated. The total serum calcium level must always be considered in its relationship to plasma protein levels, especially serum albumin. For each gram per deciliter of alteration of serum albumin above or below 4.0 mg/dL, there is a 0.8 mg/dL increase or decrease in protein-bound calcium, and thus, in total serum calcium levels. Total and, particularly, ionized calcium levels are influenced by various hormone systems.

Parathyroid Hormome

The parathyroid cells rely on a G-protein coupled membrane receptor, designated the calcium-sensing receptor (CASR), to regulate PTH secretion by sensing extracellular calcium levels[57] (Fig. 38-28). PTH secretion also is stimulated by low levels of 1,25-dihydroxy vitamin D, catecholamines, and hypomagnesemia. The PTH gene is located on chromosome 11. PTH is synthesized in the parathyroid gland as a precursor hormone preproPTH, which is cleaved first to

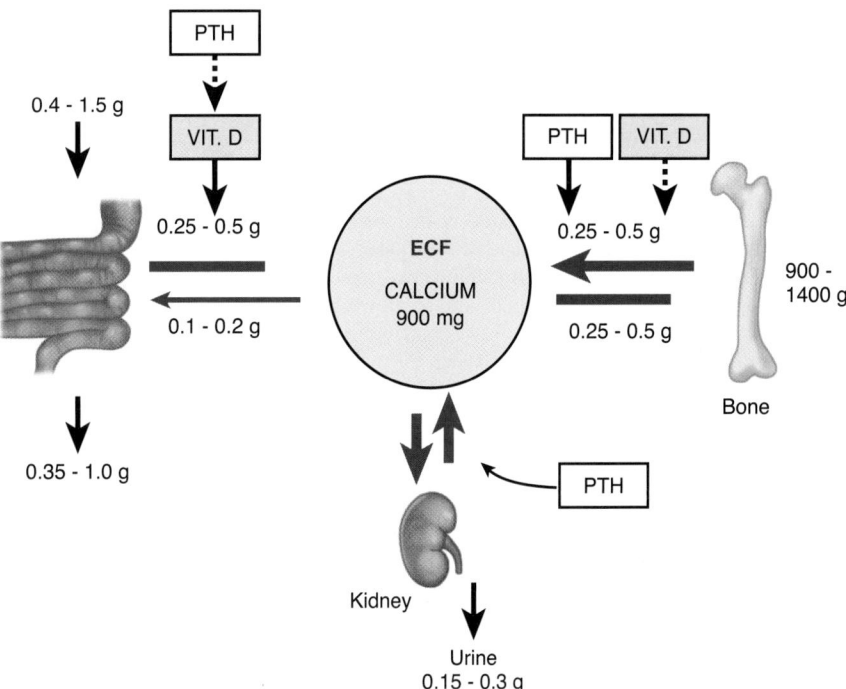

FIG. 38-27. Calcium balance and fluxes in a normal human. *Solid arrows* depict a direct effect, whereas *dashed arrows* depict an indirect effect. The thickness of the arrows is representative of the magnitude of the flux. ECF = extracellular fluid; PTH = parathyroid hormone; VIT. = vitamin. *[Reproduced with permission from Bruder J, et al: Mineral metabolism, in Felig P, Frohman L (eds):* Endocrinology and Metabolism. *New York: McGraw-Hill Publishers, Inc., 2001, p 1081.]*

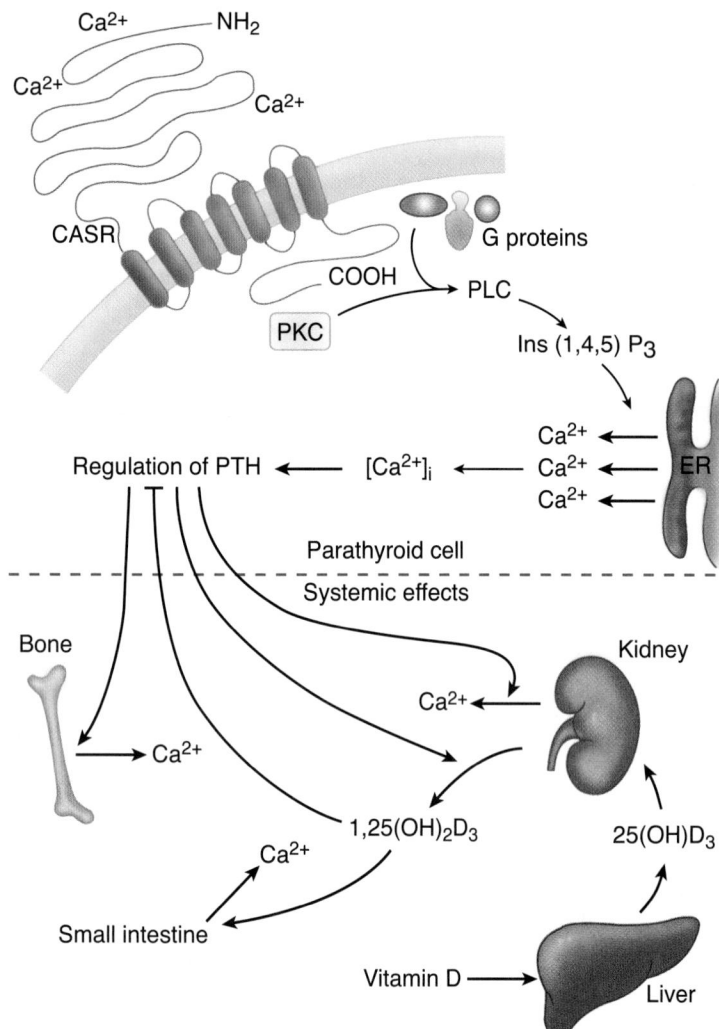

FIG. 38-28. Regulation of calcium homeostasis. The calcium-sensing receptor (CASR) is expressed on the surface of the parathyroid cell and senses fluctuations in the concentration of extracellular calcium. Activation of the receptor is thought to increase intracellular calcium levels, which, in turn, inhibit parathyroid hormone (PTH) secretion via posttranslational mechanisms. Increased PTH secretion leads to an increase in serum calcium levels by increasing bone resorption and enhancing renal calcium reabsorption. PTH also stimulates renal 1-α-hydroxylase activity, leading to an increase in 1,25-dihydroxy vitamin D, which also exerts a negative feedback on PTH secretion. PKC = protein kinase C; PLC = phospholipase C. *(Reproduced with permission from Carling T: Molecular pathology of parathyroid tumors.* Trends Endocrinol Metab *12:54, 2001. Copyright Elsevier.)*

pro-PTH and then to the final 84-amino-acid PTH. Secreted PTH has a half-life of 2 to 4 minutes. In the liver, PTH is metabolized into the active N-terminal component and the relatively inactive C-terminal fraction. The C-terminal component is excreted by the kidneys and accumulates in chronic renal failure.

PTH functions to regulate calcium levels via its actions on three target organs, the bone, kidney, and gut. PTH increases the resorption of bone by stimulating osteoclasts and promotes the release of calcium and phosphate into the circulation. At the kidney, calcium is primarily absorbed in concert with sodium in the proximal convoluted tubule, but fine adjustments occur more distally. PTH acts to limit calcium excretion at the distal convoluted tubule via an active transport mechanism. PTH also inhibits phosphate reabsorption (at the proximal convoluted tubule) and bicarbonate reabsorption. It also inhibits the Na^+/H^+ antiporter, which results in a mild metabolic acidosis in hyperparathyroid states. PTH and hypophosphatemia also enhance 1-hydroxylation of 25-hydroxyvitamin D, which is responsible for its indirect effect of increasing intestinal calcium absorption.

Calcitonin

Calcitonin is produced by thyroid C cells and functions as an antihypercalcemic hormone by inhibiting osteoclast-mediated bone resorption. Calcitonin production is stimulated by calcium and pentagastrin and also by catecholamines, cholecystokinin, and glucagon. When administered intravenously to experimental animals, it produces hypocalcemia. At the kidney, calcitonin increases phos-

phate excretion by inhibiting its reabsorption. Calcitonin plays a minimal, if any, role in the regulation of calcium levels in humans. However, it is very useful as a marker of MTC and in treating acute hypercalcemic crisis.

Vitamin D

Vitamin D refers to vitamin D_2 and vitamin D_3, both of which are produced by photolysis of naturally occurring sterol precursors. Vitamin D_2 is available commercially in pharmaceutical preparations, whereas vitamin D_3 is the most important physiologic compound and is produced from 7-dehydrocholesterol, which is found in the skin. Vitamin D is metabolized in the liver to its primary circulating form, 25-hydroxyvitamin D. Further hydroxylation in the kidney results in 1,25-dihydroxy vitamin D, which is the most metabolically active form of vitamin D. Vitamin D stimulates the absorption of calcium and phosphate from the gut and the resorption of calcium from the bone.

Hyperparathyroidism

Hyperfunction of the parathyroid glands may be classified as primary, secondary, or tertiary. PHPT arises from increased PTH production from abnormal parathyroid glands and results from a disturbance of normal feedback control exerted by serum calcium. Elevated PTH levels may also occur as a compensatory response to hypocalcemic states resulting from chronic renal failure or GI malabsorption of calcium. This secondary HPT can be reversed by correction of the underlying problem (e.g., kidney transplantation for chronic renal failure). However, chronically stimulated glands may occasionally become autonomous, resulting in persistence or recurrence of hypercalcemia after successful renal transplantation, resulting in tertiary HPT.

Primary Hyperparathyroidism

PHPT is a common disorder, affecting 100,000 individuals annually in the United States. PHPT occurs in 0.1 to 0.3% of the general population and is more common in women (1:500) than in men (1:2000). Increased PTH production leads to hypercalcemia via increased GI absorption of calcium, increased production of vitamin D_3, and reduced renal calcium clearance. PHPT is characterized by increased parathyroid cell proliferation and PTH secretion that is independent of calcium levels.

Etiology The exact cause of PHPT is unknown, although exposure to low-dose therapeutic ionizing radiation and familial predisposition account for some cases. Various diets and intermittent exposure to sunshine may also be related. Other causes include renal leak of calcium and declining renal function with age as well as alteration in the sensitivity of parathyroid glands to suppression by calcium. The latency period for development of PHPT after radiation exposure is longer than that for the development of thyroid tumors, with most cases occurring 30 to 40 years after exposure. Patients who have been exposed to radiation have similar clinical presentations and calcium levels when compared to patients without a history of radiation exposure. However, the former tend to have higher PTH levels and a higher incidence of concomitant thyroid neoplasms. Lithium therapy has been known to shift the set point for PTH secretion in parathyroid cells, thereby resulting in elevated PTH levels and mild hypercalcemia. Lithium stimulates the growth of abnormal parathyroid glands in vitro and also in susceptible patients in vivo.[58] PHPT results from the enlargement of a single gland or parathyroid adenoma in approximately 80% of cases, multiple adenomas or hyperplasia in 15 to 20% of patients, and parathyroid carcinoma in 1% of patients. Existence of two enlarged glands or double adenomas is supported by biochemical (calcium and PTH), intraoperative PTH (IOPTH), molecular, and histologic data. This entity is less common in younger patients but accounts for up to 10% of older patients with PHPT. It should be emphasized that when more than one abnormal parathyroid gland is identified preoperatively or intraoperatively, the patient has hyperplasia (all glands abnormal) until proven otherwise.

Genetics

Most cases of PHPT are sporadic. However, PHPT also occurs within the spectrum of a number of inherited disorders such as MEN1, MEN2A, isolated familial HPT, and familial HPT with jaw-tumor syndrome. All of these syndromes are inherited in an autosomal dominant fashion. PHPT is the earliest and most common manifestation of MEN1[59] and develops in 80 to 100% of patients by age 40 years old. These patients also are prone to pancreatic neuroendocrine tumors and pituitary adenomas and, less commonly, to adrenocortical tumors, lipomas, skin angiomas, and carcinoid tumors of the bronchus, thymus, or stomach. About 50% of patients develop gastrinomas, which often are multiple and metastatic at diagnosis. Insulinomas develop in 10 to 15% of cases, whereas many patients have nonfunctional pancreatic endocrine tumors. Prolactinomas occur in 10 to 50% of MEN1 patients and constitute the most common pituitary lesion. MEN1 has been shown to result from germline mutations in the *MEN1* gene, a tumor-suppressor gene located on chromosome 11q12-13 which encodes menin, a protein that is postulated to interact with the transcription factors JunD and nuclear factor κB in the nucleus, in addition to replication protein A and other proteins.[60] Most *MEN1* mutations result in a nonfunctional protein and are scattered throughout the translated nine exons of the gene. This makes presymptomatic screening for mutation carriers

difficult. *MEN1* mutations also have been found in kindreds initially suspected to represent isolated familial HPT. HPT develops in about 20% of patients with MEN2A and generally is less severe. MEN2A is caused by germline mutations of the *RET* proto-oncogene located on chromosome 10. In contrast to MEN1, genotype-phenotype correlations have been noted in this syndrome in that individuals with mutations at codon 634 are more likely to develop HPT. Patients with the familial HPT with jaw-tumor syndrome have an increased predisposition to parathyroid carcinoma. This syndrome maps to a tumor-suppressor locus *HRPT2*, on chromosome 1. Patients belonging to isolated HPT kindreds also appear to demonstrate linkage to *HRPT2*.

Approximately 25 to 40% of sporadic parathyroid adenomas and some hyperplastic parathyroid glands have LOH at 11q 13, the site of the *MEN1* gene. The parathyroid adenoma 1 oncogene (*PRAD1*), which encodes cyclin D1, a cell cycle control protein, is overexpressed in about 18% of parathyroid adenomas. This was demonstrated to result from a rearrangement on chromosome 11 that places the *PRAD1* gene under the control of the PTH promoter. Other chromosomal regions deleted in parathyroid adenomas and possibly reflecting loss of tumor-suppressor genes include 1p, 6q, and 15q, whereas amplified regions suggesting oncogenes have been identified at 16p and 19p. Sporadic parathyroid cancers are characterized by uniform loss of the tumor-suppressor gene *RB*, which is involved in cell cycle regulation, and 60% have *HRPT2* mutations. These alterations are rare in benign parathyroid tumors and may have implications for diagnosis. The *p53* tumor-suppressor gene is also inactivated in a subset (30%) of parathyroid carcinomas. Germline *HRPT2* mutations also have been detected in cases of apparently sporadic parathyroid carcinomas.[61]

Clinical Manifestations Patients with PHPT formerly presented with the "classic" pentad of symptoms (i.e., kidney stones, painful bones, abdominal groans, psychic moans, and fatigue overtones). With the advent and widespread use of automated blood analyzers in the early 1970s, there has been an alteration in the "typical" patient with PHPT. They are more likely to be minimally symptomatic or asymptomatic. Currently, most patients present with weakness, fatigue, polydipsia, polyuria, nocturia, bone and joint pain, constipation, decreased appetite, nausea, heartburn, pruritus, depression, and memory loss. Patients with PHPT also tend to score lower than healthy controls when assessed by general multidimensional health assessment tools such as the Medical Outcomes Study Short-Form Health Survey (SF-36)[62] and other specific questionnaires designed by Pasieka and associates, the Parathyroid Assessment of Symptoms (PAS score).[63] Furthermore, these symptoms and signs improve in most, but certainly not all, patients after parathyroidectomy. Truly "asymptomatic" PHPT appears to be rare, occurring in <5% of patients, as determined by prospectively administered questionnaires. Complications of PHPT are described below.

Renal Disease Approximately 80% of patients with PHPT have some degree of renal dysfunction or symptoms. Kidney stones were previously reported in up to 80% of patients but now occur in about 20 to 25%. The calculi are typically composed of calcium phosphate or oxalate. In contrast, PHPT is found to be the underlying disorder in only 3% of patients presenting with nephrolithiasis. *Nephrocalcinosis*, which refers to renal parenchymal calcification, is found in <5% of patients and is more likely to lead to renal dysfunction. Chronic hypercalcemia also can impair concentrating ability, thereby resulting in polyuria, polydipsia, and nocturia. The incidence of hypertension is variable but has been reported to occur in up to 50% of patients with PHPT. Hypertension appears to be more common in older patients and correlates with the magnitude of renal dysfunction and, in contrast to other symptoms, is least likely to improve after parathyroidectomy.

Bone Disease Bone disease, including osteopenia, osteoporosis, and osteitis fibrosa cystica, is found in about 15% of patients with PHPT. Increased bone turnover, as found in patients with osteitis fibrosa cystica, can be determined by documenting an elevated blood alkaline phosphatase level. Advanced PHPT with osteitis fibrosa cystica now occurs in <5% of patients. It has pathognomonic radiologic findings, which are best seen on x-rays of the hands and are characterized by subperiosteal resorption (most apparent on the radial aspect of the middle phalanx of the second and third fingers), bone cysts, and tufting of the distal phalanges (Fig. 38-29). The skull also may be affected and appears mottled with a loss of definition of the inner and outer cortices. Brown or osteoclastic tumors and bone cysts also may be present. Severe bone disease, resulting in bone pain and tenderness and/or pathologic fractures, is rarely observed nowadays. However, reductions of bone mineral density (BMD) with osteopenia and osteoporosis are more common. Patients with normal serum alkaline phosphatase levels almost never have clinically apparent osteitis fibrosa cystica. HPT typically results in a loss of bone mass at sites of cortical bone such as the radius and relative preservation of cancellous bone such as that located at the vertebral bodies. Patients with PHPT, however, also may have osteoporosis of the lumbar spine that improves dramatically following parathyroidectomy. Fractures also occur more frequently in patients with PHPT,

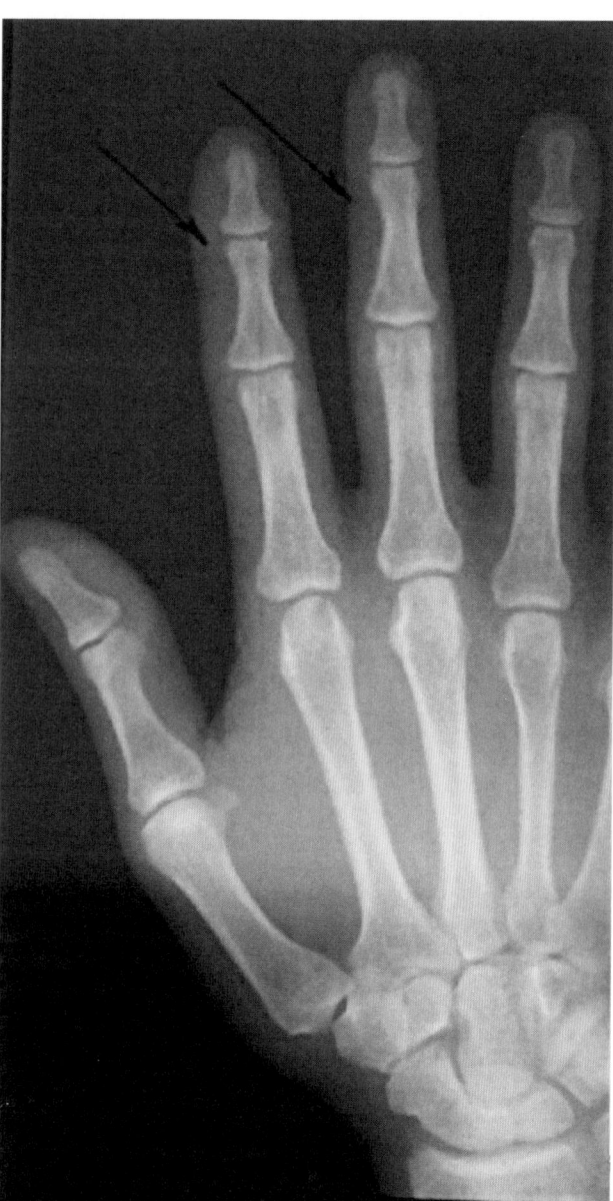

FIG. 38-29. X-ray of the hand showing subperiosteal bone resorption most apparent along the radial aspect of the middle phalanx, characteristic of osteitis fibrosa cystica.

and the incidence of fractures also decreases after parathyroidectomy. Bone disease correlates with serum PTH and vitamin D levels.

Gastrointestinal Complications PHPT has been associated with peptic ulcer disease. In experimental animals, hypergastrinemia has been shown to result from PTH infusion into blood vessels supplying the stomach, independent of its effects on serum calcium. An increased incidence of pancreatitis also has been reported in patients with PHPT, although this appears to occur only in patients with profound hypercalcemia ($Ca^{2+} \geq 12.5$ mg/dL). Patients with PHPT also have an increased incidence of cholelithiasis, presumably due to an increase in biliary calcium, which leads to the formation of calcium bilirubinate stones.

Neuropsychiatric Complications Severe hypercalcemia may lead to various neuropsychiatric manifestations such as florid psychosis, obtundation, or coma. Other findings such as depression, anxiety, and fatigue are more commonly observed in patients with only mild hypercalcemia. The etiology of these symptoms is not known. Studies demonstrate that levels of certain neurotransmitters (monoamine metabolites 5-hydroxyindoleacetic acid and homovanillic acid) are reduced in the cerebrospinal fluid of patients with PHPT when compared to controls. Electroencephalogram abnormalities also occur in patients with primary and secondary HPT and normalize following parathyroidectomy.

Other Features PHPT also can lead to fatigue and muscle weakness, which is prominent in the proximal muscle groups. Although the exact etiology of this finding is not known, muscle biopsy studies show that weakness results from a neuropathy, rather than a primary myopathic abnormality. Patients with HPT also have an increased incidence of chondrocalcinosis, gout, and pseudogout, with deposition of uric acid calcium pyrophosphate crystals in the joints. Calcification at ectopic sites such as blood vessels, cardiac valves, and skin also has been reported, as has hypertrophy of the left ventricle independent of the presence of hypertension. Several large studies from Europe also suggest that PHPT is associated with increased death rates from cardiovascular disease and cancer even in patients with mild HPT,[64,65] although this finding was not substantiated in North American studies.[66]

Physical Findings Parathyroid tumors are seldom palpable, except in patients with profound hypercalcemia. A palpable neck mass in a patient with PHPT is more likely to be thyroid in origin or a parathyroid cancer. Patients also may demonstrate evidence of band keratopathy, a deposition of calcium in Bowman's membrane just inside the iris of the eye. This nonspecific condition generally is caused by chronic eye diseases such as uveitis, glaucoma, and trauma but also may occur in the presence of conditions associated with high calcium or phosphate levels. Fibro-osseous jaw tumors, and or the presence of familial disease in patients with PHPT and jaw tumors, if present, should alert the physician to the possibility of parathyroid carcinoma.

Differential Diagnosis Hypercalcemia may be caused by a multitude of conditions, as listed in Table 38-9. PHPT and malignancy account for >90% of all cases of hypercalcemia. PHPT is more common in the outpatient setting, whereas malignancy is the leading cause of hypercalcemia in hospitalized patients. PHPT can virtually always be distinguished from other diseases causing hypercalcemia by a combination of history, physical examination, and appropriate laboratory investigations.

Hypercalcemia associated with malignancy includes three distinct syndromes. Although bone metastases may cause hypercalcemia, patients with solid tumors of the lung, breast, kidney, head and neck, and ovary often have humoral hypercalcemia of malignancy, without any associated bony metastases. In addition, hypercalcemia also may be associated with hematologic malignancies such as multiple myeloma. Humoral hypercalcemia of malignancy is known to be mediated primarily by PTH-related peptide (PTHrP), which also plays a role in the hypercalcemia associated with bone metastases and multiple myeloma.

TABLE 38-9 Differential diagnosis of hypercalcemia

Hyperparathyroidism
Malignancy—hematologic (multiple myeloma), solid tumors (due to PTHrP)
Endocrine diseases—hyperthyroidism, addisonian crisis, VIPoma
Granulomatous diseases—sarcoidosis, tuberculosis, berylliosis, histoplasmosis
Milk-alkali syndrome
Drugs—thiazide diuretics, lithium, vitamin A or D intoxication
Familial hypocalciuric hypercalcemia
Paget's disease
Immobilization

PTHrP = parathyroid hormone-related protein; VIP = vasoactive intestinal peptide.

Thiazide diuretics cause hypercalcemia by decreasing renal clearance of calcium. This corrects in normal patients within days to weeks after discontinuing the diuretic, but patients with PHPT continue to be hypercalcemic. Thiazide diuretics can, therefore, exacerbate underlying PHPT and can be used to unmask PHPT in patients with borderline hypercalcemia. Familial hypocalciuric hypercalcemia (FHH) is a rare autosomal dominant condition with nearly 100% penetrance and results from inherited heterozygous mutations in the CASR gene located on chromosome 3.[57] Homozygous germline mutations at this locus result in neonatal hypercalcemia, a condition that can rapidly prove fatal. Patients with FHH have lifelong hypercalcemia, which is not corrected by parathyroidectomy. Hypercalcemia also is found in approximately 10% of patients with sarcoidosis secondary to increased 25-hydroxy vitamin D 1-hydroxylase activity in lymphoid tissue and pulmonary macrophages, which is not subject to inhibitory feedback control by serum calcium. Thyroid hormone also has bone-resorption properties, thus causing hypercalcemia in thyrotoxic states, especially in immobilized patients. Hemoconcentration appears to be an important factor in the hypercalcemia associated with adrenal insufficiency and pheochromocytoma, although the latter patients may have associated parathyroid tumors (MEN2A), and some pheochromocytomas are known to secrete PTHrP. Other endocrine lesions such as vasoactive intestinal peptide-secreting tumors may be associated with hypercalcemia due to increased secretion of PTHrP. Milk-alkali syndrome requires the ingestion of large quantities of calcium with an absorbable alkali such as that used in the treatment of peptic ulcer disease with antacids. Ingestion of large quantities of vitamin D and A are infrequent causes of hypercalcemia, as is immobilization.

Diagnostic Investigations *Biochemical Studies* The presence of an elevated serum calcium and intact PTH or two-site PTH levels, without hypocalciuria establishes the diagnosis of PHPT with virtual certainty. These sensitive PTH assays use immunoradiometric or immunochemiluminescent techniques and can reliably distinguish PHPT from other causes of hypercalcemia. Furthermore, they do not cross-react with PTHrP (Fig. 38-30). In patients with metastatic cancer and hypercalcemia, intact PTH levels help to determine whether the patient also has concurrent PHPT. Although extremely rare, a patient with hypercalcemia may have a tumor that secretes PTH. FNAB of such a tumor for PTH levels or selective venous catheterization of the veins draining such tumors can help clarify the diagnosis.

Patients with PHPT also typically have decreased serum phosphate (~50%) and elevated 24-hour urinary calcium concentrations (~60%). A mild hyperchloremic metabolic acidosis also is present (80%), thereby leading to an elevated chloride to phosphate ratio (>33). Urinary calcium levels need not be measured routinely, except in patients who have not had previously documented normocalcemia or have a family history of hypercalcemia to rule out FHH. In patients with FHH, 24-hour urinary calcium excretion is characteristically low (<100 mg/d). Furthermore, the serum calcium to creatinine clearance ratio usually is <0.01 in patients with FHH,

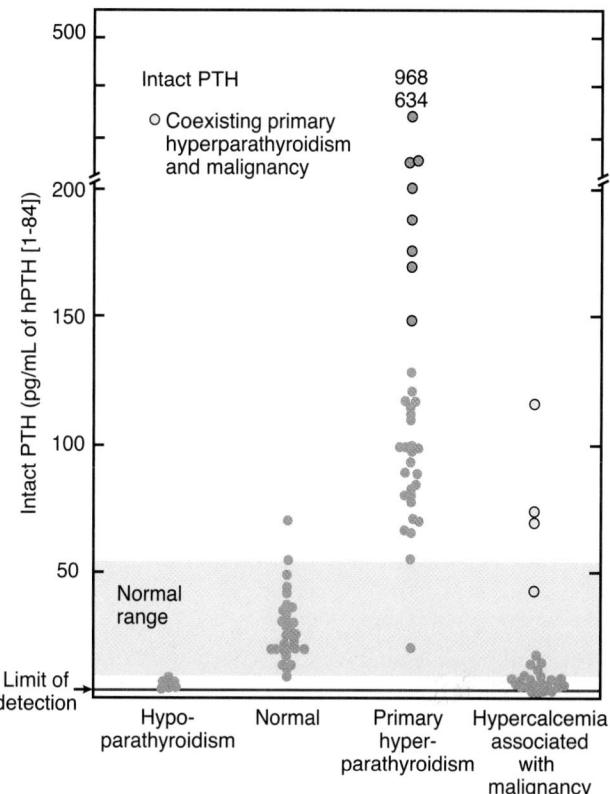

FIG. 38-30. Intact parathyroid hormone (PTH) measurement allows differentiation between the various causes of hypercalcemia. *(Reproduced with permission from Endres D, et al: Measurement of parathyroid hormone.* Endocrinol Metab Clin North Am *18:622, 1989. Copyright Elsevier.)*

whereas it is typically >0.02 in patients with PHPT. Other biochemical features of PHPT are listed in Table 38-10. Elevated levels of alkaline phosphatase may be found in approximately 10% of patients with PHPT and are indicative of high turnover bone disease. These patients are prone to developing postoperative hypocalcemia due to bone hunger. Serum and urine protein electrophoresis may be necessary to exclude multiple myeloma.

TABLE 38-10 Biochemical features of primary hyperparathyroidism

Serum Tests	Alteration
Calcium	Increased, except in normocalcemic primary hyperparathyroidism
Intact PTH	Increased or inappropriately high
Chloride	Increased or high normal
Phosphate	Decreased or low normal
Chloride:phosphate ratio	Increased (usually >33)
Magnesium	Unchanged or decreased (in patients with osteitis fibrosa cystica)
Uric acid	Normal or increased
Alkaline phosphatase	Normal or increased (in the presence of high turnover bone disease)
Acid-base status	Mild hyperchloremic metabolic acidosis
Calcium:creatinine ratio	>0.02 (vs. <0.01 in BFHH)
1,25-dihydroxy vitamin D	Normal or increased
Urine tests	
24-h urinary calcium	Normal or increased

BFHH = benign familial hypocalciuric hypercalcemia; PTH = parathyroid hormone.

Occasionally, patients present with normocalcemic PHPT due to vitamin D deficiency, a low serum albumin, excessive hydration, a high phosphate diet, or a low normal blood calcium set point. These patients have increased total PTH levels with or without increased blood ionized calcium levels and must be distinguished from patients with renal leak hypercalciuria who also have increased PTH levels due to excessive calcium loss in the urine. This can be accomplished by administering thiazide diuretics. In patients with idiopathic hypercalciuria, the urinary calcium level falls, and the secondary increase in the blood PTH level also decreases to normal whereas patients with normocalcemic HPT continue to have elevated urine calcium and blood PTH levels, and may, in fact, become hypercalcemic.

Radiologic Tests In patients with profound hypercalcemia or PHPT associated with vitamin D deficiency, hand and skull x-rays may demonstrate osteitis fibrosa cystica. BMD studies using dual energy absorptiometry are being increasingly used to assess the effects of PHPT on bone. Abdominal ultrasound examination is used selectively to document renal stones. Parathyroid localization studies are not used to confirm the diagnosis of PHPT, but rather to aid in identifying the location of the offending gland(s), as discussed below in Preoperative Localization Tests.

Treatment *Indications for Parathyroidectomy and Role of Medical Management* Most authorities agree that patients who have developed complications and have "classic" symptoms of PHPT or are younger than 50 years old should undergo parathyroidectomy. However, the treatment of patients with asymptomatic PHPT has been the subject of controversy, due, in part, to the fact that there is little agreement on what constitutes an asymptomatic patient. At the National Institutes of Health consensus conference in 1990, "asymptomatic" PHPT was defined as "the absence of common symptoms and signs of PHPT, including no bone, renal, gastrointestinal, or neuromuscular disorders." The panel advocated nonoperative management of these patients with mild PHPT based on observational studies, which suggested relative stability of biochemical parameters over time.[67] This was further substantiated by more recent work, including the study by Silverberg and colleagues.[68] In their cohort of 52 patients with asymptomatic HPT followed without surgery, levels of serum and urinary calcium, PTH, alkaline phosphatase, and vitamin D metabolites remained relatively stable over a 10-year period in most patients. However, the consensus panel considered certain patients to be candidates for surgery.[69] These guidelines were recently reassessed at a second workshop on asymptomatic PHPT held at the National Institutes of Health in 2002 as shown in Table 38-11.[70] The guidelines are essentially unchanged except for those relating to parathyroidectomy. It now is recommended for patients with smaller elevations in serum calcium levels (>1 mg/dL above the upper limit of normal) and if BMD measured at any of three sites (radius, spine, or hip) is greater than 2.5 standard deviations below

those of gender- and race-matched, not age-matched, controls (i.e., peak bone density or T score (rather than Z score) <2.5). The panel still recommends exercising caution in using neuropsychologic abnormalities, cardiovascular disease, GI symptoms, menopause, and elevated serum or urine indices of increased bone turnover as sole indications for parathyroidectomy.

To determine the best course of action for these patients, it is important to consider the natural history of untreated PHPT and the outcomes of treatment options, both medical and surgical. With respect to the former, it is important to note that, in the cohort studies mentioned in this section, a significant proportion of patients were either lost to follow-up or experienced progression of disease requiring surgery. Silverberg and associates reported development of a new indication for surgery in 14 of 52 (27%) of their asymptomatic patients and, because approximately 50% of their patients were initially treated surgically, overall, about 75% of patients were treated surgically.[68] Similarly, Scholz and Purnell[67] also reported that 23% of 147 patients in their series from the Mayo Clinic developed a new indication for parathyroidectomy during a 10-year follow-up period. Uncontrolled PHPT also leads to worsening bone, renal, and other effects, in addition to a possible effect on overall survival.

Successful parathyroidectomy results in resolution of osteitis fibrosa cystica, improved BMD (6 to 8% in the first year and up to 12 to 15% at 15 years),[68] decreased formation of new renal stones, increased muscle strength, and decreased left ventricular hypertrophy. In addition, it also improves peptic ulcer disease and a number of the nonspecific manifestations of PHPT such as fatigue, polydipsia, polyuria and nocturia, bone and joint pain, constipation, nausea, and depression in most, but not all, patients. This also has been demonstrated using symptom questionnaires and various standardized general quality-of-life assessments such as SF-36[71] and a specific parathyroidectomy assessment of symptoms scale.[63] The results were similar in a randomized controlled trial of patients with mild PHPT.[62] The increased death rate in patients with PHPT appears to be reversible by successful parathyroidectomy. Lastly, parathyroidectomy can be accomplished with >95% success rates with minimal morbidity, even in elderly patients and is the only curative treatment option for PHPT.

A number of medical therapies such as selective estrogen receptor modifiers and bisphosphonates have been used to successfully lower serum calcium and increase BMD in patients with PHPT. More recently, calcimimetics (modifiers of the sensitivity of the CASR) have been used in randomized, multicenter controlled trials and have been shown to decrease both serum calcium and PTH levels in both symptomatic and asymptomatic PHPT patients.[72] Although these therapies show promise, long-term outcome data are lacking, and their routine use is not advocated at this time. Previous investigations also have documented that parathyroidectomy is more cost-effective than medical management or follow-up. Therefore, it is recommended that parathyroidectomy should be offered to virtually all patients except those in whom the operative risks are prohibitive.

Unfortunately, to date, there are no definitive criteria to indicate which patients with mild PHPT will have progressive disease. Therefore, patients who do not undergo surgery should undergo routine follow-up consisting of biannual calcium measurements and annual measurements of BMD and serum creatinine.[70]

Preoperative Localization Tests It is important to emphasize that the diagnosis of PHPT is a metabolic one and that localization studies should not be used to make or confirm it. Localization studies may be classified into noninvasive or invasive modalities. These studies have variable performance characteristics, which, in turn, vary with experience and institutional experience, as outlined in Table 38-12.

Most endocrine surgeons agree that localization studies are mandatory and invaluable before any neck redo-parathyroid surgery, but their use before initial neck exploration continues to be controversial. Localization studies have permitted surgeons to perform more lim-

---

TABLE 38-11	Indications for parathyroidectomy in patients with asymptomatic primary HPT (2002 NIH consensus conference guidelines)

- Serum calcium >1 mg/dL above the upper limits of normal
- Life-threatening hypercalcemic episode
- Creatine clearance reduced by 30%
- Kidney stones on abdominal x-rays
- Markedly elevated 24-h urinary calcium excretion (≥400 mg/d)
- Substantially decreased bone mineral density at the lumbar spine, hip, or distal radius (>2.5 SD below peak bone mass, T score <−2.5)
- Age <50 y
- Long-term medical surveillance not desired or possible

HPT = hyperparathyroidism; NIH = National Institutes of Health; SD = standard deviation.

TABLE 38-12 Commonly used parathyroid localization studies

Study	Advantages	Disadvantages
Preoperative, noninvasive		
Sestamibi-^{99m}technetium scan	Allows planar and SPECT imaging	False-positive tests due to thyroid neoplasms, lymphadenopathy
		False-negative study more common with multiple abnormal parathyroids
Ultrasound	Identification of juxta- and intrathyroidal tumors	False-positive results due to thyroid nodules, cysts, lymph nodes, esophageal lesions
	Relatively inexpensive	False-negatives result from substernal, ectopic, and undescended tumors
		Not useful for juxta- or intrathyroidal glands
CT scan	Localization of ectopic (mediastinal) glands	False positives from lymph nodes
		Relatively high cost
		Radiation exposure
		Requires IV contrast
		Interference from shoulders and metallic clips
MRI scan	Localization of ectopic tumors	Expensive
	No radiation exposure	False positives from lymph nodes and thyroid nodules
	No IV contrast	Cannot be used in claustrophobic patients
	No metal clip artifact	
Preoperative, invasive		
FNAB	Can distinguish parathyroid tumor from lymphadenopathy using PTH assay	Experienced cytologist needed
Angiogram	Provides a road map for selective venous sampling	Expensive
	Treatment of mediastinal tumors by embolization	Experienced radiologist needed
		Neurologic complications
Venous sampling	Useful to lateralize tumor in equivocal cases or negative localization studies	Expensive, experienced radiologist needed
Intraoperative		
PTH assay	Immediate confirmation of tumor removal	Expensive
		Increased operative time, decreased accuracy in multiple gland disease

CT = computed tomography; FNAB = fine-needle aspiration biopsy; MRI = magnetic resonance imaging; PTH = parathyroid hormone; SPECT = single-photon emission computed tomography.

ited operations, some of them under local anesthesia. These "minimally invasive" procedures include unilateral and focused neck exploration, radio-guided parathyroidectomy, and several endoscopic or video-assisted approaches. The use of localization studies has been shown in some studies to be associated with lower morbidity rates (hypoparathyroidism and RLN injury) and decreased operative times, reduced duration of hospital stay and improved cosmetic outcomes; while maintaining success rates similar to those obtained with traditional bilateral neck explorations. Some studies also show that use of localization studies may be more cost effective.

There also is little consensus on which localization studies should be used. ^{99m}Tc-labeled sestamibi (Fig. 37-31A) is the most widely used and accurate modality with a sensitivity >80% for detection of parathyroid adenomas.[73] Sestamibi (Cardiolite) initially was introduced for cardiac imaging and is concentrated in mitochondria-rich tissue. It was subsequently noted to be useful for parathyroid localization due to the delayed washout of the radionuclide from hypercellular parathyroid tissue compared to thyroid tissue. Sestamibi scans generally are complemented by neck ultrasound (Fig. 38-31B), which can identify adenomas with >75% sensitivity in experienced centers,[73] and is most useful in identifying intrathyroidal parathyroids. Single-photon emission computed tomography, particularly when used with CT, has been shown to be superior to other nuclear medicine–based imaging.[74] Specifically, single-photon emission computed tomography can indicate whether an adenoma is located in the anterior or posterior mediastinum (aortopulmonary window), thus enabling the surgeon to modify the operative approach accordingly.[75] CT and MRI scans are less sensitive than sestamibi scans, but are helpful in localizing large paraesophageal and mediastinal glands. IOPTH was initially introduced in 1993 and is used to determine the adequacy of parathyroid resection (Fig. 38-32).[76] According to one commonly used criterion, when the PTH falls by 50% or greater 10 minutes after removal of a parathyroid tumor, as compared to the highest preremoval value, the test is considered positive, and the operation is terminated. IOPTH measurements, like localization studies, are less reliable in multiglandular disease.

Although preoperative localization studies and IOPTH have become widely used since their inception, the literature is lacking in studies directly comparing procedures performed with and without these studies. Furthermore, localization studies, including intraoperative PTH, are less sensitive and accurate when they are most necessary, such as in the presence of multiple gland parathyroid disease. Long-term outcome data and cost-effectiveness studies are needed before routine use of localization studies can be recommended; however, they should be used if a focused approach or reoperation is planned.[70]

Operative Approaches Unilateral parathyroid exploration was first carried out using intraoperative staining of a biopsy from the normal parathyroid gland with Sudan black dye to rule out a double adenoma. Initially, the choice of side to be explored was random, but the introduction of preoperative localization studies has enabled a more directed approach. In contrast, the focused approach identifies only the enlarged parathyroid gland, and no attempts are made to locate other normal parathyroid glands. Unilateral neck explorations have several advantages over bilateral neck exploration, including reduced operative times and complications, such as injury to the RLN and hypoparathyroidism. However, most existing studies comparing the two approaches are retrospective and do not analyze the results on an intention-to-treat basis. Another argument against a unilateral exploration is the risk of missing another adenoma on the opposite side of the neck. The incidence of double adenomas has been reported to range from 0 to 10%, with an increased incidence in elderly patients. The risk of missing a second adenoma is higher in populations with a higher incidence of multiple adenomas, such as those with familial HPT, MEN syndromes, and the elderly.

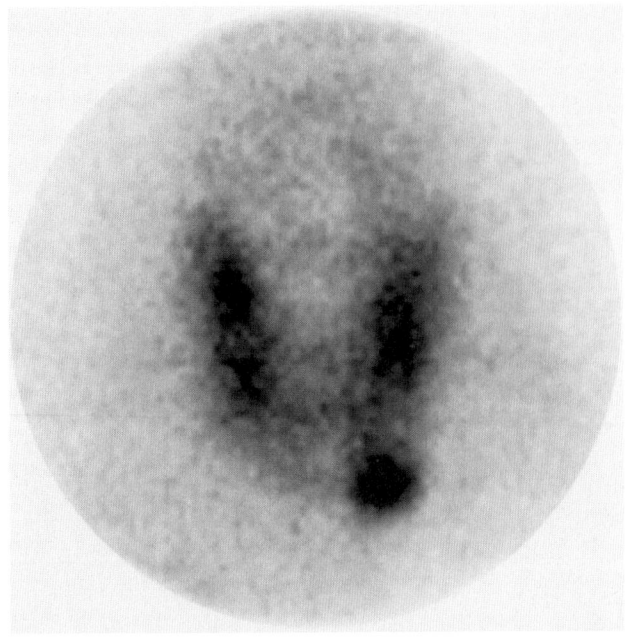

A

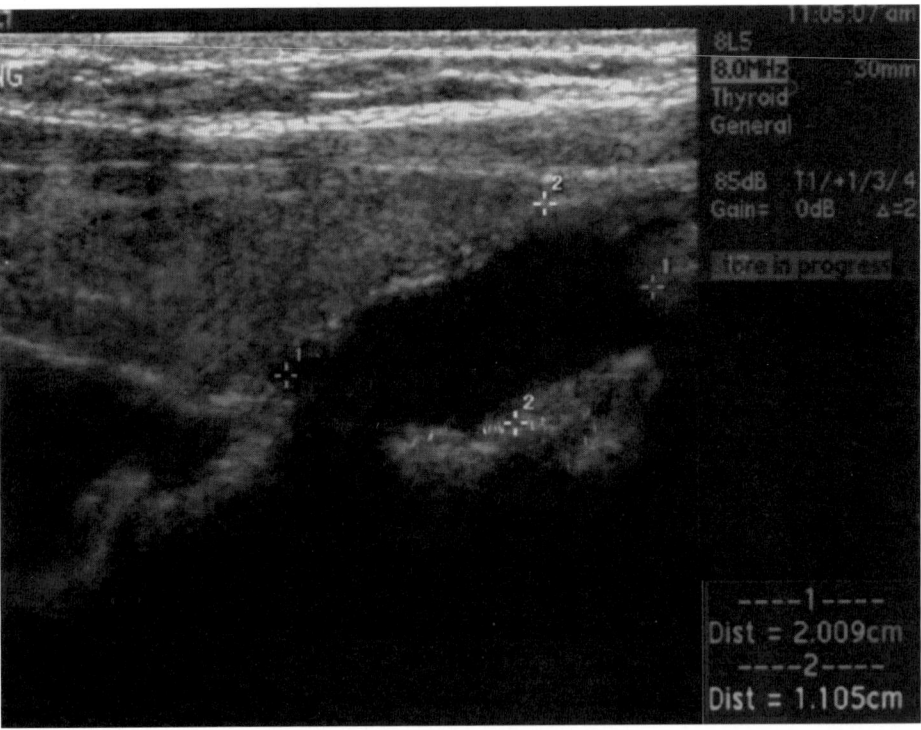

B

FIG. 38-31. **A.** Sestamibi scan in a patient with primary hyperparathyroidism showing persistent uptake suggesting a left lower hypercellular parathyroid gland. **B.** Neck ultrasound in a patient with primary hyperparathyroidism showing a left lower parathyroid adenoma.

Another difficulty inherent with unilateral exploration is the inability to discern whether the combination of an abnormal gland and a normal gland on the initial side constitute a single adenoma or asymmetric hyperplasia. A recently published update on the 5-year results of a randomized trial comparing unilateral vs. bilateral neck exploration did not note any difference in the rates of recurrent or persistent disease in the two groups of patients.[77] These issues will only be resolved by a large, prospective, multicenter study or improved molecular analytic techniques.

Radio-guided parathyroidectomy takes advantage of the ability of parathyroid tumors to retain ^{99m}Tc-sestamibi. One to two mCi of the isotope is injected before surgery and a hand-held gamma probe is used to guide the identification of the enlarged gland, taking care

to ensure the equilibration of radioactivity counts in all quadrants. Reported advantages include easier localization, particularly in reoperative cases, and the ability to perform the procedure under local anesthetic or sedation using smaller incisions. Many studies demonstrated the feasibility of this technique; however, it is rarely used now, largely because it offers little advantage over preoperative sestamibi scans and is associated with increased operative times. Like preoperative scanning, it also has reduced accuracy in the presence of multiglandular disease.

Endoscopic approaches include both video-assisted and total endoscopic techniques. Total endoscopic parathyroidectomy was first described by Gagner in 1996[78] and several other investigators have since reported on this technique. Although port placements are

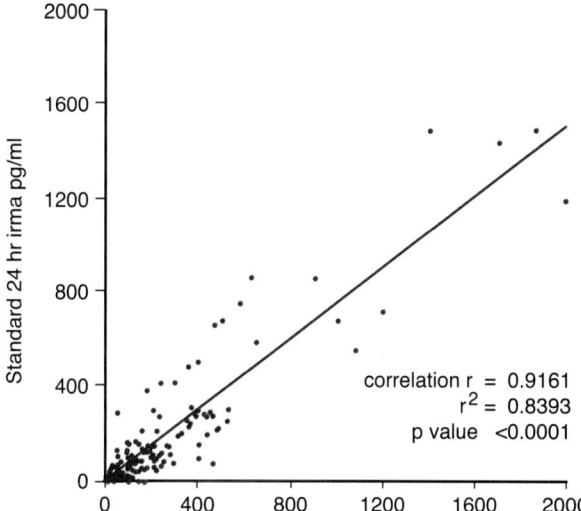

FIG. 38-32. Correlation of the 10-minute incubation time quick parathyroid hormone assay with the 24-hour immunoradiometric (irma) parathyroid hormone assay from 138 paired intraoperative samples from 38 patients undergoing parathyroidectomy. *(Reproduced with permission from Irvin G, et al: Clinical usefulness of an intraoperative "quick parathyroid hormone" assay. Surgery 114:1020, 1993. Copyright Elsevier.)*

variable, as is the case with endoscopic thyroidectomy, they all involve creation of a working space in the neck using CO_2 insufflation, with the reported advantages being superior cosmesis and excellent visualization. Although feasible, these techniques also have been associated with increased operating times, more personnel, and greater expense, and have, in general, not been useful for patients with multiglandular disease, a large thyroid mass, or previous neck surgery and irradiation. Their greatest use has been in patients with tumors at ectopic sites such as the mediastinum where thoracoscopic parathyroidectomy is an excellent alternative to sternotomy.

Studies have shown that if both sestamibi scan and neck ultrasound studies independently identify the same, enlarged parathyroid gland, and no other gland, it is indeed the abnormal gland in approximately 95% of cases. These patients with sporadic PHPT are candidates for a focused neck exploration, an approach that is most commonly referred to as *minimally invasive parathyroidectomy* and has been reported to be the method of choice for members of the International Association of Endocrine Surgeons preferring a minimal-access approach.[72] A standard bilateral neck exploration is planned if parathyroid localization studies or IOPTH are not available; if the localizing studies fail to identify any abnormal parathyroid gland or identify multiple abnormal glands, in patients with a family history of PHPT, MEN1, or MEN2A; or a concomitant thyroid disorder requires bilateral exploration. In addition, finding a minimally abnormal parathyroid gland on the side indicated by localization studies during focal exploration should prompt a bilateral exploration or at least the identification of a normal parathyroid gland on the same side. In patients with MEN1, HPT should be corrected before treatment of gastrinomas because gastrin levels decline after parathyroidectomy.

Conduct of Parathyroidectomy (Standard Bilateral Exploration)
An experienced parathyroid surgeon with a thorough knowledge of parathyroid anatomy and embryology and meticulous technique is crucial for the best surgical results. The procedure usually is performed under general anesthesia. The patient is positioned supine on the operating table with the neck extended. For a bilateral exploration, the neck is explored via a 3- to 4-cm incision just caudal to the cricoid cartilage. The initial dissection and exposure is similar to that used for thyroidectomy. After the strap muscles are separated

in the midline, one side of the neck is chosen for exploration. In contrast to a thyroidectomy, the dissection during a parathyroidectomy is maintained lateral to the thyroid, making it easier to identify the parathyroid glands and not disturb their blood supply.

Identification of Parathyroids A bloodless field is important to allow identification of parathyroid glands. The middle thyroid veins are ligated and divided, thus enabling medial and anterior retraction of the thyroid lobe, with the aid of a peanut sponge or placement of 2 to 0 silk sutures into the thyroid. The space between the carotid sheath and thyroid is then opened by gentle sharp and blunt dissection, from the cricoid cartilage superiorly to the thymus inferiorly and the RLN is identified. Approximately 85% of the parathyroid glands are found within 1 cm of the junction of the inferior thyroid artery and RLNs. The upper parathyroid glands usually are superior to this junction and dorsal (posterior) to the nerve, whereas the lower glands are located inferior to the junction and ventral (anterior) to the recurrent nerve. Because parathyroid glands are partly surrounded by fat, any fat lobule at typical parathyroid locations should be explored because the normal or abnormal parathyroid gland may be concealed in the fatty tissue. The thin fascia overlying a "suspicious" fat lobule should be incised using a sharp curved hemostat and scalpel. This maneuver often causes the parathyroid gland to "pop" out. Alternatively, gentle, blunt peanut sponge dissection between the carotid sheath and the thyroid gland often reveals a "float" sign, suggesting the site of the abnormal parathyroid gland. Normal parathyroids are light beige and only slightly darker or brown compared to adjacent fat.

Parathyroid tissue needs to be distinguished from normal or brown fat tissue, thyroid nodules, lymph nodes, and ectopic thymus. Lymph nodes generally are light beige to whitish gray in color, glassy, and multiple in number, whereas thyroid nodules generally are more vascular, firm, dark or reddish brown in color, and have a more variegated appearance. Intraoperatively, a suspicious nodule may be aspirated using a fine needle attached to a syringe containing 1 cc of saline. Very high PTH levels in the aspirate have been shown to be diagnostic in the intraoperative identification of parathyroid glands. Several characteristics such as size (>7 mm), weight, and color are used to distinguish normal from hypercellular parathyroid glands. Hypercellular glands generally are darker, more firm, and more vascular than normocellular glands. No single method is 100% reliable, and, therefore, the parathyroid surgeon must rely on experience and, at times, advice from a pathologist to help distinguish normal from hypercellular glands. Although several molecular studies have shown use in distinguishing parathyroid adenomas from hyperplasia, this determination also must be made by the surgeon intraoperatively by documenting the presence of a normal parathyroid gland.

Location of Parathyroid Glands The majority of lower parathyroid glands are found in proximity to the lower thyroid pole (Fig. 38-33A). If not found at this location, the thyrothymic ligament and thymus should be mobilized. The upper end of the cervical thymus is gently grasped with a right angle clamp, and the distal portion is bluntly dissected from perithymic fat with a peanut sponge. One can then "walk down" the thymus with successive right-angle clamps (Fig. 38-33B). Applying light tension along with a "twisting" motion helps to free the upper thymus. The carotid sheath also should be opened from the bifurcation to the base of the neck if the parathyroid tumor cannot be found. If these maneuvers are unsuccessful, an intrathyroidal gland should be sought by using intraoperative ultrasound, incising the thyroid capsule on its posterolateral surface or by performing an ipsilateral thyroid lobectomy and "bread-loafing" the thyroid lobe. Preoperative or intraoperative ultrasonography can be useful for identifying intrathyroidal parathyroid glands. Rarely, the third branchial pouch may maldescend and be found high in the neck (undescended parathymus), anterior to the carotid bulb, along with the missing parathyroid gland. Upper parathyroid glands are more

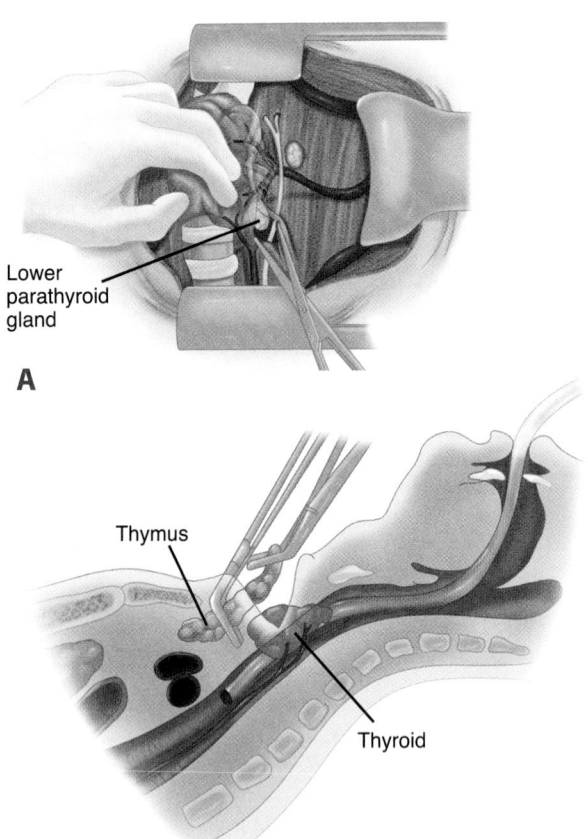

A

B

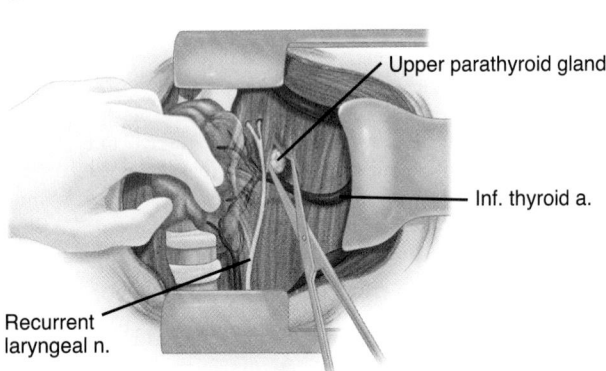

C

FIG. 38-33. Conduct of parathyroidectomy. **A.** Exposure of the lower parathyroid gland near the inferior pole of the thyroid gland and anterior to the recurrent laryngeal nerve. **B.** A thymectomy may be necessary if the lower parathyroid cannot be found in its usual location, or if the patient has familial primary hyperparathyroidism or secondary hyperparathyroidism. **C.** Exposure of the upper parathyroid gland near the insertion of the recurrent laryngeal nerve at the level of the cricothyroid muscle. a. = artery; Inf. = inferior; n. = nerve.

consistent in position and usually are found near the junction of the upper and middle thirds of the gland, at the level of the cricoid cartilage (Fig. 38-33C). Ectopic upper glands may be found in carotid sheath, tracheoesophageal groove, retroesophageal, or in the posterior mediastinum. The locations of ectopic upper and lower parathyroid glands are shown in Fig. 38-34. Every attempt must be made to identify all four glands. Treatment depends upon the number of abnormal glands.

1. A single adenoma is presumed to be the cause of a patient's PHPT if only one parathyroid tumor is identified and the other parathyroid glands are normal, a situation present in about 80% of patients with PHPT. Adenomas typically have an atrophic rim of normal parathyroid tissue but this characteristic may be absent. The adenoma is dissected free of surrounding tissue, taking care to stay immediately adjacent to the tumor, without fracturing it. The vascular pedicle is clamped, divided, and ligated. Care should be taken to not rupture the parathyroid gland to decrease the risk of parathyromatosis. If there is any question about the presumed normal glands, one of them should be biopsied and examined by frozen section.

2. If two abnormal and two normal glands are identified, the patient has double adenomas. Triple adenomas are present if three glands are abnormal and one is normal. Multiple adenomas are more common in older patients with an incidence of up to 10% in patients >60 years old. The abnormal glands should be excised, provided the remaining glands are confirmed as such, thus excluding asymmetric hyperplasia after biopsy and frozen section.

3. If all parathyroid glands are enlarged or hypercellular, patients have parathyroid hyperplasia that has been shown to occur in about 15% of patients in various series. These glands are often lobulated, usually lack the rim of normal parathyroid gland seen in adenomas, and may be variable in size. It often is difficult to distinguish multiple adenomas from hyperplasia with variable gland size. Hyperplasia may be of the chief cell (more common), mixed, or clear-cell type. Patients with hyperplasia may be treated by subtotal parathyroidectomy or by total parathyroidectomy and autotransplantation, with the choice of procedure being determined by rates of recurrence, postoperative hypocalcemia, and failure rates of autotransplanted tissue. Initial studies demonstrated equivalent cure rates and postoperative hypocalcemia for the two techniques, with the latter having the added advantage of avoiding recurrence in the neck. However, autotransplanted tissue may fail to function in about 5% of cases.

All four parathyroid glands are identified and carefully mobilized. For patients with hyperplasia, a titanium clip is placed across the most normal gland, leaving a 50-mg remnant and taking care to avoid disturbing the vascular pedicle and that the gland is resected with a sharp scalpel. If possible, it is preferable to subtotally resect an inferior gland, which is more easily accessible in case of recurrence due to its anterior location with respect to the RLN. The resected parathyroid tissue is confirmed by frozen section or PTH assay. If the remnant appears to be viable, the remaining glands are resected. If there is any question as to the viability of the initially subtotally resected gland, another gland is chosen for subtotal resection and the initial remnant is removed. Whenever multiple parathyroids are resected, it is preferable to cryopreserve tissue, so that it may be autotransplanted should the patient become hypoparathyroid. Parathyroid tissue usually is transplanted into the nondominant forearm. A horizontal skin incision is made overlying the brachioradialis muscle a few centimeters below the antecubital fossa. Pockets are made in the belly of the muscle and one to two pieces of parathyroid tissue measuring 1 mm each are placed into each pocket. A total of 12 to 14 pieces are transplanted. Autotransplanted tissue also has been reported to function when transplanted into fat.

Indications for Sternotomy A sternotomy is usually not recommended at the initial operation, unless the calcium level is >13 mg/dL. Rather, it is preferred to biopsy the normal glands and subsequently close the patient's neck and obtain localizing studies, if they were not obtained previously. Intraoperative PTH assay during the operation from large veins may be helpful. Using highly selective venous catheterization postoperatively also may be needed when noninvasive localization studies are negative, equivocal, or conflict-

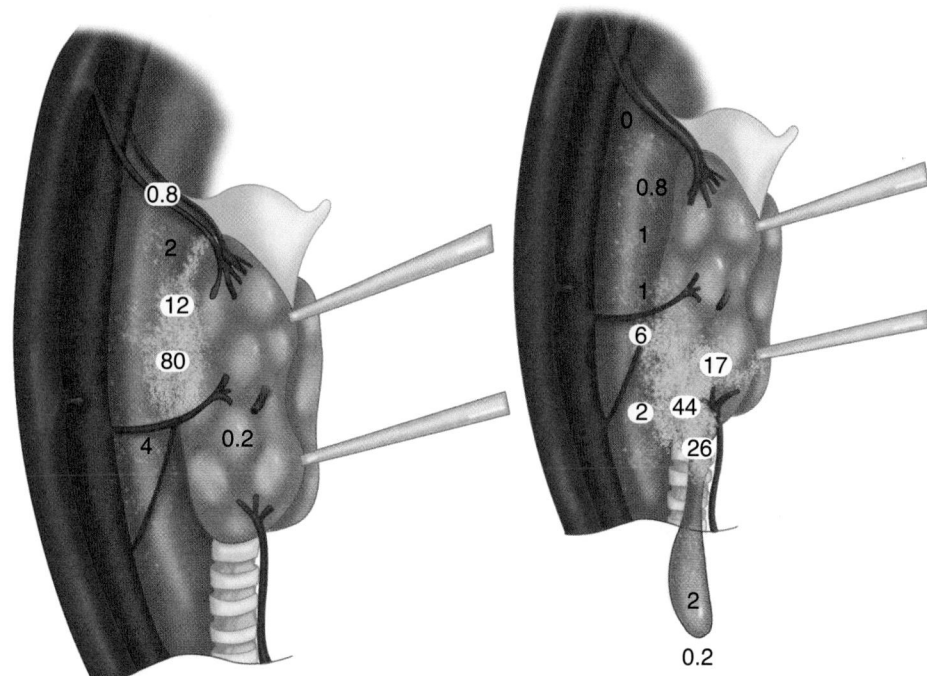

FIG. 38-34. Location of ectopic upper and lower parathyroid glands. *(Reproduced with permission from Akerström G, et al: Surgical anatomy of human parathyroid glands. Surgery 95:15, 1984. Copyright Elsevier.)*

ing. Lower parathyroid glands tend to migrate into the anterior mediastinum in the thymus or perithymic fat and usually can be approached via a cervical incision. A sternotomy is needed to deliver these tumors in approximately 5% of cases. Generally, the gland can be approached by a partial sternotomy to the third intercostal space. The midline sternotomy can be extended to the left or right side as required. Upper glands tend to migrate to the posterior mediastinum in the tracheoesophageal groove. Mediastinal glands also may be found in the aortopulmonary window or pericardium, or attached to the ascending aorta, aortic arch, or its branches.

Special Situations *Parathyroid Carcinoma* Parathyroid cancer accounts for approximately 1% of PHPT cases. It may be suspected preoperatively by the presence of severe symptoms, serum calcium levels >14 mg/dL, significantly elevated PTH levels (5 × normal), and a palpable parathyroid gland. Local invasion is most common; approximately 15% of patients have lymph node metastases and 33% have distant metastases at presentation. Intraoperatively, parathyroid cancer is suggested by the presence of a large, gray-white to gray-brown parathyroid tumor that is adherent to or invasive into surrounding tissues like muscle, thyroid, RLN, trachea, or esophagus. Enlarged lymph nodes also may be present. Accurate diagnosis necessitates histologic examination that reveals local tissue invasion, vascular or capsular invasion, trabecular or fibrous stroma, and frequent mitoses.

Treatment of parathyroid cancer consists of bilateral neck exploration, with en bloc excision of the tumor and the ipsilateral thyroid lobe. Modified radical neck dissection is recommended in the presence of lymph node metastases. Prophylactic neck dissection is not advised because it is associated with an increased risk of complications and does not appear to have a significant impact on survival. If the diagnosis is made postoperatively, a decision must be made regarding the adequacy of initial surgery based on a review of operative notes, pathology reports, localization studies, and calcium and PTH levels. If any question exists, histologic review by another experienced pathologist can be helpful. Additional procedures can then be performed accordingly. Reoperation is indicated for locally recurrent or metastatic disease to control hypercalcemia. Radiation and chemotherapy may be considered in patients with unresectable disease. Bisphosphonates have shown some effectiveness in treating hypercalcemia associated with parathyroid carcinoma. Cinacalcet

hydrochloride, a calcimimetic, can reduce PTH levels by directly binding to the CASR cells on the parathyroid gland and has been shown to be useful in controlling hypercalcemia in patients with refractory parathyroid carcinoma.[79]

Familial Hyperparathyroidism PHPT may occur as a component of various inherited syndromes such as MEN1 and MEN2A. Inherited PHPT also can occur as isolated familial HPT (non-MEN), or familial HPT with jaw tumors. The diagnosis of familial HPT is known or suspected in approximately 85% of patients preoperatively. Furthermore, patients with hereditary HPT generally have a higher incidence of multiglandular disease, supernumerary glands, and recurrent or persistent disease. Therefore, these patients warrant a more aggressive approach and are not candidates for various focused surgical approaches.

Although not absolutely necessary, preoperative sestamibi scan and ultrasound can be obtained in patients with inherited HPT to identify potential ectopic glands. A standard bilateral neck exploration is performed, along with a bilateral cervical thymectomy, regardless of the results of localization studies. Both subtotal parathyroidectomy and total parathyroidectomy with autotransplantation are appropriate and parathyroid tissue also should be cryopreserved. If an adenoma is found in patients with familial HPT, the adenoma and the ipsilateral normal parathyroid glands are resected. The normal-appearing glands on the contralateral side are biopsied and marked, so that only one side of the neck will need to be explored in the event of recurrence. Patients with MEN2A require total thyroidectomy and central neck dissection for prevention/treatment of MTC, a procedure that places the parathyroids at risk. Moreover, HPT is less aggressive in these patients. Hence, only abnormal parathyroid glands need to be resected at neck exploration. The other normal parathyroid glands should be marked with a clip.

Neonatal Hyperparathyroidism Infants with neonatal HPT present with severe hypercalcemia, lethargy, hypotonia, and mental retardation. This disorder is associated with homozygous mutations in the CASR gene. Urgent total parathyroidectomy (with autotransplantation and cryopreservation) and thymectomy is indicated. Subtotal resection is associated with high recurrence rates.

Parathyromatosis Parathyromatosis is a rare condition characterized by the finding of multiple nodules of hyper-functioning parathyroid tissue throughout the neck and mediastinum, usually following a previous parathyroidectomy. The true etiology of parathyromatosis is not known. It is postulated to arise either from overgrowth of congenital parathyroid rests (ontogenous parathyromatosis) or seeding at surgery from rupture of parathyroid tumors or subtotal resection of hyperplastic glands. Parathyromatosis represents a rare cause of persistent or recurrent HPT[80] and can be identified intraoperatively. Aggressive local resection of these deposits can result in normocalcemia but is rarely curative. Some studies suggest that these patients have low-grade carcinoma because of invasion into muscle and other structures distant from the resected parathyroid tumor.

Postoperative Care and Follow-Up Patients who have undergone parathyroidectomy are advised to undergo calcium level checks 2 weeks postoperatively, at 6 months, and then annually. Recurrence rates are rare (<1%), except in patients with familial HPT. Recurrence rates of 15% at 2 years and 67% at 8 years have been reported for MEN1 patients.

Persistent and Recurrent Hyperparathyroidism

Persistence is defined as hypercalcemia that fails to resolve after parathyroidectomy and is more common than recurrence, which refers to HPT occurring after an intervening period of at least 6 months of biochemically documented normocalcemia.[81] The most common causes for both these states include ectopic parathyroids, unrecognized hyperplasia, or supernumerary glands. More rare causes include parathyroid carcinoma, missed adenoma in a normal position, incomplete resection of an abnormal gland, parathyromatosis, or an inexperienced surgeon. The most common sites of ectopic parathyroid glands in patients with persistent or recurrent HPT are paraesophageal (28%), mediastinal (26%), intrathymic (24%), intrathyroidal (11%), carotid sheath (9%), and high cervical or undescended (2%) (Fig. 38-35).

Once the diagnosis of persistent or recurrent HPT is suspected, it should be confirmed by the necessary biochemical tests. In particular, a 24-hour urine collection should be performed to rule out FHH. In redo-parathyroid surgery, the glands are more likely to be in ectopic locations and postoperative scarring tends to make the procedure more technically demanding. Cure rates are generally lower (80 to 90% compared with 95 to 99% for initial operation) and risk of injury to RLNs and permanent hypocalcemia are higher. Therefore, an evaluation of severity of HPT and the patient's anesthetic risk (using the American Society of Anesthesiology classification of physical status or the Goldman cardiac index) is important. High-risk patients whose tumors cannot be identified by localization studies may benefit from nonoperative management such as calcimimetic drugs or angiographic embolization. The latter approach has been associated with significant complications and has not gained widespread acceptance; however, it may be helpful for poor-risk patients with ectopic glands in the mediastinum.

Preoperative localization studies are routinely performed. Noninvasive studies such as a sestamibi scan, ultrasound, and MRI (with gadolinium contrast) are recommended and have reported a combined accuracy of about 85% for these studies in cases of persistent or recurrent HPT. If these studies are negative or equivocal, highly selective venous catheterization for PTH levels is performed, which increases the accuracy to 95%. Previous operative notes and pathology reports should be carefully reviewed and reconciled with the information obtained from localization studies before any neck re-exploration. An algorithm for the treatment of patients with recurrent and persistent HPT is shown in Fig. 38-36.

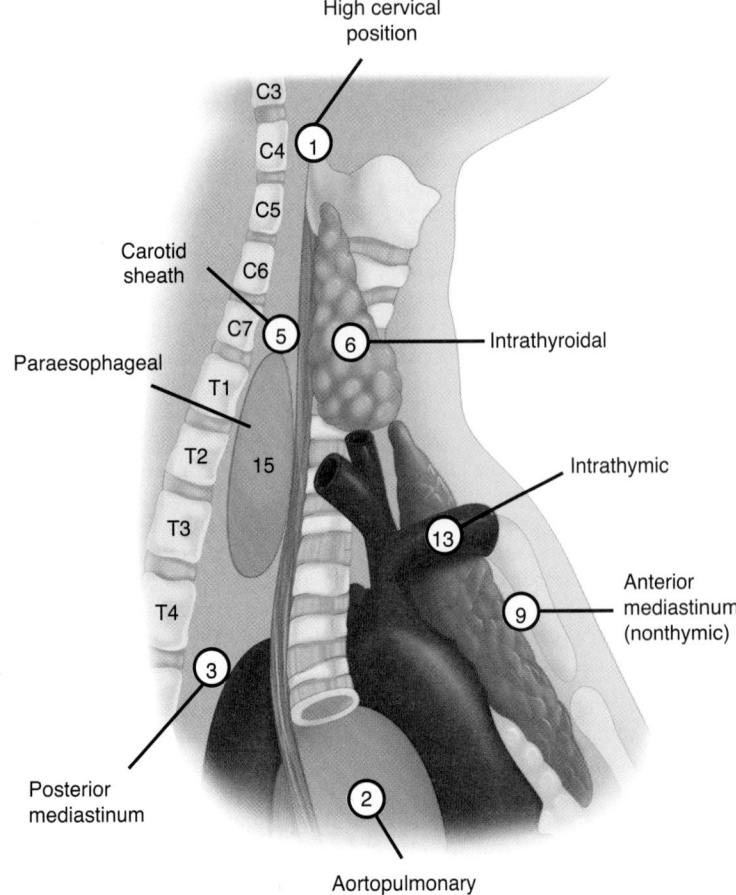

FIG. 38-35. Anatomic location of ectopic parathyroid glands. Numbers represent number of glands found in each location, with a total of 54. *(Reproduced with permission from Shen W, et al: Re-operation for persistent or recurrent primary hyperparathyroidism. Arch Surg 131:864, 1996. Copyright © 1996 American Medical Association. All rights reserved.)*

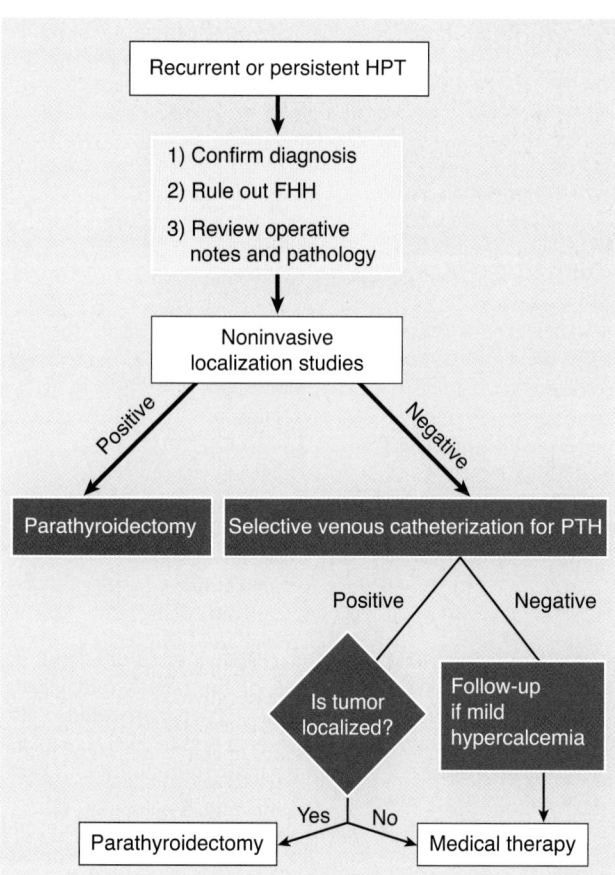

FIG. 38-36. Management of recurrent and persistent hyperparathyroidism (HPT). FHH = familial hypocalciuric hypercalcemia; PTH = parathyroid hormone.

Generally, these patients are approached with a focused exploration. The lateral approach usually is used to identify the RLN more easily. Parathyroid tissue is cryopreserved routinely.

Hypercalcemic Crisis

Patients with PHPT may occasionally present acutely with nausea, vomiting, fatigue, muscle weakness, confusion, and a decreased level of consciousness; a complex referred to as *hypercalcemic crisis*. These symptoms result from severe hypercalcemia from uncontrolled PTH

secretion, worsened by polyuria, dehydration, and reduced kidney function and may occur with other conditions causing hypercalcemia. Calcium levels are markedly elevated and may be as high as 16 to 20 mg/dL. Parathyroid glands tend to be large or multiple, and the tumor may be palpable. Patients with parathyroid cancer or familial HPT are more likely to present with hypercalcemic crisis.

Treatment consists of therapies to lower serum calcium levels followed by surgery to correct HPT. The mainstay of therapy involves rehydration with a 0.9% saline solution to keep urine output >100 cc/h. Once urine output is established, diuresis with furosemide (which increases renal calcium clearance) is begun. If these methods are unsuccessful, other drugs may be used to lower serum calcium levels as outlined in Table 38-13. Occasionally, in life-threatening cases, hemodialysis may be of benefit.

Secondary Hyperparathyroidism

Secondary HPT commonly occurs in patients with chronic renal failure but also may occur in those with hypocalcemia secondary to inadequate calcium or vitamin D intake, or malabsorption. The pathophysiology of HPT in chronic renal failure is complex and appears to be related to hyperphosphatemia (and resultant hypocalcemia), deficiency of 1,25-dihydroxy vitamin D due to loss of renal tissue, low calcium intake, decreased calcium absorption, and abnormal parathyroid cell response to extracellular calcium or vitamin D in vitro and in vivo. Patients generally are hypocalcemic or normocalcemic. Aluminum hydroxide, which often was used as a phosphate binder, has been shown to contribute to the osteomalacia observed in this disease. These patients generally are treated medically with a low-phosphate diet, phosphate binders, adequate intake of calcium and 1,25-dihydroxy vitamin D and a high calcium, low-aluminum dialysis bath. Calcimimetics have been shown to control parathyroid hyperplasia and osteitis fibrosa cystica associated with secondary HPT in animal studies and to decrease plasma PTH and total and ionized calcium levels in humans.

Surgical treatment was traditionally recommended for patients with bone pain, pruritus, and (a) a calcium-phosphate product ≥70, (b) calcium >11 mg/dL with markedly elevated PTH, (c) calciphylaxis, (d) progressive renal osteodystrophy, and (e) soft tissue calcification and tumoral calcinosis, despite maximal medical therapy. The role of parathyroidectomy in the era of calcimetics will require long-term studies; however, parathyroidectomy should be considered if PTH levels remain high despite optimal therapy.[82] Calciphylaxis is a rare, limb- and life-threatening complication of secondary HPT characterized by painful (sometimes throbbing), violaceous, and mottled lesions usually on the extremities, which often become necrotic and progress to nonhealing ulcers, gangrene, sepsis, and death. These are critically ill, high-risk patients, but successful parathyroidectomy sometimes relieves symptoms.

TABLE 38-13	Medications commonly used to treat hypercalcemia		
Medication	**Dosage and Administration**	**Mechanism Onset of Action and Duration**	**Side Effects**
Bisphosphonates (pamidronate)	60–90 mg IV over 4–24 h	Inhibits osteoclastic bone resorption; rapid onset, 2–3 d	May cause local pain and swelling, low-grade fever, lymphopenia, electrolyte abnormalities
Calcitonin	4 IU/kg SC/IM	Inhibits osteoclast function, augments renal calcium excretion; onset of action in hours; but short lived, therefore not useful as sole therapy	Transient nausea and vomiting, abdominal cramps, flushing, and local skin reaction
Mithramycin (plicamycin)	25 μg/kg per day IV for 3–4 d	Inhibits osteoclasts RNA secretion; rapid onset of action (12 h); peaks at 48–72 h and lasts days to several weeks	May cause renal, hepatic, and hematologic complications, nausea and vomiting
Gallium nitrate	200 mg/m² BSA/d IV for 5 d	Reduces urinary calcium excretion; onset of action delayed (5–7 d)	Nephrotoxicity, nausea, vomiting, hypotension, anemia, hypophosphatemia
Glucocorticoids	Hydrocortisone 100 mg IV q8h	Delayed onset of action (7–10 d); useful for hematologic malignancies, sarcoidosis, vitamin D intoxication, hyperthyroidism	Hypertension, hyperglycemia

BSA = body surface area.

Patients should undergo routine dialysis the day before surgery to correct electrolyte abnormalities. Localization studies are not necessary but can identify ectopic parathyroid glands. A bilateral neck exploration is indicated. The parathyroid glands in secondary HPT are characterized by asymmetric enlargement and nodular hyperplasia. These patients may be treated by subtotal resection, leaving about 50 mg of the most normal parathyroid gland or total parathyroidectomy and autotransplantation of parathyroid tissue into the brachioradialis muscle of the nondominant forearm. Upper thymectomy usually is performed because 15 to 20% of patients have one or more parathyroid glands situated in the thymus or perithymic fat. Bone and joint pain improve in approximately 75% of patients who undergo parathyroidectomy. Pruritus and malaise also improve in most, but not all, patients. Parathyroidectomy also has been shown to improve BMD, sexual function, muscle strength, and survival in patients with secondary HPT.

Tertiary Hyperparathyroidism

Generally, renal transplantation is an excellent method of treating secondary HPT, but some patients develop autonomous parathyroid gland function and tertiary HPT. Tertiary HPT can cause problems similar to PHPT, such as pathologic fractures, bone pain, renal stones, peptic ulcer disease, pancreatitis, and mental status changes. The transplanted kidney is also at risk. Operative intervention is indicated for symptomatic disease or if autonomous PTH secretion persists for >1 year after a successful transplant. All parathyroid glands should be identified. The traditional surgical management of these patients consisted of subtotal or total parathyroidectomy with autotransplantation and an upper thymectomy. Some authors suggest that these patients derive similar benefit from excision of only obviously enlarged glands, while avoiding the higher risks of hypocalcemia associated with the former approach. Others recommend that all parathyroid glands be identified and subtotal parathyroidectomy be performed as long-term follow-up studies show that limited excisions in these patients are associated with an up to fivefold increased risk of recurrent or persistent disease.[83]

Complications of Parathyroid Surgery

Parathyroidectomy can be accomplished successfully in >95% of patients with minimal mortality and morbidity, provided the procedure is performed by a surgeon experienced in parathyroid surgery. Specific complications include transient and permanent vocal cord palsy and hypoparathyroidism. The latter is more likely to occur in patients who undergo four-gland exploration with biopsies, subtotal resection with an inadequate remnant, or total parathyroidectomy with a failure of autotransplanted tissue. Furthermore, hypocalcemia is more likely to occur in patients with high turnover bone disease as evidenced by elevated preoperative alkaline phosphatase levels. Vocal cord paralysis and hypoparathyroidism are considered permanent if they persist for >6 months. Fortunately, these complications are rare, occurring in approximately 1% of patients undergoing surgery by experienced parathyroid surgeons.

Patients with symptomatic hypocalcemia or those with calcium levels <8 mg/dL are treated with oral calcium supplementation (up to 1 to 2 g every 4 hours). 1,25-dihydroxy vitamin D [calcitriol (Rocaltrol) 0.25 to 0.5 μg bid] may also be required, particularly in patients with severe hypercalcemia and elevated serum alkaline phosphatase levels preoperatively and with osteitis fibrosa cystica. Intravenous calcium supplementation rarely is needed, except in cases of severe, symptomatic hypocalcemia.

Hypoparathyroidism

Hypocalcemia can be the result of a multitude of conditions, which are listed in Table 38-14. The parathyroid glands may be congenitally absent in DiGeorge syndrome, which also is characterized by lack of thymic development and, therefore, a thymus-dependent lymphoid system. By far, the most common cause of hypoparathyroidism is thyroid surgery, particularly total thyroidectomy with a

TABLE 38-14	Conditions causing hypocalcemia

Hypoparathyroidism
- Surgical
- Neonatal
- Familial
- Heavy metal deposition
- Magnesium depletion

Resistance to the action of parathyroid hormone
- Pseudohypoparathyroidism
- Renal failure
- Medications—calcitonin, bisphosphonates, mithramycin

Failure of normal 1,25-dihydroxy vitamin D production
Resistance to the action of 1,25-dihydroxy vitamin D
Acute complex formation or deposition of calcium
- Acute hyperphosphatemia
- Acute pancreatitis
- Massive blood transfusion (citrate overload)
- "Hungry bones"

concomitant central neck dissection. Patients often develop transient hypocalcemia due to ischemia of the parathyroid glands; permanent hypoparathyroidism is rare. Hypoparathyroidism also may occur after parathyroid surgery, which is more likely if patients undergo a subtotal resection or total parathyroidectomy with parathyroid autotransplantation.

Acute hypocalcemia results in decreased ionized calcium and increased neuromuscular excitability. Patients initially develop circumoral and fingertip numbness and tingling. Mental symptoms include anxiety, confusion, and depression. Physical examination reveals positive Chvostek's sign (contraction of facial muscles elicited by tapping on the facial nerve anterior to the ear) and Trousseau's sign (carpopedal spasm which is elicited by occluding blood flow to the forearm with a blood pressure cuff for 2 to 3 minutes). Tetany, which is characterized by tonic-clonic seizures, carpopedal spasm, and laryngeal stridor, may prove fatal and should be avoided. Most patients with postoperative hypocalcemia can be treated with oral calcium and vitamin D supplements; IV calcium infusion is rarely required except in patients with preoperative osteitis fibrosa cystica.

ADRENAL

Historical Background

Eustachius provided the first accurate anatomic account of the adrenals in 1563. The anatomic division of the adrenals into the cortex and medulla was described much later, by Cuvier in 1805. Subsequently, Thomas Addison in 1855 described the features of adrenal insufficiency, which still bear his name. DeCreccio provided the first description of congenital adrenal hyperplasia (CAH) occurring in a female pseudohermaphrodite in 1865. Pheochromocytomas were first identified by Frankel in 1885, but were not named as such until 1912 by Pick, who noted the characteristic chromaffin reaction of the tumor cells. Adrenaline was identified as an agent from the adrenal medulla that elevated blood pressure in dogs and was subsequently named epinephrine in 1897. The first successful adrenalectomies for pheochromocytoma were performed by Roux in Switzerland, and Charles Mayo in the United States.

In 1932, Harvey Cushing described 11 patients who had moon facies, truncal obesity, hypertension, and other features of the syndrome that now bears his name. Although several individuals prepared adrenocortical extracts to treat adrenalectomized animals, cortisone was first synthesized by Kendall. Aldosterone was identified in 1952, and the syndrome resulting from excessive secretion of this mineralocorticoid was first described in 1955 by Conn.

development and include insulin-like growth factor 2; gastric inhibitory peptide; and the dosage-sensitive, sex-reversal adrenal hypoplasia (*DAX1*) gene.

Anatomy

The adrenal glands are paired, retroperitoneal organs located superior and medial to the kidneys at the level of the eleventh ribs. The normal adrenal gland measures $5 \times 3 \times 1$ cm and weighs 4 to 5 g. The right gland is pyramidal shaped and lies in close proximity to the right hemidiaphragm, liver, and inferior vena cava (IVC). The left adrenal is closely associated with the aorta, spleen, and tail of the pancreas. Each gland is supplied by three groups of vessels—the superior adrenal arteries derived from the inferior phrenic artery, the middle adrenal arteries derived from the aorta, and the inferior adrenal arteries derived from the renal artery. Other vessels originating from the intercostal and gonadal vessels may also supply the adrenals. These arteries branch into about 50 arterioles to form a rich plexus beneath the glandular capsule and require careful dissection, ligation, and division during adrenalectomy. In contrast to the arterial supply, each adrenal usually is drained by a single, major adrenal vein. The right adrenal vein is usually short and drains into the IVC, whereas the left adrenal vein is longer and empties into the left renal vein after joining the inferior phrenic vein. Accessory veins occur in 5 to 10% of patients—on the right, these vessels may drain into the right hepatic vein or the right renal vein; on the left, accessory veins may drain directly into the left renal vein. The anatomic relationships of the adrenals and surrounding structures are depicted in Fig. 38-38.

The adrenal cortex appears yellow due to its high lipid content and accounts for about 80 to 90% of the gland's volume. Histologically, the cortex is divided into three zones—the zona glomerulosa, zona fasciculata, and zona reticularis. The outer area of the zona glomerulosa consists of small cells and is the site of production of the mineralocorticoid hormone, aldosterone. The zona fasciculata is made up of larger cells, which often appear foamy due to multiple lipid inclusions, whereas the zona reticularis cells are smaller. These latter zones are the site of production of glucocorticoids and adrenal androgens. The adrenal medulla constitutes up to 10 to 20% of the gland's volume and is reddish brown in color. It produces the catecholamine hormones epinephrine and norepinephrine. The cells of the adrenal medulla are arranged in cords and are polyhedral in shape. They often are referred to as chromaffin cells because they stain specifically with chromium salts.

Adrenal Physiology

Cholesterol, derived from the plasma or synthesized in the adrenal, is the common precursor of all steroid hormones derived from the adrenal cortex. Cholesterol initially is cleaved within mitochondria to 5-δ-pregnolone, which in turn is transported to the smooth endoplasmic reticulum where it forms the substrate for various biosynthetic pathways leading to steroidogenesis (Fig. 38-39).

Mineralocorticoids

The major adrenal mineralocorticoid hormones are aldosterone, 11-deoxycorticosterone (DOC), and cortisol. Cortisol has minimal effects on the kidney due to hormone degradation. Aldosterone secretion is regulated primarily by the renin-angiotensin system. Decreased renal blood flow, decreased plasma sodium, and increased sympathetic tone all stimulate the release of renin from juxtaglomerular cells. Renin, in turn, leads to the production of angiotensin I from its precursor angiotensinogen. Angiotensin I is cleaved by pulmonary angiotensin-converting enzyme (ACE) to angiotensin II; the latter is not only a potent vasoconstrictor, but also leads to increased aldosterone synthesis and release. Hyperkalemia is another potent stimulator of aldosterone synthesis, whereas ACTH, pituitary pro-opiomelanocortin, and antidiuretic hormone are weak stimulators.

Aldosterone is secreted at a rate of 50 to 250 $\mu g/d$ (depending on sodium intake) and circulates in plasma chiefly as a complex with

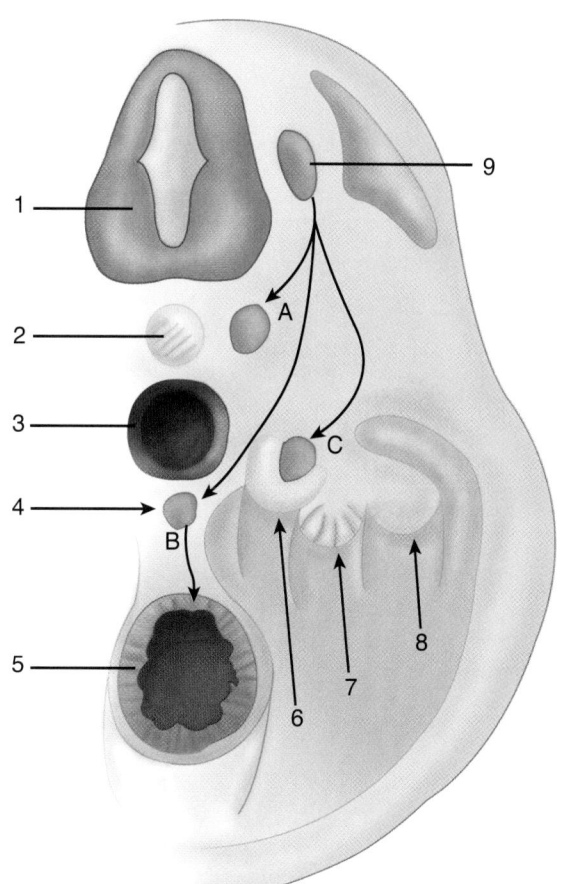

FIG. 38-37. Cross-section of the embryo depicting adrenal development (*1*) neural tube, (*2*) chorda, (*3*) aorta, (*4*) base of the mesentery, (*5*) digestive tube, (*6*) adrenal cortex, (*7*) undifferentiated gonad, (*8*) mesonephros, and (*9*) neural crest. Cells migrate from the neural crest to form the ganglia of the sympathetic trunk (*A*), sympathetic plexi (*B*), and the adrenal medulla and paraganglia (*C*). *(Reproduced with permission from Avisse C, et al: Surgical anatomy and embryology of the adrenal glands. Surg Clin North Am 80: 414, 2000. Copyright Elsevier.)*

Embryology

The adrenal or suprarenal glands are two endocrine organs in one; an outer cortex and an inner medulla, each with distinct embryologic, anatomic, histologic, and secretory features. The cortex originates around the fifth week of gestation from mesodermal tissue near the gonads on the adrenogenital ridge (Fig. 38-37). Therefore, ectopic adrenocortical tissue may be found in the ovaries, spermatic cord, and testes. The cortex differentiates further into a thin, definitive cortex and a thicker, inner fetal cortex. The latter is functional and produces fetal adrenal steroids by the eighth week of gestation, but undergoes involution after birth, resulting in a decrease in adrenal weight during the first three postpartum months. The definitive cortex persists after birth to form the adult cortex over the first 3 years of life. In contrast, the adrenal medulla is ectodermal in origin and arises from the neural crest. At around the same time as cortical development, neural crest cells migrate to the para-aortic and paravertebral areas and toward the medial aspect of the developing cortex to form the medulla. Most extra-adrenal neural tissue regresses but may persist at several sites. The largest of these is located to the left of the aortic bifurcation near the inferior mesenteric artery origin and is designated as the organ of Zuckerkandl. Adrenal medullary tissue also may be found in neck, urinary bladder, and para-aortic regions. Several factors are involved in adrenal

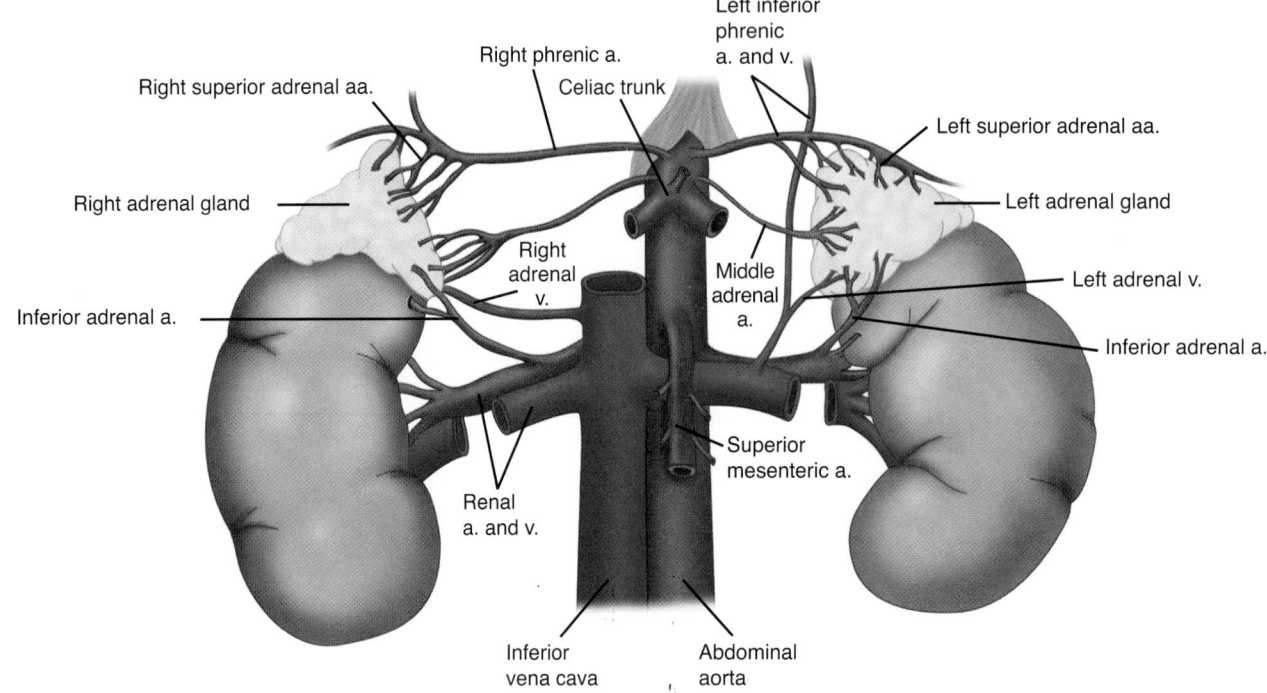

FIG. 38-38. Anatomy of the adrenals and surrounding structures. a. = artery; v. = vein.

albumin. Small amounts of the hormone bind to corticosteroid-binding globulin, and approximately 30 to 50% of secreted aldosterone circulates in a free form. The hormone has a half-life of only 15 to 20 minutes and is rapidly cleared via the liver and kidney. A small quantity of free aldosterone also is excreted in the urine. Mineralocorticoids cross the cell membrane and bind to cytosolic receptors.

The receptor-ligand complex subsequently is transported into the nucleus where it induces the transcription and translation of specific genes. Aldosterone functions mainly to increase sodium reabsorption and potassium and hydrogen ion excretion at the level of the renal distal convoluted tubule. Less commonly, aldosterone increases sodium absorption in salivary glands and GI mucosal surfaces.

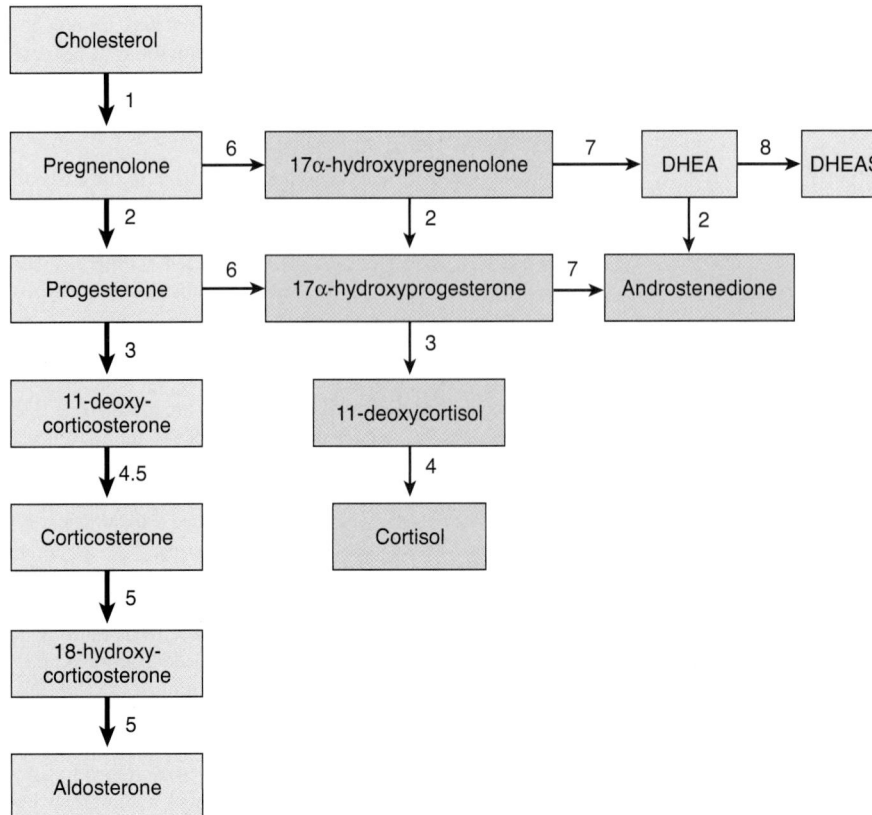

FIG. 38-39. Synthesis of adrenal steroids. The enzymes involved are (*1*) p450scc (cholesterol side chain cleavage), (*2*) 3β-hydroxysteroid dehydrogenase, (*3*) p450c21 (21β-hydroxylase), (*4*) p450c11 (11β-hydroxylase), (*5*) p450c11AS (aldosterone synthase), (*6*) p450c17 (17α-hydroxylase activity), (*7*) p450c17 (17,20-lyase/desmolase activity), and (*8*) sulfokinase. DHEAS = dehydroepiandrosterone sulfate.

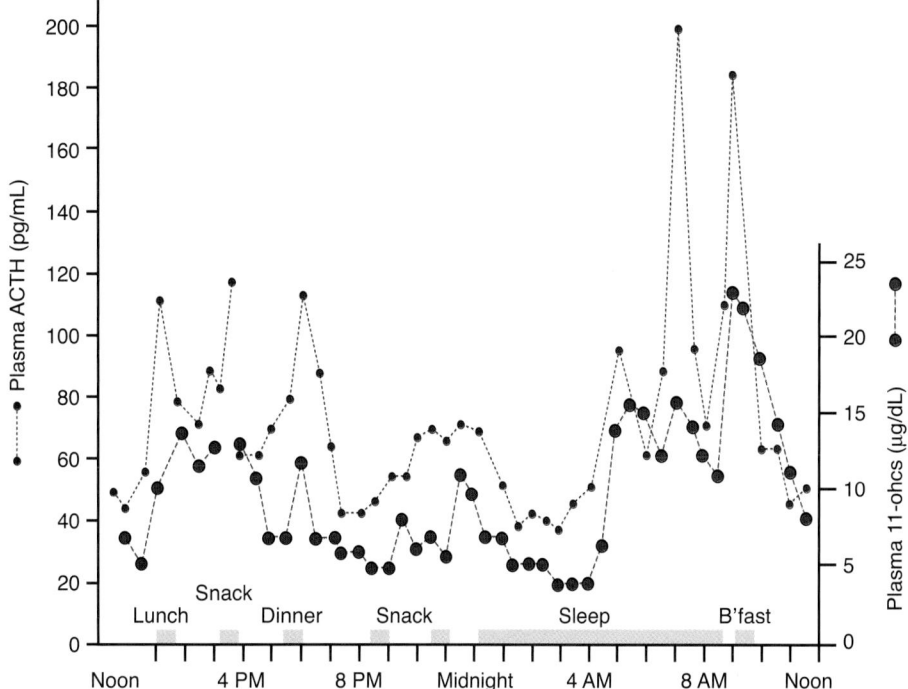

FIG. 38-40. Diurnal variation in cortisol levels as determined by half-hourly sampling in a 16-year-old girl. *(Reproduced with permission from Krieger DT, et al: Characterization of the normal temporal pattern of corticosteroid levels. J Clin Endocrinol Metab 32:269, 1971. Copyright by The Endocrine Society.)*

Glucocorticoids

The secretion of cortisol, the major adrenal glucocorticoid, is regulated by ACTH secreted by the anterior pituitary which, in turn, is under the control of corticotrophin-releasing hormone (CRH) secreted by the hypothalamus. ACTH is a 39-amino-acid protein, which is derived by cleavage from a larger precursor, pro-opiomelanocortin. ACTH is further cleaved into α-melanocyte-stimulating hormone and corticotrophin-like-intermediate peptide. ACTH not only stimulates the secretion of glucocorticoids, mineralocorticoids, and adrenal androgens, but is also trophic for the adrenal glands. ACTH secretion may be stimulated by pain, stress, hypoxia, hypothermia, trauma, and hypoglycemia. ACTH secretion fluctuates, peaking in the morning and reaching nadir levels in the late afternoon. Thus, there is a diurnal variation in the secretion of cortisol with peak cortisol excretion also occurring in the early morning and declining during the day to its lowest levels in the evening (Fig. 38-40). Cortisol controls the secretion of both CRH and ACTH via a negative feedback loop. A similar mechanism leads to the inhibition of CRH secretion by ACTH.

Cortisol is transported in plasma bound primarily to corticosteroid-binding globulin (75%) and albumin (15%). Approximately 10% of circulating cortisol is free and is the biologically active component. The plasma half-life of cortisol is 60 to 90 minutes and is determined by the extent of binding and rate of inactivation. Cortisol is converted to di- and tetrahydrocortisol and cortisone metabolites in the liver and the kidney. The majority (95%) of cortisol and cortisone metabolites are conjugated with glucuronic acid in the liver, thus facilitating their renal excretion. A small amount of unmetabolized cortisol is excreted unchanged in the urine.

Glucocorticoid hormones enter the cell and bind cytosolic steroid receptors. The activated receptor-ligand complex is then transported to the nucleus where it stimulates the transcription of specific target genes via a "zinc finger" DNA binding element. Cortisol also binds the mineralocorticoid receptor with an affinity similar to aldosterone. However, the specificity of mineralocorticoid action is maintained by the production of 11β-hydroxysteroid dehydrogenase, an enzyme that inactivates cortisol to cortisone in the kidney. Glucocorticoids have important functions in intermediary metabolism but also affect connective tissue, bone, immune, cardiovascular, renal, and central nervous systems, as outlined in Table 38-15.

Sex Steroids

Adrenal androgens are produced in the zona fasciculata and reticularis from 17-hydroxypregnenolone in response to ACTH stimulation. They include dehydroepiandrosterone (DHEA) and its sulfated counterpart (DHEAS), androstenedione, and small amounts of testosterone and estrogen. Adrenal androgens are weakly bound to plasma albumin. They exert their major effects by peripheral conversion to the more potent testosterone and dihydrotestosterone but also have weak intrinsic androgen activity. Androgen metabolites are conjugated as glucuronides or sulfates and excreted in the urine. During fetal development, adrenal androgens promote the forma-

TABLE 38-15 Functions of glucocorticoid hormones

Function/System	Effects
Glucose metabolism	Increased hepatic glycogen deposition, gluconeogenesis, decreased muscle glucose uptake and metabolism
Protein metabolism	Decreased muscle protein synthesis, increased catabolism
Fat metabolism	Increased lipolysis in adipose tissue
Connective tissue	Inhibition of fibroblasts, loss of collagen, thinning of skin, striae formation
Skeletal system	Inhibition of bone formation, increased osteoclast activity, potentiate the action of PTH
Immune system	Increases circulation of polymorphonuclear cells, decreases numbers of lymphocytes, monocytes, and eosinophils, reduces migration of inflammatory cells to sites of injury
Cardiovascular system	Increases cardiac output and peripheral vascular tone
Renal system	Sodium retention, hypokalemia, hypertension via mineralocorticoid effect, increased glomerular filtration via glucocorticoid effects
Endocrine system	Inhibits TSH synthesis and release, decreased TBG levels, decreased conversion of T_4 to T_3

PTH = parathyroid hormone; T_3 = 3,5',3-triiodothyronine; T_4 = thyroxine; TBG = thyroxine-binding globulin; TSH = thyroid-stimulating hormone.

tion of male genitalia. In normal adult males, the contribution of adrenal androgens is minimal; however, they are responsible for the development of secondary sexual characteristics at puberty. Adrenal androgen excess leads to precocious puberty in boys and virilization, acne, and hirsutism in girls and women.

Catecholamines

Catecholamine hormones (epinephrine, norepinephrine, and dopamine) are produced not only in the central and sympathetic nervous system but also the adrenal medulla. The substrate, tyrosine, is converted to catecholamines via a series of steps shown in Fig. 38-41A. Phenylethanolamine *N*-methyltransferase, which converts norepinephrine to epinephrine, is only present in the adrenal medulla and the organ of Zuckerkandl. Therefore, the primary catecholamine produced may be used to distinguish adrenal medullary tumors from those situated at extra-adrenal sites. Catecholamines are stored in granules in combination with other neuropeptides, ATP, calcium, magnesium, and water-soluble proteins called *chromogranins*. Hormonal secretion is stimulated by various stress stimuli and mediated by the release of acetylcholine at the preganglionic nerve terminals. In the circulation, these proteins are bound to albumin and other proteins. Catecholamines are cleared by several mechanisms including reuptake by sympathetic nerve endings, peripheral inactivation by catechol *O*-methyltransferase and monoamine oxidase, and direct excretion by the kidneys. Metabolism of catecholamines takes place primarily in the liver and kidneys and leads to the formation of metabolites such as metanephrines, normetanephrines, and VMA, which may undergo further glucuronidation or sulfation before being excreted in the urine (Fig. 38-41B).

Adrenergic receptors are transmembrane-spanning molecules, which are coupled to G proteins. They may be subdivided into α and β subtypes, which are localized in different tissues, have varying affinity to various catecholamines, and mediate distinct biologic effects (Table 38-16). The receptor affinities for α receptors are—epinephrine > norepinephrine >> isoproterenol; β_1 receptors—isoproterenol > epinephrine = norepinephrine; and β_2 receptors—isoproterenol > epinephrine >> norepinephrine.

Disorders of the Adrenal Cortex
Hyperaldosteronism

Hyperaldosteronism may be secondary to stimulation of the renin-angiotensin system from renal artery stenosis and to low-flow states such as congestive heart failure and cirrhosis. Hyperaldosteronism resulting from these conditions is reversible by treatment of the underlying cause. Primary hyperaldosteronism results from autonomous aldosterone secretion which, in turn, leads to suppression of renin secretion. Primary aldosteronism usually occurs in individuals between the ages of 30 to 50 years old and accounts for 1% of hypertension cases. It is associated with hypokalemia; however, more patients with Conn's syndrome are being diagnosed with normal potassium levels. Most cases result from a solitary functioning adrenal adenoma (~70%) and idiopathic bilateral hyperplasia (30%). Adrenocortical carcinoma and glucocorticoid suppressible hyperaldosteronism are rare, each accounting for <1% of cases. Glucocorticoid-suppressible hyperaldosteronism is an autosomal dominant form of hypertension in which aldosterone secretion is abnormally regulated by ACTH. This condition is caused by recombinations between linked genes encoding closely related isozymes, 11β-hydroxylase (CYP11B1), and aldosterone synthase (CYP11B2) generating a dysregulated chimeric gene with aldosterone synthase activity.

Symptoms and Signs Patients typically present with hypertension, which is long-standing, moderate to severe, and may be difficult to control despite multiple-drug therapy. Other symptoms include muscle weakness, polydipsia, polyuria, nocturia, headaches, and fatigue. Weakness and fatigue are related to the presence of hypokalemia.

Diagnostic Studies *Laboratory Studies* Hypokalemia is a common finding, and hyperaldosteronism must be suspected in any

hypertensive patient who presents with coexisting spontaneous hypokalemia (K <3.2 mmol/L), or hypokalemia (<3 mmol/L) while on diuretic therapy, despite potassium replacements. However, it is important to note that up to 40% of patients with a confirmed aldosteronoma were normokalemic preoperatively. Once the diagnosis is suspected, further tests are necessary to confirm the diagnosis. Before testing, patients must receive adequate sodium and potassium. Antihypertensive medications should be held, if possible, and spironolactone, beta blockers, ACE inhibitors, and angiotensin II receptor blockers should be avoided. Patients with primary hyperaldosteronism have an elevated plasma aldosterone concentration level with a suppressed plasma renin activity; a plasma aldosterone concentration to plasma renin activity ratio of 1:25 to 30 is strongly suggestive of the diagnosis.[84] False-positive results can occur, particularly in patients with chronic renal failure. Patients with primary hyperaldosteronism also fail to suppress aldosterone levels with sodium loading. This test can be performed by performing a 24-hour urine collection for cortisol, sodium, and aldosterone after 5 days of a high-sodium diet or alternatively giving the patient 2 L of saline while in the supine position, 2 to 3 days after being on a low-sodium diet. Plasma aldosterone levels <5 ng/dL or a 24-hour urine aldosterone <14 μg after saline loading essentially rules out primary hyperaldosteronism. Once the biochemical diagnosis is confirmed, further evaluation should be directed at determining which patients have a unilateral aldosteronoma vs. bilateral hyperplasia, because surgery is almost always curative for the former, but usually not the latter. No biochemical studies can make this distinction with 100% sensitivity, thus imaging studies are necessary.

Radiologic Studies CT scans with 0.5-cm cuts in the adrenal area can localize aldosteronomas with a sensitivity of 90%. A unilateral 0.5- to 2-cm adrenal tumor with a normal appearing contralateral gland confirms an aldosteronoma in the presence of appropriate

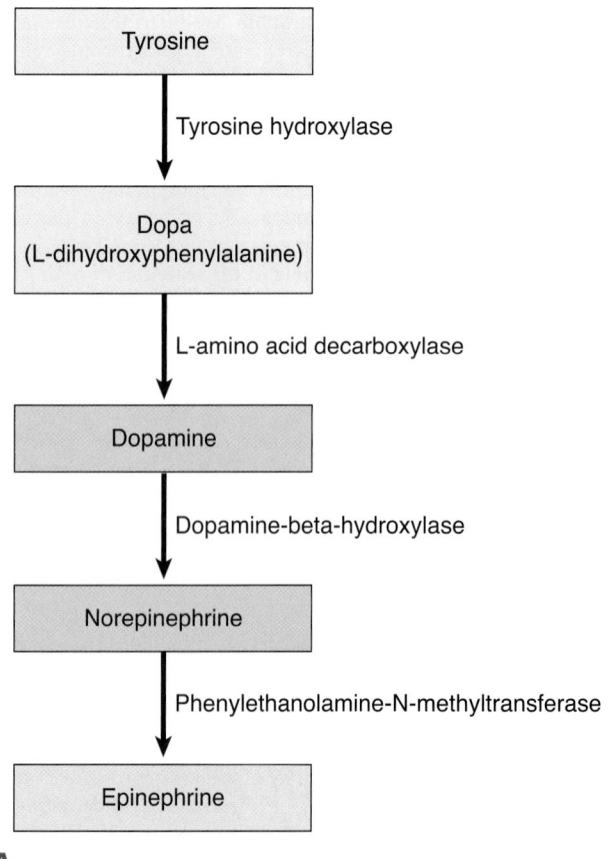

A

FIG. 38-41. **A.** Synthesis of catecholamines. (*Continued*)

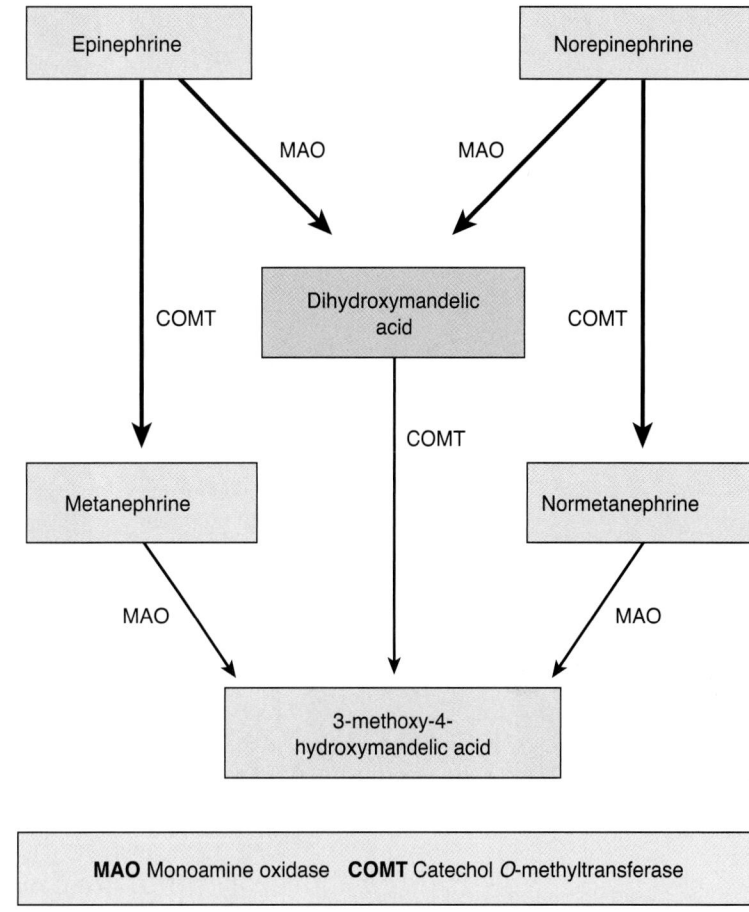

FIG. 38-41. (*Continued*) **B.** Metabolism of catecholamine hormones. **B**

biochemical parameters. MRI scans are less sensitive but more specific, particularly if opposed phase chemical shift images are obtained. MRI scans also have increased use in pregnant patients or those unable to tolerate IV contrast. If adrenal hyperplasia is suspected, the

TABLE 38-16	Catecholamine hormone receptors and effects they mediate

Receptor	Tissue	Function
α_1	Blood vessels	Contraction
	Gut	Decreased motility, increased sphincter tone
	Pancreas	Decreased insulin and glucagon release
	Liver	Glycogenolysis, gluconeogenesis
	Eyes	Pupil dilation
	Uterus	Contraction
	Skin	Sweating
α_2	Synapse (sympathetic)	Inhibits norepinephrine release
	Platelet	Aggregation
β_1	Heart	Chronotropic, inotropic
	Adipose tissue	Lipolysis
	Gut	Decreased motility, increased sphincter tone
	Pancreas	Increased insulin and glucagon release
β_2	Blood vessels	Vasodilation
	Bronchioles	Dilation
	Uterus	Relaxation

algorithm depicted in Fig. 38-42 is useful. Selective venous catheterization and adrenal vein sampling for aldosterone has been demonstrated to be 95% sensitive and 90% specific in localizing the aldosteronoma. In this procedure, the adrenal veins are cannulated and blood samples for aldosterone and cortisol are obtained from both adrenal veins and the vena cava after ACTH administration.[85] Measurement of cortisol levels is necessary to confirm proper placement of the catheters in the adrenal veins. A greater than fourfold difference in the aldosterone:cortisol ratios between the adrenal veins indicates the presence of a unilateral tumor. Some investigators use this study routinely, but it is invasive, requires an experienced interventional radiologist, and can lead to adrenal vein rupture in approximately 1% of cases. Therefore, most groups advocate use of this modality selectively in ambiguous cases, when the tumor cannot be localized and in patients with bilateral adrenal enlargement to determine whether there is unilateral or bilateral increased secretion of aldosterone. Scintigraphy with [131]I-6β-iodomethyl noriodocholesterol (NP-59) also may be used for the same purpose. Like cholesterol, this compound is taken up by the adrenal cortex, but unlike cholesterol, it remains in the gland without undergoing further metabolism. Adrenal adenomas appear as "hot" nodules with suppressed contralateral uptake, whereas hyperplastic glands show bilaterally increased uptake. This test, however, is not widely available.

Treatment Preoperatively, control of hypertension and adequate potassium supplementation (to keep K >3.5 mmol/L) are important. Patients generally are treated with spironolactone (an aldosterone antagonist), amiloride (a potassium-sparing diuretic that blocks sodium channels in the distal nephron), nifedipine (a calcium channel blocker), or captopril (an ACE inhibitor). Unilateral tumors producing aldosterone are best managed by adrenalectomy, either by a laparoscopic approach (preferred) or via a posterior open approach.

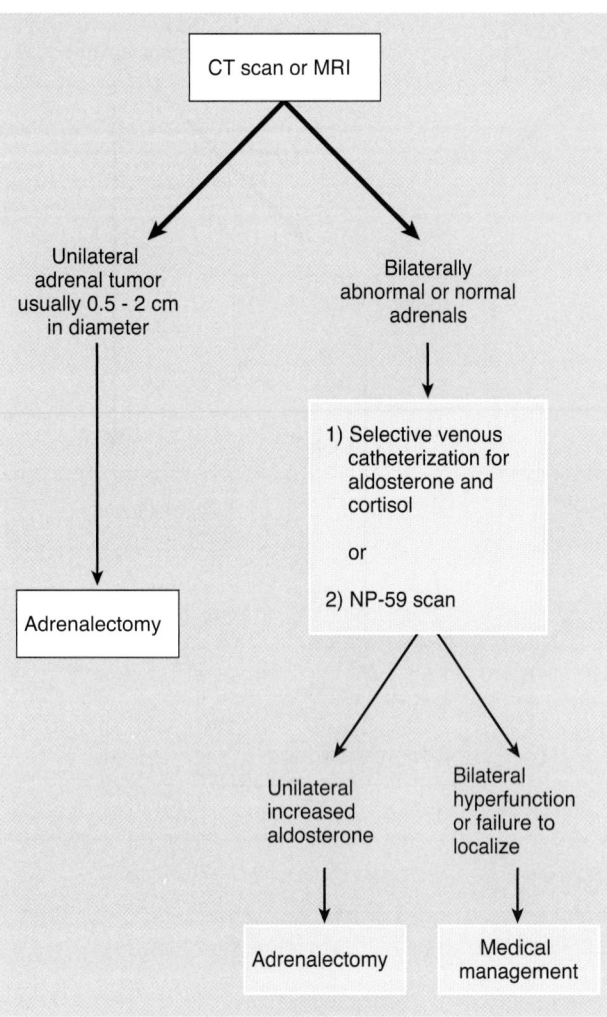

FIG. 38-42. Management of an adrenal aldosteronoma. CT = computed tomography; MRI = magnetic resonance imaging.

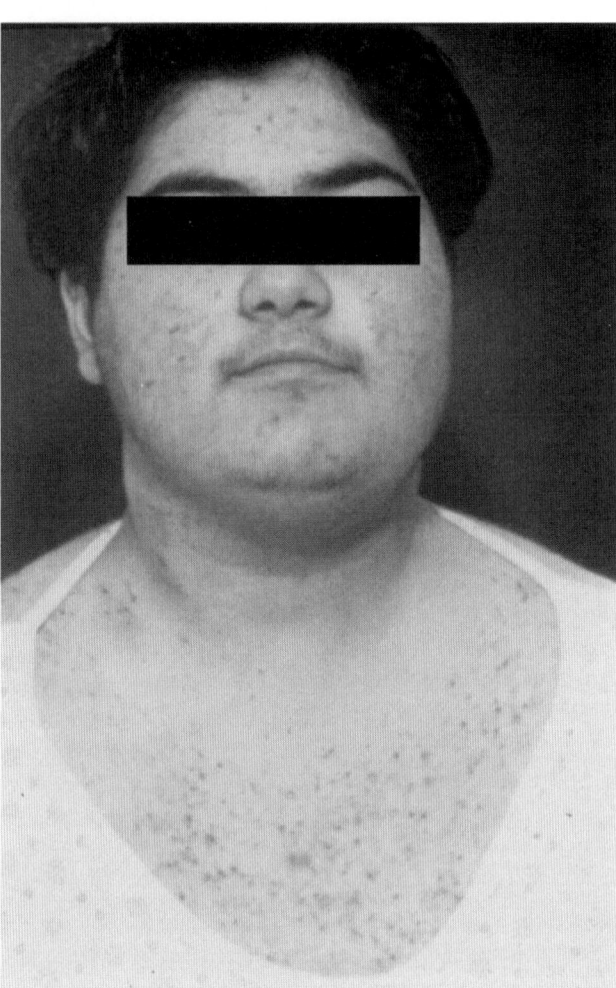

FIG. 38-43. Some characteristic features of Cushing's syndrome—moon facies, hirsutism, and acne.

If a carcinoma is suspected because of the large size of the adrenal lesion or mixed hormone secretion, an anterior transabdominal approach is preferred to permit adequate determination of local invasion and distal metastases. Only 20 to 30% of patients with hyperaldosteronism secondary to bilateral adrenal hyperplasia benefit from surgery and, as described, selective venous catheterization is useful to predict which patients will respond. For the other patients, medical therapy with spironolactone, amiloride, or triamterene is the mainstay of management. Glucocorticoid suppressible hyperaldosteronism is treated by administering exogenous dexamethasone at doses of 0.5 to 1 mg daily. Treatment with spironolactone may help decrease glucocorticoid requirements in this condition and avoid symptoms of Cushing's syndrome. Postoperatively, some patients experience transient hypoaldosteronism requiring mineralocorticoids for up to 3 months. Rarely, acute Addison's disease may occur 2 to 3 days after adrenalectomy. Adrenalectomy is >90% successful in improving hypokalemia and about 70% successful in correcting hypertension. Patients who respond to spironolactone therapy and those with a shorter duration of hypertension with minimal renal damage are more likely to achieve improvement in hypertension, whereas male patients, those >50 years old, and those with multiple adrenal nodules, are least likely to benefit from adrenalectomy.

Cushing's Syndrome

Cushing described patients with a peculiar fat deposition, amenorrhea, impotence (in men), hirsutism, purple striae, hypertension, diabetes, and other features that constitute the syndrome (Fig. 38-43).

He also recognized that several of these patients had basophilic tumors of the pituitary gland and concluded that these tumors produced hormones, which caused adrenocortical hyperplasia, thus resulting in the manifestations of the syndrome. Today, the term *Cushing's syndrome* refers to a complex of symptoms and signs resulting from hypersecretion of cortisol regardless of etiology. In contrast, *Cushing's disease* refers to a pituitary tumor, usually an adenoma, which leads to bilateral adrenal hyperplasia and hypercortisolism. Cushing's syndrome (endogenous) is a rare disease, affecting 10 in 1 million individuals. It is more common in adults but may occur in children. Women are more commonly affected (male:female ratio 1:8). Although most individuals have sporadic disease, Cushing's syndrome may be found in MEN1 families and can result from ACTH-secreting pituitary tumors, primary adrenal neoplasms, or an ectopic ACTH-secreting carcinoid tumor (more common in men) or bronchial adenoma (more common in women).

Cushing's syndrome may be classified as ACTH-dependent or ACTH-independent (Table 38-17). The most common cause of hypercortisolism is exogenous administration of steroids. However, approximately 70% of cases of endogenous Cushing's syndrome are caused by an ACTH-producing pituitary tumor. Primary adrenal sources (adenoma, hyperplasia, and carcinoma) account for about 20% of cases and ectopic ACTH-secreting tumors account for <10% of cases. CRH also may be secreted ectopically in bronchial carcinoid tumors, pheochromocytomas, and other tumors. These patients are difficult to distinguish from those with ectopic ACTH production, but can be diagnosed by determining CRH levels. Patients with

TABLE 38-17	Etiology of Cushing's syndrome

ACTH-dependent (70%)
- Pituitary adenoma or Cushing's disease (~70%)
- Ectopic ACTH production[a] (~10%)
- Ectopic CRH production (<1%)

ACTH-independent (20–30%)
- Adrenal adenoma (10–15%)
- Adrenal carcinoma (5–10%)
- Adrenal hyperplasia—pigmented micronodular cortical hyperplasia or gastric inhibitory peptide-sensitive macronodular hyperplasia (5%)

Other
- Pseudo-Cushing's syndrome
- Iatrogenic—exogenous administration of steroids

[a]From small cell lung tumors, pancreatic islet cell tumors, medullary thyroid cancers, pheochromocytomas, and carcinoid tumors of the lung, thymus, gut, pancreas, and ovary.
ACTH = adrenocorticotropic hormone; CTH = corticotrophin-releasing hormone.

TABLE 38-18	Features of Cushing's syndrome

System	Manifestation
General	Weight gain—central obesity, buffalo hump, supraclavicular fat pads
Integumentary	Hirsutism, plethora, purple striae, acne, ecchymosis
Cardiovascular	Hypertension
Musculoskeletal	Generalized weakness, osteopenia
Neuropsychiatric	Emotional lability, psychosis, depression
Metabolic	Diabetes or glucose intolerance, hyperlipidemia
Renal	Polyuria, renal stones
Gonadal	Impotence, decreased libido, menstrual irregularities

major depression, alcoholism, pregnancy, chronic renal failure, or stress also may have elevated cortisol levels and symptoms of hypercortisolism. However, these manifestations resolve with treatment of the underlying disorder, and these patients are deemed to have pseudo-Cushing's syndrome.

Primary adrenal hyperplasia may be micronodular, macronodular, or massively macronodular. Adrenal hyperplasia resulting from ACTH stimulation usually is macronodular (3-cm nodules). Primary pigmented nodular adrenocortical disease is a rare cause of ACTH-independent Cushing's syndrome, which is characterized by the presence of small (<5 mm), black adrenal nodules. Primary pigmented nodular adrenocortical disease may be associated with Carney complex (atrial myxomas, schwannomas, and pigmented nevi) and is thought to be immune related.

Symptoms and Signs The classical features of Cushing's syndrome are listed in Table 38-18. Early diagnosis of this disease requires a thorough knowledge of these manifestations, coupled with a high clinical suspicion. In some patients, symptoms are less pronounced and may be more difficult to recognize, particularly given their diversity and the absence of a single defining symptom or sign. Progressive truncal obesity is the most common symptom, occurring in up to 95% of patients. This pattern results from the lipogenic action of excessive corticosteroids centrally and catabolic effects peripherally, along with peripheral muscle wasting. Fat deposition also occurs in unusual sites, such as the supraclavicular space and posterior neck region, leading to the so-called buffalo hump. Purple striae are often visible on the protuberant abdomen. Rounding of the face leads to moon facies, and thinning of subcutaneous tissues leads to plethora. There is an increase in fine hair growth on the face, upper back, and arms although true virilization is more commonly seen with adrenocortical cancers. Endocrine abnormalities include glucose intolerance, amenorrhea, and decreased libido or impotence. In children, Cushing's syndrome is characterized by obesity and stunted growth. Patients with Cushing's disease also may present with headaches, visual field defects, and panhypopituitarism. Hyperpigmentation of the skin, if present, suggests an ectopic ACTH-producing tumor with high levels of circulating ACTH.

Diagnostic Tests The aims of diagnostic tests in the evaluation of patients suspected of having Cushing's syndrome are twofold; to confirm the presence of Cushing's syndrome and to determine its etiology (Fig. 38-44).

Laboratory Studies Cushing's syndrome is characterized by elevated glucocorticoid levels that are not suppressible by exogenous hormone administration and loss of diurnal variation. This phenomenon is used to screen patients using the overnight low-dose dexamethasone suppression test. In this test, 1 mg of a synthetic glucocorticoid (dexamethasone) is given at 11 P.M. and plasma cortisol levels are measured at 8 A.M. the following morning. Physiologically normal adults suppress cortisol levels to <3 μg/dL, whereas most patients with Cushing's syndrome do not. False-negative results may be obtained in patients with mild disease; therefore, some authors consider the test positive only if cortisol levels are suppressed to <1.8 μg/dL. False-positive results can occur in up to 3% of patients with chronic renal failure, depression, or those taking medications such as phenytoin, which enhance dexamethasone metabolism. In patients with a negative test but a high clinical suspicion, the classic low-dose dexamethasone (0.5 mg every 6 hours for eight doses, or 2 mg over 48 hours) suppression test or urinary cortisol measurement should be performed. Measurement of elevated 24-hour urinary cortisol levels is a very sensitive (95 to 100%) and specific (98%) modality of diagnosing Cushing's syndrome and is particularly useful for identifying patients with pseudo-Cushing's syndrome. A urinary cortisol-free excretion of less than 100 μg/dL (in most laboratories) rules out hypercortisolism. Recently, salivary cortisol measurements using commercially available kits also have demonstrated superior sensitivity in diagnosing Cushing's syndrome and are being increasingly used. Overall, 24-hour urinary tests for free cortisol and the overnight dexamethasone suppression test at the 5 μg/dL cutoff have the highest specificity for the diagnosis of Cushing's syndrome.[86]

Once a diagnosis of hypercortisolism is established, further testing is aimed at determining whether it is ACTH-dependent or ACTH-independent Cushing's syndrome. This is best accomplished by measurement of plasma ACTH levels (normal 10 to 100 pg/mL). Elevated ACTH levels are found in patients with adrenal hyperplasia due to Cushing's disease (15 to 500 pg/mL) and those with CRH-secreting tumors, but the highest levels are found in patients with ectopic sources of ACTH (>1000 pg/mL). In contrast, ACTH levels are characteristically suppressed (<5 pg/mL) in patients with primary cortisol-secreting adrenal tumors. The high-dose dexamethasone suppression test is used to distinguish between the causes of ACTH-dependent Cushing's syndrome (pituitary vs. ectopic). The standard test (2 mg dexamethasone every 6 hours for 2 days) or the overnight test (8 mg) may be used, with 24-hour urine collections for cortisol and 17-hydroxy steroids performed over the second day. Failure to suppress urinary cortisol by 50% confirms the diagnosis of an ectopic ACTH-producing tumor. Patients suspected of having ectopic tumors should also undergo testing for MTC and pheochromocytoma. Bilateral petrosal vein sampling also is helpful for determining whether the patient has Cushing's disease or ectopic Cushing's syndrome.

The CRH test also is helpful in determining the etiology of Cushing's syndrome. Ovine CRH (1 μg/kg) is administered intravenously, followed by serial measurements of ACTH and cortisol at 15-minute intervals for 1 hour. Patients with a primary adrenal hypercortisolism exhibit a blunted response (ACTH peak <10 pg/mL), whereas those with ACTH-dependent Cushing's syndrome demonstrate a higher elevation of ACTH (>30 pg/mL). CRH stimulation also can enhance the usefulness of petrosal vein sampling.

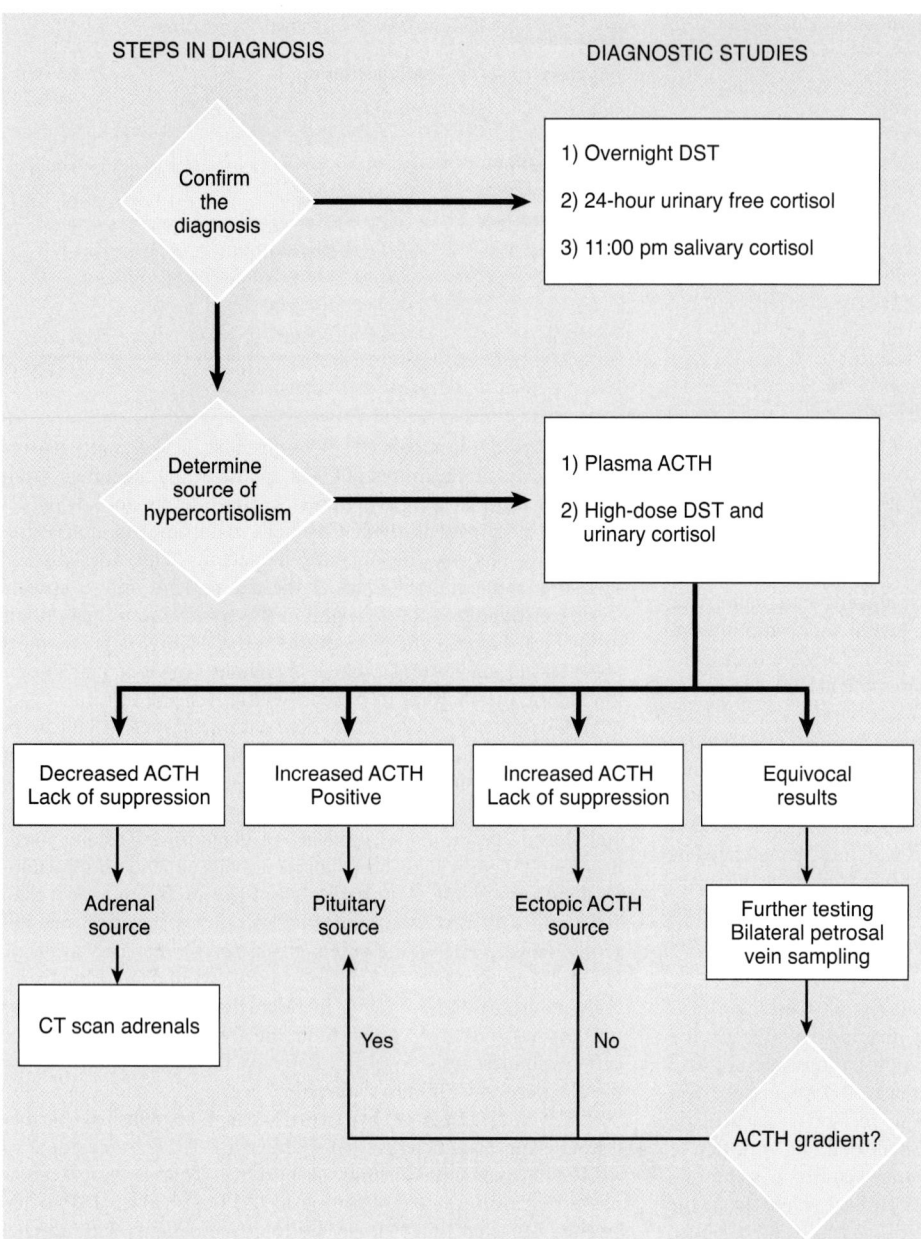

STEPS IN DIAGNOSIS

DIAGNOSTIC STUDIES

Confirm the diagnosis

1) Overnight DST
2) 24-hour urinary free cortisol
3) 11:00 pm salivary cortisol

Determine source of hypercortisolism

1) Plasma ACTH
2) High-dose DST and urinary cortisol

Decreased ACTH Lack of suppression → Adrenal source → CT scan adrenals

Increased ACTH Positive → Pituitary source

Increased ACTH Lack of suppression → Ectopic ACTH source

Equivocal results → Further testing Bilateral petrosal vein sampling → ACTH gradient?

Yes / No

FIG. 38-44. Diagnosis of Cushing's syndrome. ACTH = adrenocorticotropic hormone; CT = computed tomography; DST = dexamethasone suppression test.

Patients with pituitary tumors also have a higher peak ACTH than those with ectopic ACTH-producing tumors.

Radiologic Studies CT and MRI scans of the abdomen can identify adrenal tumors with 95% sensitivity. They also are helpful in distinguishing adrenal adenomas from carcinomas, as discussed in the subsequent section Adrenocortical Cancer. MRI scans have the added advantage of allowing assessment of vascular anatomy. Adrenal adenomas appear darker than the liver on T_2-weighted imaging. Radioscintigraphic imaging of the adrenals using NP-59 also can be used to distinguish adenoma from hyperplasia. Reports suggest that "cold" adrenal nodules are more likely to be cancerous, although this distinction is not absolute. NP-59 scanning is most useful in identifying patients with an adrenal source of hypercortisolism and primary pigmented micronodular hyperplasia.

Thin-section head CT scans are 22% sensitive and contrast-enhanced brain MRI scans are 33 to 67% sensitive at identifying pituitary tumors. Inferior petrosal sinus sampling for ACTH before and after CRH injection has been helpful in this regard and has a sensitivity approaching 100%. In this study, catheters are placed in both internal jugular veins and a peripheral vein. A ratio of petrosal to peripheral vein ACTH level of >2 in the basal state and >3 after CRH stimulation is diagnostic of a pituitary tumor. In patients suspected of having ectopic ACTH production, CT or MRI scans of the chest and anterior mediastinum are performed first, followed by imaging of the neck, abdomen, and pelvis if the initial studies are negative.

Treatment Laparoscopic adrenalectomy is the treatment of choice for patients with adrenal adenomas. Open adrenalectomy is reserved for large tumors (≥6 cm) or those suspected to be adrenocortical cancers. Bilateral adrenalectomy is curative for primary adrenal hyperplasia.

The treatment of choice in Cushing's disease is transsphenoidal excision of the pituitary adenoma, which is successful in 80% of patients. Pituitary irradiation has been used for patients with persistent or recurrent disease after surgery. However, it is associated with a high rate of panhypopituitarism, and some patients develop visual deficits. This has led to increased use of stereotactic radiosurgery, which uses CT guidance to deliver high doses of radiotherapy to the tumor (photon or gamma knife) and also bilateral laparoscopic adrenalectomy. Patients who fail to respond to either treatment are candidates for pharmacologic therapy with adrenal inhibitors (medical adrenalectomy) such as ketoconazole, metyrapone, or aminoglutethimide.

Patients with ectopic ACTH production are best managed by treating the primary tumor, including recurrences, if possible. Medical or bilateral laparoscopic adrenalectomy have been used to palliate patients with unresectable disease and those whose ectopic ACTH-secreting tumor cannot be localized.

Patients undergoing surgery for a primary adrenal adenoma secreting glucocorticoids require preoperative and postoperative steroids due to suppression of the contralateral adrenal gland. These patients are also at increased predisposition for infectious and thromboembolic complications, the latter due to a hypercoagulable state resulting from an increase in clotting factors including factor VIII and von Willebrand's factor complex, and by impaired fibrinolysis. Duration of steroid therapy is determined by the ACTH stimulation test. Exogenous steroids may be needed for up to 2 years but are needed indefinitely in patients who have undergone bilateral adrenalectomy. This latter group of patients also may require mineralocorticoid replacement therapy. Typical replacement doses include hydrocortisone (10 to 20 mg q A.M. and 5 to 10 mg q P.M.) and fludrocortisone (0.05 to 0.1 mg/day q A.M.).

Adrenocortical Cancer

Adrenal carcinomas are rare neoplasms with a worldwide incidence of two per 1 million. These tumors have a bimodal age distribution, with an increased incidence in children and adults in the fourth and fifth decades of life. The majority are sporadic, but adrenocortical carcinomas also occur in association with germline mutations of *p53* (Li-Fraumeni syndrome) and *MENIN* (multiple endocrine neoplasia type 1) genes. Loci on 11p (Beckwith-Wiedemann syndrome), 2p (Carney complex), and 9q also have been implicated.

Symptoms and Signs Approximately 50% of adrenocortical cancers are nonfunctioning.[87] The remaining secrete cortisol (30%), androgens (20%), estrogens (10%), aldosterone (2%), or multiple hormones (35%). Patients with functioning tumors often present with the rapid onset of Cushing's syndrome accompanied by virilizing features. Nonfunctioning tumors more commonly present with an enlarging abdominal mass and abdominal or back pain. Rarely, weight loss, anorexia, and nausea may be present.

Diagnostic Tests Diagnostic evaluation of these patients begins with measurement of serum electrolyte levels to rule out hypokalemia, urinary catecholamines to rule out pheochromocytomas, an overnight 1-mg dexamethasone suppression test, and a 24-hour urine collection for cortisol, 17-ketosteroids.

CT and MRI scans are useful to image these tumors (Fig. 38-45). The size of the adrenal mass on imaging studies is the single most important criterion to help diagnose malignancy. In the series reported by Copeland, 92% of adrenal cancers were >6 cm in diameter.[88] The sensitivity, specificity, and likelihood ratio of tumor size in predicting malignancy (based on Surveillance; Epidemiology, and End Results program data) was recently reported as 96%, 51%, and 2 for tumors ≥4 cm; and 90%, 78%, and 4.1 for tumors ≥6 cm.[89] Other CT imaging characteristics suggesting malignancy include tumor heterogeneity, irregular margins, and the presence of hemorrhage and adjacent lymphadenopathy or liver metastases. Moderately bright signal intensity on T_2-weighted images (adrenal mass to liver ratio 1.2:2.8), significant lesion enhancement, and slow washout after injection of gadolinium contrast also indicate malignancy, as does evidence of local invasion into adjacent structures such as the liver, blood vessels (IVC), and distant metastases. Once adrenal cancer is diagnosed, CT scans of the chest and pelvis are performed for staging. The tumor-node-metastasis (TNM) staging system for adrenocortical carcinoma is depicted in Table 38-19. Up to 70% of patients present with stage III or IV disease.

Pathology Most adrenocortical cancers are large, weighing between 100 and 1000 g. On gross examination, areas of hemorrhage and necrosis often are evident. Microscopically, cells are hyperchromatic and typically have large nuclei and prominent nucleoli. It is

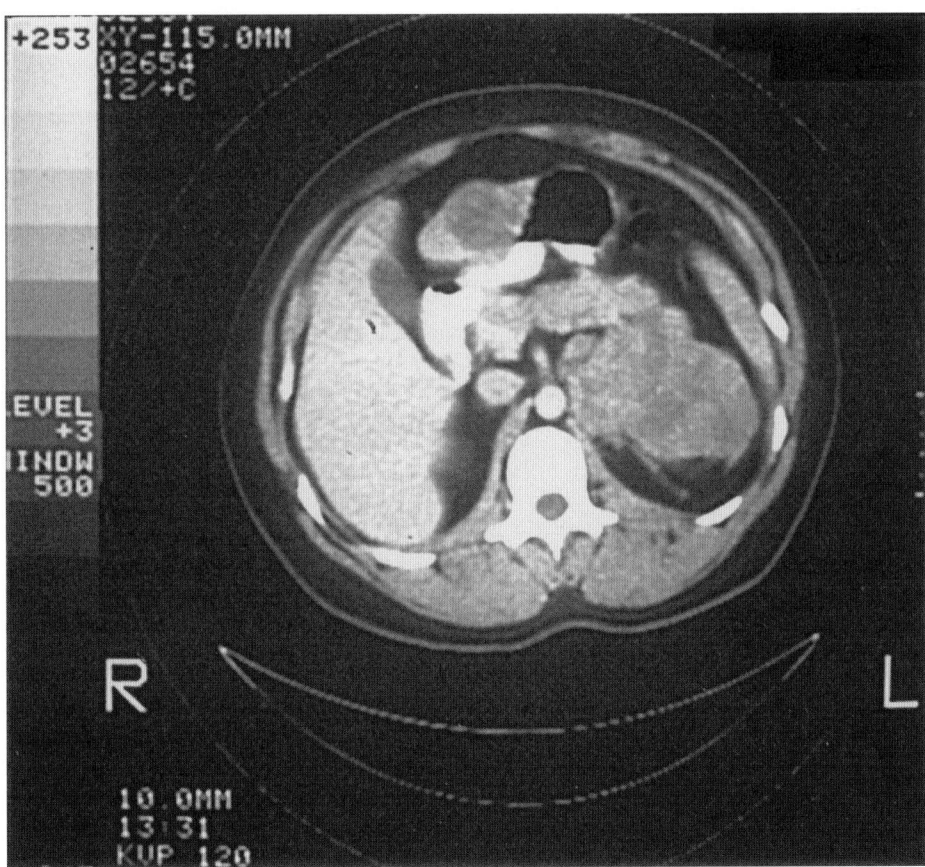

FIG. 38-45. Computed tomography scan of the abdomen showing a left adrenocortical cancer with synchronous liver metastasis.

TABLE 38-19	TNM staging for adrenocortical cancer[29]
Stage	**TNM Class**
I	T1, N0, M0
II	T2, N0, M0
III	T3, N0, M0
	T1–2, N1, M0
IV	T3–4, N1, M0
	Any T, any N, M1

Primary tumor (T): T1, size ≤5 cm without local invasion; T2, size >5 cm without local invasion; T3, any size with local invasion but no involvement of adjacent organs; T4, any size with involvement of adjacent organs.
Nodes (N): N0, no involvement of regional nodes; N1, positive regional lymph nodes.
Metastasis (M): M0, no known distal metastases, M1, distant metastases present.
Source: Used with the permission of the American Joint Committee on Cancer (AJCC), Chicago, Illinois. The original source for this material is the AJCC Cancer Staging Manual, Sixth Edition (2002) published by Springer Science and Business Media LLC, *www.springerlink.com.*

very difficult to distinguish benign adrenal adenomas from carcinomas by histologic examination alone. Capsular or vascular invasion is the most reliable sign of cancer. Weiss and associates studied a combination of nine criteria for their usefulness in distinguishing malignant from benign adrenal tumors: nuclear grade III or IV; mitotic rate greater than 5/50 high-power fields; atypical mitoses; clear cells comprising 25% or less of the tumor; a diffuse architecture; microscopic necrosis; and invasion of venous, sinusoidal, and capsular structure. Tumors with four or more of these criteria were likely to metastasize and/or recur.[90] Rarely, the diagnosis of malignancy of a completely resected adrenal tumor is often only made in retrospect by the finding of metastatic disease many years later.

Treatment The most important predictor of survival in patients with adrenal cancer is the adequacy of resection. Patients who undergo complete resection have 5-year actuarial survival rates ranging from 32 to 48%, whereas median survival is <1 year in those undergoing incomplete excision. Therefore, adrenocortical carcinomas are treated by excision of the tumor en bloc with any contiguously involved lymph nodes or organs such as the diaphragm, kidney, pancreas, liver, or IVC. This is best accomplished by open adrenalectomy via a generous subcostal incision or a thoracoabdominal incision (on the right side). The incisions should permit wide exposure, minimize chances of capsule rupture and tumor spillage, and allow vascular control of the aorta, IVC, and renal vessels, as needed.

Mitotane or o,p-DDD or 1,1-dichloro-2-(o-chlorophenyl)-2-(p-chlorophenyl) ethane, which is a derivative of the insecticide DDT, has adrenolytic activity and has been used in the adjuvant setting and for the treatment of unresectable or metastatic disease. However, the therapeutic effectiveness is conflicting, and consistent improvement in survival rates is lacking. Moreover, the drug is associated with significant GI and neurologic side effects, particularly at the effective doses of 2 to 6 g/d. Terzolo and associates retrospectively evaluated the use of mitotane in the adjuvant setting and reported significantly increased recurrence-free survival in the treatment group.[91] However, the routine use of this medication awaits evaluation in randomized, controlled trials. Determination of blood mitotane levels is helpful to ascertain whether therapeutic and nontoxic levels are present. Adrenocortical tumors commonly metastasize to the liver, lung, and bone.

Surgical debulking is recommended for isolated, recurrent disease and has been demonstrated to prolong survival. Systemic chemotherapeutic agents used in this tumor include etoposide, cisplatin, doxorubicin, and, more recently, paclitaxel, but consistent responses are rare, possibly due to the expression of the multidrug resistance gene (*MDR-1*) in tumor cells. In vitro data indicate that mitotane may be able to reverse this resistance when combined with various chemotherapeutic agents. There has been recent interest in the use of suramin, a growth factor inhibitor, as therapy for adrenocortical carcinoma; however, this requires further study, particularly because this drug may be associated with significant neurotoxicity. Gossypol, a naturally occurring insecticide (from the cotton plant *Gossypium* species), also appears to inhibit the growth of adrenocortical cancer cell lines and tumors in vivo. However, poor response rates combined with high death rates in limited clinical studies have reduced enthusiasm for this agent. Adrenocortical cancers also are relatively insensitive to conventional external beam radiation therapy. However, this modality is used in the palliation of bony metastases. Ketoconazole, metyrapone, or aminoglutethimide may also be useful in controlling steroid hypersecretion.

Sex Steroid Excess

Adrenal adenomas or carcinomas that secrete adrenal androgens lead to virilizing syndromes. Although women with virilizing tumors develop hirsutism, amenorrhea, infertility, and other signs of masculinization, such as increased muscle mass, deepened voice, and temporal balding, men with these tumors are more difficult to diagnose and, hence, usually present with disease in advanced stages. Children with virilizing tumors have accelerated growth, premature development of facial and pubic hair, acne, genital enlargement, and deepening of their voice. Feminizing adrenal tumors are less common and occur in men in the third to fifth decades of life. These tumors lead to gynecomastia, impotence, and testicular atrophy. Women with these tumors develop irregular menses or dysfunctional uterine bleeding. Vaginal bleeding may occur in postmenopausal women. Girls with these tumors experience precocious puberty with breast enlargement and early menarche.

Diagnostic Tests Virilizing tumors produce excessive amounts of the androgen precursor, DHEA, which can be measured in plasma or urine as 17-ketosteroids. Patients with feminizing tumors also have elevated urinary 17-ketosteroids in addition to increased estrogen levels. Androgen-producing tumors often are associated with production of other hormones such as glucocorticoids.

Treatment Virilizing and feminizing tumors are treated by adrenalectomy. Malignancy is difficult to diagnose histologically but is suggested by the presence of local invasion, recurrence, or distal metastases. Adrenolytic drugs such as mitotane, aminoglutethimide, and ketoconazole may be useful in controlling symptoms in patients with metastatic disease.

Congenital Adrenal Hyperplasia

CAH refers to a group of disorders, which result from deficiencies or complete absence of enzymes involved in adrenal steroidogenesis. 21-Hydroxylase (CYP21A2) deficiency is the most common enzymatic defect, accounting for >90% of cases of CAH. This deficiency prevents the production of 11-deoxycortisol and 11-DOC from progesterone precursors. Deficiency of glucocorticoids and aldosterone leads to elevated ACTH levels and overproduction of adrenal androgens and corticosteroid precursors such as 17-hydroxyprogesterone and Δ^4-androstenedione. These compounds are converted to testosterone in the peripheral tissues, thereby leading to virilization. Complete deficiency of 21-hydroxylase presents at birth with virilization, diarrhea, hypovolemia, hyponatremia, hyperkalemia, and hyperpigmentation. Partial enzyme deficiency may present at birth or later with virilizing features. These patients are less prone to the salt-wasting that characterizes complete enzyme deficiency. 11β-hydroxylase deficiency is the second most common form of CAH and leads to hypertension (from 11-DOC accumulation), virilization, and hyperpigmentation. Other enzyme deficiencies include 3β-hydroxydehydrogenase and 17-hydroxylase deficiency. Congenital adrenal lipoid hyperplasia is the most severe form of CAH, which is caused by cholesterol desmolase deficiency. It leads to the disruption of all steroid biosynthetic pathways, thus resulting in a fatal salt-wasting syndrome in phenotypic female patients.

Diagnostic Tests The particular enzyme deficiency can be diagnosed by karyotype analysis and measurement of plasma and urinary steroids. The most common enzyme deficiency, absence of 21-hydroxylase, leads to increased plasma 17-hydroxyprogesterone and progesterone levels, because these compounds cannot be converted to 11-deoxycortisol and 11-deoxycorticosterone, respectively. 11β-hydroxylase deficiency is the next most common disorder and results in elevated plasma 11-DOC and 11-deoxycortisol. Urinary 17-hydroxyprogesterone, androgens, and 17-ketosteroids also are elevated. The dexamethasone suppression test (2 to 4 mg divided qid for 7 days) can be used to distinguish adrenal hyperplasia from neoplasia. CT, MRI, and iodocholesterol scans generally are used to localize the tumors.

Treatment Patients with CAH traditionally have been managed medically, with cortisol and mineralocorticoid replacement to suppress the hypothalamic-pituitary-adrenal axis. However, the doses of steroids required often are supraphysiologic and lead to iatrogenic hypercortisolism. More recently, bilateral laparoscopic adrenalectomy has been proposed as an alternative treatment for this disease and has been successfully performed in a limited number of patients for various forms of CAH.

Disorders of the Adrenal Medulla

Pheochromocytomas

Pheochromocytomas are rare tumors with prevalence rates ranging from 0.3 to 0.95% in autopsy series and approximately 1.9% in series using biochemical screening. They can occur at any age with a peak incidence in the fourth and fifth decades of life and have no gender predilection. Extra-adrenal tumors, also called functional paragangliomas, may be found at sites of sympathetic ganglia in the organ of Zuckerkandl, neck, mediastinum, abdomen, and pelvis. Pheochromocytomas often are called the *10 percent tumor* because 10% are bilateral, 10% are malignant, 10% occur in pediatric patients, 10% are extra-adrenal, and 10% are familial.

Pheochromocytomas occur in families with MEN2A and MEN2B, in approximately 50% of patients. Both syndromes are inherited in an autosomal dominant fashion and are caused by germline mutations in the *RET* proto-oncogene. Another syndrome with an increased risk of pheochromocytomas is von Hippel-Lindau (VHL) disease, which also is inherited in an autosomal dominant manner. This syndrome also includes retinal angioma, hemangioblastomas of the central nervous system, renal cysts and carcinomas, pancreatic cysts, and epididymal cystadenomas. The incidence of pheochromocytomas in the syndrome is approximately 14%. The gene causing VHL has been mapped to chromosome 3p and is a tumor-suppressor gene. Pheochromocytomas also are included within the tumor spectrum of neurofibromatosis type 1 (NF1 gene) and other neuroectodermal disorders (Sturge-Weber syndrome and tuberous sclerosis), Carney's syndrome (gastric epithelioid leiomyosarcoma, pulmonary chondroma, and extra-adrenal paraganglioma), MEN1 syndrome, and the familial paraganglioma and pheochromocytoma syndrome caused by mutations in the succinyl dehydrogenase family of genes (SDHB, SDHC, and SDHD).[92]

Symptoms and Signs Headache, palpitations, and diaphoresis constitute the "classic triad" of pheochromocytomas. Symptoms such a anxiety, tremulousness, paresthesias, flushing, chest pain, shortness of breath, abdominal pain, nausea, vomiting, and others are nonspecific and may be episodic in nature. Cardiovascular complications such as myocardial infarction and cerebrovascular accidents may ensue. These symptoms can be incited by a range of stimuli including exercise, micturition, and defecation. The most common clinical sign is hypertension. Pheochromocytomas are one of the few curable causes of hypertension and are found in 0.1 to 0.2% of hypertensive patients. Hypertension related to this tumor may be paroxysmal with intervening normotension, sustained with paroxysms or sustained hypertension alone. Sudden death may occur in patients with undiagnosed tumors who undergo other surgeries or biopsy.

Diagnostic Tests *Biochemical Studies* Pheochromocytomas are diagnosed by testing 24-hour urine samples for catecholamines and their metabolites as well as by determining plasma metanephrine levels. Urinary metanephrines are 98% sensitive and also are highly specific for pheochromocytomas, whereas VMA measurements are slightly less sensitive and specific. False-positive VMA tests may result from ingestion of caffeine, raw fruits, or medications (α-methyldopa). Fractionated urinary catecholamines (norepinephrine, epinephrine, and dopamine) also are very sensitive but less specific for pheochromocytomas. Because extra-adrenal sites lack phenylethanolamine *N*-methyltransferase, these tumors secrete norepinephrine whereas epinephrine is the main hormone secreted from adrenal pheochromocytomas. Many physiologic and pathologic states can alter the levels of plasma catecholamines. Hence, they often are thought to be less accurate than urinary tests. Both epinephrine and norepinephrine should be measured, as tumors often secrete one or the other hormone. Sensitivities of 85% and specificities of 95% have been reported using cutoff values of 2000 pg/mL for norepinephrine and 200 pg/mL for epinephrine. Clonidine is an agent that suppresses neurogenically mediated catecholamine excess but not secretion from pheochromocytomas. A normal clonidine suppression test is defined by a decrease of basal catecholamine levels to <500 pg/mL within 2 to 3 hours after an oral dose of 0.3 mg of clonidine. Chromogranin A is a monomeric, acidic protein, which is stored in the adrenal medulla and other neuroendocrine tumors and released along with catecholamine hormones. It has been reported to have a sensitivity of 83% and a specificity of 96% and is useful in conjunction with catecholamine measurement for diagnosing pheochromocytomas. Recent studies have shown that plasma metanephrines are the most reliable tests to identify pheochromocytomas, with sensitivity approaching 100%.

Radiologic Studies Radiologic studies are useful to localize tumors and to assess the extent of spread once the diagnosis has been made with biochemical tests. CT scans are 85 to 95% sensitive and 70 to 100% specific for pheochromocytomas (Fig. 38-46A). The scans should be performed without contrast to minimize the risk of precipitating a hypertensive crisis although some recent studies suggest that IV contrast may be used. Images should include the region from the diaphragm to the aortic bifurcation so as to include the organ of Zuckerkandl. CT scans do not provide functional information and cannot definitively diagnose pheochromocytomas. MRI scans are 95% sensitive and almost 100% specific for pheochromocytomas because these tumors have a characteristic appearance on T_2-weighted images or after gadolinium. MRI is also the study of choice in pregnant women as there is no risk of radiation exposure. Metaiodobenzylguanidine (MIBG) is taken up and concentrated by vesicles in the adrenal medullar cells because its structure is similar to norepinephrine. Normal adrenal medullary tissue does not take up appreciable MIBG. ^{131}I radiolabeled MIBG is, therefore, useful for localizing pheochromocytomas (Fig. 38-46B), especially those in ectopic positions. This test has a reported sensitivity of 77 to 89% and specificity ranging from 88 to 100%.

Treatment The medical management of pheochromocytomas is aimed chiefly at blood pressure control and volume repletion. Alpha blockers such as phenoxybenzamine are started 1 to 3 weeks before surgery at doses of 10 mg twice daily, which may be increased to 300 to 400 mg/d with rehydration. Patients should be warned about orthostatic hypotension. Other alpha blockers such as prazosin and other classes of drugs such as ACE inhibitors and calcium channel blockers are also useful. Beta blockers such as propranolol at doses of 10 to 40 mg every 6 to 8 hours often need to be added preoperatively in patients who have persistent tachycardia and arrhythmias. Beta blockers should only be instituted after adequate alpha blockade and hydration to avoid the effects of unopposed alpha stimulation, (i.e., hypertensive crisis and congestive heart failure). Patients also should be volume repleted preoperatively to avoid postoperative hypotension, which ensues with the loss of vasoconstriction after tumor removal.

Adrenalectomy is the treatment of choice. The chief goal of surgery is to resect the tumor completely with minimal tumor manipulation or rupture of the tumor capsule. Surgery should be

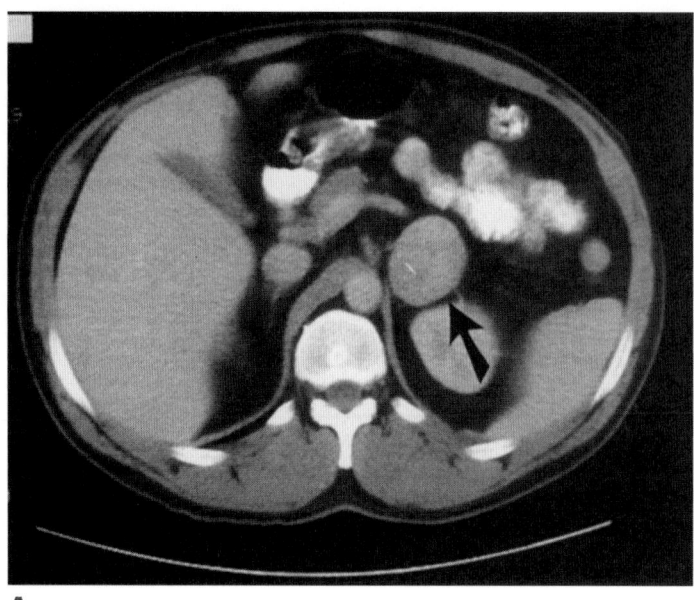

A

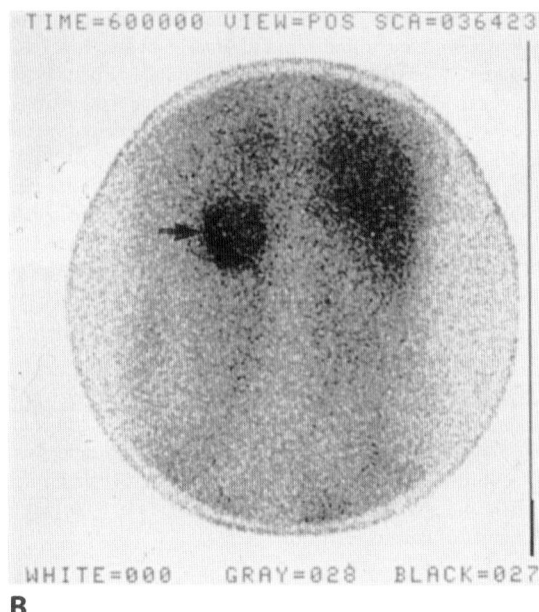

B

FIG. 38-46. A left-sided pheochromocytoma (*arrows*) imaged by a computed tomography scan of the abdomen (**A**) and a metaiodoben-zylguanidine scan viewed posteriorly (**B**).

performed with both noninvasive and invasive monitors, including an arterial line and central venous lines. In patients with congestive heart failure or underlying coronary artery disease, Swan-Ganz catheters may be necessary. Stress must be avoided during anesthesia induction, and use of inhaled agents like isoflurane and enflurane are preferred because they have minimal cardiac depressant effects. The common medications used for intraoperative blood pressure control include nitroprusside, nitroglycerin, and phentolamine. Intraoperative arrhythmias are best managed by short-acting beta blockers such as esmolol. Adrenalectomy usually was performed via an open anterior approach to facilitate detection of bilateral tumors, extra-adrenal lesions, or metastatic lesions. However, many pheochromocytomas <5 cm in diameter can be safely resected laparoscopically. Postoperatively, these patients are prone to hypotension due to loss of adrenergic stimulation and consequent vasodilatation and therefore need large volume resuscitation.

Hereditary Pheochromocytomas

Inherited pheochromocytomas tend to be multiple and bilateral. Generally, unilateral adrenalectomy is recommended in the absence of obvious lesions in the contralateral adrenal gland because of Addison disease requiring lifelong steroid replacement in patients undergoing bilateral adrenalectomy. For patients with tumors in both adrenal glands, cortical-sparing subtotal adrenalectomy may preserve adrenocortical function and avoid the morbidity of bilateral total adrenalectomy.[72] Laparoscopic subtotal adrenalectomy has been shown to provide short-term clinical results comparable to total adrenalectomy, with reduced surgical morbidity.[93] However, these patients remain at risk for recurrent pheochromocytoma, which has been reported in 20% of patients with VHL disease a median of 40 months after partial adrenalectomy, and in 33% of MEN2 patients followed for 54 to 88 months after surgery. Autotransplantation of adrenocortical tissue after total adrenalectomy may be another option for these patients and removes the risk of recurrence. However, the transplanted cortical tissue rarely provides full function, and steroid replacement usually is required.

Malignant Pheochromocytomas

Approximately 12 to 29% of pheochromocytomas are malignant, and these tumors are associated with decreased survival. There are no definitive histologic criteria defining malignant pheochromocy-

tomas. In fact, pleomorphism, nuclear atypia, and abundant mitotic figures are seen in benign tumors. Capsular and vascular invasion may be seen in benign lesions as well. Malignancy usually is diagnosed when there is evidence of invasion into surrounding structures or distant metastases. The most common sites for metastatic disease are bone, liver, regional lymph nodes, lung, and peritoneum, although the brain, pleura, skin, and muscles may also occasionally be involved. Some studies also suggest that older patient age and larger tumors are associated with a higher risk of malignancy. Although risk of malignancy increases with size for all pheochromocytomas, size does not seem to reliably predict malignancy in pheochromocytomas with local disease only.[94] Given this difficulty defining malignancy clinically (in the absence of metastatic disease), a number of other features such as DNA ploidy, tumor size, and necrosis, neuropeptide Y mRNA expression and serum neuron-specific enolase expression have been studied. Malignant pheochromocytomas are more likely to express p53 and bcl-2, and have activated telomerase. Recent data suggest that flow cytometry and molecular markers such as expression of Ki-67, tissue inhibitor of metalloproteinase, and COX-2 also have shown some use in determining malignancy. When pheochromocytomas develop in the MEN syndromes, they rarely are malignant. In contrast, patients with germline SDHB mutations appear to have a higher propensity for extra-adrenal and malignant tumors.[92]

The Adrenal Incidentaloma

Adrenal lesions discovered during imaging performed for unrelated reasons are referred to as *incidentalomas*. This definition excludes tumors discovered on imaging studies performed for evaluating symptoms of hormone hypersecretion or staging patients with known cancer. The incidence of these lesions identified by CT scans ranges from 0.4 to 4.4%.

Differential Diagnosis

The differential diagnosis of adrenal incidentalomas is shown in Table 38-20. Nonfunctional cortical adenomas account for the majority (36 to 94%) of adrenal incidentalomas in patients without a history of cancer. In a series of patients from the Mayo Clinic, no nonfunctional lesion progressed to cause clinical or biochemical abnormalities. However, other studies indicate that 5 to 20% of patients with apparently nonfunctioning cortical adenomas have

TABLE 38-20	Differential diagnosis of adrenal incidentaloma

Functioning Lesions	Nonfunctioning Lesions
Benign	Benign
Aldosteronoma	Cortical adenoma
Cortisol-producing adenoma	Myelolipoma
Sex-steroid–producing adenoma	Cyst
Pheochromocytoma	Ganglioneuroma
	Hemorrhage
Malignant	Malignant
Adrenocortical cancer	Metastasis
Malignant pheochromocytoma	Adrenocortical cancer

underlying, subtle abnormalities of glucocorticoid secretion, and a rare benign-appearing incidentaloma is a cancer.

By definition, patients with incidentalomas do not have clinically overt Cushing's syndrome, but subclinical Cushing's syndrome is estimated to occur in approximately 8% of patients. This disorder is characterized by subtle features of cortisol excess, such as weight gain, skin atrophy, facial fullness, diabetes, and hypertension, accompanied by loss of normal diurnal variation in cortisol secretion, autonomous cortisol secretion, and resistance to suppression by dexamethasone. Total cortisol produced and 24-hour urinary cortisol levels may be normal. Examination of the natural history of subclinical Cushing's syndrome indicates that, although most patients remain asymptomatic, some do progress to clinically evident Cushing's syndrome. Furthermore, cases of postoperative adrenal crisis from unrecognized suppression of the contralateral adrenal have been reported, making preoperative identification of this condition imperative, particularly in the era of early discharge following laparoscopic adrenalectomy.[95]

The adrenal is a common site of metastases of lung and breast tumors, melanoma, renal cell cancer, and lymphoma. In patients with a history of nonadrenal cancer and a unilateral adrenal mass, the incidence of metastatic disease has been reported to range from 32 to 73%. Myelolipomas are benign, biochemically nonfunctioning lesions composed of elements of hematopoietic and mature adipose tissue, which are rare causes of adrenal incidentaloma. Other less commonly encountered lesions include adrenal cysts, ganglioneuromas, and hemorrhage.

Diagnostic Investigations

The diagnostic work-up of an adrenal incidentaloma is aimed at identifying patients that would benefit from adrenalectomy, (i.e. patients with functioning tumors and those tumors at increased risk of being malignant). It is not necessary for asymptomatic patients whose imaging studies are consistent with obvious cysts, hemorrhage, myelolipomas, or diffuse metastatic disease to undergo additional investigations. All other patients should be tested for underlying hormonally active tumors by (a) low-dose (1 mg) overnight dexamethasone suppression test or 24-hour urine cortisol to rule out subclinical Cushing's syndrome and 17-ketosteroids (if sex-steroid excess is suspected), (b) a 24-hour urine collection for catecholamines, metanephrines, VMA, or plasma metanephrine to rule out pheochromocytoma, and (c) in hypertensive patients, serum electrolytes, plasma aldosterone, and plasma renin to rule out an aldosteronoma. Confirmatory tests can be performed based on the results of the initial screening studies.

Determination of the malignant potential of an incidentaloma is more difficult. The risk of malignancy in an adrenal lesion is related to its size. Lesions >6 cm in diameter have an approximate risk of malignancy of about 35%.[88] However, this size cutoff is not absolute because adrenal carcinomas also have been reported in lesions <6 cm. This has led to increased use of the imaging characteristics of incidentalomas to predict malignancy. Benign adrenal adenomas tend to be homogeneous, well encapsulated, and have smooth and regular margins. They also tend to be hypoattenuating lesions (<10 Hounsfield

units) on CT scanning. In contrast, adrenal cancers tend to be hyperattenuating (>18 Hounsfield units), inhomogeneous, have irregular borders, and may show evidence of local invasion or adjacent lymphadenopathy. On MRI T_2-weighted imaging, adenomas demonstrate low signal intensity when compared to the liver (adrenal mass to liver ratio <1.4), whereas carcinomas and metastases have moderate intensity (mass to liver ratio 1.2:2.8). Pheochromocytomas are extremely bright with mass to liver ratios >3. Unfortunately, the ranges overlap, and signal intensity is not 100% reliable for determining the nature of the lesion. Radionuclide imaging with NP-59 also has been used to distinguish between various adrenal lesions, with some investigators suggesting that uptake of NP-59 was 100% predictive of a benign lesion (adenoma) whereas absence of imaging was 100% predictive of a nonadenomatous lesion. However, the technique has not gained widespread acceptance because patients need to be given cold iodine 1 week before the study to prevent thyroid uptake, imaging needs to be delayed by 5 to 7 days after administration of the contrast, and false-positive and false-negative results occur. FNAB cannot be used to distinguish adrenal adenomas from carcinomas. This being said, FNAB is useful in the setting of a patient with a history of cancer and a solitary adrenal mass. The positive predictive value of FNAB in this situation has been shown to be almost 100%, although false-negative rates of up to 33% have been reported. Biopsies usually are performed under CT guidance and appropriate testing to rule out pheochromocytomas should be undertaken before the procedure to avoid precipitating a hypertensive crisis.

Management

An algorithm for the management of patients with incidentalomas is shown in Fig. 38-47. Patients with functional tumors or obviously malignant lesions should undergo adrenalectomy. Operative intervention also is advised in patients with subclinical Cushing's syndrome with suppressed plasma ACTH levels and elevated urinary cortisol levels because these patients are at high risk for progression to overt Cushing's syndrome. Adrenalectomy also should be considered in patients with normal ACTH and urinary free cortisol if they are <50 years old or have recent weight gain, hypertension, diabetes, or osteopenia.

For nonfunctional lesions, the risk of malignancy needs to be balanced with operative morbidity and mortality. Lesions >6 cm or those with suspicious features on imaging studies such as heterogeneity, irregular capsule, or adjacent nodes should be treated by adrenalectomy. Nonoperative therapy, with close periodic follow-up is advised for lesions <4 cm in diameter with benign imaging characteristics. However, the management of lesions 4 to 6 cm in size with benign imaging features remains controversial (i.e., this group of patients can be treated with observation or surgery). Recommendations vary from various groups of endocrine surgeons regarding this "intermediate" group of patients, with some advising adrenalectomy for tumors at cutoff sizes of 3, 4, or 5 cm. However, several important points must be considered in the management of these patients. First, size criteria for malignancy are not definitive and are derived from a selected series of patients. Second, the actual size of adrenal tumors can be underestimated by at least 1 cm by modalities such as CT and MRI scans, because tumors are larger in a cephalocaudal axis. Third, the natural history of incidentalomas is variable and depends on the underlying diagnosis, age of the study population, and the size of the mass. Older patients are more likely to have nonfunctioning adenomas. Existing data in terms of the long-term behavior of these nonfunctional lesions, although limited, indicate that malignant transformation is uncommon. Furthermore, tumors that increase in size by at least 1 cm over a 2-year follow-up period and those with subtle hormonal abnormalities appear to be more likely to enlarge. Overt hormone overproduction is more likely in tumors >3 cm and those with increased NP-59 uptake. Surgeons are more likely to operate on a 40-year-old patient with a 4-cm lesion, while electing to follow an 80-year-old patient with a similar lesion but multiple concurrent comorbidities. Based on the above considerations, our current size threshold

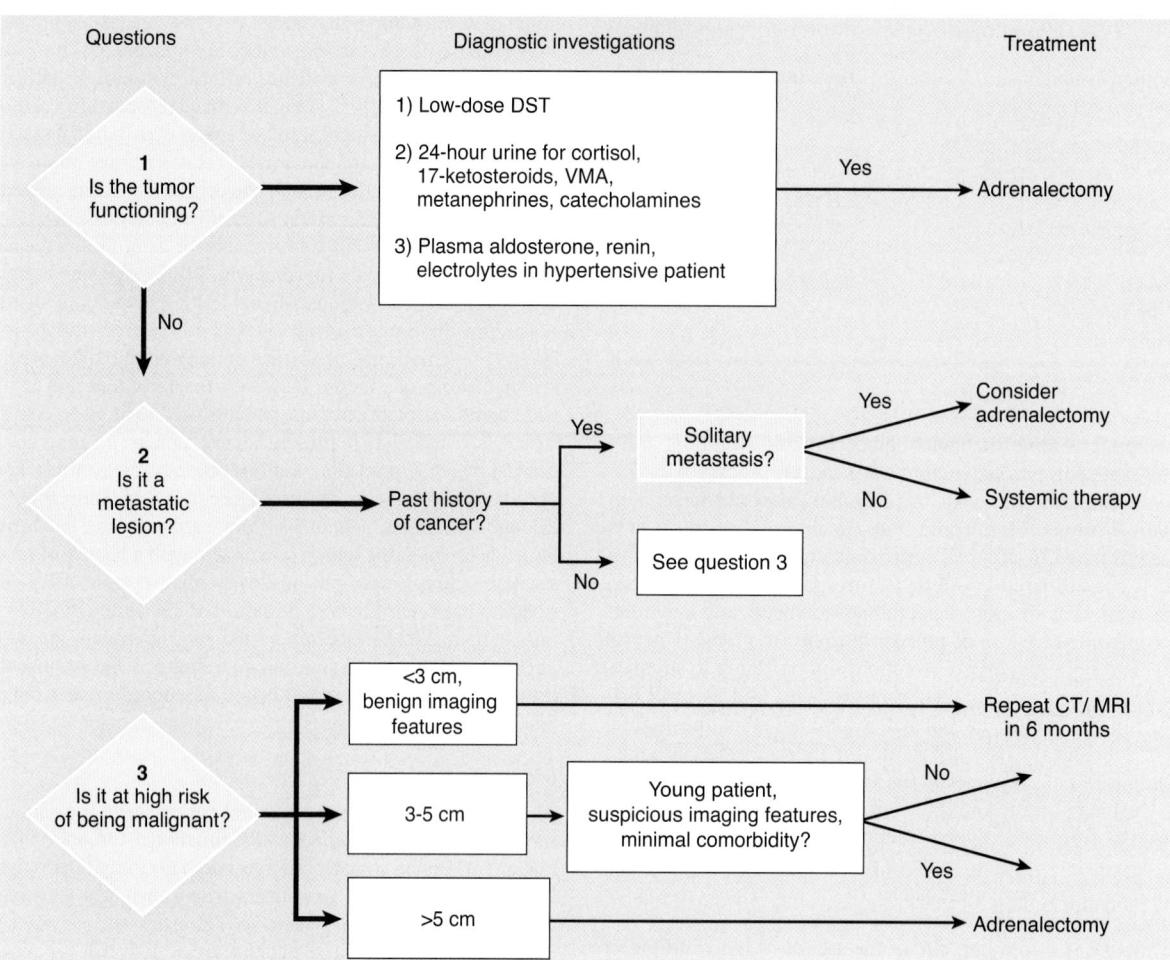

FIG. 38-47. Management algorithm for an adrenal incidentaloma. CT = computed tomography; DST = dexamethasone suppression test; MRI = magnetic resonance imaging; VMA = vanillylmandelic acid.

for adrenalectomy with a nonfunctioning homogeneous tumor is 3 to 4 cm in young patients with no comorbidities and 5 cm in older patients with significant comorbidity. Lesions that grow during follow-up also are treated by adrenalectomy. Myelolipomas generally do not warrant adrenalectomy unless there is concern regarding malignancy, which is rare, or bleeding into the lesion, which is more likely in myelolipomas >4 cm in size. These tumors, even when large, can be removed laparoscopically. Resection of solitary adrenal metastases in patients with a history of nonadrenal cancer has been demonstrated to lead to prolonged patient survival. Suspected adrenal metastases also may be resected for diagnosis or for palliation, if large and symptomatic.

Adrenal Insufficiency

Adrenal insufficiency may be primary, resulting from adrenal disease, or secondary, due to a deficiency of ACTH (Table 38-21). The most commonly encountered causes of primary adrenal insufficiency are autoimmune disease, infections, and metastatic deposits. Spontaneous adrenal hemorrhage can occur in patients with fulminant meningococcal septicemia (Waterhouse-Friderichsen syndrome). Bilateral adrenal hemorrhage also can occur secondary to trauma, severe stress, infection, and coagulopathies and, if unrecognized, is lethal. Exogenous glucocorticoid therapy with suppression of the adrenal glands is the most common cause of secondary adrenal insufficiency.

Symptoms and Signs

Acute adrenal insufficiency should be suspected in stressed patients with any of the relevant risk factors. It may mimic sepsis, myocar-

dial infarction, or pulmonary embolus and presents with fever, weakness, confusion, nausea, vomiting, lethargy, abdominal pain, or severe hypotension. Chronic adrenal insufficiency, such as that occurring in patients with metastatic tumors, may be more subtle. Symptoms include fatigue, salt-craving, weight loss, nausea, vomiting, and abdominal pain. These patients may appear hyperpigmented from increased secretion of CRH and ACTH, with increased α-melanocyte-stimulating hormone side-products.

Diagnostic Studies

Characteristic laboratory findings include hyponatremia, hyperkalemia, eosinophilia, mild azotemia, and fasting or reactive hypoglycemia. The peripheral blood smear may demonstrate eosinophilia in approximately 20% of patients. Adrenal insufficiency is diagnosed by the ACTH stimulation test. ACTH (250 μg) is infused intravenously, and cortisol levels are measured at 0, 30, and 60 minutes. Peak cortisol levels <20 μg/dL suggest adrenal insufficiency. ACTH levels also allow primary insufficiency to be distinguished from secondary causes. High ACTH levels with low plasma cortisol levels are diagnostic of primary adrenal insufficiency.

Treatment

Treatment must be initiated based on clinical suspicion alone, even before test results are obtained or the patient is unlikely to survive. Management includes volume resuscitation with at least 2 to 3 L of a 0.9% saline solution or 5% dextrose in saline solution. Blood should be obtained for electrolyte (decreased Na$^+$ and increased K$^+$) and glucose (low) and cortisol (low) levels, ACTH (increased in

TABLE 38-21	Etiology of adrenal insufficiency

Primary	Secondary
Autoimmune (autoimmune polyglandular disease type I and II)	Exogenous glucocorticoid therapy
Infectious—TB, fungi, CMV, HIV	Bilateral adrenalectomy
Hemorrhage—spontaneous (Waterhouse-Friderichsen syndrome) and secondary to stress, trauma, infections, coagulopathy, or anticoagulants	Pituitary or hypothalamic tumors
Metastases	Pituitary hemorrhage (postpartum Sheehan's syndrome)
Infiltrative disorders—amyloidosis, hemochromatosis	Transsphenoidal resection of pituitary tumor
Adrenoleukodystrophy	
Congenital adrenal hyperplasia	
Drugs—ketoconazole, metyrapone, aminoglutethimide, mitotane	

CMV = cytomegalovirus; TB = tuberculosis.

primary and decreased in secondary), and quantitative eosinophilic count. Dexamethasone (4 mg) should be administered intravenously. Hydrocortisone (100 mg IV every 8 hours) also may be used, but it interferes with testing of cortisol levels. Once the patient has been stabilized, underlying conditions such as infection should be sought, identified, and treated. The ACTH stimulation test should be performed to confirm the diagnosis. Glucocorticoids can then be tapered to maintenance doses (oral hydrocortisone 15 to 20 mg in the morning and 10 mg in the evening). Mineralocorticoids (fludrocortisone 0.05 to 0.1 mg daily) may be required once the saline infusions are discontinued.

Adrenal Surgery
Choice of Procedure

Adrenalectomy may be performed via an open or laparoscopic approach. In either approach, the gland may be approached anteriorly, laterally, or posteriorly via the retroperitoneum. The choice of approach depends on the size and nature of the lesion and expertise of the surgeon. Laparoscopic adrenalectomy has rapidly become the standard procedure of choice for the excision of most benign appearing adrenal lesions <6 cm in diameter. The role of laparoscopic adrenalectomy in the management of adrenocortical cancers is controversial. The data with respect to local tumor recurrence and intra-abdominal carcinomatosis from laparoscopic adrenalectomy for malignant adrenal tumors that were not appreciated as such, preoperatively or intraoperatively, are conflicting. Although laparo-

scopic adrenalectomy appears to be feasible and safe for solitary adrenal metastasis[96] (provided there is no local invasion and the tumor can be resected intact), open adrenalectomy or laparoscopic-assisted open adrenalectomy is the safest option for suspected or known adrenocortical cancers and malignant pheochromocytomas. Technical considerations and surgeon experience rather than absolute tumor size usually determine the size threshold for laparoscopic resection. Hand-assisted laparoscopic adrenalectomy may provide a bridge between laparoscopic adrenalectomy and conversion to an open procedure. There have been no randomized trials directly comparing open vs. laparoscopic adrenalectomy. However, studies have shown that laparoscopic adrenalectomy is associated with decreased blood loss, postoperative pain, and narcotic use; reduced length of hospital stay; and faster return to work.

Laparoscopic Adrenalectomy

The procedure is performed under general anesthesia. Arterial lines are used routinely and central lines are necessary for patients in whom massive fluid shifts are anticipated (e.g., those with large, active pheochromocytomas). A nasogastric tube and Foley catheter are recommended. Routine preoperative antibiotics are not needed, except in patients with Cushing's syndrome. The adrenals can be removed laparoscopically via a transabdominal (anterior or lateral) or retroperitoneal (lateral or posterior) approach. The lateral approach is preferred by most laparoscopic surgeons and uses gravity to aid retraction of surrounding organs. Patients, however, need to be repositioned for a bilateral procedure. The anterior transabdominal approach offers the advantage of a conventional view of the abdominal cavity and allows a bilateral adrenalectomy to be performed without the necessity of repositioning the patient. The lateral transabdominal approach is widely used and described in detail below in Lateral Transabdominal Approach.

Lateral Transabdominal Approach The patient is placed in the lateral decubitus position and the operating table is flexed at the waist to open the space between the lower rib cage and the iliac crest (Fig. 38-48). The surgeon and assistant both stand on the same side, facing the front of the patient. Pneumoperitoneum is created using a Veress needle or insufflation via a Hasson port. In general, four 10-mm trocars are placed between the midclavicular line medially and anterior axillary line laterally, one to two fingerbreadths below the costal margin (see Fig. 38-48), although additional ports may be placed, if needed. A 30° laparoscope is inserted through the second or midclavicular port. Most of the dissection is carried out via the two most lateral ports. However, the instruments and ports may be changed to provide optimum exposure, as needed.

For a right adrenalectomy, a fan retractor is inserted through the most medial port to retract the liver. An atraumatic grasper and an L-hook cautery are inserted via the two lateral ports for the dissection. The right triangular ligament is divided and the liver is rotated

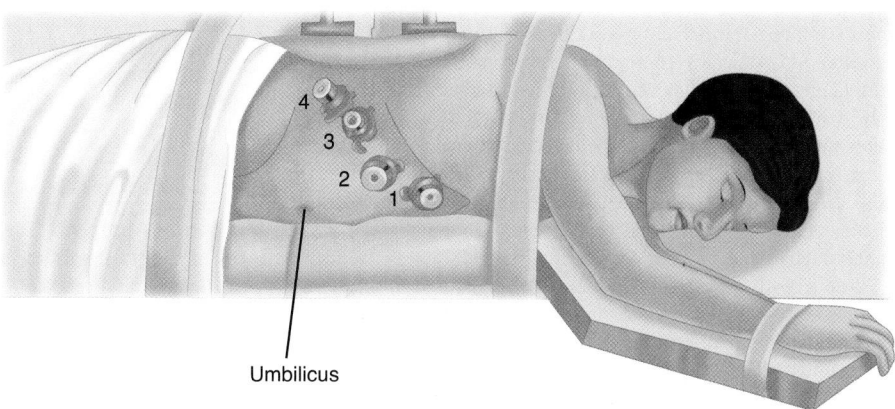

FIG. 38-48. Positioning of the patient and placement of trocars for a laparoscopic adrenalectomy. Four trocars are placed from the midclavicular to the anterior axillary line.

Umbilicus

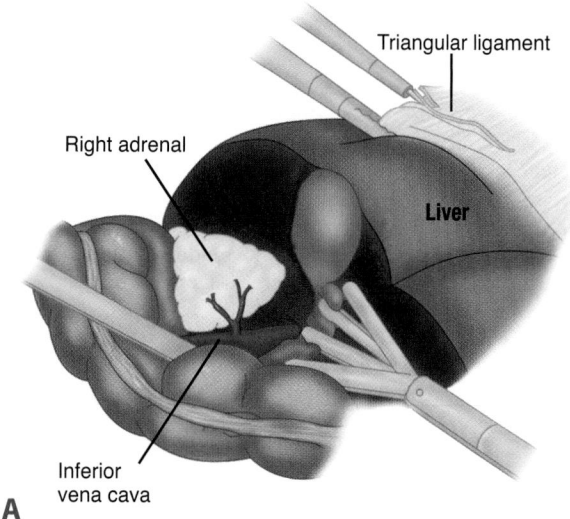

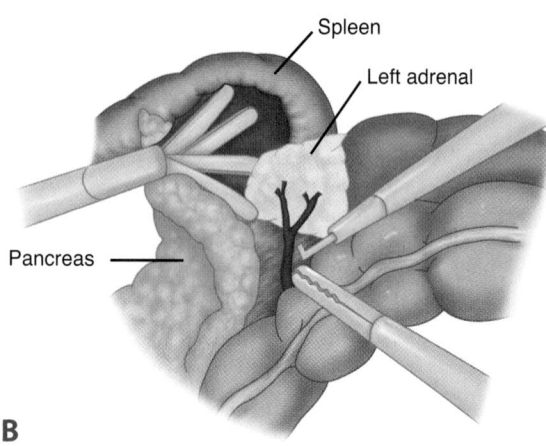

FIG. 38-49. Technique of laparoscopic adrenalectomy. Exposure of the right adrenal is facilitated by division of the triangular ligament (**A**) and dissection and reflection of the spleen and tail of the pancreas aids in identifying the left adrenal (**B**).

medially (Fig. 38-49A). Rarely, the hepatic flexure of the colon may need mobilization during a right adrenalectomy. The right kidney is identified visually and by palpation with an atraumatic grasper. The adrenal gland is identified on the superomedial aspect of the kidney. Gerota's fascia is incised with the hook cautery. Dissection of the adrenal is started superomedially and then proceeds inferiorly, dissecting around the adrenal in a clockwise manner. The periadrenal tissues are grasped or moved with a blunt grasper to facilitate circumferential dissection. The right adrenal vein is identified at its junction with the IVC, ligated with clips, and divided using endoscopic scissors. Alternatively, a vascular stapler may be used to divide the vein endoscopically. There may be a second adrenal vein on the right. Generally, two clips are left on the vena cava side. Although early identification of the adrenal vein is helpful to facilitate mobilization and prevent injury, it can be dissected whenever it is safe to do so. Early ligation of the adrenal vein makes it easier to mobilize the gland but may make subsequent dissection more difficult due to venous congestion. The arterial branches to the adrenal gland can be electrocoagulated if small or clipped and divided.

For a left adrenalectomy, the fan retractor is used to retract the spleen. The splenic flexure is mobilized early and the lateral attachments to the spleen and the tail of the pancreas are divided using the electrocautery (Fig. 38-49B). Gravity allows the spleen and the pancreatic tail to fall medially. The remainder of the dissection proceeds

similarly to that described for the right adrenal. In addition to the adrenal vein, the inferior phrenic vein, which joins the left adrenal vein medially, also needs to be dissected, doubly clipped, and divided. As with the right adrenal vein, the left-sided veins also can be divided with a vascular stapler. Once the dissection is complete, the area of the adrenal bed can be irrigated and suctioned. A drain is rarely necessary. The gland is placed in a nylon specimen bag, which is brought out via one of the ports after morcellation, if necessary.

Posterior Retroperitoneal Approach The retroperitoneal approach provides a more direct access to the adrenal gland and avoids abdominal adhesions in patients who have had previous abdominal surgery. Furthermore, bilateral adrenalectomy can be performed without repositioning the patient. Intraoperative ultrasound is helpful for identifying the adrenal but the dissection and exposure is more difficult because the working space is limited. This makes vascular control difficult and also renders it unsuitable for large (>5 cm) lesions. This technique is being increasingly used for small adenomas causing hyperaldosteronism.

The patient is placed in the prone-jackknife position, and the operating table is flexed at the waist to open the space between the posterior costal margin and the pelvis. Palpation is used to identify the position of the twelfth rib. Percutaneous ultrasound is performed to determine the outline of the underlying kidney and adrenal. When done laparoscopically, the surgeon stands on the side of the adrenal to be removed and the assistant stands on the opposite side. A 1.5-cm incision is placed 2 cm inferior and parallel to the twelfth rib, laterally at the level of the inferior pole of the kidney. Gerota's space is entered under direct vision using a 12-mm direct viewing trocar with a 0° laparoscope through the muscle layers of the posterior abdominal wall. Alternatively, blunt dissection with the surgeon's finger also can identify the space behind Gerota's fascia. The trocar is then replaced by a dissecting balloon, which is manually inflated using a hand pump under direct vision through the laparoscope. A 12-mm trocar is then reinserted into this space and CO_2 is insufflated to 12 to 15 mmHg pressure. The 0° laparoscope is replaced by a 45° laparoscope. Two additional 5- or 10-mm trocars are placed, one each on either side of the first port. Laparoscopic ultrasound then is used to help locate the adrenal gland and vessels. The adrenal dissection is begun at the superior pole and then proceeds to the lateral and inferior aspect. The medial dissection usually is performed last, and the vessels are identified and divided as described in Lateral Transabdominal Approach above.

Open Adrenalectomy

Open adrenalectomy may be performed via four approaches, each with specific advantages and disadvantages. The anterior approach allows examination of the abdominal cavity and resection of bilateral tumors via a single incision. The posterior approach avoids the morbidity of a laparotomy incision, especially in patients with cardiopulmonary disease and those prone to wound complications (Cushing's syndrome) and avoids abdominal adhesions in patients who have undergone previous abdominal surgery. Recovery time is also quicker and hospitalization shorter. However, the retroperitoneal exposure is difficult, particularly in obese patients and the small working space makes it unsuitable for tumors >6 cm in diameter. The lateral approach is best for obese patients and for large tumors because it provides a bigger working space. The thoracoabdominal approach is most useful for en bloc resection of large (>10 cm), malignant lesions. However, it is associated with significant morbidity and should be used selectively.

Anterior Approach The adrenals may be removed via a midline incision or bilateral subcostal incision (Fig. 38-50). The former allows adequate infraumbilical exposure for examination of extra-adrenal tumors, whereas the latter provides better superior and lateral exposure. For the right side, the hepatic flexure of the colon in mobilized inferiorly, the triangular ligament is incised to retract the liver medially and superiorly. A generous Kocher maneuver is used to mobilize the

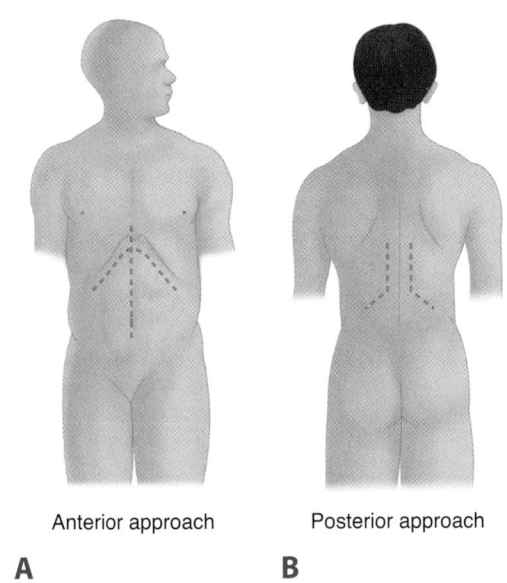

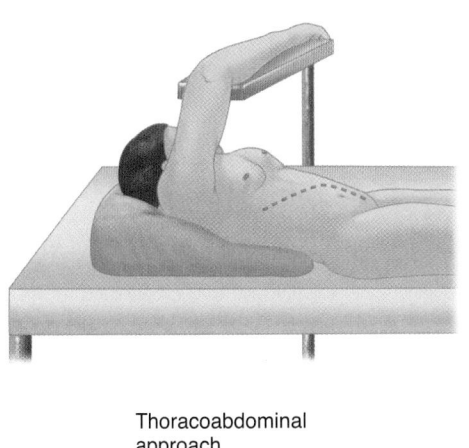

FIG. 38-50. Incisions for open adrenalectomy. Anterior approach (**A**), posterior approach (**B**), and thoracoabdominal approach (**C**).

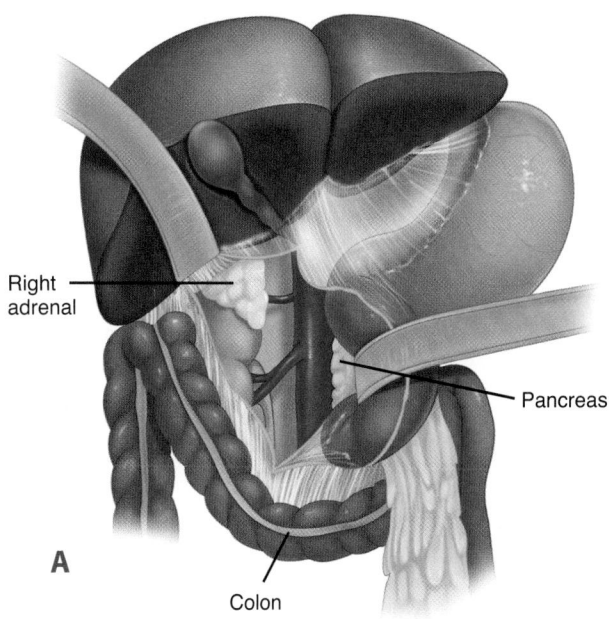

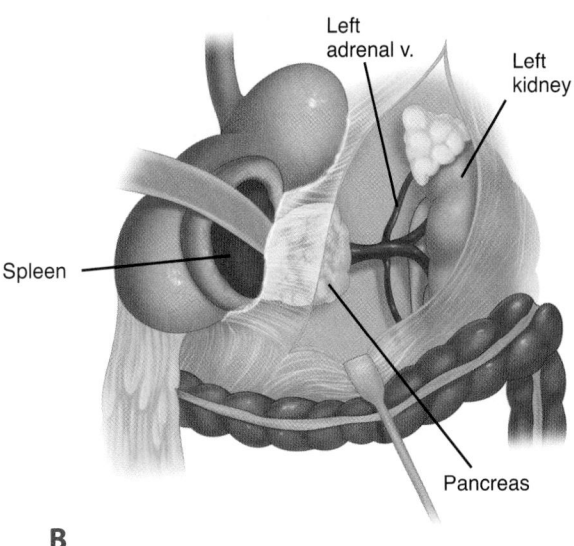

FIG. 38-51. Technique of open adrenalectomy. Exposure of the right adrenal is facilitated by a Kocher maneuver to mobilize the duodenum and upward retraction of the liver (**A**). The left adrenal can be exposed by medial visceral rotation of the spleen and pancreas (**B**). v. = vein.

duodenum anteriorly and expose the retroperitoneal fat and the IVC (Fig. 38-51A). Gerota's fascia is incised, and the gland is freed of surrounding fibro-fatty tissue and the kidney inferiorly. The lateral and superior surfaces usually are mobilized first. Then, the short, right adrenal vein is dissected, ligated, and divided, taking care not to injure the hepatic veins and IVC. On the left side, the adrenal is located cephalad to the pancreatic tail and just lateral to the aorta. For large tumors, the adrenal is best approached by medial visceral rotation to mobilize the spleen, colon, and pancreas toward the midline (Fig. 38-51B). An alternative approach is to enter the lesser sac by division of the gastrocolic ligament. The pancreas is mobilized superiorly by incision of its inferior peritoneal attachments, thus exposing the left kidney and adrenal. The gland is then mobilized as on the right side.

Posterior Approach The patient is placed prone on the operating table, similar to the laparoscopic approach. A hockey stick or curvilinear incision may be used, and extended through the latissimus dorsi and sacrospinous fascia. The twelfth rib generally is excised at its base and the eleventh rib is retracted superiorly to reveal the pleura and the lateral arcuate ligament of the liver on the right side. The pleura also is mobilized cephalad, and the adrenal and kidney are identified. The superior aspect of the gland is dissected first, and the

superior vessels are identified and ligated. This prevents superior retraction of the adrenal gland. The remainder of the gland is then dissected and the adrenal gland and tumor removed. The resulting space generally is filled with perinephric fat and closed in layers. A chest x-ray is obtained postoperatively to rule out a pneumothorax.

Lateral Approach The patient is placed in a lateral position with the table flexed and an incision is made between the eleventh and twelfth ribs or subcostally. The dissection then is performed as indicated previously in Anterior Approach.

Complications of Adrenal Surgery

Patients with Cushing's syndrome are more prone to infectious (incisional and intra-abdominal abscess) and thrombotic complications. Creation of pneumoperitoneum may result in injury to various organs from Veress needle and trocar insertion, subcutaneous emphysema, pneumothorax, and hemodynamic compromise. Excessive retraction and dissection may lead to bleeding from injury to the IVC and renal vessels, or from injury to surrounding organs such as the liver, pancreas, spleen, and stomach. Postoperative hemodynamic instability may be evident in patients with pheochromocytomas, and patients are at risk of adrenal insufficiency after bilateral adrenalectomy and sometimes after unilateral adrenalectomy (unrecognized Cushing's syndrome or, very rarely, Conn's syndrome). Long-term morbidity results mainly from injury to nerve roots during trocar insertion, which can lead to chronic pain syndromes or muscle weakness, although this is more of an issue in case of open procedures.

Approximately 30% of patients who undergo bilateral adrenalectomy for Cushing's disease are at risk of developing Nelson's syndrome from progressive growth of the pre-existing pituitary tumor. This leads to increased ACTH levels, hyperpigmentation, visual field defects, headaches, and extraocular muscle palsies. Transsphenoidal pituitary resection is the initial mode of therapy and external beam radiotherapy is used in patients with residual tumor or extrasellar invasion.

REFERENCES

Entries highlighted in bright blue are key references.

1. Plaza CP, Lopez ME, Carrasco CE, et al: Management of well-differentiated thyroglossal remnant thyroid carcinoma: time to close the debate? Report of five new cases and proposal of a definitive algorithm for treatment. *Ann Surg Oncol* 13:745, 2006.
2. Page C, Monet P, Peltier J, et al: Non-recurrent laryngeal nerve related to thyroid surgery: Report of three cases. *J Laryngol Otol* 122:757, 2008.
3. Cernea CR, Ferraz AR, Nishio S, et al: Surgical anatomy of the external branch of the superior laryngeal nerve. *Head Neck* 14:380, 1992.
4. Bouknight AL: Thyroid physiology and thyroid function testing. *Otolaryngol Clin North Am* 36:9, 2003.
5. Finkelstein SE, Grigsby PW, Siegel BA, et al: Combined [(18)F]fluorodeoxyglucose positron emission tomography and computed tomography (FDG-PET/CT) for detection of recurrent, (131)I-negative thyroid cancer. *Ann Surg Oncol* 15:286, 2008.
6. Vaidya B, Oakes EJ, Imrie H, et al: CTLA4 gene and Graves' disease: Association of Graves' disease with the CTLA4 exon 1 and intron 1 polymorphisms, but not with the promoter polymorphism. *Clin Endocrinol* 58:732, 2003.
7. Streetman DD, Khanderia U: Diagnosis and treatment of Graves disease. *Ann Pharmacother* 37:1100, 2003.
8. Hagen F, Chapman EM: Comparison of high and low dosage levels of I-131 in the treatment of thyrotoxicosis. *N Engl J Med* 277:559, 1967.
9. Singer RB: Long-term comparative cancer mortality after use of radioiodine in the treatment of hyperthyroidism, a fully reported multicenter study. *J Insur Med* 33:138, 2001.
10. Cundiff JG, Portugal L, Sarne DH: Parathyroid adenoma after radioactive iodine therapy for multinodular goiter. *Am J Otolaryngol* 22:374, 2001.
11. Muller PE, Bein B, Robens E, et al: Thyroid surgery according to Enderlen-Hotz or Dunhill: A comparison of two surgical methods for the treatment of Graves' disease. *Int Surg* 86:112, 2001.
12. Krohn K, Paschke R: Somatic mutations in thyroid nodular disease. *Mol Genet Metab* 75:202, 2002.
13. Brook I: Microbiology and management of acute suppurative thyroiditis in children. *Int J Pediatr Otorhinolaryngol* 67:447, 2003.
14. Moshynska O, Saxena A: Clonal relationship between Hashimoto's thyroiditis and thyroid lymphoma. *J Clin Pathol* 61:438, 2008.
15. Biondi B, Cooper DS: The clinical significance of subclinical thyroid dysfunction. *Endocr Rev* 29:76, 2008.
16. De M, Jaap A, Dempster J: Tamoxifen therapy in steroid-resistant Riedels disease. *Scott Med J* 47:12, 2002.
17. Knudsen N, Laurberg P, Perrild H, et al: Risk factors for goiter and thyroid nodules. *Thyroid* 12:879, 2002.
18. Ron E: Thyroid cancer incidence among people living in areas contaminated by radiation from the Chernobyl accident. *Health Phys* 93:502, 2007.
19. Kebebew E: Hereditary non-medullary thyroid cancer. *World J Surg* 32:678, 2008.
20. Bajaj Y, De M, Thompson A: Fine needle aspiration cytology in diagnosis and management of thyroid disease. *J Laryngol Otol* 120:467, 2006.
21. Nobrega LH, Paiva FJ, Nobrega ML, et al: Predicting malignant involvement in a thyroid nodule: Role of ultrasonography. *Endocr Pract* 13:219, 2007.
22. Nikiforova MN, Nikiforov YE: Molecular genetics of thyroid cancer: Implications for diagnosis, treatment and prognosis. *Expert Rev Mol Diagn* 8:83, 2008.
23. Thomas GA, Bunnell H, Cook HA, et al: High prevalence of RET/PTC rearrangements in Ukrainian and Belarussian post-Chernobyl thyroid papillary carcinomas: A strong correlation between RET/PTC3 and the solid-follicular variant. *J Clin Endocrinol Metab* 84:4232, 1999.
24. Xing M: BRAF mutation in papillary thyroid cancer: Pathogenic role, molecular bases, and clinical implications. *Endocr Rev* 28:742, 2007.
25. Lui WO, Foukakis T, Liden J, et al: Expression profiling reveals a distinct transcription signature in follicular thyroid carcinomas with a PAX8-PPAR(gamma) fusion oncogene. *Oncogene* 24:1467, 2005.
26. Roti E, Rossi R, Trasforini G, et al: Clinical and histological characteristics of papillary thyroid microcarcinoma: Results of a retrospective study in 243 patients. *J Clin Endocrinol Metab* 91:2171, 2006.
27. Hay ID, Grant CS, Taylor WF, et al: Ipsilateral lobectomy versus bilateral lobar resection in papillary thyroid carcinoma: A retrospective analysis of surgical outcome using a novel prognostic scoring system. *Surgery* 102:1088, 1987.
28. Cady B, Rossi R: An expanded view of risk-group definition in differentiated thyroid carcinoma. *Surgery* 104:947, 1988.
29. *AJCC Cancer Staging Manual*, 6th ed. New York: Springer-Verlag, 2002.
30. DeGroot LJ, Kaplan EL, McCormick M, et al: Natural history, treatment, and course of papillary thyroid carcinoma. *J Clin Endocrinol Metab* 71:414, 1990.
31. Lee JH, Lee ES, Kim YS: Clinicopathologic significance of BRAF V600E mutation in papillary carcinomas of the thyroid: A meta-analysis. *Cancer* 110:38, 2007.
32. Cady B, Sedgwick CE, Meissner WA, et al: Risk factor analysis in differentiated thyroid cancer. *Cancer* 43:810, 1979.
33. Mazzaferri EL, Jhiang SM: Long-term impact of initial surgical and medical therapy on papillary and follicular thyroid cancer. *Am J Med* 97:418, 1994.
34. Hay ID, Grant CS, Bergstralh EJ, et al: Unilateral total lobectomy: Is it sufficient surgical treatment for patients with AMES low-risk papillary thyroid carcinoma? *Surgery* 124:958; discussion 64, 1998.
35. Mazzaferri EL, Massoll N: Management of papillary and follicular (differentiated) thyroid cancer: New paradigms using recombinant human thyrotropin. *Endocr Relat Cancer* 9:227, 2002.
36. Bilimoria KY, Bentrem DJ, Ko CY, et al: Extent of surgery affects survival for papillary thyroid cancer. *Ann Surg* 246:375; discussion 81, 2007.
37. Cooper DS, Doherty GM, Haugen BR, et al: Management guidelines for patients with thyroid nodules and differentiated thyroid cancer. *Thyroid* 16:109, 2006.
38. Sivanandan R, Soo KC: Pattern of cervical lymph node metastases from papillary carcinoma of the thyroid. *Br J Surg* 88:1241, 2001.
39. Hunt JL, Yim JH, Tometsko M, et al: Loss of heterozygosity of the VHL gene identifies malignancy and predicts death in follicular thyroid tumors. *Surgery* 134:1043; discussion 7, 2003.
40. Carroll NM, Carty SE: Promising molecular techniques for discriminating among follicular thyroid neoplasms. *Surg Oncol* 15:59, 2006.
41. Weber F, Teresi RE, Broelsch CE, et al: A limited set of human MicroRNA is deregulated in follicular thyroid carcinoma. *J Clin Endocrinol Metab* 91:3584, 2006.
42. Thompson LD, Wieneke JA, Paal E, et al: A clinicopathologic study of minimally invasive follicular carcinoma of the thyroid gland with a review of the English literature. *Cancer* 91:505, 2001.
43. Short SC, Suovuori A, Cook G, et al: A phase II study using retinoids as redifferentiation agents to increase iodine uptake in metastatic thyroid cancer. *Clin Oncol (R Coll Radiol)* 16:569, 2004.
44. Keum KC, Suh YG, Koom WS, et al: The role of postoperative external-beam radiotherapy in the management of patients with papillary thyroid cancer invading the trachea. *Int J Radiat Oncol Biol Phys* 65:474, 2006.
45. Cunha N, Rodrigues F, Curado F, et al: Thyroglobulin detection in fine-needle aspirates of cervical lymph nodes: A technique for the

diagnosis of metastatic differentiated thyroid cancer. *Eur J Endocrinol* 157:101, 2007.

46. Skinner MA, Safford SD, Freemerman AJ: RET tyrosine kinase and medullary thyroid cells are unaffected by clinical doses of STI571. *Anticancer Res* 23:3601, 2003.

47. de Groot JW, Plaza Menacho I, Schepers H, et al: Cellular effects of imatinib on medullary thyroid cancer cells harboring multiple endocrine neoplasia Type 2A and 2B associated RET mutations. *Surgery* 139:806, 2006.

48. Chatal JF, Campion L, Kraeber-Bodere F, et al: Survival improvement in patients with medullary thyroid carcinoma who undergo pretargeted anti-carcinoembryonic-antigen radioimmunotherapy: A collaborative study with the French Endocrine Tumor Group. *J Clin Oncol* 24:170, 2006.

49. Brandi ML, Gagel RF, Angeli A, et al: Guidelines for diagnosis and therapy of MEN type 1 and type 2. *J Clin Endocrinol Metab* 86:5658, 2001.

50. Skinner MA, Moley JA, Dilley WG, et al: Prophylactic thyroidectomy in multiple endocrine neoplasia type 2A. *N Engl J Med* 353:1105, 2005.

51. Iagaru A, Masamed R, Singer PA, et al: Detection of occult medullary thyroid cancer recurrence with 2-deoxy-2-[F-18]fluoro-D-glucose-PET and PET/CT. *Mol Imaging Biol* 9:72, 2007.

52. Brignardello E, Gallo M, Baldi I, et al: Anaplastic thyroid carcinoma: Clinical outcome of 30 consecutive patients referred to a single institution in the past 5 years. *Eur J Endocrinol* 156:425, 2007.

53. de Perrot M, Fadel E, Mercier O, et al: Surgical management of mediastinal goiters: When is a sternotomy required? *Thorac Cardiovasc Surg* 55:39, 2007.

54. Chan WF, Lang BH, Lo CY: The role of intraoperative neuromonitoring of recurrent laryngeal nerve during thyroidectomy: A comparative study on 1000 nerves at risk. *Surgery* 140:866; discussion 72, 2006.

55. Akerström G, Malmaeus J, Bergstrom R: Surgical anatomy of human parathyroid glands. *Surgery* 95:14, 1984.

56. Gilmour J: The gross anatomy of the parathyroid glands. *J Pathol* 46:133, 1938.

57. Raue F, Haag C, Schulze E, et al: The role of the extracellular calcium-sensing receptor in health and disease. *Exp Clin Endocrinol Diabetes* 114:397, 2006.

58. Awad SS, Miskulin J, Thompson N: Parathyroid adenomas versus four-gland hyperplasia as the cause of primary hyperparathyroidism in patients with prolonged lithium therapy. *World J Surg* 27:486, 2003.

59. Doherty GM. Multiple endocrine neoplasia type 1. *J Surg Oncol* 89:143, 2005.

60. Balogh K, Racz K, Patocs A, et al: Menin and its interacting proteins: Elucidation of menin function. *Trends Endocrinol Metab* 17:357, 2006.

61. Shattuck TM, Valimaki S, Obara T, et al: Somatic and germ-line mutations of the HRPT2 gene in sporadic parathyroid carcinoma. *N Engl J Med* 349:1722, 2003.

62. Talpos GB, Bone HG 3rd, Kleerekoper M, et al: Randomized trial of parathyroidectomy in mild asymptomatic primary hyperparathyroidism: Patient description and effects on the SF-36 health survey. *Surgery* 128:1013; discussion 20, 2000.

63. Greutelaers B, Kullen K, Kollias J, et al: Pasieka Illness Questionnaire: Its value in primary hyperparathyroidism. *ANZ J Surg* 74:112, 2004.

64. Vestergaard P, Mollerup CL, Frokjaer VG, et al: Cardiovascular events before and after surgery for primary hyperparathyroidism. *World J Surg* 27:216, 2003.

65. Hedback G, Tisell LE, Bengtsson BA, et al: Premature death in patients operated on for primary hyperparathyroidism. *World J Surg* 14:829; discussion 36, 1990.

66. Wermers RA, Khosla S, Atkinson EJ, et al: Survival after the diagnosis of hyperparathyroidism: A population-based study. *Am J Med* 104:115, 1998.

67. Scholz DA, Purnell DC: Asymptomatic primary hyperparathyroidism. 10-year prospective study. *Mayo Clin Proc* 56:473, 1981.

68. Silverberg SJ, Shane E, Jacobs TP, et al: A 10-year prospective study of primary hyperparathyroidism with or without parathyroid surgery. *N Engl J Med* 341:1249, 1999.

69. Proceedings of the NIH Consensus Development Conference on diagnosis and management of asymptomatic primary hyperparathyroidism. Bethesda, Maryland, October 29–31, 1990. *J Bone Miner Res* 6:S1, 1991.

70. Bilezikian JP, Potts JT Jr., Fuleihan Gel H, et al: Summary statement from a workshop on asymptomatic primary hyperparathyroidism: A perspective for the 21st century. *J Clin Endocrinol Metab* 87:5353, 2002.

71. Sheldon DG, Lee FT, Neil NJ, et al: Surgical treatment of hyperparathyroidism improves health-related quality of life. *Arch Surg* 137:1022; discussion 6, 2002.

72. Sackett WR, Bambach CP: Bilateral subtotal laparoscopic adrenalectomy for phaeochromocytoma. *ANZ J Surg* 73:664, 2003.

73. Johnson NA, Tublin ME, Ogilvie JB: Parathyroid imaging: Technique and role in the preoperative evaluation of primary hyperparathyroidism. *AJR Am J Roentgenol* 188:1706, 2007.

74. Lavely WC, Goetze S, Friedman KP, et al: Comparison of SPECT/CT, SPECT, and planar imaging with single- and dual-phase (99m)Tc-sestamibi parathyroid scintigraphy. *J Nucl Med* 48:1084, 2007.

75. Fujii H, Kubo A: Sestamibi scintigraphy for the application of minimally invasive surgery of hyperfunctioning parathyroid lesions. *Biomed Pharmacother* 56:7s, 2002.

76. Sharma J, Milas M, Berber E, et al: Value of intraoperative parathyroid hormone monitoring. *Ann Surg Oncol* 15:493, 2008.

77. Westerdahl J, Bergenfelz A: Unilateral versus bilateral neck exploration for primary hyperparathyroidism: Five-year follow-up of a randomized controlled trial. *Ann Surg* 246:976, 2007.

78. Gagner M: Endoscopic subtotal parathyroidectomy in patients with primary hyperparathyroidism. *Br J Surg* 83:875, 1996.

79. Silverberg SJ, Rubin MR, Faiman C, et al: Cinacalcet hydrochloride reduces the serum calcium concentration in inoperable parathyroid carcinoma. *J Clin Endocrinol Metab* 92:3803, 2007.

80. Carpenter JM, Michaelson PG, Lidner TK, et al: Parathyromatosis. *Ear Nose Throat J* 86:21, 2007.

81. Caron NR, Sturgeon C, Clark OH: Persistent and recurrent hyperparathyroidism. *Curr Treat Options Oncol* 5:335, 2004.

82. Elder GJ: Parathyroidectomy in the calcimimetic era. *Nephrology* 10:511, 2005.

83. Triponez F, Kebebew E, Dosseh D, et al: Less-than-subtotal parathyroidectomy increases the risk of persistent/recurrent hyperparathyroidism after parathyroidectomy in tertiary hyperparathyroidism after renal transplantation. *Surgery* 140:990; discussion 7, 2006.

84. Schirpenbach C, Reincke M: Primary aldosteronism: Current knowledge and controversies in Conn's syndrome. *Nat Clin Pract Endocrinol Metab* 3:220, 2007.

85. Rossi GP: New concepts in adrenal vein sampling for aldosterone in the diagnosis of primary aldosteronism. *Curr Hypertens Rep* 9:90, 2007.

86. Pecori Giraldi F, Ambrogio AG, De Martin M, et al: Specificity of first-line tests for the diagnosis of Cushing's syndrome: Assessment in a large series. *J Clin Endocrinol Metab* 92:4123, 2007.

87. Rodgers SE, Evans DB, Lee JE, et al: Adrenocortical carcinoma. *Surg Oncol Clin N Am* 15:535, 2006.

88. Copeland PM: The incidentally discovered adrenal mass. *Ann Surg* 199:116, 1984.

89. Sturgeon C, Shen WT, Clark OH, et al: Risk assessment in 457 adrenal cortical carcinomas: How much does tumor size predict the likelihood of malignancy? *J Am Coll Surg* 202:423, 2006.

90. Aubert S, Wacrenier A, Leroy X, et al: Weiss system revisited: A clinicopathologic and immunohistochemical study of 49 adrenocortical tumors. *Am J Surg Pathol* 26:1612, 2002.

91. Terzolo M, Angeli A, Fassnacht M, et al: Adjuvant mitotane treatment for adrenocortical carcinoma. *N Engl J Med* 356:2372, 2007.

92. Karagiannis A, Mikhailidis DP, Athyros VG, et al: Pheochromocytoma: An update on genetics and management. *Endocr Relat Cancer* 14:935, 2007.

93. Machens A, Brauckhoff M, Gimm O, et al: Risk-oriented approach to hereditary adrenal pheochromocytoma. *Ann N Y Acad Sci* 1073:417, 2006.

94. Shen WT, Sturgeon C, Clark OH, et al: Should pheochromocytoma size influence surgical approach? A comparison of 90 malignant and 60 benign pheochromocytomas. *Surgery* 136:1129, 2004.

95. Sippel RS, Chen H: Subclinical Cushing's syndrome in adrenal incidentalomas. *Surg Clin North Am* 84:875, 2004.

96. Strong VE, D'Angelica M, Tang L, et al: Laparoscopic adrenalectomy for isolated adrenal metastasis. *Ann Surg Oncol* 14:3392, 2007.

Pediatric Surgery

David J. Hackam, Tracy C. Grikscheit,
Kasper S. Wang, Kurt D. Newman,
and Henri R. Ford

INTRODUCTION

In his classic 1953 textbook titled *The Surgery of Infancy and Childhood*, Dr. Robert E. Gross summarized the essential challenge of pediatric surgery as follows: "Those who daily operate on adults, even with the greatest of skill, are sometimes appalled—or certainly are not at their best—when called upon to operate on and care for a tiny patient. Something more than diminutive instruments or scaled-down operative manipulations are necessary to do the job in a suitable manner." To this day, surgical residents and other trainees often approach the pediatric surgical patient with the same mix of fear and anxiety, yet generally complete their pediatric surgical experience with genuine respect for the resilience of children and for the precision required in their care both in the operating room and during the perioperative period. Over the decades, the specialty of pediatric surgery has evolved considerably. Our ability to care for the smallest of

patients with surgical disorders has increased dramatically, so that even in utero surgery is now an option in certain circumstances. Similarly, our mastery of the pathophysiology of the diseases that pediatric surgeons face has increased to the point that many of these diseases are now understood at the level of molecular or cellular signaling pathways. Pediatric surgery provides the opportunity to intervene positively in a wide array of diseases and to exert a long-lasting impact on the lives of children and their grateful parents. The scope of diseases encountered in the standard practice of pediatric surgery is immense, with patients ranging in age from fetus to 18-year-olds, and includes anomalies of the head and neck, thoracic, GI, and genitourinary areas. This chapter is not designed to cover the entire spectrum of diseases a pediatric surgeon is expected to master; rather, it presents a synopsis of a handful of pediatric surgical conditions that a practicing general surgeon is likely to encounter over the course of his or her career.

PEDIATRIC SURGICAL THEMES: PITFALLS AND PEARLS

This chapter focuses on the unique considerations in the diagnosis and management of surgical diseases in the pediatric population. Many surgical trainees approach the surgical care of children with some degree of fear and trepidation. As any pediatric caregiver will attest, the surgical management of infants and children requires careful and professional interactions with their parents. The stress that the parents of sick children experience in the hospital setting can, at times, be overwhelming. It is due, in part, to the uncertainty regarding a particular prognosis, the feeling of helplessness that evolves when one is unable to care for one's child, and, in certain cases, the guilt or remorse that one feels for not seeking medical care earlier or for consenting to a particular procedure. Management of the sick child and his or her family therefore requires not only a certain set of skills but also a unique knowledge base. This section is included to summarize some important general principles in accomplishing this task.

1. Children are not little adults, but they are little people.

    In practical terms, this often-heard refrain implies that children have unique fluid, electrolyte, and medication needs. Thus, the dosage of medications and the administration of IV fluids should be based on the child's weight. The corollary of this point is that infants and young children are extremely sensitive to perturbations in their normal physiology and, because of this, may be easily tipped into fluid overload or dehydration.

2. Children whisper before they shout.

    Children with surgical diseases can deteriorate very quickly. But before they deteriorate, they often manifest subtle physical findings. These findings—referred to as *whispers*—may include signs such as tachycardia, bradycardia, hypothermia, fever, recurrent emesis, or feeding intolerance. Meticulous attention to these subtle findings may unmask the development of potentially serious, life-threatening physiologic disturbances.

3. Always listen to the mother and the father.

    Surgical diseases in children can be very difficult to diagnose because children are often minimally communicative and the information they do communicate may be confusing, conflicting, or both. In all cases, it is wise to listen to the child's parents, who have closely observed their child and know him or her best.

4. Children experience pain after surgery.

    Careful and adequate pain management must accompany surgical interventions.

5. Pediatric tissue must be handled delicately.

KEY POINTS

1. In infants with Bochdalek type congenital diaphragmatic hernia the severity of pulmonary hypoplasia and the resultant pulmonary hypertension are key determinants of survival. Barotrauma and hypoxia should be avoided.

2. During initial management of an infant with esophageal atresia and distal tracheoesophageal fistula, every effort should be made to avoid distending the gastrointestinal tract, especially when using mechanical ventilation. The patient should be evaluated for components of the VACTERL (vertebral, anorectal, cardiac, tracheoesophageal, renal, limb) anomalies. Timing and extent of surgery is dictated by the stability of the patient.

3. Although malrotation with midgut volvulus occurs most commonly within the first few weeks of life, it should always be considered in the differential diagnosis in a child with bilious emesis. Volvulus is a surgical emergency; therefore in a critically ill child, prompt surgical intervention should not be delayed for any reason.

4. When evaluating a newborn infant for vomiting, it is critical to distinguish between proximal and distal causes of intestinal obstruction utilizing both prenatal and postnatal history, physical examination and abdominal radiographs.

5. Risk factors for necrotizing enterocolitis (NEC) include prematurity, formula feeding, bacterial infection, and intestinal ischemia. Critical to the management of infants with advanced (Bell stage III) or perforated NEC is timely and adequate source control of peritoneal contamination. Early sequelae of NEC include perforation, sepsis, and death. Later sequelae include short-bowel syndrome and stricture.

6. In patients with intestinal obstruction secondary to Hirschsprung's disease a leveling ostomy or endorectal pull through should be performed using ganglionated bowel, proximal to the transition zone between ganglionic and aganglionic intestine.

7. Prognosis of infants with biliary atresia is directly related to age at diagnosis and timing of portoenterostomy. Infants with advanced age at the time of diagnosis or infants who fail to demonstrate evidence of bile drainage after portoenterostomy usually require liver transplantation.

8. Infants with omphaloceles have greater associated morbidity and mortality than infants with gastroschisis due to a higher incidence of congenital anomalies and pulmonary hypoplasia. Gastroschisis can be associated with intestinal atresia, but not with other congenital anomalies. An intact omphalocele can be repaired electively, while gastroschisis requires urgent intervention to protect the exposed intestine.

9. Prognosis for children with Wilms' tumor is defined by the stage of disease at the time of diagnosis and the histologic type (favorable vs. unfavorable). Preoperative chemotherapy is indicated for bilateral involvement, a solitary kidney, or tumor in the inferior vena cava above the hepatic veins. Gross tumor rupture during surgery automatically changes the stage to 3 (at a minimum).

10. Injury is the leading cause of death in children older than 1 year of age. Blunt mechanisms account for the majority of pediatric injuries. The central nervous system is the most commonly injured organ system and the leading cause of death in injured children.

GENERAL CONSIDERATIONS

Fluid and Electrolyte Balance

In management of the pediatric surgical patient, an understanding of fluid and electrolyte balance is critical, because the margin between dehydration and fluid overload is rather small. This is particularly true in infants, who have little reserve. Failure to pay meticulous attention to their hydration status can result in significant fluid overload or dehydration. Several surgical diagnoses, such as gastroschisis and short-bowel syndrome, are characterized by a predisposition to fluid loss. Others require judicious restoration of intravascular volume to prevent cardiac failure, as is the case in patients with congenital diaphragmatic hernia and associated pulmonary hypertension. The infant's physiologic day is approximately 8 hours in duration. Accordingly, careful assessment of the individual patient's fluid balance, including fluid intake and output for the previous 8 hours, is essential to prevent dehydration or fluid overload. Clinical signs of dehydration include tachycardia, decreased urine output, reduced skin turgor, a depressed fontanelle, absent tears, lethargy, and poor feeding. Fluid overload is often manifested by a new requirement for oxygen and the onset of respiratory distress, tachypnea, and tachycardia. The physical assessment of the fluid status of each child must include a complete head-to-toe evaluation, with emphasis on determining whether perturbations in normal physiology are present.

At 12 weeks' gestation, the total body water of a fetus is approximately 94 mL/kg. By the time the fetus reaches full term, the total body water has decreased to approximately 80 mL/kg. Total body water drops an additional 5% within the first week of life, and by 1 year of life, total body water approaches adult levels, 60 to 65 mL/kg. Parallel to the drop in total body water is the reduction in extracellular fluid. These changes are accelerated in the preterm infant, who may face additional fluid losses due to coexisting congenital anomalies or surgery. The volume of normal daily maintenance fluids for most children can be estimated using the following formula: 100 mL/kg for the first 10 kg, plus 50 mL/kg for 11 to 20 kg, plus 25 mL/kg for each additional kilogram of body weight thereafter. Because IV fluid orders are written as milliliters per hour, this can be conveniently converted to 4 mL/kg per hour up to 10 kg, plus 2 mL/kg per hour for 11 to 20 kg, and an additional 1 mL/kg per hour for each additional kilogram of body weight thereafter. For example, a 26-kg child has an estimated maintenance fluid requirement of $(10 \times 4) + (10 \times 2) + (6 \times 1) = 66$ mL/h in the absence of massive fluid losses or shock. A newborn infant with gastroschisis will manifest significant evaporative losses from the exposed bowel, so that fluid requirements will be in the range of 150 to 180 mL/kg per day.

Precise management of a neonate's fluid status requires an understanding of changes in the glomerular filtration rate (GFR) and tubular function of the kidney. The full-term newborn's GFR is approximately 21 mL/min per square meter compared with 70 mL/min per square meter in an adult. Within the first year GFR increases steadily to the point that it essentially reaches adult levels by the end of the first year of life. The capacity to concentrate urine is very limited in preterm and term infants. In comparison with an adult who can concentrate urine to 1200 mOsm/kg, infants can concentrate urine at best to 600 mOsm/kg. Although infants are capable of secreting antidiuretic hormone, the aquaporin water channel–mediated osmotic water permeability of the infant's collecting tubules is severely limited compared with that of an adult, which leads to insensitivity to antidiuretic hormone.

Sodium requirements range from 2 mEq/kg per day in term infants to 5 mEq/kg per day in critically ill preterm infants as a consequence of salt wasting. Potassium requirements range from 1 to 2 mEq/kg per day. Calcium and magnesium supplementation of IV fluids is essential to prevent laryngospasm, dysrhythmias, and tetany.

Acid-Base Equilibrium

Acute metabolic acidosis usually implies inadequate tissue perfusion and is a serious disorder in children. Potentially life-threatening causes that are specific for the pediatric population must be sought.

They include intestinal ischemia from necrotizing enterocolitis (in the neonate), midgut volvulus, and incarcerated hernia. Other causes include chronic bicarbonate loss from the GI tract and acid accumulation as in chronic renal failure. Respiratory acidosis implies hypoventilation, the cause of which should be apparent. Treatment of acute metabolic acidosis should be aimed at restoring tissue perfusion by addressing the underlying abnormality first. For severe metabolic acidemia in which the serum pH is <7.25, sodium bicarbonate should be administered using the following guideline: base deficit × weight in kilograms × 0.5 (in newborns). The last factor in the equation should be 0.4 for smaller children and 0.3 for older children. The dose should be diluted to a concentration of 0.5 mEq/mL, because full-strength sodium bicarbonate is hyperosmolar. One half the corrective dose is given, and the serum pH is measured again. During cardiopulmonary resuscitation, one half the corrective dose can be given as an IV bolus and the other half given slowly IV.

Respiratory alkalosis is usually caused by hyperventilation, which is readily correctable. Metabolic alkalosis most commonly implies gastric acid loss, as in the child with pyloric stenosis, or aggressive diuretic therapy. In the child with gastric fluid loss, administration of IV fluids with 5% dextrose, 0.5% normal saline, and 20 mEq KCl/L usually corrects the alkalosis. Potassium, however, should not be administered until adequate urine output has been established.

Blood Volume and Blood Replacement

Criteria for blood transfusion in infants and children remain poorly defined. The decision to transfuse a critically ill pediatric patient may depend on a number of clinical features that include the patient's age; the primary diagnosis; the presence of ongoing bleeding, coagulopathy, hypoxia, hemodynamic compromise, lactic acidosis, and/or cyanotic heart disease; and the overall severity of the illness. A recent survey of transfusion practices among pediatric intensivists showed that the baseline hemoglobin levels that would prompt them to recommend red blood cell (RBC) transfusion ranged from 7 to 13 g/dL. Patients with cyanotic heart disease are often transfused to higher hemoglobin values, although the threshold for transfusion in this population remains to be defined. To decrease the need for transfusion, other strategies have been considered. Studies in both critically ill adults and neonates have shown that administration of erythropoietin decreases RBC transfusion requirements. In general, there is a trend toward an avoidance of the use of RBC products whenever possible, because current studies suggest that lower hemoglobin concentrations are well tolerated by many groups of patients and that administration of RBCs may have unintended negative consequences. In addition, there is increasing evidence that transfusion of packed red blood cells (PRBCs) may have adverse effects on the host immune system in both children and adults.

A useful guideline for estimating blood volume for the newborn infant is approximately 80 mL/kg of body weight. When PRBCs are required, the transfusion requirement is usually administered in 10 mL/kg increments, which is roughly equivalent to a 500-mL transfusion for a 70-kg adult. The following formula may be used to determine the volume (in milliliters) of PRBCs to be transfused:

$$(\text{Target hematocrit} - \text{current hematocrit}) \times \text{weight (kg)} \times 80/65$$

(65 represents the estimated hematocrit of a unit of PRBCs). One transfusion from one donor is preferable to many smaller-volume transfusions. In the child, coagulation deficiencies may rapidly assume clinical significance after extensive blood transfusion. It is advisable to have fresh-frozen plasma and platelets available if >30 mL/kg has been transfused. Plasma is given in a dose of 10 to 20 mL/kg and platelets are given in a dose of 1 unit/5 kg. Each unit of platelets consists of 40 to 60 mL of fluid (plasma plus platelets). After transfusion of PRBCs to neonates with tenuous fluid balance, a single dose of a diuretic (such as furosemide 1 mg/kg) may help to facilitate excretion of the extra fluid load.

Enteral and Parenteral Nutrition

The nutritional requirements of the surgical neonate must be met for the child to grow and for surgical wounds to heal. If inadequate protein and carbohydrate calories are given, the child may not only fail to recover from surgery but may also exhibit growth failure and impaired development of the central nervous system. In general, the adequacy of growth must be assessed frequently by determining both total body weight and head circumference. Neonates with gastroschisis, intestinal atresia, or intestinal insufficiency from other causes, such as necrotizing enterocolitis, are particularly predisposed to protein-calorie malnutrition. The protein and caloric requirements for the surgical neonate are shown in Table 39-1.

Nutrition can be provided via either the enteral or parenteral route. Whenever possible, the enteral route is preferred, because it not only promotes the growth and function of the GI system but also ensures that the infant learns how to feed. Various enteral feeding preparations are available; these are listed in Table 39-2. The choice of formula is based on the individual clinical state of the child. Pediatric surgeons are occasionally faced with situations in which oral feeding is not possible. This problem can be seen in the extremely premature infant who has not yet developed the required feeding skills or in the infant with concomitant craniofacial anomalies that impair sucking, for example. In these instances, enteral feeds can be administered via either a nasojejunal or a gastrostomy tube.

When the GI tract cannot be used because of mechanical, ischemic, inflammatory, or functional disorders, parenteral alimentation must be given. Prolonged parenteral nutrition is delivered via a central venous catheter. Peripheral IV alimentation can be given using less concentrated but greater volumes of solutions. Long-term parenteral nutrition should include supplemental copper, zinc, and iron to prevent the development of trace metal deficiencies. A major complication of long-term TPN is the development of parenteral nutrition–associated cholestasis, which can eventually progress to liver failure. To prevent this major complication, concomitant enteral feedings must be instituted as soon as possible. When proximal stomas are in place, GI continuity should be restored as soon as possible. When intestinal insufficiency is associated with dilatation of the small intestine, tapering or intestinal lengthening procedures may be beneficial. Other strategies to minimize the development of TPN-related liver disease include meticulous catheter care to avoid infection, which increases cholestatic symptoms, aggressive treatment of any infection, and early cycling of parenteral nutrition in older children who can tolerate not receiving continuous dextrose solution for a limited period. Preliminary evidence in a study of 18 patients suggests the possibility that substituting omega-3 fish oil lipid emulsion for the standard soybean-based emulsions in parenteral nutritional formulas may prevent the development of TPN-related cholestasis and reverse the effects of established liver disease.

Venous Access

Obtaining reliable vascular access in an infant or child is a major responsibility of the pediatric surgeon. The goal should always be to place the catheter in the least invasive, least risky, and least painful manner, and in a location that is most accessible and facilitates long-term catheter use. In infants, central venous access may be established using a cutdown approach, either in the antecubital fossa, external jugular vein, facial vein, or proximal saphenous vein. If the internal jugular vein is used, care is taken to prevent venous occlusion. In infants >2 kg and in older children, percutaneous access of the subclavian, internal jugular, or femoral vein is possible in most cases, and central access is achieved using the Seldinger technique. The catheters are tunneled to an exit site separate from the venotomy site. Where available, peripherally inserted central catheter lines may be placed, typically via the antecubital fossa. Regardless of whether the catheter is placed by a cutdown approach or percutaneously, a chest radiograph to confirm the central location of the catheter tip and to exclude the presence of a pneumothorax or hemothorax is mandatory. When discussing the placement of central venous catheters with parents, it is important to note that the complication rate for central venous lines in children is high. The incidence of catheter-related sepsis or infection approaches 10% in many series. Superior or inferior vena caval occlusion is a significant risk after the placement of multiple lines, particularly in the smallest premature patients.

Thermoregulation

Careful regulation of the ambient environment of infants and children is crucial, because these patients are extremely thermolabile. Premature infants are particularly susceptible to changes in environmental temperature. Because they are unable to shiver and lack stores of fat, their potential for thermogenesis is impaired. This is compounded by the administration of anesthetic and paralyzing agents. Because these patients lack adaptive mechanisms to cope with the environment, the environment must be regulated. Attention to heat conservation during transport of the infant to and from the operating room is essential. Transport systems incorporating heating units are necessary for premature infants. In the operating room, the infant is kept warm by the use of overhead heating lamps, a heating blanket, warming of inspired gases, and coverage of the extremities and head with occlusive materials. During abdominal surgery, extreme care is taken to avoid wet and cold drapes. All fluids used to irrigate the chest or abdomen must be warmed to body temperature. The use of laparoscopic approaches for abdominal operations may result in more stable thermoregulation, due to decreased heat loss from the smaller wound. Constant monitoring of the child's temperature is critical in a lengthy procedure, and the surgeon should continuously communicate with the anesthesiologist regarding the temperature of the patient. The development of hypothermia in infants and children can result in cardiac arrhythmias or coagulopathy. These potentially life-threatening complications can be avoided by careful attention to thermoregulation.

TABLE 39-2 Formulas for pediatric surgical neonates

Formula	Calories (kcal/mL)	Protein (g/mL)	Fat (g/mL)	Carbohydrate (g/mL)
Human milk	0.67	0.011	0.04	0.07
Milk based				
Enfamil 20	0.67	0.015	0.038	0.069
Similac 20	0.67	0.015	0.036	0.072
Soy based				
ProSobee LIPIL	0.67	0.02	0.036	0.07
Isomil	0.67	0.018	0.037	0.068
Special				
Pregestimil LIPIL	0.67	0.019	0.028	0.091
Alimentum	0.67	0.019	0.038	0.068
Preterm				
Enfamil Premature LIPIL	0.80	0.024	0.041	0.089
Neocate	0.71	0.023	0.035	0.081

TABLE 39-1 Nutritional requirements for the pediatric surgical patient

Age	Calories (kcal/kg per day)	Protein (g/kg per day)
0–6 mo	100–120	2
6 mo–1 y	100	1.5
1–3 y	100	1.2
4–6 y	90	1
7–10 y	70	1
11–14 y	55	1
15–18 y	45	1

CHAPTER 39 Pediatric Surgery

Pain Control

All children, including neonates, experience pain. Therefore, the careful recognition and management of pediatric pain represents an important component of the perioperative management of all pediatric surgical patients. A range of pain management options are available that can improve the child's as well as the parents' comfort. The use of a pacifier, which may be dipped in sucrose, has been shown to decrease crying time and neonatal pain scores after minor procedures. Additional analgesic modalities include the use of topical anesthetic ointment (cream containing a eutectic mixture of local anesthetics) and the use of regional anesthesia, such as caudal blocks for hernias and epidural or incisional catheter infusions (On-Q system) for large abdominal or thoracic incisions. For situations in which more pain is expected, IV narcotic agents should be used. Morphine and fentanyl have an acceptable safety margin and can be administered judiciously to neonates and children. A recent randomized trial showed that administration of a morphine infusion in neonates receiving artificial ventilation decreased the incidence of intraventricular hemorrhage by 50%. In neonatal surgical patients who have been given large concentrations of narcotics over a prolonged period, transient physical dependence should not only be expected but anticipated. When narcotics are discontinued, symptoms of narcotic withdrawal may develop, including irritability, restlessness, episodes of hypertension, and tachycardia. Early recognition of these signs is essential, as is timely treatment using a thoughtful weaning schedule, appropriate assessment criteria, and administration of naloxone and other agents. In the postoperative period, patient-controlled analgesia is another excellent method of pain control. Additional means of achieving adequate pain control in children include the use of epidural analgesia and paraspinal blockade, which can be commenced at the time of surgery. By ensuring that the pediatric surgical patient has adequate analgesia, the surgeon ensures that the patient receives the most humane and thorough treatment, and provides important reassurance to all other members of the health care team and to the family that pain control is a very high priority.

NECK MASSES

The management of neck masses in children is determined by their location and the length of time that they have been present. Neck lesions are found in either the midline or lateral compartments. Midline masses include thyroglossal duct remnants, thyroid masses, thymic cysts, and dermoid cysts. Lateral lesions include branchial cleft remnants, cystic hygromas, vascular malformations, salivary gland tumors, torticollis, and lipoblastomas (a rare benign mesenchymal tumor of embryonal fat occurring in infants and young children). Enlarged lymph nodes and rare malignancies such as rhabdomyosarcoma can occur either in the midline or laterally.

Lymphadenopathy

The most common cause of a neck mass in a child is an enlarged lymph node, which typically can be found laterally or in the midline. The patient is usually referred to the pediatric surgeon for evaluation after the mass has been present for several weeks. A detailed history taking and physical examination often help determine the likely cause of the lymph node and the need for excisional biopsy. Enlarged tender lymph nodes are usually the result of a bacterial infection (staphylococcal or streptococcal). Treatment of the primary cause (e.g., otitis media or pharyngitis) with antibiotics often is all that is necessary. When the involved nodes become fluctuant, however, incision and drainage are indicated. In many North American institutions, there has been an increasing prevalence of methicillin-resistant *Staphylococcus aureus* infection of the skin and soft tissues, leading to increased staphylococcal lymphadenitis in children. More chronic forms of lymphadenitis, including infection with atypical mycobacteria, as well as cat-scratch fever, are

diagnosed based on serologic findings or the results of excisional biopsy. The lymphadenopathy associated with infectious mononucleosis can be diagnosed based on serologic testing. When the neck nodes are firm and fixed, and other enlarged nodes are present in the axillae or groin, or the history suggests lymphoma, excisional biopsy is indicated. In these cases, it is essential to obtain a chest radiograph to look for a mediastinal mass. Significant mediastinal load portends cardiorespiratory collapse due to loss of venous return and compression of the tracheobronchial tree if general anesthesia is induced. Accordingly, in such cases biopsies should be performed under local anesthesia.

Thyroglossal Duct Remnants

Pathology and Clinical Manifestations

The thyroid gland buds off the foregut diverticulum at the base of the tongue in the region of the future foramen cecum at 3 weeks of embryonic life. As the fetal neck develops, the thyroid tissue becomes more anterior and caudad until it rests in its normal position. The "descent" of the thyroid is intimately connected with the development of the hyoid bone. Residual thyroid tissue left behind during the migration may persist and subsequently present in the midline of the neck as a thyroglossal duct cyst. The mass is most commonly appreciated in the 2- to 4-year-old child when the baby fat disappears and irregularities in the neck become more readily apparent. Usually the cyst is encountered in the midline at or below the level of the hyoid bone and moves up and down with swallowing or with protrusion of the tongue. Occasionally it presents as an intrathyroidal mass. Most thyroglossal duct cysts are asymptomatic. If the duct retains its connection with the pharynx, infection may occur, and the resulting abscess will require incision and drainage. Occasionally a salivary fistula may result. Submental lymphadenopathy and midline dermoid cysts can be confused with a thyroglossal duct cyst. Rarely, midline ectopic thyroid tissue masquerades as a thyroglossal duct cyst and may represent the patient's only thyroid tissue. Therefore, if there is any question regarding the diagnosis or if the thyroid gland cannot be palpated in its normal anatomic position, it is advisable to obtain a nuclear medicine scan to confirm the presence of a normal thyroid gland. In adults the thyroglossal duct may contain thyroid tissue that can undergo malignant degeneration, although this is rarely the case in children. The presence of malignancy in a thyroglossal cyst should be suspected when the cyst grows rapidly or when ultrasonographic imaging demonstrates a complex anechoic pattern or the presence of calcification.

Treatment

If the cyst presents with an abscess, treatment should consist of drainage and administration of antibiotics. After resolution of the inflammation, resection of the cyst in continuity with the central portion of the hyoid bone and the tract connecting to the pharynx, in addition to ligation at the foramen cecum (the Sistrunk operation), is curative in >90% of patients. Lesser operations result in unacceptably high recurrence rates, and recurrence is more frequent after infection. According to a recent review, factors predictive of recurrence included more than two infections before surgery, age <2 years, and inadequate initial operation.

Branchial Cleft Anomalies

Paired branchial clefts and arches develop early in the fourth gestational week. The first cleft and the first, second, third, and fourth pouches give rise to adult organs. The embryologic communication between the pharynx and the external surface may persist as a fistula. A fistula is seen most commonly with the second branchial cleft, which normally disappears, and extends from the anterior border of the sternocleidomastoid muscle superiorly, passes inward through the bifurcation of the carotid artery, and enters the posterolateral pharynx just below the tonsillar fossa. In contrast, a third branchial cleft fistula passes posterior to the carotid bifurcation. The branchial cleft remnants may contain small pieces of cartilage and cysts, but internal fistulas are rare. A second branchial cleft sinus is suspected when clear fluid is noted draining from the external opening of the tract at the anterior border of the lower third of the sternomastoid muscle. Rarely, branchial cleft anomalies occur in association with biliary atresia and congenital cardiac anomalies, an association that is referred to as *Goldenhar's complex.*

Treatment

Complete excision of the cyst and sinus tract is necessary for cure. Dissection of the sinus tract is facilitated by passing a fine lacrimal duct probe through the external opening into the tract and using it as a guide for dissection. Injection of a small amount of methylene blue dye into the tract also may be useful. A series of two or sometimes three small transverse incisions in "stepladder" fashion is preferred to a long oblique incision in the neck, which is cosmetically undesirable. Branchial cleft cysts can present as abscesses. In these cases, initial treatment includes incision and drainage with a course of antibiotics to cover *Staphylococcus* and *Streptococcus* species, followed by excision of the cyst after the infection resolves.

Cystic Hygroma

Etiology and Pathology

Cystic hygroma (lymphangioma), occurring as a result of sequestration or obstruction of developing lymph vessels, occurs in approximately 1 in 12,000 births. Although the lesion can occur anywhere, the most common sites are in the posterior triangle of the neck, axilla, groin, and mediastinum. The cysts are lined by endothelium and filled with lymph. Occasionally unilocular cysts occur, but more often there are multiple cysts "infiltrating" the surrounding structures and distorting the local anatomy. A particularly troublesome variant of cystic hygroma is that which involves the tongue, floor of the mouth, and structures deep in the neck. Adjacent connective tissue may show extensive lymphocytic infiltration. The mass may be apparent at birth or may appear and enlarge rapidly in the early weeks or months of life as lymph accumulates; most present by age 2 years (Fig. 39-1A). Extension of the lesion into the axilla or mediastinum occurs in approximately 10% of cases and can be demonstrated preoperatively by chest radiograph, ultrasonography, or computed tomographic (CT) scan. Occasionally cystic hygromas contain nests of vascular tissue. These poorly supported vessels may

bleed and produce rapid enlargement and discoloration of the hygroma. Infection within the cysts, usually caused by *Streptococcus* or *Staphylococcus*, may occur. In the neck this can cause rapid enlargement, which may result in airway compromise. Rarely, it may be necessary to carry out percutaneous aspiration of a cyst to relieve respiratory distress.

A diagnosis of cystic hygroma by prenatal ultrasonography before 30 weeks' gestation has detected a cause of hidden mortality as well as a condition with a high incidence of associated anomalies, including abnormal karyotypes and hydrops fetalis. Occasionally, very large lesions can cause obstruction of the fetal airway. Such obstruction can result in the development of polyhydramnios by impairing the ability of the fetus to swallow amniotic fluid. In these circumstances, the airway is usually markedly distorted, which can result in immediate airway obstruction unless the airway is secured at the time of delivery. Orotracheal intubation or emergency tracheostomy while the infant remains attached to the placenta, the so-called ex utero intrapartum therapy (EXIT) procedure, may be necessary to secure the airway.

Treatment

The modern management of most cystic hygromas includes the combination of surgical excision and image-guided sclerotherapy. The initial treatment typically involves surgery in an attempt to safely remove all gross disease without damaging vital structures. Total removal of all gross disease may not be possible because of the extent of the hygroma and its proximity to, and intimate relationship with, adjacent nerves, muscles, and blood vessels (Fig. 39-1B). Radical ablative surgery is not indicated for this lesion. Conservative excision and unroofing of remaining cysts is advised, with repeated partial excision of residual hygroma and sclerotherapy if necessary and with preservation of all adjacent crucial structures. Postoperative wound drainage is important and is best accomplished by closed-suction technique. Nevertheless, fluid may accumulate beneath the surgically created flaps in the area from which the hygroma was excised, requiring multiple needle aspirations. One report notes recurrence rates of 20% after gross total resection, primarily along the surgical wound. Parents should be counseled that subtotal resections are associated with higher rates of recurrence or persistence. A combined sclerotherapy/resectional approach is particularly useful for masses that extend to the base of the tongue or the floor of the mouth.

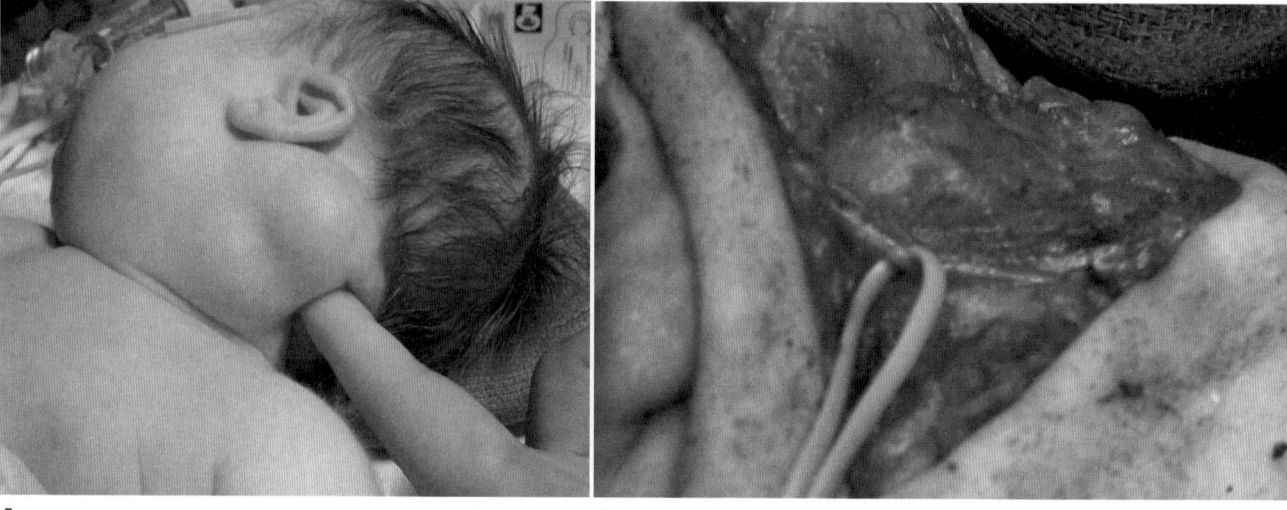

A   **B**

FIG. 39-1. A. Left cervical cystic hygroma in a 2-day-old infant. **B.** Intraoperative photograph showing a vessel loop around the spinal accessory nerve.

Torticollis

The presence of a lateral neck mass in infancy in association with rotation of the head toward the opposite side of the mass indicates the presence of congenital torticollis. This lesion results from fibrosis of the sternocleidomastoid muscle. The mass may be palpated in the affected muscle in approximately two thirds of cases. Histologically, the lesion is characterized by the deposition of collagen and fibroblasts around atrophied muscle cells. In the overwhelming majority of cases, physical therapy based on passive stretching of the affected muscle is of benefit. Rarely, surgical transection of the sternocleidomastoid muscle may be indicated.

RESPIRATORY SYSTEM

Congenital Diaphragmatic Hernia (Bochdalek's Hernia)

Pathology

The septum transversum extends to divide the pleural and coelomic cavities during fetal development. This precursor of the diaphragm normally completes separation of these two cavities at the posterolateral aspects of this mesenchymally derived structure. The most common variant of a congenital diaphragmatic hernia (CDH) is a posterolateral defect, also known as a *Bochdalek's hernia.* This anomaly is encountered more commonly on the left (80 to 90% of cases). Linkage analyses have recently implicated genetic mutations in syndromic variants of CDHs. Diaphragmatic defects allow abdominal viscera to fill the chest cavity. The abdominal cavity is small and underdeveloped and remains scaphoid after birth. Both lungs are hypoplastic, with decreased bronchial and pulmonary artery branching. Lung weight, lung volume, and DNA content are also decreased, but these findings are more striking on the ipsilateral side. In many instances, evidence suggests that a paucity of surfactant is present, which compounds the degree of respiratory insufficiency. Amniocentesis with karyotyping may show chromosomal defects, especially trisomy 18 and 21. Associated anomalies, once thought to be uncommon, are identified in 40% of these

infants, and most commonly involve the heart, brain, genitourinary system, craniofacial structures, or limbs.

Prenatal ultrasonography is successful in making the diagnosis of CDH as early as 15 weeks' gestation. Ultrasonographic findings include herniated abdominal viscera, abnormal anatomy of the upper abdomen, and mediastinal shift away from the herniated viscera (Fig. 39-2). Accurate prenatal prediction of outcome for fetuses that have CDH is very difficult. A useful index of severity for patients with left CDH is the lung-to-head ratio (LHR), which is the product of the length and the width of the right lung at the level of the cardiac atria divided by the head circumference (all measurements in millimeters). An LHR value of <1.0 is associated with a very poor prognosis, whereas an LHR of >1.4 predicts a more favorable outcome. The usefulness of the LHR in predicting outcome in patients with CDH has recently been questioned, due to the tremendous interobserver variability in calculating this ratio for a particular patient as well as the lack of reliable measures to determine postnatal disease severity.

After delivery, the diagnosis of CDH is made by chest radiograph (Fig. 39-3). The differential diagnosis includes congenital pulmonary airway malformation, in which the intrathoracic loops of bowel may be confused with multiple lung cysts. The vast majority of infants with CDH develop immediate respiratory distress, which is due to the combined effects of three factors. First, the air-filled bowel in the chest compresses the mobile mediastinum, which shifts to the opposite side of the chest, so that air exchange in the contralateral lung is compromised. Second, pulmonary hypertension develops. This phenomenon results in persistent fetal circulation, with resultant decreased pulmonary perfusion, and impaired gas exchange. Finally, the lung on the affected side is often markedly hypoplastic, so that it is essentially nonfunctional. Varying degrees of pulmonary hypoplasia on the opposite side may compound these effects. As a result, neonates with CDH are extremely sick, and the overall mortality in most series is approximately 50%.

Treatment

Significant strides have been made in the treatment of CDH through the effective application of improved methods of ventilation and

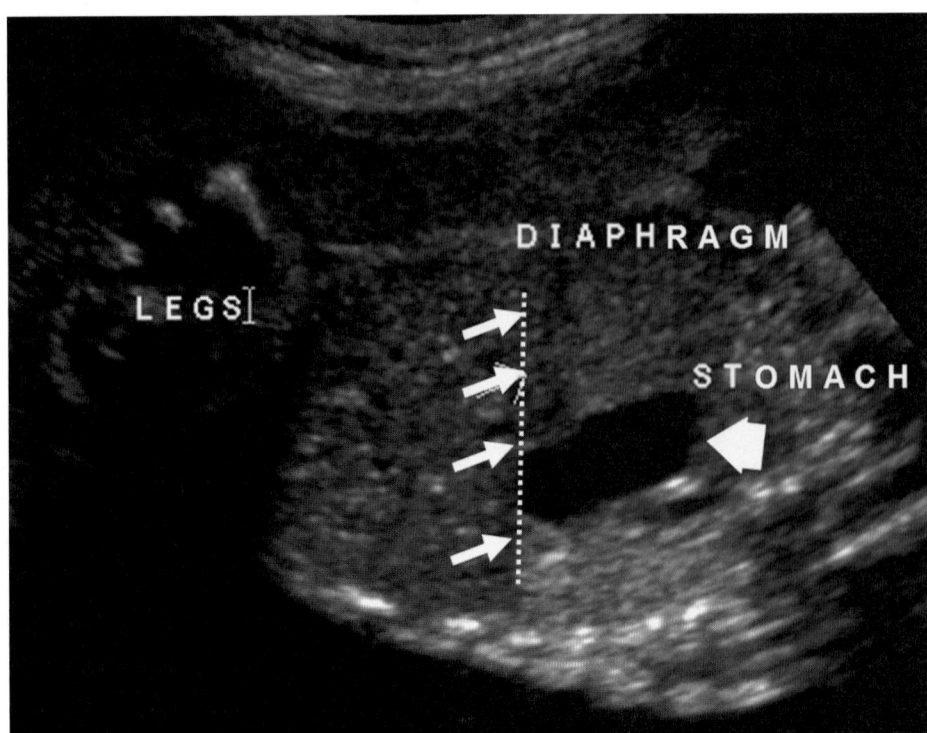

FIG. 39-2. Prenatal ultrasonographic scan of a fetus with a congenital diaphragmatic hernia. *Arrows* point to the location of the diaphragm. *Arrowhead* points to the stomach, which is in the thoracic cavity.

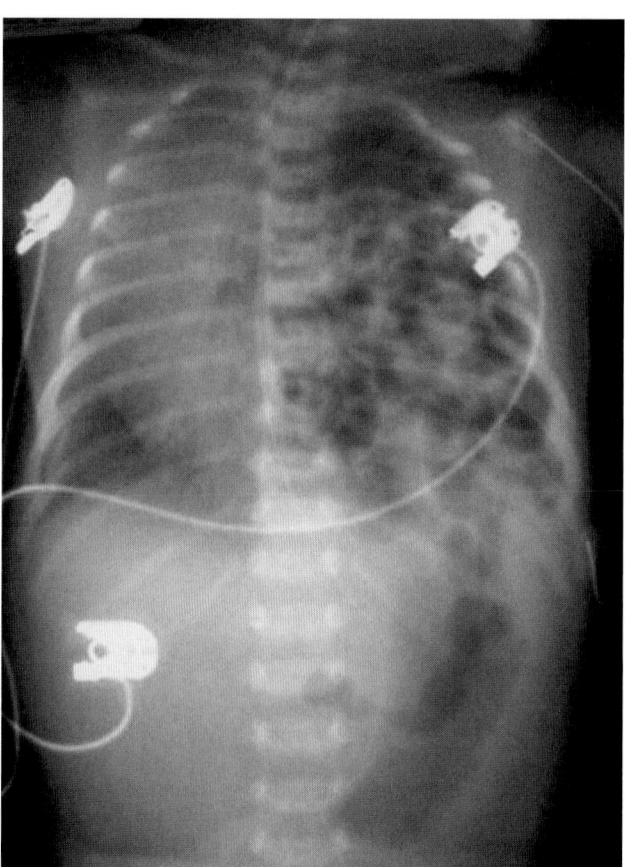

FIG. 39-3. Chest radiograph showing a left congenital diaphragmatic hernia.

timely use of extracorporeal membrane oxygenation (ECMO). Many infants are symptomatic at birth due to hypoxia, hypercarbia, and metabolic acidosis. Prompt cardiorespiratory stabilization is mandatory. It is noteworthy that the first 24 to 48 hours after birth are often characterized by a period of relative stability with high levels of partial pressure of arterial oxygen and relatively good perfusion. This has been termed the *honeymoon period*, and is followed by progressive cardiorespiratory deterioration in the majority of patients. In the past, correction of the hernia was felt to be a surgical emergency, and these patients underwent surgery shortly after birth. It is now accepted that the presence of persistent pulmonary hypertension which results in right-to-left shunting across the open foramen ovale or the ductus arteriosus and pulmonary hypoplasia are the leading causes of cardiorespiratory insufficiency. Current management therefore is directed toward preventing or reversing the pulmonary hypertension and minimizing barotrauma while optimizing oxygen delivery. To achieve this goal, infants are placed on mechanical ventilation using relatively low or "gentle" settings that prevent overinflation of the noninvolved lung. A partial pressure of arterial carbon dioxide in the range of 50 to 60 mmHg or higher is accepted as long as the pH remains ≥7.25. If these objectives cannot be achieved with conventional ventilation, high-frequency oscillatory ventilation may be used to avoid the injurious effects of conventional tidal volume ventilation. Echocardiography is used to assess the degree of pulmonary hypertension and to identify the presence of a coexisting cardiac anomaly. Minimal sedation is used, and meticulous attention to endotracheal tube patency is required. To minimize the degree of pulmonary hypertension, inhaled nitric oxide may be used. In certain patients, this agent significantly improves pulmonary perfusion, as manifested by improved oxygenation. Nitric oxide is administered into the ventilatory circuit and is used in concentrations of up to 40 parts per million. Correction of acidosis using

bicarbonate solution may minimize the degree of pulmonary hypertension. As the degree of pulmonary hypertension becomes hemodynamically significant, right-sided heart failure develops and systemic perfusion is impaired. Administration of excess IV fluid will compound the degree of cardiac failure and lead to marked peripheral edema. Inotropic support using epinephrine, dopamine, and milrinone alone or in combination may be helpful in optimizing cardiac contractility and maintaining mean arterial pressure.

Infants with CDH who remain severely hypoxic despite maximal ventilatory care may be candidates for treatment of their respiratory failure by ECMO. Venovenous or venoarterial bypass is used. Venovenous bypass is established with a single cannula through the internal jugular vein, with blood removed from and infused into the right atrium by separate ports. Venoarterial bypass is used preferentially by many centers because it provides the cardiac support that is often needed. The right atrium is cannulated by means of the internal jugular vein, and the aortic arch through the right common carotid artery. Deoxygenated blood from the right atrium is directed through the membrane oxygenator, which removes carbon dioxide from and supplies oxygen to the blood before it is returned to the infant via the carotid artery cannula. The infant is maintained on bypass until the pulmonary hypertension is reversed and lung function, as measured by compliance, is improved. This process typically occurs within 7 to 10 days, but in some infants it may take up to 3 weeks. The use of ECMO is associated with significant risk. Because patients require systemic anticoagulation, bleeding complications are the most significant, regardless of whether venoarterial or venovenous ECMO is used. Bleeding may occur intracranially or at the site of cannula insertion and can be life-threatening. Systemic sepsis is a significant problem and may necessitate decannulation. Criteria for placing infants on ECMO include the presence of normal cardiac anatomy by echocardiography, the absence of fatal chromosome anomalies, and the expectation that the infant will die without ECMO. Traditionally, a threshold of a weight of >2.5 kg and a gestational age of >34 weeks has been used to select patients for ECMO, although success has been achieved in infants with weights as low as 1.8 kg. It must be emphasized that, although ECMO may allow successful treatment of a population of neonates with refractory pulmonary hypertension, the use of this technique remains controversial. On decannulation, a decision should be made regarding whether to repair the carotid artery or not. In instances in which the child is cannulated for a brief period (≤5 days) this may be feasible. A recent study failed to show any benefit from repairing the carotid artery, although this finding remains controversial.

A strategy that does not involve the use of ECMO but instead emphasizes the use of permissive hypercapnia and the avoidance of barotrauma may provide equal overall outcome in patients with CDH. This likely reflects the fact that mortality is related to the degree of pulmonary hypoplasia and the presence of congenital anomalies, neither of which is correctable by ECMO.

The timing of diaphragmatic hernia repair remains controversial, particularly when the infant is supported on ECMO. In patients who are not placed on ECMO, repair should be performed once the hemodynamic status has been optimized. In neonates who are on ECMO, some surgeons perform early repair on bypass; others wait until the infant's lungs are fully recovered and the pulmonary hypertension has subsided, repair the diaphragm, and discontinue bypass within hours of surgery. Still others repair the diaphragm only after the infant is off bypass. Repair of the diaphragmatic hernia may be accomplished by either an abdominal or a transthoracic approach and can be performed using open or minimally invasive techniques. In the abdominal approach, through a subcostal incision, the abdominal viscera are withdrawn from the chest to expose the defect in the diaphragm. Care must be taken when reducing the spleen and liver, because bleeding from these structures can be fatal. The anterior margin is often apparent, whereas the posterior muscular rim is attenuated. If the infant undergoes heparinization on bypass, minimal dissection of the muscular margins is performed. Electrocautery is used liberally to minimize postoperative bleeding. Most infants who require ECMO support before hernia repair have large defects, often lacking the medial and posterior margins. Before the availability of ECMO therapy, most of these infants died. In about three fourths of infants who undergo repair on bypass, the use of prosthetic material is required to patch the defect, and it is sutured to the diaphragmatic remnant or around ribs or costal cartilages for large defects. If there is adequate muscle for closure, a single layer of nonabsorbable horizontal mattress suture is used to close the defect. Just before the repair is complete, a chest tube may be positioned in the thoracic cavity. The authors tend to reserve the use of chest tubes for patients who are repaired while on ECMO, because these patients are at risk for developing a hemothorax, which can significantly impair ventilation. Anatomic closure of the abdominal wall may be impossible after reduction of the viscera. Occasionally a prosthetic patch may be sutured to the fascia to facilitate closure. The patch can be removed at a later time, and the ventral hernia can be closed at that time or subsequently. In patients who are deemed to be candidates for a minimally invasive approach (stable condition, >2 kg, no pulmonary hypertension), a thoracoscopic repair may be safely performed. If the diaphragm has been repaired with the patient on ECMO, weaning and decannulation are accomplished as soon as possible. All infants are ventilated postoperatively to maintain preductal arterial oxygenation of 80 to 100 mmHg. Very slow weaning from the ventilator is necessary to avoid recurrent pulmonary hypertension.

Congenital Lobar Emphysema

Congenital lobar emphysema (CLE) is a condition manifested during the first few months of life as a progressive hyperexpansion of one or more lobes of the lung. It can be life-threatening in the newborn period, but in the older infant it causes less respiratory distress. Air entering during inspiration is trapped in the lobe. On expiration, the lobe cannot deflate and progressively overexpands, which causes atelectasis of the adjacent lobe or lobes. This hyperexpansion eventually shifts the mediastinum to the opposite side and compromises the other lung. CLE usually occurs in the upper lobes of the lung (left more often than right), followed next in frequency by the right middle lobe; however, it can occur in the lower lobes as well. It is caused by intrinsic bronchial obstruction from poor bronchial cartilage development or extrinsic compression. Approximately 14% of children with this condition have cardiac defects, with an enlarged left atrium or a major vessel causing compression of the ipsilateral bronchus.

Symptoms range from mild respiratory distress to full-fledged respiratory failure with tachypnea, dyspnea, cough, and late cyanosis. These symptoms may be static or they may progress rapidly or result in recurrent pneumonia. Occasionally, infants with CLE present with failure to thrive, which likely reflects the increased work associated with the overexpanded lung. A hyperexpanded hemithorax on the ipsilateral side is pathognomonic for CLE. Diagnosis is typically confirmed by chest radiograph, which shows a hyperlucent affected lobe with adjacent lobar compression and atelectasis. As a consequence of mass effect, the mediastinum may be shifted to the contralateral side, resulting in compression and atelectasis of the contralateral lung (Fig. 39-4). Although a chest radiograph is usually sufficient, it is sometimes important to obtain a CT scan of the chest to clearly establish the diagnosis of CLE. This should be done only in patients in stable condition. Unless foreign body or mucus plugging is suspected as a cause of hyperinflation, bronchoscopy is not advisable, because it can lead to more air trapping and cause life-threatening respiratory distress in an infant in stable condition. Treatment is resection of the affected lobe, which can be safely performed using either an open or thoracoscopic approach. Unless symptoms necessitate earlier surgery, resection can usually be performed after the infant is several months of age. The prognosis is excellent. Ongoing lung development in pediatric patients results in the generation of new alveoli in the remaining lung tissue, unlike in adult patients.

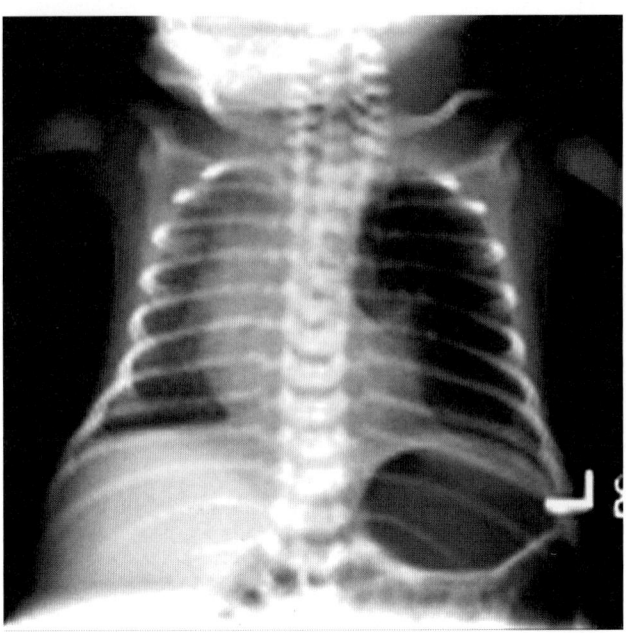

FIG. 39-4. Congenital lobar emphysema of the left upper lobe in a 2-week-old boy. Mediastinal shift is present.

Congenital Pulmonary Airway Malformation

Congenital pulmonary airway malformation (CPAM) consists of cystic proliferation of the terminal airway, which produces cysts lined by mucus-producing respiratory epithelium and elastic tissue in the cyst walls without cartilage formation. There may be a single cyst with a wall of connective tissue containing smooth muscle. Formerly known as *congenital cystic adenomatoid malformation*, CPAM may consist of a single large cyst or multiple cysts (type I), may be characterized by smaller and more numerous cysts (type II), or may resemble fetal lung without macroscopic cysts (type III). CPAMs frequently occur in the left lower lobe. However, this lesion can occur in any lobe or may occur in both lungs simultaneously. In the left lower lobe, a type I CPAM may be confused at birth with a CDH. Clinical symptoms may range from none at all to severe respiratory failure at birth. Both single and multiple cysts can produce air trapping and may be confused with CLE, pneumatoceles, or even pulmonary sequestrations. The cysts also can be involved with repeated infections and produce fever and cough in older infants and children. The diagnosis often can be made by chest radiograph. In certain cases, ultrasonographic or CT scan may be definitive (Fig. 39-5). Prenatal ultrasonography may suggest the diagnosis. In the newborn period, ultrasonography may also be useful, especially to distinguish between CPAM and CDH. Resection is curative and may need to be performed urgently in the infant with severe respiratory distress. Long term, there is a risk of malignant degeneration to pulmonary blastoma. As a result, resection of the affected lobe is usually required (Fig. 39-6). Prognosis is excellent.

Pulmonary Sequestration

In pulmonary sequestration, a mass of lung tissue, usually in the left lower chest, lacks the usual connections to the pulmonary artery or tracheobronchial tree and its blood supply is derived directly from the aorta. There are two kinds of sequestration. In extralobar sequestration a small area of nonaerated lung is separated from the main lung mass, has a systemic blood supply, and usually is located immediately above the left diaphragm. It is commonly found in cases of CDH. Intralobar sequestration more commonly occurs within the parenchyma of the left lower lobe but also can occur on the right. There is no major connection to the tracheobronchial tree, but a secondary connection may be established, perhaps through infection or via

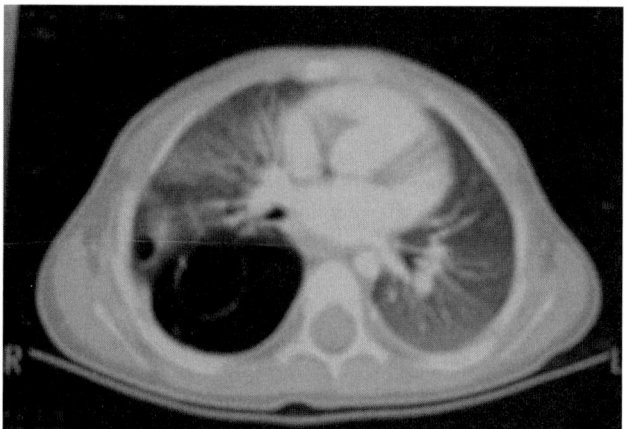

FIG. 39-5. Computed tomographic scan of the chest showing a congenital pulmonary airway malformation of the left lower lobe.

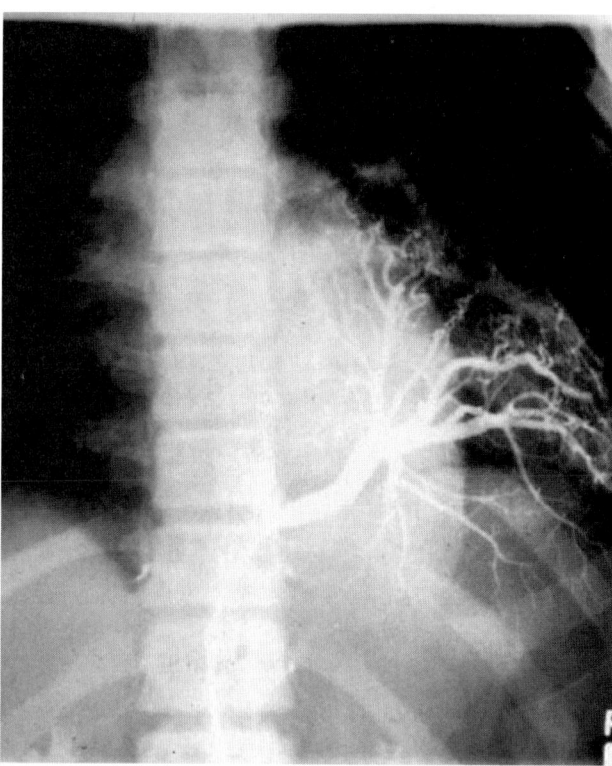

FIG. 39-7. Arteriogram showing large systemic artery supply to an intralobar sequestration of the left lower lobe.

adjacent intrapulmonary shunts. The blood supply frequently originates from the aorta below the diaphragm; multiple vessels may be present (Fig. 39-7). Venous drainage of both types can be systemic or pulmonary. The cause of sequestration is unknown but most probably involves an abnormal budding of the developing lung that picks up a systemic blood supply and never becomes connected with the bronchus or pulmonary vessels. Sequestrations may, in some cases, exhibit mixed pathology showing components consistent with CPAMs. Extralobar sequestration is asymptomatic and is usually discovered incidentally on chest radiograph. If the diagnosis can be confirmed, for example by CT scan, resection is not necessary unless the sequestration becomes symptomatic. Diagnosis of intralobar sequestration may be made prenatally and confirmed on postnatal CT scan. Alternatively, the diagnosis of intralobar sequestration may be established after repeated infections manifested by cough, fever, and consolidation in the posterior basal segment of the left lower lobe. Increasingly the diagnosis is being made in the early months of life by ultrasonography. Color Doppler ultrasonography often can be helpful in delineating the systemic arterial supply. Removal of the entire left lower lobe is usually necessary, because the diagnosis often is made late after multiple infections. Occasionally segmental resection of the sequestered part of the lung can be performed using an open, or ideally a thoracoscopic, approach. If an open approach is used, it is important to open the chest through a low intercostal space (sixth or seventh), to gain access to the vascular attachments to the aorta. These attachments may insert into the aorta below the diaphragm; in these cases division of the vessels as they traverse the thoracic cavity is essential. Prognosis is generally excellent. However, failure to obtain adequate control of these vessels may result in their retraction into the abdomen and lead to uncontrollable hemorrhage.

Bronchogenic Cyst

Bronchogenic cysts can occur anywhere along the respiratory tract from the neck to the lung parenchyma. They are probably embryonic rests of foregut origin that have been pinched off from the main portion of the developing tracheobronchial tree and are closely associated in causation with other foregut duplication cysts arising from the esophagus. For purists, foregut duplication cysts are named by their origin rather than their mucosal tissue type, therefore bronchogenic cysts may contain GI epithelium. However, although *foregut duplication cyst* is the correct terminology, it is not generally used. Bronchogenic cysts can present at any age. They may be seen on prenatal ultrasonographic scan but are discovered most often incidentally on postnatal chest radiograph. Histologically, they are hamartomatous and usually consist of a single cyst lined with respiratory epithelium, containing cartilage and smooth muscle. Although they may be completely asymptomatic, bronchogenic cysts may produce symptoms that depend on their anatomic location. In the paratracheal region of the neck they can produce airway compression and respiratory distress. In the lung parenchyma, they may become infected and present with fever and cough. In addition, they may cause obstruction of the bronchial lumen with distal atelectasis and infection. They may also cause mediastinal compression. Rarely, rupture of the cyst can occur. Chest radiograph usually shows a dense mass, and CT scan or magnetic resonance imaging (MRI) delineates the precise anatomic location of the lesion. Treatment consists of resection of the cyst, which may need to be undertaken in emergency circumstances because of airway or cardiac compression.

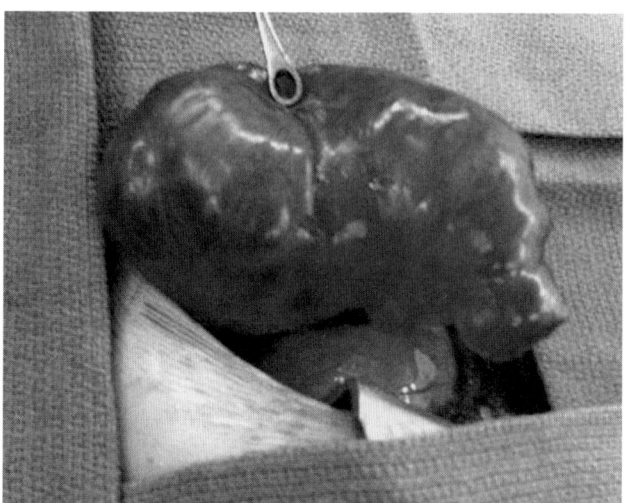

FIG. 39-6. Intraoperative photograph showing left lower lobe congenital pulmonary airway malformation seen in Fig. 39-5.

Resection can be performed either as an open procedure or, more commonly, using a thoracoscopic approach.

Bronchiectasis

Bronchiectasis is an abnormal and irreversible dilatation of the bronchi and bronchioles associated with chronic suppurative disease of the airways. Usually the children have an underlying congenital pulmonary anomaly, cystic fibrosis, or immune deficiency. Bronchiectasis also can result from chronic infection secondary to a neglected bronchial foreign body. The symptoms include a chronic cough, often productive of purulent secretions; recurrent pulmonary infection; and hemoptysis. The diagnosis is suggested by a chest radiograph that shows increased bronchovascular markings in the affected lobe. Chest CT delineates bronchiectasis with excellent resolution. The preferred treatment for bronchiectasis is medical, consisting of antibiotics, postural drainage, and bronchodilator therapy, because many children with the disease show signs of airflow obstruction and bronchial hyperresponsiveness. Lobectomy or segmental resection is indicated for localized disease that has not responded appropriately to medical therapy. In severe cases, lung transplantation may be required to replace the terminally damaged, septic lung.

Foreign Bodies

The inherent curiosity of children and their innate propensity to place new objects into their mouths to fully explore them place them at great risk for aspiration. Ingested objects can be found in the airway or in the esophagus; in both cases the results can be life-threatening.

Aspiration

Aspiration of foreign bodies most commonly occurs in the toddler age group. Peanuts are the object most frequently aspirated, although other materials (popcorn, for instance) may also be involved. A solid foreign body often will cause air trapping, with hyperlucency of the affected lobe or lung seen especially on expiration. Oil from a peanut is very irritating and may cause pneumonia. Delay in diagnosis can lead to atelectasis and infection. The most common anatomic location for a foreign body is the right main stem bronchus or the right lower lobe. The child usually will cough or choke while eating but may then become asymptomatic. Total respiratory obstruction may occur with a tracheal foreign body; however, respiratory distress is usually mild if present at all. A unilateral wheeze is often heard on auscultation. This wheeze often leads to an inappropriate diagnosis of asthma and may delay the correct diagnosis for some time. A chest radiograph will show a radiopaque foreign body, but in the case of nuts, seeds, or plastic toy parts, the only clue may be hyperexpansion of the affected lobe on an expiratory film or fluoroscopy. Bronchoscopy confirms the diagnosis and allows removal of the foreign body. It may be a very simple procedure or it may be extremely difficult, especially with a smooth foreign body that cannot be grasped easily or one that has been retained for some time. A rigid bronchoscope should be employed in all cases, and use of optical forceps facilitates grasping of the inhaled object. Epinephrine may be injected into the mucosa when the object has been present for a long period of time to minimize bleeding. Bronchiectasis may be seen as an extremely late phenomenon after repeated infections of the poorly aerated lung and may require partial or total resection of the affected lobe. The differential diagnosis of a bronchial foreign body includes an intraluminal tumor (i.e., carcinoid, hemangioma, or neurofibroma).

Caustic Ingestion and Esophageal Injury

The most common foreign body in the esophagus is a coin, followed by small toy parts. Toddlers are most frequently affected. The coin is retained in the esophagus at one of three locations: the cricopharyngeus, the area of the aortic arch, or the gastroesophageal junction, all areas of normal anatomic narrowing. Symptoms are variable depending on the anatomic position of the foreign body and the degree of obstruction. There is often a relatively asymptomatic period after ingestion. The initial symptoms are GI symptoms and include dysphagia, drooling, and vomiting. The longer the foreign body remains in the esophagus, the greater the incidence of respiratory symptoms, which include cough, stridor, and wheezing. These findings may be interpreted as signs of upper respiratory tract infections. Objects that are present for a long period of time—particularly in children who have underlying neurologic impairment—may manifest as chronic dysphagia. The chest radiograph is diagnostic in the case of an ingested coin. A contrast swallow evaluation may be required for nonradiopaque foreign bodies. Coins lodged in the upper esophagus for <24 hours may be removed using Magill forceps. In all other situations, the treatment is by esophagoscopy, rigid or flexible, for removal of the foreign body. In the case of sharp foreign bodies such as open safety pins, extreme care is required on extraction to avoid injury to the esophagus. Rarely, esophagotomy is required for removal, particularly of sharp objects. Diligent follow-up is required after removal of foreign bodies—especially batteries, which can cause liquefactive necrosis followed by strictures, and sharp objects, which can injure the underlying esophagus.

ESOPHAGUS

Esophageal Atresia and Tracheoesophageal Fistula

Repair of esophageal atresia (EA) and tracheoesophageal fistula (TEF) is an area of pediatric surgery that shows significantly better outcomes than in the past. Originally, nearly all infants born with EA and TEF died. In 1939 William E. Ladd and N. Logan Leven achieved the first successful repair by ligating the fistula, placing a gastrostomy, and reconstructing the esophagus at a later time. Subsequently, Dr. Cameron Haight in Ann Arbor, Michigan, performed the first successful primary anastomosis for EA, which remains the current approach for treatment of this condition. Despite the fact that there are several common varieties of this anomaly and the underlying cause remains obscure, a careful approach consisting of meticulous perioperative care and attention to the technical details of the operation can result in an excellent prognosis in most cases.

Anatomic Varieties

The five major varieties of EA and TEF are shown in Fig. 39-8. The most commonly seen variety is EA with distal TEF (type C), which occurs in approximately 85% of the cases in most series. The next most frequent is pure EA (type A), occurring in 8 to 10% of patients, followed by TEF without EA (type E). The latter occurs in 8% of cases and is also referred to as an *H-type fistula*, based on the anatomic similarity to that letter (Fig. 39-9). EA with fistula between both the proximal and distal ends of the esophagus and trachea (type D) is seen in approximately 2% of cases, and type B, EA with TEF between the proximal esophagus and trachea, is seen in approximately 1% of cases.

Etiology and Pathologic Presentation

The esophagus and trachea share a common embryologic origin. At approximately 4 weeks' gestation, a diverticulum forms off the anterior aspect of the proximal foregut in the region of the primitive pharynx. This diverticulum extends caudally with progressive formation of the laryngotracheal groove, which thus creates a separate trachea and esophagus. Successful development of these structures is the consequence of a complex interplay among growth and transcription factors necessary for rostral-caudal and anterior-posterior specification. The variations in clinically observed EA and TEF that result from failure of successful formation of these structures are depicted in Fig. 39-8. Although definitive genetic mutations have been difficult to identify in isolated EA-TEF, mutations

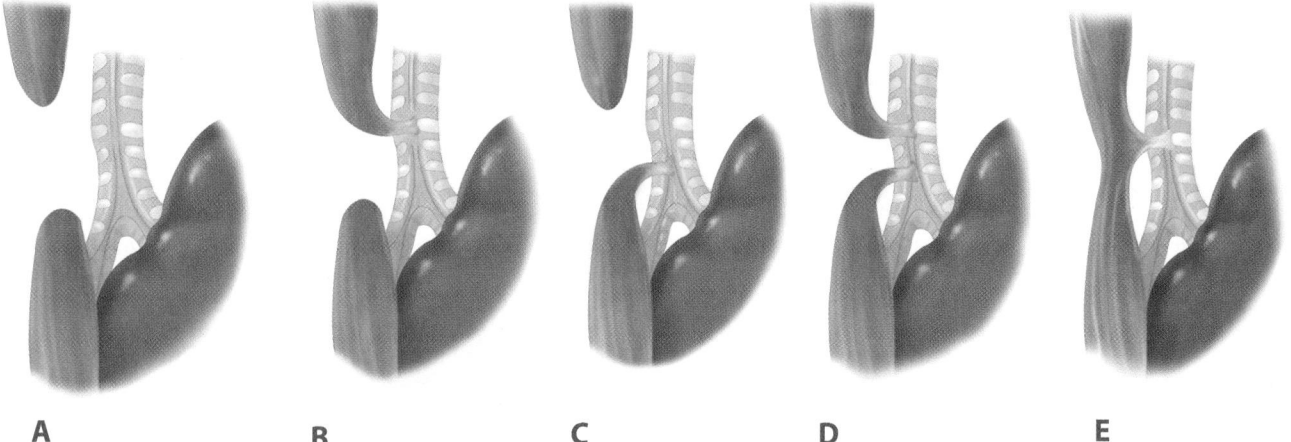

A　　**B**　　**C**　　**D**　　**E**

FIG. 39-8. The five varieties of esophageal atresia (EA) and tracheoesophageal fistula (TEF). **A.** Isolated EA. **B.** EA with TEF between the proximal segment of the esophagus and the trachea. **C.** EA with TEF between the distal esophagus and the trachea **D.** EA with fistula between both the proximal and distal ends of the esophagus and the trachea. **E.** TEF without EA (H-type fistula).

in *N-myc*, *Sox2*, and *CHD7* have been characterized in syndromic EA-TEF with associated anomalies.

Other congenital anomalies commonly occur in association with EA-TEF. For instance, VACTERL syndrome is associated with *v*ertebral anomalies (absent vertebrae or hemivertebrae), *a*norectal anomalies (imperforate anus), *c*ardiac defects, *t*racheoesophageal fistula, *r*enal anomalies (renal agenesis, renal anomalies), and *r*adial *l*imb anomalies (most often radial dysplasia). In nearly 20% of the infants born with EA, some variant of congenital heart disease occurs.

Clinical Presentation

The anatomic variant of EA-TEF in the infant predicts the clinical presentation. When the esophagus ends either as a blind pouch or as a fistula into the trachea (as in types A, B, C, and D), infants present with excessive drooling, followed by choking or coughing immediately after feeding is initiated as a result of aspiration through the fistula tract. Air in the distal intestine indicates either a patent esophagus or a fistula to the respiratory tract. In type C TEF, as the neonate coughs and cries, air is transmitted through the fistula into the stomach, which results in abdominal distention. As the abdomen distends, it becomes increasingly more difficult for the infant to breathe. This leads to further atelectasis, which compounds the pulmonary dysfunction. In patients with the C and D varieties, the regurgitated gastric juice passes through the fistula, collecting in the trachea and lungs and leading to a chemical pneumonitis, which further exacerbates the pulmonary status. In many instances, the diagnosis is actually made by the nursing staff who attempt to feed the baby and notice the accumulation of oral secretions.

The diagnosis of EA is confirmed by the inability to pass an orogastric tube into the stomach (Fig. 39-10). The dilated upper

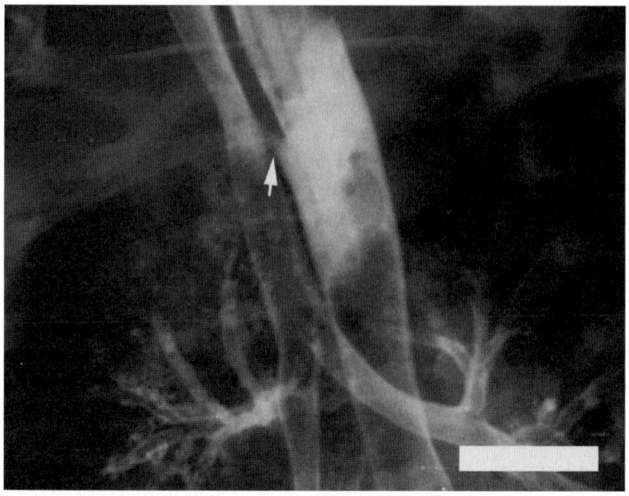

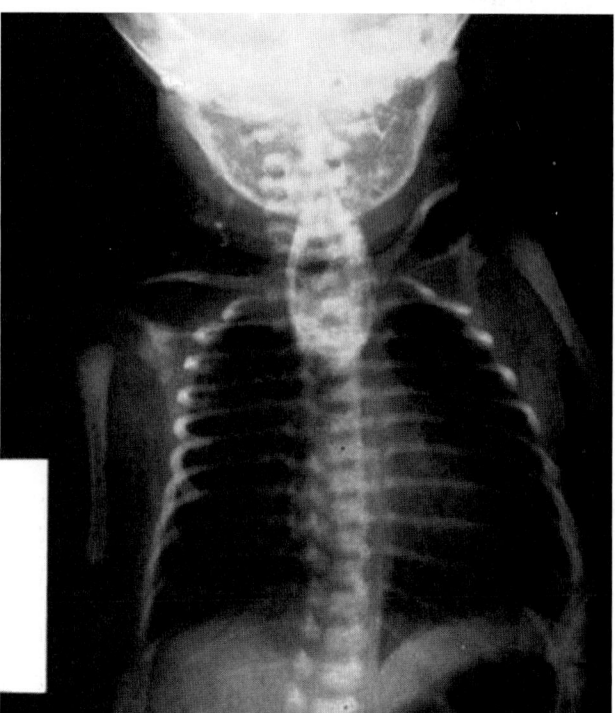

FIG. 39-10. Type C esophageal atresia with tracheoesophageal fistula. Note the catheter coiled in the upper pouch and the presence of gas below the diaphragm, which confirms the presence of the tracheoesophageal fistula.

FIG. 39-9. Barium esophagram showing an H-type tracheoesophageal fistula (*arrow*).

pouch occasionally may be seen on a plain chest radiograph. If a soft feeding tube is used, the tube will coil in the upper pouch, which provides further diagnostic certainty. An important alternative diagnosis that must be considered when an orogastric tube does not enter the stomach is that of an esophageal perforation. This problem can occur in infants after traumatic insertion of a nasogastric or orogastric tube. In this instance, the perforation classically occurs at the level of the piriform sinus, and a false passage is created that prevents the tube from entering the stomach. Whenever there is any diagnostic uncertainty, a contrast study can confirm the diagnosis of EA and occasionally document the TEF; however, the obvious risks of aspiration associated with an undrained blind pouch cannot be overstated. The presence of a TEF can be demonstrated clinically by the finding of air in the GI tract. This can be proven at the bedside by percussion of the abdomen and confirmed by plain abdominal radiograph. Occasionally, a diagnosis of EA-TEF can be suspected prenatally on ultrasonographic evaluation. Typical features include failure to visualize the stomach and the presence of polyhydramnios. These findings reflect the absence of efficient swallowing by the fetus.

In a child with EA, it is important to identify whether coexisting anomalies are present. These include cardiac defects in 38%, skeletal defects in 19%, neurologic defects in 15%, renal defects in 15%, anorectal defects in 8%, and other abnormalities in 13%. Examination of the heart and great vessels with echocardiography is important to exclude cardiac defects, because these are often the most important predictors of survival in these infants. The echocardiogram also demonstrates whether the aortic arch is left sided or right sided, which may influence the approach to surgical repair. Vertebral anomalies are assessed by plain radiography, and a spinal ultrasonographic scan is obtained. A patent anus should be confirmed clinically. The kidneys in a newborn may be assessed clinically by palpation. An ultrasonographic scan of the abdomen will demonstrate the presence of renal anomalies, which should be suspected in the child who fails to produce urine. The presence of other extremity anomalies is suspected when there are missing digits and can be confirmed by plain radiographs of the hands, feet, forearms, and legs. Rib anomalies may also be present. These may include the presence of a thirteenth rib.

Initial Management

The initial treatment of infants with EA-TEF includes attention to respiratory status, decompression of the upper pouch, and appropriate timing of surgery. Because the major determinant of poor survival is the presence of other severe anomalies, a search for other defects, including congenital cardiac disease, is undertaken. The initial strategy after the diagnosis is confirmed is to place the neonate in an infant warmer with the head elevated at least 30 degrees. A sump catheter on continuous suction is placed in the upper pouch. Both of these strategies are designed to minimize the degree of aspiration from the esophageal pouch. Acid prophylaxis is given to reduce the chemical irritation of any refluxed contents. When saliva accumulates in the upper pouch and is aspirated into the lungs, coughing, bronchospasm, and desaturation episodes can occur, which may be minimized by ensuring the patency of the sump catheter. IV antibiotic therapy is initiated, and warmed electrolyte solution is administered. When possible, the right upper extremity is avoided as a site to start an IV line, because this location may interfere with positioning of the patient during the surgical repair.

The timing of repair is influenced by the stability of the patient's condition. Definitive repair of the EA-TEF is rarely a surgical emergency. If the child is hemodynamically stable and is oxygenating well, definitive repair may be performed within 1 to 2 days after birth. This allows a careful examination for the presence of coexisting anomalies and selection of an experienced anesthetic team.

Management in the Preterm Infant

The ventilated premature neonate with EA-TEF and associated hyaline membrane disease is a patient who may develop severe, progressive cardiopulmonary dysfunction. The tracheoesophageal fistula can worsen the fragile pulmonary status as a result of recurrent aspiration through the fistula and increased abdominal distention, which impairs lung expansion. Moreover, the elevated airway pressure that is required to ventilate these patients can worsen the clinical course by forcing air through the fistula into the stomach, which exacerbates the degree of abdominal distention and compromises lung expansion. In this situation, the first priority is to minimize the degree of positive pressure needed to adequately ventilate the child. This can be accomplished using high-frequency oscillatory ventilation. If the gastric distention becomes severe, a gastrostomy tube should be placed. This procedure can be performed at the bedside under local anesthetic, if necessary. The dilated, air-filled stomach can easily be accessed through an incision in the left upper quadrant of the abdomen. Once the gastrostomy tube is placed and the abdominal pressure is relieved, the pulmonary status can paradoxically worsen. This is because the ventilation gas may pass preferentially through the fistula, which is the path of least resistance, and bypass the lungs, which thereby worsens the hypoxemia. To correct this problem, the gastrostomy tube may be placed under water seal, elevated, or intermittently clamped. If these maneuvers are to no avail, ligation of the fistula may be required. This procedure can be performed in the neonatal intensive care unit if the infant's condition is too unstable for the infant to be transported to the operating room. Some surgeons believe that division rather than ligation alone leads to reduced rates of recurrence in the initial period before definitive treatment. These interventions allow for the infant's underlying hyaline membrane disease to improve, for the pulmonary secretions to clear, and for the infant's condition to stabilize so that definitive repair can be performed.

Primary Surgical Correction

In an infant in stable condition, definitive repair is achieved through performance of a primary esophagoesophagostomy. There are two approaches to this operation: open thoracotomy and thoracoscopy. In the open approach, the infant is brought to the operating room, intubated, and placed in the lateral decubitus position with the right side up in preparation for right posterolateral thoracotomy. If a right-sided arch was determined previously to be present by echocardiography, consideration is given to performing the repair through the left chest, although most surgeons believe that the repair can be performed safely from the right side as well. Bronchoscopy may be performed to exclude the presence of additional upper pouch fistulas in cases of EA (i.e., differentiation of types B, C, and D), and to identify a laryngotracheoesophageal cleft.

The operative technique for primary repair is as described below (Fig. 39-11). A retropleural approach is generally used, because this technique prevents widespread contamination of the thorax if an anastomotic leak occurs postoperatively. The sequence of steps is the following: (a) The pleura is mobilized to expose the structures in the posterior mediastinum. (b) The fistula is divided and the tracheal opening is closed. (c) The upper esophagus is mobilized sufficiently to permit an anastomosis without tension and to determine whether a fistula is present between the upper esophagus and the trachea. Forward pressure by the anesthesia staff on the sump drain in the pouch can greatly facilitate dissection at this stage of the operation. Care must be taken when dissecting posteriorly to avoid violation of the lumen of the trachea or the esophagus. (d) The distal esophagus is mobilized. This needs to be accomplished judiciously to avoid devascularization, because the blood supply to the distal esophagus is segmental from the aorta. Most of the esophageal length is obtained by mobilizing the upper pouch, because the blood supply travels via the submucosa from above. (e) Primary esophagoesophagostomy is performed. Most surgeons create the anastomosis in a single layer using interrupted 5-0 sutures. If there is excess tension, the muscle of the upper pouch can be circumferentially incised without compromising blood supply to increase its length. Many surgeons place a transanastomotic feeding tube to institute feeds in

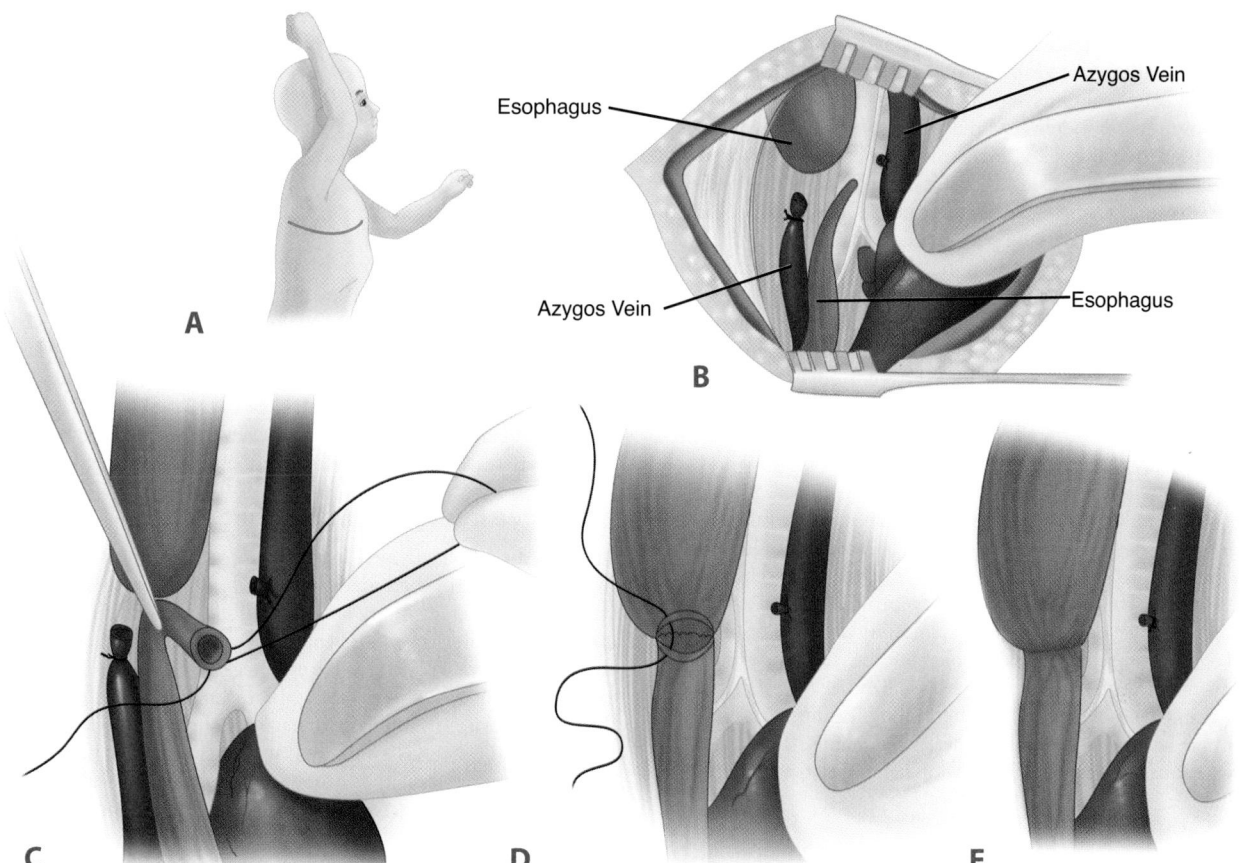

FIG. 39-11. Primary repair of type C tracheoesophageal fistula. **A.** Right thoracotomy incision. **B.** Azygous vein transected, proximal and distal esophagus demonstrated, and fistula identified. **C.** Tracheoesophageal fistula transected and defect in the trachea closed. **D.** End-to-end anastomosis between the proximal and distal esophagus. **E.** Completed anastomosis.

the early postoperative period. (f) A retropleural drain is placed, and the incision is closed in layers.

When a minimally invasive approach is selected, the patient is prepared for right-sided transthoracic thoracoscopic repair. The same steps as described earlier for the open repair are undertaken. The telescope provides excellent visualization. Identification of the fistula is performed as a first step; the fistula can be readily ligated and divided between thoracoscopically placed sutures. The anastomosis is performed in a single layer. The thoracoscopically performed TEF repair requires clear and ongoing communication between the operating surgeons and the anesthesiologist; visualization can be significantly reduced with sudden changes in lung inflation, which can potentially lead to the need to convert to an open repair. Although clear guidelines for patient selection for a thoracoscopic repair have not been established, a requirement that patients weigh >2.5 kg, be in hemodynamically stable condition, and have no comorbidities represents a reasonable starting point.

Postoperative Course

The postoperative management strategy for patients with EA-TEF is influenced to a great degree by the preference of the individual surgeon and the institutional culture. Many surgeons prefer not to leave the infants intubated postoperatively to avoid the effects of positive pressure on the site of tracheal closure. However, early extubation may not be possible in infants with preoperative lung disease, either from prematurity or pneumonia, or in infants with any vocal cord edema. When a transanastomotic tube is placed, feedings are begun slowly in the postoperative period. Some surgeons institute parenteral nutrition for several days, using a central line. The retropleural drain is assessed daily for the presence of saliva, which

indicates an anastomotic leak. Many surgeons order a contrast swallow evaluation 1 week after repair to assess the caliber of the anastomosis and to determine whether a leak is present. If there is no leak, feeding is started. The principal benefit of the thoracoscopic approach is that postoperative pain is significantly reduced, as is the requirement for postoperative narcotic analgesia.

Complications of Surgery

Anastomotic leakage occurs in 10 to 15% of patients and may be seen either in the immediately postoperative period or after several days. Early leakage (i.e., within the first 24 to 48 hours) is manifested by a new pleural effusion, pneumothorax, and sepsis, and requires immediate exploration. In these circumstances, the anastomosis may be completely disrupted, possibly due to excessive tension. Revision of the anastomosis may be possible. If not, cervical esophagostomy and gastrostomy placement is required, with a subsequent procedure to re-establish esophageal continuity. Anastomotic leakage that is detected after several days usually heals without intervention, particularly if a retropleural approach is used. Under these circumstances, administration of broad-spectrum antibiotics, pulmonary toilet, and optimization of nutrition are important. After approximately 1 week, a repeat esophagram should be taken to determine whether the leakage has resolved.

Strictures are not infrequent (10 to 20% of cases), particularly if a leak has occurred. A stricture may become apparent at any time, from the early postoperative period to months or years later. It may present as choking, gagging, or failure to thrive but often becomes clinically apparent with the transition to consumption of solid food. A contrast swallow test or esophagoscopy is confirmatory, and simple dilation is usually corrective. Occasionally, repeated dilations are required. These may be performed in a retrograde procedure in which a silk suture is placed into the oropharynx and delivered from the esophagus through a gastrostomy tube. Tucker dilators are then tied to the suture and passed in a retrograde fashion from the gastrostomy tube and delivered out of the oropharynx. Increasing sizes are used, and the silk is replaced at the end of the procedure, with one end of the silk taped to the side of the face and the other end to the gastrostomy tube. Alternatively, image-guided balloon dilation over a guidewire may be performed, with intraoperative contrast radiography used to determine the precise location of the stricture and to assess the immediate response to the dilation.

Recurrent tracheoesophageal fistula may represent a missed upper pouch fistula or a true recurrence. This may occur after an anastomotic disruption, during which the recurrent fistula may heal spontaneously. Otherwise, reoperation may be required.

Gastroesophageal reflux commonly occurs after repair of EA-TEF, potentially due to alterations in esophageal motility and the anatomy of the gastroesophageal junction. The clinical manifestations of such reflux are similar to those seen in other infants with primary gastroesophageal reflux disease. A loose antireflux procedure, such as a Nissen fundoplication, is used to prevent further reflux, but the child may have feeding problems after antireflux surgery as a result of the intrinsic dysmotility of the distal esophagus. To minimize this latter problem, some surgeons prefer to perform an incomplete wrap (such as a Toupet or a Thal wrap) rather than a 360-degree wrap. The fundoplication may be safely performed laparoscopically in experienced hands, although care should be taken to ensure that the wrap is not excessively tight.

Special Circumstances

Patients with type E TEFs (commonly referred to as *H-type*) present beyond the newborn period. Presenting symptoms include recurrent chest infections, bronchospasm, and failure to thrive. The diagnosis can be suspected from the results of barium esophagography and confirmed by endoscopic visualization of the fistula. Surgical correction is generally possible through a cervical approach after placement of a balloon catheter across the fistula and requires mobilization and division of the fistula. Outcome is usually excellent.

Patients with duodenal atresia and EA-TEF may require urgent treatment due to the presence of a closed obstruction of the stomach and proximal duodenum. In patients in stable condition, treatment consists of repair of the esophageal anomaly and correction of the duodenal atresia if the infant's condition is stable during surgery. If not, a staged approach should be used consisting of ligation of the fistula and placement of a gastrostomy tube. Definitive repair can then be performed at a later time.

Primary EA (type A) represents a challenging problem, particularly if the upper and lower ends of the esophagus are too far apart for an anastomosis to be created. Under these circumstances, treatment strategies include placing a gastrostomy tube and performing serial bougienage to increase the length of the upper pouch. This occasionally permits primary anastomosis to be performed. When the two ends cannot be brought together safely, esophageal replacement is required using either a gastric pull-up or colon interposition (see later).

Outcome

Various classification systems have been used to predict survival in patients with EA-TEF and to stratify treatment. A system devised by Waterston in 1962 was used to stratify neonates based on birth weight, the presence of pneumonia, and the identification of other congenital anomalies. In response to advances in neonatal care, surgeons at the Montreal Children's Hospital proposed a new classification system in 1993. In the Montreal experience only two characteristics were found to independently affect survival: preoperative ventilator dependence and associated major anomalies. Pulmonary disease, as defined by ventilator dependence, appeared to be a more accurate predictor than pneumonia. Spitz and col-

leagues analyzed risk factors in infants who died with EA-TEF. Two criteria were found to be important predictors of outcome: birth weight of <1500 g and the presence of major congenital cardiac disease. A new classification for predicting outcome in EA was therefore proposed: group I—birth weight of ≥1500 g without major cardiac disease, survival 97% (283 of 293); group II—birth weight of <1500 g or major cardiac disease, survival 59% (41 of 70); and group III—birth weight of <1500 g and major cardiac disease, survival 22% (2 of 9).

In general, surgical correction of EA-TEF leads to a satisfactory outcome with nearly normal esophageal function in most patients. Overall survival rates of >90% have been achieved in patients classified as in stable condition according to all the various staging systems. Infants in unstable condition have an increased mortality (40 to 60% survival) because of potentially fatal associated cardiac and chromosomal anomalies or prematurity. However, the use of a staged procedure has increased survival in even these high-risk infants.

Corrosive Injury of the Esophagus

Injury to the esophagus after ingestion of corrosive substances occurs most commonly in the toddler age group. Both strong alkalies and strong acids produce injury by liquefaction or coagulation necrosis, and because all corrosive agents are extremely hygroscopic, the caustic substance will cling to the esophageal epithelium. Subsequent strictures occur at the intrinsically narrower areas of the esophagus: the cricopharyngeus, middle esophagus, and gastroesophageal junction. A child who has swallowed an injurious substance may be symptom free but usually is drooling and unable to swallow saliva. The injury may be restricted to the oropharynx and esophagus or may extend to the stomach. There is no effective immediate antidote. Diagnosis is made by careful physical examination of the mouth and endoscopy with a flexible or rigid esophagoscope. The endoscope should be advanced only to the first level of the burn to avoid perforation. Early barium swallow testing may delineate the extent of the mucosal injury. The practitioner should be aware that the esophagus may be burned without evidence of injury to the mouth. Although previously steroids were used routinely, they have not been shown to alter stricture development or modify the extent of injury. Therefore, they are no longer part of the management of caustic injuries. Antibiotics are administered during the acute period.

The extent of injury is graded endoscopically as either mild, moderate, or severe (grade I, II or III). Circumferential esophageal injuries with necrosis have an extremely high likelihood of stricture formation. These patients should undergo placement of a gastrostomy tube once they are in clinically stable condition. A string should be inserted through the esophagus either immediately or during repeat esophagoscopy several weeks later. When established strictures are present (usually 3 to 4 weeks), dilatation is performed. The safest are retrograde dilations, in which graduated dilators are brought through the gastrostomy and advanced into the esophagus via the transesophageal string. For less severe injuries, dilatation may be attempted in antegrade fashion using either graded bougies or balloons. Management of esophageal perforation during dilation should include administration of antibiotics, irrigation, and closed drainage of the thoracic cavity to prevent systemic sepsis. If recognition is delayed or if the patient is systemically ill, esophageal diversion may be required with staged reconstruction at a later time.

Although the native esophagus can and should be preserved in most cases, severe stricture formation that does not respond to dilation is best managed by esophageal replacement. The most commonly used options for esophageal substitution are the colon (right colon or transverse/left colon) and the stomach (gastric tube or gastric pull-up). Pedicled or free grafts of the jejunum are less commonly used. The right colon graft is based on a pedicle of the middle colic artery and the left colon graft on a pedicle of the middle colic or left colic artery. Gastric tubes are fashioned from the greater curvature of the stomach based on the pedicle of the left gastroepiploic artery. When the entire stomach is used, as in gastric pull-up, the blood supply is provided by the right gastric artery. The neo-esophagus may pass (a) substernally, (b) through a transthoracic route, or (c) through the posterior mediastinum to reach the neck. A feeding jejunostomy is placed at the time of surgery and tube feedings are instituted once the postoperative ileus has resolved. In a recent review of patients treated by gastric pull-up, long-term outcome was very good. Complications included esophagogastric anastomotic leak ($n = 15$, or 36%), which uniformly resolved without intervention, and stricture formation ($n = 20$, or 49%), which responded to a course of dilation. Long-term follow up has shown that all methods of esophageal substitution can support normal growth and development, and the children enjoy reasonably normal eating habits. Because of the potential for late complications such as ulceration and stricture, follow-up into adulthood is mandatory, but complications appear to diminish with time.

Gastroesophageal Reflux

Gastroesophageal reflux (GER) occurs to some degree in all children and refers to the passage of gastric contents into the esophagus. By contrast, gastroesophageal reflux disease (GERD) describes a situation in which reflux is symptomatic. Typical symptoms include failure to thrive, bleeding, stricture formation, reactive airway disease, aspiration pneumonia, and apnea. Failure to thrive and pulmonary problems are particularly common in infants with GERD, whereas strictures and esophagitis are more common in older children and adolescents. GERD is particularly problematic in neurologically impaired children.

Clinical Manifestations

Because all infants experience occasional episodes of GER, care must be taken before labeling a child as having pathologic reflux. A history of repeated episodes of vomiting that interferes with growth and development or the presence of life-threatening events is required for the diagnosis of GERD. In older children, esophageal bleeding, stricture formation, severe heartburn, or the development of Barrett's esophagus unequivocally connotes pathologic reflux or GERD. In neurologically impaired children, vomiting due to GER must be distinguished from chronic retching.

The work-up of patients suspected of having GERD includes documentation of the episodes of reflux and evaluation of the anatomy. A barium swallow examination should be performed as an initial test. The results will indicate whether there is obstruction of the stomach or duodenum (due to duodenal webs or pyloric stenosis) and will determine whether malrotation is present. The frequency and severity of reflux should be assessed using a 24-hour pH probe study. Although this test is poorly tolerated, it provides the most accurate determination that GERD is present. Esophageal endoscopy with biopsies may identify the presence of esophagitis and is useful to determine the length of the intra-abdominal esophagus and detect the presence of Barrett's esophagus. Some surgeons order a radioisotope "milk scan" to evaluate gastric emptying, although there is little evidence to show that this test changes management when a diagnosis of GERD has been confirmed using the aforementioned modalities.

Treatment

Most patients with GERD are treated initially by conservative means. In the infant, propping up the child and thickening the formula with rice cereal are generally recommended. Some authors prefer a prone, head-up position. In the infant unresponsive to position and formula changes and the older child with severe GERD, medical therapy based on gastric acid reduction with an H_2 blocking agent and/or a proton pump inhibitor is initiated. Medical therapy is successful in most neurologically normal infants and younger children, many of whom will outgrow their need for medications. In certain patients, however, medical treatment does not provide symptomatic relief and surgery is therefore indicated. The least invasive surgical option is the placement of a nasojejunal or gastrojejunal feeding tube. Because the stomach is bypassed, food contents do not

enter the esophagus, and symptoms are often improved. As a long-term remedy, however, this therapy is associated with several problems. The tubes often become dislodged, acid reflux still occurs, and bolus feeding is generally not possible. Fundoplication provides definitive treatment for gastroesophageal reflux and is highly effective in most circumstances. The fundus may be wrapped around the distal esophagus either 360 degrees (i.e., Nissen fundoplication) or to lesser degrees (i.e., Thal or Toupet fundoplication). At present, the standard approach in most children is to perform these procedures laparoscopically whenever possible. In children with feeding difficulties and in infants <1 year of age, a gastrostomy tube should be placed at the time of surgery. Early postoperative complications include pneumonia and atelectasis, often due to inadequate pulmonary toilet and inadequate pain control with abdominal splinting. Late postoperative complications include wrap breakdown with recurrent reflux, which may require repeat fundoplication, and dysphagia due to a wrap that is too tight, which generally responds to dilation. These complications are more common in children with neurologic impairment. The keys to successful surgical management of patients with GERD include careful patient selection and meticulous operative technique.

GASTROINTESTINAL TRACT

Approach to the Vomiting Infant

The majority of infants vomit. Because infant vomiting is so common, it is important to differentiate between normal vomiting—as occurs in almost all infants, to some degree—and abnormal vomiting, which may be indicative of a potentially serious underlying disorder. The color of the emesis and the child's overall condition must be assessed. Vomit that looks like feeds and comes up immediately after a feeding is almost always *gastroesophageal reflux*. This may or may not be of concern, as described earlier. Vomiting that occurs a short while after feeding, or indeed vomiting that projects out of the baby's mouth, may be indicative of *pyloric stenosis*. By contrast, *vomit that has any green color in it is always worrisome*. This may be reflective of intestinal *volvulus*, an underlying infection, or some other cause of intestinal obstruction. A more detailed description of the management of these conditions is provided in the following sections.

Hypertrophic Pyloric Stenosis
Clinical Manifestations

The ability to provide timely diagnosis and treatment of infants with hypertrophic pyloric stenosis (HPS) is another milestone in the history of pediatric surgery. HPS occurs in approximately 1 in 300 live births and originally was believed to occur in first-born males between 3 and 6 weeks of age. Subsequent studies determined that this was a statistical error; investigators did not account for the incidence of first-born males as a group. However, children with HPS outside of this age range are commonly seen, and the cause of HPS has not been determined. Studies have shown that HPS is found in several generations of the same family, which suggests a familial link. Administration of erythromycin in early infancy was also thought to be linked to the subsequent development of HPS, but rates of HPS have not decreased with the decline in the use of erythromycin, so this may also have been an erroneous conclusion.

Infants with HPS present with nonbilious vomiting that becomes increasingly projectile over the course of several days to weeks. Eventually, the infant develops almost complete gastric outlet obstruction and is no longer able to tolerate even clear liquids. Despite the recurrent emesis, the child normally has a voracious appetite, which leads to a cycle of feeding and vomiting that invariably results in severe dehydration if the condition is untreated. Jaundice may occur in association with HPS, although the reason for this is unclear. Particularly perceptive caregivers will mention that the infant is passing less flatus, which provides a further clue that gastric outlet obstruction is complete.

Infants with HPS develop a hypochloremic, hypokalemic metabolic alkalosis. The urine pH is high initially but eventually drops because hydrogen ions are preferentially exchanged for sodium ions in the distal tubule of the kidney as the hypochloremia becomes severe. The diagnosis of pyloric stenosis usually can be made on physical examination by palpation of the typical "olive" in the right upper quadrant and the presence of visible gastric waves on the abdomen. When the olive cannot be palpated, ultrasonography can diagnose the condition accurately in 95% of patients. Criteria for ultrasonographic diagnosis include a channel length of >16 mm and pyloric thickness of >4 mm.

Treatment

Pyloric stenosis is never a surgical emergency, although the dehydration and electrolyte abnormalities may present a medical emergency. Fluid resuscitation with correction of electrolyte abnormalities and metabolic alkalosis is essential before induction of general anesthesia for operation. For most infants, administration of fluid containing 5% dextrose and 0.45% saline with 2 to 4 mEq/kg of added potassium at a rate of approximately 150 to 175 mL/kg for 24 hours will correct the underlying deficit. It is important to ensure that the child has an adequate urine output (>1 mL/kg per hour) as further evidence that rehydration has occurred. After resuscitation, a Fredet-Ramstedt pyloromyotomy is performed (Fig. 39-12). The procedure may be performed using an open or laparoscopic approach.

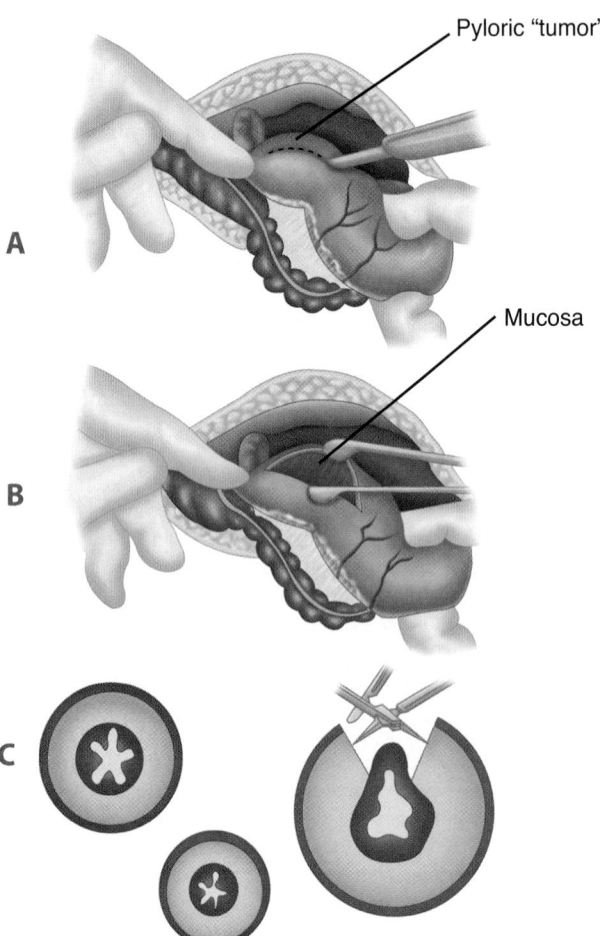

Pyloric "tumor"

Mucosa

FIG. 39-12. Fredet-Ramstedt pyloromyotomy. **A.** Pylorus delivered into wound and seromuscular layer incised. **B.** Seromuscular layer separated down to the submucosal base to permit herniation of mucosa through the pyloric incision. **C.** Cross-section demonstrating the hypertrophied pylorus, depth of incision, and spreading of muscle to permit mucosa to be herniated through the incision.

Open pyloromyotomy is performed through either an umbilical or a right upper quadrant transverse abdominal incision. The former route is cosmetically more appealing, although the transverse incision provides easier access to the antrum and pylorus. In recent years, the laparoscopic approach has gained great popularity. Two randomized trials have demonstrated that both the open and laparoscopic approaches may be performed safely with equal incidence of postoperative complications, although the cosmetic result is definitely superior after the laparoscopic approach. Whether performed using an open or laparoscopic approach, surgical treatment of pyloric stenosis involves splitting the pyloric muscle until the submucosa bulges upward. The incision begins at the pyloric vein of Mayo and extends onto the gastric antrum; it typically measures between 1 and 2 cm in length. Postoperatively, IV fluids are continued for several hours, after which an oral electrolyte solution (Pedialyte) is offered, followed by formula or breast milk, which is gradually increased to 60 mL every 3 hours. Most infants can be discharged home within 24 to 48 hours after surgery. Recently, several authors have shown that ad lib feedings are safely tolerated by the neonate and result in a shorter hospital stay.

The complications of pyloromyotomy include perforation of the mucosa (1 to 3%), bleeding, wound infection, and recurrent symptoms due to inadequate myotomy. When perforation occurs, the mucosa is repaired with a stitch that is placed to tack the mucosa down and reapproximate the serosa in the region of the tear. A nasogastric tube is left in place for 24 hours and taped securely to prevent it from reinjuring the repaired mucosa. The outcome is generally very good.

Intestinal Obstruction in the Newborn

The cardinal symptom of intestinal obstruction in the newborn is bilious emesis. Prompt recognition and treatment of neonatal intestinal obstruction can truly be lifesaving.

Intestinal obstruction can be classified as either proximal or distal, based on the clinical presentation. Proximal obstruction presents as bilious vomiting with minimal abdominal distention. In cases of complete obstruction, there may be a paucity of gas, or no distal air may be seen on the supine and upright films of the abdomen. In this case, the diagnosis of malrotation and midgut volvulus must be excluded. Distal obstruction presents with abdominal distention and bilious emesis. The physical examination will determine whether the anus is patent. Calcifications on the plain abdominal radiograph may indicate meconium peritonitis; pneumatosis and/or free abdominal air indicates necrotizing enterocolitis with or without intestinal perforation. A contrast enema study will show whether there is a microcolon indicative of jejunoileal atresia or meconium ileus. If a microcolon is not present, then the diagnoses of Hirschsprung's disease, small left colon syndrome, or meconium plug syndrome should be considered. In all cases of intestinal obstruction, it is vital to obtain abdominal films in the supine and upright (lateral decubitus) views. This is the only way to assess the presence of air-fluid levels or free air and to characterize the obstruction as proximal or distal. Moreover, unless a contrast agent is used, it is difficult to determine whether a loop of dilated bowel is part of the small or of the large intestine, because the neonatal bowel lacks typical features, such as haustra or plicae circulares, that characterize these loops in older children or adults. For this reason, care must be taken to take a complete prenatal history, to perform a thorough physical examination, and to determine the need for further contrast studies as opposed to immediate abdominal exploration.

Duodenal Obstruction

Whenever the diagnosis of duodenal obstruction is entertained, malrotation and midgut volvulus must be excluded. This topic is covered in further detail later. Other causes of duodenal obstruction include duodenal atresia, duodenal web, stenosis, annular pancreas, and duodenal duplication cyst. Duodenal obstruction is easily

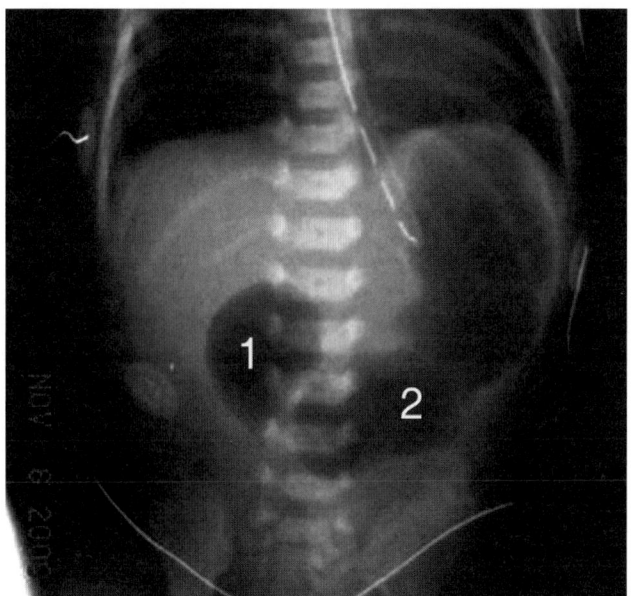

FIG. 39-13. Abdominal radiograph showing the "double bubble" sign in a newborn infant with duodenal atresia. The two bubbles are numbered.

diagnosed by prenatal ultrasonography, which demonstrates the fluid-filled stomach and proximal duodenum as two discrete cystic structures in the upper abdomen. Associated polyhydramnios is common and presents in the third trimester. In 85% of infants with duodenal obstruction, the entry of the bile duct is proximal to the level of obstruction, so that vomiting is bilious. Abdominal distention is typically not present because of the proximal level of obstruction. In those infants with obstruction proximal to the bile duct entry, the emesis is nonbilious. The classic finding on abdominal radiograph is the "double bubble" sign, which represents the dilated stomach and duodenum (Fig. 39-13). In association with the appropriate clinical picture, this finding is sufficient to confirm the diagnosis of duodenal obstruction. If there is any uncertainty, however, particularly when a partial obstruction is suspected, an upper GI series with contrast is diagnostic.

Treatment An orogastric tube is inserted to decompress the stomach and duodenum, and the infant is given IV fluids to maintain adequate urine output. If the infant appears ill, or if abdominal tenderness is present, a diagnosis of malrotation and midgut volvulus should be considered, and surgery should not be delayed. Typically, the abdomen is soft and the infant is in very stable condition. Under these circumstances, the infant should be evaluated thoroughly for other associated anomalies. Approximately one third of newborns with duodenal atresia have associated Down syndrome (trisomy 21). These patients should be evaluated for associated cardiac anomalies. Once the work-up is complete and the infant's condition is stable, he or she is taken to the operating room and the abdomen is entered through a transverse right upper quadrant supraumbilical incision under general endotracheal anesthesia. A search for associated anomalies should be performed at the time of the operation. These include malrotation, anterior portal vein, a second distal web, and biliary atresia. The surgical treatment of choice for duodenal obstruction due to duodenal stenosis or atresia or annular pancreas is a duodenoduodenostomy. This procedure can be most easily performed using a proximal transverse-to-distal longitudinal (diamond-shaped) anastomosis. In cases in which the duodenum is extremely dilated, the lumen may be tapered using a linear stapler with a large Foley catheter (24F or greater) in the duodenal lumen. It is important to emphasize that an annular pancreas is never divided. Treatment of duodenal web includes

vertical duodenotomy, partial excision of the web (to avoid injury to the inserting pancreatobiliary ducts), oversewing of the mucosa, and horizontal closure of the duodenotomy. Gastrostomy tubes are not placed routinely. Recently reported survival rates exceed 90%. Late complications from repair of duodenal atresia occur in approximately 12 to 15% of patients and include megaduodenum, intestinal motility disorders, and gastroesophageal reflux.

Intestinal Atresia

Obstruction due to intestinal atresia can occur at any point along the intestinal tract. Based on early studies in which various types of atresia were modeled in dogs by creating vascular injuries, most small intestine atresias (but not duodenal atresias) are believed to be caused by in utero mesenteric vascular accidents leading to segmental loss of the intestinal lumen. Work with transgenic mouse models currently calls this hypothesis into question, however, and suggests that atresias may be multifactorial. The incidence of intestinal atresia has been estimated to be between 1 in 2000 to 1 in 5000 live births, with equal representation of the sexes. Infants with jejunal or ileal atresia present with bilious vomiting and progressive abdominal distention. The more distal the obstruction, the more distended the abdomen and the greater the number of obstructed loops on upright abdominal films (Fig. 39-14).

In cases in which the diagnosis of complete intestinal obstruction is determined based on the clinical picture and the presence of staggered air-fluid levels on plain abdominal films, the child can be brought to the operating room after appropriate resuscitation. In these circumstances, there is little extra information to be gained by performing a barium enema study. In contrast, when diagnostic uncertainty exists, or when distal intestinal obstruction is apparent, a barium enema study is useful to establish whether a microcolon is present and to diagnose the presence of meconium plugs, small left colon syndrome, Hirschsprung's disease, or meconium ileus. Use of

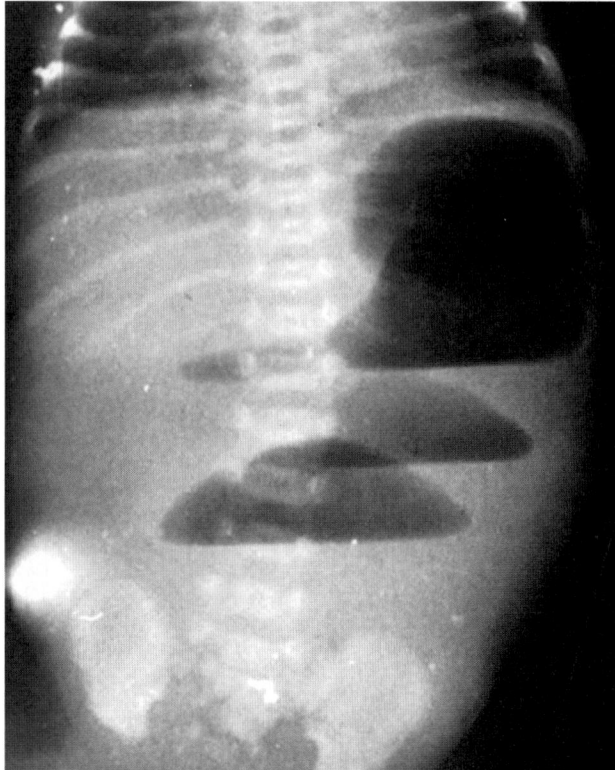

FIG. 39-14. Intestinal obstruction in the newborn showing several loops of distended bowel with air-fluid levels. This child has jejunal atresia.

barium enema testing is therefore required to safely manage neonatal intestinal obstruction, based on an understanding of the expected level of obstruction.

Surgical correction of the small intestinal atresia should be performed urgently. At laparotomy, one of several types of atresia will be encountered. In type I there is a mucosal atresia with intact muscularis. In type 1 the atretic ends are connected by a fibrous band. In type 3A the two ends of the atresia are separated by a V-shaped defect in the mesentery. Type 3B is an "apple-peel" deformity or "Christmas tree" deformity in which the bowel distal to the atresia receives its blood supply in a retrograde fashion from the ileocolic or right colic artery (Fig. 39-15). In type 4 there are multiple atresias that have a "string of sausage" or "string of beads" appearance. The disparity in lumen size between the proximal distended bowel and the small-diameter collapsed bowel distal to the atresia has led to a number of innovative techniques of anastomosis. Under most circumstances, however, an anastomosis can be performed using the end-to-back technique in which the distal, compressed loop is "fish-mouthed" along its antimesenteric border. The proximal distended loop can be tapered as described earlier. Because the distended proximal bowel rarely has normal motility, the extremely dilated portion should be resected before the anastomosis is performed.

Occasionally the infant with intestinal atresia will develop ischemia or necrosis of the proximal segment secondary to volvulus of the dilated, bulbous, blind-ending proximal bowel. Under these conditions, an end ileostomy and mucus fistula should be created, and the anastomosis should be deferred to another time after the infant stabilizes.

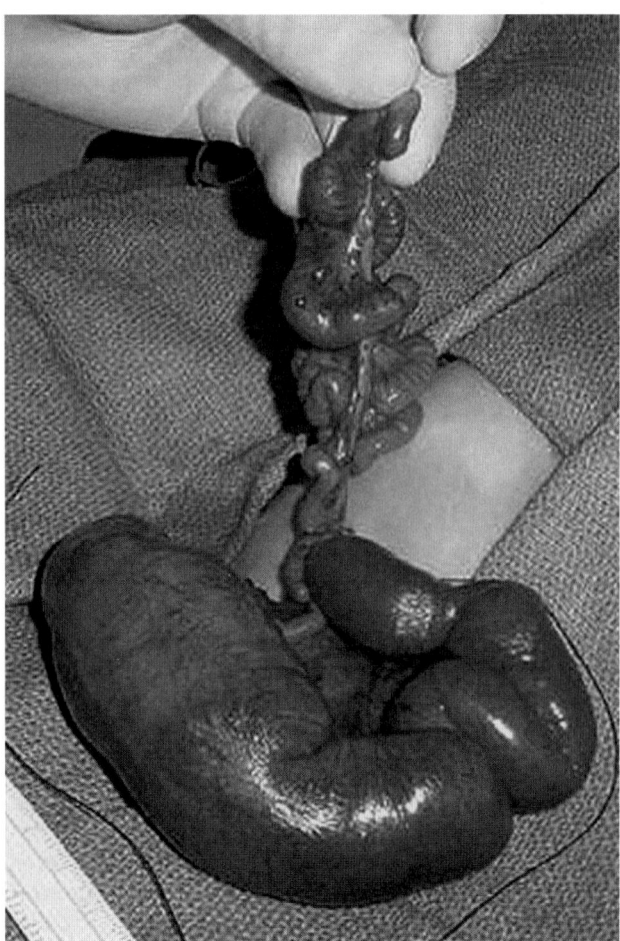

FIG. 39-15. Intraoperative photograph of newborn with "Christmas tree" type of ileal atresia.

Malrotation and Midgut Volvulus

Embryology During the sixth week of fetal development, the midgut grows too rapidly to be accommodated in the abdominal cavity and therefore prolapses into the umbilical cord. Between the tenth and twelfth weeks, the midgut returns to the abdominal cavity, undergoing a 270-degree counterclockwise rotation around the superior mesenteric artery. Because the duodenum also rotates caudal to the artery, it acquires a C loop that traces this path. The cecum rotates cephalad to the artery, which determines the location of the transverse and ascending colon. Subsequently, the duodenum becomes fixed retroperitoneally in its third portion and at the ligament of Treitz, whereas the cecum becomes fixed to the lateral abdominal wall by peritoneal bands. The takeoff of the branches of the superior mesenteric artery elongates and becomes fixed along a line extending from its emergence from the aorta to the cecum in the right lower quadrant. Although the process is not well understood, genetic mutations may predispose the host to malrotation. For instance, mutations in the gene *BCL6* resulting in absence of left-sided expression of its transcript lead to reversed cardiac orientation, defective ocular development, and malrotation. If rotation is incomplete, the cecum remains in the epigastrium, but the bands fixing the duodenum to the retroperitoneum and cecum continue to form. This results in the creation of (Ladd's) bands extending from the cecum to the lateral abdominal wall and crossing the duodenum, which creates the potential for obstruction. The mesenteric takeoff remains confined to the epigastrium, so that a narrow pedicle suspends all the branches of the superior mesenteric artery and the entire midgut. A volvulus may therefore occur around the mesentery. This twist not only obstructs the proximal jejunum but also cuts off the blood supply to the midgut. Intestinal obstruction and complete infarction of the midgut occur unless the problem is promptly corrected surgically.

Presentation and Management

Midgut volvulus can occur at any age, although it is seen most often in the first few weeks of life. Bilious vomiting is usually the first sign of volvulus, and all infants with bilious vomiting must be evaluated rapidly to ensure that they do not have intestinal malrotation with volvulus. This diagnosis should be suspected in a child with irritability and bilious emesis. If the condition is left untreated, vascular compromise of the midgut initially causes bloody stools but eventually results in circulatory collapse. Additional clues to the presence of advanced ischemia of the intestine include erythema and edema of the abdominal wall, which progresses to shock and death. It must be re-emphasized that the index of suspicion for this condition must be high, because abdominal signs are minimal in the early stages. Abdominal films show a paucity of gas throughout the intestine with a few scattered air-fluid levels (Fig. 39-16). When these findings are present, the patient should undergo immediate fluid resuscitation to ensure adequate perfusion and urine output, followed by prompt exploratory laparotomy.

Often the patient will not appear ill, and the plain films may suggest partial duodenal obstruction. Under these conditions, the patient may have malrotation without volvulus. This is best diagnosed by an upper GI series, which will show incomplete rotation with the duodenojejunal junction displaced to the right. The duodenum may show a corkscrew appearance, which is diagnostic of volvulus, or complete duodenal obstruction, with the small bowel loops entirely in the right side of the abdomen. A barium enema study may show a displaced cecum, but this sign is unreliable, especially in the small infant in whom the cecum is normally in a somewhat higher position than in the older child.

When volvulus is suspected, early surgical intervention is mandatory if the ischemic process is to be avoided or reversed. Volvulus occurs clockwise, and it is therefore untwisted counterclockwise. This can be remembered by using the memory aid "Turn back the hands of time." Subsequently, Ladd's procedure is performed. This operation does not correct the malrotation but does broaden the

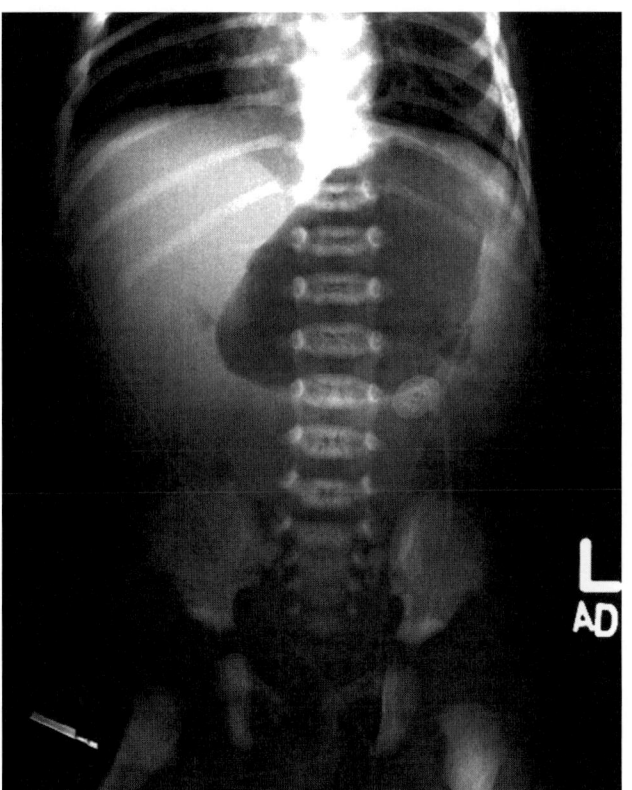

FIG. 39-16. Abdominal radiograph of a 10-day-old infant with bilious emesis. Note the dilated proximal bowel and the paucity of distal bowel gas, characteristic of a volvulus.

narrow mesenteric pedicle to prevent volvulus from recurring. This procedure is performed as follows (Fig. 39-17): The bands between the cecum and the abdominal wall and between the duodenum and terminal ileum are divided sharply to splay out the superior mesenteric artery and its branches. This maneuver brings the straightened duodenum into the right lower quadrant and the cecum into the left lower quadrant. The appendix is removed to avoid diagnostic errors in later life. No attempt is made to suture the cecum or duodenum in place. When ischemia is advanced, the volvulus is reduced without performing Ladd's procedure, and a second look is taken 24 to 36 hours later, which often shows some vascular recovery. A plastic transparent silo may be placed to facilitate constant evaluation of the intestine and to plan for the timing of re-exploration. Frankly necrotic bowel can then be resected conservatively. With early diagnosis and correction the prognosis is excellent. However, diagnostic delay can lead to mortality or to short-bowel syndrome requiring intestinal transplantation.

A subset of patients with malrotation show chronic obstructive symptoms. These symptoms may result from Ladd's bands across the duodenum or, occasionally, from intermittent volvulus. Symptoms include intermittent abdominal pain and intermittent vomiting, which may occasionally be bilious. Infants with malrotation may demonstrate failure to thrive, and they may be diagnosed initially as having gastroesophageal reflux disease. Surgical correction using Ladd's procedure as described earlier can prevent volvulus from occurring and improve symptoms in many instances. One should note, however, that volvulus can still occur after Ladd's procedure is performed, although this is uncommon.

Meconium Ileus

Pathogenesis and Clinical Presentation Infants with cystic fibrosis have characteristic pancreatic enzyme deficiencies and abnormal chloride secretion in the intestine that result in the production of viscous, water-poor meconium. Meconium ileus occurs when this thick, highly viscous meconium becomes impacted in the ileum and leads to high-grade intestinal obstruction. Meconium ileus can be either uncomplicated, in which there is no intestinal perforation, or complicated, in which prenatal perforation of the intestine has occurred or vascular compromise of the distended ileum develops. Antenatal ultrasonography may reveal the presence of intra-abdominal or scrotal calcifications, or distended bowel loops. These infants present shortly after birth with progressive abdominal distention, intermittent bilious emesis, and failure to pass meconium. Abdominal radiographs show dilated loops of intestine. Because the enteric contents are so viscous, air-fluid levels do not form, even when obstruction is complete. Small bubbles of gas become entrapped in the inspissated meconium in the distal ileum, where they produce a characteristic ground-glass appearance.

The diagnosis of meconium ileus is confirmed by a contrast enema study, which typically demonstrates a microcolon. In patients with uncomplicated meconium ileus, the terminal ileum is filled with pellets of meconium. In patients with complicated meconium ileus, intraperitoneal calcifications form, producing an eggshell pattern on plain abdominal radiograph.

Management The treatment strategy depends on whether the patient has complicated or uncomplicated meconium ileus. Patients with uncomplicated meconium ileus can be treated nonoperatively. A dilute water-soluble contrast agent is advanced through the colon under fluoroscopic control into the dilated portion of the ileum. Because these contrast agents act partially by absorbing fluid from the bowel wall into the intestinal lumen, maintaining adequate hydration of the infant during this maneuver is extremely important. The enema may be repeated at 12-hour intervals over several days until all the meconium is evacuated. Failure to reflux the contrast into the dilated portion of the ileum signifies the presence of an associated atresia or complicated meconium ileus and thus warrants exploratory laparotomy. If surgical intervention is required because of failure of contrast enemas to relieve obstruction, operative irrigation with dilute contrast agent, N-acetylcysteine (Mucomyst), or saline through a purse-string suture may be successful. Alternatively, resection of the distended terminal ileum is performed, and the meconium pellets are flushed from the distal small bowel. At this point, ileostomy and mucus fistula may be created from the proximal and distal ends, respectively. Alternatively, a Bishop-Koop anastomosis or an end-to-end anastomosis may be performed (Fig. 39-18).

Necrotizing Enterocolitis

Clinical Features Necrotizing enterocolitis (NEC) is the most frequent and lethal GI tract disorder affecting the intestine of the stressed, preterm neonate. Over 25,000 cases of NEC are reported annually. The overall mortality ranges between 10 and 50%. As a result of advances in neonatal care such as surfactant therapy as well as improved methods of mechanical ventilation, an increasing number of low-birth-weight infants are surviving neonatal hyaline membrane disease. This growing group of survivors of neonatal respiratory distress syndrome increases the number of infants at risk for developing NEC. Consequently, it is estimated that NEC soon will surpass respiratory distress syndrome as the principal cause of death in the preterm infant.

Multiple risk factors have been associated with the development of NEC. These include prematurity, initiation of enteral feeding, bacterial infection, intestinal ischemia resulting from birth asphyxia, umbilical artery cannulation, persistence of a patent ductus arteriosus, cyanotic heart disease, and maternal cocaine abuse. Nonetheless, the mechanisms by which these complex interacting causes lead to the development of NEC remain undefined. The only consistent epidemiologic precursors for NEC are prematurity and enteral alimentation, which represent the commonly encountered clinical situation of a stressed infant who is fed enterally. Of note, there is some debate regarding the importance of enteral alimenta-

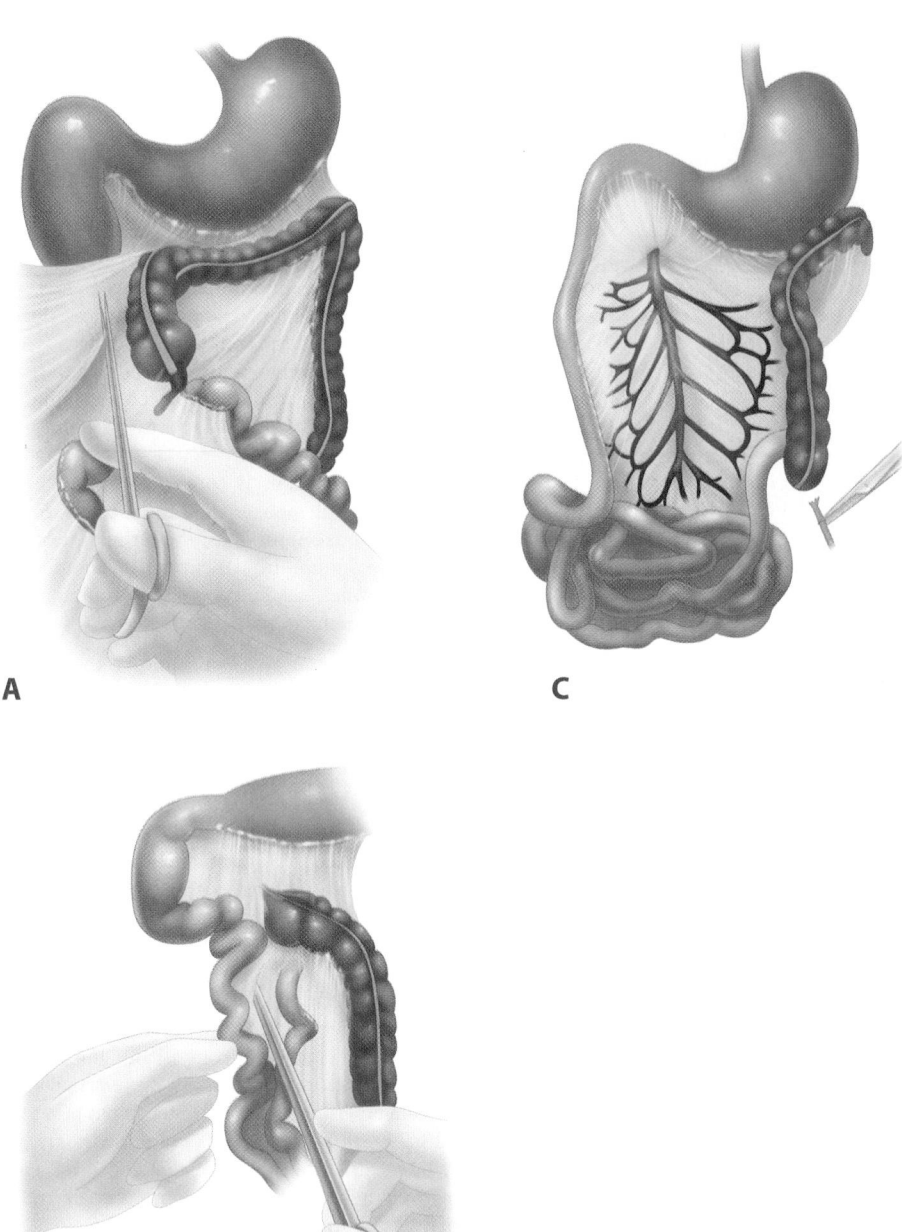

A

B

C

FIG. 39-17. Ladd's procedure for malrotation. **A.** Lysis of cecal and duodenal bands. **B.** Broadening of the mesentery. **C.** Appendectomy.

tion in the pathogenesis of NEC. A prospective randomized study showed no increase in the incidence of NEC despite adoption of an aggressive feeding strategy, and up to 10% of infants with NEC have never received any form of enteral nutrition.

The indigenous intestinal microbial flora has been postulated to play a central role in the pathogenesis of NEC. Bacterial colonization may be a prerequisite for the development of this disease, because oral prophylaxis with vancomycin or gentamicin reduces the incidence of NEC. The importance of bacteria in the pathogenesis of NEC is further supported by the finding that NEC occurs in episodic waves that can be abrogated by infection control measures and the fact that NEC usually develops at least 10 days postnatally, when the GI tract is colonized by coliforms. More recently, outbreaks of NEC have been reported in infants fed formula contaminated with *Enterobacter sakazakii*. Common bacterial isolates from the blood, peritoneal fluid, and stool of infants with advanced NEC include *Escherichia coli*, *Enterobacter*, *Klebsiella*, and occasionally coagulase-negative *Staphylococcus* species.

NEC may involve single or multiple segments of the intestine, most commonly the terminal ileum, followed by the colon. The gross findings in NEC include bowel distention with patchy areas of thinning, pneumatosis, gangrene, and frank perforation. The microscopic features include the appearance of a bland infarct characterized by full-thickness necrosis.

Clinical Manifestations Infants with NEC present with a spectrum of disease. In general, the infants are premature and may have sustained one or more episodes of stress, such as birth asphyxia, or they may have congenital cardiac disease. The clinical picture of NEC has been characterized by Bell and colleagues as progressing from a period of mild illness to a period of severe, life-threatening sepsis. Although not all infants progress through the various Bell stages, this classification scheme provides a useful format to describe the clinical picture associated with the development of NEC. In the earliest stage (Bell stage I), infants present with feeding intolerance. This is suggested by vomiting or by the presence of a

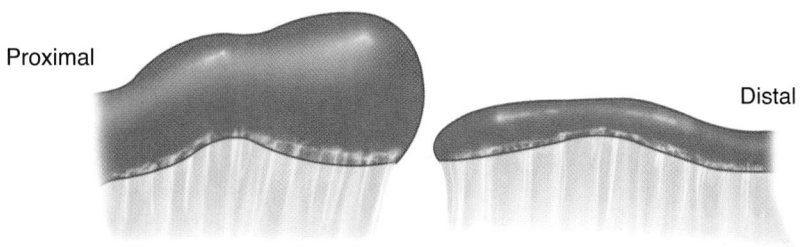

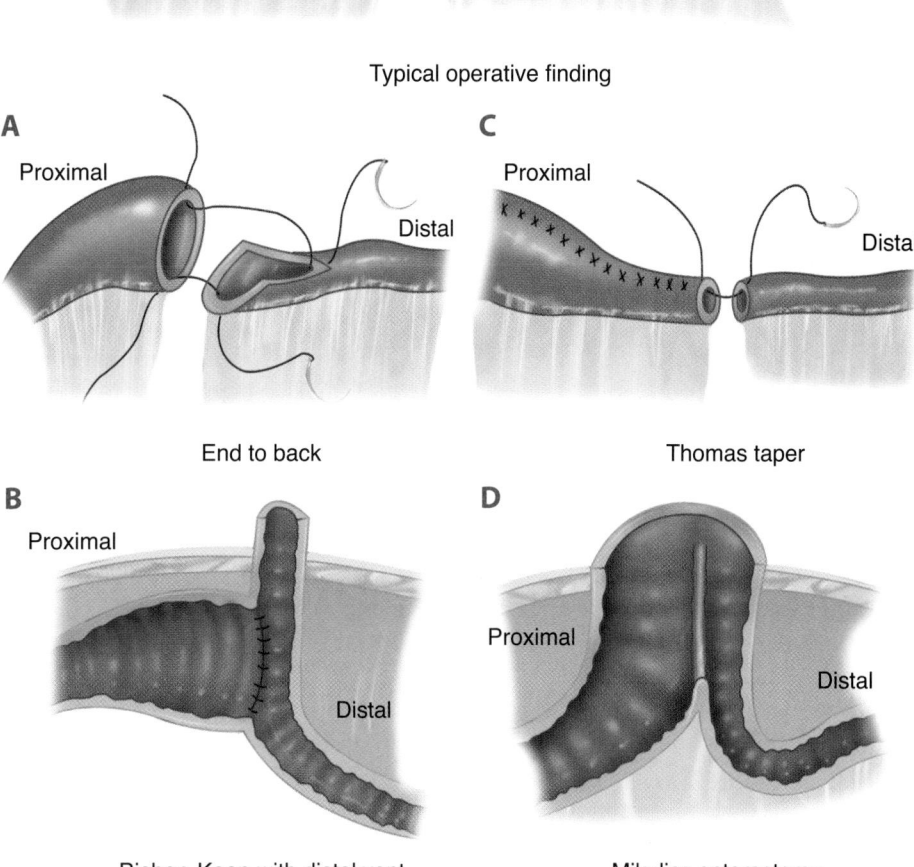

Typical operative finding

A End to back

B Bishop-Koop with distal vent

C Thomas taper

D Mikulicz enterostomy

FIG. 39-18. Techniques of intestinal anastomosis for infants with small-bowel obstruction. **A.** End-to-back anastomosis. The distal limb has been incised to create a "fish mouth" to enlarge the lumen. **B.** Bishop-Koop anastomosis. The proximal distended limb is joined to the side of the distal small bowel, which is vented by "chimney" to the abdominal wall. **C.** Tapering anastomosis. A portion of the antimesenteric wall of the proximal bowel is excised, with longitudinal closure to minimize disparity in the limbs. **D.** A Mikulicz double-barreled enterostomy is constructed by suturing the two limbs together and then exteriorizing the double stoma. The common wall can be crushed with a special clamp to create one large stoma. The stoma can be closed in an extraperitoneal manner.

large residual volume from a previous feeding in the stomach at the time of the next feeding. If they receive appropriate treatment, which consists of bowel rest and IV antibiotics, many of these infants will not progress to more advanced stages of NEC. These infants are colloquially described as experiencing a "NEC scare" and represent a population of neonates who are at risk of developing more severe NEC if a more prolonged period of stress supervenes.

Infants with Bell stage II disease have established NEC that is not immediately life-threatening. Clinical findings include abdominal distention and tenderness, bilious nasogastric aspirate, and bloody stools. These findings indicate the development of intestinal ileus and mucosal ischemia. Abdominal examination may reveal a palpable mass indicating the presence of an inflamed loop of bowel, diffuse abdominal tenderness, cellulitis, and edema of the anterior abdominal wall. The infant may appear systemically ill, with decreased urine output, hypotension, tachycardia, and noncardiac pulmonary edema. Hematologic evaluation reveals either leukocytosis or leukopenia, an increase in the number of bands, and thrombocytopenia. An increase in the blood urea nitrogen and plasma creatinine levels may be found, which signifies the development of renal dysfunction. The diagnosis of NEC may be confirmed by abdominal radiography. The pathognomonic radiographic finding in NEC is pneumatosis intestinalis, which represents invasion of the ischemic mucosa by gas-producing microbes (Fig. 39-19). Other findings include the presence of ileus or portal venous gas. The latter is a transient finding that indicates severe NEC with intestinal

necrosis. A fixed loop of bowel may be seen on serial abdominal radiographs, which suggests the possibility that a diseased loop of bowel, potentially with a localized perforation, is present. Although these infants are at risk of progressing to more severe disease, with timely and appropriate treatment, they often recover.

Infants with Bell stage III disease have the most advanced form of NEC. Abdominal radiographs often demonstrate the presence of pneumoperitoneum, which indicates that intestinal perforation has occurred. In these patients NEC may follow a fulminant course with progressive peritonitis, acidosis, sepsis, disseminated intravascular coagulopathy, and death.

Pathogenesis of Necrotizing Enterocolitis

Several theories have been proposed to explain the development of NEC. To more precisely understand the mechanisms that contribute to the pathogenesis of NEC, several groups have focused on understanding the potential clues that may be revealed by studying patients who have progressed from Bell stage I to Bell stage III disease. In general, the development of diffuse pneumatosis intestinalis—which is associated with the development of stage II NEC—is thought to be due to the presence of gas within the wall of the intestine from enteric bacteria, which suggests a causative role of bacteria in the pathogenesis of NEC. Furthermore, the development of pneumoperitoneum indicates disease progression with severe disruption of the intestinal barrier (intestinal perforation). Finally, systemic sepsis with diffuse multisystem organ dysfunction suggests

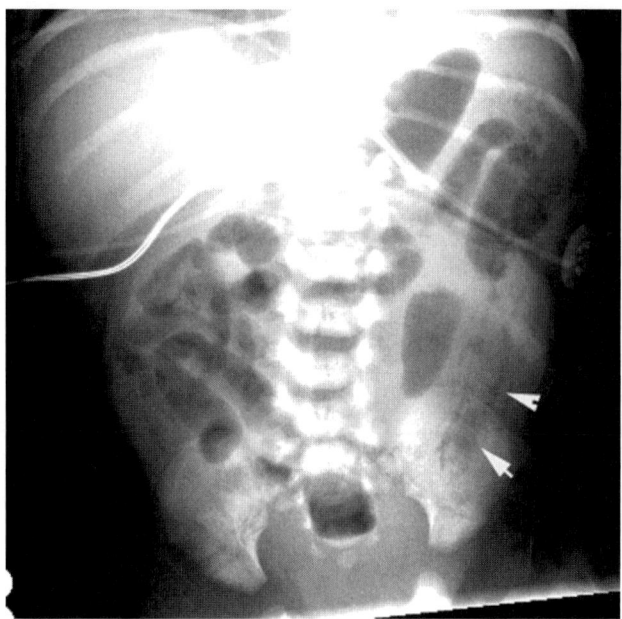

FIG. 39-19. Abdominal radiograph of infant with necrotizing enterocolitis. *Arrows* point to area of pneumatosis intestinalis.

a role for circulating proinflammatory cytokines in the pathogenesis of NEC. It has also been demonstrated that the premature intestine responds in an exaggerated fashion to bacterial products, which renders the host susceptible to barrier dysfunction and the development of NEC.

Treatment

In all infants suspected of having NEC, feedings are discontinued, a nasogastric tube is placed, and broad-spectrum parenteral antibiotics are given. The infant is resuscitated, and inotropes are administered to maintain perfusion as needed. Intubation and mechanical ventilation may be required to maintain oxygenation. TPN is started. Subsequent treatment may be influenced by the particular stage of NEC that is present. Patients with Bell stage I disease are closely monitored and generally remain on nil per os (NPO) status and are given IV antibiotics for 7 to 10 days before enteral nutrition is resumed. After this time, provided the infant fully recovers, feedings may be reinitiated.

Patients with Bell II disease merit close observation. Serial physical examinations are performed to look for the development of diffuse peritonitis, a fixed mass, progressive abdominal wall cellulitis, or systemic sepsis. If the infant fails to improve after several days of treatment, consideration should be given to exploratory laparotomy. Paracentesis may be performed, and if Gram's stain demonstrates multiple organisms and leukocytes, perforation of the bowel should be suspected, and the patient should undergo laparotomy.

In the most severe form of NEC (Bell stage III), patients have definite intestinal perforation or have not responded to nonoperative therapy. Two schools of thought exist regarding further management. One group favors exploratory laparotomy. At laparotomy, frankly gangrenous or perforated bowel is resected, and the intestinal ends are brought out as stomas. When there is massive intestinal involvement, marginally viable bowel is retained and a second-look procedure is carried out after the infant's condition stabilizes (24 to 48 hours). Patients with extensive necrosis at the second look may be managed by placing a proximal diverting stoma, resecting bowel that is definitely not viable, and leaving questionably viable bowel behind, distal to the diverted segment. If the intestine is viable except for a localized perforation without

diffuse peritonitis, and if the infant's clinical condition permits, intestinal anastomosis may be performed. In cases in which the diseased, perforated segment cannot be safely resected, drainage catheters may be left in the region of the diseased bowel, and the infant is allowed to reach stable condition.

An alternative approach to the management of infants with perforated NEC involves drainage of the peritoneal cavity. This may be performed under local anesthesia at the bedside and can be an effective means of stabilizing the desperately ill infant by relieving increased intra-abdominal pressure and allowing ventilation. When successful, this method also permits drainage of perforated bowel by establishment of a controlled fistula. Approximately one third of infants treated with drainage alone survive without requiring additional operations. Infants who do not respond to peritoneal drainage alone after 48 to 72 hours should undergo laparotomy. This procedure allows for the resection of frankly necrotic bowel and diversion of the fecal stream, and facilitates more effective drainage. It is noteworthy that a recent randomized controlled trial demonstrated that outcomes were similar in infants with NEC who were treated with primary peritoneal drainage and in those who were treated with laparotomy.

Necrotizing Enterocolitis in Older Infants

Although NEC is typically a disease that affects preterm infants, several independent groups have reported a tendency for early onset of NEC in term and near-term infants. In these patients, the pattern of disease was found to be different from that found in premature infants. Specifically, NEC in older infants typically is localized to the end of the small intestine and beginning of the colon, which suggests an ischemic pathophysiology. Four pertinent associated conditions are observed in term infants who develop NEC: congenital heart disease, in utero growth restriction, polycythemia, and perinatal hypoxic-ischemic events. As with NEC in preterm infants, NEC in older patients is also associated with formula consumption and is very rare in exclusively breastfed infants. Infants with NEC at full term typically present with bloody stools, and the disease is characterized by rapid onset of symptoms and a fulminant course. Thus, although it is true that NEC is typically a disease of premature infants, in the appropriate setting, NEC can develop at any age.

Spontaneous Intestinal Perforation vs. Necrotizing Enterocolitis

In addition to NEC, preterm infants with intestinal pathology may develop spontaneous intestinal perforation (SIP). SIP is a distinct clinical entity from NEC and is essentially a perforation in the terminal ileum. The histopathologic features of SIP are different from those of NEC. Specifically, the mucosa is not necrotic, there is no sign of ischemia, and the submucosa is thinned at the site of perforation. Unlike in NEC, in SIP pneumatosis intestinalis is absent. Moreover, the demographics of NEC and SIP are slightly different, in that infants with SIP tend to be slightly more premature, smaller, and more likely to have been receiving inotropic support. However, NEC and SIP occur with similar frequency in low-birth-weight infants. The outcome of patients in the two groups is slightly different. Because infants with SIP have isolated disease without necrosis or systemic inflammation, they tend to have a better outcome. In short, the diagnosis of SIP vs. NEC has important prognostic significance. The treatment strategies, however, are essentially the same.

Outcome Survival of patients with NEC is dependent on the stage of disease, the extent of prematurity, and the presence of associated comorbidities. Survival by stage has recently been shown to be approximately 85, 65, and 35% for infants with stages I, II, and III NEC, respectively. Strictures develop in 20% of medically or surgically treated patients, and a contrast enema study is mandatory before intestinal continuity is re-established. If all other factors are favorable, the ileostomy is closed when the child is between 2 and 2.5 kg. At the time of stoma closure, the entire intestine should be examined to search for possible strictures or other stigmata of NEC. Patients who have massive intestinal necrosis are at risk of developing short-bowel syndrome, particularly when the total length of the viable intestinal segment is <40 cm. These patients require TPN to provide adequate calories for growth and development, and may develop parenteral nutrition–associated cholestasis and hepatic fibrosis. In a significant number of these patients, transplantation of the liver and small bowel may be required.

Short-Bowel Syndrome

Short-bowel syndrome (SBS) is an expensive, morbid condition that is increasing in incidence. Congenital and perinatal conditions such as gastroschisis, malrotation, atresia, and NEC may lead to SBS. As noted previously, NEC is the most common GI emergency in neonates and occurs primarily in premature infants. As rates of prematurity are rising, so are the numbers of children with SBS and NEC. In addition, prevalence is increased for other diagnoses such as gastroschisis, which has nearly doubled. Medical and surgical treatment options carry high dollar and human costs and morbidities, including multiple infections and hospitalizations for vascular access, liver failure in conjunction with parenteral nutrition–associated cholestasis, and death. Small bowel transplantation has a reported 5-year graft survival of 48% but is attended by rejection, the morbidity of major surgery, and a lifelong need for antirejection medication. A report on 989 grafts in 923 patients by the Intestine Transplant Registry reveals improving outcomes, but *1-year* graft and patient survival rates are 65 and 77%, respectively. Preliminary data from research in a Lewis rat model of SBS indicate that transplantation of autologous cells may also aid patients someday. Tissue-engineered intestine proved an effective rescue therapy after massive small bowel resection. In the human, engineered intestine from autologous cells would avoid the problems of transplant-donor supply and immunosuppression. Because engineered small and large intestine, esophagus, stomach, and specific portions of the GI tract such as the gastroesophageal junction are formed by the same process, other intestinal deficiencies may possibly be addressed.

Intussusception

Intussusception is the leading cause of intestinal obstruction in the young child. The term refers to the condition in which a segment of intestine becomes drawn into the lumen of the more proximal bowel. The process usually begins in the region of the terminal ileum and extends distally into the ascending, transverse, or descending colon. Rarely, an intussusception may prolapse through the rectum.

The cause of intussusception is not clear, although one hypothesis suggests that hypertrophy of Peyer's patches in the terminal ileum from an antecedent viral infection acts as a lead point. Peristaltic action of the intestine then causes the bowel distal to the lead point to invaginate into itself. Idiopathic intussusception occurs in children between approximately 6 and 24 months of age. Beyond this age group, one should consider the possibility that a pathologic lead point may be present. These include polyps, malignant tumors such as lymphoma, enteric duplication cysts, and Meckel's diverticulum. Such intussusceptions are rarely reduced by air or contrast enema, and thus the lead point is identified when operative reduction of the intussusception is performed.

Clinical Manifestations Because intussusception is frequently preceded by a GI tract viral illness, the onset may not be easily determined. Typically, the infant develops paroxysms of crampy abdominal pain and intermittent vomiting. Between attacks, the infant may act normally, but as symptoms progress, increasing lethargy develops. Bloody mucus (currant jelly stool) may be passed per rectum. Ultimately, if reduction is not accomplished, gangrene of the intussusceptum occurs, and perforation may ensue. On physical examination, an elongated mass is detected in the right upper quadrant or epigastrium with an absence of bowel in the right lower quadrant (Dance's sign). The mass may be seen on plain abdominal radiograph but is more easily demonstrated on air or contrast enema.

Treatment Patients with intussusception should be assessed for the presence of peritonitis and for the severity of systemic illness. After resuscitation and administration of IV antibiotics, the child is evaluated for suitability to proceed with radiographic vs. surgical reduction. In the absence of peritonitis, the child should undergo radiographic reduction. If peritonitis is present, or if the child appears systemically ill, urgent laparotomy is indicated.

In the patient in stable condition, the air enema is both diagnostic and often curative. It constitutes the preferred method of diagnosis and nonoperative treatment of intussusception. Air is introduced with a manometer and the pressure that is administered is carefully monitored. Under most instances, this should not exceed 120 mmHg. Successful reduction is marked by free reflux of air into multiple loops of small bowel and symptomatic improvement as the infant suddenly becomes pain free. Unless both of these indications are observed, it cannot be assumed that the intussusception is reduced. If reduction is unsuccessful and the infant's condition remains stable, the infant should be brought back to the radiology suite for a repeat attempt at reduction after a few hours. This strategy has improved the success rate of nonoperative reduction in many centers. In addition, hydrostatic reduction with barium may be useful if pneumatic reduction is unsuccessful. The overall success rate of radiographic reduction varies based on the experience of the center but is typically between 60 and 90%.

If nonoperative reduction is successful, the infant may be given oral fluids after a period of observation. Failure to reduce the intussusception mandates surgery. Two approaches are used. In an open procedure, exploration is carried out through a right lower quadrant incision, with delivery of the intussuscepted mass into the wound. Reduction usually can be accomplished by gentle distal pressure, with the intussusceptum gently milked out of the intussuscipiens (Fig. 39-20). Care should be taken not to pull the bowel out, as this can cause damage to the bowel wall. The blood supply to the appendix is often compromised, and appendectomy is performed. If the bowel is frankly gangrenous, resection and primary anastomosis is performed. In experienced hands, laparoscopic reduction may be performed, even in very young infants. The procedure is carried out using a 5-mm laparoscope placed in the umbilicus and two additional 5-mm ports in the left and right lower quadrants. The bowel is inspected, and if it appears to be viable, reduction is performed by

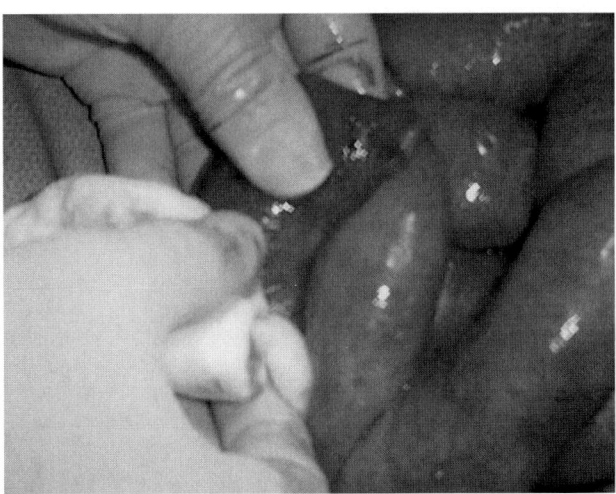

FIG. 39-20. Open reduction of intussusception. The bowel is milked backward to relieve the obstruction.

milking the bowel or using gentle traction, although this approach is normally discouraged during manual reduction. Atraumatic bowel graspers allow the bowel to be handled without injuring it.

IV fluids are continued until the postoperative ileus subsides. Patients are started on clear liquids, and the diet is advanced as tolerated. Of note, recurrent intussusception occurs in 5 to 10% of patients, independent of whether the bowel is reduced radiographically or surgically. Patients present with recurrent symptoms in the immediate postoperative period. Treatment involves repeat air enema, which is successful in most cases. In patients who experience three or more episodes of intussusception, the presence of a pathologic lead point should be suspected and carefully evaluated using contrast studies. After the third episode of intussusception, many pediatric surgeons will perform an exploratory laparotomy to reduce the bowel and to resect a pathologic lead point if identified.

Appendicitis

Presentation Correct diagnosis of appendicitis in children can be one of the most humbling and challenging tasks facing the pediatric surgeon. The classic presentation is generalized abdominal pain that localizes to the right lower quadrant followed by nausea, vomiting, fever, and peritoneal irritation in the region of the McBurney point. When children present in this manner, there should be little diagnostic delay. The child should be put on NPO status, administered IV fluids and broad-spectrum antibiotics, and brought to the operating room for an appendectomy. However, children often do not present in this manner. The coexistence of viral syndromes and the inability of young children to describe the location and quality of their pain often result in diagnostic delay. As a result, children with appendicitis, particularly those who are <5 years of age, often present with perforation. Perforation increases the length of hospital stay and makes the overall course of the illness significantly more complex.

Diagnosis of Appendicitis in Children Controversy exists regarding the role of radiographic studies in the diagnosis of acute appendicitis. Because children have less periappendiceal fat than adults, CT is less reliable in making the diagnosis. In addition, radiation exposure resulting from the CT scan may have potentially long-term adverse effects. Likewise, ultrasonography is not sufficiently sensitive or specific to allow accurate diagnosis of appendicitis, although it is very useful for excluding ovarian causes of abdominal pain. Therefore, the diagnosis of appendicitis remains largely clinical, and each clinician should develop his or her own threshold to operate or to observe the patient. A reasonable practice guideline is as follows: When the diagnosis is clinically apparent, appendectomy should be performed with minimal delay. Localized right lower quadrant tenderness associated with low-grade fever and leukocytosis in boys should prompt surgical exploration. In girls, ovarian or uterine pathology must also be considered. When there is diagnostic uncertainty, the child may be observed, rehydrated, and reassessed. In girls of menstruating age, ultrasonography may be performed to exclude ovarian pathology (cysts, torsion, or tumor). If results of all studies are negative, yet the pain persists and the abdominal findings remain equivocal, diagnostic laparoscopy may be used to determine the cause of the abdominal pain. The appendix should be removed even if it appears to be normal, unless another pathologic cause of the abdominal pain is definitively identified and the appendectomy would substantially increase morbidity.

Surgical Treatment of Appendicitis The definitive treatment for acute appendicitis is appendectomy. Before surgery, it is important that patients receive adequate IV fluids to correct the dehydration that commonly develops as a result of fever and vomiting in patients with appendicitis. Patients should also be started on antibiotics (such as a second-generation cephalosporin). Most surgeons perform a laparoscopic appendectomy, which may have some advantage over removal of the appendix through a single larger incision. During the laparoscopic appendectomy, a small incision is made at the umbilicus and two additional incisions are made in the lower abdomen.

The appendix is typically delivered through the umbilicus, and all incisions are then closed with dissolvable sutures. If the appendix is not ruptured, the patient may start drinking liquids shortly after waking up from the operation and may be advanced to a solid diet the next day. In general, the same steps are taken when appendectomy is performed through an open approach. The most common complication after appendectomy is a surgical site infection. Other complications—including bleeding and damage to other structures inside the abdomen—are extremely rare. Recovery from surgery is dependent on the individual patient. Most children go back to school approximately 1 week after surgery and usually are allowed to return to full physical activity after 2 to 3 weeks. During the recovery period, over-the-counter pain medication may be required. Older patients tend to require a longer time for full recovery.

Management of the Child with Perforated Appendicitis The signs and symptoms of perforated appendicitis can closely mimic those of gastroenteritis and include abdominal pain, vomiting, and diarrhea. Alternatively, the child may present with symptoms of intestinal obstruction. An abdominal mass may be present in the lower abdomen. When the symptoms have been present for longer than 4 or 5 days and an abscess is suspected, it is reasonable to obtain a CT scan of the abdomen and pelvis with IV, oral, and rectal contrast to visualize the appendix and look for an associated abscess, phlegmon, or fecalith (Fig. 39-21).

An individualized approach is necessary for the child who presents with perforated appendicitis. When there is evidence of generalized peritonitis, intestinal obstruction, or systemic toxicity, the child should undergo appendectomy. This should be delayed only for as long as is required to ensure adequate fluid resuscitation and administration of broad-spectrum antibiotics. The operation can be performed using an open or a laparoscopic approach. One distinct advantage of the laparoscopic approach is that it provides excellent visualization of the pelvis and all four quadrants of the abdomen. At the time of surgery, adhesions are gently lysed, abscess cavities are drained, and the appendix is removed. Drains are seldom used, and the skin incisions can be closed primarily. If a fecalith is identified outside the appendix on CT, every effort should be made to retrieve it and to remove it along with the appendix, if at all possible. Often, the child in whom symptoms have been present for longer than 4 or 5 days will present with an abscess without evidence of generalized peritonitis. Under these circumstances, it is appropriate to perform image-guided percutaneous drainage of the abscess followed by

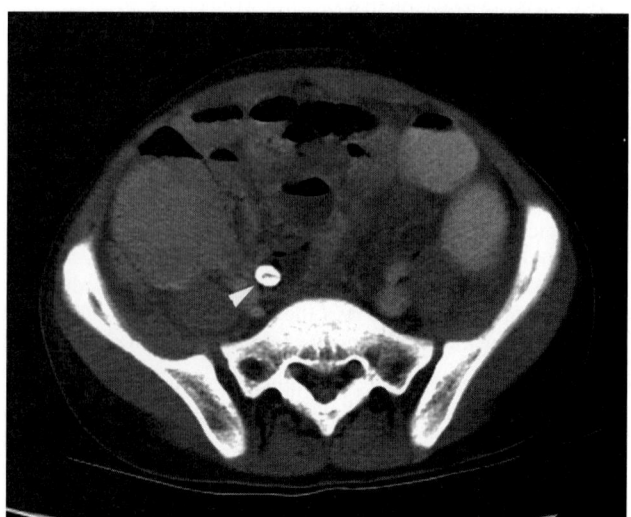

FIG. 39-21. Computed tomographic scan of the abdomen showing the presence of a ruptured appendix with pelvic fluid and a fecalith (*arrow*).

broad-spectrum antibiotic therapy. The inflammation will generally subside within several days, and the appendix can be safely removed on an outpatient basis 6 to 8 weeks later. If the child's symptoms do not improve, or if the abscess is not amenable to percutaneous drainage, then laparoscopic or open appendectomy and abscess drainage is required. Patients who present with a phlegmon in the region of a perforated appendix may be managed in a similar manner. In general, children who are younger than 4 or 5 years of age do not respond as well to an initially nonoperative approach, because their bodies do not localize or isolate the inflammatory process. Thus, these patients are more likely to require early surgical intervention. Patients who have had symptoms of appendicitis for no more than 4 days should probably undergo early appendectomy, because the inflammatory response is not as excessive during that initial period and the procedure can be performed safely.

If appendicitis isn't causing the pain, what could be causing it? As mentioned earlier, appendicitis can be one of the most difficult diagnoses to establish in children with abdominal pain, in part because of the large number of diseases that present in a similar fashion. Patients with urinary tract infection can have signs and symptoms similar to those of patients with appendicitis. However, patients with urinary tract infection are less likely to present with vomiting and are likely also to experience difficulty with urination, characterized by pressure, burning, and frequency. Constipation is commonly confused with appendicitis in its earliest stages. However, patients with constipation rarely have fever, and abnormalities will not be seen in the results of their blood work. Ovarian torsion can mimic appendicitis, given the severe abdominal pain that accompanies this condition. However, patients with ovarian torsion are generally asymptomatic until the acute onset of severe pain. By contrast, patients with appendicitis generally experience gradual onset of pain associated with nausea and vomiting. Finally, children and young adults are always at risk for the development of gastroenteritis. Unlike patients with appendicitis, however, patients with gastroenteritis generally present with persistent vomiting and occasionally diarrhea, which precedes the onset of the abdominal pain.

Intestinal Duplications

Intestinal duplications are mucosa-lined structures that are in continuity with the GI tract. Although they can occur at any level in the GI tract, duplications are found most commonly in the ileum within the leaves of the mesentery. Duplications may be long and tubular, but usually are cystic masses. In all cases, they share a common wall with the intestine. Symptoms associated with enteric duplication cysts include recurrent abdominal pain, emesis from intestinal obstruction, and hematochezia. Such bleeding typically results from ulceration in the duplication or in the adjacent intestine if the duplication contains ectopic gastric mucosa. On examination, a palpable mass is often identified. Children may also develop intestinal obstruction. Torsion may produce gangrene and perforation.

The ability to make a preoperative diagnosis of enteric duplication cyst usually depends on the presentation. CT, ultrasonography, and technetium pertechnetate scanning can be very helpful. Occasionally, a duplication can be seen on small bowel follow-through or barium enema study. For short duplications, resection of the cyst and adjacent intestine with end-to-end anastomosis can be performed. If resection of long duplications would compromise intestinal length, multiple enterotomies and mucosal stripping can be performed in the duplicated segment, which will allow the walls to collapse and become adherent. An alternative method is to divide the common wall using a linear cutting stapler to form a common lumen. Patients with duplications who undergo complete excision without compromise of the length of remaining intestine have an excellent prognosis.

Meckel's Diverticulum

Meckel's diverticulum is a remnant of a portion of the embryonic omphalomesenteric (vitelline) duct. It is located on the antimesen-

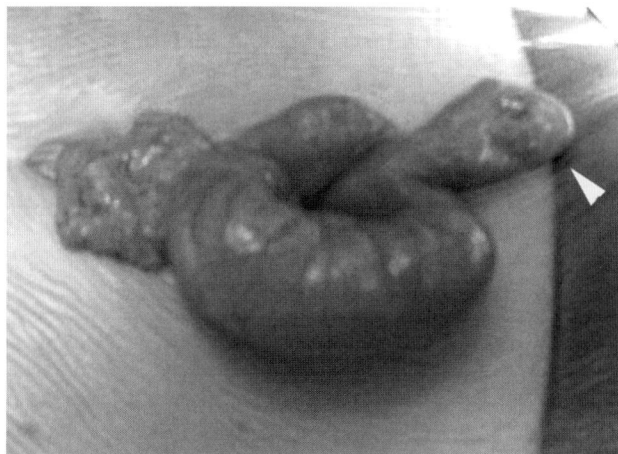

FIG. 39-22. Intraoperative photograph showing the presence of Meckel's diverticulum (*arrow*).

teric border of the ileum, usually within 2 ft of the ileocecal valve (Fig. 39-22). It may be found incidentally at surgery or may present with inflammation masquerading as appendicitis. Perforation of Meckel's diverticulum may occur if the outpouching becomes impacted with food, which leads to distention and necrosis. Occasionally, bands of tissue extend from the diverticulum to the anterior abdominal wall, and these may represent lead points around which internal hernias may develop. This is an important cause of intestinal obstruction in the older child who has a scarless abdomen. As with intestinal duplications, ectopic gastric mucosa may produce ileal ulcerations that bleed and lead to the passage of maroon stools. Pancreatic mucosa may also be present. Diagnosis may be made by technetium pertechnetate scans when the patient presents with bleeding. Treatment is surgical. If the base is narrow and there is no mass present in the lumen of the diverticulum, a wedge resection of the diverticulum with transverse closure of the ileum can be performed. A linear stapler is especially useful in this circumstance. When a mass of ectopic tissue is palpable, when the base is wide, or when there is inflammation, a resection of the involved bowel followed by end-to-end ileoileostomy is preferable.

Mesenteric Cysts

Mesenteric cysts are similar to duplications in their location within the mesentery. However, they do not contain any mucosa or muscular wall. Chylous cysts may result from congenital lymphatic obstruction. Mesenteric cysts can cause intestinal obstruction or may present as an abdominal mass. The diagnosis may be made by abdominal ultrasonography or CT. Treatment is surgical excision. This may require resection of the adjacent intestine, particularly for extensive, multicystic lesions. In cases in which complete excision is not possible due to the close proximity of the cyst to vital structures, partial excision or marsupialization should be performed.

Hirschsprung's Disease

Pathogenesis In his classic textbook entitled *Pediatric Surgery*, Dr. Orvar Swenson, who is eponymously associated with one of the classic surgical treatments for Hirschsprung's disease, described this condition as follows: "Congenital megacolon is caused by a malformation in the pelvic parasympathetic system which results in the absence of ganglion cells in Auerbach's plexus of a segment of distal colon. Not only is there an absence of ganglion cells, but the nerve fibers are large and excessive in number, indicating that the anomaly may be more extensive than the absence of ganglion cells." This description of Hirschsprung's disease is as accurate today as it was >50 years ago and summarizes the essential pathologic features of this disease: absence of ganglion cells in Auerbach's plexus and hypertrophy of associated nerve trunks. The cause of Hirsch-sprung's disease remains incompletely understood, although cur-rent thinking is that the disease results from a defect in the migration of neural crest cells, which are the embryonic precursors of the intestinal ganglion cell. Under normal conditions, the neural crest cells migrate into the intestine from cephalad to caudad. The process is completed by the twelfth week of gestation, but the migration from midtransverse colon to anus takes 4 weeks. During this latter period, the fetus is most vulnerable to defects in migration of neural crest cells. This may explain why most cases of aganglion-osis involve the rectum and rectosigmoid. The length of the agangli-onic segment of bowel is therefore determined by the most distal region that the migrating neural crest cells reach. In rare instances, total colonic aganglionosis may occur.

Recent studies have shed light on the molecular basis for Hirsch-sprung's disease. Patients with Hirschsprung's disease have an increased frequency of mutations in several genes, including *GDNF*, its receptor *Ret*, and its coreceptor *Gfra-1*. Moreover, mutations in these genes also lead to aganglionic megacolon in mice, which provides the opportunity to study the function of the encoded proteins. Initial investigations indicate that *GDNF* promotes the survival, proliferation, and migration of mixed populations of neural crest cells in culture. Other studies have revealed that *GDNF* is expressed in the gut in advance of migrating neural crest cells and is chemoattractive for neural crest cells in culture. These findings raise the possibility that mutations in the *GDNF* or *Ret* genes could lead to impaired neural crest migration in utero and the develop-ment of Hirschsprung's disease.

Clinical Presentation The incidence of sporadic Hirschsprung's disease is 1 in 5000 live births. There are reports of increased frequency of Hirschsprung's disease in multiple generations of the same family, especially in families with long-segment Hirschsprung's disease. Occasionally, such families have mutations in the genes described earlier, including the *Ret* gene. Because normal peristalsis cannot occur in the aganglionic colon, children with Hirschsprung's disease present with a functional distal intestinal obstruction. In the newborn period, the most common symptoms are abdominal disten-tion, failure to pass meconium, and bilious emesis. Any infant who does not pass meconium by 48 hours from birth must be investigated for the presence of Hirschsprung's disease. Occasionally, infants present with a dramatic complication of Hirschsprung's disease called *enterocolitis*. This pattern of presentation is characterized by abdominal distention and tenderness, and is associated with manifes-tations of systemic toxicity that include fever, failure to thrive, and lethargy. Infants are often dehydrated and demonstrate leukocytosis or an increase in circulating band forms on hematologic evaluation. On rectal examination, forceful expulsion of foul-smelling liquid feces is typically observed and represents the accumulation of stool under pressure in an obstructed distal colon. Treatment includes rehydration, systemic antibiotics, nasogastric decompression, and rectal irrigations while the diagnosis of Hirschsprung's disease is being confirmed. In children who do not respond to nonoperative management, a decompressive stoma is required. The surgeon must ensure that this stoma is placed in ganglion-containing bowel, and this must be confirmed by frozen-section analysis of bowel tissue performed at the time of stoma creation.

In approximately 20% of cases, the diagnosis of Hirschsprung's disease is made beyond the newborn period. These children have severe constipation, which has usually been treated with laxatives and enemas. Abdominal distention and failure to thrive may also be present at diagnosis.

Diagnosis The definitive diagnosis of Hirschsprung's disease is made by rectal biopsy. Samples of mucosa and submucosa are ob-tained at 1 cm, 2 cm, and 3 cm from the dentate line. In the neonatal period this biopsy can be performed at the bedside without anesthesia, because samples are taken in bowel that does not have somatic

innervation and thus the procedure is not painful to the child. In older children, the procedure should be performed as an open rectal biopsy using IV sedation. The histopathologic features of Hirschsprung's disease are the absence of ganglion cells in the myenteric plexuses, increased acetylcholinesterase staining, and the presence of hypertro-phied nerve bundles.

A barium enema examination should be performed in children in whom the diagnosis of Hirschsprung's disease is suspected. This test may demonstrate the location of the transition zone between the dilated ganglionic colon and the distal constricted aganglionic rectal segment. The authors' practice is to order this test before instituting rectal irrigations if possible, so that the difference in size between the proximal and distal bowel is preserved. Although a barium enema study can only suggest the diagnosis of Hirsch-sprung's disease, and not reliably establish it, the test is very useful in excluding other causes of distal intestinal obstruction. These include small left colon syndrome (as occurs in infants of diabetic mothers), colonic atresia, meconium plug syndrome, and the un-used colon observed in infants after the administration of magne-sium or tocolytic agents. In cases of total colonic aganglionosis, the barium enema study may reveal a markedly shortened colon. Some surgeons have found the use of rectal manometry helpful, particu-larly in older children, although the results are relatively inaccurate.

Treatment A diagnosis of Hirschsprung's disease requires surgery in all cases. The classic surgical approach consisted of a multiple-stage procedure. This included a colostomy in the newborn period, followed by a definitive pull-through operation after the child weighed >10 kg. There are three viable options for the definitive pull-through procedure that are currently used. Although individ-ual surgeons may advocate one procedure over another, studies have demonstrated that the outcome after each type of operation is similar. For each of the operations that is performed, the principles of treatment include confirming the location in the bowel where the transition zone between ganglionic and aganglionic bowel exists, resecting the aganglionic segment of bowel, and performing an anastomosis of ganglionated bowel to either the anus or a cuff of rectal mucosa (Fig. 39-23).

It is now well established that a primary pull-through procedure can be performed safely, even in the newborn period. This approach follows the same treatment principles as a staged procedure and saves the patient from an additional operation. Many surgeons perform the intra-abdominal dissection using the laparoscope. This approach is especially useful in the newborn period, because it provides excellent visualization of the pelvis. In children with significant colonic distention, it is important to allow for a period of decompression using a rectal tube if a single-staged pull-through is to be performed. In older children with a very distended, hypertro-phied colon, it may be prudent to perform a colostomy to allow the bowel to decompress, before performing a pull-through procedure. However, one should emphasize that there is no upper age limit for performing a primary pull-through.

Of the three pull-through procedures performed for Hirsch-sprung's disease, the first is the original Swenson's procedure. In this operation, the aganglionic rectum is dissected in the pelvis and removed down to the anus. The ganglionic colon is then anasto-mosed to the anus via a perineal approach. In the Duhamel procedure, dissection outside the rectum is confined to the retrorec-tal space, and the ganglionic colon is anastomosed posteriorly just above the anus. The anterior wall of the ganglionic colon and the posterior wall of the aganglionic rectum are anastomosed using a stapler. Although both of these procedures are extremely effective, they are limited by the possibility of damage to the parasympathetic nerves that are adjacent to the rectum. To circumvent this potential problem, the Soave procedure calls for dissection entirely within the rectum. The rectal mucosa is stripped from the muscular sleeve, and the ganglionic colon is brought through this sleeve and anasto-mosed to the anus. This operation may be performed completely

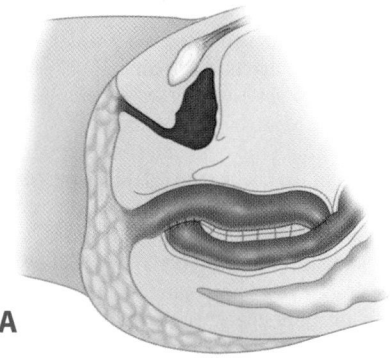

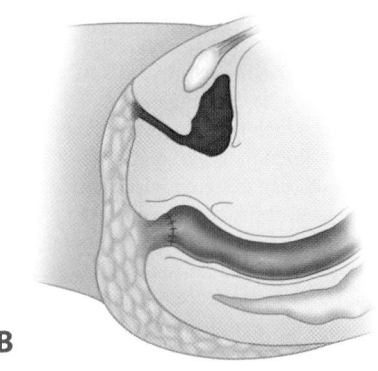

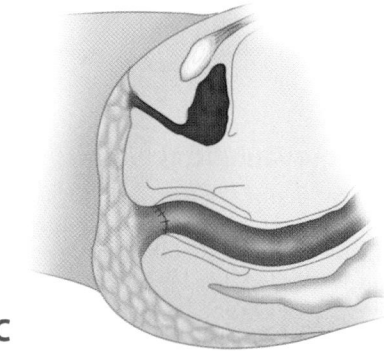

FIG. 39-23. Three operations for surgical correction of Hirschsprung's disease. **A.** The Duhamel procedure leaves the rectum in place and brings ganglionic bowel into the retrorectal space. **B.** Swenson's procedure is a resection with end-to-end anastomosis performed by exteriorizing bowel ends through the anus. **C.** In the Soave operation endorectal dissection is performed and mucosa is removed from the aganglionic distal segment. The ganglionic bowel is then brought down to the anus within the seromuscular tunnel.

from below. In all cases, it is critical that the level at which ganglionated bowel exists be determined. Most surgeons believe that the anastomosis should be performed at least 5 cm from the point at which ganglion cells are found. This avoids performing a pull-through in the transition zone, which is associated with a high incidence of complications due to inadequate emptying of the pull-through segment. Up to one third of patients who undergo a transition zone pull-through will require a reoperation.

The main complications of all procedures include postoperative enterocolitis, constipation, and anastomotic stricture. As mentioned earlier, long-term results for the three procedures are com-

parable and are generally excellent in experienced hands. These three procedures also can be adapted for total colonic aganglionosis in which the ileum is used for the pull-through segment.

Anorectal Malformations

Anatomic Description Anorectal malformations are a spectrum of congenital anomalies that include imperforate anus and persistent cloaca. Anorectal malformations occur in approximately 1 in 5000 live births and affect males and females almost equally. The embryologic basis includes failure of descent of the urorectal septum. The level to which this septum descends determines the type of anomaly that is present, which subsequently influences the surgical approach.

In patients with imperforate anus, the rectum fails to descend through the external sphincter complex. Instead, the rectal pouch ends blindly in the pelvis, above or below the levator ani muscle. In most cases, the blind rectal pouch communicates more distally with the genitourinary system or with the perineum through a fistulous tract. Traditionally, the anatomic description of imperforate anus has characterized it as either "high" or "low" depending on whether the rectum ends above the levator ani muscle complex or partially descends through this muscle (Fig. 39-24). Based on this classification system, in male patients with high imperforate anus the rectum usually ends as a fistula into the membranous urethra. In females, high imperforate anus often occurs in the context of a persistent cloaca. In both males and females, low lesions are associated with a fistula to the perineum. In males, the fistula connects with the median raphe of the scrotum or penis. In females, the fistula may end within the vestibule of the vagina, which is located immediately outside the hymen, or at the perineum.

Because this classification system is somewhat arbitrary, Peña proposed a classification system that specifically and unambiguously describes the location of the fistulous opening. In males the fistula may communicate with (a) the perineum (cutaneous perineal fistula), (b) the lowest portion of the posterior urethra (rectourethral bulbar fistula), (c) the upper portion of the posterior urethra (rectourethral prostatic fistula), or (d) the bladder neck (rectovesicular fistula). In females, the urethra may open to the perineum between the female genitalia and the center of the sphincter (cutaneous perineal fistula) or into the vestibule of the vagina (vestibular fistula) (Fig. 39-25). In both sexes, the rectum may end in a completely blind fashion (imperforate anus without fistula). In rare cases, patients may have a normal anal canal yet there may be total atresia or severe stenosis of the rectum.

In males the most frequent defect is imperforate anus with rectourethral fistula, followed by rectoperineal fistula, then rectove-

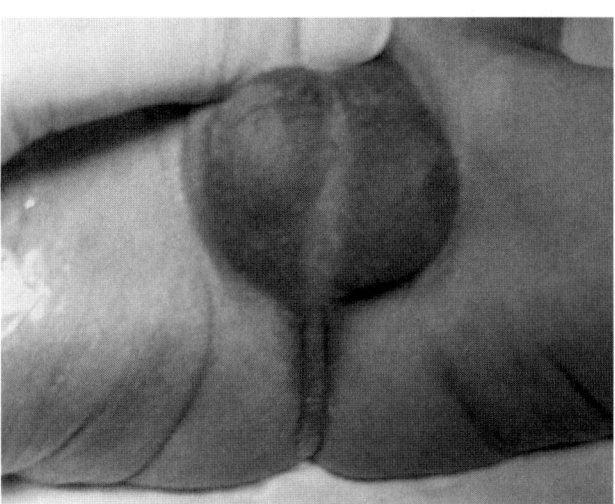

FIG. 39-24. Low imperforate anus in a male. Note the well-developed buttocks. The perineal fistula was found at the midline raphe.

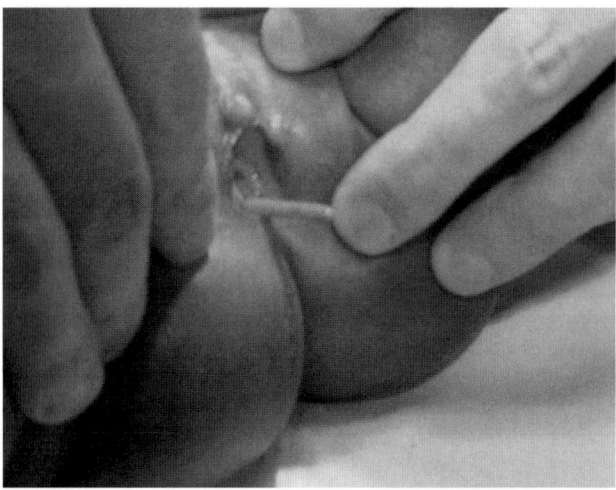

FIG. 39-25. Imperforate anus in a female. A catheter has been placed into the fistula, which is in the vestibule of the vagina.

sicular or recto–bladder neck fistula. In females, the most frequent defect is rectovestibular defect, followed by cutaneous perineal fistula. The third most common defect in females is persistent cloaca. The latter lesion represents a wide spectrum of malformations in which the rectum, vagina, and urinary tract meet and fuse into a single common channel. On physical examination, a single perineal orifice is observed, located at the place where the urethra normally opens. Typically, the external genitalia are hypoplastic.

Associated Malformations Approximately 60% of patients with an anorectal malformation have another associated malformation. The most common is a urinary tract defect, which occurs in approximately 50% of patients. Skeletal defects are also seen, and the sacrum is most commonly involved. Spinal cord anomalies, especially tethered cord, are common, particularly in children with high lesions. GI tract anomalies occur, most commonly esophageal atresia. Cardiac anomalies may be noted, and occasionally patients present with a constellation of defects as part of the VACTERL syndrome (described earlier).

Management of Patients with Imperforate Anus Patients with imperforate anus are usually in stable condition, and the diagnosis is readily apparent. Despite the obstruction, the abdomen initially is not distended, and there is rarely any urgency to intervene. The principles of management center around diagnosing the type of defect that is present (high vs. low) and evaluating for the presence of associated anomalies. It may take up to 24 hours before the presence of a fistula on the skin is noted, and thus the neonate should be observed for some period before definitive surgery is undertaken. All patients should therefore have an orogastric tube placed and should be monitored for the appearance of meconium in or around the perineum, or in the urine. Investigation for associated defects should include ultrasonography of the abdomen to assess for the presence of a urinary tract anomaly. Other tests should include an echocardiogram and spinal radiographs. Ultrasonography of the spine should be performed to look for the presence of a tethered cord. To further classify the location of the fistula as either high or low, a lateral abdominal radiograph can be obtained with a radiopaque marker on the perineum. Placing the infant in the inverted position allows the distance between the most distal extent of air in the rectum and the perineal surface to be measured. This study is imprecise, however, and may add little to the overall management of these patients.

The surgical management of infants with imperforate anus is determined by the anatomic defect. In general, when a low lesion is present, only a perineal operation is required without a colostomy. Infants with a high lesion require a colostomy in the newborn

period, followed by a pull-through procedure at approximately 2 months of age. When a persistent cloaca is present, the urinary tract needs to be carefully evaluated at the time of colostomy formation to ensure that normal emptying can occur and to determine whether the bladder needs to be drained by means of a vesicostomy. If there is any doubt about the type of lesion, it is safer to perform a colostomy rather than jeopardize the infant's long-term chances for continence by an injudicious perineal operation.

The type of pull-through procedure favored by most pediatric surgeons today is the posterior sagittal anorectoplasty, as described by Peña and DeVries. In this procedure, the patient is placed in the prone jackknife position, the levator ani and external sphincter complex is divided in the midline posteriorly, the communication between the GI tract and the urinary tract is divided, and the rectum is brought down after sufficient length is achieved. The muscles are then reconstructed and sutured to the rectum. The outcome for 1192 patients who underwent this procedure was recently reviewed by Peña and Hong. Seventy-five percent of patients were found to have voluntary bowel movements, and nearly 40% were considered totally continent. As a rule, the incidence of incontinence is increased in patients with high lesions, whereas those with low lesions are more likely to be constipated. Management of the patient with high imperforate anus can be greatly facilitated by the use of a laparoscopically assisted approach, in which the patient is operated on in the supine position and the rectum is mobilized down to the fistulous connection to the bladder neck. This fistulous connection is then divided, and the rectum is completely mobilized to below the peritoneal reflection. The operation then proceeds at the perineum, and the location of the muscle complex is determined using a nerve stimulator. A Veress needle is then advanced through the skin at the indicated site, with the laparoscope providing guidance to the exact intrapelvic orientation. Dilators are then placed over the Veress needle, the rectum is pulled through this peritoneal opening, and an anoplasty is performed.

JAUNDICE

Approach to the Jaundiced Infant

Jaundice is present during the first week of life in 60% of term infants and 80% of preterm infants. There is usually an accumulation of unconjugated bilirubin, but there may also be deposition of direct bilirubin. During fetal life, the placenta is the principal route of elimination of unconjugated bilirubin. In the newborn infant, bilirubin is conjugated through the activity of *glucuronyl transferase*. In the conjugated form, bilirubin is water soluble, which results in its excretion into the biliary system and then into the GI tract. Newborns have a relatively high level of circulating hemoglobin and relative immaturity of the conjugating machinery. This results in a transient accumulation of bilirubin in the tissues, which is manifested as jaundice. Physiologic jaundice is evident by the second or third day of life and usually resolves within approximately 5 to 7 days. By definition, jaundice that persists beyond 2 weeks is considered pathologic.

Pathologic jaundice may be due to biliary obstruction, increased hemoglobin load, or liver dysfunction. The work-up of the jaundiced infant therefore should include a search for the following possibilities: (a) obstructive disorders, including biliary atresia, choledochal cyst, and inspissated bile syndrome; (b) hematologic disorders, including ABO incompatibility, Rh incompatibility, and spherocytosis; (c) metabolic disorders, including alpha$_1$-antitrypsin deficiency, galactosemia, and pyruvate kinase deficiency; and (d) congenital infection, including syphilis and rubella.

Biliary Atresia
Pathogenesis

Biliary atresia is a rare disease associated with significant morbidity and mortality. This disease is characterized by a fibroproliferative obliteration of the biliary tree that progresses toward hepatic fibrosis, cirrhosis, and end-stage liver failure. The incidence of this disease is approximately 1 in 5000 to 1 in 12,000. The etiology of biliary atresia is likely multifactorial. In the classic textbook *Abdominal Surgery of Infancy and Childhood*, Ladd and Gross described the cause of biliary atresia as an "arrest of development during the solid stage of bile duct formation." Previously proposed theories of the cause of biliary atresia have focused on defects in hepatogenesis, prenatal vasculogenesis, immune dysregulation, infectious agents, and exposure to toxins. More recently, genetic mutations in the *cfc1* gene, implicated in left-right axis determinations, were identified in patients with biliary atresia–splenic malformation syndrome. In addition, the finding of a higher incidence of maternal microchimerism in the livers of males with biliary atresia has led to the suggestion that consequent expression of maternal antigens may lead to an autoimmune process that results in inflammation and obliteration of the biliary tree. Recent animal studies strongly implicate perinatal exposure to reovirus or rotavirus. Such viral exposure may lead to periportal inflammation mediated by interferon-γ and other cytokines.

Clinical Presentation

Infants with biliary atresia present with jaundice at birth or shortly thereafter. The diagnosis of biliary atresia is frequently not entertained by pediatricians, in part because physiologic jaundice of the newborn is so common and biliary atresia is so uncommon. For this reason, a delay in diagnosis is not unusual. However, infants with biliary atresia characteristically have acholic, pale gray stools, secondary to obstructed bile flow. With further passage of time, these infants manifest progressive failure to thrive and, if untreated, develop stigmata of liver failure and portal hypertension, particularly splenomegaly and esophageal varices.

The obliterative process of biliary atresia involves the common duct, cystic duct, one or both hepatic ducts, and the gallbladder, in a variety of combinations. Histopathologic findings for patients with biliary atresia include inflammatory changes in the parenchyma of the liver as well as fibrous deposition at the portal plates observed on trichrome staining of frozen tissue sections. In certain cases, bile duct proliferation may be seen, a relatively nonspecific marker of liver injury. Approximately 25% of patients with biliary atresia have coincidental malformations that are often associated with polysplenia and may include intestinal malrotation, preduodenal portal vein, and intrahepatic vena cava.

Diagnosis

In general, the diagnosis of biliary atresia is made using a combination of studies, because no single test is sufficiently sensitive or specific. Fractionation of the serum bilirubin is performed to determine if the associated hyperbilirubinemia is conjugated or unconjugated. Work-up commonly includes the analysis of TORCH (*t*oxoplasmosis, *o*ther infections, *r*ubella, *c*ytomegalovirus infection, and *h*erpes simplex) infection titers as well as tests for viral hepatitis. Typically ultrasonography is performed to assess for the presence of other causes of biliary tract obstruction, including choledochal cyst. The absence of a gallbladder is highly suggestive of the diagnosis of biliary atresia. However, the presence of a gallbladder does not exclude the diagnosis of biliary atresia, because in approximately 10% of biliary atresia patients, the distal biliary tract is patent and a gallbladder may be visualized, even though the proximal ducts are atretic. One should note that the intrahepatic bile ducts are never dilated in patients with biliary atresia. In many centers, a nuclear medicine scan using technetium TC 99m disofenin, performed after pretreatment of the patient with phenobarbital, has proven to be an accurate and reliable study. If radionuclide appears in the intestine, the biliary tree is patent and the diagnosis of biliary atresia is excluded. If radionuclide is concentrated by the liver but is not excreted despite treatment with phenobarbital, and results of the metabolic screen, particularly alpha$_1$-antitrypsin level, are normal,

the presumptive diagnosis is biliary atresia. Percutaneous liver biopsy findings might potentially distinguish between biliary atresia and other sources of jaundice such as neonatal hepatitis. When the results of these tests point to or cannot exclude the diagnosis of biliary atresia, surgical exploration is warranted. At surgery, a cholangiogram may be performed if possible, using the gallbladder as a point of access. This may be accomplished using a laparoscope. The cholangiogram demonstrates the anatomy of the biliary tree, reveals whether extrahepatic bile duct atresia is present, and indicates whether there is distal bile flow into the duodenum. The cholangiogram may demonstrate hypoplasia of the extrahepatic biliary system. This condition is associated with hepatic parenchymal disorders that cause severe intrahepatic cholestasis, including alpha$_1$-antitrypsin deficiency and biliary hypoplasia (Alagille syndrome). Alternatively, a cursory assessment of the extrahepatic biliary tree may clearly delineate the atresia.

Inspissated Bile Syndrome The term *inspissated bile syndrome* is applied to patients with normal biliary tracts who have persistent obstructive jaundice. Increased viscosity of bile and obstruction of the canaliculi are implicated as causes. The condition has been seen in infants receiving parenteral nutrition, but it is also encountered in patients with disorders associated with hemolysis and in patients with cystic fibrosis. In some instances, no etiologic factors can be defined. Cholangiography is both diagnostic and therapeutic in inspissated bile syndrome.

Neonatal Hepatitis *Neonatal hepatitis* may present in a similar fashion to biliary atresia. This disease is characterized by persistent jaundice due to acquired biliary inflammation without obliteration of the bile ducts. There may be a viral cause. The disease is usually self-limited.

Treatment

If the diagnosis of biliary atresia is confirmed intraoperatively, then surgical treatment is undertaken during the same procedure. Currently, first-line therapy consists of creation of a hepatoportoenterostomy, as described by Kasai. The purpose of this procedure is to promote bile flow into the intestine. The procedure is based on Kasai's observation that the fibrous tissue at the porta hepatis invests microscopically patent biliary ductules that, in turn, communicate with the intrahepatic ductal system (Fig. 39-26). Transecting this fibrous tissue at the portal plate, which is invariably encountered cephalad to the bifurcating portal vein, opens these channels and establishes bile flow into a surgically constructed intestinal conduit, usually a Roux-en-Y limb of jejunum (Fig. 39-27). Some authors believe that an intussuscepted antireflux valve is useful in preventing retrograde bile reflux, although the data suggest that it does not influence outcome. A liver biopsy is performed at the time of surgery to determine the degree of hepatic fibrosis that is present. The diameter of bile ducts at the portal plate is predictive of the likelihood of long-term success of biliary drainage through the portoenterostomy. Numerous studies also suggest that the likelihood of surgical success is inversely related to the age at the time of portoenterostomy. Infants treated before 60 days of age are more likely to achieve successful and long-term biliary drainage than are older infants. Although the outlook is less favorable for patients after the twelfth week, it is reasonable to proceed with surgery even beyond this point, because the alternative is certain liver failure. It is noteworthy that a significant number of patients have had favorable outcomes after undergoing portoenterostomy despite advanced age at the time of diagnosis.

Bile drainage is anticipated when the operation is carried out early; however, bile flow does not necessarily imply cure. Approximately one third of patients remain symptom free after portoenterostomy; the remainder require liver transplantation due to progressive liver failure. Independent risk factors that predict failure of the procedure include bridging liver fibrosis at the time of surgery and postoperative cholangitic episodes. A recent review of

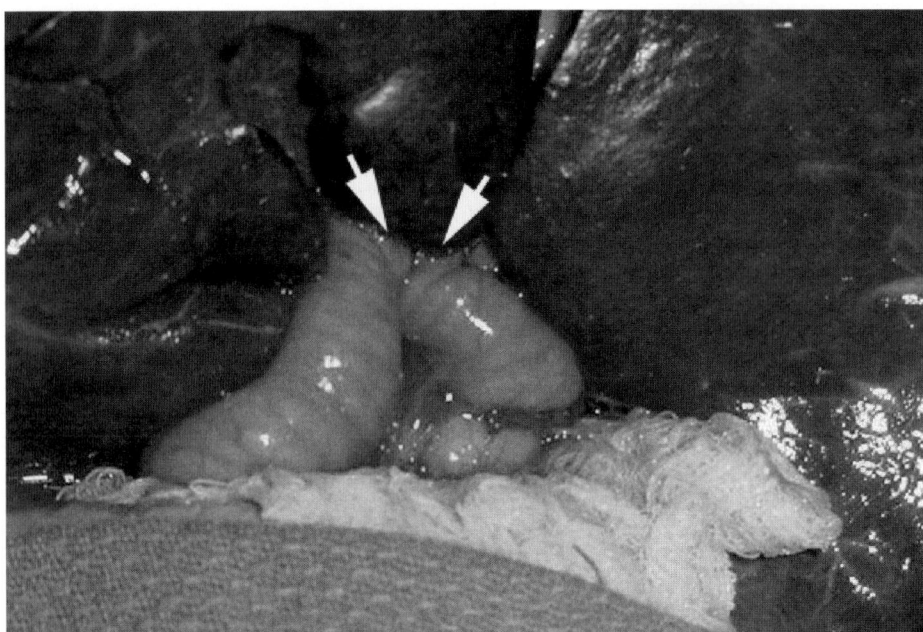

FIG. 39-26. Intraoperative photograph showing a Kasai portoenterostomy. *Arrows* denote the site of the anastomosis. Note the engorged liver.

the data of the Japanese Biliary Atresia Registry, which includes the results for 1381 patients, showed that the 10-year survival rate was 53% without transplantation and 66.7% with transplantation. A common postoperative complication is cholangitis. There is no effective strategy to completely eliminate this complication, and the

effectiveness of long-term prophylactic antibiotics has not been fully resolved. In 2002, the National Institutes of Health–supported multicenter Biliary Atresia Research Consortium (BARC) was established to investigate the etiology of biliary atresia and to identify factors that affect outcome after portoenterostomy. BARC has previously reported that rapid normalization of serum bilirubin levels and weight gain are predictive of survival with the native liver. In a prospective randomized controlled trial, BARC is currently analyzing the efficacy of corticosteroids in promoting sustained bile flow after hepatoportoenterostomy.

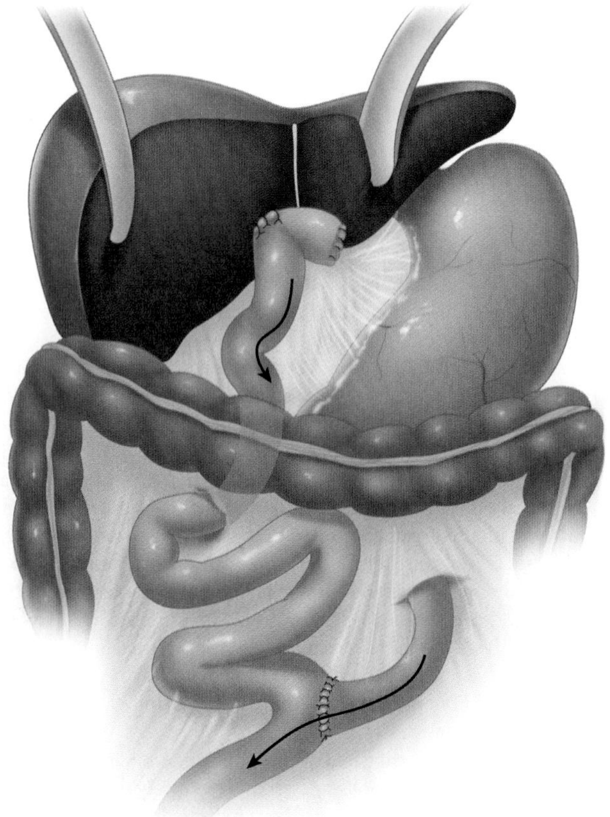

Choledochal Cyst
Classification

The term *choledochal cyst* refers to a spectrum of congenital biliary tract disorders that were previously grouped under the name *idiopathic dilatation of the common bile duct.* Based on the classification system proposed by Alonso-Lej, five types of choledochal cyst are described. Type I cysts are characterized by fusiform dilatation of the bile duct. This type is the most common and is found in 80 to 90% of cases. Type II choledochal cysts appear as an isolated diverticulum protruding from the wall of the common bile duct. The cyst may be joined to the common bile duct by a narrow stalk. Type III choledochal cysts arise from the intraduodenal portion of the common bile duct and are also known as *choledochoceles.* Type IVA cysts consist of multiple dilatations of the intrahepatic and extrahepatic bile ducts. Type IVB choledochal cysts are multiple dilatations involving only the extrahepatic bile ducts. Type V cysts (Caroli's disease) consist of multiple dilatations limited to the intrahepatic bile ducts.

Choledochal cyst is most appropriately considered the predominant feature in a constellation of pathologic abnormalities that can occur within the pancreatobiliary system. Frequently associated with choledochal cyst is an anomalous junction of the pancreatic and common bile ducts. The etiology of choledochal cyst is controversial. Babbit proposed an abnormal pancreatic and biliary duct junction, with the formation of a "common channel" into which pancreatic enzymes are secreted. This process results in weakening of the bile duct wall by gradual enzymatic destruction, which leads to dilatation, inflammation, and finally cyst formation. Not all patients with choledochal cyst demonstrate an anatomic common channel, which raises questions regarding the accuracy of this model.

FIG. 39-27. Schematic illustration of the Kasai portoenterostomy for biliary atresia. An isolated limb of jejunum is brought to the porta hepatis and anastomosed to the transected ducts at the liver plate.

Clinical Presentation

Choledochal cyst is more common in females than in males (4:1). Typically these cysts present in children beyond the toddler age group. The classic symptom triad consists of abdominal pain, mass, and jaundice. However, this complex is actually encountered in fewer than half of patients. The more usual presentation is that of episodic abdominal pain, often recurring over the course of months or years and generally associated with only minimal jaundice that may escape detection. If the disorder is left undiagnosed, patients may develop cholangitis or pancreatitis. Cholangitis may lead to the development of cirrhosis and portal hypertension. Choledochal cyst can present in the newborn period, with symptoms very similar to those of biliary atresia. Often neonates have an abdominal mass at presentation.

Diagnosis

Choledochal cyst is frequently diagnosed in the fetus during screening prenatal ultrasonography. In the older child or adolescent, abdominal ultrasonography may reveal a cystic structure arising from the biliary tree. CT will confirm the diagnosis. These studies show the dimensions of the cyst and define its relationship to the vascular structures in the porta hepatis, as well as the intrahepatic ductal configuration. Endoscopic retrograde cholangiopancreatography is reserved for cases in which confusion remains regarding the diagnosis after evaluation by less invasive imaging modalities. Magnetic resonance cholangiopancreatography may provide a more detailed depiction of the anatomy of the cyst and its relationship to the bifurcation of the hepatic ducts and to the pancreatic duct.

Treatment

The cyst wall is composed of fibrous tissue and is devoid of mucosal lining. As a result, the treatment of choledochal cyst is surgical excision followed by biliary-enteric reconstruction. There is no role for internal drainage by cystenterostomy, which leaves the cyst wall intact and leads to the inevitable development of cholangitis. Rarely, choledochal cyst can lead to the development of a biliary tract malignancy. This provides a further rationale for complete cyst excision.

Resection of the cyst requires circumferential dissection. The posterior plane between the cyst and portal vein must be carefully dissected to accomplish removal. The pancreatic duct, which may enter the distal cyst, is vulnerable to injury during distal cyst excision but can be prevented by avoiding entry into the pancreatic parenchyma. In cases in which the degree of pericystic inflammation is dense, it may be unsafe to attempt complete cyst removal. In this instance, it is reasonable to dissect within the posterior wall of the cyst, which allows the inner lining of the back wall to be dissected free from the outer layer that directly overlies the portal vascular structures. The lateral and anterior cyst, as well as the internal aspect of the back wall, is removed, but the outer posterior wall remains behind. Cyst excision is accomplished, and the proximal bile duct is anastomosed to the intestinal tract, typically via a Roux-en-Y limb of jejunum. More recently, laparoscopically assisted resections of choledochal cysts have been described. In these cases, the end-to-side jejunojejunostomy is performed extracorporeally, but the remainder of the procedure is completed using minimally invasive techniques.

The prognosis for children who have undergone complete excision of choledochal cyst is excellent. Complications include anastomotic stricture, cholangitis, and intrahepatic stone formation. These complications may develop a long time after surgery has been completed.

DEFORMITIES OF THE ABDOMINAL WALL

Embryology of the Abdominal Wall

The abdominal wall is formed by four separate embryologic folds—cephalic, caudal, and right and left lateral folds—each of which is composed of somatic and splanchnic layers. Each of the folds develops toward the anterior center portion of the coelomic cavity, joining to form a large umbilical ring that surrounds the two umbilical arteries, the vein, and the yolk sac or omphalomesenteric duct. These structures are covered by an outer layer of amnion, and the entire unit composes the umbilical cord. Between the fifth and tenth weeks of fetal development the intestinal tract undergoes rapid growth outside the abdominal cavity within the proximal portion of the umbilical cord. As development is completed, the intestine gradually returns to the abdominal cavity. Contraction of the umbilical ring completes the process of abdominal wall formation.

Failure of the cephalic fold to close results in sternal defects such as congenital absence of the sternum. Failure of the caudal fold to close results in exstrophy of the bladder and, in more extreme cases, exstrophy of the cloaca. Interruption of central migration of the lateral folds results in omphalocele. Gastroschisis, originally thought to be a variant of omphalocele, probably results from a fetal accident in the form of intrauterine rupture of a hernia of the umbilical cord.

Umbilical Hernia

Failure of the umbilical ring to close results in a central defect in the linea alba. The resulting umbilical hernia is covered by normal umbilical skin and subcutaneous tissue, but the fascial defect allows protrusion of abdominal contents. Hernias less than a centimeter in size at the time of birth usually will close spontaneously by 4 years of life. Sometimes the hernia is large enough that the protrusion is disfiguring and disturbing to both the child and the family. In such circumstances early repair may be advisable (Fig. 39-28).

Umbilical hernias are generally asymptomatic protrusions of the abdominal wall. They are generally noted by parents or physicians on physical examination, and these patients are referred for a surgical opinion due to concern for possible incarceration. Although incarceration is rarely seen in an umbilical hernia, it can happen. Children present with abdominal pain, bilious emesis, and a tender, hard mass protruding from the umbilicus. This constellation of symptoms mandates immediate exploration and repair of the hernia. In these cases, a knuckle of ischemic or necrotic bowel may be found that requires resection. More commonly, the child is asymptomatic and treatment is governed by the size of the defect,

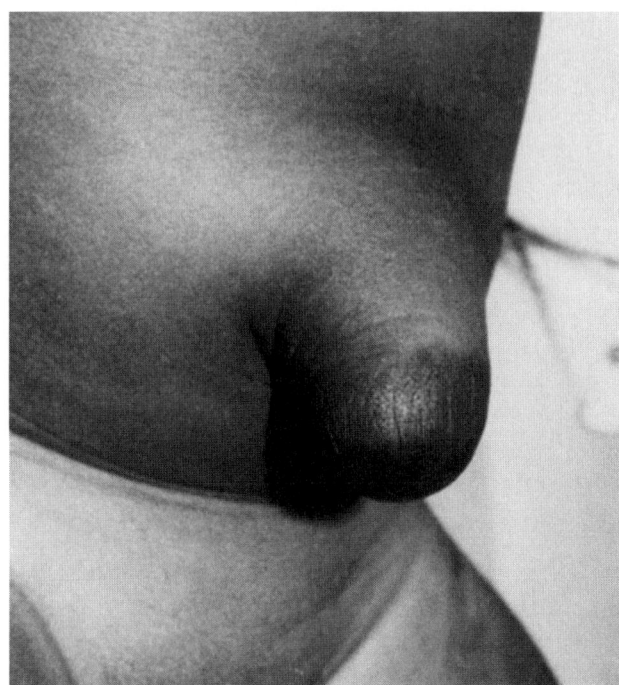

FIG. 39-28. Umbilical hernia in a 1-year-old female.

the age of the patient, and the concerns of the child and family regarding the cosmetic appearance of the abdomen. When the defect is small and spontaneous closure is likely, most surgeons will delay surgical correction until 4 or 5 years of age. If closure does not occur by this time, it is reasonable to repair the hernia. If a younger child has an extremely large hernia, or if the family or child is bothered by the cosmetic appearance, then repair is indicated.

Repair of uncomplicated umbilical hernia is performed under general anesthesia as an outpatient procedure. A small curved incision that fits into the skin crease of the umbilicus is made, and the sac is dissected free from the overlying skin. The fascial defect is repaired with permanent or long-lasting absorbable, interrupted sutures that are placed in a transverse plane. The cosmetic appearance of the umbilicus is restored by tacking the undersurface of the umbilical skin to the reapproximated fascia. The skin is closed using subcuticular sutures. The postoperative recovery is typically uneventful, and recurrence is rare.

Patent Urachus

During the development of the coelomic cavity, there is free communication between the urinary bladder and the abdominal wall through the urachus, which exits adjacent to the omphalomesenteric duct. Persistence of this tract results in a communication between the bladder and the umbilicus. The first sign of a patent urachus is moisture or urine flow from the umbilicus. Recurrent urinary tract infection can result. The urachus may be partially obliterated, with a remnant remaining beneath the umbilicus in the extraperitoneal position as an isolated cyst that may be identified by ultrasonography. Such a cyst usually presents as an inflammatory mass inferior to the umbilicus. Initial treatment is drainage of the infected cyst followed by cyst excision as a separate procedure once the inflammation has resolved.

In the child with a persistently draining umbilicus, a diagnosis of patent urachus should be considered. The differential diagnosis includes an umbilical granuloma, which generally responds to local application of silver nitrate. The diagnosis of patent urachus is confirmed by umbilical exploration. The urachal tract is excised and the bladder is closed. A patent vitelline duct may also present with umbilical drainage. In this circumstance, there is a communication with the small intestine, often at the site of Meckel's diverticulum. Treatment includes umbilical exploration with resection of the involved bowel (Fig. 39-29).

Omphalocele

Presentation

Omphalocele refers to a congenital defect of the abdominal wall in which the bowel and solid viscera are covered by peritoneum and

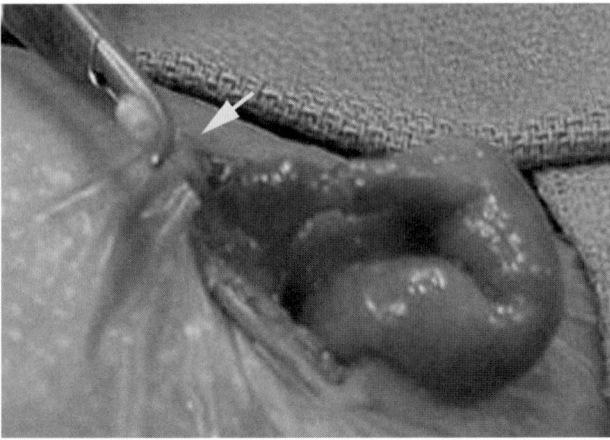

FIG. 39-29. Patent vitelline duct. Note the communication between the umbilicus and the small bowel at the site of a Meckel's diverticulum.

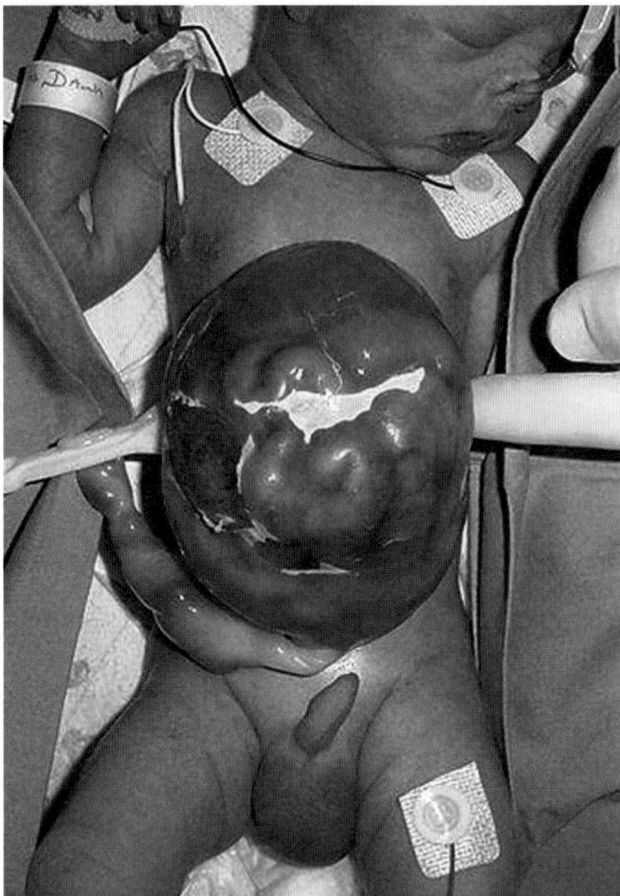

FIG. 39-30. Giant omphalocele in a newborn male.

amniotic membrane (Fig. 39-30). The umbilical cord inserts into the sac. The abdominal wall defect measures ≥4 cm in diameter. Omphalocele has an incidence of approximately 1 in 5000 live births and occurs in association with special syndromes such as exstrophy of the cloaca (vesicointestinal fissure), the Beckwith-Wiedemann constellation of anomalies (macroglossia, macrosomia, hypoglycemia, visceromegaly, and omphalocele) and the Cantrell pentalogy (lower thoracic wall malformations such as cleft sternum, ectopia cordis, epigastric omphalocele, anterior midline diaphragmatic hernia, and cardiac anomalies). The defect may be very small or large enough that it contains most of the abdominal viscera. There is a 60 to 70% incidence of associated anomalies, especially cardiac anomalies (20 to 40% of cases) and chromosomal abnormalities. Chromosomal anomalies are more common in children with smaller defects. Omphalocele is associated with prematurity (10 to 50% of cases) and intrauterine growth restriction (20% of cases).

Treatment

Immediate treatment of an infant with omphalocele consists of attending to the vital signs and maintaining body temperature. The omphalocele should be covered with saline-soaked gauze and the trunk should be wrapped circumferentially. No pressure should be placed on the omphalocele sac in an effort to reduce its contents, because this maneuver may increase the risk of rupture of the sac or may interfere with abdominal venous return. Prophylactic antibiotics should be administered in case of rupture. The subsequent treatment and outcome are determined by the size of the omphalocele. In general, small- to medium-sized defects have a significantly better prognosis than extremely large defects in which the liver is present. In these cases, not only is the management of the abdominal wall defect a significant challenge, but these patients often have concomitant pulmonary insufficiency that can lead to significant morbidity and mortality. Whenever possible, a primary repair of the omphalocele should be undertaken. This involves resection of the omphalocele membrane and closure of the fascia. A layer of prosthetic material may be required to achieve closure. In infants with a giant omphalocele (defect >7 cm in diameter, liver present within the sac), the defect cannot be closed primarily because there is simply no room to reduce the viscera into the abdominal cavity (see Fig. 39-30). Other infants may have associated congenital anomalies that complicate surgical repair. Under these circumstances, a nonoperative approach can be used. The omphalocele sac can be treated with desiccating substances such as povidone-iodine (Betadine), silver sulfadiazine (Silvadene), or sulfasalazine. Typically 2 to 3 months are required before re-epithelialization occurs. In the past, mercury compounds were used, but their use has been discontinued because of associated systemic toxicity. After epithelialization has occurred, attempts should be made to achieve closure of the anterior abdominal wall. Such procedures typically require extensive measures to achieve skin closure, including the use of biosynthetic materials. It is noteworthy that the abdominal vasculature is typically easily mobilized, due to the absence of adhesions to the sac. In cases of giant omphalocele, prolonged hospitalization is typical.

Gastroschisis
Presentation

Gastroschisis is a congenital anomaly characterized by a defect in the anterior abdominal wall through which the intestinal contents freely protrude. Unlike with omphalocele, there is no overlying sac and the size of the defect is much smaller (<4 cm). The abdominal wall defect is located at the junction of the umbilicus and normal skin and is almost always to the right of the umbilicus (Fig. 39-31). The umbilicus becomes partly detached, which allows free communication with the abdominal cavity. The appearance of the bowel provides some information with respect to the in utero timing of the defect. The intestine may be normal in appearance, which suggests that the rupture occurred relatively late during the pregnancy. More commonly, however, the intestine is thick, edematous, discolored, and covered with exudate, which implies a more longstanding process.

Unlike in infants born with omphalocele, in infants with gastroschisis the associated anomalies consist mostly of intestinal atresia. This defect can readily be diagnosed on prenatal ultrasonography (Fig. 39-32). There is no advantage to performing a cesarian section rather than a vaginal delivery. The delayed onset of intestinal function in children with gastroschisis has led some to postulate an injurious effect of amniotic fluid on the exposed bowel. This has led to consideration in some centers of early delivery to minimize intestinal damage and improve outcome. In a decade-long retro-

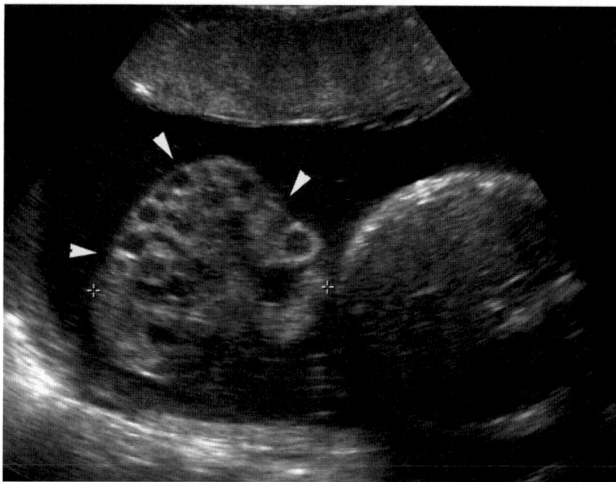

FIG. 39-32. Prenatal ultrasonographic scan showing gastroschisis in a fetus at 30 weeks' gestational age. *Arrows* point to the bowel outside within the amniotic fluid.

spective review, early delivery did not affect the thickness of bowel peel, but infants delivered before 36 weeks had a significantly longer length of hospital stay and time to enteral feeds. Based on these findings, fetal well-being should be the primary determinant of delivery for gastroschisis, as opposed to considerations regarding possible injurious effects of prolonged gestation on the bowel.

Treatment

All infants born with gastroschisis require urgent surgical treatment. Of equal importance, these infants require vigorous fluid resuscitation on the order of 160 to 190 mL/kg per day to replace significant evaporative fluid losses. In many instances, the intestine can be returned to the abdominal cavity, and a primary surgical closure of the abdominal wall is performed. Techniques that facilitate primary closure include mechanical stretching of the abdominal wall, thorough orogastric suctioning with foregut decompression, and rectal irrigation and evacuation of all the meconium. Care must be taken to prevent increased abdominal pressure during the reduction, which would lead to compression of the inferior vena cava and respiratory embarrassment, and result in abdominal compartment syndrome. To avoid this complication, it is helpful to monitor the bladder or airway pressure during reduction. In infants whose intestine has become thickened and edematous, it may be impossible to reduce the bowel into the peritoneal cavity in the immediately postnatal period. Under such circumstances, a plastic spring-loaded silo can be placed onto the bowel and secured beneath the fascia. The silo covers the bowel and allows for graduated reduction on a daily basis as the edema in the bowel wall decreases (Fig. 39-33). Surgical closure can usually be accomplished within approximately 1 week. A piece of prosthetic material may be required to bring the edges of the fascia together. If an atresia is noted at the time of closure, it is prudent to reduce the bowel at the first operation, then return after several weeks once the edema has resolved to correct the atresia. Intestinal function does not typically return for several weeks in patients with gastroschisis. This is especially true if the bowel is thickened and edematous. As a result, these patients require central line placement and institution of TPN to grow.

Prune-Belly Syndrome
Clinical Presentation

Prune-belly syndrome is a disorder that is characterized by a constellation of symptoms including extremely lax lower abdominal musculature, dilated urinary tract including the bladder, and bilateral undescended testes (Fig. 39-34). The term *prune-belly syndrome* appropriately describes the wrinkled appearance of the anterior

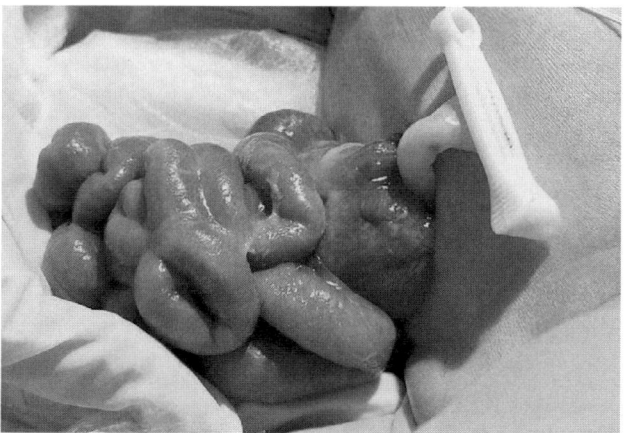

FIG. 39-31. Gastroschisis in a newborn. Note the location of the umbilical cord as well as the edematous, thickened bowel.

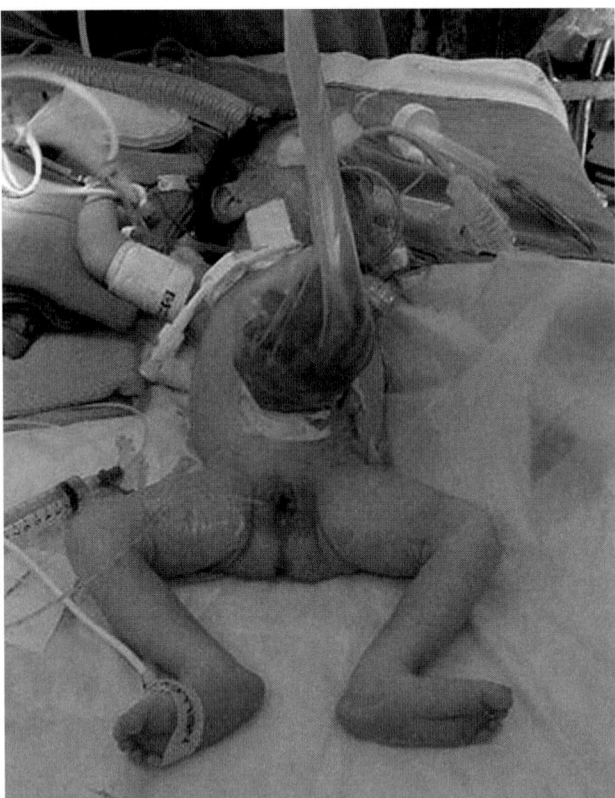

FIG. 39-33. Use of a silo in an infant with gastroschisis to allow the bowel wall edema to resolve so as to facilitate closure of the abdominal wall.

become more dilated distally. Ureteric obstruction is rarely present. The dilatation is thought to be caused by decreased smooth muscle and increased collagen in the ureters. Approximately 80% of affected individuals have some degree of vesicoureteral reflux, which can predispose to urinary tract infection. Despite the marked dilatation of the urinary tract, most children with prune-belly syndrome have adequate renal parenchyma for growth and development. Factors associated with the development of long-term renal failure include the presence of abnormal kidneys on ultrasonographic or renal scan and persistent pyelonephritis.

Treatment

Despite the ureteric dilatation, ureteric surgery currently has no role unless an area of obstruction develops. The testes are invariably intra-abdominal, and bilateral orchidopexy can be performed in conjunction with abdominal wall reconstruction at 6 to 12 months of age. Even with orchiopexy, fertility in a male with prune-belly syndrome is unlikely because spermatogenesis over time is insufficient. Deficiencies in the production of prostatic fluid and a predisposition to retrograde ejaculation contribute to infertility. Abdominal wall repair is accomplished through an abdominoplasty, which typically requires a transverse incision in the lower abdomen extending into the flanks.

Inguinal Hernia

An understanding of the management of pediatric inguinal hernias is a central component of modern pediatric surgical practice. Inguinal hernia repair represents one of the most common operations performed in children. The presence of an inguinal hernia in a child is an indication for surgical repair. The operation is termed a *herniorrhaphy* because it involves closing off the patent processus vaginalis. This is to be contrasted with the hernioplasty that is performed in adults, which requires a reconstruction of the inguinal floor.

Embryology

To understand how to diagnose and treat inguinal hernias in children, one must understand their embryologic origin. It is very useful to describe these events to the parents, who often are under the misconception that the hernia was somehow caused by their inability to console their crying child or the child's high activity level. Inguinal hernia results from a failure of closure of the processus vaginalis, a finger-like projection of the peritoneum that accompanies the testicle as it descends into the scrotum. Closure of the processus vaginalis normally occurs a few months before birth. This explains the high incidence of inguinal hernias in premature infants. When the processus vaginalis remains completely patent, a communication persists between the peritoneal cavity and the groin, resulting in a hernia. Partial closure can result in entrapped fluid, which leads to the presence of a hydrocele. A *communicating hydrocele* is a hydrocele that is in communication with the peritoneal cavity and can therefore be thought of as a hernia. When the classification system that is typically applied to adult hernias is used, all congenital hernias in children are by definition indirect inguinal hernias. Children also present with direct inguinal and femoral hernias, although these are much less common.

Clinical Manifestation

Inguinal hernias occur more commonly in males than in females (10:1) and are more common on the right side than the left. Infants are at high risk for incarceration of an inguinal hernia because of the narrow inguinal ring. Patients most commonly present with a groin bulge that is noticed by the parents as they change the infant's diapers (Fig. 39-35). Older children may notice the bulge themselves. On examination, the cord on the affected side will be thicker, and pressure on the lower abdomen usually will display the hernia on the affected side. The presence of an incarcerated hernia is indicated by a firm bulge that does not spontaneously resolve and may be associated with fussiness and irritability in the child. The infant with a strangulated inguinal hernia will have an edematous,

abdominal wall that characterizes these patients. Prune-belly syndrome is also known as *Eagle-Barrett syndrome* and the *triad syndrome* because of its three major manifestations. The incidence is significantly higher in males. Patients manifest a variety of comorbidities. The most significant is pulmonary hypoplasia, which can lead to death in the most severe cases. Skeletal abnormalities include dislocation or dysplasia of the hip and pectus excavatum.

The major genitourinary manifestation in prune-belly syndrome is ureteral dilatation. The ureters are typically long and tortuous, and

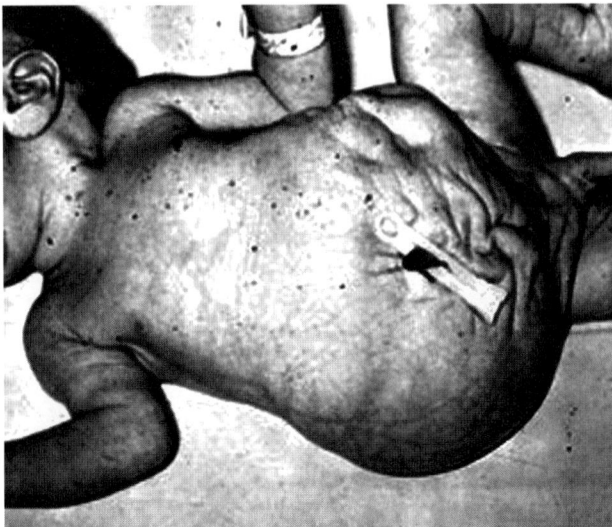

FIG. 39-34. Prune-belly (Eagle-Barrett) syndrome. Notice the flaccid abdomen.

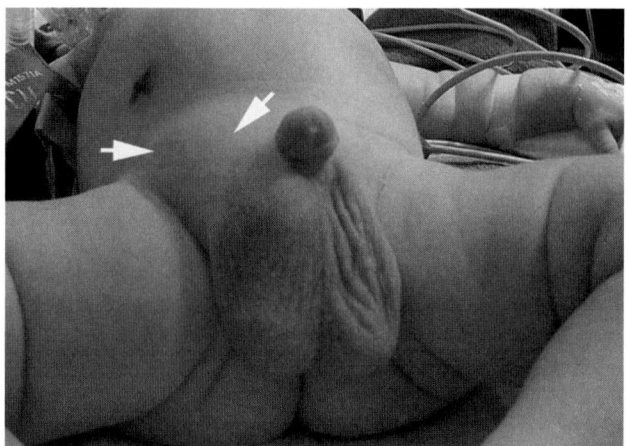

FIG. 39-35. Right inguinal hernia in a 4-month-old male. *Arrows* point to the bulge in the right groin.

tender bulge in the groin, occasionally with overlying skin changes. The child will eventually develop intestinal obstruction, peritonitis, and systemic toxicity.

Usually an incarcerated hernia can be reduced. Occasionally this may require light sedation. Gentle pressure is applied on the sac from below in the direction of the internal inguinal ring. After reduction of the incarcerated hernia, the child may be admitted for observation, and herniorrhaphy is performed within the next 24 hours to prevent recurrent incarceration. Alternatively, the child may be scheduled for surgery at the next available time slot. If the hernia cannot be reduced, or if evidence of strangulation is present, emergency operation is necessary. This may require a laparotomy and bowel resection.

When the diagnosis of inguinal hernia is made in an otherwise normal child, operative repair should be planned. Spontaneous resolution does not occur, and therefore a nonoperative approach cannot ever be justified. An inguinal hernia in a female infant or child frequently contains an ovary rather than intestine. Although the gonad usually can be reduced into the abdomen by gentle pressure, it often prolapses in and out until surgical repair is carried out. In some patients, the ovary and fallopian tube constitute one wall of the hernial sac (sliding hernia), and in these patients the ovary can be reduced effectively only at the time of operation. If the ovary is irreducible, prompt hernia repair is indicated to prevent ovarian torsion or strangulation.

When a hydrocele is diagnosed in infancy and there is no evidence of a hernia, observation is the proper therapy until the child is >12 months of age. If the hydrocele has not disappeared by 12 months, invariably there is a patent processus vaginalis, and operative hydrocelectomy with excision of the processus vaginalis is indicated. When the first signs of a hydrocele are seen after 12 months of age, the patient should undergo elective hydrocelectomy, which in a child is always performed through a groin incision. Aspiration of hydroceles is discouraged, because almost all without a patent processus vaginalis will resorb spontaneously, and those with a communication to the peritoneum will recur and require operative repair eventually.

Surgical Repair

The repair of a pediatric inguinal hernia can be extremely challenging, particularly in the premature child with incarceration. A small incision is made in a skin crease in the groin directly over the internal inguinal ring. Scarpa's fascia is seen and divided. The external oblique muscle is dissected free from overlying tissue, and the location of the external ring is confirmed. The external oblique aponeurosis is then opened along the direction of the external ring. The undersurface of the external oblique is then cleared from surrounding tissue. The

cremasteric fibers are separated from the cord structures and hernia sac, and these are then elevated into the wound. Care is taken not to grasp the vas deferens. The hernia sac is then dissected up to the internal ring and doubly suture ligated. The distal part of the hernia sac is opened widely to drain any hydrocele fluid. When the hernia is very large and the patient very small, tightening of the internal inguinal ring or even formal repair of the inguinal floor may be necessary, although the overwhelming majority of children do not require any treatment beyond high ligation of the hernia sac.

Controversy exists regarding the need for exploration of an asymptomatic opposite side in a child with an inguinal hernia. Several reports indicate that frequency of a patent processus vaginalis on the side opposite the obvious hernia is approximately 30%, although this figure decreases with increasing age of the child. Management options include never exploring the opposite side or exploring only under certain conditions, such as in premature infants or in patients in whom incarceration is present. The opposite side may be readily examined laparoscopically. To do so, a blunt 3-mm trocar is placed into the hernia sac of the affected side. The abdominal cavity is insufflated, and a 2.7-mm 70-degree camera is placed through the trocar to visualize the opposite side. The status of the processus vaginalis on the opposite side can be determined. However, the presence of a patent processus vaginalis by laparoscopy does not always imply the presence of a hernia.

Several authors have now reported a completely laparoscopic approach to the management of inguinal hernias in children. This technique requires insufflation through the umbilicus and the placement of an extraperitoneal suture to ligate the hernia sac. Proponents of this procedure emphasize the fact that no groin incision is required and that the chance of injuring cord structures is decreased. The long-term results of laparoscopic treatment remain to be established.

Inguinal hernias in children recur in <1% of patients, and recurrences usually result from missed hernia sacs at the first procedure, a direct hernia, or a missed femoral hernia. In all children, local anesthetic should be administered either by caudal injection or by direct injection into the wound. In preterm infants spinal anesthesia carries a lower risk of postoperative apnea than general anesthesia.

GENITALIA

Undescended Testis

Embryology

The term *undescended testicle* (cryptorchidism) refers to the interruption of the normal descent of the testis into the scrotum. The testicle may reside in the retroperineum, in the internal inguinal ring, in the inguinal canal, or even at the external ring. The testicle begins as a thickening on the urogenital ridge in the fifth to sixth week of embryologic life. In the seventh and eighth months the testicle descends along the inguinal canal into the upper scrotum, and with its progress the processus vaginalis is formed and pulled along with the migrating testicle. At birth, approximately 95% of infants have the testicles normally positioned in the scrotum.

A distinction should be made between an undescended testicle and an ectopic testicle. An ectopic testis, by definition, is one that has passed through the external ring in the normal pathway and then has come to rest in an abnormal location either overlying the rectus abdominis or external oblique muscle, overlying the soft tissue of the medial thigh, or behind the scrotum in the perineum. A congenitally absent testicle results from failure of normal development or an intrauterine accident leading to loss of blood supply to the developing testicle.

Clinical Presentation

The incidence of undescended testes is approximately 30% in preterm infants and 1 to 3% in term infants. For diagnosis, the child should be examined in the supine position, where visual inspection may reveal a hypoplastic or poorly rugated scrotum. Usually a unilateral undescended testicle can be palpated in the inguinal canal or in the upper scrotum. Occasionally, the testicle will be difficult or impossible to palpate, which indicates either an abdominal testicle or congenital absence of the gonad. If the testicle is not palpable in the supine position, the child should be examined with his legs crossed while seated. This maneuver diminishes the cremasteric reflex and facilitates detection of the location of the testicle.

It is now established that cryptorchid testes show an increased predisposition to malignant degeneration. In addition, fertility is decreased when the testicle is not in the scrotum. For these reasons, surgical placement of the testicle in the scrotum (orchidopexy) is indicated. This procedure does improve the fertility potential, although it is never normal. Similarly, the testicle is still at risk of malignant change, although its location in the scrotum facilitates potentially earlier detection of a testicular malignancy. Other reasons to consider orchidopexy include the risk of trauma to a testicle located at the pubic tubercle, increased incidence of torsion, and the psychologic impact of an empty scrotum in a developing male. The reason for malignant degeneration has not been established, but the evidence points to an inherent abnormality of the testicle that predisposes it to incomplete descent and malignancy rather than malignancy as a result of an abnormal environment.

Treatment

Males with bilateral undescended testicles are often infertile. When the testicle is not within the scrotum, it is subjected to a higher temperature, which results in decreased spermatogenesis. Mengel and coworkers studied 515 undescended testicles by histologic analysis and demonstrated a decreasing presence of spermatogonia after 2 years of age. Consequently it is now recommended that an undescended testicle be surgically repositioned by 2 years of age. Nevertheless, the incidence of infertility is approximately two times higher in men who underwent unilateral orchidopexy than in men with normal testicular descent.

The administration of chorionic gonadotropin occasionally may be effective in patients with bilateral undescended testes, which suggests that these patients are more likely to have a hormone insufficiency than children with unilateral undescended testicle. If there is no testicular descent after a month of endocrine therapy, operative correction should be undertaken. A child with unilateral cryptorchidism should undergo surgical correction of the problem. The operation is typically performed through a combined groin and scrotal incision. The cord vessels are fully mobilized, and the testicle is placed in a dartos pouch within the scrotum. An inguinal hernia often accompanies an undescended testis. This should be repaired at the time of orchidopexy.

Patients with a nonpalpable testicle present a challenge in management. The current approach involves laparoscopy to identify the location of the testicle. If the spermatic cord is found to traverse the internal ring or the testis is found at the ring and can be delivered into the scrotum, a groin incision is made and an orchidopexy is performed. If an abdominal testis is identified that is too far away to reach the scrotum, a two-stage Fowler-Stephens approach is used. In the first stage, the testicular vessels can be clipped via laparotomy or laparoscopically. This promotes neovasculogenesis along the vas deferens. Several months later, the second stage is performed during which the intra-abdominal testis is mobilized along with a swath of peritoneum with collateralized blood supply along the vas. This may be done laparoscopically as well. Preservation of the gubernacular attachments with their collaterals to the testicle confers improved testicular survival after orchidopexy in >90% of cases. It is nonetheless preferable to preserve the testicular vessels whenever possible and complete mobilization of the testicle with its vessels intact. Some surgeons advocate aggressive mobilization of testicular vessels up to the renal hilum if the intra-abdominal testis is within 1 or 2 cm of the internal ring. Other surgeons feel

that the staged approach to orchidopexy is superior. To date, no large-scale trial has been performed to answer this question. In either case, meticulous mobilization of the intra-abdominal testis is critical for its survival and successful orchidopexy.

Vaginal Anomalies

Surgical diseases of the vagina in children are either congenital or acquired. Congenital anomalies include a spectrum of disorders that range from simple defects (imperforate hymen) to more complex forms of vaginal atresia, including distal atresia, proximal atresia, and, the most severe, complete atresia. These defects are produced by abnormal development of the müllerian ducts and/or urogenital sinus. The diagnosis is made most often by physical examination. Secretions into the obstructed vagina produce hydrocolpos, which may present as a large, painful abdominal mass. The anatomy may be defined using ultrasonography. Pelvic MRI provides the most thorough and accurate assessment of the pelvic structures. Treatment is dependent on the extent of the defect. For an imperforate hymen, division of the hymen is curative. More complex forms of vaginal atresia require mobilization of the vaginal remnants and creation of an anastomosis at the perineum. Laparoscopy can be extremely useful in mobilizing the vagina, in draining hydrocolpos, and in evaluating the internal genitalia. Complete vaginal atresia requires the construction of skin flaps or the creation of a neovagina using a segment of colon.

The most common acquired disorder of the vagina is the straddle injury. This often occurs as young girls fall on blunt objects that cause a direct injury to the perineum. Typical manifestations include vaginal bleeding and inability to void. Unless the injury is extremely superficial, patients should be examined in the operating room where the lighting is optimal and sedation can be administered. Vaginal lacerations are repaired using absorbable sutures, and the proximity to the urethra should be carefully assessed. Before hospital discharge, the patient must be able to void spontaneously. In all cases of vaginal trauma, it is essential that the patient be assessed for the presence of sexual abuse. In cases in which abuse is suspected, early contact with the sexual abuse or child protection service is necessary, so that the appropriate microbiologic and photographic evidence can be obtained.

Ovarian Cysts and Tumors

Pathologic Classification

Ovarian cysts and tumors may be classified as non-neoplastic or neoplastic. Nonneoplastic lesions include cysts (simple, follicular, inclusion, paraovarian, or corpus luteum), endometriosis, and inflammatory lesions. Neoplastic lesions are categorized based on the three primordia that contribute to the ovary: mesenchymal components of the urogenital ridge, germinal epithelium overlying the urogenital ridge, and germ cells migrating from the yolk sac. The most common variety is germ cell tumors. Germ cell tumors are classified based on the degree of differentiation and the cellular components involved. The least differentiated tumors are the dysgerminomas, which share features similar to those of seminomas in males. Although these are malignant tumors, they are extremely sensitive to radiation and chemotherapy. The most common lesions are the teratomas, which may be mature, immature, or malignant. The degree of differentiation of the neural elements of the tumor determines the degree of immaturity. The sex cord stromal tumors arise from the mesenchymal components of the urogenital ridge. These include granulosa-theca cell tumors and Sertoli-Leydig cell tumors. These tumors often produce hormones that result in precocious puberty or hirsutism, respectively. Epithelial tumors, although rare, do occur in children. These include serous and mucinous cystadenomas.

Clinical Presentation

Children with ovarian lesions usually present with abdominal pain. Other signs and symptoms include a palpable abdominal mass, evidence of urinary obstruction, symptoms of bowel obstruction, and endocrine imbalance. The surgical approach depends on the appearance of the mass at operation (i.e., whether it is benign appearing or is suspicious for malignancy). In the case of a simple ovarian cyst, surgery depends on the size of the cyst and the severity of symptoms it causes. In general, large cysts (over 4 to 5 cm) should be resected, because they are unlikely to resolve, may be at risk of torsion, and may mask an underlying malignancy. Resection may be performed laparoscopically, and ovarian tissue should be spared in all cases.

Surgical Management

If an ovarian lesion appears malignant, levels of tumor markers, including alpha-fetoprotein (teratomas), lactate dehydrogenase (dysgerminomas), beta human chorionic gonadotrophin (choriocarcinomas), and cancer antigen 125 (epithelial tumors), should be measured. Although the diagnostic sensitivity of these markers is variable, they provide information for postoperative follow-up and indicate the response to therapy. When a malignancy is suspected, the patient should undergo a formal cancer operation. This procedure is performed through either a midline incision or a Pfannenstiel approach. Ascites fluid and peritoneal washings should be collected for cytologic study. The liver and diaphragm are inspected carefully for metastatic disease. An omentectomy is performed if there is any evidence of tumor present. Pelvic and para-aortic lymph nodes are biopsied, and the primary tumor is resected completely. Finally, the contralateral ovary is carefully inspected and, if a lesion is seen, it is biopsied. Dysgerminomas and epithelial tumors are bilateral in up to 15% of cases. It is occasionally possible to preserve the ipsilateral fallopian tube. More radical procedures are not indicated.

Ovarian Cysts in the Newborn

An increasing number of ovarian cysts are being detected by prenatal ultrasonography. In the past, surgical excision was recommended for all cysts >5 cm in diameter because of the perceived risk of ovarian torsion. It has now become apparent from serial ultrasonographic examinations that many of these lesions will resolve spontaneously. Therefore, asymptomatic, simple cysts may be observed, and surgery can be performed only when the cysts fail to decrease in size or become symptomatic. Typically, resolution occurs by approximately 6 months of age. A laparoscopic approach is preferable when simple cysts must be removed. By contrast, complex cysts of any size require surgical intervention at presentation.

Ambiguous Genitalia

Embryology

Normal sexual differentiation occurs in the sixth fetal week. In every fetus, wolffian (male) and müllerian (female) ducts are present until the onset of sexual differentiation. Normal sexual differentiation is directed by the sex-determining region of the Y chromosome (SRY). This is located on the distal end of the short arm of the Y chromosome. SRY provides a genetic switch that initiates gonadal differentiation in the mammalian urogenital ridge. Secretion of müllerian inhibiting substance (MIS) by the Sertoli cells of the seminiferous tubules results in regression of the müllerian duct, the anlage of the uterus, fallopian tubes, and upper vagina. The result of MIS secretion therefore is a phenotypic male. In the absence of SRY in the Y chromosome, MIS is not produced, and the müllerian duct derivatives are preserved. Thus, the female phenotype prevails.

For the male phenotype to develop, the embryo must have a Y chromosome, the SRY must be normal without point mutations or deletions, testosterone and MIS must be produced by the differentiated gonad, and the tissues must respond to these hormones. Any disruption of the orderly steps in sexual differentiation may be reflected clinically as variants of the intersex syndromes, which are currently referred to as disorders of sex development (DSDs).

DSDs may be classified as (a) ovotesticular DSD (with both ovarian and testicular gonadal tissue present; previously known as *true hermaphroditism*); (b) 46,XY DSD, characterized by undervirilization or undermasculinization of an XY male (only testicular tissue present; previously known as *male pseudohermaphroditism*); (c) 46,XX DSD, characterized by overvirilization or masculinization of an XX female (ovarian tissue only; female pseudohermaphroditism); and (d) 46,XY complete gonadal dysgenesis (usually underdeveloped or imperfectly formed gonads).

Ovotesticular Disorder of Sex Development (True Hermaphroditism)

Ovotesticular DSD is the rarest form of ambiguous genitalia. Patients have both normal male and normal female gonads, with an ovary on one side and a testis on the other. Occasionally, an ovotestis is present on one or both sides. The majority of these patients have a 46,XX karyotype (46,XX testicular DSD). Both the testis and the testicular portion of the ovotestis should be removed.

46,XY Disorder of Sex Development (Male Pseudohermaphroditism)

The condition of 46,XY DSD occurs in infants with an XY karyotype but deficient masculinization of the external genitalia. Bilateral testes are present, but the duct structures differentiate partly as phenotypically female. The causes of the disorder include inadequate testosterone production due to biosynthetic error, inability to convert testosterone to dihydrotestosterone due to 5α-reductase deficiency, or deficiencies in androgen receptors. The latter disorder is termed *testicular feminization syndrome*. Occasionally, the diagnosis in these children is made during routine inguinal herniorrhaphy in a phenotypic female, at which time testes are found. The testes should be resected due to the risk of malignant degeneration, although this should be done only after a full discussion with the family has occurred.

46,XX Disorder of Sex Development (Female Pseudohermaphroditism)

The syndrome of 46,XX DSD is characterized by overvirilization or masculinization of an XX female. The most common cause of this female condition is congenital adrenal hyperplasia. These children have a 46,XX karyotype but have been exposed to excessive androgens in utero. Common enzyme deficiencies include 21-hydroxylase deficiency, 11β-hydroxylase deficiency, and 3β-hydroxysteroid dehydrogenase deficiency. These deficiencies lead to overproduction of intermediary steroid hormones, which results in masculinization of the external genitalia of the XX fetus. These patients are unable to synthesize cortisol. In 90% of cases, deficiency of 21-hydroxylase causes adrenocorticotropic hormone to stimulate the secretion of excessive quantities of adrenal androgen, which masculinizes the developing female (Fig. 39-36). These infants are prone to salt loss and require cortisol replacement. Those with mineralocorticoid deficiency also require fludrocortisone replacement.

Mixed Gonadal Dysgenesis

Mixed gonadal dysgenesis is characterized by dysgenetic gonads and retained müllerian structures. The typical karyotype is mosaic, usually 45XO,46XY. The incidence of malignant tumors in the dysgenetic gonads, most commonly gonadoblastoma, is high. Therefore, they should be removed.

Management

In the differential diagnosis of patients with DSD, the following diagnostic steps are necessary: (a) evaluation of the genetic background and family history; (b) assessment of the anatomic structures by physical examination and/or ultrasonography; (c) chromosome analysis; (d) determination of biochemical factors in serum and urine to evaluate for the presence of an enzyme defect; and (e) laparoscopy for gonadal biopsy. Treatment should include correction of electrolyte

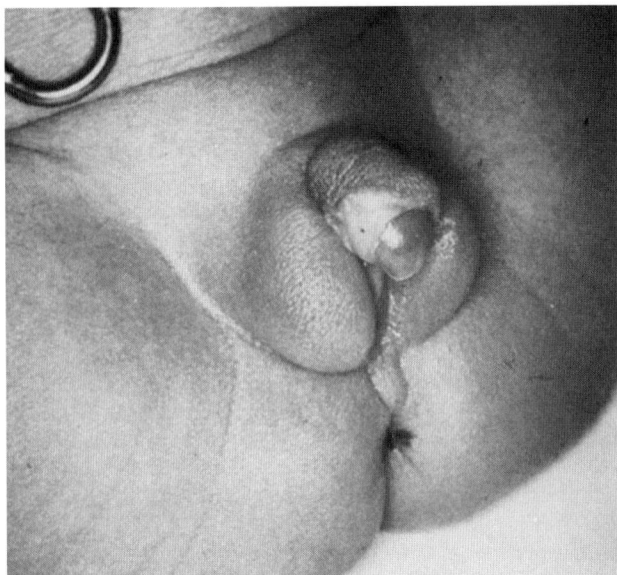

FIG. 39-36. Ambiguous genitalia manifest as enlarged clitoris and labioscrotal folds in an infant with adrenogenital syndrome.

and volume losses in cases of congenital adrenal hyperplasia and replacement of hormone deficiency. Surgical assignment of gender should never be done at the first operation. Although historically female gender had been assigned, there is abundant and convincing evidence that raising a genotypic male as a female has devastating consequences, not only anatomically but also psychosocially. This is particularly relevant given the role of prenatal and postnatal hormones on gender imprinting and identity. In general, surgical reconstruction should be performed after a full genetic work-up and with the involvement of pediatric endocrinologists, pediatric plastic surgeons, and ethicists with expertise in gender issues. Discussion with the family also plays an important role. This approach reduces the anxiety associated with these disorders and helps to ensure the normal physical and emotional development of these patients.

PEDIATRIC MALIGNANCY

Cancer is the second leading cause of death in children after trauma and accounts for approximately 11% of all pediatric deaths in the United States. Several features distinguish pediatric from adult cancers, including the presence of tumors that are predominantly seen in children, such as neuroblastomas and germ cell tumors, and the favorable response to chemotherapy observed for many pediatric solid malignancies, even in the presence of metastases.

Wilms' Tumor
Clinical Presentation

Wilms' tumor is the most common primary malignant tumor of the kidney in children. Approximately 500 new cases are seen annually in the United States, and most are diagnosed in children between 1 and 5 years of age with the peak incidence at age 3. Advances in the care of patients with Wilms' tumor have resulted in an overall cure rate of roughly 90%, even in the presence of metastatic spread. The tumor usually develops in otherwise healthy children as an asymptomatic mass in the flank or upper abdomen. Frequently, the mass is discovered by a parent while bathing or dressing the child. Other symptoms include hypertension, hematuria, obstipation, and weight loss. Occasionally the mass is discovered after blunt abdominal trauma.

Genetics of Wilms' Tumor

Wilms' tumor can arise from both germline and somatic mutations, and can occur in the presence or absence of a family history. Nearly

97% of Wilms' tumors are sporadic in that they occur in the absence of a heritable or congenital cause or risk factor. When a heritable risk factor is identified, the affected children often present at an earlier age and the disease is frequently bilateral. Most of these tumors are associated with germline mutations. It is well established that there is a genetic predisposition to Wilms' tumor in the WAGR syndrome, which consists of Wilms' tumor, *a*niridia, *g*enitourinary abnormalities, and mental *r*etardation. In addition, there is an increased incidence of Wilms' tumor in certain overgrowth conditions, particularly Beckwith-Wiedemann syndrome and hemihypertrophy. WAGR syndrome has been shown to result from the deletion of one copy each of the Wilms' tumor gene *WT1* and the adjacent aniridia gene *PAX6* on chromosome band 11p13. Beckwith-Wiedemann syndrome is an overgrowth syndrome that is characterized by visceromegaly, macroglossia, and hyperinsulinemic hypoglycemia. It arises from mutations at the 11p15.5 locus. There is evidence to suggest that analysis of the methylation status of several genes in the 11p15 locus could predict the individual risk for the development of Wilms' tumor. Importantly, however, most patients with Wilms' tumor do not have mutations at these genetic loci.

Surgical Treatment

Before operation, all patients suspected of having Wilms' tumor should undergo abdominal and chest CT. These studies characterize the mass, identify the presence of metastases, and provide information on the opposite kidney (Fig. 39-37). CT scanning also reveals the presence of nephrogenic rests, which are precursor lesions to Wilms' tumor. Abdominal ultrasonography should be performed to evaluate for the presence of renal vein or vena caval extension.

The management of patients with Wilms' tumor has been carefully analyzed within the context of large studies involving thousands of patients. These studies have been coordinated by the National Wilms Tumor Study Group (NWTSG) in North America and by the International Society of Paediatric Oncology (SIOP), mainly in European countries. Significant differences in the approach to patients with Wilms' tumor have been highlighted by these studies. The NWTSG supports a strategy of surgery followed by chemotherapy in most instances, whereas the SIOP approach is to shrink the tumor using preoperative chemotherapy. In some circumstances preoperative chemotherapy is supported by both groups, including in cases of bilateral involvement or inferior vena cava involvement that extends above the hepatic veins and involvement of a solitary kidney by Wilms' tumor. The NWTSG proponents argue that preoperative therapy in other instances results in a loss of important staging information and therefore places patients at higher risk for recurrence or, alternatively, may lead to overly aggressive treatment in some cases and greater morbidity. However,

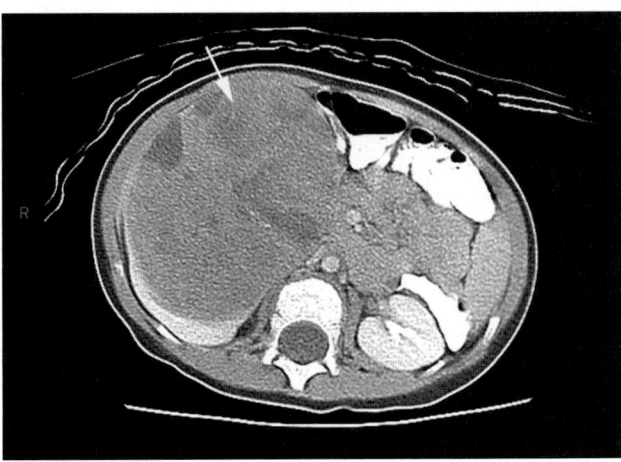

FIG. 39-37. Wilms' tumor of the right kidney (*arrow*) in a 3-year-old girl.

the overall survival rates are no different for patients treated using the NWTSG and SIOP approaches.

The goal of surgery is complete removal of the tumor. It is crucial to avoid tumor rupture or injury to contiguous organs. A sampling of regional lymph nodes should be included, and all suspicious nodes should be excised or biopsied. Typically a transverse abdominal incision is made, and a transperitoneal approach is used. The opposite side is carefully inspected to ensure that no disease is present. Although historically this involved the complete mobilization of the contralateral kidney, current evidence indicates that preoperative high-resolution CT scanning is sufficiently accurate to detect clinically significant lesions if they are present. Provided only unilateral disease is present, a radical nephroureterectomy is then performed with control of the renal pedicle as an initial step. If there is spread above the hepatic veins, an intrathoracic approach may be required. If bilateral disease is encountered, chemotherapy is administered, followed by a nephron-sparing procedure. Biopsy may be required if the patient does not respond to the initial chemotherapy.

Chemotherapy

After nephroureterectomy for Wilms' tumor, the need for chemotherapy and/or radiation therapy is determined by the histologic features and clinical stage of the tumor. Essentially, patients who have disease confined to one kidney that is completely excised surgically receive a short course of chemotherapy, and for this group a 97% 4-year survival is expected, with tumor relapse rare after that time. Patients who have more advanced disease or tumors with unfavorable histologic features receive more intensive chemotherapy and radiation therapy. Even in patients with stage IV disease, cure rates of 80% are achieved. The survival rates are worse in the small percentage of patients whose tumors are considered to be of unfavorable histologic type.

Neuroblastoma
Clinical Presentation

Neuroblastoma is the third most common pediatric malignancy and accounts for approximately 10% of all childhood cancers. The overwhelming majority of patients have advanced disease at the time of presentation, and unlike in patients with Wilms' tumor, the overall survival rate is <30%. Over 80% of cases present before the age of 4 years, and the peak incidence is 2 years of age. Neuroblastomas arise from the neural crest cells and show different levels of differentiation. The tumor originates most frequently in the adrenal glands, posterior mediastinum, neck, or pelvis but can arise in any sympathetic ganglion. The clinical presentation depends on the site of the primary and the presence of metastases.

Two thirds of these tumors are first noted as an asymptomatic abdominal mass. The tumor may cross the midline, and a majority of patients already show signs of metastatic disease. Occasionally, children may experience pain from the tumor mass or from bony metastases. Proptosis and periorbital ecchymosis may occur due to the presence of retrobulbar metastasis. Because neuroblastomas originate in paraspinal ganglia, they may invade through neural foramina and compress the spinal cord, causing muscle weakness or sensory changes. Rarely, children may have severe watery diarrhea due to the secretion of vasoactive intestinal peptide by the tumor or show paraneoplastic neurologic findings, including cerebellar ataxia or opsoclonus/myoclonus.

Diagnostic Evaluation

Because these tumors derive from the sympathetic nervous system, catecholamines and their metabolites are produced at increased levels. Elevated levels of serum catecholamines (dopamine, norepinephrine) or the urine catecholamine metabolites vanillylmandelic acid and homovanillic acid are seen. Measurement of vanillylmandelic acid and homovanillic acid in serum and urine aids in making the diagnosis and in monitoring for treatment adequacy and recurrence. The minimum criterion for a diagnosis of neuroblastoma is the presence of one of the following: (a) an unequivocal pathologic diagnosis made from tumor tissue by light microscopy (with or without immunohistologic analysis, electron microscopy, or increased levels of serum catecholamines or urinary catecholamine metabolites); or (b) the combination of bone marrow aspirate or biopsy specimen containing unequivocal tumor cells and increased levels of serum catecholamines or urinary catecholamine metabolites as described earlier.

The patient should be evaluated by abdominal CT, which may show displacement and occasionally obstruction of the ureter of an intact kidney (Fig. 39-38). Before the institution of therapy, a complete staging work-up should be performed. This includes radiograph of the chest, bone marrow biopsy, and radionuclide scans to search for metastases. Any abnormality on chest radiograph should be followed up with CT of the chest.

Prognostic Indicators

A number of biologic variables have been studied in children with neuroblastoma. An open biopsy is often required to provide sufficient tissue for analysis. The presence of hyperdiploid tumor DNA is associated with a favorable prognosis, whereas *N-myc* amplification is associated with a poor prognosis regardless of patient age. The Shimada classification describes tumors as having either favorable or unfavorable histologic features based on the degree of differentiation, the mitosis-karyorrhexis index, and the presence or absence of schwannian stroma. In general, children of any age with localized neuroblastoma and infants <1 year of age with advanced disease and favorable disease characteristics have a high likelihood of disease-free survival. By contrast, older children with advanced disease have a significantly decreased chance for cure even with intensive therapy. For example, aggressive multiagent chemotherapy has resulted in a 2-year survival rate of approximately 20% in older children with stage IV disease. Neuroblastoma in the adolescent has a worse long-term prognosis regardless of stage or site and, in many cases, a more prolonged course.

Surgery

The goal of surgery is complete resection. However, this is often not possible due to the extensive locoregional spread of the tumor at the time of presentation. Under these circumstances, a biopsy is performed and preoperative chemotherapy is provided based on the stage of the tumor. After neoadjuvant treatment has been administered, surgical resection is performed. The principal goal of surgery

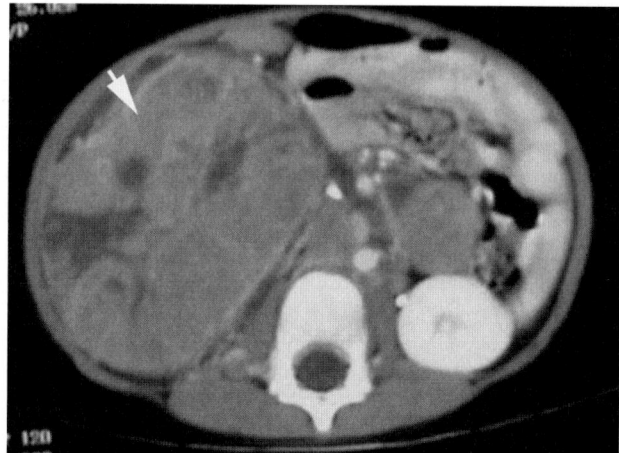

FIG. 39-38. Abdominal neuroblastoma arising from the right retroperitoneum (*arrow*).

is to obtain at least 95% resection, without compromising major structures. Abdominal tumors are approached through a transverse incision. Thoracic tumors may be approached through a posterolateral thoracotomy or through a thoracoscopic approach. An intraspinal component may be present. In all cases of intrathoracic neuroblastoma, particularly those at the thoracic inlet, it is important to be aware of the possibility that Horner's syndrome (anhidrosis, ptosis, meiosis) may develop. This typically resolves, although it may take many months to do so.

Neuroblastoma in Infants

Spontaneous regression of neuroblastoma has been well described in infants, especially in those with stage 4S disease. Regression generally occurs only in tumors with a near triploid number of chromosomes that also lack *N-myc* amplification and loss of chromosome arm 1p. Recent studies indicate that in infants with asymptomatic, small, low-stage neuroblastoma detected by screening, tumors may spontaneously regress. These patients may be observed safely without surgical intervention or tissue diagnosis.

Rhabdomyosarcoma

Rhabdomyosarcoma is a primitive soft tissue tumor that arises from mesenchymal tissues. The most common sites of origin are the head and neck (36%), extremities (19%), genitourinary tract (21%), and trunk (9%), although the tumor can arise virtually anywhere. The clinical presentation of the tumor depends on the site of origin. The diagnosis is confirmed by the findings of incisional or excisional biopsy after evaluation by MRI, CT of the affected area and the chest, and bone marrow biopsy. The tumor grows locally into surrounding structures and metastasizes widely to lung, regional lymph nodes, liver, brain, and bone marrow. The staging system for rhabdomyosarcoma is based on the tumor, nodes, and metastasis (TNM) system as established by the Soft Tissue Sarcoma Committee of the Children's Oncology Group. It is shown in Table 39-3. Surgery is an important component of the staging strategy and involves biopsy of the lesion and evaluation of lymphatics. Primary resection should be undertaken when complete excision can be performed without causing disability. If this is not possible, the lesion is biopsied and intensive chemotherapy is administered. It is important to plan the biopsy so that it does not interfere with subsequent resection. After the tumor has decreased in size, resection of gross residual disease should be performed. Radiation therapy is effective in achieving local control when microscopic or gross residual disease exists after initial treatment. Patients with completely resected tumors of embryonal histologic type do well without radiation therapy, but radiation therapy benefits patients with group I tumors of alveolar or undifferentiated histologic type.

TABLE 39-3	Staging of rhabdomyosarcoma
Stage 1	Localized disease involving the orbit or head and neck (excluding parameningeal sites), or genitourinary region (excluding bladder/prostate sites), or biliary tract (favorable sites).
Stage 2	Localized disease of any other primary site not included in the stage 1 category (unfavorable sites). Primary tumors must be ≤5 cm in diameter, and there must be no clinical regional lymph node involvement by tumor.
Stage 3	Localized disease of any other primary site. These patients differ from stage 2 patients by having primary tumors >5 cm and/or regional node involvement.
Stage 4	Metastatic disease at diagnosis.

Source: From Lawrence W Jr., Gehan EA, Hays DM, et al: Prognostic significance of staging factors of the UICC staging system in childhood rhabdomyosarcoma: A report from the Intergroup Rhabdomyosarcoma Study (IRS-II). *J Clin Oncol* 5:46, 1987; and Lawrence W Jr., Anderson JR, Gehan EA, et al: Pretreatment TNM staging of childhood rhabdomyosarcoma: A report of the Intergroup Rhabdomyosarcoma Study Group. Children's Cancer Study Group. Pediatric Oncology Group. *Cancer* 80:1165, 1997.

Prognosis

The prognosis for rhabdomyosarcoma is related to the site of origin, resectability, presence of metastases, number of metastatic sites, and histopathologic features. Primary sites associated with more favorable prognoses include the orbit and nonparameningeal head and neck, paratestis and vagina (nonbladder, nonprostate genitourinary), and the biliary tract. Patients with tumors <5 cm in size have better survival than children with larger tumors, and children with metastatic disease at diagnosis have the poorest prognosis. Tumor histologic type influences prognosis; the embryonal variant is a favorable type, whereas the alveolar type has an unfavorable prognosis.

Teratoma

Teratomas are tumors composed of tissue from all three embryonic germ layers. They may be benign or malignant, may arise in any part of the body, and are usually found in midline structures. Thoracic teratomas usually present as an anterior mediastinal mass. Ovarian teratomas present as an abdominal mass, often with symptoms of torsion, bleeding, or rupture. Retroperitoneal teratomas may present as a flank or abdominal mass.

Mature teratomas usually contain well-differentiated tissues and are benign, whereas immature teratomas contain varying amounts of immature neuroepithelium or blastemal tissues. Immature teratomas can be graded from 1 to 3 based on the amount of immature neuroglial tissue present. Tumors of higher grade are more likely to have foci of yolk sac tumor. Malignant germ cell tumors usually contain frankly neoplastic tissues of germ cell origin (i.e., yolk sac carcinoma, embryonal carcinoma, germinoma, and choriocarcinoma). Yolk sac carcinomas produce alpha-fetoprotein and choriocarcinomas produce beta human chorionic gonadotrophin, so that elevations of these substances in the serum can serve as tumor markers. Germinomas can also produce elevation of serum beta human chorionic gonadotrophin, but not to the levels associated with choriocarcinoma.

Sacrococcygeal Teratoma

Sacrococcygeal teratoma usually presents as a large mass extending from the sacrum in the newborn period. Diagnosis may be established by prenatal ultrasonography. In fetuses with evidence of hydrops and a large sacrococcygeal teratoma, prognosis is poor; thus prenatal intervention has been advocated in such patients. The mass may be as small as a few centimeters in diameter or as massive as the size of the infant (Fig. 39-39). The tumor has been classified based on the location and degree of intrapelvic extension. Lesions that grow predominantly into the presacral space often present later in childhood. The differential diagnosis consists of neural tumors, lipoma, and myelomeningoceles.

Most tumors are identified at birth and are benign. Malignant yolk sac tumor histology occurs in a minority of these tumors. Complete resection of the tumor as early as possible is essential. The rectum and genital structures are often distorted by the tumor but usually can be preserved in the course of resection. Perioperative complications of hypothermia and hemorrhage can occur with massive tumors and may prove lethal. These are of particular concern in small, preterm infants with large tumors. The cure rate is excellent if the tumor is excised completely. The majority of patients who develop recurrent disease can be treated successfully with subsequent platinum-based chemotherapy.

Liver Tumors

More than two thirds of all liver tumors in children are malignant. There are two major histologic subgroups: hepatoblastoma and hepatocellular carcinoma. The age of onset of liver cancer in children is related to the histologic type of the tumor. Hepatoblastoma is the most common malignancy of the liver in children, with most of these tumors diagnosed before 4 years of age. Hepatocellu-

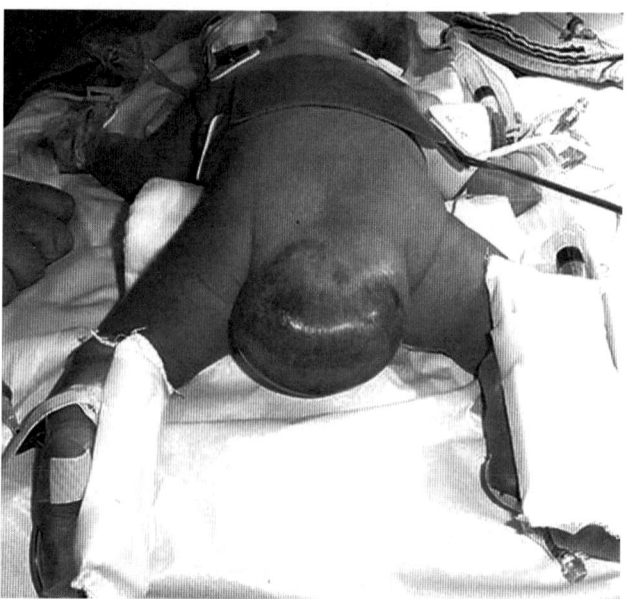

FIG. 39-39. Sacrococcygeal teratoma in a 2-day-old boy.

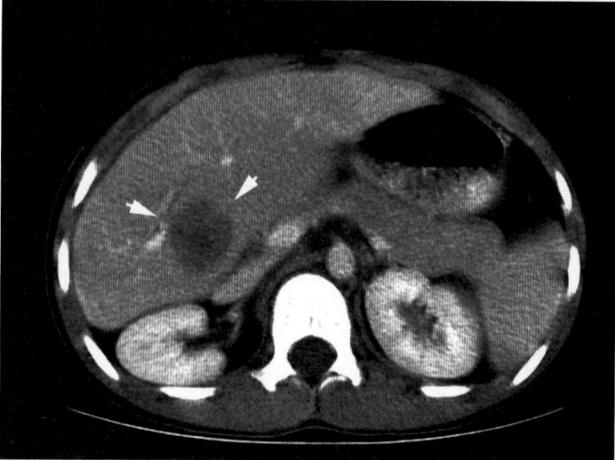

FIG. 39-40. Computed tomographic scan of the abdomen showing hepatocellular carcinoma (*arrows*) in a 12-year-old boy.

lar carcinoma is the next most common, with a peak incidence between 10 and 15 years of age. Malignant mesenchymomas and sarcomas are much less common and constitute the remainder of the malignancies. The finding of a liver mass does not necessarily imply that a malignancy is present. Nearly 50% of all masses are benign; hemangiomas are the most common lesion.

Most children with a liver tumor have an abdominal mass that is usually painless and that is discovered by the parents while changing the child's clothes or while bathing the child. Patients are rarely jaundiced but may show anorexia and weight loss. Most liver function test results are normal. Alpha-fetoprotein levels are increased in 90% of children with hepatoblastomas but are elevated much less commonly in children with other liver malignancies. Radiographic evaluation of these children should include an abdominal CT scan to identify the lesion and to determine the degree of local invasiveness (Fig. 39-40). For lesions that appear malignant, a biopsy should be performed unless the lesion can be completely resected easily. Hepatoblastoma is most often unifocal, whereas hepatocellular carcinoma is often extensively invasive or multicentric. If a hepatoblastoma is completely removed, the majority of patients survive; however, only a minority of patients have lesions amenable to complete resection at diagnosis.

A staging system based on postsurgical extent of tumor and surgical resectability is shown in Table 39-4. The overall survival rate for children with hepatoblastoma is 70%, in contrast to only 25% for those with hepatocellular carcinoma. Children diagnosed with stage I and II hepatoblastoma have a cure rate of >90% compared with 60% for those with stage III tumors and approximately 20% for those with stage IV disease. Among children diagnosed with hepatocellular carcinoma, those with stage I tumors have a good outcome, whereas those with stage III or IV tumors usually do not survive. The fibrolamellar variant of hepatocellular carcinoma may have a better prognosis.

Surgery

The abdominal CT scan usually indicates the resectability of the lesion, although occasionally this can be determined only at the time of exploration. Complete surgical resection of the tumor is the primary goal and is essential for cure. For tumors that are unresectable, preoperative chemotherapy should be administered to reduce the size of the tumor and improve the possibility for complete removal. Chemotherapy is more successful for hepatoblastoma than

for hepatocellular carcinoma. Areas of locally invasive disease, such as the diaphragm, should be resected at the time of surgery. For unresectable tumors, liver transplantation may be offered to select patients. The fibrolamellar variant of hepatocellular carcinoma may have a better outcome with liver transplantation than other hepatocellular carcinomas.

TRAUMA IN CHILDREN

Injury is the leading cause of death among children >1 year of age. In fact, trauma is responsible for almost half of all pediatric deaths—more than cancer, congenital anomalies, pneumonia, heart disease, homicide, and meningitis combined. Death from unintentional injuries accounts for 65% of all injury-related deaths in children <19 years. Motor vehicle collisions are the leading cause of death in individuals aged 1 to 19 years, followed by homicide or suicide (predominantly with firearms) and drowning. Each year, approximately 20,000 children and teenagers die as a result of injury in the United States. For every child who dies from an injury, it is calculated that 40 others are hospitalized and 1120 are treated in emergency departments. An estimated 50,000 children acquire permanent disabilities each year, most of which are the result of head injuries. Thus, pediatric trauma continues to be one of the major threats to the health and well-being of children.

Specific considerations apply to trauma in children that influence management and outcome. These relate to the mechanisms of injury, the anatomic variations in children compared with adults, and the physiologic responses of children.

TABLE 39-4	Staging of pediatric liver cancer
Stage I	No metastases, tumor completely resected
Stage II	No metastases, tumor grossly resected with microscopic residual disease (i.e., positive margins); or tumor rupture or tumor spill at the time of surgery
Stage III	No distant metastases, tumor unresectable or resected with gross residual tumor, or positive lymph nodes
Stage IV	Distant metastases regardless of the extent of liver involvement

Mechanisms of Injury

Most pediatric trauma is blunt. Penetrating injuries are seen in the setting of gun violence, falls onto sharp objects, or penetration by glass after falling through windows. Age and gender significantly influence the patterns of injury. Male children <16 years are exposed to contact sports and drive motor vehicles. As a result, they have a different pattern of injury than younger children, characterized by higher injury severity scores. In the infant and toddler age group, falls are a frequent cause of severe injury. Injuries in the home are extremely common. These include falls, near-drownings, caustic ingestion, and nonaccidental injuries.

Initial Management

The goals of managing the pediatric trauma patient are similar to those of managing the adult trauma patient and conform to the Advanced Trauma Life Support guidelines as established by the American College of Surgeons Committee on Trauma. Airway control is the first priority. In a child, respiratory embarrassment can proceed quickly to cardiac arrest. One must be aware of the anatomic differences between the airway of the child and that of the adult. The child has a shorter neck, smaller and more anterior larynx, floppy epiglottis, short trachea, and large tongue. The child's fifth digit can provide an estimate of the required size of the endotracheal tube. Alternatively, the formula (age + 16)/4 may be used. Uncuffed endotracheal tubes should be used in children <8 years of age to minimize tracheal trauma. After the airway is evaluated, breathing is assessed. Gastric distention from aerophagia can severely compromise respirations. A nasogastric tube should therefore be placed early during the resuscitation. Pneumothorax or hemothorax should be treated promptly. When evaluating the circulation, one should recognize that tachycardia is usually the earliest measurable response to hypovolemia. Other signs of impending hypovolemic shock in children include changes in mentation, delayed capillary refill, skin pallor, and hypothermia. IV access should be rapidly secured once the patient arrives in the trauma bay. The first approach should be to use the antecubital fossae. If this is not possible, a cutdown to the saphenous at the groin can be performed quickly and safely. Intraosseous cannulation can provide temporary access in infants until IV access is established. The use of percutaneous neck lines should generally be avoided. Blood is drawn for cross-matching and measurement of liver enzyme, lipase, and amylase levels and hematologic profile after the IV lines are placed.

In patients who show signs of volume depletion, a 20-mL/kg bolus of saline or lactated Ringer's solution should be given promptly. If the patient does not respond to three boluses, blood should be transfused (10 mL/kg). The source of bleeding should be established. Common sites include the chest, abdomen, pelvis, extremity fractures, or large scalp wounds. These should be carefully sought. Care is taken to avoid hypothermia by infusing warmed fluids and by using external warming devices.

Evaluation of Injury

Radiographs of the cervical spine, chest, and abdomen with pelvis should be obtained for all patients. All extremities that are suspicious for fracture should also be evaluated by radiography. This is preferable to performing routine CT scanning of the neck in the child, because radiographs provide sufficient anatomic detail in children to diagnose clinically significant cervical spine injuries while subjecting the child to significantly less radiation than CT scans. Screening blood tests that include levels of aspartate aminotransferase, alanine aminotransferase, amylase, and lipase are useful for the evaluation of liver and pancreatic injuries. Significant elevations in the levels of these enzymes require further evaluation by CT scanning. The child with significant abdominal tenderness and a mechanism of injury that could cause intra-abdominal injury should undergo abdominal CT scanning with IV and oral contrast

in all cases. Diagnostic peritoneal lavage has a limited role as a screening test in children. However, occasionally it can be useful for a child who is brought emergently to the operating room for management of significant intracranial hemorrhage. At the time of craniotomy, diagnostic peritoneal lavage can be performed concurrently to detect abdominal bleeding. Although focused abdominal ultrasonography is extremely useful in the evaluation of adult abdominal trauma, it has not been widely accepted in the management of pediatric blunt abdominal trauma. In part this relates to the widespread use of nonoperative treatment for most solid organ injuries, which would result in a positive finding on abdominal ultrasonographic scan.

Injuries to the Central Nervous System

The central nervous system (CNS) is the most commonly injured system, and CNS trauma is the leading cause of death among injured children. In the toddler age group, nonaccidental trauma is the most common cause of serious head injury. Findings suggestive of abuse include the presence of retinal hemorrhage on funduscopic evaluation and intracranial hemorrhage without evidence of external trauma (indicative of a shaking injury) as well as fractures at different stages of healing on skeletal survey. In older children, CNS injury occurs most commonly after falls and bicycle and motor vehicle collisions. The initial head CT scan often underestimates the extent of injury in children. Criteria for performing head CT include any loss of consciousness or amnesia for the trauma and inability to assess CNS status, as in the intubated patient. Patients with mild, isolated head injury (Glasgow Coma Scale score of 14 or 15) and negative results on CT scans can be discharged if their neurologic status is normal after 6 hours of observation. Young children and those in whom there is multisystem involvement should be admitted to the hospital for overnight observation. Any change in the neurologic status warrants neurosurgical evaluation and repeat CT scanning. In patients with severe head injury (Glasgow Coma Scale score of ≤8), urgent neurosurgical consultation is required. These patients are evaluated to determine whether intracranial pressure monitoring or craniotomy is necessary.

Thoracic Injuries

The pediatric thorax is pliable due to incomplete calcification of the ribs and cartilages. As a result, blunt chest injury commonly results in pulmonary contusion, although rib fractures are infrequent. Diagnosis is made by chest radiograph, and severe hypoxia requiring mechanical ventilation may be present. Pulmonary contusion usually resolves with careful ventilator management and judicious volume resuscitation. Children who have sustained massive blunt thoracic injury may develop traumatic asphyxia. This is characterized by cervical and facial petechial hemorrhages or cyanosis associated with vascular engorgement and subconjunctival hemorrhage. Management includes ventilation and treatment of coexisting CNS or abdominal injuries. Penetrating thoracic injuries may result in damage to the lung or major disruption of the bronchi or great vessels.

Abdominal Injuries

In children, the small rib cage and minimal muscular coverage of the abdomen can result in significant injury after seemingly minor trauma. The liver and spleen in particular are relatively unprotected and are often injured after direct abdominal trauma. Duodenal injuries are usually the result of blunt trauma, which may arise from child abuse or injury from a bicycle handlebar. Duodenal hematomas usually resolve without surgery. Small intestine injury usually occurs in the jejunum in the area of fixation by the ligament of Treitz. These injuries are generally caused by rapid deceleration when a lap belt is worn. There may be a hematoma on the anterior abdominal wall caused by the lap belt, the so-called seat belt sign (Fig. 39-41A). This should alert the caregiver to the possibility of an

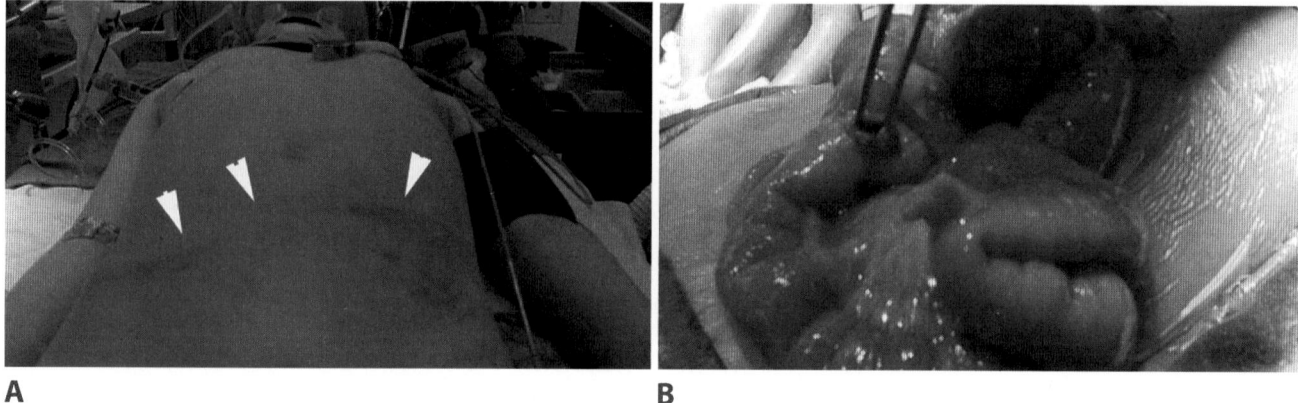

FIG. 39-41. Photographs of a patient who sustained a lap belt injury. **A.** *Arrowheads* denote bruising across the abdomen from the lap belt. **B.** At laparotomy, a perforation of the small bowel was identified.

underlying small bowel injury (Fig. 39-41B) as well as to a potential lumbar spine injury (Chance fracture).

The spleen is injured relatively commonly in blunt abdominal trauma in children. The extent of injury to the spleen is graded (Table 39-5), and management is governed by the injury grade. Current treatment involves a nonoperative approach in most cases, even for grade IV injuries, assuming the patient is hemodynamically stable. This approach avoids surgery in most cases. All patients should be placed in a monitored unit, and type-specific blood should be available for transfusion. When nonoperative management is successful, as it is in most cases, an extended period of bedrest is prescribed. This optimizes the chance for healing and minimizes the likelihood of reinjury. A typical guideline is to keep the child on extremely restricted activity for 2 weeks longer than the grade of spleen injury (i.e., a child with a grade IV spleen injury is prescribed 6 weeks of restricted activity). When the child has an ongoing fluid requirement or when a blood transfusion is necessary, exploration should not be delayed. At surgery, the spleen can often be salvaged. If a splenectomy is performed, prophylactic antibiotics and immunizations should be administered to protect against overwhelming postsplenectomy sepsis.

The liver is also commonly injured in blunt abdominal trauma. A grading system is used to characterize hepatic injuries (Table 39-6), and nonoperative management is usually successful (Fig. 39-42). Recent studies have shown that associated injuries are more significant predictors of outcome in children with liver injuries than the actual injury grade. Criteria for surgery are similar to those for splenic injury and primarily involve hemodynamic instability. The

intraoperative considerations in the management of massive hepatic injury are similar in children and adults.

Renal contusions may occur in significant blunt abdominal trauma. Nonoperative management is usually successful, unless the patient's condition is unstable due to active renal bleeding. The presence of a normal contralateral kidney should be confirmed at the time of surgery.

FETAL INTERVENTION

One of the most exciting developments in the field of pediatric surgery has been the emergence of fetal surgery. In general, performance of a fetal intervention may be justified when a defect is present that would cause devastating consequences to the infant if left uncorrected. For the overwhelming majority of congenital anomalies, postnatal surgery is the preferred modality. However, in specific circumstances, fetal surgery may offer the best possibility for a successful outcome. The decision to perform a fetal intervention requires careful patient selection as well as the availability of a multidisciplinary center that is dedicated to the surgical care of the fetus and the mother. Patient selection is dependent in part on highly accurate prenatal imaging, which includes ultrasonography and MRI. Performance of a fetal surgical procedure may be associated with significant risks to both the mother and the fetus. From the maternal viewpoint, open fetal surgery may lead to uterine bleeding due to the uterine relaxation required during the procedure. The long-term effects on subsequent pregnancies remain to be established. For the fetus, in utero surgery carries the risk of premature labor and amniotic fluid leak. As a result, these procedures are performed only when the expected benefit of fetal intervention outweighs the risk to the fetus of standard postnatal care. Currently, open fetal intervention may be efficacious in certain cases of large congenital lung lesions with hydrops, large teratomas with

TABLE 39-5	Grading of splenic injuries
Grade I	Subcapsular hematoma, <10% surface area capsular tear, <1 cm in depth
Grade II	Subcapsular hematoma, nonexpanding, 10–50% surface area; intraparenchymal hematoma, nonexpanding, <2 cm in diameter; capsular tear, active bleeding, 1–3 cm, does not involve trabecular vessel
Grade III	Subcapsular hematoma, >50% surface area or expanding; intraparenchymal hematoma, >2 cm or expanding; laceration >3 cm in depth or involving trabecular vessels
Grade IV	Ruptured intraparenchymal hematoma with active bleeding; laceration involving segmental or hilar vessels producing major devascularization (>25% of spleen)
Grade V	Shattered spleen; hilar vascular injury that devascularizes spleen

TABLE 39-6	Liver injury grading system
Grade I	Capsular tear <1 cm in depth
Grade II	Capsular tear 1–3 cm in depth, <10 cm in length
Grade III	Capsular tear >3 cm in depth
Grade IV	Parenchymal disruption 25–75% of hepatic lobe or one to three Couinaud's segments
Grade V	Parenchymal disruption >75% of hepatic lobe or more than three Couinaud's segments within a single lobe; injury to retrohepatic vena cava

Source: Reproduced with permission from Moore EE, Cogbill TH, Malangoni MA, et al: Organ injury scaling. *Surg Clin North Am* 75:293, 1995. Copyright Elsevier.

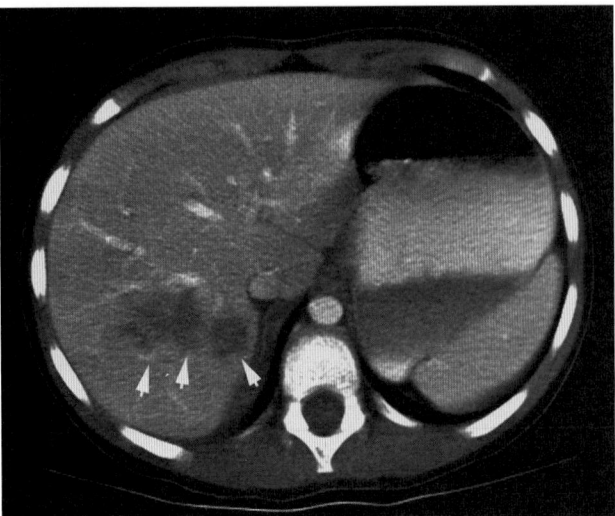

FIG. 39-42. Abdominal computed tomographic scan of a child showing a grade III liver laceration (*arrows*).

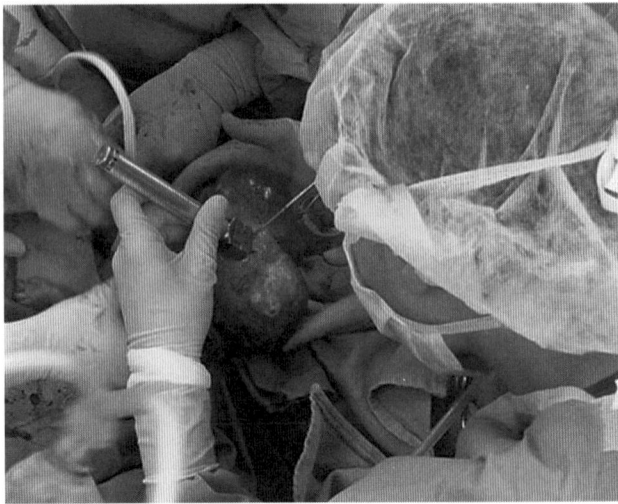

FIG. 39-43. Performance of the ex partum intrauterine treatment procedure in an infant of 34 weeks' gestational age with a large cervical teratoma. Intubation is being carried out while the fetus is on placental support.

hydrops, twin-twin transfusion syndrome, some types of congenital lower urinary tract obstruction, and myelomeningocele. This list of diagnoses that potentially may benefit from a fetal intervention is significantly shorter than that of a decade ago, due in part to improvements in the outcomes of several diseases that are managed in the postnatal period and also to the recognition of the relative lack of benefit of fetal surgery for many conditions.

Fetal Surgery for Lower Urinary Tract Obstruction

Lower urinary tract obstruction refers to a group of diseases characterized by obstruction of the distal urinary system. Common causes include the presence of posterior urethral valves and urethral atresia, as well as other anomalies of the urethra and bladder. The pathologic effects of lower urinary tract obstruction lie in the resultant massive bladder distention that occurs, which can lead to reflux hydronephrosis. This may result in oligohydramnios and cause limb contractures, facial anomalies (Potter facies), and pulmonary hypoplasia. Carefully selected patients with lower urinary tract obstruction may benefit from vesicoamniotic shunting. With relief of the obstruction and improvement in renal function, fetal growth and lung development may be preserved.

Fetal Surgery for Congenital Diaphragmatic Hernia

Given the high mortality associated with the most severe cases of congenital diaphragmatic hernia (CDH), tremendous efforts have been made to determine whether fetal intervention could improve the outcome of this disease. In 1990, Harrison and colleagues reported the first open fetal repair of CDH. The high morbidity associated with the open technique led to the development of fetal tracheal occlusion as a therapeutic approach. This was based on the observation that tracheal occlusion could lead to increased lung growth and reduction of the intrathoracic viscera in animal models. Tracheal occlusion can be achieved in utero by the placement of clips that are removed at the time of delivery. Despite initial enthusiasm for this approach, a recent randomized trial that compared fetal tracheal occlusion with standard postnatal care for left-sided CDH showed no improvement in survival for patients treated with tracheal occlusion.

Fetal Surgery for Myelomeningocele

Myelomeningocele refers to a spectrum of anomalies in which portions of the spinal cord are not covered by the spinal column. This leaves the neural tissue exposed to the injurious effects of the amniotic fluid as well as to trauma from contact with the uterine wall. Nerve damage ensues, resulting in varying degrees of lower extremity paralysis as well as bowel and bladder dysfunction. Initial observations indicated that the amount of injury increased throughout the pregnancy, which provided the rationale for fetal intervention. The current in utero approach for the fetus with myelomeningocele focuses on obtaining coverage of the exposed spinal cord. The efficacy of in utero treatment compared with postnatal repair remains to be determined.

Ex Utero Intrapartum Therapy Procedure

The ex utero intrapartum therapy (EXIT) procedure is used in circumstances in which airway obstruction is predicted at the time of delivery due to the presence of a large neck mass, such as a cystic hygroma or teratoma (Fig. 39-43), or to congenital tracheal stenosis. The success of the procedure depends on the maintenance of uteroplacental perfusion for a sufficient duration to secure the airway. To achieve this, deep uterine relaxation is obtained during a cesarian section under general anesthesia. Uterine perfusion with warmed saline also promotes relaxation and blood flow to the placenta. On average, between 20 and 30 minutes of placental perfusion can be achieved. The fetal airway is secured either by placement of an orotracheal tube or performance of a tracheostomy. Once the airway is secured, the cord is cut, and a definitive procedure may be performed to relieve the obstruction in the postnatal period. In general, infants with cystic neck masses such as lymphangiomas have a more favorable response to an EXIT procedure than infants with solid tumors such as teratomas; this is particularly true for premature infants.

BIBLIOGRAPHY

Entries highlighted in bright blue are key references.

Ahuja AT, King AD, et al: Thyroglossal duct cysts: Sonographic appearances in adults. *AJNR Am J Neuroradiol* 20:579, 1999.

Andersen B, Kallehave F, et al: Antibiotics versus placebo for prevention of postoperative infection after appendicectomy. *Cochrane Database Syst Rev* Issue 2:CD001439, 2005.

Anderson KD, Rouse TM, et al: A controlled trial of corticosteroids in children with corrosive injury of the esophagus. *N Engl J Med* 323:637, 1990.

Azarow K, Messineo A, et al: Congenital diaphragmatic hernia—a tale of two cities: The Toronto experience. *J Pediatr Surg* 32:395, 1997.

Ballance WA, Dahms BB, Shenker N, et al: Pathology of neonatal necrotizing enterocolitis: A ten-year experience. *J Pediatr* 117:S6, 1990.

Bell MJ, Ternberg JL, Feigin RD, et al: Neonatal necrotizing enterocolitis: Therapeutic decisions based upon clinical staging. *Ann Surg* 187:1, 1978.

Billmire D, Vinocur C, et al: Malignant mediastinal germ cell tumors: An intergroup study. *J Pediatr Surg* 36:18, 2001.

Bohn D: Congenital diaphragmatic hernia. *Am J Respir Crit Care Med* 166:911, 2002.

Boloker J, Bateman DA, et al: Congenital diaphragmatic hernia in 120 infants treated consecutively with permissive hypercapnia/spontaneous respiration/elective repair. *J Pediatr Surg* 37:357, 2002.

Bouchard S, Johnson MP, et al: The EXIT procedure: Experience and outcome in 31 cases. *J Pediatr Surg* 37:418, 2002.

Branstetter BF, Weissman JL, et al: The CT appearance of thyroglossal duct carcinoma. *AJNR Am J Neuroradiol* 21:1547, 2000.

Bratton S, Annich G: Packed red blood cell transfusions for critically ill pediatric patients: When and for what conditions? *J Pediatr* 142:95, 2003.

Breneman JC, Lyden E, et al: Prognostic factors and clinical outcomes in children and adolescents with metastatic rhabdomyosarcoma—a report from the Intergroup Rhabdomyosarcoma Study IV. *J Clin Oncol* 21:78, 2003.

Bruner JP, Tulipan N, et al: Fetal surgery for myelomeningocele and the incidence of shunt-dependent hydrocephalus. *JAMA* 282:1819, 1999.

Callaghan WM, MacDorman MF, Rasmussen SA, et al: The contribution of preterm birth to infant mortality rates in the United States. *Pediatrics* 118:1566, 2006.

Cassady G, Crouse DT, Kirklin JW, et al: A randomized, controlled trial of very early prophylactic ligation of the ductus arteriosus in babies who weighed 1000 g or less at birth. *N Engl J Med* 320:1511, 1989.

Chertin B, De Caluwé D, et al: Is contralateral exploration necessary in girls with unilateral inguinal hernia? *J Pediatr Surg* 38:756, 2003.

Choi RS, Vacanti JP: Preliminary studies of tissue-engineered intestine using isolated epithelial organoid units on tubular synthetic biodegradable scaffolds. *Transplant Proc* 29:848, 1997.

Cikrit D, Mastandrea J, West KW, et al: Necrotizing enterocolitis: Factors affecting mortality in 101 surgical cases. *Surgery* 96:648, 1984.

Cohen J, Schanen NC: Branchial cleft anomaly, congenital heart disease, and biliary atresia: Goldenhar complex or Lambert syndrome? *Genet Couns* 11:153, 2000.

Cohn SL, London WB, et al: MYCN expression is not prognostic of adverse outcome in advanced-stage neuroblastoma with nonamplified MYCN. *J Clin Oncol* 18:3604, 2000.

Collins SR, Griffin MR, Arbogast PG, et al: The rising prevalence of gastroschisis and omphalocele in Tennessee. *J Pediatr Surg* 42:1221, 2007.

Coppes MJ, Haber DA, et al: Genetic events in the development of Wilms' tumor. *N Engl J Med* 331:586, 1994.

Cotterill SJ, Pearson ADJ, et al: Clinical prognostic factors in 1277 patients with neuroblastoma: Results of the European Neuroblastoma Study Group "Survey" 1982–1992. *Eur J Cancer* 36:901, 2000.

Crystal P, Hertzanu Y, et al: Sonographically guided hydrostatic reduction of intussusception in children. *J Clin Ultrasound* 30:343, 2002.

Darnell CM, Thompson J, Stromberg D, et al: Effect of low-dose naloxone infusion on fentanyl requirements in critically ill children. *Pediatrics* 121:e1363, 2008. Epub April 14, 2008.

Davit-Spraul A, Baussan C, Hermeziu B, et al: CFC1 gene involvement in biliary atresia with polysplenia syndrome. *J Pediatr Gastroenterol Nutr* 46:111, 2008.

DeRusso PA, Ye W, Shepherd R, et al: Growth failure and outcomes in infants with biliary atresia: A report from the Biliary Atresia Research Consortium. *Hepatology* 46:1632, 2007.

Doné E, Gucciardo L, Van Mieghem T, et al: Prenatal diagnosis, prediction of outcome and in utero therapy of isolated congenital diaphragmatic hernia. *Prenat Diagn* 28:581, 2008.

Dunn J, Fonkalsrud E, et al: Simplifying the Waterston's stratification of infants with tracheoesophageal fistula. *Am Surg* 65:908, 1999.

Ein SH, Njere I, Ein A: Six thousand three hundred sixty-one pediatric inguinal hernias: A 35-year review. *J Pediatr Surg* 41:980, 2006.

Evans GS, Flint N, Somers AS, et al: The development of a method for the preparation of rat intestinal epithelial cell primary cultures. *J Cell Sci* 101(Pt 1):219, 1992.

Ferrari A, Bisogno G, et al: Paratesticular rhabdomyosarcoma: Report from the Italian and German Cooperative Group. *J Clin Oncol* 20:449, 2002.

Fisher JC, Jefferson RA, Arkovitz MS, et al: Redefining outcomes in right congenital diaphragmatic hernia. *J Pediatr Surg* 43:373, 2008.

Freedman AL, Johnson MP, et al: Long-term outcome in children after antenatal intervention for obstructive uropathies. *Lancet* 354:374, 1999.

Gajewski JL, Johnson VV, Sandler SG, et al: A review of transfusion practice before, during, and after hematopoietic progenitor cell transplantation. *Blood* 112:3036, 2008 [Review].

Geisler DP, Jegathesan S, et al: Laparoscopic exploration for the clinically undetected hernia in infancy and childhood. *Am J Surg* 182:693, 2001.

Geneviève D, de Pontual L, Amiel J, et al: An overview of isolated and syndromic oesophageal atresia [review]. *Clin Genet* 71:392, 2007.

Georgeson K: Laparoscopic-assisted pull-through for Hirschsprung's disease. *Semin Pediatr Surg* 11:205, 2002.

Georgeson K: Results of laparoscopic antireflux procedures in neurologically normal infants and children. *Semin Laparosc Surg* 9:172, 2002.

Gollin GA, Abarbanell AA, et al: Peritoneal drainage as definitive management of intestinal perforation in extremely low-birth-weight infants. *J Pediatr Surg* 38:1814, 2003.

Gorsler C, Schier F: Laparoscopic herniorrhaphy in children. *Surg Endosc* 17:571, 2003.

Grant D, Abu-Elmagd K, Reyes J, et al: 2003 Report of the intestine transplant registry: A new era has dawned. *Ann Surg* 241:607, 2005.

Grikscheit TC, Ochoa ER, Ramsanahie A, et al: Tissue-engineered large intestine resembles native colon with appropriate in vitro physiology and architecture. *Ann Surg* 238:35, 2003.

Grikscheit T, Ochoa ER, Srinivasan A, et al: Tissue-engineered esophagus: Experimental substitution by onlay patch or interposition. *J Thorac Cardiovasc Surg* 126:537, 2003.

Grikscheit TC, Ogilvie JB, Ochoa ER, et al: Tissue-engineered colon exhibits function in vivo. *Surgery* 132:200, 2002.

Grikscheit TC, Siddique A, Ochoa ER, et al: Tissue-engineered small intestine improves recovery after massive small bowel resection. *Ann Surg* 240:748, 2004.

Grikscheit T, Srinivasan A, Vacanti JP: Tissue-engineered stomach: A preliminary report of a versatile in vivo model with therapeutic potential. *J Pediatr Surg* 38:1305, 2003.

Grikscheit TC, Vacanti JP: The history and current status of tissue engineering: The future of pediatric surgery. *J Pediatr Surg* 37:277, 2002.

Gross RE, Ladd WE: The Field of Children's Surgery, in: Gross RE (ed): *The Surgery of Infancy and Childhood: Its Principles and Techniques.* W. B. Saunders: Philadelphia, 1953, p 1.

Gura KM, Lee S, Valim C, et al: Safety and efficacy of a fish-oil-based fat emulsion in the treatment of parenteral nutrition-associated liver disease. *Pediatrics* 121:e678, 2008.

Guthrie S, Gordon P, et al: Necrotizing enterocolitis among neonates in the United States. *J Perinatol* 23:278, 2003.

Hackam DJ, Filler R, et al: Enterocolitis after the surgical treatment of Hirschsprung's disease: Risk factors and financial impact. *J Pediatr Surg* 33:830, 1998.

Hackam DJ, Potoka D, et al: Utility of radiographic hepatic injury grade in predicting outcome for children after blunt abdominal trauma. *J Pediatr Surg* 37:386, 2002.

Hackam DJ, Reblock K, et al: The influence of Down's syndrome on the management and outcome of children with Hirschsprung's disease. *J Pediatr Surg* 38:946, 2003.

Hackam DJ, Superina R, et al: Single-stage repair of Hirschsprung's disease: A comparison of 109 patients over 5 years. *J Pediatr Surg* 32:1028, 1997.

Hamner CE, Groner JI, Caniano DA, et al: Blunt intraabdominal arterial injury in pediatric trauma patients: Injury distribution and markers of outcome. *J Pediatr Surg* 43:916, 2008.

Harrison MR: Fetal surgery: Trials, tribulations, and turf. *J Pediatr Surg* 38:275, 2003.

Harrison MR, Keller RL, et al: A randomized trial of fetal endoscopic tracheal occlusion for severe fetal congenital diaphragmatic hernia. *N Engl J Med* 349:1916, 2003.

Harrison MR, Sydorak RM, et al: Fetoscopic temporary tracheal occlusion for congenital diaphragmatic hernia: Prelude to a randomized, controlled trial. *J Pediatr Surg* 38:1012, 2003.

Hedrick H, Flake A, et al: History of fetal diagnosis and therapy: Children's Hospital of Philadelphia experience. *Fetal Diagn Ther* 18:65, 2003.

Hilton EN, Manson FD, Urquhart JE, et al: Left-sided embryonic expression of the BCL-6 corepressor, BCOR, is required for vertebrate laterality determination. *Hum Mol Genet* 16:1773, 2007. Epub May 21, 2007.

Hirschl RB, Philip WF, et al: A prospective, randomized pilot trial of perfluorocarbon-induced lung growth in newborns with congenital diaphragmatic hernia. *J Pediatr Surg* 38:283, 2003.

Johnigan RH, Pereira KD, Poole MD: Community-acquired methicillin-resistant *Staphylococcus aureus* in children and adolescents: Changing trends. *Arch Otolaryngol Head Neck Surg* 129:1049, 2003.

Johnson MP, Sutton LN, et al: Fetal myelomeningocele repair: Short-term clinical outcomes. *Am J Obstet Gynecol* 189:482, 2003.

Kalapurakal J, Li S, et al: Influence of radiation therapy delay on abdominal tumor recurrence in patients with favorable histology Wilms' tumor treated on NWTS-3 and NWTS-4: A report from the National Wilms' Tumor Study Group. *Int J Radiat Oncol Biol Phys* 57:495, 2003.

Kamata S, Ishikawa S, et al: Prenatal diagnosis of abdominal wall defects and their prognosis. *J Pediatr Surg* 31:267, 1996.

Kantarci S, Al-Gazali L, Hill RS, et al: Mutations in LRP2, which encodes the multiligand receptor megalin, cause Donnai-Barrow and facio-oculo-acoustico-renal syndromes. *Nat Genet* 39:957, 2007. Epub July 15, 2007.

Kasai M, Suzuki M: A new operation for non-correctable biliary atresia: hepatic portoenterostomy. *Shujutsu* 13:733, 1959.

Katzenstein HM, Krailo MD, Malogolowkin MH, et al: Hepatocellular carcinoma in children and adolescents: Results from the Pediatric Oncology Group and the Children's Cancer Group Intergroup Study. *J Clin Oncol* 20:2789, 2002.

Kim HB, Fauza D, Garza J, et al: Serial transverse enteroplasty (STEP): A novel bowel lengthening procedure. *J Pediatr Surg* 38:425, 2003.

Kim HB, Lee PW, et al: Serial transverse enteroplasty for short bowel syndrome: A case report. *J Pediatr Surg* 38:881, 2003.

Kliegman RM: Models of the pathogenesis of necrotizing enterocolitis. *J Pediatr* 117:S2, 1990.

Kliegman RM, Fanaroff AA: Necrotizing enterocolitis. *N Engl J Med* 310:1093, 1984.

Konkin D, O'hali W, Webber EM, et al: Outcomes in esophageal atresia and tracheoesophageal fistula. *J Pediatr Surg* 38:1726, 2003.

Kosloske AM: Indications for operation in necrotizing enterocolitis revisited. *J Pediatr Surg* 29:663, 1994.

Kosloske AM: Operative techniques for the treatment of neonatal necrotizing enterocolitis. *Surg Gynecol Obstet* 149:740, 1979.

Kosloske AM, Lilly JR: Paracentesis and lavage for diagnosis of intestinal gangrene in neonatal necrotizing enterocolitis. *J Pediatr Surg* 13:315, 1978.

Ladd WE: Foreword, in Swenson, Orvar: *Pediatric Surgery*. New York: Appleton-Century-Crofts, 1958.

Ladd WE, Gross RE: *Abdominal Surgery of Infancy and Childhood*. Philadelphia: W. B. Saunders, 1941, p 263.

Langer J, Durrant A, et al: One-stage transanal Soave pullthrough for Hirschsprung disease: A multicenter experience with 141 children. *Ann Surg* 238:569, 2003.

Levitt MA, Ferraraccio D, et al: Variability of inguinal hernia surgical technique: A survey of North American pediatric surgeons. *J Pediatr Surg* 37:745, 2002.

Lille ST, Rand RP, Tapper D, et al: The surgical management of giant cervicofacial lymphatic malformations. *J Pediatr Surg* 31:1648, 1996.

Limmer J, Gortner L, Kelsch G, et al: Diagnosis and treatment of necrotizing enterocolitis. A retrospective evaluation of abdominal paracentesis and continuous postoperative lavage. *Acta Paediatr Suppl* 396:65, 1994.

Lintula H, Kokki H, et al: Single-blind randomized clinical trial of laparoscopic versus open appendicectomy in children. *Br J Surg* 88:510, 2001.

Lipshutz G, Albanese C, et al: Prospective analysis of lung-to-head ratio predicts survival for patients with prenatally diagnosed congenital diaphragmatic hernia. *J Pediatr Surg* 32:1634, 1997.

Little D, Rescorla F, et al: Long-term analysis of children with esophageal atresia and tracheoesophageal fistula. *J Pediatr Surg* 38:852, 2003.

Loeb DM, Thornton K, Shokek O: Pediatric soft tissue sarcomas [review]. *Surg Clin North Am* 88:615, 2008.

Luig M, Lui K: Epidemiology of necrotizing enterocolitis—Part I: Changing regional trends in extremely preterm infants over 14 years. *J Paediatr Child Health* 41:169, 2005.

Lynch L, O'Donoghue D, Dean J, et al: Detection and characterization of hemopoietic stem cells in the adult human small intestine. *J Immunol* 176:5199, 2006.

Mallick IH, Yang W, Winslet MC, et al: Ischemia-reperfusion injury of the intestine and protective strategies against injury. *Dig Dis Sci* 49:1359, 2004.

Marianowski R, Ait Amer JL, et al: Risk factors for thyroglossal duct remnants after Sistrunk procedure in a pediatric population. *Int J Pediatr Otorhinolaryngol* 67:19, 2003.

Maris JM, Weiss MJ, et al: Loss of heterozygosity at 1p36 independently predicts for disease progression but not decreased overall survival probability in neuroblastoma patients: A Children's Cancer Group Study. *J Clin Oncol* 18:1888, 2000.

Martinez-Tallo E, Claure N, Bancalari E: Necrotizing enterocolitis in full-term or near-term infants: Risk factors. *Biol Neonate* 71:292, 1997.

Mengel W, Wronecki K, Schroeder J, et al: Histopathology of the cryptorchid testis. *Urol Clin North Am* 9:331, 1982.

Meyers RL, Book LS, et al: High-dose steroids, ursodeoxycholic acid, and chronic intravenous antibiotics improve bile flow after Kasai procedure in infants with biliary atresia. *J Pediatr Surg* 38:406, 2003.

Miyano T, Yamataka A, et al: Hepaticoenterostomy after excision of choledochal cyst in children: A 30-year experience with 180 cases. *J Pediatr Surg* 31:1417, 1996.

Molik KA, West KW, et al: Portal venous air: The poor prognosis persists. *J Pediatr Surg* 36:1143, 2001.

Moss R, Dimmitt R, et al: A meta-analysis of peritoneal drainage versus laparotomy for perforated necrotizing enterocolitis. *J Pediatr Surg* 36:1210, 2001.

Moss RL, Das JB, Raffensperger JG: Necrotizing enterocolitis and total parenteral nutrition–associated cholestasis. *Nutrition* 12:340, 1996.

Moyer V, Moya F, et al: Late versus early surgical correction for congenital diaphragmatic hernia in newborn infants. *Cochrane Database Syst Rev* Issue 3:CD001695, 2002.

Nadler E, Stanford A, et al: Intestinal cytokine gene expression in infants with acute necrotizing enterocolitis: Interleukin-11 mRNA expression inversely correlates with extent of disease. *J Pediatr Surg* 36:1122, 2001.

Neville HL, Andrassy RJ, et al: Lymphatic mapping with sentinel node biopsy in pediatric patients. *J Pediatr Surg* 35:961, 2000.

Nio M, Ohi R, et al: Five- and 10-year survival rates after surgery for biliary atresia: A report from the Japanese Biliary Atresia Registry. *J Pediatr Surg* 38:997, 2003.

O'Donovan DJ, Baetiong A, Adams K, et al: Necrotizing enterocolitis and gastrointestinal complications after indomethacin therapy and surgical ligation in premature infants with patent ductus arteriosus. *J Perinatol* 23:286, 2003.

Olutoye OO, Coleman BG, et al: Prenatal diagnosis and management of congenital lobar emphysema. *J Pediatr Surg* 35:792, 2000.

Ortega JA, Douglass EC, et al: Randomized comparison of cisplatin/vincristine/fluorouracil and cisplatin/continuous infusion doxorubicin for treatment of pediatric hepatoblastoma: A report from the Children's Cancer Group and the Pediatric Oncology Group. *J Clin Oncol* 18:2665, 2000.

Panesar J, Higgins K, et al: Nontuberculous mycobacterial cervical adenitis: A ten-year retrospective review. *Laryngoscope* 113:149, 2003.

Pedersen A, Petersen O, et al: Randomized clinical trial of laparoscopic versus open appendicectomy. *Br J Surg* 88:200, 2001.

Peña A: *Atlas of Surgical Management of Anorectal Malformations*. Springer, 1989.

Peña A, Guardino K, et al: Bowel management for fecal incontinence in patients with anorectal malformations. *J Pediatr Surg* 33:133, 1998.

Peña A, Hong A: Advances in the management of anorectal malformations. *Am J Surg* 180:370, 2000.

Poenaru D, Laberge J, et al: A new prognostic classification for esophageal atresia. *Surgery* 113:426, 1993.

Potoka D, Schall L, et al: Improved functional outcome for severely injured children treated at pediatric trauma centers. *J Trauma* 51:824, 2001.

Potoka DA, Schall LC, et al: Risk factors for splenectomy in children with blunt splenic trauma. *J Pediatr Surg* 37:294, 2002.

Powers CJ, Levitt MA, et al: The respiratory advantage of laparoscopic Nissen fundoplication. *J Pediatr Surg* 38:886, 2003.

Pritchard-Jones K: Controversies and advances in the management of Wilms' tumour. *Arch Dis Child* 87:241, 2002.

Puapong D, Kahng D, et al: Ad libitum feeding: Safely improving the cost-effectiveness of pyloromyotomy. *J Pediatr Surg* 37:1667, 2002.

Quinton AE, Smoleniec JS: Congenital lobar emphysema—the disappearing chest mass: Antenatal ultrasound appearance. *Ultrasound Obstet Gynecol* 17:169, 2001.

Reyes J, Bueno J, Kocoshis S, et al: Current status of intestinal transplantation in children. *J Pediatr Surg* 33:243, 1998.

Rosen NG, Hong AR, et al: Rectovaginal fistula: A common diagnostic error with significant consequences in girls with anorectal malformations. *J Pediatr Surg* 37:961, 2002.

Rothenberg S: Laparoscopic Nissen procedure in children. *Semin Laparosc Surg* 9:146, 2002.

Rothenberg SS: Thoracoscopic pulmonary surgery. *Semin Pediatr Surg* 16:231, 2007.

Samuel M, McCarthy L, et al: Efficacy and safety of OK-432 sclerotherapy for giant cystic hygroma in a newborn. *Fetal Diagn Ther* 15:93, 2000.

Sandler A, Ein S, et al: Unsuccessful air-enema reduction of intussusception: Is a second attempt worthwhile? *Pediatr Surg Int* 15:214, 1999.

Sankaran K, Puckett B, Lee DS, et al: Variations in incidence of necrotizing enterocolitis in Canadian neonatal intensive care units. *J Pediatr Gastroenterol Nutr* 39:366, 2004.

Sarioglu A, McGahren ED, Rodgers BM: Effects of carotid artery repair following neonatal extracorporeal membrane oxygenation. *Pediatr Surg Int* 16:15, 2000.

Schier F, Montupet P, et al: Laparoscopic inguinal herniorrhaphy in children: A three-center experience with 933 repairs. *J Pediatr Surg* 37:395, 2002.

Section on Hematology/Oncology: Guidelines for the pediatric cancer center and role of such centers in diagnosis and treatment. *Pediatrics* 99:139, 1997.

Shamberger R, Guthrie K, et al: Surgery-related factors and local recurrence of Wilms tumor in National Wilms Tumor Study 4. *Ann Surg* 229:292, 1999.

Shimada H, Ambros I, et al: The International Neuroblastoma Pathology Classification (the Shimada system). *Cancer* 86:364, 1999.

Shivakumar P, Campbell KM, Sabla GE, et al: Obstruction of extrahepatic bile ducts by lymphocytes is regulated by IFN-gamma in experimental biliary atresia. *J Clin Invest* 114:322, 2004.

Simons SHP, van Dijk M, et al: Routine morphine infusion in preterm newborns who received ventilatory support: A randomized controlled trial. *JAMA* 290:2419, 2003.

Soffer SZ, Rosen NG, et al: Cloacal exstrophy: A unified management plan. *J Pediatr Surg* 35:932, 2000.

Spitz L, Kiely E, et al: Oesophageal atresia: At-risk groups for the 1990s. *J Pediatr Surg* 29:723, 1994.

Strauss RA, Balu R, et al: Gastroschisis: The effect of labor and ruptured membranes on neonatal outcome. *Am J Obstet Gynecol* 189:1672, 2003.

Suzuki N, Tsuchida Y, et al: Prenatally diagnosed cystic lymphangioma in infants. *J Pediatr Surg* 33:1599, 1998.

Teich S, Barton D, et al: Prognostic classification for esophageal atresia and tracheoesophageal fistula: Waterston versus Montreal. *J Pediatr Surg* 32:1075, 1997.

Teitelbaum D, Coran A: Reoperative surgery for Hirschsprung's disease. *Semin Pediatr Surg* 12:124, 2003.

Thibeault DW, Olsen SL, et al: Pre-ECMO predictors of nonsurvival in congenital diaphragmatic hernia. *J Perinatol* 22:682, 2002.

Tolia V, Wureth A, et al: Gastroesophageal reflux disease: Review of presenting symptoms, evaluation, management, and outcome in infants. *Dig Dis Sci* 48:1723, 2003.

Tsao K, St. Peter SD, Sharp SW, et al: Current application of thoracoscopy in children. *J Laparoendosc Adv Surg Tech A* 18:131, 2008.

Tulipan N, Sutton L, et al: The effect of intrauterine myelomeningocele repair on the incidence of shunt-dependent hydrocephalus. *Pediatr Neurosurg* 38:27, 2003.

Vargas JV, Vlassov D, Colman D, et al: A thermodynamic model to predict the thermal response of living beings during pneumoperitoneum procedures. *J Med Eng Technol* 29:75, 2005.

Wang KS, Shaul DB: Two-stage laparoscopic orchidopexy with gubernacular preservation: Preliminary report of a new approach to the intraabdominal testis. *J Pediatr Endosurg Innovative Tech* 8:252, 2004.

Wenzler D, Bloom D, et al: What is the rate of spontaneous testicular descent in infants with cryptorchidism? *J Urol* 171:849, 2004.

Wildhaber B, Coran A, et al: The Kasai portoenterostomy for biliary atresia: A review of a 27-year experience with 81 patients. *J Pediatr Surg* 38:1480, 2003.

Wilson J, Lund D, et al: Congenital diaphragmatic hernia—a tale of two cities: The Boston experience. *J Pediatr Surg* 32:401, 1997.

Yang EY, Allmendinger N, Johnson SM, et al: Neonatal thoracoscopic repair of congenital diaphragmatic hernia: Selection criteria for successful outcome. *J Pediatr Surg* 40:1369, 2005.

CHAPTER 40

Urology

Jeffrey La Rochelle, Brian Shuch,
and Arie Belldegrun

ANATOMY

The anatomic structures that fall under the purview of genitourinary surgery are the kidneys, adrenals, ureters, bladder, prostate, seminal vesicles, urethra, vas deferens, and testes. They are situated mainly outside the peritoneum, but urologic surgery frequently involves intraperitoneal approaches to the kidney, bladder, and retroperitoneal lymph nodes. Furthermore, urologists must be familiar with the techniques of intestinal surgery for the purposes of urinary diversion and bladder augmentation.

Kidney and Adrenal

The kidneys are paired retroperitoneal organs that are invested in a fibro-fatty layer: Gerota's fascia. Posterolaterally, the kidneys are bordered by the quadratus lumborum and posteromedially by the psoas muscle. Anteriorly they are confined by the posterior layer of the peritoneum. On the left, the spleen lies superolaterally, separated from the kidney and Gerota's fascia by the peritoneum. On the right, the liver is situated superiorly and anteriorly and also is separated by the peritoneum. The second portion of the duodenum is in close proximity to the right renal vessels and, during right renal surgery, it must be reflected anteromedially (Kocherized) to achieve vascular control. The renal arteries, in the typical configuration, are single vessels extending from the aorta that branch into several segmental arteries before entering the renal sinus. The right renal artery passes posterior to the vena cava and is significantly longer than the left renal artery. Occasionally, the kidney is supplied by a second renal artery, typically to the lower pole. Within the kidney, there is essentially no anastomotic arterial flow, so the kidneys are prone to infarction when branch vessels are interrupted. The renal veins, which course anteriorly to the renal arteries, drain to the vena cava. The left renal vein passes anteriorly to the aorta and is much longer than the right renal vein. The left vein is in continuity with the left gonadal vein, the left inferior adrenal vein, and a lumbar vein. These veins provide adequate drainage for the left kidney in the event that drainage to the vena cava is interrupted. The right renal vein has no such collateral venous drainage.

The collecting system of the kidney is composed of several major and minor calyces that coalesce into the renal pelvis. The renal pelvis can have either a mainly intrarenal or extrarenal position. The renal pelvis tapers into the ureteropelvic junction (UPJ) where it joins with the ureter.

The adrenal glands lie superomedially to the kidneys within Gerota's fascia. There is a layer of Gerota's fascia between the adrenal and the kidney. However, in the presence of a tumor or inflammatory process, the adrenal can become very adherent to the kidney, and separation can be difficult. The arterial supply of the adrenals derives from the aorta and small branches from the renal arteries. The venous drainage on the left is mainly through the inferior phrenic vein and through the left renal vein via the inferior adrenal vein. On the right, the adrenal is drained by a very short (<1 cm) vein to the vena cava. It can be avulsed by moderate traction and can be the source of troublesome bleeding.

Ureter

The ureters are muscular structures that course anterior to the psoas muscles from the renal pelvis to the bladder. The blood supply of the proximal ureter derives from the aorta and renal artery and comes mainly from the medial direction. However, once it crosses the iliac vessels at the pelvic brim near where the iliac vessels bifurcate, it derives its blood supply laterally from branches from the iliac arteries. The blood supply has implications for managing ureteral injuries. Mobilizing the distal ureter for anastomosis requires releasing its lateral attachments, which results in ischemia, so for this reason, distal ureteral injuries are typically managed by bringing the proximal ureter to the bladder.

The ureters course along the pelvic sidewall and pass under the uterine arteries in women, making them vulnerable to injury during hysterectomy. They enter the bladder at the lateral aspect of the base. They course through the bladder musculature at an oblique angle and open into the bladder at the ureteral orifices that are relatively close to the bladder outlet.

Bladder and Prostate

The urinary bladder is situated in the retropubic space in an extraperitoneal position. A portion of the bladder dome is adjacent to the peritoneum, so ruptures at this point can result in intraperitoneal urine leakage. The anatomic relations of the bladder are dependent on the degree of filling. A very distended bladder can project above the umbilicus. At physiologic volumes (200 to 400 mL), the bladder projects modestly into the abdomen. The sigmoid colon lies superolaterally and may become adherent or fistulize to the bladder secondary to diverticulitis. The rectum lies posterior to the bladder in males, whereas the vagina and uterus are posterior in females.

In males, the prostate is in continuity with the bladder neck, and the urethra courses through it. The prostate has a significant component of smooth muscle and can provide urinary continence even in the absence of the external striated sphincter. The puboprostatic ligaments connect the prostate to the pubic symphysis, and pelvic fractures often result in proximal urethral injuries due to the traction that these ligaments provide. Between the prostate and the rectum lies Denonvilliers' fascia, which is the main anatomic barrier that prevents prostate cancer from regularly penetrating into the rectum. Just beyond the apex of the prostate is the external (voluntary) sphincter, which is part of the genitourinary diaphragm.

Penis

The penis is composed of three main bodies, along with fascia, neurovascular structures, and skin. The corpora cavernosum are the

---

KEY POINTS

1. In the surgical treatment of invasive bladder cancer, a thorough lymph node dissection is essential.

2. Patients with testicular cancer without radiographic evidence of metastasis often harbor microscopic deposits of disease and require either adjuvant treatment or very close surveillance.

3. Nephrectomy is the mainstay of treatment for localized renal cell carcinoma, and it also provides a survival benefit in the setting of metastatic disease.

4. The vast majority of renal trauma can be treated conservatively, with early surgical intervention reserved for persistent bleeding or renal vascular injuries.

5. Distal ureteral injuries should only be treated with bladder reimplantation because of the high failure rate of distal uretero-ureterostomies.

6. Extraperitoneal bladder ruptures can be treated conservatively but intraperitoneal ruptures typically require surgical repair.

7. Nearly all episodes of acute urinary retention can be treated with conservative measures such as decreasing narcotic usage and increasing ambulation.

8. Testicular torsion is an emergency where successful testicular salvage is inversely related to the delay in repair, so cases with a high degree of clinical suspicion should not wait for a radiologic diagnosis.

9. Fournier's gangrene is a potentially lethal condition that requires aggressive débridement and close follow-up due to the frequent need for repeat débridement.

10. Most small ureteral calculi will pass spontaneously, but larger stones (>6 mm) are better treated with ureteral stenting and lithotripsy.

paired, cylinder-like structures that are the main erectile bodies of the penis. Proximally, they lie along the medial aspects of the inferior pubic rami in the perineum. Distally, they fuse along their medial aspects and form the pendulous penis. The corpora cavernosum consist of a tough outer layer called the *tunica albuginea*, and spongy, sinusoidal tissue inside that fills with blood to result in erection. The two corpora cavernosum have numerous vascular interconnections, so they function as one compartment. The cavernosal arteries, which are branches of the penile artery, course through the center of the corporal sinusoidal tissue. The sinusoidal tissue is innervated by the cavernosal nerves, which are autonomic nerves that originate in the hypogastric plexus and play a critical role in erection. Before entering the penis, the cavernosal nerves travel immediately adjacent to the prostate, which explains why they often are damaged at radical prostatectomy. On the underside of the penis lies the corpus spongiosum, which surrounds the urethra. The spongiosum does not have the same tunical layers as the corpora cavernosum, so it does not exhibit the same firmness during erection. The tip of the penis, called the glans, is in continuity with the corpus spongiosum.

Surrounding all three bodies of the penis are the outer dartos fascia and the inner Buck's fascia. The dorsal nerves of the penis, which provide sensation to the penile skin, derive from the pudendal nerves and, along with the dorsal penile arteries, travel along the dorsum of the penis within Buck's fascia. The neurovascular bundle of the penis must be avoided during surgical exploration of the penis for injuries or reconstruction.

Scrotum and Testes

The scrotum is a capacious structure that contains the testes and epididymes. Because of its dependent position, significant edema can develop when a patient is fluid overloaded and bleeding can result in the accumulation of large hematomas. Beneath the skin, from superficial to deep, are the dartos, external spermatic, cremasteric, and internal spermatic fascias. These layers are not always distinct. Beneath the internal fascia are the parietal and visceral layers of the tunica vaginalis, between which hydroceles form. The visceral layer of the tunica vaginalis is adherent to the testis. The testis' noncompliant outer layer is the tunica albuginea. Inside the tunica are the seminiferous tubules. The blood supply enters the testis at the superior pole by way of the spermatic cord. In addition to the vas deferens, the cord carries three separate sources of arterial blood flow—the testicular artery that branches from the aorta below the renal artery, the cremasteric artery, and the deferential artery. Interruption of one of the arteries during vasectomy or inguinal surgery will not result in ischemia to the testis. Venous drainage parallels the arterial inflow except that the left gonadal vein drains into the renal vein rather than the vena cava. Dilation of spermatic veins is called a *varicocele* and may be palpable when a patient is standing. They are not considered pathologic unless they cause discomfort or affect fertility, which they sometimes do.

UROLOGIC MALIGNANCIES

Bladder Cancer

The most common form of bladder cancer in the United States is transitional cell carcinoma (TCC). Tobacco use, followed by occupational exposure to various carcinogenic materials such as automobile exhaust or industrial solvents are the most frequent risk factors, though many with the disease have no identifiable risks.[1] Other forms of bladder cancer, such as adenocarcinoma and squamous cell carcinoma, occur in distinct patient populations. Patients with chronic irritation from catheters, bladder stones, or schistosomiasis infection are at risk for the squamous cell variant while those with urachal remnants or bladder exstrophy have an increased risk of adenocarcinoma.

Bladder cancer can be categorized into invasive and noninvasive types. Management of TCC varies greatly, depending on the depth of invasion. A complete transurethral resection of the bladder tumor, which allows staging of the tumor, is the first step. The tumor is completely removed, if possible, along with a sampling of the muscular bladder wall underlying the tumor, because the large majority of bladder tumors grow in an exophytic pattern projecting into the bladder lumen. In females, a bimanual examination can help determine if there is fixation of the bladder to adjacent structures. Radiologic imaging of most bladder tumors is of limited benefit in determining the presence or size/stage of a bladder tumor. However, in the presence of a known bladder tumor, unilateral or bilateral hydronephrosis is an ominous sign of locally advanced disease.[2] Computed tomography (CT) scans do provide valuable information regarding metastatic involvement of pelvic lymph nodes, liver, or lung. For patients that have disease invading into bladder muscle (T2), immediate cystectomy with extended lymph node dissection offers the best chance of survival, although current long-term cure for those presenting with clinically localized disease is still only achieved in 50 to 60% of patients.[3] The addition of neoadjuvant or adjuvant chemotherapy in those without discernible metastatic spread is gaining increasing acceptance and does provide an increase in survival.[4] Patients with limited lymph node involvement may be cured with surgery alone, but those with extensive lymph node involvement have a dismal prognosis.

Patients have multiple reconstructive options, including continent and noncontinent urinary diversions. The orthotopic neobladder has emerged as a popular urinary diversion for patients without urethral involvement. This diversion type involves the detubularization of a segment of bowel, typically distal ileum, which is then refashioned into a pouch that is anastomosed to the proximal urethral. Detubularization decreases intrapouch filling pressure, which improves urinary storage capacity. The external sphincter is still intact, and voiding is achieved through sphincteric relaxation and a Valsalva's maneuver. The most common noncontinent diversion is the ileal conduit, whereby a segment of distal ileum is isolated with one end brought out through the abdominal wall as a urostomy. Ileal conduits are preferred for renal insufficiency because urine is not "stored" and therefore has less time in contact with the absorptive surface of the ileal segment. Conduits are also used when the bladder is unresectable, but urinary diversion is necessary due to intractable bleeding or severe voiding pain. Each segment of bowel that is used offers its own advantages and inherent complications.

Patients with nonmuscle invasive TCC (confined to the bladder mucosa or submucosa) can be managed with transurethral resection alone. However, patients are at risk for recurrence and progression to muscle-invasive disease. Tumor grade is extremely important in assessing the risk of disease progression. Those patients with high-grade disease or recurrent tumors can be treated with intravesical agents such as bacille Calmette-Guérin or mitomycin C. These agents decrease risk of progression and recurrence, by induction of an effective immunologic antitumor response in the case of bacille Calmette-Guérin and through direct cytotoxicity for mitomycin C. Those patients at high risk of progression that fail conservative therapy should be offered cystectomy. As upper tract recurrence is fairly common, surveillance must be performed with retrograde pyelograms or CT urograms.

Surgical Approaches and Complications

The typical surgical approach for cystectomy is a lower midline incision from just above the umbilicus to the pubic symphysis. This allows adequate exposure of the pelvic contents, iliac vessels, and lower abdominal cavity. The peritoneum between the median umbilical ligaments (urachal remnant) also is taken with the specimen. In men, the prostate is removed with the bladder. In women, the uterus, ovaries (in postmenopausal women), and anterior wall of the vagina are removed with the bladder. The vagina may be spared, depending on the location and extent of the tumor, but significantly more operative bleeding results. Robotic approaches for cystectomy are increasingly used, but the lymph node dissection and urinary diversion is still usually finished through an open incision. The benefit of the robotic portion is decreased blood loss during the pelvic dissection (due to pneumoperitoneum), and the shortening of the time that the abdomen is open.

Complications of bladder cancer surgery involve perforation during transurethral resection of the bladder tumor, which requires catheter drainage for several days if small or open repair if large and intraperitoneal, which is rare. Cystectomy and urinary diversion may result in ileus, bowel obstruction, intestinal anastomotic leak, urine leak, or rectal injury. A urine leak from the ureteroenteric anastomosis is a common cause of ileus, but may also result in intra-abdominal urinoma or abscess formation if drainage is ineffective. Deep venous thrombosis is common after cystectomy[5] due to the advanced age of most patients, proximity of the iliac veins to the resection and lymph node dissection, and the presence of malignancy.

Testicular Cancer

Testicular cancer is the most common solid malignancy in men ages 15 to 35 years of age.[6] Most men are diagnosed with an asymptomatic enlarging mass (Fig. 40-1). A major risk for the development of testicular cancer is cryptorchidism. Although the debate continues over whether early surgical intervention to bring an undescended testis into the scrotum alters the future risk of cancer, it is accepted that doing so allows much easier monitoring for the development of a testicular mass.

Most neoplasms arise from the germ cells, though nongerm cell tumors arise from Leydig's or Sertoli's cells. The nongerm cell tumors are rare and generally follow a more benign course. Germ cell cancers are categorically divided into seminomatous and nonseminomatous forms that follow different treatment algorithms.

All solid testicular masses observed on physical examination and documented on ultrasound are malignant until proven otherwise, because the vast majority are cancerous. Initial studies must include tumor markers, including alpha-fetoprotein and beta human chori-

onic gonadotrophin. Elevated tumor markers are found almost exclusively in nonseminomatous germ cell tumor, though occasionally seminomas will cause a modest rise in beta human chorionic gonadotrophin. Chest and abdominal imaging must be performed to evaluate for evidence of metastasis. The most common site of spread is the retroperitoneal lymph nodes extending from the common iliac vessels to the renal vessels, and abdominal imaging should be performed in all patients. There is no role for percutaneous biopsy of testicular masses due to the risk of seeding the scrotal wall and changing the natural retroperitoneal lymphatic drainage of the testicle, because the testes have a remarkably predictable pattern of lymphatic drainage. In cases where metastatic disease to the testicle is suspected, an open testicular biopsy by delivery of the testicle through the inguinal canal is recommended. Lymphoma may involve one or both testes, but evidence of the disease usually is present elsewhere in the body, although relapses may be isolated to the testes.

Even in the absence of enlarged lymph nodes (stage I), micrometastatic disease is often present, so adjuvant surgery or chemotherapy is offered. However, watchful waiting protocols have been gaining in popularity. Retroperitoneal lymph node dissection (RPLND) is potentially curative in the setting of limited lymph node involvement and has been the preferred adjuvant treatment of those with stage I disease; some advocate its use in stage IIa and IIb disease. Pure seminoma is exquisitely radiosensitive and stage I, IIa, and IIb disease can be treated with external beam radiation to the retroperitoneal nodes. Both forms of germ cell tumors with disseminated disease or large bulky lymph nodes are best treated with chemotherapy. However, teratoma frequently is a component of retroperitoneal lymph node metastasis, and it is not responsive to chemotherapy or radiation and can demonstrate aggressive malignant degeneration. Postchemotherapy RPLND for residual masses can be challenging. Large bulky metastases may encase the great vessels, and vascular graft placement after resection occasionally is required.

Surgical Approach and Complications

For orchiectomy, an inguinal incision is made over the external ring and carried laterally over the position of the internal ring. It is important to not violate the scrotal skin during orchiectomy due to the concern, mostly theoretical, of altering the lymphatic drainage of the testis. For RPLND, a midline incision usually is made from the xiphoid process to the pubic symphysis, although some use a thoracoabdominal approach. Laparoscopic approaches are used with increasing regularity.

Complications of testicular cancer surgery include scrotal hematoma formation, which can be prevented by meticulous hemostasis. Complications after RPLND include bowel obstruction; excessive bleeding, particularly from retrocaval lumber veins; and chylous ascites. Patients who undergo a full, bilateral RPLND often suffer from anejaculation due to the interruption of the descending postganglionic sympathetic nerve fibers that are involved in seminal emission. For this reason, right and left templates have been developed that limit dissection and preserve some of these nerves with a low risk of leaving residual microscopic cancer.[7]

Kidney Cancer

Renal cell carcinoma (RCC) is a malignancy of the renal epithelium that can arise from any component of the nephron (Fig. 40-2). In 2008, there is estimated to be 54,000 new cases in the United States, with roughly 13,000 deaths.[8] With the widespread use of imaging for many medical complaints, a stage migration has led an increased incidence of small renal masses.[9] Various histologic subtypes include clear-cell, papillary (types I and II), chromophobe, collecting duct, and unclassified forms. Collecting duct and unclassified forms have dismal prognosis and very little response to systemic therapy. Benign lesions, which are more commonly found when small tumors are removed, include oncocytomas and angiomyolipomas. Renal tumors are usually solid, but they also can be cystic. Simple cysts are very common and are not malignant, but more complex

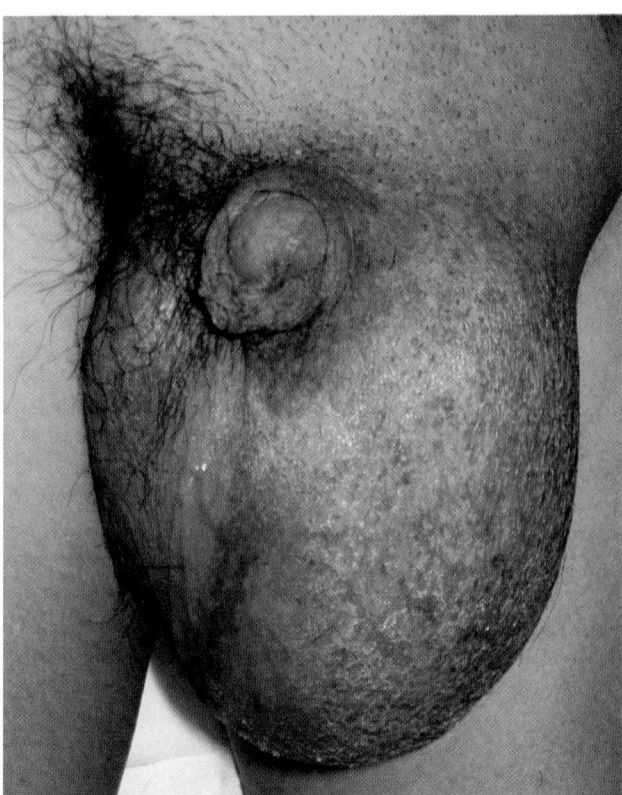

FIG. 40-1. Testicular cancer. Patients often present with advanced disease in spite of scrotal enlargement for several months.

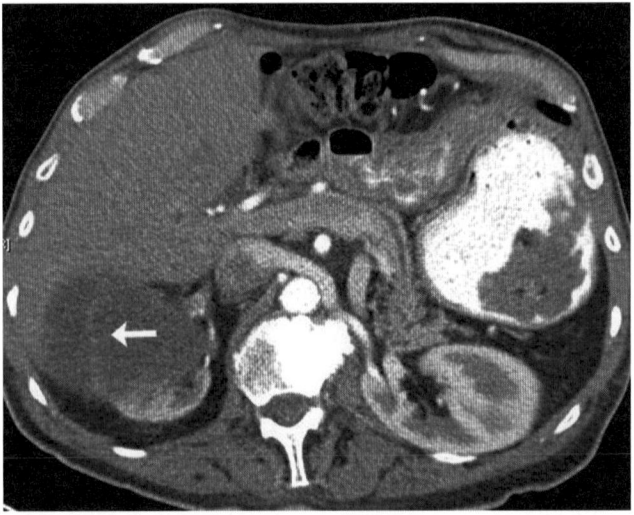

FIG. 40-2. Complex renal cyst. A right kidney with a Bosniak type 3 renal cyst. Note the enhancing septum (*arrow*). This cyst was removed and found to be a high-grade papillary renal cell carcinoma.

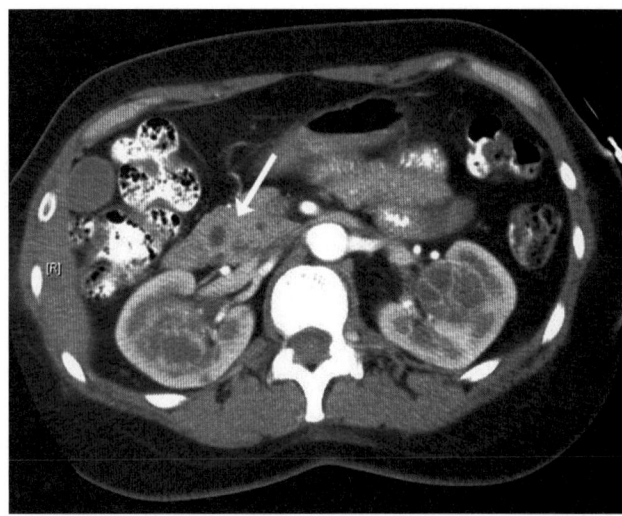

FIG. 40-3. von Hippel-Lindau disease. A computed tomography image of a patient with von Hippel-Lindau disease and bilateral kidney tumors that are predominantly intrarenal. Note the numerous cysts in the head of the pancreas (*arrow*).

cysts may be malignant. The Bosniak classification system, based on septations, calcifications, and enhancement, is used to assess the likelihood of malignancy (Table 40-1).[10]

Most cases of RCC are sporadic, but many hereditary forms have been described. These syndromes frequently involve a germline mutation in a tumor-suppressor gene. Von Hippel-Lindau disease is associated with multiple tumors including clear-cell RCC (Fig. 40-3). The involved gene, *vhl*, also frequently is mutated or hypermethylated in sporadic RCC.[11] Other rare forms include Birt-Hogg-Dubé syndrome, where patients get oncocytomas or chromophobe tumors. Patients with hereditary papillary RCC and hereditary leiomyomatosis develop papillary RCC.

The most common sites of metastasis are the retroperitoneal lymph nodes and lungs, but liver, bone, and brain also are common

sites of spread. Up to 20 to 30% of patients may present with metastatic disease, in which case, surgical debulking can improve survival, as shown in randomized controlled trials.[12,13] Patients with all but the smallest renal masses should undergo testing for the presence of metastatic disease including chest CT, bone scan, and liver function tests.

Patients with localized disease may be cured with either partial or radical nephrectomy (Fig. 40-4). The oncologic efficacy of partial nephrectomy (nephron sparing) appears to be similar to that of radical nephrectomy. However, those patients with larger tumors or with a more central tumor location may be at increased risk for surgical complications. Nephron-sparing surgery should be considered in all patients, if feasible, as those patients undergoing a radical nephrectomy are at risk for future chronic kidney disease.[14] The lack of harm from nephrectomy due to malignancy has been extrapolated from the fact that kidney donors do not routinely develop renal insufficiency. However, kidney donors are a highly selected group, and patients with renal tumors are typically older and have more comorbidities. Additionally, the risk of contralateral RCC is 2 to 3% in most series,[15] and a partial nephrectomy may prevent the future need for dialysis in case of a contralateral kidney tumor.

TABLE 40-1	Bosniak renal cyst computed tomography classification	
Category	**Description**	**Risk of Malignancy/ Management**
I	Thin-walled cyst with water density with no septations or calcifications.	0%/nonsurgical
II	Thin-walled cyst with few hairline septa that may contain fine or very limited thick calcifications. Also includes homogeneously hyperdense cysts <3 cm.	0%/nonsurgical
II F (follow)	Multiple hairline or slightly thickened septa without measurable enhancement. May contain nodular calcification. Also includes hyperdense cysts >3 cm.	~5%/should be followed for progression
III	Irregular or smooth thickened walls or septa with measurable enhancement.	~50%/surgical
IV	Same as III, but with enhancing solid components.	~100%/surgical

Source: Adapted with permission from Israel GM, Bosniak MA: An update of the Bosniak renal cyst classification system. *Urology* 66:484, 2005. Copyright Elsevier.

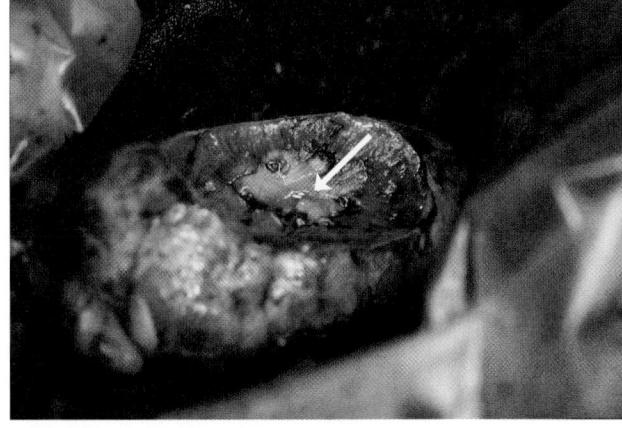

FIG. 40-4. Partial nephrectomy. A kidney after partial resection for a small renal mass. Note the visible collecting system in the base of the defect (*arrow*).

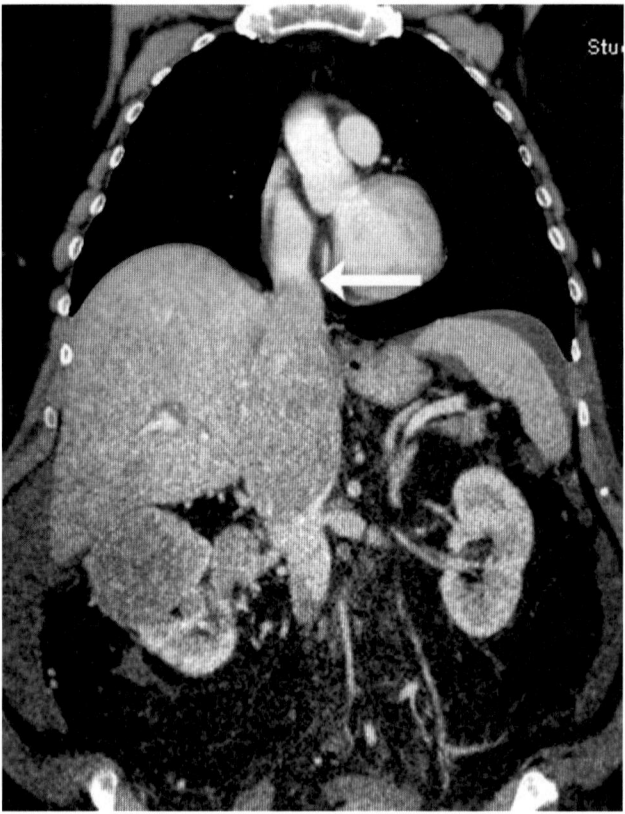

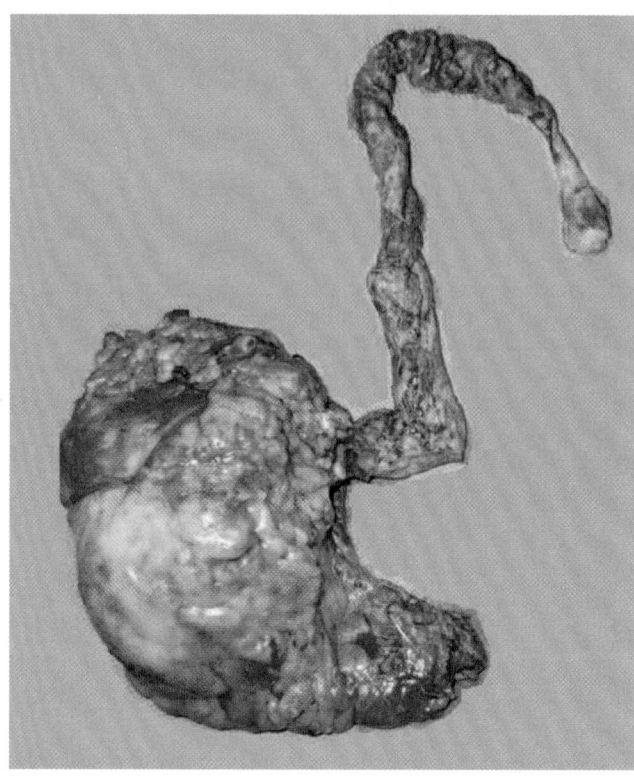

A

B

FIG. 40-5. Inferior vena cava thrombus. **A.** A multidetector computed tomographic image displaying a tumor thrombus extending above the diaphragm (*arrow*) arising from a right renal mass. **B.** An en bloc removal of a different right renal mass with a tumor thrombus that extended to the pulmonary artery. This patient is alive 6 years after surgery.

Minimally invasive techniques for renal surgery have greatly changed the field of kidney cancer. Laparoscopic radical nephrectomy allows more rapid convalescence and decreased narcotic requirements. Laparoscopic partial nephrectomy is challenging and is performed only in experienced hands due to its associated high rate of complications. Ablative techniques such as cryoablation and radiofrequency ablation have been gaining in popularity, but long-term results from these techniques are currently lacking due to their recent development. Observation also may be a viable option for small renal masses, especially in patients with multiple comorbidities or advanced age. Most small renal masses are low grade with a slow growth rate, and patients very rarely progress to metastatic disease after limited follow-up of 2 to 3 years.[16]

Up to 10% of RCC invades the lumen of the renal vein or vena cava. The degree of venous extension directly impacts the surgical approach. Patients with thrombus below the level of the liver can be managed with cross-clamping above and below the thrombus and extraction from a cavotomy at the insertion of the renal vein (Fig. 40-5A). Usually, the thrombus is not adherent to the vessel wall. However, cross-clamping the vena cava above the hepatic veins can drastically reduce cardiac preload, and therefore, bypass techniques often are necessary. For thrombus above the hepatic veins, a multidisciplinary approach with either venovenous or cardiopulmonary bypass is necessary. In cases of invasion of the wall of the vena cava or atrium, deep hypothermic circulatory arrest may be used to give a completely bloodless field. Tumor thrombus embolization to the pulmonary artery is a rare but known complication during these cases and is associated with a high mortality (Fig. 40-5B). For cases of extensive tumor thrombus, intraoperative transesophageal echocardiography should be considered for monitoring and assessment of possible thrombus embolization. If a thrombus embolization

occurs, a sternotomy/cardiopulmonary bypass with extraction of the thrombus may be life saving.

Patients undergoing resection of localized renal masses are at substantial risk of future recurrence. Many predictive features have been recognized, but the most widely accepted prognostic findings are tumor stage, grade, and size, each of which exerts an independent effect on recurrence. Surveillance strategies after nephrectomy typically involve abdominal and chest imaging at 6- to 12-month intervals for 5 to 10 years, depending on the level of risk as determined by the original lesion.[17] Isolated solitary recurrences, either local or distant, can be resected with long-term disease-free rates approaching 50%.[18]

Surgical Approach and Complications

Nephrectomy, either partial or radical, can be performed through a number of surgical approaches. Flank incisions over the eleventh or twelfth ribs from the anterior axillary line to the lateral border of the rectus muscle provide access to the kidney without entering the peritoneum. However, entry into the pleura is not uncommon. If small, the pleurotomy usually can be closed without need for a chest tube. The anterior subcostal approach also is used for nephrectomy. There is no risk for pleural entry, but this incision is transperitoneal so ileus is somewhat more likely. Laparoscopic nephrectomy is now commonplace, while laparoscopic partial nephrectomy is used less frequently. For large tumors, particularly on the right side where the liver makes exposure of the tumor more difficult, a thoracoabdominal approach is very helpful. In these cases, the flank incision is made over the tenth rib and carried further posterior and anterior than a typical flank incision. The chest and abdominal cavities are intentionally entered for maximum exposure, and the diaphragm is partially divided in a circumferential fashion, which allows cephalad retraction of the liver. A chest tube is used postoperatively. The adrenal gland is no longer routinely removed unless the tumor is adherent to it. The benefit of lymph node dissection when the nodes are not clinically involved is uncertain.

Complications of radical nephrectomy include bleeding, pneumothorax, splenic injury, liver injury, and pancreatic tail injury. Partial nephrectomy has the added risks of delayed bleeding and urine leak. Ileus is not commonplace when the peritoneal cavity is not entered.

Prostate Cancer

Prostate cancer is the most common nonskin malignancy in men, with an incidence of approximately 250,000 to 300,000 per year. Yearly screening consisting of digital rectal exam and serum prostate-specific antigen (PSA) testing starting at age 50 years old is recommended by several organizations, such as the American Cancer Society and the American Urological Association. Patients of African American descent or those with a family history of prostate cancer should be considered for screening starting at 45 years of age. Men with abnormal digital rectal exams or PSA elevation have an indication for prostate biopsy to determine the presence of the disease. With the advent of PSA screening, prostate cancer has experienced a stage migration, with most cases now discovered locally confined within the prostate. The majority of patients with prostate cancer will not die of the disease by 10 to 15 years, whether it is treated at diagnosis or not. However, those undergoing initial treatment have improved cancer-specific survival.[19]

Prostate cancer is graded according to the Gleason scoring system.[20] A primary and secondary score are assigned based on the most common and second most common histologic pattern. Grades run from 1 for the most differentiated to 5 for the least. The grades are added to give the Gleason score. In current practice, scores below 6 are almost never assigned. Gleason score, preoperative PSA level, and digital rectal exam are used to estimate the likelihood of whether the cancer is localized, locally advanced, or metastatic. Prostate cancer with high Gleason scores (8 to 10) or a high PSA level (>20) is much more likely to have spread, often at a micrometastatic level. After definitive treatment, an increasing PSA is indicative of recurrent cancer.

The most common site of spread of prostate cancer is the pelvic lymph nodes and bone. For patients with intermediate or high-risk disease based on clinical stage, grade on biopsy, and PSA level, staging includes bone scan and CT imaging to evaluate the pelvic lymph nodes. Multiple treatment options are available for men with localized disease, including radical prostatectomy (retropubic, perineal, or robotic/laparoscopic approaches), brachytherapy, and external beam radiation therapy. For low-risk disease, the efficacy of each treatment modality is thought to be similar. For low-risk disease, radical prostatectomy can be performed with unilateral or bilateral cavernosal nerve-sparing to limit postoperative erectile dysfunction (ED). For high-risk disease, either non–nerve-sparing surgery or external beam radiation therapy plus androgen deprivation may be performed. The associated morbidity of each treatment differs, and it is important to discuss the side effects with patients. Irritative voiding and bowel symptoms are common after radiation therapy, with ED being a late side effect. Radical prostatectomy is associated with early incontinence and ED (depending on nerve-sparing). Incontinence improves significantly with time, with <1% of men in experienced hands suffering severe long-term problems with urinary control. Likewise, ED improves with time. The large majority of younger men (<55 years of age) regain erectile function, often with the aid of oral medications, if both cavernosal nerves were spared.[21] Older men or those with 0 or 1 nerve spared have lower rates of erectile function.

Expectant management may be a useful strategy in men with anticipated survival of <10 years, low Gleason score (≤6), early-stage disease (cT1c), and small volume disease as determined by biopsy. Patients should be watched closely with digital rectal exam, PSA testing, and repeat biopsy at 1 year to assess the possible progression of disease. Patients, however, should be counseled that randomized controlled trials of surgery vs. observation have been shown to improve survival and lessen the risk of developing of metastatic disease.[19] Once prostate cancer has spread, it is no longer curable. Medications that lower serum testosterone or that block the androgen receptor are able to control the disease, often for years, but the cancer inevitably becomes resistant to this treatment. Nevertheless, patients with noncurable prostate cancer can live many years, and a large number die of causes other than prostate cancer.

Surgical Approach and Complications

The approach for a retropubic prostatectomy uses a lower midline incision from the pubic symphysis to approximately 5 cm below the umbilicus. The peritoneum is not entered. Lymph nodes are removed between the external iliac and obturator vessels bilaterally, although it may be omitted in cases where the probability of involvement is very low. Some regularly perform a wider dissection that may improve staging, although any therapeutic benefit is uncertain. The cavernosal nerves lay immediately posterolateral to the prostatic capsule. They may be spared if the cancer is not likely to penetrate the capsule on that side, which is a function of preoperative parameters such as biopsy results, PSA, and clinical examination. Perineal prostatectomy involves a transverse incision between the scrotum and anus. Benefits include reduced blood loss and faster convalescence, but this approach does not allow lymph node dissection and nerve-sparing is more difficult. Robotic prostatectomy has superseded laparoscopic prostatectomy due to the lower learning curve and increased agility. Benefits are lower blood loss and faster convalescence. Some claim faster return of continence and lower ED rates, but these findings have not yet been widely demonstrated.

Complications of prostatectomy depend on approach. Retropubic approaches may result in urine leaks, lymphocele, and very rarely, rectal or ureteral injury. The perineal approach has a somewhat higher rate of rectal injury. Robotic prostatectomy uses a transperitoneal approach that can occasionally result in ileus, particularly in cases of a urine leak from the vesicourethral anastomosis. All approaches carry a small risk of urinary incontinence and a more substantial risk of ED.

TRAUMA

Kidney

Renal injuries are more common during blunt trauma, accounting for 90% of injuries to the kidney. Any patient with a major deceleration injury, shock, or gross hematuria should undergo radiographic imaging of the kidneys. All patients with penetrating injuries to the flank or abdomen must undergo imaging unless unstable and requiring immediate exploration.

Renal injuries are classified by extent of damage (Table 40-2). Blunt traumatic injuries usually can be managed conservatively, while penetrating renal injuries usually require exploration. Urinary extravasation alone does not require exploration, but reimaging is necessary and, if persistent leakage is present, a stent or nephrostomy tube is indicated. All grade V vascular injuries should be considered for immediate exploration, as a delay of several hours greatly decreases the risk of renal salvage. High-grade renal injuries are associated with significant bleeding, but patients who are stable and without a pulsatile or expanding hematoma can be observed. Even in expert hands, the risk of renal loss at surgery is significant and must be considered before opening the retroperitoneum, and most grade IV injuries can be managed nonoperatively (Fig. 40-6).[22] Patients typically are placed on restricted activity until hematuria resolves. Table 40-3 lists indications for assessing surgical intervention in renal trauma patients.

If immediate operative exploration for other injuries is required, renal injury staging can be performed while in the operating room.

TABLE 40-2 American Association for the Surgery of Trauma renal injury scale

Grade	Injury Type	Description
1	Contusion	Microscopic or gross hematuria with normal imaging
	Hematoma	Subcapsular, nonexpanding without parenchymal laceration
2	Hematoma	Nonexpanding perirenal hematoma confined to renal retroperitoneum
		<1 cm in depth without urinary extravasation
3	Laceration	>1 cm in depth without collecting system rupture or urinary extravasation
4	Laceration	Parenchymal laceration through cortex, medulla, and collecting system
4	Vascular	Main renal artery or vein injury with contained hemorrhage
5	Laceration	Completely shattered kidney
5	Laceration	Avulsion of renal hilum leading to devascularized kidney

Source: Adapted with permission from Moore EE et al: Organ injury scaling. *Surg Clin North Am* 75:293, 1995. Copyright Elsevier.

If concern exists over renal injury or the presence of a retroperitoneal hematoma, a single-shot, 10-minute delayed IV pyelogram (IVP) (2 mL/kg contrast) is useful at assessing the presence of two functional kidneys and extent of injury. If the IVP is abnormal or the hematoma is pulsatile, renal exploration should be performed.

Renal exploration should begin once the renal hilum is controlled. Although rarely necessary, temporary control of the renal hilum may decrease the need for nephrectomy when a significant injury is found on exploration. Complete exposure is necessary to evaluate the extent of injury. All nonviable tissue should be débrided and segmental and intralobar arteries ligated with 4-0 chromic or polydioxanone sutures. If the collecting system is injured, it should be repaired at this time. A stent and percutaneous drain should be considered to prevent urinoma formation. A partial vascular injury to the renal vein or artery can be repaired with 5-0 or 6-0 Prolene sutures. A complete injury may require débridement, and if an end-to-end anastomosis cannot be performed, a vascular graft may be required.

Ureter

The retroperitoneal location of the ureter protects it from external trauma, and blunt injury is rare but can occur with rapid deceleration injuries. Penetrating trauma may occur but a high index of clinical suspicion is required to make the appropriate diagnosis. Any penetrating trauma involving the retroperitoneum should undergo evaluation with intraoperative inspection, IVP, or CT urogram. A retrograde pyelogram is the most sensitive test for ureteral injury, and a stent can be placed if a partial transection is observed. The ureter also is frequently injured intraoperatively, most commonly from open and laparoscopic surgical procedures including hysterectomy, low-anterior colonic resections, or aortic surgery. Endoscopic procedures such as ureteroscopy also can lead to ureteral injury such as perforation and avulsion.

Surgical repair depends on location and extent of injury. A suture in place briefly may be removed usually without consequence. Partial injuries can be primarily repaired, although all devitalized tissue must be débrided to avoid delayed tissue breakdown and urinoma formation. Ureteral stents should be placed in this situation to facilitate healing without stricture. Lower ureteral injuries (below the iliac vessels) are best treated with ureteral reimplant, as the blood supply can be tenuous, and strictures are more common with a distal uretero-ureterostomy. Midureteral level injuries can be treated with a uretero-ureterostomy if a spatulated, tension-free repair can be achieved. For longer defects, the bladder can be mobilized and

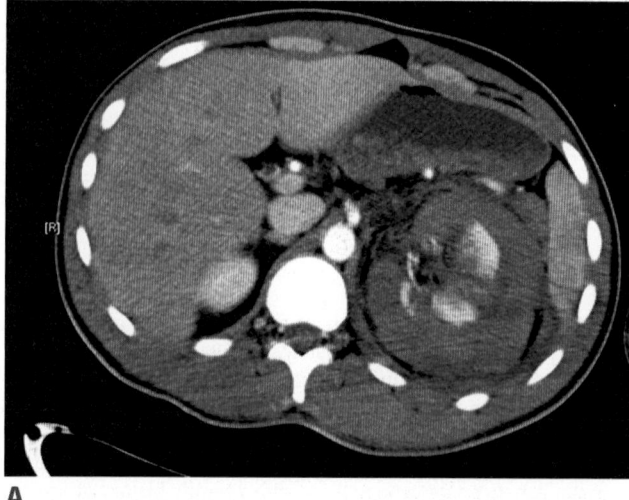

A

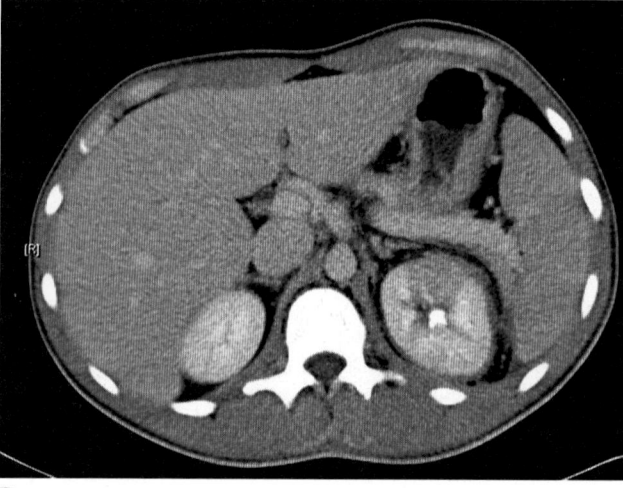

B

FIG. 40-6. Blunt renal trauma after a bicycle accident. **A.** A computed tomography image of a left kidney with several deep lacerations into the collecting system and a large perirenal hematoma. Delayed images showed urinary extravasation. This patient was managed nonoperatively. **B.** Computed tomographic image at 45 days showing significant improvement in the appearance of the kidney.

TABLE 40-3 Indications for surgical intervention for renal trauma

Absolute indications
1. Persistent, life-threatening hemorrhage from probable renal injury
2. Renal pedicle avulsion (grade V injury)
3. Expanding, pulsatile, or uncontained retroperitoneal hematoma

Relative indications
1. Large laceration of the renal pelvis or avulsion of the ureteropelvic junction
2. Coexisting bowel or pancreatic injuries
3. Persistent urinary leakage, postinjury urinoma, or perinephric abscess with failed percutaneous or endoscopic management
4. Abnormal intraoperative one-shot IV urogram
5. Devitalized parenchymal segment with associated urine leak
6. Complete renal artery thrombosis of both kidneys or of a solitary kidney when renal perfusion appears preserved
7. Renal vascular injuries after failed angiographic management
8. Renovascular hypertension

Source: Adapted with permission from Santucci RA, Wessells H, Bartsch G, et al: Evaluation and management of renal injuries: Consensus statement of the renal trauma subcommittee. *BJU Int* 93:937, 2004.

brought up to the psoas muscle (psoas hitch). For additional length, a tubularized flap of bladder (Boari flap) can be created and anastomosed to the remaining ureter. Renal mobilization with nephropexy by anchoring to the psoas muscle can provide additional length. Autotransplantation, transuretero-ureterostomy, and ileal ureter are rarely needed during an acute setting.

Bladder

Bladder injury can occur from penetrating and blunt trauma. The diagnosis should be entertained for any lower abdominal or pelvic trauma. Intraperitoneal ruptures are less common than retroperitoneal ruptures but may be seen in the setting of a full bladder before injury. Bladder injuries often are associated with pelvic fractures and may frequently occur in conjunction with urethral injuries. Nearly all patients present with gross hematuria, although occasionally microscopic hematuria is present. A delayed presentation can be associated with intoxication, but it also may occur as a result of iatrogenic injury. These patients often have electrolyte abnormalities such as metabolic derangements, azotemia, and leukocytosis from urine absorption. Patients clinically present with fevers or a prolonged ileus.

Radiographic evaluation begins with either a fluoroscopic or CT cystogram. It is vital to avoid underfilling, as it may lead to a false negative study. A preset amount can be instilled based on age calculations, which is typically approximately 300 to 400 mL in adults. The bladder can be filled under gravity by raising the Foley catheter to 15 cm above the pubic ramus. The contrast material should be allowed to fill to the natural capacity of the bladder. It is important to have a postdrainage film to assess for persistent contrast which may indicate a rupture.

Extraperitoneal bladder injuries can typically be managed with catheter drainage for 7 to 10 days. If intraoperative exploration is to occur for other injuries, repair can be performed at that time. For patients with pelvic injuries that require an open operation with placement of metal hardware, repair of the bladder rupture should be performed if possible. Intraperitoneal bladder injuries should be explored immediately and repaired. However, for cases of a missed intraperitoneal injury, patients often do well with catheter drainage only. For large ruptures after repair, a suprapubic tube is recommended, but a large urethral catheter is sufficient for smaller injuries. All injuries, especially those managed nonoperatively, should be followed up by a cystogram to document healing before catheter removal.

Urethra

Urethral injuries can be divided by anterior (penile and bulbar urethra) and posterior (membranous and prostatic) location. Any patient with blunt pelvic trauma, blood present at the urethral meatus, hematuria, inability to void, or perineal hematoma should be considered to have a urethral injury until proven otherwise. Urethral injuries should be anticipated with pubic ramus fractures and occur in 10% of unilateral and 20% of bilateral injuries.[23]

Staging is performed by retrograde urethrography. This study can be easily performed in the trauma suite with the patient in an oblique position and a 12F catheter placed in the urethral meatus. With the penis placed on traction, 30 mL of contrast is instilled while an X-ray is obtained during filling. The addition of fluoroscopy is a valuable addition to the procedure but can be omitted if not available. A partial or complete disruption can be diagnosed based on extravasation or filling of the proximal urethra. Patients with partial urethral injuries can have an attempt at catheter placement. Those with complete disruptions should have a placement of suprapubic tube.

Anterior injuries often are related to blunt straddle injuries and penetrating trauma. Blunt anterior urethral injury can be managed in multiple ways and only small series are available in the literature to compare methods. Immediate surgical repair is not recommended in the acute setting with the exception of low velocity

penetrating injuries. If the patient is stable with minimal hematoma formation, repair should be considered. In this setting of a 1- to 2-cm defect, the urethra can be débrided, spatulated, and anastomosed in an end-to-end, watertight fashion. Large defects should have treatment deferred, as grafts or flaps may be required for repair and the success may diminish with infections. For most cases, catheter drainage is recommended. Many advocate avoiding a placement of a urethral catheter, as it may convert a partial tear to a complete dissection. However, a single gentle passage performed by a urologist is safe. For a complete disruption, the placement of a suprapubic tube is recommended; however, a stricture at the site of injury may ensue.

Posterior urethral injuries usually result from pelvic crush injuries and shearing forces causing a prostatomembranous disruption. The patient's other injuries dictate urologic management. Initial open surgical exploration or the urethral injury should be avoided due to altered anatomy, risk of bleeding, and high likelihood of incontinence and ED from injury of adjacent nerves. Patients can be managed with suprapubic tube and delayed repair or with delayed primary realignment. Primary endoscopic realignment, when possible, leads to decreased rates of strictures without increasing adverse outcomes.[24,25]

Urethral strictures can be caused by trauma or inflammatory conditions. They should be staged with either a retrograde urethrography or voiding cystourethrogram (VCUG). Patients with short defects may be amenable to dilatation or cystoscopic urethrotomy. Depending on location, length, and severity, open repairs may be required. Long defects may require grafting to avoid significant penile shortening. Young patients should be considered for open surgical management to definitely repair the stricture due to the tendency of strictures to recur when treated with simple dilation.

Testes

Testicular injury most commonly occurs with blunt injuries when the testicle is forcibly compressed against the thigh or pubic bone with enough force to rupture the tunica albuginea. For patients with scrotal trauma, ultrasound is the preferred modality for staging the extent of injury. Ultrasound can evaluate the testicular blood flow, the presence of testicular contusions, intratesticular hematomas, hematoceles, or a disrupted tunica albuginea. The presence of a hematocele should increase suspicion for testicular rupture because ultrasound may not detect the tunical defect in this setting.[26]

The goal of surgery is to salvage as much parenchyma as possible and to avoid delayed complications such as ischemic atrophy or abscess formation. A large hematocele, if not evacuated, could lead to ischemic atrophy, and drainage should be considered. A ruptured tunica albuginea can be repaired primarily and nonviable parenchyma may need to be débrided. For penetrating trauma, immediate exploration is recommended for accurate staging and repair. Frequently, these injuries result in major devascularization and nonviable tissue (especially gunshot wounds). Although salvage may be possible, an orchiectomy usually is required.

Penis

Penile fractures are rare injuries that involve a traumatic rupture of the tunica albuginea, usually occurring during sexual intercourse. The engorged penile corporal bodies can rupture if sufficient force is generated against the partner's pubic symphysis or perineum (Fig. 40-7). Men may notice an immediate audible "pop" and experience rapid penile detumescence. Immediate swelling develops. If Buck's fascia is disrupted, swelling and ecchymosis can be noted throughout the perineum ("butterfly sign"). At presentation, a classic "eggplant" appearance of the penis is often, although not always, seen. Exploration by a circumcising incision and repair of the defect offers the best chance at avoiding permanent ED and penile deformity while also minimizing the risk of infection.[27] A retrograde urethrogram should be performed to rule out urethral injury at the time of surgery. Alternatively, the urethra can be

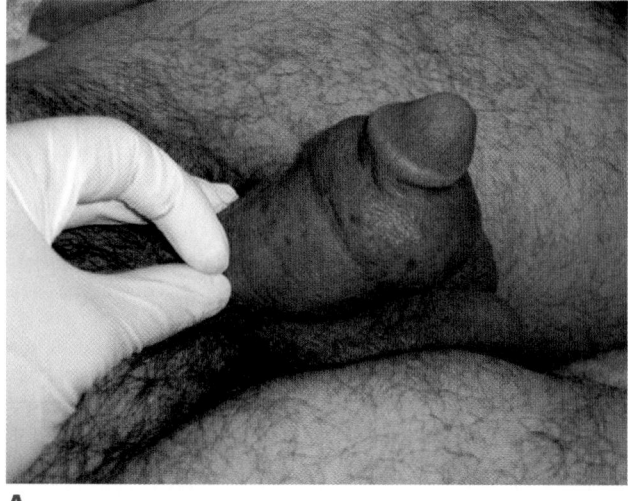

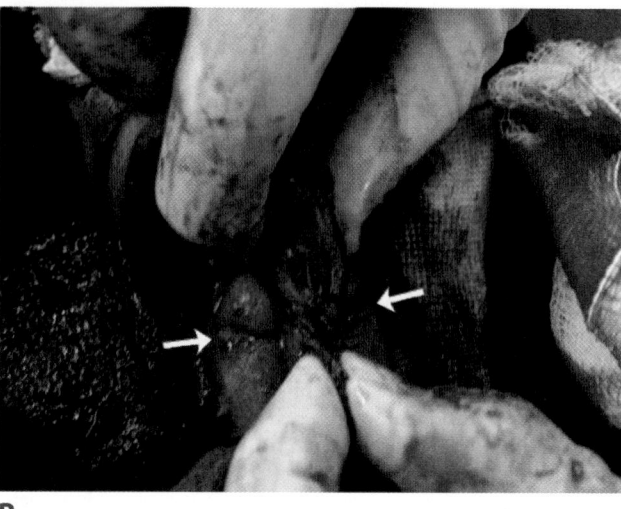

A

B

FIG. 40-7. Penile fracture. **A.** A patient with a penile fracture that was suspected based on history and examination. Note the lack of skin discoloration that is often present. **B.** Intraoperative finding of bilateral corporal body ruptures (*arrows*) along the ventral penile surface. The urethra, which is between the surgeon's fingers, surprisingly escaped injury.

manually occluded intraoperatively at the penoscrotal junction and a dilute methylene blue solution injected under pressure into the urethral meatus with a catheter-tip syringe. Leakage should be visualized if there is a urethral disruption. If present, the urethra should be repaired, taking care not to significantly narrow the lumen. A Foley catheter is left in place for several days after surgery. Any penetrating injury to the penis must undergo exploration to repair any injuries to the corporal bodies or the urethra.

EMERGENCIES

Acute Urinary Retention

Acute urinary retention (AUR) can happen in men or women and results from a variety of causes, although it most commonly occurs in men with benign prostatic hyperplasia (BPH). Other chronic causes of poor bladder emptying, such as diabetic neuropathy, urethral stricture, multiple sclerosis, or Parkinson's disease, can result in episodes of complete urinary retention, often when the bladder becomes overdistended. This frequently occurs in the hospital setting when patients have limited mobility and are receiving medications that decrease bladder contractility, including opiates or anticholinergics. Constipation, a common side effect of those medications, can itself worsen urinary retention. Significant hematuria can result in the formation of blood clots, which may block the urethra and cause retention.

Although some patients receiving large doses of narcotics or those with chronically decompensated bladders may not experience discomfort, most patients with AUR have significant pain. If the urinary retention has lasted several days (often accompanied by overflow incontinence), patients may be in renal failure. Treatment should be the placement of a urethral catheter as quickly as possible. However, BPH or urethral strictures often make the placement of a catheter difficult. For men with BPH, a coude (French for *curved*) catheter is helpful in negotiating past the angulation in the prostatic urethra (Fig. 40-8A). The curved portion (which is angled in line with the balloon port) is maintained at the 12 o'clock position as it is passed through the urethra (Fig. 40-8B). A common mistake is to use a smaller catheter to bypass the enlarged prostate. However, a larger (18F to 20F) catheter is less flexible and is more likely to push into the bladder rather than curl in the prostatic urethra. Smaller catheters are useful for bypassing a urethral stricture. A urethral stricture should be suspected when the catheter meets resistance

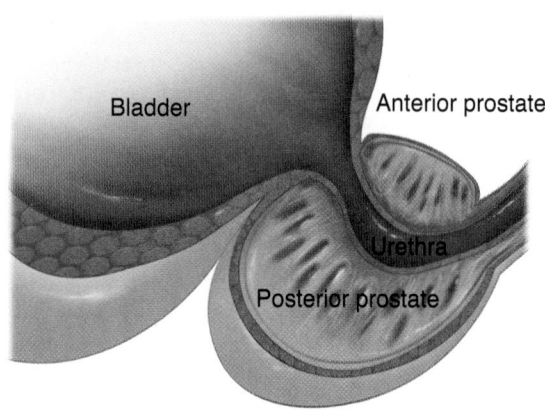

A

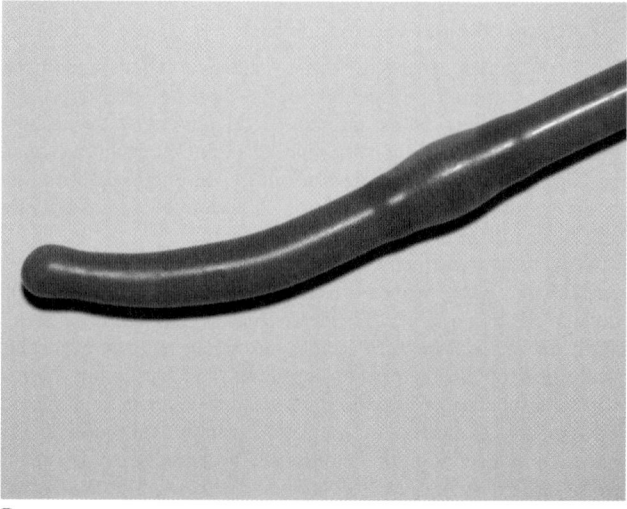

B

FIG. 40-8. Coude catheter. **A.** A schematic drawing of a lateral view of the prostatic urethra showing the upward angulation at the bladder neck, which a coude catheter is helpful in negotiating. **B.** The tip of a coude catheter. Note the curved tip, which should always point to 12 o'clock when inserted.

closer to the meatus, as many strictures occur in the distal urethra, which is narrower than the proximal portion. Using a 12F or 14F catheter often will allow the passage of the catheter into the bladder. If catheter placement is not successful, a suprapubic tube should be placed approximately two finger breadths above the pubic symphysis. Aspiration with a finder needle should be used first to localize the bladder and avoid intra-abdominal contents, although bowel injury is unlikely with a distended bladder filling the pelvis. If hematuria is the cause of retention, continuous bladder irrigation often is necessary to prevent clot formation. This is done through a large three-way catheter that has an additional port for fluid inflow. Fluid is infused by gravity only because the use of higher pressure could result in bladder rupture if outflow is occluded.

A urinalysis should be checked because a poorly emptying bladder is prone to infection. Renal function also should be assessed for those in AUR by checking the creatinine level. An elevated creatinine level suggests that AUR has resulted in renal dysfunction, and these patients are at risk for postobstructive diuresis. These patients must be closely watched for excessive urine output, often caused by an osmotic diuresis due to retained nitrogenous waste products or a temporary renal concentrating defect. Fluid and electrolytes must be replaced if the urine output exceeds 200 mL/h, especially if hemodynamic instability or electrolyte imbalances are seen. Fluid replacement typically is 0.5 mL of 0.45 normal saline for every 1 mL of urine output above 200 mL in 1 hour, although sodium and potassium supplementation requirements depend on the electrolyte status of the patient.

Once the bladder is adequately drained, the cause of AUR should be addressed. For men with suspected BPH, an alpha blocker such as tamsulosin should be started. Finasteride or dutasteride, which shrink the prostate, work over several months and will not provide significant benefit in the short term. Narcotics should be tapered as tolerated, and constipation should be treated. Acute spinal cord compression, which is accompanied by saddle paresthesias, is a neurologic emergency that requires neurosurgical or orthopedic consultation. In most cases, except severe neurologic injuries, patients will be able to resume voiding, and the catheter can be removed after 1 to 2 days. Postvoid residuals should be checked with a portable ultrasound device or by "straight" catheterization to determine the residual amount of urine left after the patient tries to empty their bladder. The inability to void or a postvoid residual over 150 to 200 mL is concerning for the development of another episode of AUR. Patients may be given the option of an indwelling catheter for another few days with a subsequent voiding trial, or learning the self intermittent catheterization technique, whereby, after predetermined intervals (4 to 6 hours) or after voiding attempts, the patient passes a catheter into their bladder and empties. This is the preferred method, as it reduces the likelihood of infections from indwelling catheters and may improve bladder functionality. However, most patients are resistant to this approach.

Testicular Torsion

The differential diagnosis of acute scrotal pain includes testicular torsion. This usually occurs in neonates or adolescent males but may be observed in other age groups. The blood supply to the testicle is compromised due to twisting of the spermatic cord within the tunica vaginalis resulting in ischemia to the epididymis and the testis. In newborns, an extravaginal torsion also can occur with twisting of the tunica vaginalis and spermatic cord together. Risk factors for torsion include undescended testis, testicular tumor, and a "bell-clapper" deformity with poor gubernacular fixation of the testicles to the scrotal wall.

Clinical history is vital for diagnosis. Patients describe a sudden onset of pain at a distinct point in time, with subsequent swelling. Physical examination may demonstrate a swollen, asymmetric scrotum with a tender, high-riding testicle. Children normally have a brisk cremasteric reflex that usually is lost in the setting of torsion. The diagnosis is made by clinical history and examination, but can be supported by a Doppler ultrasound which typically shows decreased intratesticular blood flow relative to the contralateral testis. If an ultrasound is not promptly available, timely surgical exploration should ensue if there is reasonable suspicion of torsion. However, besides ruling out other pathologies, an ultrasound can rule out an associated testicular neoplasm that would necessitate tumor serum marker evaluation and an inguinal, rather than a scrotal, incision.

Immediate surgical exploration can salvage an ischemic testes. More than 80% of testes can be salvaged if surgery is performed within 6 hours, which decreases to 20% or less as time progresses beyond 12 hours.[28] At the time of surgery, the contralateral testes also must be explored and fixed to the dartos fascia due to the possibility that the same anatomic defect allowing torsion exists on the contralateral side. Midline or bilateral transverse scrotal incisions are made. Once the testis is detorsed, it should be assessed for viability after being given time for normal blood flow to resume. The testes are fixed to the dartos fascia with a small, nonabsorbable suture on their medial and lateral aspects, taking care to ensure that the spermatic cord is not twisted before doing so. An orchiectomy should be performed to avoid later risk of abscess formation only if the testis is clearly necrotic because overall testicular function may be improved with testicular preservation in cases of moderately delayed (15 hours) presentation.[29]

Fournier's Gangrene

Fournier's gangrene is a necrotizing fasciitis of the male genitalia and perineum that can be rapidly progressing and fatal if not treated promptly (Fig. 40-9A). Mortality has been reported as high as 30 to 40%.[30] Risk factors for Fournier's include urethral strictures, perirectal abscesses, poor perineal hygiene, diabetes, cancer, HIV, and other immunocompromised states.[31] The infection spreads along the dartos, Scarpa's, and Colles' fascias. Clinical signs include fevers, perineal and scrotal pain, and associated indurated tissue. Cellulitis, eschars, necrosis, flaking skin, and crepitus may all be observed. The diagnosis is made on largely clinical suspicion, and significantly less on laboratory or radiographic findings. Classically, the patient describes pain out of proportion to the physical findings.

Prompt débridement of nonviable tissue and broad-spectrum antibiotics is necessary to prevent further spread (Fig. 40-9B). If there is damage to the external sphincter, patients may require a colostomy.[31] As the testes have a separate blood supply, they are usually not threatened and do not need to be removed. They may be tucked subcutaneously into the thigh ("thigh pouch") to ease postoperative management. Patients may frequently require return trips to the operating room for further débridement. Tight glucose control and adequate nutrition are necessary to facilitate wound healing. The large tissue defect should be initially treated with frequent dressing changes. Reconstructive strategies involving skin grafting are needed when large tissue defects result from extensive tissue damage.

Priapism

Priapism is a persistent erection for greater than 4 hours unrelated to sexual stimulation. Priapism is divided into two types, based on the underlying pathophysiology. The most common type—low flow/ischemic priapism—is a medical emergency. On examination, the penis is very tender and both cavernosal bodies will be rigid while the glans will be flaccid. Decreased venous outflow with persistent inflow results in increased intracorporal pressure and tumescence, which is the normal process of erection. Diminished arterial inflow due to elevated intrapenile pressure usually is brief under normal circumstances. Priapism is essentially a compartment syndrome.[32] With prolonged erection (priapism), the sustained decrease in arterial inflow ultimately causes tissue hypoxia, acidosis, and edema and results in long-term fibrosis and impotence, and sometimes frank necrosis. Risk factors include sickle cell disease or trait, malignancy, medications, cocaine abuse, certain antidepressants, and total parenteral nutrition.[33-35] If a cause is not identified,

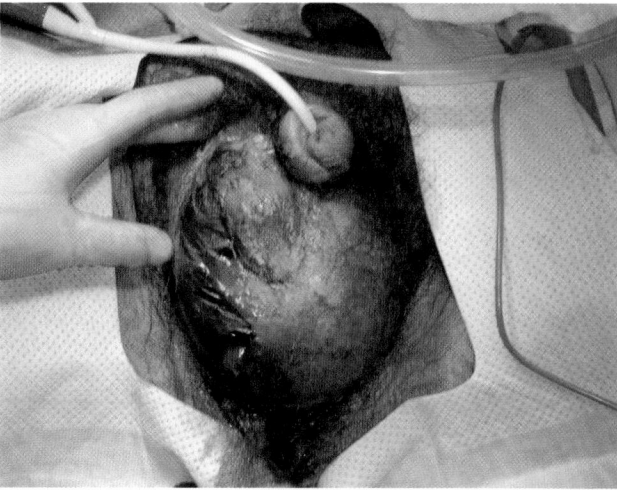

A

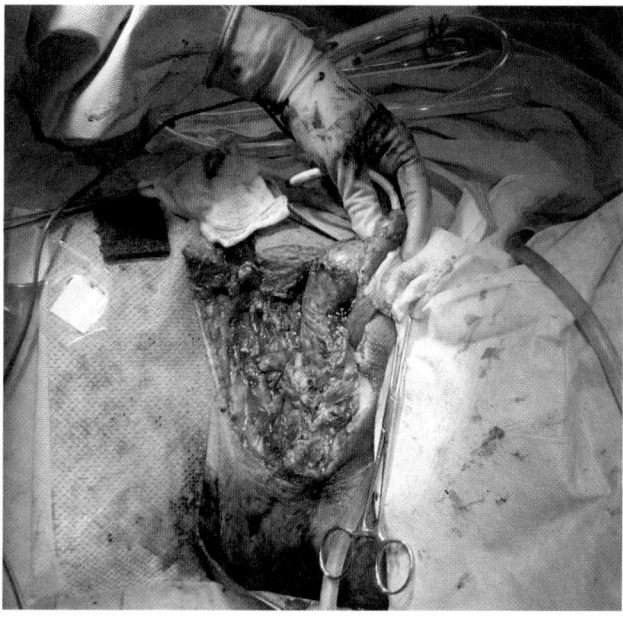

B

FIG. 40-9. Fournier's gangrene. **A.** Necrotic scrotal skin from Fournier's gangrene. **B.** Débridement of gangrenous tissue. Note the extensive débridement, which is commonly required. The right testicle required removal in this case (the left is wrapped in gauze), but typically the testes are not involved with the necrotic process.

a hematologic work-up is necessary to rule out malignancy or blood dyscrasias.

The management of priapism is rapid detumescence with the goal of preservation of future erectile function. The ability to achieve normal erections is directly related to length of the episode of priapism.[32] Low-flow priapism can be confirmed with a penile blood gas of the cavernosal bodies demonstrating hypoxic, acidotic blood. Initial management can include oral agents such as pseudoephedrine or baclofen, but more aggressive measures usually are necessary to achieve rapid detumescence. Insertion of a large gauge needle (18 gauge) into the lateral aspect of one corporal body allows thorough aspiration and irrigation of both corporal bodies because of widely communicating channels. Injection of phenylephrine (up to 200 mg in 20 mL normal saline) into the corporal bodies may be required. For those with sickle cell disease, hydration and oxygen administration should be performed first, as that is sometimes successful in this group.[36]

A surgical shunt is sometimes necessary to resolve the episode. Distal shunts should be performed first, as they can be done quickly in the emergency room with a True-Cut needle (Winter shunt). If this fails, an operative distal shunt can be performed (Al-Ghorab). Proximal shunts such as Grayhack's (coporal-saphenous vein) or Quackel's (proximal cavernosum-spongiosum) shunts may be required in refractory cases.

The other form, high flow/traumatic priapism, is rare and is related to penile or perineal trauma resulting in a cavernous artery–corporal body fistula. This form is not painful as it is not related to ischemia and can be managed conservatively. Many cases will resolve with time; those that do not can undergo selective arterial embolization.[37]

Paraphimosis

Foreskin emergencies occur in uncircumcised men. Paraphimosis is a common problem that represents a true medical emergency. When foreskin is retracted for prolonged periods, constriction of the glans penis may ensue. This is particularly likely in hospitalized patients who are confined to bed or who have altered mentation. Edema often forms in the genitals of supine patients due to the dependent position of that area. Patients with diminished consciousness will not be aware of the penile pain from paraphimosis, which may delay recognition of the problem until too late. Delay can be catastrophic as penile necrosis may occur due to ischemia.[38] Penile blocks, pain medication, and sedation are sometimes necessary before manual reduction. It is useful to apply firm pressure to the edematous distal penis for several minutes. Although painful, this reduction in penile edema can be the key to success. With the fingers pulling the constricting band distally, the thumbs can push the glans penis back into normal location. If the foreskin cannot be manually reduced, surgical intervention is required.

Emphysematous Pyelonephritis

Emphysematous pyelonephritis is a life-threatening infection that results from complicated pyelonephritis by gas-producing organisms. It is an acute necrotizing infection of the kidney that occurs predominantly in diabetic patients.[39] Patients frequently present with sepsis and ketoacidosis. *Escherichia coli* appears to be the most frequent organism responsible for this infection.[40]

Patients require supportive care, IV antibiotics, and relief of any urinary tract obstruction. Emphysematous pyelonephritis can be subdivided based on extent of infection. Those with gas confined to the parenchyma frequently can be managed conservatively with placement of a nephrostomy tube to allow drainage of purulent material. Patients with extensive involvement of the perirenal tissue may not respond to conservative management, and strong consideration should be given to expeditious nephrectomy, particularly if the patient is displaying signs of sepsis.[41]

INFECTIONS

Cystitis

Cystitis is an infection in the bladder with common symptoms of dysuria, and urinary frequency and urgency. Urinary culture (10^5 colony-forming units) is necessary to make a definitive diagnosis, although lower thresholds are meaningful if clinical suspicion is high. Urinalysis can assist with the diagnosis, as leukocyte esterase is a marker of inflammation, and nitrites are formed from bacterial reduction of nitrates. Risk factors include female gender, urinary instrumentation, urinary obstruction, diabetes, and neurologic bladder dysfunction.

An uncomplicated episode of cystitis requires a 3-day course of antibiotics. Those with complicated cystitis require 7 days of antibiotics and possible imaging studies. Asymptomatic bacteriuria does not necessarily need to be treated except if found in a pregnant women, before a planned urinary tract surgery, or with associated urinary tract obstruction. Patients undergoing nonurologic surgery also should be considered for treatment, especially those involving cardiac valves or orthopedic hardware.

Pyelonephritis

Pyelonephritis is a bacterial infection of the kidney that usually manifests itself by fevers and flank tenderness. It is frequently attributed to ascending bacteria along the path of the ureters and rarely due to hematogenous bacterial spread. Patients typically present with flank pain and fevers. However, very young or elderly patients may not demonstrate these symptoms but rather irritability, poor appetite, or altered mental status. Urinary tract imaging is not required unless urinary obstruction or stones are suspected or if the patient is not responding to antibiotics. Patients who are not septic and can tolerate fluids can be discharged home on a 2-week course of oral antibiotics. Otherwise, they should be hospitalized for IV antibiotics. Fevers from pyelonephritis may take 24 to 48 hours to subside in the setting of effective antibiotic therapy. Pyelonephritis can result in renal scarring that is accelerated in the setting of urinary obstruction. Emphysematous pyelonephritis can be a life-threatening condition with a mortality of up to 30% (see Emphysematous Pyelonephritis in the Emergencies section).

Occasionally, pyelonephritis can develop into an abscess that can be located within the renal parenchyma (renal abscess) or between the capsule and Gerota's fascia (perinephric abscess). Any patient that is not properly responding to antibiotic therapy after 72 hours should undergo imaging with CT scan to rule out an abscess or obstruction. Treatment consists of broad-spectrum IV antibiotics and percutaneous drainage.

Prostatitis

Acute prostatitis is a bacterial infection in the prostate gland, most commonly by urinary pathogens. Patients present with fevers, dysuria, and perineal or back discomfort. A digital rectal examination may indicate an indurated and tender gland. However, a brisk digital rectal examination should be avoided, as it is extremely uncomfortable for patients and is thought to cause bacteremia. Patients require a 4- to 6-week course of antibiotic therapy, typically a quinolone. Those that continue to have no improvement in 48 hours should be considered for imaging to rule out a prostatic abscess. If present, large abscesses can be managed with transurethral unroofing or percutaneous drainage.

Chronic prostatitis presents with continued lower urinary tract symptoms and pelvic pain. Chronic prostatitis may be bacterial or nonbacterial, which can be distinguished by culturing pre- and postprostatic massage urine. The bacterial form is a frequent cause of recurrent urinary tract infections in men and can be treated with a prolonged course of antibiotics. Chronic nonbacterial prostatitis does not respond to antibiotics or most other medications. Biofeedback, physical therapy, and other nonprostate-specific treatments may be effective in the treatment of this challenging clinical entity.[42]

Epididymo-Orchitis

Epididymo-orchitis is typically the result of bacterial infection originating in the urinary tract. However, most men will not show evidence of urinary tract infection. Symptoms are unilateral painful swelling of the epididymis and/or testis, often with fever. The scrotum may be erythematous on the side of involvement. The white blood cell (WBC) count often is elevated. The onset is fairly rapid, but not as sudden as torsion. An ultrasound may provide supporting evidence such as increased blood flow to the epididymis. A reactive hydrocele may be present. Intratesticular infection can result in ischemic orchitis, and reduced testicular blood flow can be seen on ultrasound. Although the clinical history of gradual onset may point to an infectious etiology, scrotal exploration is necessary when blood flow is reduced to rule out torsion unless other signs such as pyuria, elevated WBC count, or fevers are present.

Treatment is with oral antibiotics if the patient is not markedly febrile and is otherwise stable. Hospitalization and parenteral antibiotics are required if the patient has high fevers, significantly elevated WBC, or hemodynamic instability, as sepsis from epididymo-orchitis is possible. Intratesticular abscesses may form, and usually result in orchiectomy. The tunica albuginea of the testis is not compliant, so elevated pressures from intratesticular inflammation can result in ischemic necrosis of the parenchyma.

LOWER URINARY TRACT OBSTRUCTION

Benign Prostatic Hyperplasia

BPH is a clinical diagnosis describing urinary symptoms attributable to obstruction by the prostate, although some patients with BPH have minimally enlarged glands, and some with large prostates have no symptoms. The symptoms of BPH are urinary frequency, urgency, hesitancy, slow stream, and/or nocturia. These symptoms are not specific and may be caused by infection, urethral strictures, or neurologic dysfunction from diabetes, Parkinson's disease, multiple sclerosis, stroke, or spinal cord injury. Besides voiding symptoms, consequences of BPH include gross hematuria, infections due to incomplete emptying, bladder calculi, and AUR. Over time, incomplete emptying may lead to chronic bladder overdistension that can result in a defunctionalized bladder, sometimes permanently.

Medical treatment of BPH is usually the first step. Alpha blockers act on alpha receptors in the smooth muscle of the prostate and decrease its tone. 5α-Reductase inhibitors, which block the conversion of testosterone to the more potent dihydrotestosterone, shrink the prostate over several months. Both are used either singly or in combination as medical therapy for BPH. If medications are ineffective at alleviating urinary symptoms or other consequences of BPH, surgical intervention is indicated. Transurethral resection of the prostate is the mainstay of endoscopic surgical BPH treatment. It is extremely effective at improving flow and decreasing residual urine. Complications are rare but include incontinence and excessive fluid absorption of the hypotonic irrigating solution used during resection, resulting in the transurethral resection syndrome. It is due to hyponatremia and fluid overload, and although rare, can result in death. Mental status changes and pulmonary edema are managed by diuresis and sodium supplementation with hypertonic saline in severe cases. Because of these rare, but potentially dangerous side effects, laser vaporization of the prostate has grown popular. It is associated with very limited fluid absorption, and saline can be used because there is no electrocautery. There also is less bleeding. Urinary outcomes appear to be similar to transurethral resection of the prostate.[43] When the prostate is very enlarged (>100 g), endoscopic management is less effective and open surgical procedures can be used. Suprapubic (simple) prostatectomy involves enucleation of the majority of the prostate, but the capsule is left so there is minimal effect on continence and erectile function.

Urethral Stricture

The voiding symptoms of urethral stricture are very similar to BPH. Strictures may result from scarring due to infectious urethritis, prior instrumentation, trauma, or cancer. Urethral carcinoma is very rare, particularly in males, so most strictures are due to benign causes. Diagnosis is by retrograde urethrogram or cystoscopy. They may be treated with dilation or transurethral incision, but they have a tendency to recur after treatment. Open surgical excision is preferred for long or recalcitrant strictures, and long-term success rates are excellent.[44]

UPPER URINARY TRACT OBSTRUCTION

The hallmark of partial or complete upper urinary tract obstruction is hydroureteronephrosis (HN), with the ureteral dilation extending

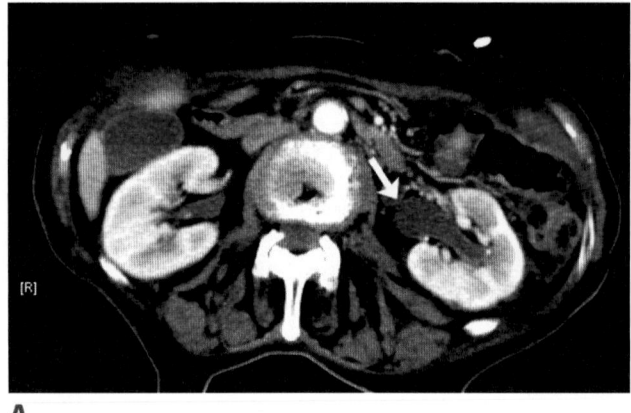 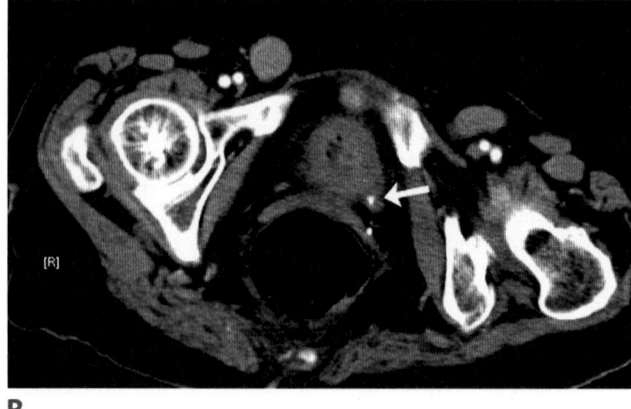

A   **B**

FIG. 40-10. Hydronephrosis and ureteral calculus. **A.** Left hydronephrosis from distal obstruction (*arrow*). **B.** A 4-mm calculus at the ureterovesical junction (*arrow*).

to the level of the obstruction (Fig. 40-10). HN may be seen on CT imaging or ultrasound, and it may range from very mild to severe, with associated parenchymal thinning in chronic cases. In the acute setting, the degree of HN does not necessarily correlate with the degree of obstruction, as it may take time for severe HN to develop. The obstruction may be intrinsic, as with calculi or ureteral tumors, or due to extrinsic compression due to varied causes, such as an intra-abdominal tumor, iliac aneurysm, or gravid uterus. Serum creatinine may be elevated, but the contralateral kidney will compensate so serum chemistries may not indicate renal impairment. Normal renal function makes intervention less urgent, but even partial obstruction may result in permanent loss of function on the affected side if not alleviated within several weeks.[45] Complete occlusion can cause permanent dysfunction within 2 weeks.[46]

Treatment of ureteral obstruction is by endoscopic placement of a ureteral stent, which is a temporary plastic tube with curls on each end to prevent migration. Stents allow flow both through the lumen and around it. When chronic stenting is required, it must be changed every 3 months to prevent severe encrustation with urinary sediments. Stents commonly become colonized with bacteria, but symptomatic infections are less common.[47] Once a stent is in place, mild residual HN often will persist due to ureteral aperistalsis and urinary reflux, but unless severe, does not represent residual obstruction.

When stent placement is unsuccessful or fails to provide adequate drainage due to severe extrinsic compression, a percutaneous nephrostomy (PCN) should be placed. This is the preferred approach when a patient is unstable because it requires less anesthesia and provides more rapid and reliable decompression of the renal collecting system.

Urolithiasis

Urolithiasis, or urinary calculus disease, may affect up to 10% of the population over the course of a lifetime.[48] Calculi are crystalline aggregates of one or more components, most commonly calcium oxalate. They also may contain calcium phosphate, magnesium ammonium phosphate (struvite), uric acid, or cystine. Calcium and struvite-containing stones often are visible on plain radiographs, but CT scans will demonstrate all calculi except those composed of crystalline-excreted indinavir, an antiretroviral medication.[49] For this reason noncontrast CT scans have become the study of choice to evaluate for urolithiasis.

Several underlying causes exist for the formation of urinary calculi. Hypercalciuria due to hyperparathyroidism, sarcoidosis, "renal leaks," or idiopathic overabsorption can lead to calcium-containing stones. Patients often will develop calculi after gastric bypass, which has been attributed to increased oxalate excretion in the

urine.[50] After bypass, dietary calcium is bound by unabsorbed dietary fats (saponification), preventing it from binding dietary oxalate, thereby making oxalate more available for intestinal absorption. Patients with gout are at risk for uric acid stones due to increased urinary uric acid and decreased urine pH, which diminishes uric acid solubility.

Urinary calculi may occur anywhere in the urinary tract. They usually are asymptomatic in the renal pelvis or bladder, but they are a very common cause of symptomatic ureteral obstruction. The obstruction may be partial or complete. Smaller stones (up to 6 mm) may cause severe symptoms, such as flank pain and nausea, but typically pass without intervention beyond supportive care.[51] Alpha blockers, which relax the distal ureter, may be given to reduce renal colic.[52] Calculi ≥7 mm are more likely to become impacted or to have a prolonged passage through the ureter. For this reason, intervention at the time of presentation is preferred for larger stones (except cases where the calculus is in the very distal ureter) due to the likelihood of repeat emergency room visits for severe symptoms.

Several methods for treating urinary calculi are available, depending on location. Obstructing stones often are temporized with stent placement, which allows proximal collecting system decompression. When urinary infection coexists with an obstructing stone, a stent can be placed, but a PCN is preferable if the patient demonstrates any instability. Definitive treatment of renal or ureteral calculi (lithotripsy) is through ureteroscopy, percutaneous nephrostolithotomy (PCNL), or extracorporeal shock wave lithotripsy (ESWL). Ureteroscopy is performed with a flexible or semirigid device that is passed to the level of the calculus. Under direct visualization, a laser fiber is passed through the scope, and energy is delivered to fragment the calculus. Fragments are extracted, although they usually will pass spontaneously. PCNL is performed through a percutaneous tract into the kidney, where a larger scope and various energy sources (laser, ultrasound) are used to fragment large renal calculi. This approach is well suited to staghorn calculi. ESWL is completely noninvasive and uses a device that delivers convergent shock-wave energy to the calculus under fluoroscopic guidance.

Complications of lithotripsy are specific to the technique used. Ureteroscopy may occasionally lead to strictures due to scarring from trauma to the ureter. If performed in the setting of infection, endoscopic irrigation can force bacteria into the renal parenchyma and result in sepsis. PCNL can cause significant bleeding, and if the tract used to access the kidney traverses the lower aspect of the pleura, large amounts of irrigating fluid can result in a significant hydrothorax. ESWL can occasionally cause renal hematomas, and splenic rupture has been seen after the treatment of a left-sided stone.[53,54]

Patients with recurrent stones benefit from stone composition analysis and metabolic work-up to determine the underlying cause if not apparent from the clinical history. Better hydration is useful for all etiologies. Patients with calcium-containing stones do not benefit from a reduction in dietary calcium unless they have absorptive hypercalciuria, which most do not. In fact, patients with higher dietary calcium have, on average, fewer episodes of urolithiasis.[55]

Retroperitoneal Fibrosis

Retroperitoneal fibrosis is a process resulting in encasement of the ureters, along with the great vessels, in a dense fibrotic mass. Many patients present in acute renal failure, and imaging demonstrates medially displaced ureters with a homogeneous, plaque-like mass in the retroperitoneum. The cause may occasionally be a neoplastic process such as histiocytosis or lymphoma—which must be ruled out—but most are idiopathic.[56] Many medications such as the ergot derivative methysergide, methyldopa, and beta blockers have been implicated as precipitating factors for the inflammatory process.[57]

Bilateral ureteral stent or PCN placement provides temporary relief of the obstruction. Corticosteroids may be given to reverse the inflammatory process, but surgical ureterolysis still usually is required to free the ureters from retroperitoneal encasement. They are brought into the peritoneum and wrapped in omentum to prevent re-entrapment.

PEDIATRIC UROLOGY

Ureteropelvic Junction Obstruction

UPJ obstruction is the most common cause of hydronephrosis found on prenatal ultrasound. UPJ obstruction also is commonly observed in children and young adults. Intrinsic and extrinsic causes of UPJ obstruction exist and can be determined by presentation. Intrinsic UPJ obstruction occurs in neonates due to an adynamic or stenotic segment of proximal ureter. This impairs flow of urine into the ureter, particularly during times of high flow, and causes dilatation of the collecting system. Over time, elevated renal pelvic pressures and recurrent infections can injure renal parenchyma. Abnormal lower pole renal arteries may be a secondary cause of UPJ obstruction by kinking the proximal ureter. Nuclear scans (mercaptoacetyltriglycine or ^{99m}Tc diethylene-triamine-penta-acetic acid) have replaced the IVP as the diagnostic modality of choice. Delayed clearance of contrast or radiotracer implies obstruction. Invasive pressure-flow examinations (Whitaker test) rarely are performed.

Not every case of UPJ obstruction requires operative intervention. Many children with hydronephrosis due to an apparent UPJ obstruction are not highly obstructed and will improve with time. However, patients with infections or impaired renal function require repair to improve drainage. Open pyeloplasty is considered the gold standard approach, especially in infants. In older children or adults, laparoscopic or robotic approaches for pyeloplasty can speed convalescence and diminish postoperative pain. An endoscopic approach, endopyelotomy, is also an option in older children and adults. Surgery involves ureteroscopy and a full-thickness lateral incision into the affected ureteral segment with a laser or knife taking care not to injure the renal hilar vessels.

Vesicoureteral Reflux

Vesicoureteral reflux (VUR) is the second most common cause of hydronephrosis after UPJ obstruction. Up to two thirds of infants presenting with urinary tract infections may be found with VUR.[58] The majority of cases occur in females. Primary reflux is a congenital anomaly caused by insufficient intramural tunneling of the distal ureter, although bladder outlet obstruction may cause unilateral or bilateral secondary reflux when the ureters are anatomically normal. The primary danger of VUR is the development of recurrent episodes of pyelonephritis, which can cause cumulative renal damage through scarring.

Neonates with hydronephrosis detected on prenatal ultrasound or infants or children experiencing a urinary tract infection should be evaluated for VUR with a VCUG. VUR is graded according to the International Classification System. Spontaneous resolution of VUR, which is the norm, is a function of the grade of VUR.[59] The large majority of low-grade (1 to 2) reflux will spontaneously resolve, while 30 to 50% of grades III and IV reflux and 9% of grade V reflux will resolve.[59,60] The initial management of VUR is controversial, particularly for moderate degrees. Surgical repair with ureteral reimplantation is effective, but may be overtreatment for those destined to resolve spontaneously. However, conservative management, consisting of antibiotic prophylaxis, may result in breakthrough infections with resistant organisms. A newer endoscopic technique, the submucosal injection of bulking agents at the ureteral orifice, is making this debate less important. It is a minimally invasive technique that may, in some patients, obviate the need for open surgical repair or long-term suppressive antibiotics. Submucosal bulking is not effective in every case, and patients with severe reflux may still need reimplantation.

Ureteroceles

A ureterocele is a cystic dilation of the terminal ureter thought to result from a persistent membrane between the ureteral bud and the urogenital sinus. Most patients will have associated genitourinary anomalies such as duplicated collecting systems or an ectopic ureteral location. Patients frequently present during childhood and can present in multiple ways depending on size and degree of obstruction. Patients may have hydronephrosis and pyelonephritis. A large, prolapsing ureterocele can cause bladder outlet obstruction, and rarely, a large ureterocele can present as an intralabial mass in a newborn child. Diagnosis can be confirmed with cystoscopy, VCUG, or IVP.

Patients with a functioning renal moiety can undergo endoscopic incision of the ureterocele; however, VUR is common postoperatively. A ureterocele in a nonfunctioning duplicated system may require a heminephrectomy to avoid infections.

Posterior Urethral Valve

Posterior urethral valves can be a particularly damaging cause of bilateral hydronephrosis in a newborn boy. The "valves," which are tissue folds located in the prostatic urethra, cause bladder outlet obstruction. Diagnosis is established with a VCUG, which may show poor bladder emptying and a dilated posterior urethra. A Foley catheter should be placed in the bladder to decompress the urinary system to allow renal function to potentially recover. Treatment involves cystoscopic ablation or resection of the valve. Even after ablation of the valves and elimination of the urethral obstruction, patients with posterior urethral valves are at significant risk of renal failure, depending on the degree of prenatal obstruction.[61] Bladders frequently suffer damage and become partially defunctionalized from prolonged prenatal obstruction, and normal voiding patterns often are not established. The most serious outcome of posterior urethral valves is pulmonary hypoplasia due to intrauterine oligohydramnios, and efforts have been made prenatally to transplacentally decompress the urinary bladder and prevent this dreaded development.

REFERENCES

Entries highlighted in bright blue are key references.

1. Wynder EL, Goldsmith R: The epidemiology of bladder cancer: A second look. *Cancer* 40:1246, 1977.
2. Canter D, Guzzo TJ, Resnick MJ, et al: Hydronephrosis is an independent predictor of poor clinical outcome in patients treated for muscle-invasive transitional cell carcinoma with radical cystectomy. *Urology* 72:379, 2008.
3. Stein JP, Cai J, Groshen S, et al: Risk factors for patients with pelvic lymph node metastases following radical cystectomy with en bloc pelvic lymphadenectomy: Concept of lymph node density. *J Urol* 170:35, 2003.
4. Grossman HB, Natale RB, Tangen CM, et al: Neoadjuvant chemotherapy plus cystectomy compared with cystectomy alone for locally advanced bladder cancer. *N Engl J Med* 349:859, 2003.
5. Lawrance WT, Rumohr JA, Chang SS, et al: Contemporary open radical cystectomy: Analysis of perioperative outcomes. *J Urol* 179:1313, 2008.

6. Bosl GJ, Motzer RJ: Testicular germ-cell cancer. *N Engl J Med* 337:242, 1997.

7. Donohue JP, Thornhill JA, Foster RS, et al: Retroperitoneal lymphadenectomy for clinical stage A testis cancer (1965 to 1989): Modifications of technique and impact on ejaculation. *J Urol* 149:237, 1993.

8. American Cancer Society: *Cancer Facts & Figures 2008.* Atlanta: American Cancer Society, 2008.

9. Hollingsworth JM, Miller DC, Daignault S, et al: Rising incidence of small renal masses: A need to reassess treatment effect. *J Natl Cancer Inst* 98:1331, 2006.

10. Israel GM, Bosniak MA: Follow-up CT of moderately complex cystic lesions of the kidney (Bosniak category IIF). *AJR Am J Roentgenol* 181:627, 2003.

11. Linehan WM, Walther MM, Zbar B: The genetic basis of cancer of the kidney. *J Urol* 170:2163, 2003.

12. Flanigan RC, Salmon SE, Blumenstein BA, et al: Nephrectomy followed by interferon alfa-2b compared with interferon alfa-2b alone for metastatic renal cell cancer. *N Engl J Med* 345:1655, 2001.

13. Mickisch GHJ, Garin A, van Poppel H, et al: Radical nephrectomy plus interferon-alfa-based immunotherapy compared with interferon alfa alone in metastatic renal cell carcinoma: a randomized trial. *Lancet* 358:966, 2001.

14. Huang WC, Levey AS, Serio AM, et al: Chronic kidney disease after nephrectomy in patients with renal cortical tumors: A retrospective cohort study. *Lancet Oncol* 7:735, 2006.

15. Rabbani F, Herr HW, Almahmeed T, et al: Temporal change in risk of metachronous contralateral renal cell carcinoma: Influence of tumor characteristics and demographic factors. *J Clin Oncol* 20:2370, 2002.

16. Bosniak MA, Birnbaum BA, Krinsky GA, et al: Small renal parenchymal neoplasms: Further observations on growth. *Radiology* 197:589, 1995.

17. Chin AI, Lam JS, Figlin RA, et al: Surveillance strategies for renal cell carcinoma patients following nephrectomy. *Rev Urol* 8:1, 2006.

18. Kavolius JP, Mastorakos DP, Pavlovich C, et al: Resection of metastatic renal cell carcinoma. *J Clin Oncol* 16:2261, 1998.

19. Bill-Axelson A, Holmberg L, Filen F, et al: Radical prostatectomy versus watchful waiting in localized prostate cancer: The Scandinavian Prostate Cancer Group-4 Randomized Trial. *J Natl Cancer Inst* 100:1144, 2008.

20. Gleason DF, Mellinger GT (Veterans Administration Cooperative Research Group): Prediction of prognosis for prostatic adenocarcinoma by combined histologic grading and clinical staging. *J Urol* 111:58, 1974.

21. Walsh PC, Marschke P, Ricker D, et al: Patient-reported urinary continence and sexual function after anatomic radical prostatectomy. *Urology* 55:58, 2000.

22. Buckley JC, McAninch JW: Selective management of isolated and nonisolated grade IV renal injuries. *J Urol* 176:2498, 2006.

23. Koraitim MM: Pelvic fracture urethral injuries: The unresolved controversy. *J Urol* 161:1433, 1999.

24. Moudouni SM, Patard JJ, Manunta A, et al: Early endoscopic realignment of post-traumatic posterior urethral disruption. *Urology* 57:628, 2001.

25. Mouraviev V, Coburn M, Santucci R: The treatment of posterior urethral disruption associated with pelvic fractures: Comparative experience of early realignment versus delayed urethroplasty. *J Urol* 173:873, 2005.

26. Corrales JG, Corbel L, Cipolla B, et al: Accuracy of ultrasound diagnosis after blunt testicular trauma. *J Urol* 150:1834, 1993.

27. Sawh SL, O'Leary MP, Ferreira MD, et al: Fractured penis: A review. *Int J Impot Res* 20:366, 2008.

28. Donohue RE, Utley WLF: Torsion of the spermatic cord. *J Urol* 40:33, 1978.

29. Taskinen S, Taskinen M, Rintala R: Testicular torsion: Orchiectomy or orchiopexy? *J Pediatr Urol* 4:210, 2008.

30. Tahmaz L, Eredemir F, Kibar Y, et al: Fournier's gangrene: Report of 33 cases and a review of the literature. *Int J Urol* 13:960, 2006.

31. Verit A, Verit FF: Fournier's gangrene: The development of a classical pathology. *BJU Int* 100:1218, 2007.

32. Pryor J, Akkus E, Alter G, et al: Priapism. *J Sex Med* 1:116, 2004.

33. Ekstrom B, Olsson AM: Priapism in patients treated with total parenteral nutrition. *Br J Urol* 59:170, 1987.

34. Dent LA, Brown WC, Murney JD: Citalopram-induced priapism. *Pharmacotherapy* 22:538, 2002.

35. Pecknold JC, Langer SF: Priapism: Trazodone versus nefazodone. *J Clin Psychiatry* 57:547, 1996.

36. Miller ST, Rao SO, Dunn EK, et al: Priapism in children with sickle cell disease. *J Urol* 154:844, 1995.

37. Hellstrom WJ, Derosa A, Lang E: The use of transcatheter superselective embolization to treat high flow priapism (arteriocavernosal fistula) caused by straddle injury. *J Urol* 178:1059, 2007.

38. Williams JC, Morrison PM, Richardson JR: Paraphimosis in elderly men. *Am J Emerg Med* 13:351, 1995.

39. Huang JJ, Tseng CC: Emphysematous pyelonephritis: Clinicoradiological classification, management, prognosis, and pathogenesis. *Arch Int Med* 160:797, 2000.

40. Aswathaman K, Gopalakrishnan G, Gnanaraj L, et al: Emphysematous pyelonephritis: Outcome of conservative management. *Urology* 71:1007, 2008.

41. Abdul-Halim H, Kehinde EO, Abdeen S, et al: Severe emphysematous pyelonephritis in diabetic patients: Diagnosis and aspects of surgical management. *Urol Int;* 75:123, 2005.

42. Capodice JL, Bemis DL, Buttyan R, et al: Complementary and alternative medicine for chronic prostatitis/chronic pelvic pain syndrome. *Evid Based Complement Alternat Med* 2:495, 2005.

43. Spaliviero M, Araki M, Wong C: Short-term outcomes of Greenlight HPS laser photoselective vaporization prostatectomy (PVP) for benign prostatic hyperplasia (BPH). *J Endourol* 22:2341, 2008.

44. Andrich DE, Mundy AR: What is the best technique for urethroplasty? *Eur Urol* 54:1031, 2008.

45. Leahy AL, Ryan PC, McEntree GM: Renal injury and recovery in partial ureteric obstruction. *J Urol* 142:199, 1989.

46. Vaughan ED, Gillenwater JY: Recovery following complete chronic unilateral ureteral occlusion: Functional, radiographic, and pathologic alterations. *J Urol* 106:27, 1971.

47. Paick SH, Park HK, Oh SJ, et al: Characteristics of bacterial colonization and urinary tract infection after indwelling of double-J ureteral stent. *Urology* 62:214, 2003.

48. Johnson CM, Wilson DM, O'Fallon WM, et al: Renal stone epidemiology: A 25-year study in Rochester, Minnesota. *Kidney Int* 16:624, 1979.

49. Daudon M, Estepa L, Kebede M, et al: Urinary calculi and crystalluria in HIV+ patients treated with indinavir sulfate. *Presse Med* 26:1612, 1997.

50. Cryer PE, Garber AJ, Hoffsten P, et al: Renal failure after small intestinal bypass for obesity. *Arch Intern Med* 135:1610, 1975.

51. Ueno A, Kawamure T, Ogawa A, et al: Relation of spontaneous passage of ureteral calculi to size. *Urology* 10:544, 1977.

52. Sayed MA, Abolysor A, Abdalla MA, et al: Efficacy of tamsulosin in medical expulsive therapy for distal ureteral calculi. *Scand J Urol Nephrol* 42:59, 2008.

53. Rashid P, Steele D, Hunt J: Splenic rupture after extracorporeal shock wave lithotripsy. *J Urol* 156:1756, 1996.

54. Marcuzzi D, Gray R, Wesley-James T: Symptomatic splenic rupture following extracorporeal shock wave lithotripsy. *J Urol* 145:547, 1991.

55. Curhan GC, Willett WC, Rimm EB, et al: A prospective study of dietary calcium and other nutrients and the risk of symptomatic kidney stones. *N Engl J Med* 328:833, 1993.

56. Koep L, Zuidema GD: The clinical significance of retroperitoneal fibrosis. *Surgery* 81:250, 1977.

57. Srinivas V, Dow D: Retroperitoneal fibrosis. *Can J Surg* 27:111, 1984.

58. Smellie JM, Normand IC: Clinical features and significance of urinary tract infection in children. *Arch Dis Child* 43:468, 1968.

59. Duckett JW: Vesicoureteral reflux: A "conservative" analysis. *Am J Kidney Dis* 3:139, 1983.

60. Arant BS: Medical management of mild and moderate vesicoureteral reflux: Follow up studies of infants and young children. A preliminary report of the Southwest Nephrology Group. *J Urol* 148:1683, 1992.

61. Kousidis G, Thomas DF, Morgan H, et al: The long-term outcome of prenatally detected posterior urethral valves: A 10 to 23-year follow-up. *BJU Int* 102:1020, 2008.

Gynecology

Joanna M. Cain, Wafic M. ElMasri,
Tom Gregory, and Elise C. Kohn

PATHOPHYSIOLOGY AND MECHANISMS OF DISEASE

The female reproductive tract is a unique component of the body with a multitude of tightly regulated functions. Many of the activities normally ongoing, such as angiogenesis and physiologic invasion, are necessary for the reproductive organs to fulfill their purpose, and are usurped in disease. Immune surveillance is modified by multiple mechanisms under investigation, regulated in a different fashion, to allow implantation, placentation, and development of the fetus. How this potential disruption of the normal immune barriers is involved in pathologic events is incompletely understood. The ongoing rupture, healing, angiogenesis, and regrowth of the ovarian capsule and endometrium during the menstrual cycle uses the same series of biologic and biochemical events that are also active in pathologic events such as endometriosis and endometriomas, mature teratomas, dysgerminomas, and progression to malignancy. Genetic abnormalities, both germline and somatic, that may cause competence and/or promote disease are now being uncovered, especially in the progression to malignancy, in pharmacogenomics, and in surgical risks such as bleeding and clotting. Incorporation of genetic and genomic information in disease diagnosis and assessment is a wave for the near future and may alter how we consider who is at risk, how diseases are diagnosed and followed, and even what drugs or therapies we use for an individual patient. These points will be incorporated with surgical approaches into discussions of anatomy, diagnostic workup, infection, surgical and medical aspects of the obstetric patient, pelvic floor dysfunction, and neoplasms.

ANATOMY

The outlet of the bony pelvis is defined by the ischiopubic ramus anteriorly and the coccyx and sacrotuberous ligaments posteriorly.[1] This outlet can be subdivided into anterior and posterior triangles, which share a common base via a line between the ischial tuberosities. The soft tissues of the anterior triangle are layered in a fashion similar to the anterior abdominal wall. The most superficial layer is a skin and adipose layer (vulva) that overlies a fascial layer (perineal membrane) that is, in turn, superficial to a muscular layer (levator ani).

Vulva

The labia majora form the cutaneous boundaries of the lateral vulva and represent the female homologue of the male scrotum (Fig. 41-1). The labia majora are fatty folds covered by hair-bearing skin in the adult. They fuse anteriorly over the anterior prominence of the symphysis pubis, the mons pubis. The deeper portions of the adipose layers are called Colles' fascia and insert onto the inferior margin of the perineal membrane, limiting spread of superficial hematomas inferiorly. Adjacent and medial to the labia majora are the *labia minora*, smaller folds of connective tissue covered laterally by non–hair-bearing skin and medially by vaginal mucosa. The anterior fusion of the labia minora forms the *prepuce and frenulum of the clitoris*; posteriorly, the labia minora fuse to create the *fossa navicularis* and posterior fourchette. The term *vestibule* refers to the area medial to the labia minora bounded by the fossa navicularis and the clitoris. Both the urethra and the vagina open into the vestibule. Skene's glands lie lateral and inferior to the urethral meatus. Cysts, abscesses, and neoplasms may arise in these glands.

Erectile tissues and associated muscles are in the space between the perineal membrane and the vulvar subcutaneous tissues (Fig. 41-2). The clitoris is formed by two crura and is suspended from the pubis. Overlying the crura are ischiocavernosus muscles that run along the inferior surfaces of the ischiopubic rami. Extending medially from the inferior end of the ischiocavernosus muscles are the superficial transverse perinei muscles. These terminate in the midline in the perineal body, caudal and deep to the posterior fourchette. Vestibular bulbs lie just deep to the vestibule and are covered laterally by bulbocavernosus muscles. These originate from

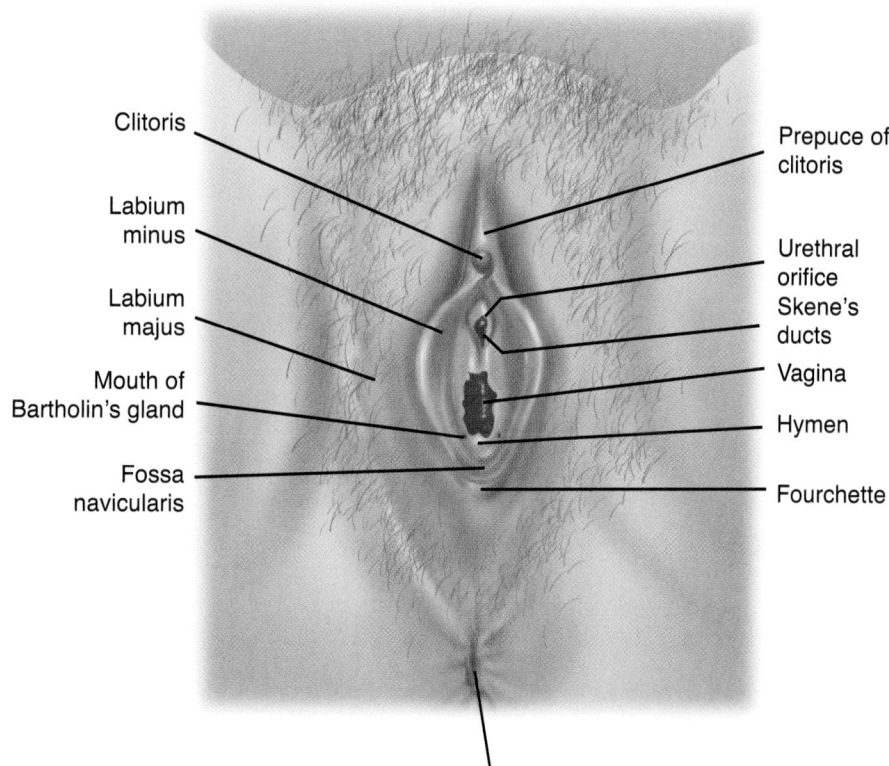

Clitoris

Labium minus

Labium majus

Mouth of Bartholin's gland

Fossa navicularis

Prepuce of clitoris

Urethral orifice
Skene's ducts

Vagina

Hymen

Fourchette

Anus

FIG. 41-1. External genitalia. *(Reproduced with permission from Rock J, Jones HW: TeLinde's Operative Gynecology, 9th ed. Philadelphia, PA: Lippincott, Williams & Wilkins, 2003, Fig. 5-1, p 70.)*

the perineal body and insert into the body of the clitoris. At the inferior end of the vestibular bulbs are Bartholin's glands, which connect to the vestibular skin by ducts.

Musculature of the Pelvic Floor

The opening of the pelvis is spanned by the muscles of the pelvic diaphragm (Fig. 41-3). These muscles contract tonically. Most anatomy textbooks fail to give a true picture of the horizontal nature of the pelvic floor musculature (due to embalming artifact). These muscles include, from anterior to posterior, bilaterally, the *pubococcygeus, puborectalis, iliococcygeus,* and *coccygeus* muscles. The first two of these muscles contribute fibers to the fibromuscular perineal body. The *urogenital hiatus* is bordered laterally by the pubococcygeus muscles and anteriorly by the *symphysis pubis*. It is through this muscular defect that the urethra and vagina pass, and it is the focal point for the study of disorders of pelvic support such as cystocele, rectocele, and uterine prolapse.

KEY POINTS

1. The general gynecology examination must incorporate the whole physical examination to adequately diagnose and treat gynecologic disorders.

2. Gynecologic causes of acute abdomen include: pelvic inflammatory disease and tubo-ovarian abscess, ovarian torsion, ruptured ectopic pregnancy, and septic abortion. Pregnancy must be ruled out early in assessment of reproductive age patients presenting with abdominal or pelvic pain.

3. Pregnancy confers important changes to both the cardiovascular system and the coagulation cascade. Trauma in pregnancy must be managed with these changes in mind.

4. Pelvic floor dysfunction (pelvic organ prolapse, urinary and fecal incontinence) is common; 11% of women will undergo a reconstructive surgical procedure at some point in their lives.

5. It is critical that abnormal lesions of vulva, vagina, and cervix are biopsied for diagnosis before any treatment is planned; postmenopausal bleeding should always be investigated to rule out malignancy. Early-stage cervical cancer is managed surgically whereas chemoradiation is preferred for stages IB and above.

6. Risk-reducing salpingo-oophorectomy should be considered in women with *BRCA1* or *BRCA2* mutations; risk-reducing salpingo-oophorectomy and complete hysterectomy should be considered in women with hereditary nonpolyposis coli cancer.

7. Complete debulking for epithelial ovarian cancer is a critical element in patient response and survival. The preferred primary therapy for optimally debulked advanced-stage ovarian epithelial ovarian cancer in women without significant intra-abdominal adhesions is intraperitoneal chemotherapy.

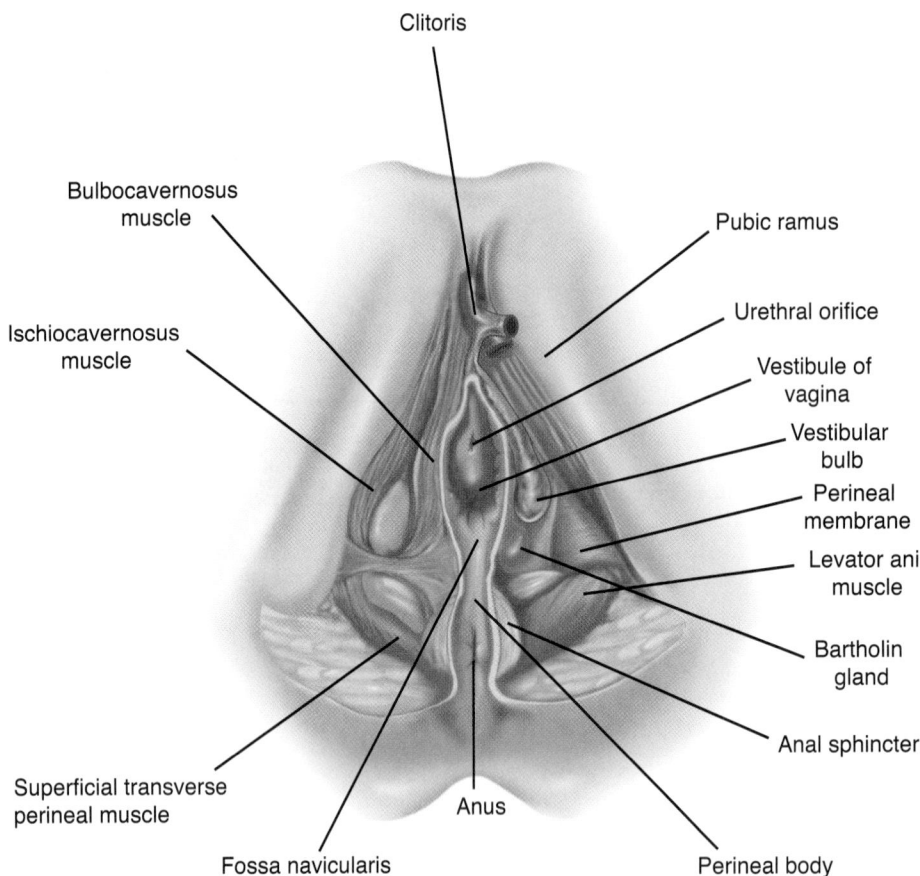

Clitoris

Bulbocavernosus muscle

Ischiocavernosus muscle

Superficial transverse perineal muscle

Fossa navicularis

Anus

Pubic ramus

Urethral orifice

Vestibule of vagina

Vestibular bulb

Perineal membrane

Levator ani muscle

Bartholin gland

Anal sphincter

Perineal body

FIG. 41-2. Superficial compartment and perineal membrane. *(Reproduced with permission from Rock J, Jones HW: TeLinde's Operative Gynecology, 9th ed. Philadelphia, PA: Lippincott, Williams & Wilkins, 2003, Fig. 5-2, p 71.)*

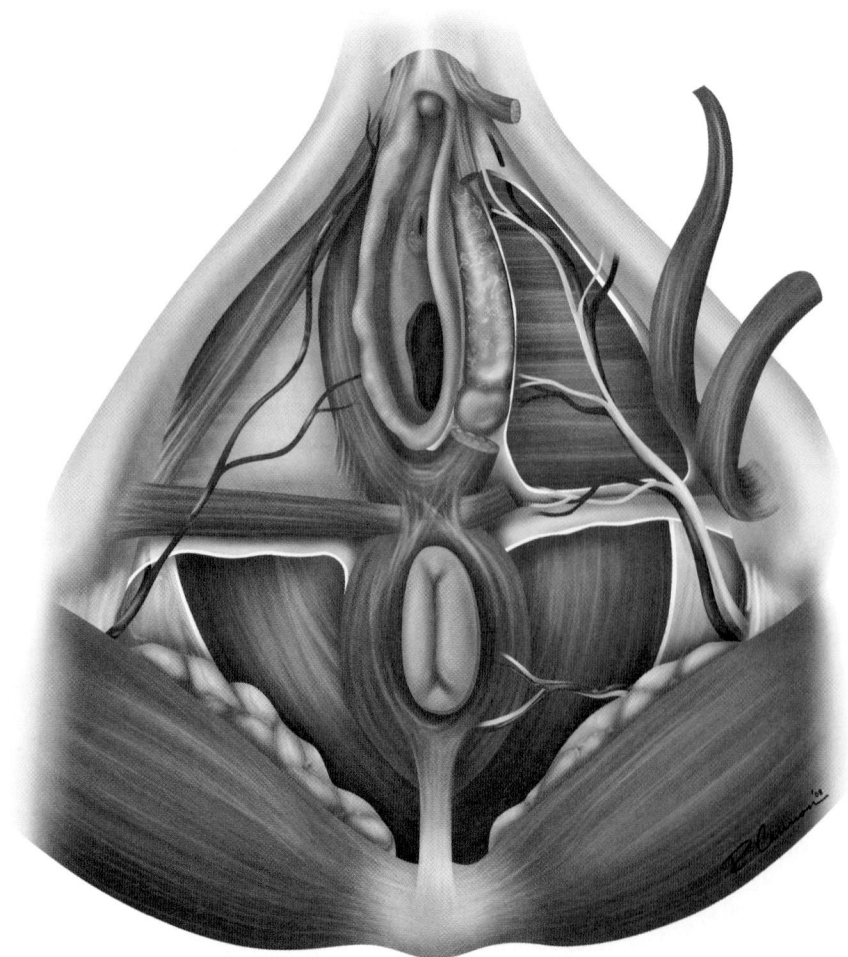

FIG. 41-3. Deeper muscles and nerves of the pelvic floor.

Nerves of the Pelvic Floor

The pudendal nerve arises from S2 to S4, travels laterally, exiting the greater sciatic foramen, hooking around the ischial spine and sacrospinous ligament, and returning via the greater sciatic foramen (Fig. 41-4). It travels through Alcock's canal and becomes the sensory and motor nerve of the perineum. The motor neurons originate in Onuf's nucleus in the sacral spinal cord and serve the tonically contracting urethral and anal sphincter. Direct branches from the S2 to S4 nerves serve the levator ani muscles. During childbirth and other excessive straining, this tethered nerve (along with the levator ani muscles) is subject to stretch injury, and at least partially responsible for many female pelvic floor disorders.

Internal Genitalia

Figure 41-5 is a view of the internal genitalia as one would approach the pelvis from a midline abdominal incision. The central uterus and uterine cervix are supported by the pelvic floor muscles. They are suspended by the lateral fibrous cardinal, or *Mackenrodt's ligament* and the uterosacral ligaments, which insert into the paracervical fascia medially and into the muscular sidewalls of the pelvis laterally. Posteriorly, the uterosacral ligaments provide support for the vagina and cervix as they course from the sacrum lateral to the rectum and insert into the paracervical fascia.

The bilateral fallopian tubes arise from the upper lateral *cornua* of the uterus and course posterolaterally. Each widens in the distal third, or *ampulla*. The ovaries are attached to the uterine cornu by the *proper ovarian ligaments*. Emanating from the uterine cornu and traveling through the inguinal canal are the round ligaments, eventually attaching to the subcutaneous tissue of the mons pubis. The ovaries are suspended from the lateral pelvis by their vascular pedicles, the *infundibulopelvic ligaments*. The peritoneum enfolding the *adnexa* (tube, round ligament, and ovary) is referred to as the *broad ligament*, although it is no more ligamentous than the peritoneum overlying the ovarian artery and vein.

The peritoneal recesses in the pelvis anterior and posterior to the uterus are referred to as the *anterior* and *posterior cul-de-sacs*. The latter is also called the *pouch* or *cul-de-sac of Douglas*. On transverse

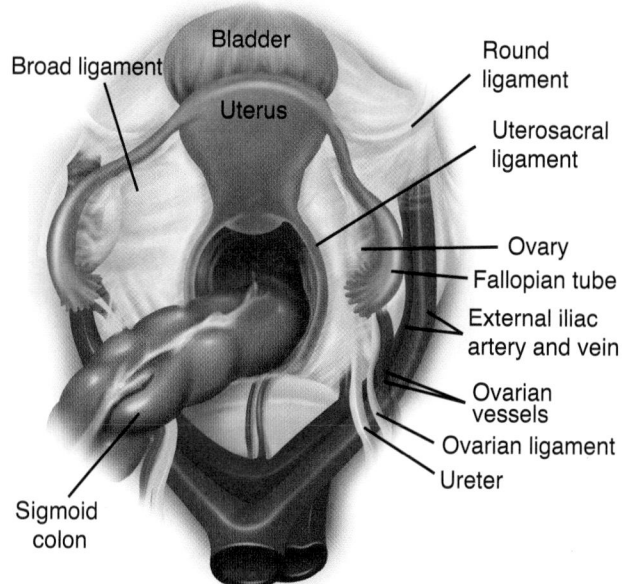

FIG. 41-5. Internal pelvic anatomy, from above.

section, several avascular, and therefore important, surgical planes can be identified (Fig. 41-6). These include the lateral paravesical and pararectal spaces, and from anterior to posterior, the retropubic or prevesical space of Retzius and the vesicovaginal, rectovaginal, and retrorectal or presacral spaces. The pelvic brim demarcates the obstetric, or true, from the false pelvis contained within the iliac crests.

The muscles of the pelvic sidewall include the iliacus, the psoas, and the obturator internus muscle (Fig. 41-7). Except for the middle sacral artery originating at the aortic bifurcation, and the ovarian arteries originating from the abdominal aorta, the blood supply to the pelvis arises from the internal iliac arteries. The internal iliac, or hypogastric arteries divide into anterior and posterior branches. The latter supply lumbar and gluteal branches. From the anterior division of the hypogastric arteries arise the obturator, uterine, pudendal, middle rectal, along with superior and middle vesical arteries. The nerves found in the pelvis are the sciatic, obturator, and femoral nerves (see Fig. 41-4). Sympathetic fibers course along the major arteries and parasympathetics form the superior and inferior pelvic plexus. The ureters enter the pelvis as they cross the distal common iliac arteries laterally and then course inferior to the

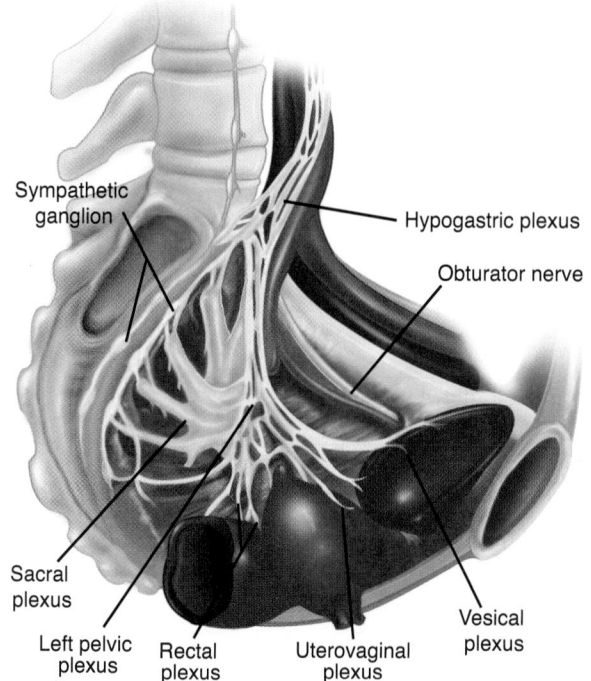

FIG. 41-4. The nerve supply of the female pelvis.

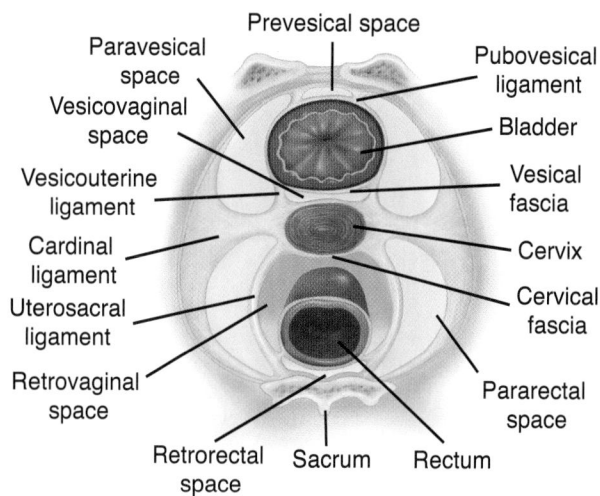

FIG. 41-6. The avascular spaces of the female pelvis.

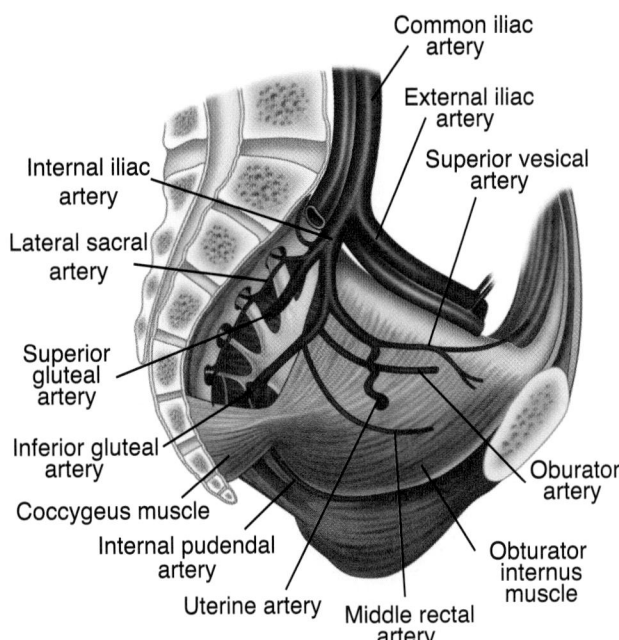

FIG. 41-7. The muscles and vasculature of the pelvis.

ovarian arteries and veins until crossing under the uterine arteries just lateral to the cervix. After traveling to the cervix, the ureters course downward and medially over the anterior surface of the vagina before entering the base of the bladder.

DIAGNOSIS

Elements of Gynecologic History

A complete history is a seminal part of any assessment (Table 41-1). Many gynecologic diseases can present with broad constitutional symptoms, occur secondary to other conditions, or be related to medications. A full history should include particular attention to family history, organ system history, including breast, GI, and urinary tract symptoms, and a careful anesthesia and surgical history. The key elements of a focused gynecologic history include the following:

- Age at menarche and menopause
- Present and past menstrual status
- Obstetrical history
- History of pelvic assessments, including cervical smear results
- History of pelvic infections and HIV status if indicated, and
- Prior gynecologic surgery(s).

Gynecologic Examination

Many women use their gynecologist as their primary care physician. When that is the case, it is necessary that a full medical and surgical history be taken and that, in addition to the pelvic examination, a minimum additional examination should include: thyroid, breast, cardiac, and pulmonary examinations. The pelvic examination starts with a full abdominal examination. Inguinal node evaluation is performed before placing the patient's legs in the dorsal lithotomy position (in stirrups). A flexible, focused light source is essential and vaginal instruments including speculums of variable sizes and shapes including pediatric sizes (Graves and Pederson) are required to assure that the patient's anatomy can be fully and comfortably viewed.

The external genitalia are inspected, noting the distribution of pubic hair, the skin color and contour, the Bartholin's and Skene's glands, and perianal area. Abnormalities are documented, and a map with measurements of abnormalities drawn. A warmed lubricated speculum is inserted into the vagina and gently opened to identify the cervix if present, or the vaginal apex if not. If there is a concern that a malignancy is present, careful digital assessment of a vaginal mass and location may be addressed before speculum placement to avoid abrading a vascular lesion and inducing hemorrhage. The speculum would then be inserted just short of the length to the mass to view that area directly before advancing. An uncomplicated speculum examination includes examination of the vaginal sidewalls, assessment of secretions including culture if necessary, and collection of the cervical cytologic specimen. Cervical cytology is performed by use of a brush placed into the cervical os, rotation of the brush, and then placement of the brush into liquid medium or spread and fixed on a glass slide, depending on the evaluation methods in use.

A bimanual examination is performed by placing two fingers in the vaginal canal; one finger may be used if patient has had prior radiation with stenosis or chemo- or other therapy with associated vaginal atrophy (Fig. 41-8). Carefully and sequentially assess the size and shape of the uterus by moving it against the abdominal hand, the adnexa by carefully sweeping the abdominal hand down the side of the uterus. The rectovaginal examination, one finger in the vagina and one in the rectal vault, is used to further examine and

Issue	Elements to Explore	Associated Issues
Menstrual history	Age at menarche, menopause Bleeding pattern, postmenopausal bleeding, spotting between periods Any medications (Coumadin, heparin, aspirin, herbals, others) or personal or family history that might lead to prolonged bleeding times	Identifies abnormal patterns related to endocrine, structural, infectious, and oncologic etiologies
Obstetrical history	Number of pregnancies, dates, type of deliveries, pregnancy loss, abortion, complications	Identifies predisposing pregnancy for gestational trophoblastic disease, possible surgical complications
Infectious diseases	Sexually transmitted diseases and treatment and/or testing for these	Also need to explore history of other GI diseases that may mimic sexually transmitted diseases (Crohn's, diverticulitis)
Contraceptive history	Present contraception if appropriate, prior use, type, and duration	Concurrent pregnancy with procedure or complications of contraceptives
Cytologic screening	Frequency, results (normal, prior abnormal Papanicolaou), any prior surgery or diagnoses, human papillomavirus testing history	Prolonged intervals increase risk of cervical cancer. Relationship to anal, vaginal, vulvar cancers.
Prior gynecologic surgery	Type (laparoscopy, vaginal, abdominal); diagnosis (endometriosis?, ovarian cysts?, tubo-ovarian abscess?); actual pathology if possible.	Assess present history against this background (for example, granulosa cell pathology, is it now recurrent?)
Pain history	Site, location, relationship (with urination, with menses, with intercourse at initiation or deep penetration?, with bowel movements?), referral?	Assesses relationship to other organ systems, and potential involvement of these with process. Common examples presenting as pelvic pain, ureteral stone, endometriosis with bowel involvement, etc.

TABLE 41-1 Key elements of the gynecologic history

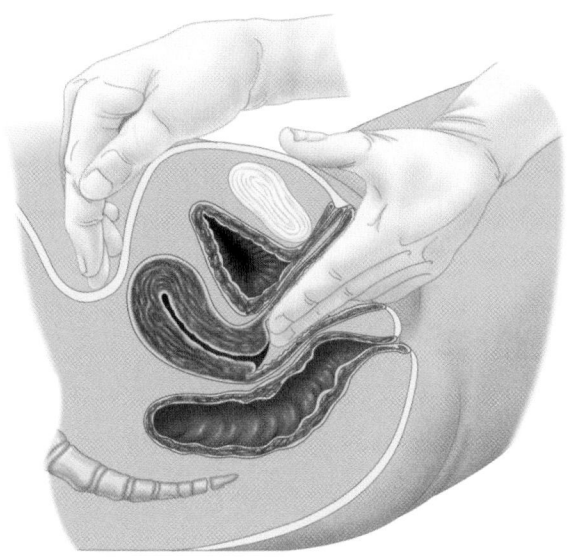

FIG. 41-8. Bimanual abdominovaginal palpation of the uterus.

characterize the location, shape, fixation, size, and complexity of the uterus, adnexa, cervix, and anterior and posterior cul de sacs. The rectovaginal exam also allows examination of the uterosacral ligaments from the back of the uterus sweeping lateral to the rectal finger to the sacrum.

It is critical that presurgical assessment include a full general examination. This is particularly important with potentially oncologic diagnoses or infectious issues to assure that the proposed surgery is both safe and appropriate. Complications such as sites of metastatic cancer or infection, associated bleeding and/or clotting issues and history, and drug exposure, allergies, and current medications must be addressed.

Screening Procedures
Cervical Cytology

The present guidelines for cervical cytology recommend annual evaluation for all sexually active women up to the age of 30 years old. After age 30, cervical cytology may be extended to every 2 to 3 years if cytology has remained negative and/or testing for human papillomavirus (HPV) high-risk types have been negative. This can be achieved with either liquid techniques or the older smear technique, recognizing that the accepted approach is moving to liquid techniques as they allow for reflex testing of HPV high-risk subtypes as appropriate. It is beyond the scope of the chapter to describe in detail the complex patterns that vary by age and prior history for following abnormal cytology findings. These must be addressed before any surgery, other than diagnostic, involving the cervix is planned. The diagnostic approach for abnormal Pap smears is detailed in Fig. 41-9.

Human Papillomavirus Testing

If liquid-based cytology is used, HPV testing for high-risk types can be done using the same specimen collected for cervical cytology.[2] HPV testing is useful to triage atypical cells of undetermined significance cytology results to either colposcopy or observation in patients beyond adolescence. Approximately half of atypical cells of undetermined significance cases will test positive for high-risk HPV subtypes and need colposcopy; those with negative tests can be followed routinely with cervical cytology. HPV testing is indicated in particular for planning intervals of cervical screening after age 30 years old. In these patients, if HPV testing is combined with cytology and both test negative, screening intervals can be spaced to every 3 years. Patients with low-grade squamous intraepithelial lesions have a high likelihood of testing positive, and as such high-risk HPV testing is not cost effective for triage; all should go to colposcopy.

Vaginal Discharge and Cultures

See section on Lower Genital Tract Infections.

Beta Human Chorionic Gonadotrophin Testing

Quantitative urinary pregnancy tests for beta human chorionic gonadotrophin (beta-hCG) are standard before any surgery in a woman of reproductive age and potential, regardless of contraception history. In addition, serum beta-hCG testing is appropriate for evaluation of suspected ectopic pregnancy, gestational trophoblastic disease (GTD), or ovarian mass in a young woman. In the case of ectopic pregnancy, serial levels are required when a pregnancy cannot be identified in the uterine cavity. As a general rule, there should be at least a 66% rise in the beta-hCG level over 48 hours if there is a viable intrauterine pregnancy.

Common Office Procedures for Diagnosis
Vulvar Biopsy

Any abnormal lesion including skin color changes, raised lesions, or ulcerations should be biopsied. Local infiltration of a longer acting anesthetic is followed by punch biopsy appropriate to the lesion. The specimen is elevated with Adson forceps and cut from its base with iris scissors.

Vaginal Biopsy

This biopsy follows the same principles as vulvar biopsy but often is difficult to perform because of the angle of the lesion. After injection with local anesthetic, traction of the area with Allis forceps and direct resection of the lesion with a Metzenbaum scissors or cervical biopsy instrument (Schubert, Kevorkian, etc.) can achieve an adequate biopsy.

Cervical biopsy topical 4% lidocaine may be adequate for the many cervical biopsies that can be done without a tenaculum. The maintenance of sharp cervical biopsy forceps is critical to success. A loop electrosurgical excision procedure (LEEP) can be performed if the lesion is more extensive or vascular and allows the ball tip to be used for cautery.

Cauterization of all of the above lesions can be performed with silver nitrate, Monsel's solution, or direct electrical cauterization as required. If not adequate, suture should suffice to provide hemostasis.

Endometrial Biopsy

An endometrial sampling should be performed before planned hysterectomy if there is a history of abnormal bleeding, defined as bleeding between periods, spotting other than midcycle, heavy bleeding, frequent bleeding, or postmenopausal bleeding. A patient with the potential for pregnancy should have a pregnancy test before the procedure. Topical 4% lidocaine can be applied under direct visualization to the anterior cervix where a tenaculum might be placed, and then in the endocervical canal with a cotton-tipped applicator. A Pipelle is inserted after cervical cleaning and the depth noted; a tenaculum is placed if the cervix is too mobile or the uterus too flexed. The specimen is obtained by pulling on the central end, creating a small amount of suction in the uterine cavity, and moving it within the cavity to access all sides.[3] Additional passes may be made if the specimen is not initially adequate.

Evaluation for Fistulae

Common office procedures to evaluate for the presence of vesicovaginal fistulae include placement of a vaginal tampon before the procedure, and then insertion of sterile milk or sterile dye into the bladder through a transurethral catheter. Evaluation of suspected ureteral fistula is best done with radiologic imaging, and when confirmed, IV injection of dye may allow for direct visualization if the site is not obvious. Rectal fistula can be identified in a similar fashion using a large Foley catheter placed in the distal rectum through which dye may be injected or with the use of an oral charcoal slurry and timed examination. Common areas for fistulae

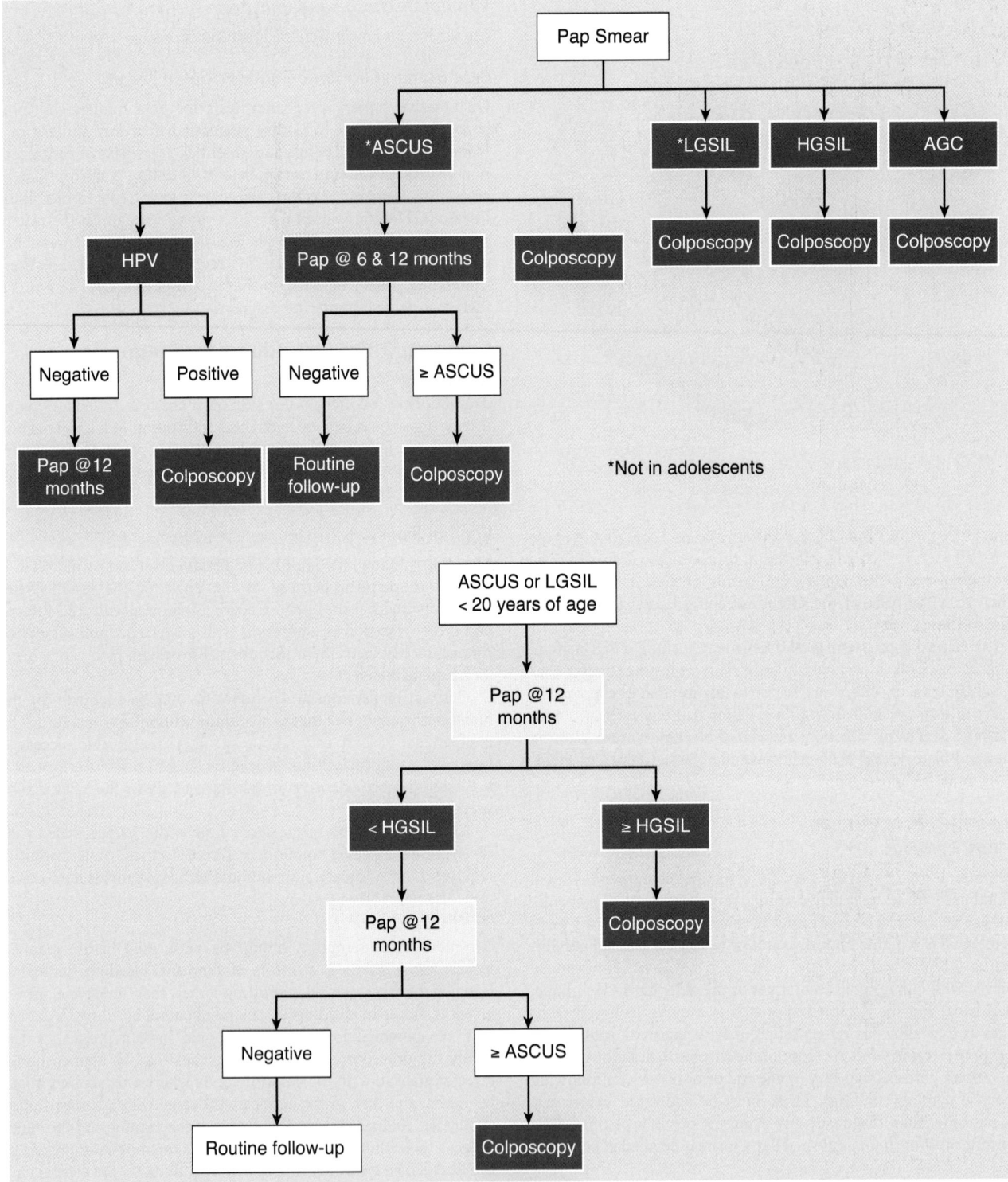

FIG. 41-9. Diagnostic approach for cervical dysplasia. AGC = atypical glandular cells; ASCUS = atypical cells of undetermined significance; HGSIL = high-grade squamous intraepithelial lesion; HPV = human papillomavirus; LGSIL = low-grade squamous intraepithelial lesion; Pap = Papanicolaou.

are at the vaginal apex, at the site of a surgical incision, or around the site of a prior episiotomy or perineal repair after a vaginal delivery.

GYNECOLOGIC INFECTIONS

Lower Genital Tract Infections

Vulvovaginal symptoms are extremely common, accounting for >10 million office visits per year in the United States. The causes of vaginal complaints are commonly infectious in origin but they include a number of noninfectious causes, such as chemicals or irritants, hormone deficiency, foreign bodies, systemic diseases, and malignancy. Symptoms are commonly nonspecific and include abnormal vaginal discharge, pruritus, irritation, burning, odor, dyspareunia, bleeding, and ulcers.

Cultures

The two most important cultures of vaginal secretions are for gonorrhea and chlamydia. A purulent discharge from the cervix should always raise suspicion of these infections even in the absence

TABLE 41-2 Features of common causes of vaginitis

	Bacterial Vaginosis	Vulvovaginal Candidiasis	Trichomoniasis
Pathogen	Anaerobic organisms	*Candida albicans*	*Trichomonas vaginalis*
% of Vaginitis	40	30	20
pH	>4.5	<4.5	>4.5
Signs and symptoms	Malodorous, adherent discharge	White discharge, vulvar erythema, pruritus, dyspareunia	Malodorous purulent discharge, vulvovaginal erythema, dyspareunia
Wet mount	Clue cells	Pseudohyphae or budding yeasts in 40% of cases	Motile trichomonads
KOH mount		Pseudohyphae or budding yeasts in 70% of cases	
Amine test	+	–	–
Treatment	Metronidazole 500 mg bid × 7 d or 2 g single dose, metronidazole or clindamycin vaginal cream	Oral fluconazole 150 mg single dose, vaginal antifungal preparations	Metronidazole 2 g single dose and treatment of partner

+ = positive; – = negative; KOH = potassium hydroxide.

of pelvic pain or other signs. These cultures are obtained by removing ectocervical discharge or blood and then with a sterile swab obtaining an endocervical swab that is then placed in carrier media for later culture on Thayer-Martin medium, and/or for enzyme linked immunosorbent assay or direct fluorescent antibody testing.

Vaginitis

Normal vaginal discharge is white or transparent, thick, and mostly odorless. It increases during pregnancy, with use of estrogen-progestin contraceptives, or at midcycle around the time of ovulation. Complaints of foul odor and abnormal vaginal discharge should be investigated. Candidiasis, bacterial vaginosis (BV), and trichomoniasis account for 90% of cases of vaginitis (Table 41-2). The initial workup includes pelvic examination, vaginal pH testing, microscopy, and,

less commonly, vulvovaginal and cervical cultures.[4] The pH of the normal vaginal secretions is 3.8 to 4.4, which is hostile to growth of pathogens. pH of 4.9 or greater is indicative of a bacterial or protozoal infection. Vaginal pH is obtained by dipping a pH tape into vaginal secretions collected on the speculum. Microscopy requires preparing wet and potassium hydroxide (KOH) mounts by adding a drop of normal saline or 10% KOH solutions to a specimen of the discharge. Microscopic examination of the wet mount may reveal motile trichomonads indicative of trichomoniasis or the characteristic clue cells of BV. KOH lyses cellular material and allows the clinician to appreciate the presence of mycelia characteristic of candidiasis. Treatment of vaginal infection before anticipated surgery is appropriate, particularly for BV, which may be associated with a higher risk for vaginal cuff infections. Figure 41-10 summarizes the diagnostic and treatment approach for common causes of vulvovaginitis.

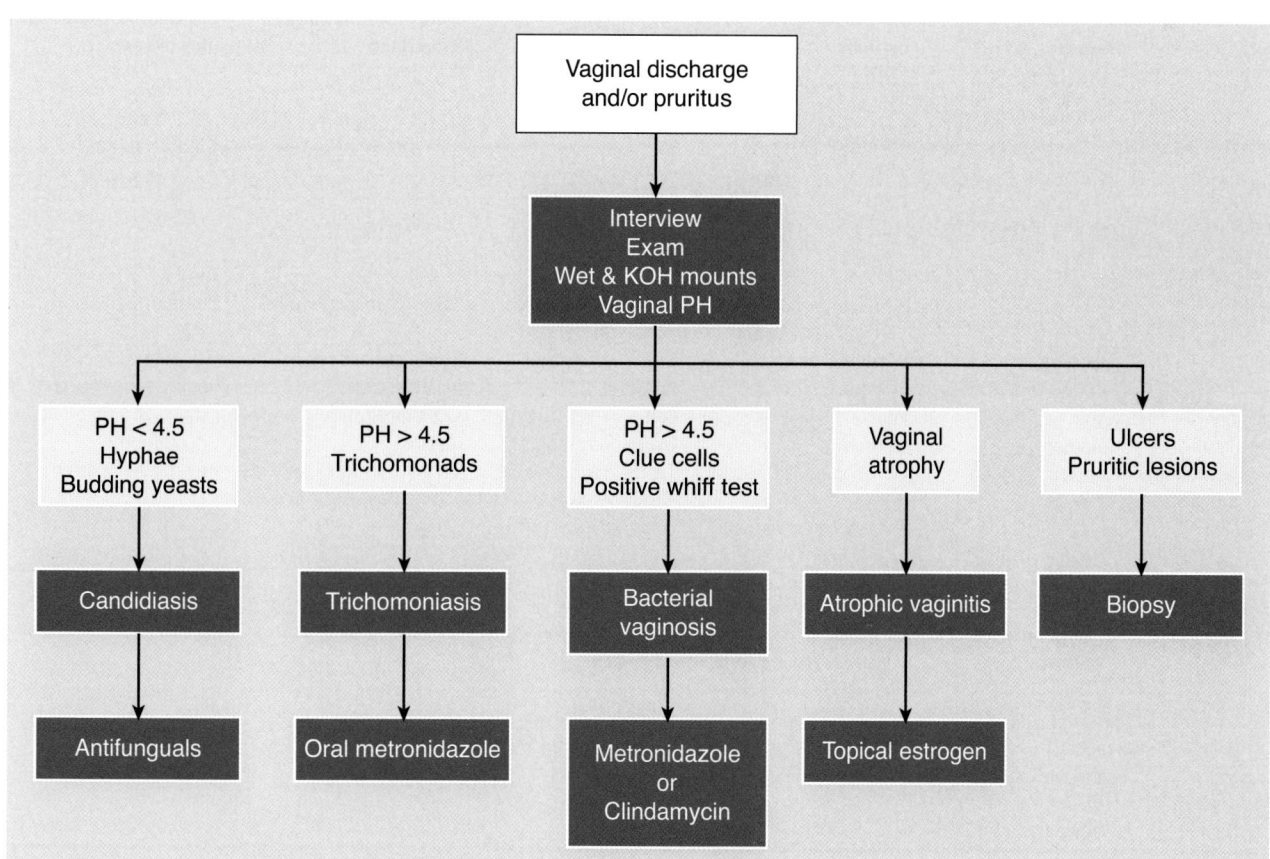

FIG. 41-10. Treatment algorithm for vulvovaginitis. KOH = potassium hydroxide.

Bacterial Vaginosis

BV is the most common cause of vaginal discharge, accounting for 50% of cases. It results from reduction in concentration of the normally dominant lactobacilli and increase in concentration of anaerobic organisms like *Gardnerella vaginalis*, *Mycoplasma hominis*, *Bacteroides* spp, and others.[5,6] Patient presentation, symptoms, cause, diagnostics, and interventions are shown in Table 41-2. Diagnosis is made by microscopy and involves recognition of clue cells, which are epithelial cells studded with adherent bacteria causing their margins to be obliterated. The discharge typically produces a fishy odor upon addition of KOH (amine or Whiff test).

Vulvovaginal Candidiasis

Vulvovaginal candidiasis is the most common cause of vulvar pruritus. It generally is caused by *Candida albicans* and occasionally by other *Candida* spp. It is common in pregnancy, in diabetics, in patients taking antibiotics, and in the immunocompromised. Seventy-five percent of women will experience one episode, with 40 to 50% having two or more. Diagnosis is confirmed by observation of pseudohyphae or yeasts on microscopy.

Trichomonas Vaginalis

Trichomonas vaginalis causes primarily a vaginal infection; however, the copious discharge results in a secondary vulvitis. Diagnosis is made with saline wet mount demonstrating motile protozoans.

Genital Ulcer Syndromes

The frequency of the infectious etiologies of genital ulcers varies by geographic location. In the United States, the most common causes of sexually transmitted genital ulcers in young adults are, in descending order of prevalence: herpes simplex virus (HSV), syphilis, and chancroid.[7] Others infectious causes of genital ulcers include lymphogranuloma venereum and granuloma inguinale. Noninfectious etiologies include Behçet's disease, neoplasms, and trauma. Establishing a diagnosis requires knowledge of the characteristics of genital ulcer syndromes and a rational approach to the evaluation of patients to guide therapy at the time of the initial encounter (Table 41-3). Confirmation of the established diagnosis requires the use of appropriate diagnostic tests.[8]

Genital Herpes

Herpes is a recurrent, incurable, sexually transmitted disease that has reached epidemic proportions. At least one in five individuals has had genital herpes in the United States. Herpes simplex infection is highly contagious and is caused by HSV-II and, less commonly, by HSV-I. Primary infection is a genital and systemic disease. Patients usually present with multiple painful vesicles that coalesce to form shallow superficial ulcers involving the vulva, vagina, and cervix.[9] Other possible symptoms include dysuria, fever, malaise, tender inguinal lymphadenopathy, and headaches. Less commonly, the infection can be subclinical and entirely asymptomatic. Once a patient is infected, there is a tendency for outbreaks at various intervals for life. Between outbreaks, the herpes virus resides dormant in the dorsal root ganglia of S2–4. Recurrent genital herpes is a local disease and characteristically less severe than the primary infection and of shorter duration. A common feature of recurrence is as prodromal phase of vulvar burning, tenderness, and pruritus lasting from a few hours up to a few days. Diagnosis is made by simple inspection of the lesions, cytology is helpful (Tzanck smear), and culture is confirmatory. Treatment is outlined in Table 41-3; alternative antiviral medications include famciclovir and valacyclovir. Vaginal delivery is contraindicated in pregnant patients presenting in labor with active genital herpes. Cesarean section is indicated and aims to prevent a potentially devastating neonatal infection.[10,11]

TABLE 41-3 Clinical features of genital ulcer syndromes

	Herpes	Syphilis	Chancroid	Lymphogranuloma Venereum	Granuloma Inguinale (Donovanosis)
Pathogen	HSV type II and, less commonly, HSV type I	*Treponema palladium*	*Haemophilus ducreyi*	*Chlamydia trachomatis* L1–L3	*Calymmatobacterium granulomatis*
Incubation period	2–7 d	Typically 2–4 wk (can range from 1–12 wk)	1–14 d	3 d–6 wk	1–4 wk (up to 6 mo)
Primary lesion	Vesicle	Papule	Papule or pustule	Papule, pustule, or vesicle	Papule
Number of lesions	Multiple, may coalesce	Usually one	Usually multiple, may coalesce	Usually one	Variable
Diameter (mm)	1–2	5–15	2–20	2–10	Variable
Edges	Erythematous	Sharply demarcated, elevated, round, or oval	Undermined, ragged, irregular	Elevated, round, or oval	Elevated, irregular
Depth	Superficial	Superficial or deep	Excavated	Superficial or deep	Elevated
Base	Serous, erythematous	Smooth, nonpurulent	Purulent	Variable	Red and rough ("beefy")
Induration	None	Firm	Soft	Occasionally firm	Firm
Pain	Common	Unusual	Usually very tender	Variable	Uncommon
Lymphadenopathy	Firm, tender, often bilateral	Firm, nontender, bilateral	Tender, may suppurate, usually unilateral	Tender, may suppurate, loculated, usually unilateral	Pseudoadenopathy
Treatment	Acyclovir 400 mg PO tid × 7–10 d for primary infection and 400 mg PO tid × 5 d for episodic management	Primary, secondary, and early latent (<1 y): benzathine PCN-G 2.4 million U IM × 1 Late latent (>1 y) and latent of unknown duration: benzathine PCN-G 2.4 million units IM qwk × 3	Azithromycin 1 g PO or ceftriaxone 250 mg IM × 1 *or* Ciprofloxacin 500 mg PO bid × 3 d *or* Erythromycin base 500 mg PO tid × 7 d	Doxycycline 100 mg PO bid × 21 d *or* Erythromycin base 500 mg PO qid × 21 d	Doxycycline 100 mg PO bid × 3 wk until all lesions have healed
Suppression	Acyclovir 400 mg PO bid for those with frequent outbreak	—	—	—	—

HSV = herpes simplex virus; PCN-G = penicillin.
Source: Adapted from Stenchever M, Droegemueller W, Herbst A, et al: *Comprehensive Gynecology*, 4th ed. St Louis: Mosby, 2001.

Syphilis

Syphilis is a chronic, systemic, sexually transmitted disease and is the second most common cause of genital ulcers and is caused by *Treponema pallidum*, an anaerobic spirochete.[12] In the United States, >36,000 cases of syphilis were reported in 2006, including 9756 cases of primary and secondary syphilis. The incidence was highest in women 20 to 24 years of age. Clinically, syphilis is divided into primary, secondary, tertiary, and congenital. The primary stage is marked by the appearance of a single ulcer (chancre). The chancre usually is firm, round, painless, may be accompanied by regional adenopathy, and develops at the site of entry of the bacterium. It lasts 3 to 6 weeks, and it heals without treatment. However, without treatment, the primary infection progresses to secondary syphilis and eventually to tertiary disease in 30% of cases, after a variable latent phase that usually lasts for years. During pregnancy, syphilis can be transmitted to the fetus and may result in the varied manifestations of congenital syphilis syndrome, which may results in fetal hydrops and intrauterine fetal demise. The diagnosis of syphilis is typically made by examination and serologic testing. Nonspecific nontreponemal tests such as rapid plasma reagin and Venereal Disease Research Laboratories are used for screening, and specific treponemal tests such as fluorescent-labeled treponema antibody absorption and microhemagglutination assay for antibodies to *T. pallidum* are used for confirmation.

Chancroid

Chancroid is a contagious sexually transmitted ulcerative disease of the vulva caused by *Haemophilus ducreyi*, small gram-negative rods that exhibit parallel alignment on Gram's staining ("school of fish").[13] After a short incubation period, the patient usually develops multiple painful soft ulcers on the vulva, mainly on the labia majora and, less commonly, on the labia minora or involving the perineal area. The chancroid ulcer has ragged, irregular borders and a base that bleeds easily and is covered with grayish exudates. Approximately half the patients will develop painful inguinal lymphadenitis within 2 weeks of an untreated infection, which may undergo liquefaction and presents as buboes.[14] These may rupture and discharge pus. Diagnosis is made by Gram's stain and, less commonly, by culture.

Lymphogranuloma Venereum

Lymphogranuloma venereum (LVG) is a sexually transmitted infection of lymphatic tissue caused by *Chlamydia trachomatis* serotypes L1, L2, and L3. LVG is rare in the United States.[15] In its primary stage, a genital ulcer develops at the site of inoculation after an incubation period of 3 to 30 days. The primary ulcer heals within a few days without therapy. The secondary phase of LVG develops 2 to 4 weeks later and is precipitated by direct spread to inguinal and perirectal lymph nodes. These painful, enlarged lymph nodes may result in the classic inguinal "groove sign" (double genitocrural fold) and may form buboes and rupture. Without adequate therapy, the patient will progress to the third stage marked by extensive inflammation and scarring. Clinical diagnosis is confirmed by serologic testing and culture. Complications include genital elephantiasis and colorectal fistulae and strictures. Treatment cures the infection and prevents ongoing tissue damage. Buboes occasionally require aspiration or incision and drainage.

Granuloma Inguinale

Granuloma inguinale, donovanosis, is an ulcerative bacterial infection of the vulva and perianal area that is transmitted via sexual contact in the majority of cases. It is caused by the intracellular gram-negative bacterium *Klebsiella granulomatis*. It is endemic in some tropical areas but is rarely seen in the United States. After a variable incubation period, the infection manifests as multiple nodules that ulcerate resulting in "beefy-red" ulcers covered with granulation tissue. These ulcers bleed easily and may coalesce, resulting in destruction of the vulvar architecture. The causative organism is difficult to culture, and diagnosis requires visualization of Donovan bodies on tissue crush preparation or biopsy. Donovan bodies are intracytoplasmic clusters of bacteria found in macrophages.

Molluscum Contagiosum

Molluscum contagiosum is a localized viral infection of the skin that typically spares the palms and soles. It can involve the genital area, and the lesions usually are small shiny papules with central umbilication. The condition is self-limited and resolves spontaneously. Genital lesions can be treated to prevent sexual transmission. Treatment options include curettage, cryotherapy, and laser ablation.

Bartholin's Cysts and Abscesses

Bartholin's glands (great vestibular glands) are located at the vaginal orifice at the 4 and 8 o'clock positions and they are rarely palpable in normal patients. They are lined with cuboidal epithelium and secrete mucoid material to keep the vulva moist. Their ducts are lined with transitional epithelium and their obstruction secondary to inflammation may lead to the development of a Bartholin's cyst or abscess. Bartholin's cysts range in size from 1 to 3 cm, and are detected on examination or recognized by the patient. They occasionally result in discomfort and dyspareunia and require treatment. Cysts and ducts can become infected and form abscesses. Infections are often polymicrobial; however, sexually transmitted *Neisseria gonorrhea* and *C. trachomatis* are sometimes implicated. Abscesses usually present as acutely inflamed, exquisitely tender masses. Treatment consists of incision and drainage and placement of a Word catheter, a small catheter with a balloon tip, for 2 to 3 weeks to allow for formation and epithelialization of a new duct. Appropriate antibiotic therapy should be instituted and modified based upon culture results. Recurrent cysts or abscesses are usually marsupialized, but on occasion necessitate excision of the whole gland. Marsupialization is done by incising the cyst or abscess wall and securing its lining to the skin edges with interrupted sutures.[16] Cysts or abscesses that fail to resolve after drainage and those occurring in patients >40 years of age should be biopsied to exclude malignancy.

Vulvar Condylomas

Condylomata acuminata (anogenital warts) are viral infections caused by HPV.[2] Genital infection with HPV is the most common sexually transmitted infection in the United States today. It is estimated that approximately 1% of sexually active adults currently have genital warts. There are more than 100 different types of HPV, and they differ in terms of the type of epithelium they infect. More than 30 types infect the anogenital epithelium, including the cervix, vagina, vulva, urethra, rectum, and anus. These are divided into low- and high-risk types. HPV 6 and 11 are the most common low-risk types and are implicated in 90% of cases of genital warts.[17] High-risk types can be found in association with invasive cancers.

Genital warts are skin colored or pink and range from smooth, flattened papules to verrucous, papilliform lesions. Lesions may be single or multiple and extensive. Diagnosis is made by simple inspection and should be confirmed with biopsy as verrucous and other vulvar cancers can be mistaken for condylomata.[18] Treatment modalities range from patient-applied ointments, physician-applied agents, and office procedures, to outpatient surgery. Patients may be prescribed 5% imiquimod cream to apply once at bedtime and wash off in the morning, three times a week, for up to 16 weeks. Trichloroacetic acid is a commonly used caustic agent for in office application and can be repeated weekly as necessary. Surgical modalities include cryotherapy, laser ablation, cauterization, and surgical excision depending on the severity and extent of the lesions.

Upper Genital Tract Infections

Pelvic inflammatory disease (PID) is an infection of the upper female genital tract involving the uterus, fallopian tubes, and ovaries, resulting in endometritis, salpingitis, and oophoritis. It often involves contiguous pelvic organs resulting in peritonitis, tubo-ovarian abscesses, and occasionally perihepatitis (Fitz-Hugh–Curtis syndrome). Long-term sequelae include infertility, chronic pelvic pain, and increased risk of ectopic pregnancy.[19,20] PID is mostly a sexually transmitted, ascending infection caused by *N. gonorrhea* and/or *C. trachomatis*, but numerous other organisms have been implicated, including normal vaginal flora. Screening for concomitant HIV infection is strongly recommended. Less commonly, PID may result from extension of other pelvic and abdominal infections such as appendicitis and diverticulitis, or may be precipitated by medical procedure, such as hysterosalpingography, endometrial biopsy, or dilation and curettage.

Risk factors for PID include age <25 years old, young age at first intercourse, nonbarrier contraception, previous episode of PID, other sexually transmitted diseases, and new or multiple sexual partners. Diagnosis can be challenging secondary to a wide range of presentations. Differential diagnosis includes appendicitis, cholecystitis, inflammatory bowel disease, pyelonephritis, nephrolithiasis, ectopic pregnancy, and ovarian torsion.[19,20] Common symptoms include fever, nausea and vomiting, lower abdominal pain, and purulent vaginal discharge. Clinical diagnosis is made by the triad of lower abdominal tenderness, cervical motion tenderness, and adnexal tenderness and may be confirmed by cervicovaginal cultures, transvaginal ultrasonography (TVUS), computed tomography (CT) scanning, and laparoscopy. Transvaginal ultrasound may reveal thickened, fluid-filled tubes with or without free pelvic fluid, while findings at the time of laparoscopy include exudates and swollen erythematous tubes. Criteria for hospitalization and IV antibiotic treatment include (Table 41-4)[7,21,22]:

- Pregnancy
- Febrile illness
- Severe pain
- PO intolerance secondary to nausea and vomiting
- Peritonitis and peritoneal signs
- Medication noncompliance
- Failure to respond to oral medications
- Pelvic or tubo-ovarian abscess

Surgical intervention becomes necessary if medical therapy of a tubo-ovarian abscess fails or if the abscess ruptures. Rupture of a tubo-ovarian abscess is a surgical emergency with a high mortality rate if not recognized and managed promptly. In addition to management of the septic shock state, total abdominal hysterectomy and bilateral salpingo-oophorectomy is the procedure of choice; however, conservative surgery must be considered in young patients desiring of future fertility. The abdomen should be explored for metastatic abscesses, and special attention must be paid to bowel, bladder, and ureteral safety due to the friability of the infected tissue and the adhesions commonly encountered at the time of surgery. Placement of an intraperitoneal drain and mass closure of the peritoneum, muscle, and fascia with delayed-absorbable or permanent sutures is advised. Closure of the skin and subcutaneous layer should be avoided in patients with frank pus and delayed primary closure or closure by secondary intention is recommended because of the high rate of wound infections in these patients. Conservative surgery, when feasible, may be attempted by laparoscopy and may involve unilateral salpingo-oophorectomy or drainage of the abscess and liberal irrigation of the abdomen and pelvis.

SURGICAL CONDITIONS OF THE OBSTETRIC PATIENT

Many women will undergo invasive diagnostic procedures for prenatal diagnosis. Between 0.2 and 2.2% of pregnant women will require surgery in pregnancy for issues both related and unrelated to the pregnancy.[23–26] Another 25 to 30% will have cesarean deliveries,[27] increasing the risks for associated or subsequent emergency hysterec-

TABLE 41-4	Centers for Disease Control and Prevention recommended treatment of pelvic inflammatory disease (2007)

Oral regimens
  Ceftriaxone 250 mg IM in a single dose
  plus
  Doxycycline 100 mg PO bid × 14 d
  with or without
  Metronidazole 500 mg PO bid × 14 d
  or
  Cefoxitin 2 g IM in a single dose and probenecid 1 g PO administered concurrently in a single dose
  plus
  Doxycycline 100 mg PO bid × 14 d
  with or without
  Metronidazole 500 mg PO bid × 14 d
  or
  Other parenteral third-generation cephalosporin (e.g., ceftizoxime or cefotaxime)
  plus
  Doxycycline 100 mg PO bid × 14 d
  with or without
  Metronidazole 500 mg PO bid × 14 d
Parenteral regimens
  Recommended regimen A
    Cefotetan 2 g IV every 12 h
    or
    Cefoxitin 2 g IV every 6 h
    plus
    Doxycycline 100 mg orally or IV every 12 h
  Recommended regimen B
    Clindamycin 900 mg IV every 8 h
    plus
    Gentamicin loading dose IV or IM (2 mg/kg of body weight), followed by a maintenance dose (1.5 mg/kg) every 8 h. Single daily dosing may be substituted.
  Alternative parenteral regimen
    Ampicillin/sulbactam 3 g IV every 6 h
    plus
    Doxycycline 100 mg orally or IV every 12 h

tomies with future pregnancies. Although these procedures typically are performed by obstetricians and gynecologists, occasionally a general surgeon will be consulted for assistance with postoperative or intraoperative issues. Physiologic changes due to pregnancy should be kept in mind (Table 41-5).[23]

Trauma in the obstetric patient requires stabilization of the mother, but the fetal compartment needs to be considered. Optimal maternal circulation and oxygenation is important, and when feasible, a left lateral tilt should be instituted to improve venous return because the gravid uterus often impedes blood flow to the right heart through direct pressure on the vena cava. Several coagulation factors are increased in pregnancy, increasing the likelihood for thromboembolic events, but also giving the unsuspecting surgeon false security when low-normal levels are observed during resuscitative efforts.

Procedures Performed before Viability
Amniocentesis/Chorionic Villus Sampling

Prenatal genetic diagnosis typically requires obtaining fetal tissue or cells. While newer techniques using maternal blood are currently being evaluated, the traditional methods for obtaining fetal genetic material are amniocentesis and chorionic villus sampling. Chorionic villus sampling is typically performed between 10 to 12 weeks gestation by using ultrasound to guide a flexible catheter transcervically into the trophoblastic tissue surrounding the gestational sac.

TABLE 41-5	Physiologic changes due to pregnancy

Cardiovascular changes
  Increased cardiac output
  Increased blood volume
  Decreased systemic vascular resistance
  Decreased venous return from lower extremities
Respiratory changes
  Increased minute ventilation
  Decreased functional residual capacity
GI changes
  Decreased gastric motility
  Delayed gastric emptying
Coagulation changes
  Increased clotting factors (II, V, VII, VIII, IX, X, and XII)
  Increased fibrinogen
  Increased risk for venous thromboembolism
Renal changes
  Increased renal plasma flow and glomerular filtration rate
  Ureteral dilation
  Initial increased bladder capacity

Source: Adapted with permission from Gabbe S, Niebyl J, Simpson J: *Obstetrics: Normal and Problem Pregnancies*, 4th ed. Philadelphia: Churchill Livingstone, 2001, Chap. 19, p 608. Copyright © Elsevier.

An amniocentesis is performed after about 13 weeks gestation by ultrasound-associated guidance of a 22-gauge spinal needle into the amniotic cavity. Fetal cells can be isolated, while other markers for chromosomal abnormalities and neural tube defects can be obtained from the amniotic fluid. Pregnancy loss attributable to these procedures is around 0.5%.

Pregnancy Terminations

Modern methods of contraception are highly effective, but still have a 0.5 to 5% failure rate. In addition, fetal conditions incompatible with life can result in planned termination. While the overall mortality rate related to pregnancy termination in the U.S. is around 1 per 100,000 induced abortions, rising with advanced gestational age, the maternal mortality rate for normal pregnancy and delivery is nine times that high.[28] Although legal, nonsurgical options are now available for early pregnancy, the safest and most commonly performed procedure is a cervical dilation and vacuum curettage. After the uterine cervix is grasped with a tenaculum, the cervix is forcibly dilated with tapered rods (occasionally using adjunctive prostaglandins), and an appropriately sized vacuum cannula is inserted into the uterus to remove the products of conception. Additional forceps can be used as necessary. The most common complications are infections, hemorrhage due to uterine atony, cervical lacerations, uterine perforations, and inadvertent bowel injury from the vacuum cannula or forceps.

Cerclage

A cervical cerclage may improve pregnancy outcomes in selected patients felt to have cervical incompetence. Shirodkar and McDonald techniques have been described;[29,30] both involve transvaginally placing a nonabsorbable suture at the uterocervical junction to lengthen and close the cervix. For a patient with a severely shortened or absent cervix, a laparotomy can access the abdominal portion of the lower uterine segment for an abdominal cerclage.

Ectopic Pregnancies

Extrauterine pregnancies can be located along the fallopian tubes and on the ovary. Rarely, implantation can occur primarily on other abdominal organs, or secondarily implant after tubal or uterine rupture. Historically, ectopic pregnancies were associated with high mortality rates; early diagnosis is the key to minimizing maternal morbidity and mortality. Sensitive assays for beta-hCG and improvements in ultrasound technology allow potential visualization of early gestations. Early ectopic pregnancies can be managed with methotrexate. Advanced ectopic pregnancy or a patient with unstable vital signs is managed by laparoscopy or laparotomy. Linear salpingostomy along the antimesenteric border and removal of the products of conception is a reasonable option unless the oviduct has already ruptured and a large hemoperitoneum already exists, in which case removal of the tube should be performed.

Procedures Performed after Viability
Obstetric Lacerations and Repair

The mean biparietal diameter of a term infant approaches 10 cm. The measured hiatus of the nulliparous vaginal introitus is approximately 2 cm. As a result, at the time of vaginal delivery, perineal lacerations, and with decreasing frequency, episiotomies are quite common. These lacerations involve, in varying degrees, the vaginal mucosa, the muscular elements inserting onto the perineal body, the levator ani, and in 4 to 5% of vaginal deliveries, the anal sphincter or anorectal mucosa. Although these are typically straightforward layered closures, knowledge of the anatomy is important. Incomplete reconstruction can contribute to future pelvic floor disorders as well as the development of fistulae.

Cesarean Deliveries

An increasing proportion of children are born by cesarean delivery. In 2004, 1.2 million or 29% of live births in the United States were cesarean deliveries, and this rate is increasing.[27] Current typical indications for cesarean delivery include: nonreassuring fetal status, breech or other malpresentations, triplet and higher order gestations, cephalopelvic disproportion, failure to progress, placenta previa, and active genital herpes. Previous low transverse cesarean delivery is not a contraindication to subsequent vaginal birth after cesarean; however, much of the increase in cesarean delivery in the past decade is attributable to planned repeat cesareans. Because there is decreased blood loss, and the subsequent uterine rupture rate with future pregnancies is about 0.5%, cesarean deliveries typically are performed via a lower anterior (caudal) uterine transverse incision (Fig. 41-11). Abdominal access is obtained by a Pfannenstiel or Maylard incision. Once the abdomen is entered, a vesicouterine reflection is created if a low transverse uterine incision is planned. The uterine incision is then made and extended laterally, avoiding

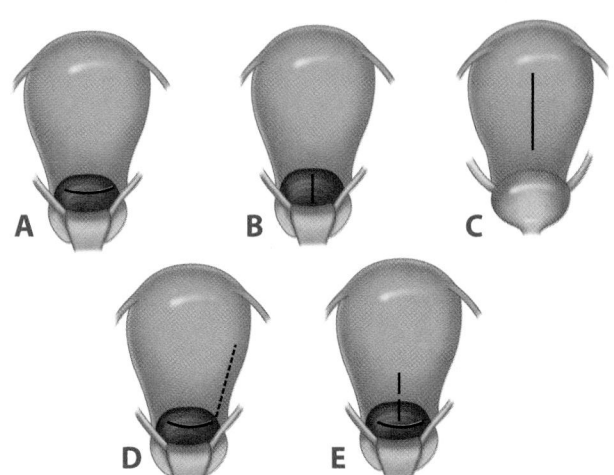

FIG. 41-11. Uterine incisions for cesarean delivery. **A.** Low transverse incision. **B.** Low vertical incision. **C.** Classical incision. **D.** J incision. **E.** T incision. (*Reproduced with permission from Gabbe S, Niebyl J, Simpson J:* Obstetrics: Normal and Problem Pregnancies, *5th ed. Philadelphia: Churchill Livingstone, 2007, Fig 19-3. Copyright © Elsevier.*)

the uterine vessels. After amniotomy, the baby is delivered, and the uterus closed. Approximately 1000 mL of blood typically is lost during a cesarean delivery. Along with rapid closure of the uterine incision, uterotonics such as IV oxytocin are administered. In certain very early viable gestations, or in the case of certain transverse lies, a classical (vertical) uterine incision is made. Following classical cesarean deliveries, future pregnancies have an 8% or greater risk of uterine rupture, and this is an absolute indication for a planned repeat cesarean delivery. Infection, excessive blood loss due to uterine atony, and urinary tract and bowel injuries are potential complications at the time of cesarean delivery, and are increased following labor. Moreover, with each subsequent cesarean delivery, the risk of those injuries, as well as abnormal placentation (placenta accreta, increta, and percreta), rises. Bleeding can only be controlled in some instances by performing a cesarean hysterectomy.

Peripartum Hysterectomy

A cesarean or postpartum (if a cesarean delivery has not previously occurred) hysterectomy involves the same steps as in a nonpregnant patient, but is distinctly different due to the engorged vessels and the pliability of the tissues. If a cesarean section has been performed, occasionally the incision can be used for traction to keep the vessels and tissues attenuated. Vascular pedicles should be secured with clamps, but not ligated until both uterine arteries have been secured to fully control bleeding. Lack of typical anatomic landmarks requires careful identification of the ureters and the dilated cervix visually or by palpation to separate from the bladder and vagina (Fig 41-12). As this procedure is often done for life-threatening hemorrhage, appropriate blood products, including packed red blood cells, fresh-frozen plasma, and fibrinogen, should be on call and usually are required. Because fibrinogen is typically elevated in a pregnant woman, a low-normal fibrinogen level can be cause for alarm and further fibrinogen may be required before any consumptive coagulopathy reverses. A massive transfusion protocol often is helpful.

Gestational Trophoblastic Disease[31,32]

GTD is an important gynecologic entity to consider when uterine size is significantly greater than expected for date in pregnancy, bleeding occurs in pregnancy, or in abnormal bleeding after pregnancy loss, abortion, or full-term delivery. Diagnosis is by ultrasound and measurement of serum beta-hCG, followed by pathologic examination of curettage specimens. There are two subtypes of GTD: complete, containing no fetal tissue and diploid on karyotype; and partial, containing fetal tissue and triploid. The chromosome pattern suggests paternal origin. These can be associated with theca lutein ovarian cysts often >6 cm in diameter that are fragile and generally should be followed without any surgical intervention as they resolve with removal or treatment of the GTD. Metastatic GTD can present on the cervix, vagina, liver, or lung and should not be managed surgically, as chemotherapy is the primary therapy and the incidence of bleeding complications is significant.

Primary surgery for diagnosis and initial therapy is a suction dilatation and curettage. Oxytocin is started either before anesthesia or immediately as the cervix is being dilated. The largest suction catheter possible (12 mm preferred) is gently inserted through the cervix and suction turned on, to allow the tissue to be removed and the uterus to rapidly decrease, with less blood loss. Following this, a sharp curettage of the uterus is done with a larger curette associated with a higher risk for perforation. Following diagnosis, beta-hCG is followed weekly until normal for 3 weeks, then monthly for at least 6 months. Any increase in beta-hCG may trigger further evaluation and consideration of chemotherapy.

PELVIC FLOOR DYSFUNCTION

Pelvic floor disorders can be categorized, from a urogynecologic perspective, into three main topics: female urinary incontinence

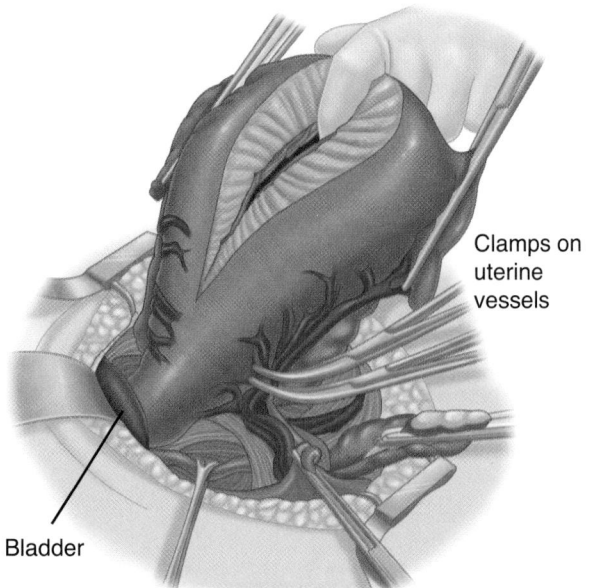

Clamps on uterine vessels

Bladder

Ureter identified

FIG. 41-12. Demonstration of location of distal ureter and bladder, and their relationship to uterine vessels. *(Reproduced with permission from Nichols DH:* Gynecology and Obstetric Surgery, *Vol. I., 1993, Fig. 68-5, p 1130. Copyright © Elsevier.)*

and voiding dysfunction, pelvic organ prolapse, and disorders of defecation.[33] Approximately 11% of women will undergo surgery for incontinence or prolapse.[34] The normal functions of support, storage, and evacuation can be altered by derangements in neuromuscular function both centrally and peripherally, and through acquired changes in connective tissue. Reconstructive surgeons aim to repair or compensate for many of these losses.

Evaluation

Diagnostic evaluations, in addition to the history and examinations described above under Gynecologic Examination, can aid in the diagnosis of many pelvic floor disorders. Cystoscopy, multichannel urodynamics, and/or fluoroscopic evaluation of the urinary tract can be obtained for patients with urinary incontinence or voiding dysfunction.[35] Defecography, anal manometry, and endorectal ultrasound may be useful for diagnosis of defecatory dysfunction. A standardized examination called the *pelvic organ prolapse quantification*[35] helps to clarify which vaginal compartment, and therefore, which specific structure, has lost its anatomic integrity in women with uterovaginal prolapse. Finally, dynamic magnetic resonance imaging (MRI) and pelvic floor electromyography have growing use for all three disorders.

SURGERY FOR PELVIC ORGAN PROLAPSE

Vaginal Procedures[36]

Many factors are important in determining which reconstructive operation is optimal for a given patient with pelvic organ prolapse. Surgical decisions often are based on case series and expert opinions that may not have universal applicability. However, the few reports with the highest level of evidence suggest that failure rates for prolapse reconstruction may be twice as high using the vaginal approach when compared with the abdominal route.[36,37]

Colporrhaphy

Anterior colporrhaphy begins with incision of the anterior vaginal epithelium in a midline sagittal direction. The epithelium is dissected away from the underlying vaginal muscularis. Although many surgical descriptions refer to plication of the "endopelvic" or "pubocervical" fascia, such structures have not been shown to exist as histologically distinct layers. The vaginal muscularis is plicated with interrupted delayed absorbable stitches, after which the epithelium is trimmed and reapproximated. The vaginal canal is therefore shortened and narrowed proportionately to the amount of removed epithelium. Posterior colporrhaphy is performed in a similar manner, often including the distal pubococcygeus muscles in the plication. In addition to the vaginal shortening and neuropathy that may be induced by these dissections, levator plication is associated with a significant risk of postoperative dyspareunia. These factors influence the selection of appropriate patients for colporrhaphy procedures.

Sacrospinous Fixation

The sacrospinous ligament is used as a unilateral fixation point for the vaginal apex. The procedure begins with entry into the rectovaginal space, usually by incising the posterior vaginal wall at its attachment to the perineal body. The space is developed to the level of the vaginal apex, and the rectal pillar is penetrated to gain access to the pararectal space. The sacrospinous ligament is found embedded in and continuous with the coccygeus muscle, which extends from the ischial spine to the lateral surface of the sacrum. A long-ligature carrier is used to place sutures medial to the ischial spine, through the substance of the ligament-muscle complex. Structures at risk in this procedure include the pudendal neurovascular bundle, the inferior gluteal neurovascular bundle, lumbosacral plexus, and sciatic nerve. After the stitches are placed, the free ends are sewn to the undersurface of the vaginal cuff. The sacrospinous stitches are tied to firmly approximate the vagina to the ligament without suture bridging. The epithelial incision is closed.

Uterosacral Ligament Suspension

Both sacrospinous fixation and suspension of the vaginal apex to the uterosacral ligaments may be performed immediately following vaginal hysterectomy or applied to posthysterectomy vaginal vault prolapse. The procedure is based on the concept that the natural support structures for the apical vagina and cervix are the uterosacral ligaments. When using the uterosacral ligaments for repair of prolapse, it is important to recall that these structures are not "ligaments" in the true sense of the word, but rather condensations of smooth muscle, collagen, and elastin. The integrity and strength of these structures may vary greatly from patient to patient. The repair uses the middle third of the ligament, which allows firm tissue-to-tissue approximation to the vagina and does not divert the ureter medially. Several support stitches are placed, such that the lateral-most portion of the vaginal cuff is attached to the distal-most part of the ligament and the medial cuff to the proximal ligament. Intraoperative evaluation of the lower urinary tract is important to confirm the absence of ureteral compromise.

Colpocleisis

A colpocleisis removes part or all of the vaginal epithelium. This obliterates the vaginal vault, leaving the external genitalia unchanged. Colpocleisis is reserved for patients who are elderly, who do not wish to retain coital ability, and for whom there is good reason not to perform a more extensive reconstructive operation. The main benefits of colpocleisis operations are their simplicity, speed, and high efficacy. The LeFort colpocleisis technique, done for complete uterovaginal prolapse, involves denudation of a rectangular portion of vaginal epithelium on both the anterior and posterior walls followed by suture reapproximation of the exposed submucosal surfaces. The uterus is left in situ. Lateral drainage canals remain for drainage of uterine secretions. By contrast, total colpocleisis involves hysterectomy, if applicable, followed by excision of the entire anterior and posterior epithelium. Successive purse-string sutures through the vaginal muscularis are used to reduce the prolapsed organs to above the level of the levator plate.

The bladder neck is displaced posteriorly by the repair, placing the patient at risk for postoperative stress incontinence; a concomitant procedure to stabilize the urethrovesical junction is recommended. This may involve plication of the anterior vaginal muscularis (Kelly plication), pubourethral ligament plication, or a sling procedure, depending on preoperative urodynamic findings.

Abdominal Procedures

Sacrocolpopexy

Pelvic reconstructive surgery by the abdominal approach has, as its main advantage, the use of graft material for support of the vaginal apex. The natural apical support structure, the cardinal–uterosacral ligament complex, is often damaged and attenuated. The use of graft material to compensate for defective vaginal support structures is well described.[38] Apical support defects rarely exist in isolation. Therefore, the sacrocolpopexy may be modified to include the anterior and posterior vaginal walls as well as the perineal body in the suspension. Sacrocolpopexies can be performed via laparotomy as well as via laparoscopy. Like rectopexies and low anterior resections, deep pelvic access is needed. Significant suturing at varied angles is required. The advent of the da Vinci robotic laparoscopic system has made visualization and adequate placement of the mesh and sutures easier to perform when using the minimally invasive approach.

A rigid stent is placed into the vagina to facilitate its dissection from the overlying bladder and rectum, and to allow the graft material to be spread evenly over its surface. A strip of synthetic mesh is fixed to the anterior and posterior vaginal wall. The peritoneum overlying the presacral area is opened, extending to the posterior cul-de-sac. The sigmoid colon is retracted medially and the anterior surface of the sacrum is skeletonized. Two to four permanent sutures are placed through the anterior longitudinal ligament in the midline, starting at the S2 level and proceeding distally. The sutures are passed through the graft at an appropriate location to support the vaginal vault without tension. The peritoneum is then closed with an absorbable running suture. The most dangerous potential complication of sacrocolpopexy is life-threatening sacral hemorrhage.

SURGERY FOR STRESS URINARY INCONTINENCE

There are a multitude of studies addressing the efficacy of different surgical procedures for urinary incontinence. The interpretation of this literature is often difficult because of a lack of standardized definitions or standardized procedures. Stress incontinence is believed to be caused by lack of urethrovaginal support (urethral hypermobility) or intrinsic sphincter deficiency (ISD). *ISD* is a term applied to a subset of stress-incontinent patients who have particularly severe symptoms, including urine leakage with minimal exertion. This condition often is recognized clinically as the low pressure or "drainpipe" urethra. The urethral sphincter mechanism in these patients is severely damaged, limiting coaptation of the urethra. There are no set specific or objective criteria that define ISD, although urodynamic criteria often are used to support it. Standard surgical procedures used to correct stress incontinence share a common feature: partial urethral obstruction that achieves urethral closure under stress. Despite older literature to the contrary, this objective does not require that the bladder neck be "elevated to a high retropubic location."[39]

Needle Suspension

The transvaginal needle suspension was first described in 1959 by Pereyra.[40] Variations on this technique include the Stamey, Gittes, and Raz procedures. After an anterior colpotomy is made, the vaginal epithelium is dissected and mobilized to the level of the descending pubic rami. The space of Retzius is entered bilaterally using a blunt clamp or closed heavy Mayo scissors to penetrate the perineal membrane along the inferior aspect of the descending pubic ramus. A long, angled needle is passed through a small transverse suprapubic incision, through the rectus fascia, through the space of Retzius, to bring up the ends of a suture that has been secured to the periurethral vaginal muscularis. Variations exist in the way in which the suture is attached to the periurethral tissue and the method of abdominal wall fixation. Long-term studies of needle procedures have shown evidence of steadily increasing failure rates, likely a result of suture pullout from the periurethral vaginal tissue.

Retropubic Colposuspension

The space of Retzius is approached extraperitoneally, from an abdominal approach, allowing the bladder to be mobilized from the surrounding adipose tissue and lateral pelvis. Overlying fat and blood vessels in the area of the vesical neck are cleared away.

Marshall-Marchetti-Krantz Procedure

In the Marshall-Marchetti-Krantz procedure, a permanent suture is placed lateral to the urethra bilaterally and tied to the periosteum of the pubic ramus or perichondrium of the symphysis pubis. The surgical objective is to appose the urethra to (or within 1 to 2 cm of) the posterior surface of the symphysis pubis. Osteitis pubis is a rare, but serious, potential complication that can result from trauma and devascularization of the symphysis. This and suture pullout from the symphysis has prompted the search for improved techniques.

Burch Procedure

The most quoted description of the Burch procedure is that of Tanagho in 1976.[41] Two pairs of large-caliber delayed-absorbable suture are placed through the periurethral vaginal wall, one pair at the midurethra and one at the urethrovesical junction. Each stitch is then anchored to the ipsilateral Cooper's (iliopectineal) ligament. The sutures are tied with the operator's nondominant hand placed vaginally to give preferential support to the urethrovesical junction relative to the anterior vaginal wall without overcorrection. Long-term outcome studies up to 10 years have shown the Burch procedure yields cure rates of 80 to 85%.

Suburethral Sling

A variety of organic and synthetic graft materials have been used to construct suburethral slings. Synthetic materials fell out of favor after a high incidence of postoperative urinary retention and urethral damage were found to be associated with their use. Currently, the most commonly used sling materials include autografts of rectus fascia and processed cadaveric allografts (fascia lata). The procedure is performed by a combined abdominovaginal approach, using a small transverse suprapubic skin incision. The anterior vaginal epithelium is incised in the midline from the midurethra to just proximal to the urethrovesical junction, as identified by the bulb of an indwelling urethral catheter. The epithelium is dissected from the underlying muscularis using sharp dissection bilaterally. The space of Retzius is entered using a blunt clamp or closed heavy Mayo scissors to penetrate the perineal membrane along the inferior aspect of the descending pubic ramus. Maintenance of the proper angle of penetration is important to minimize the risk of injury to the obturator neurovascular bundle or ilioinguinal nerve laterally, and urethra or bladder medially. A Bozeman clamp or long-angled ligature carrier is used to perforate the rectus fascia two fingerbreadths superior to the pubic bone just medial to the pubic tubercle, and the instrument is guided along the back of the pubic bone through the space of Retzius and into the vaginal incision to retrieve one arm of the sling. After bringing up the other side of the sling, and confirming the absence of urinary tract injury, the sling arms are tied. Most often the sling arms are sutured to the rectus fascia or to one another, although procedures using pubic bone anchors also have been described. The base of the sling is positioned at the urethrovesical junction. Cure rates range from 75 to 95% for the many different types of sling procedures. Slings are associated with higher complication rates than most other incontinence procedures, most frequently involving voiding dysfunction, urinary retention, new-onset urge incontinence, and foreign-body erosion.

Tensionless Sling

The tension-free vaginal tape is a modified sling that uses a strip of polypropylene mesh. Unlike traditional sling procedures, the mesh is positioned at the midurethra, not the urethrovesical junction, and is not sutured or otherwise fixed into place. Advantages of tension-free vaginal tape include the ability to perform the procedure under local anesthesia and on an outpatient basis. Small subepithelial tunnels are made bilaterally to the descending pubic rami through an anterior vaginal wall incision. A specialized conical metal needle coupled to a handle is used to drive one end of the sling through the perineal membrane, space of Retzius, and through one of two small suprapubic stab incisions. The tape is set in place without any tension after bringing up the other end of the tape through the other side. Recently, multiple modifications have been made to carry the tape through the bilateral medial portions of the obturator space. Risks of the procedure include visceral injury from blind introduction of the needle, bleeding, and nerve and muscle injury in the obturator space. Additionally, voiding dysfunction and delayed erosion of mesh into the bladder or urethra has been seen.

Collagen

Bulking agent injection is indicated for patients with urodynamically proven stress incontinence that meets criteria for ISD, but is negative for urethral hypermobility. Glutaraldehyde cross-linked bovine dermal collagen has since become the most widely used injectable agent. Use of other materials, including silicone polymers (Macroplastique) and carbon-coated zirconium beads (Durasphere), also has been described. Anesthesia is easily obtained by using intraurethral 2% lidocaine jelly and/or transvaginal injection of the periurethral tissues with 5 mL of 1% lidocaine. A transurethral or periurethral technique may be used, using a 30° operating female cystourethroscope to directly visualize the injection. The material is injected underneath the urethral mucosa at the bladder neck and proximal urethra, usually at the 4 and 8 o'clock positions, until mucosal apposition is seen. Patients must demonstrate a negative reaction to a collagen skin test before injection. The long-term cure rate is 20 to 30%, with an additional 50 to 60% of patients demonstrating improvement.[31] Repeat injections frequently are necessary because of migration and dissolution of the collagen material.

PELVIC NEOPLASMS

Vulvaginal Lesions

Benign Vulvar Lesions

Many women suffer with undiagnosed symptoms of vulvar disease. They endure vulvar itching and pain and eventually seek medical help only to be commonly misdiagnosed and treated with repeated courses of antifungals. Vulvar conditions like contact dermatitis, atrophic vulvovaginitis, lichen sclerosis, lichen planus, lichen chronicus simplex, Paget's disease, Bowen's disease, and invasive vulvar cancer are not uncommon. Systemic disease like psoriasis, eczema, Crohn's disease, Behçet's disease, vitiligo, and seborrheic dermatitis may also involve the vulvar skin. Patients presenting with chronic vulvar symptoms should be carefully interviewed, examined, and a vulvar biopsy obtained whenever the diagnosis is in question, the patient is not responding to treatment, or premalignant and malignant disease is suspected.

Atrophic Vulvovaginitis This is common in postmenopausal patients and causes thinning and atrophy of the vaginal mucosa and vulvar skin secondary to inadequate estrogenation. Patients may be asymptomatic or present with vulvar itching, burning, and/or dyspareunia. This condition is commonly managed with vaginal estrogen preparations used once or twice weekly.

Vulvar Contact Dermatitis This dermatitis is a common cause of acute or chronic vulvar pruritus and can be irritant or allergic.[42] Irritant dermatitis usually results from overzealous hygiene habits such as the use of harsh soaps and frequent douching, but is also common in patients with urinary or fecal incontinence, especially the elderly and the disabled. Allergic vulvar dermatitis is caused by a variety of allergens such as fragrances and topical antibiotics. The mainstay of treatment is to identify and discontinue the offending agent or practice, or providing a skin barrier in the case of incontinence.

Leukoplakias There are three types of leukoplakia, a flat white abnormality. *Lichen sclerosis* is the most common cause of leukoplakia.[42] It affects women 30 to 40 years of age. Classically, it results in a figure-of-eight pattern of white epithelium around the anus and vulva, resulting in variable scarring and itching, and, less commonly, pain. Diagnosis is confirmed with biopsy and treatment consists of steroids such as clobetasol 0.05% ointment daily for up to 12 weeks. *Lichen planus* is a cause of leukoplakia with an onset in the fifth and sixth decade of life. Lichen planus, in contrast to lichen sclerosis, which is limited to the vulva and perianal skin, can involve the vagina and oral mucosa, and erosions occur in the majority of patients leading to a variable degree of scarring. Patients usually have a history of dysuria and dyspareunia and complain of a burning vulvar pain. Histology is not specific, and biopsy is recommended. Treatment is with steroid ointments. Systemic steroids are indicated for severe and/or unresponsive cases. *Lichen simplex chronicus* is the third cause of leukoplakia, but is distinguished from the other lichen diseases by epidermal thickening, absence of scarring, and a severe intolerable itch.[42] Intense scratching is not uncommon and contributes to the severity of the symptoms and predisposes the cracked skin to infections. Treatment consists of cessation of the scratching that sometimes requires sedation, elimination of any allergen or irritant, suppression of inflammation with potent steroid ointments, and treatment of any coexisting infections.

Paget's Disease of the Vulva Paget's disease of the vulva is an intraepithelial disease of unknown etiology that affects mostly white postmenopausal women in their sixth decade of life. It causes chronic vulvar itching and is sometimes associated with an underlying invasive vulvar adenocarcinoma or invasive cancers of the breast, cervix, or GI tract. Grossly, the lesion is variable but usually confluent, raised, erythematous to violet, and waxy in appearance. Biopsy is required for diagnosis; the disease is intraepithelial and characterized by Paget's cells with large pale cytoplasm. Treatment is assessment for other potential concurrent adenocarcinomas and then surgical removal by wide local resection of the involved area with a 2-cm margin. Free margins are difficult to obtain because the disease usually extends beyond the clinically visible area.[43,44] Intraoperative frozen section of the margins can be done to ensure complete resection. Unfortunately, Paget's vulvar lesions have a high likelihood of recurrence even after securing negative resection margins.

Vulvar Intraepithelial Neoplasia

Vulvar intraepithelial neoplasia (VIN) is similar to its cervical intraepithelial neoplasia (CIN) counterpart and is graded on the degree of epithelial involvement as mild (VIN I), moderate (VIN II), severe (VIN III), or vulvar carcinoma in situ (Bowen's disease).[45] Risk factors include HPV infection, prior VIN, HIV infection, immunosuppression, smoking, vulvar dermatoses such as lichen sclerosis, CIN, and cervical cancer. VIN can be unifocal or multifocal. Unifocal lesions commonly affect postmenopausal women and lack a clear association with HPV, while multifocal disease mostly affects younger reproductive age females and has a strong association with HPV infection. Fifty percent of patients are asymptomatic, with vulvar pruritus being the most common complaint in those with symptoms. Lesions may be vague or raised, and velvety with sharply demarcated borders. Diagnosis is made with a vulvar skin

biopsy and multiple biopsies are sometimes necessary. Colposcopy with application of 5% acetic acid and identification of the acetowhite lesions of VIN is a valuable diagnostic tool for subtle lesions and will help guide the biopsy. Evaluation of the perianal and anal area is important as the disease may involve these areas, particularly in immunocompromised and nicotine-addicted women. Once invasive disease is ruled out, treatment usually involves wide surgical excision; however, the initial treatment approach may include 5% imiquimod cream, carbon dioxide laser ablation, or cavitational ultrasonic surgical aspiration and depends on the number of lesions and their severity. When laser ablation is used, a 1-mm depth in hair-free areas is usually sufficient, while hairy lesions require ablation to a 3-mm depth because the hair follicles' roots can reach a depth of 2.5 mm. Unfortunately, VIN tends to recur in up to 30% of cases and high-grade lesions (VIN III, carcinoma in situ) progress to invasive disease in approximately 10% of patients if left untreated.[46]

Vulvar Cancer

Vulvar cancer is the fourth most common gynecologic cancer and is responsible for 4% of the female reproductive cancers and 0.6% of all cancers in women.[47] It mostly affects postmenopausal women, and the mean age at diagnosis is 65 years old. Risks factors are similar to those for VIN with persistent infection with high-risk HPV types being responsible for the majority of cases. Patients usually present with a vulvar ulcer or mass. Pruritus is a common complaint, and vulvar bleeding or enlarged inguinal lymph nodes are signs of advanced disease. Careful evaluation of the patient is necessary to rule out concurrent lesions of the vagina and cervix. Biopsy is required and should be sufficient to allow evaluation of the extent of stromal invasion. Vulvar carcinomas are squamous in 90% of cases. Other less common histologies include melanoma (5%), basal cell carcinoma (2%), and soft tissue sarcomas (1 to 2%).

Spread of the vulvar carcinomas is by direct local extension and via lymphatic microembolization. Hematogenous spread is uncommon except for vulvar melanoma. Lymphatic spread seems to follow a stepwise, predictable pattern (Fig. 41-13): (a) the superficial inguinal lymph nodes, which lie in the subcutaneous tissue overlying the inguinal ligament; (b) the deep inguinal lymph nodes, which lie along the course of the round ligament in the inguinal canal; (c) the superficial femoral lymph nodes, grouped around the saphenous vein just superficial to the fossa ovalis; (d) the deep femoral lymph nodes, including the most cephalad node of Cloquet or Rosenmüller; and ultimately, (e) the external iliac lymph nodes.[48–50] The node of Cloquet is an important sentinel node situated in the route of spread to the pelvic lymph nodes. Vulvar cancer is staged

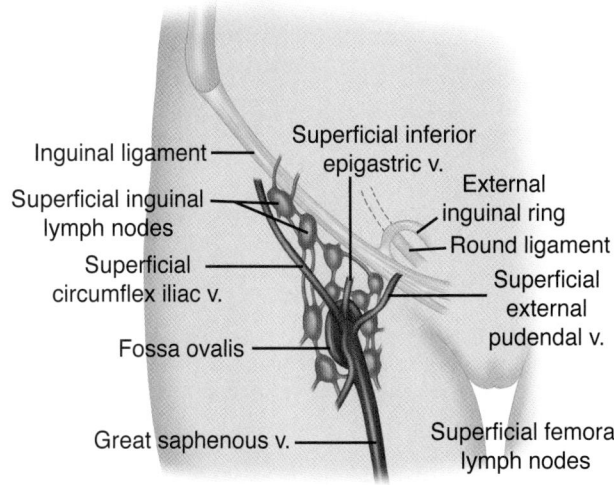

FIG. 41-13. Lymphatic drainage of the vulva delineated by Stanley Way. v. = vein.

TABLE 41-6	International Federation of Gynecology and Obstetrics staging of vulvar carcinoma
Stage	
0	Carcinoma in situ, intraepithelial carcinoma
IA	Tumor confined to the vulva or perineum, ≤2 cm in greatest dimension, negative nodes, stromal invasion ≤1 mm
IB	Tumor confined to the vulva or perineum, ≤2 cm in greatest dimension, negative nodes, stromal invasion >1 mm
II	Tumor confined to the vulva and/or perineum, >2 cm in greatest dimension, negative nodes
III	Tumor of any size with adjacent spread to the lower urethra or anus and/or unilateral regional lymph node metastasis
IVA	Tumor invades any of the following: upper urethra, bladder or rectal mucosa, pelvic bone, or bilateral regional node metastasis
IVB	Any distant metastasis including pelvic lymph nodes

surgically with the inguinofemoral lymph node status being the most important prognostic factor. The International Federation of Gynecology and Obstetrics staging system for vulvar cancer is widely used and provides a schema in which prognosis and therapy are closely linked to stage (Table 41-6).[51] Patients with early-stage disease have a favorable prognosis with approximately 90% 5-year survival rates for stage I disease; stages III and IV disease carry a poor prognosis with 5-year survival rates ranging from 15 to 30%. The exception is melanoma for which the pathologic staging by depth of invasion of the primary tumor and then known metastases is more likely to identify risk for recurrence.

Treatment is individualized, especially with early-stage disease. Surgical resection is the mainstay of treatment for early stages. The most conservative procedure should be performed in view of the high morbidity of aggressive surgical management.[48–50] The historical single-stage en bloc radical vulvectomy championed by Way and Taussig (Fig. 41-14) has been largely abandoned and replaced by the modified radical vulvectomy and bilateral inguinofemoral lymphadenectomy performed through three separate incisions. Stage IA can be adequately treated with an excisional biopsy with a 1-cm disease-free margin. Stages IB and II disease require radical

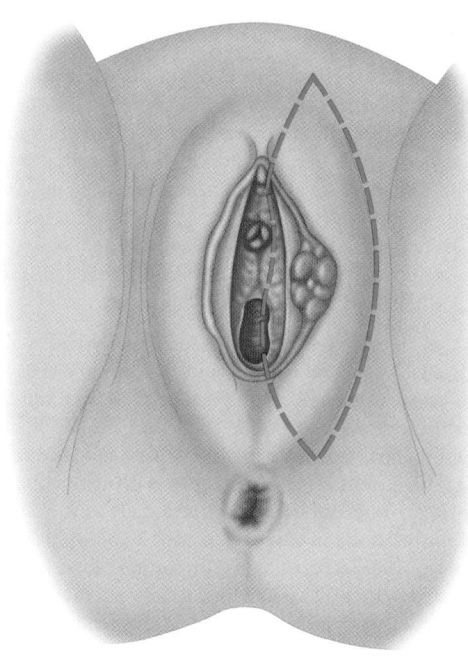

FIG. 41-15. Extent of modified radical hemivulvectomy for stages I and II squamous cancer of the vulva.

wide excision with a 2-cm margin, but modified radical hemivulvectomy also is used (Fig. 41-15).

Treatment options for stage III and IV disease include: (a) chemoradiation followed by limited resection if needed, (b) radical vulvectomy, and (c) radical vulvectomy coupled with pelvic exenteration. Recently, external beam radiotherapy combined with radiosensitizing chemotherapy of cisplatin and 5-fluorouracil is emerging as the preferred initial management of advanced disease followed by limited surgical resection of residual disease.[52,53] Reconstruction of the vulva and groin, if needed, can be accomplished by using myocutaneous flaps based on the gracilis, sartorius, or tensor fasciae latae muscles.

The need for inguinal lymphadenectomy (Figs. 41-16 and 41-17) is dictated by the extent of the disease and is essential for planning therapy to provide a better opportunity for cure. Nodal involvement is rare in stage IA, and hence, lymphadenectomy is not needed. Inguinal lymphadenectomy is indicated beyond stage IA and unilateral is recommended for lateralized lesions or bilateral for central lesions that cross the midline or those involving the periclitoral area. The extent of dissection varies from superficial in the case of clinically negative

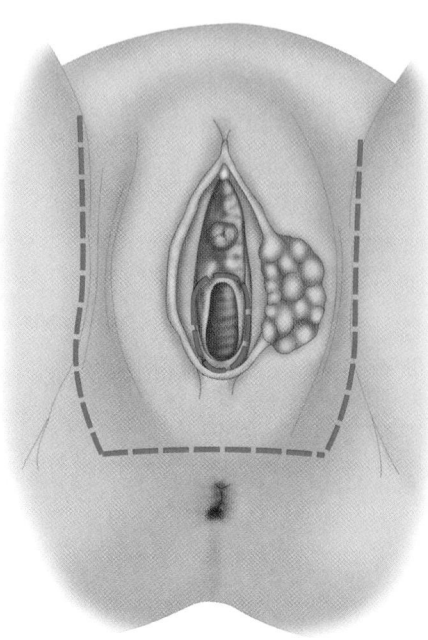

FIG. 41-14. En bloc radical vulvectomy outlined by Way and Taussig.

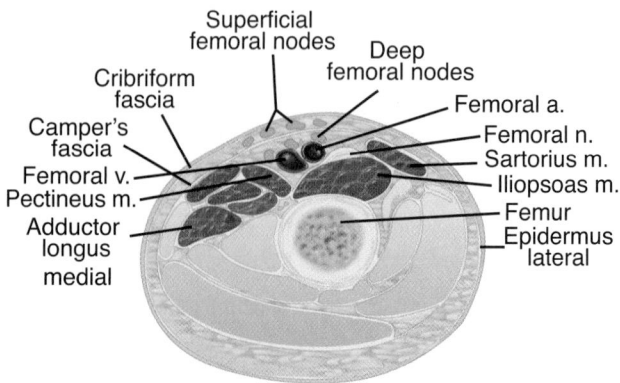

FIG. 41-16. Superficial inguinal lymphadenectomy. a. = artery; m. = muscle; n. = nerve.

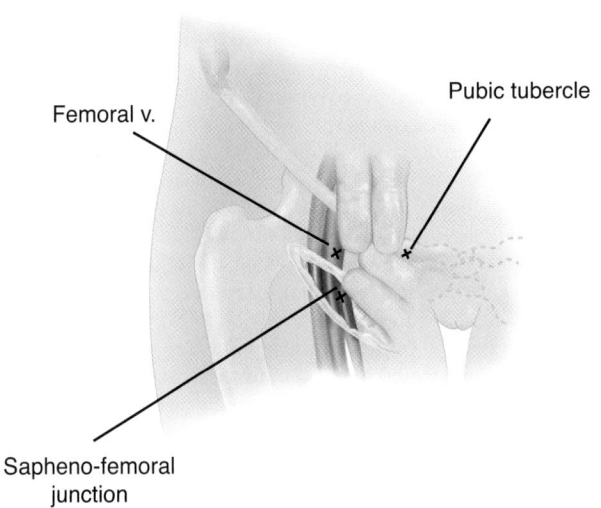

FIG. 41-17. Incision recommended for superficial inguinal lymph-adenectomy. v. = vein.

nodes, resection of gross-only disease, to full groin dissection. Vulvar sentinel lymph node biopsy is under investigation by the Gynecologic Oncology Group (GOG). This concept is widely used in breast cancer and melanoma and involves peritumor injection of isosulfan blue dye, a radioactive tracer, or a combination of both to facilitate intraoperative identification of involved sentinel nodes in the majority of patients. Preliminary data are encouraging and may allow patients with negative sentinel nodes to avoid complete groin dissection and its attendant morbidity such as lower extremity lymphedema.

Nodal failure in the groin and pelvis is difficult to treat successfully, and attention to primary management of these areas is key. Postoperative adjuvant inguinal and pelvic radiotherapy is indicated when inguinal lymph nodes are positive, and is superior to pelvic lymphadenectomy, which has been largely abandoned. It also is indicated when the vulvectomy margins are positive or close positive for disease and further surgical management is not anatomically feasible.

Vaginal Cancer

Vaginal carcinoma is a rare gynecologic malignancy and accounts for only about 2 to 3% of cancers affecting the female reproductive system.[54] Squamous cell carcinomas account for 85 to 90% of cases, while adenocarcinomas, malignant melanomas, and soft tissue sarcomas make up the remaining 10 to 15%. More than two thirds of vaginal cancers are diagnosed in women 60 years of age or older. Risk factors include vaginal intraepithelial neoplasia (VAIN), persistent HPV infection with high-risk types, VIN, CIN and cervical cancer, diethylstilbestrol (DES) exposure in utero, smoking, HIV infection, and immunosuppression. Patients with vaginal cancer usually present with postmenopausal and/or postcoital bleeding and may also complain of vaginal discharge, vaginal mass, dysuria, hematuria, rectal bleeding, or pelvic pain which may be indicative of advanced disease. Diagnosis is made via biopsy of suspicious lesions, which may require colposcopic guidance.

DES is a drug used in the past in the management of patients with recurrent miscarriages. It was removed from the market in 1971 secondary to reports linking its in utero exposure to the development of clear-cell adenocarcinoma of the cervix and vagina in the exposed daughters, as well as a variety of vaginal, cervical, and uterine anomalies.[55,56] The risk of clear-cell adenocarcinoma is one in 1000 of those exposed with an average age at diagnosis of 19 years (7 to 33 years). The incidence of vaginal clear-cell adenocarcinoma is in decline as most DES-exposed daughters are now older than 35 years, and beyond the risk range.

Vaginal Intraepithelial Neoplasia VAIN is similar to VIN and is classified based on the degree of epithelial involvement as mild (I), moderate (II), severe (III), or carcinoma-in-situ.[45] Upward of 65 to 80% of VAIN or vaginal cancers are associated with HPV infection. The majority of lesions are located in the upper one third of the vagina. Lesions are usually asymptomatic and found incidentally on cytologic screening. Diagnosis is made via guided biopsy of acetowhite lesions at the time of colposcopy. Lesions may appear flat or raised white with sharply demarcated borders and may show vascular changes. The presence of aberrant vessels with marked branching is suggestive of invasive disease. VAIN is treated with laser ablation, surgical excision, or topical 5-fluorouracil therapy.

Vaginal Carcinoma Vaginal cancer is staged clinically by pelvic exam, chest x-ray, cystoscopy, and proctoscopy (Table 41-7).[51] Studies such as IV pyelogram, barium enema, and CT scans also may be used as needed to define the extent of disease. Vaginal cancer spreads by local extension to adjacent pelvic structures, by lymphatic embolization to regional lymph nodes, and, less commonly, via the hematogenous route to distant organs such as the lungs and liver. Lesions in the upper vagina drain directly into the pelvic lymph nodes and onto the para-aortic nodes, while lesions involving the lower third drain initially to the inguinofemoral lymph nodes from which they then spread to the pelvic nodes.

Treatment of stage I disease, involving the upper vagina, may be achieved with surgery or via intracavitary radiation therapy.[48–50] Surgery consists of a radical hysterectomy, upper vaginectomy, and bilateral pelvic lymphadenectomy. Stage I disease in the mid- to lower vagina usually is treated with radiation and concurrent chemotherapy. External beam pelvic radiation is the mainstay of treatment for stages II–IV and may be followed by intracavitary and/or interstitial brachytherapy. With treatment, prognosis for early-stage disease is excellent with >90% 5-year survival rates. Advanced-stage disease, however, carries a poor prognosis with only 15 to 40% 5-year survival rates for stage III–IV disease.

Lesions of the Cervix

Benign Cervical Lesions

Benign lesions of the cervix include endocervical polyps, nabothian cysts (clear, fluid-filled cysts with smooth surfaces), posttrauma (such as delivery-related cervical tear, or prior cervical surgery) malformation of the cervix, and cervical condylomata. If small, office biopsy is appropriate if the diagnosis is not clear. For endocervical polyps, exploration of the base of the polyp with a cotton swab tip to identify that it is cervical and not uterine, and to identify the stalk characteristics, can help identify the appropriate surgical approach. If small, and the base is identified, simply grasping it with ring forceps and slowly rotating it until separated from the base may be adequate. Use of LEEP is appropriate for larger lesions or for specimens of areas identified as abnormal by colposcopy or visual

TABLE 41-7	International Federation of Gynecology and Obstetrics staging of vaginal carcinoma
Stage	
0	Carcinoma in situ; intraepithelial neoplasia grade 3
I	Tumor limited to the vaginal wall
II	Tumor has involved the subvaginal tissue but has not extended to the pelvic wall
III	Tumor extends to the pelvic wall
IV	Tumor has extended beyond the true pelvis or has involved the mucosa of the bladder or rectum
IVA	Tumor invades bladder and/or rectal mucosa and/or direct extension beyond the true pelvis
IVB	Distant metastasis

inspection. For condylomata proven by biopsy, LEEP or laser ablation is appropriate.

Cervical Cancer

Cervical cancer accounts for about 17,000 cases per year and over 5000 deaths in the United States. It is a major killer worldwide with 250,000 deaths annually. Cervical screening is correlated with early identification and treatment of preinvasive disease.[57] Cervical cancer is most common in women with long intervals between screening, or with no prior screening. The presence of inherited genetic variations that increase the likelihood of developing cervical cancer when exposed to oncogenic subtypes of HPV is likely and under active investigation.

The oncogenes of high-risk HPV are both initiating and promoting for cervical cancer. Other correlates with disease include concurrent active HIV infection with immunosuppression, smoking, and probably other genetic factors. It is anticipated that early vaccination, before infection, will function as primary prevention for cervical cancer. It is expected to reduce both the risk and frequency of high-grade CIN, but also translate to marked reduction in actual invasive cancer, requiring 20 to 40 years to see full impact. However, not all high-risk HPV subtypes are covered in the two vaccines available in 2009. Thus, vaccination will likely prevent approximately 70% of cancers in the United States, depending on regional area distribution of oncogenic subtypes. Vaccines are approved for girls ages 9 to 26, but are recommended preferentially for the younger girls as there was a stronger immunologic response seen.

Staging and Management The diagnosis of cervical cancer is made by cervical biopsy, either of a gross lesion or a colposcopically identified lesion. The majority of the histology is squamous, with adenocarcinoma comprising about 20% of cases, and occasional rare and aggressive variants such as neuroendocrine tumors. Staging is clinical, not surgical, and follows the International Federation of Gynecology and Obstetrics guidelines, which mesh with TNM staging. Staging and management options are outlined in Table 41-8.

Surgical Management *Radical Hysterectomy* This procedure generally is performed through an abdominal incision, either vertical or transverse muscle cutting, although laparoscopic and robotic-assisted radical hysterectomy is increasing.[58] The key elements are dissection of the pelvic and periaortic nodes, and the dissection of the parametrium from the pelvic sidewall to allow en bloc removal

with the uterus. Two areas of dissection account for the unique risks of this procedure. The dissection of the ureter out of the tunnel below the uterine arteries, allowing the uterine arteries to be ligated near the internal iliac artery, has a small increase in risk for ureterovaginal fistula equivalent to that of primary radiation. The dissection of the uterosacral ligaments around the rectum and development of the rectal space inferiorly carries an increased likelihood of constipation. These two key elements of the radical hysterectomy are illustrated in Fig. 41-18. Both laparoscopic and open radical hysterectomies allow for the maintenance of the ovaries because the incidence of metastases to this area is very low, providing a clear advantage over radiation therapy.

Initial evaluation of the abdomen and palpation of nodal areas and parametrium should be done to further assess the presence or absence of metastatic disease before proceeding with a radical hysterectomy and node dissection. Access to the retroperitoneum is obtained through opening the round ligaments at their lateral insertion to the pelvic wall (see Fig. 41-18C) and extending the peritoneal incision lateral to the infundibulopelvic ligaments bilaterally and contiguously over the bladder peritoneum. The paravesical space is opened using blunt dissection that follows the contour of the pelvic floor in the shape of a bowl down and medially around the bladder. A similar dissection, again following the bowl shape of the posterior pelvis, is used to dissect the pararectal space (see Fig. 41-18E), leaving the parametria between these two spaces for palpation for disease and dissection. The infundibulopelvic ligament or utero-ovarian ligament, depending on whether the patient is retaining ovaries, is identified separately from the ureter and separated at this point. The ureter is identified on the medial leaf of the broad ligament, dissected free, and suspended with vessel loops for traction as needed for full dissection through the canal under the uterine artery and into the bladder. The parametria is further dissected by lateral retraction of the superior vesicle artery and identification of the uterine artery and vein coursing in the parametria over the ureter. The ureter is dissected below with a right angle to allow for direct visualization when the artery and vein are clamped lateral to this, and then dissected medially over the ureter. This dissection should continue until the ureter is separated from the parametria down to the level of the ureter's bladder insertion. Posteriorly, the peritoneal incision is continued over the cul-de-sac and the medial peritoneum separated from the ureter. The rectovaginal space is developed bluntly, by opening this cul-de-sac area and then blunt dissection parallel to the vagina (parallel to the floor). The uterosacral ligaments are identified between the pararectal and rectovaginal spaces which can then be

---

TABLE 41-8 International Federation of Gynecology and Obstetrics cervical cancer staging and management options

Stage	Description	Options for Management
0	Carcinoma-in-situ	Adenocarcinoma in situ: hysterectomy, although some may be followed for preservation if all margins negative on cone Squamous-in-situ: local excision with loop electrosurgical excision procedure or cone or laser ablation
I	Confined to the cervix A1: minimal invasion A2: <5 mm from base of epithelium and ≤7 mm lateral spread B1: More than A2 and <4 cm total diameter B2: >4 cm total diameter	A1 and some A2: fertility preservation through large cone followed by close monitoring, followed by hysterectomy B1 and B2: radical hysterectomy or chemoradiation; radical trachelectomy with uterine preservation for childbearing is under investigation for highly selected patients
II	Involvement of the upper two thirds of the vagina, without parametrial involvement (A) or with parametrial involvement (B)	For some IIA radical hysterectomy may be considered IIA and B: chemoradiation is preferred
III	A. Involvement of the lower third of the vagina B. Involvement of a parametria to the sidewall or obstruction of one or both ureters on imaging	Chemoradiation
IV	A. Local involvement of the bladder or rectum B. Distant metastases	A. Chemoradiation B. Chemotherapy with palliative radiation as indicated

ligated with an ENDO GIA or serial clamps. Further dissection anteriorly frees the bladder from the vagina and the vaginal tissue is then clamped and cut. Lymphadenectomy can be performed either before the radical hysterectomy or after and includes the external and internal iliac chains distally to the level of the circumflex vein, the obturator fossa (with direct visualization of the obturator nerve), and para-aortic chains as appropriate.

Radical Trachelectomy with Intact Uterus Interest in fertility preservation with stage IA1 and 2, and stage IB1 lesions has led to the development of methods of radical trachelectomy with uterine preservation. This procedure depends on an adequate blood supply to the uterus from the ovarian anastomoses, as the cervical portion is removed. The lower uterine segment is closed with a cerclage and attached directly to the vaginal cuff. The rates of recurrence, pregnancy outcomes, and the best surgical candidates for this surgery are still under development.

Radical Trachelectomy after Prior Supracervical Hysterectomy With the increase in supracervical hysterectomies, the incidence of trachelectomy and radical trachelectomy also is increasing. The procedure follows the same precepts of a radical hysterectomy, but with scarring, and the risk for ureteral, bladder, or bowel injury is higher. Even so, for younger women, this is preferable to primary radiation.

Pelvic Exenteration for Recurrent Disease Cervical cancer recurrences after primary surgical management are treated with radiation. Surgery may be a consideration in selected patients with recurrent cervical cancer who have received maximal radiation therapy. If the recurrence is locally confined with no evidence of spread or metastatic disease, then pelvic exenteration may be considered. This procedure is becoming less frequent because of the increased local control achieved with chemoradiation, and the frequency of the presence of metastatic disease upon recurrence. Attempted exenteration procedures are aborted intraoperatively if metastatic disease is found. Exenteration is tailored for the disease size and location and may be supralevator or extend below the levator ani muscle and require vulvar resection as well (Fig. 41-19). Reconstruction of the pelvis may require a continent urinary pouch (if radiation enteritis is limited) or ileal conduit and colostomy, as well as rebuilding the pelvic floor and vagina with gracilis or other grafts.

Uterine Corpus
Benign Uterine Diseases

The average age of menarche, first menstrual period, in the United States is 12 years and 5 months. Duration of normal menstruation is between 2 to 7 days, with a flow of <80 mL, and cycles of 21 to 35 days. Various female reproductive disorders such as dysfunctional uterine bleeding (DUB), miscarriages, leiomyomas, uterine polyps, adenomyosis, endometrial hyperplasia, and uterine cancer have in common abnormally heavy uterine bleeding as a frequent manifestation.[59] Nonpregnant patients, who present with heavy bleeding and are 35 years of age and older or have risk factors for endometrial cancer, must be ruled out for malignancy as the first step in their management. Abnormal uterine bleeding is described based on the bleeding pattern:

- Menorrhagia: prolonged (>7 days) or excessive (>80 mL daily) menstrual cycles occurring at regular intervals
- Metrorrhagia: menstrual cycles occurring at irregular intervals and more frequently
- Menometrorrhagia: prolonged or excessive menstrual cycles occurring at irregular and more frequent intervals

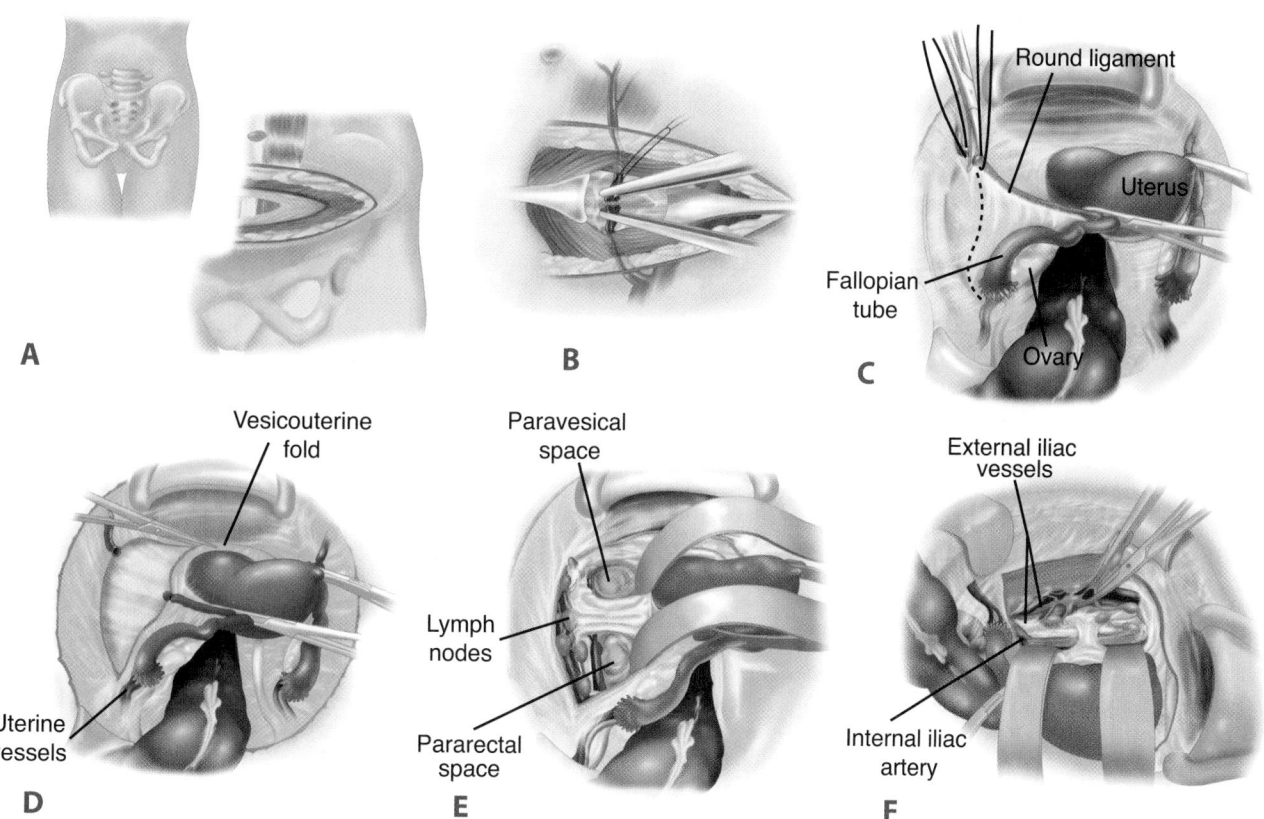

FIG. 41-18. Radical hysterectomy. **A.** Exposure of the inferior epigastric vessels before transection of the rectus muscles. **B.** Ligation of the inferior epigastric vessels before transection of the rectus muscles. **C.** Ligation and division of the round ligaments opens the pelvic retroperitoneum. **D.** First peritoneal incision lateral to the ovarian vessels and across the vesicouterine fold. **E.** Narrow malleable retractors (Indiana retractors) are placed into the paravesical and pararectal spaces to provide excellent access to the lateral pelvic sidewall and pelvic lymph nodes. **F.** Pelvic lymphadenectomy (external and internal iliac vessels). *(Continued)*

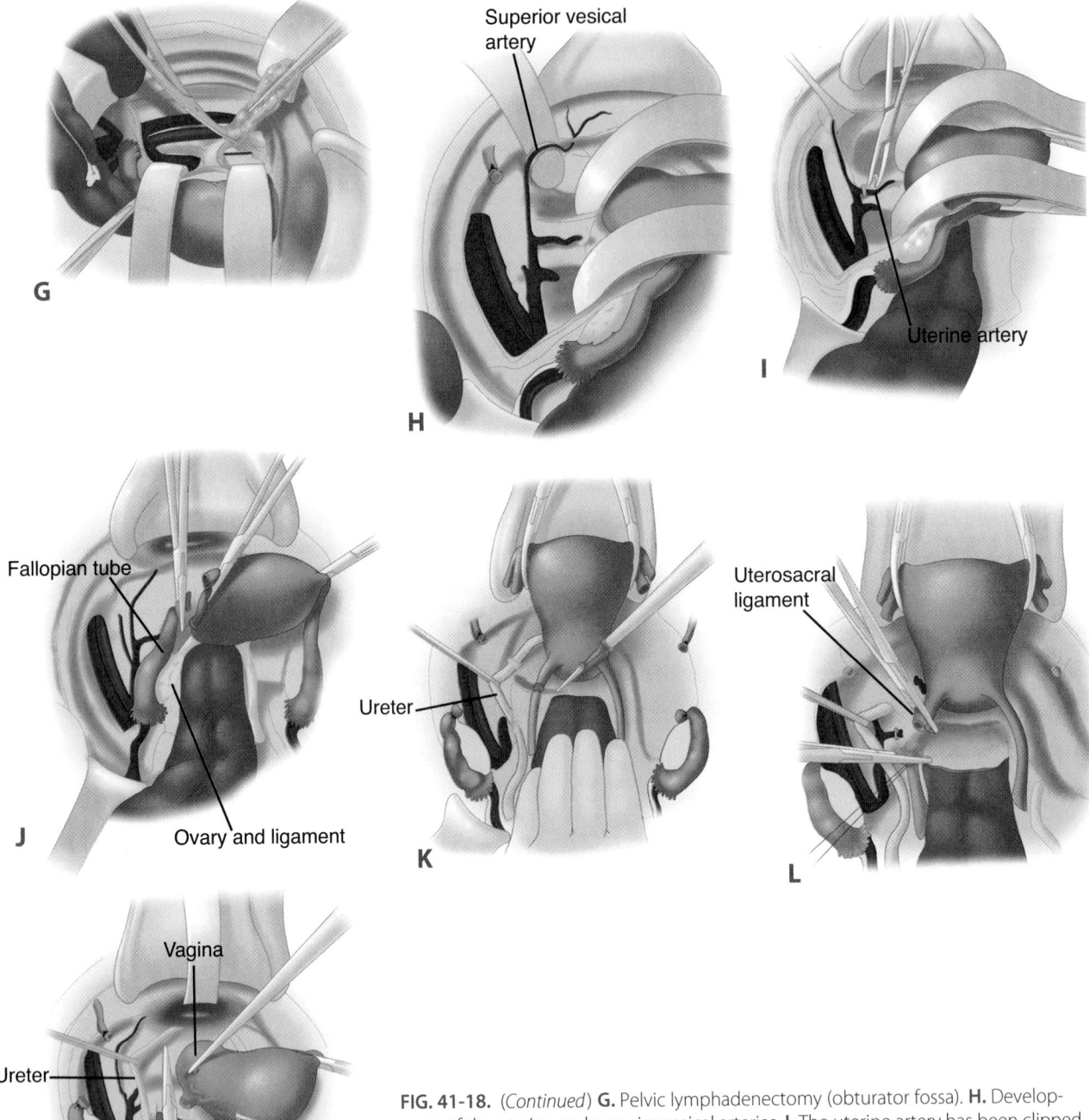

FIG. 41-18. (*Continued*) **G.** Pelvic lymphadenectomy (obturator fossa). **H.** Development of the uterine and superior vesical arteries. **I.** The uterine artery has been clipped and divided near its origin. **J.** The proper ovarian ligament and proximal fallopian tube are clamped and divided if the ovary is to be preserved. **K.** The ureters have been detached from the posterior peritoneum of the broad ligament and are retracted laterally. The rectovaginal space is developed using blunt finger dissection. **L.** Transection of the uterosacral ligaments. **M.** Clamps are placed on the lateral vagina, taking care to remove 3 to 4 cm of the upper vagina.

- Intermenstrual bleeding (spotting): bleeding of variable amounts occurring between regular menstrual cycles
- Polymenorrhea: menstrual cycles occurring at regular intervals of <21 days
- Oligomenorrhea: menstrual cycles occurring at intervals of >35 days
- Amenorrhea: absence of uterine bleeding for 6 months or a period equivalent to three missed cycles

Dysfunctional Uterine Bleeding DUB is the most common cause of abnormal uterine bleeding during the reproductive years. DUB is defined as uterine bleeding not explained by an identifiable anatomic or structural cause such as polyps or fibroids. It is common in adolescents and in perimenopausal women and manifests as menorrhagia or menometrorrhagia with intervening periods of oligomenorrhea or complete amenorrhea. Bleeding can at times be severe, and patients may present with anemia and hypovolemia-related symptoms necessitating blood transfusions. The most common cause of DUB is anovulatory cycles that often can be managed by cycling patients on oral contraceptive pills (OCPs) or insertion of a progestin-releasing intrauterine device (Mirena IUD).

Endometrial Polyps Endometrial polyps are localized hyperplastic growth of endometrial glands and stroma around a vascular core forming sessile or pedunculated projections from the surface of the endometrium.[60] They may be single or multiple. Many are asymp-

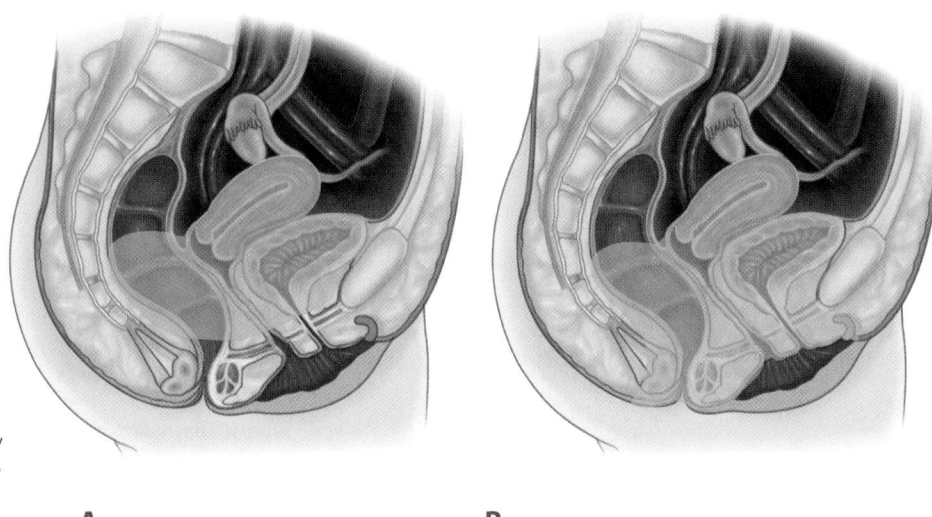

FIG. 41-19. Pelvic exenteration may be limited to the supralevator space (**A**) or can extend below the levator ani muscle (*shaded area*) (**B**).

A

B

tomatic; however, they are responsible for about 25% of cases of abnormal uterine bleeding, usually metrorrhagia. Polyps are common in patients on tamoxifen therapy (30%) and in perimenopausal and postmenopausal women. Endometrial polyps are rarely neoplastic (<1%). Up to 30% may harbor foci of endometrial hyperplasia. Diagnosis can be made with saline infused hysterosonography, hysterosalpingography, or by direct visualization at the time of hysteroscopy. Treatment, in the absence of malignancy, involves resection with an operative hysteroscope or by sharp curettage.

Adenomyosis *Adenomyosis* refers to ectopic endometrial glands and stroma situated within the myometrium. When diffuse, it results in globular uterine enlargement secondary to hyperplasia and hypertrophy of the surrounding myometrium. Adenomyosis is very common, tends to occur in parous women, and is frequently an incidental finding at the time of surgery. Adenomyosis causes heavy painful menses when symptomatic. Diagnosis is suspected in a parous woman with menorrhagia, dysmenorrhea, and diffuse globular uterine enlargement. MRI may reveal islands within the myometrium with increased signal intensity.[61] Definitive diagnosis is made by pathologic examination of the hysterectomy specimen, and hysterectomy is the only definitive treatment for this condition.

Endometriosis Endometriosis is the finding of ectopic endometrial glands and stroma outside the uterus. It a common condition affecting 10% of the general population, and it is an incidental finding at the time of laparoscopy in >20% of asymptomatic women. It is especially prevalent in patients suffering from chronic pelvic pain (80%) and infertility (20 to 50%).[59] The pathophysiology of endometriosis is poorly understood, and etiologic theories explaining dissemination of endometrial glands include retrograde menstruation, lymphatic and vascular spread of endometrial glands, and coelomic metaplasia. Endometriosis commonly involves the ovaries, pelvic peritoneal surfaces, and uterosacral ligaments. Other possible sites include the rectovaginal septum, sigmoid colon, intraperitoneal organs, retroperitoneal space, ureters, incisional scars, umbilicus, and even the thoracic cavity. Involvement of the fallopian tubes may lead to scarring, blockage, and subsequent infertility. Ovarian involvement varies from superficial implants to large complex ovarian masses called *endometriomas* ("chocolate cysts"). Endometriomas are found in approximately one third of women with endometriosis and often are bilateral.

Endometriosis can be totally asymptomatic, and symptoms, when present, vary from mild dyspareunia and cyclic dysmenorrhea to debilitating chronic pelvic pain with acute exacerbations at the time of menses. Less common manifestations include painful defecation, hematochezia, and hematuria if there is bowel and/or

bladder involvement. Pelvic examination in symptomatic patients typically demonstrates generalized pelvic tenderness, nodularity of the uterosacral ligaments, and, at times, a pelvic mass may be appreciated if an endometrioma is present. The severity of symptoms does not correlate with the degree of clinical disease present. Endometriosis also can cause increase in serum CA 125, a biomarker used to monitor response of epithelial ovarian cancer to therapy. CA 125 is neither strongly sensitive nor specific for ovarian cancer and can be elevated with other inflammatory and neoplastic pathologies involving the female reproductive tract and those that irritate the peritoneal and/or serosal surfaces. It can be elevated beyond the normal range (<35 U/mL) in women with ovarian and other sites of endometriosis and does not signify that there is an underlying ovarian cancer. Definite diagnosis of endometriosis usually requires laparoscopy and visualization of the pathognomonic endometriotic implants. These appear as blue, brown, black, white, or yellow lesions that can be raised and, at times, puckered, giving them a "gunpowder" appearance. Biopsy is not routinely done but should be obtained if the diagnosis is in doubt.

Treatment is guided by severity of the symptoms and whether preservation of fertility is desired and varies from expectant, medical, to surgical.[62,63] Expectant management is appropriate in asymptomatic patients. Those with mild symptoms can be managed successfully with cyclic or continuous OCPs combined with the as-needed use of analgesics such as NSAIDs. Moderate symptoms are treated with medroxyprogesterone acetate 10 to 20 mg orally daily or 150 mg IM injection every 3 months. Its use should be limited to 2 years or less because of its negative effects on bone density. Severe symptoms are treated with either danazol or gonadotropin-releasing hormone (GnRH) agonists to induce medical pseudomenopause. Danazol has been largely abandoned secondary to its marked androgenic side effects, such as acne and hirsutism. GnRH agonists act by suppressing the release of gonadotropins (luteinizing and follicle-stimulating hormones) from the pituitary gland and are available in injections or nasal spray preparations. Common side effects include hot flashes and vaginal dryness secondary to the hypoestrogenic state. They also result in decreased bone density, and their use should not exceed 6 months. Conservative surgical therapy is a popular option because it can be done at the time of the diagnostic laparoscopy and usually involves lysis of adhesions, ablation of endometriotic implants using carbon dioxide laser or electrocautery, and/or resection of deep endometriotic implants.[62] Patients with moderate to severe symptoms are commonly placed on GnRH agonists for 6 months following the surgery, which usually results in longer remissions. Endometriomas rarely respond to medical therapy, and surgical intervention is indicated and usually involves cystectomy with complete resection of the cyst wall. Medical therapy is no better than expectant management on subsequent pregnancy rates in patients infertile due to endometriosis. Conservative surgical therapy in patients with patent fallopian tubes results in pregnancy in about 50% of cases. Unfortunately, endometriosis is a chronic disease and conservative therapy, medical or surgical, provides only temporary relief, with the majority of patients relapsing within 1 to 2 years. In patients with severe debilitating symptoms who do not desire future fertility and have not responded to conservative management, extirpative surgery to remove the uterus, ovaries, and fallopian tubes is curative and should be considered.

Uterine Leiomyomas Leiomyomas, also known colloquially as *fibroids*, are the most common female pelvic tumor and represent growth of the uterine smooth muscle cells (myometrium). They are common in the reproductive years and by age 50 years old, at least 60% of white and up to 80% of black women are or have been affected. Leiomyomas vary in size, location, number, and effect and are described according to their anatomic location (Fig. 41-20) as intramural, subserosal, submucosal, pedunculated, cervical, and can rarely be ectopic.[59] Most are asymptomatic; however, abnormal uterine bleeding caused by leiomyomas is the most common indication for hysterectomy in the United States. Other manifestations include pain, pregnancy complications, and infertility. Pain generally results from degenerating myomas that outgrew their blood supply or from compression of other pelvic organs such as the bowel, bladder, and ureters. High levels of pregnancy hormones frequently cause significant enlargement of pre-existing myomas, which may lead to significant distortion of the uterine cavity, resulting in recurrent miscarriages, fetal malpresentations, intrauterine growth restriction, obstruction of the birth canal, and the subsequent need for cesarean delivery, abruption, preterm labor, and pain from degeneration.

Bleeding is usually heavy and irregular (menometrorrhagia) and can be severe at times, requiring hospitalization. Examination reveals an enlarged, irregular uterus and, in severe cases, a large, solid pelvic mass extending to the upper abdomen. Diagnosis is usually made by TVUS, although CT and MRI can be used. Hysterosalpingography or saline-infused hysterosalpingography can be especially useful in the cases of submucosal and intrauterine myomas. Most are benign, and malignant degeneration occurs in <1% of cases and is usually encountered in the menopausal years. A postmenopausal patient presenting with vaginal bleeding and a rapidly enlarging uterine mass must be ruled out for uterine leiomyosarcoma. Management options of leiomyomas are tailored to the individual patient, depending on her age and desire for fertility and the size, location, and symptoms of the myomas. Conservative management

options include OCPs, medroxyprogesterone acetate, GnRH agonists, uterine artery embolization, and myomectomy.[64–66] Uterine artery embolization is contraindicated in patients planning future pregnancy and frequently results in acute degeneration of myomas requiring hospitalization for pain control. Myomectomy is indicated in patients with infertility and those who wish to preserve their reproductive capabilities and can be done by laparoscopy, hysteroscopy, or laparotomy.

Unfortunately, medical management provides only temporary relief, and myomas tend to recur after surgery either de novo or from growth and enlargement of smaller myomas that were undetectable at the time of the initial surgery. The only definitive curative therapy is hysterectomy, which can be done vaginally, abdominally, or by laparoscopy. In anemic patients, treatment with GnRH agonists for 3 months before the surgery may allow them time to normalize their hematocrit and avoid transfusions, decreases blood loss at the time of hysterectomy, and shrinks the myomas by an average of 30%, possibly making the preferred vaginal surgical approach more feasible.

Endometrial Hyperplasia and Endometrial Intraepithelial Neoplasia

Endometrial hyperplasia is caused by a chronic unopposed hyperestrogenic state (relative absence of progesterone) and is characterized by proliferation of endometrial glands resulting in increased gland-to-stroma ratio. It can be asymptomatic or, more commonly, results in abnormal vaginal bleeding. It is a histologic diagnosis made upon endometrial biopsy and is classified as simple or complex with and without atypia (World Health Organization classification)[67]:

- Simple hyperplasia: cystically dilated glands
- Complex hyperplasia: crowded, back-to-back, branching glands with minimal intervening stroma
- Atypical hyperplasia: presence of nuclear atypia

Untreated endometrial hyperplasia progresses to malignancy in 1%, 3%, 8%, and 29% of cases of simple hyperplasia, complex hyperplasia, simple hyperplasia with atypia, and complex hyperplasia with atypia, respectively.[68] Simple and complex hyperplasias can be treated with progestins such as medroxyprogesterone acetate 10 to 20 mg/d for 14 days and followed up with endometrial sampling. Atypical hyperplasia is considered a premalignant condition and is ideally treated with simple hysterectomy. However, if preservation of fertility is desired or surgery contraindicated, treatment with high doses of progestins such as megestrol acetate 40 to 160 mg/d usually reverses these lesions. Close follow-up and repeated sampling are necessary.

Modern molecular precancer diagnostic advances have allowed detection of preclinical disease and have provided a deeper insight into endometrial carcinogenesis. Sporadic, initiating mutations such as the loss of the phosphatase and tensin homologue tumor suppressor function occur frequently and early in the process. Once the mutant clone expands and accumulates additional genetic damage, the lesion can subsequently become recognizable as the earliest morphologic abnormality detectable, endometrial intraepithelial neoplasia (EIN).[69,70] The diagnostic criteria for EIN are:

- Presence of cytological demarcation
- Glandular crowding (volume percentage of stroma <55%)
- Size of at least 1 mm
- Exclusion of cancer, polyps, mimics, and artifacts

EIN can result from all the hyperplasias, with progression to EIN fueled, in part, by an unopposed estrogenic state.

Endometrial Cancer

Endometrial cancer is the most common gynecologic malignancy and fourth most common cancer in women. It is most common in menopausal women in the fifth decade of life; up to 15 to 25% of cases occur before menopause and 1 to 5% before age 40 years old. Risk

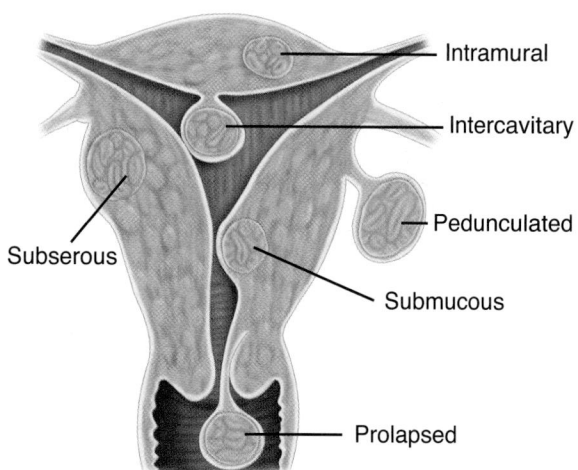

FIG. 41-20. Types of uterine myomas.

Intramural

Intercavitary

Pedunculated

Subserous

Submucous

Prolapsed

factors include unopposed estrogen, obesity, nulliparity, chronic anovulation, late menopause, hypertension, diabetes, hyperplasia with atypia, Lynch II syndrome, and prolonged use of tamoxifen. Protective factors include smoking and use of combination OCPs. Adenocarcinomas are the most prevalent histologic type. Sarcomas are rare; prior pelvic radiation and use of tamoxifen are known risk factors for sarcomas.

Hereditary Nonpolyposis Coli Cancer Hereditary nonpolyposis coli cancer, a cancer family syndrome, also known as Lynch II syndrome, is an autosomal dominant inherited predisposition to develop colo-rectal carcinoma and other extracolonic cancers, predominantly including tumors of the uterus and ovaries, with rare but defined inclusion of breast cancer.[71] The risk of colorectal carcinoma is as high as 75% by age 75 years old. Affected female patients have a 40% and 10% lifetime risk of developing uterine and ovarian cancers, respectively. Surveillance has not been proven to identify disease in early stage for these patients but is (informally) recommended and should include annual cervical cytology, mammography, TVUS, CA 125 measurements, and an endometrial biopsy.

Endometrial adenocarcinomas are divided into type I and type II. Type I tumors are estrogen-dependent endometrioid histology and have a relatively favorable prognosis. Women at highest risk are those with morbid obesity (body mass index >30) or abdominal obesity of metabolic syndrome. Type II endometrial cancers are estrogen-independent, aggressive, and characterized by nonen-dometrioid histology, the most common of which is papillary serous adenocarcinoma. Postmenopausal bleeding is the most common presentation of type I disease and permits diagnosis in early stages of the disease, which explains the relatively favorable prognosis of endometrioid endometrial carcinoma. Abnormal bleeding should prompt endometrial evaluation and sampling, which is usually done with an office endometrial biopsy and at times requires curettage or diagnostic hysteroscopy. TVUS often reveals a thickened endome-trial stripe. An endometrial stripe measuring 5 mm or more in a postmenopausal patient raises concern and should be followed by endometrial sampling; patients with stripe of 4 mm or less rarely have occult malignancy, and TVUS may thus be used to triage patients before invasive endometrial sampling. Uterine cancer is surgically staged and is graded based on the degree of histologic differentiation of the glandular components (Table 41-9).[51]

Treatment is surgical and involves a laparotomy, total abdomi-nal hysterectomy, bilateral salpingo-oophorectomy, peritoneal cy-tology, pelvic and para-aortic lymph node sampling, and resection of any gross disease.[48–50] The need for postoperative adjuvant radiation or chemotherapy is individualized based on the histology and stage of the disease. For example, stage IA grade 1 or 2 disease requires no further therapy, patients with stage IB grade 1 or 2 disease often receive intravaginal brachytherapy to decrease the incidence of vaginal cuff recurrence, stage IIC requires pelvic radiation, and for advanced-stage papillary serous histology chemo-therapy (carboplatin) often is advocated. Finally, lymph nodal status negatively impacts survival, and patients with positive para-aortic lymph nodes should receive extended-field radiation.

COMMON UTERINE SURGICAL PROCEDURES

Dilatation and Curettage

At one time dilatation of the cervix and curettage of the endometrial cavity was among the most common surgical procedures performed in this country. Simple office biopsy and medical means of dealing with abnormal bleeding have largely replaced the need for diagnos-tic dilatation and curettage. In some cases curettage is necessary for the relief of profuse uterine hemorrhage. It is indicated for removal of endometrial polyp or therapeutic termination of pregnancy and for retained placental tissue following abortion or obstetric delivery.

The patient is placed on the operating table in a lithotomy position, and the vagina and cervix are prepared as for any vaginal

TABLE 41-9	International Federation of Gynecology and Obstetrics staging of carcinoma of the uterine corpus

Stages	Characteristics
IA G123	Tumor limited to endometrium
IB G123	Invasion to $<\frac{1}{2}$ myometrium
IC G123	Invasion to $>\frac{1}{2}$ myometrium
IIA G123	Endocervical glandular involvement only
IIB G123	Cervical stromal invasion
IIIA G123	Tumor invades serosa or adnexa or positive peritoneal cytology
IIIB G123	Vaginal metastases
IIIC G123	Metastases to pelvic or para-aortic lymph nodes
IVA G123	Tumor invasion to bladder and/or bowel mucosa
IVB	Distant metastases including intra-abdominal and/or inguinal lymph node

Histopathology—Degree of Differentiation

Cases should be grouped by the degree of differentiation of the adeno-carcinoma:

G1	5% or less of a nonsquamous or nonmorular solid growth pattern
G2	6–50% of a nonsquamous or nonmorular solid growth pattern
G3	>50% of a nonsquamous or nonmorular solid growth pattern

Notes on Pathologic Grading

Notable nuclear atypia, inappropriate for the architectural grade, raises the grade of a grade I or grade II tumor by I. In serous adenocarcinomas, clear-cell adenocarcinomas, and squamous cell carcinomas, nuclear grading takes precedence. Adenocarcinomas with squamous differen-tiation are graded according to the nuclear grade of the glandular component.

Rules Related to Staging

Because corpus cancer is now surgically staged, procedures previously used for determination of stages are no longer applicable, such as the finding of fractional dilatation and curettage to differentiate between stage I and II. It is appreciated that there may be a small number of patients with corpus cancer who will be treated primarily with radia-tion therapy. If that is the case, the clinical staging adopted by the International Federation of Gynecology and Obstetrics in 1971 would still apply, but designation of that staging system would be noted. Ideally, width of the myometrium should be measured along with the width of tumor invasion.

operation. The cervix is grasped on the anterior lip with a tenacu-lum. Some traction on the cervix is necessary to straighten the cervical canal and the uterine cavity. A uterine sound is inserted into the uterine cavity, and the depth of the uterus is noted. The cervical canal is then systematically dilated beginning with a small cervical dilator. Most operations can be performed after the cervix is dilated to accommodate a number 8 or 9 Hegar dilator or its equivalent. Dilatation is accomplished by firm, constant pressure with a dilator directed in the axis of the uterus (Fig. 41-21).

After the cervix is dilated to admit the curette, the endocervical canal should be curetted and the sample submitted separate from the endometrial curettings. The endometrial cavity is then systemi-cally scraped with a uterine curette. After the uterus has been thoroughly curetted, a ureteral stone forceps may be used to explore the endometrial cavity, searching for polyps or pedunculated neo-plasms. When the procedure is complete, the tenaculum is re-moved; the tenaculum site is evaluated for bleeding.

The major complication of dilatation and curettage is perfora-tion of the uterus, diagnosed when the operator finds no resistance to a dilator or curette. Laparoscopy to identify any damage to vessels or bowel may be required to assess the perforation. Curettage of the

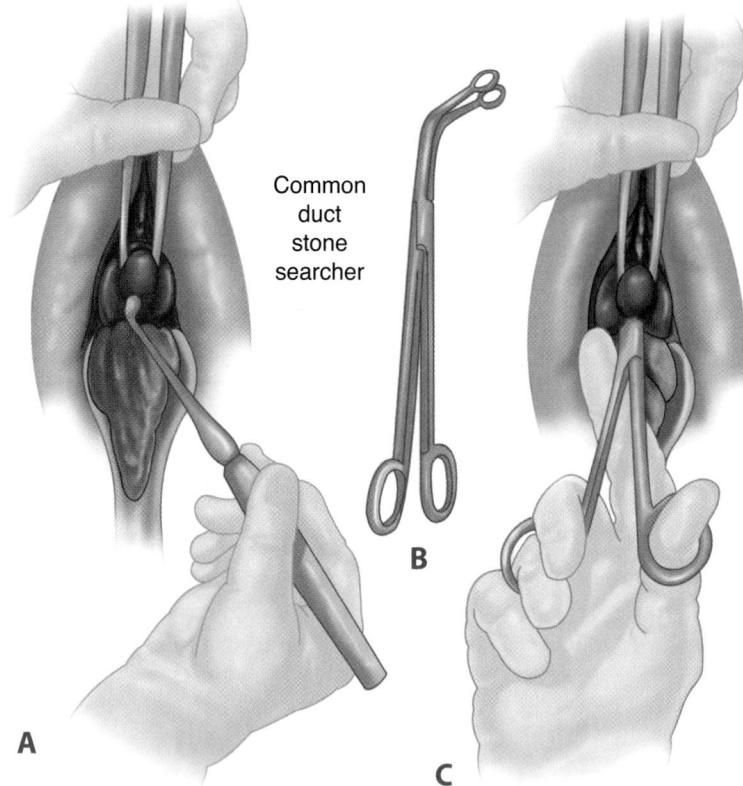

Common duct stone searcher

A

B

C

FIG. 41-21. **A** through **C.** Dilatation and curettage of the uterus.

postabortal uterus must be approached carefully because the uterus is extremely soft and perforation can occur with very little warning. Using the largest curette available or suction curettage is a safer choice than a small curette, which tends to cause perforation with less pressure.

Hysteroscopy

Hysteroscopy, like laparoscopy, has gained widespread support as a very useful technique for both diagnosis and treatment of intrauterine pathology and for ablation of the endometrium as an alternative to hysterectomy for the treatment of abnormal uterine bleeding.

General Hysteroscopic Techniques

Type of Instruments Hysteroscopes can be divided into the categories of diagnostic, operative, and hysteroresectoscope. The lens for all three is identical. This is usually a fiber-optic lens and light source with an outside diameter of 3 mm and an objective lens that is offset up to 30° from the long axis of the instrument. In contrast, the sleeves for the three types of hysteroscopes vary considerably. The diagnostic sleeve usually has an external diameter of 5 mm and a single-direction flow. Because outflow is limited, bleeding may impede a clear intrauterine view. The operative sleeve, with an external diameter usually <10 mm, has a flow-through design with separate channels for input and outflow of distention media. A separate channel is available for placement of operating instruments. The final type of sleeve is the hysteroresectoscope. This is also of a flow-through design and has an integral unipolar resecting loop identical to a urologic resectoscope. The loop can be replaced with a roller ball for endometrial ablation.

Distention Media and Pumps Several distention media have found widespread use for hysteroscopy. For operative hysteroscopy, one of the first fluid media used was 30% dextran and 70% dextrose. This syrup-like substance usually is introduced by hand with a large syringe. The advantage is simplicity and low cost. The view is excellent in the absence of bleeding. The disadvantage is the diffi-

culty in completely removing the substance from the instruments. More recently, aqueous solutions with pressure-controlled pumps have been used. For operative hysteroscopy, where electrosurgery is not being used, it is safest to use a balanced salt solution. Moderate fluid intravasation will be of no consequence in a healthy individual. However, intravasation of larger volumes can result in fluid overload, especially in a patient with any cardiac compromise. To minimize this risk, the use of a fluid-medium pump is recommended rather than gravity or a pressure cuff to limit pressure to <80 mmHg. When electrosurgery is used for hysteroresectoscope excision of leiomyomas or roller-ball endometrial ablation, a nonconducting solution such as glycine must be used. Significant vascular intravasation can cause hyponatremia, potentially resulting in cerebral edema, coma, or even death. For this reason, protocols must be followed rigorously to detect and treat significant intravasation whenever these solutions are used. Intraoperatively, differences in distention medium input and output should be calculated every 15 minutes. If the difference is >500 mL, a diuretic should be given and the source of the loss identified. If the difference is >1000 mL, the procedure also should be terminated immediately. Whenever significant intravasation is suspected, serum sodium level should be checked immediately postoperatively and a few hours later because later hyponatremia, presumably due to transperitoneal absorption, has been reported.

Hysteroscopic Procedures

Diagnostic Hysteroscopy After determining the position of the uterus, the anterior cervix is grasped with a tenaculum and traction placed to straighten the cervical canal. The lens and diagnostic sleeve are placed into the cervix, and distention medium is introduced with a pressure of 80 to 90 mmHg. The hysteroscope is advanced slowly and carefully toward the fundus, using tactile and visual cues to avoid perforation. The entire uterine cavity is inspected, and any abnormal anatomy is documented. As the hysteroscope is withdrawn, the uterocervical junction and the endocervix are examined.

Directed Endometrial Biopsy If a focal abnormality of the endometrium is observed, directed biopsy may be more accurate than a simple uterine curettage. The cervix is dilated to allow passage of an 8- to 10-mm flow-through operating hysteroscope, and a balanced salt solution is used for distention. Once the hysteroscope is positioned in the uterine cavity, the area of interest is biopsied under direct visualization.

Polypectomy If an intrauterine polyp is discovered, the base of the polyp is incised with hysteroscopic scissors, and the polyp is grasped with grasping forceps. The hysteroscope, sleeve, and polyp are removed simultaneously, because most polyps will not fit through the operating channel. Extremely large polyps may have to be removed piecemeal. Any residual base of the polyp may be removed with biopsy forceps.

Uterine Septum Resection A septum may be resected with scissors, electrosurgery, or laser. Scissors are used most commonly in light of the minimal vascularity of septa and the decreased potential for bowel injury should inadvertent uterine perforation occur. An operating hysteroscope is placed into the uterine cavity, which will appear to be two tubular structures rather than the broad uterine fundus usually encountered. The septum is then evenly divided toward the fundus. If scissors are used, rather than a power cutting instrument, the presence of bleeding indicates that the level of resection is shifting from the avascular septum to the vascular myometrium.

Removal of Intrauterine Synechiae The removal of synechiae is performed in a manner similar to that described above for a uterine septum in the Uterine Septum Resection section, except that the anatomy, and thus the visual cues for location of normal uterine wall, are completely unpredictable from patient to patient. In difficult cases, simultaneous transabdominal ultrasound is extremely helpful in guiding the direction and limits of resection. Standby laparoscopy should be available in the event of perforation. Following surgery, some type of intrauterine splint, such as an intrauterine device or a balloon catheter, is often placed to avoid synechia reformation. Patients usually are placed on estrogen supplementation for a month and prophylactic antibiotics until the intrauterine splint is removed 1 to 2 weeks later.

Intrauterine Myomectomy Pedunculated or submucosal leiomyoma can be removed safely hysteroscopically with subsequent improvement in both abnormal uterine bleeding and infertility. Because myoma tissue is relatively dense, a power cutting instrument is required. The choices are either laser or, more commonly, electrosurgery. Both pedunculated and submucosal fibroids are shaved into small pieces with either the laser fiber or the hysterorectoscope. In the case of a pedunculated fibroid, the urge to simply transect the stalk as a first step should be resisted unless the fibroid is 10 mm or less in size. Fibroids that are larger than this are difficult to remove in one piece without excessive cervical dilatation. Morcellation is much easier when the stalk is still attached for stability.

Endometrial Ablation A common treatment for abnormal uterine bleeding in the absence of endometrial hyperplasia is ablation of the endometrium. In the recent past, this was performed with an operative hysteroscope using a laser fiber or with a resectoscope using an electrosurgical "roller barrel or ball." As described previously for myoma resection, under Distention Media and Pumps, a balanced salt solution is used for laser resection, and an electrolyte-free solution is used for electrosurgery. For both techniques, the endometrium is destroyed down to the myometrium in a systematic fashion starting at the cornua and ending in the lower uterine segment. More recently, hysteroscopic endometrial ablation has been widely supplanted by variations of balloon thermal ablation. For this procedure, a probe with attached balloon is blindly placed into the uterus. Heated saline is circulated in the balloon to coagulate the endometrium. Balloon ablation requires less technical skill and appears to have less risk of complication than the hysteroscopic approaches. Both hysteroscopic and balloon ablation techniques result in amenorrhea in approximately half the patients and decreased menstruation in another third of the patients over the first year of therapy.

Myomectomy

Myomectomy can be performed either with open laparotomy or laparoscopic approaches. Hemostasis for the procedure can be aided by direct injection near the base of the fibroid with dilute vasopressin or through the placement of a Penrose drain (Fig. 41-22) around the base of the uterus and pulled through small perforations in the broad ligament lateral to the uterine blood supply on either side and clamped to form a tourniquet for uterine blood flow.

An incision is made through the uterine musculature into the myoma. The pseudocapsule surrounding the tumor is identified and the tumor is bluntly or sharply dissected. After the myoma is freed of its lateral attachments, it can often be twisted to expose a pedicle that frequently contains its major blood supply. On occasion, several myomas may be removed through a single incision. The uterine wounds are closed with absorbable sutures to obliterate the dead space and provide hemostasis. The uterine serosa is closed with a 3-0 absorbable suture placed subserosally if possible. A patch of Interceed to cover the uterine incision may prevent adhesion formation.

Hysterectomy for Benign Disease: Abdominal Hysterectomy

The abdomen is entered through an appropriate incision. The upper abdomen is examined for evidence of extrapelvic disease, and a suitable retractor is placed in the abdominal wound. The uterus is grasped at either cornu with Kocher clamps and pulled up into the wound (Fig. 41-23). The round ligament is identified and divided. If the ovaries are to be removed, the peritoneal incision is extended from the round ligament lateral to the infundibulopelvic ligament for approximately 2.5 cm. The retroperitoneal space is bluntly opened. The ureter is identified on the medial leaf of the broad ligament. The infundibulopelvic ligament is isolated, clamped, and cut, and the suture ligated. A similar procedure is carried out on the opposite side. In the event that the ovaries are not to be removed, the ureter is identified and an opening below the utero-ovarian ligament and fallopian tube created. The fallopian tube and ovarian ligament are divided. The peritoneum is opened over the bladder fold between the divided round ligaments. The bladder is mobilized by sharply dissecting it free of the anterior surface of the uterus and cervix. The peritoneum on the posterior surface of the uterus is dissected free of the uterus and then cut. Clamps are placed on the uterine vessels at the cervicouterine junction, cut, and ligated. The cardinal ligaments are then serially clamped, cut, and ligated. Following division of the remaining cardinal ligaments, the uterus is elevated, and the vagina clamped or opened directly, and then the cervix removed from the vagina with scissors or a knife. Sutures are placed at each lateral angle of the vagina. The remainder of the vagina is closed anterior to posterior with a running absorbable suture. Pelvic reperitonealization is not necessary.

Vaginal Hysterectomy

Vaginal hysterectomy is an acceptable approach in those patients in whom the uterus descends, the bony pelvis allows vaginal operation, the uterine tumors are small enough to permit vaginal removal, and the patient is amenable to vaginal operation. In the presence of large myomas, pretreatment with GnRH analogues may allow vaginal operation that would have been impossible previously. The patient is placed in a lithotomy position. A bladder catheter can be placed before the procedure. A weighted vaginal speculum is placed in the posterior vagina, and the cervix is grasped with a tenaculum and pulled in the axis of the vagina (Figs. 41-24 and 41-25). Injection of the cervix and paracervical tissue with analgesic with epinephrine may be helpful in defining planes and decreasing obscuring bleeding.

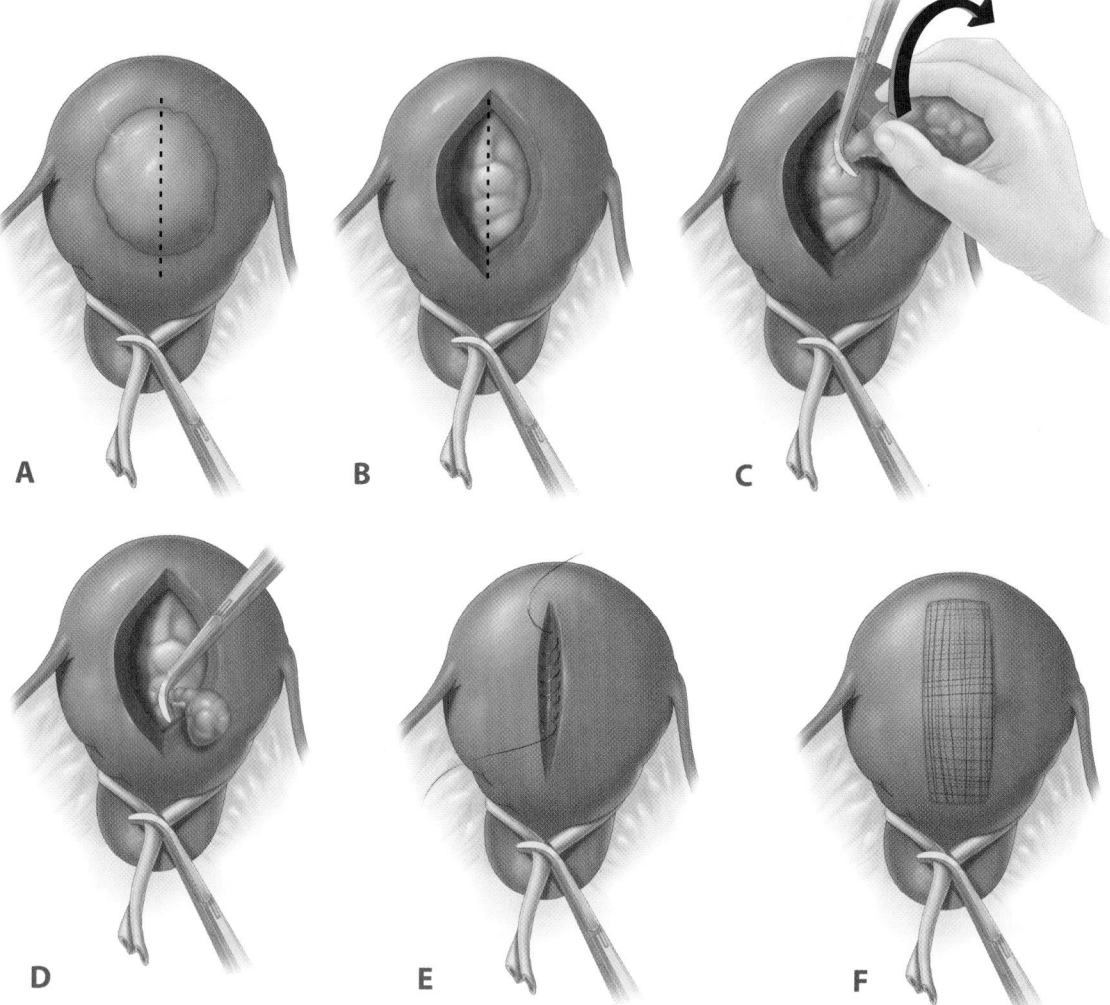

FIG. 41-22. Myomectomy. **A.** Hemostatic "tourniquet'" in place before myomectomy. **B.** Uterine incision for myomectomy. **C.** Removal of myoma. **D.** Several myomas may be removed through a single incision. **E.** The uterine wound is closed with an absorbable suture. **F.** The uterine wound covered with mesh to retard adhesions.

A circumferential incision may be made with a scalpel or scissors. The posterior cul-de-sac is identified and entered with scissors. The weighted speculum is then placed in this cavity. Mayo scissors are used to dissect down to the pubocervical-vesical fascia. The vaginal mucosa and the bladder are sharply and bluntly dissected free of the cervix and the lower portion of the uterus. When the peritoneum of the anterior cul-de-sac is identified, it is entered with the scissors, and a retractor is placed in the defect. The uterosacral ligaments are identified, doubly clamped, cut, and ligated. Serial clamps are placed on the parametrial structures above the uterosacral ligament; these pedicles are cut, and ligated. At the cornu of the uterus, the tube, round ligament, and suspensory ligament of the ovary are doubly clamped and cut. The procedure is carried out usually concurrently on the opposite side, and the uterus is removed. The pelvis is inspected for hemostasis; all bleeding must be meticulously controlled at this point.

The pelvic peritoneum is closed with a running purse-string suture incorporating those pedicles which were held, the uterosacral and ovarian pedicles. This exteriorizes those areas which might tend to bleed. The sutures attached to the ovarian pedicles are cut. The vagina may be closed with interrupted mattress stitches, incorporating the uterosacral ligaments into the corner of the vagina with each lateral stitch. On occasion, the uterus, which is initially too large to remove vaginally, may be reduced in size by morcellation. After the uterine vessels have been clamped and ligated, serial wedges are taken from the central portion of the uterus to reduce the uterine mass. This procedure will allow the vaginal delivery of even very large uterine leiomyomas.

Endoscopic Surgery

Placement of the Veress Needle and Primary Trocar

The standard method for gynecologic laparoscopy follows the same methodology as all minimally invasive surgery generally with four ports: umbilical, two lateral, and one suprapubic. After transillumination to locate the superficial vessels, an attempt is made to laparoscopically locate the inferior epigastric vessels. Secondary trocars are placed under laparoscopic visualization either 3 to 4 cm above the symphysis pubis in the midline, or 8 cm above the symphysis pubis approximately 8 cm lateral to the midline. This location approximates McBurney's point on the right side of the abdomen. At the end of the procedure, the sleeves are removed and the sites observed for signs of hemorrhage. Any trocar site >5 mm should be closed with a full-thickness suture (to include both the anterior and posterior rectus abdominus fascia) to prevent herniation through the defect.

Diagnostic Laparoscopy

This common procedure involves the placement of a 5- or 10-mm lens through an intraumbilical port, often with a 5-mm port placed

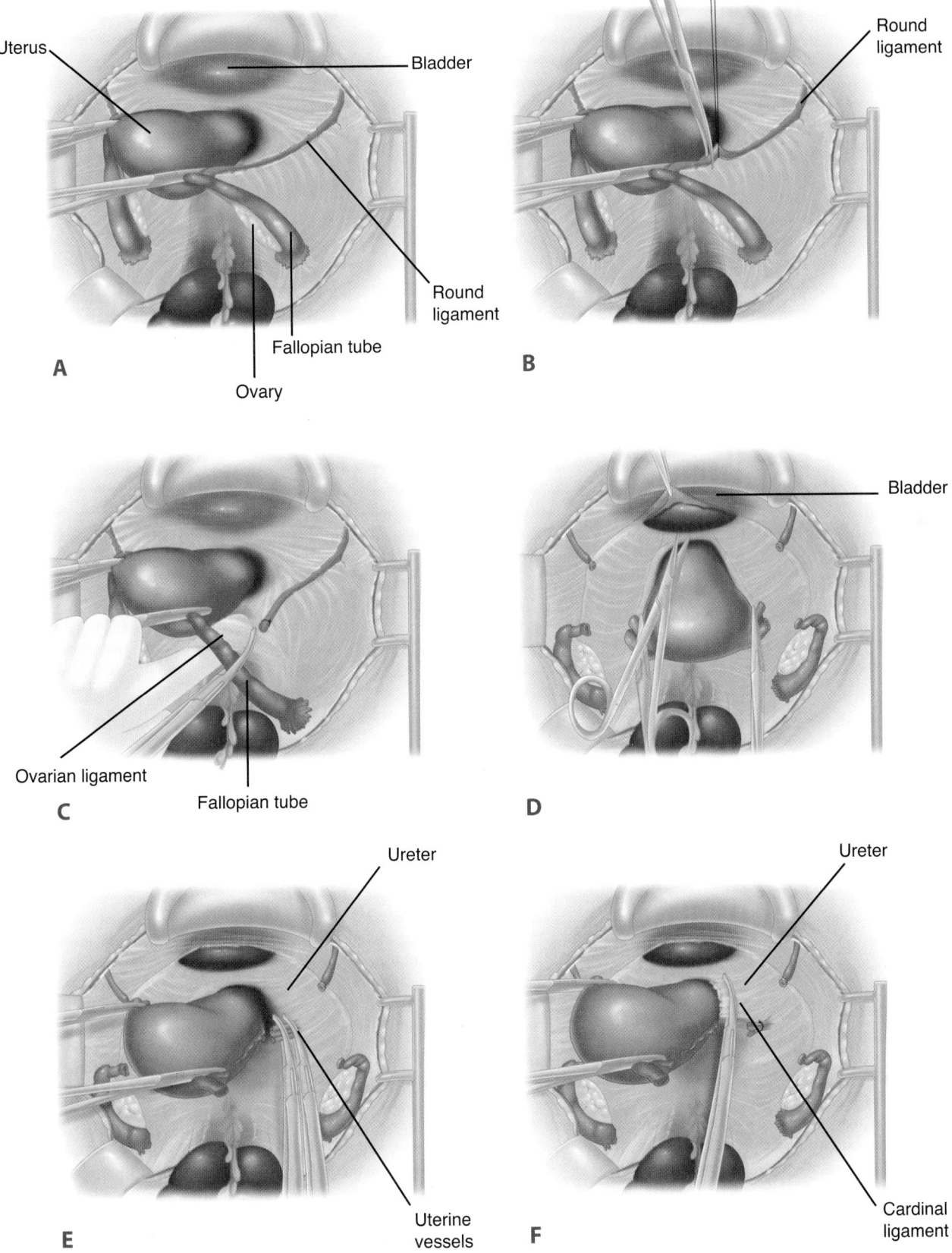

FIG. 41-23. Hysterectomy. **A.** The uterus grasped at the cornua. **B.** The round ligament is cut. **C.** The ovarian ligament and fallopian tube are isolated. **D.** The bladder is mobilized. **E.** The uterine vessels are clamped. **F.** The cardinal ligaments are clamped. (*Continued*)

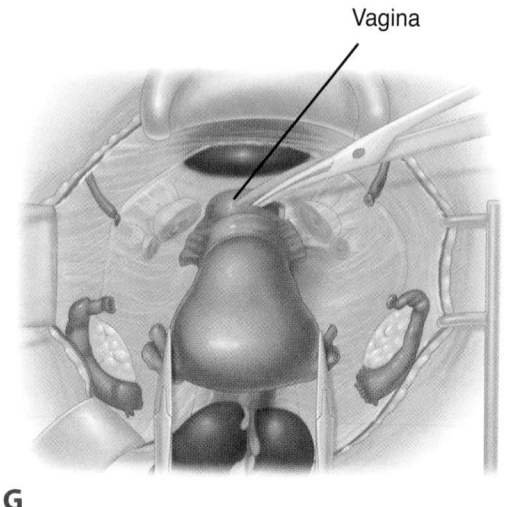

G

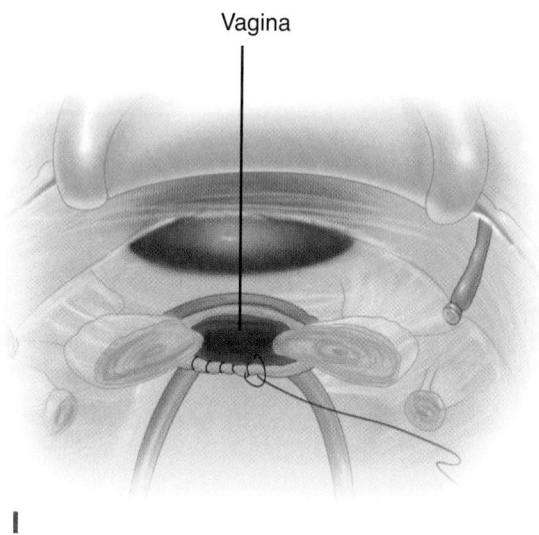

I

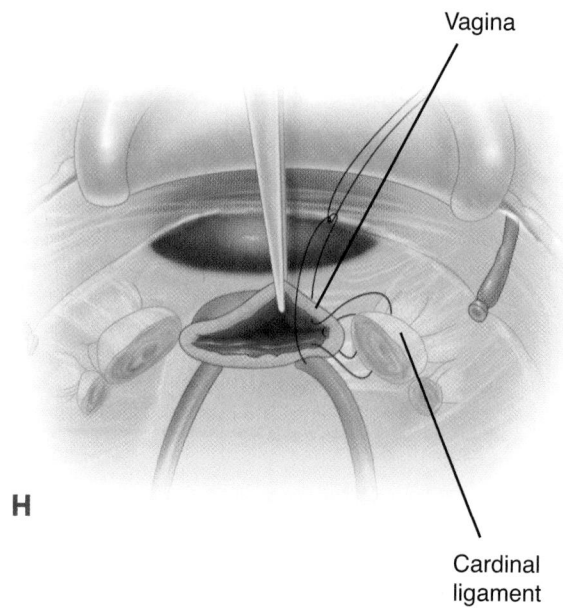

H

FIG. 41-23. (*Continued*) **G.** The vagina is entered. **H.** The cardinal ligaments are sutured to the vagina. **I.** The vagina is "closed open."

above the symphysis for manipulation with a wand or Babcock graspers. Pelvic organs are closely inspected in a systematic fashion for signs of disease, and if tubal patency is an issue, a dilute dye solution is injected transcervically (chromopertubation).

Tubal Sterilization Procedures

As in diagnostic laparoscopy, a one- or two-port technique can be used. Tubes are occluded in the midisthmic section (approximately 3 cm from the cornua) using clips, elastic bands, or bipolar electrosurgery. With electrosurgery, approximately 2 cm of tube should be desiccated. Pregnancy rates after any of these techniques have been reported in the range of three per 1000 women.

Lysis of Adhesions

Pelvic adhesions usually are related to previous surgery, endometriosis, or infection, the latter of which can be either genital (i.e., PID) or extragenital (e.g., ruptured appendix) in origin. Adhesions can be lysed mechanically with scissors if not vascular, or harmonic scissors or any of the power techniques discussed in the minimally invasive surgery section. Some degree of adhesion reformation is unavoidable. Adhesion reformation can be minimized by achieving good hemostasis using discrete application of electrosurgery. Postoperatively, barrier methods have been shown to decrease adhesion formation in both animal and human studies but have not been demonstrated to improve outcome in terms of either subsequent pregnancies or pain relief.

Ovarian Cystectomy

The laparoscopic removal of ovarian cysts <6 cm in diameter in premenopausal women has become common. Using a multiple-port technique, the peritoneal cavity is inspected for signs of malignancy, including ascites, peritoneal or diaphragmatic implants, and liver involvement or unexpected malignant appearance of the ovary. In the absence of signs of malignancy, pelvic washings are obtained, and the ovarian capsule is excised with scissors or a power instrument. The cyst is shelled out carefully and placed in a bag, intact if possible. The bag opening is brought through the lower port incision along with the 10-mm port. The cyst may need to be drained to facilitate removal, but only after the bag edges are firmly out of the abdomen assuring no leakage within the abdomen. Hemostasis of the ovary is achieved with bipolar electrocoagulation, but the ovary usually is not closed, because this may increase postoperative adhesion formation. Except in the obvious cases of simple cysts, endometriomas, or dermoid cysts, the cyst wall should be sent for frozen section to verify the absence of the malignancy. If malignancy is detected, immediate definitive surgery, usually by laparotomy, is recommended. All cyst walls are sent for permanent section and pathologic diagnosis. If a cyst should rupture before removal, the cyst contents are thoroughly aspirated, and the cyst wall is removed and sent for pathologic evaluation. The peritoneal cavity is copiously rinsed with Ringer's lactate solution. This is especially important when a dermoid cyst is ruptured, because the

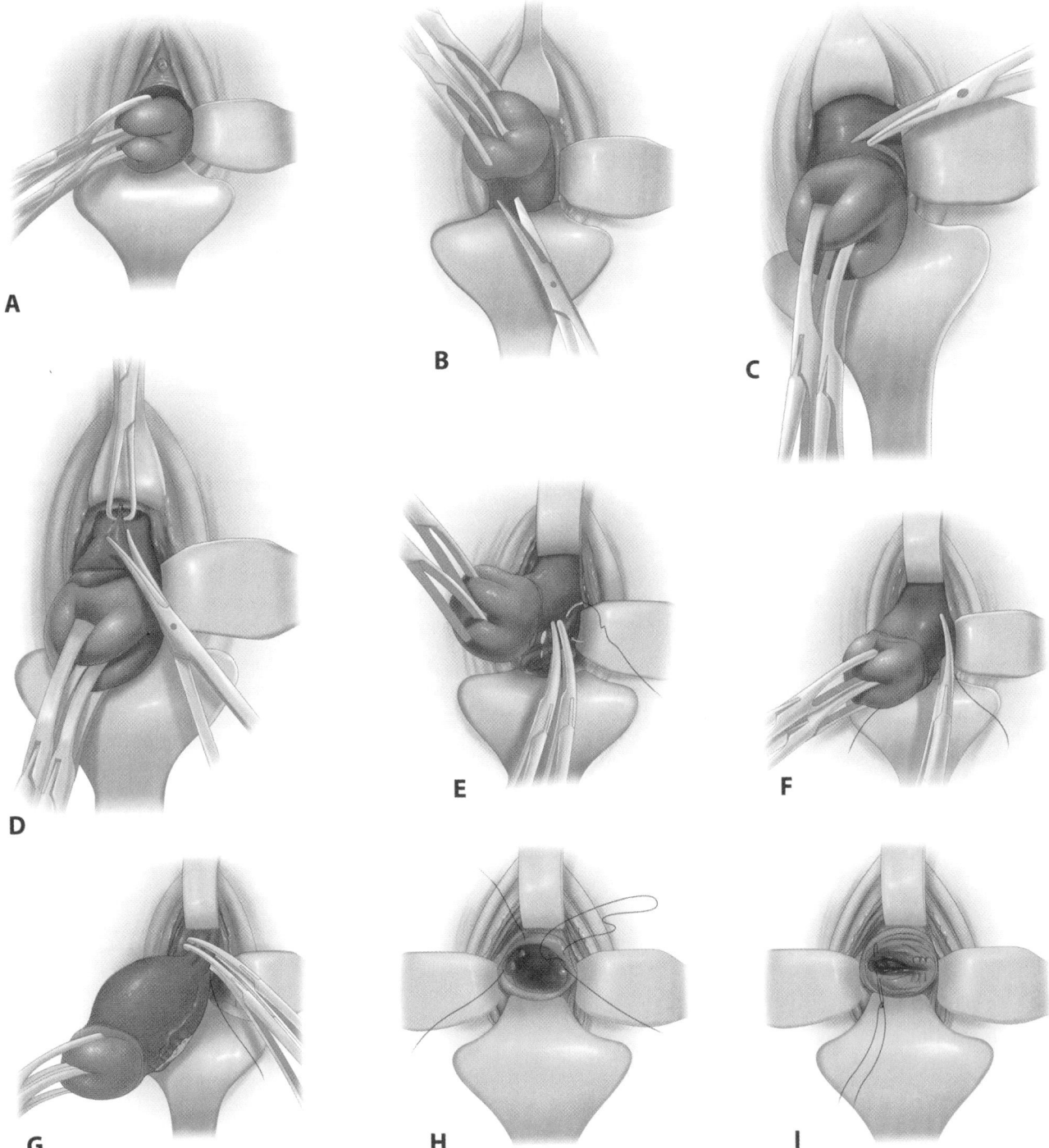

FIG. 41-24. Vaginal hysterectomy. **A.** Traction is placed on the uterus. **B.** The posterior cul-de-sac is entered. **C.** The vaginal mucosa is circumcised. **D.** The anterior cul-de-sac is entered. **E.** The uterosacral ligaments are clamped. **F.** The uterosacral ligaments are tied. **G.** The fallopian tube, round ligament, and ovarian ligament are ligated. **H.** The peritoneum is closed. **I.** The vaginal mucosa is closed.

sebaceous material can cause a chemical peritonitis unless all the visible oily substance is carefully removed.

Although malignancies are not commonly encountered using the guidelines outlined in this chapter, there has been concern that rupture may worsen the patient's prognosis and increase risk for port-site metastases. When a malignancy is diagnosed, the timing of definitive surgical treatment is important and would preferably be immediately with the diagnosis at laparoscopy, which lessens the risk for port-site metastases. Ovarian cysts >6 cm and those discovered in postmenopausal women also can be removed laparoscopi-

cally. Because of the increased risk of malignancy associated with these situations, laparotomy is more commonly used. Laparoscopy may be a reasonable alternative in select patients if standard methods for staging are used in conjunction with appropriate frozen-section evaluation and expedient definitive therapy when indicated.

Removal of Adnexa

Using a multiple-port technique, the vascular supply to the tissue can first be desiccated with bipolar cautery and then divided with harmonic scissors. Special care must be taken to identify and avoid

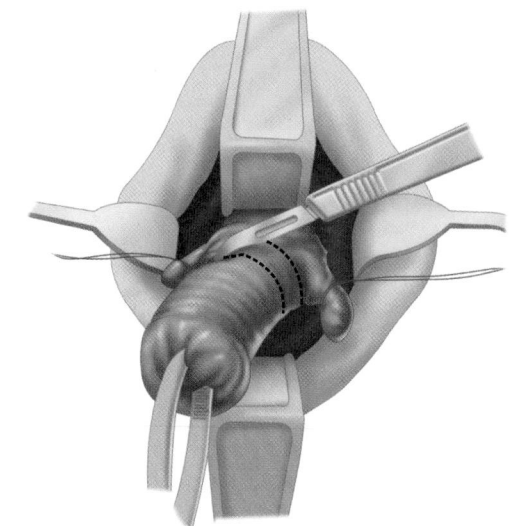

FIG. 41-25. Uterine morcellation through the vagina.

the ureter, which lies retroperitoneally as it crosses the ovarian vessels and courses along the ovarian fossa (Fig. 41-26). Direct identification of the ureter and visualization before cauterization of the infundibulopelvic ligament is required. The periovarian peritoneum is dissected toward the uterus with power scissors and the connection to the uterus (or in the absence of a uterus, the old round ligament, and cardinal ligament tissue) cauterized and separated as appropriate.

Once the adnexa has been excised and hemostasis is achieved, attention is turned to removing the tissue from the peritoneal cavity. Small specimens can be removed using a retrieval bag via a 12-mm port. The port is removed with the sack, and the fascial incision is enlarged, if required.

For larger specimens, the opening of the sack is exposed outside the abdomen while the specimen remains in the abdomen. A cyst can be aspirated, and the remaining specimen can be removed piecemeal, taking care not to allow intraperitoneal spillage. In difficult cases, the specimen can be removed via a vaginal colpotomy incision. For this procedure, a 12-mm port is placed through the posterior cul-de-sac under direct visualization. A retrieval sack is placed through the port, and the port and specimen in the sack are removed together. The distensible peritoneum and vaginal wall will allow the removal of a large specimen through a relatively small defect, which can then be closed with a running suture vaginally. Prophylactic antibiotics may decrease the risk of infection.

Myomectomy

Uterine leiomyomas often are approachable via the laparoscope. Hemostasis is assisted by intrauterine injection of dilute vasopressin (10 U in 50 mL) at the site of incision. Pedunculated leiomyomas can be excised at the base using scissors or a power instrument. Intramural leiomyomas require deep dissection into the uterine tissue, which must be closed subsequently with laparoscopic suturing techniques. Because myomectomies are associated with considerable postoperative adhesion formation, barrier techniques are used to decrease adhesion formation. Removing the specimen often requires morcellation and power morcellators have been developed that significantly expedite this technique.

Hysterectomy

Laparoscopy has been used to augment vaginal hysterectomy to avoid laparotomy in patients with known pelvic adhesions, endometriosis, or in whom the uterus is enlarged by leiomyoma. Although multiple variations in technique exist, there are three basic laparoscopic approaches for hysterectomy: laparoscopic-assisted vaginal hysterectomy, laparoscopic hysterectomy (LH), and laparoscopic supracervical hysterectomy (LSH). The technically simplest, and probably the most widely applied, is the laparoscopic-assisted vaginal hysterectomy. For this procedure, a multiple-port approach is used to survey the peritoneal cavity, and any pelvic adhesions are lysed. The round

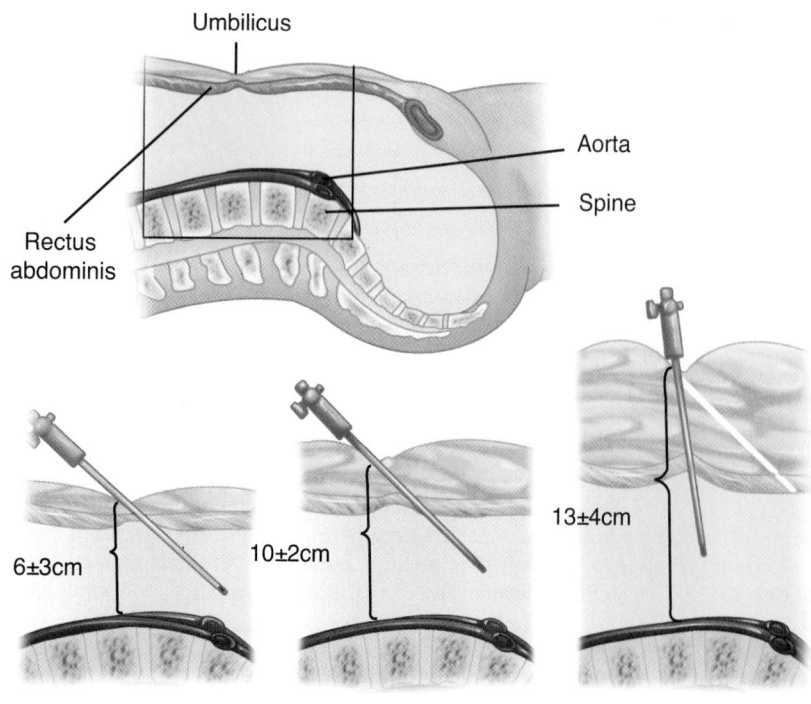

FIG. 41-26. Changes in the anterior abdominal wall anatomy with weight.

Umbilicus

Aorta

Spine

Rectus abdominis

6±3cm

10±2cm

13±4cm

Non-obese

Overweight

Obese

ligaments are then occluded and divided, and the uterovesical peritoneum and peritoneum lateral to the ovarian ligament are incised. The course of the ureter and any adhesions or implants such as endometriosis that might place the ureter in the way of the surgical dissection are carefully dissected. Next, the proximal uterine blood supply is dissected for identification and then occluded and divided often with cauterization and then power scissors to complete the separation. When the ovaries are removed, the infundibulopelvic ligaments (containing the ovarian vessels) are divided. If the ovaries are conserved, the utero-ovarian ligament and blood vessels are divided and occluded. In many cases, the posterior cul-de-sac also is incised laparoscopically and the uterosacral ligaments separated with coagulation and power scissors. The amount of dissection that is done before the vaginal portion depends on the individual patient characteristics, and may include as little as the ovarian and adhesion management to full dissection including the bladder dissection with only the last vaginal incision done by the vaginal approach, which would be a LH. This procedure is used for the indications listed above and also when lack of uterine descent makes the vaginal approach impossible.

The third common laparoscopic approach is the LSH. This procedure has been advocated for all benign indications for hysterectomy. Technically, it is begun in a manner identical to the first two approaches. However, after the proximal vessels are divided and the bladder is dissected from the anterior uterus, the ascending branches of the uterine arteries are occluded and the entire uterine fundus is removed from the cervix. The endocervix is either cauterized or cored out. The fundus is then morcellated and removed through a 12-mm abdominal port or through a special transcervical morcellator. The end result is an intact cervix and cuff, with no surgical dissection performed near the uterine artery and adjacent ureter. This approach avoids both a large abdominal incision and a vaginal incision. According to its advocates, this approach minimizes operating time, recovery time, and risk of both infection and ureteral injury. LSH has yet to be widely applied, in part out of concern for the subsequent risk of developing cancer in the residual cervical stump. In addition, women may develop bleeding from the remaining lower uterine segment that can be bothersome, even if preventive measures have been taken.

Injury to Abdominal Wall Vessels

Abdominal wall vessel injuries have become more common with the development of more complicated operative laparoscopic procedures that use lateral trocar placement and larger trocars. These vessels include the inferior ("deep") epigastric vessels, the superficial epigastric vessels, and the superficial circumflex iliac vessels (Fig. 41-27). Injury to the inferior epigastric artery can result in life-threatening hemorrhage. Injury to these or other vessels can result in significant hematoma or postoperative blood loss if unrecognized.

The primary methods to avoid vessel injury are knowledge of the vessels at risk and visualization of them before trocar placement when possible. The superficial vessels often can be seen and avoided by transillumination of the abdominal wall with the laparoscope. In contrast, the larger inferior epigastric vessels cannot be seen by transillumination because of their deeper location. But these vessels often can be seen laparoscopically and avoided as they course along the peritoneum between the lateral umbilical fold of the bladder and the insertion of the round ligament into the inguinal canal.

Because the vessels may not be visible in some patients either by transillumination or laparoscopically, it is important to know their most likely location and place lateral trocars accordingly. Although the traditional location used for lateral trocar placement was approximately 5 cm from the midline, a safer location may be 8 cm or more above the symphysis pubis and 8 cm from the midline, because both the superficial and inferior epigastric arteries are located approximately 5.5 cm from the midline (see Fig. 41-27).

Anatomic variation and anastomoses between vessels make it impossible to know the exact location of all the abdominal wall vessels. For this reason, other strategies also should be used to avoid

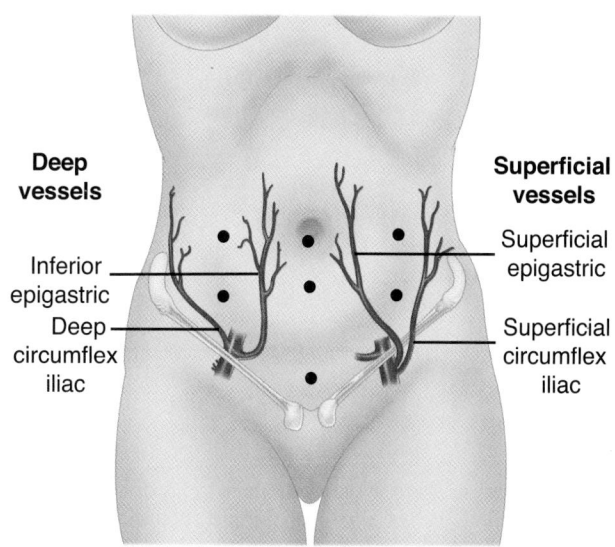

FIG. 41-27. Location of anterior abdominal wall blood vessels.

vessel injury, including the use of trocars with conical tips rather than pyramid tips, and the use of the smallest trocars possible lateral to the midline.

Intestinal Injury

Another potentially serious complication of laparoscopic surgery is injury to either small or large intestines. An unrecognized bowel injury may occur at the time of trocar insertion, especially if the patient has had previous abdominal procedures that often result in bowel adhesions to the anterior abdominal wall peritoneum. To minimize the risk of bowel injury in patients who have undergone previous laparotomy, an open technique for placement of the first port is advocated.

Because of the limited field of view, some bowel injuries may not be seen during surgery. These injuries usually manifest 1 to 3 days after surgery, well after the patient has been released following these primarily outpatient procedures and any patient concerns in this time period should be addressed seriously and rapidly.

Urologic Injuries

Bladder injury is an uncommon laparoscopic injury, most commonly occurring as a result of retroperitoneal perforation during lower trocar placement or during sharp dissection of the bladder from the lower uterine segment during hysterectomy. The latter of these two situations is usually recognized intraoperatively; the first sign of the former may be postoperative hematuria or lower-port incisional drainage. Once diagnosed, large defects require layered closure, whereas smaller defects usually close spontaneously within days or weeks with the aid of transurethral catheter drainage.

Ureteral injury may occur as a result of any procedure that requires dissection or ligation of sidewall vessels, such as removal of an adnexa, because the ureter is adjacent to the pelvic peritoneum in the area of the ovarian fossa (see Fig. 41-5). This complication also has been reported after fulguration of endometriosis on the pelvic sidewall.

Another common cause of ureteral injury is hysterectomy, because the ureter often is located <2 cm from the cervix. This type of injury appears to be increased during LH when compared to abdominal or vaginal hysterectomy, apparently because of the modification of the standard techniques required for the laparoscopic approach.

Ureteral injuries, including complete ligation, partial resection, or thermal injuries, usually will manifest within hours to days of

TABLE 41-10	Ovarian cancer symptom index (2007) and ACOG guidelines for patient referral to gynecologic oncology

Ovarian Cancer Symptom Index	ACOG Guidelines for Referral of Premenopausal Women with Mass Suspicious for Ovarian Cancer	ACOG Guidelines for Referral of Postmenopausal Women with Mass Suspicious for Ovarian Cancer

Development of, change in, and/or persistence in:
  Bloating
  Pelvic or abdominal pain
  Difficulty eating or feeling full quickly
  Urinary symptoms of urgency or frequency
	One or more of:
	  CA 125 > 200 U/mL
	  Ascites
	  Evidence of abdominal or distant metastasis
	  Family history of one or more first-degree
	    relatives with ovarian or breast cancer
		One or more of:
		  Elevated CA 125
		  Ascites
		  Nodular or fixed pelvic mass
		  Evidence of abdominal or distant metastasis
		  Family history of one or more first-degree
		    relatives with ovarian or breast cancer

ACOG = American College of Obstetricians and Gynecologists.

surgery. Complete obstruction most often manifests as flank pain, whereas the first sign of partial or complete transection may be symptoms of intra-abdominal irritation caused by urine leakage. Transperitoneal thermal injuries resulting from fulguration of endometriosis may be similar to those after transection, but the appearance of symptoms may be delayed several days until tissue necrosis occurs.

EPITHELIAL FALLOPIAN TUBE AND OVARIAN MALIGNANCY

Presentation and Screening of Tubal and Epithelial Ovarian Neoplasms

There were an estimated 22,400 new cases and 15,280 deaths due to ovarian cancers in 2007, yielding a fractional death rate of 68% and making this the most deadly of gynecologic cancers.[72,73] Developing a method for early and accurate diagnosis can and will save lives. Gynecologic neoplasms can present with symptoms, although these symptoms are neither sensitive nor specific to the pathologic process. Common symptoms for either benign or malignant ovarian tumors include pelvic discomfort, cramping, pain, fullness, headache, backache, and others. These are all symptoms that can be attributed to a variety of pathology from infection to pregnancy to irritable bowel syndrome to cancer. Recent work has identified an ovarian cancer symptom index (Table 41-10), now adopted/supported by the Ovarian Cancer National Alliance, the Gynecologic Cancer Foundation, the Society of Gynecologic Oncologists, and the American Cancer Society. It is based on a 2007 publication by Goff and colleagues, and describes symptoms of bloating, pelvic or abdominal pain, difficulty eating or feeling full quickly, and urinary symptoms of urgency or frequency.[74] These are symptoms that women with ovarian cancer report as newly developed and persistent, or representing a distinct change from their personal norm. The consensus statement says that if the symptom(s) persist for more than a few weeks, the woman should seek medical care. This medical attention should include an evaluation specifically targeted for identification of gynecologic malignancy.

A reliable, highly specific and highly sensitive format for early diagnosis of ovarian and tubal cancers does not exist. CA 125 is used commonly but has only been approved by the U.S. Food and Drug Administration for use as a biomarker to follow response to therapy for ovarian and tubal cancer patients.[75] Longitudinal studies are ongoing looking at changes in CA 125 over time as a trigger to advance to transvaginal ultrasound and subsequent diagnostics.[76] CA 125, for endometriosis, cannot reliably differentiate benign and malignant disease, nor can it reliably identify early-stage disease where patients with ovarian cancer may realize potential for cure of their disease. The ability to identify those women with a high likelihood of malignant ovarian disease, and especially early-stage malignant disease, is needed.

Triage to the proper professional for intervention of women with masses related to the ovary and fallopian tube is a point of concern. Current American College of Obstetrics and Gynecology recommendations do not support direct referral of a patient with undiagnosed pelvic/ovarian mass to a gynecologic oncologist (see Table 41-10). A recent study indicates that the American College of Obstetrics and Gynecology referral guidelines were 93% sensitive and 60% specific with a positive predictive value of 64% for postmenopausal women, but only 80% sensitive and 70% specific with a positive predictive value of 40% in premenopausal women. This suggests that there are a number of women, especially premenopausal women, who may have benefited from early referral to a gynecologic oncologist.[77] Multiple studies have shown that only 25 to 33% of women with ovarian/tubal cancers have their diagnostic and debulking surgical procedure done by gynecologic oncologists; the remainder are seen by general surgeons and general gynecologists. These studies show inferior patient outcome for women who have had primary surgical attention by nongynecologic oncologists. Development of reliable tools to guide triage of patients to gynecologic oncologists remains important; the utility of the ovarian cancer symptom index needs to be validated prospectively. Criteria strictly based upon lesion size are neither logical nor optimal for ovarian/tubal cancer diagnosis.

Risk Factors

No common risk factors have been identified for most benign ovarian and tubal masses or neoplasms of low malignant potential (LMP or borderline). Ovarian endometriosis can mimic ovarian/tubal cancer symptoms and also can be associated with an increase in CA 125. It has been associated with an increased risk of malignant ovarian disease of endometrioid and clear-cell histology with reported relative risks in the range of 1.4. The cause of endometriosis and how it is a risk for ovarian malignancy remains a point of study. Risk factors for malignancy are presented in Table 41-11. No risk factors have been found that are applicable to LMP disease.

TABLE 41-11	Risk and protective factors for epithelial ovarian and fallopian tube cancers

Protective Factors	Risks
Oral contraceptive use, especially >5 y	Primary and secondary infertility
Tubal ligation	Nulliparity
Lactation	*BRCA1/2* mutation and HNPCC syndrome
Pregnancy	Family history without genetic risk
Oophorectomy, salpingectomy	Endometriosis
	Personal history of breast cancer or first-degree relative with breast cancer
	? Hormone replacement therapy

HNPCC = hereditary nonpolyposis colorectal cancer.

Family history of breast and/or epithelial ovarian cancer is one of the strongest factors for lifetime risk of having breast or epithelial ovarian cancer. Approximately 90% of ovarian cancer is sporadic; of the remaining 10% of cases, 75% of hereditary ovarian cancers has been attributed to mutations in the *BRCA1* and *BRCA2* genes, 7% to hereditary nonpolyposis colorectal cancer syndrome, and the remainder to familial cancer of undefined genetic origin.[78] The lifetime risk of ovarian cancer in *BRCA1* mutation carriers range has been estimated at 40 to 60%, and it is 15 to 45% in *BRCA2* carriers. Controversy exists as to the protective effect of oral contraception pills. The only confirmed prevention is risk-reducing salpingo-oophorectomy (RRSO).[79,80] The risk of ovarian or tubal malignancy is reduced to approximately 5% with RRSO, the resultant cancer presenting as a primary peritoneal cancer. A RRSO procedure must include, at a minimum, the complete resection of the ovaries and extrauterine fallopian tubes bilaterally. In the absence of hysterectomy, an intrauterine remnant of tube is left behind, raising concerns regarding the risk of cancer development in this portion of the tube. This procedure can be done readily by laparoscopy with the smallest morbidity to the patient barring other surgical risks for the laparoscopic approach. Current evolving data suggest that the risk of tumor arises predominantly from the fimbria, suggesting that this less aggressive surgery may be adequate for most patients. Some patients still undergo total abdominal hysterectomy and bilateral salpingo-oophorectomy as a definitive procedure. Postoperative estrogen replacement therapy is controversial. Retrospective data suggest that it may remove some of the breast-cancer protective effect of the surgery but is unlikely to affect ovarian/tubal cancer risk.

Types of Epithelial Tubal and Ovarian Neoplasms
Benign Neoplasms

Benign tubal and ovarian neoplasms have been described. However, the progression of benign tumors to invasive malignant disease remains unclear. Cystic masses are the most common benign findings and include follicular cysts, endometriomas, and cystadenomas or cystadenofibromas. These appear to arise from the surface epithelium, inclusion cyst epithelium, and or epithelium of endometriosis; their advancement to frank malignancy is a point of contention. These lesions present most commonly as incidental findings of hyperechogenic simple cystic masses, predominantly in younger women.

Tubal Intraepithelial Neoplasia

Data to support progressive development of tubal and epithelial ovarian malignancies, similar to what is now recognized in colorectal and lung carcinomas, are limited. No clear consensus defining a precursor lesion has emerged. The ovary contains limited epithelium, the single-cell thick-surface epithelial layer and the epithelium lining inclusion cysts. Transition zones within the surface epithelium have been identified in early-stage disease and LMP tumors suggesting the surface epithelium may be a cell source. The fallopian tube contains the largest surface area of epithelium in the gynecologic organs. This epithelium is organized in a serous papillary pattern, one that is seen in well-differentiated ovarian and tubal neoplasms and is aggravated with worsening differentiation.

Recent studies suggest that the fallopian tube may be the source of the serous cancers of women with *BRCA1/2* mutations, and by extension, perhaps all serous cancers.[81] Convention in pathology is to call a serous cancer of the adnexa ovarian in origin if a clear separation of tubal and ovarian origin cannot be made. This commonly occurs with advanced disease where the integrity of the local adnexa is disrupted. Careful pathologic review of the RRSO specimens has revealed transition zones and shown carcinoma-in-situ and progression to invasion in microscopic lesions. Molecular analysis has identified a p53 signature that can be seen in purportedly benign cells maintained through progression to tubal intraepithelial neoplasia, consisting of p53 mutation, evidence of DNA damage by expression of gamma-H2AX, increasing MiB1 index,

changes in epithelial polarity, and development of pseudostratification leading to intraepithelial neoplasm. Studies suggest that tubal intraepithelial neoplasia may be a precursor to aggressive and highly disseminated disease.

Low Malignant Potential Tumor

LMP tumor, also known as *borderline tumor*, is histologically different from true malignancy. It is seen in the ovary with case reports of occurrences in fallopian tubes and accounts for approximately 15% of ovarian neoplasms. The World Health Organization defines LMP tumors as characterized by epithelial proliferation greater than seen in benign tumors and lack of destructive (ovarian) stromal invasion. This entity has an earlier median age of onset, up to two decades earlier than epithelial malignant tumors. Presentation is predominantly stage I and II, and histology includes all subtypes identified for frank malignancy: papillary serous, mucinous, clear-cell, endometrioid, and transitional or Brenner tumor.[82,83] Surgical intervention is the recommendation of choice. Stages I and II LMP tumors have a 10-year survival of nearly 100%.

A subset of LMP papillary tumor, micropapillary, has been identified.[84,85] Micropapillary tumors have a profusion of micropapillary tufts, sometimes with destruction of architecture. A controversy exists as to whether or not this is further down the progression toward malignancy or just another presentation of a serous neoplasm. In 2004, a consensus review occurred from which criteria for diagnosis were developed and from which the position was taken that this histology does not portend a worse prognosis, and therefore, should not be subject to postsurgical treatment. There are series published indicating a potentially worse outcome; the controversy is whether or not these academic center series are a biased presentation of the subset of LMP disease.

LMP and micropapillary LMP may have sites of dissemination, consistent with the observation of stage II and III disease. Ovarian and tubal neoplasms spread to the peritoneal cavity, and an early site of deposit is on serosal surfaces. Sites of LMP dissemination do not have single-cell or clustered cell invasion nor do they induce a desmoplastic response in the secondary site. They are thus called implants rather than actual invasive metastases. There is a subset of LMP that has true microinvasion and controversy exists as to postsurgical intervention. Microinvasive LMP involves invasion into the ovarian stroma, through either the capsule for surface LMP disease, or through the epithelial basement membrane from inclusion cyst sources. There is greater consensus that microinvasion is a risk factor for a worse prognosis. Other potential poor prognostic factors include nodal involvement, aneuploidy, and residual disease after debulking surgery. Chemotherapy is not routinely advocated and is addressed on a case-by-case basis.

Invasive Tubal and Epithelial Ovarian Cancers

Malignancy of the fallopian tube is predominantly papillary serous in histology. Epithelial ovarian cancer includes (papillary) serous, endometrioid, clear-cell, transitional, and mucinous histotypes. There are differences in gene expression patterns of the different histotypes, but not driving identification of different initial cells of origin. Surgery is used in epithelial ovarian and fallopian tube cancers in five settings:

- Initial staging and cytoreduction (Tables 41-12 and 41-13)
- Interval debulking
- Second look procedures
- Secondary cytoreduction
- Palliation of disease complications

Interval debulking is surgical intervention done after several cycles of chemotherapy; this chemotherapy may have been neoadjuvant or after initial diagnostic and staging laparotomy. It is usually done in situations where the gynecologic oncologist cannot safely cytoreduce the patient. The Gynecologic Oncology Group (GOG)-152 study did not show a survival benefit for interval debulking in

TABLE 41-12	International Federation of Gynecology and Obstetrics staging of epithelial ovarian cancer

Stage	Characteristic
I	Growth limited to the ovaries
IA	Growth limited to one ovary; no ascites; no tumor on the external surfaces, capsule intact
IB	Growth limited to both ovaries; no ascites; no tumor on the external surfaces, capsule intact
IC	Tumor either stage IA or stage IB but with tumor on the surface of one or both ovaries, or with capsule ruptured, or with ascites containing malignant cells or with positive peritoneal washings
II	Growth involving one or both ovaries on pelvic extension
IIA	Extension or metastases to the uterus or tubes
IIB	Extension to other pelvic tissues
IIC	Tumor either stage IIA or IIB with tumor on the surface of one or both ovaries, or with capsule(s) ruptured, or with ascites containing malignant cells or with positive peritoneal washings
III	Tumor involving one or both ovaries with peritoneal implants outside the pelvis or positive retroperitoneal or inguinal nodes; superficial liver metastases equals stage III; tumor is limited to the true pelvis but with histologically verified malignant extension to small bowel or omentum
IIIA	Tumor grossly limited to the true pelvis with negative nodes but with histologically confirmed microscopic seeding of abdominal peritoneal surfaces
IIIB	Tumor of one or both ovaries; histologically confirmed implants of abdominal peritoneal surfaces, none exceeding 2 cm in diameter; nodes negative
IIIC	Abdominal implants >2 cm in diameter or positive retroperitoneal or inguinal nodes
IV	Growth involving one or both ovaries with distant metastases; if pleural effusion is present, there must be positive cytologic test results to allot a case to stage IV; parenchymal liver metastases equals stage IV

Source: From the International Federation of Gynecology and Obstetrics, with permission.

TABLE 41-13	Components of comprehensive surgical staging and debulking of epithelial ovarian cancer

Vertical abdominal incision adequate to visualize the diaphragms
Evacuation of ascites
Peritoneal washings of each pelvic gutter and diaphragm
En bloc hysterectomy and bilateral salpingo-oophorectomy
Supracolic omentectomy
Retroperitoneal and pelvic lymph node dissection
Examination of the entire bowel
Random biopsies of apparently uninvolved areas of peritoneum, pericolic gutters, diaphragm

disease, and evidence of nodal disease immediately upstages a patient to stage III disease and is important in subsequent treatment planning.

Primary Debulking Surgery

The primary goal of the initial surgical intervention for a suspected ovarian malignancy is complete dissection and removal of the primary and metastatic implants of ovarian carcinoma. When epithelial ovarian cancer is identified on frozen section, node dissection is also indicated (see Table 41-13). Decisions about the benefits and risks of radical debulking for individual presentations and diverse pathology depend on the age and medical stability of the patient as well as the pathologic type of the cancer. Conservative, fertility-sparing surgery can be considered only for likely stage I grade 1 or 2 epithelial ovarian cancer or for germ cell malignancies with no obvious metastases. It is the decision making related to the underlying pathology and understanding of the disease process that determines the extent and type of procedure more so than the surgical techniques themselves.

Standard primary debulking of epithelial ovarian cancer includes removal of the uterus, tubes, ovaries, and omentum. Dissection of pelvic and periaortic lymph nodes is required if no gross intraperitoneal disease (>2 cm in longest diameter) is seen, if the patient is eligible for and interested in a cooperative group trial where surgical practice is normalized across the group, or if there are enlarged nodes that require removal to complete debulking in a situation where clinical trial does not so dictate. Hysterectomy and bilateral salpingo-oophorectomy are usually completed with standard techniques, although extensive dissection of the peritoneum to remove disease over the bladder peritoneum or cul-de-sac or radical parametrial dissection to achieve debulking may be required. The retroperitoneum usually is spared, allowing dissection from the underside of the peritoneum throughout the cul-de-sac, gutters, and the pelvic peritoneum for debulking. Omentectomy is usually supracolic, performed after separation of the avascular posterior leaf of the omentum over the transverse colon and then dissection of the lesser sac separating the mesentery from the anterior portion of the omentum. This is particularly important when bulky disease is present, to assure that dissection of the omentum is separated from any mesenteric or bowel adhesions or disease process that would be addressed separately if feasible. This is then serially dissected with ligation of the right and left gastroepiploic vessels and the short gastrics as they course through the omentum. Radical resection of disease may require splenectomy, bowel, liver, and/or diaphragm resection, which is appropriate based on likelihood of complete debulking at the end of the surgery and the overall health status of the patient, as it is directly related to significant morbidity and mortality.

Placement of Intraperitoneal Port for Intraperitoneal Chemotherapy

If surgical resection has resulted in complete debulking and no significant residual adhesions preventing complete intra-abdominal spread of fluid are present, and the patient has been counseled and

patients undergoing maximal initial cytoreduction followed by platinum/taxane therapy.[86] There are situations where the management of the individual leads to use of this route. Second-look surgery, which is done after the completion of adjuvant chemotherapy to assess residual disease or benefit of therapy, is now less commonly done. The amount of residual disease after completion of chemotherapy has long been known to have prognostic importance. The advent of more sensitive noninvasive imaging has further reduced the frequency of second-look operations. Secondary cytoreduction is debulking surgery done upon recurrence of disease after an initial postchemotherapy remission. Patients who have had a disease-free period of at least 12 months following initial therapy, who, on examination and imaging, have no evidence of carcinomatosis or miliary spread, and have localized disease, are considered optimal candidates. Retrospective studies have suggested a possible survival advantage of secondary debulking under these circumstances. A prospective randomized trial is ongoing to confirm this hypothesis. Debulking done after subsequent relapses has not been shown to result in an outcome benefit. Finally, surgery is used to palliate disease complications. The most common cause of palliative surgery is bypass of bowel obstruction.

Ovarian cancer does not progress logically following the same format as other gynecologic cancers. Local dissemination to pelvic organs and side walls are seen and define stage II disease; this disease presents in stage III or IV in >75% of cases, intraperitoneal dissemination or beyond. Common sites of dissemination include along the pericolic gutters, on the peritoneal surface of the diaphragms, on serosal surfaces, and in periaortic and pelvic lymph nodes. Negative pelvic lymph nodes do not rule out periaortic

TABLE 41-14 Standards of care for adjuvant therapy of epithelial ovarian or tubal carcinoma

	Platinum	Taxane	No. of Cycles
Early stage	Carboplatin AUC 5–7.5 IV	Paclitaxel 175 mg/m² over 3 h IV	3–6
Optimally debulked <1 cm residual	Carboplatin AUC 5–7.5 IV	Paclitaxel 175 mg/m² over 3 h IV	6
	or	*or*	
	See Table 41-15 for intraperitoneal therapy	Docetaxel 75 mg/m² over 1 h	
Suboptimally debulked	Carboplatin AUC 5–7.5 IV	Paclitaxel 175 mg/m² over 3 h IV	6
		or	
		Docetaxel 75 mg/m² over 1 h	

AUC = area under curve using the Calvert formula.

CHAPTER 41 Gynecology

agrees to intraperitoneal therapy, then placement of an intraperitoneal port is appropriate. This is usually a 9.6F venous port, with the port placed over the right or left lower abdominal wall and tunneled to an insertion through the fascia in the lower abdomen. The tip should be placed in the right or left pelvis. If done secondarily, this will require two incisions, one for the port pocket and one for the direct visualization of the placement through the fascia and peritoneum to assure a tight but not constricting seal with sutures in this lower incision.

Postsurgical Adjuvant Therapy and Therapy of Recurrent Disease
Postsurgical Treatment of Early-Stage Disease

Early-stage tubal and epithelial ovarian cancers, stage I disease specifically, have an excellent outcome. Stages IA and B, restricted to one or both ovaries or one or both of the fallopian tubes (see Table 41-12), and of low grade can be cured in up to 90 to 95% of cases by a complete surgical staging procedure. The prevailing position in the United States is that women with stage IA or IB, grade 1 or 2 disease do not benefit from chemotherapy. This stems in part from the GOG-7601 study, showing no benefit of melphalan adjuvant therapy compared with observation.[87] The standard of care for women with stages IC and II and all women with grade 3 or clear-cell histology is adjuvant chemotherapy. The current treatment recommendations are found in Table 41-14, three to six cycles of carboplatin in combination with paclitaxel or docetaxel (stages IC and II for the latter). The GOG-157 study was a randomization of three vs. six cycles of carboplatin and paclitaxel and yielded no significant difference in progression-free or overall survival.[88] The subsequent study, GOG-175, a randomization between three cycles of carboplatin and paclitaxel with or without 6 months of weekly paclitaxel at 40 mg/m² is maturing and has not yet been reported. Natural history and delayed intervention studies from Europe suggest that withholding therapy until recurrence in stage I patients can have a good outcome.[89,90] Treatment with a platinum agent upon recurrence is associated with potential for cure but not to the

level seen with adjuvant treatment. The GOG has now recommended that stage II patients be considered for advanced-stage clinical trials.

Adjuvant Therapy of Advanced-Stage Tubal and Ovarian Cancers

Defining Optimal and Suboptimal Disease Completeness of initial staging and debulking surgery is important as a prognostic indicator in addition to defining stage of disease. Data since the mid-1970s have consistently confirmed that the more completely resected a patient, the better her outcome. This led to segregating patients into subsets of optimally and suboptimally debulked disease for treatment purposes. The initial definition of optimal debulking was residual disease where no lesion had a diameter >2 cm; note the summation of disease or estimate of total bulk residual has not been used in ovarian cancer. Since GOG-111,[91] the study that introduced paclitaxel into epithelial ovarian cancer treatment, the definition of optimal disease has been no residual lesion >1 cm in diameter. Recent GOG studies have segregated patient entry by optimal and suboptimal disease residual using this definition.

Intraperitoneal Therapy for Optimally Cytoreduced Stage III Patients In 2006, the National Cancer Institute issued a Clinical Alert indicating that intraperitoneal administration of adjuvant chemotherapy should be considered first line for all women with optimally cytoreduced epithelial ovarian cancer. This Clinical Alert occurred in response to the completion and analysis of three independent randomized clinical trials, all of which showed a significant survival advantage for intraperitoneal therapy. It recommended all optimally cytoreduced patients be treated with intraperitoneal cisplatin 100 mg/m² with a taxane, following the GOG-172 study (Table 41-15).[92,93] Patients who are not good candidates for intraperitoneal therapy should receive the IV standard of care applied to all other advanced-stage ovarian cancer patients. Intraperitoneal therapy can be administered through a variety of means. These include Tenckhoff catheter and intraperitoneal Port-A-Cath type catheters. However, the use of vascular ports is preferred due

TABLE 41-15 Seminal clinical trials of intraperitoneal therapy in optimally cytoreduced ovarian cancer patients

Trial	No. of Patients	Disease-Free Survival	Overall Survival
SWOG-8501/GOG-104ᵃ	654		41 vs. 49 mo
C 100 mg/m² IV + CTX 600 mg/m² IV vs. C 100 mg/m² IP + CTX 600 mg/m² IV			P = .02, HR 0.76
GOG-114	462	22 vs. 28 mo P = .02,	52 vs. 63 mo
P 135 mg/m² IV over 24 h, C 75 mg/m² IV d2 vs. Carb AUC 9 IV × two cycles followed by C 100 mg/m² IP + P 135 mg/m² IV over 24 h		RR 0.78	P = .05, RR 0.81
GOG-172	415	18.2 vs. 23.8 mo	49.7 vs. 65.6 mo
P 135 mg/m² IV over 24 h, C 75mg/m² IV d2 vs. P 135 mg/m² IV over 24 h, C 100 mg/m² IP d2 and P 60 mg/m² IP d8		RR 0.8, P = .05	RR 0.75, P = .03

ᵃAllowed optimal patients defined as <2 cm residual disease.
AUC = area under curve using the Calvert formula; C = cisplatin; Carb = carboplatin; CTX = cyclophosphamide; GOG = Gynecologic Oncology Group; HR = hazard ratio; IP = intraperitoneal; P = paclitaxel; RR = relative risks; SWOG = Southwest Oncology Group.

to decreased incidence of bowel and adhesive complications compared to intraperitoneal catheters with multiple holes on the end, such as a Tenckhoff. It is further recommended that the intraperitoneal access device be consented for and placed at initial surgery when the diagnosis of ovarian cancer is made pre- or intraoperatively and there is high likelihood of complete debulking. These devices can be removed with minimal trauma at the bedside or with outpatient surgery should an alternative therapy be selected.

Chemotherapy for Advanced-Stage Disease Patients who have suboptimally debulked disease and/or who are not candidates for intraperitoneal therapy should receive IV adjuvant chemotherapy. Randomized clinical trials of the past decade support use of a platinum compound and a taxane as the standard of care (see Table 41-14). Although eight cycles of therapy were administered in the international intergroup study, GOG-182, a five-arm trial with carboplatin/paclitaxel as the control arm, the recommended standard is six cycles. The arms incorporating a third agent as a triplet, alternating doublet/triplet, or sequential doublets showed no improvement over the control arm, and at present, no additional agents are standard for initial therapy. In addition, there are no randomized data to validate the use of drug sensitivity testing to select adjuvant therapy. Data suggest that the normalization of CA 125 by the third treatment cycle may be prognostic for later recurrence. The role of targeted therapies in the treatment of newly diagnosed ovarian and tubal cancer patients is under investigation. The GOG-218 study includes arms in which bevacizumab is included in adjuvant therapy and/or in a postadjuvant maintenance phase, given at a dose of 15 mg/kg; a similar cooperative group study is ongoing in Europe using bevacizumab at 7.5 mg/kg.

Intervention in Recurrent Disease Chemotherapy is the mainstay of therapy for recurrent tubal and epithelial ovarian cancers. Treatment approaches are based upon platinum sensitivity[94] (Table 41-16). Exceptions include recurrence after a >12-month disease-free interval with isolated resectable disease, late recurrence with sites of disease causing organ risk, and palliation for disease-related complications. Radiation therapy, while very effective against tubal and ovarian cancer, is not commonly used in the United States except for isolated sites of recurrence and in situations where surgical palliation may not be feasible. Referral to an oncologist with specific expertise in chemotherapeutic treatment of ovarian cancer and access to clinical trials is important. In determining secondary and subsequent therapy, consideration of prior therapies, sites of disease, organs at risk from cancer, organs sustaining injury from prior therapy, and quality of life desires of the patient should be taken into consideration.

TABLE 41-16	Definitions of platinum resistance and guidelines for treatment of recurrent disease

Platinum Sensitivity	Definition	Intervention
Refractory	Progression while receiving a platinum	Nonplatinum-based chemotherapy
		Platinum with gemcitabine
Resistant	Progression within 6 mo of completing treatment	Nonplatinum-based chemotherapy
		Platinum with gemcitabine
Sensitive	Progression beyond 6 mo of completing treatment	Consider secondary debulking if >12 mo since treatment
		Consider platinum ± taxane
		Nonplatinum-based chemotherapy

NONEPITHELIAL CANCERS OF THE OVARY AND FALLOPIAN TUBE

Germ Cell Tumors

Germ cell tumors occur most commonly in women under age 30 years old, grow and disseminate rapidly, and are symptomatic. The rapid growth may be accompanied by torsion producing an acute abdomen and need for emergent intervention. Most common are the benign forms of teratomas; within the malignant category, the most common malignant form is dysgerminoma, which is made up of pure undifferentiated germ cells. Bilaterality occurs in up to 15% of patients and elevated beta-hCG may occur. Staging, including removal of the involved ovary, biopsy of any suspicious areas, node dissection, and omentectomy, should be done initially but does not require hysterectomy or removal of the second ovary if fertility preservation is of concern and no extension of disease is observed. Evidence of extraovarian spread, such as nodal metastases, requires adjuvant therapy. Chemotherapy is the most common adjuvant intervention, although radiation therapy, the previous standard, may be considered. The cure rate remains high, near 90% with metastatic disease; recurrent disease is more difficult to eradicate.

Less common are immature teratomas, endodermal sinus or yolk sac tumors, mixed tumors, malignant teratomas (embryonal carcinomas), and choriocarcinomas. Endodermal sinus tumors may have elevated alpha-fetoprotein levels in the blood and, in the case of mixed germ cell tumors, beta-hCG may also be elevated. Both markers are useful to follow during definitive therapy. Early spread of these tumors occurs and other than completely resected stage I, grade 1 immature teratoma, all others require adjuvant therapy with a platinum-containing regimen. In addition, women of older age than the usual germ cell malignancy (>30 years old) can have midline (mediastinal) germ cell tumors. These are treated with chemotherapy after careful assessment for a pelvic primary. The success of therapy for this germ cell presentation does not carry the positive prognosis that the pelvic germ cell cancer does.

Sex Cord-Stromal Cell Tumors

Although rare, stromal cell tumors can present with symptoms referable to endocrine activity of the tumor. These include combinations of the mesenchymal (fibromas, sarcomas) and sex cord cell components (granulosa, theca, Sertoli, Leydig). Granulosa cell tumors are the most common in this group and are a low-grade malignancy treated with conservative surgery similar to germ cell in young women as <3% are bilateral. Debulking surgery is the primary means of management if more extensive. These tumors and the thecomas in the same class often stimulate estrogen production and can be found in association with endometrial hyperplasia and cancer (5%) as well. Granulosa cell tumors can recur over a prolonged period given their low rate of proliferation and tendency for local or intraperitoneal recurrence. Inhibin has been shown to be elaborated by these tumors and often is followed to identify recurrence of the disease. The Sertoli/Leydig cell tumors can present with virilization as a primary symptom. Evaluation of the ovary when this symptom is found is always of value. For the most part, these are benign and unilateral tumors and removal alone is adequate.

REFERENCES

Entries highlighted in bright blue are key references.

1. Anson B: *Atlas of Human Anatomy.* Philadelphia: WB Saunders, 1950.
2. Stanley M: Genital human papillomavirus infections—current and prospective therapies. *J Natl Cancer Inst Monogr* 31:117, 2003.
3. Mutch DG, Powell MA, Allsworth JE, et al: How accurate is Pipelle sampling: A study by Huang et al. *Am J Obstet Gynecol* 196:280, 2007.
4. Anderson MR, Klink K, Cohrssen A: Evaluation of vaginal complaints. *JAMA* 291:1368, 2004.
5. Eschenbach DA, Davick PR, Williams BL, et al: Prevalence of hydrogen peroxide-producing Lactobacillus species in normal women and women with bacterial vaginosis. *J Clin Microbiol* 27:251, 1989.

6. Hill GB: The microbiology of bacterial vaginosis. *Am J Obstet Gynecol* 169:450, 1993.

7. Workowski KA, Berman SM: Sexually transmitted diseases treatment guidelines, 2006. *MMWR Recomm Rep* 55:1, 2006.

8. Morse SA, Trees DL, Htun Y, et al: Comparison of clinical diagnosis and standard laboratory and molecular methods for the diagnosis of genital ulcer disease in Lesotho: Association with human immunodeficiency virus infection. *J Infect Dis* 175:583, 1997.

9. Kimberlin DW, Rouse DJ: Clinical practice. Genital herpes. *N Engl J Med* 350:1970, 2004.

10. Brown ZA, Wald A, Morrow RA, et al: Effect of serologic status and cesarean delivery on transmission rates of herpes simplex virus from mother to infant. *JAMA* 289:203, 2003.

11. Stone KM, Brooks CA, Guinan ME, et al: National surveillance for neonatal herpes simplex virus infections. *Sex Transm Dis* 16:152, 1989.

12. Hook EW 3rd, Marra CM: Acquired syphilis in adults. *N Engl J Med* 326:1060, 1992.

13. Morse SA: Chancroid and Haemophilus ducreyi. *Clin Microbiol Rev* 2:137, 1989.

14. Ernst AA, Marvez-Valls E, Martin DH: Incision and drainage versus aspiration of fluctuant buboes in the emergency department during an epidemic of chancroid. *Sex Transm Dis* 22:217, 1995.

15. Mabey D, Peeling RW: Lymphogranuloma venereum. *Sex Transm Infect* 78:90, 2002.

16. Downs MC, Randall HW Jr. The ambulatory surgical management of Bartholin duct cysts. *J Emerg Med* 7:623, 1989.

17. Habel LA, Van Den Eeden SK, Sherman KJ, et al: Risk factors for incident and recurrent condylomata acuminata among women. A population-based study. *Sex Transm Dis* 25:285, 1998.

18. Brodell LA, Mercurio MG, Brodell RT: The diagnosis and treatment of human papillomavirus-mediated genital lesions. *Cutis* 79:5, 2007.

19. Bernstein R, Kennedy WR, Waldron J: Acute pelvic inflammatory disease: A clinical follow-up. *Int J Fertil* 32:229, 1987.

20. Chow JM, Yonekura ML, Richwald GA, et al: The association between Chlamydia trachomatis and ectopic pregnancy. A matched-pair, case-control study. *JAMA* 263:3164, 1990.

21. Update to CDC's sexually transmitted diseases treatment guidelines, 2006: Fluoroquinolones no longer recommended for treatment of gonococcal infections. *MMWR Morb Mortal Wkly Rep* 56:332, 2007.

22. Ness RB, Soper DE, Holley RL, et al: Effectiveness of inpatient and outpatient treatment strategies for women with pelvic inflammatory disease: Results from the Pelvic Inflammatory Disease Evaluation and Clinical Health (PEACH) Randomized Trial. *Am J Obstet Gynecol* 186:929, 2002.

23. Gabbe S, Niebyl J, Simpson J: *Obstetrics: Normal and Problem Pregnancies*, 4th ed. Philadelphia: Churchill Livingstone, 2002.

24. Allen JR, Helling TS, Langenfeld M: Intraabdominal surgery during pregnancy. *Am J Surg* 158:567, 1989.

25. Brodsky JB: Anesthesia and surgery during early pregnancy and fetal outcome. *Clin Obstet Gynecol* 26:449, 1983.

26. Brodsky JB, Cohen EN, Brown BW Jr., et al. Surgery during pregnancy and fetal outcome. *Am J Obstet Gynecol* 138:1165, 1980.

27. National Institutes of Health state-of-the-science conference statement: Cesarean delivery on maternal request March 27–29, 2006. *Obstet Gynecol* 107:1386, 2006.

28. Jones R: Abortion in the United States: Incidence and access to services, 2005. *Perspect Sex Reprod Health* 40:6, 2008.

29. McDonald IA: Suture of the cervix for inevitable miscarriage. *J Obstet Gynaecol Br Emp* 64:346, 1957.

30. Shirodkar V: New method of operative treatment for habitual abortions in the second trimester of pregnancy. *The Antiseptic* 52:299, 1955.

31. Shih IeM: Gestational trophoblastic neoplasia—pathogenesis and potential therapeutic targets. *Lancet Oncol* 8:642, 2007.

32. Garner EI, Goldstein DP, Feltmate CM, et al: Gestational trophoblastic disease. *Clin Obstet Gynecol* 50:112, 2007.

33. Walters M, Karram M: *Urogynecology and Reconstructive Pelvic Surgery*, 3rd ed. Philadelphia: Mosby, 2007.

34. Olsen AL, Smith VJ, Bergstrom JO, et al: Epidemiology of surgically managed pelvic organ prolapse and urinary incontinence. *Obstet Gynecol* 89:501, 1997.

35. Bump RC, Mattiasson A, Bo K, et al: The standardization of terminology of female pelvic organ prolapse and pelvic floor dysfunction. *Am J Obstet Gynecol* 175:10, 1996.

36. Benson JT, Lucente V, McClellan E: Vaginal versus abdominal reconstructive surgery for the treatment of pelvic support defects: A prospective randomized study with long-term outcome evaluation. *Am J Obstet Gynecol* 175:1418; discussion 21, 1996.

37. Maher CF, Qatawneh AM, Dwyer PL, et al: Abdominal sacral colpopexy or vaginal sacrospinous colpopexy for vaginal vault prolapse: A prospective randomized study. *Am J Obstet Gynecol* 190:20, 2004.

38. Nygaard IE, McCreery R, Brubaker L, et al: Abdominal sacrocolpopexy: A comprehensive review. *Obstet Gynecol* 104:805, 2004.

39. Rock J, Jones H: *TeLinde's Operative Gynecology*, 10th ed. Philadelphia: Lippincott, Williams and Wilkins, 2008.

40. Pereyra AJ: A simplified surgical procedure for the correction of stress incontinence in women. *West J Surg Obstet Gynecol* 67:223, 1959.

41. Tanagho EA: Colpocystourethropexy: The way we do it. *J Urol* 116:751, 1976.

42. Margesson LJ: Vulvar disease pearls. *Dermatol Clin* 24:145, 2006.

43. Fanning J, Lambert HC, Hale TM, et al: Paget's disease of the vulva: Prevalence of associated vulvar adenocarcinoma, invasive Paget's disease, and recurrence after surgical excision. *Am J Obstet Gynecol* 180:24, 1999.

44. Tebes S, Cardosi R, Hoffman M: Paget's disease of the vulva. *Am J Obstet Gynecol* 187:281; discussion 83, 2002.

45. Cardosi RJ, Bomalaski JJ, Hoffman MS: Diagnosis and management of vulvar and vaginal intraepithelial neoplasia. *Obstet Gynecol Clin North Am* 28:685, 2001.

46. Modesitt SC, Waters AB, Walton L, et al: Vulvar intraepithelial neoplasia III: Occult cancer and the impact of margin status on recurrence. *Obstet Gynecol* 92:962, 1998.

47. Beller U, Quinn MA, Benedet JL, et al: Carcinoma of the vulva. FIGO 6th Annual Report on the Results of Treatment in Gynecological Cancer. *Int J Gynaecol Obstet* 95:S7, 2006.

48. Berek J, Hacker N: *Practical Gynecologic Oncology*, 4th ed. Philadelphia: Lippincott, Williams and Wilkins, 2004.

49. Disaia P, Creasman W: *Clinical Gynecologic Oncology*. St Louis: Elsevier Mosby, 2007.

50. Hoskins W, Perez C, Young R. *Principles and Practice of Gynecologic Oncology*. Philadelphia: Lippincott, Williams and Wilkins, 2000.

51. Benedet JL, Bender H, Jones H 3rd, et al: FIGO staging classifications and clinical practice guidelines in the management of gynecologic cancers. FIGO Committee on Gynecologic Oncology. *Int J Gynaecol Obstet* 70:209, 2000.

52. Montana GS, Thomas GM, Moore DH, et al: Preoperative chemoradiation for carcinoma of the vulva with N2/N3 nodes: A Gynecologic Oncology Group study. *Int J Radiat Oncol Biol Phys* 48:1007, 2000.

53. Moore DH, Thomas GM, Montana GS, et al: Preoperative chemoradiation for advanced vulvar cancer: A phase II study of the Gynecologic Oncology Group. *Int J Radiat Oncol Biol Phys* 42:79, 1998.

54. Beller U, Benedet JL, Creasman WT, et al: Carcinoma of the vagina. FIGO 6th Annual Report on the Results of Treatment in Gynecological Cancer. *Int J Gynaecol Obstet* 95:S29, 2006.

55. Herbst AL, Ulfelder H, Poskanzer DC: Adenocarcinoma of the vagina. Association of maternal stilbestrol therapy with tumor appearance in young women. *N Engl J Med* 284:878, 1971.

56. Herbst AL, Ulfelder H, Poskanzer DC, et al: Adenocarcinoma of the vagina. Association of maternal stilbestrol therapy with tumor appearance in young women. 1971. *Am J Obstet Gynecol* 181:1574, 1999.

57. Wright TC Jr., Massad LS, Dunton CJ, et al: 2006 consensus guidelines for the management of women with cervical intraepithelial neoplasia or adenocarcinoma in situ. *J Low Genit Tract Dis* 11:223, 2007.

58. Pikaart DP, Holloway RW, Ahmad S, et al: Clinical-pathologic and morbidity analyses of Types 2 and 3 abdominal radical hysterectomy for cervical cancer. *Gynecol Oncol* 107:205, 2007.

59. Stenchever M, Droegemueller W, Herbst A, et al: *Comprehensive Gynecology*, 4th ed. St Louis: Mosby, 2001.

60. Van Bogaert LJ: Clinicopathologic findings in endometrial polyps. *Obstet Gynecol* 71:771, 1988.

61. Byun JY, Kim SE, Choi BG, et al: Diffuse and focal adenomyosis: MR imaging findings. *Radiographics* 19:S161, 1999.

62. Boing C, Kimmig R: [Surgical management of endometriosis—an overview]. *Gynakol Geburtshilfliche Rundsch* 47:124, 2007.

1514

CHAPTER 41

Gynecology

63. Petta CA, Matos AM, Bahamondes L, et al: Current practice in the management of symptoms of endometriosis: A survey of Brazilian gynecologists. *Rev Assoc Med Bras* 53:525, 2007.

64. Filicori M, Hall DA, Loughlin JS, et al: A conservative approach to the management of uterine leiomyoma: Pituitary desensitization by a luteinizing hormone-releasing hormone analogue. *Am J Obstet Gynecol* 147:726, 1983.

65. Matsuo H, Maruo T: [GnRH analogues in the management of uterine leiomyoma]. *Nippon Rinsho* 64:75, 2006.

66. Szabo E, Nagy E, Morvay Z, et al: [Uterine artery embolization for the conservative management of leiomyoma]. *Orv Hetil* 142:675, 2001.

67. Mutter GL: Diagnosis of premalignant endometrial disease. *J Clin Pathol* 55:326, 2002.

68. Kurman RJ, Kaminski PF, Norris HJ: The behavior of endometrial hyperplasia. A long-term study of "untreated" hyperplasia in 170 patients. *Cancer* 56:403, 1985.

69. Mutter GL: Endometrial intraepithelial neoplasia (EIN): Will it bring order to chaos? The Endometrial Collaborative Group. *Gynecol Oncol* 76:287, 2000.

70. Mutter GL, Zaino RJ, Baak JP, et al: Benign endometrial hyperplasia sequence and endometrial intraepithelial neoplasia. *Int J Gynecol Pathol* 26:103, 2007.

71. Aarnio M, Mecklin JP, Aaltonen LA, et al: Life-time risk of different cancers in hereditary non-polyposis colorectal cancer (HNPCC) syndrome. *Int J Cancer* 64:430, 1995.

72. Heintz AP, Odicino F, Maisonneuve P, et al: Carcinoma of the ovary. FIGO 6th Annual Report on the Results of Treatment in Gynecological Cancer. *Int J Gynaecol Obstet* 95:S161, 2006.

73. Bhoola S, Hoskins WJ: Diagnosis and management of epithelial ovarian cancer. *Obstet Gynecol* 107:1399, 2006.

74. Goff BA, Mandel LS, Drescher CW, et al: Development of an ovarian cancer symptom index: Possibilities for earlier detection. *Cancer* 109:221, 2007.

75. Bast RC, Klug TL, St. John E, et al: A radioimmunoassay using a monoclonal antibody to monitor the course of epithelial ovarian cancer. *N Engl J Med* 309:883, 1983.

76. Jacobs IJ, Skates SJ, Macdonald N, et al: Screening for ovarian cancer: A pilot randomised controlled trial. *Lancet* 354:509, 1999.

77. Dearking AC, Aletti GD, McGree ME: How relevant are ACOG and SGO guidelines for referral of adnexal mass? *Obstet Gynecol* 110:841, 2007.

78. Lu KH: Hereditary gynecologic cancers: Differential diagnosis, surveillance, management and surgical prophylaxis. *Fam Cancer* 7:53, 2008.

79. Kauff ND, Satagopan JM, Robson ME, et al: Risk-reducing salpingo-oophorectomy in women with a BRCA1 or BRCA2 mutation. *N Engl J Med* 346:1609, 2002.

80. ACOG Practice Bulletin No. 89. Elective and risk-reducing salpingo-oophorectomy. *Obstet Gynecol* 111:231, 2008.

81. Callahan MJ, Crum CP, Medeiros F, et al: Primary fallopian tube malignancies in BRCA-positive women undergoing surgery for ovarian cancer risk reduction. *J Clin Oncol* 25:3985, 2007.

82. Seidman JD, Kurman RJ: Ovarian serous borderline tumors: A critical review of the literature with emphasis on prognostic indicators. *Hum Pathol* 31:539, 2000.

83. Bell DA, Longacre TA, Prat J, et al: Serous borderline (low malignant potential, atypical proliferative) ovarian tumors: Workshop perspectives. *Hum Pathol* 35:934, 2004.

84. Ayhan A, Guvendag Guven ES, Guven S, et al: Recurrence and prognostic factors in borderline ovarian tumors. *Gynecol Oncol* 98:439, 2005.

85. Deavers MT, Gershenson DM, Tortolero-Luna G, et al: Micropapillary and cribriform patterns in ovarian serous tumors of low malignant potential: A study of 99 advanced-stage cases. *Am J Surg Pathol* 26:1129, 2002.

86. Secondary surgical cytoreduction in advanced ovarian carcinoma: A Gynecologic Oncology Group study. *N Engl J Med* 351:2489, 2004.

87. Young RC, Walton LA, Ellenberg SS, et al: Adjuvant therapy in stage I and stage II epithelial ovarian cancer. *N Engl J Med* 322:1021, 1990.

88. Bell J, Brady MF, Young RC, et al: Randomized phase III trial of three versus six cycles of adjuvant carboplatin and paclitaxel in early-stage epithelial ovarian carcinoma: A Gynecologic Oncology Group study. *Gynecol Oncol* 102:432, 2006.

89. Trimbos JB, Parmar M, Vergote I, et al: International Collaborative Ovarian Neoplasm trial 1 and Adjuvant ChemoTherapy In Ovarian Neoplasm trial: Two parallel randomized phase III trials of adjuvant chemotherapy in patients with early-stage ovarian carcinoma. *J Natl Cancer Inst* 95:105, 2003.

90. Colombo N, Guthrie D, Chiari S, et al: International Collaborative Ovarian Neoplasm trial 1: A randomized trial of adjuvant chemotherapy in women with early-stage ovarian cancer. *J Natl Cancer Inst* 95:125, 2003.

91. McGuire WP, Hoskins WJ, Brady MF, et al: Cyclophosphamide and cisplatin compared with paclitaxel and cisplatin in patients with stage III and stage IV ovarian cancer [see comments]. *N Engl J Med* 334:1, 1996.

92. Armstrong DK, Bundy BN, Wenzel L, et al: Intraperitoneal cisplatin and paclitaxel in ovarian cancer. *N Engl J Med* 354:34, 2006.

93. Walker JL, Armstrong DK, Huang HQ, et al: Intraperitoneal catheter outcomes in a phase III trial of intravenous versus intraperitoneal chemotherapy in optimal stage III ovarian and primary peritoneal cancer: A Gynecologic Oncology Group Study. *Gynecol Oncol* 100:27, 2006.

94. Markman M, Reichman B, Hakes T, et al: Responses to second-line cisplatin-based intraperitoneal therapy in ovarian cancer: Influence of a prior response to intravenous cisplatin. *J Clin Oncol* 9:1801, 1991.

Neurosurgery

Michael L. Smith, Joel A. Bauman,
and M. Sean Grady

OVERVIEW

Neurologic surgery is a discipline of medicine and the specialty of surgery that provides the operative and nonoperative management (i.e., prevention, diagnosis, evaluation, treatment, critical care, and rehabilitation) of disorders of the central, peripheral, and autonomic nervous systems (ANSs). This includes their supporting structures and vascular supply; the evaluation and treatment of pathologic processes that modify the function or activity of the nervous system, including the hypophysis; and the operative and nonoperative management of pain. Such disorders include those of the brain, meninges, skull and skull base, and their blood supply, including surgical and endovascular treatment of disorders of the intracranial and extracranial vasculature supplying the brain and spinal cord; disorders of the pituitary gland; disorders of the spinal cord, meninges, and vertebral column, including those that may require treatment by fusion, instrumentation, or endovascular techniques; and disorders of the cranial and spinal nerves throughout their distribution.

An accurate history is the first step toward neurologic diagnosis. A history of trauma or of neurologic symptoms is of obvious interest, but general constitutional symptoms are also important. Neurologic disease may have systemic effects, while diseases of other systems may affect neurologic function. The patient's general medical ability to withstand the physiologic stress of anesthesia and surgery should be understood. A detailed history from the patient and/or family, along with a reliable physical examination, will clarify these issues.

NEUROANATOMY

An understanding of neuroanatomy is the foundation of comprehensive neurologic examination and diagnosis. Salient features will be considered, from cephalad to caudad. The cerebral hemispheres (or telencephalon) consist of the cerebral cortex, underlying white matter, the basal ganglia, hippocampus, and amygdala. The cerebral cortex is the most recently evolved part of the nervous system. Its functions are mapped to discrete anatomic areas. The frontal areas are involved in executive function, decision making, and restraint of emotions. The motor strip, or precentral gyrus, is the most posterior component of the frontal lobes, and is arranged along a homunculus with the head inferior and lateral to the lower extremities superiorly and medially. The motor speech area (Broca's area) lies in the left posterior inferior frontal lobe in almost all right-handed people and in up to 90% of left-handed people. The parietal lobe lies between the central sulcus anteriorly and the occipital lobe posteriorly. The postcentral gyrus is the sensory strip, also arranged along a homunculus. The rest of the parietal lobe is involved with awareness of one's body in space and relative to the immediate environment, body orientation, and spatial relationships. The occipital lobes are most posterior. The visual cortex is arrayed along the apposing medial surfaces of the occipital lobes. The left occipital lobe receives and integrates data from the left half of each retina. A left occipital lesion would therefore result in inability to see objects right of center. The temporal lobes lie below the sylvian fissures. The hippocampus, amygdala, and lower optic radiations (Meyer's loops) are important components of the temporal lobe and are involved in memory, emotion, and visual pathways, respectively. The receptive speech area (Wernicke's area) lies in the area of the posterior superior temporal lobe and the inferior parietal lobe, usually on the left. The basal ganglia include the caudate, putamen, and the globus pallidus. Basal ganglia structures are involved with modulation of movement via inhibition of motor pathways.

Lying deep to the cerebral hemispheres is the diencephalon, which includes the thalamus and hypothalamus. The thalamus is a key processor and relay circuit for most motor and sensory information going to or coming from the cortex. The hypothalamus, at the base of the brain, is a key regulator of homeostasis, via the autonomic and neuroendocrine systems.

The brain stem consists of the midbrain (mesencephalon), pons (metencephalon), and medulla (myelencephalon). Longitudinal fibers run through the brain stem, carrying motor and sensory information between the cerebral hemispheres and the spinal cord. The corticospinal tract is the major motor tract, while the medial lemniscus and the spinothalamic tracts are the major sensory tracts. The nuclei of cranial nerves III through XII are also located within the brain stem. These nerves relay the motor, sensory, and special sense functions of the eye, face, mouth, and throat. The cerebellum arises from the dorsal aspect of the brain stem. It integrates somatosensory, vestibular, and motor information for coordination and timing of movement. Midline, or vermian, lesions lead to truncal ataxia. Lateral, or hemispheric, lesions lead to tremor and dyscoordination in the extremities.

The ventricular system is a cerebrospinal fluid (CSF)–containing contiguous space inside the brain, continuous with the subarachnoid space outside the brain. The paired lateral ventricles consist of temporal, occipital, and frontal horns, as well as the main body. CSF travels from each lateral ventricle through the foramina of Monroe to the third ventricle, located between the left and right thalami. CSF then drains through the cerebral aqueduct to the fourth ventricle in the brain stem. The foramen of Magendie (midline) and paired foramina of Luschka (lateral) drain to the subarachnoid space. Choroid plexus creates the CSF, mostly in the lateral ventricles. The average adult has an approximate CSF volume of 150 mL and creates approximately 500 mL per day.

The spinal cord starts at the bottom of the medulla and extends through the spinal canal down to approximately the first lumbar vertebra. Motor tracts (efferent pathways) continue from the brain stem down via the lateral and anterior corticospinal tracts to anterior horn cells, and then exit via ventral nerve roots. Sensory information (afferent pathways) enters via dorsal nerve roots, travels up the dorsal columns (proprioception and fine touch) or the spinothalamic tract (pain and temperature), and into the brain stem. Paired nerves exit the spinal cord at each level. There are 31 pairs: 8 cervical, 12 thoracic, 5 lumbar, 5 sacral, and 1 coccygeal.

The dorsal and ventral nerve roots at each level fuse to form mixed motor-sensory spinal nerves and spread through the body to provide innervation to muscles and sensory organs. The C5–T1 spinal nerves intersect in the brachial plexus and divide to form the main nerve branches to the arm, including the median, ulnar, and radial nerves. The L2–S4 spinal nerves intersect in the lumbosacral plexus and divide to form the main nerve branches to the leg, including the common peroneal, tibial, and femoral nerves.

The principal motor tract is the corticospinal tract. It is a two-neuron path, with an upper motor neuron and a lower motor neuron. The upper motor neuron cell body is located within the motor strip of the cerebral cortex. The axon travels through the internal capsule to the brain stem, decussates at the brain stem–spinal cord junction, and travels down the contralateral corticospinal tract to the lower motor neuron in the anterior horn at the appropriate level. The lower motor neuron axon then travels via peripheral nerves to its target muscle. Damage to upper motor neurons results in hyperreflexia and mild atrophy. Damage to lower motor neurons results in flaccidity and significant atrophy.

The two major sensory tracts are three-neuron pathways. Fine touch and proprioceptive signals enter the spinal cord via the dorsal root ganglia and then ascend ipsilaterally via the dorsal columns. They then synapse and decussate in the lower medulla, travel up the contralateral medial lemniscus to make a second synapse in the thalamus, and then finally ascend to the sensory cortex. Pain and temperature fibers first synapse in the dorsal horn of the spinal cord at their entry level, decussate, and then travel up the contralateral

CHAPTER 42

Neurosurgery

KEY POINTS

1. Neurologic surgery specializes in primarily surgical management of central, peripheral, and autonomic nervous system disorders.

2. Although clinical examination is paramount, neurosurgical diagnosis and treatment are aided largely by a variety of modalities, such as magnetic resonance imaging and intracranial pressure monitoring.

3. The common treatment goals for traumatic brain and spinal injury are aimed at preventing secondary insults of hypoxia and hypotension.

4. Aneurysmal subarachnoid hemorrhage remains one of the most morbid and intensive neurosurgical diseases. Endovascular therapy is a growing technology that allows for safer securing of ruptured aneurysms.

5. Brain tumors can arise from primary or metastatic tissues. Treatment typically involves resection, followed by radiation and/or chemotherapy, depending on the type and grade of tumor.

6. Degenerative spine disease affects mainly the cervical and lumbar regions. Narrowing of the canal in the cervical spine may cause myelopathy or radiculop-

athy, while narrowing in the lumbar spine results in radiculopathy, neurogenic claudication, or cauda equina syndrome.

7. Spinal instrumentation is used for surgical stabilization of many types of spinal instability, including traumatic, infectious, oncologic, and degenerative.

8. Infection of the nervous system is a serious and prevalent medical problem. Operative management is indicated for most conditions in which there is symptomatic compression of neural structures.

9. Functional neurosurgery via device implantation is a rapidly evolving discipline that has already become the standard of care in treating medically refractory Parkinson's disease and essential tremor. A wider variety of deep brain stimulation targets will treat additional neuropsychiatric diseases.

10. Stereotactic radiosurgery is a powerful treatment option for intracranial disease, whether it is primary or adjunct. Gamma knife surgery can be used to treat tumors, vascular malformations, and cranial neuralgias.

spinothalamic tracts to the thalamus. The second synapse occurs in the thalamus, and the output axons ascend to the sensory cortex.

The aforementioned motor and sensory tracts together constitute the somatic nervous system. In addition to this system, the ANS is the other constituent of the nervous system. The ANS carries messages for homeostasis and visceral regulation from the central nervous system (CNS) to target structures such as arteries, veins, the heart, sweat glands, and the digestive tract.[1] CNS control of the ANS arises particularly from the hypothalamus and the nucleus of the tractus solitarius. The ANS is divided into the sympathetic, parasympathetic, and enteric systems. The sympathetic system drives the "fight or flight" response, using epinephrine to increase heart rate, blood pressure, blood glucose, and temperature, as well as to dilate the pupils. It arises from the thoracolumbar spinal segments. The parasympathetic system promotes the "rest and digest" state, and uses acetylcholine to maintain basal metabolic function under nonstressful circumstances. It arises from cranial nerves III, VII, IX, and X, and from the second to fourth sacral segments. The enteric nervous system controls the complex synchronization of the digestive tract, especially the pancreas, gallbladder, and small and large bowels. It can run autonomously but is regulated by the sympathetic and parasympathetic systems.

NEUROLOGIC EXAMINATION

The neurologic examination is divided into several components and generally is done from head to toe. First assess mental status. A patient may be awake, lethargic (will follow commands and answer questions, but then returns to sleep), stuporous (difficult to arouse at all), or comatose (no purposeful response to voice or pain). Cranial nerves may be thoroughly tested in the awake patient, but pupil reactivity, eye movement, facial symmetry, and gag are the most relevant when mental status is impaired. Motor testing is based on maximal effort of major muscle groups in those able to follow commands, while assessing for amplitude and symmetry of movement to deep central pain may be all that is possible for stuporous patients. Table 42-1 details scoring for motor assessment tests. Characteristic motor reactions to pain in patients with depressed mental status include withdrawal from stimulus, localization to stimulus, flexor (decorticate) posturing, extensor (decerebrate) posturing, or no reaction (in order of worsening pathology). Figure 42-1 diagrams the clinical patterns of posturing. This forms the basis of determining the Glasgow Coma Scale (GCS) motor score, as detailed in Table 42-2. Light touch, proprioception, temperature, and pain testing may be useful in awake patients but is often impossible without good cooperation. It is critical to document sensory patterns in spinal cord injury (SCI) patients. Muscle stretch reflexes should be checked. Often comparing left to right or upper extremity to lower extremity reflexes for symmetry is the most useful for localizing a lesion. Check for ankle-jerk clonus or up-going toes (Babinski's test). Presence of either is pathologic and signifies upper motor neuron disease.

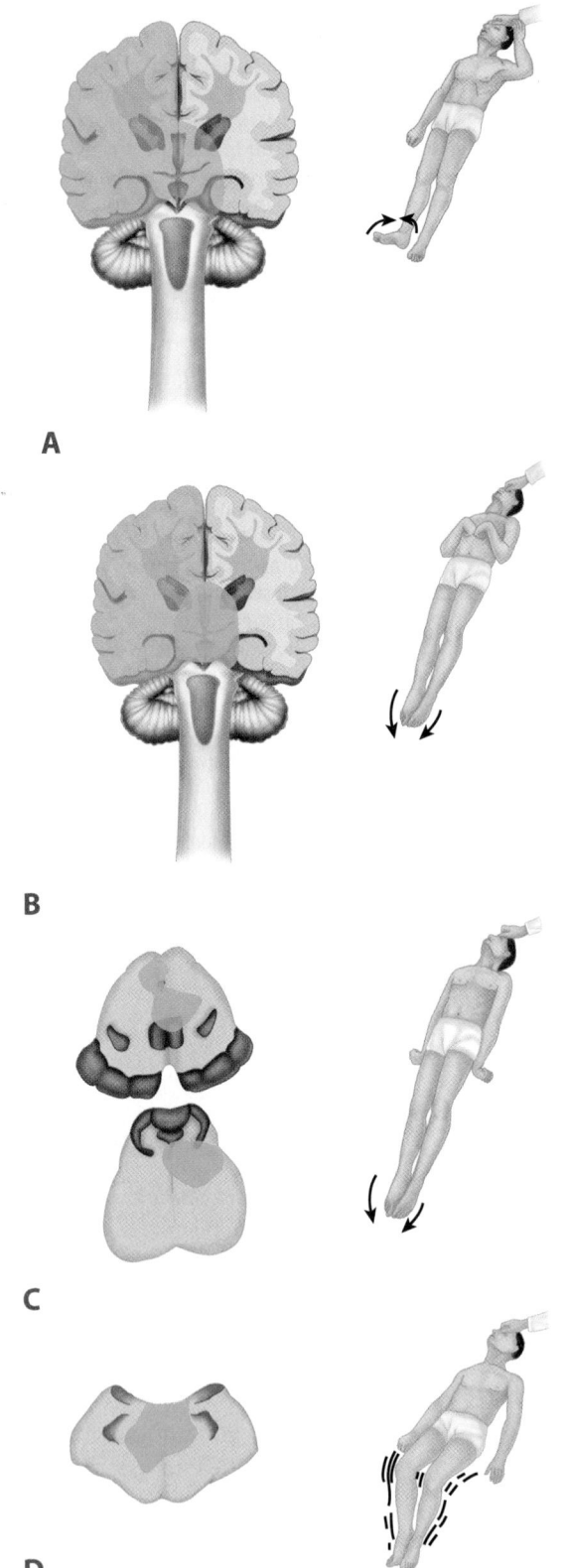

FIG. 42-1. Patterns of motor responses associated with various lesions. **A.** Left hemispheric lesion with right hemiplegia and left localization. **B.** Deep cerebral/thalamic lesion with bilateral flexor posturing. **C.** Midbrain or pontine lesion with bilateral extensor posturing. **D.** Medullary lesion with general flaccidity. *[Adapted with permission from Rengachary SS: Impaired consciousness, in Rengachary SS, Ellenbogen RG (eds):* Principles of Neurosurgery, *2nd ed. Edinburgh: New York, Elsevier Mosby, 2005, p 87. Copyright Elsevier.]*

TABLE 42-1	Motor scoring system

Grade	Description
0	No muscle contraction
1	Visible muscle contraction without movement across the joint
2	Movement in the horizontal plane, unable to overcome gravity
3	Movement against gravity
4	Movement against some resistance
5	Normal strength

TABLE 42-2	The Glasgow Coma Scale score[a]						
Motor Response		**Verbal Response**		**Eye-Opening Response**	
Obeys commands	6	Oriented	5	Opens spontaneously	4
Localizes to pain	5	Confused	4	Opens to speech	3
Withdraws from pain	4	Inappropriate words	3	Opens to pain	2
Flexor posturing	3	Unintelligible sounds	2	No eye opening	1
Extensor posturing	2	No sounds	1		
No movement	1				

[a]Add the three scores to obtain the Glasgow Coma Scale (GCS) score, which can range from 3 to 15. Add "T" after the GCS if intubated and no verbal score is possible. For these patients, the GCS can range from 3T to 10T.

Diagnostic Studies

Plain Films

Plain x-rays of the skull may demonstrate fractures, osteolytic or osteoblastic lesions, or pneumocephaly (air in the head). The use of skull plain films has decreased given the rapid availability and significantly increased detail of head computed tomography (CT) scans. Plain films of the cervical, thoracic, and lumbar spine are used to assess for evidence of bony trauma or soft tissue swelling suggesting fracture. Spinal deformities and osteolytic or osteoblastic pathologic processes also will be apparent. The shoulder girdle usually poses problems in visualizing the cervicothoracic junction clearly.

Computed Tomography

The noncontrast CT scan of the head is an extremely useful diagnostic tool in the setting of new focal neurologic deficit, decreased mental status, or trauma. It is rapid and almost universally available in hospitals in the United States. Its sensitivity allows for the detection of acute hemorrhage. A contrast-enhanced CT scan will help show neoplastic or infectious processes. In the current era, contrast CT generally is used for those patients who cannot undergo magnetic resonance imaging (MRI) scanning due to pacemakers or metal in the orbits. Fine-slice CT scanning of the spine is helpful for defining bony anatomy and pathology, and is usually done after an abnormality is seen on plain films, or because plain films are inadequate (especially to visualize C7 and T1 vertebrae). Finally, high-speed multislice scanners, combined with timed-bolus contrast injections, allow CT angiography. A thin-slice axial scan is obtained during the passage of contrast through the cerebral arteries and reconstructed in three dimensions to assess for vascular lesions. CT angiography does not reliably detect lesions, such as cerebral aneurysms <3 mm across, but can provide detailed morphologic data of larger lesions. Newer, multislice scanner technology is approaching the resolution of conventional angiography.

Magnetic Resonance Imaging

MRI provides excellent imaging of soft tissue structures in the head and spine. It is a complex and evolving science. Several of the most clinically useful MRI sequences are worth describing. T1 sequences made before and after gadolinium administration are useful for detecting neoplastic and infectious processes. T2 sequences facilitate assessment of neural compression in the spine by the presence or absence of bright T2 CSF signals around the cord or nerve roots. Diffusion-weighted images can detect ischemic stroke earlier than CT. Fine-slice time-of-flight axial images can be reformatted in three dimensions to build MRI angiograms and MRI venograms. MRI angiograms can detect stenosis of the cervical carotid arteries or intracranial aneurysms >3 mm in diameter. MRI venograms can assess the dural venous sinuses for patency or thrombosis.

Angiography

Transarterial catheter-based angiography remains the gold standard for evaluation of vascular pathology of the brain and spine.

The current state of the art is biplanar imaging to reduce dye load and facilitate interventional procedures. Digital subtraction technologies minimize bony interference in the resultant images. Bilateral carotid arteries and bilateral vertebral arteries may be injected and followed through arterial, capillary, and venous phases for a complete cerebral angiogram.

Electromyography and Nerve Conduction Studies

Electromyography and nerve conduction studies (EMG/NCS) are useful for assessing the function of peripheral nerves. EMG records muscle activity in response to a proximal stimulation of the motor nerve. NCS record the velocity and amplitude of the nerve action potential. EMG/NCS typically is performed approximately 3 to 4 weeks after an acute injury, as nerves distal to the injury continue to transmit electrical impulses normally until degeneration of the distal nerve progresses.

Invasive Monitoring

There are several methods of monitoring intracranial physiology. The three described here are bedside intensive care unit (ICU) procedures and allow continuous monitoring. All three involve making a small hole in the skull with a hand-held drill. They generally are placed in the right frontal region to minimize the neurologic impact of possible complications such as hemorrhage. The most reliable monitor, *always*, is an alert patient with a reliable neurologic examination. If a reliable neurologic examination is not possible due to the presence of brain injury, sedatives, or paralytics, and if there is active and unstable intracranial pathology, then invasive monitoring is required.

External Ventricular Drain

An external ventricular drain is also known as a *ventriculostomy*. A perforated plastic catheter is inserted into the frontal horn of the lateral ventricle. An uninterrupted fluid column through a rigid tube allows transduction of intracranial pressure (ICP). CSF also can be drained to reduce ICP or sampled for laboratory studies.

Intraparenchymal Fiber-Optic Pressure Transducer

An intraparenchymal fiber-optic pressure transducer is commonly referred to as a *bolt*. Again, a small hole is drilled in the skull. A threaded post locks securely into the skull and holds the fiber-optic catheter in place. A bolt allows ICP monitoring only, but it is smaller and less invasive than a ventriculostomy, and may be associated with fewer complications, although the data do not clearly support this.

Brain Tissue Oxygen Sensors

The brain tissue oxygen sensor is a recent development that has already demonstrated a mortality benefit in traumatic brain injury patients.[2] The device is screwed into the skull in the same manner as the bolt; however, the sensor catheter is an electrochemical oxygen–tension sensitive membrane. A single bolt can be designed to accept a pressure sensor, oxygen sensor, and brain temperature sensor. Patients with severe brain injury due to trauma or aneurysmal hemorrhage may benefit from placement of these three sensors and a ventriculostomy to drain CSF for control of ICP. This treatment requires two twist-drill holes, which may be placed on adjacent or opposite sides of the head.

NEUROLOGIC AND NEUROSURGICAL EMERGENCIES

Raised Intracranial Pressure

ICP normally varies between 4 and 14 mmHg. Sustained ICP levels above 20 mmHg can injure the brain. The Monro-Kellie doctrine states that the cranial vault is a rigid structure, and therefore, the total volume of the contents determines ICP. The three normal contents of the cranial vault are brain tissue, blood, and CSF. The brain's contents can expand due to swelling from traumatic brain injury (TBI), stroke, or reactive edema. Blood volume can increase by extravasation to form a hematoma, or by reactive vasodilation in a hypoventilating, hypercarbic patient. CSF volume increases in the setting of hydrocephalus. Figure 42-2 demonstrates classic CT findings of hydrocephalus. Addition of a fourth element, such as a tumor or abscess, also will increase ICP. The pressure-volume curve depicted in Fig. 42-3 demonstrates a compensated region with a small ΔP/ΔV, and an uncompensated region with large ΔP/ΔV. In the compensated region, increased volume is offset by decreased volume of CSF and blood.

Increased ICP can injure the brain in several ways. Focal mass lesions cause shift and herniation. Temporal lesions push the uncus medially and compress the midbrain. This phenomenon is known as *uncal herniation*. The posterior cerebral artery (PCA) passes between the uncus and midbrain and may be occluded, leading to occipital infarct. Masses higher up in the hemisphere can push the cingulate gyrus under the falx cerebri. This process is known as *subfalcine herniation*. The anterior cerebral artery (ACA) branches run along the medial surface of the cingulate gyrus and may be occluded, leading to medial frontal and parietal infarcts. Diffuse

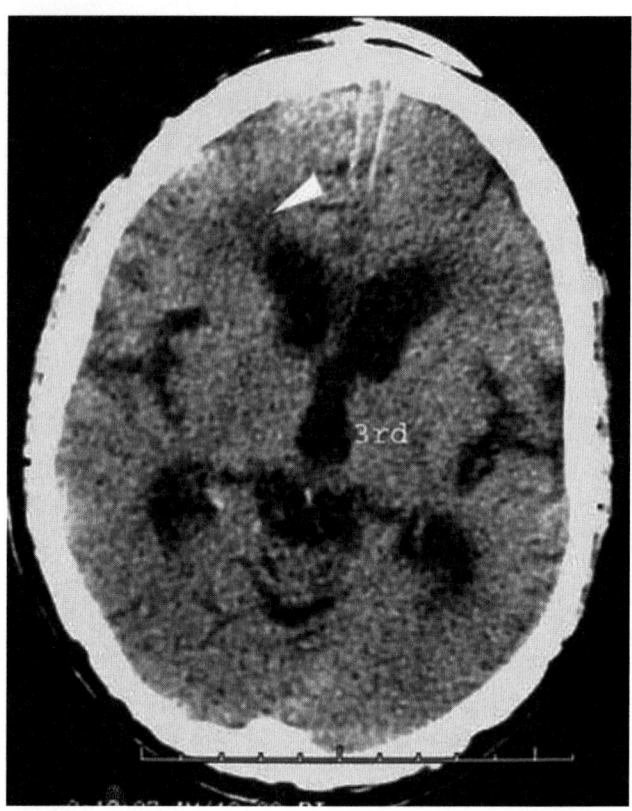

FIG. 42-2. Head computed tomography scan demonstrating hydrocephalus. The third ventricle (*3rd*) is widened and rounded, the anterior horns of the lateral ventricles are plump, and pressure-driven flow of cerebrospinal fluid into brain parenchyma adjacent to the ventricles is seen (*arrowhead*). This is known as *transependymal flow of cerebrospinal fluid.*

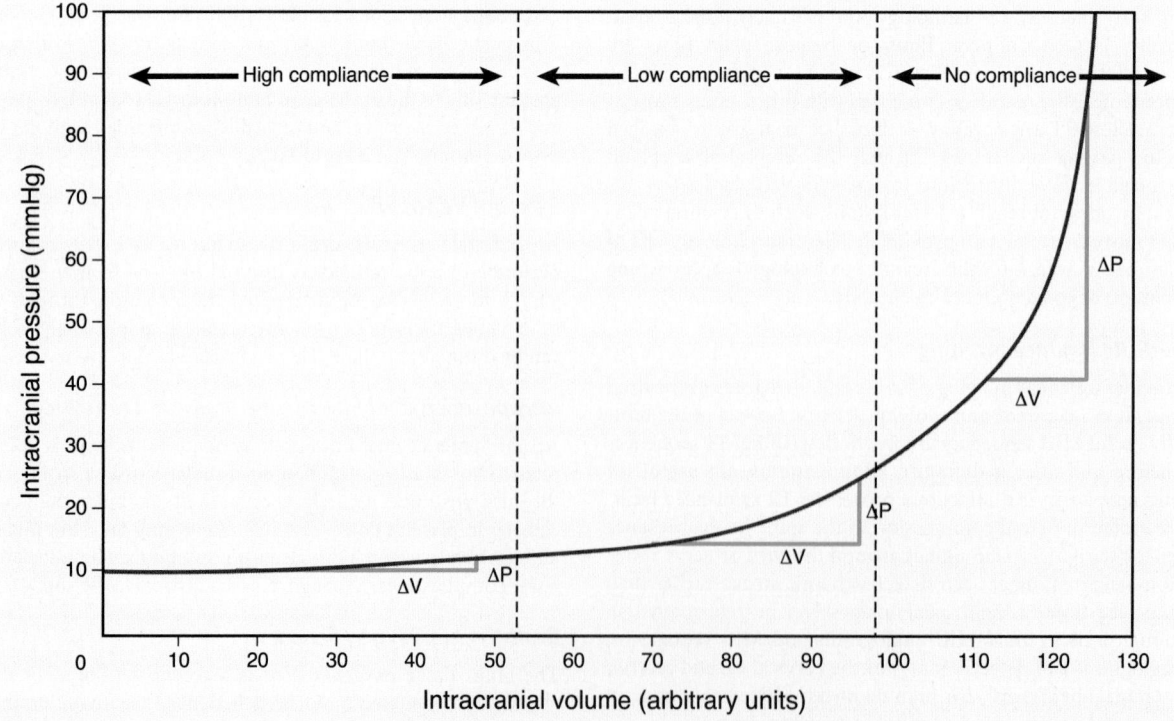

FIG. 42-3. Pressure-volume curve demonstrating the effect of changing the volume of intracranial contents on intracranial pressure. Note the compensated zone, with little change of pressure with change of volume, and the uncompensated zone, with significant change of pressure with change of volume. [*Adapted with permission from Rengachary SS: Intracranial pressure, in Rengachary SS, Ellenbogen RG (eds): Principles of Neurosurgery, 2nd ed. Edinburgh; New York: Elsevier Mosby, 2005, p 67. Copyright Elsevier.*]

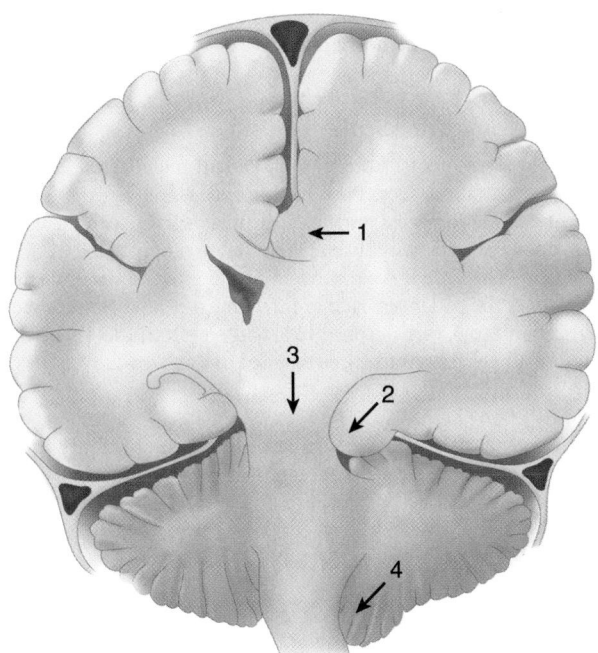

FIG. 42-4. Schematic drawing of brain herniation patterns. *1.* Subfalcine herniation. The cingulate gyrus shifts across midline under the falx cerebri. *2.* Uncal herniation. The uncus (medial temporal lobe gyrus) shifts medially and compresses the midbrain and cerebral peduncle. *3.* Central transtentorial herniation. The diencephalon and midbrain shift caudally through the tentorial incisura. *4.* Tonsillar herniation. The cerebellar tonsil shifts caudally through the foramen magnum. *[Reproduced with permission from Cohen DS, Quest DO: Increased intracranial pressure, brain herniation and their control, in Wilkins RH, Rengachary SS (eds):* Neurosurgery, *2nd ed. New York: McGraw Hill, 1996, p 349.]*

PaCO$_2$ to roughly 35 mmHg can reverse the process and save the patient's life.

Brain Stem Compression

Disease in the posterior fossa (brain stem and cerebellum) requires special consideration. The volume of the posterior fossa is small. Hemorrhage or stroke in the posterior fossa that causes mass effect can rapidly kill the patient in two ways. Occlusion of the fourth ventricle causes acute obstructive hydrocephalus, leading to raised ICP, herniation, and then death. The mass effect can also lead directly to brain stem compression (Fig. 42-5). Symptoms of brain stem compression include agitation, progressive obtundation, and hypertension, followed rapidly by brain death. A patient exhibiting any of these symptoms needs an emergent neurosurgical evaluation for possible ventriculostomy or suboccipital craniectomy (removal of the bone covering the cerebellum). This situation is especially critical, as expeditious decompression can lead to significant functional recovery of patients who present near brain death.

Stroke

Patients presenting with acute focal neurologic deficits at a clearly defined time of onset (i.e., when the patient was last seen in a normal state of health) must be evaluated as rapidly as possible. An emergent head CT scan should be done. The study is often normal, because CT changes from ischemic stroke may take up to 24 hours to appear (Fig. 42-6). A patient with a clinical diagnosis of acute stroke <3 hours old, without hemorrhage on CT, may be a candidate for thrombolytic therapy with tissue plasminogen activator (tPA). Emergent MRI is helpful but not diagnostically necessary.

Seizure

A seizure is defined as an uncontrolled synchronous organization of neuronal electrical activity. A new-onset seizure often signifies an irritative mass lesion in the brain, particularly in adults, in whom

increases in pressure in the cerebral hemispheres can lead to central, or transtentorial, herniation. Increased pressure in the posterior fossa can lead to upward central herniation or downward tonsillar herniation through the foramen magnum. Uncal, transtentorial, and tonsillar herniation can cause direct damage to the very delicate brain stem. Figure 42-4 diagrams patterns of herniation.

Patients with increased ICP, also called intracranial hypertension (ICH), often will present with headache, nausea, vomiting, and progressive mental status decline. Cushing's triad is the classic presentation of ICH: hypertension, bradycardia, and irregular respirations. This triad is usually a late manifestation. Focal neurologic deficits such as hemiparesis may be present if there is a focal mass lesion causing the problem. Patients with these symptoms should undergo head CT as soon as possible.

Initial management of ICH includes airway protection and adequate ventilation. A bolus of mannitol up to 1 g/kg causes free water diuresis, increased serum osmolality, and extraction of water from the brain. The effect is delayed by about 20 minutes and has a transient benefit. Driving serum osmolality above 300 mOsm/L is of indeterminate benefit and can have deleterious cardiovascular side effects, such as hypovolemia that leads to hypotension and decreased brain perfusion. Cases of ICH typically require rapid neurosurgical evaluation. Ventriculostomy, craniotomy, or craniectomy may be needed for definitive decompression.

It is critical to note that lethargic or obtunded patients often have decreased respiratory drive. This causes the partial pressure of arterial carbon dioxide (PaCO$_2$) to increase, resulting in cerebral vasodilation and worsening of ICH. This cycle causes a characteristic "crashing patient," who rapidly loses airway protection, becomes apneic, and herniates. Emergent intubation and ventilation to reduce

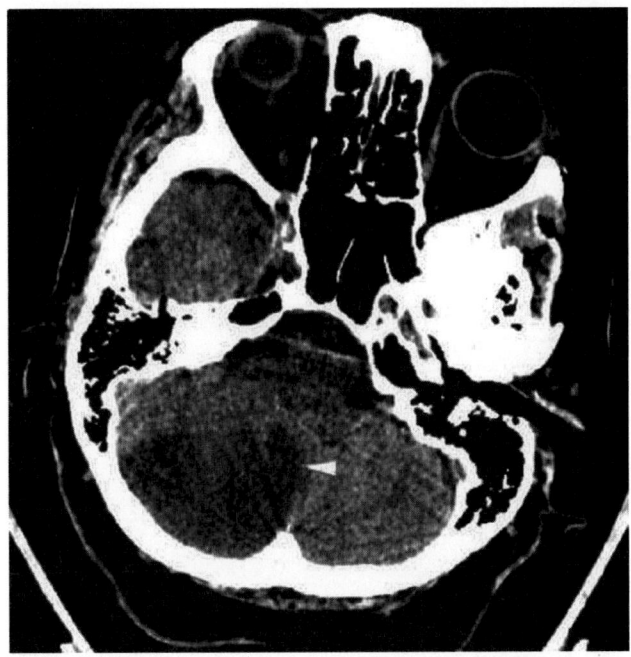

FIG. 42-5. Maturing cerebellar stroke seen as a hypodense area in the right cerebellar hemisphere (*arrowhead*) on head computed tomography in a patient with rapidly progressing obtundation 2 days after the initial onset of symptoms. Swelling of the infarcted tissue causes posterior fossa mass effect. The fourth ventricle is obliterated and not visible, and the brain stem is being compressed.

tumors commonly present with seizure. Patients with traumatic intracranial hemorrhage are at risk for seizure. In addition to airway and ventilatory problems, a seizing patient is also at risk for neural excitotoxicity if the activity is prolonged, such as in *status epilepticus*. Any patient with a new-onset seizure should have imaging of the brain, such as a head CT scan, after the seizure is controlled and the patient is resuscitated.

TRAUMA

Trauma is the leading cause of death in children and young adults; however, the incidence of death and disability from trauma has been slowly decreasing. This decline is partly attributable to increased awareness of safety devices such as seat belts and motorist helmets. Nonetheless, trauma remains a major cause of morbidity and mortality, and it can affect every major organ system in the body. The three main areas of neurosurgical focus are: TBI, spine and SCI, and peripheral nerve injury.

Head Trauma

Glasgow Coma Scale Score

The initial assessment of the trauma patient includes the primary survey, resuscitation, secondary survey, and definitive care. Neurosurgical evaluation begins during the primary survey with the determination of the GCS score (usually referred to simply as the *GCS*) for the patient. The GCS is determined by adding the scores of the best responses of the patient in each of three categories. The motor score ranges from 1 to 6, verbal from 1 to 5, and eyes from 1 to 4. The GCS therefore ranges from 3 to 15, as detailed in Table 42-2.

Scalp Injury

Blunt or penetrating trauma to the head can cause injury to the densely vascularized scalp, and significant blood loss can occur.

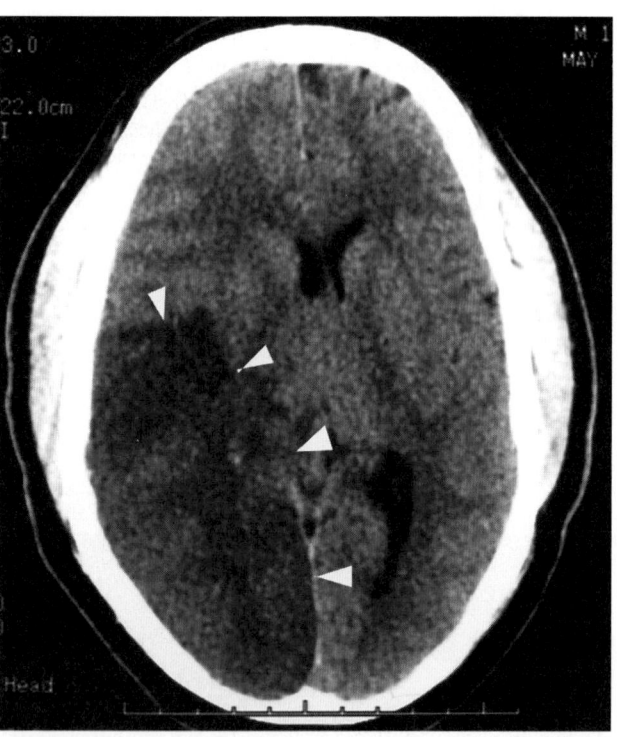

A

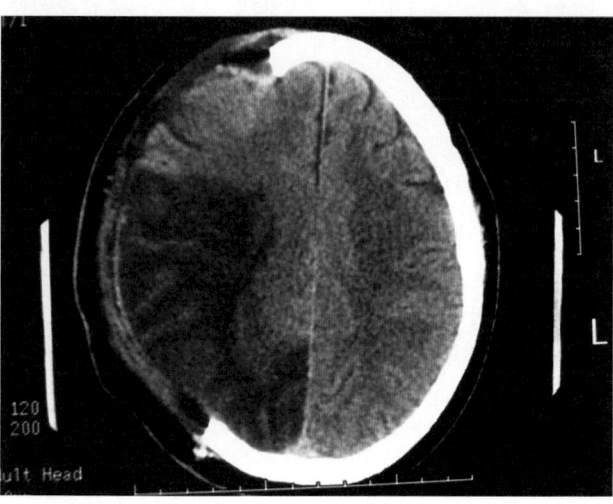

B

FIG. 42-6. A. Head computed tomography scan of a patient with a 4-day-old stroke that occluded the right middle cerebral and posterior cerebral arteries. The infarcted tissue is the hypodense (*dark*) area indicated by the *arrowheads*. The patient presented with left-sided weakness and left visual field loss, but then became less responsive, prompting this head computed tomography. Note the right-to-left midline shift. **B.** Same patient status post decompressive right hemicraniectomy. Note the free expansion of swollen brain outside the normal confines of the skull. **C.** Patient with a right middle cerebral artery ischemic stroke with areas of hemorrhagic conversion, seen as hyperdense (*bright*) areas within the infarcted tissue. This patient also required hemicraniectomy for severe mass effect. Note the lack of midline shift postoperatively.

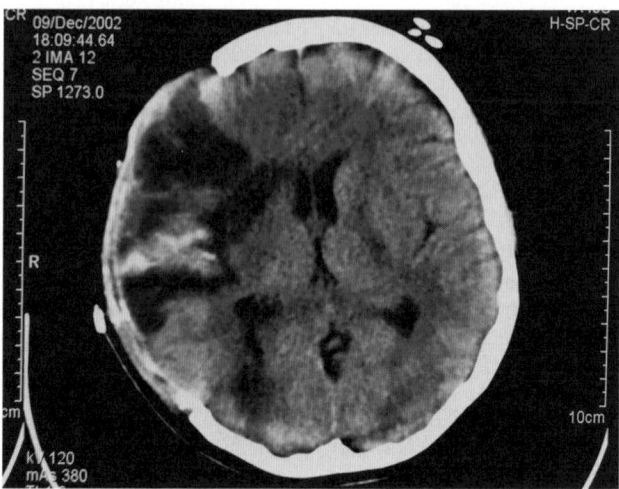

C

Direct pressure initially controls the bleeding, allowing close inspection of the injury. If a simple laceration is found, it should be copiously irrigated and closed primarily. If the laceration is short, a single-layer percutaneous suture closure will suffice. If the laceration is long or has multiple arms, the patient may need débridement and closure in the operating room (OR), with its superior lighting and wider selection of instruments and suture materials. Careful reapproximation of the galea will provide a more secure closure and better hemostasis. Blunt trauma also can cause crush injury with subsequent tissue necrosis. These wounds require débridement and consideration of advancement flaps to cover the defect.

Skull Fractures

The usual classification system for bone fractures may be applied to the skull. The fracture may be characterized by skull x-rays or head CT.[3] A closed fracture is covered by intact skin. An open, or compound, fracture is associated with disrupted overlying skin. The fracture lines may be single (linear); multiple and radiating from a point (stellate); or multiple, creating fragments of bone (comminuted). Closed skull fractures do not normally require specific treatment. Open fractures require repair of the scalp and operative débridement. Indications for craniotomy include depression greater than the cranial thickness, intracranial hematoma, and frontal sinus involvement.[4] Skull fractures generally indicate that a significant amount of force was transmitted to the head and should increase the suspicion for intracranial injury. Fractures that cross meningeal arteries can cause rupture of the artery and subsequent epidural hematoma (EDH) formation.

Depressed skull fractures may result from a focal injury of significant force. The inner and outer cortices of the skull are disrupted, and a fragment of bone is pressed in toward the brain in relation to adjacent intact skull. The fragment may overlap the edge of intact bone, or may plunge completely below the level of adjacent normal skull. The inner cortex of the bone fragments often has multiple sharp edges that can lacerate dura, brain, and vessels. Craniotomy is required to elevate the fracture, repair dural disruption, and obtain hemostasis in these cases (Fig. 42-7). However, fractures overlying dural venous sinuses require restraint. Surgical exploration can lead to life-threatening hemorrhage from the lacerated sinus.

Fractures of the skull base are common in head-injured patients, and they indicate significant impact. They are generally apparent on routine head CT, but should be evaluated with dedicated fine-slice coronal-section CT scan to document and delineate the extent of the fracture and involved structures. If asymptomatic, they require no treatment. Symptoms from skull base fractures include cranial nerve deficits and CSF leaks. A fracture of the temporal bone, for instance, can damage the facial or vestibulocochlear nerve, resulting in vertigo, ipsilateral deafness, or facial paralysis. A communication may be formed between the subarachnoid space and the middle ear, allowing CSF drainage into the pharynx via the eustachian tube or from the ear (otorrhea). Extravasation of blood results in ecchymosis behind the ear, known as *Battle's sign*. A fracture of the anterior skull base can result in anosmia (loss of smell from damage to the olfactory nerve), CSF drainage from the nose (rhinorrhea), or periorbital ecchymoses, known as *raccoon eyes*.

Copious clear drainage from the nose or ear makes the diagnosis of CSF leakage obvious. Often, however, the drainage may be discolored with blood or small in volume if some drains into the throat. The halo test can help differentiate. Allow a drop of the fluid to fall on an absorbent surface such as a facial tissue. If blood is mixed with CSF, the drop will form a double ring, with a darker center spot containing blood components surrounded by a light halo of CSF. If this test is indeterminate, the fluid can be sent for beta-transferrin testing, which will only be positive if CSF is present.

Many CSF leaks will heal with elevation of the head of the bed for several days. A lumbar drain can augment this method. A lumbar

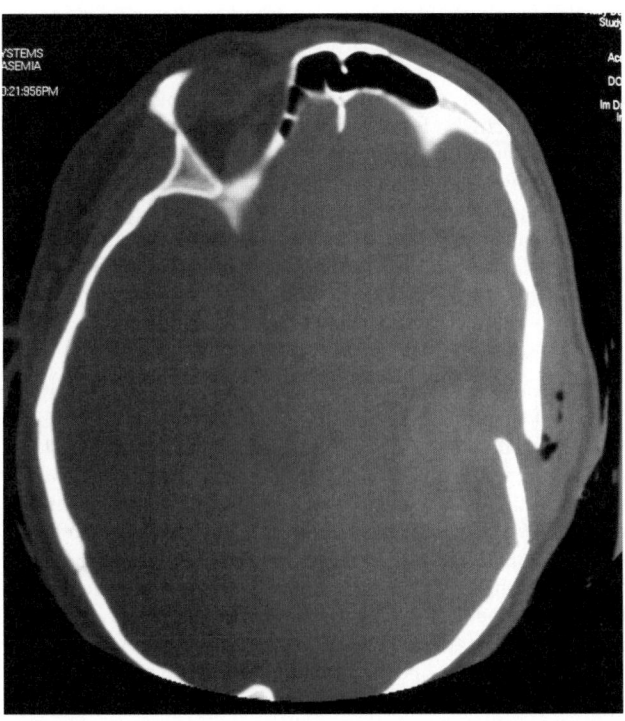 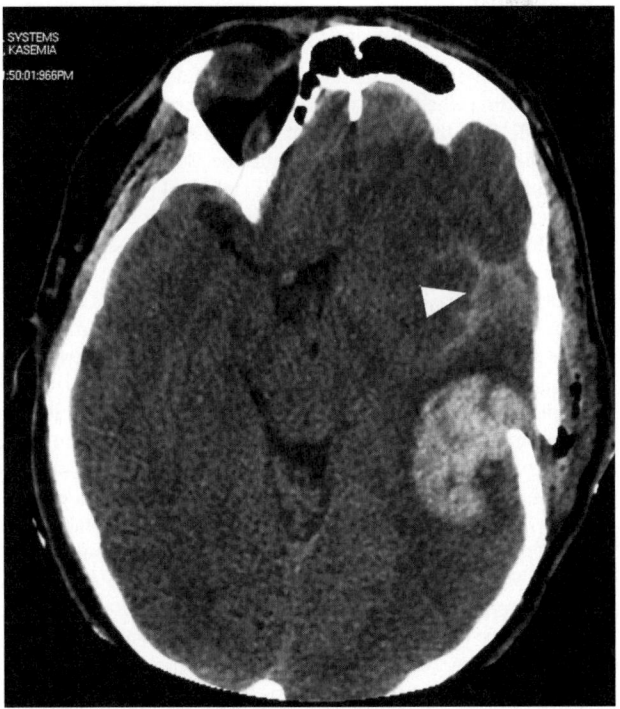

A **B**

FIG. 42-7. A. Bone-window axial head computed tomography (CT) of a patient who presented aphasic after being struck with the bottom of a beer bottle. CT demonstrates a depressed skull fracture in the left posterior temporoparietal area. **B.** Brain-window axial head CT demonstrating intraparenchymal hematoma caused by laceration of cortical vessels by the edge of the fractured bone. *Arrowhead* indicates traumatic subarachnoid hemorrhage in the sylvanian fissure.

drain is a catheter placed in the lumbar CSF cistern to decompress the cranial vault and allow the defect to heal by eliminating normal hydrostatic pressure. There is no proven efficacy of antibiotic coverage for preventing meningitis in patients with CSF leaks.

Traumatic cranial neuropathies generally are managed conservatively, with documentation of the extent of impairment and signs of recovery. Patients with traumatic facial nerve palsies may benefit from a course of steroids, although their benefit is unproven. Patients with facial nerve palsy of abrupt onset, who do not respond to steroids within 48 to 72 hours, may be considered for surgical decompression of the petrous portion of the facial nerve. Patients also may present with delayed-onset facial nerve palsy. Again, steroids are used and surgery is considered, with mixed results.

Closed Head Injury

Closed head injury (CHI) is the most common type of TBI and a significant cause of morbidity and mortality in the United States. There are two important factors that affect the outcome in CHI and TBI in general. The initial impact causes the *primary injury*, defined as the immediate injury to neurons from transmission of the force of impact. The long, delicate axons of the neurons can shear as they undergo differential acceleration or deceleration along their projecting pathways. Prevention strategies, such as wearing helmets, remain the best means to decrease disability from primary injury. Subsequent neuronal damage due to the sequelae of trauma is referred to as *secondary injury*. Hypoxia, hypotension, hydrocephalus, intracranial hypertension, and intracranial hematoma are all mechanisms of secondary injury. The focus of basic research in brain trauma, critical care medicine, and neurosurgical intervention is to decrease the effects of secondary injury.

The Brain Trauma Foundation's most recent summary of management recommendations for brain-injured patients was published in 2007 and is endorsed by the American Association of Neurological Surgeons, Congress of Neurological Surgeons, and the World Health Organization. The guidelines standardize the care of these patients with the hope of improving outcomes. Some of the common patterns of CHI, including concussion, contusion, and diffuse axonal injury, are discussed below in Types of Closed Head Injury.[5]

Initial Assessment The initial evaluation of a trauma patient remains the same whether or not the primary surveyor suspects head injury. The first three elements of the ABCDs of resuscitation—*a*irway, *b*reathing, and *c*irculation—must be assessed and stabilized. Hypoxia and hypotension worsen outcome in TBI (due to secondary injury), making cardiopulmonary stabilization critical. Patients who cannot follow commands require intubation for airway protection and ventilatory control. The fourth element, assessment of "D," for *d*isability, is undertaken next. Motor activity, speech, and eye opening can be assessed in a few seconds and a GCS score assigned.

The following is an example of how a primary surveyor may efficiently assess disability and GCS: Approach the patient and enter his or her field of view. Observe whether the patient is visually attentive. Clearly command: "Tell me your name." Then ask the patient to lift up two fingers on each side sequentially, and wiggle the toes. A visually or verbally unresponsive patient should be assessed for response to peripheral stimuli such as nail-bed pressure, or deep central painful stimulation, such as a firm, twisting pinch of the sensitive supraclavicular skin. Watch for eye opening and movement of the extremities, whether purposeful or reflexive. Assess the verbal response. The motor, verbal, and eye-opening scores may be correctly assigned using this rapid examination. An initial assessment of the probability of significant head injury can be made, assuming that pharmacologic and toxic elements have not obscured the examination. The surveyor must also take note of any external signs of head injury, including bleeding from the scalp, nose, or ear, or deformation of the skull or face.

Medical Management Several medical steps may be taken to minimize secondary neuronal injury and the systemic consequences of head injury. Patients with a documented CHI and evidence of

intracranial hemorrhage or depressed skull fracture should receive a 17-mg/kg phenytoin loading dose, followed by 1 week of therapeutic maintenance phenytoin, typically 300 to 400 mg/d. Phenytoin prophylaxis has been shown to decrease the incidence of early posttraumatic seizures.[6] There is no evidence to support longer-term use of prophylactic antiepileptic agents. Blood glucose levels should be closely monitored by free blood sugar checks and controlled with sliding scale insulin. Fevers also should be evaluated and controlled with antipyretics, as well as source-directed therapy when possible. Hyperglycemia and hyperthermia are toxic to injured neurons and contribute to secondary injury. Head-injured patients have an increased prevalence of peptic ulceration and GI bleeding. Peptic ulcers occurring in patients with head injury or high ICP are referred to as Cushing's ulcers, and may be related to hypergastrinemia. Ulcer prophylaxis should be used. Compression stockings or athrombic pumps should be used when the patient cannot be mobilized rapidly.

Classification Head injury can be classified as mild, moderate, or severe. For patients with a history of head trauma, classification is as follows: severe head injury if the GCS score is 3 to 8, moderate head injury if the GCS score is 9 to 12, and mild head injury if the GCS score is 13 to 15. Many patients present to emergency rooms and trauma bays with a history of head trauma. A triage system must be used to maximize resource utilization while minimizing the chance of missing occult or progressing injuries.

Head trauma patients who are asymptomatic, who have only headache, dizziness, or scalp lacerations, and who did not lose consciousness have a low risk for intracranial injury and may be discharged home without a head CT scan.[7,8] Head-injured patients who are discharged should be sent home with reliable family or friends who can observe the patient for the first postinjury day. Printed discharge instructions, which describe monitoring for confusion, persistent nausea, weakness, or speech difficulty, should be given to the caretaker. The patient should return to the emergency department for evaluation of such symptoms.

Patients with a history of altered consciousness, amnesia, progressive headache, skull or facial fracture, vomiting, or seizure have a moderate risk for intracranial injury and should undergo prompt head CT. If the CT is normal, and the neurologic examination has returned to baseline (excluding amnesia of the event), then the patient can be discharged to the care of a responsible adult, again with printed criteria for returning to the emergency room. Otherwise the patient must be admitted for a 24-hour observation period.

Patients with depressed consciousness, focal neurologic deficits, penetrating injury, depressed skull fracture, or changing neurologic examination have a high risk for intracranial injury. These patients should undergo immediate head CT and admission for observation or intervention as needed.

Types of Closed Head Injury

Concussion A concussion is defined as temporary neuronal dysfunction following nonpenetrating head trauma. The head CT is normal, and deficits resolve over minutes to hours. Definitions vary; some require transient loss of consciousness, while others include patients with any alteration of mental status. Memory difficulties, especially amnesia of the event, are very common. Concussions may be graded. One method is the Colorado grading system.[9] Head trauma patients with confusion only are grade 1, patients with amnesia are grade 2, and patients who lose consciousness are grade 3. Studies have shown that the brain remains in a hypermetabolic state for up to a week after injury. The brain is also much more susceptible to injury from even minor head trauma in the first 1 to 2 weeks after concussion. This is known as second-impact syndrome, and patients should be informed that, even after mild head injury, they might experience memory difficulties or persistent headaches.

Contusion A *contusion* is a bruise of the brain, and occurs when the force from trauma is sufficient to cause breakdown of small vessels and extravasation of blood into the brain. The contused areas appear

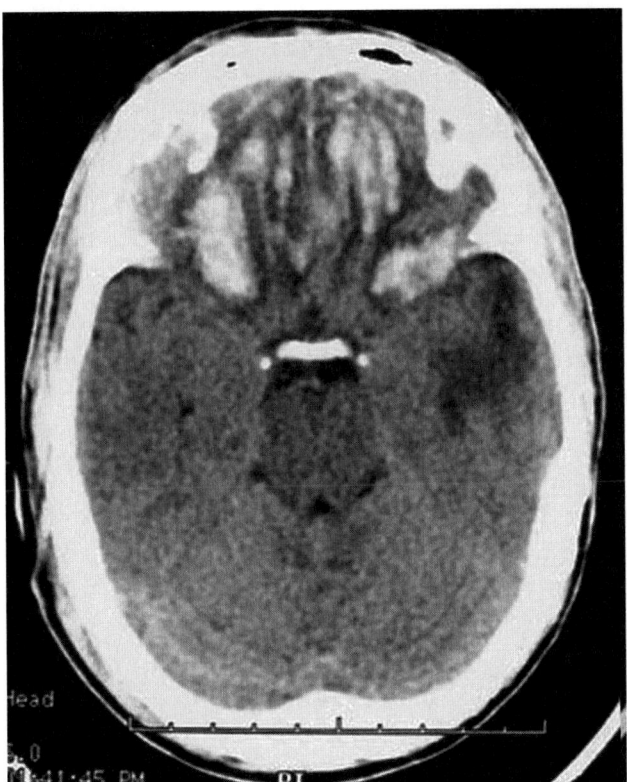

FIG. 42-8. Severe bilateral contusions in the basal aspect of the frontal lobes, caused by the brain moving over the rough, irregular skull base during sudden cranial acceleration.

Traumatic Intracranial Hematomas

The various traumatic intracranial hematomas contribute to death and disability secondary to head injury. Hematomas can expand rapidly and cause brain shifting and subsequent herniation. Emergent neurosurgical evaluation and intervention often are necessary.

Epidural Hematoma EDH is the accumulation of blood between the skull and the dura. EDH usually results from arterial disruption, especially of the middle meningeal artery. The dura is adherent to bone, and some pressure is required to dissect between the two. EDH has a classic three-stage clinical presentation that is probably seen in only 20% of cases. The patient is initially unconscious from the concussive aspect of the head trauma. The patient then awakens and has a lucid interval while the hematoma subclinically expands. As the volume of the hematoma grows, the decompensated region of the pressure-volume curve is reached, ICP increases, and the patient becomes lethargic and herniates. Uncal herniation from an EDH classically causes ipsilateral third nerve palsy and contralateral hemiparesis.

On head CT the clot is bright, biconvex (lentiform), and has a well-defined border that usually respects cranial suture lines. The clot generally forms over the convexities but may rarely occur in the posterior fossa as well.

Open craniotomy for evacuation of the congealed clot and hemostasis generally is indicated for EDH. Patients who meet all of the following criteria may be managed conservatively: clot volume <30 cm³, maximum thickness <1.5 cm, and GCS score >8.[10] Prognosis after successful evacuation is better for EDH than subdural hematoma (SDH). EDHs are associated with lower-energy trauma with less resultant primary brain injury. Good outcomes may be seen in 85 to 90% of patients, with rapid CT scan and intervention.[11]

Acute Subdural Hematoma An acute SDH is the result of an accumulation of blood between the arachnoid membrane and the dura. Acute SDH usually results from venous bleeding, typically from tearing of a bridging vein running from the cerebral cortex to the dural sinuses. The bridging veins are subject to stretching and tearing during acceleration/deceleration of the head, because the brain shifts in relation to the dura, which firmly adheres to the skull. Elderly and alcoholic patients are at higher risk for acute SDH formation after head trauma due to the greater mobility of their atrophied brains within the cranial vault.

On head CT scan, the clot is bright or mixed-density, crescent-shaped (lunate), may have a less distinct border, and does not cross the midline due to the presence of the falx. Most SDHs occur over the cerebral hemispheres, but they may also occur between the hemispheres or layer over the tentorium.

Open craniotomy for evacuation of acute SDH is indicated for any of the following: thickness >1 cm, midline shift >5 mm, or GCS drop by two or more points from the time of injury to hospitalization. Nonoperatively managed hematomas may stabilize and eventually reabsorb, or evolve into chronic SDHs.[12] This management requires frequent neurologic examinations until stabilization of the clot as proven by serial head CT scans.

The prognosis for functional recovery is significantly worse for acute SDH than EDH because it is associated with greater primary injury to brain parenchyma from high-energy impacts. Prompt recognition and intervention minimizes secondary injury. The elderly, patients with low admission GCS, or high postoperative ICP do poorly, with as few as 5% attaining functional recovery.[13]

Chronic Subdural Hematoma Chronic SDH is a collection of blood breakdown products that is at least 2 to 3 weeks old. Acute hematomas are bright white (hyperdense) on CT scan for approximately 3 days, after which they fade to isodensity with brain, and then to hypodensity after 2 to 3 weeks. A true chronic SDH will be as dark as CSF on CT. Traces of white are often seen due to small hemorrhages into the collection. These small bleeds may expand the collection enough to make it symptomatic. This phenomenon is referred to as

bright on CT scan, as seen in Fig. 42-8. The frontal, occipital, and temporal poles are most often involved. The brain sustains injury as it collides with rough, bony surfaces. Contusions themselves rarely cause significant mass effect as they represent small amounts of blood in injured parenchyma rather than coherent blood clots. Edema may develop around a contusion, causing mass effect. Contusions may enlarge or progress to frank hematoma, particularly during the first 24 hours. Contusions also may occur in brain tissue opposite the site of impact. This is known as a *contre-coup injury*. These contusions result from deceleration of the brain against the skull.

Diffuse Axonal Injury Diffuse axonal injury is caused by damage to axons throughout the brain, due to rotational acceleration and then deceleration. Axons may be completely disrupted and then retract, forming axon balls. Small hemorrhages can be seen in more severe cases, especially on MRI. Hemorrhage is classically seen in the corpus callosum and the dorsolateral midbrain.

Penetrating Injury These injuries are complex and must be evaluated individually. The two main subtypes are missile (e.g., due to bullets or fragmentation devices) and nonmissile (e.g., due to knives or ice picks). Some general principles apply. If available, skull x-rays and CT scans are useful in assessing the nature of the injury. Cerebral angiography must be considered if the object passes near a major artery or dural venous sinus. Operative exploration is necessary to remove any object extending out of the cranium, as well as for débridement, irrigation, hemostasis, and definitive closure. Small objects contained within brain parenchyma are often left in place to avoid iatrogenic secondary brain injury. Antibiotics are given to decrease the chances of meningitis or abscess formation. High-velocity missile injuries (from high-powered hunting rifles or military weapons) are especially deadly, because the associated shock wave causes cavitary tissue destruction of an area that is much larger than the projectile itself. Projectiles that penetrate both hemispheres or traverse the ventricles are almost universally fatal.

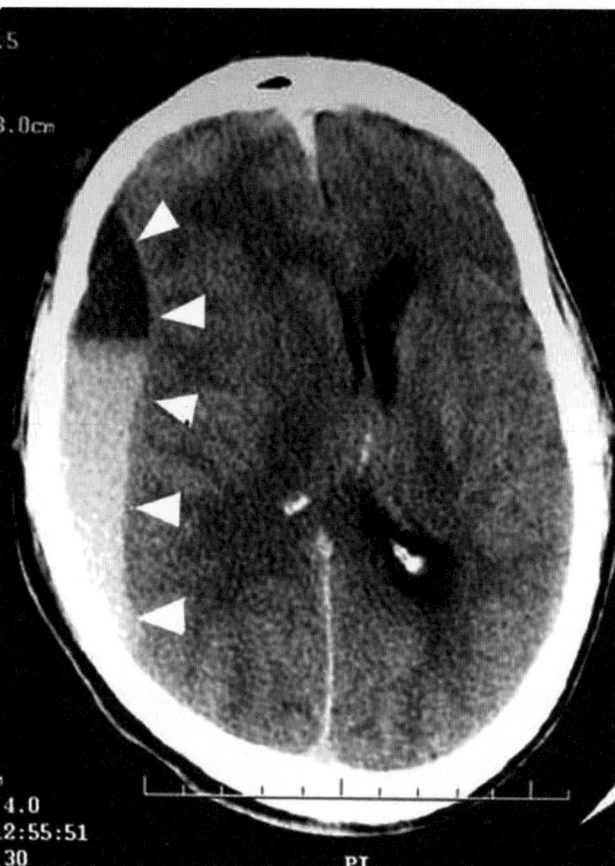

FIG. 42-9. Head computed tomography scan of an elderly patient with progressing left hemiplegia and lethargy, demonstrating an acute-on-chronic subdural hematoma. History revealed that the patient sustained a fall 4 weeks before presentation. *Arrowheads* outline the hematoma. The acute component is slightly denser and is seen as the hyperdense area in the dependent portion.

an *acute-on-chronic SDH.* Figure 42-9 demonstrates the CT appearance of an acute-on-chronic SDH. Vascularized membranes form within the hematoma as it matures. These membranes may be the source of acute hemorrhage.

Chronic SDHs often occur in patients without a clear history of head trauma, as they may arise from minor trauma. Alcoholics, the elderly, and patients on anticoagulation are at higher risk for developing chronic SDH. Patients may present with headache, seizure, confusion, contralateral hemiparesis, or coma.

A chronic SDH >1 cm or any symptomatic SDH should be surgically drained. Unlike acute SDH, which consists of a thick, congealed clot, chronic SDH typically consists of a viscous fluid, with a texture and the dark brown color reminiscent of motor oil. A simple burr hole can effectively drain most chronic SDHs. However, the optimal treatment of chronic SDH remains controversial.[14] Most authorities agree that burr hole drainage should be attempted first to obviate the risks of formal craniotomy. A single burr hole placed over the dependent edge of the collection can be made, and the space copiously irrigated until the fluid is clear. A second, more anterior burr hole can then be placed if the collection does not drain satisfactorily due to containment by membranes. The procedure is converted to open craniotomy if the SDH is too congealed for irrigation drainage, the complex of membranes prevents effective drainage, or persistent hemorrhage occurs that cannot be reached with bipolar cautery through the burr hole. The required surgical prepping and draping are always performed to allow simple conversion to craniotomy, and the incisions and burr holes are placed to allow easy incorporation into question mark–shaped craniotomy flaps.

There are various strategies to prevent reaccumulation of blood. Subdural or subgaleal drains may be left in place for 1 to 2 days. Mild hydration and bedrest with the head of the bed flat may encourage brain expansion. High levels of inspired oxygen may help draw nitrogen out of the cavity. Regardless of the strategy used, follow-up head CT scans are required postoperatively and approximately 1 month later to document resolution.

Intraparenchymal Hemorrhage Isolated hematomas within the brain parenchyma are more often associated with hypertensive hemorrhage or arteriovenous malformations (AVMs). Bleeding may occur in a contused area of brain. Mass effect from developing hematomas may present as a delayed neurologic deficit. Delayed traumatic intracerebral hemorrhage is most likely to occur within the first 24 hours. Patients with contusion on the initial head CT scan should be reimaged 24 hours after the trauma to document stable pathology. Indications for craniotomy include: any clot volume >50 cm³ or a clot volume >20 cm³ with referable neurologic deterioration (GCS 6–8) and associated midline shift >5 mm or basal cistern compression.[15]

Vascular Injury

Trauma to the head or neck may cause damage to the carotid or vertebrobasilar systems. Generally, *dissection* refers to violation of the vessel wall intima. Blood at arterial pressure can then open a plane between the intima and media, within the media, or between the media and adventitia. The newly created space within the vessel wall is referred to as the *false lumen.* Tissue or organs supplied by dissected vessels may subsequently be injured in several ways. Expansion of the hematoma within the vessel wall can lead to narrowing of the true vessel lumen and reduction or cessation of distal blood flow. Slow-flowing or stagnant blood within the false lumen exposed to thrombogenic vessel wall elements may thrombose. Pieces of thrombus may then detach and cause distal embolic arterial occlusion. Also, the remaining partial-thickness vessel wall may rupture, damaging adjacent structures.

Traumatic dissection may occur in the carotid artery (anterior circulation) or the vertebral or basilar arteries (posterior circulation). Dissections may be extradural or intradural. Intradural dissection can present with subarachnoid hemorrhage (SAH), whereas extradural dissection cannot.

Traditional angiography remains the basis of diagnosis and characterization of arterial dissection. Angiographic abnormalities include stenosis of the true lumen, or "string-sign," visible intimal flaps, and the appearance of contrast in the false lumen. Four-vessel cerebral angiography should be performed when suspicion of dissection exists.

Historically, patients with documented arterial dissection have been anticoagulated with heparin and then warfarin to prevent thromboembolic stroke. Trauma patients often have concomitant absolute or relative contraindications to anticoagulation, complicating management. Antiplatelet therapy is often implemented in lieu of full anticoagulation, however, there is no randomized clinical trial comparing the two therapies.[16] Consider surgical intervention for persisting embolic disease and for vertebral dissections presenting with SAH. Surgical options include vessel ligation and bypass grafting. Interventional radiology techniques include stenting and vessel occlusion. Occlusion techniques depend on sufficient collateral circulation to perfuse the vascular territory previously supplied by the occluded vessel.

Carotid Dissection Carotid dissection may result from neck extension combined with lateral bending to the opposite side, or trauma from an incorrectly placed shoulder belt tightening across the neck in a motor vehicle accident. Extension or bending stretches the carotid over the bony transverse processes of the cervical vertebrae, while seat belt injuries cause direct trauma. Symptoms of cervical carotid dissection include contralateral neurologic deficit from brain ischemia, headache, and ipsilateral Horner's syndrome from disruption of the sympathetic tracts ascending from the stellate ganglion on the surface of the carotid artery. The patient may complain of hearing or feeling a bruit.

Traumatic vessel wall injury to the portion of the carotid artery running through the cavernous sinus may result in a carotid-cavernous fistula (CCF). This creates a high-pressure, high-flow pathophysiologic blood flow pattern. CCFs classically present with pulsatile proptosis (the globe pulses outward with arterial pulsation), retro-orbital pain, and decreased visual acuity or loss of normal eye movement (due to damage to cranial nerves III, IV, and VI as they pass through the cavernous sinus). Symptomatic CCFs should be treated to preserve eye function. Fistulae may be closed by balloon occlusion using interventional neuroradiology techniques. Fistulae with wide necks are difficult to treat and may require total occlusion of the parent carotid artery.

Vertebrobasilar Dissection Vertebrobasilar dissection may result from sudden rotation or flexion/extension of the neck, chiropractic manipulation, or a direct blow to the neck. Common symptoms are neck pain, headache, and brain stem stroke or SAH. The risks and benefits of aspirin therapy are unclear when a vertebral dissection extends intracranially. The theoretically increased friability of the vessel wall may increase the risk of SAH when coupled with an antiplatelet agent. Consultation of a stroke neurologist is recommended in this situation.

Brain Death

Brain death occurs when there is an absence of signs of brain stem function or motor response to deep central pain in the absence of pharmacologic or systemic medical conditions that could impair brain function.

Clinical Examination A neurologist, neurosurgeon, or intensivist generally performs the clinical brain death examination. Two examinations consistent with brain death 12 hours apart, or one examination consistent with brain death followed by a consistent confirmatory study generally is sufficient to declare brain death (see below). Hospital regulations and local laws regarding documentation should be followed closely.

Establish the absence of complicating conditions before beginning the examination. The patient must be normotensive, euthermic, and oxygenating well. The patient may not be under the effects of any sedating or paralytic drugs.

Documentation of no brain stem function requires the following: nonreactive pupils; lack of corneal blink, oculocephalic (doll's eyes), oculovestibular (cold calorics) reflexes; and loss of drive to breathe (apnea test). The apnea test demonstrates no spontaneous breathing even when $PaCO_2$ is allowed to rise above 60 mmHg.

Deep central painful stimuli are provided by bilateral forceful twisting pinch of the supraclavicular skin and pressure to the medial canthal notch. Pathologic responses such as flexor or extensor posturing are *not* compatible with brain death. Spinal reflexes to peripheral pain, such as triple flexion of the lower extremities, are compatible with brain death.

Confirmatory Studies Confirmatory studies are performed after a documented clinical examination consistent with brain death. A study consistent with brain death may obviate the need to wait 12 hours for a second examination. This is especially important when the patient is a potential organ donor, as brain-dead patients often have progressive hemodynamic instability. Lack of cerebral blood flow consistent with brain death may be documented by cerebral angiography or technetium radionuclide study. A "to-and-fro" pattern on transcranial Doppler ultrasonography indicates no net forward flow through the cerebral vasculature, consistent with brain death. An electroencephalogram (EEG) documenting electrical silence has been used, but it generally is not favored because there is often artifact or noise on the recording. EEG may confuse the situation and is especially difficult for families to understand.

Spine Trauma

The spine is a complex biomechanical and neural structure. The spine provides structural support for the body as the principal component of the axial skeleton, while protecting the spinal cord and nerve roots. Trauma may fracture bones or cause ligamentous disruption. Often, bone and ligament damage occur together. Damage to these elements reduces the strength of the spine and may cause instability, which compromises both supportive and protective functions. Spine trauma may occur with or without neurologic injury. Neurologic injury from spine trauma is classified as either incomplete or complete. If there is some residual motor or sensory neurologic function below the level of the lesion, as assessed by clinical examination, the injury is incomplete.[17] A patient with complete neurologic dysfunction persisting 24 hours after injury has a very low probability of return of function in the involved area.

Neurologic injury from spine trauma may occur immediately or in delayed fashion. Immediate neurologic injury may be due to direct damage to the spinal cord or nerve roots from penetrating injuries, especially from stab wounds or gunshots. Blunt trauma may transfer sufficient force to the spine to cause acute disruption of bone and ligament, leading to subluxation, which is a shift of one vertebral element in relation to the adjacent level. Subluxation decreases the size of the spinal canal and neural foramina and causes compression of the cord or roots. Such neural impingement can also result from retropulsion of bone fragments into the canal during a fracture. Transection, crush injury, and cord compression impairing perfusion are mechanisms leading to SCI. Delayed neurologic injury may occur during transportation, examination of an improperly immobilized patient, or during a hypotensive episode.

The Mechanics of Spine Trauma

Trauma causes a wide variety of injury patterns in the spine due to its biomechanical complexity. A mechanistic approach facilitates an understanding of the patterns of injury, as there are only a few types of forces that can be applied to the spine. Although these forces are discussed individually, they often occur in combination. Several of the most common injury patterns are then presented to illustrate the clinical results of these forces applied at pathologically high levels.

Flexion/Extension Bending the head and body forward into a fetal position flexes the spine. Flexion loads the spine anteriorly (the vertebral bodies) and distracts the spine posteriorly (the spinous process and interspinous ligaments). High flexion forces occur during front-end motor vehicle collisions, and backward falls when the head strikes first. Arching the neck and back extends the spine. Extension loads the spine posteriorly and distracts the spine anteriorly. High extension forces occur during rear-end motor vehicle collisions (especially if there is no headrest), frontward falls when the head strikes first, or diving into shallow water.

Compression/Distraction Force applied along the spinal axis (axial loading) compresses the spine. Compression loads the spine anteriorly and posteriorly. High compression forces occur when a falling object strikes the head or shoulders, or when landing on the feet, buttocks, or head after a fall from height. A pulling force in line with the spinal axis distracts the spine. Distraction unloads the spine anteriorly and posteriorly. Distraction forces occur during a hanging, when the chin or occiput strikes an object first during a fall, or when a passenger submarines under a loose seat belt during a front-end motor vehicle collision.

Rotation Force applied tangential to the spinal axis rotates the spine. Rotation depends on the range of motion of intervertebral facet joints. High rotational forces occur during off-center impacts to the body or head or during glancing automobile accidents.

Patterns of Injury

Certain patterns of injury resulting from combinations of the above mentioned forces occur commonly and should be recognized during plain film imaging of the spine. Always completely evaluate the spine. A patient with a spine injury at one level has a significant risk for additional injuries at other levels.

Cervical The cervical spine is more mobile than the thoracolumbar spine. Stability comes primarily from the multiple ligamentous connections of adjacent vertebral levels. Disruption of the cervical ligaments can lead to instability in the absence of fracture. The mass of the head transmits significant forces to the cervical spine during abrupt acceleration or deceleration, increasing risk for injury.

Jefferson Fracture Jefferson fracture is a bursting fracture of the ring of C1 (the atlas) due to compression forces. There are usually two or more fractures through the ring of C1. The open-mouth odontoid view may show lateral dislocation of the lateral masses of C1. The rule of Spence states that 7 mm or greater combined dislocation indicates disruption of the transverse ligament. The transverse ligament stabilizes C1 with respect to C2. Jefferson fractures dislocated <7 mm usually are treated with a rigid collar, while those dislocated 7 mm or greater usually are treated with a halo vest. Surgical intervention is not indicated.

Odontoid Fractures The odontoid process, or dens, is the large ellipse of bone arising anteriorly from C2 (the axis) and projecting up through the ring of C1 (the atlas). Several strong ligaments connect the dens to C1 and to the base of the skull. Odontoid fractures usually result from flexion forces. Odontoid fractures are classified as type I, II, or III. A type I fracture involves the tip only. A type II fracture passes through the base of the odontoid process. A type III fracture passes through the body of C2. Types II and III are considered unstable and should be externally immobilized by a halo vest or fused surgically. Surgery often is undertaken for widely displaced fractures (poor chance of fusing) and for those that fail external immobilization. Type I fractures usually fuse with external immobilization only.

Hangman's Fracture Traditionally considered a hyperextension/distraction injury from placement of the noose under the angle of the jaw, hangman's fractures also may occur with hyperextension/compression, as with diving accidents, or hyperflexion. The injury is defined by bilateral C2 pars interarticularis fractures. The pars interarticularis is the bone between superior and inferior facet joints. Thus, the posterior bony connection between C1 and C3 is lost. Hangman's fractures heal well with external immobilization. Surgery is indicated if there is spinal cord compression or after failure of external immobilization.

Jumped Facets—Hyperflexion Injury The facet joints of the cervical spine slope forward. In a hyperflexion injury, the superior facet can "jump" pathologically up and forward over the inferior facet if the joint capsule is torn. Hyperflexion/rotation can cause a unilateral jumped facet, whereas hyperflexion/distraction leads to bilateral jumped facets. Patients with a unilateral injury usually are neurologically intact, while those with bilateral injury usually have spinal cord damage. The anteroposterior diameter of the spinal canal decreases more with bilateral injury, leading to spinal cord compression (Fig. 42-10).

Thoracolumbar The thoracic spine is stabilized significantly by the rib cage. The lumbar spine has comparatively large vertebrae. Thus, the thoracolumbar spine has a higher threshold for injury than the cervical spine. A three-column model is useful for categorizing thoracolumbar injuries.[18] The anterior longitudinal ligament and the anterior half of the vertebral body constitute the anterior column. The posterior half of the vertebral body and the posterior longitudinal ligament constitute the middle column. The pedicles, facet joints, laminae, spinous processes, and interspinous ligaments constitute the posterior column.

Compression Fracture Compression fracture is a compression/flexion injury causing failure of the anterior column only. It is stable and not associated with neurologic deficit, although the patient may still have significant pain (Fig. 42-11).

Burst Fracture Burst fracture is a pure axial compression injury causing failure of the anterior and middle columns. It is unstable, and perhaps half of patients have neurologic deficit due to compression of the cord or cauda equina from bone fragments retropulsed into the spinal canal.

Chance Fracture Chance fracture is a flexion-distraction injury causing failure of the middle and posterior columns, sometimes with anterior wedging. Typical injury is from a lap seat-belt hyperflexion with associated abdominal injury. It often is unstable and associated with neurologic deficit.

Fracture-Dislocation Fracture-dislocation is failure of the anterior, middle, and posterior columns caused by flexion/distraction, shear, or compression forces. Neurologic deficit can result from retropulsion of middle column bone fragments into the spinal canal, or from subluxation causing decreased canal diameter (Fig. 42-12).

Initial Assessment and Management

The possibility of a spine injury must be considered in all trauma patients. A patient with no symptoms referable to neurologic injury, a normal neurologic examination, no neck or back pain, and a known mechanism of injury unlikely to cause spine injury is at minimal risk for significant injury to the spine. Victims of moderate or severe trauma, especially those with injuries to other organ systems, usually fail to meet these criteria or cannot be assessed adequately. The latter often is due to impaired sensorium or significant pain. Because of the potentially catastrophic consequences of missing occult spine instability in a neurologically intact patient, a high level of clinical suspicion should govern patient care until completion of clinical and radiographic evaluation.

The trauma patient should be kept on a hard flat board with straps and pads used for immobilization. A hard cervical collar is kept in place. These steps minimize forces transferred through the spine, and therefore decrease the chance of causing dislocation, subluxation, or neural compression during transport to the trauma bay. The patient is then moved from the board to a flat stretcher. The primary survey and resuscitation are completed. Physical examination and initial x-rays follow.

For the examination, approach the patient as described in the section on Neurologic Examination earlier in this chapter. Evaluation for spine or SCI is easier and more informative in awake patients. If the patient is awake, ask if he or she recalls details of the nature of the trauma, and if there was loss of consciousness, numbness, or inability to move any or all limbs. Assess motor function by response to commands or pain, as appropriate. Assess pinprick, light touch, and joint position, if possible. Determining the anatomically lowest level of intact sensation can pinpoint the level of the lesion along the spine. Testing sensation in an ascending fashion will allow the patient to better discern the true stimulus as opposed to determine when it is extinguished. Document muscle stretch reflexes, lower sacral reflexes (i.e., anal wink and bulbocavernosus), and rectal tone.

American Spinal Injury Association Classification The American Spinal Injury Association provides a method of classifying patients with spine injuries. The classification indicates completeness and level of the injury and the associated deficit. A form similar to that shown in Fig. 42-13 should be available in the trauma bay and completed for any spine injury patient. The association also has worked to develop recommendations and guidelines to standardize the care of SCI patients in an effort to improve the quality of care.

Neurologic Syndromes

Penetrating, compressive, or ischemic cord injury can lead to several characteristic presentations based on the anatomy of injury. The neurologic deficits may be deduced from the anatomy of the long sensory and motor tracts and understanding of their decussations

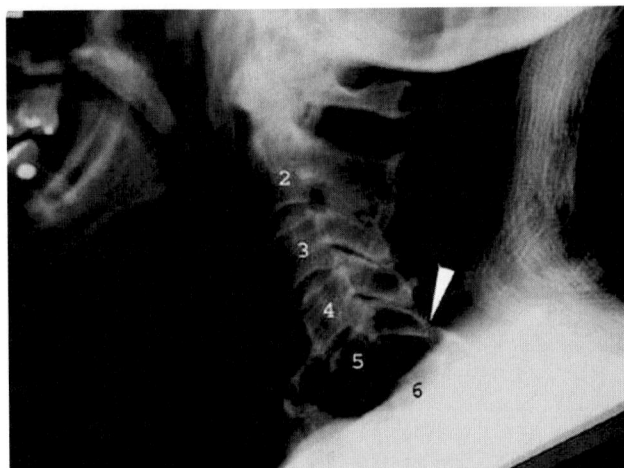

A

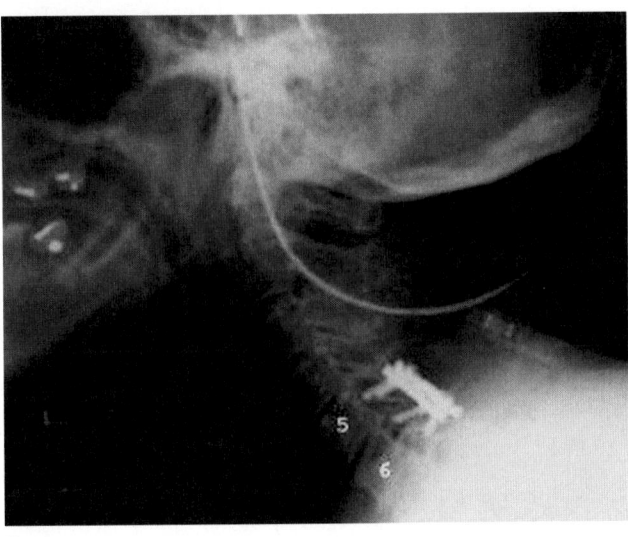

C

D

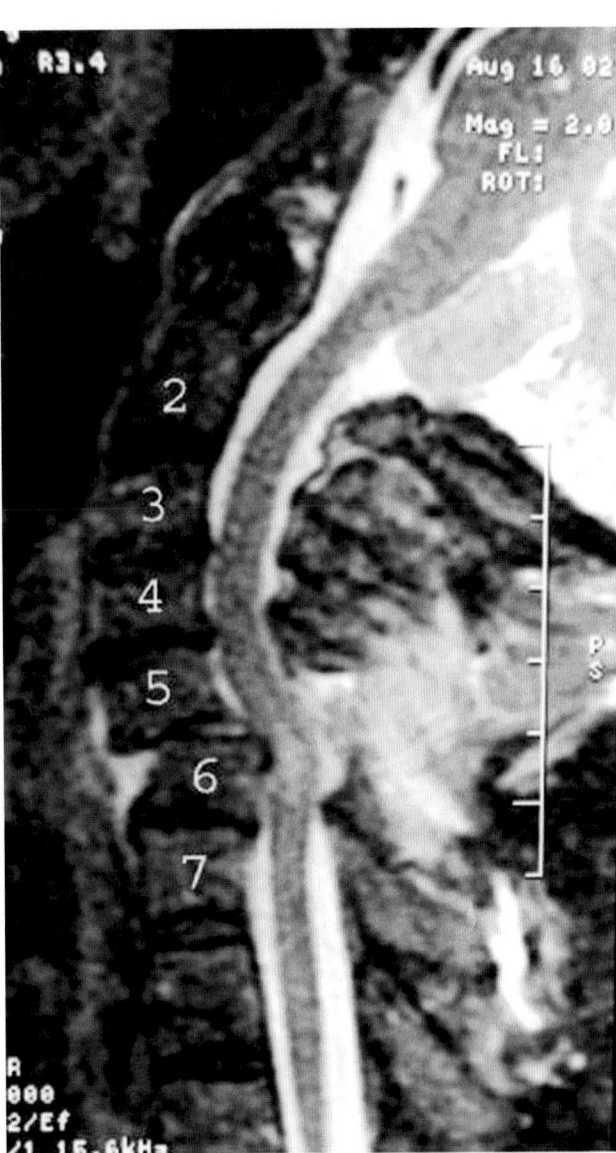

B

FIG. 42-10. A. Lateral cervical spine x-ray of an elderly woman who struck her head during a backward fall. *Arrowhead* points to jumped facets at C5–C6. Note the anterior displacement of the C5 body with respect to the C6 body. **B.** Sagittal T2-weighted magnetic resonance imaging of the same patient, revealing compromise of the spinal canal and compression of the cord. Note the bright signal within the cord at the level of compression, indicating spinal cord injury. **C.** Lateral cervical spine x-ray of same patient after application of cervical traction and manual reduction. Note restoration of normal alignment. **D.** Lateral cervical spine x-ray after posterior cervical fusion to restabilize the C5–C6 segment of the spine.

(Fig. 42-14). Four patterns are discussed. First, injury to the entire cord at a given level results in anatomic or functional cord transection with total loss of motor and sensory function below the level of the lesion. The typical mechanism is severe traumatic vertebral subluxation reducing spinal canal diameter and crushing the cord. Second, injury to half the cord at a given level results in Brown-Séquard syndrome, with loss of motor control and proprioception ipsilaterally and loss of nociception and thermoception contralater-

ally. The typical mechanism is a stab or gunshot wound. Third, injury to the interior gray matter of the cord in the cervical spine results in a central cord syndrome, with upper extremity worse than lower extremity weakness and varying degrees of numbness. The typical mechanism is transient compression of the cervical cord by the ligamentum flavum buckling during traumatic neck hyperextension. This syndrome occurs in patients with pre-existing cervical stenosis. Fourth, injury to the ventral half of the cord results in the

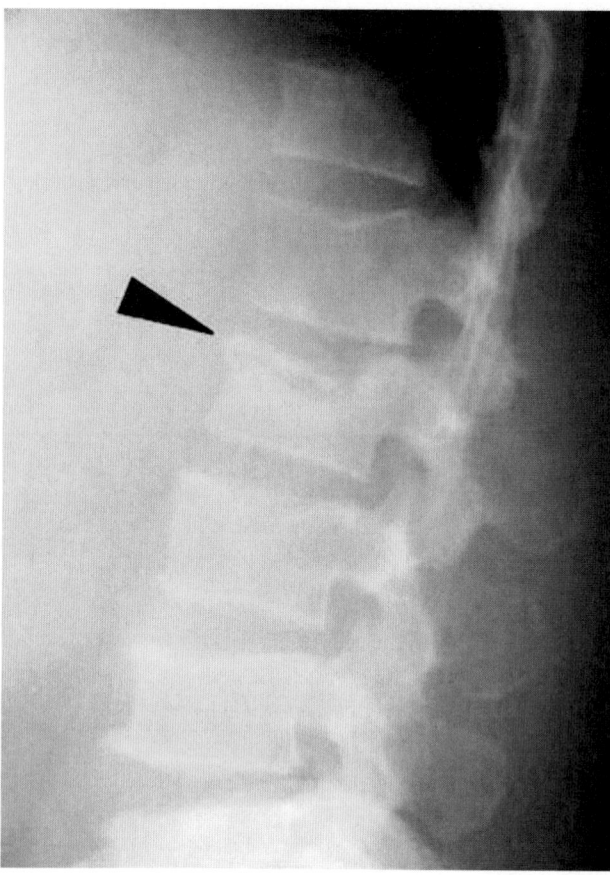

A

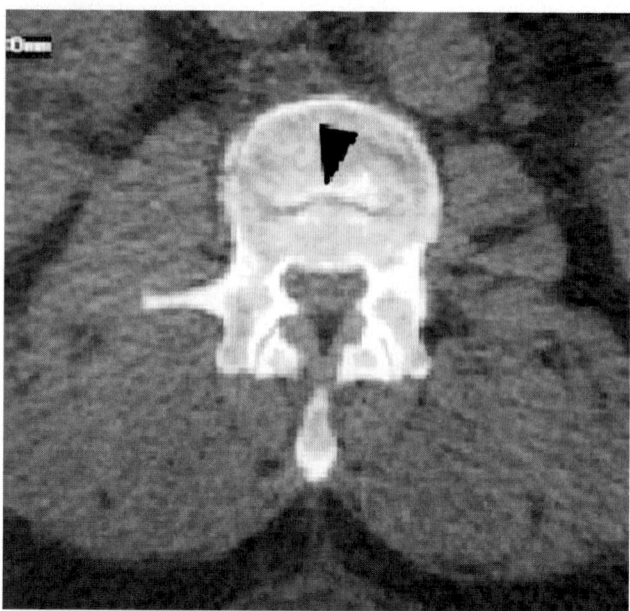

B

FIG. 42-11. A. Lateral lumbar spine x-ray showing a compression fracture of L2. *Arrowhead* points to anterior wedge deformity. Note the posterior wall of the vertebral body has retained normal height and alignment. **B.** Axial computed tomography scan through the same fracture. *Arrowhead* demonstrates a transverse discontinuity in the superior endplate of the L2 body.

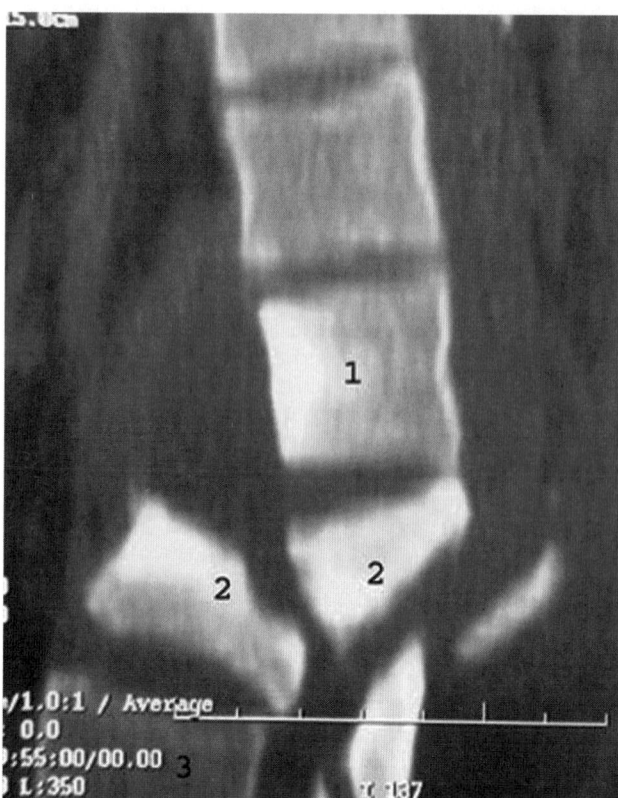

FIG. 42-12. Sagittal reconstruction of an axial fine-slice computed tomography scan through the lumbar spine demonstrating a severe fracture-dislocation through the body of L2.

anterior cord syndrome, with paralysis and loss of nociception and thermoception bilaterally. The typical mechanism is an acute disc herniation or ischemia from anterior spinal artery occlusion.

Studies

Anteroposterior and lateral plain films provide a rapid survey of the bony spine. Plain films detect fractures and dislocations well. Adequate visualization of the lower cervical and upper thoracic spine often is impossible because of the shoulder girdle. Complete plain film imaging of the cervical spine includes an open-mouth view to assess the odontoid process and the lateral masses of C1. Fine-slice CT scan with sagittal and coronal reconstructions provides good detail of bony anatomy and is good for characterizing fractures seen on plain films, as well as visualizing C7–T1 when not well seen on plain films. MRI provides the best soft tissue imaging. Canal compromise from subluxation, acute disc herniations, or ligamentous disruption is clearly seen. MRI also may detect EDHs or damage to the spinal cord itself, including contusions or areas of ischemia.

Definitive Management

Spinal-Dose Steroids The National Acute Spinal Cord Injury studies (NASCIS I and II) provide the basis for the common practice of administering high-dose steroids to patients with acute SCI. A 30-mg/kg IV bolus of methylprednisolone is given over 15 minutes, followed by a 5.4-mg/kg per hour infusion begun 45 minutes later. The infusion is continued for 23 hours if the bolus is given within 3 hours of injury, or for 47 hours if the bolus is given within 8 hours of injury. The papers indicate greater motor and sensory recovery at 6 weeks, 6 months, and 1 year after acute SCI in patients who received methylprednisolone.[19,20] However, the NASCIS trial data have been extensively criticized, as many argue that the selection criteria and study design were flawed, making the results ambiguous. Patients

ASIA IMPAIRMENT SCALE

☐ **A = Complete:** No motor or sensory function is preserved in the sacral segments S4-S5.

☐ **B = Incomplete:** Sensory but not motor function is preserved below the neurological level and includes the sacral segments S4-S5.

☐ **C = Incomplete:** Motor function is preserved below the neurological level, and more than half of key muscles below the neurological level have a muscle grade less than 3.

☐ **D = Incomplete:** Motor function is preserved below the neurological level, and at least half of key muscles below the neurological level have a muscle grade of 3 or more.

☐ **E = Normal:** motor and sensory function are normal

CLINICAL SYNDROMES

☐ Central Cord
☐ Brown-Sequard
☐ Anterior Cord
☐ Conus Medullaris
☐ Cauda Equina

ASIA

STANDARD NEUROLOGICAL CLASSIFICATION OF SPINAL CORD INJURY

MOTOR — KEY MUSCLES

C5 Elbow flexors
C6 Wrist extensors
C7 Elbow extensors
C8 Finger flexors (distal phalanx of middle finger)
T1 Finger abductors (little finger)

0 = total paralysis
1 = palpable or visible contraction
2 = active movement, gravity eliminated
3 = active movement, against gravity
4 = active movement, against some resistance
5 = active movement, against full resistance
NT = not testable

L2 Hip flexors
L3 Knee extensors
L4 Ankle dorsiflexors
L5 Long toe extensors
S1 Ankle plantar flexors

Voluntary anal contraction (Yes/No)

TOTALS ☐ + ☐ = ☐ **MOTOR SCORE**
(MAXIMUM) (50) (50) (100)

SENSORY — KEY SENSORY POINTS

0 = absent
1 = impaired
2 = normal
NT = not testable

Any anal sensation (Yes/No)

TOTALS { ☐ + ☐ } = ☐ **PIN PRICK SCORE** (max: 112)
= ☐ **LIGHT TOUCH SCORE** (max: 112)
(MAXIMUM) (56) (56) (56) (56)

*Key Sensory Points

NEUROLOGICAL LEVEL	R	L	COMPLETE OR INCOMPLETE?	☐	ZONE OF PARTIAL PRESERVATION	R	L
The most caudal segment with normal function	SENSORY		Incomplete = Any sensory or motor function in S4-S5		Caudal extent of partially innervated segments	SENSORY	
	MOTOR		**ASIA IMPAIRMENT SCALE** ☐			MOTOR	

This form may be copied freely but should not be altered without permission from the American Spinal Injury Association. 2000 Rev.

FIG. 42-13. The American Spinal Injury Association system for categorizing spinal cord injury patients according to level and degree of neurologic deficit.

who receive such a large corticosteroid dose have increased rates of medical and ICU complications, such as pneumonias, which have a deleterious effect on outcome. A clear consensus on the use of spinal-dose steroids does not exist.[21] A decision to use or not use spinal-dose steroids may be dictated by local or regional practice patterns, especially given the legal liability issues surrounding SCI. Patients with gunshot or nerve root (cauda equina) injuries, or those who are pregnant, <14 years old, or on chronic steroids were excluded from the NASCIS studies and should not receive spinal-dose steroids. In addition to steroids, hypothermia for SCI has also received attention. There is even less evidence supporting the use of this treatment, and thus, it is not recommended.[22]

Orthotic Devices Rigid external orthotic devices can stabilize the spine by decreasing range of motion and minimizing stress transmitted through the spine. Commonly used rigid cervical orthoses include Philadelphia and Miami-J collars. Cervical collars are inadequate for C1, C2, or cervicothoracic instability. Cervicothoracic orthoses brace the upper thorax and the neck, improving stabilization over the cervicothoracic region. Minerva braces improve high cervical stabilization by bracing from the upper thorax to the chin and occiput. Halo-vest assemblies provide the most external cervical stabilization. Four pins are driven into the skull to lock the halo ring in position. Four posts arising from a tight-fitting rigid plastic vest immobilize the halo ring. Lumbar stabilization may be pro-

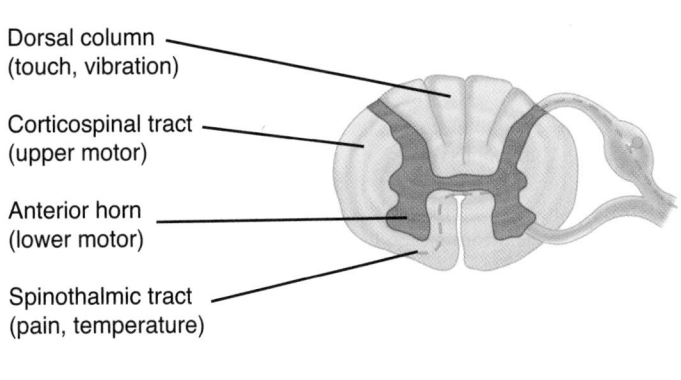

Dorsal column (touch, vibration)

Corticospinal tract (upper motor)

Anterior horn (lower motor)

Spinothalmic tract (pain, temperature)

FIG. 42-14. Spinal cord injury patterns. a. = artery. (*Adapted with permission from Hoff J, Boland M: Neurosurgery, from* Principles of Surgery, *7th ed. New York: McGraw-Hill, 1999, p 1837.*)

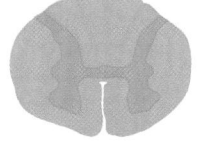
Transection

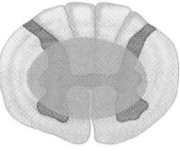
Central cord

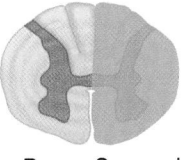
Brown-Sequard

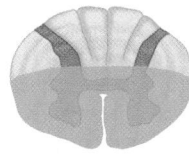
Anterior spinal a.

vided by thoracolumbosacral orthoses. A variety of companies manufacture lines of spinal orthotics. A physician familiar with the technique should fit a halo-vest. Assistance from a trained orthotics technician improves fitting and adjustment of the other devices.

Surgery Neurosurgical intervention has two goals. First is the decompression of the spinal cord or nerve roots in patients with incomplete neurologic deficits. These patients should be decompressed expeditiously, especially if there is evidence of neurologic deterioration over time. Second is the stabilization of injuries judged too unstable to heal with external immobilization only. Spine trauma patients with complete neurologic deficit, without any signs of recovery, or those without any neurologic deficits who have bony or ligamentous injury requiring open fixation, may be medically stabilized before undergoing surgery. Surgical stabilization may be indicated for some injuries that would eventually heal with conservative treatment. Surgical stabilization can allow early mobilization, aggressive nursing care, and physical therapy. Solid surgical stabilization may also allow a patient to be managed with a rigid cervical collar who would otherwise require halo-vest immobilization.

Continued Care

Regional SCI centers with nurses, respiratory therapists, pulmonologists, physical therapists, physiatrists, and neurosurgeons specifically trained in caring for these patients may improve outcomes. Frequently encountered ICU issues include hypotension and aspiration pneumonia. Chronically, prevention and treatment of deep venous thrombosis, autonomic hyperreflexia, and decubitus ulcer formation are important. Many patients with cervical or high thoracic cord injuries require prolonged ventilatory support until the chest wall becomes stiff enough to provide resistance for diaphragmatic breathing. Patients with high cervical cord injuries (C4 or above) will often require permanent ventilatory support. Patients should be transferred to SCI rehabilitation centers after stabilization of medical and surgical issues.

Peripheral Nerve Trauma

The peripheral nervous system extends throughout the body and is subject to injury from a wide variety of trauma. Peripheral nerves transmit motor and sensory information between the CNS and the body. An individual nerve may have pure motor, pure sensory, or mixed motor and sensory functions. The key information-carrying structure of the nerve is the axon. The axon transmits information from the neuronal cell body and may measure from <1 mm to >1 m in length. Axons that travel a significant distance are often covered with myelin, which is a lipid-rich, electrically insulating sheath formed by Schwann cells. Myelinated axons transmit signals much more rapidly than unmyelinated axons because the voltage shifts and currents that define action potentials effectively jump from gap to gap over the insulated lengths of the axon.

Axons, whether myelinated or unmyelinated, travel through a collagenous connective tissue known as *endoneurium*. Groups of axons and their endoneurium form bundles known as *fascicles*. Fascicles run through a tubular collagenous tissue known as *perineurium*. Groups of fascicles are suspended in mesoneurium. Fascicles and their mesoneurium run through another tubular collagenous tissue known as *epineurium*. The epineurium and its contents form the nerve.

There are four major mechanisms of injury to peripheral nerves. Nerves may be lacerated, stretched, compressed, or contused. Knives, passing bullets, or jagged bone fractures may lacerate nerves. Adjacent expanding hematomas or dislocated fractures may stretch nerves. Expanding hematomas, external orthoses such as casts or braces, or blunt trauma over a superficial nerve may compress or crush nerves. Shock waves from high-velocity bullets may contuse nerves. These mechanisms of injury cause damage to the various anatomic components of the nerve. The patterns of damage are categorized below.

Certain nerve segments are particularly vulnerable to injury. The following four characteristics make a nerve segment more vulnerable: proximity to a joint, superficial course, passage through a confined space, and being fixed in position.

Types of Injury

The traditional classification system for peripheral nerve injury is the Seddon classification. Seddon described three injury patterns as defined below in the Neurapraxia, Axonotmesis, and Neurotmesis sections. The Seddon classification provides a simple, anatomically based approach to peripheral nerve injury.[23]

Neurapraxia Neurapraxia is defined as the temporary failure of nerve function without physical axonal disruption. Axon degeneration does not occur. Return of normal axonal function occurs over hours to months, often in the 2- to 4-week range.

Axonotmesis Axonotmesis is the disruption of axons and myelin. The surrounding connective tissues, including endoneurium, are intact. The axons degenerate proximally and distally from the area of injury. Distal degeneration is known as *Wallerian degeneration*. Axon regeneration within the connective tissue pathways can occur, leading to restoration of function. Axons regenerate at a rate of 1 mm per day. Significant functional recovery may occur for up to 18 months. Scarring at the site of injury from connective tissue reaction can form a neuroma and interfere with regeneration.

Neurotmesis Neurotmesis is the disruption of axons and endoneurial tubes. Peripheral collagenous components, such as the epineurium, may or may not be intact. Proximal and distal axonal degeneration occurs. The likelihood of effective axonal regeneration across the site of injury depends on the extent of neuroma formation and on the degree of persisting anatomic alignment of the connective tissue structures. For instance, an injury may damage axons, myelin, and endoneurium, but leave perineurium intact. In this case, the fascicle sheath is intact, and appropriate axonal regeneration is more likely to occur than if the sheath is interrupted.

Management of Peripheral Nerve Injury

The sensory and motor deficits should be accurately documented. Deficits are usually immediate. Progressive deficit suggests a process such as an expanding hematoma and may warrant early surgical exploration. Clean, sharp injuries may also benefit from early exploration and reanastomosis. Most other peripheral nerve injuries should be observed. EMG/NCS studies should be done 3- to 4 weeks postinjury if deficits persist. Axon segments distal to the site of injury will conduct action potentials normally until Wallerian degeneration occurs, rendering EMG/NCS before 3 weeks uninformative. Continued observation is indicated if function improves. Surgical exploration of the nerve may be undertaken if no functional improvement occurs over 3 months. If intraoperative electrical testing reveals conduction across the injury, continue observation. In the absence of conduction, the injured segment should be resected and end-to-end primary anastomosis attempted. However, anastomoses under tension will not heal. A nerve graft may be needed to bridge the gap between the proximal and distal nerve ends. The sural nerve often is harvested, as it carries only sensory fibers and leaves a minor deficit when resected. The connective tissue structures of the nerve graft may provide a pathway for effective axonal regrowth across the injury.

Patterns of Injury

Brachial Plexus The brachial plexus may be injured in a variety of ways. Parturition or a motorcycle accident can lead to plexus injury due to dislocation of the glenohumeral joint. Attempting to arrest a fall with one's hands can lead to a stretch injury of the plexus due to abrupt movement of the shoulder girdle. An apical lung (Pancoast) tumor can cause compression injury to the plexus. There are many patterns of neurologic deficits possible with injury to the various components of the brachial plexus, and understanding them all would require extensive neuroanatomic discussion. Two well-known eponymous syndromes are Erb's palsy and Klumpke's palsy. Injury high in the plexus to the C5 and C6 roots resulting from glenohumeral dislocation causes Erb's palsy with the characteristic "bellhop's tip" position. The arm hangs at the side, internally rotated. Hand movements are not affected. Injury low in the plexus, to the C8 and T1 roots, resulting from stretch or compression injury, causes Klumpke's palsy with the characteristic "claw hand" deformity. There is weakness of the intrinsic hand muscles, similar to that seen with ulnar nerve injury.

Radial Nerve The radial nerve courses through the axilla, then laterally and posteriorly in the spiral groove of the humerus. Improper crutch use can cause damage to the axillary portion. The section of the nerve traversing the spiral groove can be damaged by humerus fractures or pressure from improper positioning during sleep. This classically occurs when the patient is intoxicated and is called "Saturday night palsy." The key finding is wrist drop (i.e., weakness of hand and finger extensors). Axillary (proximal) injury causes triceps weakness in addition to wrist drop.

Common Peroneal Neuropathy The common peroneal nerve forms the lateral half of the sciatic nerve (the medial half being the tibial nerve). It receives contributions from L4, L5, S1, and S2. It emerges as a separate nerve in the popliteal fossa and laterally wraps around the fibular neck, after which it splits to form the deep and superficial peroneal nerves. The superficial, fixed location at the fibular neck makes the common peroneal nerve susceptible to compression. The classic cause of traumatic peroneal neuropathy is crush injury from a car bumper striking the lateral aspect of the leg at the knee. Symptoms of common peroneal neuropathy include foot drop (weakness of the tibialis anterior), eversion weakness, and numbness over the anterolateral surface of the lower leg and dorsum of the foot. In contrast, a foot drop due to L5 radiculopathy spares eversion because the S1 fibers are intact. Surgical exploration of a common peroneal crush lesion is typically a low yield endeavor. Rare cases may be due to compressive fibers or adhesions that may be lysed, with the possibility of return of function.

CEREBROVASCULAR DISEASE

Cerebrovascular disease is the most frequent cause of new, rapid-onset, nontraumatic neurologic deficit. It is far more common than seizures or tumors. Vascular structures are subject to a variety of chronic pathologic processes that compromise vessel wall integrity. Diabetes, high cholesterol, high blood pressure, and smoking are risk factors for vascular disease. These conditions can lead to vascular damage by such mechanisms as atheroma deposition causing luminal stenosis, endothelial damage promoting thrombogenesis, and weakening of the vessel wall resulting in aneurysm formation or dissection. These processes may coexist. For instance, a vessel containing an atheromatous plaque will have a decreased luminal diameter. The plaque also may have compromised endothelium, providing the opportunity for thrombus formation, which can lead to acute total occlusion of the remaining lumen. Aneurysms and dissection often occur in atheromatous vessels. Specific patterns of disease relevant to the cerebrovascular system include atheromatous and thrombotic carotid occlusion, brain ischemia from proximal embolic disease, vessel wall rupture leading to hemorrhage, and rupture of abnormal, thin-walled structures, specifically aneurysms and AVMs.

Ischemic Diseases

Ischemic stroke accounts for approximately 85% of acute cerebrovascular events. Symptoms of acute ischemic stroke vary based on the functions of the neural tissues supplied by the occluded vessel, and the presence or absence of collateral circulation. The circle of Willis provides extensive collateral circulation, as it connects the right and left carotid arteries to each other and each to the vertebrobasilar system. Patients with complete occlusion of the carotid artery proximal to the circle of Willis may be asymptomatic if the blood flow patterns can shift and provide sufficient circulation to the ipsilateral cerebral hemisphere from the contralateral carotid and the basilar artery. However, the anatomy of the circle of Willis is highly variable. Patients may have a hypoplastic or missing communicating artery with resultant bilateral ACA supply by one carotid; or the PCA may be supplied by the carotid artery rather than the basilar. Similarly, one vertebral artery is often dominant and the other is hypoplastic. These variations may make disease in a particular vessel more neurologically devastating than in a patient with full collateral circulation. Occlusion distal to the circle of Willis generally results in a stroke in the territory supplied by that particular artery.

Neurologic deficit from occlusive disease may be temporary or permanent. A patient with sudden-onset focal neurologic deficit that resolves within 24 hours has had a transient ischemic attack. A patient with permanent deficit has had a completed stroke.

Thrombotic Disease

The most common area of neurologically significant vessel thrombosis is the carotid artery in the neck. Disease occurs at the carotid bifurcation. Thrombosis of a carotid artery chronically narrowed by atheroma can lead to acute carotid occlusion. As discussed above, this can be asymptomatic. The more common concern is thromboembolus. Intracranial arterial occlusion by local thrombus formation may occur, but it is rare compared to embolic occlusion.

Management

Complete occlusion of the carotid artery without referable neurologic deficit requires no treatment. A patient with new neurologic deficit and an angiographically confirmed complete carotid occlusion contralateral to the symptoms should be considered for emergent carotid endarterectomy.[24] Surgery should be performed within 2 hours of symptom onset. This time restriction significantly reduces the number of candidates. Surgery should not be performed on obtunded or comatose patients. This time restriction significantly reduces the number of candidates.

Embolic Disease

Emboli causing strokes may originate from a number of sources, including: the left atrium, during atrial fibrillation, a hypokinetic left ventricular wall segment, valvular vegetations, an atheromatous aortic arch, stenotic/atheromatous carotid bifurcations, or from the systemic venous system in the presence of a right-to-left shunt, such as a patent foramen ovale. The majority of emboli enter the anterior (carotid) circulation rather than the posterior (vertebrobasilar) circulation. Characteristic clinical syndromes result from embolic occlusion of the various vessels.

Common Types of Strokes

Anterior Cerebral Artery Stroke The ACA supplies the medial frontal and parietal lobes, including the motor strip, as it courses into the interhemispheric fissure. ACA stroke results in contralateral leg weakness.

Middle Cerebral Artery Stroke The MCA supplies the lateral frontal and parietal lobes and the temporal lobe. MCA stroke results in contralateral face and arm weakness. Dominant-hemisphere MCA stroke causes language deficits. Proximal MCA occlusion with ischemia and swelling in the entire MCA territory can lead to significant intracranial mass effect and midline shift (see Fig. 42-6).

Posterior Cerebral Artery Stroke The PCA supplies the occipital lobe. PCA stroke results in a contralateral homonymous hemianopsia (see Fig. 42-6).

Posterior Inferior Cerebellar Artery Stroke The PICA supplies the lateral medulla and the inferior half of the cerebellar hemispheres. PICA stroke results in nausea, vomiting, nystagmus, dysphagia, ipsilateral Horner's syndrome, and ipsilateral limb ataxia. The constellation of symptoms resulting from PICA occlusion is referred to as the *lateral medullary* or *Wallenberg's syndrome*.

Management

Ischemic stroke management has two goals: reopen the occluded vessel and maintain blood flow to ischemic "penumbra" tissues bordering the vascular territory. Reopening the vessel may be attempted with recombinant tPA.[25] tPA administration within 3 hours of the onset of neurologic deficit improves outcome at 3 months. In the setting of suspected ischemic stroke, a head CT must be performed immediately to differentiate ischemic from hemorrhagic stroke. Intracranial hemorrhage, major surgery within the previous 2 weeks, GI or genitourinary hemorrhage in the previous 3 weeks, platelet count less than $100,000/\mu L$, and systolic blood pressure >185 mmHg are among the contraindications to tPA therapy.

Patients not eligible for tPA require hemodynamic optimization and neurologic monitoring. Admit such patients to the ICU stroke service for blood pressure management and frequent neurologic checks. Permissive hypertension allows for maximal cerebral perfusion. Systolic blood pressure >180 mmHg may require treatment, but the optimal mean arterial pressure goal is between 100 to 140 mmHg. Give normal saline solution without glucose (which could injure neurons in the penumbra), and aim for normovolemia. A stroke patient who worsens clinically should undergo repeat head CT to evaluate for hemorrhage or increasing mass effect from swelling, which typically peaks 3 to 5 days after the stroke. Significant swelling from an MCA or cerebellar strokes may cause herniation and brain stem injury. A decompressive hemicraniectomy or suboccipital craniectomy can be a life-saving intervention for these select stroke patients.

Hemorrhagic Diseases

Intracranial hemorrhage from abnormal or diseased vascular structures accounts for approximately 15% of acute cerebrovascular events. Hypertension and amyloid angiopathy account for most intraparenchymal hemorrhages, although AVMs, aneurysms, venous thrombosis, tumors, hemorrhagic conversion of ischemic infarct, and fungal infections also may be the cause. The term *intracranial hemorrhage* frequently is used to mean intraparenchymal hemorrhage and will be used here. Intracranial hemorrhage causes local neuronal injury and dysfunction and also may cause global dysfunction due to mass effect if sufficiently large. AVM or aneurysm rupture results in SAH because the major cerebral and cortical blood vessels travel in the subarachnoid space, between the pia and the arachnoid membrane. SAH can cause immediate concussive-like neuronal dysfunction by exposure of the brain to intra-arterial pressure pulsations during the hemorrhage; it can cause delayed ischemia from cerebral arterial vasospasm. Patients presenting with intracranial hemorrhages that do not follow typical patterns should undergo angiography or MRI to evaluate for possible underlying lesions, such as AVM or tumor.

Hemorrhagic stroke typically occurs within the basal ganglia or cerebellum. The patient is usually hypertensive on admission and has a history of poorly controlled hypertension. Such patients are more likely to present with lethargy or obtundation, compared to those who suffer an ischemic stroke. Depressed mental status results from brain shift and herniation secondary to mass effect from the hematoma in deep structures. Ischemic stroke does not cause mass effect acutely; and therefore, patients are more likely to present with normal consciousness and a focal neurologic deficit. Hemorrhagic strokes tend to present with a relatively gradual decline in neurologic function as the hematoma expands, rather than the immediately maximal symptoms caused by ischemic stroke. Table 42-3 provides a listing of relative incidences of intracranial hemorrhage by anatomic distribution.

TABLE 42-3	Anatomic distribution of intracranial hemorrhages and correlated symptoms	
% of Intracranial Hemorrhages	**Location**	**Classic Symptoms**
50	Basal ganglia (putamen, globus pallidus), internal capsule	Contralateral hemiparesis
15	Thalamus	Contralateral hemisensory loss
10–20	Cerebral white matter (lobar)	Depends on location (weakness, numbness, partial loss of visual field)
10–15	Pons	Hemiparesis; may be devastating
10	Cerebellum	Lethargy or coma due to brain stem compression and/or hydrocephalus
1–6	Brain stem (excluding pons)	Often devastating

Hypertension

Hypertension increases the relative risk of intracranial hemorrhage by approximately fourfold, likely due to chronic degenerative vasculopathy. Hypertensive hemorrhages often present in the basal ganglia, thalamus, or pons, and result from breakage of small perforating arteries that branch off of much larger parent vessels (Fig. 42-15).

Most hypertensive hemorrhages should be medically managed. The hematoma often contains intact, salvageable axons because the blood dissects through and along neural tracts, and surgical clot evacuation destroys these axons. Factors potentially favoring surgery include: superficial clot location, young age, nondominant hemisphere, rapid deterioration, and significant mass effect. However, the most comprehensive randomized clinical trials to date did not show an overall improved outcome in surgically evacuated intracranial hemorrhage, except for the subgroup of patients with clot <1 cm from the cortical surface.[26] Medical management includes moderate blood pressure control, normalizing platelet and clotting function, phenytoin, and electrolyte management. Intubate patients who cannot clearly follow commands to prevent aspiration and hypercarbia. Follow and document the neurologic examination and communicate with the family regarding appropriateness for rehabilitation vs. withdrawal of care.

Amyloid Angiopathy

The presence of pathologic amyloid deposition in the media of small cortical vessels compromises vessel integrity and tends to cause more superficial (lobar) hemorrhages than hypertensive intracranial hemorrhage. Amyloid laden vessels may hemorrhage multiple times. The superficial location of amyloid hemorrhages may make surgical evacuation less morbid compared to typical deep hypertensive hemorrhages. Nonetheless, medical management and family counseling should be approached similarly to patients with hypertensive hemorrhages.

Cerebral Aneurysm

An aneurysm is a focal dilatation of the vessel wall and is most often a balloon-like outpouching, but may also be fusiform. Aneurysms usually occur at branch points of major vessels (e.g., internal carotid artery bifurcation), or at the origin of smaller vessels (e.g., posterior communicating artery or ophthalmic artery). Approximately 85% of aneurysms arise from the anterior circulation (carotid) and 15% from the posterior circulation (vertebrobasilar). Table 42-4 shows the percentage distribution of cerebral aneurysms by location. Aneurysms are thin walled and at risk for rupture. The major cerebral vessels, and

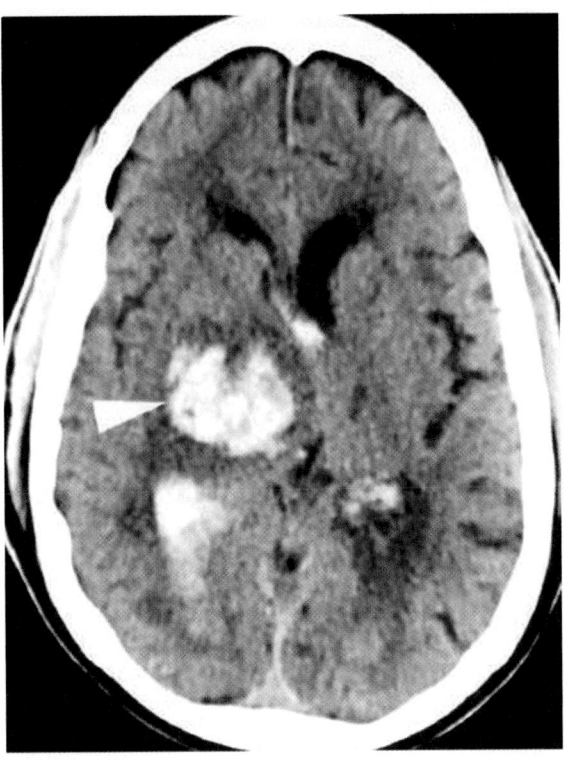

A

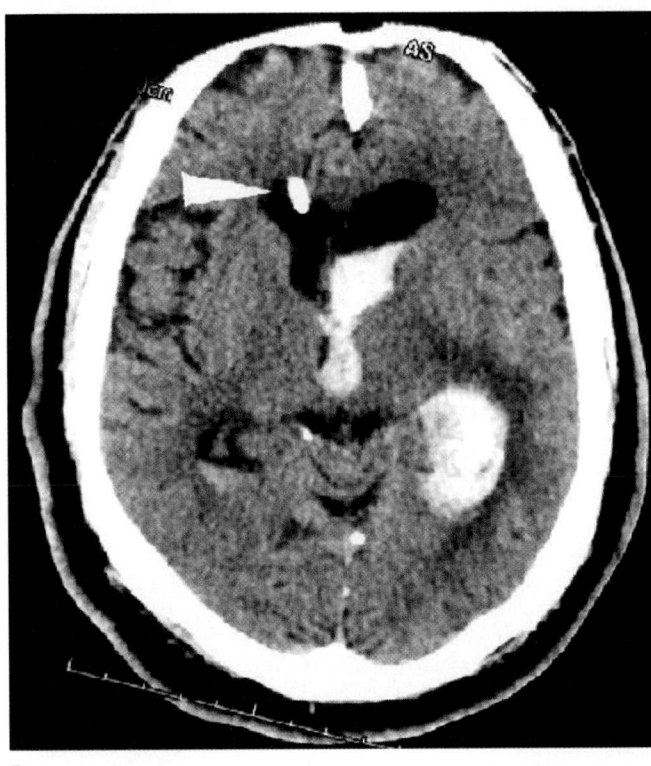

B

FIG. 42-15. A. Head computed tomography scan of a patient with left-sided weakness and progressive lethargy reveals a right basal ganglia hemorrhage (*arrowhead*). The blood clot is bright white. Hypodensity around the clot represents cerebral edema. There is blood within the ventricular system. **B.** Another patient with intraventricular extension of a basal ganglia hemorrhage. The patient developed right-sided weakness and then lethargy. Head computed tomography indicated hydrocephalus. A ventriculostomy was placed for cerebrospinal fluid drainage (*arrowhead* indicates cross-sectional view of the catheter entering the anterior horn of the right lateral ventricle).

therefore aneurysms, lie in the subarachnoid space. Rupture results in SAH. The aneurysmal tear may be small and seal quickly, or it may not. SAH may consist of a thin layer of blood in the CSF spaces, or thick layers of blood around the brain and extending into brain parenchyma, resulting in a clot with mass effect. Because the meningeal linings of the brain are sensitive, SAH usually results in a sudden, severe "thunderclap" headache. A patient will classically describe "the worst headache of my life." Presenting neurologic symptoms may range from mild headache to coma to sudden death. The Hunt-Hess grading system categorizes patients clinically (Table 42-5).

Patients with symptoms suspicious for SAH should have a head CT immediately. Acute SAH appears as a bright signal in the fissures and CSF cisterns around the base of the brain, as shown in Fig. 42-16. CT is rapid, noninvasive, and approximately 95% sensitive. In patients with suspicious symptoms but negative head CT, a

lumbar puncture (LP) should be performed. An LP with xanthochromia and high red blood cell counts (usually 100,000/mL), which do not decrease between tubes 1 and 4, is consistent with SAH. Negative CT and LP essentially rules out SAH. Patients diagnosed with SAH require four-vessel cerebral angiography within 24 hours to assess for aneurysm or other vascular malformation. Catheter angiography remains the gold standard for assessing the patient's cerebral vasculature, relevant anomalies, and presence, location, and morphology of the cerebral aneurysms. Figure 42-17A and 42-17B demonstrate the typical digital subtraction angiographic view of a cerebral aneurysm. Figure 42-17C shows the anatomy of the circle of Willis in a simplified graphic representation to assist in visualizing the locations of various cerebral aneurysms.

SAH patients should be admitted to the neurologic ICU. Hunt-Hess grade 4 and 5 patients require intubation and hemodynamic

TABLE 42-4	Prevalence of cerebral aneurysm by location
Prevalence	**Aneurysm Location (Vernacular Name)**
Anterior circulation 85%	30% Anterior communicating artery (A-Comm)
	25% Posterior communicating artery (P-Comm)
	20% Middle cerebral artery bifurcation
	10% Other
Posterior circulation 15%	10% Basilar artery, most frequently at the basilar tip
	5% Vertebral artery, usually at the posterior inferior cerebellar artery

TABLE 42-5	The Hunt-Hess clinical grading system for subarachnoid hemorrhage
Hunt-Hess Grade	**Clinical Presentation**
0	Asymptomatic; unruptured aneurysm
1	Awake; asymptomatic or mild headache; mild nuchal rigidity
2	Awake; moderate to severe headache, cranial nerve palsy (e.g., cranial nerve III or IV), nuchal rigidity
3	Lethargic; mild focal neurologic deficit (e.g., pronator drift)
4	Stuporous; significant neurologic deficit (e.g., hemiplegia)
5	Comatose; posturing

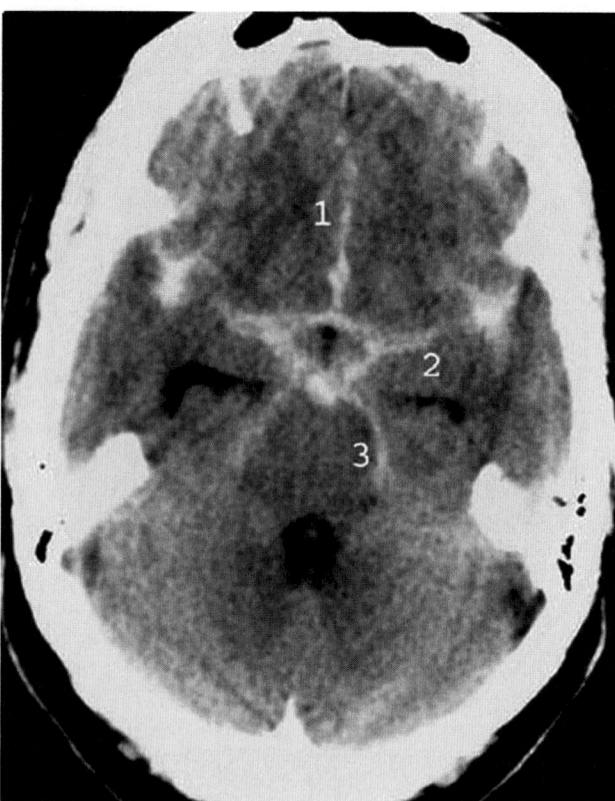

FIG. 42-16. Head computed tomography scan of a patient who experienced a sudden, severe headache. Subarachnoid hemorrhage is visible as hyperdense signal in the interhemispheric fissure (*1*), bilateral sylvian fissures (*2* shows the left fissure), and in the ambient cisterns around the midbrain (*3*). This gives the classic five-pointed-star appearance of a subarachnoid hemorrhage. Visible temporal tips of the lateral ventricles indicate hydrocephalus.

includes maintenance of optimal perfusion with hypertension and mild hypervolemia, as well as administration of nimodipine, a calcium channel blocker that may decrease the incidence and degree of spasm. Neurointerventional options for treating symptomatic vasospasm include intra-arterial papaverine or nicardipine, and balloon angioplasty for larger caliber vessels.

Aneurysmal SAH has an approximate mortality rate of 50% in the first month. Approximately one third of survivors return to pre-SAH function, and the remaining two thirds have mild to severe disability. Most require rehabilitation after hospitalization.

Arteriovenous Malformations

AVMs are abnormal, dilated arteries and veins without an intervening capillary bed. The nidus of the AVM contains a tangled mass of vessels but no neural tissue. AVMs may be asymptomatic or present with SAH or seizures. Small AVMs present with hemorrhage more often than large AVMs, which tend to present with seizures. Headache, bruit, or focal neurologic deficits are less common symptoms. AVMs hemorrhage at an average rate of 2 to 4% a year. Figure 42-18 demonstrates the angiographic appearance of an AVM in arterial and venous phases.

There are several management differences for SAH due to AVM vs. aneurysm. Definitive therapy for the AVM usually is delayed 3 to 4 weeks to allow the brain to recover from acute injury. There is less risk of devastating early rebleeding from AVMs, and vasospasm is less relevant. Adjacent brain may be hyperemic after removal of the high-flow arteriovenous shunt, making hypertension and hypervolemia harmful rather than beneficial. Three therapeutic modalities for AVMs are currently in common use: microsurgical excision, endovascular glue embolization, and stereotactic radiosurgery (SRS). AVMs that are large, near eloquent cortex, or that drain to deep venous structures are considered high grade and more difficult to surgically resect without causing significant neurologic deficit. Radiosurgery can treat these lesions, although it is limited to lesions <3 cm in diameter and has a 2-year lag time (i.e., the AVM may bleed in the interval). Embolization reduces flow through the AVM. It is usually considered adjunctive therapy, but it may serve as the sole treatment for deep, inaccessible lesions.

TUMORS OF THE CENTRAL NERVOUS SYSTEM

A wide variety of tumors affect the brain and spine. Primary benign and malignant tumors arise from the various elements of the CNS, including neurons, glia, and meninges. Tumors metastasize to the CNS from many primary sources. Presentation varies widely depending on relevant neuroanatomy. Prognosis depends on histology and anatomy. Modern brain tumor centers use team approaches to CNS tumors, as patients may require a combination of surgery, radiation therapy, chemotherapy, SRS, and research protocol enrollment. Tumors affecting the peripheral nervous system are discussed in the Peripheral Nerve section.

Intracranial Tumors

Intracranial tumors can cause brain injury from mass effect, dysfunction or destruction of adjacent neural structures, swelling, or abnormal electrical activity (seizures). Supratentorial tumors commonly present with focal neurologic deficit, such as contralateral limb weakness, visual field deficit, headache, or seizure. Infratentorial tumors often cause increased ICP due to hydrocephalus from compression of the fourth ventricle, leading to headache, nausea, vomiting, or diplopia. Cerebellar hemisphere or brain stem dysfunction can result in ataxia, nystagmus, or cranial nerve palsies. Infratentorial tumors rarely cause seizures.

All patients with symptoms concerning for brain tumor should undergo MRI with and without gadolinium. Initial management of a patient with a symptomatic brain tumor generally includes dexamethasone for reduction of vasogenic edema and phenytoin if the

monitoring and stabilization. The current standard of care for ruptured aneurysms requires early aneurysmal occlusion. There are two options for occlusion. The patient may undergo craniotomy with microsurgical dissection and placement of a titanium clip across the aneurysm neck to exclude the aneurysm from the circulation and reconstitute the lumen of the parent vessel. The second option is to "coil" the aneurysm via an endovascular approach. The patient is taken to the interventional neuroradiology suite for placement of looped titanium coils inside the aneurysm dome. The coils support thrombosis and prevent blood flow into the aneurysm. Factors favoring craniotomy and clipping include young age, good medical condition, and broad aneurysm necks. Factors favoring coiling include age, medical comorbidities, and narrow aneurysm necks. Due to coil migration or compaction over time, surgical clipping is believed to result in a more definitive cure. The decision to clip or coil is complex and should be fully explored. The International Subarachnoid Aneurysm Trial researchers suggested that endovascular occlusion resulted in better outcomes for certain types of cerebral aneurysms, although this trial was marred by poor selection and randomization techniques, and the validity of its conclusions have been questioned.[27] Long-term outcomes may be better in younger patients with clipped aneurysms.[28] Debate also continues regarding optimal care for unruptured intracranial aneurysms.[29]

SAH patients often require 1 to 3 weeks of ICU care after aneurysm occlusion for medical complications that accompany neurologic injury. In addition to routine ICU concerns, SAH patients are also at risk for cerebral vasospasm. In vasospasm, cerebral arteries constrict pathologically and can cause ischemia or stroke from 4 to 21 days after SAH. Current vasospasm prophylaxis

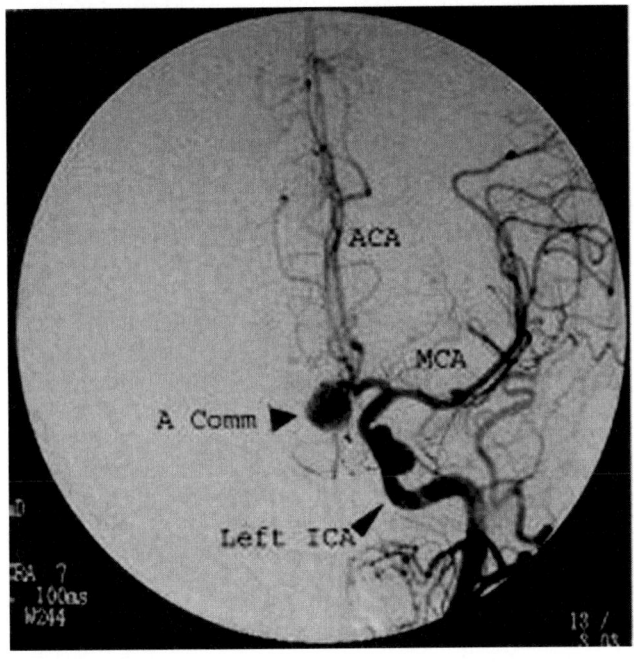

A

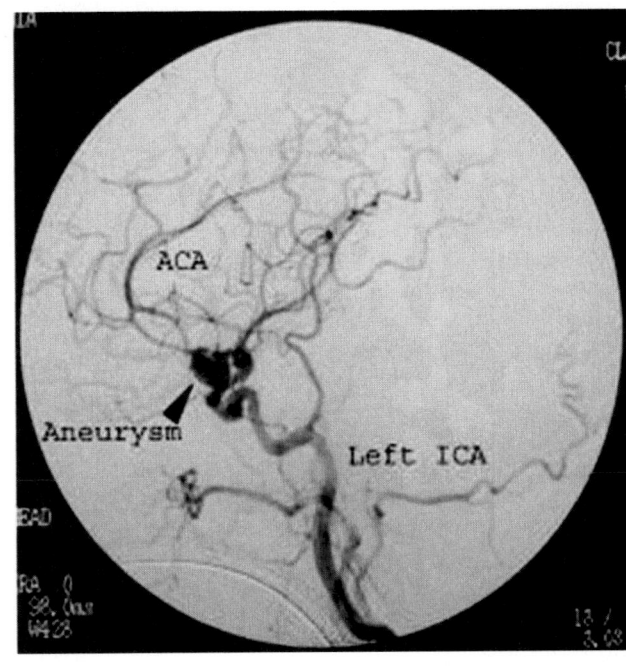

B

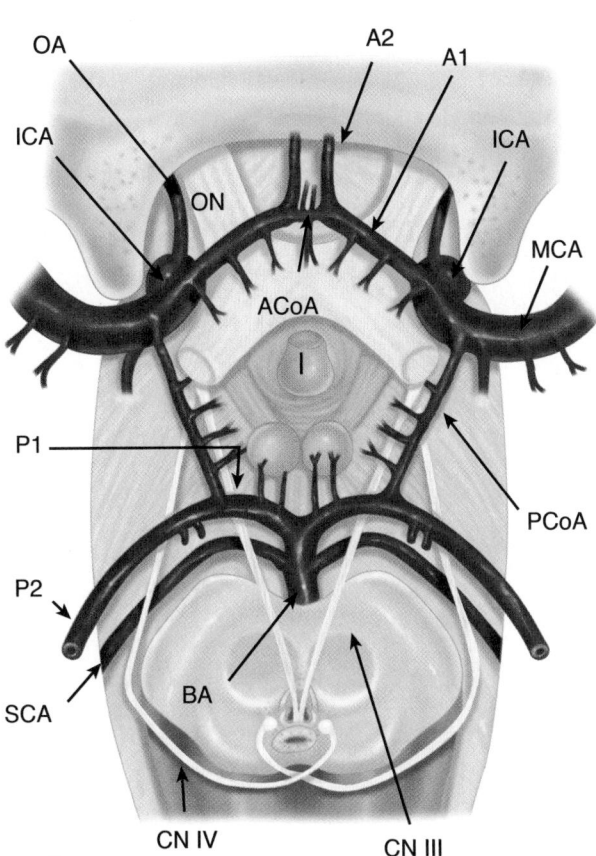

C

FIG. 42-17. A. Anteroposterior view after injection of contrast dye in the left internal carotid artery demonstrates a 13-mm diameter anterior communicating artery aneurysm (*A Comm*). The left internal carotid, middle carotid, and anterior cerebral arteries are clearly seen. **B.** Lateral view of the same injection again demonstrates the aneurysm. **C.** Figure depicting the anatomy of the circle of Willis in relation to key structures on the base of the brain. A1 = first section of anterior cerebral artery, before anterior communicating artery; A2 = second section of anterior cerebral artery, after anterior communicating artery; ACA = anterior cerebral artery; ACoA = anterior communicating artery; BA = basilar artery; CN III = third cranial nerve (oculomotor nerve); CN IV = fourth cranial nerve (trochlear nerve); I = infundibulum (the attachment of the pituitary stalk); ICA = internal cerebral artery; MCA = middle cerebral artery; OA = ophthalmic artery; ON = optic nerve; P1 = first section of posterior cerebral artery, before the posterior communicating artery; P2 = second section of the posterior cerebral artery, after the posterior communicating artery; PCA = posterior cerebral artery; PCoA = posterior communicating artery; SCA = superior cerebellar artery. (*Reproduced with permission from Osborn AG, Jacobs JM:* Diagnostic Cerebral Angiography, *2nd ed. Philadelphia: Lippincott, Williams & Wilkins, 1998, p 108.*)

patient has seized. Patients with significant weakness, lethargy, or hydrocephalus should be admitted for observation until definitive care is administered.

Metastatic Tumors

Prolonged cancer patient survival and improved CNS imaging have increased the likelihood of diagnosing cerebral metastases. The sources of most cerebral metastases are (in decreasing frequency): lung, breast, kidney, GI tract, and melanoma. Lung and breast cancers account for more than half of cerebral metastases. Metastatic cells usually travel to the brain hematogenously and frequently seed the gray-white junction. Other common locations are the cerebellum and the meninges. Meningeal involvement may result in carcinomatous meningitis, also known as *leptomeningeal carcinomatosis*. MRI pre- and postcontrast administration is the study of choice for evaluation. Figure 42-19 demonstrates bilateral cerebellar metastases. These lesions are typically well circumscribed, round, and

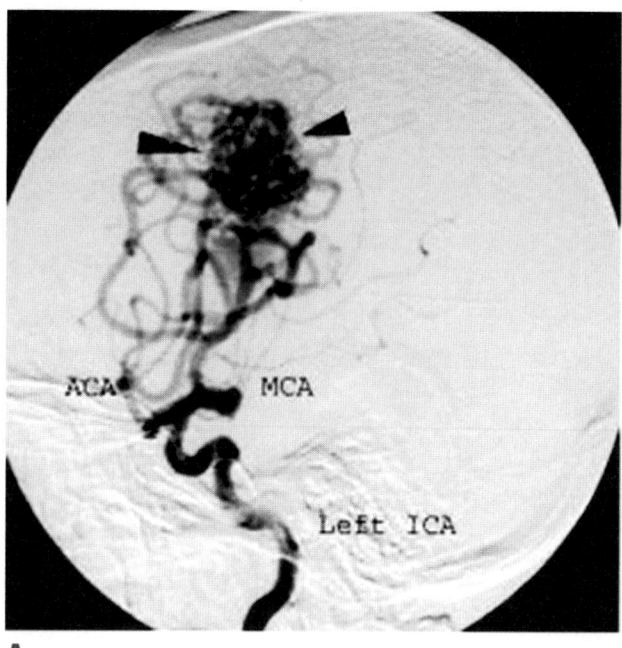

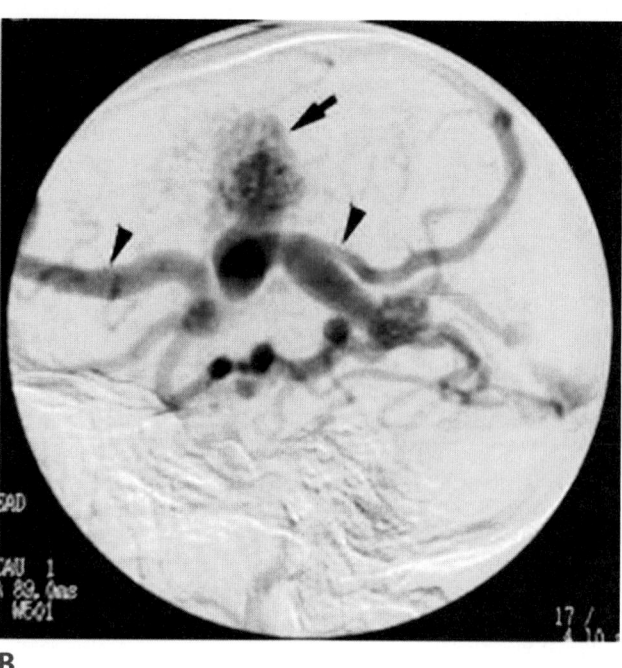

A

B

FIG. 42-18. A. Lateral view after injection of contrast dye in the left internal carotid artery demonstrates a 3 × 4 cm left frontal arteriovenous malformation indicated by *arrowheads*. This image was taken 1.06 seconds after dye injection, and is referred to as an *arterial phase image*. **B.** Same view taken 4.10 seconds after dye injection, providing a *venous phase image*. The *arrow* points to the arteriovenous malformation nidus. The *arrowheads* indicate two pathologically enlarged draining veins. ACA = anterior cerebral artery; ICA = internal carotid artery; MCA = middle cerebral artery.

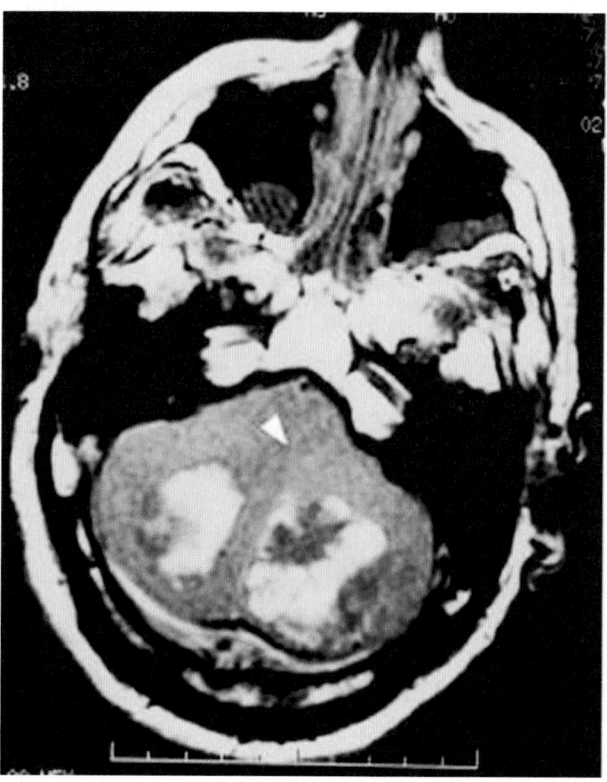

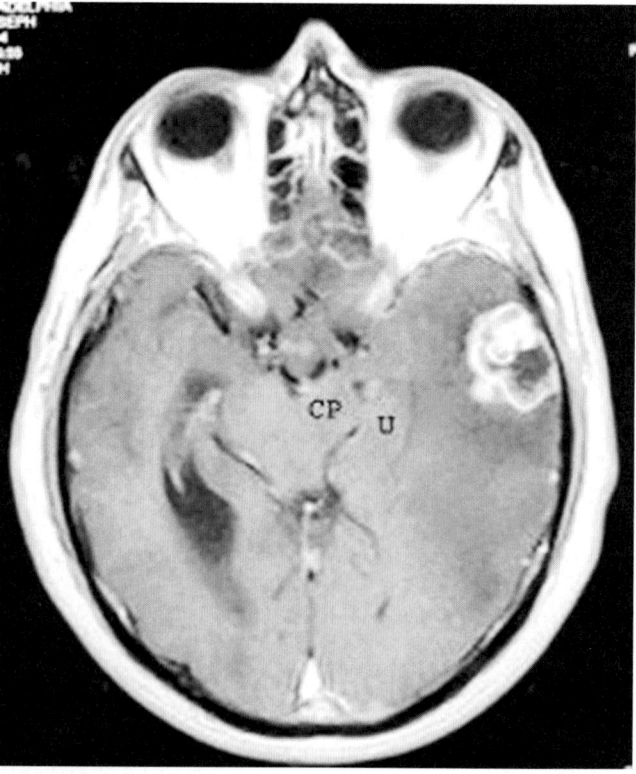

A

B

FIG. 42-19. A. Precontrast T1-weighted axial magnetic resonance imaging demonstrating bilateral hemorrhagic cerebellar metastases. Patient presented with ataxia and then lethargy progressing to deep coma. This patient has total effacement of the fourth ventricle and severe brain stem compression. The fourth ventricle cerebrospinal fluid space should be at the tip of the *arrowhead*. Patient recovered to normal mental status after emergent posterior fossa craniotomy. **B.** Postcontrast T1-weighted axial magnetic resonance imaging demonstrating a ring-enhancing lesion in the lateral left temporal lobe with moderate edema. The uncus (*U*) is compressing the left cerebral peduncle (*CP*) and displacing the brain stem to the right.

multiple. Such findings should prompt a metastatic work-up, including CT scan of the chest, abdomen, and pelvis, and a bone scan.

Management largely depends upon the primary tumor, overall tumor burden, patient's medical condition, and location and number of metastases. The patient's and family's beliefs regarding aggressive care must be considered. Craniotomy plus whole-brain radiation therapy (WBRT) has been shown to benefit patients with a single surgically accessible metastatic lesion, compared to radiation therapy alone. Median survival increased from 15 to 40 weeks in one randomized trial.[30] Postoperative radiotherapy may not increase overall survival but it does significantly reduce original lesion recurrence.[31] Studies do not support craniotomy unless all detectable metastases can be resected. Recent data suggest that SRS (e.g., gamma knife) may be applied to multiple metastases in one session with improved outcome.[32]

Glial Tumors

Glial cells provide the anatomic and physiologic support for neurons and their processes in the brain. The several types of glial cells give rise to distinct primary CNS neoplasms.

Astrocytoma

Astrocytoma is the most common primary CNS neoplasm. The term *glioma* often is used to refer to astrocytomas specifically, excluding other glial tumors. Astrocytomas are graded from I to IV. Grades I and II are referred to as low-grade astrocytoma, grade III as anaplastic astrocytoma, and grade IV as glioblastoma multiforme (GBM). Prognosis varies significantly between grades I/II, III, and IV, but not between I and II. Median survival is 8 years after diagnosis with a low-grade tumor, 2 to 3 years with an anaplastic astrocytoma, and

roughly 1 year with a GBM. GBMs account for almost two thirds of all astrocytomas, anaplastic astrocytomas account for two thirds of the rest, and low-grade astrocytomas the remainder. Figure 42-20 demonstrates the typical appearance of a GBM.

The great majority of astrocytomas infiltrate adjacent brain. Juvenile pilocytic astrocytomas and pleomorphic xanthoastrocytomas are exceptions. These tumors are circumscribed, low grade, and associated with a good prognosis. Histologic features associated with higher grade include hypercellularity, nuclear atypia, and endovascular hyperplasia. Necrosis is present only with GBMs; it is required for the diagnosis.

Gross total resection should be attempted for suspected astrocytomas. Motor cortex, language centers, deep or midline structures, or brain stem location may make this impossible without unacceptable, devastating neurologic deficit. Such lesions may be limited to stereotactic needle biopsy. Gross total resection followed by radiation therapy improves survival for all grades, although radiation therapy may be delayed until recurrence in low-grade tumors. Chemotherapy such as temozolomide is of limited efficacy and typically is reserved for GBM. There are various ongoing research studies for GBM adjuvant therapy; these should be discussed with the patient and family. Other options include Iotrex-containing balloons for conformal radiation brachytherapy (Glia-Site), placed in the resection cavity at the time of surgery for recurrence. Adjuvant therapy remains marginally effective; survival has changed little over the last several decades.

Oligodendroglioma

Oligodendroglioma accounts for approximately 10% of gliomas. They often present with seizures. Calcifications and hemorrhage on CT or MRI suggest the diagnosis. Oligodendrogliomas are also

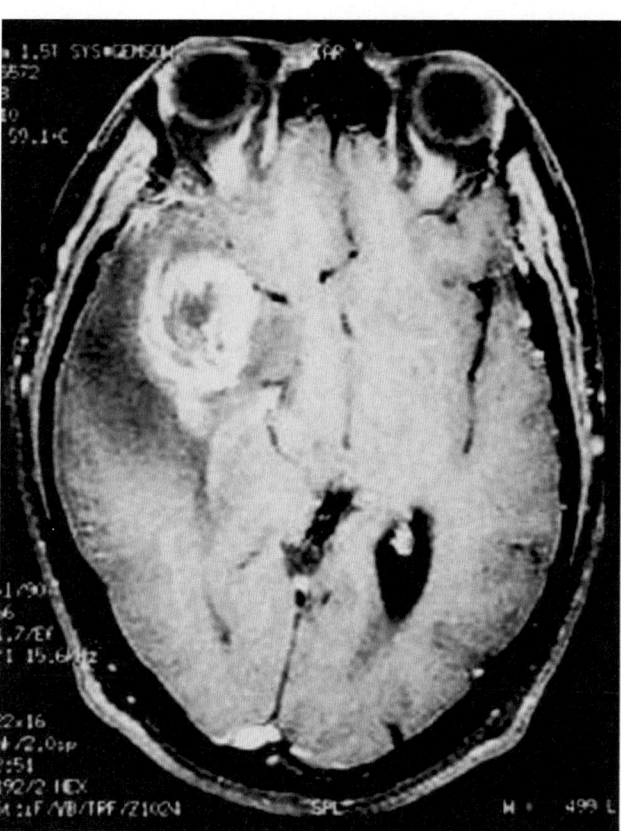

A

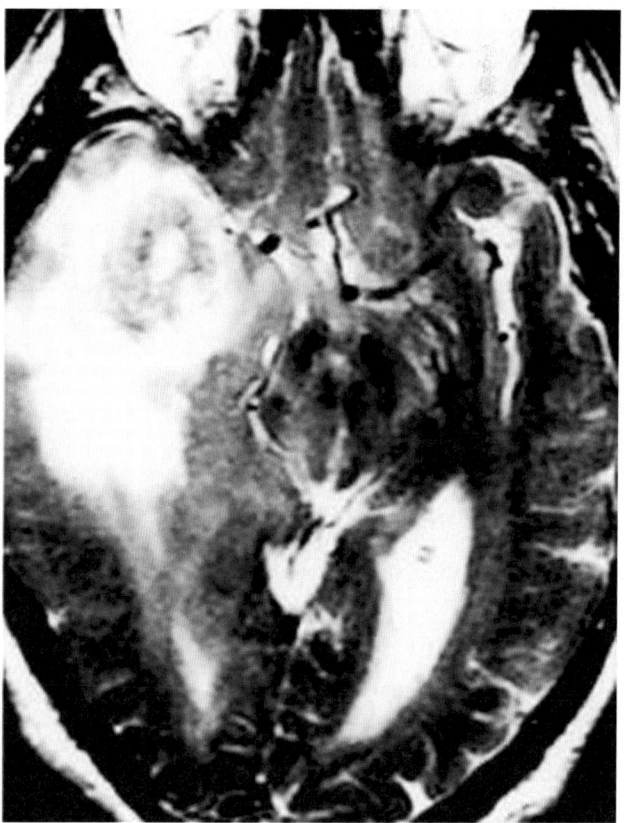

B

FIG. 42-20. A. Postcontrast T1-weighted axial magnetic resonance imaging demonstrating a ring-enhancing lesion in the anteromedial right temporal lobe with central necrosis (*dark area*) consistent with glioblastoma multiforme. **B.** T2-weighted axial magnetic resonance imaging with extensive bright signal signifying peritumoral edema seen with glioblastoma multiformes.

graded from I to IV; grade portends prognosis. Prognosis is better overall than for astrocytomas. Median survival ranges from 2 to 7 years for highest and lowest grade tumors, respectively. Aggressive resection improves survival. Many oligodendrogliomas will respond to procarbazine, lomustine (CCNU), vincristine (PCV) chemotherapy. A particular chromosomal deletion, 1p19q, has been associated with robust response to the chemotherapeutic agent temozolomide. Radiation has not been clearly shown to prolong survival.

Ependymoma

The lining of the ventricular system consists of cuboidal/columnar ependymal cells from which ependymomas may arise. Although most pediatric ependymomas are supratentorial, two thirds of adult ependymomas are infratentorial. Supratentorial ependymomas arise from the lateral or third ventricles. The infratentorial tumors arise from the floor of the fourth ventricle (i.e., off the posterior brain stem). The most common symptoms are headache, nausea, vomiting, or vertigo, secondary to increased ICP from obstruction of CSF flow through the fourth ventricle. The tumors may grow out the foramina of Luschka to form a cerebellopontine angle mass. They may also spread through the CSF to form "drop mets" in the spinal canal. The two main histologic subtypes are papillary and anaplastic, the latter characterized by increased mitotic activity and areas of necrosis. Gross total resection often is impossible because the tumor arises from the brain stem. The goal of surgery is to achieve maximal resection without injuring the very delicate brain stem. Suboccipital craniotomy and midline separation of the cerebellar hemispheres allows access to tumors in the fourth ventricle. Postoperative radiation therapy significantly improves survival. Patients with CSF spread documented by LP or contrast MRI should also have whole-spine radiation plus focused doses to visualized metastases.

Choroid Plexus Papilloma

The choroid plexus is composed of many small vascular tufts covered with cuboidal epithelium. It represents part of the interface between blood and brain. The choroid cells create CSF from blood and release it into the ventricular system. Choroid plexus papillomas and choroid plexus carcinomas (rare, mostly pediatric) may arise from these cells. Papillomas usually occur in infants (typically supratentorial in the lateral ventricle) but also occur in adults (usually infratentorial in the fourth ventricle). Papillomas are well circumscribed and vividly enhance due to extensive vasculature. Like ependymomas, adult choroid plexus papillomas usually present with symptoms of increased ICP. Treatment is surgical excision. Total surgical excision is curative; recurrent papillomas should be re-resected. Radiation or chemotherapy are not indicated for papillomas. Radiation is adjunctive to aggressive surgery for carcinomas, but the results are generally poor.

Neural Tumors and Mixed Tumors

Neural and mixed tumors are a diverse group that includes tumors variously containing normal or abnormal neurons and/or normal or abnormal glial cells. Primitive neuroectodermal tumors arise from bipotential cells, capable of differentiating into neurons or glial cells.

Medulloblastoma

Primitive neuroectodermal tumor is the most common type of medulloblastoma. Most occur in the first decade of life, but there is a second peak around age 30. Medulloblastoma is the most common malignant pediatric brain tumor. They are usually midline. Most occur in the cerebellum and present with symptoms of increased ICP. Histologic characteristics include densely packed small round cells with large nuclei and scant cytoplasm. They are generally not encapsulated, frequently disseminate within the CNS, and should undergo surgical resection followed by radiation therapy and chemotherapy.

Ganglioglioma

Ganglioglioma is a mixed tumor in which both neurons and glial cells are neoplastic. They occur in the first three decades of life, often in the medial temporal lobe, as circumscribed masses that may contain cysts or calcium and may enhance. The presenting symptom is usually a seizure, due to the medial temporal location. Patients have a good prognosis after complete surgical resection.

Neural Crest Tumors

Multipotent neural crest cells develop into a variety of disparate cell types, including smooth muscle cells, sympathetic and parasympathetic neurons, melanocytes, Schwann cells, and arachnoid cap cells. They migrate in early development from the primitive neural tube throughout the body.

Miscellaneous Tumors
Meningioma

Meningiomas are derived from arachnoid cap cells of the arachnoidea mater. They appear to arise from the dura mater grossly and on MRI and are commonly referred to as *dural-based tumors*. The most common intracranial locations are along the falx (Fig. 42-21), the convexities (i.e., over the cerebral hemispheres), and the sphenoid wing. Less common locations include the foramen magnum, olfactory groove, and inside the lateral ventricle. Most are slow growing, encapsulated, benign tumors. Aggressive atypical or malignant meningiomas may invade adjacent bone or cerebral cortex. Previous cranial irradiation increases the incidence of meningio-

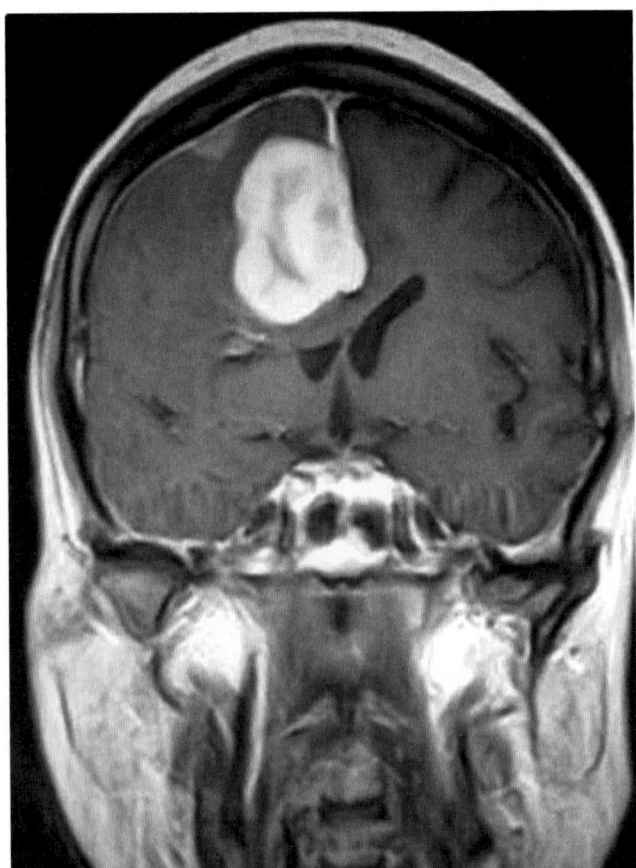

FIG. 42-21. Postcontrast T1-weighted coronal magnetic resonance imaging demonstrating a brightly enhancing lesion arising from the falx cerebri with moderate edema and mass effect on the right lateral ventricle. This is a falcine meningioma. Note also the small separate meningioma arising from the dura over the cerebral convexity.

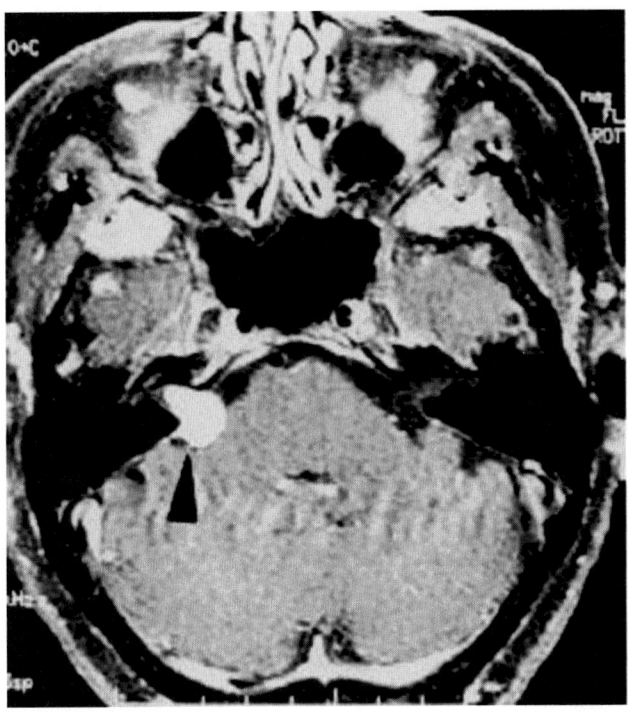

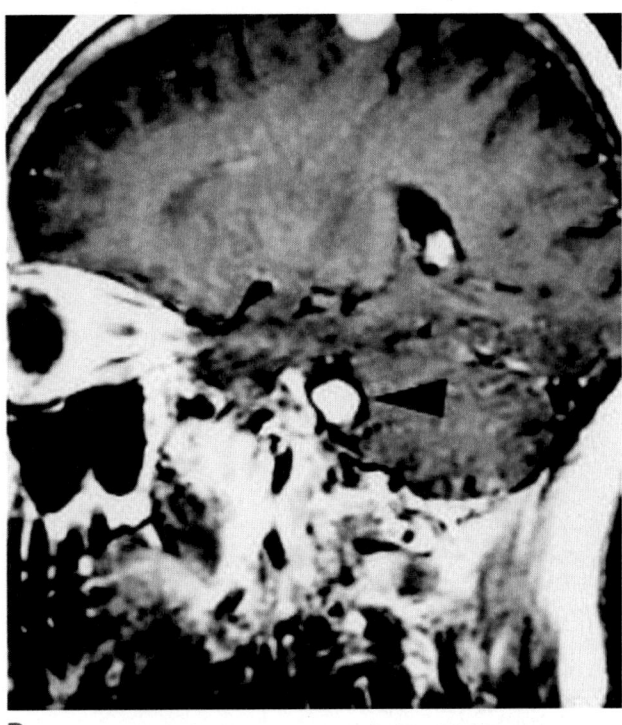

A   **B**

FIG. 42-22. A. Postcontrast T1-weighted axial magnetic resonance imaging demonstrating a brightly enhancing mass on the right vestibular nerve with an enhancing tail going into the internal auditory canal (*arrowhead*). Pathology demonstrated vestibular schwannoma. **B.** Postcontrast T1-weighted sagittal magnetic resonance imaging of the same lesion, indicated by the *arrowhead*. Note small incidental meningioma at the top of the scan.

mas. Approximately 10% of patients with a meningioma have multiple meningiomas. Total resection is curative, although involvement with small perforating arteries or cranial nerves may make total resection of skull base tumors impossible without significant neurologic deficit. Small, asymptomatic meningiomas can be followed until symptomatic or until significant growth is documented on serial imaging studies. Atypical and malignant meningiomas may require postoperative radiation. Patients may develop recurrences from the surgical bed or distant de novo tumors.

Vestibular Schwannoma (Acoustic Neuroma)

Vestibular schwannomas arise predominantly from the superior half of the vestibular portion of the vestibulocochlear nerve (cranial nerve VIII) (Fig. 42-22). Commonly, patients present with progressive hearing loss, tinnitus, or balance difficulty. Large tumors may cause brain stem compression and obstructive hydrocephalus. Bilateral acoustic neuromas are pathognomonic for neurofibromatosis type 2 (NF2), a syndrome resulting from a chromosome 22 mutation. NF2 patients have an increased incidence of spinal and cranial meningiomas and gliomas.

Vestibular schwannomas may be treated with microsurgical resection or conformal SRS (gamma knife or linear accelerator technology). The main complication with treatment is damage to the facial nerve (cranial nerve VII), which runs through the internal auditory canal with the vestibulocochlear nerve. Risk of facial nerve dysfunction increases with increasing tumor diameter.

Pituitary Adenoma

Pituitary adenomas arise from the anterior pituitary gland (adenohypophysis). Tumors <1 cm diameter are considered microadenomas; larger tumors are macroadenomas. Pituitary tumors may be functional (i.e., secrete endocrinologically active compounds at pathologic levels) or nonfunctional (i.e., secrete nothing or inactive compounds).

Functional tumors are often diagnosed when quite small, due to endocrine dysfunction. The most common endocrine syndromes are Cushing's disease, due to adrenocorticotropic hormone secretion, Forbes-Albright syndrome, due to prolactin secretion, and acromegaly, due to growth hormone secretion. Nonfunctional tumors are typically diagnosed as larger lesions causing mass effects such as visual field deficits due to compression of the optic chiasm or panhypopituitarism due to compression of the gland. Figure 42-23 demonstrates a large pituitary adenoma. Hemorrhage into a pituitary tumor causes abrupt symptoms of headache, visual disturbance, decreased mental status, and endocrine dysfunction. This is known as *pituitary apoplexy.*

Symptomatic pituitary tumors should be decompressed surgically to eliminate mass effect and/or to attempt an endocrine cure. However, prolactin-secreting tumors (prolactinomas) usually shrink with dopaminergic therapy alone, namely bromocriptine, which inhibits production and secretion of prolactin. Consider surgery for prolactinomas with persistent mass effect or endocrinologic dysfunction in spite of adequate dopamine agonist therapy. Most pituitary tumors are approached through the nose via the transsphenoidal approach. Minimally invasive endoscopic sinus surgery techniques are being used increasingly.

Hemangioblastoma

Hemangioblastomas occur almost exclusively in the posterior fossa. Twenty percent occur in patients with von Hippel-Lindau (VHL) disease, a multisystem neoplastic disorder. Other tumors associated with VHL are renal cell carcinoma, pheochromocytoma, and retinal angiomas. Many appear as cystic tumors with an enhancing tumor on the cyst wall known as the *mural nodule.* Surgical resection is curative for sporadic (non-VHL associated) tumors. Pathology reveals abundant thin-walled vascular channels; internal debulking may be bloody. En bloc resection of the mural nodule alone, leaving the cyst wall, is sufficient.

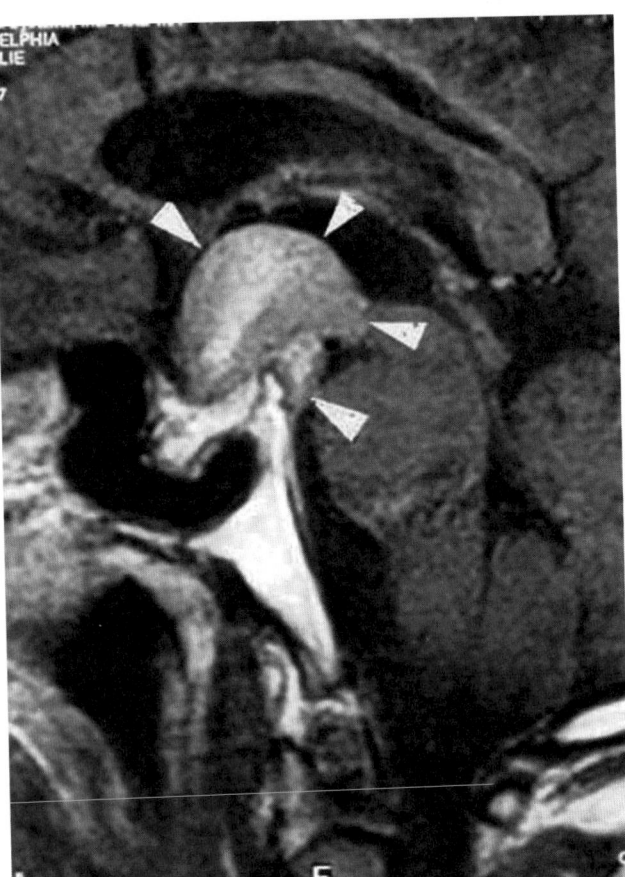

FIG. 42-23. Postcontrast T1-weighted sagittal magnetic resonance imaging demonstrating a large sellar/suprasellar lesion (*arrowheads*) involving the third ventricle superiorly and abutting the midbrain and pons posteriorly. The patient presented with progressive visual field and acuity loss. Pathology and lab work revealed a nonfunctioning pituitary adenoma.

Lymphoma

CNS lymphoma may arise either primarily in the CNS or secondarily from systemic disease. Recent rising incidence may be due to growing transplant and AIDS populations. Presenting symptoms include mental status changes, headache due to increased ICP, and cranial nerve palsy due to lymphomatous meningitis (analogous to carcinomatous meningitis). Often, lymphoma appears hyperdense on CT due to dense cellularity, and most lesions typically enhance with contrast. Surgical excision is not indicated. Stereotactic needle biopsy usually confirms the diagnosis. Subsequent treatment includes steroids, whole-brain radiation, and chemotherapy. Intrathecal methotrexate is an option.

Embryologic Tumors

Embryologic tumors result from embryonal remnants that fail to involute completely or differentiate properly during development.

Craniopharyngioma

Craniopharyngiomas are benign cystic lesions that occur most frequently in children. There is a second peak of incidence around 50 years of age. Calcification occurs in all pediatric and roughly half of adult craniopharyngiomas. Symptoms result from compression of adjacent structures, especially the optic chiasm. Pituitary or hypothalamic dysfunction or hydrocephalus may develop. Treatment is primarily surgical. Excision is somewhat easier in children, as the tumor is often soft and easily suctioned. Adult tumors are often firm and adherent to adjacent vital structures. Visual loss, pituitary endocrine

hypofunction, diabetes insipidus, and cognitive impairment from basal frontal injury are common complications.

Epidermoid

Epidermoid tumors are cystic lesions with stratified squamous epithelial walls from trapped ectodermal cell rests that grow slowly and linearly by desquamation into the cyst cavity. The cysts contain keratin, cholesterol, and cellular debris (Fig. 42-24). They occur most frequently in the cerebellopontine angle and may cause symptoms due to brain stem compression. Recurrent bouts of aseptic meningitis may occur due to release of irritative cyst contents into the subarachnoid space (Mollaret's meningitis). Treatment is surgical drainage and removal of the cyst wall. Intraoperative spillage of cyst contents can lead to severe chemical meningitis and must be avoided by containment and aspiration.

Dermoid

Dermoids are less common than epidermoid tumors. They contain hair follicles and sebaceous glands in addition to a squamous epithelium. Dermoids may be found anywhere along the craniospinal axis. They are more commonly midline structures and are associated with more anomalies than epidermoids. They may be traumatic, as from a LP that drags skin structures into the CNS. Bacterial meningitis may occur when associated with a dermal sinus tract to the skin along the spine. Treatment of symptomatic lesions is surgical resection, again with care to control cyst contents.

Teratoma

Teratomas are germ cell tumors that arise in the midline, often in the pineal region (the area behind the third ventricle, above the mid-

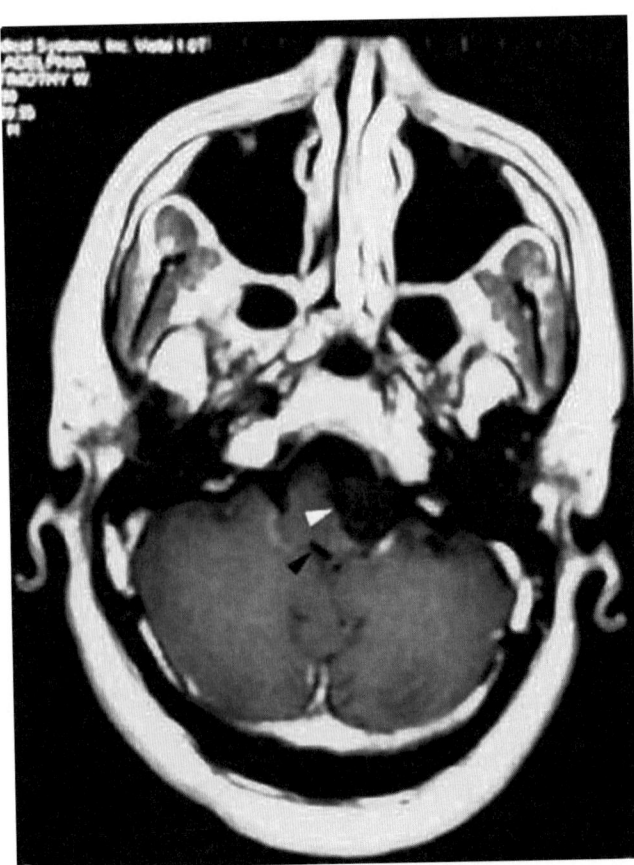

FIG. 42-24. Postcontrast T1-weighted axial magnetic resonance imaging demonstrating a nonenhancing mass in the left cerebellopontine angle with brain stem compression. *White arrowhead* indicates interface of tumor and brain stem. *Black arrowhead* indicates deformed fourth ventricle. Pathology revealed epidermoid tumor.

brain and cerebellum). They contain elements from all three embryonal layers: ectoderm, mesoderm, and endoderm. Teratomas may contain skin, cartilage, GI glands, and teeth. Teratomas with more primitive features are more malignant, while those with more differentiated tissues are more benign. Surgical excision may be attempted. However, prognosis for malignant teratoma is very poor.

Spinal Tumors

A wide variety of tumors affect the spine. Approximately 20% of CNS tumors occur in the spine. Unlike cranial tumors, the majority of spinal tumors are histologically benign. Understanding two major spinal concepts—stability and neural compression—facilitates an understanding of the effects of spinal tumors. Destruction of bones or ligaments can cause spinal instability, leading to deformities such as kyphosis, subluxation, or possible subsequent neural compression. Tumor growth in the spinal canal or neural foramina can cause direct compression of the spinal cord or nerve roots and cause pain and loss of function. Classically, the pain is worse at night. Anatomic categorization provides the most logical approach to these tumors. Certain tumors present in characteristic locations. An understanding of the anatomy leads to an understanding of the clinical presentation and possible therapeutic options.

Extradural Tumors

Extradural tumors account for approximately 55% of spinal tumors. This category includes tumors arising within the bony vertebral structures and from within the epidural space. Destruction of the bone can lead to instability and fractures, causing pain and/or deformity. Epidural expansion can lead to spinal cord or nerve root compression with myelopathy, radiculopathy, or a combination thereof.

Metastatic Tumors Metastatic tumors are the most common extradural tumors. Spinal metastases most commonly occur in the thoracic and lumbar vertebral bodies because the greatest volume of red bone marrow is found in these regions. The most common primary sources of spine metastasis are lymphoma, lung, breast, and prostate. Other sources include renal, colon, thyroid, sarcoma, and melanoma. Most spinal metastases create osteolytic lesions. Osteoblastic, sclerotic lesions suggest prostate cancer in men and breast cancer in women.

Patients with progressive neurologic dysfunction due to a metastatic lesion should undergo urgent surgery followed by radiation therapy.[33] Patients with debilitating pain may undergo radiation therapy with close observation for neurologic deterioration. Preoperative neurologic function correlates with postoperative function. Patients may lose function over hours. These patients should be given high-dose IV dexamethasone, taken immediately to MRI, and then to the OR or radiation therapy suite. Indications for surgery include failure of radiation therapy, spinal instability, recurrence after radiation therapy, and the need for diagnosis in cases of unknown primary tumors. Most cases with significant bone involvement require both decompression and fusion. Bony fusion usually takes 2 to 3 months. Prognosis governs operative decisions. Surgery is unlikely to improve quality of life for patients with a life expectancy of 3 months or less, but it is likely to improve quality of life for patients with life expectancy of 6 months or more. Benefit for patients with 3- to 6-months life expectancy is unclear and requires frank discussion with the patient and family. Patients who are unlikely to tolerate general anesthesia, are already completely paralyzed, or who have very radiosensitive tumors such as multiple myeloma and lymphoma, should not generally undergo surgery.

Primary Tumors Hemangiomas are benign tumors found in 10% of people at autopsy. They occur in the vertebral bodies of the thoracolumbar spine and are frequently asymptomatic. They are often vascular and may hemorrhage, causing pain or neurologic deficit. Large hemangiomas can destabilize the spine and predispose to fracture. Osteoblastic lesions include osteoid osteoma and osteoblastoma. The latter tends to be larger and more destructive.

Aneurysmal bone cysts are non-neoplastic, expansile, lytic lesions containing thin-walled blood cavities that usually occur in the lamina or spinous processes of the cervicothoracic spine. They may cause pain or sufficiently weaken the bone to cause a fracture. Cancers arising primarily in the bony spine include Ewing's sarcoma, osteosarcoma, chondrosarcoma, and plasmacytoma.

Intradural Extramedullary Tumors

Intradural extramedullary tumors constitute approximately 40% of spinal tumors and arise from the meninges or nerve root elements. They may compress the spinal cord, causing myelopathy, or the nerve roots, causing radiculopathy. The most common intradural extramedullary tumors are typically benign, slow growing, and well circumscribed. Rare benign epidural masses include arachnoid cysts, dermoids, and epidermoids. Rare malignant epidural tumors include metastases and high-grade gliomas, or "drop" metastases from posterior fossa gliomas.

Meningioma Meningiomas arise from the arachnoidea mater. They appear to be dural based and enhance on MRI. An enhancing "dural tail" may be seen. They occur most commonly in the thoracic spine (Fig. 42-25) but also arise in the cervical and lumbar regions. Some

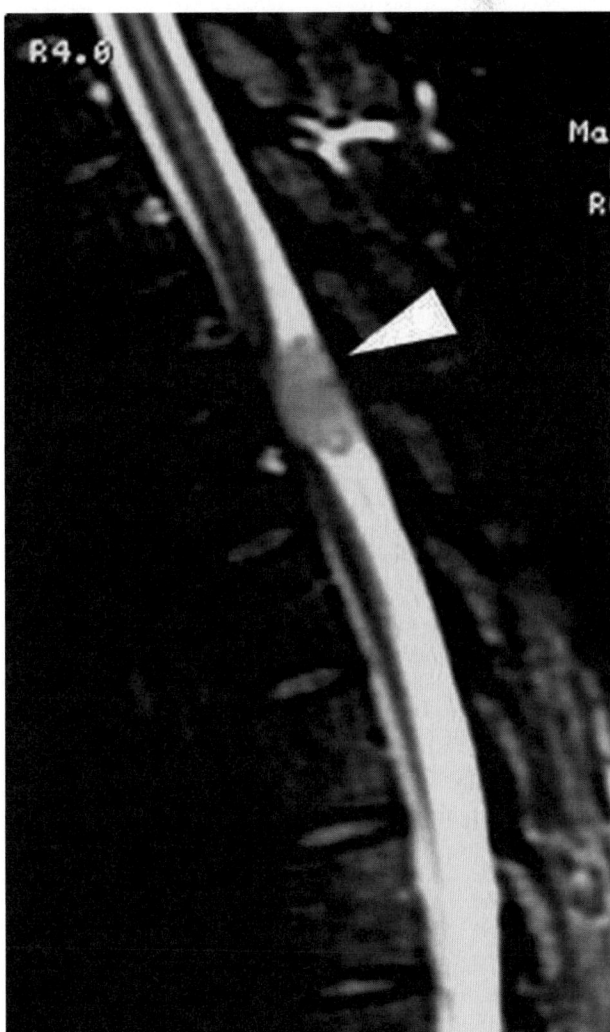

FIG. 42-25. T2-weighted sagittal magnetic resonance imaging of the midthoracic spine demonstrating a well-encapsulated tumor arising from the dura posteriorly and compressing the spinal cord. *Arrowhead* points to dorsal location of the mass. The patient presented with worsening gait and lower extremity spasticity. Pathology demonstrated meningioma.

spinal meningiomas grow into the epidural space. Growth causes cord compression and progressive myelopathy with hyperreflexia, spasticity, and gait difficulties. Surgical excision is the treatment of choice. The surgeon often finds a clean margin between the tumor, dura, and spinal cord, allowing en bloc resection without damage to the cord.

Schwannoma Schwannomas are derived from peripheral nerve sheath Schwann cells. They are benign, encapsulated tumors that rarely undergo malignant degeneration. Two thirds are entirely intradural, one sixth are entirely extradural, and one sixth have a classic "dumbbell" shape from intradural and extradural components. Symptoms result from radiculopathy, often presenting as pain or myelopathy. Symptomatic lesions should be surgically resected. The parent nerve root usually can be preserved. Patients with multiple schwannomas likely have NF2. In these patients, a careful neurologic examination is needed to determine which lesions are symptomatic and require resection.

Neurofibroma In contrast to schwannomas, neurofibromas tend to appear more fusiform and to grow within the parent nerve, rather than forming an encapsulated mass branching off the nerve. Neurofibromas are benign but not encapsulated. They present similarly to schwannomas, and the two may be difficult to differentiate on imaging. Salvage of the parent nerve is more challenging with neurofibromas. To improve the likelihood of total resection, thoracic and high cervical nerve roots may be sacrificed with minimal deficit. Patients with multiple neurofibromas likely have NF1, also known as *von Recklinghausen's neurofibromatosis*. Resection for symptomatic lesions should be offered.

Intramedullary Tumors

Intramedullary tumors constitute approximately 5% of spinal tumors. They arise from within the parenchyma of the spinal cord. Common presenting symptoms are local dysesthesia, burning pain, radicular pain, sensory loss, weakness, or sphincter dysfunction. Patients with such symptoms should undergo MRI of the entire spine with and without enhancement.

Ependymoma Ependymomas are the most common intramedullary tumors in adults. There are several histologic variants. The myxopapillary type occurs in the conus medullaris or the filum terminale in the lumbar region and has the best prognosis after resection. The cellular type occurs more frequently in the cervical cord. Many spinal ependymomas have cystic areas and may contain hemorrhage. Surgical removal can improve function. A distinct tumor margin often exists, allowing safer excision. Postoperative radiation therapy after subtotal resection may prolong disease control.

Astrocytoma Astrocytomas are the most common intramedullary tumors in children, although they also occur in adults. They may occur at all levels, although more often in the cervical cord. The tumor may interfere with the CSF-containing central canal of the spinal cord, leading to a dilated central canal, referred to as *syringomyelia* (*syrinx*). Spinal astrocytomas are usually low grade, but complete excision is rarely possible due to the nonencapsulated, infiltrative nature of the tumor. As a result, patients with astrocytomas fare worse overall than patients with ependymomas.

Other Tumors

Other types of rare tumors include high-grade astrocytomas, dermoids, epidermoids, teratomas, hemangiomas, hemangioblastomas, and metastases. Patients usually present with pain. Prognosis generally depends on preoperative function and the histologic characteristics of the lesion.

SPINE: BASIC CONCEPTS

The spine is a complex structure and is subject to an extensive array of pathologic processes, including degeneration, inflammation, infection, neoplasia, and trauma. Discussions of spine trauma, tumor, and infection are addressed separately in this chapter in the Infection—Spine, Spinal Tumors, and Spine Trauma sections. General concepts, common patterns of disease, and basic operative interventions are presented here.

The spine consists of a series of stacked vertebrae, intervening discs, and longitudinal ligaments. The vertebrae consist of the vertebral body anteriorly and the pedicles, articular facets, laminae, and spinous processes posteriorly. The intervertebral discs have two components. The tough, fibrous ring that runs around the outer diameter of the two adjacent vertebral bodies is known as the annulus fibrosus. The spongy material inside the ring of the annulus is known as the *nucleus pulposus*. The annulus and the nucleus provide a cushion between adjacent vertebral bodies, absorb forces transmitted to the spine, and allow some movement between the vertebral bodies. The ligaments stabilize the spine by limiting the motion of adjacent vertebrae.

Stability and neural compression are the two concepts critical to understanding the mechanics and pathologic processes affecting the spine.

Stability

The spinal column is the principal structural component of the axial spine, and it must bear significant loads. The vertebrae increase in size from the top to the bottom of the spine, correlating with the increased total loads that the more caudal elements must bear. The cervical spine is the most mobile. Cervical stability depends greatly on the integrity of the ligaments that run from level to level. The thoracic spine is the least mobile, due to the stabilizing effect of the rib cage. The lumbar spine has relatively massive vertebrae, supports heavy loads, and has intermediate mobility. The sacral spine is fused together and has no intrinsic mobility. The load borne by the lumbar spine is transmitted to the sacrum, and then the pelvis through the sacroiliac joints. The coccyx is the most inferior segment of the spine and has no significant contribution to load bearing or mobility.

A stable spine is one that can bear normally experienced forces resulting from body mass, movement, and muscle contraction, while maintaining normal structure and alignment. An unstable spine will shift or sublux under these forces. The determinants of spinal stability vary throughout the cervical, thoracic, and lumbar portions. In elementary form, stability depends on the structural integrity of the hard, bony elements of the vertebral column, as well as the tensile integrity and security of the supporting ligamentous attachments. Plain x-rays and CT scans are sensitive for detecting bony defects such as fractures or subluxation, while MRI better detects disruptions of the soft tissues, including ligaments and intervertebral discs. Specific patterns of abnormalities seen on imaging studies may suggest or diagnose spinal instability.

A common form of nontraumatic spinal instability is lumbar spondylolisthesis, which is typically a forward slippage of a lumbar vertebra relative to the lower vertebra on which it rests. This results from congenital or degenerative disruption of the pars interarticularis, the critical bridge of bone that spans adjacent facet joints. In the setting of a pars defect, there is no solid bony connection between the adjacent vertebrae. The spine is unstable and anterior listhesis (slippage) may result. Patients typically present with severe low back pain that is exacerbated with movement and load bearing (mechanical low back pain). Radiculopathy in this setting indicates neuroforaminal compression. Figure 42-26 demonstrates an L4 and L5 spondylolisthesis.

Neural Compression

Besides providing a stable central element of the body's support structure, the spine also must protect the spinal cord as it descends in the central canal and the nerve roots as they pass from the central canal out the neural foramina to form the peripheral nervous system. In a healthy spine, the spinal cord and nerve roots are suspended in CSF, free of mechanical compression. Pathologic processes that can lead to CSF space impingement and neural compression include: hypertrophic degenerative changes in the

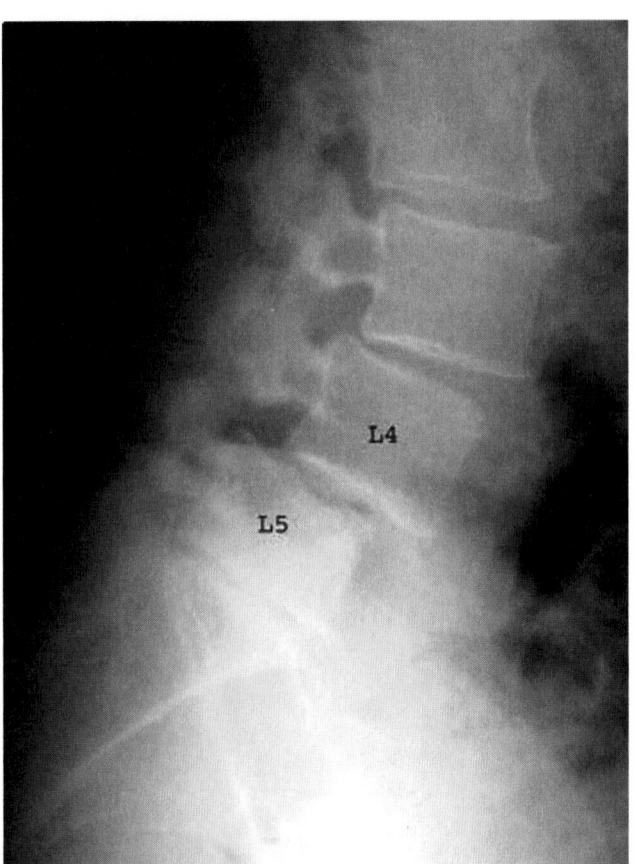

FIG. 42-26. Lateral lumbar spine x-ray demonstrates a 25% anterior slippage of L4 on L5 due to a defect in the L4 pars interarticularis. This is called *spondylolisthesis.*

intervertebral discs and facet joints, expansion of epidural masses such as tumors or abscesses, and subluxation (i.e., slippage) of adjacent vertebral bodies. Subluxation may be due to trauma that exceeds the spine's load-bearing capabilities and leads to structural failure, or chronic structural degradation by degenerative disease, infection, or tumor. Subluxation reduces the cross-sectional area of the central canal and the neural foramina (see Fig. 42-10B). Reduced central canal area can lead to myelopathy. Reduced neural foraminal area can lead to radiculopathy.

Myelopathy

Compression of the spinal cord can cause a disturbance of function known as *myelopathy.* This dysfunction may be secondary to the direct effects of compression, cord ischemia due to reduced perfusion, or pathologic changes due to repeated cord trauma. These mechanisms lead to demyelination of the corticospinal tracts, which are long descending motor tracts. Corticospinal tract damage leads to upper motor neuron signs and symptoms, including hyperreflexia, spasticity, and weakness. These mechanisms also cause dam-

age to the dorsal columns, which carry ascending proprioception, vibration, and two-point discrimination information. Loss of proprioception makes fine motor tasks and ambulation difficult.

Radiculopathy

Compression of the nerve roots causes disturbance of root function, known as *radiculopathy.* Characteristic features of radiculopathy include lower motor neuron signs and symptoms (hyporeflexia, atrophy, and weakness) and sensory disturbances such as numbness or tingling sensations (paresthesias), burning sensations (dysesthesias), and shooting (radicular) pain. Myelopathy and radiculopathy often present together in diseases that involve the central canal and the neural foramina. This combination can lead to lower motor neuron dysfunction at the level of disease, and upper motor neuron dysfunction below that level.

Patterns of Disease
Cervical Radiculopathy

The cervical nerve roots exit the central canal above the pedicle of the same-numbered vertebra and at the level of the higher adjacent intervertebral disc. For example, the C6 nerve root passes above the C6 pedicle at the level of the C5–C6 discs. The cervical nerve roots may be compressed acutely by disc herniation, or chronically by hypertrophic degenerative changes of the discs, facets, and ligaments. Table 42-6 summarizes the effects of various disc herniations. Most patients with acute disc herniations will improve without surgery. NSAIDs or cervical traction may help alleviate symptoms. Patients whose symptoms do not resolve or who have significant weakness should undergo decompressive surgery. The two main options for nerve root decompression are anterior cervical discectomy and fusion (ACDF) and posterior cervical foraminotomy (keyhole foraminotomy). ACDF allows more direct access to and removal of the pathology (anterior to the nerve root). However, the procedure requires fusion because discectomy causes a collapse of the interbody space and instability will likely occur. Figure 42-27 demonstrates a C6–C7 ACDF with the typical interposed graft and plating system. Keyhole foraminotomy allows for decompression without requiring fusion, but it is less effective for removing centrally located canal pathology.

Cervical Spondylotic Myelopathy

The term *spondylosis* refers to diffuse degenerative and hypertrophic changes of the discs, intervertebral joints, and ligaments, which collectively result in spinal stenosis. Spinal cord dysfunction (myelopathy) due to cord compression from cervical spinal degenerative disease is therefore referred to as cervical spondylotic myelopathy (CSM). CSM classically presents with spasticity and hyperreflexia due to corticospinal tract dysfunction, upper extremity weakness and atrophy from degeneration of the motor neurons in the anterior horns of the spinal gray matter, and loss of lower extremity proprioception due to dorsal column injury. Figure 42-28 demonstrates typical findings. Patients complain of difficulty buttoning shirts, using utensils, and ambulating. Spondylosis is usually diffuse, so the usual treatment for CSM is multilevel (usually C3–C7) cervical laminectomy, although patients with disease localized over one to three levels may be candidates for anterior decompression and

Level	Frequency (%)	Root Injured	Reflex	Weakness	Numbness
C4–C5	2	C5	—	Deltoid	Shoulder
C5–C6	19	C6	Biceps	Biceps brachii	Thumb
C6–C7	69	C7	Triceps	Wrist extensors (wrist drop)	Second and third digits
C7–T1	10	C8	—	Hand intrinsics	Fourth and fifth digits

TABLE 42-6 Cervical disc herniations and symptoms by level

Source: Adapted with permission from Greenberg MS: *Handbook of Neurosurgery,* 6th ed. New York: Thieme Medical Publishers, 2005, Table 14.14, p 318.

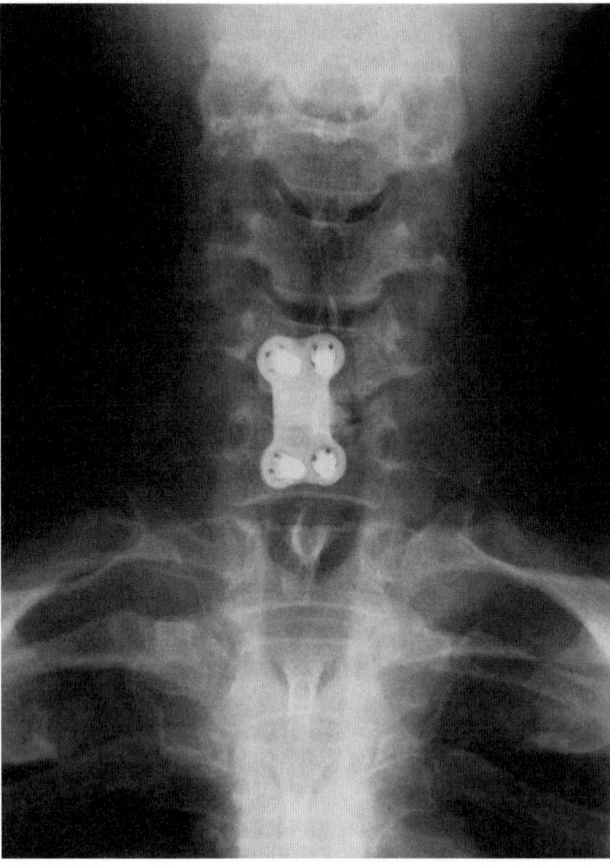

A

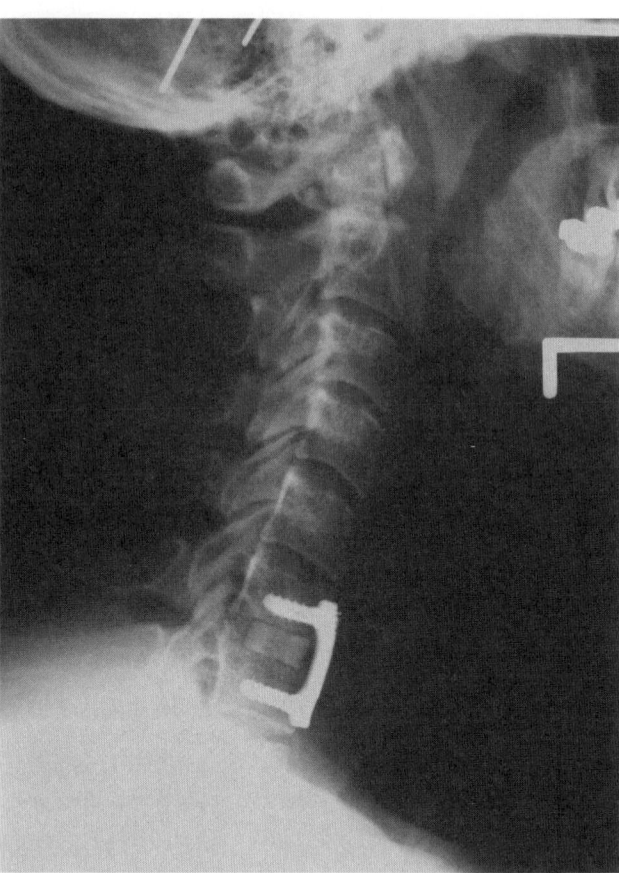

B

FIG. 42-27. A. Anteroposterior cervical spine x-ray showing the position of an anterior cervical plate used for stabilization after C6–C7 discectomy. Patient presented with right triceps weakness and dysesthesias in the right fifth digit. Magnetic resonance imaging revealed a right paracentral C6–C7 herniated disc compressing the exiting C7 nerve root. **B.** Lateral cervical spine x-ray of the same patient clearly demonstrates the position of the plate and screws. The allograft bone spacer placed in the drilled-out disc space is also apparent.

fusion. Figure 42-29 demonstrates the postoperative appearance of a vertebral corpectomy and fusion for CSM. Thorough cervical laminectomy decompresses the cord posteriorly. Patients often have slow recovery due to the extensive chronic changes in the cervical cord and may benefit from rehabilitation programs. The other disease that classically presents with combined upper and lower motor neuron symptoms is amyotrophic lateral sclerosis (ALS). Care must be taken to avoid offering cervical laminectomy to a patient with undiagnosed ALS. Two findings help differentiate CSM from ALS: cranial nerve dysfunction such as dysphagia (not typically caused by cervical spine disease) and sensory disturbance (not found in ALS).

Thoracic Disc Herniation

Thoracic disc herniation accounts for <1% of herniated discs. A patient may present with radicular pain or sensorimotor changes in the lower extremities due to cord compression. A posterior approach via midline incision and laminectomy should be avoided because of the high incidence of cord injury from manipulation and retraction. Anterior approaches via thoracotomy minimize risk to the cord and allow excellent access to the disc. The radicular arteries running from the aorta to the thoracic cord should be spared, when possible, to avoid ischemia. Alternatively, a posterolateral approach is possible via resection of the rib head and facet joint. Finally, a transpedicular approach may be attempted for lateral disc herniations.[34]

Lumbar Radiculopathy

Lumbar nerve roots exit the thecal sac, pass over the higher adjacent disc space, and exit the canal under the pedicle of the same-numbered vertebra. Therefore, the L5 nerve root passes over the L4–L5 disc space and exits under the L5 pedicle (Fig. 42-30). Lumbar discs may herniate with or without a history of trauma or straining. They normally cause lancinating (radicular) pain down the leg (Table 42-7). Most acute herniated lumbar discs improve symptomatically without surgery. Surgery is indicated for symptoms persisting more than 6 to 8 weeks, progressive motor deficit (e.g., foot drop), or for patients with incapacitating pain not manageable with analgesics. Discectomy is performed using a midline incision, partial removal of the overlying laminae (hemilaminectomy or laminotomy), identification of the thecal sac and nerve root, and extraction of disc fragments. Free-floating disc fragments may be found. Often, however, the herniated disc material is still contained within the annulus, requiring incision of the posterior longitudinal ligament and curettage of the disc space. After lumbar discectomy, approximately two thirds of patients will have complete relief of pain, and up to 85% will have significant improvement.

Neurogenic Claudication

Neurogenic claudication is characterized by low back and leg pain that occurs while walking and is relieved by stopping, leaning forward, or sitting. It is normally caused by degenerative lumbar stenosis causing compression of the cauda equina. Neurogenic claudication must be distinguished from vascular claudication, which tends to resolve quickly with cessation of walking. There is typically no need to change position, and the pain follows a stocking distribution rather than a dermatomal distribution. Pallor and coldness of the feet, and normal neurologic examination are also

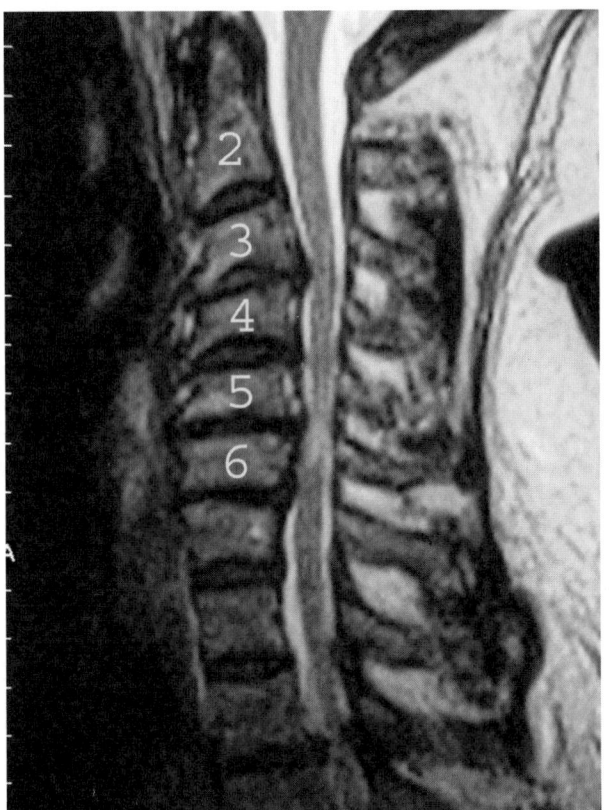

FIG. 42-28. T2-weighted sagittal magnetic resonance imaging of the cervical spine showing multilevel degenerative changes causing spinal stenosis that is worst at C5–C6. Note the bright signal within the cord at that level, consistent with myelopathy.

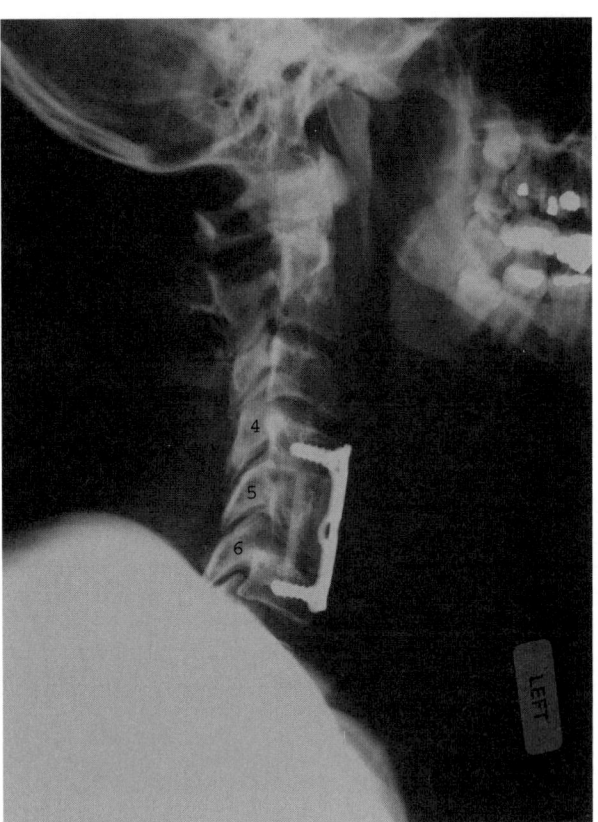

FIG. 42-29. Lateral cervical spine x-ray status post C5 corpectomy for cervical spondylotic myelopathy. This involves removal of the C4–C5 disc, C5 vertebral body, and C5–C6 disc, decompressing at two levels. A bone strut is visible bridging C4 to C6. The plate and screws stabilize the segments.

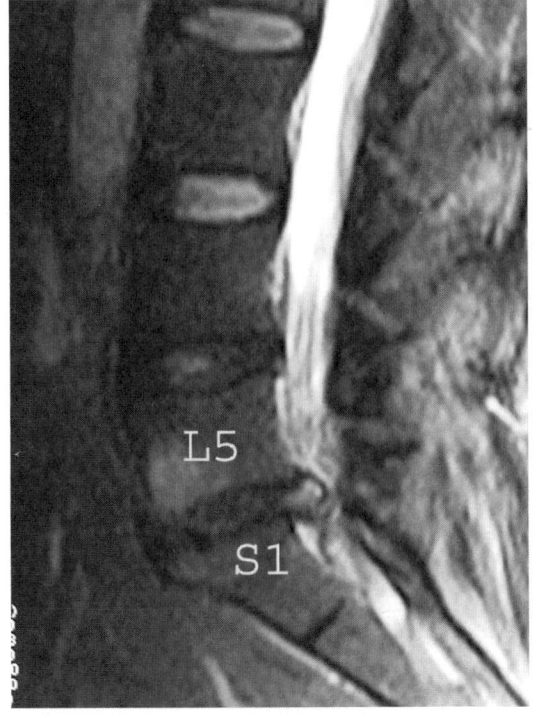

A

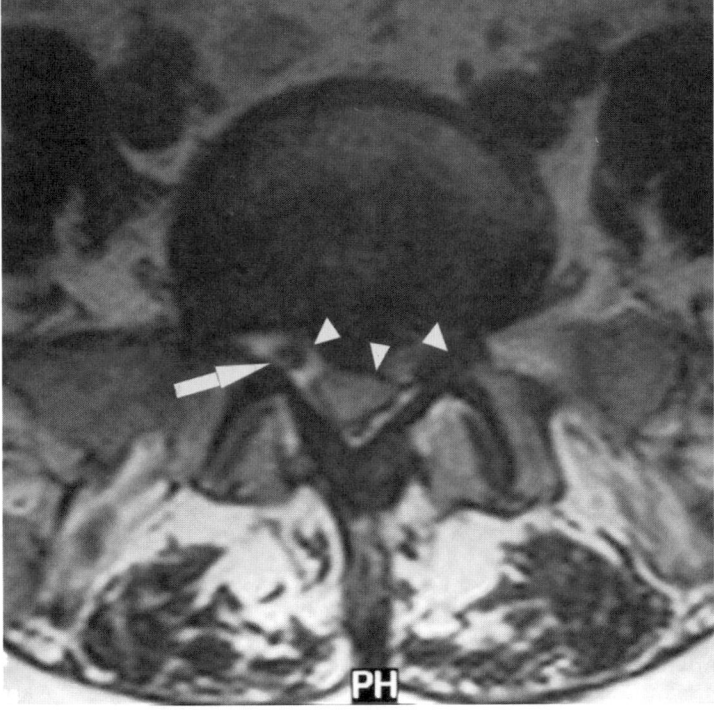

B

FIG. 42-30. **A.** T2-weighted sagittal magnetic resonance imaging shows an L5–S1 disc herniation causing significant canal compromise and displacement of nerve roots. **B.** T2-weighted axial magnetic resonance imaging of the same patient shows the large left paracentral disc herniation at L5–S1. *Arrowheads* delineate the extent of the herniation. The *arrow* indicates the right S1 nerve root passing through free of compression. The left S1 nerve root is under severe compression and is not seen.

TABLE 42-7	Lumbar disc herniations and symptoms by level				
Level	**Frequency (%)**	**Root Injured**	**Reflex**	**Weakness**	**Numbness**
L3–L4	5	L4	Patellar	Quadriceps	Anterior thigh
L4–L5	45	L5	—	Tibialis anterior (foot drop)	Great toe
L5–S1	50	S1	Achilles	Gastrocnemius	Lateral foot

Source: Adapted with permission from Greenberg MS: *Handbook of Neurosurgery*, 6th ed. New York: Thieme Medical Publishers, 2005, Table 14.9, p 304.

typical, though diabetic patients may present a challenge with microvascular neuropathy. Patients with neurogenic claudication have a slowly progressive course and may be surgical candidates when their pain interferes with their lifestyle. The usual surgery is an L3 to L5 lumbar laminectomy to decompress the nerve roots.

Cauda Equina Syndrome

Cauda equina syndrome is due to compression of the cauda equina and may result from massive disc herniation, EDH, epidural abscess, tumor, or subluxation from trauma. Patients with cauda equina compression often present with urinary retention, saddle anesthesia, or progressing leg weakness. Saddle anesthesia is numbness in the perineum, genitals, buttocks, and upper inner thighs. Patients with suspected cauda equina syndrome should undergo immediate MRI of the lumbar spine to evaluate for a surgical lesion. Mass lesions should be removed urgently via laminectomy to preserve sphincter function and ambulation.

Spine Fusion Surgery

Fusion surgery is often required for patients with spinal instability resulting from disease, surgical intervention, or both. Fusion procedures lock adjacent vertebrae together. Fusion occurs when the body forms a solid mass of bone incorporating the adjacent vertebrae, eliminating normal intervertebral movement. Stabilization and immobilization promote bony fusion. Internal instrumentation and external orthoses are often used to stabilize and immobilize the fused spinal segments.

Spinal Instrumentation

Internal fixation devices for spinal segmental immobilization have been developed for all levels of the spine. Most spinal instrumentation constructs have two elements. The first element is a device that solidly attaches to the vertebral bodies. Options include wires wrapped around laminae or spinous processes, hooks placed under the lamina or around the pedicles, or screws placed in the pedicles or the vertebral bodies. The second element is a device that traverses vertebral segments. Options include rods and plates that lock directly to the wires, hooks, or screws at each vertebral level. Spinal instrumentation devices are available for anterior and posterior fusion in the cervical, thoracic, and lumbar regions. Most modern spinal instrumentation devices are made of titanium to minimize problems with future MRI scanning (Fig. 42-31). All spinal instrumentation constructs will eventually fail by loosening or breaking if bony fusion does not occur.

Arthrodesis

Arthrodesis refers to the obliteration of motion or instability by incorporating the relevant components into a solid mass of bone. Arthrodesis must occur in any fused segment to have long-term stability. Failure of arthrodesis results in failed fusion, often in the form of a fibrous nonunion. The rates of successful fusion are higher in the cervical spine than the lumbar spine. Arthrodesis requires ingrowth of new bone formed by the patient's osteoblasts across the unstable defect. Inserting graft material, such as autograft or allograft, into the defect provides a bridge for osteoblasts and promotes fusion. The term *autograft* refers to the patient's own

bone, often harvested from the iliac crest. Iliac crest bone graft is a source of both cortical and cancellous bone. Cortical bone provides structural support, while cancellous bone provides a matrix for bony ingrowth. The term *allograft* refers to sterilized bone from human tissue banks. Allografts also may be cortical, cancellous, or both. Allograft lacks the array of osteoinductive endogenous compounds intrinsic to autograft, although supplemental products such as demineralized bone matrix paste can be added to encourage new bone formation. Other techniques for increasing the rates of successful fusion are being developed, including the integration of osteoinductive bone morphogenetic proteins, known as *BMPs*, into the fusion constructs.

Dynamic stabilization refers to the creation of spinal stability without achieving a bony fusion. The concept applies to both cervical and lumbar motion segments. Artificial lumbar and cervical disc replacement therapies are recent developments in degenerative spine disease that address this concept. However, their use is limited to very select cases. Another motion preservation technique that may hold promise is segmental "soft" stabilization.[35] In cases of degenerative spondylolisthesis, such systems in the lumbar spine allow for decompressive laminectomy without increasing slippage. In theory, adjacent level facets and discs are spared the stresses of a neighboring bony fusion moment arm.

PERIPHERAL NERVE

Common pathologic processes that compromise function of the peripheral nervous system include mechanical compression, ischemia, inflammation, and neoplasia.

Peripheral Nerve Tumors

Most peripheral nerve tumors are benign and grow slowly. Significant pain increases the likelihood that the patient has a malignant tumor. Treatment for peripheral nerve tumors is surgical resection to establish diagnosis and evaluate for signs of malignancy. These tumors have various degrees of involvement with the parent nerve. Some can be resected with minimal or no damage to the nerve. Tumors that grow within the nerve often contain functioning fascicles. Total excision of these tumors requires sacrifice of the parent nerve. The choice of subtotal resection, nerve preservation, and observation, vs. total resection with nerve sacrifice depends on tumor histology and the function of the parent nerve.

Schwannoma

Schwannomas are the most common peripheral nerve tumors, also referred to as *neurilemomas* or *neurinomas*. Most occur in the third decade of life. These benign tumors arise from Schwann cells, which form myelin in peripheral nerves. The most characteristic presentation is a mass lesion with point tenderness and shooting pains on direct palpation. Spontaneous or continuous pain suggests malignancy. Schwannomas tend to grow slowly and eccentrically on parent nerves. The eccentric location and discrete encapsulated nature of these tumors often allow total resection without significant damage to the parent nerve. Subtotal resection and observation is reasonable for schwannomas entwined in important nerves, as the incidence of malignant transformation is extremely low.

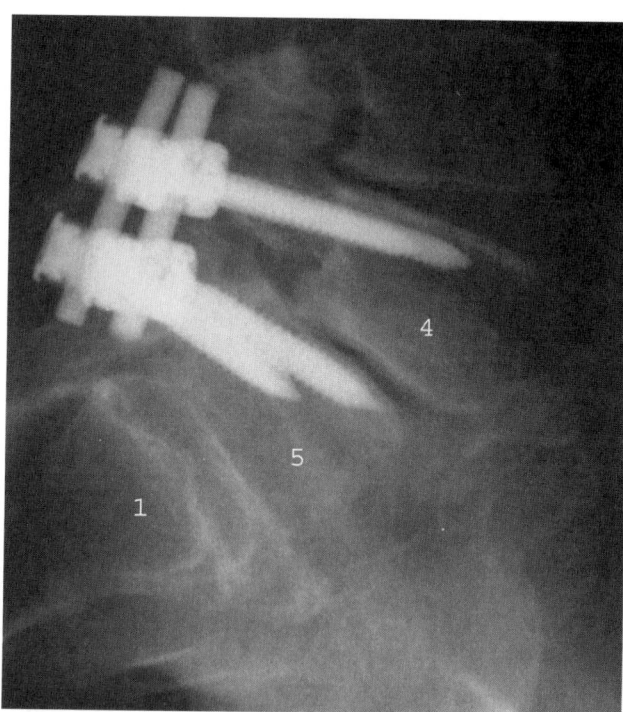
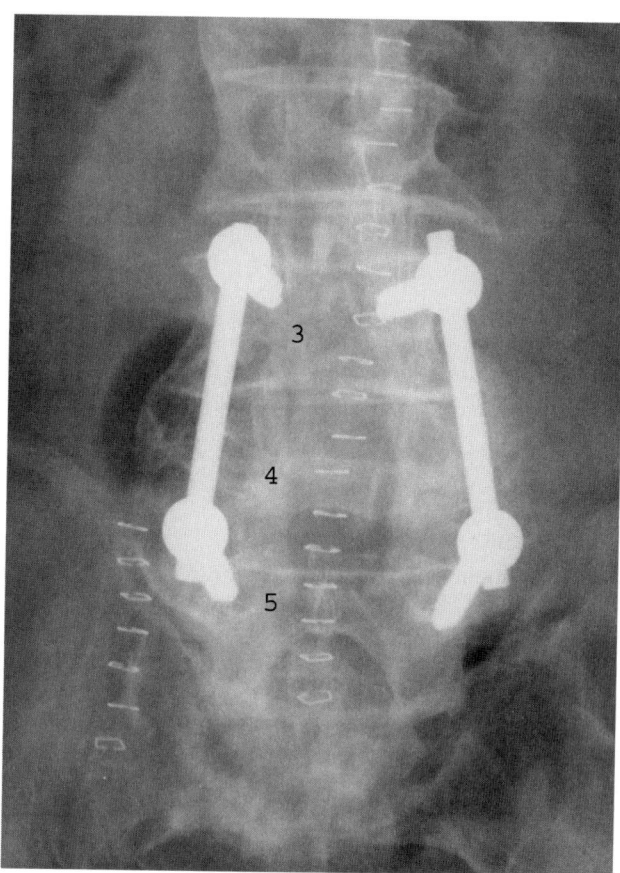

A

B

FIG. 42-31. A. Lateral lumbar spine x-ray showing pedicle screws and connecting rods used to stabilize L4 with respect to L5. This instrumentation was placed as part of a fusion operation to stabilize progressive L4–L5 spondylolisthesis with intractable low back pain. **B.** Anteroposterior lumbar spine x-ray showing L3 to L5 instrumentation with pedicle screws and connecting rods. The patient had previously sustained an L4 burst fracture. Note the significant loss of height of the L4 body compared to adjacent levels. The small row of staples to the right delineates the incision over the iliac crest used to harvest cancellous bone as a nonstructural osteoinductive autograft fusion designed to induce formation of a solid bone bridge from L3 to L5 (arthrodesis).

Neurofibroma

Neurofibromas arise within the nerve and tend to be fusiform masses, unlike schwannomas, which tend to grow out of the nerve. Neurofibromas often present as a mass that is tender to palpation. They usually lack the shooting pains characteristic of schwannomas. Neurofibromas are often difficult to resect completely without sacrifice of the parent nerve. Neurofibromas have a higher incidence of malignant transformation; therefore, patients with known residual tumors require close observation. Patients with NF1 often have multiple neurofibromas. These patients should be offered resection for symptomatic tumors. Risk of malignant degeneration is up to 10%. Malignant neurofibromas have the histologic characteristics of sarcoma.

Malignant Nerve Sheath Tumors

Malignant nerve sheath tumors include solitary sarcomas, degenerated neurofibromas, and neuroepitheliomas. Patients with malignant peripheral nerve tumors typically complain of constant pain, rather than pain only on palpation, and are more likely to have motor and sensory deficits in the distribution of the parent nerve. Treatment for these tumors is radical excision. This often requires sacrifice of the parent nerve. Invasion of nearby soft tissues may occur and necessitate wide resection or amputation in an attempt to prevent systemic metastasis.

Entrapment Neuropathies

Entrapment neuropathy is neurologic dysfunction in nerves passing through a pathologically small, fixed space. Nerve dysfunction may result directly from chronic, repetitive pressure on the nerve, or from ischemic damage due to impaired perfusion.[36] Entrapment causing dysfunction of nerve signaling may cause numbness, paresthesias, weakness, or muscle atrophy. By far the two most common sites of entrapment neuropathy are the ulnar nerve at the medial aspect of the elbow and the median nerve at the wrist. EMG/NCS usually demonstrate slowing across the entrapped segment of nerve. Mechanical peripheral nerve disorders resulting from trauma (brachial plexus disruption, radial nerve damage from humerus fractures, and common peroneal nerve crush injuries) are discussed in the section on Trauma.

Ulnar Neuropathy

The ulnar nerve has contributions from the C7, C8, and T1 nerve roots, arises from the medial cord of the brachial plexus, and supplies most of the intrinsic hand muscles (interossei and third and fourth lumbricals), and sensation to the fourth and fifth digits. It passes posteriorly to the medial epicondyle at the elbow in the condylar groove. This segment is superficial and subject to external compression and repetitive minor impacts. Patients with ulnar entrapment at the elbow present with numbness and tingling in the medial palm, as well as the fourth and fifth digits. Motor deficits include weakness and wasting of the intrinsic hand muscles. Treatment for symptomatic ulnar entrapment neuropathy is surgical exploration and incision of the fibrous aponeurotic arch that overlies the nerve. A 6-cm curvilinear incision centered between the medial epicondyle and the olecranon allows exploration of up to 10 cm of nerve and lysis of compressive tissues.

Carpal Tunnel Syndrome

The median nerve has contributions from the C5 to T1 nerve roots, arises from the medial and lateral cords of the brachial plexus, and supplies the muscles of wrist and finger flexion and sensation to the palmar aspect of the first, second, and third digits. The median nerve passes through the carpal tunnel in the wrist, lying superficial to the four deep and four superficial flexor tendons. The transverse carpal ligament is a tough, fibrous band that forms the roof of the carpal tunnel. The ligament attaches to the pisiform and hamate medially and the trapezium and scaphoid laterally. Patients complain of numbness and tingling in the supplied digits, clumsiness, and worsening with sleep or repetitive wrist movement. Patients may notice wasting of the thenar eminence. Treatment for symptomatic carpal tunnel syndrome unresponsive to splinting, analgesics, and rest is surgical division of the flexor retinaculum. This often provides prompt relief of pain symptoms and slow recovery of numbness and strength.

Autoimmune and Inflammatory Disorders

These are not surgical diseases, but merit brief mention as they are included in the differential diagnosis for new-onset weakness. Their characteristic presentations help distinguish them from weakness due to structural lesions.

Guillain-Barré Syndrome

Guillain-Barré syndrome is an acute inflammatory demyelinating polyradiculopathy often occurring after viral infection, surgery, inoculations, or mycoplasma infections. Patients classically present with weakness ascending from the legs to the body, arms, and even cranial nerves. Symptoms usually progress over 2 to 4 weeks and then resolve. Care is supportive. Respiratory weakness may require ventilatory support.

Myasthenia Gravis

Myasthenia gravis is an autoimmune process in which antibodies form to the acetylcholine receptors of muscles, leading to fluctuating weakness. Most patients have either thymic hyperplasia or thymoma. The most common symptoms are diplopia, ptosis, dysarthria, and dysphagia. More severe cases have limb or respiratory involvement. Weakness worsens with repetitive movement. Treatment is with acetylcholinesterase inhibitors and possible thymectomy.

Eaton-Lambert Syndrome

Eaton-Lambert syndrome is an autoimmune process with antibodies to the presynaptic calcium channels. This is a paraneoplastic syndrome most commonly associated with oat cell carcinoma. Patients have weakness of proximal limb muscles that improves with repetitive movement. This diagnosis must prompt oncologic evaluation.

INFECTION

CNS infections of interest to neurosurgeons include those that cause focal neurologic deficit due to mass effect, require surgical aspiration or drainage because antibiotic therapy alone is insufficient, cause mechanical instability of the spine, or occur after neurosurgical procedures.

Cranial

Osteomyelitis

The skull is highly vascular and resistant to infections. Osteomyelitis of the skull may develop by contiguous spread from pyogenic sinus disease or from contamination by penetrating trauma. *Staphylococcus aureus* and *S. epidermidis* are the most frequent causative organisms. Patients usually present with redness, swelling, and pain. Contrast head CT aids diagnosis and shows the extent of involved bone, along with associated abscesses or empyema. Osteomyelitis

treatment entails surgical débridement of involved bone followed by 2 to 4 months of antibiotics. Craniotomy wound infections are a special concern because performing a craniotomy creates a devascularized free bone flap susceptible to infection and not penetrated by antibiotics. These wounds must be débrided and the bone flaps removed and discarded. Subsequent care involves appropriate antibiotic therapy, observation for signs of recurrent infection off antibiotics, and return to the OR for titanium or methylmethacrylate cranioplasty 6 to 12 months later.

Subdural Empyema

Subdural empyema is a rapidly progressive pyogenic infection. The subdural space lacks significant barriers to the spread of the infection, such as compartmentalization or septations. Subdural empyema usually occurs over the cerebral convexities. Potential infectious sources include sinus disease, penetrating trauma, and otitis. Streptococci and staphylococci are the most frequently found organisms. Presenting symptoms include fever, headache, neck stiffness, seizures, or focal neurologic deficit. Neurologic deficit results from inflammation of cortical blood vessels, leading to thrombosis and stroke. The most common deficit is contralateral hemiparesis. Patients with suggestive symptoms should undergo rapid contrast CT scan. LP frequently fails to yield the offending organism and risks herniation due to mass effect. Typical treatment is wide hemicraniectomy, dural opening, and lavage. The pus may be thick or septated, making burr hole drainage or small craniotomy insufficient. Patients then require 1 to 2 months of antibiotics. Subdural empyema has 10 to 20% mortality risk and common chronic sequelae, including seizure disorder and residual hemiparesis. However, many patients make a good recovery.

Brain Abscess

Brain abscess is encapsulated infection within the brain parenchyma. It may spread hematogenously in patients with endocarditis or intracardiac or intrapulmonary right-to-left shunts, by migration from the sinuses or ear, or via direct seeding by penetrating trauma. Disorganized cerebritis often precedes formation of the organized, walled-off abscess. Patients may present with nonspecific symptoms such as headache, nausea, or lethargy, or with focal neurologic deficit such as hemiparesis. Alternatively, patients may present in extremis if the abscess ruptures into the ventricular system. Abscesses appear as well-demarcated, ring-enhancing, thin-walled lesions on CT scan and MRI, and often have associated edema and mass effect. Patients require antibiotic therapy after needle aspiration or surgical evacuation. Antibiotic therapy without surgical evacuation may be considered for patients with small, multiple, or critically located abscesses. Abscesses that are large, cause mass effect, decreased mental status, or that fail to decrease in size after 1 week of antibiotics, should be evacuated. Nonsurgical management still requires aspiration or biopsy for organism culture and sensitivities. Blood and CSF cultures rarely give definitive diagnosis. Removal of an encapsulated abscess significantly shortens the length of antibiotic therapy required to eliminate all organisms. Common chronic sequelae after successful treatment include seizures or focal neurologic deficit.

Spine

Pyogenic Vertebral Osteomyelitis

Pyogenic vertebral osteomyelitis is a destructive bacterial infection of the vertebrae, usually of the vertebral body. Vertebral osteomyelitis frequently results from hematogenous spread of distant disease, but may occur as an extension of adjacent disease, such as psoas abscess or perinephric abscess. *S. aureus* and *Enterobacter* spp. are the most frequent etiologic organisms. Patients usually present with fever and back pain. Diabetics, IV drug abusers, and dialysis patients have increased incidence of vertebral osteomyelitis. Epidural extension may lead to compression of the spinal cord or nerve roots with resultant neurologic deficit. Osteomyelitis presents a lytic picture on imaging and must be distinguished from neoplastic disease. Adjacent intervertebral disc involvement occurs frequently with pyogenic osteomyelitis, but rarely with neoplasia. Plain films and CT help assess the extent of bony destruction or deformity such as kyphosis. MRI shows adjacent soft tissue or epidural disease. Most cases can be treated successfully with antibiotics alone, although the organism must be isolated to steer antibiotic choice. Blood cultures may be positive. Surgical intervention may be required for débridement when antibiotics alone fail, or for stabilization and fusion in the setting of instability and deformity.

Tuberculous Vertebral Osteomyelitis

Tuberculous vertebral osteomyelitis, also known as *Pott's disease*, occurs most commonly in underdeveloped countries and in immuno-compromised people. Several features differentiate tuberculous osteo-myelitis from bacterial osteomyelitis. The infection is indolent and symptoms often progress slowly over months. Tuberculosis rarely involves the intervertebral disc. The involved bodies may have sclerotic rather than lytic changes. Multiple nonadjacent vertebrae may be involved. The upper lumbar and lower thoracic vertebrae are most commonly affected. Diagnosis requires documentation of acid-fast bacilli. Treatment involves long-term antimycobacterial drugs. Patients with spinal instability or neural compression from epidural inflamma-tory tissue should undergo débridement and fusion as needed.

Discitis

Primary infection of the intervertebral disc space, or discitis, is most commonly secondary to postoperative infections. Spontaneous dis-citis occurs more commonly in children. *S. epidermidis* and *S. aureus* account for most cases. The primary symptom is back pain. Other signs and symptoms include radicular pain, fevers, paraspinal muscle spasm, and localized tenderness to palpation. Many cases will resolve without antibiotics, which generally are given for positive blood or biopsy cultures or persistent constitutional symp-toms. Most patients will have spontaneous fusion across the in-volved disc and do not need débridement or fusion.

Epidural Abscess

Epidural abscesses may arise from or spread to the adjacent bone or disc, so distinguishing between vertebral osteomyelitis or discitis and a spinal epidural abscess may be difficult. The most common presenting signs and symptoms are back pain, fever, and tenderness to palpation of the spine. The most significant risk of epidural abscess is weakness progressing to paralysis due to spinal cord or nerve root damage. Cord and root damage may be due to direct compression or to inflammatory thrombosis resulting in venous infarction. *S. aureus* and *Streptococcus* spp. are the most common organisms. Methicillin-resistant *S. aureus* now constitutes a signifi-cant proportion of these infections, as high as 40%.[37] The source may be hematogenous spread, local extension, or operative contamina-tion. MRI best demonstrates the epidural space and degree of neural compromise. Patients with spinal epidural abscess and neurologic compromise should undergo surgical débridement for decompres-sion and diagnosis, followed by culture-directed antibiotic therapy. Relative contraindications to surgery include prohibitive comorbid-ities or total lack of neurologic function below the involved level. Patients with no neurologic deficits and an identified organism may be treated with antibiotics alone and very close observation. How-ever, this management strategy remains somewhat controversial because these patients can undergo rapid and irreversible neurologic decline. Most epidural abscesses can be accessed via laminectomy without fusion. Collections predominantly anterior to the cervical or thoracic cord may require anterior approach and fusion.

FUNCTIONAL NEUROSURGERY

Epilepsy Surgery

Seizures result from uncontrolled neuronal electrical activity. Sei-zures may result from irritative lesions in the brain, such as tumors

or hematomas, or from physiologic or structural abnormalities. Seizures may involve a part of the brain (focal) or the entire brain (generalized). Focal seizures may be associated with normal con-sciousness (simple) or decreased consciousness (complex). All gen-eralized seizures cause loss of consciousness. Focal seizures may secondarily generalize. Patients with multiple unprovoked seizures over time are considered to have epilepsy. The type of epilepsy depends on such factors as type of seizures, electroencephalo-graphic (EEG) findings, associated syndromes, and identifiable etiologies. All patients with unexplained seizures (i.e., no obvious cause such as head trauma or alcohol withdrawal) require thorough neurologic evaluation, including imaging to evaluate for a mass lesion. Antiepileptic drugs (AEDs) form the first line of therapy for epilepsy, initially as monotherapy, then as combination therapy. Epilepsy patients who have failed satisfactory trials of several AED combination regimens may be candidates for surgical intervention. Lack of seizure control or patient intolerance of the medications may constitute failure. Epilepsy surgery can decrease the frequency of seizures by resection of the electrical source of the seizures, or decrease the severity of seizures by disconnecting white matter tracts through which the abnormal electrical activity spreads. Three types of epilepsy surgery are discussed. Epilepsy surgery appears to be extremely underused, given the relatively low risk of the proce-dures, and the crippling social and economic effects of uncontrolled or partially controlled epilepsy.[38] Patients with symptoms, imaging abnormalities, and EEG analysis compatible with a specific seizure focus are most likely to have good results from epilepsy surgery.

Anterior Temporal Lobectomy

Medial temporal lobe structural abnormalities can lead to complex partial seizures (CPS). Many patients with CPS have poor seizure control on medications. Patients with CPS may have significant reduction in seizure frequency or cessation of seizures after resection of the anterior temporal lobe. The amygdala and the head of the hippocampus are removed as part of the lobectomy. Resection may be taken back approximately 4.5 cm from the temporal tip in the language-dominant hemisphere, and 6 cm from the temporal tip in the language nondominant hemisphere, with low risk of significant deficits.[39] Two main risks of anterior temporal lobectomy are mem-ory problems and visual problems. Removal of the hippocampus in a patient with an atrophied or nonfunctional contralateral hippocam-pus causes a global memory deficit. Interruption of the optic radia-tions, which carry visual signals from the contralateral superior visual quadrants of both eyes, causes a contralateral superior quadrantano-pia, known as a *pie in the sky* field deficit.

Corpus Callosotomy

Patients with generalized seizures, atonic seizures associated with drop attacks, or absence seizures, who are found to have bilaterally coordinated pathologic cortical discharges on EEG and who fail AED therapy, may be candidates for corpus callosotomy. The corpus callosum is a large white matter tract that connects the cerebral hemispheres. Loss of consciousness requires simultaneous seizure activity in both hemispheres. Focal or partial seizures may spread via the corpus callosum to the contralateral hemisphere, causing general-ization and loss of consciousness. Division of the corpus callosum can interrupt this spread. Patients may have decreased numbers of sei-zures and/or fewer episodes of lost consciousness. Usually only the anterior half or two thirds of the corpus callosum is divided, as more extensive division increases the risk of disconnection syndrome. Patients with disconnection syndrome are unable to match objects in the opposite visual hemifields, to identify objects held in one hand with the other hemifield, and to write with the left hand or name objects held in the left hand (in left hemisphere–dominant patients).

Hemispherectomy

Children with intractable epilepsy, structural anomalies in one hemi-sphere, and contralateral hemiplegia, may have improved seizure control after resection of the hemisphere (anatomic hemispherectomy) or disruption of all connections to the hemisphere (functional hemispherectomy). Functional hemispherectomy often is preferred over anatomic hemispherectomy because of the high incidence of complications such as hematoma formation and ventriculoperitoneal shunt dependence associated with the latter.

Deep Brain Stimulation

Patients with essential tremor and medically refractory Parkinson's disease have abnormal activity in the nuclei of the basal ganglia. The basal ganglia are extrapyramidal structures that modulate and regulate signals in the corticospinal (pyramidal) tracts. Abnormal extrapyramidal activity leads to the loss of the normal modulation of movement and thus the clinical manifestations of the diseases. Fine electrical leads placed in these deep basal ganglia nuclei and connected to pulse generators modify the pathologic signals. The pulse generators are usually placed in the chest in a manner similar to cardiac pacemakers. Connector wires travel from the generators in the subcutaneous space up the neck and in the subgaleal space in the head, to connect the pulse generators to the electrical leads. Proper lead placement is accomplished with stereotactic guidance. A frame is rigidly fixed to the patient's head, and an MRI is obtained with the frame in place. Calculation of the coordinates of the millimeter-sized deep brain nuclei is performed in relation to the three-dimensional space defined by the fixed frame, allowing for accurate targeting of the fine electrical leads (Fig. 42-32). Postoperatively, the pulse generators can be interrogated and adjusted with hand-held, transcutaneous, noninvasive devices as needed for symptom control.

Essential Tremor

Essential tremors are action tremors of 4 to 8 Hz rhythmic oscillation that often affect one arm or the head. Essential tremor often starts in the third or fourth decade of life, and increases in frequency and amplitude with age. Beta blockers decrease symptoms. Patients with poor medical control and significant functional impairment can benefit significantly from placement of a deep brain stimulator in the contralateral ventralis intermediate nucleus of the thalamus. Placement of ventralis intermediate nucleus stimulators for essential tremor

appears to result in durable symptom control with good postoperative neuropsychologic outcomes in properly selected patients.[40,41]

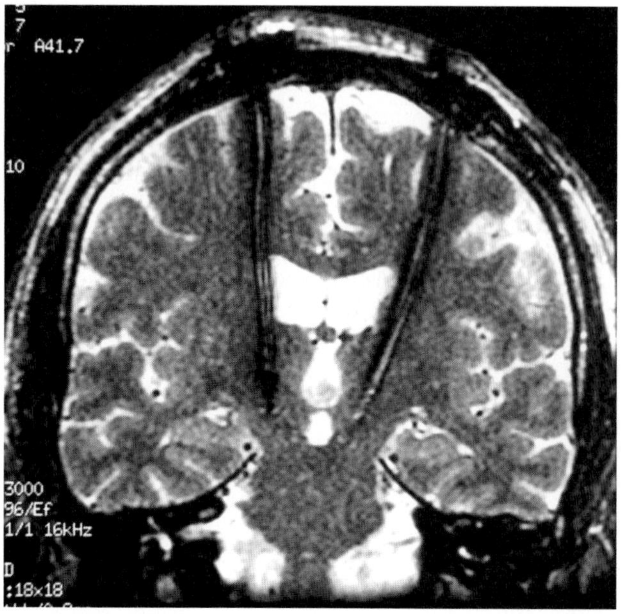

Parkinson's Disease

Parkinson's disease is a progressive disorder characterized by rigidity, bradykinesia, and resting tremor, due to loss of dopamine-secreting neurons in the substantia nigra and locus ceruleus. It is also known as *paralysis agitans*. Dopaminergic agents such as levodopa/carbidopa and anticholinergic agents such as amantadine and selegiline form the basis of medical therapy. Patients with poor medical control or significant drug side effects may benefit significantly from placement of bilateral deep brain stimulators in the subthalamic nuclei. Although the globus pallidus interna has also been a widely targeted area, the subthalamic nuclei is now the most accepted target in deep brain stimulation for Parkinson's disease.[42] Deep brain stimulation provides durable symptom relief with good postoperative neuropsychologic function in properly selected patients.[43]

Trigeminal Neuralgia

Trigeminal neuralgia, also known as *tic douloureux*, is characterized by repetitive, unilateral, sharp, and lancinating pains in the distribution of, typically, the second, but sometimes third, branch of cranial nerve V, the trigeminal nerve. The patient may describe a "trigger point," an area on the face that elicits the pain when touched. A current leading etiologic hypothesis for trigeminal neuralgia is irritation and pulsatile compression of the root entry zone of the nerve by an artery in the posterior fossa, usually a loop of the superior cerebellar artery. The pain is excruciating and can be debilitating. Medical therapy, including carbamazepine and amitriptyline, may reduce the frequency of events. Options for medically refractory cases include percutaneous injection of glycerol into the path of the nerve, peripheral transection of the nerve branches, SRS, and microvascular decompression (MVD).

MVD involves performing a small posterior fossa craniotomy on the side of the symptoms, retraction of the cerebellar hemisphere, and exploration of cranial nerve V. If an artery is found near the nerve, the vessel is freed of any adhesions and nonabsorbable material is placed between the nerve root and the artery. MVD remains the first definitive management option because SRS is associated with a substantial incidence of facial numbness.[44,45]

STEREOTACTIC RADIOSURGERY

The term *stereotactic radiosurgery* (SRS) refers to techniques that allow delivery of high-dose radiation that conforms to the shape of the target and has rapid isodose fall-off, minimizing damage to adjacent neural structures. The two most common devices used for conformal SRS for intracranial lesions are the LINAC (linear accelerator) and the gamma knife. LINAC delivers a focused beam of x-ray radiation from a port that arcs part way around the patient's head. Linear accelerators are commonly used to provide fractionated radiation for lesions outside the CNS. They are found in most radiation oncology departments. SRS can be performed with these existing units, after upgrades to the software and collimators. The gamma knife delivers 201 focused beams of gamma radiation from cobalt sources through a specially designed colander-like helmet. Gamma knife units are used only for intracranial disease and cost up to $5 million; thus, they are most appropriate in high patient–volume centers. There is ongoing debate in the literature regarding the two technologies.[46-48] Both continue to evolve, allowing more precise and complex isodose conformation to complex lesions. Most lesions can be treated equally well with either technology. Lesions abutting the medulla or the spinal cord should not be treated with SRS, because these structures do not tolerate the radiation dose delivered to structures within millimeters of the target. Also, medullary or spinal cord compression can result from swelling of the lesion after the radiosurgery dose, resulting in devastating neurologic deficit.

FIG. 42-32. Fast spin echo coronal magnetic resonance imaging demonstrating position of deep brain stimulator leads in the subthalamic nuclei bilaterally. The electrodes appear thick and wavy due to magnetic susceptibility artifact.

Proton beam is an evolving SRS technology that may play a specialized role in treatment of lesions where posttarget exiting radiation limits photon-based therapies.[49] For example, the physical properties of photons cause destruction upon entry and exit from tissue, which can be particularly harmful to skull-base or clival lesions such as chordoma, in which the exiting pathway travels through the brain stem. Proton beam therapy uses accelerated protons, which dissipate energy upon impact and do not cause additional exiting damage. Currently, there are very few centers using this technology.

CyberKnife is another radiosurgery system that has neurosurgical application. It is a frameless, robotic, LINAC-based system that allows for targeting of spinal neoplasms with higher resolution than conventional external beam radiotherapy.[50] Using imaging tracking in real time, the CyberKnife is able to adjust to breathing artifact and patient movement. The application of this technology is rapidly growing.

Arteriovenous Malformations

SRS has been found to be an effective stand-alone therapy for AVMs up to 3 cm in diameter. SRS is best for lesions that are difficult to access surgically due to high likelihood of postoperative neurologic deficit. SRS is not effective for lesions >3 cm. Effective obliteration and elimination of the risk of hemorrhage takes 2 to 3 years. Overall, there is an approximately 2% annual incidence of AVM hemorrhage,[51] although one study found a 50% decrease in hemorrhage rate during the latency period before angiographic obliteration.[52] Nonetheless, surgical excision remains the preferred therapeutic modality, while SRS is reserved for cases deemed very high-risk for surgery due to location or patient factors.[53] Some patients with large AVMs who undergo surgery will have unresectable residual lesions. SRS may be used as an effective adjunctive therapy in these patients.

Vestibular Schwannomas

SRS has been introduced as a therapeutic alternative to microsurgical resection for vestibular schwannomas up to 2.5 cm in maximum diameter. SRS provides high rates of tumor growth arrest and possible reduction in size with low rates of facial nerve palsy. Patients with functional ipsilateral preprocedure hearing may be more likely to retain functional hearing postprocedure than with microsurgery. The limitations of SRS include inability to treat tumors >2.5 cm, the possibility of radiation-induced malignant transformation of these benign tumors, and lack of long-term follow-up. SRS centers are accumulating experience with these tumors and accumulating data on long-term results.[54,55] The indications for microsurgery and SRS will continue to evolve. Either approach should be undertaken at a high-volume center, as studies show the patient outcomes improve with increased surgeon experience.[56]

Intracranial Metastases

Patients with solitary or multiple intracranial metastases may be treated primarily with SRS.[57] Patients have improved survival after SRS compared to no treatment or WBRT, and similar survival to patients undergoing total surgical resection. Patients with lesions >3 cm in diameter or evidence of ICH should undergo surgical decompression rather than SRS. Some studies show improved survival with up to seven intracranial masses. Patients with multiple intracranial masses have almost zero long-term survival, and most will die of their intracranial disease. Patients with intracranial metastases live 3 to 6 months on average with medical care and WBRT. This can be extended to 9 to 16 months with SRS or surgery, depending on tumor type, age, and patient condition.[58]

CONGENITAL AND DEVELOPMENTAL ANOMALIES

Dysraphism

Dysraphism describes defects of fusion of the neural tube involving the neural tube itself, or overlying bone or skin. Dysraphism may occur in the spine or the head. Neural tube defects are among the most common congenital abnormalities. Prenatal vitamins, especially folic acid, reduce the incidence of neural tube defects.

Spina Bifida Occulta

Spina bifida occulta is congenital absence of posterior vertebral elements. The spinous process is always missing, the laminae may be missing to various degrees, but the underlying neural tissues are not involved. Spina bifida occulta is found in 25% of the general population, and is asymptomatic unless associated with other developmental abnormalities.

Spina Bifida with Myelomeningocele

Spina bifida with myelomeningocele describes the congenital absence of posterior vertebral elements with protrusion of the meninges through the defect, with underlying neural structural abnormalities. Common findings include weakness and atrophy of the lower extremities, gait disturbance, urinary incontinence, constipation, and deformities of the foot. Myelomeningoceles arising from the high lumbar cord usually cause total paralysis and incontinence, while those arising from the sacral cord may have only clawing of the foot and partial urinary function loss. Myelomeningocele patients often have hydrocephalus and a Chiari II malformation, an abnormal downward herniation of the cerebellum and brain stem through the foramen magnum. Patients with abnormal protrusion of meninges through the bony defect without abnormalities of the underlying neural tissue have a meningocele. Most of these patients are neurologically normal.

Encephalocele

Herniation of brain encased in meninges through the skull that forms an intracranial mass is referred to as *encephalocele*. Herniation of meninges without brain tissue is referred to as a *meningocele*. Most occur over the convexity of the skull. More rarely, the tissue protrudes through the skull base into the sinuses. Treatment involves excision of the herniated tissue and closure of the defect. Most patients with encephaloceles and meningoceles have impaired cognitive development. Patients with greater amounts of herniated neural tissue tend to have more severe cognitive deficits.

Craniosynostosis

Craniosynostosis is the abnormal early fusion of a cranial suture line with resultant restriction of skull growth in the affected area and compensatory bulging at the other sutures. Skull growth occurs at the cranial sutures for the first 2 years of life, at the end of which the skull has achieved >90% of its eventual adult size. Fusion of the sagittal suture, or sagittal synostosis, results in a boat-shaped head, known as *scaphocephaly*. Unilateral coronal synostosis results in ipsilateral forehead flattening and outward deviation of the orbit, known as *plagiocephaly*. The contralateral normal forehead appears to bulge by comparison. Bilateral coronal synostosis results in a broad, flattened forehead, known as *brachycephaly*, and is often associated with maxillary hypoplasia and proptosis. Unilateral or bilateral lambdoid synostosis results in flattening of the occiput. Occipital flattening can result from abnormal suture fusion (synostosis), or from physical remolding of the skull caused by always placing the baby in the supine position for sleep (known as *positional plagiocephaly*). Placing the baby in the prone position or tilted onto the contralateral side may restore near-normal skull shape in most cases of lambdoid synostosis, avoiding surgery. Treatment for synostoses in general is surgical, involving resection of the fused suture, or more complex reconstructive techniques for severe or refractory cases.

Hydrocephalus

Excess CSF in the brain that results in enlarged ventricles is known as *hydrocephalus*. The adult forms approximately 500 mL of CSF per day, much of it in the lateral ventricles. CSF flows from the

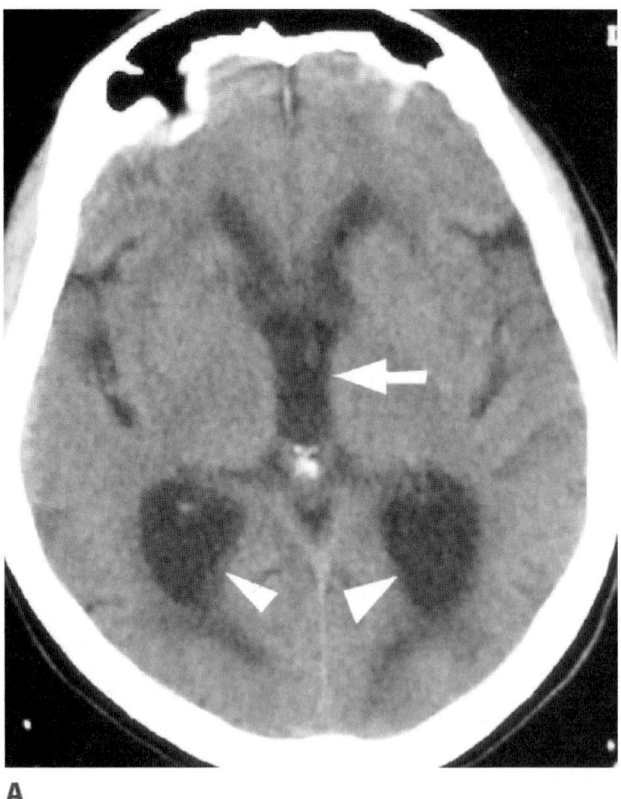

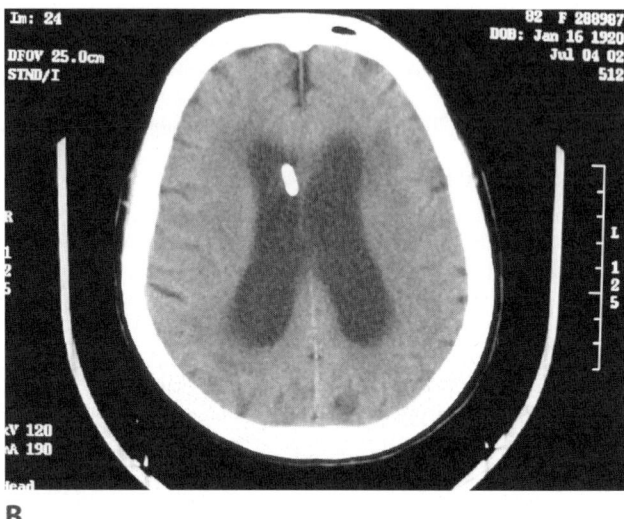

A   **B**

FIG. 42-33. A. Axial head computed tomography scan revealing dilated ventricular system. Note dilated atria of the lateral ventricles (*arrowheads*) and rounded third ventricle (*arrow*). The large size of the ventricles and lack of transependymal flow indicate a chronic process (contrast to Fig. 42-2). The patient had normal-pressure hydrocephalus and had improved ambulation after placement of a ventriculoperitoneal shunt. **B.** Higher cut from same scan showing ventricular catheter in place in the frontal horn of the right lateral ventricle.

ventricles to the subarachnoid space and is then absorbed into the venous blood through the arachnoid granulations. Hydrocephalus may be classified as communicating or obstructive (outlined in the next two sections), and congenital or acquired. Congenital lesions associated with or causing hydrocephalus include stenosis of the cerebral aqueduct, Chiari malformation, myelomeningocele, and intrauterine infection. Acquired hydrocephalus may result from occlusion of arachnoid granulations by meningitis, germinal matrix hemorrhage, or SAH. CSF pathways may be occluded by adjacent tumors (Fig. 42-33).

Communicating Hydrocephalus

Obstruction at the level of the arachnoid granulations constitutes communicating hydrocephalus. This usually causes dilation of the lateral, third, and fourth ventricles equally. The most common causes in adults are meningitis and SAH. Hydrocephalus may be transient after SAH, with re-establishment of normal CSF absorption after the protein content of the CSF returns to normal and the granulations reopen.

Obstructive Hydrocephalus

Obstruction of CSF pathways is known as *obstructive hydrocephalus*. Ventricles proximal to the obstruction dilate, while those distal to the obstruction remain normal in size. Typical patterns include dilation of the lateral ventricles due to a colloid cyst occluding the foramen of Monro, dilation of the lateral and third ventricles due to a tectal (midbrain) glioma or pineal region tumor occluding the cerebral aqueduct, or dilation of the lateral and third ventricles with obliteration of the fourth ventricle by an intraventricular tumor of the fourth ventricle. Obstructive hydrocephalus may present precipitously and require urgent shunting to prevent herniation.

Chiari I Malformation

Chiari I malformation is the caudal displacement of the cerebellar tonsils below the foramen magnum. It may be seen as an incidental

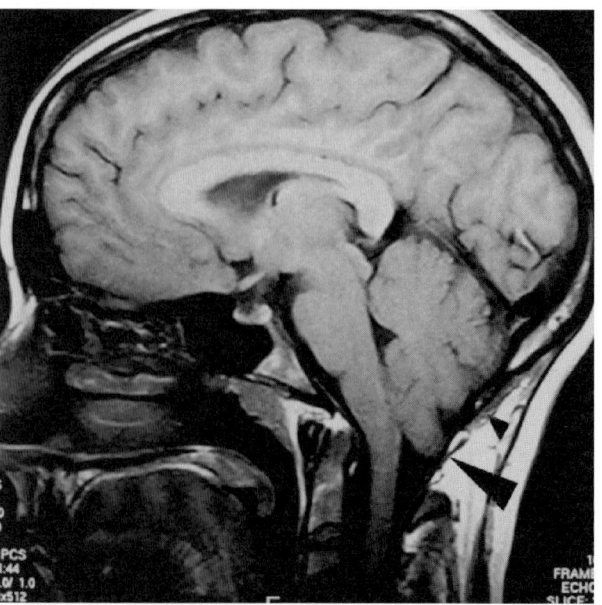

FIG. 42-34. T1-weighted sagittal magnetic resonance imaging of a patient with a Chiari I malformation. The *large arrowhead* points to the cerebellar tonsils. The *small arrowhead* points to the posterior arch of the foramen magnum.

finding on MRI scans in asymptomatic patients. Symptomatic patients usually present with headache, neck pain, or symptoms of myelopathy, including numbness or weakness in the extremities. A syrinx may be associated, but the brain stem and lower cranial nerves are normal in Chiari I malformations. Chiari II malformations are more severe and involve caudal displacement of the lower brain stem and stretching of the lower cranial nerves. Symptomatic patients may be treated with suboccipital craniectomy to remove the posterior arch of the foramen magnum, along with removal of the posterior ring of C1. Removal of these bony structures relieves the compression of the cerebellar tonsils and cervicomedullary junction, and may allow re-establishment of normal CSF flow patterns. Figure 42-34 demonstrates typical MRI appearance of a Chiari I malformation.

REFERENCES

Entries highlighted in bright blue are key references.

1. Kandel E, Schwartz J, Jessell T: *Principles of Neural Science*, 4th ed. New York: McGraw-Hill Professional, 2000.
2. Stiefel MF, Spiotta A, Gracias VH, et al: Reduced mortality rate in patients with severe traumatic brain injury treated with brain tissue oxygen monitoring. *J Neurosurg* 103:805, 2005.
3. Masters SJ, McClean PM, Arcarese JS, et al: Skull x-ray examinations after head trauma. Recommendations by a multidisciplinary panel and validation study. *N Engl J Med* 316:84, 1987.
4. Bullock MR, Chesnut R, Ghajar J, et al: Surgical management of depressed cranial fractures. *Neurosurgery* 58:S56, 2006.
5. Brain Trauma Foundation, American Association of Neurological Surgeons, Congress of Neurological Surgeons. Guidelines for the management of severe traumatic brain injury. *J Neurotrauma* 24:S1, 2007.
6. Temkin NR, Dikmen SS, Wilensky AJ, et al: A randomized, double-blind study of phenytoin for the prevention of post-traumatic seizures. *N Engl J Med* 323:497, 1990.
7. Ingebrigtsen T, Romner B: Routine early CT-scan is cost saving after minor head injury. *Acta Neurologica Scandinavica* 93:207, 1996.
8. Stein SC, Ross SE: The value of computed tomographic scans in patients with low-risk head injuries. *Neurosurgery* 26:638, 1990.
9. Kelly JP, Nichols JS, Filley CM, et al: Concussion in sports. Guidelines for the prevention of catastrophic outcome. *JAMA* 266:2867, 1991.
10. Bullock MR, Chesnut R, Ghajar J, et al: Surgical management of acute epidural hematomas. *Neurosurgery* 58:S7, 2006.
11. Jones NR, Molloy CJ, Kloeden CN, et al: Extradural haematoma: Trends in outcome over 35 years. *Br J Neurosurg* 7:465, 1993.
12. Bullock MR, Chesnut R, Ghajar J, et al: Surgical management of acute subdural hematomas. *Neurosurgery* 58:S16, 2006.
13. Howard MA 3rd, Gross AS, Dacey RG Jr, et al: Acute subdural hematomas: An age-dependent clinical entity [see comment]. *J Neurosurg* 71:858, 1989.
14. Hamilton MG, Frizzell JB, Tranmer BI: Chronic subdural hematoma: The role for craniotomy reevaluated. *Neurosurgery* 33:67, 1993.
15. Bullock MR, Chesnut R, Ghajar J, et al: Surgical management of traumatic parenchymal lesions. *Neurosurgery* 58:S25, 2006.
16. Lyrer P, Engelter S: Antithrombotic drugs for carotid artery dissection. *Stroke* 35:613, 2004.
17. Maynard FM Jr, Bracken MB, Creasey G, et al: International standards for neurological and functional classification of spinal cord injury. American Spinal Injury Association. *Spinal Cord* 35:266, 1997.
18. Denis F: The three column spine and its significance in the classification of acute thoracolumbar spinal injuries. *Spine* 8:817, 1983.
19. Bracken MB, Shepard MJ, Collins WF, et al: A randomized, controlled trial of methylprednisolone or naloxone in the treatment of acute spinal-cord injury. Results of the second national acute spinal cord injury study [see comment]. *N Engl J Med* 322:1405, 1990.
20. Bracken MB, Shepard MJ, Collins WF Jr, et al: Methylprednisolone or naloxone treatment after acute spinal cord injury: 1-year follow-up data. Results of the second national acute spinal cord injury study [see comment]. *J Neurosurg* 76:23, 1992.
21. Hugenholtz H, Cass DE, Dvorak MF, et al: High-dose methylprednisolone for acute closed spinal cord injury—only a treatment option. *Can J Neurol Sci* 29:227, 2002.

22. Resnick DK, Kaiser MG, Fehlings M, et al: *Hypothermia and Human Spinal Cord Injury: Position Statement and Evidence Based Recommendations from the AANS/CNS Joint Section on Disorders of the Spine and the AANS/CNS Joint Section on Trauma*. Washington, DC: AANS/CNS Joint Section of Disorders of the Spine and Peripheral Nerves, 2007.
23. Seddon HJ. Three types of nerve injury. *Brain* 66:237, 1943.
24. Anonymous. Beneficial effect of carotid endarterectomy in symptomatic patients with high-grade carotid stenosis. North American Symptomatic Carotid Endarterectomy Trial Collaborators [see comment]. *N Engl J Med* 325:445, 1991.
25. Anonymous. Tissue plasminogen activator for acute ischemic stroke. The National Institute of Neurological Disorders and Stroke rt-PA Stroke Study Group [see comment]. *N Engl J Med* 333:1581, 1995.
26. Mendelow AD, Gregson BA, Fernandes HM, et al: Early surgery versus initial conservative treatment in patients with spontaneous supratentorial intracerebral haematomas in the International Surgical Trial in Intracerebral Haemorrhage (STICH): A randomised trial. *Lancet* 365:387, 2005.
27. Molyneux A, Kerr R, Stratton I, et al: International Subarachnoid Aneurysm Trial (ISAT) of neurosurgical clipping versus endovascular coiling in 2143 patients with ruptured intracranial aneurysms: A randomised trial [see comment] [reprint in *J Stroke Cerebrovasc Dis* 11:304, 2002]. *Lancet* 360:1267, 2002.
28. Mitchell P, Kerr R, Mendelow AD, et al: Could late rebleeding overturn the superiority of cranial aneurysm coil embolization over clip ligation seen in The International Subarachnoid Aneurysm Trial? *J Neurosurg* 108:437, 2008.
29. Raftopoulos C, Goffette P, Vaz G, et al: Surgical clipping may lead to better results than coil embolization: Results from a series of 101 consecutive unruptured intracranial aneurysms. *Neurosurgery* 52:1280; discussion 1287, 2003.
30. Patchell RA, Tibbs PA, Walsh JW, et al: A randomized trial of surgery in the treatment of single metastases to the brain. *N Engl J Med* 322:494, 1990.
31. Patchell RA, Tibbs PA, Regine WF, et al: Postoperative radiotherapy in the treatment of single metastases to the brain: A randomized trial. *JAMA* 280:1485, 1998.
32. Aoyama H, Shirato H, Tago M, et al: Stereotactic radiosurgery plus whole-brain radiation therapy vs stereotactic radiosurgery alone for treatment of brain metastases: A randomized controlled trial. *JAMA* 295:2483, 2006.
33. Patchell RA, Tibbs PA, Regine WF, et al: Direct decompressive surgical resection in the treatment of spinal cord compression caused by metastatic cancer: A randomised trial. *Lancet* 366:643, 2005.
34. Le Roux PD, Haglund MM, Harris AB: Thoracic disc disease: Experience with the transpedicular approach in twenty consecutive patients. *Neurosurgery* 33:58, 1993.
35. Mulholland RC, Sengupta DK: Rationale, principles and experimental evaluation of the concept of soft stabilization. *Eur Spine J* 11:S198, 2002.
36. Dawson D, Hallett M, Wilbourn A. *Entrapment Neuropathie*, 3rd ed. Baltimore: Lippincott Raven, 1999.
37. Darouiche RO: Spinal epidural abscess. *N Engl J Med* 355:2012, 2006.
38. Benbadis SR, Heriaud L, Tatum WO, et al: Epilepsy surgery, delays and referral patterns—are all your epilepsy patients controlled? *Seizure* 12:167, 2003.
39. Rausch R, Kraemer S, Pietras CJ, et al: Early and late cognitive changes following temporal lobe surgery for epilepsy [see comment]. *Neurology* 60:951, 2003.
40. Fields JA, Troster AI, Woods SP, et al: Neuropsychological and quality of life outcomes 12 months after unilateral thalamic stimulation for essential tremor. *J Neurol Neurosurg Psychiatry* 74:305, 2003.
41. Rehncrona S, Johnels B, Widner H, et al: Long-term efficacy of thalamic deep brain stimulation for tremor: Double-blind assessments. *Mov Disord* 18:163, 2003.
42. Kleiner-Fisman G, Herzog J, Fisman DN, et al: Subthalamic nucleus deep brain stimulation: Summary and meta-analysis of outcomes. *Mov Disord* 21:S290, 2006.
43. Perozzo P, Rizzone M, Bergamasco B, et al: Deep brain stimulation of the subthalamic nucleus in Parkinson's disease: Comparison of pre- and postoperative neuropsychological evaluation. *J Neurol Sci* 192:9, 2001.
44. Barker FG 2nd, Jannetta PJ, Bissonette DJ, et al: The long-term outcome of microvascular decompression for trigeminal neuralgia. *N Engl J Med* 334:1077, 1996.

CHAPTER 42 Neurosurgery

45. Kondo A: Microvascular decompression surgery for trigeminal neuralgia. *Stereotact Funct Neurosurg* 77:187, 2001.

46. Bova FJ, Goetsch SJ: Modern linac stereotactic radiosurgery systems have rendered the gamma knife obsolete. *Medical Physics* 28:1839, 2001.

47. Konigsmaier H, de Pauli-Ferch B, et al: The costs of radiosurgical treatment: Comparison between gamma knife and linear accelerator. *Acta Neurochirurgica* 140:1101; discussion 1110, 1998.

48. Suh JH, Barnett GH, Miller DW, et al: Successful conversion from a linear accelerator-based program to a gamma knife radiosurgery program: The Cleveland Clinic experience. *Stereot Funct Neurosurg* 72:159, 1999.

49. Chen CC, Chapman P, Petit J, et al: Proton radiosurgery in neurosurgery. *Neurosurg Focus* 23:E5, 2007.

50. Gerszten PC, Ozhasoglu C, Burton SA, et al: CyberKnife frameless stereotactic radiosurgery for spinal lesions: Clinical experience in 125 cases. *Neurosurgery* 55:89; discussion 98, 2004.

51. Karlsson B, Lax I, Soderman M: Risk for hemorrhage during the 2-year latency period following gamma knife radiosurgery for arteriovenous malformations. *Int J Radiat Oncol Biol Phys* 49:1045, 2001.

52. Maruyama K, Kawahara N, Shin M, et al: The risk of hemorrhage after radiosurgery for cerebral arteriovenous malformations. *N Engl J Med* 352:146, 2005.

53. Pan DH, Guo WY, Chung WY, et al: Gamma knife radiosurgery as a single treatment modality for large cerebral arteriovenous malformations. *J Neurosurg* 93:113, 2000.

54. Regis J, Pellet W, Delsanti C, et al: Functional outcome after gamma knife surgery or microsurgery for vestibular schwannomas. *J Neurosurg* 97:1091, 2002.

55. Shin M, Ueki K, Kurita H, et al: Malignant transformation of a vestibular schwannoma after gamma knife radiosurgery. *Lancet* 360:309, 2002.

56. Elsmore AJ, Mendoza ND: The operative learning curve for vestibular schwannoma excision via the retrosigmoid approach. *Br J Neurosurg* 16:448, 2002.

57. Gerosa M, Nicolato A, Foroni R, et al: Gamma knife radiosurgery for brain metastases: A primary therapeutic option. *J Neurosurg* 97:515, 2002.

58. Pollock BE, Brown PD, Foote RL, et al: Properly selected patients with multiple brain metastases may benefit from aggressive treatment of their intracranial disease. *J Neurooncol* 61:73, 2003.

Michael H. Heggeness, Francis H. Gannon, Jacob
Weinberg, Peleg Ben-Galim, and Charles A. Reitman

GROWING SPECIALTY

Orthopedic surgery is a broad and actively growing surgical specialty. It concerns the nonoperative and operative treatment of disorders of the musculoskeletal system including bones, joints, muscles, tendons, ligaments, and nerves. The orthopedic surgeon must be familiar with the normal growth and development of the musculoskeletal system, as well as disorders that can arise from genetic or developmental abnormalities, trauma, infection, inflammatory processes, the degenerative process, and neoplasm. In every patient, the orthopedic surgeon will work hard to find nonsurgical solutions for the patient's condition. However, surgical treatments are often necessary to preserve or restore musculoskeletal function, assist in healing, or palliate pain.

Anatomy of Long Bones

Much of an orthopedic surgeon's practice concerns treatment of the "long bones." Long bones generally consist of an epiphysis (the portion of the bone on either end which usually contains an articular surface). The *epiphysis* is formed from an epiphyseal ossification center at either end of most long bones separated from the *metaphysis* of the long bone by the growth plate (Fig. 43-1). After skeletal maturity, the ends of bones continue to be referred to as the *epiphyseal region*. The metaphysis of a long bone is the region immediately below the growth plate or its remnant. The metaphysis tapers to become the shaft or *diaphysis* of the long bone.

Long bones are composed of one or more articular surfaces, covered with hyaline cartilage, thick durable cortex of dense bone, and an interior region of trabecular bone and marrow. It is important to know that all bone is subject to turnover with resorption and new bone formation, occurring in both the trabecular bone and the cortex. Cortical bone does turn over considerably slower than trabecular bone, however, by a factor of approximately seven or eight (Fig. 43-2). Another major function of the bone, in addition to its mechanical function, is the regulation of serum calcium levels. Hematopoiesis also occurs in the marrow.

The cells that synthesize bone matrix (osteoid) are the *osteoblasts*. Essentially all surfaces of the bone are covered with osteoblasts or osteocytes. Osteoblasts, which are active in bone synthesis, are noted histologically to be large with abundant cytoplasm. Quiescent osteoblasts are thin and "flat."

Joint Anatomy

Mobile joints are called *diarthrodial joints*. In such joints, there is no direct bone to bone contact. Instead, weight bearing and motion are accomplished through intervening surfaces or hyaline (articular) cartilage. Stability of the joints is accomplished through musculotendinous action and limited and guided by the presence of ligaments and the joint capsule itself. The joint capsule also serves to enclose the lubricating synovial fluid, which provides nutrition to the chondrocytes in the articular cartilage and facilitates gliding motions between the two cartilage surfaces.

Muscle Anatomy

Skeletal muscle is, by weight, the single largest tissue in the body. The structure of skeletal muscle is indicated in Fig. 43-3. Muscle contraction is accomplished by adenosine triphosphate driven sliding motions between actin and myosin filaments, driven by the adenosine triphosphatase of the myosin molecule. Precisely arranged, actin and myosin containing sarcomeres form the basic contractile apparatus, the *myofiber*. Multiple myofibers compose a muscle fiber and multiple muscle fibers compose the *fascicle*. In turn, multiple fascicles form a muscle.

Basic Biomechanics

An understanding of basic biomechanics is critical to an orthopedic surgeon. Bone generally is considered to be a rather static rigid structure; however, this is a misconception. Not only are the cells

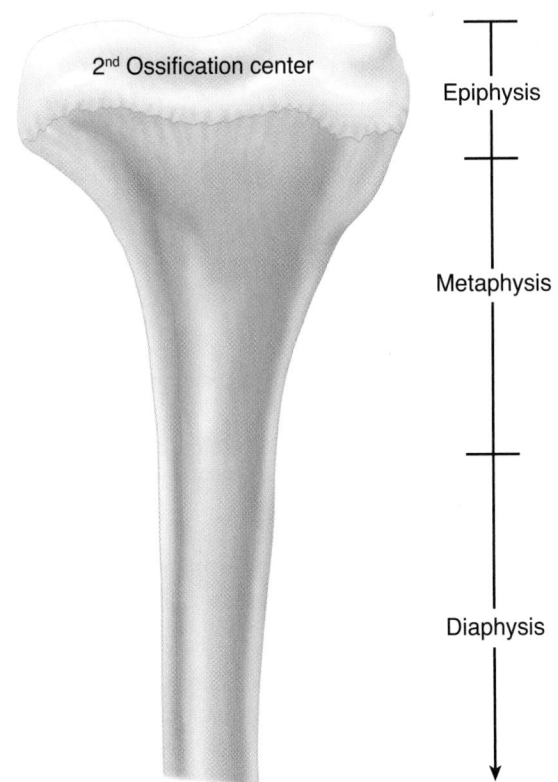

FIG. 43-1. Long bones have three sections. The end is the epiphysis or secondary ossification center, the adjacent area is the metaphysis, and the middle of the bone is the diaphysis. The metaphysis is broader than the diaphysis, has a thin cortex, and is composed of primarily cancellous bone.

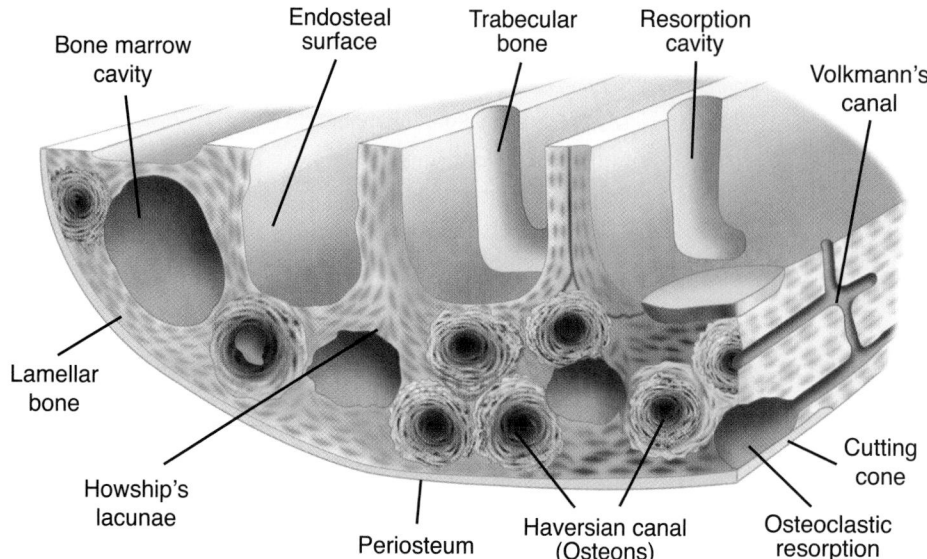

FIG. 43-2. The cellular and structural organization of bone.

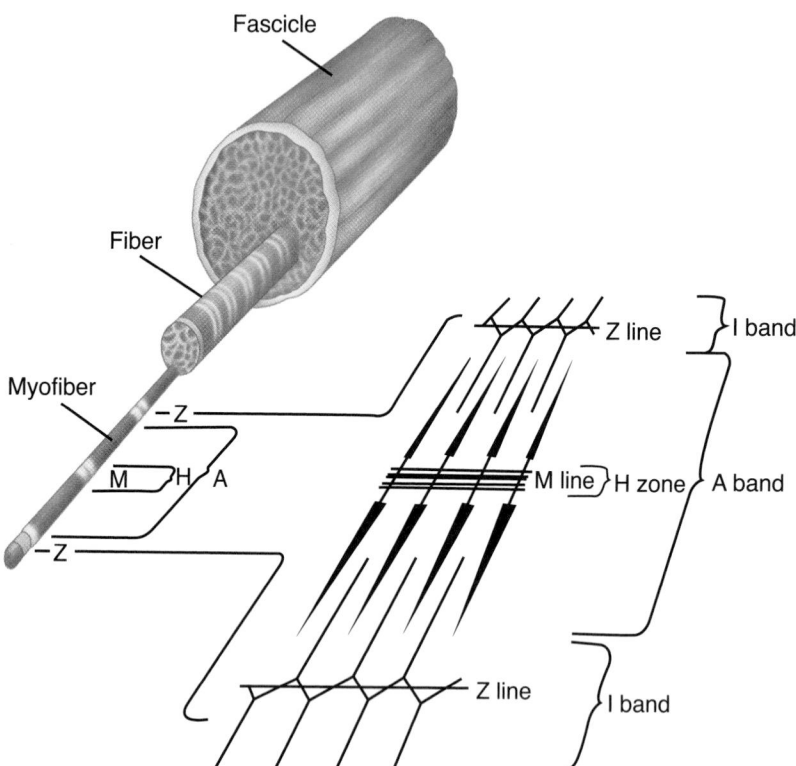

FIG. 43-3. Organization of skeletal muscle from the microscopic to the macrostructural level. *[Reproduced with permission from Simon SR (ed): Orthopaedic Basic Science. Rosemont, IL: American Academy of Orthopaedic Surgeons, 1994, p 91.]*

KEY POINTS

1. The assessment of any patient with a musculoskeletal complaint or injury must include a careful history and a physical examination that includes the neurologic, vascular, and muscular bony assessment.

2. Fractures frequently involve significant soft tissue as well as bony injury.

3. Open fractures (fractures where the fracture hematoma extends to a wound in the skin) require urgent operative irrigation and débridement.

4. The majority of fractures can be managed nonoperatively, with a cast or a brace.

5. Orthopedic injuries in pediatric patients are managed differently than in adults. Injury to the physis (growth plate) are common and require special management. Bone injury in young patients heal so quickly that prompt treatment and close follow-up is critical.

and matrix of the bone subject to regular turnover, the bone itself normally flexes and bends to a surprising degree.

Biomechanical engineers use the words *stress* and *strain* to describe the material properties of bone, and tissue, as well as orthopedic implants. The word *stress* refers to force exerted per unit area. The word *strain* is used to define deformation of a material when placed under stress. The mechanical properties of most materials can be displayed in a stress/strain curve. The *stiffness* of a material is expressed by the slope of such a curve. Strain in a bone or other material is usually elastic (or completely reversible) under low levels of stress. When the exerted force causes reversible changes to the material, plastic deformation or mechanical failure (fracture) is said to occur.

The mechanical behaviors of a substance can be changed substantially by the presence of focal defects in the material. For example, a bone will break much more easily at or near a small defect of the bone. This is due to concentration of stress forces in this area, a so-called *stress riser*. This can occur at the site of a destructive lesion, such as a tumor, or more importantly, can result from surgical intervention with the creation of screw holes (Fig. 43-4).

Biomechanics of Skeletal Motion

The joints move by the action of muscles on the bone through their tendinous attachments. The effect of a muscle contraction depends on its origin and insertion and on the constraints and geometry of the intervening joint or joints. The effect of most muscles can be usefully viewed as a *lever arm*. The amount of force needed to move an object is heavily influenced by the length of the level arm (Fig. 43-5). Contraction of a muscle unit with a short lever arm results in a large application of force, generally at a low speed. A longer lever arm will diminish the amount of effective force that can be exerted, but can result in a great rapidity of motion. Thus, because of the lever arms present at the elbow and shoulder, one can move the hand and throw an object at a rate many times faster than the maximal rate of muscle contraction.

TRAUMATIC BONE LESIONS

Fracture Repair

The biologic and histologic events in fracture repair can be divided into three general stages. The duration and classification of each

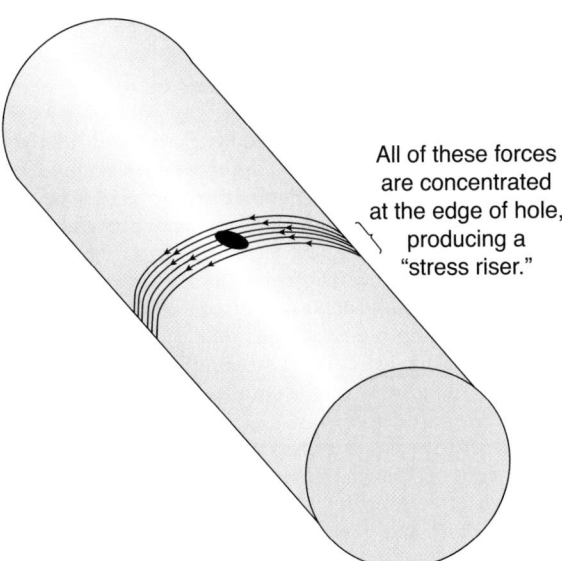

FIG. 43-4. A stress riser is a hole or defect in a material that produces a concentration of forces. This increases the risk of the material failing under conditions that, without the stress riser, would not lead to failure of the material.

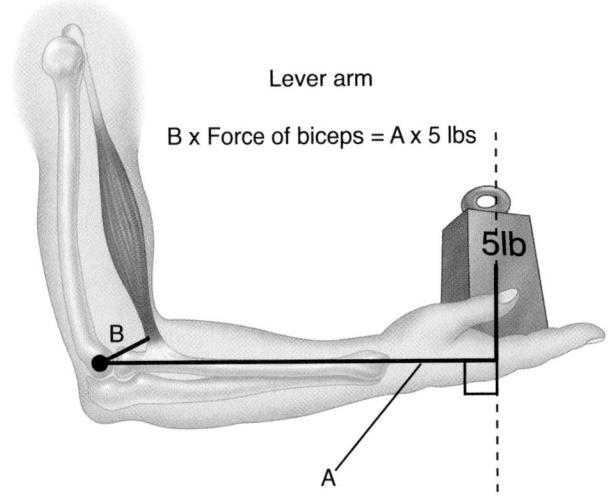

Lever arm

B x Force of biceps = A x 5 lbs

5lb

FIG. 43-5. The biceps muscle with its insertion to the bicipital tuberosity of the radius has a short lever arm compared to the length of the forearm that is the lever arm for the weight in the hand. The biceps force must be much greater than the weight of the ball because of the difference between the two lever arms.

stage is variable based on age, general health, and other factors. Additionally, these stages can overlap, as there are no definitive features to suggest progression of one stage to another. The three stages are (a) circulatory, which includes closure of any wound and primary callus formation, (b) metabolic, the stage where the primary callus is reinforced leading to clinical union, and (c) mechanical, the stage in which the united bone is remodeled along the lines of stress.

Once a fracture has occurred, the surrounding muscle, vessels, and other soft tissues are damaged as well. A cellular response, with inflammatory cells and undifferentiated mesenchymal cells, is prominent in the first 3 to 5 days.

The biologic events that lead to fracture healing are complex, and as yet, incompletely understood. Most fractures heal by way of callus formation. In some unusual instances, when fractured fragments are in close physical contact, bone healing involves direct osteonal penetration from across the fracture site, a process called *primary bone healing*. In normal long-bone fracture healing, the clinical process has been described in four stages: inflammation, soft callus, hard callus, and bone remodeling.

These mesenchymal cells are the hallmark of the circulatory stage of fracture repair and lead to the appearance of chondrocytic, osteoblastic, and vascular cells. These components form the structure of the primary callus. The hematoma is invaded from the periphery by granulation tissue that adds to and aids in the callus formation.

The cellular phase is followed by the vascular phase. The hematoma gradually is replaced by a cellular and vascular bed. With this comes a passive hyperemia and decreased oxygen tension that is conducive for cartilage formation. While this occurs, there is an osteoclastic response to remove the previously damaged bone and make way for the newly formed bone. With enough cartilage formation and the subsequent endochondral ossification, the primary callus is formed. Changes also occur in the periosteum adjacent to the fracture. The periosteal cells adjacent to the fracture become active and produce a matrix that elevates the periosteum and adds to the primary callus. This brings the *circulatory stage* to a close.

The second stage is primarily concerned with reinforcement of the callus. The initial callus is remodeled by the removal and replacement of the woven bone into a more mature lamellar bone. The lamellar bone provides the strength and support at this stage. The necrotic debris and inflammation is gone by this point, and the callus is primarily defined by the bone formation and remodeling.

The metabolic phase leads into the mechanical stage with remodeling and realignment of bone and callus along the lines of stress. This process continues and will last up to 2 years, depending on a number of factors.

As this process continues, a defined cortex will emerge with a lamellar Haversian structure. The healed area of the fracture itself also will have a cancellous interior with normal marrow contents including fat and hematopoietic elements.

Early in the healing process, the cartilage initially synthesized by chondrocytes within the callus is reflected by the presence of significant amounts of chondroitin sulfate and dermatan sulfate as well as type II cartilage. As healing continues, synthesis of type I collagen will predominate over other types, and the amounts of collagen matrix proteins also will decrease.

Growth Factors

Since the original description of bone morphogenic proteins by Marshall Urist in 1974, the existence of several small protein and polypeptide growth factors have been identified. At present, these growth factors are under intense study because of their potential application to the manipulation of the bone healing process. It is likely that the normal biologic functions of these proteins control and regulate the bone formation and resorption. Bone morphogenic protein is a low molecular weight protein that can influence the differentiation of mesenchymal cells into mature osteoblasts.

Other protein factors that can affect fracture healing include insulin-like growth factor, transforming growth factor beta, and platelet-derived growth factor (PDGF). Insulin-like growth factor stimulates bone cell proliferation and the production of cartilage matrix. Transforming growth factor beta induces the synthesis of cartilage, proteoglycans, and type II collagen. PDGF stimulates proliferation of osteoblasts and increases the rate of synthesis of type I collagen. PDGF is also known to be a chemotactic agent and induces the migration of inflammatory cells into the callus. This process is distinct from the process of primary bone healing in long bones with the extension of cutting cones across areas of firm bony contact with direct extension of new Haversian canals that span the two opposed surfaces. Osteoclasts at the front of such a cutting cone resorb cylindrical channels from the bone that are subsequently filled in by concentric layers of lamellar bone with a central vascular channel.

TREATMENT OF FRACTURES AND DISLOCATIONS

The majority of fractures are managed nonsurgically. Optimal treatment depends on multiple factors, including the location and type of fracture. In some instances (such as a minimally displaced fracture of the middle phalanx of one of the lesser toes) no treatment at all other than those for symptoms of pain generally are necessary (Fig. 43-6). In most other fractures, some form of immobilization is the treatment of choice, this might involve a simple sling (as for a midshaft clavicle fracture) or a more robust splint or brace. When more complete immobilization is desired, immobilization in a circumferential plaster or fiberglass cast is often ideal.

The technical aspects of creating a cast often are underestimated. A proper cast is carefully constructed to immobilize the fractured bone in question and avoid the complications of loss of reduction, neurovascular compromise, pressure ulceration of skin, or the creation of joint contractures. Nondisplaced fractures generally are treated by simple casting. Should the fracture be unacceptably displaced, a closed reduction (applying force by direct pressure, traction, or other maneuvers) to realign the bones precedes the application of the cast. This often requires local, regional, or systemic anesthesia. To construct a cast, the affected limb is often, but not always, first covered with a cloth sleeve or stocking. Critically, the limb is then covered with a generous amount of cast padding. Those inexperienced with casting almost always apply far

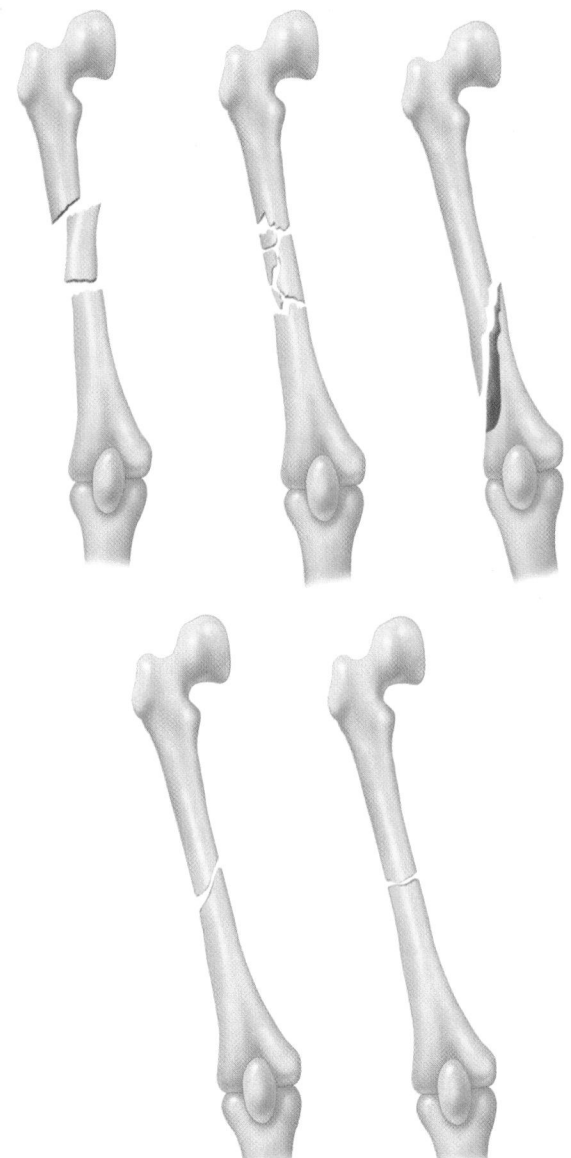

FIG. 43-6. Types of fracture. *Top row*: segmental, comminuted, and spiral. *Bottom row*: oblique and transverse.

too little padding. Insufficient padding, particularly overlying a bony prominence, can cause skin erosion within the immobilizing cast, a potentially devastating complication.

After adequate padding is in place, plaster or fiberglass is gently rolled on to the limb. The cast material is applied wet and will generate heat while hardening. This exothermic reaction is sometimes underestimated. Patients can sustain burns during application of thick casts or splints. Several minutes are required, and for this reason, it is applied in layers while maintaining reduction of the fracture. The process can be both technically demanding and tiring.

An alternative to plaster is fiberglass cast tape. This is superior to plaster in terms of strength to weight ratio and has largely replaced plaster for many casting applications. Fiberglass tape itself, however, is a bit elastic and creates an extra potential hazard of creating a cast too tight. This can lead to excessive compression to the limb.

Finally, swelling of the injured limb beneath the plaster cast can be a significant and dangerous issue. In many minimally displaced fractures, a circumferential plaster or fiberglass cast can be safely applied immediately. For many other injuries, definitive casts are applied 24 to 72 hours after the acute injury because of the potential for ongoing swelling beneath the cast, which all too frequently results in skin problems or neurovascular compromise.

Generally, the cast application, particularly if the casting involves reduction maneuvers, are followed by immediate postprocedure x-ray imaging, to verify a satisfactory alignment of the fracture fragments. It also is customary to repeat imaging through the cast during the course of healing to ensure that the cast is successfully maintaining a satisfactory reduction.

Internal Fixation

Internal fixation refers to any device placed surgically to directly hold bones in position. These can include sutures, wires and screws, plates, rods, or nails. General principles of internal fixation, however, will be detailed below in Simple Screw Fixation and Intramedullary Internal Fixation.

Simple Screw Fixation

Many times simply fixing two fractured bones together using individual screws can be effective. The technical challenge of screw fixation often is underestimated. The surgeon must choose an appropriate sized screw and place it correctly with good purchase on the bone. Bone screws come in a variety of designs to address specific fracture fixation problems. A *cortical screw* is a screw with a large inner diameter and shallow screw threads. This screw is designed to have a high breaking strength for its total diameter, and the screws threads are intended to engage cortical bone. Purchase of shallow screw threads in cortical bone can be excellent.

Cancellous screws have a deeper thread pattern and a smaller inner shaft diameter. They are designed to obtain fixation in less dense cancellous bone. *Lag screws* also are commonly used. These are screws in which only the distal portion of the screw length is threaded. These screws penetrate one bone fragment without thread fixation. When a second fracture fragment is engaged by the threaded portion of the screw, turning the screw head tight down to the cortex of the first bony fragment will pull or "lag" the distal fragment toward the screw head. Compression of the fractured bones is the result.

Intramedullary Internal Fixation

Fractures of the shaft of long bones often are managed by intramedullary rods or nails. A metal rod is inserted into the medullary canal to obtain a tight and secure fit to immobilize the fracture. Often, as in the femur, the medullary canal is sequentially reamed over a guidewire to allow insertion of a stout rod. Frequently, the rod is further stabilized by inserting "locking screws" that transfix the bone cortex and pass through appropriate holes in the rod either distal, proximal, or both.

Open Fractures

Fortunately, fractures of the bone usually do not occur with penetration of the skin. When a fracture occurs, and the fracture hematoma is not in continuity with a wound of the skin, the fracture is said to be closed. Such a fracture hematoma may become secondarily infected, but such events are uncommon.

A more serious condition exists when the fracture hematoma communicated with a wound of the skin. Such injuries are called *open fractures*. The fractured ends of the bone are frequently driven through the skin at the moment of injury, often leaving deceptively small wounds. Penetrating trauma also can lead to open fractures, and bacterial contamination must be assumed to be present in all such cases. All such injuries carry a serious risk of infection and osteomyelitis.

Except in unusual circumstances, all open fractures are initially treated by a formal irrigation and débridement procedure performed in the operating room.[1] Depending on the circumstances of each individual injury, the initial débridement can be followed by simple splinting, or external fixation (with definitive operative treatment performed at a later date), or by definitive internal fixation. In severe injuries, with extensive soft tissue injury, the fracture treatment usually is performed in stages.[2] It must be stressed, however, that urgent débridement of open fractures is a critical step in the treatment of these patients.

Compartment Syndrome

A compartment syndrome is a clinical emergency and describes a clinical situation where muscle tissue compartment edema constrained by the investing muscle fascia results in increased muscle compartment pressures sufficient to stop small vessel flow of blood. Severe problems arise when the profusion pressure in the capillary bed is approached or exceeded by the intracompartmental pressure. In this situation, perfusion of the muscle is compromised and muscle necrosis results. The diagnosis of a compartment syndrome is a clinical one, based on complaints of local pain out of proportion to the apparent injury, in association with pain, on passive stretch of the involved muscles. This situation can arise after a period of ischemia, after local blunt trauma, and, frequently, in the presence of an acute fracture. Measurement of compartment pressures, using one of a number of commercially available devices, involves inserting a needle into the suspected muscle compartments to measure pressure. Pressure measurements alone are not reliable to absolutely rule in or rule out the diagnosis, but they can be a useful adjunct to clinical assessment, particularly valuable in obtunded or unconscious patients. Pressure measurements that are greater than 30 mmHg or within 30 mmHg of the diastolic blood pressure are consistent, but not absolutely diagnostic with the presence of a compartment syndrome. The diagnosis is a clinical one. Treatment of a compartment syndrome is always surgical and involves extensive skin incisions and fascial release of all suspected muscle compartments.

An untreated compartment syndrome will result in necrosis of involved muscle compartments with subsequent contracture and severe loss of function in the affected limb.

FRACTURES OF THE CALCANEUS

Fractures of the calcaneus are common and frequently are associated with falls from a height. In assessing patients presenting with a fractured calcaneus, the orthopedist should always consider a possible concurrent fracture of the spine, as these injuries frequently occur together (Fig. 43-7).

Fractures of the calcaneus can be extra-articular. More frequently, calcaneal fractures involve the subtalar joint or the calcaneal cuboid, and sometimes, calcaneal navicular joints. Often, a practitioner will need computed tomography (CT) scan imaging as well as plain x-ray images to fully document the extent of injury in a calcaneal fracture.

Extra-Articular Calcaneal Fractures

Fracture of the posterior third of the calcaneus without articular involvement can result from falls or crush injuries. Other extra-articular calcaneal fractures are avulsion injuries to the insertional area of the Achilles tendon. In all such cases, final clinical judgment and experience are important, but in general, if fragments are large and displaced, internal fixation using screws is often a consideration (Fig. 43-8). Screw fixation within the calcaneus can be technically challenging, as unfortunately the cortex of this bone often is surprisingly thin and the trabecular bone often is disappointingly porous.

Calcaneal Fractures Involving the Subtalar Joint

Calcaneal fractures involving the subtalar joint usually are best assessed by CT scan as well as plain x-ray images. Displaced fractures of the calcaneus involving the subtalar joint usually are

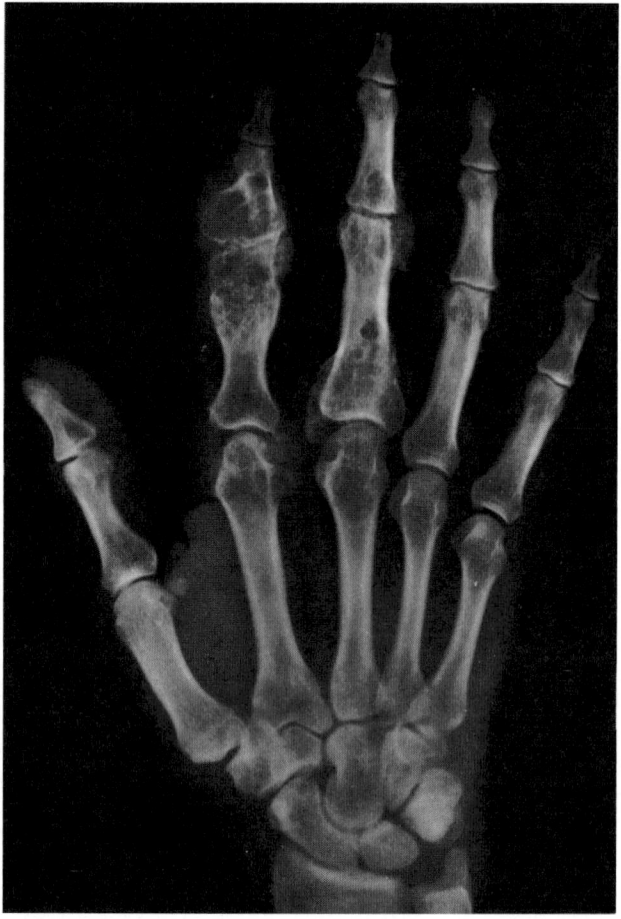

FIG. 43-7. Multiple enchondromas of the hand.

best managed by open reduction and internal fixation, using screws and screw-plate devices.

Fractures of the Talus

Fractures of the talus are common and frequently the result of forced dorsal flexion of the foot and ankle. As with most fractures of the tarsal bones, complete assessment of the injury often requires the use of CT scan images as well as plain x-ray views. The surface of the talus itself is covered by large areas of articular cartilage from the tibiotalar articulation to the talocalcaneal articulation (the subtalar joint) and the talonavicular joints. The blood supply to the bone is, therefore, a bit tenuous. Accordingly, many fractures of the talus are complicated by avascular necrosis. The main vascular supply to the bone of the talar neck is through the branches of the dorsalis pedis and of the peroneal arteries. The arteries of the tarsal canal are the main source of blood for the talar body. Displaced fractures of the talus are, therefore, at very high risk of avascular necrosis. Avascular necrosis osteonecrosis also can occur from nondisplaced fractures. Nondisplaced fractures of the body of the talus usually are treated nonoperatively through bracing or casting. Displaced fractures of the talar body generally are treated by open reduction and internal fixation.

Fractures of the Talar Neck

Fractures of the talar neck also may be managed nonoperatively with casting or bracing and strict nonweightbearing. Nondisplaced fractures of the talar neck carry approximately 14% of the incidents of avascular necrosis. Displaced talar neck fractures are essentially always treated by careful open reduction followed by internal fixation.[3] Reported avascular necrosis rates for displaced talar neck fractures range from 30 to 100%.

Midfoot Trauma Fractures of the Tarsal Bones

The tarsal bones (the navicular, the cuboid, and the three cuneiform bones) link the hind foot to the metatarsals. The precise arrangements of these bones provide mechanical stability to the arch of the foot. The large articular surfaces of these bones, however, also make avascular necrosis a potential complication with any fracture. Isolated fractures of the tarsal bones are uncommon. The force needed to fracture these bones is usually quite high. Such injuries are associated with trauma to adjacent structures, frequently including dislocations of the tarsometatarsal joints. The articulation between the tarsal bones and the metatarsals is referred to as *Lisfranc's joint.* Fracture dislocations in this area of the foot are generally the results of large torsional forces delivered to the foot while the foot is held in dorsiflexion. Such dislocations can be associated with multiple fractures and can involve any number of the metatarsals. Displaced dislocations to any of these joints almost always are managed operatively by internal fixation (Fig. 43-9).

Fractures of the Metatarsals

Fracture of the base of the metatarsals can occur by similar mechanisms to the Lisfranc fracture/dislocation, but are not associated with signifi-

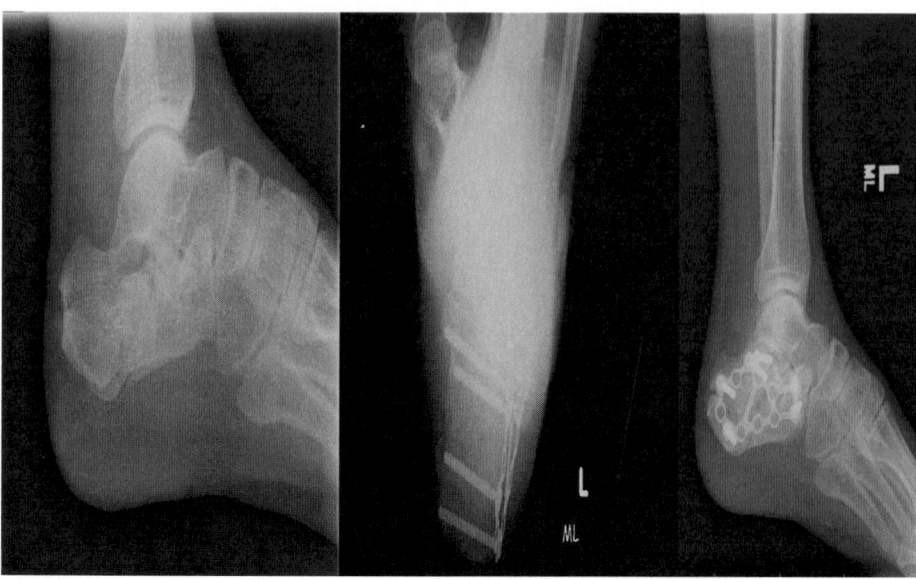

FIG. 43-8. X-ray images of a comminuted intra-articulation calcaneus fracture, before and after open reduction and internal fixation.

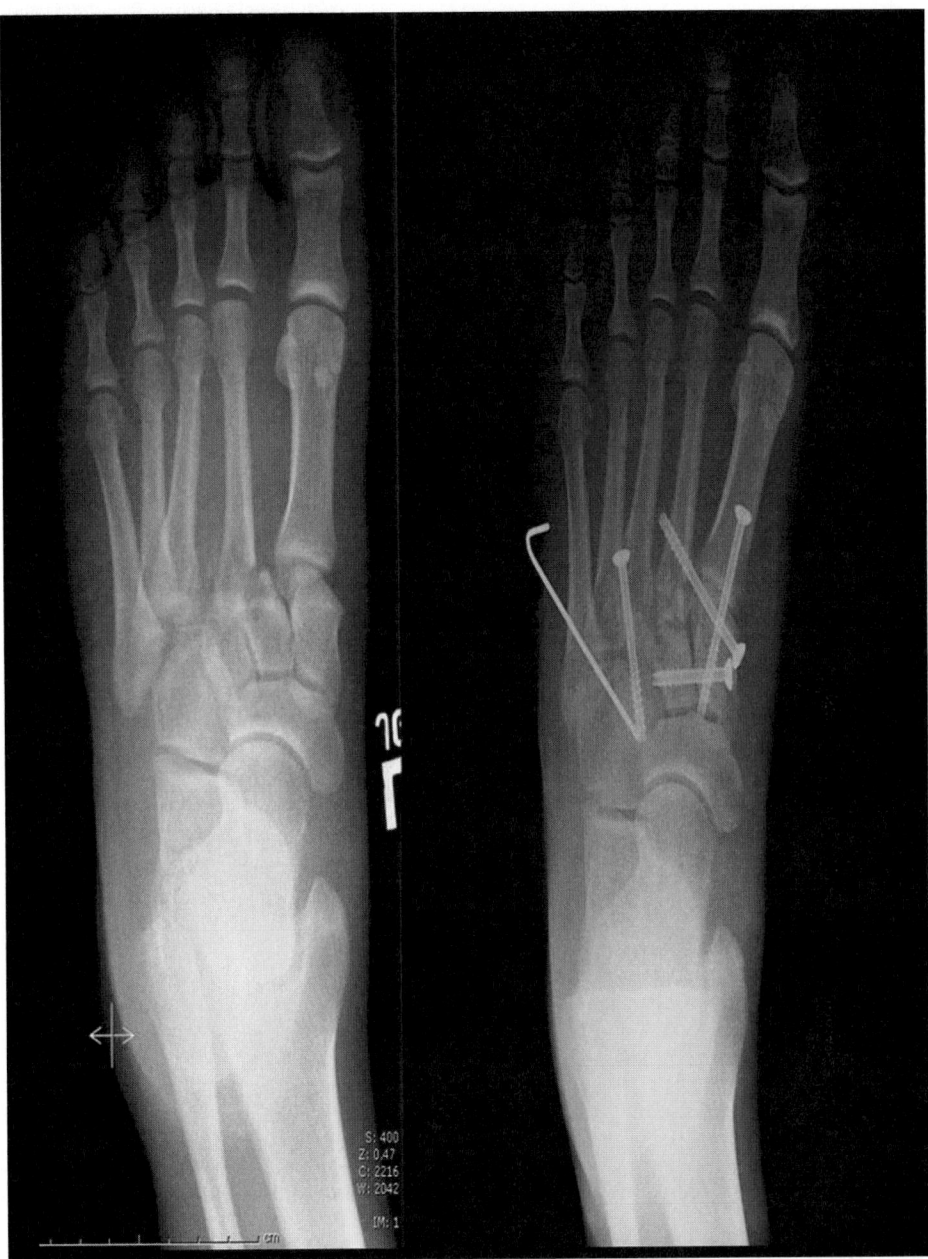

FIG. 43-9. X-ray images of a patient with a fracture dislocation of the tarsometatarsal joints of the foot, before and after reduction and internal fixation.

cant joint deformities. These usually are successfully managed by simple immobilization. Distal fractures of the metatarsal shaft, particularly the first metatarsal, are more often treated directly by internal fixation to ensure proper alignment of the weightbearing portion of these bones.

Fractures of the Fifth Metatarsal

Fractures of the fifth metatarsal merit special discussion. The very proximal fracture of the posterolateral tuberosity of the fifth metatarsal is usually the result of an avulsion mechanism. Such fractures do not traverse the shaft of the metatarsal and are successfully treated by simple immobilization. Slightly more distal fractures of the proximal metatarsal, however, require closer follow-up because malunions and nonunions are frequently a result and sometimes require internal fixation.

Fractures of the Metatarsal-Phalangeal Joints

Fractures of the metatarsal-phalangeal joints are common and usually are the result of direct trauma. Injuries to the metatarsalphalangeal joints and the proximal phalanx frequently are managed by "buddy taping" of the involved digit to an uninjured neighboring

toe. Injuries to the first metatarsal-phalangeal joint often are best treated with a rigid-soled shoe. Injuries to the first metatarsalphalangeal joint that involve injury to the articular surfaces are sometimes best treated by open reduction and internal fixation.

Fractures of the Ankle

Fractures of the ankle are extremely common. These fractures are always intra-articular. Because the ankle joint is a major weightbearing joint subject to large rotational loads, precise reconstruction of the joint is a very high priority.[4]

Anatomy of the Ankle

The ankle joint is comprised of the talus, tibia, and fibula. The talus normally fits immediately beneath the distal tibia and is restrained medially by the buttress that the medial malleolus provides. Laterally, the talus is restrained by the articular surface of the fibula which, in precise alignment with the distal tibia, allows for flexion and extension of the ankle. Ligamentous stability of the medial ankle is provided by the "deltoid" ligament that attaches to the medial malleolus of the tibia and talus. Stability of the talofibular joint is provided by the anterior talofibular ligament (a common site for sprains of the ankle), the calcaneal-fibular ligament, and the posterior talofibular ligaments.

Dislocations of the Ankle

Dislocations of the ankle are common. They usually occur in combination with significant fractures of the tibia or fibula. A much more rare injury would be a purely ligamentous injury that may allow either an anterior or posterior dislocation.

With or without an associated fracture, a dislocation of the ankle joint threatens the blood supply to the foot and requires prompt neurovascular evaluation. Whether or not an acute neurologic deficit or vascular compromise is identified, prompt relocation of the talus in its anatomic position beneath the tibia should be done as soon as possible. An ankle joint that remains dislocated puts the patient at risk for an evolving neurovascular injury and a possible compartment syndrome.

Ankle dislocation without associated fracture can be managed either operatively (with primary repair of the major stabilizing ligaments), or nonoperatively by immobilization as determined by physical examination, imaging, and the demonstrated stability of the talus beneath the tibia after relocation.

Lateral Malleolus Fractures

An isolated distal fibula fracture, often referred to as a *lateral malleolus fracture*, should be anatomically reduced whenever possible. This often can be accomplished by closed reduction and casting (Figs. 43-10 and 43-11).

If closed reduction maneuvers do not result in an anatomic or near-anatomic restoration of the anatomy of the ankle, precise open reduction and internal fixation is indicated. Even a disruption of as little as 1 mm in the position of the lateral malleolus can result in a

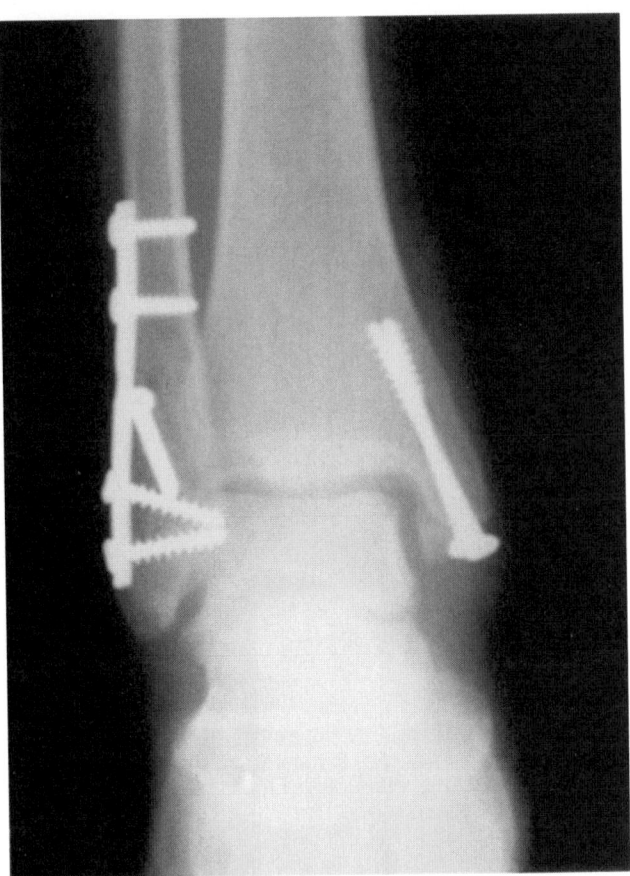

FIG. 43-11. Anteroposterior radiograph of a patient who has an open reduction and internal fixation of the bimalleolar ankle fracture.

lateral shift of the talus and a decreased contact area between the tibia and talus of almost 50% and can markedly accelerate degenerative arthritis. Surgical exposure of the distal fibula is by a lateral incision. Fracture fragments are precisely aligned and fixed in place generally using a screw and plate device. With accurate reduction and internal fixation, excellent function can result.

Isolated Medial Malleolar Fractures

An isolated fracture of the medial malleolus is caused in most cases by an avulsion of the malleolus. If the fracture is not displaced, or if it can be anatomically reduced by closed means, casting or bracing may be adequate and appropriate treatment. Surgical treatment of an isolated medial malleolus generally consists of exposure of the bones through a medial approach, precise anatomical alignment, and fixation using screws inserted from distal to proximal. Postoperative management will generally include postoperative casting or bracing.

Bimalleolar Fractures

The bimalleolar fracture is an injury that includes fracture of both the distal fibula and distal tibia. Such injuries often are accompanied by significant subluxation or even complete dislocation of the tibiotalar joint. Prompt reduction of the dislocation is indicated. Almost all such fractures are treated operatively to allow the best possible realignment of the fracture fragments and the joint anatomy.[5]

Posterior Malleolus Fracture

The posterior portion of the distal tibia (the posterior third of the tibiotalar articular surface) often is referred to as the *posterior malleolus*. Isolated fractures of the posterior malleolus are rare, but fractures of this weightbearing surface of the tibiotalar joint are frequently found in patients with fracture of both malleoli. This

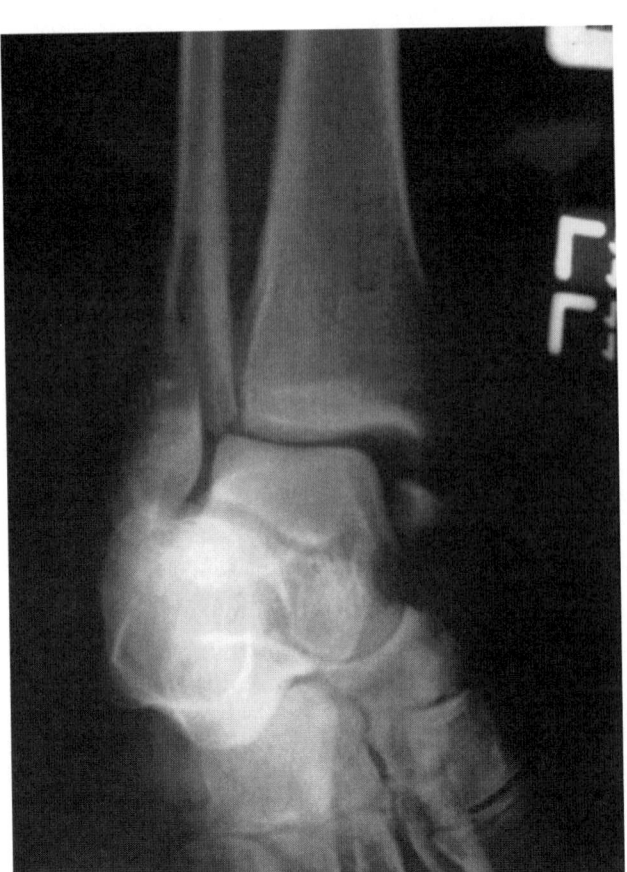

FIG. 43-10. Anteroposterior radiograph of a patient with a bimalleolar fracture.

injury can be called a *trimalleolar fracture*. If the fracture comprises more than one third of the tibiotalar joint or if such fractures have significant displacement, internal fixation of this posterior malleolar fracture fragment may be indicated.

Ankle Syndesmosis

The precise alignment of the tibia and the fibula are important to the function of the ankle joint. A robust ligamentous attachment of the two bones, the *ankle syndesmosis* is an important stabilizer of the ankle and generally extends at least 4 cm above the joint. Quite frequently, injuries to the tibiotalar joint also disrupt the syndesmosis, causing a splaying or widening of the tibia and fibula. Such injuries generally are managed with a "syndesmotic screw" inserted from lateral to medial, transfixing both fibula and tibia. Ligamentous healing generally is slower than bone healing, and such screws are, therefore, usually left in place for 8 to 12 weeks. Elective screw removal at that time is common, but the consequence of leaving the screw in place beyond 3 months is screw breakage. The possible morbidity caused by a broken screw in this area is minimal.

Acute Rupture of the Achilles Tendon

The gastrocsoleus muscle complex acting on the calcaneus through the Achilles tendon can result in very high forces, particularly with sporting activities that involve jumping or rapid changes of direction while running. The Achilles tendon can rupture.[6] This is apparent clinically as weakness in plantar flexion. The patient often notes an audible "pop" at the time of injury. Open reconstruction of the tendon is frequently performed, often using augmenting material (cadaver tendon or the autologous plantaris tendon). Operative reconstruction of this tendon does, however, have a significant and troublesome rate of wound complication such as local infection or skin necrosis. Accordingly, many practitioners manage this injury nonoperatively with casting or bracing. Either approach is reasonable.

Fractures of the Tibial Plafond: Pilon Fractures

High-energy fractures of the distal tibia and fibula that involve both the distal shaft of the tibia and the weightbearing surface are called *tibial plafond fractures* or, more commonly, *pilon fractures*. Due to the subcutaneous nature of these high energy fractures, skin complications, compartment syndromes, wound healing problems, and

nonunions frequently complicate the care of patients with pilon fractures, which represent one of the most difficult challenges in the entire field of orthopedic trauma (Fig. 43-12).

Pilon fractures almost always are displaced and are almost universally associated with significant soft tissue damage. Treatment nearly always involves open reduction and internal fixation of the bone fragments with as meticulous reconstruction of the ankle joint as possible. Immediate reconstructive surgery rarely is undertaken, however, because of the extremely high incidence of soft tissue complications. In most cases, the lower limb is stabilized by external fixation often with limited open reduction and internal fixation of the fibula to help establish and maintain anatomic length. A definitive reconstruction procedure on the tibia often is postponed until the acute swelling has resolved. This approach has been shown to lessen the incidence of soft tissue complications. With or without appropriate stabilization and timing, wound complications are common. Wound breakdown is seen in >10% of such injuries. The incidence of wound infection is high as are nonunion of the distal fragments. Posttraumatic arthritic joints are distressingly common.

Fractures of the Tibial Shaft

Fractures of the tibial shaft usually result from direct blows or torsional mechanisms.[7] The nearly subcutaneous position of the bone means that open fractures are commonly seen. Thus, inspection of the skin, particularly the anterior leg, is critically important. Fractures that result from a direct blow usually result in a transverse or oblique tibia injury often sparing the fibula. Torsional injury (frequent in skiers) will often lead to a spiral fracture of the tibia, often with associated fibular injury at the knee or the ankle. High-energy trauma to the limb can lead to comminuted fracture and extensive soft tissue injury.

Management of tibial shaft fracture can be accomplished by a simple closed reduction and long leg cast immobilization. Advancing the patient to a functional brace within 4 to 6 weeks often is recommended. Nonunion of fractures managed closed is a significant problem, and cast immobilization, when used, usually is necessary for approximately 3 to 4 months. Intramedullary nailing of the tibia is now commonly performed and, indeed, is the preferred form of treatment more often than not. An intramedullary nail is inserted across the fracture site, proceeding proximal to distal. Small diameter nails ("nonreamed nails") can be impacted across the fracture site

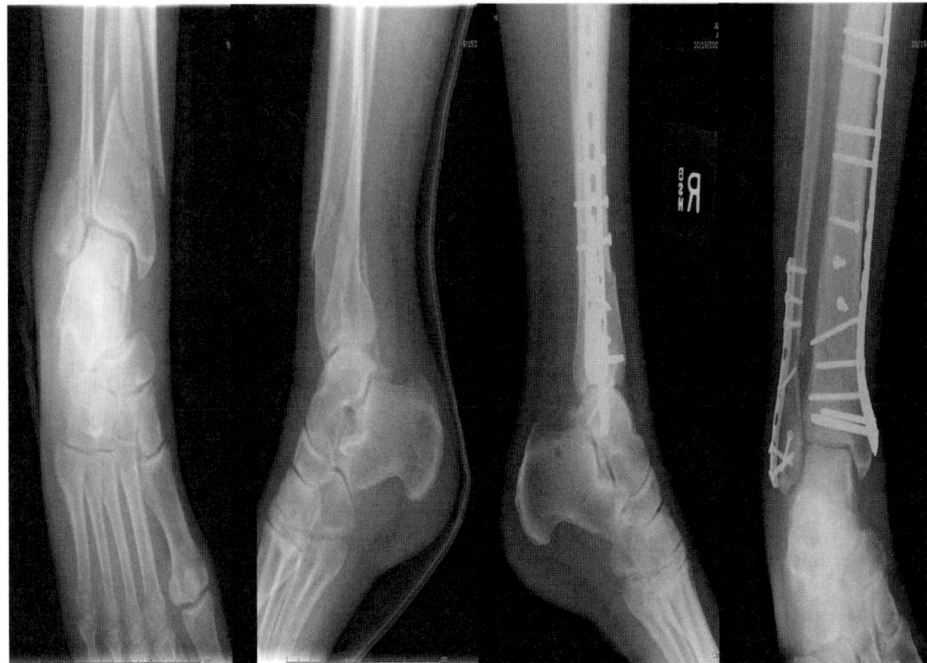

FIG. 43-12. Radiographs of a severe fracture of the distal tibia and fibula, before and after open reduction and internal fixation. High-energy trauma to the distal leg can frequently lead to neurovascular injury, compartment syndrome, and wound healing problems.

directly. Another alternative, particularly with more unstable fractures, is a rigid intramedullary nail where reaming devices of graduated diameter are passed across the fracture site, before inserting a larger nail. These larger nails often are manufactured with screw holes positioned distal and proximal to accept transfixing distal and proximal interlocking screws to assist in controlling length and rotation.

Fractures of the Tibia Plateau

The upper surface of the tibia, which articulates with the condyles of the femur, has a relatively flat surface and is usually referred to as the *tibia plateau*.[8] Fractures of this large articular surface can represent a challenge. The weightbearing demands of this surface are high, and the fractures are often accompanied by crushing and impaction of the cartilage menisci and the underlying cancellous bone, making reconstruction particularly challenging as several of the many pieces of this three dimensional puzzle can be partially crushed (Fig. 43-13). Fractures can involve the medial or the lateral plateau or both and often are accompanied by a significant angular deformity. Minimally displaced fractures can be managed nonoperatively with a cast or a brace. Criteria for nonoperative treatment include <3 mm of documented articular step-off and ligamentous stability of the knee when held in extension. More severe fractures with displaced articular fragments generally are managed operatively by anterior, medial, lateral, or combined surgical approaches and direct internal fixation of the fracture fragments. This can be done by transfixing screws or screw-plate devices or, most often, a combination. Because of crushing of the metaphyseal bone, bone grafting (local, iliac crest, or allograft) often is necessary to reconstruct the original anatomy. Reconstruction of ligaments and menisci also sometimes is indicated.

Fracture involving this large articular weightbearing surface often leads to chronic stiffness of the joint or early arthritis. The treating surgeon must be alert for associated injures such as compartment syndrome of the leg or associated peroneal nerve injury.

Dislocation of the Knee

A dislocation of the knee (dislocation of the joint between the femur and the tibia should not to be confused with a dislocation of the patella) is a devastating injury, and is nearly always the result of a high-energy injury mechanism. Massive ligamentous injury is necessary to allow a dislocation, which can happen in any direction (anterior, posterior, medial, lateral, or rotatory). This injury often is initially unappreciated as after a knee dislocation a spontaneous reduction, or relocation by the initial treating personnel may delay the diagnosis.

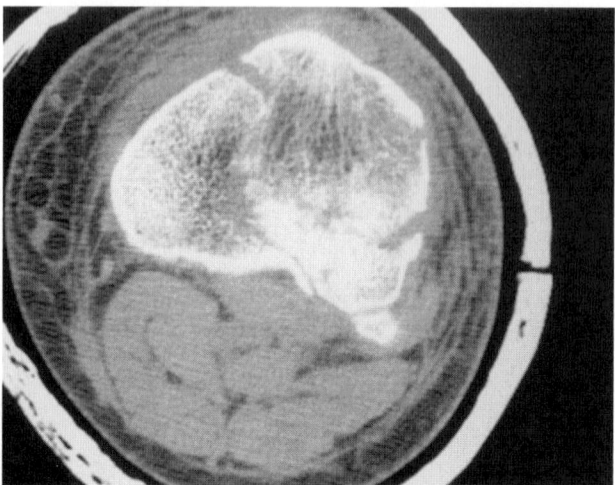

FIG. 43-13. Computed tomography image of a proximal tibial fracture. The details of the fracture are more easily seen with a computed tomography scan. This improves preoperative surgical planning.

Nonetheless, immediate prompt relocation of the knee is a high priority in the emergency management of this condition. Dislocation of the knee has a high associated incidence of neurovascular injury and compartment syndrome. Even if a frank arterial injury is not present, kinking or compression of the vessel and intimal flap tears due to the dislocation can limit the blood flow to the limb. After relocation, immediate assessment of pulses is necessary. Prompt radiographic visualization of the arterial supply to the lower limb is indicated when pulses are deficient. Close attention to the possibility of an evolving compartment syndrome is necessary as well. Depending on clinical assessment and on the extent of the ligamentous injuries, on some occasions, nonoperative management using immobilization is reasonable. In most cases, however, repair of the ligamentous structures with special attention to the posterior capsule is undertaken.

Late stiffness of the knee, and, occasionally, late instability of the knee, are potential complications of this devastating injury. If close attention is not paid to the strong possibility of arterial injury or compartment syndrome, death of the limb can result.

Dislocation of the Patella

Dislocation of the patella, usually in the lateral direction, is a relatively common injury in adolescents, particularly adolescent athletes. Treatment consists of manual reduction of the patella, generally performed with the knee in full extension. Initial treatment is immobilization in extension for an approximate 6-week interval. The most common complication of this injury is recurrent dislocation.

Fractures of the Patella

Fractures of the patella can result from failure of the patella under tension, which usually leads to a nondisplaced or mildly displaced simple transverse fracture. Avulsion fractures of the upper pole also are possible. Direct blows to the knee as from a dashboard to a nonrestrained automobile passenger often lead to comminuted fractures that can involve large areas of the articular surface. Minimally displaced fractures can be managed nonoperatively with a brace in extension. Comminuted fractures, particularly with displaced fragments, may be best managed by open reduction and internal fixation.

Fractures of the Distal Femur

Fractures of the distal femur can present a variety of challenges to the orthopedic trauma surgeon. Simple transverse fractures of the metaphysis do occur without intra-articular involvement (Fig. 43-14). These are less common, however, than are injuries that involve one or both condyles of the femur. As with all intra-articular fractures, great effort is extended to anatomically reduce the fracture fragments and precisely reconstruct and realign the joint surfaces. In most such injuries, fractures are managed with internal fixation, most commonly with transfixing screws combined with either medial or lateral plate fixation. As with all intra-articular fractures, complications can include loss of reduction, nonunion, or malunion. The most common late complication is osteoarthritis.

Fractures of the Femoral Shaft

Fractures of the femoral shaft more frequently are caused by high-energy trauma. It is common for such patients to have associated injuries. Almost all femoral shaft injuries are managed surgically, usually by intramedullary nailing.[9] Intramedullary nails are inserted usually after sequential reaming. They usually are inserted proximal to distal through an entry point immediately medial to the greater trochanter or the proximal femur (Fig. 43-15). In some situations, it is preferable to use a "retrograde" approach where a similar rod is inserted distal to proximal with an entry point within the knee joint (this procedure requires a knee arthrotomy). Intramedullary nails often are sufficient to control length and rotation. In severely comminuted fractures, another situation where additional stability is desired, many available intramedullary rod systems have proximal and distal holes to allow transfixing "locking" screws to be inserted

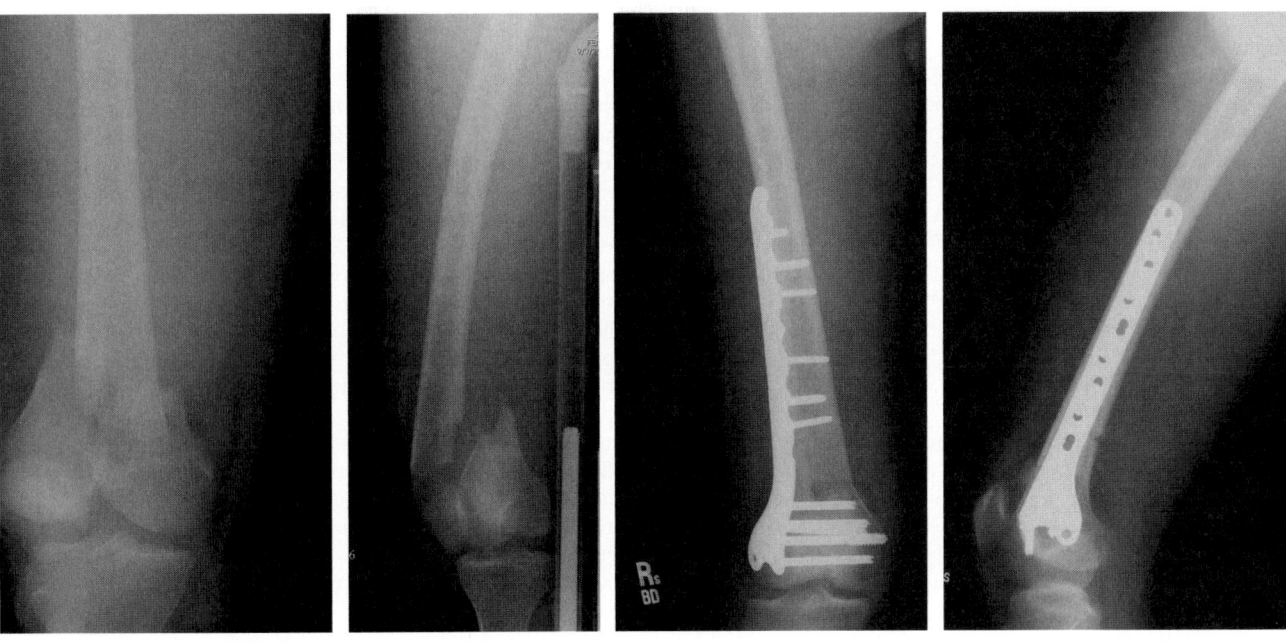

FIG. 43-14. Radiographic images of a supracondylar femur fracture, before and after open reduction and internal fixation. Note that the fracture cleaved the femoral condyle apart, requiring reconstruction of the distal articular surface.

in a bicortical manner to transfix the whole intramedullary rod. This provides outstanding rotational and axial control.

In some unusual cases, the use of an external fixator may be indicated in treating a femoral shaft fracture. The usual indication for this is a polytrauma patient with other severe life-threatening injuries where stability of the limb is of lesser priority than other surgical procedures. External fixation may also be a good treatment choice for patients with severe open fractures of the femoral shaft that require wound care or access. Finally, external fixation also is considered in patients who have major ipsilateral vascular injuries.

Fractures of the Hip

Fractures of the hip (proximal femur) are extremely common. They are major injuries with significant risk of morbidity and mortality. It is

important for all of the physicians involved in treating a patient with an acute hip fracture that the severity of the injury not be underestimated. The acute survival rate from this injury is approximately 90%. Various authors have reported that the mortality rate for patients sustaining a hip fracture can be as high as 25 to 50% when assessed 1-year postinjury.

As is well known, hip fractures are strongly associated with antecedent osteoporosis. Osteoporosis, the advanced age of many of the patients, and associated medical comorbidities make survival from this injury a concern for every such patient. Physicians taking care of these patients must include careful medical assessment and follow-up on medical comorbidities. Such concerns must also extend to the social welfare of the patient after hospital discharge. Decreased mobility, pain, and disruption of routine can lead to deep vein thrombosis, pneumonia, pressure ulcers, and depression. It is also important to understand that a hip fracture is often a precipitating life event, in that a patient so

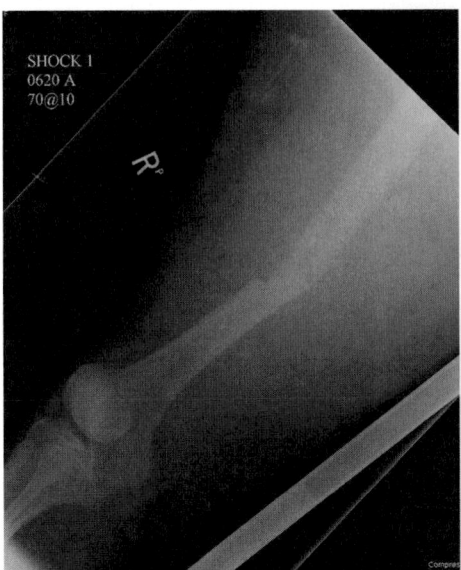
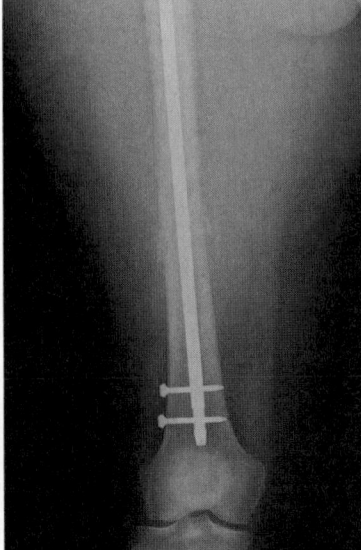
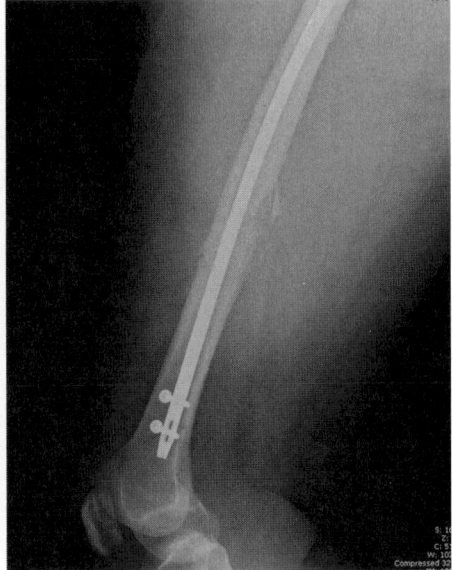

FIG. 43-15. An oblique fracture of the shaft of the femur, before and after reamed intramedullary fixation with a stout nail and interlocking screws. This treatment allows near immediate ambulation for the patient.

afflicted may transition from independent living to assisted living or nursing home situations.

Although not necessarily part of the immediate acute management, essentially all patients sustaining a hip fracture should be evaluated for osteoporosis and treated appropriately for their mineral densities postoperatively.

CLASSIFICATION OF FRACTURES OF THE HIP

Fractures of the hip generally are classified as three distinct types: femoral neck fractures, intertrochanteric fractures, and subtrochanteric fractures.

Femoral Neck Fractures

Fractures of the femoral neck comprise approximately one half of all fractures of the proximal femur. They are most common in elderly patients. The anatomy of the hip joint is an important consideration in the management of this fracture. The hip joint capsule extends from the rim of the acetabulum to the base of the neck of the femur. Fractures of the femoral neck are, therefore, entirely intrascapular. The blood supply to the femoral neck is accordingly quite precarious. In some adult patients, there is a limited blood supply from the ligamentum teres of the acetabulum, which contains a small branch of the obturator artery. The major route for blood supply to the femoral head in all patients (the only blood supply to the femoral head in most patients) is derived from vessels within and along the surface of the bone of the femoral neck.

Femoral neck fractures, as they are entirely within the joint capsule, usually are not associated with hemodynamically significant blood loss. Fracture hematomas are contained within the hip capsule. When the femoral neck fracture is displaced, disruption of the blood flow to the femoral head is virtually certain. Accordingly, osteonecrosis of the femoral head in displaced fractures is nearly inevitable.[10] It is often better for the patient to proceed directly to prosthetic replacement of the femoral head. This operation is called a *hemiarthroplasty* and involves replacing the femoral neck and head with a metal and plastic prosthesis that will fit within the native acetabulum. This generally is done by a posterior approach to the hip, exposure and entry into the joint capsule, removal of the doomed femoral head, resection of the residual femoral neck to allow reaming of the proximal medullary canal, and insertion of an appropriately sized prosthesis. After placement of the prosthesis, the artificial head is relocated into the native acetabulum, tissues are opposed, and the skin closed. Although this technique allows near immediate weightbearing on the involved limb, it has a significant physiologic stress for the patients. The secure placement of the femoral component within the proximal shaft of the femur can be done using polymethylmethacrylate bone cement that creates a mantle about the shaft of the prosthesis. This has the advantage of immediate, secure fixation of the femoral component. A disadvantage of this technique is that the polymethylmethacrylate cement is an attractive substrate for bacterial biofilms should the patient acquire a perioperative infection. An alternative to the use of polymethylmethacrylate cement is the use of a "press fit" prosthesis. In such noncemented techniques, more precisely shaped protheses are impacted into the proximal femur to obtain a tight interference fit. One disadvantage of this prosthesis type in treatment of a hip fracture is that obtaining a tight "press fit" of the prosthesis does involve some risk of an iatrogenic femur fracture (Fig. 43-16).

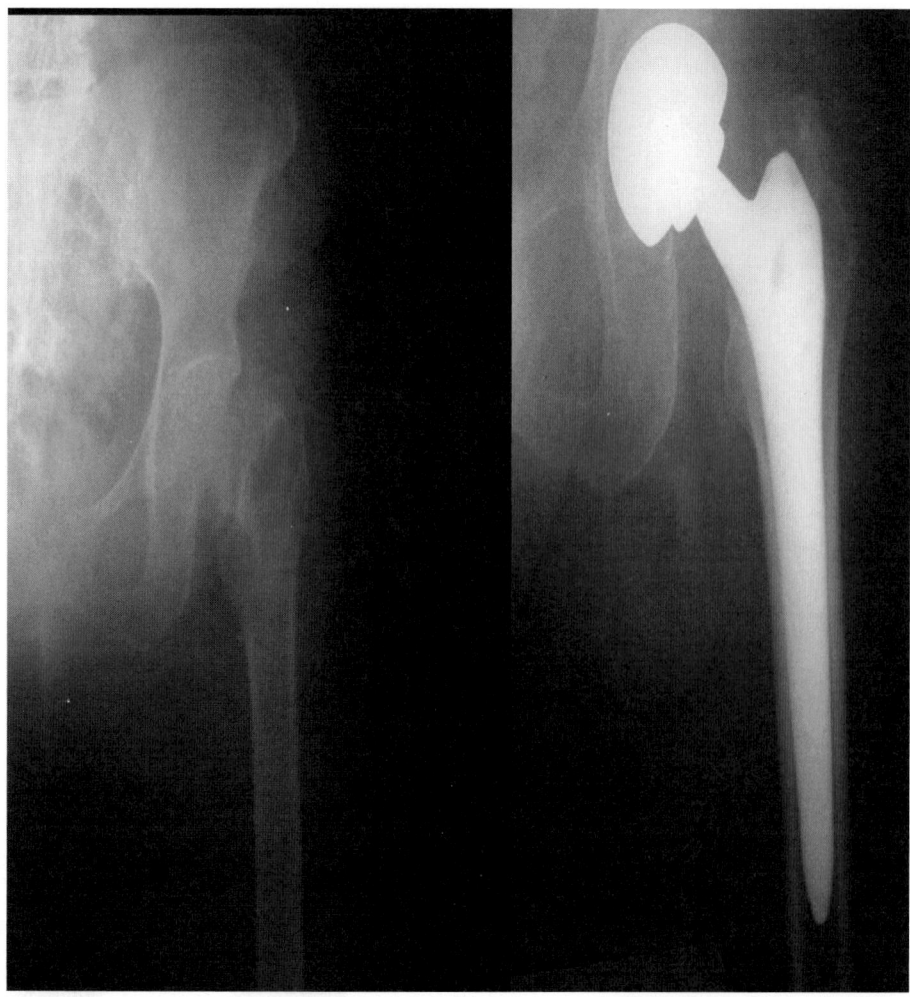

FIG. 43-16. A displaced fracture of the femoral neck. This injury so predictably leads to osteonecrosis of the femoral head that it is best managed (as shown) by hemiarthroplasty. In this case, a noncemented implant was selected.

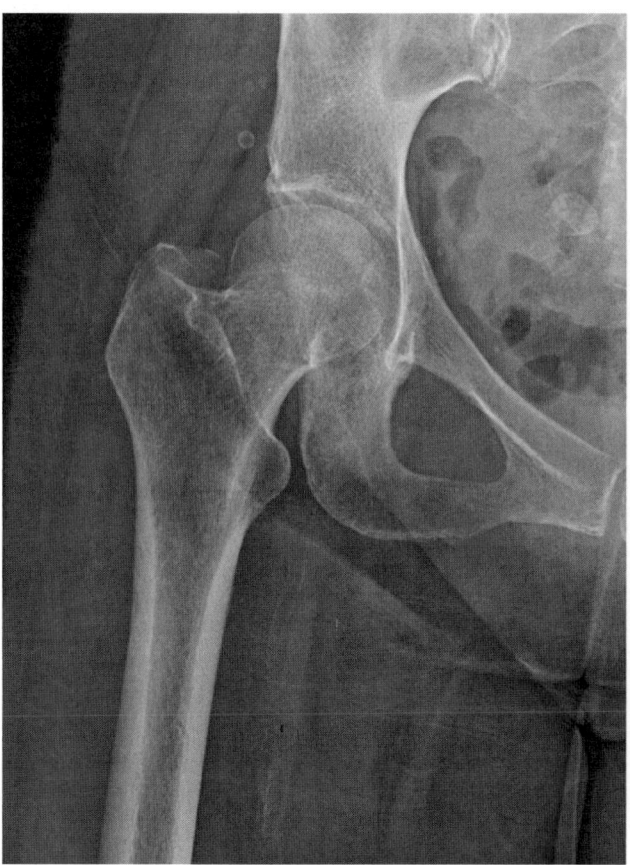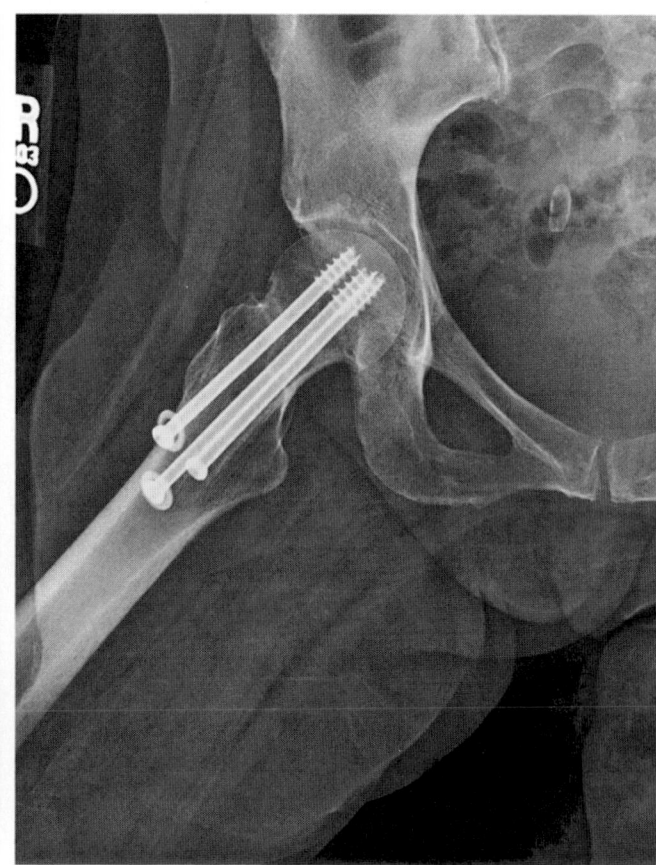

FIG. 43-17. Pre- and postoperative radiographs of a patient with a displaced fracture of the femoral neck and pre-existing severe arthritic change in the acetabulum. The patient was managed by performing a total hip replacement, with replacement of both the acetabular surface and the femoral head and neck.

The placement of the arthroplasty prosthesis to replace the proximal femur is a good option for the patient only if the acetabular side of the joint is healthy. If the acetabular side of the joint is severely arthritic, wear of the prosthetic femoral head on the acetabulum is predicted to be unacceptably painful. Accordingly, in patients with significant osteoarthritic change that preceded their femoral neck fracture event, proceeding directly to a total hip arthroplasty with replacement of both the femoral and acetabular sides of the joint may be the best choice for the patient. Discussion of the technique is found in the Total Hip Arthroplasty section of this chapter.

Nondisplaced or impacted fractures of the femoral head can occur without critical disruption of the blood supply to the femoral head. Accordingly, such fractures most frequently are managed by internal fixation in situ using three or four screws (Fig. 43-17) inserted through the cortex of the lateral proximal femur, which transfix the fracture site and engage the femoral head. Placement of such screws can be done through very small skin incisions and, in most cases, do not require any direct exposure of the bone. These procedures result in minimal blood loss and often can lead to a very rapid postoperative recovery.

Intertrochanteric Fractures of the Hip

Fractures of the hip also frequently occur in the region between the greater and the lesser trochanters. Such fractures are referred to as *intertrochanteric fractures of the hip*. They may represent a single fracture line, or several discrete fragments may be created. A discrete fragment representing the lesser trochanter is a common result. Unlike femoral neck fractures, fractures of the trochanteric region of the femur usually result in substantial blood loss that may have hemodynamic consequences for the patient. Monitoring the patient's hemodynamic indices and hematocrit are important in any patient with an intertrochanteric fracture. Like fractures of the

femoral neck, almost all fractures of the intertrochanteric region are managed operatively, because nonoperative treatment has an extremely high incidence of complication. Treatment of the intertrochanteric fracture essentially always involves internal fixation. This can be done using a fracture table whereby the alignment of the lower limb can be mechanically held in a reduced position while surgery is performed. Alternatively, it can be performed in a supine position on a radiolucent table using manual reduction methods.

In most cases, a lateral approach to the hip is made and fixation of the fracture is achieved by transfixing the trochanter and the femoral neck and head with a large screw. This can be placed in conjunction with a screw and plate device (together called a *sliding hip screw*). Another alternative is a cephalomedullary device where fixed angle screws engage a short intramedullary nail inserted proximal to distal through the proximal region of the trochanter or through the piriformis fossa. With placement of either device (the choice of which usually is dictated by the fracture morphology), the patient is capable of near immediate postoperative weightbearing.

Subtrochanteric Fractures and Femoral Shaft Fractures

Subtrochanteric fractures of the hip are generally the result of higher-energy injury mechanisms than femoral neck or intertrochanteric fractures. They are, accordingly, more likely to occur with other bone or soft tissue injuries. In most cases, subtrochanteric fractures are managed by an intramedullary device, which may be inserted with or without reaming. As muscle attachments to the proximal fragments result in forceful displacement of the fragments, open resection often is necessary. Almost all fractures of the diaphysis of the femur are managed with the use of an intramedullary rod. These are placed after sequential reaming. In

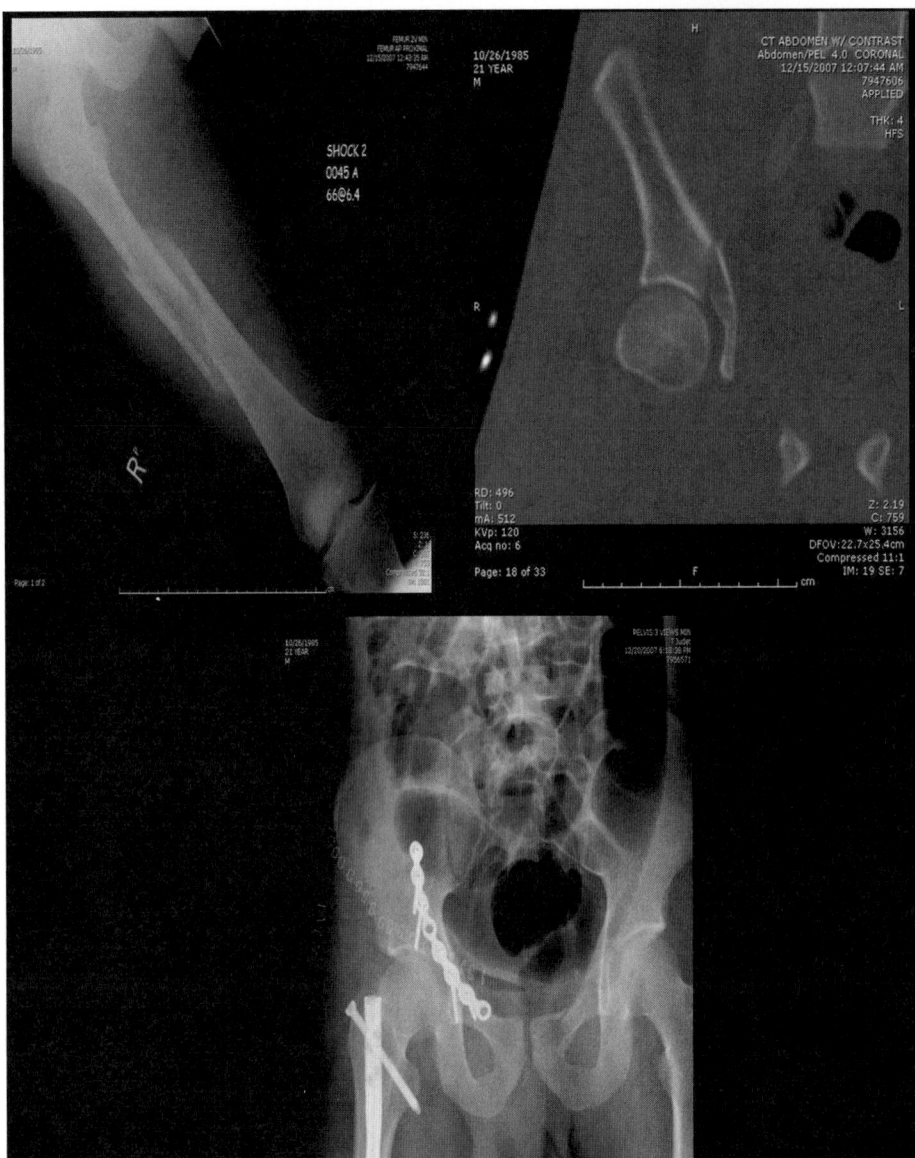

FIG. 43-18. Computed tomographic image (*top*) and x-ray (*bottom*) of a patient with a spiral fracture of the right femur with an ipsilateral acetabular fracture. X-ray images postoperatively demonstrate the reamed nail with locking screw that internally fixes the femur, as well as the acetabular plate fixation. Note also the pubic ramus fracture that did not require surgical treatment.

many cases, the intramedullary device is augmented by either locking screws or a transfixing screw that engages the femoral neck. In most cases, immediate postoperative weightbearing is possible.

Hip Dislocation

Hip dislocation is a severe, high-energy injury that frequently is associated with multitrauma patients. Most dislocations of the hip occur in the posterior direction. Such injuries frequently result in neurovascular compromise. Indeed, an isolated hip dislocation may represent a life-threatening injury. Emergent reduction is strongly indicated. This usually can be accomplished closed. If this is unsuccessful, prompt open reduction is recommended.

Hip dislocations often are associated with acetabular fractures and, less commonly but significantly, with fractures of the femoral head (Fig. 43-18). Obviously, a fracture of the femoral head with associated acetabular injury and/or femoral head fracture is a very serious injury indeed. Common complications with any of these injuries are posttraumatic arthritis, osteonecrosis, and recurrent dislocation. Associated neurovascular injuries are common.[11] Acetabular fractures can occur with or without frank hip dislocation. Acetabular fractures frequently are seen in association with other fractures of the pelvis (Fig. 43-19). Significant blood loss from bone bleeding is a major concern with these injuries.

Operative treatment of the acetabular fracture is directed at reconstruction and internal fixation of the original acetabular anatomy and the creation of a stable hip joint.[12] The acetabulum can be exposed through an anterior, lateral, or posterior approach depending on the osseous injury. Surgical treatment of an acetabular fracture is a major undertaking, requiring special training and experience.

PELVIC TRAUMA

Pubic Ramus Fractures

Pubic ramus fractures usually are seen after minor trauma in older patients with osteoporosis. Such fractures usually present with diffuse anterior pelvic pain and may or may not occur with an identifiable traumatic event. Tenderness to gentle lateral compression can be a useful physical examination maneuver. Pubic ramus fractures are frequently associated with concurrent sacral fractures. Vertical fractures through the sacral ala often involving multiple sacral foramina frequently occur with this injury. Interestingly, the sacral fractures are often quite nondisplaced and may be difficult or impossible to see on plain x-ray images. Nondisplaced fractures of the sacrum and minimally displaced fractures of the pelvic rami usually are managed with analgesics and mobilization. These injuries are compatible with full weightbearing. An apparent slight pelvic

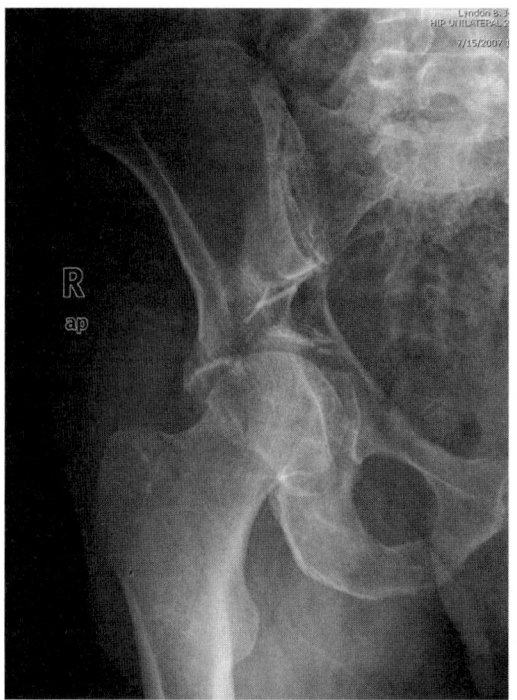
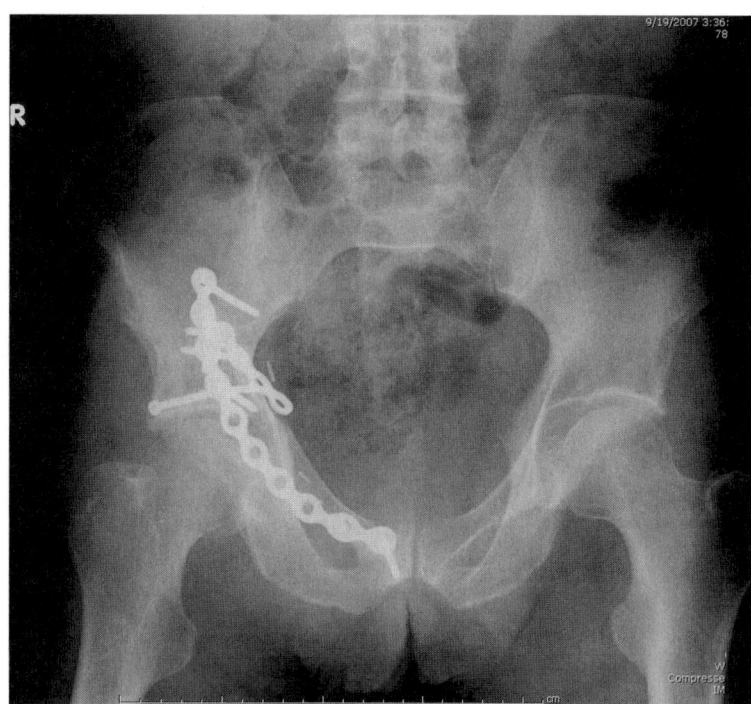

FIG. 43-19. X-ray images of a patient with a right acetabulum fracture, before and after operative reconstruction. Note the protrusion of the head of the femur into the pelvis before surgery.

fracture in a young patient without osteoporosis, however, should trigger a more robust search for associated injuries or malignancy.

Fractures of the Pelvic Ring

Fractures of the pelvic ring are an unfortunate but frequent consequence of high-energy trauma.[13,14] Vertical fractures through the posterior elements of the pelvis or sacrum associated with anterior ring injury may result in "open booking" of the pelvis. Vertical translation of large portions of the pelvis with such injuries are all too often associated with major visceral injury and potentially catastrophic blood loss. Injuries to the bladder, ureter, urethra, and kidney also frequently occur in association with these injuries. Any associated hematuria must be aggressively investigated. Unfortunately, patients with such injuries frequently present with hemodynamic difficulties due to hypovolemia and blood loss. Sometimes, this can be improved by the urgent application of an external fixator to engage the ilia bilaterally. Compression and stabilization of the pelvis can help limit bone bleeding. Reconstruction of major pelvic disruption of this kind is a major undertaking and usually is performed 3 to 10 days after the initial injury to allow bone bleeding to stabilize.[15] These reconstructive procedures are clinically challenging and must be extremely well planned. They should only be undertaken by orthopedic surgeons with special training and experience with this injury (Fig. 43-20).

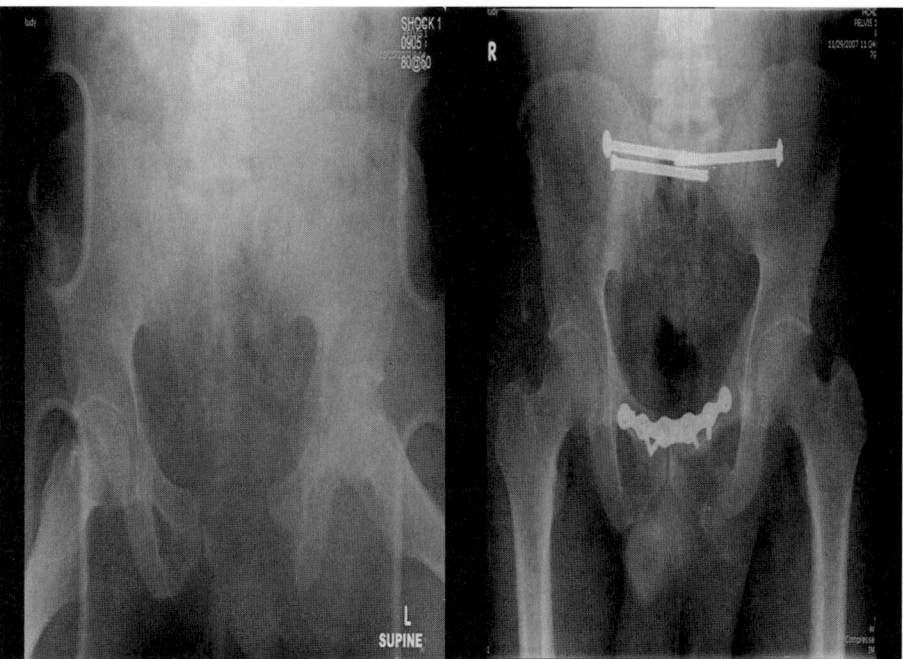

FIG. 43-20. Pre- and postoperative image of a patient with displaced fractures of the pubis and the sacro-iliac joint. Such injuries are the result of high-energy trauma and are frequently associated with visceral injury and severe blood loss.

FRACTURES OF THE SHOULDER

Fractures of the Clavicle

Fractures of the medial third of the clavicle are rare. Often what appears to be a fracture of the medial clavicle is actually a dislocation of the sternoclavicular joint. When anteriorly displaced, this injury, while painful, requires only symptomatic treatment. In contrast, posterior dislocation of the sternoclavicular joint can impinge the great vessels and may be managed by closed reduction. With general anesthesia, the arm is abducted and a lateral force is applied, and a towel, clip, or bone holding clamp can be used to apply anterior forces on the clavicle that can relocate this joint. These maneuvers should be undertaken only when a surgeon is available for any associated great vessel injury. Fortunately, such injuries are rare (Fig. 43-21).

Fractures of the middle third of the clavicle are quite common. Indeed, they are one of the most commonly seen fractures in an orthopedic practice. A fracture of the clavicle often is apparent on visual inspection, as the middle third of the clavicle is virtually subcutaneous. Fortunately, such injuries are rarely associated with skin penetration. Nonunions of the midshaft of the clavicle do occur, although they are rare. Accordingly, symptomatic treatment with mild analgesic medication and a sling is usually sufficient treatment.

Fractures of the Distal Clavicle

Fractures of the distal third of the clavicle can be more troublesome. When such fractures are displaced, it is frequently the result of concomitant rupture of the coracoclavicular ligaments. A significantly displaced clavicle may impinge the shoulder musculature and interposed soft tissue may result in nonunion. Accordingly, closed reduction, pinning, and/or open reduction and internal fixation of distal clavicle fractures often is recommended. In any surgical treatment of the clavicle, the proximity of the lung, the great vessel, and the brachial plexus must be kept in mind.

Fractures of the Scapula

Fractures of the scapula can result from direct blows to the shoulder or from falls onto the arm. Most scapula fractures are managed conservatively with exceptions made for those that have significant involvement of the glenoid. In such cases, open reduction and internal fixation using screws and small plates generally is recommended. These procedures usually are performed through a posterior approach.

Fractures of the Proximal Humerus

Fractures of the proximal humerus are common.[16] This is a frequent event in older individuals with osteoporosis but can result from significant trauma to younger individuals as well.

Minimally displaced fracture or impacted fractures of the femoral neck are best managed by immobilization with a shoulder immobilizer brace, a sling, or a sling and swath. Displaced fractures of the neck and humerus without a great deal of comminution often are managed by intramedullary internal fixation inserted from distal to proximal. This approach can be difficult in patients with osteoporosis, as the metaphyseal bone of the humerus is often quite porous.

Fractures of the proximal humerus, which involve the humeral head, are a particularly difficult problem. A large portion of the humeral head is covered with articular cartilage, and fracture events often will lead to up to four discrete fragments as classified by Dr. Neer.[17] When there is significant displacement of these fragments, leaving large pieces of articular bone without blood supply, avascular necrosis (osteonecrosis) is likely to occur. Accordingly, such fractures with displaced interarticular fragments are usually most appropriately managed by hemiarthroplasty; the humeral head is replaced with a prosthesis affixed to the humeral shaft with an intramedullary extension. Unfortunately, hemiarthroplasty procedures do not completely restore normal strength and range of motion to the shoulder; however, it generally gives a very functional result and is certainly preferable to the complications that ensue from an osteonecrosis of the humeral head.

Fractures of the Humeral Shaft

Fractures of the humeral shaft can result from falls or from direct trauma. They are most usually managed by open reduction and internal fixation with a stout screw-plate device. Intramedullary fixation is also an option, but insertion of an intramedullary device is more challenging in the humerus than in other long bones because of the specific anatomy of the elbow and shoulder (Fig. 43-22).

Any treatment plan for a diaphyseal fracture of the humerus must take into consideration the anatomy of the radial nerve that spirals down the arm in contact with the humerus. Thus, the radial

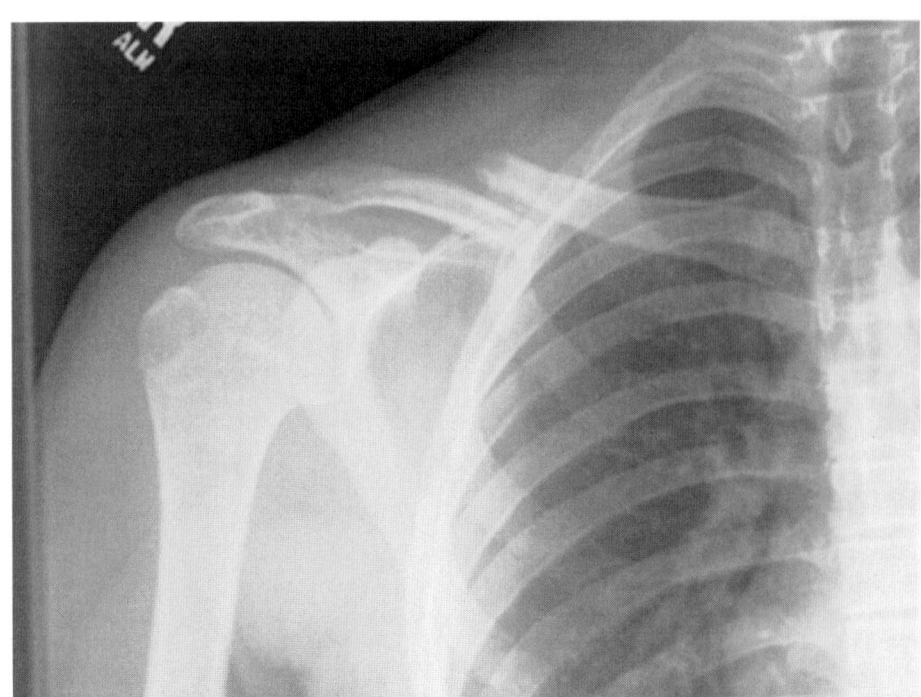

FIG. 43-21. Anteroposterior radiograph of a patient with a fractured clavicle. As usual, there is elevation of the medial fragment and shortening of the clavicle. This fracture will heal, and the function will be excellent with closed treatment. The patient can be treated with a sling.

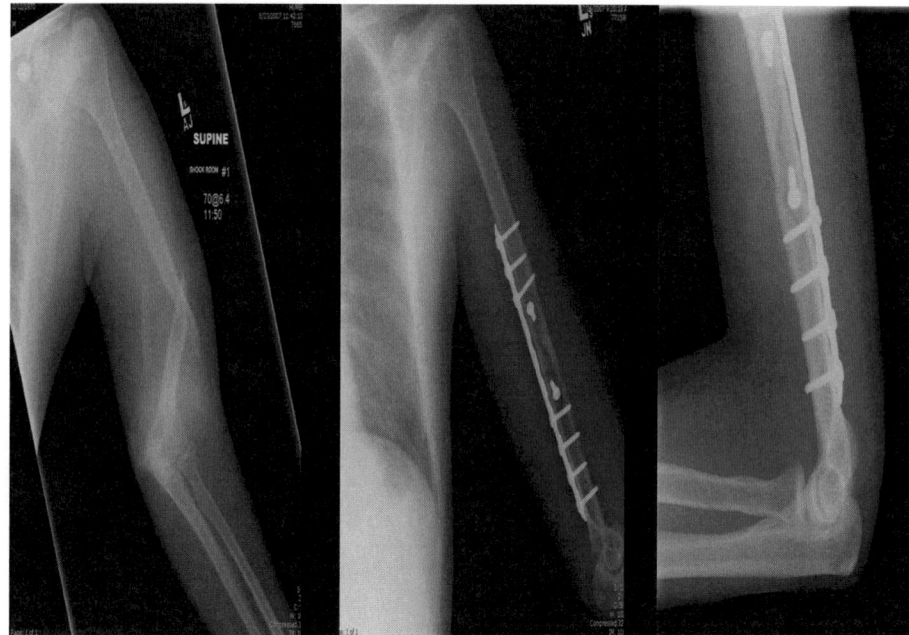

FIG. 43-22. X-ray images of a comminuted spiral fracture of the shaft of the humerus, before and after open reduction and internal fixation using a plate and screws. This injury is frequently associated with neurovascular compromise; particularly at risk is the radial nerve.

nerve is at great risk for injury both at the time of the injury and at the time of surgical treatment.[18] Careful attention to the neurovascular status of the limb, particularly of the radial nerve, is a strong concern in the management of these injuries.[19]

FRACTURES OF THE ELBOW AND FOREARM

Fractures of the Distal Humerus

Fractures of the distal humerus in adult patients thankfully do not involve the articular surface of the humerus nearly as often as those seen in pediatric practice. An extra-articular supracondylar humeral fracture in favorable cases can be managed by immobilization, although, to ensure good control of these fracture fragments and to prevent subsequent displacement, such fractures most often are managed by internal fixation. This can be accomplished by either a posterior medial or lateral surgical approach, depending on fracture morphology. With extensive comminution, combined approaches may be considered. When such fractures have an intra-articular component, precise reconstruction of the joints is, of course, a high priority. The elbow joint, formed by three long bones, the radius, ulna, and humerus, can present the surgeon with a difficult reconstructive problem. In most cases, it is useful to reconstruct the articular surface by separately and precisely placing screws to restore the articular anatomy. Once this is done, the distal fragments can then be affixed to the humeral shaft by appropriate screw-plate devices.

It should be noted that, in some difficult cases of articular fractures of the distal humerus, an olecranon osteotomy (deliberate creation of an olecranon fracture) can be a good way to visualize the trochlea to assist the surgeon in reconstructing an intra-articular fracture of the distal humerus. When this is accomplished, the olecranon then can be fixed as discussed in Fractures of the Olecranon below.

Fractures of the Olecranon

The proximal ulna and the olecranon fossa articulate with the trochlea of the distal humerus. This joint provides much of the bony stability of the joint. Fractures of the olecranon are common and may result from avulsion mechanisms, falls, or in rare cases, blows to the elbow. Very small and minimally displaced fracture fragments of the olecranon may be successfully managed by immobilization alone. In many cases, reconstruction of the joint can be accomplished with a single leg screw inserted from proximal to distal or a cerclage wire and with pins. In some cases with severe

comminution, simple excision of the fracture fragment may also yield a highly functional elbow. Even where properly placed, the olecranon fixation devices are often symptomatic due to its subcutaneous location. Accordingly, hardware removal procedures after fractures have healed is often a consideration.

Fractures of the Radial Head

Fractures of the radial head are common injuries. In many cases, a single fracture line is present, and one or two transfixing screws inserted through a lateral approach can provide adequate fixation. Where reconstruction is difficult, excision of the radial head can be considered. Removal of the radial head may, in some individuals, lead to proximal migration of the radius. In some unfortunate patients, wrist symptoms can develop as a result. Reconstruction of the radial head and/or replacement with one of a number of prosthetic devices is now receiving more attention. Some controversy does surround this specific issue.

Fractures of the Ulnar Shaft

Fractures of either the radius or the ulna within the forearm can represent significant diagnostic and treatment challenges. Careful evaluation of both the elbow and the wrist is essential when assessing these injuries. It must be kept in mind that the precise anatomy of the shafts of these bones also is necessary for pronation and supination of the forearm. It is very common for a radial or an ulnar fracture to be associated with a concomitant wrist or elbow injury or a subtle fracture or dislocation of its neighboring long bone.

Fractures of the ulnar shaft are common and usually result from a direct blow to the ulnar forearm. The ulna in the forearm is subcutaneous and vulnerable to blows. The name *night stick fracture* is applied to the diaphyseal fractures of the ulna that result from a direct blow. They are due to one common mechanism, that of a direct blow by a club or night stick.

Such fractures in the ulna shaft usually are managed nonsurgically with the use of a cast. Proximal ulnar shaft fractures or those with significant angulation may be managed by open reduction and internal fixation.

Fracture of the Ulna and the Radius (Fracture of Both Bones of the Forearm)

Fractures of the shafts of both bones of the forearm are common injuries, sometimes associated with high-energy mechanisms

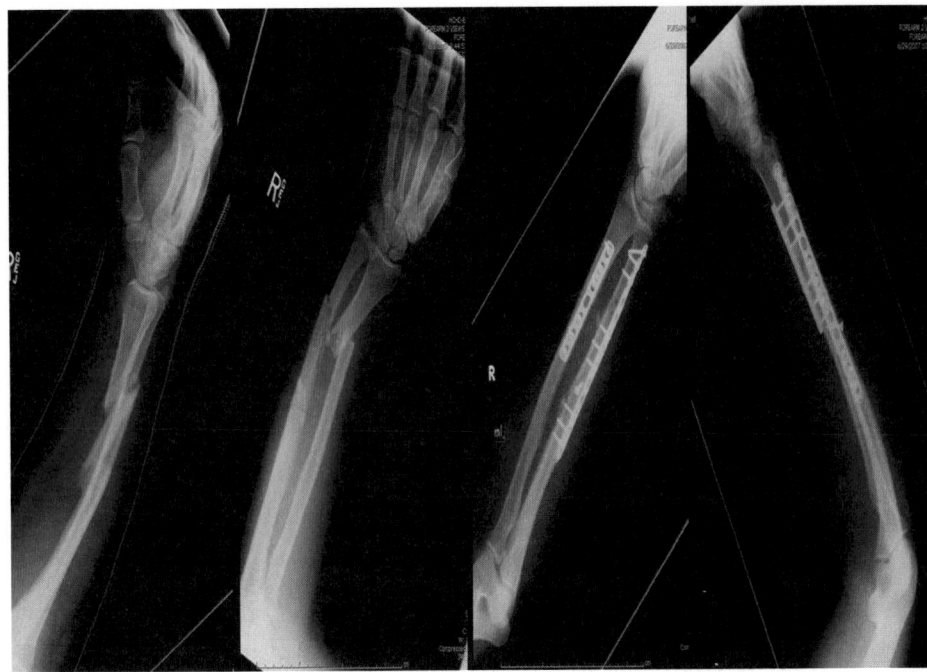

FIG. 43-23. X-ray images of a patient with fractures of both bones of the forearm before and after open reduction and internal fixation. Note that the ulna fracture is segmental. Precise alignment of the radial and ulnar shafts is important for pronation and supination.

(Fig. 43-23). In pediatric patients, the high potential for bony remodeling nonoperative treatment often is appropriate in very young individuals. In adults, however, precise reconstruction of the alignment and contour of the shafts of these bones is important to maintain pronation and supination function. Accordingly, fractures of both bones of the forearm within the shaft are most commonly treated by open reduction and internal fixation using screw-plate devices for each bone.

Fractures of the Proximal Ulna with Radial Head Dislocation (Monteggia Fracture Dislocation)

This particular injury pattern is relatively common, and unfortunately, the dislocation of the radial head sometimes is unrecognized.[20] In almost every case, an internal fixation of the ulna is indicated with closed reduction of the radial head. The treating surgeon must be alert to possible neurovascular injury and compartment syndrome. Late complications to this injury can include heterotopic ossification and redislocation of the radial head.

Fractures of the Shaft of the Radius with Radial Ulnar Dislocation (Galeazzi Fracture or Piedmont Fracture)

Radial shaft fractures often are associated with ligamentous injury to the distal radioulnar joint.[21] This injury, which may escape detection of the unwary, could lead to instability of the wrist. The radioulnar joint injury may be purely ligamentous or may be accompanied by a fracture of the ulnar styloid. The treating surgeon must be alert for widening of the distal radioulnar joint. The stability of this joint may need to be addressed surgically to avoid a chronically painful wrist.

Fractures of the Wrist and Hand

Fractures of the distal radius and ulna, and fractures of the wrist and hand are discussed in Chap. 44.

MUSCULOSKELETAL INFECTIONS

Infections of the Bone

Infections of the bone (osteomyelitis) frequently can represent diagnostic challenges. Infections of the bone can occur to a wide variety of organisms, ranging from gram-positive and gram-negative bacteria to microbacteria and even fungi. Immunocompromised patients (particularly those on immunosuppressive medications, corticosteroids, or suffering from HIV infection) can present with bone infections caused by very unusual pathogens. Accordingly, when a bone infection is suspected, biopsy for culture is nearly always necessary. Indeed, bony changes caused by bone infection quite often mimic the appearance of tumor. Accordingly, it is recommended during any biopsy procedure of a presumptive infection that tissue samples be sent for histopathology. Likewise, it is strongly recommended that anytime a suspected tumor of the bone is biopsied, specimens also are obtained and sent for culture.

Osteomyelitis is an inflammation of the bone, usually the result of infection, which involves both the local bone tissue and the surrounding marrow and is located in the intramedullary canal. Infections of the subperiosteal space are termed *periostitis*. The morphologic features are similar to infections occurring in other organ systems and the same cells are involved.

Although osteomyelitis is similar to infections in other organs, the process is unique in that the cortical bone prevents release of the increased local pressure that normally accompanies inflammations. In soft tissues, this pressure can be dissipated into the surrounding tissue, but in the intramedullary canal, the pressure change produces infarction of the marrow fat by compressing the capillary and sinusoidal beds that supply it. This marrow infarction results in coagulative necrosis initially and then is replaced by a myxofibrous stroma. Cancellous trabeculae also are infarcted by the collapse of the vessels and also undergo necrosis. These necrotic segments of bone often are not resorbed and are termed *sequestrae*. These will calcify and remain centrally located, and they appear radiologically as very dense areas within the lytic portion of the process. Reactive, viable bone often will form around a sequestrum; this bone is called an *involucrum*.

Given the increased pressure, there is an increased osteoclastic response with resorption at the endosteal surfaces and within the necrotic trabeculae. However, the pressure, if the underlying infection is left untreated or undiagnosed, often will outstrip the ability of the osteoclasts to effectively remodel the intramedullary space. This leads to a penetration of the cortex (via Volkmann's canals) by the inflammation that reached the periosteum. This will result in new bone formation by the periosteal disruption that will be noted radiologically. The periosteal reaction can be quite dramatic radiographically and can mimic a malignancy, especially in children.

In patients with acute osteomyelitis, the radiologic features do not appear until 1 to 14 days after the onset of symptoms. The initial x-ray appearance is a vague, localized osteoporosis as a result of the removal of the dead trabecular bone and initial stages of endosteal resorption. This transforms to a mottled appearance on the plain film as more bone is resorbed, with the end result of a lytic area with or without a sequestrum.

As the infection progresses, the radiologic and morphologic features transform as the inflammation becomes chronic. The marrow gradually is replaced by fibrous tissue, and the inflammatory cells are composed of mononuclear cells (i.e., lymphocytes and plasma cells). Radiologically, this appears as patchy sclerosis in the intramedullary space. A sinus tract may be appreciated especially on CT and magnetic resonance imaging (MRI). The periosteal reaction becomes more compact and often can appear lamellated.

The causative organisms on biopsy often are not visualized histologically, even with special stains. Microbiologic culture is the preferred method for demonstrating the causative agent.

Hematogenous Osteomyelitis

Hematogenous spread of bacteria to the bone is a common event.[22] It is seen most frequently in children, likely due to the vascular anatomy at the epiphyseal growth plate, although it is also commonly seen in patients after illnesses involving bacteremias. It may also arise, apparently spontaneously, after incidental seeding of the bone without identifiable antecedent illness. Bone infections are frequently painful, and indeed, usually cause severe pain. Afflicted pediatric patients may be less likely to express the symptom clearly.

Focal Osteomyelitis of the Bone

Antibiotic treatment for severe bone infections generally is not nearly as successful as antibiotic treatment for most soft tissue infections. Thus, prolonged IV therapy often is indicated (6 weeks or more), and most severe bone infections also are débrided surgically. When possible, the sequestrum is removed entirely. Bone infections in children are almost all due to *Staphylococcus aureus* and, on many occasions, pediatric patients are well treated by antibiotics specifically directed to this organism. In contrast, in adult patients with osteomyelitis, a huge variety of infective organisms have been identified, and it is strongly recommended that, whenever possible, antibiotic treatment be postponed until after tissue biopsy from the infected focus is obtained for culture and sensitivity analysis.

Many patients are immunocompromised due to various causes, which can include chronic corticosteroid use, HIV infection, chemotherapy for cancers, and immunosuppression after organ transplant. In any patient, particularly those who are immunocompromised, the variety of organisms causing osteomyelitis is wide indeed. It is imperative to culture for aerobic organisms, anaerobic organisms, acid microbacteria, and fungus in all such cases. It is speculated that the frequent presentation of pediatric patients with metaphyseal osteomyelitis may be due to the anatomy of the metaphyseal growth plate. Large vessels, particularly veins, supply the growth plate as a site of high metabolic activity and bone synthesis. These large vessels frequently demonstrate a "hairpin turn" at the physis, and studies have shown that the flow of blood, particularly in these veins, may be slow. It is speculated that bacteria may lodge here due to low flow rates. The possibility that local transient thrombosis of these veins may provide a focus for infection also has been raised. At any event, the area of bone immediately adjacent to the physis is a frequent focus for infection.

Chronic osteomyelitis may lead to a fistula or chronically draining sinus. This is a commonly seen problem in diabetic patients, but may arise in any incompletely treated osteomyelitis. Successful treatment of this problem is challenging. Once the chronic infection is established, it is then amply demonstrated that culture of the

sinus itself is very unreliable at revealing the causative organism in the deep tissues. When definitive treatment is undertaken, an adequate culture from the deep tissues is mandatory.

An interesting, if unfortunate observation in patients with chronic osteomyelitis with draining sinuses is that malignancy, particularly squamous cell carcinomas, can arise within the chronically inflamed tissue. This possibility must be kept in mind when treating patients with chronic osteomyelitis.

Granulomatous Osteomyelitis

A *granuloma* is a chronic inflammatory process with central giant cells and macrophages with a peripheral cuff of lymphocytes and plasma cells. Plain radiographs generally are notable for ossification and calcification with variable degrees of lucency. The histology demonstrates granuloma formation that is identical to that seen in other locations. The most common granulomatous condition in the skeletal system is due to tuberculosis.

Tuberculosis more commonly manifests as an arthritis rather than osteomyelitis. However, when it does manifest in bone, typically it occurs in the spine. Deformity as a result of the infection may be severe due to the destruction of the vertebra or vertebrae. In the adult, the infection more often begins beneath the periosteum and may spread under the anterior longitudinal ligament and involve the vertebrae some distance away. The histologic features are those of chronic osteomyelitis, with fibrosis, bone destruction, and prominent caseous necrosis.

Septic Arthritis

Septic arthritis, as the name implies, is an infection of a diarthrodial joint. Organisms, usually bacteria, proliferate within the joint cavity, and in almost every case, cause marked limitation of joint motion, and severe pain with joint loading or motion. Patients with septic arthritis often demonstrate high fever, leukocytosis, and severe malaise. The involved joint typically becomes tensely swollen, warm, and exquisitely tender. Spontaneous septic arthritis can and does occur in all age groups, but it is most common in children. It generally is believed that most cases of acute septic arthritis in children derive from foci of acute osteomyelitis of the metaphysis that "breaks through" into the joint. Joints where the growth plate is enclosed by the joint capsule are common sites for this event (humerus, proximal femur). An infection in the joint typically puts the articular cartilage at risk for irreversible damage. Accordingly, prompt recognition of this entity and initiation of treatment is essential. It also must be recognized that some noninfectious processes can mimic the presentation of an infected joint. Such common clinical entities include acute gouty arthritis, an acute flare of an inflammatory arthritis such as rheumatoid arthritis, or an acute hemarthrosis. Generally, the first step in the evaluation of a patient suspected of septic arthritis is aspiration of the joint. The joint fluid is examined for cells, blood, and the presence of uric acid or calcium pyrophosphate crystals.

In the presence of a leucocytosis and no other firm diagnosis, treatment involves prompt irrigation and débridement of the joint. In some easily accessible joints, such as the knee, the irrigation and débridement can be carried out with an arthroscope. In many other joints, there is a need for an open arthrotomy with surgical exploration débridement and aggressive irrigation of the joint. After such procedure, the selection of the antibiotic regimen and its duration generally are decided after consultation with an infectious disease specialist. The antibiotic regimen is tailored to the infective organism and clinical situation of the individual patient.

DISORDERS OF THE FOOT AND ANKLE

Osseous Anatomy

The distal tibia and fibula combine with the talus to form the ankle joint. Primary motion of the ankle joint is flexion and extension and a normal arch of motion is approximately 60°, 20° of dorsiflexion, and 40° of plantar flexion. This tibiotalar joint bears very large loads during gait and especially during vigorous activity. Underneath the talus, the talocalcaneal joint, also called the *subtalar joint*, is the site of significant inversion and eversion (normally between 5° and 20°). The metatarsal-phalangeal joints normally move very little. Metatarsal-phalangeal joints and interphalangeal joints principally move in flexion and extension.

Evaluation of the Patient

Physical Examination

Gait abnormalities should be noted. The presence of edema or skin lesions should be recorded as signs of vascular insufficiency or inflammatory disease.

The dorsalis pedis and the tibialis anterior pulses usually are readily located. Scars, consistent with previous wound healing problems, can indicate chronic disease.

Tenderness of the joints can indicate degenerative arthritis or inflammatory disease. Significant joint deformity often is characteristic of inflammatory joint disease such as rheumatoid arthritis. The major ligaments of the ankle can be palpated; frequently of specific interest is the anterior talofibular ligament and the tibial calcaneal ligaments. Both are frequently injured during ankle sprains. The range of motion of the joints should be assessed. Chronic talofibular ligament injuries are common and can be demonstrated by an anterior drawer sign by drawing the hind foot forward at the tibiotalar joint. In acute sprains, this maneuver will be acutely painful, in the chronic sprain it will not.

Radiographic Examinations

A study of the foot would include specific views including the anteroposterior (AP) lateral and oblique as well as AP lateral and mortis views of the ankle. The mortis view is a particularly useful view of the ankle that is taken in a slightly oblique AP direction to display the ankle joint space with the talus in alignment with the ankle joint. This allows assessment of the joint space of the tibiotalar and fibulotalar joints. In the diagnosis and treatment of many foot and ankle disorders, CT scans, MRI scans, bone scans, venous and arterial vascular studies, and other radiographic techniques are used with a specific purpose.

Common Degenerative Conditions of the Ankle

Hallux valgus is a common deformity in the foot characterized by valgus angulation to the first metatarsal-phalangeal joint. There are numerous factors that influence the development of hallux valgus, but overwhelmingly, the most common culprit is tight shoe ware that puts extra pressure on the first toe in a valgus direction. A lifetime of narrow, high-heeled shoe wear can create substantial, painful, and unsightly first toe deformities. Once hallux valgus is present, angulation of the first ray is such that eventually bowstringing the tendons crossing the joint acts to increase the deformity. Most notable is a plantar and lateral shift of the abductor hallucis tendon. Lesser toe deformities frequently accompany this condition, usually with identical risk factors. Frequently, skin problems develop due to contact between adjacent rays.

Treatment

Conservative treatment for degenerative arthritis and associated deformities will often suffice. This generally consists of shoe modifications. Such measures are always the first choice of treatment.

Surgical treatment of hallux valgus generally is satisfying in the relief of cosmetic issues and pain.[23] A successful operation must address several issues that contribute to the problem. Specifically, valgus deviation of the great toe must be corrected, and frequently, a varus deviation of the first metatarsal also must be addressed. Reconstruction of the flexor apparatus and relocation of the sesamoid bones is also important (to relieve deforming forces and prevent recurring deformity). Usually excision or resection of the medial bony eminence (medial osteophytes from the metatarsal-phalangeal joint) also is performed. The reconstruction often consists of reefing the capsule and adjusting the position of tendons that cross the joint. Often, a metatarsal osteotomy is performed, which can be done by a variety of means.

Hallux Rigidus

Hallux rigidus is a common condition that frequently affects athletes or patients who are accustomed to wearing high-heeled shoes. The condition is a painful loss of motion, particularly in dorsal flexion of the metatarsal-phalangeal joint of the first toe, usually accompanied by exuberant osteophytes on the dorsal surfaces of both joints. When accompanied by significant degenerative change, this condition is sometimes addressed by fusion and bone grafting of the involved joint.

Deformities of the Lesser Toes

Angular deformities of the lesser toes generally are categorized as "crossover toe" deformities. The causes are usually shoe wear related to the pathophysiology of hallux valgus. Such angular deformities often also present in hallux valgus patients and are often concurrent. Also commonly symptomatic are the mallet toe, the hammer toe, and the claw toe deformities, all of which are related to flexion deformities of the individual digits. Multiple claw toe deformities are frequently seen in neurologic disease and their presence may indicate more significant systemic neurologic pathology. In general, conservative treatments centering on appropriate footwear generally are helpful. In severe intractable cases, surgical treatment generally involves resection of the extensor digitorum brevis or lengthening of the extensor digitorum brevis tendon, occasionally accompanied by lengthening or tenotomy of the extensor digitorum longus. On rare occasion, surgical resection or ablation of the interphalangeal joints can be effective treatment.

Nerve Entrapment Syndromes

Morton's neuroma is a common and painful condition of the common digital nerve of the foot, most frequently in the first, second, or third web space. Although the word *neuroma* is commonly used, it may be better described as degenerative disease of the nerve. Repetitive microtrauma and chronic compression may be contributing factors. Morton's neuroma is most common in females. Diagnosis is by physical examination, specifically, reproduction pain with mediolateral compression of the foot and local tenderness. Conservative treatment consists of wide-toed shoes with a firm sole. A metatarsal pad worn inside the shoe to support the more proximal metatarsals can be useful. When conservative treatments fail, excision of the nerve (leaving the patient with some small sensory deficits) can be appropriate treatment.

Tarsal Tunnel Syndrome

The space between the medial malleolus and adjacent surface of the calcaneus is referred to as the *tarsal tunnel*. Beneath the dense layer of ligaments, the tarsal tunnel contains the tendons of the flexor hallus longus and flexor digitorum longus, as well as the tibialis posterior tendon and a neurovascular bundle. Rather analogous to carpal tunnel syndrome, nerve compression can cause significant discomfort. The symptoms often are felt distal to the site of compression and at times outside of the normal distribution of the posterior tibial nerve. This diagnosis almost always is associated with tenderness over the tarsal tunnel. Symptoms may be due to identifiable neuromas, inflammatory disease, or the effects of old trauma. The true etiology is often debated. Electrodiagnostic studies are occasionally used. Shoe modification including immobilization in a brace can be useful, but many of these patients do undergo surgical treatment, which involves exploration of the tunnel and release of the flexor retinaculum and of the fascia.

Rheumatoid Arthritis of the Foot

The foot and ankle frequently are involved in patients with systemic inflammatory diseases such as rheumatoid arthritis. As in the hand and wrist, the effects of inflammatory disease can manifest in erosive disease of the ligaments and tendons (including rupture) as well as erosive disease of the bones and joints.[24]

The feet are the major source of disability for patients with rheumatoid arthritis. Indeed, with the incidents of rheumatoid arthritis known to be approximately 1% in North America, the orthopedic surgeon must be alert to the characteristic signs of inflammatory disease in the foot (exuberant articular enlargement, joint deformity, and synovitis), and often, it will be up to the orthopedic surgeon to make the initial diagnosis of rheumatoid arthritis.

Inflammatory disease in the foot most frequently begins in the metatarsal-phalangeal joints and leads to subluxation or even frank dislocation at the base of the proximal phalanges. Deformity and pain beneath the metatarsal heads also can be presenting complaints; often physical examination will reveal significant soft tissue reactions on the plantar surface of the hind foot. A valgus deformity of the hind foot is seen in inflammatory disease due to involvement of the talocalcaneal joints and ligaments. Valgus angulation and lateral subluxation of the joint result and may cause the loss of the longitudinal arch of the foot. Mild to moderate cases of rheumatoid disease of the foot can be managed by medications and modified shoe ware. Hindfoot valgus deformities often are treated by bony fusion (often a triple arthrodesis: a fusion of the talus, calcaneus, and navicular).

Heel Pain Syndrome—Plantar Fasciitis

Heel pain syndrome is a relatively common condition that can cause severe and sometimes near disabling pain. Pain generally is felt on the plantar surface of the foot immediately anterior to the calcaneus. This area of the foot is tender to palpation, and the patient will report severe pain upon first arising from a bed or a chair with the first few minutes of weightbearing on the foot being extremely painful. In general, the severe pain with the initiation of weightbearing abates with continued weightbearing but will return after any short interval of rest. There is controversy over the exact pathophysiology underlying the symptoms. Irritation and inflammation of the plantar fascia generally is agreed to be the underlying cause. In some patients, entrapment of the first branch of the lateral plantar nerve can be identified. On such an occasion, release of the deep fascia adjacent to this nerve can provide substantial relief.

Posterior Heel Pain

Pain in the region of the Achilles tendon insertion on the calcaneus is common. This can be due to a bursitis, either posterior or anterior to the Achilles tendon, which most commonly presents with local posterior heel pain exacerbated by exertion. Physical examination will reveal tenderness anterior to the Achilles tendon. This usually can be managed nonoperatively with immobilization (walking boot) and anti-inflammatory medications.

Insertional Achilles tendonitis (tendinosis) of the Achilles tendon most frequently is seen in patients >40 years of age, and often is associated with a tight heel cord. Tendinosis can be disabling and generally is treated with immobilization and rest, stretching of the gastrocsoleus and Achilles region, and shoe modification. When severe and persistent, this condition is treated operatively by débridement of the tendon involved. If the tendon insertional area on the calcaneus is severely attenuated, operative reconstruction of the tendon may be necessary.

SPORTS MEDICINE

Athletic injury can, of course, encompass many areas in the musculoskeletal system. The orthopedic subspecialty of "sports medicine" has developed in response to a very high incidence of soft tissue injuries (ligament, tendon, and cartilage) in patients who are active in exercise and athletics. The most problematic joints in this regard are the knee and the shoulder. Orthopedic treatment for such injuries involves careful history, physical examination, and close attention to the need and desires of the individual patient. Surgical intervention for ligament and cartilage injuries in such patients most frequently is done using arthroscopic technique.

Anatomy of the Knee

The principal mechanical function of the knee is that of a hinge joint, but the knee does bear tremendous axial loads as well as torsional and sheer forces. The major stabilizing structures within the knee unfortunately are frequently injured. The anterior cruciate ligament (ACL) is a very stout ligament that is situated centrally within the knee. Its mechanical functions are complex, but the most important is to restrain the tibia from forward excursion below the femur. The posterior cruciate ligament (PCL) lies immediately behind the ACL. The PCL undoubtedly has multiple functions, the most important and most easily assessed is its function to restrain posterior sliding movements of the tibia beneath the femur. The medial collateral ligament (MCL) is located outside of the joint capsule and restrains the knee from bending in a valgus direction. The lateral collateral ligament is analogous to the MCL and joins the lateral femoral epicondyle to the fibular head. The function of the lateral collateral ligament is to restrain the joint from varus angulation. All of these ligaments are vulnerable to injury.

Menisci

Within the joint, the two large articular surfaces of the condyles articulate with the cartilage of the tibial plateau. Crescent-shaped fibrocartilage menisci lie medially and laterally within the joint and serve to guide the femoral condyles' motion and to more evenly distribute loads across the joint. The menisci are important stabilizing structures. The fibrocartilaginous menisci are vascularized only in their outer third. Because of their significant mechanical function, they are subject to both acute traumatic tears (acute tears) as well as progressive degeneration (degenerative tears).

The medial meniscus is torn more frequently than the lateral. Tears of either the medial or the lateral meniscus may be clinically silent or they may cause significantly disabling symptoms. Tears of the menisci have been reported in virtually all portions of the meniscus. Radial and longitudinal tears are common.[25] A special type of a longitudinal tear is the "bucket handle tear," which parallels the C-shaped contour of the meniscus and can create a significant and problematic flap if it displaces.

Symptoms caused by a meniscal tear can include local pain and intermittent swelling of the knee, as well as pain on weightbearing. Displaced meniscal tears may cause interference with joint motion and, on some occasions, can frankly prevent the knee from full extension, a so-called *locked knee*. The locked knee joint does occasionally yield to manipulation to reduce the meniscal tear. More frequently, such patients require timely surgery to excise or repair the flap.

Options for treatment of a meniscal tear include resection and reshaping of the torn area, generally preferred for small tears (Fig. 43-24).[26] Very large tears in young active patients usually are treated by primary meniscal repair, generally using arthroscopic technique (Fig. 43-25). Complete excision of a torn meniscus, once quite popular, is now recommended only rarely because of loss of the meniscal load distributing function that can accelerate osteoarthritic change in the knee.[27] On some occasions, badly injured menisci in young active patients can be successfully treated by allograft replacement of the meniscus from a cadaver source. The long-term results of this approach are not yet clear.

Ligamentous Injuries of the Knee

MCL injury will occur after excessive valgus stress of the knee. Unfortunately, it is sometimes associated with a meniscal injury.

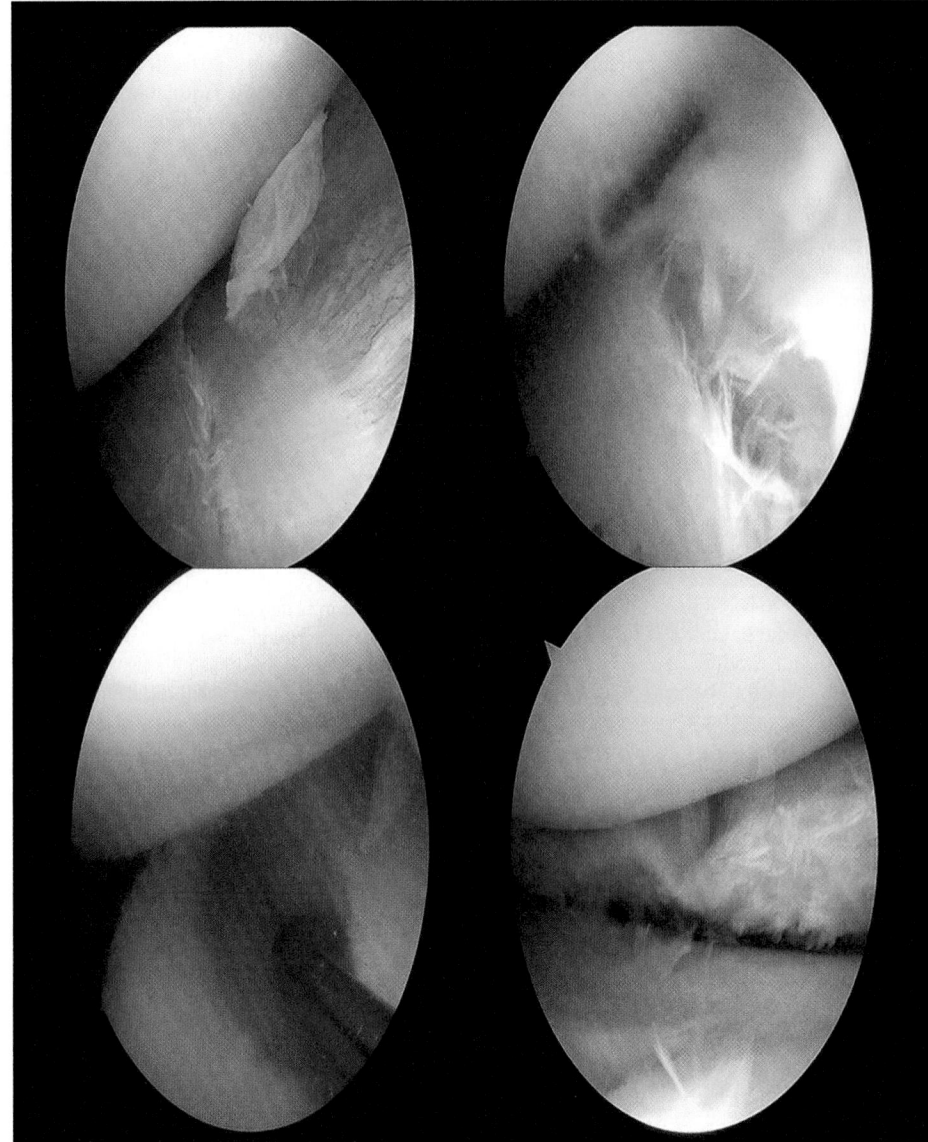

FIG. 43-24. Arthroscopic images of a tear of the medial meniscus of the knee before (*top*) and after (*bottom*) arthroscopic débridement. (*Courtesy of Dr. David Green.*)

Nonoperative treatment is preferred for an isolated MCL injury. In most cases, full return of function is anticipated.

Lateral collateral ligament injuries are much less common than MCL ligament injuries. Similarly, however, they are most often managed nonoperatively. ACL injuries can be isolated injuries, but often are seen in combination with MCL rupture and medial or lateral meniscal tear. The triad of MCL, medial meniscus, and ACL tears is most common in contact sports (e.g., football) or jumping sports (e.g., basketball).

Anterior Cruciate Ligament Injury

A functioning ACL is not necessary for most individual's activities and daily living.[26] Indeed, many competitive athletes can function at a high level of competition with an ACL deficient knee as well, presumably due to secondary soft tissue constraints, muscle activities, and individual effort. Unfortunately, many individuals with an ACL-deficient knee due to traumatic failure of the ligament find themselves unable to compete because of instabilities of the knee. Accordingly, in patients for whom athletic endeavor is an important part of their life, reconstruction of the intercruciate ligament is a useful procedure that has prolonged many patients' athletic participation (Fig. 43-26).[28]

Evaluation of the patient for possible ACL injury involves a Lachman test: manual passive assessment of the AP stability of the knee, which is held in slight extension. Diagnosis of the ACL rupture and other associated internal joints of the knee usually is confirmed by an MRI image of the affected joint. Various techniques for the reconstruction of the cruciate ligament are described, which generally involve autograft or allograft tissues placed through tunnels within the tibia and the femur.[29] A central slip of the patellar tendon, including a portion of the bony attachment from both the tibial eminence and of the patella itself, is popular, as are woven grafts from hamstring tendons. Other graft sources also have found favor. Accurate placement of the bony tunnels for the graft and proper tensioning of the graft are critical portions of this procedure. Following the procedure, a lengthy rehabilitation process generally is necessary.

The PCL is less frequently injured than the ACL. A rupture of the PCL is, in general, better tolerated than is an ACL-deficient knee. A useful examination maneuver to test for PCL function is a posterior drawer test, which is essentially the reverse of the Lachman test where a slightly flexed knee is tested for the stability of the tibia beneath the femur by passive manipulation. PCL reconstruction is less commonly performed than ACL reconstruction, although, when functional deficits result from this injury, surgical treatment may be rewarding for athletic patients.[30] Chronic PCL-deficient knees are thought to have an increased incidence of osteoarthritis, particularly in the patellofemoral and medial knee compartments.

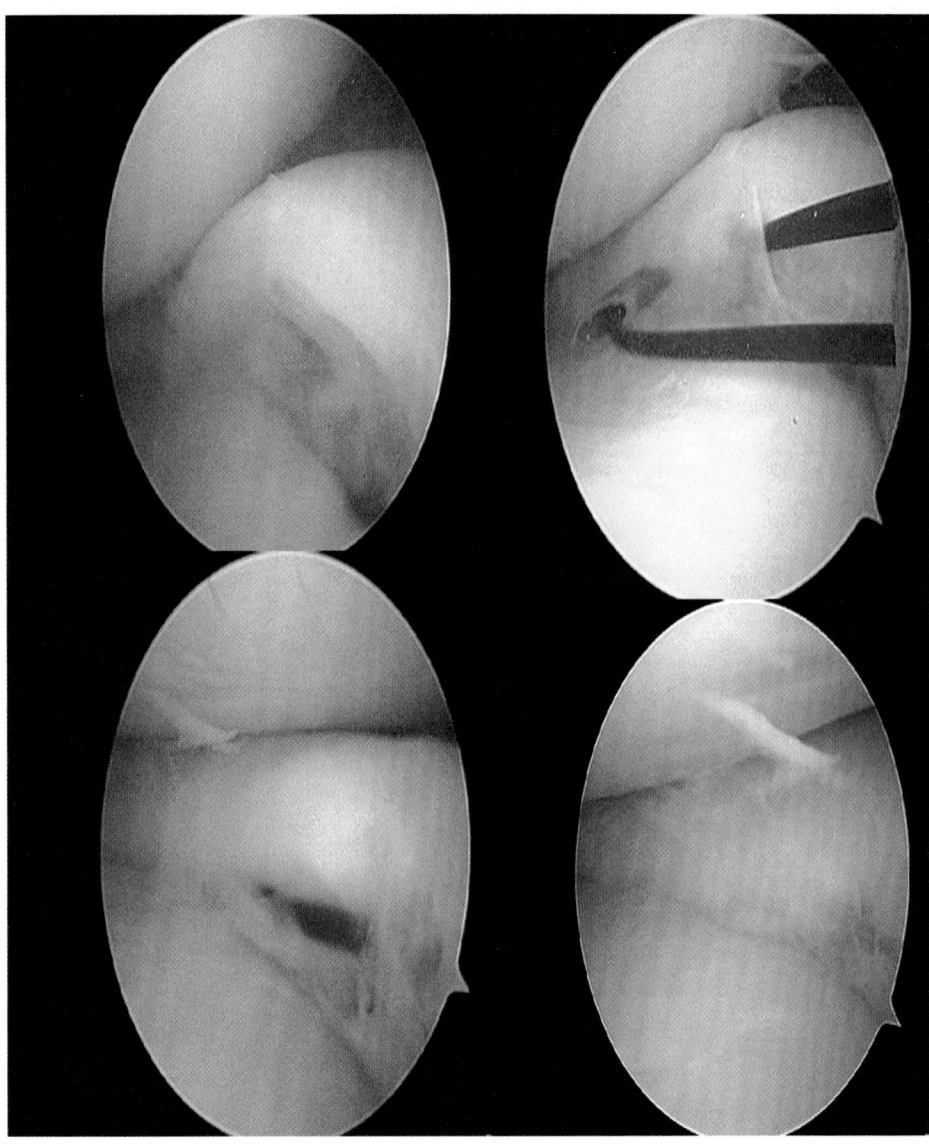

FIG. 43-25. Arthroscopic images of a horizontal tear of the medial meniscus. The tear is repaired using a "buried suture" technique. *(Courtesy of Dr. David Green.)*

THE SHOULDER

Shoulder Dislocation and Shoulder Instability

The glenohumeral joint is a ball and socket joint. Some stability for the very shallow socket of the glenoid is provided by the glenoid labrum, but this very mobile large joint is the most frequently dislocated joint in the human body. Dislocations can result from major or minor trauma. Although the dislocation can occur in the posterior or inferior directions, the most common direction for dislocation is anterior. A patient with an anterior dislocation will complain of local pain and will present with an internally rotated shoulder. The anterior position of the humeral head in such dislocation can make the radiographic diagnosis challenging. An AP x-ray, a glenoid (axillary) view, and a Y view of the shoulder is recommended in assessing this injury. Associated neurovascular injury is possible but rare. When carefully assessed, it often is found to be a transient axillary nerve palsy (≥30%). Relocation of the shoulder is generally accomplished with the patient supine by subjecting the arm to gentle traction in a position of slight abduction. Some sedation before the maneuver is helpful. After relocation of shoulder dislocation, the patient generally is provided a sling for comfort. Prolonged immobilization of the shoulder (as was done in years past) is not recommended.[31] Prolonged immobilization will often lead to substantial stiffness in the shoulder and does not appreciably decrease the redislocation rate. Unfortunately, after an anterior

dislocation, many patients will experience recurrent dislocations.[32] When these become multiple events, surgical stabilization of the shoulder is considered. Numerous procedures for reconstructing and tightening the shoulder capsule are described, many of which now are accomplished arthroscopically.

Impingement Syndromes

After minor trauma, repetitive injury, and sometimes without an identifiable inciting event, many patients experience symptoms of shoulder pain. Pain from a shoulder impairment syndrome often is reported in the anterior shoulder and is exacerbated by abduction of the shoulder, which can be due to irritation of the tissues in the subacromial space.

Shoulder impingement syndromes represent a broad spectrum of disease ranging from simple bursitis to tendonitis of the long head of the biceps or supraspinatus tendon.[33] In many cases, this impingement syndrome can progress to a frank tear of the supraspinatus tendon, the most cephalad of the rotator cuff tendons. The diagnosis is confirmed by documenting leakage of contrast in a shoulder arthrogram. MRI imaging also can be definitive, and ultrasonography is readily available and quite accurate.

Interestingly, patients with rotator cuff tears frequently are asymptomatic, and many have excellent use of the shoulder without apparent pain or difficulty. On the other hand, many patients with such tears report with severe disabling pain, and many are unable to

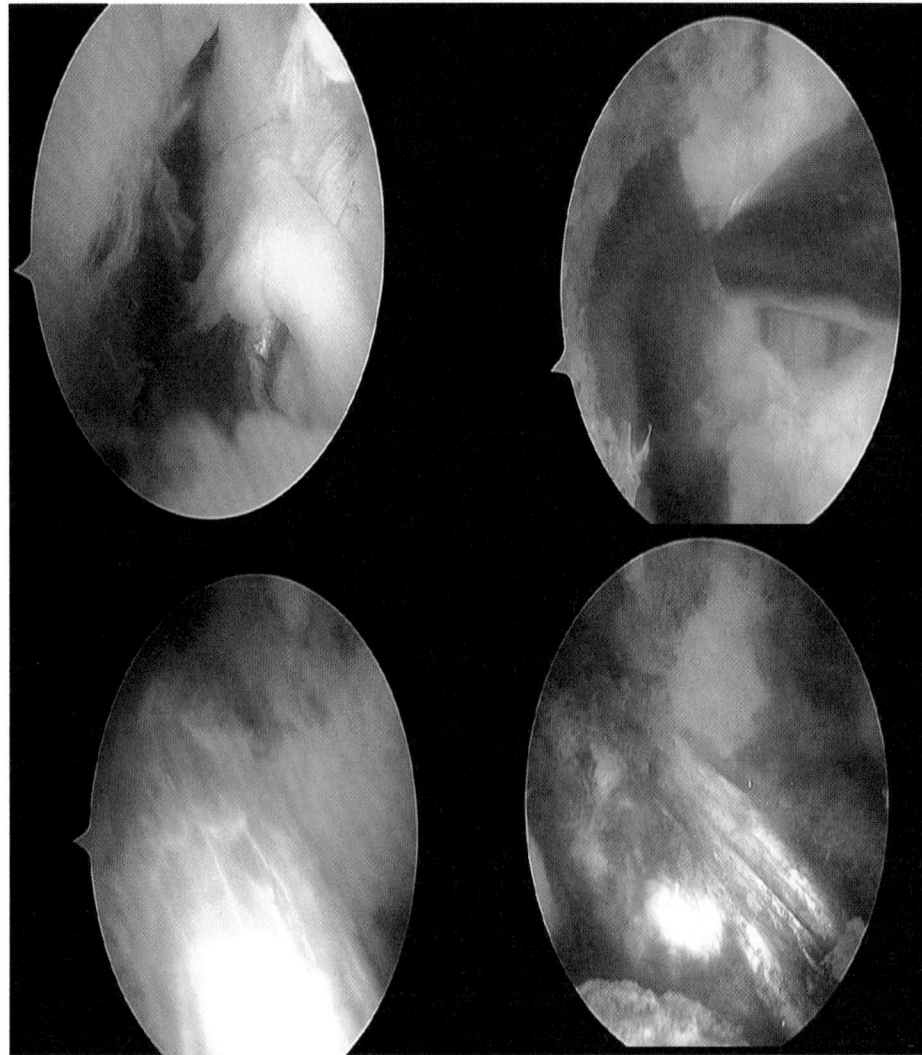

FIG. 43-26. Arthroscopic images of a patient with a rupture of the anterior cruciate ligament before *(top)* and after *(bottom)* reconstruction with a tendon graft. *(Courtesy of Dr. David Green.)*

pursue sporting activities as a result. Accordingly, surgical repair of a rotator cuff injury is often indicated to restore function. Primary repair of the rotator cuff is accomplished, in most cases, arthroscopically.[34] The procedure sometimes is accompanied by a bony resection of the inferior portion of the acromion.

The Acromioclavicular Joint

The acromioclavicular joint is stout and not very mobile. This joint is vulnerable to ligament injuries (sprains), particularly in athletic endeavors where blows to the shoulder or falls onto the shoulder are common. Such injuries range from simple partial thickness injures (grade 1 sprains) to frank tearing of the acromial-clavicular and acromioclavicular coracoacromial ligaments causing displacement of the joint. Such injuries are common in contact sports such as football, and are particularly common in athletes playing ice hockey. An acromioclavicular sprain is referred to as a *shoulder separation* and is not to be confused with a glenohumeral dislocation. Treatment for such a shoulder separation (acromial-clavicular sprain) usually is symptomatic. Significantly displaced injuries involving frank tearing of the coracoclavicular ligaments sometimes are reconstructed surgically.

THE SPINE

Spinal Trauma

The treatment of spinal trauma is one of the most challenging areas in orthopedic surgery. Situations at times are extremely challenging because many patients who have sustained significant spinal trauma also have concomitant visceral and other musculoskeletal injuries as well. Prioritizing treatment in these situations can be challenging. In patients with an isolated spinal cord injury, the major concerns for the treating orthopedic surgeon are the neurologic status of the patient, the possible presence of ongoing spinal cord compression, and the stability of the spine and the possible need for stabilization.[35]

Assessment of the neurologic status of the patient is covered in Chap. 42 on Neurosurgery. A detailed physical examination in search for other injuries as well as the thorough assessment for any neurologic deficits should be done early in the evaluation of these patients.[36] Priorities of care follow the primary concerns of airway, ventilation, and circulation. If the patient is neurologically intact, then the primary concern is assessment of the spinal stability to know whether or not mobilization of the patient (often necessary for other treatments) is safe and whether successful healing of the spinal injury is likely without surgical intervention.

In patients with significant neurologic deficits, the immediate question is asked whether or not there is ongoing compression of the spinal cord or the nerve root for which a decompressive procedure would be indicated. In most spinal cord injury situations, prompt decompression of ongoing neural compression is performed whenever possible. Unfortunately, the true benefits of such interventions are very difficult to objectively assess. There is a growing body of evidence that suggests that prompt decompression in spinal cord injury can make a detectable and measurable difference in the acute and semiacute neurologic function. Whether patients so treated are truly better 6 months or a year after their injury is a question that is still debated.

Extensive laboratory investigation using animal models with spinal cord injury suggested that very prompt decompression of a localized spinal cord leads to objective and measurable differences in recovery. The optimal time for this decompression in humans is not yet known. A body of animal data suggests that early intervention is better than late intervention.

Occipital Cervical Dislocation

Dislocation of the occiput on the occipital condyles of the atlas (C1) is a common injury after high-energy trauma, particularly motor vehicle trauma. Unfortunately, only a tiny fraction of the patients with this injury survive, as it is almost always accompanied by a high cervical spine or brain stem injury. For the rare patients who survive this injury, traction on the spine is contraindicated. Definitive treatment consists of stabilization and fusion in situ using a screw-plate or rod screw device spanning from the occiput to the midcervical spine.[37]

Fractures of C1 (Jefferson Fracture)

The Jefferson fracture, eloquently discussed by Dr. Jefferson in 1920, is a fracture of the C1 ring.[38] The C1 vertebra does not have a true anterior body as do all of the rest of the vertebrae. The rather thin anterior and posterior rings are subject to fracture, particularly with axial load injuries. The Jefferson fracture results in a lateral spread of the lateral masses of C1, which are visible on an AP (through the mouth) x-ray image of the upper cervical spine. This injury actually results in an increase in the size of the spinal canal, and thus, rarely is associated with neurologic injury. Fortunately, the bony fractures heal quite reliably. The treatment of choice in Jefferson fractures is bracing with either a cervicothoracic orthosis or a halo ring and vest.

Fractures of C2 (Odontoid Fracture)

The odontoid is a peg of bone that arises off the central body of the C2 vertebra and articulates with the anterior ring of the C1 vertebra. The articulation between the odontoid (or dens) in the C1 vertebra and the atlantoaxial facet joint is the site where half of normal cervical rotational movement occurs. The odontoid is a relatively small structure, however, and it is vulnerable to fracture. The types of odontoid fracture are eloquently discussed by Anderson and D'Alonzo in their classic paper, which describes a generally benign "type I" fracture that consists of an avulsion fracture off the very tip of the odontoid.[39] These type I fractures are thought to arise from the alar ligaments that span from the tip of the odontoid to the skull (bypassing the C1 vertebra). Such isolated avulsion fractures, although they may be painful, do not represent any danger to the patient. Type I fractures generally are managed symptomatically with expected satisfactory outcomes.

A fracture through the base of the odontoid, at the level of the articular surfaces of the facet joints, is classified as a "type II" injury in the Anderson and D'Alonzo classification scheme (Fig. 43-27). These fractures result from oblique or lateral loading forces on the odontoid. The rather small fracture surface created by this and the small surface of cancellous bone within the odontoid may be reasons why this particular variety of odontoid fracture heals poorly. When such fractures are immobilized in cervicothoracic orthosis or halo vest, nonunion rates ranging from 20 to 80% have been reported. Accordingly, treatment of a type II odontoid fracture is most usually operative. Stabilization of the fracture can be accomplished through an anterior approach by directly transfixing the odontoid with a screw initiated at the anterior/inferior border of the C2 body and inserted across the fracture site and up into the odontoid. This is a technically demanding screw placement and is only done with the availability of excellent intraoperative imaging techniques. An alternative to direct fixation of this fracture is a posterior stabilization and fusion of C1 on C2. This can be done by sublaminar wiring cable techniques or by posterior screw fixation. The anterior odontoid screw fixation does allow the potential for

continued rotational movement between C1 and C2. The posterior fusion of C1 and C2, while restoring safety and stability, also results in a markedly diminished range of motion of the cervical spine.

Anderson and D'Alonzo type III fractures are described as those that extend into the body of C2, below the bone of the odontoid. The fractures' surfaces are large and well vascularized. Type III fractures heal reliably with halo brace, or other brace designs. Surgical intervention rarely is needed.

Hangman's Fractures of C2

Hangman's fractures or traumatic spondylolisthesis of C2 are fractures that occur through the pars interarticularis of C2 (the segment of the posterior elements between the superior and inferior facets of C2). This fracture results from sudden extension forces on the neck causing a fracture through this area of C2, which is one of the thinner portions of the posterior elements of this vertebra. This fracture, in most cases, does not result in any narrowing of the spinal canal. The overwhelming majority of patients with minimally displaced hangman's fractures are neurologically intact. Treatment for this injury is almost always nonoperative employing simple immobilization using a cervicothoracic orthosis or a halo vest. With higher-energy injuries (such as those intentionally created in judicial hangings), more severe extension forces can create dislocation of the C2–3 facet complex and injury of the C2–3 disc. Such displaced fractures can and do compromise the spinal canal. When significant displacement occurs, death can result due to compromise of respiration. Infrequently encountered are neurologically intact patients who have significantly displaced hangman's fractures. These patients are managed by internal fixation and bone grafting between C2 and C3 (Fig. 43-28).

Compression Fracture of the Cervical Spine

Compression fractures of the cervical spine refer to an axial load injury with failure of the end plate, but preservation of the posterior cortex of the vertebral body. This will occur in the vertebrae of C3 to C7 and may or may not be associated with a fracture of the anterior cortex. In either case, with the posterior cortex of the vertebral body intact, no compromise of the neural elements results. The healing potential for these fractures is very high, and such patients generally are managed nonoperatively. Analgesics are prescribed as is a cervical brace for comfort.

Burst Fractures of the Cervical Spine

Burst fractures of the cervical spine arise as a result of failure under axial loads. Unrestrained motor vehicle occupants striking a windshield and diving accidents are common injury mechanisms. The burst fracture is distinct from the compression fracture, however, in that the posterior cortex of the vertebral body is fractured. This frequently results in displacement (retropulsion) of bony fragments into the canal, which can cause neurologic injury and dysfunction. Very high-energy burst fractures can result in fractures of the posterior elements as well; however, this is less commonly seen. A burst fracture noted in the neurologically intact patient can be managed conservatively by bed rest and traction. This can be appropriate treatment for a cooperative teenage patient who has potential to heal a fracture within a very short interval. Far more commonly, these occur in adult patients, for whom prolonged bed rest is not only inconvenient but risky. Accordingly, the overwhelming majority of such patients are managed operatively by anterior débridement of the fracture (necessary should there be neurologic compromise) and reconstruction using a bone graft strut and the application of a screw and plate device. Plate fixation after strut grafting and decompression generally will allow immediate mobilization of the patient. Patients are restrained from rigorous activities until after fracture healing is confirmed in 6 to 15 weeks.

Unilateral and Bilateral Facet Dislocation

A forceful flexion with distraction forces (such as can happen in an automobile accident with a restrained driver) can result in forward

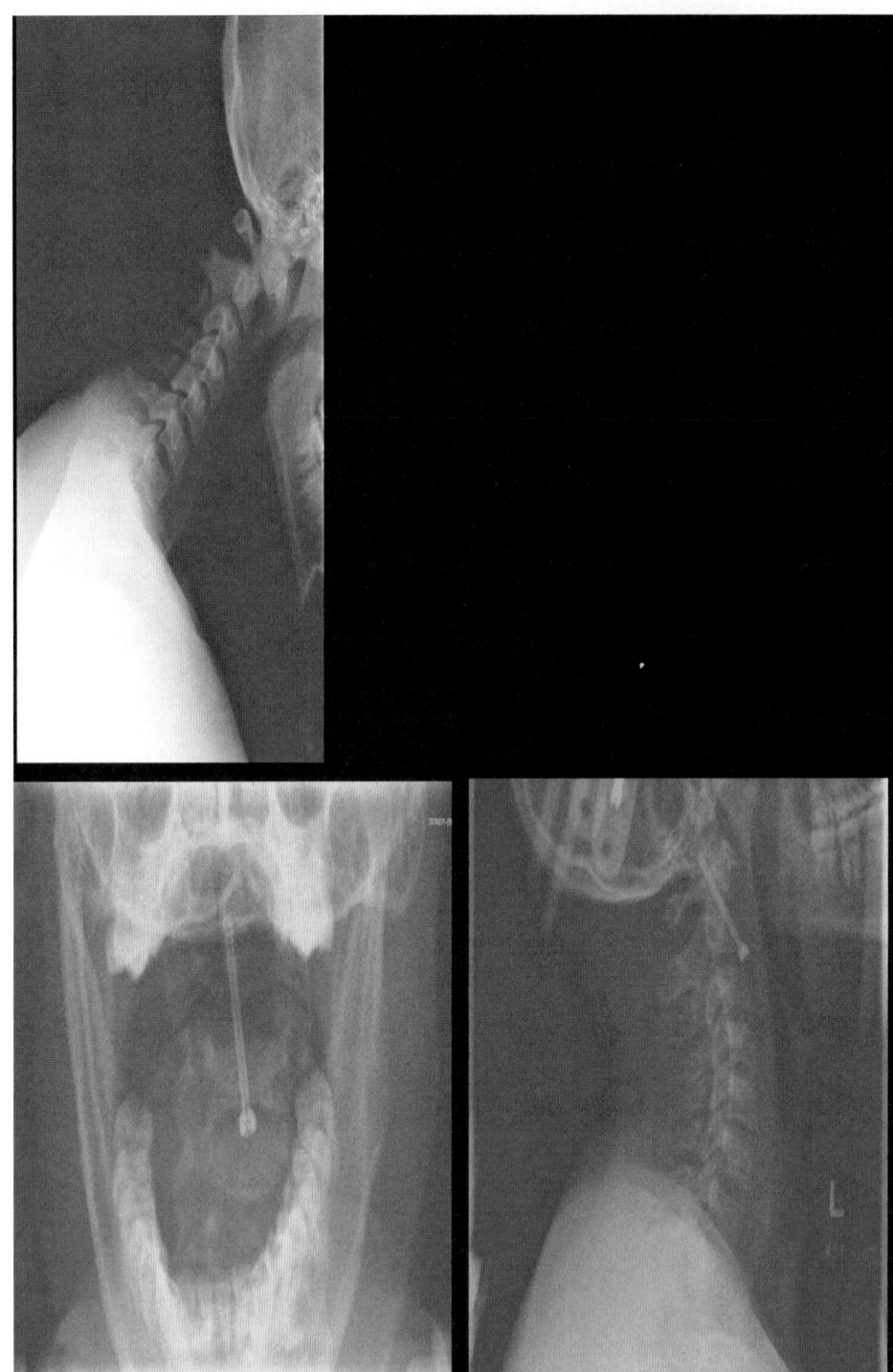

FIG. 43-27. X-ray images of a displaced fracture of the odontoid process of C2, before and after reduction and internal fixation. Transverse fracture at the bone of the odontoid (type II) has a high nonunion rate when managed nonoperatively.

subluxation of the cervical vertebrae on a subjacent neighbor with dislocation of one or both of the facet joints. Interestingly, the diagnosis usually can be made with confidence by examination of a lateral x-ray image, as dislocation of one facet joint predictably will result in an anterior displacement of precisely 50% of the AP diameter of the involved vertebral body.

Bilateral facet dislocation typically is caused by an anterior displacement of 50%. On occasion, fractures of the facet joint occur in association with the dislocation. A unilateral facet dislocation rarely results in spinal cord injury; however, bilateral facet dislocations frequently do. Radicular symptoms following unilateral or bilateral dislocation are common, as the dislocated facet can narrow the exit foramen and impinge the intervening nerve roots. Treatment for this injury consists of axial traction, usually exerted after placement of

cranial tongs, followed by graduated application of weight and periodic x-rays. This always is done with the patient awake because of safety concerns. When successful reduction is attained, the risk of recurrent dislocation is so high that most patients are then taken to surgery for posterior fusion procedures of the involved vertebrae. This can be done with interspinous process wiring or by a screw-plate or screw-rod device, with screws inserted into the lateral masses. Postoperative stabilization with a cervical collar is at the discretion of the treating surgeon. Excellent long-term results are generally expected.

Clay Shoveler's Injury

Clay shoveler's injury is a common, but often missed injury to the spinous process of a lower cervical vertebra or the upper thoracic

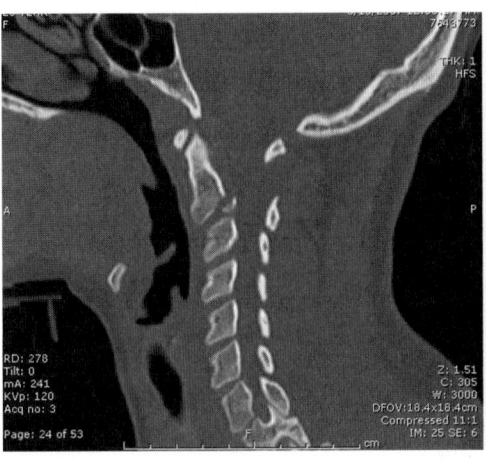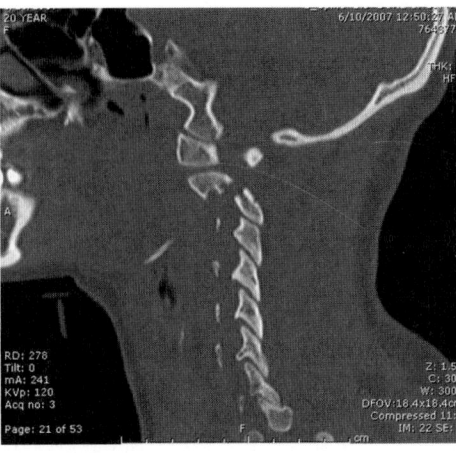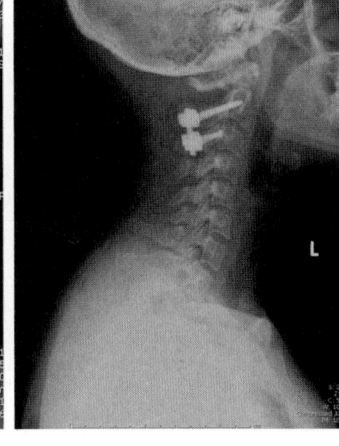

FIG. 43-28. Preoperative computed tomography images and a postoperative X-ray of a patient with a displaced hangman's fracture of C2 (traumatic spondylolisthesis). Most hangman's fractures are managed nonoperatively, but in severely displaced fractures, reduction and stabilization with bone grafting is indicated. This can be done with either an anterior or (as shown) posterior procedure.

vertebrae. It is most common at the levels of C6, C7, T1, and T2, and is the result of avulsion fracture of the spinous process by the paraspinal muscle forces. The injury was originally described in convicts involved with shoveling clay and soil. This is most commonly seen today after motor vehicle trauma. These fractures are at times difficult to see on x-ray images (because of the density shadow cast by the patient's shoulder). The fracture itself generally requires only symptomatic treatment (analgesics with or without a soft collar for comfort); however, it behooves the treating physician to look for such injuries when they are suspected.

FRACTURES OF THE THORACIC AND LUMBAR SPINE

Thoracic Lumbar Spine Injury

Thoracic and lumbar fractures generally are discussed together because the mechanism fracture of these distinct anatomic areas is similar. Fractures of the thoracic spine are generally more stable than similar injuries in the lumbar spine because of the stability afforded by the ribs. Also, of course, neurologic injury patterns are different in the thoracic and proximal lumbar spine because of the presence of the spinal cord, which normally ends at the L2 level. Accordingly, injuries that compromise the spinal canal are more likely to cause neurologic deficits in the thoracic spine than in the lumbar spine. Nonetheless, general patterns of injury and their treatments are very similar.

Compression Fracture

Acute compression fracture in the thoracic and lumbar spine is a relatively common event. Traumatic compression fractures in patients with normal bone densities may involve a fracture of the superior or, less frequently, inferior end plate with or without associated posterior cortical failure. The zone of injury for the compression fracture is confined to the "anterior column" as defined by Dr. Francis Denis[40] in his classic paper in 1983 (Fig. 43-29). Isolated injuries to the anterior column do not result in neurologic deficit, because the posterior cortex of the vertebral body, and thus, the borders of the spinal canal remain intact; these injuries are not at all likely to lead to instability. Treatment is generally symptomatic with the use of braces for comfort and analgesics. In most cases, the fracture is noted to have successfully healed with resolution of pain within 4 to 10 weeks.

Burst Fracture

Burst fracture, caused by more severe axial load forces, is common following falls and motor vehicle trauma. A burst fracture involves fracture of one or both end plates and the anterior cortex of a thoracal

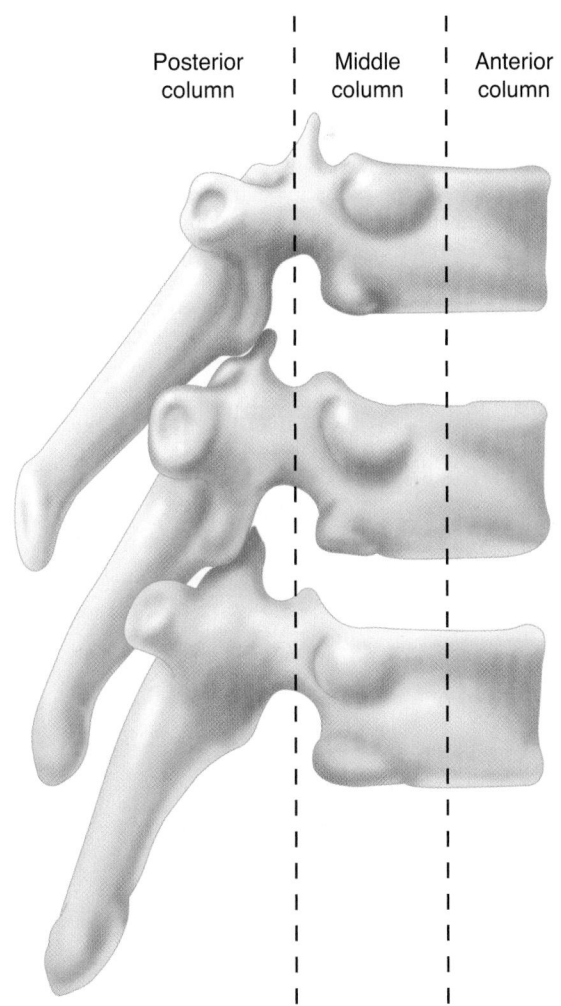

FIG. 43-29. The spine can be thought of as three columns. Two of three can maintain stability.

lumbar vertebra with an associated failure of the posterior cortex. Frequently, the posterior cortical fracture results in retropulsion of bone into the canal, which can cause compromise of the neural elements and acute neurologic deficit. The retropulsed fragment in a burst fracture injury typically has a trapezoidal shape, which reflects the trabecular anatomy in the area at the base of the pedicles where failure occurs.[41] On occasion, with even more severe injury loads, posterior element fractures can occur, most frequently, the vertical fracture of the lamina caused by forces exerted through the facet causing a spreading force on the posterior elements. Such vertical lamina fractures are particularly important because, quite frequently, this fracture will contain an invaginated segment of the dura mater, sometimes with accompanying nerve roots. Surgical intervention posteriorly on such fracture can result in an iatrogenic dural tear and/ or root injury.

Neurologically intact patients with burst fractures usually are managed quite successfully by nonoperative means using a rigid orthosis and analgesics. When significant neurologic injury is noted, surgical treatment usually is recommended. Most commonly, this consists of an anterior exposure of the fractured vertebrae and removal of the fractured anterior elements. This procedure is called a *corpectomy*. Concomitant with this (as in cervical spine burst fractures), both adjacent discs are excised to expose the bony end plates. A strut graft is placed; this can be either autograft or allograft or manufactured struts of titanium or ceramic. Generally, a laterally placed rod or plate system also is inserted to afford stability. The anterior approach allows direct decompression of the spinal canal and removal of any retropulsed fragments.

Another alternative is the posterior approach to the spine, which may or may not involve laminectomy and direct exposure of the neural elements. Because the offending compression is directed anteriorly, good visualization of the intraspinal fragments can be difficult from this approach, and usually, decompression is sought by distraction instrumentation. Hooks and screws are placed into vertebrae above and below the fractured segment and longitudinal stretching forces are applied through an attached rod. This usually results in partial reduction of the neurologic compression. When the posterior longitudinal ligament becomes tight, it will exert a corrective force encouraging the fragments in the canal to migrate back closer to their normal anatomic position. Predictable decompression of the spinal canal using posterior distracting techniques is not absolute. On average, this will result in improvement of the canal diameter, but in some cases, despite a technically well performed procedure, ongoing compression may persist.

Seatbelt Injuries (Flexion Distraction Injuries)

Flexion distraction injuries result from distractive forces on the spine. The mechanism for this is acute forward flexion of the trunk and anterior restraint such as a lap belt type seat belt. As the pelvis and upper torso moves forward, a fulcrum is created that can create a failure of the spine under tension beginning with the posterior elements and extending through the spine. Failure can take place through the soft tissues with tearing of the dorsal fascia, the interspinous ligament, dislocation of the facets, and tearing of the discs. It also may occur through the bone with frank failure in tension of the bone of the spinous process, the lamina, the pedicles, and the body. This "all bone" variant carries the name *Chance fracture*, named not for its unique morphology, but in deference to Dr. Chance who first described this injury in 1958.[42]

Fortunately, flexion distraction injuries usually do not result in neurologic injury as the spinal neural elements are generally much more tolerant of distractive forces than they are of compression. Unfortunately, when the flexion distraction injury occurs predominantly through soft tissue, reliable healing of the soft tissue is not expected and posterior stabilization using internal fixation and an associated bone graft generally is indicated to restore stability to the spine.

Interestingly, because of the rough irregular surfaces of the bone, fractures of the all bone variant (Chance fracture) are usually quite stable. Bracing is recommended, but the "all bone" Chance injury generally is quite successfully managed nonoperatively.

Fracture Dislocations of the Spine

Fracture dislocations of the spine are severe injuries associated with displaced injury of the bony elements, with either a translational or rotational component. By necessity, the presence of a translational or rotational deformity will result in canal compromise. The majority of patients sustaining these severe injuries do have a neurologic deficit, which is frequently profound (Fig. 43-30).

Reduction of the displaced bones generally is indicated and is usually the best way to improve the canal dimensions. The prognosis for neurologic recovery in a patient with a neurologically complete injury is dismal. Patients with partial preservation of function often can make remarkable neurologic recoveries. Patients

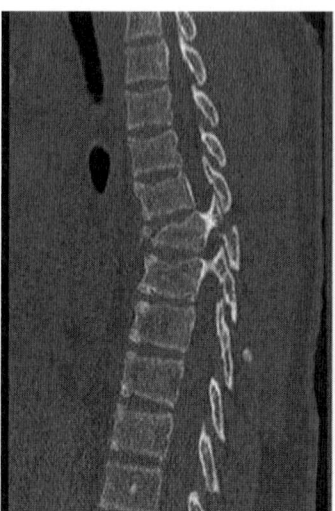
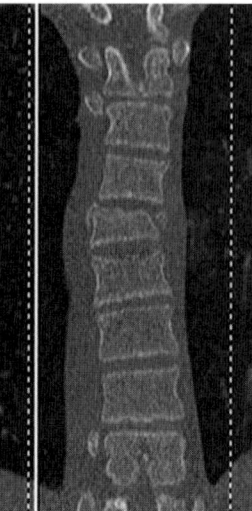
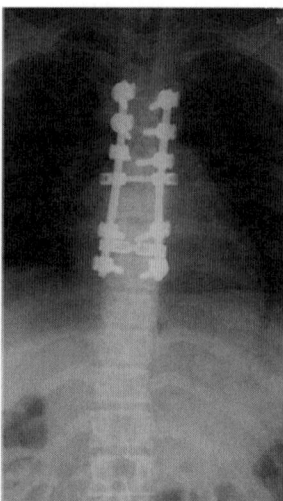
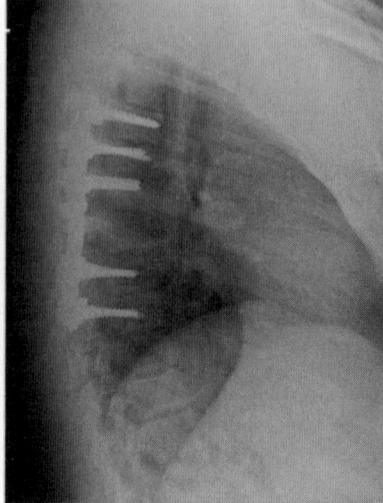

FIG. 43-30. Preoperative computed tomography images and postoperative x-ray images of a patient with fractures of T5 and T6 and an "incomplete" spinal cord injury. The spinal canal was decompressed and the fractures stabilized using pedicle screw instrumentation.

with fracture dislocations of the spine are essentially always managed operatively to stabilize the spine, to safeguard any neurologic function that might remain, or to allow mobilization of the patient and early initiation of rehabilitation.

Disc Herniation

Disc herniation is an extremely common event generally seen between the ages of 20 and 50 years old. It can occur in the cervical, thoracic, or the lumbar spine. It consists of a tear or an attritional failure of the annulus of the intervertebral disc, allowing the nucleus pulposus material to penetrate through the annulus and enter the canal. The incidence of this phenomenon is impressive. Fortunately, the majority of such events are minimally symptomatic. A majority of the population will have a disc herniation during a normal lifetime. Classically, disc herniations present with axial pain either in the neck or in the lumbar area, which over 1 to 14 days progresses to include a radicular pain in the upper or lower extremity. Nerve root impingements can occur, depending on the location of the herniation, of traversing nerve root or the exiting nerve root at any given level. Large herniations may impinge both of these nerve roots. In the cervical spine, potential for spinal cord compression also is noted, although this is not particularly common. When a disc herniation is causing myelopathic symptoms, it should be treated aggressively.

The expected natural history of disc herniations is that of spontaneous resolution of symptoms. This is presumed to occur through natural accommodation of the nerve root to the compression and to the resolution of the acute inflammatory process that may accompany the acute annular injury. Several studies have demonstrated that the extruded nucleus pulposus material actually undergoes a significant amount of resorption over time as well. Accordingly, at least approximately 90% of radiculopathies due to disc herniation do resolve or substantially improve within 8 weeks. Thus, surgical intervention even for severe radiculopathies is not recommended in this initial 6- to 8-week interval.[43] Should significant symptoms persist beyond this point in time, the decision is made between the surgeon and the patient about options for surgery. Should surgery be elected, excision of the involved disc and decompression of the nerve roots can be performed with an excellent prognosis. Thus, the great majority of patients express satisfaction with the results.

Surgical treatment for a cervical disc herniation usually consists of an anterior approach to the spine with dissection through a transverse incision on the anterior neck. Dissection is carried lateral to the trachea and esophagus and medial to the carotid sheath to expose the bones and discs of the anterior cervical spine. The disc is removed in total from anterior to posterior; this allows direct visualization of the dura and the extruded disc. In most cases, the disc space is then bone grafted to effect a fusion between the involved vertebrae. In most cases, a low profile titanium plate is then affixed to the involved vertebrae by locking screws. The advantage of the anterior approach is that it allows visualization of the disc material, including any central component.

An alternative surgical approach is a posterior decompression and laminectomy. Dissection is carried through the midline to expose the posterior elements of the spine. A portion of the lamina at the involved level is removed to allow access into the canal. This is an excellent option for foraminal impingements or for very lateral disc herniations. It is not possible from a posterior approach to visualize an exposed central disc herniation because of the presence of the spinal cord, which cannot be safely touched or manipulated. An advantage to the posterior approach is that this can be done without the need for fusion or instrumentation.

The surgical approach for a disc herniation of the lumbar spine is similar to the posterior approach just described in the cervical spine. A midline incision is created with exposure of the posterior elements of the spine. Portions of the lamina are removed until good visualization of the lateral recess is possible. Unlike the cervical spine, gentle retraction of the dura is possible in the lower lumbar spine, allowing visualization of the traversing nerve roots as

well as of the disc fragment. Thus, even a central disc fragment can be removed under excellent direct visualization of the lumbar spine. This can be done from a very small incision, and in nearly every case, without the need for fusion or instrumentation.

Spinal Stenosis

Spinal stenosis is an acquired narrowing of the spinal canal and can occur in the cervical, thoracic, or lumbar spines. This generally is due to a combination of degenerative changes in the spine , loss of disc height, and bulging of both of the annular tissue as well as the ligamentum flavum; both will contribute to narrowing of the canal. The larger culprit is often hypertrophic changes in the facet joints with osteophyte formation, which can contribute to significant nerve impingement. Cervical stenosis can cause progressive myelopathic symptoms of hyperreflexia, ataxia, balance problems, and four quadrant weakness. On occasion, concomitant root compression also can cause upper extremity radicular pains.

In the lumbar spine, a more common picture is that of "neurogenic claudication." Patients are asymptomatic at rest, but with ambulation, they experience progressive discomfort, weakness, and at times, numbness in the lower extremities. The lower extremity symptoms, resulting from lumbar spinal stenosis, generally resolve very promptly with sitting or forward flexion of the body. It can be demonstrated that increasing lumbar lordosis (as with standing or walking) will cause further narrowing of the canal due to bulging of the ligamentum flavum and positioning of the arthritic facets.

Temporary relief for spinal stenosis in both the cervical and lumbar spine can result from epidural administration of corticosteroids. Definitive treatment for disabling symptoms consists of decompressive surgery, specifically removal of the offending laminae and resection of hypotrophic bone from the involved facets.[44] If extensive bony resection is performed, particularly in the cervical spine, stabilization using bone grafts and internal fixation (rods or plates) may be indicated.

Spinal stenosis is a clinical entity most common in patients >50 years of age and occasionally, substantially older. Unfortunately, the same patient group often has acquired spinal deformities of degenerative spondylolisthesis or degenerative scoliosis.[45] The presence of significant symptoms of spinal stenosis in the presence of a deformity such as spondylolisthesis or scoliosis can create a difficult management problem. Simple decompression in the face of a spondylolisthesis or a significant scoliosis may lead to abrupt, precipitous, and problematic progression of the patient's spinal deformity. Accordingly, when decompressive procedures are planned for patients with deformity, in most cases, concomitant fusion procedures with instrumentation are recommended. Unfortunately, these are large and potentially morbid surgical procedures that often are contraindicated for patients with debilitating comorbidities.

Back Pain and Degenerative Disc Disease

Causes for low back pain are myriad, and unfortunately, for many patients, such pains become chronic and disabling. Complaints of low back pain should always alert the physician to the possibility of a dire process such as a malignancy. Metastatic disease is present in the spine with a frightening frequency.

Degenerative disease of the spine is common and clearly can cause disabling low back pain. One enduring mystery, thus far, has been the limited correlation between degenerative disease demonstrated on imaging studies and levels of clinical back pain. Many patients with severe degenerative changes have no pain at all, while others with only mild degenerative disease on imaging studies complain of disabling symptoms. Evaluation and treatment of these patients remains an area of great controversy. One option in the management of disabling low back pain in the presence of degenerative disease is to consider fusion operations of the spine.

Fusion procedures for painful degenerative osteoarthritic joints have historically been very successful in the extremities. Although fusion of the hip and knee for these indications has largely been supplanted by joint replacement procedures, it is recognized that knee fusion and hip fusion, as well as wrist, elbow, and shoulder fusion, can represent very effective pain relieving procedures. Unfortunately, the observed clinical results when fusion operations are applied to the spine are clearly less successful. Complicating issues of secondary gain, psychiatric issues, and the difficult diagnostic questions of which portions of the axial elements are causing the pain fuel the controversy.

Many surgeons advocate the use of *discography*, a provocative test done on an awake patient wherein a needle is inserted percutaneously into a disc space and contrast is injected. Flow of the contrast through the disc and annulus in an abnormal way is interpreted to document degenerative changes within the disc. Simultaneous provocation of "typical" pain by the injection is thought to confirm the anatomic location of the offending pain. Unfortunately, even with the use of discography, the success rate with such fusion procedures is controversial at best. Documentation of small numbers of unmyelinated nerve fibers within the outer annulus of the disc has been widely accepted by many as the true source of such back pain. Recently, the documentation of extensive innervation of the epidural space, and indeed of the vertebral bone itself, has raised other questions about possible pain sources in these patients. Work on this subject is continuing.

A newer option for the management of degenerative disc disease is the use of an intervertebral disc replacement prosthesis. Several designs are now in use throughout the world. Substantial controversy surrounds their use, having to do with their true effectiveness, their potential for loosening, the potential creation of wear debris, and the difficulty associated with a future revision surgery. These prostheses are placed in close proximity to the contents of the spinal canal and to the great vessels. Future management of this challenging clinical problem is presently unclear.

Scoliosis

Scoliosis is a term used to describe a lateral curve of the bones of the spine. This can easily be documented on x-ray images. Because of the anatomy of the spine, lateral bending deformity will always be accompanied by an associated rotational deformity as well, a phenomenon called *coupling*. Thus, the scoliosis curve will always have a rotational component. Scoliosis is a three-dimensional entity.

The description of scoliotic curves is the topic for extensive mechanical and anatomic study, and several good schemes to measure and define the curves are in use. The most common one and most convenient is the Cobb method, after Dr. Cobb's description in 1948.[46] Lines are drawn along the end plates of the vertebral bodies at either end of the curve and the angle from where these lines intersect is taken as the "magnitude" of the curve. This technique does not take into account the rotational component of the deformities, which are measured by other means.

Scoliosis curves are not only classified by their magnitude, but by their etiology. Scoliotic curves are classified as congenital (developmental abnormal shapes of the involved bones), degenerative (a curve caused by degenerative changes in the joints of the spine), metabolic (caused by generalized genetic metabolic disease such as mucopolysaccharidosis), neurogenic (spinal deformities caused by primary neurologic insult such as cerebral palsy or spinal cord injury), and myogenic curves (those curves associated with primary muscle problems). Such myogenic curves commonly are seen in muscular dystrophy patients. Idiopathic curves are the most common form of scoliosis. It is now emerging that idiopathic scoliosis actually represents a spectrum of genetic disease due to several different genes with variable penetrance. This chapter will limit the majority of discussion to degenerative curves and idiopathic curves.

Degenerative curves generally are seen in patients over the age of 50 years old. At times, it is impossible to distinguish a primary degenerative curve from an idiopathic curve with associated degenerative disease. In any event, adults with scoliosis and progressive painful arthritic spines often have disabling symptoms, not only of

axial pain, but of imbalance in posture due to these curves. Symptomatic measures using medications, therapy, and activity modification are, at times, rather unsatisfying. In severe cases, where objective deformity is noted and the patient's medical condition warrants, surgical intervention to apply corrective forces by the use of internal fixation with rod and screw constructs can result in substantial improvement and quality of life. These operations are undertaken only after careful forethought, meticulous informed consent, patient education, and careful preoperative and perioperative medical attention. These are challenging surgical procedures with a high rate of complication.

Idiopathic Scoliosis

Idiopathic scoliosis has infantile, juvenile, and adolescent forms. The overwhelming majority of the patients acquire their curves during adolescence. These curves, apparently due to a spectrum of genetic disorders with variable penetrance, generally manifested during early adolescence and may progress rapidly during periods of skeletal growth. Generally speaking, significant progression of these curves is arrested after skeletal maturity. During active skeletal growth, however, rapidly progressive deformity can arise. Initial management may consist of simple observation. Curves that are progressing at a rate likely to lead to significant deformity often are treated by the use of braces. Braces are applied to the trunk to hold the spine in a corrected position. Braces cannot result in permanent correction of a curve, but often are effective in slowing or arresting progression of a curve. Brace treatment for a patient with idiopathic scoliosis is generally most effective for curves between 20° and 40° as measured by the Cobb technique. If bracing is ineffective, or for patients with large curves, surgical intervention may be appropriate. Surgical treatment consists of using rods for instrumentation of the spine in an improved position with grafting and fusion, and can result in dramatic correction of these curves (Fig. 43-31). Such procedures also have the potential for significant complications and always result in markedly diminished truncal motion. The decision for surgery in an adolescent with scoliosis is always carefully considered and generally is undertaken only in the presence of unabated progression. It is a combined decision among the surgeon, parents, and patient.

Neuromuscular Scoliosis

Scoliosis due to neurogenic cause generally is noted early in life. There are hundreds of neurologic conditions that can lead to scoliosis, such as polio and cerebral palsy. Such curves are usually uncompensated, meaning that the patient is unable to lean with his upper body to restore balance. Accordingly, these curves often make standing, and even sitting, unbalanced (Fig. 43-32). Nonambulatory patients often undergo scoliosis correction surgery to facilitate sitting balance and to avoid skin breakdown caused by pelvic obliquity.

ORTHOPEDIC PATHOLOGY AND ONCOLOGY

Introduction

The orthopedic surgeon quite frequently is asked to deal with both benign and malignant tumors. Given the complexity of these entities, an approach to diagnosing and treating these lesions requires the collaboration of the surgeon, radiologist, and pathologist; ideally with discussion both before and after biopsy and definitive treatment among all three. Failure to allow for adequate communication between all concerned often leads to misdiagnosis or worse.

The most commonly encountered tumor problem facing orthopedic surgeons is that of metastatic disease to the bone. Many carcinomas, most notably lung, prostate, thyroid, breast, and kidney, quite frequently metastasize to the bone. Such skeletal metastases are often painful and may weaken the bone to the point where a

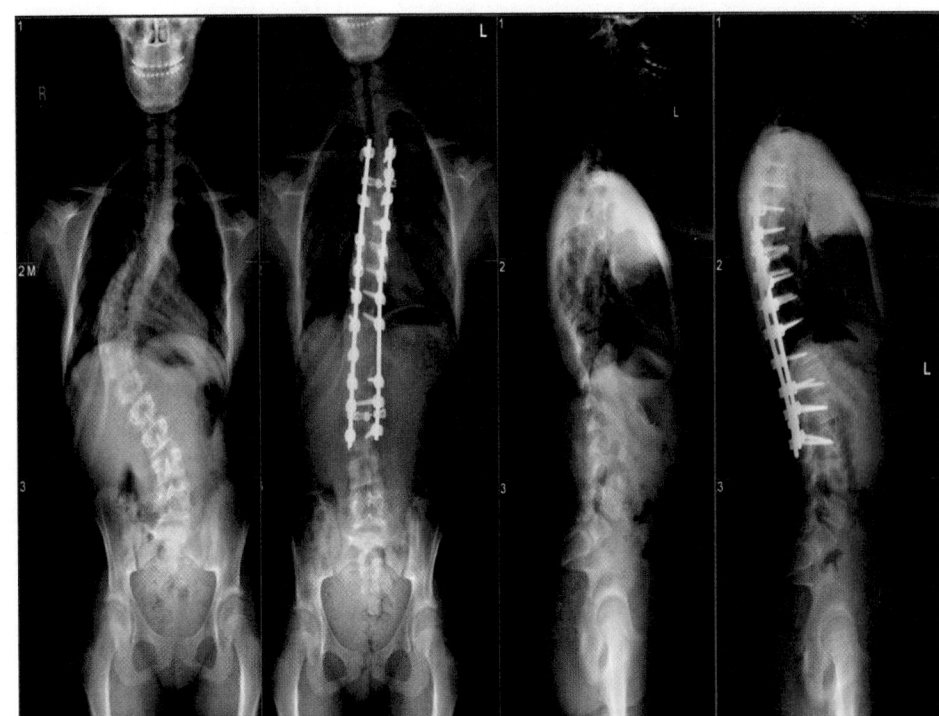

FIG. 43-31. Preoperative and post-operative images of a 13-year-old patient with progressive idiopathic scoliosis that was not controlled by bracing. Excellent correction was obtained with posterior instrumentation and fusion. *(Courtesy of Dr. Darrell Hanson.)*

pathologic fracture occurs. Unfortunately, the orthopedist is quite frequently the physician who makes the initial diagnosis of metastatic disease, as such painful lesions or associated fractures can be the presenting event for many patients with such cancer.

When first evaluating a patient with a bony lesion, the orthopedist will use imaging studies, always to include plain x-ray images, and often other imaging techniques such at MRI, CT scan, and bone scan. Laboratory studies and patient history also are always considered.

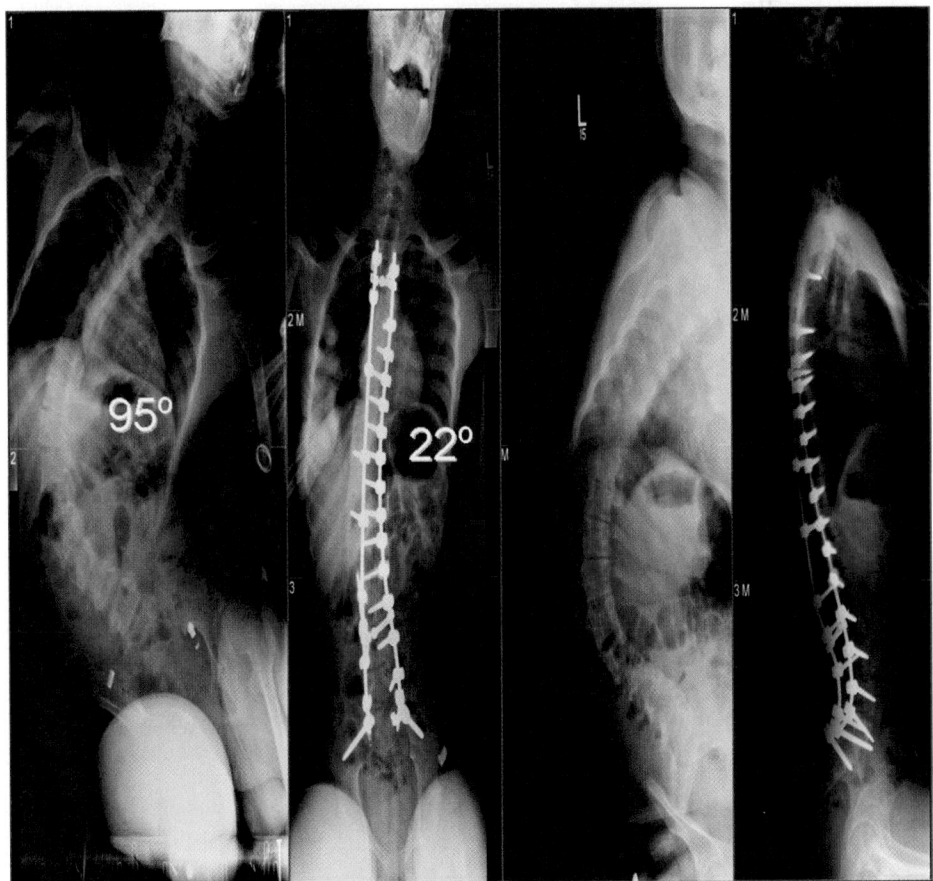

FIG. 43-32. Pre- and postoperative images of a 14-year-old patient with a progressive scoliosis associated with cerebral palsy. This curve was causing progressive problems with sitting balance that were successfully overcome with surgical correction and fusion. *(Courtesy of Dr. Darrel Hanson.)*

Bone lesions are notoriously challenging to identify. The possibility of malignancy or infection must be kept in mind in approaching any abnormal tissue in the bone. The orthopedic oncologist should always consider the possibility that the lesion in question could be a metastatic focus with a distant primary, may represent a focus of infection, may represent a non-neoplastic or developmental lesion, may represent a benign lesion, or may represent a lymphoma or myeloma. Finally, it could represent a primary malignancy of the mesenchymal tissues (a sarcoma).

In patients with suspected metastatic disease, laboratory studies, x-rays, physical examination, and history will quite frequently reveal a primary source of tumor. Generally, the treatment rendered for the osseous metastases is nonsurgical. Unfortunately, a large metastatic lesion within the bone will frequently weaken the bone to the point of fracture. If a fracture has already occurred at the time of presentation, surgical treatment for stabilization and palliation of pain usually is indicated. Prevention is often recommended, as bone healing in the phase of metastatic disease is reliable. Restoring function to the patient is a high priority in such lesions that are frequently treated by internal fixation and sometimes with bone grafting.

There are a number of non-neoplastic lesions of bone that mimic neoplasms. In the majority of cases, the first concern is that of accurate diagnosis. A malignant bone neoplasm, if misdiagnosed, can lead to disaster.

Benign non-neoplasms of the bone are relatively common. They must be differentiated from malignant lesions. Benign lesions may be indolent, but some benign neoplasms are locally aggressive and destructive. Certain aggressive benign lesions, when occurring in difficult locations such as the spine, may result in paralysis or death.

Bone Neoplasms

Sarcomas are the result of malignant transformation of cells of mesenchymal lineage. Some sarcomas are slow growing, while others are rapidly progressive. They are discussed here individually.

Metastatic Diseases

Unfortunately, pathologic fractures are common. Any surgery on a lesion of this kind will be accompanied by an intraoperative biopsy of the abnormal tissue. Another frequently encountered problem is that of patients with metastatic disease that have large bony lesions that have not yet resulted in fracture.[47] Recognizing these lesions can be surprisingly difficult. As much as 50% of a long bone substance may be destroyed by tumor before such lesions are visible on routine x-rays (Fig. 43-33). A large lesion occupying a significant portion of the shaft or long bone should be considered for prophylactic internal fixation. Procedures often can be done without opening the fracture site by inserting rods or nails from a distal site to traverse the lesion. Such internal fixation procedures can actually protect the bone from fracture and can spare the patient a much more involved surgery.

Management of Patients with Sarcomas of the Bone

The initial step in managing patients with bone sarcomas is a complete medical evaluation, including laboratory studies, investigation of the chest for possible metastatic lesions, and an assessment for other possible bony lesions (Fig. 43-34). In almost every case, initial biopsy is performed as a separate step before any surgical intervention.[48] It is imperative that surgical planning and procedures be executed by an experienced tumor surgeon. The biopsy incision is carefully planned to traverse a minimum number of tissue planes so that the entire area of the biopsy dissection including the skin incision may be excised should the patient subsequently undergo a definitive resection of the tumor.[49,50] Accordingly, incisions are as small as possible and oriented longitudinally.[51,52] Discussion of the biopsy with the interpreting pathologist is strongly encouraged before performing the biopsy.[53] Whenever possible, biopsy tissue is obtained for "permanent" pathology analysis as well as culture and

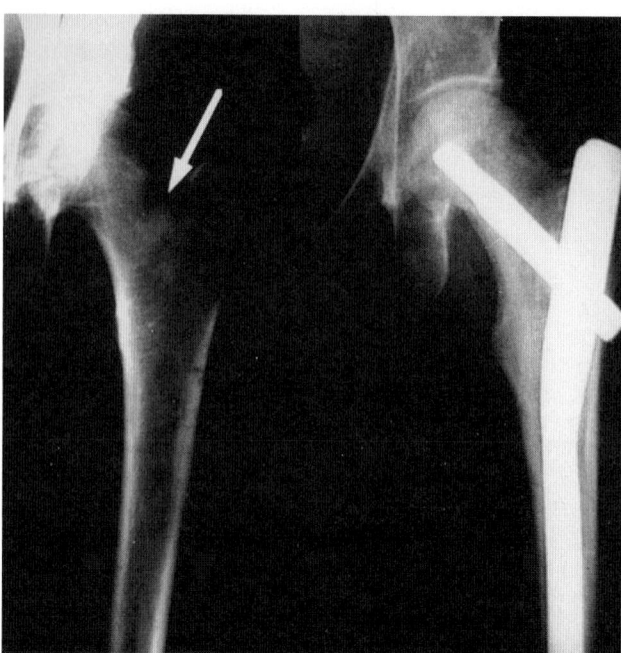

FIG. 43-33. Impending fracture of the proximal femur (*arrow*) from metastatic breast carcinoma. Internal fixation using an intramedullary device (Zickel nail) with subsequent radiation therapy allows local control of the tumor and healing of the fracture.

frozen section (Fig. 43-35). The frozen section is performed intraoperatively whenever possible.[54] The purpose of the frozen section is not to provide a diagnosis; indeed, frozen section examination of sarcoma lesions is rarely definitive. The purpose of the frozen section is to ensure that the obtained tissue represents a reasonable sampling of the abnormal tissue. The critical information sought with the frozen section analysis is to ensure that the biopsy has been taken "within the lesion." Following this, the incision is closed. No further surgical treatment is undertaken until the final diagnosis has been established.

Metastatic Sarcomas

Metastases from sarcomas can arise in many different tissues, but the most common site of initial metastatic disease is the lung. When a sarcoma is suspected, physical examination and imaging of the chest is an early and important consideration.

Chemotherapy in the Treatment of Sarcomas

Use of chemotherapy before definitive surgical resection neoadjuvant treatment is now commonly a part of the management of many, if not most, sarcomas.[55] Effective therapeutic agents have been developed over the last 30 years that are often effective in causing a reduction in the size of the malignant lesions. Chemotherapy alone is not successful in affecting a cure of any sarcoma; however, combined combinations of chemotherapy and surgery can lead to gratifying long-term survival rates and cures.

Bone-Forming Tumors—Osteoid Osteoma (Benign)

Osteoid osteoma is a benign bone-forming lesion of uncertain etiology that presents with a central radiolucent nidus (<1.5 cm) and dense surrounding sclerosis. This lesion occurs in patients under the age of 20 years old (usually under the age of 12) but can occasionally occur in older patients. They are predominantly intracortical in location except when they occur in the small bones of the hands and feet where they are intramedullary. Radiologically, they

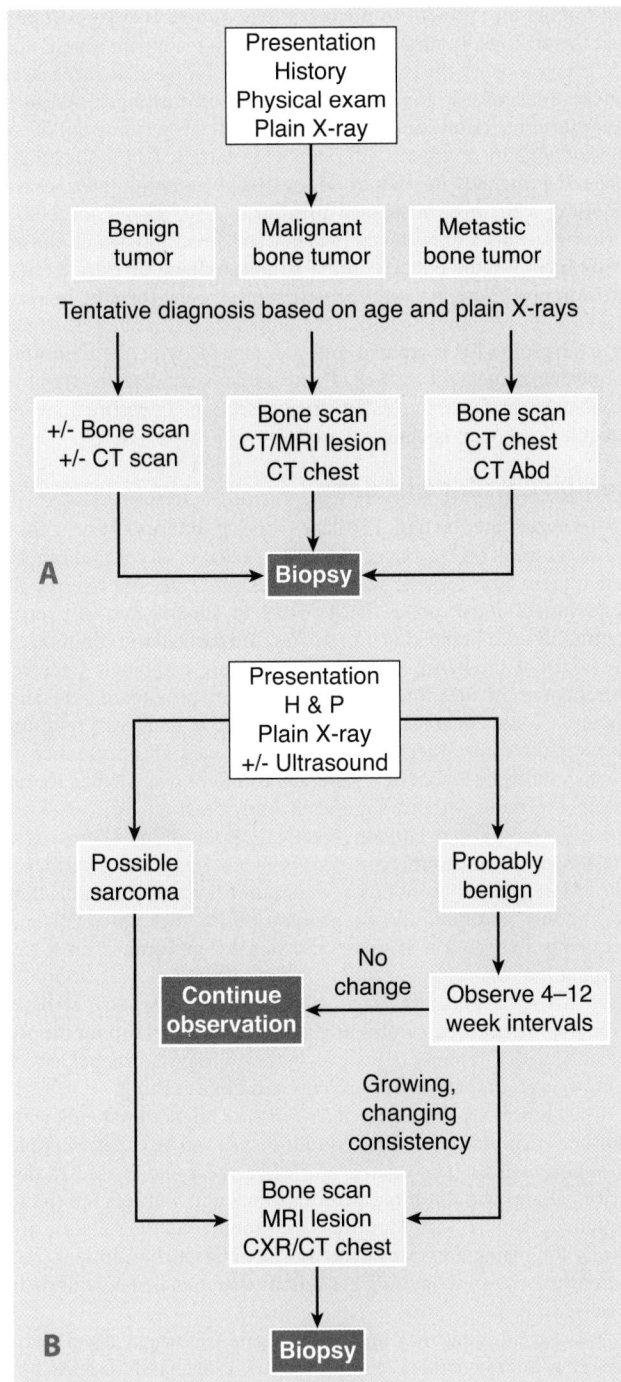

FIG. 43-34. Staging algorithms for (**A**) bone tumors and (**B**) soft tissue tumors. Abd = abdomen; CT = computed tomography; CXR = chest x-ray; H&P = history and physical examination; MRI = magnetic resonance imaging. [Modified with permission from Kasser JR (ed): Orthopaedic Knowledge Update 5. Rosemont, IL: American Academy of Orthopaedic Surgeons, 1996, p 136.]

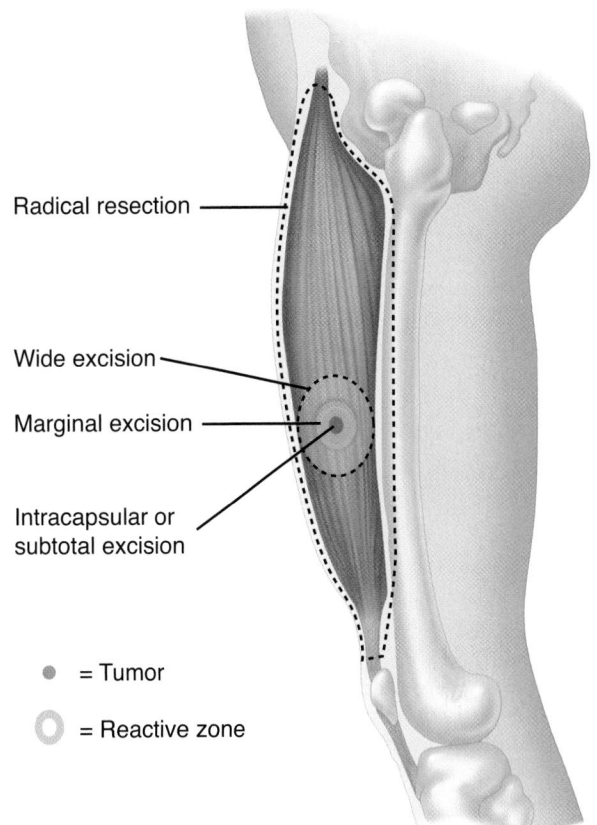

FIG. 43-35. Definitions of surgical margins for bone and soft tissue sarcomas. (Modified with permission from Enneking WF et al: A system for the surgical staging of musculoskeletal sarcoma. Clin Orthop 153:106, 1980.)

which in a significant proportion of cases spontaneously regress, usually after a period of 1 to 7 years. Should more aggressive treatment be contemplated, an accessible lesion can be treated by percutaneous radiofrequency ablation (heat administered through high frequency alternating currents). On other occasions, it can be treated by surgical excision.

Osteoblastoma (Benign)

Osteoblastoma is a relatively rare bone-producing tumor that can grow locally to large size although it does not metastasize. Patients may present with local pain, or on occasion, a mass. The histologic appearance of the lesions consists of cells with regularly shaped nuclei often seen with areas of hemorrhagic tissue and irregularly deposited osteoid.

Osteoblastoma is, by definition, >1.5 cm and has histologic features identical to the nidus of the osteoid osteoma. Although these lesions can occur anywhere, they have a propensity to develop in the posterior elements of the spine where they can mimic a malignancy radiologically. The radiologic appearance is of a purely lytic lesion with occasional internal matrix production. In smaller or thinner bones, the osteoblastoma will often "break out" into the surrounding soft tissue mimicking a malignant lesion. Histologically, an osteoblastoma will show new bone formation in irregular distributions with a rich fibrovascular stroma. Mitotic figures can be noted, especially if the lesion has been fractured or during pregnancy, but malignant transformation is rare. Osteoblastomas generally are managed by excision or local curettage.

Osteogenic Sarcoma

Osteogenic sarcomas are malignant. There are an array of subtypes of osteogenic sarcomas that display varying degrees of potential for metastases. Osteogenic sarcoma tumors are distinguished by the direct syn-

are noted to be a dense cortical sclerosis on plain film. The nidus can be difficult to observe, and CT often is helpful in this regard. Histologically, the nidus is a dense fibrovascular proliferation with abundant new bone formation and active osteoblastic and osteoclastic activity. The surrounding sclerosis is very dense and approaches that seen in the normal cortex.

The pain produced by this tumor can be quite intense. Interestingly, this pain is predictably dramatically responsive to aspirin or a NSAID medication. Indeed, regular medication with anti-inflammatories often can present definitive treatment for these lesions

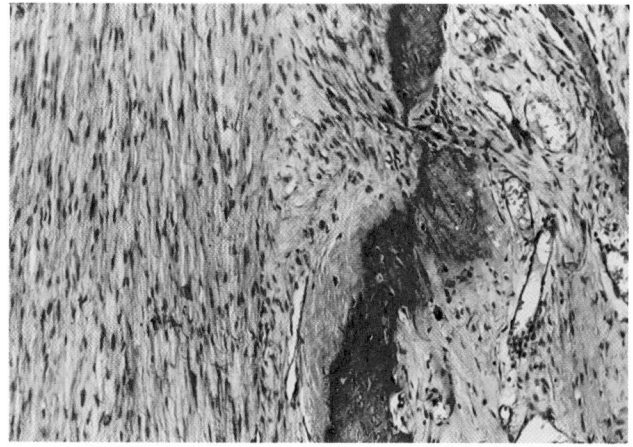

FIG. 43-36. Low-power photomicrograph reveals cartilage matrix that entraps and destroys bone. The myxoid nature to the matrix suggests a grade II lesion.

thesis of osteoid by the tumor cells. A low-grade variant of the osteogenic sarcoma is the periosteal osteogenic sarcoma. This is a slow-growing tumor and predictably occurs on the external surface of a long bone cortex. It is very common on the posterior aspect of the distal femur. Periosteal osteogenic sarcoma generally appears to be a large, circumscribed, densely sclerotic mass arising from the cortex. It generally is adherent to or continuous with the bone. Treatment for a periosteal osteogenic sarcoma (after confirmation by a carefully planned biopsy) is surgical excision with a wide margin. Adjunctive radiation therapy or chemotherapy may be indicated for periosteal osteogenic sarcomas with good levels of cure. Long-term survival from a periosteal osteogenic sarcoma after a successful wide local excision can be >90%.

Classic Osteosarcoma (Malignant)

High-grade *osteogenic sarcomas* generally take origin from within the medullary cavity of the bone and are the most common type of osteogenic sarcoma (Fig. 43-36). It is the most common bone malignancy in children and is especially common in the distal femur, proximal tibia, and proximal humerus. Osteogenic sarcomas may contain focal areas of cartilage formation; occasionally other mesenchymal tissues such as fat or muscle may be seen. The presence of any bone formation by the tumor cells, however, establishes the diagnosis of osteogenic sarcoma.

Treatment for high-grade osteogenic sarcomas nearly always involves preoperative and postoperative chemotherapy as well as a wide excision of the lesion.[56] Frequently, this necessitates amputation. In some cases, it is possible to resect large segments of a long bone, such as the tibia or the fibula, and reconstruct the limb. This is a highly specialized area of orthopedic surgery with the use of specific protheses (generally custom designed). The use of large osteochondral allografts often can be very helpful to preserve function in these patients. Chemotherapy and local radiation is frequently used. Long-term survival after the successful local resection of a high-grade osteogenic sarcoma can be >60%.

Osteosarcoma, although predominantly seen in young patients, can be seen in older patients as a result of previous radiation or chemotherapy or underlying conditions such as Paget's disease. Unfortunately, the osteosarcomas that arise in these conditions are uniformly high grade.

CARTILAGE-FORMING TUMORS

Cartilage-Forming Neoplasms

Cartilage-forming neoplasms are another clinical challenge. As one might expect, there are both benign and malignant cartilage-form-

ing tumors that present in the bone. When there is any possibility that the orthopedic surgeon is dealing with a malignant lesion, it is obligatory to work the patient up adequately for possible metastases before undertaking any definitive biopsy or treatment. As with bone-forming lesions, special attention is placed on ruling out other sites of bone involvement and possible metastatic foci in the lungs. General principles for biopsy of a cartilage containing lesion are identical with those discussed previously (Fig. 43-44) for bone-forming lesions. Care is taken to plan a small incision, which can be easily incorporated entirely into a large debulking or extralesional excision procedure. As with the treatment of bone-forming lesions, it is strongly recommended that the biopsy procedure be performed by a surgeon who is trained and comfortable with the definitive surgical management as well. Preoperative consultation with the pathologist and intraoperative frozen section to ensure that an adequate specimen is obtained are important steps.

Benign Cartilage Lesions

Chondromas are benign cartilage-forming tumors. When they occur centrally on the bone, they are referred to as *enchondromas*. When these lesions occur in the cortical bone, they are referred to as *periosteal chondromas*. Both forms of chondromas are most commonly seen in the long bones. They are particularly common in the bones of the hand, where they can cause pathologic fracture. Other common sites for chondromas are the proximal femur and humerus. Most enchondromas are identified as incidental findings on x-ray taken for other purposes. The radiographic appearance of an enchondroma is that of a generally round or oval-shaped lesion within the bone without significant bony reaction. All cartilage-forming tumors can contain areas of calcification. Microscopic analysis of an enchondroma reveals normal appearing cartilage. The lesion generally contains a small number of cartilage cells that do not show proliferation or pleiomorphism. The enchondroma frequently has such a familiar and benign appearance on x-ray imaging that management often consists of simple observation. In cases where lesions are large, painful, or display any atypical radiographic features, careful investigation and work-up for biopsy are indicated. On many occasions, biopsy (always accompanied by culture) is accompanied by curettage and bone grafting.

The clinical syndrome of *Ollier's disease* refers to patients with multiple enchondromas. This condition also can be called *multiple enchondromatosis*. The related *Maffucci's syndrome* is used to describe patients with multiple enchondromas and multiple soft tissue angiomas. Patients with Maffucci's syndrome or Ollier's disease are at risk for malignant transformation of their enchondromas and therefore do require ongoing periodic evaluations throughout their lives (see Fig. 43-7).

Endochondromas may involve any bone that originates in cartilage. They are frequently seen in the bones of the hands and feet but can be seen in the long bones and the pelvis. Endochondromas are thought to arise from islands of cartilage that are left behind as the growth plate moves away from them. These islands can grow independently and slowly increase in size. The longer they are present, the more they will mature through endochondral ossification and calcify, which appears as arcs and rings on plain films. In the hands and feet, endochondromas can thin the cortex, increasing the chance for fracture.

Osteochondroma

Osteochondromas are benign cartilage-forming lesions that arise within the cortex of the bone, usually in the metaphyseal region. The lesions arise from abnormalities in the epiphysial growth plate. Lesions have a cartilage "cap" that proliferates and can form a substantial-sized mass beneath the cartilage in histologically normal bone. Osteochondromas may be broad based (sessile), or on some occasions, have a defined, discrete stalk. Such osteochondromas are called *pedunculated*. For lesions with a characteristic appearance, observation alone can suffice. In some patients, however, the lesions

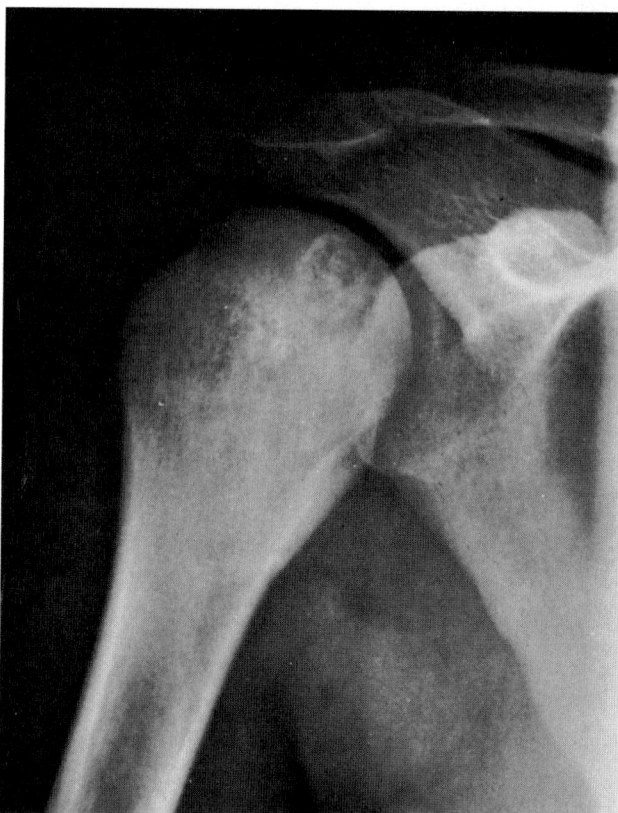

FIG. 43-37. Benign chondroblastoma (Codman's tumor) of the humerus.

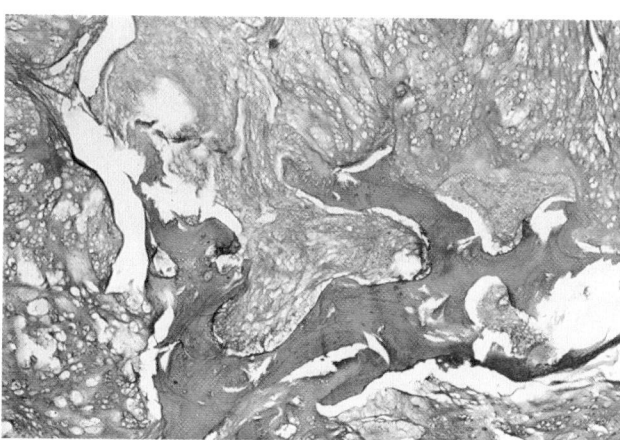

FIG. 43-39. High-power photomicrograph demonstrates the increased cellularity of a grade III chondrosarcoma.

portion of the lesion and may represent chondroblasts. A small, but significant percentage of chondroblastomas are capable of metastases. Generally, they are managed by curettage and bone grafting.

Chondrosarcomas

Chondrosarcoma is a malignant neoplasm of cartilage (Figs. 43-38 and 43-39). It is most common in adults and is commonly seen in the pelvis, spine, proximal humerus, and the knee. Most frequently, the presenting symptom is that of local pain. X-ray images show an expansive destructive lesion of the bone frequently with focal areas of calcification within the tumor (Figs. 43-40 and 43-41). It is important to differentiate the x-ray finding of calcification within cartilage tumors from that of ossification within a bone-forming tumor such as osteogenic sarcoma. The cartilage present in a chondrosarcoma is visualized on an x-ray as a disorganized density without cortication or trabecularization. Chondrosarcomas too often present challenging problems with management. Many of the tumors are within the spine or pelvis skeleton, making ablative surgery or amputation difficult or impossible. Further, many, if not most, chondrosarcomas are slow growing and are, thus, often less susceptible to chemotherapy and radiation therapy than many other sarcomas.

can become painful, usually because of mechanical problems. In such cases, they can be surgically resected. Any painful osteochondroma should be taken seriously, however, as there is a described incidence (approximately 1%) of malignant transformation.

Chondroblastoma

Chondroblastomas are benign cartilage-forming tumors nearly always found in the epiphysis area of a young patient usually before skeletal maturity. It is common for patients with chondroblastomas to present with pain. Generally, plain x-ray images of the joint reveal a focus of bone lysis or resorption surrounded by a rim of sclerotic, reactive bone (Fig. 43-37). Proliferating cells are seen within the lytic

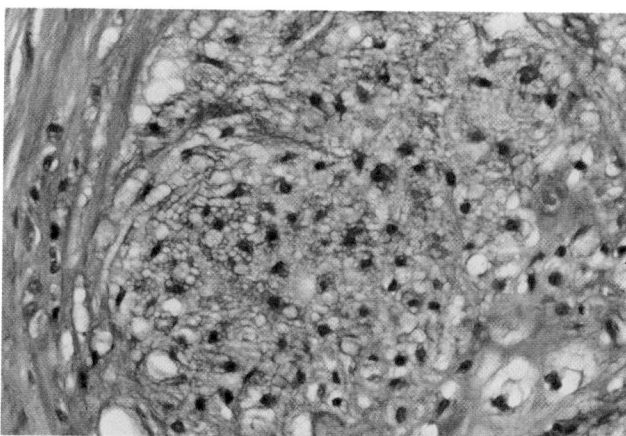

FIG. 43-38. Medium power photomicrograph demonstrates an atypical bone-producing lesion with spindled cells.

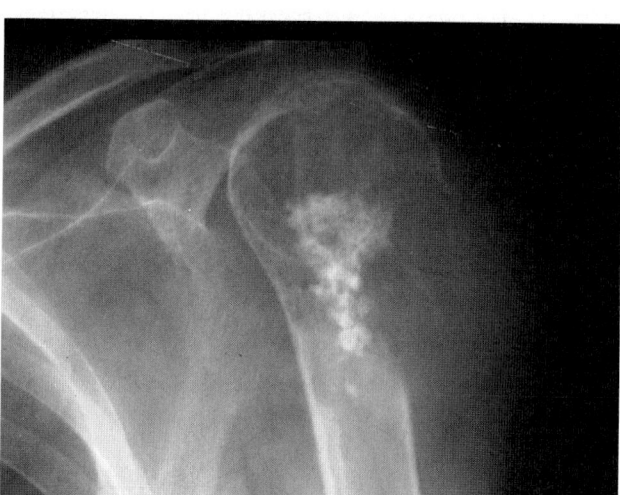

FIG. 43-40. Plain film of the proximal humerus demonstrates a metaphyseal matrix-producing lesion with arc- and ring-like formations consistent with cartilage formation. The lateral aspect of the lesion shows destruction of the cortex with soft tissue mass in keeping with the diagnosis of dedifferentiated chondrosarcoma.

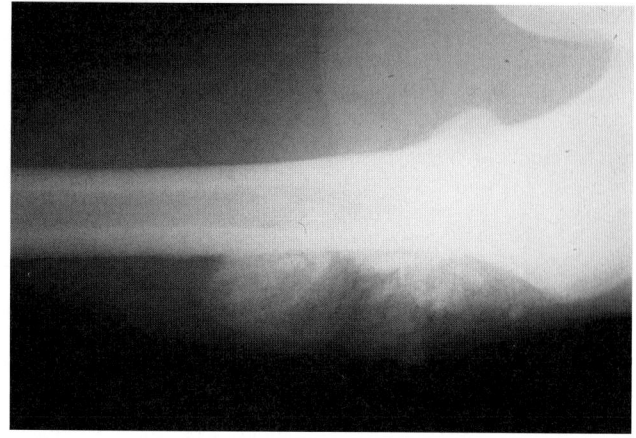

FIG. 43-41. Plain film of the proximal humerus demonstrates an ivory-like lesion of the proximal diaphysis with sunburst type periosteal reaction.

Treatment of a chondrosarcoma generally consists of a wide surgical resection alone.

FIBROUS LESIONS OF THE BONE

Aneurysmal Bone Cysts

An aneurysmal bone cyst is a reactive condition not thought to represent a neoplasm, which consists of a cyst. It can present after a pathologic fracture or due to complaints of local pain with an associated mass. Histology reveals large, blood-filled spaces with a true endothelial lining, foreign-body–type giant cells, and occasional woven bone formation. Care must be taken to examine the lesion adequately as secondary aneurysmal change is quite common and many lesions diagnosed as aneurysmal bone cyst are actually caused by another lesion with associated extensive cyst formation. Small lesions may be followed with simple observation, however, because risk of pathologic fracture means that the majority is treated by local curettage and bone grafting.

Unicameral Bone Cyst

Unicameral bone cyst is a benign lesion, most commonly found in the metaphyseal regional of long bones (frequently the humerus of growing children). This lesion can present after pathologic fracture, but also is occasionally noted due to local pain or a mass. The cause for this condition is unknown. Radiographic appearance is generally that of a large, single, cystic structure within the bone. The histologic appearance of the lesion is that of a fluid-filled cystic area within the bone. The lining of the unicameral bone cyst is composed of fibrous tissue with occasional giant cells. Small lesions may be managed by simple observation, whereas larger lesions, in which fracture risk is significant, are managed by a local curettage and bone grafting.

Fibrous Dysplasia (Fibro-Osseous Dysplasia)

Fibrous dysplasia is a commonly seen lesion in children. It is usually an isolated, slow-growing hematoma consisting of mixed bone and fibrous tissue. Fibrous dysplasia is a lesion composed of a spindle-shaped, mononuclear stroma with woven bone formation. This lesion may involve one bone (monostotic) or multiple bones (polystotic). The radiologic features usually demonstrate areas of radiolucency with a hazy and diffuse internal matrix production often termed *ground glass*. The histologic features show a bland spindle cell proliferation with irregularly shaped woven bone formation. The bone arises directly out of the background stroma. Occasional giant cells, hemorrhage, and myxoid degeneration can occur, espe-

cially if the lesion is fractured. It most frequently is asymptomatic but, unfortunately in some patients, large metaphyseal lesions can lead to focal growth disturbance and bone deformity. Pathologic fracture also is sometimes seen. In the absence of fracture or deformity, the lesions usually are painless and asymptomatic and they are most commonly diagnosed as incidental findings on radiographs. When present in the proximal femur, successive fracture events may lead to a characteristic "Shepherd's crook" appearance to the proximal femur. Plain radiographs often are diagnostic and small lesions may be managed by simple observation. When lesions cause significant symptoms or when pathologic fracture is considered likely, curettage and internal fixation bone grafting often are offered as treatment.

Non-Ossifying Fibroma

Non-ossifying fibroma is one of the most common bone lesions and can be found commonly as incidental lesions and in autopsy series. It presents as an eccentrically located, radiolucent lesion of the metaphysis with a lobulated or soap-bubble appearance. These proliferations have a dense peripheral sclerosis and may or may not have a fracture associated with it. Histologically, these lesions are composed of bland spindle stromal cells in a storiform pattern with admixed giant cells and xanthoma cells. Hemosiderin can be noted if the lesion is fractured. These lesions usually are treated conservatively. If a fracture is present, it can be curetted and grafted.

VASCULAR LESIONS OF BONE

Hemangiomas of Bone

Hemangiomas of bone are benign conditions that represent foci of dilated vascular venous structures within the bone. Hemangiomas are not neoplasms. Hemangiomas are commonly seen in the vertebral bodies where characteristic appearance of sclerosis is accompanied by coarse vertical striations within the bone. This characteristic appearance generally is adequate to establish the diagnosis. Hemangiomas rarely require treatment.

Tumors of Hematopoetic Tissue

Tumors of the hematopoietic tissues include lymphomas and myelomas. Surgical treatment of lymphomas are discussed in Chap. 10.

Myeloma is a malignancy that results from the transformation of cells of the plasma-cell lineage. Multiple myeloma is usually a systemic disease. Proliferating, malignant, antibody-producing plasma cells infiltrate the marrow in multiple bones. This can result in focal areas of bone resorption, often with a patchy distribution, creating an appearance of "moth-eaten" bones. Frequently, the process is diffuse and systemic, leading to diffuse nonfocal loss of bone in a condition that nearly exactly mimics osteoporosis in its radiographic presentation. Presenting symptoms are often systemic complaints such as weakness, lethargy, or weight loss. Commonly, the condition may manifest as a pathologic fracture.

Myeloma is most common in patients >50 years of age and can present in patients in their eighth and ninth decades of life. On this basis, any patient with clinical signs of diminished mineral density, particularly those who sustain a fracture, may have an underlying multiple myeloma. The diagnosis most commonly is made by laboratory studies.

Plasma cells will produce a monoclonal spike on serum protein electrophoresis in the majority of cases. The presence of a characteristic monoclonal spike may establish the diagnosis. In some patients, the secreted antibody [which may be from any antibody group—immunoglobulin (IG) G, IgA, IgM] may be apparent and rapidly cleared from the blood and can almost always be seen on a urine protein electrophoresis study. Frequently in such patients, the erythrocyte sedimentation rate is elevated as the result of the altered serum protein composition.

Solitary Myeloma (Plasmacytoma)

In some patients, the presence of a myeloma is limited to a single solitary osseous lesion: a plasmacytoma. When a patient evaluation indicates the likelihood that a solitary bone lesion is the sole focus of the myeloma, local radiation may be appropriate. Treatment for all of these myelomas generally centers around chemotherapy, often using multiple agents.

Chordoma

Chordomas are slow-growing malignancies derived from embryonic notochord cells. Chordomas nearly always arise in the axial skeleton and most commonly involve the occiput or the sacrum. They can be found in the vertebrae. Chordomas are not found in the extremities.

About one third of these tumors arise intracranially (skull base), about half are found in the sacrum, with the rest in the spine. Radiographically, cranial chordomas occur in the midline of the base of the skull and produce destruction of the spheno-occipital and hypophyseal areas. Sacrococcygeal chordomas take on an oval or circular appearance as they break out of the sacrum and grow into the pelvis. Microscopically, the hallmark is the large physaliferous cell, whose vacuolated cytoplasm gives it a soap-bubble appearance. These lesions are biphasic with the second population of polyhedral cells with an eosinophilic cytoplasm.

Chordoma patients usually present with local pain and, given their proximity to the spine, often present with radicular or myelopathic symptoms. Sacral tumors may present rectal or urinary sphincter dysfunction, and occasionally, GI obstructive symptoms. Plain radiographs will often, but certainly not always, reveal the lesion. A central area of bony destruction with a soft tissue mass is characteristic. Chordomas are frequently fatal, however, because without local control, these centrally located tumors can threaten vital functions. The mainstay of treatment is wide local resection with a wide surgical margin. On rare occasions, radiation therapy may be indicated. In general, chordomas are not responsive to chemotherapy.

Chordomas are malignant tumors that are slow growing, locally destructive and invasive, and late to metastasize.

Giant Cell Tumor of Bone

Giant cell tumor of bone is a benign neoplasm of bone that can be very aggressive and destructive locally. The cellular origin for this tumor is unknown. Giant cell tumor of bone is most frequently seen in the long bones and is rare in children. Diagnosis is generally made following patient complaints of local pain. X-ray images reveal a lytic expansile lesion of the bone that is most frequently localized in the metaphysis of a long bone. Histologic analysis shows a mixture of round, oval, and spindle-shaped cells and numerous multinucleic giant cells. Treatment of giant cell tumor of bone involves aggressive and complete local resection. An incomplete resection frequently results in recurrence and may result in significant functional impairment and even amputation.

Giant cell tumors of bone are locally aggressive and destructive lesions that arise in the metaphysic of long bones in skeletally mature individuals. Giant cell tumors of bone are commonly found around the knee but can be seen in many locations. Plain films will show an eccentrically located metaphyseal lesion that is radiolucent. Most of the lesions will show cortical breakout with an associated soft tissue mass. Morphologically, these lesions consist of rounded mononuclear cells with admixed giant cells, hemosiderin, and new bone formation. These lesions have a high tendency to recur.

Ewing's Sarcoma of Bone

Ewing's sarcoma of bone, or Ewing's tumor, is a small, round cell sarcoma most common in children and younger adults. Ewing's sarcoma is most common in the long bones, especially the metaphyseal regions of the femur, tibia, and humerus. Patients present with complaints of local pain, interestingly, often accompanied by fever.

Ewing's sarcoma is an undifferentiated tumor occurring in children and primarily involves the diaphysis of long bones. Radiographically the early Ewing's tumor may be relatively inconspicuous. The tumor appears as an ill-defined area of "moth-eaten" osteolytic destruction. It becomes more pronounced as the tumor progresses and often will show an aggressive periosteal reaction. The usual microscopic picture is that of sheets and geographic areas of small round blue cells with pale nuclei. There is no matrix production within these tumors unless there is an associated fracture. These cells are loaded with glycogen and a periodic acid–Schiff histochemical stain will be positive. These tumors have a characteristic 11:22 translocation that can be very helpful in making the correct diagnosis (Fig. 43-42).

Treatment of Ewing's sarcoma begins with a carefully planned biopsy. Definitive treatment may or may not involve surgical resection, but multiagent chemotherapy and radiation are the mainstays of treatment.

Subungual Exostosis

Subungual exostosis is a subperiosteal, osteochondral proliferation usually in the distal toes, but it can be located in the fingers. The x-ray will show a mineralized formation, usually the distal phalanx with a soft tissue swelling and occasionally ulcer formation. Additionally, there is no communication with the underlying medullary canal that

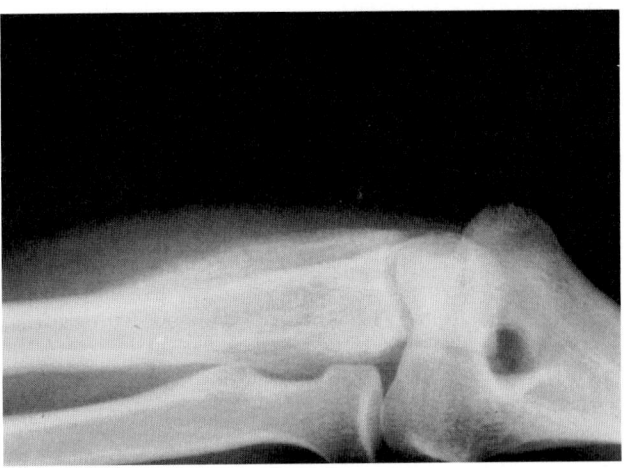

A

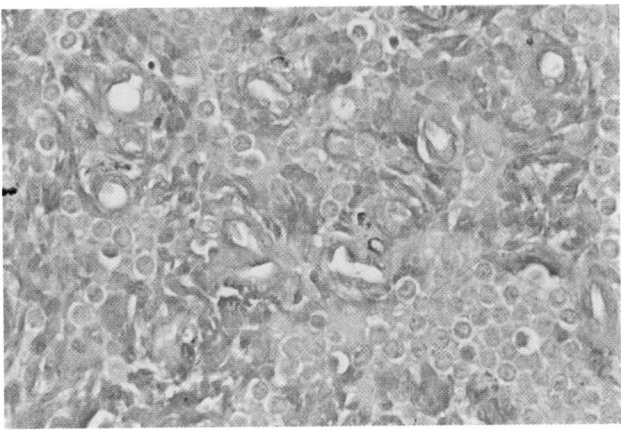

B

FIG. 43-42. A. Plain film of the elbow shows a permeative lesion of the ulna with a periosteal response in an "onion skin" pattern. **B.** A medium power photomicrograph reveals bland, small, round, blue cells and vessels characteristic of Ewing's sarcoma (hematoxylin-eosin, original magnification × 40).

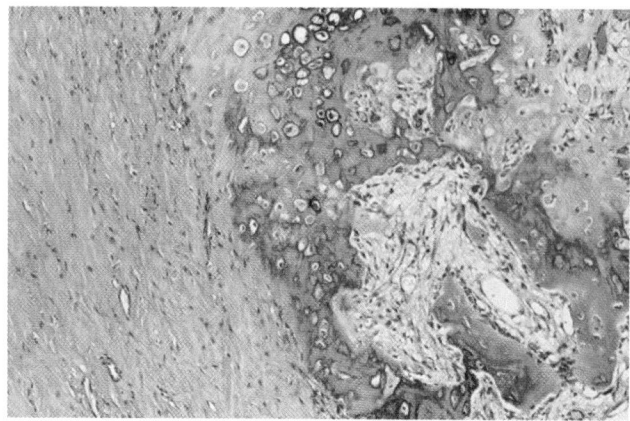

FIG. 43-43. Medium-power photomicrograph shows maturing bone intimately associated with soft tissue (hematoxylin-eosin, original magnification × 100).

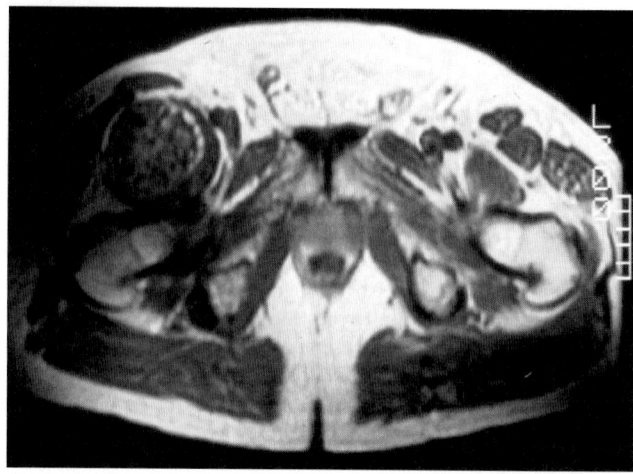

A

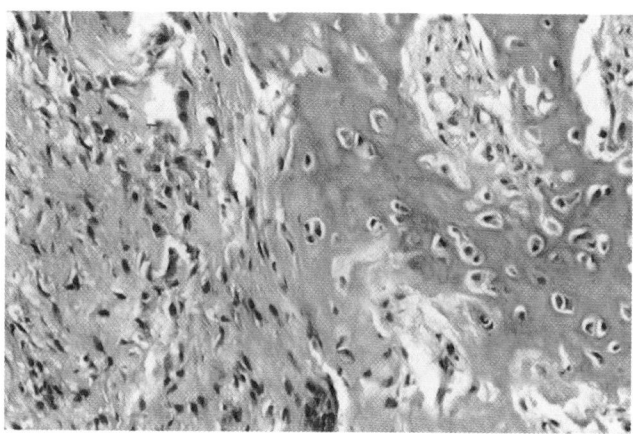

B

FIG. 43-44. A. Magnetic resonance imaging of the hips demonstrates a large, soft tissue mass anterior to the right hip with heterogeneous signal and a sharp demarcation from the surrounding tissue. **B.** A medium-power photomicrograph demonstrates cartilage and bone maturing in an endochondral mechanism with delicate vessels that merges with the surrounding soft tissue (hematoxylin-eosin, original magnification × 100).

separates this from a true osteochondroma. Histologically, these lesions are composed of chondro-osseous matrix that emerges into the surrounding soft tissue. The cellular proliferation can be quite reactive and misinterpreted as a more aggressive process. Definitive treatment is surgical resection. These lesions often can recur if the overlying fibrous cap is not entirely removed (Figs. 43-43 and 43-44).

Myositis Ossificans

Myositis ossificans is the result of posttraumatic ossification of a hematoma in the soft tissue. It most often occurs in muscle but can occur in fascia, tendon, joint capsule, and occasionally, fat. In cases of myositis ossificans, the endochondral bone formation follows essentially the same process as that of fracture callus formation. The damaged soft tissue is removed and the hematoma begins to organize with mesenchymal cells that differentiate into chondroblastic, osteoblastic, and vascular-type cells. Radiologically, these lesions are noted in the soft tissue and show an arrangement of bone and cartilage at the periphery of the lesion and interior soft tissue. This results in an "egg shell" calcification/ossification. Histologically, the features are bone and cartilage at the periphery of the lesion and a fibrovascular core. Over time, the outer endochondral ring will remodel to lamellar bone with an interior fibro-fatty center.

Paget's Disease

Paget's disease is a relatively common condition of bone, most frequently seen in patients >40 years of age. Paget's disease may be mono-ostotic, or it may be seen in multiple bones. It is most commonly seen in the pelvis and spine but may also frequently occur in the humerus, femur, and tibia. The lesion results from abnormalities in the bone in the remodeling process, felt to be due to abnormalities in the osteoclasts. X-ray images of pagetic bone show characteristic sclerosis with coarsened trabeculae, cortical thickening, and often, cortical expansion of the bone. The appearance of the bone may also contain lytic as well as sclerotic areas.

Microscopic appearance of pagetic bone shows broad irregular trabeculae, often with visible lines (indicating incomplete mineralization). On occasion, the striking appearance of "mosaic bone" is seen, which refers to large areas of incompletely mineralized bone that creates an appearance reminiscent of mosaic tile. The critical histologic feature of Paget's disease is not the partial mineralized bone, however; it is the presence of large osteoclasts with abnormally large numbers of nuclei. Normal osteoclasts will have from two to four nuclei, in pagetic bone it is common to see osteoclasts with from five to 50 or more nuclei.

It is speculated that the large abnormal osteoclasts result from late effects of a pre-existing paramyxovirus infection. It is believed that increased bony resorption by these abnormal osteoclasts causes

local lysis of bone. The rapid healing process that follows leads to the disorganized and coarse bony texture.

Bones involved with advanced Paget's disease can be subject to pathologic fracture. Bony abnormalities surround joints and often lead to accelerated arthritic change. Paget's disease is common in the spine, particularly in the lumbar spine. The characteristic bony expansion and arthritic change in the spine frequently results in the clinical syndrome of spinal stenosis.

Treatment of Paget's disease generally is nonsurgical with the use of antiresorptive medicine such as bisphosphonates and/or calcitonin. Such medical treatment is usually sufficient for most patients with Paget's disease. Neglected Paget's or resistant cases will occasionally go to surgery for lumbar decompressive laminectomy (for spinal stenosis) or for joint replacement. Surgical treatment for patients with Paget's disease must be preceded by antiresorptive therapy as arteriovenous shunting in pagetic bone is frequently encountered. Bone bleeding can be a major problem in Paget's patients who are not medically treated.

Stress Fracture

Stress fractures are a result of an active remodeling as a result of stress that most often is noticed in an episode of sudden increase in physical activity. This is very common in military recruits during basic training, but this can be seen in anyone with a sudden increase in athletic activity. Localized pain and tenderness is typical, and the skin can be locally red. X-ray examination may be unrevealing early on; however, subsequent films may show a periosteal reaction to increase suspicion for this condition. The most common location for stress fractures is the proximal tibia, but they can occur anywhere. As the fracture develops, films will show a lucent line perpendicular to the long axis of the involved bone. Histologically, this process is composed of aggregates of the osteoclasts removing bone with paucity of osteoblastic response and a variable amount of periosteal response.

JOINT RECONSTRUCTION

The Surgical Treatment of Arthritis

One of the most challenging problems facing the orthopedic surgeon is the treatment of degenerative and inflammatory diseases of joints. In all cases, the primary objectives are to relieve pain and to preserve motion and function. In the treatment of any joint complaint, a thorough evaluation of the patient's symptoms, history, and a thorough physical examination are essential. The orthopedic surgeon must distinguish between inflammatory disease and degenerative disease. The laboratory and imaging studies are also tremendously useful. It is always hoped that a nonsurgical means can be used to help the patient. Medications, physical therapy, rest, braces, and time are often all that is needed to assist the patient with an arthritic joint. On frequent occasion, however, more invasive treatments are necessary.

Injection of Joints

For several decades, the treatment options for painful joints have included the injection of various substances. Local anesthetic agents can be injected into a joint for diagnostic purposes. Corticosteroids are frequently injected into joints for symptomatic relief (this can be done for both inflammatory disease and osteoarthritis). The use of intra-articular corticosteroid injections is controversial. This often provides short-term relief of pain and swelling symptoms; however, the long-term consequences of this technique are debated.

More recently, injections of high-molecular-weight, polysaccharide molecules such as hyaluronic acid have become popular in the treatment of degenerative disease of large joints. The utility of this technique is not yet quite clear in the evidence-based literature, but it does appear that at least some patients get substantial and somewhat lasting relief from these techniques.

Synovectomy

Synovectomy is the surgical removal of substantial portions of the synovial lining of a joint. This is another procedure that can, on occasion, help a patient. The technique frequently has been applied to joints damaged by hemophilia. In severely symptomatic disease, intra-articular synovectomy also can be of benefit to patients with inflammatory disease such as rheumatoid arthritis.

Periarticular Osteotomy

Arthritic joints often develop angular deformities. This can be from selective loss of cartilage from areas of high wear. It also can be from malalignments, either congenital or acquired after injury. It is quite common, for example, for osteoarthritis of the knee to be severe in the medial tibial-femoral portion of the joint and relatively mild in the lateral compartment. An osteotomy of the proximal tibia to selectively transfer weight to the healthier cartilage can often provide a prolonged period of relief to such patients. In a similar way, young adults with malaligned hips can often benefit from osteotomies of the proximal femur to create better femoral acetabular articulation.

Fusion

Many arthritic joints can be surgically treated by bony arthrodesis fusion instead of joint replacement. This is most frequently per-

formed in joints where motion is not critical. Fusion of certain joints of the foot (including painful degenerative arthritis of the first metacarpal and numerous bones of the midfoot) can be satisfactorily managed by applying bone grafts across the involved joint, transfixing the joint with internal fixation, screws, or periarticular plates.

The arthritic wrist frequently is managed by fusion procedures, as the mobility of the shoulder, elbow, and fingers will usually allow preservation of excellent useful function.

Arthrodesis of the shoulders is less frequently performed than arthroplasty of the shoulder, but it is an established and reasonably successful procedure. Nonetheless, fusion of the glenohumeral joints often allows satisfactory function, particularly in heavy laborers because of the compensatory motion of the trunk, scapulothoracic joints, elbow, and wrist.

Joint Arthroplasty—(Joint Replacement)

Patients with severe intractable joint pain can be treated with prosthetic replacement of the diseased joint with an artificial joint composed of metal and plastic. This technique was successfully introduced by Sir John Charnley in the 1960s who successfully developed and first performed total joint replacement procedures on the hip. The genius of Dr. Charnley has been amply demonstrated as this procedure continues to remain one of the most successful operative interventions.[57]

A joint prosthesis, in nearly all cases, involves a mobile surface, most commonly composed of high-molecular-weight polyethylene (the original material chosen by Dr. Charnley), which is affixed to metal components that are anchored to the involved native bone. The metal components of a joint prosthesis can be affixed to native bone by precise carpentry and impaction (impaction fit). Such metal implants often are surfaced with porous metals that allow bony ingrowth (porous coated implants). In Dr. Charnley's original procedure, a polymer of methylmethacrylate was used to cement the metal components in place. Polymethylmethacrylate cement material continues in common use today, although the majority of hip and knee replacements are now performed with noncemented technique.

Total Hip Arthroplasty

Images of a total hip replacement procedure are displayed in Figs. 43-6, 43-13, 43-33, and 43-45 through 43-50. The patient has a

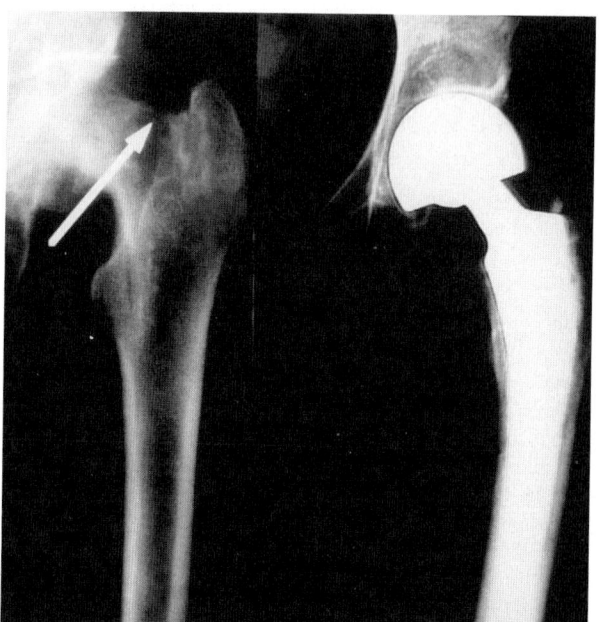

FIG. 43-45. Pathologic fracture of the femoral neck (*arrow*), treated by femoral head excision and endoprosthetic hip replacement. In cases with acetabular involvement, the acetabulum must also be replaced.

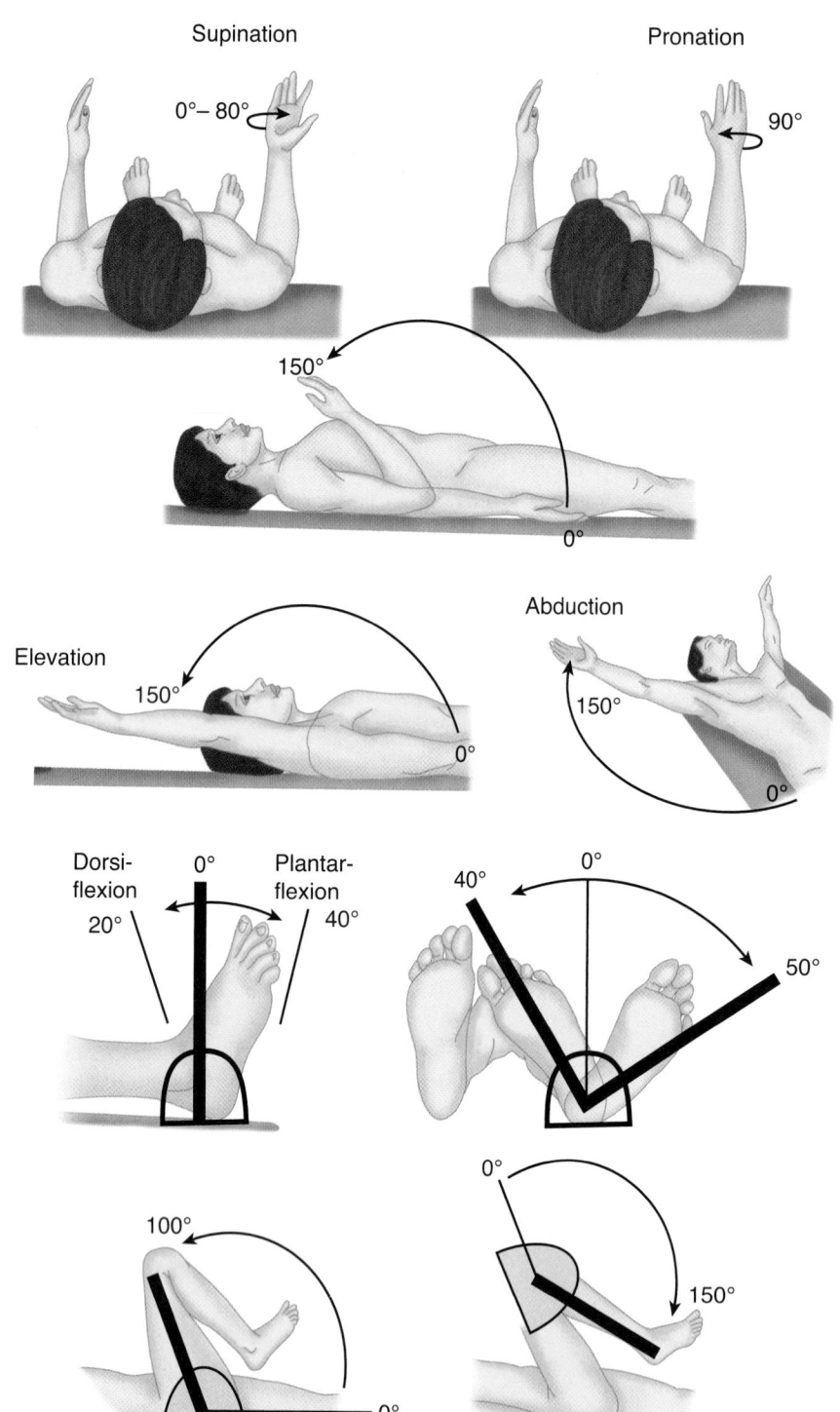

FIG. 43-46. Range of motion is measured in degrees. Each joint has a normal range and, when examining a patient with a joint or extremity disorder, the involved joint's range of motion should be measured and recorded.

severely arthritic joint surface with sclerosis and cystic changes in both the femoral and acetabular articular surfaces. The patient was experiencing severe pain with essentially all activities of daily living and had lost the ability to move about normally. After the failure of conservative care to improve function, the patient can be taken to surgery for replacement of the hip.

The hip joints can be exposed through a variety of surgical approaches. The most commonly performed is the posterior approach to the hip. The incision is made through the skin and fascia of the lateral proximal thigh, and dissection is continued deeper to expose the posterolateral portion of the proximal femur, the greater trochanter, and associated muscles. The short rotators are dissected away from the proximal trochanter, and the femoral neck is exposed

by entering the hip capsule. Removal of the femoral head is accomplished by transecting the femoral neck with a power saw and dislocating the femoral head. The proximal femur is prepared by successive removal of bone from the medullary cavity. Specially shaped reamers and rasps are inserted to create an appropriate space for the stem of the femoral prosthesis. Similarly, any remaining articular cartilage is removed from the acetabulum using sequentially sized reamers to the level of good cancellous bone. The acetabular portion of the prosthesis, which contains the high–molecular-weight polyethylene articular surface, is attached to a metal cup. The prosthesis (usually metal or ceramic) is then impacted into place. The joint is then relocated, and the wound is closed.

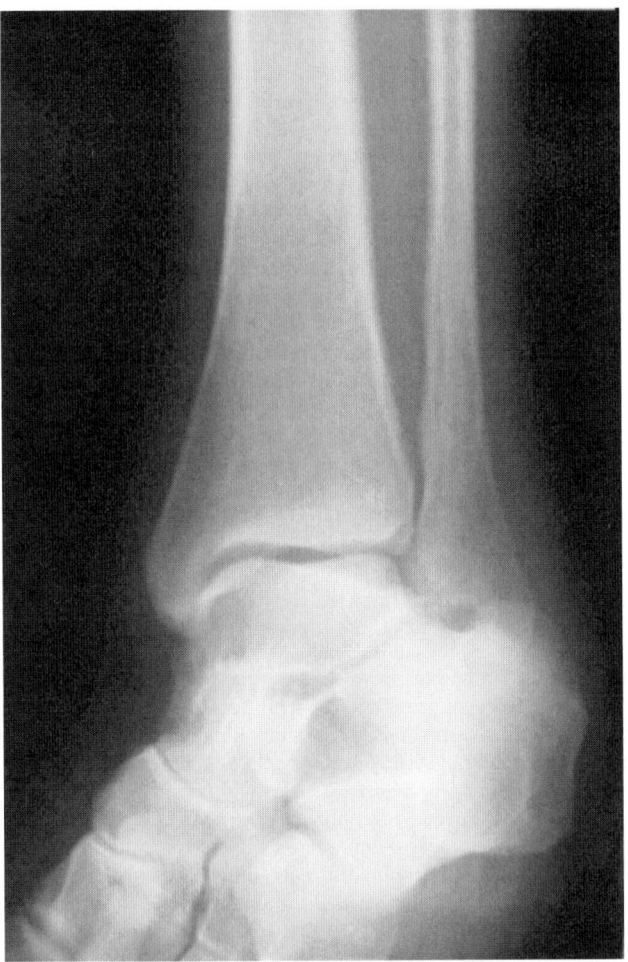

FIG. 43-47. A mortise view of a normal ankle. This view allows visualization of the relationship between the distal tibia and fibula.

Great care is taken during the performance of this surgery to attain a functional anatomic position for both the femoral and acetabular components. Malposition of either component can lead to rotational deformity, premature wear, or dislocation. As is readily apparent, during the surgical exposure, many of the intrinsic stabilizers of the hip joint are divided during the dissection needed to perform the surgery. Accordingly, following a total hip replacement procedure, restrictions are placed on the patient's range of motion until an adequate amount of scar is formed to help preserve long-term stability of the joint.

Total Knee Arthroplasty

Total knee replacement involves resecting the native articular surface and subchondral bone from the femur, tibia, and the patella. Analogous to hip replacements, the distal femur generally is reconstructed with a large metal weightbearing surface shaped to mimic the femoral condyles. The tibial plateau is replaced by a high-molecular-weight polyethylene surface usually attached to a flat metal surface, which is then affixed to the distal tibia by a stem, or screws, or both. The patella surface generally is reconstructed with a high-molecular-weight polyethylene articular surface.

As with the hip, these components may be affixed to the bone using polymethylmethacrylate cement, although press fit components using various surface treatments to promote adhesion and bone ingrowth also are commonly used.

A total knee replacement generally is accomplished through an anterior peripatellar approach, with the knee widely exposed; the articular surfaces are resected using precise saw cuts, guided by

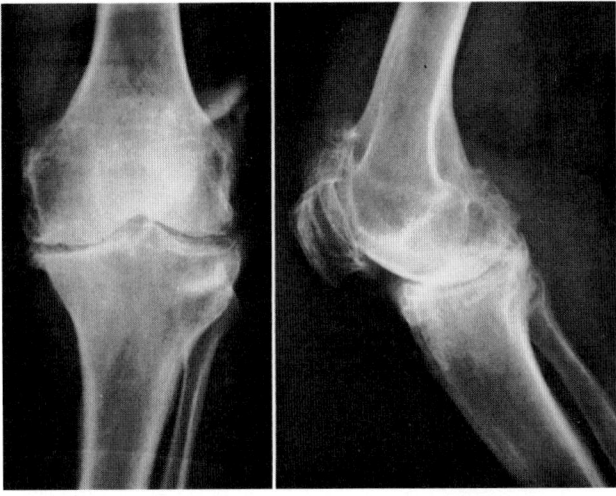

FIG. 43-48. Primary osteoarthritis of the knee. Anteroposterior and lateral radiographs showing varus deformity of the knee with joint space narrowing and osteophyte production on medial, lateral, and posterior aspects of the tibia, on anterior aspects of the femoral condyles, and on upper and lower poles of the patella. There is minimal cyst formation and sclerosis of subchondral bone of the medial joint space.

templates and jigs. Appropriate alignment of the components is essential for a successful result. Also critical is ligamentous balancing of the knee, such that medial and lateral stabilizing ligaments and the patellar tendon can function normally. Knee replacements can be performed with implants designed to make use of the normal cruciate ligaments. Other total knee designs accommodate these stabilizing functions as well and involve resection of these ligaments.

Complications of Total Joint Arthroplasty

Artificial joints are used to replace worn out and damaged natural joints. Sadly, the artificial joints themselves are also subject to wear and damage and can fail by a variety of mechanisms. Total joint replacement components can loosen, fracture, or disassemble.

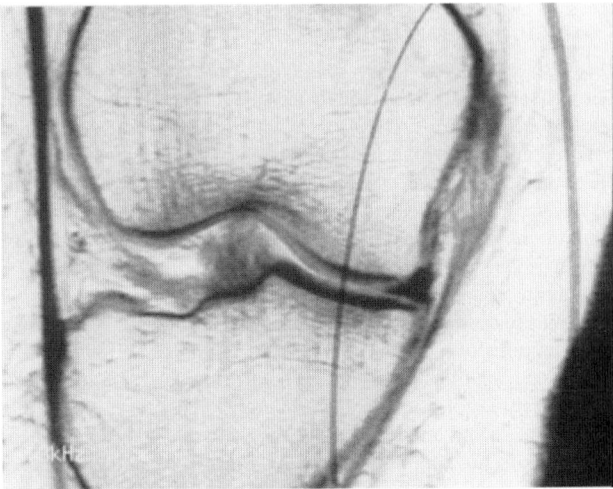

FIG. 43-49. Coronal magnetic resonance imaging of a knee. The meniscus is easily seen as a dark (no signal) triangular structure between the femoral condyle and tibia. The medial collateral ligament is disrupted. Magnetic resonance imaging is a valuable tool to evaluate injuries to the soft tissues of the extremities.

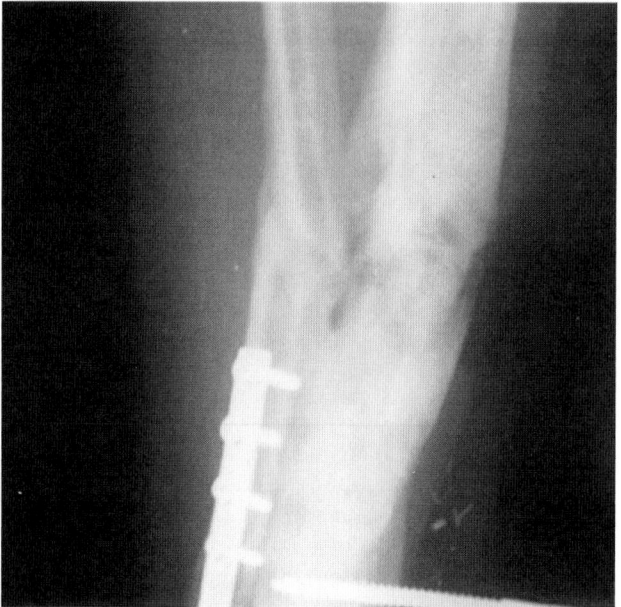

FIG. 43-50. Anteroposterior radiograph of a patient with chronic osteomyelitis. The patient had a compound (open) fracture of his tibia treated with an open reduction and internal fixation. He has developed a chronic infection. The plate that was on his tibia has been removed. The bone is denser than normal, and the medullary canal cannot be seen well. This suggests that there is sequestered (necrotic) bone that needs to be débrided if the infection is to be controlled.

Artificial joints can be damaged by virtue of corrosion or simply "wear out." Other complications include infection (acute, delayed, or chronic), contracture, and periprosthetic fracture.

As arthritis and osteoporosis are both disease processes most common in older patients, they often occur together. Insertion of a prosthetic joint in a patient with osteoporosis requires special care to prevent intraoperative fractures. The purpose of an artificial joint creates a stress riser at the interface between prosthesis and bone. Unfortunately, fractures adjacent to total joint implants are not uncommon. Treatment for this problem is individualized and may involve internal fixation, replacement of the prosthesis, or both.

Corrosion, Wear, and Osteolysis

Osteolysis is a major concern to the total knee replacement surgeon. The term *osteolysis* can be used to describe virtually any form of bony resorption, including that associated with metastatic disease or infection. In joint replacement, it generally refers to one of two unwanted phenomena. Osteolysis is a term that is used to describe focal bony resorption at the immediate interface between the prosthesis and the bone or the cement mantle and the bone. The motion of a loose implant on the bone prosthesis interface is such that bony resorption can occur, and unfortunately, without surgical revision, there is frequent progression of bone resorption to the point where mechanical symptoms of hip pain or knee pain result. The presence of an increasing zone of osteolysis in the periprosthetic region becomes a strong relative indication for revision of the implant.

A more serious and problematic form of osteolysis is that caused by a noninfectious inflammatory reaction to wear debris. Wear of the high-molecular-weight polyethylene articular surface can generate and disperse microscopic particles of high-molecular-weight polyethylene, which often cause a focal tissue inflammatory reaction. Reticuloendothelial cell proliferation and the action of other inflammatory cells may result at times in very aggressive rates of bony resorption. The process often is painful. When extensive osteolysis of

this type is allowed to proceed for substantial lengths of time, serious and problematic loss of periarticular bone can result, adding additional difficulty to revision surgery. Particulate methylmethacrylate cement debris also can play a role in this form of osteolysis.

Due to this problem of osteolysis, joint prosthesis designers have focused a great deal of attention on precisely engineering the articular surfaces and exploring options for other bearing surfaces materials. Metal on metal bearing surfaces and the use of other plastics or ceramics are areas of intense ongoing study.

All total joint replacement prostheses have the potential to wear out or loosen. Accordingly, they are rarely indicated for young active patients, who will place a high mechanical demand on the prosthetic joint, although joint replacement may be very appropriate for "low demand" patients with systemic inflammatory disease.

Revision or replacement of a loose infected or "worn out" joint prosthesis is an involved and technically challenging procedure. Such surgeries often involve extensive and difficult cement removal, and may involve the need for extensive bone grafting. For some difficult clinical challenges, custom-made revision prosthesis is used.

PEDIATRIC ORTHOPEDIC SURGERY

The treatment of musculoskeletal pathology in pediatric patients is different in many ways from the treatment of adult patients. The orthopedic surgeon treating pediatric patients must be aware of numerous congenital and developmental conditions. Further, the skeletal system is growing. Preservation of normal growth is a significant priority in the management of this patient group.

The pediatric orthopedic surgeon must be able to recognize and treat a large number of inherited congenital conditions, which include inherited metabolic disorders, inherited neurologic conditions, and inherited musculoskeletal anatomic abnormalities. The diagnosis and treatment of these inherited syndromes and disorders are beyond the scope of this chapter.

Birth Injuries Causing Neurologic Impairment
Brachial Plexus Palsy

Injury of the brachial plexus during delivery was once a commonly encountered management problem. Patient with associated plexus injuries can present with mild, moderate, or severe impairment of the involved upper extremity, which can, on occasion, involve upper or lower roots and trunks of the plexus. Modern obstetrical practice has markedly decreased the incidence of this problem, which unfortunately still occurs in approximately 0.2% of all births. Such injuries are associated with large birth weight, forceps delivery, breech presentation, and prolonged labor. A plexus injury may represent a stretch injury or, on some occasions, a frank avulsion of nerve roots. In most patients, nonsurgical management is pursued with aggressive therapy and passive exercise to preserve motor motion in the shoulder while awaiting return of neurologic function. In unusual cases, surgical repair of injured roots and trunks of the plexus is performed.

Cerebral Palsy

Cerebral palsy is a nonprogressive neuromuscular disorder, which usually is recognized before age 2 years old. It is considered to take origin from an injury to the developing brain. Usually, the specific cause is not identifiable. There is a wide variation in the consequences for cerebral palsy that may or may not be associated with mental impairment. Cerebral palsy is classified in physiologic and anatomic categories as spastic (the most common), athetotic, ataxic, and mixed. The majority of cerebral palsy patients are hyperreflexic with increased muscle tone and spasm. Such patients also are classified as having hemiplegia (upper and lower extremities) or diplegia where low extremity problems are greater than those in the upper extremity. Patients with cerebral palsy frequently develop spinal deformities, which is discussed separately in the Scoliosis section. Orthopedic treatments center on maintaining function and preserving range of motion. Tendon lengthening procedures, release of contractures, and tendon transfers can be helpful both in upper and lower extremities. Gait disorders are the focus of a great deal of attention, and often, major improvements in walking ability can be accomplished by well-planned tendon lengthening procedures and contracture releases.

Because of unbalanced muscle forces due to associated spasticity, hip dysfunction, unfortunately, which frequently leads to hip dislocation or subluxation, is a significant problem for many cerebral palsy patients. Initial treatment often consists of abductor tendon releases that can be very rewarding. In some cases where a diagnosis is made late, or where soft tissue releases are unsuccessful, tendon balancing procedures may be combined with open reduction of a hip joint, sometimes augmented by acetabular reconstruction or osteotomy of the proximal femur.

Knee contracture due to hamstring tightness is another commonly seen problem. Hamstring lengthening and other muscular tendon releases can be helpful.

Foot and ankle deformities can also result from a cerebral palsy and usually are treated, even in nonambulatory patients, to facilitate shoe wear. Maintaining normal foot anatomy is essential in an ambulatory patient. The most common foot deformity caused by cerebral palsy is an equinovalgus foot, which is caused by heel cord contracture and peroneal spasm. Tendon balancing can be helpful. In severe cases, bony reconstruction also can be indicated.

Skeletal Growth

Acquired musculoskeletal disorders in the pediatric patient cover a wide spectrum of disease, which includes injury, inflammatory disease, and developmental disorders. In all of these conditions, the treating surgeon must remember that immature bones are actively growing; preserving bone growth is a high priority of treatment (Fig. 43-51). In addition, the immature skeleton is incompletely ossified. Accurate diagnosis of an injury or musculoskeletal condition can be much more difficult because large portions of the skeleton are still cartilaginous and may be invisible radiographically with plain film. As can be seen, the epiphysis, generally containing an articular surface, is positioned at the ends of the long bone with an intervening physis or growth plate. The normal epiphysis is the site of longitudinal growth of a long bone. It is wide enough to be readily visible on clinical x-rays. The physis has specific layers or zones defined histologically adjacent to the epiphyseal bone known as the *reserve zone* of pluripotential cells. Proceeding from the reserve zone is the *zone of differentiation*, where differentiation of cartilage is first demonstrated. Below the zone of differentiation is the *zone of proliferation*, characterized by extensive cell division. Beneath the zone of proliferation is the *zone of maturation*, where more mature chondrocyte morphology is manifest. Beneath the zone of maturation is the *hypertrophic zone* where cells increase in size. Cell death and calcification of the cartilage matrix then occurs in the *zone of calcification*.

Preservation of normal growth in this area is important. Injury or insult to the growth plate can lead to premature growth arrest or angular deformity of the limb and a significant cosmetic and functional problem. Surrounding the metaphyseal and diaphyseal bone is the periosteal layer. The periosteum in immature individuals is far more thick and cellular than in adults. This metabolically active periosteum is responsible for the synthesis of new bone onto the diaphyseal and metaphyseal bone and is responsible for the circumferential growth of the bones. In very young patients, the metaphysis and epiphysis may be completely unossified.

Ossification centers in the epiphysis and will appear in a very predictable order. An understanding of the expected sequence of ossification and its expected chronology are critical for the appropriate treatment of young patients. It must also be noted that some bones, particularly those of the spine, normally manifest multiple distinct ossification centers.

General Considerations in Pediatric Fractures

The treatment of a fractured bone in a pediatric patient involves all of the issues present in adult injuries. In a child, however, treating physicians and surgeons are also much concerned with the status of the growth plate. Unfortunately, the epiphyseal growth plate is a very common site of fracture, as this unossified area of the bone is naturally weak and prone to fracture. Careful treatment of the injured growth plate is a high priority of treatment, and it must be kept in mind that reduction of fracture fragments through and across the growth plate must be done with great care.

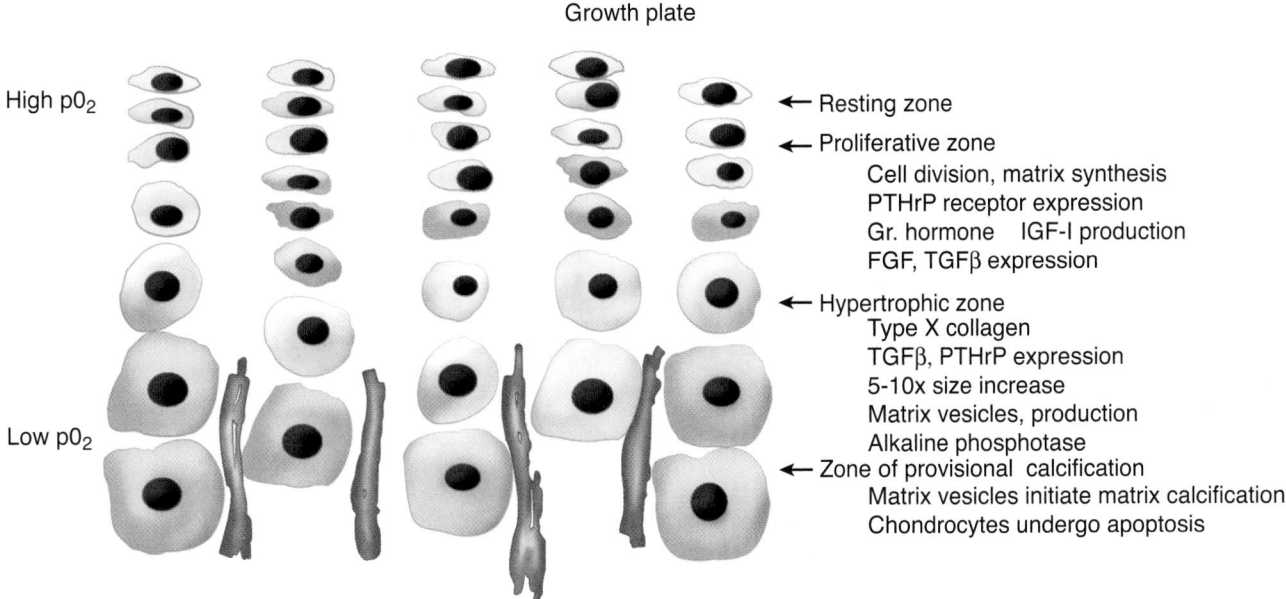

Growth plate

High pO₂ — Resting zone

← Proliferative zone
  Cell division, matrix synthesis
  PTHrP receptor expression
  Gr. hormone   IGF-I production
  FGF, TGFβ expression

← Hypertrophic zone
  Type X collagen
  TGFβ, PTHrP expression
  5-10x size increase
  Matrix vesicles, production
  Alkaline phosphotase

Low pO₂ — Zone of provisional calcification
  Matrix vesicles initiate matrix calcification
  Chondrocytes undergo apoptosis

FIG. 43-51. Structure and function relationships of the growth plate. Calcified cartilage bars form scaffold for osteoblasts to deposit new bone; osteoclast-like cells reabsorb calcified cartilage through remodeling. FGF = fibroblast growth factor; Gr. = growth; IGF-I = insulin-like growth factor I; PTHrP = parathyroid hormone-related peptide; TGF*β* = transforming growth factor beta.

Classification of Growth Plate Injuries

Classification of growth plate injuries has important implications as doctors communicate about the treatment of a patient. The exact type of physeal injury is important for the prognosis and treatment of the fracture. Salter and Harris described a very useful classification of growth plate injuries.[58] A type I injury is a simple transverse failure of the physis without involvement of the ossified epiphysis or metaphysis. A Salter-Harris type II fracture contains a component of fracture through the growth plate in continuity with a fracture of the metaphysis. Salter-Harris type III fracture occurs partially through the epiphysis and partially through the growth plate. These fractures are essentially always intra-articular. A Salter-Harris type IV injury is one which has a fracture line extending through the physis extending from the metaphysis through into the epiphysis. Finally, a Salter-Harris type V injury is a subtle injury where the physis itself is injured but not displaced.

Treatment of pediatric injuries that involve the growth plate are centered around precise and accurate reduction of the fragments and growth plate. Internal fixation of growth plate injuries is performed with great care to assist in the accurate positioning of the fragments for optimal healing. When possible, effort is made to avoid placing hardware that extends through the growth plate for fear of increasing the chance of premature growth plate closure.

Diaphyseal Injuries in a Pediatric Patient

Fractures of the diaphysis of the long bones of pediatric patients are often treated closed. Interestingly, precise and accurate reduction of such fractures is, at times, less critical in pediatric patients than it is in adult patients because of the extensive remodeling that pediatric patients are capable of. An angular deformity within the plane of an adjacent joint is often completely remodeled by the accommodating growth of the child. When internal fixation of a diaphyseal fracture is performed on a child, the physis is avoided whenever possible.

Fractures of the Pediatric Hip

Pediatric hip fractures carry a high potential for growth arrest and deformity. Very young patients with hip fractures are frequently treated by casting. A large cast encompassing the abdomen, lower back, pelvis, and lower limb is often a good choice. Such "spica" casts are well tolerated by very young patients, to some degree, because the period of immobilization can be relatively short in a very young patient because of their rapid healing potential. Displaced fractures of the hip in somewhat older patients are frequently managed operatively. If the displacement is mild, it may be managed with a spica cast. In some cases, a screw is inserted through a very small skin incision through the trochanteric region of the femur and traverse to fracture physis and engage the femoral head. It is necessary to do this with direct fluoroscopic image guidance. Careful attention to the screw position in these two planes is essential to make sure there is no penetration of the femoral head.

Fractures of the Intratrochanteric Region in the Pediatric Hip

In very young patients, this injury may be managed with a spica cast. In older patients, internal fixation may also be used.

Fractures of the Femoral Shaft

In children, femur fractures are usually low-energy injuries in contrast to adult femur fractures. Fractures of the femoral shaft in pediatric patients <6 years old may be managed with a spica cast. Minor degrees of angular deformity are acceptable and will remodel. More major degrees of angular deformities (up to 30° in the sagittal plane) may be acceptable because of the growth potential in these very young patients. Fractures in patients >6 years of age can be managed by limited internal fixation (Fig. 43-52). Flexible intramedullary nails are popular in the treatment of this injury.[59] A patient who is approaching skeletal maturity (14 years or older)

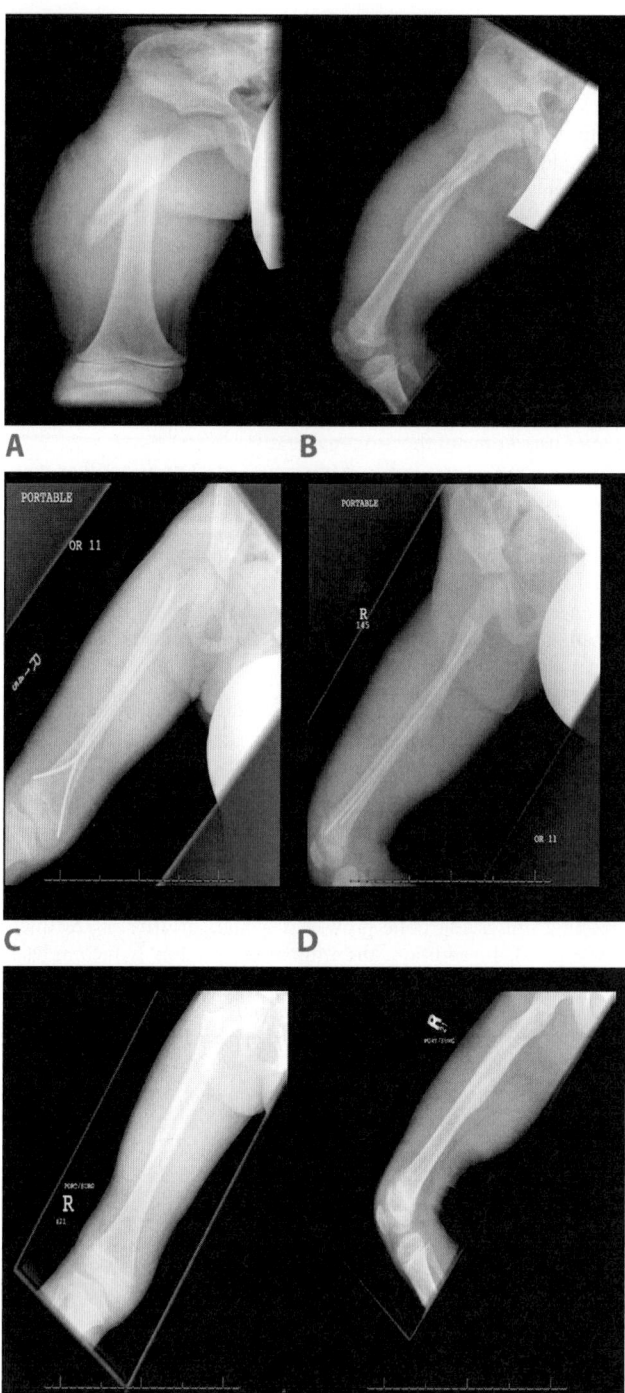

FIG. 43-52. A spiral fracture of the shaft of the femur in a child. **A** and **B** document the displaced fracture. **C** and **D** demonstrate the x-ray appearance after closed reduction and the insertion of flexible rods. **E** and **F** demonstrate the healed bone, after hardware removal, with preservation of the growth plate.

may be managed by a rigid intramedullary reamed nail, much as would be used in an adult. Extra-articular fractures of the distal femur or of the proximal tibia are generally managed in a long leg cast, unless there is excessive displacement or angulation.

Fractures of the Pediatric Ankle

Fractures of the ankle in pediatric patients virtually always involve the growth plate. Salter-Harris I and II injuries (without physeal fractures) are generally managed by simple casting (Fig. 43-53). Intra-articular

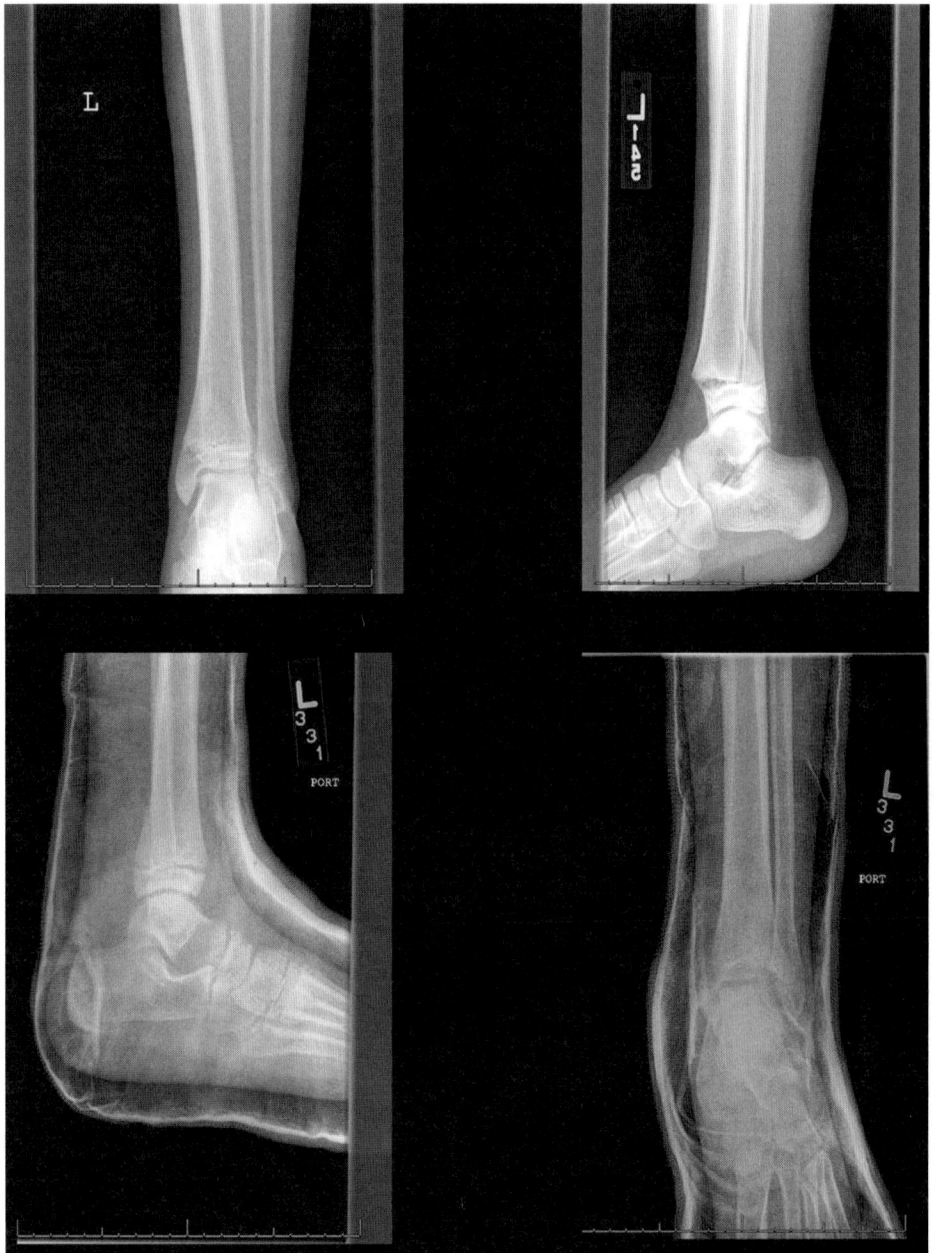

FIG. 43-53. Anteroposterior and lateral x-ray images of a Salter-Harris type II fracture of the distal tibia in a child. The displaced fracture involving the physis was reduced and immobilized in a cast.

fractures (Salter-Harris III or IV) are usually managed by closed reduction and internal fixation using percutaneous pins or screw fixation. In general, smooth nonthreaded pins are used, and care is taken not to traverse the physis unless absolutely necessary for stability.

Usually, the medial portion of the distal tibial physis fuses before the lateral. In such patients, an interesting fracture called a *juvenile Tillaux* fracture can occur. This Salter-Harris type II fracture involves a fracture through the lateral epiphysis and lateral physis. For these patients with the growth plate in the process of closing, open reduction and precise internal fixation generally is recommended. Another challenging physeal injury in pediatric patients is the so-called *triplane fracture*. This is a complex Salter-Harris type IV fracture involving fractures to the physis, metaphysis, and epiphysis. Usually the three fractures occur in three orthogonal planes. This injury is usually managed by closed reduction with or without percutaneous pinning. This fracture often requires CT imaging to assess degree of joint line displacement.

Fractures of the Pediatric Elbow

Fractures of the pediatric elbow create a special anxiety in the treating orthopedic surgeon. The elbow is a complex joint with

articulation between the distal humerus and both the radius and ulna. In addition, there are separate ossification centers for the radial head: the olecranon as well as the medial and lateral epiphysis of the humerus. In very young patients, a fracture through the distal humeral epiphysis is often mistaken for a dislocation of the elbow (an injury that is extremely rare) (Fig. 43-54). A complete understanding of the ossification centers of the elbow as well as the timing of their appearance is essential to the confident diagnosis of the exact injury. Such fractures that also involve injury to the shafts of the radius or ulna are the pediatric equivalent of the Monteggia and Galeazzi fractures described previously in Fractures of the Ulnar Radius. Reduction and accurate alignment of the articular surfaces and accurate positioning of the radial head (often dislocated in these injuries) are high priorities in treatment. In general, closed reduction and percutaneous pin placement (often by necessity traversing the growth plate) is usually the most appropriate treatment option.[60]

In assessment and treatment to these injuries, great attention must be placed to the neurovascular anatomy about the elbow. Associated injury to the brachial artery, to the traversing radial ulna and medial nerves are common. Assessment of the neurovascular function is essential before, during, and after treatment. Even after

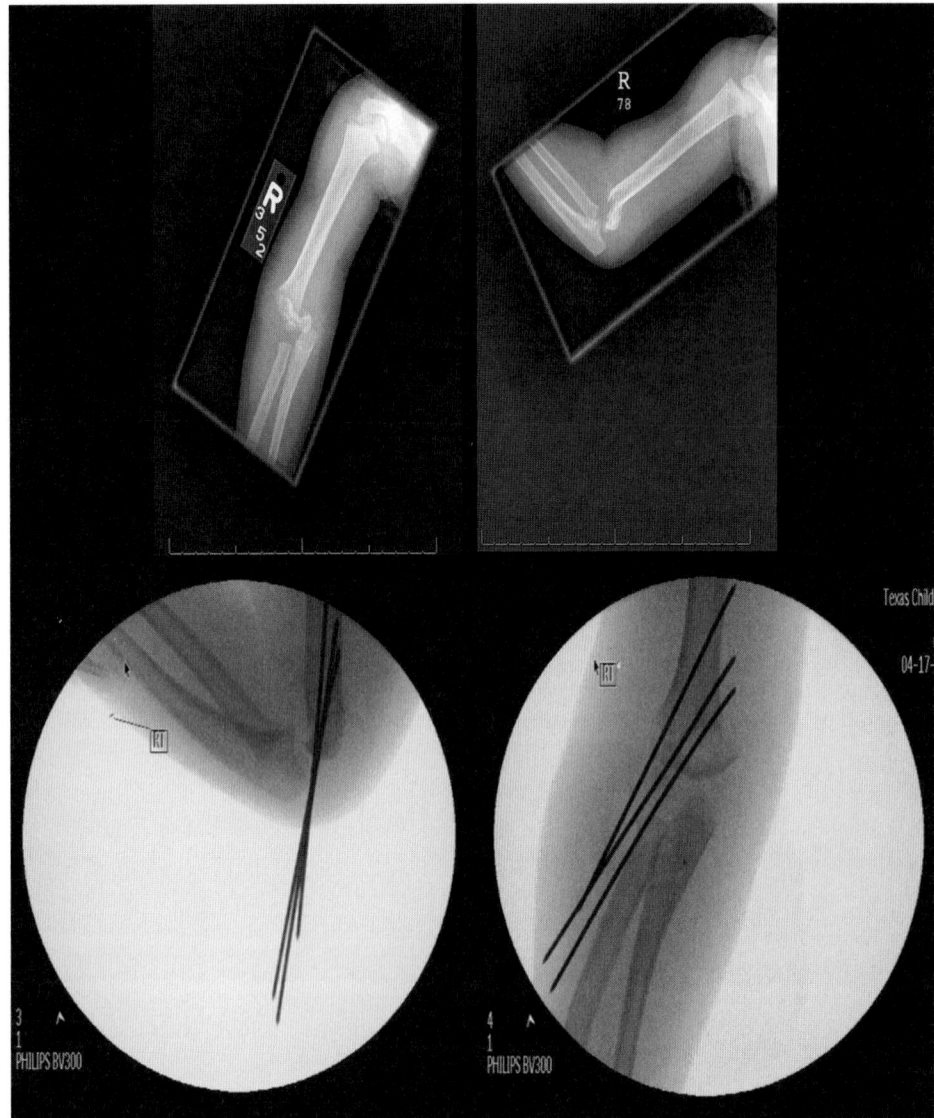

FIG. 43-54. A displaced supracondylar fracture in a child is shown before and after reduction and percutaneous pin fixation.

successful closed reduction, pinning, and immobilization, close meticulous follow-up for maintenance of reduction and of neurovascular status of the limb is important.

DEVELOPMENTAL DISEASE IN CHILDREN

Developmental Dysplasia of the Hip

Developmental dysplasia of the hip (DDH) was previously called *congenital dysplasia of the hip*. The disorder is characterized by instability of the developing hip and may progress to frank, chronic dislocation of the hip. DDH is seen most frequently in newborns with a positive family history, who have breech positioning in utero, who are female, or who are firstborn.[61–63] The disorder does not appear to have a strong genetic component.

The most unfortunate situation in patients with DDH is in those who are diagnosed late. A chronically dislocated hip is a challenging problem for clinical management. Such untreated dislocations lead eventually to contracted hip musculature, a dysplastic acetabulum, and the formation of a fibrous "pulvinar," which can occupy the acetabulum and prevent reduction. As these are potential serious consequences, effort is put into early diagnosis of DDH. Newborns, generally within the first 3 days of life, are examined for hip instability. Two maneuvers are performed, one of which is Ortolani's test, which consists of gentle elevation and abduction of the femur.

With the abduction maneuver, a palpable click or pop will signify the relocation of a dislocated hip. Another maneuver, Barlow's test, is performed by gentle adduction and depression of the femur (posterior pressure), which can cause a similar palpable click or pop as a hip in its normal position slips into a dislocated position. It is important that these maneuvers be performed gently and only after proper training. Infants with a dislocated or dislocatable hip will sometimes seem to have leg discrepancies of the femur when the hip is positioned in 90°. It also is possible to make a tentative diagnosis based on the appearance of the skinfolds of the buttock. X-ray images can be helpful, but in the case of newborn children, the relevant portions of the acetabulum and femoral head are not yet ossified and x-ray diagnosis is a bit unreliable. More helpful is the use of ultrasound to image the hips. A skilled ultrasonographer can often demonstrate an impressive amount of detail in a dislocated or dislocatable hip. When the diagnosis is made promptly, treatment can, in most cases, result in an essentially normal hip joint. If the diagnosis is made later, prognosis may not be as favorable. Treatment of undiagnosed patients after they attain walking age (9 to 14 months) can be very challenging.

Treatment of Developmental Dysplasia of the Hip

Treatment of a newborn who has a dislocated or dislocatable hip generally is based on achieving proper positioning of the femoral head in the acetabulum and maintaining a concentric reduction. In

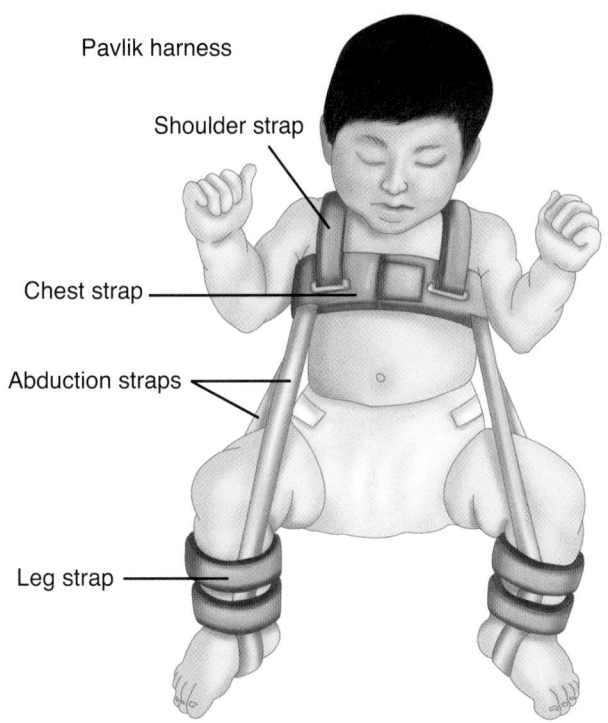

Pavlik harness
Shoulder strap
Chest strap
Abduction straps
Leg strap

FIG. 43-55. Pavlik harness used to treat newborns with hip dysplasia. (Reproduced with permission from *http://www.musckids.com/health_library/hrnewborn/ddh.htm.*)

most cases with a dislocatable hip, the child is placed in a Pavlik harness, which maintains the hips in flexion and mild abduction. Extremes of abduction must be avoided, as maintaining hip in significant abduction can lead to avascular necrosis of the head (Fig. 43-55). With 1 to 3 months of treatment, the Pavlik harness is generally successful. In some patients, with more severe disease, selective tenotomies of some of the adductor muscles may be indicated.

In neglected or undiagnosed DDH, when the patient reaches walking age without achieving a stable hip, open reduction is often

necessary (Fig. 43-56). In such cases, an anterior approach to the hip generally is performed. Any pulvinar within the acetabulum is removed, and the femoral head is located. Often, these procedures are combined with capsular releases and adductor tenotomies. In cases with significant muscular contraction, femoral shortening (osteotomy to shortening of the femur) may be indicated. Following open reduction of osteonecrosis of the femoral head can occur. Restoration of the full pain-free motion of the hip is not always possible. In rare cases where open reduction does not produce a stable hip, some patients with severe DDH may be managed by pelvic osteotomy, where acetabular reconstruction or the creation of an acetabular shelf is performed.[63] In some cases, a varus osteotomy of the proximal femur also may be considered.

Legg-Calvé-Perthes Disease

Legg-Calvé-Perthes disease, also known as *coxa plana*, is a condition of the pediatric hip characterized by a flattened, misshapen femoral head.[64] The etiology of the problem is related to osteonecrosis of the proximal femoral epiphysis and is thought to result from vascular compromise.[65] Legg-Calvé-Perthes disease generally presents in children, usually males, between the ages of 4 and 8 years old. Presenting symptoms generally include groin or knee pain, decreased hip range of motion, and a limp. The Trendelenburg gait (tilting of the pelvis) is also commonly seen. Symptomatic treatment with traction, physical therapy, abduction exercise, crutches, and occasionally, femoral and pelvic osteotomies, are all offered as treatments. Unfortunately, a good solution for Legg-Calvé-Perthes disease has been elusive thus far.

Slipped Capital Femoral Epiphysis

A *slipped capital femoral epiphysis* (SCFE) is an acquired disorder of the epiphysis thought to be associated with weakness in the perichondrial ring of the growth plate.[66] Children within the ages of 10 to 16 years old are noted to have the displacement of the epiphysis on the femoral neck. In most cases, there is no identifiable trauma history. It is not known whether this is acquired insidiously or acutely (Fig. 43-57). It is associated with African American heritage, obesity, and is somewhat more common in boys than in girls. Twenty-five percent of cases are bilateral. SCFE usually is diagnosed in patients who complain of pain. It is important to know that the pain caused by this pathology is usually located in the groin and proximal anterior thigh. It is also quite common for patients to

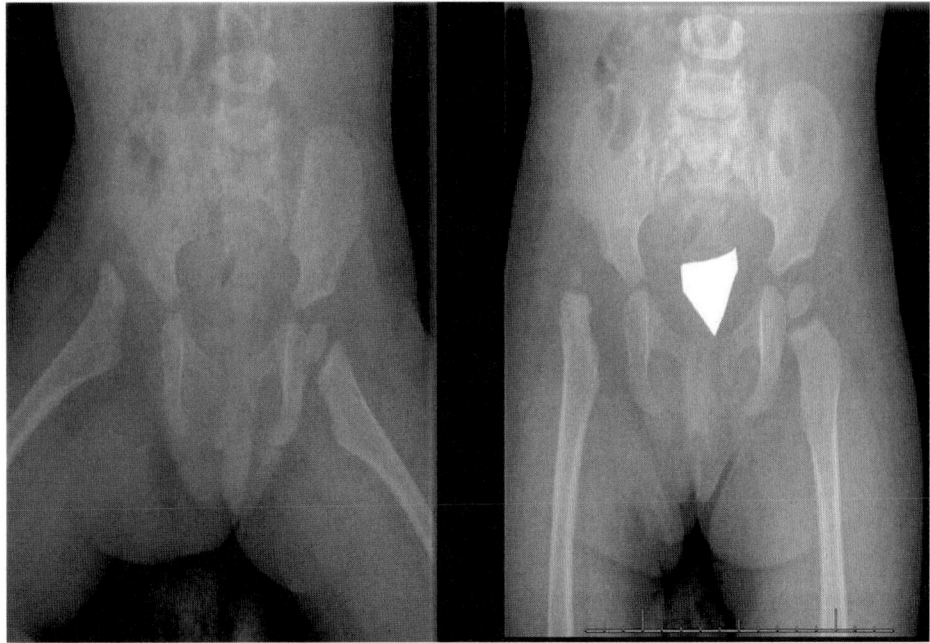

FIG. 43-56. X-ray images of a child with developmental dysplasia of the hip. Note that the right hip is dislocated and that the right acetabulum is shallow and malformed.

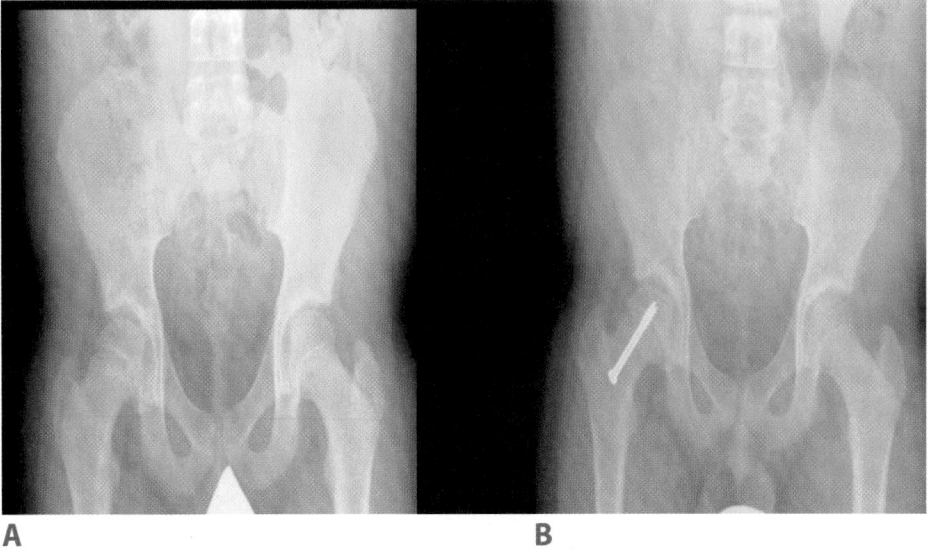

FIG. 43-57. Radiographic images of a young patient with a slipped capital femoral epiphysis, before (**A**) and after (**B**) screw fixation.

complain of pain about the knee. In pediatric patients with complaints of knee pain, an effort should always be made to assess the ipsilateral hip as well.

Treatment for virtually all SCFE patients is percutaneous screw fixation. The procedure is done through a small skin incision; a screw is inserted through the femoral neck to engage the epiphysis. Reduction of the slipped epiphysis is contraindicated because of an increased risk of avascular necrosis. Most practitioners find one screw to be adequate to prevent further slip.

Lower Extremity Rotational Abnormalities

The pediatric patients with lower extremity rotational abnormalities present with abnormal rotation of the lower extremities often resulting in "intoeing" stance and gait. The diagnosis of femoral anteversion, tibial torsion, and metatarsus adductus are used to describe rotational abnormalities at these respective anatomic locations. It should be noted that most children do have a mild degree of intoeing as a normal developmental stage.

Excessive rotation in internal rotation in the femur, most commonly seen in children age 3 to 7 years old, will usually correct by age 8. Severe degrees of rotation with functional impairment that do not correct after age 10 or 11 years old may be managed by rotational femoral osteotomy.

Tibial torsion is the most common cause of an intoeing gait. This is most frequently noted in 1- and 2-year-old children. This is often bilateral. Although occasionally intoeing can be marked, pediatric tibial torsion will completely resolve without treatment in almost every case.

Metatarsus adductus is a condition of forefoot adduction, generally seen in infants. Of note, this may be associated with DDH of the hip. As with most rotational abnormalities, the overwhelming majority of these cases also resolve spontaneously.

Congenital Talipes Equinovarus

Congenital talipes equinovarus, unfortunately frequently called *club foot*, is a common problem in pediatric orthopedic surgery (Fig. 43-58).[67] In involved patients, this disorder, which is slightly more common in males than females, is associated with contractures of the medial tendons of the foot, often associated with a tight Achilles tendon.[68] Contractures of the joint capsules of the ankle, hindfoot, and midfoot are also noted. Such feet are evaluated by radiographs before, during, and after treatment.[69] In most cases, the problem can be corrected by meticulous sequential corrective casting of the foot. A successful program of casting may be complete in from 1 to 5 months and can often yield an essentially normal foot

before walking age. In patients with more severe disease or in those who initiate treatment later, surgical release of contracted soft tissues may be necessary.[70] In most cases, such surgical releases are not contemplated before 6 to 8 months of age.[71]

Osgood-Schlatter Disease

Osgood-Schlatter disease is a very common problem most often seen in athletically active adolescents. This disorder is characterized by ossification in the distal patellar tendon at the point of its insertion onto the tibial apophysis. This disorder is thought to result from mechanical stress on the tendinous insertional area. X-ray views of the involved knee show a characteristic irregularity in the insertional area and often show separately discrete ossicles within the tendon itself. The disease will present with severe local pain and exquisite tenderness in the area of the tibial tubercle.

Effective treatment for the disease can be obtained by activity restriction, which is generally quite unwelcomed by the patient. If the symptoms are improved, athletic participation can be reasonable. In almost every case, symptoms do regress after skeletal maturity or the discontinuance of active athletic participation. In rare cases, persistive symptoms into adulthood can occur. Moderate success can be obtained by surgical excision of ossicles within the tendon of adults.

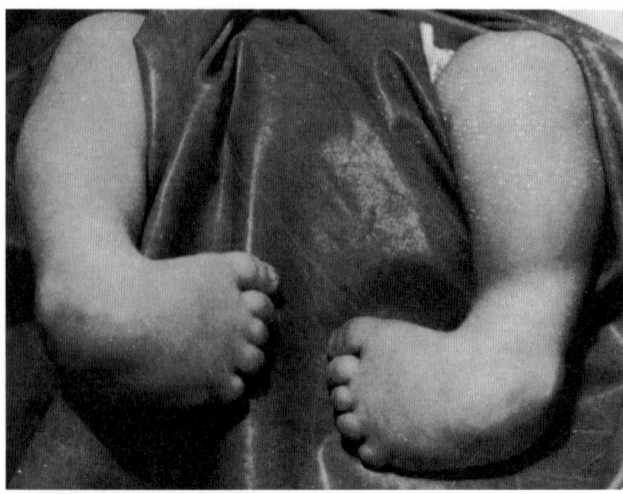

FIG. 43-58. Characteristic deformities of talipes equinovarus, or club foot.

The Future of Orthopedic Surgery

The treatment of musculoskeletal disease is progressing at a rapid pace. There is a very strong trend toward the use of less invasive surgical techniques, and the technology necessary for minimally invasive surgery is advancing rapidly.

During the next decade, application of molecular medicine techniques to numerous musculoskeletal problems are likely. The use of molecular genetic techniques to enhance or even replace many of our present surgical treatments.

REFERENCES

Entries highlighted in bright blue are key references.

1. Gustilo RB, Anderson JT: Prevention of infection in the treatment for one thousand and twenty-five open fractures of long bones. *J Bone Joint Surg Am* 58:453, 1976.

2. Weiland AJ, Moore FR, Daniel RK: The efficacy of free tissue transfer in the treatment of osteomyelitis. *J Bone Joint Surg Am* 66:181, 1984.

3. Hawkins LG: Fractures of the neck of the talus. *J Bone Joint Surg Am* 52:991, 1970.

4. Lauge-Hansen N: Fractures of the ankle. II. Combined experimental-surgical and experimental-roentgenologic investigations. *Arch Surg* 60:957, 1950.

5. Tejwani NC, McLaurin TM, Walsh M, et al: Are outcomes of bimalleolar fractures poorer than those of lateral malleolar fractures with medial ligamentous injury? *J Bone Joint Surg Am* 89:1438, 2007.

6. Saltzman C, Terusch DS: Achilles tendon injuries. *J Am Acad Orthop Surg* 6:316, 1998.

7. Nicoll EA: Fractures of the tibial shaft: A survey of 705 cases. *J Bone Joint Surg Br* 46:373, 1964.

8. Schatzker J, McBroom R, Bruce D: The tibial plateau fracture: The Toronto Experience 1968–1975. *Clin Orthop* 138:94, 1979.

9. Winquist RA, Hansen ST, Clawson K: Closed intramedullary nailing of femoral fractures: A report of five hundred and twenty cases. *J Bone Joint Surg Am* 66:259, 1984.

10. Garden RS: Malreduction and avascular necrosis in subcapital fractures of the femur. *J Bone Joint Surg Br* 53:183, 1971.

11. Shin SS: Circulatory and vascular changes in the hip flowing traumatic hip dislocation. *Clin Orthop* 140:255, 1979.

12. Letournel E: Acetabulum fractures: Classification and management. *Clin Orthop* 151:81, 1980.

13. Burgess AR, Eastridge BJ, Young JWR, et al: Pelvic ring disruptions: Effective classification system and treatment protocols. *J Trauma* 30:848, 1990.

14. Tile M: Acute pelvic fracture: I. Causation and classification. *J Am Acad Orthop* 4:143, 1996.

15. Tile M: Acute pelvic fracture II. Principles of management. *J Am Acad Orthop* 4:152, 1996.

16. Rockwood CA, Matsen FA: *The Shoulder*, 2nd ed. Vol. 1. Philadelphia: WB Saunders, 1998, p 495.

17. Neer CS II: *Shoulder Reconstruction*. Philadelphia: WB Saunders, 1990.

18. Holstein A, Lewis GB: Fractures of the humerus with radial nerve paralysis. *J Bone Joint Surg Am* 45:1382, 1963.

19. Sarmiento A, Kinman PB, Galvin EG, et al: Functional bracing of fractures of the shaft of the humerus. *J Bone Joint Surg Am* 59:596, 1977.

20. Ring D, Jupiter JB, Simpson NS: Monteggia fractures in adults. *J Bone Joint Surg Am* 80:1733, 1998.

21. Mikic ZDJ: Galeazzi fracture-dislocations. *J Bone Joint Surg Am* 57:1071, 1975.

22. Trueta J: Acute hematogenous osteomyelitis: Its pathology and treatment. *Bull Hosp Jt Dis* 14:5, 1953.

23. Richardson EG, Donley BG: Disorders of hallux, in Canale ST (ed): *Campbell's Operative Orthopaedics*, 10th ed. St. Louis: CV Mosby, 2003.

24. Krause JO, Brodsky JW: Peroneus brevis tendon tears: Pathophysiology, surgical reconstruction, and clinical results. *Foot Ankle Int* 19:271, 1998.

25. Mackenzie R, Palmer CR, Lomas DJ, et al: Magnetic resonance imaging of the knee: Diagnostic performance studies. *Clin Radiol* 51:251, 1996.

26. Shirakura K, Terauchi M, Kizuki S, et al: The natural history of untreated anterior cruciate ligaments tears in recreational athletes. *Clin Orthop* 317:227, 1995.

27. Fairbank TJ: Knee joint changes after meniscectomy. *J Bone Join Surg Br* 30:664, 1948.

28. Clancy WG, Ray JM, Zoltan DJ: Acute tears of the anterior cruciate ligament: Surgical versus conservative treatment. *J Bone Joint Surg Am* 70:1483, 1988.

29. Fu FH, Bennett CH, Lattermann C, et al: Current trends in anterior cruciate ligament reconstruction, Part I. *Am J Sports Med* 27:821, 1999.

30. Harner CD, Hoher J: Current concepts: Evaluation and treatment of posterior cruciate ligament injuries. *Am J Sports Med* 26:471, 1998.

31. Goldberg BA, Scarlet MM, Harryman DT II: Management of the stiff shoulder. *J Orthop Sci* 4:462, 1999.

32. Silliman JF, Hawkins RJ: Classification and physical diagnosis of instability of the shoulder. *Clin Orthop* 291:7, 1993.

33. Bigliani LU, Levine WN: Current concepts review: Subacromial impingement syndrome. *J Bone Joint Surg* 79:1854, 1997.

34. Gartsman, GM: Arthroscopic management of rotator cuff disease. *J Am Acad Orthop Surg* 6:259, 1998.

35. Cotler JM, Silveri CP, An HS, et al: *Surgery of Spinal Trauma*. Philadelphia: Lippincott, Williams and Wilkins, 2000.

36. Vaccaro AR: *Fractures of the Cervical, Thoracic, and Lumbar Spine.* New York: Marcel Dekker, 2003.

37. Ben-Galim PJ, Sibai T, Hipp JA, et al: Internal decapitation: Survival after head to neck dissociation injuries. *Spine* 33:16, 2008.

38. Jefferson G: Fracture of the atlas vertebra: Report of four cases and a review of those previously recorded. *Br J Surgery* 7:407, 1920.

39. Anderson LD, D'Alonzo RT: Fractures of the odontoid process of the axis. *J Bone Joint Surg Am* 86:2081, 2004.

40. Denis F: The three column spine and its significance in the classification of acute thoracolumbar spinal injuries. *Spine* 8:817, 1983.

41. Heggeness MH, Doherty BJ: The trabecular anatomy of thoracolumbar vertebrae: Implications for burst fractures. *J Anat* 191:309, 1997.

42. Chance GQ: Note on a type of flexion fracture of the spine *Br J Radiol* 21:452, 1948.

43. Weinstein JN, Tosteson TD, Lurie JD, et al: Surgical vs nonoperative treatment for lumbar disk herniation. *JAMA* 296:2441, 2006.

44. Katz JN, Lipson SJ: Seven to ten year outcome of decompressive surgery for degenerative lumbar spinal stenosis. *Spine* 21:92, 1996.

45. Herkowitz HN, Kurz LT: Degenerative lumbar spondylolisthesis with spinal stenosis: A prospective study comparing decompression with decompression and intertransverse process arthrodesis. *J Bone Joint Surg Am* 73:802, 1991.

46. Cobb JR: Outline for the study of scoliosis, in *The American Academy of Orthopaedic Surgeons: Instructional Course Lectures*, Vol. 5. Ann Arbor: J.W. Edwards, 1948, p 261.

47. Snyder BD, Hauser-Kara DA, Hipp JA, et al: Predicting fracture through benign skeletal lesions with quantitative computed tomography. *J Bone Joint Surg Am* 88:55, 2006.

48. Simon MA, Finn HA: Diagnostic strategy for bone and soft-tissue tumors. *J Bone Joint Surg Am* 75:6222, 1993.

49. Bell RS, O'Sullivan B, Liu FF, et al: The surgical margin in soft tissue sarcoma. *J Bone Joint Surg Am* 71:370, 1989.

50. Simon MA: Current concepts review: Limb salvage for osteosarcoma. *J Bone Joint Surg Am* 70:301, 1988.

51. Mankin HJ, Lange TA, Spanier SS: The hazards of biopsy in patients with malignant primary bone and soft tissue tumors. *J Bone Joint Surg Am* 64:1121, 1982.

52. Mankin HJ, Mankin DJ, et al: The hazards of the biopsy, revisited. Members of the Musculoskeletal Tumor Society. *J Bone Joint Surg Am* 78:656, 1996.

53. Heare TC, Enneking WF, Heare MJ: Staging techniques and biopsy of bone tumors. *Orthop Clin North Am* 20:273, 1989.

54. Simon MA, Bierman JS: Biopsy of bone and soft tissue lesions. *J Bone Joint Surg Am* 75:616, 1993.

55. Yasko AW, Lane JM: Current concepts review: Chemotherapy for bone and soft-tissue sarcoma of the extremities. *J Bone Joint Surg Am* 73:1263, 1991.

56. Enneking WF, Spanier SS, et al: A system for the surgical staging of musculoskeletal sarcoma. *Clin Orthop* 153:106, 1980.

57. Charnley J: *Low Friction Arthroplasty: Theory and Practice*. London: Churchill-Livingstone, 1979.

58. Salter RB, Harris WR: Injuries involving the epiphyseal plate. *J Bone Joint Surg Am* 45:587, 1963.

59. Bone LB, Johnson KD, Weigelt J, et al: Early vs. delayed stabilization of femoral fractures. A prospective randomized study. *J Bone Joint Surg Am* 71:336, 1989.

60. Skaggs DL, et al: Operative treatment of supracondylar fractures of the humerus in children. The consequences of pin placement. *J Bone Joint Surg Am* 3:735, 2001.

61. Weinstein SL, Mubarak SJ, Wenger DR: Developmental hip dysplasia and dislocation. Part I. *J Bone Joint Surg Am* 85:1824, 2003.

62. Weinstein SL, Mubarak SJ, Wenger DR: Developmental hip dysplasia and dislocation. Part II. *J Bone Joint Surg Am* 85:2024, 2003.

63. Willis RB: Developmental dysplasia of the hip: Assessment and treatment before walking age. *Instr Course Lect* 50:541, 2001.

64. Herring JS, Neustadt JB, William JJ, et al: The lateral pillar classification of Legg-Calvé-Perthes disease. *J Pediatr Orthop* 12:143, 1992.

65. Catterall A: The natural history of Perthes' disease. *J Bone Joint Surg Br* 53:37, 1971.

66. Crawford AH: Current concepts review: Slipped capital femoral epiphysis. *J Bone Joint Surg Am* 70:1422, 1988.

67. Lichtblau S: A medial and lateral release operation for clubfoot: A preliminary report. *J Bone Joint Surg Am* 55:1377, 1973.

68. Cummings RJ, Davidson RS, Armstrong PF, et al: Congenital clubfoot. *J Bone Joint Surg Am* 84:290, 2002.

69. Ponseti IV: *Congenital Clubfoot. Fundamentals for Treatment.* Oxford: Oxford University Press, 1996.

70. Turco VJ: Surgical correction of the resistant clubfoot: One-stage posteromedial release with internal fixation: A preliminary report. *J Bone Joint Surg Am* 53:477, 1971.

71. Cummings, RJ, Davidson RS, Armstrong PF, et al: Congenital clubfoot. *Instr Course Lect* 51:385, 2002.

Surgery of the Hand and Wrist

Scott D. Lifchez and Subhro K. Sen

TREATMENT PRINCIPLES

The highly mobile, functional, and strong hand is a major distinguishing point between human beings and the nonhuman primates. The hand is an essential participant for activities of daily living, vocation, and recreational activities. The hand is even adaptable enough to read for the blind and speak for the mute. The underlying goal of all aspects of hand surgery is to maximize mobility, sensibility, stability, and strength while minimizing pain. These goals are then maximized to the extent possible given the patient's particular pathology.

Bones

The hand is highly mobile in space to allow maximum flexibility in function. As such, a number of directions particular to the hand are necessary to properly describe position, motion, etc.[1] *Palmar* (or volar) refers to the anterior surface of the hand in the anatomic position; *dorsal* refers to the posterior surface in the anatomic position. The hand can rotate at the wrist level; rotation to bring the palm down is called *pronation*, to bring the palm up is called *supination*. Because the hand can rotate in space, the terms medial and lateral are avoided. Radial and ulnar are used instead as these terms do not vary with respect to the rotational position of the hand. Abduction and adduction, when used on the hand, refer to movement of the digits away from and toward the middle finger, respectively (Fig. 44-1).

The hand is comprised of 19 bones arranged in five rays.[2] A ray is defined as a digit (finger or thumb) from the metacarpal (MC) base to the tip of the digit (Fig. 44-2A). The rays are numbered 1 through 5, beginning with the thumb. By convention, however, they are referred to by name: thumb, index, middle, ring, and small. There are five metacarpals, comprising the visible palm of the hand. Each digit has a proximal and a distal phalanx, but only the fingers have a middle phalanx as well. The metacarpophalangeal (MP) joint typically allows 90° of flexion with a small amount of hyperextension. In addition, the fingers can actively abduct (move away from the middle finger) and adduct (move toward the middle finger). The thumb, in contrast, moves principally in the flexion-extension arc at the MP joint. Although there can be laxity in the radial and ulnar direction, the thumb cannot actively move in these directions at the MP level. The proximal interphalangeal (PIP) joint is the critical joint for finger mobility. Normal motion is 0 to 95° (full extension to flexion). The distal interphalangeal (DIP) joint also moves only in a flexion-extension plane from 0 to 90° on average. The thumb interphalangeal (IP) joint also moves only in a flexion-extension plane. Its normal motion is highly variable between individuals, but averages 0 to 80°.

Each of the MP and IP joints has a radial and ulnar collateral ligament to support it. The IP joint collateral ligaments are on tension with the joint fully extended. For the fingers, the MP joint collateral ligaments are on tension with the joint bent 90°. Collateral ligaments have a tendency to contract when not placed on tension; this becomes relevant when splinting the hand (see Trauma section on splinting below).

The wrist consists of eight carpal bones divided into two rows (see Fig. 44-2B).[2] The proximal row consists of the scaphoid, lunate, and triquetrum. The lunate is the principal axis of motion of the hand onto the forearm. It bears approximately 35% of the load of the wrist onto the forearm. The scaphoid is an oddly shaped bone, which bears

55% of the load of the hand onto the forearm, but also serves as the principal link between the proximal and distal rows, allowing for motion while maintaining stability. Both the scaphoid and the lunate articulate with the radius. The triquetrum resides ulnar to the lunate. It does not interact with the ulna proximally; rather it interacts with a cartilage suspended between the ulnar styloid and the distal radius called the *triangular fibrocartilage complex* (see Fig. 44-2B). The remaining 10% of load of the hand onto the forearm is transmitted through the triangular fibrocartilage complex.[3]

The distal row consists of four bones. The trapezium resides between the scaphoid and the thumb MC. Distally, it has a saddle-shaped surface, which interacts with a reciprocally saddle-shaped base of the thumb MC to allow for high mobility of the thumb carpometacarpal (CMC) joint in radial-ulnar and palmar-dorsal directions and opposition (see Fig. 44-1B). The trapezoid rests between the scaphoid and the index finger MC. The capitate, the largest carpal bone and first to ossify in a child, lies between the lunate and the middle finger MC but also interacts with the scaphoid on its proximal radial surface. The index and middle finger CMC joints are highly stable and have minimal mobility. The hamate is the ulnar-most bone in the distal row, sitting between the triquetrum proximally and the ring and small finger metacarpals distally. The ring and small finger CMC joints are mobile, but principally in the flexion-extension direction.

The pisiform is a carpal bone only by geography. It is a sesamoid bone within the flexor carpi ulnaris (FCU) tendon (see below under Muscles Affecting the Hand and Wrist). It does not bear load, and can be excised, when necessary, without consequence.

Muscles Affecting the Hand and Wrist

The wrist is moved by multiple tendons that originate from the forearm and elbow. The digits of the hand are moved by both intrinsic (originating within the hand) and extrinsic (originating proximal to the hand) muscles. All of these muscles are innervated by the median, radial, or ulnar nerves (or their branches) (Fig. 44-3).

Three muscles flex the wrist, all of which originate from the medial epicondyle of the humerus. The flexor carpi radialis (FCR, median nerve) inserts on the base of the volar index finger MC. The FCU (ulnar nerve) also originates from the proximal ulna and inserts on the volar base of the small finger MC. The palmaris longus tendon does not insert on a bone; it inserts on the palmar fascia, located deep to the skin in the central proximal palm, and is absent in up to 15% of patients. The FCR tends also to deviate the wrist radially, the FCU ulnarly.

All three wrist extensors are innervated by the radial nerve or its branches. The extensor carpi radialis longus (ECRL) originates from the distal shaft of the humerus and inserts on the dorsal base of the index finger MC. The extensor carpi radialis brevis (ECRB) originates from the lateral epicondyle of the humerus and inserts on the dorsal base of the middle finger MC. The extensor carpi ulnaris (ECU) originates from the lateral epicondyle of the humerus and inserts on the dorsal base of the small finger MC. The ECRL tends to deviate the wrist radially; the ECU ulnarly.

The long flexors of the fingers all originate from the medial epicondyle of the humerus. The flexor digitorum superficialis (FDS) inserts on the base of the middle phalanx of each finger and primarily flexes the PIP joint. The flexor digitorum profundus (FDP) inserts on the base of the distal phalanx and primarily flexes the DIP

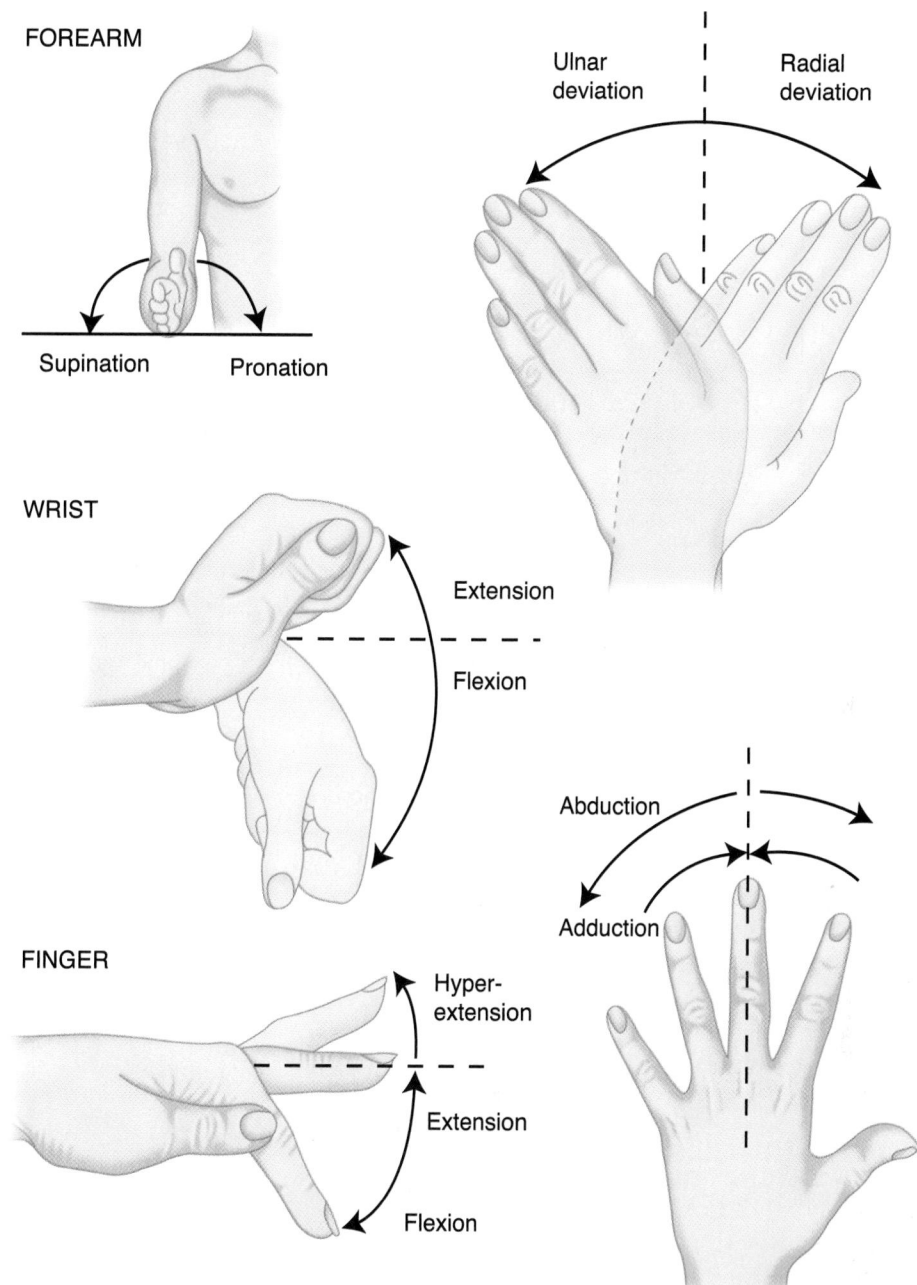

FIG. 44-1. Terminology of common hand motions. *[Reproduced with permission from American Society for Surgery of the Hand (ed): The Hand: Examination and Diagnosis, 3rd ed. Copyright © Elsevier, 1990.] (Continued)*

KEY POINTS

1. Surgery of the hand is a regional specialty, integrating components of neurologic, orthopedic, plastic, and vascular surgery.

2. Understanding hand anatomy is the key to proper diagnosis of injury, infection, and degenerative disease of the hand.

3. After evaluation and/or treatment, patients should be splinted to protect the injured digits and keep the collateral ligaments of the injured joints on tension (metacarpophalangeal joints flexed, interphalangeal joints extended).

4. Clinical examination, particularly noting the area of greatest tenderness and/or inflammation, is the most useful diagnostic tool for hand infections.

5. If a patient managed conservatively for "cellulitis" does not improve within 24 to 48 hours of appropriate IV antibiotics, abscess must be suspected.

6. Vascular injuries producing warm ischemia (incomplete amputations or direct vessel trauma with compromised distal perfusion) must be addressed urgently to prevent irreversible tissue loss.

7. Healing of an injured or diseased structure in the hand is not the endpoint of treatment; the goal of any intervention must be to obtain structural healing, relief of pain, and maximization of function.

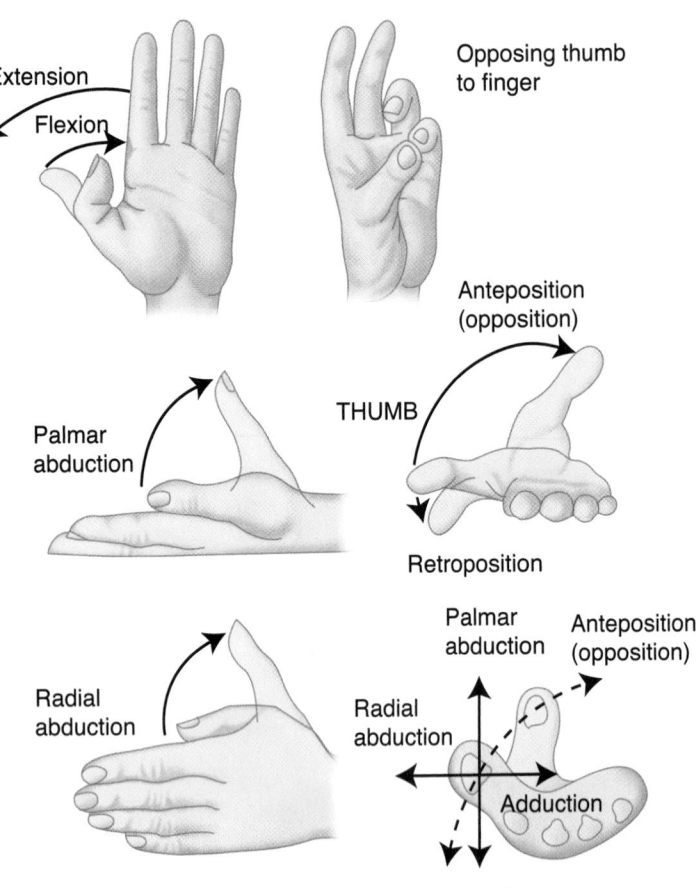

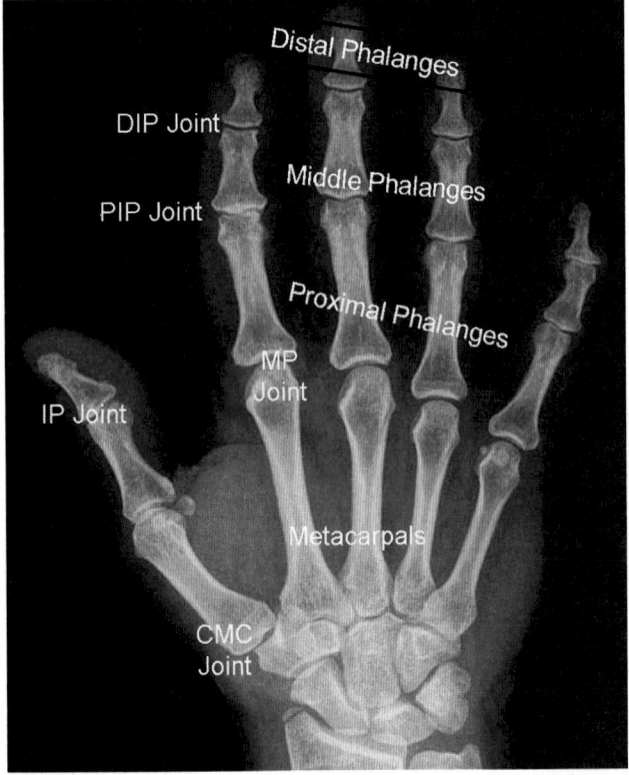

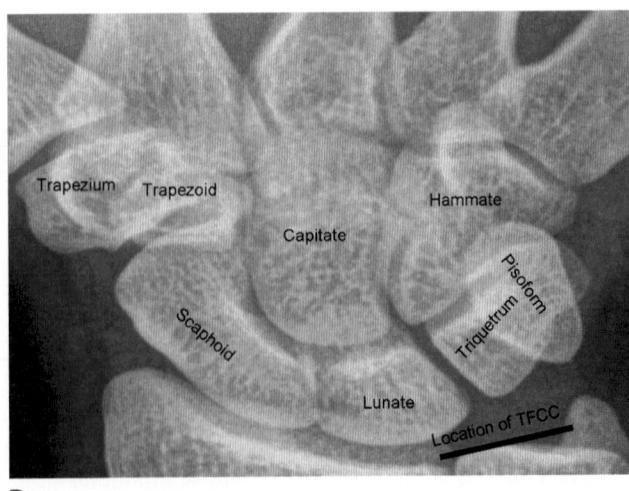

A

B

FIG. 44-2. Bony architecture of the hand and wrist. **A.** Bones of the hand and digits. All rays have metacarpophalangeal (MP) joints. The fingers have proximal and distal interphalangeal (PIP and DIP) joints, but the thumb has a single IP joint. **B.** Bones of the wrist: the proximal row consists of the scaphoid, lunate, and capitate. The distal row bones articulate with the metacarpals: the trapezium with the thumb, the trapezoid with the index, the capitate with the middle, and the hamate with the ring and small. The pisiform bone is a sesamoid within the flexor carpi ulnaris tendon. It overlaps the triquetrum and hamate but does not contribute to a carpal row. CMC = carpometacarpal; TFCC = triangular fibrocartilage complex.

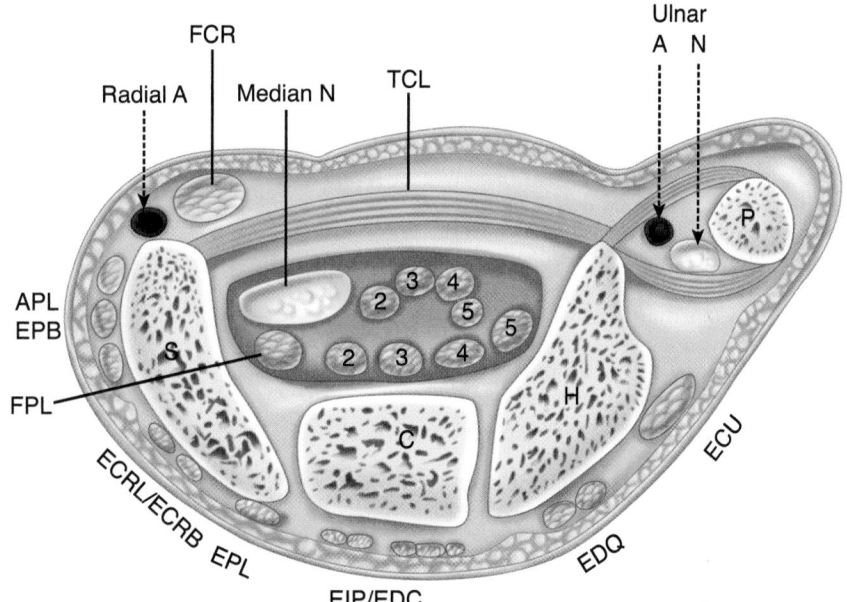

FIG. 44-3. Cross-section of the wrist at the midcarpal level. The relative geography of the neurologic and tendinous structures can be seen. The transverse carpal ligament (TCL) is the roof of the carpal tunnel, passing volar to the median nerve and long flexor tendons. The TCL is also the floor of the ulnar tunnel, or Guyon's canal, passing dorsal to the ulnar artery and nerve. The wrist and digital extensor tendons are also seen, distal to their compartments on the distal radius and ulna. Bones: C = capitate; H = hamate; P = pisiform; S = scaphoid. Tendons (flexor digitorum superficialis is volar to flexor digitorum profundus within the carpal tunnel): 2 = index finger; 3 = middle finger; 4 = ring finger; 5 = small finger. A = artery; APL = abductor pollicis longus; ECRB = extensor carpi radialis brevis; ECRL = extensor carpi radialis longus; ECU = extensor carpi ulnaris; EDC = extensor digitorum communis; EDQ = extensor digiti quinti; EIP = extensor indices proprius; EPB = extensor pollicis brevis; EPL = extensor pollicis longus; FCR = flexor carpi radialis; FPL = flexor pollicis longus; N = nerve.

joint. The flexor pollicis longus (FPL) originates more distally, from the ulna, radius, and interosseous membrane between them in the forearm. It inserts on the base of the distal phalanx of the thumb and primarily flexes the IP joint. All of these tendons can also flex the more proximal joint(s) in their respective rays. All of these muscles are innervated by the median nerve (or its branches) except the FDP to the ring and small finger, which are innervated by the ulnar nerve.

The extrinsic extensors of the fingers and thumb are all innervated by the PIN (branch of the radial nerve). The extensor digitorum communis (EDC) originates from the lateral epicondyle of the humerus and extends the MP joints of the fingers. It is somewhat unusual in its insertion in that it does not insert on the dorsal base of the proximal phalanx, but rather into a soft tissue sling called the *sagittal hood* that surrounds the proximal phalanx base and pulls up on the volar surface in a hammock-like manner. More distally in the dorsal forearm, the extensor indices proprius (EIP) and extensor digiti quinti (EDQ) originate from the ulna, radius, and posterior interosseous membrane and insert on the sagittal hood of the index and small fingers, respectively.

The thumb has three separate extrinsic extensors. All of these originate from the dorsal ulna in the mid-forearm and are innervated by the PIN. The abductor pollicis longus (APL) inserts on the radial base of the thumb MC to produce some extension, but mostly abduction. The extensor pollicis brevis (EPB) inserts on the base of the thumb proximal phalanx. The extensor pollicis longus (EPL) inserts on the base of the thumb distal phalanx.

The intrinsic muscles of the hand are what allow human beings fine, subtle movements of the hand. Microsurgery, typing, and even video gaming would be difficult, if not impossible, without them.

The thenar muscles originate from the volar radial surface of the scaphoid and trapezium and the flexor retinaculum. The abductor pollicis brevis inserts on the radial base of the thumb proximal phalanx and abducts the thumb in a radial and volar direction. The opponens pollicis (OP) inserts on the radial distal aspect of the thumb MC and draws the thumb across the palm toward the small finger. The flexor pollicis brevis (FPB) inserts on the base of the thumb proximal phalanx and flexes the thumb MP joint. The abductor pollicis brevis, OP, and superficial head of the FPB are all innervated by the thenar motor branch of the median nerve.

The lumbrical muscles are unique in the body in that they originate from a tendon. Each finger's lumbrical originates from the FDP tendon in the palm. The lumbrical tendon passes along the radial aspect of the digit to flex the MP and extend the IP joints. The index and middle lumbricals are median nerve innervated, and the ring and small finger lumbricals are ulnar nerve innervated.

The hypothenar muscles originate from the pisiform, hamate, and flexor retinaculum and insert on the ulnar base of the small finger proximal phalanx. The abductor digiti quinti abducts the small finger. The opponens digiti quinti brings the small finger across the palm in reciprocal motion to the OP. The flexor digiti quinti flexes the small finger MC. All these muscles are innervated by the ulnar nerve.

The interosseous muscles occupy the space between the MC bones. Their tendons insert on the bases of the proximal phalanges. All act to flex the MP joints and extend the IP joints. The three palmar interosseous muscles adduct the fingers. The four dorsal interosseous muscles abduct the fingers. The adductor pollicis originates from the middle finger MC and inserts on the ulnar base of the thumb proximal phalanx. It acts to adduct the thumb. All of these muscles, as well as the deep head of the FPB, are innervated by the ulnar nerve.

Tendons and Pulleys

Multiple pulleys pass over or surround the extrinsic tendons en route to or within the hand. Their purpose is to prevent bow stringing of the tendon, which would decrease the efficiency of its force transmission.

The most well known of the wrist level pulleys is the flexor retinaculum, also known as the *transverse carpal ligament*. It attaches to the scaphoid tubercle and trapezium radially, and the hook of the hamate bone and pisiform ulnarly. Deep to this ligament, between the scaphoid (radially) and the hamate (ulnarly), pass the FDS, FDP, and FPL tendons as well as the median nerve. This area is also known as the *carpal tunnel* (see Fig. 44-3).

On the dorsum of the wrist, the extensor retinaculum is divided into six compartments. Beginning on the radial aspect of the radius, the first compartment contains the APL and EPB tendons. The second holds the ECRL and ECRB tendons. The EPL passes through the third compartment. The fourth compartment contains the EIP and EDC tendons; the fifth, the EDQ, and the sixth, the ECU. The sixth compartment is located on the ulnar aspect of the distal ulna. Although the compartments end at the radiocarpal/ulnocarpal joints, the relative geography of the tendons is preserved over the carpal bones (see Fig. 44-3).

In the hand, the pulleys maintain the long flexor tendons in close apposition to the fingers and thumb. There are no extensor pulleys within the hand. Each finger has five annular and three cruciate pulleys (Fig. 44-4). The second and fourth (A2 and A4) pulleys are the critical structures that prevent bowstringing of the finger.[4] The remaining pulleys can be divided as needed for surgical exposure or to relieve a stricture area.

Vascular

Two major arteries serve the hand. The radial artery travels under the brachioradialis muscle in the forearm. At the junction of the middle and distal thirds of the forearm, the artery becomes superficial and palpable, passing just radial to the FCR tendon. At the wrist level, the artery splits into two branches. The smaller, superficial branch passes volarly into the palm to contribute to the superficial palmar arch. The larger branch passes dorsally over the scaphoid bone, under the EPL and EPB tendons (known as the *anatomic snuffbox*), and back volarly between the proximal thumb and index finger metacarpals to form the superficial palmar arch.

The ulnar artery travels deep to the FCU muscle in the forearm. When the FCU becomes tendinous, the ulnar artery resides deep and slightly radial to it. At the wrist, the artery travels between the hamate and pisiform bones superficial to the transverse carpal ligament (known as *Guyon's canal*) into the palm. The larger, superficial branch forms the superficial palmar arch. The deeper branch contributes to the deep palmar arch (Fig. 44-5A). In 97% of

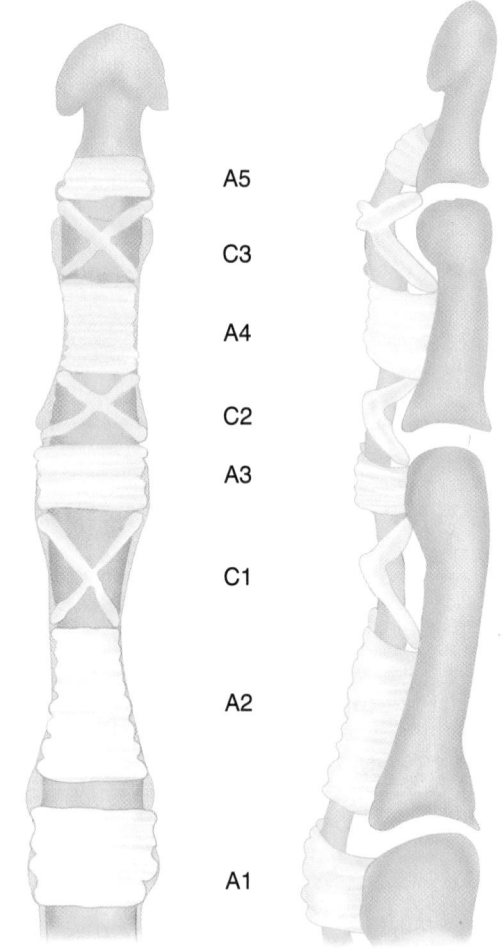

FIG. 44-4. Drawing of anteroposterior and lateral view of the pulley system.

patients, at least one of the deep or superficial palmar arches is intact, allowing for the entire hand to survive on the radial or ulnar artery.[5]

Each digit receives a radial and ulnar digital artery. For the thumb, the radial digital artery may come from the deep palmar

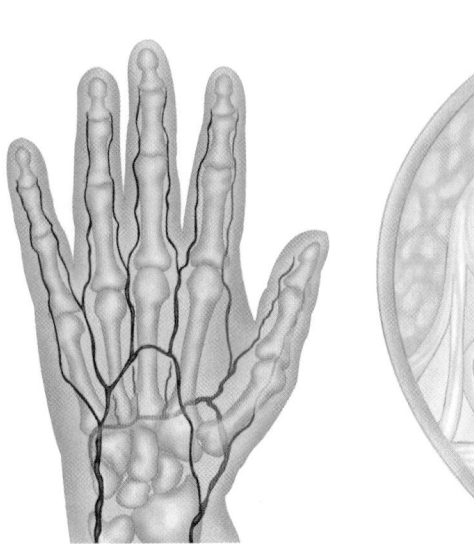
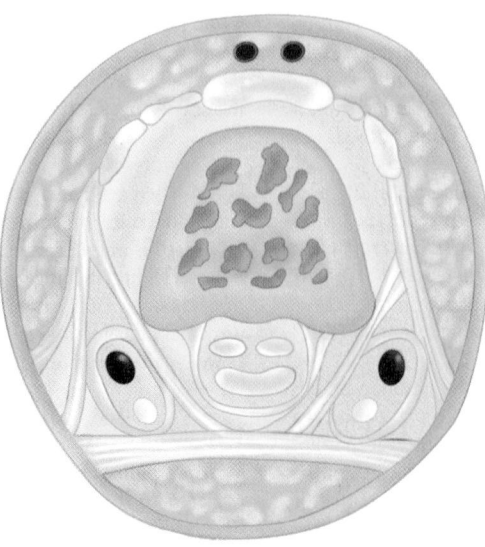

A **B**

FIG. 44-5. Arteries of the hand and finger. **A.** Relative position of the superficial and deep palmar arches to the bony structures and each other; note the radial artery passes dorsal to the thumb metacarpal base, through the first web space, and anterior to the index metacarpal base as it forms the deep arch. **B.** The neurovascular bundles lay volar to the midaxis of the digit with the artery dorsal to the nerve; Grayson's ligament (volar) and Cleland's ligament (dorsal) connect the bone to the skin surrounding the bundle.

arch or the main body of the radial artery. The larger ulnar digital artery comes off the deep arch as either a single unit, the princeps pollicis artery, or less frequently, as the first common digital artery, which then splits into the radial digital artery to the index finger and the ulnar digital artery to the thumb. The second, third, and fourth digital arteries typically branch off the superficial palmar arch and pass between the index/middle, middle/ring, and ring/small fingers respectively, ultimately dividing into two proper digital arteries each. The ulnar digital artery of the small finger comes off as a separate branch from the superficial arch. Within the finger, the proper digital arteries travel lateral to the bones and tendons, just palmar to the midaxis of the digit, but dorsal to the proper digital nerves (see Fig. 44-5B).

Nerve

Three principal nerves serve the forearm, wrist, and hand: the median, radial, and ulnar nerves. The most critical of these from a sensory standpoint is the median nerve. The median nerve begins as a terminal branch of the medial and lateral cords of the brachial plexus. It receives fibers from C5–T1. The palmar cutaneous branch of the median nerve serves the proximal, radial-sided palm. The main body of the median nerve splits into several branches after the carpal tunnel: a radial digital branch to the thumb, an ulnar digital nerve to the thumb, and a radial digital nerve to the index finger (sometimes beginning as a single first common digital nerve); the second common digital nerve that branches into the ulnar digital nerve to the index finger and the radial digital nerve to the middle finger; and a third common digital nerve that branches into the ulnar digital nerve to the middle finger and a radial digital nerve to the ring finger. The digital nerves provide volar-sided sensation from the MC head level to the tip of the digit. They also, through their dorsal branches, provide dorsal-sided sensation to the digits from the midportion of the middle phalanx distally via dorsal branches. The thenar motor branch of the median nerve most commonly passes through the carpal tunnel and then travels in a recurrent fashion back to the thenar muscles. Less commonly, the nerve passes through or proximal to the transverse carpal ligament en route to its muscles.

In the forearm, the median nerve gives motor branches to all of the flexor muscles except the FCU, and the ring and small finger portions of the FDP. Distal median motor fibers (with the exception of those to the thenar muscles) are carried through a large branch called the *anterior interosseous nerve*.

The ulnar nerve is a terminal branch of the medial cord of the brachial plexus. It receives innervation from C8 and T1 roots. The FCU and FDP (ring/small) receive motor fibers from the ulnar nerve. In the distal forearm, 5 cm above the head of the ulna, the nerve gives off a dorsal sensory branch. Once in the hand, the nerve splits into the motor branch and sensory branches. The motor branch curves radially at the hook of the hamate bone to innervate the intrinsic muscles as described above in Muscles Affecting the Hand and Wrist. The sensory branches become the ulnar digital nerve to the small finger and the fourth common digital nerve which splits into the ulnar digital nerve to the ring finger and the radial digital nerve to the small finger. The sensory nerves provide distal dorsal sensation similar to the median nerve branches.

The radial nerve is the larger of two terminal branches of the posterior cord of the brachial plexus. It receives fibers from C5–T1 nerve roots. It innervates all of the extensor muscles of the forearm and wrist, principally through its PIN branch. The major exception to this is the ECRL, which is innervated by the main body of the radial nerve in the distal upper arm. Unlike on the flexor surface, there is no ulnar nerve contribution to extension of the wrist, thumb, or finger MP joints. As noted above in Muscles Affecting the Hand and Wrist, the ulnar innervated intrinsic hand muscles are the principal extensors of the finger interphalangeal joints, although the long finger extensors (EDC, EIP, EDQ) make a secondary contribution to this function.

In the proximal dorsal forearm, the superficial radial nerve (SRN) is the other terminal branch of the radial nerve. It travels deep to the brachioradialis muscle until 6 cm proximal to the radial styloid, where it becomes superficial. The SRN provides sensation to the dorsal hand and the radial three and one half digits up to the level of the mid-middle phalanx (where the dorsal branches of the proper digital nerves take over, as described earlier in this section). The dorsal branch of the ulnar nerve provides sensation to the ulnar one and one half digits and dorsal hand in complement to the SRN.

HAND EXAMINATION

Emergency Room/Inpatient Consultation

A common scenario in which the hand surgeon will be introduced to the patient is in trauma or other acute situations. The patient is evaluated by inspection, palpation, and provocative testing. Upon inspection, one should first note the position of the hand. The resting hand has a normal cascade of the fingers, with the small finger flexed most and the index finger least (Fig. 44-6). Disturbance of this suggests a tendon or skeletal problem. Also note any gross

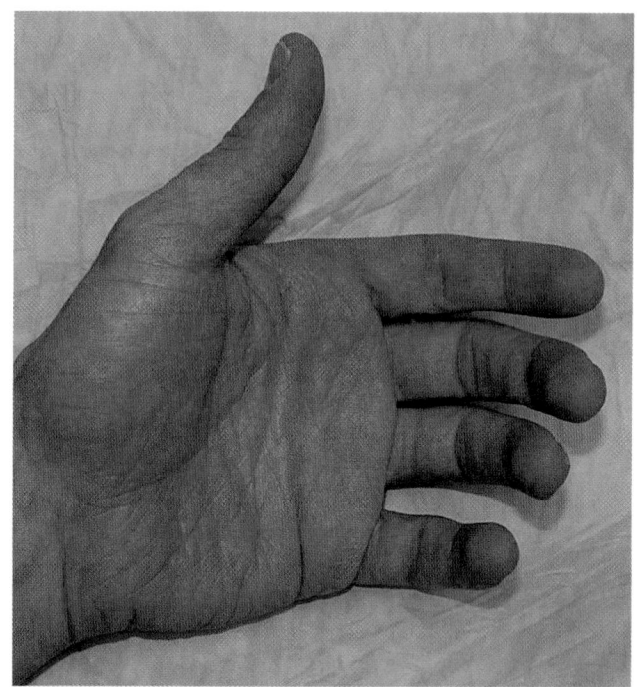

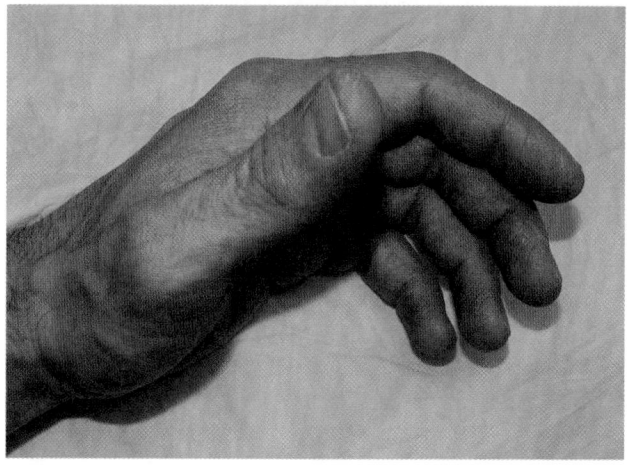

FIG. 44-6. In the normal resting hand, the fingers assume a slightly flexed posture from the index finger (least) to the small finger (most).

deformities or wounds, and what deeper structures, if any, are visible in such wounds. Observe for abnormal coloration of a portion or all of the hand (this can be skewed by ambient temperature or other injuries), gross edema, and/or clubbing of the fingertips.

Palpation typically begins with the radial and ulnar artery pulses at the wrist level. Pencil Doppler examination can supplement this and evaluate distal vessels. A pulsatile signal is normally detectable by pencil Doppler in the pad of the finger at the center of the whorl of creases. Discrepancies between digits should be noted. If all other tests are inconclusive, pricking the involved digit with a 25-gauge needle should produce bright red capillary bleeding. If an attached digit demonstrates inadequate or absent blood flow (warm ischemia), the urgency of completing the evaluation and initiating treatment markedly increases.

Sensation must be evaluated before any administration of local anesthetic. At a minimum, light and sharp touch sensation should be documented for the radial and ulnar aspects of the tip of each digit. Beware of writing "sensation intact" at the conclusion of this evaluation. Medicolegally, intact means perfect and can be a liability if the sensation is measured more thoroughly after an intervention and noted not to be perfect. Rather, one should document what was tested (e.g., "light and sharp touch sensation present and symmetric to the tips of all digits of the injured hand"). In the setting of a sharp injury, sensory deficit implies a lacerated structure until proven otherwise. Once sensation has been evaluated and documented, the injured hand can be anesthetized for patient comfort during the remainder of the examination (see below under Local Anesthesia).

Ability to flex and extend the wrist and digital joints is typically examined next. At the wrist level, the FCR and FCU tendons should be palpable during flexion. The wrist extensors are not as readily palpated due to the extensor retinaculum. Ability to flex the DIP joint (FDP) is tested by blocking the finger at the middle phalanx level. To test the FDS to each finger, hold the remaining three fingers in slight hyperextension and ask the patient to flex the involved digit (Fig. 44-7). This maneuver makes use of the fact that the FDP tendons share a common muscle belly. Placing the remaining fingers in extension prevents the FDP from firing, and allows on the FDS, which has a separate muscle belly for each tendon, to fire. Strength in grip, finger abduction, and thumb opposition is tested and compared

to the uninjured side. Range of motion (ROM) for the wrist, MP, and IP joints should be noted and compared to the opposite side.

If there is suspicion for closed space infection, the hand should be evaluated for erythema, swelling, fluctuance, and localized tenderness. The dorsum of the hand does not have fascial septae, thus dorsal infections can spread more widely than palmar ones. The epitrochlear and axillary nodes should be palpated for enlargement and tenderness. Findings for specific infectious processes will be discussed in the Infections section.

Additional examination maneuvers and findings, such as those for office consultations, will be discussed with each individual disease process covered later in this chapter.

HAND IMAGING

Plain X-Rays

Almost every hand evaluation should include plain x-rays of the injured/affected part. A standard, anteroposterior, lateral, and oblique view of the hand or wrist (as appropriate) is rapid, inexpensive, and usually provides sufficient information about the bony structures to achieve a diagnosis in conjunction with the symptoms and findings.[6]

Lucencies within the bone should be noted. Most commonly, these represent fractures, but they can, on occasion, represent neoplastic or degenerative processes. Great care should be taken to evaluate the entire x-ray, typically beginning away from the area of the patient's complaint. Additional injuries can be missed that might affect the treatment plan selected and eventual outcome.

Congruency of adjacent joints also should be noted. The MP and IP joints of the fingers should all be in the same plain on any given view. Incongruency of the joint(s) of one finger implies fracture with rotation. At the wrist level, the proximal and distal edge of the proximal row and proximal edge of the distal row should be smooth arcs,[7] known as Gilula's arcs (Fig. 44-8A). Disruption of these implies ligamentous injury or possibly dislocation (see Fig. 44-8B).

Computed Tomography

CT scanning of the hand and wrist can provide additional bony information when plain x-rays are insufficient. Comminuted fractures of the distal radius can be better visualized for number and orientation of fragments. Scaphoid fractures can be evaluated for displacement and comminution preoperatively as well as for the presence of bony bridging postoperatively (Fig. 44-9). CT scans are also useful for CMC fractures of the hand where overlap on a plain x-ray lateral view may make diagnosis difficult.

Unlike the trunk and more proximal extremities, CT scans with contrast are less useful to demonstrate abscess cavities.

Ultrasonography

Ultrasonography has the advantages of being able to demonstrate soft tissue structures and being available on nights and weekends. Unfortunately, it is also highly operator dependent. In the middle of the night, when magnetic resonance imaging (MRI) is not available, ultrasound may be able to demonstrate a large deep infection in the hand but is rarely more useful than a thorough clinical examination.

Magnetic Resonance Imaging

MRI provides the best noninvasive visualization of the soft tissue structures. With contrast, MRI can demonstrate an occult abscess. Unfortunately, it usually is not available on nights and weekends when this information is often needed. MRI also can demonstrate soft tissue injuries such as cartilage or ligament tears or tendonitis (usually by demonstrating edema in the area in question). It can demonstrate occult fractures that are not sufficiently displaced to be seen on x-ray or CT (again, by demonstrating edema). MRI also can demonstrate vascular disturbance of a bone, as with the patient with avascular necrosis of the scaphoid shown in Fig. 44-10.

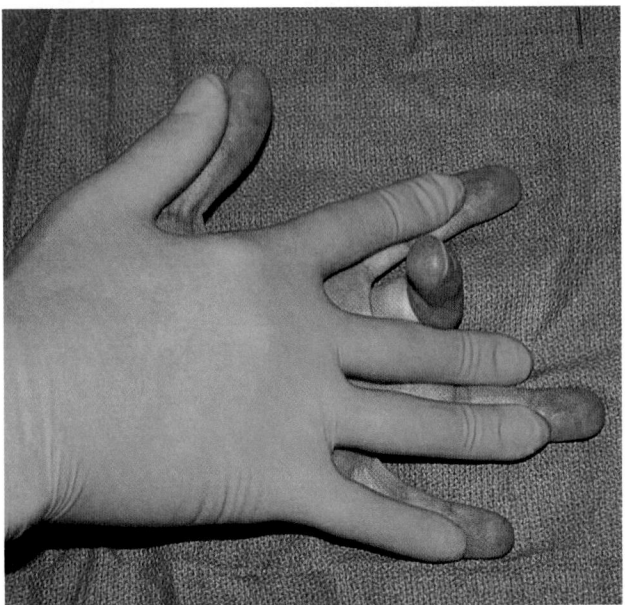

FIG. 44-7. The examiner holds the untested fingers in full extension, preventing contracture of the flexor digitorum profundus. In this position, the patient is asked to flex the finger, and only the flexor digitorum superficialis will be able to fire.

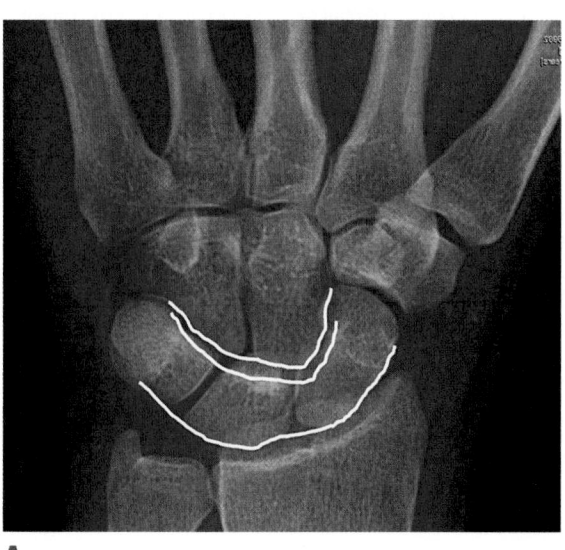

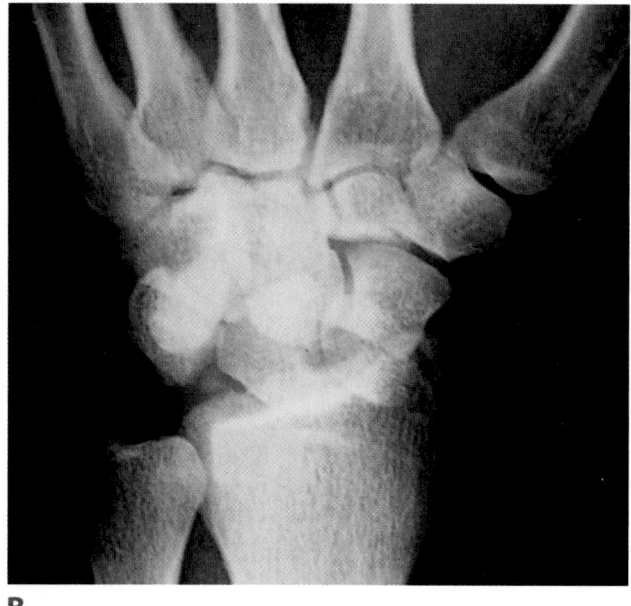

FIG. 44-8. Gilula's arcs are seen shown in this normal patient (**A**) and in a patient with a scaphoid fracture and perilunate dislocation (**B**).

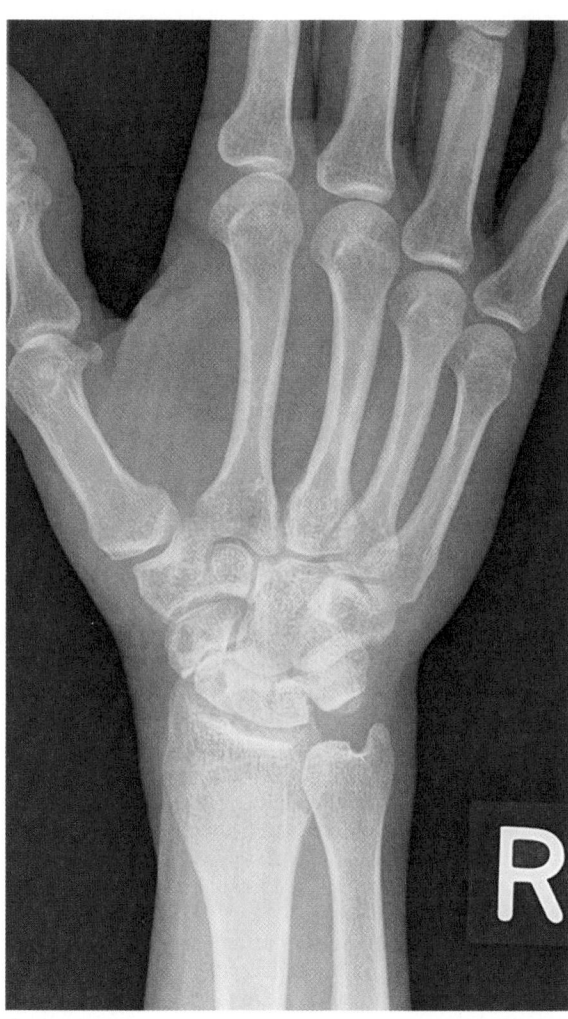

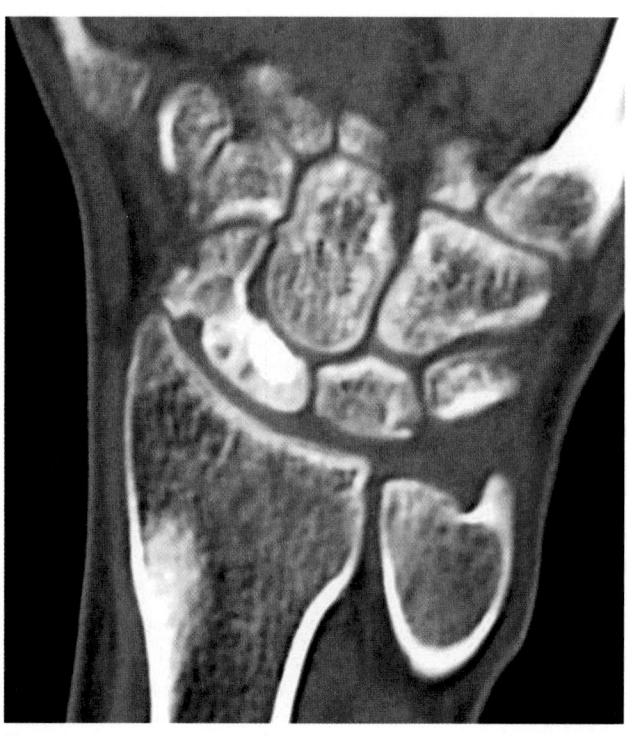

FIG. 44-9. A. Preoperative images demonstrate a nonunion of a scaphoid fracture sustained 4 years earlier. **B.** Postoperatively, cross-sectional imaging with a computed tomography scan in the coronal plan demonstrates bone crossing the previous fracture line. This can be difficult to discern on plain x-rays due to overlap of bone fragments.

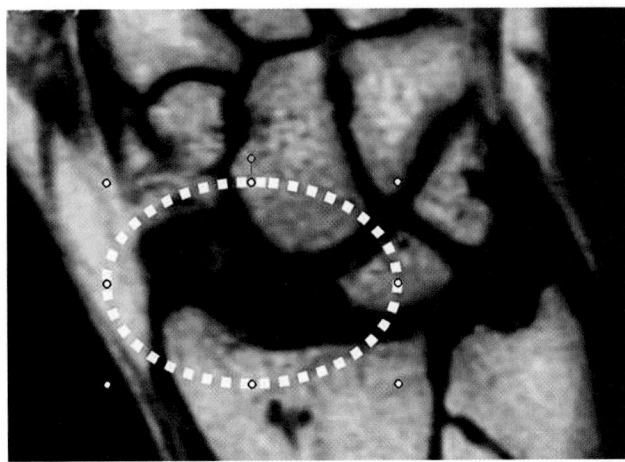

FIG. 44-10. T1-weighted magnetic resonance imaging (seen here) shows perfused bone as *white*. In this patient, there is the absence of whiteness where the scaphoid should be (*dashed circle*), consistent with avascular necrosis.

Angiography

Angiography of the upper extremity is rarely used. Magnetic resonance angiography and computed tomography angiography in many centers provide sufficient resolution of the vascular structures to make it necessary. Also, primary vascular disease of the upper extremity is relatively uncommon. In the trauma setting, vascular disturbance usually mandates exploration and direct visualization of the structures in question, and angiography is thus obviated.

For a patient with vascular disease of the upper extremity, angiography of the upper extremity is usually performed through a femoral access much like with the leg. An arterial catheter can be used to deliver thrombolytic drugs to treat an occlusive process.

TRAUMA

The upper extremity–injured patient may have additional injuries to other parts of the body. All injured patients should receive an appropriate trauma survey to look for additional injuries. Although the hand provides critical function to the patient, treatment of life or more proximal limb-threatening injuries takes precedence.

The patient with upper extremity trauma is evaluated as described in the Hand Examination section. Perform an appropriate sensory examination early. Once sensory status has been documented, administration of local anesthesia can provide comfort to the patient during the remainder of the evaluation and subsequent treatment. Patients should receive tetanus toxoid for penetrating injuries if more than 5 years have passed since the last vaccination.

Local Anesthesia

Anesthetic blockade can be administered at the wrist level, digital level, or with local infiltration, as needed. Keep in mind that all local anesthetics are less effective in areas of inflammation. The agents most commonly used are lidocaine and bupivacaine. Lidocaine has the advantage of rapid onset while bupivacaine has the advantage of long duration (average 6 to 8 hours).[8] Although bupivacaine can produce irreversible heart block in high doses, this is rarely an issue given the amounts typically used in the hand. For pediatric patients, the tolerated dose is 2.5 mg/kg. This can be easily remembered by noting that when using 0.25% bupivacaine, 1mL/kg is acceptable dosing.

A commonly held axiom is that epinephrine is unacceptable to be used in the hand. Several recent large series have dispelled this myth.[9] Epinephrine should not be used in the fingertip, and not in concentrations higher than 1:100,000 (i.e., what is present in commercially available local anesthetic with epinephrine). Beyond that, its use is acceptable and may be useful in an emergency room (ER) where tourniquet control may not be available. Also, as most ER procedures are done under pure local anesthesia, many patients will not tolerate the discomfort of the tourniquet beyond 30 minutes.[10] Not only will epinephrine provide hemostasis, it also prolongs the effect of the local anesthetic.

Simple lacerations, particularly on the dorsum of the hand, can be anesthetized with local infiltration. This is performed in the standard fashion.

Blocking of the digital nerves at the MC head level is useful for volar injuries distal to this point and for dorsal injuries beyond the midpoint of the middle phalanx (via dorsal branches of the proper digital nerves). Fingertip injuries are particularly well anesthetized by this technique. There are two principal ways to anesthetize a digit (Fig. 44-11A and 44-11B). The flexor sheath technique introduces the needle in the slightly more sensitive volar skin at the MC head level; the intermetacarpal technique introduces the needle in the slightly less sensitive web space skin, but requires two injections for a single digit.

Blocking one or more nerves as they cross the wrist can provide several advantages: anesthesia for multiple injured digits, avoiding areas of inflammation where the local anesthetic agent may be less effective, and avoiding injection where the volume of fluid injected may make treatment harder (such as fracture reduction). Four major nerves cross the wrist: the median nerve, SRN, ulnar nerve, and dorsal sensory branch of the ulnar nerve (see Fig. 44-11C, 44-11D, and 44-11E). When blocking the median and ulnar nerves, beware of intraneural injection, which can cause irreversible neural scarring. If the patient complains of severe paresthesias with injection, or high resistance is encountered, the needle should be repositioned.

Fractures and Dislocations

For dislocations and displaced fractures, a visible deformity is often present. Nondisplaced fractures may not show a gross deformity, but will have edema and tenderness to palpation at the fracture site. The fracture should be described for its displacement, rotation, and angulation. The fracture should also be described in terms of comminution, the number and complexity of fracture fragments. Displacement is described as a percentage of the diameter of the bone; rotation is described in degrees of supination or pronation with respect to the rest of the hand; angulation is described in degrees. To avoid confusion, it is useful to describe in which direction the angle of the fracture points. All injuries should be evaluated for nearby wounds (open) that may introduce bacteria into the fracture site or joint space (Fig. 44-12).

Once the initial force on the fracture ceases, the tendons passing beyond the fracture site provide the principal deforming force. Their force is directed proximally and, to a lesser extent, volarly. Based on this, the stability of a fracture can be determined by the orientation of the fracture with respect to the shaft of the bone. Transverse fractures are typically stable. Oblique fractures typically shorten. Spiral fractures typically rotate as they shorten and thus require surgical treatment.

Fractures of the tuft of the distal phalanx are commonly seen. Slamming of a finger in a door is a common causative mechanism. These fractures are often nondisplaced and do not require treatment beyond protection of the distal phalanx from additional trauma while the fracture heals.

Displaced transverse fractures of the phalanges can usually be reduced with distraction. The distal part is pulled away from the main body of the hand, then pushed in the direction of the proximal shaft of the finger, then distraction is released. Postreduction x-rays should always be performed to document satisfactory reduction. Oblique and spiral fractures usually are unstable after reduction. The involved digit(s) should be splinted until appropriate surgical intervention can be performed.

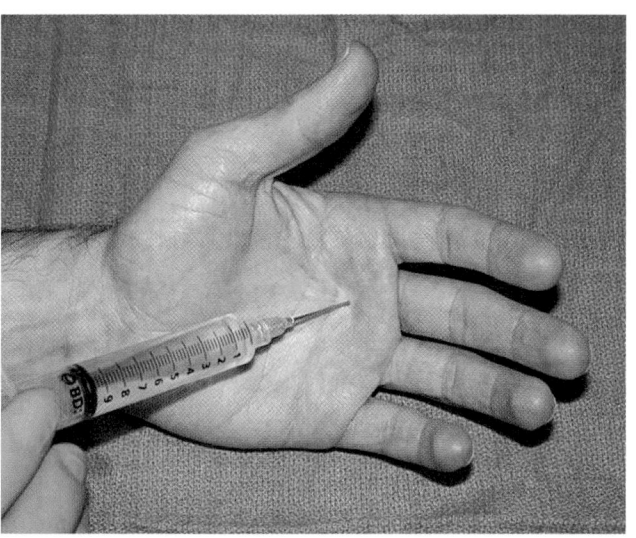

A

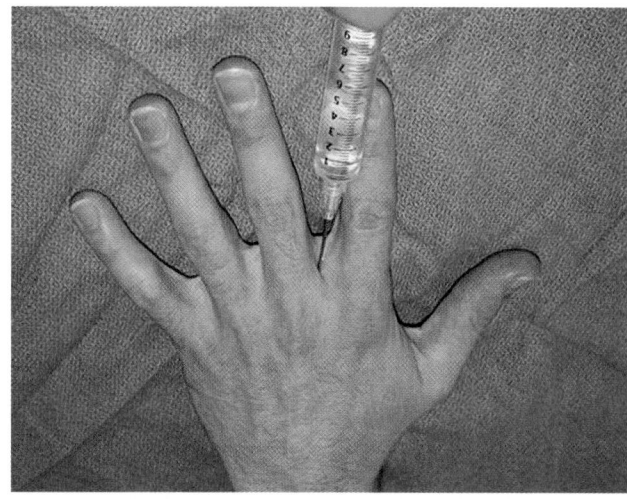

B

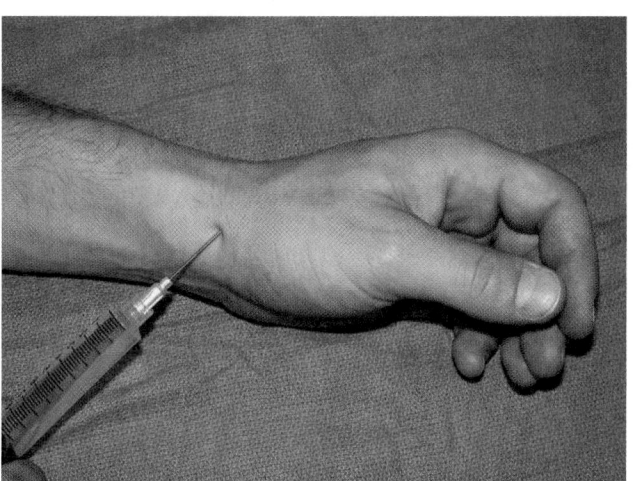

C

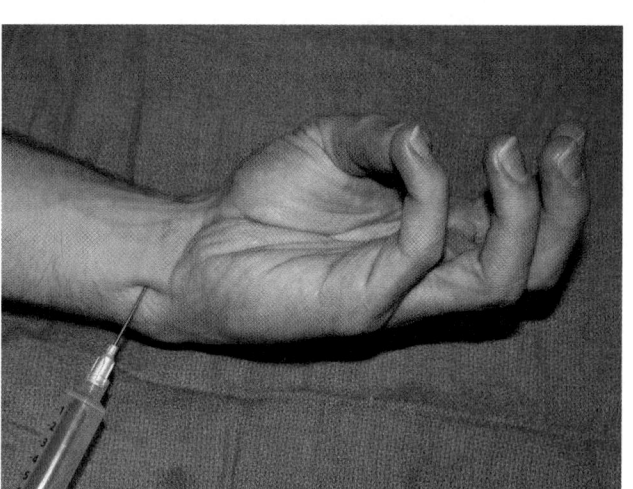

D

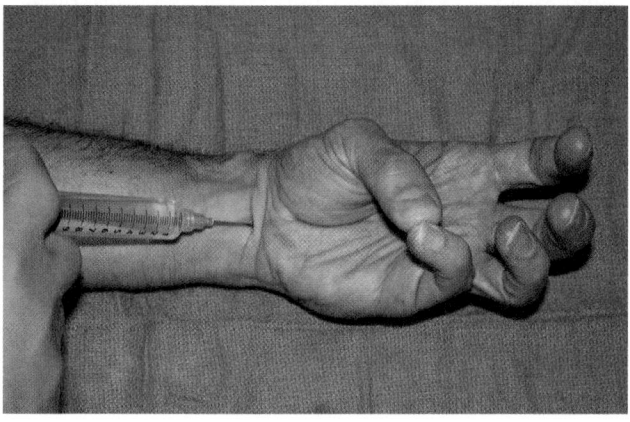

E

FIG. 44-11. Local anesthesia can be administered at the digital or the wrist level. **A.** A single injection into the flexor tendon sheath at the metacarpal head level provides complete anesthesia for the digit. **B.** Alternatively, one can inject from a dorsal approach into the web space on either side. **C.** The superficial radial nerve is blocked by infiltrating subcutaneously over the distal radius from the radial artery pulse to the distal radioulnar joint. The dorsal sensory branch of the ulnar nerve is blocked in similar fashion over the distal ulna. **D.** To block the ulnar nerve, insert the needle parallel to the plane of the palm and deep to the flexor carpi ulnaris tendon; aspirate to confirm the needle is not in the adjacent ulnar artery. **E.** To block the median nerve, insert the needle just ulnar to the palmaris longus tendon into the carpal tunnel. One should feel two points of resistance: one when piercing the skin, the second when piercing the antebrachial fascia.

Articular fractures of the interphalangeal and MPs are worrisome because they may compromise motion. Chip fractures must be evaluated for instability of the collateral ligaments. If the joint is stable, the patient should initially be splinted for comfort. Motion therapy should be instituted early (ideally within the first week) to prevent stiffness. For larger fractures, the patient should be splinted until surgical treatment can be performed. In surgery, the fracture is typically internally fixated to allow for early motion, again with the goal of preventing stiffness.[11]

Dislocations of the PIPs produce traction on the neurovascular structures but usually do not lacerate them. In general, the patient should not be sent home with a joint that remains dislocated. Most commonly, the distal part is dorsal to the proximal shaft and sits in a hyperextended position. For this patient, the examiner gently applies pressure to the base of the distal part until it passes beyond the head of the proximal phalanx. Once there, the relocated PIP joint is gently flexed, confirming the joint is, in fact, reduced. The joint is splinted in slight flexion to prevent redislocation. On occasion, the

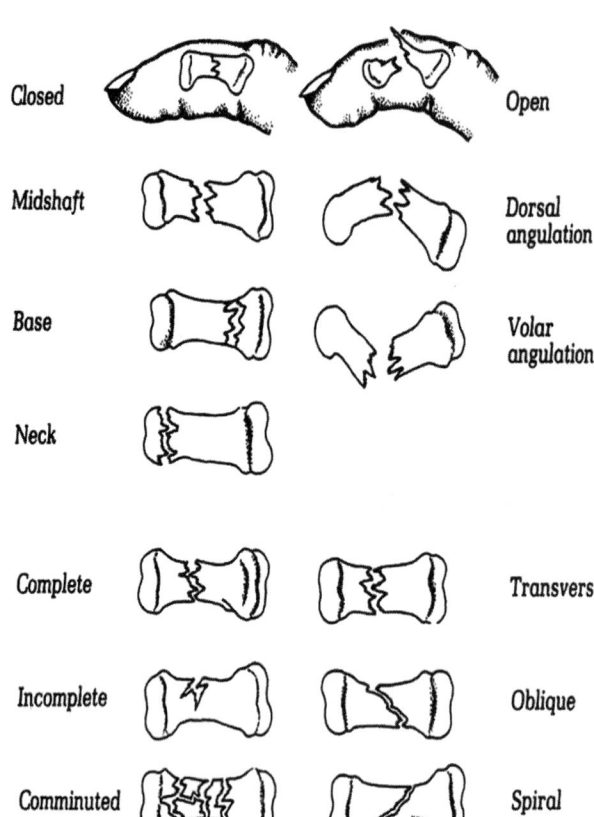

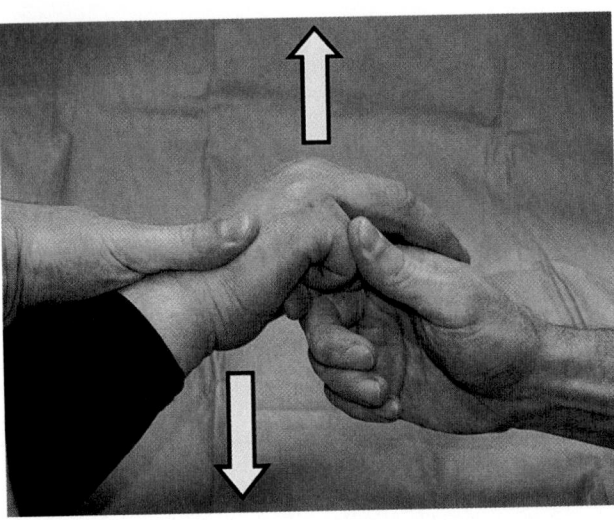

FIG. 44-13. The Jahss maneuver. The surgeon fully flexes the patient's small finger into the palm and secures it in his distal hand. The proximal hand controls the wrist and places the thumb on the patients fracture apex (the most prominent dorsal point). The examiner distracts the fracture, pushes dorsally with the distal hand (*up arrow*) and resists dorsal motion with the proximal hand (*down arrow*).

FIG. 44-12. Schematic representation of types of fractures by presence/absence of nearby wound, location within the bone, complexity, and orientation. *[Reproduced with permission from American Society for Surgery of the Hand (ed): The Hand: Examination and Diagnosis, 3rd ed. Copyright © Elsevier 1990.]*

head of the proximal phalanx may pass between the two slips of the FDS tendon. For these patients, the joint cannot be reduced in a closed fashion.

Angulated fractures of the small finger MC ("boxer's fracture") are another common injury seen in the ER. Typical history is that the patient struck another individual or rigid object with a hook punch. These often are stable after reduction using the Jahss maneuver (Fig. 44-13).

Fractures of the base of the thumb MC base often are unstable. The Bennett fracture displaces the volar-ulnar base of the bone. The remainder of the articular surface and the shaft typically dislocate dorsoradially and shorten. The thumb often appears grossly shortened, and the proximal shaft of the MC may reside at the level of the trapezium or even the scaphoid on x-ray. In a Rolando fracture, a second fracture line occurs between the remaining articular surface and the shaft. These fractures nearly always require open reduction and internal fixation.

In general terms, most nondisplaced fractures do not require surgical treatment. The scaphoid bone of the wrist is a notable exception to this rule. Due to peculiarities in its vascular supply, particularly vulnerable at its proximal end, nondisplaced scaphoid fractures can fail to unite in up to 20% of patients, even with appropriate immobilization. Recent developments in hardware and surgical technique have allowed stabilization of the fracture with minimal surgical exposure. One prospective randomized series of scaphoid waist fractures demonstrated shortening of time to union by up to 6 weeks in the surgically treated group, but no difference in rate of union.[12] Surgical treatment for nondisplaced scaphoid fractures is not indicated for all patients, but may be useful in the younger, more active patient who would benefit from an earlier return to full activity.

Ligament injuries of the wrist can be difficult to recognize. Patients often present late and may not be able to localize their pain. In severe cases, the ligaments of the wrist can rupture to the point of dislocation of the capitate off the lunate, or even the lunate off the radius. Mayfield and colleagues classified the progression of this injury into four groups.[13] In the most severe group, the lunate dislocates off the radius into the carpal tunnel. In some circumstances, the scaphoid bone may break rather than the scapholunate ligament rupturing. Attention to the congruency or disruption of Gilula's arcs will help the examiner to recognize this injury. For patients with the type 4 (most severe) and some with the type 3 injury, the examiner should also evaluate for sensory disturbance in the median nerve distribution, as this may indicate acute carpal tunnel syndrome (CTS) and necessitate more urgent intervention.

After reduction of fractures and dislocations (as well as after surgical repair of these and many other injuries), the hand must be splinted in a protected position. For the fingers, MP joints should be splinted 90°, the IPs at 0° (called the *intrinsic plus position*). The wrist is generally splinted at 20° extension, as this puts the hand in a more functional position. This keeps the collateral ligaments on tension and helps prevent secondary contracture. In general, one of three splints should be used for the ER patient (Fig. 44-14). The ulnar gutter splint uses plaster around the ulnar border of the hand. It is generally appropriate for small finger injuries only. Dorsal plaster splints can be used for injuries of any of the fingers. Plaster is more readily contoured to the dorsal surface of the hand than the volar surface, particularly in the setting of trauma-associated edema. For thumb injuries, the thumb spica splint is used to keep the thumb radially and palmarly abducted from the hand. For injuries involving the thumb MP joint or distal, the IP joint should be included in the splint. For more proximal injuries, it need not be included.

Tendons

Injuries to the flexor and extensor tendons compromise the mobility and strength of the digits. On inspection, injury normally is suspected by loss of the normal cascade of the fingers. The patient should be examined as described above in Emergency Room/Inpatient Consultation to evaluate for which tendon motion is deficient. If the patient is unable to cooperate, extension of the wrist will produce passive flexion of the fingers and also demonstrate a deficit. This is referred to as the *tenodesis maneuver*.

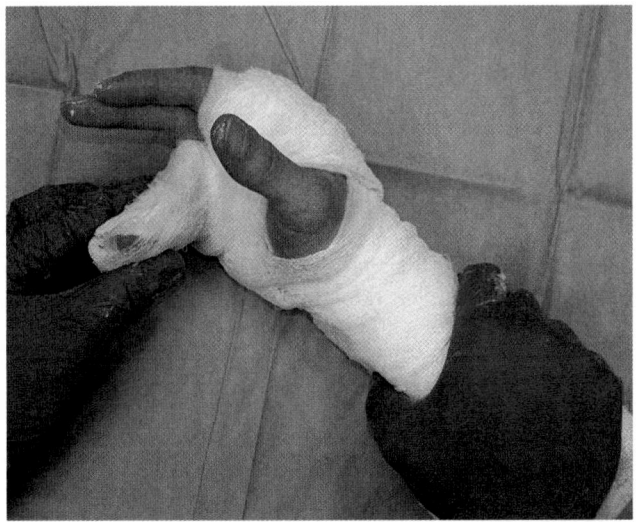

A

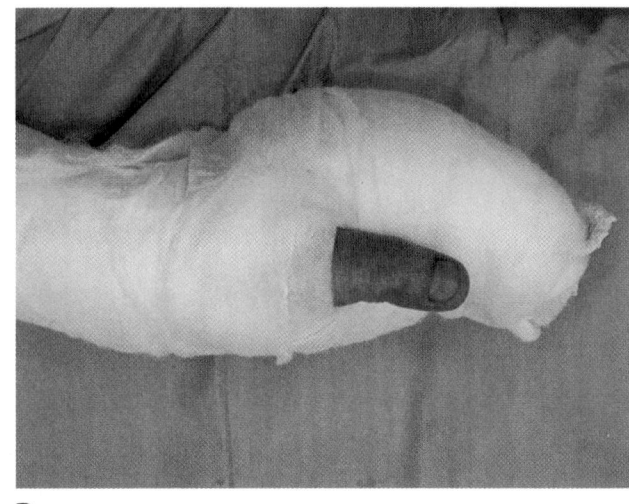

B

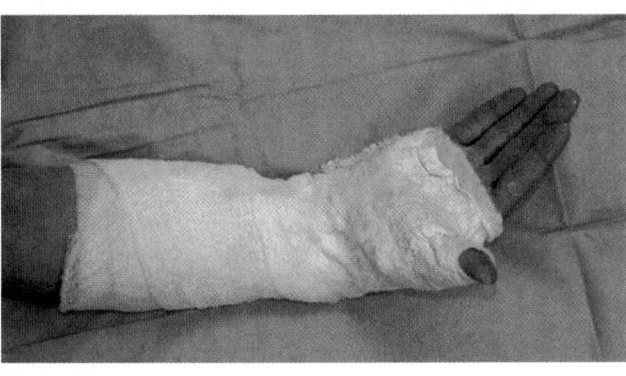

C

FIG. 44-14. Common splints used for hand injuries/surgeries. **A.** Ulnar gutter splint. The ring and small fingers are included. The surgeon pushes on the dorsum of the fingers with the distal hand to produce interphalangeal (IP) joint extension and metacarpophalangeal joint flexion to 90° while the proximal hand controls wrist position. **B.** Dorsal four-finger splint. As with the ulnar gutter splint, finger metacarpophalangeal joints are flexed to 90° with IP joints kept fully extended. **C.** Thumb spica splint. One easy method to fabricate is to place one slab of plaster radially over the wrist and thumb with a second square of plaster over the thenar eminence that joins the first. In this patient the IP joint was not included. For injuries at, or distal to, the metacarpophalangeal joint, the IP should be included in the splint.

Flexor tendon injuries are described based on zones (Fig. 44-15). Up until 40 years ago, zone 2 injuries were always reconstructed and never repaired primarily due to concern that the bulk of repair within the flexor sheath would prevent tendon glide. The work of Dr. Kleinert and colleagues at the University of Louisville changed this "axiom" and established the principle of primary repair and early controlled mobilization postoperatively.[14] Flexor tendon injuries should always be repaired in the OR. Although they do not need to be repaired on the day of injury, the closer to the day of injury they are repaired, the easier it will be to retrieve the retracted proximal end. The laceration should be washed out and closed at the skin level only using permanent sutures. The hand should be splinted as described above in Fractures and Dislocations; one notable difference is that the wrist should be splinted at slight flexion (about 20°) to help decrease the retracting force on the proximal cut tendon end.

Extensor tendons do not pass through a sheath in the fingers. As such, bulkiness of repair is less of a concern. With proper supervision/experience and equipment, primary extensor tendon repair can be performed in the ER.

Very distal extensor injuries near the insertion on the dorsal base of the distal phalanx may not have sufficient distal tendon to hold a suture. Closed injuries, called *mallet fingers*, can be treated with extension splinting of the DIP joint for 6 continuous weeks. For patients with open injuries, a dermatotenodesis suture is performed. A 2-0 or 3-0 suture is passed through the distal skin, tendon remnant, and proximal tendon as a mattress suture. Be sure to use a suture of a different color than the skin closing sutures to help prevent removing the dermatotenodesis suture(s) too soon. The DIP joint is splinted in extension.

More proximal injuries are typically repaired with a 3-0 braided polyester suture. Horizontal mattress or figure-of-eight sutures should be used, two per tendon if possible. Great care should be used to ensure matching the appropriate proximal and distal tendon ends. The patient is splinted with IP joints in extension and the wrist in extension per usual. MP joints should be splinted in 45° flexion, sometimes less. Although this position is not ideal for MP collateral ligaments, it is important for taking tension off the tendon repairs. The patient should be seen within 1 week of repair to initiate hand therapy.

Nerve Injuries

In the setting of a sharp injury, a sensory deficit implies a nerve laceration until proven otherwise. For blunt injuries, even displaced fractures and dislocations, nerves often are contused but not lacerated and are managed expectantly. Nerve repairs require appropriate microsurgical equipment and suture; they should not be performed in the ER. As with tendons, nerve injuries do not require immediate exploration. However, earlier exploration will allow for easier identification of structures. Earlier exploration also will allow for less scar tissue to be present; the nerve must be resected back to healthy nerve fascicle before repair. Delay between injury and repair can thus make a difference between the ability to repair a nerve primarily or the need to use a graft. The injured hand should be splinted with MPs at 90° and IPs at 0°, as described above in Fractures and Dislocations.

Vascular Injuries

Vascular injuries have the potential to be limb or digit threatening. A partial laceration of an artery at the wrist level can potentially even cause exsanguinating hemorrhage. Consultations for these injuries must be evaluated urgently.

Initial treatment for an actively bleeding wound should be direct local pressure for no less than 10 continuous minutes. If this is

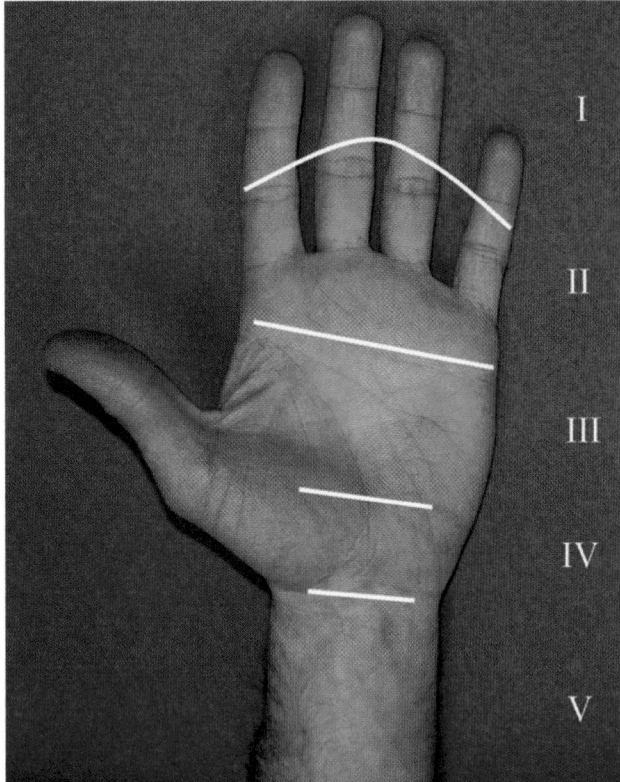

FIG. 44-15. The zones of flexor tendon injury: *I.* Flexor digitorum superficialis insertion to the flexor digitorum profundus insertion. *II.* Start of the A1 pulley to the flexor digitorum superficialis insertion. *III.* End of the carpal tunnel to the start of the A1 pulley. *IV.* Within the carpal tunnel. *V.* Proximal to the carpal tunnel.

gent guidelines have been established regarding what should be replanted. Indications for replantation include amputations of the thumb, multiple digit amputations, and amputations in children. Relative contraindications to replantation include crush injuries, injuries to a single digit distal to the PIP joint, and patients who are unable to tolerate a long surgical procedure. As with all guidelines, one should evaluate the particular needs of the injured patient. In East Asian cultures, a greater emphasis has been placed on salvaging all digits if at all possible due to the societal association of hand integrity with character integrity. In these settings, distal single digit amputations often will be replanted.

In preparation for replantation, the amputated part and proximal stump should be appropriately treated. The amputated part should be wrapped in moistened gauze and placed in a sealed plastic bag. This bag should then be placed in an ice water bath. Do not use dry ice and do not allow the part to contact ice directly; frostbite can occur in the amputated part, which will decrease its chance of survival after replantation. Bleeding should be controlled in the proximal stump by as minimal a means as necessary, and the stump dressed with a nonadherent gauze and bulky dressing.

For digital amputations deemed unsalvageable, revision amputation can be performed in the ER if appropriate equipment is available. Bony prominences should be smoothed off with a rongeur and/or rasp. Great care must be taken to identify the digital nerves and resect them back as far proximally in the wound as possible; this helps decrease the chance of painful neuroma in the skin closure. Skin may be closed with permanent or absorbable sutures; absorbable sutures will spare the patient the discomfort of suture removal several weeks later. For more proximal unsalvageable amputations, revision should be preformed in the OR to maximize vascular and neural element control.

Prostheses can be made for amputated parts. The more proximal the amputation, the more important to function the prosthesis is likely to be. Although finger level prostheses generally are considered cosmetic, those patients with multiple finger amputations proximal to the DIP have demonstrable functional benefit from their prostheses as well.[16]

Fingertip Injuries

Fingertip injuries are among the most common pathologies seen in an ER. The usual history is that a door closed on the finger (commonly the middle, due to its increased length) or something heavy fell on the finger.

Initial evaluation should include: wound(s) including the nail bed, perfusion, sensation, and presence and severity of fractures. For the common scenario, complex lacerations with minimally displaced fracture(s) and no loss of perfusion, the wound is cleansed, closed, and splinted in the ER. To properly assess the nail bed, the nail plate (hard part of the nail) should be removed. A Freer periosteal elevator is well suited for this purpose. Lacerations are repaired with 6-0 fast gut suture. Great care must be taken when suturing as excessive traction with the needle can further lacerate the tissue. After repair, the nail folds are splinted with the patient's own nail plate (if available) or with aluminum foil from the suture pack. This is done to prevent scarring from the nail folds down to the nail bed that would further compromise healing of the nail.

In some situations, tissue may have been avulsed in the injury and be unavailable for repair. Choice of treatment options depends on the amount and location of tissue loss (Fig. 44-16). For wounds <1 cm² with no exposed bone, secondary intention will produce excellent functional and aesthetic results. For larger wounds or wounds with bone exposed, one must decide if the finger is worth preserving at the current length or if shortening to allow for primary closure is a better solution. A useful guideline is the amount of fingernail still present; if greater than 50% is present, local or regional flap coverage may be a good solution.

If sufficient local tissue is present, homodigital V-Y flaps can be considered. If volar skin is in excess, a volar V-Y flap can be raised and advanced distally. If not, bilateral V-Y flaps can be raised and

unsuccessful, an upper extremity tourniquet inflated to 100 mmHg above the systolic pressure should be used. It should be noted that one should keep this tourniquet time to <2 hours to avoid tissue necrosis. Once bleeding is controlled well enough to evaluate the wound, it may be cautiously explored to evaluate for bleeding points. One must be very cautious if attempting to ligate these to ensure that adjacent structures such as nerves are not included in the ligature.

The hand must be evaluated for adequacy of perfusion to the hand as a whole as well as the individual digits. Capillary refill, turgor, Doppler signal, and bleeding to pinprick all provide useful information regarding vascular status. The finger or hand with vascular compromise requires urgent operative exploration. Unlike the complete amputation, in which the amputated part can be cold preserved (see below in Amputations and Replantation), devascularization without amputation produces warm ischemia, which is tolerated only for a matter of hours.

For the noncritical vascular injury, two treatment options exist. Simple ligation will control hemorrhage. At least one of the palmar arterial arches are intact in 97% of patients,[5] so this will usually not compromise hand perfusion. Each digit also has two arterial inflows and can survive on one (see Amputations and Replantation section below). In the academic hospital setting, however, consideration should be given to repairing all vascular injuries. Instructing a resident in vascular repair in the noncritical setting will produce a more skilled and prepared resident for when a critical vascular injury does arise.

SPECIAL CONSIDERATIONS

Amputations and Replantation

After replantation was first reported,[15] replantation was attempted for nearly all amputations. Over the ensuing decades, more strin-

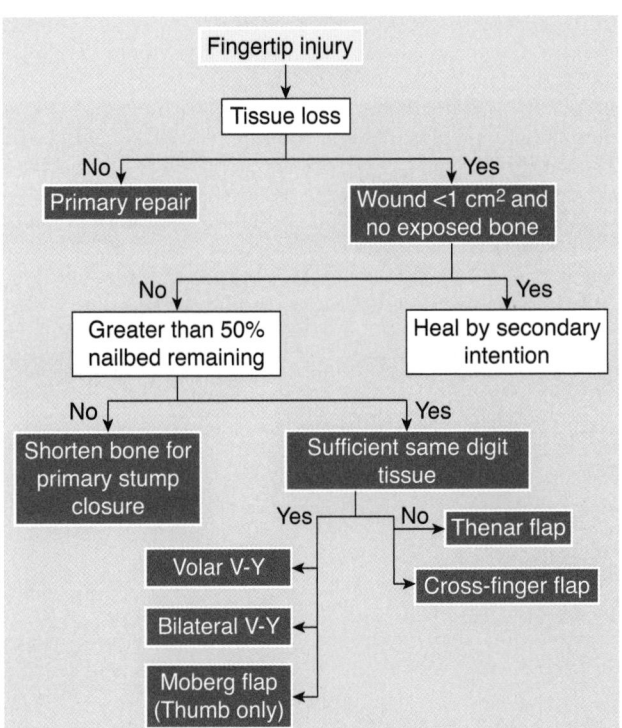

FIG. 44-16. Treatment algorithm for management of fingertip injuries. See text for description of flaps.

advanced distally to meet in the midline. Both of these flaps allow for full-thickness tissue to be brought distally. The proximal apex of the donor site should not cross the DIP flexion crease. Common postoperative complaints include hypersensitivity at the tip and cold intolerance.[17] For the thumb only, the entire volar skin including both neurovascular bundles can be raised and advanced distally up to 1.5 cm.[18] The thumb receives separate vascularity to its dorsal skin from the radial artery. This flap is not advisable for the fingers. Patients retain full sensibility in the advanced skin and can be mobilized within days of surgery (Fig. 44-17A, 44-17B, and 44-17C).

For wounds too large to cover with homodigital tissue, regional flaps can be considered. The skin from the distal radial thenar eminence can be raised as a random pattern flap (see Fig. 44-17D, 44-17E, and 44-17F). The finger is maintained in flexion for 14 to 21 days until division of the flap pedicle and inset of the flap. Some authors have reported prolonged stiffness in patients over 30 years old, but careful flap design helps minimize this complication.[19] Alternatively, the skin from the dorsum of the middle phalanx of an adjacent digit can be raised as a flap to cover the volar P3 (see Fig. 44-17G, 44-17H, and 44-17I). The flap is inset at 14 to 21 days. Long-term studies have shown this flap develops sensation over time.[20]

Patients with fingertip injuries must be assessed for the possibility of salvage of the injured digit(s) taken within the context of the patient's recovery needs and goals. The surgeon then matches the available options to the particular patient's needs (see Fig. 44-16).

High-Pressure Injection Injuries

High-pressure devices are commonly used for cleaning and applications of liquids such as lubricants and paint. Most commonly, the inexperienced worker accidentally discharges the device into his nondominant hand at the base of the digit. Severity of injury depends on the amount and type of liquid injected; hydrophobic compounds cause greater damage.

These injuries are typically quite innocuous to inspection. They are, however, digit threatening emergencies. The patient should be informed of the severity of the injury, and exploration is ideally performed within 6 hours of injury. Up to 50% of such injuries

result in loss of the digit, although recent studies with early recognition and treatment have decreased this number.[21] Early, frank discussion with the patient and initiation of appropriate treatment produce the best results and medicolegal protection.

Compartment Syndromes

Compartment syndromes can occur in the forearm and/or the hand. As in other locations, these are potentially limb-threatening issues. Principal symptoms are pain in the affected compartments, tense swelling, tenderness to palpation over the compartment, and pain with passive stretch of the muscles of the compartment.[22] Pulse changes are a late finding; normal pulses do not rule out compartment syndrome.

There are three compartments in the forearm and four groups of compartments in the hand. The volar forearm is one compartment. On the dorsum of the forearm, there is the dorsal compartment as well as the mobile wad compartment, beginning proximally over the lateral epicondyle. In the hand, the thenar and hypothenar muscle wads each behave as a separate compartment. The seven interosseous muscles each behave as a separate compartment.

Compartment syndrome can be caused by intrinsic and extrinsic causes. Intrinsic causes include edema and hematoma due to fracture. Extrinsic causes include splints and dressings that are circumferentially too tight and IV infiltrations. Infiltrations with hyperosmolar fluids such as x-ray contrast and dextrose-50 are particularly dangerous because additional water will be drawn in to neutralize the hyperosmolarity.

Measurement of compartment pressures can be a useful adjunct to assessment of the patient. The Stryker pressure measurement device or a similar device is kept in many operating rooms for this purpose. The needle is inserted into the compartment in question, a gentle flush with 0.1 to 0.2 mL of saline clears the measurement chamber, and a reading is obtained. Studies have disagreed whether the criteria is a pressure (30 to 45 mmHg, depending on the series), or within a certain amount of the diastolic blood pressure.[23]

Compartment releases are performed in the OR under tourniquet control. Release of the volar forearm compartment includes release of the carpal tunnel. As the incision travels distally, it should pass ulnarly and then curve back radially just before the carpal tunnel. This avoids a linear incision across a flexion crease and also decreases the chance of injury to the palmar cutaneous branch of the median nerve. One dorsal forearm incision can release the dorsal compartment and the mobile wad. In the hand, the thenar and hypothenar compartments are released each with a single incision. The interosseous compartments are released with incisions over the index and ring MC shafts. Dissection then continues radial and ulnar to the index and ring finger metacarpal shafts to release all of the interosseous muscle compartments. Any dead muscle is débrided. Incisions are left open and covered with a nonadherent dressing. The wrist and hand are splinted in the protected position as described above in Fractures and Dislocations. The wounds are re-explored in 2 to 3 days to assess for muscle viability. Often, the incisions can be closed primarily, but a skin graft may be needed for the forearm.

If the examiner feels the patient does not have a compartment syndrome, elevation and serial examination are mandatory. When in doubt, it is better to release an early compartment syndrome than wait to release and risk muscle necrosis. Progression of compartment syndrome can lead to Volkmann's ischemic contracture with muscle loss, and scarring that may compress nerves and other critical structures. Medicolegally, it is far easier to defend releasing an early compartment syndrome than delaying treatment until the process has progressed to necrosis and/or deeper scarring.

COMPLICATIONS

Nonunion

Any fractured bone has the risk of failing to heal. Fortunately, in the fingers and hand, this is a rare problem. Tuft injuries, where soft

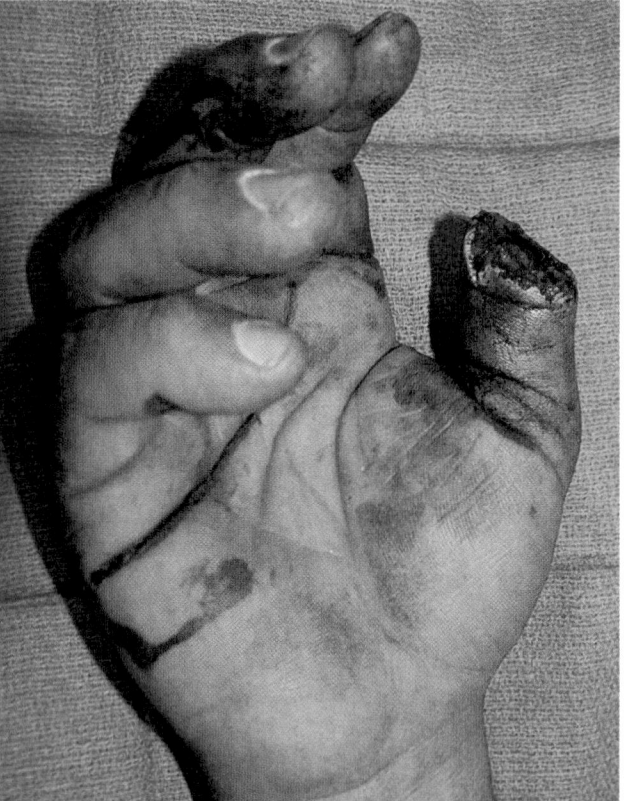

A

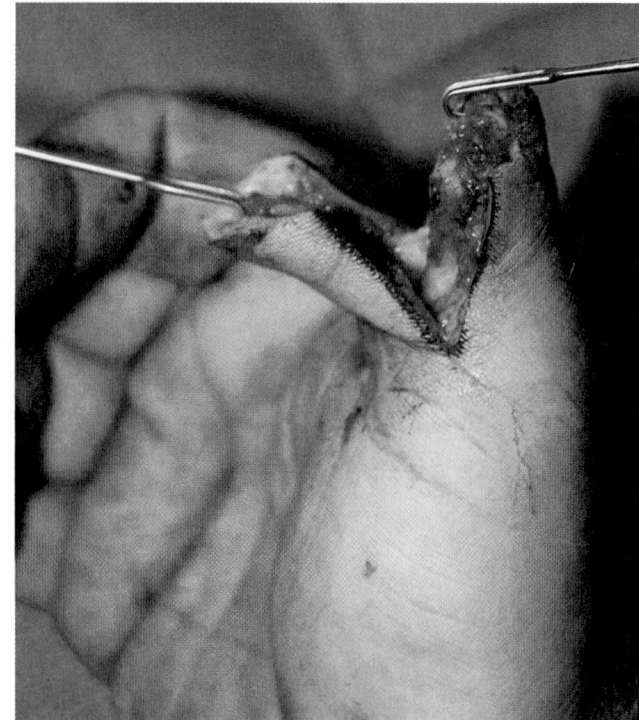

B

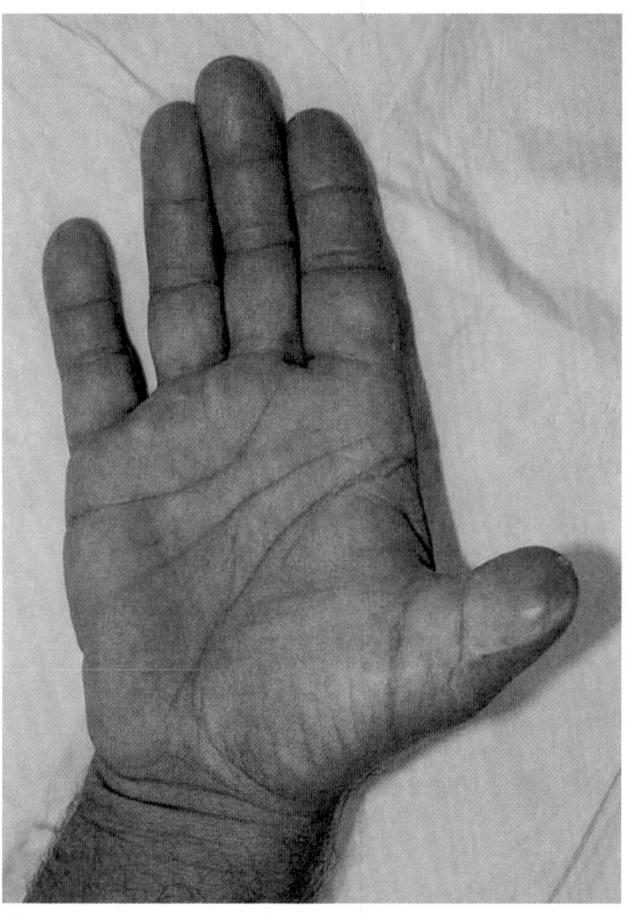

C

FIG. 44-17. Local flaps for digital tip coverage. **A** through **C.** For thumb injuries, Moberg described elevation of the entire volar skin with both neurovascular bundles for distal advancement. Sensation to the advanced skin is maintained. (*Continued*)

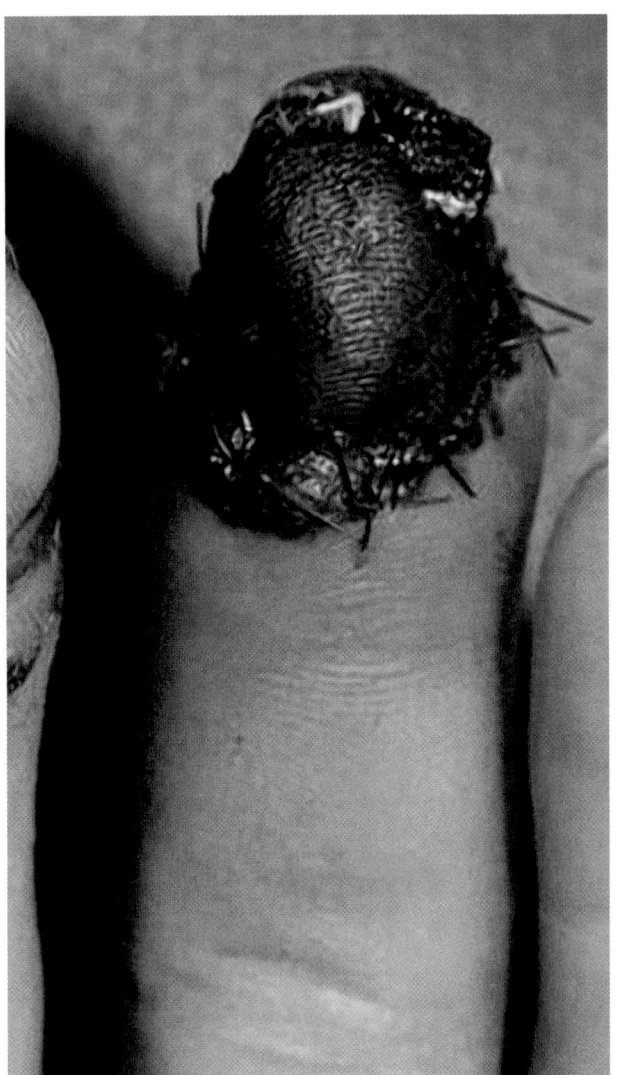

D

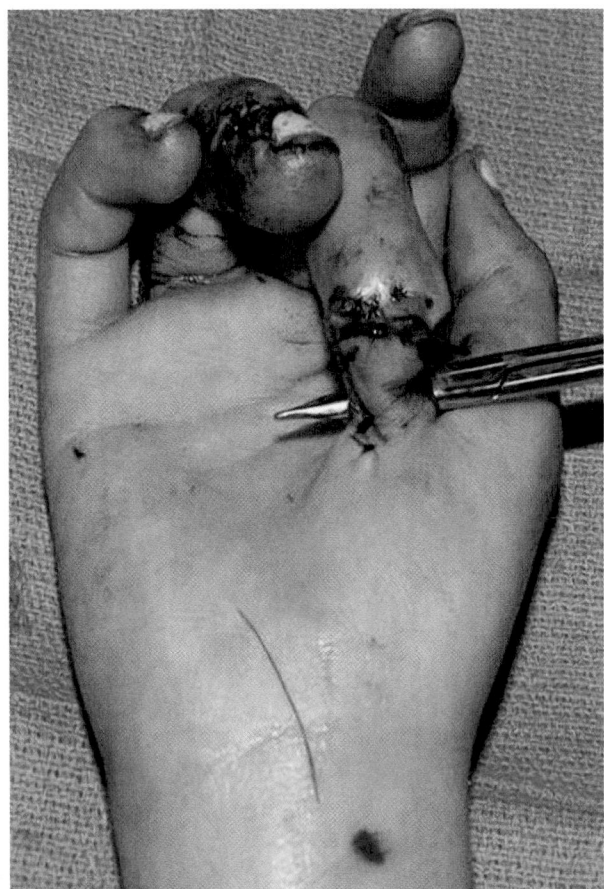

E

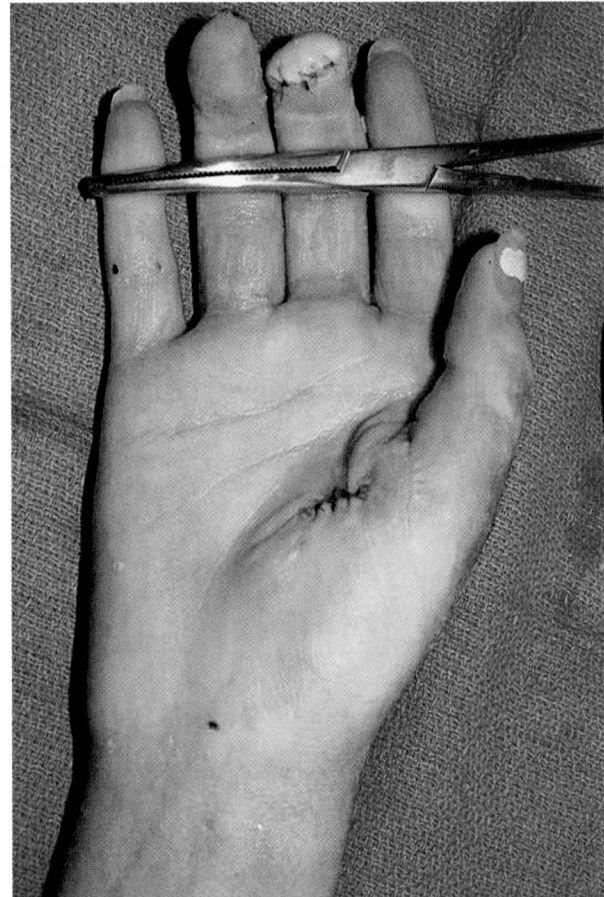

FIG. 44-17. (*Continued*) **D** through **F.** An 8-year-old girl underwent fingertip replantation that did not survive. A thenar flap was transferred to cover the defect. Some authors advise against its use in patients >30 years old. (*Continued*)

F

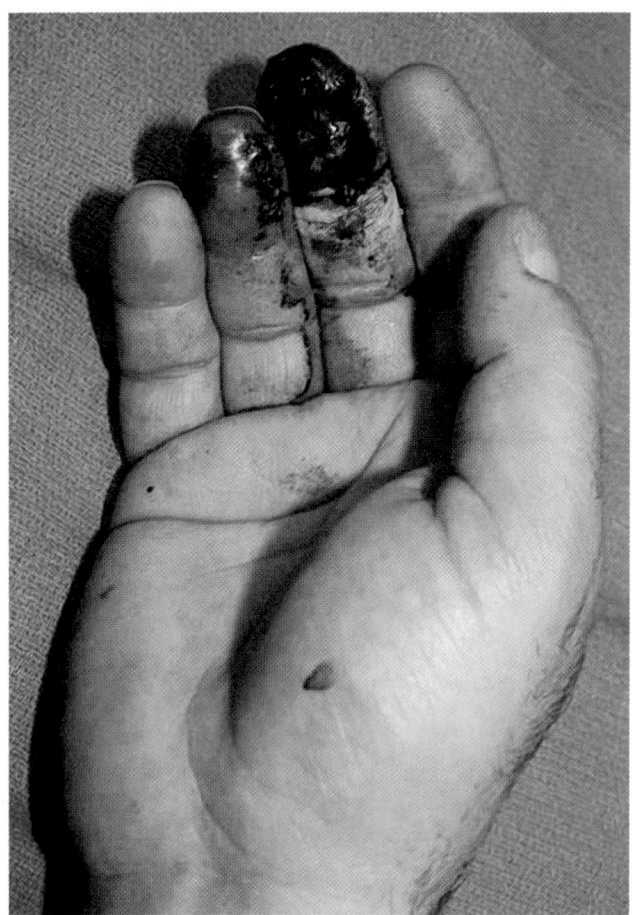

G

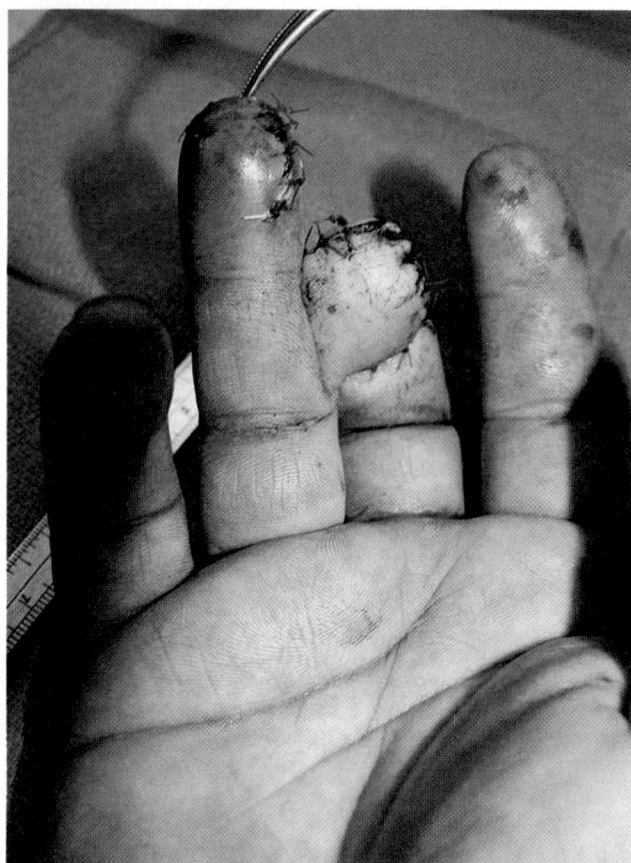

H

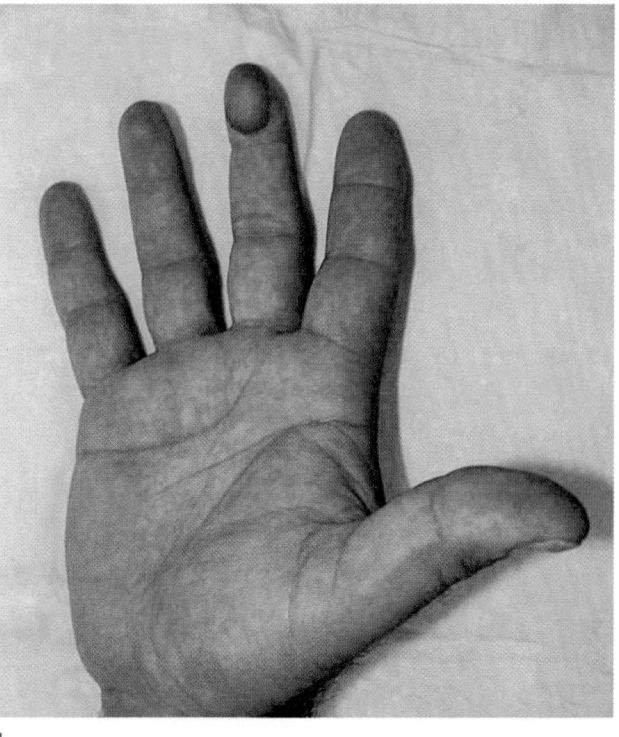

I

FIG. 44-17. (*Continued*) **G** through **I.** In this 45-year-old man, the entire skin of P3 of the long finger was avulsed and unrecoverable. A cross-finger flap was transferred and provides excellent, durable coverage. The border of the flap and surrounding skin is still apparent 4.5 months after surgery.

tissue interposes between the fracture fragments, have a relatively higher risk of this problem. The nonunited tuft can be treated with débridement and bone grafting, or revision amputation, depending on the needs and goals of the patient. Phalangeal and MC nonunions

are also quite rare. They can similarly be treated with débridement of the nonunion, grafting, and rigid fixation.[24] More proximally, the scaphoid bone of the wrist has a significant risk of nonunion even if nondisplaced (see Fig. 44-9A). Any patient suspected of a scaphoid injury, namely those with tenderness at the anatomic snuffbox, should be placed in a thumb spica splint and re-evaluated within 2 weeks, even if initial x-rays show no fracture. Scaphoid nonunions can be quite challenging to repair,[25] and immobilization at the time of injury in a thumb spica splint is essentially always warranted.

Stiffness

The desired outcome of any hand injury is a painless, mobile, functional hand. Multiple factors can contribute to decreased mobility: complex injuries of soft tissue and bone, noncompliance of the patient with postoperative therapy, and inappropriate splinting. The surgeon performing the initial evaluation can greatly impact this last factor. Again, the goal of splinting is to keep the collateral ligaments on tension (MPs at 90°, IP joints straight). For severe cases of stiffness, mobilization surgeries such as tenolyses and capsulotomies[26] can be performed, but these rarely produce normal ROM. Prevention of joint contractures with appropriate splinting and early, protected mobilization are the best options to maximize mobility at the end of healing.

Neuroma

Any lacerated nerve will form a neuroma. A neuroma consists of a ball of scar and axon sprouts at the end of the injured nerve.[27] In unfavorable circumstances, this neuroma can become quite painful. The SRN is particularly notorious for this problem. By providing proximal axon sprouts a target, nerve repair is an excellent preventive technique. In some circumstances, such as injuries requiring amputation, this is not possible. As mentioned above in Amputations and Replantation, the surgeon should resect the nerve stump as far proximally in the wound as possible to avoid the nerve stump healing in the cutaneous scar to minimize this risk.

For the patient who develops a painful neuroma, nonsurgical treatments are initiated first. The neuroma can be identified by the presence of a Tinel's sign. Therapy techniques of desensitization, ultrasound, and electrical stimulation have all proven useful. Corticosteroid injection to the neuroma also has proven useful in some hands.

When these techniques fail, surgery is contemplated. The neuroma can be resected, but a new one will form to replace it. The nerve ending can be buried in muscle or even bone to prevent the neuroma from residing in a superficial location where it may be impacted frequently.

Regional Pain Syndromes

Injuries to the upper extremity can occasionally result in the patient experiencing pain beyond the area of initial injury. *Reflex sympathetic dystrophy* and *sympathetic mediated pain* are two terms that have been used in the past to describe this phenomenon. Both are inaccurate, as the sympathetic nervous system is not always involved. Current terminology for this condition is *complex regional pain syndrome* (CRPS). Type I occurs in the absence of a documented nerve injury; type II occurs in the presence of one.[28]

CRPSs manifest as pain beyond the area of initial injuries. There is often associated edema and changes in hair and/or sweat distribution. Comparison to the unaffected side is useful to better appreciate these findings. Multiple imaging modalities have been evaluated as potential diagnostic tests for CRPS. At this time, there are no imaging studies that can be considered diagnostic for CRPS.[29]

For the patient in whom the diagnosis of CRPS is not clear, no definitive diagnostic study exists. Patients suspected of CRPS should be referred for aggressive hand therapy. Brief trials of oral corticosteroids have been successful in some series. Referral to a pain management specialist for a trial of stellate ganglion blocks also is frequently used.

NERVE COMPRESSION

Nerves conduct signals along their axonal membranes toward their end organs. Sensory axons carry signals from distal to proximal; motor axons from proximal to distal. Myelin from Schwann cells allows faster conduction of signals. Signals jump from the start of one Schwann cell to the end of the cell (a location called a *gap junction*) and only require the slower membrane depolarization in these locations.

Nerve compression creates a mechanical disturbance of the nerve.[30] In early disease, the conduction signal is slowed across the area of compression. When compression occurs to a sufficient degree for a sufficient time, individual axons may die off. On a nerve conduction study, this manifests as a decrease in amplitude. Muscles receiving motor axons may show electrical disturbance on electromyogram when sufficiently deprived of their axonal input.

Compression of sensory nerves typically produces a combination of numbness, paresthesias (pins and needles), and pain. Knowledge of the anatomic distribution of the peripheral nerves can aid in diagnosis. Sensory disturbance outside an area of distribution of a particular nerve (e.g., volar and dorsal radial-sided hand numbness for median nerve) makes compression of that nerve less likely. Diseases that cause systemic neuropathy (e.g., diabetes) can make diagnosis more difficult.

Nerve compression can theoretically occur anywhere along a peripheral nerve's course. The most common sites of nerve compression in the upper extremity are median nerve at the carpal tunnel, ulnar nerve at the cubital tunnel, and ulnar nerve at Guyon's canal. Other, less common locations of nerve compression are described as well. In addition, a nerve can become compressed in scar due to a previous trauma.

Carpal Tunnel Syndrome

The most common location of upper extremity nerve compression is the median nerve at the carpal tunnel, CTS. The carpal tunnel is bordered by the scaphoid bone radially, the lunate and capitate bones dorsally, and the hook of the hamate bone ulnarly (see Fig. 44-3). The transverse carpal ligament, also called the *flexor retinaculum*, is its superficial border. The FPL, four FDS, and four FDP tendons pass through the carpal tunnel along with the median nerve. Of these 10 structures, the median nerve is relatively superficial and radial to the other nine.

An estimated 53 per 10,000 working adults have evidence of CTS. The National Institute for Occupational Safety and Health website asserts "There is strong evidence of a positive association between exposure to a combination of risk factors (e.g., force and repetition, force and posture) and CTS".[31] There is disagreement among hand surgeons regarding whether occurrence of CTS in a patient who does repetitive activities at work represents a work-related injury.

Initial evaluation of the patient consists of symptom inventory: location and character of the symptoms, sleep disturbance due to symptoms, history of dropping objects, and difficulty manipulating small objects such as buttons, coins, or jewelry clasps.

Physical examination should begin with inspection. Look for evidence of wasting of the thenar muscles. Tinel's sign should be tested over the median nerve from the volar wrist flexion crease to the proximal palm. Phalen's test (maximal flexion of the wrist for 1 minute) and reverse Phalen's (maximal extension) are tested. Applying pressure over the carpal tunnel while flexing the wrist has been shown in one series to have the highest sensitivity as compared to Phalen's and Tinel's signs.[32] Strength of the thumb in opposition also should be tested.

Early treatment of CTS consists of conservative management. The patient is given a splint to keep the wrist at 20° extension worn at nighttime. Many patients can have years of symptom relief with this management. As a treatment and diagnostic modality, corticosteroid injection of the carpal tunnel is often used. Mixing local anesthetic into the solution provides the benefit of early symptom relief (corticosteroids often take 3 to 7 days to provide noticeable benefit), and report of postinjection anesthesia in the median nerve distribution confirms the injection went into the correct location. Multiple authors have shown a strong correlation to relief of symptoms with corticosteroid injection and good response to carpal tunnel release.[33]

When lesser measures fail or are no longer effective, carpal tunnel release is indicated. Open carpal tunnel release is a time-tested procedure with documented long-term relief of symptoms. A direct incision is made over the carpal tunnel, typically in line with where the ring finger pad touches the proximal palm in flexion. Skin is divided followed by palmar fascia. The carpal tunnel contents are visualized as they exit the carpal tunnel. The transverse carpal ligament is divided with the median nerve visualized and protected at all times. Skin typically is closed in a single layer, and a volar wrist splint is applied. Improvement in symptoms is typically noted by the first postoperative visit, although symptom relief may be incomplete for patients with long-standing disease or systemic nerve-affecting diseases such as diabetes.

In recent years, endoscopic techniques have been devised to address CTS. All involve avoidance of incising the skin directly over the carpal tunnel. Patients are typically allowed to cautiously move their wrist immediately after surgery. In experienced hands, endoscopic carpal tunnel release provides the same relief of CTS with less intense and shorter lasting postoperative pain. After 3 months, however, the results are equivalent to open release.[34] In inexperienced hands, there may be a higher risk of injury to the median nerve with the endoscopic techniques; this procedure is not for the occasional carpal tunnel surgeon.

Cubital Tunnel Syndrome

The second most common location of upper extremity nerve compression is the ulnar nerve where it passes behind the elbow at the cubital tunnel. The cubital tunnel retinaculum passes between the medial epicondyle of the humerus and the olecranon process of the ulna. It stabilizes the ulnar nerve in this location during elbow motion. Over time, or sometimes after trauma, the ulnar nerve can become less stabilized in this area. Motion of the elbow then produces trauma to the nerve as it impacts the retinaculum and medial epicondyle.

Cubital tunnel syndrome may produce sensory and motor symptoms.[35] The small finger and ulnar half of the ring fingers may have numbness, paresthesias, and/or pain. Unlike the median nerve, volar and dorsal symptoms in these digits are explained by ulnar neuropathy at the elbow. The patient also may report weakness in grip due to effects on the FDP tendons to the ring and small fingers and the intrinsic hand muscles. Patients with advanced disease may complain of inability to fully extend the ring and small finger IPs.

Physical examination for cubital tunnel syndrome begins with inspection. Look for wasting in the hypothenar eminence and the interdigital web spaces. When the hand rests flat on the table, the small finger may rest in abduction with respect to the other fingers; this is called *Wartenberg's sign*. Tinel's sign often is present at the cubital tunnel. Elbow flexion test (holding the elbow maximally flexed for 1 minute) often will be positive. Grip strength and finger abduction strength should be compared to the unaffected side. Froment's paper sign can be tested by placing a sheet of paper between the thumb and index finger and instructing the patient to hold on to the paper while the examiner pulls it away without flexing the finger or thumb (this tests the strength of the adductor pollicis and first dorsal interosseous muscles). If the patient must flex the index finger and/or thumb (FDP-index and FPL, both median nerve supplied) to maintain traction on the paper, this is a positive response.

Early treatment of cubital tunnel syndrome begins with avoiding maximal flexion of the elbow. Splints often are used for this purpose. Corticosteroid injection rarely is done for this condition; unlike in the carpal tunnel, there is very little space within the tunnel outside of the nerve. Injection in this area runs a risk of intraneural injection that can cause permanent scarring of the nerve and dysfunction.

When conservative management fails, surgery has been contemplated. Simple release of the cubital tunnel retinaculum, with or without removal of the medial epicondyle, is reported, but is less commonly done. Most commonly, surgery for ulnar nerve com-

pression at the elbow involves transposition of the nerve anterior to the elbow. For heavier patients with lower demand arms, the nerve often is kept in the subcutaneous plane. Great care must be taken to avoid creating a new constriction point with any fascial sling used to keep the nerve anterior. For thinner patients and/or those with higher demand arms, the nerve usually is placed in a pocket within the flexor-pronator muscle mass. The superficial fascia is incised in a stair step fashion. Dissection then proceeds into the muscle mass. All septae within the muscle are incised or excised as appropriate. The nerve is then transposed into the muscle pocket. The fascia is then closed in a z-lengthened fashion to prevent compression on the nerve. The wound is closed in layers, and the arm is splinted with the elbow flexed at 90°. Some surgeons splint the wrist and fingers as well. Therapy, with an initial emphasis on recovering ROM, usually is begun within the first week after surgery.

Other Sites of Nerve Compression

All nerves crossing the forearm have areas described where compression can occur.[35] The median nerve can be compressed as it passes under the pronator teres. The anterior interosseous branch of the median nerve can be compressed more distally with isolated motor (no sensory) deficits. The ulnar nerve can be compressed as it passes through Guyon's canal. The radial nerve, or its posterior interosseous branch, can be compressed as it passes through the radial tunnel (distal to the elbow where the nerve divides and passes under the arch of the supinator muscle). The SRN can be compressed distally in the forearm as it emerges from under the brachioradialis tendon, called *Wartenberg's syndrome*. As mentioned at the beginning of the Nerve Compression section, any nerve can become compressed in scar at the site of a previous trauma.

DEGENERATIVE JOINT DISEASE

As with other joints on the body, the joints of the hand and wrist can develop degenerative changes. Symptoms typically begin in the fifth decade of life. Symptoms consist of joint pain and stiffness, and often are exacerbated with changes in the weather. Any of the joints can become involved. As the articular cartilage wears out, pain typically increases and ROM decreases. The patient should always be asked to what degree symptoms are impeding activities.

Physical findings are documented in serial fashion from the initial visit and subsequent visits. Pain with axial loading of the joint may be present. Decreased ROM may be a late finding. Instability of the collateral ligaments of the joint typically is not found in the absence of inflammatory arthritis.

Plain x-rays are typically sufficient to demonstrate arthritis. Initially, the affected joint has a narrower radiolucent space between the bones. As joint degeneration progresses, the joint space further collapses. Bone spurs, loose bodies, and cystic changes in the bone adjacent to the joint all may become apparent. X-ray findings do not always correlate with patient symptoms. Patients with advanced x-ray findings may have minimal symptoms, and vice versa. Treatment is initiated and progressed based on the patient's symptoms, regardless of imaging findings.

Initial management begins with rest of the painful joint. Splints often are useful but may significantly impair the patient in activities and thus are frequently used at nighttime only. Oral NSAID medications such as ibuprofen and naproxen also are useful. Patients on blood thinners may not be able to take these, and some patients simply do not tolerate the gastric irritation side effect even if they take the medication with food.

For patients with localized disease affecting only one or a few joints, corticosteroid injection may be contemplated. Needle insertion can be difficult because these joint spaces are quite narrow even before degenerative disease sets in. Also, corticosteroid injections are suspensions, not solutions; injected corticosteroid will remain in the joint space and can be seen as a white paste if surgery is performed on a joint that has been previously injected. For this reason, it is unwise to ever inject any joint more than two to three times.

Small Joints (Metacarpophalangeal and Interphalangeal)

When conservative measures fail, two principal surgical options exist: arthrodesis and arthroplasty. The surgeon and patient must decide together as to whether conservative measures have failed. Surgery for arthritis, whether arthrodesis or arthroplasty, is performed for the purpose of relieving pain. Arthrodesis, fusion of a joint, provides excellent relief of pain and is durable over time. However, it comes at the price of total loss of motion.

Silicone implant arthroplasty has been available for over 40 years.[36] Rather than a true replacement of the joint, the silicone implant acts as a spacer between the two bones adjacent to the joint. This allows for motion without bony contact that would produce pain. Long-term studies have shown that all implants fracture over time, but usually continue to preserve motion and pain relief.[37]

In the past 10 years, resurfacing implant arthroplasties have become available for the small joints of the hand. Metals, ceramics, and pyrolytic carbon compounds have all been used to fabricate such implants. These are designed to behave as true joint resurfacers (as knee and hip arthroplasty implants are), and have shown good outcomes in short- and intermediate-term studies.[37] Neither the silicone nor the resurfacing arthroplasties preserve (or restore) full motion of the MP or PIP joints. This must be considered before any implant arthroplasty.

Wrist

The CMC joint of the thumb, also called the *basilar joint*, is another common location of arthritis pain. Pain in this joint is particularly disturbing of function as the CMC joint is essential for opposition and cylindrical grasp. Patients will typically complain of pain with opening a tight jar or doorknob, and strong pinch activities such as knitting. Conservative management is used first, as described at the beginning of the Degenerative Joint Disease section. Prefabricated, removable thumb spica splinting can provide excellent relief of symptoms for many patients.

Multiple surgical options exist for thumb CMC arthritis. Many resurfacing implants have been used in the past; often, they have shown good short- and intermediate-term results and poor long-term results. Resection of the arthritic trapezium provides excellent relief of pain; however, most authors feel that stabilization of the thumb MC base is necessary to prevent shortening and instability.[38] Recently, one author has demonstrated excellent long-term results from resection of the trapezium without permanent stabilization of the MC base.[39] For both of these operations, the thumb base may not be sufficiently stable to withstand heavy labor. For these patients, fusion of the thumb CMC in opposition provides excellent pain relief and durability. The patient must be warned preoperatively that he will not be able to lay his hand flat after the surgery. This loss of motion can be problematic when the patient attempts to tuck in clothing or reach into a narrow space.

Degenerative change of the radiocarpal and midcarpal joints is often a consequence of scapholunate ligament injury. Often, the initial injury goes untreated, with the patient believing it is merely a "sprain;" the patient is first diagnosed with the initial injury when he presents years later with degenerative changes.

Degenerative wrist changes associated with the scapholunate ligament follow a predictable pattern over many years, called *scapholunate advanced collapse* or *SLAC wrist*.[40] Because of this slow progression, patients usually can be treated with a motion-sparing procedure (Fig. 44-18A). If there is truly no arthritic change present, the scapholunate ligament can be reconstructed.

If arthritis is limited to the radiocarpal joint, two motion-sparing options are available. The proximal carpal row (scaphoid, lunate, and triquetrum) can be removed (proximal row carpectomy). The lunate facet of the radius then articulates with the base of the

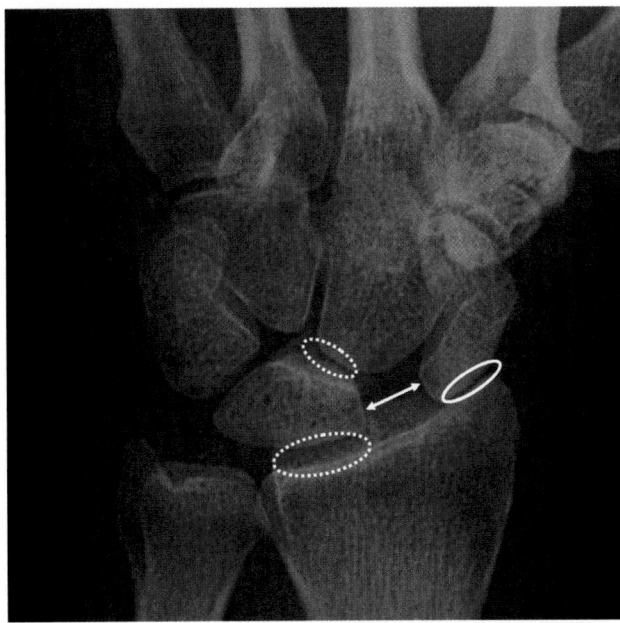

A

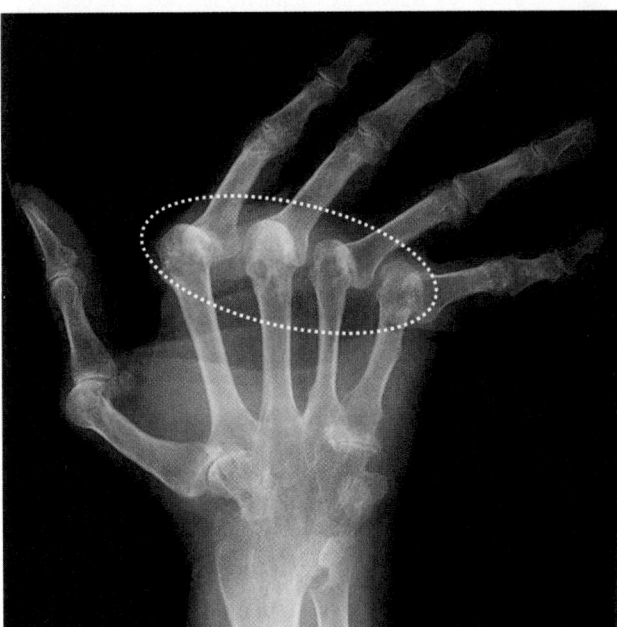

B

FIG. 44-18. Arthritis of the hand and wrist. **A.** This patient injured her scapholunate ligament years before presentation. The scapholunate interval is widened (*double arrow*), and the radioscaphoid joint is degenerated (*solid oval*), but the radiolunate and lunocapitate joint spaces are well preserved (*dashed ovals*). **B.** This patient has had rheumatoid arthritis for decades. The classic volar subluxation of the metacarpophalangeal joints of the fingers (*dashed oval*) and radial deviation of the fingers are apparent.

capitate, whose articular surface is similar in shape to that of the base of the lunate. Most series show maintenance of about 66% of wrist motion and 66% of hand strength or more, as compared to the opposite side.[41] Alternatively, the scaphoid can be excised and four-bone fusion (lunate, capitate, hamate, triquetrum) can be performed. This maintains the full length of the hand and the lunate in the lunate facet of the radius. Some series have shown better strength but less mobility with this technique; others have shown equivalent results to the proximal row carpectomy.[42] The four-bone fusion does appear to be more durable for younger patients and/or those who perform heavy labor.

If the patient presents with pancarpal arthritis, or motion-sparing measures have failed to alleviate pain, total wrist fusion is the final surgical option. The distal radius is fused through the proximal and distal carpal rows to the third MC, typically with a dorsal plate and screws. Multiple, long-term studies have shown excellent pain relief and durability; this comes at the exchange of total loss of wrist motion. This is surprisingly well tolerated in most patients, especially if the other hand/wrist is unaffected. The only activity of daily life that cannot be done with a fused wrist is personal toileting.

Rheumatoid Arthritis

Rheumatoid arthritis (RA) is an inflammatory arthritis that can affect any joint in the body. Inflamed synovium causes articular cartilage breakdown with pain and decreased ROM. The goals of hand surgery for the RA patient are relief of pain, improvement of function, slowing progression of disease, and improvement in appearance.[43] In addition, swelling of the joint due to the inflammation can cause laxity and even failure of the collateral ligaments supporting the joints. Recent advances in the medical care of RA have made the need for surgical care of these patients far less common than in previous decades.

MP joints of the fingers are commonly affected. The base of the proximal phalanx progressively subluxates and eventually dislocates volarly with respect to the MC head. The collateral ligaments, particularly on the radial side, stretch out and cause the ulnar deviation of the fingers characteristic of the rheumatoid hand. Early in the disease, synovectomy with extensor centralization can be attempted. In more advanced cases, the joint may not be salvageable (see Fig. 44-18B). For these patients, implant arthroplasty is the mainstay of surgical treatment. Silicone implants have been used for >40 years with good results.[44] The silicone implant acts as a spacer between proximal and distal bone, rather than as a true resurfacing arthroplasty. The radial collateral ligament must be repaired to appropriate length to correct the preoperative ulnar deviation of the MP joint. Extensor tendon centralization is then performed, as needed, at the end of the procedure.

For MP joint and PIP joint disease, fusion is an option. However, because RA usually affects multiple joints, fusion is typically avoided due to impaired function of adjacent joints, which would leave a severe motion deficit to the finger.

Failure of the support ligaments of the distal radio-ulnar joint (DRUJ) leads to the *caput ulnae* posture of the wrist with the ulnar head prominent dorsally. As this dorsal prominence becomes more advanced, the ulna head, denuded of its cartilage to act as a buffer, erodes into the overlying extensor tendons. Extensor tenosynovitis, followed ultimately by tendon rupture, begins ulnarly and proceeds radially. Rupture of the ECU tendon may go unnoticed due to the intact ECRL and ECRB tendons to extend the wrist. EDQ rupture may go unnoticed if a sufficiently robust EDC tendon to the small finger exists. Once the fourth compartment (EDC) tendons begin to fail, the motion deficit is unable to be ignored by the patient.

Surgical solutions must address the tendon ruptures as well as the DRUJ synovitis and instability and ulna head breakdown that led to them.[43] Excision of the ulna head removes the bony prominence. The DRUJ synovitis also must be resected. Finally, the remaining distal ulna must be stabilized. Multiple techniques have been described using portions of FCU, ECU, wrist capsule, and combinations thereof.

The ruptured extensor tendons typically are degenerated over a significant length. Primary repair is almost never possible, and the frequent occurrence of multiple tendon ruptures makes repair with graft less desirable due to the need for multiple graft donors. Feldon and colleagues[43] recommend the following for increasing numbers of extensor tendon ruptures: for a single finger tendon rupture (most commonly to the small finger), EIP transfer; for two fingers (ring and small fingers), EIP transfer to the small finger and end-to-side repair of the ring finger to the intact middle finger extensor; for

three fingers, EIP transfer to ring and small with middle finger end-to-side to the index or FDS (middle or ring finger) transfer to ring and small (if EIP unavailable) and middle finger end-to-side to the index; for rupture of all four finger extensors, FDS (ring) is transferred to the ring and small extensors and FDS (middle) is transferred to the index and middle extensors.

Strict compliance with postoperative therapy is essential to maximizing the surgical result. Due to the chronic inflammation associated with RA, tendon and ligament repairs will be slower to achieve maximal tensile strength. Prolonged nighttime splinting, usually for months, helps prevent recurrence of extensor lag. Finally, the disease may progress over time. Reconstructions that were initially adequate may stretch out or fail over time.

DUPUYTREN'S CONTRACTURE

In 1614, a Swiss surgeon named Felix Plater first described contracture of multiple fingers due to palpable, cord-like structures on the volar surface of the hand and fingers. The disease state he described would ultimately come to be known as *Dupuytren's contracture*. Dupuytren's name came to be associated with the disease after he performed an open fasciotomy of a contracted cord before a class of medical students in 1831.[45]

The palmar fascia consists of collagen bundles in the palm and fingers. These are primarily longitudinally oriented, and reside as a layer between the overlying skin and the underlying tendons and neurovascular structures. There are also connections from this layer to the deep structures below and the skin above. Much is known about the progression of these structures from their normal state (called bands) to their contracted state, but little is known about how or why this process begins.

The Dupuytren's nodule represents the basic unit of disease.[46] Increased collagen deposition leads to a palpable nodule in the palm. Over time, there is increased deposition distally into the fingers. This collagen becomes organized and linearly oriented. These collagen bundles, with the aid of myofibroblasts, contract down to form the cords that are the hallmark of the symptomatic patient. Detail of the molecular and cellular biology of Dupuytren's disease is beyond the scope of this chapter, but is available in multiple hand surgery texts.[47]

Most nonoperative management techniques will not delay the progression of disease. Corticosteroid injections may soften nodules and decrease discomfort associated with them, but are ineffective against cords. Splinting similarly has been shown not to retard disease progression. Injectable clostridial collagenase has shown promise in clinical trials[48] but has not yet been reported in large or long-term series. It also is not yet commercially available.

For patients with advanced disease, including contractures of the digits that limit function, surgery is the mainstay of therapy. Although rate of progression should weigh heavily in the decision of whether or not to perform surgery, general guidelines are MP contracture of 30° or more and/or PIP contracture of 20° or more.[49]

Surgery consists of an open approach through the skin down to the involved cords. Skin is elevated off the underlying cords. Great care must be taken to preserve as much as possible of the subdermal vascular plexus with the elevated skin flaps to minimize postoperative skin necrosis. All nerves, tendons, and blood vessels in the operative field should be identified. Once this is done, the involved cord is resected while keeping the critical deeper structures under direct vision. Skin is then closed, with local flap transpositions as needed, to allow for full extension of the fingers that have been released (Fig. 44-19).

Dermatofasciectomy is an alternative to simple fasciectomy as described in the preceding paragraph. In dermatofasciectomy, overlying skin is resected along with the Dupuytren's cord. The wound is then typically closed with a skin graft. Dermatofasciectomy should only be performed if the skin cannot be separated from the underlying cords. Skin grafting should only be performed if the remaining skin after resection cannot be rearranged with local flaps to cover the wounds without the need for skin grafting.

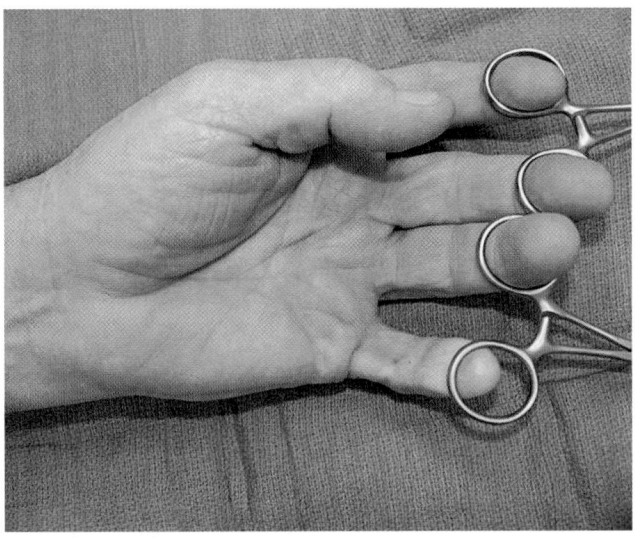

A

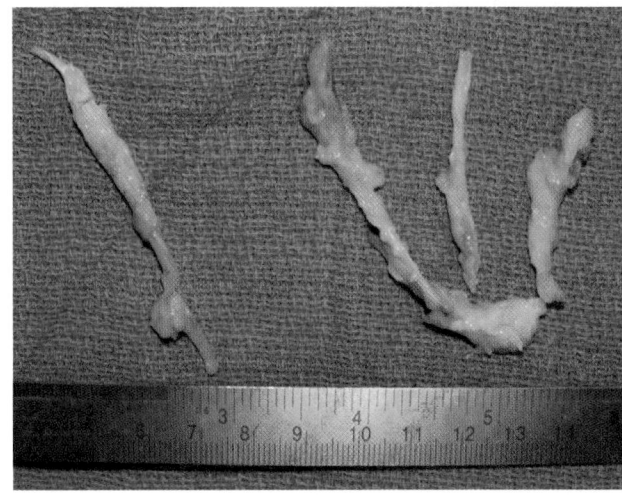

B

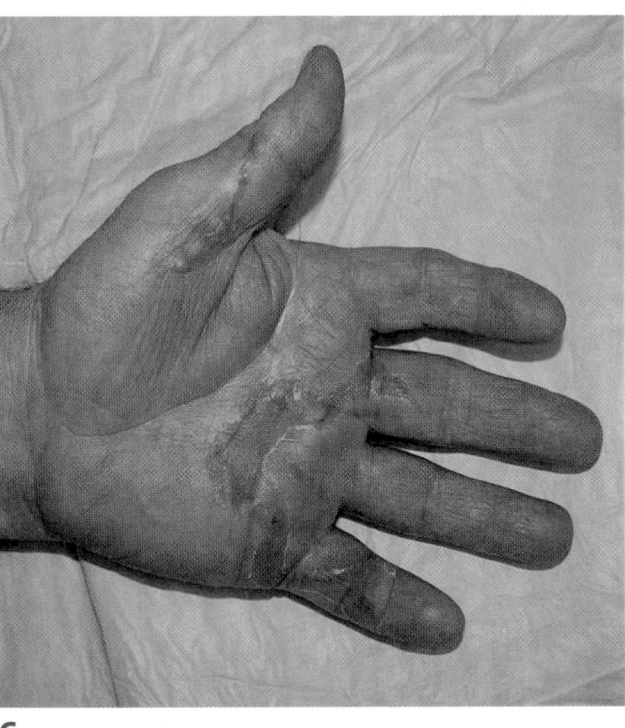

C

FIG. 44-19. Dupuytren's disease. **A.** This patient has cords affecting the thumb, middle, ring, and small fingers. **B.** The resected specimens are shown. **C.** Postoperatively, the patient went on to heal all his incisions and, with the aid of weeks of hand therapy, recovered full motion.

In the past, some authors have advocated total fasciectomy of the hand with the idea that recurrence/extension of disease could be prevented. Unfortunately, recurrences still occurred in these patients, and revision surgery became much more difficult.

Complications of surgical treatment of Dupuytren's disease occur as often as 17%.[50] Problems include: digital nerve laceration, digital artery laceration, buttonholing of the skin, hematoma, swelling, and pain including some patients with CRPS (see above section on Regional Pain Syndromes). Digital nerve injury can be quite devastating, producing annoying numbness at best or a painful neuroma in worse situations. Although the surgeon goes into the operation knowing that he/she must identify the nerves and other critical structures, a fascial cord can be mistaken for a nerve and vice versa. It is best to identify the nerve proximal to the area involved with Dupuytren's disease and track it distally into the affected area.

The hand is splinted in full extension at the end of surgery. Hand therapy typically is instituted within 1 week of surgery to begin mobilization of the fingers and edema control. The therapist also can identify any early wound problems as he/she will see the patient more frequently than the surgeon. Extension hand splinting is maintained for 4 to 6 weeks with nighttime splinting continued for an additional 6 to 8 weeks. After this point, the patient is serially followed for evidence of recurrence or extension of disease.

TENDONITIS/TENOSYNOVITIS

Trigger Finger

Stenosing tenosynovitis of the flexor tendon sheath, also known as *trigger finger* (TF), is one of the most common upper limb problems to be encountered in hand surgery practice. The condition starts with discomfort in the palm during movements of the involved digits. Gradually, the flexor tendon causes painful popping or snapping as the patient flexes and extends the digit. The patient often will present with a digit locked in a flexed position, which may require gentle passive manipulation to regain full extension.

The phenomenon is due to a difference in size of the affected flexor tendon and the retinacular pulley. The mismatch is due to formation of a nodule in the FDS tendon, where it passes under the A1 pulley in the region of the MC head (see Fig. 44-4). In rare instances, a nodule distal to it in the tendon of the FDP also can be responsible.

The most common etiology of TF is idiopathic formation of a nodule on the flexor tendon that obstructs gliding underneath the A1 pulley. The differential diagnosis includes localized swelling due to a partially lacerated flexor tendon catching against the A1 pulley, a nodule in the FDS that catches against the A3 pulley, locking caused by abnormal MC head shape preventing normal collateral ligament motion (staghorn lesion), foreign body in the MP joint, ganglion cyst of the tendon sheath, and sagittal band rupture causing the EDC to subluxate off the MC head and snap back in extension.

Several studies demonstrate a correlation between TF and activities that require exertion of pressure in the palm while performing powerful grip or repetitive forceful digital flexion. Proximal phalangeal flexion in power-grip activities causes high loads at the distal edge of the A1 pulley.[51] Some have suggested that bunching of the interwoven flexor tendon fibers causes the reactive intratendinous nodule observed at surgery.[52]

Stenosing tenosynovitis is much more common in women than men.[51] In several series, peak incidence of trigger digit occurred in the fifth to sixth decades of life. The dominant hand is more affected, and involvement of several fingers is not unusual. The most commonly affected digit is the thumb, followed by the ring, long, small, and index fingers.[53]

Signs and symptoms include palpable popping, clicking or snapping sensation over the A1 pulley, locking in flexion (in later stages, passive manipulation is needed to extend the digit), stiffness of the digit, tenderness over the A1 pulley, flexion deformity or joint contracture in late presentations, especially the PIP joint.

The goal of treatment for trigger digits is to eliminate the locking and allow full movement of the finger or thumb without discomfort. Swelling around the flexor tendon and tendon sheath must be reduced to allow smooth gliding of the tendon.

Nonoperative treatment includes limiting the activities that aggravate the condition. Splinting and/or oral anti-inflammatory medication may help. If symptoms continue, a corticosteroid injection into the tendon sheath at the pulley is often effective in relieving the trigger digit. The authors prefer triamcinolone acetonide (40 mg/mL) mixed with 0.5% plain bupivacaine. The needle is inserted at the MC head, advanced until bone is encountered, and then withdrawn approximately 0.5 mm until resistance gives way, allowing the medication to be injected. Approximately 1 mL is deposited in the tendon sheath. The needle is withdrawn and pressure is applied. Fingers with irreducible flexion contractures should be treated with surgery, not steroid injection.

Several studies advocate the use of percutaneous trigger release, in which the bevel of a needle is used to section the A1 pulley in an office procedure. This technique has been reported to be a safe alternative to open techniques.[54] Gilberts and associates compared the results from open vs. percutaneous technique and found similar efficacy but quicker recovery in the percutaneous group.[55] No serious complications have been reported with this technique, although there is a risk of incomplete pulley release, especially in severe cases. The use of this technique is not recommended in the thumb.

If nonsurgical forms of treatment do not relieve the symptoms, surgery is indicated. This surgery is performed as an outpatient, usually with simple local anesthesia. The goal of surgery is to divide the A1 pulley at the base of the finger so that the tendon can glide more freely. A 10- to 15-mm incision is made over the affected MC head. Blunt dissection is used to spread the subcutaneous tissue and palmar fascia to expose the flexor tendon and sheath. The A1 pulley is identified and sharply transected longitudinally. Care should be taken to identify the demarcation between the A1 and A2 pulleys so that the A2 pulley is not violated. At completion, the finger is

ranged to ensure that there is no residual triggering. Gentle traction on the flexor tendons also confirms that the A1 pulley has been completely released. Occasionally, a reduction tenoplasty may need to be performed if a large nodule is present (e.g., in RA). The skin incision is closed and a soft dressing is applied.

Active motion of the finger generally begins immediately after surgery. Normal use of the hand usually can be resumed once comfort and pain control permits. Occasionally, hand therapy is required after surgery to regain better use.

Nonoperative management is felt to be very safe without the risk of major complications. With the open technique, prolonged tenderness over the incision may occur. Infrequent complications include nerve injury, recurrence, and bowstringing of the flexor tendons due to sectioning of the A2 pulley.

De Quervain's Tenosynovitis

De Quervain's disease, described in 1895 by Swiss surgeon Fritz de Quervain, is a stenosing tenosynovitis that causes tendon entrapment of the first dorsal compartment of the wrist. It is a common cause of wrist and hand pain, particular during thumb motion.

The tendons of APL and EPB muscles pass through the first dorsal compartment. These tendons are secured tightly against the radial styloid by the extensor retinaculum. Frequent abduction of the thumb with ulnar deviation of the wrist is thought to create tension and eventual friction along the tendon sheath surrounding the APL and EPB. This friction leads to irritation and swelling of the sheath as well as thickening of the tendon that resists gliding.

The differential diagnosis includes: ganglion of the extensor retinaculum, osteoarthritis of thumb CMC joint, degenerative arthritis at the radioscaphoid joint, CTS, SRN neuropathy at the wrist, scaphoid fracture, and intersection syndrome (see the Intersection Syndrome section).

The average age of presentation is in the fifth and sixth decades, and the condition has been reported to be up to six times more common in women than men.[51] The disease also seems to affect pregnant or recently postpartum women and is thought to be due to repetitive lifting of infants. The wrist is usually affected bilaterally.[56] De Quervain's also is seen in association with inflammatory conditions such as rheumatoid disease.

Patients usually present with complaints of pain, several weeks to months in duration, along the radial aspect of the wrist aggravated by thumb motion. The most common symptoms are pain when grasping or pinching and tenderness at the first dorsal compartment, where the abductor policis longus and extensor policis brevis pass over the wrist joint (see Fig. 44-3). In some patients, a lump or thickened mass can be felt in the area 1 to 2 cm proximal to the radial styloid. Severe, sharp pain can be elicited by having the patient flex the thumb across the palm, make a fist, and then ulnarly deviate the wrist (Finkelstein's test) (Fig. 44-20).[57] There should be no tenderness in the forearm proximal to the first dorsal compartment. Axial loading of the thumb should not elicit tenderness and pain, unless there is concomitant CMC joint arthritis.

If treated early, some cases improve with short periods of rest in a thumb spica splint, followed by stretching exercises designed to improve tendon gliding. The patient should also modify activity to avoid motions that trigger symptoms. Compliance with splinting can be an issue; symptoms tend to recur after the splint is removed and the causative activities are resumed. Oral NSAID medications are of some benefit.

If splinting and NSAIDs fail, corticosteroid injection is the next line of treatment. The technique is similar to that used in TF. Injection into the tendon sheath of the first dorsal compartment has been shown to reduce tendon thickening and inflammation.[58] Corticosteroid injection has been reported to be effective in 50 to 80% of patients after one to two injections.[51]

With corticosteroid injections, possible complications of note include: transient anesthesia of the SRN at the first web space of the

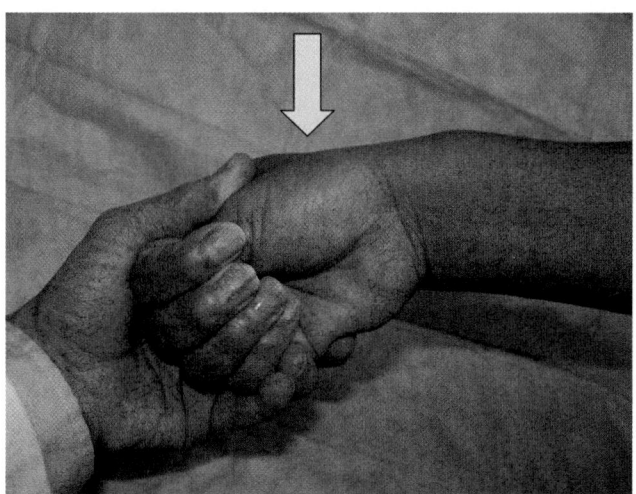

FIG. 44-20. Finkelstein's test. The patient places the thumb in the palm and makes a loose fist. The examiner then ulnarly deviates the patient's wrist (as indicated by the *arrow*). Pain at the first dorsal compartment with this maneuver is a positive response.

dorsal hand, direct injection injury to the radial nerve causing persistent pain (cheiralgia paresthetica), skin hypopigmentation in dark-skinned individuals, subcutaneous tissue atrophy, tendon weakening, and rupture (rare).

More severe cases or those that do not respond to conservative treatment may require surgery to release the first dorsal compartment. In this procedure, a transverse incision is made over the first dorsal compartment approximately 1 cm proximal to the radial styloid. Longitudinal blunt dissection is used to expose the roof of the first dorsal compartment. Sharp or transverse dissection in this area increases the likelihood of injury to the SRN, which runs superficial to the ligament. The ligament covering the compartment is then sharply opened longitudinally along its dorsal margin. Attention must be paid to the variant anatomy in this region.[59] Frequently, there is a septum between the EPB and APL tendons;[60] if this septum is identified, it must also be released, or symptoms will not be relieved. The skin incision is closed and a soft dressing is applied.

Although the surgical management of de Quervain's tenosynovitis is straightforward, complications can be bothersome. Persistent symptoms from an incompletely released first dorsal compartment can necessitate surgical re-exploration. Volar or dorsal subluxation of the tendons is possible; if symptomatic, reconstruction of the sheath with a slip of brachioradialis or a strip of adjacent dorsal retinaculum can be performed. Injury to the SRN is a rare, but serious complication. Laceration or retraction injury to the nerve can cause neuritis or a painful neuroma. The complication is avoided by careful blunt dissection and gentle retraction. Controversy still exists regarding the optimal management of an iatrogenic lacerated radial sensory nerve.

Intersection Syndrome

Intersection syndrome is tenosynovitis in which the tendons in the second dorsal compartment, radial wrist extensors ECRL and ECRB, cross over the tendons of the first dorsal compartment, EPB and APL. Intersection syndrome is characterized by pain in the distal dorsoradial forearm due to irritation of the affected tendons. The pain is proximal and ulnar to that of de Quervain's tenosynovitis and may be associated with localized swelling.[61]

Although this condition occurs at the intersection of the tendons of the first and second extensor compartments (proximal to the extensor retinaculum), many contend that the condition is a tenosynovitis of the ECRL and ECRB tendons. Intersection syndrome also can be caused by direct trauma to the second dorsal compartment. The differential diagnosis includes de Quervain's tenosynovitis,

thumb CMC arthritis, radial sensory nerve irritation (Wartenberg's syndrome), and EPL tendonitis.

Intersection syndrome is thought to be associated with activities that require repetitive wrist flexion and extension. Weightlifters, rowers, and other athletes are particularly prone to this condition.

Patients with intersection syndrome complain of dorsal radial wrist or forearm pain. Symptoms are exacerbated by repetitive wrist flexion and extension associated with thumb motion. On examination, a focal swelling at the area of intersection often is present. Active or passive wrist motion may produce a characteristic crepitus in severe cases.

Conservative treatment includes immobilization, activity modification, and pharmacologic intervention. A thumb spica splint effectively immobilizes the wrist extensors and thumb extensors. Several weeks of immobilization, followed by gradual splint weaning, usually is recommended. Activity modification at home and/or work also is critical. NSAIDs help alleviate pain and inflammation.

In recalcitrant cases, a corticosteroid injection into the second dorsal compartment is effective. Once the symptoms are under control, a program of supervised hand therapy leads to long-term recovery.

Surgery can be effective in cases that do not respond to conservative measures. The second extensor compartment is approached through a dorsal longitudinal incision, beginning over the wrist and continuing proximally 3 to 4 cm to the inflamed area.[62] The dorsal forearm fascia is divided longitudinally. Branches of the radial sensory nerve are identified and protected. The ECRL and ECRB tendons are released by longitudinally incising the extensor retinaculum over the second dorsal compartment. A thorough tenosynovectomy may be performed while elevating and protecting the tendons. The extensor retinaculum is not repaired. Skin is closed routinely, and the hand is placed in a volar thumb spica splint, maintaining the wrist at 15 to 20° of extension for 1 week. This is followed by early wrist ROM exercises.

No large series documenting treatment outcomes exist in the literature. There are reports that approximately 60% of patients respond to conservative management while 100% of patients who require surgery obtain long-term symptomatic relief.[62] Release of the second dorsal compartment could theoretically lead to bowstringing of the ECRL and ECRB tendons in extreme wrist extension; however, this complication has not been reported in the literature.

INFECTIONS

The most common cause of hand infections is trauma. Other predisposing conditions include diabetes and neuropathies. Ninety percent of infections are caused by gram-positive organisms *Staphylococcus aureus*, *Streptococcus viridans*, Group A *Streptococcus*, and *S. epidermis*. Infection in the hand, as in most areas of the body, can be localized by five cardinal signs: rubor (redness), calor (heat), tumor (swelling), dolor (pain), and loss of function. Treatment of any hand infection focuses on drainage, antibiotics, splint immobilization, and elevation.[63]

Cellulitis

Cellulitis of the hand is a nonsuppurative inflammation of the subcutaneous tissues. It is characterized by erythema, swelling, induration and warmth, and pain and tenderness. The most common pathogenic organisms are *Staphylococcus* and *Streptococcus*. Mainstays of treatment are elevation, splint immobilization, and judicious use of antibiotics. By definition, a diagnosis of cellulitis means that no purulence is present. If the patient does not improve within 24 to 48 hours, an abscess must be suspected.

Paronychia

Paronychia is an infection of the nail bed or the periungual soft tissue. It sometimes begins as a hangnail and often presents as a small

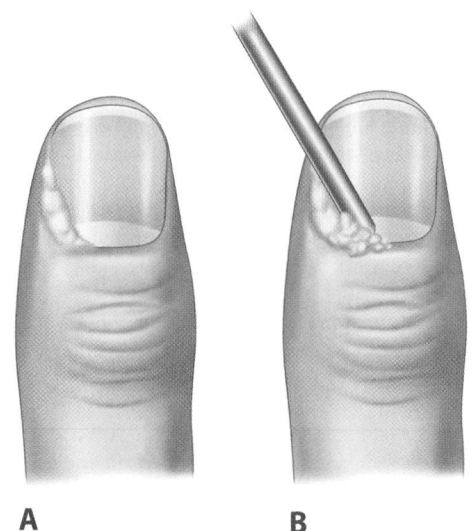

FIG. 44-21. Paronychia. **A.** Fluctuance in the nail fold is the hallmark of this infection. **B.** Technique of drainage between the nail plate and nail fold.

collection of purulent material at the side of the nail bed. In acute paronychia, the causative organisms are usually *S. aureus* or streptococci, less commonly *Pseudomonas* or *Proteus* species. Organisms enter through a break in the epidermis frequently due to nail biting or aggressive manicuring. In chronic paronychia, infection (usually *Candida* species) enters via the hand receiving prolonged exposure to a moist environment, such as those used as dishwashers.

Paronychia develops along the nail margin (lateral and proximal nail folds), manifesting over hours to days with pain, warmth, redness, and swelling. Pus usually develops along the nail margin, less commonly beneath the nail. Rarely, infection penetrates deep into the finger and may produce infectious flexor tenosynovitis (FTS).

Early treatment is warm compresses or soaks and an antistaphylococcal antibiotic. First-generation cephalosporins have traditionally been used, but the increasing prevalence of methicillin-resistant *S. aureus*[64] has led the authors to begin empiric treatment with vancomycin. Fluctuant swelling or visible pus should be drained with a Freer elevator or the bevel of an 18-gauge needle inserted between the nail and nail fold (Fig. 44-21). If the abscess resides under the eponychial fold, then a proximally based flap of eponychium can be reflected up to allow for better drainage. An abscess that extends below the nail necessitates partial removal of the nail plate. A thin gauze wick should be inserted for 24 to 48 hours to maintain patency of the drainage tract.

Felon

A felon is a closed-space, purulent infection of the fingertip pulp. It is usually extremely painful, and if left untreated, can lead to ischemia and necrosis. The thumb and index finger are the most commonly affected digits.

The fingertip pulp is divided into numerous small compartments by vertical septa that connect the distal phalanx bone to the overlying skin. Infection in these compartments can lead to abscess formation, tremendous edema, and rapid development of increased pressure in a closed space. The increased pressure may compromise blood flow and lead to necrosis of the skin and pulp.

Wooden splinters or minor cuts are common predisposing causes; however, in half of patients, the condition is idiopathic. Initial minor injury causes inflammation, which is first confined by the tough fibrous septa within the pulp. Early infection causes pain and tenderness. At this stage, infection may resolve spontaneously with antibiotics. If resolution does not occur, increasing swelling and throbbing pain herald abscess formation.

Felons are characterized by marked throbbing pain, tension, and edema of the fingertip pulp. *S. aureus* is the most common causative organism. More and more community-acquired methicillin-resistant *S. aureus* infections are being reported. Gram-negative organisms have been reported in immunosuppressed patients and diabetics. Fingertip blood glucose measurements have been implicated as an etiology. *Eikenella corrodens* infections have been reported in persons with diabetes who bite their fingernails.[63]

Adequate early treatment can prevent abscess formation. Tetanus should be updated. Antibiotics with activity against staphylococcal and streptococcal organisms should be administered. In cases where significant tension is present, the fingertip must be decompressed to preserve venous flow, whether or not a frank abscess has formed. The drained fluid should be sent for culture.

The procedure to drain a felon is straightforward (Fig. 44-22). A digital block is performed. This is followed by a short skin incision. Only the skin is incised. Pus is evacuated using a blunt instrument to decrease the chance of severing a digital nerve or entering the tendon sheath. Gauze is loosely packed into the wound to prevent skin closure. A loose dressing and finger splint is applied. The hand is elevated and splinted.

There is some debate regarding the choice of incision. A longitudinal incision over the area of maximal fluctuance (see Fig. 44-22) is effective and avoids the serious iatrogenic complications associated with other described incisions such as a transverse incision or an incision on the lateral aspect of the finger. The incision should not cross the DIP flexion crease to prevent formation of a flexion contracture. Probing is not carried out proximally to avoid extension of infection into the flexor tendon sheath. Lateral incisions, volar transverse incisions, and hockey stick and fish-mouth incisions have been suggested; however, these incisions offer no benefit and increase the potential for serious injury. In particular, the traditional lateral incision can causes ischemia and anesthesia by injuring one or both neurovascular bundles. The fish-mouth incision can lead to an unstable painful fingertip.

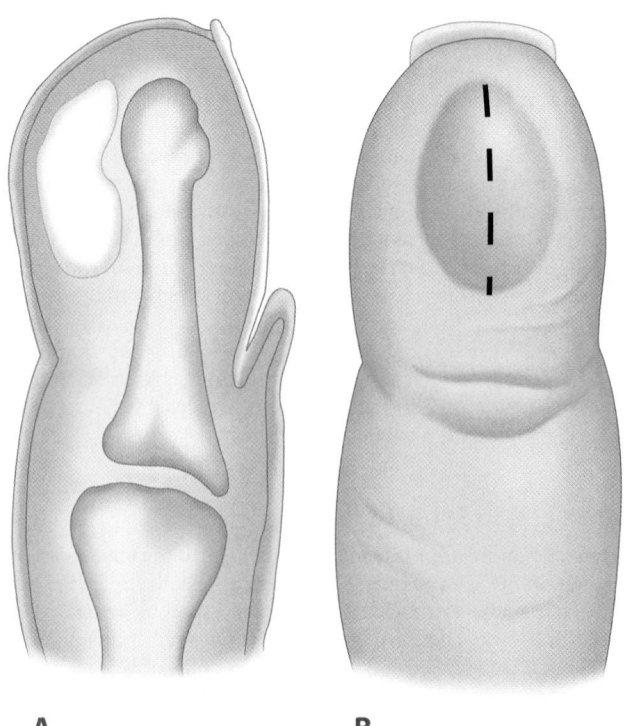

FIG. 44-22. A and **B.** The area of purulence in a felon is located in the pad of the distal phalanx as shown. **B.** A longitudinally oriented incision is made over the area of maximal fluctuance; this incision should not cross the distal interphalangeal joint crease. See text for additional details.

Untreated or incompletely treated infections can lead to osteomyelitis, tenosynovitis, and septic arthritis.

Bites

Human bites to the hand may lead to serious infections from any of the numerous organisms found in the oral cavity. Inoculation typically occurs during an altercation in which the skin and tendons over the MP and/or PIP joints are abraded and lacerated from an opponent's tooth. The initial clinical appearance of these "fight bites" often is deceptively benign, leading to delays in seeking care and more severe infection on presentation.

Human bites require aggressive evaluation and treatment. It is important to understand the mechanism of injury: the skin and joint capsule are trapped between a tooth and underlying bone. A 3-mm penetration can inoculate a joint in the hand. Treatment of these penetrating injuries includes irrigation and débridement of any purulence or devitalized structure(s). The hand should be immobilized and elevated. The patient should be placed on broad-spectrum antibiotics to cover *Staphylococcus, Streptococcus*, and anaerobic bacteria, such as amoxicillin/clavulanic (again recent trends in sensitivities have made penicillins less effective against *Staphylococcus*). *E. corrodens* is an organism commonly isolated from human fight bites. Skin lacerations should be left open to heal secondarily. Dog, cat, and other animal bites are treated similarly.

HERPETIC WHITLOW

Herpetic whitlow is a self-limited herpes simplex virus (HSV) infection of the distal finger. In the United States, HSV infection of the hand occurs in 2.4 cases per 100,000 population per year.[65] It is the most common viral infection of the hand and infections by HSV1 or HSV2 are clinically indistinguishable. Direct inoculation of the virus into a wound is usually the mechanism of infection. Herpetic whitlow often is found in adult women with genital herpes, children with coexistent herpetic gingivostomatitis, and health care workers exposed to orotracheal secretions.

The infection usually involves a single finger that is painful, erythematous, and swollen. It is characterized by vesicles early in the disease process. After about 2 weeks, the vesicles coalesce, and the infection may be mistaken for a paronychia or felon.

Diagnosis usually is made by a careful history and physical. On examination, tenderness is present but is less severe than that found in bacterial infections. The distinction is very important to make because performing an incision and drainage on a herpetic whitlow can lead to secondary bacterial infection as well as spread of the herpes virus. If the vesicle is unroofed, fluid obtained can be sent for a Tzanck smear and/or viral culture to confirm the diagnosis. Most commonly, however, diagnosis can be made without intervention on the involved digit.

Herpetic whitlow usually resolves spontaneously in 2 to 3 weeks. The main goals of treatment are to prevent both oral inoculation and spread of the infection, as well as to obtain symptomatic relief. The involved digit should be kept covered with a dry dressing. Some authors recommend treatment with oral acyclovir for 10 days if the diagnosis is made early in symptom onset, although acyclovir has not been demonstrated to shorten the course of this self-limited infection. Stronger evidence exists to recommend oral acyclovir for recurrent infections during the prodromal stage, as well as in immunocompromised patients. Infection can recur in 30 to 50% of patients, but the initial infection is typically the most severe.

FLEXOR TENOSYNOVITIS

FTS is a severe pathophysiologic state causing disruption of normal flexor tendon function in the hand. A variety of etiologies are responsible for this process. Most acute cases of FTS are due to purulent infection. FTS also can occur secondary to chronic inflammation as a result of diabetes, RA, crystalline deposition, overuse syndromes, amyloidosis, psoriatic arthritis, systemic lupus erythematosus, and sarcoidosis.

Suppurative FTS has the ability to rapidly destroy a finger's functional capacity and is considered a surgical emergency.

Much of the original work on infectious FTS was done in the early 1900s.[66] In the 1940s, postoperative sheath irrigation was suggested.[67] Besser, Carter, Burman, and Nevaiser have described multiple techniques of closed continuous irrigation and/or débridement as early as the 1960s.[68]

Suppurative FTS results from bacteria multiplying in the closed space of the flexor tendon sheath and culture-rich synovial fluid medium. Natural immune response mechanisms cause swelling and migration of inflammatory cells and mediators. The septic process and this inflammatory reaction within the tendon sheath quickly erode the paratenon, leading to adhesions and scarring. The ultimate consequences are tendon necrosis, disruption of the tendon sheath, and digital contracture.

The primary mechanism of infectious FTS usually is penetrating trauma. Most infections are caused by skin flora, including both *Staphylococcus* and *Streptococcus* species. Bacteria involved vary by etiology of the infection: bite wounds (*Pasteurella multocida*—cat, *E. corrodens*—human); *Bacteroides, Fusobacterium, Haemophilus* species, gram-negative organisms—diabetic patients; hematogenous spread (*Mycobacterium tuberculosis, Neisseria gonorrhea*); water-related punctures (*Vibrio vulnificus, M. marinum*). Infection in any of the fingers may spread proximally into the wrist, carpal tunnel, and forearm, also known as *Parona's space*.[69]

With the accumulation of purulence in the flexor tendon sheath, pressure can increase within the closed space and inhibit the inflammatory response. The increased pressure also inhibits blood flow and adds to the destructive process. Tendon ischemia increases the likelihood of tendon necrosis and rupture.

Patients with infectious FTS present with complaints of pain, redness, and fever. Physical examination reveals Kanavel's "cardinal" signs of flexor tendon sheath infection,[66] which are finger held in slight flexion, fusiform swelling, tenderness along the flexor tendon sheath, and pain over the flexor sheath with passive extension of the digit (Fig. 44-23A).

Kanavel's signs may be absent in patients who are immunocompromised, have early manifestations of infection, have recently received antibiotics, or have a chronic, indolent infection. The differential diagnosis includes inflammatory (nonsuppurative) FTS, herpetic whitlow, pyogenic arthritis, gout, fracture, degenerative arthritis or RA, sesamoiditis, and angiolipoma (found in case reports masquerading as FTS).

If a patient presents with suspected infectious FTS, empiric IV antibiotics should be initiated. Prompt medical therapy in early cases may prevent the need for surgical drainage. For healthy individuals, empiric antibiotic therapy should cover *Staphylococcus* and *Streptococcus*. For immunocompromised patients (including diabetics) or infections associated with bite wounds, empiric treatment should include coverage of gram-negative organisms as well.

Adjuncts to antibiotics include splint immobilization (intrinsic plus position preferred) and elevation until infection is under control. Hand rehabilitation (i.e., ROM exercises and edema control) should be initiated once pain and inflammation are under control.

If medical treatment alone is attempted, then inpatient observation for a minimum of 48 hours is indicated. Surgical intervention is necessary if no obvious improvement has occurred within 12 to 24 hours. In addition, for patients who are immunocompromised or have diabetes, surgery is warranted.

Several surgical approaches can be used to drain infectious FTS. The method used is based upon the extent of the infection. Michon developed a classification scheme[70] that can be useful in guiding surgical treatment:

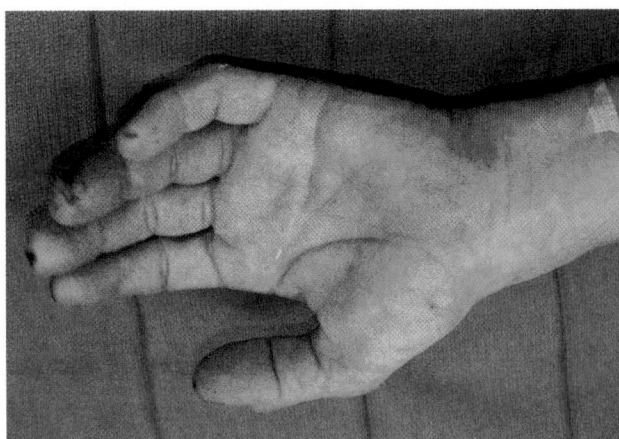

A

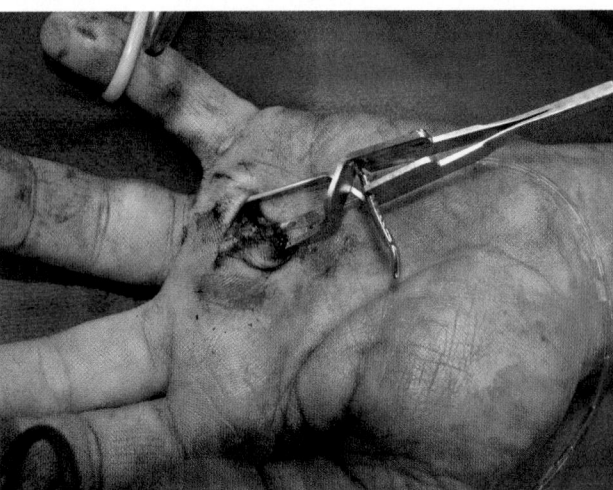

B

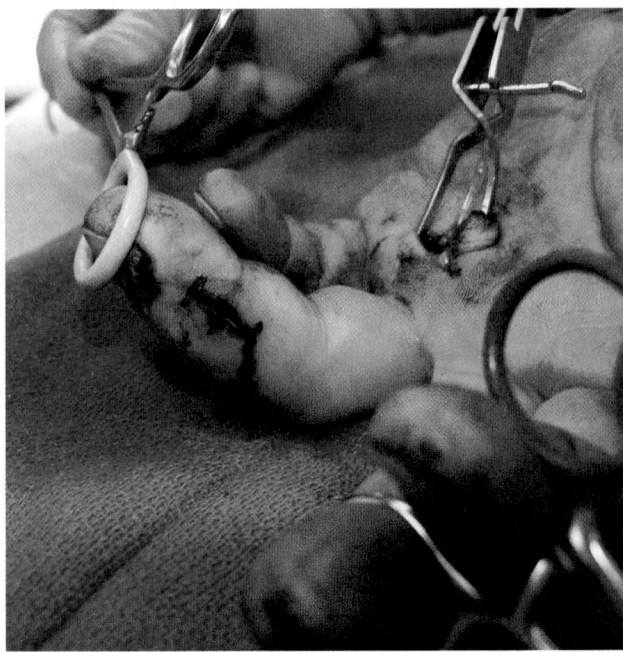

C

FIG. 44-23. Suppurative flexor tenosynovitis of the ring finger. **A.** The finger demonstrates fusiform swelling and flexed posture. **B.** Proximal exposure for drainage. **C.** Distal drainage incision.

Stage I. Findings: Increased fluid in sheath, mainly a serous exudate

Treatment: Catheter irrigation

Stage II. Findings: Purulent fluid, granulomatous synovium

Treatment: Minimal invasive drainage ± indwelling catheter irrigation

Stage III. Findings: Necrosis of the tendon, pulleys, or tendon sheath

Treatment: Extensive open débridement and possible amputation

Current recommendations for stage and I and II infections advocate proximal and distal incisions for adequate drainage and irrigation. A proximal incision is made over the A1 pulley (see Fig. 44-23B). In the digit, either a volar zigzag (Brunner) incision or a midaxial incision may be used distally. This distal incision is made over the region of the A5 pulley (see Fig. 44-23C). A Brunner incision allows better initial exposure but may yield difficulties with tendon coverage if skin necrosis occurs. If used, the midaxial incision should be dorsal to the neurovascular bundle. A 16-gauge catheter or 5F pediatric feeding tube then is inserted into the tendon sheath through the proximal incision. The sheath is copiously irrigated with normal saline. Excessive fluid extravasation into the soft tissue of the digit should be avoided because the resulting increase in tissue pressure can lead to necrosis of the digit. The catheter is removed after irrigation. A small drain is placed in the distal incision, and the wounds are left open. Some surgeons prefer a continuous irrigation technique for a period of 24 to 48 hours. The catheter is sewn in place, and a small drain is placed at the distal incision site. Continuous or intermittent irrigation every 2 to 4 hours with sterile saline can then be performed through the indwelling catheter.

Indications for open tendon sheath débridement include stage III infections, chronic infections, or infections caused by atypical mycobacteria. To expose the tendon sheath, a Brunner incision or a longitudinal midaxial incision is made along the length of the digit. The thumb and small fingers are approached from the radial side, and the remaining digits are approached from the ulnar side. The incision begins distally at the level of the A5 pulley, or just beyond the distal flexion crease, and is extended proximally to the web space. For extensive infections, the sheath is opened at all of the cruciate pulleys while preserving the A2 and A4 pulleys. The purulent fluid should be sent for aerobic, anaerobic, fungal, acid-fast bacilli, and atypical acid-fast bacilli cultures. In cases of known mycobacterial infection, extensive tenosynovectomy may be necessary. If the small finger or thumb is involved and there is evidence of palmar bursae involvement, an additional incision proximal to the transverse carpal ligament is made to ensure adequate drainage of the radial and ulnar bursae. The sheath is copiously irrigated, and the wounds are left open with drains in place.

After surgery, an intrinsic plus splint is applied, the hand is elevated, and the appropriate empiric antibiotic coverage is instituted while awaiting culture results. The hand is re-examined the following day. Whirlpool therapy and ROM are begun. Drains are removed before discharge from the hospital. The wounds are left open to heal by secondary intention. In severe cases, repeat irrigation and operative débridement may be required.

The length of IV antibiotic treatment is determined by the culture and sensitivity results and specific patient factors. The transition from IV to oral antibiotics should be based not only on the culture results but also on the clinical progress. Oral antibiotics should be continued for 7 to 14 days. Follow-up should continue until the infection has resolved, all wounds are closed, and pain-free full motion has returned.

Patients with infectious FTS that present early and have no comorbidities have a good prognosis. Patients that present with fulminant infection, have chronic infections, or are immunocompromised have increased risks of long-term complications and impairment. The most common complication is finger stiffness secondary to intrasheath adhesions. If loss of functional motion persists, tenolysis is considered 4 months postoperatively. The second major complication is soft tissue necrosis, which is more commonly seen in patients who have diabetes[71] or who present late in the disease process.

Joint Space Infections

The joints of the fingers are easily violated by penetrating trauma. Dorsally, they are only covered by skin and extensor tendon, and laterally, the collateral ligaments lie directly beneath the skin. As a result, sharp objects can readily inoculate the joint with infectious organisms. The common cause of septic arthritis is human or animal bite injuries to the MP joints. Septic arthritis can occur after trauma to the joint with teeth, needles, or thorns, or concomitant with tenosynovitis or osteitis. The symptoms are localized pain, tenderness, and swelling of the joint. Passive movement and axial loading of the joint are very painful. In the early stage, x-rays may demonstrate a slightly widened joint space. Joint destruction may be detected several weeks later. In these cases, osteomyelitis is most likely present. Early surgical treatment is most important to drain the infection and prevent the sequelae of septic arthritis.

Treatment of septic arthritis depends on which joint is involved. For the IP joints, the surgeon incises dorsally and opens the joint just lateral to the terminal extensor tendon (DIP joints) or between the central slip and a lateral band (PIP joints). The joint is irrigated and the skin is left open. For the MP joints, a dorsal incision is made. The extensor tendon is split longitudinally. The joint capsule is incised and partially resected, and the joint irrigated thoroughly. The capsule and skin are left open, but the extensor tendon is closed with a running, locking, absorbable suture. Even in patients treated early, arthritis and fibrous ankylosis cannot always be avoided.

In patients suspected of pyogenic wrist arthritis vs. crystalline arthropathy, arthrocentesis can be attempted before considering surgical intervention. Lister's tubercle (the bony prominence on the dorsal distal radius that serves as a pulley for the EPL) is palpated. An 18-gauge needle is inserted approximately 1 cm distal to this, angled 10° proximal (rather than true perpendicular) to the skin. Aspirated fluid should be sent for Gram's stain, crystal analysis, and culture. If a "dry tap" yields no fluid, 3 mL of sterile saline should be instilled and then aspirated, and sent for the same studies.

If Gram's stain or culture comes back positive, or the patient's clinical course is compelling for intervention, surgical drainage of the wrist is performed. A longitudinal incision is made between the tendons of the third (EPL) and fourth (EDC and EIP) compartments. The wrist capsule is opened at the scapholunate interval over the radiocarpal joint. Great care is taken to avoid injuring the ligament connecting the scaphoid and lunate bones. A Penrose drain is placed and the skin is left open. The wrist is splinted and the hand elevated. Whirlpool and ROM therapy are begun on postoperative day 1.

Web Space Infections

The second, third, and fourth web spaces are potential sites for infection. Within the web lies a fascial support structure called the *natatory ligament.* This can become contracted in Dupuytren's disease, but in the case of a web space infection, it serves as a partial separation between the volar and dorsal web space. Infection typically occurs as dorsal and volar pus pockets with a narrow connection through the natatory ligament, thus the term *collar button abscess.* On examination, patients typically have pain, swelling, and fluctuance on the palmar and/or dorsal web space surface. The adjacent fingers rest in abduction (Fig. 44-24A) and forced adduction causes pain. These infections are drained through separate dorsal and volar incisions. Great care is taken to leave a skin bridge >1 cm intact in the web. A Penrose drain is placed across both incisions (see Fig. 44-24B) and is removed before discharge from the hospital.

Palmar Space Infections

The deep palmar spaces may develop abscesses after puncture wounds. These infections may cause erythema, fluctuance, and

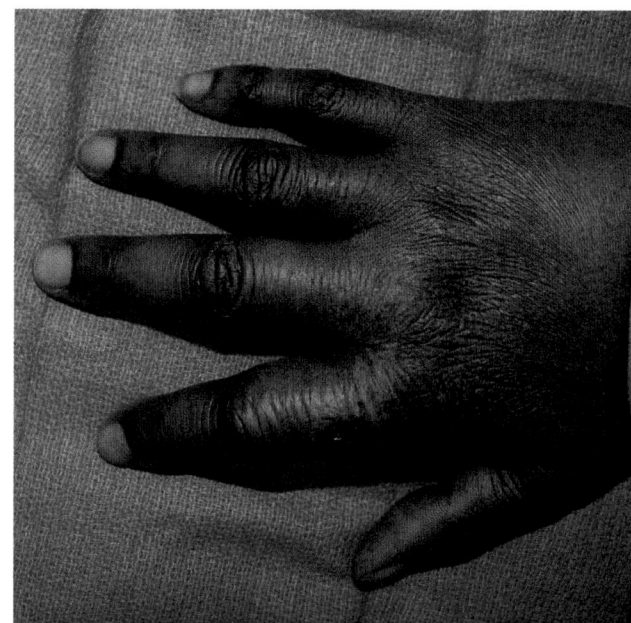

A

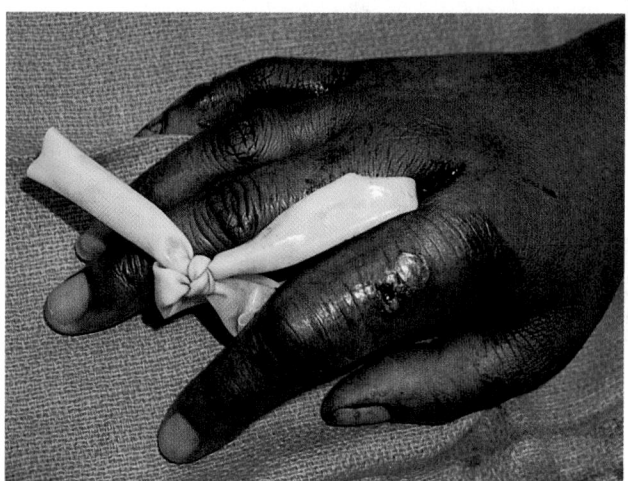

B

FIG. 44-24. A. The fingers surrounding the involved (second) web space rest in greater abduction than the other fingers. **B.** Dorsal and volar drainage incision are made, separated by a bridge of intact web skin; a Penrose drain prevents the skin from closing too early.

pain. The deep fascial spaces of the hand are potential spaces and consist of the hypothenar, midpalmar, and thenar spaces. The hypothenar space begins at the radial border of the hypothenar muscle fascia and passes over the ulnar border of the hand. The midpalmar space is demarcated by the palmar interosseous muscles dorsally and the flexor tendons of the fingers volarly. Lastly, the thenar space consists of the area between the adductor pollicis muscle dorsally and the flexor tendon of the second digit ventrally. In some patients, thenar space infection may spread distally to the first web and then dorsally over the first dorsal interosseous muscle, referred to as a *pantaloon abscess.*

These compartments are susceptible to infection by direct penetrating trauma, spread from a neighboring compartment, or hematogenous seeding. Because of the dorsal location of the hand lymphatics, erythema and swelling commonly appear over the dorsum of the hand, even when the injury is of palmar origin. Treatment involves careful incision and drainage and the usual postoperative modalities. For pantaloon abscesses, a second incision is necessary

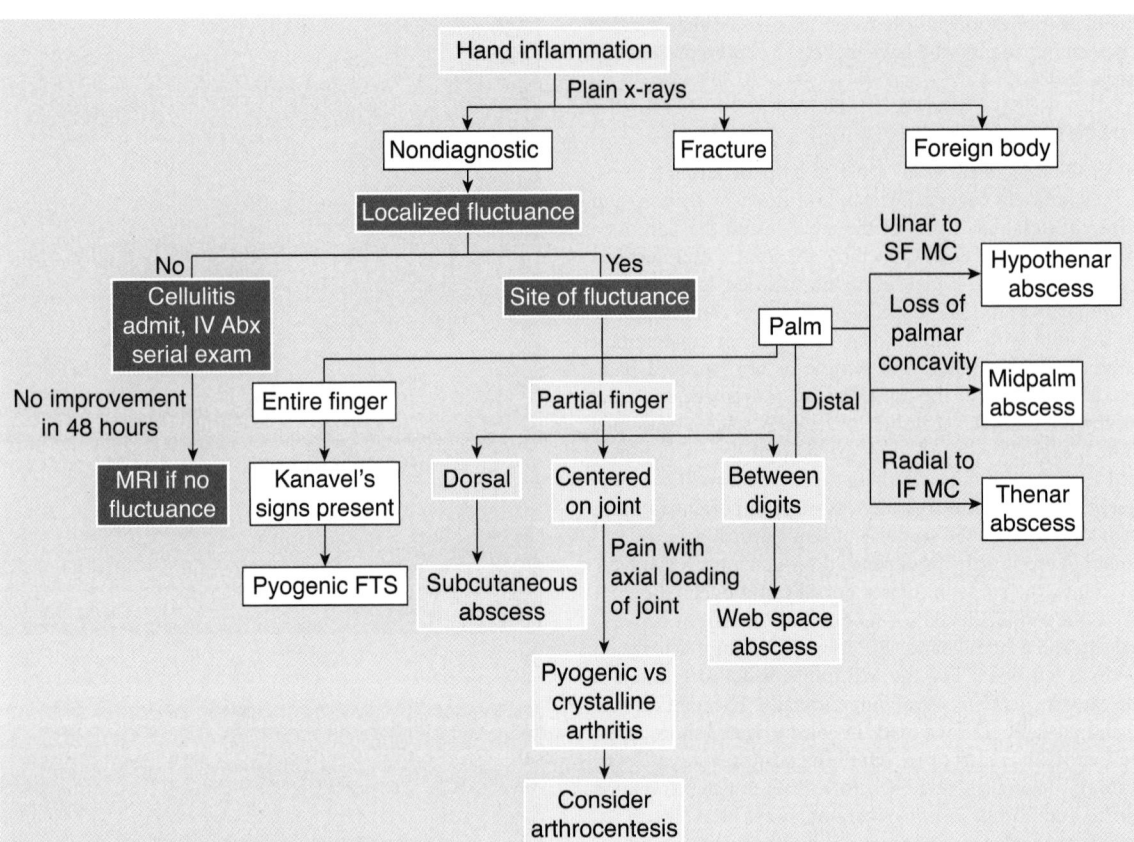

FIG. 44-25. Diagnostic algorithm. Diagnostic work-up for a patient with hand inflammation to evaluate for infection. See text for details about particular infectious diagnoses. Abx = antibiotics; FTS = flexor tenosynovitis; IF MC = index finger metacarpal; MRI = magnetic resonance imaging; SF MC = small finger metacarpal.

dorsal to the web space. A bridge of web skin must be left intact to prevent the risk of postoperative web space contracture. A Penrose drain is used similar to treatment for a collar button abscess.

For the patient with inflammation of the hand and suspicion for infection, clinical examination is the most useful diagnostic tool. Plain x-rays are useful to exclude fracture and foreign body. For each abscess location, clinical examination findings can be used to support or exclude a particular diagnosis (Fig. 44-25).

TUMORS

Abnormal lumps and bumps, considered to be tumors, are extremely common on the hand. They may vary from benign growths that are simply unsightly to malignant masses that require urgent treatment. Fortunately, most tumors on the hand are benign. Diagnosis usually can be made from the history given by the patient and examination of the lesion. Pathologic examination of tissue provides the final diagnosis.

Tumors may arise from any of the bones or soft tissues. The majority of lesions can be cured by removal but this often can be difficult for anatomic reasons. Tumors can lie close to important structures in the hand, such as nerves and vessels, which must be identified and carefully protected intraoperatively.

Tumors in the hand can be broadly categorized as being benign or malignant; the most common lesions are described below in Benign Lesions and Malignant Tumors.

Benign Lesions

Ganglion cysts are the most common soft tissue tumors in the hand.[72] These lesions can be painful and usually are found on the dorsal wrist,

followed by the volar wrist, flexor tendon sheath, and the dorsal DIP joint (the mucous cyst). These non-neoplastic, mucinous, fluid-filled pseudocysts arise from synovial linings of irritated and inflamed joints, ligaments, and tendon sheaths. As they have no epithelial lining, the focus of treatment is the site of production or leakage of the synovial fluid, rather than the cyst itself. Cysts may be aspirated; the sudden decrease in cyst pressure may allow the two sides of the stalk to coapt and close. Definitive therapy is surgical excision of the stalk and débridement of the synovial origin. In the common dorsal wrist ganglion, débridement of the dorsal wrist capsule over the scapholunate ligament is felt to be the most important aspect in achieving a low recurrence rate. Volar wrist ganglions arise at the radioscaphocapitate ligament along the radioscaphoid joint. Excision requires complete dissection and protection of the adjacent radial artery and branches of the SRN. For excision of ganglions arising from the flexor tendon sheath, the underlying annular pulleys and adjacent proper digital neurovascular bundles must be protected during dissection.

Lipomas are very common tumors of the body. However, despite their benign nature, the growth of lipomas in the hand can cause neurologic changes by compressing nearby peripheral nerves. They can compress the median nerve and cause symptoms similar to that seen in CTS. Lipomas also can cause sensory deficits from compression of the ulnar nerve and SRN in the hand.[73]

Enchondromas arise from cartilage and are the most common primary bone tumors of the hand.[74] These lesions account for >90% of bone tumors seen in the hand.[75] The proximal phalanges are the most common sites of occurrence, followed by the MC bones. On radiographs, an enchondroma usually is seen as a well-defined radiolucent lesion in the diaphysis or metaphysis and also may have a well-defined sclerotic rim. Although these tumors are benign, local bony destruction can lead to pathologic fracture.

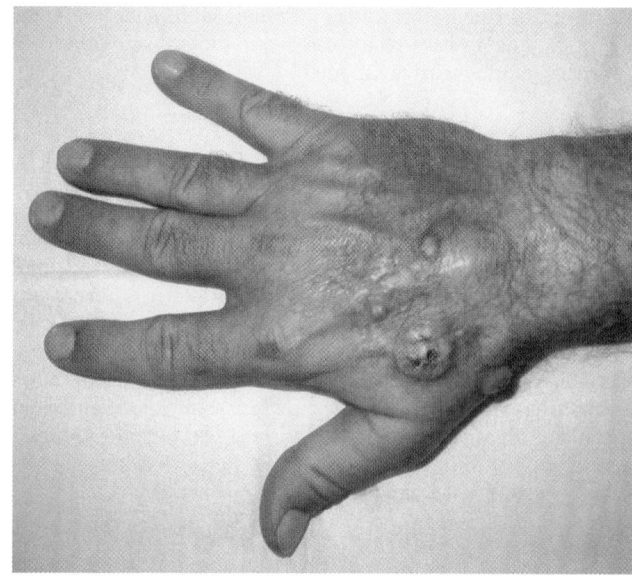

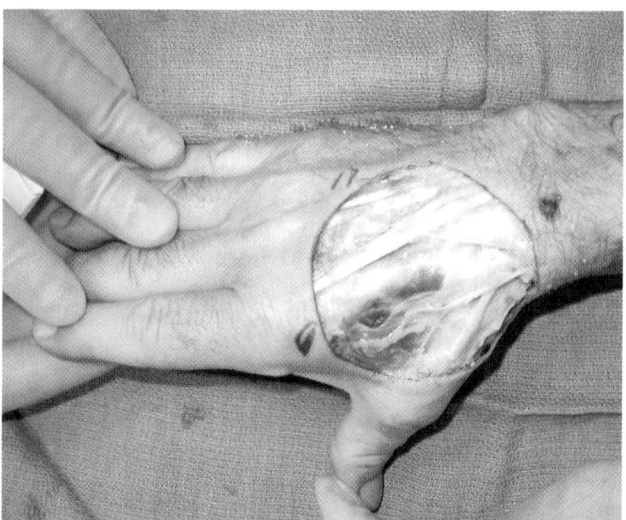

Giant cell tumor of the tendon sheath is the second most common tumor of the hand. This tumor arises from the tendon sheath and includes discrete, nodular, or polypoid masses that affect the digits. The etiology is generally unknown, although a widely accepted explanation describes a reactive hyperplasia associated with an inflammatory process.[76] The tumor is usually painless and asymptomatic, except for occasional distal numbness if it compresses a nearby digital nerve. Typically, these masses occur along the volar aspect of the hand and fingers and are most commonly adjacent to the DIP joint. The tumors are firm, lobulated, slow-growing masses that are firmly fixed to the underlying structures. The overlying skin often is freely mobile over proximal masses in the fingers. Pressure exerted by the tumors can cause cortical erosion of adjacent bony structures. The treatment of choice is marginal excision of the giant cell tumor.

Giant cell tumor of bone most frequently is found in patients in their second to fourth decades of life. Jaffe provided the current clinical description and grading system used today.[77] It is characterized by the pathologic presence of multinucleated giant cells. Pain is frequently the primary symptom.[78] An expanding mass, primarily in the epiphysis, leads to cortical destruction and eventual pathologic fracture. Giant cell tumors are seen in the distal radius, and less commonly, in the phalanges. Nonsurgical treatment includes radiation and embolization. Surgical options include intralesional curettage, although this has been associated with a significant rate of recurrence. Currently, adjuvant therapy such as cryosurgery and bone cement packing has decreased the rate of recurrence following intralesional curettage.[79]

Pyogenic granulomas may occur in the skin as solitary, raised lesions with hyperemic and ulcerated features. Trauma with superimposed infection and/or inflammation is considered to be the most probable cause of these lesions, which are not true neoplasms. Vascular causes have also been described.[80] Definitive treatment of pyogenic granulomas involves excision with a generous margin of surrounding normal tissue. An alternative effective treatment is to shave off the lesion flush with the skin and coagulate the base.

Malignant Tumors

Squamous cell carcinoma (SCC) is the most common primary malignant tumor of the hand, accounting for 75 to 90% of malignancies.[81] It is two to five times more prevalent in males. Risk factors include sun exposure, x-ray exposure, chronic ulcers, immunosuppression, xeroderma pigmentosa, and actinic keratosis. Solar radiation is the most modifiable risk factor for SCC. Ulcers that develop within old burn or traumatic scars may undergo malignant change (Marjolin's ulcers), representing a more aggressive SCC. Transplant patients on immunosuppressive therapy have a fourfold increased risk of developing skin cancer while patients with xeroderma pigmentosum have a 1000-fold increase in the development of nonmelanotic SCC. These cancers often manifest as small, firm nodules or plaques with indistinct margins. The surface of the lesions may have various irregularities ranging from smooth to verruciform to ulcerated (Fig. 44-26). Scaling, bleeding, and crusting are often seen. Typically, SCC is only locally invasive; however, metastatic rates of up to 20% have been reported in radiation beds and burn scars. Treatment options include curettage and electrodesiccation, cryotherapy, and radiotherapy. Standard treatment is excision with 0.5- to 1-cm margins.[81]

Basal cell carcinoma (BCC) accounts for 3 to 12% of hand malignancies. Risk factors are similar to those for SCC and include chronic sun exposure, light complexion, and immunosuppression. Other associated conditions include inorganic arsenic exposure and Gorlin's syndrome. BCC classically presents on the hand as a small, well-defined nodule with a translucent, pearly border with overlying telangiectasias. Metastasis are extremely rare. Treatment options for BCC include curettage with electrodesiccation, cryosurgery, and radiation. Standard therapy is surgical excision with 0.5-cm margins. Although performed routinely for facial BCC, Mohs micrographic surgery rarely is indicated for lesions of the hand.

FIG. 44-26. Squamous cell cancer on the dorsal hand. **A.** The patient had a previous excision of squamous cell carcinoma with recurrence along the incision. **B.** Intraoperative defect after resection with 1-cm margins. Paratenon is intact. The wound was temporarily covered with allograft; once final margins were negative, a split-thickness sheet skin was placed.

Melanoma accounts for approximately 3% of primary malignant hand tumors, although this incidence is rising.[82] Risk factors include long-term sun exposure, previous dysplastic nevi, fair complexion, family history of melanoma, and congenital nevi. Lesions with increased growth, change in color or shape, irregular borders, and accelerated growth are suggestive of melanoma. A pigmented lesion under the nail bed must be aggressively pursued with biopsy because of the concern for subungual melanomas. Survival is related to the Breslow thickness of the lesion. The principal treatment is surgical excision or amputation, with 1-cm margins for lesions up to 1 mm in depth, and 2-cm margins for thicker lesions.[83] Clinically palpable nodes should be removed to allow staging. Although there is little role for elective lymph node dissections, sentinel lymph node status has been shown to be a valuable prognostic factor. Isolated limb perfusion may offer hope for salvage therapy of metastatic disease.

Subungual melanomas are treated with amputation at the level of the DIP joint. Studies have reported a 5-year survival rate of 66% in patients with subungual melanoma.[84]

BURNS

Even though the palm of the hand comprises only 1% of total body surface area, burns of the hand can represent a serious short- or long-term disability. Hand burns are considered to be severe injuries requiring specialized treatment at a burn center. The management of hand burns is multidisciplinary and requires the expertise of hand surgeons, nurses, and occupational therapists. The multidisciplinary treatment of hand burns begins on the day of injury and may be carried out simultaneously with resuscitation and other treatment. Management objectives include edema control, avoidance of prolonged immobilization, prevention of infection, preservation of viable tissue, and prevention of contractures.

Acute Management

After airway and breathing concerns are addressed in the primary survey, circulation to the hand needs to be assessed. Evaluation of radial, ulnar, and palmar arch pulses should be undertaken by palpation or Doppler ultrasound at initial evaluation and frequently thereafter. Objective evidence of inadequate perfusion (i.e., deteriorating clinical examination with changes in or loss of pulse or Doppler signal) indicates the need for escharotomy, especially in the setting of full-thickness circumferential hand and/or arm burns. Escharotomy may be performed at bedside using a scalpel or electrocautery under local anesthesia and/or IV sedation. In the forearm, axially oriented midradial and midulnar incisions are made for the entire extent of the full-thickness burn. Escharotomy should progress distally (wrist, hand, then digits) as necessary to restore perfusion. Digital escharotomies are achieved via midaxial incisions over the radial aspects of the thumb and small finger, and the ulnar aspect of the index, middle, and ring fingers.[85] This incision location on the digits is preferred to avoid scars that may be painful on the pinch and contact surfaces of the digits.

Edema formation in burned hands hinders motion and may be a factor in later contracture formation. The hands must be elevated above the level of the heart to minimize edema formation. This is the most important initial step in the management of hand burns and can be done in any sized burn without hindering resuscitation, pulmonary, or other critical care management.

After initial débridement of devitalized tissue, burned hands should be cleansed twice daily. Burns that are clearly partial to full thickness may be managed with silver sulfadiazine cream. Some centers also use mafenide acetate in conjunction with silver sulfadiazine. A number of dressings are available for the treatment of clean partial-thickness burns. Allograft (human cadaver skin), although expensive, provides an excellent temporary dressing. Another option is Biobrane biosynthetic wound dressing (Bertek Pharmaceuticals, Morgantown, WVa), a bilayer semisynthetic dressing consisting of an elastic nylon fabric bonded to a semipermeable silastic membrane and coated with collagen polypeptides. Gloves manufactured from this material are available in a variety of sizes and are ideal dressings for clean partial-thickness burns of the hands. Cultured autologous keratinocytes also have been found to be useful in wound coverage.

A burned hand that is not properly positioned, splinted, or ranged will develop debilitating contractures. These contractures represent major disabilities that are difficult to correct with subsequent reconstructive surgery. A typical contracture is an "intrinsic minus" position where the MP joints are fixed in hyperextension and the PIP joints are fixed in a position of flexion.[86] The collateral ligaments of the MP joint are the most important structures of the burned hand. For this reason, positioning of the burned hand should place the MP joints at maximum flexion to maximally stretch these collateral ligaments. The ideal anatomic position for splinting is the intrinsic plus position with the thumb fully abducted. An orthoplastic splint may be fashioned and secured to the forearm over burn dressings; Velcro straps allow the splint to be loosened to compensate for progressive edema. In special cases, burned hands can be maintained in a safe functional position by temporary Kirshner wire arthrodesis of unstable MP and IP joints.

Occupational therapy has a major impact on hand function following burn injury. Early attention from occupational therapy can minimize the need for later reconstruction.[87] Re-establishment of function is the ultimate goal for the patient and is directly dependent upon patient effort expended during occupational therapy sessions. Some clinicians feel that the function present at 1-year postinjury represents that plateau of rehabilitation potential.

In many cases, with good wound care, skin will heal spontaneously without the need for operative intervention. In other cases, surgical excision of the burn with split-thickness skin grafting will be necessary. Grafting should be undertaken as soon as it becomes obvious that wound healing will not be complete by postburn day 14.

Considerable controversy surrounds the need, timing, and method of grafting of burned hands. Several prospective studies show that final surgical management vs. nonoperative care does not impact functional outcome of burned hands. Likewise, function is not affected by the choice of sheet graft over meshed graft, and some claim that cosmetic result is similar with meshed and unmeshed grafts to the hands. The timing of hand graft application is also controversial. For burn patients, the first goal of skin grafting is survival, the second is function, and the third is aesthetics.[88] This should be taken into account when planning skin grafting to the burned hand. The complete coverage of two burned hands with sheet grafts will likely require harvest of several large autografts. These same autografts, when meshed, could cover a larger area on the trunk, thereby reducing the total burn size. However, it makes little sense to leave a burn survivor with nonfunctional hands because grafting was deferred until the remainder of the skin was healed. A balance between survival and function must be struck.[89]

Tangential excision of burned hands should be performed under tourniquet to minimize potentially significant blood loss. Skin grafts are secured with skin staples, suture, or fibrin glue. Some surgeons will place the hand into a splint before grafting is commenced to minimize shearing. The splint is removed within 1 week, and gentle therapy is initiated. The patient is encouraged to use the hands for activities of daily living, and active ROM exercises are prescribed.

Vacuum-assisted closure devices (V.A.C., KCI, San Antonio, Tex) have advanced wound care, in general, and have particular usefulness in the hand. A sponge specifically designed for the hand is available and is currently used at many centers in the treatment of hand burns (Fig. 44-27). Studies are underway that investigate whether burn progression is limited and edema is reduced by the early application of vacuum therapy. The hand V.A.C. sponge also provides an excellent method of splinting the burned hand in a position of function.

Reconstruction

The most common upper extremity deformities requiring reconstruction after burns are dorsal hand and web space contractures. Ideally, proper positioning prevents dorsal hand contractures. If the initial excision was tangential rather than fascial, such that some remnant dorsal subcutaneous fat remains, a scar release can be performed. The released scar will slide distally, and a skin graft can fill in the defect created behind it. Any release must result in complete ROM of the MP joints. Web space contractures can be minimized by proper early surgery and compression gloves supplemented with web space conformers. In the normal web space, the leading edge of the volar aspect of the web is distal to the dorsal aspect. In the typical dorsal web space contracture, this is reversed, with dorsal syndactyly.

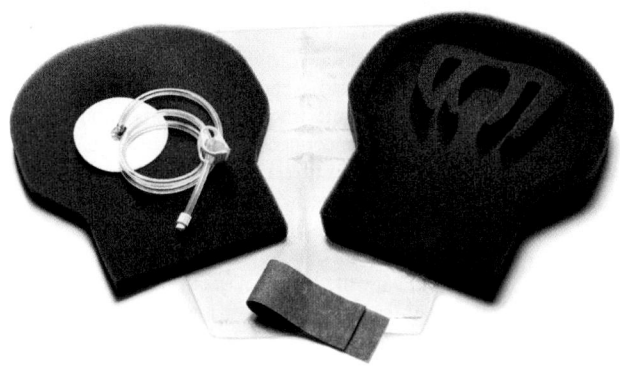

FIG. 44-27. V.A.C. GranuFoam Hand Dressing. *(Courtesy of KCI Licensing, Inc., 2008, used with permission.)*

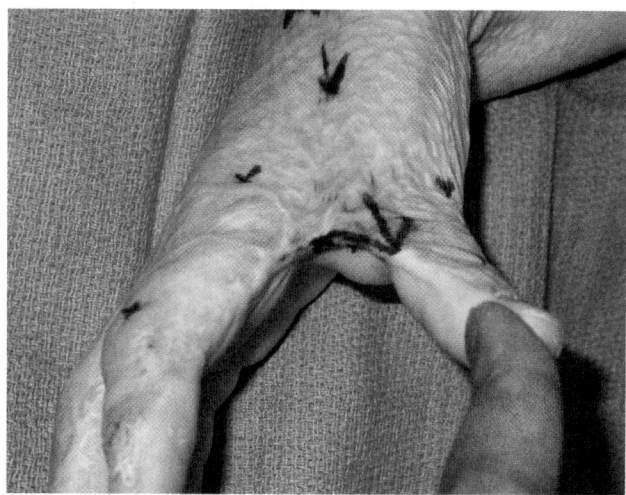

A

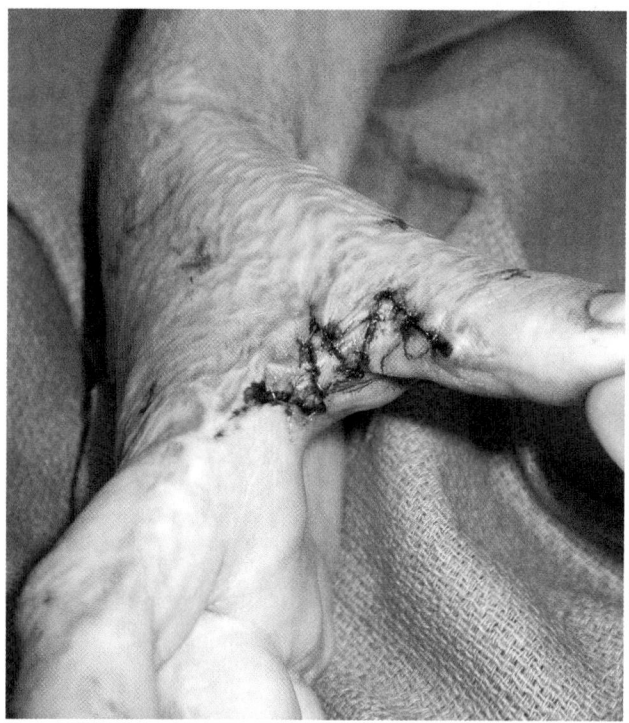

B

FIG. 44-28. Z-plasty release of web space contracture. **A.** First web space burn contracture. **B.** Immediate postoperative result.

When severe, abduction of the digits is limited. Repair can be achieved with local flaps and Z-plasties (Fig. 44-28).

When burns of the hands are deep, initial débridement may result in exposure of viable tendon or joints. Flap coverage is then required. A local flap of choice is the reversed radial forearm flap. Extensive injury may require free-tissue transfer such as a free anterolateral thigh flap (Fig. 44-29) or free lateral arm flap. In cases where local flaps are unavailable due to extent of injury and free tissue transfer is contraindicated because of overall medical condition or vascular insufficiency, other pedicle flaps have been used, such as the groin flap. Recently, dermal substitutes have been used when a flap or full-thickness skin graft would have been necessary but was unavailable or unwise for the patient.[90]

Special Situations

Chemical burns of the hands are continuously flushed with water until the pain significantly decreases or stops. Acid burns may require 20 minutes of irrigation while alkali burns may require several hours of irrigation. Hydrofluoric acid burns are a special consideration. This type of burn is marked by slow onset of severe pain as the compound reaches deeper tissues. Hydrofluoric acid avidly binds tissue and circulating calcium, resulting in hypocalcemia that can lead to cardiac arrhythmia and arrest. Following water irrigation, a mixture of calcium gluconate in an aqueous jelly is placed into a surgical glove, which is then used to cover the burned hand. Effectiveness of treatment is assessed by relief of pain. If topical therapy does not relieve pain, then locally injected intra-arterial calcium may be necessary.[91]

As electrical current passes through tissue, heat is generated in the intervening muscle and bone, leading to damage and necrosis of these tissues. The skin itself tends to dissipate heat externally and may remain uninjured. The examiner must have a high index of suspicion for deeper pathology, including compartment syndrome and rhabdomyolysis of the forearm muscles. Criteria for performing fasciotomy are similar for other circumstances of compartment syndrome, although some surgeons perform fasciotomy empirically based on mechanism of injury. In the upper extremity, fasciotomy should include the volar, mobile wad, and dorsal compartments of the forearm via two incisions placed 180° to each other. Carpal tunnel release is performed as part of the forearm release. Fasciotomy of the thenar, hypothenar, and interosseous compartments of the hand also may be performed depending on site of current entry and clinical examination.

VASCULAR DISEASE

Vascular disorders encompass a broad spectrum of pathophysiologic states that results in aberrant microvascular perfusion, poten-tially threatening the viability of the hand or digits. Vascular disorders of the upper extremity and hand can be classified into acute or chronic categories.

Acute vascular injury to the hand can be due to trauma or iatrogenic causes. Traumatic vascular injury is discussed earlier in this chapter under Vascular Injuries. Iatrogenic causes include radial artery catheterization or drug injection. Acute vessel thrombosis may ensue, which may produce distal ischemia. The hand is assessed for perfusion within the injured adequacy of perfusion distally. Clinical examination and pencil Doppler evaluation may provide sufficient information. When these do not, contrast angiography remains the gold standard evaluation for vessel patency. It also can be used to direct localized thrombolytic therapy or as guidance for balloon embolectomy or vascular bypass, when indicated.

Chronic vascular disorders tend to develop more slowly and are seen in an older population. This category includes atherosclerosis,

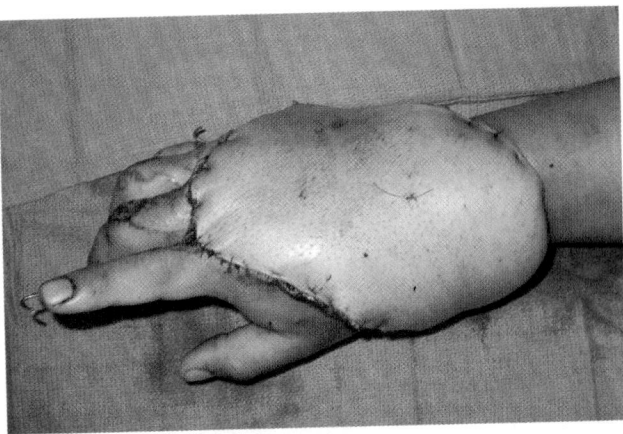

FIG. 44-29. Free anterolateral thigh flap reconstruction of a large dorsal hand wound. Once wound coverage is stable, this flap will need to be surgically revised to achieve proper contour.

progressive thrombosis (including hypothenar hammer syndrome), thromboangiitis obliterans (Buerger's disease), embolism, and vasospastic disease.

Atherosclerosis of the brachial, radial, or ulnar artery with acute thrombosis may require surgical exploration, thrombectomy, and possible saphenous vein interposition grafting. Although angioplasty is often used to treat atherosclerotic lesions in other vascular beds, radial and ulnar artery arteriosclerosis is best treated by surgery. Frequently, both radial and ulnar arteries are affected by disease, and hence, the patient presents with symptoms. The presence of a complete palmar arterial arch with good distal runoff may allow good results with repair of only the radial or the ulnar artery. Atherosclerotic changes in the hand and finger arteries are difficult to treat and often associated with severe systemic disease and diabetes. Distal vessels that can receive a bypass graft must be present on angiography to consider a bypass procedure. Amputation may be the best option in cases where pain or gangrene is sufficiently severe. Aneurysms can be resected and repaired primarily with interpositional vein grafts.

Hypothenar Hammer Syndrome

Aneurysmal thrombosis of the ulnar artery at the hook of the hamate is a common type of vascular occlusion in the hand. It is known as *hypothenar hammer syndrome* because it is often the result of repetitive trauma to the ulnar side of the palm associated with pounding as performed by laborers.[92] Symptoms present may include pain, numbness and tingling, weakness of grip, discoloration of the fingers, and even gangrene or ulcers of the fingertips. Thrombosis of the ulnar artery can dislodge, leading to embolism in the palmar arch or digital vessels.

If acute in onset, proximal occlusions may be embolectomized with a balloon catheter, or sometimes, under direct vision via an arteriotomy. Very distal embolism may require infusion of thrombolytics to dissolve clots and allow reperfusion. Large-vessel acute embolism and reperfusion may result in edema and compartment syndrome, requiring fasciotomy. A high index of suspicion must be maintained.

For the more common scenario of chronic, progressive occlusion, the involved segment of ulnar artery should be resected. There is disagreement in the literature regarding whether simple ligation and excision is sufficient for patients with sufficient distal flow or if all patients should undergo vascular reconstruction.[93] The authors' personal preference is to reconstruct all patients.

Vasospastic Disease

Raynaud's phenomenon results from excessive sympathetic nervous system stimulation. Perfusion is diminished and fingers often become cyanotic. Although the onset of the symptoms is benign, chronic episodes can result in atrophic changes and painful ulceration or gangrene of the digits. Raynaud's disease is present when Raynaud's phenomenon occurs without another associated disease. This disease predominately affects young women and is often bilateral. In contrast, Raynaud's syndrome occurs when Raynaud's phenomenon is associated with an underlying connective tissue disorder, such as scleroderma. Arterial stenosis is present due to disease changes in blood vessels as a result of the specific medical disorder.

Scleroderma is an autoimmune connective tissue disorder resulting in fibrosis and abnormal collagen deposition in tissue. Many organs can be affected, with the skin most commonly and noticeably involved. In this disease, blood vessels are injured by intimal fibrosis leading to microvascular disease. The vessels become subject to Raynaud's phenomenon and patients develop painful, ulcerated, and sometimes necrotic digits.

Sympathectomy can provide pain relief and healing of ulcers for patients with scleroderma and Raynaud's phenomenon. In this procedure, adventitia is stripped from the radial artery, ulnar artery, superficial palmar arch, and digital arteries in various combinations based on which digits are most affected. The decrease in sympathetic tone allows for vasodilation and increased blood flow. Patients being considered for sympathectomy typically undergo a trial of lidocaine infiltration near the vessels one intends to sympathectomize. If the patient notes significant distal pain relief and/or previously ischemic tissue improves in color, sympathectomy may provide the same results in a long-term fashion.[94]

CONGENITAL DIFFERENCES

Congenital differences in a newborn can be particularly disabling as the child learns to interact with the environment through the use of his/her hands. The degree of anomaly can range from minor, such as a digital disproportion, to severe, such as total absence of a bone. In recent years, increasing knowledge of the molecular basis of embryonic limb development has significantly enhanced the understanding of congenital differences. Congenital hand differences have an incidence of 1:1500 births. The two most common differences encountered are syndactyly and polydactyly.[95]

There are numerous classification systems for hand differences. The Swanson classification, adopted by the American Society for Surgery of the Hand, delineates seven groups (headers in bold below), organized based on anatomic parts affected by types of embryonic failures.[96]

Failure of Formation of Parts

The failure of the formation of parts is a group of congenital differences that forms as a result of a transverse or longitudinal arrest of development. Conditions in this group include radial club hand, a deformity that involves some or all of the tissues on the radial side of the forearm and hand, or ulnar club hand, which involves underdevelopment or absence of the ulnar-sided bones.

Failure of Separation of Parts

The failure of the separation of parts comprises conditions where the tissues of the hand fail to separate during embryogenesis. Syndactyly, in which two or more fingers are fused together, is the most common congenital hand deformity. Syndactyly occurs in seven out of every 10,000 live births. There is a familial tendency to develop this deformity. This deformity often involves both hands, and males are more often affected than females. Surgical release of syndactyly requires the use of local flaps to create a floor for the interdigital web space and to partially surface the adjacent sides of the separated digits (Fig. 44-30). Residual defects along the sides of the separated fingers are covered with full-thickness skin grafts. Surgery is indicated when the webbing occurs distal to the usual point of separation of the fingers and the webbing prohibits full use of the fingers. Surgery usually is performed at 6 to 12 months of age.

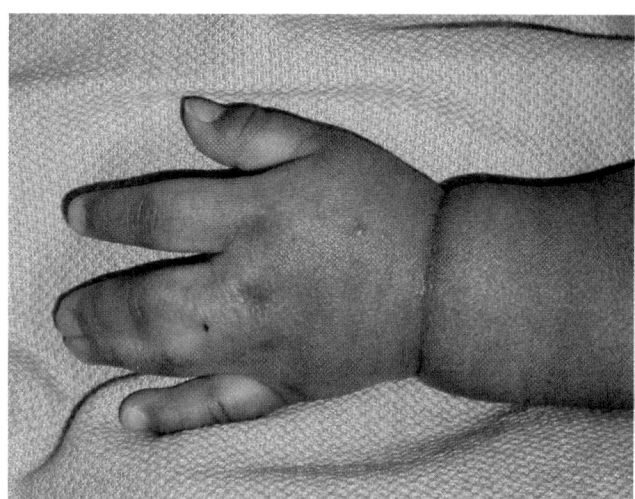

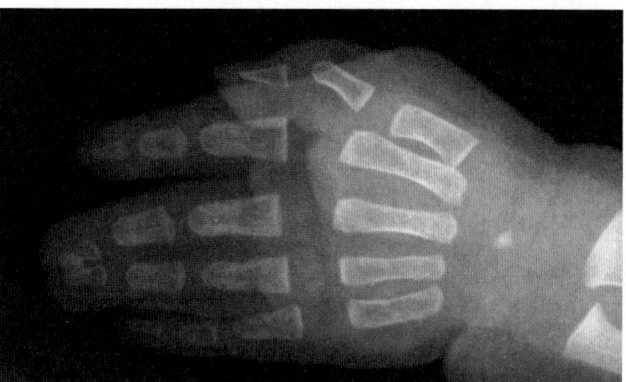

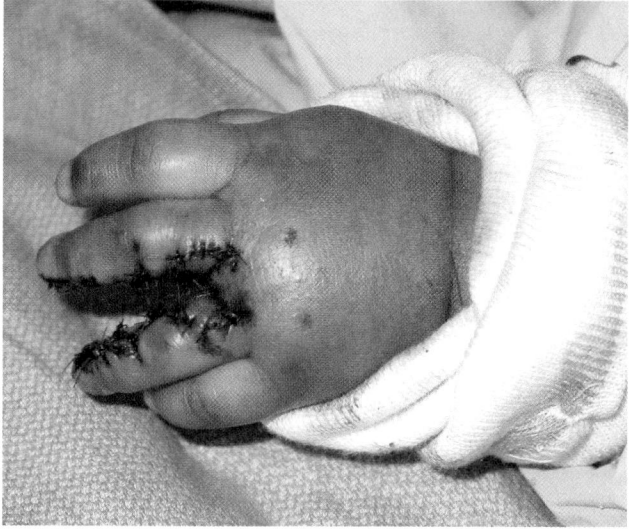

FIG. 44-30. Syndactyly. Hand of a 1-year-old patient with complex syndactyly between the long and ring finger. *Complex syndactyly* refers to fingers joined by bone or cartilaginous union, usually in a side-to-side fashion at the distal phalanges. The syndactyly is divided with interdigitating full-thickness flaps, a dorsal trapezoidal-shaped flap to resurface the floor of the web space, and full-thickness skin grafts. Note the skin grafts on the ulnar and radial sides of the new web space.

Duplications of Parts

Duplication of digits is also known as *polydactyly*. Radial polydactyly is usually manifest as thumb duplication. Wassel described a classification system for thumb duplications based on the level of bifurcation.[97] When two thumbs are present in the same hand, they are rarely both normal in size, alignment, and mobility. In the most common form of thumb duplication, a single broad MC supports two proximal phalanges, each of which support a distal phalanx. Optimal reconstruction requires merging of elements of both component digits. Usually the ulnar thumb is maintained. If the duplication occurs at the MP joint, the radial collateral ligament is preserved with the MC and attached to the proximal phalanx of the ulnar thumb. Surgery is usually performed at 6 to 12 months of age. Ulnar-sided polydactyly, may usually be treated by simple excision.

Overgrowth of Parts

Overgrowth of digits also is known a *macrodactyly*, which causes an abnormally large digit. In this situation, the hand and the forearm also may be involved. In this rare condition, all parts of a digit are affected; however, in most cases, only one digit is involved, and it is usually the index finger. This condition is more commonly seen in males. Surgical treatment of this condition is complex, and the outcomes may be less than desirable. Sometimes, amputation of the enlarged digit is recommended.

Undergrowth of Parts

Underdeveloped fingers or thumbs are associated with many congenital hand deformities. Surgical treatment is not always required to correct these deformities. Underdeveloped fingers may include the following: small digits (brachydactyly), missing muscles, underdeveloped or missing bones, or absence of a digit.

Constriction Band Syndrome

Constriction band syndrome is a set of congenital differences that occurs when a tissue band forms around the digit(s) arm in utero, causing problems that can affect blood flow and normal growth. This condition may be associated with other problems such as clubfoot, cleft lip, cleft palate, or other craniofacial anomalies. The cause of the ring constrictions is unknown. Some theories suggest that folds or bands in the amniotic membrane may be responsible for this condition.

Generalized Skeletal Problems and Syndromes

This is a rare and complex group of unclassified problems.

Treatment

In addition to the managements described above, treatments for congenital anomalies may include limb manipulation and stretching, splinting of the affected limbs, tendon transfers, external appliances (to help realign misshapen digits or hands), physical therapy (to help increase the strength and function of the hand), correction of contractures, skin grafts, and prosthetics.[98]

REFERENCES

Entries highlighted in bright blue are key references.

1. American Society for Surgery of the Hand, in: *The Hand: Examination and Diagnosis*, 3rd ed. New York: Churchill Livingstone, 1990, p 5.
2. Moore KL: The upper limb, in Moore KL (ed): *Clinically Oriented Anatomy*, 3rd ed. Baltimore, Md: Williams & Wilkins, 1992, p 501.
3. Schuind F, Cooney WP, Linscheid RL, et al: Force and pressure transmission through the normal wrist. A theoretical two-dimensional study in the posteroanterior plane. *J Biomech* 28:587, 1995.
4. Doyle JR: Anatomy of the flexor tendon sheath and pulley system: A current review. *J Hand Surg [Am]* 14:349, 1989.
5. Dumanian GA, Segalman K, Buehner JW, et al: Analysis of digital pulse-volume recordings with radial and ulnar artery compression. *Plast Reconstr Surg* 102:1993, 1998.
6. Green DP: General principles, in Green DP, Hotchkiss RN, Pedersen WC, et al (eds): *Green's Operative Hand Surgery*, 5th ed. Philadelphia, Pa: Churchill Livingstone, 2005, p 3.
7. Gilula LA: Carpal injuries: Analytic approach and case exercises. *AJR Am J Roentgenol* 133:503, 1979.

8. Cousins MJ, Mather LE: Clinical pharmacology of local anaesthetics. *Anaesth Inten Care* 8:257, 1980.

9. Lalonde D, Bell M, Benoit P, et al: A multicenter prospective study of 3,110 consecutive cases of elective epinephrine use in the fingers and hand: The Dalhousie Project clinical phase. *J Hand Surg [Am]* 30:1061, 2005.

10. Yousif NJ, Grunert BK, Forte RA, et al: A comparison of upper arm and forearm tourniquet tolerance. *J Hand Surg [Br]* 18:639, 1993.

11. Hastings H 2nd, Carroll C 4th: Treatment of closed articular fractures of the metacarpophalangeal and interphalangeal joints. *Hand Clin* 4:203, 1988.

12. Bond CD, Shin AY, McBride MT, et al: Percutaneous screw fixation or cast immobilization for nondisplaced scaphoid fractures. *J Bone Joint Surg [Am]* 83:483, 2001.

13. Mayfield JK, Johnson RP, Kilcoyne RF: The ligaments of the wrist and their functional significance. *Anat Rec* 186:417, 1976.

14. Kleinert HE, Kutz JE, Atasoy E, et al: Primary repair of flexor tendons. *Orthop Clin North Am* 4:865, 1973.

15. Komatsu S, Tamai S: Successful replantation of a completely cut-off thumb: Case report. *Plast Reconstr Surg* 42:374, 1968.

16. Lifchez SD, Marchant-Hanson J, Matloub HS, et al: Functional improvement with digital prosthesis use after multiple digit amputations. *J Hand Surg [Am]* 30:790, 2005.

17. Frandsen PA: V-Y plasty as treatment of finger tip amputations. *Acta Orthop Scand* 49:255, 1978.

18. Moberg E: The treatment of mutilating injuries of the upper limb. *Surg Clin North Am* 44:1107, 1964.

19. Melone CP Jr., Beasley RW, Carstens JH Jr.: The thenar flap—an analysis of its use in 150 cases. *J Hand Surg [Am]* 7:291, 1982.

20. Johnson RK, Iverson RE: Cross-finger pedicle flaps in the hand. *J Bone Joint Surg Am* 53:913, 1971.

21. Bekler H, Gokce A, Beyzadeoglu T, et al: The surgical treatment and outcomes of high-pressure injection injuries of the hand. *J Hand Surg Eur Vol* 32:394, 2007.

22. Mubarak SJ, Hargens AR: Acute compartment syndromes. *Surg Clin North Am* 63:539, 1983.

23. Gulgonen A: Compartment syndrome, in Green DP, Hotchkiss RN, Pedersen WC, et al (eds): *Green's Operative Hand Surgery*, 5th ed. Philadelphia, Pa: Churchill Livingstone, 2005, p 1985.

24. Wray RC Jr., Glunk R: Treatment of delayed union, nonunion, and malunion of the phalanges of the hand. *Ann Plast Surg* 22:14, 1989.

25. Munk B, Larsen CF: Bone grafting the scaphoid nonunion: A systematic review of 147 publications including 5,246 cases of scaphoid nonunion. *Acta Orthop Scand* 75:618, 2004.

26. Curtis RM: Capsulectomy of the interphalangeal joints of the fingers. *J Bone Joint Surg Am* 36:1219, 1954.

27. Nath RK, Mackinnon SE: Management of neuromas of the hand. *Hand Clin* 12:745, 1996.

28. Stanton-Hicks M, Jänig W, Hassenbusch S, et al: Reflex sympathetic dystrophy: Changing concepts and taxonomy. *Pain* 63:127, 1997.

29. Schürmann M, Zaspel J, Löhr P, et al: Imaging in early posttraumatic complex regional pain syndrome: A comparison of diagnostic methods. *Clin J Pain* 23:449, 2007.

30. Mackinnon SE: Pathophysiology of nerve compression. *Hand Clin* 18:231, 2002.

31. *http://www.cdc.gov/niosh/docs/97-141/ergotxt5a.html*: National Institutes for Occupational Safety and Health. Hand/Wrist Musculoskeletal disorders (Carpal Tunnel Syndrome, Hand/Wrist Tendinitis, and Hand/Arm Vibration Syndrome): Evidence for Work-Relatedness. NIOSH Publication No. 97-141 [accessed Feb. 11, 2009].

32. Williams TM, Mackinnon SE, Novak CB, et al: Verification of the pressure provocative test in carpal tunnel syndrome. *Ann Plast Surg* 29:8, 1992.

33. Green DP: Diagnostic and therapeutic value of carpal tunnel injection. *J Hand Surg [Am]* 9:850, 1984.

34. Trumble TE, Diao E, Abrams RA, et al: Single-portal endoscopic carpal tunnel release compared with open release: A prospective, randomized trial. *J Bone Joint Surg Am*; 84:1107, 2002.

35. Mackinnon SE, Novak CB: Compression neuropathies, in Green DP, Hotchkiss RN, Pedersen WC, et al (eds): *Green's Operative Hand Surgery*, 5th ed. Philadelphia, Pa: Churchill Livingstone, 2005, p 999.

36. Swanson AB: Implant resection arthroplasty of the proximal interphalangeal joint. *Orthop Clin North Am* 4:1007, 1973.

37. Branam BR, Tuttle HG, Stern PJ, et al: Resurfacing arthroplasty versus silicone arthroplasty for proximal interphalangeal joint osteoarthritis. *J Hand Surg [Am]* 32:775, 2007.

38. Burton RI, Pellegrini VD Jr.: Surgical management of basal joint arthritis of the thumb. Part II. Ligament reconstruction with tendon interposition arthroplasty. *J Hand Surg [Am]* 11:324, 1986.

39. Gray KV, Meals RA: Hematoma and distraction arthroplasty for thumb basal joint osteoarthritis: minimum 6.5 year follow-up evaluation. *J Hand Surg [Am]* 32:23, 2007.

40. Watson HK, Ballet FL: The SLAC wrist: Scapholunate advanced collapse patter of degenerative arthritis. *J Hand Surg [Am]* 9:358, 1984.

41. Stern PJ, Agabegi SS, Kiefhaber TR, et al: Proximal row carpectomy. *J Bone Joint Surg Am* 87:166, 2005.

42. Goldfarb CA, Stern PJ, Kiefhaber TR: Palmar midcarpal instability: The results of treatment with 4-corner arthrodesis. *J Hand Surg [Am]* 29:258, 2004.

43. Feldon P, Terrono AL, Nalebuff EA, et al: Rheumatoid arthritis and other connective tissue disorders, in Green DP, Hotchkiss RN, Pedersen WC, et al (eds): *Green's Operative Hand Surgery*, 5th ed. Philadelphia, Pa: Churchill Livingstone, 2005, p 2049.

44. Swanson AB: Finger joint replacement by silicone rubber implants and the concept of implant fixation by encapsulation. *Ann Rheum Dis* 28:47, 1969.

45. Elliot D, Ragoowansi R: Dupuytren's disease secondary to acute injury, infection or operation distal to the elbow in the ipsilateral upper limb—a historical review. *J Hand Surg [Br]* 30:148, 2005.

46. Luck JV: Dupuytren's contracture: A new concept of the pathogenesis correlated with surgical management. *J Bone Joint Surg Am* 41:635, 1959.

47. McGrouther DA. Dupuytren's contracture, in Green DP, Hotchkiss RN, Pedersen WC, et al (eds): *Green's Operative Hand Surgery*, 5th ed. Philadelphia, Pa: Churchill Livingstone, 2005, p 159.

48. Badalamente MA, Hurst LC: Efficacy and safety of injectable mixed collagenase subtypes in the treatment of Dupuytren's contracture. *J Hand Surg [Am]* 32:767, 2007.

49. Saar JD, Grothaus PC: Dupuytren's disease: An overview. *Plast Reconstr Surg* 106:125, 2000.

50. Prosser R, Conolly WB: Complications following surgical treatment for Dupuytren's contracture. *J Hand Ther* 9:344, 1996.

51. Wolfe SW: Tenosynovitis, in: Green DP, Hotchkiss RN, Pederson WC, et al (eds): *Green's Operative Hand Surgery*, 5th ed. Philadelphia, Pa: Churchill Livingstone, 2005, p 2137.

52. Hueston JT, Wilson WF: The aetiology of trigger finger explained on the basis of intratendinous architecture. *Hand* 4:257, 1972.

53. Fahey JJ, Bollinger JA: Trigger-finger in adults and children. *J Bone Joint Surg Am* 36:1200, 1954.

54. Eastwood DM, Gupta KJ, Johnson DP: Percutaneous release of the trigger finger: An office procedure. *J Hand Surg [Am]* 17:114, 1992.

55. Gilberts EC, Beekman WH, Stevens HJ, et al: Prospective randomized trial of open versus percutaneous surgery for trigger digits. *J Hand Surg [Am]* 26:497, 2001.

56. Moore JS: De Quervain's tenosynovitis: Stenosing tenosynovitis of the first dorsal compartment. *J Occup Environ Med* 39:990, 1997.

57. Finkelstein H: Stenosing tendovaginitis at the radial styloid process. *J Bone Joint Surg* 12:509, 1930.

58. Weiss AP, Akelman E, Tabatabai M: Treatment of de Quervain's disease. *J Hand Surg [Am]* 19:595, 1994.

59. Jackson WT, Viegas SF, Coon TM: Anatomical variations in the first extensor compartment of the wrist. A clinical and anatomical study. *J Bone Joint Surg [Am]* 68:923, 1986.

60. Littler JW, Freedman DM, Malerich MM: Compartment reconstruction for de Quervain's disease. *J Hand Surg [Br]* 27:242, 2002.

61. Hanlon DP, Luellen JR: Intersection syndrome: A case report and review of the literature. *J Emerg Med* 17:969, 1999.

62. Grundberg AB, Reagan DS: Pathologic anatomy of the forearm: Intersection syndrome. *J Hand Surg [Am]* 10:299, 1985.

63. Hausman MR, Lisser SP: Hand infections. *Orthop Clin North Am* 23:171, 1992.

64. Bach HG, Steffin B, Chhadia AM, et al: Community-associated methicillin-resistant *Staphylococcus aureus* hand infections in an urban setting. *J Hand Surg [Am]* 32:380, 2007.

65. Gill MJ, Arlette J, Buchan KA: Herpes simplex virus infection of the hand. A profile of 79 cases. *Am J Med* 84:89, 1988.

66. Kanavel AB: The treatment of acute suppurative tenosynovitis—discussion of technique, in: *Infections of the Hand; A Guide to the Surgical Treatment of Acute and Chronic Suppurative Processes in the Fingers, Hand, and Forearm*, 5th ed. Philadelphia: Lea and Farbinger, 1925, p 985.

67. Dickson-Wright A: Tendon sheath infections. *Proc Roy Soc Med* 37:504, 1943.

68. Gosain AK, Markison RE: Catheter irrigation for treatment of pyogenic closed space infections of the hand. *Br J Plast Surg* 44:270, 1991.

69. Boles SD, Schmidt CC: Pyogenic flexor tenosynovitis. *Hand Clin* 14:567, 1998.

70. Michon J: Phlegmon of the tendon sheaths. *Ann Chir* 28:277, 1974.

71. Kour AK, Looi KP, Phone MH, et al: Hand infections in patients with diabetes. *Clin Orthop Relat Res* 331:238, 1996.

72. Nelson CL, Sawmiller S, Phalen GS: Ganglions of the wrist and hand. *J Bone Joint Surg [Am]* 54:1459, 1972.

73. Leffert RD: Lipomas of the upper extremity. *J Bone Joint Surg [Am]* 54:1262, 1972.

74. Athanasian EA: Principles of diagnosis and management of musculoskeletal tumors, in Green DP, Hotchkiss RN, Pederson WC, et al (eds): *Green's Operative Hand Surgery*, 3rd ed. New York, NY: Churchill Livingstone, 1993, p 2206.

75. Bauer RD, Lewis MM, Posner MA: Treatment of enchondromas of the hand with allograft bone. *J Hand Surg [Am]* 13:908, 1988.

76. Jaffe HL, Lichtenstein HL, Elsutro CJ: Pigmented villonodular synovitis, bursitis, and tenosynovitis. *Arch Pathol* 31:731, 1941.

77. Jaffe HL, Lichtenstein L, Portis RB: Giant cell tumor of bone. Its pathologic appearance, grading, supposed variants and treatment. *Arch Pathol* 30:993, 1940.

78. Campanacci M: Giant cell tumor, in: *Bone and Soft Tissue Tumors: Clinical Features, Imaging, Pathology and Treatment*, 2nd ed. New York, NY: Springer-Verlag, 1999, p 99.

79. Cottalorda J, Bourelle S, Stephan JL, et al: Radiologic case study. Giant-cell tumor of the wrist in a skeletally immature girl. *Orthopedics* 25:550, 2002.

80. Witthaut J, Steffens K, Koob E: Reliable treatment of pyogenic granuloma of the hand. *J Hand Surg [Br]* 19:791, 1994.

81. TerKonda SP, Perdikis G: Non-melanotic skin tumors of the upper extremity. *Hand Clin* 20:293, 2004.

82. Glat PM, Shapiro RL, Roses DF, et al: Management considerations for melanonychia striata and melanoma of the hand. *Hand Clin* 11:183, 1995.

83. Balch CM, Soong SJ, Smith T, et al: Long-term results of a prospective surgical trial comparing 2 cm vs. 4 cm excision margins for 740 patients with 1-4 mm melanomas. *Ann Surg Oncol* 8:101, 2001.

84. Heaton KM, El-Naggar A, Ensign LG, et al: Surgical management and prognostic factors in patients with subungual melanoma. *Ann Surg* 219:197, 1994.

85. Sheridan RL: Acute hand burns in children: Management and long-term outcome based on a 10-year experience with 698 injured hands. *Ann Surg* 229:558, 1999.

86. Robson MC, Smith DJ: Burned hand, in Jurkiewicz MJ (ed): *Plastic Surgery: Principles and Practices*. St Louis, Mo: C.V. Mosby Co, 1990.

87. Achauer BM: *Burn Reconstruction*. New York, NY: Thieme Medical Publishers, 1991.

88. Sheridan RL: Comprehensive management of burns. *Curr Prob Surg* 38:641, 2001.

89. Goodwin CW, McGuire MS, McManus WF, et al: Prospective study of burn wound excision of the hands. *J Trauma* 23:510, 1983.

90. Haslik W, Kamolz LP, Nathschläger G, et al: First experiences with the collagen-elastin matrix Matriderm as a dermal substitute in severe burn injuries of the hand. *Burns* 33:364, 2007.

91. Hatzifotis M, Williams A, Muller M, et al: Hydrofluoric acid burns. *Burns* 30:156, 2004.

92. Conn J Jr., Bergan JJ, Bell JL: Hypothenar hammer syndrome: Posttraumatic digital ischemia. *Surgery* 68:1122, 1970.

93. Zimmerman NB, Zimmerman SI, McClinton MA, et al: Long-term recovery following surgical treatment for ulnar artery occlusion. *J Hand Surg [Am]* 19:17, 1994.

94. Ruch DS, Holden M, Smith BP, et al: Periarterial sympathectomy in scleroderma patients: Intermediate-term follow-up. *J Hand Surg [Am]* 27:258, 2002.

95. Giele H, Giele C, Bower C, et al: The incidence and epidemiology of congenital upper limb anomalies: A total population study. *J Hand Surg [Am]* 26:628, 2001.

96. Swanson AB: A classification for congenital limb malformations. *J Hand Surg [Am]* 1:8, 1976.

97. Wassel HD: The results of surgery for polydactyly of the thumb. A review. *Clin Orthop Relat Res* 64:175, 1969

98. McCarroll HR: Congenital anomalies: A 25-year overview. *J Hand Surg [Am]* 25:1007, 2000.

Plastic and Reconstructive Surgery

Joseph E. Losee, Michael Gimbel, J. Peter Rubin,
Christopher G. Wallace, and Fu-Chan Wei

HISTORICAL BACKGROUND

The field of plastic surgery focuses on the restoration of form and function to those who have congenital and acquired deformities. Plastic surgery routinely addresses new problems and challenges; therefore, the plastic surgeon must have an expert knowledge of anatomy and surgical technique to address new challenges.

The word *plastic* is derived from the Greek *plastikos*, meaning "to mold." Although the term *plastic surgery* can be found in several medical writings from the eighteenth and nineteenth centuries, it was John Staige Davis who established the name of the specialty with the 1919 publication of his book *Plastic Surgery—Its Principles and Practice.*

Certainly, for centuries plastic surgery operations have been performed. One of the earliest accounts of reconstructive surgery can be found in the *Sushruta Samhita*, an early text from the sixth or seventh century B.C. by the practitioner Sushruta. In this writing, the reconstruction of an amputated nose with a pedicled forehead flap and the reconstruction of the ear with cheek flaps was described. In addition, in the first century A.D., the Roman physicians Aulus Cornelius Celsus and Paulus Aegineta described operations for traumatic injuries of the face.

The first textbook of plastic surgery is believed to be Gaspara Tagliacozzi's 1597 publication *De Curtorum Chirurgia per Insitionem.* This text describes the reconstruction of the nose with a pedicled arm flap. The nineteenth century saw advances in reconstructive surgery, including Giuseppe Baronio's successful grafting of sheepskin. The techniques for perfecting human skin grafting followed in the later part of the century.

Great advances in plastic surgery occurred as a result of the first and second world wars. Out of the fields of dental surgery, otolaryngology, ophthalmology, and general surgery, the discipline of plastic surgery was established. The founders of the field include Sir Harold Gillies, an otolaryngologist, who established a center for the treatment of maxillofacial injuries in England; V. H. Kazanjian, a dental surgeon from Boston, who established a center in France for the treatment of facial injuries incurred in World War II; and Vilray P. Blair, from St. Louis, who established centers for the treatment of soft tissue and maxillofacial reconstruction for the U.S. Army. With the onset of World War II, centers of excellence for hand reconstruction appeared as well.

In the last 50 years, advances in the field of plastic surgery have included the transplantation of both autologous and allogeneic tissue, tissue expansion, techniques of moving tissues regionally within the body as muscle and myocutaneous flaps, the distant transfer of free flaps using microsurgery, replantation of traumatically amputated extremities and digits, and the emergence of the field of craniofacial surgery. The future of plastic surgery will likely see further advances in the realms of regenerative medicine, fetal surgery, and reconstructive transplantation with composite tissue allotransplants.

GENERAL PRINCIPLES

Skin Incisions

Human skin exists in a state of tension created by internal and external factors. Externally, skin and underlying subcutaneous tissue are acted on by gravity and clothing. Internally, skin is subjected to forces generated by underlying muscles, joint extension and flexion, and tethering of fibrous tissues from zones of adherence. As a result, when skin is incised linearly it gapes to variable degrees. When a circular skin excision is performed, the skin defect assumes an elliptical configuration paralleling the lines of greatest tension. Carl Langer, an anatomist from Vienna, first fully described these tension lines in the mid-1800s based on his studies of fresh cadavers.[1] A. F. Borges described another set of skin lines that, different from Langer's lines, reflect the vectors of relaxed skin tension.[2] Although the term *Langer's lines* often is used interchangeably with the term *relaxed skin tension lines*, the former lines describe skin tension vectors observed in the stretched integument of cadavers exhibiting rigor mortis, whereas the latter lines lay perpendicular to and more accurately reflect the action of underlying muscle.[2] Kraissl's lines, which run along natural wrinkles and skin creases, tend also to follow the relaxed skin tension lines (Fig. 45-1). Relaxed skin tension lines may be exploited to create incisions and reconstructions that minimize anatomic distortion and improve cosmesis. In areas of anatomic mobility, such as the neck or over joints, incisions are oriented less for aesthetic reasons and more with the goal of avoiding scar contractures and subsequent functional compromise. In general, incisions are placed perpendicular to the action of the joint.

There are situations, however, in which the direction of the incision has been pre-established, as in acute lacerations, burns, or old contracted and distorting scars. In these circumstances the principles of proper incision placement can be combined with simple surgical techniques to reorient the scar and lessen the deformity. The Z-plasty technique uses the transposition of random skin flaps both to break up a linear scar and to release a scar contracture through lengthening (Fig. 45-2; Table 45-1).

W-plasty is the technique of scar excision and reconstruction in zigzag fashion to camouflage the resulting scar. In areas where pressure or shearing forces are expected, as in weightbearing areas, incision planning should be performed carefully to minimize the effect of antagonistic forces on the healing incision. This point is discussed further in "Pressure Sore Treatment."

Wound Healing

The fundamentals of plastic surgery are based on wound-healing physiology. Wound repair consists of an exquisitely regulated symphony of molecular and cellular instruments that act in concert to restore the local tissue environment to prewound conditions. Metabolic imbalances in the wound milieu drive this orchestration and continue to direct it until healing resolves the mechanical and meta-

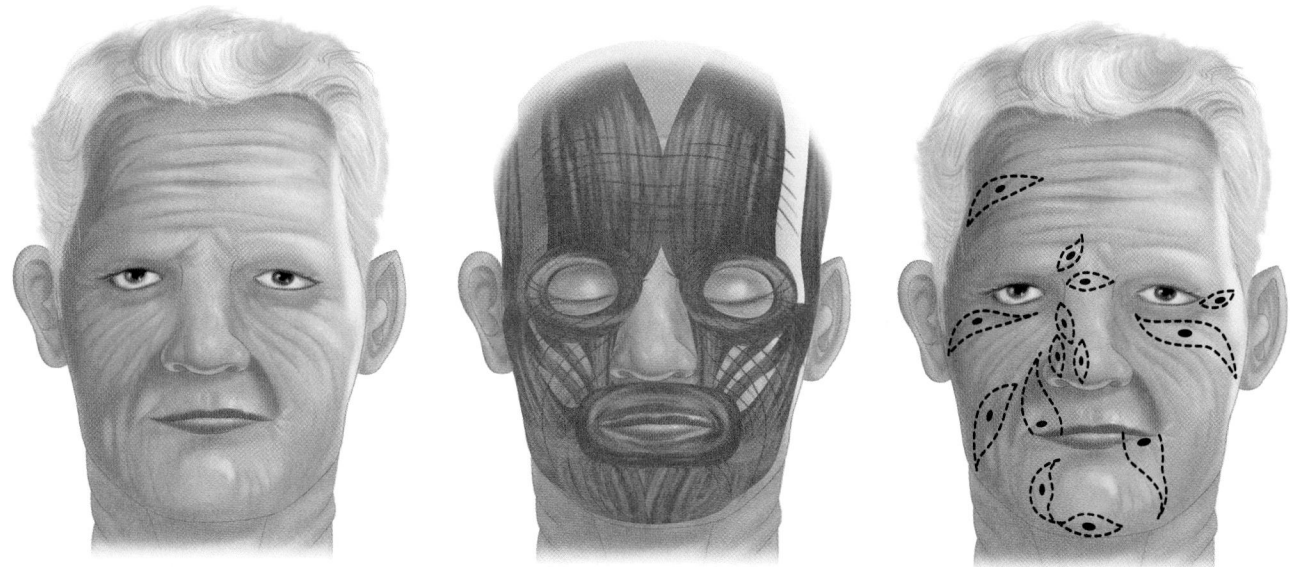

FIG. 45-1. Relaxed skin tension lines. (*Reprinted with permission from Wilhelmi et al.[1]*)

bolic problems. Although a detailed review of wound physiology is presented elsewhere in this text, it is useful to emphasize several points.

Tissue injury, be it mechanical or metabolic, profoundly and instantly disrupts the tissue microenvironment and sets into motion a cascade of events that combine to re-establish the environmental status quo. Disrupted blood vessels fill the wound space with red blood cells and plasma. Injured cells release factor III (thromboplastin), which accelerates the clotting cascade. Clotting factors in the plasma are activated, and the coagulation cascade forms thrombin and eventually fibrin. Simultaneously, the complement system activates and produces chemoattractive complement protein fragments. Platelets, activated by thrombin and exposed collagen, release a number of growth factors and cytokines. Traumatized vessels contract in response to both direct physical stimulation (mediated by the autonomic nervous system) and prostaglandins released by platelets. Intact local microvasculature vasodilates and leaks plasma in response to inflammatory mediators such as histamine, kinins, and serotonin. These early events, and others, establish hemostasis and inflammation.[3]

Platelet activation initiates the first major escalation in the inflammatory response. Within minutes platelets release a number of signaling molecules from their α-granules to attract macro-

phages, polymorphonuclear cells (PMNs), fibroblasts, and vascular endothelial cells. Within a few hours of injury, PMNs and macrophages invade the wound space and begin to remove tissue debris, coagulation proteins, and bacteria. Although both PMNs and macrophages begin to marginate early, PMNs dominate during the first few days. PMNs also constitute the primary defense against invading organisms that have breached the epithelial barrier. PMNs and macrophages, in concert with the complement system, form the basis of "natural" or "nonspecific" immunity. If there is no infection or foreign material, the neutrophil population quickly diminishes by the second day, whereas macrophages continue to amass.[3]

Macrophages become the major population by the third day after injury. These cells then dominate the wound region for days to weeks. Macrophages are thought to be the "masterminds" behind the complicated and finely tuned array of repair events that characterizes the proliferative phase of healing. Like neutrophils, activated macrophages continue the task of wound débridement. They are a rich source of degradative enzymes that process the extracellular matrix to make room for remodeling. Tightly coordinated release of the many growth factors, colony-stimulating factors, interleukins, interferons, and cytokines gives the macrophage the ability to regu-

KEY POINTS

1. Plastic surgery is the field of surgery that addresses congenital and acquired defects, striving to return form and function.

2. Children diagnosed with cleft and craniofacial anomalies benefit from interdisciplinary care at a specialized center focusing on team care. Long-term follow-up during growth and development is critical for optimal outcomes.

3. Reconstructive surgery attempts to restore form and function through techniques that include skin grafting, use of muscle flaps, bone grafting, tissue expansion, free tissue transfer with microsurgery, and replantation.

4. Aesthetic surgery is surgery performed to reshape the normal structure of the body to improve the patient's appearance and self-esteem. Patients undergoing aesthetic surgery present a unique challenge. The most important outcome parameter is patient satisfaction, and therefore a thorough understanding of the patient's motivations, goals, and expectations is critical.

5. Plastic surgery has been a field of innovation. The future of the specialty likely includes advancements in the areas of regenerative medicine, fetal surgery, and reconstructive transplantation with composite tissue allotransplants.

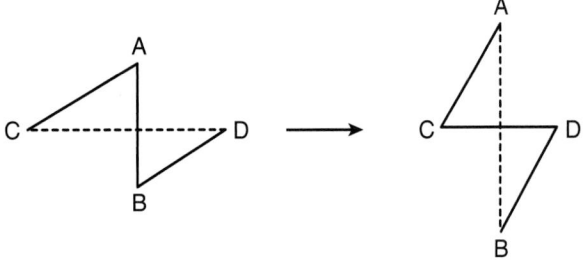

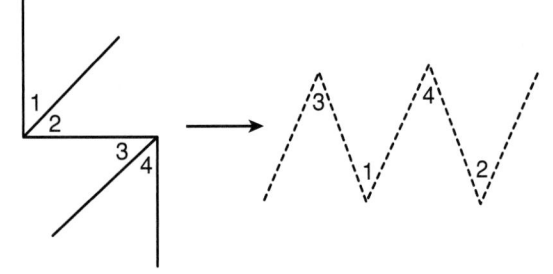

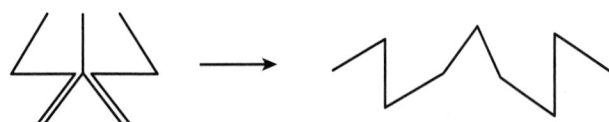

FIG. 45-2. Schematic of the Z-plasty technique. *Top:* Simple Z-plasty. *Middle:* Four-flap Z-plasty. *Bottom:* Five-flap Z-plasty. *(Modified with permission from Hudson DA: Some thoughts on choosing a Z-plasty: The Z made simple.* Plast Reconstr Surg *106:665, 2000.)*

late migration, proliferation, and specific protein synthesis of multiple cell lines. Macrophages lead the characteristic procession of new tissue into the wound dead space. Immature, replicating fibroblasts follow the macrophages. Mature fibroblasts then advance into the wound space and are, in turn, followed by newly forming capillary buds, the last cells in the procession.[3]

As previously mentioned, injury perturbs the microenvironment and leads to the autoamplifying inflammatory phase. As a result of these processes, three changes occur in the wound: the environment becomes hypoxic, acidotic, and hyperlactated. There is at least one biochemical pathway by which this low redox potential state can signal cells to take biologic action—the adenosine diphosphoribose (ADPR) system. Specifically, recent evidence has shown that alterations of the polyADPR system affect regulation of collagen and vascular endothelial growth factor (VEGF) transcription.[3] Thus, the metabolic state that is so deranged in the wound microenvironment is intimately linked to altered cellular function, which leads to reparative cell phenotypes.

TABLE 45-1	Tissue lengthening with Z-plasty

Type of Z-Plasty	Increase in Length of Central Limb (%)
Simple 45-degree	50
Simple 60-degree	75
Simple 90-degree	100
Four-flap with 60-degree angles	150
Double-opposing	75
Five-flap	125

Source: Modified with permission from Hudson DA: Some thoughts on choosing a Z-plasty: The Z made simple. *Plast Reconstr Surg* 106:665, 2000.

TABLE 45-2	Preoperative management

- Assess and optimize cardiopulmonary function; correct hypertension.
- Treat vasoconstriction: attend to blood volume, thermoregulatory vasoconstriction, pain, and anxiety.
- Assess recent nutrition and provide treatment as appropriate.
- Treat existing infection.
- Assess wound risk using the SENIC index.
- Start administration of vitamin A in patients taking glucocorticoids.
- Maintain tight blood glucose control.

SENIC = Study on the Efficacy of Nosocomial Infection Control.
Source: Modified with permission from Hunt TK, Hopf HW: Wound healing and wound infection: What surgeons and anesthesiologists can do. *Surg Clin North Am* 77:587, 1997. Copyright Elsevier.

After inflammation has begun, fibroblasts are attracted by many stimuli and then proliferate and migrate into the site of injury. Fibroblasts are the major producers of collagen in the repair response. Substances that increase collagen deposition and maturation include lactate, oxygen, and growth factors. Lack of these agents and steroid treatments decrease collagen in wounds.

Macrophages also usher along angiogenesis, largely through the release of VEGF. VEGF production is upregulated by the same wound metabolic environment that stimulates collagen production. Also like collagen synthesis, VEGF release is increased by hyperoxia. As neovascularization takes place, many of the conditions that signaled the start of the inflammatory and proliferative phases are resolved, and the wound-healing response recedes.

Epidermal cells are attracted to the healing wound by the same cytokines that attract other wound cells. Epithelialization proceeds best in a moist environment with high oxygen tension.[3]

Preoperative, intraoperative, and postoperative interventions may be taken by the surgeon to minimize infection and optimize wound healing (Tables 45-2 to 45-4). These measures all draw on what we understand of the physiologic wound-healing process.

Skin Grafts and Skin Substitutes

Discussion of skin grafting requires a basic review of skin anatomy. Skin is comprised of 5% epidermis and 95% dermis. The dermis contains sebaceous glands, whereas sweat glands and hair follicles are located in the subcutaneous tissue. The dermal thickness and concentration of skin appendages vary widely from one location to another on the body. The skin vasculature is superficial to the superficial fascial system and parallels the skin surface. The cutaneous vessels branch at right angles to penetrate subcutaneous tissue and arborize in the dermis, finally forming capillary tufts between dermal papillae.[4]

TABLE 45-3	Intraoperative management

- Administer appropriate prophylactic antibiotics at start of procedure. Keep antibiotic levels high during long operations.
- Keep patient warm.
- Maintain gentle surgical technique with minimal use of ties and cautery.
- Keep wounds moist.
- Perform irrigation in cases of contamination.
- Elevate tissue oxygen tension by increasing the level of inspired oxygen.
- Delay closure of heavily contaminated wounds.
- Use appropriate sutures (and skin tapes).
- Use appropriate dressings.

Source: Modified with permission from Hunt TK, Hopf HW: Wound healing and wound infection: What surgeons and anesthesiologists can do. *Surg Clin North Am* 77:587, 1997. Copyright Elsevier.

TABLE 45-4 Postoperative management

- Keep patient warm.
- Provide analgesia to keep patient comfortable, if not pain free.
- Keep up with third-space losses. Remember that fever increases fluid losses.
- Assess perfusion and react to abnormalities.
- Avoid diuresis until pain is gone and patient is warm.
- Assess losses (including thermal losses) if wound is open.
- Assess need for parenteral/enteral nutrition and respond.
- Continue to control hypertension and hyperglycemia.

Source: Modified with permission from Hunt TK, Hopf HW: Wound healing and wound infection: What surgeons and anesthesiologists can do. *Surg Clin North Am* 77:587, 1997. Copyright Elsevier.

Skin grafting dates back >3000 years to India, where forms of the technique were used to resurface nasal defects in thieves who were punished for their crimes with nose amputation. Modern skin grafting methods include split-thickness grafts, full-thickness grafts, and composite tissue grafts (Table 45-5). Each technique has advantages and disadvantages. Selection of a particular technique depends on the requirements of the defect to be reconstructed, the quality of the recipient bed, and the availability of donor site tissue.

Split-Thickness Grafts

Split-thickness skin grafting represents the simplest method of superficial reconstruction in plastic surgery. Many of the characteristics of a split-thickness graft are determined by the amount of dermis present. Less dermis translates into less primary contraction (the degree to which a graft shrinks in dimensions after harvesting and before grafting), more secondary contraction (the degree to which a graft contracts during healing), and better chance of graft survival. Thin-split grafts have low primary contraction, high secondary contraction, and high reliability of graft take, often even in imperfect recipient beds. Thin grafts, however, tend to heal with abnormal pigmentation and poor durability compared with thick-split grafts and full-thickness grafts. Thick-split grafts have more primary contraction, show less secondary contraction, and may take less hardily. Split grafts may be meshed to expand the surface area that can be covered. This technique is particularly useful when a large area must be resurfaced, as in major burns. Meshed grafts usually also have enhanced reliability of engraftment, because the fenestrations allow for egress of wound fluid and excellent contour matching of the wound bed by the graft. The fenestrations in meshed grafts re-epithelialize by secondary intention from the surrounding graft skin. The major drawbacks of meshed grafts are poor cosmetic appearance and high secondary contraction. Meshing ratios used usually range from 1:1.5 to 1:6, with higher ratios associated with magnified drawbacks.

Full-Thickness Grafts

By definition full-thickness skin grafts include the epidermis and the complete layer of dermis from the donor skin. The subcutaneous

TABLE 45-5 Classification of skin grafts

Type	Description	Thickness (in)
Split thickness	Thin (Thiersch-Ollier)	0.006–0.012
	Intermediate (Blair-Brown)	0.012–0.018
	Thick (Padgett)	0.018–0.024
Full thickness	Entire dermis (Wolfe-Krause)	Variable
Composite tissue	Full-thickness skin with additional tissue (subcutaneous fat, cartilage, muscle)	Variable

Source: Modified with permission from Andreassi A, Bilenchi R, Biagioli M, et al: Classification and pathophysiology of skin grafts. *Clin Dermatol* 23:332, 2005. Copyright Elsevier.

tissue is carefully removed from the deep surface of the dermis to maximize the potential for engraftment. Full-thickness grafts are associated with the least secondary contraction upon healing, the best cosmetic appearance, and the highest durability. Because of this, they are frequently used in reconstructing superficial wounds of the face and the hands. These grafts require pristine, well-vascularized recipient beds without bacterial colonization, previous irradiation, or atrophic wound tissue.

Graft Take

Skin graft take occurs in three phases, imbibition, inosculation, and revascularization. Plasmatic imbibition refers to the first 24 to 48 hours after skin grafting, during which time a thin film of fibrin and plasma separates the graft from the underlying wound bed. It remains controversial whether this film provides nutrients and oxygen to the graft or merely a moist environment to maintain the ischemic cells temporarily until a vascular supply is re-established. After 48 hours a fine vascular network begins to form within the fibrin layer. These new capillary buds interface with the deep surface of the dermis and allow for transfer of some nutrients and oxygen. This phase, called *inosculation*, transitions into revascularization, the process by which new blood vessels either directly invade the graft or anastomose to open dermal vascular channels and restore the pink hue of skin. These phases are generally complete by 4 to 5 days after graft placement. During these initial few days the graft is most susceptible to deleterious factors such as infection, mechanical shear forces, and hematoma or seroma.[4]

Composite Grafts

Composite tissue grafts are donor tissue containing more than just epidermis and dermis. They commonly include subcutaneous fat, cartilage and perichondrium, and muscle. Although less common than skin grafts, grafts of this type are particularly useful in select cases of nasal reconstruction. Excision of the thick skin of the nasal lobule may create too deep a defect to reconstruct with a full-thickness skin graft. The ear lobe composite graft provides thicker coverage with good color match and a fairly inconspicuous donor site (Fig. 45-3). Similarly, the root of the helix of the ear may be used to reconstruct the alar rim, providing skin coverage, cartilaginous support, and internal lining in a single technique.

Flaps

A flap is a vascularized block of tissue that is mobilized from its donor site and transferred to another location, adjacent or remote, for reconstructive purposes. The difference between a graft and a flap is that a graft brings no vascular pedicle and derives its blood flow from recipient site revascularization, whereas a flap arrives with its blood supply intact.

Random Pattern Flaps

Random pattern flaps have a blood supply based on small, unnamed blood vessels in the dermal-subdermal plexus, as opposed to the discrete, well-described, directional vessels of axial pattern flaps (Fig. 45-4). Random flaps are typically used to reconstruct relatively small, full-thickness defects that are not amenable to skin grafting. Unlike axial pattern flaps, random flaps are limited by their geometry. The generally accepted reliable length:width ratio for a random flap is 3:1. Exceptions to this rule abound, however. There are many different types of random cutaneous flaps that differ in geometry and mobility. A *transposition flap* is rotated about a pivot point into an adjacent defect (Fig. 45-5). A *Z-plasty* is a type of transposition flap in which two flaps are rotated, each into the donor site of the other, to achieve central limb lengthening (see Fig. 45-2). Another common transposition flap is the *rhomboid (Limberg) flap* (Fig. 45-6). The *bipedicle flap* is comprised of two mirror-image transposition flaps that share their distal, undivided margin. *Rotational flaps* are similar to transpositional flaps but differ in that they are semicircular (Fig. 45-7). *Advancement flaps* slide forward or backward along the

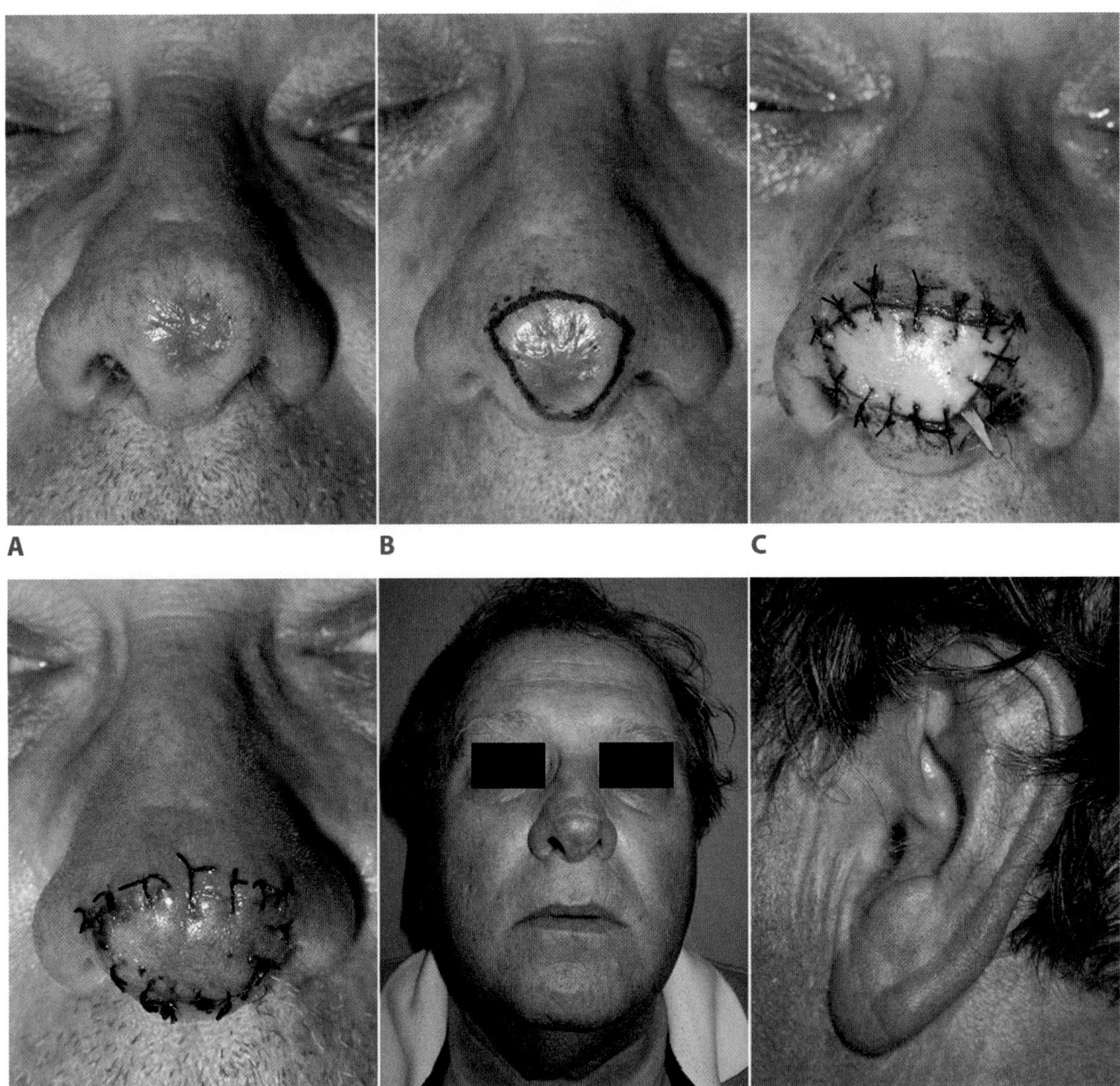

FIG. 45-3. Composite graft reconstruction of nasal lobule. **A.** Scarred lobule from previous lesion excision. **B.** Scar excision markings. **C.** Insetting of composite ear lobe skin and subcutaneous fat graft. **D.** Postoperative day 3; note the pink hue of revascularization. **E.** Appearance at 5 weeks postoperatively. **F.** Donor site at 5 weeks postoperatively.

flap's long axis. Two common variants include the rectangular advancement flap and the V-Y advancement flap (Fig. 45-8). Like transposition flaps, *interpolation flaps* rotate about a pivot point. Unlike transposition flaps, they are inset into defects near, but not adjacent, to the donor site. An example of an interpolation flap is the thenar flap for fingertip reconstruction (Fig. 45-9).

Fasciocutaneous and Myocutaneous Flaps

The *composition* of a flap is its tissue components. For example, a cutaneous flap contains skin and a variable amount of subcutaneous tissues. A fasciocutaneous flap contains skin, fascia, and intervening subcutaneous tissues. A muscle flap contains muscle only, whereas a myocutaneous flap contains muscle with its overlying skin and intervening tissues. An osseous flap contains vascularized bone

only, whereas an osteomyocutaneous flap contains in addition muscle, skin, and subcutaneous tissues.

The *contiguity* of a flap describes its source. Local flaps are transferred from a position adjacent to the defect. Regional flaps are from the same anatomic region of the body as the defect (e.g., the lower extremity region or the head and neck region). Distant flaps are transferred from a different anatomic region to the defect. Local, regional, and distant flaps may be pedicled, in that they remain attached to the blood supply at their source. Distant flaps may also be transferred as *free flaps* by microsurgical techniques; these are completely detached from the body, and their blood supply is reinstated by anastomoses to recipient vessels close to the defect.

Axial pattern flaps are based on an anatomically defined configuration of vessels.[6] Arising from the aorta are arteries that supply the internal viscera and other deep vessels that divide to form the main

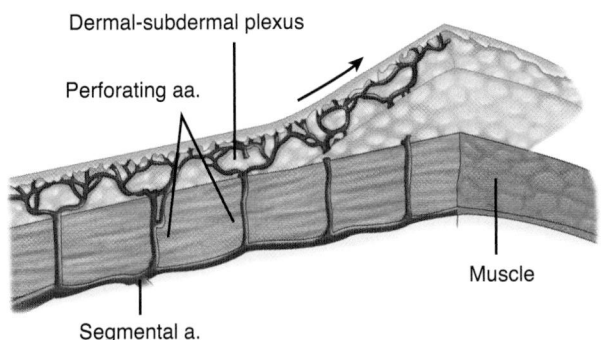

FIG. 45-4. Random pattern flap architecture. a. = artery. *(Reproduced with permission from Aston et al.[5])*

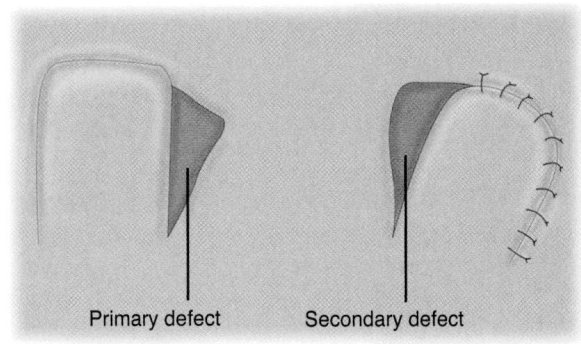

FIG. 45-5. Random pattern transposition flap.

arterial supplies to the trunk, head, and extremities. They ultimately feed interconnecting vessels that supply the vascular plexuses of the fascia, subcutaneous tissue, and skin. These interconnecting vessels reach the skin via either fasciocutaneous (also called *septocutaneous*) vessels that traverse fascial septae, musculocutaneous perforators that penetrate muscle bellies, or direct cutaneous vessels that traverse neither muscle bellies nor fascial septae.[7] Axial pattern flaps, incorporating suprafascial tissues, are supplied by these fasciocutaneous (septocutaneous), musculocutaneous, or direct cutaneous arteries.

The internal viscera are also a source of axial pattern flaps, such as the jejunum flap and omentum flap. The circulation of bone- and muscle-containing flaps also is mainly axial in pattern. It also is possible to design local flaps, such as V-Y advancements and rhomboid flaps, as axial pattern flaps. The volume of tissue reliably supplied by the arterial input (and venous drainage) of an axial pattern flap defines its limits, not length:breadth ratios. This can be clarified conceptually. The arterial tree can be described in terms of angiosomes, territories (anatomic, dynamic, and potential), and

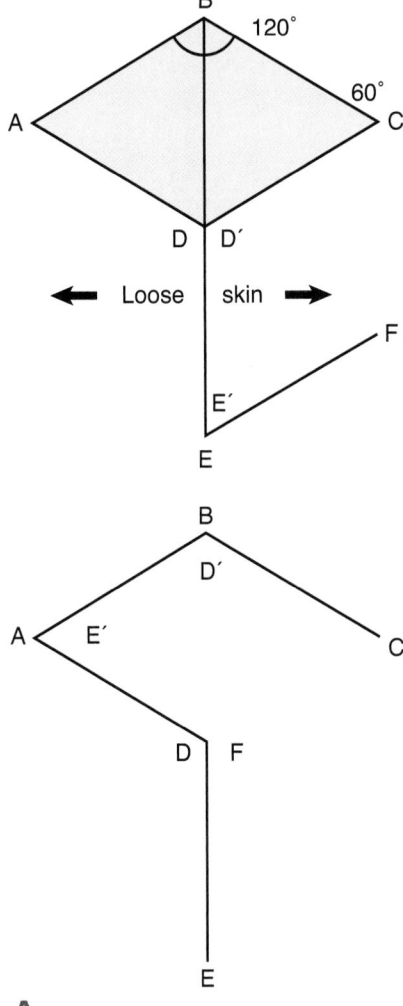

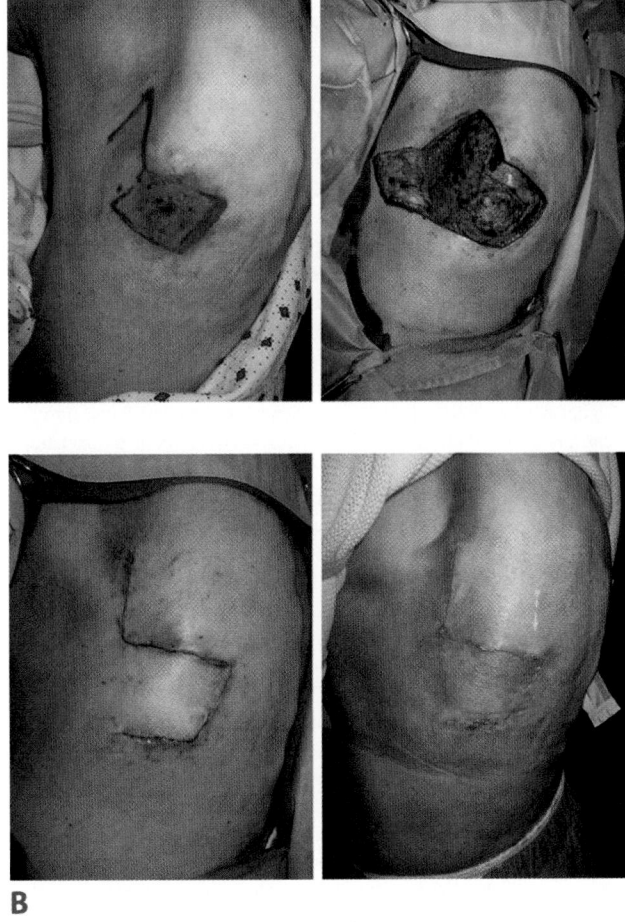

FIG. 45-6. A and **B.** Random pattern transposition flap, the rhomboid flap. *(Photographs reproduced with permission from M. Gimbel.)*

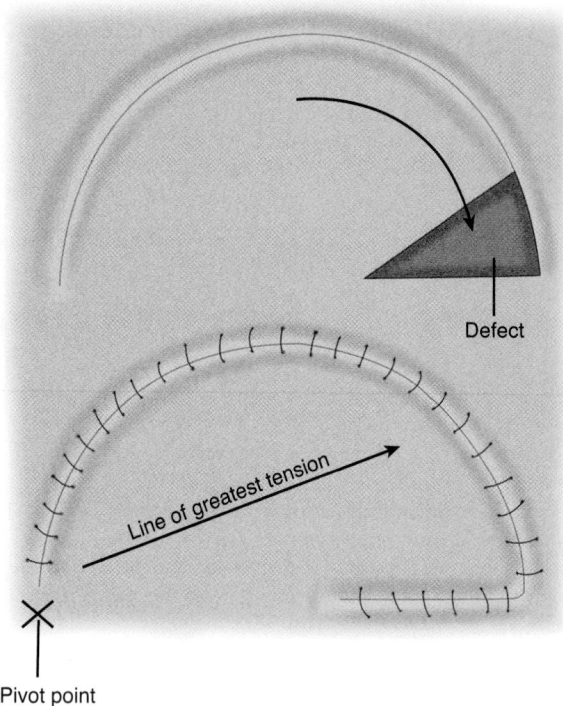

FIG. 45-7. Random pattern rotational flap. *(Reproduced with permission from Aston et al.[5])*

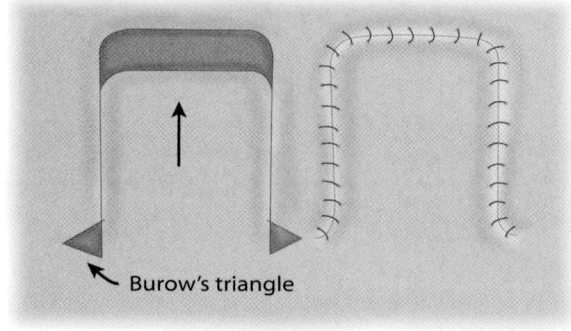

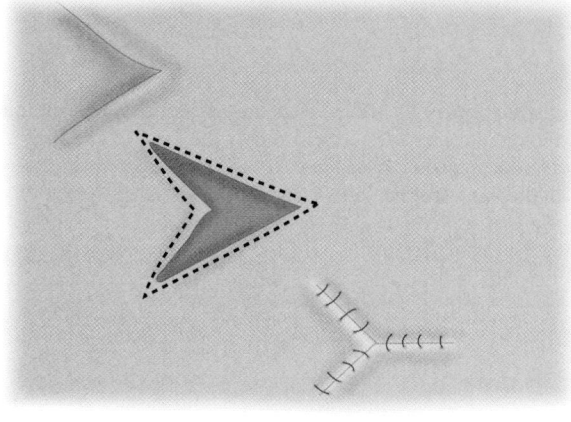

FIG. 45-8. Random pattern advancement flap. **A.** Rectangular advancement flap with Burow's triangle excision. **B.** V-Y advancement flap. *(Reproduced with permission from Aston et al.[5])*

choke vessels.[8] Each artery supplies a block of tissue called an *angiosome*; neighboring angiosomes overlap. The anatomic territory of an artery is defined by the limits of its ramifications, where it forms anastomoses with neighboring anatomic territories. The vessels that pass between anatomic territories are called *choke vessels*. The dynamic territory of an artery is the volume of tissue stained by an intravascular administration of fluorescein into that artery. The *potential territory* of an artery is the volume of tissue that can be included in a flap that has undergone conditioning. Both the dynamic and potential territories extend beyond the anatomic territory of an artery. Although these territories of the artery supplying an axial pattern flap provide some guidance to the limits of such a flap harvest, there remains no quantifiable method to predict these safe limits exactly. By virtue of their defined blood supply, the contiguity of axial pattern flaps, unlike that of random pattern flaps, may be local, regional, or distant, and pedicled or free. Axial pattern flaps may also possess some areas with random pattern circulation, usually located at the flap periphery.

Conditioning refers to any procedure that increases the reliability of a flap. Invoking the delay phenomenon, for example, has improved the survival of flaps whose use is frequently complicated by unpredictable partial necrosis, such as the pedicled transverse rectus abdominis myocutaneous (TRAM) flap. The procedure can be particularly useful in patients at higher risk, such as those who are obese, smoke, or have received radiotherapy. One method of delay for the pedicled TRAM flap is to divide a major portion of its blood supply, the deep inferior epigastric artery on both sides, approximately 2 weeks before transfer. In response, blood from the anatomic angiosome of the superior epigastric artery appears to flow into that of the interrupted deep inferior epigastric artery via intervening choke vessels. As a result, the flap becomes conditioned to rely on the superior epigastric artery. The TRAM flap can then be transferred based on the superior epigastric artery with less risk of its distal portions' becoming ischemic and possibly necrotic. Several theories have been proposed to explain the delay phenomenon, including metabolic compensatory responses to relative ischemia and dilatation of choke vessels; however, its mechanisms remain incompletely understood.[9]

Further subclassifications of flap circulation have been introduced for muscular and fasciocutaneous flaps.[10] Individual muscles have been classified by Mathes and Nahai into five types (I to V) according to their blood supply (Table 45-6). This classification is also applied to the respective myocutaneous flaps. Fasciocutaneous flaps also have been classified by Nahai and Mathes into types A, B, and C (Table 45-7). The inclusion of muscle in a flap may serve to increase flap bulk (so as to obliterate dead space) or to provide a functioning component with the harvest of its motor nerve for coaptation to a recipient motor nerve. The purported advantages of muscle-containing flaps over fasciocutaneous flaps for use in previously infected tissue beds or for fracture healing have been debated.

With progressive advancements in flap transfer techniques and an understanding of microvascular flap anatomy, plastic surgeons have steadily increased the number and variety of available flaps, thereby improving the results of flap reconstructions. In addition, this knowledge has reduced the morbidity associated with flap harvest. Perhaps the most important advancement in flap surgery within the last two decades has been the introduction of the perforator flap.[11] Perforator flaps evolved from the observation that the muscle component of myocutaneous flaps served only as a passive carrier of blood supply to the overlying fasciocutaneous tissues (fascia, skin, and intervening subcutaneous tissues). Previous to this, it had been deemed necessary to include the muscle for reliable harvest of fasciocutaneous tissues supplied by its musculocutaneous perforators, even if it was not necessary to include that muscle for the reconstruction. This unfortunately caused an unnecessary muscular deficit at the donor site, and for this reason these flaps were sometimes abandoned. The introduction of intramuscular retrograde dissection techniques, however, allowed the skeletonization of a musculocutaneous perforator from its encasement within a muscle belly, which spared that muscle from flap harvest

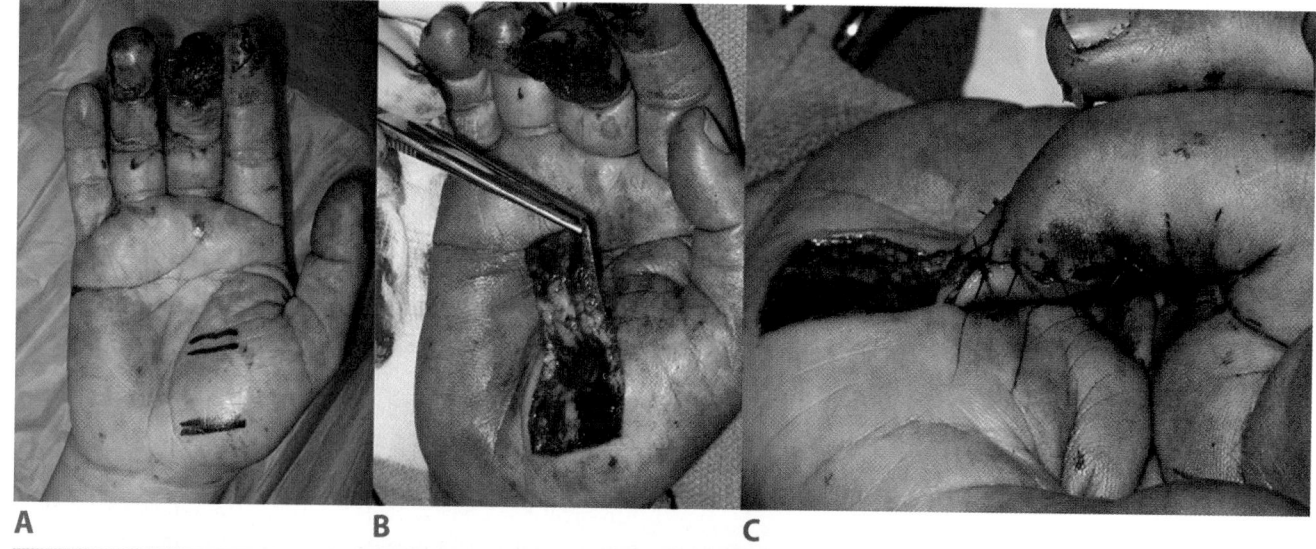

A   B   C

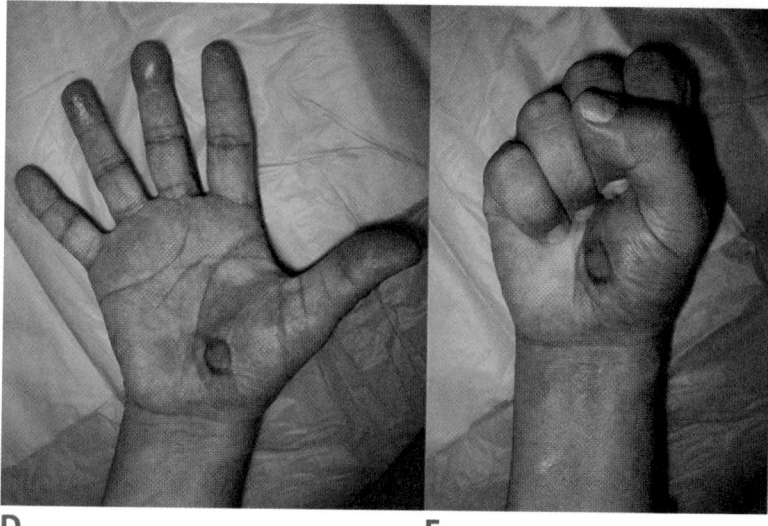

D   E

FIG. 45-9. Random pattern interpolation flap—the thenar flap. **A.** Middle fingertip injury with exposed bone and tendon. **B.** Elevation of distally based random pattern thenar flap. **C.** Insetting. **D** and **E.** Function and form at 3 months, after skin grafting of donor site. (*Photographs reproduced with permission from M. Gimbel.*)

and preserved its donor site function.[7,11] Further refinement of this concept gave rise to the harvest of cutaneous flaps based on any vessel that penetrated the fascia, which preserved the muscle (when the vessel was a musculocutaneous perforator) as well as the fascia (by suprafascial dissection). Within the last decade, free-style flap harvest has also been introduced.[12] With a handheld Doppler ultrasound probe, the surgeon is able to identify an arterial supply to almost any area of skin with the desired reconstructive characteristics and trace that pedicle in retrograde fashion along whatever direction it takes, preserving donor site fascia and muscle as necessary. Although the exact definition of what a perforator flap is remains contentious, its advantages remain clear: reduced donor site morbidity, reduced flap bulk, and increased flexibility in choosing desired flap components for reconstruction. The circulation of perforator flaps is axial in pattern; consequently, they can be transferred as pedicled island flaps or by microvascular free tissue transfer.

TABLE 45-6 Mathes-Nahai classification of muscular flaps

Classification	Vascular Supply	Example
Type I	One vascular pedicle	Gastrocnemius
Type II	Dominant and minor pedicles (the flap cannot survive based only on the minor pedicles)	Gracilis
Type III	Two dominant pedicles	Rectus abdominis
Type IV	Segmental pedicles	Sartorius
Type V	One dominant pedicle with secondary segmental pedicles (the flap can survive based only on the secondary pedicles)	Pectoralis major

TABLE 45-7 Nahai-Mathes classification of fasciocutaneous flaps

Classification	Vascular Supply	Example
Type A	Direct cutaneous vessel that penetrates the fascia	Temporoparietal fascial flap
Type B	Septocutaneous vessel that penetrates the fascia	Radial artery forearm flap
Type C	Musculocutaneous vessel that penetrates the fascia	Transverse rectus abdominis myocutaneous flap

Free Tissue Transfer

A free tissue transfer (or transplantation), often referred to as a *free flap* procedure, is an autogenous transplantation of vascularized tissues. Any axial pattern flap with pedicle vessels of a suitable diameter can be transferred as a free flap. This involves three main steps: (a) complete detachment of the flap, with devascularization, from the donor site; (b) revascularization of the flap with anastomoses to blood vessels in the recipient site; and (c) an intervening period of flap ischemia. Flap circulation must be restored within a tolerable ischemia time.

Given the small diameter of most flap pedicle vessels (usually between 0.8 and 4.0 mm), these anastomoses are usually performed using an operative microscope that provides dedicated illumination and between 6× and 40× magnification. Any surgery performed with the aid of an operative microscope is termed *microsurgery*; such anastomoses are therefore termed *microvascular anastomoses*. High-magnification surgical loupes are usually used for flap harvest, especially for dissecting the flap pedicle, because they allow greater operator freedom. Aside from microvascular anastomosis, microsurgical techniques include microneural coaptation, microlymphatic anastomosis, and microtubular anastomosis.

The first successful free tissue transfer in humans was transfer of a jejunal free flap for cervical esophagus reconstruction performed in 1957; however, the surgeons did not use microvascular surgery for the anastomoses. The first *microvascular* free tissue transfers in humans were carried out during the late 1960s and early 1970s. Free flaps were initially considered to be a last-resort option to reconstruct the most complex defects. However, as a result of improved microsurgical techniques and microinstrumentation, as well as proper patient and free flap selection and effective postoperative monitoring methods, the success rates have increased to exceed 95%.[13] Today, free tissue transfer is often the first-choice treatment for many defects and is no longer considered the last-ditch effort. It is now ubiquitously used in appropriate patients by reconstructive plastic surgeons worldwide.

The predetermining factor in free flap failure is occlusion of its anastomotic lifeline blood supply due to thrombosis. As enumerated by Virchow's triad, any factors that alter normal laminar blood flow, cause endothelial damage, or change the constitution of blood (producing hypercoagulability) increase the risk of thrombosis (Table 45-8).[14] Avoidance of this complication therefore begins with a thorough patient evaluation for the presence of acquired or inherited thrombophilic tendencies. The patient's hemodynamic status influences that of the free flap and should be optimized. The effect of

tobacco smoking on free flap success has been debated, with some larger retrospective studies reporting no difference in thromboembolic complications; however, smoking is well known to affect wound healing.[13,15] Smoking, and the use of potentially vasoconstrictive agents, such as caffeine, should be avoided for several weeks before a free flap procedure. The restoration of normal laminar blood flow and avoidance of endothelial damage are addressed principally by careful flap insetting and meticulous microvascular surgical technique.

Planning a free flap goes beyond a simple calculation of matching flap and defect dimensions and tissue characteristics. The surgeon must, in addition, consider several important technicalities: what flap pedicle length and size are required (affected by flap choice), which recipient vessels to use, how to orient anastomoses (end to end or end to side), how to deal with mismatched donor and recipient vessel dimensions, how to overcome unhealthy donor and/or recipient vessels (e.g., traumatic dissection, scarred surgical field due to previous operation or radiotherapy), how to inset flap tissues (to maximize functional and cosmetic results without detriment to flap circulation), how to route the pedicle (to restore normal blood flow without pedicle kinking, twisting, or compression), how to position the patient (especially if the flap is to be inset over mobile soft tissue or joints), how to place postoperative dressings (so as to produce no compression of the flap or pedicle), and what donor site morbidity will likely result (there is a risk-benefit decision between defect severity and flap choice).[16] In addition, the surgeon must have a suitable backup plan to overcome intraoperative troubles; for example, insufficient pedicle length can be addressed with an interpositional vein graft adjoining the donor and recipient vessels, and iatrogenic vessel injury or severely aberrant anatomy may necessitate use of a backup flap or backup recipient vessels.[13]

A clear understanding of the blood supply to the free flap and its tissue components is a prerequisite to harvesting a viable free flap. Pedicle vessels must be identified and protected, and handled minimally and atraumatically to avoid thrombogenic factors (see Table 45-8). Meticulous technique also reduces the risk of vasospasm, but the latter can be ameliorated by topical lidocaine or papaverine should it occur. Critical vessels connecting flap components must also be recognized and preserved. Under microscope magnification, the donor and recipient vessels should be dissected back to health. The presence of, for example, venous valves, atherosclerotic plaques, intimal trauma, and intraluminal prolapse of adventitial tissue at or adjacent to the anastomosis site increases the risk of thrombosis. The vessel ends should be cleared of periadventitial tissues for 3 to 5 mm with sharp dissection under the microscope. Periadventitial dissection should be limited to this extent, so as to avoid potential devascularization of the vessel wall by removal of the vasa vasorum and prevent the subsequent delayed development of a perianastomotic pseudoaneurysm. Adventitiectomy also helps relieve vasospasm by increasing compliance of the vessel wall and by inducing a local sympathectomy effect. The vessel ends usually are stabilized with a double approximating microvascular clamp for anastomosis. Interrupted sutures or, less commonly, continuous sutures can accomplish the anastomosis. The microneedle typically has a three eighths circle curvature and is between 30 and 150 μm in size. Its monofilament microsuture is usually between 9-0 and 11-0 caliber. The dimensions of the vessels to be anastomosed define the choice of microneedle and microsuture. Less commonly, suture alternatives such as fibrin adhesives or laser welding (these remain largely experimental) and mechanical anastomotic devices (e.g., venous couplers) may be used. Triangulating or bisecting suturing techniques can help to achieve an even placement of sutures. Normally, each suture should include the full thickness of both vessel walls, none should catch the opposite vessel wall (which causes disastrous luminal occlusion and intimal trauma), and the size of each bite should approximate the vessel wall thickness. The configuration of the anastomosis can be either end to end (Fig. 45-10), if the distal circulation can be adequately preserved, or end to side (Fig. 45-11) if the distal circulation must be preserved, as in the case of an

TABLE 45-8	Thrombogenic factors that can affect free flap pedicles and anastomoses

Altered Laminar Blood Flow	Endothelial Damage	Hypercoagulability
Tension or intimal malalignment at the anastomosis site; twisting, kinking, compression, or vasospasm of pedicle vessels	Iatrogenic damage (e.g., back-walled anastomotic suture, poor vessel handling, too many sutures)	Acquired thrombophilic tendency (e.g., pregnancy, paraneoplastic Trousseau's syndrome, antiphospholipid antibody syndromes)
Nearby intraluminal structures (e.g., atherosclerotic plaque, venous valves, back-walled anastomotic suture)	Previous vessel damage (e.g., atherosclerosis, trauma)	Hereditary thrombophilias (e.g., activated protein C resistance, protein C/protein S deficiency, hyperhomocysteinemia)

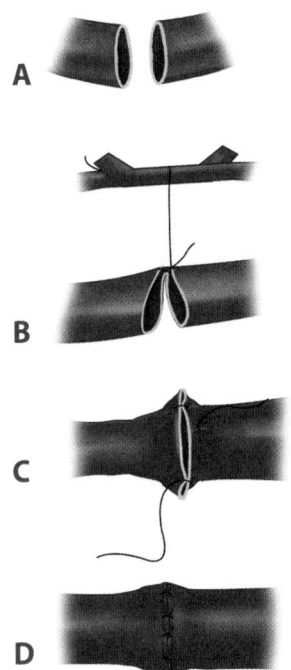

FIG. 45-10. **A** through **D.** End-to-end anastomosis.

arterially compromised extremity supplied by one dominant vessel. An end-to-side orientation may also be useful to overcome dramatically mismatched donor-recipient vessel dimensions. Whatever the method chosen, microanatomic differences between the vessels should be respected so as to achieve accurately approximated intimal surfaces in a tension-free anastomosis, devoid of redundancy that might promote kinking.[13]

The clinical monitoring of a free flap should start during flap harvest, especially before its pedicle is divided. A free flap that is struggling to maintain normal perfusion characteristics during harvest most likely has insufficient circulation, which may be due to arterial or venous compromise, or a combination of both (Table 45-9). Flap

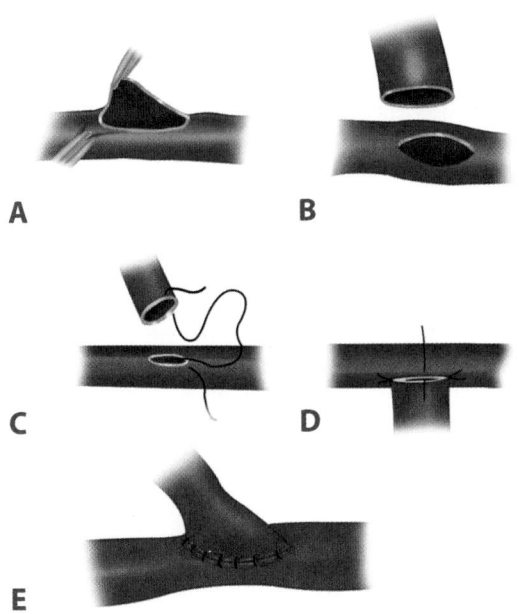

FIG. 45-11. **A** through **E.** End-to-side anastomosis.

TABLE 45-9 Clinical signs of arterial and venous compromise in a free flap[a]

Clinical Sign	Arterial Compromise	Venous Compromise
Color	Becoming paler	Increasingly reddish or purplish
Temperature	Becoming cooler	Becoming warmer
Tissue turgor	Reducing	Increasing
Capillary refill time	Becoming slower	Becoming faster
Pinprick bleeding	Increasingly sluggish	Quickening (and darkening)

[a]Note that venous and arterial compromise may coexist, and one may lead to the other.

compromise may be due to reversible factors such as pedicle kinking, tensioning, or twisting; patient hemodynamic compromise; or an overly large flap harvest for the chosen pedicle vessels. If poor flap perfusion continues despite the absence or correction of all these factors, an inherent flap problem or a critical vascular injury to the flap or its pedicle must be considered, and it may not be safe to continue its harvest. This is one clear example of a situation in which a backup plan may require execution.

Clinical flap monitoring continues after successful restoration of arterial inflow and venous outflow. The mainstay of postoperative free flap monitoring is clinical assessment (see Table 45-9), although supplementary instrument monitoring also can be helpful. Doppler ultrasound assessment of arterial and venous signals is useful for monitoring buried or concealed flaps. If flap perfusion was healthy before division of its donor site pedicle, then poor perfusion after anastomoses is likely due to either a technical error or insufficient systemic hemodynamics. The latter usually is correctable by ensuring that the patient and the patient's environment are suitably warm and by initiating IV colloid challenge or, if indicated, blood transfusion. Numerous potential technical errors, which have been described in the earlier paragraphs on planning and anastomosis technique, may occur. Routine postoperative patient monitoring includes measurement of total fluid inputs, urinary catheter output (which should be >1 mL/kg per hour), core temperature, and arterial blood pressure (systolic pressure should be >100 mmHg), as well as pulse oximetry. The patient and free flap are best monitored in an intensive care setting by experienced staff until both are stable enough for routine ward assessments.[13]

Occlusion of the anastomosis most commonly arises from internal thrombosis or from external compression of the pedicle, such as from surrounding tissues, fluid accumulation (e.g., hematoma and tissue edema), or overly tight dressings or skin sutures. Because there is a threshold of ischemia beyond which a flap will sustain irreversible tissue and/or microcirculatory damage, it is important that the early signs of flap circulatory compromise be recognized as quickly as possible and the underlying problem diagnosed and corrected promptly if flap health is to be restored successfully. Different tissues tolerate differing durations of ischemia in correlation with their tissue-specific basal metabolic rate. Although cooling free flaps (to reduce basal metabolic rate) has a variably protective effect in experimental settings, it appears that this practice contributes little to improving free flap success in the clinical setting as long as warm ischemia times are kept to <4 hours for most tissues; exceptions include bowel flaps, which are more susceptible to ischemia.[13]

Given that the predisposing factor for free flap failure is thrombosis formation, it is understandable that plastic surgeons have looked to anticoagulant therapies in an effort to improve success rates. The routine use of anticoagulants remains controversial. Although such drugs, including the dextrans, aspirin, heparin, and also some fibrinolytics, appear beneficial in experimental settings, large clinical trials have failed to show any conclusive associations between their use and either free flap success or failure rates.[17] It seems intuitive to use these drugs for failing free flaps as an adjunctive measure alongside operative re-exploration and surgical intervention. The surgeon must be aware of their contraindications and recognize that their side effects, apart from bleeding, are occasionally serious. Venous congestion may be addressed by surgical measures as well as by application of medicinal *Hirudo medicinalis* leeches (with concomitant *Aeromonas hydrophilia* prophylaxis) or by chemical "leeching" (topical heparin combined with dermal punctures).

Unfortunately, the "no-reflow" phenomenon is occasionally witnessed and leads to irreversible flap failure. This describes a situation in which no venous return drains into the pedicle vein of the flap, even though adequate arterial inflow passes the arterial anastomoses and is seen to enter the flap tissues. The no-reflow phenomenon sometimes follows an extended ischemic insult and appears to be a self-perpetuating cycle of endothelial cellular swelling, inflammatory vasoconstriction, impaired microcirculatory flow, stasis, microcirculatory thromboses, progressive ischemia, and flap failure.[13]

Despite these potential problems, free flap success rates exceed 95% in experienced hands.[18] There is no doubt that increasing microsurgical experience is critical to improving free flap success rates. The laboratory setting is an excellent environment in which to progress beyond the early portion of one's learning curve through supervised microsurgical training and execution of microvascular anastomoses and microvascular free flap procedures in small animals.

Tissue Expansion

Although skin grafts and local flaps are very useful in reconstructing many superficial defects, they are not without their drawbacks. Both leave donor site defects with cosmetic and/or functional sequelae. Grafts are limited in color match and durability, whereas local flaps may supply insufficient tissue and produce contour irregularities. The advent of tissue expansion has created the potential to greatly increase the amount of local, well-matched tissue that can be advanced or transposed as a flap while decreasing donor site morbidity.

The most common method of skin expansion involves the placement of an inflatable silicon elastomer balloon with an integrated or remote port beneath the skin and subcutaneous tissue followed by serial inflation with saline. After completion of expansion, usually over weeks to months, the expander is removed and the redundant overlying skin may be advanced into an adjacent defect. Expanders are now available in a multitude of shapes and sizes that can be tailored to the reconstruction. In breast reconstruction the tissue expander is replaced with a permanent implant instead of using the tissue as a flap to re-create the volume of the breast mound. Histologically, expanded skin demonstrates thickened dermis with enhanced vasculature and diminished subcutaneous fat. Studies have shown that the skin expansion is due not merely to stretch or creep but also to actual generation of new tissue.[19]

The technique of tissue expansion comes with its share of potential complications, including infection, hematoma, seroma, expander extrusion, implant failure, skin necrosis, pain, and neurapraxia. Furthermore, an inflated expander is certainly a very visible, albeit temporary, deformity that may cause patients much distress.

Despite these imperfections, tissue expansion has become a major treatment modality in the management of giant congenital nevi, secondary reconstruction of extensive burn scars, scalp reconstruction, and breast reconstruction. The technique has permitted the plastic surgeon to perform reconstructions with tissue of similar color, texture, and thickness with minimal donor site morbidity.

PEDIATRIC PLASTIC SURGERY

Cleft Lip and Palate

Orofacial clefting is the most common congenital anomaly and is known to occur in 1 in 500 live white births.[20] The incidence is lower in African Americans and higher in Native Americans and Asians. Clefting of the lip and/or palate is felt to occur around the eighth week of embryogenesis, either by failure of fusion of the medial nasal process and the maxillary prominence or by failure of mesodermal migration and penetration between the epithelial bilayer of the face. The cause of orofacial clefting is felt to be multifactorial. Factors that likely increase the incidence of clefting include increased parental age, drug use and infections during pregnancy, smoking during pregnancy, and a family history of orofacial clefting. The increased chance of clefting when there is an affected parent is approximately 4%.

The *primary palate* is defined as all tissue anterior to the incisive foramen, including the anterior hard palate (premaxilla), alveolus, lip, and nose. The secondary palate includes everything posterior to the incisive foramen, including the majority of the hard palate and the soft palate (velum). Clefting can involve the lip and nose, with or without a palatal cleft. Clefts of the lip and/or palate are first classified as unilateral or bilateral, and then as complete or incomplete (Fig. 45-12). Complete clefts of the lip affect the entire lip and extend up into the nose. Incomplete clefts affect only a portion of the lip and contain a bridge of tissue connecting the central and lateral lip elements, referred to as *Simonart's band.*

Treatment Protocol

Considerable controversy remains over the details of the timing, technique, and protocol for treating children with orofacial clefting. The treatment protocol described in this chapter is accepted at many large cleft centers around the United States. All infants born with cleft-craniofacial anomalies benefit from care by a specialized team dedicated to the treatment of congenital anomalies. Today, this is widely accepted as the standard of care. Often, patients are seen prenatally after a diagnosis is made using sophisticated antenatal ultrasonography. The prenatal consultation has proven to be beneficial to parents, serving to dispel fears and uncertainties, and assuring them that treatment exists. After the infant's birth, a team evaluation occurs, and input is obtained from the surgeon, speech and language pathologist, social worker, craniofacial orthodontist, geneticist, otorhinolaryngologist, and pediatrician. For infants born with orofacial clefting, initial concerns relate to successful feeding and breathing. Infants with palatal clefts cannot generate negative pressure when suckling and therefore need milk dispensed into their mouths from a specialized nurser when they make suckling motions. Once adequate nutrition and a safe airway are ensured, attention is turned to the cleft anomaly. Attempts to lessen the deformity and set the stage for the surgical repair of the lip and nose begin with a process known as *presurgical infant orthopedics (PSIO)*, which includes procedures such as nasoalveolar molding (NAM) (Fig. 45-13). NAM repositions the neonatal alveolar segments, brings the lip elements into close approximation, stretches the deficient nasal components, and turns wide complete clefts into the morphology of narrow "incomplete" clefts. After PSIO with NAM, the definitive single-stage cleft lip and nose repair is performed at 3 to 6 months of age. With this initial operation, the lip deformity is repaired and a primary nasoplasty reconstructs the cleft lip nasal deformity. If the family does not have access to PSIO or have the resources for this time-intensive therapy, a cleft lip adhesion can be performed as an initial stage in the repair. The preliminary cleft lip adhesion unites the upper lip and nasal sill, truly converting complete clefts into incomplete clefts. A cleft lip adhesion is performed in the first or second month of life, and the definitive cleft lip and nose repair follows at 4 to 6 months. After the definitive cleft lip and nose repair, the cleft palate is repaired in a single stage at 9 to 12 months of age.

Unilateral Cleft Lip

The unilateral cleft lip is classically associated with a cleft lip nasal deformity. The cleft lip nasal deformity includes lateral, inferior, and posterior displacement of the alar cartilage. This results from the deficient and clefted underlying skeleton as well as the unopposed pull of the clefted orbicularis oris muscle abnormally inserted on the alar

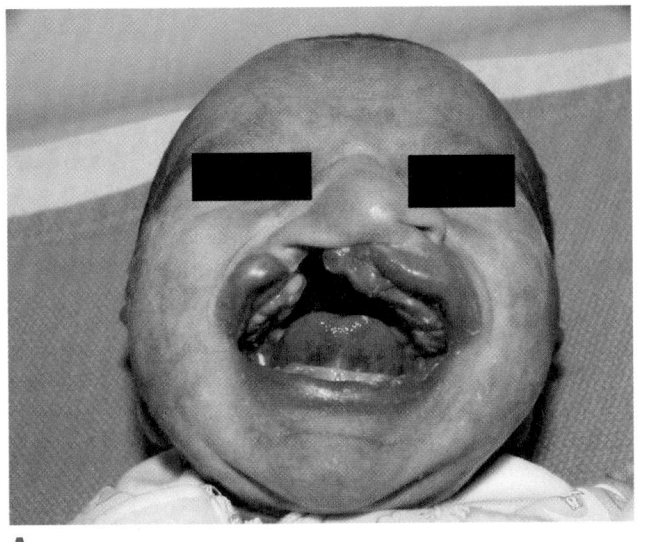

A

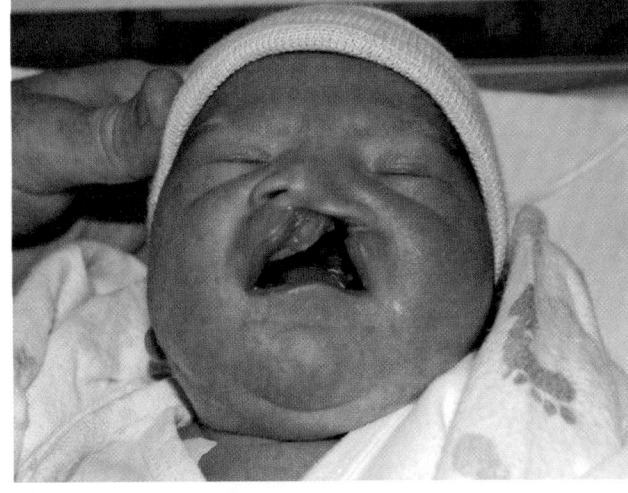

A

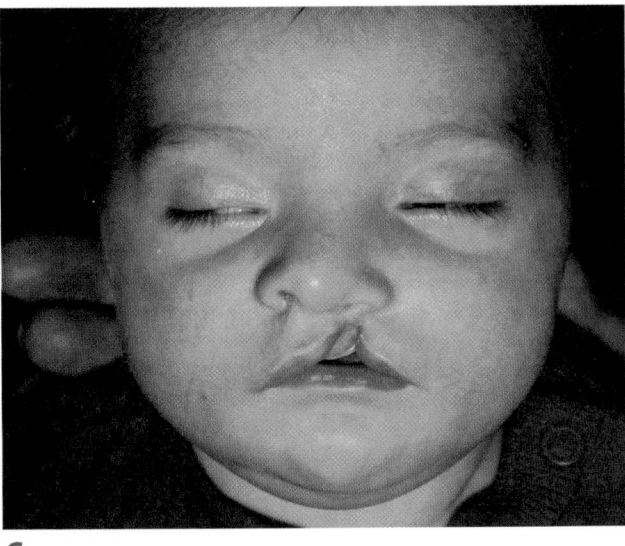

B

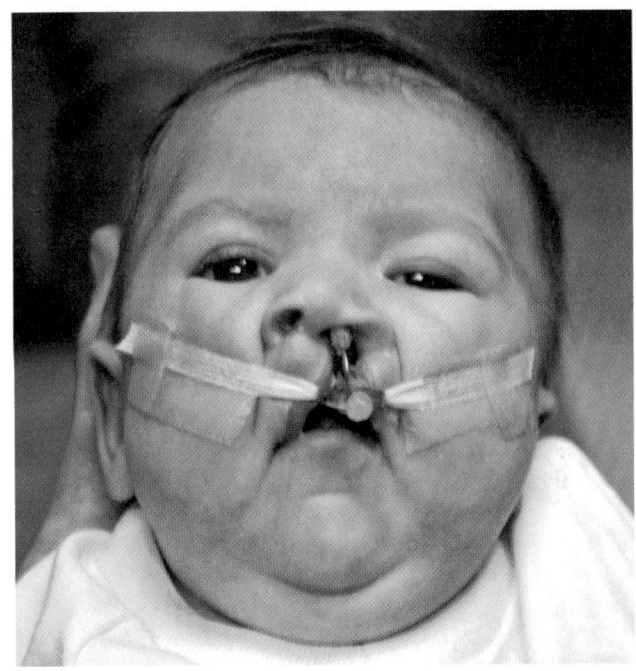

B

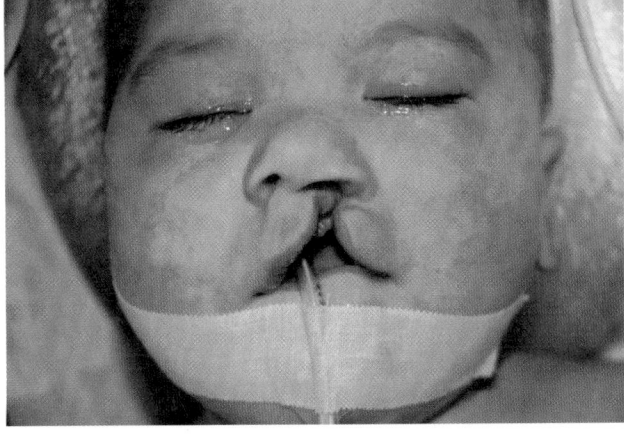

C

C

FIG. 45-12. A. Unilateral cleft lip and palate. **B.** Bilateral cleft lip and palate. **C.** Incomplete unilateral cleft lip.

FIG. 45-13. A. Complete left-sided cleft lip, nose, and palate. **B.** Nasoalveolar molding. **C.** After nasoalveolar molding, preoperative appearance before cleft lip and nose repair. *(Continued)*

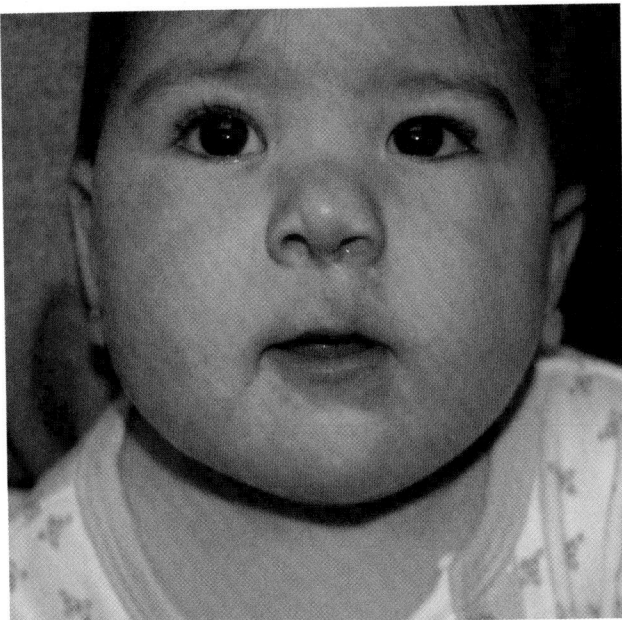

D

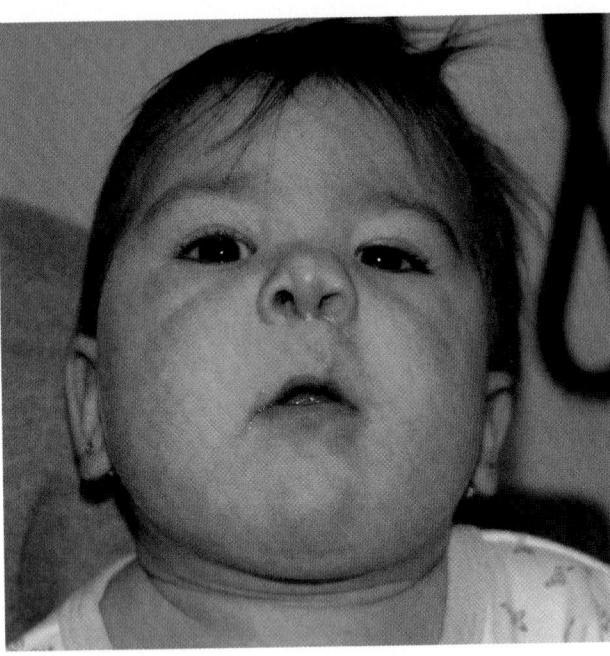

E

FIG. 45-13. (*Continued*) **D.** Frontal view after cleft lip and nose repair. **E.** Worm's-eye view after cleft lip and nose repair.

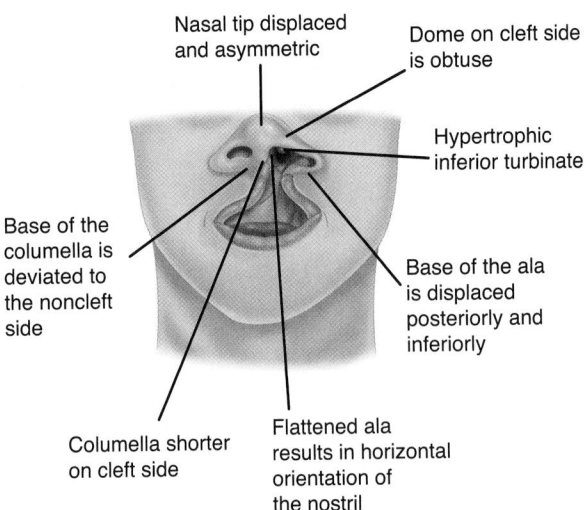

Nasal tip displaced and asymmetric

Dome on cleft side is obtuse

Hypertrophic inferior turbinate

Base of the columella is deviated to the noncleft side

Base of the ala is displaced posteriorly and inferiorly

Columella shorter on cleft side

Flattened ala results in horizontal orientation of the nostril

A

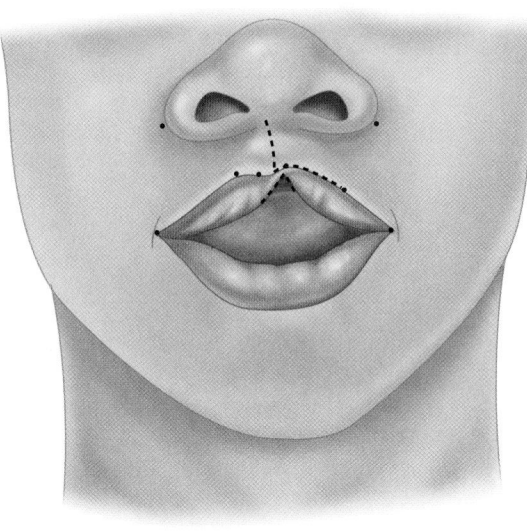

B

FIG. 45-14. **A.** Unilateral cleft lip and nose deformity. **B.** The rotation-advancement repair.

base (Fig. 45-14A). The maxillary minor segment (the smaller alveolar/maxillary segment on the clefted side) is collapsed medially. The process of unilateral cleft lip repair can be thought of as "philtral subunit reconstruction." The goal of the operation is to level Cupid's bow and reconstruct the central philtrum of the lip, ideally placing the incision and subsequent scar as close to the normal philtral column as possible. The surgical repair is performed under general anesthesia, and local anesthesia containing epinephrine is used. Many different techniques of cleft lip and nose repair have been proposed; however, most of the commonly used procedures are variations of a "rotation-advancement" procedure.[21] The rotation-advancement procedure, as championed by Millard (Fig. 45-14B), rotates the philtral subunit of the central lip downward to level Cupid's bow as the lateral lip element is advanced into the defect created by the downward rotation of the

philtrum. Some surgeons choose to perform primary closure of the alveolar cleft at the time of primary lip and nose repair, called a *gingivoperiosteoplasty*. If the alveolar cleft is to be repaired, the gingivoperiosteoplasty is performed by raising mucoperiosteal flaps within the alveolar cleft margin and reapproximating them across the alveolar cleft defect. This creates a bony tunnel closed with periosteal flaps and facilitates the generation of bone in the alveolar defect. It is accepted today that some form of primary nasoplasty should be performed at the time of primary definitive lip repair. Techniques to release and reposition the nasal tip cartilages, as well as the ala, are performed with variations of tip rhinoplasties using suture methods. Some surgeons choose to use postoperative internal and/or external splints to maintain the nasal correction achieved at surgery during the healing process.

Bilateral Cleft Lip

In the complete bilateral cleft lip and nose deformity, the central lip element, called the *prolabium*, is entirely separate from the rest of the upper lip. The prolabium is displaced on top of the central alveolar segment, called the *premaxilla*, containing the unerupted four central incisors. Often, the premaxilla and prolabium are

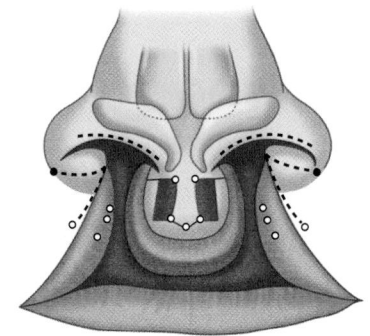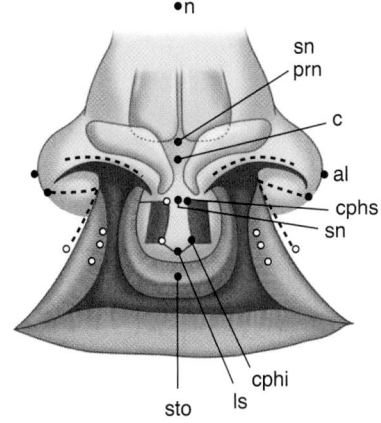

FIG. 45-15. Mulliken bilateral cleft lip and nose repair. al = ala nasi; c = highest point of columella nasi; cphi = crista philtri inferior; cphs = crista philtri superior; ls = labiale superius; n = nasion; prn = pronasale; sn = subnasale; sto = stomion.

outwardly displaced. This is referred to as a *flyaway premaxilla.* For the child with a complete bilateral cleft lip and nose, PSIO is a very important step in preparing the child for definitive lip and nose surgery by retracting the premaxilla into the maxillary arch, repositioning the lip segments, and stretching the rudimentary columella. Bilateral cleft lip and nose repairs often are versions of straight-line repairs, with the Mulliken technique being the more commonly performed (Fig. 45-15). In the bilateral cleft lip deformity, the new philtrum is made from the prolabium and is united to the lateral lip elements on top of the repaired orbicularis oris muscle.[22]

Cleft Palate

During the eighth to twelfth weeks of gestation, the mandible becomes more prognathic, the tongue drops from beneath the clefted lateral palatine processes, and the palatal shelves migrate upward into a more horizontal position and fusion occurs. A cleft palate results from the failure of fusion of the two palatal processes. As with labial clefting, isolated clefts of the palate are multifactorial in etiology, and isolated clefts of the palate are more likely to be associated with other anomalies. Between 8 to 10% of isolated clefts of the palate are associated with the 22q deletion of velocardiofacial syndrome.[23]

The main goal of cleft palate surgery is to help the patient attain normal speech, which results from velopharyngeal competence. During speech, the soft palate, or velum, is moved posteriorly and superiorly, primarily by the levator palatini muscle sling that suspends the velum from the skull base. Velopharyngeal competence is obtained during attempted speech when the velum approximates the posterior pharyngeal wall, preventing air and liquid from regurgitating into the nasal cavity. Velopharyngeal competence allows intraoral pressure to be built up for speech sounds. A cleft palate precludes this from occurring and results in velopharyngeal incompetence, or VPI. Because it is impossible for the oral and nasal cavities to be partitioned in the patient with a cleft palate, it is also difficult for the patient to develop negative intraoral pressure for an effective suck. Therefore, specialized nursers are used to dispense liquid into the infant's mouth during the suckling motions. Children with clefts of the palate have an increased incidence of otitis media; this may be related to the abnormality of the velar musculature and ineffective function of the eustachian tube. The increased incidence of otitis media can result in hearing loss if not treated appropriately. In addition, VPI and nasal air escape during speech results in hypernasal speech.

As with the repair of cleft lip and nose, the timing, technique, and protocols for cleft palate repair are controversial. Most agree that palate repair should be performed before the development of speech. The cleft palate usually is repaired when the infant is between 6 and 18 months of age. Cleft palate repair also is performed under general anesthesia, with the head slightly hyperextended and a retractor, such as the Dingman mouth gag, placed intraorally to retract the tongue and endotracheal tube. An epinephrine solution is injected into the palate. Techniques of hard palate closure include the use of unipedicled hard palate mucoperiosteal flaps as in the Wardill-Veau-Kilner repair or bipedicled hard palate mucoperiosteal flaps as in the von Langenbeck repair. Both the unipedicled and bipedicled hard palate palatoplasty techniques rely on the greater palatine neurovascular pedicle. Soft palate or velar closure techniques are divided into straight-line and Z-plasty procedures. With either a straight-line or Z-plasty velar repair, the levator palatini muscle should be independently repaired; this is called an *intravelar veloplasty.* The clefted levator is identified coursing sagittally in an anterior-posterior direction, abnormally inserted onto the posterior edge of the hard palate. In intravelar veloplasty, it is released from the posterior edge of the hard palate in the midline and dissected free from abnormal attachments to the aponeurosis of the tensor veli palatini muscle and superior constrictor laterally. After its complete release, the levator palatini muscle is united in the midline, with reconstruction of the levator muscle sling that suspends the velum from the skull base and aids in velopharyngeal competence.

The authors prefer the double opposing Z-plasty technique of soft palate or velar reconstruction known as the *Furlow palatoplasty.*[24] The procedure uses four triangular flaps, two oral and two nasal, with the posteriorly based flaps containing the released levator muscles. The Z-plasty lengthens the soft palate, prevents longitudinal scarring from a straight-line repair, and produces a secondary pharyngoplasty effect by narrowing the velopharyngeal port (Fig. 45-16).

Complications of palatoplasty include wound-healing problems resulting in a breakdown of the suture line and the development of a fistula. The literature reports fistula rates ranging from approximately 1 to 20%. Treatment of palatal fistulae is particularly challenging, because the recurrence rates have been noted to approach 96%. The second most common complication of palatoplasty is the incomplete correction of speech and the development of postoperative VPI. The literature reports postoperative VPI rates ranging from 10 to 40%. Some of the best rates of velopharyngeal competence have been reported with the Furlow double opposing Z-plasty palatoplasty. Postoperative VPI is treated with pharyngoplasty: either a posterior pharyngeal flap pharyngoplasty or a sphincter pharyngoplasty. A posterior pharyngeal flap is a static flap formed from the posterior pharyngeal wall including mucosa and a portion of the superior constrictor muscle. The midline superiorly based pharyngeal flap is inset into the posterior free edge of the soft palate, permanently attaching it to the posterior pharyngeal wall. The sphincter pharyngoplasty has been reported to involve creation of a dynamic sphincter made with the bilateral posterior tonsillar pillars containing the palatopharyngeus muscle. The superiorly based tonsillar pillars are elevated from the lateral pharynx and inset into

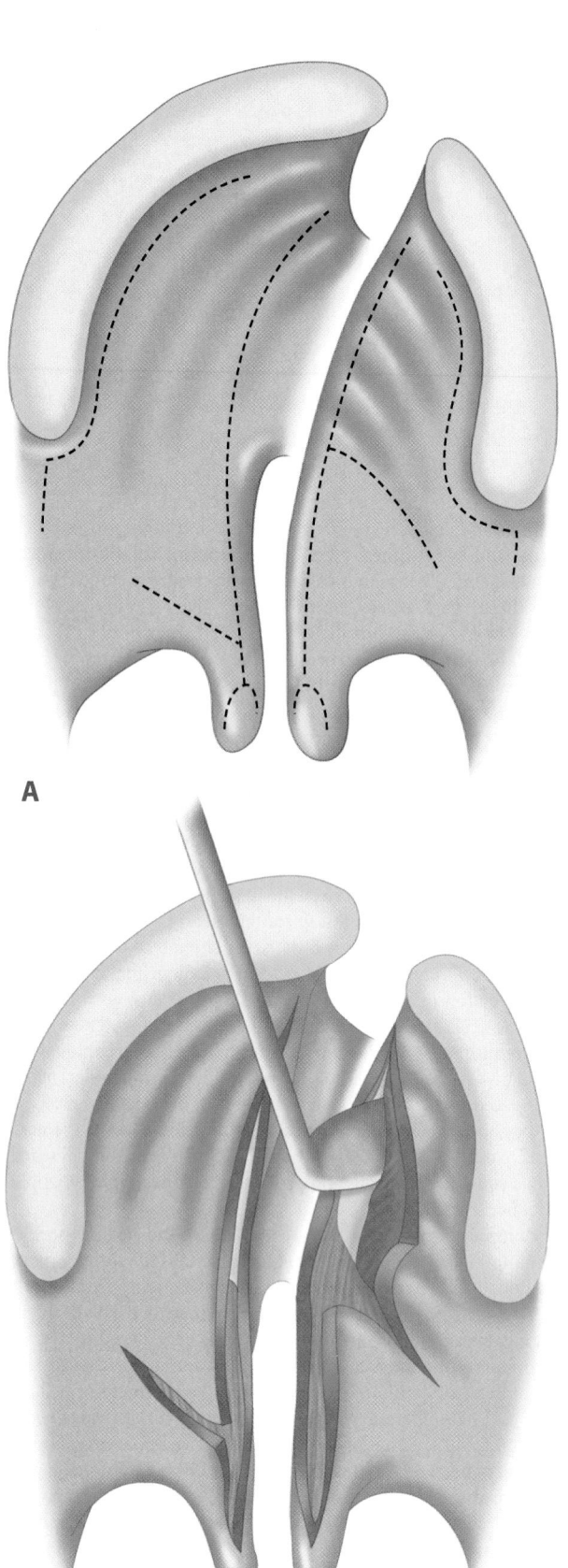

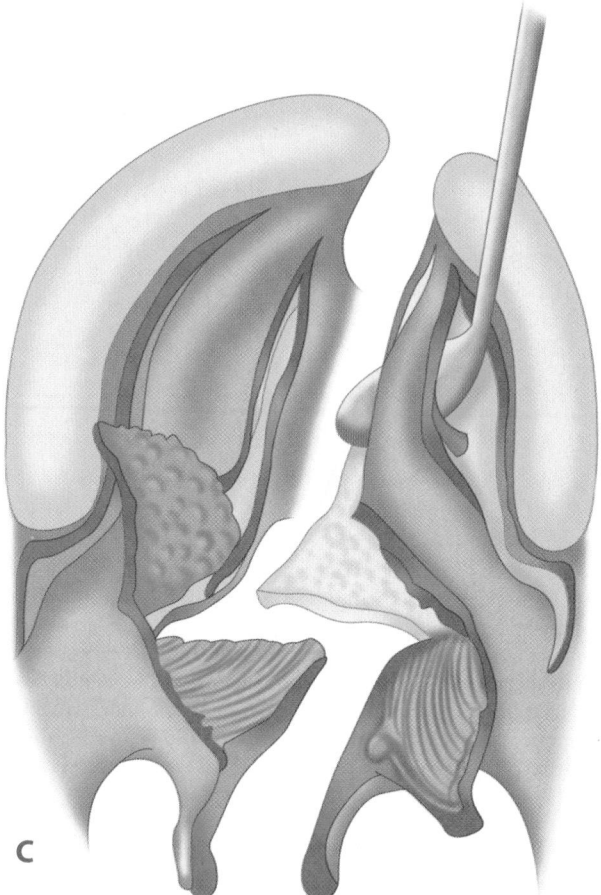

FIG. 45-16. A. Markings for the Furlow double opposing Z-plasty palatoplasty. **B.** Raising the oral flaps in a Furlow palatoplasty. **C.** The complete dissection of a Furlow palatoplasty.

a horizontal incision on the posterior pharyngeal wall at the level of the adenoid pad.

Craniofacial Anomalies
History, Overview, and Classification System

Craniofacial surgery is the subspecialty of plastic surgery dealing with hard and soft tissue deformities of the craniofacial skeleton, treating the congenital, developmental, and acquired defects of the cranial and/or facial skeleton. Craniofacial surgery addresses the functional and equally important appearance-related issues surrounding these deformities. Attempting to separate the functional impairment from the appearance-related issues is arbitrary, because it can be argued that the most important function of a face is to look like a face.[25] Numerous studies have established the importance of facial form and the significant emotional impact that facial deformities have on a person's life and sense of self.

The field of craniofacial surgery finds its origins in the aftermath of the world wars and the need to treat massive facial injuries. In 1967, Dr. Paul Tessier, now recognized as the father of craniofacial surgery, first publicly presented his concepts of using wide exposure and a transcranial route to treating craniofacial deformities with large segmental movements of bone. An American disciple of Dr. Tessier, Dr. Linton Whitaker of the Children's Hospital of Philadelphia, working with the Committee on Nomenclature and Classification of Craniofacial Anomalies of the American Cleft Palate-Craniofacial Association, presented a simple and practical classification system for craniofacial anomalies (Table 45-10).

It is the standard of care today that an interdisciplinary team of experts with specialized knowledge and training in treating children with craniofacial anomalies care for children who have such anomalies. The preoperative work-up and evaluation must be thorough and should include imaging (computed tomography, or CT; magnetic resonance imaging, or MRI; cephalography), photography, blood work, anesthesia consultation, and other components as the condition dictates. Craniofacial procedures are often long, complicated surgeries of significant magnitude, with an attendant risk of blood loss, serious morbidity, and even mortality. Significant blood loss is a realistic possibility, and preparation for blood conservation and transfusion must be made. The routine surgical approach to the craniofacial skeleton can be via a coronal incision, and after a bifrontal craniotomy, the orbital and facial skeleton can be addressed. Bone grafts for reconstruction can be split calvarial grafts or, alternatively, grafts from the ribs or iliac crest. Rigid fixation is obtained with bioresorbable plates, screws, and sutures. Despite the magnitude of the procedures, significant morbidity (blindness, brain injury, significant infection, cerebrospinal fluid leak, intracranial hematoma) or mortality is rare.

Craniofacial Clefts

The rare craniofacial clefts have been subclassified by Tessier (Fig. 45-17). The Tessier classification of craniofacial clefts considers the orbit as the center around which the clefts radiate as the spokes of a wheel, numbered from 0 to 14. The facial clefts (0 to 7) and their

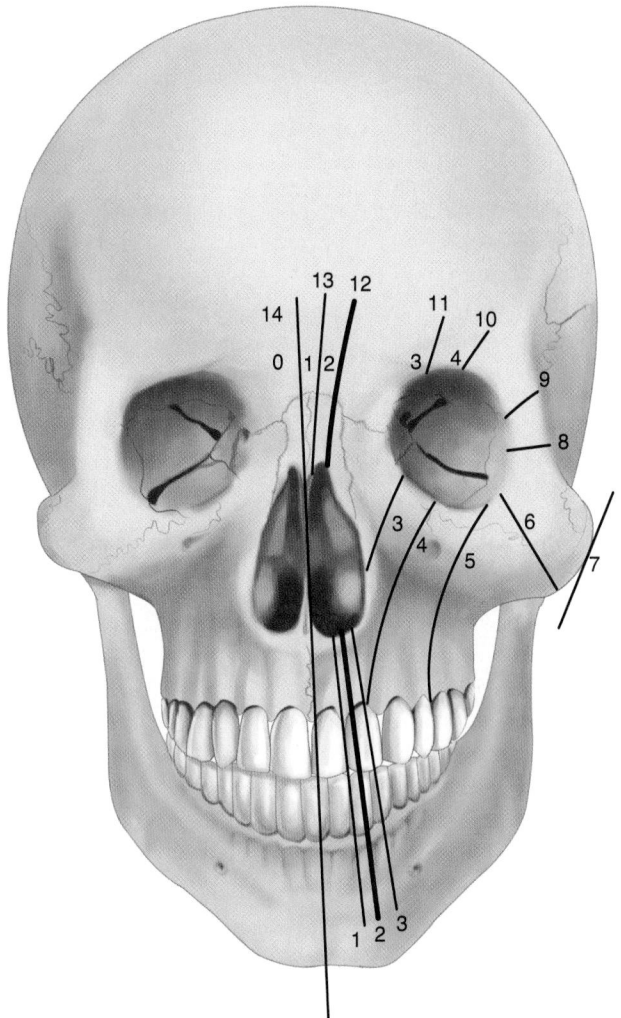

FIG. 45-17. Tessier's classification of craniofacial clefts.

cranial extensions (8 to 14) are often associated and total 14 (Fig. 45-18). Treacher Collins syndrome (Fig. 45-19), also known as *mandibulofacial dysostosis*, is a type of craniofacial clefting disorder representing bilateral 6-7-8 clefts. This autosomal dominant disorder with variable penetrance has the following manifestations: hypoplasia of the zygomas, asymmetry and hypoplasia of the mandible, ear anomalies, and colobomas of the lower eyelids. Craniofacial microsomia, also known as *hemifacial microsomia*, can be classified as a form of clefting as well (Fig. 45-20). Manifestations of this anomaly usually involve the hard and soft tissue of one half of the craniofacial skeleton. Deformities range in severity from complete absence of an affected facial component (globe, mandible, ear) to mild asymmetries. Ear deformities range from complete absence of the ear to only preauricular skin tags. Similarly, the eye deformities range from complete absence of the globe to various anomalies including epibulbar dermoids. Hypoplasia of the temporal skull, maxilla and zygoma, and orbit are seen in varying degree and affect the underlying skeleton as well as the overlying soft tissues. The classical deformity of hemifacial microsomia affects the mandible. Hypoplasia of the hemimandible, as well as the maxilla, results in dental malocclusions (Fig. 45-20C). Mandibular hypoplasia may range from minor underdevelopment of otherwise normal components to complete absence of the condyle, ramus, and proximal body. Treatment of hemifacial microsomia includes management of the airway and attention to other functional conditions. Treatment of the mandibular deformity includes distraction osteogenesis during growth and orthognathic procedures at skeletal maturity. Ear deformities are reconstructed

TABLE 45-10	Classification of craniofacial anomalies

I. Clefts
    a. Centric
    b. Acentric
II. Synostoses
    a. Symmetric
    b. Asymmetric
III. Atrophy, hypoplasia
IV. Neoplasia, hypertrophy, hyperplasia
V. Unclassified

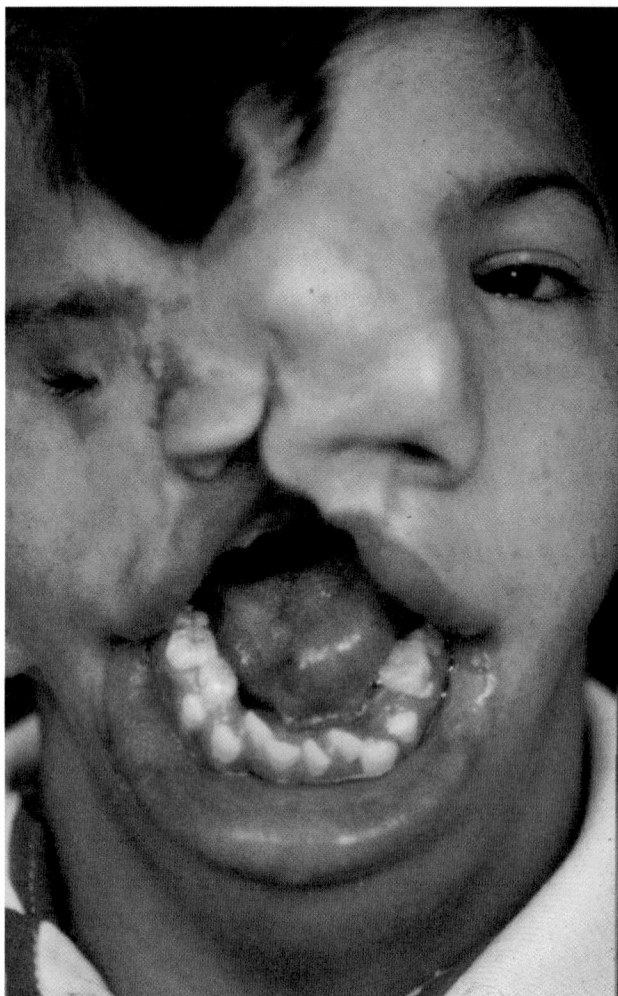

FIG. 45-18. Craniofacial cleft. *[Reproduced with permission from Losee J, Kirschner R (eds): Comprehensive Cleft Care, 1st ed. New York: McGraw-Hill Professional, 2008, Chap. 27, Fig. 3.]*

synostosis, important functional aspects include the potential for intracranial hypertension, which may result from brain growth restricted by an unyielding skull. The chances of intracranial hypertension increase with the number of sutures affected. Blindness and mental deficiencies secondary to an increase in intracranial pressure can likely be prevented by the surgical expansion of the cranium to release the fused suture, correct the abnormal head shape, and remodel the skull. The standard procedure used today in the correction of these synostotic deformities is fronto-orbital advancement. Fronto-orbital advancement, performed using a transcranial approach, includes a frontal craniotomy and orbital repositioning. The complex or multisutural synostoses are often syndromic, resulting from gain-in-function mutations of the fibroblast growth factor receptors (FGFR1, FGFR2, FGFR3). These syndromes of craniosynostosis include the Apert, Crouzon, Pfeiffer, and Saethre-Chotzen syndromes. The syndromic craniosynostoses not only in-

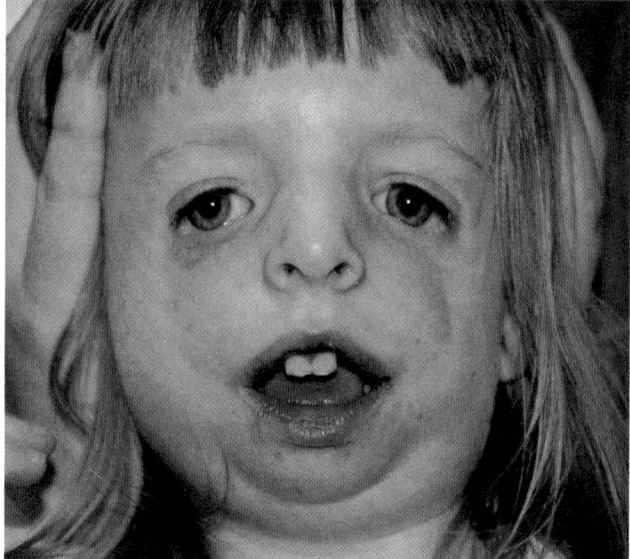

A

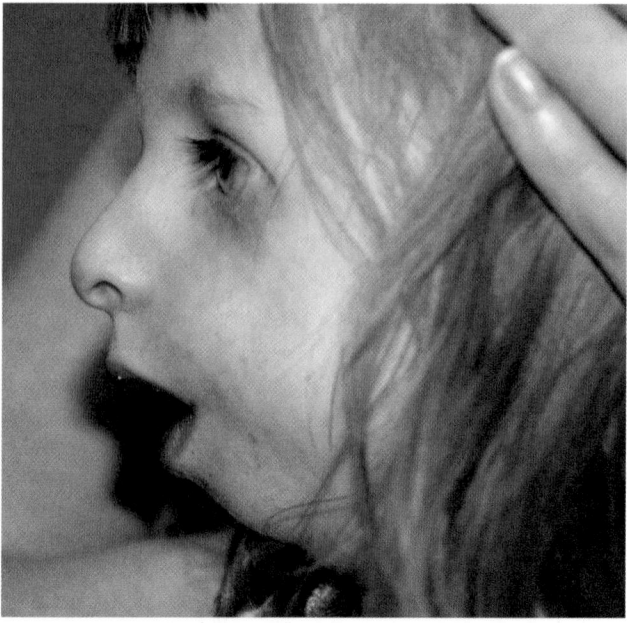

B

FIG. 45-19. Child with Treacher Collins syndrome. **A.** Frontal view. **B.** Lateral view. (*Continued*)

with techniques using costal cartilage and local soft tissue. Soft tissue deficiencies of the hemiface can be treated with fat injections, dermal-fat grafts, or free tissue transfer. Orbital hypertelorism is yet another type of midline craniofacial (0-14) clefting. *Orbital hypertelorism* is defined as a lateralization of the entire orbit, increasing the intraorbital distance and resulting from midline conditions such as encephaloceles, frontonasal dysplasia, and syndromic craniosynostosis. The treatment of severe orbital hypertelorism includes a transcranial approach to four-wall orbital box osteotomies, resection or treatment of the abnormal midline process, mobilization, medialization of the orbital complexes, and nasal reconstruction with a cantilever nasal bone graft.

Craniosynostosis

The craniosynostoses are a group of disorders that result from the abnormal obliteration or premature fusion of the cranial sutures. The craniosynostoses can be subdivided into simple or single-suture craniosynostoses, and complex, syndromic, or multiple-suture craniosynostoses. The cranial sutures allow for the normal growth of the skull, and therefore the classic presentation of craniosynostosis is an abnormal head shape. The resultant abnormal head shapes are secondary to an inhibition of skull growth at right angles to the fused suture and a compensatory overexpansion of the skull perpendicular to the fused suture into areas with open sutures. These abnormal head shapes provide a basis for the classification of craniosynostoses. In addition to appearance-related deformities resulting from cranio-

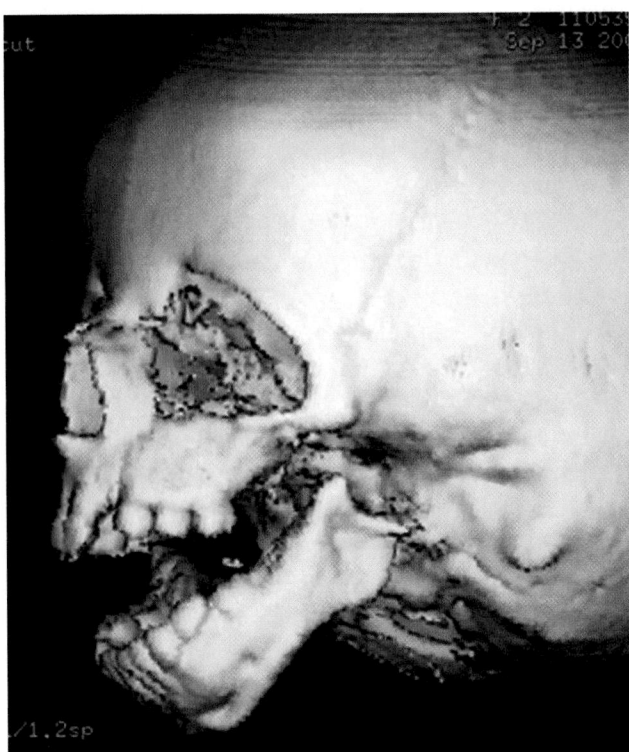

C

FIG. 45-19. (*Continued*) **C.** Three-dimensional computed tomographic scan of the craniofacial skeleton.

clude bicoronal synostosis but also involve the midface with resulting exorbitism and midface hypoplasia. Multilevel airway anomalies, obstructive sleep apnea, corneal exposure, intracranial hypertension, feeding difficulties, and severe malocclusion are some of the associated anomalies found in children with syndromic craniosynostoses. In addition to fronto-orbital advancement, facial osteotomies (i.e., Le Fort III craniofacial dysjunction) are required to treat the orbital, midfacial, and occlusal deformities.

Atrophy and Hypoplasia

The categories of craniofacial atrophy and hypoplasia encompass many conditions such as Pierre Robin sequence and Romberg's progressive hemifacial atrophy. Pierre Robin sequence is characterized by three pathognomonic findings: microretrognathia, glossoptosis, and respiratory distress. Pierre Robin sequence may or may not be associated with a palatal cleft. It is thought by some to occur secondary to a fixed and flexed fetal head position that inhibits mandibular growth and results in micrognathia. The micrognathia prevents the natural caudal migration of the tongue from between the clefted palatal shelves, and the resulting deformity as described earlier. The functional consequences include intermittent respiratory obstruction and obstructive sleep apnea that may affect feeding, growth, and safety of the airway. Treatment of a child mildly affected with Pierre Robin sequence may include simply positioning the child prone until the child "grows out" of the condition. However, if the child is severely affected and unable to feed adequately or has an unsafe airway, surgical intervention is required. For decades, tracheotomy was the initial and definitive treatment of choice; however, today many initially attempt a tongue-lip adhesion, treating the glossoptosis and alleviating respiratory obstruction by suturing the tongue tip to the lower lip. The tongue-lip adhesion is taken down at the time of palatoplasty. Should the tongue-lip adhesion not adequately correct the obstruction, then neonatal mandibular distrac-

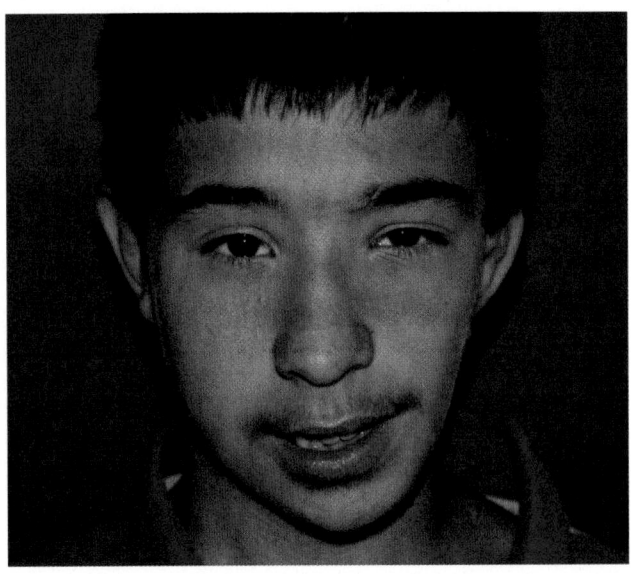

A

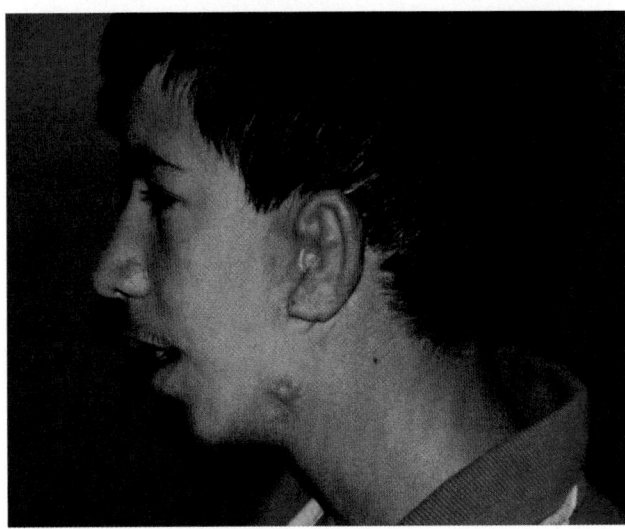

B

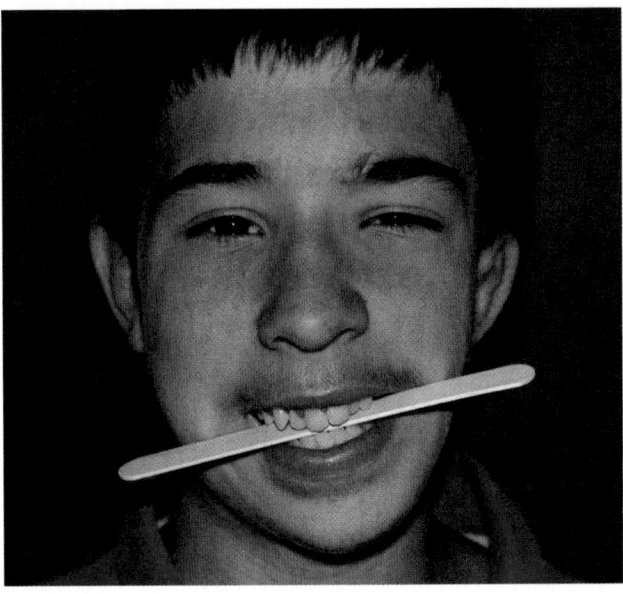

C

FIG. 45-20. Child with left-sided craniofacial/hemifacial microsomia. **A.** Frontal view. **B.** Lateral view. **C.** Bite plane.

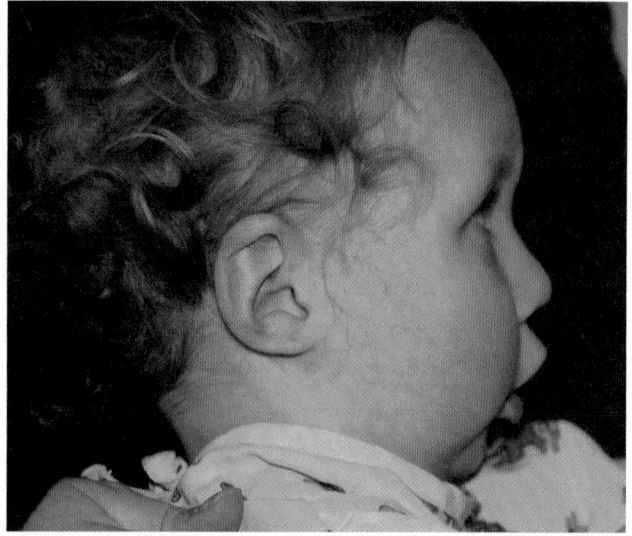

A

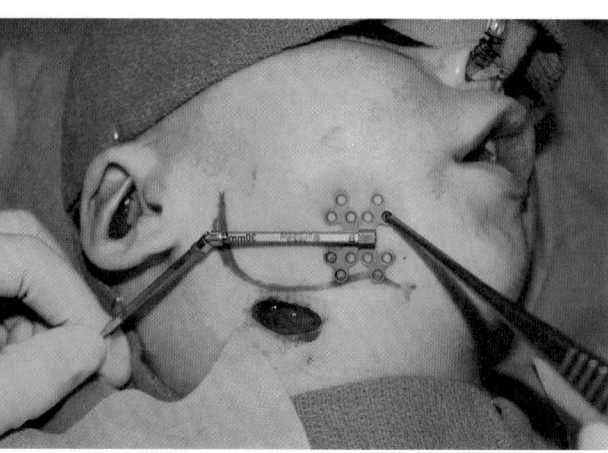

B

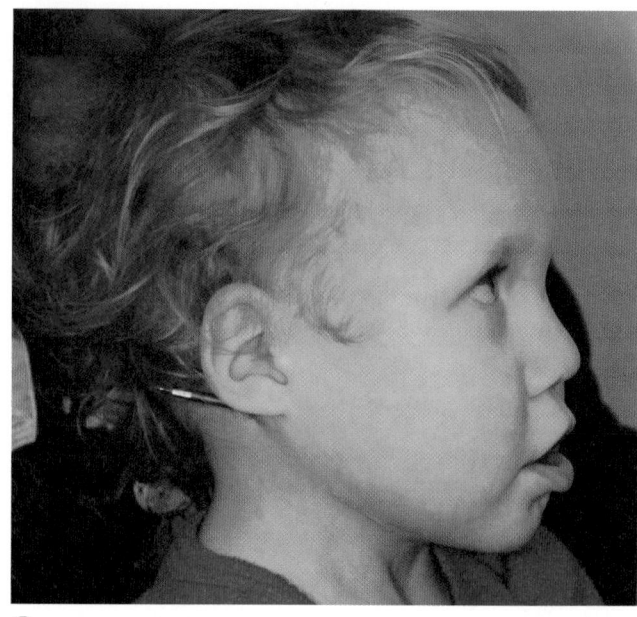

C

FIG. 45-21. A. Lateral view of a child with Pierre Robin sequence and mandibular microretrognathia. **B.** Intraoperative photo of a submandibular incision and planning for the placement of a buried mandibular distractor. **C.** Lateral view of the child after mandibular distraction with slight overcorrection of retrognathia. The distractor is still in place as evident from the activating rod seen exiting the skin retroauricularly.

tion can be used to correct the underlying microretrognathia and relieve the obstructive symptoms (Fig. 45-21). Another syndrome of atrophy and hypoplasia is Romberg's progressive hemifacial atrophy, also known as *Parry-Romberg syndrome* (Fig. 45-22). Romberg's disease is a disorder of unknown etiology, beginning in childhood or adolescence, in which hemifacial atrophy of the skin, subcutaneous fat, muscle, bone, and cartilage progresses for a variable period of time before spontaneously ceasing or "burning out" 2 to 10 years after beginning. Most believe treatment should be delayed until at least 1 year after the process of atrophy has ceased. Some hematologists and oncologists have treated the early presentation of Romberg's disease with chemotherapy. After the cessation of atrophy, reconstruction of the craniofacial skeleton and soft tissues may begin with bone and/or cartilage grafts, alloplastic implants, dermal-fat grafts, fat grafting, and possibly free tissue transfers.

Hyperplasia, Hypertrophy, and Neoplasia

The categories of craniofacial hyperplasia, hypertrophy, and neoplasia encompass a wide variety of conditions affecting the craniofacial skeleton. These include vascular anomalies (discussed later in this chapter), neurofibromatosis, hemifacial hypertrophy, and bony conditions such as osteomas and fibrous dysplasia. Fibrous dysplasia can be monostotic, affecting a single location, or polyostotic, affecting more than a single location in the skeleton; it may be associated with skin pigmentation abnormalities and endocrine involvement, and be termed *polyostotic* or *McCune-Albright syn-*

drome. Treatment of fibrous dysplasia of the craniofacial skeleton includes block resection and reconstruction with bone grafts. If extensive involvement exists and block resection is not possible or feasible, partial resection and contouring of the affected bone is possible, as long as there is the understanding that long-term outcomes and the behavior of the disease are unpredictable.

Vascular Anomalies

Vascular anomalies are vascular birthmarks that all appear similar: flat or raised, in various shades of red and purple.[26] For centuries, they have been named by similarly colored food and drink (i.e., strawberry hemangioma, port-wine stain). Today these vascular birthmarks have been biologically classified as either *hemangiomas* or *vascular malformations*. The Greek suffix -*oma* means "swelling" or "tumor" and today connotes a lesion characterized by hyperplasia. Hemangiomas are congenital vascular anomalies that undergo a phase of rapid growth followed by slow regression, based on endothelial cell kinetics. Malformations are abnormal vascular channels lined with quiescent endothelium, usually are seen at birth, never regress, and have the potential to expand. The differential diagnosis of vascular anomalies is routinely made by a detailed accurate history and clinical examination. For deep lesions, radiographic studies may help determine the diagnosis. Biopsy is used if the diagnosis is uncertain or there is concern over the potential of malignancy.

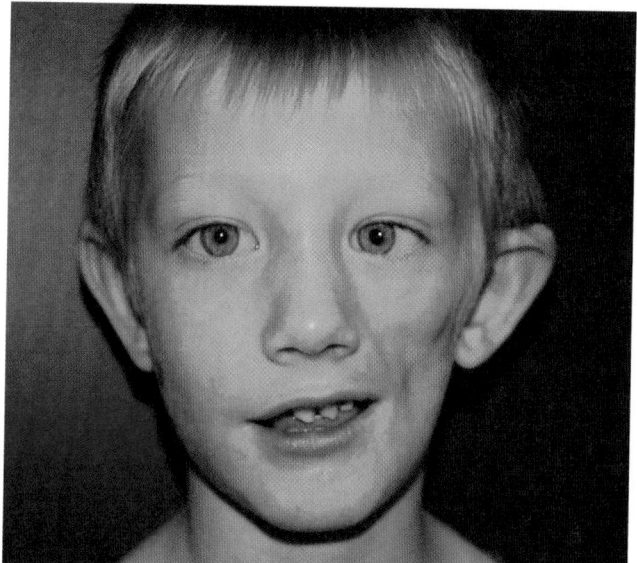

FIG. 45-22. Frontal view of a child with left-sided Romberg's progressive hemifacial atrophy.

Hemangiomas

The infantile hemangioma is the most common birthmark, affecting 10 to 12% of whites, with a 3-5:1 predilection for females and an increased incidence in preterm infants (23%) (Fig. 45-23). Hemangiomas are solitary in 80% of cases and multiple in 20%. In children with multiple (more than three) cutaneous hemangiomas, abdominal ultrasound is suggested to rule out hemangiomatosis with visceral involvement. Hemangiomas do not cause bleeding disorders; however, more invasive lesions such as kaposiform hemangioendothelioma can result in Kasselbach-Merritt syndrome, characterized by platelet trapping and disordered bleeding. Hemangiomas are usually first noted around 2 weeks of life as a flat pink spot, often confused with a superficial scratch. Around the second month of life they enter the *proliferating phase* in which rapid growth is seen caused by plump, rapidly dividing endothelial cells. If the hemangioma is superficial, the skin becomes crimson and raised; if the lesion is deep, a dark blue or purple color is noted with less superficial swelling. Hemangioma growth frequently peeks before the first year, and then the lesions enter the *involuting phase* in which growth is commiserate with the child. The involuting phase is characterized by diminishing endothelial activity and luminal enlargement. The lesion begins to "gray," losing its intense reddish color and taking on a purple-gray shade with overlying "crepe paper" skin. The involution phase continues until 5 to 10 years of age. Regression of the lesion is then complete. The *involuted phase* begins in 50% of children by 5 years of age and in 70% by 7 years. If there was cutaneous ulceration during the proliferative phase, a cutaneous scar may persist, along with the yellow-gray crepe paper–like skin with fibro-fatty deposition. In 50% of children, near-normal skin is restored. The treatment of hemangiomas is largely observational, with reassurance of parents that regression and involution will occur. Cutaneous ulceration secondary to a proliferating hemangioma occurs in 5% of cases and more frequently with lip or urogenital lesions. Local wound care, topical application of lidocaine for pain, and laser cauterization may be beneficial treatment modalities. Problematic or endangering hemangiomas (i.e., periocular lesions threatening amblyopia, airway lesions, facially disfiguring lesions) occur in 10% of cases. The first-line treatment for problematic hemangiomas is systemic corticosteroid therapy, which is particularly effective (85% response rate). Second-line therapies include interferon and vincristine, each with its own attendant effectiveness and morbidity. Laser therapy has been claimed by some to be effective in the treatment of early hemangiomas; however, there has been no conclusive proof that

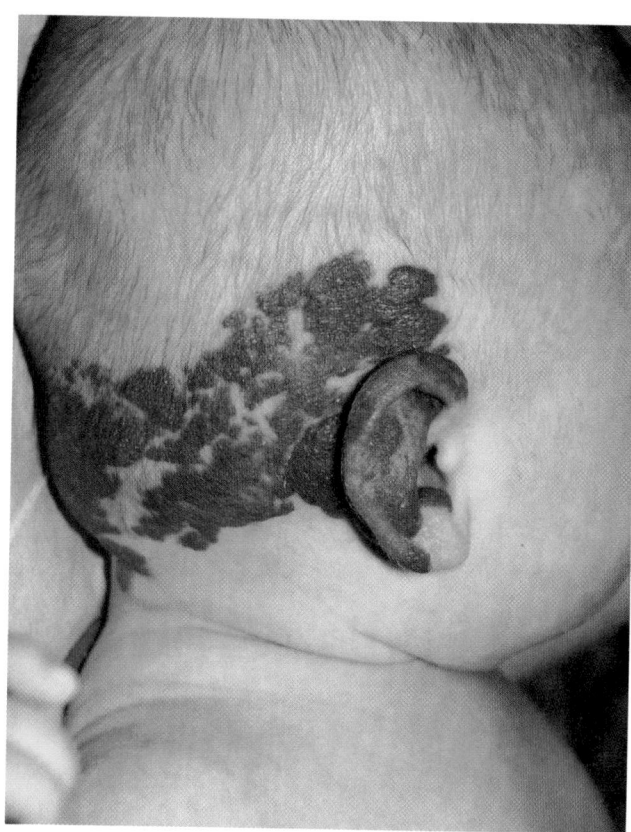

FIG. 45-23. Hemangioma of the ear and retroauricular region.

laser therapy either diminishes lesion bulk or induces involution. Laser therapy has been effective in lightening affected skin. Surgery for hemangiomas in the proliferating phase is largely limited to treatment of problematic lesions (i.e., eyelid lesions threatening amblyopia). Hemangioma surgery usually is reserved for the treatment of secondary deformities and residual fibro-fatty depositions, among other indications.

Vascular Malformations

Vascular malformations are subclassified by vessel type, such as lymphatic, capillary, venous, or arterial, and by rheologic characteristics, such as slow flow and fast flow. Slow-flow lesions include capillary malformations (CMs) and telangiectasias, lymphatic malformations (LMs), and venous malformations (VMs). Fast-flow lesions include arterial malformations (AMs) and arteriovenous malformations (AVMs). In addition, there are combined malformations. One such combined lesion occurs in Klippel-Trénaunay syndrome in which CMs, LMs, and VMs are found and may be associated with soft tissue and skeletal hypertrophy in one or more of the limbs (Fig. 45-24A).

CMs are pink-red macular vascular stains that are present at birth and persist throughout life. These lesions tend to become more verrucous and darker throughout life. CMs are effectively treated with a pulsed-dye laser, and the results often are better with treatment in infancy and young childhood. Laser therapy often is repetitive and prolonged. CMs of the head and neck, historically called *port-wine stains*, may be associated with Sturge-Weber syndrome, which includes vascular involvement of the leptomeninges and ocular pathology (Fig. 45-24B).

LMs are anomalous lymphatic channels that never regress and have the potential to affect underlying muscle and bone, causing significant swelling and bony overgrowth. They have historically been called *lymphangiomas* or *cystic hygromas* (Fig. 45-24C). LMs can be classified as microcystic, macrocystic, or both. LMs expand or contract with the flow of lymph, infection, or intralesional hemorrhage.

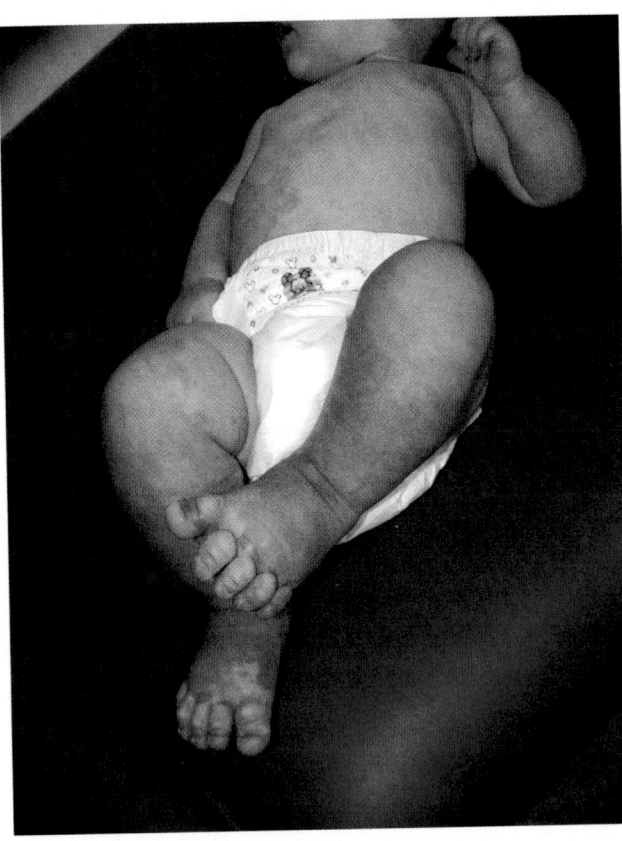

A

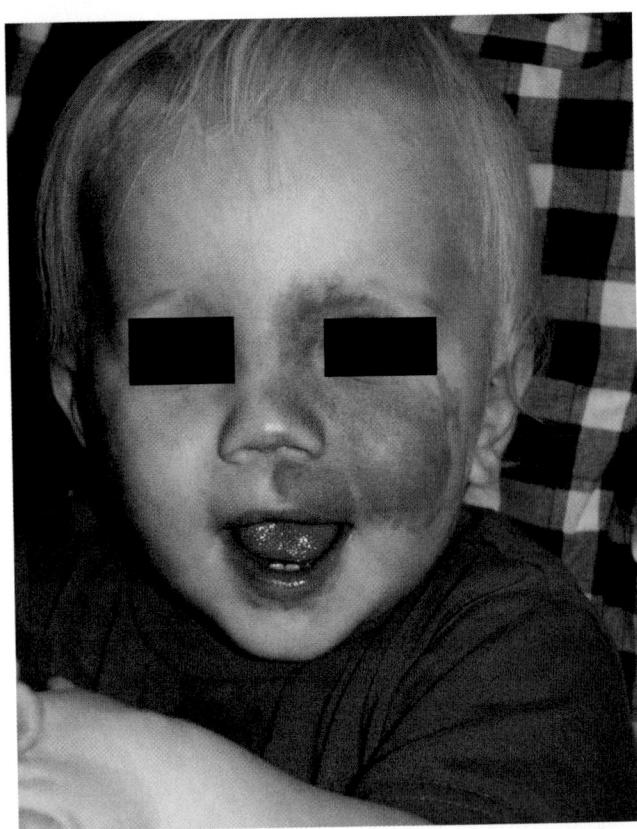

B

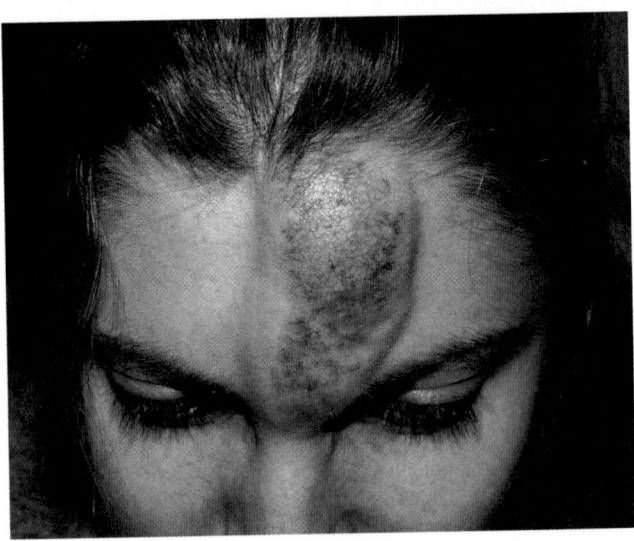

C

D

FIG. 45-24. A. Klippel-Trénaunay syndrome, with combined vascular anomaly (capillary malformation, lymphatic malformation, venous malformation) of the leg. **B.** Sturge-Weber syndrome, with V1 and V2 capillary malformation of the left face. **C.** Lymphatic malformation of the neck, previously referred to as *cystic hygroma*. **D.** Venous malformation of the forehead.

Superficial LMs that affect the skin often produce cutaneous vesicles that may coalesce and weep lymph fluid. Sclerotherapy remains a major treatment modality for LMs, and lesions that are macrocystic can be aspirated before sclerotherapy. Although surgery rarely removes the entire lesion, surgical resection is the only possibility for cure. These resections often are challenging, lengthy, and associated with significant blood loss, and the potential exists for regeneration of lymph channels and recurrence of the LMs postoperatively.

VMs are frequently bluish, soft, and compressible, and swell when dependent (Fig. 45-24D). VMs grow with the child, expand slowly, and may enlarge during puberty. Patients often complain about stiffness and pain with thrombosis. VMs can affect the skin, muscle, and bone. MRI is the modality of choice for imaging these lesions. Preoperative sclerosis followed by surgical extirpation is the treatment of choice for VMs that cause functional or appearance-related disability. VMs have the tendency to recanalize and re-expand. Use of elastic support stocking and low-dose aspirin therapy are important adjunctive treatment modalities for VMs involving the legs.

Pure AMs are rare and more commonly present as AVMs. AVMs appear as red violaceous skin with a palpable mass beneath. Local warmth, bruit, and thrill are frequently present. AVMs have the likely consequences of ischemic changes, ulceration, intractable pain, and intermittent bleeding. The natural history of AVMs has been described as consisting of four stages: quiescence, expansion, destruction, and decompensation. Usually, treatment for AVM is initiated when signs and symptoms of ischemic pain, ulceration, bleeding, or hemodynamic instability (stages 3 and 4) are evident. Surgical treatment includes arterial embolization to temporarily occlude the nidus 24 to 72 hours before surgical extirpation. The nidus and overlying affected skin must be widely excised, and reconstruction can be performed afterward.

Congenital Melanocytic Nevi

Congenital melanocytic nevi (CMNs) contain nevus cells and are usually present at birth. Lesions are frequently light to dark brown and round or oval, and vary greatly in size, pattern, and anatomic location. The most common location of CMNs is the trunk, followed by the extremities and head and neck. Frequently, larger lesions are associated with multiple smaller satellite lesions. Over time, these lesions may become less (or sometimes more) pigmented and develop hypertrichosis and a variegated texture, including nodularity. Small CMNs are <1.5 cm in diameter, and large ones are >10 cm. Giant CMNs usually are >20 cm in their greatest dimension in adulthood, and this correlates with a 9-cm scalp lesion or a 6-cm trunk lesion in an infant. All CMNs should be monitored for worrisome changes that indicate the need for biopsy, including ulceration, uneven pigmentation, change in shape, and nodularity. There is controversy over the actual incidence of malignant transformation of CMNs; however, most experts believe that melanoma may arise directly from a CMN. No convincing study to date has proven

that excision of a CMN reduces the rate of malignant transformation to melanoma; however, many clinicians feel that excision serves at least to debulk the lesion. The reported lifetime risk for melanoma arising in small or large CMNs is between 0 and 5%; the risk for giant CMNs is estimated to be between 5 and 10%.[27] In addition to being at risk for melanoma, patients with large or giant CMNs are at risk for neurocutaneous melanocytosis (leptomeningeal melanosis), and this condition includes collections of melanocytes in the leptomeninges. Neurocutaneous melanocytosis carries a lifetime non-reducible risk of central nervous system melanoma and other morbidity and mortality from seizures, hydrocephalus, and other central nervous system conditions. MRI screening for infants born with large or giant CMNs is recommended to make the diagnosis of neurocutaneous melanocytosis.

Many different treatments have been advocated for the child with CMN; however, the overwhelming goals are to remove (or at least reduce) the risk of malignant transformation, preserve function, and improve cosmesis. Dermabrasion, chemical peels, and laser therapy have been reported to improve the appearance; however, none of these modalities completely removes nevus cells. To address malignant potential, only complete excision is a possible solution, and this is difficult, because nevus cells may extend beyond the skin and into the deep subcutaneous tissue and even the underlying muscle. The surgical options include direct excision and primary closure, serial excision, excision and skin grafting, and staged tissue expansion with subsequent lesion excision and lap reconstruction (Fig. 45-25). Treatment options have particular indications with respect to the location of the nevus. Scalp lesions are best treated with tissue expansion. Full-thickness skin grafting is best used for ear and eyelid reconstruction. Tissue expansion is associated with increased morbidity in lower extremity reconstruction, and therefore excision and grafting, even with previously expanded full-thickness skin grafts, is often the treatment of choice. In summary, CMNs often are treated surgically to decrease the risk of malignant degeneration to melanoma as well as to correct the significant appearance-related deformity.

RECONSTRUCTIVE SURGERY

Facial Reconstruction after Fracture
General Principles

As technologic advances raise the level of energy involved in modern systems of transportation, recreation, and weaponry, so follow in-

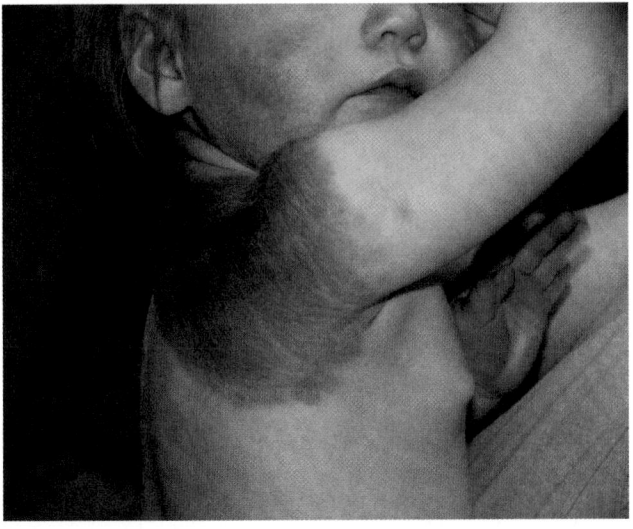
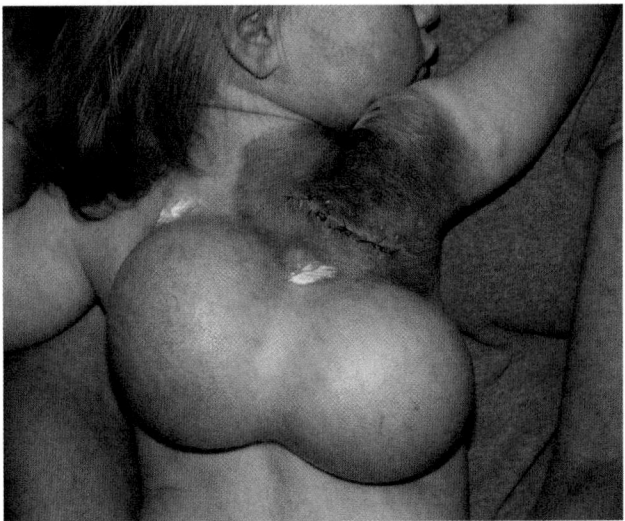

A **B**

FIG. 45-25. A. Congenital melanocytic nevus (CMN) of the posterior shoulder. **B.** Treatment of CMN of the posterior shoulder with tissue expansion. (*Continued*)

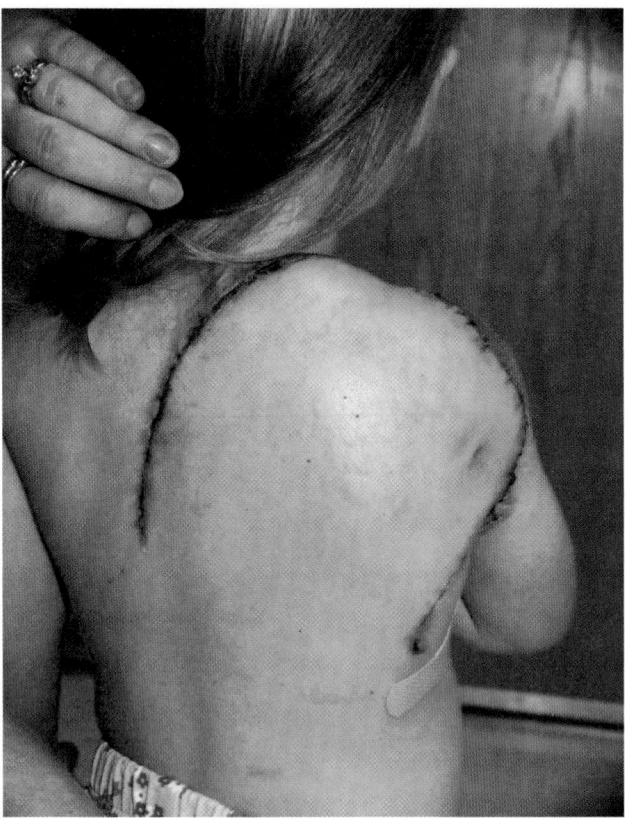

C

FIG. 45-25. (*Continued*) **C.** Appearance of the posterior shoulder after removal of tissue expanders, excision of the CMN, and flap coverage.

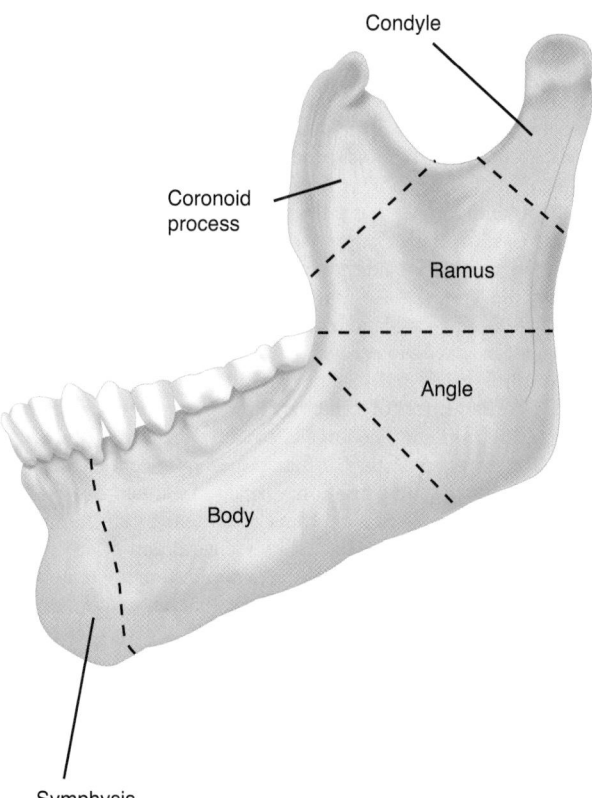

FIG. 45-26. Mandibular anatomy. (*Reproduced with permission from Thornton J, Hollier L: Facial fractures II: Lower third. Selected Readings Plast Surg 9:1, 2002.*)

creases in the degree of maxillofacial destruction related to misadventures with this technology. The first phase of care for the patient with maxillofacial trauma is activation of the advanced trauma life support protocol. Concomitant injuries beyond the face are the rule rather than the exception. The most common life-threatening considerations in the facial trauma patient are airway maintenance, control of bleeding, identification and treatment of aspiration, and identification of other injuries. Once the patient's condition has been stabilized and life-threatening injuries treated, attention is directed to diagnosis and management of craniofacial injuries.

Physical examination of the face with attention to lacerations, bony step-offs, instability, tenderness, ecchymosis, facial asymmetry, and deformity guides the examiner to underlying hard tissue injuries. Traditional specialized radiography has largely been replaced by widely available high-resolution CT. Coronal, sagittal, and three-dimensional reconstructions of images further elucidate complex injuries.

Mandible Fractures

Mandibular fractures are common injuries that may lead to permanent disability if not diagnosed and properly treated. The mandibular angle, ramus, coronoid process, and condyle are points of attachment for the muscles of mastication, including the masseter, temporalis, lateral pterygoid, and medial pterygoid muscles (Fig. 45-26). Fractures are frequently multiple, and disturbances in dental occlusion reflect the forces of the many muscles of mastication on the fracture segments. Dental occlusion is perhaps the most important basic relationship to understand about fracture of the midface and mandible. The Angle classification system describes the relationship of the maxillary teeth to the mandibular teeth. Class I is normal occlusion, with the mesial buccal cusp of the first maxillary molar

fitting into the intercuspal groove of the mandibular first molar. Class II malocclusion is characterized by anterior (mesial) positioning, and class III malocclusion is posterior (distal) positioning of the maxillary teeth with respect to the mandibular teeth (Fig. 45-27).

Nonsurgical treatment may be used in situations in which there is minimal to no displacement, preservation of the pretraumatic occlusive relationship, and normal range of motion. The goals of surgical treatment include restoration of pretraumatic dental occlusion, reduction and stable fixation of the fracture, and repair of soft tissue. Operative repair involves seating of the condyles within the glenoid fossa, achievement of maxillary-mandibular fixation with arch bars or intermaxillary screws to establish proper dental occlusion, and intraoral, extraoral, or combination surgical exposure of fracture lines. The mandibular plating approach follows one of two schools of thought: rigid fixation as espoused by the Association of Internal Fixation group (AO/ASIF) and less rigid but functionally stable fixation (Champy technique). Regardless of the stabilization approach, one of the postoperative objectives is release from maxillary-mandibular fixation and resumption of range of motion as soon as possible to minimize the risk of ankylosis. Other potential complications include infection, nonunion, malunion, malocclusion, facial nerve branch injury, infra-alveolar or mental nerve injury, and dental fractures.

Orbital Fractures

Treatment of all but the simplest orbital injuries should include evaluation by an eye specialist to assess visual acuity and rule out globe injury. Orbital fractures may involve the orbital roof, floor, or lateral or medial walls. The most common orbital fracture is the orbital floor blow-out fracture caused by direct pressure to the globe and sudden increase in intraorbital pressure. Because the medial floor

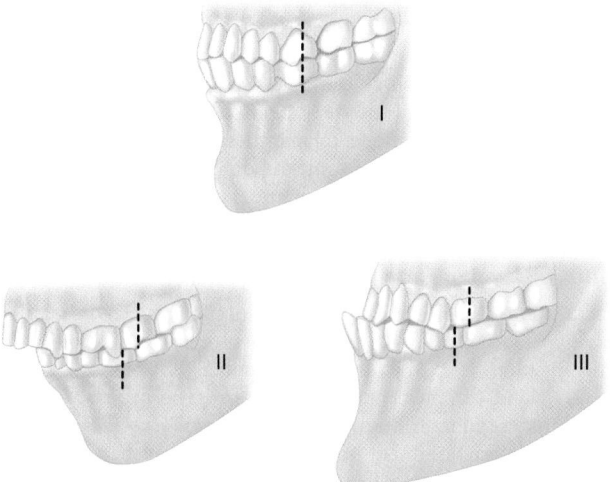

FIG. 45-27. Angle classification. Class I: The mesial buccal cusp of the maxillary first molar fits into the intercuspal groove of the mandibular first molar. Class II: The mesial buccal cusp of the maxillary first molar is mesial to the intercuspal groove of the mandibular first molar. Class III: The mesial buccal cusp of the maxillary first molar is distal to the intercuspal groove of the mandibular first molar. *(Reproduced with permission from Thornton J, Hollier L: Facial fractures II: Lower third.* Selected Readings Plast Surg *9:1, 2002.)*

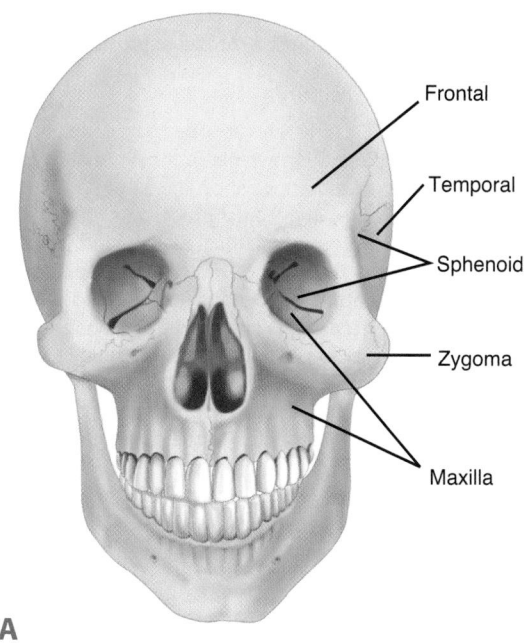

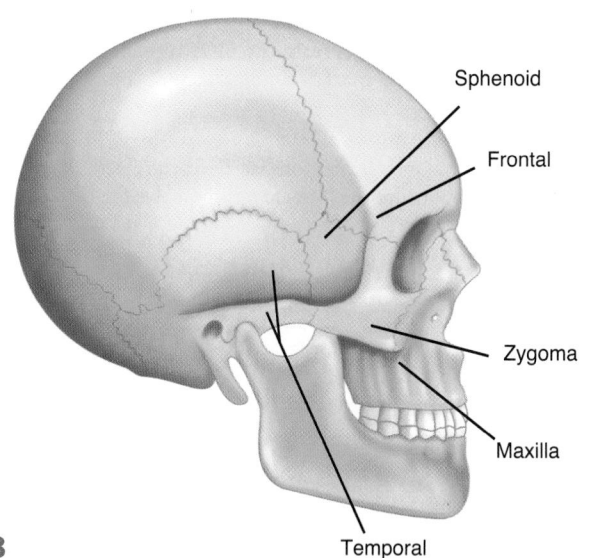

FIG. 45-28. Facial bone anatomy. *(Reproduced with permission from Hollier et al.[28])*

and inferior medial wall are made of the thinnest bone, fractures occur most frequently at these locations. These injuries may be treated expectantly if they are sufficiently small and without complication. However, larger blow-out fractures and those associated with enophthalmos (increased intraorbital volume), entrapment of inferior orbital tissues (diagnosed via the forced duction test), or diplopia lasting >2 weeks generally require surgical treatment.[28] There are many approaches to the orbital floor, including the transconjunctival, subciliary, and lower blepharoplasty incisions. All provide access to the orbital floor and allow for repair with a multitude of different autogenous and synthetic materials. Late complications include persistent diplopia, enophthalmos, ectropion, and entropion.

Lateral and inferior orbital rim fractures also are not uncommon and are often associated with the zygomaticomaxillary complex fracture pattern, as discussed later.

Special mention should be made of two uncommon complications after orbital fracture. Superior orbital fissure syndrome results from compression of structures contained in the superior orbital fissure in the posterior orbit. These include cranial nerves III, IV, and VI, and the first sensory division of cranial nerve V. Compression of these structures leads to symptoms of eyelid ptosis, globe proptosis, paralysis of the extraocular muscles, and anesthesia in the cranial nerve V1 distribution. If the optic nerve (cranial nerve II) is also involved, symptoms include blindness and the syndrome is dubbed *orbital apex syndrome.* Both of these syndromes are medical emergencies, and steroid therapy or surgical decompression is considered.

Zygoma and Zygomaticomaxillary Complex Fractures

The zygoma forms the lateral and inferior borders of the orbit. It articulates with the sphenoid bone in the lateral orbit, the maxilla medially and inferiorly, the frontal bone superiorly, and the temporal bone laterally (Fig. 45-28). Zygoma fractures may involve the arch alone or many of its bony relationships. Isolated arch fractures manifest as a flattened, wide face with associated edema and ecchymosis. Nondisplaced fractures may be treated nonsurgically, whereas displaced and comminuted arch fractures may be reduced and stabilized indirectly (Gilles approach) or, for more complicated fractures, directly through a coronal incision.

The zygomaticomaxillary complex (ZMC) fracture involves disruption of the zygomatic arch, the inferior orbital rim buttress, the zygomaticomaxillary buttress, the lateral orbital wall, and the zygomaticofrontal buttress. The fracture segment tends to rotate laterally and inferiorly, creating an expanded orbital volume, limited mandibular excursion, an inferior cant to the palpebral fissure, and a flattened malar eminence. ZMC fractures are almost always accompanied by numbness in the infraorbital nerve distribution and subconjunctival hematoma. Displaced fractures are treated by exposure through multiple incisions to gain access to all of the buttresses requiring fixation. These include the upper eyelid incision (zygomaticofrontal buttress and lateral orbital wall), the subtarsal or transconjunctival incision (orbital floor and infraorbital rim), and the maxillary gingivobuccal sulcus incision (zygomaticomaxillary buttress). Again, significantly complex zygomatic fractures require wide exposure through a coronal approach.[5]

Naso-Orbital-Ethmoid Fractures

Naso-orbital-ethmoid (NOE) fractures are often part of a constellation of panfacial fractures and intracranial injuries. Anatomically, the fracture pattern involves the medial orbits, nasal bones, nasal processes of the frontal bone, and frontal processes of the maxilla. These injuries result in severe functional deficit and cosmetic deformity from collapse of the nose, ethmoids, and medial orbits; displacement of medial canthal ligament fixation; and nasolacrimal apparatus disruption. Telecanthus is produced by splaying apart of the nasomaxillary buttresses to which the medial canthal ligaments are attached. Treatment typically involves plating or wiring all bone fragments meticulously, potentially with primary bone grafting, to restore their normal configuration. Key to the successful repair of an NOE fracture is the careful re-establishment of the nasomaxillary buttress and restoration of the pretrauma fixation points of the medial canthal ligaments. If comminution is severe, this may be achievable using transnasal wiring of the ligaments.

Frontal Sinus Fractures

The region of the frontal sinus is a relatively weak structural point in the upper face. For this reason, it is a common location for fracture in facial trauma. The paired sinuses each have an anterior bony table that determines the contour of the forehead and a posterior table that separates the sinus from the dura. Each sinus drains through the medial floor into its frontonasal duct, which empties into the middle meatus within the nose. Treatment of a frontal sinus fracture depends on the fracture characteristics (Fig. 45-29).

Nasal Fractures

The nose is the most common facial fracture site due to its prominent location, and such fracture can involve the cartilaginous nasal septum, the nasal bones, or both. It is important to perform an intranasal examination to determine whether a septal hematoma is present. If present, a septal hematoma must be incised, drained, and packed to prevent pressure necrosis of the nasal septum and long-term midvault collapse. Closed reduction of nasal fractures may be performed under local or general anesthesia. Unfortunately, many, if not most, show some deformity upon final healing, requiring rhinoplasty if airway obstruction is present or if improved appearance is desired.

Panfacial Fractures

Fractures of multiple bones in various locations fall into the category of panfacial fracture. These may involve frontal and maxillary sinus fractures, NOE fractures, orbital and ZMC fractures, palatal fractures, and complex mandible fractures. The difficulty in the repair of these injuries lies not in the technical aspects of fixation but in the re-establishment of normal relationships between facial features in the absence of all pretraumatic reference points. Without proper correction of bony fragment relationships, facial width is exaggerated and facial projection is lost. The key point in approaching the patient with a panfacial fracture is first to reduce and repair the zygomatic arches and frontal bar to establish the frame and width of the face. The nasomaxillary and zygomaticomaxillary buttresses may then be repaired within this correct frame. Next, the maxilla may be reduced to this framework, followed by palatal fixation if needed. Finally, now that the midface relationships have been corrected, maxillary-mandibular fixation can be applied with the mandible in correct occlusion followed by plating of any mandibular fractures.[29]

Ear Reconstruction

Acquired defects of the auricle have many causes, and many different choices for reconstruction are available. Reconstructive approach often is determined by the size and location of the defect. Small helical

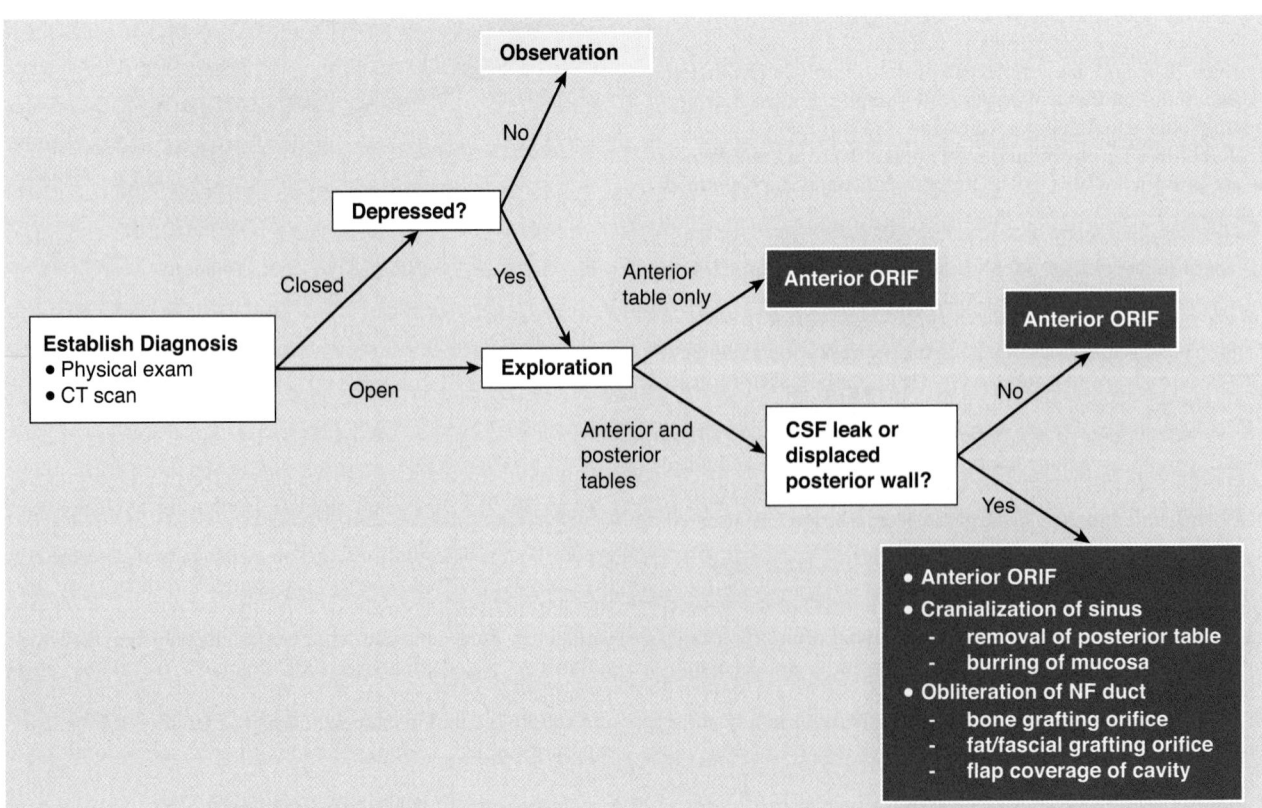

FIG. 45-29. Algorithm for the treatment of frontal sinus fracture. CSF = cerebrospinal fluid; CT = computed tomography; NF = nasofrontal; ORIF = open reduction, internal fixation.

lesions may be simply excised as a wedge and closed primarily. Larger defects of the upper and middle thirds of the ear may use antihelical and conchal cartilage reduction patterns to reduce the circumference of the helix to allow primary closure. When helical defects are too large for this solution, local flaps may be used to close or re-create the missing tissue. Postauricular flaps created in staged procedures may be manipulated to create a skin tube mimicking the furled helix and bridging the gap of a defect. Alternatively, use of an Antia-Buch chondrocutaneous advancement flap combined with cartilaginous reduction allows for closure of defects[30] (Fig. 45-30). Even larger defects of the upper and middle thirds of the ear may be reconstructed with large local skin flaps combined with contralateral cartilage grafts or contralateral composite grafts. Although ear lobe defects are relatively simple to close primarily, lower third auricular

defects that involve more than just the lobe are complex and require cartilaginous support, often combined with local skin flaps.

Nasal Reconstruction

Reconstruction of the nose requires appreciation of the nine aesthetic subunits that are defined by normal anatomic contours and lighting patterns (Fig. 45-31). In general, if a defect involves ≥50% of a subunit, the remainder of the subunit should be excised and included in the reconstruction. The nose can be thought of as being composed of three layers: skin cover, structural support, and mucosal lining. When a defect or anticipated defect is evaluated, it is useful to consider what layers of tissue will be missing so that a reconstruction can be devised that replaces each layer. Nasal reconstruction

CHAPTER 45 Plastic and Reconstructive Surgery

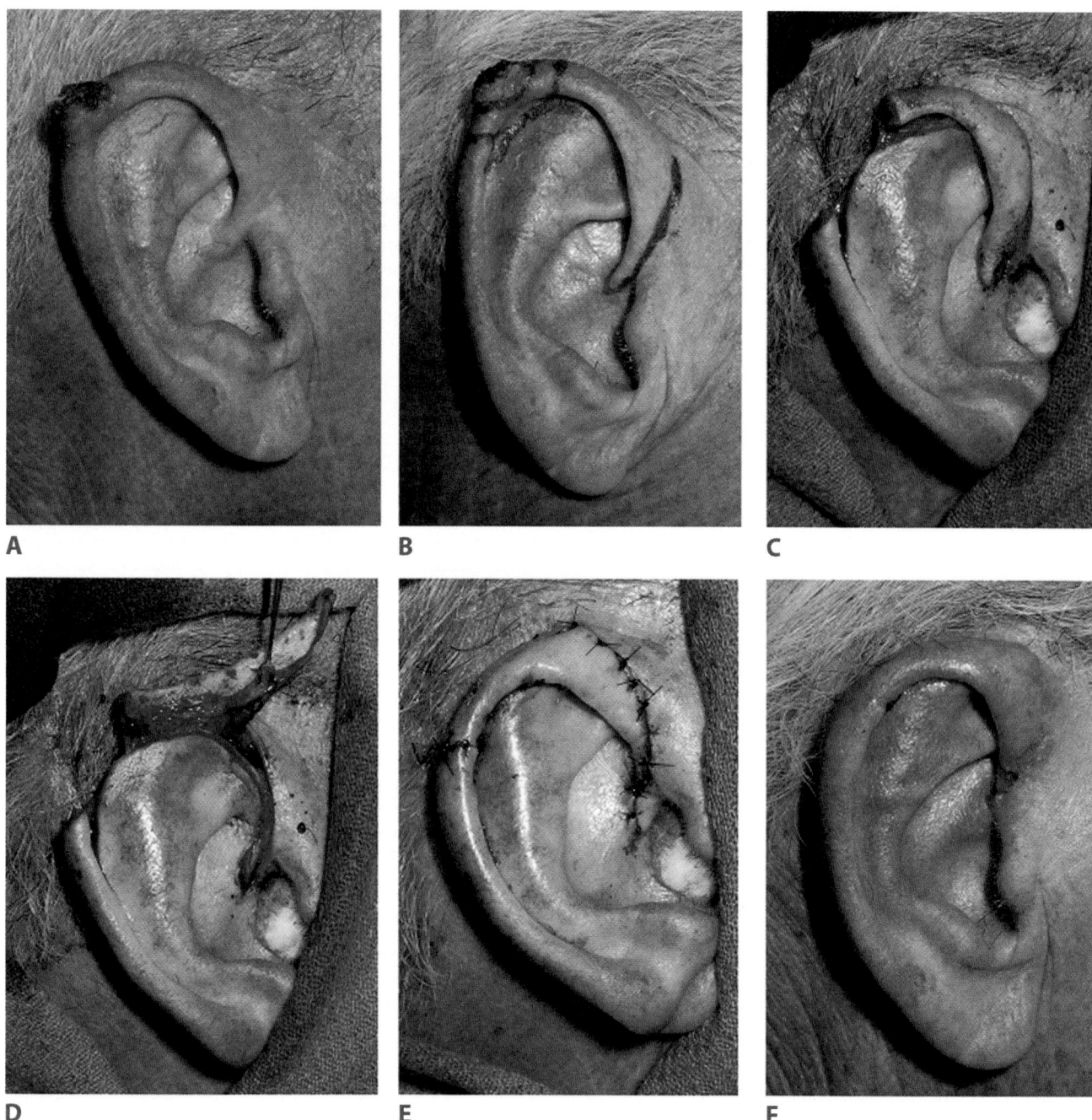

FIG. 45-30. Modified Antia-Buch ear reconstruction. **A.** Superior helix lesion. **B.** Excision pattern and reconstruction markings. **C.** Defect, flap elevation, and cartilage reduction. **D.** V-Y advancement of the flap. **E.** Flap insetting. **F.** Appearance at 1 month after surgery. *(Photographs reproduced with permission from M. Gimbel.)*

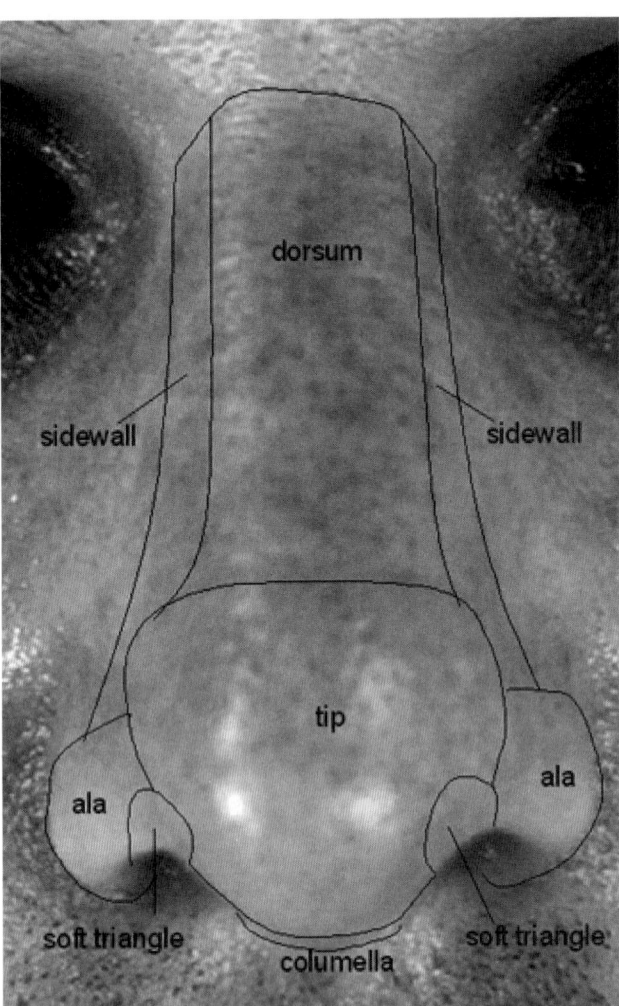

FIG. 45-31. Nasal aesthetic subunits. *(Photograph reproduced with permission from M. Gimbel.)*

methods draw on the full arsenal of reconstructive techniques. Healing by secondary intention is successfully used in concavities such as the alar groove. Split- or full-thickness skin grafts may be used for superficial defects of the nasal dorsum or sidewall. Composite grafts may be used for the nasal tip or alar rim (see Fig. 45-3). Local random pattern flaps are useful in closing small defects of the dorsum and tip, and may be combined with cartilage grafts if structural support is needed. Axial pattern flaps are commonly used for larger defects. These flaps have the advantage of being able to cover and revascularize underlying cartilage grafts and enjoy a close color match to surrounding skin. Workhorse flaps often used in nasal reconstruction include the nasolabial flap and the paramedian forehead flap (Fig. 45-32). Even larger defects may require scalping flaps or free radial forearm flaps. Split calvarial cantilever bone grafts may provide the nasal dorsum support. Lining is generally achieved with scar tissue turnover flaps, mucoperichondrial flaps from within the nasal vestibule, or skin grafting of the underside of transposed flaps.

Lip Reconstruction

The lips are important for articulate speech, eating and maintenance of oral competence, facial expression, and aesthetic harmony of the lower face. Three layers of tissue form the upper and lower lips: skin, muscle, and mucosa. Blood supply is through the facial artery and its branches to the lip, the superior and inferior labial arteries. Lip defects can arise from trauma, burns, neoplasms, congenital lesions, clefts, or infection. The most common malignancy in the upper lip is

basal cell carcinoma, and the most common in the lower lip is squamous cell carcinoma. As with almost all types of reconstruction, choice of technique is heavily dependent on defect size, location, and deficient structures. The goals of lip reconstruction are restoration of the competent oral sphincter with vermilion apposition, preservation of sensation, and avoidance of microstomia, all while preserving a near-normal static and dynamic appearance. In the upper and lower lip, vermilion-only defects can be corrected with advancement of the labial mucosa, often called a *lip shave*. In defects of less than one third the horizontal length, enough redundancy is present to allow primary closure. More complex decisions must be made for defects that are between one third and two thirds of the total lip length. The two categories of lip flap technique are transoral cross-lip flaps and circumoral advancements flaps. Cross-lip flaps include the Abbé flap and the Estlander flap. The Abbé flap was originally designed to reconstruct central upper lip (tubercle) defects with lower lip full-thickness tissue vascularized by one of the labial arteries (Fig. 45-33). The technique requires a second-stage procedure for division of the pedicle. The Estlander flap is similar in principle but is based laterally at the oral commissure and is used to reconstruct lateral upper or lower lip lesions. Both the Estlander and Abbé flaps are denervated, but sensation and perhaps even motor function return over months.[31] The Karapandzic technique is an advancement-rotation flap technique designed for central lower lip defects. Although good function, sensation, and mobility are preserved, a side effect is reduction in the size of the oral aperture. The Webster-Bernard technique uses cheek tissue advancement flaps to replace defects with full-thickness or partial-thickness cheek incisions extended laterally from the commissure (Fig. 45-34). When performed bilaterally, both the Karapandzic and the Webster-Bernard methods can be used to reconstruct a complete upper or lower lip.

In addition, microvascular free tissue transfer reconstruction may be necessary in cases where there is no remaining lip. The radial forearm free flap is the most commonly used for this purpose, usually transferred with the palmaris longus tendon for lip support.

Eyelid Reconstruction

The eyelids protect the eye from exposure and are another crucial aesthetic structure of the face. They consist of an anterior lamella (skin and orbicularis oculi muscle) and a posterior lamella (tarsus and conjunctiva). The eyelid blood supply is robust, and ischemia is rarely a concern in reconstruction.

Upper Eyelid

Defects comprising <25% of the upper eyelid can generally be closed primarily in pentagonal approximating fashion (Fig. 45-35). For defects involving 25 to 50% of the upper eyelid, lateral canthotomy (release of the lateral canthal tendon) and cantholysis (release of the superior limb of the lateral palpebral tendon) can be performed to allow advancement and are often combined with use of a lateral semicircular flap (Fig. 45-36). Defects larger than 50% of the upper eyelid may be reconstructed with a Cutler-Beard full-thickness advancement flap or a modified Hughes tarsoconjunctival advancement flap (Fig. 45-37).

Lower Eyelid

Lower eyelid reconstruction considerations parallel those for the upper eyelid. In addition, special attention must be given to the prevention of scleral visibility and ectropion, which can arise from excessive vertical tension due to either technique or scarring. Similar reconstructive methods may be used, including direct closure, semicircular flaps and canthal release, and advancement flaps. Grafts may also be used if the defect is partial thickness. Full-thickness contralateral upper eyelid skin grafts are suitable for replacing the anterior lamella. The posterior lamella requires sturdy, nonkeratinized graft tissue, such as cartilage (tarsal, ear, or nasal septal) or hard palate mucosal grafts, to allow globe apposition.[32]

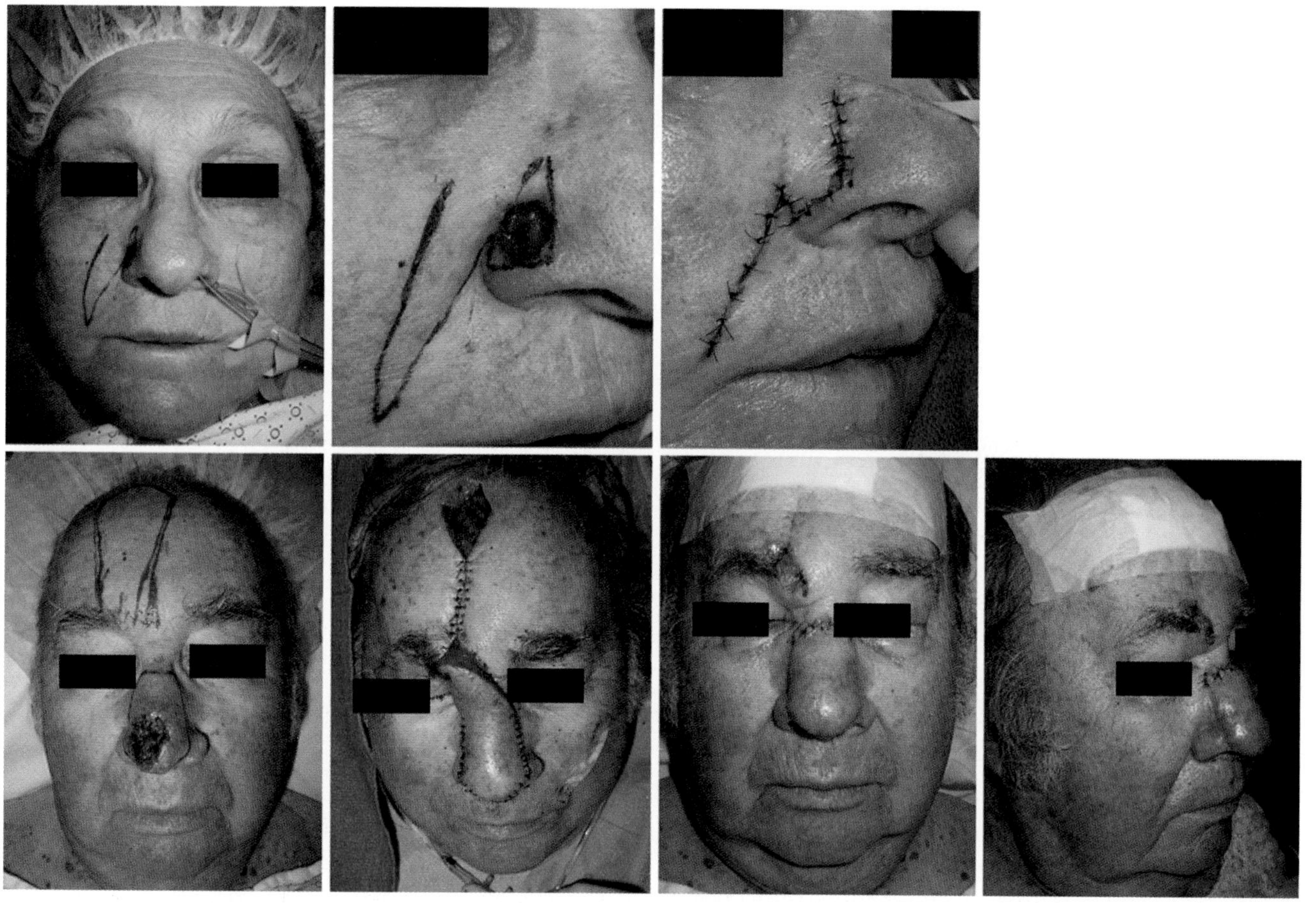

FIG. 45-32. Nasal reconstruction with axial pattern flaps. *Top row:* Nasolabial flap reconstruction of an alar defect. *Bottom row:* Paramedian forehead flap reconstruction of the nasal lobule. *(Photographs reproduced with permission from M. Gimbel.)*

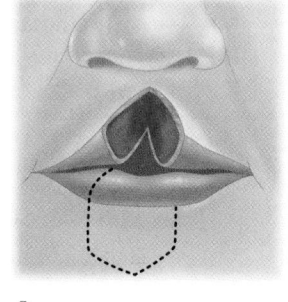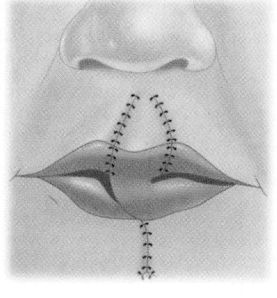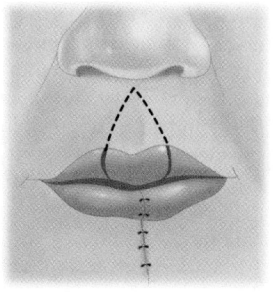

FIG. 45-33. Abbé flap upper lip reconstruction. **A.** Defect and flap design. **B.** Rotation of the flap and primary closure of the donor site. **C.** Division of the pedicle (after 2 to 3 weeks) and final insetting.

Ptosis

In the normal eyelid, the orbicularis oculi muscle, Müller's muscle, and levator palpebrae muscle act in concert to open and close the palpebral aperture and to maintain the level of the upper eyelid with respect to the pupil. Eyelid ptosis is created by derangement of this cooperative action. Ptosis may be congenital or acquired. Congenital ptosis is caused by lid anomalies, ophthalmoplegia, and synkinesis, whereas acquired ptosis can be neurogenic, myogenic, or traumatic in nature. Horner's syndrome is a form of neurogenic ptosis caused by interrupted sympathetic innervation that leads to ptosis, miosis, and anhydrosis. A thorough evaluation of the ptotic patient includes a general eye and visual acuity examination, attention to signs of exposure or irritation, measurement of marginal-reflex distance, observation of the height of the supratarsal fold, and assessment of levator function. Severity of ptosis and degree of levator dysfunction are critical in deciding the appropriate corrective procedure (Table 45-11). Mild ptosis may be addressed with the Fasanella-Servat procedure, which involves excision of the superior tarsal edge, conjunctiva, and levator aponeurosis, and mullerectomy. Other corrections of mild ptosis usually involve variations on this procedure. Moderate ptosis with fair to good levator function may be treated with some form of a levator aponeurosis shortening procedure. Severe ptosis with poor levator function requires use of an alternate eyelid motor. The frontalis muscle fascial sling technique, which uses strips of fascial grafts sutured to the frontalis muscle, is one such solution.

Skull and Scalp Reconstruction
Scalp Reconstruction

The scalp is formed of five layers: *S*kin, sub*C*utaneous tissue, galea *A*poneurotica, *L*oose areolar tissue, and *P*ericranium (SCALP). The

CHAPTER 45 Plastic and Reconstructive Surgery

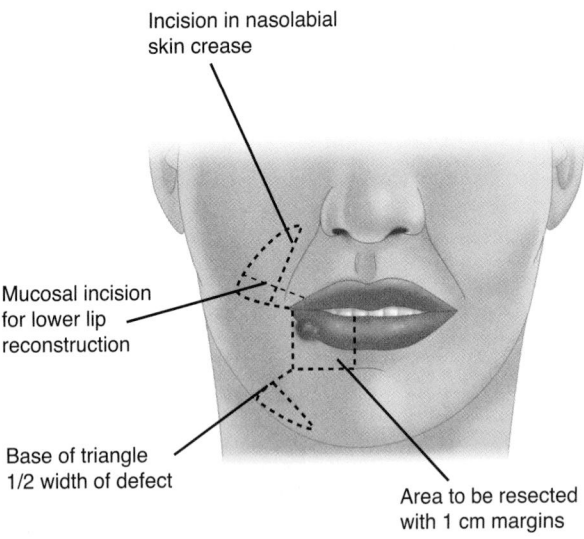

Incision in nasolabial skin crease

Mucosal incision for lower lip reconstruction

Base of triangle 1/2 width of defect

Area to be resected with 1 cm margins

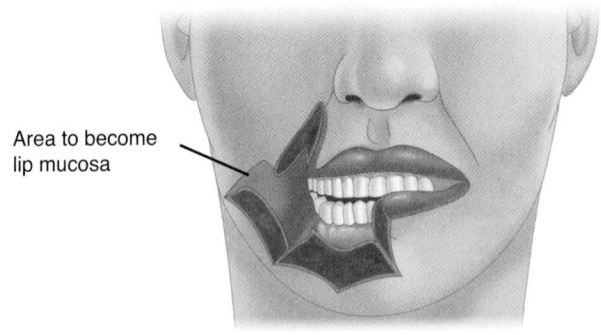

Area to become lip mucosa

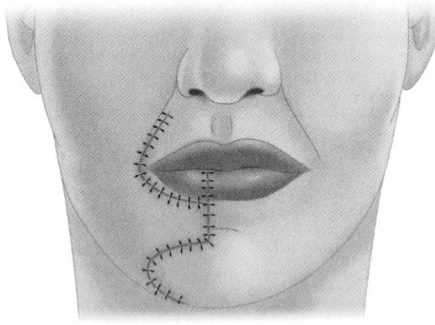

FIG. 45-34. Webster-Bernard lip reconstruction technique. *(Reproduced with permission from Closmann JJ, Pogrel A, Schmidt BL: Reconstruction of perioral defects following resection for oral squamous cell carcinoma. J Oral Maxillofac Surg 64:367, 2006. Copyright Elsevier.)*

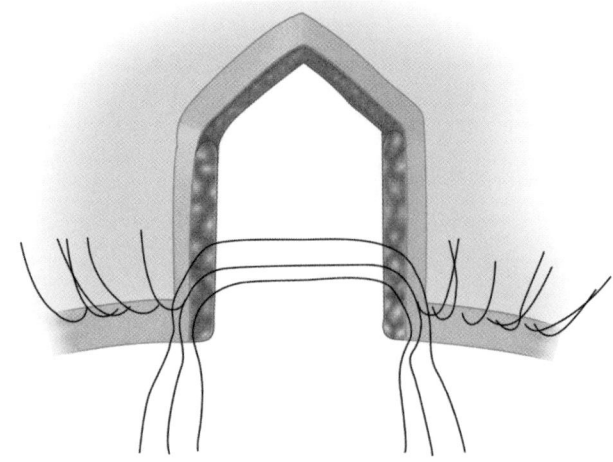

FIG. 45-35. Upper eyelid defect of <25%. Primary closure. *(Reproduced with permission from Pham RT: Reconstruction of the upper eyelid. Otolaryngol Clin North Am 38:1023, 2005. Copyright Elsevier.)*

scalp is well vascularized bilaterally by branches of the external carotid artery, including the superficial temporal arteries, the occipital arteries, and the posterior auricular arteries. In addition, the bilateral supraorbital and supratrochlear arteries contribute to the forehead and anterior scalp blood supply. These vessels run in the subcutaneous tissue layer, just superficial to the galea. Because of this rich blood supply, scalp lacerations can lead to dramatic blood loss, an event that usually can be curtailed by a simple running/locking suture closure.

Partial-thickness scalp loss due to trauma usually occurs at the level of the loose areolar tissue plane and is treated initially with débridement of devitalized tissue. If a partial-thickness defect is small enough, primary closure or skin graft can be used. Although the cosmetic result is often less than desirable, all layers of the scalp will accept a skin graft, including the calvaria if it is burred down to its diploë. Grafted areas may be reconstructed later with hair-bearing scalp skin through the use of flaps or tissue expansion. Because the scalp is relatively inelastic, scoring of the galeal layer often facilitates closure of full-thickness defects, but care must be taken to avoid lacerating the blood vessels just superficial to the galea. Larger areas of loss (4 to 8 cm) may be covered with large scalp flaps, as classically described by Orticochea.[33] Grafting of defects or donor sites leaves a visible area of alopecia. Tissue expansion has been very successful in replacing scarred or grafted regions with hair-bearing skin. Defects larger than 8 to 10 cm are best treated with microsurgical free tissue transfer. Total or subtotal scalp avulsions are rare injuries that usually occur when a person's long hair becomes caught in rotating machinery. These potentially devastating injuries are ideally treated by scalp replantation, because the avulsed segment usually has preserved vessels (Fig. 45-38).

Calvarial Reconstruction

Autogenous bone remains the material of choice for reconstruction of skull defects. Its advantages include resistance to infection and ability to heal with strength. All autogenous bone sources have the disadvantage of donor site morbidity. Bone grafts can be harvested from a normal area of the calvaria, of which the outer table may be used as a graft for defects of limited size. Care must be taken during harvest to avoid compromise of the inner table. Rib bone may also be used, either as a split-rib graft or as a microsurgical free osseous flap. Unfortunately, use of ribs to reconstruct the skull may give an unappealing "washboard" appearance to the scalp. Another disadvantage of bone grafts, although not flaps, is graft resorption over time.

Alternative materials to autogenous bone exist for calvarial reconstruction, including methyl methacrylate, titanium, and hydroxyapatite (with or without bone morphogenic protein). Although they have the advantage of no donor site, these plastics and metals are associated with a higher risk of infection necessitating removal. Various formulations of calcium phosphate hydroxyapatites are being actively studied as bone replacement materials.

Head and Neck Reconstruction

The head and neck region has a compact arrangement of critical and complex structures encasing the essential access routes to the GI and respiratory systems. The tissues of the face, mouth, and

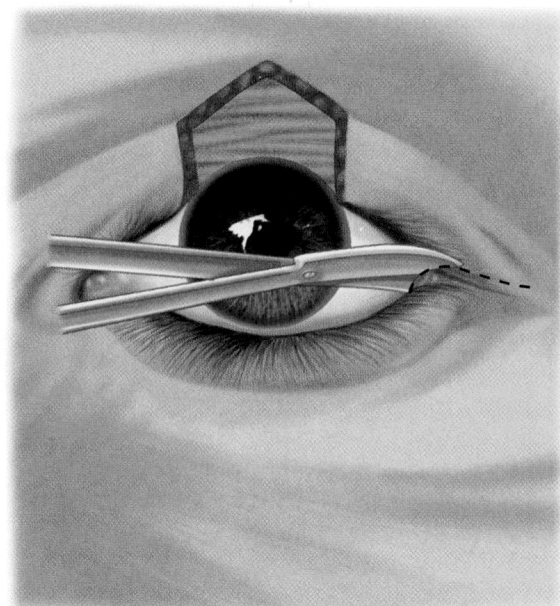

A

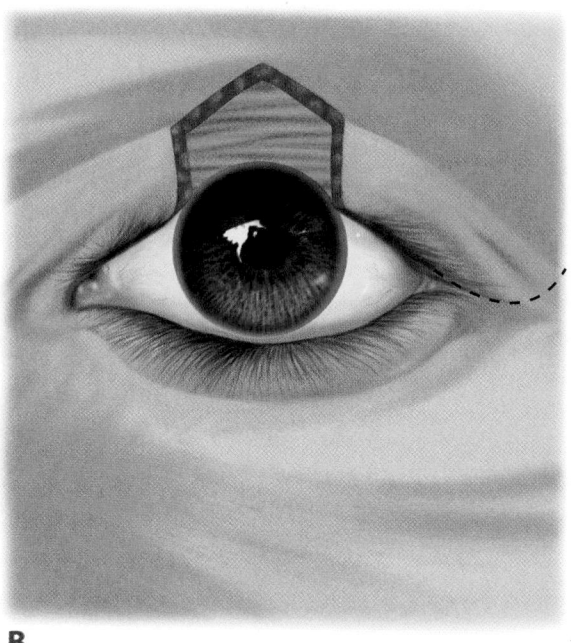

B

FIG. 45-36. Upper eyelid defect of 25 to 50%. **A.** Lateral canthotomy. **B.** Semicircular flap. *(Reproduced with permission from Pham RT: Reconstruction of the upper eyelid. Otolaryngol Clin North Am 38:1023, 2005. Copyright Elsevier.)*

cavities serve as a primary communication interface with the external environment through facial and verbal expression. Therefore, cancer resections with adequate safety margins can be severely and multiply debilitating. The management of head and neck cancer patients demands an integrated multidisciplinary team approach that includes the skills of ablative and reconstructive surgeons, medical and radiation oncologists, pathologists, nutritionists, and functional and psychologic rehabilitation specialists.

Tumor-Ablative Surgery

The freedom available to the ablative surgeon to completely excise a tumor is limited, at least partly, by the capability of the reconstructive surgeon to restore anatomic continuity and achieve successful

wound healing. A neck dissection to remove cervical lymphatics and nodes may be performed for prophylactic or curative intent, for more accurate prognostication by operative staging, and/or for solidification of plans for adjunctive treatments. It is important to be familiar with the tumor, nodes, and metastases (TNM) classification and staging of head and neck cancers. The N and M parameters are fairly constant for most head and neck cancers, whereas the T parameter varies according to tumor location.

Principles of Reconstruction

The reconstructive surgeon aims to restore lost anatomic components adequately. Residual deficits, seemingly inconsequential, may progress to psychologic morbidity, societal malacceptance, and social withdrawal. Uncomplicated and timely wound healing is important to allow radiotherapy when indicated and smooth discharge to home and occupation.

Each defect can be addressed by a number of methods, but the technique must be decided for each individual patient. Although a more complex reconstruction might offer improved outcomes, it may bring an increased risk of complications. Some patients may therefore benefit from use of a simpler method with more acceptable anesthetic and operative risk rather than a gold-standard reconstruction. Such an approach may be appropriate, for example, for an elderly patient with an advanced T4 cancer and short life expectancy. Reconstruction is impossible for some functional losses, such as the enucleation of an eye, but replacement by a reasonably aesthetic prosthesis may be achievable.[34]

Reconstructive Options by Region

Before the 1970s, autogenous tissue reconstructions were largely restricted to local or regional pedicled flaps, including the trapezius, pectoralis, and deltopectoral workhorse flaps. With microvascular free tissue transplantation, defects that were previously deemed nearly impossible to reconstruct can now be addressed in a single operation. Consequently, head and neck cancers that were historically unresectable have become more operable.

Intraoral Structures The reconstructive choice for mouth floor, tongue, and other intraoral defects is dictated by the dimension of the defect, the volume of tissue lost, and residual tongue mobility. The tongue and adjacent mucosal surfaces heal exceptionally well, so small defects may be treated by primary closure or even left to heal spontaneously. Smaller defects, less than one fourth glossectomy, may be treated with a skin graft or perhaps primary closure if tongue mobility is preserved. Larger defects, more than one third glossectomy, call for reconstruction by free tissue transfer, commonly a free radial forearm or anterolateral thigh flap for smaller- or larger-volume defects, respectively. Total glossectomy defects are a major challenge, and there exists no ideal method to restore tongue motor functions. The primary goal is to protect the airway from aspiration. Swallowing and articulation are often suboptimal after total glossectomy reconstructions. Options include bulkier myocutaneous free flaps harvested from the anterolateral thigh, the back (latissimus dorsi), or the abdomen (rectus abdominis), or pedicled regional flaps (e.g,. latissimus dorsi).[35]

The reconstructive choice for other intraoral soft tissue defects should also take into consideration the specific characteristics of the defect, such as its thickness and dimensions, and involvement of the oral commissure, facial skin, and/or neck. Buccal defects, for example, may be adequately treated with a radial forearm free flap or a thin anterolateral thigh flap. Thicker defects may be more appropriately reconstructed with a fasciocutaneous anterolateral thigh free flap. Those that extend through the full thickness of the cheek to involve the external facial skin may be reconstructed with a cutaneous or myocutaneous anterolateral thigh free flap that has been folded to address the internal mucosal, external skin, and intervening soft tissue defects simultaneously.[36] When the contour of the neck is sunken and asymmetric after a neck dissection, it is possible

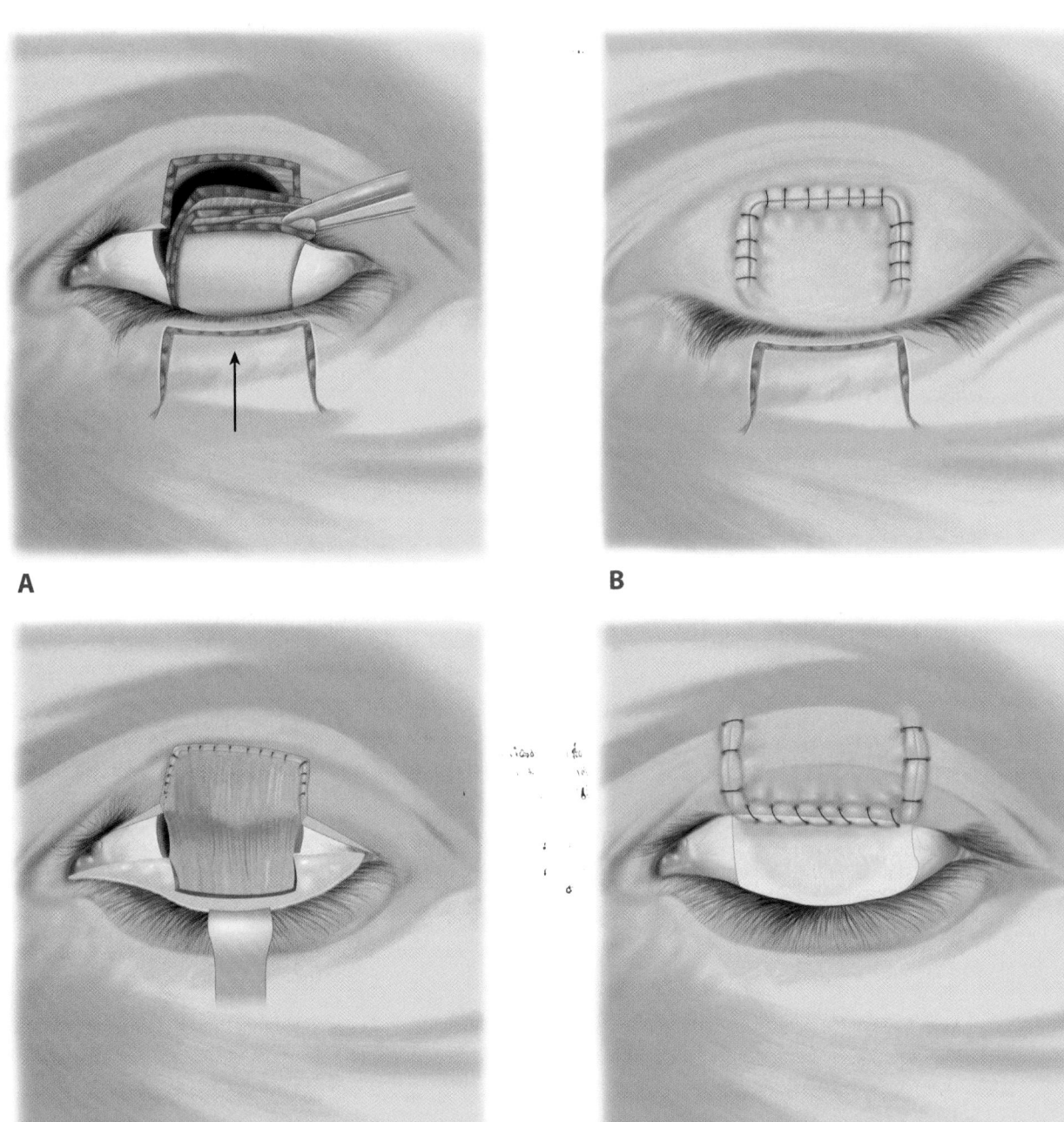

FIG. 45-37. Upper eyelid defect of >50%. **A** and **B.** Cutler-Beard full-thickness lower eyelid advancement flap. **C** and **D.** Hughes lower eyelid tarsoconjunctival advancement flap. *(Reproduced with permission from Pham RT: Reconstruction of the upper eyelid. Otolaryngol Clin North Am 38:1023, 2005. Copyright Elsevier.)*

to improve symmetry by insetting part of the flap into the neck. This maneuver also obliterates dead space and helps protect the adjacent major neurovascular structures.

Mandible and Midface Mandibular defects may arise from the ablation of tumors involving the bone itself or from the need to satisfy clearance margins for adjacent soft tissue tumors. Segmental mandibular defects can be classified as isolated bone defects, compound defects (bone and oral lining *or* skin), composite defects (bone, oral lining, *and* skin), or extensive composite defects (bone, oral lining, skin, and soft tissues).[37] The primary goals of mandibular reconstruction are to restore bony continuity, masticatory (with

TABLE 45-11	Eyelid ptosis classification
Classification of ptosis severity	
Mild	1–2 mm
Moderate	3 mm
Severe	4+ mm
Classification of levator function	
Excellent	12–15 mm
Good	8–12 mm
Fair	5–7 mm
Poor	2–4 mm

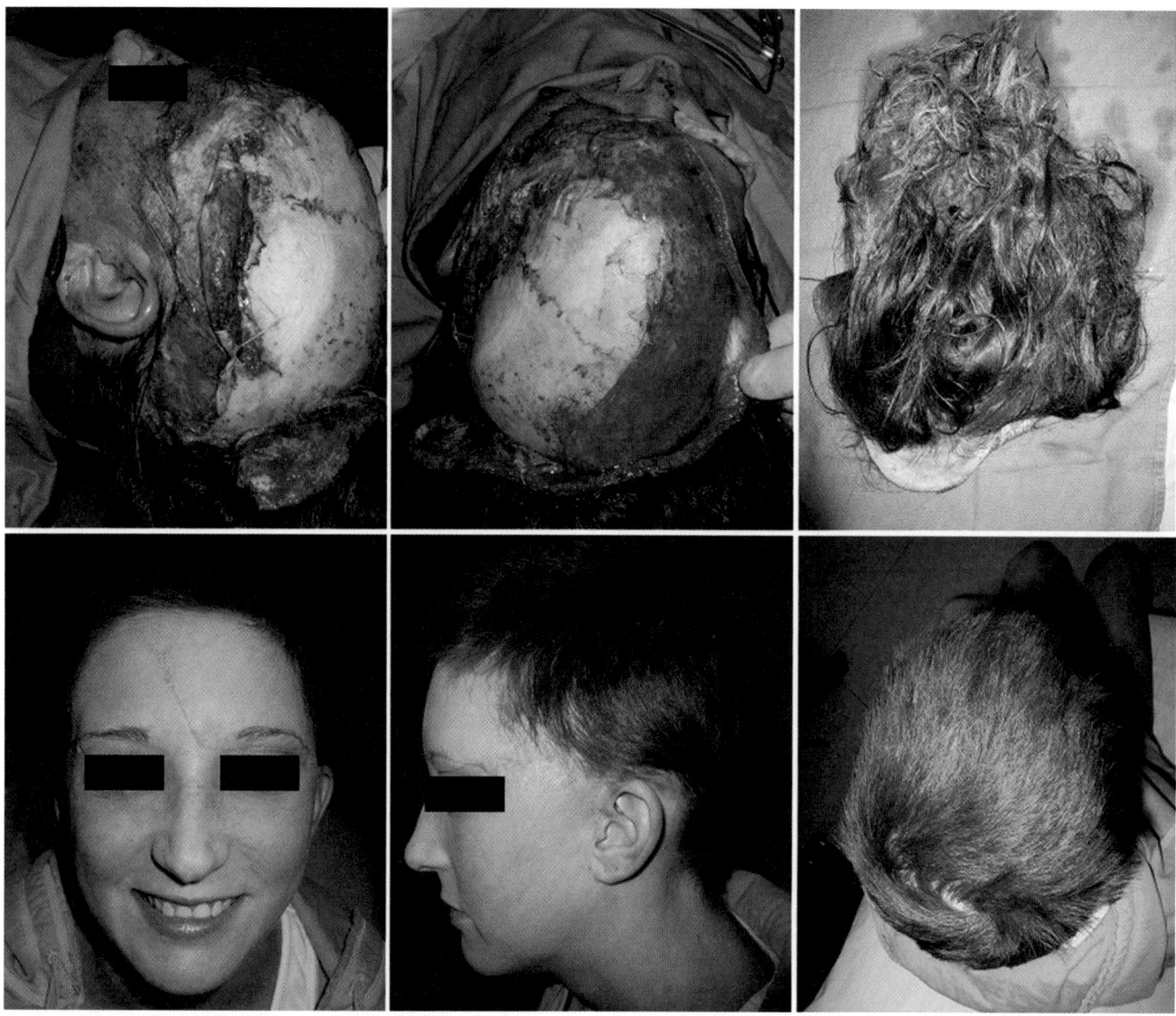

FIG. 45-38. Twenty-five-year-old woman with 70% scalp avulsion after a pedestrian-automobile accident. *Top row:* Defect and specimen intraoperatively. *Bottom row:* Appearance 9 weeks after microsurgical scalp replantation. *(Photographs reproduced with permission from M. Gimbel.)*

accurate dental occlusion) and speech functions, and facial contour, and to maintain tongue mobility. Early mandibular reconstructions involved the use of various prosthetic materials, with or without conventional bone grafts, and accompanying local or regional soft tissue flaps. Although small segmental defects are still reconstructible using autogenous bone grafts, they are not vascularized and therefore may fail, especially if radiotherapy is administered. The best option for most mandibular defects is the fibula bone free flap with an adjoined skin island supplied by reliable septocutaneous vessels (occasionally musculocutaneous perforators) from the peroneal artery and vein; this is termed a *fibula osteoseptocutaneous free flap* (Fig. 45-39).[38] Its many desirable characteristics include (a) the ability to withstand multiple osteotomies (as long as the periosteal blood supply is not interrupted) so that the bone can be folded to re-create the contour of any mandibular region, (b) an unmatched supply of sturdy bone length (22 to 26 cm in the adult) sufficient to reconstruct even angle-to-angle mandibular defects, (c) a bicortico-cancellous structure that can tolerate the incorporation of osseointegrated dental implants, (d) acceptable donor site morbidity when the flap is appropriately harvested, and (e) a donor site location that allows a two-team approach for simultaneous tumor ablation and flap harvest.[39,40] Reasonable alternatives include vascularized bone flaps from the iliac crest, radius, or ribs. Extensive composite man-

dibular defects may demand more than one free flap (such as one anterolateral thigh free flap with one fibula osteoseptocutaneous free flap) to reconstruct the entire anatomy in one operation.[41] These principles are also applicable to other bony defects in the head and neck region, including maxillary and other midfacial defects. The goals of midface reconstruction include the restoration of facial contour and projection, achievement of accurately occlusive maxillary dentition, provision of appropriate infraocular support, and sealed separation of adjacent nasal and oral cavities.

Esophagus and Hypopharynx The goals of reconstruction for esophageal and hypopharyngeal defects, which may be circumferential or partial, are to maintain luminal patency, restore speech and swallowing, and avoid strictures, fistulas, and GI anastomotic leaks. Reconstructive options for partial defects include primary closure, if luminal narrowing is insignificant, and skin (or dermal) grafts for partial-lining defects. A regional muscle flap may be useful for patching small full-thickness defects, but larger defects call for free tissue transfer of a jejunal flap or a tubed fasciocutaneous flap.[42] The jejunal flap procedure was the first successful free tissue transfer in humans, performed in 1957 for reconstruction of the cervical esophagus. It has since become a robust option for this purpose. A proximal segment is harvested based on its mesenteric blood supply and inset into the neck in the isoperistaltic direction. Disadvantages of the jejunal flap include halitosis, slow swallowing transit times, and a "wet" voice. Tubed fasciocutaneous free flap options, including the anterolateral thigh and radial forearm flaps, are also popular; however, they may have a greater risk of stricturing than the free jejunal flap. Nevertheless, proponents of such flaps favor the resultant vocal qualities and faster transit times.

Recipient Vessels in the Head and Neck for Free Flaps Commonly used recipient arteries for free tissue transfer in the head and neck include the ipsilateral superior thyroid, lingual, facial, superficial temporal, and transverse cervical arteries. End-to-side anastomosis with the carotid artery is associated with potentially lethal carotid blow-out injury. Anastomoses with contralateral vessels are useful when ipsilateral vessels are not available, such as in patients with recurrent cancer who have undergone previous free flap procedures or in patients who have an otherwise difficult ipsilateral neck.[7,12,17,22] Vein grafts may occasionally be necessary to overcome insufficient pedicle length. For venous drainage, tributaries of the superficial and deep jugular systems are convenient. Finally, protection of the major vessels and nerves of the neck is possible after neck dissection by overlaying residual free flap tissues. This also aids in improving the contour and symmetry of the neck for aesthetic purposes and obliterates any dead space.

Complications Apart from the general complications that may be encountered with any major operation or prolonged anesthesia, there exist several specific potential complications of head and neck

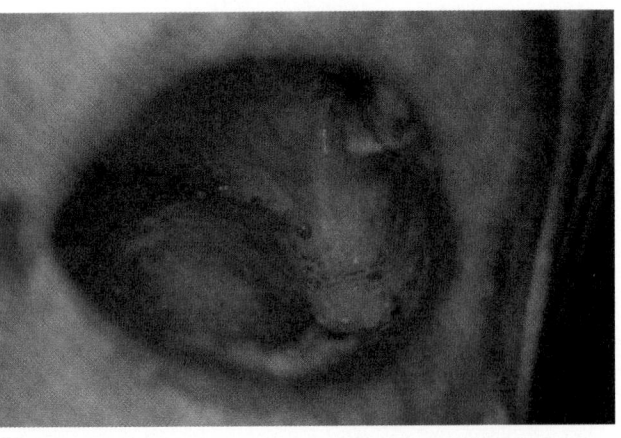

A

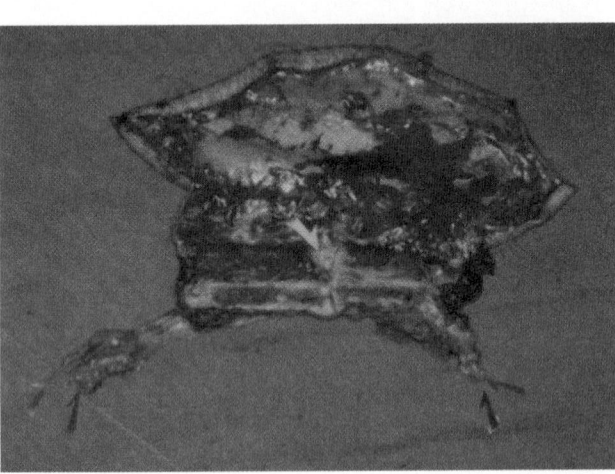

C

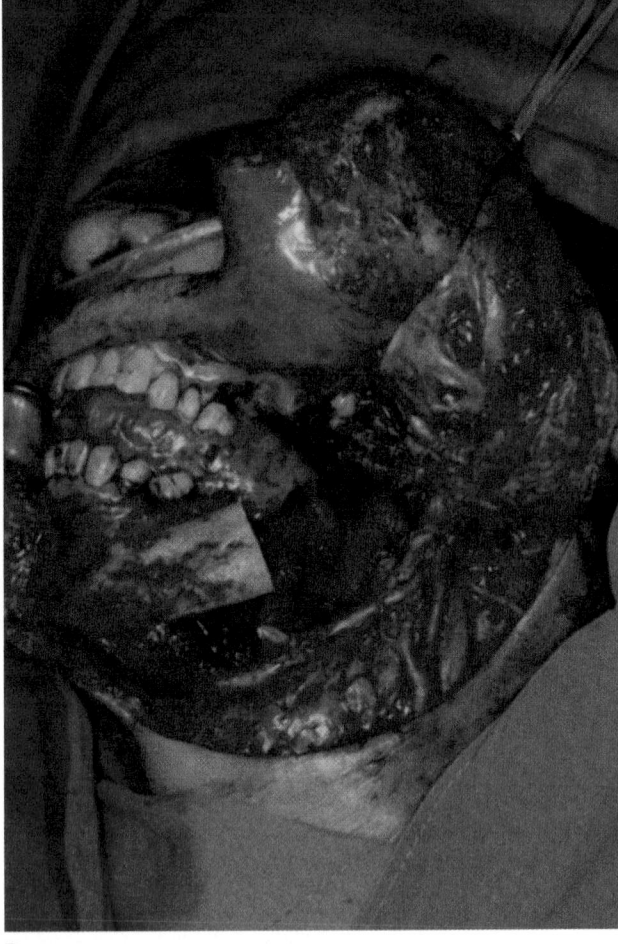

B

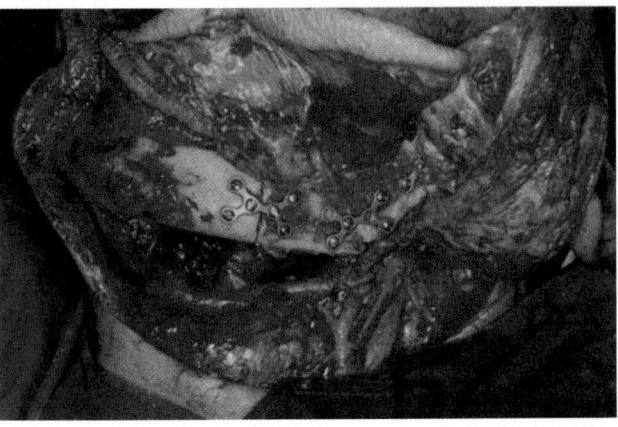

D

FIG. 45-39. Soft tissue and bony reconstruction of a compound segmental mandibular defect using a fibula osteoseptocutaneous free flap. **A.** Squamous cell carcinoma seen arising from the left buccal mucosa. **B.** Compound segmental left mandibular defect resulting from wide local excision of the neoplasm, which invaded the bone and local soft tissues. **C.** Fibula osteoseptocutaneous free flap; the pedicle artery (*red arrows*), pedicle vein (*blue arrows*), and osteotomy site (*yellow arrow*) are indicated. **D.** After contouring and miniplate fixation, the fibula osteoseptocutaneous free flap was inset into the left mandibular defect, with the skin paddle used to reconstruct the intraoral soft tissues. (*Continued*)

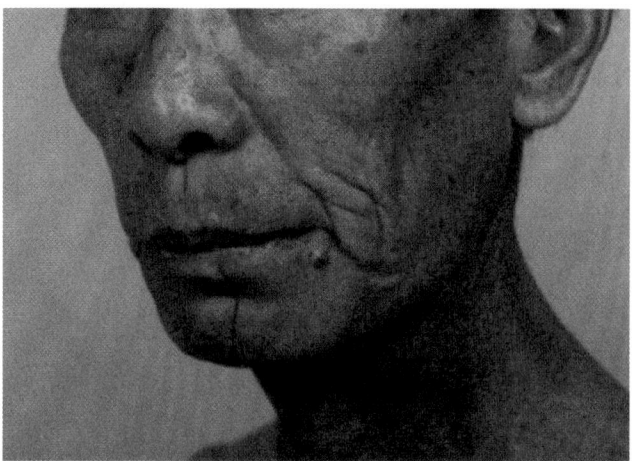

E

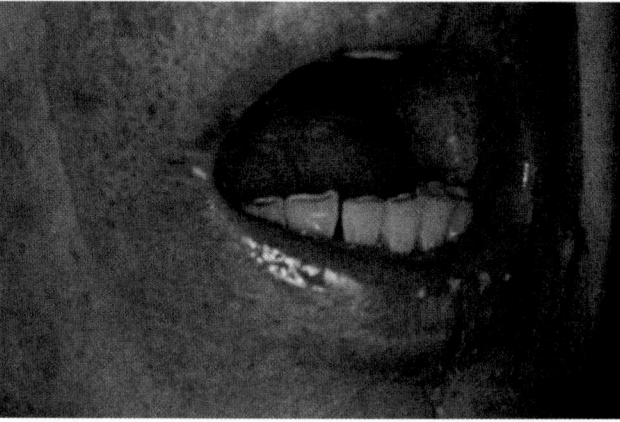

F

FIG. 45-39. (*Continued*) **E** and **F.** Four months after reconstruction the patient had good mouth opening and good cosmesis; note the skin paddle of the free flap visible intraorally.

ablative and reconstructive surgery. Specific intraoperative complications include air embolus, pneumothorax, and injuries to important vessels, lymphatics, or cranial nerves. Specific perioperative complications include carotid artery blow-out, flap necrosis, infections, saliva or chyle leakage, airway problems, and acute psychiatric disturbances. Examples of later complications are prolonged pain syndromes, fistulas, scar contractures, and problems associated with radiotherapy such as flap shrinkage (potentially with metalwork exposure) and osteoradionecrosis.

Facial Reanimation

Facial nerve paralysis is a debilitating and emotionally depressing condition that presents many functional and aesthetic problems. Loss of mimetic muscle activity leads to poor articulation and drooling from oral incompetence, exposure keratopathy from dysfunctional lacrimation and paralytic ectropion, and impaired socialization from facial disfigurement and difficulty expressing emotion. Facial nerve dysfunction has a number of possible causes, including oncologic resection, temporal bone or skull base surgery, trauma, congenital conditions (Möbius' syndrome), and idiopathic origin. The main considerations in treatment are management of forehead and brow symmetry, eyelid closure, oral competence and symmetry, and smile dynamics. The long-term goals include normal static appearance, symmetry with movement, and restoration of voluntary muscular control. Although the best results usually require multistaged, complex surgeries, the elderly patient is better served by a single-stage procedure that provides immediate improvement.

Neural Techniques

Traumatic injuries to the facial nerve without segmental nerve loss are best treated with primary end-to-end neurorrhaphy of the facial nerve stumps. The success of this repair depends on accurate approximation of nerve ends and achievement of a tension-free epineural repair with fine sutures, usually 8-0 nylon or finer. In segmental facial nerve loss due to trauma or oncologic resection, interpositional nerve grafts lead to the most successful reconstruction and may approach the results of primary repair. Grafting ideally is performed at the time of the injury rather than in delayed fashion. Donor nerves include the cervical plexus, great auricular nerve, and sural nerve. Timing of reanimation after nerve repair depends on distance of the repair from the motor end plates. Axonal regeneration proceeds at approximately 1 mm/d, whereas motor end plates deteriorate at approximately 1% per week and are gone by 2 to 3 years. In general, facial tone returns approximately 6 months after repair and voluntary motion a few months later.[43] Problems associated with facial nerve repair and grafting are weakness, mass movement (synkinesia), and dyskinesia. If the proximal facial nerve stump is available but the distal stumps are not, the cervical plexus can be harvested and proximally anastomosed to the facial nerve stump and distally implanted into the mimetic muscles to allow neurotization and partial restoration of function.

Nerve transfer techniques borrow other local cranial nerves to innervate the distal facial nerve stump if grafting cannot be done. This requires the availability of distal facial nerve or nerve branch stumps. Typically used donor nerves include the ipsilateral hypoglossal nerve, spinal accessory nerve, and cross-face sural nerve graft from a contralateral facial nerve branch (redundant buccal or zygomatic branch). Disadvantages of this technique include those of nerve repair or grafting plus loss of donor nerve function and facial hypertonia. Transfer of the complete hypoglossal nerve creates ipsilateral tongue paralysis and hemitongue atrophy with mild to moderate intraoral dysfunction.[43]

Muscle Transposition Techniques

All of the aforementioned neural techniques rely on the presence of a functional distal neuromuscular unit. When the distal neuromuscular unit is deficient, as in congenital facial paralysis or in situations in which reconstruction is not undertaken until 2 to 3 years after the original insult, muscle transposition is considered. Muscle transposition techniques require intense muscular retraining to achieve the intended dynamics. A classic muscle dynamic facial sling uses the temporalis muscle, innervated by the trigeminal nerve and perfused by the deep temporal branch of the internal maxillary artery. The muscle is released along with its aponeurosis from the temporal fusion line, reflected inferomedially, and attached to the modiolus at the oral commissure, the nasolabial fold, and potentially the orbicularis oculi. Disadvantages include lack of spontaneous movement, temporomandibular joint dysfunction, and soft tissue fullness over the zygomatic arch. Other transferable muscle units include the masseter muscle and the anterior belly of the digastric muscle. The latter is useful in restoring depressor function of the lower lip in cases of isolated paralysis of the marginal mandibular branch of the facial nerve.[43]

Innervated Free Tissue Transfer

Microsurgical free innervated muscle transfer may be considered in the same situations as local muscle transfers but is especially appropriate when concomitant soft tissue augmentation is needed. Muscles described for this purpose include the gracilis, latissimus dorsi, serratus anterior, and pectoralis minor muscles. The procedure may be performed in a single stage if the proximal facial nerve stump is available for anastomosis or if a long enough donor muscle nerve is present to reach the contralateral facial nerve branches. Often, however, it is a staged procedure beginning with establishment of a local neural source via cross-facial nerve grafting. The extent of axonal regeneration through the graft is monitored using Tinel's test. After sufficient axonal progression, approximately 6 to 12 months, the free muscle transfer is performed via vascular anastomoses to the superfi-

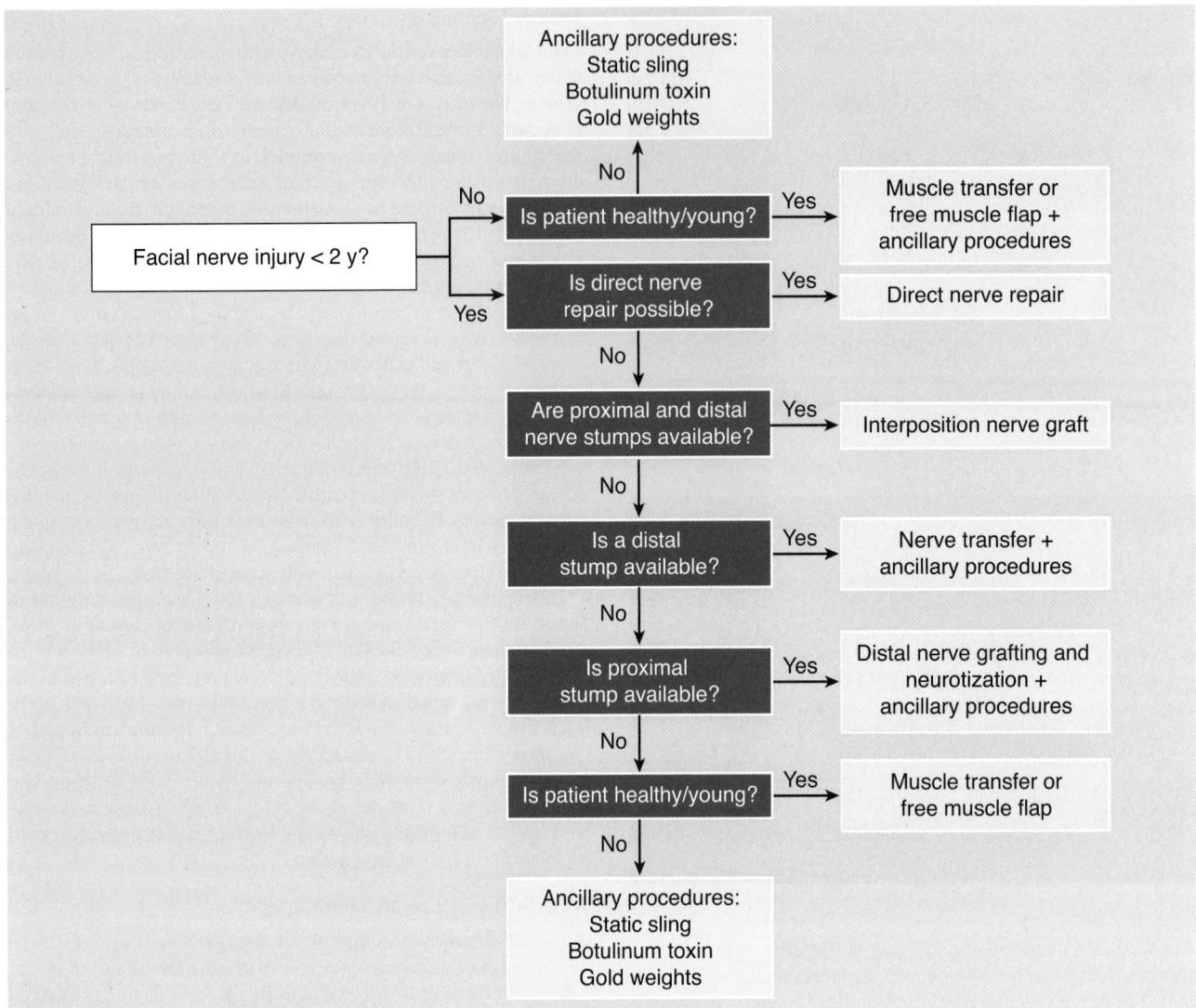

FIG. 45-40. Facial reanimation treatment algorithm.

cial temporal or facial vessels, recipient and donor nerve coaptation, and fixation of the muscle to the zygoma superolaterally and to the nasolabial fold, upper lip orbicularis, and lower lip orbicularis inferomedially. Disadvantages of free muscle transfer include donor site morbidity, lengthy surgical times, and the need for specialized microsurgical skills.

Ancillary Procedures

One of the most important goals of treatment for facial paralysis is rehabilitation of the periocular region. This objective may be simply achieved with implantation of gold or platinum upper eyelid weights, which allows gravity to assist with lid closure. Static fascial slings are used to improve symmetry when comorbid conditions preclude more extensive and staged surgeries. Sling materials include tensor fasciae latae, Gore-Tex, and human acellular dermal allograft. Nonsurgical techniques play a significant role in improving facial symmetry, both as a primary intervention and an adjunct to surgery. Contralateral mimetic muscle hypertonicity is tempered with botulinum toxin injections. Finally, soft tissue rejuvenative techniques such as cervicofacial rhytidectomy, blepharoplasty, browlift, and midface lift can improve the soft tissue effects of facial nerve paralysis (Fig. 45-40).

Breast Reconstruction

Breast cancer is the most common malignancy and the second leading cause of cancer-related death among women in the United States. One

in eight women will develop breast cancer sometime during her life (overall lifetime risk). Breast reconstruction began as a means to reduce chest wall complications and deformities from mastectomy. Reconstruction has now been shown to benefit women in terms of psychologic well-being and quality of life.[44] The goal of breast reconstruction is to re-create form and symmetry while avoiding delay in adjuvant cancer treatment. A number of studies have shown that breast reconstruction, both immediate and delayed, does not impede standard oncologic treatment, does not delay detection of recurrent cancer, and does not change the overall mortality associated with the disease.[3,45–47]

Preoperative counseling of the breast cancer patient regarding reconstruction options should include discussion of the timing and type of reconstruction, alternatives to surgical reconstruction, and realistic expectations. The plastic surgeon and surgical oncologist must maintain close communication to achieve optimal results.

Timing of Reconstruction

Immediate reconstruction is defined as initiation of the breast reconstructive process at the time of the ablative surgery. This is usually done in patients with early-stage disease for whom there is low expectation of postoperative radiation therapy. Immediate reconstruction takes advantage of the preserved, supple skin envelope made possible by the skin-sparing mastectomy approach. In general, this allows a more aesthetically pleasing and symmetric reconstruction. It is also psychologically advantageous to the patient to avoid living with the mastectomy deformity, as the patient must with delayed reconstruction. Furthermore, the cost to the medical system is less with immediate reconstruction, because fewer operations are required than for staged procedures. Disadvantages include the potential delay of adjuvant therapy due to surgical site complication, partial necrosis of mastectomy skin flaps, and the possibility that unanticipated postoperative radiation therapy is recommended based on pathology information. Breast reconstructions by all techniques are adversely affected by radiation therapy, and many surgeons feel reconstruction should be delayed until at least 6 months after treatment.

Delayed breast reconstruction is initiated at least 3 to 6 months after mastectomy. This approach avoids mastectomy flap unreliability and radiation therapy unpredictability. However, the patient is subjected to an additional operative procedure, and overall cosmetic result is often worse (especially with autologous tissue reconstruction).

Partial Breast Reconstruction

Over the last decade many women have chosen breast conservation therapy (BCT) consisting of segmental mastectomy with sentinel lymph node biopsy and/or axillary lymph node dissection combined with postoperative whole-breast irradiation. Although this less invasive cancer treatment is quite beneficial to many women, significant breast deformity can result from the tissue removal and radiation-induced changes, especially in women with small breasts. *Oncoplastic surgery* refers to the set of techniques developed to lessen breast deformity from partial mastectomy, both in the delayed and the immediate settings. One of the most common methods of minimizing defect visibility in large-breasted women is to rearrange the breast parenchyma at the time of tumor extirpation using reduction mammoplasty techniques. Dermatoglandular pedicles supporting the nipple-areolar complex can be designed in any number of orientations to avoid the defect location. This procedure, combined with traditional contralateral breast reduction, can result in excellent cosmetic outcomes, often better than preoperative

appearance (Fig. 45-41). The lateral thoracodorsal flap, based on the lateral intercostal perforators at the inframammary fold, is particularly useful in correcting lateral breast defects[48] (Fig. 45-42).

One drawback of these oncoplastic techniques when performed at the time of segmental mastectomy is the chance that, if the specimen margins are not clear, the reconstruction must be taken down to allow for re-excision. The oncologic implications of reusing the flap in this setting are unclear. Another shortcoming is the potential for fat necrosis, especially distally, in these nonaxial pattern flaps.

Implant-Based Reconstruction

By necessity or patient choice many women undergo mastectomy for local control of breast cancer. In fact, recently in response to the increased recognition of multifocal disease and experience with poor aesthetic results after BCT in small-breasted patients, some women have chosen mastectomy despite being candidates for BCT. The simplest method of reconstructing the breast is placement of an implant into the mastectomy defect. Occasionally an implant may be placed at the time of mastectomy as a one-stage mound reconstruction. Usually, however, the first stage involves placement of a silicone shell tissue expander under the chest wall musculature (pectoralis major, serratus anterior, superior rectus sheath), followed by expansion of the skin and pocket weekly over the following 3 months. The patient then returns to the operating room for removal of the expander and placement of a saline or silicone breast implant (Figs. 45-43, 45-44). After exhaustive investigation, silicone implants have been proven as safe and effective as saline implants in breast augmentation and reconstruction. After another 3 months, the nipple is reconstructed, usually under local anesthesia.

The advantages of the tissue expander/implant–based reconstruction are absence of donor site morbidity, short operative times, and short recovery periods. The disadvantages include the need for more reconstructive stages and longer cumulative time to completion of

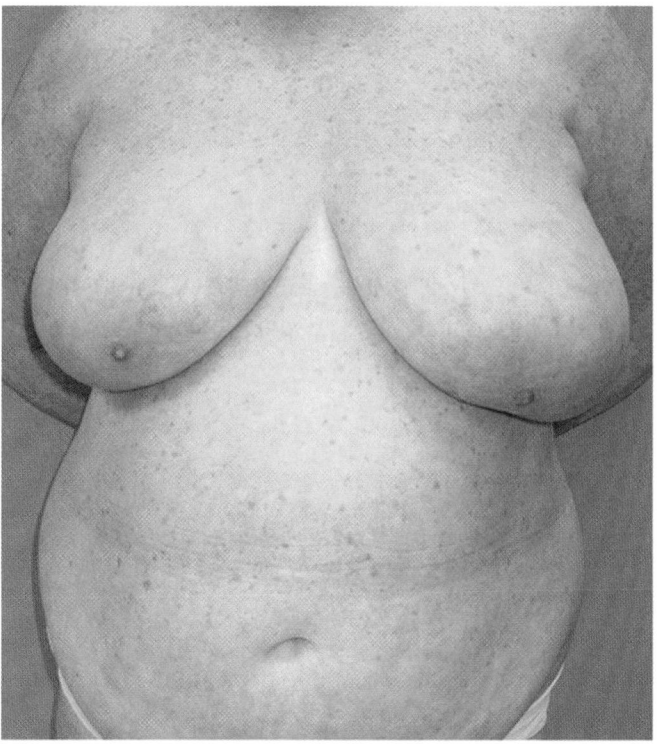

A

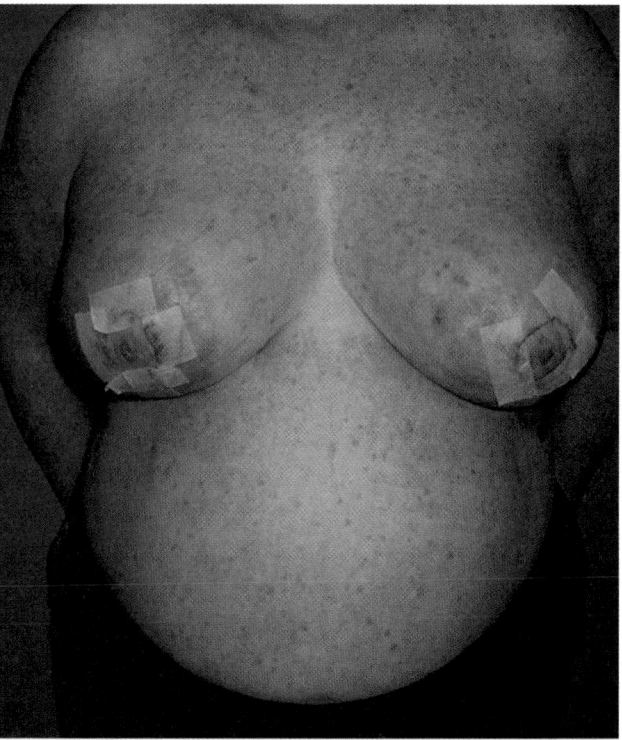

B

FIG. 45-41. Preoperative (**A**) and 1-week postoperative (**B**) photos of a 52-year-old patient with cancer at the 6 o'clock position of the left breast. Oncoplastic superomedial pedicle reduction on the left breast was performed simultaneously with a left segmental mastectomy of the lesion and a contralateral symmetrization reduction. *(Photographs reproduced with permission from M. Gimbel.)*

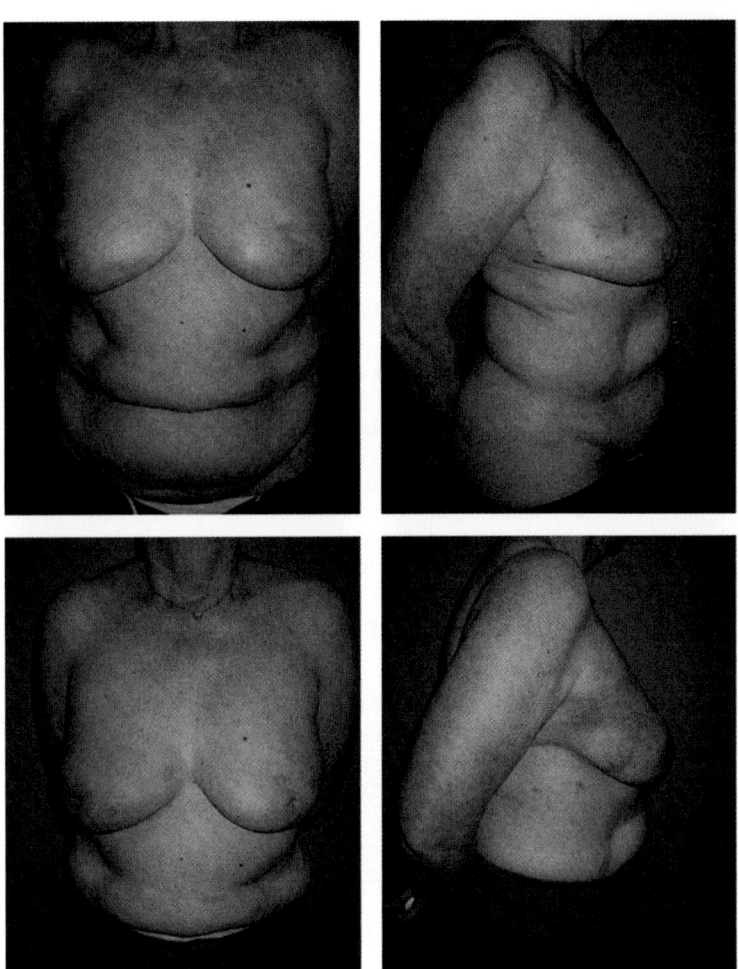

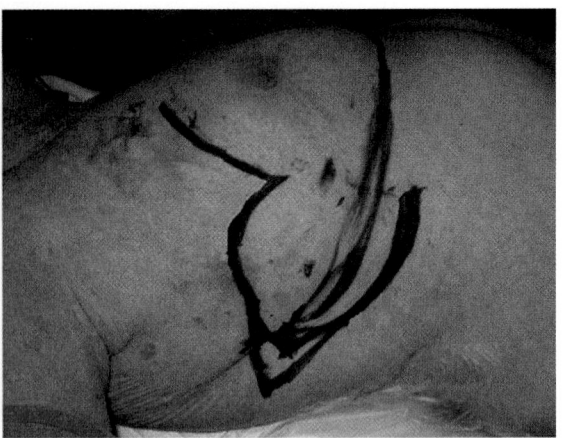

FIG. 45-42. Preoperative, intraoperative, and 4-month postoperative photos of a 66-year-old woman with right breast cancer at the 10 o'clock position. Oncoplastic lateral thoracodorsal flap reconstruction was performed simultaneously with a right breast segmental mastectomy of the lesion. *(Photographs reproduced with permission from M. Gimbel.)*

reconstruction. Implant breast reconstructions tend to lack the natural breast feel and ptotic appearance. This is particularly noticeable in unilateral reconstructions. Complications related to the tissue expander or implant include infection, malposition, hematoma, seroma, and rupture and deflation. Long term the most common problem requiring reoperation is the formation of dense scarring around the implant (capsular contracture) causing firmness, visible deformity,

and even discomfort. In addition, implants are medical devices that undergo mechanical wear, which ultimately leads to leakage and deflation. When all reasons are taken into account, the chance that a patient will need additional surgery on her reconstructed breast within 5 years of implant-based reconstruction is approximately 35%.[49] The results worsen and the rate of complication increases further when implants are placed in an irradiated chest wall, regardless of whether the radiation therapy occurs before or after reconstruction. The use of implants in such cases generally is discouraged.

Total Autologous Tissue Reconstruction

An entirely different way to reconstruct the breast mound avoids the placement of implants in favor of using only the patient's own redundant tissue. Indications for total autologous breast reconstruction are many and varied, including patient preference, previous or anticipated chest wall radiation treatment, a ptotic contralateral breast, and previous failed implant reconstruction. Contraindications are lack of a suitable donor site due to scarring or minimal adiposity, morbid obesity, and serious comorbidities that preclude a longer surgery and recovery period.

The most commonly used donor site is the abdomen. Most women in the breast cancer patient population have redundant skin and fat in the lower abdomen that may be transferred to the chest wall and fashioned into a breast mound. Many techniques have been developed to transfer this tissue, both as pedicled myocutaneous flaps and as free flaps. The workhorse abdominal flap for breast reconstruction is the pedicled transverse rectus abdominis myocutaneous (TRAM) flap. This flap is based on the superior epigastric vessels that run on the undersurface of the rectus abdominis muscle. A transversely oriented skin paddle with underlying fat is isolated based on its perforating

FIG. 45-43. Tissue expansion and implant-based breast reconstruction. *(Illustrations reproduced with permission from M. Gimbel.)*

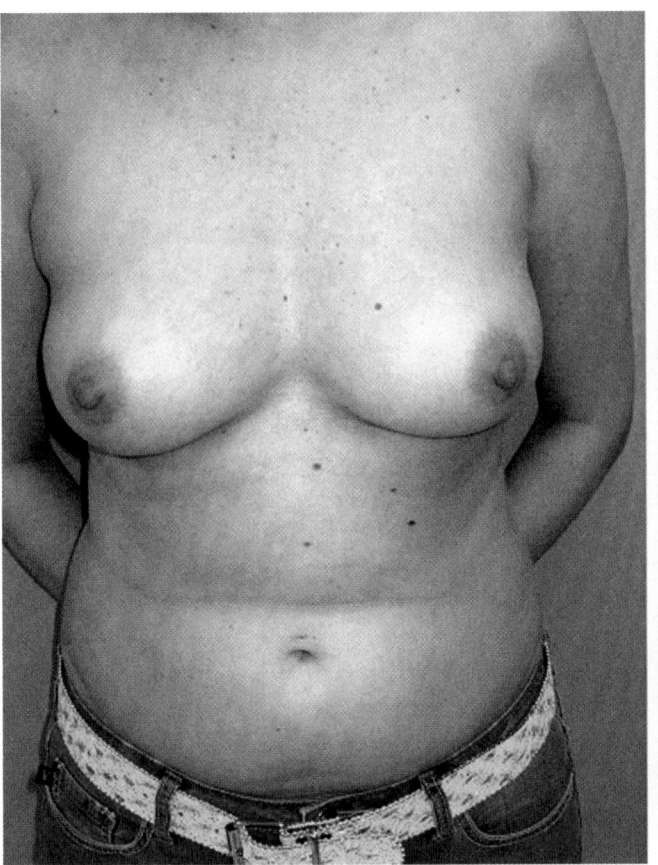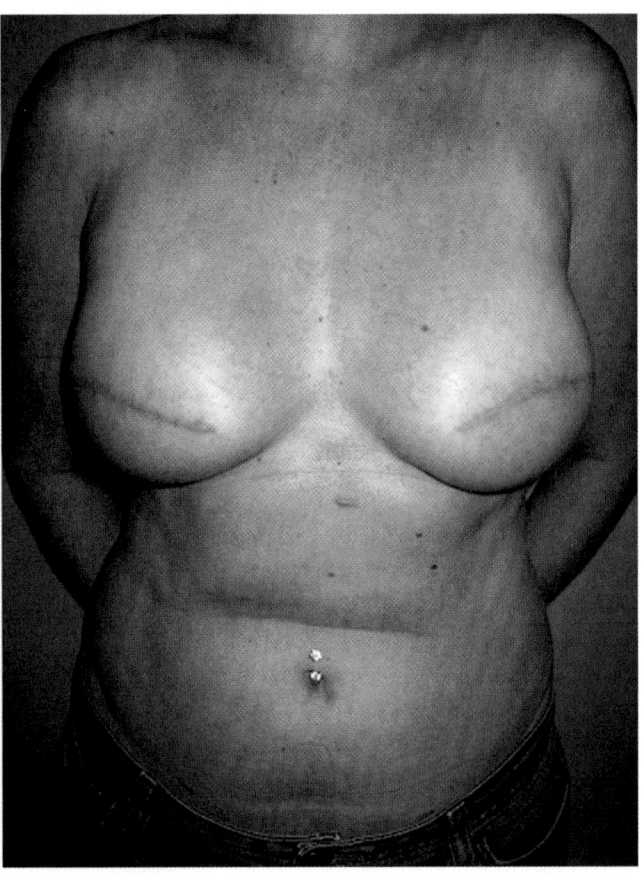

A   **B**

FIG. 45-44. Bilateral tissue expander/implant–based breast reconstruction. Appearance preoperatively (**A**) and 2 months after saline implant exchange (**B**). *(Photographs reproduced with permission from M. Gimbel.)*

vessels that course through the rectus muscle to join the main superior epigastric pedicle. The flap, along with the rectus muscle and blood supply, is tunneled under the anterior chest wall and delivered into the mastectomy defect, where it is then shaped into a breast mound. The donor site is closed in a manner similar to an abdominoplasty. The advantages of this and all total autologous reconstruction techniques are creation of a breast that looks and feels natural, that changes volume along with the patient's weight (and the contralateral natural breast), and that avoids the potential complications of breast implants. In addition, patients are often pleased to have the side benefits of an abdominoplasty. The pedicled TRAM flap procedure is also relatively quick for a total autologous reconstruction. Downsides include the potential for partial or complete flap failure, fat necrosis, fullness in the upper abdomen from the tunneled pedicle, abdominal wall bulge or hernia, and abdominal wall weakness.

The free TRAM flap was introduced to improve on the sometimes limited volume of tissue that can be carried by the relatively indirect blood supply of the pedicled TRAM's superior epigastric vessels. The free TRAM flap is similar to the pedicled TRAM flap but is based on the deep inferior epigastric vessels, which are the dominant blood supply to the lower abdomen. The flap is harvested as a free flap and the deep inferior epigastric artery and vein are anastomosed to recipient vessels in the chest, usually the internal mammary or the thoracodorsal vessels. A refinement to this method is the muscle-sparing free TRAM flap procedure, in which less fascia and rectus abdominis muscle is harvested with the flap to minimize donor site morbidity. The ultimate muscle-sparing free TRAM flap is the deep inferior epigastric perforator flap (Fig. 45-45). In this case, the fascia is opened but no muscle is included with the flap, and the perforating vessels of the deep inferior epigastric system are dissected between the muscle fibers to join the main pedicle. When patients are carefully selected,

muscle-sparing techniques decrease abdominal wall morbidity and increase useful pedicle length for microsurgery without significantly compromising flap perfusion[50] (Fig. 45-46A and 45-46B). Finally, in some patients the lower abdominal tissue may be transferred to the breast as a free flap without violating the abdominal wall fascia at all. The superficial inferior epigastric artery is capable of supporting enough abdominal tissue volume to reconstruct the breast. Because this artery and its accompanying vein do not traverse the anterior rectus sheath, the flap can be harvested with no more abdominal wall morbidity than an abdominoplasty. Unfortunately this artery is frequently absent or too diminutive in size to ensure a reliable anastomosis. Despite the many advantages of microsurgical total autologous breast reconstruction, it is associated with longer operative times than pedicled TRAM procedures, requires expertise in microsurgery, and has the potential for complete flap failure due to microvascular thrombosis.

Implant and Autologous Tissue Reconstruction

The pedicled latissimus dorsi myocutaneous flap procedure is a straightforward, reliable method used for breast reconstruction. It is often reserved for reconstructing breasts when other methods have previously failed. The latissimus flap is relegated to second-choice status because it carries the major disadvantage of autologous tissue reconstruction (donor site morbidity) as well as all of the potential complications associated with breast implants. That aside, the latissimus flap/implant–based reconstruction can produce excellent cosmetic results with relatively low donor site morbidity (Fig. 45-47). The latissimus dorsi muscle with overlying skin paddle is elevated based on its thoracodorsal vessel pedicle, tunneled through the axilla, and delivered into the mastectomy site. After partial insetting, either a tissue expander or permanent implant is placed behind the

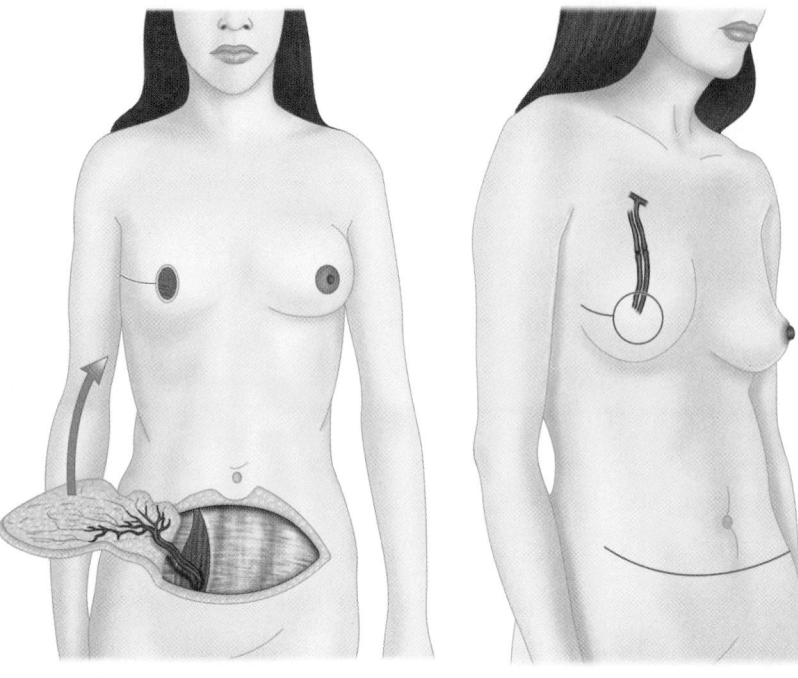

FIG. 45-45. Deep inferior epigastric perforator flap breast reconstruction. *(Illustrations reproduced with permission from M. Gimbel.)*

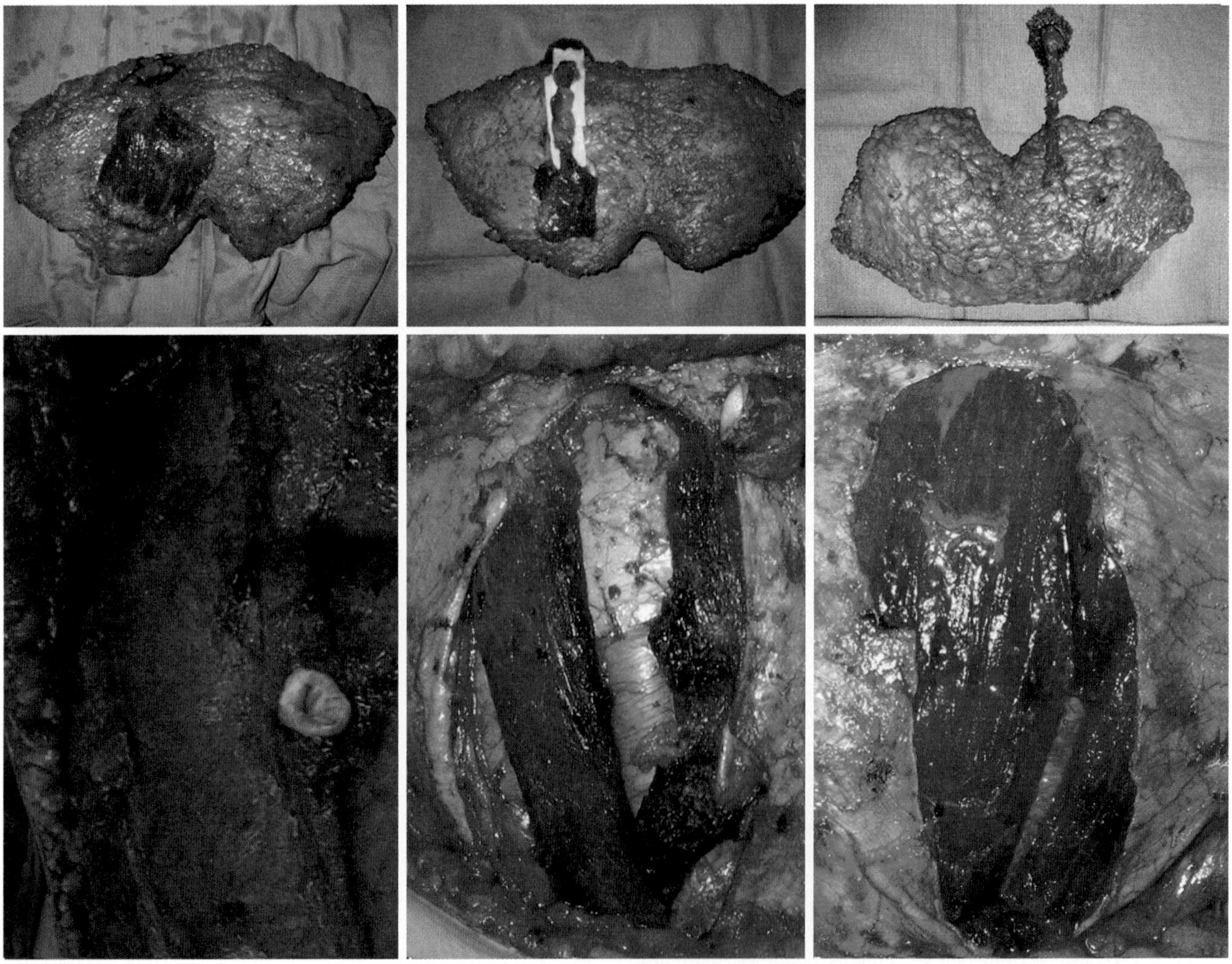

A

FIG. 45-46. A. *Left upper and lower panels:* Free transverse rectus abdominis myocutaneous (FTRAM) flap and its donor site defect. *Middle upper and lower panels*: Muscle-sparing FTRAM flap and its donor site defect. *Right upper and lower panels*: Deep inferior epigastric perforator flap and its donor site defect. *(Continued)*

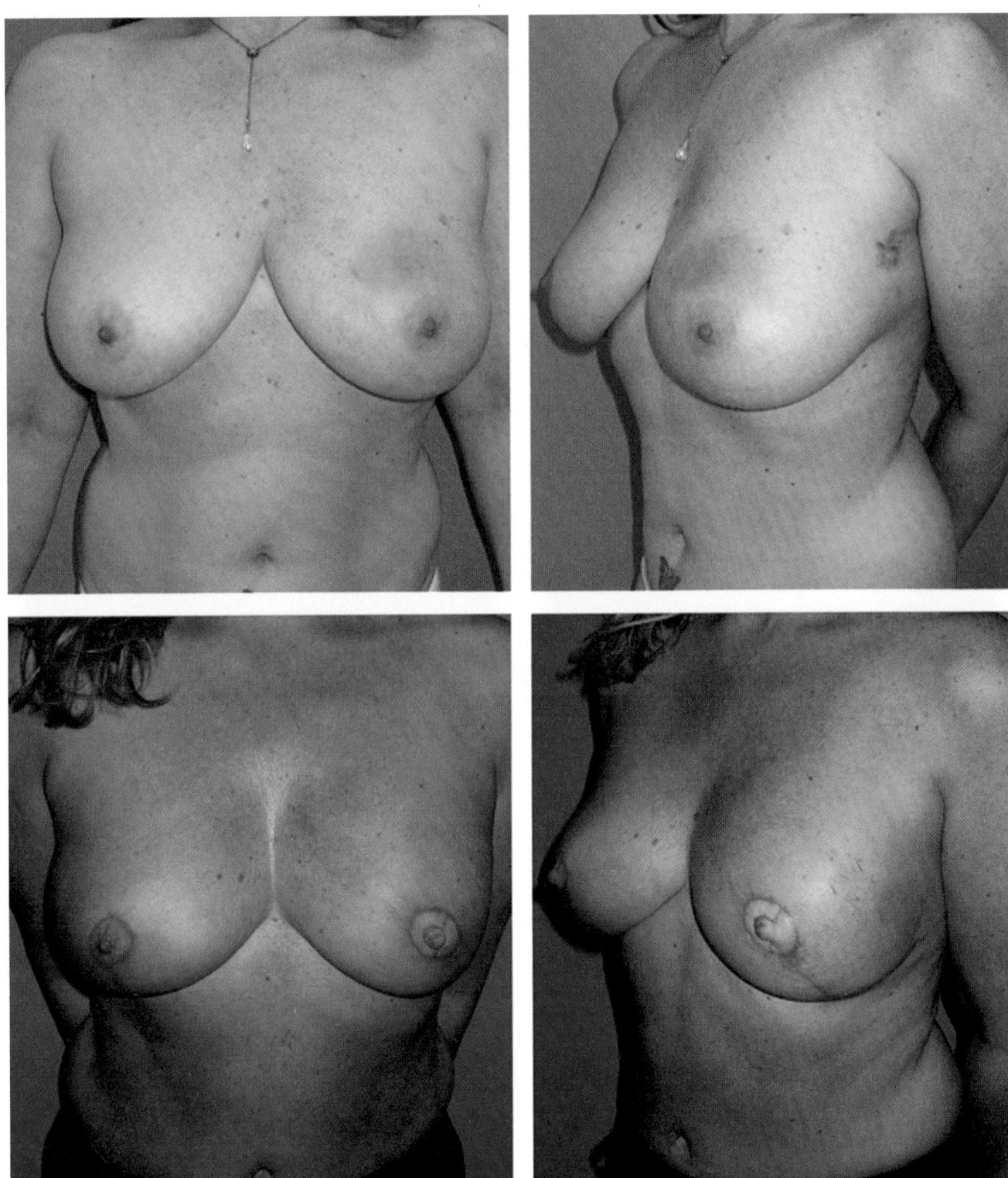

B

FIG. 45-46. (*Continued*) **B.** Preoperative and postoperative photos of a 43-year-old woman with a left muscle-sparing FTRAM breast reconstruction and right symmetrization reduction mammoplasty. (*Photographs reproduced with permission from M. Gimbel.*)

muscle to give adequate volume to the reconstruction (Fig. 45-48). Drawbacks specific to this method include contour irregularity of the back, high rate of postoperative seroma, and noticeable weakness in the shoulder (uncommon).

Accessory Procedures

After creation of the breast mound, refinements and accessory procedures are performed after approximately 3 months. These

may include mound revision via liposuction or direct excision, scar revisions, fat grafting, and nipple-areola complex reconstruction. Scores of methods have been described for reconstructing the nipple. These include local flap techniques (e.g., star flap, skate flap, C-V flap), grafting techniques (contralateral nipple/areola sharing, groin skin, labia skin), and tattooing. Nipple reconstructions are initially purposefully overprojected in anticipation of approximately 50% loss of projection over the first 6 months.

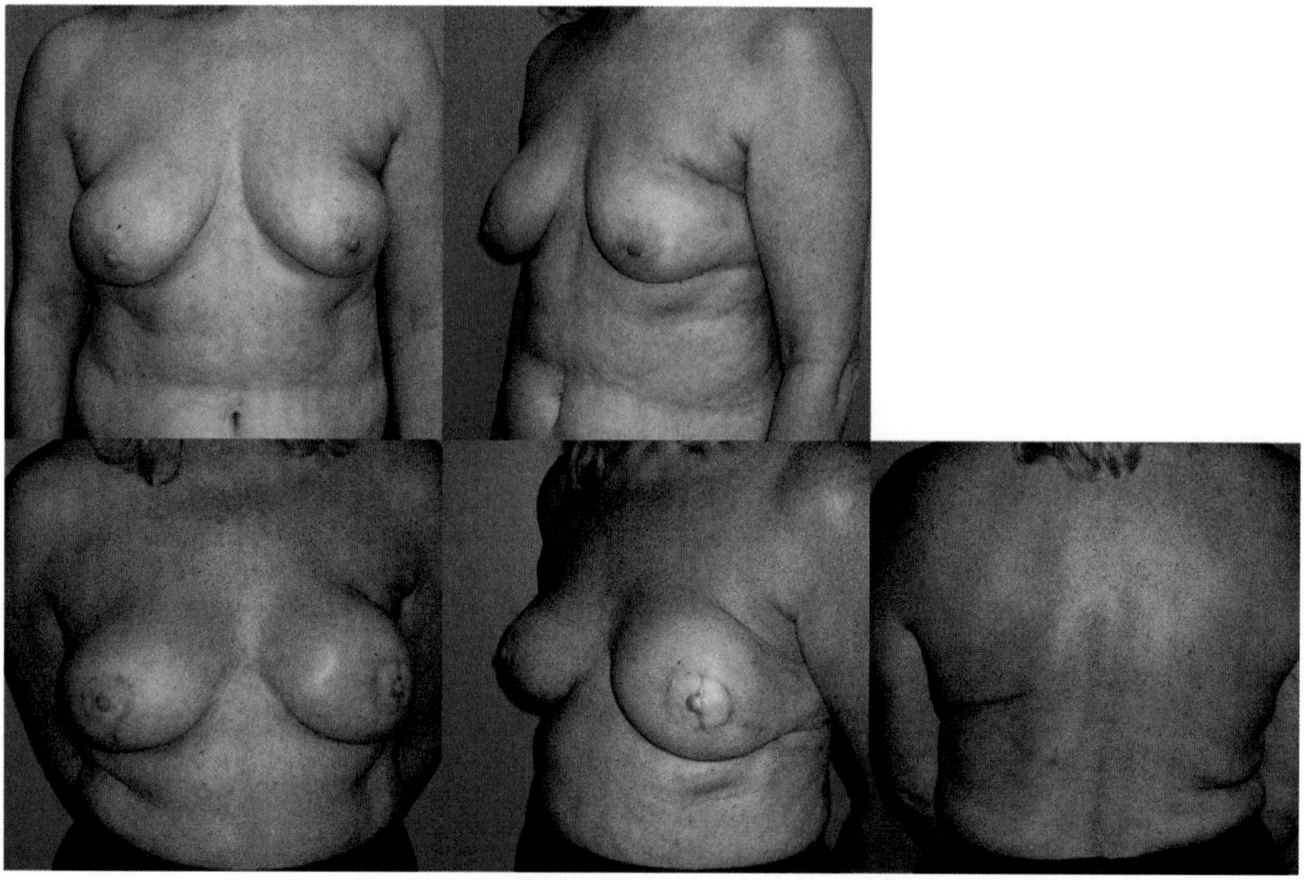

FIG. 45-47. Preoperative and postoperative photos of a 58-year-old woman with a left latissimus dorsi flap/silicone implant breast reconstruction and right symmetrization mastopexy. *(Photographs reproduced with permission from M. Gimbel.)*

Radiation-Related Considerations

With some notable exceptions, most surgeons advocate avoidance of implant-based breast reconstruction in chest walls that have previously received radiation or are likely to receive radiation due to the relatively high rate of complications and disappointing results. Delayed total

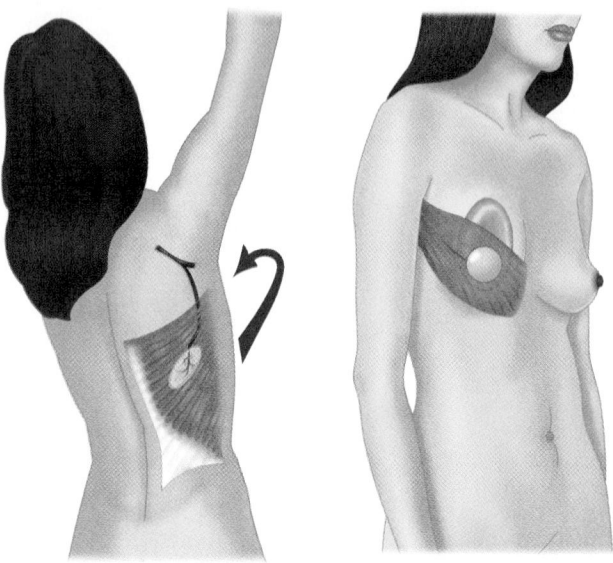

FIG. 45-48. Latissimus dorsi flap/implant–based breast reconstruction. *(Illustrations reproduced with permission from M. Gimbel.)*

autologous reconstructions bring healthy nonirradiated tissue to replace the damaged fibrotic tissue and are the preferred mode of breast reconstruction in this setting. Similarly, latissimus dorsi/implant reconstructions replace much of the irradiated skin, which probably explains to some degree why, in the face of previous irradiation, implants fair better with an overlying latissimus flap than without.

The question of whether total autologous reconstructions should be done before or after anticipated radiation therapy is still controversial. Those in favor of delaying the reconstruction argue that an irradiated flap will exhibit shrinkage and fibrosis that subtracts from the overall aesthetic result. Those in favor of performing immediate reconstruction in this setting feel that, because immediate reconstructions have inherently better aesthetics, the imperfect result due to irradiation it is still comparable to the result of delayed reconstruction without the additional operation. To date no prospective study has been performed comparing the two approaches.

Trunk and Abdominal Reconstruction

In the trunk, as in most areas of the body, choice of reconstructive method is determined by the location and size of the defect, and the properties of the deficient tissue. A distinction is made between partial-thickness and full-thickness defects in deciding between grafts, flaps, synthetic materials, or a combination of techniques. Unlike the head and the lower leg, the trunk harbors a relative wealth of regional transposable axial pattern flaps that allow sturdy reconstruction, only rarely requiring distant free tissue transfer. Indeed, the trunk serves as the body's arsenal, providing its most robust flaps to rebuild its largest defects.

Thoracic Wall

The chest wall is a rigid framework designed to resist both the negative pressure associated with respiration and the positive pressure from coughing and from transmitted intra-abdominal forces. Furthermore, it protects the heart, lungs, and great vessels from external trauma. Reconstructions of chest wall defects must emulate these functions.

The pectoralis major muscle is the workhorse pedicled flap for coverage of the sternum, upper chest, and neck. It is a type of V flap with one dominant pedicle (pectoral branch of the thoracoacromial artery) and several secondary segmental pedicles (intercostal perforators and the pectoral branch of the lateral thoracic artery).[51] The muscle may be advanced or transposed on its dominant pedicle or used as a turnover flap based on its internal mammary perforators. Both methods are useful in covering the sternum after dehiscence or infection. Before the turnover flap is elevated previous operative notes should be reviewed carefully to determine whether the internal mammary artery is still a viable perfusion source; the artery, especially the left, is frequently used for heart revascularization. The muscle may also be used for obliteration of intrathoracic dead space infections and as a myocutaneous flap for head and neck reconstruction. Although it is a reliable flap, the loss of the pectoralis major muscle results in upper extremity weakness and cosmetic deformity from loss of the anterior axillary fold.[52]

The rectus abdominis muscle is a type III axial pattern flap that can be based on the superior epigastric vessels or the deep inferior epigastric vessels.[51] When elevated as a myocutaneous flap it can be designed with a transverse (TRAM) or vertical skin paddle. Although the vertical rectus abdominis muscle flap has better vascularized skin due to its multiple longitudinally oriented perforators, the TRAM flap provides a larger area of donor skin that can be primarily closed with an easily concealable scar. The rectus abdominis muscle is frequently used for lower sternum reconstruction when the pectoralis muscle is insufficient. It can also be used in pedicle or free flap configuration for repair of large chest wall defects from cancer resection (Fig. 45-49).

The latissimus dorsi myocutaneous flap is probably the most widely used flap in nonsternal chest wall reconstructions due to its broad size, location, reliability, and pedicle length. The flap is based on the thoracodorsal vessels arising from the subscapular system. Its secondary blood supply comes from the posterior intercostal and lumbar vessels.[51] The arc of rotation of this flap can extend to most areas on the ipsilateral torso as well as to the abdomen, head and neck, and upper arm. The serratus anterior muscle can be included on the same vascular pedicle to further increase its surface area. Use of this donor site is relatively well tolerated, but shoulder weakness can be significant. The major drawbacks of the latissimus flap are its conspicuous scar and the high risk of seroma.[52]

The trapezius muscle flap, based on the transverse cervical vessels, is generally used as a pedicled flap to cover the upper midback, base of neck, and shoulder. The superior portion of the muscle along with the acromial attachment and spinal accessory nerve are preserved to maintain shoulder elevation function. Other useful flaps of the thoracic region include the scapular/parascapular fasciocutaneous flap, the external oblique flap, the medially or laterally based thoracoepigastric skin flaps, and the omental flap.

When a full-thickness defect of the chest wall involves more than two adjacent ribs, the inherent rigidity of soft tissue flaps may

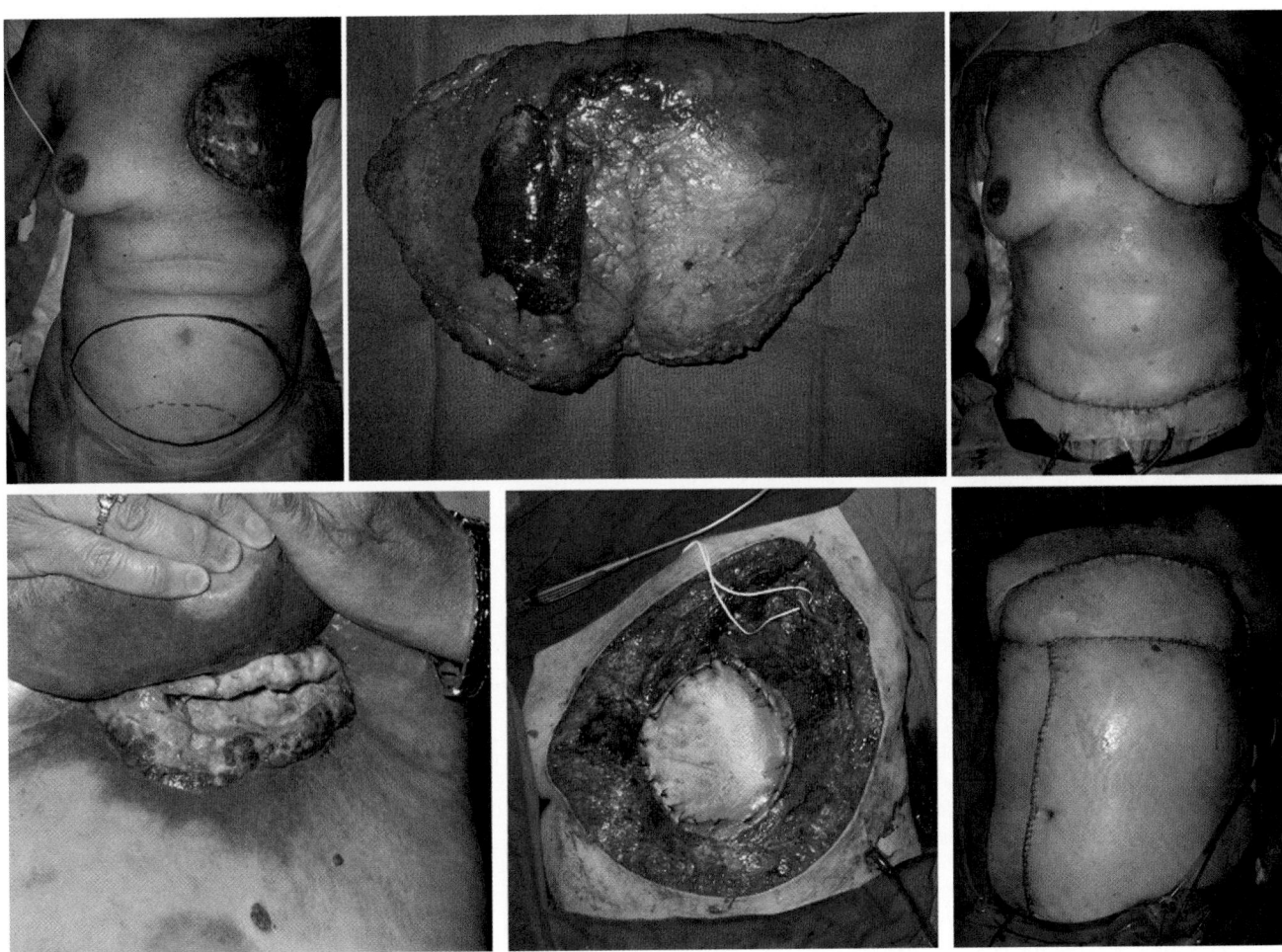

FIG. 45-49. *Top row:* Free transverse rectus abdominis muscle reconstruction of a large partial-thickness chest wall defect. *Bottom row:* Full-thickness chest wall defect reconstructed in two layers with human acellular dermal allograft and overlying pedicled vertical rectus abdominis muscle flap. *(Photographs reproduced with permission from M. Gimbel.)*

provide insufficient chest wall integrity. Although cadaveric bone and autologous bone grafts have been used in the past to lend structural support, the availability of well-tolerated synthetic and biologic materials has become more common. These materials include polypropylene (Prolene), polyethylene (Marlex), and polytetrafluoroethylene (Gore-Tex) meshes, methyl methacrylate, and acellular dermal allograft. Even if these avascular foreign bodies must be removed due to chronic infection, often a thick fibrous layer of tissue will have formed that can maintain chest wall stability.[52]

Abdominal Wall

The abdominal wall also protects the internal vital organs from trauma, but with layers of strong torso-supporting muscles and fascia rather than with osseous structures. The goals of reconstruction are restoration of structural integrity, prevention of visceral eventration, and provision of dynamic muscular support. Defects in the abdominal wall may arise from trauma, oncologic resection, congenital deformities, and infection. By far the most common reason for abdominal wall deficiency, however, is incisional fascial dehiscence and herniation after laparotomy. When a reconstruction plan is being formulated, careful physical examination and review of the medical history will help prevent selection of an otherwise sound strategy that, because of previous incisions and trauma, is destined for failure.

Partial Defects of the Abdominal Wall

Large defects of the abdominal skin and subcutaneous tissue are usually easily controlled with skin grafts, local advancement flaps, or tissue expansion. Myofascial defects are more difficult to manage. The abdominal wall fascia requires a minimal-tension closure to avoid dehiscence, recurrent incisional hernia formation, or abdominal compartment syndrome.[53] Prosthetic meshes are frequently used to replace the fascia in clean wounds and in operations that create myofascial defects. When the area of fascial deficiency is contaminated, as in infected mesh reconstructions, enterocutaneous fistulas, or viscous perforations, prosthetic mesh is avoided because of the risk of infection. A delayed reconstruction can be performed by insetting a resorbable polyglactin (Vicryl) mesh that will eventually granulate to allow skin grafting. The ensuing hernia is repaired later with prosthetics under cleaner conditions. The separation-of-components procedure has enjoyed much success in closing large midline defects without resorting to mesh. This procedure involves advancement of bilateral myofascial flaps consisting of the anterior rectus fascia/rectus abdominis/internal oblique/transversus abdominis muscle complex. Mobility of this myofascial unit is created by release of the external oblique muscle at the semilunate line. Midline defects measuring up to 10 cm superiorly, 18 cm centrally, and 8 cm inferiorly can be closed using separation of components.[54] This technique is less effective in closing lateral defects, for which regional muscle and fascial flaps are usually better suited (rectus abdominis flap, internal oblique flap, external oblique flap).[53]

Full-thickness abdominal defects and large myofascial defects require large robust pedicled flaps or free flaps for closure. The tensor fasciae latae pedicled flap, based on the ascending branch of the lateral circumflex femoral vessels, is useful in reconstructing the lower two thirds of the abdomen. Bilateral flaps can be used for very large defects, although the skin-grafted donor site is unsightly. The rectus femoris flap and the vastus lateralis flap can be used for smaller lower abdominal defects. The "mutton-chop" flap, which is an extended rectus femoris flap with fascia lata included distally, has been used successfully in closing massive defects.[55,56] Large defects of the upper abdominal wall may be repaired with pedicled extended latissimus dorsi flaps with attached pregluteal fascia. Very large full-thickness defects, especially superiorly, are best treated with free tissue transfer of large myofascial units such as the latissimus dorsi or the tensor fasciae latae. These can also be innervated flaps to re-establish contractile force and strength in the abdominal wall.

Extremity Reconstruction
Posttraumatic Reconstruction

Historically, significant advances in the treatment of traumatic wounds have occurred during those times of greatest need—wars. World War I was closely predated by the beginnings of aseptic surgery and anesthesia, and marked a turning point in wound management and trauma surgery. With the beginnings of modern orthopedic and plastic surgery; improvements in the understanding of anesthesia, trauma resuscitation, and infection; and the availability of early antibiotics, these times witnessed a move away from amputation for all compound extremity fractures toward an increase in attempts at limb salvage. The introduction and maturation of microsurgical techniques brought increasingly successful distal extremity replantations and free flap reconstructions. Soft tissue reconstruction thus advanced alongside evolving techniques of bone fixation, joint reconstruction, and general vascular surgery. Current lower extremity reconstruction incorporates the use of vascularized bone, composite tissues, and functioning muscle transfers tailored to the given defect.[57] The future may behold the use of tissue-engineered vascularized composite tissue constructs and cadaveric composite tissue allotransplantation.

Common causes of high-energy lower extremity trauma, outside of wartime, include road traffic accidents, falls from a height, direct blows, sports injuries, and gunshots. Understanding the anatomy of the lower limb compartments, nerve and vascular supplies, muscle functions, skeletal structure, and mechanics is essential for accurate bony and soft tissue restoration for function and appearance. Several limb-salvage scoring systems have been suggested to aid in the decision regarding whether to amputate or attempt limb salvage, but their routine use remains controversial; nevertheless, they can provide guidance during this life-altering decision process.[58] Open (compound) fractures are often classified according to the system devised by Gustilo and colleagues (Table 45-12).[59]

In addition to following standard multiple trauma evaluation and resuscitation guidelines, the multidisciplinary team must assess the peripheral neurovascular status, soft tissue defects, and configuration of fractures.[57,60] Bony stabilization may be critical to controlling fracture hemorrhage. Angiography or Doppler ultrasound examination may help assess vascular integrity. Compartment syndrome must be monitored for, and fasciotomies performed when necessary. Antitetanus vaccine and antibiotics should be provided as soon as possible according to contemporary guidelines.[61] An evaluation of the patient as a whole allows treatment to be planned within the context of comorbidities, socioeconomic considerations, and rehabilitative potential. The loss of plantar sensation may favor below-knee amputation. Revascularization of a mangled major extremity brings a risk of massive reperfusion injury and multiple organ failure.

TABLE 45-12	Gustilo and Anderson classification of compound fractures
Classification	**Description**
Grade I	Wound <1 cm; minimal contamination, comminution, and soft tissue damage
Grade II	Wound >1 cm; moderate soft tissue damage and minimal periosteal stripping
Grade IIIa	Substantial contamination and severe soft tissue damage but adequate fracture coverage; usually due to high-energy trauma
Grade IIIb	Substantial contamination, periosteal stripping, severe soft tissue damage, and inadequate fracture coverage; usually due to high-energy trauma
Grade IIIc	Any open fracture with an associated arterial injury requiring repair

In terms of surgical management, the order of repair is fracture stabilization followed by vascular repair and reconstruction of a stable soft tissue envelope. The choice of method for soft tissue coverage is determined by the location and extent of the injury (Table 45-13). Coverage for weightbearing areas should be durable, stable (non-shearing), and sensate. Properly fitted footwear provides essential protection against pressure-related complications. Split-thickness skin grafts are reasonable for coverage of exposed healthy muscle or soft tissue. Local flaps may be used to cover smaller defects. Free tissue transplantation is preferred for larger or more complex defects with bony exposure, particularly in the middle and lower thirds of the leg where limited local soft tissues are available for reconstruction. Free flaps need not be limited to providing only soft tissue coverage; incorporation of vascularized bone, such as of fibula or iliac crest, can aid in fracture management. Chimeric flap configurations can improve flap insetting into composite defects. Flow-through designs, such as the anterolateral thigh flow-through free flap, can be used to bridge segmental vascular defects to revascularize the distal extremity. Muscular flaps can be motor innervated to restore lost muscle functions at the recipient site (Fig. 45-50).[62–64] Other techniques, such as tissue expansion and vacuum-assisted closure, may be indicated in select circumstances. Traditional cross-leg flaps are almost never used nowadays; they cause complete immobilization and increase the risk of deep vein thrombosis and contracture formation.

With the availability of microvascular free tissue transplantation, radical débridements can be adequate even for the largest wounds.

TABLE 45-13	Some lower extremity reconstructive options for soft tissue coverage after fracture
Area of Defect	**Reconstructive Options**
Femur	Sartorius muscle/MC flap (anterior defects)
	TFL muscle/MC flap (posterior defects)
	Vastus lateralis/medialis muscle/MC (mid to lower thigh defects)
	ALT for fasciocutaneous flap
	Free osseous flaps useful for segmental femur defects
Knee and proximal third of tibia	Gastrocnemius muscle (medial or lateral head, or both) with SSG
	Distally based ALT flap
	Free tissue transfer for larger defects
Middle third of tibia	Soleus muscle with SSG
	Gastrocnemius head(s) with SSG
	Flexor digitorum longus muscle
	Tibialis anterior muscle "book flap" (preserves function)
	Free tissue transfer for larger defects
Distal third of tibia	Free tissue transfer usually the first choice
	Reversed sural artery flap
	Peroneal perforator fasciocutaneous flap
	Local muscle flaps for smaller defects

ALT = anterolateral thigh; MC = myocutaneous; SSG = split-thickness skin graft; TFL = tensor fasciae latae.

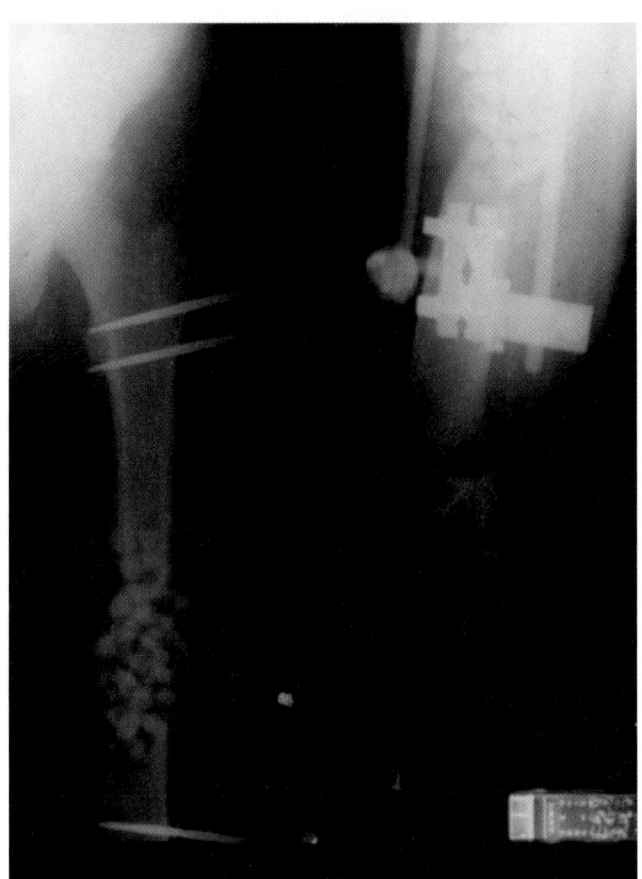

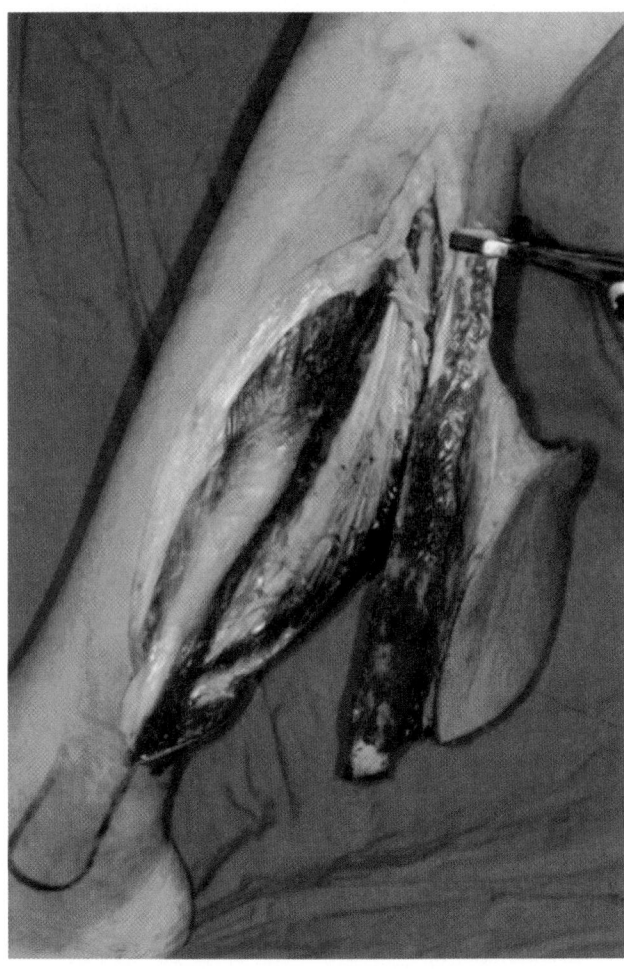

A

B

FIG. 45-50. Soft tissue and bony reconstruction of a Gustilo IIIb open segmental fracture of the right femur using a double-barreled fibula osteoseptocutaneous free flap. **A.** Antibiotic-impregnated beads were placed as a temporary spacer in the segmental femur bone gap after primary débridement; an external fixator is in place. **B.** Two weeks later, a free left fibula osteoseptocutaneous flap was harvested, osteotomized into a double-barreled configuration, and transferred as a microvascular free flap to the contralateral limb. (*Continued*)

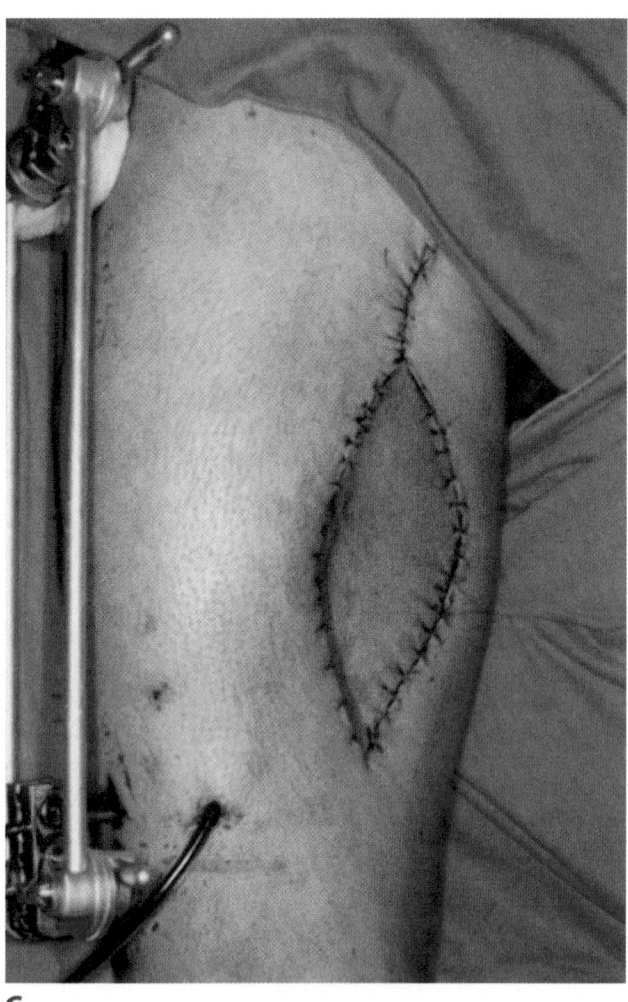

C

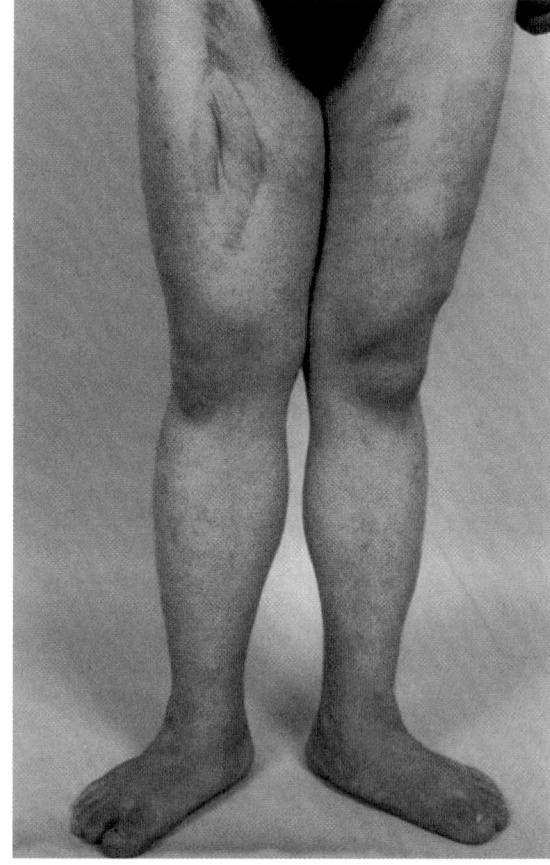

D

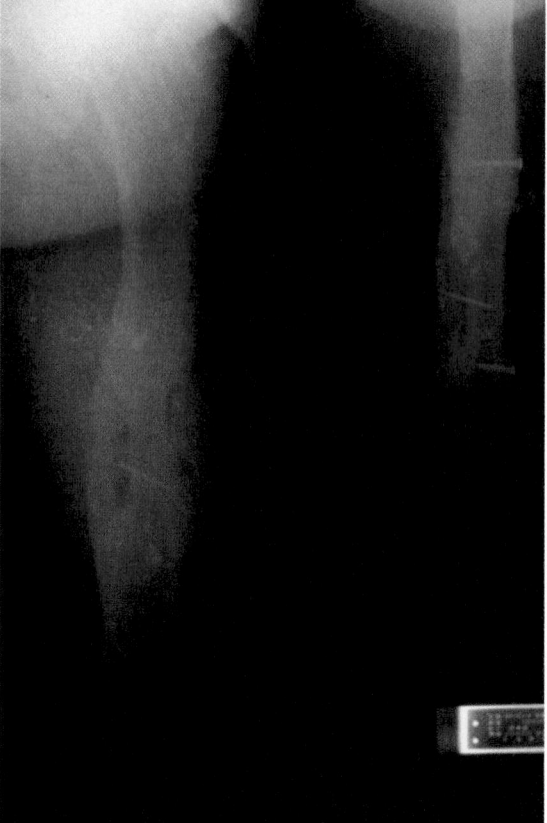

E

FIG. 45-50. (*Continued*) **C.** The skin paddle of the free flap provides a useful means for postoperative clinical monitoring of the viability of the underlying fibula bone. **D** and **E.** The patient is shown fully weightbearing without assistance 20 months after reconstruction; hypertrophy of the double-barreled fibula was noted on the radiographs.

Early one-stage wound coverage and bony reconstruction is generally advocated whenever possible.[2,57,60,61] It is reasonable for reconstruction to be deferred briefly, however, if there remain tissues of questionable viability, so that these can be reassessed and débrided as required. Temporary placement of a biologic dressing is one method to assess the viability and cleanliness of questionable tissues; a skin graft will fail if laid onto an unhealthy graft bed. If débridement produces an irregular dead space that cannot be completely obliterated, or if débridement remains questionable even after a second look, the resultant cavity may be filled with antibiotic-impregnated beads or available vascularized soft tissues to act as a spacer until definitive reconstruction is possible. This applies also to segmental bone losses within a soft tissue envelope of doubtful viability. In these situations, soft tissue coverage preferably is still achieved early; bony reconstruction can be completed at a later date, when both the bone and soft tissue envelope are stable and healthy. Although it remains debated whether fasciocutaneous or muscular (musculocutaneous or muscle alone) flaps are superior for treating compound fractures, it is critical to obliterate dead space with fresh tissue, and this is often more easily achieved using muscle.

Osteomyelitis often complicates inadequately débrided compound leg fractures. Delayed coverage also appears to increase the risk of this dreaded complication. Generous irrigation, débridement, removal of dead bone (even in a segment), expedient antibiotic therapy, and healthy soft tissue coverage are important in both acute compound fracture and established posttraumatic osteomyelitis. Large segmental bone losses can be addressed with microvascular free transplantation of osseous flaps or distraction lengthening.[57,60]

When limb salvage either is not possible or is not in the best interests of the patient, attention is directed to providing soft tissue stump coverage suitable for weightbearing and allowing ambulation with a properly fitted prosthesis. Ideally, local tissues are used; however, when they are unavailable or inadequate, the amputated part can be a useful source of skin grafts or tissues for microvascular free transfers to the stump, which preserves length and avoids a more proximal amputation.

Reconstruction after Oncologic Resection

The refinements in surgical ablation techniques, in adjuvant radiation therapy and chemotherapy, and in limb reconstruction methods have opened the possibility for curative limb-sparing treatments instead of amputation. Extensive soft tissue and segmental long bone defects from radical tumor resection and radiation-compromised wound healing can often be reconstructed nowadays by liberal importation of fresh tissues through microvascular free tissue transplantation tailored to the defect.

Diabetic Ulceration

The pathophysiology of primary diabetic lower limb complications has three main components: peripheral neuropathy (motor, sensory, and autonomic), peripheral vascular disease, and immunodeficiency. Altered foot biomechanics and gait caused by painless collapse of ligamentous support, foot joints, and foot arches change weightbearing patterns. Blunted pain allows cutaneous fissuring and ulceration to progress. Multiflora infections are established amid local immunodeficiency and microvasculopathy. Frank neuroarthropathic Charcot's foot deformities may ultimately result. Cutaneous ulcerations may chronically deteriorate relatively painlessly, involving deeper tissues, including bone. Persistent soft tissue infection and osteomyelitis, worsened by peripheral vascular compromise and immunodeficiency, traditionally ends in gangrene and amputation. Previously, 50 to 70% of lower extremity amputations performed for nontraumatic causes were due to diabetes.[13,31] Improved patient education and medical management, timelier detection of diabetic foot problems and referral for treatment, and the use of more refined techniques for wound management have helped increase the chances of limb preservation.

Diabetic patients with lower limb disease often have significant multisystemic comorbidities that must be optimized for surgery;

strict perioperative control of blood glucose levels is mandatory. Clinical examination must include documentation of sensory deficits, vascular insufficiencies, and evidence of osteomyelitis. Plain radiographs, MRI, nuclear bone scans, and angiography or duplex imaging may be indicated. A patient with significant vascular disease may be a candidate for lower extremity bypass. Nerve conduction studies may diagnose surgically reversible neuropathies at compressive sites and aid in decisions about whether to perform sensory nerve transfers to restore plantar sensibility. Antibiotic and fungal therapies should be guided by tissue culture results.

Plastic surgical management starts with thorough débridement of devitalized or infected tissues, purulent cavities, and osteomyelitic bone. Methods of wound closure are dictated by the extent and location of the postdébridement defect (Table 45-14). Vacuum-assisted closure may be appropriate for superficial defects. Skin grafts should be used cautiously and not in weightbearing areas. Local and regional flaps can be used after careful evaluation of their vascularity given concurrent peripheral vascular disease and possible recent distal vascular bypass procedures. Microvascular free tissue transfers are appropriate when defects are large or when local flaps are not available. Combination lower extremity bypass and free flap coverage has proved beneficial for the treatment of the diabetic foot in terms of healing and reduction of disease progression. Orthopedic surgeons should be consulted to improve foot biomechanics and address bony prominences to reduce the risk of recurrent ulceration. Proper footwear (including orthotic devices and off-loading shoe inserts), hygiene, and toenail and skin care are essential.[65]

Lymphedema

The lymphatic system provides a high-volume transport mechanism, clearing proteins and lipids from the interstitial space to the systemic vasculature by means of differential pressure gradients. Factors that contribute to circulatory lymphatic flow include segmental lymphangion contractility, skeletal muscle activity, and one-way valves that prevent backflow.[66,67] The lymphatics course throughout the body alongside the venous system, into which they eventually drain via the major thoracic and cervical ducts. With lymphatic obstruction, abnormal connections form between the superficial and deep lymphatics and between the lymphatic and venous systems. Lymphatic stagnation, hypertension, and valvular incompetence contribute to edema, inflammatory fibrovascular proliferation, and collagen depo-

TABLE 45-14	Some reconstructive options for the diabetic foot
Area of Defect	**Reconstructive Options**
Forefoot	V-Y advancement
	Toe island flap
	Single toe amputation
	Lisfranc's amputation
Midfoot	V-Y advancement
	Toe island flap
	Medial plantar artery flap
	Free tissue transfer
	Transmetatarsal amputation
Hindfoot	Lateral calcaneal artery flap
	Reversed sural artery flap
	Medial plantar artery flap ± flexor digitorum brevis
	Abductor hallucis muscle flap
	Abductor digiti minimi muscle flap
	Free tissue transfer
	Syme's amputation
Foot dorsum	Supramalleolar flap
	Reversed sural artery flap
	Thinner free flaps (e.g., temporoparietal fascia, radial forearm, groin flaps)

sition, causing firm, nonpitting swelling with peau d'orange cutaneous changes. Lymphoscintigraphy reveals the lymphatic anatomy and quantifies lymphatic flow. MRI provides anatomic information regarding lymphatic trunks, nodes, and obstructive lesions. It is essential to rule out neoplastic lymphatic invasion, especially after oncologic ablation, as a cause of secondary lymphedema. Lymphangiosarcoma is a rare cause of lymphedema that is deadly if diagnosed late.[68]

Primary lymphatic obstruction may arise from congenital malformations of the lymphatic system such as lymphatic hypoplasia, functional insufficiency, or absence of lymphatic valves. Identified genetic causes include the autosomal dominant Milroy disease. Lymphedema praecox accounts for >90% of cases of primary lymphedema, generally appears during puberty but sometimes as late as the third decade, and occurs more commonly in females. It is usually unilateral and limited to the foot and calf. Lymphedema tarda appears after the age of 35 years and is relatively rare. Secondary (acquired) lymphedema is much more common, with filariasis being the leading cause worldwide. In Western countries, secondary lymphedema is more commonly the result of neoplasms and their surgical treatments and radiotherapy.[13,67]

The mainstay of treatment for lower extremity lymphedema is nonsurgical measures, including one or more of the following: use of external compressive garments and devices, limb elevation, administration of antibiotics for episodes of cellulitis, and specialized complex physical therapy.[69] The efficacy of available surgical options is generally poor, and these are reserved for cases in which aggressive nonsurgical measures have failed. The classic Charles procedure involved radical excision of lymphedematous fascial and suprafascial tissues with skin grafting for coverage; cosmetic outcomes were often disastrous, and functional problems arose due to high rates of contracture, wound breakdown, and ulcerations. This method was later modified into multiple staged excisions of subcutaneous tissues. Other techniques include liposuction and bridging procedures. Microsurgical lymphatic-lymphatic, lymphatic-venous, lymphatic-venous-lymphatic, and lymph node–venous anastomoses have all been tried to relieve obstructive lymphedema, and all techniques show some efficacy early on; however, longer-term results are highly variable.[70] Nonsurgical techniques can be, and usually are, combined with any of the surgical methods.

Pressure Sore Treatment

A *pressure ulcer* is defined as tissue injury, usually over a bony prominence, due to pressure or a combination of pressure and shear forces. These wounds occur in patients debilitated by age, illness, immobilization from orthopedic injuries, or spinal cord injury. Prevention of pressure ulcers first requires identification of susceptible patients. Once such patients are identified, measures to prevent development of ulceration include frequent position changes (by both the patient and caretakers), use of pressure reduction equipment (low air loss mattresses and seat cushions, heel protectors), nutritional optimization, hygienic control of incontinence, and medical and/or surgical treatment of muscle spasm and joint contracture. Once an ulcer has developed these same factors must be carefully evaluated and deficiencies corrected before embarking on a complex reconstructive treatment plan. Successful reconstruction also requires a medically stable, cooperative, motivated patient with adequate social support.

Pressure ulcers are described by their stage, based on depth of tissue injury (Table 45-15).[71] Stage I and II ulcers are treated conservatively with dressing changes and basic pressure ulcer prevention strategies as already discussed. Patients with stage III or IV ulcers should be evaluated for surgery. The wound is examined for soft tissue infection or abscess, osteomyelitis, and involvement of deeper structures or spaces (e.g., joint space, urethra, spinal canal) to determine the urgency and specific requirements of the problem. Blood laboratory work and imaging studies are performed to help establish whether soft tissue or bone infection is present. Radiographs are

TABLE 45-15	National Pressure Ulcer Advisory Panel staging system
Classification	**Description**
Stage I	Intact skin with nonblanchable redness
Stage II	Partial-thickness loss of dermis; may present as blister
Stage III	Full-thickness loss of dermis with visible subcutaneous fat (no deeper structures exposed)
Stage IV	Full-thickness loss of dermis with exposed bone, tendon, or muscle
Unstageable	Full-thickness loss of dermis with ulcer base obscured by eschar

usually adequate to rule out osteomyelitis; CT and MRI are helpful when plain films are equivocal. Wet gangrenous tissue and abscesses should be surgically débrided without delay to prevent or treat sepsis. In patients who do not meet the strict reconstruction criteria, débridement to healthy tissue without subsequent reconstruction may be the optimal treatment. If bone is present at the wound base, it should be débrided only to bleeding bone and left with a smooth contour. Complete ischiectomy should not be performed for ischial decubitus ulcers, because removal of one ischium only transfers subsequent pressure trauma to the contralateral ischium or the perineum. If osteomyelitis is present, which is best proven by culture of specimens obtained by intraoperative bone biopsy, long-term antibiotic therapy guided by microorganism sensitivity is indicated. A special note should be made regarding surgical treatment of spinal cord injury patients with T5 or higher injuries. In these patients, manipulation of a pressure ulcer and even simple urinary retention can trigger autonomic hyperreflexia. This dangerous condition is characterized by critically high blood pressure elevation and sympathetic discharge. Effective management is immediate recognition and reversal of trigger factors along with prompt administration of pharmacologic agents to prevent complications such as intracranial and retinal hemorrhage, seizure, cardiac irregularities, and death.

Direct closure of a pressure ulcer is rarely performed because it usually creates tension in the healing tissues already stressed by nonphysiologic external pressure, predisposing the closure to breakdown. Skin grafting is useful for shallow ulcers with well-vascularized beds that are not subjected to high mechanical shear. Unfortunately, these requirements remove most pressure ulcers from skin graft candidacy. The mainstay of deep pressure ulcer reconstruction is coverage with well-vascularized local flaps. There is debate over whether myocutaneous flaps are better than fasciocutaneous flaps for resurfacing regions prone to excess pressure and shear. Although myocutaneous flaps have excellent bulk and blood supply, muscle has low tolerance for ischemic injury. From an anatomic viewpoint there is no pressure point on the human body where bone is padded by muscle. On the other hand, although fasciocutaneous flaps provide reasonable bulk and are teleologically appropriate, some argue that subcutaneous fat and fascia have low resistance to pressure and shear forces, and have less robust perfusion than muscle.[72]

The anatomic location of the pressure ulcer naturally has a profound impact on flap choice. Regardless of the wound site, however, the flap design should be very large, more than needed for closure, so that if the ulcer recurs the flap can be readvanced. In addition, care should be taken to place suture lines, the weakest part of the reconstruction, away from pressure points. Over the last few decades, patterns have developed in the selection of particular flaps for particular pressure sores. Sacral decubiti are well treated with gluteus maximus myocutaneous flaps (Fig. 45-51). In ambulatory patients, either the superior or the inferior gluteus muscle is spared to preserve hip extension function. The downside of using the gluteal muscle is the relatively bloody dissection. A common alternative is

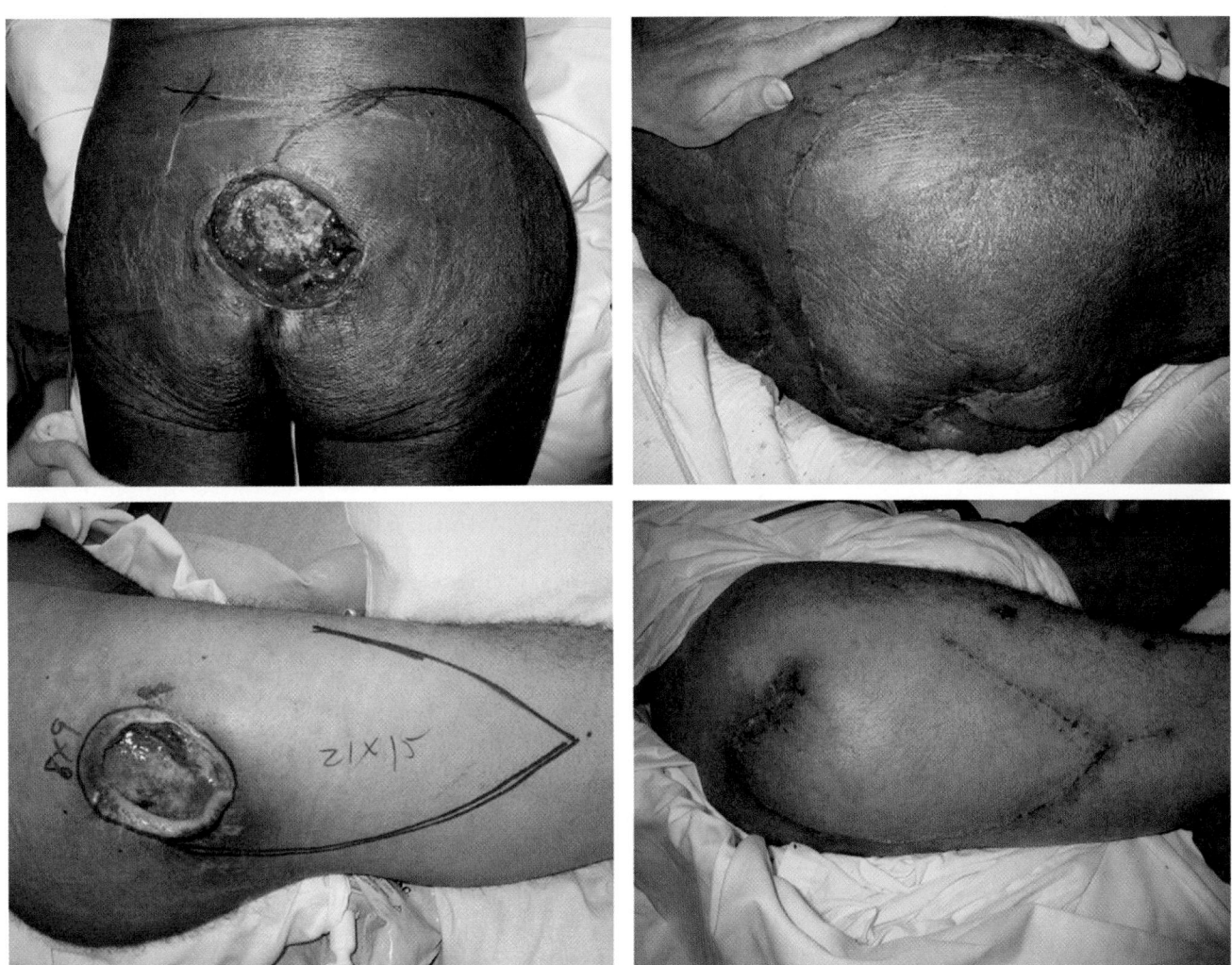

FIG. 45-51. Flap reconstruction of pressure ulcers. *Top row:* Preoperative and 1-month postoperative photos of a stage IV sacral decubitus ulcer treated with a myocutaneous gluteus maximus flap. *Bottom row:* Preoperative and 1-month postoperative photos of a stage IV trochanteric ulcer treated with a myocutaneous V-Y tensor fasciae latae flap. *(Photographs reproduced with permission from M. Gimbel.)*

the gluteal fasciocutaneous advancement or rotational flap. Ischial pressure sores are generally due to sitting in a wheelchair with improper cushioning or insufficient position changes. A good first-choice flap for ischial wound reconstruction is the hamstring V-Y myocutaneous flap. The gluteus maximus flap may also be transposed inferiorly to cover this wound. A fasciocutaneous alternative is the posterior thigh flap, based on the continuation of the inferior gluteal artery. Trochanteric ulcers develop from prolonged positioning in the lateral decubitus position or from poorly fitting seat or wheelchair equipment. The tensor fasciae latae myocutaneous flap is an expendable muscle unit in ambulatory patients that has a reliable blood supply. It can be advanced superiorly or transposed on its long arc of rotation (see Fig. 45-51). Good second-choice flaps are the rectus femoris muscle flap and the vastus lateralis myocutaneous flap. When pressure sores are neglected they can become confluent, forming large areas of deep tissue destruction. This dire situation may require hip disarticulation and use of the upper leg soft tissue as a total thigh flap for coverage.

The postoperative care after flap reconstruction of pressure ulcers is as important for success as the surgery itself. The authors recommend transfer of the patient from the operating room table onto an air-fluidized bed, where the patient will remain for the next 7 to 10 days in the hospital. Meticulous instructions must be given to the nursing staff and therapists regarding the positioning and rolling of the patient to prevent stressing the suture lines during

these maneuvers. Nutrition and muscle spasm control are carefully maintained. The posthospitalization care plan, which should have been arranged preoperatively, is confirmed to avoid lapses in proper care. Patients with ischial sores are advised to abstain from sitting for 6 weeks to allow for sufficient healing. Care of the pressure ulcer patient is a labor-intensive process that requires attention to detail by the surgeon, nurses, therapists, caseworkers, and family. Unfortunately, small gaps in care inevitably lead to large gaps in the debilitated patient's integument.

Reconstructive Transplant Surgery

Composite tissue allotransplantation (CTA), such as hand and face transplantation, has become a clinical reality and offers enormous potential for many reconstructive problems, including amputation of extremities. However, as with solid organ transplantation, there remains the issue of allograft rejection. In contrast to visceral organ transplantation, which involves homogeneous tissues, CTA may involve a combination of skin, subcutaneous tissue, nerve, blood vessels, muscle, tendon, and bone, and thus carry the antigenicities of all these tissue types. The basic principles of immunosuppression for solid organ transplantation have been applied to CTA and include therapy with a variety of combinations of T-cell–depleting agents, monoclonal antibodies, calcineurin inhibitors, antimetabolites, and rapamycin. The complications associated with immuno-

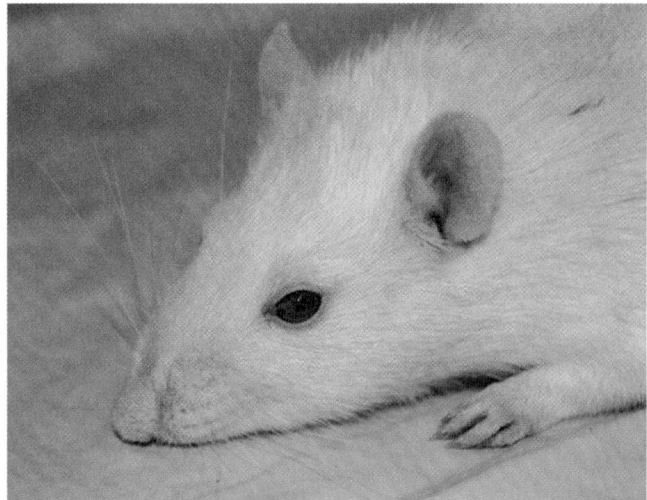
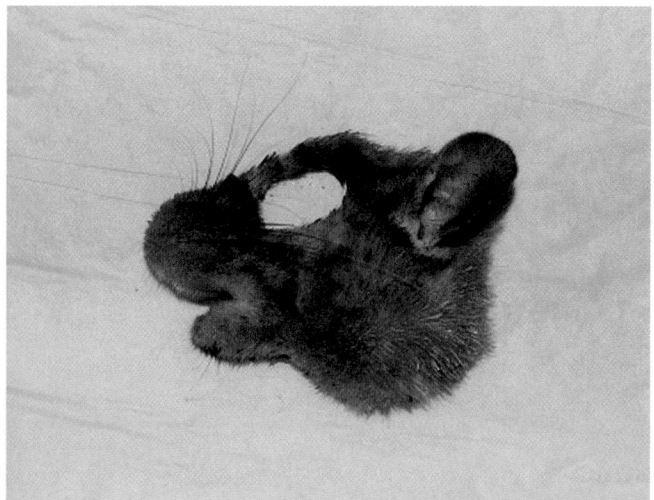
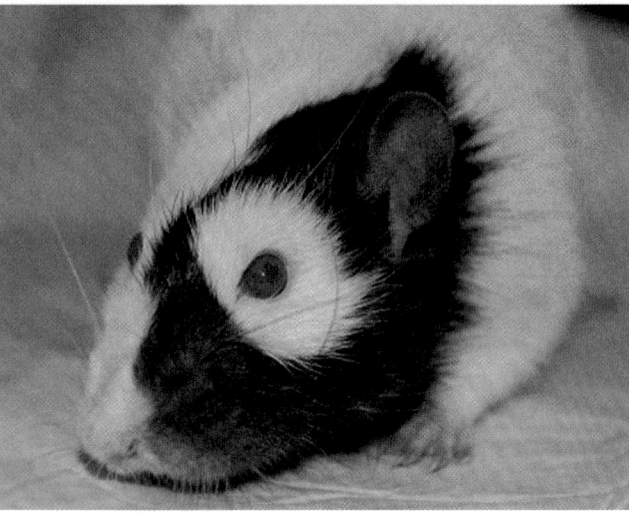

FIG. 45-52. Hemifacial composite tissue allotransplantation in a rat model. *(Photographs reproduced with permission from K. McLean.)*

suppression are well known, including opportunistic infections, metabolic disturbances, and malignancies. Patients selected to undergo CTA, specifically hand transplantation, are young and healthy and therefore more resistant to immunosuppressive side effects than typically less robust solid organ recipients.

As with any surgical procedure the benefits, success rate, and complications must be understood. Unlike solid organ transplantation, CTA is not a lifesaving procedure. There remains much debate over the risks associated with lifelong administration of potentially dangerous immunosuppressive agents to patients who have no life-threatening illness. The ultimate goal in CTA research is immune tolerance in which the recipient of the allograft remains fully immunocompetent yet does not mount an immunologic response to the transplanted allograft. Accomplishment of this goal would allow the decrease or possible elimination of immunosuppressive medications. If immune tolerance is achieved, CTA clinical applications will broaden dramatically as they become the next frontier in reconstructive surgery[73] (Fig. 45-52).

AESTHETIC SURGERY

The American Medical Association defines *cosmetic surgery* as "surgery performed to reshape normal structures of the body to improve the patient's appearance and self-esteem." *Reconstructive surgery* is performed on structures of the body that are abnormal due to congenital defects, developmental abnormalities, trauma, infection, tumors, or disease. It is generally performed to improve function but may also be done to approximate a normal appearance.[74] In practical terms, there are both reconstructive and cosmetic elements to almost every plastic surgery case, and the definition of "normal" structure is sometimes unclear. Nevertheless, there are patients for whom it is a priority to make surgical changes to their bodies in the clear absence of a functional deformity. Aesthetic surgery patients present a unique challenge to the plastic surgeon, because the most important outcome parameter is not truly appearance, but patient satisfaction. Optimally, a good cosmetic outcome will be associated with a high level of patient satisfaction. For this to be the case, the plastic surgeon must do a careful analysis of the patient's motivations for wanting surgery, along with the patient's goals and expectations. The surgeon must make a reasonable assessment that the improvements that can be achieved through surgery will meet the patient's expectations. The surgeon must appropriately counsel the patient about the magnitude of the recovery process, the exact location of scars, and potential complications. If complications do occur, the surgeon must manage these in a manner that preserves a positive doctor-patient relationship.

Assessment of Facial Aesthetics

A thorough evaluation of the patient who presents for facial aesthetic surgery should start with elicitation of the patient's chief complaint, and the examination should be focused on that region. Physical examination of the entire face should note skin quality as well as the presence of redundant skin on the neck, jowls, and eyelids. Depth of the nasolabial folds and the presence of "marionette" lines on the chin should be noted. Brow position should be evaluated, along with the distance from brow to hairline. Bulging fat in the lower eyelid region and the presence of a "tear trough" deformity, or deep fold at the lid-cheek junction, should be evaluated. Facial fat atrophy and descent, a hallmark of facial aging, should be noted.

Blepharoplasty and Browlift

Excess skin and adipose deposits of the upper eyelid are approached through an incision based on the supratarsal crease. Careful attention to marking will avoid the complication of overresection. A strip of orbicularis muscle is often excised to accentuate the supratarsal fold. Fat deep to the orbital septum is resected selectively. In the lower lid, excess skin is removed through a subciliary incision. Lower eyelid fat may be either excised or repositioned. Complications can include hematoma, lower lid retraction, and injury to ocular muscles. If a hematoma forms in the retro-orbital region, a true surgical emergency exists. Permanent vision loss can occur if it is not immediately decompressed. Brow ptosis, judged relative to the superior orbital rim, can be corrected through a number of incisions (Fig. 45-53).[75]

Facelift

Correction of jowls, nasolabial folds, and redundant neck skin can be accomplished with a facelift procedure that both removes skin and tightens the superficial musculoaponeurotic system (SMAS) layer. The SMAS lies deep to the subcutaneous tissue and contains the muscles of facial expression. The facial nerves are in a plane just deep to the SMAS. The SMAS can be simply plicated or a portion of it excised and closed. A sub-SMAS dissection technique can help to elevate and develop this layer in separate fashion, with care being taken to avoid injury to the underlying facial nerves. The incisions for most facelift techniques are preauricular with extension into the temporal hairline superiorly and into the retroauricular region posteriorly and inferiorly (Figs. 45-54, 45-55). The platysmal layer is continuous with the SMAS layer and can be plicated through a small

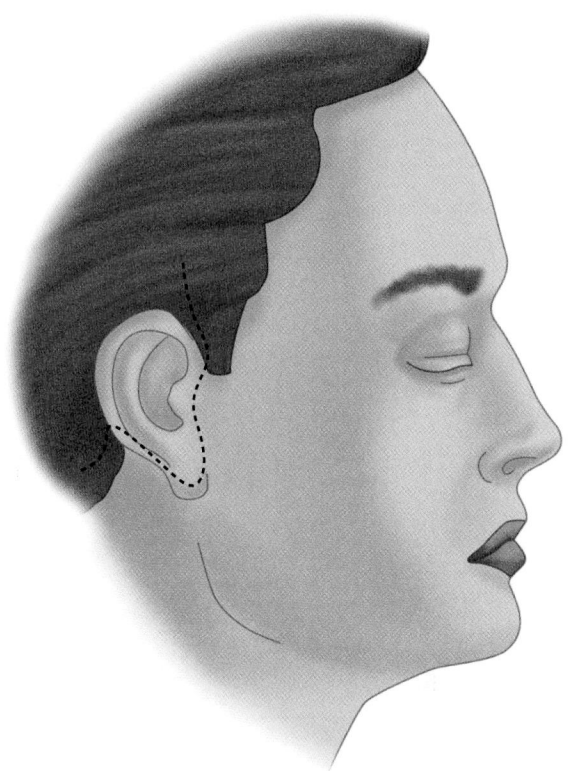

FIG. 45-54. Incisions for cervicofacial rhytidectomy.

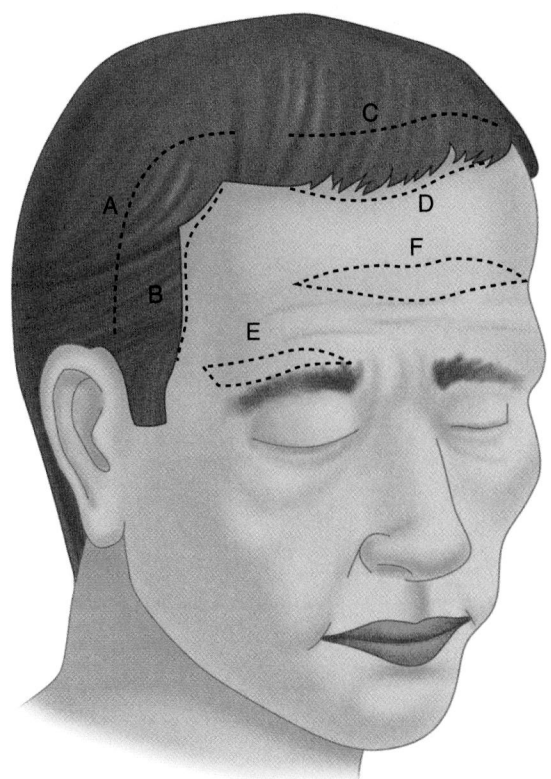

FIG. 45-53. Incisions for browlift. *A,* Temporal scalp incision; *B,* temporal hairline incision; *C,* midline scalp incision; *D,* mid-hairline incision; *E,* direct eyebrow incision; *F,* direct forehead incision.

neck incision to eliminate the appearance of vertical bands along the muscle edge. The most common facelift complication is hematoma, which may require operative drainage to prevent skin flap necrosis. Injury to facial nerves, most often temporal branch and marginal mandibular branch, is seen in approximately 1% of cases.[76]

Rhinoplasty

The key to understanding rhinoplasty is appreciating the complex nasal anatomy (Fig. 45-56) and the way in which altering this framework will impact the appearance of the nose. Evaluation of the rhinoplasty patient not only should include the aesthetic complaints, but also should consider the function of the nasal airways. Nasal airway obstruction can occur from several structural problems. A deviated septum can severely impede airflow, as can problems with the internal nasal valve. Obstruction at the internal nasal valve, which is the junction of the upper lateral cartilage and septum, can be identified by applying lateral traction on the cheek skin to open the valve and observing whether airflow improves (Cottle sign). Airway obstruction can be addressed surgically at the time of rhinoplasty. Aesthetic deformities of the dorsum of the nose are treated by a combination of osteotomies, which serve to reposition the nasal bones, and rasping of the bone. Aesthetic deformities of the tip of the nose are treated by reducing the width of the lower lateral cartilages and/or sewing the cartilages together to reduce tip width. Small tips can be augmented with cartilage grafts harvested from septum or auricle (Fig. 45-57). Complications of rhinoplasty include induction of new nasal airway obstruction and a variety of aesthetic deformities.[77]

Suction Lipectomy

Liposuction involves the removal of adipose tissue through minimal incisions using a hollow suction cannula. Although the scarring is quite innocuous, a key principle of liposuction is that fat is being removed without skin tightening. Therefore, one relies on the patient's inherent skin elasticity to provide retraction over the treated adipose depot. Assessment of skin tone is a vital part of the patient evaluation.

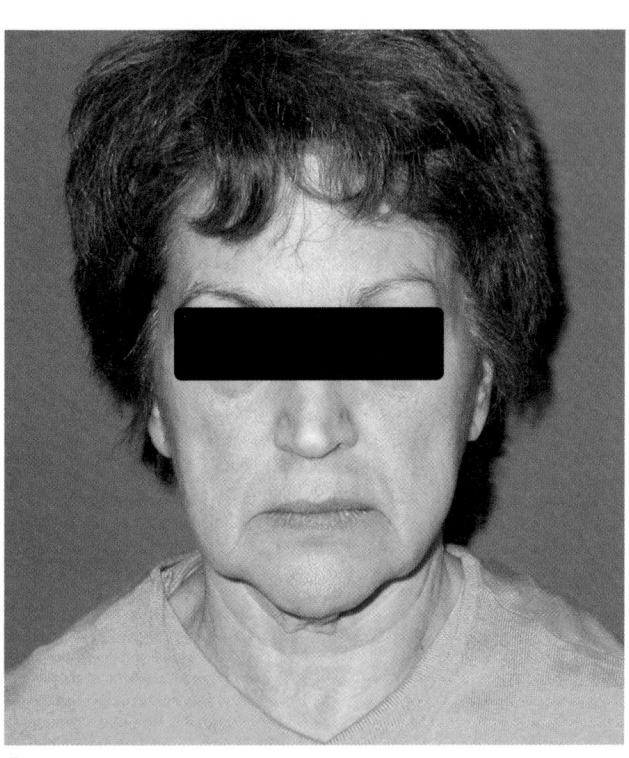
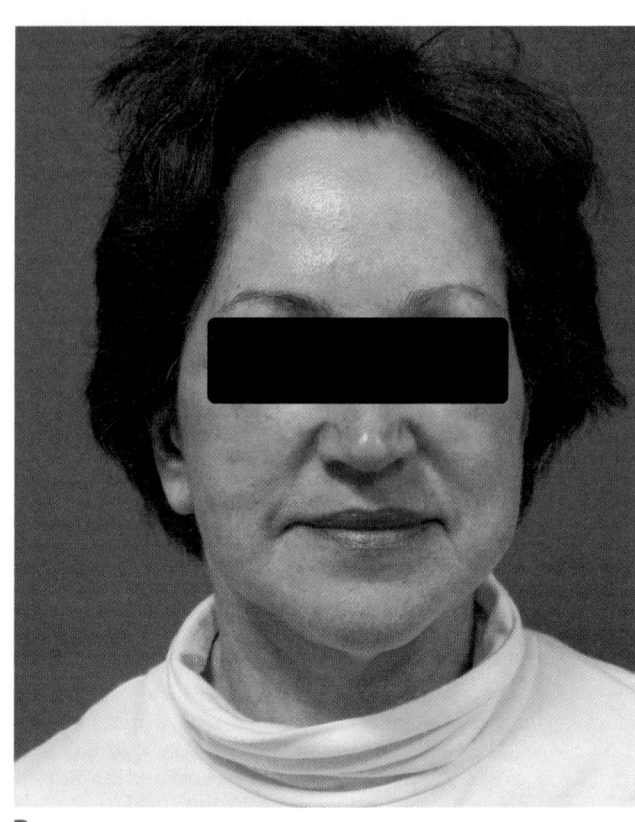

A **B**

FIG. 45-55. Facelift. **A.** Preoperative appearance. **B.** Postoperative appearance.

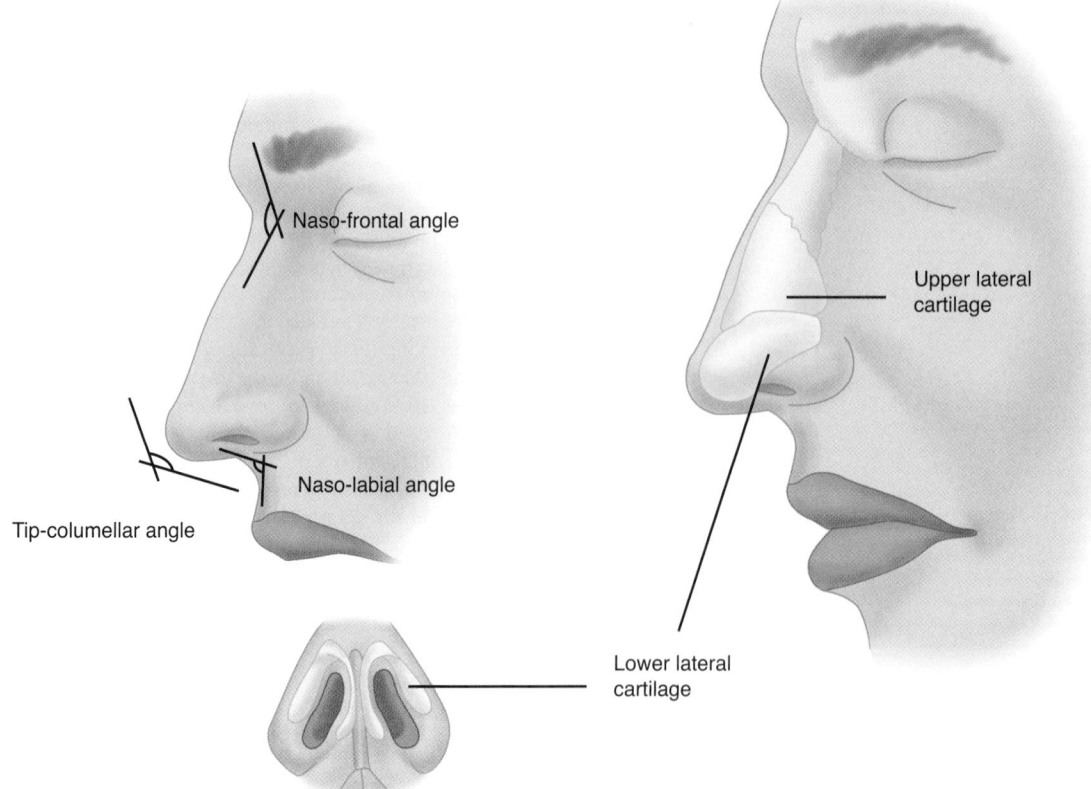

Naso-frontal angle

Naso-labial angle

Tip-columellar angle

Upper lateral cartilage

Lower lateral cartilage

FIG. 45-56. Rhinoplasty anatomy.

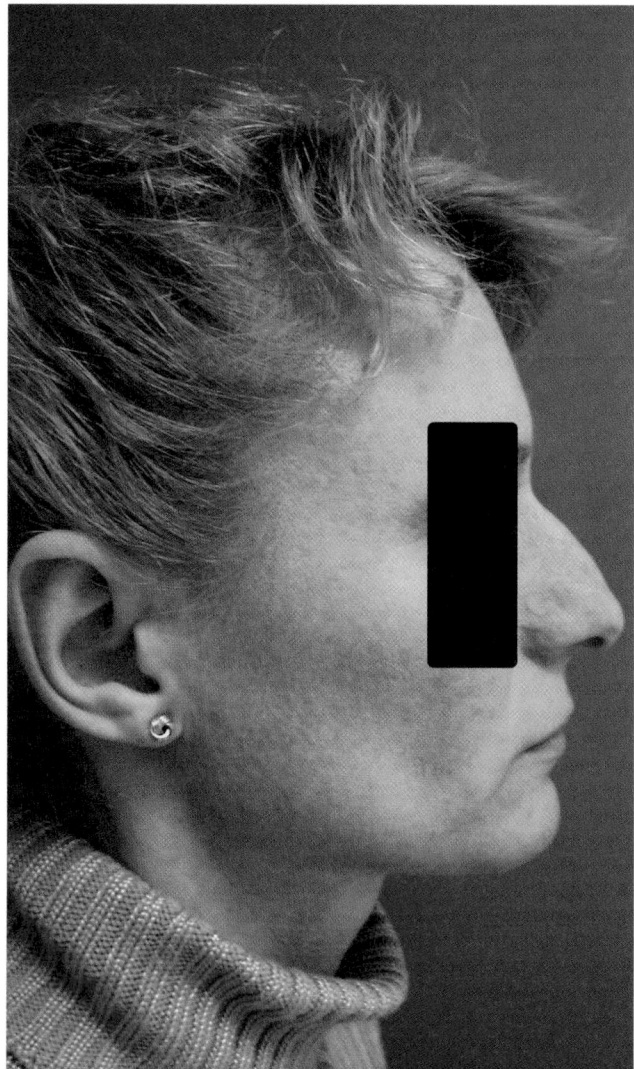

A

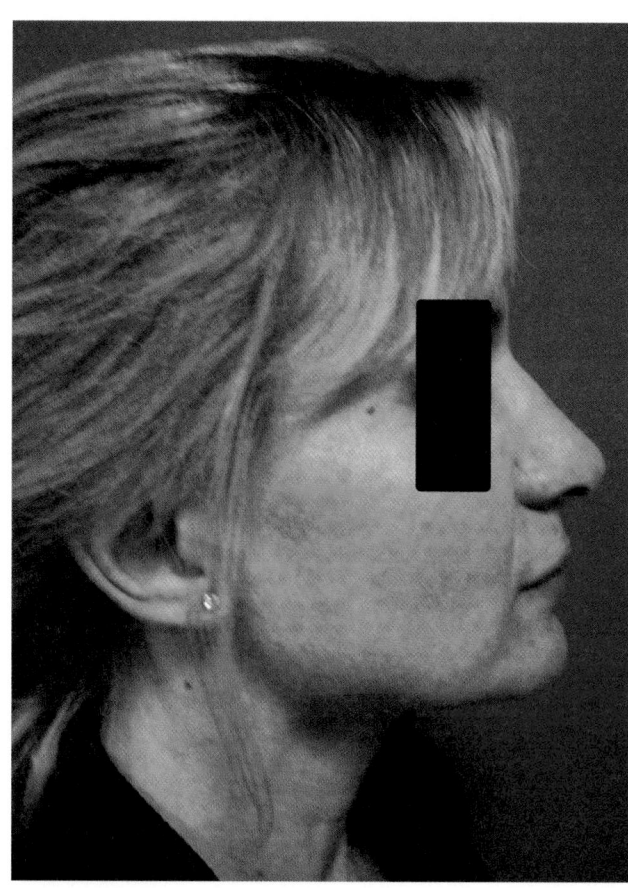

B

FIG. 45-57. Rhinoplasty. **A.** Preoperative appearance. **B.** Postoperative appearance.

If there is skin laxity in the area to be treated, it may worsen after liposuction. Importantly, liposuction should be used as a tool for contouring prominent adipose depots and is not considered a weight loss treatment. The best candidates for liposuction are individuals who are close to their goal weight and have focal adipose deposits that are resistant to diet and exercise (Fig. 45-58). The suction cannula removes fat by avulsing small parcels of adipose tissue into small holes at the cannula tip. With standard suction lipectomy, fat is removed only when the cannula is actively moved through the tissue planes. Minimal tissue effects are seen when the cannula is stationary. In general, larger-diameter cannulas remove adipose tissue at a faster rate but carry a higher risk of causing contour irregularities such as grooving and uneven removal of fat. Newer liposuction technology uses an ultrasonic probe to emulsify the fat via cavitation before suction. Advocates of ultrasonic liposuction report that the technique provides a more even and uniform removal of adipose tissue. Recognizing that no one technique is best for all patients and all anatomic regions, many surgeons use ultrasonic energy selectively.

A major advance in the field of liposuction was the development of tumescent local anesthesia. This method involves the infiltration of very dilute lidocaine and epinephrine (lidocaine 0.05% and epinephrine 1:1,000,000) in large volumes throughout the subcutaneous tissues. Tumescent volumes may range from one to three times the anticipated aspirate volume. The dilute lidocaine provides sufficient anesthesia to allow the liposuction to be performed without additional agents, although many surgeons prefer to use sedation or even

general anesthetic when large volumes of fat are to be removed. When general anesthesia is used, the lidocaine dose may be reduced or even eliminated. With tumescent anesthesia, the absorption of the dilute lidocaine from the subcutaneous tissue is very slow, with peak plasma concentrations occurring approximately 10 hours after the procedure.[78] Therefore, the standard lidocaine dosing limit of 7 mg/kg may be safely exceeded. Current recommendations suggest a limit of 35 mg/kg of lidocaine with tumescent anesthesia.[79] A very important component of the tumescent anesthetic solution is the dilute epinephrine, which limits blood loss during the procedure.

Safety issues are paramount for liposuction because of potential fluid shifts postoperatively and hypothermia. If ≥5000 mL of aspirate is to be removed, the procedure should be performed in an accredited acute care hospital facility. After the procedure, vital signs and urinary output should be monitored overnight in an appropriate facility by qualified and competent staff who are familiar with perioperative care of the liposuction patient.[79]

Excisional Body Contouring

When significant skin laxity is present, improvement in contour can be achieved only through skin excision. Therefore, all body-contouring surgery represents a trade of excess skin for scar, and this must be emphasized during patient consultation. The patient willing to accept scars in exchange for improved contour is likely to be satisfied with the procedures. With the increased number of bariatric surgery proce-

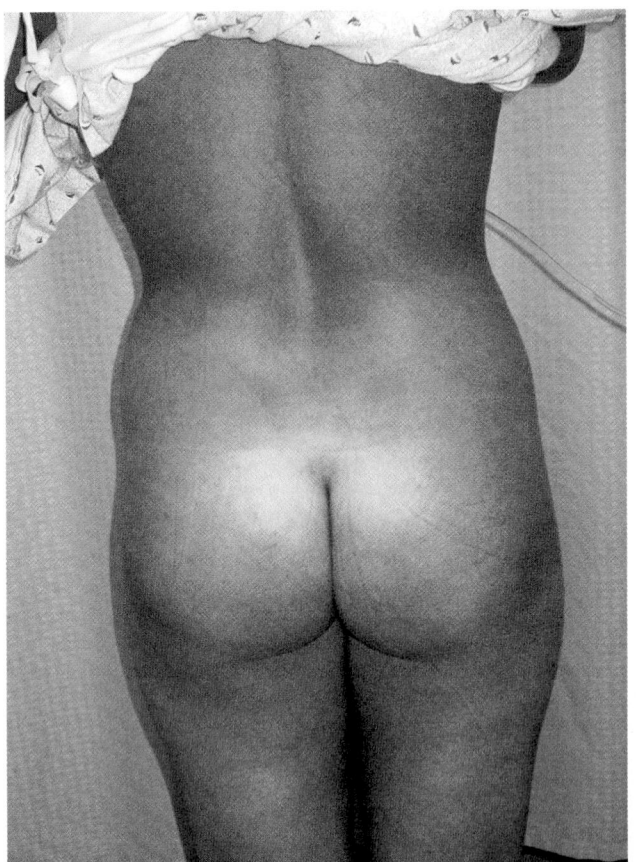

A

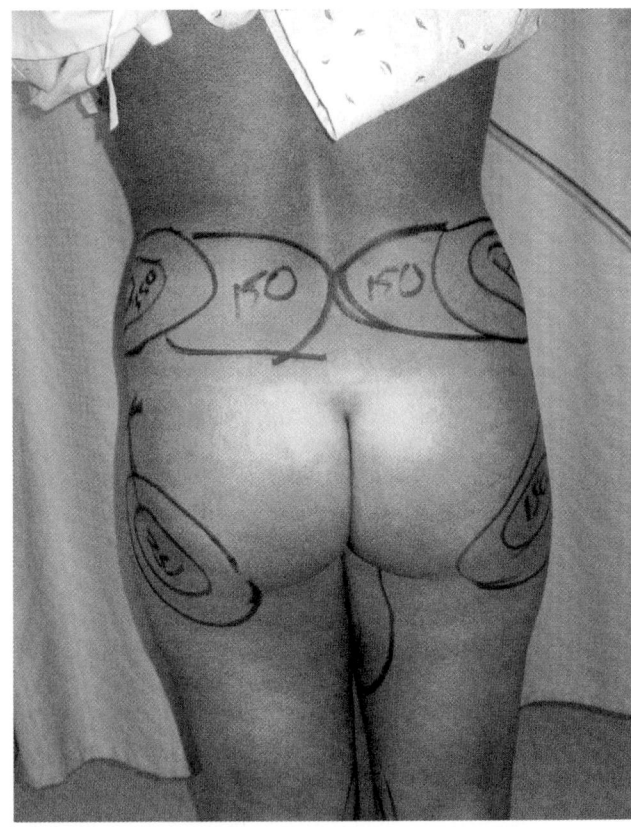

B

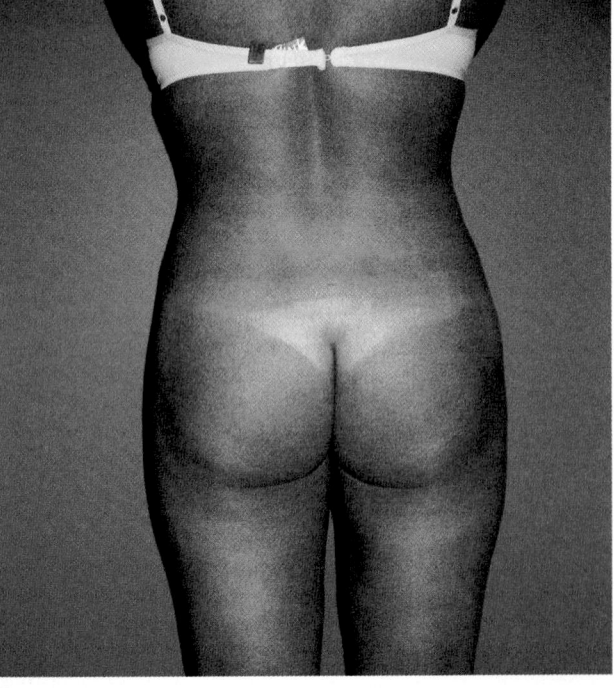

C

FIG. 45-58. **A** and **B.** Preoperative photos of a 22-year-old woman with focal adipose deposits on the trunk and extremities. **C.** Patient 3 months after surgery.

dures over the past decade, body-contouring surgery has become very popular and is emerging as a new subspecialty of plastic surgery.

Abdominoplasty/Panniculectomy

Abdominoplasty/panniculectomy is the most common body-contouring procedure and can range from a limited-incision skin re-

moval in the lower abdomen to a major skin excision with transposition of the umbilicus and placation of the rectus muscles to further enhance contour.[80] Some patients may benefit from a concurrent vertical incision to remove skin in two vectors (Fig. 45-59). Possible complications include skin necrosis, persistent paresthesias of the abdominal wall, seroma, and wound separation. Necrosis of

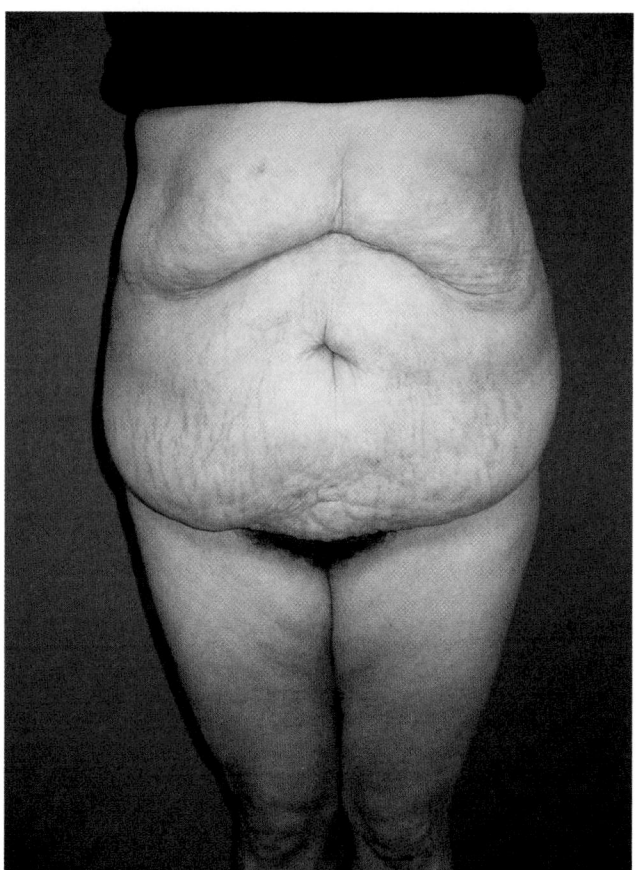

A

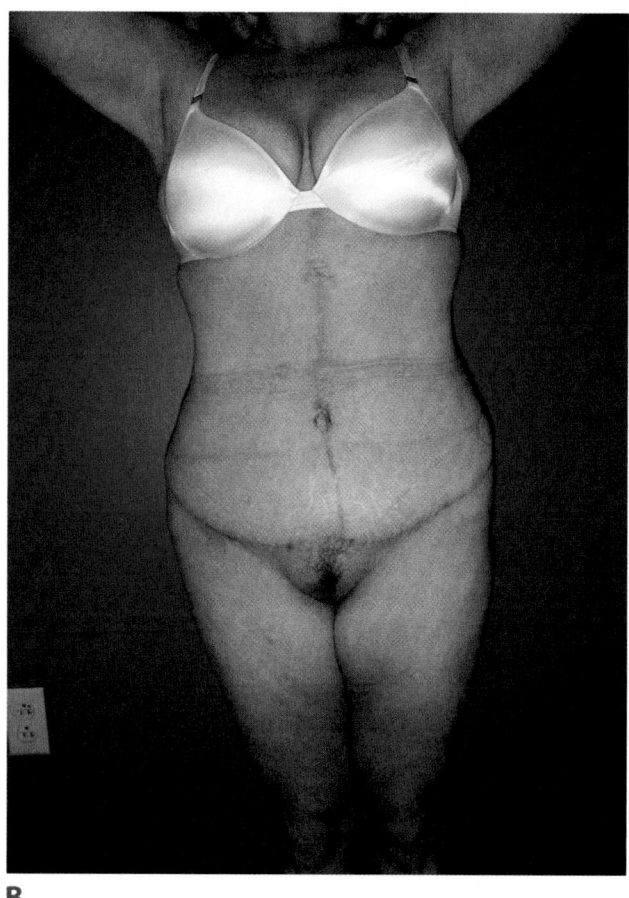

B

FIG. 45-59. A. Preoperative photo of 35-year-old woman after gastric bypass and massive weight loss. **B.** Patient 12 months after a fleur-de-lis abdominoplasty.

the umbilicus may complicate preservation of that structure if the stalk is excessively long or an umbilical hernia is repaired. Adding a vertical resection increases the incidence of skin necrosis, especially at the confluence of scars in the lower abdomen.

Brachioplasty (Arm Lift)

Brachioplasty, or arm lift, leaves a visible longitudinal scar on the upper arm. Therefore, it is reserved for patients with excessive skin in that region. The patient willing to accept the scar can be happy with the results. Complications include distal seroma and wound separation. Paresthesias in the upper arm and forearm may occur secondary to injury of sensory nerves passing through the resection area, although this rarely affects function. Scar contracture in the axilla may limit shoulder excursion in rare cases and require revision.

Thigh and Buttock Lift

Treatment of loose skin on the thighs and buttocks involves a spectrum of operations customized to the individual patient. The outer thighs can be lifted at the same time that an abdominoplasty is performed with one continuous scar along the belt line. The same scar can be continued all the way around the back to lift the buttocks as well. This combination of abdominoplasty, thigh lift, and buttock lift is commonly referred to as a *circumferential lower body lift*. The inner thighs can be contoured by lifting the skin and placing the incisions along the groin crease. Firmly anchoring the deep thigh fascia to Colles' fascia is essential to help prevent spreading of the labia. In cases of severe excess skin on the inner thighs, a long vertical incision is necessary. Complications of thigh and buttock lift include seroma, wound separation, skin necrosis, and change in the shape of

the genital region (with possible sexual dysfunction). Blood loss during the procedure may necessitate transfusion.

Reduction Mammaplasty

Breast reduction is performed to treat symptoms of macromastia, most commonly consisting of the triad of upper back pain, bra strap grooving, and rashes under the fold of the breasts. Although this procedure has reconstructive indications, the aesthetic outcome is of considerable importance. Fundamental to the success of the procedure is the establishment of symmetric and proper nipple position. Nipple ptosis is graded by the nipple position relative to the inframammary fold (IMF). Grade 1 ptosis describes a nipple ≤1 cm below the IMF. Grade 2 ptosis describes a nipple 1 to 3 cm below the IMF. Grade 3 ptosis describes a nipple position >3 cm below the IMF. *Pseudoptosis* or *bottoming out* is a term used to describe the descent of the breast tissue below the nipple and is a potential long-term complication of breast reduction. In addition to classification of nipple ptosis, a thorough preoperative evaluation also includes measurement of the distance from sternal notch to nipple bilaterally, as well as measurement of the distance from nipple to IMF. The base width of the breast should also be considered. Many patients are found to have significant baseline asymmetries in these measurements. Preoperative breast cancer screening consistent with current American Cancer Society guidelines should be performed for all patients undergoing elective breast reshaping surgery. The planned new nipple position should be symmetrical at the IMF along the breast meridian. There are many technical variations of the breast reduction procedure, but nearly all of them have common elements of reshaping the skin envelope in three dimensions and moving the nipple to a new location on a vascularized

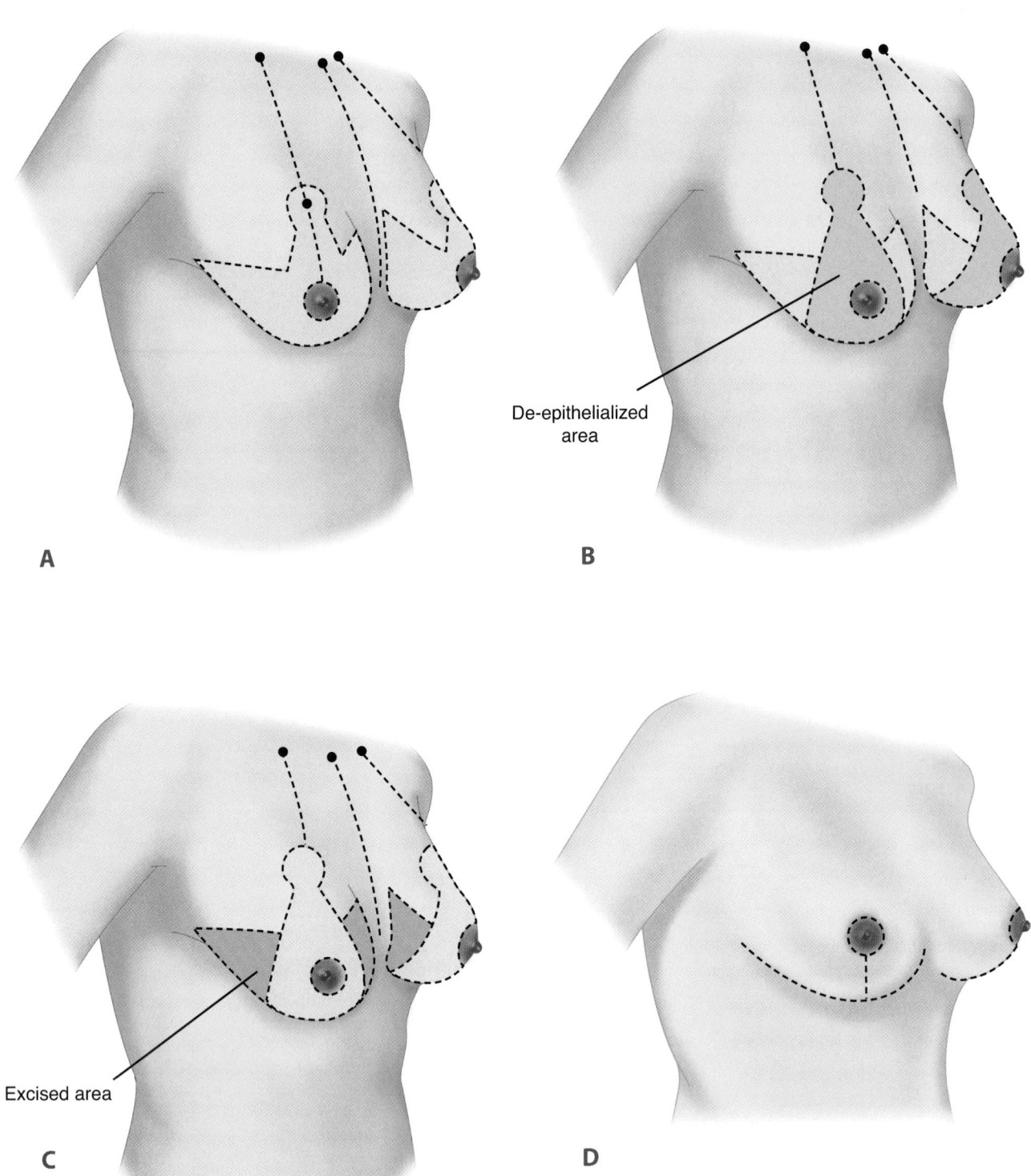

A

B

De-epithelialized area

C

Excised area

D

FIG. 45-60. Inferior pedicle reduction mammaplasty. **A.** Markings for Wise pattern reduction. **B.** Purple area is region to be de-epithelialized. **C.** Dark blue region is area to be resected. A segment of the inferior pedicle is de-epithelialized. The inferior pedicle is dissected straight down to the chest wall, with maintenance of an 8- to 10-cm pedicle width. Lateral and medial segments are resected. After this is accomplished, the superior flap is dissected to the clavicle. Breast subcutaneous tissue and parenchyma are resected from the superior pole. The vertical limbs are brought together and to the meridian of the inframammary fold. The nipple is then set in its new superior position. **D.** T-shaped incision on final closure.

tissue pedicle. The pedicle is de-epithelialized to preserve the subdermal vascular plexus. Figure 45-60 shows the classic "keyhole" Wise pattern reduction technique. The skin resection is designed to create a conical shape, and the nipple is transposed on an inferiorly based pedicle.[81] This results in an inverted T–shaped scar. Figure 45-61 shows a patient treated using this technique. All breast reduction

techniques keep the scars on the lower half of the breast so they are covered by clothing. Techniques have been designed to minimize scar length and even eliminate the horizontal component in the IMF. Figure 45-62 depicts a vertical scar skin resection pattern with the nipple preserved on a superior pedicle.[82,83] For excessively large breasts, the required pedicle length may be too long to provide

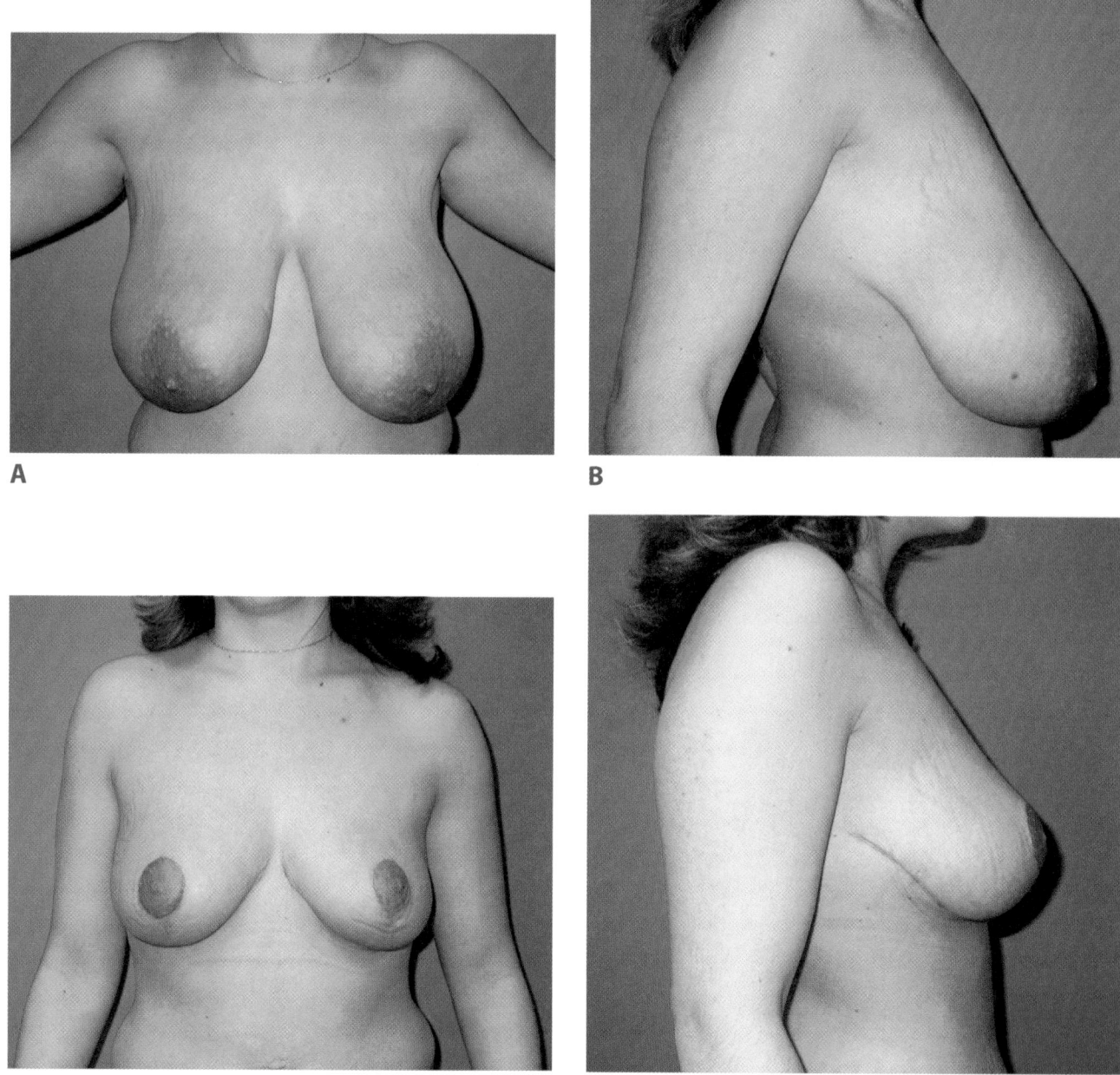

A **B** **C** **D**

FIG. 45-61. **A** and **B.** Preoperative photos of a 25-year-old woman with symptoms of upper back pain, bra strap grooving, and rashes under the folds of her breasts treated with a Wise pattern inferior pedicle reduction. **C** and **D.** Patient 6 months after surgery.

adequate blood supply to the nipple. In such cases, the nipple is removed and replaced onto a viable tissue bed as a full-thickness skin graft. Complications of breast reduction include decreased nipple sensation, nipple loss (rare), skin necrosis, hematoma, and fat necrosis. This last complication can result in a firm mass of scar within the breast that may need careful evaluation and follow-up to distinguish it from a neoplastic mass. Long-term complications include inability to breastfeed and pseudoptosis, as mentioned earlier.

Mastopexy

In contradistinction to breast reduction, in which patients are treated for symptoms related to heavy breasts, mastopexy is a three-dimensional reshaping of the breast performed with no or minimal volume removal. The principles are the same, however: The skin envelope is

contoured and the nipple location optimized. Because the degree of ptosis may be less severe than in breast reduction cases, the patterns of skin resection can vary widely. Minimal patterns may involve excision of just a crescent of skin from above the areola or a periareolar ("donut") resection. The Wise keyhole pattern can be used for larger skin excisions.

Augmentation Mammaplasty

Although the use of prosthetic implants can successfully increase breast size, the surgeon must fully understand both the risks of the biomaterials and the way in which a specific implant of given shape and size can be surgically integrated into the existing breast mound to achieve the desired result.[84] To address the latter point, the surgeon must first consider the possible surgical approaches for implant

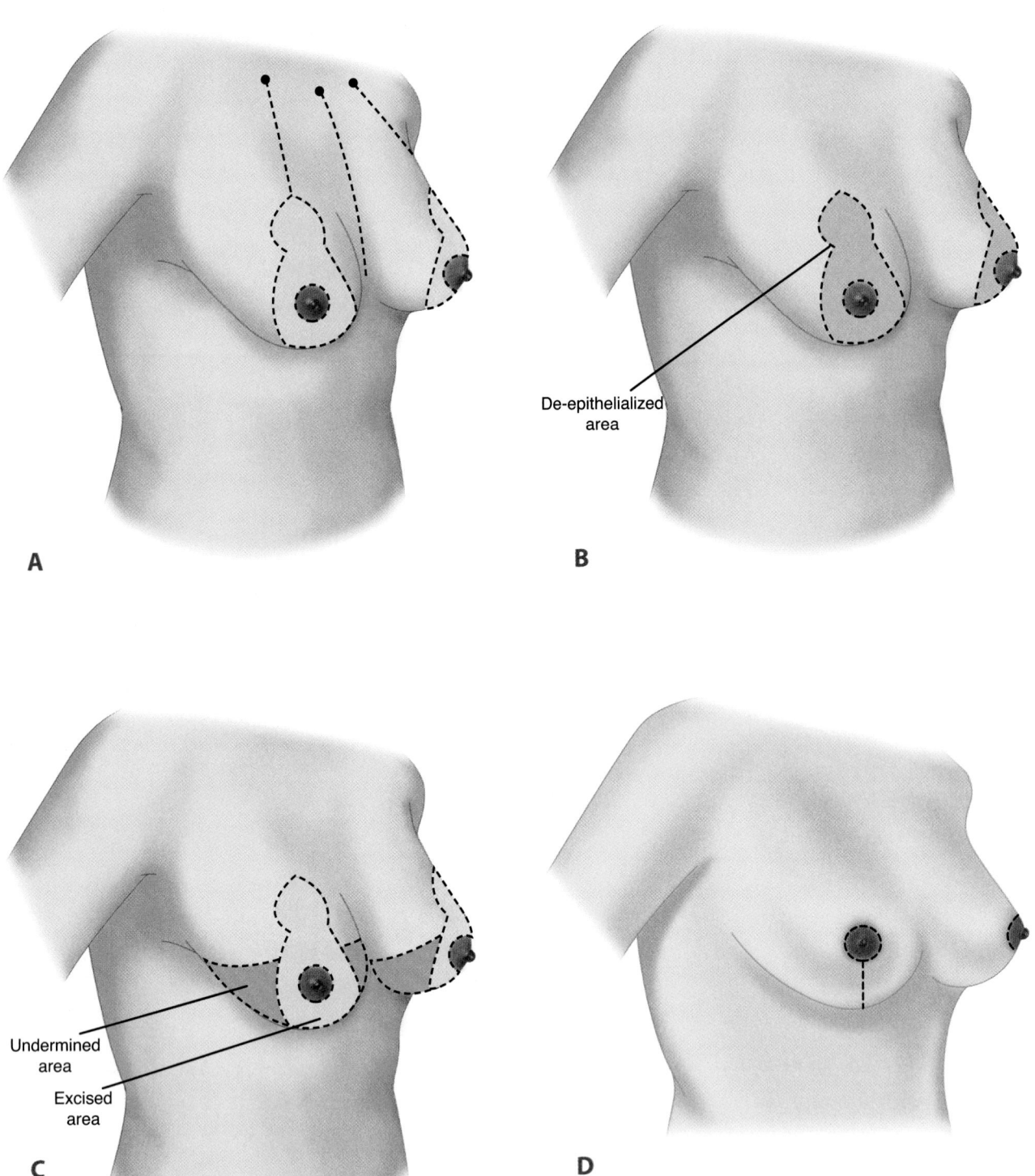

A

B

De-epithelialized area

C

Undermined area

Excised area

D

FIG. 45-62. Vertical reduction mammaplasty, Lejour technique. **A.** Markings for vertical reduction. **B.** Purple area is region to be de-epithelialized. **C.** Dark blue region represents inferior pole to be resected. The shaded regions are the lateral and medial segments that are to be undermined; these areas can also be liposuctioned. The superior pedicle is de-epithelialized and dissected to the chest wall. The tissue and parenchyma from the inferior pole are resected. The pillars from the lateral and medial segments are sewn together. The nipple is transposed on its pedicle to its new position. **D.** Closure of the vertical mammaplasty. There is bunching up of skin and tissue along the vertical limb that will resolve over time; in addition, the new inframammary fold will declare itself superior to the original one.

placement. The three commonly used incisions for placement of cosmetic breast implants are inframammary, periareolar, and axillary (Fig. 45-63).[85] A transumbilical breast augmentation technique has been advocated by some surgeons more recently, but critics of this approach point out that there is poor control over the dissection of

the implant pocket and that direct access to the tissues of the breast is inadequate to control bleeding vessels. In addition, only saline implants can be used with transumbilical breast augmentation because the prefilled silicone implants are too large to pass through the incision and narrow tunnel. The implants may be placed in a subglan-

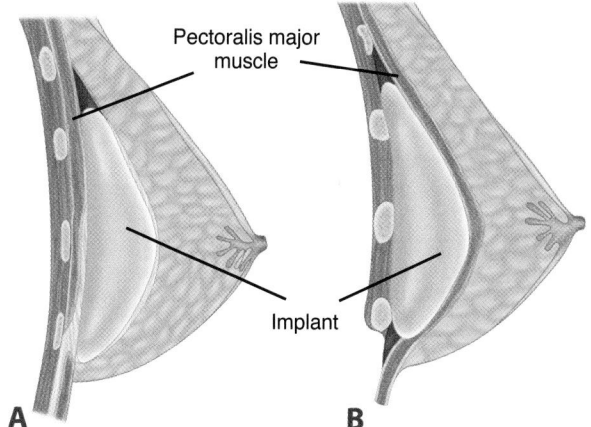

FIG. 45-64. Placement of breast implant. **A.** Subglandular. **B.** Subpectoral.

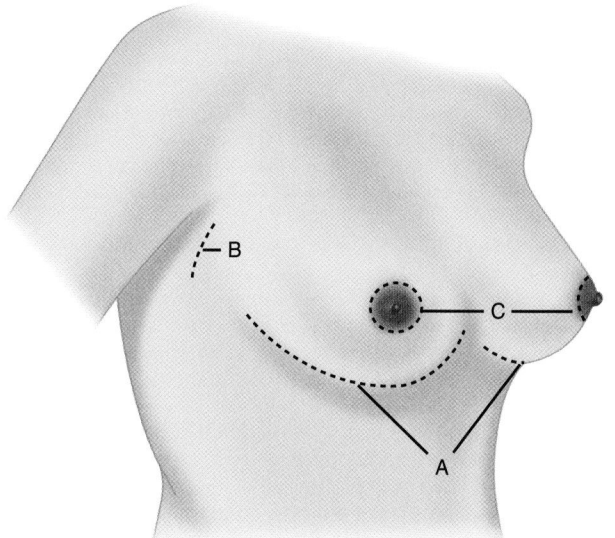

FIG. 45-63. Incisions for augmentation mammaplasty. *A,* Inframammary; *B,* axillary; *C,* periareolar.

dular or subpectoral position (Fig. 45-64). Many surgeons prefer the subpectoral placement because it provides greater soft tissue coverage in the upper pole of the breast and can hide contour irregularities related to the implant. This soft tissue coverage is especially important with saline implants, because visible rippling can occur. The next issue to consider is existing nipple position. If a patient has mild ptosis, the sheer volume of the implant may raise the nipple to an acceptable level. For more severe ptosis, a concurrent mastopexy is necessary. Some surgeons advocate performing the mastopexy as a second stage after the implant has settled into position.

Potential complications related to the implant itself are numerous, and the patient must be fully informed of these possibilities before undergoing surgery. One important point is that there is a high likelihood that the patient will require a second operation to address an implant problem. The implant complications are essentially all local. Although there was concern in the past that implants might be associated with systemic connective tissue disorders, large epidemiologic studies have not supported such a link. The fears over implant safety were so strong that the Food and Drug Administration (FDA) declared a moratorium on the use of silicone gel implants in 1992. At that time, saline-filled implants were still allowed for general cosmetic use. Data were compiled on silicone gel implants, and these devices were approved by the FDA for general use in 2006.[86] Potential implant complications include rupture of the device. For saline implants, this results in rapid deflation. For silicone gel implants, the rupture may be not be obvious and can be confirmed by MRI. Another complication is capsular contracture, which results in a tight envelope of scar that can distort the shape of the implant and cause pain in severe cases. A complication more common to saline devices is the appearance of rippling in the upper pole of the device. Implant malposition can also distort the breast shape and require reoperation. Safety data printed on the official FDA-approved package insert from one of the device manufacturers show the incidence of reoperation to be 29.9% over 7 years in a study of 901 women undergoing primary breast augmentation with saline-filled implants (postapproval study). The rate of severe capsular contracture (grade 3 or 4 on a 4-point scale) was 15.7%, and the rate of implant rupture was 9.8%.[87] For silicone gel–filled implants, the reoperation rate was observed to be 23.5% over 4 years in a study of 455 women undergoing primary breast augmentation. The rate of severe capsular contracture (grade 3 or 4 on a 4-point scale) was 13.2%, and the rate of implant rupture (evaluated by MRI) was 2.7%.

The three most common reasons for operation, in order, were capsular contracture (28.9%), implant malposition (15.6%), and ptosis (14.1%). For secondary augmentation, complication rates were much higher, with the reoperation rate over 4 years rising to 35.2%. The rate of capsular contracture was 17.0%, and the rate of implant rupture was 4.0%.[88]

Another concern regarding breast implants is the issue of whether adequate mammography can be performed after augmentation. Displacement techniques can be used by the mammographer to view the breast tissue. Although patients are advised that implants may affect mammography, a study surveying women who did and did not undergo breast augmentation found no statistical difference in survival or detection of carcinoma between the two cohorts.[89]

Gynecomastia

Male breast excess or gynecomastia can be caused by a host of medical diseases and pharmacologic agents. Medical conditions associated with gynecomastia include liver dysfunction, endocrine abnormalities, Klinefelter's syndrome, renal disease, testicular tumors, adrenal or pituitary adenomas, secreting lung carcinomas, and male breast cancer. Causative pharmacologic agents include marijuana, digoxin, spironolactone, cimetidine, theophylline, diazepam, and reserpine. Although these numerous causes must be considered, a majority of patients present with either idiopathic enlargement of the breast parenchyma (more common in teenagers) or simple skin ptosis and excess adipose deposits on the chest wall (considered pseudogynecomastia; more common in adult males). To obtain a flat chest, both liposuction and/or skin excision techniques can be used.[90]

REFERENCES

Entries highlighted in bright blue are key references.

1. Wilhelmi BJ, Blackwell SJ, Phillips LG: Langer's lines: To use or not to use. *Plast Reconstr Surg* 104:208, 1999.
2. Borges AF: *Elective Incisions and Scar Revision,* vol. 1. Boston: Little, Brown, 1973, p 2.
3. Gimbel ML, Hunt TK: Wound healing and hyperbaric oxygen, in Kindwall EP, Whelan HT (eds): *Hyperbaric Medicine Practice,* 2nd ed. Flagstaff, Ariz: Best Publishing Company, 1999, p 169.
4. Kelton PL: Skin grafts and skin substitutes. *Selected Readings Plast Surg* 9:1, 1999.
5. Aston JS, Beasley RW, Thorne CHM (eds): *Grabb and Smith's Plastic Surgery,* 5th ed. Philadelphia: Lippincott–Raven Publishers, 1997.
6. McGregor IA, Morgan G: Axial and random pattern flaps. *Br J Plast Surg* 26:202, 1973.
7. Wei FC, Jain V, Suominen S, et al: Confusion among perforator flaps: What is a true perforator flap? *Br J Plast Surg* 107:874, 2001.

8. Taylor GI, Palmer JH: The vascular territories (angiosomes) of the body: Experimental study and clinical applications. *Br J Plast Surg* 40:113, 1987.

9. Ghali S, Butler PE, Tepper OM, et al: Vascular delay revisited. *Plast Reconstr Surg* 119:1735, 2007.

10. Mathes SJ, Nahai F: *Reconstructive surgery: Principles, anatomy, and technique,* 1st ed, vol. 1. New York: Churchill Livingstone, 1997.

11. Koshima I, Soeda S: Inferior epigastric artery skin flaps without rectus abdominis muscle. *Br J Plast Surg* 42:645, 1989.

12. Wei FC, Mardini S: Free-style free flaps. *Plast Reconstr Surg* 114:910, 2004.

13. Wei FC, Souminen S: Principles and techniques of microvascular surgery, in Mathes SJ (ed): *Plastic Surgery,* 2nd ed. Philadelphia: Elsevier, 2006, p 507.

14. Widmaier EP, Raff H, Strang KT: Cardiovascular physiology, in *Vander, Sherman, and Luciano's Human Physiology—the Mechanisms of Body Function,* 9th ed. New York: McGraw-Hill, 2004, p 375.

15. Chang DW, Reece GP, Wang B, et al: Effect of smoking on complications in patients undergoing free TRAM flap breast reconstruction. *Plast Reconstr Surg* 105:2374, 2000.

16. Lutz BS, Wei FC: Microsurgical workhorse flaps in head and neck reconstruction. *Clin Plast Surg* 32:421, 2005.

17. Kroll SS, Miller MJ, Reece GP, et al: Anticoagulants and hematomas in free flap surgery. *Plast Reconstr Surg* 96:643, 1995.

18. Kildal M, Wei FC, Chang YM: Free vascularized bone grafts for reconstruction of traumatic bony defects of mandible and maxilla. *World J Surg* 25:1067, 2001.

19. Kayser MR: Surgical flaps. *Selected Readings Plast Surg* 9:1, 1999.

20. Centers for Disease Control and Prevention: Improved national prevalence estimates for 18 selected major birth defects—United States, 1999–2001. *MMWR Morb Mortal Wkly Rep* 54:1301, 2006.

21. Salyer KE, Marchac A, Chang MS, et al: Unilateral cleft lip/nose repair, in Losee JE, Kirschner RE (eds): *Comprehensive Cleft Care.* New York: McGraw-Hill Professional, 2008.

22. Mulliken JB: Mulliken bilateral cleft nasolabial repair, in Losee JE, Kirschner RE (eds): *Comprehensive Cleft Care.* New York: McGraw-Hill Professional, 2008.

23. McDonald-McGinn D, Zackai EH: 22q11.2 deletion syndrome, in Losee JE, Kirschner RE (eds): *Comprehensive Cleft Care.* New York: McGraw-Hill Professional, 2008.

24. LaRossa D, Kirschner RE: Modified Furlow cleft palate repair, in Losee JE, Kirschner RE (eds): *Comprehensive Cleft Care.* New York: McGraw-Hill Professional, 2008.

25. Whitaker LA, Barlett SP: Craniofacial anomalies, in Jurkiewicz MJ, Krizek TJ, Mathes SJ, et al (eds): *Plastic Surgery: Principles and Practice,* vol. 1. St. Louis: Mosby, 1990, p 99.

26. Mulliken JB: Vascular anomalies, in Thorne CH (ed): *Grabb and Smith's Plastic Surgery,* part III. Philadelphia: Lippincott Williams & Wilkins, 2007, p 191.

27. Jenson J, Gosain A: Congenital melanocytic nevi, in Thorne CH (ed): *Grabb and Smith's Plastic Surgery,* part II. Philadelphia: Lippincott Williams & Wilkins, 2007, p 120.

28. Hollier L, Thornton J: Facial fracture I: Upper two-thirds. *Selected Readings Plast Surg* 9:1, 2002.

29. Gruss JS, Bubak PJ, Egbert MA: Craniofacial fractures: An algorithm to optimize results. *Clin Plastic Surg* 19:195, 1992.

30. Antia NH, Buch MS: Chondrocutaneous advancement flap for the marginal defect of the ear. *Plast Reconstr Surg* 39:472, 1967.

31. Anvar BA, Evans BC, Evans GR: Lip reconstruction. *Plast Reconstr Surg* 120:57e, 2007.

32. Chandler DB, Gausas RE: Lower eyelid reconstruction. *Otolaryngol Clin North Am* 38:1033, 2005.

33. Orticochea M: New three-flap reconstruction technique. *Br J Plast Surg* 24:184, 1971.

34. Tanner PB, Mobley SR: External auricular and facial prosthetics: A collaborative effort of the reconstructive surgeon and anaplastologist. *Facial Plast Surg Clin North Am* 14:137, 2006.

35. Yu P, Robb GL: Reconstruction for total and near-total glossectomy defects. *Clin Plast Surg* 32:411, 2005.

36. Wei FC, Jain V, Celik N, et al: Have we found an ideal soft-tissue flap? An experience with 672 anterolateral thigh flaps. *Plast Reconstr Surg* 109:2219, 2002.

37. Daniel R: Mandibular reconstruction with vascularized iliac crest: A 10-year experience [discussion]. *Plast Reconstr Surg* 82:802, 1988.

38. Wei FC, Chen HC, Chuang CC, et al: Fibular osteoseptocutaneous flap: Anatomic study and clinical application. *Plast Reconstr Surg* 78:191, 1986.

39. Wei FC, Santamaria E, Chang YM, et al: Mandibular reconstruction with fibular osteoseptocutaneous free flap and simultaneous placement of osseointegrated dental implants. *J Craniofac Surg* 8:512, 1997.

40. Wei FC, Seah CS, Tsai YC, et al: Fibula osteoseptocutaneous flap for reconstruction of composite mandibular defects. *Plast Reconstr Surg* 93:294, 1994.

41. Wei FC, Yazar S, Lin CH, et al: Double free flaps in head and neck reconstruction. *Clin Plast Surg* 32:303, 2005.

42. Archibald S, Young JE, Thoma A: Pharyngo-cervical esophageal reconstruction. *Clin Plast Surg* 32:339, 2005.

43. Tate JR, Tollefson TT: Advances in facial reanimation [review]. *Curr Opin Otolaryngol Head Neck Surg* 14:242, 2006.

44. Wilkins EG, Cederna PS, Lowery JC, et al: Prospective analysis of psychosocial outcomes in breast reconstruction: One-year postoperative results from the Michigan Breast Reconstruction Outcome Study. *Plast Reconstr Surg* 106:1014, 2000.

45. Alderman AK, Wilkins EG, Kim HM, et al: Complications in postmastectomy breast reconstruction: Two-year results of the Michigan Breast Reconstruction Outcome Study. *Plast Reconstr Surg* 109:2265, 2002.

46. Wilson CR, Brown IM, Weiller-Mithoff E, et al: Immediate breast reconstruction does not lead to a delay in the delivery of adjuvant chemotherapy. *Eur J Surg Oncol* 30:624, 2004.

47. Newman LA, Kuerer HM, Hunt KK, et al: Presentation, treatment, and outcome of local recurrence after skin-sparing mastectomy and immediate breast reconstruction. *Ann Surg Oncol* 5:620, 1998.

48. Munhoz AM, Montag E, Arruda EG, et al: The role of the lateral thoracodorsal fasciocutaneous flap in immediate conservative breast surgery reconstruction. *Plast Reconstr Surg* 117:1699, 2006.

49. Handel N, Cordray T, Gutierrez J, et al: A long-term study of outcomes, complications, and patient satisfaction with breast implants. *Plast Reconstr Surg* 117:757; discussion 768, 2006.

50. Nahabedian MY, Manson PN: Contour abnormalities of the abdomen after transverse rectus abdominis muscle flap breast reconstruction: A multifactorial analysis. *Plast Reconstr Surg* 109:81, 2002.

51. Mathes SJ, Nahai F: *Reconstructive Surgery: Principles, Anatomy, and Technique.* New York: Churchill Livingstone, 1997.

52. Skoracki RJ, Chang DW: Reconstruction of the chest wall and thorax. *J Surg Oncol* 94:455, 2006.

53. Rohrich RJ, Lowe JB, Hackney FL, et al: An algorithm for abdominal wall reconstruction. *Plast Reconstr Surg* 105:202, 2000.

54. Shestak KC, Edington HJ, Johnson RR: The separation of anatomic components technique for the reconstruction of massive midline abdominal wall defects: Anatomy, surgical technique, applications, and limitations revisited. *Plast Reconstr Surg* 105:731, 2000.

55. Brown DM, Sicard GA, Flye MW, et al: Closure of complex abdominal wall defects with bilateral rectus femoris flaps with fascial extensions. *Surgery* 114:112, 1993.

56. Dibbell DG, Mixter RC, Dibbell DG Sr.: Abdominal wall reconstruction (the "mutton chop" flap). *Plast Reconstr Surg* 87:60, 1991.

57. MacKenzie DJ, Seyfer AE: Reconstructive surgery: Lower extremity coverage, in Mathes SJ (ed): *Plastic Surgery,* 2nd ed. Philadelphia: Elsevier, 2006, p 1355.

58. Bosse MJ, MacKenzie EJ, Kellam JF, et al: An analysis of outcomes of reconstruction or amputation after leg-threatening injuries. *N Engl J Med* 347:1924, 2002.

59. Gustilo RB, Merkow RL, Templeman D: The management of open fractures. *J Bone Joint Surg Am* 72:299, 1990.

60. Harvey EJ, Levin LS: Reconstructive surgery: Skeletal reconstruction, in Mathes SJ (ed): *Plastic Surgery,* 2nd ed. Philadelphia: Elsevier, 2006, p 1383.

61. Crowley DJ, Kanakaris NK, Giannoudis PV: Débridement and wound closure of open fractures: The impact of the time factor on infection rates. *Injury* 38:879, 2007.

62. Tseng WS, Chen HC, Hung J, et al: "Flow-through" type free flap for revascularization and simultaneous coverage of a nearly complete amputation of the foot: Case report and literature review. *J Trauma* 48:773, 2000.

63. Lin CH, Wei FC, Lin YT, et al: Lateral circumflex femoral artery system: Warehouse for functional composite free-tissue reconstruction of the lower leg. *J Trauma* 60:1032, 2006.

64. Yazar S, Lin CH, Wei FC: One-stage reconstruction of composite bone and soft-tissue defects in traumatic lower extremities. *Plast Reconstr Surg* 114:1457, 2004.

65. Colen LB, Uroskie T: Foot reconstruction, in Mathes SJ (ed): *Plastic Surgery*, 2nd ed. Philadelphia: Elsevier, 2006, p 1403.

66. Szuba A, Rockson SG: Lymphedema: Anatomy, physiology and pathogenesis. *Vasc Med* 2:321, 1997.

67. Szuba A, Rockson SG: Lymphedema: Classification, diagnosis and therapy. *Vasc Med* 3:145, 1998.

68. Chung KC, Kim HJ, Jeffers LL: Lymphangiosarcoma (Stewart-Treves syndrome) in postmastectomy patients. *J Hand Surg [Am]* 25:1163, 2000.

69. Beahm EK, Walton RL, Lohman RF: Vascular insufficiency of the lower extremity: Lymphatic, venous, and arterial, in Mathes SJ (ed): *Plastic Surgery*, 2nd ed. Philadelphia: Elsevier, 2006, p 1455.

70. Gloviczki P: Principles of surgical treatment of chronic lymphoedema. *Int Angiol* 18:42, 1999.

71. Black J, Baharestani MM, Cuddigan J, et al: National Pressure Ulcer Advisory Panel's updated pressure ulcer staging system. *Adv Skin Wound Care* 20:269, 2007.

72. Sorensen JL, Jorgensen BJ, Gottrup F: Surgical treatment of pressure ulcers. *Am J Surg* 188:42S, 2004.

73. Hettiaratchy S, Randolph MA, Petit F, et al: Composite tissue allotransplantation—a new era in plastic surgery? *Br J Plast Surg* 57:381, 2004.

74. American Medical Association: H-475.992 definitions of "cosmetic" and "reconstructive" surgery. Chicago: American Medical Association, 2002. Available at *http://www.ama-assn.org/* [accessed January 15, 2008].

75. Paul MD: The evolution of the brow lift in aesthetic plastic surgery. *Plast Reconstr Surg* 108:1409, 2001.

76. Thorne CM, Aston SG: Aesthetic surgery of the aging face, in Aston SG, Beasley RW, Thorne CH (eds): *Grabb and Smith's Plastic Surgery*, 5th ed. Philadelphia: Lippincott–Raven Publishers, 1997, p 633.

77. Sheen JH: *Aesthetic Rhinoplasty*. St. Louis: Mosby, 1987.

78. Rubin JP, Bierman C, Rosow CE, et al: The tumescent technique for local anesthesia: The effect of high tissue pressure and dilute epinephrine on absorption of lidocaine. *Plast Reconstr Surg* 103:990, 1999.

79. Iverson RE, Lynch DJ: Practice advisory on liposuction. *Plast Reconstr Surg* 113:1478, 2004.

80. Ramirez OM: Abdominoplasty and abdominal wall rehabilitation: A comprehensive approach. *Plast Reconstr Surg* 105:425, 2000.

81. Courtiss EH, Goldwyn RM: Reduction mammaplasty by the inferior pedicle technique. *Plast Reconstr Surg* 59:64, 1977.

82. Lassus C: A 30-year experience with vertical mammaplasty. *Plast and Reconstr Surg* 97:373, 1996.

83. Lejour M: Vertical mammaplasty without inframammary scar and with breast liposuction. *Perspect Plast Surg* 4:64, 1990.

84. Tebbetts JB: A system for breast implant selection based on patient tissue characteristics and implant–soft tissue dynamics. *Plast Reconstr Surg* 109:1396, 2002.

85. Hidalgo DA: Breast augmentation: Choosing the optimal incision, implant, and pocket plane. *Plast Reconstr Surg* 105:2202, 2000.

86. *http://www.fda.gov/cdrh/breastimplants/index.html*: Breast Implants Home Page, 2006, U.S. Food and Drug Administration [accessed January 15, 2008].

87. Allergan saline-filled breast implants [package insert]. Santa Barbara, Calif: Allergan, 2007.

88. Allergan silicone-filled breast implants [package insert]. Santa Barbara, Calif: Allergan, 2007.

89. Miglioretti DL, Rutter CM, Geller BM, et al: Effect of breast augmentation on the accuracy of mammography and cancer characteristics. *JAMA* 291:442, 2004.

90. Braunstein GD: Gynecomastia. *N Engl J Med* 328:490, 1993.

CHAPTER 46

Surgical Considerations in the Elderly

Rosemarie E. Hardin and Michael E. Zenilman

GENERAL CONSIDERATIONS

The old pediatric surgery adage that children are not just "small people" holds true for the other end of the age spectrum, the growing geriatric surgery population. With the aging and expanding U.S. population, a dramatic increase is anticipated in the number of geriatric patients that will require various surgical interventions. By 2030, people >65 years of age will account for 20% of the overall population.[1] Furthermore, half of all Americans currently alive can expect to reach the ninth decade of life.[2] Elderly patients represent a unique surgical challenge due to the complexity of comorbid conditions and physiologic changes that occur with aging. These physiologic changes, inherent to the aging process, result in decline of physiologic reserve, development of cognitive and functional impairments, and, not uncommonly, development of multiple comorbid conditions. Physiologic age is of greater importance in perioperative management of elderly surgical patients than chronologic age because it takes into account the burden of comorbid disease. It is, therefore, an accurate predictor of postoperative morbidity and mortality. The hallmark of physiologic aging or "senescence" is

decreased functional reserve of critical organ systems, resulting in the decreased ability of these systems to cope with challenge, with surgical stress being a prime example. The age of 70 years typically is accepted as the start of senescence because age-related organ dysfunction and development of comorbid conditions sharply increases between ages 70 and 75 years.[3] With improved technologies and expanded criteria for surgical interventions in extremely aged patients, increased awareness of the special needs of this population is required to ensure a comprehensive preoperative assessment, delivery of optimal surgical care, and minimization of postoperative complications. Most importantly, the ability to perform an intervention must be balanced with retention of postoperative physical and cognitive function. It is, therefore, crucial to deliver quality surgical care to an elderly patient using a multidisciplinary approach involving the patient and their family, geriatric medical physician, surgeon, and at times, intensivists.

It is estimated that, by the year 2030, there will be 70 million people >65 years old, a stark increase over the 35 million in 2000.[4] This ever growing elderly population will increasingly require surgical consultation and intervention. Patients >65 years old account for approximately 60% of the current general surgeon's workload.[5] Patients >65 years old account for approximately 50% of all emergent operations and 75% of operative mortality.[4] These statistics challenge a surgeon to have an in-depth understanding of the careful perioperative evaluation required in elderly patients and the tailoring of surgical interventions based on unique changes in physiologic reserve of the patients and comorbid conditions that make elderly patients more susceptible to postoperative complications. After all, elderly patients may tolerate the surgical interventions but not the complications. Therefore, the careful perioperative assessment will lead to improved outcomes in progressively older age cohorts, thereby increasing the upper age limits of surgical candidacy.

The importance of this chapter is to highlight salient management strategies for aged surgical patients to provide optimal care and reduce postoperative complications. A particular problem in the elderly population is the potential delay in surgical treatment either from missing a diagnosis secondary to atypical presentations or postponing elective operations because of the misconception that elderly patients will suffer increased complications and poor outcomes as a result of advanced age alone. For example, elective inguinal and umbilical hernia repairs are often postponed due to age bias; these can lead to potentially devastating consequences of bowel ischemia, gangrene, and perforation, to which elderly patients respond poorly (Fig. 46-1). Emergency hernia repairs are one of the most common procedures performed in older patients. Approximately 40% of hernia repairs are performed for incarceration or bowel obstruction in patients >65 years old.[5] Emergency repair of hernias is associated with an increased morbidity rate of approximately 50% and a mortality rate ranging between 8 to 14%; a significant increase from the 2% mortality rate following elective repair.[5] One can argue that proper preoperative assessment and timely intervention would have prevented the complicated course that is marked by a need for intensive care resuscitation for intra-abdominal sepsis, a prolonged hospital course, and a requirement for physical rehabilitation secondary to progressive debilitation from prolonged immobilization. This chapter explores the physiologic changes associated with aging and the importance of the perioperative assessment and the tailored management of specific surgical diseases in this population.

PHYSIOLOGY OF AGING

Elderly surgical patients are a heterogeneous cohort with varying degrees of functional impairments and comorbid burdens. The "young old patient" may lead an active lifestyle with few, if any,

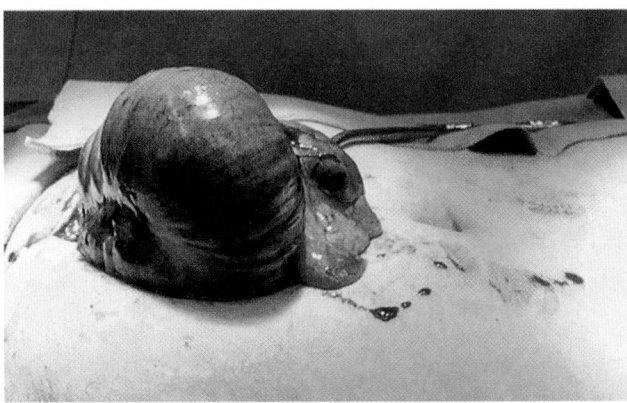

FIG. 46-1. Timely surgical intervention for a medically optimized elderly surgical candidate cannot be overemphasized. Elective procedures can be carried out safely in elderly patients avoiding the potentially devastating consequences of emergency surgery: ischemia, perforation, or death. This is an example of an umbilical hernia resulting in bowel strangulation in an elderly patient with devastating consequences. *(Courtesy of David Ford, M.D.)*

comorbid conditions. But even for this seemingly healthy group, it is crucial to remember that there are inherent physiologic changes that occur with aging and affect every organ system. These physiologic changes may become more apparent and clinically consequential with the additional stressor of major illness and operative interventions. Therefore, chronologic age is rarely an accurate predictor of morbidity and mortality from surgical interventions. It is, however, an accurate marker for declining physiologic reserve and the presence of comorbid conditions. These, in turn, place elderly patients at higher risk because of impaired cardiac, pulmonary, renal, and neurological reserves, thereby increasing the morbidity and mortality of surgical interventions. Physiologic age, in addition to comorbid conditions, more accurately predicts surgical outcomes in the elderly than chronologic age. The physiologic changes of aging are summarized in Table 46-1.

SURGERY IN THE ELDERLY

It is critical in the assessment of an elderly surgical candidate to evaluate physiologic age and to maintain a high index of suspicion

KEY POINTS

1. Emergency surgery in the elderly carries a mortality rate that is 3–4 times that seen after elective surgery.

2. Physiologic age, not chronologic age, is the consequence of diminished functional reserve due to comorbid conditions, and is the major predictor of perioperative morbidity and mortality in the elderly.

3. Impaired cardiac function is responsible for more than half of the postoperative deaths in elderly patients, so careful attention must be paid to intravascular volume status in the perioperative period.

4. In addition to cardiac impairment, deficiencies in pulmonary, renal, nutritional, and cognitive function are major factors in the development of postoperative complications in the elderly.

5. In elderly patients with acute appendicitis or acute cholecystitis, one third lack fever, one third lack an elevated white blood cell count, and one third lack physical findings of peritonitis.

6. Laparoscopic approaches to surgical management, including the use of exploratory laparoscopy to rule out surgical disease, is associated with fewer complications and more rapid recovery in the elderly.

7. Analgesic doses should be reduced and titrated carefully in the elderly to avoid delirium; meperidime (Demerol R) should not be used for pain control in elderly patients.

8. The goal of palliative care is to relieve symptoms and preserve physical and mental well-being.

TABLE 46-1	Physiologic limitations of aging, their clinical consequences, and "best practices" in the elderly surgical patient	
Age-Related Changes	**Clinical Consequences**	**Best Practices**
Body composition		
Significantly decreased muscle mass, accounting for much of decreased lean tissue mass Increased fat mass	Erosion of muscle mass during acute illness may result in strength rapidly falling below important clinical thresholds (e.g., impaired coughing, decreased mobility, increased risk of venous thrombosis) Altered volumes of drug distribution	Maintain physical function through effective pain relief, avoiding tubes, drains, and other "restraints," early mobilization, and assistance with mobilization. Minimize fasting, provide early nutritional supplementation or support (both protein-calorie and micronutrient). Adjust drug dosages for volume of distribution.
Respiratory		
Decreased vital capacity Increased closing volume Decreased airway sensitivity and clearance Decreased partial pressure of oxygen	Less effective cough Predisposition to aspiration Increased closure of small airways during tidal respiration, especially postoperatively and when supine, leading to increased atelectasis and shunting Predisposition to hypoxemia	Provide early mobilization, assumption of upright rather than supine position. Ensure effective pain relief to allow mobilization, deep breathing. Provide routine supplemental oxygen in the immediate postoperative period, and then, as needed. Minimize use of nasogastric tubes.
Cardiovascular		
Decreased maximal heart rate, cardiac output, ejection fraction Reliance on increased end-diastolic volume to increase cardiac output Slowed ventricular filling, increased reliance on atrial contribution Decreased baroreceptor sensitivity Thermoregulation Diminished sensitivity to ambient temperature and less efficient mechanisms of heat conservation, production, and dissipation Febrile responses to infection may be blunted in frail or malnourished elderly and those at extreme old age.	Greater reliance on ventricular filling and increases in stroke volume (rather than ejection fraction) to achieve increases in cardiac output Intolerant of hypovolemia Intolerant of tachycardia, dysrhythmias, including atrial fibrillation Predisposition to hypothermia (e.g., decline in body temperature during surgery is more marked unless preventive measures are taken) If there is hypothermia, shivering may result, associated with marked increases in oxygen consumption and cardiopulmonary demands. Fever may be absent despite serious infection, especially in frail elderly.	Use vigorous fluid resuscitation to achieve optimal ventricular filling. Nonvasoconstricting inotropes and afterload reduction may be more effective, if pharmacologic support is required. Use active measures to maintain normothermia during surgical procedures and to rewarm after trauma: warmed IV fluids, humidified gases, warm air. Maintaining intraoperative normothermia reduces wound infections, adverse cardiac events, and length of hospital stay. Be aware of hypothermia in trauma resuscitation.
Renal function, fluid-electrolyte homeostasis		
Decreased sensitivity to fluid, electrolyte perturbations Decreased efficiency of solute, water conservation, and excretion Decreased renal mass, renal blood flow, and glomerular filtration rate Increased renal glucose threshold	Predisposition to hypovolemia Predisposition to electrolyte disorders, (e.g., hyponatremia) Predisposition to hyperglycemia Predisposition to hyperosmolar states	Pay meticulous attention to fluid and electrolyte management. Recognize that a "normal" serum creatinine value reflects decreased creatinine clearance because muscle mass (i.e., creatinine production) is decreased concurrently. Select drugs carefully: Avoid those that may be nephrotoxic (e.g., aminoglycosides) or adversely affect renal blood flow (e.g., NSAIDs). Adjust drug dosages as appropriate for altered pharmacokinetics.

Source: Reproduced with permission from Watters JM: Surgery in the elderly. *Can J Surg* 45:106, 2002.

for surgical pathology, keeping in mind that elderly patients often present with atypical symptoms and can present with vague abdominal examinations that may effectively mask intra-abdominal catastrophe. This is worsened by coexistent medical problems and altered mentation that may be the result of organic brain disease such as dementia, drugs, infection, or dehydration. Acute appendicitis and acute cholecystitis are examples of common acute surgical pathologies with which elderly patients present late or have delayed diagnosis or misdiagnosis. This often leads to higher rates of perforation and complications that adversely affect morbidity and mortality.[6] In fact, biliary tract disease, including acute cholecystitis, is the most common indication for surgical intervention in the elderly. This is likely related to age-related changes within the biliary system, specifically increased lithogenicity of bile and increased prevalence of cholelithiasis.[7] Delayed diagnosis may lead to complications such as ascending cholangitis and gallstone ileus.

Elderly patients may not present with typical symptoms of acute abdominal pain, fever, or leukocytosis, likely secondary to depressed immune response of elderly patients. A careful assessment is crucial to timely operative intervention. In fact, in older patients presenting with acute appendicitis, the initial diagnosis is correct in less than half of the patients.[7]

Assessment of an elderly patient presenting with abdominal pain should begin with assuring stable hemodynamics and initiating appropriate resuscitation, as these patient are often profoundly dehydrated. As with most initial evaluations, airway, breathing, and circulation are initial priorities. A careful history and physical examination should follow and provide invaluable clues to the underlying disease process. The chief complaint should be elicited as well as a history of previous admissions, which may alert to recurrent diseases such as acute diverticulitis or previous operations that may draw focus to adhesive small-bowel obstruction. It is also important to obtain a detailed history regarding comorbid conditions and current medications. Initial evaluation may include electrocardiogram to rule out coronary ischemia and chest x-ray to rule out congestive heart failure (CHF) or pneumonia. Basic laboratory evaluation will help to rule out common medical etiologies for abdominal pain, such as coronary ischemia, acute pancreatitis, hepatitis, or urinary tract infections. Then careful referral for radiographic imaging will help to confirm the diagnosis and allow timely operative intervention. Regardless, the importance of a high degree of clinical suspicion cannot be overemphasized.

PREOPERATIVE ASSESSMENT

Surgical risk increases with advancing age as a consequence of physiologic decline and the development of comorbid conditions that make the elderly surgical patient more susceptible to postoperative complications. These complications are, in turn, poorly tolerated because of decreased physiologic reserve. Comorbid illness serves as the basis for the American Society of Anesthesiologists' (ASA's) physical status classification[8] (Table 46-2). This is a valuable tool for identifying elderly patients who are at high risk for postoperative complications because it is based on organ system dysfunction and severity of functional impairment. It helps to identify subgroups of patients in whom appropriate measures should be taken to reduce the risk of adverse outcomes. Importantly, it also identifies emergency surgery as a dangerous risk factor for perioperative morbidity and mortality. The physiologic changes that occur with normal aging result in increased risks associated with anesthesia and surgery, but careful assessment of potential problems in the perioperative period combined with implementation of preventative measures can significantly reduce complications associated with general anesthesia in the elderly patient.[9] Adequate control and understanding of the potential negative impact of comorbid conditions on surgical outcomes allows an appropriate preoperative evaluation that, in turn, leads to acceptable morbidity and mortality. A useful algorithm for the preoperative assessment of an elderly surgical patient is provided in Fig. 46-2.

Cardiac complications are the leading cause of perioperative complications and death in surgical patients of all age groups, but particularly among the elderly. This is because they likely have existing cardiac dysfunction, combined with normal physiologic decline and poor functional reserve. The combined effect of depletion of intravascular volume, age-related impairment of response to catecholamines, and increased myocardial relaxation time adversely affects the functioning of an elderly patient under stress in the perioperative period.[10] Aging has been demonstrated to cause a decrease in cardiac output by approximately 1% per year. Older individuals fail to augment heart rate to the same extent as younger individuals. More importantly, the ability to increase cardiac output with aging is dependent on ventricular dilatation, which is determined by preload.[11] This is precisely the reason that careful attention

must be paid to volume status in the perioperative period. Dehydration or poor resuscitation may occur in elderly surgical patients for a variety of reasons, and both are poorly tolerated. Over one half of all postoperative deaths in elderly patients and 11% of postoperative complications are a result of impaired cardiac function under physiologic stress. Incomplete emptying of the ventricle at end systole and subsequent reduction in ejection fraction is characteristic of the aging heart.[10] Reduced distensibility (i.e., preload), in addition to acute stressors, could lead to impaired coronary perfusion and cardiac ischemia.

As a result, the physiologic stress of general anesthesia and surgical interventions can unmask the limited cardiac reserve of the elderly patient. For example, poor reserve may become evident with increased myocardial oxygen demand resulting from tachycardia or loss of vascular tone from the vasodilatory effects of many general anesthetic agents.[1] Another important predictor of surgical outcomes and cardiac complications in the elderly is the presence of CHF. CHF is present in approximately 10% of patients >65 years old and is the leading cause of postoperative morbidity and mortality.[12] This number will likely rise over the next few years as percutaneous intervention and statin drugs prevent and prolong survival from acute myocardial infarction. Therefore, identifying correctable and uncorrectable cardiovascular disease is critical before elective surgical interventions. Simple steps such as maintaining proper fluid balance and limiting myocardial work will aid in minimizing complications.

Pulmonary complications are a major source of morbidity and mortality in elderly surgical patients. The result of the changes that occur with the respiratory system with aging limits the maximal breathing capacity by age 70 to 50% of the capacity present at age 30.[12] In addition, there is a decline in the forced expiratory volume in 1 second (FEV1) with advancing age. It is estimated that humans lose 35 mL of their FEV1 per year over the age of 35 years old. There is a slow decline between ages 35 and 65 years old followed by a much more progressive decline at approximately 75 years of age.[13] Pulmonary complications account for up to 50% of postoperative complications and 20% of preventable deaths.[14] Risk factors for pulmonary complications include a positive smoking history, presence of shortness of breath, or clinical evidence of chronic obstructive pulmonary disease. All elderly patients undergoing major surgical interventions should have a baseline chest radiograph. Screening spirometry can be performed to determine forced vital capacity and FEV1. A baseline arterial blood gas measurement also will help to identify hypoxemia and hypercapnia, both of which may increase postoperative complications. If abnormalities are found, perioperative use of bronchodilators and incentive spirometry may be invaluable. When possible, regional anesthetic techniques may provide excellent analgesia while helping to reduce the postoperative pulmonary complications associated with general anesthesia and endotracheal intubation.

Elderly surgical patients are also at increased risk of renal compromise in the perioperative period. Renal size and volume decrease with age, accompanied by intrarenal vascular changes. There is a decrease in the number of glomeruli and nephron mass, resulting in decreased filtration area. Subsequently, serum creatinine concentration is an insensitive indicator of renal function in the elderly.[10] The physiologic changes in renal function in elderly patients increase susceptibility to renal ischemia as well as to nephrotoxic agents. Age-related changes in renal function result from progressive glomerulosclerosis and reduction in renal mass resulting in decreased creatinine clearance and glomerular filtration rate. This is worsened by a decline in cardiac output with increasing age and subsequent decrease in renal blood flow. It has been shown that patients with impaired glomerular filtration rate are more susceptible to volume changes that occur in the perioperative period. Furthermore, decreased drug elimination can potentiate the effects of nephrotoxic drugs and prolong the sedative effects of anesthetics and narcotic used for postoperative pain management.[12] Acute renal failure is proven to dramatically increase morbidity and mortality in elderly

TABLE 46-2	American Society of Anesthesiologists' Physical Status Classification ASA Risk Stratification of Anesthetic/Surgical Risk
Class 1	Healthy patient
Class 2	Mild systemic disease
Class 3	Severe (but not incapacitating) systemic disease
Class 4	Severe systemic disease posing a constant threat to life
Class 5	Moribund with life expectancy <24 h, independent of operation
Class 6	Organ donor

Note: Suffix "e" is added to the class for emergency operations.
Source: Adapted with permission from Muravchick S: Preoperative assessment of the elderly patient. *Anesthesiol Clin North America* 18:71, 2000.

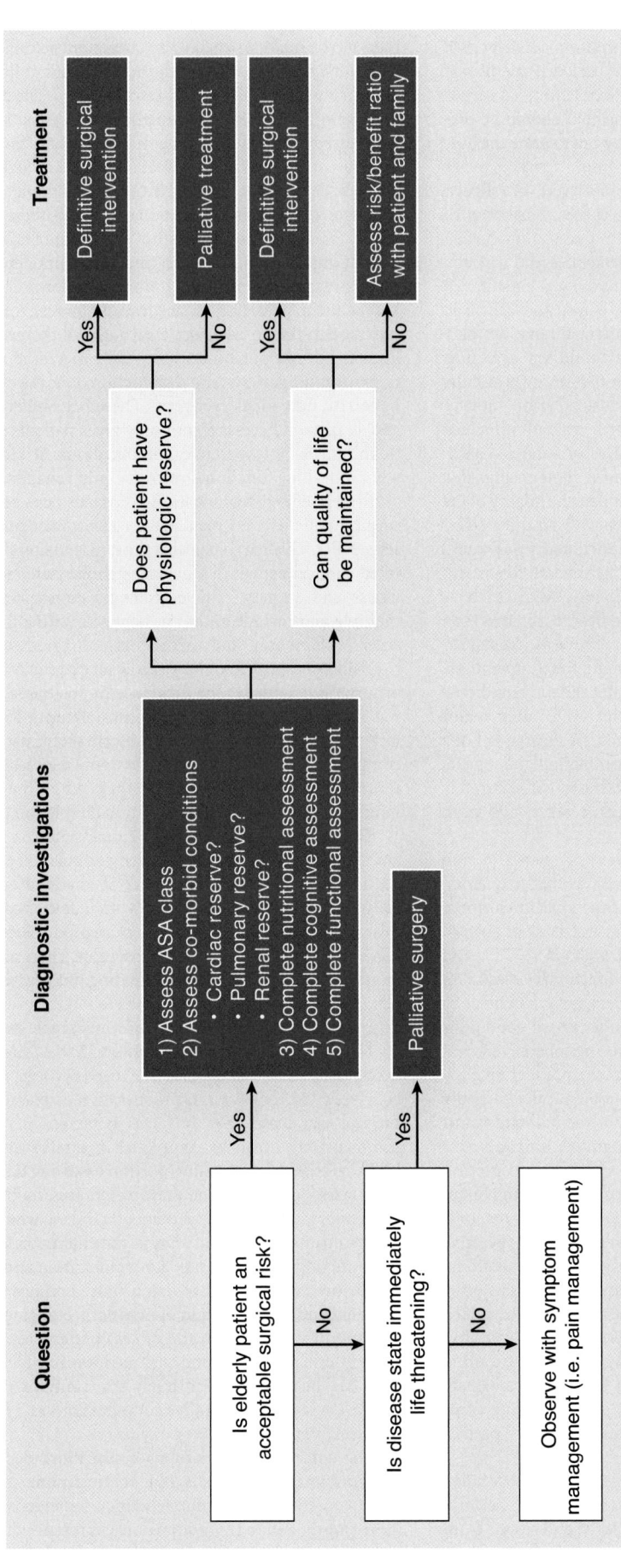

FIG. 46-2. Useful preoperative algorithm to determine elderly patient's suitability for definitive surgical intervention balancing therapeutic goals, physiologic reserve, and quality of life with palliative treatment and surgery as viable options. ASA = American Society of Anesthesiologists.

patients. The mortality of perioperative renal failure is approximately 50% and may be even higher in elderly patients. Therefore, careful management of fluid and electrolyte status is prudent to avoid imbalances and limit exposure to nephrotoxic diagnostic studies and medications in the perioperative period. Patients >70 years old may be susceptible to the nephrotoxic effects of certain drugs, including certain anesthetic agents, and thus should be protected by hydration and diuresis, as long as they can tolerate the fluid load.[10] Prompt recognition of renal compromise, marked by an elevation of blood urea nitrogen or creatinine levels, or oliguria requires aggressive correction of underlying causes. Furthermore, electrolyte imbalances can lead to potentially devastating cardiac complications, specifically, conduction abnormalities and arrhythmias.[12] Although not routinely advocated in younger patients, elderly patients should have routine electrolyte panels and urinalysis before all surgical interventions to identify potential renal dysfunction.[15] Underlying causes of abnormalities found on screening should be corrected before surgery and necessitate intravascular volume repletion to ensure adequate renal perfusion perioperatively.

It is important that a thorough preoperative evaluation include an accurate assessment of the functional status of surgical candidates as well as their cognitive level of functioning. This ensures that operative intervention will not significantly impair the quality of life of an elderly surgical candidate. The ability to withstand the stress of surgical interventions is dependent on functional reserve and ability to build an appropriate response to perioperative stress.[10] The ability to perform activities of daily living (ADL) such as feeding, dressing, bathing, and toileting have been correlated with postoperative morbidity and mortality. Preoperative functional assessment can be measured by hand grip strength, timed up and go, and functional reach tests. All of these tests independently predicted better recovery and shorter time to recover ADL after major surgery. In addition, these tests provide an accurate assessment of a patient's muscle mass, nutritional status, coordination, gait speed, balance, and mobility.[5] Proper functional assessment will accurately predict rehabilitation needs, estimate biologic reserve, and even signal complications.[10]

The functional status of an elderly patient is related to and predictive of pulmonary and cardiac complications that may ensue following surgical interventions. For example, functional impairment often leads to immobility, which can lead to increased risk of postoperative atelectasis, pneumonia, deep vein thrombosis (DVT), and pulmonary embolism. Furthermore, proper functional assessment has been shown to improve diagnostic and therapeutic outcomes as well as lead to identification of previously undiagnosed conditions that may be treatable preoperatively or managed perioperatively.[10]

Cognitive function often is overlooked in the preoperative assessment of patients, because patients are not typically formally evaluated before surgical intervention (i.e., mini-mental state examination). However, knowledge of baseline cognitive function provides invaluable information because subtle changes in cognition often herald postoperative complications, such as underlying infection. Cognitive impairment including delirium and confusion commonly occur in the elderly patient during the early postoperative period and can result in increased morbidity, delayed functional recovery, and prolonged hospitalizations. The etiology of this postoperative cognitive dysfunction may be multifactorial. Advanced age, history of alcohol abuse, baseline cognitive disturbance, hypoxia, and hypotension have all been shown to be contributing factors.[16] It is crucial that careful attention be paid to adequate postoperative analgesia to improve recovery while avoiding compromise of cognitive function. Finally, dementia is a known predictor of poor long-term survival.

Formal nutritional assessment is invaluable in the perioperative assessment of elderly patients. Poor nutritional status in elderly patients is more common than previously believed and results from the interplay between physiologic, psychosocial, and economic changes that accompany the aging process. Elderly patients may

have poor nutritional status because of either poor intake from the underlying illness or pre-existing comorbid conditions. It is estimated that approximately 9 to 15% of persons >65 years old are found to be malnourished in an outpatient setting. This increases to 12 to 50% and 25 to 60% in the acute inpatient hospital setting and chronic institutional settings, respectively.[17] The cycle of frailty that occurs with chronic undernutrition or malnutrition can lead to progressive functional decline, loss of muscle mass, and decreased oxygen consumption and metabolic rate among several other potentially debilitating consequences to this population.[17] Therefore, adequate assessment of nutritional status of these patients preoperatively and the prompt institution of nutritional support is of utmost importance. This is an integral component of the preoperative assessment, considering that nutritional status is a proven independent predictor of surgical outcomes. Allowing a patient's nutritional state to deteriorate throughout the perioperative period leads to adverse outcomes, specifically increased nosocomial infections, multiorgan system dysfunction, poor wound healing, and impaired functional recovery. Therefore, nutritional assessment and support, if necessary, not only gives patients additional reserve to minimize postoperative complications, it aids in appropriate wound healing, functional recovery, and rehabilitation.

Protein energy malnutrition (PEM) also can result from keeping surgical patients who may already have inadequate nutritional reserve NPO. This may occur in a short period in the elderly, malnourished surgical patient in a hypermetabolic state induced by stress of illness and surgery. The physiologic consequences of PEM are multiple and include anorexia, hepatic dysfunction, decreased mucosal proliferation, and sarcopenia.[17] A good marker of PEM is hypoalbuminemia , also shown to be an extremely accurate predictor of surgical outcomes. The incidence of postoperative complications was increased in patients with serum albumin levels <3.5 g/L.[17] In fact, current recommendations indicate that if patients demonstrate compromise of nutritional status as defined by >10% weight loss and serum albumin level <2.5 g/dL, they should be considered for a minimum of 7 to 10 days of nutritional repletion prior to surgery.[10]

The significant impact of nutritional status on surgical outcomes and functional recovery in the elderly population after surgical intervention underscores the importance of an accurate assessment preoperatively. In busy surgical practices, the question arises as to whether this can be done in a fairly easy, quick, reproducible, and cost-effective manner while obtaining vital information. There are several methods of assessing nutritional status including anthropomorphic measures (i.e., body mass index), biochemical laboratory values (i.e., transferring, albumin and prealbumin), and clinical assessments.[17]

The Mini Nutritional Assessment (MNA) is a validated nutritional assessment tool that has been used for several years, which can be a valuable tool for the preoperative assessment of the elderly surgical candidate. The MNA is depicted in Fig. 46-3, and as demonstrated, it can be completed in a relatively short time. The MNA consists of a screening portion assessing the patient's current body mass index, food intake and weight loss, mobility, and presence of stressors, depression, or dementia, all of which can exacerbate undernutrition or malnutrition in the elderly patient. This is aimed at identifying patients at risk for malnutrition and subsequent need for further evaluation involving a more complete psychosocial assessment and determination of mode of feedings, as well as objective measurements of midarm and calf circumferences. This tool helps to identify undernutrition and malnutrition in older individuals, >65 years old, helping to direct timely interventions. This, in turn, may help to decrease postoperative complications and result in improved functional recovery in these patients.

The combined effects of poor nutrition, decreased cognition, and immune impairments due to nutritional or pharmacologic factors create a treacherous tendency for elderly patients to have more poorly defined symptoms or to present with more advanced disease. In acute abdominal conditions, such as acute appendicitis and acute cholecystitis, one third of elderly patients will lack an

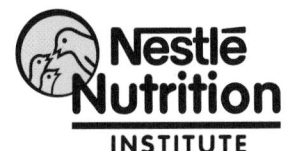

Mini Nutritional Assessment
MNA®

Last name:	First name:	Sex:	Date:

Age:	Weight, kg:	Height, cm:	I.D. Number:

Complete the screen by filling in the boxes with the appropriate numbers.
Add the numbers for the screen. If score is 11 or less, continue with the assessment to gain a malnutrition indicator score.

Screening

A Has food intake declined over the past 3 months due to loss of appetite, digestive problems, chewing or swallowing difficulties?
0 = severe loss of appetite
1 = moderate loss of appetite
2 = no loss of appetite

B Weight loss during the last 3 months
0 = weight loss greater than 3 kg (6.6 lbs)
1 = does not know
2 = weight loss between 1 and 3 kg (2.2 and 6.6 lbs)
3 = no weight loss

C Mobility
0 = bed or chair bound
1 = able to get out of bed/chair but does not go out
2 = goes out

D Has suffered psychological stress or acute disease in the past 3 months
0 = yes   2 = no

E Neuropsychological problems
0 = severe dementia or depression
1 = mild dementia
2 = no psychological problems

F Body Mass Index (BMI) (weight in kg) / (height in m²)
0 = BMI less than 19
1 = BMI 19 to less than 21
2 = BMI 21 to less than 23
3 = BMI 23 or greater

Screening score (subtotal max. 14 points)
12 points or greater Normal – not at risk – no need to complete assessment
11 points or below Possible malnutrition – continue assessment

Assessment

G Lives independently (not in a nursing home or hospital)
0 = no   1 = yes

H Takes more than 3 prescription drugs per day
0 = yes   1 = no

I Pressure sores or skin ulcers
0 = yes   1 = no

J How many full meals does the patient eat daily?
0 = 1 meal
1 = 2 meals
2 = 3 meals

K Selected consumption markers for protein intake
• At least one serving of dairy products
   (milk, cheese, yogurt) per day   yes ☐   no ☐
• Two or more servings of legumes
   or eggs per week   yes ☐   no ☐
• Meat, fish or poultry every day   yes ☐   no ☐
0.0 = if 0 or 1 yes
0.5 = if 2 yes
1.0 = if 3 yes

L Consumes two or more servings
of fruits or vegetables per day?
0 = no   1 = yes

M How much fluid (water, juice, coffee, tea, milk…)
is consumed per day?
0.0 = less than 3 cups
0.5 = 3 to 5 cups
1.0 = more than 5 cups

N Mode of feeding
0 = unable to eat without assistance
1 = self-fed with some difficulty
2 = self-fed without any problem

O Self view of nutritional status
0 = views self as being malnourished
1 = is uncertain of nutritional state
2 = views self as having no nutritional problem

P In comparison with other people of the same age,
how does the patient consider his/her health status?
0.0 = not as good
0.5 = does not know
1.0 = as good
2.0 = better

Q Mid-arm circumference (MAC) in cm
0.0 = MAC less than 21
0.5 = MAC 21 to 22
1.0 = MAC 22 or greater

R Calf circumference (CC) in cm
0 = CC less than 31   1 = CC 31 or greater

Assessment (max. 16 points)	
Screening score	
Total assessment (max. 30 points)	

Malnutrition indicator score
17 to 23.5 points   at risk of malnutrition
Less than 17 points   malnourished

Ref. Vellas B, Villars H, Abellan G, et al. Overview of the MNA® - Its History and Challenges. J Nutr Health Aging 2006;10:456-465.
Rubenstein LZ, Harker JO, Salva A, Guigoz Y, Vellas B. Screening for Undernutrition in Geriatric Practice: Developing the Short-Form Mini Nutritional Assessment (MNA-SF). J. Geront 2001;56A: M366-377.
Guigoz Y. The Mini-Nutritional Assessment (MNA®) Review of the Literature - What does it tell us? J Nutr Health Aging 2006;10:466-487.

© Nestlé, 1994, Revision 2006. N67200 12/99 10M
For more information : www.mna-elderly.com

FIG. 46-3. A reproduction of the validated Mini Nutritional Assessment, a quick and easy, validated assessment tool that is invaluable for the accurate nutritional assessment of the elderly surgical candidate. *(Reproduced with permission from Nestle USA, Inc.)*

elevated white blood cell count, one third will lack fever, and one third will lack physical findings of localized peritonitis. These deficits contribute to a threefold higher rate of perforated appendicitis and gangrene of the gallbladder in elderly patients compared to young patients. An "unimpressive" physical exam in an elderly patient with acute onset of abdominal symptoms should never be taken as a sign of the absence of surgical disease.

SPECIFIC CONSIDERATIONS

Cardiovascular

It is estimated that approximately 40% of the projected 25 million octogenarians comprising the U.S. population by the year 2025 will have serious cardiovascular symptoms.[18] With the aging of the population, undoubtedly, many patients will require cardiovascular surgical interventions. With advances in cardiopulmonary bypass technique, myocardial protection, and improved perioperative care, coronary artery bypass grafting (CABG) and valve replacement operations can be safely performed in elderly patients. Senile calcific aortic stenosis is common within this population, and referral for aortic valve replacement is increasing, encompassing many patients who are extremely aged, >75 years old (Fig. 46-4). Interestingly, despite some degree of age bias in referral patterns for elderly patients to undergo major cardiac surgery, advanced age alone is not a predictor of poorer outcomes or increased mortality when compared to younger patients. It has been demonstrated that emergency operations, preoperative New York Heart Association (NYHA) functional class 3 or greater, and chronic renal failure were the main predictors of increased operative mortality.[18] In one study, preoperative renal dysfunction, cerebrovascular disease, valve surgery, and catastrophic state were independent predictors of increased mortality in elderly patients.[19] Elderly patients with nondialysis-dependent renal dysfunction had a 60% chance of death during a 5-year follow-up period compared to 25% in elderly patients without a history of renal dysfunction. Similarly, the presence of cerebrovascular disease resulted in a twofold increase in mortality among elderly patients.[19] Even patients who were 80 years of age or more did not have any significant increase in surgical risk and within this population, the 4-year actuarial survival was 70.5% with an event-free survival of approximately 60.6%.[19]

There has been a significant trend in providing definitive operative intervention to elderly patients requiring CABG. Although older patients have higher morbidity and mortality rates after cardiac surgery than do younger patients, these rates are significantly decreasing. The Society of Thoracic Surgeons reports perioperative mortality rates ranging from 1.6% in patients 51 to 60 years of age to 7.7% in those 81 to 90 years of age.[20] This decline in morbidity and mortality rates likely reflects better preoperative assessment and patient selection. Furthermore, this decline has occurred despite the advancing age of cardiac patients at time of referral, advanced disease, and greater comorbid disease burden. Elderly patients are more likely to have significant triple-vessel disease accompanied by poor ejection fraction, left ventricular hypertrophy, significant valvular disease, and previous history of myocardial infarction than are younger patients.[20] Elderly patients also are more likely to be classified as NYHA functional class 3 or higher and are more likely to present on an emergent basis, in part because of reluctance to provide elective intervention in these patients because of presumptive poorer outcome. Despite the increased risk of morbidity and mortality compared to younger patients, elderly patients, including those >80 years old, can undergo CABG with acceptable mortality risk. The overall mortality rate is approximately 7 to 12% for elderly patients, including those CABGs performed under emergency conditions. This figure decreases to approximately 2.8% when CABG is performed electively with careful preoperative evaluation.[21]

Valve Replacement

There also is an increasing percentage of the geriatric population presenting with symptomatic valvular disease requiring intervention. The most common valvular abnormality present in elderly patients is calcific aortic stenosis, which can lead to angina and syncope.[22] The operative mortality from aortic valve replacement is estimated to be between 3 and 10%, with an average of approximately 7.7%.[20] If aortic stenosis is allowed to progress without operative intervention, CHF will ensue. The average survival of these patients is approximately 1.5 to 2 years. If a patient is a candidate for operative intervention, age should not be a deterrent, especially considering the potential to increase life expectancy. It has been recommended that the minimally symptomatic octogenarian with aortic stenosis should be considered a low-risk patient and expected to experience an uneventful operative course and expedient recovery, especially with carefully selected patients. More importantly, if these elective procedures are delayed until symptoms or left ventricular dysfunction develop, patients may suffer from unnecessary increased operative risk and mortality.[18] Furthermore, there is a demonstrable improvement in quality of life in these patients, with many improving their NYHA functional classification.

Elderly patients require surgery for mitral valve disease when ischemic regurgitation is present. Surgery for mitral valve disease carries a higher morbidity and mortality than for aortic intervention, with an estimated mortality rate as high as 20%.[20] Left ventricular function usually is compromised in patients requiring intervention, leading to a poorer outcome in these patients. The surgical outcome for mitral valve procedures depends on the extent of the disease, age of the patient, presence of pulmonary hypertension, and extent of coronary artery disease. The presence of comorbid conditions combined with the emergent nature of surgery in a large percentage of elderly patients further worsens the outcome. Therefore, a decision regarding management of mitral valve disease should be individualized to each patient with the above factors considered. Another concern regarding elderly patients who require surgery for valve disease is the additional requirement for coronary revascularization. This increases the morbidity and mortality from surgical intervention. An elderly patient with many comorbid conditions in need of a combined procedure should only have critically stenosed vessels bypassed.[22] Therefore, advanced age is not a contraindication to performing combined procedures; however, a higher mortality rate should be expected. Neurologic complications from valve surgery are particularly common in elderly patients. It has been estimated that approximately 30% of patients >70 years old who undergo valve

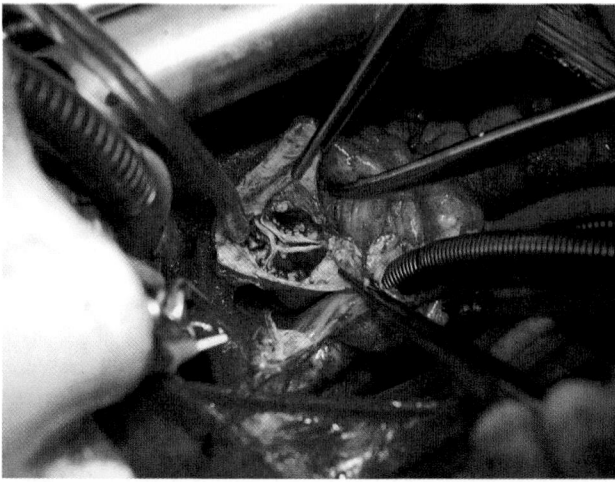

FIG. 46-4. Intraoperative photograph of aortic annulus of an elderly patient with moderate aortic calcific stenosis as seen during replacement with a prosthetic aortic valve. Calcific deposits are readily apparent. *(Courtesy of Robert Lowery, M.D.)*

procedures develop either transient or permanent neurologic dysfunction.[22] This often is a result of embolism from debris dislodged from the valve during the procedure or from a formed thrombus in the right atrium.

An important consideration in valve replacement procedures in elderly patients is the type of prosthesis to be used. Elderly patients are at increased risk from bleeding-associated anticoagulation complications. This is especially significant in patients who have experienced falls and minor trauma that have resulted in significant intracranial hemorrhage. To avoid the lifelong requirement for anticoagulants, bioprosthetic valves should be used in place of mechanical valves whenever possible.[22] Although the bioprosthetic valves are not as durable as mechanical valves, studies demonstrate excellent structural integrity 10 years postprocedure, making it an appropriate choice in an elderly patient.

Kidney Transplantation

The number of patients requiring treatment for end-stage renal disease (ESRD) continues to dramatically increase, with a disproportionate increase in older ESRD patients. In 2000, more than 51% of hemodialysis patients in the United States were ≥65 years old.[23] Although there is currently no age limitation for access to transplantation within the United States, there has been a hesitancy to transplant kidneys from older donors as well as to transplant scarce organs to elderly patients for fear of increased graft loss. Therefore, there have been limited data on short- and long-term outcomes of renal transplantation in elderly patients until recently.

Successful kidney transplantation is preferred treatment for ESRD and long-term patient survival is higher in elderly patients who have been transplanted compared to those that remain on hemodialysis. The projected life span for patients currently on the transplant waiting list who are age 60 to 74 years old is approximately 6 years. This increases to 10 years posttransplantation.[23] For comparison, the expected life span of a 70-year-old patient in the general population is 13.4 years. Kidney transplantation affords all patients, including those in the elderly cohorts, improved quality of life with greater longevity without a significant difference in overall patient morbidity, mortality, or graft survival. Among dialysis patients ages 70 years and older, renal transplantation was associated with a 41% lower risk of death compared to age matched wait-listed patients. A clear survival advantage also has been demonstrated in carefully selected patients 75 years and older. A benefit is observed among patients whose life expectancy is expected to exceed 1.8 years.[24] Although the literature on long-term outcomes is still inconclusive, it has been demonstrated that there is no statistically significant difference in short-term outcomes, specifically, primary nonfunction, delayed graft function, inhospital mortality, and length of stay, among elderly patients undergoing renal transplantation.[23]

In the last decade, there has been a shift favoring the transplantation of kidneys from older donors as well as transplantation of donor grafts to older recipients. A new strategy is the use of "extended criteria donors" (ECDs) for elderly recipients, using dual kidney transplantation to increase the net total nephron mass, resulting in favorable outcomes. One such patient was a 70-year-old male who received a dual ECD renal transplant with return of creatine to normal levels shortly after surgery (Fig. 46-5). There has been a progressive increase in the use of ECD kidneys, which accounted for 16% of all transplants from deceased donors in 2003; approximately 33% of these organs were used for transplantation in elderly recipients. The adoption of dual kidney donation from elderly patients with depressed renal function expanded the donor population to patients >75 years of age, >15% of whom demonstrated evidence of glomerulosclerosis.[25] The increased nephron mass achieved with dual kidney transplantation compensated for the possible decreased renal function with advancing age. The net result is that recipients demonstrate similar postoperative graft function when compared to single kidney transplantation. Elderly recipients of ECD kidneys

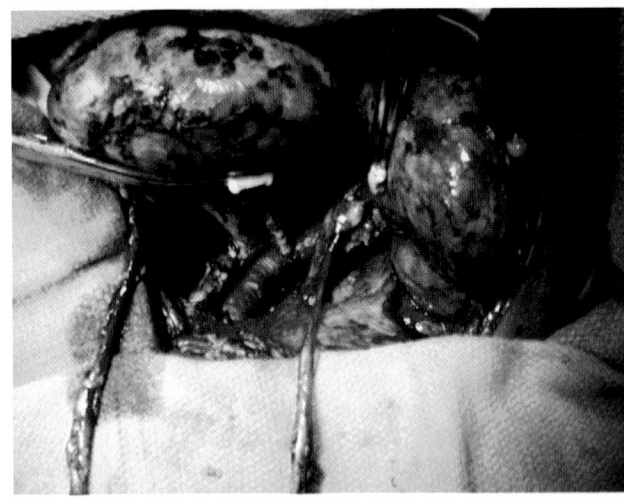

FIG. 46-5. Intraoperative photograph of dual extended criteria donor renal transplant in an elderly patient who subsequently had return of creatinine levels to normal shortly after surgery. (*Courtesy of Dale Distant, M.D.*)

demonstrated a 25% decrease in risk of mortality compared to wait-listed patients on hemodialysis.[24]

Elderly patients have better graft function, with decreased incidence of delayed graft function and fewer episodes of acute rejection, than do younger patients. This may be the result of decreased immune competence with aging. With the lower occurrence of both acute and chronic rejection in elderly patients, it has been suggested that elderly patients would benefit from lower doses of immunosuppressive agents. However, this decreased competence is balanced by the increased incidence of infections from viruses such as herpes zoster, cytomegalovirus and Epstein-Barr, as well as posttransplant neoplasia, including lymphoproliferative disorders.

Interestingly, graft loss in the elderly population is mostly attributable to the patient's death, primarily secondary to cardiovascular disease. Pre-existing cardiovascular disease may be worsened by the use of corticosteroids and calcineurin inhibitors, both of which are essential to the antirejection regimen posttransplantation. It must be kept in mind, however, that age-related mortality due to cardiovascular disease is double for patients on the transplant list compared to those who receive a transplant. Other main causes of patient death posttransplantation with graft survival are infection and malignancy. The decreased immune competence with advanced age combined with powerful immunosuppressive drugs places the elderly patient at greater susceptibility to infection and increased risk of morbidity and mortality. However, modification of current immunosuppression regimens may lead to a decrease in infection complications among elderly patients.[23] Careful preoperative assessment for these conditions minimizes postoperative complications and graft loss in this population.

Cancer

The incidence of most cancers is age dependent, and the exponentially expanding aged population is rapidly increasing the number of elderly patients requiring multimodal therapy for various oncologic diseases, primarily lung, breast, pancreas, esophagus, stomach, and colorectal malignancies. Approximately 50% of cancer diagnoses are currently made in patients aged 70 years or older.[10] According to predicted estimations, the increase in the elderly population will account for up to a 51% increase in the number of patients undergoing oncologic procedures by the year 2020.[1] The increased life expectancy of the geriatric patient coupled with the increasing incidence of cancer with advancing age will most definitely lead to an increased prevalence of malignant disease amendable to surgical intervention within this population. This is an area of great interest given that randomized clinical trials to determine the outcomes of elderly patient undergoing curative resections as well as neoadjuvant and adjuvant chemotherapy and radiation are lacking. In addition, rarely are elderly patients included in clinical trials; therefore, treatment decisions often are based on surgeon experience that may be flawed with inherent biases regarding the outcome of complete oncologic resections in elderly patients. Given the sparse outcomes data, many surgeons also may be reluctant to expose older patients to the toxic effects of chemotherapy and radiation without proven efficacy in this geriatric population. This highlights the need for research targeting the specific needs of elderly patients with malignancy to aid in the development of specific treatment guidelines for various cancers within this age cohort. In fact, the oncogeriatric population may be undertreated for malignant diseases and not receive curative resections as well as neoadjuvant and adjuvant therapies afforded to younger patients.[11] Potential reasons include poorer functional status compared to younger patients, patient and family preference, age bias, life expectancy, and concerns regarding quality of life after major operative interventions.[26] Surgeons will be challenged to decide whether major surgery is justified in elderly patients, especially those with limited life expectancy. Effectiveness of oncologic surgery in elderly patients depends on whether a cure can be achieved safely without compromise to functional status or quality of life. Postoperative life expectancy should be improved by surgery, or, at the very least, not diminished. A useful treatment algorithm is

provided in Fig. 46-6. A study undertaken using the Surveillance, Epidemiology and End Results database assessing cancer-directed surgery (CDS) for localized disease for solid malignancies found that the rates of CDS declined with increasing age for all cancers, especially noted for the aged elderly >70 years old. In addition, CDS was less likely to occur with patients found to have lung, esophagus, stomach, liver, or pancreatic cancer.[1] A careful assessment of the general and cancer-related condition of the patient is crucial to planning the best surgical intervention and postoperative adjuvant therapy.

Formulating a comprehensive, multimodal treatment plan for an elderly patient with a malignancy amendable to surgical intervention is based on careful consideration of the patient's expected life span, specifically if the life span is expected to exceed survival from the malignancy. Additionally, considerations include the patient's ability to tolerate the surgery and any complications that may ensue, as well as the likelihood that the patient would suffer a complication from the cancer which would adversely impact quality of life.[27] There is an ongoing international study that is titled "Preoperative Assessment of Cancer in the Elderly (PACE)" that is attempting to determine a scoring system that aids in assessing the oncogeriatric patient for surgical intervention. The PACE study incorporates several validated instruments that assess the functional and physiologic status of patients including the Mini Mental State Examination, ADL, Geriatric Depression Scale, and the ASA classification among other useful instruments. Interestingly, the PACE assessment also includes The

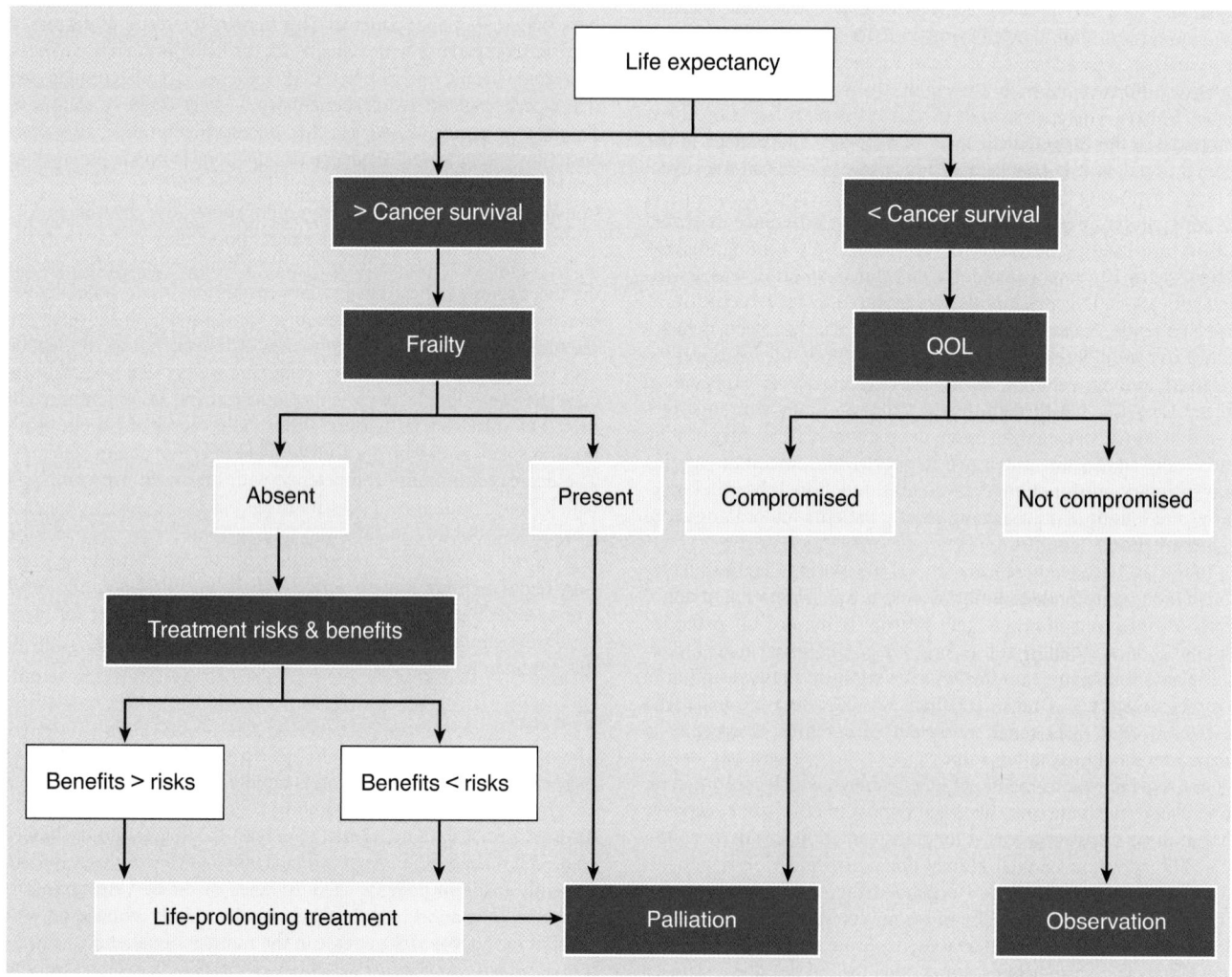

FIG. 46-6. A useful treatment algorithm to illustrate the effectiveness of oncologic surgery depends on the balance between achieving cure and maintaining functional quality of life (QOL). *(Reproduced with permission from Balducci L, Beghe C: Cancer Control: Journal of the Moffitt Cancer Center 6:466, 1999.)*

Physiological and Operative Severity Score for enumeration of Mortality and Morbidity, which has been shown to predict morbidity and postoperative mortality in general surgery and in patients with lung and colorectal malignancy. This score factors in the age of the patient and gives consideration to operative factors, including the type of surgical procedure used, the presence and extent of malignancy, and the timing of the operation (i.e., planned elective procedure or an emergency intervention).[10] Palliative interventions are a part of the therapeutic armamentarium; however, a surgeon must weigh these variables carefully to determine if surgical intervention is appropriate.

Breast

It is projected that there will be a 72% increase in the number of elderly women diagnosed with breast cancer in the United States by 2025. Furthermore, 50% of breast cancers occur after the age of 65 years old and 25% after the age of 75 years old.[28] The estimated risk for development of new breast cancer is one in 14 women aged 60 to 79 years old compared to one in 24 in women aged 40 to 59 years old.[28] Mortality rates following breast cancer surgery in elderly women is <1%, and therefore, surgical interventions remain the cornerstone of therapy for breast cancer in elderly women. However, as expected, the presence of comorbid conditions affects clinical outcomes in elderly patients with breast cancer. A recent study demonstrated the presence of comorbid conditions in patients with breast cancer rose to as high as 55% in patients >80 years of age, with cardiovascular disease, diabetes, and previous cancer being most common.[29] As expected, the resulting 5-year survival rate was lower in patients with two or more comorbid conditions.

A recent study on risk factors for breast cancer in patients >75 years of age showed similarity to younger women and included obesity, nulliparity, family history, and advanced age at menopause.[30] Interestingly, although breast cancer presentation in elderly patients may be diagnosed at more advanced stages, both clinical and pathologic data demonstrate less aggressive disease in elderly women with more favorable biologic characteristics. Elderly breast cancer patients are more likely to have estrogen-positive tumors and increasing endocrine responsiveness.[30] Large percentages of elderly women are not offered conventional therapies for breast cancer, and the management of the axilla is frequently omitted. For example, elderly patients who are offered breast conservation surgery for breast cancer are less likely to have axillary dissection, postoperative radiation, and chemotherapy. This will undoubtedly influence surgical outcomes in elderly patients with breast cancer considering that local recurrence rates after conservative surgery without radiotherapy are reported from as low as 3% to as high as 47%. Advancing age has been demonstrated to be an independent predictor of concordance with treatment guidelines for definitive surgical therapy and adjuvant chemotherapy, as well as hormonal therapy. A study demonstrated that the odds of receiving a recommendation for chemotherapy decreased by 22% for each year of advancing patient age.[26] The concept of nonsurgical management of breast cancer in elderly patients is falling out of favor because there is currently no rationale for denying surgical therapy for elderly breast cancer patients. Surgery and hormonal therapy were the best options for overall survival, breast cancer–specific survival, and disease-free survival. A Cochrane Review concluded that treatment with tamoxifen alone is not the best option because of higher local progression of disease; 81% compared to 38% with surgical intervention. Furthermore, the response rate only lasts for approximately 18 to 24 months.[26] The final conclusion is that surgery remains the standard of care for elderly patients with breast cancer. Alternative therapies should be reserved for patients who have multiple comorbid conditions leading to poor candidacy for operative intervention, those who are frail, or those who refuse surgery.

A timely study comparing the mortality after breast-conserving surgery (BCS) alone, BCS plus radiation therapy, mastectomy, and the receipt of adjuvant tamoxifen in elderly breast cancer patients determined less than standard treatment for these patients resulted in increased mortality. Elderly women receiving BCS without radiotherapy have more than twice the rate of breast cancer mortality compared to women undergoing mastectomy. In addition, in older women with estrogen receptor and progesterone receptor positive tumors receiving tamoxifen, the rate of breast cancer death increased substantially with the decreasing duration of tamoxifen use.[31] The standard of treatment for elderly patients with breast cancer should be the same as younger patients; BCS plus radiotherapy when indicated. If patients decline postoperative radiotherapy or are medically unfit for radiotherapy, mastectomy should be performed. Furthermore, elderly patients with tumor size <2 to 3 cm and no clinical evidence of axillary involvement should be offered sentinel node biopsy.[32]

One of the most interesting controversies surrounding breast cancer in elderly women is the appropriate age limits of screening. A retrospective study demonstrated a decline in cancer-related mortality among women who underwent regular screening mammography up to 75 years of age.[30] Women who underwent at least two mammographic examinations between the ages of 70 to 79 years experienced a two-and-one-half–fold reduction in breast cancer mortality compared to elderly women who did not undergo screening.[26] Current recommendations are to offer yearly mammography to women up to age 75, which should be continued after age 75 in women without severe comorbid conditions. In women with multiple comorbidities, the decision to perform screening should be based on estimated life expectancy. Screening benefits depend on life expectancy. People with <5 to 10 years of life expectancy are unlikely to benefit from screening. The American Geriatric Society recommends that screening should be individualized rather than set by age-specific guidelines. The current recommendation is that no upper age limit for screening be set as long as the estimated life expectancy is 4 or more years.

Colorectal

The incidence of colorectal cancer (CRC) increases with advancing age, similar to most other malignant conditions. Approximately 90% of cases of CRC are diagnosed in patients >55 years old.[33] Of concern is the increased postoperative morbidity and mortality following extensive surgical resections in elderly patients, with a significant increase in patients >70 years old. In fact, inhospital mortality for patients >85 years old undergoing surgery for colorectal malignancy is estimated to be ninefold greater than for younger patients.[33] Furthermore, elderly patients often have decreased cancer-specific survival when compared to younger patients. It has been proven that the 5-year cancer-specific survival for CRC is similar among the age cohorts. Therefore, age is not an independent factor accounting for the decreased survival among elderly patients. It is rather a consequence of comorbid conditions and impaired physical capacity necessary for recovery from perioperative physiological stress.[33] This leads to bias regarding poorer outcomes in elderly patients. For this reason, many elderly patients are receiving suboptimal cancer therapy and limited resections resulting in decreased survival rates and poorer outcomes. With the ever aging population, this must be addressed and clinical modifications implemented to improve outcomes of elderly patients undergoing surgical interventions for colorectal malignancies. Elderly patients should have continued, aggressive screening for colorectal malignancy and strict adherence to accepted surgical and adjuvant treatment guidelines.

One of the most important aspects to delivering appropriate care to elderly patients with CRC is to consider the patient's wishes as well as expectations from the surgical intervention. In this respect, functional outcomes and quality of life take precedence in treating elderly patients, especially the aged elderly. Of patients >75 years old who underwent elective surgery, few demonstrated protracted decline in ADL and most experienced significant improvement in quality of life.[34] Approximately 10% of elderly patients >80 years old have protracted postoperative disability. Estimation of physical ability and surgical stress is useful for predicting decline in ADL and postoperative disability. It has been shown that, in patients <80 years of age, a complete resection for cure is most important, whereas in patients >80 years old, avoidance of a stoma becomes paramount. These are important considerations for the geriatric surgeon.[33]

A prospective study was recently undertaken to specifically evaluate the epidemiology and risk of surgical intervention for CRC in elderly patients. A large cohort of 47,455 patients was divided based on age <75 years old and >75 years old.[33] It was determined that a significant portion of elderly CRC patients are female, with multiple comorbidities leading to advanced ASA levels of 3 and above. The study determined that elderly patients underwent surgical interventions less often than younger patients (81% vs. 88% respectively, P <.001), more frequently required urgent or emergency operations, and were more likely to have operative procedures in which the primary cancer was not resected. Obstructive tumors are significantly more common in patients >70 years old, and elderly patients are still presenting far too commonly with surgical emergencies resulting from obstruction and perforation in up to 40% of the cases.[11] In addition, elderly patients had higher postoperative mortality than younger patients (10.6% vs. 3.8%, respectively). Right-sided resections, Hartmann's procedures, transanal endoscopic microsurgery, and transanal resection of tumors were more common in elderly patients, whereas formal resections, including low anterior and abdominoperineal resections, were more common in younger patients.[33] Elderly patients are less likely to undergo CDS; with each half a decade increase in age >70 years old, the odds of receiving cancer-directed surgery were reduced by 44%. Interestingly, many of these patients presented with lower-stage Duke classification lesions. However, this was not secondary to earlier presentations as one might assume, but rather secondary to understaging from surgical treatment. Accurate staging may not be possible with local resections, limiting the number of lymph nodes available for proper staging.[35] Elderly patients also are less likely to undergo preoperative irradiation and neoadjuvant chemotherapy, reducing the likelihood of curative resection.[33]

Liver resection for CRC liver metastases in properly selected elderly patients 70 years of age or greater is feasible with older patients having similar operative survival to younger patients. Palliative surgery remains a viable option for elderly patients with disseminated CRC and should be aimed at the reduction of symptoms such as pain, obstruction, or hemorrhage. Bowel obstruction can be relieved with intestinal bypass or a diverting colostomy. The most common site of disseminated disease is the liver, and uncontrolled liver metastases are responsible for pain, abdominal distention, jaundice, and inferior vena caval obstruction. Elderly patients with metastatic disease who are not candidates for curative resection may be considered for ablation of the lesions by local destruction, cryotherapy, or radiofrequency ablation. More traditional means such as chemotherapy, which can be administered via the hepatic artery or radiation, also may be used.[36]

Similar to breast cancer, an upper age limit for CRC has not been clearly established. Screening for CRC may not lead to an observed survival benefit until 5 years or longer after screening had occurred. This would limit the benefit of screening in aged populations with limited life expectancy. An interesting way of looking at this controversy is from a recent study that determined that the number of screening colonoscopies needed to prevent one CRC-related death (NNS) increased as with increasing age and comorbidities. For example, in healthy men and women aged 75 to 79 years old, the NNS was 50. The corresponding NNS in patients 90 years and older was 279 in women and 482 in men.[37] Consideration for continued screening in very elderly patients should take into account age and predicted life expectancy, comorbid burden, expected duration of the protective effect of screening, risk for cancer, results of previous screening colonoscopies, and patient preference.[37]

Lung

Lung cancer is the leading cause of cancer-related deaths in the United States for patients >70 years old. National Cancer Institute statistics show that the peak incidence of lung cancer is between 75 and 79 years of age. Elderly lung cancer patients also have a higher mortality rate, and therefore, the peak mortality rate is between ages 75 and 84 years.[38] Non–small cell lung cancer accounts for roughly 80% of all lung cancer cases, and >50% of these patients are >65 years of age. Interestingly, approximately 30% of these patients are 70 years or older at diagnosis.[39] Lung cancer is highly prevalent among elderly patients, so much so that a 2-cm, asymptomatic, solitary pulmonary nodule in a 70-year-old male smoker has a >70% chance of being an occult lung cancer.[2] Squamous cell carcinomas are more common among elderly patients than among younger patients, and these tumors are associated with a higher incidence of local disease, tend to have lower recurrence rates, and have longer survival times than nonsquamous cancers.[38] In cases of resectable primary lung cancer, surgery remains the treatment of choice independent of age.[11]

The estimated life expectancy of untreated lung cancer is approximately 9 months. This can increase to as high as 18 months with palliative chemotherapy and radiation. However, the life expectancy of an elderly patient who has undergone a successful operative resection is estimated to be as high as 31 months, making this the preferred option when feasible.[13] However, despite this and the fact that more elderly patients present with stage I disease, elderly patients are offered curative surgery less frequently than younger counterparts. The same holds true for chemotherapy and radiation.

Advanced age is an independent risk factor for death after thoracotomy, with significantly increased mortality after age 65. These reasons are multifactorial partly due to the physiologic debilitation that occurs with division of the intrathoracic muscles that aid in respiratory function and the loss of lung volume after resections.[13] One study demonstrated that patients 70 years of age or older who underwent thoracotomy for lung cancer had an operative mortality rate of 14%, which is directly related to the extent of the pulmonary resection. In one of the largest prospective, multi-institutional trials conducted, The Lung Cancer Study Group, increasing age led to a significant increase in 30-day mortality for patients undergoing thoracotomy and lung resection.[13] They found overall mortality to be approximately 3.5% in patients <65 years old, which rose to 7.3% for patients 70 years or older and as high as 8.1% for octogenarians. However, with improved surgical options, including minimally invasive video-assisted thoracic surgery (VATS) in the past decade, the mortality rate has ranged from 3% to 5% in carefully selected patients.[2] In a recent study conducted to determine if VATS resulted in lower morbidity in the elderly population in comparison to open, rib-spreading thoracotomy, the overall morbidity for minimally invasive surgery was 28%; this increased to 45% with traditional open procedures.[39] Furthermore, elderly patients undergoing VATS tended to have less severe complications compared to patients undergoing thoractomy.[39] Limited resections (segmentectomies) may be a consideration in elderly patients with limited life expectancy or poor cardiac and pulmonary reserve who may not tolerate a more extensive procedure. Some studies have shown that limited resections may provide a comparable survival rate to lobectomies in elderly patients as long as the resection includes all foci of tumors and provides a microscopically free margin. The most striking finding was that any survival difference between treatment modalities disappeared after 71 years of age. Interestingly, even smaller resections such as VATS and wedge resection may be a viable oncologic option in an elderly patient with resectable disease but limited life expectancy.[13] This is limited to very small tumors <7 mm in diameter and not yet proven to be clinically efficacious. Of particular interest is that VATS procedures may result in lower rates of postoperative confusion in elderly patients and this may be secondary to the decreased physiologic stress of minimally invasive procedures, faster recovery rates, and decreased narcotic requirement for pain control.[13] Careful preoperative selection and optimization combined with aggressive postoperative care and rehabilitation make surgical intervention for resectable disease feasible in aged populations.

Trauma

Patients >65 years of age currently account for approximately 23% of total hospital trauma admissions—many of which are multisystem and life threatening.[40] Geriatric trauma will continue to challenge surgeons in understanding the physical and physiologic impact of various mechanisms of injury, the need for careful assessment of comorbid conditions with particular attention to medication regimens, the rehabilitative capacity of an elderly trauma patient, and the knowledge of specific interventions that help to minimize morbidity and mortality in this population following traumatic injury.

The current geriatric population has fewer disabilities and is considerably more active than previous generations, which predisposes them to traumatic injuries. The most common type of trauma is blunt injury resulting from falls and motor vehicle collisions or pedestrian accidents. Falls currently account for 20% of severe injuries in elderly patients. Many underlying chronic and acute diseases common to elderly patients place them at increased risk for falls. These diseases include postural hypotension, leading to syncopal "drop attacks"; dysrhythmias from sick sinus syndrome; autonomic dysfunction; polypharmacy with improper dosage of antihypertensives and oral hypoglycemic agents resulting in hypotension; and hypoglycemia, respectively.[41]

Elderly patients also can fall victim to penetrating trauma, especially in elderly patients who may have underlying depression and suicidal ideations or are victims of elder abuse. It is estimated that approximately 40% of all trauma patients by 2050 will be >65 years old.[42] With the expanding elderly population, this will be an increasing source of morbidity and mortality; the risk of death after major trauma with multi-system and life-threatening injuries rises steeply after age 45 years old and doubles by age 75 years old. In contrast to what is observed for abdominal and thoracic surgery, even after controlling for injury severity and pre-existing medical conditions, patients aged 65 years and older sustaining traumatic injury were 4.6 times more likely to die than younger patients.[42] Of note, there are several interesting aspects of care of the acutely injured elderly patient that must be kept in mind. First, physiologic reserve can be challenged by trauma. For example, previously unknown disease such as cardiac impairment may be acutely unmasked. Secondly, medications common to elderly patients, such as beta blockers and anticoagulation, can not only inhibit the physiologic response to stress but may even worsen injury. Finally, elderly patients with impaired functional status posttrauma are more likely to lose their ability to function independently without the support of a nursing home.

Elderly patients are particularly susceptible to trauma due to changes that occur with aging, specifically, gait instability, decreased hearing and visual acuity, presence of confusion or dementia, underlying comorbid conditions, and poor reserve to tolerate the physiologic stress of traumatic injuries. Pre-existing medical conditions increase the risk of death after trauma significantly (up to threefold).[40] This is worsened when combined with an elderly patient's decreased functional reserve for handling physiologic abnormalities accompanying major trauma, such as hypotension and hypoxia. It is important to consider a trauma patient's age, as patients aged 65 to 80 years old have a 6.6% overall mortality rate after traumatic injury, which rises to 10% in patients 80 years or older.[42]

Despite the increased risk of morbidity and mortality after traumatic injury, it is interesting to note that there is currently an under-triaging of elderly patients to level 1 trauma centers despite high injury severity scores.[42] In one study, elderly patients >65 years old were five times more likely to be under-triaged to nondesignated trauma hospitals than younger counterparts.[42] However, a reduction in morbidity and mortality and posttraumatic complications as well as faster rehabilitation can result from better triaging practices. In one particular study involving acutely injured octogenarians with injury severity scores between 21 to 45, inhospital survival was as high as 56% in trauma centers, and this dramatically decreased to 8% in those treated at nontrauma hospitals.[42]

It is important to determine the medication regimen of elderly trauma patients. Medications such as beta blockers, calcium channel blockers, diuretics, and afterload reduction agents may impair critical augmentation of myocardial function in trauma patients, especially if they are hypovolemic. Approximately 20% of the elderly population with coronary artery disease and 10% of those with hypertension are currently on beta blocker therapy.[42] Therefore, tachycardia, one of the most valued signs of continued hypovolemia from either ongoing blood volume loss or underresuscitation, is lost in the elderly patient on beta blocker therapy. This makes interpretation of hemodynamic parameters in elderly patients inaccurate and, at times, misleading, which could lead to delays in appropriate interventions and resuscitation. However, it is important to keep in mind that, to date, evidence supporting early hemodynamic monitoring in elderly patients is lacking.

The other medication class that can be detrimental to an elderly, acutely injured patient is anticoagulation, ranging from aspirin and clopidogrel (Plavix) to warfarin, which may, at times, be supratherapeutic. Massive intracranial hemorrhages resulting from minor falls from standing in elderly patients are demonstrated in Fig. 46-7. Both patients subsequently had extremely poor prognosis. Warfarin therapy may be used in patients with atrial fibrillation, DVT, and prosthetic heart valves. The mortality rate of elderly patients on warfarin with a traumatic intracranial hemorrhage was 48% compared with 10% in an age-matched cohort not on anticoagulation therapy.[42] One of the most important caveats to treating elderly patients on anticoagulation with blunt head injury is the potential for significant, life-threatening intracranial hemorrhage despite initial normal head (computed tomography) CT scans. In one study, >70% of patients with minor mechanisms and negative CT scan, admitted for observation subsequently, clinically deteriorated within 12 hours of admission with a Glasgow Coma Scale of <10 and were subsequently found to have significant intracranial hemorrhages.[42] Therefore, prompt reversal of anticoagulation, particularly if supratherapeutic, is warranted to reduce morbidity and mortality following blunt head injury. In addition to increased risk of mortality in elderly patients sustaining blunt head trauma, a significant portion fail to resume functional independence after traumatic injury. It is estimated that approximately 20 to 25% of elderly trauma patients require discharge to a skilled nursing facility for long-term care and rehabilitation.[40] Poor functional outcome has been attributed to several factors among which are age >75 years old, presence of shock on admission, severe head injury, and development of infectious complications.

A particular concern in elderly patients sustaining blunt trauma is pelvic and extremity fractures (Fig. 46-8). Elderly patients are particularly susceptible to these injuries secondary to underlying medical conditions such as osteoporosis. Furthermore, these injuries, in particular, can not only increase the mortality of elderly trauma patients but also can predispose them to complications resulting from immobility leading to pneumonia and atelectasis, DVT, and pulmonary embolism. These injuries also predispose to functional impairment. Pelvic fractures are the most serious skeletal injury in the elderly.[43] Timely surgical intervention for extremity fractures in elderly patients is crucial to prompt recovery and helps to minimize mortality and morbidity from such injuries. In one study, a delay in providing surgical treatment for hip fractures by more than 2 days was associated with greater than double the risk of death within the first postoperative year.[42]

MINIMALLY INVASIVE SURGERY

Laparoscopy

Open abdominal procedures may require more intensive postoperative care, longer hospital stays, and an increased need for postoperative rehabilitation and possible institutionalization for elderly patients with limited reserve. However, the increasing experience

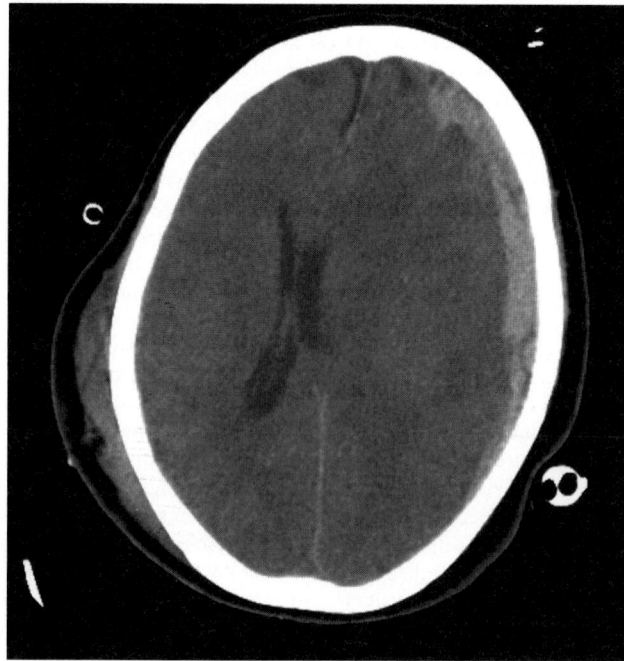
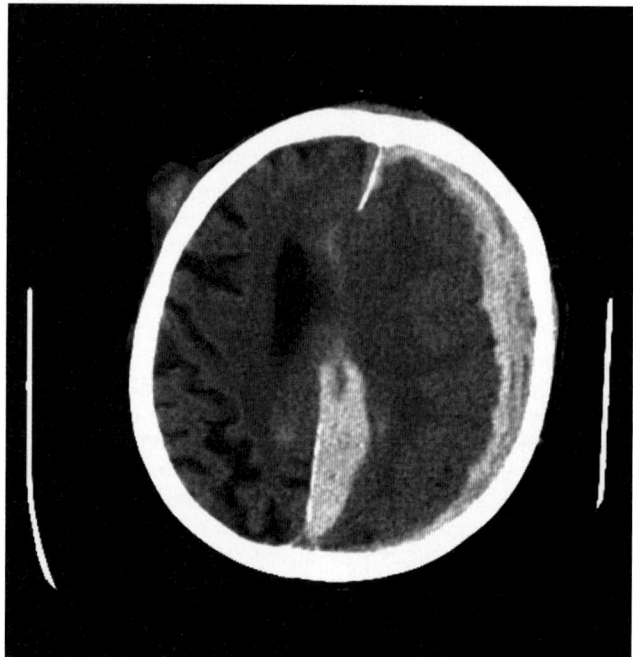

FIG. 46-7. Massive intracranial hemorrhage resulting from seemingly minor trauma. The importance of immediate reversal of anticoagulation in elderly patients cannot be overestimated.

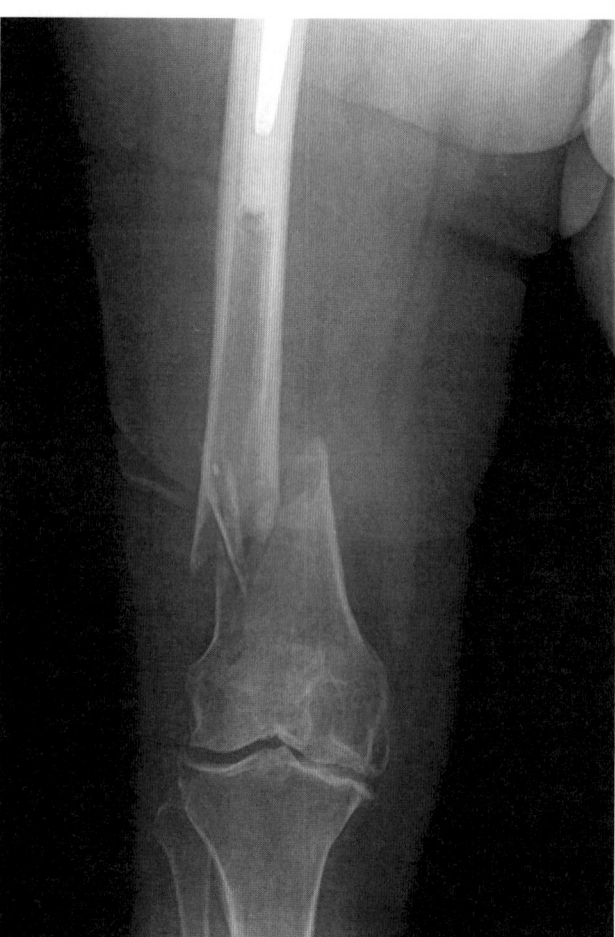

FIG. 46-8. Elderly patients are extremely susceptible to long bone fractures due to underlying medical conditions such as osteoporosis, leading to death or debilitation. Interestingly, this patient who suffered a traumatic long bone fracture had previously undergone a hip replacement a few months prior following a simple fall.

with laparoscopic techniques, combined with minimized pain, decreased length of hospital stay, and low morbidity and mortality rates, has led to the increased use of minimal access procedures among elderly patients. It has expanded from cholecystectomies to more complex procedures including colon resections, gastrectomies, and cardiac surgery.

Laparoscopic surgery reduces common postoperative complications such as atelectasis, GI ileus, and wound infections. In elderly surgical patients, these complications easily progress to pneumonia, DVT, and metabolic and electrolyte disturbances.[43] Decreased postoperative pain from smaller incisions leads to faster return to a preoperative level of functioning including early ambulation, which decreases complications from prolonged bed rest, such as DVT and pneumonia from compromised pulmonary mechanics. The latter is especially important for elderly patients because deconditioning occurs with long hospital stays, which depresses their ability to return to preoperative functional status. Laparoscopic surgery also provides the added benefit of reduction of the inflammatory, hormonal, and metabolic stress induced by major open surgical operations. However, these benefits must be balanced against the potential adverse effects of carbon dioxide (CO_2) insufflation and hemodynamic alterations induced by pneumoperitoneum and increased intra-abdominal pressure with concomitant decrease in venous return.[44] Therefore, decisions to perform minimal access procedures in the elderly must be individualized to the patient with careful consideration of the impact of comorbid conditions and the potential for poor cardiopulmonary reserves. This helps to provide the optimal circumstance for intervention resulting in improved surgical outcomes.

The cardiopulmonary effects induced by pneumoperitoneum are secondary to CO_2 insufflation and increased intra-abdominal pressure.[44] CO_2 insufflation is associated with hypercarbia and acidosis, both of which are proven direct myocardial depressants.[44] Hypercarbia is reported to be problematic in patients with pre-existing pulmonary disease with chronic CO_2 retention, but this is rarely observed. In patients without pre-existing disease, these alterations can be minimized by increasing minute ventilation during the procedure. The increased intra-abdominal pressure during insufflation can lead to increased afterload, increased peripheral vascular resistance and mean systemic pressure, and decreased preload.[44] This can result in depressed myocardial function, which is of potentially serious consequence in an elderly patient with poor physiologic reserve.

It is important to maintain tight control over the intra-abdominal pressure applied during the laparoscopic procedure. For example, pressures up to 20 mmHg are associated with increased filling pressures and cardiac output. However, further increased elevations result in decreased central venous pressures and cardiac output, which can be life threatening in a patient with pre-existing cardiac dysfunction and poor functional reserve.

Although the occurrence of these serious consequences are rare, adequate preoperative knowledge of the physiologic changes induced by laparoscopic techniques, as well as the changes that occur with advancing age, leads to better control of the variables that lead to adverse outcomes. Maintenance of adequate preload (i.e., adequate IV fluid administration) and intraoperative volume control, and careful mechanical ventilation to control hypercarbia and acidosis are basic concepts that allow the safe application of minimally invasive techniques in the elderly. It also is important to remember that elderly patients undergoing laparoscopic procedures must be closely monitored for any evidence of respiratory or hemodynamic compromise resulting from the pneumoperitoneum. If such changes do occur, it is crucial to immediately decompress the abdomen and allow the patient time to recover.

Studies have demonstrated that both advanced age >70 years old and an ASA classification of 3 or 4 are associated with higher conversion rates for laparoscopic cholecystectomy to open cholecystectomy.[45] These additional challenges, however, are not a contraindication to attempting the less invasive approach because conversion to an open procedure does not adversely impact the overall morbidity and mortality of the patient.

A particularly useful application of minimally invasive techniques is to rule out a surgical abdomen in an elderly patient presenting with acute abdominal pain. Vague, poorly localized pain, further obscured by several underlying confounding comorbid conditions, as is the case with ischemic colitis and mesenteric ischemia, may subject an elderly patient with poor reserve to the risk of general anesthesia and a negative exploratory laparotomy. Analysis of several studies directed at the application of laparoscopic techniques for the patient with acute abdominal pain demonstrated that approximately 41% had pathology necessitating open laparotomy, 10% had pathology amenable to laparoscopic intervention (i.e., acute cholecystitis), and 48% had nonsurgical disease that was subsequently managed nonoperatively, avoiding a negative exploration.[45] Therefore, laparoscopic evaluation of abdominal pain in the critically ill elderly patient may prove to be a valuable tool.

ENDOVASCULAR SURGERY

Abdominal aortic aneurysm (AAA) is a disease that primarily affects the elderly male patient. With increasing use of screening abdominal CT scans and ultrasounds for evaluation of various abdominal complaints, AAAs are being identified with greater frequency, most of which are diagnosed in elderly patients, given the increased prevalence of AAA with increasing age. In fact, the percentage of AAA rises from about 1% at age 55 to 60 years to approximately 10% in patients 80 years of age or older.[46] Elderly patients, and octogenarians in particular, were deemed poor operative candidates for the traditional open repair given the frequent presence of comorbid conditions and limited cardiopulmonary reserve to tolerate a major operation or the many hours of required operative time and general anesthesia. Elderly patients had an increased perioperative morbidity and mortality following open aortic surgery in comparison to younger cohorts. However, the introduction of endovascular techniques for repair of AAA has shifted the risk-benefit ratio for operative intervention, allowing

greater life expectancy for the elective repair of this potentially life-threatening condition with the benefits of minimally invasive techniques as described above.

Studies have demonstrated that endovascular aortic repair (EVAR) is feasible and efficacious in elderly patients, including those previously considered unfit for open repair. EVAR is a minimally invasive technique in which a prosthetic graft is introduced into the aortic lumen via the common femoral artery to exclude the aortic aneurysm sac. EVAR significantly reduces operative and anesthesia times, blood loss, intensive care needs, length of stays, and major postoperative morbidity associated with open AAA repair. The most common complication following EVAR in elderly patients is renal impairment. Typically, patients are discharged 1 to 2 days following surgery and the graft is deployed via small bilateral groin incisions, obviating the need for a major laparotomy incision. Figure 46-9 demonstrates the endovascular repair of AAA and right iliac artery aneurysm via bilateral groin access in an 82-year-old man who was discharged from the hospital on postoperative day 2. This procedure also can be done using epidural anesthesia for high-risk candidates who may tolerate general anesthesia poorly. Endovascular repair has even been described under local anesthesia in patients at extreme high risk of rupture and death or after rupture and hemodynamic instability precluding the ability to tolerate general anesthesia.[47] This was a reportable circumstance and obviously not the current standard of care.

Careful consideration of the life expectancy and the risk of rupture dictate the necessity for intervention. EVAR remains a viable option in elderly patients. Nonoperative management is justified in frail elderly patients with multiple comorbidities and reduced life expectancy whose operative risks outweigh the risk of rupture and in those who are unlikely to survive long enough to benefit from the repair.

THYROID AND PARATHYROID SURGERY

The prevalence of thyroid disease increases with advancing age. The etiologies, risk factors, and presentations of thyroid disease are similar across all ages, and therefore, are not discussed in detail. Of note, however, is that elderly patients more often present with cardiac manifestations of hyperthyroidism, such as atrial fibrillation, than do their younger counterparts. A common finding requiring evaluation in elderly patients is the presence of a thyroid nodule, usually detected by physical examination. These nodules usually are single and four times more common in women, making them a particular concern for postmenopausal elderly women. Indications for surgical intervention for thyroid nodules are dependent on the characteristics of the nodule (i.e., whether it is benign or malignant, or whether the patient is euthyroid or thyrotoxic). In addition, surgical intervention becomes necessary if the nodule enlarges, producing compressive symptoms.

Papillary carcinoma in elderly patients tends to be sporadic with a bell-shaped distribution of age at presentation, occurring primarily in patients aged 30 to 59 years old. The incidence of papillary carcinoma decreases in patients >60 years of age.[48] However, patients >60 years of age have increased risk of local recurrence and for the development of distant metastases. Metastatic disease may be more common in this population secondary to delayed referral for surgical intervention because of the misconception that the surgeon will be unwilling to operate on an elderly patient with thyroid disease. Age is also a prognostic indicator for patients with follicular carcinoma. There is a 2.2 times increased risk of mortality from follicular carcinoma per 20 years of increasing age.[49] Therefore, prognosis for elderly patients with differentiated thyroid carcinomas is worse when compared to younger counterparts. The higher prevalence of vascular invasion and extracapsular extension among older patients is, in part, responsible for the poorer prognosis in geriatric patients. Advancing age

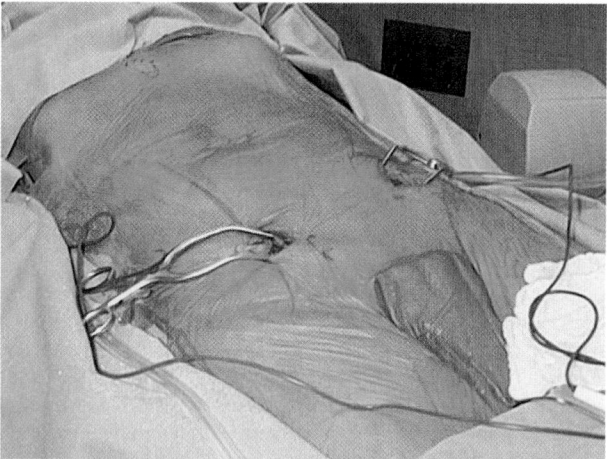

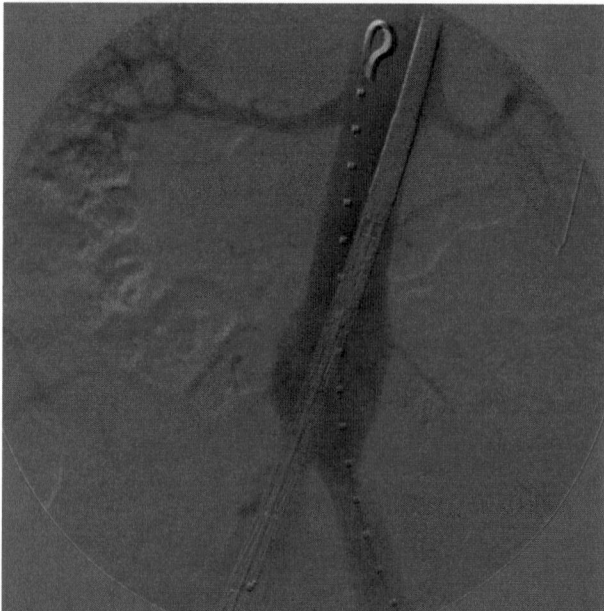

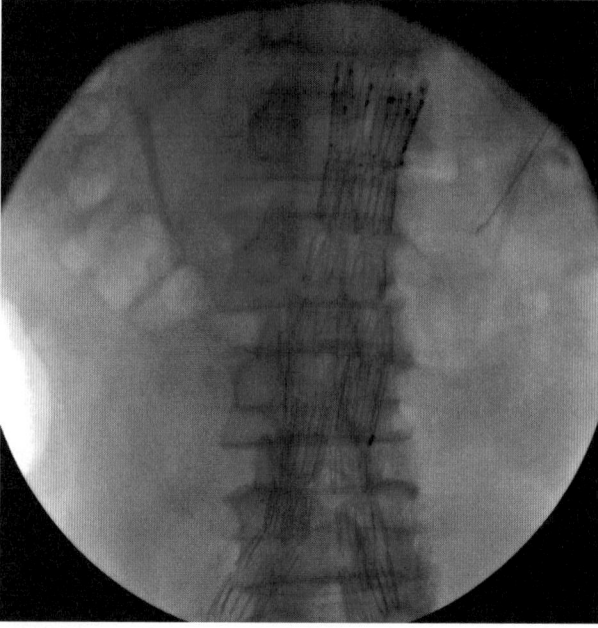

FIG. 46-9. Endovascular repair of abdominal aortic aneurysms (AAAs) is gaining favor for suitable elderly patients to prevent rupture. Through minimal groin incisions, this 82-year-old patient underwent repair of an AAA and right iliac artery aneurysm and was discharged on postoperative day 2.

leads to increased mortality risk for patients with thyroid cancer and is demonstrated by the AMES (*age, metastases, extent of primary tumor, and size of tumor*) classification system developed by the Lahey Clinic.

Anaplastic carcinoma is a highly aggressive form of thyroid carcinoma with dismal prognosis. It accounts for approximately 1% of all thyroid malignancies; however, it occurs primarily in elderly patients.[50] This poorly differentiated tumor rapidly invades local structures, leading to clinical deterioration and eventually tracheal obstruction. These patients may present with a painful, rapidly enlarging neck mass accompanied by dysphagia and cervical tenderness. This leads to respiratory compromise and impingement of the airway. Unfortunately, because of the aggressive nature of the disease and the dismal prognosis, surgical resection of the tumor is not attempted for cure. Furthermore, radiation therapy and chemotherapy offer little benefit. Airway blockage, however, may necessitate surgical palliation or permanent tracheostomy to alleviate symptoms of respiratory distress.

PARATHYROID SURGERY

Approximately 2% of the geriatric population, including 3% of women 75 years of age or older, will develop primary hyperparathyroidism.[51] Geriatric patients are usually referred to surgery only when advanced disease is present because of concerns regarding the risks of surgery, but low rates of morbidity and negligible mortality combined with high cure rates of approximately 95 to 98% make parathyroidectomy safe and effective. Convincing evidence of the benefit of surgery is the usual marked symptomatic improvement, which greatly improves the quality of life for most patients. The National Institutes of Health Consensus Development Statement recommends curative therapy after diagnosis of primary hyperthyroidism is established in a patient regardless of age. Specific indications for operative intervention regardless of age include a 30% decrease in creatinine clearance, 24-hour urinary calcium excretion >400 mg, and decreased bone density.[52,53]

Elderly patients are especially prone to developing mental manifestations of hyperparathyroidism that may be severe enough to produce a dementia-like state. There often is a significant improvement in mental status after parathyroidectomy. Another specific symptom of hyperparathyroidism that may easily be mistaken for osteoporosis and can be present in postmenopausal, elderly women is orthopedic disease; specifically back pain, and possibly, the occurrence of vertebral fractures. This pain can be of moderate intensity, leading to impaired mobility and severely affecting the quality of life of elderly patients. The decreased bone density observed in elderly patients with hyperparathyroidism tends to improve during the first 2 years after successful parathyroid surgery.

Limited parathyroidectomies with minimal dissection in geriatric patients are an effective alternative. This is a viable option in patients with multiple comorbid conditions in whom the increased risk of surgical intervention or general anesthesia remains a concern. One study demonstrated that preoperative localization of the hyperfunctioning gland with the aid of ^{99m}Tc-sestamibi nuclear scanning, as well as intraoperative parathyroid hormone (PTH) assays to rapidly confirm that all hypersecreting glands have been removed, allows limited parathyroidectomy to be performed with accuracy in elderly patients (Fig. 46-10).[51] This procedure is described as "limited" because bilateral neck dissection for identification and biopsy of the remaining glands to determine if they are hypersecreting becomes unnecessary. The half-life of intact PTH is approximately 3 to 4 minutes. Therefore, a drop in the intraoperative PTH level at approximately 10 minutes after resection of the suspect hypersecreting gland suggests a 98% probability that the patient will return to normocalcemic levels postoperatively.[51]

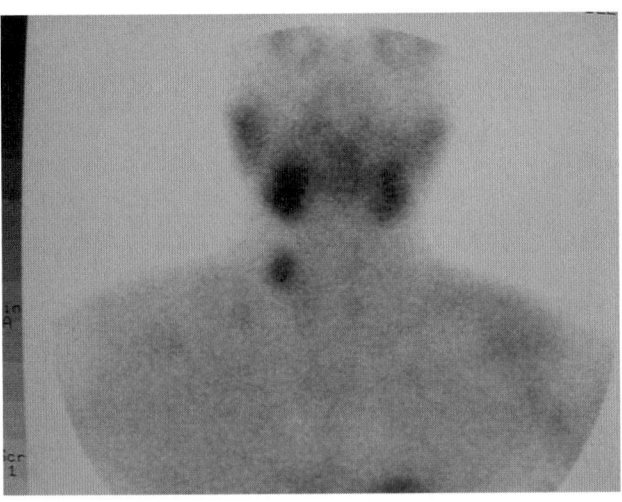

A

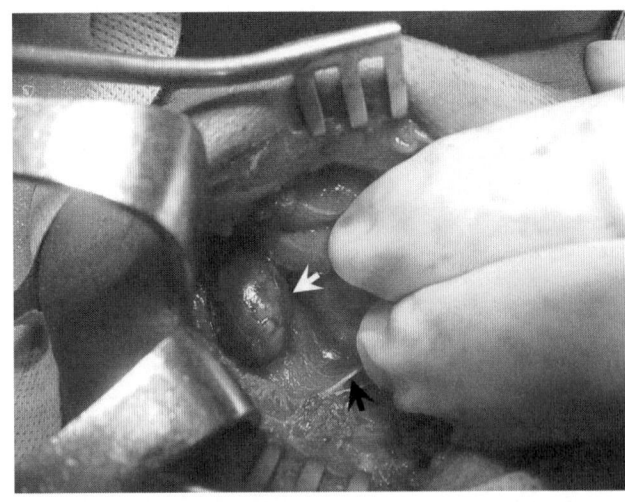

B

FIG. 46-10. Parathyroid adenoma in an elderly patient with high calcium levels and elevated parathyroid hormone levels. **A.** Sestamibi scan showed right-upper-gland adenoma facilitating a directed incision. **B.** One-g pituitary adenoma was easily identified intraoperatively (*white arrow*). *Black arrow* points to the recurrent laryngeal nerve.

PALLIATIVE SURGERY

Palliative surgery is defined as surgical intervention targeted to alleviate a patient's symptoms, thus improving the patient's quality of life despite minimal impact on the patient's survival (see Chap. 48).[54] With an increasing number of aging surgical patients who often present with advanced disease, surgeons must be familiar with the concept of palliation to control disease. This concept focuses on providing the maximal benefit to the patient using the least-invasive intervention. Ultimately, this leads to symptom relief and preservation of the quality of life in terminal disease states. The uses of palliative surgery can range from extensive debulking operations aimed at aiding in the effectiveness of chemotherapy and radiation, to less complex operations to alleviate symptoms such as intractable vomiting, severe pain, cachexia, and anorexia that are common to terminal disease states. The success of palliative surgery is a careful balance between achieving symptom relief while ensuring that the development of new symptoms from the palliative intervention itself does not occur.

Palliative care in the treatment of advanced disease often is associated with age bias; older patients are more prone to be offered palliative care in comparison to younger patients. In a recent survey, two surgical scenarios were presented to a panel of surgeons.[35] The first patient was an 85-year-old woman with excellent functional status presenting for evaluation of back pain, jaundice, weight loss, and vomiting. Appropriate studies were completed with CT scan that demonstrated a mass in the head of the pancreas with invasion into the portal vein. The patient in the second scenario experienced identical symptoms, but was significantly younger. Most of the surgeons selected major surgical intervention for the younger patient, while only one third of the panel offered the same intervention for the older patient. The majority offered only palliative care for the older patient. It is important to note that those surgeons who offered operative intervention based their decision on the functional status of the patient preoperatively. When transitioning from curative therapy to palliation, the risks and benefits of the proposed surgical intervention should be examined, as well as the intended impact to the patient's quality of life.

There currently is no evidence to support that palliative surgery is less effective for elderly patients with surgically unresectable disease. Younger patients undergoing palliative interventions do not have a demonstrated improved outcome when compared to disease-matched older patients. Therefore, it is important to recognize that age is not a limitation to surgical intervention, and that all interventions should be individualized based on the severity of symptoms and the predicted benefit.

Surgical palliative care can range from nonoperative management of malignant obstructions by percutaneous methods (Fig. 46-11) to laparoscopic surgery for the treatment of life-threatening illness by minimally invasive technique (Fig. 46-12). An interesting challenge in palliative care is the determination of the actual cause of a patient's symptoms to offer the most beneficial, but least invasive, intervention. Treatment of malignant pleural effusions, for example, should be tailored to the source of the symptoms, not the effusion. Effusions should be treated only when they cause significant distress for patients with terminal disease.[35] Dyspnea in a terminal patient can be the result of chest wall restriction, pulmonary fibrosis from previous radiation treatment, infiltration of the primary cancer, or early airway obstruction from mediastinal spread of the primary tumor.[35] If it is determined that a patient's dyspnea is largely secondary to a malignant pleural effusion, the goal of palliative intervention is lung expansion, preferably with permanent pleurodesis. Permanent control can be achieved via thoracoscopy or by more invasive thoracotomy with chemical pleurodesis.[35] The latter intervention is highly effective for permanent resolution, and therefore, may be more invasive than necessary for patients with late-stage terminal disease. In these patients, medical pleurodesis with intrapleural injection of a sclerosant via thoracostomy tube placement is a better alternative.[35] For surgical therapy, minimally invasive procedures such as VATS may be an appropriate method to assess the apposition of pleural surfaces and may allow for talc pleurodesis or insertion of a pleuroperitoneal shunt.[35]

Palliative intervention for symptom relief and prevention of complications can be demonstrated in the management of terminal pancreatic cancer and metastatic CRC. Two thirds of patients with pancreatic cancer present with advanced disease, which often is diagnosed after evaluation of obstructive jaundice. Despite advanced disease, surgical intervention improves quality of life through relief of biliary obstruction. Percutaneous transhepatic stenting has emerged as a viable alternative to surgical bypass, achieving similar results and lowering mortality rates with the occurrence of fewer early complications. Endoscopic stenting is yet another option. If a patient does not have multiple comorbidities with good functional status, surgical intervention then can provide

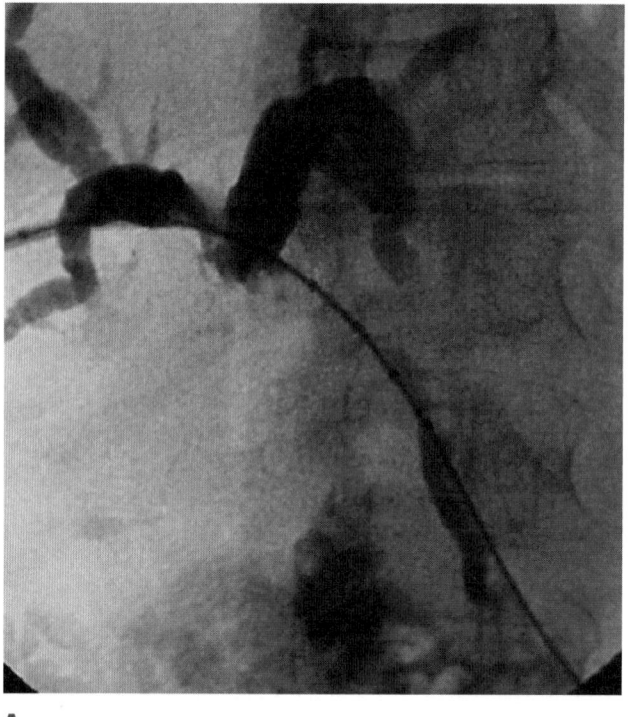

A

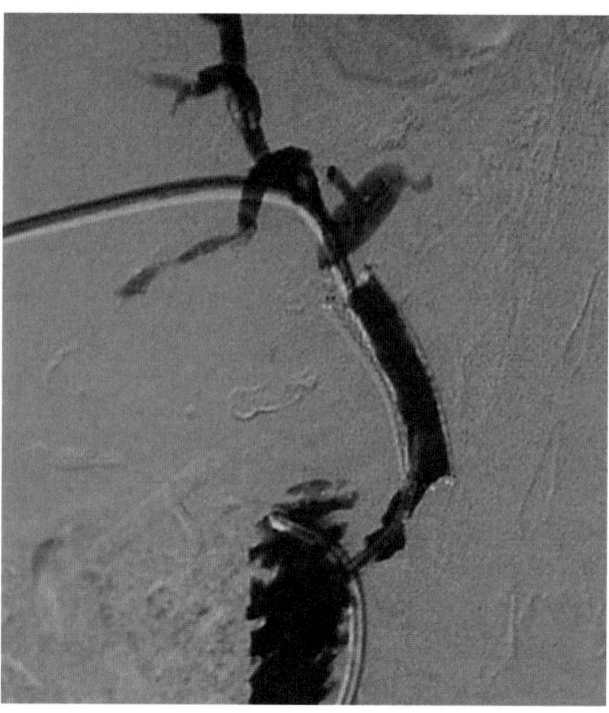

B

FIG. 46-11. Palliative care in an 82-year-old woman with obstructive jaundice from unresectable cholangiocarcinoma. Computed tomography scan showed metastatic disease to the liver. **A.** A percutaneous drainage of the biliary system with a stent placed across the obstruction from the hilum to the distal common bile duct. **B.** Two days later, a covered permanent metallic wall stent was placed across the obstruction.

a definitive diagnosis and permanent biliary decompression and gastric drainage. In addition, an important palliative intervention that can be provided to patients with the open procedure is chemical splanchnicectomy, which is infiltration of the celiac plexus with an agent such as alcohol for effective relief of intractable pain from tumor invasion of the celiac plexus.[35] A gastroenterostomy drainage procedure is effective protection against gastric outlet obstruction, which inevitably develops in 30% of patients.

Palliative surgery for disseminated CRC should be aimed at the reduction of symptoms such as pain, obstruction, or hemorrhage. Bowel obstruction can be relieved with intestinal bypass or a diverting colostomy. The most common site of disseminated disease is the liver. Uncontrolled liver metastasis is responsible for pain, abdominal distention, jaundice, and inferior vena caval obstruction. Many patients with liver metastasis are not candidates for resection, and therefore may be considered for ablation of the lesions by local destruction, cryotherapy, or radiofrequency ablation. More traditional means, such as chemotherapy, which can be administered via the hepatic artery or radiation, also may be used. Systemic corticosteroid therapy can be used in patients with advanced metastatic disease to reduce pain caused by swelling of the liver capsule. If bone metastases are present, pain may be controlled by irradiation, and prophylactic fixation of long bones may be considered to decrease pain as well as morbidity from pathologic fractures.[35] Similarly, cerebral irradiation and high-dose steroid therapy may help to decrease intracranial pressure from metastatic disease as well as delay the onset of neurologic symptoms and cognitive impairment, which are essential to maintain quality of life of the patient.[35]

SPECIFIC SYMPTOM MANAGEMENT

Gastrointestinal Disturbances

The distressing symptoms often faced by terminally ill patients either result from the disease process or as a side effect of treatment. The causes of nausea and vomiting in terminally ill patients are multifactorial and can be attributed to various medications or chemotherapy treatments, gastric stasis, obstruction of the GI tract, mesenteric metastases, irritation of the GI tract, raised intracranial pressure from cerebral metastasis, or anxiety-induced emesis. Treatment should be focused on prevention of dehydration and malnutrition from poor oral intake. Antiemetics may be administered for control of nausea and vomiting. The oral route of administration is the best option for prophylaxis before chemotherapy treatments. However, other preparations such as suppositories or injections can be appropriate for patients who are unable to tolerate oral medications.

Diarrhea and constipation also are common GI disturbances in terminal patients. Constipation is particularly common in patients receiving chronic narcotic medications. Constipation also can be caused by such events as tumor invasion leading to intestinal obstruction, metabolic abnormalities such as hypercalcemia from metastatic disease, and dehydration. Because constipation may be worsened by dehydration, adequate fluid intake often helps to alleviate symptoms. Constipation can lead to fecal impaction, nausea, and colicky abdominal pain. If there is difficulty distinguishing between constipation and early bowel obstruction, diagnostic tests are useful, but should be kept to a minimum in terminal patients. Patients can be treated with stool softeners and stimulant agents. Laxatives with peristalsis-stimulating action, such as senna or bisacodyl, should be used with caution because of the potential for causing intestinal colic.

The occurrence of diarrhea also is multifactorial and can be caused by medications, overload incontinence with fecal impaction, from the disease process itself, malignant bowel obstruction, or improper laxative therapy. Radiation therapy can cause diarrhea by damage of the intestinal mucosa, which results in the release of prostaglandins and the malabsorption of bile salts that increases peristalsis. Once the underlying causes are identified and appropriately managed, patients can be given bulk-forming agents and opiate derivatives to aid in symptomatic improvement.

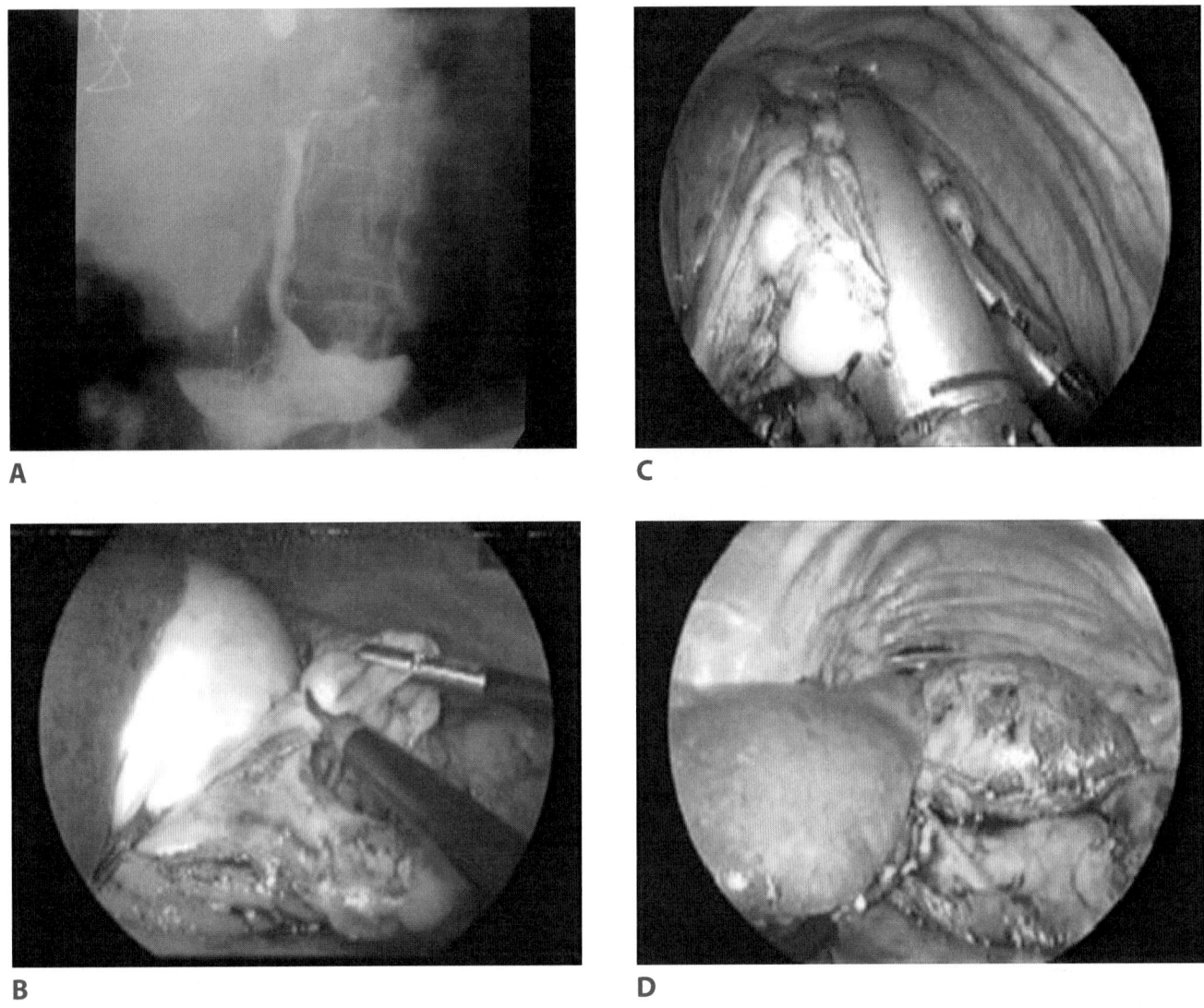

FIG. 46-12. An 85-year-old man with dementia presenting with a bleeding GI stromal tumor in the fundus of the stomach, treated with laparoscopic gastrectomy. **A.** The upper GI series delineating the tumor. **B.** Laparoscopic division of short gastric artery with harmonic scalpel. **C.** Division of stomach with Endo-GIA stapler. **D.** Resection of the mass before removal from abdomen via an endobag.

DEPRESSION AND ASTHENIA

Asthenia is a condition of reduced energy levels accompanied by fatigue and generalized weakness without the presence of physical or mental exertion.[55] In a study by Hinshaw and associates, asthenia was present in approximately 90% of patients and was more prevalent than pain, leading to the potential for impaired quality of life.[55] Both of these symptoms commonly affect the terminally ill patient. However, if identified, appropriate interventions can be provided in an effort to improve quality of life and enhance the patient's functional status. In cancer patients, overactivity of the hypothalamic-pituitary-adrenal axis and elevation of interleukin-6 levels have been reported in patients suffering with depression. Natural killer cell activity has been demonstrated to decline in patients with depression, causing an immunosuppressive effect and weakening the patient's response to tumor.[55] Poorly controlled pain and complications from disease progression also can cause terminal patients to develop depression. These complications include somnolence and depression that can occur with hypercalcemia from bony metastases with lung and breast cancer. These must be controlled as much as possible before the consideration of pharmacologic therapy to alleviate symptoms of depression.

Appropriate therapy for depression and asthenia must be individualized. If a patient has good functional status with a predicted survival time of several months, the initiation of standard antidepressants is appropriate. However, if there is an expected short survival period with progression of depressive symptoms impairing quality of life, then a psychostimulant is more appropriate because of its immediate effect, better short-term efficacy, and the tendency for development of tolerance, usually within 3 months.[55] Psychostimulants such as amphetamine and methylphenidate also increase appetite at lower doses and help to reduce sedation that may result from treatment with narcotic medications for pain management.[55] Psychostimulants also are effective in the management of asthenia, which shares a common clinical presentation with depression. However, pharmacologic therapy for asthenia should be provided only after treatable causes of this symptom, such as medications (including narcotics), the presence of pain, anemia, dehydration, and infection, as well as metabolic abnormalities, such as hyponatremia, hypokalemia, and hypercalcemia, have been assessed and corrected.[55]

Cachexia and Anorexia

Cachexia refers to catabolic changes associated with progressive wasting that is present in patients with advanced illness; prominent symptoms include anorexia, weight loss, and asthenia.[56] A subsequent loss of muscle and fat leading to anemia, hypoalbuminemia, and hypoproteinemia also is common. This is a chronic form of malnutrition and is not reversible with short-term nutritional support and hyperalimentation.[56] Malnourished cancer patients with cachexia have reduced response to antineoplastic medications, radiation, and chemotherapy, as well as decreased survival rates.[35] The mechanism of cachexia is poorly understood, but hypotheses include actions of interleukin-6, tumor necrosis factor, and interferon-mediating metabolic changes in chronic illness.[56]

Management of cachexia begins with the identification of correctable causes. Patients may have underlying metabolic derangements, as well as dehydration, that must be appropriately treated. Poorly controlled pain, anemia, and sleep disturbances also may exacerbate symptoms of cachexia, leading to malnutrition and wasting. Patients with terminal disease additionally often suffer from GI disturbances, such as constipation and nausea, which may lead to anorexia. Malabsorption is common in patients with pancreatic cancer, and supplementation of pancreatic enzymes may improve absorption and help to improve nutritional status. Nausea and vomiting should be appropriately managed. It is important to rule out mechanical causes of malnutrition that can effectively be treated with nonoperative management such as bowel rest and nasogastric tube compression or operative intervention.

If no underlying correctable abnormalities are identified, patients may benefit from pharmacologic intervention with dexamethasone and prednisone, which increase appetites in patients with advanced cancer, leading to improved quality of life.[56] The onset of effect is rapid but short-lived, and thus should be reserved for patients at terminal stages of disease. Other agents, such as progestational drugs, namely megestrol acetate (Megace), also stimulate appetite and cause weight gain in cachexia patients.[56]

Malignant Bowel Obstruction

Patients with malignant bowel obstruction typically present with cramping abdominal pain, nausea, and vomiting, which may be a common complication of advanced terminal disease secondary to GI malignancy or from extrinsic compression of bowel loops from progressive tumor burden. Conservative management can be effective and includes NPO, IV hydration, and nasogastric decompression. However, long-term management often is difficult. Medical management with pharmacologic agents such as somatostatin analogues to decrease GI output may also be considered for symptom alleviation, along with analgesics and antiemetics. Octreotide effectively decreases the volume of GI secretions via inhibition of intestinal hormones and growth hormone and is 70% effective in patients suffering with bowel obstruction with the added effect of decreasing colic and nausea.[56] However, surgical palliation via bypass procedures, decompressing, or diverting ostomies may be required.

Surgical intervention may provide permanent alleviation of obstruction and eliminate the need for repeated nasogastric decompressions that can limit patient comfort. In one study, approximately 40 to 70% of patients reported relief of symptoms of obstruction after surgical intervention.[56] This must be balanced against the risk of perioperative mortality from surgical intervention, which ranges from approximately 12 to 20%, as well as the potential for mortality from wound infection, poor wound healing, and fistula formation.[56] Patients in whom the risk of surgical intervention outweighs the benefit of palliation include patients who have ascites or multiple sites of obstruction accompanied by poor functional status and poor nutrition with serum albumin levels <3 g/dL.[56] Should conservative management fail in a patient who is unfit to undergo surgical intervention, alternatives include a venting gastrostomy or jejunostomy, which can be inserted percutaneously.[35]

Pain Management

Intractable pain is one of the most distressing symptoms affecting a terminally ill patient. Nociceptive pain can be categorized as somatic, visceral, or deafferentation pain.[57,58] Visceral pain frequently is sec-

ondary to tumor involvement of sympathetically innervated organs by either direct invasion or compression that leads to stretching or distention of the affected viscera. Typical examples are metastatic invasion of organs such as with distention of the liver capsule by tumor or pain that occurs with pancreatic cancer from invasion of nerve roots or plexus. This pain typically is poorly localized and difficult to describe. Somatic pain results from the activation of somatic nociceptors and typically is well localized and constant. A common example is bone metastasis. Deafferentation pain, also known as *neuropathic pain*, results from injury to the nervous system from tumor compression or infiltration. This pain often is severe and leads to functional impairment such as that which occurs with invasion of the lumbosacral or brachial plexus.

Drugs that are commonly used in pain management are nonopioid compounds such as acetaminophen and nonsteroidal compounds.[56] These drugs often can be combined with opioids to improve analgesia. Opioids are the other class of familiar drugs useful in pain management and include codeine or stronger agents such as morphine, oxycodone, methadone, hydromorphone (Dilaudid), and fentanyl. Adjuvant agents such as corticosteroids, antidepressants, muscle relaxants, and certain anticonvulsants may be used in combination with opioid and nonopioid compounds for synergistic effects. The initial assessment of the patient should attempt to assess the pain in regard to severity, alleviating/aggravating factors, and other qualitative features often used to describe pain. The best therapy for the individual patient then should be determined. It is important to keep patient comfort in mind and to address comorbid conditions that will affect treatment. For example, dysphagia leads to difficulty in swallowing, making oral medications either painful or impossible; diaphoresis may alter the effect of transdermal patches because of an inability to stay in place; and muscle wasting and cachexia will make intramuscular and subcutaneous routes of administration extremely painful. If a patient is vomiting or has had profuse diarrhea, oral and rectal medications are inappropriate. The most common method to administer medications is the oral route, but buccal and sublingual approaches to medication administration are particularly useful in patients who suffer with dysphagia.[56] Liquid forms are easier as well. IV administration, as well as other more intrusive methods of drug administration, also can be used.

For most postoperative pain regimens, medications have been dosed on an as-needed basis. However, terminal patients with chronic, constant, debilitating pain require more regimental administration with around-the-clock dosing, sustained-release medications, or immediate-release medications used for breakthrough pain management. A useful method currently used for pain management is the use of long-acting narcotics with extended analgesic effect. Transdermal fentanyl (Duragesic) patches that reduce the requirement for frequent dosing with excellent control of pain are particularly helpful in chronic pain management. One patch may be applied every 72 hours, but frequency can be increased to every 48 hours for more severe, chronic pain.

Medication dosing should constantly be evaluated and adjusted according to the patient's pain scale. On the typical scale of one to 10 in increasing severity, if a patient rates pain between three and six despite the current regimen, then dosages should be increased by 25 to 50%; if a patient rates pain between seven and 10, dosages may be increased by 50 to 100%.[56]

NSAIDs are effective in managing mild to moderate somatic pain and pain associated with inflammation. NSAIDs such as aspirin, ibuprofen, and naproxen, as well as acetaminophen, are particularly effective for managing pain from bony metastases. These medications do have a "ceiling effect," meaning the drug ceases to provide analgesia above a certain dosage.[59] These drugs also should be used with caution in elderly populations because of the potential to cause delirium as well as other toxic side effects, such as GI bleeding and renal failure. Opioids such as codeine can be added to NSAIDs for an increased analgesic effect. If pain remains poorly controlled, stronger opioids, such as morphine, hydromorphone, and fentanyl, can be administered.

Short-acting medications, such as Demerol, which has a half-life of approximately 2.5 to 3 hours, should be avoided in the management of chronic pain.[56] Demerol, for example, does not have many administration options and is given only by injection because it is ineffective by oral administration. Furthermore, it has toxic intermediates that lead to central nervous system toxicity, resulting in tremors, confusion, or seizure activity. These intermediates may also lower the threshold for seizure activity.[56]

Many side effects can occur with administration of pain medications on a chronic basis, the most common being GI symptoms. For example, the most common side effect of opioid administration is constipation, secondary to decreased peristaltic activity and increased absorption.[56] Consequently, all patients who are administered opioids also should be placed on a stool softener to avoid constipation. It is important to note that some patients may require an increase in their pain medication regimen at particular times, such as before aggressive wound care or during transport.

Respiratory depression is often a concern when prescribing high doses of opioids. This is far less common in patients who have been on a constant regimen of opioid compounds for >36 hours.[56] Tolerance to the respiratory-depressant effect of opioids develops within 36 hours of administration, leading to relatively safe administration in terminally ill patients.[56] Addiction to pain medication should not be a deterrent to providing adequate pain management. Addiction is defined as the preoccupation and seeking of medications, despite known harm, for a reason other than pain management. Terminally ill patients require pain medication for control of severe intractable pain to improve their quality of life but rarely demonstrate symptoms of addiction.

Ethical Considerations

Ethical considerations and end-of life care dilemmas have gained prominent focus in the care of elderly patients, especially in the terminal stages of illness. This is a particularly important issue given the increasing effectiveness of modern therapies and sophisticated intensive care available to patients with the technical ability to sustain life indefinitely. It is, therefore, critical to begin to address these issues early in the course of disease to properly interact with patients and family members regarding prognosis, treatment options, alternatives, and plan of care in terminal stages. Development of a definitive plan of care for a terminally ill patient eases the transition from curative therapy to palliation. Open discussions regarding end-of-life care, withholding or withdrawal of life support, and medical futility are critical issues for patients, family, and caregivers and should be held as soon as is appropriate.

Defining medical futility remains controversial in respect to both practical definitions and clinical determinants. The American Thoracic Society has stated that "a life-sustaining intervention is futile if reasoning and experience indicate that the intervention would be highly unlikely to result in meaningful survival for the patient," with attention paid to both the duration of the survival as well as quality of life.[55] Table 46-3 summarizes the goals for ethical decision making in the elderly surgical patient.

In actual clinical practice, it is difficult to predict whether a particular therapy will, in fact, be futile. Prognostic scales have been developed to better define medical futility based on objective patient data. For example, the Acute Physiology and Chronic Health Evaluation score can be used as a quantitative prognosis tool. However, this is a general scoring system and, although predictive of gross mortality, it is difficult to individualize for patients. However, this system could help clarify a patient's wishes regarding life-sustaining treatment via advance directives, living wills, and do not resuscitate (DNR) orders to avoid unnecessary prolongation of futile treatment.

Physicians are not required to provide life-sustaining treatments that are deemed medically futile. This can override requests by patients or family members to continue aggressive therapy. It is important to realize that palliation is different from euthanasia and is

TABLE 46-3 Goals for ethical decision making in elderly surgical patient

1. Acknowledge medical futility; physicians are not required to provide life-sustaining treatment that is deemed medically futile.
2. Clarify patients' wishes regarding life-sustaining therapies in accordance with Patient Self-Determination Act (i.e., advance directives, living wills, do not intubate/resuscitate orders).
3. Respect patient autonomy: right to accept and refuse treatment despite consequences of decision.
   - Ensure mental competency before establishing autonomy.
   - May appoint surrogate decision maker in case of incapacitation.

protected by the law, even if it hastens the occurrence of death by the principle of double effect. Double effect is defined as an act with good intention that produces a secondary effect that is harmful.[56] Therefore, physicians should not fear legal retribution from families in disagreements regarding treatment plans.

The governing principle in end-of-life decision making is patient autonomy, which takes precedence over physicians' judgment of what is the most appropriate care. A patient has a right to refuse treatment, even if it delays appropriate treatment or results in the patient's death.[56] However, these preferences need to be documented during a time of mental competency. Surrogate decision making is tantamount to a patient's wishes, giving surrogates complete decision-making responsibilities. Physicians are not required to provide futile care. The Patient Self-Determination Act allows a patient to document preferences for life-sustaining interventions and resuscitation before undergoing treatments in the form of advance directives and living wills.[54] These documents define the patient's wishes regarding life-support measures. In addition, a surrogate for decision making can be appointed by the patient to make decisions regarding plan of care in the event the patient becomes mentally incapacitated.[54] Despite the availability of such documentation, few patients make necessary arrangements before clinical decompensation. Furthermore, this issue is rarely addressed by the physician with the patient and family until recovery is unlikely. Unfortunately, most DNR orders are written only within days of a patient's death. This issue should always be addressed with patients before operative intervention. It is important to also acknowledge that DNR orders can be temporarily suspended in the operating room, placing both the surgeon and patient at ease. This practice is appropriate because most adverse events that occur in the operating room are secondary to acute, reversible events and are immediately detectable with careful monitoring. Necessary interventions can be instituted immediately in a controlled setting with excellent results, unlike events that may occur outside the operating room.

To summarize, the four goals of surgical care of elderly patients are as follows:

1. Provide timely diagnosis of disease processes followed by appropriate intervention without the bias of ageism and the false assumption that elderly patients will suffer increased morbidity and mortality.
2. Provide a careful preoperative assessment, taking into consideration the physiologic changes that occur with aging, to optimize an elderly patient for surgical interventions, thereby improving outcomes.
3. Provide interventions that maximize a patient's life span without comprising quality of life and independent function.
4. Relieve suffering with palliation when surgical care is not achievable.

The challenge for a surgeon, therefore, is to improve perioperative care of the elderly surgical patient with careful patient selection, accurately assess risk factors to reduce postoperative morbidity and mortality, and deliver quality surgical interventions without compromising functional vitality.

REFERENCES

Entries highlighted in bright blue are key references.

1. O'Connell JB, Maggard MA, Ko CY: Cancer-directed surgery for localized disease: Decrease utilization in the elderly. *Ann Surg Oncol* 11:962, 2004.
2. Jaklitsch MT, Bueno R, Swanson SJ, et al: New surgical options for elderly lung cancer patients. *Chest* 116:480, 1999.
3. Asmis TR, Ding K, Seymour L et al: Age and comorbidity as independent factors in the treatment of non-small cell lung cancer: A review of National Cancer Institute of Canada Clinical Trials Group Trials. *J Clin Oncol* 26:54, 2008.
4. Richardson J, Cocanour C, Kern J, et al: Perioperative risk assessment in the elderly and high risk patients. *J Am Coll Surg* 199:133, 2004.
5. Williams SL, Jones PB, Pofahl WE: Preoperative management of the older patient—A surgeon's perspective: Part 1. *Clin Geriatr* 14:24, 2006.
6. Zenilman ME: Surgery in the elderly. *Curr Probl Surg* 35:99, 1998.
7. Lyon C, Clark DC: Diagnosis of acute abdominal pain in older patients. *Am Fam Physician* 74:1537, 2006.
8. Muravchick S: Preoperative assessment of the elderly patient. *Anesthesiol Clin North Am* 18:71, 2000.
9. Hazen SE, Larsen PD, Martin JL: General anesthesia and elderly surgical patients. *AORN J* 65:819, 1997.
10. Pasetto LM, Lise M, Monfardini S: Preoperative assessment of elderly cancer patients. *Crit Rev Oncol Hematol* 64:10, 2007.
11. Ramesh HS, Pope D, Gennari R, et al: Optimising surgical management of elderly cancer patients. *World J Surg Oncol* 3:17, 2005.
12. Loran DB, Zwischenberger JB, et al: Thoracic surgery in the elderly. *J Amer Coll Surg* 199:773, 2004.
13. Jaklitsch MT, et al: Thoracoscopic surgery in elderly lung cancer patients. *Crit Rev Oncol Hematol* 49:169, 2004.
14. Ergina PL: Preoperative care of the elderly surgical patient. *World J Surg* 17:192, 1993.
15. Beck LH: Perioperative renal, fluid, and electrolyte management. *Clin Geriatr Med* 6:557, 1990.
16. Chen X, Xhao M, White PF, et al: The recovery of cognitive function after general anesthesia in elderly patients: a comparison of desflurane and sevoflurane. *Anesth Analg* 93:1489, 2001.
17. Rosenthal RA: Nutritional concerns in the older surgical patient. *J Am Coll Surg* 199:785, 2004.
18. Cerillo AG, Kodami AA, Solinas M, et al: Aortic valve surgery in the elderly patient: A retrospective review. *Interact Cardiovasc Thorac Surg* 6:308, 2007.
19. Srinivasan AK, Oo AY, Grayson AD, et al: Mid-term survival after cardiac surgery in elderly patients: Analysis of predictors for increased mortality. *Interact Cardiovasc Thorac Surg* 3:289, 2004.
20. Davis EA, Gardner TJ, Gillinov AM, et al: Valvular disease in the elderly: Influence on surgical results. *Ann Thorac Surg* 55:333, 1993.
21. Richmond TS, Kaunder D, Strumpf N, et al: Characteristics and outcomes of serious traumatic injury in older adults. *J Am Geriatr Soc* 50:215, 2002.
22. Aziz S, Grover FL: Cardiovascular surgery in the elderly. *Cardiol Clin* 17:213, 1999.
23. Fabrizii V, Winkelmayer WC, Klauser R, et al: Patient and graft survival in older kidney transplant recipients: Does age matter? *J Am Soc Nephrol* 15:1052, 2004.
24. Rao PS, Merion RM, Ashby VB, et al: Renal transplantation in elderly patients older than 70 years of age: Results from the Scientific Registry of Transplant Recipients. *Transplantation* 83:1069, 2007.
25. Andres A, Morales JM, et al: Double versus single renal allografts from aged donors. *Transplantation* 69:2060, 2000.
26. Giordano SH, Hortobagyi GN, Kau SC, et al: Breast cancer treatment guidelines in older women. *J Clin Oncol* 23: 783, 2005.
27. Hoekstra HJ: Cancer surgery in the elderly. *Eur J Cancer* 37:S235, 2001.
28. Dellapasqua S, Colleoni M, Castiglione M, et al: New criteria for selecting elderly patients for breast cancer adjuvant treatment studies. *Oncologist* 12:952, 2007.
29. Scalliet P, Kirkove C: Breast cancer in elderly women: Can radiotherapy be omitted? *Eur J Cancer* 43:2264, 2007.
30. Gennari R: Breast cancer in elderly women. Optimizing the treatment. *Breast Cancer Res Treat* 110:199, 2008.
31. Yood MU, Owusu C, Buist DSM, et al: Mortality impact of less than standard treatment in older breast cancer patients. *J Amer Coll Surg* 206:66, 2008.
32. Wildiers H, Kunkler I, Biganzoli L, et al: Management of breast cancer in elderly individuals: Recommendations of the International Society of Geriatric Oncology. *Lancet Oncol* 8:1101, 2007.
33. Tan E, Tilney H, Thompson M, et al: The United Kingdom National Bowel Cancer Project: Epidemiology and surgical risk in the elderly. *Eur J Cancer* 43:2285, 2007.
34. Amemiya T, Oda K, Ando M, et al: Activities of daily living and quality of life of elderly patients after elective surgery for gastric and colorectal cancers. *Ann Surg* 246:222, 2007.
35. Chang GJ, Skibber JM, Feig BW: Are we undertreating rectal cancer in the elderly? *Ann Surg* 246:215, 2007.
36. McCahill LE, Krouse RS, Chu DZ, et al: Decision making in palliative surgery. *J Am Coll Surg* 195:411, 2002.
37. Kahi CJ, et al: Survival of elderly persons undergoing colonoscopy: Implications for colorectal cancer screening and surveillance. *Gastrointest Endosc* 66:544, 2007.
38. Mery CM, Pappas AN, Bueno R et al: Similar long-term survival of elderly patients with non-small cell lung cancer treated with lobectomy or wedge resection within the surveillance, epidemiology and end results database. *Chest* 28:237, 2005.
39. Cattaneo SM, Park BJ, Wilton AS, et al: Use of video-assisted thoracic surgery for lobectomy in the elderly results in fewer complications. *Ann Thoracic Surg* 85:231, 2008.
40. Richmond TS, Kaunder D, et al: Characteristics and outcomes of serious traumatic injuries in older adults. *J Am Geriatr Soc* 50:215, 2002.
41. Rubenstein LZ, Josephson KR: The epidemiology of falls and syncope. *Clin Geriatr Med* 18:141, 2002.
42. Chang TT, Schecter WP: Injury in the elderly and end-of-life decisions. *Surg Clin North Am* 87:229, 2007.
43. Stewart BT, Stitz RW, Lumley JW: Laparoscopically assisted colorectal surgery in the elderly. *Br J Surg* 86:938, 1999.
44. Ballista-Lopez C, Cid JA, Poves I, et al: Laparoscopic surgery in the elderly patient: Experience of a single laparoscopic unit. *Surg Endosc* 17:333, 2003.
45. Rosenthal RA, Zenilman ME, Katlic MR (eds): *Principles and Practice of Geriatric Surgery*. New York: Springer-Verlag, 2001.
46. Biebl M, Lau LL, Hakaim AG, et al: Midterm outcomes of endovascular abdominal aortic aneurysm repair in octogenarians: A single institution's experience. *J Vasc Surg* 40:435, 2004.
47. Morales JP, Irani FG, Junes KG, et al: Endovascular repair of a ruptured aortic aneurysm under local anesthesia. *Brit J Radiol* 78:62, 2005.
48. McConahey WM, Hay ID, Wodner LB, et al: Papillary thyroid cancer treated at the Mayo Clinic, 1946–1970: Initial manifestations, pathologic findings, therapy and outcome. *Mayo Clin Proc* 61:978, 1986.
49. Mueller-Gaertner H, Brzac HT, Rehpenning W: Prognostic indices for tumor relapse and tumor mortality in follicular thyroid carcinoma. *Cancer* 67:1903, 1991.
50. Har-El G, Sidi J, Segal K, et al: Thyroid cancer in patients 70 years of age or older. *Ann Otol Rhinol Laryngol* 96:403, 1987.
51. Irvin GL, Carneiro DM: "Limited" parathyroidectomy in geriatric patients. *Ann Surg* 233:612, 2001.
52. Sheldon DG, Lee FT, Neil NJ, et al: Surgical treatment of hyperparathyroidism improves health related quality of life. *Arch Surg* 137:1022, 2002.
53. Consensus Development Conference Panel: NIH conference. Diagnosis and management of asymptomatic primary hyperparathyroidism: Consensus development conference statement. *Ann Intern Med* 114:593, 1991.
54. Sullivan DJ, Hansen-Flaschen J: Termination of life support after major trauma. *Surg Clin North Am* 80:1055, 2000.
55. Hinshaw DB, Carnahan JM, Johnson DL: Depression, anxiety, and asthenia in advanced illness. *J Am Coll Surg* 195:271, 2002.
56. Dunn GP, Milch RA, Mosenthal AC, et al: Palliative care by the surgeon. *J Am Coll Surg* 194:509, 2002.
57. Conner SR: *Hospice: Practice, Pitfalls and Promise*. Washington: Taylor and Francis, 1988.
58. Sheehan DC, Forman WB: *Hospice and Palliative Care Concepts and Practice*. Boston: Jones and Bartlett, 1996.
59. Breen CM, Abernethy AP, Abbott KM, et al: Conflict associated with decisions to limit life-sustaining treatment in intensive care units. *J Gen Intern Med* 16:283, 2001.

CHAPTER 47

Anesthesia of the Surgical Patient

Robert S. Dorian

TRUE COLLABORATION

The discipline of anesthesia embodies control of three great concerns of humankind: consciousness, pain, and movement. The field of anesthesiology combines the administration of anesthesia with the perioperative management of the patient's concerns, pain management, and critical illness. The fields of surgery and anesthesiology are truly collaborative and continue to evolve together, enabling the care of sicker patients and rapid recovery from outpatient and minimally invasive procedures.

BRIEF HISTORY OF ANESTHESIA

The discovery of anesthesia is one of the seminal American contributions to the world. Along with infection control and blood transfusion, anesthesia has enabled surgery to occupy its fundamental place in medicine. Before the advent of modern anesthesia in the 1840s, many substances and methods were tried in the search for pain relief and better operating conditions. Opium, alcohol, exposure to cold, compression of peripheral nerves, constriction of the carotid arteries to produce unconsciousness, and hypnosis (mesmerism) all proved less than satisfactory and dictated rapid and crude surgical procedures. Patients had to be restrained by several attendants, and only the most stoic could tolerate the screams heard in the operating theater. Charles Darwin, who witnessed two such operations, "rushed away before they were completed. Nor did I ever attend again, for hardly any inducement would have been strong enough to make me do so; this being long before the blessed days of chloroform. The two cases fairly haunted me for many a long year."[1]

Modern Beginnings

In 1842, Crawford Long (1815–1878), a physician in rural Georgia, used diethyl ether to induce surgical anesthesia for the removal of two small neck tumors. Diethyl ether had been known for over 800 years but was not used for analgesic purposes. It became an inexpensive and popular recreational drug in the mid-nineteenth century and was used by American medical students at "ether frolics." Although Long did experiments to verify the analgesic effects of ether, he did not publish his work until 1848, in the *Southern Medical Journal*, too late to be the unquestioned discoverer of anesthesia.[2]

Although Humphrey Davy (1778–1829) suggested using nitrous oxide for the relief of pain in surgical procedures in 1800, this was not pursued until 1844 by dentist Horace Wells (1815–1848). Wells astutely observed that a man who was injured after inhaling nitrous oxide during an exhibition of the "laughing gas" displayed no awareness of pain. After experimenting on himself, Wells attempted to demonstrate the analgesic effects of nitrous oxide for a dental procedure at Harvard Medical School in 1845. The public demonstration was a failure because nitrous oxide has analgesic properties but does not suffice as the sole anesthetic agent in every patient. Wells never recovered from his humiliating experience and eventually committed suicide. But he does hold a place in history as the

first person to recognize and use the only anesthetic from the 1800s that is still in use today—nitrous oxide.

Ether Day

William Morton (1819–1868) was a dentist and partner of Horace Wells. After taking a course in anesthesia from Wells, Morton left the partnership in Hartford, Conn, and established himself in Boston. He continued his interest in anesthesia, but with diethyl ether replacing nitrous oxide. Ether proved a good choice, as it supports respiration and the cardiovascular system at analgesic levels and is potent enough to administer in room air without hypoxia. He practiced the administration of ether on a dog and then used it when extracting teeth from patients in his office. On October 16, 1846, Morton gave the first public demonstration of ether as an anesthetic for Johns Collins Warren, distinguished surgeon and a founder of Massachusetts General Hospital. In attendance in the surgical amphitheater were several surgeons, medical students, and a newspaper reporter. After anesthesia was induced using a makeshift inhaler, Warren successfully removed a vascular mass from the patient's neck with no ill effects. Warren was an originator of the *Boston Medical and Surgical Journal* (now *The New England Journal of Medicine*), and by November 1846, the demonstration was published in an article by Henry J. Bigelow.[3] The stature of Warren and Bigelow lent considerable credence to the advent of surgical anesthesia; as news spread rapidly, surgeons around the world were quick to adopt this "American invention." Massachusetts General Hospital has restored and preserved the original amphitheater where the demonstration took place, now called the *Ether Dome*. It is designated as a Registered National Historic Landmark commemorating the first public demonstration, rather than discovery, of the use of ether as an anesthetic.

The First Anesthesiologists

John Snow (1813–1858) made science out of the art of anesthesia. He was a respected London physician who applied a scholarly, scientific method to investigate the clinical properties and pharmacology of ether, chloroform, and other anesthetic agents. Snow was an astute observer and published a detailed account of the five degrees of etherization in 1847. He vastly improved the apparatus for administering ether and mastered the clinical techniques of anesthetizing patients. As the leading anesthetist of his day, he gave anesthetics to the royal family, including chloroform during labor to Queen Victoria for the birth of Prince Leopold. The Queen's endorsement of "that blessed chloroform" removed the moral and social stigma against relieving pain during childbirth and brought

KEY POINTS

1. The incremental interchange of ideas across the specialties of anesthesia and surgery demonstrates the collaborative nature of science in general, and medicine in particular. Many surgeons contributed to the growth in anesthesia; more comprehensive anesthesia, in turn, allowed more complex surgery to develop.

2. The role of the anesthesiologist has expanded to become the perioperative physician. The anesthesiologist evaluates the patient preoperatively, provides the anesthetic, and is involved in postoperative pain relief.

3. The specialties of critical care medicine and pain medicine have grown out of the expanded field of

anesthesiology. The postanesthesia care unit gave rise to the intensive care unit; the treatment of acute and chronic pain syndromes by anesthesiologists contributed to the growth of pain medicine as a specialty.

4. New and improved airway and intubation devices, such as the laryngeal mask airway and the video laryngoscope, along with the American Society of Anesthesiologists' airway management algorithm, have led to improved management and control of routine and difficult airways.

5. The study of proteomics will lead to anesthetics tailored to individuals, maximizing effects and reducing side effects of various anesthetic drugs.

anesthesia into public awareness. Chloroform, popularized in England by James Simpson (1811–1870), had a narrow therapeutic index and placed great clinical demands on the anesthetist. Ether, with its ability to maintain the cardiovascular and respiratory systems, remained in common use in the United States and often was administered by house staff, medical students, or nurses. Snow encouraged the administration of anesthesia by a physician and felt that a physician dedicated specifically to that purpose was appropriate and necessary. Snow and other exceptional British physicians specializing in anesthesia [Joseph Clover (1825–1882) and Sir Frederick Hewitt (1857–1916)] created a standard of excellence in the latter half of the nineteenth century. This atmosphere of professionalism led to the formation of anesthesia societies and the publication of papers in the prestigious *British Medical Journal and Lancet* in England years before such organizations existed in America.[4]

Cocaine: The First Local Anesthetic

The ancient Incas chewed coca leaves as a stimulant and may have been aware of its local anesthetic properties, allegedly facilitating trephination of the skull by chewing a clump of coca leaves and dripping the resultant saliva into the wound. The active alkaloid of the coca leaf was synthesized in 1860 and called *cocaine* by German chemist Albert Niemann, who noted that it "benumbs the nerves of the tongue, depriving it of feeling."[5] Sigmund Freud (1856–1939) of Vienna received a supply of cocaine from Merck, studied its properties, and wrote the famous monograph "Uber Coca" in 1884. Freud was primarily interested in the stimulant and euphoric effects of cocaine and attempted to use it to treat morphine addiction. Freud and Karl Koller (1857–1944), an ophthalmologic intern, began to perform physiologic experiments with cocaine, measuring its effects on muscle strength. Although they both noted that the drug caused numbness of the tongue when swallowed, it was Koller who first instilled it into his own cornea; report of its use as a local anesthetic galvanized the medical world. Soon after, young American surgeons William Halsted (1852–1922) and Richard Hall described intradermal injection of cocaine and were the first to use it for regional blocks of the facial nerves, brachial plexus, and the internal pudendal and posterior tibial nerves.[6] Halstead later became the first professor of surgery and chief surgeon at Johns Hopkins University, where he remained for >30 years. One of the founding fathers of modern surgery, he pioneered radical mastectomy with lymphadenectomy and the use of rubber gloves. While experimenting on themselves, Halstead and other early researchers became addicted to cocaine.[7] Its toxic effects were the stimulus to find other local anesthetics—procaine was synthesized in 1905 and lidocaine in 1943.

The New York neurologist Leonard Corning (1855–1923) observed the regional blocks of Halstead and Hall, analytically studied local anesthesia effects on dogs, applied his knowledge to humans, and published the first textbook on local anesthesia in 1886. After experimenting on the spinal nerves of a dog, he intradurally injected a solution of cocaine into a patient, called it *spinal anesthesia*, and commented that it might be useful in surgery. His suggestion went unheeded for >10 years, until August Bier (1861–1949), a prominent German surgeon, gave the first deliberate spinal anesthetic.[8] This incremental interchange of ideas and advances across the Atlantic and across the specialties of anesthesia and surgery demonstrates the collaborative nature of science in general, and medicine in particular. The development of surgery and anesthesia exemplify the dichotomy of two fledgling specialties that are mutually dependent, yet increasingly autonomous.

Twentieth Century

Developments in anesthesia on both sides of the Atlantic progressed rapidly in the twentieth century. The convergence of technologies that produced the hollow needle and syringe, coupled with the synthesis of barbiturates, gave rise to IV anesthesia in the early 1900s. Barbital, followed by hexobarbital and thiopental in 1934, produced rapid and more pleasant induction of anesthesia than the inhaled gases. The concept of "balanced anesthesia" began in 1925, when John Lundy (1894–1973) proposed the use of thiopentone for induction, followed by inhaled agents for maintenance of anesthesia. Lundy directed the department of anesthesiology at the Mayo Clinic for 28 years. He established the first recovery room and blood bank, authored the first textbook on modern anesthesia, and helped found the American Board of Anesthesiology.

Nitrous oxide, diethyl ether, and chloroform, all discovered fortuitously by observation, remained the dominant inhalation agents until the accidental discovery of cyclopropane's anesthetic properties in 1923. Although rapid acting and pleasant smelling, cyclopropane was limited by its flammability and cardiac irritability. Because it was known that fluorination would reduce or eliminate flammability of chemical compounds, British chemist Charles Suckling set out to synthesize an anesthetic that was stable, potent, volatile, and not flammable. He successfully produced halothane in 1953. Introduced into clinical practice in 1956 after extensive testing in Manchester, England, and paired with an accurate calibrated vaporizer, halothane quickly became the most widely used fluorinated anesthetic. Enflurane and isoflurane, synthesized in the United States by Ross Tyrell, were introduced into clinical practice in 1972 and 1981, respectively. The newest agents, desflurane and sevoflurane, were introduced into clinical practice in the early 1990s. They possess a low solubility and are characterized by rapid onset and recovery, making them particularly well suited to outpatient surgery.

The motto of the American Society of Anesthesiologists (ASA) is "vigilance," and to that end, there has been continued progress in objective mechanical measurement of patient well-being. The early anesthesiologists used clinical signs such as patient color, depth of respiration, and pulse rate to monitor depth of anesthesia and patient well-being. Harvey Cushing, who eventually became Moseley Professor of Surgery at the Peter Bent Brigham Hospital, began the first anesthesia records or "ether charts" in 1895 while a medical student. They recorded pulse, respiratory rates, pupillary diameter, and the amounts of ether and other drugs administered. He later introduced the use of the portable sphygmomanometer of Riva-Rocci to measure blood pressure, and the precordial stethoscope to monitor breath and heart sounds. Monitoring has since progressed to its current state with incremental developments in electrocardiography, pulse oximetry, and mass spectrometry, all mandatory for the safe administration of any anesthetic.

The control of the patient's airway and respiration as the purview of the anesthesiologist evolved with techniques of endotracheal intubation as pioneered by Sir Ivan Magill (1888–1986), and the invention of the cuffed endotracheal tube by Arthur Guedel (1883–1965). This later merged with the invention of mechanical ventilation and its introduction to the operating room as the embodiment of today's anesthesia machine. It was this expertise at control of respiration that paved the way for the most revolutionary modern development in anesthesia—the use of muscle relaxants. Curare, a nondepolarizing muscle relaxant, was popularized by Harold Griffith of Montreal. His report of the successful use of curare was a galvanizing event that revolutionized the practice of anesthesia, as the relaxation of abdominal muscles could be controlled to facilitate surgery.[9] The depolarizing relaxant succinylcholine was introduced in 1949, and research has continued to provide the newer nondepolarizing drugs mivacurium, pancuronium, rocuronium, atracurium, and cisatracurium.

Anesthesiology Today— The Perioperative Physician

The specialty of anesthesia is no longer limited to the operating room. It is natural that anesthesiology, born out of the quest to relieve pain, gave rise to the field of acute and chronic pain medicine. The anesthesiologist consulting on the acute pain service may recommend oral, IM, or IV analgesia with a variety of agents, or patient-controlled analgesia. Postsurgical patients also may be treated with nerve blocks: regional (e.g., brachial plexus, popliteal, and femoral) or neuraxial (epidural or intrathecal). The discipline of chronic pain addresses patients who suffer for months or years with cancer or other debilitating diseases. Treatment modalities escalate from orally administered drugs, to diagnostic and therapeutic nerve blocks, to more invasive measures like dorsal column nerve stimulators, and radiofrequency or cryosurgical nerve ablation.

Daily management of the airway, fluids and transfusions, ventilation, drug delivery, monitoring, and caring for the sickest patients in the postanesthesia care unit prepared anesthesiologists to become major contributors to the development of critical care medicine. Out of the 28 founding members of the Society of Critical Medicine, 10 were anesthesiologists.[10]

The American Board of Anesthesiology became an independent board in 1941, and since then, has granted board certification to >25,000 diplomates. Certificates in Anesthesia Pain Management and Anesthesia Critical Care Medicine are granted to those completing additional postgraduate training. The ASA has >35,000 members, and its official journal, *Anesthesiology*, has a monthly circulation of 40,000 worldwide.

BASIC PHARMACOLOGY

Pharmacokinetics

Pharmacokinetics or the *time dependency* of a drug describes the relationship between the dose of a drug and its plasma or tissue concentration. It is what the body does to the drug. It relates to absorption, distribution, metabolism, and elimination. The route of administration, metabolism, protein binding, and tissue distribution all affect the pharmacokinetics of a particular drug.

Administration, Distribution, Metabolism, and Elimination

Administration of a drug affects its pharmacokinetics, as there will be different rates of drug entry into the circulation. For example, the oral and IV routes are subject to first-pass effect of the portal circulation; this can be bypassed with the nasal or sublingual route. Other routes of drug administration include transdermal, intramuscular, subcutaneous, or inhalation.

Distribution is the delivery of a drug from the systemic circulation to the tissues. Once a drug has entered the systemic circulation, the rate at which it will enter the tissues depends on several factors:

Molecular size of the drug, capillary permeability, polarity, and lipid solubility. Small molecules will pass more freely and quickly across cell membranes than large ones, but capillary permeability is variable and results in different diffusion rates. Renal glomerular capillaries are permeable to almost all non–protein-bound drugs; capillaries in the brain are fused (i.e., they have tight junctions) and are relatively impermeable to all but the tiniest molecules (the blood-brain barrier). Un-ionized molecules pass more easily across cell membranes than charged molecules; diffusibility also increases with increasing lipid solubility.

Plasma protein and tissue binding. Many drugs bind to circulating proteins like albumin, glycoproteins, and globulins. Disease, age, and the presence of other drugs will affect the amount of protein binding; drug distribution is affected because only the unbound free portion of the drug can pass across the cell membrane. Drugs also bind reversibly to body tissues; if they bind with high affinity, they are said to be sequestered in that tissue (e.g., heavy metals are sequestered in bone).[11]

The fluid volume in which a drug distributes is termed the *volume of distribution* (Vd). This mathematically derived value gives a rough estimation of the overall physical distribution of a drug in the body. A general rule for volume distribution is that the greater the Vd, the greater the diffusibility of the drug. Because drugs have variable ionization rates and bind differently to plasma proteins and tissues, the Vd is not a good predictor of the actual concentration of the drug after administration.

Determining the apparent Vd (dose/concentration) is an attempt to more accurately ascertain the drug dose administered and its final concentration.

Metabolism is the permanent breakdown of original compounds into smaller metabolites. Drug elimination varies widely; some drugs are excreted unchanged by the body, some decompose via plasma enzymes, and some are degraded by organ-based enzymes in the liver. Many drugs rely on multiple pathways for elimination (i.e., metabolized by liver enzymes then excreted by the kidney). When a drug is given orally, it reaches the liver via the portal circulation and is partially metabolized before reaching the systemic circulation. This is why an oral dose of a drug often must be much higher than an equally effective IV dose. Some drugs (e.g., nitroglycerine) are hydrolyzed presystemically in the gut wall and must be administered sublingually to achieve an effective concentration.

It is important to remember that the response to drugs varies widely. The disposition of drugs is affected by age; weight; sex; pregnancy; disease states; and the concomitant use of alcohol, tobacco, and other licit and illicit drugs. Genetic polymorphism, or variations in genes which cause differing drug effects, is another explanation of varying drug response. This will be discussed later in the Future Direction of Anesthesia section on proteomics. This as yet unpredictable response to drugs underscores the importance of the most important monitor in the operating room—the anesthesiologist, who continuously assesses the patient's vital signs and adjusts the doses of anesthetic agents to match the surgical stimulus.

Pharmacodynamics

Pharmacodynamics, or how the plasma concentration of a drug translates into its effect on the body, depends on biologic variability, receptor physiology, and clinical evaluations of the actual drug. It is what the drug does to the body. An *agonist* is a drug that causes a response. A *full agonist* produces the full tissue response, and a *partial agonist* provokes less than the maximum response induced by a full agonist. An antagonist is a drug that does not provoke a response itself, but blocks agonist-mediated responses. An *additive effect* means that a second drug acts with the first drug and will produce an effect that is equal to the algebraic summation of both drugs. A *synergistic effect* means that two drugs interact to produce an effect that is greater than expected from the two drugs' algebraic summation.[12]

Hyporeactivity means a larger than expected dose is required to produce a response, and this effect is termed *tolerance, desensitization*, or *tachyphylaxis*. Tolerance usually results from chronic drug exposure, either through enzyme induction (e.g., alcohol) or depletion of neurotransmitters (e.g., cocaine).

Potency, Efficacy, Lethal Dose, and Therapeutic Index

The *potency* of a drug is the dose required to produce a given effect, such as pain relief or a change in heart rate. The average sensitivity to a particular drug can be expressed through the calculation of the effective dose; ED_{50} would have the desired effect in 50% of the general population. The *efficacy* of any therapeutic agent is its power to produce a desired effect. Two drugs may have the same efficacy but different potencies. The difference in potency of the two drugs is described by the ratio $ED_{50}b/ED_{50}a$, where *a* is the less potent drug. If the $ED_{50}b$ equals 4 and the $ED_{50}a$ equals 0.4, then drug *a* is 10 times as potent as drug *b*. For example, 10 mg of morphine produces analgesia equal to that of 1 mg of hydromorphone. They are equally effective, but hydromorphone is 10 times as potent as morphine.

Dose-response curves show the relationship between the dose of a drug administered (or the resulting plasma concentration) and the pharmacologic effect of the drug. The pharmacologic effect might be secretion of a hormone, a change in heart rate, or contraction of a muscle. Between 20 and 80% of the maximum effect, the logarithm of the dose and its response has a linear relationship. The

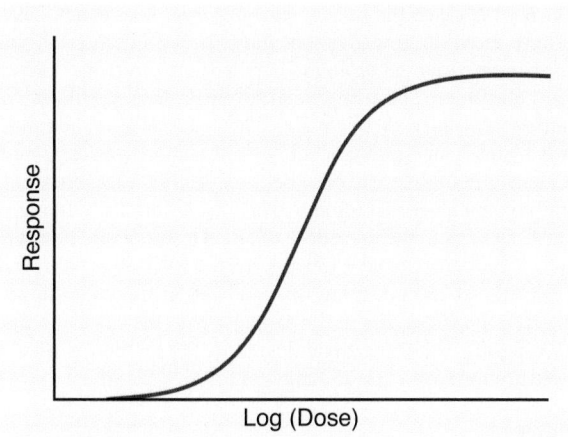

FIG. 47-1. Basic dose-response curve.

term *dose* only applies to the amount administered and not the actual concentration. If the concentration of an antagonist is increased (in the presence of a fixed concentration of agonist), the dose-response curve will be shifted to the right, and a higher agonist concentration will be required to achieve the desired effect. A basic dose-response curve is shown in Fig. 47-1.

The *lethal dose* (LD_{50}) of a drug produces death in 50% of animals to which it is given. The ratio of the lethal dose and effective dose, LD_{50}/ED_{50}, is the *therapeutic index*. A drug with a high therapeutic index is safer than a drug with a low or narrow therapeutic index.

ANESTHETIC AGENTS

Anesthesia can be *local*, *regional*, or *general* (Table 47-1). Local anesthesia is accomplished using a local anesthetic drug that can be injected intradermally and is used for the removal of small lesions or to repair traumatic injuries. Local anesthesia is the most frequent anesthetic administered by surgeons and may be accompanied by IV sedation to improve patient comfort.

Local Anesthetics

Local anesthetics are divided into two groups based on their chemical structure: the amides and the esters. In general, the amides are metabolized in the liver and the esters are metabolized by plasma cholinesterases, which yield metabolites with slightly higher allergic potential than the amides (Table 47-2).

Amides

Lidocaine, bupivacaine, mepivacaine, prilocaine, and ropivacaine have in common an amide linkage between a benzene ring and a hydrocarbon chain that, in turn, is attached to a tertiary amine. The benzene ring confers lipid solubility for penetration of nerve membranes, and the tertiary amine attached to the hydrocarbon chain makes these local anesthetics water soluble. Lidocaine has a more rapid onset and is shorter acting than bupivacaine; however, both are widely used for tissue infiltration, regional nerve blocks, and spinal and epidural anesthesia. Ropivacaine is the most recently introduced local anesthetic. It is clinically similar to bupivacaine in that it has a slow onset and a long duration, but is less cardiotoxic. All amides are 95% metabolized in the liver, with 5% excreted unchanged by the kidneys.

TABLE 47-1	Anesthetic agents, their actions, and their clinical uses					
Effect	**Monitor**	**IV Drugs**	**Potent Gases**	**Weak Gases**	**Local Anesthetics**	
Unconsciousness Amnesia Anxiolysis	Electroencephalogram Clinical signs	Benzodiazepines Midazolam Diazepam Lorazepam Barbiturates Propofol Etomidate Ketamine[a]	Sevoflurane Desflurane Isoflurane Enflurane Halothane	Nitrous oxide	—[c]	
Analgesia	Heart rate Blood pressure Respiratory rate Clinical signs	Opioids Morphine Meperidine Hydromorphone Fentanyl NSAIDs Ketorolac Parecoxib	Sevoflurane Desflurane Isoflurane Enflurane Halothane	Nitrous oxide	Amides Lidocaine Bupivacaine Mepivacaine Prilocaine Ropivacaine Regional peripheral nerve blocks	Esters Cocaine Procaine Chloroprocaine Tetracaine Benzocaine
Muscle relaxation Paralysis	Nerve stimulator Tidal volume Hand grip 5-second head lift Clinical signs	Depolarizing agent Succinylcholine Nondepolarizing agents Pancuronium Vecuronium Rocuronium Atracurium *Cis*-atracurium Mivacurium	Sevoflurane Desflurane Isoflurane Enflurane Halothane	—[b]	Brachial plexus Sciatic Femoral Cervical plexus Regional central nerve blocks Spinal Epidural	

[a]Note that the IV agents are quite specific in their effects, except for ketamine, which has both amnestic and analgesic qualities.
[b]The potent inhalational anesthetics contribute to all three components of anesthesia, but nitrous oxide has weak amnestic and analgesic properties and provides no muscle relaxation at all.
[c]The local anesthetics produce excellent analgesia and muscle relaxation, but contribute nothing to amnesia or anxiolysis; these anesthetics must be supplemented with an IV sedative. General anesthesia entails all three elements of anesthesia (amnesia, analgesic, and muscle relaxation).

TABLE 47-2	Biologic properties of commonly used local anesthetics		

Agent	Equianesthetic Concentration (%)	Approximate Anesthetic Duration (min)	Site of Metabolism
Esters			
Procaine	2	50	Plasma
Chloroprocaine	2	45	Plasma
Tetracaine	0.25	175	Plasma
Amides			
Prilocaine	1	100	Liver/lung
Lidocaine	1	100	Liver
Mepivacaine	1	100	Liver
Bupivacaine	0.25	175	Liver
Ropivacaine	0.3	150	Liver
Etidocaine	0.25	200	Liver

Source: Reproduced with permission from Mather LE, Tucker GT: Properties, absorption, and disposition of local anesthetic agents, in Cousins MJ, Bridenbaugh PO (eds): *Cousins and Bridenbaugh's Neural Blockade in Clinical Anesthesia and Pain Medicine*, 4th ed. Philadelphia: Lippincott Williams & Wilkins, 2009, p 49.

Esters

Cocaine, procaine, chloroprocaine, tetracaine, and benzocaine have an ester linkage in place of the amide linkage mentioned above in the Amides section. Unique among local anesthetics, cocaine occurs in nature, was the first used clinically, produces vasoconstriction [making it useful for topical application (e.g., for intranasal surgery)], releases norepinephrine from nerve terminals resulting in hypertension, and is highly addictive. Cocaine is a Schedule II drug. Procaine, synthesized in 1905 as a nontoxic substitute for cocaine, has a short duration and is used for infiltration. Tetracaine has a long duration and is useful as a spinal anesthetic for lengthy operations. Benzocaine is for topical use only. The esters are hydrolyzed in the blood by pseudocholinesterase. Some of the metabolites have a greater allergic potential than the metabolites of the amide anesthetics, but true allergies to local anesthetics are rare.

The common characteristic of all local anesthetics is a reversible block of the transmission of neural impulses when placed on or near a nerve membrane. Local anesthetics block nerve conduction by stabilizing sodium channels in their closed state, preventing action potentials from propagating along the nerve. The individual local anesthetic agents have different recovery times based on lipid solubility and tissue binding, but return of neural function is spontaneous as the drug is metabolized or removed from the nerve by the vascular system.

Toxicity of local anesthetics results from absorption into the bloodstream or from inadvertent direct intravascular injection. Toxicity manifests first in the more sensitive central nervous system (CNS), and then the cardiovascular system.

Central Nervous System

As plasma concentration of local anesthetic rises, symptoms progress from restlessness to complaints of tinnitus. Slurred speech, seizures, and unconsciousness follow. Cessation of the seizure via administration of a benzodiazepine or thiopental and maintenance of the airway is the immediate treatment. If the seizure persists, the trachea must be intubated with a cuffed endotracheal tube to guard against pulmonary aspiration of stomach contents.

Cardiovascular System

With increasingly elevated plasma levels of local anesthetics, progression to hypotension, increased P-R intervals, bradycardia, and cardiac arrest may occur. Bupivacaine is more cardiotoxic than other local anesthetics. It has a direct effect on ventricular muscle, and because it is more lipid soluble than lidocaine, it binds tightly to sodium

channels (it is called the *fast-in, slow-out local anesthetic*). Patients who have received an inadvertent intravascular injection of bupivacaine have experienced profound hypotension, ventricular tachycardia and fibrillation, and complete atrioventricular heart block that is extremely refractory to treatment. The toxic dose of lidocaine is approximately 5 mg/kg; that of bupivacaine is approximately 3 mg/kg.

Calculation of the toxic dose before injection is imperative. It is helpful to remember that for any drug or solution, 1% = 10 mg/mL. For a 50-kg person, the toxic dose of bupivacaine would be approximately 3 mg/kg, or $3 \times 50 = 150$ mg. A 0.5% solution of bupivacaine is 5 mg/mL, so 150 mL/5 mg/mL = 30 mL as the upper limit for infiltration. For lidocaine in the same patient, the calculation is 50 kg × 5 mg/mL = 250 mg toxic dose. If a 1% solution is used, the allowed amount would be 250 mg/10 mg/mL = 25 mL.

Additives

Epinephrine has one physiologic and several clinical effects when added to local anesthetics. Epinephrine is a vasoconstrictor, and by reducing local bleeding, molecules of the local anesthetic remain in proximity to the nerve for a longer time period. Onset of the nerve block is faster, the quality of the block is improved, the duration is longer, and less local anesthetic will be absorbed into the bloodstream, thereby reducing toxicity. Although epinephrine 1:200,000 (5 μg/mL) added to a local anesthetic for infiltration will greatly lengthen the time of analgesia, epinephrine-containing solutions should not be injected into body parts with end-arteries, such as toes or fingers, as vasoconstriction may lead to ischemia or loss of a digit. When added to the local anesthetic, sodium bicarbonate will raise the pH, favoring the non-ionized uncharged form of the molecule. This speeds the onset of the block, especially in local anesthetics that are mixed with epinephrine. The pH of such solutions is around 4.5; therefore, the addition of sodium bicarbonate results in a relatively large increase in pH.[13]

Regional Anesthesia

Peripheral

Local anesthetic can be injected *peripherally*, near a large nerve or plexus, to provide anesthesia to a larger region of the body. Examples include the brachial plexus for surgery of the arm or hand, blockade of the femoral and sciatic nerves for surgery of the lower extremity, ankle block for surgery of the foot or toes, intercostal block for analgesia of the thorax postoperatively, or blockade of the cervical plexus, which is ideal for carotid endarterectomy. Risks of peripheral regional nerve blocks are dependent on their location. For example, nerve blocks injected into the neck risk puncture of the carotid or vertebral arteries, intercostal nerves are in close proximity to the vascular bundle and have a high rate of absorption of local anesthetic, and nerve blocks of the thorax run the risk of causing pneumothorax. All peripheral nerve blocks may be supplemented intraoperatively with IV sedation and/or analgesics.

Central

Local anesthetic injected *centrally* near the spinal cord—spinal or epidural anesthesia—provides anesthesia for the lower half of the body. This is especially useful for genitourinary, gynecologic, inguinal hernia, or lower-extremity procedures. Spinal and epidural anesthesia block the spinal nerves as they exit the spinal cord. Spinal nerves are mixed nerves; they contain motor, sensory, and sympathetic components. The subsequent block will cause sensory anesthesia, loss of motor function, and blockade of the sympathetic nerves from the level of the anesthetic distally to the lower extremities. Subsequent vasodilation of the vasculature from sympathetic block may result in hypotension, which is treatable with IV fluids and/or pressors.

Spinal Anesthesia

Local anesthetic is injected directly into the dural sac surrounding the spinal cord. The level of injection is usually below L1 to L2, where the spinal cord ends in most adults. Because the local anesthetic is injected directly into the cerebrospinal fluid surrounding the spinal cord, only a small dose is needed, the onset of anesthesia is rapid, and the blockade thorough. Lidocaine, bupivacaine, and tetracaine are commonly used agents of differing durations; the block wears off naturally via drug uptake by the cerebrospinal fluid, bloodstream, or diffusion into fat. Epinephrine as an additive to the local anesthetic will significantly prolong the blockade.

Possible complications include hypotension, especially if the patient is not adequately prehydrated; high spinal block requires immediate airway management; and postdural puncture headache sometimes occurs. Spinal headache is related to the diameter and configuration of the spinal needle, and can be reduced to approximately 1% with the use of a small 25- or 27-gauge needle.

Cauda equina syndrome is injury to the nerves emanating distal to the spinal cord resulting in bowel and bladder dysfunction, and lower-extremity sensory and motor loss. It has mainly been seen in cases in which indwelling spinal microcatheters and high (5%) concentrations of lidocaine were used. Indwelling spinal catheters are no longer used.

Epidural Anesthesia

Epidural anesthesia could also be called *extradural anesthesia*, because local anesthetics are injected into the epidural space surrounding the dural sac of the spinal cord. Much greater volumes of anesthetic are required than with spinal anesthesia, and the onset of the block is longer—10 to 15 minutes. As in spinal anesthesia, local anesthetic bathes the spinal nerves as they exit the dura; the patient achieves analgesia from the sensory block, muscle relaxation from blockade of the motor nerves, and hypotension from blockade of the sympathetic nerves as they exit the spinal cord. Note that regional anesthesia, whether peripheral or central, provides only two of the three major components of anesthesia—analgesia and muscle relaxation. Anxiolysis, amnesia, or sedation must be attained by supplemental IV administration of other drugs (e.g., the benzodiazepines or propofol infusion).

Complications are similar to those of spinal anesthesia. Inadvertent injection of local anesthetic into a dural tear will result in a high block, manifesting as unconsciousness, severe hypotension, and respiratory paralysis requiring immediate aggressive hemodynamic management and control of the airway. Indwelling catheters are often placed through introducers into the epidural space, allowing an intermittent or continuous technique, as opposed to the single-shot method of spinal anesthesia. By necessity, the epidural-introducing needles are of a much larger diameter (17- or 18-gauge) than spinal needles, and accidental dural puncture more often results in a severe headache that may last up to 10 days if left untreated.

General Anesthesia

General anesthesia describes a triad of three major and separate effects: unconsciousness (and amnesia), analgesia, and muscle relaxation (see Table 47-1). IV drugs usually produce a single, discrete effect, while most inhaled anesthetics produce elements of all three. General anesthesia is achieved with a combination of IV and inhaled drugs, each used to its maximum benefit. The science and art of anesthesia is a dynamic process. As the amount of stimulus to the patient changes during surgery, the patient's vital signs are used as a guide and the quantity of drugs is adjusted, maintaining an equilibrium between stimulus and dose. General anesthesia is what patients commonly think of when they are to be "put under," and can be a cause of considerable preoperative anxiety.[14]

Intravenous Agents

Unconsciousness and Amnesia The IV agents that produce unconsciousness and amnesia are frequently used for the induction of general anesthesia. They include barbiturates, benzodiazepines, propofol, etomidate, and ketamine. Except for ketamine, the following agents have no analgesic properties, nor do they cause paralysis or muscle relaxation.

Barbiturates The most common barbiturates are thiopental, thiamylal, and methohexital. The mechanism of action is at the γ-aminobutyric acid (GABA) receptor, where they inhibit excitatory synaptic transmission. They produce a rapid, smooth induction within 60 seconds, and wear off in about 5 minutes. In higher doses and in patients with intravascular depletion, they cause hypotension and myocardial depression. The barbiturates are anticonvulsants and protect the brain during neurosurgery by reducing cerebral metabolism.

Propofol Propofol is an alkylated phenol that inhibits synaptic transmission through its effects at the GABA receptor. With a short duration, rapid recovery, and low incidence of nausea and vomiting, it has emerged as the agent of choice for ambulatory and minor general surgery. Additionally, propofol has bronchodilatory properties that make its use attractive in asthmatic patients and smokers. Propofol may cause hypotension, and should be used cautiously in patients with suspected hypovolemia and/or coronary artery disease (CAD), the latter of which may not tolerate a sudden drop in blood pressure. It can be used as a continuous infusion for sedation in the intensive care unit setting. Propofol is an irritant and frequently causes pain on injection.

Benzodiazepines The most important uses of the benzodiazepines are for reduction of anxiety and to produce amnesia. Frequently used IV benzodiazepines are diazepam, lorazepam, and midazolam. They all inhibit synaptic transmission at the GABA receptor, but have differing durations of action. The benzodiazepines can produce peripheral vasodilatation and hypotension, but have minimal effects on respiration when used alone. They must be used with caution when given with opioids; a synergistic reaction causing respiratory depression is common. The benzodiazepines are excellent anticonvulsants and only rarely cause allergic reactions.

Etomidate Etomidate is an imidazole derivative used for IV induction. Its rapid and almost complete hydrolysis to inactive metabolites results in rapid awakening. Like the above IV agents, etomidate acts on the GABA receptor. It has little effect on cardiac output and heart rate, and induction doses usually produce less reduction in blood pressure than that seen with thiopental or propofol. Etomidate is associated with pain on injection and more nausea and vomiting than thiopental or propofol.

Ketamine Ketamine differs from the above IV agents in that it produces analgesia as well as amnesia. Its principal action is on the *N*-methyl-D-aspartate receptor; it has no action on the GABA receptor. It is a dissociative anesthetic, producing a cataleptic gaze with nystagmus. Patients may associate this with delirium and hallucinations while regaining consciousness. The addition of benzodiazepines has been shown to prevent these side effects. Ketamine can increase heart rate and blood pressure, which may cause myocardial ischemia in patients with CAD. Ketamine is useful in acutely hypovolemic patients to maintain blood pressure via sympathetic stimulation, but is a direct myocardial depressant in patients who are catecholamine depleted. Ketamine is a bronchodilator, making it useful for asthmatic patients, and rarely is associated with allergic reactions.

Analgesia

The IV analgesics most frequently used in anesthesia today have little effect on consciousness, amnesia, or muscle relaxation. The most important class is the *opioids*, so called because they were first isolated from opium, with morphine, codeine, meperidine, hydromorphone, and the fentanyl family being the most common. The most important *nonopioid* analgesics are ketamine (discussed above in the Ketamine section) and ketorolac, an IV NSAID.

Opioid Analgesics The commonly used opioids—morphine, codeine, oxymorphone, meperidine, and the fentanyl-based compounds—act centrally on μ-receptors in the brain and spinal cord. The main side effects of opioids are euphoria, sedation, constipation, and respiratory depression, which also are mediated by the same μ-receptors in a dose-dependent fashion. Although opioids have differing potencies required for effective analgesia, *equianalgesic doses of opioids result in equal degrees of respiratory depression.* Thus, there is no completely safe opioid analgesic. The synthetic opioids fentanyl, and its analogues sufentanil, alfentanil, and remifentanil, are commonly used in the operating room. They differ pharmacokinetically in their lipid solubility, tissue binding, and elimination profiles, and therefore have differing potencies and durations of action. Remifentanil is remarkable in that it undergoes rapid hydrolysis that is unaffected by sex, age, weight, or renal or hepatic function, even after prolonged infusion. Recovery is within minutes, but there is little residual postoperative analgesia.

Naloxone and the longer-acting naltrexone are pure opioid *antagonists.* They can be used to reverse the side effects of opioid overdose (e.g., respiratory depression), but the analgesic effects of the opioid also will be reversed.

Nonopioid Analgesics *Ketamine*, an *N*-methyl-D-aspartate receptor antagonist, is a potent analgesic, but is one of the few IV agents that also causes significant sedation and amnesia. Unlike the μ-receptor agonists, ketamine supports respiration. It can be used in combination with opioids, but the dysphoric effects must be masked with the simultaneous use of sedatives, usually a benzodiazepine like midazolam.

Ketorolac is a parenteral NSAID that produces analgesia by reducing prostaglandin formation via inhibition of the enzyme cyclooxygenase (COX). Intraoperative use of ketorolac reduces postoperative need for opioids. Two forms of COX have been identified: COX-1 is responsible for the synthesis of several prostaglandins as well as prostacyclin, which protects gastric mucosa, and thromboxane, which supports platelet function. COX-2 is induced by inflammatory reactions to produce more prostaglandins. Ketorolac (as well as many oral NSAIDs, aspirin, and indomethacin) inhibits both COX-1 and COX-2, which causes the major side effects of gastric bleeding, platelet dysfunction, and hepatic and renal damage. Parecoxib is a parenteral COX-2 NSAID now being tested that would presumably produce analgesia and reduce inflammation without causing GI bleeding or platelet dysfunction.

Neuromuscular Blocking Agents

Neuromuscular blocking agents have no amnestic, hypnotic, or analgesic properties; patients must be properly anesthetized *before* and *in addition to* the administration of these agents. A paralyzed but unsedated patient will be aware, conscious, and in pain, yet be unable to communicate their predicament. Inappropriate administration of a neuromuscular blocking agent to an awake patient is one of the most traumatic experiences imaginable. Neuromuscular blockade is not a substitute for adequate anesthesia, but is rather an adjunct to the anesthetic. Depth of neuromuscular blockade is best monitored with a nerve stimulator to ensure patient immobility intraoperatively, and to confirm a lack of residual paralysis postoperatively.[15]

Unlike the local anesthetics, which affect the ability of nerves to conduct impulses, the neuromuscular blockers have no effect on either nerves or muscles, but act primarily on the *neuromuscular junction.*

There is one commonly used *depolarizing* neuromuscular blocker—succinylcholine. This agent binds to acetylcholine receptors on the postjunctional membrane in the neuromuscular junction and causes depolarization of muscle fibers.

Although the rapid onset (<60 seconds) and rapid offset (5 to 8 minutes) make succinylcholine ideal for management of the airway in certain situations, total body muscle fasciculations can cause postoperative aches and pains, an elevation in serum potassium levels, and an increase in intraocular and intragastric pressure. Its use in patients with burns or traumatic tissue injuries may result in a high enough rise in serum potassium levels to produce arrhythmias and cardiac arrest. Unlike other neuromuscular blocking agents, the

effects of succinylcholine cannot be reversed. Succinylcholine is rapidly hydrolyzed by plasma cholinesterase, also referred to as *pseudocholinesterase.* There are many reasons for a patient to have low pseudocholinesterase levels, such as liver disease, concomitant use of other drugs, pregnancy, and cancer. These factors are usually not clinically problematic, delaying return of motor function only by several minutes. Some patients have a genetic disorder manifesting as atypical plasma cholinesterase; the atypical enzyme has less-than-normal activity, and/or the patient has extremely low levels of the enzyme. The incidence of the homozygous form is approximately one in 3000; the effects of a single dose of succinylcholine may last several hours instead of several minutes. Treatment is to keep the patient sedated and unaware he or she is paralyzed, continue mechanical ventilation, test the return of motor function with a peripheral nerve stimulator, and extubate the patient only after he or she has fully regained motor strength. Two separate blood tests must be drawn: *pseudocholinesterase level* to determine the amount of enzyme present, and *dibucaine number*, which indicates the quality of the enzyme. Patients with laboratory-confirmed abnormal pseudocholinesterase levels and/or dibucaine numbers should be counseled to avoid succinylcholine as well as mivacurium, which is also hydrolyzed by pseudocholinesterase. First-degree family members should also be tested. Succinylcholine is the only IV triggering agent of malignant hyperthermia (MH) (discussed below in the Malignant Hyperthermia section).

There are several competitive *nondepolarizing* agents available for clinical use. The longest acting is *pancuronium*, which is excreted almost completely unchanged by the kidney. Intermediate-duration neuromuscular blockers include *vecuronium* and *rocuronium*, which are metabolized by both the kidneys and liver, and *atracurium* and cis-*atracurium*, which undergo breakdown in plasma known as *Hofmann elimination.* The agent with shortest duration is *mivacurium*, the only nondepolarizer that is metabolized by plasma cholinesterase, and like succinylcholine, is subject to the same prolonged blockade in patients with plasma cholinesterase deficiency. All nondepolarizers reversibly bind to the postsynaptic terminal in the neuromuscular junction and prevent acetylcholine from depolarizing the muscle. Muscle blockade occurs without fasciculation and without the subsequent side effects seen with succinylcholine. The most commonly used agents of this type and their advantages and disadvantages are listed in Table 47-3.

The reversal of neuromuscular blockade is not a true reversal of the drug, as with protamine reversal of heparinized patients. Neuromuscular blocking reversal agents, usually neostigmine, edrophonium, or pyridostigmine, increase acetylcholine levels by inhibiting acetylcholinesterase, the enzyme that breaks down acetylcholine. The subsequently increased circulating levels of acetylcholine pre-

---

TABLE 47-3 Advantages and disadvantages to common nondepolarizing neuromuscular blocking agents

Agent	Duration (h)	Advantages	Disadvantages
Pancuronium	>1	No histamine release	Tachycardia; slow onset; long duration
Vecuronium	<1	No cardiovascular effects	Intermediate onset
Rocuronium	<1	Fast onset; no cardiovascular effects	—
Mivacurium	<1	Fast onset; short duration & histamine release	—

Source: Adapted with permission from Rutter TW, Tremper KK: Anesthesiology and pain management, in Greenfield LJ (ed): *Greenfield's Surgery: Scientific Principles and Practice*, 4th ed. Philadelphia: Lippincott & Williams, 2006, p 452.

TABLE 47-4	Advantages and disadvantages of common inhalational agents		
Agent	**MAC (%)**	**Advantages**	**Disadvantages**
Nitrous oxide	105	Analgesia; minimal cardiac and respiratory depression	Sympathetic stimulation; expansion of closed air space
Halothane	0.75	Effective in low concentrations; minimal airway irritability; inexpensive	Cardiac depression and arrhythmia hepatic necrosis; slow elimination
Enflurane	1.68	Muscle relaxation No effect on cardiac rate or rhythm	Strong smell; seizures
Isoflurane	1.15	Muscle relaxation; no effect on cardiac rate or rhythm	Strong smell
Desflurane	6	Rapid induction and emergence	Coughing; high cost
Sevoflurane	1.71	Rapid induction and emergence; pleasant smell; ideal for mask induction	High cost; metabolized by liver

MAC = minimum alveolar concentration.

Source: Adapted with permission from Rutter TW, Tremper KK: Anesthesiology and pain management, in Greenfield LJ (ed): *Greenfield's Surgery: Scientific Principles and Practice*, 4th ed. Philadelphia: Lippincott & Williams, 2006, p 450.

vail in the competition for the postsynaptic receptor, and motor function returns. Use of the peripheral nerve stimulator is required to follow depth and reversal of motor blockade, but it is essential to correlate data from the nerve stimulator with clinical signs that indicate return of motor function, including tidal volume, vital capacity, hand grip, and 5-second sustained head lift.

Inhalational Agents

Unlike the IV agents, the inhalational agents provide all three characteristics of general anesthesia: unconsciousness, analgesia, and muscle relaxation. However, it would be impractical to use an inhalation-only technique in larger surgical procedures, because the doses required would cause unacceptable side effects, so IV adjuncts such as opioid analgesics and neuromuscular blockers are added to optimize the anesthetic. All inhaled anesthetics display a dose-dependent reduction in mean arterial blood pressure except for nitrous oxide, which maintains or slightly raises the blood pressure. Nitrous oxide, although not potent enough to use alone, provides partial anesthesia and allows a second agent to be used in smaller doses, reducing side effects.

Minimum alveolar concentration (MAC) is a measure of anesthetic potency. It is the ED_{50} of an inhaled agent (i.e., the dose required to block a response to a painful stimulus in 50% of subjects). The higher the MAC, the less potent an agent is. The potency and speed of induction of inhaled agents correlates with their lipid solubility and is known as the *Meyer-Overton rule*. Nitrous oxide has a low solubility and is a weak anesthetic agent, but has the most rapid onset and offset. The "potent" gases (e.g., desflurane, sevoflurane, enflurane, and halothane) are more soluble in blood than nitrous oxide and can be given in lower concentrations, but have longer induction and emergence characteristics.

Sevoflurane and desflurane are the two most recently introduced inhalational agents in common use. Because of their relatively lower tissue and blood solubility, induction and recovery are more rapid than with isoflurane or enflurane.

All of the potent inhalational agents (e.g., halothane, isoflurane, enflurane, sevoflurane, and desflurane), as well as the depolarizing agent succinylcholine, are triggering agents for MH. Table 47-4 lists the advantages and disadvantages of each agent.

ANESTHESIA MANAGEMENT

Preoperative Evaluation and Preparation

The ASA has adopted basic standards for the evaluation of patients before surgery. These standards require the anesthesiologist to determine the medical status of the patient by developing a plan of anesthetic care and to discuss this plan with the patient and/or legal guardian.

The preoperative visit results in a summary of all pertinent findings, including a detailed medical history, current drug therapy, complete physical examination, and laboratory and specific testing results. Based on these findings, the anesthesiologist may find that the patient is not in optimal medical condition to undergo elective surgery. These findings and opinions are then discussed with the patient's primary physician, and the surgery may be delayed or cancelled until the patient's medical condition is further tested and optimized.

The detailed medical history obtained at the preoperative visit should include the patient's previous exposure and experience with anesthesia, as well as any family history of problems with anesthesia. History of atopy (medication, foods, or environmental) is an important aspect of this evaluation in that it may predispose patients to form antibodies against antigens that may be represented by agents administered during the perioperative period. A careful review of major organ systems and their function also should be performed.

The physical examination is targeted primarily at the CNS, cardiovascular system, lungs, and upper airway. Specific areas to investigate are shown in Table 47-5.

Concurrent medications must be fully explored, and adverse interactions with agents administered during the perioperative period need to be considered. However, concurrent medications that produce desired effects (i.e., beta blockade, antihypertensive, and antiasthma medications) can and should be continued throughout the perioperative period; patients should be counseled to continue these medications up to and including the morning of surgery. Careful documentation will allow the anesthesiologist to make informed decisions about the perioperative selection of drugs and therapy as well as monitoring techniques.

Preoperative laboratory data and specific testing for elective surgery should be patient- and situation-specific. Examples include: serum potassium for a patient on diuretics, glucose in a diabetic

TABLE 47-5	Preoperative physical examination		
Central Nervous System	**Cardiovascular System**	**Respiratory System**	**Oral Airway**
Consciousness; neurocognition; peripheral sensory	Blood pressure; standing and sitting, bilateral; peripheral pulses; heart auscultation; heart rate; murmur; rhythm	Auscultation of lungs; wheezes; rales	Cervical spine mobility; visualize uvula; artificial teeth; thyromental distance

TABLE 47-6	American Society of Anesthesiologists physical status classification system
P1	A normal healthy patient
P2	A patient with mild systemic disease
P3	A patient with severe systemic disease
P4	A patient with severe systemic disease that is a constant threat to life
P5	A moribund patient who is not expected to survive without the operation
P6	A declared brain-dead patient whose organs are being removed for donor purposes

TABLE 47-7	American Society of Anesthesiologists physical status and mortality

Score	Mortality (%)
P1	0.1
P2	0.2
P3	1.8
P4	7.8
P5	9.4

Source: Reproduced with permission from Aitkenhead AR, Rowbotham D, Smith G (eds): *Textbook of Anesthesia*, 4th ed. Churchill Livingstone, 2001, p 288.

patient, or hemoglobin concentration in any surgery with a high risk of blood loss. Coagulation tests are not necessary if the patient is not receiving anticoagulants or has no signs or symptoms of abnormal clotting. Otherwise healthy patients usually do not need preoperative laboratory testing, and tests performed within the previous 6 months are usually sufficient.[16] Other tests that should be generated by history and physical examination include chest radiograph if there is evidence of chest disease, and pulmonary function tests in patients who are morbidly obese, severe asthmatics, or patients undergoing pulmonary resection surgery. An electrocardiogram should be performed in all symptomatic patients, and in asymptomatic men age 45 years or older and asymptomatic women age 50 years or older. Urine pregnancy testing should be performed on the day of surgery in all women of childbearing age.

Risk Assessment

An integral part of the preoperative visit is for the anesthesiologist to assess patient risk. Risk assessment encompasses two major questions: (a) Is the patient in optimal medical condition for surgery? and (b) Are the anticipated benefits of surgery greater than the surgical and anesthetic risks associated with the procedure?

Research into quantifying preoperative factors that correlate with the development of postoperative morbidity and mortality has recently gained great interest. Originally designed as a simple classification of a patient's physical status immediately before surgery, the ASA physical status scale is one of the few prospective scales that correlate with the risk of anesthesia and surgery (Table 47-6).

Criticism of the ASA scale is primarily due to its exclusion of age and difficulty of intubation (discussed later in this chapter). Cullen and associates examined 1095 patients undergoing total hip replacement, prostatectomy, or cholecystectomy, and found that both age and ASA scale accurately predicts postoperative morbidity and mortality[17] (Table 47-7). The ASA scale remains useful and should be applied to all patients during the preoperative visit.

Evaluation of the Airway

The airway examination is an effort to identify those patients in whom management of the airway and conventional endotracheal intubation may be difficult. It is vitally important to recognize such patients before administering medications that induce apnea.

Mallampati Classification

The amount of the posterior pharynx one can visualize preoperatively is important and correlates with the difficulty of intubation. A large tongue (relative to the size of the mouth) that also interferes with visualization of the larynx on laryngoscopy will obscure visualization of the pharynx. The Mallampati classification (Fig. 47-2, Table 47-8) is based on the structures visualized with maximal mouth opening and tongue protrusion in the sitting position.

Other predictors of difficult intubation include obesity, immobility of the neck, interincisor distance <4 cm in an adult, a large overbite, or the inability to shift the lower incisors in front of the upper incisors. The thyromental distance [i.e., the distance from the thyroid cartilage to the mentum (tip of the chin)] should be >6.5 to 7 cm.

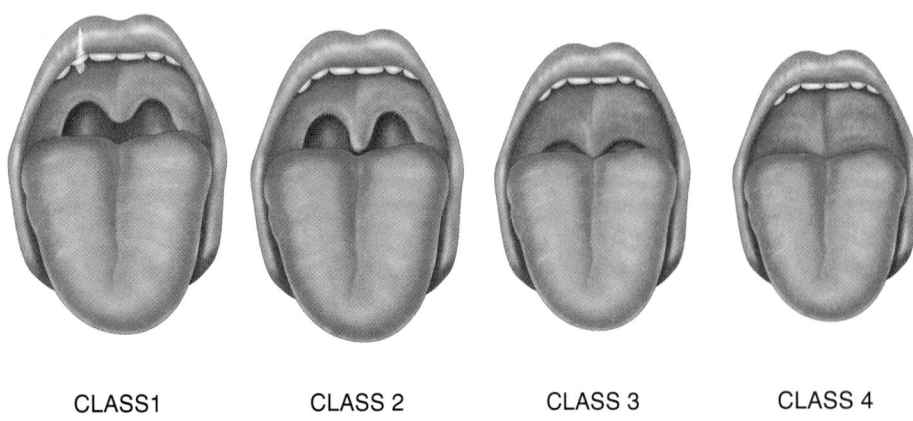

CLASS 1   CLASS 2   CLASS 3   CLASS 4

MALLAMPATI CLASSIFICATION

CLASS 1: Soft palate, fauces, uvula, pillars
CLASS 2: Soft palate, fauces, portion of uvula
CLASS 3: Soft palate, base of uvula
CLASS 4: Hard palate only

FIG. 47-2. The Mallampati classification.

TABLE 47-8	Mallampati classification

Class I: soft palate, fauces, uvula, pillars
Class II: soft palate, fauces, portion of uvula
Class III: soft palate, base of uvula
Class IV: hard palate only

Consideration of Patients with Comorbidities

A thorough knowledge of the pathophysiology of concurrent medical conditions regardless of the reason for surgery is essential for optimal perioperative care. Optimal anesthesia extends beyond pharmacology and technical procedures. Specifically, ischemic heart disease, renal dysfunction, pulmonary disease, metabolic and endocrine disorders, CNS diseases, and diseases of the liver and biliary tract can have major impact on the management of anesthesia.

Ischemic Heart Disease

Ischemic heart disease is the result of the heart demanding more oxygen (O_2) than its supply can provide. A supply problem may be due to many factors, including hypoxia, anemia, hypotension and coronary artery atherosclerosis, thrombosis, or spasm. Additionally, the problem may be an increase in myocardial O_2 demand (tachycardia). In the vast majority of cases, the most responsible lesion is a reduction in the luminal area of coronary arteries due to atherosclerosis.

An estimated 14 million people in the United States have ischemic heart disease. Of these, as many as 4 million have few or no symptoms and are unaware that they are at risk for angina pectoris, myocardial infarction, or sudden death.

An important goal of the preoperative visit is for the anesthesiologist to ascertain the patient's severity, progression, and functional limitations induced by ischemic heart disease. Furthermore, this visit can elucidate the possibility of previously undiagnosed ischemic heart disease. A thorough investigation of risk factors for ischemic heart disease is essential during the preoperative visit. The risk of perioperative death due to myocardial infarction in patients without ischemic heart disease is approximately 1%.[18] In contrast, the risk in patients with known or suspected ischemic heart disease is approximately 3%,[18] and in patients undergoing surgery for peripheral vascular disease, the combined risk of death due to cardiac causes is 29%.[19]

Major Risk Factors for Coronary Artery Disease

The risk of *hypercholesterolemia* is proportional to the increased serum level of low-density lipoprotein cholesterol. Reduction achieved via decreased dietary fat or pharmacotherapy reduces risk.

Hyperlipidemia may be familial, and thus may account for the fact that a strong family history of premature CAD is a significant risk factor. High-density lipoprotein cholesterol is protective.

Although definitely a risk factor, hypertension alone probably does not cause plaques. Rather, it may act synergistically with hypercholesterolemia by first causing mechanical wall stress and damage.

Smoking causes endothelial damage, and therefore promotes plaque thrombosis. Cessation greatly reduces the risk of CAD.

Diabetes mellitus is a strong independent risk factor. A hypothesis is that glycosylation products cause release of growth factors that stimulate smooth muscle proliferation.

Other Risk Factors

Hyperhomocysteinemia is becoming an established independent risk factor, but is still under evaluation. Reduction of levels by folate therapy may be beneficial.

Advanced age, male sex, obesity, and a sedentary lifestyle can also put a person at risk for developing ischemic heart disease.[20]

Drugs used for the medical management of patients with ischemic heart disease should be continued throughout the perioperative period. Withdrawal of an antihypertensive drug or suspension of beta blockade can induce unwanted increases in sympathetic nervous system activity.[12]

Induction of anesthesia in patients with ischemic heart disease can be safely accomplished with a number of IV drugs. As many as 45% of patients have been shown to have myocardial ischemia during the stress of tracheal intubation, and direct laryngoscopy should be used for the shortest time possible to minimize the magnitude of stimulation.[21]

The intraoperative anesthetic technique should allow for the prompt control of hemodynamic variables; the maintenance of the balance between myocardial O_2 delivery and myocardial O_2 demand is probably the single most important factor in managing patients with ischemic heart disease. In this regard, muscle relaxants with minimal to no effects on heart rate and blood pressure, such as vecuronium and rocuronium, are attractive choices for neuromuscular blockade. Additionally, controlled myocardial depression using a volatile anesthetic in patients with a normal left ventricular ejection fraction may help to minimize the stimulation of the sympathetic nervous system and subsequent increases in myocardial O_2 requirements. In patients with impaired left ventricular function, continued myocardial depression with volatile anesthetics may not be tolerated; the addition of short-acting opioids such as fentanyl is beneficial. In cardiac surgical patients, it is not uncommon for high-dose opioids to be used as the predominant anesthetic.

Pulmonary Disease

Chronic pulmonary disease has developed into a worldwide public health problem. Chronic obstructive pulmonary disease (COPD), distinguished from asthma that is characterized by reversible airway smooth muscle constriction, is a progressive disease that leads to the destruction of the lung parenchyma.

Infection, noxious particles, and gases can exacerbate COPD. Historically, certain lung function parameters (i.e., significantly abnormal spirometry or arterial blood gas analysis) were once considered contraindications for anesthesia. However, anesthetic techniques have improved, and it has been shown that patients with severe lung disease can safely undergo anesthesia.[22] Zollinger and Pasch found no specific parameters of lung function that were predictive of postoperative lung complications. The highest predictive parameter found was upper abdominal surgery and thoracic surgery.[23]

General anesthesia can be performed safely in patients with pulmonary disease.[24] Inhaled anesthetics are often used due to their bronchodilating properties.[25] Some authors have advocated pretreatment with salbutamol, a long-acting beta agonist, which may prevent bronchoconstriction during anesthetic induction.[26,27]

Regional and local anesthesia have the benefit of avoiding tracheal irritation and stimulating bronchospasm. However, patients with COPD may become hypoxic while lying strictly supine, and sensory levels of anesthetic above T10 are associated with the impairment of respiratory muscle activity necessary for patients with COPD to maintain adequate ventilation.[12]

Intraoperatively, mechanical ventilation using a slow breathing rate (at eight breaths per minute) should be used to allow for passive exhalation in the presence of increased airway resistance. This slow breathing, facilitated by high inspiratory flow rate, may allow for improved maintenance of normal partial pressure of arterial oxygen (PaO_2) and partial pressure of arterial carbon dioxide (CO_2) levels. Patients should also be well hydrated during the procedure with adequate crystalloid/colloid volume therapy, which may allow for less viscous pulmonary secretions following surgery.

Renal Disease

Five percent of the adult population may have pre-existing renal disease that could contribute to perioperative morbidity.[28] In addition, the risk of acute renal failure is increased by certain events or patient characteristics independent of pre-existing renal disease, such as hypovolemia and obstructive vascular disease. Ischemic tubular damage (i.e., acute tubular necrosis) is the most likely cause of acute renal failure in the perioperative period, reflecting events that cause an imbalance of O_2 supply to O_2 demand in the medullary ascending tubular cells.

Virtually all anesthetic drugs and techniques are associated with decreases in renal blood flow, the glomerular filtration rate, and urine output, reflecting multiple mechanisms such as decreased cardiac output, altered autonomic nervous system activity, neuroendocrine changes, and positive pressure ventilation. Renal blood flow (15 to 25% of the cardiac output) far exceeds renal O_2 needs, but ensures optimal clearance of wastes and drugs. Prehydration and the depth of anesthesia may influence the renal response to anesthesia.

Management of anesthesia in patients with chronic renal disease requires attention to intraoperative fluid management and tight control of ventilation, as respiratory alkalosis will shift the oxyhemoglobin dissociation curve, and respiratory acidosis could raise serum potassium to dangerous levels. Because of decreased excretion by the kidney, doses of opioids and neuromuscular blocking agents must be attenuated.

Hepatobiliary Disease

Management of anesthesia for the patient with liver disease requires an understanding of the many physiologic functions of the liver: synthesis of albumin and coagulation factors, metabolism of drugs, glucose homeostasis, and the production of bilirubin. Data from the 1970s suggested that approximately 1 in every 700 adult patients who are scheduled for elective surgical procedures has unknown liver disease or is in the prodromal phase of viral hepatitis. Severe hepatic necrosis following surgery and anesthesia is most often due to decreased hepatic O_2 delivery rather than the anesthetic.

Regional anesthesia may be useful in patients with advanced liver disease, assuming coagulation status is acceptable. When general anesthesia is selected, administration of modest doses of volatile anesthetics with or without nitrous oxide or fentanyl often is recommended. Selection of nondepolarizing muscle relaxants should consider clearance mechanisms for these drugs. For example, patients with hepatic cirrhosis may be hypersensitive to mivacurium because of the lowered plasma cholinesterase activity. Perfusion to the liver is maintained by administering fluids (guided by filling pressures) and maintaining adequate systemic pressure and cardiac output.

The coexisting presence of liver disease may influence the selection of volatile anesthetics. Halothane is the anesthetic most studied regarding possible hepatotoxicity. Halothane hepatitis occurs rarely (approximately 1:25,000 patients) and may have an immune-mediated mechanism stimulated by repeated exposures to halothane.[29] Halothane, enflurane, isoflurane, and desflurane all yield a reactive oxidative trifluoroacetyl halide and may be cross-reactive, but the magnitude of metabolism of the volatile anesthetics is a probable factor in the ability to cause hepatitis.[30] Halothane is metabolized 20%, enflurane 2%, isoflurane 0.2%, and desflurane 0.02%; desflurane probably has the least potential for liver injury. Sevoflurane does not yield any trifluoroacetylated metabolites and is unlikely to cause hepatitis.

An estimated 15 to 20 million adults in the United States have biliary tract disease. Treatment of gallbladder disease by open or laparoscopic cholecystectomy is most often performed with general anesthesia supplemented with muscle relaxants. Complete biliary tract obstruction could interfere with the clearance of some muscle relaxants dependent on liver metabolism, such as vecuronium and pancuronium. Anesthetic considerations for laparoscopic cholecystectomy are similar to those for other laparoscopic procedures. Insufflation of the abdominal cavity with CO_2 results in increased intra-abdominal pressure that may interfere with the ease of ventilation and venous return. During laparoscopic cholecystectomy, placement of the patient in the reverse Trendelenburg position favors movement of abdominal contents away from the operative site and may improve ventilation. However, this position may further interfere with venous return and reduce cardiac output,

emphasizing the need to maintain intravascular fluid volume. Mechanical ventilation of the lungs is recommended to ensure adequate ventilation in the presence of increased intra-abdominal pressure and to offset the effects of systemic absorption of CO_2 used during insufflation of the abdominal cavity. High intra-abdominal pressure may increase the risk of passive reflux of gastric contents. Tracheal intubation with a cuffed tube is advised to minimize the risk of pulmonary aspiration.

Metabolic and Endocrine Disease

Metabolic and endocrine disorders encompass a wide range of diseases. These diseases may be the primary reason for surgery or can exist in patients requiring surgery for other unrelated disorders. Preoperative evaluation of endocrine function consists of relevant medical history, glucose or protein in the urine, vital signs, history of fluctuations in body weight, survey of sexual function, and concomitant medications. The three metabolic and endocrine conditions that are most prevalent in patients undergoing surgery are diabetes mellitus, hypothyroidism, and obesity. The prevalence of all three conditions, either alone or in combination, in the general population has been steadily rising throughout the world for the past 20 to 30 years.[12,31] The aging population and changes in the diagnostic criteria for diabetes mellitus are sure to continue this trend.[12,32]

Patients with diabetes are at an increased risk for perioperative myocardial ischemia, stroke, renal dysfunction or failure, and increased mortality.[33] Increased wound infections and impairment of wound healing also is associated with the pre-existence of diabetes in patients undergoing surgery.[34]

The stress response to surgery is associated with hyperglycemia in nondiabetic patients due to increased secretion of catabolic hormones, and a combination of reduced insulin secretion and increased insulin resistance.[35,36] Improved glycemic control in diabetic patients undergoing major surgery has been shown to improve perioperative morbidity and mortality; avoidance of hypoglycemia and hyperglycemic events is the standard of care in these patients.[32,37–39]

Anesthetic techniques in the diabetic patient can modulate the secretion of catabolic hormones.[40] However, regional anesthesia may carry greater risks to the diabetic patient with autonomic neuropathy, and the hypotension associated with regional anesthesia may be deleterious to the diabetic patient with co-existing CAD.[32] There is no evidence that regional anesthesia or general anesthesia, either alone or in combination, offers any benefit to the diabetic surgical patient in terms of morbidity or mortality.[32]

Hypothyroidism is a deficiency in the secretion of the thyroid hormones, thyroxine and 3,5',3-triiodothyronine, by the thyroid gland. More than 5 million Americans have this common medical condition, and as many as 10% of women may have some degree of thyroid hormone deficiency. Controlled clinical trials have not shown an increase in risk when patients with mild to moderate hypothyroidism undergo surgery.[41] Nevertheless, close monitoring of these patients for adverse effects of anesthesia, including delayed gastric emptying, adrenal insufficiency, and hypovolemia, is warranted.[42]

The prevalence of significant obesity continues to rise both in developed and developing countries and is associated with an increased incidence of a wide spectrum of medical and surgical pathologies[43] (Table 47-9). In the United States, one-third of people have a body weight more than 20% above their ideal weight.[44] Body mass index (BMI) is calculated by dividing the weight in kilograms by the square of the height in meters. In the United States, the prevalence of a BMI >25 kg/m^2 is 59.4% for men, 50.7% for women, and 54.9% for adults overall. Patients with a BMI >28 have increased perioperative morbidity over the general population.

Anesthetic management of the obese patient is problematic, and tasks such as establishing IV access, applying monitoring equipment, managing the airway, and transporting the patient are more difficult. Ventilation may be a particular problem because of obstructive sleep apnea or because obesity itself imposes a restrictive ventilatory state with decreased expiratory reserve and vital capac-

TABLE 47-9	Disease conditions associated with obesity
Category	**Examples**
Cardiovascular disease	Sudden death, cardiomyopathy, hypertension, coronary artery disease, peripheral vascular disease
Respiratory disease	Restrictive lung disease, sleep apnea
Endocrine disease	Diabetes mellitus, hypothyroidism
GI disease	Hernia, gallstones
Malignancy	Breast, prostate, colorectal cancer
Musculoskeletal	Osteoarthritis, back pain

Source: Reproduced with permission from Adams JP, Murphy PG: Obesity in anaesthesia and intensive care. *Br J Anaesth* 85:91, 2000. By permission of Oxford University Press.

ity.[12] Induction of anesthesia is particularly challenging in the obese patient, as there is increased risk of pulmonary aspiration, and the increased mass of soft tissue about the head and neck make establishing and maintaining a patent airway difficult.

The impact of obesity on the pharmacokinetics of anesthetic drugs is variable. For example, blood volume is often increased in obese patients, which can decrease predicted concentrations of drugs, but adipose tissue has low blood flow, which could elevate blood concentrations of these agents. It is prudent to calculate the first dose of anesthetic based on ideal body weight, and base subsequent dosages on the patient's responsiveness.[12,45]

Central Nervous System Disease

Diseases of the CNS present unique situations for the anesthesiologist and require an understanding of the relationship between intracranial pressure (ICP), cerebral blood flow (CBF), and cerebral metabolic rate of O_2 consumption ($CMRO_2$). Preoperative assessment of ICP is difficult, as symptoms of headache, nausea, and vomiting are nonspecific, and signs of retinal changes do not occur acutely. A midline shift on computed tomography scanning or magnetic resonance imaging may indicate an expanding lesion in the brain.

Provision of anesthesia for intracranial procedures must balance hemodynamic factors such as fluid volume, mean arterial pressure, ICP, and CBF. For intracranial tumors, the mass effect of the tumor makes control of ICP and CBF critical. In intracranial aneurysm surgery, the goal of the anesthetic is to prevent sudden increases in systemic blood pressure that could rupture the aneurysm, especially during the stress of laryngoscopy and endotracheal intubation.

The relationship between mean arterial pressure, ICP, and CBF is affected by pharmacologic agents. Inhalational agents in high concentrations (>0.6 MAC) cause dilation of the cerebral vasculature, decreasing cerebral vascular resistance. CBF is therefore increased in a dose-dependent fashion, despite decreases in $CMRO_2$.[12]

Propofol decreases CBF, ICP, and $CMRO_2$.[46] Propofol may also decrease systemic blood pressure, resulting in a decrease in cerebral perfusion pressure; however, propofol does not alter the autoregulation of CBF.[47] Etomidate is a potent cerebral vasoconstrictor that reduces CBF and ICP and should be used with caution in patients with epilepsy due to its excitatory effects seen on electroencephalograms.[48]

Opioids decrease CBF and may also decrease ICP under certain conditions. However, Sperry and associates have reported increases in ICP with the administration of fentanyl in head trauma patients.[49] Additionally, opioids have a depressant effect on consciousness and ventilation that may increase ICP if accompanied by an increase in partial pressure of arterial CO_2; opioids should be used with caution in head trauma patients.

Regardless of the drugs or technique selected, maintenance of stable hemodynamics is optimal. Recovery from anesthesia should be smooth, avoiding pain, coughing, and straining, all of which can increase blood pressure and ICP and cause bleeding at the surgical site.

Fluid therapy can increase cerebral edema and ICP when administered in large quantities, resulting in hypervolemia. Euvolemia should be the goal in head trauma patients, while hypervolemia may be beneficial for patients with intracranial aneurysms, to reduce vasospasm.

INTRAOPERATIVE MANAGEMENT

Induction of General Anesthesia

During induction of anesthesia, the patient becomes unconscious and rapidly apneic, myocardial function is usually depressed, and vascular tone abruptly changes. The induction of general anesthesia is the most critical component of practicing anesthesia, as the majority of catastrophic anesthetic complications occur during this phase. There are several different techniques used for the induction of general anesthesia, each with significant advantages and disadvantages (Fig. 47-3). Each patient must be carefully evaluated during the preoperative period to ensure that the most efficacious and safe technique is used.

IV induction, used primarily in adults, is smooth and is associated with a high level of patient satisfaction. The addition of opioids will blunt the response of laryngoscopy and intubation to avoid hypertension and tachycardia.

In a patient with a full stomach, the standard induction technique may result in vomiting and pulmonary aspiration of stomach contents. The goal of *rapid sequence induction* is to achieve secure protection of the airway with a cuffed endotracheal tube while preventing vomiting and aspiration.

Rapid sequence induction is performed as follows:

Proceed only after evaluation of the airway predicts an uncomplicated intubation.

Preoxygenate the patient.

Rapidly introduce an IV induction agent (e.g., propofol).

An assistant to the anesthesiologist presses firmly down on the cricoid cartilage to block any gastric contents from being regurgitated into the trachea, and

A muscle relaxant is injected, and the trachea is quickly intubated. The assistant is instructed not to release pressure on the cricoid cartilage until the cuff of the endotracheal tube is inflated and the position of the tube is confirmed.

Patients undergoing *inhalation induction* progress through three stages: (a) awake, (b) excitement, and (c) surgical level of anesthesia. Adult patients are not good candidates for this type of induction, as the smell of the inhalation agent is unpleasant and the excitement stage can last for several minutes, which may cause hypertension, tachycardia, laryngospasm, vomiting, and aspiration. Children, however, progress through stage 2 quickly and are highly motivated for inhalation induction as an alternative to the IV route. The benefit of postinduction IV cannulation is the avoidance of many presurgical anxieties, and inhalation induction is the most common technique for pediatric surgery.

Management of the Airway

After induction of anesthesia, the airway may be managed in several ways, including by face mask, with a laryngeal mask airway (LMA), or, most definitively, by endotracheal intubation with a cuffed endotracheal tube. Nasal and oral airways can help establish a patent airway in a patient being ventilated with a mask by creating an air passage behind the tongue (Fig. 47-4).

The LMA is a cuffed oral airway that sits in the oropharynx. It is passed blindly, and the cuff is inflated to push the soft tissues away from the laryngeal inlet. Because it does not pass through the vocal cords, it does not fully protect against aspiration. It should not be used in patients with a full stomach (Fig. 47-5; lower left).

The accurate placement of an endotracheal tube requires skill and proper equipment and conditions. Usually, the patient is unconscious and immobile (including paralysis of the muscles of respiration). Intubation is typically performed under direct visualization by looking through the mouth with a laryngoscope directly at the vocal cords

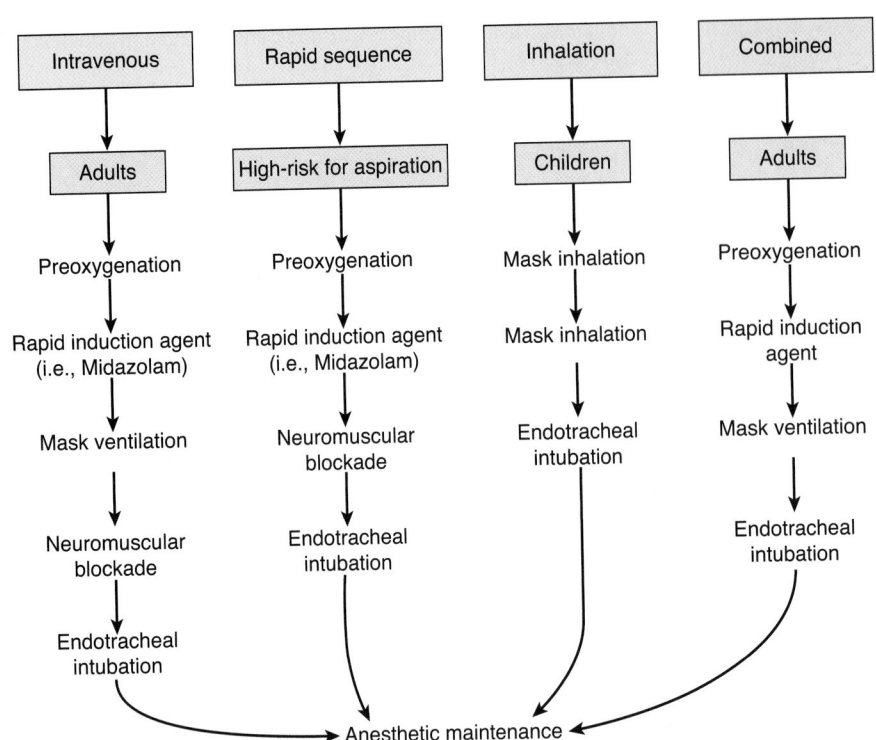

FIG. 47-3. Techniques for the induction of general anesthesia.

(direct laryngoscopy), and watching the endotracheal tube pass through the cords into the trachea. To obtain a direct line of sight, the patient is placed in the sniffing position. The neck is flexed at the lower cervical spine and extended at the atlanto-occipital joint. This flexion and extension are amplified during laryngoscopy. Laryngoscope handles contain batteries and can be fitted with curved (Macintosh) or straight (Miller) blades (see Fig. 47-5, top row).

Some patients have physical characteristics or a history suggesting difficulty in placing an endotracheal tube. A short neck, limited neck mobility, small interincisor distance, short thyromental distance, and Mallampati class IV may all represent a challenge to endotracheal intubation. Several devices have been developed to assist in management of the difficult airway. The Bullard rigid fiberoptic laryngoscope is a self-contained device that can be passed through a mouth with a narrow opening (Fig. 47-6). The head and

neck also can be kept in a neutral position, as a direct line of sight needed with a standard laryngoscope is not necessary. Another new intubating device is the Glide scope, which allows visualization of the vocal cords on a screen (Fig. 47-7).

The intubating laryngeal mask airway (ILMA) is an advanced form of LMA designed to maintain a patent airway as well as facilitate tracheal intubation with an endotracheal tube. The ILMA can be placed in anticipated or unexpectedly difficult airways as an airway rescue device and as a guide for intubating the trachea. An endotracheal tube can be passed blindly through the ILMA into the larynx, or the ILMA can be used as a conduit for a flexible fiberoptic scope (Fig. 47-8).

The flexible fiberoptic intubation scope is the gold standard for difficult intubation. It is indicated in difficult or compromised airways where neck extension is not desirable, or in cases with risk

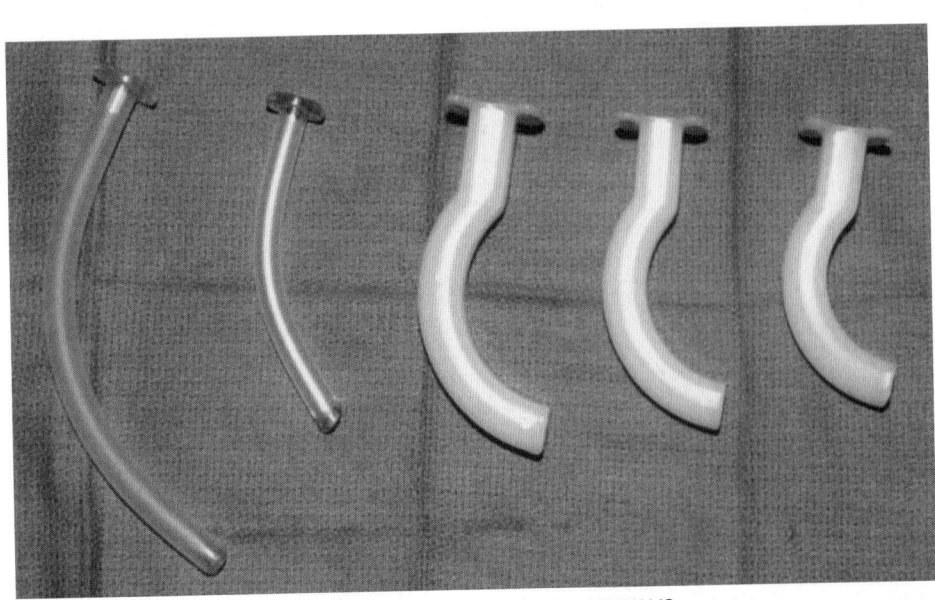

NASAL AIRWAYS   ORAL AIRWAYS

FIG. 47-4. From left to right: two nasal airways and three oral airways.

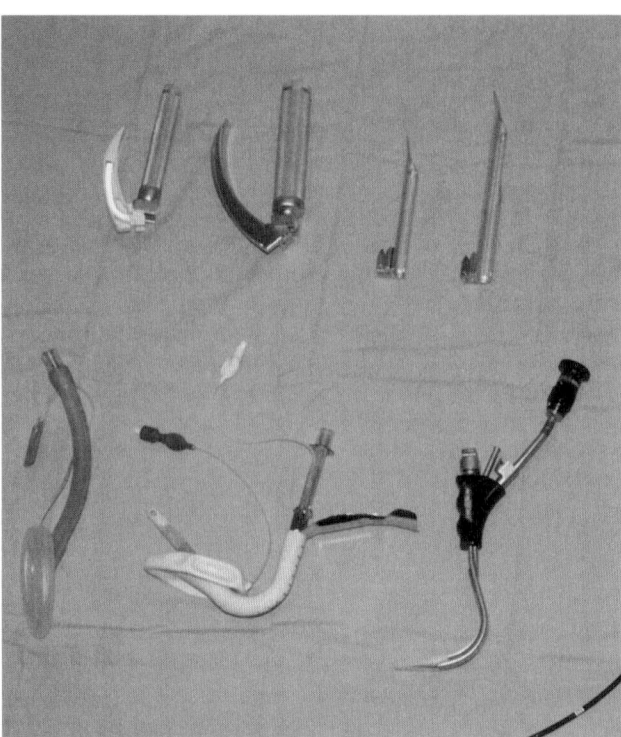

FIG. 47-5. (*Top*) Laryngoscopes with curved straight blades; (*Bottom*) laryngomask airway, intubating laryngomask airway, and Bullard rigid fiberoptic laryngoscope.

of dental damage. The scope is constructed of fiberoptic bundles and cables encased in a sheath. The cables permit manipulation of the tip of the scope by adjustments made at the operating end of the device. There is a port for suction and/or insufflation of O₂. The scope gives excellent visualization of the airway with minimal hemodynamic stress when used properly. It can be used nasally or

orally in an awake, spontaneously ventilating patient, whose airway has been treated with topical anesthetic. It requires skill for proper use, is expensive, and requires careful maintenance (Fig. 47-9).

The ASA has developed algorithms for management of the difficult airway.[50] These are shown in Figs. 47-10 and 47-11.

Fluid Therapy

Numerous preparations of IV fluid are available for the replacement of perioperative fluid losses in patients undergoing surgery. Different fluid preparations may influence clinical parameters (e.g., platelet function) and may also affect postoperative outcome.

Traditionally, IV fluids have been classified according to whether they are crystalloid or colloid in nature. *Crystalloid fluids* comprise electrolyte solutions with or without a bicarbonate precursor such as acetate or lactate. The *colloids* contain a complex sugar or protein suspended in an electrolyte solution. A further distinction between IV fluid types may be based on the nature of the solution. Normal saline-based (0.9% sodium chloride) preparations (crystalloid or colloid) contain no electrolytes other than sodium and chloride. In contrast, balanced salt-based fluids such as lactated Ringer's solution contain other electrolytes, with or without a bicarbonate precursor.

Several types of colloids are available, but three are most commonly used—hydroxyethyl starch (HES), gelatin, and albumin. The HES preparations differ from one another according to their concentration, molecular weight, and extent of hydroxyethylation or substitution, with resultant varying physiochemical properties. HES solutions most often are described according to their weight-averaged mean molecular weight in kilodaltons (kDa): high-molecular-weight (450 kDa), middle-molecular-weight (200 kDa, 270 kDa), and low-molecular-weight (130 kDa, 70 kDa). HES 450 kDa solutions are available in a normal saline solution (HES 450/NS) and in a lactated, balanced salt solution (HES 450/BS). Although all of these colloids are used in Europe, gelatins are not available in the United States, and the only HES preparations approved by the U.S. Food and Drug Administration are the 6% high-molecular-weight (450 kDa) formulations.

The administration of a large volume of any type of IV fluid will cause dilution of platelets and coagulation factors and may lead to coagulopathy (i.e., dilutional coagulopathy). In addition, fluids can

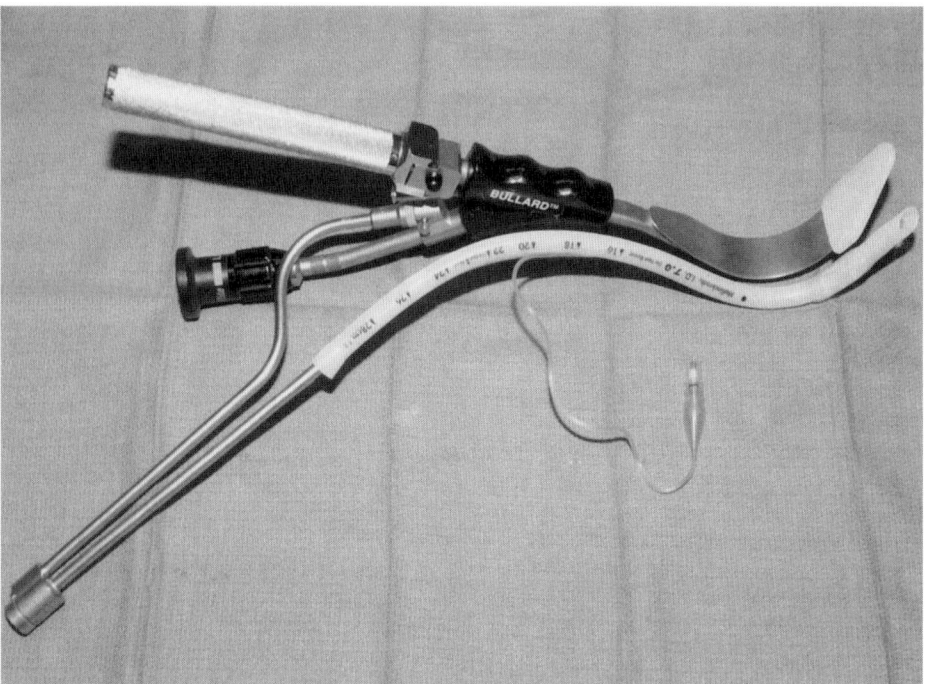

FIG. 47-6. The Bullard rigid fiberoptic laryngoscope with endotracheal tube.

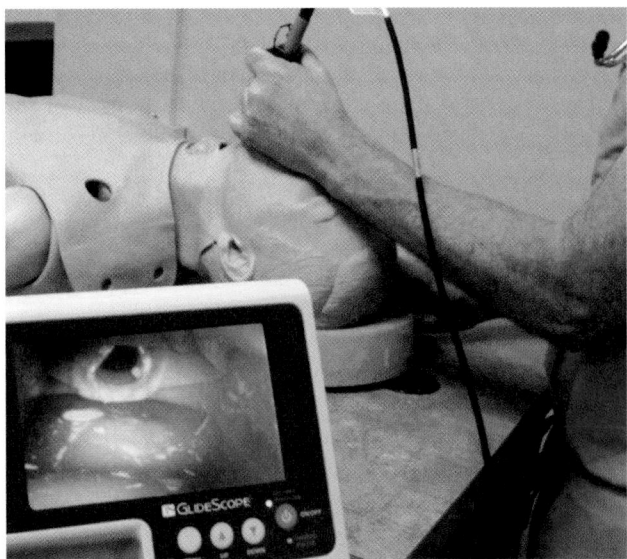

FIG. 47-7. Video laryngoscope.

have a direct impact on blood clotting through effects on circulating components of the coagulation cascade or by altering platelet function.

Recent evidence suggests that the nature of the solution itself may influence coagulation and bleeding. HES 450/NS may be associated with more bleeding than other fluids. HES 450 in a balanced salt solution appears to be equivalent to 5% albumin with respect to bleeding outcomes.[51–53] Waters and colleagues reported that patients undergoing abdominal aortic aneurysm repair who received lactated Ringer's solution received smaller volumes of platelets and had less blood product exposure than those treated with normal saline.[54]

It is possible that certain fluids may induce hypercoagulability that may be reflected not only by less bleeding, but also by an increased incidence of postoperative thrombotic complications (e.g., deep vein thrombosis and cerebrovascular accident). There are laboratory data[55] to suggest that IV fluid administration may induce a hypercoagulable state, but the clinical significance of this remains unclear.

The type of fluid administered intraoperatively to a patient can have a significant impact on renal function. The administration of HES/NS or normal saline to critically ill patients or elderly patients undergoing major surgery was associated with the development of renal dysfunction.[56–58]

The administration of adequate IV fluids during the perioperative period results in a lower incidence of nausea, vomiting, and antiemetic use after minor or day case surgery.[59] In major noncardiac surgical patients, the administration of HES 450 (in a BS or NS solution, or a combination of balanced crystalloid and colloid) has been associated with less postoperative nausea, vomiting, and antiemetic use, and earlier return of postoperative bowel function as reflected by first consumption of solid food, than the administration of 5% albumin, lactated Ringer's solution, or normal saline alone.[60]

Studies of patients undergoing ambulatory surgery have shown that perioperative IV fluid administration decreases the incidence of dizziness, drowsiness, thirst, and headache.[61] In a randomized crossover study of healthy volunteers, subjective deterioration in mental status (lassitude and difficulty in abstract thinking) was reported only by individuals who received 0.9% sodium chloride, and not by those who received lactated Ringer's solution.[62] The possible effect of different IV fluid preparations on CNS function has not yet been fully explored.

The relative impact of crystalloids and/or colloids on pulmonary function has been the subject of long-standing debate. No difference in postoperative pulmonary function was seen in cardiac surgery patients, orthopedic patients, or urologic surgery patients treated intraoperatively with different colloids.[56,63,64] In a number of studies in major surgical patients that compared crystalloid (lac-

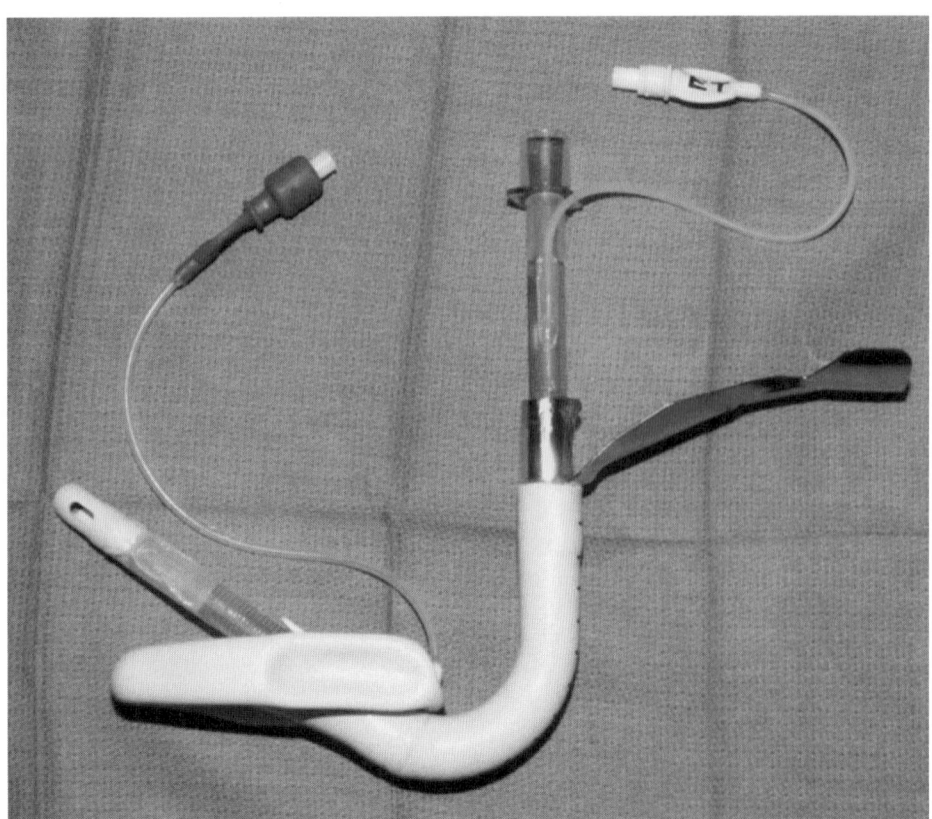

FIG. 47-8. Intubating laryngeal mask airway with endotracheal tube.

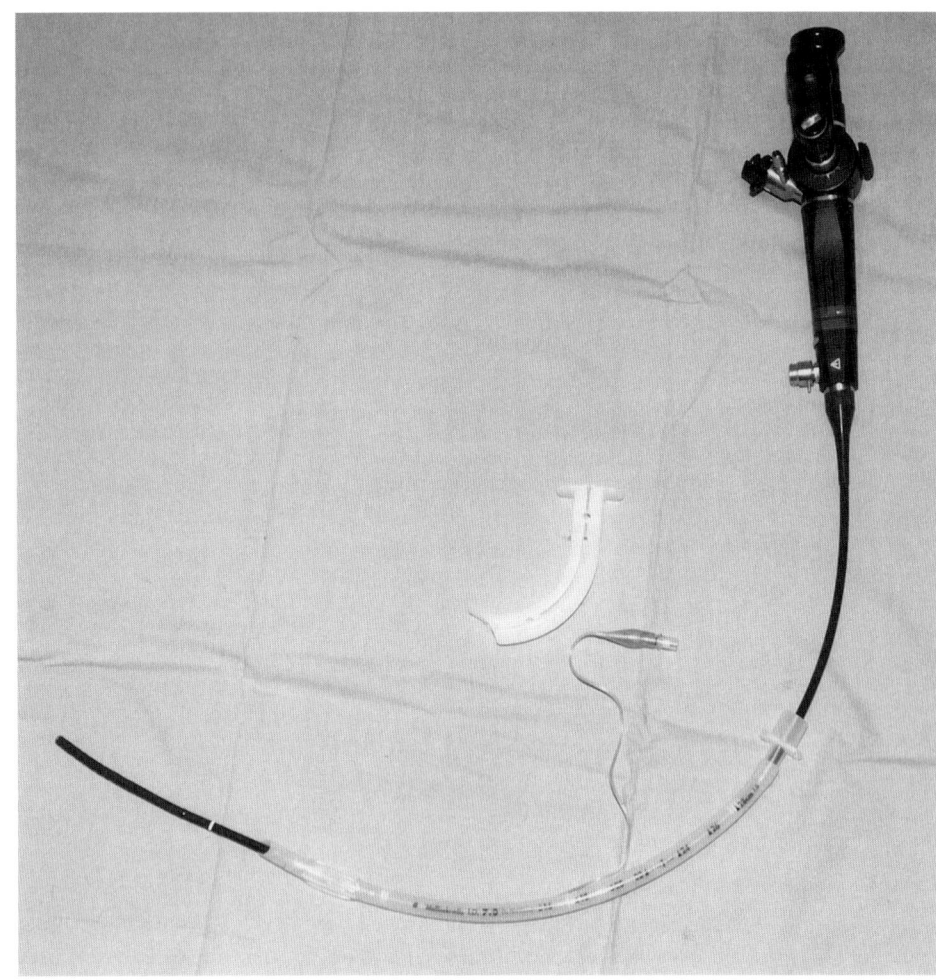

FIG. 47-9. Flexible fiberoptic intubation scope with endotracheal tube.

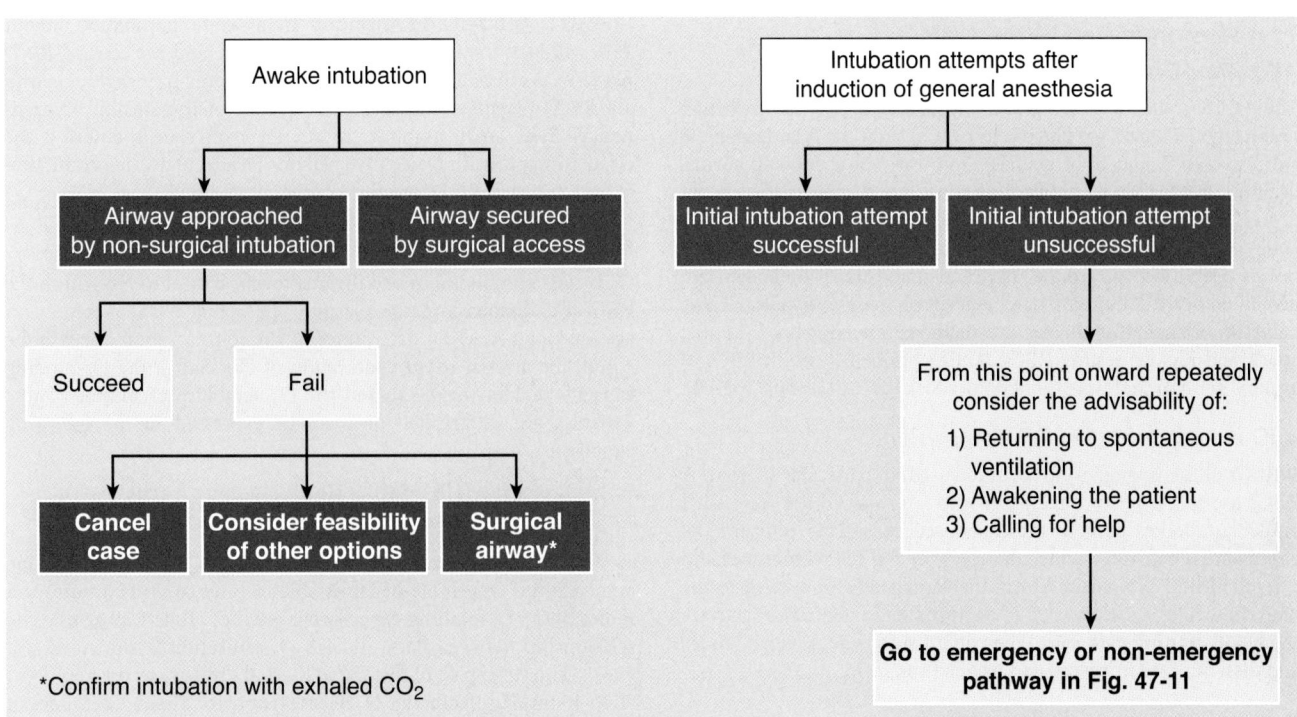

FIG. 47-10. American Society of Anesthesiologists airway management algorithm, Part I. CO_2 = carbon dioxide. *(Reproduced with permission from Practice guidelines for management of the difficult airway: An updated report by the American Society of Anesthesiologists Task Force on Management of the Difficult Airway. Anesthesiology 98:1269, 2003.)*

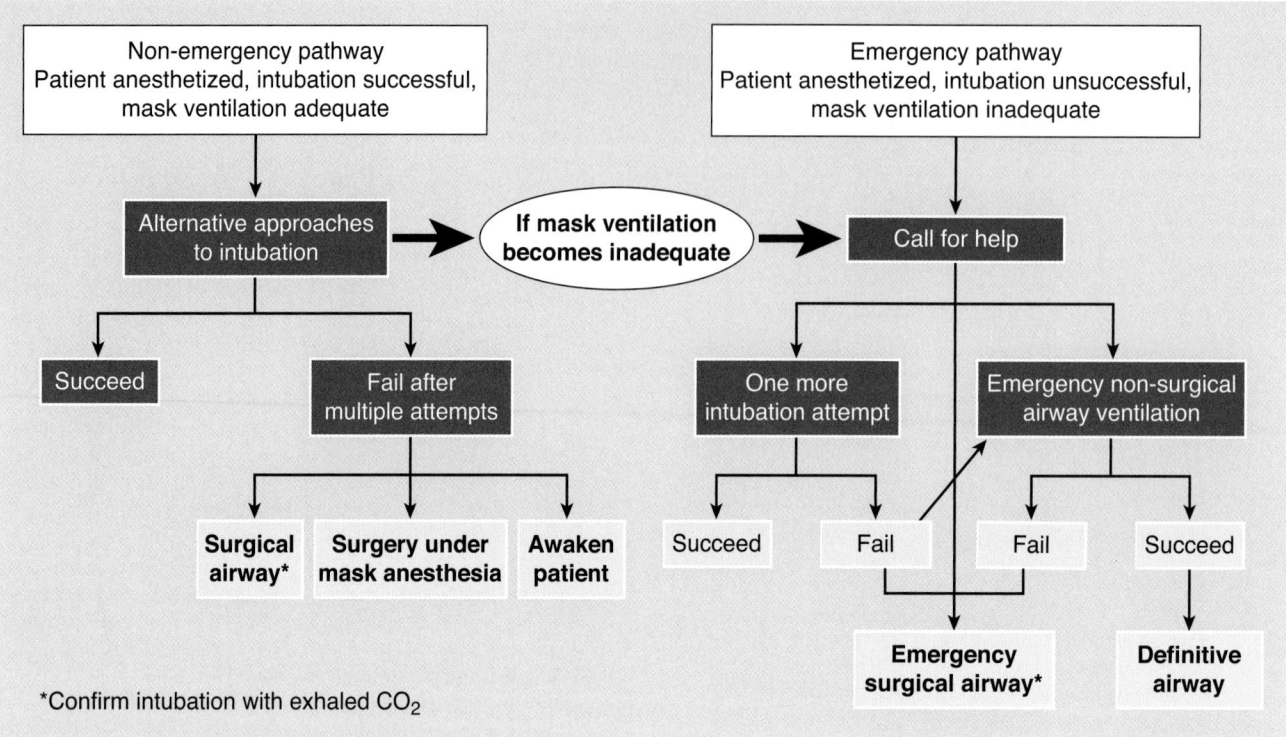

FIG. 47-11. American Society of Anesthesiologists airway management algorithm, Part II. CO_2 = carbon dioxide. *(Reproduced with permission from Practice guidelines for management of the difficult airway: An updated report by the American Society of Anesthesiologists Task Force on Management of the Difficult Airway. Anesthesiology 98:1269, 2003.)*

tated Ringer's solution) with colloid (HES 130/NS, HES 450/NS, 5% albumin/BS),[65–67] no difference was seen in the incidence or duration of mechanical ventilation or other indices of respiratory function. These findings suggest that the intraoperative administration of crystalloids does not have a detrimental effect on pulmonary function compared with the administration of colloids.

Transfusion of Red Blood Cells

ABO Blood Groups

There are four different ABO groups, which are determined by whether or not an individual's red blood cells (RBCs) carry the A antigen, the B antigen, both A and B, or neither. From early in childhood, normal healthy individuals make antibodies against A or B antigens that are not expressed on their own cells. People who are group A have anti-B antibodies in their plasma, people who are group B have anti-A antibodies, people who are group O have anti-A and anti-B antibodies, and people who are group AB have neither of these antibodies. These naturally occurring antibodies are mainly immunoglobulin M that attack and rapidly destroy RBCs. Anti-A antibodies attack RBCs of group A (or AB), and anti-B antibodies attack RBCs of group B (or AB).

ABO-Incompatible Red Cell Transfusion

If RBCs of the wrong group are transfused, in particular if group A RBCs are infused into a recipient who is group O, the recipient's anti-A antibodies bind to the transfused cells. This activates the complement pathways, which damages the red cell membranes and lyses the RBCs. Hb released from the damaged RBCs is toxic to the kidneys, while the fragments of ruptured cell membranes activate the blood-clotting pathways. The patient suffers acute renal failure and disseminated intravascular coagulation.

Basics of Red Blood Cell Compatibility

Ensuring that the right blood group is transfused is imperative. It is essential to ensure that no ABO-incompatible RBC transfusion is ever given. This avoidable accident is likely to kill or harm the patient.

Procedures in which compatibility is determined by establishing both transfusion recipient and donor blood ABO types via crossmatch analysis have evolved over years of clinical and laboratory experience to minimize the risk of this disastrous error. These procedures will continue to evolve as improved computerized systems are introduced to help staff avoid errors in blood administration.

Rhesus D Antigen and Antibody In a white population, about 15% will lack the Rhesus D (Rh D) antigen, and are termed *Rh D negative*. Antibodies to Rh D antigen occur only in individuals who are Rh D negative, and as a consequence of transfusion or pregnancy. Even small amounts of Rh D positive cells entering the circulation of an Rh D negative person can stimulate the production of antibodies to Rh D, usually immunoglobulin G.

Physiologic Response and Tolerance of Anemia

O_2 is carried in blood in two distinct forms: bound to Hb within the RBC and dissolved in the plasma. The actual oxygen content of arterial blood (CaO_2) is determined by the concentration of Hb in the blood, the arterial oxygen saturation of Hb (SaO_2), the O_2-binding capacity of Hb, the PaO_2, and the O_2 solubility of plasma. These variables are interrelated and can be expressed in the following equation:

$$CaO_2 = (Hb \times SaO_2 \times Hb \ O_2 \ binding \ capacity) + (PaO_2 \times plasma \ O_2 \ solubility).$$

Adult Hb consists of four protein chains, each carrying one heme group. One mole of Hb is able to bind to a maximum of 4 moles of O_2. O_2-binding capacity per gram of Hb is 1.39 g/mL. The relationship between PaO_2 and Hb O_2 saturation is shown in Fig. 47-12. The steep part of this curve [partial pressure of oxygen (PO_2) 20 to 40 mmHg] facilitates O_2 release from Hb. Tissue PO_2 values of different organs are also shown in Fig. 47-12 and lie on this steep part of the curve, facilitating O_2 release from Hb.

Mild anemia is compensated by a shift in the Hb-O_2 dissociation curve. The impact of more severe anemia may be physiologically

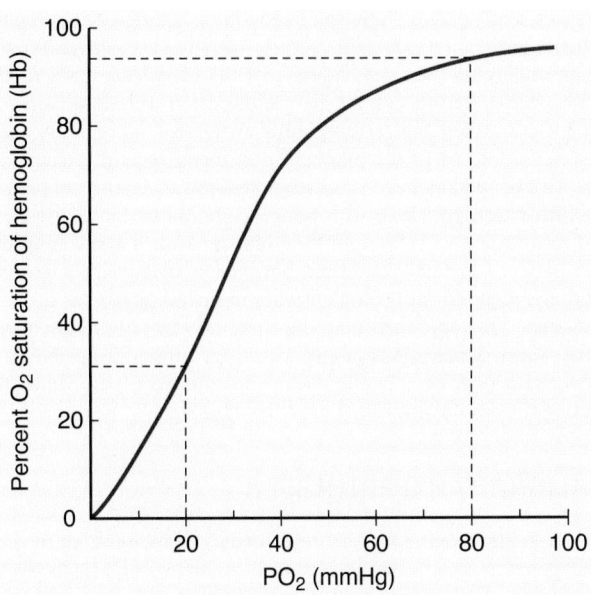

FIG. 47-12. Oxygen hemoglobin dissociation curve. O_2 = oxygen; PO_2 = partial pressure of oxygen.

modulated by an increase in cardiac output, which will increase tissue perfusion and cause a decrease in peripheral vascular resistance and decreases in whole blood viscosity.[68,69]

Anemia not only decreases the O_2 content of blood but also decreases blood viscosity, promoting an increase in regional blood flow. Moreover, this increase in blood flow augments the perfused capillary area by an increase in filling pressures and microvasculature vasodilation that results in an increase in O_2 uptake by the tissue beds.[70] The effects of blood transfusion on O_2 uptake are not as optimal as increasing blood flow, because the rise in hematocrit increases blood viscosity, which alters regional microvascular blood flow (i.e., perfusion).[55]

In normal animals undergoing acute hemodilution, cardiovascular function is maintained until the Hb level reaches between 3 and 5 g/dL, at which point ischemic changes then begin to appear on endocardial electrocardiogram leads (i.e., ST-segment changes).[71,72]

Hemodilution and Critical Hematocrit

The intentional dilution of blood volume often is referred to as *acute normovolemic hemodilution (ANH) anemia.* ANH is a technique in which whole blood is removed from a patient, while the circulating blood volume is maintained with acellular fluid. Blood is collected via central lines with simultaneous infusion of crystalloid or colloid solutions. Collected blood is reinfused after major blood loss has ceased, or sooner, if indicated. Blood units are reinfused in the reverse order of collection.

Under conditions of ANH, the increased plasma compartment becomes an important source of O_2, which is delivered to the tissues. Oxygenation is maintained by increased cardiac output and increased O_2 extraction by the tissues, and when these compensatory mechanisms fail to match the O_2 needs of the tissues, the "critical hematocrit" is said to have been reached. The critical hematocrit has been a source of debate for many years. A theoretical model was developed that describes the relation between hematocrit, myocardial O_2 demand, and the required coronary blood flow during progressive hemodilution.[73] Using this model, the determinants of critical hematocrit and the limits of ANH can be calculated based on the limits of coronary reserve. Because the critical hematocrit varies with O_2 consumption and degree of CAD, a fixed critical hematocrit as a transfusion trigger is not appropriate in most patients. Rather,

the indication for blood transfusions must individually take into account the specific circumstances of the patient, such as expected blood loss and required O_2 transport capacity reserves, hemodynamic stability, CAD, and systemic O_2 consumption.

RECOVERY FROM ANESTHESIA

Reversal of Neuromuscular Blockade

The elimination of neuromuscular blocking agents from the body and subsequent resumption of neuromuscular transmission takes a considerable amount of time, even with drugs such as vecuronium that have relatively short half-lives. Additionally, it is time consuming to wait for complete spontaneous recovery at the end of a surgical procedure. Therefore, it has become routine to antagonize the neuromuscular block pharmacologically with the use of reversal agents. Reversal agents raise the concentration of the neurotransmitter acetylcholine to a higher level than that of the neuromuscular blocking agent. This is accomplished by the use of anticholinesterase agents, which reduce the breakdown of acetylcholine. The most commonly used agents are neostigmine, pyridostigmine, and edrophonium.

The common side effects of these three anticholinesterase agents are bradycardia, bronchial and intestinal smooth muscle contractions, and excessive secretions from salivary and bronchial glands. These effects are primarily mediated by effects on muscarinic receptors, which are effectively blocked by the concomitant use of antimuscarinic drugs such as atropine or glycopyrrolate. To ensure adequate ventilation postoperatively, it is important that the neuromuscular blocking agents are fully reversed, as assessed by monitoring twitch strength with a nerve stimulator and clinically correlating this with signs such as grip strength or 5-second head lift.

The Postanesthesia Care Unit

It is of primary importance that all patients awakening from anesthesia are followed in a recovery room, as approximately 10% of all anesthetic accidents occur in the recovery period. As more serious surgeries are performed on older and sicker patients, the number of patients requiring postoperative ventilation and medications to support their circulation increases with age. The new trend for postoperative pain control with continuous epidural administration of local anesthetics and narcotics demands close observation, because respiratory depression can occur. In most hospitals, the number of intensive care beds is too small to accommodate the increasing number of these patients. What originally began as the recovery room now must function as an intensive care unit setting for short stays. The name "recovery room" has been changed to postanesthetic care unit (PACU).

A variety of physiologic disorders that can affect different organ systems need to be diagnosed and treated in the PACU during emergence from anesthesia and surgery. Postoperative nausea and vomiting (PONV), airway support, and hypotension requiring pharmacologic support have been observed to be the most frequent complications in the PACU.[74] However, abnormal bleeding, hypertension, dysrhythmia, myocardial infarction, and altered mental status are not uncommon.[74]

Postoperative Nausea and Vomiting

PONV typically occurs in 20 to 30% of surgical cases,[75] with considerable variation in frequency reported between studies (range 8 to 92%).[76] PONV is generally considered a transient, unpleasant event carrying little long-term morbidity; however, aspiration of emesis, gastric bleeding, and wound hematomas may occur with protracted or vigorous retching or vomiting. Troublesome PONV can prolong recovery room stay and hospitalization, and is one of the most common causes of hospital admission following ambulatory surgery. Published evidence suggests that prophylactic administration of antiemetics is not cost-effective in the surgical setting.[77]

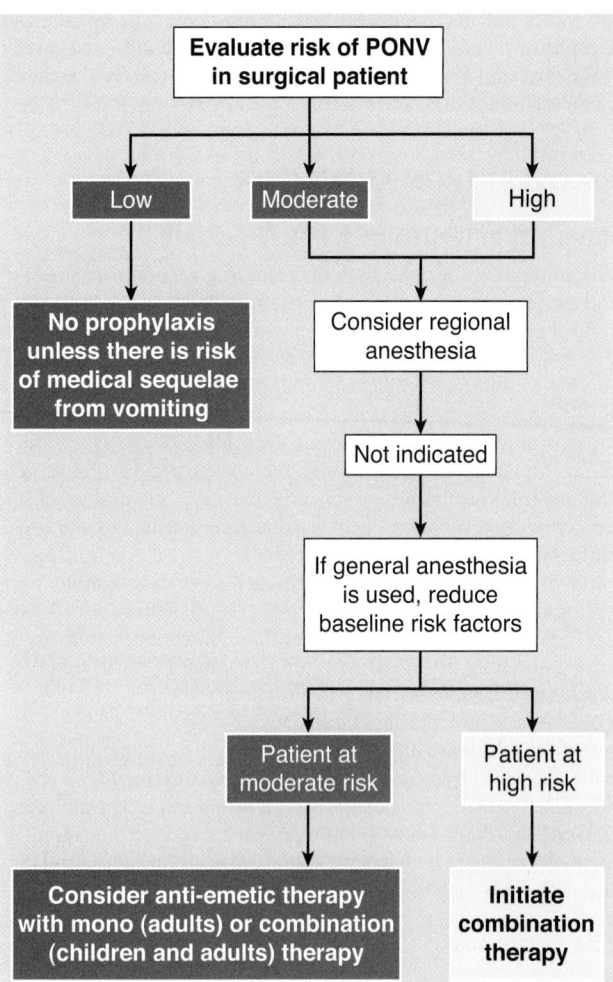

FIG. 47-13. Algorithm for the management of postoperative nausea and vomiting (PONV). *(Reproduced with permission from Gan TJ, Meyer T, Apfel CC, et al: Consensus guidelines for managing postoperative nausea and vomiting.* Anesth Analg *97:62, 2003.)*

Recent consensus guidelines using data from systematic reviews, randomized trials and studies, and data from logistic regression models have been published.[77] An algorithm showing these guidelines is shown in Fig. 47-13.

Agents usually administered for PONV are the serotonin receptor antagonists ondansetron, dolasetron, granisetron, and tropisetron. The safety and efficacy of the compounds, when given at the end of surgery, are virtually identical.[77,78] Metoclopramide, when used in the standard dose of 10 mg, is ineffective for PONV.[79] Although some studies have shown higher doses (20 mg) to have some effect on PONV, most evidence suggests that the serotonin receptor antagonists are the most efficacious choice.

Pain: The Fifth Vital Sign

Analgesic research methodology has been enhanced since the 1960s through the use of graduated and visual analog scales, tools that permit the standardization of pain scores. One frequently used graduated scale is a four-point measure of pain intensity (0 = no pain, 1 = mild pain, 2 = moderate pain, and 3 = severe pain) and a five-point measure of relief (0 = no relief, 1 = a little relief, 2 = some relief, 3 = a lot of relief, and 4 = complete relief).

Acute postoperative pain and its treatment (or prophylaxis) are significant challenges for the health care professional. Despite the recent development of new nonnarcotic analgesics and a better understanding of the side effects associated with pain medication of

all types, acute postoperative pain remains a significant concern for patients and represents an extremely negative experience for patients undergoing surgery. Many patients experience pain in the postoperative period despite the use of potent techniques such as patient-controlled analgesia, epidural analgesia, and regional anesthesia. The culture of acceptance of postoperative pain is changing. The American Pain Society has advocated the assessment of pain as the fifth vital sign, along with temperature, pulse, blood pressure, and respiratory rate. The four vital signs provide a quick snapshot of a patient's general condition, but pain management advocates claim the picture is not complete without including pain as the fifth vital sign. This approach may improve the efficacy of pain treatment. Many departments of anesthesiology support an active pain service and provide consultation for postoperative pain relief, including the administration of nerve blocks (Fig. 47-14).

MALIGNANT HYPERTHERMIA

MH is a life-threatening, acute disorder, developing during or after general anesthesia. The clinical incidence of MH is about 1:12,000 in children and 1:40,000 in adults. A genetic predisposition and one or more triggering agents are necessary to evoke MH. Triggering agents include all volatile anesthetics (e.g., halothane, enflurane, isoflurane, sevoflurane, and desflurane), and the depolarizing muscle relaxant succinylcholine. Volatile anesthetics and/or succinylcholine cause a rise in the myoplasmic calcium concentration in susceptible patients, resulting in persistent muscle contraction. The classic MH crisis entails a hypermetabolic state, tachycardia, and the elevation of end-tidal CO_2 in the face of constant minute ventilation. Respiratory and metabolic acidosis and muscle rigidity follow, as well as rhabdomyolysis, arrhythmias, hyperkalemia, and sudden cardiac arrest. A rise in temperature is often a late sign of MH.

Treatment must be aggressive and begin as soon as a case of MH is suspected:

Call for help.
Stop all volatile anesthetics and give 100% O_2.
Hyperventilate the patient up to three times the calculated minute volume.
Begin infusion of dantrolene sodium, 2.5 mg/kg IV. Repeat as necessary, titrating to clinical signs of MH. Continue dantrolene for at least 24 hours after the episode begins.

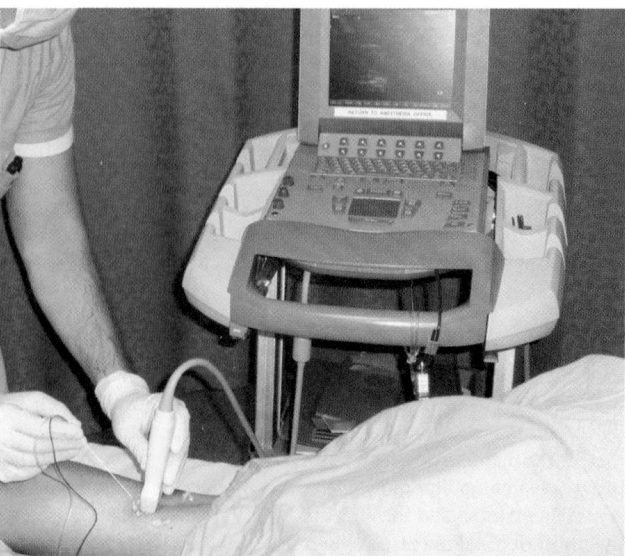

FIG. 47-14. Popliteal ultrasound.

Give bicarbonate to treat acidosis if dantrolene is ineffective.

Treat hyperkalemia with insulin, glucose, and calcium.

Avoid calcium channel blockers

Continue to monitor core temperature.

Call the MH hotline to report the case and get advice: 1-888-274-7899.

FUTURE DIRECTION OF ANESTHESIA

The general mantra of "gene therapy is the future of medicine" must be more specifically related to how those genes create, shape, and regulate proteins. The study of how proteins manifest their activity and/or concentration, is called *proteomics* (from proteome—a fusion of "protein" and "genome").

As the technology advances to biologically identify individual proteins, studies of individual levels of proteomes will allow the study of disease processes on the molecular level, directly aiding diagnosis and therapeutics.[80]

Specifically to the field of anesthesiology, the technology of proteomics will be used to elucidate the actual mechanism of action of our anesthetic drugs and how these drugs have differing effects on different individuals. There will be a day when a buccal swab in the preoperative clinic will become routine; the results telling us which opioids carry the fewest side effects for that particular patient, for example, or which antiemetics are most effective, or which postoperative analgesics to use—a tailored anesthetic. Recent studies in mice have examined the $\alpha 5$ subunit of the GABA receptor, which appears to regulate memory. The human genome is polymorphic for the $\alpha 5$ gene; because each variant may manifest in different amounts of memory/amnesia, proteomics may someday lead to tests that determine the propensity of a particular patient to experience awareness and allow us to tailor the anesthetic even further.[81]

REFERENCES

Entries highlighted in bright blue are key references.

1. Darwin F, Darwin C: *The Autobiography of Charles Darwin.* Kallista, Victoria, Australia: Totem Books, 2003, p 12.
2. Calverly RK: Anesthesia as a specialty: Past, present, and future, in Barash PG, Cullen BF, Stoelting RK (eds): *Clinical Anesthesia.* Philadelphia: Lippincott-Raven, 1996, p 6.
3. Bigelow HJ: Insensibility during surgical operations produced by inhalation. *Boston Med Surgical J* 35:356, 1846.
4. Vandam LD: History of anesthetic practice, in Miller RD (ed): *Anesthesia.* Philadelphia: Churchill Livingstone, 2000, p 7.
5. Meade RH: *An Introduction to the History of General Surgery.* Philadelphia: WB Saunders Co, 1968, p 78.
6. Rushman GB, Davies NJH, Atkinson RS: *A Short History of Anaesthesia.* Oxford: Butterworth-Heinemann, 1998, p 140.
7. Hall RJ: Hydrochlorate of cocaine. *NY Med J* 40:643, 1884.
8. Rushman GB, Davies NJH, Atkinson RS: *A Short History of Anaesthesia.* Oxford: Butterworth-Heinemann, 1998, p 145.
9. Griffith HR, Johnson GE: The use of curare in general anesthesia. *Anesthesiology* 3:418, 1942.
10. Stoelting RK, Miller RD: *Basics of Anesthesia.* Philadelphia: Churchill-Livingstone, 2000, p 436.
11. Hull CJ: Principles of pharmacokinetics, in Hemmings H, Hopkins PM (eds): *Foundations of Anesthesia.* London: Mosby, 2000, p 77.
12. Stoelting RD, Dierdorf SF: *Stoelting's Anesthesia and Co-Existing Disease,* 5th ed. Philadelphia: Saunders, 2008.
13. Butterworth JF IV: Local anesthetics and regional anesthesia, in Hemmings H, Hopkins PM (eds): *Foundations of Anesthesia.* London: Mosby, 2000, p 298.
14. Royston D, Cox F: Anaesthesia: The patient's point of view. *Lancet* 362:1648, 2003.
15. Savarese JJ, Caldwell JE, Lien CA, et al: Pharmacology of muscle relaxants and their antagonists, in Miller RD (ed): *Anesthesia.* Philadelphia: Churchill Livingstone, 2000, p 414.
16. Kaplan EB, Sheiner LB, Boeckmann AJ, et al: The usefulness of preoperative laboratory screening. *JAMA* 253:3576, 1985.
17. Cullen DJ, Apolone G, Greenfield S, et al: ASA physical status and age predict morbidity after three surgical procedures. *Ann Surg* 220:3, 1994.
18. Mangano DT, Goldman L: Preoperative assessment of patients with known or suspected coronary disease. *N Engl J Med* 333:1750, 1995.
19. Wong T, Detsky AS: Preoperative cardiac risk assessment for patients having peripheral vascular surgery. *Ann Intern Med* 116:743, 1992.
20. Lee TH, Marcantonio ER, Mangione CM, et al: Derivation and prospective validation of a simple index for prediction of cardiac risk of major noncardiac surgery. *Circulation* 100:1043, 1999.
21. Kleinman B, Henkin RE, Glisson SN, et al: Qualitative evaluation of coronary flow during anesthetic induction using thallium-201 perfusion scans. *Anesthesiology* 64:157, 1986.
22. Smetana GW: Preoperative pulmonary evaluation. *N Engl J Med* 340:937, 1999.
23. Zollinger AH, C Pasch T: Preoperative pulmonary evaluation: Facts and myths. *Curr Opinion Anesthesiol* 14:59, 2002.
24. Warner DO, Warner MA, Offord KP, et al: Airway obstruction and perioperative complications in smokers undergoing abdominal surgery. *Anesthesiology* 90:372, 1999.
25. Mutlu GM, Factor P, Schwartz DE, et al: Severe status asthmaticus: Management with permissive hypercapnia and inhalation anesthesia. *Crit Care Med* 30:477, 2002.
26. Scalfaro P, Sly PD, Sims C, et al: Salbutamol prevents the increase of respiratory resistance caused by tracheal intubation during sevoflurane anesthesia in asthmatic children. *Anesth Analg* 93:898, 2001.
27. Groeben H, Schlicht M, Stieglitz S, et al: Both local anesthetics and salbutamol pretreatment affect reflex bronchoconstriction in volunteers with asthma undergoing awake fiberoptic intubation. *Anesthesiology* 97:1445, 2002.
28. Byrick RJ, Rose DK: Pathophysiology and prevention of acute renal failure: The role of the anesthetist. *Can J Anaesth* 37:457, 1990.
29. Elliott RH, Strunin L: Hepatotoxicity of volatile anaesthetics. *Br J Anaesth* 70:339, 1993.
30. Njoku D, Laster MJ, Gong DH, et al: Biotransformation of halothane, enflurane, isoflurane, and desflurane trifluoroacetylated liver proteins: Association between protein acylation and hepatic injury. *Anesth Analg* 84:173, 1997.
31. Eldridge AJ, Sear JW: Peri-operative management of diabetic patients. Any changes for the better since 1985? *Anaesthesia* 51:45, 1996.
32. McAnulty GR, Robertshaw HJ, Hall GM: Anaesthetic management of patients with diabetes mellitus. *Br J Anaesth* 85:80, 2000.
33. Risum O, Abdelnoor M, Svennevig JL, et al: Diabetes mellitus and morbidity and mortality risks after coronary artery bypass surgery. *Scand J Thorac Cardiovasc Surg* 30:71, 1996.
34. Zacharias A, Habib RH: Factors predisposing to median sternotomy complications. Deep vs. superficial infection. *Chest* 110:1173, 1996.
35. Halter JB, Pflug AE: Effects of anesthesia and surgical stress on insulin secretion in man. *Metabolism* 29:1124, 1980.
36. Thorell A, Nygren J, Hirshman MF, et al: Surgery-induced insulin resistance in human patients: Relation to glucose transport and utilization. *Am J Physiol* 276:E754, 1999.
37. Das UN: Is insulin an endogenous cardioprotector? *Crit Care* 6:389, 2002.
38. Das UN: Insulin and inflammation: Further evidence and discussion. *Nutrition* 18:526, 2002.
39. Das UN: Insulin and the critically ill. *Crit Care* 6:262, 2002.
40. Hall GM: The anaesthetic modification of the endocrine and metabolic response to surgery. *Ann R Coll Surg Engl* 67:25, 1985.
41. Weinberg AD, Brennan MD, Gorman CA, et al: Outcome of anesthesia and surgery in hypothyroid patients. *Arch Intern Med* 143:893, 1983.
42. Murkin JM: Anesthesia and hypothyroidism: A review of thyroxine physiology, pharmacology, and anesthetic implications. *Anesth Analg* 61:371, 1982.
43. Adams JP, Murphy PG: Obesity in anaesthesia and intensive care. *Br J Anaesth* 85:91, 2000.
44. Rosenbaum M, Leibel RL, Hirsch J: Obesity. *N Engl J Med* 337:396, 1997.
45. Bouillon T, Shafer SL: Does size matter? *Anesthesiology* 89:557, 1998.
46. Pinaud M, Lelausque JN, Chetanneau A, et al: Effects of propofol on cerebral hemodynamics and metabolism in patients with brain trauma. *Anesthesiology* 73:404, 1990.

47. Strebel S, Kaufmann M, Guardiola PM, et al: Cerebral vasomotor responsiveness to carbon dioxide is preserved during propofol and midazolam anesthesia in humans. *Anesth Analg* 78:884, 1994.

48. Reddy RV, Moorthy SS, Dierdorf SF, et al: Excitatory effects and electroencephalographic correlation of etomidate, thiopental, methohexital, and propofol. *Anesth Analg* 77:1008, 1993.

49. Sperry RJ, Bailey PL, Reichman MV, et al: Fentanyl and sufentanil increase intracranial pressure in head trauma patients. Anesthesiology 77:416, 1992.

50. Practice guidelines for management of the difficult airway: An updated report by the American Society of Anesthesiologists Task Force on Management of the Difficult Airway. *Anesthesiology* 98:1269, 2003.

51. Bennett-Guerrero EFR, Mets B, Manspeizer HE, et al: Impact of normal saline based versus balanced salt intravenous fluid replacement on clinical outcomes: A randomized blinded trial. *Anesth Analg* 95:A147, 2001.

52. Gan T: Randomized comparison of coagulation profile when Hextend or 5% albumin is used for intraoperative fluid resuscitation. *Anesth Analg* 95:A193, 2001.

53. Petroni KG, Brimingham S: Hextend is a safe alternative to 5% albumin for patients undergoing elective cardiac surgery. *Anesth Analg* 95:A198, 2001.

54. Waters JH, Gottlieb A, Schoenwald P, et al: Normal saline versus lactated Ringer's solution for intraoperative fluid management in patients undergoing abdominal aortic aneurysm repair: An outcome study. *Anesth Analg* 93:817, 2001.

55. Gan TJ, Bennett-Guerrero E, Phillips-Bute B, et al: Hextend, a physiologically balanced plasma expander for large volume use in major surgery: A randomized phase III clinical trial. Hextend Study Group. *Anesth Analg* 88:992, 1999.

56. Gallandat Huet RC, Siemons AW, Baus D, et al: A novel hydroxyethyl starch (Voluven) for effective perioperative plasma volume substitution in cardiac surgery. *Can J Anaesth* 47:1207, 2000.

57. Cittanova ML, Leblanc I, Legendre C, et al: Effect of hydroxyethylstarch in brain-dead kidney donors on renal function in kidney-transplant recipients. *Lancet* 348:1620, 1996.

58. Schortgen F, Lacherade JC, Bruneel F, et al: Effects of hydroxyethylstarch and gelatin on renal function in severe sepsis: A multicentre randomised study. *Lancet* 357:911, 2001.

59. Elhakim M, el-Sebiae S, Kaschef N, et al: Intravenous fluid and postoperative nausea and vomiting after day-case termination of pregnancy. *Acta Anaesthesiol Scand* 42:216, 1998.

60. Gan TJ, Soppitt A, Maroof M, et al: Goal-directed intraoperative fluid administration reduces length of hospital stay after major surgery. *Anesthesiology* 97:820, 2002.

61. Yogendran S, Asokumar B, Cheng DC, et al: A prospective randomized double-blinded study of the effect of intravenous fluid therapy on adverse outcomes on outpatient surgery. *Anesth Analg* 80:682, 1995.

62. Williams EL, Hildebrand KL, McCormick SA, et al: The effect of intravenous lactated Ringer's solution versus 0.9% sodium chloride solution on serum osmolality in human volunteers. *Anesth Analg* 88:999, 1999.

63. Vogt NH, Bothner U, Lerch G, et al: Large-dose administration of 6% hydroxyethyl starch 200/0.5 total hip arthroplasty: Plasma homeostasis, hemostasis, and renal function compared to use of 5% human albumin. *Anesth Analg* 83:262, 1996.

64. Vogt N, Bothner U, Brinkmann A, et al: Peri-operative tolerance to large-dose 6% HES 200/0.5 in major urological procedures compared with 5% human albumin. *Anaesthesia* 54:121, 1999.

65. Lang K, Boldt J, Suttner S, et al: Colloids versus crystalloids and tissue oxygen tension in patients undergoing major abdominal surgery. *Anesth Analg* 93:405, 2001.

66. Marik PE, Iglesias J, Maini B: Gastric intramucosal pH changes after volume replacement with hydroxyethyl starch or crystalloid in patients undergoing elective abdominal aortic aneurysm repair. *J Crit Care* 12:51, 1997.

67. Virgilio RW, Rice CL, Smith DE, et al: Crystalloid vs. colloid resuscitation: Is one better? A randomized clinical study. *Surgery* 85:129, 1979.

68. Murray JF, Escobar E, Rapaport E: Effects of blood viscosity on hemodynamic responses in acute normovolemic anemia. *Am J Physiol* 216:638, 1969.

69. Woodson RD, Auerbach S: Effect of increased oxygen affinity and anemia on cardiac output and its distribution. *J Appl Physiol* 53:1299, 1982.

70. Messmer K: *Blood Rheology Factors and Capillary Blood Flow*. Berlin: Springer-Verlag, 1991, p 312.

71. Wilkerson DK, Rosen AL, Sehgal LR, et al: Limits of cardiac compensation in anemic baboons. *Surgery* 103:665, 1988.

72. Hagl S, Heimisch W, Meisner H, et al: The effect of hemodilution on regional myocardial function in the presence of coronary stenosis. *Basic Res Cardiol* 72:344, 1977.

73. Hoeft A, Wietasch JK, Sonntag H, et al: Theoretical limits of "permissive anemia." *Zentralbl Chir* 120:604, 1995.

74. Hines R, Barash PG, Watrous G, et al: Complications occurring in the postanesthesia care unit: A survey. *Anesth Analg* 74:503, 1992.

75. Watcha MF, White PF: Postoperative nausea and vomiting. Its etiology, treatment, and prevention. *Anesthesiology* 77:162, 1992.

76. Camu F, Lauwers MH, Verbessem D: Incidence and aetiology of postoperative nausea and vomiting. *Eur J Anaesthesiol* 9:25, 1992.

77. Gan TJ, Meyer T, Apfel CC, et al: Consensus guidelines for managing postoperative nausea and vomiting. *Anesth Analg* 97:62, 2003.

78. Sun R, Klein KW, White PF: The effect of timing of ondansetron administration in outpatients undergoing otolaryngologic surgery. *Anesth Analg* 84:331, 1997.

79. Henzi I, Walder B, Tramer MR: Metoclopramide in the prevention of postoperative nausea and vomiting: A quantitative systematic review of randomized, placebo-controlled studies. *Br J Anaesth* 83:761, 1999.

80. Atkins JH, Johansson JS: Technologies to shape the future: Proteomics applications in anesthesiology and critical care medicine. *Anesth Analg* 102:1207, 2006.

81. Orser BA, Mazer CD, Baker AJ: Awareness during anesthesia. *CMAJ* 178:185, 2008.

Ethics, Palliative Care, and Care at the End of Life

Daniel E. Hall, Peter Angelos, Geoffrey P. Dunn,
Daniel B. Hinshaw, and Timothy M. Pawlik

Dedicated to the advancement of surgery along its scientific and moral side.

> June 10, 1926, dedication on the Murphy Auditorium,
> the first home of the American College of Surgeons

WHY ETHICS MATTER

Ethical concerns involve not only the interests of patients, but also the interests of surgeons and society. Surgeons choose among the options available to them because they have particular opinions regarding what would be good (or bad) for their patients. Aristotle described practical wisdom (Greek: *phronesis*) as the capacity to choose the best option from among several imperfect alternatives (Fig. 48-1).[1] Frequently, surgeons are confronted with clinical or interpersonal situations in which there is incomplete information, uncertain outcomes, and/or complex personal and familial relationships. The capacity to choose wisely in such circumstances is the challenge of surgical practice.

DEFINITIONS

Biomedical ethics is the system of analysis and deliberation dedicated to guiding surgeons toward the "good" in the practice of surgery. One of the most influential ethical "systems" in the field of biomedical ethics is the principlist approach as articulated by Beauchamp and Childress.[2] In this approach to ethical issues, moral dilemmas are deliberated by using four guiding principles: autonomy, beneficence, nonmaleficence, and justice.[2]

The principle of autonomy respects the capacity of individuals to choose their own destiny, and it implies a right for individuals to make those choices. It also implies an obligation for physicians to permit patients to make autonomous choices about their medical care. Beneficence requires that proposed actions aim at and achieve something good whereas nonmaleficence aims at avoiding concrete harm: *primum non nocere*.* Justice requires a fairness where both the benefits and burdens of a particular action are distributed equitably.

---

*"First do no harm."

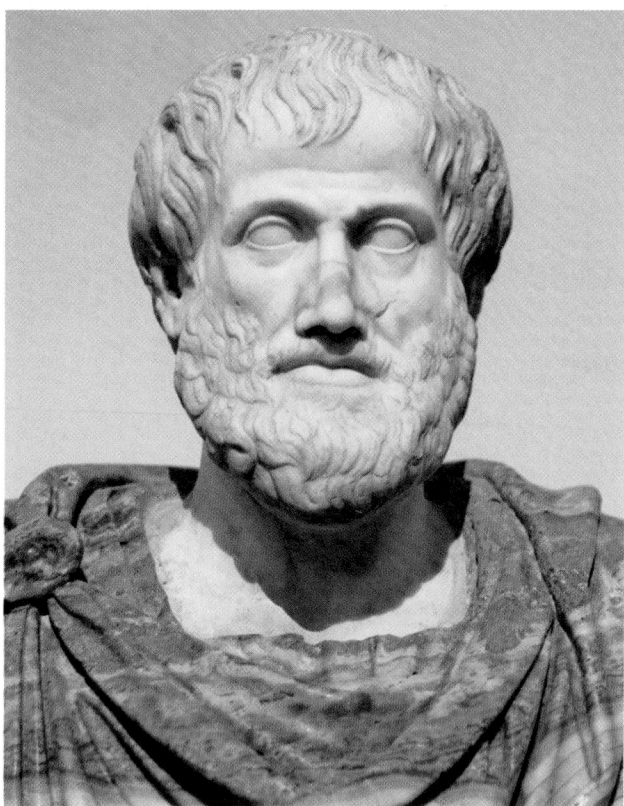

FIG. 48-1. Bust of Aristotle. Marble, Roman copy after a Greek bronze original by Lysippos from 330 B.C. *[From* http://en.wikipedia. org/wiki/File:Aristotle_Altemps_Inv8575.jpg*: Ludovisi Collection, Accession number Inv. 8575, Palazzo Altemps, Location Ground Floor, Branch of the National Roman Museum. Photographer/source Jastrow (2006) from Wikipedia (accessed March 8, 2009).]*

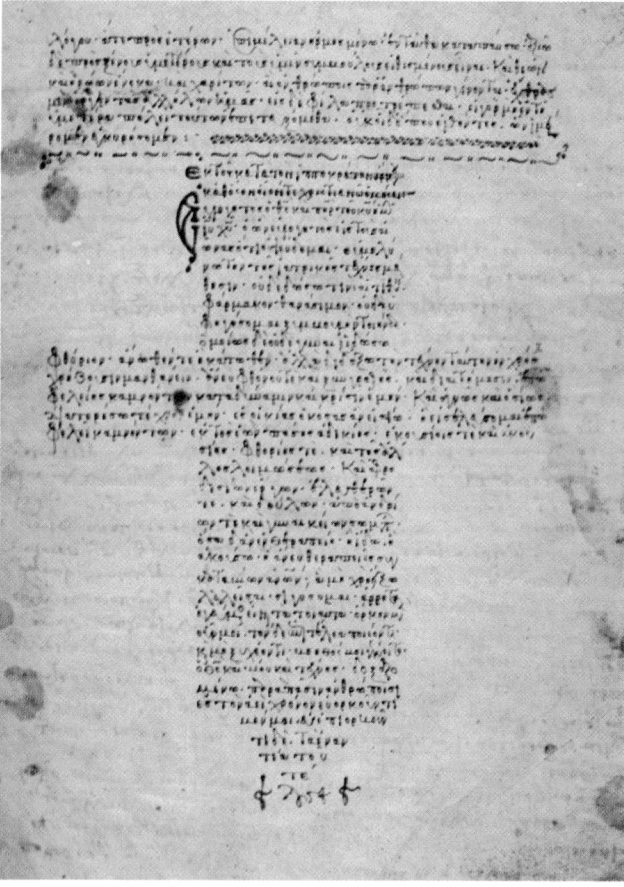

FIG. 48-2. Twelfth-century Byzantine manuscript. The Hippocratic oath was written out in the form of a cross from the Folio Biblioteca Vaticana. *[From* http://en.wikipedia.org/wiki/File:HippocraticOath.jpg*: Rutkow IM: Surgery: An Illustrated History 1993, p 27, from Wikipedia (accessed March 8, 2009).]*

BIOMEDICAL ETHICS: AN OVERVIEW

The history of medical ethics has its origins in antiquity. The Hippocratic Oath along with other professional codes has guided the actions of physicians for thousands of years (Fig. 48-2). The modern practice of medicine is therefore rooted in the Hippocratic tradition, but the growing technical powers of modern medicine raise new questions that were inconceivable in previous generations. Life support, dialysis, and modern drugs, as well as organ and cellular transplantation, have engendered new moral and ethical

KEY POINTS

1. The physician should document that the patient or surrogate has the capacity to make a medical decision.

2. The physician discloses to the patient details regarding the diagnosis and treatment options sufficient for the patient to make an informed consent.

3. Living wills are written to anticipate treatment options and choices in the event that a patient is rendered incompetent by a terminal illness.

4. The durable power of attorney for health care identifies surrogate decision makers and invests them with the authority to make health care decisions on a patient's behalf in the event that patients are unable to speak for themselves.

5. Surgeons should encourage their patients to clearly identify their surrogates early in the course of treatment.

6. Seven requirements for the ethical conduct of clinical trials have been articulated: value, scientific validity, fair subject selection, favorable risk-benefit ratio, independent review, informed consent, and respect for enrolled subjects.

7. The Association of American Medical Colleges stresses three key points regarding potential conflict of interest: full disclosure, aggressive monitoring, and misconduct management.

8. Disclosure of error is consistent with recent ethical advances in medicine toward more openness with patients and the involvement of patients in their care.

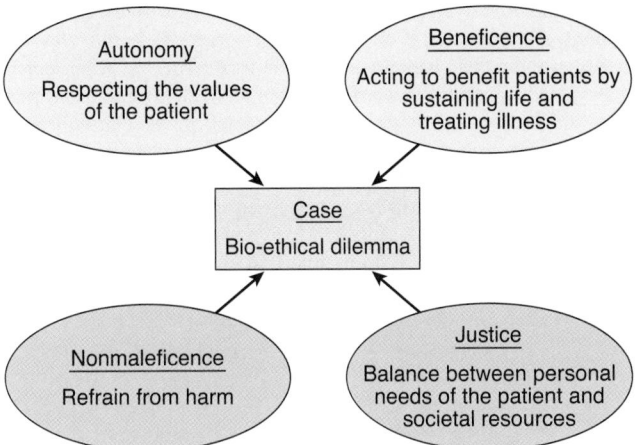

FIG. 48-3. The four principles of the care-based paradigm.

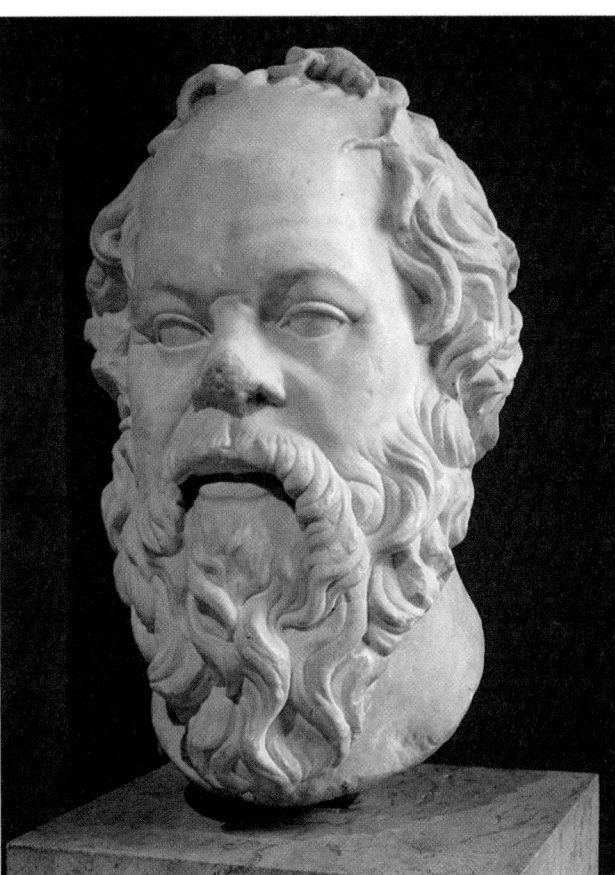

FIG. 48-4. Portrait of Socrates. Marble, Roman artwork (1st century), speculated to be a copy of a lost bronze statue made by Lysippos. [From http://en.wikipedia.org/wiki/File:Socrates_Louvre.jpg: Old fund. Accession number Ma 59 (MR 652) Location Department of Greek, Etruscan and Roman Antiquities, Sully wing, ground floor, room 17. Photographer/source Eric Gaba (User:Sting), July 2005. Wikipedia (accessed March 8, 2009). The photographer has licensed this photo under the Creative Commons Attribution ShareAlike 2.5 License. Official license: http://creativecommons.org/licenses/by-sal/2.5/]

dilemmas. As such, the ethical challenges faced by the surgeon have become more complex and require greater attention.

The case-based paradigm for bioethics is used when a difficult clinical situation confronts the clinical team and questions with apparently conflicting values or principles are raised (Fig. 48-3). The first step is to clarify the relevant principles (e.g., autonomy, beneficence, nonmaleficence, and justice) and values (e.g., self-determination, quality of life, etc.) at stake. After identifying the principles and values that are affecting the situation, a proposed course of action is considered given the circumstances.

Much of the discourse in bioethics adopts this "principlist" approach in which the relevant principles are identified, weighted and balanced, and then applied to formulate a course of action. This approach to bioethics is a powerful technique for thinking through moral problems, as the four principles define the dimensions of the ethical dilemma and provide a means for assessing the impact or extent of each value and principle at stake.

The concept of *virtue ethics* was born with Socrates (Fig. 48-4) and raised in Plato's *Republic* where the four cardinal virtues of courage, justice, temperance, and practical wisdom are discussed.[3–5] Practical wisdom is developed and acquired through experience. As such, the apprenticeship model of surgical residency teaches much more than technical mastery but moral training as well. In fact, the sociologist Charles Bosk argues that the "postgraduate training of surgeons is above all things an ethical training."[6]

SPECIFIC ISSUES IN SURGICAL ETHICS

Informed Consent

Although a relatively recent development, the doctrine of informed consent is one of the most widely established tenets of modern biomedical ethics. During the nineteenth and early twentieth centuries, most physicians practiced a form of benign paternalism whereby patients were rarely involved in the decision-making process regarding their medical care, relying instead on the beneficence of the physician. Consensus among the wider public eventually changed such that surgeons are now expected to have an open discussion about diagnosis and treatment with the patient to obtain informed consent. In the United States, the legal doctrine of *simple* consent dates from the 1914 decision in *Schloendorff v The Society of New York Hospital* regarding a case in which a surgeon removed a diseased uterus after the patient had consented to an examination under anesthesia, but with the express stipulation that no operative excision should be performed. The physician argued that his decision was justified by the beneficent obligation to avoid the risks of a second anesthetic. However, Justice Benjamin Cardozo stated:

Every human being of adult years and sound mind has a right to determine what shall be done with his body; and a surgeon who performs an operation without his patient's consent commits an assault, for which he is liable in damages . . . except in cases of emergency, where the patient is unconscious, and where it is necessary to operate before consent can be obtained.[7]

Having established that patients have the right to determine what happens to their bodies, it took some time for the modern concept of *informed* consent to emerge from the initial doctrine of *simple* consent. The initial approach appealed to a *professional practice standard* whereby physicians were obligated to disclose to patients the kind of information that experienced surgeons customarily disclosed.[8] However, this disclosure was not always adequate for patient needs. In another landmark case, *Canterbury v Spence*, the court rejected the professional practice standard in favor of the *reasonable person standard* whereby physicians are obliged to disclose to patients all information regarding diagnosis, treatment options, and risks that a "reasonable patient" would want to know in a similar situation. Rather than relying on the practices or consensus of the medical community, the reasonable person standard empowers the public (reasonable persons) to determine how much information should be disclosed by physicians to ensure that consent is truly informed. The court did recognize, however, that there are practical limits on the amount of information that can be communicated or assimilated.[8] Subsequent litigation has revolved around what reasonable people expect to be disclosed in the consent process to include the nature and frequency of potential complications, the prognostic life expectancy,[9] and the surgeon-specific success rates.[7] Despite the litigious environment of medical practice, it is difficult to prosecute a case of inadequate informed consent so long as the clinician has made a concerted and documented effort to involve the patient in the decision-making process.

Adequate informed consent entails at least four basic elements: (a) The physician documents that the patient or surrogate has the capacity to make a medical decision; (b) The surgeon discloses to the patient details regarding the diagnosis and treatment options sufficiently for the patient to make an informed choice; (c) The patient demonstrates understanding of the disclosed information before (d) authorizing freely a specific treatment plan without undue influence (Fig. 48-5). These goals are aimed at respecting each patient's prerogative for autonomous self-determination. To accomplish these goals, the surgeon needs to engage in a discussion about the causes and nature of the patient's disease, the risks and benefits of available treatment options, as well as details regarding what patients can expect after an operative intervention.[10–17]

Informed consent can be challenging in certain clinical settings. For example, obtaining consent for emergency surgery, where decisions are often made with incomplete information, can be difficult. Emergency consent requires the surgeon to consider if and how possible interventions might save a patient's life, and if successful, what kind of disability might be anticipated. Surgical emergencies are one of the few instances where the limits of patient autonomy are freely acknowledged, and surgeons are empowered by law and ethics to act promptly in the best interests of their patients according to the surgeon's judgment. Most applicable medical laws require physicians to provide the standard of care to incapacitated patients, even

if it entails invasive procedures without the explicit consent of the patient or surrogate. If at all possible, surgeons should seek the permission of their patients to provide treatment, but when emergency medical conditions render patients unable to grant that permission, and when delay is likely to have grave consequences, surgeons are legally and ethically justified in providing whatever surgical treatment the surgeon judges necessary to preserve life and restore health.[7] This justification is based on the social consensus that most people would want their lives and health protected in this way, and this consensus is manifest in the medical profession's general orientation to preserve life. It may be that subsequent care may be withdrawn or withheld when the clinical prognosis is clearer, but in the context of initial resuscitation of injured patients, incomplete information makes clear judgments about the patient's ultimate prognosis or outcome impossible.

The process of consent can also be challenging in the pediatric population. For many reasons, children and adolescents cannot participate in the process of giving informed consent in the same way as adults. Depending on their age, children may lack the cognitive and emotional maturity to participate fully in the process. In addition, depending on the child's age, their specific circumstances, as well as the local jurisdiction, children may not have legal standing to fully participate on their own independent of their parents. The use of parents or guardians as surrogate decision makers only partially addresses the ethical responsibility of the surgeon to involve the child in the informed consent process. The surgeon should strive to augment the role of the decision makers by involving the child in the process. Specifically, children should receive age-appropriate information about their clinical situation and therapeutic options so that the surgeon can solicit the child's "assent" for treatment. In this manner, while the parents or surrogate decision makers formally give the informed consent, the child remains an integral part of the process.

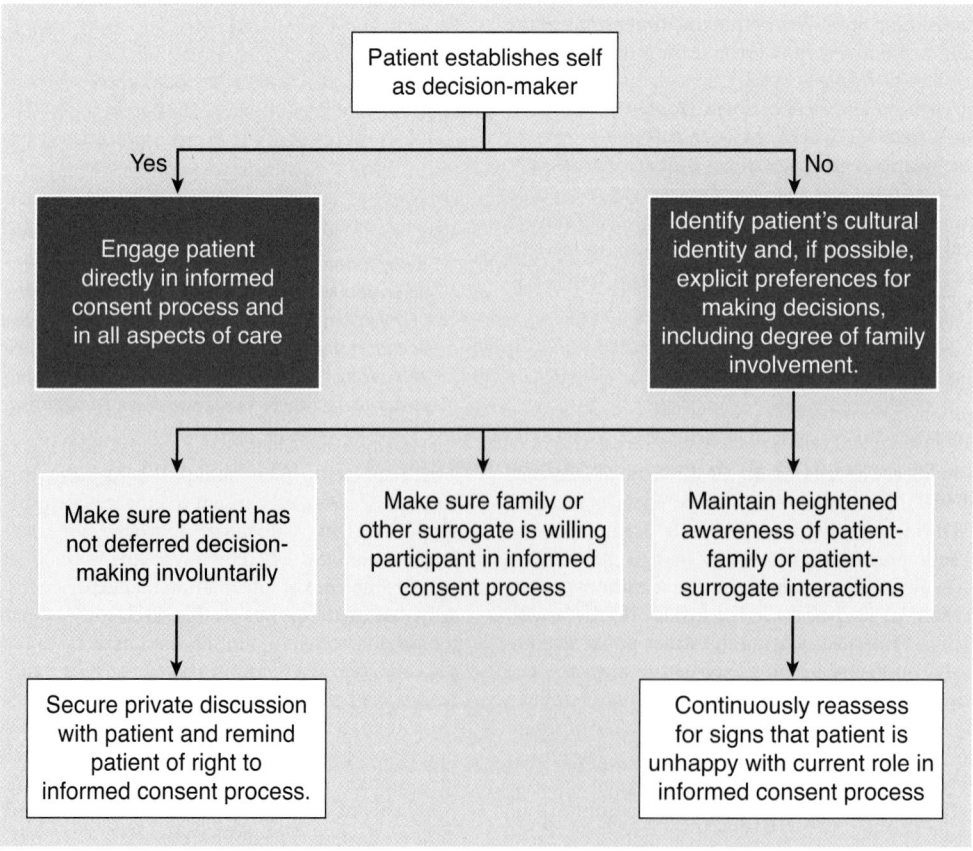

FIG. 48-5. Algorithm for navigating the process of informed consent. *(From Childers R, Lipsett A, Pawlik T: Informed consent and the surgeon.* J Am Coll Surg *E-pub Jan. 21, 2009. Copyright 2009, with permission from Elsevier.)*

Certain religious practices can present difficulties in treating minor children in need of life-saving blood transfusions; however, case law has made clear the precedent that parents, regardless of their held beliefs, may not place their minor children at mortal risk. In such a circumstance, the physician should seek counsel from the hospital medicolegal team, as well as from the institutional ethics team. Legal precedent has, in general, established that the hospital or physician can proceed with providing all necessary care for the child.

Obtaining "consent" for organ donation deserves specific mention.[18] Historically, discussion of organ donation with families of potential donors was performed by transplant professionals, who were introduced to families by intensivists after brain death had been confirmed and the family had been informed of the fact of death. In other instances, consent might be obtained by intensivists caring for the donor, as they were assumed to know the patient's family and could facilitate the process. However, issues of moral "neutrality" as part of end-of-life care in the intensive care unit have caused a shift in how obtaining "consent" for organ donation is handled. Responsibility for obtaining consent from the donor family is now vested in trained "designated requestors" (or "organ procurement coordinators")[19] or by "independent" intensivists who do not have a therapeutic clinical relationship with the potential donor.[20] In this way, the donor family can be allowed to make the decision regarding donation in a "neutral" environment without erosion of the therapeutic relationship with the treating physician.

The process of informed consent also can be limited by the capacity of patients to assimilate information in the context of their illness. For example, despite the best efforts of surgeons, evidence suggests that patients rarely retain much of what is disclosed in the consent conversation, and they may not remember discussing details of the procedure that become relevant when postoperative complications arise.[21] It is important to recognize that the doctrine of informed consent places the most emphasis on the principle of autonomy precisely in those clinical situations when, because of their severe illness or impending death, patients are often divested of their autonomy.

The Boundaries of Autonomy: Advanced Directives and Powers of Attorney

Severe illness and impending death can often render patients incapable of exercising their autonomy regarding medical decisions. One approach to these difficult situations is to make decisions in the "best interests" of patients, but because such decisions require value judgments about which thoughtful people frequently disagree, ethicists, lawyers. and legislators have sought a more reliable solution. Advanced directives of various forms have been developed to carry forward into the future the autonomous choices of competent adults regarding health care decisions. Furthermore, the courts often accept "informal" advanced directives in the form of sworn testimony about statements the patient made at some time previous to their illness. When a formal document expressing the patient's advanced directives fails to exist, surgeons should consider the comments patients and families make when asked about their wishes in the setting of debilitating illness.

Living wills are written to anticipate treatment options and choices in the event that a patient is rendered incompetent by a terminal illness. In the living will, the patient indicates which treatments she wishes to permit or prohibit in the setting of terminal illness. The possible treatments addressed often include mechanical ventilation, cardiopulmonary resuscitation, artificial nutrition, dialysis, antibiotics, or transfusion of blood products. Unfortunately, living wills are often too vague to offer concrete guidance in complex clinical situations, and the language ("terminal illness," "artificial nutrition") can be interpreted in many ways. Furthermore, by limiting the directive only to "terminal" conditions, it does not provide guidance for common clinical scenarios like advanced dementia, delirium, or persistent vegetative states where the patient is unable to make decisions, but is not "terminally" ill. Perhaps even more problematic is the evidence that demonstrates that healthy patients cannot reliably predict their preferences when they are actually sick. For example, the general public estimates the health-related quality of life (HRQoL) score of patients on dialysis at 0.39, although dialysis patients themselves rate their HRQoL at 0.56.[22] Similarly, patients with colostomies rated their HRQoL at 0.92, compared to a score of 0.80 given by the general public for patients with colostomies.[22] For these and other reasons, living wills are often unable to provide the extent of assistance they promise.[23]

An alternative to living wills is the durable power of attorney for health care in which patients identify surrogate decision makers and invest them with the authority to make health care decisions on their behalf in the event that they are unable to speak for themselves. Proponents of this approach hope that the surrogate will be able to make decisions that reflect the choices that the patients themselves would make if they were able. Unfortunately, several studies demonstrate that surrogates are not much better than chance at predicting the choices patients make when the patient is able to state a preference.[7,23,24] These data reveal a flaw in the guiding principle of surrogate decision making: Surrogates do not necessarily have privileged insight into the autonomous preferences of patients. However, the durable power of attorney at least allows patients to choose the person who will eventually make prudential decisions on their behalf and in their best interests; therefore, respecting the judgment of the surrogate is a way of respecting the self-determination of the incapacitated patient.[25]

There is continuing enthusiasm for a wider use of advanced directives. In fact, the 1991 Patient Self Determination Act requires all U.S. health care facilities to (a) inform patients of their rights to have advanced directives, and (b) to document those advanced directives in the chart at the time any patient is admitted to the health care facility.[7] However, only a minority of patients in U.S. hospitals have advanced directives despite concerted efforts to teach the public of their benefits. For example, the ambitious SUPPORT trial used specially trained nurses to promote communication between physicians, patients, and their surrogates to improve the care and decision making of critically ill patients. Despite this concerted effort, the intervention demonstrated "no significant change in the timing of do not resuscitate (DNR) orders, in physician-patient agreement about DNR orders, in the number of undesirable days (patients experiences), in the prevalence of pain, or in the resources consumed."[26]

Some of the reluctance around physician-patient agreement about DNR orders may reflect patient and family anxiety that DNR orders equate to "do not treat." Patients and families should be assured, when appropriate, that declarations of DNR/do not intubate will not necessarily result in a change in ongoing routine clinical care. The issue of temporarily rescinding DNR/do not intubate orders around the time of an operative procedure may also need to be addressed with the family.

Patients should be encouraged to clearly identify their surrogates, both formally and informally, early in the course of treatment, and before any major elective operation. Often, around the time of surgery or at the end of life, there are limits to patient autonomy in medical decision making. Seeking an advanced directive or surrogate decision maker requires time that is not always available when the clinical situation deteriorates. As such, these issues should be clarified as early as possible in the patient-physician relationship.

Withdrawing and Withholding Life-Sustaining Therapies

The implementation of various forms of life support technology raise a number of legal and ethical concerns about when it is permissible to withdraw or withhold available therapeutic technology. There is general consensus among ethicists that there are no philosophic differences between withdrawing (stopping) or withholding (not starting) treatments that are no longer beneficial.[27] However, the right to refuse, withdraw, and withhold beneficial treatments was not established before the landmark case of Karen Ann Quinlan. In 1975, Ms. Quinlan lapsed into a persistent vegetative state requiring ventilator support. After several months without clinical improvement, Ms. Quinlan's parents asked the hospital to withdraw ventilator support. The hospital refused, fearing prosecution for euthanasia. The case was appealed to the New Jersey Supreme Court where the justices ruled that it was permissible to withdraw ventilator support.[28] This case established a now commonly recognized right to withdraw "extraordinary" life-saving technology if it is no longer desired by the patient or the patient's surrogate.

The difference between "ordinary" and "extraordinary" care, and whether there is an ethical difference in withholding or withdrawing "ordinary" vs. "extraordinary" care, has been an area of much contention. The 1983 Nancy Cruzan case highlighted this issue. In this case, Ms. Cruzan had suffered severe injuries in an automobile crash that rendered her in a persistent vegetative state. Ms. Cruzan's family asked that her tube feeds be withheld, but the hospital refused. The case was appealed to the U.S. Supreme Court, which ruled that the tube feeding could be withheld if her parents demonstrated "clear and convincing evidence" that the incapacitated patient would have rejected the treatment.[29] In this ruling, the court essentially ruled that there was no legal distinction between "ordinary" vs. "extraordinary" life-sustaining therapies.[30] In allowing the feeding tube to be removed, the court accepted the principle that a competent person (even through a surrogate decision maker) has the right to decline treatment under the Fourteenth Amendment of the U.S. Constitution. The court noted, however, that there has to be clear and convincing evidence of the patient's wishes (principle of autonomy) and that the burdens of the medical intervention should outweigh its benefits (consistent with the principles of beneficence and nonmaleficence).

In deliberating the issue of withdrawing vs. withholding life-sustaining therapies, the principle of "double effect" is often mentioned. According to the principle of "double effect," a treatment (e.g., opioid administration in the terminally ill) that is intended to help and not harm the patient (i.e., relieve pain) is ethically acceptable even if an unintended consequence (side effect) of its administration is to shorten the life of the patient (e.g., by respiratory depression). Under the principle of double effect, a physician may withhold or withdraw a life-sustaining therapy if the surgeon's *intent* is to relieve suffering, not to hasten death. The classic formulation of double effect has four elements (Fig. 48-6).

Withholding or withdrawing of life-sustaining therapy is ethically justified under the principle of double effect if the physician's intent is to relieve suffering, not to kill the patient. Thus, in managing the distress of the dying, there is a fundamental ethical difference between titrating medications rapidly to achieve relief of distress and administering a very large bolus with the intent of causing apnea. It is important to note, however, that although the use of opioids for pain relief in advanced illness is frequently cited as the classic example of the double effect rule, opioids can be used safely without significant risk. In fact, if administered appropriately, in the vast majority of instances the rule of double effect need not be invoked when administering opioids for symptom relief in advanced illness.[31]

In accepting the ethical equivalence of withholding and withdrawing of life-sustaining therapy, surgeons can make difficult treatment decisions in the face of prognostic uncertainty.[27] In light of this, some important principles to consider when considering withdrawal of life-sustaining therapy include: (a) Any and all treatments can be withdrawn. If circumstances justify withdrawal of one therapy (e.g., IV pressors, antibiotics), they may also justify withdrawal of others. (b) Be aware of the symbolic value of continuing some therapies (e.g., nutrition, hydration) even though their role in palliation is questionable. (c) Before withdrawing life-sustaining therapy, ask the patient and family if a spiritual advisor (e.g., pastor, imam, rabbi, or priest) should be called. (d) Consider requesting an ethics consult.

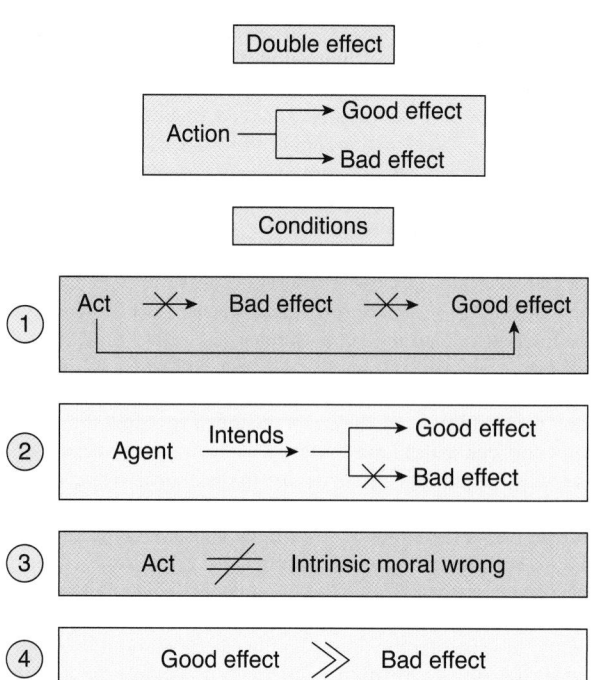

FIG. 48-6. The four elements of the double effect principle: 1) The good effect is produced directly by the action and not by the bad effect. 2) The person must intend only the good effect, even though the bad effect may be foreseen. 3) The act itself must not be intrinsically wrong, or needs to be at least neutral. 4) The good effect is sufficiently desirable to compensate for allowing the bad effect.

Although the clinical setting may seem limited, a range of options usually exists with respect to withdrawing or withholding treatment, allowing for an incremental approach, for example (a) continuing the current regimen without adding new interventions or tests; (b) continuing the current regimen but withdrawing elements when they are no longer beneficial; and (c) withdrawing and withholding all treatments that are not targeted to relieve symptoms and maximize patient comfort.[32]

The surgeon might consider discussing the clinical situation with the patient or proxy decision maker, identify the various therapeutic options, and delineate the reasons why withholding or withdrawing life-sustaining therapy would be in the patient's best interest. If the patient (or designated proxy decision maker) does not agree with withholding or withdrawing life-sustaining therapy, the surgeon should consider or recommend a second medical opinion. If the second opinion corroborates that life-sustaining therapy should be withheld or withdrawn but the patient/family continues to disagree, the surgeon should consider assistance from institutional resources such as the ethics committee and hospital administration. Although the surgeon is not ethically obligated to provide treatment that he or she believes is futile, the surgeon is responsible for continued care of the patient, which may involve transferring the patient to a surgeon who is willing to provide the requested intervention.[27]

PALLIATIVE CARE

General Principles of Palliative Care

Palliative care is a coordinated, interdisciplinary effort that aims to relieve suffering and improve quality of life for patients and their families in the context of serious illness.[33] It is offered simultaneously with all other appropriate medical treatment, and its indication is not limited to situations associated with a poor prognosis for survival. Palliative care strives to achieve more than symptom control, but it should not be confused with noncurative treatment.

The World Health Organization defines palliative care as "an approach that improves the quality of life of patients and their families facing the problems associated with life-threatening illness, through the prevention and relief of suffering by means of early identification and impeccable assessment and treatment of pain and other problems, physical, psychosocial, and spiritual."[34] Palliative care is both a philosophy of care and an organized, highly structured system for delivering care.

Palliative care includes the entire spectrum of intervention for the relief of symptoms and the promotion of quality of life. No specific therapy, including surgical intervention, is excluded from consideration. Therefore, surgeons have valuable contributions to make to palliative care. Furthermore, *surgical palliative care* can be defined as the treatment of suffering and the promotion of quality of life for seriously or terminally ill patients under the care of surgeons.[35] The standard of palliative treatment lies in the agreement between patient and physician that the expected outcome is relief from distressing symptoms, lessening of pain, and improvement of quality of life. The decision to intervene is based on the treatment's ability to meet the stated goals, rather than its impact on the underlying disease.

The fundamental elements of palliative care consist of pain and nonpain symptom management, communication among patients, their families, and care providers, and continuity of care across health systems and through the trajectory of illness. Additional features of system-based palliative care are team-based planning that includes patient and family; close attention to spiritual matters; and psychosocial support for patients, their families, and care providers, including bereavement support.

Indications for palliative care consultation in surgical practice include: (a) patients with conditions that are progressive and life-limiting, especially if characterized by burdensome symptoms, functional decline, and progressive cognitive deficits; (b) assistance in clarification or reorientation of patient/family goals of care; (c) assistance in resolution of ethical dilemmas; (d) situations in which a patient/surrogate declines further invasive or curative treatments with stated preference for comfort measures only; (e) patients who are expected to die imminently or shortly after hospital discharge; and (f) provision of bereavement support for patient care staff, particularly after loss of a colleague under care[35] (Table 48-1).

Palliative Care: History and Philosophy

Palliative care, by virtue of its diverse goals, practices, and practitioners, has many origins, but it would not have emerged as a comprehensive philosophy of care without the seminal contributions of Dame Cicely Saunders (Fig. 48-7). Her life's work began at the bedside of an individual patient, but it ultimately led to the modern hospice movement, spawned a new medical specialty, initiated extensive scientific and social research, and has changed the perception of death and dying for millions of patients and families.

Saunders was a registered nurse, a medical social worker, and ultimately, a physician who was inspired by the needs of suffering

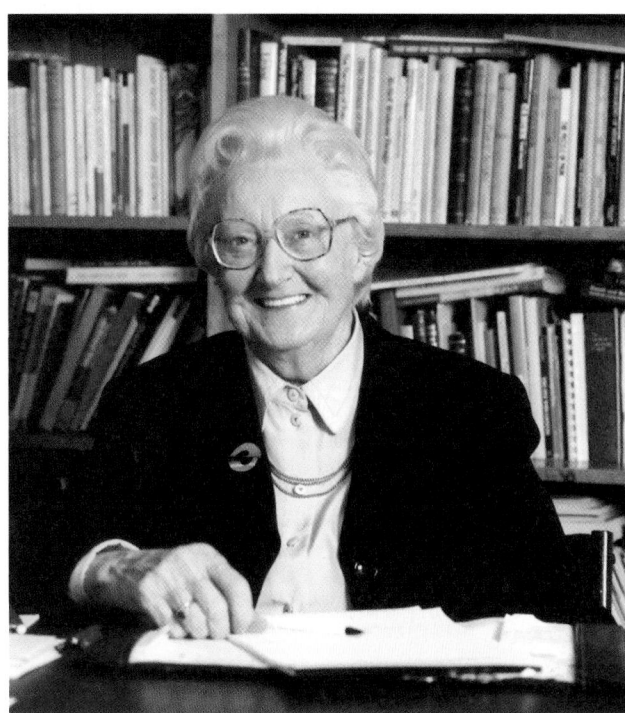

FIG. 48-7. Dame Cicely Mary Strode Saunders. *(Courtesy of St. Christopher's Hospice.)*

soldiers in World War II. Her mentor, thoracic surgeon Howard Barrett, ultimately convinced her to become a physician to increase the credibility of her ideas in the physician-dominated health care system of that time. Saunders made three seminal contributions to the emerging field of palliative care: (a) She observed that the quality of life for patients with pain from advanced cancer is improved with scheduled dosing of opioids; (b) she developed the concept of Total Pain[41] to include physiologic, spiritual, and existential dimensions of pain; and (c) she founded St. Christopher's Hospice in 1967. Each of these contributions illustrates principles that have become the salient themes of all palliative care: the emphasis on symptom control that correlates with enhanced quality of life, the recognition of the spiritual and existential dimensions of health and illness, and the insistence on teamwork as the operational model for delivery of care. Nathan Cherny (Fig. 48-8), another pioneer of palliative care, echoes these themes in his definition of palliative care: "[it] is concerned with three things: the quality of life, the value of life, and the meaning of life."[33] Therefore, it is *existence*, not death, that is the focus of palliative care.

Surgeons have had an integral role in palliative care as it has evolved, and surgical procedures have been part of the armamentarium for symptom relief. For example, although mastectomy, gastrectomy, pancreaticoduodenectomy, and the Blalock-Taussig shunt are thought of as curative, or at least definitive, operations, the initial rationale for developing these procedures was their efficacy as palliative treatment.[37,38] The official report from Massachusetts General Hospital of its experience treating victims of the Coconut Grove fire presciently identified psychologic and social care as major components for the total care the burn victims received.[39]

In addition to developing procedures with palliative utility, surgeons have also made important contributions to the philosophy of palliative care. For example, in 1975, shortly after the hospice concept was established, the distinguished surgeon-educator J. Englebert Dunphey addressed the concept of nonabandonment of terminally ill patients in a landmark lecture that deeply shaped the developing specialty of palliative care.[40]

TABLE 48-1 | Indications for palliative care consultation

Patients with conditions that are progressive and life-limiting, especially if characterized by burdensome symptoms, functional decline, and progressive cognitive deficits

Assistance in clarification or reorientation of patient/family goals of care

Assistance in resolution of ethical dilemmas

Situations in which patient/surrogate declines further invasive or curative treatments with stated preference for comfort measures only

Patients who are expected to die imminently or shortly after hospital discharge

Provision of bereavement support for patient care staff, particularly after loss of a colleague under care

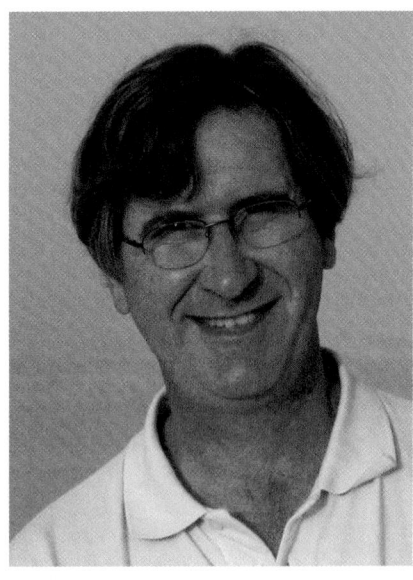

FIG. 48-8. Nathan Cherny, a pioneer for palliative care.

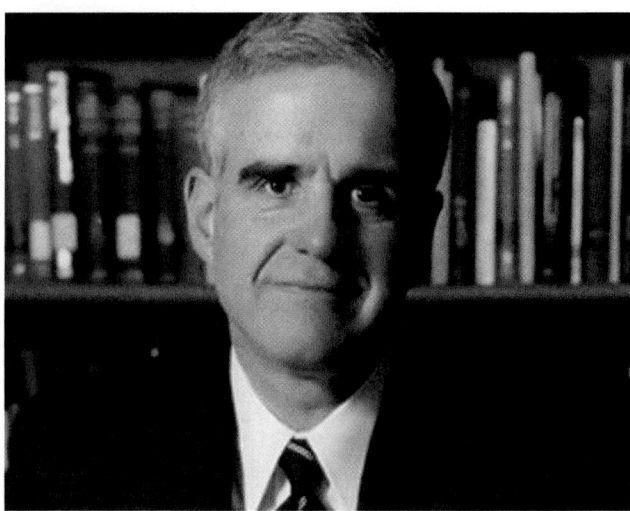

FIG. 48-9. Balfour Mount. *(With permission from McGill University.)*

The term *palliative care* was coined by a Canadian surgeon, Balfour Mount (Fig. 48-9), in 1975 on the opening of the first hospital-based palliative care program in North America. Surgeons were active in the establishment of many community hospice programs in the United States and have contributed popular professional and lay books on the subject.[41–43]

Over the past decade, the American College of Surgeons has issued several statements of principles outlining standards of palliative and end-of-life care in addition to its support of programs disseminating information to surgeons about the principles and

practices of palliative care.[44–46] The Royal College of Surgeons has acknowledged palliative care as a domain of expected competence for Fellowship for over a decade, and since 2002, the American Board of Surgery has included palliative care as a domain of expected knowledge for its qualifying exam.

Over the last 40 years, hospice and palliative care have become established components of health care systems in varying degrees in most countries of the world. Table 48-2 shows a comparison of palliative care and hospice. Both have received repeated endorsements by the World Health Organization,[47] medical societies,[44] and

TABLE 48-2	Comparison of palliative and hospice care	
	Palliative Care	**Hospice (Medicare Benefit)**
Eligibility	• May be initiated by physician referral at time of diagnosis of any serious illness regardless of prognosis • No renewal criteria because of lack of prognosis requirement • All illnesses, ages	• Patient is eligible for Medicare Part A • Patient certified (two physicians) to have probable survival of 6 mo or less if disease, untreated, pursues its natural course • Patient (surrogate if patient not competent) must sign form electing hospice benefit • Eligibility may be renewed as long as patient continues to meet admission criteria • All terminal illnesses • Medicare benefit does not require Do Not Resuscitate for eligibility • Medicare benefit does not require primary caregiver in the home • Hospice care must be provided by a Medicare-certified hospice program
Venues of service	• Hospitals including Veteran's Administration hospitals • Health care clinics • Assisted living facilities • Nursing homes • Home	• Majority cared for at home • Hospitals, including Veteran's Administration hospitals • Assisted living facilities • Nursing homes
Treatments	• Palliative and disease-directed therapies such as chemotherapy and dialysis	• Palliative only • Some hospice programs will authorize continued dialysis, total parenteral nutrition, tube feedings, and chemotherapy
Insurance	• Some treatments and medications covered by Medicare, Medicaid, and private insurers	• More defined and comprehensive than palliative care reimbursement • Medicare covers all expenses related to hospice care: medications, procedures, consultant's fees, durable medical equipment, home nursing visits, bereavement services up to 1 y after the date of death • Medicaid benefit similar to Medicare in almost all states • Most insurance plans have a hospice benefit
Team composition	• Interdisciplinary • Composition flexible depending on clinical setting	• Interdisciplinary • Medicare requires physician, nurse, social worker, and a volunteer as core team members • Patient may retain primary physician or be followed by hospice medical director

medical specialty boards.[48] More than just a philosophy of care, hospice and palliative care have emerged as a medical specialty that provides a standard medical practice to patients in institutional settings and in patient homes. Palliative medicine was recognized as a medical subspecialty by the Royal College of Medicine in 1987 and by the American Board of Medical Specialties in 2006. Many insurers now reimburse these services as a standard benefit, and in the United States, the Medicare hospice benefit provides a per diem in support of nursing, social services, nurse aides, physician oversight, volunteers, chaplain support, durable medical equipment, and the cost of medications for symptom control.

Although all patients, regardless of prognosis, may benefit from the services of a palliative care physician with expertise in relieving intractable symptoms, hospice care[49] is a specific form of palliative care intended for patients who have an estimated prognosis of 6 months or less to live, usually certified by two physicians (the attending physician and hospice medical director). Initially, there are two certification periods of 3 months each, followed by recertification every 60 days thereafter. Continued services may continue well beyond the original 6 months of estimated survival, and they are based on ongoing disease progression, further functional decline, and persistent symptom burden. The goal of hospice is to provide holistic care at the end of life focused on relief of the patient's suffering. Most Americans indicate a preference to die at home, but nearly 75% die in an institutional setting (half in acute hospitals and another one fourth in nursing homes). Of the one fourth that do die at home, hospice services can help make that experience better for both patient and surviving loved ones. Earlier referral and wider use of the hospice benefit may help more patients achieve their goal of dying at home.

Concepts of Suffering, Pain, Health, and Healing

Palliative care addresses specifically the individual patient's experience of suffering due to illness. Indeed, the philosophical origins of palliative care began with attention to suffering and the existential questions suffering engenders. More than mere technologic evolution in the management of symptoms, the early proponents of palliative care sought a revolution in the moral foundations of medicine that challenged the assumptions that so often seemed to result in futile invasive intervention, and identified many of the problems that were subsequently taken up by medical ethicists. This reorientation of the goals of medical care from a focus on disease and its management to the patient's experience of illness focuses attention on the purpose of medicine and the meaning of health and healing.

Over the past half century, several concepts and theories about the nature of pain, suffering, and health have been proposed in service of the evolving conceptual framework of palliative care. For example, while considering the differences between disease-oriented and illness-oriented approaches to the care of seriously ill patients, psychiatrist Arthur Kleinman wrote, "There is a moral core to healing in all societies. [Healing] is the central purpose of medicine . . . the purpose of medicine is both control of disease processes and care for the illness experience. Nowhere is this clearer than in the relationship of the chronically ill to their medical system: For them, the control of disease is by definition limited; care for the life problems created by the disorder is the chief issue."[50]

The relief of pain has been the clinical foundation for hospice and palliative care. It has been defined by the International Association for the Study of Pain as "An unpleasant sensory and emotional experience associated with actual or potential tissue damage, or described in terms of such damage."[51] For purposes of interdisciplinary palliative care, Saunders's concept of "Total Pain"[36] is a more useful definition and is frequently used as the basis for palliative assessments. Total Pain is the sum total of four principal domains of pain: physical, psychologic, social or socioeconomic, and spiritual. Each of these contributes to, but is not synonymous with, suffering.

Persons suffer when their individual integrity or personhood is threatened: "Bodies do not suffer, only persons do."[52] Personhood

entails a transcendent dimension that often can frame the existential threat of death in some broader sense of meaning. As such, issues related to a person's past history and future legacy become compellingly more central as physical decline becomes increasingly pronounced. As argued by Cassell, if physicians understand suffering in only its physical dimension (attention to laboratory values, x-rays, etc.), they may ignore the psychologic and spiritual pain that accompanies dying; such neglect may not only fail to relieve suffering, but actually compound it.[52] Saunders's taxonomy of pain and Cassell's portrayal of the mechanism of suffering collectively represent the structure and function of the human psyche in the context of life-threatening illness.

Frankl[53] contributed to the philosophy of palliative care the notion that the willingness to survive is related to the capacity to make sense out of suffering, giving suffering a sense of meaning. Brody described suffering as the sense of anguish that besets an individual near the end of his life when his personal narrative is fragmented to the point of incoherence. This fragmentation prevents the individual from transforming his personal narrative into a legacy that will endure after death. Brody challenges physicians caring for severely ill patients to consider how their participation in the care of patients might best assist those patients in transforming a "broken story" into a "transcendent legacy."[54]

Finally, the developmental framework for the end of life proposed by Byock[55] views the last phases of life not so much as an arena for suffering, but as a natural phase of life with its own developmental tasks, which, when achieved, result in deeply satisfying personal growth that reciprocates with the growth of those sharing this experience. Byock's four developmental tasks of the dying include: (a) renewal of a sense of personhood and meaning, (b) bringing closure to personal and community relationships, (c) bringing closure to worldly affairs, and (d) acceptance of the finality of life.

Effective Communication and Negotiating the Goals of Care

Changing the goals of care from cure to palliation near the end of life is both emotionally and clinically challenging, and it depends on a clear prognosis and effective communication. Unfortunately, prognostication can be notoriously difficult and inaccurate in advanced illness, and Christakis has argued that, to a large degree, physicians have abdicated their traditional responsibility to provide clear prognosis regarding incurable disease and approaching death.[56] However, there are validated tools for prognosis in critical illness (APACHE, MODS, etc.), and with most advanced diseases, functional status is the most powerful predictor of survival. For example, patients with advanced metastatic cancer who are resting/sleeping for 50% or more of normal waking hours and require some assistance with activities of daily living (ADL) have a projected survival of weeks, and patients who are essentially bedfast and dependent for ADL have a projected survival of days to a week or two at best. Table 48-3 shows a simple prognostic tool to aid clinicians in recognizing patients nearing the end of life.

Alternatively, the Karnofsky Performance Scale is a scale of functional status ranging from 100 (high level of function) to 0 (death). It is commonly used in palliative care to roughly assess patient anticipated needs as well as prognosis. The Palliative Performance Scale[57] is a validated[58] expansion of the Karnofsky Performance Scale that includes five palliative-focused domains, including ambulation, activity level, self-care, intake, and level of consciousness, in addition to evidence of disease. The Missoula-Vitas Quality of Life Index is a 25-question scale specifically for palliative care and hospice patients that scores symptoms, function, interpersonal relationships, well being, and spirituality. Updates and Spanish versions are available.[55]

Regardless of the prognostic tool used, the prognosis should be conveyed to the patient and family. If done well, communication and negotiation with patients and families about advanced terminal illnesses can potentially avoid great psychologic harm and help

TABLE 48-3	Simple prognostication tool in advanced illness (especially cancer)		
Functional Level		**Performance Status (ECOG)**	**Prognosis**
Able to perform all basic ADLs independently and some IADLs		2	Months
Resting/sleeping up to 50% or more of waking hours and requiring some assistance with basic ADLs		3	Weeks to a few months
Dependent for basic ADLs and bed to chair existence		4	Days to a few weeks at most

These observations apply to patients with advanced, progressive, incurable illnesses (e.g., metastatic cancer refractory to treatment).
Basic ADL = activities of daily living (e.g., transferring, toileting, bathing, dressing, and feeding oneself); IADL = instrumental activities of daily living (e.g., more complex activities such as meal preparation, performing household chores, balancing a checkbook, shopping, etc.); ECOG = Eastern Cooperative Oncology Group functional (performance) status.

make a difficult transition easier. To communicate effectively and compassionately, it is helpful to pursue an organized process similar to the structured history and physical central to the evaluation of any patient. One such structured approach to delivering unfavorable news proposes six steps that can be easily learned by clinicians: (a) getting started by selection of the appropriate setting, introductions, and seating; (b) determining what the patient or family knows; (c) determining what the patient or family wants to know; (d) giving the information; (e) expressing empathy; and (f) establishing expectations, planning, and aftercare (Table 48-4).[59] Success with this approach to breaking bad news is critically dependent upon the clinician's ability to empathically respond to the patient's (and family's) reaction to the news.[60] The empathic response does not require the surgeon to share the same emotions of the patient, but it does require the surgeon to identify the patient's emotion and accurately reflect that awareness back to the patient. Patient assessment in these conversations should give the highest priority to identifying and responding to the most immediate source of distress. Relieving a pressing symptom is prerequisite for a more thorough search for other potential sources of suffering, and the assessment process, itself, can be therapeutic if conducted in a respectful and gentle manner.

CARE AT THE END OF LIFE

The process of dying and the care of a patient at the time of death is a distinct clinical entity that demands specific skills from physicians. The issues specific to dying and the available tools for compassionate care at the end of life are addressed in this section.

TABLE 48-4	Communicating unfavorable news: Important principles

- Setting: Find a quiet, private place to meet. Sit down close to the patient.
- Listen: Clarify the patient's and/or the family's understanding of the situation.
- "Warning shot": Prepare patient and family and obtain their permission to communicate bad news (e.g., "I'm afraid I have bad news.").
- Silence: Pause after giving bad news. Allow patient/family to absorb/react to the news.
- Encourage: Convey hope that is realistic and appropriate to the circumstances (e.g., patient will not be abandoned; symptoms will be controlled).

The Syndrome of Imminent Demise[32,61]

In a patient who has progressed to the terminal stage of an advanced illness (e.g., cancer), a number of signs provide evidence of imminent death. As terminally ill patients progress toward death, they become increasingly bedbound, requiring assistance for all basic ADL. There is a steady decrease in desire and requests for food and fluids. More distressing to the dying patient is a progressively dry mouth that may be confused by the treating team as thirst. It is often exacerbated by anticholinergic medications, mouth breathing, and supplemental oxygen (O_2) administered without humidification.

With progressive debility, fatigue, and weight loss, it is common for terminally ill patients to experience increasing difficulty swallowing. This may result in aspiration episodes and an inability to swallow tablets, requiring alternative routes for medication administration (e.g., IV, SC, PR, sublingual, buccal, or transdermal). In addition to the increased risk of aspiration, patients near death develop great difficulty clearing oropharyngeal and upper airway secretions, leading to noisy breathing or the so-called "death rattle." As death approaches, the respiratory pattern may change to increasingly frequent periods of apnea often following a Cheyne-Stokes pattern of rapid, progressively longer breaths leading up to an apneic period. As circulatory instability develops near death, patients may exhibit cool and mottled extremities. Periods of confusion are often accompanied by decreasing urine output and episodes of fecal and urinary incontinence.

A number of cognitive changes occur as death approaches. Patients who are in the last days of life may demonstrate some signs of confusion or delirium. Agitated delirium is a prominent feature of a difficult death. Other cognitive changes that may be seen include a decreased interest in social interactions, increased somnolence, reduced attention span, disorientation to time (often with altered sleep-wake cycles), and an altered dream life, including vivid "waking dreams" or visual hallucinations. Reduced hearing and visual acuity may be an issue for some patients; however, patients who appear comatose may still be aware of their surroundings. Severely cachectic patients may lose the ability to keep their eyes closed during sleep because of loss of the retro-orbital fat pad.

Common Symptoms at the End of Life and Their Management[32,61,62]

The three most common, major symptoms that threaten the comfort of dying patients in their last days are respiratory distress, pain, and cognitive failure. General principles that are applicable to symptom management in the last days of life include: (a) anticipating symptoms before they develop; (b) minimizing technologic interventions (usually manage symptoms with medications); and (c) planning alternative routes for medications in case the oral route fails. It may be possible to cautiously reduce the dose of opioids and other medications as renal clearance decreases near the end of life, but it is important to remember that increased somnolence and decreasing respirations are prominent features of the dying process independent of medication side effects. Sudden cessation of opioid analgesics near the end of life could precipitate withdrawal symptoms, and therefore, medications should not be stopped for increasing somnolence or slowed respirations.

The principles of pharmacotherapy for pain and nonpain symptoms in the palliative care setting are outlined in Table 48-5. The World Health Organization,[34] the United States Agency for Health Care Policy and Research,[63] the Academy of Hospice and Palliative Medicine,[64] and many other agencies have endorsed a "step ladder" approach to cancer pain management that can predictably result in satisfactory pain control in most patients (Table 48-6). More refractory pain problems require additional expertise, and occasionally, more invasive approaches (Tables 48-7 and 48-8).

The primary treatment of dyspnea (air hunger) in the dying is opioids, which should be cautiously titrated to increase comfort and reduce tachypnea to a range of 15 to 20 breaths/min. Air movement

TABLE 48-5	Principles of pharmacotherapy in palliative care

- Believe patient report of symptoms.
- Modify pathologic process when possible and appropriate.
- In terminally ill, avoid medications not directly linked to symptom control.
- Use a multidisciplinary approach.
- Consider nonpharmacologic approaches whenever possible.
- Engage participation of clinical pharmacist in treatment plan.
- Select drugs that can multitask (i.e., use haloperidol for agitated delirium and nausea).
- For pain, use adjuvant medications when possible (see Table 48-8).
- When using opioids, spare when possible (adjuvant medication, local or regional anesthetics, surgical interventions, etc.).
- Avoid fixed combination drugs.
- Avoid excessive cost.
- Select agents with minimum side effects.
- Anticipate and prophylax against side effects.
- For the elderly, the hypoproteinemic, the azotemic: "Start low and go slow."
- Oral route whenever possible and practical.
- No IM injections.
- Scheduled dosing, not prn, for persistent symptoms.
- Stepwise approach. (See the World Health Organization Analgesic Ladder for pain. See Table 48-6.)
- Reassess continuously and titrate to effect.
- Use equianalgesic doses when changing opioids (see Table 48-6).
- Assess patient/family's comprehension of management plan.

across the face generated by a fan can sometimes be quite helpful. If this is not effective, empiric use of supplemental O_2 by nasal cannula (2 to 3 L/min) may bring some subjective relief, independent of observable changes in pulse oximetry. Supplemental O_2 should be humidified to avoid exacerbation of dry mouth. Typical starting doses of an immediate release opioid for breathlessness should be one half to two thirds of a starting dose of the same agent for cancer pain. For patients already on opioids for pain, a 25 to 50% increment in the dose of the current immediate release agent for breakthrough pain often will be effective in relieving breathlessness in addition to breakthrough pain.

The availability and variety of drugs should not prevent consideration of nonpharmacologic therapy. Massage therapy, music therapy, art therapy, guided imagery, hypnosis, physical therapy, pet therapy, and others play a constructive role not only for the relief of symptoms, but for promoting a sense of hope through improving function, aesthetic pleasure, and social connectedness. Talents and capacities neglected during the treatment and progression of disease can be recovered even in the most advanced stages of illness.

Pain is often less of a problem in the last days of life because the reduced activity level is associated with lower incident pain. This, combined with lower renal clearance of opioids, may result in greater potency of the prescribed agents. Severe pain crises are fortunately rare, but when they are inadequately addressed, can

TABLE 48-6	The World Health Organization three-step ladder for control of cancer pain[34]

Step 1 mild pain (visual analogue scale, 1–3)
   Nonopioid ± adjuvant medication
Step 2 moderate pain (visual analogue scale, 4–6)
   Opioid for mild to moderate pain and nonopioid ± an adjuvant
Step 3 severe pain (visual analogue scale, 7–10)
   Opioid for moderate to severe pain ± nonopioid ± an adjuvant

cause great and lasting distress (complicated grief) for loved ones who witness the final hours or days of agony. Such situations may require continuous administration of parenteral opioids. As death approaches and patients become less verbal, it is important to assess pain frequently, including the use of close observation for nonverbal signs of distress (e.g., grimacing, increased respiratory rate). Adequate dosing of opioid analgesics may require alternate route(s) of administration as patients become more somnolent or develop swallowing difficulties. Opioids should not be stopped abruptly, even if the patient becomes nonresponsive because sudden withdrawal can cause severe distress.[65,66]

Cognitive failure at the end of life is manifested in most patients by increasing somnolence and delirium. Gradually increasing somnolence can be accompanied by periods of disorientation and mild confusion, and it may respond to the reassuring presence of loved ones and caregivers with minimal need for medications. A more distressing form of delirium also can develop, manifested by increasing agitation that may require the use of neuroleptic medications. Increasing amounts of opioids and/or benzodiazepines may exacerbate the delirium (especially in the elderly).

Pronouncing Death[67]

If the body is hypothermic or has been hypothermic, such as a drowning victim pulled from the water in the winter, the physician should not declare death until warming attempts have been made. In the hospital, hospice, or home setting, the declaration of death becomes part of the medical or legal record of the event. There are a number of physical signs of death a physician should look for in confirming the patient's demise: complete lack of responsiveness to verbal or tactile stimuli, absence of heart beat and respirations, fixed pupils, skin color change to a waxen hue as blood settles, gradual poikilothermia, and sphincter relaxation with loss of urine and feces. For deaths in the home with patients who have been enrolled in hospice, the hospice nurse on call should be contacted immediately. In some states, deaths at home may require a brief police investigation and report. For deaths in the hospital, the family must be notified (in person, if possible). A coroner or medical examiner may need to be contacted under specific circumstances (e.g., deaths in the operating room), but most deaths do not require their services. However, the pronouncing physician will need to complete a death certificate according to local regulations. Survivors may also be approached, if appropriate, regarding potential autopsy and organ donation. Finally, it is important to accommodate religious rituals that may be important to the dying patient or the family. *Bereavement* is the experience of loss by death of a person to whom one is attached. *Mourning* is the process of adapting to such a loss in the thoughts, feelings, and behaviors that one experiences after the loss.[68] Although grief and mourning are accentuated in the immediate period around death, it is important to note that patients and families may begin the process of bereavement well before the time of death as patients and families grieve incremental losses of independence, vitality, and control. In addition to the surviving loved ones, it is important to acknowledge that caregivers also experience grief for the loss of their patients.[69,70]

PROFESSIONAL ETHICS: CONFLICT OF INTEREST, RESEARCH, AND CLINICAL ETHICS

Conflict of Interest

Conflicts of interest for surgeons can arise in many situations in which the potential benefits or gains to be realized by the surgeon are, or are perceived to be, in conflict with the responsibility to put the patient's interests before the surgeon's own. Conflicts of interest for the surgeon can involve actual or perceived situations in which the individual stands to gain monetarily by his or her role as a physician or investigator. In the academic community, monetary gain may not be the primary factor. Instead, motivators such as power, tenure, or

TABLE 48-7 Analgesics for persistent pain

Drug	Initial Dosing (Adult, >60 kg)	Comments
Mild persistent pain, visual analogue scale (VAS) 1–3		
Acetaminophen (Tylenol)	325–650 mg PO qid Maximum = 3200 mg/24 h	Use <2400 mg if other potentially hepatotoxic drugs taken. Acetaminophen contained in concurrent nonprescription medications can easily exceed maximum daily allowable dose.
Aspirin	600–1500 mg PO qid	Gastric bleeding, platelet dysfunction
Choline magnesium trisalicylate (Trilisate)	750–1500 mg PO bid	Useful for avoiding platelet dysfunction
Ibuprofen (Advil, Motrin)	200–400 mg PO qid Maximum = 3200 mg/24 h	Gastropathy, nephropathy, decreased platelet aggregation
Naproxen (Naprosyn)	250 mg PO bid Maximum = 1300 mg/24 h	Available as a transcutaneous gel
Moderate persistent pain, VAS 4–6		
Hydrocodone (Vicodin, Lortab)	5–7.5 mg PO q4h	Most prescribed drug in the United States Acetaminophen in compounded drug limits use to moderate pain.
Oxycodone	5 mg PO q4h	Sold as single agent or compounded with aspirin or acetaminophen. Slow release form available (Oxycontin)
Severe persistent pain, VAS 7–10		
Morphine	10 mg PO q2–4h 2–4 mg IV q4h	Standard drug for comparison to alternative opioids. Avoid or caution when giving to the elderly, patients with diminished glomerular filtration rate, or liver disease. Slow release PO form available (MS Contin).
Hydromorphone	1–3 mg PO, PR q4h 1 mg IV, SC q4h	Suppository form available Oral dose forms limited to 4 mg maximum
Fentanyl, transdermal	12 μg/h patch q72h	Not for acute pain management. Do not use on opioid-naive patients. Absorption unpredictable in cachectic patients.
Methadone	**Consultation with pain management, clinical pharmacists, or palliative care/ hospice services skilled in methadone use is recommended for those inexperienced in prescribing methadone.**	Not a first-line agent, although very effective, especially for pain with a neuropathic component Very inexpensive Can be given PO, IV, SC, PR, sublingually, and vaginally Its long half-life makes dosing more difficult than alternative opioids and close monitoring is required when initiating Numerous medications, alcohol, and cigarette smoking can alter its serum levels **Physicians who write methadone prescriptions for pain should specify this indication.** Methadone use for drug withdrawal treatment requires special licensure.

Risk factors for NSAID-induced nephropathy include: advanced age, decreased glomerular filtration rate, congestive heart failure, hypovolemia, pressors, hepatic dysfunction, concomitant nephrotoxic agents. Dose reduction and hydration reduce risk.
Opioids compounded with aspirin or acetaminophen are limited to treatment of moderate persistent pain because of dose-limiting toxicities of acetaminophen and aspirin.
Slow-release preparations of morphine and oxycodone may be given rectally.
Timed-release tablets or patches should never be crushed or cut.
Opioid analgesics are the agents of choice for severe cancer-related pain. Sedation is a common side effect when initiating opioid therapy. Tolerance to this usually develops within a few days. If sedation persists beyond a few days, a stimulant (methylphenidate 2.5–5 mg PO bid) can be given.
Initiate bowel stimulant prophylaxis for constipation when prescribing opioids unless contraindicated.
Adjuvant or coanalgesic agents are drugs that enhance analgesic efficacy of opioids, treat concurrent symptoms that exacerbate pain, or provide independent analgesia for specific types of pain (e.g., a tricyclic antidepressant for treatment of neuropathic pain). Coanalgesics can be initiated for persistent pain at any visual analogue scale level. Gabapentin is commonly used as an initial agent for neuropathic pain.
No place for meperidine (Demerol), propoxyphene [Darvon, Darvocet, or mixed agonist-antagonist agents (Stadol, Talwin)] in management of persistent pain.
Always consider alternative approaches (axial analgesia, operative approaches, etc.) when managing severe persistent pain.
NOTE: These are not recommendations for specific patients. The inter- and intraindividual variability to opioids requires individualizing dosing and titration to effect.
Source: Adapted, with permission from Dunn GP: Surgical palliative care, in Cameron JL (ed): *Current Surgical Therapy*, 9th ed. Philadelphia: Elsevier, 2008. Copyright Elsevier.

authorship on a publication may serve as potential sources of conflict of interest. For example, the accrual of subjects in research studies or patients in surgical series may ensure surgeons better authorship or more financial gains. The dual-role of the surgeon-scientist therefore needs to be considered because the duty as surgeon can conflict with the role of scientist or clinical researcher.

Research Ethics

Over the last three decades in the United States, the ethical requirements for the conduct of human subject research have been formalized and widely accepted. Although detailed informed consent is a necessary condition for the conduct of ethically good human subject research, other factors also determine whether research is designed and conducted ethically. Emanuel and colleagues[71] described seven requirements for all clinical research studies to be

ethically sound: (a) value—enhancement(s) of health or knowledge must be derived from the research; (b) scientific validity—the research must be methodologically rigorous; (c) fair subject selection—scientific objectives, not vulnerability or privilege, and the potential for and distribution of risks and benefits, should determine communities selected as study sites and the inclusion criteria for individual subjects; (d) favorable risk-benefit ratio—within the context of standard clinical practice and the research protocol, risks must be minimized, potential benefits enhanced, and the potential benefits to individuals and knowledge gained for society must outweigh the risks; (e) independent review—unaffiliated individuals must review the research and approve, amend, or terminate it; (f) informed consent—individuals should be informed about the research and provide their voluntary consent; and (g) respect for enrolled subjects—subjects should have their privacy protected, the opportunity to withdraw, and their well-being monitored.[71]

TABLE 48-8	Examples of adjuvant medications for treatment of neuropathic, visceral, and bone pain[a]	
Drug Class	**Initial Dosing (Adult, >60 kg)**	**Comments**

Tricyclic antidepressants
  Best for continuous burning or tingling pain and allodynia
  Efficacy for pain not due to antidepressant effect
	Amitriptyline 10–25 mg PO qhs	Sedating properties may be useful for relief of other concurrent symptoms. Side effects may precede benefit. Avoid in the elderly due to anticholinergic side effects.

Dose generally less than that required for antidepressant effect	Nortriptyline 10–25 mg PO qd	Less anticholinergic effect
Dose titrated up every few days until effect. Pain may respond to alternative antidepressants if no response to initial agent.	Doxepin 10–25 mg PO qhs Imipramine 10–25 mg PO qd	
Anticonvulsants For shooting, stabbing pain	Gabapentin 100–300 mg PO qd. Titrate up rapidly as needed. Max: 1800 mg qd	Commonly used first-line agent. Generally well tolerated. Does not require blood level monitoring.
	Carbamazepine 200 mg PO q12h	Effective. Well studied. Requires blood monitoring.
	Valproic acid 250 mg PO tid	
Local anesthetics Systemic use requires monitoring. Nebulized local anesthetics (lidocaine, bupivacaine) can be used for severe, refractory cough.	Lidocaine transdermal patch 5%. Apply to painful areas. Max: 3 simultaneous patches over 12 h (each patch contains 700 mg lidocaine).	Systemic toxicity can result from applying more than recommended number per unit time and in patients with liver failure. Effective for postherpetic neuralgia.
	Lidocaine/prilocaine topical. Apply to painful areas.	
Miscellaneous	Bisphosphonates (pamidronate, zoledronic acid)	For bone pain and reduced incidence of skeletal complications secondary to malignancy—best results in myeloma and breast cancer. Contraindicated in renal failure.
	Calcitonin nasal spray	Refractory bone pain
	Dexamethasone	For bone pain, acute nerve compression, visceral pain secondary to tumor infiltration or luminal obstruction by reducing inflammatory component of tumor
	Radionuclides (Sr-89)	For malignant bone pain secondary to osteoclastic activity. 4–6 wk delay in benefit. Requires adequate bone marrow reserve. For prognosis of more than 3 mo.
	Octreotide	Reduces GI secretions that contribute to visceral pain

[a]Recommendations are based on experience of practitioners of hospice and palliative medicine and in some instances do not reflect current clinical trials.
Source: Adapted, with permission from Dunn GP: Surgical palliative care, in Cameron JL (ed): *Current Surgical Therapy*, 9th ed. Philadelphia: Elsevier, 2008. Copyright Elsevier.

Special Concerns in Surgical Research

A significant issue for clinical surgical research is that it is often analyzed in a retrospective manner and not commonly undertaken in a prospective double-blind, randomized fashion. For a randomized trial to be undertaken, the researchers should be in a state of equipoise—that is, there must be a state of genuine uncertainty on the part of the clinical investigator or the expert medical community regarding the comparative therapeutic merits of each arm in a trial.[72] To randomize subjects to receive two different treatments, a researcher must believe that the existing data are not sufficient to conclude that one treatment strategy is better than another. In designing surgical trials, surgeons usually have biases that one treatment is better than another and often have difficulty maintaining the state of equipoise. As such, it is frequently difficult to demonstrate that a randomized trial is necessary or feasible, and treatment options that question the validity of clinical tenets are difficult to accept. Meakins has suggested that a slightly different hierarchy of evidence applies to evidence-based surgery.[73]

A second major issue for surgical trials is whether it is ethically acceptable to have a placebo-controlled surgical trial. Some commentators have argued that sham surgery is always wrong because, unlike a placebo medication that is harmless, every surgical procedure carries some risk.[74] Others have argued that sham operations are essential to the design of a valid randomized clinical trial because, without a sham operation, it is not possible to know if the surgical intervention is the cause of improvement in patient symptoms or whether the improvement is due to the effect of having

surgery.[75,76] Most surgeons readily agree that designing an appropriately low-risk sham surgical procedure would create problems for the surgeon-patient relationship in that the surgeon would need to keep the sham a secret.[77] In this sense, a sham surgical arm of a trial is very different from a placebo medication in that there cannot be blinding of the surgeon as to which procedure was undertaken. As a result, to have a sham surgery arm in a clinical trial, the interactions between the surgeon and the subject must be limited and the surgeon performing the procedure should not be the researcher who follows the subject during the trial. Despite difficulties with designing a surgical trial in which the surgeon could ethically perform a sham operation, there are specific circumstances that allow for placebo operations to be conducted, so long as certain criteria are met and are analyzed on a case by case basis.[78,79]

Surgical Innovation and Surgical Research

An important issue is whether surgical innovation should be treated as research or as standard of care. Many of the advances in surgical technique and surgical technology have resulted from the innovations that individual surgeons have discovered or created during the course of challenging operations. As every patient is different and the surgeon is always trying to determine the best way to complete an operation, innovations have developed that have often moved the field of surgery forward.[80] In the Korean and Vietnam wars, the military guidelines for the treatment of vascular injuries recommended ligation and amputation rather than interposition grafting of vascular injuries. Individual surgeons chose to ignore those guidelines and subsequently demonstrated the value of reconstructive techniques that ultimately became the standard of care. It is debated whether modifications in an accepted surgical technique based on the circumstances of an individual patient and the skill and judgment of an individual surgeon should require the same type of prior approval that enrollment in a clinical trial would warrant.[81] However, if a surgeon decides to use a new technique on several occasions and to study the outcomes, Institutional Review Board approval and all other ethical requirements for research are necessary. These situations require strict oversight as well as explicit consent by the patient.[82] In particular, when developing new and innovative techniques, the surgeon should work in close consultation with his or her senior colleagues, including the chairperson of the department. Frequently, more senior individuals can provide sage ethical advice regarding what constitutes minor innovative changes in a technique vs. true novel research.

When compared to the formalized process for new drug approval by the Food and Drug Administration, the process for a surgeon developing an innovative operation is relatively unregulated and unsupervised.

Clinical Ethics: Disclosure of Errors

Disclosure of error—either in medical or research matters—is important, but often difficult (see Chap. 12). Errors of judgment, errors in technique, and system errors are responsible for most errors that result in complications and deaths. Hospitals are evaluated based on the number of complications and deaths that occur in surgical patients, and surgeons traditionally review their complications and deaths in a formal exercise known as the *mortality and morbidity conference*, or *M&M*. The exercise places importance on the attending surgeon's responsibility for errors made, whether he or she made them themselves, and the value of the exercise is related to the effect of "peer pressure"—the entire department knows about the case—on reducing repeated occurrences of such an error. Although a time-honored ritual in surgery, the M&M conference is nonetheless a poor method for analyzing causes of error and for developing methods to prevent them. Moreover, the proceedings of the M&M conference are protected from disclosure by the privilege of "peer review," and the details are rarely shared with patients or those outside of the department.

A report from the United States Institute of Medicine titled "To Err Is Human" highlighted the large number of medical errors that occur and encouraged efforts to prevent patient harm.[83] Medical errors are generally considered to be "preventable adverse medical events."[84] Given that medical errors clearly occur with some frequency, the question becomes what and how should patients be told of medical errors and what is the surgeon's ethical responsibility for this disclosure.[85]

Disclosure of error is consistent with the ethical tenets of openness with patients and the involvement of patients in their care. In contrast, failing to disclose errors to patients undermines public trust in medicine and potentially compromises the treatment of the consequences of errors. In addition, failure to self-disclose medical errors can be construed as a breach of professional ethics, as it is a failure to act solely for the patient's best interests. Patients require information regarding medical errors so that additional harm can be avoided. In addition, information regarding a medical error may be needed so that patients can make independent and well-informed decisions about future aspects of their care. The principles of autonomy and justice dictate that surgeons need to respect individuals by being fair in providing accurate information about all aspects of their care—even the medical errors.

Disclosing one's own errors is therefore part of the ethical standard of honesty and putting the patient's interests above one's own. Disclosing the errors of others is more complicated and may require careful consideration and consultation. Surgeons sometimes discover that a prior operation has included an apparent error; an injured bile duct or a stenotic anastomosis may lead to the condition for which the surgeon is now treating the patient. Declaring a finding as an "error" may be inaccurate, however, and a nonjudgmental assessment of the situation is usually advisable. When clear evidence of a mistake is at hand, the surgeon's responsibility is defined by his or her obligation to act as the patient's agent.

REFERENCES

Entries highlighted in bright blue are key references.

1. Aristotle: Nichomachean Ethics, Book VI, in Ackrill J (ed): *A New Aristotle Reader.* Princeton, NJ: Princeton University Press, 1987, p 416.
2. Beauchamp TL, Childress JF: *Principles of Biomedical Ethics*, 3rd ed. New York: Oxford University Press, 1989.
3. Pellegrino ED: Toward a virtue-based normative ethics for the health professions. *Kennedy Inst Ethics J* 5:253, 1995.
4. Pellegrino ED: Professionalism, profession and the virtues of the good physician. *Mt. Sinai J Med* 69:378, 2002.
5. *http://plato.stanford.edu/archives/fall2007/entries/ethics-virtue*: Hursthouse R: Virtue Ethics, Fall 2007, The Stanford Encyclopedia of Philosophy [accessed January 8, 2008].
6. Bosk C: *Forgive and Remember*, 2nd ed. Chicago: University of Chicago Press, 2003 (1979).
7. McCullough LB, Jones JW, Brody BA, (eds): *Surgical Ethics.* New York: Oxford University Press, 1998.
8. Faden RR, Beauchamp TL: *A History and Theory of Informed Consent.* New York: Oxford University Press, 1986.
9. Bernat JL, Peterson LM: Patient-centered informed consent in surgical practice. *Arch Surg* 141:86, 2006.
10. Schneider CE: *The Practice of Autonomy: Patients, Doctors, and Medical Decisions.* New York: Oxford University Press, 1998.
11. Robb A, Etchells E, Cusimano MD, et al: A randomized trial of teaching bioethics to surgical residents. *Am J Surg* 189:453, 2005.
12. Steinemann S, Furoy D, Yost F, et al: Marriage of professional and technical tasks: A strategy to improve obtaining informed consent. *Am J Surg* 191:696. 2006.
13. Guadagnoli E, Soumerai SB, Gurwitz JH, et al: Improving discussion of surgical treatment options for patients with breast cancer: Local medical opinion leaders versus audit and performance feedback. *Breast Cancer Res Treat* 61:171, 2000.
14. Braddock CH 3rd, Edwards KA, Hasenberg NM, et al: Informed decision making in outpatient practice: Time to get back to basics. *JAMA* 282:2313, 1999.
15. Leeper-Majors K, Veale JR, Westbrook TS, et al: The effect of standardized patient feedback in teaching surgical residents informed consent: Results of a pilot study. *Curr Surg* 60:615, 2003.
16. Courtney MJ: Information about surgery: What does the public want to know? *ANZ J Surg* 71:24, 2001.
17. Newton-Howes PA, Dobbs B, Frizelle F: Informed consent: What do patients want to know? *N Z Med J* 111:340, 1998.
18. Streat S: Clinical review: Moral assumptions and the process of organ donation in the intensive care unit. *Crit Care* 8:382, 2004.
19. Williams MA, Lipsett PA, Rushton CH, et al: The physician's role in discussing organ donation with families. *Crit Care Med* 31:1568, 2003.
20. Pearson IY, Zurynski Y: A survey of personal and professional attitudes of intensivists to organ donation and transplantation. *Anaesth Intensive Care* 23:68, 1995.
21. Sulmasy DP, Lehmann LS, Levine DM, et al: Patients' perceptions of the quality of informed consent for common medical procedures. *J Clin Ethics* 5:189, 1994.
22. Ubel PA, Loewenstein G, Jepson C: Whose quality of life? A commentary exploring discrepancies between health state evaluations of patients and the general public. *Qual Life Res* 12:599, 2003.
23. Schneider CE: After autonomy. *Wake Forest Law Review* 41:411, 2006.
24. Sulmasy DP, Terry PB, Weisman CS, et al: The accuracy of substituted judgments in patients with terminal diagnoses. *Ann Intern Med* 128:621, 1998.
25. Sulmasy DP, Hughes MT, Thompson RE, et al: How would terminally ill patients have others make decisions for them in the event of decisional incapacity? A longitudinal study. *J Am Geriatr Soc* 55:1981, 2007.

26. SUPPORT Principle Investigators. A controlled trial to improve care for seriously ill hospitalized patients. The study to understand prognoses and preferences for outcomes and risks of treatments (SUPPORT). The SUPPORT Principal Investigators. *JAMA* 274:1591, 1995.

27. Pawlik TM: Withholding and withdrawing life-sustaining treatment: A surgeon's perspective. *J Am Coll Surg* 202:990, 2006.

28. In re *Quinlan*. 355 A2d 647 (JN). Vol 429 US 9221976.

29. *Cruzan vs. Director, Missouri Dept of Health*, 497(1990).

30. Annas GJ: Nancy Cruzan and the right to die. *N Engl J Med* 323:670, 1990.

31. Sykes N, Thorns A: The use of opioids and sedatives at the end of life. *Lancet Oncol* 4:312, 2003.

32. Nelson KA, Walsh D, Behrens C, et al: The dying cancer patient. *Semin Oncol* 27:84, 2000.

33. Doyle D, Hanks G: Introduction, in *Oxford Textbook of Palliative Medicine*, 3rd ed. New York: Oxford University Press, 2004.

34. *www.who.int/cancer/palliative/definition/en/print.html*: WHO Definition of Palliative Care, 2008, World Health Organization [accessed March 25, 2009].

35. Dunn G: Surgical palliative care, in Mosby (ed): *Current Surgical Therapy*, 9th ed. Philadelphia: Elsevier, 2008.

36. Saunders C: The challenge of terminal care, in Symington T, Carter R (eds): *Scientific Foundations of Oncology*. London: Heineman, 1976 p 673.

37. Billroth T: Open letter to Dr. L Wittleshöfer. *Wiener Medizinische Wochenschrift* 31:162, 1881.

38. Whipple A: Present day surgery of the pancreas. *N Engl J Med* 226:515, 1942.

39. Aub JC, Beecher HK, Cannon B, et al: *Management of the Coconut Grove Burns at the Massachusetts General Hospital*. Philadelphia, PA: JB Lippincott Co, 1943.

40. Dunphy JE: Annual discourse—on caring for the patient with cancer. *N Engl J Med* 295:313, 1976.

41. Zimmerman J: *Hospice—Complete Care for the Terminally Ill*. Baltimore: Urban and Schwarzenberg, 1981.

42. Nuland S: *How We Die: Reflections on Life's Final Chapter*. New York: Alfred A. Knopf, 1994.

43. Chen P: *Final Exam*. New York: Alfred K. Knopf, 2007.

44. Task Force on Surgical Palliative Care, Committee on Ethics: Statement of principles of palliative care. *Bull Am Coll Surg* 90:34, 2005.

45. American College of Surgeons: Principles guiding care at end of life. *Bull Am Coll Surg* 83:46, 1998.

46. Surgeons Palliative Care Workgroup: Report from the Field. *J Am Coll Surg* 197:661, 2003.

47. Cancer pain relief and palliative care. Report of a WHO Expert Committee. *World Health Organ Tech Rep Ser* 804:1, 1990.

48. American Board of Internal Medicine Committee on Evaluation of Clinical Competence. *Caring for the Dying: Identification and Promotion of Physician Competency—Education Resource Document*. Philadelphia: American Board of Internal Medicine, 1996.

49. Storey P, Knight C: *UNIPAC One: The Hospice/Palliative Medicine Approach to End-of-Life Care*. American Academy of Hospice and Palliative Medicine. Dubuque, IA: Kendall/Hunt Publishing Co, 1998.

50. Kleinman A: *The Illness Narratives. Suffering, Healing & the Human Condition*. New York: Basic Books, 1988.

51. International Association for the Study of Pain, Subcommittee on Taxonomy. Part II. Pain Terms: A current list with definitions and notes on usage. *Pain* 6:249, 1979.

52. Cassell E: *The Nature of Suffering and the Goals of Medicine*. New York: Oxford University, 1991.

53. Frankl V: *Man's Search for Meaning*. New York: Washington Square Press, 1985.

54. Brody H: "My story is broken; can you help me fix it?" Medical ethics and the joint construction of narrative. *Lit Med* 13:79, 1994.

55. Byock IR, Merriman MP: Measuring quality of life for patients with terminal illness: The Missoula-VITAS quality of life index. *Palliat Med* 12:231, 1998.

56. Christakis NA, Lamont EB: Extent and determinants of error in doctors' prognoses in terminally ill patients: Prospective cohort study. *BMJ* 320:469, 2000.

57. Anderson F, Downing GM, Hill J, et al: Palliative performance scale (PPS): A new tool. *J Palliat Care* 12:5, 1996.

58. Morita T, Tsunoda J, Inoue S, et al: Validity of the palliative performance scale from a survival perspective. *J Pain Symptom Manage* 18:2, 1999.

59. Buckman R: *How to Break Bad News. A Guide for Health Care Professionals*. Baltimore: Johns Hopkins University Press, 1992.

60. Kubler-Ross E: *On Death and Dying*. London: Routledge, 1973.

61. Twycross R, Lichter I: The terminal phase, in Doyle D, Hanks G, MacDonald N (eds): *Oxford Textbook of Palliative Medicine*. New York, NY: Oxford University Press, 1998, p 977.

62. Hinshaw DB: Spiritual issues in surgical palliative care. *Surg Clin North Am* 85:257, 2005.

63. Jacox A, Carr D, Payne R, et al: Management of cancer pain. *AHCPR Publication No. 94-052: Clinical Practice Guideline No. 9*. Rockville, MD: US Department of Health and Human Services, Public Health Service, 1994.

64. Storey P, Knight C: *UNIPAC Three: Assessment and Treatment of Pain in the Terminally Ill*, 2nd ed. New York, NY: Mary Ann Liebert, Inc, 2003.

65. Rubenfeld GD, Crawford SW: Principles and practice of withdrawing life-sustaining treatment in the ICU, in Curtis JR, Rubenfeld GD (eds): *Managing Death in the Intensive Care Unit*. New York: Oxford University Press, 2001.

66. Rousseau P: Existential distress and palliative sedation. *Anesth Analg* 101:611, 2005.

67. The EPEC-O Project, Educating Physicians in End-of-Life Care-Oncology: *Module 6: Last Hours of Living*. Bethesda, MD: National Cancer Institute, 2007.

68. Worden J: *Bereavement Care*. Philadelphia: Lippincott Williams and Wilkins, 2002.

69. Bishop JP, Rosemann PW, Schmidt FW: Fides ancilla medicinae: On the ersatz liturgy of death in biopsychosociospiritual medicine. *The Heythrop Journal* 49:20, 2008.

70. Schroeder-Sheker T: *Transitus: A Blessed Death in the Modern World*. Mt. Angel, Oregon: St. Dunstan's Press, 2001.

71. Emmanuel EJ, Wendler D, Grady C: What makes clinical research ethical? *JAMA* 283:2701, 2000.

72. Freedman B: Equipoise and the ethics of clinical research. *N Engl J Med* 317:141, 1987.

73. Meakins J: Innovation in surgery: The rules of evidence. *Am J Surg* 183:399, 2002.

74. Lefering R, Neugebauer E: Problems of randomized controlled trials in surgery. Paper presented at: Nonrandomized Comparative Clinical Studies 1997, Heidelberg.

75. Flum DR: Interpreting surgical trials with subjective outcomes: Avoiding UnSPORTsmanlike conduct. *JAMA* 296:2483, 2006.

76. Moseley JB, O'Malley K, Petersen NJ, et al: A controlled trial of arthroscopic surgery for osteoarthritis of the knee. *N Engl J Med* 347:81, 2002. Summary for patients in: *J Fam Pract* 51:813, 2002.

77. Angelos PA: Sham surgery in research: A surgeon's view. *Am J Bioeth* 3:65, 2003.

78. Miller FG: Sham surgery: An ethical analysis. *Sci Eng Ethics* 10:157, 2004.

79. Angelos P: Sham surgery in clinical trials. *JAMA* 297:1545; author reply 1546, 2007.

80. Riskin DJ, Longaker MT, Gertner M, et al: Innovation in surgery: A historical perspective. *Ann Surg* 244:686, 2006.

81. Biffl WL, Spain DA, Reitsma AM, et al: Responsible development and application of surgical innovations: A position statement of the Society of University Surgeons (draft statement of 2/19/08).

82. McKneally MF, Daar AS: Introducing new technologies: Protecting subjects of surgical innovation and research. *World J Surg* 27:930, 2003.

83. Kohn LT, Corrigan JM, Donaldson MS: *To Err Is Human: Building a Safer Health System*. Washington: National Academy Press, 2000.

84. Brennan TA, Leape LL, Laird NM, et al: Incidence of adverse events and negligence in hospitalized patients. Results of the Harvard Medical Practice Study I. *N Engl J Med* 324:370, 1991.

85. Hebert PC, Levin AV, Robertson G: Bioethics for clinicians: 23. Disclosure of medical error. *CMAJ* 164:509, 2001.

CHAPTER 1

5. *http://www.acgme.org/acWebsite/downloads/RRC_progReq/440general surgery01012008.pdf*: ACGME Program Requirements for Graduate Medical Education in Surgery, 2007, Accreditation Council for Graduate Medical Education [accessed January 15, 2008].
14. Scott DJ, Dunnington GL: New ACS/APDS skills curriculum: Moving the learning curve out of the operating room. *J Gastrointest Surg* 12:213, 2008. Epub October 10, 2007.
17. Dunnington GL, Williams RG: Addressing the new competencies for residents' surgical training. *Acad Med* 78:14, 2003.
93. *http://www.acgme.org/acwebsite/portfolio/cbpac_faq.pdf*: ACGME Learning Portfolio: A Professional Development Tool, 2008, Accreditation Council for Graduate Medical Education [accessed June 18, 2008].

CHAPTER 2

2. Lowry SF: Human endotoxemia: A model for mechanistic insight and therapeutic targeting. *Shock* 24 Suppl 1:94, 2005.
3. Borovikova LV, Ivanova S, Zhang M, et al: Vagus nerve stimulation attenuates the systemic inflammatory response to endotoxin. *Nature* 405:458, 2000.
8. Dellinger RP, Levy MM, Carlet JM, et al: Surviving Sepsis Campaign: International guidelines for management of severe sepsis and septic shock: 2008. *Crit Care Med* 36:296, 2008.
41. Agnese DM, Calvano JE, Hahm SJ, et al: Human toll-like receptor 4 mutations but not CD14 polymorphisms are associated with an increased risk of gram-negative infections. *J Infect Dis* 186:1522, 2002.
82. Lowry SF: A new model of nutrition influenced inflammatory risk. *J Am Coll Surg* 205(4 Suppl):S65, 2007.

CHAPTER 3

29. Lucas CE: The water of life: A century of confusion. *J Am Coll Surg* 192:86, 2001.
42. Shires GT, Williams J, Brown F: Acute changes in extracellular fluids associated with major surgical procedures. *Ann Surg* 154:803, 1961.
43. Shires GT, Jackson DE: Postoperative salt tolerance. *Arch Surg* 84:703, 1962.
44. Shires GT III, Peitzman AB, Albert SA, et al: Response of extravascular lung water to intraoperative fluids. *Ann Surg* 197:515, 1983.

CHAPTER 4

7. Baldwin ZK, Spitzer AL, Ng VL, et al: Contemporary standards for the diagnosis and treatment of heparin-induced thrombocytopenia (HIT). *Surgery* 143:305, 2008.
23. Brohi K, Cohen MJ, Ganter MT, et al: Acute coagulopathy of trauma: Hypoperfusion induces systemic anticoagulation and hyperfibrinolysis. *J Trauma* 64:1211, 2008.
34. Kearon C, Hirsh J: Management of anticoagulation before and after elective surgery. *N Engl J Med* 336:1506, 1997.
57. Herbert PC, Wells GW, Blajchman MA, et al: A multicenter, randomized, controlled clinical trial of transfusion requirement in critical care. *N Engl J Med* 340:409, 1999.
73. Holcomb JB, Wade CE, Michalek JE, et al: Increased plasma and platelet to RBC ratios improve outcome in 466 massively transfused civilian trauma patients. *Ann Surg* 248:447, 2008.

CHAPTER 5

20. Nathan C: Points of control in inflammation. *Nature* 420:846, 2002.
62. Holcomb JB: Damage control resuscitation. *J Trauma* 62(6 Suppl):S36, 2007.
71. Borgman MA, Spinella PC, Perkins JG, et al: The ratio of blood products transfused affects mortality in patients receiving massive transfusions at a combat support hospital. *J Trauma* 63:805, 2007.
78. Dellinger RP, Levy MM, Carlet JM, et al: Surviving Sepsis Campaign: International guidelines for management of severe sepsis and septic shock. *Crit Care Med* 36:296, 2008.

CHAPTER 6

28. Chastre J, Wolff M, Fagon JY, et al: Comparison of 8 vs 15 days of antibiotic therapy for ventilator-associated pneumonia in adults: A randomized trial. *JAMA* 290:2588, 2003.
30. Stone HH, Bourneuf AA, Stinson LD: Reliability of criteria for predicting persistent or recurrent sepsis. *Arch Surg* 120:17, 1985.
57. Solomkin JS, Mazuski JE, Baron EJ, et al: Infectious Diseases Society of America: Guidelines for the selection of anti-infective agents for complicated intra-abdominal infections. *Clin Infect Dis* 37:997, 2003.
66. Nathens AB, Curtis JR, Beale RJ, et al: Management of the critically ill patient with severe acute pancreatitis. *Crit Care Med* 32:2524, 2004.
87. Dellinger RP, Levy MM, Carlet JM, et al: Surviving Sepsis Campaign: International guidelines for management of severe sepsis and septic shock: 2008. *Crit Care Med* 36:296, 2008.

CHAPTER 7

3. Feliciano DV, Mattox KL, Moore EE (eds): *Trauma*, 6th ed. New York: McGraw-Hill, 2008.
6. American College of Surgeons: *Advanced Trauma Life Support*, 7th ed. Chicago: American College of Surgeons, 2004.
13. Brain Trauma Foundation, American Association of Neurological Surgeons, Congress of Neurological Surgeons: Guidelines for the management of severe traumatic brain injury. *J Neurotrauma* 24(Suppl):S1, 2007.

CHAPTER 8

1. Baxter CR, Shires T: Physiological response to crystalloid resuscitation of severe burns. *Ann N Y Acad Sci* 150:874, 1968.
5. Klein MB, Nathens AB, Emerson D, et al: An analysis of the long-distance transport of burn patients to a regional burn center. *J Burn Care Res* 28:49, 2007.
41. Friedrich JB, Sullivan SR, Engrav LH, et al: Is supra-Baxter resuscitation in burn patients a new phenomenon? *Burns* 30:464, 2004.
95. Curreri PW, Richmond D, et al: Dietary requirements of patients with major burns. *J Am Diet Assoc* 65:415, 1974.

118. Engrav LH, Heimbach DM, Reus JL, et al: Early excision and grafting vs. nonoperative treatment of burns of indeterminant depth: A randomized prospective study. *J Trauma* 23:1001, 1983.

CHAPTER 9

40. Thornton FJ, Barbul A: Healing in the gastrointestinal tract. *Surg Clin North Am* 77:549, 1997.

86. Hopf HW, Ueno C, Aslam R, et al: Guidelines for the treatment of arterial insufficiency ulcers. *Wound Repair Regen* 14:693, 2006.

87. Hopf HW, Ueno C, Aslam R, et al: Guidelines for the prevention of lower extremity arterial ulcers. *Wound Repair Regen* 16:175, 2008.

88. Robson MC, Cooper DM, Aslam R, et al: Guidelines for the treatment of venous ulcers. *Wound Repair Regen* 14:649, 2006.

89. Flour M: Venous ulcer management: Has research led to improved healing for the patient? in Cherry G (ed): *The Oxford European Wound Healing Course Handbook.* Oxford: Positif Press, 2002, p 33.

91. Steed DL, Attinger C, Colaizzi T, et al: Guidelines for treatment of diabetic ulcers. *Wound Repair Regen* 14:680, 2006.

94. Steed DL, Attinger C, Brem H, et al: Guidelines for the prevention of diabetic ulcers. *Wound Repair Regen* 16:169, 2008.

95. Whitney J, Phillips L, Aslam R, et al: Guidelines for the treatment of pressure ulcers. *Wound Repair Regen* 14:663, 2006.

96. Eaglstein WH, Falanga V: Chronic wounds. *Surg Clin North Am* 77:689, 1997.

101. Mustoe TA: Evolution of silicone therapy and mechanism of action in scar management. *Aesthetic Plast Surg* 32:82, 2008.

CHAPTER 10

1. Jemal A, Siegel R, Ward E, et al: Cancer statistics, 2007. *CA Cancer J Clin* 57:43, 2007.

4. Hanahan D, Weinberg RA: The hallmarks of cancer. *Cell* 100:57, 2000.

6. Fearon ER, Vogelstein B: A genetic model for colorectal tumorigenesis. *Cell* 61:759, 1990.

70. *http://monographs.iarc.fr/ENG/Classification/index.php:* IARC Monographs on the Evaluation of Carcinogenic Risks to Humans, Complete List of Agents Evaluated and Their Classification, International Agency for Research on Cancer (IARC) [accessed January 16, 2008].

74. *http://monographs.iarc.fr/ENG/Classification/crthgr01.php:* IARC Monographs on the Evaluation of Carcinogenic Risks to Humans, Overall Evaluations of Carcinogenicity to Humans: Group 1: Carcinogenic to Humans, International Agency for Research on Cancer (IARC) [accessed January 16, 2008].

83. Smith RA, Cokkinides V, Brawley OW. Cancer screening in the United States, 2009: a review of current American Cancer Society guidelines and issues in cancer screening. *CA Cancer J Clin* 59:27, 2009. Review.

CHAPTER 11

6. Murray JE, Merrill JP, Harrison JH, et al: Prolonged survival of human-kidney homografts by immunosuppressive drug therapy. *N Engl J Med* 268:1315, 1963.

15. Matas AJ, Kandaswamy R, Gillingham K, et al: Prednisone free maintenance immunosuppression—a 5 year experience. *Am J Transplant* 5:2473, 2005.

59. Sutherland DE, Gruessner RW, Dunn DL, et al: Lessons learned from more than 1000 pancreas transplants at a single institution. *Am Surg* 233:463, 2001.

62. Freeman RB Jr., Wiesner RH, Roberts JP, et al: Improving liver allocation: MELD and PELD. *Am J Transplant* 4 Suppl 9:114, 2004.

95. Patel R, Paya CV: Infections in solid-organ transplant recipients: *Clin Microbiol Rev* 10:86, 1997.

CHAPTER 12

3. Kohn KT, Corrigan JM, Donaldson MS: *To Err Is Human: Building a Safer Health System.* Washington, DC: National Academy Press, 1999.

17. Christian CK, Gustafson ML, Roth EM, et al: A prospective study of patient safety in the operating room. *Surgery* 139:159, 2006.

18. Makary MA, Sexton JB, Freischlag JA, et al: Operating room teamwork among physicians and nurses: Teamwork in the eye of the beholder. *J Am Coll Surg* 202:746, 2006.

20. Makary MA, Mukherjee A, Sexton JB, et al: Operating room briefings and wrong-site surgery. *J Am Coll Surg* 204:236, 2007.

41. Michaels RK, Makary MA, Dahab Y, et al: Achieving the National Quality Forum's "Never Events": Prevention of wrong site, wrong procedure, and wrong patient operations. *Ann Surg* 245:526, 2007.

113. Van den Berghe G, Wouters P, Weekers F, et al: Intensive insulin therapy in the critically ill patients. *N Engl J Med* 345:1359, 2001.

CHAPTER 13

13. Gattinoni L, Brazzi L, Pelosi P, et al: A trial of goal-oriented hemodynamic therapy in critically ill patients. SVo2 Collaborative Group. *N Engl J Med* 333:1025, 1995.

15. Rivers EP, Ander DS, Powell D: Central venous oxygen saturation monitoring in the critically ill patient. *Curr Opin Crit Care* 7:204, 2001.

30. Shah MR, Hasselblad V, Stevenson LW, et al: Impact of the pulmonary artery catheter in critically ill patients: Meta-analysis of randomized clinical trials. *JAMA* 294:1664, 2005

35. Shoemaker WC, Appel PL, Kram HB, et al: Prospective trial of supranormal values of survivors as therapeutic goals in high-risk surgical patients. *Chest* 94:1176, 1988.

76. Ventilation with lower tidal volumes as compared with traditional tidal volumes for acute lung injury and the acute respiratory distress syndrome. The Acute Respiratory Distress Syndrome Network. *N Engl J Med* 342:1301, 2000.

CHAPTER 14

80. Marescaux J, Dallemagne B, Perretta S, et al: Surgery without scars: Report of transluminal cholecystectomy in a human being. *Arch Surg* 142:823; discussion 826, 2007.

88. Fleshman J, Sargent DJ, Green E, for The Clinical Outcomes of Surgical Therapy Study Group: Laparoscopic colectomy for cancer is not inferior to open surgery based on 5-year data from the COST Study Group trial. *Ann Surg* 246:655; discussion 662, 2007.

89. Fried GM, Clas D, Meakins JL: Minimally invasive surgery in the elderly patient. *Surg Clin North Am* 74:375, 1994.

95. Anvari M: Telesurgery: Remote knowledge translation in clinical surgery. *World J Surg* 31:1545, 2007.

CHAPTER 15

1. Alberts B, Johnson A, Lewis J, et al: *Molecular Biology of the Cell,* 4th ed. New York: Garland Science, 2002.

2. Watson JD, Crick FH: Molecular structure of nucleic acids; a structure for deoxyribose nucleic acid. *Nature* 171:737, 1953.

5. Wolfsberg TG, Wetterstrand KA, Guyer MS, et al: A user's guide to the human genome. *Nature Genetics* Supplement, 2002. (Also see the Nature website: *http://www.nature.com/nature/supplements/collections/humangenome/.*)

22. Mullis K, Faloona F, Scharf S, et al: Specific enzymatic amplification of DNA in vitro: The polymerase chain reaction. *Cold Spring Harb Symp Quant Biol* 51:263, 1986.

26. Hannon GJ: *RNAi, A Guide To Gene Silencing.* New York: Cold Spring Harbor Laboratory Press, 2003.

CHAPTER 16

3. Nemes Z, Steinert PM: Bricks and mortar of the epidermal barrier. *Exp Mol Med* 31:5, 1999.

60. Marler JJ, Mulliken JB: Vascular anomalies: Classification, diagnosis, and natural history. *Facial Plast Surg Clin North Am* 9:495, 2001.

74. Balch CM, Buzaid AC, Soong SJ, et al: Final version of the American Joint Committee on Cancer staging system for cutaneous melanoma. *J Clin Oncol* 16:3635, 2001.

CHAPTER 17

71. Saslow D, et al: American Cancer Society guidelines for breast screening with MRI as an adjunct to mammography. *CA Cancer J Clin* 57:75, 2007.

99. Breast, in Greene FL, et al (eds): *AJCC Cancer Staging Manual*, 6th ed. New York: Springer-Verlag, 2002, p 223.

128. Paik S, et al: A multigene assay to predict recurrence of tamoxifen-treated, node-negative breast cancer. *N Engl J Med* 351:2817, 2004.

136. Effects of radiotherapy and surgery in early breast cancer. An overview of the randomized trials. Early Breast Cancer Trialists' Collaborative Group. *N Engl J Med* 333:1444, 1995.

160. Krag DN, et al: Technical outcomes of sentinel-lymph-node resection and conventional axillary-lymph-node dissection in patients with clinically node-negative breast cancer: Results from the NSABP B-32 randomised phase III trial. *Lancet Oncol* 8:881, 2007.

201. Effects of chemotherapy and hormonal therapy for early breast cancer on recurrence and 15-year survival: An overview of the randomised trials. *Lancet* 365:1687, 2005.

CHAPTER 18

8. Lanza DC, Kennedy DW: Adult rhinosinusitis defined. *Otolaryngol Head Neck Surg* 117:S1, 1997.

66. Wolf GT, Hong WK, Fischer SG, et al: Induction chemotherapy plus radiation compared with surgery plus radiation in patients with advanced laryngeal cancer. *N Engl J Med* 324:1685, 1991.

80. Eicher SA, Weber RS: Surgical management of cervical lymph node metastases. *Curr Opin Oncol* 8:215, 1996.

90. Urken ML, Buchbinder D, Costantino PD, et al: Oromandibular reconstruction using microvascular composite flaps: Report of 210 cases. *Arch Otolaryngol Head Neck Surg* 124:46, 1998.

CHAPTER 19

13. Swanson SJ, Herndon JE 2nd, D'Amico TA, et al: Video-assisted thoracic surgery lobectomy: Report of CALGB 39802—a prospective, multi-institution feasibility study. *J Clin Oncol* 25:4993, 2007.

14. Demmy TL, James TA, Swanson SJ, et al: Troubleshooting video-assisted thoracic surgery lobectomy. *Ann Thorac Surg* 79:1744; discussion 1753, 2005.

48. Colice GL, Shafazand S, Griffin JP, et al: Physiologic evaluation of the patient with lung cancer being considered for resectional surgery: ACCP evidenced-based clinical practice guidelines (2nd edition). *Chest* 132(3 Suppl):161S, 2007.

52. Groome PA, Bolejack V, Crowley JJ, et al: The IASLC Lung Cancer Staging Project: Validation of the proposals for revision of the T, N, and M descriptors and consequent stage groupings in the forthcoming (seventh) edition of the TNM classification of malignant tumours. *J Thorac Oncol* 2:694, 2007.

85. Ilowite J, Spiegler P, Chawla S: Bronchiectasis: New findings in the pathogenesis and treatment of this disease. *Curr Opin Infect Dis* 21:163, 2008.

179. Tremblay A, Michaud G: Single-center experience with 250 tunnelled pleural catheter insertions for malignant pleural effusion. *Chest* 129:362, 2006.

CHAPTER 20

20. Kouchoukos NT, Blackstone EH, Doty DB, et al: Congenital aortic stenosis, in Kouchoukos NT, Blackstone EH, Doty DB, et al (eds): *Kirklin/Barrat-Boyes Cardiac Surgery*, 3rd ed. Philadelphia: Churchill Livingstone, 2003, p 1269

27. Ross DN: Replacement of aortic and mitral valves with a pulmonary autograft. *Lancet* 57:956, 1967

52. Karamlou T, Bernasconi A, Jaeggi E, et al: Factors associated with arch reintervention and growth of the aortic arch after coarctation repair in neonates weighing less than 2.5 kg. *J Thorac Cardiovasc Surg*, 2009 (in press).

57. McCrindle BW, Jones TK, Morrow WR, et al: Acute results of balloon angioplasty of native coarctation versus recurrent aortic obstruction are equivalent. Valvuloplasty and Angioplasty of Congenital Anomalies (VACA) Registry Investigators. *J Am Coll Cardiol* 28:1810, 1996.

83. Karamlou T, Gurofsky R, Al Sukhni E, et al: Factors associated with mortality and reoperation in 377 children with total anomalous pulmonary venous connection. *Circulation* 115:1591, 2007.

95. deLeval MR, Kilner P, Gerwillig M, et al: Total cavopulmonary connection: A logical alternative to atriopulmonary connection for complex Fontan operations. *J Thorac Cardiovasc Surg* 96:682, 1988

148. Karamlou T, McCrindle BW, Williams WG: Surgery insight: Late complications following repair of tetralogy of Fallot and related surgical strategies for management. *Nature Cardiovasc Med* 3:611, 2006.

CHAPTER 21

1. Libby P. Braunwald's Heart Disease: *A Textbook of Cardiovascular Medicine*, 8th ed. Philadelphia: Saunders Elsevier, 2007.

7. Eleven-year survival in the Veterans Administration randomized trial of coronary bypass surgery for stable angina. The Veterans Administration Coronary Artery Bypass Surgery Cooperative Study Group. *N Engl J Med* 311:1333, 1984.

13. Comparison of coronary bypass surgery with angioplasty in patients with multivessel disease. The Bypass Angioplasty Revascularization Investigation (BARI) Investigators. *N Engl J Med* 335:217, 1996.

17. Hannan EL, Racz MJ, Walford G, et al: Long-term outcomes of coronary-artery bypass grafting versus stent implantation. *N Engl J Med* 352:2174, 2005.

33. Jamieson WR, von Lipinski O, Miyagishima RT, et al: Performance of bioprostheses and mechanical prostheses assessed by composites of valve-related complications to 15 years after mitral valve replacement. *J Thorac Cardiovasc Surg* 129:1301, 2005.

40. Carpentier A. Cardiac valve surgery--the "French correction." *J Thorac Cardiovasc Surg* 86:323, 1983.

41. Bonow RO, Carabello BA, Kanu C, et al: ACC/AHA 2006 guidelines for the management of patients with valvular heart disease: A report of the American College of Cardiology/American Heart Association Task Force on Practice Guidelines (writing committee to revise the 1998 Guidelines for the Management of Patients With Valvular Heart Disease): Developed in collaboration with the Society of Cardiovascular Anesthesiologists: Endorsed by the Society for Cardiovascular Angiography and Interventions and the Society of Thoracic Surgeons. *Circulation* 114:e84, 2006.

50. Mohty D, Orszulak TA, Schaff HV, et al: Very long-term survival and durability of mitral valve repair for mitral valve prolapse. *Circulation* 104:I1, 2001.

85. Acker MA, Bolling S, Shemin R, et al: Mitral valve surgery in heart failure: Insights from the Acorn Clinical Trial. *J Thorac Cardiovasc Surg* 132:568, 577.e1, 2006.

89. Athanasuleas CL, Stanley AW Jr., Buckberg GD, et al: Surgical anterior ventricular endocardial restoration (SAVER) in the dilated remodeled ventricle after anterior myocardial infarction. RESTORE group. Reconstructive Endoventricular Surgery, returning Torsion Original Radius Elliptical Shape to the LV. *J Am Coll Cardiol* 37:1199, 2001.

96. Rose EA, Gelijns AC, Moskowitz AJ, et al: Long-term mechanical left ventricular assistance for end-stage heart failure. *N Engl J Med* 345:1435, 2001.

CHAPTER 22

1. Johnston KW, Rutherford RB, Tilson MD, et al: Suggested standards for reporting on arterial aneurysms. Subcommittee on Reporting Standards for Arterial Aneurysms, Ad Hoc Committee on Reporting Standards, Society for Vascular Surgery and North American Chapter, International Society for Cardiovascular Surgery. *J Vasc Surg* 13:452, 1991.

2. Bickerstaff LK, Pairolero PC, Hollier LH, et al: Thoracic aortic aneurysms: A population-based study. *Surgery* 92:1103, 1982.

25. Elefteriades JA: Natural history of thoracic aortic aneurysms: Indications for surgery, and surgical versus nonsurgical risks. *Ann Thorac Surg* 74:S1877, 2002.

43. Gott VL, Cameron DE, Alejo DE, et al: Aortic root replacement in 271 Marfan patients: A 24-year experience. *Ann Thorac Surg* 73:438, 2002.

71. Coselli JS, LeMaire SA, Köksoy C, et al: Cerebrospinal fluid drainage reduces paraplegia after thoracoabdominal aortic aneurysm repair: Results of a randomized clinical trial. *J Vasc Surg* 35:631, 2002.

CHAPTER 23

24. Kita MW: Carotid endarterectomy in symptomatic carotid stenosis: NASCET comparative results at 30 months of follow-up. *J Insur Med* 24:42, 1992.

25. Warlow CP: Symptomatic patients: The European Carotid Surgery Trial (ECST). *J Mal Vasc* 18:198, 1993.

52. Greenhalgh RM, Brown LC, Kwong GP, et al: Comparison of endovascular aneurysm repair with open repair in patients with abdominal aortic aneurysm (EVAR trial 1), 30-day operative mortality results: Randomised controlled trial. *Lancet* 364:843, 2004.

53. Prinssen M, Verhoeven EL, Buth J, et al: A randomized trial comparing conventional and endovascular repair of abdominal aortic aneurysms. *N Engl J Med* 351:1607, 2004.

90. Hansen KJ, Cherr GS, Craven TE, et al: Management of ischemic nephropathy: Dialysis-free survival after surgical repair. *J Vasc Surg* 32:472; discussion 481, 2000.

106. Dormandy JA, Rutherford RB: Management of peripheral arterial disease (PAD). TASC Working Group. TransAtlantic Inter-Society Concensus (TASC). *J Vasc Surg* 31:S1, 2000.

CHAPTER 24

25. Kearon C, Kahn SR, Agnelli G, et al. Antithrombotic therapy for venous thromboembolic disease: American College of Chest Physicians Evidence-Based Clinical Practice Guidelines (8th edition). *Chest* 133:454S, 2008.

67. Geerts WH, Bergqvist D, Pineo GF, et al: Prevention of venous thromboembolism: American College of Chest Physicians Evidence-Based Clinical Practice Guidelines (8th edition). *Chest* 133:381S, 2008.

60. Eklof B, Kistner RL, Masuda EM: Surgical treatment of acute iliofemoral deep venous thrombosis, in Gloviczki P, Yao JST (eds): *Handbook of Venous Disorders*. New York: Arnold, 2001, p 202.

112. Gloviczki P, Bergan JJ, Rhodes JM, et al: Mid-term results of endoscopic perforator vein interruption for chronic venous insufficiency: Lessons learned from the North American Subfascial Endoscopic Perforator Surgery registry. The North American Study Group. *J Vasc Surg* 29:489, 1999.

CHAPTER 25

Akiyama H, Tsurumaru M: Radical lymph node dissection for cancer of the thoracic esophagus. *Ann Surg* 220:364, 1994.

Bonavina L, Nosadinia A, et al: Primary treatment of esophageal achalasia: Long-term results of myotomy and Dor fundoplication. *Arch Surg* 127:222, 1992.

Castel DW, Richter J (eds): *The Esophagus*. Boston: Little, Brown & Co., 1999.

Chang EY, Morris CD, Seltman AK, et al: The effect of antireflux surgery on esophageal carcinogenesis in patients with Barrett's esophagus: A systematic review. *Ann Surg* 246:11, 2007.

Clark GW, Ireland AP, Peters JH, et al: Short segments of Barrett's esophagus: A prevalent complication of gastroesophageal reflux disease with malignant potential. *J Gastrointest Surg* 1:113, 1997.

Csendes A, Braghetto I, et al: Late results of a prospective randomized study comparing forceful dilatation and oesophagomyotomy in patients with achalasia. *Gut* 30:299, 1989.

Cunningham D, Allum WH, Stenning SP, et al: Perioperative chemotherapy versus surgery alone for resectable gastroesophageal cancer. *N Engl J Med* 6;355:11, 2006.

DeMeester SR, DeMeester TR: Columnar mucosa and intestinal metaplasia of the esophagus: Fifty years of controversy. *Ann Surg* 231:303, 2000.

DeMeester TR, Johansson KE, et al: Indications, surgical technique, and long-term functional results of colon interposition or bypass. *Ann Surg* 208:460, 1988.

DeMeester TR, Johnson LF, et al: Patterns of gastroesophageal reflux in health and disease. *Ann Surg* 184:459, 1976.

DeMeester TR, Lafontaine E, et al: The relationship of a hiatal hernia to the function of the body of the esophagus and the gastroesophageal junction. *J Thorac Cardiovasc Surg* 82:547, 1981.

Eckardt V, Aignherr C, Bernhard G: Predictors of outcome in patients with achalasia treated by pneumatic dilation. *Gastroenterology* 103:1732, 1992.

Farrell TM, Richardson WS, Trus TL, et al: Response of atypical symptoms of gastroesophageal reflux antireflux surgery. *Br J Surg* 88:1649, 2001.

Fass R: Epidemiology and pathophysiology of symptomatic gastroesophageal reflux disease. *Am J Gastroenterol* 98:S2, 2003.

Gebski V, Burmeister B, Smithers BM, et al: Survival benefits from neoadjuvant chemoradiotherapy or chemotherapy in oesophageal carcinoma: A meta-analysis. *Lancet* 8:226, 2007.

Gouge TH, Depan HJ, Spencer FC: Experience with the Grillo pleural wrap procedure in 18 patients with perforation of the thoracic esophagus. *Ann Surg* 209:612, 1989.

Gurski RR, Peters JH, Hagen JA, et al: Barrett's esophagus can and does regress following antireflux surgery: A study of prevalence and predictive features. *J Am Coll Surg* 196:706, 2003.

Hagen JA, DeMeester TR, Peters JH, et al: Curative resection for esophageal adenocarcinoma analysis of 100 en bloc esophagectomies. *Ann Surg* 234:520, 2001.

Helm JF, Dodds WJ, et al: Effect of esophageal emptying and saliva on clearance of acid from the esophagus. *N Engl J Med* 310:284, 1984.

Hill LD, Kozarek RA, et al: The gastroesophageal flap valve. In vitro and in vivo observations. *Gastrointest Endosc* 44:541, 1996.

Hofstetter WA, Peters JH, DeMeester TR, et al: Long term outcome of antireflux surgery in patients with Barrett's esophagus. *Ann Surg* 234:532, 2001.

Hulscher JB, Van Sandick JW, de Boer AG, et al: Extended transthoracic resection compared with limited transhiatal resection for adenocarcinoma of the esophagus. *N Engl J Med* 347:1662, 2002.

Johnson LF, DeMeester TR: Development of 24-hour intraesophageal pH monitoring composite scoring. *J Clin Gastroenterol* 8:52, 1986.

Kahrilas PJ, Wu S, et al: Attenuation of esophageal shortening during peristalsis with hiatus hernia. *Gastroenterology* 109:1818, 1995.

Kelsen DP, Winter KA, Gunderson LL, et al: Long-term results of RTOG trial 8911 (USA Intergroup 113): A random assignment trial comparison of chemotherapy followed by surgery compared with surgery alone for esophageal cancer. *J Clin Oncol* 25:3719, 2007.

Lagergren J, Bergstrom R, Lindgren A, et al: Symptomatic gastroesophageal reflux as a risk factor for esophageal adenocarcinoma. *N Engl J Med* 340:825, 1999.

Law S, Kwong DL, Kwok KF, et al: Improvement in treatment results and long term survival of patients with esophageal cancer: Impact of chemoradiation and change in treatment strategy. *Ann Surg* 238:339, 2003.

Leuketich JD, Alvelo-Rivera M, Buenaventura PO, et al: Minimally invasive esophagectomy: Outcomes in 222 patients. *Ann Surg* 238:486, 2003.

Liebermann-Meffert DM, Meier R, Siewert JR: Vascular anatomy of the gastric tube used for esophageal reconstruction. *Ann Thorac Surg* 54:1110, 1992.

Lundell L, Miettinen P, Myrvold HE, et al: Long-term management of gastro-oesophageal reflux disease with omeprazole or open antireflux surgery: Results of a prospective randomized trial. *Eur J Gastroenterol Hepatol* 12:879, 2000.

Oelschlager BK, Chang L, Pellegrini CA: Improved outcome after extended gastric myotomy for achalasia. *Arch Surg* 138:490, 2003.

Oelschlager BK, Pellegrini CA, Hunter J, et al: Biologic prosthesis reduces recurrence after laparoscopic paraesophageal hernia repair: A multicenter, prospective, randomized trial. *Ann Surg* 244:481, 2006.

Omloo JM, Lagarde SM, Hulscher JB, et al: Extended transthoracic resection compared with limited transhiatal resection for adenocarcinoma of the mid/distal esophagus: Five year survival of a randomized clinical trial. *Ann Surg* 246:992, 2007.

Orringer MB, Marshall B, Chang AC, et al: Two thousand transhiatal esophagectomies: changing trends, lessons learned. *Ann Surg* 246:363; discussion 372, 2007.

Patti MG, Fisichella PM, Peretta S, et al: Impact of minimally invasive surgery on the treatment of esophageal achalasia: A decade of change. *J Am Coll Surg* 196:698, 2003.

Patti MG, Goldberg HI, et al: Hiatal hernia size affects LES function, esophageal acid exposure, and the degree of mucosal injury. *Am J Surg* 171:182, 1996.

Pearson FG, Cooper JD, et al: Gastroplasty and fundoplication for complex reflux problems. *Ann Surg* 206:473, 1987.

Peters JH, Clark GWB, et al: Outcome of adenocarcinoma arising in Barrett's esophagus in endoscopically surveyed and non-surveyed patients. *J Thorac Cardiovasc Surg* 108:813, 1994.

Reid BJ, Weinstein WM, et al: Endoscopic biopsy can detect high-grade dysplasia or early adenocarcinoma in Barrett's esophagus without grossly recognizable neoplastic lesions. *Gastroenterology* 94:81, 1988.

Richards WO, Torquati A, Holzman MD, et al: Heller myotomy versus Heller myotomy with Dor fundoplication for achalasia: A prospective randomized double-blind clinical trial. *Ann Surg* 240:405; discussion 412, 2004.

Salo JA, Isolauri JO, et al: Management of delayed esophageal perforation with mediastinal sepsis. Esophagectomy or primary repair? *J Thorac Cardiovasc Surg* 106:1088, 1993.

Smith CD, McClusky DA, Rajhad MA, et al:When fundoplication fails: Redo? *Ann Surg* 241:861, 2005.

Sontag SJ, O'Connell S, Khandelwal S, et al: Asthmatics with gastroesophageal reflux: Long term results of a randomized trial of medical and surgical antireflux therapies. *Am J Gastroenterol* 98:987, 2003.

Stein HJ, Barlow AP, et al: Complications of gastroesophageal reflux disease: Role of the LES, esophageal acid and acid/alkaline exposure, and duodenogastric reflux. *Ann Surg* 216:35, 1992.

Trus TL, Bax T, Richardson WS, et al: Complications of laparoscopic paraesophageal hernia repair. *J Gastrointest Surg* 1:221; discussion 228, 1997.

Trus TL, Laycock WS, Waring JP, et al: Improvement in quality of life measures after laparoscopic antireflux surgery. *Ann Surg* 229:331, 1999.

Urschel JD, Ashiku S, Thurer R, et al: Salvage or planned esophagectomy after chemoradiation for locally advanced esophageal cancer: A review. *Dis Esophagus* 16:60, 2003.

Zaninotto G, Annese V, Costantini M, et al: Randomized controlled trial of botulinum toxin versus laparoscopic Heller myotomy for esophageal achalasia. *Ann Surg* 239:364, 2004.

Zaninotto G, DeMeester TR, et al: Esophageal function in patients with reflux-induced strictures and its relevance to surgical treatment. *Ann Thorac Surg* 47:362, 1989.

CHAPTER 26

26. Cummings DE, Overduin J: Gastrointestinal regulation of food intake. *J Clin Invest* 117:13, 2007.
54. Fox JG, Wang TC: Inflammation, atrophy, and gastric cancer. *J Clin Invest* 117:60, 2007.
67. Harbison SP, Dempsey DT: Peptic ulcer disease. *Curr Probl Surg* 42:346, 2005.
98. Dicken BJ, Bigam DL, Cass C, et al: Gastric adenocarcinoma: Review and considerations for future directions. *Ann Surg* 241:27, 2005.
108. Gold JS, DeMatteo RP: Combined surgical and molecular therapy: The gastrointestinal stromal tumor model. *Ann Surg* 244:176, 2006.

CHAPTER 27

36. Nguyen NT, Goldman C, Rosenquist CJ, et al: Laparoscopic versus open gastric bypass: A randomized study of outcomes, quality of life, and costs. *Ann Surg* 234:279, 2001.
54. Dixon JB, O'Brien PE, Playfair J, et al: Adjustable gastric banding and conventional therapy for type 2 diabetes. A randomized controlled trial. *JAMA* 299:316, 2008.
58. Buchwald H, Avidor Y, Braunwald E, et al: Bariatric surgery. A systematic review and meta-analysis. *JAMA* 292:1724, 2004.

74. Schauer PR, Ikramuddin S, Gourash W, et al: Outcomes after laparoscopic Roux-en-Y gastric bypass for morbid obesity. *Ann Surg* 232:515, 2000.
80. Christou NV, Sampalis JS, Liberman M, et al: Surgery decreases long-term mortality, morbidity, and health care use in morbidly obese patients. *Ann Surg* 240:416, 2004.
107. Sjostrom L, Narbro K, Sjostron CD, et al: Effects of bariatric surgery on mortality in Swedish obese subjects. *N Engl J Med* 357:741, 2007.
108. Adams TD, Gress RE, Smith SC, et al: Long-term mortality after gastric bypass surgery. *N Engl J Med* 357:753, 2007. Another important article documenting that bariatric surgery decreases mortality in the severely obese population.
109. Rubino F, Marescaux J: Effect of duodenal-jejunal exclusion in a nonobese animal model of type 2 diabetes: A new perspective for a old disease. *Ann Surg* 239:1, 2004.

CHAPTER 28

3. Thomson ABR, Keelan M, Thiesen A, et al: Small bowel review: Normal physiology part 2. *Dig Dis Sci* 46:2588, 2001.
23. Foster NM, McGory ML, Zingmond DS, et al: Small bowel obstruction: A population-based appraisal. *J Am Coll Surg* 203:170, 2006.
44. Evenson AR, Shrikhande G, Fischer JE: Abdominal abscess and enteric fistula, in Zinner MJ, Ashley SW (eds): *Maingot's Abdominal Operations*, 11th ed. New York: McGraw Hill, 2007, p 184.

CHAPTER 29

9. Lynch HT, Lynch JF, Lynch PM, et al: Hereditary colorectal cancer syndromes: Molecular genetics, genetic counseling, diagnosis and management. *Fam Cancer* 7:27, 2008.
15. Tjandra JJ, Dykes SL, Kumar RR, et al: Practice parameters for the treatment of fecal incontinence. *Dis Colon Rectum* 50:1497, 2007.
75. Sauer R, Becker H, Hohenberger W, et al: Preoperative versus postoperative chemoradiation for rectal cancer. *N Engl J Med* 351:1731, 2004.

CHAPTER 30

4. Radford-Smith GL, Edwards JE, Purdie DM, et al. Protective role of appendicectomy on onset and severity of ulcerative colitis and Crohn's disease. *Gut* 51:808, 2002.
92. Yamini D, Vargas H, Klein S, et al: Perforated appendicitis: Is it truly a surgical urgency? *Am Surg* 64:970, 1998.
93. Owen A, Moore O, Marven S, et al: Interval laparoscopic appendectomy in children. *J Laparoendosc Adv Surg Tech A* 16:308, 2006.

CHAPTER 31

51. Schwartz M, Roayaie S, Konstadoulakis M: Strategies for the management of hepatocellular carcinoma [review]. *Nat Clin Pract Oncol* 4:424, 2007.
76. Pawlik TM, Schulick RD, Choti MA: Expanding criteria for resectability of colorectal liver metastases [review]. *Oncologist* 13:51, 2008.
95. Mazzaferro V, Chun YS, Poon RT, et al: Liver transplantation for hepatocellular carcinoma [review]. *Ann Surg Oncol* 15:1001, 2008.
159. Adam R, Miller R, Pitombo M, et al: Two-stage hepatectomy approach for initially unresectable colorectal hepatic metastases. *Surg Oncol Clin N Am* 16:525, 2007.
174. Koffron AJ, Auffenberg GB, Kung RD, et al: Evaluation of 300 minimally invasive liver resections at a single institution: Less is more. *Ann Surg* 246:385; discussion, 392, 2007.

CHAPTER 32

10. Woods CM, Mawe GM, Saccone GTP: The sphincter of Oddi: Understanding its control and function. *Neurogastroenterol Motil* 17(Supp 1):31, 2005.
57. Hunter JG: Acute cholecystitis revisited: Get it while it's hot. *Ann Surg* 227:468, 1998.

75. Way LW, Stewart L, Gantert W, et al: Causes and prevention of laparoscopic bile duct injuries: Analysis of 252 cases from a human factors and cognitive psychology perspective [Comment]. *Ann Surg* 237:460, 2003.

96. Mulholland MW, Yahanda A, Yeo CJ: Multidisciplinary management of perihilar bile duct cancer. *J Am Coll Surg* 193:440, 2001.

CHAPTER 33

25. Pandol SJ, Saluja AK, Imrie CW, et al: Acute pancreatitis: Bench to the bedside. *Gastroenterology* 133:1056 e1, 2007.

31. Whitcomb DC, Gorry MC, Preston RA, et al: Hereditary pancreatitis is caused by a mutation in the cationic trypsinogen gene. *Nat Genet* 14:141, 1996.

149. Lankisch PG, Lohr-Happe A, Otto J, et al: Natural course in chronic pancreatitis. Pain, exocrine and endocrine pancreatic insufficiency and prognosis of the disease. *Digestion* 54:148, 1993.

166. Andersen DK: Mechanisms and emerging treatments of the metabolic complications of chronic pancreatitis. *Pancreas* 35:1, 2007.

185. Aspelund G, Topazian MD, Lee JH, et al: Improved outcomes for benign disease with limited pancreatic head resection. *J Gastrointest Surg* 9:400, 2005.

198. Nealon WH, Walser: Duct drainage alone is sufficient in the operative management of pancreatic pseudocyst in patients with chronic pancreatitis. *Ann Surg* 237:614, discussion 620, 2003.

228. Nealon WH, Thompson JC: Progressive loss of pancreatic function in chronic pancreatitis is delayed by main pancreatic duct decompression. A longitudinal prospective analysis of the modified puestow procedure. *Ann Surg* 217:458, discussion 466, 1993.

263. Beger HG, Schlosser W, Friess HM, et al: Duodenum-preserving head resection in chronic pancreatitis changes the natural course of the disease: A single-center 26-year experience. *Ann Surg* 230:512, discussion 519, 1999.

265. Frey CF, Smith GJ: Description and rationale of a new operation for chronic pancreatitis. *Pancreas* 2:701, 1987.

270. Ho HS, Frey CF: The Frey procedure: Local resection of pancreatic head combined with lateral pancreaticojejunostomy. *Arch Surg* 136:1353, 2001.

271. Farkas G, Leindler L, Daroczi M, et al: Organ-preserving pancreatic head resection in chronic pancreatitis. *Br J Surg* 90:29, 2003.

274. Koninger J, Seiler CM, Sauerland S, et al: Duodenum-preserving pancreatic head resection—a randomized controlled trial comparing the original Beger procedure with the Berne modification (ISRCTN No. 50638764). *Surgery* 143:490, 2008.

277. Strate T, Bachmann K, Busch P, et al: Resection vs drainage in treatment of chronic pancreatitis: Long-term results of a randomized trial. *Gastroenterology* 134:1406, 2008.

304. Biankin AV, Kench JG, Dijkman FP, et al: Molecular pathogenesis of precursor lesions of pancreatic ductal adenocarcinoma. *Pathology* 35:14, 2003.

CHAPTER 34

80. Cassar K, Munro A: Iatrogenic splenic injury. *J R Coll Surg Edinb* 47:731, 2002.

111. Winslow E, Brunt M: Perioperative outcomes of laparoscopic versus open splenectomy: A meta-analysis with an emphasis on complications. *Surgery* 134:647, 2003.

112. Taylor MD, Genuit T, Napolitano LM: Overwhelming postsplenectomy sepsis and trauma: Time to consider revaccination? *J Trauma* 59:1482, 2005.

CHAPTER 35

Anthony T, Bergen PC, Kim LT, et al: Factors affecting recurrence following incisional herniorrhaphy. *World J Surg* 24:95, 2000.

Duchene DA, Winfield HN, Cadeddu JA, et al: Multi-institutional survey of laparoscopic ureterolysis for retroperitoneal fibrosis. *Urology* 69:1017, 2007.

Kelly JK, Hwang WS: Idiopathic retractile (sclerosing) mesenteritis and its differential diagnosis. *Am J Surg Pathol* 13:513, 1989.

Luijendijk RW, Hop WC, van den Tol MP, et al: A comparison of suture repair with mesh repair for incisional hernia. *N Engl J Med* 343:392, 2000.

Pierce RA, Spitler JA, Frisella MM, et al: Pooled data analysis of laparoscopic vs. open ventral hernia repair: 14 years of patient data accrual. *Surg Endosc* 21:378, 2007.

Saborido BP, Romero CJ, Medina ME, et al: Idiopathic segmental infarction of the greater omentum as a cause of acute abdomen. Report of two cases and review of the literature. *Hepatogastroenterology* 48:737, 2001.

CHAPTER 36

51. Rosenberg SA, Tepper J, Glatstein E, et al: The treatment of soft-tissue sarcomas of the extremities: Prospective randomized evaluations of (1) limb-sparing surgery plus radiation therapy compared with amputation and (2) the role of adjuvant chemotherapy. *Ann Surg* 196:305, 1982.

62. Yang JC, Chang AE, Baker AR, et al: Randomized prospective study of the benefit of adjuvant radiation therapy in the treatment of soft tissue sarcomas of the extremity. *J Clin Oncol* 16:197, 1998.

73. O'Sullivan B, Davis AM, Turcotte R, et al: Preoperative versus postoperative radiotherapy in soft-tissue sarcoma of the limbs: A randomised trial. *Lancet* 359:2235, 2002.

90. Adjuvant chemotherapy for localised resectable soft-tissue sarcoma of adults: Meta-analysis of individual data. Sarcoma Meta-analysis Collaboration. *Lancet* 350:1647, 1997.

CHAPTER 37

19. Rutkow IM, Robbins AW: "Tension-free" inguinal herniorrhaphy: A preliminary report on the "mesh plug" technique. *Surgery* 114:3, 1993.

37. Fitzgibbons RJ Jr, Giobbie-Harder A, Gibbs JO, et al: Watchful waiting vs repair of inguinal hernia in minimally symptomatic men: A randomized clinical trial. *JAMA* 295:285, 2006.

41. Lichtenstein IL, Shulman AG, Amid PK: Use of mesh to prevent recurrence of hernias. *Postgrad Med* 87:155, 160. 1990.

47. Neumayer L, Giobbie-Harder A, Jonasson O, et al: Open mesh versus laparoscopic mesh repair of inguinal hernia. *N Engl J Med* 350:1819, 2004.

53. Collaboration EH: Laparoscopic compared with open methods of groin hernia repair: Systematic review of randomized controlled trials. *Br J Surg* 87:860, 2000.

CHAPTER 38

33. Mazzaferri EL, Jhiang SM: Long-term impact of initial surgical and medical therapy on papillary and follicular thyroid cancer. *Am J Med* 97:418, 1994.

37. Cooper DS, Doherty GM, Haugen BR, et al: Management guidelines for patients with thyroid nodules and differentiated thyroid cancer. *Thyroid* 16:109, 2006.

70. Bilezikian JP, Potts JT Jr., Fuleihan Gel H, et al: Summary statement from a workshop on asymptomatic primary hyperparathyroidism: A perspective for the 21st century. *J Clin Endocrinol Metab* 87:5353, 2002.

CHAPTER 39

Bell MJ, Ternberg JL, Feigin RD, et al: Neonatal necrotizing enterocolitis: Therapeutic decisions based upon clinical staging. *Ann Surg* 187:1, 1978.

Bouchard S, Johnson MP, et al: The EXIT procedure: Experience and outcome in 31 cases. *J Pediatr Surg* 37:418, 2002.

DeRusso PA, Ye W, Shepherd R, et al: Growth failure and outcomes in infants with biliary atresia: A report from the Biliary Atresia Research Consortium. *Hepatology* 46:1632, 2007.

Grant D, Abu-Elmagd K, Reyes J, et al: 2003 Report of the intestine transplant registry: A new era has dawned. *Ann Surg* 241:607, 2005.

Grikscheit TC, Vacanti JP: The history and current status of tissue engineering: The future of pediatric surgery. *J Pediatr Surg* 37:277, 2002.

Gross RE, Ladd WE: The Field of Children's Surgery, in: Gross RE (ed): *The Surgery of Infancy and Childhood: Its Principles and Techniques.* W. B. Saunders: Philadelphia, 1953, p 1.

Hackam DJ, Potoka D, et al: Utility of radiographic hepatic injury grade in predicting outcome for children after blunt abdominal trauma. *J Pediatr Surg* 37:386, 2002.

Hackam DJ, Reblock K, et al: The influence of Down's syndrome on the management and outcome of children with Hirschsprung's disease. *J Pediatr Surg* 38:946, 2003.

Hackam DJ, Superina R, et al: Single-stage repair of Hirschsprung's disease: A comparison of 109 patients over 5 years. *J Pediatr Surg* 32:1028, 1997

Harrison MR: Fetal surgery: Trials, tribulations, and turf. *J Pediatr Surg* 38:275, 2003.

Katzenstein HM, Krailo MD, Malogolowkin MH, et al: Hepatocellular carcinoma in children and adolescents: Results from the Pediatric Oncology Group and the Children's Cancer Group Intergroup Study. *J Clin Oncol* 20:2789, 2002.

Langer J, Durrant A, et al: One-stage transanal Soave pullthrough for Hirschsprung disease: A multicenter experience with 141 children. *Ann Surg* 238:569, 2003.

Levitt MA, Ferraraccio D, et al: Variability of inguinal hernia surgical technique: A survey of North American pediatric surgeons. *J Pediatr Surg* 37:745, 2002.

Mengel W, Wronecki K, Schroeder J, et al: Histopathology of the cryptorchid testis. *Urol Clin North Am* 9:331, 1982.

Pena A, Guardino K, et al: Bowel management for fecal incontinence in patients with anorectal malformations. *J Pediatr Surg* 33:133, 1998.

Shimada H, Ambros I, et al: The International Neuroblastoma Pathology Classification (the Shimada system). *Cancer* 86:364, 1999.

Spitz L, Kiely E, et al: Oesophageal atresia: At-risk groups for the 1990s. *J Pediatr Surg* 29:723, 1994.

Thibeault DW, Olsen SL, et al: Pre-ECMO predictors of nonsurvival in congenital diaphragmatic hernia. *J Perinatol* 22:682, 2002.

Wilson J, Lund D, et al: Congenital diaphragmatic hernia—a tale of two cities: The Boston experience. *J Pediatr Surg* 32:401, 1997.

CHAPTER 40

3. Stein JP, Cai J, Groshen S, et al: Risk factors for patients with pelvic lymph node metastases following radical cystectomy with en bloc pelvic lymphadenectomy: Concept of lymph node density. *J Urol* 170:35, 2003.

12. Flanigan RC, Salmon SE, Blumenstein BA, et al: Nephrectomy followed by interferon alfa-2b compared with interferon alfa-2b alone for metastatic renal cell cancer. *N Engl J Med* 345:1655, 2001.

14. Huang WC, Levey AS, Serio AM, et al: Chronic kidney disease after nephrectomy in patients with renal cortical tumors: A retrospective cohort study. *Lancet Oncol* 7:735, 2006.

19. Bill-Axelson A, Holmberg L, Filen F, et al: Radical prostatectomy versus watchful waiting in localized prostate cancer: The Scandinavian Prostate Cancer Group-4 Randomized Trial. *J Natl Cancer Inst* 100:1144, 2008.

22. Buckley JC, McAninch JW: Selective management of isolated and nonisolated grade IV renal injuries. *J Urol* 176:2498, 2006.

55. Curhan GC, Willett WC, Rimm EB, et al: A prospective study of dietary calcium and other nutrients and the risk of symptomatic kidney stones. *N Engl J Med* 328:833, 1993.

CHAPTER 41

23. Gabbe S, Niebyl J, Simpson J: *Obstetrics: Normal and Problem Pregnancies*, 4th ed. Philadelphia: Churchill Livingstone, 2002.

33. Walters M, Karram M: *Urogynecology and Reconstructive Pelvic Surgery*, 3rd ed. Philadelphia: Mosby, 2007.

48. Berek J, Hacker N: *Practical Gynecologic Oncology*, 4th ed. Philadelphia: Lippincott, Williams and Wilkins, 2004.

50. Hoskins W, Perez C, Young R. *Principles and Practice of Gynecologic Oncology.* Philadelphia: Lippincott, Williams and Wilkins, 2000.

59. Stenchever M, Droegemueller W, Herbst A, et al: *Comprehensive Gynecology*, 4th ed. St Louis: Mosby, 2001.

CHAPTER 42

5. Brain Trauma Foundation, American Association of Neurological Surgeons, Congress of Neurological Surgeons. Guidelines for the management of severe traumatic brain injury. *J Neurotrauma* 24:S1, 2007.

18. Denis F: The three column spine and its significance in the classification of acute thoracolumbar spinal injuries. *Spine* 8:817, 1983.

24. Anonymous. Beneficial effect of carotid endarterectomy in symptomatic patients with high-grade carotid stenosis. North American Symptomatic Carotid Endarterectomy Trial Collaborators [see comment]. *N Engl J Med* 325:445, 1991.

27. Molyneux A, Kerr R, Stratton I, et al: International Subarachnoid Aneurysm Trial (ISAT) of neurosurgical clipping versus endovascular coiling in 2143 patients with ruptured intracranial aneurysms: A randomised trial [see comment] [reprint in *J Stroke Cerebrovasc Dis* 11:304, 2002]. *Lancet* 360:1267, 2002.

30. Patchell RA, Tibbs PA, Walsh JW, et al: A randomized trial of surgery in the treatment of single metastases to the brain. *N Engl J Med* 322:494, 1990.

CHAPTER 43

1. Gustilo RB, Anderson JT: Prevention of infection in the treatment for one thousand and twenty-five open fractures of long bones. *J Bone Joint Surg Am* 58:453, 1976.

40. Denis F: The three column spine and its significance in the classification of acute thoracolumbar spinal injuries. *Spine* 8:817, 1983.

43. Weinstein JN, Tosteson TD, Lurie JD, et al: Surgical vs nonoperative treatment for lumbar disk herniation. *JAMA* 296:2441, 2006.

58. Salter RB, Harris WR: Injuries involving the epiphyseal plate. *J Bone Joint Surg Am* 45:587, 1963.

63. Willis RB: Developmental dysplasia of the hip: Assessment and treatment before walking age. *Instr Course Lect* 50:541, 2001.

CHAPTER 44

1. American Society for Surgery of the Hand, in: *The Hand: Examination and Diagnosis*, 3rd ed. New York: Churchill Livingstone, 1990, p 5.

6. Green DP: General principles, in Green DP, Hotchkiss RN, Pedersen WC, et al (eds): *Green's Operative Hand Surgery*, 5th ed. Philadelphia, Pa: Churchill Livingstone, 2005, p 3.

9. Lalonde D, Bell M, Benoit P, et al: A multicenter prospective study of 3,110 consecutive cases of elective epinephrine use in the fingers and hand: The Dalhousie Project clinical phase. *J Hand Surg [Am]* 30:1061, 2005.

CHAPTER 45

13. Wei FC, Souminen S: Principles and techniques of microvascular surgery, in Mathes SJ (ed): *Plastic Surgery,* 2nd ed. Philadelphia: Elsevier, 2006, p 507.

16. Lutz BS, Wei FC: Microsurgical workhorse flaps in head and neck reconstruction. *Clin Plast Surg* 32:421, 2005.

25. Whitaker LA, Barlett SP: Craniofacial anomalies, in Jurkiewicz MJ, Krizek TJ, Mathes SJ, et al (eds): *Plastic Surgery: Principles and Practice*, vol. 1. St. Louis: Mosby, 1990, p 99.

38. Wei FC, Chen HC, Chuang CC, et al: Fibular osteoseptocutaneous flap: Anatomic study and clinical application. *Plast Reconstr Surg* 78:191, 1986.

53. Rohrich RJ, Lowe JB, Hackney FL, et al: An algorithm for abdominal wall reconstruction. *Plast Reconstr Surg* 105:202, 2000.

CHAPTER 46

24. Rao PS, Merion RM, Ashby VB, et al: Renal transplantation in elderly patients older than 70 years of age: Results from the Scientific Registry of Transplant Recipients. *Transplantation* 83:1069, 2007.

26. Giordano SH, Hortobagyi GN, Kau SC, et al: Breast cancer treatment guidelines in older women. *J Clin Oncol* 23: 783, 2005.

30. Gennari R: Breast cancer in elderly women. Optimizing the treatment. *Breast Cancer Res Treat* 110:199, 2008.

38. Mery CM, Pappas AN, Bueno R et al: Similar long-term survival of elderly patients with non-small cell lung cancer treated with lobectomy or wedge resection within the surveillance, epidemiology and end results database. *Chest* 28:237, 2005.

39. Cattaneo SM, Park BJ, Wilton AS, et al: Use of video-assisted thoracic surgery for lobectomy in the elderly results in fewer complications. *Ann Thoracic Surg* 85:231, 2008.

42. Chang TT, Schecter WP: Injury in the elderly and end-of-life decisions. *Surg Clin North Am* 87:229, 2007.

CHAPTER 47

11. Hull CJ: Principles of pharmacokinetics, in Hemmings H, Hopkins PM (eds): *Foundations of Anesthesia*. London: Mosby, 2000, p 77.

12. Stoelting RD, Dierdorf SF: *Stoelting's Anesthesia and Co-Existing Disease*, 5th ed. Philadelphia: Saunders, 2008.

50. Practice guidelines for management of the difficult airway: An updated report by the American Society of Anesthesiologists Task Force on Management of the Difficult Airway. *Anesthesiology* 98:1269, 2003.

77. Gan TJ, Meyer T, Apfel CC, et al: Consensus guidelines for managing postoperative nausea and vomiting. *Anesth Analg* 97:62, 2003.

80. Atkins JH, Johansson JS: Technologies to shape the future: Proteomics applications in anesthesiology and critical care medicine. *Anesth Analg* 102:1207, 2006.

CHAPTER 48

2. Beauchamp TL, Childress JF: *Principles of Biomedical Ethics*, 3rd ed. New York: Oxford University Press, 1989.

8. Faden RR, Beauchamp TL: *A History and Theory of Informed Consent*. New York: Oxford University Press, 1986.

35. Dunn G: Surgical palliative care, in Mosby (ed): *Current Surgical Therapy*, 9th ed. Philadelphia: Elsevier, 2008.

36. Saunders C: The challenge of terminal care, in Symington T, Carter R (eds): *Scientific Foundations of Oncology*. London: Heineman, 1976 p 673.

37. Billroth T: Open letter to Dr. L Wittleshöfer. *Wiener Medizinische Wochenschrift* 31:162, 1881.

46. Surgeons Palliative Care Workgroup: Report from the Field. *J Am Coll Surg* 197:661, 2003.

47. Cancer pain relief and palliative care. Report of a WHO Expert Committee. *World Health Organ Tech Rep Ser* 804:1, 1990.

62. Hinshaw DB: Spiritual issues in surgical palliative care. *Surg Clin North Am* 85:257, 2005.

63. Jacox A, Carr D, Payne R, et al: Management of cancer pain. *AHCPR Publication No. 94-052: Clinical Practice Guideline No. 9*. Rockville, MD: US Department of Health and Human Services, Public Health Service, 1994.

INDEX

Note: Page numbers followed by *t* indicate tables; those followed by *f* indicate figures.